SECOND EDITION

HEART DISEASE

A Textbook of Cardiovascular Medicine

Edited by

EUGENE BRAUNWALD, M.D.

Hersey Professor of the Theory and Practice of Physic;
Herrman Ludwig Blumgart Professor of Medicine, Harvard Medical School;
Chairman, Department of Medicine,
Brigham and Women's and Beth Israel Hospitals, Boston

W. B. SAUNDERS COMPANY

PHILADELPHIA · LONDON · TORONTO · MEXICO CITY · RIO DE JANEIRO · SYDNEY · TOKYO

W. B. Saunders Company: West Washington Square
Philadelphia, PA 19105

1 St. Anne's Road
Eastbourne, East Sussex BN21 3UN, England

1 Goldthorne Avenue
Toronto, Ontario M8Z 5T9, Canada

Apartado 26370 — Cedro 512
Mexico 4, D.F., Mexico

Rua Coronel Cabrita, 8
Sao Cristovao Caixa Postal 21176
Rio de Janeiro, Brazil

9 Waltham Street
Artarmon, N.S.W. 2064, Australia

Ichibancho, Central Bldg., 22-1 Ichibancho
Chiyoda-Ku, Tokyo 102, Japan

Library of Congress Cataloging in Publication Data
Main entry under title:

Heart disease.

Includes bibliographical references and index.
1. Heart—Diseases. I. Braunwald, Eugene.
[DNLM: 1. Heart diseases—Complications. WG 200
H4364]
RC681.H362 1984 616.1'2 83-2850
ISBN 0-7216-1938-X (single v.)
ISBN 0-7216-1939-8 (v. 1)
ISBN 0-7216-1940-1 (v. 2)
ISBN 0-7216-1941-X (set)

ISBN: SINGLE VOLUME 0-7216-1938-X
ISBN: VOLUME 1 0-7216-1939-8
ISBN: VOLUME 2 0-7216-1940-1
ISBN: SET 0-7216-1941-X

HEART DISEASE

Last digit is the print number: 9 8 7 6 5 4

Dedicated to the memory of my father,

WILLIAM BRAUNWALD

CONTRIBUTORS

JOSEPH S. ALPERT, M.D.

Professor of Medicine, University of Massachusetts Medical School. Director, Division of Cardiovascular Medicine, University of Massachusetts Medical Center, Worcester, Massachusetts.

Pulmonary Hypertension; Congenital Heart Disease in the Adult; Acute Myocardial Infarction: Pathological, Pathophysiological, and Clinical Manifestations

MURRAY G. BARON, M.D.

Professor of Radiology, Emory University School of Medicine. Associate Chairman of Radiology, Emory University Hospital, Atlanta, Georgia.

Radiological and Angiographic Examination of the Heart

WILLIAM H. BARRY, M.D.

Associate Professor of Medicine, Harvard Medical School. Director, Cardiac Catheterization Laboratory, Brigham and Women's Hospital, Boston, Massachusetts.

Cardiac Catheterization

EUGENE H. BLACKSTONE, M.D.

Cardiovascular Surgical Research Professor, The University of Alabama School of Medicine, University of Alabama, Birmingham, Alabama.

General Principles of Cardiac Surgery

KENNETH M. BOROW, M.D.

Associate Professor of Medicine, Cardiology, University of Chicago. Director, Cardiac Noninvasive Imaging Laboratory, University of Chicago Hospitals and Clinics, Chicago, Illinois.

Congenital Heart Disease in the Adult

EUGENE BRAUNWALD, M.D.

Hersey Professor of the Theory and Practice of Physic, and Herrman Ludwig Blumgart Professor of Medicine, Harvard Medical School. Chairman, Department of Medicine, Brigham and Women's and Beth Israel Hospitals, Boston, Massachusetts.

The History; The Physical Examination; Contraction of the Normal Heart; Pathophysiology of Heart Failure; Assessment of Cardiac Function; Clinical Manifestations of Heart Failure; The Management of Heart Failure; Pulmonary Edema: Cardiogenic and Noncardiogenic; Pulmonary Hypertension; Congenital Heart Disease in the Adult; Valvular Heart Disease; Coronary Blood Flow and Myocardial Ischemia; Acute Myocardial Infarction: Pathological, Pathophysiological, and Clinical Manifestations; The Management of Acute Myocardial Infarction; Chronic Ischemic Heart Disease; The Cardiomyopathies and Myocarditides; Primary Tumors of the Heart; Pericardial Disease; Traumatic Heart Disease; Cor Pulmonale and Pulmonary Thromboembolism; Hematologic-Oncologic Disorders and Heart Disease; Endocrine and Nutritional Disorders and Heart Disease; Renal Disorders and Heart Disease; General Anesthesia and Noncardiac Surgery in Patients with Heart Disease

MICHAEL S. BROWN, M.D., D.Sc. (Hon.)

Professor, Department of Molecular Genetics, and Director, Center for Genetic Diseases, University of Texas Health Science Center at Dallas. Senior Attending Physician, Parkland Memorial Hospital, Dallas, Texas.

Genetics and Cardiovascular Disease

PETER F. COHN, M.D.

Professor of Medicine and Chief of Cardiology Division, State University of New York Health Sciences Center, Stony Brook, New York.

Chronic Ischemic Heart Disease; Traumatic Heart Disease

WILSON S. COLUCCI, M.D.

Assistant Professor of Medicine, Harvard Medical School. Associate Physician, Brigham and Women's Hospital, Boston, Massachusetts.

Primary Tumors of the Heart

ERNEST CRAIGE, M.D.

Henry A. Foscue Distinguished Professor of Cardiology, University of North Carolina School of Medicine. Director, Cardiac Graphics Laboratory, North Carolina Memorial Hospital, Chapel Hill, North Carolina.

Heart Sounds; Echophonocardiography and Other Noninvasive Techniques to Elucidate Heart Murmurs

ROMAN W. DE SANCTIS, M.D.

Professor of Medicine, Harvard Medical School. Physician and Director of Clinical Cardiology, Massachusetts General Hospital, Boston, Massachusetts.

Diseases of the Aorta

EDWIN G. DUFFIN, Ph.D.

Clinical Research Manager, Pacing Division, Medtronic, Inc., Minneapolis, Minnesota.

Cardiac Pacemakers

HARVEY FEIGENBAUM, M.D.

Distinguished Professor of Medicine, Indiana University School of Medicine. Senior Research Associate, Krannert Institute of Cardiology, Indianapolis, Indiana.

Echocardiography

MANNING FEINLEIB, M.D., Dr. P.H.

Clinical Professor, Georgetown University of Medicine, Washington, D.C. Visiting Lecturer on Epidemiology, Harvard School of Public Health, Boston, Massachusetts. Associate, Johns Hopkins University, Baltimore, Maryland. Director, National Center for Health Statistics, Hyattsville, Maryland.

Risk Factors for Coronary Artery Disease and Their Management

CHARLES FISCH, M.D.

Distinguished Professor of Medicine, Indiana University School of Medicine. Director, Krannert Institute of Cardiology and Division of Cardiology, Indiana University School of Medicine, Indianapolis, Indiana.

Electrocardiography and Vectorcardiography

WILLIAM F. FRIEDMAN, M.D.

J. H. Nicholson Professor of Pediatric Cardiology, University of California, Los Angeles, School of Medicine. Professor and Chairman, Department of Pediatrics, U.C.L.A. Center for Health Sciences, Los Angeles, California.

Congenital Heart Disease in Infancy and Childhood; Acquired Heart Disease in Infancy and Childhood

GOFFREDO G. GENSINI, M.D.

Clinical Professor of Medicine, State University of New York Upstate Medical Center College of Medicine. Director, Monseigneur Toomey Cardiovascular Laboratory and Research Department, Saint Joseph Hospital Health Center, Syracuse, New York.

Coronary Arteriography

JOSEPH L. GOLDSTEIN, M.D., D.Sc. (Hon.)

Paul J. Thomas Professor and Chairman, Department of Molecular Genetics, University of Texas Health Science Center at Dallas. Senior Attending Physician, Parkland Memorial Hospital, Dallas, Texas.

Genetics and Cardiovascular Disease

MICHAEL N. GOTTLIEB, M.D.

Assistant Clinical Professor of Medicine, Harvard Medical School. Associate Physician, Brigham and Women's Hospital, Boston, Massachusetts.

Renal Disorders and Heart Disease

WILLIAM GROSSMAN, M.D.

Professor of Medicine, Harvard Medical School. Chief, Cardiovascular Division, Beth Israel Hospital, Boston, Massachusetts.

Cardiac Catheterization; High–Cardiac Output States; Pulmonary Hypertension

THOMAS P. HACKETT, M.D.

Eben S. Draper Professor of Psychiatry, Harvard Medical School. Chief of Psychiatry, Massachusetts General Hospital, Boston, Massachusetts.

Emotion, Psychiatric Disorders, and the Heart

ROBERT I. HANDIN, M.D.

Associate Professor of Medicine, Harvard Medical School. Director, Hematology Division, Brigham and Women's Hospital, Boston, Massachusetts.

Hematologic-Oncologic Disorders and Heart Disease

B. LEONARD HOLMAN, M.D.

Professor of Radiology, Harvard Medical School. Director, Clinical Nuclear Medicine Services, Brigham and Women's Hospital, Boston, Massachusetts.

Nuclear Cardiology

ROLAND H. INGRAM, Jr., M.D.

Parker B. Francis Professor of Medicine, Harvard Medical School. Director, Respiratory Divisions, Brigham and Women's and Beth Israel Hospitals, Boston, Massachusetts.

Pulmonary Edema: Cardiogenic and Noncardiogenic; Relationship Between Diseases of the Heart and Lungs

NORMAN M. KAPLAN, M.D.

Professor of Internal Medicine, University of Texas Southwestern Medical School. Chief, Hypertension Section, Parkland Memorial Hospital, Dallas, Texas.

Systemic Hypertension: Mechanisms and Diagnosis; Systemic Hypertension: Therapy

JAMES K. KIRKLIN, M.D.

Assistant Professor of Surgery, University of Alabama School of Medicine. Staff Physician, Department of Surgery, University of Alabama Medical Center, Birmingham, Alabama.

General Principles of Cardiac Surgery

JOHN W. KIRKLIN, M.D.

Professor of Surgery, University of Alabama School of Medicine. Director, Division of Cardiothoracic Surgery, Department of Surgery, and Director, Alabama Congenital Heart Disease Diagnosis and Treatment Center, University of Alabama Medical Center, Birmingham, Alabama.

General Principles of Cardiac Surgery

ROBERT I. LEVY, M.D.

Vice President for Health Sciences, Columbia University College of Physicians and Surgeons, New York, New York.

Risk Factors for Coronary Artery Disease and Their Management

BEVERLY H. LORELL, M.D.

Assistant Professor of Medicine, Harvard Medical School. Co-Director, Hemodynamic Research Laboratory, and Attending Cardiologist, Beth Israel Hospital, Boston, Massachusetts.

Pericardial Disease

BERNARD LOWN, M.D.

Professor of Cardiology, Harvard School of Public Health. Senior Physician, Brigham and Women's Hospital, Boston, Massachusetts.

Cardiovascular Collapse and Sudden Cardiac Death

E. REGIS McFADDEN, Jr., M.D.

Associate Professor of Medicine, Harvard Medical School. Director of Research, Shipley Institute of Medicine, Brigham and Women's Hospital, Boston, Massachusetts.

Cor Pulmonale and Pulmonary Thromboembolism; Relationship Between Diseases of the Heart and Lungs

ALBERT OBERMAN, M.D., M.P.H.

Professor and Chairman, Department of Preventive Medicine, The University of Alabama School of Medicine. Active Medical Staff, University of Alabama Hospitals, Birmingham, Alabama.

Rehabilitation of Patients with Coronary Artery Disease

JOSEPH K. PERLOFF, M.D.

Professor of Medicine and Pediatrics, University of California, Los Angeles, School of Medicine. Attending Physician, U.C.L.A. Center for Health Sciences, Los Angeles, California.

Neurological Disorders and Heart Disease; Pregnancy and Cardiovascular Disease

GERALD M. POHOST, M.D.

Associate Professor of Medicine, Harvard Medical School. Director of Nuclear Cardiology, Cardiac Unit, Massachusetts General Hospital, Boston, Massachusetts.

Nuclear Magnetic Resonance Imaging of the Heart

ADAM V. RATNER, B.A.

Special Fellow in Cardiac NMR, Massachusetts General Hospital, Boston, Massachusetts. Fellow, Stanley J. Sarnoff Society of Fellows for Cardiovascular Research, Medical Student, University of Texas Southwestern Medical School, Dallas, Texas.

Nuclear Magnetic Resonance Imaging of the Heart

ROBERT ROBERTS, M.D.

Professor of Medicine, Baylor College of Medicine. Chief of Cardiology, The Methodist Hospital, Houston, Texas.

Hypotension and Syncope

JERROLD F. ROSENBAUM, M.D.

Assistant Professor of Psychiatry, Harvard Medical School. Chief, Clinical Psychopharmacology Unit, Massachusetts General Hospital, Boston, Massachusetts.

Emotion, Psychiatric Disorders, and the Heart

DAVID S. ROSENTHAL, M.D.

Associate Professor of Medicine, Harvard Medical School. Clinical Director, Hematology Division, Brigham and Women's Hospital, Boston, Massachusetts.

Hematologic-Oncologic Disorders and Heart Disease

JOHN ROSS, Jr., M.D.

Professor of Medicine, University of California, San Diego, School of Medicine. Cardiologist, University of California Medical Center, San Diego, California.

Contraction of the Normal Heart

L. THOMAS SHEFFIELD, M.D.

Professor, Department of Medicine, The University of Alabama School of Medicine. Director, ECG Laboratory and Allison Laboratory of Exercise Electrophysiology, University Hospital. Attending Cardiologist, University Hospital and Veterans Administration Hospital, Birmingham, Alabama.

Exercise Stress Testing

EVE E. SLATER, M.D.

Assistant Professor of Medicine, Harvard Medical School. Chief, Hypertension Unit, Massachusetts General Hospital, Boston, Massachusetts.

Diseases of the Aorta

THOMAS W. SMITH, M.D.

Professor of Medicine, Harvard Medical School. Chief, Cardiovascular Division, Brigham and Women's Hospital, Boston, Massachusetts.

The Management of Heart Failure

BURTON E. SOBEL, M.D.

Professor of Medicine and Director of Cardiovascular Division, Washington University School of Medicine. Cardiologist-in-Chief, Barnes Hospital, St. Louis, Missouri.

Cardiac and Noncardiac Forms of Acute Circulatory Failure (Shock); Hypotension and Syncope; Coronary Blood Flow and Myocardial Ischemia; The Management of Acute Myocardial Infarction

EDMUND H. SONNENBLICK, M.D.

Professor of Medicine, The Albert Einstein College of Medicine. Chief, Division of Cardiology, Hospital of the Albert Einstein College of Medicine and The Bronx Municipal Hospital Center, Bronx, New York.

Contraction of the Normal Heart

GENE H. STOLLERMAN, M.D.

Professor of Medicine, Boston University School of Medicine. Attending Physician, University Hospital, Boston, Massachusetts.

Rheumatic and Heritable Connective Tissue Diseases of the Cardiovascular System

LOUIS WEINSTEIN, M.D., Ph.D.

Lecturer in Medicine, Harvard Medical School. Physician and Director of the Clinical Services of the Division of Infectious Disease, Department of Medicine, Brigham and Women's Hospital, Boston, Massachusetts.

Infective Endocarditis

GORDON H. WILLIAMS, M.D.

Professor of Medicine, Harvard Medical School. Chief, Endocrinology-Hypertension Service, Brigham and Women's Hospital, Boston, Massachusetts.

Endocrine and Nutritional Disorders and Heart Disease

ROBERT W. WISSLER, Ph.D., M.D.

Donald N. Pritzker Distinguished Service Professor of Pathology, The Pritzker School of Medicine of the University of Chicago. Physician, University of Chicago Medical Center, Chicago, Illinois.

Principles of the Pathogenesis of Atherosclerosis

MARSHALL A. WOLF, M.D.

Associate Professor of Medicine, Harvard Medical School, Associate Physician-in-Chief, Brigham and Women's Hospital, Boston, Massachusetts.

General Anesthesia and Noncardiac Surgery in Patients with Heart Disease

JOSHUA WYNNE, M.D.

Assistant Professor of Medicine, Harvard Medical School. Director, Noninvasive Cardiac Laboratory, and Associate Physician, Brigham and Women's Hospital, Boston, Massachusetts.

The Cardiomyopathies and Myocarditides

DOUGLAS P. ZIPES, M.D.

Professor of Medicine, Indiana University School of Medicine. Senior Research Associate, Krannert Institute of Cardiology. Attending Physician, University Hospital, Veterans Administration Medical Center, and Wishard Memorial Hospital, Indianapolis, Indiana.

Genesis of Cardiac Arrhythmias: Electrophysiological Considerations; Management of Cardiac Arrhythmias; Specific Arrhythmias: Diagnosis and Treatment; Cardiac Pacemakers

PREFACE TO THE SECOND EDITION

The rates at which the various branches of medicine progress are by no means uniform. To even the most casual observer, it is evident that cardiology is now moving ahead at an unprecedented velocity. Because of the enormous advances in clinical cardiology and cardiovascular science that have occurred in the four years since publication of the first edition, preparation of the second edition of *Heart Disease* has been a task that has been both more challenging and more intellectually invigorating than I had anticipated. Although the basic format of the book has remained the same, the new edition incorporates extensive changes. Eight entirely new chapters have been added or substituted: Electrocardiography and Vectorcardiography by Charles Fisch; Nuclear Magnetic Resonance Imaging by Adam V. Ratner and Gerald M. Pohost; Genesis of Cardiac Arrhythmias, Management of Cardiac Arrhythmias, Diagnosis and Management of Specific Cardiac Arrhythmias, and The Use of Cardiac Pacemakers, all by Douglas P. Zipes; Rehabilitation of Patients with Coronary Artery Disease by Albert Oberman; Diseases of the Pericardium by Beverly Lorell and Eugene Braunwald; and General Principles of Cardiac Surgery by John W. Kirklin, Eugene H. Blackstone, and James K. Kirklin.

Many new and important areas have been covered, including the use of newly developed imaging techniques—specifically CAT scanning, digital radiography, and nuclear magnetic resonance imaging and much greater emphasis on the applications of two-dimensional echocardiography in cardiovascular diagnosis; the use of intracoronary administration of thrombolytic agents in the treatment of evolving myocardial infarction; the application of Bayesian analysis in the diagnosis of ischemic heart disease by exercise electrocardiography; the use of newer inotropic agents, cardiac transplantation, and mechanical circulatory assistance in the treatment of congestive heart failure; the application of electrophysiological testing in the diagnosis of patients with cardiac arrhythmias; the use of newer antiarrhythmic drugs, electrical stimulation, and surgery in the treatment of previously intractable arrhythmias; current approaches to patients resuscitated from ventricular fibrillation; implications of the results of recent trials relative to the treatment of patients with mild essential hypertension; newer considerations in the selection of artificial heart valves; the role of surgery in the management of infective endocarditis; the basic pharmacology of calcium-channel blocking agents and their use in the treatment of various forms of cardiovascular disease; the role of prostaglandins in thrombosis; and the use of exercise testing in the early postinfarction period for the selection of candidates for coronary artery bypass grafting.

Considerable revisions have been made in both galley and page proofs to accommodate information about the most recent advances in the field; particular emphasis has been placed on insuring a comprehensive and up-to-date bibliography; and several hundred references to publications that appeared in 1983 have been inserted. There are more than 570 new figures and tables.

To the extent that this textbook proves useful to those who wish to broaden their knowledge of cardiovascular medicine and thereby aids in the care of patients afflicted with heart disease, credit must be given to the many talented and dedicated persons involved in its preparation. I offer my deepest appreciation to my fellow contributors for their professional expertise, knowledge, and devoted scholarship, which have so enriched this book. It has been a personal pleasure for me to deal with the W. B. Saunders Company. Mr. John Hanley, President, and Mr. Dereck Jeffers, Medical Editor, have been particularly helpful, as has been their effective production team—Ms. Lorraine Kilmer, Ms. Donna Kennedy, and Mr. Frank Polizzano. Ms. Diane Q. Forti, Special Editor for the first edition, continued to provide outstanding editorial support, while Ms. Patricia Higgins in my office rendered most capable secretarial and editorial services.

Without question, this edition could not have become a reality were it not for the skill and dedication of several very special persons. My responsibilities to the Harvard Medical School and the Brigham and Women's and Beth Israel Hospitals during my leave of absence were shouldered most effectively by my colleagues, Drs. Marshall Wolf, Stephen Robinson, and Steven Come, who provided the Department of Medicine with exemplary leadership. My administrative assistants, Mrs. Mary Jackson at the Brigham and Ms. Judith Walls at the Beth Israel, were enormously helpful in maintaining the orderly flow of activity essential to a busy Department of Medicine. I am deeply indebted to them as well as to Dr. Daniel C. Tosteson, Dean of the Harvard Medical Schoool; Dr. Richard Nesson, President of the Brigham and Women's Hospital; and Dr. Mitchell T. Rabkin, President of the Beth Israel Hospital, for graciously allowing me the freedom to devote myself to this task. My wife, Dr. Nina S. Braunwald, my mother, Mrs. Clare Braunwald, and my children, Karen Gail, Denise Allison, and Adrienne Jill, provided the personal support, encouragement, and understanding so essential for one who adds a task of this dimension to an already crowded professional life.

EUGENE BRAUNWALD

FROM THE PREFACE TO THE FIRST EDITION

Today cardiovascular disease is the greatest scourge afflicting the population of the industrialized nations. As with previous scourges—bubonic plague, yellow fever, and smallpox—cardiovascular disease not only strikes down a significant fraction of the population without warning but causes prolonged suffering and disability in an even larger number. In the United States alone, despite recent encouraging declines, cardiovascular disease is still responsible for almost one million fatalities each year, well over half of all deaths, and almost 5 million persons afflicted with cardiovascular disease are hospitalized each year. The cost of this disease in terms of human suffering is almost incalculable; direct annual costs approximate $18 billion, and indirect annual costs due to morbidity amount to over $10 billion.

Fortunately, research focusing on the causes, diagnosis, treatment, and prevention of heart disease is moving ahead rapidly. In the last 25 years, in particular, we have witnessed an explosive expansion of our understanding of the structure and function of the cardiovascular system—both normal and abnormal—and of our ability to evaluate these parameters in the living patient, sometimes by means of techniques that require penetration of the skin but also, with increasing accuracy, by noninvasive methods. Simultaneously, remarkable progress has been made in preventing and treating cardiovascular disease by medical and surgical means. Indeed, in the United States, the aforementioned steady reduction in mortality from cardiovascular disease during the past decade suggests that the effective application of this increased knowledge is beginning to prolong man's life span—the most valued resource on earth.

An attempt to summarize our present understanding of heart disease in a comprehensive textbook for the serious student of this subject is a formidable undertaking. Following the untimely death of Dr. Charles K. Friedberg, whose masterful text served as a bible to me and to a whole generation of cardiologists during the 1950's and 1960's, the W.B. Saunders Company invited me to accept this responsibility. Younger colleagues, particularly cardiology fellows and medical residents at the Brigham, convinced me of the need for such a book.

Since the early part of this century, clinical cardiology has had a particularly strong foundation in the basic sciences of physiology and pharmacology. More recently, the disciplines of molecular biology, genetics, developmental biology, biophysics, biochemistry, experimental pathology, and bioengineering have also begun to provide critically important information about cardiac function and malfunction. Although it was decided that *Heart Disease: A Textbook of Cardiovascular Medicine* was to be primarily a clinical treatise and not a textbook of fundamental cardiovascular science, an effort has been made to explain, in some detail, the scientific basis of cardiovascular diseases.

Heart Disease is divided into four parts: Part I deals with the examination of the patient in the broadest sense, including clinical findings and the theory and application of modern invasive and noninvasive techniques used to elicit information about the heart and the circulation. Part II is concerned with the pathophysiology, diagnosis, and treatment of the principal abnormalities of circulatory function, including heart failure, shock, arrhythmias, and abnormalities of arterial pressure. Part III consists of descriptions of the principal congenital and acquired diseases affecting the heart, pericardium, aorta, and pulmonary vascular bed in adults and children. Primary disease of other organ systems, such as the nervous, hematopoietic, endocrine, renal, and pulmonary systems, is frequently accompanied by important cardiac complications. Patients with these conditions present particularly challenging problems to both cardiac and noncardiac specialists. Accordingly, Part IV discusses the manner in which diseases of other organ systems affect the circulation and vice versa.

In order to provide a comprehensive, authoritative text in a field that has become as broad and deep as cardiovascular medicine, I chose to enlist contributions from a number of able colleagues. However, it was hoped that my personal involvement in the writing of about half the book would make it possible to eliminate the fragmentation, gaps, inconsistencies, organizational difficulties, and impersonal tone that sometimes plague multiauthored texts. I sought a compromise between a book that is too lengthy (and therefore expensive) as a result excessive repetition and one in which all duplication is eliminated, resulting in fragmented coverage of certain subjects. To help achieve this objective, extensive cross references have been provided within the text.

EUGENE BRAUNWALD

CONTENTS

PART I
EXAMINATION OF THE PATIENT

PART I

EXAMINATION OF THE PATIENT

1 THE HISTORY

by Eugene Braunwald, M.D.

IMPORTANCE OF THE HISTORY: THE PHYSICIAN'S ROLE

Specialized examinations of the cardiovascular system, presented in Chapters 3 to 11, provide a large portion of the data base required to establish a specific anatomical diagnosis of cardiac disease and to determine the extent of functional impairment of the heart. Although the development of these methods represents one of the triumphs of modern medicine, their appropriate use is *to supplement but not to supplant* a careful clinical examination, which remains the cornerstone of the assessment of the patient with known or suspected cardiovascular disease. There is a temptation in cardiology, as in many other areas of medicine, to carry out expensive, uncomfortable, and occasionally even hazardous procedures to establish a diagnosis when a detailed and thoughtful history and physical examination may be sufficient. Obviously, it is undesirable to subject patients to the unnecessary risks and expenses inherent in many specialized tests when a diagnosis can be made based on an adequate clinical examination or when their management will not be altered significantly as a result of these tests.[1] Intelligent selection of investigative procedures from the broad array now available requires more sophisticated decision-making than was necessary when the choices were limited to the electrocardiogram and chest roentgenogram. The history and physical examination provide the critical information necessary for these decisions.

The Role of the History. The overreliance on laboratory tests has increased as physicians attempt to utilize their time more efficiently by delegating responsibility for taking the history to a physician's assistant or nurse or even by issuing a questionnaire—an approach that I consider to be an undesirable trend insofar as the patient with known or suspected heart disease is concerned. First of all, it must be appreciated that the history remains the richest source of information concerning the patient's illness, and any practice that might diminish the quality of information provided by the history could ultimately impair the quality of care. Second, the physician's attentive and thoughtful taking of a history establishes a bond with the patient that may be valuable later in securing the patient's compliance in following a complex treatment plan, undergoing hospitalization for an intensive diagnostic work-up or a hazardous operation, and, in some instances, accepting that heart disease is not present at all. It is largely through the direct contact established between the patient and physician during the clinical examination that this confidence can best be established.

Taking a history also permits the physician to evaluate the results of diagnostic tests that have strong subjective components, such as the determination of exercise capacity (see p. 272). Perhaps most importantly, a careful history allows the physician to evaluate the impact of the disease, or the fear of the disease, on the patient's total life and to assess the patient's personality, emotion, and stability; often it provides a glimpse of the patient's responsibilities, fears, aspirations, and threshold for discomfort as well as the likelihood of compliance with one or another therapeutic regimen. Whenever possible, the physician should question not only the patient but also relatives or close friends in order to obtain a clearer understanding of the extent of the patient's disability and a broader perspective concerning the impact of the disease on both the patient and the family. (For example, the patient's spouse is more likely than the patient to provide a history of Cheyne-Stokes [periodic] respiration.)

In interpreting the history obtained from a patient with known or suspected heart disease, it must be appreciated that the combination of the widespread fear of cardiovascular disorders and the deep-seated emotional, symbolic, and sometimes even religious connotations concerning this organ's function may, on the one hand, provoke symptoms that mimic those of organic heart disease in persons with normal cardiovascular systems or, on the other, cause so much fear that serious symptoms are repressed or denied by patients with organic heart disease. Functional complaints referable to the cardiovascular system may also develop in patients with organic heart disease. The unraveling of symptoms and signs due to organic heart disease from those which are unrelated is an important and challenging task, and the history is the most valuable tool in carrying out this task.

Technique. Several approaches can be employed successfully in obtaining a medical history. I believe that the patient should first be given the opportunity to relate his or her experiences and complaints. Although time-consuming and likely to include much seemingly irrelevant information, this technique has the advantage of providing considerable information concerning the patient's intelligence and emotional make-up. After the patient has given an account of the illness, the physician should obtain information concerning the onset and chronology of symptoms; their location, quality, and intensity; the precipitating, aggravating, and relieving factors; and the response to therapy.

Of course, a detailed general medical history including the personal past history, occupational history, nutritional history, and review of systems must be obtained. Concern should focus on a past history of rheumatic fever, chorea, venereal disease or exposure to it, thyroid disease, recent dental extractions or manipulations, earlier examinations that showed abnormalities of the cardiovascular system as reflected in restriction from physical activity at school and in rejection for life insurance, employment, or military service. Personal habits such as exercise, cigarette smoking, alcohol intake, and parenteral use of drugs—illicit and otherwise—should be ascertained, and the exact nature of the patient's work should be assessed. The increasing appreciation of the importance of genetic influences in many forms of heart disease (Chap. 47) underscores the importance of the family history. Details of obtaining the family history in a patient with a possible genetic disorder involving the heart are presented on p. 1611.

A cardinal principle of cardiovascular evaluation is that myocardial or coronary function that may be adequate at rest may be inadequate during exertion; therefore, specific attention should be directed to the influence of activity on the patient's symptoms. Thus, a history of chest pain or discomfort and/or undue shortness of breath that appears only during activity is characteristic of heart disease, whereas the opposite pattern, i.e., the appearance of symptoms at rest and their remission during exertion, is observed only rarely in patients with organic heart disease but is more characteristic of functional disorders. In attempting to assess the severity of functional impairment, the extent of activity and the rate at which it is performed before symptoms develop should be determined and related to a detailed consideration of the therapeutic regimen. For example, the complaint of exertional dyspnea after walking slowly up a flight of stairs in a patient on maximal treatment for heart failure denotes far more severe functional disability than does a similar symptom occurring in an untreated patient who has run up a flight of stairs. It is often useful to ask the patient whether a specific activity that now is difficult, such as climbing two flights of stairs, could be accomplished more easily 3, 6, and 12 months earlier.

As the patient relates the history, important nonverbal clues are often provided. The physician should observe the patient's attitude, reactions, and gestures while being questioned, as well as his or her choice of words or emphasis. Tumulty has likened obtaining a meaningful clinical history to playing a game of chess: "The patient makes a statement and based upon its content, and mode of expression, the physician asks a counter-question. One answer stimulates yet another question until the clinician is convinced that he understands precisely all of the circumstances of the patient's illness."

PRINCIPAL SYMPTOMS OF HEART DISEASE

The principal symptoms of heart disease include dyspnea, chest pain or discomfort, syncope, palpitation, edema, cough, hemoptysis, and excess fatigue. Cyanosis is more often a sign rather than a symptom, but it may be a key feature of the history, particularly of patients with congenital heart disease. Without doubt, history-taking is the most valuable technique available for determining whether or not these symptoms are caused by heart disease. Examples of the manner in which these symptoms may serve as a guide to diagnosis are given in the following pages, and reference is made to other portions of the book that contain more detailed information.

DYSPNEA (see also pp. 492 and 1789)

Dyspnea is defined as an abnormally uncomfortable awareness of breathing; it is one of the principal symptoms of cardiac and pulmonary disease.[2] Since dyspnea can be caused by strenuous exertion in healthy subjects and only moderate exertion in those who are normal but unaccustomed to exercise, it should be regarded as abnormal only when it occurs at rest or at a level of physical activity not expected to cause this symptom. Dyspnea is associated with a wide variety of diseases of the heart and lungs, chest wall, and respiratory muscles as well as with anxiety; the history is the most valuable means of establishing the etiology.

The *sudden* development of dyspnea suggests pulmonary embolism, pneumothorax, acute pulmonary edema, pneumonia, or obstruction of a major airway. In contrast, in most forms of *chronic* heart failure, dyspnea progresses slowly over weeks or months. It should be recognized that such a protracted course may also occur in a variety of other unrelated conditions, including obesity, pregnancy, and bilateral pleural effusions. Inspiratory dyspnea suggests obstruction of the upper airways, whereas dyspnea during expiration characterizes obstruction of the lower airways. Exertional dyspnea suggests the presence of organic diseases, such as left ventricular failure or chronic obstructive lung disease, whereas dyspnea developing at rest may occur in pneumothorax or pulmonary embolism or may be functional. Dyspnea that occurs *only* at rest and is absent on exertion is almost invariably functional. A functional origin is suggested when dyspnea, or simply a heightened awareness of breathing, is accompanied by brief stabbing pain in the region of the cardiac apex or prolonged (more than 2 hours) dull chest pain, and is associated with difficulty in getting enough air into the lungs, claustrophobia, or sighing respirations that are relieved by exertion, by taking a few deep breaths, or by sedation. A history of relief of dyspnea by bronchodilators and corticosteroids suggests asthma as the etiology, whereas relief of dyspnea by rest, digitalis, and diuretics suggests left heart failure.

In patients with *heart failure,* dyspnea is a clinical expression of pulmonary venous and capillary hypertension. It occurs either during exertion or, in resting patients, in the recumbent position and is relieved promptly by sitting upright or standing (orthopnea). The *sudden* occurrence of dyspnea in a patient with a history of rheumatic heart disease suggests the development of atrial fibrillation, rupture of chordae tendineae, or pulmonary embolism.

Paroxysmal nocturnal dyspnea is due to interstitial pulmonary edema secondary to left ventricular failure (p. 493). This condition, beginning usually 2 to 5 hours after the onset of sleep and often associated with sweating and wheezing, is frightening to the patient. Paroxysmal nocturnal dyspnea is relieved by the patient's sitting on the side of the bed or getting out of bed. However, a positional change lasting approximately 20 or more minutes may be required to relieve this symptom, whereas simple orthopnea may be relieved in less than 5 minutes after the patient sits upright. Although paroxysmal nocturnal dyspnea secondary to left ventricular failure is usually accompanied by coughing, a careful history often discloses that the dyspnea *precedes* the cough, not vice versa. In contrast, patients with *chronic pulmonary disease* may also awaken at night, but cough and expectoration often precede the dyspnea. These patients also often have a long history of smoking and a chronic cough with sputum production and wheezing and may be able to breathe more easily while leaning forward. Nocturnal dyspnea in patients with pulmonary disease is usually relieved after the patient rids himself of secretions rather than specifically by sitting up. Details of the value and limitations of the history of dyspnea in differentiating between primary diseases of the heart and lungs[2a] are presented on p. 494 and 1790.

Patients with *pulmonary embolism* usually experience sudden dyspnea that may be associated with apprehension, palpitation, hemoptysis, or pleuritic chest pain. The development or intensification of dyspnea, sometimes associated with a feeling of faintness, may be the only complaint of the patient with pulmonary emboli. Dyspnea accompanying thoracic pain occurs in *acute myocardial infarction.* Occasionally dyspnea is an "*anginal equivalent*" (p. 1337), i.e., a symptom secondary to myocardial ischemia that occurs in place of typical anginal discomfort. This form of dyspnea may be closely associated with a sensation of tightness in the chest, is present on exertion or emotional stress, is relieved by rest but not recumbency, has a duration similar to angina (i.e., 2 to 10 minutes), and is usually responsive to nitroglycerin but not to digitalis. The sudden development of dyspnea in the sitting rather than in the lying position, or in any particular position, suggests the possibility of a *myxoma* (p. 1416) or *ball-valve thrombus* in the left atrium. When dyspnea is relieved by squatting, it is caused most commonly by tetralogy of Fallot or a variant thereof (p. 990).

CHEST PAIN OR DISCOMFORT

(Table 1–1; see also pp. 1335 to 1338)

Although chest pain or discomfort is one of the cardinal manifestations of cardiac disease, it is critical to recognize that it may originate not only in the heart but also in (1) a variety of noncardiac intrathoracic structures, such as the aorta, pulmonary artery, bronchopulmonary tree, pleura, mediastinum, esophagus, and diaphragm; (2) the tissues of the neck or thoracic wall, including the skin, thoracic muscles, cervicodorsal spine, costochondral junctions, breasts,

TABLE 1–1 DIFFERENTIAL DIAGNOSIS OF EPISODIC CHEST PAIN RESEMBLING ANGINA PECTORIS

	Duration	Quality	Provocation	Relief	Location	Comment
Effort angina	5–15 minutes	Visceral (pressure)	During effort or emotion	Rest, nitroglycerin	Substernal radiates	First episode vivid
Rest angina	5–15 minutes	Visceral (pressure)	Spontaneous (? with exercise)	Nitroglycerin	Substernal radiates	Often nocturnal
Mitral prolapse	Minutes to hours	Superficial (rarely visceral)	Spontaneous (no pattern)	Time	Left anterior	No pattern, variable character
Esophageal reflux	10 minutes to 1 hour	Visceral	Recumbency, lack of food	Food, antacid	Substernal epigastric	Rarely radiates
Esophageal spasm	5–60 minutes	Visceral	Spontaneous, cold liquids, exercise	Nitroglycerin	Substernal radiates	Mimics angina
Peptic ulcer	Hours	Visceral, burning	Lack of food, "acid" foods	Foods, antacids	Epigastric substernal	
Biliary disease	Hours	Visceral (wax and wane)	Spontaneous, food	Time, analgesia	Epigastric ? radiates	Colic
Cervical disc	Variable (gradually subsides)	Superficial	Head and neck movement, palpation	Time, analgesia	Arm, neck	Not relieved by rest
Hyperventilation	2–3 minutes	Visceral	Emotion tachypnea	Stimulus removal	Substernal	Facial paresthesia
Musculoskeletal	Variable	Superficial	Movement palpation	Time, analgesia	Multiple	Tenderness
Pulmonary	30 minutes +	Visceral (pressure)	Often spontaneous	Rest, time, bronchodilator	Substernal	Dyspneic

Reproduced with permission from Christie, L. G., Jr., and Conti, C. R.: Systematic approach to the evaluation of angina-like chest pain. Am. Heart J. *102*:897, 1981.

sensory nerves, or spinal cord; and (3) subdiaphragmatic organs such as the stomach, duodenum, pancreas, and gallbladder.[3-5] Factitious pain or pain of functional origin may also occur in the chest. Although a wide variety of laboratory tests are available to aid in the differential diagnosis of chest pain, the history is without any question the most valuable mode of examination. In obtaining the history of a patient with chest pain, it is helpful to have a mental checklist and to ask the patient to describe the location, radiation, and character of the pain; what causes and relieves the pain; time relationships, including the duration, frequency, and pattern of recurrence of the pain; and associated symptoms. It is also particularly useful to observe the patient's gestures. Clenching the fist in front of the chest while describing the sensation (Levine's sign) is a strong indication of an ischemic origin for the pain.

Quality. It is important to recognize that angina means *choking*, not pain. Thus, the discomfort of angina often is described not as pain at all but rather as an unpleasant sensation; "pressing," "squeezing," "strangling," "constricting," "bursting," and "burning" are some of the adjectives commonly used to describe this sensation. "A band across the chest" and "a weight in the center of the chest" are other frequent descriptions. Often with severe attacks the discomfort may radiate from the chest to the shoulders, extremities, neck, jaws, and teeth. It is characteristic of angina that the intensity of effort required to incite it seems to vary from day to day and throughout the day in the same patient, but often a careful history will uncover explanations for this, such as meals ingested, weather, emotions, and the like. Patients note frequently that activities that may cause angina in the morning or when first undertaken do not do so later in the day. When the threshold for angina is quite variable and defies any pattern, the possibility that myocardial ischemia is caused by coronary spasm should be considered (p. 1336). Thus, a careful history may indicate not only the cause of the pain (i.e., myocardial ischemia) but can even provide a clue to the mechanism of the ischemia (spasm vs. organic obstruction).

When dyspnea is an "anginal equivalent," the patient may describe the midchest as the site of the shortness of breath, whereas true dyspnea is usually not as well localized. Other anginal equivalents are discomfort limited to areas that are ordinarily sites of secondary radiation, such as the ulnar aspect of the left arm and forearm, lower jaw, teeth, neck, or shoulders, and the development of gas and belching, nausea, "indigestion," dizziness, and diaphoresis. Anginal equivalents above the mandible or below the umbilicus are quite uncommon.

The chest discomfort of *pulmonary hypertension* may be identical to that of typical angina; it is caused either by dilatation of the pulmonary arteries or by right ventricular ischemia. The chest discomfort of *unstable angina* and *acute myocardial infarction* (p. 1278) is similar qualitatively to that of angina pectoris in location and character; however, it usually radiates more widely than does angina and is more severe and therefore is generally referred to as pain by the patient. The discomfort generally develops unrelated to unusual effort or emotional stress, often with the patient at rest, or even sleeping. Usually nitroglycerin does not provide complete or lasting relief.

Acute pericarditis (p. 1474) is frequently preceded by a history of a viral upper respiratory infection. The inflammation causes pain that is sharper than is anginal discomfort, is more left-sided than central, and is often referred to the neck or flank. The pain of pericarditis lasts for hours and is little affected by effort but often aggravated by breathing, turning in bed, swallowing, or twisting the body; unlike angina, the pain may lessen when the patient sits up and leans forward.

Aortic dissection (p. 1548) is suggested by persistent pain with radiation to the back and into the lumbar region in an individual with a history of hypertension. An expanding *thoracic aortic aneurysm* may erode the vertebral bodies and cause localized, severe, boring pain that is usually worse at night. An aneurysmally enlarged left atrium in patients with mitral valve disease rarely causes chest pain; instead, patients commonly complain of discomfort in the back or right side of the chest that intensifies on exertion.

Chest-wall pain may be due to *costochondritis* or *myositis* with local costochondral or muscle tenderness, which may be aggravated by moving or coughing. It may also accompany or follow herpes zoster, chest injury, or *Tietze's syndrome* (i.e., discomfort localized in swelling of the costochondral and costosternal joints, which are painful on palpation).

Functional or *psychogenic chest pain* may be one feature of an anxiety state, also called Da Costa's syndrome or neurocirculatory asthenia. It is localized typically to the area of the cardiac apex and consists of a dull, persistent ache that lasts for hours and is often accentuated by or alternates with attacks of sharp, lancinating stabs of inframammary pain of one or two seconds' duration. The condition may occur with emotional strain and fatigue, bears little relation to exertion, and may be accompanied by precordial tenderness. Attacks are usually associated with palpitation, hyperventilation, dyspnea, generalized weakness, and other signs of emotional instability or depression. The pain may not be completely relieved by any medication other than analgesics, but it is partially attenuated by many types of interventions, including rest, exertion, tranquilizers, and placebos. Therefore, in contrast to ischemic pain, functional pain is more likely to show variable responses to interventions on different occasions. Since functional chest pain is often preceded by hyperventilation, which in turn may cause increased muscle tension and be responsible for diffuse chest tightness, some instances of so-called functional chest pain may, in fact, have an organic basis. Chest pain is common in patients with *prolapse of the mitral valve* (p. 1091). The pain varies considerably among patients; it may be similar to that of classic angina pectoris or may resemble the chest pain of neurocirculatory asthenia described above.

Patients who have angina pectoris or have suffered a myocardial infarction often become "heart conscious" and become acutely aware of every kind of chest discomfort. It is particularly challenging to separate organic from functional chest pain in these patients, and the history provides the principal means of determining the extent to which these patients are limited by myocardial ischemia.

Location. Embryonically the heart is a midline viscus; thus, cardiac ischemia produces anginal symptoms that are characteristically felt across both sides of the chest or chiefly substernally. Occasional patients complain of discomfort only to the left or rarely right of the midline. If the pain or discomfort can be localized to the skin or superficial structures, it generally arises from the chest wall. Thus, if the patient can point directly to the site of discomfort, it is usually not angina pectoris, which, like other symptoms arising in deeper structures, tends to be diffuse and eludes precise localization. Pain under or in the region of the left nipple is usually noncardiac in origin and may be functional or due to osteoarthritis, gaseous distention of the stomach, or the splenic flexure syndrome. Although pain due to myocardial ischemia often radiates to the left arm or left shoulder, such radiation also occurs in pericarditis and disorders of the cervical spine. Chest pain that radiates to the neck and jaw occurs in pericarditis as well as in myocardial ischemia. Dissection of the aorta or enlargement of an aortic aneurysm produces pain in the *back* rather than in the front of the chest.

Duration. The duration of the pain is important in determining its etiology. Anginal pain is relatively short, usually lasting from 2 to 10 minutes. However, if the pain is very brief, i.e., a momentary, lancinating, sharp pain, or discomfort that lasts less than 30 seconds, angina can usually be excluded; such a short duration points instead to musculoskeletal pain, pain due to hiatal hernia, or functional pain. Chest pain lasting hours may be seen with acute myocardial infarction, pericarditis, aortic dissection, musculoskeletal disease, herpes zoster, and anxiety.

Precipitating and Aggravating Factors. Angina pectoris occurs characteristically on exertion, particularly when hurrying or walking on an upgrade. Thus, the development of chest discomfort or pain when walking, typically in the cold and against a wind, and after a heavy meal, is characteristic of angina pectoris. An exception is *Prinzmetal's (variant) angina,* which characteristically occurs at rest (p. 1360) and may or may not be affected by exertion; however, it must be remembered that classic (nonvariant) angina, although most often precipitated by effort, not uncommonly may be experienced at rest, as in unstable angina; exertion intensifies the discomfort. Emotional stress also may precipitate angina. Chest pain that occurs after protracted vomiting may be due to the *Mallory-Weiss syndrome,* i.e., a tear in the lower portion of the esophagus. Pain that occurs while bending over is often radicular and may be associated with *osteoarthritis* of the cervical or upper thoracic spine. Chest pain occurring when moving the neck may be due to a *herniated intervertebral disk,* whereas substernal and epigastric discomfort during swallowing may be due to *esophageal spasm. Esophagitis* with or without a hiatal hernia may also be associated with substernal or epigastric burning pain that is brought on by eating or lying down after meals and that may be relieved with antacids; it is often accompanied by acid reflux into the mouth (water brash). Chest pain aggravated by swallowing may also be due to acute pericarditis, whereas pain intensified by coughing may be due to pericarditis, bronchitis, or pleurisy or may be of radicular origin. Pain that occurs when the patient is exhausted is often functional. *Congenital absence of the pericardium* (p. 1517) produces chest pain that is relieved by changing position in bed, is brought on by lying on the left side, and lasts a few seconds. Pain due to the *scalenus anticus (thoracic outlet) syndrome* may be confused with angina because it is often associated with paresthesias along the ulnar distribution of the arm and forearm. However, in contrast to angina, not only is it typically precipitated by abduction of the arm, lifting a weight, or working with the hands above the shoulders, but it is not brought on by walking.

Relief of Pain. Nitroglycerin and rest characteristically relieve the discomfort of angina in approximately 2 to 5 minutes. If more than 10 minutes transpire before relief, the diagnosis of chronic stable angina becomes questionable and instead suggests unstable angina, acute myocardial infarction, or pain not caused by myocardial ischemia at all. Although nitroglycerin commonly relieves the pain of angina pectoris, the discomfort of esophageal spasm and esophagitis may also be relieved by this drug. Angina pectoris is alleviated by quiet standing or sitting; the recumbent position may not relieve angina. Chest pain secondary to *acute pericarditis* is characteristically relieved by leaning forward, whereas pain that is relieved by food or antacids may be due to *peptic ulcer disease* or esophagitis. Pain that is alleviated by holding the breath in deep expiration is commonly due to *pleurisy.* Some patients with highly nonspecific angina pectoris as well as others with upper gastrointestinal disease or anxiety report relief of symptoms after belching.

Accompanying Symptoms. The physician should always be respectful of the patient who reports the presence of chest pain and profuse sweating. This combination of symptoms frequently signals a serious disorder, often acute myocardial infarction. Severe chest pain accompanied by nausea and vomiting is also often due to myocardial infarction. The latter diagnosis, as well as pneumothorax or pulmonary embolism, is suggested when pain is associated with shortness of breath. Chest pain accompanied by palpitation may be due to the acute myocardial ischemia that results from a tachyarrhythmia-induced increase in myocardial oxygen consumption in the presence of coronary artery disease. Chest pain accompanied by hemoptysis suggests pulmonary embolism with infarction or lung tumor, whereas pain accompanied by fever occurs in pneumonia, pleurisy, and pericarditis. Functional pain is commonly accompanied by frequent sighing, anxiety, or depression.

CYANOSIS (see also p. 949)

Cyanosis is a bluish discoloration of the skin and mucous membranes resulting from an increased amount of reduced hemoglobin or of abnormal hemoglobin pigments in the blood perfusing these areas. There are two principal forms of cyanosis: (1) *central cyanosis,* characterized by decreased arterial oxygen saturation due to right-to-left shunting of blood or impaired pulmonary function, and (2) *peripheral cyanosis,* most commmonly secondary to cutaneous vasoconstriction due to a low cardiac output or exposure to cold air or water; if peripheral cyanosis is localized to an extremity, arterial or venous obstruction should be suspected. A history of cyanosis localized to the hands suggests *Raynaud's phenomenon.* Central cyanosis due to congenital heart disease or pulmonary disease characteristically worsens during exertion, whereas the resting peripheral cyanosis of congestive heart failure may be accentuated only slightly, if at all, during exertion.

Cyanosis usually becomes apparent at a mean capillary concentration of 4 gm/dl reduced hemoglobin (or 0.5 gm/dl methemoglobin). In general, a history of cyanosis in Caucasians is rarely elicited unless arterial saturation is 85 per cent or less; in pigmented races arterial saturation has to drop far lower before cyanosis is perceptible. Cyanosis generally occurs in patients with *congenital heart disease* when the volume of a right-to-left shunt exceeds 25 percent of the left ventricular output. Since it is the *absolute* quantity of reduced hemoglobin in the blood that is responsible for cyanosis, the higher the total hemoglobin content, the greater the tendency toward cyanosis; thus, patients with marked polycythemia become cyanotic at higher levels of arterial oxygen saturation than do patients with normal hematocrit values, and cyanosis may be absent in patients with severe anemia despite marked arterial desaturation.

Although a history of cyanosis beginning in infancy suggests a congenital cardiac malformation with a right-to-left shunt, *hereditary methemoglobinemia* is another, albeit rare, cause of congenital cyanosis; the diagnosis of this condition is supported by a family history of cyanosis in the absence of heart disease.

A history of cyanosis limited to the neonatal period suggests the diagnosis of atrial septal defect with transient right-to-left shunting or, more commonly, pulmonary parenchymal disease or central nervous system depression. Cyanosis beginning at age 1 to 3 months may be reported when spontaneous closure of a patent ductus arteriosus unmasks the reduction of pulmonary blood flow in the presence of right-sided obstructive cardiac anomalies (p. 995). If cyanosis appears at age 6 months or later in childhood, it may be due to the development or progression of obstruction to right ventricular outflow in patients with ventricular septal defect. Development of cyanosis between ages 5 and 15 years suggests an Eisenmenger's reaction with right-to-left shunting as a consequence of a progressive increase in pulmonary vascular resistance (p. 964).

SYNCOPE (see also p. 932)

Syncope, which may be defined as a loss of consciousness, results most commonly from reduced perfusion of the brain. This, in turn, may be due to a reduction of systemic vascular resistance, an elevation of cerebrovascular resistance, hypovolemia, a variety of arrhythmias, and any other condition that causes a sudden reduction of cardiac output and therefore of cerebral blood flow. It should be distinguished from emotional disturbances in which hyperventilation, anxiety, and hysterical fainting are prominent and from seizure disorders, especially petit mal epilepsy.

The history is extremely valuable in the differential diagnosis of syncope (Table 28–1, p. 929). Several daily attacks of loss of consciousness suggest (1) Stokes-Adams attacks, i.e., transient asystole or ventricular fibrillation in the presence of atrioventricular block; (2) other cardiac arrhythmias (Chap. 21); or (3) epilepsy. These diagnoses are suggested when the loss of consciousness is abrupt and occurs over 1 or 2 seconds; a more gradual onset suggests vasodepressor syncope (i.e., the common faint), syncope due to hyperventilation or, much less commonly, hypoglycemia. Cardiac syncope is often of gradual onset without aura, and is usually *not* associated with convulsive movements, urinary incontinence, and a postictal confusional state. Patients with epilepsy often have a prodromal aura preceding the seizure. Injury from falling is common, as is urinary incontinence and a postictal confusional state, associated with headache and drowsiness. Unconsciousness for a few seconds suggests vasodepressor syncope or syncope secondary to postural hypotension, whereas a longer period suggests aortic stenosis or hyperventilation. *Hysterical fainting* is usually not accompanied by any untoward display of anxiety or change in pulse, blood pressure, or skin color, and there may be a question about whether any true loss of consciousness occurred. It is often associated with paresthesias of the hands or face, hyperventilation, dyspnea, chest pain, and feelings of acute anxiety.

Syncope independent of body position suggests Stokes-Adams attacks, hyperventilation, or epilepsy, whereas syncope of other etiologies usually occurs in the upright position. Syncope occurring upon bending, leaning, or assuming a particular body position should raise the possibility of a left atrial myxoma (p. 1460) or a ball-valve thrombus. Since syncope is an unusual feature of mitral stenosis, when it does occur in a patient thought to have this condition, the possibility of left atrial *myxoma* or *ball-valve thrombus* should be considered. Syncope occurring during or immediately following exertion suggests *aortic stenosis, hypertrophic obstructive cardiomyopathy,* or *primary pulmonary hypertension.* Syncope is rare in patients with angina pectoris unless the latter is secondary to aortic stenosis or hypertrophic obstructive cardiomyopathy. Syncope following insulin administration suggests a hypoglycemic etiology; syncope several hours after eating is characteristic of reactive hypoglycemia. Loss of consciousness following an emotional stress suggests that it is vasodepressor syncope or secondary to hyperventilation.

Patients with *vasodepressor syncope* often have a long history of fainting, commonly associated with emotional or painful stimuli. This, the most usual form of syncope, may be precipitated by the sight or loss of blood or by physical or emotional stress; it can be averted by promptly lying down, and it is characteristically preceded by symptoms of autonomic hyperactivity such as dim vision, giddiness, yawning, sweating, and nausea (p. 934). Syncope secondary to *cerebrovascular disturbance* is often preceded by aphasia, unilateral weakness, or confusion. A history of fainting following sudden movements of the head, shaving the neck, or wearing a tight collar suggests carotid sinus syncope (p. 932). Syncope associated with chest pain may be secondary to massive acute myocardial infarction or infarction associated with arrhythmias; occasionally, following recovery of consciousness, the associated chest pain may be forgotten, and the infarction may be recognized only by means of characteristic changes in serum enzymes and the electrocardiogram.

Consciousness is regained quite promptly in syncope of cardiovascular origin but more slowly with epilepsy. When consciousness is regained after vasodepressor syncope, the patient is usually pale and diaphoretic with a slow heart rate, whereas after a Stokes-Adams attack, the face is often flushed and there may actually be cardiac acceleration. Patients who sustain an injury when falling to the ground during a fainting spell usually have epilepsy or occasionally syncope of cardiac origin, but they rarely have sustained physical damage during reported unconsciousness related to emotional disturbance.

A *family history of syncope* or near syncope can often be elicited in patients with hypertrophic obstructive cardiomyopathy or ventricular tachyarrhythmias associated with Q-T prolongation (pp. 727 and 1626). A family history of epilepsy is positive in approximately 4 per cent of patients with convulsive disorders. Syncope associated with progressive intensification of cyanosis in an infant or child with cyanotic congenital heart disease is likely to be due to cerebral anoxia as a consequence of an increase in the right-to-left shunt, secondary to an increase in the obstruction to right ventricular outflow or a reduction in systemic vascular resistance (p. 950). A history of syncope during childhood suggests the possibility of a cardiovascular anomaly obstructing left ventricular outflow—valvular, supravalvular, or subvalvular aortic stenosis. In patients with hypertrophic obstructive cardiomyopathy, syncope is often post-tussive and occurs in the erect position, when arising suddenly, after standing erect for long periods, and during or immediately after cessation of exertion.

Patients with syncope secondary to *orthostatic hypotension* often have a history of drug therapy for hypertension or of abnormalities of autonomic function, such as impotence, disturbances of sphincter function, peripheral neuropathy, and anhidrosis (p. 930). When syncope is secondary to hypovolemia, there is often a history of melena, anemia, menorrhagia, or treatment with anticoagulants. Syncope associated with *cerebrovascular insufficiency* is frequently associated with a history of unilateral blindness, weakness, paresthesias, or memory defects.

PALPITATION

This common symptom is defined as an unpleasant awareness of the beating of the heart. It may be brought about by a variety of disorders involving changes in cardiac rhythm or rate, including all forms of tachycardia, ectopic beats, compensatory pauses, augmented stroke volume due to valvular regurgitation, hyperkinetic (high–cardiac output) states, and the sudden onset of bradycardia. In the case of premature contractions the patient is more commonly aware of the postextrasystolic beat than of the premature beat itself, and it appears that it is the motion of the heart within the chest that is perceived rather than the increase in cardiac contractility. This explains why palpitation is not a characteristic feature of aortic or pulmonic stenosis or of severe systemic or pulmonary hypertension, conditions characterized by an increased force of cardiac contraction.

When episodes of palpitation last for an instant, they are described as "skipped beats" or a "flopping sensation" in the chest and most commonly are due to extrasystoles. On the other hand, the sensation that the heart has "stopped beating" often correlates with the compensatory pause following a premature contraction. Palpitation characterized by a slow heart rate may be due to atrioventricular block or sinus node disease. When palpitation begins and ends abruptly, it is often due to a paroxysmal tachycardia such as paroxysmal atrial or junctional tachycardia, atrial flutter, or fibrillation, whereas a gradual onset and cessation of the attack suggest sinus tachycardia and/or an anxiety state. A history of chaotic rapid heart action suggests the diagnosis of atrial fibrillation; fleeting and repetitive palpitation suggests multiple ectopic beats. A history of multiple paroxysms of tachycardia, followed by palpitation that occurs only with effort or excitement suggests paroxysmal atrial fibrillation that has become permanent —the palpitation being experienced only when the ventricular rate rises. Some patients have taken their pulse during palpitation or have asked a companion to do so. A rate between 100 and 140 beats/min suggests sinus tachycardia, a rate of approximately 150 beats/min suggests *atrial flutter,* and a rate exceeding 160 beats/min suggests *paroxysmal supraventricular tachycardia.*

A history of palpitation during or after strenuous physical activities is normal, whereas palpitation during mild exertion suggests the presence of heart failure, anemia, or thyrotoxicosis, or that the individual is severely "out of condition." A feeling of forceful heart action accompanied by throbbing in the neck suggests aortic regurgitation. When palpitation can be relieved suddenly by stooping, breathholding, or induced gagging or vomiting, i.e., by vagal maneuvers, the diagnosis of paroxysmal supraventricular tachycardia is suggested. A history of syncope following an episode of palpitation suggests either asystole or severe bradycardia following the termination of a tachyarrhythmia or a Stokes-Adams attack. A history of palpitation associated with anxiety, a lump in the throat, dizziness, and tingling in the hands and face suggests sinus tachycardia accompanying an anxiety state with hyperventilation. Tachycardia associated with angina suggests myocardial ischemia that has been precipitated by increased oxygen demands induced by the rapid heart rate.

As an adjunct to the history, it may be possible to ascertain the rhythm responsible for the palpitation by tapping the finger on the patient's chest in a variety of rhythms and asking the patient to identify the pattern which most closely resembles the abnormal feeling.

In many individuals no obvious cause for palpitation emerges despite careful work-up, including a correlation between episodes of palpitation with a simultaneously recorded ambulatory electrocardiogram (p. 632) or an electrocardiogram recorded by transtelephonic transmission. Anxiety is responsible for the symptom in many such patients, but some of them have known heart disease and may be receiving a vasodilator for the treatment of hypertension or nifedipine for the treatment of myocardial ischemia. In these patients palpitation may be due to postural hypotension resulting in reflex cardiac acceleration.

EDEMA (see also p. 497)

Localization of edema is helpful in elucidating its etiology. Thus a history of edema of the legs that is most pronounced in the evening is characteristic of heart failure or bilateral chronic venous insufficiency. In most patients any visible edema of both lower extremities is preceded by a weight gain of at least 7 to 10 lb. As cardiac edema progresses, it usually ascends to involve the legs, thighs, genitals, and abdominal wall. In patients with heart failure who remain chiefly in bed, the edema localizes particularly in the sacral area. Edema located in both the abdomen

often associated with a history of postural hypotension and peripheral neuropathy. *Hypertrophic cardiomyopathy* (p. 1409), which is generally transmitted as an autosomal dominant trait, is often associated with a family history of this condition and sometimes with a family history of sudden death. The characteristic symptoms are angina, dyspnea, and syncope, which are often intensified paradoxically by digitalis and which occur during or immediately after exercise.

HIGH-OUTPUT HEART FAILURE

Patients with symptoms of heart failure (breathlessness and excess fluid accumulation) with warm extremities often have *high-output heart failure* (Chap. 24). They should be questioned about a history of anemia and of its common causes and accompaniments, such as menorrhagia, melena, peptic ulcer, hemorrhoids, sickle cell disease, and the neurological manifestations of vitamin B_{12} deficiency. Also, in such patients an attempt should be made to elicit a history of thyrotoxicosis (p. 1727) (weight loss, polyphagia, diarrhea, diaphoresis, heat intolerance, nervousness, breathlessness, muscle weakness, and goiter). Patients with beriberi heart disease responsible for high-output heart failure often present with a history characteristic of peripheral neuritis, alcoholism, poor eating habits, diet fads, or upper gastrointestinal surgery.

Patients with chronic *cor pulmonale* (see Chap. 46) frequently have a history of smoking, chronic cough and sputum production, dyspnea, and wheezing relieved by bronchodilators. Alternatively, they may present with a history of pulmonary emboli, phlebitis, and the sudden development of dyspnea at rest with palpitations, pleuritic chest pain, and, in the case of massive infarction, syncope.

PERICARDITIS AND ENDOCARDITIS

In patients in whom *pericarditis* or *cardiac tamponade* is suspected (Chap. 43), an attempt should be made to elicit a history of chest trauma, neoplastic disease of the chest with or without extensive radiation, myxedema, scleroderma, a recent viral infection, tuberculosis, or contact with tuberculous patients. The sequence of development of abdominal swelling, ankle edema, and dyspnea should be determined, since ascites often precedes edema, which in turn may precede exertional dyspnea in patients with chronic constrictive pericarditis. A history of joint symptoms with a face rash suggests the possibility of systemic lupus erythematosus (SLE), an important cause of pericarditis, and it should be recalled that procainamide, hydralazine, and isoniazid can produce an SLE-like syndrome (p. 1660).

The diagnosis of *infective endocarditis* is suggested by a history of fever, severe night sweats, anorexia and weight loss, and embolic phenomena expressed as hematuria, back pain, petechiae, tender finger pads, and a cerebrovascular accident (p. 1149).

Drug-Induced Heart Disease. The increasing appreciation that a wide variety of cardiac abnormalities can be induced by drugs makes a meticulous history of drug intake of great importance.[6] Catecholamines, whether administered exogenously or when secreted by a pheochromocytoma (p. 1734), may produce a myocarditis and arrhythmias. Digitalis glycosides can be responsible for a variety of tachy- and bradyarrhythmias as well as gastrointestinal, visual, and central nervous system disturbances (p. 525). Quinidine may cause Q-T prolongation, ventricular tachycardia of the *torsade de pointes* variety, syncope, and sudden death, presumably due to ventricular fibrillation (p.

TABLE 1–2 A COMPARISON OF THREE METHODS OF ASSESSING CARDIOVASCULAR DISABILITY

Class	New York Heart Association Functional Classification	Canadian Cardiovascular Society Functional Classification	Specific Activity Scale
I	Patients with cardiac disease but without resulting limitations of physical activity. Ordinary physical activity does not cause undue fatigue, palpitation, dyspnea, or anginal pain.	Ordinary physical activity, such as walking and climbing stairs, does not cause angina. Angina with strenuous or rapid or prolonged exertion at work or recreation.	Patients can perform to completion any activity requiring ≥ 7 metabolic equivalents, e.g., can carry 24 lb up eight steps; carry objects that weigh 80 lb; do outdoor work (shovel snow, spade soil); do recreational activities (skiing, basketball, squash, handball, jog/walk 5 mph).
II	Patients with cardiac disease resulting in slight limitation of physical activity. They are comfortable at rest. Ordinary physical activity results in fatigue, palpitation, dyspnea, or anginal pain.	Slight limitation of ordinary activity. Walking or climbing stairs rapidly, walking uphill, walking or stair climbing after meals, in cold, in wind, or when under emotional stress, or only during the few hours after awakening. Walking more than two blocks on the level and climbing more than one flight of ordinary stairs at a normal pace and in normal conditions.	Patient can perform to completion any activity requiring ≥ 5 metabolic equivalents but cannot and does not perform to completion activities requiring ≥ 7 metabolic equivalents, e.g., have sexual intercourse without stopping, garden, rake, weed, roller skate, dance fox trot, walk at 4 mph on level ground.
III	Patients with cardiac disease resulting in marked limitation of physical activity. They are comfortable at rest. Less than ordinary physical activity causes fatigue, palpitation, dyspnea, or anginal pain.	Marked limitation of ordinary physical activity. Walking one to two block on the level and climbing more than one flight in normal conditions.	Patient can perform to completion any activity requiring ≥ 2 metabolic equivalents but cannot and does not perform to completion any activities requiring ≥ 5 metabolic equivalents, e.g., shower without stopping, strip and make bed, clean windows, walk 2.5 mph, bowl, play golf, dress without stopping.
IV	Patient with cardiac disease resulting in inability to carry on any physical activity without discomfort. Symptoms of cardiac insufficiency or of the anginal syndrome may be present even at rest. If any physical activity is undertaken, discomfort is increased.	Inability to carry on any physical activity without discomfort—anginal syndrome *may be* present at rest.	Patient cannot or does not perform to completion activities requiring ≥ 2 metabolic equivalents. *Cannot* carry out activities listed above (Specific Activity Scale, Class III).

Reproduced by permission of the American Heart Association, Inc., from Goldman L. et al. Comparative reproducibility and validity of systems for assessing cardiovascular functional class: Advantages of a new specific activity scale. Circulation *64*: 1227, 1981.

7. *Inherited connective tissue disord*
syndrome (p. 1665), osteogenesis in
Ehlers-Danlos syndrome (p. 1668), pse
cum (p. 1669), associated with aortic
and regurgitation, mitral valve prola
disease, and pericarditis; Hurler's sy
disorders of mucopolysaccharide meta
sociated with arrhythmias, valvular di
ure.

8. *Collagen vascular diseases:* system
sus (p. 1660) (valvulitis, myocarditis, a
kylosing spondylitis (p. 1656) (diseas
aortic valve), rheumatoid arthritis (p
and valve disease), vasculitis (p. 1660
and myocarditis), polymyositis (p.
pericarditis, and myocarditis).

9. *Sarcoidosis* (p. 1426) associated wi
myopathy and arrhythmias.

10. *Chronic hemolytic anemia* (p. 16
dilatation and myocarditis secondary
mosiderosis.

In patients in whom these and relate
are present or suspected, the physical
be conducted so as to allow recognit
disorder and evaluation of the presence
diovascular involvement.

THE GENERAL EXAMIN

Although one can employ a variety
rying out the physical examination, I
with an assessment of the general ap
tient and then employing the regiona
with the head and ending with the lo
desirable, whenever possible, to exami
examining table or bed whose head se
Examination in a quiet room at a com
and in daylight is optimal.

GENERAL APPEARAN

An assessment of the patient's ge
usually begun with a detailed inspecti
the history is being obtained.[1,1a] The g
pearance of the patient, the skin color,
pallor or cyanosis should be noted, as
of shortness of breath, orthopnea,
Stokes) respiration (p. 499), and dis
veins. If the patient is in pain, is he c
(typical of angina pectoris); moving ab
more comfortable position (characteris
dial infarction); or most comfortable s
failure) or leaning forward (pericarditis
will also reveal whether the patient's
with each heart beat and whether
(bounding arterial pulsations, as oc
stroke volume of severe aortic regurgi
fistula, or complete atrioventricular b
the head, neck, and upper extremities.
malnutrition, and cachexia, which occ

729). Paradoxically the administration of antiarrhythmic drugs is one of the major causes of serious cardiac arrhythmias.[7]

Disopyramide (p. 659), beta-adrenergic blockers (p. 1349), and the calcium channel blocker verapamil (p. 1351) may depress ventricular performance, and in patients with ventricular dysfunction these drugs may intensify heart failure. Alcohol is also a potent myocardial depressant and may be responsible for the development of a cardiomyopathy (p. 1406), arrhythmias, and possibly sudden death. Tricyclic antidepressants may cause orthostatic hypotension and arrhythmias (p. 1838). Lithium, also used in the treatment of psychiatric disorders, can aggravate preexisting cardiac arrhythmias, particularly in patients with heart failure in whom the renal clearance of this ion is impaired.

The anthracycline compounds doxorubicin (Adriamycin) and daunorubicin, which are widely used because of their broad spectrum of activity against various tumors, may cause or intensify left ventricular failure, arrhythmias, myocarditis, and pericarditis (p. 1690). Cyclophosphamide, an antineoplastic alkylating agent, may also cause left ventricular dysfunction. Although not a drug, radiation may cause acute and chronic pericarditis (p. 1509), a pancarditis (p. 1445), and coronary artery disease; further, it may enhance the aforementioned cardiotoxic effects of the anthracyclines.

ASSESSING CARDIOVASCULAR DISABILITY
(Table 1–2)

One of the greatest values of the history is in categorizing the *degree* of cardiovascular disability, so that a given patient's status can be followed over time, the effects of a therapeutic intervention assessed, and patients compared with one another. The Criteria Committee of the New York Heart Association have provided a widely used classification that relates symptoms to "ordinary" activity.[8] The term "ordinary," of course, is subject to varying interpretation, as are terms such as "undue fatigue" that are used in this classification, and this has limited its accuracy and reproducibility. Somewhat more detailed and specific criteria were provided by the Canadian Cardiovascular Society,[9] but this classification and grading is limited to patients with angina pectoris. Recently, Goldman et al.[10] have developed a new specific activity scale in which classification is based on the estimated metabolic cost of various activities. Although this specific activity scale has not yet been widely used, it appears to be more reproducible and to be a better predictor of exercise tolerance than either the New York Heart Association Classification or the Canadian Cardiovascular Society Criteria.

References

1. Sandler, G.: The importance of the history in the medical clinic and the cost of unnecessary tests. Am. Heart J. *100*:928, 1980.
2. Fishman, A. P.: The first approach to the patient with respiratory signs and symptoms. *In* Fishman, A. P. (ed.): Pulmonary Diseases and Disorders. New York, McGraw-Hill Book Co., 1980, pp. 3–28.

2a. Loke, J.: Distinguishing cardiac versus pulmonary limitation in exercise performance. Chest *83*:441, 1983.

3. Levene, D. L., Billings, R. F., Davies, G. M., Edmeads, J., and Saibil, F. G. (eds.): Chest Pain: An Integrated Diagnostic Approach. Philadelphia, Lea and Febiger, 1977.
4. Levine, H. J.: Difficult problems in the diagnosis of chest pain. Am. Heart J. *100*:108, 1980.
5. Christie, L. G., and Conti, C. R.: Systematic approach to the evaluation of angina-like chest pain. Am. Heart J. *102*:897, 1981.
6. Bristow, M. R. (ed.): Drug-Induced Heart Disease. Amsterdam, Elsevier, 1980, 476 pp.
7. Velebit, V., Podrid, P., Lown, B., Cohen, B. M., and Graboys, T. B.: Aggravation and provocation of ventricular arrhythmias by antiarrhythmic drugs. Circulation *65*:880, 1982.
8. The Criteria Committee of the New York Heart Association: Diseases of the Heart and Blood Vessels; Nomenclature and Criteria for Diagnosis, 6th ed. Boston, Little, Brown and Co., 1964.
9. Campeau, L.: Grading of angina pectoris. Circulation *54*:522, 1975.
10. Goldman, L., Hashimoto, B., Cook, E. F., and Loscalzo, A.: Comparative reproducibility and validity of systems for assessing cardiovascular functional class: Advantages of a new specific activity scale. Circulation *64*:1227, 1981.

GENERAL REFERENCES

Braunwald, E.: Alterations in circulatory and respiratory function. *In* Petersdorf, R. G., et al. (eds.): Harrison's Principles of Internal Medicine, 10th ed. New York, McGraw-Hill Book Co., 1983, pp. 155–181.

Constant, J.: The evolving check list in history-taking. *In* Bedside Cardiology, 2nd ed. Boston, Little, Brown and Co., 1976, pp. 1–22.

Dressler, W.: Clinical Aids in Cardiac Diagnosis. New York, Grune and Stratton, 1970.

Fowler, N. O.: The history in cardiac diagnosis. *In* Fowler, N. O. (ed.): Cardiac Diagnosis and Treatment, 3rd ed. Hagerstown, Md., Harper and Row, 1980, pp. 23–29.

Kraytman, J.: Cardiorespiratory system. *In* The Complete Patient History. New York, McGraw-Hill Book Co., 1979, pp. 11–112.

Oram, S.: Clinical examination. *In* Clinical Heart Disease, 2nd ed. London, William Heinemann, 1981, pp. 45–60.

Parkinson, J.: Cardiac symptoms. Ann. Intern. Med. *35*:499, 1951.

Tumulty, P. A.: Obtaining the history. *In* The Effective Clinician. Philadelphia, W. B. Saunders Co., 1973, pp. 17–28.

White, P. D.: Clues in the Diagnosis and Treatment of Heart Disease. Springfield, Ill., Charles C Thomas, 1955.

Wood, P.: The chief symptoms of heart failure. *In* Diseases of the Heart and Circulation, 3rd ed. Philadelphia, J. B. Lippincott, 1968, pp. 1–25.

2

T

E

THE GENERAL EXAMINA

Two of the most common pitfalls in cine are the failure by the cardiologis fects of systemic illnesses on the cardi the failure by the noncardiologist to manifestations of systemic illnesses th on other organ systems. In order to patients known to have or suspected ease require not only a detailed exami vascular system but a meticulou examination as well. For example, the with previously stable rheumatic valv tery disease may suddenly deteriorate progression of the underlying cardiac because of the development of an unr as a bleeding peptic ulcer or a maligna change in the patient's cardiac conditi sification of angina or dyspnea, ma presence of the other disorder.

The presence of cardiac disease sho search for frequent noncardiac concor riosclerosis of the cerebral vessels and lower extremities and aorta in patients

Editor's Note: Examination of the cardiova spection and palpation of the arterial and veno as well as auscultation of the heart. The findin amination can be aided enormously by graphic carrying out the cardiovascular examination an findings are presented in this chapter and in chapter focuses on the findings elicited by ph Chapters 3 and 4 deal primarily with the graph ings. The three chapters should be considered a covered are similar and the material does not separation between physical and graphic modes gree of overlap in content among these chapters

In *Down's syndrome* (mongolism, trisomy 21), which is often associated with congenital heart disease (p. 1613), there is mental deficiency, a prominent medial epicanthus, and a large, often protruding tongue, low-set ears, a poorly formed nasal bridge, and hypoplastic mandible. Adenoma sebaceum of the face may be accompanied by a cardiac *rhabdomyoma* (p. 1461). Approximately 5 per cent of infants with congenital heart disease (most commonly ventricular septal defect) have the so-called cardiofacial syndrome, characterized by unilateral partial lower facial weakness, which may become apparent only when the patient cries.[5] In the so-called *velocardiofacial syndrome*,[6] a cleft of the secondary palate, a long vertical face, and deep overbite with retruded mandible accompany congenital heart disease, most commonly a ventricular septal defect.

Hypertelorism (widely set eyes) is observed in patients with *Noonan's syndrome*,[7] who often have pulmonic stenosis (Figure 47–1, p. 1615); *Turner's syndrome*, often accompanied by coarctation of the aorta (p. 1614); the *multiple lentigines syndrome* (also termed LEOPARD syndrome) (Figure 47–3, p. 1616), often associated with pulmonic stenosis and hypertrophic cardiomyopathy;[8] and *Hurler's syndrome* (arrhythmias and valvular regurgitation) (p. 1670). The facies of one group of patients with a nonfamilial type of *supravalvular aortic stenosis* and mental retardation is quite characteristic (see Figure 29–31, p. 981) and includes hypertelorism; a broad, high forehead; strabismus and epicanthal folds; low-set ears; upturned nose; a long upper lip and wide mouth; and hypoplasia of the mandible, with a pointed chin, small teeth, and dental deformities[9] (p. 982). Patients with *stenosis of the pulmonary artery* and/or its branches often have an unusual facial appearance characterized by a large mouth, a blunt upturned nose, wide-set eyes, internal strabismas, and malformed teeth.[1]

Scleroderma, which can cause several forms of heart disease (p. 1663), can often be recognized in the face, where skin becomes firm, thickened, and leathery in texture and is tightly bound to the underlying subcutaneous tissues. In the late stages of this disease the skin is atrophic, and there is immobility, particularly around the mouth. Patients with *systemic lupus erythematosus* (p. 1660) may present with a butterfly rash on the face. *Acromegaly* (p. 1722) is associated with enlargement of the head, coarse facial features, prognathism, and macroglossia. *Cushing's syndrome*, in which hypertension is often present (p. 1732), is characterized by a moon facies, hirsutism, and acne. *Paget's disease* of bone, which may be associated with a high cardiac output state (p. 817), is characterized by enlargement of the skull. Episodic facial flushing occurs in patients with *carcinoid tumors* (p. 1430) and *pheochromocytoma* (p. 1734). A high, arched palate, prominent ears, and shimmering irides are characteristic of *Marfan syndrome* (p. 1665).

The *muscular dystrophies*, the cardiac manifestations of which are described in Chapter 50, may also affect facial appearance profoundly. Patients with *myotonic dystrophy* (p. 1708) exhibit a dull, expressionless face, with ptosis due to weakness of the levator muscles; the forehead is furrowed, and the temporalis and sternocleidomastoid muscles are atrophied. In the *facioscapulohumeral type* of *muscular dystrophy* (Landouzy-Déjerine) (p. 1708), nearly all the facial muscles are weak, particularly the orbicularis oris, preventing the patients from puckering the mouth and whistling; weakness of the orbicularis oculi, diffuse fattening of the face, and facial asymmetry (particularly around the mouth) are also characteristic.

In patients with *Werner's syndrome*, who are at high risk of developing premature coronary and arterial atherosclerosis, there is premature graying of the hair, frontal baldness, beaking of the nose, cataract formation, and proptosis. Myotonic muscular dystrophy (p. 1708) may also cause premature graying of the hair, frontal thinning or baldness, and early cataracts.

EYES

External ophthalmoplegia and ptosis due to muscular dystrophy of the extraocular muscles occur in the *Kearns-Sayre syndrome*, which may be associated with complete heart block and myocardial failure[10] (p. 1714).

Exophthalmos and stare occur not only in hyperthyroidism, which can cause high-output cardiac failure (p. 1727), but also in advanced congestive heart failure, in which there is severe pulmonary venous hypertension and weight loss (p. 496).[11] The stare is probably due to lid retraction caused by the increased adrenergic tone that accompanies heart failure. Severe tricuspid regurgitation[12] and a carotid artery–cavernous sinus fistula can also cause pulsatile exophthalmos.

Attention should be directed to the *iris* to look for an arcus, a circumferential light ring around the iris. When this ring begins inferiorly, leaving a rim peripherally, and occurs in a young person, it is frequently associated with hypercholesterolemia (Fig. 2–1), xanthelasma (small yellowish deposits of cholesterol on the eyelids), and premature atherosclerosis. (In blacks, an arcus often does not reflect hypercholesterolemia.) Iridodonesis (tremulous iris), in which the iris is not properly supported by the lens because of dislocation or weakness of the suspensory free ligament, occurs in Marfan syndrome. Gray-white spots (Brushfield's spots) in the iris occur in Down's syndrome. Iridocyclitis and enlargement of the lacrimal glands are seen in sarcoidosis, which may be associated with cardiomyopathy (p. 1426).

Blue scleras may be seen in patients with Marfan syndrome (p. 1665), Ehlers-Danlos syndrome (p. 1668), and osteogenesis imperfecta (p. 1668)—disorders that may be associated with aortic dilatation, regurgitation, and dissection and with prolapse of the mitral valve. *Argyll Robertson pupils* (small, irregular, unequal pupils that do not dilate properly on administration of mydriatic drugs and that fail to react to light but constrict on accommodation) are diagnostic of central nervous system syphilis; this may be associated with cardiovascular syphilis, characterized by aneurysm of the ascending aorta, coronary ostial stenosis, and aortic regurgitation (p. 1562). The *cornea* may be clouded in Hurler's syndrome. *Cataracts* are associated with the so-called rubella syndrome, in which a variety of congenital cardiac malformations occur; premature cataracts also occur in Refsum's disease and in myotonic muscular dystrophy, both of which may be associated with cardiomyopathy (p. 1708); *vitreous opacities* are frequent in

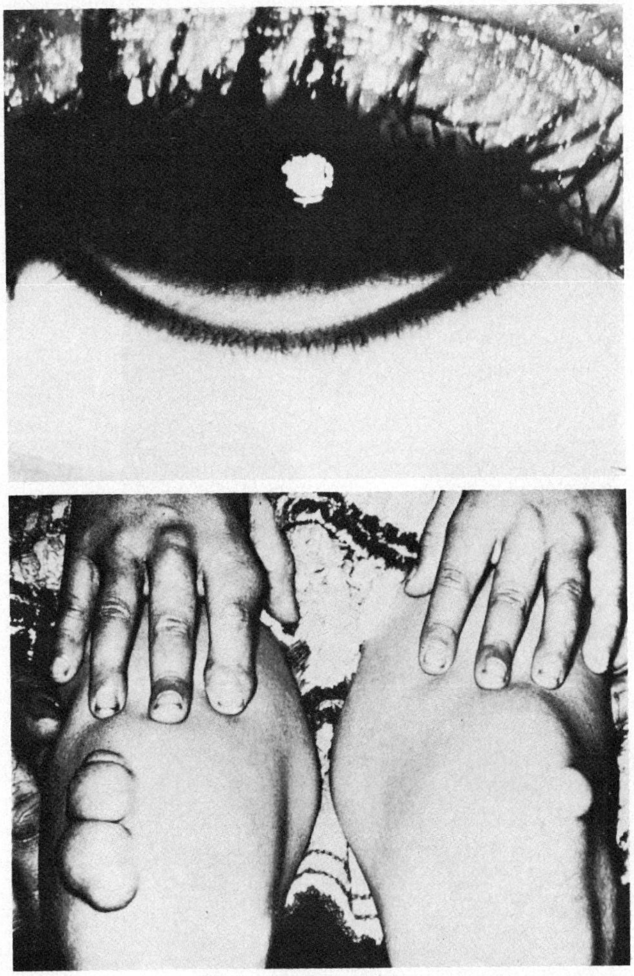

FIGURE 2–1 Arcus juvenilis and xanthelasma of the lids (*top*) and tendinous xanthomas of the knees (*bottom*) in a patient with familial hypercholesteremia. The patient was a 10-year-old girl with a serum cholesterol level of 665 mg per 100 ml. Several other members of the family had a similar syndrome. (From Cogan, D. G.: Ophthalmic Manifestations of Systemic Vascular Disease. Philadelphia, W. B. Saunders Co., 1974, pp. 14 and 15.)

patients with familial amyloidosis, in whom a restrictive cardiomyopathy may be present.

Fundi. Examination of the *fundi* allows classification of arteriolar disease in patients with hypertension (Fig. 2–2*A*) and may be helpful in the recognition of arteriosclerosis. Beading of the retinal artery may be present in patients with hypercholesteremia (Fig. 2–2*B*), and wreathlike arteriovenous anastomoses around the disk are characteristic of Takayasu's disease (p. 1558) (Fig. 2–2*C*). Hemorrhages near the disks with white spots in the center (Roth's spots) occur in infective endocarditis (p. 1151) (Fig. 2–2*D*). Embolic retinal occlusions may occur in patients with rheumatic heart disease, left atrial myxoma, and atherosclerosis of the aorta or arch vessels. Papilledema is present not only in patients with malignant hypertension (Chap. 26) but also in cor pulmonale with severe hypoxia. In coarctation of the aorta, the retinal arteries are particularly tortuous but may not show other changes characteristic of hypertensive retinopathy.[13] In patients with cyanosis and polycythemia, the retinal veins are particularly dilated and edema and retinal papilledema are occasionally present.

SKIN AND MUCOUS MEMBRANES

Central cyanosis (due to intracardiac or intrapulmonary right-to-left shunting) is observed in warm sites, including the conjunctivae and the mucous membranes of the oral cavity, while peripheral cyanosis (due to reduction of peripheral blood flow, such as occurs in heart failure and peripheral vascular disease) is characteristically observed in cool, exposed areas such as the extremities, particularly the nailbeds and nose. Polycythemia can often be suspected from inspection of the conjunctivae, lips, and tongue, which in anemia are pale and in polycythemia are darkly congested.[14] A blotchy cyanotic tinge to the skin associated with episodic flushing, particularly of the face, occurs in patients with *carcinoid tumors,* which may be associated with valvular heart disease (p. 1430).

Bronze pigmentation of the skin and loss of axillary and pubic hair occur in *hemochromatosis* (which may result in cardiomyopathy owing to iron deposits in the heart) (p. 1425). Jaundice may be observed in patients following pulmonary infarction as well as in patients with congestive hepatomegaly or cardiac cirrhosis. *Lentigines,* i.e., small brown macular lesions on the neck and trunk that begin at about age 6 and do not increase in number with sunlight, are observed in patients with pulmonic stenosis and hypertrophic cardiomyopathy[8] (p. 1409).

The skin is ruddy in patients with polycythemia and Cushing's syndrome; sallow and yellowish in both myxedema and in uremia; fine and silky in thyrotoxicosis; coarse and dry in myxedema and acromegaly; thickened and yellow (particularly in the neck and antecubital region) in pseudoxanthoma elasticum; smooth and glossy in longstanding Raynaud's syndrome; and warm and moist in anemia, beriberi, and other high-output states (Chap. 24). Increased sweating, most commonly a cold sweat in the palms, is observed in patients with neurocirculatory asthenia. *Erythema marginatum* (evanescent lesions confined primarily to the trunk) and *subcutaneous nodules* (which occur on the extensor surface of the elbows or over bony prominences such as the spine or skull) may be present in acute rheumatic fever (p. 1648). *Petechiae* occur in infective endocarditis; café-au-lait spots, freckles, and cutaneous neurofibromas occur in patients with pheochromocytoma (p. 1734), while *symmetric vitiligo* of the extremities is seen in patients with hyperthyroidism. Bluish pigmentation of the ear and nose cartilage is characteristic of *ochronosis,* which can produce serious valvular deformities (Chap. 32). Large areas of *psoriasis* or *exfoliative dermatitis* may be responsible for high-output heart failure (p. 820).

Several types of xanthomas, i.e., cholesterol-filled nodules, are found either subcutaneously or over a tendon in patients with hyperlipoproteinemia (Chap. 35). Premature atherosclerosis frequently develops in these individuals. *Tuberoeruptive xanthomas,* present subcutaneously or on the extensor surfaces of the extremities, and *xanthoma striatum palmare,* which produces yellowish, orange, or pink discoloration of the palmar and digital creases, occur most commonly in patients with type III hyperlipoproteinemia (p. 1215). Patients with *xanthoma tendinosum* (Fig. 2–1), i.e., nodular swellings of the tendons, especially of the elbows, extensor surfaces of the hands, and Achilles' tendons, usually have type II hyperlipoproteinemia (p. 1214).

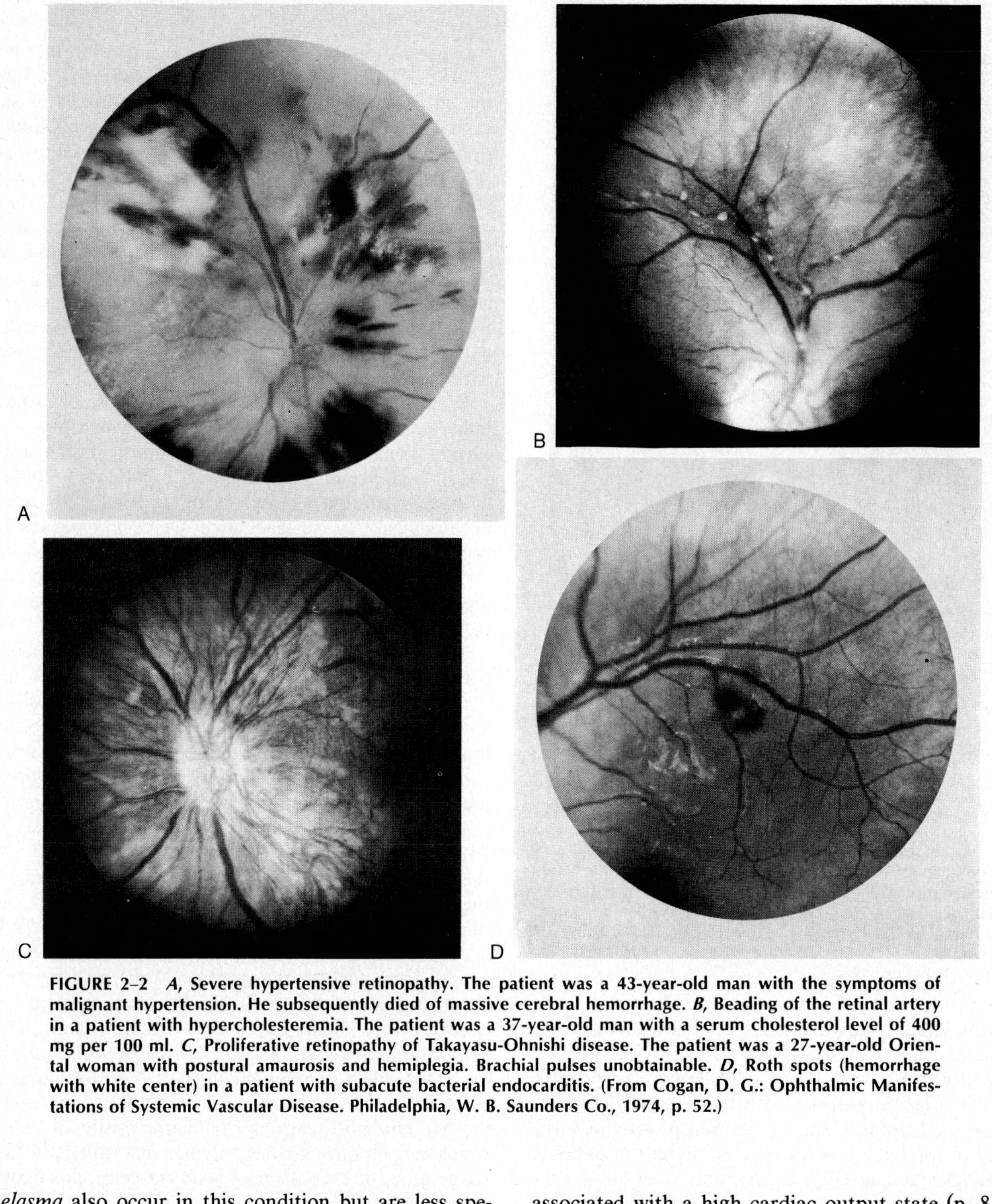

FIGURE 2–2 *A*, Severe hypertensive retinopathy. The patient was a 43-year-old man with the symptoms of malignant hypertension. He subsequently died of massive cerebral hemorrhage. *B*, Beading of the retinal artery in a patient with hypercholesteremia. The patient was a 37-year-old man with a serum cholesterol level of 400 mg per 100 ml. *C*, Proliferative retinopathy of Takayasu-Ohnishi disease. The patient was a 27-year-old Oriental woman with postural amaurosis and hemiplegia. Brachial pulses unobtainable. *D*, Roth spots (hemorrhage with white center) in a patient with subacute bacterial endocarditis. (From Cogan, D. G.: Ophthalmic Manifestations of Systemic Vascular Disease. Philadelphia, W. B. Saunders Co., 1974, p. 52.)

Xanthelasma also occur in this condition but are less specific (Fig. 2–1). *Eruptive xanthomas* are tiny, yellowish nodules, 1 to 2 mm in diameter on an erythematous base, which may present anywhere on the body and are associated with hyperchylomicronemia and are therefore often found in patients with type I and type V hyperlipoproteinemia (p. 1216).

Hereditary telangiectasia are multiple capillary hemangiomas occurring in the skin, nasal mucosa, and upper respiratory and gastrointestinal tracts that resemble the spider nevi seen in patients with liver disease. When present in the lung, they are associated with pulmonary arteriovenous fistulas and cause central cyanosis. Spider nevi on the face occur in patients with *chronic liver disease,* which may be associated with a high cardiac output state (p. 819). Nicotine staining of the fingers suggests excessive cigarette smoking, an important risk factor for the development of coronary artery disease (p. 1216).

EXTREMITIES

A variety of congenital and acquired cardiac malformations are associated with characteristic changes in the extremities. Among the congenital lesions, short stature, cubitus valgus, and medial deviation of the extended forearm is characteristic of *Turner's syndrome* (p. 1614). Patients with the *Holt-Oram syndrome* (Table 29–2, p. 943), i.e., atrial septal defect with skeletal deformities, often have a thumb with an extra phalanx, a so-called "fingerized thumb," which lies in the same plane as the fingers, making it difficult to appose the thumb and fingers. In addition, they may exhibit deformities of the radius and ulna, causing difficulty in supination and pronation. There is often asymmetry of skeletal involvement, with the left side more severely affected.[15] Polydactyly and hypoplastic fingernails are part of the *Ellis–van Creveld syndrome* (chondroectodermal dysplasia), a disorder frequently associated with atrial or ventricular septal defect (p. 1617). Arachnodactyly is characteristic of the *Marfan syndrome* (p. 1665). Normally, when a fist is made over a clenched thumb, the latter does not extend beyond the ulnar side of the hand, but it usually does so in Marfan's syndrome. When the wrist is encircled by the thumb and little finger of the opposite hand, the little finger will overlap the thumb by at least 1 cm in more than three-fourths of patients with Marfan's syndrome but will rarely do so in individuals without this syndrome.[16] In *osteogenesis imperfecta*, hyperextensibility of the joints is common, but arachnodactyly is not.[17] In patients with *homocystinuria*, the extremities may be elongated and other skeletal abnormalities, such as kyphoscoliosis and pectus carinatum, may be present. Ulnar deviation of the fourth and fifth fingers and flexion at the metacarpophalangeal joints occur in *Jaccoud's arthritis*,[18] a rare concomitant of rheumatic heart disease. In *Down's syndrome*, there is a Simian palm crease, increased space between the fourth and fifth fingers, and a short fifth finger that is curved inward, while in Turner's syndrome the fingers tend to be short.

Raynaud's phenomenon, which sometimes occurs in association with primary pulmonary hypertension (p. 836), scleroderma (p. 1663), and coronary spasm (p. 1360), is characterized by intermittent pallor and/or cyanosis of the extremities precipitated by exposure to cold. With the passage of time, the skin overlying the fingers and under the nails becomes atrophic. Cold, pale or blue hands accompanied by collapse of the forearm veins signifies peripheral vasoconstriction, which may be a normal response to cold, anxiety, or a low cardiac output. In patients with peripheral vascular disease, the ischemic foot typically exhibits paleness on elevation and rubor on dependency.

High cardiac output states (Chap. 24) produce warm, pink hands associated with distention of the forearm veins (signs of vasodilatation). Redness of the palmar eminences may be a sign of severe liver disease, while a fine tremor of the outstretched hands suggests thyrotoxicosis. Peripheral *arteriovenous fistula* or *Paget's disease* of bone may cause local warmth and excessive growth of the affected limb. Systolic flushing of the nailbeds, which can be readily detected by pressing a flashlight against the terminal digits (Quincke's sign), is a sign of aortic regurgitation and of other conditions characterized by a greatly widened pulse pressure. *Differential cyanosis*, in which the hands and fingers (especially on the right side) are pink and the feet and toes are cyanotic, is indicative of patent ductus arteriosus with reversed shunt due to pulmonary hypertension (p. 955); this finding can often be brought out by exercise. On the other hand, *reversed differential cyanosis*, in which cyanosis of the fingers exceeds that of the toes, suggests transposition of the great arteries, pulmonary hypertension, preductal narrowing of the aorta, and reversed flow through a patent ductus arteriosus.[19]

Clubbing of the fingers and toes[20] (Fig. 2–3). Clubbing of the extremities is characteristic of central cyanosis (cyanotic congenital heart disease or pulmonary disease with hypoxia). It may also appear within a few weeks of the development of infective endocarditis but usually develops after two or three years of central cyanosis. Clubbing is also observed in a variety of suppurative pulmonary lesions and carcinoma of the lung as well as in gastrointestinal disorders, including biliary cirrhosis and regional enteritis; occasionally, it is a harmless familial condition. The earliest forms of clubbing are characterized by increased glossiness and cyanosis of the skin at the root of the nail.[21] Following obliteration of the normal angle between the base of the nail and the skin, the soft tissue of the pulp becomes hypertrophied, the nail root floats freely, and its loose proximal end can be palpated. In the more severe forms of clubbing, bony changes occur, i.e., *hypertrophic pulmonary osteoarthropathy*; these changes involve the terminal digits and in rare instances even the wrists, ankles, elbows, and knees. *Unilateral clubbing* of the fin-

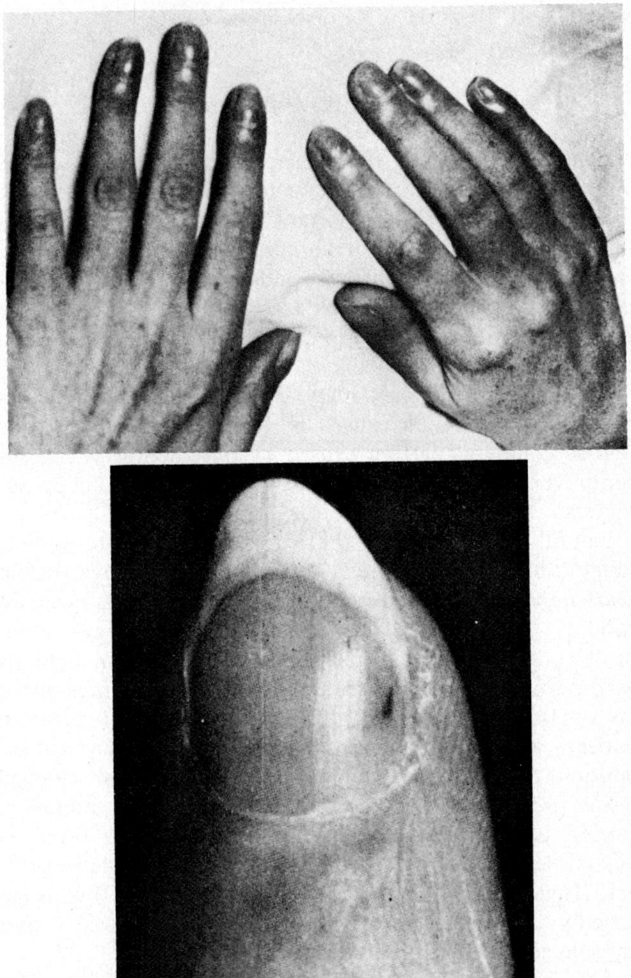

FIGURE 2–3 *Top*, Clubbing of fingers in subacute infective endocarditis. *Bottom*, Splinter hemorrhages due to subacute infective endocarditis. (From Oram, S.: Clinical Heart Disease. London, William Heinemann Medical Books, Ltd., 1971, pp. 289 and 290.)

gers is rare but can occur when an aortic aneurysm interferes with the arterial supply to one arm. Not to be confused with clubbing are the subungual fibromas of the fingers that occur in tuberous sclerosis, a condition often associated with cardiac rhabdomyoma.[22]

Osler's nodes are small, tender, erythematous skin lesions due to infected emboli and occurring most frequently in the pads of the fingers or toes and in the palms of the hands or soles of the feet, whereas *Janeway lesions* are slightly raised, nontender hemorrhagic lesions in the palms of hands and soles of the feet; both these lesions as well as petechiae occur in infective endocarditis (p. 1151). When the latter occur under the nailbeds, they are termed *splinter hemorrhages* (Fig. 2–3).

Edema of the extremities is a common finding in congestive heart failure; however, if it is present in only one leg, it is more likely due to venous obstructive disease than to heart failure. Firm pressure on the pretibial region for 10 to 20 seconds may be necessary for the detection of edema in ambulatory patients. In patients confined to bed, edema appears first in the sacral region. Edema may involve the face in children with heart failure of any etiology and in adults with heart failure associated with marked elevation of systemic venous pressure (e.g., constrictive pericarditis and tricuspid valve disease).

CHEST AND ABDOMEN

Examination of the thorax should begin with observations of the respiratory rate, effort, and regularity. The shape of the chest is important as well; thus, a barrel-shaped chest with low diaphragms suggests emphysema, bronchitis, and possibly cor pulmonale. In chronic obstructive pulmonary disease, accessory muscles are used during inspiration, while expiration is prolonged and often accompanied by wheezing.

Inspection of the chest may reveal a bulging to the right of the upper sternum caused by an aortic aneurysm or a venous collateral pattern caused by obstruction of the superior vena cava, which may also be caused by aortic aneurysm.

Painful enlargement of the *liver* may be due to venous congestion; the tenderness disappears in longstanding heart failure. Hepatic systolic expansile pulsations occur in patients with severe tricuspid regurgitation (Fig. 15–4, p. 497), and presystolic pulsations can be felt in patients with pure tricuspid stenosis and sinus rhythm. Transmitted (as opposed to intrinsic) pulsations of the liver occur in patients with right ventricular enlargement, aneurysmal dilatation of the upper abdominal aorta, and a widened pulse pressure. When firm pressure over the abdomen causes cervical venous distention, i.e, when there is *abdominojugular reflux,* right heart failure is usually present. *Ascites* is also characteristic of heart failure, but is especially characteristic of tricuspid valve disease and chronic constrictive pericarditis.

Splenomegaly may occur in the presence of severe congestive hepatomegaly, most frequently in patients with constrictive pericarditis or tricuspid valve disease. The spleen may be enlarged and painful in infective endocarditis as well as following splenic embolization. Splenic infarction is frequently accompanied by an audible friction rub.

Both *kidneys* may be palpably enlarged in patients with hypertension secondary to polycystic disease. Auscultation of the abdomen should be carried out in all patients with hypertension; a systolic bruit secondary to renal artery stenosis may be audible near the umbilicus or in the flank (p. 880).

Atherosclerotic aneurysms of the abdominal aorta are usually readily detected on palpation (p. 1543), except in markedly obese patients. In patients with *coarctation of the aorta,* no abdominal pulsations are palpable despite the presence of prominent arterial pulses in the neck and upper extremities; arterial pulses in the lower extremities are reduced or absent.

THE JUGULAR VENOUS PULSE

Important information concerning the dynamics of the right side of the heart can be obtained by inspection of the jugular venous pulse.[23,24] Since the venous valves between the superior vena cava and external jugular veins may interfere with pressure estimation in the latter, the *internal* jugular vein is ordinarily employed in the examination. The venous pulse can be analyzed more readily on the right than on the left side of the neck, because the right innominate and jugular veins extend cephalad in an almost straight line along with the superior vena cava, thus favoring transmission of hemodynamic changes from the right atrium, while the left innominate vein may be kinked or compressed by a variety of normal structures, by a dilated aorta, or by an aneurysm.

The patient should be lying comfortably during the examination; clothing should be removed from the neck and upper thorax, and although the head should rest on a pillow, it must not be elevated at a sharp angle from the trunk. The jugular venous pulse may be examined effectively by shining a light tangentially across the neck. Most patients with heart disease are examined most effectively in the 45-degree position, but in patients in whom venous pressure is high, a greater inclination (60 or even 90 degrees) is required to obtain visible pulsations, while in those in whom jugular venous pressure is low, a lesser inclination (30 degrees) is desirable. In order to amplify the pulsations of the jugular veins, it may be helpful to place the patient in the supine position and try to increase venous return by elevating the patient's legs.

The internal jugular vein is located deep within the neck, where it is covered by the sternocleidomastoid muscle and is therefore not usually visible as a discrete structure, except in the presence of severe venous hypertension. However, its pulsations are transmitted to the skin of the neck, where they are usually easily visible. Sometimes considerable difficulty may be experienced in differentiating between the carotid and jugular venous pulses in the neck, particularly when the latter exhibits prominent *v* waves, as occurs in patients with tricuspid regurgitation. However, there are several helpful clues: (1) The arterial pulse is a sharply localized rapid movement that may not be readily visible but that strikes the palpating fingers with considerable force; in contrast, the venous pulse, while more readily visible, often disappears when the palpating finger is placed on the pulsating area. (2) The arterial pulsations do not change when the patient is in the upright position, whereas venous pulsations usually disappear, unless the venous pressure is greatly elevated. (3) Compression of the root of the neck does not affect the arterial pulse but usually abolishes venous pulsations, except in the presence of extreme venous hypertension.

Two principal observations can usually be made from examination of the neck veins: the level of venous pressure and the type of venous wave pattern. In order to estimate jugular venous pressure, the height of the oscillating top of the distended proximal portion of the internal jugular vein, which reflects right atrial pressure, should be determined. The upper limit of normal is 4 cm above the sternal angle, which corresponds to a central venous pressure of approximately 9 cm H_2O, since the right atrium is approximately 5 cm below the sternal angle. When the veins in the neck collapse in a subject in the horizontal position, it is likely that the central venous pressure is subnormal. When obstruction of veins in the lower extremities is responsible for edema, pressure in the neck veins is not elevated and the abdominal-jugular reflux is negative.

The *abdominal-jugular reflux* can be tested by applying firm pressure to the periumbilical region for 30 to 60 seconds with the patient breathing quietly while the jugular veins are observed; increased respiratory excursions or strain should be avoided. In normal subjects jugular venous pressure rises only transiently, while pressure is continued, whereas in right ventricular failure the jugular venous pressure remains elevated.

Pattern of the Venous Pulse. The events of the cardiac cycle, shown in Figure 12–25, p. 431, provide an explanation for the details of the jugular venous pulse pattern (Figs. 2–4 and 3–34, p. 63). The *a* wave in the venous pulse results from venous distention due to right atrial systole, while the *x* descent is due to atrial relaxation; the *c* wave, which occurs simultaneously with the carotid arterial pulse,[25] is an inconstant wave in the jugular venous pulse and may be due in part to forceful closure of the tricuspid valve; sometimes it is an artifact produced by the adjacent carotid arterial pulse. It is followed by the *x'* descent, caused by the pulling down of the floor of the atrium (descent of the base) by ventricular contraction. (Many investigators refer to this wave as the *x* descent.) The *v* wave results from the rise in right atrial pressure when blood flows into the right atrium during ventricular systole when the tricuspid valve is shut, and the *y* descent, i.e., the downslope of the *v* wave, is related to the decline in right atrial pressure when the tricuspid valve reopens. While all or most of these events can usually be recorded, they are not readily distinguishable on inspection. The descents or downward collapsing movements of the jugular veins are more rapid, produce larger excursions, and are therefore more prominent to the eye than are the ascents (Fig. 2–4). The normal dominant jugular venous descent, the *x'* descent, occurs just prior to the second heart sound, while the *y* descent ends after the second heart sound. With an increase in central venous pressure, the *v* wave becomes higher and the *y* collapse becomes more prominent. The *a* wave can be recognized when it is abnormally prominent; it occurs just before the first heart sound or carotid pulse and has a sharp rise and fall. The *v* wave occurs just after the arterial pulse and has a slower, undulating pattern.

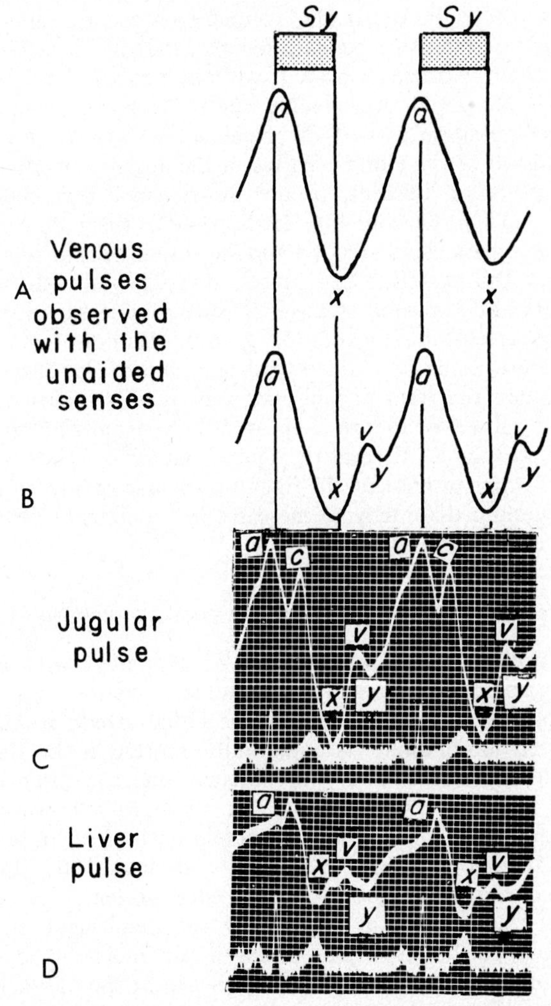

FIGURE 2–4 *A* and *B*, Tracings of the normal venous pulse observed with the unaided eyes. *A*, The outstanding feature is the systolic collapse (*x*), which alternates with a high peak (*a*). *B*, Sometimes in normal subjects a second peak is seen in early diastole (*v*), which is followed by a trough (*y*) that is shallower than the systolic dip (*x*).

C, The graph of the jugular pulse shows, similar to tracing *B*, two peaks (*a* and *v*) and two troughs (*x* and *y*). In addition, a small peak (*c*) interrupts the *x* descent. The *c* wave cannot be perceived with the unaided eye.

D, The most prominent feature of the hepatic pulse, like the jugular pulse, is a systolic dip (*x*). The *a* wave is small. (From Dressler, W.: Clinical Aids in Cardiac Diagnosis. New York, 1970, p. 195, by permission of Grune and Stratton.)

Alterations in Disease. Elevation of jugular venous pressure reflects an increase in right atrial pressure and occurs in heart failure, reduced compliance of the right ventricle, pericardial disease, hypervolemia, and obstruction of the superior vena cava. During inspiration, the jugular venous pressure normally declines but the *amplitude* of the pulsations increases. *Kussmaul's sign* is a paradoxical rise in the height of the jugular venous pressure during inspiration, which occurs frequently in patients with chronic constrictive pericarditis and sometimes in congestive heart failure and tricuspid stenosis. The *x* descent may be prominent in patients with enlarged *a* waves, as well as in patients with right ventricular volume overload (atrial septal defect). Constrictive pericarditis (p. 1488) is characterized by a rapid and deep *y* descent without a prominent *v* wave (Fig. 3–38, p. 65); occasionally, the *x*′ descent is prominent in this condition as well. A prominent *v* wave or *cv* wave, i.e., fusion of the *c* and *v* waves in the absence or attenuation of an *x*′ descent, occurs in tricuspid regurgitation (Fig. 3–37, p. 64, and Fig. 15–5, p. 497); the *y* descent is gradual in tricuspid stenosis and steep in tricuspid regurgitation. Tall *a* waves are present in patients with sinus rhythm and tricuspid stenosis or atresia or right ventricular hypertension (Fig. 3–35, p. 63). Cannon (giant) *a* waves are noted in patients with atrioventricular dissociation when the right atrium contracts against a closed tricuspid valve (see Figure 3–36, p. 64). In atrial fibrillation, the *a* wave and *x* descent disappear, and the *x*′ descent becomes more prominent. In right ventricular failure and sinus rhythm, there may be increases in prominence of both the *a* and *v* waves.

INDIRECT MEASUREMENT OF BLOOD PRESSURE

Systolic arterial pressure can be estimated without a sphygmomanometer cuff by gradually compressing the brachial artery while palpating the radial artery; the force required to obliterate the radial pulse represents the systolic blood pressure, and with practice, one can often estimate this level within 20 mm Hg. Ordinarily, however, a sphygmomanometer is used to obtain an indirect measurement of blood pressure.[26,27] The cuff should fit snugly around the arm, with its lower edge at least one inch above the antecubital space, and the diaphragm of the stethoscope should be placed close to or under the edge of the sphygmomanometer cuff. The width of the cuff selected should be at least 40 per cent of the circumference of the limb to be used. The standard size, with a 5-inch-wide cuff, is designed for adults with an arm of average size. When this cuff is applied to a large upper arm or a normal adult thigh, arterial pressure will be overestimated;[28] when it is applied to a small arm, the pressure will be underestimated. The cuff width should be approximately 1½ inches in infants and small children, 3 inches in young children (2 to 5 years), and 8 inches in obese adults. The bag should be long enough to extend at least halfway around the limb (10 inches in adults). Mercury manometers are, in general, more accurate and reliable than the aneroid type.

In order to measure arterial pressure in the upper extremity, the patient should be seated or lying comfortably and relaxed, the arm should be slightly flexed and at heart level, and the cuff should be inflated rapidly to approximately 30 mm Hg above the anticipated systolic pressure.[29] These maneuvers, which diminish the volume of blood in the venous bed, decrease the tissue pressure distal to the cuff and thereby increase the flow into the occluded brachial artery. The cuff is then deflated slowly; the pressure at which the brachial pulse can be palpated is close to the systolic pressure. The cuff should be deflated rapidly after the diastolic pressure is noted and a full minute allowed to elapse before pressure is remeasured in the same limb.

To measure pressure in the legs, the patient should lie on his or her abdomen, an 8-inch-wide cuff should be applied with the compression bag over the posterior aspect of the midthigh and should be rolled diagonally around the thigh to keep the edges snug against the skin, and auscultation should be carried out in the popliteal fossa. In order to measure pressure in the lower leg, an arm cuff is placed over the calf, and auscultation is carried out over the posterior tibial artery. Regardless of where the cuff is applied, care must be taken to avoid letting the rubber part of the balloon of the cuff extend beyond its covering and to avoid placing the cuff on so loosely that central ballooning occurs.

Korotkoff sounds. There are five phases of Korotkoff sounds, i.e., sounds produced by the flow of blood as the constricting blood pressure cuff is gradually released. The first appearance of clear, tapping sounds (phase I) represents the systolic pressure. These sounds are replaced by soft murmurs during phase II and by louder murmurs during phase III, as the volume of blood flowing through the constricted artery increases. The sounds suddenly become muffled in phase IV, when constriction of the brachial artery diminishes as arterial diastolic pressure is approached. Korotkoff sounds disappear in phase V, which is usually within 10 mm Hg of phase IV. Diastolic pressure measured directly through an intraarterial needle and external manometer corresponds closely to phase V. In severe aortic regurgitation, however, when the disappearance point is extremely low, sometimes 0 mm Hg, the sound of muffling (phase IV) is much closer to the intraarterial diastolic pressure than is the disappearance point (phase V). When there is a sizable difference between phases IV and V of the Korotkoff sounds (>10 mm Hg), both pressures should be recorded (e.g., 142/54/10 mm Hg). Korotkoff sounds may be difficult to hear and arterial pressure difficult to measure when arterial pressure rises at a slow rate (as in aortic stenosis), when the vessels are markedly constricted (as in hypovolemic shock), and when the stroke volume is reduced (as in severe heart failure). Very soft or inaudible Korotkoff sounds can often be accentuated by dilating the blood vessels of the upper extremities simply by opening and closing the fist repeatedly. In states of shock, the indirect method of measuring blood pressure is unreliable, and arterial pressure should be measured through an intraarterial needle.

The *auscultatory gap* is a silence that sometimes separates the first appearance of the Korotkoff sounds from their second appearance at a lower pressure. This phenomenon tends to occur when there is venous distention or reduced velocity of arterial flow into the arm, as occurs in severe aortic stenosis. If the first muffling of sounds is considered to be the diastolic pressure, it will be overestimated. If the second appearance is taken as the systolic pressure, it will be underestimated. On the other hand, sounds transmitted through the arterial tree from prosthetic aortic valves may be responsible for falsely high readings.

In order to determine arterial pressure in the basal condition, the patient should have rested in a quiet room for 15 minutes. It is desirable to record the arterial pressure in both arms at the time of the initial examination; differences in systolic pressure exceeding 15 mm Hg between the two arms when measurements are made in rapid sequence suggest obstructive lesions involving the aorta or the origin of the innominate and subclavian arteries, or supravalvular aortic stenosis (p. 982). In patients with vertebral-basal artery insufficiency, a difference in pressure between the arms may signify that a subclavian steal is responsible for the cerebrovascular symptoms.[30] In order to determine whether orthostatic hypotension is present, arterial pressure should be determined with the patient in both the supine and the erect positions. However, regardless of the patient's posture, the brachial artery should be at the level of the heart to avoid superimposition of the effects of gravity on the recorded pressure.

Normally, the systolic pressure in the legs is up to 20 mm Hg higher than in the arms, but the diastolic pressure is usually virtually identical. The recording of a higher diastolic pressure in the legs than in the arms suggests that the thigh cuff is too small. When systolic pressure in the popliteal artery exceeds that in the brachial artery by more than 20 mm Hg (Hill's sign), aortic regurgitation is usually present.[31] Blood pressure should be measured in the lower extremities in patients with hypertension to detect coarctation of the aorta or when obstructive disease of the aorta or its immediate branches is suspected.

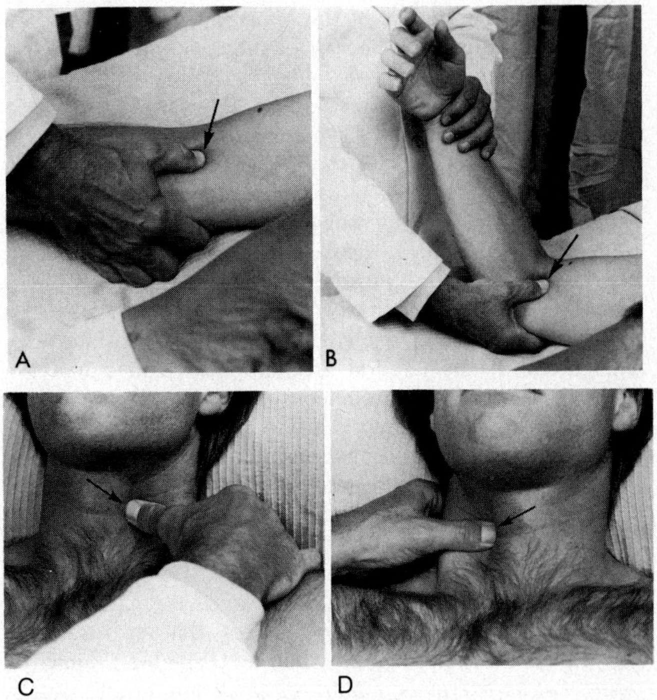

FIGURE 2–5 *A,* Palpation of the right brachial pulse with the thumb while the patient's arm lies at the side with the palm up. *B,* Palpation of the right brachial pulse with the patient's elbow resting in the palm of the examiner's hand. The thumb explores the antecubital fossa (*arrow*), while the patient's forearm is passively raised and lowered to achieve maximum relaxation of muscles around the elbow. *C* and *D,* Palpation of the carotid pulse. The examiner places the right thumb (*arrow*) on the patient's left carotoid artery (*C*). The left thumb (*arrow*) is then applied separately to the right carotid (*D*). (Reproduced with permission from Perloff, J. K. (Ed.): *Physical Examination of the Heart and Circulation,* Philadelphia, W. B. Saunders Co., 1982, pp. 58 and 60.

THE ARTERIAL PULSE

The arterial pulse is determined by a combination of factors, including the left ventricular stroke volume, the ejection velocity, the relative compliance and capacity of the arterial system, and the pressure waves that result from the antegrade flow of blood and reflections of the arterial pressure pulse returning from the peripheral circulation.[32] Bilateral palpation of the carotid, radial, brachial, femoral, popliteal, dorsalis pedis, and posterior tibial pulses should be part of the examination of all cardiac patients. The frequency, regularity, and shape of the pulse wave and the character of the arterial wall should be determined.[33] The carotid pulse (Fig. 2–5*A*) provides the most accurate representation of the central aortic pulse[33a]. The brachial artery is the vessel ordinarily most suitable for appreciating the rate of rise of the pulse and the contour, volume, and consistency of the peripheral vessels. This artery is located at the medial aspect of the elbow, and it may be helpful to flex the arm in order to palpate it; palpation of the artery should be carried out with the thumb exerting pressure on the artery until its maximal movement is detected (Fig. 2–5*B*). A normal rate of rise of the arterial pulse suggests that there is no obstruction to left ventricular outflow, whereas a pulse wave of small amplitude with normal configuration suggests a reduced stroke volume.

THE NORMAL PULSE. The pulse in the ascending aorta normally rises rapidly to a rounded dome;[34] this initial rise reflects the peak velocity of blood ejected from the left ventricle. A slight anacrotic notch or pause is frequently recorded, but only occasionally felt, on the ascending limb of the pulse. The descending limb of the central aortic pulse is less steep than is the ascending limb, and it is interrupted by the incisura, a sharp downward deflection related to closure of the aortic valve (Fig. 3–21, p. 54, and Fig. 4–3, p. 70). Immediately thereafter, the pulse wave rises slightly and then declines gradually throughout diastole. As the pulse wave is transmitted to the periphery, its upstroke becomes steeper, the systolic peak becomes higher, the anacrotic shoulder disappears, and the sharp incisura is replaced by a smoother, later dicrotic notch followed by a dicrotic wave. Normally, the height of this dicrotic wave diminishes with age, hypertension, and arteriosclerosis. In the central arterial pulse (central aorta and innominate and carotid arteries), the rapidly transmitted shock of left ventricular ejection results in a peak in early systole, referred to as the *percussion wave*; a second, smaller peak, the *tidal wave*, presumed to represent a reflected wave from the periphery, can often be recorded but is not normally palpable. However, in older subjects, particularly those with increased peripheral resistance, as well as in patients with arteriosclerosis and diabetes, the tidal wave may be somewhat higher than the percussion wave; i.e., the pulse reaches a peak in late systole. In peripheral arteries, the pulse wave normally has a single sharp peak.

ABNORMAL PULSES. When vascular resistance and arterial stiffness are increased, as in hypertension, there is an increase in pulse wave velocity, and the pulse contour has a more rapid upstroke and greater amplitude. Reduced or unequal carotid arterial pulsations occur in patients with carotid atherosclerosis and with diseases of the aortic arch, including aortic dissection, aneurysm, and Takayasu's disease (Chap. 45). In *supravalvular aortic stenosis* there is a streaming of the jet toward the innominate artery, and the carotid and brachial arterial pulses are stronger on the right than on the left side, and pressures are higher in the right than in the left arm (Fig. 4–6, p. 72, and p. 982). The pulses of the upper extremity may be reduced or unequal in a variety of other conditions, including arterial embolus or thrombosis, anomalous origin or aberrant path of the major vessels, and cervical rib or scalenus anticus syndrome. Asymmetry of right and left popliteal pulses is characteristic of iliofemoral obstruction. Weakness or absence of radial, posterior tibial, or dorsalis pedis pulses on one side suggests arterial insufficiency. In *coarctation of the aorta* the carotid and brachial pulses are bounding, rise rapidly, and have large volumes, while in the lower extremities, the systolic and pulse pressures are reduced, their rate of rise is slow, and there is a late peak. This delay in the femoral arterial pulses can usually be readily detected by simultaneous palpation of the femoral and radial arterial pulses.

In patients with fixed obstruction to left ventricular outflow, the carotid pulse rises slowly (*pulsus tardus*); the upstroke is frequently characterized by a thrill (the *carotid shudder*); and the peak is reduced, occurs late in systole, and is sustained (Figs. 3–22, p. 56; 4–4, p. 70; and 4–7, p. 72). There is a notch on the upstroke of the carotid pulse (anacrotic notch) that is so distinct that two separate waves can be palpated in what is termed an *anacrotic pulse. Pulsus parvus* is a pulse of small amplitude, usually because of a reduction of stroke volume. *Pulsus parvus et tardus* refers to a small pulse with a delayed systolic peak, which is characteristic of severe aortic stenosis. This type of pulse is more readily appreciated by palpating the carotid rather than a more peripheral artery. Patients with severe aortic stenosis and heart failure usually exhibit simply a reduced pulse amplitude, i.e., *pulsus parvus,* and the delay in the upstroke is not readily apparent. However, this delay is readily recorded. In elderly patients with inelastic peripheral arteries, the pulse may rise normally despite the presence of aortic stenosis.

The carotid arterial pulse may be prominent or exaggerated in any condition in which pulse pressure is increased, including anxiety or other high cardiac output states (Chap. 24), as well as in bradycardia, and peripheral arteriosclerosis with loss of arterial distensibility. In patients with *mitral regurgitation* or *ventricular septal defect,* the forward stroke volume (from the left ventricle into the aorta) is usually normal, but the fraction ejected during early systole is greater than normal; hence, the arterial pulse is of normal volume (the pulse pressure is normal), but the pulse may rise abnormally rapidly.[35] Exaggerated or bounding arterial pulses may be observed in patients with an elevated stroke volume, with sympathetic hyperactivity, and in patients with a rigid, sclerotic aorta. In *aortic regurgitation,*[31] there is a very brisk rate of rise with an increased pulse pressure (Fig. 3–24, p. 57). The *Corrigan or water-hammer pulse* of aortic regurgitation consists of an abrupt upstroke (percussion wave) followed by rapid collapse later in systole, but no dicrotic notch. Corrigan's pulse reflects a low resistance in the reservoir into which the left ventricle rapidly discharges an abnormally elevated stroke volume, and it can be exaggerated by raising the patient's arm. In *acute* aortic regurgitation, the left ventricle may not be greatly dilated, and premature closure of the mitral valve may occur and limit the volume of aortic reflux;[36] therefore, the aortic diastolic pressure may *not* be very low, the arterial pulse *not* bounding, and the pulse pressure *not* widened despite a serious abnormality of valve function (p. 1109). "Pistol-shot" sounds heard over the femoral artery when the stethoscope is placed on it (*Traube's sign*), a systolic murmur heard over the femoral artery when it is gradually compressed proximally and a diastolic murmur when the artery is compressed distally (*Duroziez's sign*[31,37]) and Quincke's sign (p. 1110) are also characteristic of severe, chronic aortic regurgitation; of these, Duroziez's sign is the most predictive. Bounding arterial pulses are also present in patients with patent ductus arteriosus or large arteriovenous fistulas; in hyperkinetic states such as thyrotoxicosis, pregnancy, fever, and anemia; in severe bradycardia; and in vessels proximal to a coarctation of the aorta.

In the presence of atrioventricular dissociation, when atrial activity is irregularly transmitted to the ventricles, the strength of the peripheral arterial pulse depends on the time interval between atrial and ventricular contractions. In a patient with rapid heart action, the presence of such variations is suggestive of ventricular tachycardia; with an equally rapid rate, an absence of variation of pulse strength suggests a supraventricular mechanism.

BISFERIENS PULSE. A bisferiens pulse is characterized by two systolic peaks, the percussion and tidal waves, separated by a distinct midsystolic dip; the peaks may be equal or either may be larger. This type of pulse may be detected most readily by palpation of the carotid and less commonly of the radial arteries. It occurs in conditions in which a large stroke volume is ejected rapidly from the left ventricle[38] and is observed most commonly in patients with pure aortic regurgitation (Fig. 3–24, p. 57) and with a combination of aortic regurgitation and stenosis; it may disappear as heart failure supervenes.

A bisferiens pulse is also noted in patients with *hypertrophic obstructive cardiomyopathy*[39] (Figs. 3–23, p. 56, and 4–9, p. 73), but the bifid nature may only be recorded, not palpated; on palpation there may merely be a rapid upstroke. In these patients the initial prominent percussion wave is associated with rapid ejection of blood into the aorta during early systole, followed by a rapid decline as obstruction becomes manifest in midsystole and by a tidal (reflected) wave. The bisferiens pulse of hypertrophic obstructive cardiomyopathy must be distinguished from the anacrotic pulse palpable in some patients with pure aortic stenosis; in both groups of patients with obstruction to left ventricular outflow a double pulse may be palpable. However, in patients with fixed obstruction the pulse rises slowly and the tidal wave is the higher of the two, while in hypertrophic obstructive cardiomyopathy, the pulse rises rapidly and the percussion wave is dominant. In some patients with hypertrophic cardiomyopathy with no or little obstruction to left ventricular outflow, the arterial pulse is normal in the basal state, but obstruction and a bisferiens pulse can be elicited by means of the Valsalva maneuver or inhalation of amyl nitrite. Occasionally, a bisferiens pulse is observed in hyperkinetic circulatory states, and very rarely it occurs in normal individuals.

DICROTIC PULSE. Not to be confused with a bisferiens pulse, in which both peaks occur in systole, is a dicrotic pulse, in which the normally small wave that follows aortic valve closure (i.e., the dicrotic notch) is exaggerated and measures more than 50 per cent of the pulse pressure on direct pressure recordings and in which the dicrotic notch is low (i.e., near the diastolic pressure) (Fig.

3–25, p. 57). It may be present in normal hypotensive subjects with reduced peripheral resistance, as occurs in fever, and it may be elicited or exaggerated by inspiration or the inhalation of amyl nitrite. Rarely, a dicrotic pulse may be noted in healthy adolescents or young adults, but it usually occurs in conditions such as cardiac tamponade, severe heart failure, and hypovolemic shock, in which a low stroke volume is ejected into a soft elastic aorta. A dicrotic pulse is rarely present when systolic pressure exceeds 130 mm Hg.

PULSUS ALTERNANS. Mechanical alternans is a sign of severe depression of myocardial function (p. 1484). Although more readily recognized on sphygmomanometry, when the systolic pressure alternates by more than 20 mm Hg it can be detected by palpation of a peripheral (femoral or radial) pulse or by the recording of an indirect carotid pulse tracing (Fig. 3–26, p. 58). Palpation should be carried out with light pressure and with the patient's breath held in midexpiration to avoid the superimposition of respiratory variation on the amplitude of the pulse. Pulsus alternans is generally accompanied by alternation in the intensity of the Korotkoff sounds and occasionally by alternation in intensity of the heart sounds. Rarely, alternans is so marked that the weak beat is not perceived at all. Aortic regurgitation, systemic hypertension, and reducing venous return by head-tilting or nitroglycerin all exaggerate pulsus alternans and assist in its detection. Pulsus alternans, which is frequently precipitated by a premature ventricular contraction (Fig. 15–7, p. 499), is characterized by a regular rhythm and must be distinguished from pulsus bigeminus (see below), which is usually regularly irregular.

PULSUS BIGEMINUS. A bigeminal rhythm is caused by the occurrence of premature contractions, usually ventricular, occurring after every other beat and results in alternation of the strength of the pulse, which can be confused with pulsus alternans. However, in contrast to the latter, in which the rhythm is regular, in pulsus bigeminus the weak beat always follows the shorter interval. In normal persons or in patients with fixed obstruction to left ventricular outflow, the compensatory pause following a premature beat is followed by a stronger-than-normal pulse. However, in patients with hypertrophic obstructive cardiomyopathy, the postpremature ventricular contraction beat is weaker than normal because of increased obstruction to left ventricular outflow[40] (p. 1418).

PULSUS PARADOXUS. This is a reduction in the strength of the arterial pulse during inspiration or an exaggerated inspiratory fall in systolic pressure (more than 10 mm Hg during quiet breathing). When marked, i.e., an inspiratory reduction of pressure greater than 20 mm Hg, it can be detected simply by careful palpation of the radial or brachial arterial pulse. Milder degrees of a paradoxical pulse can be readily detected on sphygmomanometry: the cuff is inflated to suprasystolic levels and is deflated slowly at a rate of about 2 mm Hg per heart beat; the peak systolic pressure during expiration is noted. The cuff is then deflated even more slowly, and the pressure is again noted when Korotkoff sounds become audible throughout the respiratory cycle. Normally, the difference between the two pressures should not exceed 8 mm Hg during quiet respiration. (Pulsus alternans can also be detected by this maneuver by noting whether peak systolic pressure or the intensity of the Korotkoff sounds alternates when respiration is held.)

Pulsus paradoxus represents an exaggeration of the normal decline in systolic arterial pressure with inspiration, which results from the reduced left ventricular stroke volume and the transmission of negative intrathoracic pressure to the aorta. It is a frequent finding in patients with cardiac tamponade (p. 1481), occurs less frequently (in about half) in patients with chronic constrictive pericarditis (p. 1489), and is also observed in patients with emphysema and bronchial asthma (who have wide respiratory swings of intrapleural pressure),[41] as well as in hypovolemic shock, pulmonary embolus, pregnancy, and extreme obesity. Aortic regurgitation tends to prevent the development of pulsus paradoxus despite the presence of cardiac tamponade. *Reversed* pulsus paradoxus (an inspiratory rise in arterial pressure) can occur in hypertrophic obstructive cardiomyopathy.[42]

EXAMINATION OF THE HEART

INSPECTION

The cardiac examination proper should commence with inspection of the chest, which can best be accomplished with the examiner standing at the foot of the bed or examining table. Respirations—their frequency, regularity, and depth—as well as the relative effort required during inspiration and expiration, should be noted (p. 496). Simultaneously, one should search for cutaneous abnormalities, such as spider nevi (seen in hepatic cirrhosis and Osler-Weber-Rendu disease). Dilation of veins on the anterior chest wall with caudal flow suggests obstruction of the superior vena cava, while cranial flow occurs in patients with obstruction of the inferior vena cava. Precordial prominence is most striking if cardiac enlargement developed before puberty, but it may also be present, although to a lesser extent, in patients in whom cardiomegaly developed in adult life, after the period of thoracic growth.[43,44]

A heavy muscular thorax, contrasting with less developed lower extremities, suggests coarctation of the aorta, in which visible collateral arteries may be present in the axillae and along the lateral chest wall. The upper portion of the thorax exhibits symmetrical bulging in children with stiff lungs in whom the inspiratory effort is increased. An emphysematous-appearing chest or anterior bulge in the area of the manubrium in a child suggests pulmonary hypertension. A "shield chest" is a broad chest in which the angle between the manubrium and the body of the sternum is greater than normal and is associated with widely separated nipples; it is frequently observed in Turner's and Noonan's syndromes. Careful note should be made of other deformities of the thoracic cage, such as *kyphoscoliosis,* which may be responsible for cor pulmonale (p. 1596); *ankylosing spondylitis,* sometimes associated with aortic regurgitation (p. 1656); and *pectus carinatum* (pigeon chest), which may be associated with Marfan syndrome but does not directly affect cardiovascular function.

Pectus excavatum, a condition in which the sternum is displaced posteriorly, is commonly observed in Marfan syndrome (p. 1665), homocystinuria, Ehlers-Danlos syndrome (p. 1668), Hunter-Hurler syndrome (p. 1670), and a small fraction of patients with mitral valve prolapse (p.

1091). This thoracic deformity rarely compresses the heart or elevates the systemic and pulmonary venous pressures, and the signs of heart disease are more often apparent rather than real. Displacement of the heart into the left thorax, prominence of the pulmonary artery, and a parasternal midsystolic murmur all may falsely suggest the presence of organic heart disease. It may be associated with palpitation, tachycardia, fatigue, mild dyspnea, and some impairment of cardiac function.[45,46] Lack of normal thoracic kyphosis, i.e., the *straight back* syndrome,[1] is often associated with expiratory splitting of the second heart sound, a parasternal midsystolic murmur, and enlargement of the pulmonary artery on x-ray; therefore, it may be confused with atrial septal defect.[47,48]

Cardiovascular pulsations should be looked for on the entire chest but specifically in the regions of the cardiac apex, the left parasternal region, and the third left and second right intercostal spaces. Prominent pulsations in these areas suggest enlargement of the left ventricle, right ventricle, pulmonary artery, and aorta, respectively. A thrusting apex exceeding 2 cm in diameter suggests left ventricular enlargements; systolic retraction of the apex may be visible in constrictive pericarditis. Normally, cardiac pulsations are not visible lateral to the midclavicular line; when present there, they signify cardiac enlargement unless there is thoracic deformity or congenital absence of the pericardium. Shaking of the entire precordium with each heart beat may occur in patients with severe valvular regurgitation, large left-to-right shunts, complete AV block, hypertrophic obstructive cardiomyopathy, and various hyperkinetic states. Aortic aneurysms may produce visible pulsations of one of the sternoclavicular joints of the right anterior thoracic wall.

PALPATION (Table 2–1)

Pulsations of the heart and great vessels that are transmitted to the chest wall are best appreciated when the examiner is positioned on the right side of a supine patient. In order to palpate the movements of the heart and great vessels, the examiner should utilize the fingertips or the area just proximal thereto. Precordial movements should be timed by using the simultaneously palpated carotid pulse or auscultated heart sounds.[49] The examination should be carried out with the trunk elevated to 30 degrees, both with the patient supine and in the partial left lateral decubitus positions; the latter increases the amplitude of the left ventricular impulse. Rotating the patient into the left lateral decubitus position causes the heart to move laterally and increases the palpability of both normal and pathological thrusts of the left ventricle. Indeed, it converts the normal systolic retraction of the apex to an outward expansion. Obese, muscular, and emphysematous persons may have weak or undetectable cardiac pulsations in the absence of cardiac abnormality, while thoracic deformities (e.g., kyphoscoliosis, pectus excavatum) can alter the pulsations transmitted to the chest wall. In the course of cardiac palpation, precordial tenderness may be detected; this important finding (p. 1338) may result from trauma, costochondritis, or Tzietse's syndrome and may be an important indication that chest pain is not due to myocardial ischemia.

THE LEFT VENTRICLE. The *apex beat,* also referred to as the cardiac impulse and the apical thrust, is usually produced by left ventricular contraction and is the lowest and most lateral point on the chest at which the cardiac impulse can be appreciated; normally it is medial

TABLE 2–1 CHARACTERISTICS OF PRECORDIAL MOTION IN VARIOUS CARDIAC ABNORMALITIES

Aortic Regurgitation	Atrial Septal Defect	Congestive Cardiomyopathy	Coronary Artery Disease
Apex impulse hyperdynamic in mild to moderate AR Severe AR: LV dilatation results in sustained impulse which is displaced laterally and downward (especially chronic AR) Systolic retraction medial to PMI Palpable *a* wave may be present	Hyperdynamic parasternal impulse PA impulse may be present RV impulse may be sustained if pulmonary hypertension is present and occasionally with large L to R shunt without elevated PA pressure	Sustained and displaced LV impulse, usually felt over 2 interspaces Palpable *a* wave (S_4) and S_3 common Parasternal lift, midsystolic bulge common	Usually normal at rest unless prior MI Palpable S_4 in left decubitus position Ectopic LV bulge thrust if dyssynergy or LV aneurysm. May have transient abnormalities (e.g., bulge, heave) during acute infarction or attack of angina
Hypertrophic Cardiomyopathy	**Mitral Regurgitation**	**Mitral Stenosis**	**Valvar Aortic Stenosis**
Systolic thrill superior, medial to apex impulse Vigorous LV apical impulse, often sustained Large palpable *a* wave, especially in left decubitus position Occasional mid- or late systolic bulge—"triple ripple"	Apical systolic thrill in severe MR Apex impulse hyperdynamic Severe and/or chronic MR: apex is displaced laterally, sustained with amplitude Can have late parasternal impulse with severe MR without pulmonary hypertension Parasternal (RV) heave if significant pulmonary hypertension S_3 visible and palpable if severe MR S_4 palpable with acute onset MR	Small or impalpable apex impulse but S_1 typically palpable Opening snap palpable medial to apex Apical diastolic thrill in left decubitus position Parasternal lift is common; suggests pulmonary hypertension at rest or with effort	Systolic thrill—aortic area, 2 LICS. Or occasionally at apex Sustained and forceful LV apical impulse Little lateral (leftward) displacement of apex unless LV dilatation has occurred Palpable *a* wave (S_4) is common and indicates severe aortic obstruction

AR = aortic regurgitation; LV = left ventricular; PA = pulmonary artery; RV = right ventricle; MI = myocardial infarction; MR = mitral regurgitation. (Reproduced with permission from Abrams, J.: Examination of the precordium: Primary Cardiol. *8*:156–158, 1982.)

and superior to the intersection of the left midclavicular line and the fifth intercostal space. Although displacement of the apex beat outside the midclavicular line is almost always associated with cardiac enlargement, thoracic deformities—particularly scoliosis, straight back, and pectus excavatum—can result in the lateral displacement of a normal-sized heart. Although the apex beat is also often the point of maximal impulse (PMI), this is not always the case, since the pulsations produced by other structures, e.g., an enlarged right ventricle, a dilated pulmonary artery, or an aneurysm of the aorta, may be more powerful than the apex beat.

The apex cardiogram (p. 58), which traces the movement of the chest wall, often represents the pulsation of the entire left ventricle, not only the movement of the apex itself. Therefore, its contour differs from what is perceived on palpation of the chest or what is recorded by the kinetocardiogram, a device in which the motion of specific points on the chest wall are recorded relative to a fixed point in space,[50] and which therefore presents a more faithful graphic registration of the movements of the palpating finger on the chest wall.

Systolic Motion. During isovolumetric contraction, the heart normally rotates counterclockwise (as one faces the patient), and the lower anterior portion of the left ventricle strikes the anterior chest wall, causing a brief outward motion followed by retraction of the left ventricle and the adjacent chest wall during ejection. The segment of the left ventricle responsible for the apex beat is usually medial to the actual cardiac apex, identified on radiological or angiographic examination. For timing purposes it is useful to correlate pulsations while simultaneously listening to heart sounds; a convenient way to do this is to correlate the observed motion of the stethoscope, placed at the apex, with the auscultatory events.

The peak outward motion of the apex impulse is brief and occurs simultaneously with, or just after, aortic valve opening; then the left ventricular apex moves inward. In asthenic persons, in patients with mild left ventricular enlargement, and in subjects with a normal left ventricle but an augmented stroke volume, as occurs in anxiety and other hyperkinetic states, the cardiac impulse may be overactive; i.e., the outward thrust during systole is exaggerated in amplitude, but it is not sustained during ejection. With moderate or severe left ventricular enlargement, the outward systolic thrust persists throughout ejection, often lasting up to the second heart sound (Figs. 2–6 and 2–7), and this motion may be accompanied by retraction of the left parasternal region. This rocking motion can often be appreciated by placing the index finger of one hand on the apex beat and that of the other hand in the parasternal region and by observing the simultaneous outward motion of the former with retraction of the latter. The left ventricular heave or lift, which is more prominent in left ventricular dilatation than in concentric hypertrophy, is characterized by a sustained outward movement of an area that is larger than the normal apex, i.e., more than 2 cm by 2 cm. An *aneurysm of the left ventricle* also produces a larger-than-normal area of pulsation of the left ventricular apex. Alternatively, it may produce a sustained systolic bulge several centimeters superior to the left ventricular impulse. In patients with *left ventricular dyskinesia*, as occurs in acute myocardial ischemia or following myocardial infarction, there may be two distinct impulses separated from each

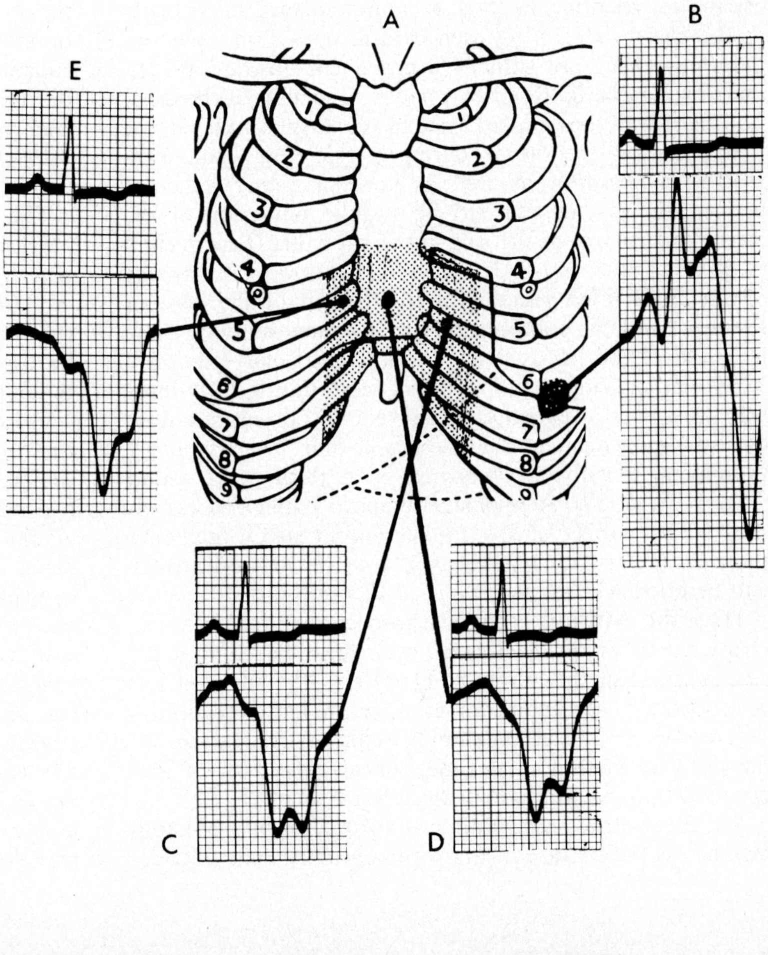

FIGURE 2–6 A large area of systolic retraction is indicated on the chest wall diagram (*A*) by light shading. Graphs taken from three points of this area (*C, D,* and *E*) show a sweeping downward movement during systole as evidence of retraction. The apex beat, felt in the 6th intercostal space, is indicated by an area of heavy shading. A graph of the apical thrust (*B*) shows a sustained upward movement, indicative of a left ventricular overload. The patient was a 40-year-old man with marked rheumatic aortic regurgitation. (From Dressler, W.: Clinical Aids in Cardiac Diagnosis. New York, 1970, p. 83, by permission of Grune and Stratton.)

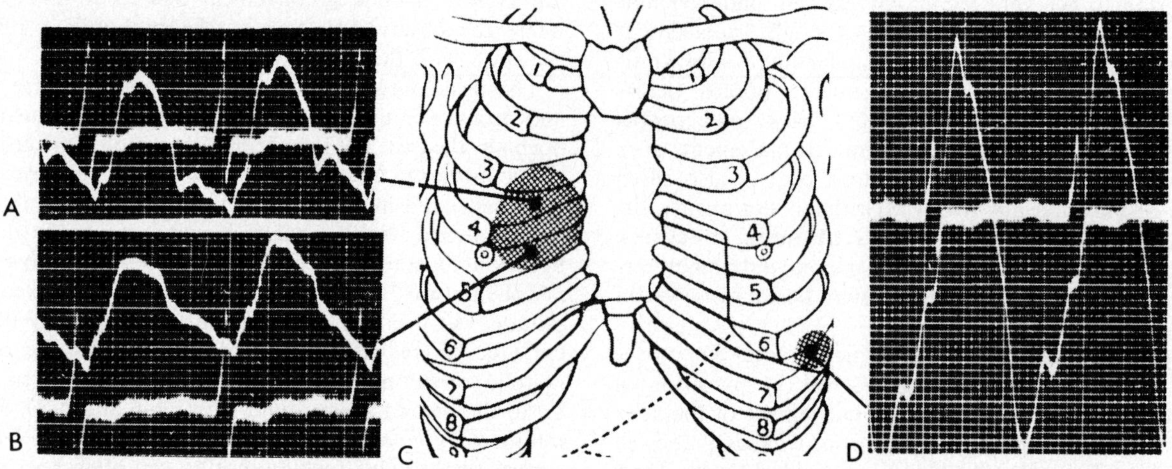

FIGURE 2–7 Diagram of the anterior wall (*C*) showing two areas of heaving pulsation (indicated by heavy shading). The area on the left side of the chest represents the apical thrust of a hypertrophied ventricle, as is shown on a graph (*D*). The curve rises 0.05 sec after onset of QRS and forms a broad, high peak during systole. Another area of systolic outward movement is present on the right side of the chest. Two recordings taken from this area (*A* and *B*) show curves that differ distinctly from that of the apical thrust. They rise 0.12 sec after QRS and resemble an arterial pulse. The pulsation on the right half of the chest was caused by a dissecting aneurysm of the ascending aorta. (From Dressler, W.: Clinical Aids in Cardiac Diagnosis. New York, 1970, p. 91, by permission of Grune and Stratton.)

other by several centimeters. In *mitral stenosis* there may be a brief prominent apical tap owing to an accentuated first sound, which must be distinguished from the apical thrust of an enlarged left ventricle.

A double systolic outward thrust of the left ventricle is occasionally present in patients with prolapse of the mitral valve (Fig. 3–31, p. 61) and is characteristic of patients with hypertrophic obstructive cardiomyopathy (Fig. 3–30, p. 60) who also often exhibit a typical presystolic cardiac expansion, resulting in three separate outward movements of the chest wall during each cardiac cycle.[39] In *aortic regurgitation* the apex exhibits a prominent outward thrust, but this may be followed by systolic retraction of the anterior chest wall as a consequence of the large stroke volume that evacuates the thorax during systole (Fig. 2–6). *Constrictive pericarditis* (as well as nonconstricting adherent pericarditis) is characterized by systolic retraction of the chest, particularly of the ribs in the left axilla (Broadbent's sign) (Figs. 2–8 and 3–33, p. 62). This inward movement results from interference with the descent of the base of the heart and the compensatory exaggerated motion of the free wall of the left ventricle during ventricular ejection.[51] When left ventricular filling is very rapid during early diastole, as occurs in patients with severe mitral regurgitation, outward movement of the chest wall may be particularly prominent, usually accompanied by a third heart sound (Fig. 3–28, p. 59). A hypokinetic apical impulse is associated with a variety of low cardiac output states, including those secondary to hypovolemia, constrictive pericarditis, and pericardial effusion.

Diastolic Motion. The outward motion of the apex characteristic of rapid left ventricular diastolic filling is accentuated when the inflow of blood into the left ventricle is accelerated, as occurs, for example, in mitral regurgitation or when the left ventricular ejection fraction is reduced. This motion is the mechanical equivalent of and occurs simultaneously with a third heart sound.

When the atrial contribution to ventricular filling is augmented, as occurs in patients with concentric left ventricular hypertrophy, myocardial ischemia, and myocardial fibrosis, a presystolic pulsation (usually accompanying a fourth heart sound) is palpable, resulting in a double outward movement of the left ventricular impulse (Fig. 3–29, p. 60, and 4–4, p. 70). This presystolic expansion is most readily discernible during expiration, when the patient is in the left lateral decubitus position, and it can be confirmed by detecting the motion of the stethoscope placed over the left ventricular impulse or by observing the motion of the tip of a pencil or tongue depressor when the proximal portion is placed near the left ventricular impulse. It can be enhanced by sustained hand grip. Presystolic expansion of the right ventricle occurs in right ventricular hypertrophy and pulmonary hypertension. It may be appreciated by subxiphoid palpation of the right ventricle during inspiration.

The Right Ventricle. A palpable anterior systolic movement (replacing systolic retraction) in the left parasternal region (Fig. 2–9*A*) usually represents *right ventricular enlargement,* which, in the absence of associated left ventricular enlargement, may be accompanied by reciprocal systolic retraction of the apex. Exaggerated motion of the entire parasternal area usually reflects increased right ventricular recoil due to augmented stroke volume, as occurs in patients with atrial septal defect, while a sustained left parasternal outward thrust reflects right ventricular hypertrophy due to pressure overload, as occurs in pulmonic stenosis. With marked right ventricular enlargement, this chamber occupies the apex and the left ventricle is displaced posteriorly. When both ventricles are enlarged, both the left parasternal and the apical areas may rise with systole, but an area of systolic retraction between them can sometimes be appreciated. In patients with emphysema, an enlarged right ventricle is sometimes detected most readily in the subxiphoid region by palpating the epigastrium and pointing the finger upward (Fig. 2–9*B*). With marked isolated right ventricular enlargement, the heart may rotate in a clockwise manner, and the right ventricle may form the cardiac apex, producing findings that may

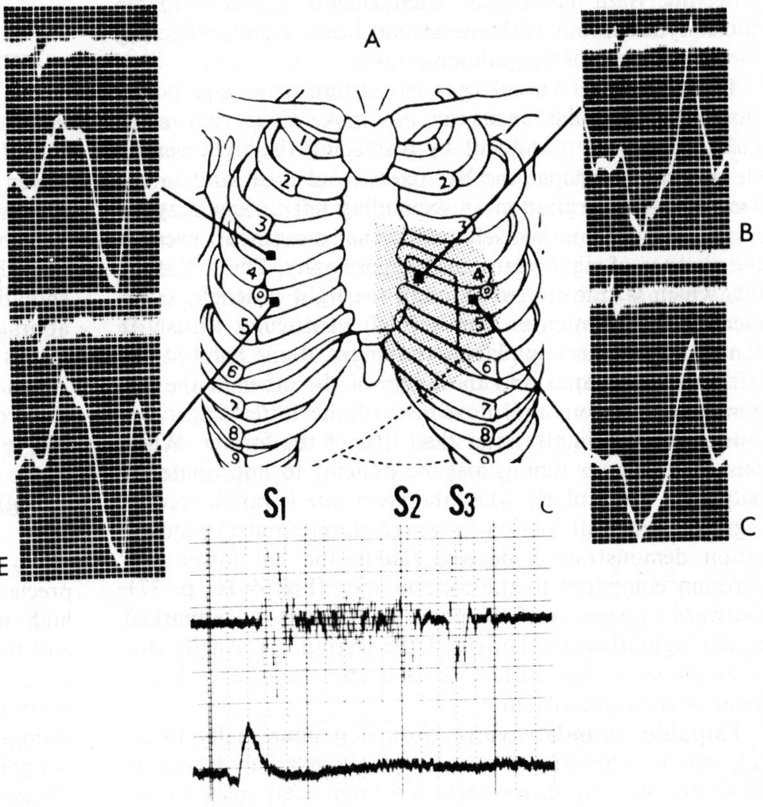

FIGURE 2-8 The chest diagram (*A*) shows an extensive area of systolic retraction on the left side (indicated by light shading). Graphs *B* and *C* were taken from two points of the pulsating area. During systole, both curves move briskly downward and then rise to a sharp peak in early diastole (rebound). Graphs *D* and *E*, taken from two points in the right midclavicular line, show pulsations of opposite direction. The curves move upward during systole and sharply downward during early diastole. The phonocardiogram (*bottom*) shows a holosystolic murmur and a third heart sound "pericardial knock." The tracings are from a 56-year-old woman who suffered from constrictive pericarditis confirmed on postmortem examination. (From Dressler, W.: Clinical Aids in Cardiac Diagnosis. New York, 1970, p. 87, by permission of Grune and Stratton.)

be confused with those of left or biventricular enlargement. When acute myocardial ischemia or myocardial infarction causes dyskinetic movement of the ventricular septum, there may be a transient left parasternal impulse not caused by right ventricular enlargement.

Pulmonary hypertension and/or increased pulmonary blood flow frequently produces a prominent systolic pulsation of the pulmonary artery in the second intercostal space just to the left of the sternum. This pulsation is often associated with a prominent left parasternal impulse,

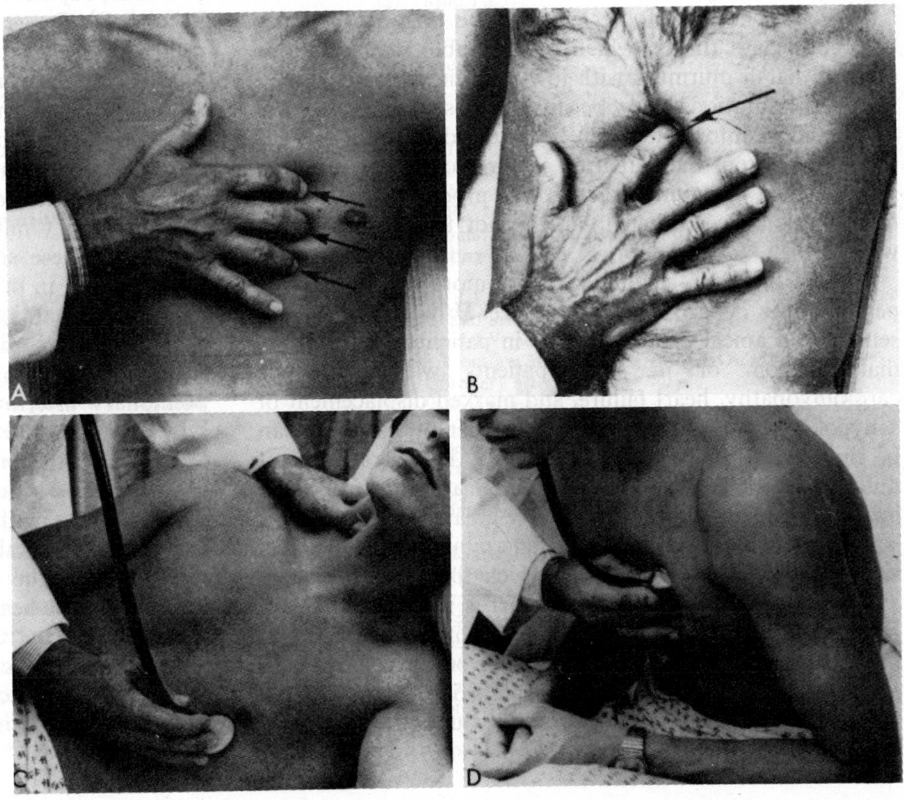

FIGURE 2-9 *A*, Palpation of the anterior wall of the right ventricle by applying the tips of three fingers in the third, fourth, and fifth interspaces, left sternal edge, during full held exhalation. Patient is supine with the trunk elevated 30 degrees. *B*, Palpation of the inferior wall of the right ventricle in the epigastrium. The flat of the hand is directed upward and toward the left shoulder. The tip of the index finger (arrow) palpates the right ventricle as it descends during full held inspiration. The patient is supine with trunk elevated 30 degrees. *C*, The stethoscope is applied to the cardiac apex while the patient lies in a partial left lateral decubitus position. The examiner's free left hand is used to palpate the carotid artery for timing purposes. *D*, The soft-high frequency early diastolic murmur of either aortic regurgitation or pulmonary hypertensive pulmonary regurgitation is best elicited by applying the stethoscopic diaphragm very firmly to the mid-left sternal edge. The patient leans forward with breath held in full exhalation. (Reproduced with permission from Perloff, J. K. (Ed.): Physical Examination of the Heart and Circulation. Philadelphia, W. B. Saunders Co., 1982.)

late, and whether it is high-pitched (such as a systolic click) or low-pitched (such as a third or fourth heart sound, i.e., S_3 or S_4) (Fig. 2–11). When two heart sounds are heard at the time of S_1, it is often difficult to differentiate between a split S_1, a combination of S_4 and S_1, and a combination of S_1 and an ejection click.[64] The S_4 is usually audible only at the apex and often in the left lateral decubitus position; it is usually low-pitched, associated with palpable presystolic distention of the left ventricle, and attenuated by increased pressure on the bell of the stethoscope. It is rarely heard at the lower left sternal border, where splitting of S_1 is most easily detected. The ejection click is usually louder than the second component of a split S_1 and is often audible at the base of the heart, while splitting of S_1 is rarely heard in this area.

Ejection sounds, which coincide with the full opening of the semilunar valves, are high-pitched and clicking and are heard best with the diaphragm of the stethoscope. Aortic ejection sounds are heard best in the second right interspace and at the apex and are not notably affected by respiration, while pulmonic ejection sounds are heard best in the second left interspace and often diminish in intensity during inspiration. Mid- to late systolic clicks are heard in mitral valve prolapse (p. 1091), are of high frequency, and are also heard best with the diaphragm.

Diastolic Sounds. Opening snaps (of the mitral or tricuspid valve) indicate that the valve is mobile. These high-pitched sounds are heard best through the diaphragm.

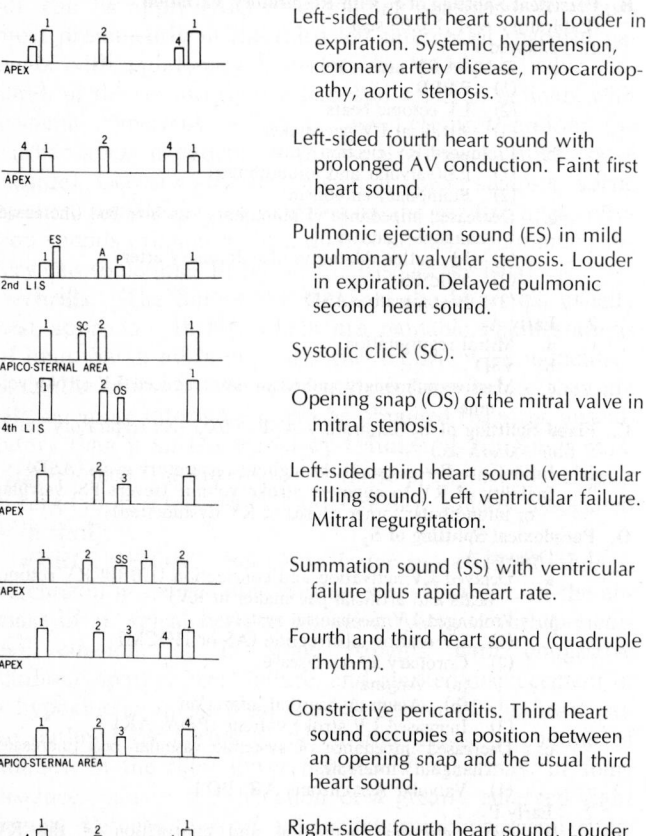

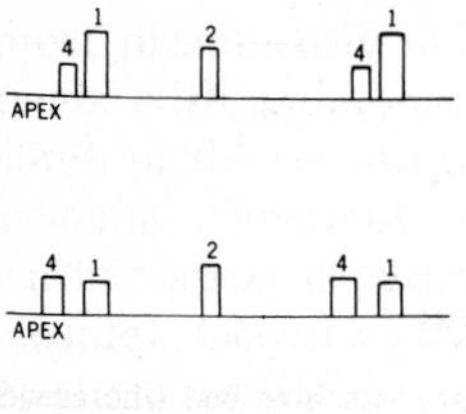

Left-sided fourth heart sound. Louder in expiration. Systemic hypertension, coronary artery disease, myocardiopathy, aortic stenosis.

Left-sided fourth heart sound with prolonged AV conduction. Faint first heart sound.

Pulmonic ejection sound (ES) in mild pulmonary valvular stenosis. Louder in expiration. Delayed pulmonic second heart sound.

Systolic click (SC).

Opening snap (OS) of the mitral valve in mitral stenosis.

Left-sided third heart sound (ventricular filling sound). Left ventricular failure. Mitral regurgitation.

Summation sound (SS) with ventricular failure plus rapid heart rate.

Fourth and third heart sound (quadruple rhythm).

Constrictive pericarditis. Third heart sound occupies a position between an opening snap and the usual third heart sound.

Right-sided fourth heart sound. Louder in inspiration. Pulmonary hypertension, large left-to-right shunt at atrial level.

FIGURE 2–11 Interpretation of extra sounds. 1, 2, 3, and 4 refer to the first, second, third, and fourth sounds. A and P refer to the aortic and pulmonic valve closure sounds, respectively. LIS = left intercostal space; LSB = left sternal border. (From Ravin, A., et al.: Auscultation of the Heart. Chicago, Year Book Medical Publishers, 1977, p. 80.)

The diastolic sound during passive filling which occurs during the *y* descent of the atrial pressure pulse is termed the third heart sound (S_3), while the sound which occurs during ventricular filling caused by atrial contraction is called the fourth heart sound (S_4).[68] When S_3 and S_4 are abnormal, they are referred to as third or fourth heart sound "gallops." S_3 may be normal in children and young adults but when heard in men over the age of 40 years and women over the age of 50 years, they are generally abnormal. Healthy adults may have an S_4, but when heard in the young, this sound is usually abnormal. Since S_3 and S_4 (whether normal or not) are produced by rapid ventricular filling, they are absent in the presence of mitral or tricuspid stenosis. Third and fourth heart sounds are best heard with the bell of the stethoscope, are intensified by the recumbent position and by exercise, such as a few sit-ups, or sustained hand-grip. Inspiration enhances third or fourth heart sounds originating from the right ventricle, but has little detectable effect on such sounds originating from the left ventricle.

S_3 occurs as active ventricular relaxation (reflected in the decline in ventricular pressure) ends and passive filling (reflected in a diastolic rise in ventricular pressure) begins.[67a] It is intensified by rapid early diastolic filling, an elevated atrial pressure, and increased or abnormal diastolic distensibility of the ventricle. Conditions causing ventricular diastolic overload with atrial hypertension are often responsible for an S_3 which is audible in states of increased cardiac output, such as during the third trimester of pregnancy, after exertion, or in anxiety-related tachycardia. It also occurs with impaired left ventricular function of any cause. In the presence of coronary artery disease, an S_3 strongly suggests left ventricular dyskinesia or aneurysm. In patients with aortic regurgitation it usually signifies a reduced ejection fraction and elevated end-systolic volume[69] and in patients with reduced cardiac reserve it correlates well with the response to digitalis.[70]

An S_4 is generally associated with an elevated ventricular end-diastolic pressure and a high ratio of left ventricular wall thickness–to–cavity diameter. As left ventricular distensibility decreases, atrial systole becomes responsible for more than 25 per cent of ventricular filling, and an S_4 may become prominent. Vigorous atrial contraction is necessary to produce an audible S_4, which can be recorded phonocardiographically in about 50 per cent of normal adults, but it is extremely low in intensity and usually not audible. However, a loud, palpable S_4 is almost always abnormal. The common denominators are left ventricular hypertrophy, increased left ventricular end-diastolic pressure, and some restriction to diastolic filling. An S_4 is characteristic of aortic stenosis with a significant left ventricular–aortic pressure gradient, hypertrophic cardiomyopathy, and acute mitral regurgitation. Reduced left ventricular compliance following myocardial infarction often results in an audible S_4. A right ventricular S_4 is common in pulmonary hypertension and pulmonary stenosis.

MURMURS AND OTHER ADVENTITIOUS SOUNDS

Cardiac murmurs should be timed, and their length in the cardiac cycle and their shape, i.e., their intensity (or loudness) as a function of time, should be noted. The *intensity* of a murmur is determined by the quantity and velocity of blood flow across the sound-producing area, by its distance from the stethoscope, and by the transmission qualities of the tissue between the origin of the murmur and the stethoscope.[71] Murmurs are accentuated in thin persons and diminished in patients who are obese, in emphysema, and in the presence of pleural or pericardial fluid.[53] They are accentuated in hyperdynamic states and reduced in hypodynamic states. It is helpful to grade the intensity of murmurs; six grades, as described by Levine, are commonly distinguished.[72] A *Grade 1/6* murmur is the faintest that can be detected, often only after close concentration and adjustment of the stethoscope. A *Grade 2/6* murmur is a faint murmur but can be detected immediately. A *Grade 3/6* murmur is moderately loud, and a *Grade 4/6* murmur is loud. A *Grade 5/6* murmur is a very loud murmur but requires placement of the stethoscope on the chest to be audible. A *Grade 6/6* murmur is so loud that it can be heard even without placing the stethoscope on the chest. The *length* of a murmur depends upon the duration of the events, such as a pressure gradient responsible for it, while the *radiation* of a murmur is determined by its site of origin, its intensity, the direction of the blood flow responsible for the murmur, and the physical characteristics of the chest.[71] The *quality* of murmurs should be described using adjectives such as blowing, harsh, rumbling, musical, and high- or low-pitched. Murmurs with mixed high and medium frequencies sound harsh or rasping, while those with a narrow frequency range, often owing to vibration of an intracardiac structure such as a valve leaflet, are musical or honking in quality.

The interpretation of heart murmurs is based equally on their characteristics (timing, intensity, duration, location, quality, and pitch) and the accompanying auscultatory features, such as the character of the splitting of S_2 as well as the presence of ejection sounds and of S_3 and S_4. The etiology of various murmurs is presented in Table 2–3, and Figures 2–12 and 2–13 illustrate a variety of murmurs and sounds. A discussion of the most important heart murmurs is presented in Chapter 4.

Pericardial friction rubs are the sounds made by two inflamed layers of the pericardium sliding over one another, but they may be present even when there is considerable pericardial effusion. Friction rubs are generally described as scratching, grating, crunching, and creaking; they seem close to the ear and may vary in distribution from a site that is sharply localized to a small area of the precordium to the entire left hemithorax.[73,74] Usually they are most readily audible along the left sternal edge using the diaphragm with firm pressure and are often better heard during deep inspiration and with the patient leaning forward or in the prone position and propped up by the elbows.[75] The sounds are commonly "to and fro" and have either one or two diastolic components. In some patients, however, only a systolic component is audible. Friction rubs may be confused with the to-and-fro murmurs of combined aortic stenosis and regurgitation. Pleural-pericardial friction rubs are caused by the inflamed pleura against the parietal pericardium and are usually heard only during inspiration.

Acute mediastinal emphysema produces loud, bizarre, crunching sounds over the precordium, mainly during systole; these are audible most prominently near the apex and sometimes only with the patient in the left lateral recumbent position.[57] *Diaphragmatic flutter* produces regular sounds that are independent of the pulse and are audible over the entire thorax, even in the right axilla, far removed from the heart.[57]

A *cervical venous hum* is a continuous murmur heard best with the stethoscopic bell in the lateral portion of the

TABLE 2–3 PRINCIPAL CAUSES OF HEART MURMURS

- **A. Organic Systolic Murmurs**
  - 1. Midsystolic (Ejection)
    - a. AORTIC
      - (1) Obstructive
        - (a) Supravalvular—supraaortic stenosis, coarctation of the aorta
        - (b) Valvular—AS and sclerosis
        - (c) Infravalvular—HOCM
      - (2) Increased flow, hyperkinetic states, AR, complete heart block
      - (3) Dilatation of ascending aorta, atheroma, aortitis, aneurysm of aorta
    - b. PULMONARY
      - (1) Obstructive
        - (a) Supravalvular—pulmonary arterial stenosis
        - (b) Valvular—pulmonic valve stenosis
        - (c) Infravalvular—infundibular stenosis
      - (2) Increased flow, hyperkinetic states, left-to-right shunt (e.g., ASD, VSD)
      - (3) Dilatation of pulmonary artery
  - 2. Pansystolic (Regurgitant)
    - a. Atrioventricular valve regurgitation (MR, TR)
    - b. Left-to-right shunt to ventricular level
- **B. Early Diastolic Murmurs**
  - 1. Aortic regurgitation (see also Table 32–11, p. 1106)
    - a. Valvular: rheumatic deformity; perforation post-endocarditis, post-traumatic, post-valvulotomy
    - b. Dilatation of valve ring: aortic dissection, annuloectasia, cystic medial necrosis, hypertension
    - c. Widening of commissures: syphilis
    - d. Congenital: bicuspid valve, with ventricular septal defect
  - 2. Pulmonic regurgitation (see also p. 1122)
    - a. Valvular: post-valvulotomy, endocarditis, rheumatic fever, carcinoid
    - b. Dilatation of valve ring: pulmonary hypertension; Marfan's syndrome
    - c. Congenital: isolated or associated with tetralogy of Fallot, VSD, pulmonic stenosis
- **C. Mid-diastolic Murmurs**
  - 1. Mitral stenosis
  - 2. Carey-Coomb's murmur (mid-diastolic apical murmur in acute rheumatic fever)
  - 3. Increased flow across nonstenotic mitral valve (e.g., MR, VSD, PDA, high-output states, and complete heart block)
  - 4. Tricuspid stenosis
  - 5. Increased flow across nonstenotic tricuspid valve (e.g., TR, ASD, and anomalous pulmonary venous return)
  - 6. Left and right atrial tumors
- **D. Continuous Murmurs**
  - 1. Patent ductus arteriosus
  - 2. Coronary AV fistula
  - 3. Ruptured aneurysm of sinus of Valsalva
  - 4. Aortic septal defect
  - 5. Cervical venous hum
  - 6. Anomalous left coronary artery
  - 7. Proximal coronary artery stenosis
  - 8. Mammary souffle
  - 9. Pulmonary artery branch stenosis
  - 10. Bronchial collateral circulation
  - 11. Small (restrictive) ASD with MS
  - 12. Intercostal AV fistula

AR = aortic regurgitation; AS = aortic stenosis; ASD = atrial septal defect; AV = arteriovenous; HOCM = hypertrophic obstructive cardiomyopathy; MR = mitral regurgitation; MS = mitral stenosis; PDA = patent ductus arteriosus; TR = tricuspid regurgitation; VSD = ventricular septal defect. (*A* and *C* modified from Oram, S. (ed.): Clinical Heart Disease. London, William Heinemann Medical Books, Ltd., 1981; *D* modified from Fowler, N. O. (ed.): Cardiac Diagnosis and Treatment. Hagerstown, Harper and Row, 1980.)

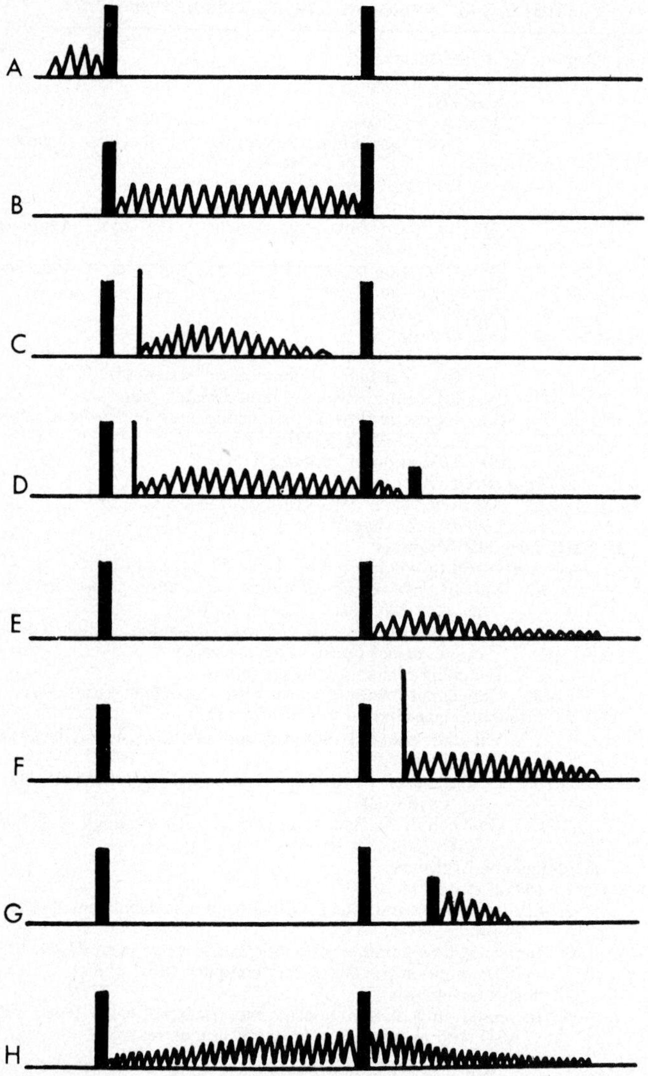

FIGURE 2–12 Diagram depicting principal heart murmurs:

A, Presystolic murmur of mitral or tricuspid stenosis.

B, Pansystolic murmur of mitral or tricuspid incompetence or of ventricular septal defect.

C, Aortic ejection murmur beginning with an ejection click and fading before the second heart sound.

D, Systolic murmur in pulmonic stenosis spilling through the aortic second sound, pulmonic valve closure being delayed.

E, Aortic pulmonary diastolic murmur.

F, Long diastolic murmur of mitral stenosis following the opening snap.

G, Short mid-diastolic inflow murmur following a third heart sound.

H, Continuous murmur of patent ductus arteriosus.

(From Wood, P.: Diseases of the Heart and Circulation. Philadelphia, J. B. Lippincott Co., 1968, p. 75.)

right supraclavicular fossa with the patient sitting or standing and can be confused with the murmur produced by a patent ductus arteriosus.[76] It is due to the rapid downward flow of blood through a jugular vein that becomes artificially stenosed when the patient is in the upright position, and it disappears when the jugular vein is compressed or when the patient assumes the recumbent position. A venous hum can be intensified by tilting the chin upward and can be abolished by pressure over the upper part of the jugular vein. It is common in normal children and in conditions in which the circulation is hyperkinetic such as anemia, thyrotoxicosis, or pregnancy.

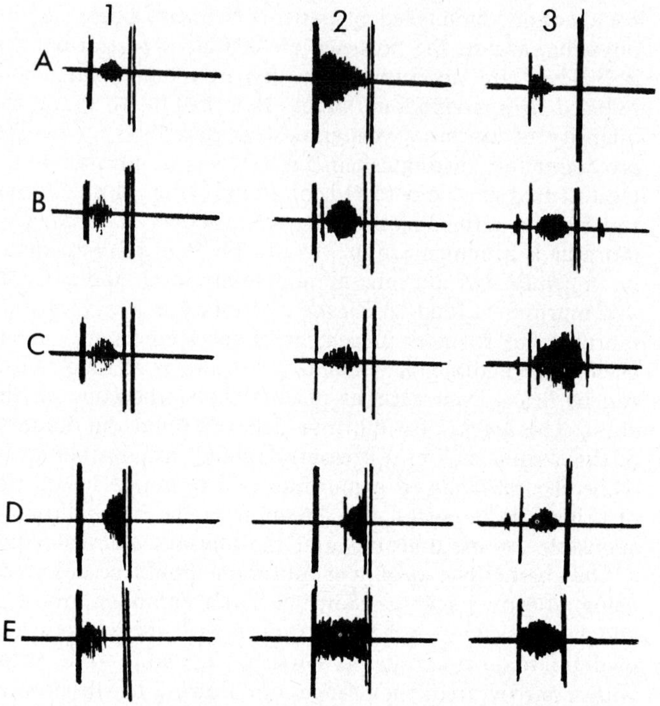

FIGURE 2–13 Sketches of various murmurs and heart sounds.

A–1, Short, midsystolic murmur, with normal aortic and pulmonic components of S_2—findings consistent with an innocent murmur.

A–2, Holosystolic murmur that decreases in the latter part of systole—a configuration observed in acute mitral regurgitation.

A–3, An ejection sound and a short early systolic murmur, plus accentuated, closely split S_2—consistent with pulmonary hypertension, as with Eisenmenger's ventricular septal defect.

B–1, Early to midsystolic murmur with vibratory component—typical of an innocent murmur.

B–2, An ejection sound followed by a diamond-shaped murmur and wide splitting of S_2 that may be present with atrial septal defect or mild pulmonic stenosis; an ejection sound is more likely with valvular pulmonic stenosis.

B–3, Crescendo-decrescendo systolic murmur, not holosystolic; S_3 and S_4 are present—findings consistent with mitral systolic murmur heard in congestive cardiomyopathy or coronary artery disease with papillary muscle dysfunction and cardiac decompensation.

C–1, Longer, somewhat vibratory crescendo-decrescendo systolic murmur with wide splitting of S_2 sound. If S_2 becomes fused with expiration, atrial septal defect is less likely; if the remainder of the cardiovascular evaluation is normal, this finding is consistent with an innocent murmur.

C–2, Midsystolic murmur and wide splitting of S_2 that was "fixed"—findings typical of atrial septal defect.

C–3, Prolonged diamond-shaped systolic murmur masking A_2 with delayed P_2, S_4, and ejection sound—findings typical of valvular pulmonic stenosis of moderate severity.

D–1, Late apical systolic murmur of prolapsing mitral valve leaflet.

D–2, Systolic click–late apical systolic murmur of prolapsing mitral leaflet syndrome.

D–3, S_4 and midsystolic murmur consistent with mitral systolic murmur of cardiomyopathy or ischemic heart disease.

E–1, Early crescendo-decrescendo systolic murmur ending in midsystole consistent with innocent murmur and small ventricular septal defect.

E–2 and *E–3*, Holosystolic murmurs consistent with mitral or tricuspid regurgitation and ventricular septal defect. (From Harvey, W. P.: Innocent vs. significant murmurs. Curr. Probl. Cardiol. Vol. 1, No. 8, 1976.)

A *mammary souffle* is a systolic or continuous murmur sometimes heard over the breasts of pregnant or lactating women[77] that can be confused with continuous murmurs produced by pulmonary arteriovenous fistula, patent ductus arteriosus, and other forms of congenital heart disease (Table 2–3*D*). It is presumably caused by the increased flow of blood through the engorged breast, generally commences just after the first heart sound, is best heard with the patient supine and may disappear in the upright position or with pressure from the stethoscope.

Cardiorespiratory murmurs are systolic (rarely continuous) murmurs heard on inspiration but not when the breath is held or during expiration, and they may result from the movement of air in the bronchial tree during systole and inspiration.[78]

DYNAMIC AUSCULTATION

This is the technique of altering circulatory dynamics by means of a variety of physiological and pharmacological maneuvers and determining their effects on heart sounds and murmurs.[79] As outlined in Figure 2–10 and Tables 2–4 and 2–5, an appreciation of the effects of these interventions can be of great value in the interpretation of a variety of auscultatory findings. The interventions most commonly employed in dynamic auscultation include respiration, postural changes, the Valsalva maneuver, premature ventricular contractions, isometric exercise, and vasoactive agents—amyl nitrite, methoxamine, and phenylephrine.

Respiration

SPLITTING OF S_2. The splitting of S_2 can usually be appreciated best along the left sternal border and is audible when A_2 and P_2 are separated by more than 0.02 sec. During inspiration A_2 ordinarily becomes softer in part because of the increased volume of lung that becomes interposed between the heart and chest wall; P_2 becomes louder because of increased flow into the pulmonary artery. A_2 normally occurs less than 0.02 sec after the pressure in the left ventricle falls below that in the aorta, while P_2 occurs 0.03 to 0.09 sec after the decline of pressure in the right ventricle below that in the central pulmonary artery; these intervals have been termed the "hang-out" intervals, and their durations are inversely proportional to the impedance to blood flow in the aortic and pulmonic circuits.[80] The lower capacitance and higher resistance of the systemic compared to the pulmonary circulation result in a shorter hang-out interval in the aorta than in the pulmonary artery, and this difference contributes to the normal delay in P_2 compared to A_2 and therefore to the splitting of S_2. As the impedance to pulmonary flow increases with progressive pulmonary hypertension, the hang-out interval in the pulmonary artery shortens (Fig. 2–10*D*), and there is a reduction in the width of splitting of S_2, so that in severe pulmonary hypertension S_2 may become fused. Several factors play a role in the normal widening of the separation between A_2 and P_2 during inspiration.

During inspiration, venous return to the right side of the heart is augmented, resulting in a higher right ventricular stroke volume and lengthening of the duration of right ventricular ejection. When the respiratory rate is normal, these changes are accompanied by a reduced return of blood to the left side of the heart and a lower left ventricular stroke volume and shorter ejection time. In part, the difference in the effects of respiration on the stroke volumes of the two ventricles is due to the delay in transmission of the augmented right ventricular stroke volume through the pulmonary vascular bed, so that it reaches the left ventricle three or four cardiac cycles later, i.e., during the following expiration.[81] The greater delay in P_2, which accounts for about 75 per cent of the widening of the splitting,[59] results from the increased right ventricular stroke volume and ejection time and an inspiratory decline in pulmonary vascular impedance, with further prolongation of the hang-out interval. The pooling of blood in the lungs during inspiration, with decreased venous return to the left heart, is responsible for shortening of left ventricular systole; earlier occurrence of A_2 accounts for about 25 per cent of the inspiratory augmentation of the width of splitting of S_2.

In normal adults, A_2 and P_2 are separated by 0.04 to

TABLE 2–4 PHYSIOLOGICAL AND PHARMACOLOGICAL MANEUVERS USEFUL IN DIFFERENTIAL DIAGNOSIS OF SIMILAR AUSCULTATORY FINDINGS

Auscultatory Problems	Helpful Maneuvers*
Systolic murmur of valvular aortic stenosis vs. hypertrophic subaortic stenosis	Sudden squatting, Valsalva maneuver
Systolic murmur of valvular aortic stenosis vs. mid- to late systolic mitral valve dysfunction	Sudden standing, amyl nitrite
Systolic murmur of valvular aortic stenosis vs. mitral regurgitation	Amyl nitrite, phenylephrine, variation in cycle length
Diastolic rumble of mitral stenosis vs. Austin Flint murmur	Amyl nitrite
Diastolic murmur of mitral stenosis vs. tricuspid stenosis	Respiration
Systolic murmur of mitral regurgitation vs. tricuspid regurgitation	Respiration
Supraclavicular bruit vs. aortic stenosis	Extension of shoulder, compression of subclavian artery
Ejection sound in pulmonic stenosis vs. aortic stenosis	Respiration
Small ventricular septal defect vs. pulmonic stenosis	Amyl nitrite, phenylephrine
Large ventricular septal defect with fixed vs. hyperkinetic pulmonary hypertension	Amyl nitrite
Systolic murmur of pulmonic stenosis vs. tetralogy of Fallot	Amyl nitrite
Continuous murmur of patent ductus arteriosus vs. cervical venous hum	Compression of neck veins
Fourth sound plus first sound vs. separation of two components of first heart sound	Respiration, sudden standing, lying with passive leg-raising
Second sound plus opening snap vs. wide separation of second heart sound components	Respiration, phenylephrine, sudden standing

*See Table 2–5 for typical response. (From Criscitiello, M. G.: Physiologic and pharmacologic aids in cardiac auscultation. *In* Fowler, N. O. (ed.): Cardiac Diagnosis and Treatment. Hagerstown, Harper and Row, 1980, p. 89.)

TABLE 2–5 RESPONSE OF MURMURS AND HEART SOUNDS TO PHYSIOLOGICAL AND PHARMACOLOGICAL INTERVENTIONS

Clinical disorder	Intervention and Response
SYSTOLIC MURMURS	
Aortic outflow obstruction	
Valvular aortic stenosis	Louder with passive leg-raising, with sudden squatting, with Valsalva release (after five to six beats), following a pause induced by a premature beat, or after amyl nitrite; fades during Valsalva strain and with isometric handgrip
Hypertrophic obstructive cardiomyopathy	Louder with standing, during Valsalva strain, or with amyl nitrite; fades with sudden squatting, recumbency, or isometric handgrip
Pulmonic stenosis	Midsystolic murmur increases with amyl nitrite except with marked right ventricular hypertrophy; also increases during first few beats after Valsalva release
Mitral regurgitation	
Rheumatic	Murmur louder with sudden squatting, isometric handgrip, or phenylephrine; softens with amyl nitrite
Mitral valve prolapse	Midsystolic click moves toward S_1 and late systolic murmur starts earlier with standing, Valsalva strain, and amyl nitrite; click may occur earlier on inspiration; murmur starts later and click moves toward S_2 during squatting, with recumbency, and often after pause induced by a premature beat
Papillary muscle dysfunction	Late systolic murmur generally softer after a pause induced by a premature beat; response to amyl nitrite variable, depending on acute or chronic nature of this disorder
Tricuspid regurgitation	Murmur increases during inspiration, with passive leg-raising, and with amyl nitrite
Ventricular septal defect	
Small defect with pulmonary hypertension	Fades with amyl nitrite; increases with isometric handgrip or phenylephrine
Large defect with hyperkinetic pulmonary hypertension	Louder with amyl nitrite; fades with phenylephrine
Large defect with severe pulmonary vascular disease	Little change with any of above interventions
Tetralogy of Fallot	Murmur softens with amyl nitrite
Supraclavicular bruit	Altered by compression of subclavian artery; may be eliminated by extension of ipsilateral shoulder
DIASTOLIC MURMURS	
Aortic regurgitation	
Blowing diastolic murmur	Increases with sudden squatting, isometric handgrip, or phenylephrine
Austin Flint murmur	Fades with amyl nitrite
Pulmonary regurgitation	
Congenital	Early or mid-diastolic rumble increases on inspiration and with amyl nitrite
Pulmonary hypertension	High-frequency blowing murmur not altered by above interventions
Mitral stenosis	Mid-diastolic and presystolic murmurs louder with exercise, left lateral position, coughing, isometric handgrip, or amyl nitrite; phenylephrine widens A_2-OS interval; inspiration produces sequence of A_2-P_2-OS
Tricuspid stenosis	Mid-diastolic and presystolic murmurs increase during inspiration, with passive leg-raising, and with amyl nitrite
CONTINUOUS MURMURS	
Patent ductus arteriosus	Diastolic phase amplified with isometric handgrip or phenylephrine; diastolic phase fades with amyl nitrite
Cervical venous hum	Obliterated by direct compression of jugular veins or by Valsalva strain
ADDED HEART SOUNDS	
Gallop rhythm	
Ventricular gallop (S_3) and atrial gallop (S_4)	Accentuated by lying flat with passive leg-raising; decreased by standing or during Valsalva; right-sided gallop sounds usually increase during inspiration; left-sided during expiration.
Summation gallop	Separates into ventricular gallop (S_3) and atrial gallop (S_4) sounds when heart rate slowed by carotid sinus massage
Ejection sounds	Ejection sound in pulmonary stenosis fades and occurs closer to the first sound during inspiration

From Criscitiello, M. G.: Physiologic and pharmacologic aids in cardiac auscultation. *In* Fowler, N. O. (ed.): Cardiac Diagnosis and Treatment. Hagerstown, Harper and Row, 1980, p. 88).

0.05 sec during inspiration, with a single S_2 heard during expiration (split ≤ 0.02 sec). Occasionally there may be residual audible splitting in expiration (0.03 to 0.04 sec) in the supine position, but in normal adults auditory expiratory splitting disappears in the sitting or standing position. Expiratory splitting heard in both the supine and upright positions is uncommon in normal subjects of any age. Expiratory splitting of ≥ 0.03 sec, with an increase of ≤ 0.015 sec in the width of splitting, is considered to be "fixed" splitting.

There are four types of abnormal splitting of S_2: (1) Absent splitting (single S_2), (2) splitting that is persistent during expiration, (3) fixed splitting, and (4) paradoxical splitting. The major causes of each are presented in Table 2–2, and further discussion of this subject can be found on pp. 45–47.

S_3, S_4, AND EJECTION SOUNDS. When third and fourth sounds originate from the left ventricle, they are characteristically augmented during expiration and diminished during inspiration, whereas they exhibit the opposite response when they originate from the right side of the heart. Like other left-sided events, the opening snap of the mitral valve may become softer during inspiration and louder during expiration owing to respiratory alterations in venous return, whereas the opening snap of the tricuspid valve behaves in the opposite fashion. Inspiration also diminishes the intensity of valvular pulmonic ejection sounds, since the elevation of right ventricular diastolic pressure causes partial presystolic opening of the pulmonic valve and therefore less upward motion of the valve during systole. On the other hand, respiration does not affect the intensity of nonvalvular pulmonic ejection sounds or of aortic ejection sounds.

MURMURS. Respiration exerts more pronounced and consistent alterations on murmurs originating from the right than the left side of the heart. During inspiration, the diastolic murmurs of tricuspid stenosis and pulmonic regurgitation, the systolic murmurs of tricuspid regurgitation[82] and of mild or moderate pulmonic stenosis, and the pre-systolic murmur of Ebstein's anomaly are all accentuated. During expiration, the increased venous return to the left side of the heart may result in mild accentuation of the diastolic murmur of mitral stenosis and the systolic murmurs of mitral regurgitation, ventricular septal defect, and valvular aortic stenosis. The inspiratory reduction in left ventricular size in patients with mitral valve prolapse increases the redundancy of the mitral valve and therefore the degree of valvular prolapse; consequently, the midsystolic click and the systolic murmurs occur earlier during systole and frequently become accentuated[83] (p. 1092). The effects of inspiration on auscultatory findings may be accentuated by the use of the Müller maneuver, i.e., forced inspiration against a closed glottis. Deep, maintained expiration tends to accentuate soft, early diastolic murmurs of aortic or pulmonic regurgitation.

Postural Changes

Assumption of the lying from the standing or sitting position results in an increase in venous return, which augments first right ventricular and, several cardiac cycles later, left ventricular stroke volume. The principal auscultatory changes include widening of the splitting of S_2 in all phases of respiration and augmentations of right-sided S_3 and S_4 and, several cardiac cycles later, left-sided S_3 and S_4.[84] The systolic murmurs of valvular pulmonic and aortic stenosis, the systolic murmurs of mitral and tricuspid regurgitation and ventricular septal defect, and most functional systolic murmurs are augmented. On the other hand, since left ventricular end-diastolic volume rises, the systolic murmur of hypertrophic obstructive cardiomyopathy is diminished, and the midsystolic click and systolic murmur associated with mitral valve prolapse are delayed and sometimes attenuated.[79,83]

Sudden standing or sitting up from a lying position has the opposite effect; in patients in whom there is relatively wide splitting of S_2 during expiration—a finding that may be confused with fixed splitting—the width of the splitting is reduced, so that a normal pattern emerges during the respiratory cycle. No change in splitting occurs in patients with true fixed splitting.

SQUATTING. A change from standing to squatting increases venous return and systemic resistance simultaneously. Stroke volume and arterial pressure rise, and the latter may induce a transient reflex bradycardia. The auscultatory features include augmentation of S_3 and S_4 (from both ventricles) and as a consequence of an increased in stroke volume, the systolic murmurs of aortic and pulmonic stenosis and the diastolic murmurs of mitral and tricuspid stenosis become louder.[79] The elevation of arterial pressure increases blood flow through the right ventricular outflow tract of patients with the tetralogy of Fallot and increases the volume of mitral regurgitation and of the left-to-right shunt through a ventricular septal defect, thereby increasing the intensity of the systolic murmur in these conditions. Also, the diastolic murmur of aortic regurgitation is augmented consequent to an increase in aortic reflux. The combination of elevated arterial pressure and increased venous return increases left ventricular size, which reduces the obstruction to outflow and therefore the intensity of the systolic murmur of hypertrophic obstructive cardiomyopathy;[85] the midsystolic click of mitral valve prolapse and the systolic murmur are delayed.

Assumption of the left lateral recumbent position accentuates the intensity of S_1, S_3, and S_4 originating from the left side of the heart; the opening snap and the murmurs associated with mitral stenosis and regurgitation; the midsystolic click and late systolic murmur of mitral valve prolapse; and the Austin Flint murmur associated with aortic regurgitation. Sitting up and leaning forward make the diastolic murmurs of aortic and pulmonic regurgitation more readily audible.

THE VALSALVA MANEUVER. During phase I, the initial phase of the Valsalva maneuver, intrathoracic pressure rises, producing a transient increase in left ventricular output. During phase II, the straining phase, systemic venous return declines; filling of the right and then of the left side of the heart are reduced; and the stroke volume and mean arterial and pulse pressures fall and heart rate increases. As a consequence, S_3 and S_4 become attenuated and the A_2–P_2 interval narrows.[59] As stroke volume and arterial pressure fall, the systolic murmurs of aortic and pulmonic stenosis and of mitral and tricuspid regurgitation, and the diastolic murmurs of aortic and pulmonic regurgitation and of tricuspid and mitral stenosis all diminish. However, as left ventricular volume is reduced, the systolic murmur of hypertrophic obstructive cardiomyopathy becomes louder,[86] and the systolic click and murmur of mitral valve prolapse commence earlier. During phase III, the release of the Valsalva maneuver, the aortic and pulmonic components of S_2 normally become more widely separated.[59,87] During the first few beats of phase IV, the overshoot following release of the Valsalva murmurs and filling sounds (S_3 and S_4) originating from the right side of the heart return to normal and may be transiently accentuated. Filling sounds and murmurs originating from the left side of the heart also return to pre-Valsalva levels after six to eight beats and then may be transiently augmented.

An abnormal "square-wave" response to the Valsalva maneuver (see Figure 15–9, p. 501) occurs in patients with atrial septal defect, mitral stenosis, and heart failure of any etiology. With such a response, the above-described changes in hemodynamics and therefore in the auscultatory findings do *not* occur.

POSTPREMATURE VENTRICULAR CONTRACTIONS. When a premature contraction is followed by a significant pause, both an increase in ventricular filling and an augmentation of cardiac contractility occur. Consequently, during the postpremature beat, the systolic murmurs of aortic and pulmonic stenosis and of hypertrophic obstructive cardiomyopathy are augmented,[40] while the systolic murmurs of rheumatic mitral regurgitation and of ventricular septal defect are not altered significantly. The systolic murmur of tricuspid regurgitation and the diastolic murmur of aortic regurgitation become louder consequent to increased right ventricular filling and an elevated arterial pressure, respectively. The increase in left ventricular size delays the systolic click and the systolic murmur of mitral valve prolapse. Similar auscultatory changes follow prolonged diastolic pauses in atrial fibrillation and sinus arrhythmia.

ISOMETRIC EXERCISE. This can be carried out

simply and reproducibly using a calibrated handgrip device, but isometric exercise should be avoided in patients with ventricular arrhythmias and myocardial ischemia. Handgrip should be sustained for 20 to 30 seconds, but a Valsalva maneuver during the handgrip must be avoided. Isometric exercise results in significant increases in systemic vascular resistance, arterial pressure, heart rate, cardiac output, left ventricular filling pressure, and heart size. As a consequence, (1) S_3 and S_4 originating from the left side of the heart become accentuated, (2) the systolic murmur of aortic stenosis is diminished as a result of a reduction of the pressure gradient across the aortic valve, (3) the diastolic murmur of aortic regurgitation and the systolic murmurs of rheumatic mitral regurgitation and ventricular septal defect increase, (4) the diastolic murmur of mitral stenosis becomes louder consequent to the increase in cardiac output, and (5) the systolic murmur of hypertrophic obstructive cardiomyopathy and the systolic click and murmur secondary to mitral valve prolapse are delayed because of the increased left ventricular volume.

Pharmacological Agents

Inhalation of *amyl nitrite* for 10 to 15 seconds produces marked vasodilatation, resulting first in a reduction of systemic arterial pressure, then in a reflex tachycardia, followed in turn by an increase in stroke volume and in venous return.[88–91] S_1 is augmented and A_2 is diminished. The opening snaps of the mitral and tricuspid valves become louder, and as arterial pressure falls, the A_2-opening snap interval shortens. An S_3 originating in either ventricle is augmented, owing to greater rapidity of ventricular filling, but since mitral regurgitation is reduced, the S_3 associated with this lesion is diminished. The systolic murmurs of valvular aortic stenosis, pulmonic stenosis, hypertrophic obstructive cardiomyopathy, and functional systolic murmurs are all accentuated because of the increase in left ventricular contractility and stroke volume. The reduction of arterial pressure increases the right-to-left shunt and decreases the blood flow from the right ventricle to the pulmonary artery and diminishes the systolic ejection murmur in patients with tetralogy of Fallot.[92] The increase in cardiac output augments the diastolic murmurs of mitral and tricuspid stenosis and of pulmonary regurgitation and the systolic murmur of tricuspid regurgitation. However, as a result of the fall in systemic arterial pressure, the systolic murmurs of mitral regurgitation and ventricular septal defect, the diastolic murmurs of aortic regurgitation, and the Austin Flint murmur as well as the continuous murmurs of patent ductus arteriosus and of systemic arteriovenous fistula are all diminished.[93] The reduction of cardiac size results in an earlier appearance of the midsystolic click and systolic murmur of mitral valve prolapse; the intensity of the systolic murmur exhibits a variable response.

Methoxamine and *phenylephrine* increase systemic arterial pressure. In general, methoxamine, 3 to 5 mg intravenously, elevates arterial pressure by 20 to 40 mm Hg for 10 to 20 minutes, but phenylephrine is preferred because of its shorter duration of action; 0.5 mg of phenylephrine administered intravenously elevates systolic pressure by approximately 30 mm Hg for only 3 to 5 minutes.[89] Both drugs cause a reflex bradycardia and decreased contractility and cardiac output. The intensity of S_1 is usually reduced, A_2 becomes softer, and the A_2-mitral opening snap interval becomes prolonged. The responses of S_3 and S_4 are variable. As a result of the increased arterial pressure, the diastolic murmur of aortic regurgitation; the systolic murmurs of mitral regurgitation, ventricular septal defect, and tetralogy of Fallot; and the continuous murmur of patent ductus arteriosus and systemic arteriovenous fistula all become louder.[93,94] On the other hand, as a consequence of the increase in left ventricular size, the systolic murmur of hypertrophic obstructive cardiomyopathy becomes softer, and the click and murmur of mitral valve prolapse syndrome are delayed. The reduction in stroke volume diminishes the systolic murmur of valvular aortic stenosis.[79]

References

1. Perloff, J. K.: Physical examination of the heart and circulation. Philadelphia, W. B. Saunders Co., 1982.

1a. Silverman, M. E.: Causes of valve disease: Visual clues. J. Cardiovasc. Med. *8*: 340, 1983.

2. Greenwood, R. D., Rosenthal, A., Parisi, L., Flyer, D. C., and Nadas, A. S.: Extracardiac abnormalities in infants with congenital heart disease. Pediatrics *55*:485, 1975.

3. Shoenfeld, Y., Mor, R., Weinberger, A., Avidor, I., and Pinkhas, J.: Diagonal ear lobe crease and coronary risk factors. J. Am. Geriatr. Soc. *28*:184, 1980.

4. Wood, P.: Diseases of the Heart and Circulation. 3rd ed. Philadelphia, J. B. Lippincott, 1968, p. 625.

5. Cayler, G. G., Blumenfeld, C. M., and Anderson, R. L.: Further studies of patients with the cardiofacial syndrome. Chest *60*:161, 1971.

6. Young, D., Shprintzen, R. J., and Goldberg, R. B.: Cardiac malformations in the velocardiofacial syndrome. Am. J. Cardiol. *46*:643, 1980.

7. Noonan, J. A.: Hypertelorism with Turner phenotype. Am. J. Dis. Child. *116*: 373, 1968.

8. St. John Sutton, M. G., Tajik, A. J., Giuliani, E. R., Gordon, H., and Su, W. P. D.: Hypertrophic obstructive cardiomyopathy and lentiginosis: A little known neural ectodermal syndrome. Am. J. Cardiol. *47*:214, 1981.

9. Beuren, A. J., Schultze, C., Eberle, P., Harmjanz, D., and Aptiz, J.: The syndrome of supravalvular aortic stenosis, peripheral pulmonary stenosis, mental retardation and similar facial appearance. Am. J. Cardiol. *13*:471, 1964.

10. Clark, D. S., Myerburg, R. J., Morales, A. R., Befeler, B., Hernandez, F. A., and Gelband, H.: Heart block in Kearns-Sayre syndrome. Chest *68*:727, 1975.

11. Cogan, D. G.: Ophthalmic Manifestations of Systemic Vascular Disease. Philadelphia, W. B. Saunders Co., 1974.

12. Earnest, D. L., and Hurst, J. W.: Exophthalmos, stare, increase in intra-ocular pressure and systolic propulsion of the eyeballs due to congestive heart failure. Am. J. Cardiol. *26*:351, 1970.

13. Walker, G. L., and Stanfield, T. F.: Retinal changes associated with coarctation of the aorta. Trans. Am. Ophthalmol. Soc. *50*:407, 1952.

14. Fishman, A. P.: Cyanosis. *In* Fishman, A. P. (ed.): Pulmonary Diseases and Disorders. New York, McGraw-Hill Book Co., 1980, pp. 78 and 79.

15. Smith, A. T., Sack, G. H., Jr., and Taylor, G. J.: Holt-Oram syndrome. J. Pediatr. *95*:538, 1979.

16. Walker, B. A., and Murdoch, J. L.: The wrist sign. Arch. Intern. Med. *126*:276, 1970.

17. Criscitiello, M. G., Ronan, J. A., Besterman, E. M., and Schoenwetter, W.: Cardiovascular abnormalities in osteogenesis imperfecta. Circulation *31*:255, 1965.

18. Zvaifler, N. J.: Chronic postrheumatic fever (Jaccoud's) arthritis. N. Engl. J. Med. *267*:10, 1962.

19. Buckley, M. J., Mason, D. T., Ross, J., Jr., and Braunwald, E.: Reversed differential cyanosis with equal desaturation of the upper limbs. Syndrome of complete transposition of the great vessels with complete interruption of the aortic arch. Am. J. Cardiol. *15*:111, 1965.

20. Finger clubbing. Lancet *1*:1285, 1975.

21. Lanken, P. N., and Fishman, A. P.: Clubbing and hypertrophic osteoarthropathy. *In* Fishman, A. P. (ed.): Pulmonary Diseases and Disorders. New York, McGraw-Hill Book Co., 1980, pp. 84–91.

22. Pomerleau, O. F., and Schwarz, H. J.: Tuberous sclerosis with unusual findings: A case report. J. Maine Med. Assoc. *60*:137, 1969.

23. Constant, J.: Arterial and venous pulsations in cardiovascular diagnosis. J. Cardiovasc. Med. *5*:973, 1980.

24. Swartz, M. H.: Jugular venous pressure pulse: Its value in cardiac diagnosis. Primary Cardiol. *8*:197, 1982.

25. Rich, L. L., and Tavel, M. E.: The origin of the jugular C wave. N. Engl. J. Med. *284*:1309, 1971.

26. Bordley, J., III, Connor, C. A. R., Hamilton, W. F., Kerr, W. J., and Wiggers, C. J.: Recommendations for human blood pressure determinations by sphygmomanometers. Circulation *4*:503, 1951.

27. London, S. B., and London, R. E.: Critique of indirect diastolic end point. Arch. Intern. Med. *119*:39, 1967.

28. Maxwell, M. H., Schroth, P. C., Waks, A. U., Karam, M., and Dornfeld, L.

P.: Error in blood-pressure measurement due to incorrect cuff size in obese patients. Lancet 2:33, 1982.
29. Kirkendall, W. M., Burton, A. C., Epstein, F. H., and Freis, E. D.: Recommendations for human blood pressure determination by sphygmomanometers. Circulation *36*:980, 1967.
30. Sproul, G.: Basilar artery insufficiency secondary to obstruction of left subclavian artery. Circulation *28*:259, 1963.
31. Sapira, J. D.: Quincke, de Musset, Duroziez, and Hill: Some aortic regurgitations. South. Med. J. *74*:459, 1981.
32. Abrams, J.: The arterial pulse. Primary Cardiol., *8*:138, 1982.
33. Schlant, R. C., and Feiner, J. M.: The arterial pulse—clinical manifestations. Curr. Probl. Cardiol. Vol. 1, No. 5, 1976, 50 pp.
33a. Perloff, J. K.: The physiologic mechanisms of cardiac and vascular physical signs. J. Am. Coll. Cardiol. *1*:184, 1983.
34. Marshall, H. W., Helmholz, H. F., Jr., and Wood, E. H.: Physiological consequences of congenital heart disease. *In* Hamilton, W. F., and Dow, P. (eds.): Handbook of Physiology. Section 2, Circulation. Vol. I. Washington, D.C., American Physiological Society, 1962, pp. 417–487.
35. Elkins, R. C., Morrow, A. G., Vasko, J. S., and Braunwald, E.: The effects of mitral regurgitation on the pattern of instantaneous aortic blood flow. Clinical and experimental observations. Circulation *36*:45, 1967.
36. Kelly, E. R., Morrow, A. G., and Braunwald, E.: Catheterization of the left side of the heart: A key to the solution of some perplexing problems in cardiovascular diagnosis and management. N. Engl. J. Med. *262*:162, 1960.
37. Rowe, G. G., Afonso, S., Castillo, C. A., and McKenna, D. H.: The mechanism of the production of Duroziez's murmur. N. Engl. J. Med. *272*:1207, 1965.
38. Fleming, P. R.: The mechanism of the pulsus bisferiens. Br. Heart J. *19*:519, 1957.
39. Braunwald, E., Lambrew, C. T., Rockoff, S. D., Ross, J., Jr., and Morrow, A. G.: Idiopathic hypertrophic subaortic stenosis. I. A description of the disease based upon an analysis of 64 patients. Circulation *30* (Suppl. 4):3, 1964.
40. Brockenbrough, E. C., Braunwald, E., and Morrow, A. G.: A hemodynamic technic for the detection of hypertrophic subaortic stenosis. Circulation *23*:189, 1961.
41. Rebuck, A. S., and Pengelly, L. D.: Development of pulsus paradoxus in the presence of airways obstruction. N. Engl. J. Med. *288*:66, 1973.
42. Massumi, R. A., Mason, D. T., Zakauddin, V., Zelis, R., Otero, J., and Amsterdam, E. A.: Reversed pulsus paradoxus. N. Engl. J. Med. *289*:1272, 1973.
43. Davies, H.: Chest deformities in congenital heart disease. Br. J. Dis. Chest *53*:151, 1959.
44. Perloff, J. K.: Diagnostic inferences drawn from observation and palpation of the precordium with special reference to congenital heart disease. Adv. Cardiopulm. Dis. *4*:13, 1969.
45. Reusch, C. S.: Hemodynamic studies in pectus excavatum. Circulation *24*:1143, 1961.
46. Beiser, G. D., Epstein, S. E., Stampfer, M., Goldstein, R. E., Noland, S. P., and Levitsky, S.: Impairment of cardiac function in patients with pectus excavatum. N. Engl. J. Med. *287*:267, 1972.
47. deLeon, A. C., Perloff, J. K., Twigg, H. L., and Majd, M.: The straight back syndrome. Clinical cardiovascular manifestations. Circulation *32*:193, 1965.
48. Siegel, J. S., and Schechter, E.: The straight back syndrome. Am. J. Med. *42*:309, 1967.
49. Abrams, J.: Examination of the precordium. Primary Cardiol. *8*:156, 1982.
50. Bancroft, W. H., Jr., Eddleman, E. E., Jr., and Larkin, L. N.: Methods and physical characteristics of the kineto-cardiographic and apex cardiographic systems for recording low-frequency precordial motion. Am. Heart J. *73*:756, 1967.
51. Dressler, W.: Clinical Aids in Cardiac Diagnosis. New York, Grune and Stratton, 1970, 246 pp.
52. Counihan, T. B., Rappaport, M. B., and Sprague, H. B.: Physiologic and physical factors that govern the clinical appreciation of cardiac thrills. Circulation *4*:716, 1951.
53. Rappaport, M. B., and Sprague, H. B.: Physiologic and physical laws that govern auscultation, and their clinical application: The acoustic stethoscope and the electrical amplifying stethoscope and stethograph. Am. Heart J. *21*:257, 1941.
54. Faber, J. J., and Burton, A. C.: Spread of heart sounds over chest wall. Circ. Res. *11*:96, 1962.
55. Stein, P. D.: A Physical and Physiological Basis for the Interpretation of Cardiac Auscultation. Mt. Kisco, N.Y., Futura Publishing Co., 1981, 288 pp.
56. Leatham, A.: Auscultation of the Heart and Phonocardiography. Edinburgh, Churchill Livingstone, 1975, p. 181.
57. Levine, S. A., and Harvey, W. P.: Clinical Auscultation of the Heart. 2nd ed. Philadelphia, W. B. Saunders Co., 1959, 657 pp.
58. Luisada, A. A., and Portaluppi, F.: The Heart Sounds. New York, Praeger Publishers, 1982, 246 pp.
59. Aygen, M. M., and Braunwald, E.: The splitting of the second heart sound in normal subjects and in patients with congenital heart disease. Circulation *25*:328, 1962.
60. Beck, W., Schrire, V., and Vogelpoel, L.: Splitting of the second heart sound in constrictive pericarditis, with observations on the mechanism of pulsus paradoxus. Am. Heart J. *64*:765, 1962.
61. Leatham, A.: The second heart sound: Key to auscultation of the heart. Acta Cardiol. *19*:395, 1964.
62. Yurchak, P. M., and Gorlin, R.: Paradoxical splitting of the second heart sound in coronary heart disease. N. Engl. J. Med. *269*:741, 1963.
63. Leatham, A.: Auscultation of the heart since Laennec. Thorax *36*:95, 1981.
64. Abrams, J.: The first heart sound. Primary Cardiol. *8*:15, 1982.
65. O'Toole, J. D., Reddy, S. P., Curtiss, E. I., Griff, F. W., and Shaver, J. A.: The contribution of tricuspid valve close to the first heart sound: An intracardiac micromanometer study. Circulation *53*:752, 1976.
66. Shaver, J. A., and O'Toole, J. D.: The second heart sound: Newer concepts. Part I: Normal and wide physiological splitting. Mod. Concepts Cardiovasc. Dis. *46*:7, 1977.
67. Shaver, J. A., and O'Toole, J. D.: The second heart sound: Newer concepts. Part II: Paradoxical splitting and narrow physiological splitting. Mod. Concepts Cardiovasc. Dis. *46*:13, 1977.
67a. Oxawa, Y., Smith, D., and Craige, E.: Origin of the third heart sound. II. Studies in hyman subjects. Circulation. *67*:399, 1983.
68. Abrams, J.: The third and fourth heart sounds. Primary Cardiol. *8*:47, 1982.
69. Abdulla, A. M., Frank, M. J., Erdin, R. A., Jr., and Canedo, M. I.: Clinical significance and hemodynamic correlates of the third heart sound gallop in aortic regurgitation: A guide to optimal timing of cardiac catheterization. Circulation *64*:463, 1981.
70. Lee, D. C-S., Johnson, R. A., Bingham, J. B., Leahy, M., Dinsmore, R. E., Goroll, A. H., Newell, J. B., Strauss, H. W., and Haber, E.: Heart failure in outpatients: A randomized trial of digoxin versus placebo. N. Engl. J. Med. *306*:699, 1982.
71. Rushmer, R. F., and Morgan, C.: Meaning of murmurs. Am. J. Cardiol. *21*:722, 1968.
72. Freeman, A. R., and Levine, S. A.: The clinical significance of the systolic murmur. A study of 1000 consecutive "noncardiac" cases. Ann. Intern. Med. *6*:1371, 1933.
73. Holldack, K., Heller, A., and Groth, W.: The pericardial friction rub in the phonocardiogram. Am. J. Cardiol. *4*:351, 1959.
74. Harvey, W. P.: Auscultatory findings in diseases of the pericardium. Am. J. Cardiol. *7*:15, 1961.
75. Dressler, W.: Effect of respiration on the pericardial friction rub. Am. J. Cardiol. *7*:130, 1961.
76. Fowler, N. O., and Gause, R.: The cervical venous hum. Am. Heart J. *67*:135, 1964.
77. Tabatznik, B., Randall, T. W., and Hersch, C.: The mammary souffle of pregnancy and lactation. Circulation *22*:1069, 1960.
78. Harvey, W. P.: Innocent versus significant murmurs. Curr. Probl. Cardiol. Vol. 1., No. 8, 1976, 51 pp.
79. Delman, A. J., and Stein, E.: Dynamic Cardiac Auscultation and Phonocardiography: A Graphic Guide. Philadelphia, W. B. Saunders Co., 1979, pp. 559–792.
80. Shaver, J. A., O'Toole, J. D., Curtiss, E. I., Thompson, M. E., Reddy, P. S., and Leon, D. F.: Second heart sound. *In* Physiologic Principles of Heart Sounds and Murmurs. New York, American Heart Association, Monograph No. 46, 1975, pp. 58–67.
81. Goldblatt, A., Harrison, D. C., Glick, G., and Braunwald, E.: Studies on cardiac dimensions in intact, unanesthetized man. II. Effects of respiration. Circ. Res. *13*:455, 1963.
82. Rios, J. C., Massumi, R. A., Breesmen, W. T., and Sarin, R. K.: Auscultatory features of acute tricuspid regurgitation. Am. J. Cardiol. *23*:4, 1969.
83. Fontana, M. E., Wooley, C. F., Leighton, R. F., and Lewis, R. P.: Postural changes in left ventricular and mitral valvular dynamics in the systolic click-late systolic murmur syndrome. Circulation *51*:165, 1975.
84. Rodin, P., and Tabatznik, B.: The effect of posture on added heart sounds. Br. Heart J. *25*:69, 1963.
85. Nellen, M., Gotsman, M. S., Vogelpoel, L., Beck, W., and Schrire, V.: Effect of prompt squatting on the systolic murmur in idiopathic hypertrophic obstructive cardiomyopathy. Br. Med. J. *3*:140, 1967.
86. Braunwald, E., Oldham, H. N., Jr., Ross, J., Jr., Linhart, J. W., Mason, D. T., and Fort, L., III: The circulatory response of patients with idiopathic hypertrophic subaortic stenosis to nitroglycerin and to the Valsalva maneuver. Circulation *29*:422, 1964.
87. van der Hauwaert, L. G.: The effect of the Valsalva maneuver on the splitting of the second sound. Acta Cardiol. *19*:518, 1964.
88. Barlow, J., and Shillingford, J.: The use of amyl nitrite in differentiating mitral and aortic systolic murmurs. Br. Heart J. *20*:162, 1958.
89. Beck, W., Schrire, V., Vogelpoel, L., Nellen, M., and Swanepoel, A.: Hemodynamic effects of amyl nitrite and phenylephrine on the normal human circulation and their relation to changes in cardiac murmurs. Am. J. Cardiol. *8*:341, 1961.
90. Schrire, V., Vogelpoel, L., Beck, W., Nellen, M., and Swanepoel, A.: The effects of amyl nitrite and phenylephrine on the intracardiac murmurs of small ventricular septal defects. Am. Heart J. *62*:225, 1961.
91. Vogelpoel, L., Schrire, V., Nellen, M., and Swanepoel, A.: The use of amyl nitrite in the differentiation of Fallot's tetralogy and pulmonary stenosis with intact ventricular septum. Am. Heart J. *57*:803, 1959.
92. Vogelpoel, L., Schrire, V., Nellen, M., and Swanepoel, A.: The use of phenylephrine in the differentiation of Fallot's tetralogy from pulmonary stenosis with intact ventricular septum. Am. Heart J. *59*:489, 1960.
93. Criscitiello, M.: Physiologic and pharmacologic aids in cardiac auscultation. *In* Fowler, N. O. (ed.): Cardiac Diagnosis and Treatment. 3rd ed. Hagerstown, Harper and Row, 1980, pp. 77–90.
94. Crevasse, L.: The use of a vasopressor agent as a diagnostic aid in auscultation. Am. Heart J. *58*:821, 1959.

3

HEART SOUNDS:

PHONOCARDIOGRAPHY; CAROTID, APEX, AND JUGULAR VENOUS PULSE TRACINGS; AND SYSTOLIC TIME INTERVALS

by Ernest Craige, M.D.

Phonocardiography, or the graphic representation of heart sounds and murmurs, has been practiced since the turn of the century.[1] As commonly used, the term phonocardiography also embraces pulse tracings—carotid, apex, and jugular venous—so that a relatively complete graphic reproduction of auscultatory, visible, and palpable signs of cardiac origin can be provided.[2–6] With the addition of echocardiography to the armamentarium of noninvasive techniques it has become possible to display the echo signal in conjunction with the older graphic methods of multichannel records, the result being an enormously increased diagnostic potential. The combined method is called *echophonocardiography.*[7,8]

In this chapter we will describe the technique of recording phonocardiograms with carotid, apex, and jugular venous pulsations and will discuss the utility of the combined method—echophonocardiography—in the identification and interpretation of heart sounds. In Chapter 4 the role of echophonocardiography in studies of heart murmurs will be considered. The techniques, usefulness, and limitations of echocardiography are presented in Chapter 5.

CARDIAC VIBRATIONS AND THEIR REGISTRATION BY GRAPHIC METHODS

Contraction and relaxation of the heart produces vibrations over the precordium which are perceived by auscultation and palpation, as discussed in Chapter 2. The spectrum of vibrations reaching the chest wall is dominated by the very low frequencies perceived at the bedside as palpable phenomena.[2] A recording that would represent the cardiac vibrations exactly as received and without filtration would not be useful, since the enormous size of the low-frequency vibrations would preclude an adequate representation of the less intense higher frequencies, appreciated acoustically as heart sounds and murmurs. Therefore the recording apparatus, like the human ear itself, must be provided with a system of filters, so that the resulting graphic record may more nearly approximate the sound spectrum perceived by the ear.[9,10]

The principal energy of the palpable movements of the heart emanates from very low-frequency vibrations, i.e., at the lower end of the 0 to 30 cps range.[11] The lower threshold of audibility, although variable, is approximately at 30 cps and extends up to several thousand cycles per second. However, most vibrations of cardiac origin that appear to be of diagnostic importance are in the spectrum of 30 to 1000 cps.[12] Thus, the phonocardiograph should be able to filter out the very low-frequency vibrations which can be represented as a displacement tracing or apexcardiogram. The remaining higher frequency vibrations can then be suitably amplified, so that the resulting graphic records may simulate the phenomena appreciated by auscultation. By a selective filtration system, the lower frequencies in the audible range may be permitted to dominate the tracing, such as might be useful in recording third and fourth heart sounds and low-frequency rumbling murmurs. Alternatively, suppression of low frequencies and amplification of high-frequency vibrations results in optimal presentation of the first and second heart sounds, ejection sounds, opening snaps, and murmurs such as those of mitral and aortic regurgitation.[2]

PHONOCARDIOGRAPHIC TECHNIQUE

Facilities and Equipment. One of the main reasons for disappointment with phonocardiograms is the inadequacy of tracings due to faulty technique or poor recording conditions. The room must be quiet or sound-conditioned, with a sound-absorbent ceiling and wall covering, drapes over the windows, and a carpet, and mechanical noises, such as humming and rattling of air conditioners or fans, must be eliminated in order to obtain tracings free of background noise. To avoid a confusion of wires, transducers should be hung from racks appropriately located on the wall near the patient's head.

The bed should be comfortable, allow elevation of the patient's head, and be high enough so that the examiner can conveniently auscultate and apply the necessary transducers. Usually the patient is supine, with the head elevated for comfort or as required for optimal visualization or registration of venous or carotid pulsations. During recording of the carotid pulse, a pillow should be placed beneath the patient's shoulders in order to hyperextend the neck and thereby thrust the carotid artery forward, supported firmly by the transverse processes of the cervical spine. It may be necessary for the patient to assume the left lateral decubitus position to enhance auscultatory and palpable phenomena at the cardiac apex.

Paper speed is usually set at 100 mm/sec, which is optimal for measurement of systolic time intervals[13] as well as for observation of the relationship of heart sounds and valvular and ventricular events. However, slower paper speeds may be preferable for displaying the effects of respiration or other physiological or pharmacological maneuvers or in scanning the heart by means of the accompanying echocardiogram.

Although a variety of microphones for heart-sound registration is available, we prefer the air-coupled type, attached to the lightly lubricated chest wall by means of a rubber suction bulb.* Any excess hair that might interfere with the firm, air-tight attachment of the microphone should be removed. Smaller transducers are essential for infants and small children and are also useful where prominent ribs preclude adequate contact with the microphone rim.

Transducers for pulse tracings—carotid, apex, or venous—are commonly of the piezoelectric crystal type. A funnel or tambour is applied to the pulsation under study, and changes in air pressure are conducted via a rubber tube to the crystal device for conversion to electrical signals. The transducer-recording system must have an adequate time constant of 3.0 sec or more. With some of the older equipment, too short a time constant resulted in distortion of the curves and subtle temporal displacement of important landmarks in the carotid and apex tracings.[11,14,15] The principles of physics pertinent to this subject are beyond the scope of this chapter; however, a simple test of one's apparatus for the adequacy of the duration of the time constant consists merely of observing the effect on the oscilloscope of sustained pressure applied to the funnel or tambour of the transducer. If after a rapid rise of the signal on the oscilloscope, there is an immediate (0.3 sec or so) fall to the baseline, despite continued pressure on the sensing head of the transducer, then obviously the apparatus will yield a systematic distortion of the pulsatile phenomena being recorded. This distortion is equivalent to a partial differentiation of the signal.[16] A plateau will appear as an inverted V, and a shallow trough may become a deep crevasse. Besides these morphological alterations, the timing of landmarks (which constitutes one of the principal uses of pulsatile records) may be disturbed, resulting in erroneous interpretations. A time constant of 3.0 sec or more is adequate for recording carotid, apex, and venous pulsations. An infinite time constant may be theoretically superior but is usually impractical, owing to the wide swings of the baseline associated with respiration that make interpretation difficult.

Respiration can be monitored by means of a nasal thermistor probe. This produces a satisfactory curve that can be superimposed on the other parameters of a multichannel tracing. Alternatively, a strain-gauge device that reponds to chest expansion may be employed, but this has the disadvantage that the expansile belt may interfere with placement of the transducers on the chest wall. The technique and equipment required for echocardiography are described in Chapter 5.

A number of satisfactory recorders are available, and the choice depends on such factors as obtaining satisfactory phonocardiograms and echocardiograms, price, availability of service, and size and portability of the equipment. The recorder should be capable of multichannel registration at a variety of paper speeds. Some recorders provide immediate processing, although this may sacrifice the vivid contrast of black and white tracings. The latter usually require a separate photographic developer.

Recording Technique. In view of the many possible combinations of transducers and chest-wall locations, the registration of graphic tracings must be preceded by a bedside assessment of the problem. Ideally, the clinician should be present in the noninvasive

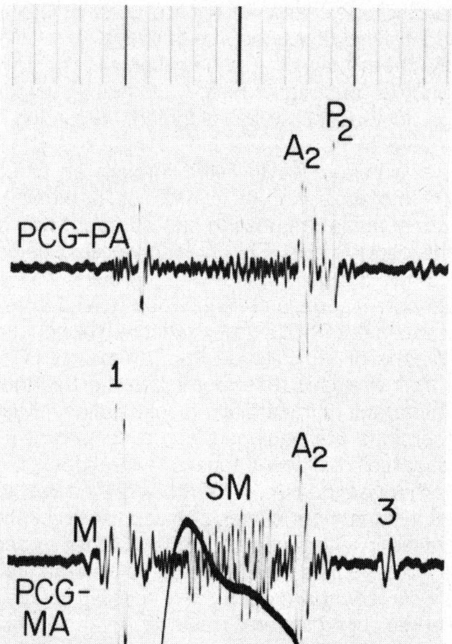

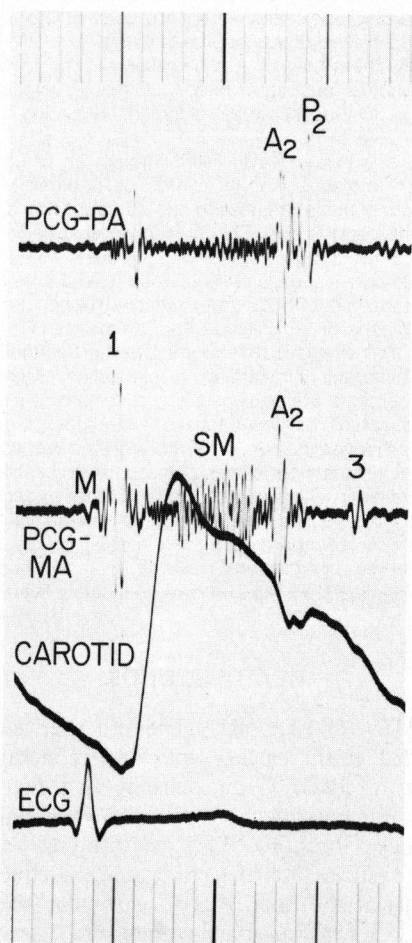

FIGURE 3–1 Phonocardiogram in mild mitral regurgitation. Two phonocardiograms are taken simultaneously, one at the second left intercostal space (PCG-PA) and one at the cardiac apex (PCG-MA). This demonstrates the wide transmission of the aortic component of the second heart sound (A_2) while the pulmonic component (P_2) is confined to the upper left sternal edge. A late systolic murmur (SM) and third sound (3) are best seen at the apex. Also, the initial low-frequency component (M) of the first sound (1) is seen at the same location. In the illustrations in this chapter, the following symbols will be used to indicate location of the microphones on the chest wall: AA = second right intercostal space; PA = second left intercostal space; LSE = lower left sternal edge (third or fourth left intercostal space); MA = cardiac apex. (Time lines = 0.04 sec.)

*Leatham microphone, Irex Company, Ramsey, New Jersey.

laboratory to supervise application of the microphones to the most informative locations on the chest wall. If this is not possible, the areas best suited for registration can be designated with a mark, or at least the problem should be indicated clearly, so that laboratory personnel can make the most appropriate choices. It must be emphasized that informative tracings cannot be provided by a technician applying transducers to the chest wall in a routine, unsupervised manner. Phonocardiograms thus recorded are more often misleading than helpful in cardiac diagnosis. In general, it is preferable to record from two microphones simultaneously in order to clarify the transmission of certain sounds such as P_2 and to separate such sounds from others occurring in close temporal proximity, such as opening snaps, third sounds, and the like (Fig. 3–1).[17]

The most commonly used sites for application of the microphones are those generally employed in auscultation: the second right interspace, often called the "aortic area"; the second left interspace, or the "pulmonary area"; the lower left sternal edge and xiphoid region, or the "tricuspid area"; and the cardiac apex, or the "mitral area." The designation of these anatomical locations on the thoracic wall as "valve areas" is an oversimplification that may be misleading, since there is no exclusive transmission of acoustical events from any particular valve to a certain area on the chest wall. Thus the designations "AA," "MA," and other similar symbols for second right interspace, cardiac apex, and so on are used in the illustrations in Chapters 3 and 4 simply for economy of space.

Occasionally, there may be a competition for chest-wall space between microphones and ultrasound transducers, especially in children. In such instances, some judgment regarding priorities for positions will have to be exercised. Following the application of the microphones, it is imperative to listen through an amplifying stethoscope plugged into the recorder in order to determine whether the auscultatory phenomena in question can be heard and adequately visualized on the oscilloscope. This precaution also helps to eliminate artifacts due to hair or poor contact with the chest wall and to identify artifacts due to bowel sounds or percussion noises from hyperdynamic chest-wall movement. All these extraneous sounds are more easily identified by means of auscultation than by means of a graphic record, in which their rhythmic recurrence with the heartbeat may simulate some important intracardiac manifestation. Most phonocardiographic recordings are equipped with a system of filters that can be used to suppress the low-frequency vibrations of cardiac origin which would otherwise dominate the tracing. The resultant spectrum of vibrations simulates more closely the sounds perceptible to the human ear. A choice of filters can be made in order to accentuate low-frequency diastolic sounds and rumbles or, alternatively, the higher frequency valvular sounds (i.e., S_1, S_2, opening snaps) or murmurs (e.g., that of aortic regurgitation). However, even the best equipment commercially available will fail to record adequately faint, high-pitched murmurs.

HEART SOUNDS

FIRST HEART SOUND. The first heart sound (S_1) is best recorded at the cardiac apex and is identified by its relationship to the ECG and carotid upstroke (Fig. 3–1). It consists phonocardiographically of an initial inaudible low-frequency vibration, "M," occurring at the onset of ventricular systole, then two intense high-frequency bursts of vibrations at the time of atrioventricular valve closure, followed by a few variable low-intensity vibrations (Fig. 3–2).[18,19]

The genesis of heart sounds, particularly the origin of S_1, has been a controversial issue since the early part of the nineteenth century. Arguments have centered on the question of whether or not the atrioventricular valves make a significant contribution to sound genesis. The classic theory relates the principal high-frequency vibrations of S_1 to mitral and tricuspid closure, respectively.[20–22] An alternative hypothesis attributes the high-frequency elements of S_1 to the movement and acceleration of blood in early systole, the first element being related to left ventricular dP/dt

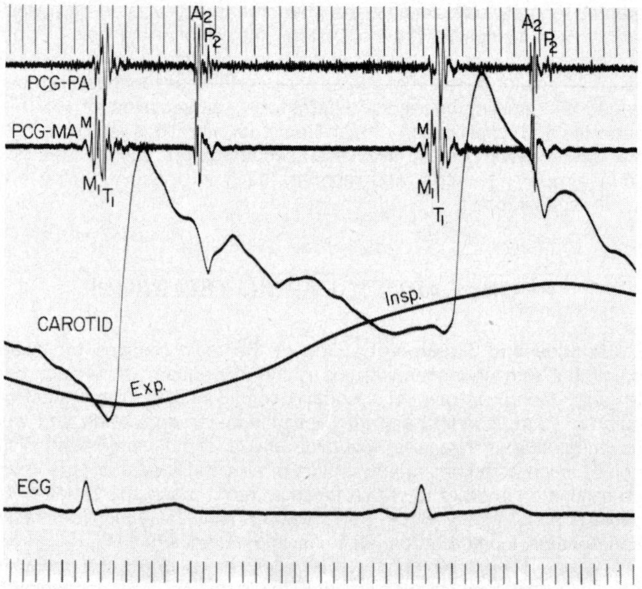

FIGURE 3–2 Normal phonocardiogram. The first heart sound is best seen at the cardiac apex (PCG-MA) and consists of a low-frequency component (M), followed by two high-frequency bursts of vibrations (M_1, T_1), and finally a few low-intensity, low-frequency vibrations in early systole. Normal widening of the A_2- P_2 interval with inspiration is demonstrated.

and the second to ejection of blood into the root of the aorta.[23,24] In the past this problem was studied by means of hemodynamic investigations with catheterization of the relevant heart chambers combined with phonocardiography. The delay occasioned by the transmission of pressure pulses through fluid-filled catheters makes routine catheterization unsuitable for such observations. High-fidelity tracings obtained via catheter-tipped micromanometers demonstrate the pressure crossover points between left atrium and ventricle, signaling the moment of *onset* of valve closure that inevitably must precede final closure by an appreciable interval.[25–28]

The technique of echophonocardiography is particularly applicable to studies of this problem,[29,30] since valvular and acoustical events are transmitted from their source to graphic registration with essentially no time delay, thereby facilitating the accumulation of data necessary for resolution of the problems associated with the origin of heart sounds (Fig. 3–3). Variation in intensity of the major elements of S_1 has been studied in cases of complete heart block[31,32] and ventricular premature beats.[33] The relative contribution of the velocity of mitral valve closure as opposed to the force of left ventricular contraction in the determination of the intensity of S_1 has been investigated in a rapidly fluctuating situation such as atrial fibrillation, and velocity of mitral valve closure was found to have the dominant role. These studies are consistent with the classic theory that presumes that atrioventricular closure and the ensuing tension of valvular structures are associated with the initiation of vibrations appreciated acoustically as S_1.[8,29,30,32] The observation of Traill and Fortuin of a loud "presystolic first heart sound" in diastole simultaneous with premature closure of the mitral valve in severe aortic regurgitation provides additional evidence favoring the valvular origin of S_1.[34]

Normal Splitting of S_1. The two major components of S_1 are separated by a narrow interval of 0.02 to 0.03 sec in most normal subjects.[22] This degree of separation is difficult to perceive by means of auscultation, and phonocardiography may record the two elements of S_1 blurring into a continuum of vibrations. Normal splitting is recorded most satisfactorily in the pediatric age group. The mitral component, M_1, is the louder and is best recorded at the cardiac apex. The tricuspid component, T_1, that immediately follows is best recorded at the left lower sternal border.

Abnormal Splitting of S_1. Abnormal splitting of S_1 may result from either electrophysiological or hemodynamic changes that alter the timing of atrioventricular valve closure.

Electrical Factors. These include abnormalities associated with bundle branch block,[35,36] ectopic ventricular beats, ventricular tachycardia, idioventricular rhythm, preexcitation, and ventricular pacing.[37] Wide splitting with preservation of the normal sequence (M_1 to T_1) may be recorded in right bundle branch block, ectopic beats or idioventricular rhythms originating in the left ventricle, pacing from the left ventricle, or preexcitation patterns that result in left ventricular contraction before right. Reversed splitting may occur with the opposite of the above situations, i.e., ectopic rhythms and paced beats originating in the right ventricle. It does not follow, however, that reversed splitting necessarily occurs in left bundle branch block (LBBB), since the *onset* of the left ventricular pressure rise often starts on time despite the *delay* in the completion of depolarization of the left side, which causes the characteristic electrocardiographic pattern.[38] Burggraf has shown that in LBBB there may be a normal sequence (M_1 followed by T_1) or a simultaneous M_1T_1 or a reversal of the two elements.[39] Typically, the low amplitude of S_1 in LBBB makes identification of individual components more difficult.

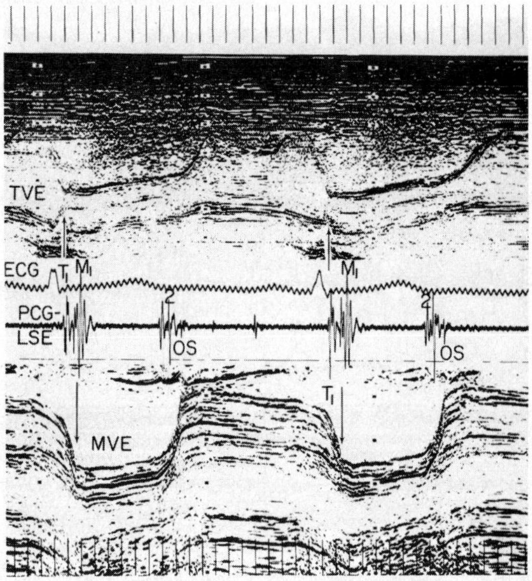

FIGURE 3–4 Reversed splitting of S_1 in mitral stenosis. A dual echophonocardiogram shows a widely split S_1 with T_1 identified by its coincidence with tricuspid valve closure (↑) preceding M_1, which occurs at the time of mitral valve closure (↓). An opening snap (OS) follows S_2 and is identified by its occurrence at the time of full opening of the mitral valve in early diastole.

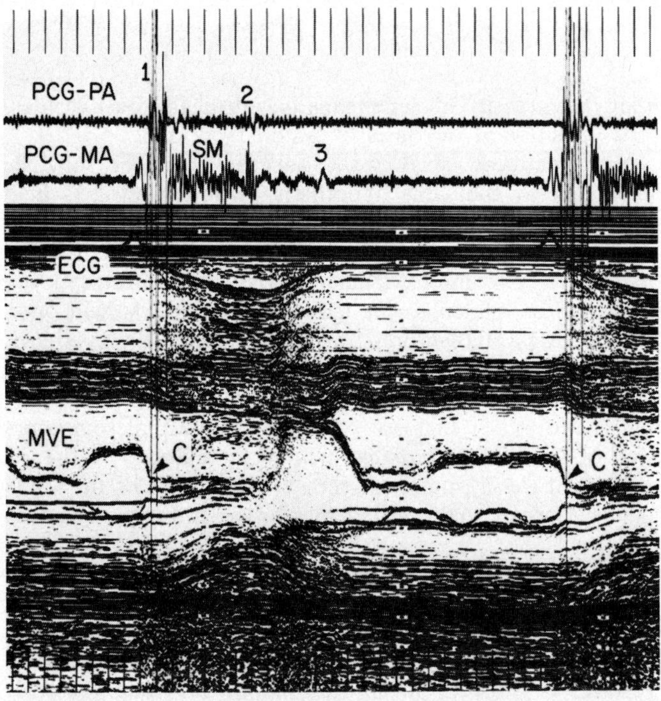

FIGURE 3–3 An echophonocardiogram showing the relationship between mitral valve closure and a very loud first heart sound (1). PCG at the cardiac apex (MA) shows a holosystolic murmur of mild mitral regurgitation. The C points indicate apposition of the leaflets of the mitral valve on the mitral valve echogram (MVE).

Hemodynamic Factors. Hemodynamic abnormalities that result in alteration in the timing of M_1 and T_1 include mitral stenosis and left atrial myxoma. In mitral stenosis, pressure in the left ventricle must rise to higher than normal levels before pressure in the left atrium is exceeded and the mitral valve starts to close.[40] In severe cases the delay in the timing of mitral valve closure, and therefore of M_1, may result in reversed splitting of S_1 (Fig. 3–4). Similarly, in left atrial myxoma, M_1 is delayed as the result of a hemodynamic situation simulating that of mitral stenosis. With extrusion of the tumor from ventricle to atrium, a loud, late S_1 is audible and usually palpable.

Mixed Electrical and Hemodynamic Factors. In Ebstein's anomaly (pp. 996 and 1040) the combination of right bundle branch block (RBBB) and an unusually large, deformed tricuspid valve results in a greatly delayed T_1.[41] Closure of the large anterior tricuspid leaflet in association with a loud, high-frequency sound as long as 0.14 sec after closure of the mitral valve provides a characteristic echophonocardiographic picture (Fig. 3–5).[41,42] The diagnostic specificity of these findings obviates cardiac catheterization in most instances.

Intensity of S_1. Several factors are of importance in determining the intensity of the major components of S_1, and these include the ability of the atrioventricular valves to close, their mobility, the velocity of their closing movement, and the strength of ventricular systole. "Closure" of the atrioventricular valves as perceived echocardiographically occurs at the "*c*-point," where the leaflets are seen to approximate each other in early systole. Echocardiography cannot distinguish between *apposition* of the leaflets and the *tension* on the bellies of the leaflets which immediately follows. Presumably it is the latter event that is associated with vibrations perceived as sound.

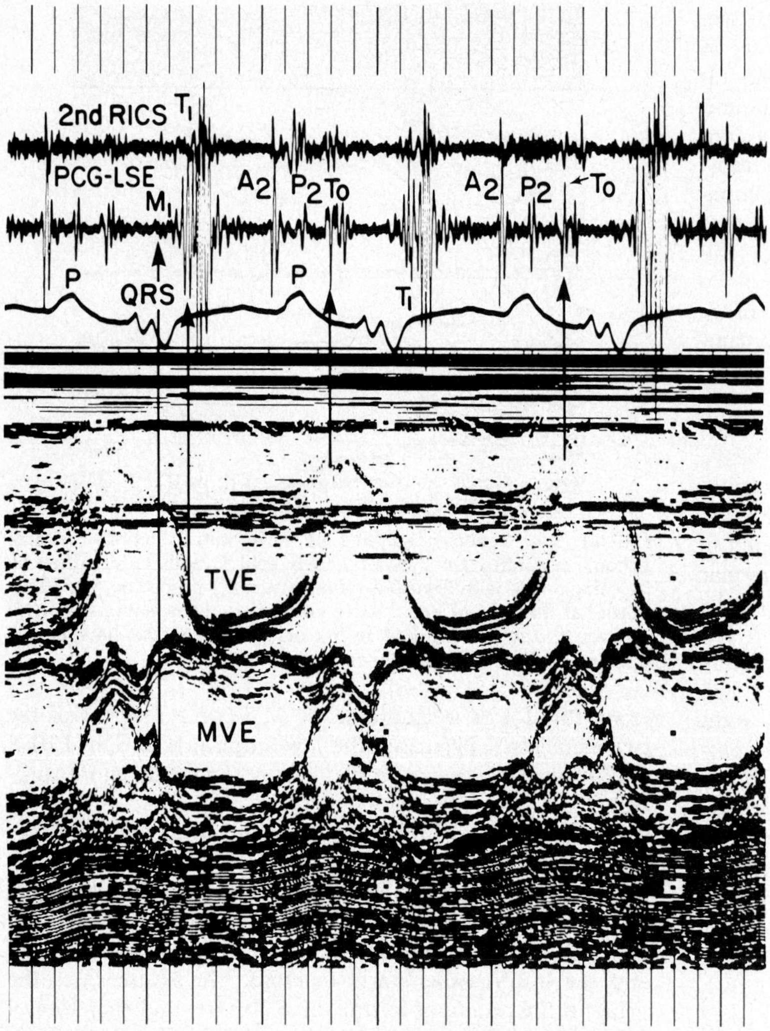

FIGURE 3–5 Ebstein's anomaly. Echophonocardiogram of the tricuspid valve (TVE) and mitral valve (MVE) showing delayed closure of the large tricuspid valve 0.12 sec from onset of the QRS complex. Closure of the tricuspid valve is associated with a very loud T_1 or "sail sound," which dwarfs the mitral component of S_1 (M_1). Additional sounds include tricuspid opening (T_0) synchronous with the E-point of the tricuspid echo.

Ability of the AV Valves to Close. In mitral regurgitation, in which closure of the valve is ineffectual, S_1 may be soft. This is best illustrated in rheumatic valvular disease, in which shortening and thickening of the chordae tendineae preclude normal closure. In prolapse of the mitral valve, however, the valve may seat normally in early systole, an event associated with a loud S_1 (Fig. 3–1), although prolapse of the valve and regurgitation may occur later in systole.[43]

Mobility of the Valve. A calcified valve that is completely immobilized is associated with a soft or absent S_1.

Velocity of Closure. This is the most important factor in determining the intensity of S_1. Clinical observations pertinent to this subject have indicated that the velocity of closure of the mitral valve varies on a beat-to-beat basis. Such opportunities for study are afforded by cases of complete heart block[31,32] and atrial fibrillation.[8] A high velocity of closure has been found to correlate with a loud S_1 and a slow velocity of closure with a soft S_1. When the valve is completely closed at the onset of ventricular systole, as with a long P-R interval[32] or with severe, acute aortic regurgitation,[44] S_1 may be silent or, occasionally, audible in diastole,[34] depending on the velocity of the closing movement. These observations support the clinical teaching of Wolferth and Margolies, who many years ago proposed that the intensity of S_1 depends on mitral (atrioventricular) valve position at the onset of systole.[45]

The loudness of T_1 in atrial septal defect may be explained by the same hypothesis, since the valve is held open by the augmented flow from right atrium to right ventricle, until final closure occurs with right ventricular systole.[46,47] The loud M_1 characteristic of mitral stenosis may also be related to the fact that the valve is held open by the transvalvular pressure gradient until a very sharp, high-velocity closing movement of the valve apparatus is effected by ventricular systole (Fig. 3–4). If a loud M_1 is present in mitral stenosis, one may assume that some portion of the valve is capable of moving (bulging) in the direction of the atrium even though the mouth of the valve may be largely immobilized by fibrosis and even calcification.

Strength of Ventricular Systole. Although obviously closure of the AV valves is dependent on ventricular systole, the contribution of the *force of ventricular contraction* to the intensity of S_1 is less than that of the *velocity of valve closure.*[8,48] Thus, in atrial fibrillation, the long diastoles which, according to the Starling principle, should lead to the most forceful contractions are not necessarily followed by the loudest first heart sounds.[8] In fact a sound may at times be observed when the mitral valve closes precocious-

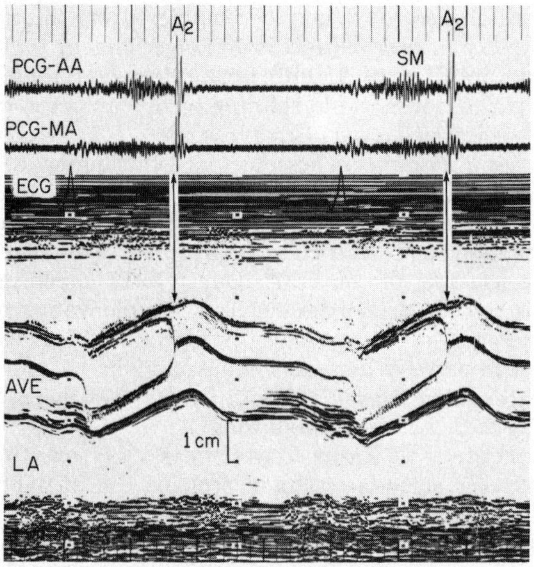

FIGURE 3–6 Echophonocardiogram illustrating the relationship between closure of the aortic valve and onset of the high-frequency vibrations of A_2. An ejection systolic murmur (SM) is noted in the phonocardiogram from the second right intercostal space. AVE = aortic valve echo; LA = left atrium.

ly in diastole when no ventricular contraction at all has taken place.[34,49] In left bundle branch block a variety of factors may contribute to the characteristic softness of S_1, including extracardiac abnormalities such as emphysema in older subjects, impaired ventricular contraction due to myocardial disease, and partial closure of the valve prior to ventricular systole owing to a long P-R interval plus a further delay between onset of the QRS complex and initiation of ventricular systole in some cases of LBBB.[36,39]

SECOND HEART SOUND. The classic explanation of the origin of the two components of the second heart sound relates these events to closure of the aortic and pulmonic valves, respectively, thus warranting the designations "A_2" and "P_2."[20,22,50] The coincidence of the onset of A_2 and aortic valve closure is clearly demonstrable in combined echophonocardiographic recordings (Fig. 3–6). In vitro studies of Stein and associates utilizing high-speed cinematographic techniques have confirmed and delineated in precise detail the role of valvular vibrations in the origin and intensity of A_2.[51,52] Careful investigations by Hirschfeld et al. utilizing high-fidelity aortic root pressure tracings in conjunction with echo- and phonocardiograms demonstrate the simultaneous occurrence of aortic valve closure, the onset of A_2, and the incisura in the pressure record.[53] These observations reinforce the traditional concept of the role of the aortic valve in the genesis of A_2.[54]

The pulmonic component of the second heart sound (P_2) is generally attributed to closure and tensing of the pulmonic valve.[20,22,50] This relationship is more difficult to demonstrate by echophonocardiography than the analogous events on the left side of the heart, because one can rarely visualize more than one cusp of the pulmonic valve and therefore the exact moment of closure cannot be accurately pinpointed. In Figure 3–7, however, from a patient with chronic rheumatic heart disease, the closing point of the valve cusps can be seen and is synchronous with P_2.

By auscultation or phonocardiography the two elements of the second heart sound are best appreciated in the pulmonary area or second left intercostal space where normal splitting is demonstrated on inspiration. The aortic component of S_2 can be identified by its occurrence just before the incisura of the carotid pulse tracing and by its wide transmission to the cardiac apex. P_2, on the other hand, is usually recorded only at the upper left sternal edge, unless it is of abnormal intensity.

Therefore the method recommended above, of utilizing two sound transducers simultaneously, is ideally suited for recording the timing, relative intensity, transmission, and behavior in conjunction with respiration of the two elements of S_2.[22] Quiet deep breathing with the mouth open is the best method of producing the desired physiological alterations, since it will be relatively free from obscuring artifacts.

Normal Splitting of S_2. In newborn infants S_2 is initially single.[55] However, during the first day of life, with falling resistance in the pulmonary circuit, the inspiratory separation of A_2 and P_2 becomes perceptible phonocardiographically. Normally, thereafter, fusion of the elements of S_2 occurs with expiration, and separation varying from 0.02 to 0.06 sec occurs with inspiration.[56]

In older subjects in whom auscultation and phonocardiographic observations may be obscured by emphysema,

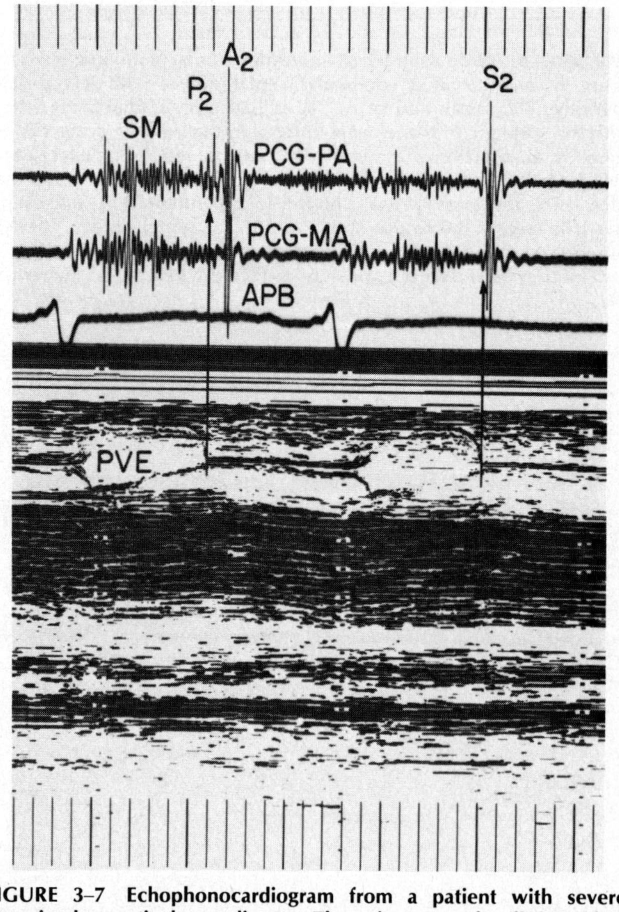

FIGURE 3–7 Echophonocardiogram from a patient with severe chronic rheumatic heart disease. There is reversed splitting of S_2 such that P_2 precedes A_2 in the first beat. In the second beat, which is premature (APB), the two elements of S_2 fuse. A simultaneous echo of the pulmonary valve (PVE) shows that P_2 occurs coincident with closure of the two visible cusps.

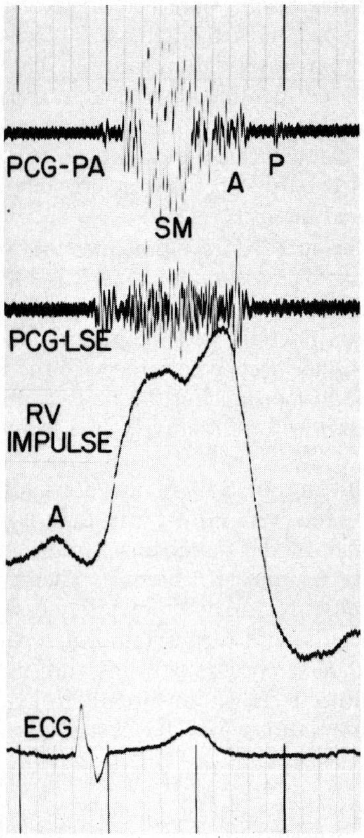

FIGURE 3–8 Wide splitting of S_2 in infundibular pulmonic stenosis. There is an associated ventricular septal defect with left-to-right shunting. The separation of A_2- P_2 is 0.08 sec, a figure consistent with the systemic pressures encountered in the right ventricle (RV).[57] There is an ejection murmur in the second left intercostal space (PA) from the RV outflow obstruction, whereas at the lower sternal edge (LSE), the murmur has a holosystolic configuration, suggesting that it is largely the result of the ventricular septal defect. The RV impulse recorded at LSE shows a prominent *a* wave (A) and a sustained systolic thrust consistent with right ventricular hypertrophy.

only one element of S_2 may by audible, giving the erroneous impression that splitting is no longer present.

Wide Splitting of S_2 with Respiratory Variation. As with splitting of S_1, wide splitting of S_2 may occur for either electrical or hemodynamic reasons.

Electrical Factors. Those factors contributing to prolongation of the interval between A_2 and P_2 include right bundle branch block, pacing of the left ventricle, preexcitation, and ventricular premature beats originating on the left side of the heart. Under these circumstances graphic records demonstrate a further prolongation of the A_2-P_2 interval with inspiration, even though this is usually difficult to perceive by means of auscultation.

Hemodynamic Factors. Those factors that increase the splitting of S_2 include the following.

OBSTRUCTION TO RIGHT VENTRICULAR OUTFLOW. Valvular pulmonic stenosis results in prolongation of right ventricular systole, with delay and diminution of P_2. The magnitude of the separation of A_2-P_2 can be used to estimate the severity of the stenosis, being greater with higher right ventricular pressures (Fig. 3–8).[57] With infundibular stenosis, a similar separation of the components of S_2 is seen.

SHORTENING OF LEFT VENTRICULAR EJECTION TIME. In severe mitral regurgitation, the left ventricular ejection time is abnormally short and A_2 is early, resulting in a prolongation of the interval between A_2 and P_2. Respiratory variation is preserved.

Broad Fixed Splitting of S_2. In atrial septal defect there is, in most instances, broad and fixed splitting of S_2 (Fig. 3–9).[58] Fixed separation of A_2-P_2 is defined as a gap that varies no more than 0.01 sec with inspiration and expiration. The mechanism for the broad and fixed characteristics of the second heart sound has been studied in Murgo's laboratory by means of carefully monitored beat-to-beat simultaneous measurements of flow, pressure, and systolic time intervals in the right and left heart.[59] These

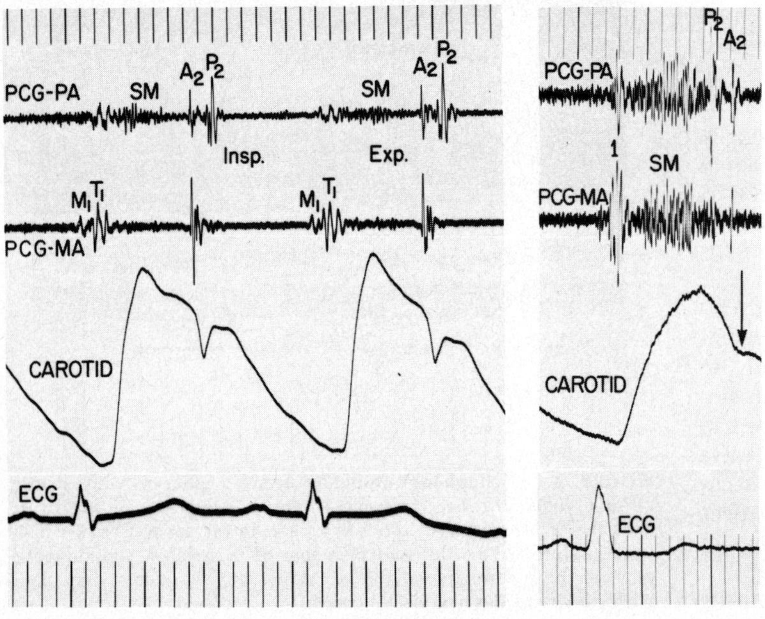

FIGURE 3–9 *Left,* Atrial septal defect showing a midsystolic murmur (SM) and "fixed" splitting of S_2 in the second left intercostal space (PCG-PA). The separation of A_2 and P_2 is 0.06 sec in inspiration and expiration. The first heart sound shows a relatively loud tricuspid component (T_1). *Right,* Aortic stenosis, with reversed splitting of S_2. There is a prominent midsystolic murmur. A_2 is identified by its occurrence immediately prior to the incisura (arrow) on the carotid pulse tracing. P_2 is seen to fall still earlier by 0.04 sec. The carotid upstroke is slow and is shattered by coarse vibrations.

investigators have shown that during expiration the right heart ejection dynamics in patients with atrial septal defect are normal and the wide expiratory split is explained by an abnormally shortened left ventricular ejection time. During inspiration, P_2 is delayed in patients with atrial septal defect and in normal subjects. However, unlike in normal subjects, A_2 does not move to an earlier position during inspiration in patients with atrial septal defect. A_2 thus retains a relatively constant interval with P_2. These findings are consistent with the 1960 phonocardiographic studies Shafter.[60]

Paradoxical Splitting of S_2. Reversal in the normal sequences of A_2-P_2 can occur from either electrical or hemodynamic causes.

Electrical Factors. Electrical disturbances that alter the normal sequence of depolarization of the ventricles include left bundle branch block (Fig. 3–10) and ectopic beats, paced beats, or idioventricular rhythm originating on the right side of the heart. Preexcitation may also result in a precedence of right ventricular systole and reversal of S_2.

Hemodynamic Factors. Mechanical factors that are associated with prolongation of left ventricular ejection time include outflow obstruction of the left ventricle, as in aortic stenosis (Fig. 3–9), or hypertrophic obstructive cardiomyopathy (HOCM). Paradoxical splitting of S_2 is found only in the most severe cases. In patent ductus arteriosus, the increased stroke volume of the left ventricle may also lengthen left ventricular ejection time, resulting in a reversal of A_2-P_2. However, the accentuation of the murmur at

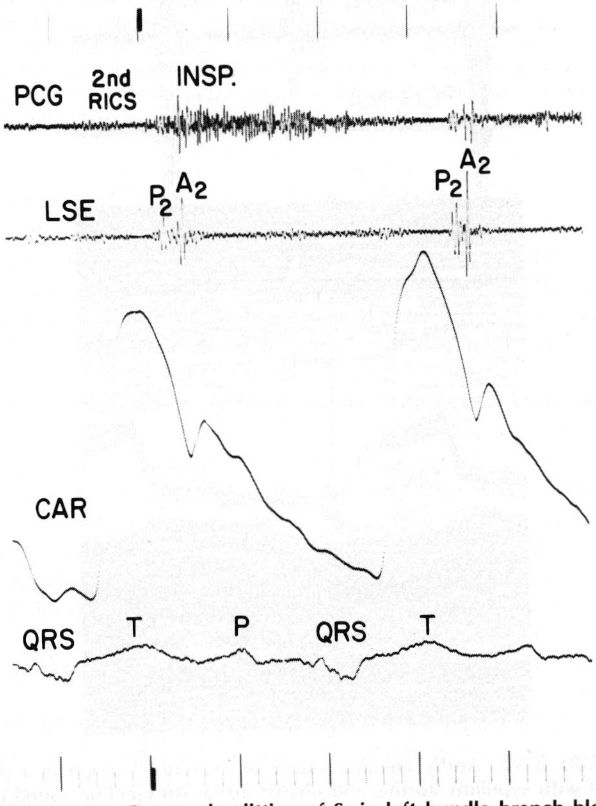

FIGURE 3–10 Reversed splitting of S_2 in left bundle branch block. PCG at left sternal edge (LSE) shows P_2 before A_2, the latter being identified by its occurrence immediately before the incisura in the carotid pulse tracing. With inspiration the gap between P_2 and A_2 narrows, illustrating the physical sign that would permit the detection of reversed splitting by auscultation.

the time of S_2, which is characteristic of this defect, obscures the details of S_2 both on auscultation and on the phonocardiogram.

Single S_2. The second sound may seem to be single on auscultation or on the phonocardiogram because (1) it is indeed single, (2) one of its two elements is inaudible, or (3) both components occur simultaneously. The most common cause for an *apparently* single S_2 is inability to hear or record the fainter of the two elements of the sound (usually P_2) due to emphysema, obesity, or other technical problems. A truly single S_2, however, is seen in tetralogy of Fallot or pulmonary atresia, in which A_2 is loud and is usually easily recorded, whereas pulmonary closure is so soft that it escapes detection. Fusion of the two elements of S_2 resulting in a very loud single S_2 occurs with ventricular septal defect with pulmonary hypertension.

Intensity of S_2. Recording the two elements of S_2 is best accomplished with the microphone at the upper left sternal border. Although P_2 is best appreciated in this location and is poorly transmitted elsewhere, it ordinarily does not exceed A_2 in intensity in normal subjects, even at the upper left sternal edge. When it is shown by graphic records to exceed A_2 in amplitude or to be unusually widely transmitted, such as to the cardiac apex, one must suspect pulmonary hypertension or atrial septal defect.[61] An exaggerated P_2 is, however, only a crude indicator of pulmonary hypertension. In atrial septal defect, P_2 may be accentuated and widely transmitted even when the pulmonary arterial pressure is normal.

A diminished P_2 is found in pulmonic stenosis, either valvular or infundibular, since this obstructing lesion results in low pressure in the pulmonary artery and therefore a diminished force effecting closure of the valve (Fig. 3–8).

Accentuation of A_2, like other phonocardiographic observations of heart-sound intensity, is usually a subjective assessment owing to variations in thickness of the chest wall and other technical factors that make quantitation virtually impossible. Nevertheless, an increase in A_2 can frequently be noted in systemic hypertension, coarctation of the aorta, and corrected transposition of the great arteries.

Reduction in intensity of A_2 occurs in aortic stenosis in adults, in whom the valve is often immobilized by calcification. In children with congenitally deformed but still mobile valve cusps, the intensity of A_2 is usually normal. A soft A_2 may be found in aortic regurgitation. Sabbah et al. attribute this to (1) the lower diastolic pressure in the aorta that results in a diminished rate of change in the driving pressure, i.e., the diastolic pressure gradient between the aorta and the left ventricle that effects valve closure; and (2) a diminished ability of the abnormal valve to become tense and vibrate after closure.[62]

EJECTION SOUNDS. Ejection sounds of aortic origin are of high frequency and occur early in systole, usually 0.12 to 0.14 sec after the Q wave of the electrocardiogram. These sounds are most prominent in association with a deformed aortic valve, as in congenital aortic stenosis, bicuspid configuration (Fig. 3–11),[63–65] or rheumatic heart disease. A mobile valve is necessary for sound production, since with heavy calcification and immobilization of the valve the ejection sound disappears. Aortic ejection sounds from deformed valves are widely

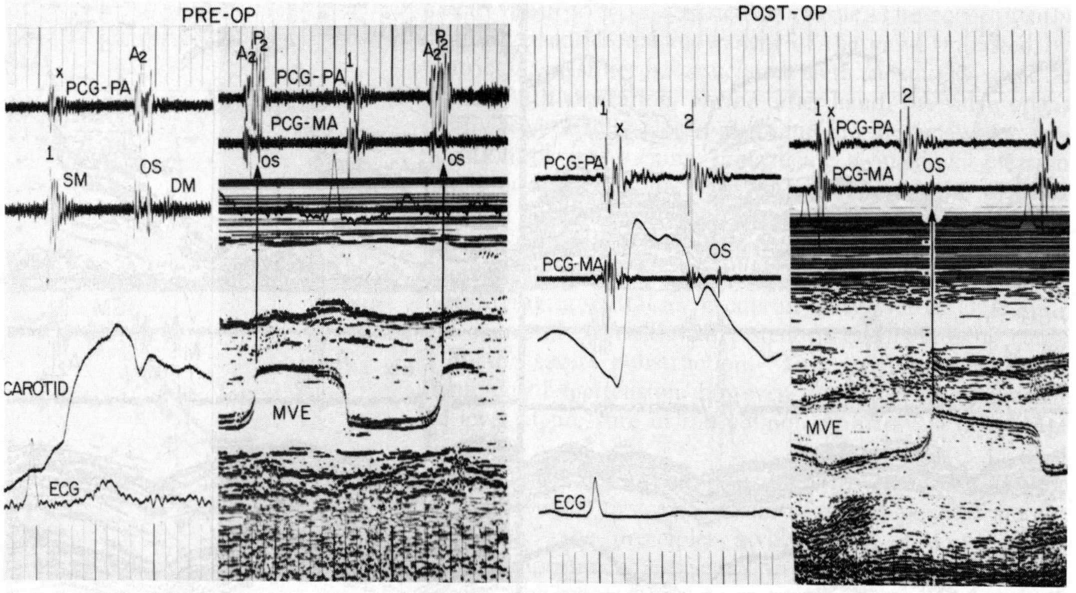

FIGURE 3–14 Mitral stenosis. The two left panels (pre-op) illustrate an opening snap (OS) occurring 0.04 sec after A_2, its identity confirmed by coincidence with full opening of the mitral valve (arrow). P_2 is visible only in the phonocardiogram at PA, occupying the space between A_2 and OS. An ejection sound (x) is seen in the tracing from the second left interspace (PA), reflecting pulmonary hypertension. Following successful valvulotomy (post-op), the OS moves out to 0.10 sec from A_2. The differences in carotid pulse wave contour in the two tracings are accounted for by technical imperfections in the pre-op record, since there was no evidence of aortic valve disease.

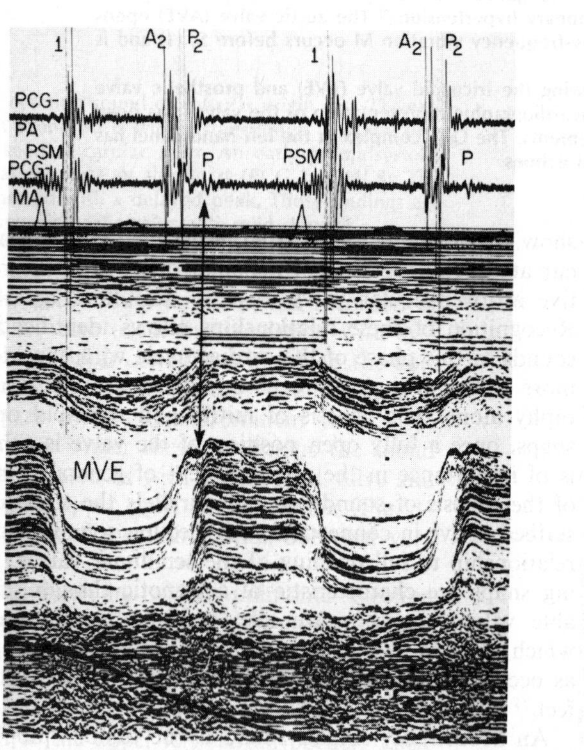

FIGURE 3–15 Left atrial myxoma. A young woman with a large myxoma resulting in symptoms of pulmonary congestion. S_1 is accentuated and delayed and is preceded by a brief "presystolic" crescendo murmur (PSM) occurring as the tumor mass (dense echoes in MVE) is thrust by ventricular contraction into the orifice of the mitral valve, thereby obstructing inflow from the atrium. P_2 is accentuated because of pulmonary hypertension and is widely transmitted to the cardiac apex (MA). It is followed by a tumor "plop" (P), which occurs 0.10 sec from A_2 and is coincident with completion of the ventricular excursion of the tumor mass (arrow).

shown to coincide with the time of maximal valve prolapse (Fig. 3–31).[75] This observation is consistent with the thesis advanced above that high-frequency sounds of cardiac origin occur when a valve has moved in response to hemodynamic forces and is suddenly checked in its course.

THIRD AND FOURTH HEART SOUNDS. In contrast to S_1, S_2, ejection sounds, and opening snaps, which are predominantly of high frequency, third (S_3) and fourth (S_4), or atrial, sounds are of low frequency. The left-sided S_3 occurs in association with rapid filling of the ventricle, as in normal youthful subjects, mitral regurgitation (Fig. 3–1), or thyrotoxicosis.[76] In other pathological conditions, such as left ventricular failure, the term "gallop" is applied to the analogous sound,[77] but once again its pathogenesis is related to ventricular filling in early diastole. In pericardial constriction, ventricular filling is also confined to early diastole and terminates with a sharp S_3 or pericardial "knock" (Fig. 3–16).[78] In all these situations, the phonocardiogram records a low-frequency vibration (S_3) simultaneously with the peak of the rapid filling wave of the apex cardiogram. The echocardiographic correlation, however, is less helpful than with the high-frequency sounds discussed above. The third sound may be associated with a change in the E–F slope of mitral valve closure, but this probably reflects a change in the pattern of ventricular filling rather than being indicative of a direct causative relationship. The onset of the third heart sound has been reported to bear a close relationship to halting of the rapid posterior motion of the left ventricular wall in early diastole,[79] although this relationship has been questioned by other investigators.[80] Recent studies by Ozawa et al.[80a] attribute the sound to a sudden inherent limitation in the long axis filling movement of the left ventricle, a view consistent with traditional concepts dating from Potain in the nineteenth century.

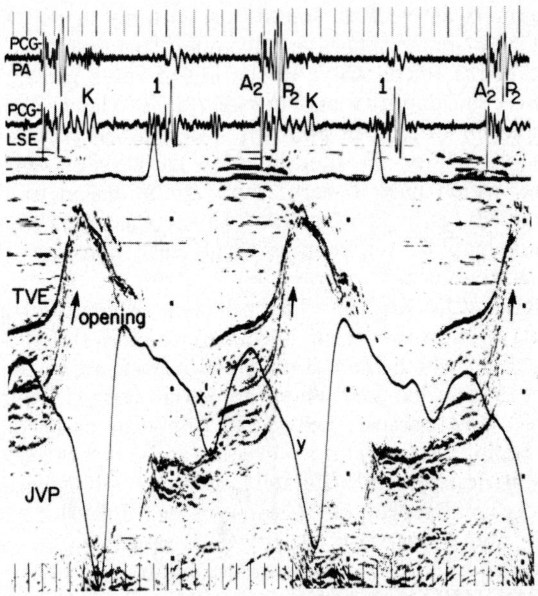

FIGURE 3–16 Pericardial knock. The relationship of the third sound or knock (K) associated with constrictive pericarditis to the jugular venous pulse (JVP) and movements of the tricuspid valve TVE is shown. The valve opens completely (arrows) before the knock. The latter, however, is closely related temporally to the nadir of the *y* descent of the JVP. P_2 is accentuated and widely transmitted, consistent with the pulmonary hypertension that was found at cardiac catheterization.

Fourth sounds, or atrial sounds, occur under circumstances of altered compliance of the ventricle, either left or right.[81] Thus, in coronary heart disease, HOCM, aortic stenosis, and systemic hypertension, a left-sided S_4 is a common feature (Fig. 3–17). A right-sided S_4 may be found under analogous circumstances, as in pulmonary hypertension or pulmonic valve stenosis.[82]

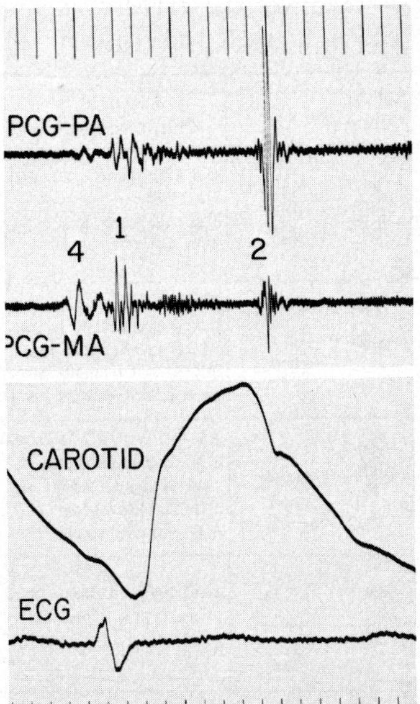

FIGURE 3–17 Fourth heart sound (4) in association with systemic hypertension and left ventricular hypertrophy. The low frequency of S_4 is apparent, compared with S_1 and S_2.

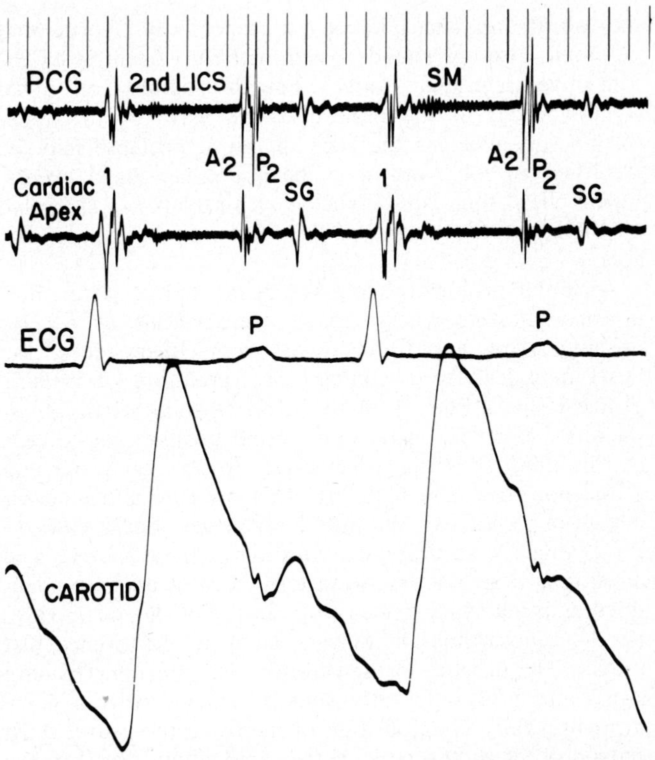

FIGURE 3–18 Summation sound, often called summation gallop, (SG) in a young woman with second-degree AV block characterized by Wenckebach periods. Atrial systole occurs in early diastole owing to the long P-R interval, and the augmented left ventricular filling results in a summation sound.

Identification of S_4 in a graphic tracing is best accomplished by noting its coincidence with the peak of the *a* wave in the accompanying apexcardiogram.[83] The echophonocardiogram is also less useful here than in identification of the high-frequency sounds discussed previously. The left-sided S_4 occurs during the phase of atrial reopening of the mitral valve and is temporally related to the *a* point of the mitral valve motion. The combination of a long P-R interval and a rapid heart rate may result in telescoping of diastolic events in such a way that third and fourth sounds may merge to form a loud summation sound (Fig. 3–18).[84]

ECHOPHONOCARDIOGRAPHY FOR THE IDENTIFICATION OF HEART SOUNDS. The finding on auscultation of two discrete sounds in quick succession at the onset of systole presents a common auscultatory problem. This combination could be due to normal splitting of S_1, with both mitral (M_1) and tricuspid (T_1) elements being well heard, as in normal youthful subjects (Figs. 3–2, 3–4, and 3–5), atrial septal defect, or right bundle branch block. Alternatively, a somewhat similar combination of sounds could be produced by S_4-S_1 or by S_1 and an ejection sound, as with a bicuspid aortic valve or valvular pulmonic stenosis (Figs. 3–11 to 3–14, and 3–17). A sequence of S_1 and an early systolic click of mitral origin can also present in this fashion. Although the associated findings, on physical examination, x-ray, and electrocardiogram may clarify this problem, one may wish to resort to echophonocardiography for a more certain solution. M_1 and T_1 can be identified by their coincidence with full closure of the mitral and tricuspid valves, respectively. Aortic and pulmonic ejection sounds occur with full opening of the respective semilunar valve. Fourth sounds, or atrial sounds, occur at the peak of the *a* wave of the apexcardiogram, whereas the click of mitral prolapse may be identified as occurring after the above-mentioned events. Mitral clicks sometimes coincide with prolapse of the valve on the echocardiogram, but this relationship is not invariable.

A similar problem often exists at the end of systole and in early diastole when various combinations of A_2, P_2, opening snaps, and third sounds from either side of the heart may lead to a confused interpretation of bedside physical signs (Figs. 3–14 to 3–16). Opening of the prosthetic valve in the mitral or tricuspid position also occurs in this phase of the cardiac cycle. A very early opening snap, indicative of a high left atrial pressure and a severe degree of stenosis of the mitral valve, may occur close to P_2, so that the accurate identification of these sounds is of more than academic importance. A_2 is most precisely identified as being synchronous with closure of the aortic valve on the echocardiogram as well as by its occurrence just prior to the incisura in the carotid artery tracing. Opening snaps and prosthetic valve sounds coincide with achievement of a fully open position of the respective valve; third sounds occur at the peak of the rapid filling wave on the apexcardiogram. P_2, then, is often identified by exclusion because of the difficulty in delineating closure of the pulmonic valve echocardiographically.

CONCEPTS OF THE GENESIS OF HEART SOUNDS. From the observations summarized in the preceding pages, we offer the following hypotheses to explain the origin of heart sounds that may be divided into high- and low-frequency categories. Of the high-frequency sounds, the first and second heart sounds are causally related to completed closure of the atrioventricular and similunar valves, respectively. High-frequency sounds occur at the time of complete opening of these valves and are recognized as ejection sounds or opening snaps. A high-frequency sound occurs at the time of completion of prolapse of the mitral valve in the mitral valve prolapse syndrome. The majority and possibly all of these sounds are valvular in origin. In contrast, low-frequency sounds are probably related to alterations in patterns of ventricular filling, which may in turn cause alterations in motion of the atrioventricular valves. Thus, the high-frequency sounds may be regarded as "valvular" and the low-frequency sounds as "ventricular."

FRICTION RUBS. The principal elements of a pericardial friction rub occur during those phases of the cardiac cycle in which there is maximal movement of the heart in the pericardial sac. These are atrial systole, ventricular systole, and passive ventricular filling in early diastole. This timing of auscultatory events can be portrayed graphically if desired. Unfortunately, however, phonocardiography does not reproduce the unique auscultatory quality of a rub, and therefore it usually adds nothing to a bedside assessment made by a competent examiner.

PROSTHETIC VALVE SOUNDS. Surgical implantation of prosthetic valves and pacemakers has resulted in a whole array of new auscultatory phenomena. The sounds produced by prostheses vary, depending on their location, their manner of opening and closing, and their constituents—plastic, steel, or biological tissues.[84a] In general, the metal balls used in Starr-Edwards valves produce the loudest, most distinctive sounds on both opening and closing.[85] Tilting disk valves (e.g., Björk-Shiley or Lillehei-Kaster) produce loud, crisp sounds on closing but little or no sound on opening.[86] Porcine heterograft valves produce a sound similar to that of a normal valve on closing, but they may open silently.[87] The timing of prosthetic valve movements may occasionally provide information regarding malfunction, since the movements of prostheses are in response to rapidly fluctuating pressures in adjacent heart chambers. For example, the expected time of opening of most of the currently used prostheses in the mitral posi-

Prosthesis type	Mitral Prosthesis	Acoustic Characteristics	Aortic Prosthesis	Acoustic Characteristics
Ball Valves	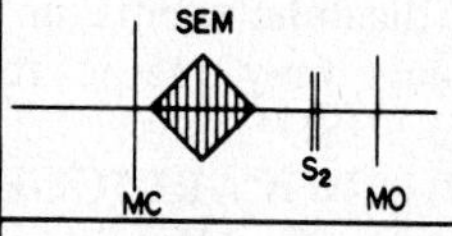	1) A_2–MO interval 0.07–0.11 sec. 2) MO > MC 3) II–III/VI Systolic ejection murmur (SEM) 4) No diastolic murmur	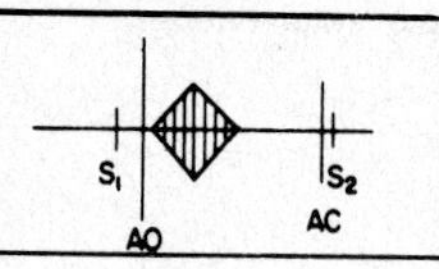	1) S_1–AO interval 0.07 sec. 2) AO > AC 3) II/VI harsh SEM 4) No diastolic murmur
Disc Valves	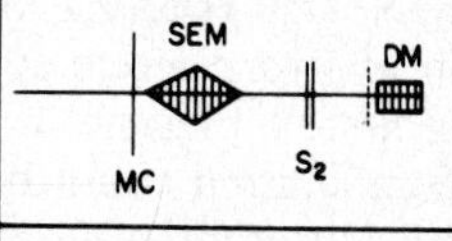	1) A_2–MO interval 0.05–0.09 sec. 2) MO is rarely heard 3) II/VI SEM is usually heard 4) I–II/VI diastolic rumble is usually heard	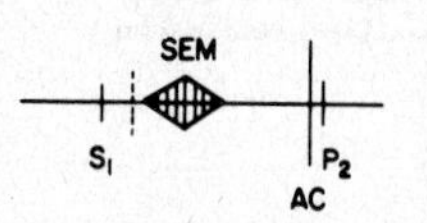	1) S_1–AO interval 0.04 sec. 2) AO is uncommonly heard, AC is usually heard 3) II/VI SEM is usually heard 4) Occasional diastolic murmur
Porcine Valves	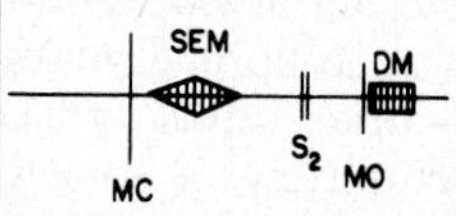	1) A_2–MO interval 0.1 sec. 2) MO is audible 50% 3) I–II/VI apical SEM 50% 4) Diastolic rumble ½–⅔	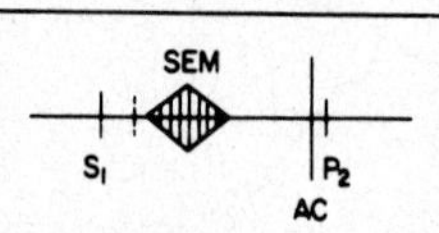	1) S_1–AO interval 0.03–0.08 sec. 2) AO is uncommonly heard, AC is usually heard 3) II/VI SEM in most 4) No diastolic murmur
Bileaflet Valve (St. Jude)			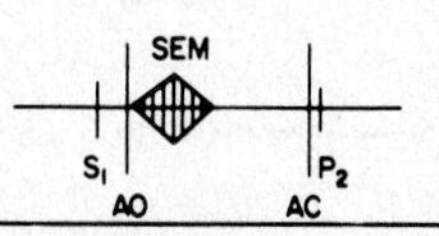	1) AO and AC commonly heard 2) A soft SEM is common

FIGURE 3–19 Summary of the acoustic characteristics of each valve prosthesis according to type and location. SEM = systolic ejection murmur; DM = diastolic murmur; S_1 = first heart sound; S_2 = second heart sound; P_2 = pulmonic second sound; A_2 = aortic second sound; AO = aortic valve opening sound; AC = aortic valve closure sound; MO = mitral valve opening sound; MC = mitral valve closure sound. (Reproduced with permission from Smith, N. D., Raizada, V., and Abrams, J.: Auscultation of the normally functioning prosthetic valve. Ann. Intern. Med. *95*:594, 1981.)

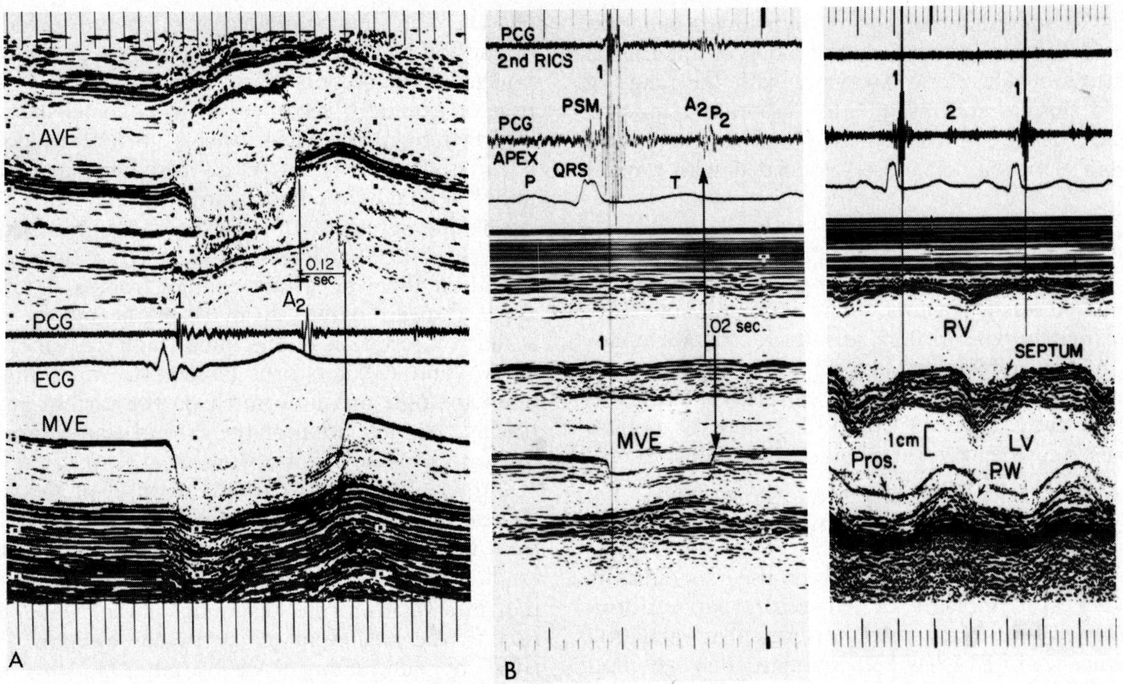

FIGURE 3–20 *A,* **Echophonocardiogram from a patient with a normally functioning Lillihei-Kaster prosthesis in the mitral position. The dual echo shows the aortic valve above (AVE) and mitral prosthesis below (MVE). A_2 is coincident with aortic valve closure and is followed after 0.12 sec by full opening of the prosthesis.**

B, ***Left,*** **A Starr-Edwards prosthesis in the mitral position, malfunctioning due to thrombosis causing obstruction. The valve closes with a loud sound (1) preceded by a presystolic crescendo murmur (PSM) resembling that of mitral stenosis. The prosthesis opens only 0.02 sec after A_2, indicating an extremely short isovolumetric relaxation time, which in turn suggests a high left atrial pressure.**

Right, **In the same patient the echo shows a dilated right ventricle (RV) with paradoxical septal movement consistent with the clinically evident tricuspid regurgitation. The left ventricle (LV) is relatively small, a point discounting paravalvular leak and favoring obstruction at the valve level as an explanation for the suspected left atrial hypertension.**

tion is approximately 0.08 sec following the aortic component of S_2 (Figs. 3–19 and 3–20A).[85–87] This period reflects the isovolumetric relaxation time of the left ventricle, and a major factor determining its length is left atrial pressure. Obstruction of the prosthesis by a thrombus or a paravalvular leak will produce elevation of left atrial pressure, and isovolumetric relaxation time will be abbreviated.[88] Once one has established that there may be malfunction of the prosthesis, differential diagnosis of mitral obstruction due to thrombosis from mitral regurgitation resulting from paravalvular leak requires a further step—examination of the left ventricular chamber by echocardiography. Obstruction of the valve simulates mitral stenosis, and one would expect to find no increase in ventricular size from control records and no evidence of hyperdynamic ventricular wall movements (Fig. 3–20B). With paravalvular leak, however, the stroke volume of the left ventricle will be augmented, resulting in exaggerated movements of the posterior wall of the left ventricle and normalization of the septal movements, which are ordinarily hypokinetic or even paradoxical following open-heart prosthetic valve surgery (Chap. 5).[89,90]

For an analysis of prosthetic valve function by the method described above, a combination of echo-and phonocardiography is necessary, since A_2 is detected on the sound record, and the opening of many of the valves in current use is silent and must be documented by a simultaneous echocardiogram.[88]

PACEMAKER SOUNDS. A sharp, high-frequency sound of very brief duration is occasionally audible overlying a transvenous pacemaker placed in the right ventricle. This sound, which may be accompanied by a slight twitch of skeletal muscle in the underlying area of the chest wall, is coincident with the pacemaker spike and is believed to arise from the stimulation of intercostal muscle.[91]

CAROTID PULSE TRACINGS

The carotid pulse is recorded by placement of the transducer firmly over the arterial pulsation, previously identified by palpation. As noted above, its prominence can be enhanced by hyperextension of the neck.

NORMAL CAROTID PULSE. The normal carotid pulse tracing (Figs. 3–1 and 3–2) has a rapid, smooth upstroke, beginning approximately 0.12 to 0.15 sec from the onset of the QRS complex in adults; it reaches a peak within 0.12 sec. Following the period of rapid ejection of blood from the left ventricle, the pulse wave declines to the dicrotic notch, or incisura, which is caused by aortic valve closure. Owing to the transmission time of the pulse wave from the aortic root to the site of application of the transducer over the carotid artery, there is a variable delay from the aortic closure sound, A_2, to the incisura of approximately 0.02 to 0.03 sec (Figs. 3–1 and 3–2). During diastole, the carotid pulse wave usually falls gently until the next systolic pulse. The shape of carotid pulse curves varies widely among different normal individuals and even in the same subject, depending on the mode of application of the transducer. Therefore experience with the range of normality in this, as well as in other laboratory tests, is necessary in order to appreciate truly abnormal curves and also to avoid erroneous diagnoses associated with normal variants.

APPLICATIONS OF CAROTID PULSE TRACINGS

Timing of Acoustic Events. The incisural notch occurs approximately 0.02 to 0.03 sec after aortic valve closure and A_2. Therefore the carotid pulse tracing is a reliable marker for this important auscultatory and phonocardiographic event (Figs. 3–1 and 3–2) and is a most valuable basic ingredient in the phonocardiographic examination.

Systolic Time Intervals

Systolic time intervals (STI) have been used sporadically for a century as a measure of left ventricular performance.[92–95] It is only in recent years however, that validation of the significance of STI has been obtained through comparative studies with various invasive indices of ventricular function (Chap. 14). This has led to widespread acceptance of STI as a simple, inexpensive, and nontraumatic method of estimating left ventricular performance and following the patient's progress over time. Many investigators have contributed to our rapidly increasing knowledge of the significance and utility of STI in clinical medicine. In particular, Weissler, Lewis, and associates have been responsible for popularization of this noninvasive method, and the reader is referred to their extensive publications for further details on the subject.[13,96–105,107,110]

The three basic STI are the preejection period (PEP), the left ventricular ejection time (LVET), and the total electromechanical interval (QS_2) (Fig. 3–21). In order to avoid misleading errors, the technique of recording must be carried out with meticulous attention to detail. STI are obtained from simultaneous fast-speed (100 mm/sec) recordings of the electrocardiogram, the phonocardiogram, and the carotid pulsation.[13] The ECG lead that most clearly displays the onset of left ventricular depolarization is chosen. The phonocardiogram must provide a clear view of the initial high-frequency vibrations of the aortic component of the second heart sound (A_2). The carotid pulsation is generally recorded with a funnel-shaped pick-up attached by polyethylene tubing to a transducer with an adequate time constant, as discussed earlier in this chapter under Technique in Phonocardiography. For clear and accurate measurement of STI, one should employ tracings with the following characteristics: (1) a clear initial depolarization force departing acutely from a flat baseline on the electrocardiogram, to mark the beginning of QRS; (2) a sharp inscription of the initial high-frequency vibrations of A_2; and (3) a clearly discernible rapid upstroke and pointed single incisural notch on the carotid arterial pulse tracing. Amplification of the carotid signal should be adequate to provide a pulse wave of at least 5 cm in height.[98]

The QS_2 is measured from the onset of the QRS to the earliest high-frequency vibrations of A_2. LVET is measured from the beginning upstroke to the trough of the incisural notch of the carotid pulse tracing (Fig. 3–21). The PEP is that interval from the beginning of ventricular depolarization to the beginning of ventricular ejection. PEP is derived by subtracting LVET from QS_2, this step being necessary in order to eliminate the delay in transmission of the arterial pulse from the aortic root to the position on the carotid artery of the transducer. The PEP is made up of the electromechanical interval plus the isovolumetric contraction time. The electromechanical interval is relatively constant in most individuals, except where there is left ventricular conduction delay, as in left bundle branch block. Therefore, variations in isovolumetric contraction time constitute the principal information of physiological significance in measurements of the PEP.

In applying STI measurements, correction must be made for differences in heart rate. When heart rate is derived from the R-R interval, a simple linear equation best describes the relationship of STI to rate. The regression equations of Weissler have been generally adopted (Table 3–1) for this purpose.

In applying STI clinically, derivations from normal regressions can be indicated by expressing each of the systolic time intervals as an "index" value, as shown in Table 3–1. By calculating the index value, one obtains an estimate

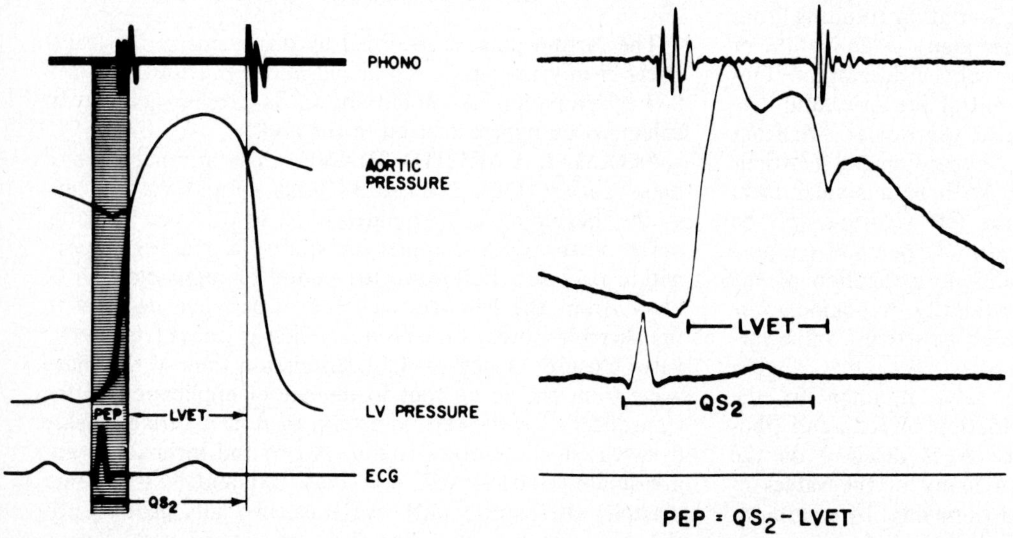

Figure 3–21 On the left is a diagram of the left ventricular events which constitute the STI. On the right is a recording of a phonocardiogram, external carotid pulse, and electrocardiogram at 100 mm/sec paper speed. The subintervals of the STI are indicated on both. (From Lewis, R. P., et al.: A critical review of the systolic time intervals. Circulation *56*:146, 1977. By permission of the American Heart Association, Inc.)

TABLE 3–1 CALCULATION OF STI INDEX VALUES FROM RESTING REGRESSION EQUATIONS

Sex	Equation	Normal Index (msec)	SD
M	$QS_2I = 2.1\ hr + QS_2$	546	14
F	$QS_2I = 2.0\ hr + QS_2$	549	14
M	LVETI = 1.7 hr + LVET	413	10
F	LVETI = 1.6 hr + LVET	418	11
M	PEPI = 0.4 hr + PEP	131	10
F	PEPI = 0.4 hr + PEP	133	10

Key: I=index; SD=standard deviation; M=male; F=female; hr=heart rate.
From Weissler, A.M., et al.: Bedside technics for the evaluation of ventricular function in man. Am. J. Cardiol. *23*:577, 1969.

of the deviation from normal that cannot be explained by the heart rate. Thus, for example, a QS_2 index (QS_2I) of 506 msec in a man is easily recognized as being 40 msec shorter than the expected normal value of 546 msec.

At rates below 110 beats/min, the PEP and LVET shorten proportionately as heart rate increases. Therefore, a simple and increasingly popular method of expressing variations in STI in the normal range of heart rates is by the ratio of PEP/LVET. This ratio may identify left ventricular dysfunction when either the PEPI or the LVETI or both are still within the limits of normal. Since in many types of left ventricular dysfunction PEP lengthens and LVET shortens, higher ratios for PEP/LVET are abnormal. The PEP/LVET ratio is normally approximately 0.34 to 1,[98] with the upper limit being 0.42 to 1.[100]

Factors Influencing the STI. Factors known to influence the PEP and LVET are listed in Table 3–2. With left ventricular failure, regardless of cause, PEPI lengthens and LVETI shortens. Prolongation of PEPI is principally due to a reduced rate of left ventricular pressure rise during isovolumetric systole (LV dP/dt).[13] PEPI can also be prolonged by delayed electrical activation, as in LBBB. Under these circumstances, obviously a prolongation of PEPI cannot be used as an indicator of diminished left ventricular performance, since the problem may be simply due to electrical delay. An estimate of the delay can be obtained from the apexcardiogram.[96]

TABLE 3–2 FACTORS INFLUENCING SYSTOLIC TIME INTERVALS

	Increase (↑)	Decrease (↓)
PEP	LV muscle failure Left bundle branch block ↓Preload Negative inotropic agents	Aortic valve disease ↓LV isovolumic pressure Positive inotropic agents
LVET	Aortic valve disease ↓Afterload	LV muscle failure ↓Preload Positive inotropic agents Negative inotropic agents
QS_2	Left bundle branch block Aortic valve disease	Positive inotropic agents

From Lewis, R.P., et al.: A critical review of the systolic time intervals. Circulation *56*:146, 1977, by permission of the American Heart Association, Inc.

The shortening of LVETI that occurs with heart failure is a complex result of alterations in the rate and extent of fiber shortening of the left ventricle as well as delay in the onset of ejection due to prolongation of PEPI. Of these several factors, probably the most influential is a diminished extent of fiber shortening.[99] Thus, a shortened LVETI or abnormally elevated PEP/LVET ratio may be found in the presence of a diminished stroke volume. It is of interest to note that the absolute size of the stroke volume does not determine LVET, but rather the size of the stroke volume relative to the end-diastolic volume.[99] Studies relating the PEP/LVET ratio to left ventricular ejection fraction determined by quantitative angiography have shown a close correlation.[101] The relationship has been obtained in patients having valvular and nonvalvular heart disease with a wide variation in functional impairment.

The duration of systole (QS_2I) is remarkably constant for any individual patient. Many types of heart disease result in directionally opposite changes in PEPI and LVETI. QS_2I may therefore be relatively unaffected.[102] However, with inotropic stimulation, such as with digitalis or catecholamines, QS_2I is shortened.[103]

Clinical Applications of Systolic Time Intervals

Evaluation of Left Ventricular Performance in Chronic Myocardial Disease. In a wide variety of heart diseases involving the left ventricle, including myocarditis, cardiomyopathy, coronary artery disease, hypertensive heart disease, and mitral valve disease, a deterioration in left ventricular performance may be manifest in an elevated PEP/LVET ratio. As mentioned above, this ratio correlates best with the angiographic ejection fraction.[100,101,104] Frequently, when overt manifestations of heart failure have been eliminated with diuretics, the persisting severe left ventricular dysfunction continues to be reflected in an abnormal PEP/LVET ratio.[105] On the other hand, a fundamental change such as a subsidence of myocarditis or relief of a reversible cardiomyopathy can be monitored by means of a gradually falling PEP/LVET ratio in serial observations. The STI have been used to estimate prognosis in patients following healed myocardial infarction, with an abnormal PEP/LVET ratio being found to indicate a significantly worse prognosis over a 5-year period.[100] These results are consistent with the generally agreed upon observation that left ventricular function is a major prognostic factor in coronary artery disease.

Aortic Valve Disease. In aortic valve disease, either stenosis or regurgitation, there is a shortening of PEPI and a lengthening of LVETI such that the PEP/LVET ratio tends to fall.[98] The PEPI is short in aortic stenosis owing to the rapid dP/dt and low aortic diastolic pressure. Significant outflow tract obstruction lengthens LVETI. This observation has led to the use of STI as an additional noninvasive parameter for estimating severity of aortic stenosis.[106] Where left ventricular dysfunction has complicated the course of aortic stenosis, opposing trends are found, with PEPI lengthening and LVETI shortening. The net result is that PEP/LVET cannot be reliably used to assess left ventricular function in aortic stenosis.

In aortic regurgitation there is also a shortening of PEPI because of the low diastolic pressure and a lengthening of

LVETI.[98] Although a tendency can be found for PEP/LVET to fall with severe aortic regurgitation, the quantitative value of such a measurement has not been established.

Use of STI in Clinical Pharmacology. One of the most promising areas for the use of STI in the future is in clinical pharmacology. Extensive studies have been performed demonstrating the effects of digitalis glycosides on STI.[107–109] These show that QS_2I responds by shortening in the presence of inotropic stimulation. Propranolol, on the other hand, has been shown to lengthen QS_2I when excessive adrenergic tone is present, and it has been suggested that the STI may become a useful measure for determining the adequacy of beta blockade of angina pectoris.[110] Similarly, the STI can be used to measure the cardiotoxic effect of antineoplastic agents[111,112] and of antiarrhythmic agents and the cardiostimulatory effects of dobutamine and of various vasodilators.

In summary, studies in the past 20 years have established that externally derived systolic time intervals accurately reflect their invasively determined counterparts. The STI have been shown to correlate well with widely accepted measures of left ventricular function, such as the ejection fraction, in a great variety of clinical disorders. The effects of an increasing array of pharmacological agents on the STI are being carefully evaluated, and results are being made available for clinical use. Therefore, STI have become a valuable adjunct to the clinical evaluation of patients and in following their course over prolonged periods, since the measurements are harmless and inexpensive. The method, like any laboratory test, can be abused if performed indiscriminately or with less than impeccable techniques and instrumentation. Only temporal data are obtained by STI. Therefore, the method is not useful in differential diagnosis, since heart diseases of a variety of etiologies have similarly disturbed measurements. Valvular disease such as aortic stenosis or regurgitation affects the STI profoundly and often in a direction opposite to the effects of myocardial disease. The same is true of certain drugs and catecholamines. Therefore, these deceptively simple measurements actually require a very sophisticated overall appreciation of the entire clinical and pharmacological situation if they are to be used effectively and in the patient's best interest.

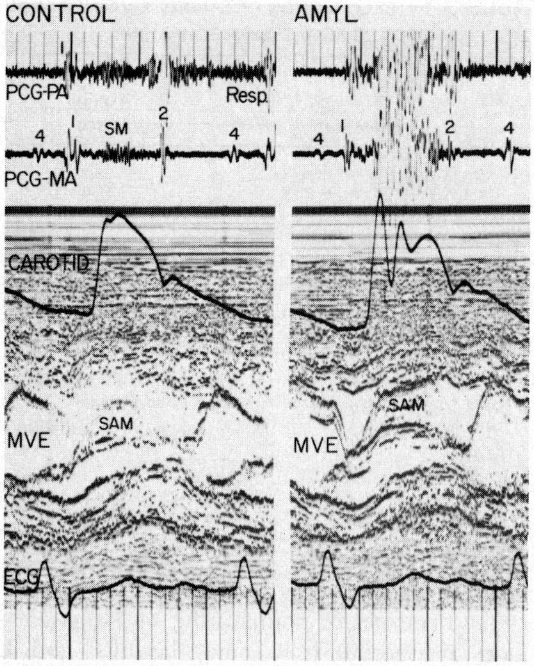

FIGURE 3–23 Hypertrophic obstructive cardiomyopathy (HOCM). ***Left,*** **The control echophonocardiogram shows a fourth sound (4) at MA. The PCG-PA is obscured by a respiratory artifact (Resp). A midsystolic ejection murmur coincides with systolic anterior movement of the MVE (SAM). The carotid pulse contour is within normal limits.** ***Right,*** **Following inhalation of amyl nitrate (AMYL) the murmur becomes louder and the carotid pulse becomes deformed with a spike-and-dome pattern characteristic of HOCM. These changes are coincident with a more prominent SAM, which appears to be in contact with the interventricular septum.**

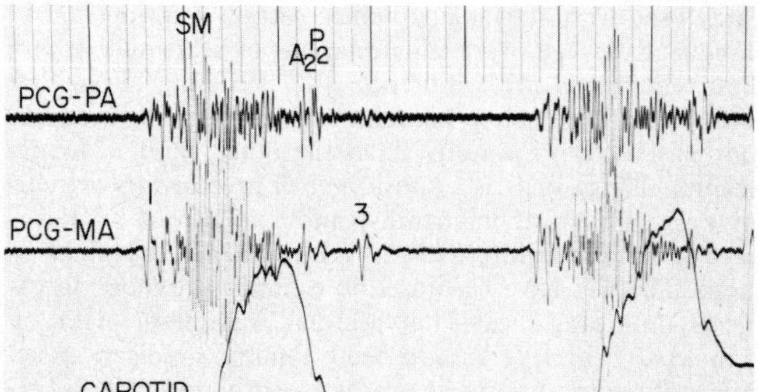

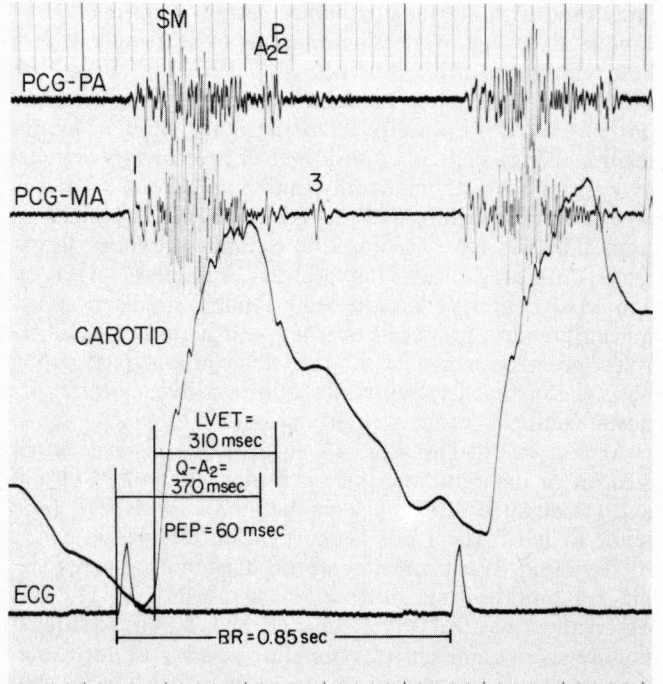

FIGURE 3–22 Valvular aortic stenosis in an 11-year-old boy with moderately severe obstruction (gradient=50 to 60 mm Hg across the aortic valve). A loud midsystolic murmur is seen in all valve areas. The carotid upstroke is delayed and shattered by coarse vibrations. A_2 is well preserved. A third sound (3) is present, probably a normal finding in this youthful subject. The STI indicate a short PEP and prolonged LVET.[13]

CAROTID PULSE CONTOUR PATTERNS

Variability in morphological and temporal details of the carotid pulse may result from technical aspects of the recording, including the choice and application of transducers.[13] In spite of these problems, however, a considerable amount of qualitative information can be derived from alterations in carotid pulse wave tracings in various disease states. A slowly rising carotid pulse deformed by a shudder—the graphic representation of a thrill—is characteristic of valvular or subvalvular diaphragmatic aortic stenosis (Fig. 3–22). Unfortunately, efforts to quantitate the severity of aortic stenosis by the contour of the carotid pulse, the rapidity of its upstroke, or the achievement of its peak[106] have been disappointing.[113] In elderly patients with arteriosclerotic and therefore inelastic peripheral vasculature, the upstroke of the carotid pulse may be relatively swift despite severe obstruction. Conversely, in some cases of severe aortic regurgitation without any systolic gradient across the valve, the physical and graphic signs during systole may nevertheless simulate those of aortic stenosis.

A spike-and-dome pattern characterizes the carotid pulse wave of HOCM (Fig. 3–23). A bisferiens pulse is characteristic of aortic regurgitation or mixed aortic stenosis and regurgitation (Fig. 3–24). A large dicrotic wave is sometimes seen in cardiomyopathy and other low-output conditions such as postoperatively in valve replacement for aortic or mitral regurgitation (Fig. 3–25).[114,115] Further examples of the use of carotid pulse tracings in combination with other noninvasive techniques, including echocardiograms, are illustrated in Chapter 4.

Abnormalities of Pulse Frequency, Regularity, and Amplitude

Inequality of Pulses. By using two pulse-sensitive transducers simultaneously, one can document inequality of the carotid pulses in arteriosclerotic occlusive disease, dissecting aneurysm, or supravalvular aortic stenosis. Diminished amplitude and delay in the femoral arterial pulse in coarctation of the aorta can be demonstrated by the simultaneous recording of the femoral and the brachial or carotid pulses.

Changes in Amplitude with Normal Rhythm. The reduction in amplitude of the pulse on inspiration characteristic of *paradoxical pulse* is readily documented by carotid pulse recording performed in conjunction with a pneumogram. The patient should be instructed to breathe slowly and more deeply than usual during the registration of this phenomenon.

Pulsus alternans can also be confirmed by arterial pulse tracings and is often accentuated during the first few beats following a premature ventricular beat (Fig. 3–26). Since the peripheral pulses are more sensitive for the detection of pulsus alternans than is the carotid pulse, one may find it useful to apply the pulse transducer over the femoral artery. The graphic record demonstrates not only the alternating height of the pulse waves but also a beat-to-beat alteration in the rate of rise of the pulse wave as well as in systolic time intervals. The stronger beats display a shorter PEP and longer LVET and therefore a lower PEP/LVET ratio than do the weaker beats, reflecting the higher level of the contractile state in the former.[116]

Ectopic Rhythms. With ventricular tachycardia, variations in the amplitude of the pulse from beat to beat reflect the rapidly changing sequence of atrial and ventricular systole and the results of more effective ventricular contraction when fortuitously there is a properly timed atrial systole. The totally irregular rhythm and beat-to-beat changes in the amplitude of the pulse characteristic of atrial fibrillation can be documented by carotid pulse tracings. Similarly, the ineffective systoles occasioned by premature beats are easily demonstrable.

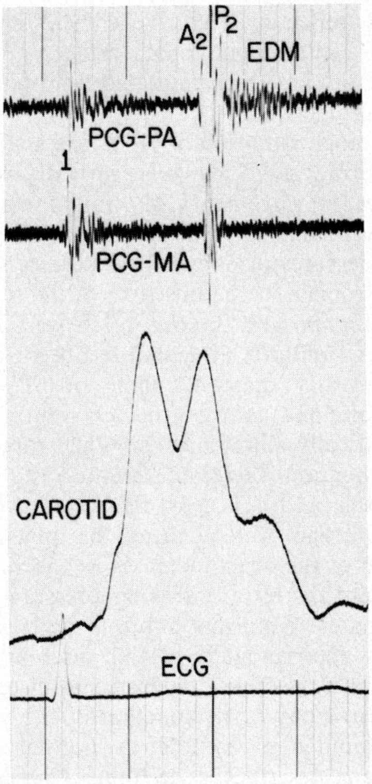

FIGURE 3–24 Pulsus bisferiens in aortic regurgitation. The carotid pulse is bifid, and there is a large excursion reflecting the wide pulse pressure. The phonocardiogram establishes that both humps of the carotid pulse are systolic in time (i.e., prior to A_2), thus separating the bisferiens pulse from a large dicrotic wave (Fig. 3–27), with which it may be confused at the bedside. There is no incisura, owing to aortic incompetence. EDM = early diastolic murmur.

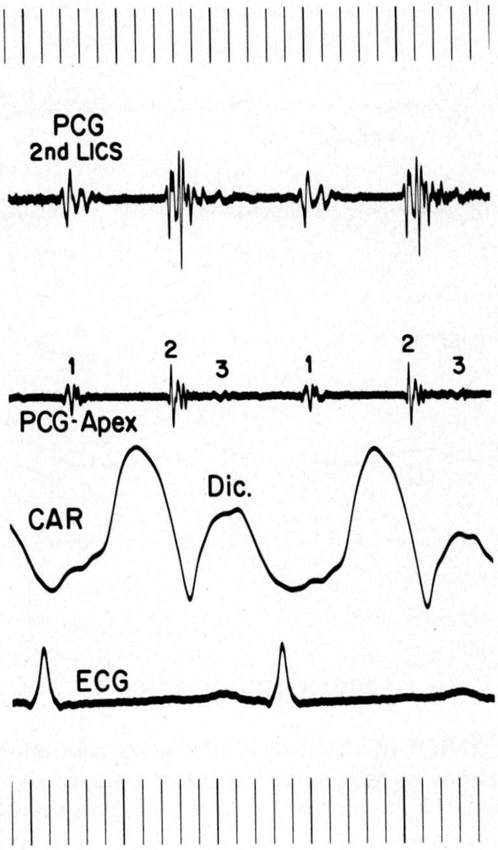

FIGURE 3–25 Dicrotic wave (Dic.) in the pulse tracing of a man with cardiomyopathy.

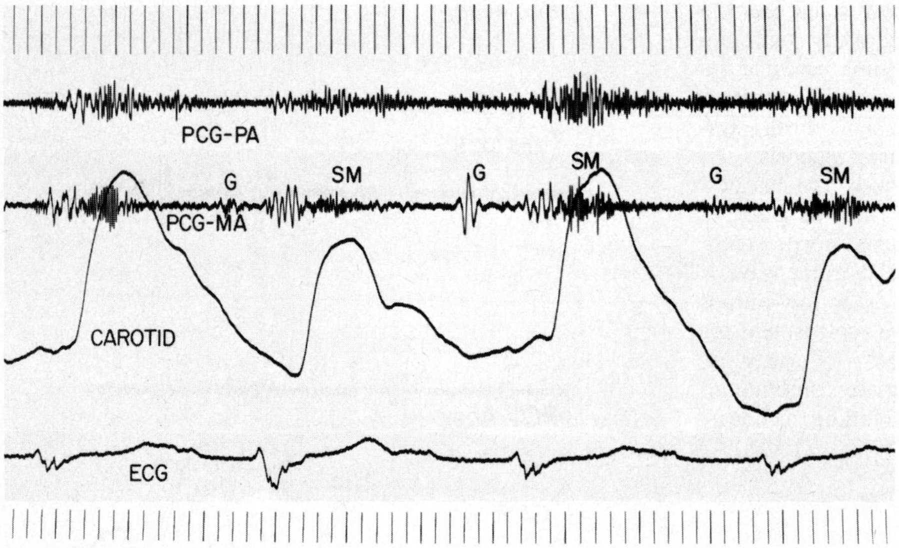

FIGURE 3–26 Pulsus alternans in a man with aortic stenosis and left ventricular failure. The first and third beats are of greater amplitude than are the second and fourth beats. The stronger beats are also marked by a louder murmur (SM) and less abnormality of STI. The diastolic sound (G) is louder after the second (weak) beat. It is a summation sound caused by merging of S_3 and S_4, resulting from the combined effect of a rapid heart rate and a prolonged P-R interval.

APEXCARDIOGRAPHY[117]

TECHNIQUE. The apex impulse is best appreciated on palpation as well as for recording purposes by having the patient lie in a partial left lateral decubitus position. A triangular supporting pillow beneath the back promotes comfort and relaxation. The optimal registration of the apexcardiogram may require that the patient hold his breath in partial exhalation. The transducer funnel or tambour may be held by hand over the left ventricular apex. Alternatively, a strap can be used to hold the transducer in place, but this technique makes it more difficult to keep the device in proper position. The transducer used in apexcardiography senses the *relative* position of the diaphragm of the transducer with respect to its rim. (With a funnel device, the skin serves as a diaphragm.) Thus, ordinarily the rim of the sensing head of the transducer rests on the ribs, and its diaphragm moves with the soft tissues in the intercostal space. Reproducibility in recording the apexcardiogram is adversely affected by differences in the patient's position, the pressure with which the transducer is applied, and, most of all, failure to place the transducer precisely over the point of maximum impulse. Other methods of recording precordial motion include kinetocardiography[118] and cardiokymography.[119] These methods avoid the problem of relative movement of the chest wall with respect to the rim of the transducer mentioned above and record, instead, absolute movement. Kinetocardiography accomplishes this by attaching the transducer to a fixed point in space, a technique that is useful but too cumbersome for routine use. Cardiokymography employs a capacitance transducer that is held slightly separated from the chest wall.[119] The apparatus is light and easily applied and has recently been found to be of value in detecting wall-motion abnormalities after exercise in patients with ischemic heart disease.[120] Although each of these techniques is useful, space does not permit a discussion of the normal patterns and variations observed in disease states. The following paragraphs therefore will deal with apexcardiography, which is the most widely used method of recording precordial movement.

NORMAL APEXCARDIOGRAM. The apexcardiogram is a graphic representation of precordial movement. As the name implies, it is usually recorded over the left ventricular apex.[117] However, the same technique and equipment can be used to record movements at the left sternal edge, reflecting right ventricular hypertrophy or pulsations of a dilated pulmonary artery.[82,121] The heave resulting from an anteriorly situated ventricular aneurysm can also be appreciated.

The physiological correlations of the major landmarks of the apexcardiogram have been carefully worked out by Willems et al.[122,123] by means of simultaneous registration of the left ventricular apexcardiogram and high-fidelity left ventricular pressures in dogs. These studies showed a very precise synchronism in the upstroke of the systolic wave of the apexcardiogram and the rise in left ventricular pressure (Fig. 3–27). A similar relationship has been reported in humans.[124] The early diastolic nadir or "0"-point in the apexcardiogram and that in the left ventricular pressure are also practically simultaneous.[122] The rapid upstroke of the apexcardiogram therefore initiates the isovolumetric phase of systole and is largely completed during this portion of the cardiac cycle. During this phase the external circumference of the heart increases as the ventricle changes its shape and the intraventricular pressure rises. The upstroke terminates in normal subjects with the "E"-point, which occurs approximately at the onset of ejection. The E-point, however, is often obliterated in disease states that result in hypertrophy or dysfunction of the ventricle. During the remainder of systole in normal subjects, the apexcardiogram describes a declining plateau as the volume of the heart diminishes. A more abrupt decline begins to occur just before the second heart sound. A nadir or 0-point is reached in early diastole at approximately the time of opening of the mitral valve. This is followed by a rapid filling wave and a slow filling wave, reflecting analogous events in the left ventricular pressure curve. In late diastole, the *a* wave is recorded, reflecting movement of a small amount of blood into the left ventricle as a result of atrial systole. In normal subjects the *a* wave is of modest height, usually less than 15 per cent in amplitude with respect to the total height of the apexcardiogram.

In a combined tracing, with phonocardiograms and carotid pulse tracing, the systolic upstroke of the apexcardiogram can be used to divide the preejection period into its two major components—the electromechanical interval and the isovolumetric contraction time (Fig. 3–27). Such a division would be useful in LBBB, in which the electromechanical interval might constitute a disproportionate part of the PEP. The 0-point in early diastole should not be used as a marker for mitral valve opening, since its relation to this event is only an approximation, and a more accurate reflection of valve movement is provided by the echocardiogram (Figs. 3–4 and 3–14). The diastolic waves of the apexcardiogram, i.e., the rapid filling wave and the *a* wave, are the low-frequency counterparts of the third and fourth, or atrial, sounds, respectively. Therefore the apexcardiogram can be used to identify diastolic auscultatory events (Figs. 3–28 and 3–30).

APEXCARDIOGRAPHY IN DISEASE. The systolic portion of the apexcardiogram has only a limited number of patterns of diagnostic utility. These can be broadly classified as (1) *normal* (described above), (2) *hyperdynamic*, and (3) *sustained*.[125]

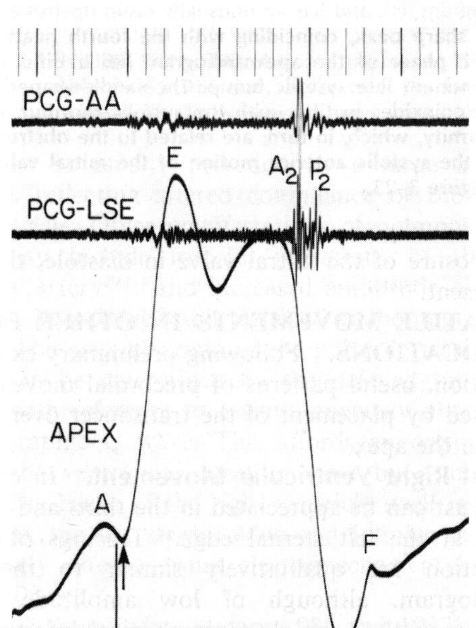

FIGURE 3–27 **Normal apexcardiogram. A low-amplitude *a* wave (A) in presystole follows the P wave of the ECG, which is not visible in this lead. The onset of the QRS (downward arrow) is followed after a brief electromechanical interval (0.02 sec) by the onset of the swift upward movement of the apex tracing (upward arrow), culminating in the E point at approximately the time of beginning ejection into the aorta. A generally declining curve during systole ends with an abrupt downward fall at the time of A_2. The nadir (0) is reached at approximately the time of mitral valve opening. The rapid filling wave (F) occurs during early diastolic filling of the left ventricle.**

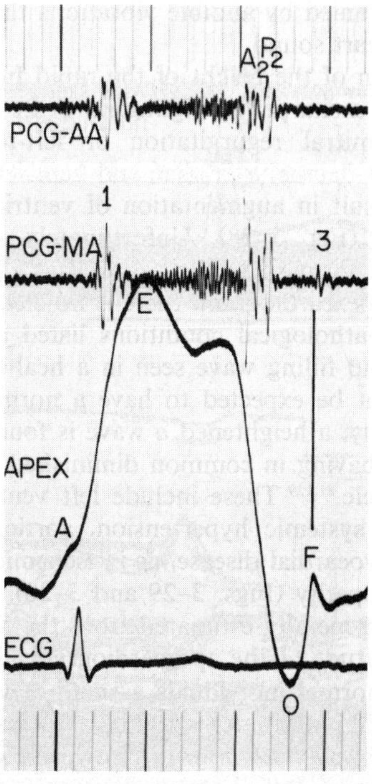

FIGURE 3–28 **Hyperdynamic apexcardiogram in mitral regurgitation. The configuration of the tracing in systole is qualitatively similar to a normal curve, although the amplitude was clearly exaggerated by palpation. The rapid filling wave (F) is higher than normal and terminates in a sharp point coincident with its audible counterpart, the third heart sound (3).**

Hyperdynamic movement is perceived at the bedside as a thrust of exaggerated height but one which falls away immediately from the palpating fingers. It is found in conditions characterized by an increased stroke volume such as in normal subjects after exercise, in thyrotoxicosis, or in mitral regurgitation (Fig. 3–28).[125,126] The graphic tracing shows a systolic wave of normal shape but of increased amplitude (although this is difficult to measure) and a prominent rapid filling wave.

The *sustained* impulse is the graphic equivalent of a heave or thrust, as may be found in left ventricular hypertrophy, such as that associated with hypertension or aortic stenosis (Fig. 3–29). The systolic portion of a sustained apical impulse is characterized by a plateau or a dome-shaped or rising curve, in contrast to the gentle systolic decline seen in the normal or hyperdynamic tracing. An accompanying finding is a prominent *a* wave. A somewhat similar heave is found in cardiomyopathy or chronic ischemic heart disease. A variant of the sustained impulse occurs in HOCM, in which the systolic portion may be bifid in configuration preceded by a large *a* wave, thus giving a triple-humped appearance (Fig. 3–30).

In the mitral prolapse or click murmur syndrome, a collapse or deep notch in the apex impulse may occasionally be noted coinciding with the click as recorded on an accompanying phonocardiogram (Fig. 3–31).[127] Left atrial myxoma may cause a very deep notch on the systolic upstroke of the apexcardiogram. This notch occurs at the time of extrusion of the tumor from ventricle to atrium

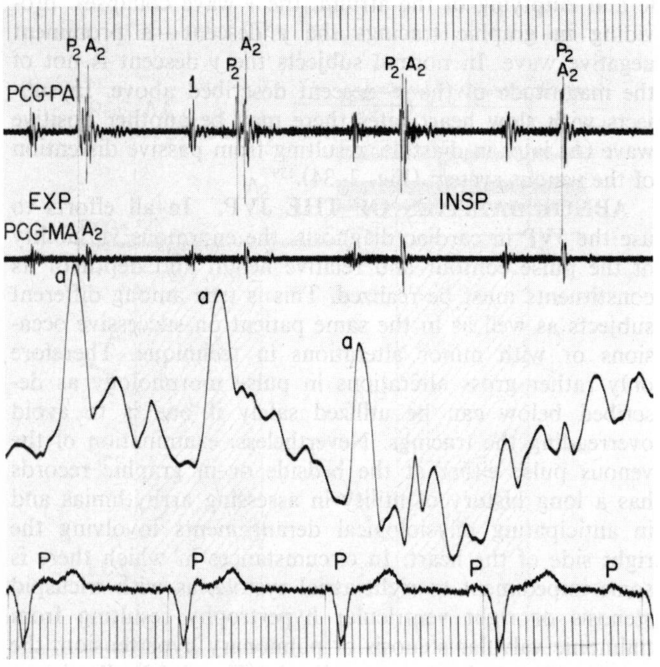

FIGURE 3–36 Jugular venous pressure (JVP) showing "cannon" *a* waves in a patient with a transvenous pacemaker in the right ventricle. In the first three cycles, atrial systole coincides with ventricular systole, so that the right atrium is contracting against a closed tricuspid valve. There is reversed splitting of S_2, with P_2 preceding A_2 in expiration (EXP), but narrowing of separation occurs with inspiration (INSP).

36). An intermittent accentuation of the *a* wave in ventricular tachycardia indicates that atria and ventricles are out of phase, and it may therefore be of some help in certain clinical circumstances in distinguishing ventricular tachycardia from atrial tachycardia with bundle branch block. A prominent *a* wave may be found in association with *left* ventricular hypertrophy, presumably reflecting encroachment by the hypertrophied interventricular septum on the right ventricle—the Bernheim effect.

In tricuspid regurgitation, the *v* wave is unusually prominent, the *x'* descent becomes shallower, and with increasing hemodynamic deterioration the *c* and *v* waves merge to form a prominent ascending plateau (Fig. 3–37). Under these circumstances the *v* wave no longer reflects merely the normal passive accumulation of blood in the right atrium and venous system while the tricuspid valve is closed in systole; rather, it is due to a massive retrograde wave through an incompetent valve into the great veins. Unfortunately, the time-honored custom of using the letter *v* for both the normal systolic peak and the abnormal regurgitant wave when the valve is incompetent has interfered with understanding the genesis of these waves of the JVP in health and disease.

The *x* descent that results from atrial relaxation is seldom of any prominence and can reach significant proportions only when atrial and ventricular systoles are separated, as with a long P-R interval or in complete heart block.

The *x'* descent is normally one of the most prominent features of the JVP. It becomes shallow or is eliminated in tricuspid regurgitation. It may be deep in some cases of constrictive pericarditis.[143]

The *y* descent is less steep in tricuspid stenosis. Unfortunately, this assessment must be subjective, since the waves of the JVP cannot be quantitated and the relative swiftness of their movements is dependent on apparatus, technique, and paper speed. In constrictive pericarditis, however, a rapid, deep *y* descent interrupting an otherwise high plateau of the venous pulse provides a pattern familiar to hemodynamicists, since it simulates the "square-root sign" recorded in diastolic pressure tracings from all the heart chambers (Fig. 3–38).

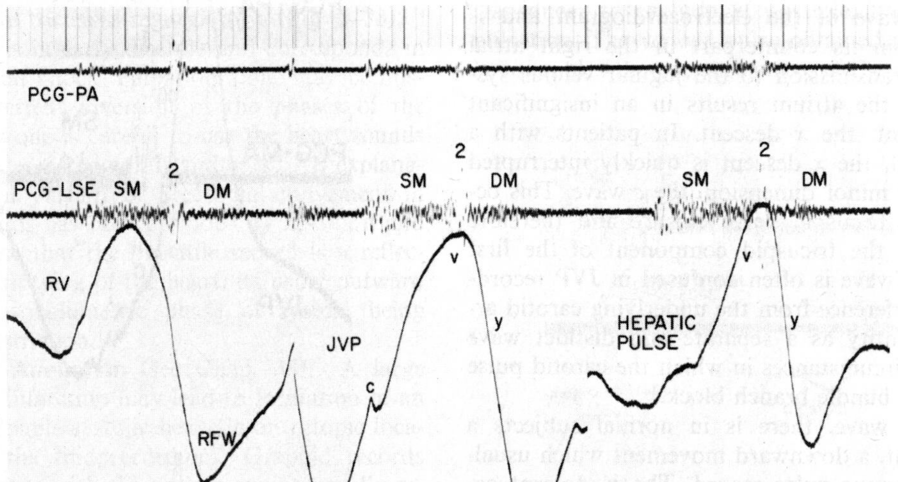

FIGURE 3–37 Tricuspid regurgitation secondary to mitral stenosis and pulmonary hypertension. *Left,* RV impulse showing a sustained heave, palpable at the left sternal edge. The PCG shows systolic and diastolic murmurs of tricuspid regurgitation at the left sternal edge (LSE). This right ventricular heave is a consequence of right ventricular hypertrophy secondary to pulmonary hypertension and is in contrast to the inward systolic movement seen in tricuspid regurgitation due to intrinsic abnormality of the tricuspid valve, with normal RV pressures as seen in Figure 3–32. *Center,* JVP shows an enormous *v* wave due to tricuspid regurgitation and retrograde flow. *Right,* Hepatic pulse is similar to JVP, although its ascent is slightly delayed.

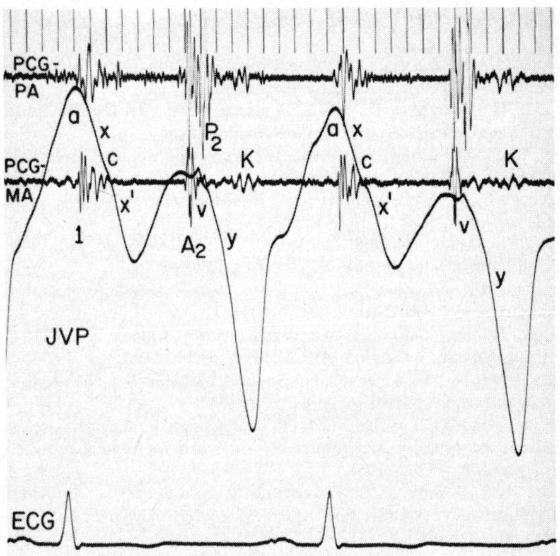

FIGURE 3–38 Jugular venous pressure (JVP) in constrictive pericarditis. In this severe and longstanding case, the *x′* descent has become very shallow and the *y* descent is the principal feature, indicating that antegrade flow from the venous system to the right heart is now limited to early diastole.[142] A pericardial knock (K) is seen at approximately the nadir of the *y* descent.

SUMMARY

Phonocardiograms and pulse-wave tracings of carotid, apex, and venous origin have a number of uses which may be summarized as follows:

1. *As an objective record of physical signs.* Although descriptions and diagrams in patients' charts are helpful in evaluating changes occurring over time, a more accurate and detailed collection of data can be provided by graphic records of sounds, murmurs, and pulsatile phenomena. These are often valuable in studying the progression of disease or the effects of pharmacological and surgical interventions.
2. *To determine temporal relationships*:
   a. Systolic time intervals as ordinarily measured require a combination of phonocardiogram, carotid pulse tracing, and electrocardiogram.
   b. Other temporal relationships such as A_2-OS time can be only roughly estimated by auscultation but can be accurately determined by phonocardiography.
3. *In the identification of heart sounds.* Difficulties may be encountered in determining the identity of sounds clustered around the beginning or end of systole. Such problems can be clarified by phonocardiography in combination with other graphic methods. In particular, the major elements of S_1, ejection sounds, opening snaps, and low-frequency sounds (S_3, S_4) can be accurately identified by combined multichannel tracings.
4. *In affording clues to specific diagnoses from distinctive heart-sound or pulse-wave patterns.* Although many phonocardiographic and pulse-wave patterns lack specificity, they may be quite useful in confirming suspected diagnoses such as aortic stenosis, HOCM, constrictive pericarditis, and so on, as outlined above.
5. *In teaching bedside diagnostic skills.* The utility of graphic methods, either "live" on an oscilloscope or in permanent form on paper, is well established as a powerful tool in facilitating the acquisition and enhancement of skills in physical diagnosis at all levels of training.

Phonocardiography is *not* useful as a means of determining the presence or absence of barely detectable murmurs. Very soft murmurs often merge with background vibrations in the tracing and therefore cannot be identified with any more certainty than by auscultation.

Acknowledgments

The author is indebted to his colleague Dr. Peter Mills and many others who collaborated in the collection from our own laboratory of data used in this chapter. Dr. Mills is the coauthor of a paper on this subject[8] that has been freely quoted in this and the following chapter. Dr. Richard P. Lewis has been very helpful with the section on systolic time intervals. I am also very grateful for the technical assistance of Ms. Sally Moos and Ms. Carla Wolfe of the Cardiac Graphics Laboratory at North Carolina Memorial Hospital, Chapel Hill, North Carolina, who are responsible for the records used as illustrations in Chapters 3 and 4.

References

1. Einthoven, W., and Geluk, M. A. J.: Die Registrierung der Herztöne. Pflüger's Arch. Physiol. *57*:617, 1894.
2. McKusick, V. A.: Cardiovascular Sound in Health and Disease. Baltimore, Williams and Wilkins, 1958.
3. Fishleder, B. L.: Exploración cardiovascular y fono mecanocardiografía clínica. México, La Prensa Médica Mexicana, 1966.
4. Tavel, M. E.: Clinical phonocardiography and external pulse recording, 3rd ed. Chicago, Year Book Publishers, 1978.
5. Esper, R. J., and Madoery, R. J.: Progresos en auscultación y fono mecanocardiografía. Buenos Aires, López Libreros, 1974.
6. Leatham, A.: Auscultation of the Heart and Phonocardiography. London, Churchill Livingstone, 1975.
7. Craige, E.: On the genesis of heart sounds: Contributions made by echocardiographic studies. Circulation *53*:207, 1976.
8. Mills, P., and Craige, E.: Echophonocardiography. Prog. Cardiovasc. Dis. *20*: 337, 1978.
9. Zalter, R., Hodara, H., and Luisada, A. A.: Phonocardiography. I. General principles and problems of standardization. Am. J. Cardiol. *4*:3, 1959.
10. Lewis, D. H.: Phonocardiography. *In* Hamilton, W. F., and Dow, P. (eds.): Handbook of Physiology. Section 2, Circulation. Vol. I. Washington, D. C., American Physiological Society, 1962, p. 685.
11. Kesteloot, H., Willems, J., and Van Vollenhoven, E.: On the physical principles and methodology of mechanocardiography. Acta Cardiol. *24*:147, 1969.
12. Butterworth, J. S., Chassin, M. R., McGrath, R., and Reppert, E. H.: Cardiac Auscultation. New York, Grune and Stratton. 1960.
13. Lewis, R. P., Rittgers, S. E., Forester, W. F., and Boudoulas, H.: A critical review of the systolic time intervals. Circulation *56*:146, 1977.
14. Craige, E., and Schmidt, R. E.: Precordial movements over the right ventricle in normal children. Circulation *32*:232, 1965.
15. Mashimo, K., Tanabe, T., Kinoshita, S., Sakamoto, S., and Tsushima, N.: An instrumental aspect of apexcardiography: Decay characteristic of transducers and its clinical implication. Jap. Heart J. *7*:536, 1966.
16. Leech, G.: The apexcardiogram: Recording technique and relation to cardiac function. Application notes for cardiovascular instrumentation. Vol. 1, No. 4. Irex Medical Systems, Upper Saddle River, New Jersey, 1973.
17. Leatham, A.: Phonocardiography. Br. Med. Bull. *8*:333, 1952.
18. Rappaport, M. B., and Sprague, H. B.: The graphic registration of the normal heart sound. Am. Heart J. *23*:591, 1942.
19. Armstrong, T. G., and Gotsman, M. S.: Initial low frequency vibrations of the first heart sound. Br. Heart J. *35*:691, 1973.
20. Rouanet, J.: Analyse des bruits du coeur. Thesis No. 252, Paris, 1832. (Reprinted in reference 2 above.)
21. Dock, W.: Mode of production of the first heart sound, Arch. Intern. Med. *51*: 737, 1933.
22. Leatham, A.: Splitting of the first and heart sounds. Lancet *2*:607, 1954.
23. Luisada, A. A., MacCanon, D. M., Kumar, S., and Feigen, L. P.: Changing views on the mechanism of the first and second heart sounds. Am. Heart J. *88*: 503, 1974.
24. Di Bartolo, G., Nunez-Dey, D., Muiesan, G., MacCanon, D. M., and Luisada, A. A.: Hemodynamic correlates of the first heart sound. Am. J. Physiol. *201*: 888, 1961.

25. Laniado, S., Yellin, E. L., Miller, H., and Frater, R. W. M.: Temporal relation of the first heart sound to closure of the mitral valve. Circulation *47*:1006, 1973.
26. Lakier, J. B., Fritz, V. U., Pocock, W. A., and Barlow, J. B.: The mitral components of the first heart sound. Br. Heart J. *34*:160, 1972.
27. Lakier, J. B., Bloom, K. R., Pocock, W. A., and Barlow, J. B.: Tricuspid component of first heart sound. Br. Heart J. *35*:1275, 1973.
28. O'Toole, J. D., Reddy, P. S., Curtiss, E. L., Griff, F. W., and Shaver, J. A.: The contribution of tricuspid valve closure to the first heart sound. An intracardiac micromanometer study. Circulation *53*:752, 1976.
29. Waider, W., and Craige, E.: The first heart sound and ejection sounds: Echophonocardiographic correlation with valvular events. Am. J. Cardiol. *35*:346, 1975.
30. Craige, E.: Echocardiography in studies of the genesis of heart sounds and murmurs (Chapter 2). *In* Yu, P., and Goodwin, J. (eds.): Progress in Cardiology. Vol. 4. Philadelphia, Lea and Febiger, 1975.
31. Shah, P. M., Kramer, D. H., and Gramiak, R.: Influence of the timing of atrial systole in mitral valve closure and on the first heart sound in man. Am. J. Cardiol. *26*:231, 1970.
32. Burggraf, G. W., and Craige, E.: The first heart sound in complete heart block. Circulation *50*:17, 1974.
33. Kostis, J. B.: Mechanisms of heart sounds. Am. Heart J. *89*:546, 1975.
34. Traill, T. A., and Fortuin, N. J.: Presystolic mitral closure sound in aortic regurgitation with left ventricular hypertrophy and first degree heart block. Br. Heart J. *48*:78, 1982.
35. Brooks, N., Leech, G., and Leatham, A.: Complete right bundle branch block: Echophonocardiographic study of first heart sound and right ventricular contraction tones. Br. Heart J. *41*:637, 1979.
36. Hultgren, H. N., Craige, E., and Bilisoly, J.: The late first heart sound in left bundle branch block. Circulation *64* (Suppl. 4):27, 1981.
37. Haber, E., and Leatham, A.: Splitting of heart sounds from ventricular asynchrony in bundle-branch block, ventricular ectopic beats, and artificial pacing. Br. Heart J. *27*:691, 1965.
38. Braunwald, E., and Morrow, A. G.: Origin of heart sounds as elucidated by analysis of the sequence of cardiodynamic events. Circulation *18*:971, 1958.
39. Burggraf, G. W.: The first heart sound in left bundle branch block: An echophonocardiographic study. Circulation *63*:429, 1981.
40. Wooley, C. F.: Intracardiac phonocardiography; intracardiac sound and pressure in man. Circulation *57*:1039, 1978.
41. Crews, T. L., Pridie, R. B., Benham, R., and Leatham, A.: Auscultatory and phonocardiographic findings in Ebstein's anomaly. Correlation of first heart sound with ultrasonic records of tricuspid valve movement. Br. Heart J. *34*: 681, 1972.
42. Tajik, A. J., Gau, G. T., Giuliani, E. R., Ritter, D. G., and Schattenberg, T. T.: Echocardiogram in Ebstein's anomaly with Wolff-Parkinson-White preexcitation syndrome, type B. Circulation *47*:813, 1973.
43. Dashkoff, N., Fortuin, N. J., and Hutchins, G. M.: Clinical features of severe mitral regurgitation due to floppy mitral valve. Circulation *50* (Suppl. 3):60, 1974.
44. Mann, T., McLaurin, L., Grossman, W., and Craige, E.: Acute aortic regurgitation due to infective endocarditis, N. Engl. J. Med. *293*:108, 1975.
45. Wolferth, C. C., and Margolies, A.: Certain effects of auricular systole and prematurity of beat on the intensity of the first heart sound. Trans. Am. Assoc. Physicians *45*:44, 1930.
46. Leatham, A., and Gray, I.: Auscultatory and phonocardiographic signs of atrial septal defect. Br. Heart J. *18*:193, 1956.
47. Lopez, J. F., Linn, H., and Shaffer, A. B.: The apical first heart sound as an aid in the diagnosis of atrial septal defect. Circulation *26*:1296, 1962.
48. Stept, M. E., Heid, C. E., Shaver, J. A., Leon, D. F., and Leonard, J. J.: Effect of altering P-R interval on the amplitude of the first heart sound in the anesthetized dog. Circ. Res. *25*:255, 1969.
49. Mills, P. G., Chamusco, R. F., Moos, S., and Craige, E.: Echophonocardiographic studies of the contribution of the atrioventricular valves to the first heart sound. Circulation *54*:944, 1976.
50. Lewis, J. K., and Dock, W.: The origin of the heart sounds and their variations in myocardial disease. J.A.M.A. *110*:271, 1938.
51. Sabbah, H. N., and Stein, P. D.: Investigation of the theory and mechanism of the origin of the second heart sound. Circ. Res. *29*:874. 1976.
52. Stein, P. D: A Physical and Physiological Basis for the Interpretation of Cardiac Auscultation: Evaluations Based Primarily on the Second Heart Sound and Ejection Murmurs. Mount Kisco, N.Y., Futura Publishing Co., 1981.
53. Hirschfeld, S., Liebman, J., Borkat, G., and Bormuth, C.: Intracardiac pressure-sound correlates of echocardiographic aortic valve closure. Circulation *55*:602, 1977.
54. Potain, P. C.: Note sur les dédoublements normaux des bruits du coeur. Bull. Mém. Soc. Méd. Hôp. (Paris) *3*:138, 1866.
55. Craige, E., and Harned, H. S.: Phonocardiographic and electrocardiographic studies in normal newborn infants. Am. Heart J. *65*:180, 1963.
56. Harris, A., and Sutton, G. C.: Second heart sound in normal subjects. Br. Heart J. *30*:739, 1968.
57. Leatham, A., and Weitzman, D.: Auscultatory and phonocardiographic signs of pulmonary stenosis. Br. Heart J. *19*:303, 1957.
58. Leatham, A., and Gray, I.: Auscultatory and phonocardiographic signs of atrial septal defect. Br. Heart J. *18*:193, 1956.
59. Damore, S., Murgo, J. P., Bloom, K. R., and Rubal, B. J.: Second heart sound dynamics in atrial septal defect. Circulation *64*(Suppl. 4):28, 1981.
60. Shafter, H. A.: Splitting of the second heart sound. Am. J. Cardiol. *6*:1013, 1960.
61. Perloff, J. K.: Auscultatory and phonocardiographic manifestations of pulmonary hypertension. Prog. Cardiovasc. Dis. *9*:303, 1967.
62. Sabbah, H. N., Khaja, F., Anbe, D. T., and Stein, P. D.: The aortic closure sound in pure aortic insufficiency. Circulation *56*:859, 1977.
63. Ross, R. S., and Criley, J. M.: Cineangiocardiographic studies of the origin of cardiovascular physical signs. Circulation *30*:255, 1964.
64. Hancock, E. W.: The ejection sound in aortic stenosis. Am. J. Med. *40*:569, 1966.
65. Leech, G., Mills, P., and Leatham, A.: The diagnosis of a non-stenotic biscuspid aortic valve. Br. Heart J. *40*:941, 1978.
66. Leatham, A., and Vogelpoel, L.: Early systolic sound in dilatation of the pulmonary artery. Br. Heart J. *16*:21, 1954.
67. Minhas, K., and Gasul, B. M.: Systolic clicks: Clinical phonocardiographic and hemodynamic evaluation. Am. Heart J. *57*:49, 1959.
68. Hultgren, H. N., Reeve, R., Cohn, K., and McLeod, R.: The ejection click of valvular pulmonic stenosis. Circulation *40*:631, 1969.
69. Mills, P., Amara, I., McLaurin, L. P., and Craige, E.: Noninvasive assessment of pulmonary hypertension from right ventricular isovolumic contraction time. Am. J. Cardiol. *46*:272, 1980.
70. Curtiss, E. I., Reddy, P. S., O'Toole, J. D., and Shaver, J. A.: Alterations of right ventricular systolic time intervals by chronic pressure and volume overloading. Circulation *53*:997, 1976.
71. Mills, P. G., Brodie, B., McLaurin, L. P., Schall, S., and Craige, E.: Echocardiographic and hemodynamic relationships of ejection sounds. Circulation *56*:430, 1977.
72. Margolies, A., and Wolferth, C. C.: The opening snap in mitral stenosis. Am. Heart J. *7*:443, 1932.
73. Craige, E.: Editorial. On the genesis of heart sounds: Contribution made by echocardiographic studies. Circulation *53*:207, 1976.
74. Millward, D. K., McLaurin, L. P., and Craige, E.: Echocardiographic studies to explain opening snaps in presence of nonstenotic mitral valves. Am. J. Cardiol. *31*:64, 1973.
75. Criley, J. M., Lewis, K. B., Humphries, J. O., and Ross, R. S.: Prolapse of the mitral valve: Clinical and cine-angiocardiographic findings. Br. Heart J. *28*: 488, 1966.
76. Nixon, P. G. F.: The genesis of the third heart sound. Am. Heart J. *65*:712, 1963.
77. Harvey, W. P., and Stapleton, J.: Clinical aspects of gallop rhythm with particular reference to diastolic gallops. Circulation *18*:1017, 1958.
78. Tyberg, T. I., Goodyer, A. V. N., and Langou, R. A.: Genesis of pericardial knock in constrictive pericarditis. Am. J. Cardiol. *46*:570, 1980.
79. Sakamoto, T., Ichiyasu, H., Hayashi, T., Kawarakani, H., Amano, K., and Hada, Y.: Genesis of the third heart sound. Jap. Heart J. *17*:150, 1976.
80. Prewitt, T., Gibson, D., Brown, D., and Sutton, G.: The "rapid filling wave" of the apex cardiogram: its relation to echocardiographic and cineangiographic measurements of ventricular filling. Br. Heart J. *37*:1256, 1975.
80a. Ozawa, Y., Smith, D., and Craige. E.: Localization of the origin of the third heart sound. Circulation *66* (Suppl. 2):210, 1982.
81. Gibson, T. C., Madry, R., Grossman, W., McLaurin, L. P., and Craige, E.: The A wave of the apexcardiogram and left ventricular diastolic stiffness. Circulation *49*:441, 1974.
82. Kesteloot, H., and Willems, J.: Relationship between the right apexcardiogram and the right ventricular dynamics. Acta Cardiol. *22*:64, 1967.
83. Craige, E.: The fourth heart sound. *In* Leon, D. F., and Shaver, J. A. (eds.): Physiologic Principles of Heart Sounds and Murmurs. New York, American Heart Association Monograph, No. 46, 1975, p. 74.
84. Shah, P. M., and Jackson, D.: Third heart sound and summation gallop. *In* Leon, D. F., and Shaver, J. A. (eds.): Physiologic Principles of Heart Sounds and Murmurs. New York, American Heart Association Monograph No. 46, 1975, p. 79.
84a. Smith, N. D., Raizada, V., and Abraus, J.: Auscultation of the normally functioning prosthetic valve. Ann. Intern. Med. *95*:594, 1981.
85. Hultgren, H. N., and Hubis, H.: A phonocardiographic study of patients with the Starr-Edwards mitral valve prosthesis. Am. Heart J. *69*:306, 1965.
86. Gibson, T. C., Starek, P. J. K., Moos, S., and Craige, E.: Echocardiographic and phonocardiographic characteristics of the Lillehei-Kaster mitral valve prosthesis. Circulation *49*:434, 1974.
87. Smith, N. D., Raizada, V., and Abrams, J.: Auscultation of the normally functioning prosthetic valve. Ann. Intern. Med. *95*:594, 1981.
88. Brodie, B. R., Grossman, W., McLaurin, L. P., Starek, P. J. K., and Craige, E.: Diagnosis of prosthetic mitral valve malfunction with combined echophonocardiography. Circulation *53*:93, 1976.
89. Miller, H. C., Gibson, D. G., and Stephens, J. D.: Role of echocardiography and phonocardiography in diagnosis of mitral paraprosthetic regurgitation with Starr-Edwards protheses. Br. Heart J. *35*:1217, 1973.
90. Burggraf, G. W., and Craige, E.: Echocardiographic studies of left ventricular wall motion and dimensions after valvular heart surgery. Am. J. Cardiol. *35*: 473, 1975.
91. Harris, A.: Pacemaker "heart sound." Br. Heart J. *29*:608, 1967.
92. Garrod, A. H.: On some points connected with the circulation of the blood, arrived at from a study of the sphygmograph-trace. Proc. R. Soc. Lond. *23*: 140, 1874–1875.
93. Bowen, W. P.: Changes in heart rate, blood pressure and duration of systole resulting from bicycling. Am. J. Physiol. *11*:59, 1904.

94. Wiggers, C. J.: Studies on the consecutive phases of the cardiac cycle. II. The laws governing the relative durations of ventricular systole and diastole. Am. J. Physiol. *56*:439, 1921.
95. Lombard, W. P., and Cope, O. M.: The duration of the systole of the left ventricle of man. Am. J. Physiol. *77*:263, 1926.
96. Lewis, R. P., Leighton, R. F., Forester, W. F., and Weissler, A. M.: Systolic time intervals. *In* Weissler, A. M. (ed.): Noninvasive Cardiology. New York, Grune and Stratton, 1974, p. 301.
97. Weissler, A. M.: Current concepts in cardiology. Systolic time intervals. N. Engl. J. Med. *296*:321, 1977.
98. Lewis, R. P., Diagnostic value of systolic time intervals in man. *In* Fowler, N.O. (ed.): Diagnostic Methods in Cardiology. Philadelphia, F.A. Davis Co., 1975, pp. 245–264.
99. Lewis, R. P.: The use of systolic time intervals for evaluation of left ventricular function. *In* Noble, O., and Fowler, N. O (ed.): Noninvasive Diagnostic Methods in Cardiology. Philadelphia, F. A. Davis, 1983.
100. Weissler, A. M., O'Neill, W. W., Sohn, Y. H., Stack, R. S., Chew, P. C., and Reed, A. H.: Prognostic significance of systolic time intervals after recovery from myocardial infarction. Am. J. Cardiol. *48*:995, 1981.
101. Garrard, C. L., Jr., Weissler, S. M., and Dodge, H. T.: The relationship of alterations in systolic time intervals to ejection fraction in patients with cardiac disease. Circulation *42*:455, 1970.
102. Weissler, A. M., Harris, W. S., and Schoenfeld, C. D.: Systolic time intervals in heart failure in man. Circulation *37*:149, 1968.
103. Lewis, R. P., Boudoulas, H., Forester, W. F., and Weissler, A. M.: Shortening of electromechanical systole as a manifestation of excessive adrenergic stimulation in acute myocardial infarction. Circulation *46*:856, 1972.
104. Lewis, R. P., Boudoulas, H., Welch, T. G., and Forester, W. F.: Usefulness of systolic time intervals in coronary artery disease. Am. J. Cardiol. *37*:787, 1976.
105. Unverferth, D. V., Lewis, R. P., Leier, C. V., Magorien, R. D., and Fulkerson, P. K.: The use of echocardiography and systolic time intervals in monitoring therapy of congestive heart failure. J. C. U. *8*:479, 1980.
106. Bonner, J. A., Sacks, H. N., and Tavel, M. E.: Assessing the severity of aortic stenosis by phonocardiography and external carotid pulse recordings. Circulation *48*:247, 1973.
107. Weissler, A. M., Snyder, J. R., Schoenfeld, C. D., and Cohen, S.: Assay of digitalis glycosides in man. Am. J. Cardiol. *17*:768, 1966.
108. Carliner, N. H., Gilbert, C. A., Pruitt, A. W., and Goldbert, L. I.: Effect of maintenance digoxin therapy on systolic time intervals and serum digoxin concentrations. Circulation *50*:94, 1974.
109. Forester, W. F., Lewis, R. P., Weissler, A. M., and Wilke, T. A.: The onset and magnitude of the contractile response to commonly used digitalis glycosides in normal subjects. Circulation *49*:517, 1974.
110. Boudoulas, H., Beaver, B. M., Kates, R. E., and Lewis, R. P.: Pharmacodynamics of inotropic and chronotropic responses to oral propranolol. Studies in normal subjects and in patients with angina. Chest *73*:146, 1978.
111. Bristow, M. R., Mason, J. W., Billingham, M. E., and Daniels, J. R.: Doxorubicin cardiomyopathy: Evaluation by phonocardiography, endomyocardial biopsy and cardiac catheterization. Ann. Intern. Med. *88*:168, 1978.
112. Al-Israil, S. A. D., and Whittaker, J. A.: Systolic time interval as index of schedule-dependent doxorubicin cardiotoxicity in patients with acute myelogenous leukemia. Br. Med. J. *1*:1392, 1979.
113. Ichiyasu, H., and Craige, E.: Assessment of the severity of aortic stenosis from the carotid pulse tracing. Jap. Heart J. *21*:465, 1980.
114. Orchard, R. C., and Craige, E.: Dicrotic pulse after open heart surgery. Circulation *62*:1107, 1980.
115. Ewy, G. A., Rios, J. C., and Marcus, F. I.: The dicrotic arterial pulse. Circulation *39*:655, 1969.
116. Hada, Y., Wolfe, C., and Craige, E.: Pulsus alternans determined by biventricular simultaneous systolic time intervals. Circulation *65*:617, 1982.
117. Craige, E.: Apexcardiography. *In* Weissler, A. M. (ed.): Noninvasive Cardiology. New York, Grune and Stratton, 1974, p. 1.
118. Eddleman, E. E.: Ultra low frequency precordial movements—kinetocardiograms. Am. J. Cardiol. *4*:649, 1959.
119. Vas, R., Diamond, G. A., Wyatt, H. L., Protasio, L., da Luz, P. L., Swan, H. J. C., and Forrester, J. S.: Noninvasive analysis of regional myocardial wall motion: Cardiokymography. Am. J. Physiol. *233*:700, 1977.
120. Silverberg, R. A., Diamond, G. A., Vas, R., Tzivoni, D., Swan, H. J. C., and Forrester, J. S.: Noninvasive diagnosis of coronary artery disease: The cardiokymographic stress test. Circulation *61*:579, 1980.
121. Sakamoto, T., Matsuhisa, M., Inoue, K., Hayashi, T., and Ito, U.: Clinical and hemodynamic observation of indirect pulmonary artery pulse tracing. Cardiovasc. Sound Bull. *3*:127, 1973.
122. Willems, J. L., Kesteloot, H., and De Geest, H.: Influence of acute hemodynamic changes on the apexcardiogram in dogs. Am. J. Cardiol. *29*:504, 1972.
123. Willems, J. L., De Geest, H., and Kesteloot, H.: On the value of apexcardiography for timing intracardiac events. Am. J. Cardiol. *28*:59, 1971.
124. Bush, C. A., Lewis, R. P., Leighton, R. F., Fontana, M. E., and Weissler, A. M.: Verification of systolic time intervals and true isovolumic contraction time from the apexcardiogram by mitromanometer catheterization of the left ventricle and aorta. Circulation *41* (Suppl. 3):121, 1970.
125. Sutton, G. C., Prewitt, T. A., and Craige, E.: Relationship between quantitated precordial movement and left ventricular function. Circulation *41*:179, 1970.
126. Sutton, G. C., Craige, E., and Grizzle, J. E.: Quantitation of precordial movement. II. Mitral regurgitation. Circulation *35*:483, 1967.
127. Lucardie, S. M., and Durrer, D.: The late systolic murmur. Arch. Kreislaufforsch. *53*:174, 1967.
128. Algary, W. P., and Craige, E.: Left atrial myxoma. Diagnosis with the help of the phonocardiogram and apexcardiogram. Arch. Intern. Med. *129*:470, 1972.
129. Voigt, G. C., and Friesinger, G. C.: The use of apexcardiography in the assessment of left ventricular diastolic pressure. Circulation *41*:1015, 1970.
130. DiMattéo, J., LaFont, H., Hui Bon Hoa, F., et al.: La courbe méchanique ventriculaire dans l'insuffisance aortique. Arch. Mal. Coeur *60*:1320, 1967.
131. Fortuin, N. J., and Craige, E.: On the mechanism of the Austin Flint murmur. Circulation *45*:558, 1972.
132. Schmidt, R. E., and Craige, E.: Precordial movements over the right ventricle in children with pulmonary stenosis. Circulation *32*:241, 1965.
133. Armstrong, T. G., and Gotsman, M. S.: The left parasternal lift in tricuspid incompetence. Am. Heart J. *88*:183, 1974.
134. Mounsey, J. P. D.: Inspection and palpation of the cardiac impulse. Prog. Cardiovasc. Dis. *10*:187, 1967.
135. El-Sherif, A., and El-Said, G.: Jugular, hepatic, and praecordial pulsations in constrictive pericarditis. Br. Heart J. *33*:305, 1971.
136. Craige, E., and Fortuin, N. J.: Noninvasive measurement of ventricular function in chronic ischemic heart disease. *In* Likoff, W., Segal, B. L., Insull, W., and Moyer, J. H. (eds.): Atherosclerosis and Coronary Heart Disease. New York, Grune and Stratton, 1972, p. 221.
137. Basta, L. L., Wolfson, P., Eckbert, D. L., and Abboud, F. M.: The value of left parasternal impulse recordings in the assessment of mitral regurgitation. Circulation *48*:1055, 1973.
138. Manolas, J., Wirz, P., and Rutihauser, W.: Relationship between duration of systolic upstroke of apexcardiogram and internal indexes of myocardial function in man. Am. Heart J. *91*:726, 1976.
139. Constant, J.: The x' descent in jugular contour nomenclature and recognition. Am. Heart J. *88*:372, 1974.
140. Benchimol, A., and Tippit, H. C.: The clinical value of the jugular and hepatic pulses. Prog. Cardiovasc. Dis. *10*:159, 1967.
141. Rich, L. L., and Tavel, M. E.: The origin of the jugular C wave. N. Engl. J. Med. *284*:1309, 1971.
142. Sivaciyan, V., and Ranganathan, N.: Transcutaneous Doppler jugular venous flow velocity recording: Clinical and hemodynamic correlates. Circulation *57*:930, 1978.
143. Kesteloot, H., and Denef, B.: Value of reference tracings in the diagnosis and assessment of constrictive epi- and pericarditis. Br. Heart J. *32*:675, 1970.

4 ECHOPHONOCARDIOGRAPHY AND OTHER NONINVASIVE TECHNIQUES TO ELUCIDATE HEART MURMURS

by Ernest Craige, M.D.

Most cardiac murmurs are believed to arise from disturbances of blood flow manifest as turbulence. Turbulence is defined as an irregular condition of motion in which velocity and pressure show a random variation in relation to time and space coordinates.[1] Fluctuating velocities and pressures due to turbulence presumably produce local vibrations at the wall of the vessel or heart chamber which then are transmitted to the chest wall and perceived as murmurs.[2] Maximum turbulence is found in the recipient vessel or chamber, such as, for example, in the root of the great vessels in aortic or pulmonic stenosis, in the left atrium in mitral regurgitation, and in the cavity of the left ventricle in aortic regurgitation.[3] Noninvasive cardiac diagnostic methods—specifically echophonocardiography—can be used to illustrate the common types of heart murmurs encountered in clinical practice.

SYSTOLIC MURMURS[4,5]

CLASSIFICATION OF SYSTOLIC MURMURS. The convenient classification of systolic murmurs into two main categories—*ejection* and *regurgitant*—as popularized by Leatham, has improved our understanding of pathogenetic mechanisms as well as facilitated communication among observers.[4] In general, "ejection murmurs" are midsystolic in timing and are the result of ejection of blood into the root of one of the great vessels. A classic example of an ejection murmur is that associated with stenosis of one of the semilunar valves (Fig. 4–1). The term "regurgitant murmur" has been used to describe a holosystolic murmur that may be found when the pressure relationships between the donor chamber (ventricle) and the recipient chamber (atrium, or lower pressure ventricle) fa-

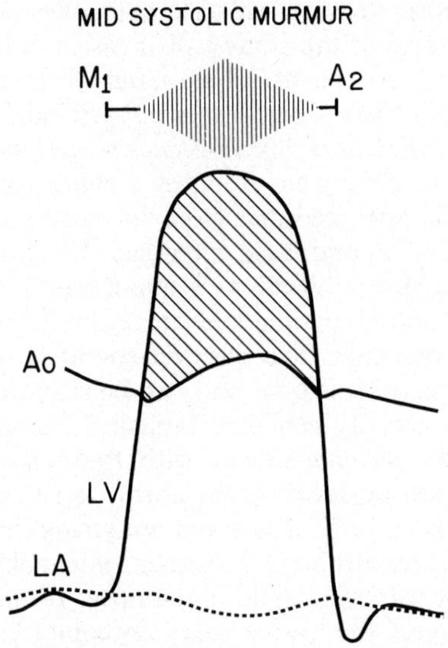

FIGURE 4–1 Midsystolic murmur in aortic stenosis, with pressure records from left ventricle (LV), left atrium (LA), and aorta (A_o). In early systole, LV pressure rises swiftly and opens the aortic valve, whereupon ejection into the root of the aorta can begin; only then does the midsystolic or ejection murmur start, peaking at the time of maximum gradient across the valve (shaded area). At the end of systole, the falling pressure in the LV results in diminishing flow across the aortic valve, and the murmur fades away before A_2.

vor retrograde flow *throughout* systole (Fig. 4–2). With improved understanding of variations in the hemodynamic patterns of mitral valve disease, it has become apparent that the physical signs associated with mitral regurgitation may also vary greatly. For instance, in acute mitral regurgitation, the murmur may be prominent in early and midsystole but may terminate before the second heart sound. In mitral valve prolapse, on the other hand, the murmur may be confined to late systole. These alterations from the classic pattern are readily explicable on the basis of known information concerning the anatomical and physiological derangements in these conditions. Thus, efforts to describe these abbreviated murmurs within the framework of the "ejection" and "regurgitant" terminology has led to a confusing misuse of terms, such as "ejection-type" murmur to describe a murmur that results from regurgitation but is less than holosystolic in duration.

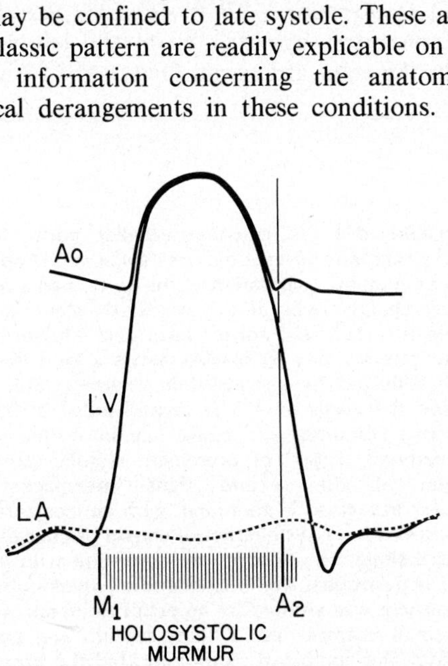

FIGURE 4–2 Holosystolic murmur. In mitral regurgitation LV pressure rises and immediately exceeds LA pressure. Thus the regurgitant murmur begins with M_1, continues throughout systole, and may continue even slightly beyond A_2, because the falling pressure in the LV still exceeds that of the LA, thus favoring continuing regurgitation.

Therefore, in this chapter, simple descriptive terms, such as "early systolic," "late systolic," "holosystolic," and "midsystolic," will be used to indicate the position of systolic murmurs in the cardiac cycle. Murmurs that begin with the first heart sound and proceed to the second sound on their side of origin are called holosystolic. A murmur that begins with the first heart sound and finishes in either mid- or late systole but well before the second heart sound on its side of origin is designated an early systolic murmur. Conversely, with a late systolic murmur, early systole is silent, the murmur generally beginning in mid- to late systole and proceeding to the second heart sound on its side of origin. If the murmur begins at an interval after the first heart sound and ends before the second, and both early and late systole are murmur-free, the murmur is designated "midsystolic."

MIDSYSTOLIC MURMURS

Physiological Murmurs. The commonest murmur is soft, midsystolic in time, and not associated with any cardiac abnormality. Such functional or innocent murmurs are usually best heard and recorded at the left sternal edge in either the second or the third left intercostal space. Most commonly they consist phonocardiographically of random noise, i.e., vibrations of various frequencies.[6] The intensity of physiological murmurs can be magnified by physical activity, excitement, pregnancy, anemia, thyrotoxicosis, fever, and so on, presumably owing to increases in the volume and velocity of ejection. In thin subjects or individuals with a depressed sternum, proximity of the stethoscope or microphone to the source of the murmur may result in even greater intensity. The source of physiological midsystolic murmurs is thought to be the right ventricular outflow tract and root of the pulmonary artery, because their area of maximal intensity is at the left sternal edge overlying these anatomical structures. The innocent murmurs, maximal lower over the midprecordium, are often more musical or even grunting in quality and appear on the phonocardiogram in crescendo-decrescendo silhouette, with vibrations of a constant frequency rather than random noise (Fig. 4–3). Appreciation of the innocent nature of the murmurs described above is facilitated by the absence of other evidence of heart disease by means of physical examination, electrocardiogram, and chest x-ray. From a phonocardiographic point of view, the midsystolic timing of the murmur is important in differentiating it from the holosystolic murmur of an interventricular septal defect. The basal systolic murmur of an atrial septal defect, however, represents an exaggerated flow murmur in midsystole resulting from augmentation of right ventricular stroke volume. It therefore resembles an innocent murmur. Attention to the details of the second heart sound, however, should clarify this problem, since the wide, fixed splitting of S_2, which is characteristic of atrial septal defect (see Figure 3–9*A*, p. 46), would not be found with an innocent or physiological murmur. Other causes of midsystolic murmurs resulting from ejection across deformed or

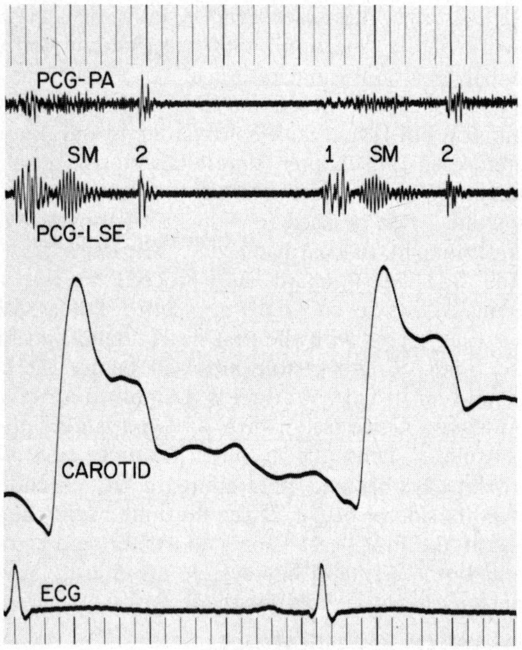

FIGURE 4–3 **Functional murmur in a healthy 20-year-old man. The midsystolic timing of the murmur and vibratory appearance are characteristic of many innocent murmurs. The phonocardiogram is otherwise normal, as is the carotid pulse tracing. PCG-PA =phonocardiogram in second left intercostal space; PCG-LSE =phonocardiogram at left sternal edge.**

obstructing outflow tracts and semilunar valves are described in the following paragraphs.

Obstruction to Left Ventricular Outflow.[7,8] Midsystolic murmurs are characteristically found in patients with obstruction of the outflow tract. Combined phono- and echocardiographic studies are particularly useful in determining the underlying pathological condition in these cases, although conventional M-mode echocardiography alone may be of very limited value. Echophonocardiography may also provide valuable guidelines when difficult decisions regarding the timing of invasive studies must be made. It may also be useful in serial observations of patients in whom the obstruction is not critical.

Congenital Valvular Aortic Stenosis (see also Chaps. 29 and 30). This condition produces a characteristic midsystolic murmur best recorded from its position of maximal intensity in the second right interspace or aortic area (Fig. 4–4). In youthful subjects, this abnormality is almost invariably associated with an aortic ejection sound, which initiates the murmur. The ejection sound is widely transmitted over the precordium and can be recorded at the mitral area. Its identity can be established echophonocardiographically by its coincidence with the achievement of a maximally open position by the aortic valve (see Figure 3–11, p. 48). A_2 is well preserved in young individuals in whom the valve, although deformed, is capable of closing and being set into vibration at the onset of diastole.[9] With advancing age, the valve may become calcified and immobilized, with diminution or obliteration of both the ejection sound and A_2. The murmur itself is of little help in determining the severity of the valvular abnormality. There is a tendency for the murmur to peak later in systole with severe stenosis.[10] The loudness of the murmur is not proportional to the severity of the obstruction. A loud murmur may occur merely with sclerosis of the valve where there is no significant gradient across it. Conversely, in a moribund patient with the most severe stenosis, the murmur may become faint or disappear entirely as the left ventricular stroke volume declines. More useful information indicating a severe degree of stenosis may be provided as follows: (1) prolongation of left ventricular ejection time (LVET) may be determined from an accompanying carotid pulse tracing (Fig. 4–5)[10]; (2) paradoxical splitting of S_2 may appear, owing to a delay in A_2, associated with the long LVET (see Figure 3–9*B*, p. 46); (3) there may be evidence of concentric hypertrophy of the left ventricle, as manifest in the echocardiogram (Fig. 4–4); (4) the *a* wave

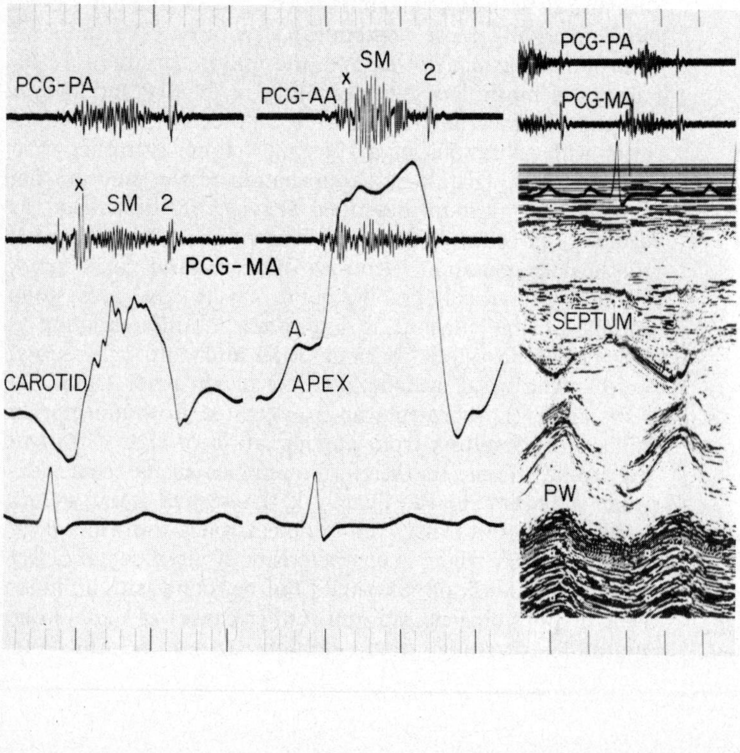

FIGURE 4–4 **Congenital valvular aortic stenosis. An asymptomatic 10-year-old boy, successfully operated upon in infancy for coarctation of the aorta, had a residual murmur characteristic of valvular aortic stenosis presumably due to a bicuspid aortic valve. *Left,* Phonocardiogram at the cardiac apex (PCG-MA) shows a loud ejection sound (X) followed by a midsystolic murmur (SM) transmitted from the aortic area. The carotid pulse is shattered with coarse vibrations and peaks late in systole. *Center,* The "diamond shape" or prominent systolic murmur is best seen at the second right interspace (AA). The apexcardiogram is abnormal, with an exaggerated *a* wave followed by a systolic heave shown graphically by an upward slope. The findings are consistent with left ventricular hypertrophy. *Right,* Concentric hypertrophy of the left ventricle was verified by an echocardiogram which shows a small chamber but a thick septum and posterior wall (PW). The combined study indicated the presence of significant aortic stenosis despite absence of symptoms. At catheterization a systolic gradient of 80 mm Hg was demonstrated.**

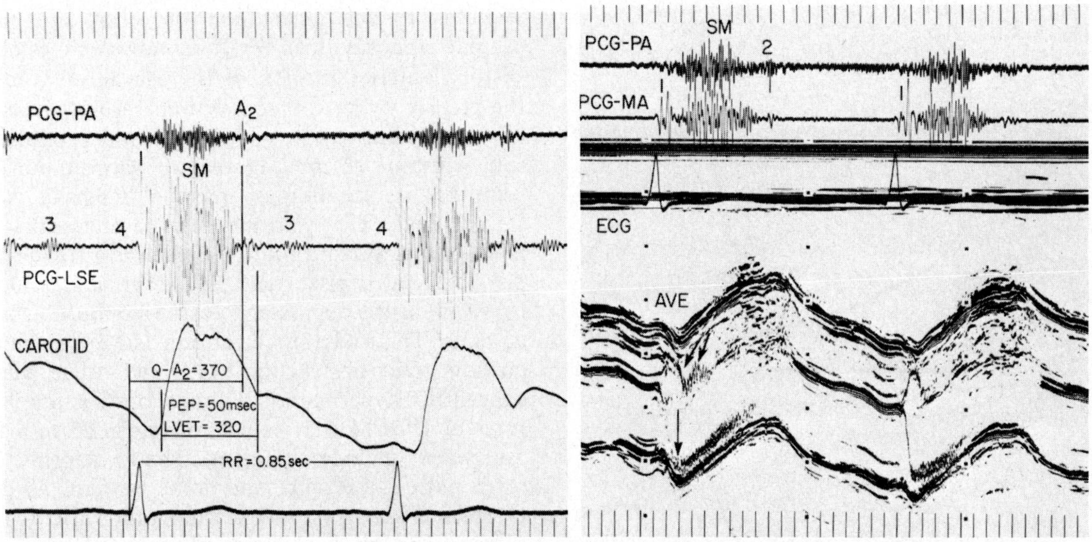

FIGURE 4–5 **Subvalvular aortic stenosis. A 12-year-old boy with a loud midsystolic murmur maximal at the left sternal edge. *Left,* Phonocardiogram illustrating the murmur. The carotid pulse tracing is deformed by coarse vibrations coincident with the murmur. Left ventricular ejection time (LVET) is prolonged for the heart rate. Soft third and fourth heart sounds (S_3 and S_4) are also recorded. *Right,* Echophonocardiogram showing the auscultatory findings in conjunction with an aortic valve echo (AVE). The valve partially closes in early systole and vibrates at the time of the murmur (slanting arrows). The posterior cusp opens fully (vertical arrow), and there is no ejection sound, which, if present, would be manifest by discrete vibrations synchronous with full opening of the valve. Diagnosis of thick fibrous subvalvular aortic stenosis was confirmed by catheterization with a peak valve gradient of 75 mm Hg.**

in the apexcardiogram may be exaggerated, and the appearance of its auscultatory counterpart, the S_4, may also provide an indirect indication of increased left ventricular mass and loss of compliance (Fig. 4–4)[11,12]; and (5) the jugular venous pulse may become abnormal in severe, longstanding aortic stenosis of any variety. One may note an unusually prominent *a* wave reflecting altered filling characteristics of the right ventricle, possibly due to encroachment by the hypertrophied interventricular septum—the so-called Bernheim syndrome.[13] A point system utilizing a combination of variables has recently been found useful by Nakamura et al.[14] in increasing the sensitivity and specificity of the noninvasive assessment of the severity of aortic stenosis.

Fibrous Subaortic Stenosis (see also p. 980). This condition is congenital in origin and is associated with a murmur identical to that of valvular stenosis, although its focus of maximal intensity may be over the midprecordium rather than the aortic area. The carotid pulse is also similar to that in valvular stenosis. However, two observations are of value in differential diagnosis by echophonocardiographic methods: (1) the absence of an ejection sound at the time of full aortic valve opening in the patient with fibrous or diaphragmatic subaortic stenosis (Fig. 4–5),[15] and (2) partial closure and fluttering of the aortic valve in early systole (Fig. 4–5).[16] This curious behavior of the valve is not peculiar to fibrous subaortic stenosis but may occur in hypertrophic obstructive cardiomyopathy (HOCM) as well as, to a minor degree, in normal individuals. However, the combination of the midsystolic murmur, absence of an ejection sound, partial closure and fluttering of the aortic valve in early systole, and absence of poststenotic dilatation on the x-ray should permit a reasonably confident diagnosis of fibrous or diaphragmatic subaortic stenosis. An early diastolic murmur of mild aortic regurgitation may be found in association with fibrous subvalvular stenosis. An estimate of severity may be provided by the same criteria as those listed above, under Congenital Valvular Aortic Stenosis.

Supravalvular Aortic Stenosis (see also Chap. 29). The midsystolic murmur in this congenital abnormality is similar to that of valvular and subvalvular stenosis.[7,15] It is usually of great intensity over the aortic area, to the right of the upper sternum, and is well transmitted over the vessels of the neck. Graphic tracings can be used to display the murmur, but such records are of little value in localizing the obstruction or determining its severity. A simultaneous recording of both carotid pulses, however, may disclose an inequality in amplitude and slope, apparently resulting from the direction of the jet of blood that has traversed the stenotic area (Fig. 4–6). This usually leads to inequality of the carotid and brachial pulses, which are more prominent on the right side (p. 982). An ejection sound is usually not present in supravalvular aortic stenosis,[17] and aortic regurgitation is most unusual.

Valvular Aortic Stenosis of Rheumatic Origin (see also Chap. 32). The findings here are similar to those found in the congenital variety, although the ejection sound is only rarely seen and, when present, is inconspicuous, especially later in the natural history, when the valve has calcified. The presence of associated valvular lesions may be helpful in establishing the etiology.

Atypical Presentation of Aortic Stenosis. In older patients, particularly those suffering from complicating conditions such as emphysema, the presentation of aortic stenosis may differ markedly from that of congenital stenosis in childhood. In elderly patients, the murmur of valvular aortic stenosis, regardless of etiology, is some-

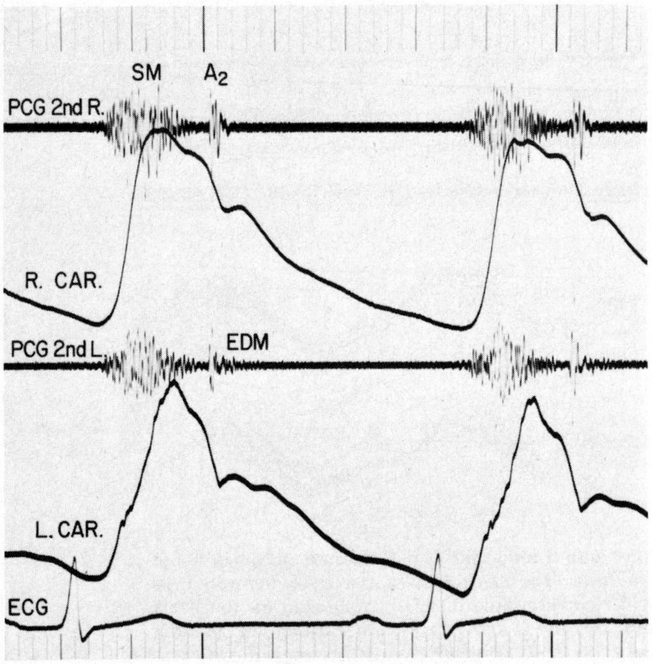

FIGURE 4–6 Supravalvular aortic stenosis. A loud midsystolic murmur was recorded in the right and left second intercostal spaces and was audible over the whole upper chest. Right and left carotid pulse tracings recorded simultaneously illustrate differences in their contours; note the more delayed upstroke in the left compared with the right carotid pulse. At catheterization a gradient of 95 mm Hg was recorded between left ventricle and aorta beyond the obstruction. The early diastolic murmur (EDM) of slight aortic regurgitation is unusual in this condition.

times heard best, if not exclusively, at the mitral area (Fig. 4–7).[18-20] Under these circumstances identification of the murmur as being ejection in character and presumably of aortic origin may be made by an experienced auscultator by noting the midsystolic peaking of the murmur and its termination before S_2. This latter sign may be obscured, however, by the faintness or absence of the second sound. The ejection sound is also faint or usually absent, because of the inevitable calcification of the valve. Clarification of this problem may be gained by noting the behavior of the murmur with an arrhythmia such as premature beats or atrial fibrillation, and confirmation by phonocardiography may be very helpful (Fig. 4–8). The ejection murmur of aortic stenosis fluctuates remarkably in intensity with the strength of left ventricular systole, whereas the murmur of mitral regurgitation is much less affected.[18] Other graphic records which may be helpful in differentiating aortic stenosis from mitral regurgitation include the carotid pulse tracing and systolic time intervals. The carotid upstroke is characteristically sharp in mitral regurgitation, but it is slow-rising and shattered in aortic stenosis (see Figure 3–22, p. 56, and Figure 4–4). PEP is prolonged in mitral regurgitation and LVET is shortened, giving an abnormally high PEP/LVET ratio. In aortic stenosis, the reverse is found—PEP is abbreviated and LVET is prolonged.[21]

Hypertrophic Obstructive Cardiomyopathy (HOCM) (see also p. 1409). The presence or absence of left ventricular outflow obstruction in patients with HOCM was an early stimulus to the correlation of echo- and phonocardiographic abnormalities.[22,23] It is now well established that systolic anterior motion of the mitral valve impinging on the grossly hypertrophied septum results in obstruction to left ventricular outflow (Chap. 5) and produces a midsystolic murmur resembling that of valvular obstruction except that its location of maximal intensity is at the left sternal edge. The murmur may be augmented by an element of mitral regurgitation, which is a frequent additional physiological derangement. However, it is seldom possible to distinguish a separate holosystolic murmur at the cardiac apex. The midsystolic murmur suggests the presence of outflow tract obstruction[24] but may occur where there is concentric hypertrophy without obstruction.[25] Other features of HOCM that can be documented in a noninvasive assessment include the characteristic deformity of the carotid pulse—the spike-and-dome pattern, as described in Chapter 3—and the apexcardiogram with its exaggerated *a* wave and bifid or saddle-shaped appearance in systole (see Figure 3–30, p. 60). The cusps of the aortic valve can be seen, in an accompanying echo, to close partially at the time of the systolic anterior movement of the mitral leaflet and the onset of the murmur.[26] A combined study utilizing all these parameters with echocardiography is useful, therefore, in demonstrating the simultaneity and presumed physiological relationship of the systolic anterior movement of the mitral valve impinging on the hypertrophied septum and the dramatic array of auscultatory and pulsa-

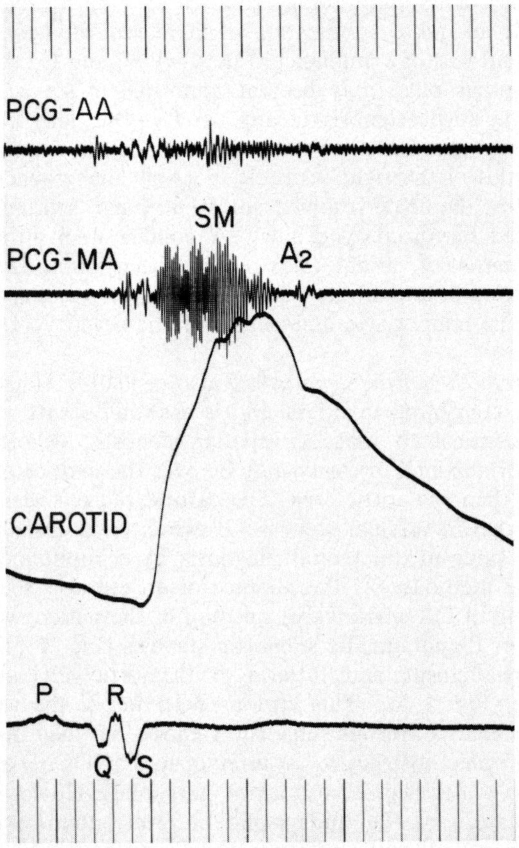

FIGURE 4–7 Aortic stenosis in an elderly man. The murmur is faint in the second right interspace (PCG-AA) but is prominent at the cardiac apex (MA). The carotid upstroke is delayed and demonstrates coarse vibrations.

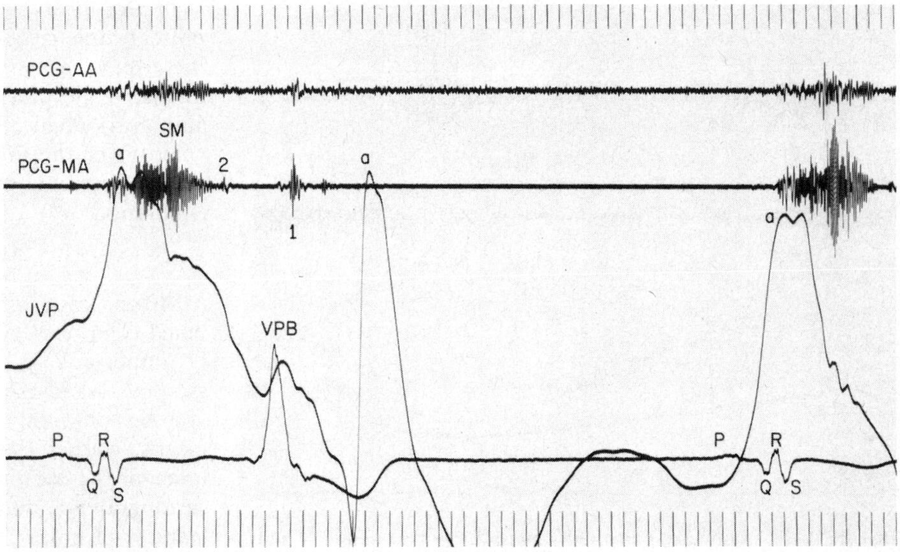

FIGURE 4–8 Aortic stenosis (same patient as in Figure 4–7). The weak ventricular premature beat (VPB) fails to produce a murmur, but the postextrasystolic beat results in accentuation of the murmur. The JVP demonstrates a prominent *a* wave in the conducted beats and a "cannon wave" with the VPB, owing to contraction of the right atrium against a closed tricuspid valve.

tile events that ensue (Fig. 4–9). In addition, the modifications in these signs produced by pharmacological and physical maueuvers, as described in Chapter 2, can be documented by echophonocardiography.

Ejection Through a Normal Valve into a Dilated Aortic Root. In hypertension, arteriosclerosis, and other conditions associated with aortic dilatation, a midsystolic murmur may be recorded over the aortic area. It is usually less intense than that associated with obstructive lesions and terminates earlier in systole. The upstroke of the carotid

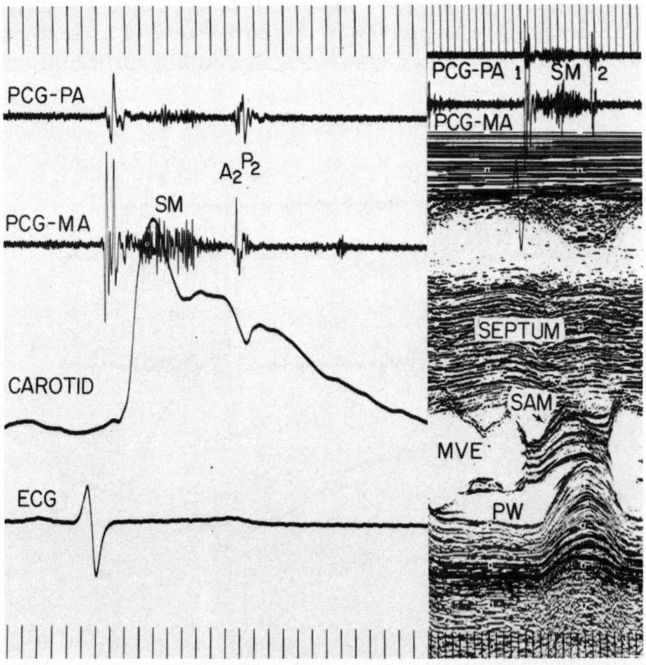

FIGURE 4–9 Hypertrophic obstructive cardiomyopathy (HOCM). *Left,* Carotid tracing illustrating a swift upstroke with a dip at the time of the midsystolic murmur, followed by a second hump during systole. *Right,* Echophonocardiogram showing the relationship between the murmur and the outflow tract obstruction resulting from the systolic anterior movement of the mitral valve (SAM), which appears to appose itself closely to the enormously hypertrophied septum.

pulse is normal, and there is no prolongation of left ventricular systole manifest by lengthening of LVET and reversed splitting of S_2.

Obstruction to Right Ventricular Outflow (see also Chaps. 29 and 30). The physiological principles underlying the echophonocardiographic findings in obstruction to left ventricular outflow also apply to the right side of the heart. On the right side, however, the effect of inspiration in augmenting ventricular filling represents an additional factor.

Pulmonic Valve Stenosis. The murmur of pulmonic valvular stenosis is intense and of a harsh quality. It is maximal in the second left interspace and diminishes in all directions from this point. The murmur is midsystolic. However, more so than with the murmur of aortic stenosis, the timing of peak intensity can be used as an indicator of severity, being delayed in those patients with more severe obstruction. In the most severe cases, the murmur may peak late in systole and continue to or even *through* A_2, thus appearing to be holosystolic. Under these circumstances, however, since P_2 becomes further delayed with prolongation of right ventricular systole, the murmur remains *midsystolic* with respect to *right*-sided events of the cardiac cycle.[27] (See also Chap. 3.) The murmur is initiated by a pulmonary ejection sound which is also localized to the upper left sternal border and is loudest in *expiration* (Fig. 4–10).[28] Echophonocardiography can be very helpful in identifying an ejection sound by its exact coincidence with the achievement of a maximally open position by the pulmonary valve. The characteristic fluctuations of the sound with respiration can be readily documented. The phonocardiogram is also useful in displaying the increased separation of A_2-P_2, which is roughly proportional to the severity of the obstruction and the resultant rise in right ventricular systolic pressure.[27] The apexcardiographic transducer can be used to register the right ventricular heave, which marks the more severe examples of pulmonic valve stenosis.[29] The jugular venous pulse displays a prominent *a* wave in the presence of a thickened, hypertrophied, and noncompliant ventricle.

Subpulmonic (Infundibular) Stenosis. When this obstructive condition is found in isolation, i.e., without an as-

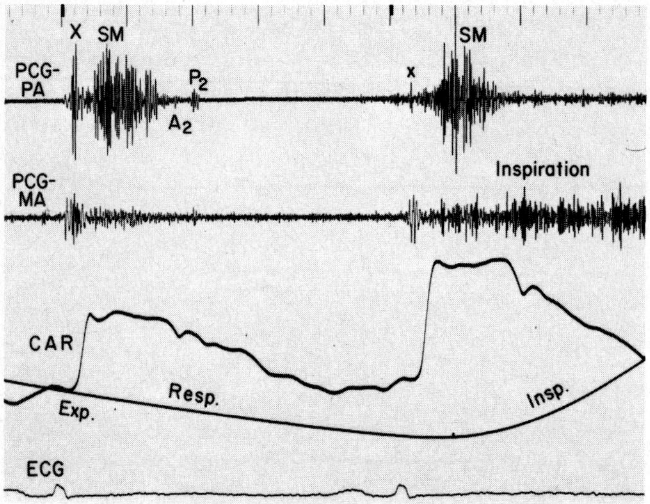

FIGURE 4–10 Valvular pulmonic stenosis. The first sound is not visible. The loud sound "X" at the beginning of systole is an ejection sound that is maximal in the second left interspace (PA). It is loud in expiration and diminishes with inspiration. The ejection sound is followed by a midsystolic murmur (SM). P_2 is diminutive and delayed.

sociated interventricular septal defect, the murmur is identical with that described earlier for valvular pulmonic stenosis,[30] although the location of its maximal intensity is lower along the left sternal border, in the third interspace. The ejection sound is lacking, however, as is the poststenotic dilatation on x-ray. Echocardiography reveals an early partial closing movement and fluttering of the pulmonary valve.[31] More often than in isolation, infundibular pulmonary stenosis occurs in conjunction with an interventricular septal defect, in which situation a whole spectrum of combinations of murmurs and heart sounds can be recorded as determined by the relative severity of the two major pathophysiological factors—the outflow obstruction and the interventricular defect.[32] At the one extreme, when the infundibular stenosis is mild, the physical signs as recorded phonocardiographically are dominated by the loud pansystolic murmur of the interventricular septal defect, upon which is superimposed the ejection murmur resulting from the stenosis. Frequently the silhouette of the murmur in the phonocardiogram taken low along the left sternal edge is holosystolic with a more or less constant intensity, whereas in the pulmonary area there is a definite midsystolic peak reflecting the obstructive lesion. There is no ejection sound. S_2 is widely split, as in valvular pulmonic stenosis, but P_2 is louder, probably reflecting the augmented flow through the pulmonary artery and higher pressures in the pulmonary artery as a result of the left-to-right shunt.

In cases in which the degree of infundibular stenosis is more severe, right-to-left shunting occurs through the ventricular septal defect, i.e., the classic tetralogy of Fallot. Under these circumstances the murmur from the ventricular defect disappears. The midsystolic murmur in the pulmonary area, however, can still be recorded, but its duration and intensity are lessened.[32] P_2 becomes inaudible and can rarely be recorded, even under ideal conditions. Thus the second sound (A_2) is single. An ejection sound of aortic origin is frequently audible and can be recorded widely over the precordium.

In the most extreme cases, when pulmonary atresia is present, the right-sided systolic murmur disappears, but there may be a short, early to midsystolic murmur resulting from ejection into a dilated aortic root. S_2 is single, and an aortic ejection sound can usually be recorded. Elsewhere over the thorax one can occasionally hear and record the continuous murmur from the bronchial collateral circulation.

Holosystolic Murmurs

Mitral Regurgitation[4,33,34] (see also Chap. 31). Combined echo- and phonocardiographic studies are particularly important in assessing patients with mitral regurgitation. Although the presence of the characteristic holosystolic murmur suggests the diagnosis by noninvasive means, neither the etiology nor the hemodynamic importance of the condition is usually apparent from the phonocardiographic findings alone. The echocardiographic features of mitral regurgitation are often nonspecific, but a useful index of the severity of the regurgitation is provided by the hyperdynamic left ventricular wall motion, left ventricular cavity dimensions, and left atrial enlargement (Chap. 5). Thus, whereas auscultation and phonocardiography establish the diagnosis, echocardiography is used to assess the severity of the regurgitation and, on occasion, its pathogenesis.

Mitral Regurgitation due to Rheumatic Heart Disease. The holosystolic murmur is best recorded at the cardiac apex (Fig. 4–11). It immediately follows S_1, which may be of reduced intensity unless there is a mixed lesion of stenosis and regurgitation. The murmur continues to or at times slightly beyond A_2. The second sound is normally split or may be more widely split than normal. However, variation with respiration is preserved. A third sound is a common accompaniment of moderate to severe mitral regurgitation,

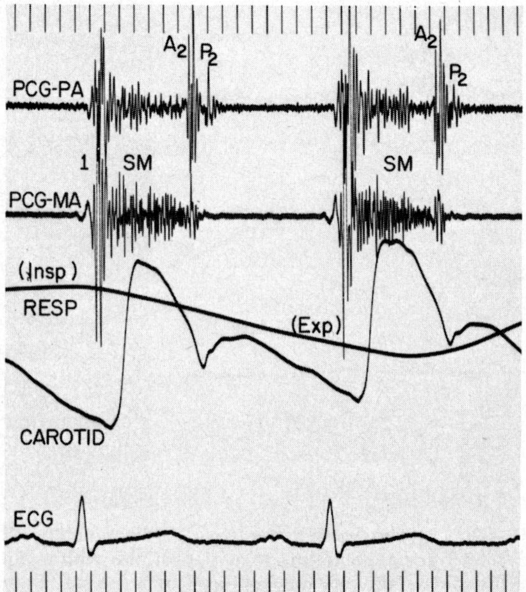

FIGURE 4–11 Mitral regurgitation due to rheumatic heart disease in a 25-year-old man with no symptoms and a small heart. The holosystolic murmur is most prominent at the cardiac apex (PCG-MA). S_1 is unusually loud, suggesting the possibility of early mitral stenosis, although there is no diastolic murmur.

and in the more severe cases a mid-diastolic rumble may be recorded in the mitral area.[35]

The echocardiographic appearance of rheumatic mitral regurgitation comprises a spectrum of mitral valve motion ranging from an apparently normal pattern to one in which the features of mitral stenosis are prominent. The combination of a holosystolic murmur and an echocardiogram consistent with mitral stenosis indicates the presence of mitral valvular disease with a rheumatic basis.

Mitral Regurgitation Secondary to Cardiomyopathy. Phonocardiography is of little help in the important differential diagnosis of severe diffuse cardiomyopathy as opposed to that of primary valvular disease. In cardiomyopathy, the murmur is holosystolic as in rheumatic heart disease, and there may be a prominent third sound that is also nonspecific, since it is a feature common to both cardiomyopathy and severe mitral regurgitation, regardless of pathogenesis. Systolic time intervals display similar abnormalities—prolongation of PEP and shortening of LVET, with a resulting increase in the PEP/LVET ratio (p. 54).[21] However, the echocardiogram may be most helpful in this differential diagnosis, since the dilated inert left ventricle of cardiomyopathy[36] contrasts sharply with

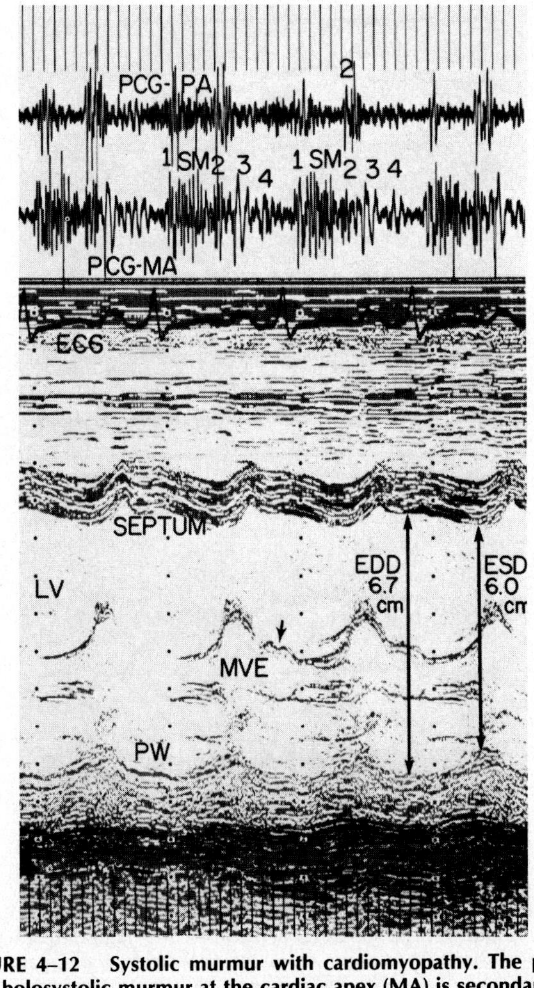

FIGURE 4–12 Systolic murmur with cardiomyopathy. The prominent holosystolic murmur at the cardiac apex (MA) is secondary to a severe diffuse alcoholic cardiomyopathy. There is very little difference between the left ventricular diameter in diastole (EDD) and that in systole (ESD). Additional phonocardiographic findings include gallop sounds (3 and 4). Arrow points to B notch on mitral valve echo, suggesting elevated left ventricular end-diastolic pressure. (Paper speed = 50 mm/sec.)

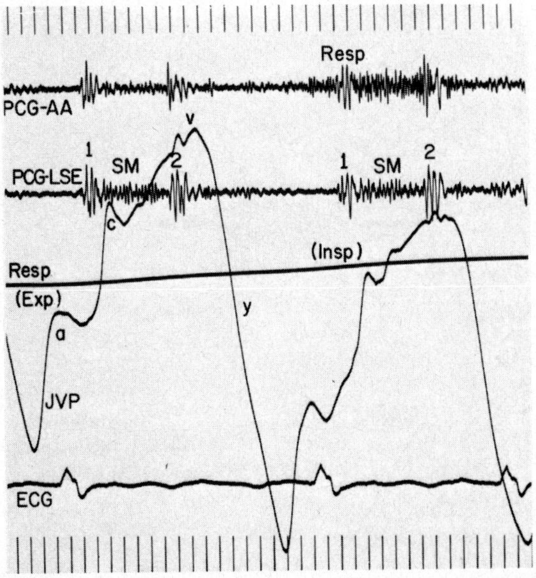

FIGURE 4–13 Tricuspid regurgitation, secondary to cor pulmonale resulting from thromboembolic disease. The phonocardiogram shows a holosystolic murmur at the left sternal edge (LSE). In this example the intensity of the murmur is not affected by inspiration. The accompanying JVP is abnormal with a very prominent *cv* plateau and *y* descent. The *x'* descent, which would normally follow the *c* wave, has been eliminated. Although the patient is in atrial flutter, there is an *a* wave in presystole which can be ascribed to atrial contraction.

the hyperdynamic movements of the septum and posterior wall in severe mitral regurgitation of rheumatic origin (Fig. 4–12).

Tricuspid Regurgitation Secondary to Pulmonary Hypertension.[37] Although noninvasive methods are useful in the diagnosis of tricuspid regurgitation, the graphic registration of the murmur may be disappointing (Fig. 4–13). Even more than with mitral regurgitation, the intensity of the murmur fails to correlate with the severity of the hemodynamic abnormality.[38,39] It is often overshadowed by the murmurs of accompanying valvular disease, since tricuspid regurgitation is most often a complication of left-sided disease that has resulted in pulmonary hypertension. The murmur is classically recorded best at the left lower sternal edge. With dilatation of the right ventricle, its point of maximal intensity may be shifted toward the left to the usual location of mitral murmurs. This can lead to an erroneous impression of *mitral* regurgitation, when tricuspid insufficiency has developed as a late result of severe mitral stenosis with pulmonary hypertension. Accentuation of the murmur with inspiration (Carvallo's sign) is a well-known feature of tricuspid regurgitation[40] that can be documented phonocardiographically. An accompanying venous pulse tracing will illustrate the parallel accentuation of *cv* waves with inspiration. Carvallo's sign, however, is not invariably present[41] and can be abolished by the onset of right ventricular failure, which prevents the inspiratory augmentation of right ventricular stroke volume responsible for intensification of the murmur. A third sound and mid-diastolic flow rumble of right-sided origin are seen with the more severe cases of tricuspid regurgitation,[37] as in the analogous situation on the left side of the heart. Precordial movement at the left sternal edge consists

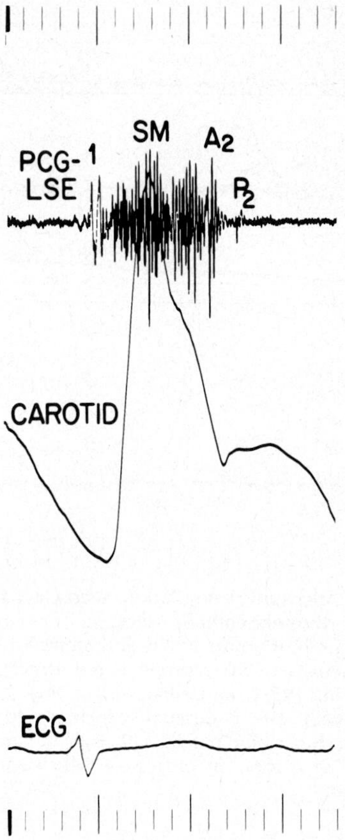

FIGURE 4–14 Ventricular septal defect with a large left-to-right shunt. A loud holosystolic murmur is seen, with accentuation in midsystole.

of a systolic heave of right ventricular hypertrophy when tricuspid regurgitation occurs as a consequence of right ventricular failure secondary to pulmonary hypertension.[42] The echocardiogram demonstrates a dilated right ventricular chamber and paradoxical movement of the interventricular septum (see Chap. 5). When tricuspid regurgitation occurs as a consequence of isolated damage to the valve itself rather than secondary to pulmonary hypertension, the physical signs and their graphic representation may be quite different (Chap. 31). The murmur may have a decrescendo configuration and be confined to early and midsystole.[43] This variant is discussed below, under Early Systolic Murmurs.

Ventricular Septal Defect (see also Chaps. 29 and 30). The murmur of a ventricular septal defect (VSD) is holosystolic, since in its typical expression (Roger's murmur)[44] it arises from the passage of blood throughout systole from the high-pressure left ventricle to the relatively low-pressure right ventricle through the defect. Thus the hemodynamic situation favors a holosystolic timing of the shunt as well as the murmur, which arises from the turbulence generated in the recipient chamber, the right ventricle. The murmur is quite intense and is located maximally in the third and fourth left interspaces, from which focus it diminishes centrifugally (Fig. 4–14).[45,46] The second heart sound is usually normal, although the degree of splitting may be somewhat exaggerated. However, respiratory variation is maintained.

In the smaller defects which characterize the classic Roger type of ventricular septal defect, the volume of the shunt is determined by the size of the septal aperture. The variations in hemodynamic patterns, which are conditioned by the size of the defect and the level of pulmonary arterial pressure, are roughly reflected in modifications in the graphic signs.[45] With larger shunts, the auscultatory and phonocardiographic signs of increased diastolic flow across the mitral valve may be manifest in an S_3 and mid-diastolic rumbling murmur. The apexcardiogram displays a hyperdynamic pattern—a systolic movement of normal shape but exaggerated amplitude and a prominent rapid filling wave. Although it is not usually possible to visualize the defect in the septum by M-mode echocardiography, one can detect indirect signs of the magnitude of the shunt in the size of the left-sided heart chambers and mobility of the left ventricular walls.

With pulmonary hypertension (the Eisenmenger type of VSD), the physical (Chap. 28) and graphic signs are remarkably altered (Fig. 4–15). The volume and direction of

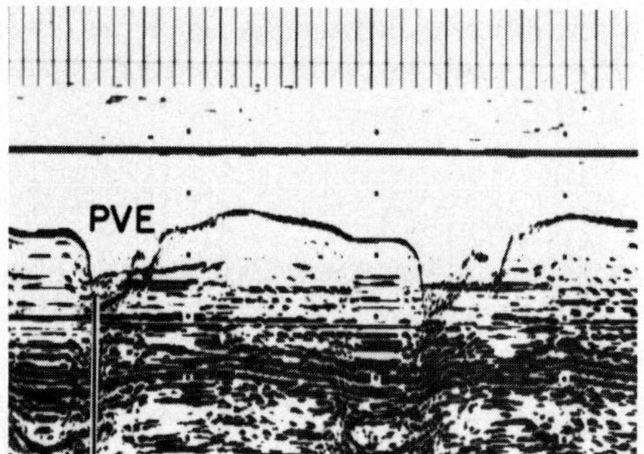

FIGURE 4–15 Dual echophonocardiogram in Eisenmenger's syndrome. A loud second sound (2) is followed by a high-frequency decrescendo diastolic murmur (edm) of pulmonary regurgitation. In the latter part of diastole, this merges with a lower frequency right-sided Austin Flint murmur (AFM). The loud ejection sound (X) is of pulmonary valve origin, as shown by the vertical line. The simultaneous echo of the aortic valve shows a tendency to closure in the latter half of systole, reflecting a dwindling stroke volume in this very ill patient.

shunting are now regulated by the relative resistances of the pulmonary and systemic circuits. As pressures in the two ventricles equilibrate in systole and as bidirectional shunting ensues owing to the large size of the defect, the systolic murmur resulting from the shunt disappears.[45] There remains a brief early to midsystolic ejection murmur resulting from flow into the dilated root of the pulmonary artery. This murmur is initiated by an ejection sound occurring at the time of full opening of the cusps of the pulmonic valve (Chap. 3). The timing of the ejection sound is delayed with pulmonary hypertension, owing to prolongation of the isovolumetric contraction time.[46] The second sound is very intense and is often palpable and results from the simultaneous closure of A_2 and an accentuated P_2. Accompanying murmurs that may be recorded in the more severe and longstanding cases of the Eisenmenger variant of ventricular septal defect include those of pulmonary regurgitation (Graham Steell), tricuspid regurgitation,[47] and, on occasion, a right-sided Austin Flint murmur.[48]

EARLY SYSTOLIC MURMURS

Acute Mitral Regurgitation (see also Chap. 32). Acute mitral regurgitation constitutes a syndrome that has been increasingly identified in recent years. Although less common than the chronic variety, acute mitral regurgitation is important because of its severity and reversibility in many instances, if it is accurately and promptly diagnosed. It occurs in association with rupture of the chordae tendineae or papillary muscle or with a severe damage to the valve itself, such as from trauma or infective endocarditis. Acute mitral regurgitation requires special consideration, since its auscultatory and phonocardiographic manifestations are unusual for mitral regurgitation—often resembling those of aortic stenosis. The murmur is usually pansystolic but tapers in intensity in late systole and in extreme cases may terminate before A_2.[49] The reason for the decrescendo character of the murmur is the unusual hemodynamic situation resulting from regurgitation of a large volume of blood during systole into a small, previously normal left atrium. The impact of the regurgitant bolus on a relatively noncompliant atrium results in an extraordinarily high *v* wave in late systole. Thus ventricular and atrial pressures (Fig. 4–16)[50,51] may equilibrate in late systole, with throttling of the regurgitant stream and suppression of the murmur. Despite its shortened duration, the murmur can be seen in a combined echophonocardiogram to be initiated at the time of mitral valve closure or well before the opening of the aortic valve, thus distinguishing it from a midsystolic murmur, which would also diminish in intensity in late systole but which would not start until after the aortic valve had opened. Other phonocardiographic signs include an S_3, as in the more usual types of mitral regurgitation. An S_4 may be recorded in acute mitral regurgitation[52] as well as its palpable counterpart, an *a* wave on the apexcardiogram. This is an important feature of the syndrome, which, like the unusual murmur described above, would not be expected in chronic mitral regurgitation. In the more severe cases a precordial heave that peaks in late systole can be recorded (Fig. 4–16). Its graphic configuration is qualitatively similar to the *v* wave of the left atrial pressure pulse, and it is thought to originate from the action of the whole heart being pushed against the chest wall, caused by sudden expansion during systole of the posteriorly located left atrium.[53]

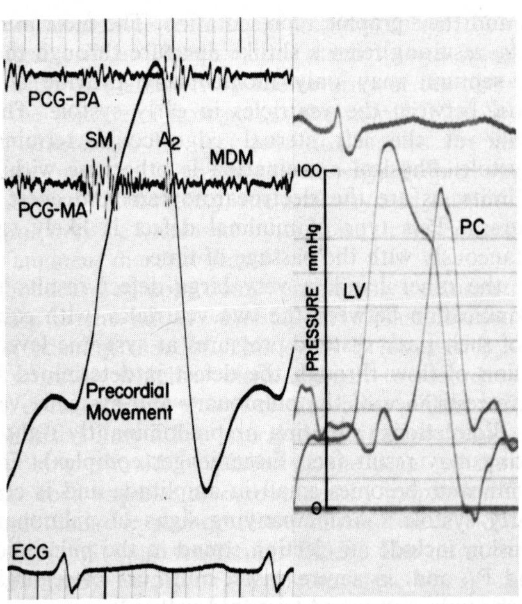

FIGURE 4–16 Acute mitral regurgitation in a young man with infective endocarditis. *Left,* Phonocardiogram at the cardiac apex (PCG-MA); an early systolic murmur (SM) begins with the onset of systole and terminates in mid- to late systole. *Right,* Pressure tracings from left ventricular (LV) and pulmonary capillary (PC) wedge positions. The high pressure (> 90 mm Hg) achieved in the left atrium in late systole results in equilibrium of pressures in LV and LA and termination of the systolic murmur. The unusual precordial movement pattern in the left-hand panel resembles the *v* wave in the PC wedge pressure and presumably reflects a forward thrust of the heart, resulting from massive left atrial expansion during systole. The mid-diastolic murmur (MDM) is a ventricular filling murmur or flow rumble.

Tricuspid Regurgitation due to Isolated Disease of the Valve (see also Chap. 32). When tricuspid regurgitation occurs owing to isolated disease of the valve itself rather than secondary to pulmonary hypertension, the phonocardiographic "silhouette" of the systolic murmur may be altered, so that it is decrescendo and terminates before the second heart sound. Isolated damage to the valve may occur from infective endocarditis or trauma. Under those circumstances, pressures in the right ventricle may be virtually normal. However, the high *v* wave generated in the right atrial pressure pulse by the regurgitant stream may lead to equalization of ventricular and atrial pressures in the latter part of systole, with diminution or suppression of the murmur. This occurs in a manner analogous to the alteration of the systolic murmur in acute mitral regurgitation, described above. Unfortunately, neither the timing nor the intensity of the murmur can be used to estimate the severity of the leak. Precordial movement in severe tricuspid regurgitation with normal right ventricular pressure may consist of an inward movement during systole and an expansion in diastole, reflecting massive volume changes in the underlying right ventricle.[54]

Congenital Heart Disease with Pulmonary Hypertension (see also Chaps. 29 and 30). Although the classic murmur of a ventricular septal defect is holosystolic, circumstances occur at both ends of the spectrum of severity of this condition that may drastically modify the physical

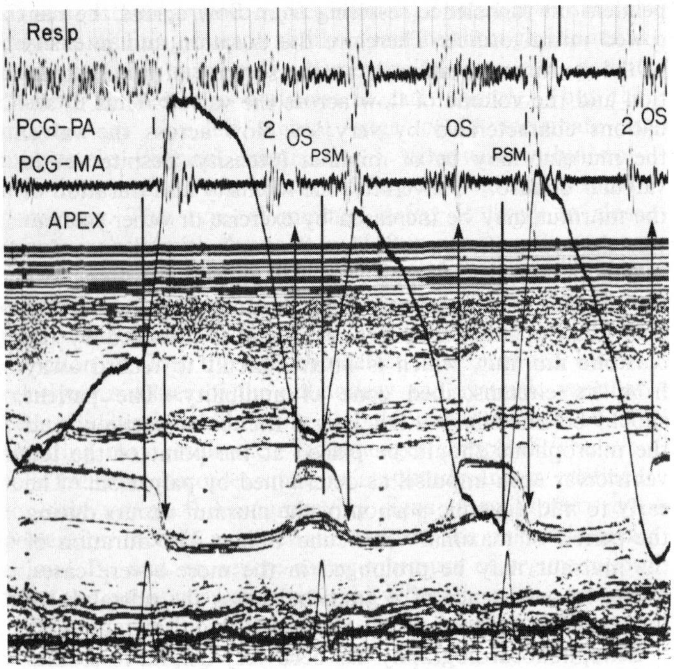

FIGURE 4–18 Mitral stenosis in atrial fibrillation. Echophonocardiogram illustrating a "presystolic" murmur (PSM) occurring only after the short diastoles. There is no PSM with the first cycle, which followed a longer diastole. The PSM is associated with the closing movement of the mitral valve (downward arrows). This, in turn, is initiated by ventricular systole, the onset of which is marked by the upstroke of the apex (heavy vertical lines). The relationship of the opening snap (OS) to opening of the mitral valve is shown by the upward arrows.

Tricuspid Stenosis. Tricuspid stenosis is a relatively rare condition occurring principally in association with far advanced rheumatic heart disease with mitral stenosis (p. 1115). Therefore the phonocardiographic signs may be overshadowed by those of the accompanying valvular disease.[76] Since most patients in the later stages of rheumatic heart disease will be in atrial fibrillation, the murmur of tricuspid stenosis will be found in early to mid-diastole, wh en there is a maximal gradient across the valve and a high velocity flow.[77] In normal sinus rhythm, the murmur may be confined to presystole and can be attributed to flow across the obstructing valve resulting from right atrial systole.[76] Maximal intensity of the murmur is at the left lower sternal edge.

Since the graphic signs described above could easily be confused with those of mitral stenosis, it is necessary to observe and record the effects of respiration on the intensity of the murmur.[78] A dramatic increase in intensity of the murmur with inspiration is very helpful, since this occurs with tricuspid but not with mitral stenosis. Simultaneous registration of the jugular venous pulse usually demonstrates enormous *a* waves in patients in normal sinus rhythm,[78] owing to retrograde flow in the venous system while the right atrium is contracting against a stenotic valve.[79] The echocardiogram may disclose alterations in the movements of the tricuspid valve in diastole similar to those of mitral stenosis. However, this valve is considerably more difficult to record by echo than is the mitral.

Left Atrial Myxoma (see also p. 1460). Murmurs associated with left atrial myxoma simulate those of mitral valve disease, but both the character and the intensity of the murmurs may change profoundly on successive examinations or with alterations in position. The systolic murmur results from mitral regurgitation due to damage to the valve from trauma inflicted by the movable tumor mass[80] or from interference with apposition of the valve leaflets. A diastolic murmur is often present and is usually confined to late diastole or presystole. The pathogenesis of this murmur is probably analogous to that of the final crescendo phase of the presystolic murmur of mitral stenosis,[74] as can be demonstrated by combined echophonocardiographic observation (Fig. 4–20). Thus it can be shown that the "presystolic" crescendo actually occurs with the onset of ventricular systole at a time when the rising pressure in the ventricle is forcing the movable tumor back through the mitral orifice against the stream of blood that is still flowing from atrium to ventricle. The crescendo phase of the murmur culminates in the loud delayed first sound, related to the completed excursion of the tumor toward the atrium.[81]

Atrioventricular Flow Rumbles

Mitral Regurgitation Rapid flow across atrioventricular valves in early to mid-diastole often results in low-pitched rumbling murmurs simulating the physical sign of mitral stenosis. The most common example of this type of murmur is in mitral regurgitation, in which an increased volume of blood is moving from atrium to ventricle during passive ventricular filling. It is interesting that the flow rumble does not occur when the mitral valve has first

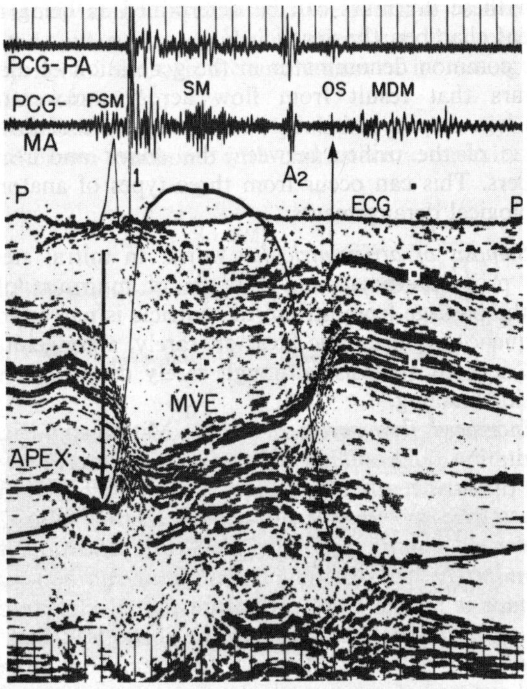

FIGURE 4–19 Mitral stenosis in a 49-year-old woman with a history of mitral commissurotomy 16 years previously with a good result. Sinus rhythm remains normal. An echophonocardiogram is combined with an apexcardiogram to show the relationship of the onset of LV systole to the presystolic crescendo murmur (PSM) (see text). The opening snap of the mitral valve (OS) occurs with full opening of the mitral valve (light arrow) and is followed by a mid-diastolic murmur (MDM). Mild accompanying aortic valve disease accounts for the crescendo-decrescendo systolic murmur transmitted to the mitral area (SM).

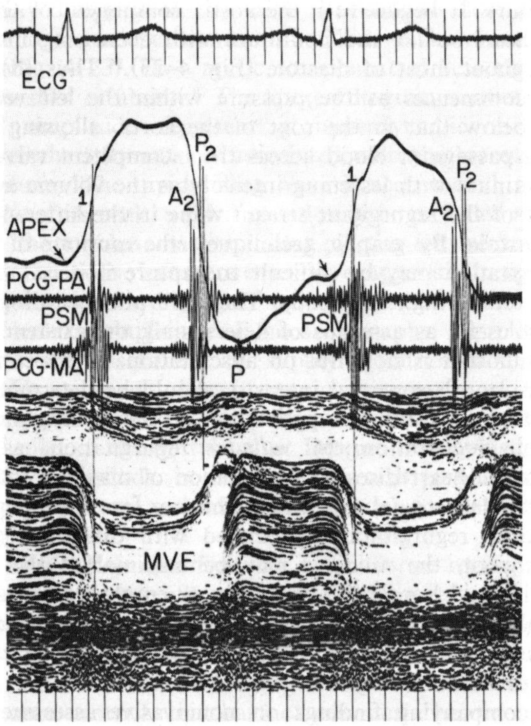

FIGURE 4–20 Left atrial myxoma. Echophonocardiogram illustrating the relationship between the presystolic murmur (PSM) and movement of the tumor mass through the mitral valve and into the atrium under the impact of ventricular systole. Timing of ventricular systole is provided by the apexcardiogram, the upstroke of which is indicated by an arrow.

opened and is most widely open with presumably maximal flow.[82,83] Rather it begins a few hundredths of a second later. Echophonocardiographic studies have clarified the relationship between valve motion and generation of the murmur.[74] These observations show that after opening widely in early diastole, the mitral valve makes a partial closing movement while presumably a high volume of blood is still moving antegrade across its closing orifice. This results, in effect, in a functional mitral stenosis, in which too large a volume of blood is moving across the valve for the dimensions of the aperture. A mid-diastolic pressure gradient may be demonstrated under these circumstances.[84,85]

Left-to-Right Shunts. A similar pathogenetic mechanism probably occurs in left-to-right shunts, such as patent ductus arteriosus or ventricular septal defect, in which there is augmented flow across a normal mitral valve.[86] On the right side of the heart, diastolic flow rumbles occur with atrial septal defect or anomalous pulmonary venous drainage in a manner analogous to the left-sided murmurs noted above. In atrial septal defect, a combined echophonocardiographic examination shows a closing movement of the tricuspid valve in early to mid-diastole at a time when a very large flow is taking place from atrium to ventricle (Fig. 4–21). The location of maximal intensity of the murmur by intracardiac phonocardiography is in the right ventricular inflow tract.[87]

Austin Flint Murmur. The apical rumbling diastolic murmur occurring in pure aortic regurgitation was first described by the renowned American clinician Austin Flint.[88] He attributed the murmur to functional mitral stenosis resulting from impingement of the regurgitant stream on the anterior leaflet of the mitral valve. Although a number of alternative hypotheses to explain the genesis of the murmur have been advanced since Flint's time, modern studies combining echo- and phonocardiography support his original contention.[89] The mitral valve can be seen to effect a premature partial closing movement in early to mid-diastole and again following atrial systole while atrial contents are moving in an antegrade direction across the mitral orifice. Thus conditions exist for a functional type of mitral stenosis and the genesis of a murmur simulating organic obstruction. The murmur may be confined to late diastole (presystolic) in the milder cases, but in moderately severe aortic regurgitation there may be both mid-diastolic and late diastolic components, giving an hourglass configuration to the murmur on the phonocardiogram. The Flint murmur has been thought by some to be related to the vibrations of the anterior leaflet of the mitral valve, a characteristic echocardiographic feature of aortic regurgitation. These vibrations are the result, however, of the play on the leaflet of the regurgitating cascade of blood from the aortic root. The mitral valvular vibrations are therefore coincident in time with the early diastolic murmur of aortic regurgitation and *not* the Flint murmur, the timing of which is mid- and/or late diastolic.

In the most severe cases, such as in acute aortic insufficiency resulting from infective endocarditis, the Flint murmur may be confined to mid-diastole. This variant of the murmur is explained by the highly abnormal pressure relationships resulting from massive aortic regurgitation and generation of very high pressures in end diastole in the left

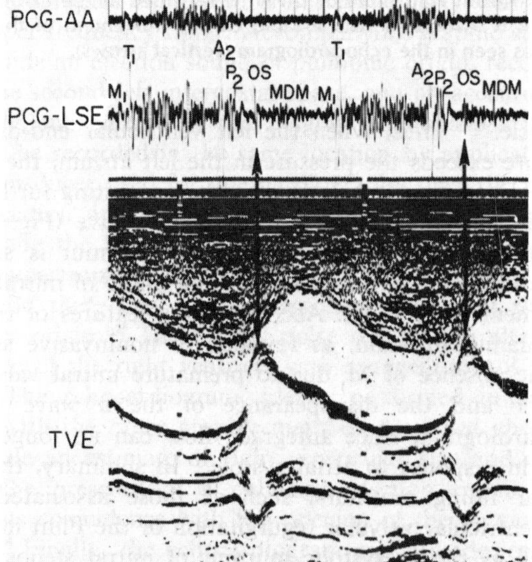

FIGURE 4–21 Mid-diastolic rumble in atrial septal defect. Echophonocardiogram demonstrating a mid-diastolic murmur (MDM) at the left sternal edge. The tricuspid valve is closing sharply during this phase of diastole while antegrade flow is occurring across it. Other phonocardiographic features of ASD include an accentuated T_1, an opening snap (OS) of tricuspid origin (arrow), and an ejection systolic murmur. The movements of the valve in systole are not well recorded.

5 ECHOCARDIOGRAPHY

by Harvey Feigenbaum, M.D.

PRINCIPLES OF ECHOCARDIOGRAPHY

Creation of Image Using Pulsed Reflected Ultrasound

The term *echocardiography* refers to a group of tests that utilize ultrasound to examine the heart and record information in the form of echoes, i.e., reflected sonic waves. The upper limit for audible sound is 20,000 cycles/second, or 20 kiloHertz (kHz = 1000 cycles/second[1] The sonic frequency used for echocardiography ranges from 1 to 7 million cycles/second, or 1 to 7 megaHertz (MHz).[2] In adults the frequencies commonly employed are 2 to 3.5 MHz, while in children they are usually higher, ranging from 3.5 to 7.0 MHz. The *resolution* of the recording, which is the ability to distinguish two objects that are spatially close together, varies directly with the frequency and inversely with the wave length. High-frequency (short wave length) ultrasound can identify separate objects that are less than 1 mm apart. Beams having lower frequencies and longer wave lengths have poorer resolution. However, the degree of *penetration,* which is the ability to transmit sufficient ultrasonic energy into the chest to provide a satisfactory recording, is inversely proportional to the frequency of the signal. Since a high-frequency ultrasonic beam (i.e., 3 or 5 MHz) is unable to penetrate a thick chest wall, lower frequency ultrasonic beams are used in adults. While this permits penetration through the chest wall, it partially sacrifices resolution; however, even with a transducer producing a beam of 2.25 MHz, which is commonly used in adult echocardiography, it is still possible to resolve objects that are 1 to 2 mm apart.

Although diagnostic ultrasound, including echocardiography, is an imaging technique, there are many fundamental differences between ultrasound and other techniques used to create an image of an internal structure. Examinations that use ionizing radiation, whether in the form of an x-ray beam or a radioactive isotope, usually record the *shadow* of a structure, while ultrasound creates an image using *reflected* energy. Visualization of a structure using light relies on the reflection of energy off the object in question and its capture in the eye or on photographic film; ultrasonic imaging utilizes the same basic principle. It should be recalled that imaging with both light and ultrasound is utilized in nature; indeed, several mammalian species, including bats, dolphins, and whales, rely on ultrasound instead of vision. The technology necessary to create ultrasonic images has been available for many years, and medical diagnostic ultrasound is an outgrowth of both industrial nondestructive testing of materials and naval sonar.[1-3]

The principles by which ultrasound creates an image are depicted in Figure 5–1. The transducer at the side of the beaker of water has a piezoelectric element that vibrates very rapidly and produces ultrasound when activated by an electrical field.[3] The original piezoelectric material used was quartz, but a variety of different ceramics are now used for this purpose. If a burst of electrical energy is imparted to the transducer, it will emit a burst of ultrasound, which travels through the beaker. As long as the medium through which the sound travels is homogeneous, the ultrasonic waves will travel in a straight line. When the ultrasound strikes an interface between two media which have different acoustical properties, the sound behaves according to the laws of reflection and refraction,[1,2] analogous to light. Whether or not ultrasound is reflected by an interface depends upon the difference in the acoustical impedances of the two media. Although acoustical impedance is the product of the density of the object and the velocity of sound through that object, for all practical purposes one can consider the acoustical impedance to be a function of density. Thus, if the interface is between a liquid and a solid, the ultrasonic wave will generally be reflected. If the interface is between two solids of different densities, the quantity of reflected ultrasound is usually less. Thus, the quantity of energy reflected is directly proportional to the difference in the acoustical impedances (or densities) of the object and its surrounding media and to the angle at which the

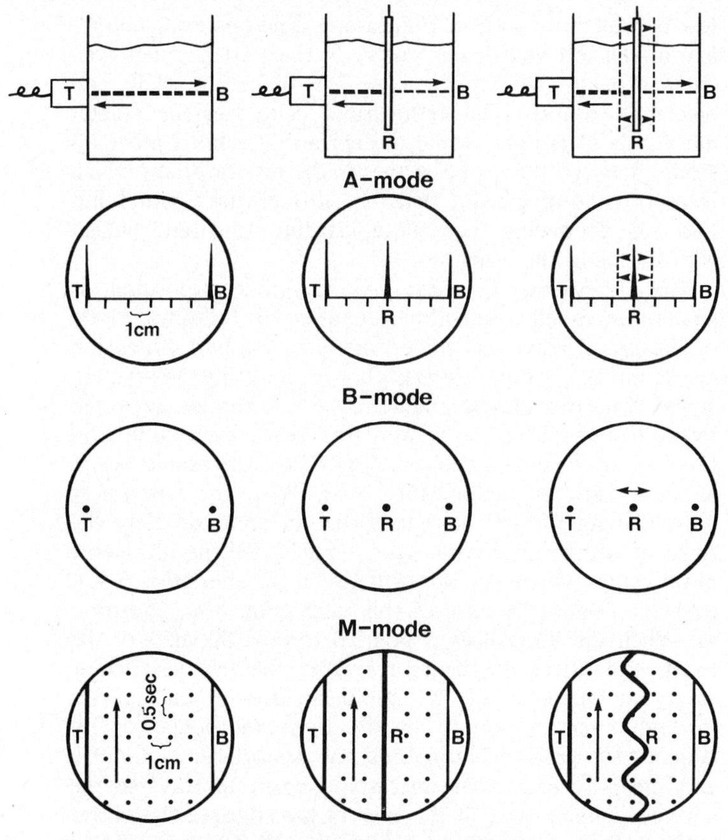

FIGURE 5–1 Diagrams illustrating the principles of acoustic imaging using pulsed reflected ultrasound (see text for details). T = transducer, B = beaker, R = rod. (Modified from Feigenbaum, H., and Zaky, A.: Use of diagnostic ultrasound in clinical cardiology. J. Indiana State Med. Assoc. *59*:140, 1966.)

beam strikes the object; i.e., the more perpendicular the beam is to the object, the lower the percentage of reflected energy.

The left panel of Figure 5–1 shows diagrammatically an ultrasonic beam, which consists of individual bursts of ultrasound that leave the transducer, travel through the fluid, strike the far side of the beaker, are reflected by this interface, retrace their original path, and again strike the transducer. The piezoelectric element in the transducer not only converts electrical energy into ultrasonic impulses but also converts ultrasound back to electrical energy. Thus, when the reflected ultrasound (echo) strikes the piezoelectric element in the transducer, an electrical signal is produced. If the time it takes for (a) the ultrasound to leave the transducer and return and (b) the velocity of sound through the medium are both known, the distance between the transducer and the reflected interface can be calculated. By calibrating the echograph (ultrasonoscope) for a velocity of sound in the medium under examination, the time that it takes for the ultrasound to leave and return as an echo can be automatically converted to distance. Thus, the far wall of the beaker is depicted on the oscilloscope as being 6 cm from the transducer.

If a rod is placed in the water so that it transects the ultrasonic beam, part of the energy will strike and be reflected by the rod before the beam strikes the far side of the beaker. Thus, the returning ultrasonic energy or echo from the rod will strike the transducer sooner than that returning from the far side of the beaker, and the corresponding electrical signal produced by the echo from the rod will be closer to the transducer than will that from the beaker. Also, since some of the ultrasonic energy is reflected by the rod, less energy will remain to strike the far wall of the beaker, and the magnitude of the echo (Fig. 5–1, center panel) will be reduced. There are adjustments in ultrasonic instrumentation which provide depth compensation and thereby correct for this loss of ultrasonic energy from distant or far objects. From examination of the A-mode echo ("A" refers to amplitude) in Figure 5–1 (center panel), one could deduce that the far wall of the beaker is 6 cm from the transducer and that an echo-reflecting object is present in the center of the beaker, 3 cm from the transducer.

If the rod were moving back and forth as in the right panel of Figure 5–1, the ultrasonic examination would differ. The transducer functions as a transmitter of ultrasound for a very short period of time, just over one μsec in commercial echocardiographs. During the remaining time the transducer functions as a receiver, waiting for echoes to be converted into electrical signals. The rapidity or the repetition rate with which the transducer fires the 1 μsec impulses varies depending upon the design of the instrument. Commercial M-mode instruments commonly pulse the transducer 1000 times/sec with 1 μsec impulses. Thus, the transducer functions as a receiver during approximately 999 μsec of each msec.

In the left and center panels of Figure 5–1, the wall of the beaker and the rod are not moving. All the ultrasonic impulses firing at a rate of 1000/sec take the same time to leave the transducer and return as echoes. Therefore, the signals or echoes seen on the oscilloscope are static. In the right panel, the object moves constantly and therefore the time required for the ultrasound to leave the transducer and return as an echo varies correspondingly and the echo signal on the oscilloscope moves. In the A-mode presentation the echo from the rod moves back and forth within the center of the beaker. To record the motion of the rod, one could make a movie or television recording of the moving echo on the oscilloscope. A more practical method of recording this echo motion is to convert the amplitude of the echo to brightness, which changes the display from the A-mode to the B-mode (the "B" refers to brightness), in which the returning echoes are displayed on the oscilloscope as dots rather than as spikes. Stronger signals are therefore taller on the A-mode and brighter on the B-mode presentation. Since the echoes are now dots instead of spikes, a dimension becomes available, and the element of time can be introduced by sweeping the oscilloscope. On the M-mode presentation ("M" refers to motion) displayed in Figure 5–1, the oscilloscope sweeps from bottom to top. In the left and center panels the structures are fixed, and therefore the M-mode presentation shows simply a series of parallel lines. In the right panel the rod moves back and forth in a regular manner, its echo inscribing a sinusoidal curve on the M-mode oscilloscope.

Thus, the M-mode presentation permits recording of amplitude and of the rate of motion of moving objects with great accuracy; the sampling rate is essentially 1000 pulses/second, the repetition rate of the transducer. Since electrocardiograms and other cardiac parameters are conventionally displayed on the oscilloscope together with the echocardiograph, the oscilloscope usually sweeps from left to right rather than from bottom to top; therefore, the transducer is generally displayed at the top of the oscilloscopic image rather than on the left side, as depicted in Figure 5–1.

M-Mode Echocardiography

Technique. The ultrasonic transducer is ordinarily placed on the surface of the chest, usually along the left sternal border (Fig. 5–2), and the ultrasonic beam is directed toward the part of the heart to be examined. In Figure 5–3 the ultrasound is depicted as passing through a small portion of the right ventricle, the interventricular septum, and the cavity and posterior wall of the left ventricle. This diagram is analogous to Figure 5–1 except that the transducer is now at the top rather than at the side. Therefore, on the echocardiogram, time is displayed on the abscissa and distance on the ordinate. The various structures which transect the ultrasonic beam produce echoes on the oscilloscope; the first object through which the beam travels is the chest wall, which produces a series of echoes. Since these echoes do not move with the cardiac cycle, they are displayed as a series of straight horizontal lines. The ultrasonic beam then strikes the anterior wall of the right ventricle, which may or may not be well imaged, depending upon the configuration of the patient's thoracic cage and the frequency of the beam; in this particular tracing the anterior wall of the right ventricle is indistinct.

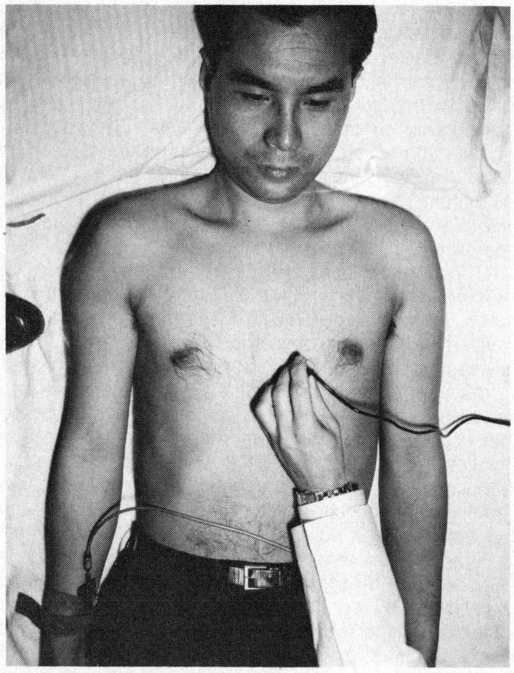

FIGURE 5–2 Placement of the ultrasonic echocardiographic transducer on the chest along the left sternal border. (From Feigenbaum, H., et al.: Left ventricular wall thickness measured by ultrasound. Arch. Intern. Med. *121*:391, 1968. Copyright 1968, American Medical Association.)

The next area recorded on the echocardiogram is a relatively echo-free space between the anterior right ventricular wall and the right side of the interventricular septum, which represents a portion of the right ventricular cavity. The echoes which make up the interventricular septum consist of echoes from the right and left sides of the septum. Posterior to the septal echoes is the relatively echo-free space of the left ventricular cavity. This cavity frequently has echoes from the mitral valve apparatus, only a few of which are seen in Figure 5–3. The posterior boundary of the left ventricular cavity is the posterior left ventricular wall, which is made up of endocardial and epicardial echoes. The endocardial echo has the greater amplitude of motion, while the epicardial echo is more intense. Between these two echoes is the myocardium, which is more echo-producing than the intracavitary blood but less echo-producing than the epicardium and lung, which is posterior to the heart.

The M-Mode Tracing. An M-mode recording is sometimes called a one-dimensional or an "ice-pick" view of the heart. However, since time is the second dimension on M-mode tracings, this display is not truly one-dimensional. One can greatly augment the information provided by an isolated M-mode view of the heart, such as in Figure 5–3, by changing the direction of the ultrasonic beam, as in an arc or sector (Fig. 5–4). With the transducer placed along the left sternal border in approximately the third or fourth intercostal space (Fig. 5–2), the ultrasonic beam can be swept in a sector between the apex (Fig. 5–4*A*, position 1) and the base of the heart (Fig. 5–4*A*, position 4). When the transducer is pointed toward the apex of the heart, the ultrasonic beam traverses the left ventricular cavity at the level of the papillary muscles and passes through a small portion of the right ventricular cavity (Fig. 5–4*B*, position 1). Tilting the transducer superiorly and medially causes the ultrasonic beam to traverse the left ventricular cavity at the level of the edges of the mitral valve leaflets or the chordae (position 2). The beam again passes through a small portion of the right ventricle. By directing the transducer more superiorly and medially (position 3), more of the anterior leaflet of the mitral valve can be recorded and the beam may traverse part of the left atrial cavity. Further tilting of the transducer superiorly and medially (position 4) directs the beam through the root of the aorta, the leaflets of the aortic valve, and the body of the left atrium.

Figure 5–5 is a diagram of an echocardiographic record-

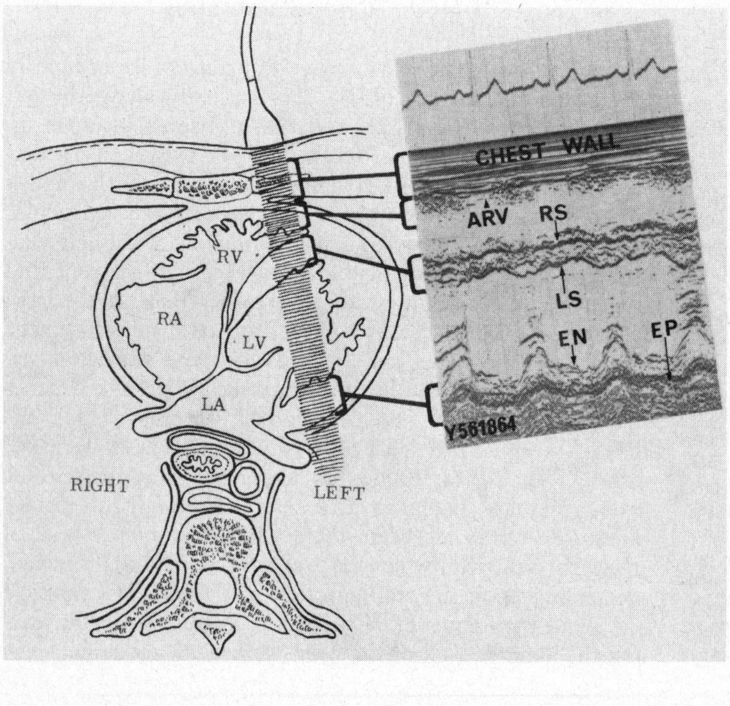

FIGURE 5–3 Diagrammatic cross-section of the heart and corresponding echocardiogram showing the cardiac structures transected by an ultrasonic beam directed toward the left ventricle. The ultrasound passes through the chest wall, the anterior right ventricular wall (ARV), a small portion of the right ventricular cavity, the interventricular septum, the cavity of the left ventricle, and the posterior left ventricular wall. RS = right side of interventricular septum, LS = left side of interventricular septum, EN = posterior left ventricular endocardium, EP = posterior left ventricular epicardium. (Modified from Popp, R. L., et al.: Estimation of right and left ventricular size by ultrasound. A study of the echoes from the interventricular septum. Am. J. Cardiol. *24*:523, 1969.)

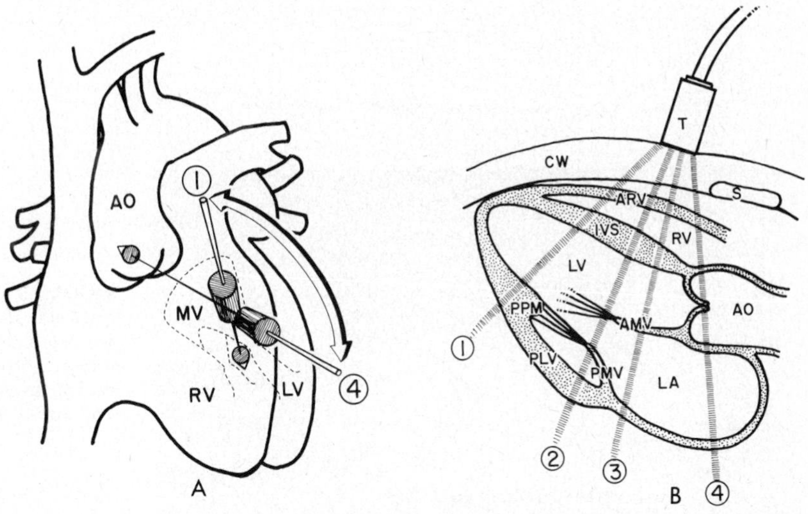

FIGURE 5–4 Diagram demonstrating how the ultrasonic transducer is commonly directed in an arc or sector between the base of the heart and the apex (*A*). *B*, Cross-section of the heart parallel to the long axis of the left ventricle showing the structures through which the ultrasound beam passes as it is directed from the apex toward the base of the heart, as shown in *A*. T = transducer, S = sternum, ARV = anterior right ventricular wall, RV = right ventricular cavity, IVS = interventricular septum, LV = left ventricle, PPM = posterior papillary muscle, PLV = posterior left ventricular wall, AMV = anterior mitral valve, PMV = posterior mitral valve, AO = aorta, LA = left atrium, MV = mitral valve. (From Feigenbaum, H.: Clinical applications of echocardiography. Progr. Cardiovasc. Dis. *14*:531, 1972, by permission of Grune and Stratton.)

ing as the transducer is swept in a sector from the apex toward the base of the heart, the areas between the dotted lines in Figure 5–5 corresponding to the directions of the beam shown in Figure 5–4. An electrocardiogram helps to identify the events of the cardiac cycle. Beginning on the left side of Figure 5–5 (position 1), the chest wall echoes are recorded, followed by those of the anterior wall of the right ventricle. The right ventricular cavity is then recorded as an echo-free space. The next structure is the interventricular septum, with the right side of the septum frequently represented as a double or triple line and the left side as a single echo. Frequently, a mass of echoes originating from the posterior papillary muscle is evident posterior to the left ventricular cavity. Even further posterior is the posterior wall of the left ventricle. The intense echoes behind the heart originate from the lung. In transducer position 2 the principal change in the echogram is that parts of the mitral valve apparatus, either chordae or edges of the leaflets, are recorded within the left ventricular cavity. In this position the ultrasonic beam also traverses more of the body of the left ventricle, and the diameter of the left ventricular cavity, i.e., the distance between the left side of the interventricular septum and the posterior left ventricular endocardium, is greatest.

As the transducer is tilted slightly superiorly and medially, the anterior and posterior leaflets of the mitral valve are recorded. Tilting the transducer even further toward the base of the heart (position 3) causes the echoes produced by the posterior leaflet to drop out, and only the anterior leaflet of the mitral valve is recorded. The beam now passes through the posterior wall of the left atrium instead of that of the left ventricle. The posterior wall of the atrium moves posteriorly, i.e., away from the chest wall, during systole, while the posterior wall of the left ventricle moves anteriorly. When the transducer is directed toward the base of the heart (position 4), the beam passes through the anterior wall of the aorta (rather than the interventricular septum) and the posterior wall of the aortic root, which also constitutes the anterior wall of the left atrium (rather than the anterior leaflet of the mitral valve). Echoes from two or more leaflets of the aortic valve can frequently be recorded from between the two aortic walls.

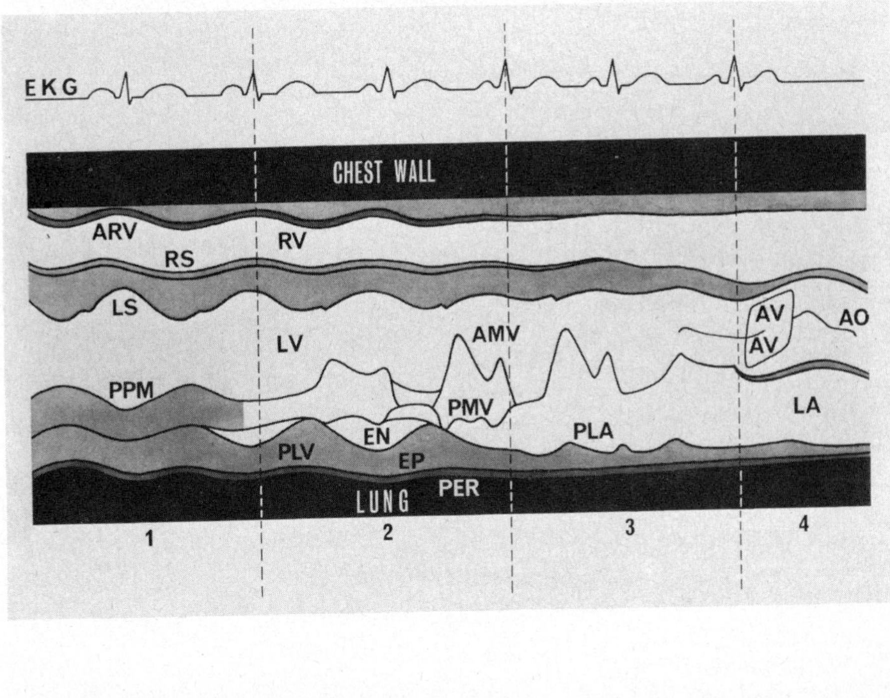

FIGURE 5–5 Diagrammatic presentation of an M-mode echocardiogram as the transducer is directed from the apex (position 1) to the base of the heart (position 4). Areas between the dotted lines correspond to the transducer position, as depicted in Figure 5–4. EN = endocardium of the left ventricle, EP = epicardium of the left ventricle, PER = pericardium, PLA = posterior left atrial wall. Other abbreviations as in Figure 5–4. (From Feigenbaum, H.: Clinical applications of echocardiography. Progr. Cardiovasc. Dis. *14*:531, 1972, by permission of Grune and Stratton.)

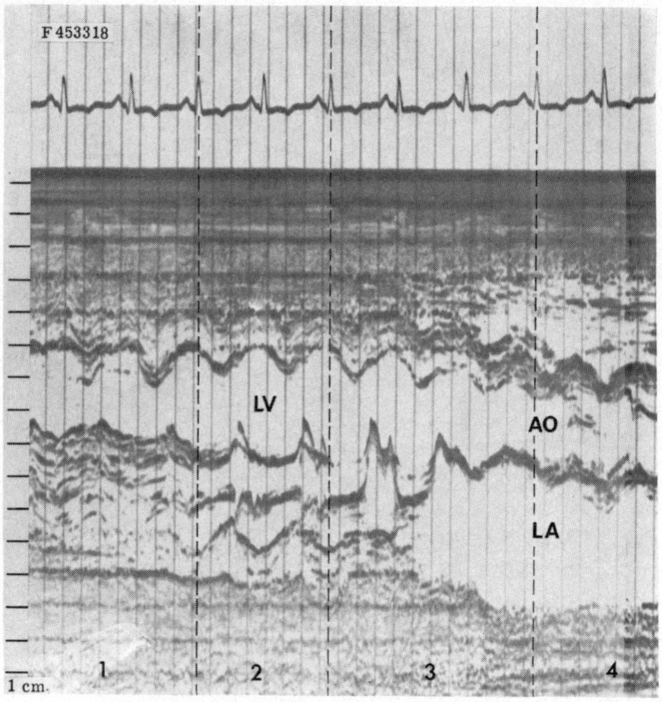

FIGURE 5–6 M-mode echocardiographic scan of the heart. Areas between the dotted lines correspond to those similarly designated in Figure 5–5. LV = left ventricular cavity, AO = aorta, LA = left atrium. (From Feigenbaum, H.: Clinical applications of echocardiography. Progr. Cardiovasc. Dis. *14*:531, 1972, by permission of Grune and Stratton.)

The leaflets separate and form a boxlike structure during systole and come together as a single line in diastole; the left atrial cavity lies behind the aorta.

Figure 5–6 is an actual M-mode scan on which many of the structures shown diagrammatically in Figure 5–5 can be recognized. However, the right ventricular cavity is not visible in positions 1 and 2; frequently, this cavity can be visualized only when the gain is turned down to record fewer echoes close to the transducer. In position 1, the posterior papillary muscle is recorded as a mass of somewhat ill-defined echoes approximately 2 to 3 cm from the left side of the interventricular septum. In position 2, echoes having a pattern of motion characteristic of the leaflets of the mitral valve become apparent. This pattern is best noted by the rapid motion of the echoes in early diastole when the anterior leaflet moves anteriorly and the posterior leaflet posteriorly. A clearly defined endocardial echo behind the posterior leaflet of the mitral valve is recorded. In position 3, an echo from the anterior leaflet of the mitral valve is recorded, but the posterior leaflet has dropped out, and as the transducer is tilted further superiorly, the posterior wall of the left atrium replaces that of the left

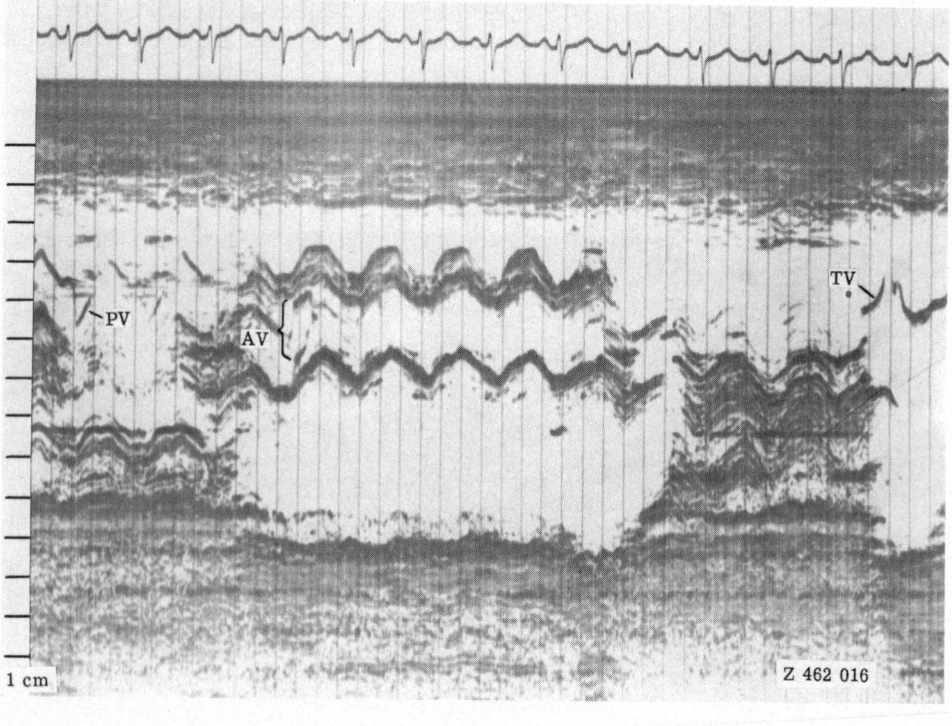

FIGURE 5–7 M-mode scan recording echoes from a pulmonic valve (PV), aortic valve (AV), and tricuspid valve (TV). (From Feigenbaum, H.: Echocardiography. 2nd ed. Philadelphia, Lea and Febiger, 1976.)

ventricle. In position 4, echoes from the aorta and the body of the left atrium are recorded, and echoes from the aortic valve leaflets are apparent in the last two cardiac cycles. These leaflets appear as thin echoes and form a box-like configuration during ventricular systole.

Figure 5–7 shows echoes from the aorta and aortic valve; by tilting the transducer medially from the aortic valve, it is possible to record the anterior leaflet of the tricuspid valve, which is similar in appearance to the recording from the anterior leaflet of the mitral valve. When the transducer is directed superiorly and laterally from the aortic valve, a posterior leaflet of the pulmonary valve can be recorded (Fig. 5–7).

Two-Dimensional Echocardiography

M-mode echocardiography, the original ultrasonic technique developed for cardiac examination, has proved to be extremely valuable, especially in recording the motion of cardiac structures parallel to the ultrasonic beam. However, there are significant limitations to this method of examination; it does not permit effective evaluation of the shape of cardiac structures nor can it depict lateral motion, i.e., motion perpendicular to the ultrasonic beam. Real-time, cross-sectional, or two-dimensional echocardiography, officially designated two-dimensional echocardiography by the American Society of Echocardiography, has become popular because it provides information not available in M-mode echocardiography. By moving the ultrasonic beam very rapidly, two-dimensional echocardiography can depict cardiac shape and lateral motion, which are otherwise difficult or impossible to evaluate with M-mode echocardiography. Such recordings are displayed on movie film or videotape.

The principle of two-dimensional or cross-sectional echocardiography is depicted in Figure 5–8, in which the object of interest is a sphere on a wire which oscillates in a liquid medium. An M-mode examination of such an object would record the motion with great accuracy at a rapid sampling rate. However, as the ball moved upward it would leave the path of the stationary ultrasonic beam, and its image would therefore not be recorded during those instants. The M-mode tracing would record only that component of the motion that is parallel to the ultrasonic beam and obviously only while the ball is within the path of the beam. Thus, the full excursion would not be appreciated, and the shape of the object could not be recognized. However, if the ultrasonic beam were to move rapidly through an angle, a sector scan of the moving sphere would be obtained (Fig. 5–8*B*).

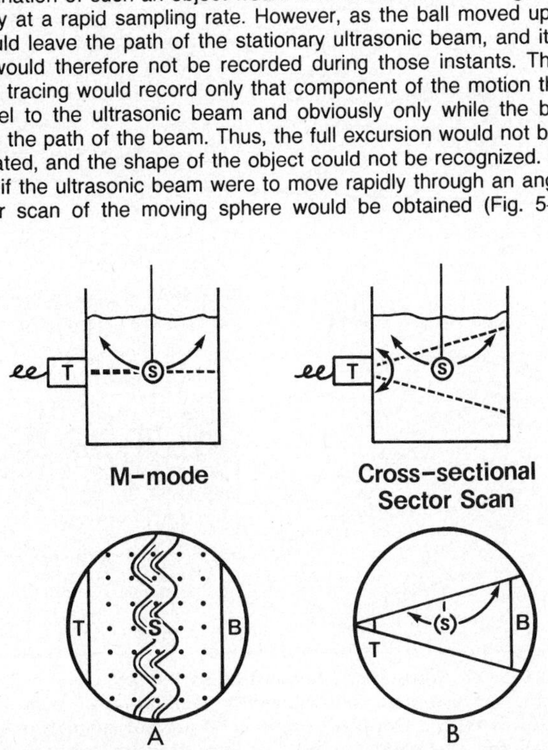

FIGURE 5–8 Diagrams demonstrating how the M-mode and cross-sectional examinations would record the motion of a moving sphere (S) in a beaker of water. The M-mode recording would show a series of wavy lines as the moving ball cuts across the ultrasonic beam (*A*). The cross-sectional recording would show a spatially correct spherical object moving within the pie-shaped sector image (*B*).

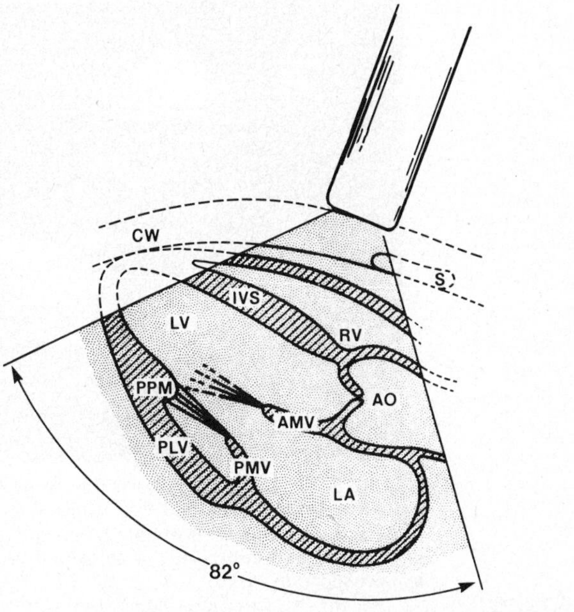

FIGURE 5–9 Diagram showing how to obtain a cross-sectional or two-dimensional image of the heart parallel to the long axis of the left ventricle. CW = chest wall. Other abbreviations as in Figure 5–4.

Each of the B-mode lines is laid down in a position on the oscilloscope which reflects the position of the ultrasonic beam. As the beam is directed upward, the echocardiographic B-mode lines would be laid down at a similar angle on the oscilloscope. Spatial orientation is now introduced into the recording and a reasonable facsimile of the spherical object becomes evident. In addition, almost the entire pendular motion of the ball can be appreciated by recording motion that is lateral as well as perpendicular to the ultrasonic beam. One disadvantage of this method is that the recording is on videotape, and the sampling rate therefore is usually reduced by 30 to 60 frames/second or less rather than the 1000 impulses/second recorded with the M-mode examination.

The type of examination diagrammed in Figure 5–8*B* is termed a "real-time, cross-sectional, or two-dimensional sector scan." The tip of the transducer is essentially stationary, and the beam can be moved in an arc, mechanically by oscillating a single transducer or by rotating a series of transducers.[4,5] The ultrasound can also be steered electronically using the so-called *phased array* principle, in which multiple ultrasonic elements are utilized to make up the beam and in which the firing sequence of the elements is controlled.[6] A computer or microprocessor is necessary to control the firing of the elements and the direction of the beam. There are many technical differences between a mechanical sector scanner and a phased array scanner.[2,7] The technology in two-dimensional echocardiography is still evolving, so the advantages and disadvantages of the two systems are constantly changing. Irrespective of which type of sector scanner one uses, the two-dimensional images are essentially similar. As might be anticipated, the phased-array scanners are generally more expensive than the mechanical scanners.

Since the patient is usually examined in the recumbent position, as with M-mode echocardiography, the standard orientation for two-dimensional echocardiography is for the transducer and anterior chest wall to be displayed at the top of the picture. Figure 5–9 shows a diagram of how a two-dimensional image of the heart might be obtained, and in Figure 5–10 are shown two individual frames representing stop-action sequences from a videotape recording of a normal heart in which the mitral and aortic valves and parts of the left ventricle, left atrium, and aorta are imaged. It must be recalled that all these structures do not lie in the same plane. For example, it is not ordinarily possible to include both the long axis of the apex and the aorta in a single picture; this is not the case with angiography. Since these two-dimensional echograms are displayed on videotape, they superficially resemble cineangiocardiograms. However, the latter display intracavitary contrast material, while the two-dimensional images represent individual "slices" of the heart.

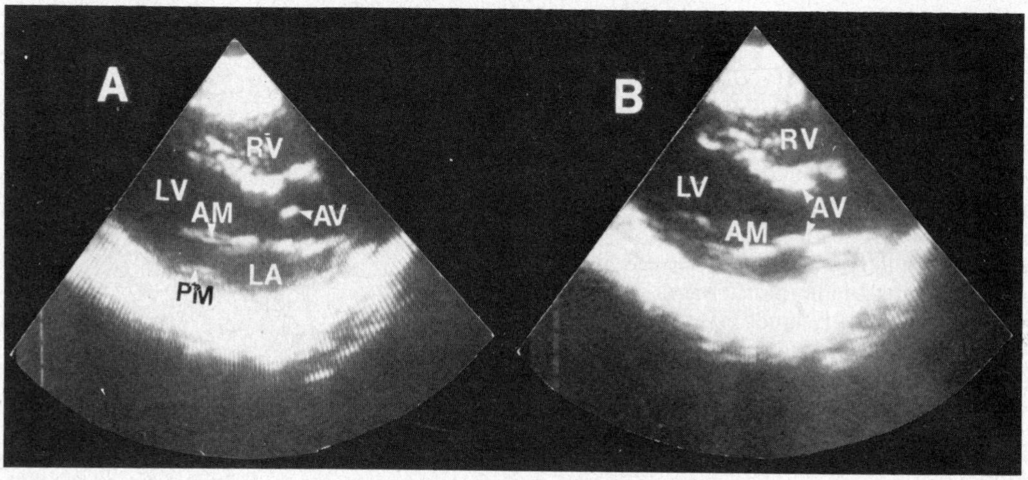

FIGURE 5–10 Long-axis cross-sectional echographic images of the left ventricle (LV), right ventricle (RV), mitral valve, aortic valve, and left atrium (LA) during diastole (*A*) and systole (*B*). During diastole the anterior (AM) and posterior (PM) mitral leaflets are apart and the aortic valve leaflets (AV) come together as a single echo in the midportion of the aorta (*A*). With systole, the mitral leaflets come together and the aortic valve leaflets separate (*B*).

Doppler Echocardiography

According to the Doppler principle, when an ultrasonic wave is reflected from a moving object, the frequency of the reflected ultrasound is altered and the difference in frequency between the ultrasound emitted and that received depends on the velocity of the reflecting interface and the angle at which the beam strikes the object. This change in frequency is often referred to as the *Doppler shift*. In order to calculate the actual velocity, the angle which the object in question makes with respect to the ultrasonic beam must be known. Although the moving target could be a cardiac valve or wall, Doppler ultrasound is used most often to examine the velocity of blood flow, the ultrasonic energy being reflected by the red blood cells. Since the frequency difference (Doppler shift) coming from the stream of moving blood is in the audible range, the frequency of which is related to the velocity of the moving object, the ultrasound energy is sent in a continuous wave and is therefore commonly called *continuous wave* or *CW Doppler*.

Doppler ultrasound has been used primarily to evaluate blood flow in superficial arteries and veins[8–11] and has proved to be useful in detecting obstructions in peripheral arteries[11] and venous thrombosis.[10] Recording the velocity of blood flow in the central aorta or major central arteries, such as the common carotid artery, has been used to reflect changes in aortic blood flow,[12–17] but *absolute* measurements of blood flow by this technique are quite difficult to accomplish. The pattern of blood flow in the central arteries is altered in conditions such as hypertrophic obstructive cardiomyopathy (HOCM)[18,19] and aortic regurgitation[20,21]; reverse flow during diastole has been noted in the latter, and it has been suggested that a semiquantitative estimate of the regurgitant fraction can be derived from a ratio of the reverse to the forward flow velocity on the Doppler recording.

Instrumentation has become available that combines the Doppler principle with standard pulsed ultrasound used for cardiac imaging.[22,23] By using pulsed instead of continuous wave ultrasound, it is now possible both to image the heart and to obtain a Doppler signal from some area within it.[24] Figure 5–11 demonstrates how a pulsed Doppler examination could be obtained from the root of the aorta. By gating the Doppler sample in the root of the aorta either on an M-mode or a two-dimensional echocardiogram, one will receive the Doppler signal from that area of the heart. There are three principal techniques for recording the resultant Doppler signal.[22] Since the returning sound is in the audible range, one will hear the Doppler shift during the examination. One can make the diagnosis by interpreting the sound generated from the Doppler examination either in real time during the actual examination or from an audio tape recording. There are also two methods of recording the Doppler signal on hard copy. The first technique utilizes the "time-interval histogram."[25,26] By using a zero-crossing technique to analyze the frequencies of the returning sound, such a recording plots the frequencies of the sound against time. The direction of the flow is also indicated on the tracing; flow toward the transducer is plotted above the baseline and flow away from the transducer below the baseline. This particular technique is

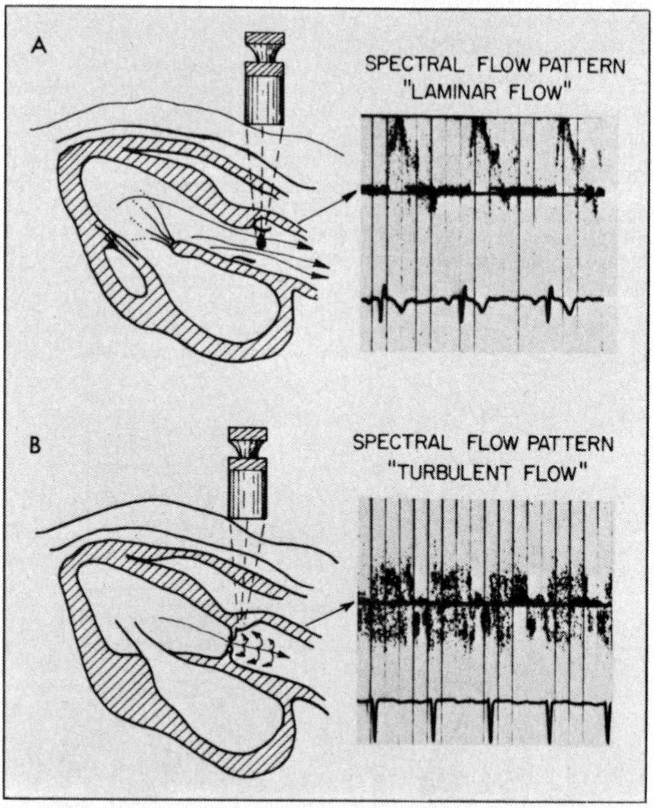

FIGURE 5–11 Illustration demonstrating the principle of how a time-interval histogram can distinguish "laminar flow" from "turbulent flow." With a Doppler sample in an area of laminar or normal flow, all dots that comprise the time interval histogram are close together, since all velocities at a given instant are relatively equal (*A*). With turbulent or disturbed flow (*B*) there are multiple velocities and directions of flow, and thus the Doppler signals are scattered above and below the baseline. (From Baker, D.W., Rubenstein, S.A., and Lorch, G.S.: Pulsed Doppler echocardiography: Principles and applications. Am. J. Med. *63*:69, 1977).

very useful in differentiating normal or "laminar flow" from abnormal or "turbulent or disturbed flow." Figure 5–11 demonstrates the time-interval histogram of laminar flow (*A*) and turbulent flow (*B*). If the sampling volume is recording an area of laminar blood flow, all returning frequencies are relatively homogeneous and the dots being plotted are close together. The recording would indicate that all the blood being sampled is moving in the same direction and at approximately the same frequencies. If the sampling volume is in an area of turbulent or disturbed flow, then a different time-interval histogram pattern is recorded. There will be multiple Doppler signals of differing frequencies and directions. Thus, on the time-interval histogram one sees multiple dots displayed, indicating variations in both frequency and direction. The ability to distinguish laminar from turbulent blood flow is one of the principal diagnostic uses for Doppler echocardiography.

Figure 5–12 is a Doppler echocardiographic recording of a patient with rheumatic mitral regurgitation. The M-mode echocardiogram is seen in the upper half of the recording. The site of the sample volume is indicated by a line on the M-mode tracing. The time-interval histogram is in the lower half of the recording. During systole the mitral regurgitant jet generates a turbulent signal with multiple frequencies, most of which are moving away from the transducer (arrow).

Because of the spatial orientation inherent in two-dimensional echocardiography, it is advantageous to obtain the Doppler signal by first placing the Doppler sampling volume on the two-dimensional echocardiogram.

There are many limitations to the time-interval histogram technique for recording the Doppler signal.[22,26] The principal advance has been to record a fast Fourier tracing of the Doppler signal. This method of analyzing the signal is far more accurate with regard to correct measurement of velocity recorded from the moving column of blood. All of the newer Doppler instruments have switched to some form of Fourier analysis of the Doppler signal. Figure 5–13 demonstrates a fast Fourier display of the Doppler signal from a patient with tricuspid regurgitation. The disturbed or turbulent flow (arrow) is recorded on this Doppler echocardiogram. The sampling volume (Doppler probe) is displayed on the M-mode echocardiogram posterior to the tricuspid valve (TV).

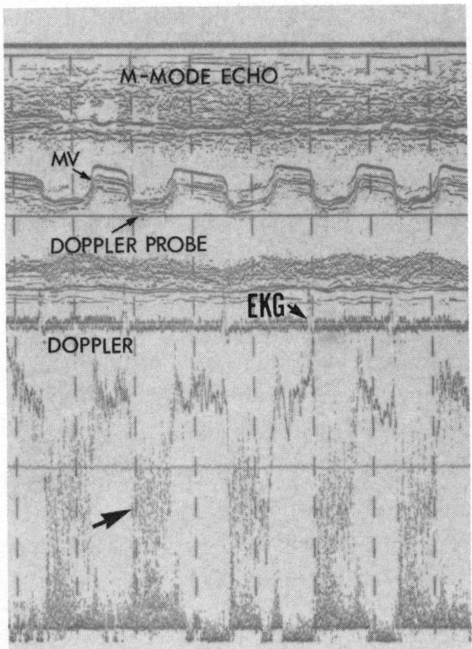

FIGURE 5–12 Doppler echocardiographic study of a patient with rheumatic mitral stenosis and insufficiency. The Doppler probe or sampling site is within the left atrium behind the mitral valve (MV). The Doppler signal generated by the regurgitant blood leaking into the left atrium can be as seen as a band of downward displaced dots on the Doppler tracing (arrow). The line in the middle of the Doppler tracing is a baseline or zero reference.

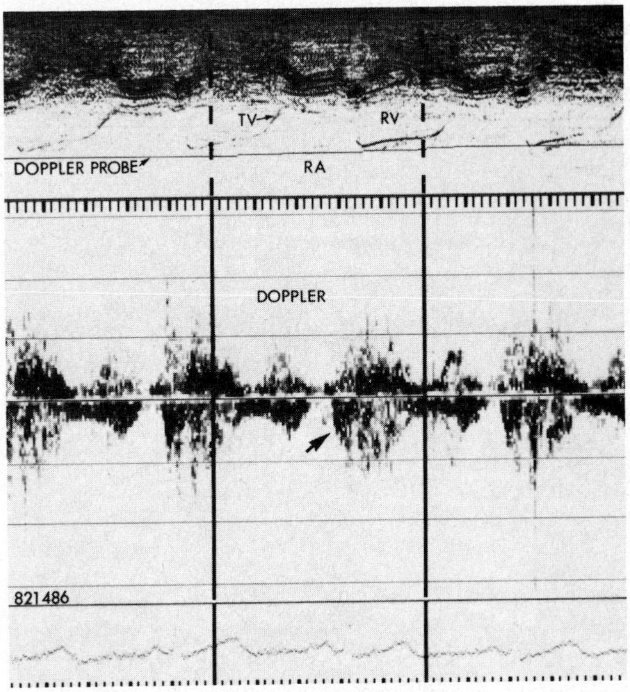

FIGURE 5–13 Doppler echocardiographic examination of a patient with tricuspid regurgitation using a fast Fourier recording of the Doppler signal. The disturbed or turbulent flow (arrow) is readily recognized. The Doppler probe is located within the right atrium (RA) posterior to the tricuspid valve (TV). RV = right ventricle.

Although the popularity of Doppler echocardiography has been increasing rapidly, there are still many difficulties with this type of examination.[22] Pulsed Doppler has a limitation in the maximum velocity that can be recorded with this technique. If the velocity is so great that the frequency of the returning sound wave is higher than the sampling rate of the pulsed Doppler, then "aliasing" will occur whereby the system will be unable to identify the frequency of the returning sound. Continuous-wave ultrasound does not have this problem, but it is difficult to localize the Doppler signal using continuous ultrasound. There are many continuing attempts to quantitate the Doppler signal both for blood flow and for quantitation of abnormal blood flow patterns, but all of these techniques still have their difficulties. It is possible to use multiple Doppler gates or sampling sites to display the blood flow patterns directly on the M-mode recording.[27] It is also theoretically possible that the Doppler blood flow patterns could be displayed on the two-dimensional echocardiogram.[28] However, these multiple gating Doppler techniques are still investigational.

Another limitation of pulsed Doppler echocardiography is that the depth of the examination is limited by the available frequency. With the frequency in the range of 3.0 to 3.5 MHz, it is difficult to obtain a Doppler signal from distances beyond 12 or 13 cm from the transducers. The pulse repetition rate must be reduced when examining distances this far from the transducer, and the ability to record high velocity flow is lost.

Contrast Echocardiography

Ultrasound is an extremely sensitive detector of intravascular bubbles. The injection of almost any liquid into the intravascular spaces will introduce many microbubbles that appear as a cloud of echoes on the echocardiogram. Figure 5–14 demonstrates an M-mode echocardiogram of a patient with a right-to-left shunt at the ventricular level. The contrast can be seen initially in the right ventricle. It then traverses the interventricular septum and appears in the left ventricle. As will be noted later, this technique is obviously a sensitive method of detecting right-to-left shunts. The contrast agents that have been used include the patient's blood, saline, dextrose in water, and indocyanine green dye.[29-31] In all cases the contrast effect originates from suspended microbubbles in the fluid. Injection of small quantities of carbon dioxide gas have also been used for contrast

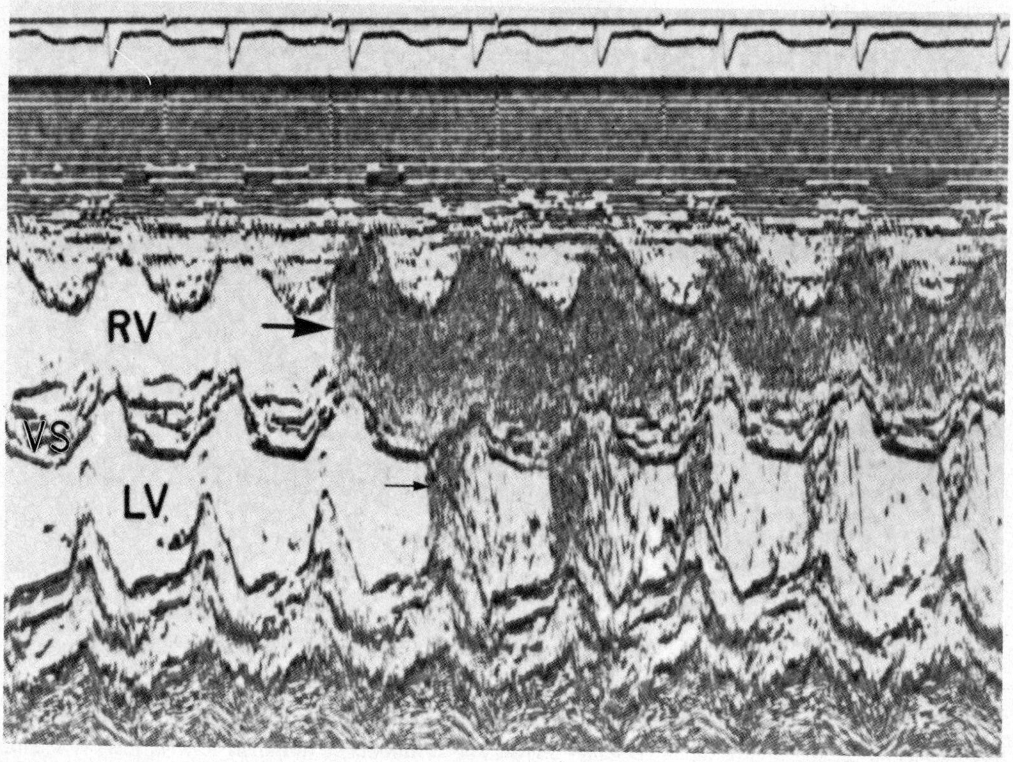

FIGURE 5–14 A contrast M-mode echocardiogram in a patient with a right-to-left shunt at the ventricular level. The dark mass of echoes from the injected contrast (large arrow) is initially seen in the right ventricular cavity (RV) and next is seen (small arrow) in the left ventricle (LV) above the mitral valve. Normally the contrast should not appear on the left side of the heart at all. If the shunt were at the atrial level, contrast would appear in the left and right ventricles simultaneously and would be seen posterior to the mitral valve. VS = ventricular septum. (From Seward, J. B., et al.: Echocardiographic contrast studies: Initial experience. Mayo Clin. Proc. *50*: 163, 1975.)

echocardiography.[32] Hydrogen peroxide will give a strong contrast effect by producing tiny intravascular bubbles of oxygen.[33] Commercially manufactured microbubbles may be available soon. The potential clinical uses for contrast echocardiography are numerous. There is much ongoing research in this area.

Technical Limitations

There are many technical difficulties inherent in ultrasound examinations of the heart. The principal problem is posed by the poor transmission of ultrasound through bony structures or through air-containing lungs, and the examiner must try to avoid these structures. A variety of techniques have been developed to circumvent this problem. The subxiphoid or subcostal examination was one of the first approaches shown to be useful, especially in patients with hyperinflated lungs and a low diaphragm.[34] Placing the transducer at the cardiac apex has also proved to be useful[35-37]; placing it into the suprasternal notch also avoids the lungs and bony thorax and allows imaging of the arch of the aorta, the left pulmonary artery, and the left atrium.[38] When this view is enlarged using the two-dimensional technique, a larger portion of the arch of the aorta, some of the arch vessels, and the descending aorta can be visualized.[39-40]

Despite improvements in echocardiographic techniques and instrumentation, there are still some patients in whom it is difficult to record satisfactory echocardiograms.[41] Patients with large, thick chest walls and small hearts represent the most difficult patients to examine, and chest deformities can occasionally be troublesome. The success rate for technically satisfactory echocardiograms is usually highest in younger patients. Another problem is that the echoes are recorded most effectively if the transducer is perpendicular or almost perpendicular to the structure in question. Small changes in angulation can decrease the quality of the recording. As a result, the examiner must be able to angle the probe as accurately as possible. Whether the heart is examined with a single-dimensional probe, as with M-mode echocardiography, or with two-dimensional device, proper direction of the ultrasonic beam is critical. Echocardiographic controls can also influence the image profoundly, and the operator must be skilled to make certain that artifacts and distortions are not introduced through improper use of the gain controls. Thus, although the echocardiographic examination is quite simple and painless for the patient, it can be extremely difficult to perform, so that a well-trained individual is required for both the examination and the interpretation of results.

EXAMINATION OF THE NORMAL HEART

M-Mode Echocardiogram

Echocardiograms can be extremely confusing to physicians not familiar with this technique. For example, many physicians are not aware of the fact that the mitral valve closes in mid-diastole, and thus the fact that the motion of its anterior leaflet resembles the letter "M" in diastole is not perfectly obvious. However, with a thorough knowledge of cardiac anatomy, physiology, and hemodynamics, it is not difficult to understand how an M-mode echocardiographic tracing is recorded and how the various structures should appear on such a recording. Figure 5–15 *A* shows an M-mode scan that encompasses the full length of the mitral valve apparatus. The echoes from this structure are striking and are readily identified. The anterior leaflet of the mitral valve shows a downward motion in mid-diastole, and the characteristic "M" pattern is recorded. The posterior mitral leaflet is essentially a mirror-image of the anterior leaflet, except the amplitude of its motion is less.

Figure 5–15*B* is an M-mode examination of a normal mitral valve. The end of systole, just prior to the opening of the valve, is designated "D." The maximum excursion of the anterior leaflets is designated "E" and the nadir of the initial diastolic closing wave "F." The diastolic closing rate, or the "E to F slope," is indicated by the line drawn on Figure 5–15*B*. This slope is frequently not straight but curved. With atrial systole, blood is propelled through the mitral orifice and the leaflets reopen. The peak of this reopening of the mitral valve is designated "A"; with atrial relaxation, the valve begins to close again. Ventricular systole begins during the downward slope of the mitral leaflet and may produce a slight interruption of the closure wave,

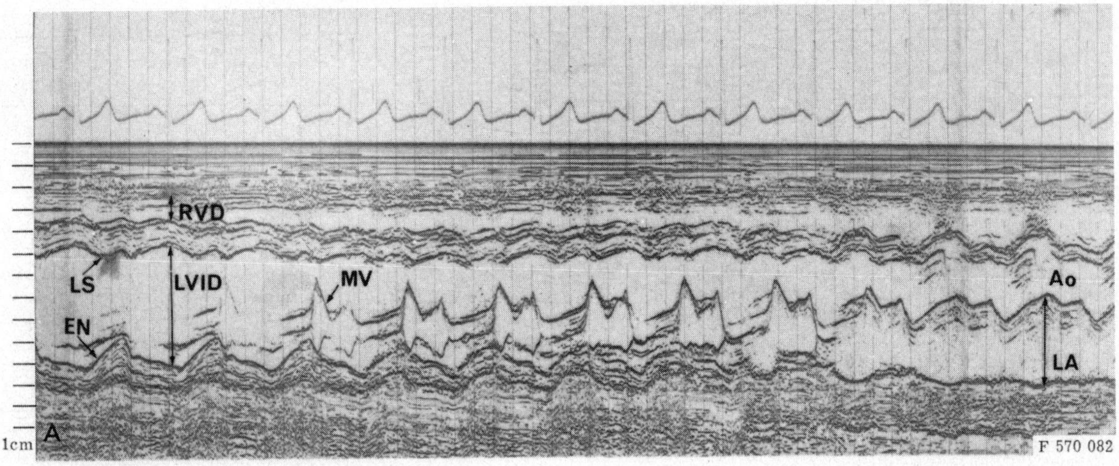

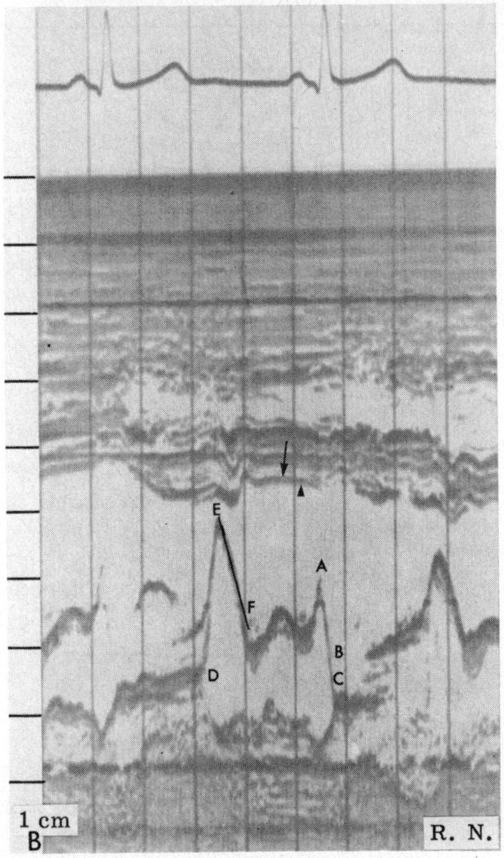

FIGURE 5–15 *A*, M-mode scan from the left ventricle to the aorta (AO) and left atrium (LA) in a normal subject. RVD = right ventricular dimension. LVID = left ventricular internal dimension, LS = left septal echoes, EN = posterior left ventricular endocardial echoes, MV = mitral valve. (From Chang, S.: M-mode Echocardiographic Techniques and Pattern Recognition. Philadelphia, Lea and Febiger, 1976.)

B, M-mode echocardiogram of a normal mitral valve. The letters A through F denote various portions of the anterior leaflet motion. The arrow indicates the leading edge of the echo from the left side of the interventricular septum; the arrowhead denotes the trailing edge of that echo (From Feigenbaum, H.: Echocardiography. 2nd ed. Philadelphia, Lea and Febiger, 1976.)

at point "B." (This is not always evident and is not so in Figure 5–15*B*.) Complete closure occurs following the onset of ventricular systole at "C."

The left ventricular cavity is bordered by the interventricular septum anteriorly and the posterior left ventricular wall posteriorly. Both walls move toward each other during systole, so that the diameter of the cavity decreases with systole. Both walls are approximately 1 cm thick in diastole, and the thickness increases during systole. A small portion of the right ventricular cavity lies anterior to the interventricular septum, and the anterior wall of the right ventricle is shown at the top of the tracing; the latter structure cannot always be imaged, especialy in adults.

As the ultrasonic beam is swept superiorly and medially toward the base of the heart, the posterior leaflet of the mitral valve drops out and the posterior left atrial wall is seen to lie behind the anterior leaflet of the mitral valve. At the junction between the left atrium and ventricle the ultrasonic beam traverses both chambers during a given cardiac cycle. Because the atrioventricular junction moves in a superoinferior direction during each cycle, the stationary ultrasonic beam may record the left atrial wall during systole and the left ventricular wall during diastole. As the beam is directed more superiorly into the body of the left atrium, the relatively stationary posterior wall of the left atrium is imaged. The aorta, represented by two parallel moving echoes which move anteriorly during systole and posteriorly during diastole, lies anterior to the left atrium. The anterior wall of the aorta is in continuity with the echoes from the interventricular septum, and the posterior wall of the aorta is in continuity with the echoes of the anterior leaflet of the mitral valve. The aortic valve leaflets

TABLE 5–1 NORMAL VALUES OF ECHOCARDIOGRAPHIC MEASUREMENTS IN ADULTS

	Range (cm)	Mean (cm)	Number of Subjects
Age (years)	13 to 54	26	134
Body surface area (M^2)	1.45 to 2.22	1.8	130
RVD—flat	0.7 to 2.3	1.5	84
RVD—left lateral	0.9 to 2.6	1.7	83
LVID—flat	3.7 to 5.6	4.7	82
LVID—left lateral	3.5 to 5.7	4.7	81
Posterior LV wall thickness	0.6 to 1.1	0.9	137
Posterior LV wall amplitude	0.9 to 1.4	1.2	48
IVS wall thickness	0.6 to 1.1	0.9	137
Mid IVS amplitude	0.3 to 0.8	0.5	10
Apical IVS amplitude	0.5 to 1.2	0.7	38
Left atrial dimension	1.9 to 4.0	2.9	133
Aortic root dimension	2.0 to 3.7	2.7	121
Aortic cusps' separation	1.5 to 2.6	1.9	93
Percentage of fractional shortening*	34% to 44%	36%	20%
Mean rate of circumferential shortening (Vcf),** or mean normalized shortening velocity	1.02 to 1.94 circ/sec	1.3 circ/sec	38

$* \ \frac{\text{LVIDd} - \text{LVIDs}}{\text{LVIDd}}$ $** \ \frac{\text{LVIDd} - \text{LVIDs}}{\text{LVIDd} \times \text{Ejection time}}$

RVD = Right ventricular dimension
LVID = Left ventricular internal dimension; d = end diastole; s = end systole
LV = Left ventricle
IVS = Interventricular septum

lie within the root of the aorta; only the anterior aortic valve leaflet is recorded in Figure 5–15, although both valve leaflets are better visualized in Figure 5–6. Two of the leaflets, probably the right coronary leaflet and the noncoronary leaflet, make up the boxlike configuration observed during systole as the aortic valve opens. As the leaflets come together in diastole a *single* echo is commonly recorded.

M-Mode Echocardiographic Measurements

Numerous measurements have been suggested for M-mode echocardiography. Figure 5–16 demonstrates some of the measurements that can be obtained from an M-mode echocardiogram. Most of these measurements involve the left ventricle, the aortic root, and the left atrium. The American Society of Echocardiography has standardized the common measurements used in M-mode echocardiography.[42] A key consideration in these measurements is that the leading edge of an echo, i.e., that portion of the echo closest to the transducer, is more readily identified and precisely measured than is the trailing edge. The arrow in Figure 5–15*B* denotes the leading edge of the echo from the left side of the interventricular septum, while the arrowhead in the same figure indicates the trailing edge. The precise location of the leading edge of an echo is easily accomplished and involves little error; however, the width of an individual echo, and therefore the identification of the trailing edge, varies depending on how the signal is processed in an individual instrument. Also, because of variations in instruments, the onset of the QRS complex in standard lead II is taken as denoting the end of diastole. The American Society of Echocardiography also recommends that the M-mode measurements be averaged from three or four cardiac cycles and preferably at end-expiration. The timing and location of the various measurements are indicated in Figure 5–16. The left ventricular dimension should be taken just beyond the mitral valve or at

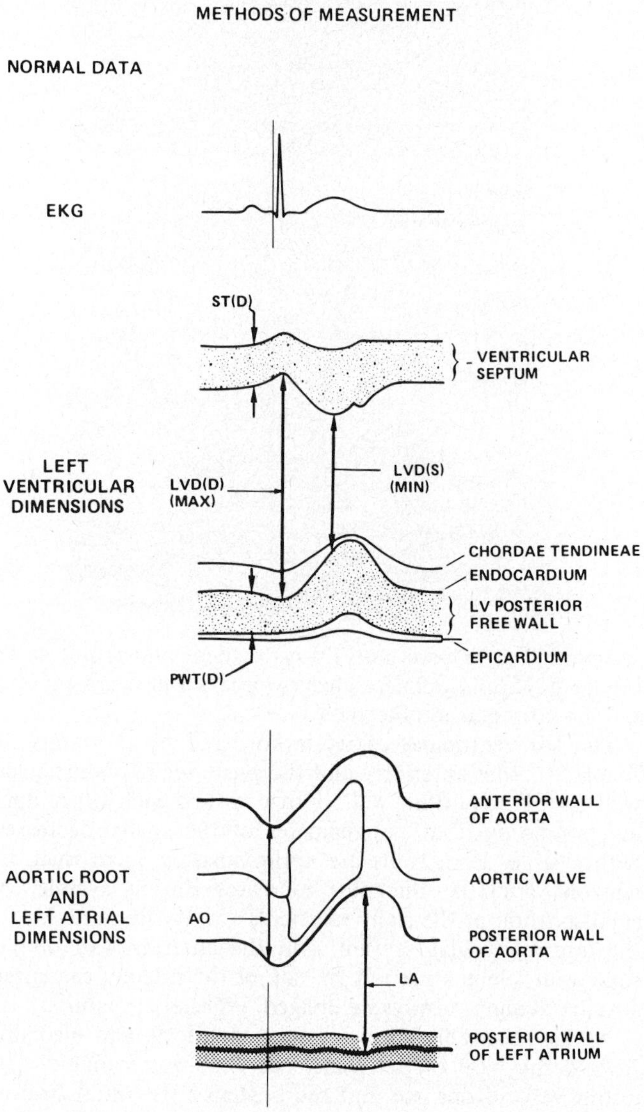

FIGURE 5–16 Methods for obtaining M-mode echocardiographic measurements. ST(D) = diastolic septal thickness; LVD(D) and LVD(S) = diastolic and systolic left ventricular diameter; PWT(D) = diastolic posterior wall thickness; AO = aorta; LA = left atrium. (From Henry, W.L., Gardin, J.M., and Ware, J.H.: Echocardiographic measurements in normal subjects from infancy to old age. Circulation *62*:1054, 1980.)

the chordae tendineae. In infants and young children, left ventricular dimensions are probably best recorded at the level of the mitral valve. The end-diastolic dimension is taken at the onset of the QRS complex, while end-systolic measurement is obtained at the instant of maximum posterior (downward) position of the interventricular septum, which usually precedes the peak anterior (upward) position of the posterior left ventricular wall. When septal motion is abnormal, the instant of peak upward position of the posterior ventricular endocardium may be taken at end-systole. A true right ventricular dimension can be obtained only when the anterior right ventricular wall is well delineated; otherwise, only an estimate of this dimension can be made.

Wall thickness is also measured from leading edge to leading edge, and the width of the interventricular septum is the distance from the anterior surface of the right to the anterior surface of the left septal echo. The thickness of the posterior left ventricular wall is measured from the anterior surface of the posterior left ventricular endocardial echo to that from the anterior surface of the posterior left ventricular epicardium.

Although mitral valve measurements have been made since the onset of echocardiography in the 1950's, these measurements are of limited value. The closing velocity or E to F slope is very non-specific and has relatively little diagnostic value. The amplitude of excursion of the mitral valve is still used for judging pliability of the valve. The American Society of Echocardiography decided that the D to E amplitude should be used to judge the excursion of the mitral valve rather than the C to E amplitude as recommended by some investigators (Fig. 5–15B).

Table 5–1 provides some normal values for commonly used M-mode echocardiographic measurements. These data represent approximations and do not conform in all instances to the criteria developed by the American Society of Echocardiography. Nor do they take into account that some changes in measurements occur during aging.[43] Normal values for children can be quite complex. The reader is encouraged to refer to some of the references, since more exhaustive normal values have been obtained.[2]

Two-Dimensional Echocardiographic Views

One could essentially obtain an infinite number of slices of the heart using two-dimensional echocardiography. In the early development of this technique investigators were utilizing many different approaches in examining the heart with this ultrasonic technique.[44] The American Society of Echocardiography has attempted to standardize and simplify the many two-dimensional examinations described.[45] The Society felt that all views could be categorized into three orthogonal planes, as illustrated in Figure 5–17. These planes are the long-axis, short-axis, and four-chamber. The long-axis plane is the imaging plane that transects the heart perpendicular to the dorsal and ventral surfaces of the body and parallel to the long axis of the heart. The plane transecting the heart perpendicular to the dorsal and ventral surfaces of the body, but perpendicular to the long axis of the heart, is defined as the short-axis plane. The plane that transects the heart approximately parallel to the dorsal and ventral surfaces of the body is referred to as the four-chamber plane. It should be emphasized that these views or planes are with reference to the heart and not to the thorax or body.

These ultrasonic planes or views can be obtained from more than one transducer location. Figure 5–18*A* demonstrates that one can obtain the long-axis view with the transducer in the apical position, in the parasternal position (left sternal border), or in the suprasternal notch. A short-axis view (Fig. 5–18*B*) cuts across the heart so that the left ventricle looks like a circle. The right ventricle can be seen curving around the left ventricle. Such an examination can be obtained with the transducer in the parasternal position or in the subcostal (subxiphoid) position. The four-chamber view is depicted in Figure 5–18*C*. Such a view permits the examination of all four cardiac chambers simultaneously. This type of examination can be obtained with the transducer over the cardiac apex or with the transducer in the subcostal position.

Table 5–2 lists the various two-dimensional echocardiographic examinations categorized according to the location of the transducer, the plane of the examination, and the cardiac structure being examined.

Figure 5–10 is an example of a parasternal long-axis examination

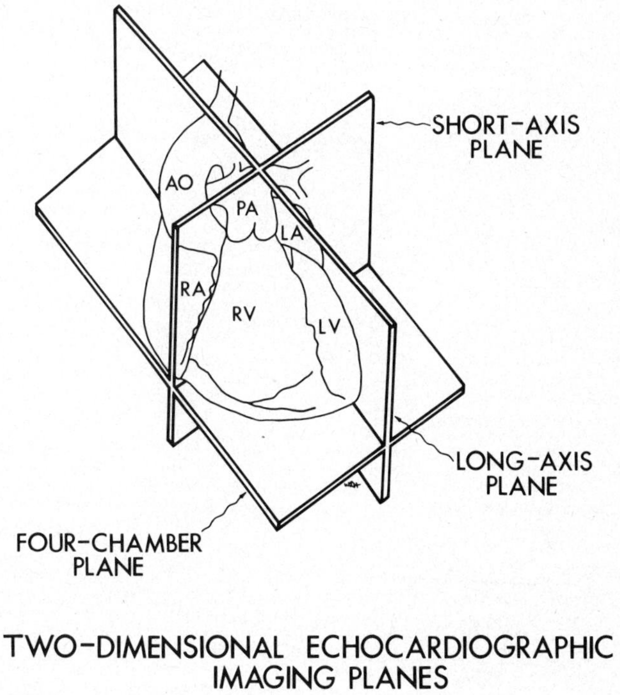

FIGURE 5–17 **Diagram demonstrating the three orthogonal planes for two-dimensional echocardiographic imaging. AO = aorta; PA = pulmonary artery; LA = left atrium; RA = right atrium; RV = right ventricle; LV = left ventricle. (From Henry, W.L., et al.: Report of the American Society of Echocardiography Nomenclature and Standards in Two-dimensional Echocardiography. Circulation *62*:212, 1980.)**

through the left ventricle. The right ventricle, right atrium, and tricuspid valve can also be recorded with the transducer in the parasternal position (Fig. 5–19). The plane of the transducer does not exactly fit either the long axis or short axis. However, the plane is closer to that of the long axis than that of the short axis and thus is categorized as a long-axis study. Figure 5–20 shows the right ventricular inflow tract and right atrium by way of such a parasternal examination.

TABLE 5–2 TWO-DIMENSIONAL ECHOCARDIOGRAPHIC EXAMINATION

Parasternal Approach
Long-axis plane
Root of aorta: aortic valve, left atrium, left ventricular outflow tract
Body of left ventricle, mitral valve
Left ventricular apex
Right ventricular inflow tract–tricuspid valve
Short-axis plane
Root of the aorta, aortic valve, pulmonary valve, tricuspid valve, right ventricular outflow tract, left atrium, pulmonary artery, coronary arteries
Left ventricle, mitral valve
Left ventricle, papillary muscles
Left ventricle, apex
Apical Approach
Four-chamber plane
Four chamber
Four chamber with aorta
Long-axis plane
Two chamber: left ventricle, left atrium
Two chamber with aorta
Subcostal Approach
Four-chamber plane
Short-axis plane
Left ventricle
Right ventricle
Inferior vena cava
Suprasternal Approach
Four-chamber plane: arch of aorta–descending aorta
Long-axis plane: arch of aorta–pulmonary artery, left atrium

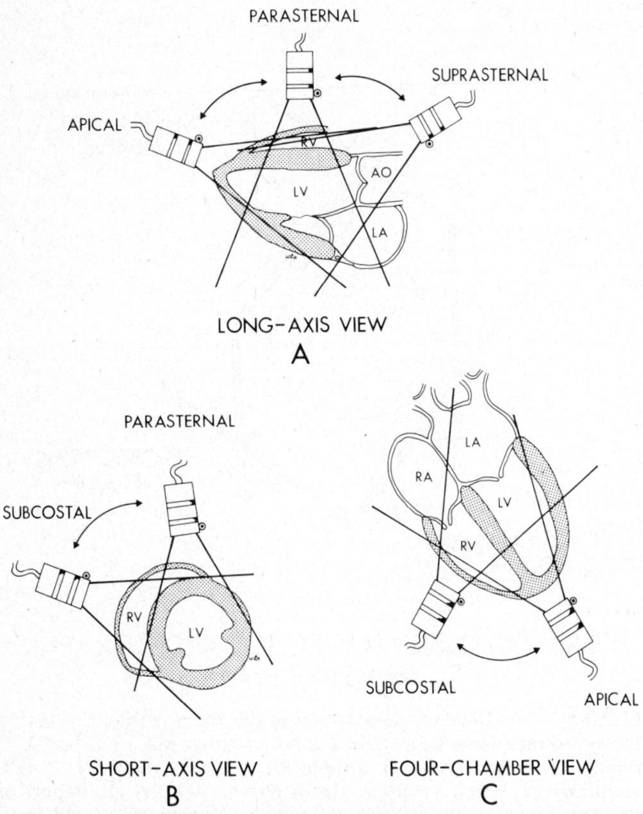

FIGURE 5–18 Diagrams demonstrating how one can obtain the various orthogonal planes from different transducer positions. (From Henry, W.L., et al.: Report of the American Society of Echocardiography Nomenclature and Standards in Two-dimensional Echocardiography. Circulation *62*:212, 1980.)

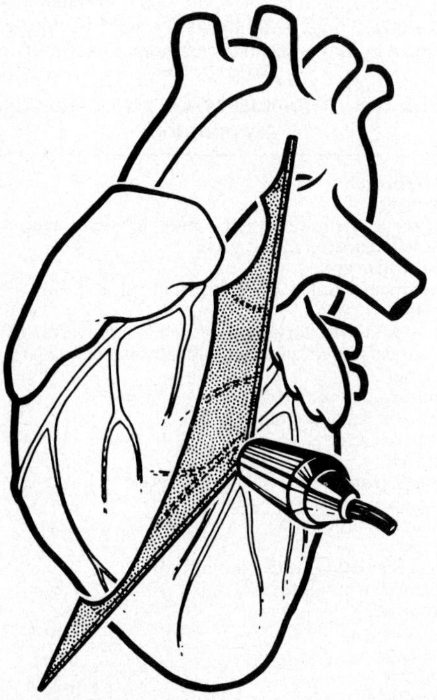

FIGURE 5–19 Transducer position for long-axis parasternal examination of the tricuspid valve, right atrium, and right ventricular inflow tract. (From Feigenbaum, H.: Echocardiography. 3rd ed. Philadelphia, Lea & Febiger, 1981.)

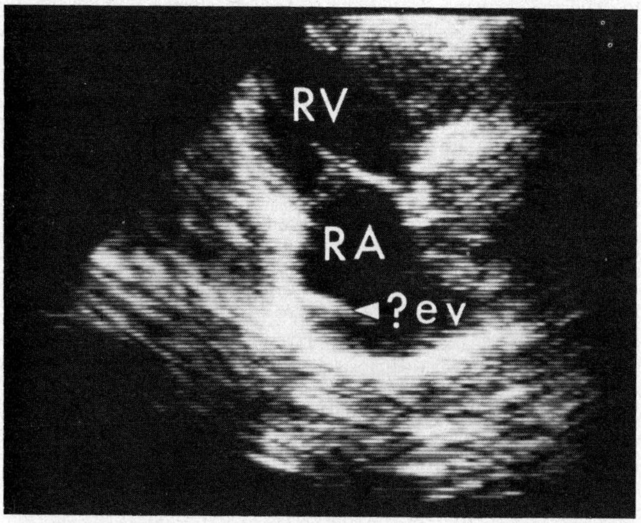

FIGURE 5–20 Two-dimensional echocardiogram of the right atrium (RA) and right ventricular inflow tract (RV). ev = eustachian valve. (From Feigenbaum, H.: Echocardiography. 3rd ed. Philadelphia, Lea & Febiger, 1981.)

Various short-axis examinations are diagrammatically illustrated in Figure 5–21. The short-axis views are commonly obtained at the level of the apex, the papillary muscles, the mitral valve, and the base of the heart. With slight variation in angulation the short-axis examination of the base of the heart can also record the pulmonary valve and the pulmonary artery with its bifurcation. It is also possible to use this examination to record the origins of the coronary arteries and the left atrial appendage.

Figure 5–22 diagrammatically illustrates the two commonly used two-dimensional echocardiographic views with the transducer placed at the cardiac apex. Plane 1 demonstrates the apical four-chamber view of the heart. Figure 5–23*A* shows an example of a four-chamber apical echocardiogram. It is possible to obtain an apical view of the long axis of the heart similar to that seen from the parasternal view. Such an examination would include portions of the right ventricle and the aorta. A more common examination is a so-called apical two-chamber view (Fig. 5–22, plane 2). This examination requires slight clockwise rotation of the transducer to avoid the right ventricle completely. Thus, one records only the left ventricle and the left atrium (Fig. 5–23*B*). This view can be considered a modification of an apical long-axis view.

The subcostal transducer location produces examinations roughly in the four-chamber and short-axis planes. The ultrasonic plane indicated in Figure 5–24*A* is similar to examining plane 1 in Figure 5–22. The resultant subcostal four-chamber echocardiogram appears in Figure 5–25*A*. Figures 5–24*B* and 5–25*B* show how the transducer can be rotated 90 degrees to provide a subcostal short-axis examination of the heart. The subcostal four-chamber view is particularly helpful in examining the interatrial and interventricular septa. By directing the transducer in a slightly modified short-axis examination, one can obtain an excellent view of the right side of the heart (Fig. 5–26*A*). The subcostal location also permits an opportunity to direct the ultrasonic beam through the inferior vena cava and hepatic vein[46] (Figs. 5–26*B* and 5–27).

The two examining planes with the transducer in the suprasternal notch are depicted in Figure 5–28. The ultrasonic view in Figure 5–28 *A* is roughly equivalent to that of a four-chamber plane, and the view in Figure 5–28*B* is somewhat comparable to that of the long-axis plane. However, it is probably best to orient the ultrasonic beam with regard to the arch of the aorta rather than to the heart, since one does not record much of the heart with the transducer in this position, especially in the adult. In addition, the planes are different than with the transducer at the apex or subcostal region. Thus, better terminology with regard to the examining plane from the suprasternal location would be parallel or perpendicular to the arch of the aorta. Figure 5–29 shows a suprasternal examination parallel to the arch of the aorta.

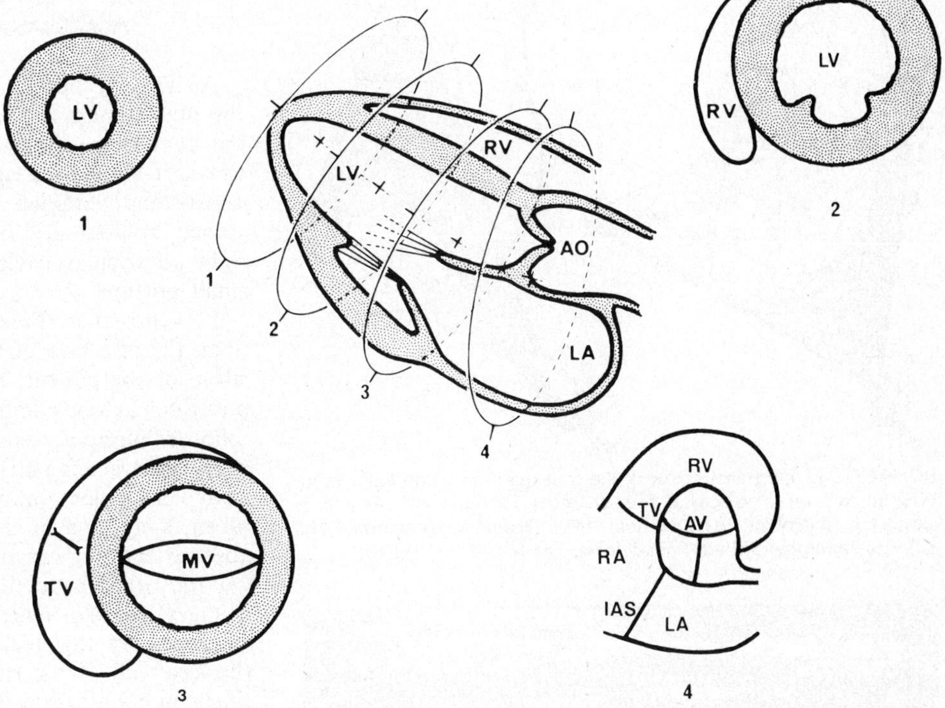

FIGURE 5–21 Diagrams showing how short-axis echographic cross-sectional images of the heart, which are perpendicular to the long axis of the left ventricle, are obtained. Diagram 1 shows a short-axis left ventricular echogram near the cardiac apex. Diagram 2 demonstrates part of the right ventricle (RV) and the circular left ventricular cavity (LV) at the level of the papillary muscles, which can be seen to bulge into the LV cavity. Diagram 3 is closer to the base of the heart and shows the left ventricle at the level of the mitral valve (MV). Diagram 4 shows a short-axis cross-section of the base of the heart with the aorta, aortic valve (AV), left atrium (LA), interatrial septum (IAS), right atrium (RA), tricuspid valve (TV), and right ventricular outflow tract (RV).

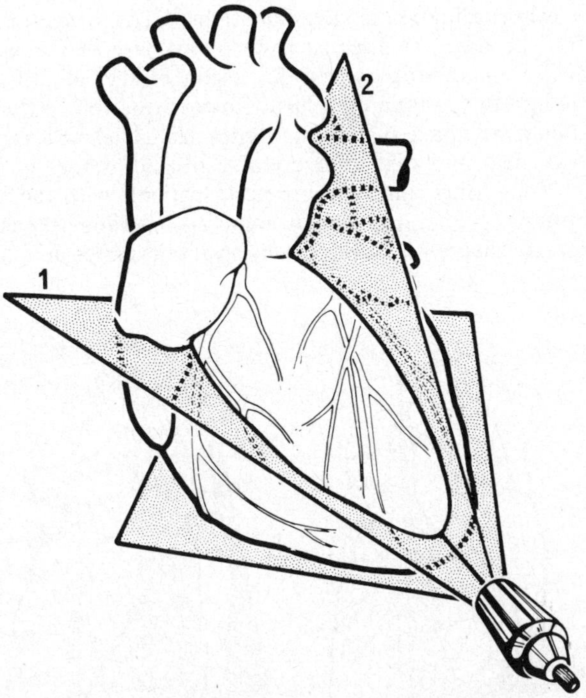

FIGURE 5–22 Transducer position and examining planes for apical two-dimensional echocardiograms. Plane 1 passes through the four chamber plane of the heart. Plane 2 represents the path of the ultrasonic beam for the two-chamber apical examination. (From Feigenbaum, H.: Echocardiography. 3rd ed. Philadelphia, Lea & Febiger, 1981.)

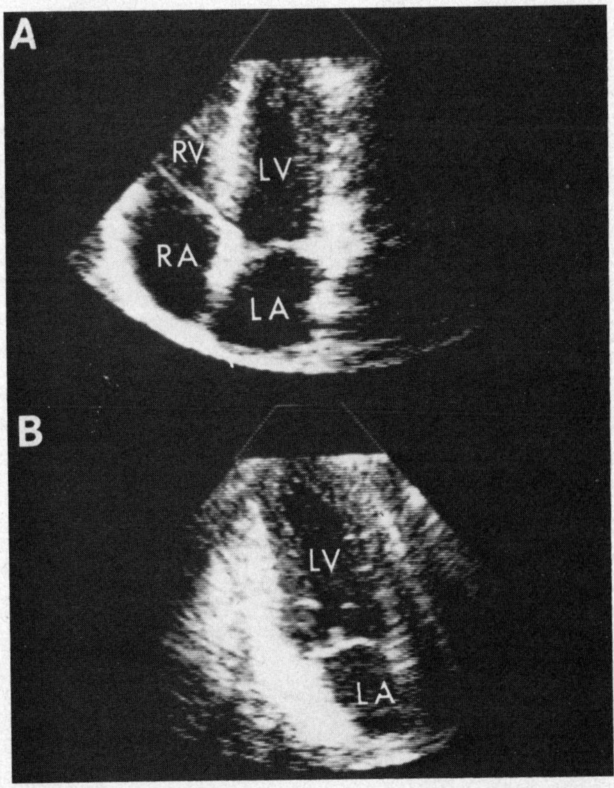

FIGURE 5–23 Four-chamber (*A*) and two-chamber (*B*) apical two-dimensional echocardiograms. RV = right ventricle; LV = left ventricle; RA = right atrium; and LA = left atrium. (From Feigenbaum, H.: Echocardiography. 3rd ed. Philadelphia, Lea & Febiger, 1981.)

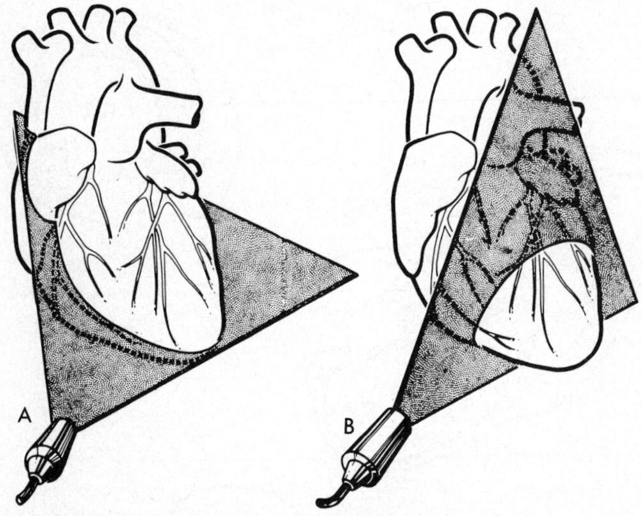

FIGURE 5–24 **Diagrams showing the transducer position and examining planes for a subcostal four-chamber examination (*A*) and a subcostal short-axis examination (*B*). (From Feigenbaum, H.: Echocardiography. 3rd ed. Philadelphia, Lea & Febiger, 1981.)**

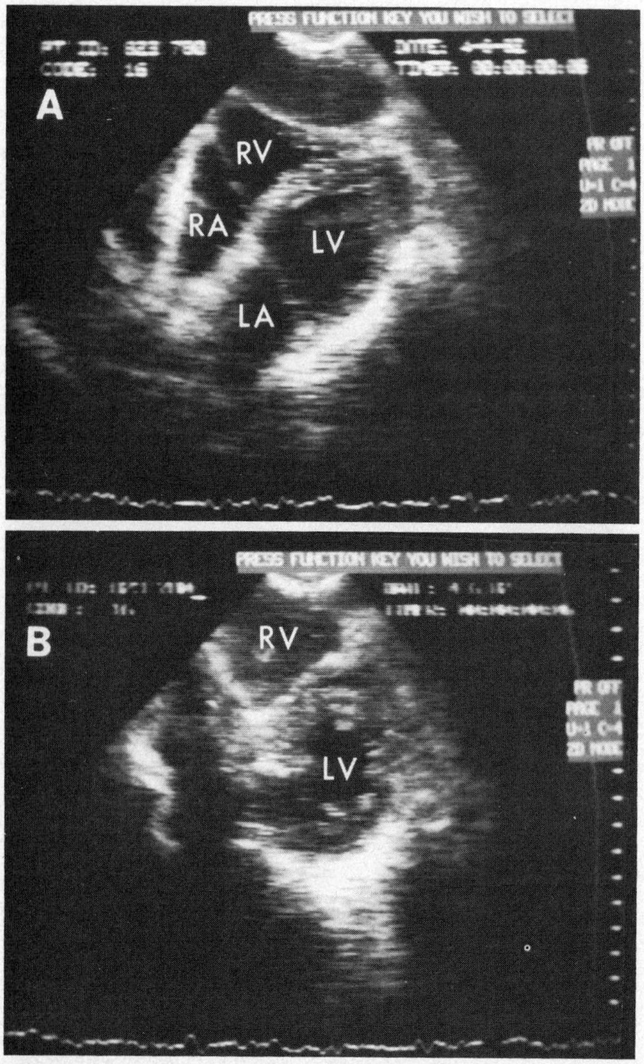

FIGURE 5–25 **Two-dimensional echocardiograms obtained with the transducer in the subcostal position. Echogram *A* represents a four-chamber view and *B* is a short-axis examination. RV = right ventricle; RA = right atrium; LA = left atrium; LV = left ventricle.**

EVALUATION OF CARDIAC PERFORMANCE

Assessment of Cardiac Chambers

As already noted, M-mode echocardiography provides the opportunity for examining the left ventricle, left atrium, root of the aorta, and a small portion of the right ventricle. It should be appreciated that the right ventricular dimensions obtained with the transducer along the left sternal boarder are subject to significant error, since the right ventricular cavity is irregular in shape and only a small portion of it is actually examined.[47] In addition, the right ventricular dimension varies significantly depending upon the direction of the ultrasonic beam and also the position of the patient. As the patient assumes a left lateral position, as is commonly done to obtain satisfactory echocardiographic examinations, right ventricular dimensions often change strikingly. As crude as measurement of right ventricular dimensions might be, it is still very helpful in many clinical situations in assessing the presence or absence of right ventricular dilatation[48] and hypoplasia.[49,50] On the other hand, it should be recognize d that subtle changes in right ventricular size can be missed or falsely suggested by this technique. Although, as already noted, the free wall of the right ventricle cannot be imaged routinely in adults, it is more accessible to measurement in children, in whom right ventricular hypertrophy is a common problem and in whom higher frequency transducers can be used. The subcostal approach has also recently been proposed for assessment of the right ventricular wall.[51]

Measurement of left atrial dimensions was one of the first echocardiographic determinations.[52] The technique in which the beam is directed toward the base of the heart provides an anteroposterior dimension of the left atrium. Although this examination has withstood the test of time,[53] it should be noted that the posterior left atrial wall is not always clear and that a variety of confusing echoes in this area of the heart can be recorded. In patients with thoracic deformities,[54] the left atrium may not assume its usual spherical shape,[55] and the anteroposterior dimension may

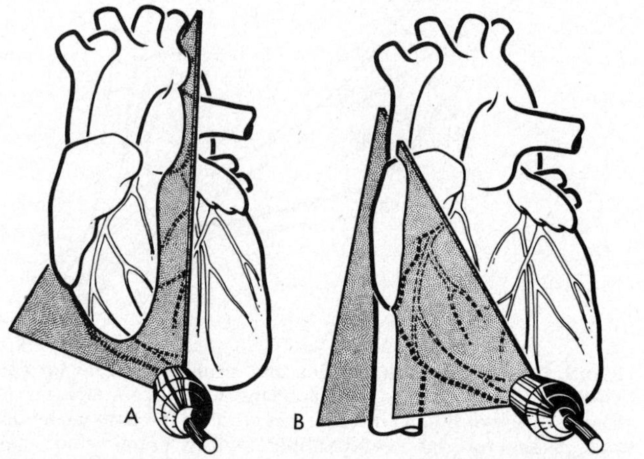

FIGURE 5–26 **Diagram demonstrating the examining planes and transducer positions for the subcostal examination for the right side of the heart (*A*) and the inferior vena cava (*B*). (From Feigenbaum, H.: Echocardiography. 3rd ed. Philadelphia, Lea & Febiger, 1981.)**

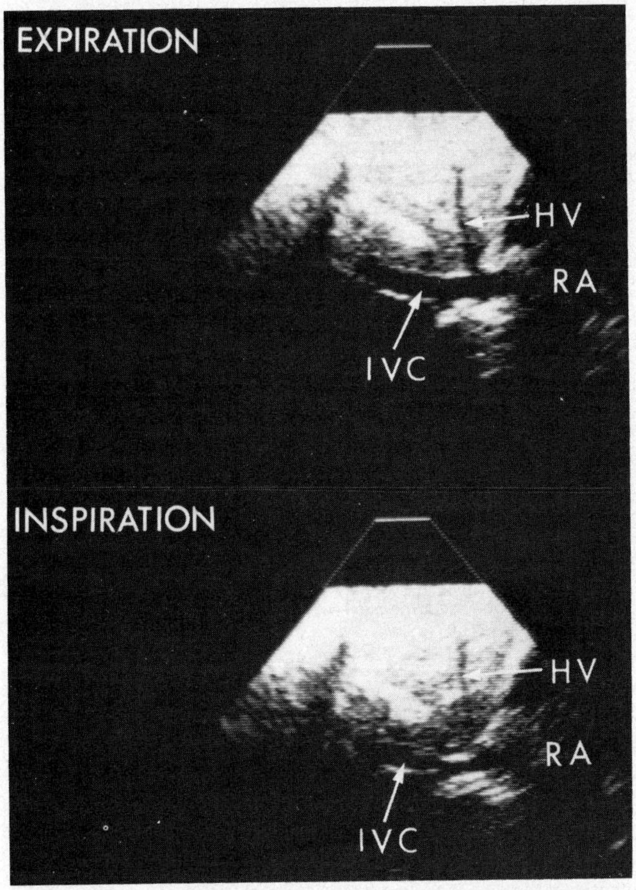

FIGURE 5–27 Subcostal two-dimensional echocardiogram of the inferior vena cava (IVC) and hepatic veins (HV). The inferior vena cava decreases in size with inspiration. RA = right atrium. (From Feigenbaum, H.: Echocardiography. 3rd ed. Philadelphia, Lea & Febiger, 1981.)

be misleading in judging its overall size. In patients with pectus excavatum the superoinferior left atrial dimension, as obtained via the suprasternal approach, may more accurately reflect the true size of this chamber.[54] Recent experience suggests that two-dimensional echocardiographic examination may improve upon the echocardiographic assessment of left atrial size.[56,57] The location and shape of the interatrial septum as seen on two-dimensional echocardiography may help in assessing the state of the left atrium.[58]

The ability to evaluate the function of the left ventricle by means of echocardiography has been one of the principal factors in the increasing application of this technique. The standard M-mode technique may be used to record a dimension of the left ventricle between the left side of the interventricular septum and the endocardial surface of the posterior left ventricular wall.[59,60] Measurements of this dimension in end-diastole and end-systole may be made, and although these dimensions can be used to estimate ventricular volume, there are many potential errors in calculations,[61] since many assumptions that are not always valid are required to obtain the volume of a three-dimensional object from measurement of a single dimension. Irrespective of whether or not M-mode echocardiography can calculate true left ventricular volumes, simple dimensions of the left ventricle can provide an estimate of the overall size

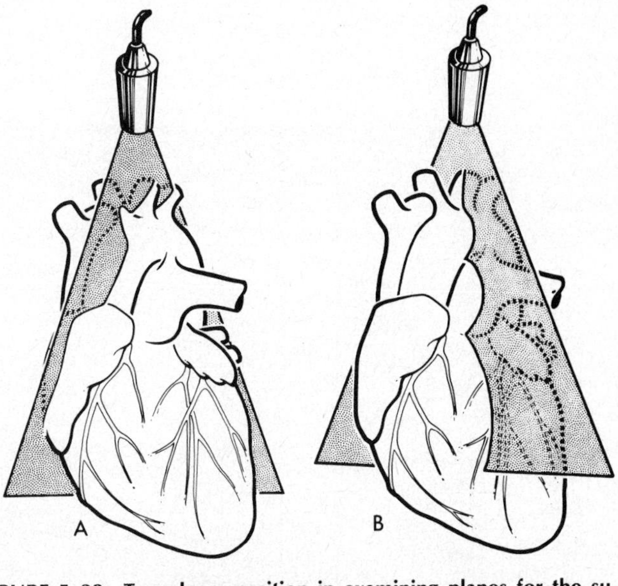

FIGURE 5–28 Transducer position in examining planes for the suprasternal examination parallel to the arch of the aorta (*A*) and perpendicular to the arch of the aorta (*B*). (From Feigenbaum, H.: Echocardiography. 3rd ed. Philadelphia, Lea & Febiger, 1981.)

and performance of the left ventricle in a large percentage of patients.[62]

The left ventricular internal dimension is usually measured at the level of the chordae tendineae or at the tips of the leaflets of the mitral valve (Fig. 5–30), where it provides a measure of the internal diameter at the upper third of the left ventricular cavity, probably including the outflow tract. The diastolic dimension correlates well with the overall size of the left ventricle and can be used to determine the presence of left ventricular dilation. The systolic dimension provides an indication of end-systolic size, and comparing systolic and diastolic dimensions provides an assessment of the myocardial shortening of the upper portion of the left ventricle. Fractional shortening, i.e., the difference between the end-diastolic and end-systolic dimensions divided by the end-diastolic dimension,[62] provides information analogous to the angiographic ejection

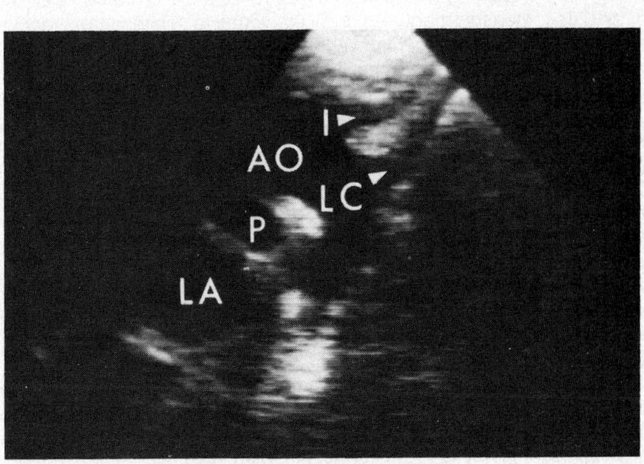

FIGURE 5–29 Suprasternal echocardiographic examination of the arch of the aorta (AO), pulmonary artery (P), and left atrium (LA). I = innominate artery; LC = left common carotid artery.

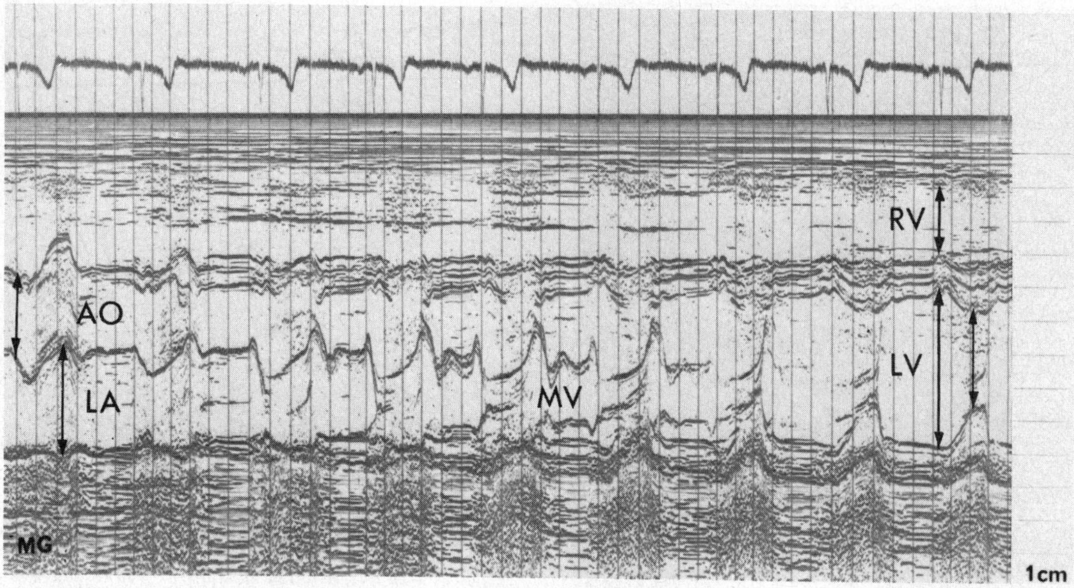

FIGURE 5–30 Normal M-mode echocardiogram showing some commonly used measurements. AO = aorta, LA = left atrium. MV = mitral valve, RV = right ventricle, LV = left ventricle.

fraction. The quotient of fractional shortening and ejection time provides the mean fractional or circumferential shortening.[63] While these measurements are useful in judging left ventricular performance, it must be appreciated that the ventricle must be contracting uniformly for them to reflect global function. These echocardiographic measurements assess the status of only the basal portion of the chamber and must be interpreted with caution in patients with segmentally diseased left ventricles.[64]

Another M-mode echocardiographic technique for assessing the status of the left ventricle is to measure the distance between the E point of the mitral valve and the left side of the interventricular septum.[65,66] Normally, the mitral E point and the left side of the septum are within a few millimeters of each other. The upper limits of normal of the mitral E point–septal separation (EPSS) is approximately 8 mm. As the left ventricular ejection fraction decreases, the EPSS increases. Although there are some limitations to the utility of this measurement, especially when there is regional left ventricular dysfunction, this measurement is useful and fairly popular. Even though the observation is principally empiric, there is some rationale behind the measurement. As the left ventricle dilates, the septum moves anteriorly. The opening of the mitral valve is largely dependent upon the volume of blood passing through that orifice. As the mitral valve flow or left ventricular stroke volume decreases, the amplitude of the E point is decreased. Thus, with a decreased stroke volume and/or left ventricular dilatation, the septum and anterior mitral leaflet would move in opposite directions. Therefore, with a decreased ejection fraction, which is stroke volume divided by diastolic volume, it is not unreasonable to expect an increase in the distance between the mitral valve E point and the interventricular septum. Naturally, if there is intrinsic valvular disease, such as mitral stenosis, then the excursion of the mitral valve is not a reliable indicator of flow through that orifice. In patients with aortic regurgitation, mitral valve flow is not an indicator of total left ventricular stroke volume, and one would not be able to provide an assessment of ejection fraction.

Most echocardiographic measurements of the cardiac chambers have been done with M-mode echocardiography. Such has been the case not only because M-mode echocardiography developed prior to two-dimensional echocardiography but also because of the convenience of having the recording on strip chart paper so that measurements can be made with simple calipers. Unfortunately, there are many theoretical limitations to the M-mode measurements. The lack of spatial orientation in the M-mode examination can distort the measurements in many individuals. This fact is true for all of the cardiac chambers.

Two Dimensional Echocardiography. The limited number of sampling sites for the M-mode dimension also curtails the clinical usefulness of these measurements. Thus, it is not surprising that there has been interest in using two-dimensional echocardiography for assessing the cardiac chambers. The hesitancy to use the two-dimensional approach has been partially because of the inconvenience associated with analyzing a recording made on videotape. With the advent of newer videotape and video disc systems, electronic calipers, bit pads, light pens, and computers, it is becoming more convenient to make the necessary measurements from the two-dimensional examination. It is hoped that the future computers will identify specific echoes and make measurements automatically.[67–69]

There have been a number of attempts to use two-dimensional echocardiography to calculate left ventricular volumes.[70–76] Several geometric formulas have been suggested.[71] These formulas include the area-length technique commonly used for angiographic volumes. The Simpson's rule formula is fairly attractive because it minimizes the effect of geometric shape for calculating volumes. An intriguing formula is that which describes the left ventricle as a bullet, which consists of a cylinder and a half of a prolate ellipse.[72] The formula for calculating left ventricular volume using the "bullet formula" is volume equals five-sixths the area of the left ventricle times the length of the left ventricle ($V = 5/6\ AL$). This formula is attractive because of its simplicity and because the area of the left ventricle and the length of the left ventricle can be easily obtained with two-dimensional echocardiography. The accuracy and reproducibility of the various techniques for calculating left ventricular volumes have not been substantiated. Thus, the calculation of left ventricular volumes is not a routine part of the echocardiographic examination at the present time. There are limitations with any technique which attempts to calculate volume from an examination that is less than truly three-dimensional.

An interesting approach to calculating left ventricular ejection fraction eliminates some of the problems with the actual calculation of volumes.[77] By obtaining multiple diameters of the left ventricle one can transform the fractional shortening of these multiple diameters into ejection fraction either by measuring the fractional change of the length or by estimating fractional length change by a qualitative assessment of apical motion. This particular approach is attractive because of its simplicity and because it obviates some of the limitations of the two-dimensional calculations for volume.

Another simplified approach to assessing the left ventricle with two-dimensional echocardiography is merely to obtain minor axis measurements using the parasternal long-axis and short-axis views. It is possible to obtain a true minor dimension using the parasternal long-axis examination. One can also obtain a short-axis area at the level of the papillary muscles. Derived indices, such as fractional shortening or fractional area change, can be obtained with this approach. Figures 5–31 and 5–32 illustrate how one can obtain the minor dimension from the parasternal long-axis examination (Fig. 5–31) and how the short-axis area can be measured at the level of the papillary muscles (Fig. 5–32).

Attempts have also been made to use two-dimensional echocardiography for calculating right ventricular[78] and left atrial[56,57] volumes. There has also been an attempt at assessing the size of the right atrium using two-dimensional echocardiography.[78] As with the left ventricular measurements, none of the two-dimensional techniques has achieved wide acceptance. However, with the increasing interest in quantitative two-dimensional echocardiography one can anticipate that chamber assessment using the two-dimensional approach should become routine in the near future.

Although echocardiography has been used almost exclusively for evaluating the cardiac chambers at rest, there is increasing interest in performing the ultrasonic examination during or immediately after exercise.[79–81] Most of these studies have utilized supine bicycle exercise. However, in some cases, upright bicycle exercise or isometric exercise has been utilized.

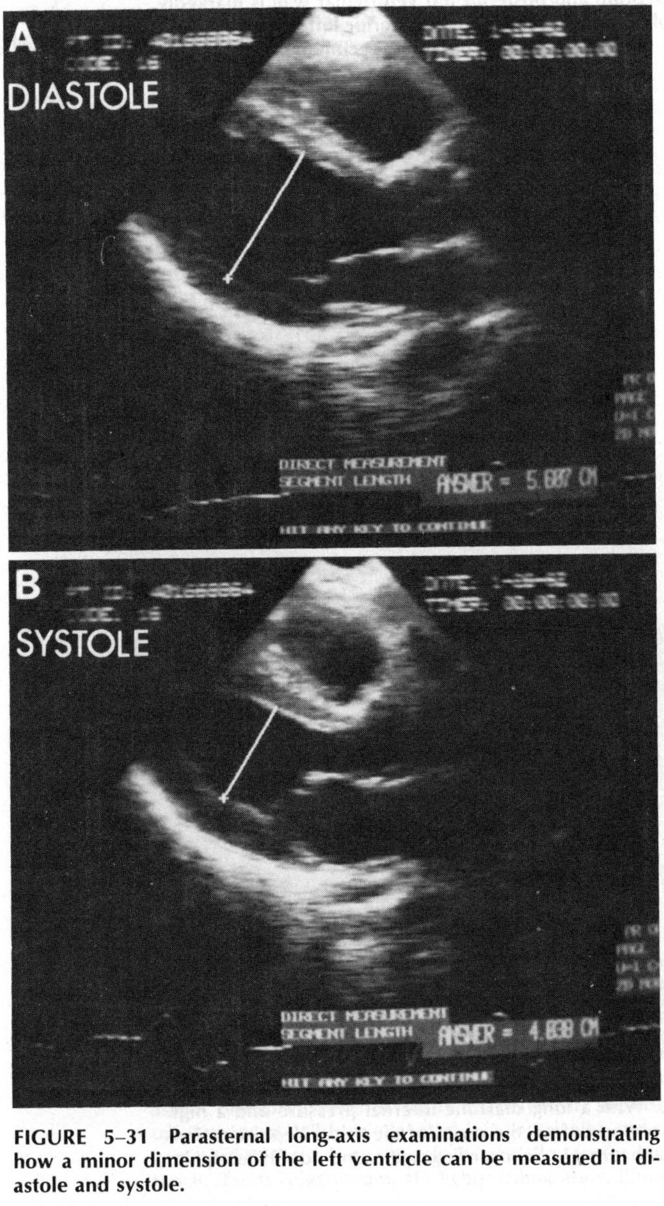

FIGURE 5–31 Parasternal long-axis examinations demonstrating how a minor dimension of the left ventricle can be measured in diastole and systole.

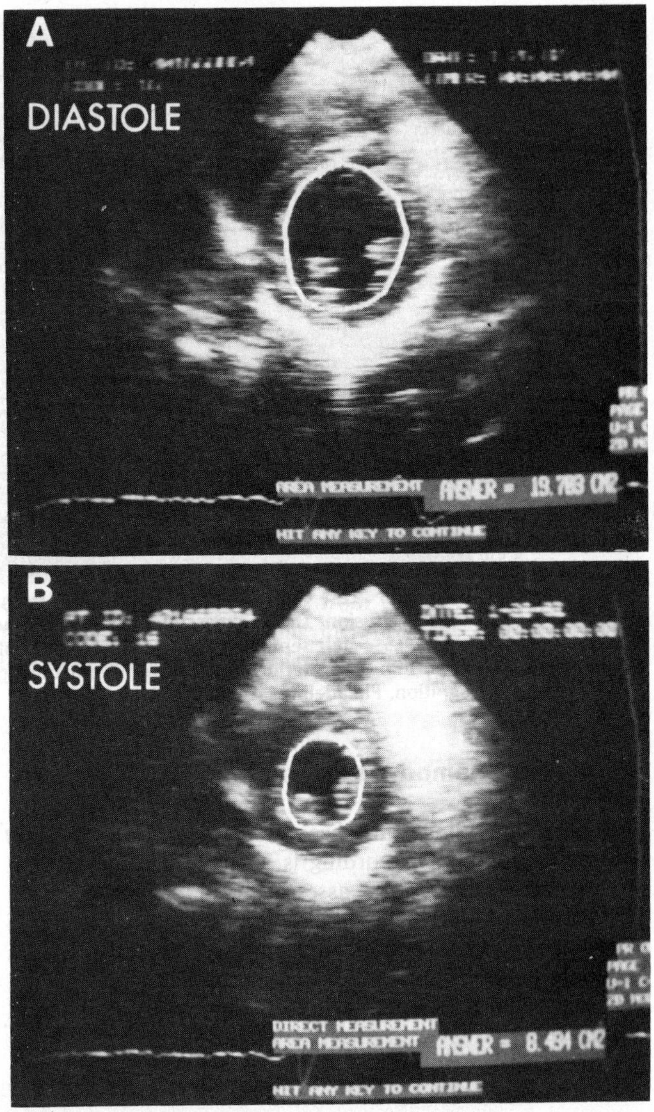

FIGURE 5–32 Short-axis two-dimensional echocardiograms demonstrating how the area of the left ventricle at the papillary muscle level can be measured in diastole and systole.

Echocardiography may also be employed to measure the thickness of the walls of the ventricle.[82–84] Although this measurement can also be made using angiography, many errors are inherent in this technique. For example, the presence of pericardial effusion invalidates the angiographic measurement of diastolic wall thickness. In addition, during systole much of the contrast material is squeezed out of the intertrabecular crevices, and the angiographically determined systolic thickness is probably too large. Echocardiography provides the opportunity for measuring left ventricular wall thickness more accurately, especially in systole. The absolute thickness of the ventricle is important in determining the presence of left ventricular hypertrophy (Fig. 5–33) and in estimating left ventricular mass.[84,85] Echocardiography also permits measurement of changes in left ventricular thickness during the cardiac cycle. Normally, the left ventricular wall thickens during systole, but in pathologic conditions this thickening decreases and actual systolic thinning has been noted in acute ischemia or myocardial infarction.[86,87]

identifying groups of patients with elevated left ventricular diastolic pressures.

A recent study has noted that the interval between the Q wave of the electrocardiogram and the mitral valve closure point or C point correlates with the left ventricular filling pressure or mean pulmonary capillary wedge pressure.[101] Also, there was an inverse relationship between these pressures and the time interval between closure of the aortic valve and opening of the mitral valve. The ratio Q=MVC/AVC=E correlated well with the mean pulmonary artery wedge pressure.

Although alterations in *tricuspid valve* flow appear to influence the tricuspid valve echogram, there has been little documentation of such a relationship. Abnormal (i.e., interrupted) closure of the tricuspid valve in patients with elevated right ventricular diastolic pressure has been noted,[2,102] and in patients with augmented flows through the tricuspid valve, as occurs with atrial septal defect, large tricuspid valves with augmented amplitudes of motion are frequently observed.[103]

Analysis of *aortic valve* motion also provides useful hemodynamic information. Thus, in patients with obstructive hypertrophic cardiomyopathy, or discrete subaortic stenosis, closure of the aortic valve occurs during midsystole as the subaortic obstruction suddenly becomes manifest (Fig. 5–36).[104–108] In patients with mitral regurgitation there may be gradual premature closure of the aortic valve late during systole as blood regurgitates into the left atrium and forward flow into the aorta diminishes.[2] This gradual late systolic closure of the aortic valve may also be seen in low cardiac output states in which the left ventricle may not be capable of sustaining a continuous flow of blood across the aortic valve, and a correlation has been observed between the amplitude and duration of separation of the aortic leaflets and the left ventricular stroke volume.[111,112] In patients with severe aortic regurgitation and markedly elevated left ventricular diastolic pressure the aortic valve may open prior to ventricular systole.[109,110]

Echograms of the *pulmonary valve* have proved to be very useful in reflecting hemodynamic events as well. Although the pulmonary valve echogram is probably influenced in part by the movement of structures to which it is attached,[113] the pressure relationship between the right ventricle and the pulmonary artery also influences the motion of the pulmonary valve (Fig. 5–37). Normally, atrial systole produces a slight downward motion of the pulmonary valve.[114–116] Whether at least part of this motion is due wholly or in part to the posterior motion of the entire base of the heart with atrial systole is not clear. However, there is evidence to suggest that the normal rise in right ventricular pressure occurring during atrial contraction may affect the position of the pulmonary valve. In pulmonic stenosis, the right ventricular systolic and end-diastolic pressures rise without any similar elevation in pulmonary artery pressure, and the atrial contribution to right ventricular pressure is exaggerated and usually sufficient to open the pulmonary valve prior to ventricular systole (Fig. 5–37).[116] This exaggerated *a* wave in the pulmonary valve

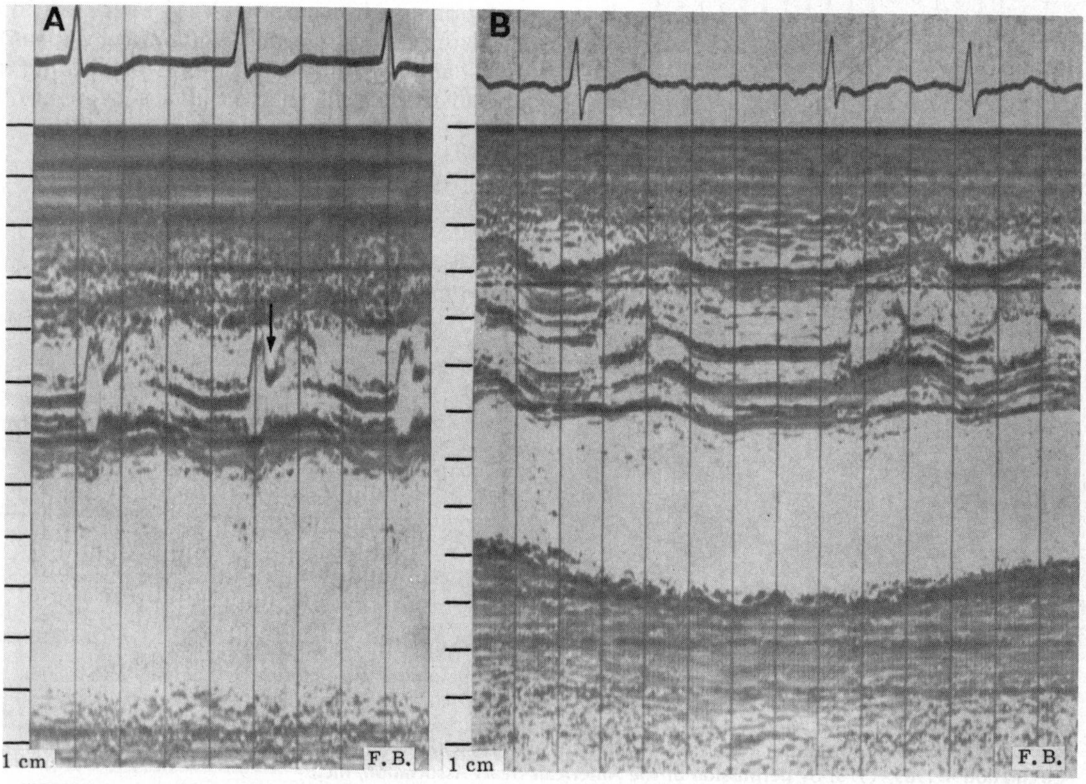

FIGURE 5–36 Aortic valve echocardiograms from a patient with hypertrophic obstructive cardiomyopathy before (*A*) and after (*B*) use of propranolol. With subvalvular obstruction here is closure of the aortic valve in early systole (arrow). This systolic closure disappears as the obstruction is relieved by the use of the beta-adrenergic blocking agent (*B*). (From Feigenbaum, H.: Clinical applications of echocardiography. Progr. Cardiovasc. Dis. *14*:531, 1972, by permission of Grune and Stratton.)

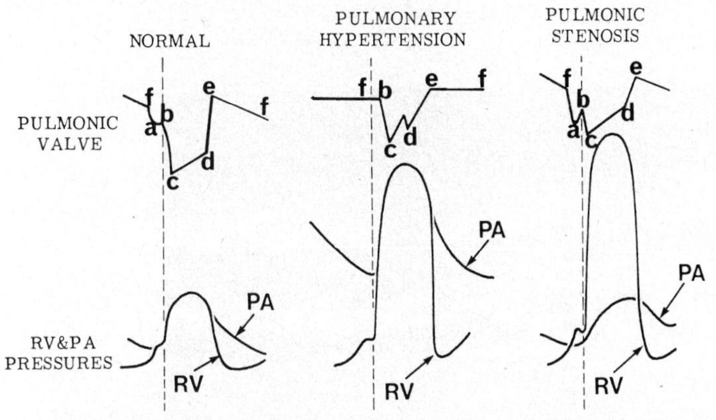

FIGURE 5–37 Diagrams demonstrating the relationship of the pulmonic valve echogram and right-heart pressure in the normal state, with pulmonary hypertension, and with pulmonic stenosis. PA = pulmonary artery pressure, RV = right ventricular pressure. (See text for details.) (From Feigenbaum, H.: Echocardiography. 2nd ed. Philadelphia, Lea and Febiger, 1976.)

echogram reflects the difference in pressures across the pulmonic valve at the end of ventricular diastole. In patients with elevated right ventricular diastolic pressure due to right ventricular failure, tricuspid regurgitation, constrictive pericarditis, or a communication between the aorta and right ventricle, the elevated pressure in the right ventricle in early diastole may cause opening of the pulmonic valve even prior to the onset of atrial systole.[117]

Pulmonary Hypertension. An increase in pulmonary artery pressure has been shown to influence pulmonary valve motion in several ways (Fig. 5-37).[118,119] One of the most consistent changes is the elimination of atrial systolic motion, and the absence or marked reduction of the pulmonary valve *a* wave is one of the echocardiographic signs of pulmonary hypertension. As might be expected, when right ventricular failure occurs in pulmonary hypertension, right ventricular diastolic pressure may rise sufficiently so that a small *a* wave may again be recorded.[2,118] Another sign of pulmonary hypertension is midsystolic closure of the pulmonary valve.[119] While this finding has not been explained, it is probably related to elevated pulmonary vascular resistance.[120] Several other less sensitive and specific signs of pulmonary hypertension have been reported using the pulmonary valve echogram. These include a flat diastolic (E-F) slope, delayed opening of the valve, and an increased velocity of opening of the valve.[118]

The pulmonary valve echogram has been used to calculate systolic time intervals (Chap. 3) of the right side of the heart,[121] and these intervals, in turn, have been used to estimate pulmonary artery pressure and the status of right ventricular performance.[122,123] The pre-ejection period is the time interval from the start of the electrocardiographic QRS to the onset of opening of the pulmonary valve, and the ejection time is the length of time that the pulmonary valve is open. The use of echocardiography for right-sided time intervals has been limited to children, primarily because in adults the closing of the pulmonary valve, which is necessary for measuring ejection time, is rarely recorded unless there is marked dilatation of the pulmonary artery.

With the two-dimensional echocardiographic examination of the inferior vena cava and hepatic vein, more information concerning right-sided hemodynamics is being obtained. This particular examination can be helpful in assessing the central venous pressure by noting the size of the venous vessels.[124]

The *Doppler echocardiogram* records the pattern and velocity of blood flow within the heart and great vessels and thus would theoretically be an ideal tool for the noninvasive assessment of cardiac hemodynamics.[125] There have been numerous attempts to use Doppler echocardiography to measure left ventricular stroke volume.[13–16,126] Most techniques utilize the recording of Doppler flow from the thoracic aorta. The ultrasonic beam can be directed at either the ascending or the descending aorta. Theoretically, if one knew the velocity of the flow in the aorta together with the cross-sectional area of the aorta one could accurately calculate the flow. Unfortunately, this possibility has yet to be substantiated by multiple investigators. Since the flow is not laminar, the velocity in the center of the aorta is different from the velocity near the edge of the aorta. Theoretically, it is necessary to record the blood velocity profile across the aorta. In addition, the measurement of the cross-sectional area of the aorta has been difficult even with two-dimensional echocardiography. Despite these limitations the flow patterns can be assessed within the aorta using Doppler echocardiography and there is some evidence that it may be possible to follow sequential changes in blood flow in a given individual.[17,125] There is also a suggestion that by calculating blood flow acceleration in the aorta, which is the first derivative of the velocity, the functional state of the left ventricle can be assessed.[126]

As a general rule, the echocardiographic signs predicting altered hemodynamics, while relatively insensitive, are fairly reliable when present. They may be helpful in individual patients, especially when serial echograms are used and progressive changes are recorded.

ACQUIRED VALVULAR HEART DISEASE

(See also Chapter 32)

Rheumatic Mitral Valve Disease

MITRAL STENOSIS. The detection of mitral stenosis was the first clinical application of echocardiography[127–129] and remains an important technique in the evaluation of patients with suspected mitral valve disease since echocardiography can allow visualization of the mitral valve in a manner not possible with any other procedure. The M-mode examination provides a sensitive assessment of the motion and thickness of the valve leaflets,[105,130,131] while the two-dimensional technique provides a spatial image of the valve and allows direct measurement of the valve orifice.[132–134]

Figure 5–38 shows an M-mode echocardiogram of a patient with calcific mitral stenosis. The motion of the mitral valve is considerably altered from the normal pattern seen in Figure 5–15; the normal "M"-shaped configuration during diastole is no longer present, since the presence of a holodiastolic atrioventricular pressure gradient (diastasis) prevents rapid closure of the valve in mid-diastole. Although sinus rhythm was present, there was no reopening of the valve with atrial contraction and no *a* wave. Thus, the echocardiographic hallmark of mitral stenosis is the absence of valve closure in mid-diastole and of reopening

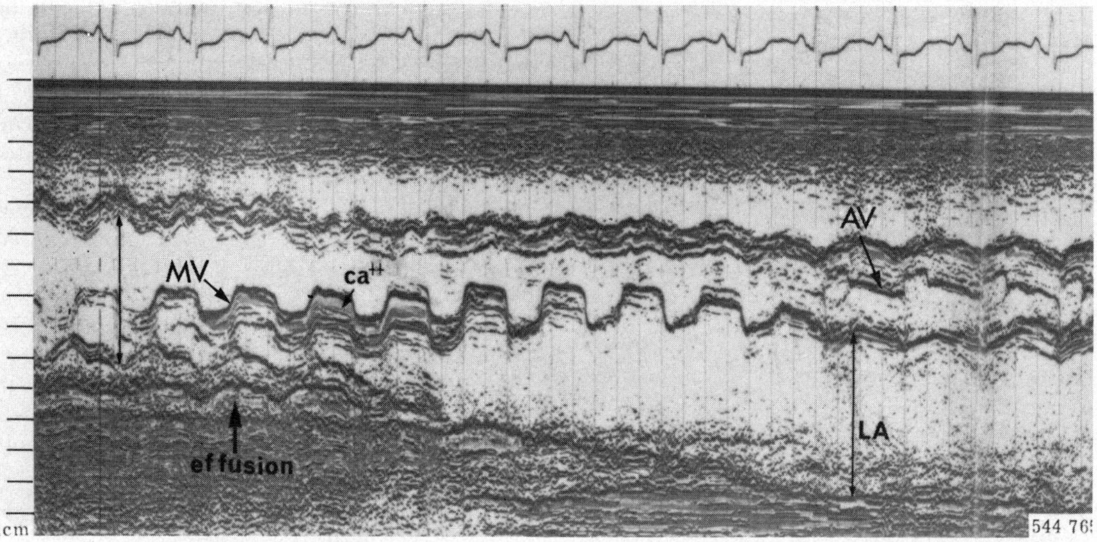

FIGURE 5–38 M-mode scan from a patient with mitral stenosis. The valve is calcified (ca^{++}) and immobile. The left atrium (LA) is dilated and there is moderate posterior pericardial effusion. AV = aortic valve. (From Chang, S.: M-Mode Echocardiographic Techniques and Pattern Recognition. Philadelphia, Lea and Febiger, 1976.)

in late diastole. Although this decreased (flat) diastolic (E-F) slope is characteristic of mitral stenosis, it is not specific.[128,129] Other conditions such as decreased left ventricular compliance or a low cardiac output may also reduce the diastolic slope of mitral valve motion.[135–137]

In addition to the change in motion of the valve, the number of echoes originating from the valve is increased when the valve is fibrotic or calcified,[131] and the second echocardiographic sign of mitral stenosis is increased thickness of the valve leaflets. (Note that the quantity of echoes originating from the mitral valve in Figure 5–38 is considerably greater than in Figure 5–15.) The third sign is inadequate separation of the anterior and posterior leaflets of the valve during diastole.[137] Normally, the two leaflets move in opposite directions during diastole, but when fused, as in mitral stenosis, they do not separate widely and may actually appear to move in the same direction (Fig. 5–38). The echocardiographic findings of reduced diastolic slope, increased thickness, and decreased separation of the valve leaflets provide a sensitive and accurate method for detection of mitral stenosis. There are relatively few conditions that can be confused with hemodynamically significant mitral stenosis echocardiographically; these include reduced compliance of the left ventricle as well as a combination of mild rheumatic mitral stenosis and a markedly reduced cardiac output.

Besides establishing (or excluding) the diagnosis qualitatively, echocardiography can also provide some quantitation of the obstruction. The original criterion for judging the severity of mitral stenosis was the diastolic (E-F) slope[128,129]—the flatter the slope, the more severe the stenosis. More recent evaluation of this sign has shown it to be less accurate than was originally thought. Hemodynamic factors such as the rate of filling of the left ventricle and its compliance can influence the diastolic slope.[135,136] However, two-dimensional echocardiography provides an opportunity to visualize and measure the flow-restricting orifice of the stenotic mitral valve directly (Fig. 5–39). A number of investigators have demonstrated that the two-dimensional quantitation of mitral stenosis is superior not only to the E-F slope on the M-mode echocardiogram,[134] but perhaps even to cardiac catheterization and Gorlin's formula in the presence of mitral regurgitation.[132]

Two-dimensional echocardiography also assists in the

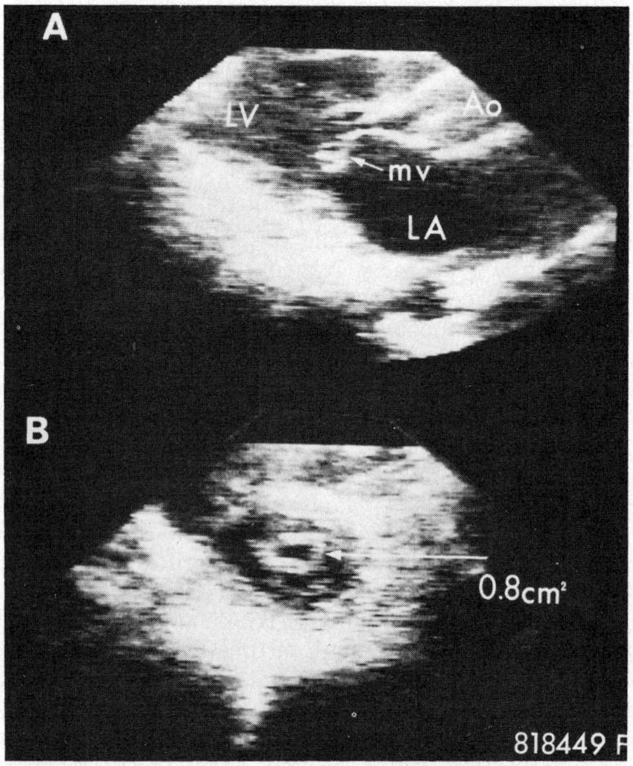

FIGURE 5–39 Two-dimensional echocardiograms of a patient with mitral stenosis. The domed mitral valve (mv) can be seen in the long-axis examination (*A*). The short-axis examination (*B*) demonstrates the orifice of the stenotic valve and provides the opportunity for determining the degree of stenosis.

qualitative diagnosis of mitral stenosis. By noting doming of the mitral leaflets (Fig. 5–39*A*) one can be assured of the valve's restricted motion. "Doming" of any valve on two-dimensional echocardiography is a characteristic sign of stenosis. The distortion in shape with opening of the valve indicates that the tips of the leaflets are restricted in their ability to open, whereas the bodies of the leaflets still wish to accommodate more blood flow. Thus the leaflets are curved or "domed." Doming is used to distinguish a valve that is truly stenotic from one that opens poorly because of low flow.

Echocardiography can also help determine whether or not a stenotic mitral valve is suitable for a commissurotomy by estimating its pliability[105,130] and degree of calcification.[131] The former is judged by measuring the greatest amplitude of motion of the mitral valve. If the anterior leaflet has an opening motion which exceeds 2 cm, the valve is considered to be pliable. Calcification or fibrosis of the valve is reflected by the number of echoes originating from the valve. Although echocardiographic evaluation is not absolutely specific for evaluating the mitral valve, it is probably more reliable than merely searching for an opening snap on auscultation or phonocardiography or for calcification on fluoroscopy.

Echocardiography is also useful for evaluating the effect of mitral stenosis on the cardiac chambers. The left atrium is almost always dilated (Fig. 5–38), and the left ventricular cavity is usually normal or reduced in size. A left atrial emptying index has been devised from the pattern of motion of the posterior aortic wall.[138,139] Normally the aortic wall echo, which is also the anterior wall of the left atrium, moves downward or posteriorly rapidly in early diastole. With mitral obstruction the early diastolic motion is reduced. The signs of pulmonary hypertension (described above) are commonly present on the pulmonary valve echogram in patients with mitral stenosis and sinus rhythm.

MITRAL REGURGITATION. Echocardiography is not as useful in the assessment of patients with rheumatic mitral regurgitation. None of the techniques using the mitral valve echogram, such as a rapid diastolic (E-F) slope[114,140,141] and wide separation of the leaflets during systole, for the detection of mitral regurgitation has proved to be reliable. Two-dimensional echocardiography, which images the regurgitant orifice in systole, has been proposed to solve this problem,[142] but its value has not yet been confirmed.

Doppler echocardiography offers a much better opportunity for the detection of mitral regurgitaton of any type.[143,144] Figure 5–12 demonstrates a Doppler examination in a patient with rheumatic mitral regurgitation. By placing the sampling gate in the left atrium behind the mitral valve, one can detect systolic turbulence indicative of the regurgitant jet. The Doppler technique appears to be reasonably sensitive; however, its ability to quantitate the degree of mitral regurgitation is still controversial.

Echocardiography is useful in evaluating the effect of regurgitation on the cardiac chambers. There is evidence of left ventricular diastolic overload, consisting of increased left ventricular end-diastolic dimensions and an augmented left ventricular stroke volume. The motion of the septum usually exceeds that of the posterior left ventricular wall; left atrial dilatation is almost invariably present in chronic mitral regurgitation, and left atrial expansion during systole can occasionally be detected.[2,57] The echocardiographic differentiation between rheumatic and nonrheumatic mitral regurgitation is based on the thickening and restriction of motion which is present in patients with rheumatic valvular disease, even in those with essentially pure regurgitation. On the other hand, the leaflets are thin and delicate and move freely in the nonrheumatic forms.

Prolapsed and Flail Mitral Valve

PROLAPSE. Echocardiography is particularly useful in the diagnosis of prolapse of the mitral valve (p. 1089). Figure 5–40 demonstrates the principal M-mode finding in this condition—a fairly abrupt posterior (downward) motion of the mitral valve apparatus in mid- or late systo-

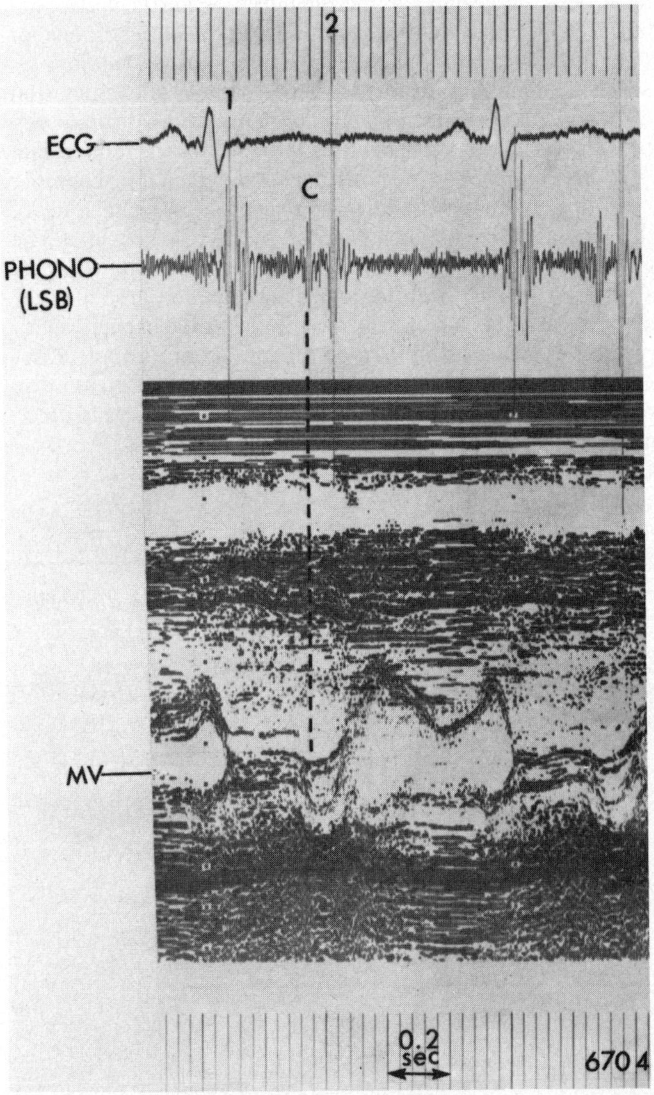

FIGURE 5–40 Phonocardiogram and M-mode echocardiogram from a patient with mitral valve prolapse. The late systolic click (C) on the phonocardiogram corresponds to late systolic posterior displacement of the mitral valve (MV). (From Tavel, M. E.: Clinical Phonocardiography and External Pulse Recordings, 3rd Ed. Chicago, Yearbook Medical Publishers, 1978.)

le.[145–147] This motion often commences simultaneously with the mid- or late systolic click (Fig. 5–40), a typical auscultatory and phonocardiographic finding in this condition (Chap. 4). Although this mid- or late systolic posterior motion of the mitral valve is a reasonably specific sign of mitral valve prolapse, it is not a very sensitive sign. Many patients with this lesion fail to show it, while in others the prolapse is a holosystolic event, i.e., there is posterior displacement of the valve throughout systole (Fig. 5–41).[148,149] Minor degrees of posterior displacement of the mitral valve can occur normally, and there is a troublesome "gray" zone in which it is difficult to determine whether the prolapse is normal or not.[150,151] Late or holosystolic prolapse, as in Figures 5–40 and 5–41, in which the leaflets move posteriorly by at least 5 mm (Fig. 5–41), is generally accepted as abnormal. However, when the holosystolic "hammocking" is less than 5 mm,[152] the diagnosis is not clear-cut.

Several findings on two-dimensional echocardiography have been suggested for the diagnosis of mitral valve prolapse,[153–155] including the recording of buckling of one or both mitral leaflets into the left atrium during systole. Figure 5–42 demonstrates a parasternal long-axis examination of a patient with mitral valve prolapse. Both leaflets can be seen buckling or herniating into the left atrium in late systole. Figure 5–43 demonstrates an apical four-chamber view of a patient with mitral valve prolapse. The level of the mitral valve annulus is noted by the dashed line. The anterior or septal mitral leaflet bulges well into the left atrium on this echocardiogram. Unfortunately, the amount of systolic prolapse noted on the two-dimensional echocardiograms also exhibits a continuum from normal to abnormal, and there may still be a problem in differentiating between prolapse and a normal variant with this technique.

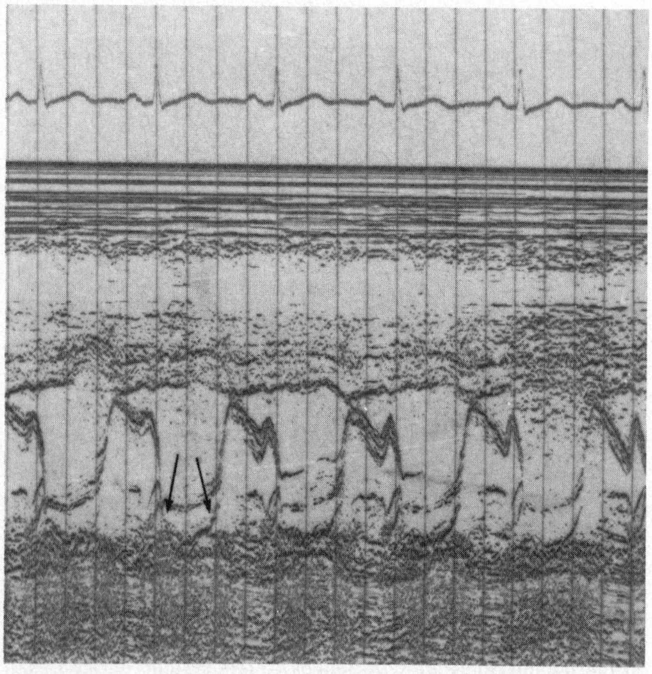

FIGURE 5–41 Mitral valve echocardiogram from a patient with holosystolic mitral prolapse (arrows). (From Feigenbaum, H.: Echocardiography. 2nd ed. Philadelphia, Lea and Febiger, 1976.)

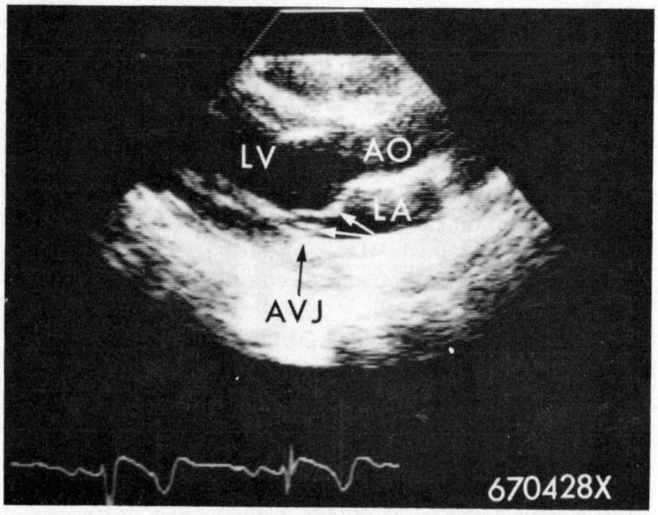

FIGURE 5–42 Two-dimensional long-axis echocardiogram of a patient with mitral valve prolapse. Both the anterior and posterior mitral leaflets (arrows) curve into the left atrium (LA). The posterior leaflet makes almost a hairpin turn as it moves to the atrial side of the atrioventricular junction (AVJ). LV = left ventricle; AO = aorta. (From Feigenbaum, H.: Echocardiography. 3rd ed. Philadelphia, Lea & Febiger, 1981.)

Secondary echocardiographic findings in patients with mitral valve prolapse include excessive amplitude of motion of the valve during diastole which can be appreciated in both M-mode and two-dimensional examinations. Some thickening of the leaflets is not uncommon and is presumably due to myxomatous degeneration; the latter is rarely confused with the thickening associated with mitral stenosis, but since valve motion is not restricted, it can be con-

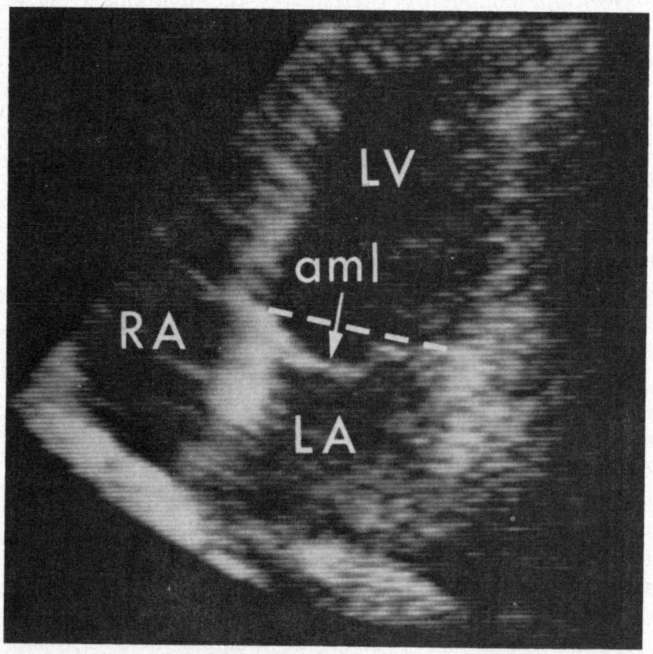

FIGURE 5–43 Apical four-chamber echocardiogram of a patient with mitral valve prolapse demonstrating a curved anterior mitral leaflet (aml) that extends beyond the plane of the mitral annulus (dashed line). LV = left ventricle; LA = left atrium; RA = right atrium. (From Feigenbaum, H.: Echocardiography. 3rd ed. Philadelphia, Lea & Febiger, 1981.)

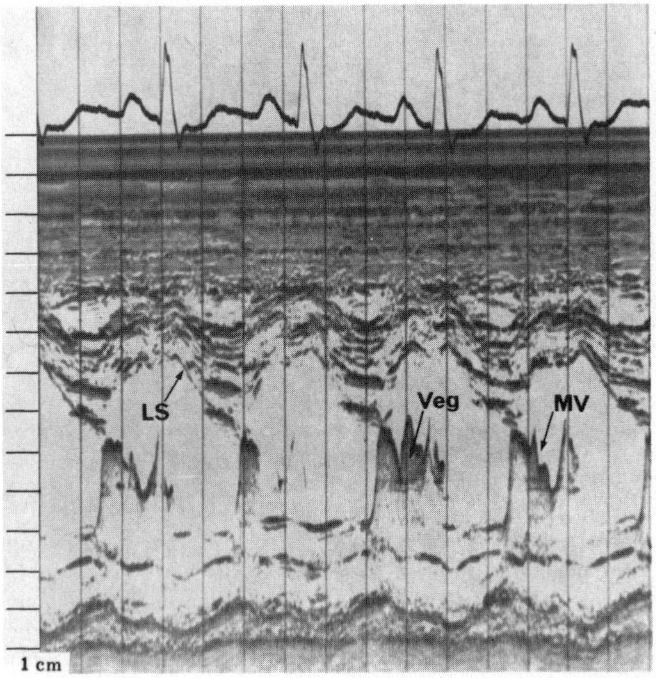

FIGURE 5–44 M-mode echocardiogram from a patient with torn chordae of the anterior mitral leaflet and vegetations (Veg) secondary to bacterial endocarditis. During diastole the anterior mitral leaflet (MV) exhibits chaotic coarse fluttering. LS = left septum. (From Feigenbaum, H.: Echocardiography. 2nd ed. Philadelphia, Lea and Febiger, 1976.)

fused with a vegetation.[156] Excessive motion of the atrioventricular ring, as determined by two-dimensional echocardiography, has been reported in patients with prolapse of the mitral valve. Also, the presence of an abnormal contraction pattern on the left ventricular echogram has been described in these patients[157,158]; the specificity and diagnostic usefulness of these findings remain to be defined.

FLAIL MITRAL VALVE. There are several reports in the literature describing the echocardiographic findings in patients with a flail mitral valve, i.e., with a leaflet that has lost its normal support and therefore flutters in the bloodstream. In many of these patients the mitral valve echogram presents an extreme form of mitral valve prolapse with marked posterior displacement of the mitral valve during systole.[2,159,160] In some patients flail valves are a consequence of infective endocarditis,[161] and vegetations can sometimes be imaged (Chap. 33). In Figure 5–44 a very coarsely fluttering anterior leaflet of the mitral valve is imaged, a motion which is characteristically chaotic, without a reproducible pattern from beat to beat.[159] This type of motion is suggestive of torn chordae tendineae inserting primarily into the anterior mitral leaflet. The principal finding in Figure 5–45, an echocardiogram of a patient with a flail mitral valve secondary to infective endocarditis, shows the echo of a structure, presumably a vegetation, attached to the mitral valve, which moves posteriorly into the left atrium during systole. Thus, the echocardiographic signs of a flail valve can be chaotic motion (as in Figure 5–44), excessive posterior motion during systole, or even recording of a portion of the mitral valve in the left atrium during systole (Fig. 5–45). These signs are all indicative of disruption of the valve but are not necessarily pathognomonic, since a vegetation without a flail valve may also be imaged in the left atrium.

Several studies of flail mitral valves have emphasized their fluttering motion during both diastole[162] and systole.[163] The systolic fluttering is probably a reliable sign of disruption of the mitral valve apparatus, but diastolic fluttering may not be specific, since other conditions such as aortic regurgitation and markedly increased flow across the mitral valve may cause the valve apparatus to flutter during diastole.

Utilizing two-dimensional echocardiography, it has also been noted in patients with ruptured chordae tendineae that a portion of the mitral valve apparatus prolapses or

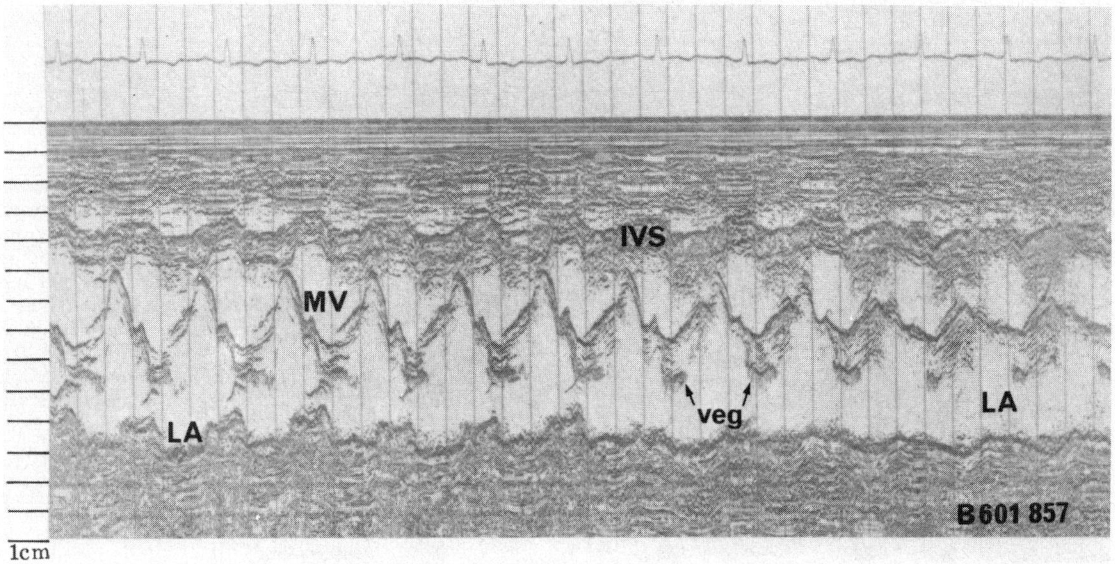

FIGURE 5–45 M-mode scan of a patient with infective endocarditis and vegetations (Veg) on the mitral valve. Echoes from the vegetations can be seen during systole within the left atrial cavity (LA). IVS = interventricular septum, MV = mitral valve. (From Chang, S.: M-Mode Echocardiographic Techniques and Pattern Recognition. Philadelphia, Lea and Febiger, 1976.)

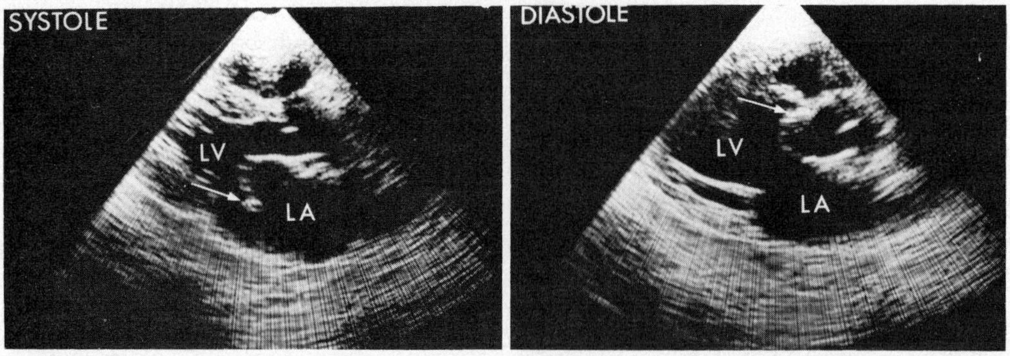

FIGURE 5–46 Long-axis echocardiogram demonstrating a mobile vegetation (arrows) on the anterior leaflet of a flail mitral valve. In systole the vegetation and leaflet protrude into the left atrium and in diastole the valve moves into the left ventricular outflow tract. LV = left ventricle, LA = left atrium. (From Feigenbaum, H.: Echocardiography. 3rd ed. Philadelphia, Lea & Febiger, 1981.)

herniates into the left atrium during systole (Fig. 5–46).[164] The differentiation between a prolapsing and a flail valve is that in the case of prolapse the body of the leaflet moves into the left atrium while the tips of the leaflets remain within the left ventricle, whereas with a flail valve the tips of the valve are displaced into the left atrium during systole.

Aortic Valve Disease

STENOSIS. The echocardiographic hallmark of aortic stenosis is thickening of the leaflets with narrowing of the orifice.[165,166] Thus, the echocardiographic signs of aortic stenosis are similar to those of mitral stenosis but are not as reliable. Figure 5–47 compares a normal and a stenotic aortic valve. There are more echoes originating from the latter, and the leaflets do not open as widely. Assessment of thickening of the valve is subjective, since even the normal valve sometimes appears to have excessive echoes, and assessing the motion of the leaflets can also be difficult at times. Thus, while standard M-mode echocardiography can be helpful in making the diagnosis of valvular aortic stenosis, both the sensitivity and the specificity of the technique leave much to be desired. For example, a noncalcified congenitally stenotic aortic valve may be totally unrecognized by M-mode echocardiography.[102] Furthermore, assessing the severity of aortic stenosis by measuring the separation of aortic valve leaflets on the M-mode tracing is quite imprecise.[166,167]

The severity of the stenosis, however, may be judged indirectly from determining any secondary effects on the left ventricle. Thus, the severity of the valvular obstruction[168–170,172] and the level of left ventricular systolic pressure[170,171] can be judged from the thickness of the left ven-

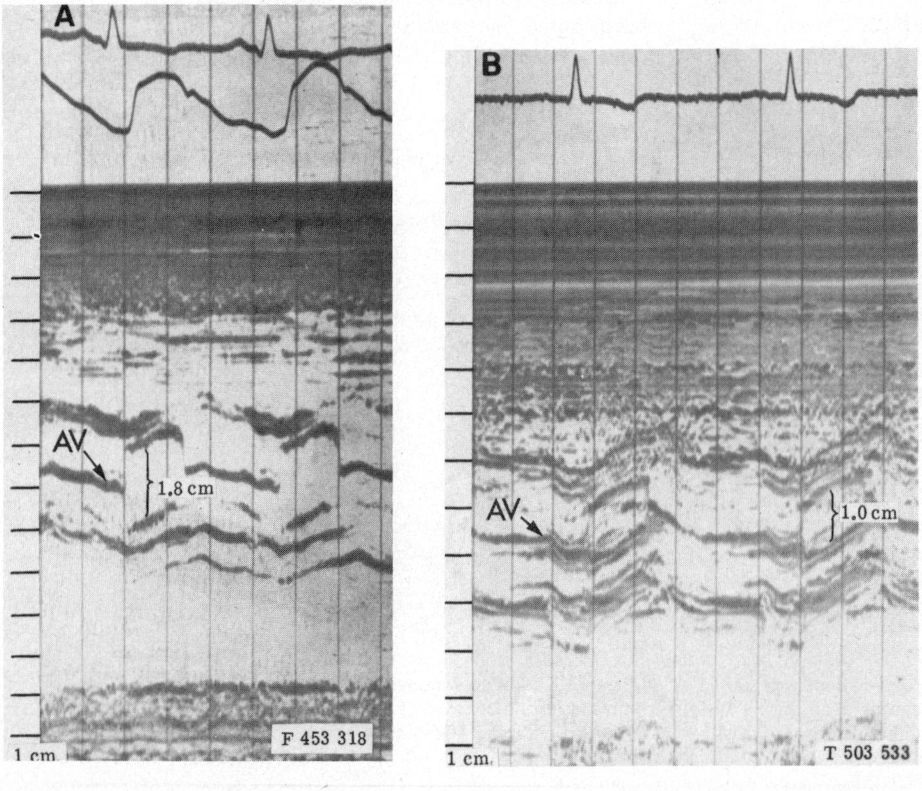

FIGURE 5–47 Aortic valve echocardiograms from a patient with a normal aortic valve (*A*) and from a patient with valvular aortic stenosis (*B*). The echoes are thinner and less echo-producing and separate more widely in the normal valve than in aortic stenosis. AV = aortic valve. (From Feigenbaum, H.: Echocardiography, 2nd ed. Philadelphia, Lea and Febiger, 1976.)

tricular wall. Unfortunately, the technique is not reliable in the presence of left ventricular dilatation. By obtaining a spatially correct image of the aortic valve using two-dimensional echocardiography, it is possible to appreciate its domed shape and to measure the diameter of the flow-restricting orifice (Fig. 5–48).[173,174] Thus, two-dimensional echocardiography has significantly improved the qualitative diagnosis of aortic stenosis, especially in the young patient. Unfortunately, there are still problems with attempting to quantitate the degree of aortic stenosis using two-dimensional echocardiography.[175] Although a diameter of the flow-restricting orifice can be obtained, its measurement has significant limitations. The diameter determined by echocardiography is probably more helpful in the young patient with a pliable aortic valve. Once the valve becomes rigid, the diameter no longer is a predictor of the orifice. Attempts at measuring the cross-sectional area of the stenotic aortic valve have not been nearly as successful as with the mitral valve. Thus, this technique is not practical. One can judge the pliability of the leaflets in short axis and gain further information concerning the severity of the stenosis.[176] Thus far, the two-dimensional technique, especially in the adult patient, can judge the extreme situations, but it is still difficult to distinguish between moderate and severe aortic stenosis.

Preliminary data suggest that Doppler echocardiography may be able to judge the pressure gradient across the aortic valve in patients with aortic stenosis, since, theoretically, at least, the velocity is a function of the pressure gradient.[177–179] These findings obviously must be confirmed before they can be used routinely in the clinical setting.

REGURGITATION. *Direct* echocardiographic examination of the aortic valve is of limited value in the detection of aortic regurgitation; however, several findings should be noted. When the aortic valve is disrupted or flail, it may flutter during diastole.[180–183] When present, this finding is quite reliable, but it is not sensitive and is rarely seen in patients with chronic aortic regurgitation. In patients with infective endocarditis and aortic regurgitation, echoes from a vegetation or a portion of the disrupted aortic valve prolapsing into the left ventricular outflow tract during diastole are commonly imaged.[180,182,184–186] However, the diagnosis of aortic regurgitation on the basis of diastolic separation of the aortic valve leaflets does not appear to be reliable.[187] The diagnosis of aortic valve prolapse with two-dimensional echocardiography has been reported.[155,188]

The most common echocardiographic finding in aortic regurgitation is fine fluttering of the anterior leaflet of the mitral valve during diastole (Fig. 5–34).[88–90] Rarely, the posterior mitral leaflet and even the left side of the interventricular septum also flutter.[189,190] These movements presumably are caused by the regurgitant jet flowing into the left ventricle. It is important to recognize that this finding is only of qualitative value in the detection of aortic regurgitation, and it is usually absent when aortic regurgitation coexists with rheumatic mitral stenosis, presumably because of the rigidity of the mitral valve under these circumstances.

Doppler echocardiography is able to detect aortic regurgitation in a high percentage of patients.[20,21,144,191] By placing the sampling volume in the left ventricular outflow tract, one can detect the high velocity turbulent flow during diastole. There is some confusion in differentiating aortic regurgitation from the turbulent diastolic flow with mitral stenosis. However, the abnormal flow from aortic regurgitation commences slightly before that from mitral stenosis, and one can help differentiate the valvular lesions by noting the onset of the turbulent flow and the opening of the mitral valve. There are also data indicating that one could judge the severity of the aortic regurgitation by the Doppler examination in the aorta.[20,21] The amount or per cent of diastolic reverse flow within the aorta has some relationship to the severity of aortic regurgitation.

Closure of the mitral valve in mid-diastole is consistent with severe, and usually acute, aortic regurgitation (Fig. 5–34).[91–93] Echocardiographic signs of left ventricular volume overload, with dilatation of the left ventricle and exaggerated motion of the interventricular septum, are helpful signs of moderate and severe aortic regurgitation. Echocardiography has been suggested as a useful method of assessing left ventricular function in patients with aortic regurgitation. A reduced fractional shortening and especially an enlarged end-systolic dimension on M-mode echocardiography have been suggested as indicators of reduced ventricular function and are useful in judging the timing for valvular surgery[192] (Chap. 32). Other investigators have suggested that exercise echocardiography can help assess left ventricular function in patients with aortic regurgitation.[193] The reliability of these techniques for timing valvular surgery for aortic regurgitation has yet to be determined.

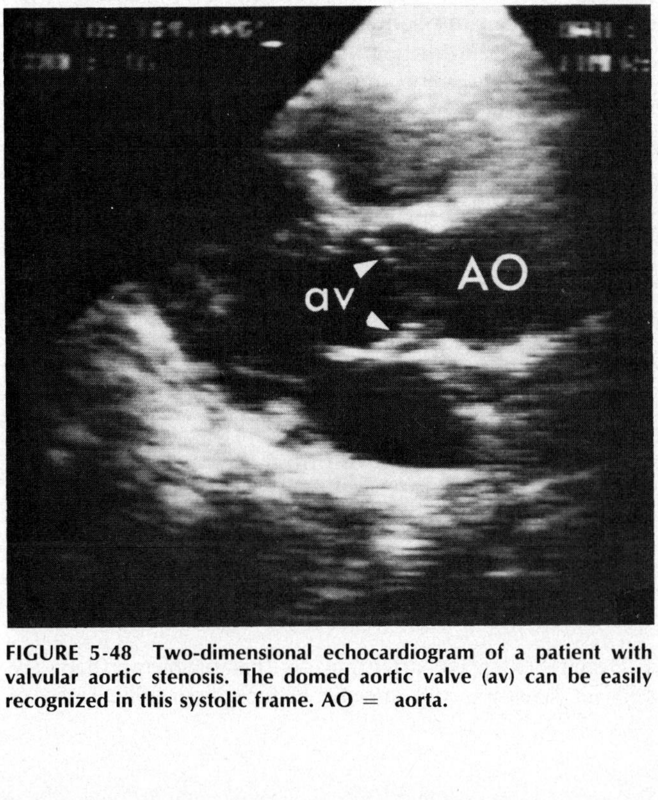

FIGURE 5-48 Two-dimensional echocardiogram of a patient with valvular aortic stenosis. The domed aortic valve (av) can be easily recognized in this systolic frame. AO = aorta.

Tricuspid Stenosis and Regurgitation

In *tricuspid stenosis,* the principal M-mode abnormality is a decrease in the diastolic slope of the anterior leaflet,[114,194] similar to that occurring in mitral stenosis. Again, as in the case of the mitral valve, a reduced diastolic slope occurs in, but is not specific for, tricuspid stenosis and may also be seen in the presence of a low cardiac output and reduced right ventricular compliance. However, a normal steep diastolic slope helps to exclude the presence of tricuspid stenosis. Thickening of the valve is not as prominent in tricuspid as it is in mitral stenosis, and this sign is not as valuable in diagnosing tricuspid valve disease. Also, since the posterior leaflet of the tricuspid valve cannot usually be imaged, reduced separation of the leaflets cannot be appreciated in the majority of patients with tricuspid stenosis.

Two-dimensional echocardiography offers a more reliable technique for the qualitative assessment of tricuspid stenosis.[195] By noting doming of the tricuspid valve the diagnosis of tricuspid stenosis can be made with fair reliability.

Aside from the diagnosis of tricuspid valve prolapse,[155,196] the M-mode and two-dimensional echocardiographic signs for *tricuspid regurgitation* are indirect. Both techniques detect a pattern indicative of a right ventricular volume overload. The M-mode echocardiogram reveals a dilated right ventricular dimension and anterior (rather than the normal posterior) motion of the interventricular septum during isovolumic contraction and sometimes during ejection.[47] Two-dimensional echocardiography notes an abnormal shape of the septum during diastole[197]; with increased diastolic flow through the tricuspid valve, as occurs in tricuspid regurgitation, atrial septal defect, and other conditions producing right ventricular volume overload, the augmented filling of the right ventricle indents the septum so that it bulges into the left ventricle during diastole.[197,198] During ejection the septum returns to its normal position, and the left ventricle again becomes spherical.

A more direct diagnosis of tricuspid regurgitation can be obtained with Doppler echocardiography or contrast echocardiography. Detecting a turbulent systolic jet in the right atrium with Doppler echocardiography is proving to be a very sensitive technique for detecting tricuspid regurgitation.[199] Because the right-sided chambers are close to the transducer, Doppler echocardiography is more reliable in detecting tricuspid regurgitation than mitral regurgitation. Contrast echocardiography is also useful in detecting tricuspid regurgitation.[200-202] With the injection of contrast into a peripheral arm vein in patients with tricuspid regurgitation, contrast echoes are recorded during systole in the inferior vena cava and hepatic veins. One can obtain some semiquantitative impression of the degree of tricuspid regurgitation using this technique.

Infective Endocarditis

(See also Chapter 33)

Echocardiography provides an opportunity for visualizing the vegetations of infective valvular endocarditis, which appear as echo-producing masses attached to the infected valve (Fig. 5–44).[184-186,203-205] Vegetations must be approximately 3 to 4 mm in diameter before they can be appreciated on the echocardiogram[203,206]; they are usually asymmetrical, commonly involving one leaflet more than another. If the vegetation is associated with destruction of the valve or if it is on a long "stalk," it can be readily imaged; its excessive motion can be appreciated on both M-mode (Fig. 5–45)[207,208] and two-dimensional echocardiography (Fig. 5–46).[209] Some very large vegetations have been described, and these seem often to involve the tricuspid valve (Fig. 5–49)[2,206,210,211] or may result from infection with *Candida albicans.*

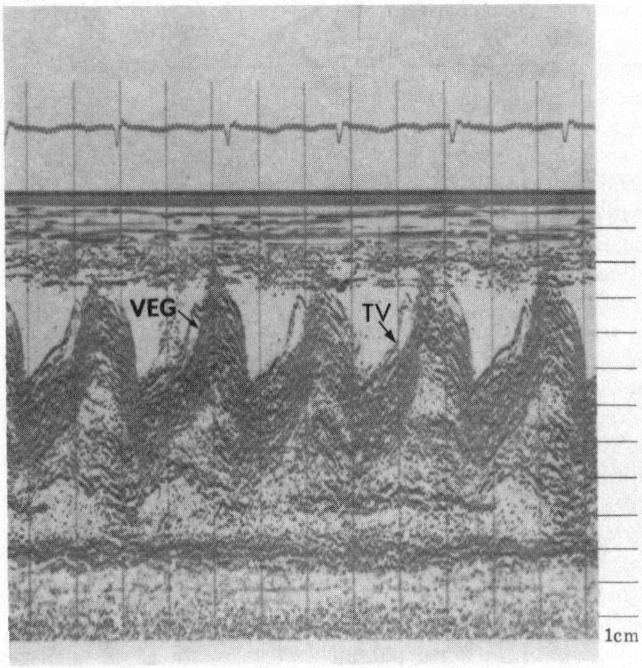

FIGURE 5–49 Echocardiogram demonstrating a large bacterial vegetation (VEG) on the tricuspid valve (TV). (From Feigenbaum, H.: Echocardiography, 2nd ed. Philadelphia, Lea and Febiger, 1976.)

Many patients with clinically proven infective endocarditis do not have recognizable vegetations on the echocardiogram,[212] especially if the involved valves remain competent.[206] In one study, only one-third of patients with proven endocarditis had vegetations that could be visualized on the echocardiogram.[212] Studies, especially using two-dimensional echocardiography,[213] have noted a much higher frequency of vegetations on the echocardiogram. However, the frequency is not 100 per cent,[214] so that a negative echocardiogram does not rule out endocarditis. When vegetations are evident, the valve frequently may be diseased to the point at which its function is significantly impaired[206] and surgical replacement may be necessary.[212,215] However, with more sensitive echocardiographic methods for detecting vegetations, principally two-dimensional echocardiography, the finding of vegetations is not as ominous as first thought.

Vegetations visualized echocardiographically need not be bacterial[216-218] or even infected.[219,220] Infected vegetations may be difficult to distinguish from myxomatous degeneration of the valve,[156,181,209,220] although this differentiation is usually readily accomplished clinically.

Prosthetic Valves

Despite extensive attention to this problem, there are still no sensitive and specific echocardiographic signs of prosthetic valve malfunction.[221–234] Most published reports of prosthetic valve malfunction represent isolated case studies, and the findings include large thrombi[229,235,236] and balls or discs that adhere to the cage intermittently or permanently.[223,225,226,231,237–243] Abnormal motion of a ball or disc usually results from thrombus[238] or ball variance.[231] A useful sign of a malfunctioning Björk-Shiley valve in the mitral position is a rounding of the E point on the M-mode echocardiogram.[245] An abnormal rocking motion of a prosthetic valve resulting from the sutures pulling loose from the annulus has been reported.[241,242] The significance of the "fine" intracavitary echoes originating from prosthetic valves in the mitral position is unclear.[243] Thickening of the porcine valve leaflets is useful in judging deterioration of this valve.[244]

An attempt has been made to assess the function of prosthetic mitral valves by noting that the motion of the prosthetic cage is reduced with obstruction. As with any other form of valvular regurgitation, when it occurs through a prosthetic valve there is evidence of ventricular volume overload. If regurgitation occurs through a prosthetic aortic valve, fluttering of the natural mitral valve may occur, just as is the case for regurgitation through the natural aortic valve. The motion of the interventricular septum is commonly abnormal for at least six months following open heart surgery.[246] Although the mechanism for this phenomenon has not been defined, if either the mitral or aortic prosthetic valve leaks significantly, the resultant left ventricular volume overload may prevent the occurrence of abnormal septal motion. Thus, *normal* septal motion in the first six months following aortic or mitral valve replacement is a sign of abnormality and suggests the presence of valvular regurgitation.[247–250] Doppler echocardiography is probably the best echocardiographic technique for evaluating prosthetic valve regurgitation.[251]

Thus, while echocardiography can record the motion of a prosthetic valve, unfortunately it is not always possible to assess its function. Thrombi, vegetations, and malfunction can occur without specific echocardiographic change. Probably, a change in serial echocardiograms is more significant in judging deterioration of prosthetic valve function than is an isolated recording, and combining echocardiography with phonocardiography for determining the timing of valve opening and closing may be helpful in evaluating prosthetic valve function, especially in the mitral position.[235,252–256]

CALCIFIED MITRAL ANNULUS

Calcification of a mitral annulus can be readily demonstrated by echocardiography.[257–264] The principal finding is a band of dense echoes between the mitral valve and the posterior left ventricular wall (Fig. 5–50).

CONGENITAL HEART DISEASE

(See also Chapters 29 and 30)

Deductive Echocardiography

"Deductive echocardiography" refers to a technique useful in the diagnosis of congenital heart disease by which an attempt is made to deduce the anatomy of the heart by identifying the atria, atrioventricular valves, ventricles, semilunar valves, and great vessels.[265,266] The chest roentgenogram is useful in identification of the atria. The loca-

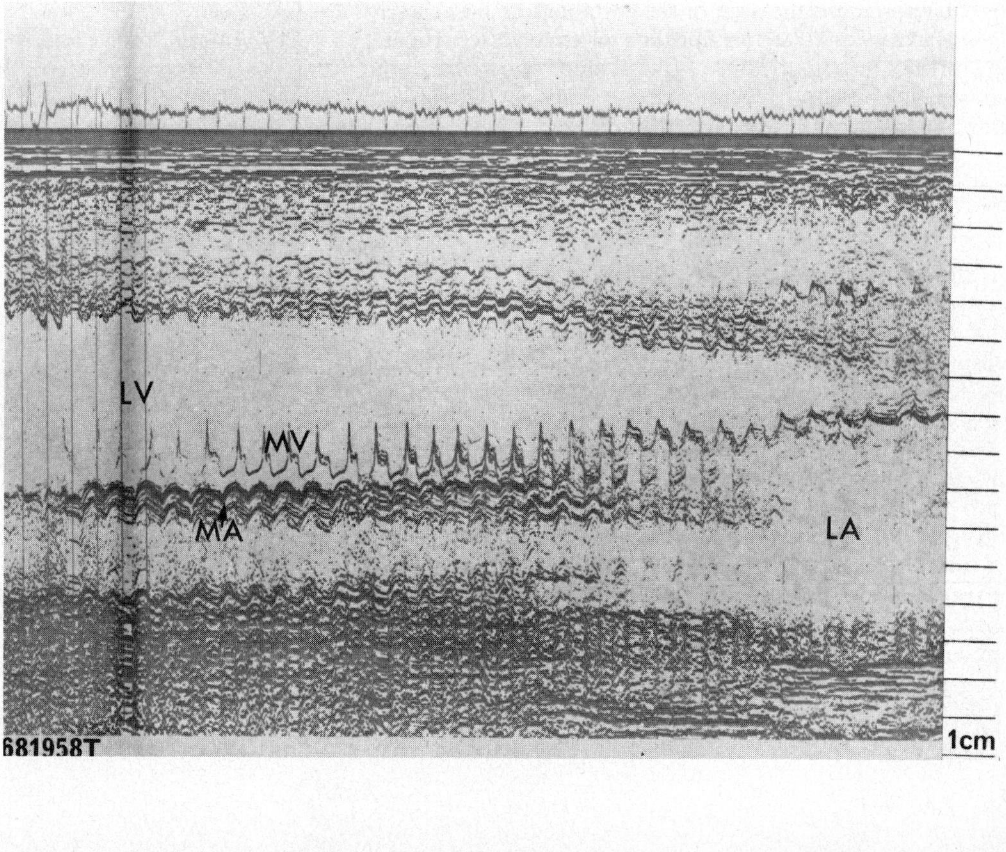

FIGURE 5–50 M-mode echocardiographic scan of a patient with a calcified mitral annulus (MA). The dark band of echoes from the annulus is posterior to the mitral valve (MV) and extends into the left ventricular cavity (LV). LA = left atrium.

tion of the trilobed lung or the stomach bubble can be used to decide whether or not the atria are in their normal position; the right atrium will be in its proper position if the lungs and the abdominal organs are also properly situated. The tricuspid valve is ordinarily in continuity with the "anatomic" right ventricle and the mitral valve with the left. Using M-mode echocardiography one can identify the mitral valve as that valve which is in direct continuity with a semilunar valve.[265,266] On the other hand, ventricular myocardium is usually interposed between the tricuspid and pulmonary valves. Thus, by using M-mode scanning to observe the relationship between an atrioventricular valve and the corresponding semilunar valve, it is possible to deduce whether it is a mitral or a tricuspid valve. Then, the anatomic ventricle to which it is connected can also be identified. Two-dimensional echocardiography is also useful for identifying the atrioventricular valves.[271] The tricuspid valve is attached to the interventricular septum closer to the apex than is the mitral valve.[267-269] The attachment of the two atrioventricular valves can be readily assessed using the apical four-chamber view.

The semilunar valves can be more difficult to differentiate, since they appear to be essentially identical on both M-mode and two-dimensional echocardiograms. Normally, the ejection time of the right ventricle exceeds that of the left, and this difference may be helpful in the differentiation of the semilunar valves. Unfortunately, the ejection time of the two valves may be similar in the presence of pulmonary hypertension. However, in such patients the administration of oxygen may lower the pulmonary artery pressure sufficiently to disclose a difference in ejection times and thereby assist in identification of the valves.[265] Two-dimensional echocardiography offers the opportunity of directly identifying the great vessels. It is possible to record the pulmonary artery bifurcation, which can be clearly differentiated from the nonbifurcating aorta.[270] It is also possible to record the arch of the aorta and its branches to help make a positive identification of that vessel. Having identified the individual valves and chambers, the echocardiographer then proceeds to localize these structures and determine their interrelationships.

Valvular Disease

The bicuspid aortic valve is probably the most common congenital anomaly (p. 976). Echocardiographic findings in this anomaly are based on the eccentric closure of the bicuspid aortic valve, so that the aortic valve echoes are no longer in the center of the aorta during diastole.[272,273] A useful though not totally reliable "eccentricity index" relates the width of the aortic lumen to the shortest distance between a cusp and the nearest margin of the aorta.[273] Two-dimensional echocardiography in patients with bicuspid aortic valves has also shown an eccentric position of the cusps in diastole.[274,275] Two-dimensional echocardiography can also identify the specific commissures in many patients. By identifying two rather than three commissures, one can make the echocardiographic diagnosis of bicuspid aortic valve.[275]

In aortic stenosis the echocardiographic findings are similar, if the valve is congenitally deformed or diseased as a result of rheumatic fever. Figure 5–48 shows a two-dimensional echocardiogram obtained from a patient with a typically domed congenitally stenotic valve. The two-dimensional technique clearly improves on the diagnosis of congenital aortic stenosis,[173] since the M-mode examination can fail to appreciate the domed nature of the valve. Estimating the severity of aortic stenosis directly is very difficult to accomplish with the M-mode examination, but this can be done indirectly by measuring the extent of left ventricular hypertrophy.[168-172] Two-dimensional echocardiography offers the possibility of measuring the separation of the stenotic aortic leaflets. Some but not all echocardiographers feel that the separation is related to the severity of the aortic stenosis.[173,174]

The echocardiographic findings in congenital mitral stenosis resemble those in rheumatic mitral stenosis in older children and adults.[276-278] However, in the young child or infant the congenitally stenotic mitral valve is more mobile and is not nearly as thickened as a rheumatic valve and the diastolic slope is not as flat.

The echocardiographic findings in *valvular pulmonic stenosis* include an accentuation of the *a* wave on the pulmonary valve echogram as noted earlier in this chapter (Fig. 5–37 and p. 108).[116] The powerful right atrial contraction increases right ventricular end-diastolic pressure above the relatively low pulmonary artery diastolic pressure, so that transmission of the atrial contraction through the right ventricle leads to premature opening of the pulmonary valve. Normally, this wave rises to a maximum of approximately 5 mm with inspiration; in pulmonic stenosis it may increase to 10 mm. While the exaggerated

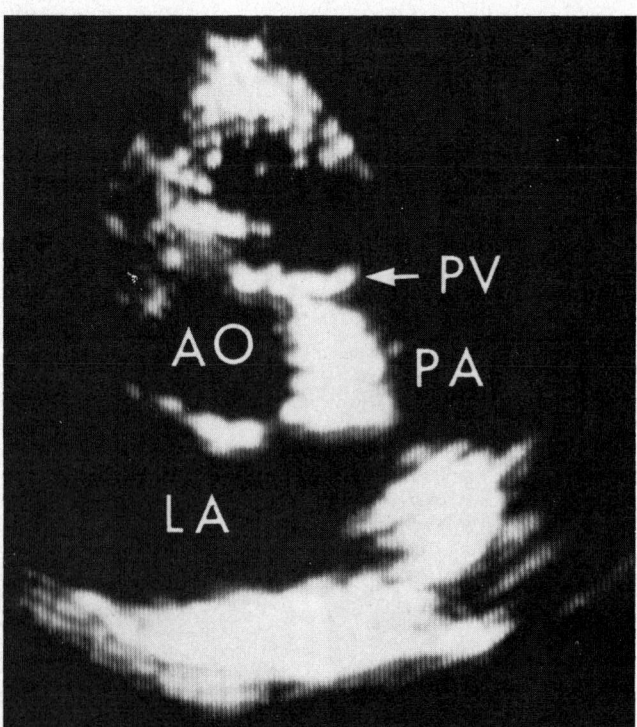

FIGURE 5–51 Two-dimensional echocardiogram of a patient with pulmonic stenosis. The domed, stenotic pulmonary valve (PV) curves into the pulmonary artery (PA) in the systolic frame. AO = aorta; LA = left atrium. (From Feigenbaum, H.: Echocardiography. 3rd ed. Philadelphia, Lea & Febiger, 1981.)

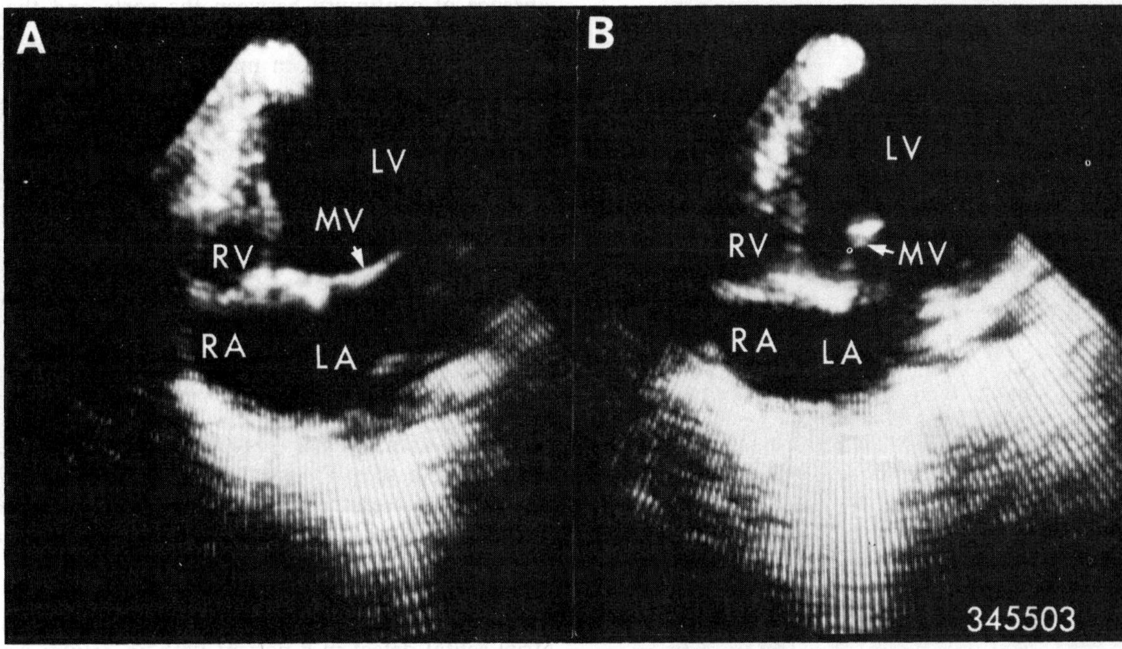

FIGURE 5–52 Apical four-chamber two-dimensional echocardiograms of a patient with tricuspid atresia. The mitral valve (MV) can be seen opening into a large left ventricular chamber (LV). The right ventricle (RV) is small and is separated from the right atrium (RA) by a dense band of linear echoes. No valvular structure could be identified in the region of the tricuspid valve. LA = left atrium. (From Feigenbaum, H.: Echocardiography. 3rd ed. Philadelphia, Lea & Febiger, 1981.)

a wave in pulmonic stenosis is a helpful sign, it must be appreciated that it is not specific, since it may also be present in patients with an elevated stroke volume, regardless of the cause.[54]

The domed stenotic pulmonary valve resembles the congenitally stenotic aortic valve on two-dimensional echocardiography.[279] Normally, the open leaflets are parallel to the wall of the pulmonary artery during systole, but when the valve is domed and stenotic, they curve away from the wall (Fig. 5–51). Though only a single leaflet of the pulmonary valve is ordinarily imaged, its domed appearance is sufficient to establish the diagnosis. The sensitivity and specificity of this technique still remain to be established.

The characteristic echocardiographic findings of *Ebstein's anomaly* of the tricuspid valve consist of increased motion, a position to the left of its usual location, varying diastolic slopes from beat to beat and, most reliably, delayed closure of the tricuspid valve.[280–282] Normally, and even in the presence of right bundle branch block, tricuspid follows mitral valve closure by less than 50 msec[283]; an interval between 50 and 70 msec should raise the suspicion of Ebstein's anomaly, and an interval greater than 70 msec strongly supports the diagnosis.

Two different approaches for the diagnosis of Ebstein's anomaly by means of two-dimensional echocardiography have been proposed:[284–286] the short-axis cross-sectional view of the tricuspid valve demonstrates the abnormally positioned tricuspid valve,[284] while with the apical approach, all four cardiac chambers can be imaged,[285,286] also allowing recognition of the malpositioned tricuspid valve.

VALVULAR ATRESIA. Atresia of cardiac valves is generally associated with hypoplasia of the ipsilateral ventricle (Chap. 29). Thus, aortic or mitral atresia is associated with a hypoplastic left ventricle,[287] while tricuspid or pulmonary atresia is associated with hypoplasia of the right ventricle.[49,50] Diminutive ventricles have been noted on M-mode tracings in patients with valvular atresia, and the atretic valves have been imaged with both M-mode[287] and two-dimensional techniques (Fig. 5–52).[288,289]

SUBVALVULAR OBSTRUCTIONS. A variety of congenital subvalvular obstructions have been detected echocardiographically. Early systolic closure of the aortic valve has been observed in patients with both *discrete* (Fig. 5–53)[107–109] and *hypertrophic obstructive cardiomyopathy* (Fig. 5–36).[104–106] In addition, systolic fluttering of the aortic valve is often exaggerated, although some degree of aortic valve fluttering may be seen normally. Although midsystolic closure and fluttering of the aortic valve are not specific findings for subaortic stenosis, they can be very helpful in differentiating valvular from subvalvular obstruction, since they do not occur in the former condition. Narrowing of the left ventricular outflow tract can sometimes also be detected by the M-mode technique in patients with discrete subaortic stenosis,[290] but this area of the heart is difficult to image using this method.

Examination of the outflow tract is easier, however, with two-dimensional echocardiography, and the subvalvular obstruction can be more readily identified directly by this technique (Fig. 5–54).[291–293] Moreover, the two-dimensional technique also permits the classification of the types of discrete obstruction into the discrete membranous and the diffuse types.[291] The ability to distinguish between them may be of considerable clinical importance, since their management may differ. The membranous form is frequently situated just below the aortic valve and may therefore be difficult to recognize at catheterization, since the short subvalvular chamber can be missed on a pull-out pressure recording. Indeed, the thin membrane can even be

Ultrasonic Examination of the Coronary Arteries

The principal value of echocardiography in patients with ischemic heart disease is determining the *consequences* of coronary obstruction, while the location of obstructions in the coronary arteries is predicted indirectly by assessing the motion of various segments of the left ventricle.[411,412] For example, abnormal motion of the interventricular septum suggests an obstruction of the proximal left anterior descending coronary artery.[412] Obviously, this is *indirect* evidence that is relatively insensitive, since the interventricular septum may move normally despite obstruction of the left anterior descending coronary artery.

Two-dimensional echocardiography can record the left main coronary artery and a small portion of the right coronary artery.[403] Obstructive lesions in the left main coronary artery have been demonstrated by several investigators.[414] Such obstructions are seen as masses of high intensity echoes in the vicinity of the left main coronary artery.[415,416] The echocardiographic technique for making this diagnosis is tedious and requires frame-by-frame analysis of the two-dimensional examination. This particular echocardiographic application has not achieved widespread acceptance, and its proper role in the management of patients has not been defined.

CARDIOMYOPATHIES

(See also Chapter 41)

Hypertrophic Obstructive Cardiomyopathy (HOCM)

Echocardiography is an important diagnostic tool in patients with HOCM and has enriched our understanding of this abnormality. The first echocardiographic abnormality to be noted was systolic anterior motion of the mitral valve (termed "SAM") (Fig. 5–69).[136,419–422] which appeared to be related to and was correlated with the presence of obstruction to left ventricular outflow.[104,423] The shorter the distance between the septum and the leaflet and the longer the duration of apposition between these two structures, the greater the degree of obstruction. This echocardiographic finding not only provided another diagnostic sign of HOCM but also demonstrated the critical importance of involvement of the mitral valve apparatus in the obstruction.[424] More recently SAM has been noted in a variety of patients, some of whom had no evidence of left ventricular hypertrophy[2,425–429]; it has been observed in patients with anemia and hypovolemia as well as in those with a hyperdynamic left ventricle.[427] It is possible that SAM is a nonspecific sign that occurs whenever the left ventricular systolic volume is reduced, either because of hypertrophy, as in HOCM, or in the presence of a hyperdynamic state.[429,430]

A second echocardiographic finding in patients with HOCM is midsystolic closure of the aortic valve (Fig. 5–36).[104–106] However, as noted earlier (p. 108), this sign is not specific for HOCM and is also present in patients with discrete subaortic stenosis. While not sensitive, this finding, when present, usually indicates a significant amount of obstruction.

Hypertrophy of the septum with abnormal organization of myocardial cells may be on e of the basic abnormalities of HOCM,[431,432] and key echocardiographic findings are disproportionate hypertrophy of the septum in relation to the posterior wall of the left ventricle, so that the ratio of thickness of septum to free wall exceeds 1.3 (Fig. 5–69),[433–435] and reduced motion of the hypertrophied septum.[436,437] It has also been shown that asymmetrical septal hypertrophy (ASH) is transmitted as an autosomal dominant trait and that there are patients with asymmetrical septal hypertrophy who do not show SAM and therefore do not have obstruction to left ventricular outflow (Fig. 5–70).[431,433,438,439] While the concept of recognizing ASH with or without obstruction to left ventricular outflow by echocardiography is an important one, there are limitations to its

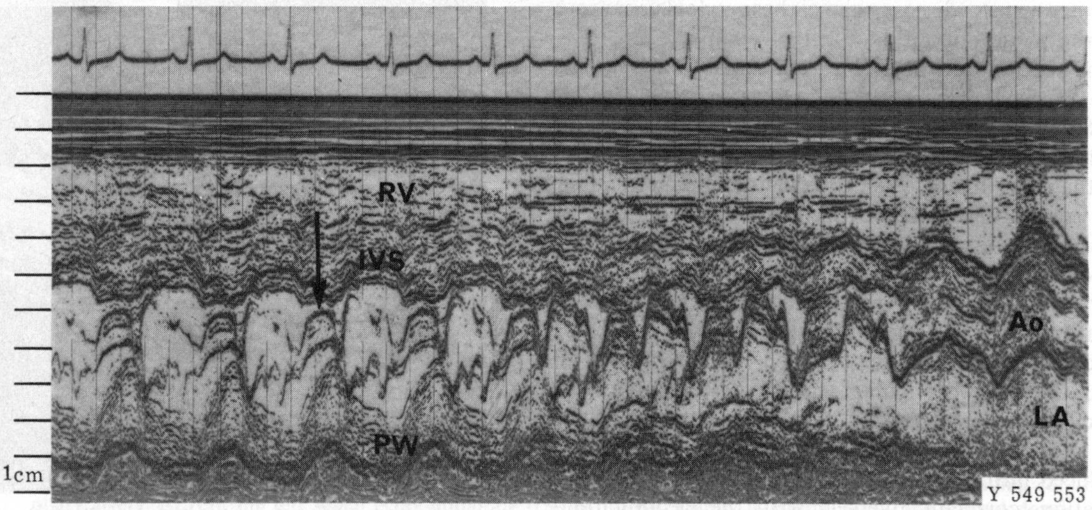

FIGURE 5–69 M-mode echocardiogram from a patient with hypertrophic subaortic stenosis demonstrating systolic anterior motion (arrow) of the mitral valve. RV = right ventricle, IVS = interventricular septum, PW = posterior left ventricular wall, Ao = aorta, LA = left atrium. (From Chang, S.: M-mode Echocardiographic Technique and Pattern Recognition. Philadelphia, Lea and Febiger, 1976.)

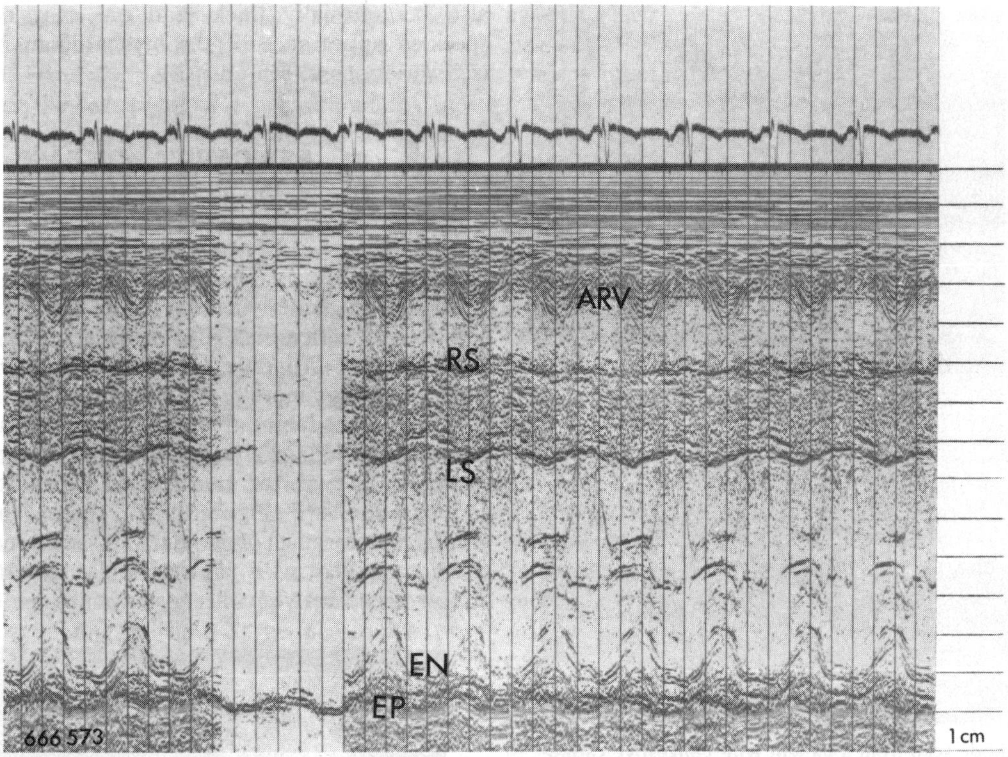

FIGURE 5–70 Echocardiogram from a patient with asymmetrical septal hypertrophy but no evidence of outflow obstruction. The distance between the right (RS) and left (LS) septal echoes is considerably greater than is the thickness of the posterior left ventricular myocardium between the endocardial (EN) and epicardial (EP) echoes.

echocardiographic diagnosis. First, the thickness of the septum may be difficult to measure echocardiographically; in Figure 5–69 the left side of the septum is clearly identified, but the right side is not as distinct and septal thickness cannot always be measured precisely. Second, it must be appreciated that ASH is not pathognomonic for HOCM and related myopathies[440,441] and can occur in a variety of other disease states (including right ventricular hypertrophy and coronary artery disease[440,442] and even in patients on chronic hemodialysis[443]) in a form which is indistinguishable echocardiographically from genetically determined ASH. In addition, some patients with HOCM may have concentric rather than asymmetrical hypertrophy, in which the septal and posterior left ventricular walls are equal in thickness.

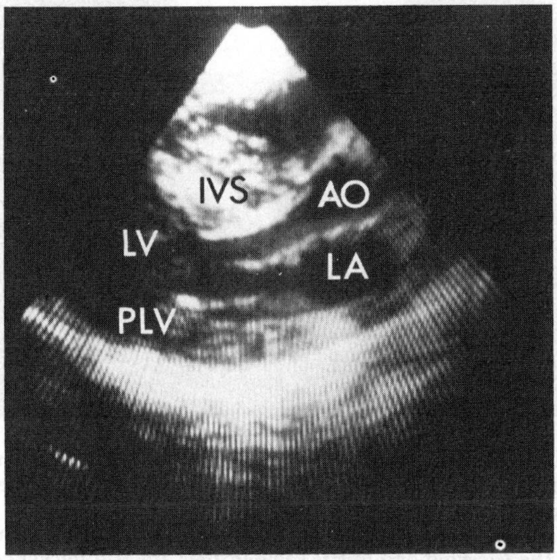

FIGURE 5–71 Cross-sectional echogram from a patient with hypertrophic subaortic stenosis with a markedly hypertrophied interventricular septum (IVS). LV = left ventricle, PLV = posterior left ventricular wall, AO = aorta, LA = left atrium.

Two-dimensional echocardiography provides additional information by indicating the shape and location of the hypertrophied septum in patients with known or suspected HOCM (Fig. 5–71).[444–448] This technique can also be used to assess the effectiveness of myotomy and myectomy.[449] An intriguing but as yet unconfirmed observation is that the echoes from the diseased septum in HOCM are denser than those from the free posterior wall.

Congestive (Dilated) Cardiomyopathy

The echocardiogram characteristically reveals a dilated, poorly contracting left ventricle in patients with congestive cardiomyopathy (Fig. 5–72).[450,451] Signs of reduced cardiac output include a poorly moving aorta, reduced opening of the mitral valve, and slow closure of the aortic valve. The left atrium is dilated, and the abnormal closure of the mitral valve indicative of elevated left ventricular diastolic pressure is frequently noted. It must be appreciated that these findings are nonspecific and may occur in patients with coronary artery disease. However, at least one portion of the left ventricle, usually the posterior wall, contin-

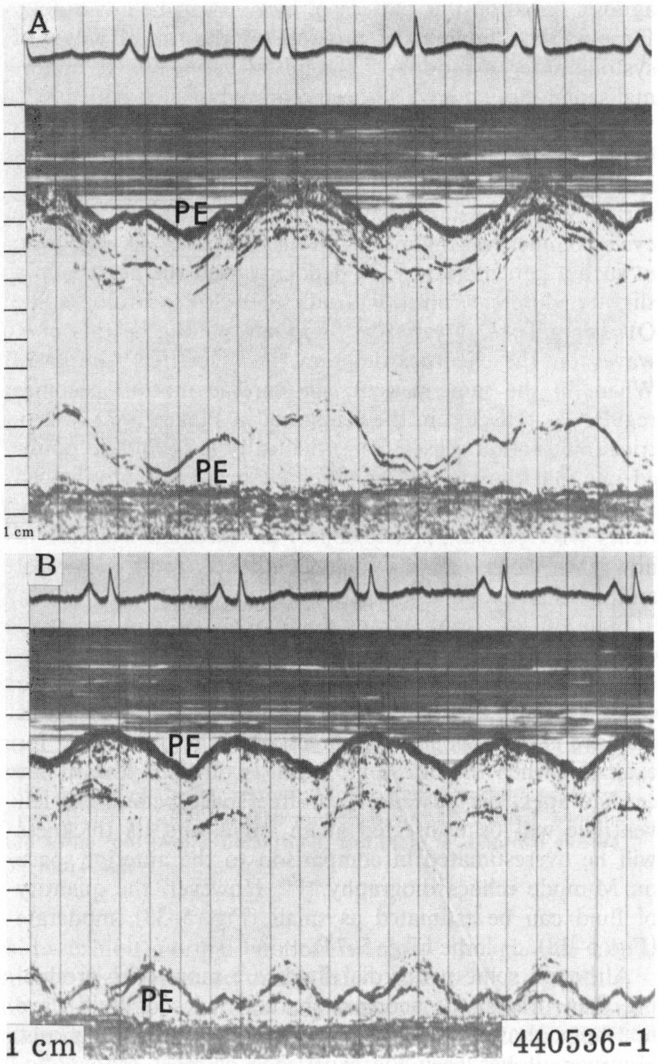

FIGURE 5–75 Echocardiograms from a patient with massive pericardial effusion (PE). *A*, Anterior right ventricular echo (ARV) and posterior left ventricular epicardial echoes move essentially in similar directions. The position of the heart differs slightly with each cardiac cycle. The corresponding electrocardiogram shows electrical alternation. Upon removal of some of the pericardial fluid (*B*), cardiac excursions are synchronous with each electrical depolarization, and electrical alternation is no longer present. (From Feigenbaum, H.: Echocardiography, 2nd ed. Philadelphia, Lea and Febiger, 1976.)

Although the diagnosis of pericardial effusion is one of the most common and important uses of echocardiography, it must be emphasized that there are technical difficulties associated with the application of this (as of every other) echocardiographic technique. Even when proper techniques are used, confusing situations can arise. For example, a retrocardiac pleural effusion can mimic a posterior pericardial effusion. However, the fact that there is usually significantly less pericardial effusion behind the left atrium than behind the ventricle can be a helpful sign. While a pleural effusion may also be less behind the left atrium, it decreases at the atrioventricular junction abruptly rather than gradually, as is the case with pericardial effusion; also, pleural effusions are not usually apparent anteriorly. Positioning the patient so that the pleural fluid no longer collects behind the heart will be helpful except where it is loculated.[467,468] A giant left atrium may produce an echo-free space behind the left ventricular wall and give the appearance of a large posterior pericardial effusion,[469] and even a retrograde hiatal hernia can present a confusing echogram.[470]

Although M-mode echocardiography is usually sufficient for the echocardiographic diagnosis of pericardial effusion, two-dimensional echocardiography also plays a role in this diagnosis. The two-dimensional approach is particularly helpful in patients with loculated effusions.[471] If there are adhesions to the point that the fluid is not evenly distributed within the pericardial cavity, then the two-dimensional approach will be superior to the M-mode examination, which might even be misleading. It is not surprising that two-dimensional echocardiography is more accurate in attempting to quantitate the degree of pericardial effusion, since this examination can record all of the fluid surrounding the heart (Fig. 5–76). The two-dimensional approach also can be helpful in distinguishing pleural from pericardial effusion. By identifying the descending aorta one can distinguish pericardial effusion, which separates the aorta from the heart, from pleural effusion, which collects posterior to the descending aorta.[472] Metastases to the pericardium have been detected with two-dimensional echocardiography as well.[473]

Once the diagnosis of pericardial effusion has been established, a number of echocardiographic criteria for the detection of cardiac tamponade have been suggested.[474–479]

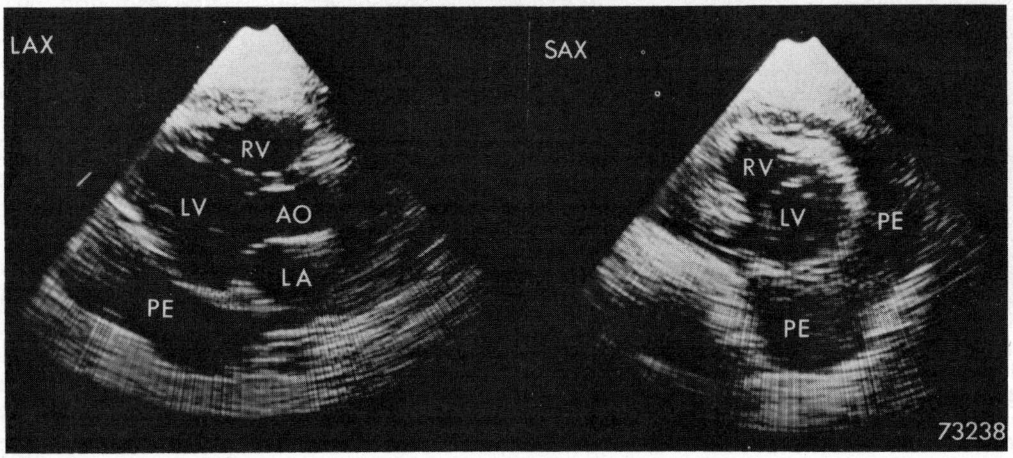

FIGURE 5–76 Long-axis (LAX) and short-axis (SAX) two-dimensional echocardiograms of a patient with a large pericardial effusion. The pericardial effusion (PE) can be seen accumulating posteriorly and laterally. RV = right ventricle; LV = left ventricle; AO = aorta; LA = left atrium. (From Feigenbaum, H.: Echocardiography. 3rd ed. Philadelphia, Lea & Febiger, 1981.)

The newest and possibly most reliable echocardiographic finding with tamponade is compression of the right ventricular free wall in early diastole. This finding is noted by a posterior displacement of the anterior free wall on the M-mode echocardiogram[477,478] (Fig. 5–77). The free wall then moves anteriorly following atrial systole. This observation has been confirmed with two-dimensional echocardiography by noting a collapse of the right ventricular free wall on the two-dimensional examination[478] (Fig. 5–78). Another study has noted a collapse of the right atrial free wall on the two-dimensional four-chamber view.[479] This right atrial sign is probably comparable to the right ventricular free wall collapse with tamponade. Both of these signs appear to be very sensitive for hemodynamic impairment secondary to the tamponade. The finding may antedate the clinical signs of tamponade. The other echocardiographic signs of tamponade, such as reduction of the size of the right ventricular cavity, flat diastolic motion of the left ventricular wall, and variations in the E to F slope of the mitral valve,[474–476] have not proved to be reliable.

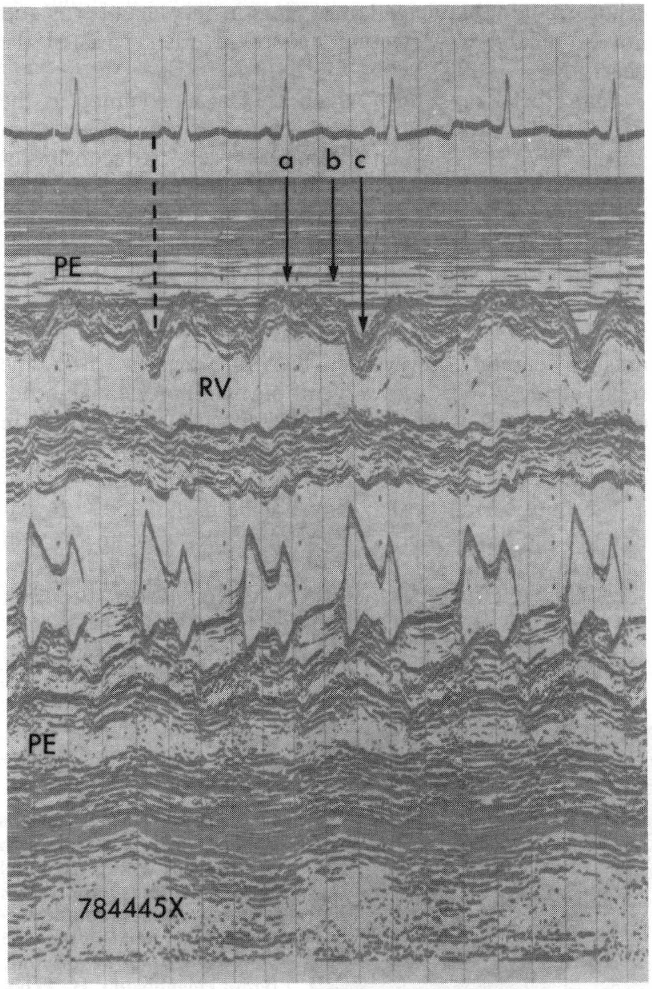

FIGURE 5–77 M-mode echocardiogram of a patient with pericardial effusion and clinical evidence of tamponade. The right ventricular free wall moves gradually posteriorly during systole (from a to b). In early diastole there is an abrupt downward or posterior motion of the right ventricular free wall (c and dashed line). PE = pericardial effusion; RV = right ventricle.

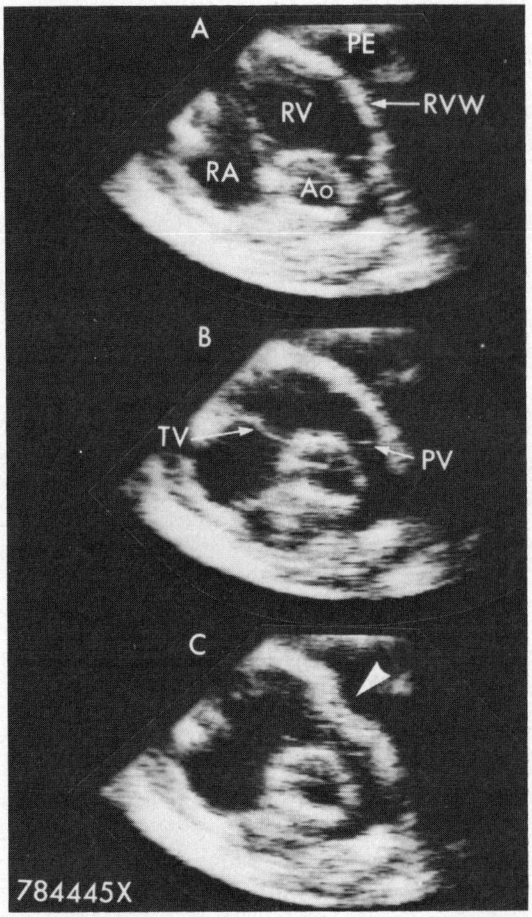

FIGURE 5–78 Parasternal short-axis two-dimensional echocardiograms in a patient with cardiac tamponade. *A* represents end-diastole. At end-systole (*B*), the right ventricle (RV) is smaller but normal in shape. Both the tricuspid valve (TV) and pulmonary valve (PV) are closed. With early diastole (*C*) the tricuspid valve has opened and the shape of the right ventricle has been distorted (large arrowhead) by collapse of the right ventricular wall (RVW). PE = pericardial effusion; RA = right atrium; AO = aorta. (From Armstrong, W.F., Schilt, B.F., Helper, D.J., Dillon, J.C., and Feigenbaum, H.: Diastolic collapse of the right ventricle with cardiac tamponade: An echocardiographic study. Circulation *65*:1491, 1982.)

Constrictive Pericarditis. Echocardiography can be of some value in the diagnosis of a thickened pericardium with constrictive pericarditis.[480–484] However, the reliability of the techniques is limited. Although a thickened pericardium can be detected in many patients,[2,480] particularly those who also have pericardial fluid, this finding by itself does not imply the presence of constriction. The echocardiographic signs of constriction include lack of diastolic motion, i.e., a flat diastolic slope of the posterior left ventricular wall,[2,487] abnormal motion of the interventricular septum,[485–487] and a very short and steep E to F slope of the mitral valve.[2] The echocardiographic signs of constriction are not very sensitive and are certainly not specific; at best they raise the suspicion of this condition.

CARDIAC TUMORS

(See also Chapter 42)

ATRIAL TUMORS. Left atrial myxoma is by far the most common cardiac tumor, and echocardiography has

References

1. Carlsen, E. N.: Ultrasound physics for the physician: A brief review. J. Clin. Ultrasound *3*:69, 1975.
2. Feigenbaum, H.: Echocardiography. 3rd ed. Philadelphia, Lea and Febiger, 1981.
3. Wells, P. N. T.: Ultrasonics in Clinical Diagnosis. 2nd ed. New York, Churchill Livingstone, 1977.
4. Griffith, J. M., and Henry, W. L.: A sector scanner for real-time two-dimensional echocardiography. Circulation *49*:1147, 1974.
5. Eggleton, R. C., Feigenbaum, H., Johnston, K. W., Weyman, A. E., Dillon, J. C., and Chang, S.: Visualization of cardiac dynamics with real-time B-mode ultrasonic scanner. *In* White, D. (ed.): Ultrasound in Medicine. New York, Plenum Press, 1975, p. 385.
6. Von Ramm, O. T., and Thurstone, F. L.: Cardiac imaging using a phased array ultrasound system. Circulation *53*:258, 1976.
7. Helak, J. W., Plappert, T., Muhammad, A., and Reichek, N.: Two dimensional echocardiographic imaging of the left ventricle: Comparison of mechanical and phased array systems in vitro. Am. J. Cardiol. *48*:728, 1981.
8. Rushmer, R. F., Baker, D. W., and Stegall, H. F.: Transcutaneous Doppler flow detection as a non-destructive technique. J. Appl. Physiol. *21*:554, 1966.
9. Lavenson, G. S., Rich, N. M., and Baugh, J. H.: Value of ultrasonic flow detection in the management of peripheral vascular disease. Am. J. Surg. *120*:522, 1970.
10. Sigel, B., Popley, G. L., Boland, J., Wagner, D. K., and Mapp, E. M.: Augmentation of flow sounds in the ultrasonic detection of venous abnormalities. Invest. Radiol. *2*:256, 1967.
11. Strandness, D. E., McCutcheon, E. P., and Rushmer, R. F.: Application of a transcutaneous Doppler flow meter in evaluation of occlusive arterial disease. Surg. Gynecol. Obstet. *122*:1039, 1966.
12. Light, L. H.: Transcutaneous observation of blood velocity in the ascending aorta in man. Biol. Cardiol. *26*:214, 1969.
13. Huntsman, L. L., Gams, E., Johnson, C. C., and Fairbanks, E.: Transcutaneous determination of aortic blood flow velocities in man. Am. Heart J. *89*:605, 1975.
14. Sequeira, R. F., Light, L. H., Gross, G., and Raftery, E. B.: Transcutaneous aortovenography. A quantitative evaluation. Br. Heart J. *38*:443, 1976.
15. Kolettis, M., Jenkins, B. S., and Webb-Peploe, M. M.: Assessment of left ventricular function by indices derived from aortic flow velocity. Br. Heart J. *38*:18, 1976.
16. Colocousis, J. S., Huntsman, L. L., and Curreri, P. W.: Estimation of stroke volume changes by ultrasonic Doppler. Circulation *56*:914, 1977.
17. Buchtal, A., Hanson, G. C., and Peisach, A. R.: Transcutaneous aortovenography. Potentially useful technique in management of critically ill patients. Br. Heart J. *38*:451, 1976.
18. Joyner, C. R., Jr., Harrison, F. S., Jr., and Gruber, J. W.: Diagnosis of hypertrophic subaortic stenosis with a Doppler velocity flow detector. Ann. Intern. Med. *74*:692, 1971.
19. Boughner, D. R., Schuld, R. L., and Persaud, J. A.: Hypertrophic obstructive cardiomyopathy. Assessment by echocardiographic and Doppler ultrasound techniques. Br. Heart J. *37*:917, 1975.
20. Thompson, P. D., Mennel, R. G., MacVaugh, H., and Joyner, C. R.: The evaluation of aortic insufficiency in humans with a transcutaneous Doppler velocity probe. Ann. Intern. Med. *72*:781, 1970.
21. Boughner, D. R.: Assessment of aortic insufficiency by transcutaneous Doppler ultrasound. Circulation *52*:874, 1975.
22. Pearlman, A. S., Stevenson, J. G., and Baker, D. W.: Doppler echocardiography: Applications, limitations and future directions. Am. J. Cardiol. *46*:1256, 1980.
23. Baker, D. W., Rubenstein, S. A., and Lorch, G. S.: Pulsed Doppler echocardiography: Principles and applications. Am. J. Med. *63*:69, 1977.
24. Johnson, S. L., Baker, D. W., Lute, R. A., and Dodge, H. T.: Doppler echocardiography: The localization of cardiac murmurs. Circulation *48*:810, 1973.
25. Lorch, G., Rubenstein, S., Baker, D., Dooley, T., and Dodge, H.: Doppler echocardiography. Use of a graphical display system. Circulation *56*:576, 1977.
26. Goldberg, S. J., Areias, J. C., Spitaels, S. E. C., and deVilleneuve, V. H.: Use of time interval histographic output from echo-Doppler to detect left-to-right atrial shunts. Circulation *58*:147, 1978.
27. Stevenson, G., Kawabori, I., and Brandestini, M.: Color-coded Doppler visualization of flow within ventricular septal defects: Implications for peak pulmonary artery disease. Am. J. Cardiol. *49*:944, 1982.
28. Bommer, W. J., and Miller, L.: Real-time two-dimensional color-flow Doppler: Enhanced Doppler flow imaging in the diagnosis of cardiovascular disease. Am. J. Cardiol. *49*:944, 1982 (Abstract).
29. Gramiak, R., Shah, P. M., and Kramer, D. H.: Ultrasound cardiography: Contrast studies in anatomy and function. Radiology *92*:939, 1969.
30. Feigenbaum, H., Stone, J. M., Lee, D. A., Nasser, W. K., and Chang, S.: Identification of ultrasound echoes from the left ventricle using intracardiac injections of indocyanine green. Circulation *41*:615, 1970.
31. Kerber, R. E., Kioschos, J. M., and Lauer, R. M.: Use of an ultrasonic contrast method in the diagnosis of valvular regurgitation and intracardiac shunts. Am. J. Cardiol. *34*:722, 1974.
32. Meltzer, R. S., Serruys, P. W., Hugenholtz, P. G., and Roelandt, J.: Intravenous carbon dioxide as an echocardiographic contrast agent. J. Clin. Ultrasound *9*:127, 1981.
33. Gaffney, F. A., Lin, J-C., Peshock, R. M., and Buja, L. M.: Hydrogen peroxide: A new, reliable 2D echocardiographic contrast agent. Am. J. Cardiol. *49*:955, 1982.
34. Chang, S., and Feigenbaum, H.: Subxiphoid echocardiography. J. Clin. Ultrasound *1*:14, 1973.
35. Weyman, A. E., Peskoe, S. M., Williams, E. S., Dillion, J. C., and Feigenbaum, H.: Detection of left ventricular aneurysms by cross-sectional echocardiography. Circulation *54*:936, 1976.
36. Silverman, N. H., and Schiller, N. B.: Apex echocardiography. A two-dimensional technique for evaluating congenital heart disease. Circulation *57*:503, 1978.
37. Hickman, H. O., Weyman, A. E., Wann, L. S., Phillips, J. F., Dillion, J. C., Feigenbaum, H., and Marshall, J.: Cross-sectional echocardiography of the cardiac apex. Circulation *56*:III-153 (Abstract), 1977.
38. Goldberg, B. B.: Suprasternal ultrasonography. J.A.M.A. *215*:245, 1971.
39. Sahn, D. J., Goldberg, S. J., McDonald, G., and Allen, H. D.: Suprasternal notch real-time cross-sectional echocardiography for imaging the pulmonary artery, aortic arch, and decending aorta. Am. J. Cardiol. *39*:266, 1977.
40. Snider, A. R., and Silverman, N. H.: Suprasternal notch echocardiography: A two-dimensional technique for evaluating congenital heart disease. Circulation *63*:165, 1981.
41. Bansal, R. C., Tajik, A. J., Seward, J. B., and Offord, K. P.: Feasibility of two-dimensional echocardiographic examination in adults. Prospective study of 200 patients. Mayo Clin. Proc. *55*:291, 1980.
42. Sahn, D. J., DeMaria, A., Kisslo, J., and Weyman, A.: Recommendations regarding quantitation in M-mode echocardiography: Results of a survey of echocardiographic measurements. Circulation *58*:1072, 1978.
43. Henry, W. L., Gardin, J. M., and Ware, J. H.: Echocardiographic measurements in normal subjects from infancy to old age. Circulation *62*:1054, 1980.
44. Tajik, A. J., Seward, J. B., Hagler, D. J., Mair, D. D., and Lee, J. T.: Two-dimensional real-time ultrasonic imaging of the heart and great vessels: Technique image orientation, structure identification, and validation. Mayo Clin. Proc. *53*:271, 1978.
45. Henry, W. L., DeMaria, A., Gramiak, R., King, D. L., Kisslo, J. A., Popp, R. L., Sahn, D. J., Schiller, N. B., Tajik, A., Teichholz, L. E., and Weyman, A. E.: Report of the American Society of Echocardiography Nomenclature and Standards in Two-dimensional Echocardiography. Circulation *62*:212, 1980.
46. Meltzer, R. S., McGhie, J., and Roelandt, J.: Inferior vena cava echocardiography. J. Clin. Ultrasound *10*:47, 1982.
47. Popp, R. L., Wolfe, S. B., Hirata, T., and Feigenbaum, H.: Estimation of right and left ventricular size by ultrasound. A study of the echoes from the interventricular septum. Am. J. Cardiol. *24*:523, 1969.
48. Diamond, M. A., Dillon, J. C., Haine, C. L., Chang, S., and Feigenbaum, H.: Echocardiographic features of atrial septal defect. Circulation *43*:129, 1971.
49. Chestler, E., Jaffe, H. S., Vecht, R., Beck, W., and Schrire, V.: Ultrasound cardiography in single ventricle and the hypoplastic left and right heart syndromes. Circulation *42*:123, 1970.
50. Meyer, R. A., and Kaplan, S.: Echocardiography in the diagnosis of hypoplasia of the left or right ventricle in the neonate. Circulation *46*:55, 1972.
51. Matsukubo, H., Matsuura, T., Endo, N., Asayama, J., Watanabe, T., Furukawa, K., Kunishige, H., Katsume, H., and Ijichi, H.: Echocardiographic measurement of right ventricular wall thickness. A new application of subxiphoid echocardiography. Circulation *56*:278, 1977.
52. Hirata, T., Wolfe, S. B., Popp, R. L., Helmen, C. H., and Feigenbaum, H.: Estimation of left atrial size using ultrasound. Am. Heart J. *78*:43, 1969.
53. Yabek, S. M., Isabel-Jones, J., Bhatt, D. R., Nakazawa, M., Marks, R. A., and Jarmakani, J. M.: Echocardiographic determination of left atrial volumes in children with congenital heart disease. Circulation *53*:268, 1976.
54. Goldberg, S. J., Allen, H. D., and Sahn, D. J.: *In* Pediatric and Adolescent Echocardiography. Chicago, Year Book Medical Publishers, 1975, pp. 34, 47, and 117.
55. Lemire, F., Tajik, A. J., and Hagler, D. J.: Asymmetric left atrial enlargement: An echocardiographic observation. Chest *69*:779, 1976.
56. Schabelman, S., Schiller, N. B., Silverman, N. H., and Ports, T. A.: Left atrial volume estimation by two-dimensional echocardiography. Cathet. Cardiovasc. Diagn. *7*:165, 1981.
57. Gehl, L. G., Mintz, G. S., Kotler, M. N., and Segal, B. L.: Left atrial volume overload in mitral regurgitation: A two dimensional echocardiographic study. Am. J. Cardiol. *49*:33, 1982.
58. Dillon, J. C., Weyman, A. E., Feigenbaum, H., Eggleton, R. C., and Johnston, K. W.: Cross-sectional echocardiographic examination of the interatrial septum. Circulation *55*:115, 1977.
59. Feigenbaum, H., Popp, R. L., Wolfe, S. B., Troy, B. L., Pombo, J. F., Haine, C. L., and Dodge, H. T.: Ultrasound measurements of the left ventricle: A correlative study with angiography. Arch. Intern. Med. *129*:461, 1972.
60. Fortuin, N. J., Hood, W. P., Jr., and Craige, E.: Evaluation of left ventricular function by echocardiography. Circulation *46*:26, 1972.
61. Teichholz, L. E., Kreulen, T., Herman, M. V., and Gorlin, R.: Problems in echocardiographic volume determinations: Echocardiographic-angiographic correlations in the presence or absence of asynergy. Am. J. Cardiol. *37*:7, 1976.
62. McDonald, I. G., Feigenbaum, H., and Chang, S.: Analysis of left ventricular wall motion by reflected ultrasound: application to assessment of myocardial function. Circulation *46*:14, 1972.

63. Quinones, M. A., Gaasch, W. H., and Alexander, J. K.: Echocardiographic assessment of left ventricular function: With special reference to normalized velocities. Circulation *50*:42, 1974.
64. Feigenbaum, H.: Echocardiographic examination of the left ventricle. Circulation *51*:1, 1975.
65. Massie, B. M., Schiller, N. B., Ratshin, R. A., and Parmley, W. W.: Mitral-septal separation: New echocardiographic index of left ventricular function. Am. J. Cardiol. *39*:1008, 1977.
66. Child, J. S., Krivokapich, J., and Perloff, J. K.: Effect of left ventricular size on mitral E point to ventricular septal separation in assessment of cardiac performance. Am. Heart J. *101*:797, 1981.
67. Skorton, D. J., McNary, C. A., Child, J. S., Newton, F. C., and Shah, P. M.: Digital image processing of two dimensional echocardiograms: Identification of the endocardium. Am. J. Cardiol. *48*:479, 1981.
68. Garcia, E., Gueret, P., Bennett, M., Corday, E., Zwehl, W., Meerbaum, S., Corday, S., Swan, H. J., and Berman, D.: Real time computerization of two-dimensional echocardiography. Am. Heart J. *101*:783, 1981.
69. Levy, R., Garcia, E., Zwehl, W., Murphy, F., Corday, S. R., Childs, W., Meerbaum, S., and Corday, E.: Objective echocardiographic quantitation of left ventricular volumes by use of automated computerized edge-detection analysis in canines and humans. Am. J. Cardiol. *49*:897, 1982.
70. Schiller, N. B., Acquatella, H., Ports, T. A., Drew, D., Goerke, J., Ringertz, H., Silverman, N. H., Carlsson, E., and Parmley, W. W.: Left ventricular volume from paired biplane two-dimensional echocardiography. Circulation *60*:547, 1979.
71. Folland, E. D., Parisi, A. F., Moynihan, P. F., Jones, D. R., Feldman, C. L., and Tow, D. E.: Assessment of left ventricular ejection fraction and volumes by real-time, two-dimensional echocardiography. Circulation *62*:760, 1979.
72. Gueret, P., Meerbaum, S., Wyatt, S., Wyatt, H. L., Uchiyama, T., Lang, T. W., and Corday, E.: Two-dimensional echocardiographic quantitation of left ventricular volumes and ejection fraction. Importance of accounting for dyssynergy in short-axis reconstruction models. Circulation *62*:1308, 1980.
73. Jacobs, L. E., Hall, J. D., Gubernick, I., Meister, S. G., and Barrett, M. J.: Axial versus lateral resolution: Inherent errors in two-dimensional echocardiography imaging. Am. J. Cardiol. *49*:1020, 1982.
74. Kan, G., Visser, C. A., Lie, K. I., and Durrer, D.: Left ventricular volumes and ejection fraction by single plane two-dimensional apex echocardiography. Eur. Heart J. *2*:339, 1981.
75. Starling, M. R., Crawford, M. H., Sorensen, S. G., Levi, B., Richards, K. L., and O'Rourke, R. A.: Comparative accuracy of apical biplane cross-sectional echocardiography and gated equilibrium radionuclide angiography for estimating left ventricular size and performance. Circulation *63*:1075, 1981.
76. Barrett, M. J., Jacobs, L., Gomberg, J., Horton, L., Wolf, N. M., and Meister, S. G.: Simultaneous contrast imaging of the left ventricle by two-dimensional echocardiography and standard ventriculography. Clin. Cardiol. *5*:208, 1982.
77. Quinones, M. A., Waggoner, A. D., Reduto, L. A., Nelson, J. G., Young, J. B., Winters, W. L., Jr., Ribeiro, L. G., and Miller, R. R.: A new, simplified and accurate method for determining ejection fraction with two-dimensional echocardiography. Circulation *64*:744, 1981.
78. Watanabe, T., Katsume, H., Matsukubo, H., Furukawa, K., and Ijichi, H.,: Estimation of right ventricular volume with two dimensional echocardiography. Am. J. Cardiol. *49*:1946, 1982.
79. Crawford, M. H., White, D. H., and Amon, K. W.: Echocardiographic evaluation of left ventricular size and performance during handgrip and supine and upright bicycle exercise. Circulation *59*:1188, 1979.
80. Weiss, J. L., Weisfeldt, M. L., Mason, S. J., Garrison, J. B., Livengood, S. V., and Fortuin, N. J.: Evidence of Frank-Starling effect in man during severe semisupine exercise. Circulation *59*:655, 1979.
81. Zwehl, W., Gueret, P., Meerbaum, S., Holt, D., and Corday, E.: Quantitative two dimensional echocardiography during bicycle exercise in normal subjects. Am. J. Cardiol. *47*:866, 1981.
82. Feigenbaum, H., Popp, R. L., Chip, J. N., and Haine, C. L.: Left ventricular wall thickness measured by ultrasound. Arch. Intern. Med. *121*:391, 1968.
83. Grossman, W., McLaurin, L. P., Moos, S. P., Stefadouros, M. A., and Young, D. T.: Wall thickness and diastolic properties of the left ventricle. Circulation *49*:129, 1974.
84. Troy, B. L., Pombo, J., and Rackley, C. E.: Measurement of left ventricular wall thickness and mass by echocardiography. Circulation *45*:602, 1972.
85. Devereux, R. B., and Reichek, N.: Echocardiographic determination of left ventricular mass in man. Anatomic validation of the method. Circulation *55*:613, 1977.
86. Sasayama, S., Franklin, D., Ross, J., Kemper, W. S., and McKown, D.: Dynamic changes in left ventricular wall thickness and their use in analyzing cardiac function in the conscious dog. A study based on a modified ultrasonic technique. Am. J. Cardiol. *38*:870, 1976.
87. Corya, B. C., Rasmussen, S., Feigenbaum, H., Knoebel, S. B., and Black, M. J.: Systolic thickening and thinning of the septum and posterior wall in patients with coronary artery disease, congestive cordiomyopathy, and atrial septal defect. Circulation *55*:109, 1977.
88. Joyner, C. R., Dyrda, I., and Reid, M. M.: Behavior of the anterior leaflet of the mitral valve in patients with the Austin-Flint murmur. Clin. Res. *14*:251 (Abstract), 1966.
89. Dillon, J. C., Haine, C. L., Chang, S., and Feigenbaum,. H.: Significance of mitral fluttering in patients with aortic insufficiency. Clin. Res. *18*:304 (Abstract), 1970.
90. Winsberg, F., Gabor, G. E., and Hernberg, J. G.: Fluttering of the mitral valve in aortic insufficiency. Circulation *41*:225 (Abstract), 1970.
91. Pridie, R. B., Beham, R., and Oakley, C. M.: Echocardiography of the mitral valve in aortic valve disease. Br. Heart J. *33*:296, 1971.
92. Botvinick, E. H., Schiller, N. B., Wickramasekaran, R., Klausner, S. C., and Getz, E.: Echocardiographic demonstration of early mitral valve closure in severe aortic insufficiency. Its clinical implications. Circulation *51*:836, 1975.
93. Mann, T., McLaurin, L., Grossman, W., and Craige, E.: Assessing the hemodynamic severity of acute aortic regurgitation due to infective endocarditis. N. Engl. J. Med. *293*:108, 1975.
94. Laniado, S., Yellin, E., Kotler, M., Levy, L., Stadler, J., and Terdiman, R.: A study of the dynamic relations between the mitral valve echogram and phasic mitral flow. Circulation *51*:104, 1975.
95. Layton, C., Gent, G., Pridïe, R., McDonald, A., and Brigden, W.: Diastolic closure rate of normal mitral valve. Br. Heart J. *35*:1066, 1973.
96. DeMaria, A. N., Lies, J. E., King, J. F., Miller, R. R., Amsterdam, E. A., and Mason, D. T.: Echographic assessment of atrial transport, mitral movement, and ventricular performance following electroversion of supraventricular arrhythmias. Circulation *51*:273, 1975.
97. Lalani, A. V., and Lee, S. J. K.: Echocardiographic measurement of cardiac output using the mitral valve and aortic root echo. Circulation *54*:738, 1976.
98. Rasmussen, S., Corya, B. C., Feigenbaum, H., Black, M. J., Lovelace, D. E., Phillips, J. F., Noble, R. J., and Knoebel, S. B.: Stroke volume calculated from the mitral valve echogram in patients with and without ventricular dyssynergy. Circulation *58*:125, 1978.
99. Konecke, L. L., Feigenbaum, H., Chang, S., Corya, B. C., and Fischer, J. C.: Abnormal mitral valve motion in patients with elevated left ventricular diastolic pressures. Circulation *47*:989, 1973.
100. Lewis, J. R., Parker, J. O., and Burggraf, G. W.: Mitral valve motion and changes in left ventricular end-diastolic pressures: A correlative study of the PR-AC interval. Am. J. Cardiol. *42*:383, 1978.
101. Askenazi, J., Koenigsberg, D. I., Ziegler, J. H., and Lesch, M.: Echocardiographic estimates of pulmonary artery wedge pressure. N. Engl. J. Med. *305*:1566, 1981.
102. Chang, S.: M-Mode Echocardiographic Techniques and Pattern Recognition. Philadelphia, Lea and Febiger, 1976.
103. Chiotellis, P., Lees, R., Goldblatt, A., Liberthson, R., and Myers, G.: New criteria for echocardiographic diagnosis of atrial septal defect. Circulation (Suppl. II) *52*:134 (Abstract), 1975.
104. Shah, P. M., Gramiak, R., Adelman, A. G., and Wigle, E. D.: Role of echocardiography in diagnostic and hemodynamic assessment of hypertrophic subaortic stenosis. Circulation *44*:891, 1971.
105. Feigenbaum, H.: Clinical applications of echocardiography. Progr. Cardiovasc. Dis. *14*:531, 1972.
106. Sabbah, H. N., and Stein, P. D.: Mechanism of early systolic closure of the aortic valve in discrete membranous subaortic stenosis. Circulation *65*:399, 1982.
107. Davis, R. A., Feigenbaum, H., Chang, S., Konecke, L. L., and Dillon, J. C.: Echocardiographic manifestations of discrete subaortic stenosis. Am. J. Cardiol. *33*:277, 1974.
108. Wong, P., Cotter, L., and Gibson, D. G.: Early systolic closure of the aortic valve. Br. Heart J. *44*:386, 1980.
109. Pietro, D. A., Parisi, A. F., Harrington, J. J., and Askenazi, J.: Premature opening of the aortic valve: An index of highly advanced aortic regurgitation. J. Clin. Ultrasound *6*:170, 1978.
110. Nathan, M. P. R., Arora, R., and Rubenstein, H.: Mid-diastolic aortic valve opening in bacterial endocarditis of aortic valve. Clin. Cardiol. *5*:294, 1982.
111. Yeh, H. C., Winsberg, F., and Mercer, E. M.: Echocardiographic aortic valve orifice dimension: Its use in evaluating aortic stenosis and cardiac output. J. Clin. Ultrasound *1*:182, 1973.
112. Corya, B. C., Rasmussen, S., Phillips, J. F., and Black, M. J.: Forward stroke volume calculated from aortic valve echograms in normal subjects and patients with mitral regurgitation secondary to left ventricular dysfunction. Am. J. Cardiol. *47*:1215, 1981.
113. Green, S. E., and Popp, R. L.: The relationship of pulmonary valve motion to the motion of surrounding cardiac structures: A two-dimensional and dual M-mode echocardiographic study. Circulation *64*:107, 1981.
114. Edler, I., Gustafson, A., Karlefors, T., and Christensson, B.: Ultrasound cardiography. Acta Med. Scand. (Suppl.)*370*:68, 1961.
115. Gramiak, R., Nanda, N. C., and Shah, P. M.: Echocardiographic detection of pulmonary valve. Radiology *102*:153, 1972.
116. Weyman, A. E., Dillon, J. C., Feigenbaum, H., and Chang, S.: Echocardiographic patterns of pulmonic valve motion in pulmonic stenosis. Am. J. Cardiol. *34*:644, 1974.
117. Wann, L. S., Weyman, A. E., Dillon, J. C., and Feigenbaum, H.: Premature pulmonary valve opening. Circulation *55*:128, 1977.
118. Nanda, N. C., Gramiak, R., Robinson, T. I., and Shah, P. M.: Echocardiographic evaluation of pulmonary hypertension. Circulation *50*:575, 1974.
119. Weyman, A. E., Dillon, J. C., Feigenbaum, H., and Chang, S.: Echocardiographic patterns of pulmonary valve motion with pulmonary hypertension. Circulation *50*:905, 1974.
120. Tahara, M., Tanaka, H., Nakao, S., Yoshimura, H., Sakurai, S., Tei, C., and Kashima, T.: Hemodynamic determinants of pulmonary valve motion during systole in experimental pulmonary hypertension. Circulation *64*:1249, 1981.
121. Hirschfeld, S., Meyer, R., Schwartz, D. C., Korfhagen, J., and Kaplan, S.:

Measurement of right and left ventricular systolic time intervals by echocardiography. Circulation *51*:304, 1975.
122. Hirschfeld, S., Meyer, R., Schwartz, D. C., Korfhagen, J., and Kaplan, S.: The echocardiographic assessment of pulmonary artery pressure and pulmonary vascular resistance. Circulation *52*:642, 1975.
123. Mills, P., Amara, I., McLaurin, L. P., and Craige, E.: Noninvasive assessment of pulmonary hypertension from right ventricular isovolumic contraction time. Am. J. Cardiol. *46*:272, 1980.
124. Reeves, W. C., Leaman, D. M., Bounocore, E., Babb, J. D., Dash, H., Schwiter, E. J., Ciotola, T. J., and Hallahan, W.: Detection of tricuspid regurgitation and estimation of central venous pressure by two-dimensional contrast echocardiography of the right superior hepatic vein. Am. Heart J. *102* :374, 1981.
125. Magnin, P. A., Stewart, J. A., Myers, S., vonRamm, O., and Kisslo, J. A.: Combined Doppler and phased-array echocardiographic estimation of cardiac output. Circulation *63*:388, 1981.
126. Elkayam, U., Gardin, J. M., Berkley, R., Hughes, C., and Henry, W. L.: Use of Doppler blood flow velocity measurements to evaluate the response of systemic vascular resistance to vasodilators in patients with congestive heart failure. Am. J. Cardiol. *49*:943, 1982.
127. Edler, I.: Ultrasound cardiogram in mitral valve disease. Acta Chir. Scand. *111*: 230, 1956.
128. Edler, I., and Gustafson, A.: Ultrasonic cardiogram in mitral stenosis. Acta Med. Scand. *159*:85, 1957.
129. Joyner, C. R., Reid, J. M., and Bond, J. P.: Reflected ultrasound in the assessment of mitral valve disease. Circulation *27*:506, 1963.
130. Effert, S.: Pre- and post-operative evaluation of mitral stenosis by ultrasound. Am. J. Cardiol. *19*:59, 1967.
131. Joyner, C. R., and Reid, J. M.: Ultrasound cardiogram in the selection of patients for mitral valve surgery. Ann. N.Y. Acad. Sci. *118*:512, 1965.
132. Henry, W. L., Griffith, J. M., Michaelis, L. L., McIntosh, C. L., Morrow, A. G., and Epstein, S. E.: Measurement of mitral orifice area in patients with mitral valve disease by real-time, two-dimensional echocardiography. Circulation *51*:827, 1975.
133. Nichol, P. M., Gilbert, B. W., and Kisslo, J. A.: Two-dimensional echocardiographic assessment of mitral stenosis. Circulation *55*:120, 1977.
134. Wann, L. S., Weyman, A. E., Dillon, J. C., and Feigenbaum, H.: Determination of mitral valve area by cross-sectional echocardiography. Ann. Intern. Med. *88*:337, 1978.
135. Zaky, A., Nasser, W. K., and Feigenbaum, H.: Study of mitral valve action recorded by reflected ultrasound and its application in the diagnosis of mitral stenosis. Circulation *37*:789, 1968.
136. Shah, P. M., Gramiak, R., and Kramer, D. H.: Ultrasound localization of left ventricular outflow obstruction in hypertrophic obstructive cardiomyopathy. Circulation *40*:3, 1969.
137. Duchak, J. M., Jr., Chang, S., and Feigenbaum, H.: The posterior mitral valve echo and the echocardiographic diagnosis of mitral stenosis. Am. J. Cardiol. *29*:628, 1972.
138. Strunk, B. L., London, E. J., Fitzgerald, J., Popp, R. L., and Barry, W. H.: The assessment of mitral stenosis and prosthetic mitral valve obstruction, using the posterior aortic wall echocardiogram. Circulation *55*:885, 1977.
139. Naccarelli, G. V., Moneir, A. M., Watts, L. E., and Zelis, R.: Echocardiographic assessment of mitral stenosis by the left atrial emptying index. Chest *76*:668, 1979.
140. Joyner, C. R., and Reid, J. M.: Application of ultrasound in cardiology and cardiovascular physiology. Progr. Cardiovasc. Dis. *5*:482, 1963.
141. Segal, B. L., Likoff, W., and Kingsley, B.: Echocardiography: Clinical application in mitral regurgitation. Am. J. Cardiol. *19*:50, 1967.
142. Wann, L. S., Feigenbaum, H., Weyman, A. E., and Dillon, J. C.: Detection of rheumatic mitral regurgitation using cross-sectional echocardiography. Am. J. Cardiol. *41*:1258, 1978.
143. Blanchard, D., Diebold, B., Peronneau, P., Foult, J. M., Nee, M., Guermonprez, J. L., and Maurice, P.: Non-invasive diagnosis of mitral regurgitation by Doppler echocardiography. Br. Heart J. *45*:589, 1981.
144. Quinones, M. A., Yung, J. B., Waggoner, A. D., Ostojic, M. C., Ribeiro, L. G. T., and Miller, R. R.: Assessment of pulsed Doppler echocardiography in detection and quantification of aortic and mitral regurgitation. Br. Heart J. *44*: 612, 1980.
145. Dillon, J. C., Haine, C. L., Chang, S., and Feigenbaum, H.: Use of echocardiography in patients with prolapsed mitral valve. Am. J. Cardiol. *43*: 503, 1971.
146. Kerber, R. E., Isaeff, D. M., and Hancock, E. W.: Echocardiographic patterns in patients with the syndrome of systolic click and late systolic murmur. N. Engl. J. Med. *284*:691, 1971.
147. Shah, P. M., and Gramiak, R.: Echocardiographic recognition of mitral valve prolapse. Circulation (Suppl. III) *42*:45 (Abstract), 1970.
148. Popp, R. L., Brown, O. R., Silverman, J. F., and Harrison, D. C.: Echocardiographic abnormalities in the mitral valve prolapse syndrome. Circulation *49*:428, 1974.
149. DeMaria, A. N., King, J. F., Bogren, H. G., Lies, J. E., and Mason, D. T.: The variable spectrum of echocardiographic manifestations of the mitral valve prolapse syndrome. Circulation *50*:33, 1974.
150. Sahn, D. J., Wood, J., Allen, H. D., Peoples, W., and Goldberg, S. J.: Echocardiographic spectrum of mitral valve motion in children with and without mitral valve prolapse: The nature of false positive diagnosis. Am. J. Cardiol. *39*:422, 1977.
151. Montella, S., Belli, C., Corallo, S., et al.: Variable aspects in mitral valve prolapse. Echocardiographic and phonocardiographic studies of 68 cases. G. Ital. Cardiol. *6*:601, 1976.
152. Markiewicz, W., Stoner, J., London, E., Hunt, S. A., and Popp, R. L.: Mitral valve prolapse in one hundred presumably healthy young females. Circulation *53*:464, 1976.
153. Sahn, D. J., Allen, H. D., Goldberg, S. J., and Friedman, W. F.: Mitral valve prolapse in children. A problem defined by real-time cross-sectional echocardiography. Circulation *53*:651, 1976.
154. Gilbert, B. W., Schatz, R. A., Von Ramm, O. T., Behar, V. S., and Kisslo, J. A.: Mitral valve prolapse. Two-dimensional echocardiographic and angiographic correlation. Circulation *54*:716, 1976.
155. Morganroth, J., Jones, R. H., Chen, C. C., and Naito, M.: Two dimensional echocardiography in mitral, aortic and tricuspid valve prolapse. The clinical problem, cardiac nuclear imaging considerations and a proposed standard for diagnosis. Am. J. Cardiol. *46*:1164, 1980.
156. Chandraratna, P. A. N., and Langevin, E.: Limitations of the echocardiogram in diagnosing valvular vegetations in patients with mitral valve prolapse, Circulation *56*:436, 1977.
157. Mathey, D. G., Decoodt, P. R., Allen, H. N., and Swan, H. J. C.: Abnormal left ventricular contraction pattern in the systolic click-late systolic murmur syndrome. Circulation *56*:311, 1977.
158. D'Cruz, I. A., Shah, S., Hirsch, L. J., and Goldberg, A. N.: Cross-sectional echocardiographic visualization of abnormal systolic motion of the left ventricle in mitral valve prolapse. Cathet. Cardiovasc. Diagn. *7*:35, 1981.
159. Duchak, J. M., Jr., Chang, S., and Feigenbaum, H.: Echocardiographic features of torn chordae tendineae. Am. J. Cardiol. *29*:260 (Abstract), 1972.
160. Sweatman, T., Selzer, A., Kamagaki, M., and Cohn, K.: Echocardiographic diagnosis of mitral regurgitation due to ruptured chordae tendineae. Circulation *46*:580, 1972.
161. Giles, T. D., Burch, G. E., and Martinez, E. C.: Value of exploratory "scanning" in the echocardiographic diagnosis of ruptured chordae tendineae. Circulation *49*:678, 1974.
162. Humphries, W. C., Hammer, W. J., McDonough, M. T., Lemole, G., McCurdy, R. R., and Spann, J. F., Jr.: Echocardiographic equivalents of a flail mitral leaflet. Am. J. Cardiol. *40*:802, 1977.
163. Meyer, J. F., Frank, M. J., Goldberg, S., and Cheng, T. O.: Systolic mitral flutter, an echocardiographic clue to the diagnosis of ruptured chordae tendineae. Am. Heart J. *94*:3, 1977.
164. Mintz, G. S., Kotler, M. N., Segal, B. L., and Parry, W. R.: Two-dimensional echocardiographic recognition of ruptured chordae tendineae. Circulation *57*: 244, 1978.
165. Gramiak, R., and Shah, P. M.: Echocardiography of the normal and diseased aortic valve, Radiology *96*:1970.
166. Winsberg, F.: Aortic valve, *In* Gramiak, R., and Waag, R. C. (eds.): Cardiac Ultrasound. St. Louis, The C. V. Mosby Co., 1975, p. 74.
167. Chang, S., Clements, S., and Chang, J.: Aortic stenosis: Echocardiographic cusp separation and surgical description of aortic valve in 22 patients. Am. J. Cardiol. *39*:499, 1977.
168. Taleno, J., Frazin, L., Stephanides, L., Croke, R., Loeb, H., and Gunnar, R.: Echocardiographic index for estimating the severity of aortic stenosis. Circulation *54*:II-233 (Abstract), 1976.
169. Johnson, G. L., Meyer, R. A., Schwartz, D. C., Korfhagen, J., and Kaplan, S.: Echocardiographic evaluation of fixed left ventricular outlet obstruction in children. Circulation *56*:299, 1977.
170. Aziz, K. U., Van Grondelle, A., Paul, M. H., and Muster, A. J.: Echocardiographic assessment of the relation between left ventricular wall and cavity dimensions and peak systolic pressure in children with aortic stenosis. Am. J. Cardiol. *40*:775, 1977.
171. Reichek, N., and Devereux, R. B.: Reliable estimation of peak left ventricular systolic pressure by M-mode echographic-determined end-diastolic relative wall thickness: Identification of severe valvular aortic stenosis in adult patients. Am. Heart J. *103*:202, 1982.
172. Blackwood, R. A., Bloom, K. R., and Williams, C. M.: Aortic stenosis in children. Experience with echocardiographic predictions of severity. Circulation *57*:263, 1978.
173. Weyman, A. E., Feigenbaum, H., Dillon, J. C., and Chang, S.: Cross-sectional echocardiography in assessing the severity of valvular aortic stenosis. Circulation *52*:828, 1975.
174. Weyman, A. E., Feigenbaum, H., Hurwitz, R. A., Girod, D. A., and Dillon, J. C.: Cross-sectional echocardiographic assessment of the severity of aortic stenosis in children. Circulation *55*:773, 1977.
175. DeMaria, A. N., Bommer, J. W., Joye, J., Lee, G., Bouteller, J., and Mason, D. T.: Value and limitations of cross-sectional echocardiography of the aortic valve in the diagnosis and quantification of valvular aortic stenosis. Circulation *62*:304, 1980.
176. Godley, R. W., Green, D., Dillon, J. C., Rogers, E. W., Feigenbaum, H., and Weyman, A. E.: Reliability of two-dimensional echocardiography in assessing the severity of valvular aortic stenosis. Chest *79*:657, 1981.
177. Hatle, L., Angelsen, B. A., and Tromsdal, A.: Non-invasive assessment of aortic stenosis by Doppler ultrasound. Br. Heart J. *43*:284, 1980.
178. Stamm, R. B., and Martin, R. P.: Use of continuous wave Doppler for evaluation of stenotic aortic and mitral valves. Am. J. Cardiol. *49*:943, 1982.
179. Cannon, S. R., Richards, K. L., and Rollwitz, W. T.: Digital Fourier techniques in the diagnosis and quantification of aortic stenosis with pulsed-Doppler echocardiography. J. Clin. Ultrasound *10* :101, 1982.

180. Wray, R. M.: Echocardiographic manifestations of flail aortic valve leaflets in bacterial endocarditis. Circulation *51*:832, 1975.
181. Estevez, C. N., Dillon, J. O., Walker, P. D., Feigenbaum, H., and Chang, S.: Echocardiographic manifestations of aortic cusp rupture in a case of myxomatous degeneration of the aortic valve. Chest *69*:544, 1976.
182. Rolston, W. A., Hirschfeld, D. S., Emilson, B. B., and Cheitlin, M. D.: Echocardiographic appearance of ruptured aortic cusp. Am. J. Med. *62*:133, 1977.
183. Fox, S., Kotler, M. N., Segal, B. L., and Parry, W.: Echocardiographic diagnosis of acute aortic valve endocarditis and its complications. Arch. Intern. Med. *137*:85, 1977.
184. Sheikh, M. U., Covarrubias, E. A., Ali, N., Sheikh, N. M., Lee, W. R., and Roberts, W. C.: M-mode echocardiographic observations in active bacterial endocarditis limited to the aortic valve. Am. Heart J. *102*:66, 1981.
185. Berger, M. Gallerstein, P. E., Benhuri, P., Balla, R., and Goldberg, E.: Evaluation of aortic valve endocarditis by two-dimensional echocardiography. Chest *80*:61, 1981.
186. Martinez, E. C., Burch, G. E., and Giles, T. D.: Echocardiographic diagnosis of vegetative aortic bacterial endocarditis. Am. J. Cardiol. *34*:845, 1974.
187. Feizi, O., Symons, C., and Yacoub, M.: Echocardiography of the aortic valve. I. Studies of normal aortic valve, aortic stenosis, aortic regurgitation and mixed aortic valve disease. Br. Heart J. *36*:341, 1974.
188. Mardelli, R. J., Morganroth, J., Naito, M., and Chen, C. C.: Cross-sectional echocardiographic detection of aortic valve prolapse. Am. Heart J. *100*:295, 1980.
189. Cope, G. D., Kisslo, J. A., Johnson, M. L., and Myers, S.: Diastolic vibration of the interventricular septum in aortic insufficiency. Circulation *51*:589, 1975.
190. Friedewald, V. E., Jr., Futral, J. E., Kinard, S. A., and Phillips, B.: Oscillations of the interventricular septum in aortic insufficiency. J. Clin. Ultrasound *2*:229 (Abstract), 1974.
191. Ciobanu, M., Abbasi, A. S., Allen, M., Hermer, A., and Spellberg, R.: Pulsed Doppler echocardiography in the diagnosis and estimation of severity of aortic insufficiency. Am. J. Cardiol. *49*:339, 1982.
192. Henry, W. L., Bonow, R. O., Borer, J. S., Ware, J. H., Kent, K. M., Redwood, D. R., McIntosh, C. L., Morrow, A. G., and Epstein, S. E.: Observations on the optimum time for operative intervention for aortic regurgitation. I. Evaluation of the results of aortic valve replacement in symptomatic patients. Circulation *61*:741, 1980.
193. Paulsen, W., Boughner, D. R., Persaud, J., and Devries, L.: Aortic regurgitation. Detection of left ventricular dysfunction by exercise echocardiography. Br. Heart J. *46*:380, 1981.
194. Joyner, C. R., Hey, B. E., Jr., Johnson, J., and Reid, J. M.: Reflected ultrasound in the diagnosis of tricuspid stenosis. Am. J. Cardiol. *19*:66, 1967.
195. Guyer, D., Gillam, L., Dinsmore, R., Clark, M. C., Block, P., Palacios, I., and Weyman, A. E.: Detection of tricuspid stenosis by two-dimensional echocardiography. Am. J. Cardiol. *49*:1041 (Abstract), 1982.
196. Inoue, D., Furukawa, K., Matsukubo, H., Watanabe, T., and Katsume, H.: Subxiphoid two-dimensional echocardiographic detection of tricuspid valve prolapse. Chest *76*:693, 1979.
197. Weyman, A. E., Wann, S., Feigenbaum, H., and Dillon, J. C.: Mechanism of abnormal septal motion in patients with right ventricular volume overload: A cross-sectional echocardiographic study. Circulation *54*:179, 1976.
198. Tanaka, H., Tei, C., Nakao, S., Tahara, M., Sakurai, S., Kashima, T., and Kanehisa, T.: Diastolic bulging of the interventricular septum toward the left ventricle. Circulation *62*:558, 1980.
199. Waggoner, A. D., Quinones, M. A., Young, J. B., Brandon, T. A., Shah, A. A., Verani, M. S., and Miller, R. R.: Pulsed Doppler echocardiographic detection of right-sided valve regurgitation. Experimental results and clinical significance. Am. J. Cardiol. *47*:271, 1981.
200. Lieppe, W., Behar, V. S., Scallion, R., and Kisslo, J. A.: Detection of tricuspid regurgitation with two-dimensional echocardiography and peripheral vein injections. Circulation *57*:128, 1978.
201. Wise, N. K., Myers, S., Fraker, T. D., Stewart, J. A., and Kisslo, J. A.: Contrast M-mode ultrasonography of the inferior vena cave. Circulation *63* :1100, 1981.
202. Meltzer, R. S., vanHoogenhuyze, D., Serruys, P. W., Haalebos, M. M., Hugenholtz, P. G., and Roelandt, J.: Diagnosis of tricuspid regurgitation by contrast echocardiography. Circulation *63*:1093, 1981.
203. Dillon, J. C., Feigenbaum, H., Konecke, L. L., Davis, R. H., and Chang, S.: Echocardiographic manifestations of valvular vegetations. Am. Heart J. *86*: 698, 1973.
204. Spangler, R. D., Johnson, M. D., Holmes, J. H., and Blount, S. G., Jr.: Echocardiographic demonstration of bacterial vegetations in active infective endocarditis. J. Clin. Ultrasound *1*:126, 1973.
205. Sharma, S., Katdare, A. D., Munsi, S. C., and Kinare, S. G.: M-mode echocardiographic detection of pulmonic valve infective endocarditis. Am. Heart J. *102*:131, 1981.
206. Andy, J. J., Sheikh, M. U., Ali, N., Barnes, B. O., Fox, L. M., Curry, C. L., and Roberts, W. C.: Echocardiographic observations in opiate addicts with active infective endocarditis. Am. J. Cardiol. *40*:17, 1977.
207. Yoshikawa, J., Tanaka, K., Owaki, T., and Kato, H.: Cord-like aortic valve vegetation in bacterial endocarditis. Circulation *53*:911, 1976.
208. Roy, P., Tajik, A. J., Giuliani, E. R., Schattenberg, T. T., Gau, G. T., and Frye, R. L.: Spectrum of echocardiographic findings in bacterial endocarditis. Circulation *53*:474, 1976.
209. Gilbert, B. W., Haney, R. S., Crawford, F., McClellan, J., Gallis, H. A., Johnson, M. L., and Kisslo, J. A.: Two-dimensional echocardiographic assessment of vegetative endocarditis. Circulation *55*:346, 1977.
210. Kisslo, J., Von Ramm, O. T., Haney, R., Jones, R., Juk, S. S., and Behar, V. S.: Echocardiographic evaluation of tricuspid valve endocarditis. An M-mode and two-dimensional study. Am. J. Cardiol. *38*:502, 1976.
211. Berger, M., Delfin, L. A., Jelveh, M., and Goldberg, E.: Two-dimensional echocardiographic findings in right-sided infective endocarditis. Circulation *61*: 855, 1980.
212. Wann, L. S., Dillon, J. C., Weyman, A. E., and Feigenbaum, H.: Echocardiography in bacterial endocarditis. N. Engl. J. Med. *295*:135, 1976.
213. Martin, R. P., Meltzer, R. S., Chia, B. L., Stinson, E. B., Rakowski, H., and Popp, R. L.: Clinical utility of two-dimensional echocardiography in infective endocarditis. Am. J. Cardiol. *46*:379, 1980.
214. Hickey, A. J., Wolfers, J., and Wilcken, D. E. L.: Reliability and clinical relevance of detection of vegetations by echocardiography in bacterial endocarditis. Br. Heart J. *46*:624, 1981.
215. Come, P. C., Isaacs, R. E., and Riley, M. F.: Diagnostic accuracy of M-mode echocardiography in active infective endocarditis and prognostic implications of ultrasound-detectable vegetations. Am. Heart J. *103*:839, 1982.
216. Gottlieb, S., Khuddus, S. A., Balooki, H., Dominquez, A. E., and Myerburg, R. J.: Echocardiographic diagnosis or aortic valve vegetations in Candida endocarditis. Circulation *50*:826, 1974.
217. Arvan, S., Cagin, N., Levitt, B., et al.: Echocardiographic findings in a patient with Candida endocarditis of the aortic valve. Chest *70*:300, 1976.
218. Gomes, J. A., Calderon, J., Lajam, F., et al.: Echocardiographic detection of fungal vegetations in *Candida parasilopsis* endocarditis. Am. J. Med. *61*:273, 1976.
219. Estevez, C. M., and Corya, B. C.: Serial echocardiographic abnomalities in nonbacterial thrombotic endocarditis of the mitral valve. Chest *69*:801, 1976.
220. Fitchett, D. H., and Oakley, C. M.: Granulomatous mitral valve obstruction. Br. Heart J.*38*:112, 1976.
221. Winters, W. L., Gimenez, J. L., and Soloff, L.: Clinical applications of ultrasound in the analysis of prosthetic ball valve function. Am. J. Cardiol. *19* :97, 1967.
222. Siggers, D. C., Srivongse, S. A., and Deuchar, D.: Analysis of dynamics of mitral Starr-Edwards valve prosthesis using reflected ultrasound. Br. Heart J. *33*: 401, 1971.
223. Johnson, M. L., Holmes, J. H., and Paton, B. C.: Echocardiographic determination of mitral disc valve excursion. Circulation *47*:1274, 1973.
224. Douglas, J. E., and Williams, G. D.: Echocardiographic evaluation of the Björk-Shiley prosthetic valve. Circulation *50*:52, 1974.
225. Chandraratna, P. A. N., Lopez, J. M., Hildner, F. J., Samet, P., Ben-Zvi, J., (with technical assistance of D. Gindlesperger): Diagnosis of Björk-Shiley aortic valve dysfunction by echocardiography. Am. Heart J. *91*:318, 1976.
226. Bernal-Ramirez, J. A., and Phillips, J. H.: Echocardiographic study of malfunction of the Björk-Shiley prosthetic heart valve in the mitral position. Am. J. Cardiol. *40*:449, 1977.
227. Smith, R. A., Kerber, R. E., and Snyder, J. W.: Noninvasive diagnostic evaluation of the normal Beall mitral prosthesis. Cathet. Cardiovasc. Diagn. *2* :289, 1976.
228. Bomba, M. A., Capella, G., Pandolfini, E., and Rossi, P.: Morphology of the echoes of the Lillehei-Kaster prosthesis in aortic and mitral sites. Boll. Soc. Ital. Cardiol. *20*:1775, 1975.
229. Bloch, W. N., Jr., Felner, J. M., Wickliffe, C., et al.: Echocardiographic diagnosis of thrombus on a heterograft aortic valve in the mitral position. Chest *70*: 399, 1976.
230. Bloch, W. N., Felner, J. M., Wickliffe, C., Symbas, P. N., and Schlant, R. C.: Echocardiogram of the porcine aortic bioprosthesis in the mitral position. Am. J. Cardiol. *38*:293, 1976.
231. Wann, L. S., Pyhel, H. J., Judson, W. E., Tavel, M. E., and Feigenbaum, H.: Ball variance in a Harken mitral prosthesis. Echocardiographic and phonocardiographic features. Chest *72*:785, 1977.
232. Bommer, W., Yoon, D., Grehl, T. M., Mason, D. T., Neumann, A., and DeMaria, A. N.: In vitro and in vivo evaluation of porcine bioprostheses by cross-sectional echocardiography. Am. J. Cardiol. *41*:405 (Abstract), 1978.
233. Schapira, J. N., Martin, R. P., Fowles, R. E., Rakowski, H., Stinson, E. B., French, J. W., Shumway, N. E., and Popp, R. L.: Two-dimensional ultrasound sector scanning for assessment of patients with bioprosthetic valves. Am. J. Cardiol. *41*:406 (Abstract), 1978.
234. Mintz, G. S., Carlson, E. B., and Kotler, M. N.: Comparison of noninvasive techniques in evaluation of the nontissue cardiac valve prosthesis. Am. J. Cardiol. *49*:39, 1982.
235. Ben-Zvi, J., Hildner, F. J., Chandraratna, P. A., and Samet, P.: Thrombosis on Björk-Shiley aortic valve prosthesis: Clinical, arteriographic, echocardiographic, and therapeutic observations in seven cases. Am. J. Cardiol. *34*: 538, 1974.
236. Raj, M. V. J., Srinivas, V., and Evans, D. W.: Thrombotic jamming of a tricuspid prosthesis. Br. Heart J. *38*:1355, 1976.
237. Kawai, N., Segal, B. L., and Linhart, J. W.: Delayed opening of Beall mitral prosthetic valve detected by echocardiography. Chest *67*:239, 1975.
238. Oliva, P. B., Johnson, M. L., Pomerantz, M., and Levine, A.: Dysfunction of the Beall mitral prosthesis and its detection by cinefluoroscopy and echocardiography. Am. J. Cardiol. *31*:393, 1973.
239. Pfeifer, J., Goldschlager, N., Sweatman, T., Gerbode, E., and Selzer, A.: Malfunction of mitral ball valve prosthesis due to thrombus. Am. J. Cardiol. *29*:95, 1972.

240. Srivastava, T. N., Hussain, M., Gray, L. A., Jr., et al.: Echocardiographic diagnosis of a stuck Björk-Shiley aortic valve prosthesis. Chest *70*:94, 1976.
241. Berndt, T. B., Goodman, D. J., and Popp, R. L.: Echocardiographic and phonocardiographic confirmation of suspected caged mitral valve malfunction. Chest *70*:221, 1976.
242. Mehta, A., Kessler, K. M., Tamer, D., Pefkaros, K., Kessler, R. M., and Myerburg, R. J.: Two-dimensional echographic observations in major detachment of a prosthetic aortic valve. Am. Heart J. *101*:231, 1981.
243. Schuchman, H., Feigenbaum, H., Dillon, J. C., and Chang, S.: Intracavitary echoes in patients with mitral prosthetic valves. J. Clin. Ultrasound *3*:111, 1975.
244. Alam, M., Goldstein, S., and Lakier, J. B.: Echocardiographic changes in the thickness of porcine valves with time. Chest *79*:663, 1981.
245. Assad-Morell, J. L., Tajik, A. J., Anderson, M. W., Tancredi, R. G., Wallace, R. B., and Giuliani, E. R.: Malfunctioning tricuspid valve prosthesis: Clinical phonocardiographic, echocardiographic and surgical findings. Mayo Clin. Proc. *42*:443, 1974.
246. Burggraf, G. W., and Craige, E.: Echocardiographic studies of left ventricular wall motion and dimensions after valvular heart surgery. Am. J. Cardiol. *35*: 473, 1975.
247. Miller, H. C., Gibson, D. G., and Stephens, J. D.: Role of echocardiography and phonocardiography in the diagnosis of mitral paraprosthetic regurgitation with Starr-Edwards prostheses. Br. Heart J. *35*:1217, 1973.
248. Miller, H. C., Stephens, J. D., and Gibson, D. G.: Echocardiographic features of mitral Starr-Edwards paraprosthetic regurgitation. Br. Heart J. *35*:560, 1973.
249. Yoshikawa, J., Owaki, T., Kato, H., and Tanaka, K.: Abnormal motion of interventricular septum in patients with prosthetic valve. Cardiovasc. Sound Bull. *5*:211, 1976.
250. Bourdillon, P. D. V., and Sharratt, G. P.: Malfunction of Björk-Shiley valve prosthesis in tricuspid position. Br. Heart J. *38*:1149, 1976.
251. Veyrat, C., Cholot, N, Abitbol, G., and Kalmanson, D.: Non-invasive diagnosis and assessment of aortic valve disease and evaluation of aortic prosthesis function using echo pulsed Doppler velocimetry. Br. Heart J. *43* :393, 1980.
252. Belenkie, I., Carr, M., Schlant, R. C., Nutter, D. O., and Symbas, P. N.: Malfunction of a Cutter-Smeloff mitral ball valve prosthesis: Diagnosis by phonocardiography and echocardiography. Am. Heart J. *86*:339, 1973.
253. Brodie, B. R., Grossman, W., McLaurin, L., Starek, P. J. K., and Craige, E.: Diagnosis of prosthetic mitral valve malfunction with combined echo-phonocardiography. Circulation *53*:93, 1976.
254. Gibson, T. C., Starek, J. K., Moos, S., and Craige, E.: Echocardiographic and phonocardiographic characteristics of the Lillehei-Kaster mitral valve prosthesis. Circulation *49*:434, 1974.
255. Griffiths, B. F., Charles, R., and Coulshed, N.: Echophonocardiography in diagnosis of mitral paravalvular regurgitation with Björk-Shiley prosthetic valve. Br. Heart J. *43*:325, 1980.
256. Waggoner, A. D., Quinones, M. A., Young, J. B., Nelson, J. G., Winters, W. L., Jr., Peterson, P. K., and Miller, R. R.: Echo-phonocardiographic evaluation of obstruction of prosthetic mitral valve. Chest *78*:60, 1980.
257. Hirschfeld, D. S., and Emilson, B. B.: Echocardiogram in calcified mitral annulus. Am. J. Cardiol. *36*:354, 1975.
258. Dashkoff, N., Karacuschansky, M., Come, P. C., and Fortuin, N. J.: Echocardiographic features of mitral annulus calcification. Am. Heart J. *94*: 585, 1977.
259. Gabor, G. E., Mohr, B. D., Goel, P. C., and Cohen, B.: Echocardiographic and clinical spectrum of mitral annular calcification. Am. J. Cardiol. *38*:836, 1976.
260. Curati, W. L., Petitclerc, R., and Winsberg, F.: Ultrasonic features of mitral annulus calcification. A report of 21 cases. Radiology *122*:215, 1977.
261. Schott, C. R., Kotler, M. N., Parry, W. R., and Segal B. L.: Mitral annular calcification. Clinical and echocardiographic correlations. Arch. Intern. Med. *137*:1143, 1977.
262. D'Cruz, I. A., Cohen, H. C., Prabhu, R. Bisla, V., and Glick, G.: Clinical manifestations of mitral annulus calcification, with emphasis on its echocardiographic features. Am. Heart J. *94*:367, 1977.
263. Meltzer, R. S., Martin, R. P., Robbins, B. S., and Popp, R. L.: Mitral annular calcification: Clinical and echocardiographic features. Acta Cardiol. *35*:189, 1980.
264. Mellino, M., Salcedo, E. E., Lever, H. M., Vasudevan, G., and Kramer, J. R.,: Echographic-quantified severity of mitral annulus calcification: Prognostic correlation to related hemodynamic, valvular, rhythm and conduction abnormalities. Am. Heart J. *103*:222, 1982.
265. Solinger, R., Elbl, F., and Minhas, K.: Deductive echocardiographic analysis in infants with congenital heart disease. Circulation *50*:1072, 1974.
266. Meyer, R. A., Schwartz, D. C., Covitz, W., and Kaplan, S.: Echocardiographic assessment of cardiac malposition. Am. J. Cardiol. *33*:896, 1974.
267. Foale, R., Stefanini, L., Rickards, A., and Somerville, J.: Left and right ventricular morphology in complex congenital heart disease defined by two dimensional echocardiography. Am. J. Cardiol. *49*:93, 1982.
268. Hagler, D. J., Tajik, A. J., Seward, J. B., Edwards, W. D., Mair, D. D., and Ritter, D. G.: Atrioventricular and ventriculoarterial discordance (corrected transposition of the great arteries). Wide-angle two-dimensional echocardiographic assessment of ventricular morphology. Mayo Clin. Proc. *56*:591, 1981.
269. Motro, M., Kishon, Y., Shem-Tov, A., and Neufeld, H. N.: Identification of a tricuspid valve in the mitral position in corrected tranposition of the great vessels by cross-sectional echocrdiography. Am. Heart J. *101*:229, 1981.
270. Houston, A. V, Gregory, N. L., and Coleman, E. N.: Echocardiographic identification of aorta and main pulmonary artery in complete transposition. Br. Heart J. *40*:377, 1978.
271. Henry, W. L., Maron, B. J., and Griffith, J. M.: Cross-sectional echocardiography in the diagnosis of congenital heart disease. Identification of the relation of the ventricles and great arteries. Circulation *56*:267, 1977.
272. Nanda, N. C., Gramiak, R., Manning, J., Mahoney, E. B., Lipchik, E. O., and DeWeese, J. A.: Echocardiographic recognition of the congenital bicuspid aortic valve. Circulation *49*:870, 1974.
273. Radford, D. J., Bloom, K. R., Izukawa, R., Moes, C. A. F., and Rowe, R. D.: Echocardiographic assessment of bicuspid aortic valves. Circulation *53*:80, 1976.
274. Nanda, N. C., and Gramiak, R.: Evaluation of bicuspid aortic valves by two-dimensional echocardiography. Am J. Cardiol. *41*:372 (Abstract), 1978.
275. Brandenburg, R. O., Jr., Tajik, A. J., Edwards, W. D., Reeder, G. S., Shub, C., and Seward, J. B.: Accuracy of two-dimensional echocardiographic diagnosis of bicuspid aortic valve: Echocardiographic-anatomic correlative study in 115 patients. Am. J. Cardiol. *49*:1040 (Abstract), 1982.
276. Lundstrom, N. R.: Echocardiography in the diagnosis of congenital mitral stenosis and an evaluation of the results of mitral valvulotomy. Circulation *46* :44, 1972.
277. Driscoll, D. J., Gutgesell, H. P., and McNamara, D. G.: Echocardiographic features of congenital mitral stenosis. Am. J. Cardiol. *42*:259, 1978.
278. Smallhorn, J., Tommasini, G., Deanfield, J., Doublas, J., Gibson, D., and Macartney, F.: Congenital mitral stenosis. Anatomical and functional assessment by echocardiography. Br. Heart J. *45*:527, 1981.
279. Weyman, A. E., Hurwitz, R. A., Girod, D. A., Dillon, J. C., Feigenbaum, H., and Green, D.: Cross-sectional echocardiographic visualization of the stenotic pulmonary valve. Circulation *56*:769, 1977.
280. Lundstrom, N. R.: Echocardiography in the diagnosis of Ebstein's anomaly of the tricuspid valve. Circulation *47*:597, 1973.
281. Tajik, A. J., Gau, G. T., Giuliani, E. R., Ritter, D. G., and Schattenberg, T. T.: Echocardiogram in Ebstein's anomaly with Wolff-Parkinson-White pre-excitation syndrome, type B. Circulation *47*:813, 1973.
282. Yuste, P., Minguez, I., Aza, V., Senor, J., Asin, E., and Martinezaabordiu, C.: Echocardiography in the diagnosis of Ebstein's anomaly. Chest *66*:273, 1974.
283. Milner, S., Meyer, R. A., Venables, A. W., Korfhagen, J., and Kaplan, S.: Mitral and tricuspid valve closure in congenital heart disease. Circulation *53* :513, 1976.
284. Henry, W.L, Sahn, D. J., Griffith, J. M., Goldberg, S. J., Maron, B. J., McAllister, H. A., Allen, H. D., and Epstein, S. E.: Evaluation of atrioventricular valve morphology in congenital heart disease by real-time cross-sectional echocardiography. Circulation (Suppl. II) *52*:120 (Abstract), 1975.
285. Ports, T. A., Silverman, N. H., and Schiller, N. B.: Two-dimensional echocardiographic assessment of Ebstein's anomaly. Circulation *58*:336, 1978.
286. Kambe, T., Ichimiya, S., Toguchi, M., Hibi, N., Fukui, Y., Nishimura, K., Sakamoto, N., and Hojo, Y.: Apex and subxiphoid approaches to Ebstein's anomaly using cross-sectional echocardiography. Am. Heart J. *100*:53, 1980.
287. Lundstrom, N. R.: Ultrasound cardiographic studies of the mitral valve region in young infants with mitral atresia, mitral stenosis, hypoplasia of the left ventricle and cor triatriatum. Circulation *45*:324, 1972.
288. Weyman, A. E., Caldwell, R. L., Hurwitz, R. A., Girod, D. A., Dillon, J. C., Feigenbaum, H., and Green, D.: Cross-sectional echocardiographic characterization of aortic obstruction. I. Supravalvular aortic stenosis and aortic hypoplasia. Circulation *57*:491, 1978.
289. Rigby, M. L., Gibson, D. G., Joseph, M. C., Lincoln, J. C. R., Shinebourne, E. A., Shore, D. F., and Anderson, R. H.: Recognition of imperforate atrioventricular valves by two dimensional echocardiography. Br. Heart J. *47* :329, 1982.
290. Popp, R. L., Silverman, J. F., French, J. W., Stinson, E. B., and Harrison, D. C.: Echocardiographic findings in discrete subvalvular aortic stenosis. Circulation *49*:226, 1974.
291. Weyman, A. E., Feigenbaum, H., Dillon, J. C., Chang, S., Hurwitz, R. A., and Girod, D. A.: Cross-sectional echocardiography in the diagnosis of discrete subaortic stenosis. Am. J. Cardiol. *37*:358, 1976.
292. DiSessa, T. G., Hagan, A. D., Isabel-Jones, J. B., Ti, C. C., Mercier, J. C., and Friedman, W. F.: Two-dimensional echocardiographic evaluation of discrete subaortic stenosis from the apical long axis view. Am. Heart J. *101*:774, 1981.
293. Wilcox, W. D., Seward, J. B., Hagler, D. J., Mair, D. D., and Tajik, A. J.: Discrete subaortic stenosis. Two-dimensional echocardiographic features with angiographic and surgical correlation. Mayo Clin. Proc. *55*:425, 1980.
294. Weyman, A. E., Dillon, J. C., Feigenbaum, H., and Chang, S.: Echocardiographic differentiation of infundibular from valvular pulmonary stenosis. Am. J. Cardiol. *36*:21, 1975.
295. Caldwell, R. L., Weyman, A. G., Hurwitz, R. A., Girod, D. A., and Feigenbaum, H.: Right ventricular outflow tract assessment by cross-sectional echocardiography in tetralogy of Fallot. Circulation *59*:395, 1979.
296. Chung, K. J., Nanda, N. C., Manning, J. A., and Gramiak, R.,: Echocardiographic findings in tetralogy of Fallot. Am. J. Cardiol. *31*:126, 1973.
297. Tajik, A. J., Gau, G. T., Ritter, D. G., and Schattenberg, T. T.: Echocardiogram in tetralogy of Fallot. Chest *64*:107, 1973.

298. Morris, D. C., Felner, J. M., Schlant, R. C., and Franch, R. H.: Echocardiographic diagnosis of tetralogy of Fallot. Am. J. Cardiol. *36*:908, 1975.
299. Seward, J. B., Tajik, A. J., Hagler, D. J., Giuliani, E. R., Gau, G. T., and Ritter, D. G.: Echocardiogram in common (single) ventricle: Angiographic-anatomic correlation. Am. J. Cardiol. *39*:217, 1977.
300. Bini, R. M., Bloom, K. R., Culham, J. A. G., Freedom, R. M., Williams, C. M., and Rowe, R. D.: The reliability and practicality of single crystal echocardiography in the evaluation of single ventricle, angiographic, and pathological correlates. Circulation *57*:269, 1978.
301. Felner, J. W., Brewer, D. B., and Franch, R. H.: Echocardiographic manifestations of single ventricle. Am. J. Cardiol. *38*:80, 1976.
302. Assad-Morell, J. L., Tajik, A. J., And Giuliani, E. R.: Aneurysm of membranous interventricular septum: Echocardiographic features. Mayo Clin. Proc. *49*:164, 1974.
303. Fast, J. H., and Moene, R. J.: Echocardiographic diagnosis of an aneurysm of the membranous ventricular septum. Acta Paediatr. Scand. *66*:521, 1977.
304. Canale, J. M., Sahn, D. J. Valdes-Cruz, L. M., Allen, H. D., Goldberg, S. J., and Ovitt, T. W.: Accuracy of two-dimensional echocardiography in the detection of aneurysms of the ventricular septum. Am. Heart J. *101*:255, 1981.
305. Cheatham, J. P., Latson, L. A., and Gutgesell, H. P.: Ventricular septal defect in infancy: Detection with two dimensional echocardiography. Am. J. Cardiol. *47*:85, 1981.
306. Piot, J. D., Lucet, P., Losay, J., Touchot, A., Petit, J., David, P., Piot, C., and Binet, J. P.: Diagnosis and localization of ventricular septal defects by two-dimensional echocardiography. 50 cases. Arch. Mal. Coeur. *74*:1001, 1981.
307. Bierman, F. Z., Fellows, K., and Williams, R. G.: Prospective identification of ventricular septal defects in infancy using subxiphoid two-dimensional echocardiography. Circulation *62*:807, 1980.
308. Rigby, M. L., Anderson, R. H., Gibson, D., Jones, O. D. H., Joseph, M. C., and Shinebourne, E. A.: Two dimensional echocardiographic categorisation of the univentricular heart. Br. Heart J. *46*:603, 1981.
309. Smallhorn, J. F., Tommasini, G., Anderson, R. H., and Macartney, F. J.: Assessment of atrioventricular septal defects by two dimensional echocardiography. Br. Heart J. *47*:109, 1982.
310. Dillon, J. C., Weyman, A. E., Feigenbaum, H., Eggleton, R. C., and Johnston, K. W.: Cross-sectional echocardiographic examination of the interatrial septum. Circulation *55*:115, 1977.
311. Lieppe, W., Scallion, R., Behar, V. S., and Kisslo, J. A.: Two-dimensional echocardiographic findings in atrial septal defect. Circulation *56*:447, 1977.
312. Nasser, F. N., Tajik, A. J., Seward, J. B., and Hagler, D. J.: Diagnosis of sinus venosus atrial septal defect by two-dimensional echocardiography. Mayo Clin. Proc. *56*:568, 1981.
313. Goldberg, S. J., Allen, H. D., and Sahn, D. J.: Echocardiographic detection and management of patent ductus arteriosus in neonates with respiratory distress syndrome: A two-and-one-half year prospective study. J. Clin. Ultrasound *5*:161, 1977.
314. Sahn, D. J., Vaucher, Y., Williams, D. E., Allen, H. D., Goldberg, S. J., and Friedman, W. F.: Echocardiographic detection of large left to right shunts and cardiomyopathies in infants and children. Am. J. Cardiol. *38*:73, 1976.
315. Baylen, B. G., Meyer, R. A., Kaplan, S., Ringenburg, W. E., and Korfhagen, J.: The critically ill premature infant with patent ductus arteriosus and pulmonary disease—an echocardiographic assessment. J. Pediatr. *86*:423, 1975.
316. Goldberg, S. J., Allen, H. D., Sahn, D. J., Friedman, W. F., and Harris, T.: A prospective 2½ year experience with echocardiographic evaluation of prematures with patent ductus arteriosus (PDA) and respiratory distress syndrome (RDS). Am. J. Cardiol. *35*:139 (Abstract), 1975.
317. Baylen, B., Meyer, R. A., Korfhagen, J., Benzing, G., Bubb, M. E., and Kaplan, S.: Left ventricular performance in the critically ill premature infant with patent ductus arteriosus and pulmonary disease. Circulation *55*:182, 1977.
318. McCann, W. D., Harbold, N. B., and Giuliani, B. R.: The echocardiogram in right ventricular overload. J.A.M.A. *221*:1243, 1972.
319. Tajik, A. J.: Echocardiographic pattern of right ventricular diastolic volume overload in children. Circulation *46*:36, 1972.
320. Paquet, M., and Gutgesell, H.: Echocardiographic features of total anomalous pulmonary venous connection. Circulation *51*:599, 1975.
321. Canedo, M. I., Stefadouros, M. A., Frank, M. J., Moore, H. V., and Cundey, D. W.: Echocardiographic features of cor triatriatum. Am. J. Cardiol. *40*:615, 1977.
322. Weindorf, S., Goldberg, H., Goldman, M., and Reitman, M.: Diagnosis of cor triatriatum by two-dimensional echocardiography. J. Clin. Ultrasound *9*:97, 1981.
323. Duff, D. F., and Gutgesell, H. P.: The use of saline or blood for ultrasonic detection of a right-to-left intracardiac shunt in the early postoperative patient. Am. Heart J. *94*:402, 1977.
324. Seward, J. B., Tajik, A. J., Spangler, J. G., and Ritter, D. G.: Echocardiographic contrast studies: Initial experience. Mayo Clin. Proc. *50*:163, 1975.
325. Seward, J. B., Tajik, A. J., Hagler, D. J., and Ritter, D. G.: Peripheral venous contrast echocardiography. Am. J. Cardiol. *39*:202, 1977.
326. Valdes-Cruz, L. M., Pieroni, D. R., Roland, A., and Varghese, P. J.: Echocardiographic detection of intracardiac right-to-left shunts following peripheral vein injections. Circulation *54*:558, 1976.
327. Funabashi, T., Toshida, H., Nakaya, S., Maeda, T., and Taniguchi, N.: Echocardiographic visualization of ventricular septal defect in infants and assessment of hemodynamic status using a contrast technique. Circulation *64*: 1025, 1981.
328. Weyman, A. E., Wann, L. S., Hurwitz, R.A., Dillon, J. C., and Feigenbaum, H.: Negative contrast echocardiography: A new technique for detecting left-to-right shunts. Circulation *56*: II-89 (Abstract), 1977.
329. Kronik, G., and Mosslacher, H.: Positive contrast echocardiography in patients with patent foramen ovale and normal right hemodynamics. Am. J. Cardiol. *49*:1806, 1982.
330. Bourdillon, P. D., Foale, R. A., and Rickards, A. F.: Identification of atrial septal defects by cross-sectional contrast echocardiography. Br. Heart J. *44*:401, 1980.
331. Sahn, D. J., Allen, H. D., George, W., Mason, M., and Goldberg, S. J.: The utility of contrast echocardiographic techniques in the care of critically ill infants with cardiac and pulmonary disease. Circulation *56*:959, 1977.
332. Sahn, D. J., Terry, R. W., O'Rourke, R., Leopold, G., and Friedman, W. F.: Multiple crystal echocardiographic evaluation of endocardial cushion defect. Circulation *50*:25, 1974.
333. Stevenson, J. G., Kawabori, I., Dooley, T. K., and Guntheroth, W. G.: Diagnosis of ventricular septal defect by pulsed Doppler echocardiography—sensitivity, specificity, limitations. Circulation *58*:322, 1978.
334. Stevenson, J. G., Kawabori, I., and Guntheroth, W.G.: Pulsed Doppler echocardiographic diagnosis of patent ductus arteriosus: Sensitivity, specificity, limitations, and technical features. Cathet. Cardiovasc. Diagn. *6*:255, 1980.
335. Williams, R. G., and Rudd, M.: Echocardiographic features of endocardial cushion defects. Circulation *49*:418, 1974.
336. Komatsu, Y., Nagai, Y., Shibuya, M., Takao, A., and Hirosawa, K.: Echocardiographic analysis of intracardiac anatomy in endocardial cushion defect. Am. Heart J. *91*:210, 1976.
337. Yoshikawa, J., Owaki, T., Kato, H., Tomita, Y., and Baba, K.: Echocardiographic diagnosis of endocardial cushion defects. Jpn. Heart J. *16*:1, 1975.
338. Beppu, S., Nimura, Y., Nagata, S., Tamai, M., Matsuo, H., Matsumoto, M., Kawashima, Y., Sakakibara, H., and Abe, H.: Diagnosis of endocardial cushion defect with cross-sectional and M-mode scanning of echocardiography. Differentiation from secundum atrial septal defect. Br. Heart J. *38*:911, 1976.
339. Hagler, D. J., Tajik, A. J., Seward, J. B., and Ritter, D. G.: Real-time phased-array 80° sector echocardiography: Atrioventricular canal defects. Circulation *56*:III-42 (Abstract), 1977.
340. Beppu, S., Nimura, Y., Sakakibara, H., Nagata, S., Park, Y-D., Baba, K., Naito, Y., Ohta, M., Kamiya, T., Koyanagi, H., and Fujita, T.: Mitral cleft in ostium primum atrial septal defect assessed by cross-sectional echocardiography. Circulation *62*:1099, 1980.
341. LaCorte, M. A., Fellows, K. E., and Williams, R. G.: Overriding tricuspid valve: Echocardiographic and angiocardiographic features. Am. J. Cardiol. *37*:911, 1976.
342. Seward, J. B., Tajik, A. J., Hagler, D. J., and Mair, D. D.: Straddling atrioventricular valve: Diagnostic two-dimensional echocardiographic features. Am. J. Cardiol. *41*:354 (Abstract), 1978.
343. Smallhorn, J. F., Tommasini, G., and Macartney, F. J.: Detection and assessment of straddling and overriding atrioventricular valves by two-dimensional echocardiography. Br. Heart J. *46*:254, 1981.
344. Usher, B. W., Goulden, D., and Murgo, J. P.: Echocardiographic detection of supravalvular aortic stenosis. Circulation *49*:1257, 1974.
345. Bolen, J. L., Popp, R. L., and French, J. W.: Echocardiographic features of supravalvular aortic stenosis. Circulation *52*:817, 1975.
346. Nasrallah, A. T., and Nihill, M.: Supravalvular aortic stenosis. Echocardiographic features. Br. Heart J. *37*:662, 1975.
347. Weyman, A. E., Feigenbaum, H., Dillon, J. C., Chang, S., Hurwitz, R. A., and Girod, D. A.: Localization of left ventricular outflow obstruction by cross-sectional echocardiography. Am. J. Med. *60*:33, 1976.
348. Sahn, D. J., Allen, H. D., McDonald, G., and Goldberg, S. J.: Real-time cross-sectional echocardiographic diagnosis of coarctation of the aorta. A prospective study of echocardiographic-angiographic correlations. Circulation *56*:762, 1977.
349. Assad-Morell, J. L., Seward, J. B., Tajik, A. J., Hagler, D. J., Giuliani, E. R., and Ritter, D. G.: Echophonocardiographic and contrast studies in conditions associated with systemic arterial trunk overriding the ventricular septum. Circulation *53*:663, 1976.
350. Chandraratna, P. A. N., Bhaduri, U., Littman, B. B., and Hildner, F. J.: Echocardiographic findings in persistent truncus arteriosus in a young adult. Br. Heart J. *36*:732, 1974.
351. Chung, K. J., Alexson, C. G., Manning, J. A., and Gramiak, R.: Echocardiography in truncus arteriosus: The value of pulmonic valve detection. Circulation *48*:281, 1973.
352. Henry, W. L., Maron, B. J., Griffith, J. M., Redwood, D. R., and Epstein, S. E.: Differential diagnosis of anomalies of the great arteries by real-time, two-dimensional echocardiography. Circulation *51*:283, 1975.
353. Houston, A. B., Gregory, N. L., and Coleman, E. N.: Two-dimensional sector scanner echocardiography in cyanotic congenital heart disease. Br. Heart J. *39*:1076, 1977.
354. Hagler, D. J., Tajik, A. J., Seward, J. B., Mair, D. D., and Titter, D. G.: Double-outlet right ventricle: Wide-angle two dimensional echocardiographic observations. Circulation *63*:419, 1981.
355. Hagler, D. J., Tajik, A. J., Seward, J. B., Mair, D. D., and Ritter, D. G.:

469. Ratshin, R. A., Smith, M. K., and Hood, W. P., Jr.: Possible false-positive diagnosis of pericardial effusion by echocardiography in presence of large left atrium. Chest *65*:112, 1974.
470. Popp, R. L., and Harrison, D. C.: Echocardiography. *In* Weissler, A. M. (ed.): Noninvasive Cardiology. New York, Grune and Stratton, 1974.
471. Martin, R. P., Rakowski, H., French, J., and Popp, R. L.: Localization of pericardial effusion with wide angle phased array echocardiography. Am. J. Cardiol. *42*:904, 1978.
472. Haaz, W. S., Mintz, G. S., Kotler, M. N., Parry, W., and Segal, B. L.: Two dimensional echocardiographic recognition of the descending thoracic aorta: Value in differentiating pericardial from pleural effusions. Am. J. Cardiol. *46*:739, 1980.
473. Chandraratna, P. A., and Aronow, W. S.: Detection of pericardial metastases by cross-section echocardiography. Circulation *63*:197, 1981.
474. D'Cruz, I. A., Cohen, H. C., Prabhu, R., and Glick, G.: Diagnosis of cardiac tamponade by echocardiography: Changes in mitral valve motion and ventricular dimensions: with special reference to paradoxical pulse. Circulation *52*:460, 1975.
475. Settle, H. P., Adolph, R. J., Fowler, N. O., Engel, P., Agruss, N. S., and Levenson, N. I.: Echocardiographic study of cardiac tamponade. Circulation *56*:951, 1977.
476. Schiller, N. B., and Botvinick, E. H.: Right ventricular compression as a sign of cardiac tamponade. An analysis of echocardiographic ventricular dimensions and their clinical implications. Circulation *56*:774, 1977.
477. Shina, S., Yaginuma, T., Kondo, K., Kawai, N., and Hosoda, S.: Echocardiographic evaluation of impending cardiac tamponade. J. Cardiogr. *9*:555, 1979.
478. Armstrong, W. F., Schilt, B. F., Helper, D. J., Dillon, J. C., and Feigenbaum, H.: Diastolic collapse of the right ventricle with cardiac tamponade: An echocardiographic study. Circulation *65*:1491, 1982.
479. Gillam, L. D., Guyer, D., King, M. E., Marshall, J., and Weyman, A. E.: Hydrodynamic compression of the right atrial free wall, a new highly-sensitive echocardiographic sign of cardiac tamponade. Am. J. Cardiol. *49*:1010, 1982.
480. Schnittger, I., Bowden, R. E., Abrams, J., and Popp, R. L.: Echocardiography: Pericardial thickening and constrictive pericarditis. Am. J. Cardiol. *42*:388, 1978.
481. Lewis, B. S.: Real time two dimensional echocardiography in constrictive pericarditis. Am. J. Cardiol. *49*:1789, 1982.
482. Pandian, N., Skorton, D., Kieso, R., Pai, A. L., and Kerber, R.: Characterization of left ventricular diastolic filling in constrictive pericarditis by two-dimensional echocardiography: Experimental and clinical studies. Circulation *64*:IV-204, 1981.
483. Elkayam, U., Kotler, M. N., Segal, B., and Parry, W.: Echocardiographic findings in constrictive pericarditis: A case report. Isr. J. Med. Sci. *12*:1308, 1976.
484. Chandraratna, P. A. N., and Imaizumi, T.: Echocardiographic diagnosis of thickened pericardium. Cardiovasc. Med. *3*:1279, 1978.
485. Gibson, T. C., Grossman, W., McLaurin, L. P., Moos, S., and Craige, E.: An echocardiographic study of the interventricular system in constrictive pericarditis. Br. Heart J. *38*:738, 1976.
486. Pool, P. E., Seagren, S. C., Abbasi, A. S., Gharuzi, Y., and Kraus, R.: Echocardiographic manifestations of constrictive pericarditis: Abnormal septal motion. Chest *68*:684, 1975.
487. Voelkel, A. G., Pietro, D. A., Folland, E. D., Fisher, M. C., and Parisi, A. F.: Echocardiographic features of constrictive pericarditis. Circulation *58*:871, 1978.
488. Effert, S., and Domanig, E.: The diagnosis of intra-atrial tumor and thrombi by the ultrasonic echo method. Germ. Med. Meth. *4*:1, 1959.
489. Wolfe, S. B., Popp, R. L., and Feigenbaum, H.: Diagnosis of atrial tumors by ultrasound. Circulation *39*:615, 1969.
490. Finegan, R. E., and Harrison, D. C.: Diagnosis of left atrial myxoma by echocardiography. N. Engl. J. Med. *282*:1022, 1970.
491. Schattenberg, T. T.: Echocardiographic diagnosis of left atrial myxoma. Mayo Clin. Proc. *43*:620, 1968.
492. Kostis, J. B., and Moghadam, A. N.: Echocardiographic diagnosis of left atrial myxoma. Chest *58*:550, 1970.
493. Abdulla, A. M., Stefadouros, M. A., Mucha, E., Moore, H. V., and O'Malley, G. A.: Left atrial myxoma: Echocardiographic diagnosis and determination of size. J.A.M.A. *238*:510, 1977.
494. Perry, L. S., King, J. F., Zeft, H. J., Manley, J. C., Gross, C. M., and Wann, L. S.: Two-dimensional echocardiography in the diagnosis of left atrial myxoma. Br. Heart J. *45*:667, 1981.
495. Tway, K. P., Shah, A. A., and Rahimtoola, S. H.: Multiple bilateral myxomas demonstrated by two-dimensional echocardiography. Am. J. Med. *71*:896, 1981.
496. Furukawa, K., Katsume, H., Matsukubo, H., and Inoue, D.: Echocardiographic findings of floating thrombus in left atrium. Br. Heart J. *44*:599, 1980.
497. Schweizer, P., Bardos, P., Erbel, R., Meyer, J., Merx, W., Messmer, B. J., and Effert, S.: Detection of left atrial thrombi by echocardiography. Br. Heart J. *45*:148, 1981.
498. Farooki, Z. Q., Green, E. W., and Arciniegas, E.: Echocardiographic pattern of right atrial tumour motion. Br. Heart J. *38*:580, 1976.
499. Atsuchi, Y., Nagai, Y., Nakamura, K., et al.: Echocardiographic diagnosis of prolapsing right atrial myxoma. Jpn. Heart J. *17*:798, 1976.
500. Riggs, T., Paul, M. H., DeLeon, S., and Ilbawi, M.: Two dimensional echocardiography in evaluation of right atrial masses: Five cases in pediatric patients. Am. J. Cardiol. *48*:961, 1981.
501. Howard, R. J., Pollick, C., Rambihar, V., Drobac, M., Martin, R. P., Popp, R. L., and Rakowski, H.: Two-dimensional echocardiographic detection of right atrial tumors. Am. J. Cardiol. *49*:1041 (Abstract), 1982.
502. Nicholson, K. G., Prior, A. L., Norman, A. G., Naik, D. R., and Kennedy, A.: Bilateral atrial myxomas diagnosed preoperatively and successfully removed. Br. Heart J. *2*:440, 1977.
503. Fitterer, J. D., Spicer, M. J., and Nelson, W. P.: Echocardiographic demonstration of bilateral atrial myxomas. Chest *70*:282, 1976.
504. Gustafson, A. G., Edler, I. G., and Dahlback, O. K.: Bilateral atrial myxomas diagnosed by echocardiography. Acta Med. Scand. *201*:391, 1977.
505. Werner, J. A., Cheitlin, M. D., Gross, B. W., Speck, S. M., and Ivey, T. D.: Echocardiographic appearance of the Chiari network: Differentiation from right-heart pathology. Circulation *63*:1104, 1981.
506. Morgan, D. L., Palazola, J., Reed, W., Bell, H. H., Kindred, L. H., and Beauchamp, G. D.: Left heart myxomas. Am. J. Cardiol. *40*:611, 1977.
507. Meller, J., Teichholz, L. E., Pichard, A. O., Matta, R., Litwak, R., Herman, M. V., and Massie, K. F.: Left ventricular myxoma. Echocardiographic diagnosis and review of the literature. Am. J. Med. *63*:816, 1977.
508. Roelandt, J., Bletter, W. B., Leuftink, E. W., vanDorp, W. G., tenCate, F., and Nauta, J.: Ultrasonic demonstration of right ventricular myxoma. J. Clin. Ultrasound *5*:191, 1977.
509. Asayama, J., Kunishige, H., Katsume, H., Watanabe, T., Matsukubo, H., Endo, N., Matsuura, T., Ijichi, H., Onouchi, Z., Tomizawa, M., Goto, M., and Nakata, K.: The ultrasound cardiographic findings of myxoma in the right ventricular wall. Cardiovasc. Sound Bull. *5*:129, 1975.
510. Roelandt, J., Bletter, W. B., Leuftink, E. W., vanDorp, W. G., tenCate, F., and Nauta, J.: Ultrasonic demonstration of right ventricular myxoma. J. Clin. Ultrasound *5*:191, 1977.
511. Krivokapich, J., Warren, S. E., Child, J. S., Kaufman, J. A., Vieweg, W. V., and Hagan, A. D.: M-mode and cross-sectional echocardiographic diagnosis of right ventricular cavity mass. J. Clin. Ultrasound *9*:5, 1981.
512. Levisman, J. A., MacAlpin, R. N., Abbasi, A. S., Ellis, N., and Eber, L. M.: Echocardiographic diagnosis of a mobile, pedunculated tumor in the left ventricular cavity. Am. J. Cardiol. *36*:957, 1975.
513. Nanda, N. C., Barold, S. S., Gramiak, R., Ong, L. S., and Heinle, R. A.: Echocardiographic features of right ventricular outflow tumor prolapsing into the pulmonary artery. Am. J. Cardiol. *40*:272, 1977.
514. Chandraratha, P. A. N., Pedro, S. S., Elkins, R. C., and Grantham, N.: Echocardiographic, angiocardiographic, and surgical correlations in right ventricular myxoma simulating valvar pulmonic stenosis. Circulation *55*:619, 1977.
515. Farooki, Z. Q., Henry, J. G., Arciniegas, E., and Green, E. W.: Ultrasonic pattern of ventricular rhabdomyoma in two infants. Am. J. Cardiol. *34*:842, 1974.
516. Milner, S., Abramowitz, J. A., and Levin, S. E.: Rhabdomyoma of the heart in a newborn infant. Diagnosis by echocardiography. Br. Heart J. *43*:623, 1980.
517. Yabek, S. M., Isabel-Jones, J., Gyepes, M. T., and Jarmakani, J. M.: Cardiac fibroma in a neonate present with severe congestive heart failure. J. Pediatr. *91*:310, 1977.
518. Ports, T. A., Schiller, N. B., and Strunk, B. L.: Echocardiography of right ventricular tumors. Circulation *56*:439, 1977.
519. Bluschke, V., Köhler, E., Ruppert, C., and Böcker, K.: Diagnosis of a cardiac metastasis of a fibrosarcoma by two-dimensional echocardiography (author's transl.). Z. Kardiol. *70*:492, 1981.
520. Koiwaya, Y., Kawachi, Y., Orita, Y., Nakamura, M., Hirata, T., Yamamota, K., and Omae, T.: Echocardiographic detection of metastatic cardiac mural tumor. J. Clin. Ultrasound *8*:443, 1980.
521. Canedo, M. I., Otken, L., and Stefadouros, M. A.: Echocardiographic features of cardiac compression by a thymoma simulating cardiac tamponade and obstruction of the superior vena cava. Br. Heart J. *39*:1038, 1977.
522. Baduini, G., Paolillo, V., and Di Summa, M.: Echocardiographic findings in a case of acquired pulmonic stenosis from extrinsic compression by a mediastinal cyst. Chest *80*:507, 1981.
523. Shah, A., and Schwartz, H.: Echocardiographic features of cardiac compression by mediastinal pancreatic pseudocyst. Chest *77*:440, 1980.
524. Farooki, Z. Q., Adelman, S., and Green, E. W.: Echocardiographic differentiation of a cystic and a solid tumor of the heart. Am. J. Cardiol. *39*:107, 1977.
525. Mintz, G. S., Kotler, M. N., Segal, B. L., and Parry, W. R.: Two dimensional echocardiographic recognition of the descending thoracic aorta. Am. J. Cardiol. *44*:232, 1979.
526. Come, P. C., Sacks, B., Vine, H., McArdle, C., Koretsky, S., and Weintraub, R.: Ultrasonic visualization of the posterior thoracic aorta in long axis: Diagnosis of a saccular mycotic aneurysm. Chest *79*:470, 1981.
527. Goldberg, B. B.: Aortosonography. Int. Surg. *62*:294, 1977.
528. Lababidi, Z., and Monzon, C.: Early cardiac manifestations of Marfan's syndrome in the newborn. Am. Heart J. *102*:943, 1981.
529. Nanda, N. C., Gramiak, R., and Shah, P. M.: Diagnosis of aortic root dissection by echocardiography. Circulation *48*:506, 1973.
530. Millward, D. K., Robinson, N. J., and Craige, E.: Dissecting aortic aneurysm diagnosed by echocardiography in a patient with rupture of the aneurysm into the right atrium. Am. J. Cardiol. *30*:427, 1972.

531. Moothart, R. W., Spangler, R. D., and Blout, S. G., Jr.: Echocardiography in aortic root dissection and dilatation. Am. J. Cardiol. *36*:11, 1975.
532. Kronzon, I., and Mehta, S. S.: Illustrative echocardiogram: Aortic root dissection. Chest *65*:88, 1974.
533. Yuste, P., Aza, V., Minguez, I., Cerezo, L., and Martinez-Bardiu, C.: Dissecting aortic aneurysm diagnosed by echocardiography. Br. Heart J. *36*: 111, 1974.
534. Brown, O. R., Popp, R. L., and Kloster, F. E.: Echocardiographic criteria for aortic root dissection. Am. J. Cardiol. *36*:17, 1975.
535. Krueger, S. K., Starke, H., Forker, A. D., and Eliot, R. S.: Echocardiographic mimics of aortic root dissection. Chest *67*:441, 1975.
536. Victor, M. F., Mintz, G. S., Kotler, M. N., Wilson A. R., and Segal, B. L.: Two dimensional echocardiographic diagnosis of aortic dissection. Am. J. Cardiol. *48*:1155, 1981.
537. Smuckler, A. L., Nomeir, A. M., Watts, L. E., and Hackshaw, B. T.: Echocardiographic diagnosis of aortic root dissection by M-mode and two-dimensional techniques. Am. Heart J. *103*:897, 1982.
538. D'Cruz, I. A., Jain, M., Campbell, C., and Goldberg, A. N.: Ultrasound visualization of aortic dissection by right parasternal scanning, including systolic flutter of the intimal flap. Chest *80*:239, 1981.
539. Nicholson, W. J., and Cobbs, B. W., Jr.: Echocardiographic oscillating flap in aortic root dissecting aneurysm, Chest *70*:305, 1976.
540. Krueger, S. K., Wilson, C. S, Weaver, W. F., Reese, H. E., Caudill, C. C., and Rourke, T.: Aortic root dissection: Echocardiographic demonstration of torn intimal flap. J. Clin. Ultrasound *4*:35, 1976.
541. Matsumoto, M., Matsuo, H., Beppu, S., Yoshioka, Y., Kawashima, Y., Nimura, Y., and Abe, H.: Echocardiographic diagnosis of ruptured aneurysms of sinus of Valsalva. Report of two cases. Circulation *53*:382, 1976.
542. Rothbaum, D. A., Dillon, J. C., Chang, S., and Feigenbaum, H.: Echocardiographic manifestation of right sinus of Valsalva aneurysm. Circulation *49*:768, 1974.
543. Engle, P. J., Held, J. S., van der Bel-Kahn, J., and Spitz, H.: Echocardiographic diagnosis of congenital sinus of Valsalva aneurysm with dissection of the interventricular septum. Circulation *63*:705, 1981.

6 RADIOLOGICAL AND ANGIOGRAPHIC EXAMINATION OF THE HEART

by Murray G. Baron, M.D.

The radiological examination of the heart provides detailed information regarding cardiac structure and function that cannot be duplicated with a similar degree of accuracy by any other diagnostic method. The appearance of the heart and lungs on ordinary chest roentgenograms often indicates the presence of heart disease and, at times, is diagnostic of a specific cardiac abnormality. Correct interpretation of the cardiac shadow in the frontal view is particularly important, because a chest roentgenogram in this projection is included as part of most routine medical examinations and provides a convenient survey method for the detection of otherwise unsuspected heart disease. In those patients with a known cardiac condition, the chest roentgenogram is of use in assessing its severity, in documenting the progress of the disease, in evaluating the presence and severity of secondary complications, and as an indicator of the efficacy of treatment. *Fluoroscopy* is of value in the detection of intracardiac and coronary arterial calcification and in the diagnosis of conditions such as pericardial effusion or atrial septal defect. Aside from such specific indications, fluoroscopy is of limited usefulness. Of all the imaging techniques, *angiocardiography* is the most comprehensive method for studying the intracardiac anatomy. Although it is an "invasive procedure" in that it is usually carried out in conjunction with cardiac catheterization (Chap. 9) (digital radiographic examinations can be carried out with intravenous injection of contrast medium [p. 191]), the risk to the patient is usually minimal, while the anatomical and hemodynamic information derived from angiocardiograms is often essential for establishing a correct diagnosis and planning a logical therapeutic approach. A special form of angiography, that of the coronary arteries (i.e., coronary arteriography), is considered in Chapter 10.

THE CARDIAC SERIES

The heart appears relatively homogeneous on a chest film because the myocardium, valves, and other cardiac structures have essentially the same radiodensity as blood, and their shadows blend imperceptibly with one another. Intracardiac lesions cannot be visualized unless they are calcified. The contours of the cardiac silhouette are clearly outlined because they contrast with the adjacent radiolucent air-containing lungs. Only those chambers and vessels that form a border on any particular view can be evaluated. However, the heart is a three-dimensional structure, and therefore multiple views are required in order to bring each of the chambers and great vessels into profile. Even then, the posterior border of the heart cannot be clearly identified unless the esophagus is filled with radiopaque material. A complete plain film study of the heart comprises four views of the chest: frontal, lateral, 60-degree right anterior oblique, and 45-degree left anterior oblique. On the first three views the patient swallows barium in order to opacify the esophagus.

Except in the more severe congenital anomalies, such as the transposition complexes or hypoplasia of the left ventricle, the chambers of the heart and great vessels always occupy the same relative position within the cardiac silhouette. *Dilatation* of each structure affects the contours of the heart in a fairly characteristic manner that is similar from case to case. However, this is not true with concentric cardiac *hypertrophy.* As the ventricular wall thickens, it tends to encroach on the cavity and may not increase the outer diameter of the chamber. Considerable myocardial hypertrophy can be present without causing a significant change in the shape of the cardiac silhouette. Even when the hypertrophy does result in cardiac enlargement, the appearance of the heart is often nonspecific.

Frontal View (Fig. 6–1)

In this view, the upper half of the right cardiac border is formed by the superior vena cava and the lower half by the right atrium. The caval portion is relatively straight, while the lateral margin of the atrium forms a gentle, con-

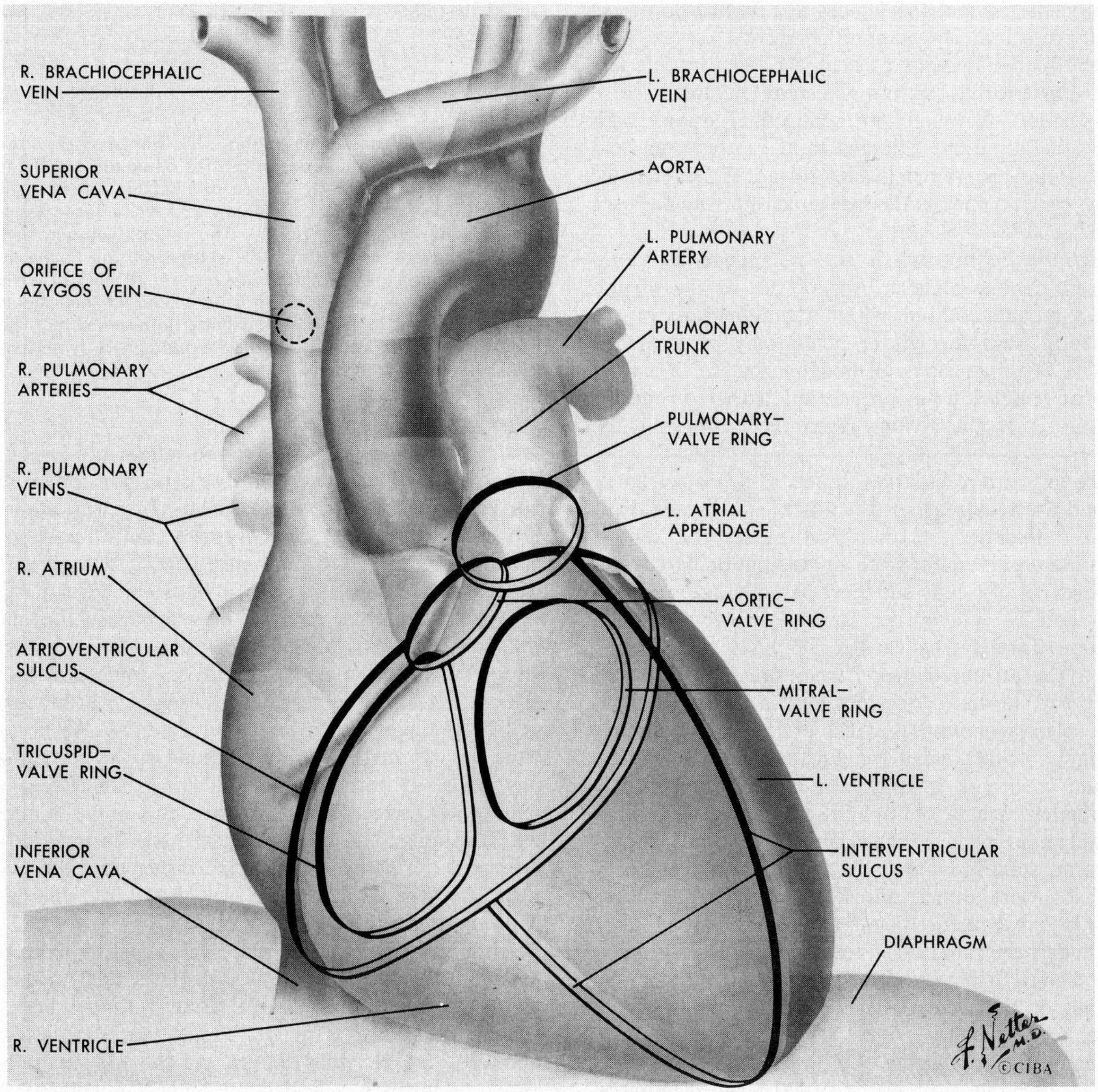

FIGURE 6–1 Frontal projection of the heart. (Reproduced with permission from The CIBA Collection of Medical Illustrations by Frank H. Netter, M.D. Vol. 5, The Heart, edited by F. Y. Yonkman. Copyright 1969, CIBA Pharmaceutical Co., Division of CIBA-GEIGY Corp. All rights reserved.)

vex curve that extends to the diaphragm. The junction of the two structures is usually indicated by a shallow angle, where their contours meet. If the patient can take a sufficiently deep inspiration, a small portion of the inferior vena cava may become visible as a triangular shadow between the diaphragm and the border of the right atrium.

The left cardiac border is composed of three distinct curvatures: The uppermost bulge is formed by the aortic knob, below which is the curve of the main pulmonary artery and sometimes a portion of the left pulmonary artery; most of the remainder of the left cardiac contour represents the anterolateral margin of the left ventricle. The left atrial appendage reaches the left border of the heart and is seen in profile as a short, straight segment between the pulmonary artery and the left ventricle. If the atrium is not enlarged, this segment cannot be delimited on plain films; however, it is identifiable fluoroscopically, because its pulsations are not in phase with those of the ventricle.

THE ATRIA. Enlargement of the *right atrium* causes broadening of the cardiac silhouette to the right, with accentuation of the curvature of the atrial contour (Fig. 6–2). Normally, the *right ventricle* does not form a border in the frontal projection and cannot be viewed directly. As the ventricle dilates, it tends to push the left ventricle laterally and posteriorly, causing widening of the cardiac shadow to the left. Especially with congenital lesions, such as tetralogy of Fallot, the enlarged right ventricle may extend beyond the left ventricle and form the left cardiac border. The cardiac apex is then elevated and rounded (see Figure 6–37, p. 172).

As the *left atrium* increases in size, its appendage bulges from the left cardiac contour, the border of the atrium may form a second contour within the right part of the cardiac shadow, and the left bronchus may be displaced upward. The last two signs, although accurate, are relatively insensitive and are not present unless there is considerable dilatation of the atrium. Even then, they may be absent.

When the left atrium enlarges, it tends to project backward beyond the remainder of the heart. This localized increase in the thickness of the heart causes the central portion of the cardiac silhouette to be abnormally dense. The increased density ends suddenly at the margins of the left atrium, and its right border can be visualized as a distinct contour through the cardiac silhouette (Fig. 6–2). However, if the atrium distends from side to side more than posteriorly, so that it does not form a localized bulge, its shadow blends in with the rest of the heart, and its borders may not be visualized. Furthermore, when the right atrium enlarges, it may also extend posteriorly, alongside the left atrium, obliterating the latter's right border. A double contour, even when present, is often difficult to visualize on standard films. Because the roentgen technique used for chest films is adjusted so that the exposure provides an optimal picture of the lungs, an enlarged heart is usually underpenetrated. The dense cardiac shadow then obscures the contour of the left atrium, although it may be quite obvious on an overexposed film or one made with a Bucky grid.

Occasionally, the confluence of the *right pulmonary veins* is visible through the right portion of the cardiac silhouette and can resemble the double density caused by left atrial enlargement. However, the lateral border of the venous shadow is relatively straight and not convex as is the contour of an enlarged left atrium. In addition, when the left atrium is enlarged, the entire central portion of the cardiac silhouette is abnormally dense. A giant left atrium can extend beyond the right atrium and form part, or all, of the right cardiac border, in which case the margin of the right atrium is seen within the cardiac silhouette. Elevation of the left main bronchus has some drawbacks as a sign of left atrial enlargement. Often, the bronchus is hidden by the hilar and mediastinal shadows. When the bronchus can be identified, it is difficult to be certain whether its course is normal or not if the displacement is not marked. Displacement of the bronchus must be interpreted with caution if the film was not made during full inspiration or if the patient was supine rather than erect. In both situations, the carinal angle is widened and the left bronchus elevated.

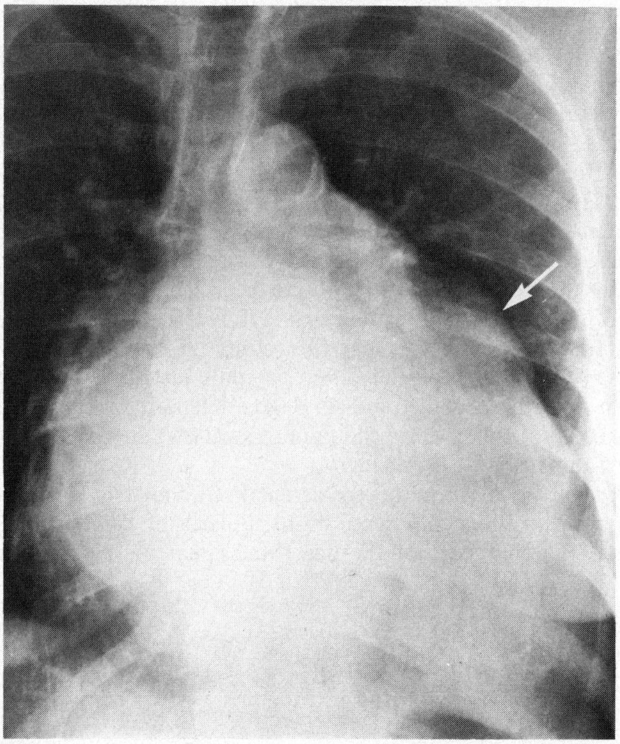

FIGURE 6–2 Enlargement of the atria, frontal view. The enlargement of the right portion of the cardiac silhouette and the increased curvature of its border are caused by dilatation of the right atrium. The left atrial appendage is dilated and forms a localized bulge (arrow) on the left cardiac border. The double contour on the right side, the increased density of the central portion of the heart, and the elevation of the left main bronchus are all signs of left atrial enlargement. The widening of the heart to the left indicates ventricular enlargement, in this case involving both ventricles. The patient had severe mitral valve disease with pulmonary hypertension and tricuspid regurgitation.

Abnormal prominence of the left atrial appendage is the most sensitive sign of left atrial enlargement in the frontal view. The appendage dilates along with the body of the atrium, and its segment on the left heart border, which is normally flat, becomes convex. As the appendage becomes larger, it forms a well-defined bulge immediately beneath the pulmonary artery segment. An aneurysm of the antero-

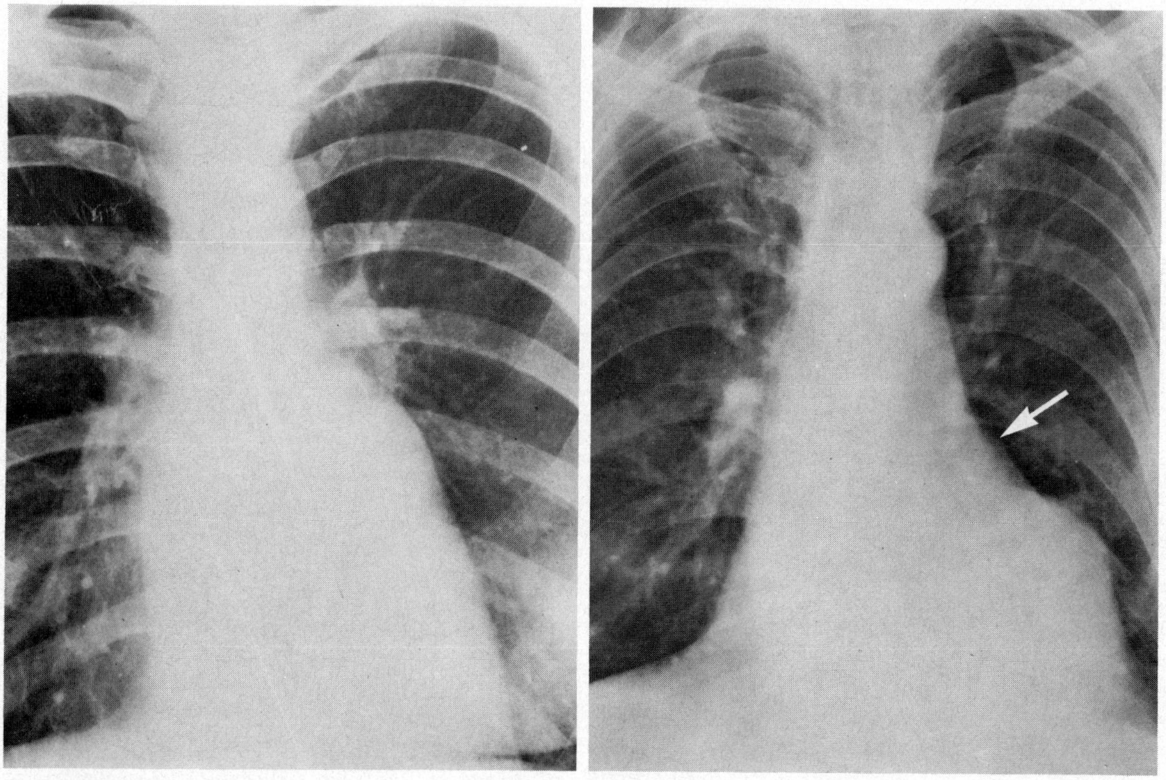

FIGURE 6–3 Dilatation of the left atrial appendage—differential diagnosis. *A*, Mitral stenosis. The only sign of left atrial enlargement is dilatation of its appendage, which forms a bulge on the left cardiac contour immediately beneath the pulmonary artery segment. *B*, Ventricular aneurysm. In this case, the bulge on the left cardiac contour is separated from the pulmonary artery segment. The intervening portion of the heart border is formed by the left atrial appendage (arrow) and the basal portion of the anterolateral left ventricular wall.

lateral wall of the left ventricle can cause a similar bulge but at a lower level on the cardiac contour, some distance below the pulmonary artery (Fig. 6–3).

THE LEFT VENTRICLE. The shape of an enlarged *left ventricle* depends, to some extent, on the underlying cause. When the dilatation results from a diastolic overload, particularly in aortic regurgitation, the chamber enlarges mainly along its long axis. The cardiac apex is displaced downward and to the left (Fig. 6–4*A*). Although this axis of the ventricle is elongated when the dilatation is due to myocardial disease, the width of the chamber is also significantly increased, so that the dilated ventricle assumes a more globular shape (Fig. 6–4*B*).

As the left ventricle enlarges, it becomes more difficult to evaluate the size of the left atrium on the frontal film. Widening of the cardiac silhouette to the left tends to minimize, or even mask, the prominence of a dilated left atrial appendage (see Figures 6–8 and 6–11). In order to judge the size of the two chambers properly, it is usually necessary to obtain other views of the heart, particularly the left oblique projection (see Figure 6–14*C*). When both the left atrium and the left ventricle are enlarged, the relative degrees of dilatation of the chambers have diagnostic importance. Left atrial enlargement does not necessarily indicate disease of the mitral valve but can occur in response to elevation of the left ventricular end-diastolic pressure. In the latter case, the degree of enlargement of the left atrium will be less than that of the left ventricle, while the opposite is usually true when the chambers are dilated because of mitral valve disease.

CARDIAC VALVES. The frontal view is of limited usefulness for the detection of *valve calcification.* The aortic valve is projected over the left border of the spine, and calcific deposits on the valve cusps are usually obscured by the vertebral bodies. The mitral valve lies below and to the left of the aortic valve within the densest portion of the cardiac shadow, and only relatively coarse calcific deposits can be visualized. Valve calcifications are easier to recognize by means of fluoroscopy. As the heart beats, the mitral valve describes a shallow, elliptical trajectory, with its long axis oriented to the left and slightly downward, while the aortic valve moves in a vertical direction.

Lateral View (Fig. 6–5)

The anterior border of the cardiac shadow is formed by the body and the outflow tract of the right ventricle, the supravalvular portion of the main pulmonary artery, and the aorta. The normal ventricle abuts the lower third of the sternum. Because lung is interposed between the sternum and the cardiac structures, the upper retrosternal space is radiolucent. As the right ventricle dilates, its outflow portion extends anteriorly toward the sternum and encroaches on the retrosternal clear space. However, this is not always a reliable sign of right ventricular enlargement,

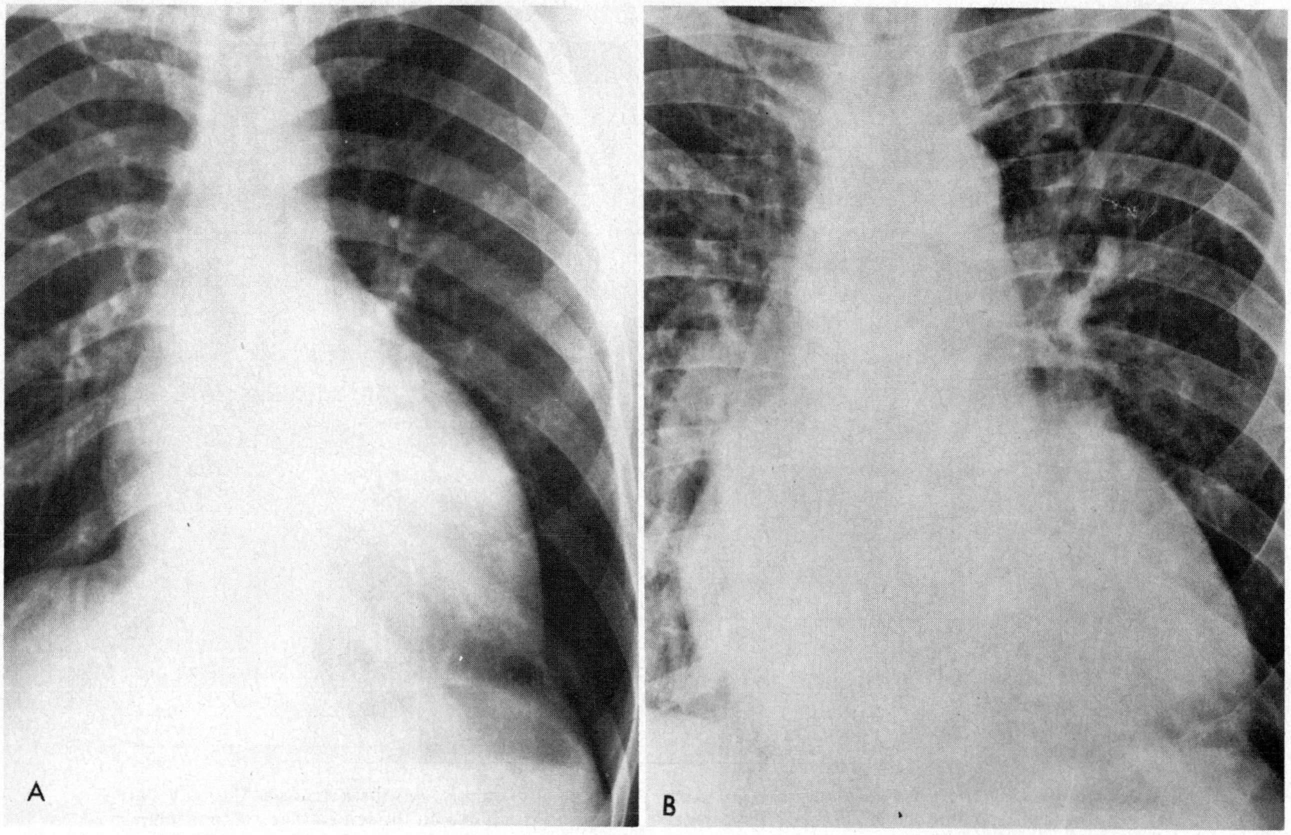

FIGURE 6–4 Enlargement of the left ventricle, frontal view. *A*, Aortic regurgitation. Enlargement of the left ventricle has occurred mainly along its long axis, so that the cardiac apex is displaced downward and to the left. This shape of the cardiac silhouette is characteristic of the type of ventricular dilatation associated with regurgitation of the aortic valve. (From Donoso, E., and Gorlin, R. [eds.]: Current Cardiovascular Topics. Vol. 3, Angina Pectoris. New York, Stratton Intercontinental Medical Book Co., 1977.) *B*, Ischemic heart disease with significant impairment of myocardial function. The long and short axes of the ventricle are more or less evenly elongated, causing the chamber to have a globular shape.

because it depends upon the shape of the chest as well as upon the size of the heart. In a patient with a narrow chest, as in the "straight back" syndrome, the retrosternal space is often obliterated by a normal-sized heart simply because there is no space for it in the thorax. Conversely, in a patient with pulmonary emphysema and a barrel-shaped chest, the heart can be considerably enlarged and still barely reach the sternum.

The posterior border of the heart is formed by the posterior aspect of the left atrium and the left ventricle. On a film made during deep inspiration, the supradiaphragmatic portion of the inferior vena cava and a small part of the right atrium may be uncovered. The ventricular border is usually clearly seen as it is outlined by adjacent air-containing lung. However, the left atrial component of the posterior cardiac border merges with the shadow of the mediastinum and is not well delineated. The esophagus lies directly behind the heart and, when filled with opaque material, can be used to evaluate left atrial size. The normal atrium, in the erect position, does not affect the esophagus, but as it enlarges, it indents the anterior wall of the esophagus and displaces it posteriorly (Fig. 6–6*A*). The indentation caused by an enlarged atrium begins immediately below the carina and involves the midportion of the esophagus. The lower esophagus lies below the atrium and is adjacent to the left ventricle. When only the atrium is enlarged, the supradiaphragmatic portion of the esophagus remains in its normal postion and shows no indentation.

The portion of the esophagus immediately above the diaphragm may be indented by an enlarged left ventricle (Fig. 6–6*B*). More commonly, the dilated ventricle extends laterally as well as posteriorly and bypasses the esophagus (Fig. 6–7). When both the left atrium and the left ventricle are dilated, the esophagus is usually displaced posteriorly in one continuous sweep, beginning just below the carina and continuing down to the diaphragm (Fig. 6–8).

On occasion, the appearance of the esophagus in the lateral view can be misleading. If there are tertiary contractions of the esophagus or if it is not well distended with barium, no indentation or displacement will be seen even though the left atrium is of considerable size. Furthermore, because the esophagus is not fixed to the heart, it may slide medially as the heart enlarges and will not appear displaced when viewed from the side. On the other hand, the esophagus is loosely attached to the descending aorta and can be pulled backward when this vessel is tortuous, the displacement being almost identical to that caused by an enlarged atrium. The correct cause of the displacement can be recognized because the curve of the esophagus exactly parallels that of the aorta.

The relationship between the shadow of the inferior vena cava and the posterior border of the heart in the lat-

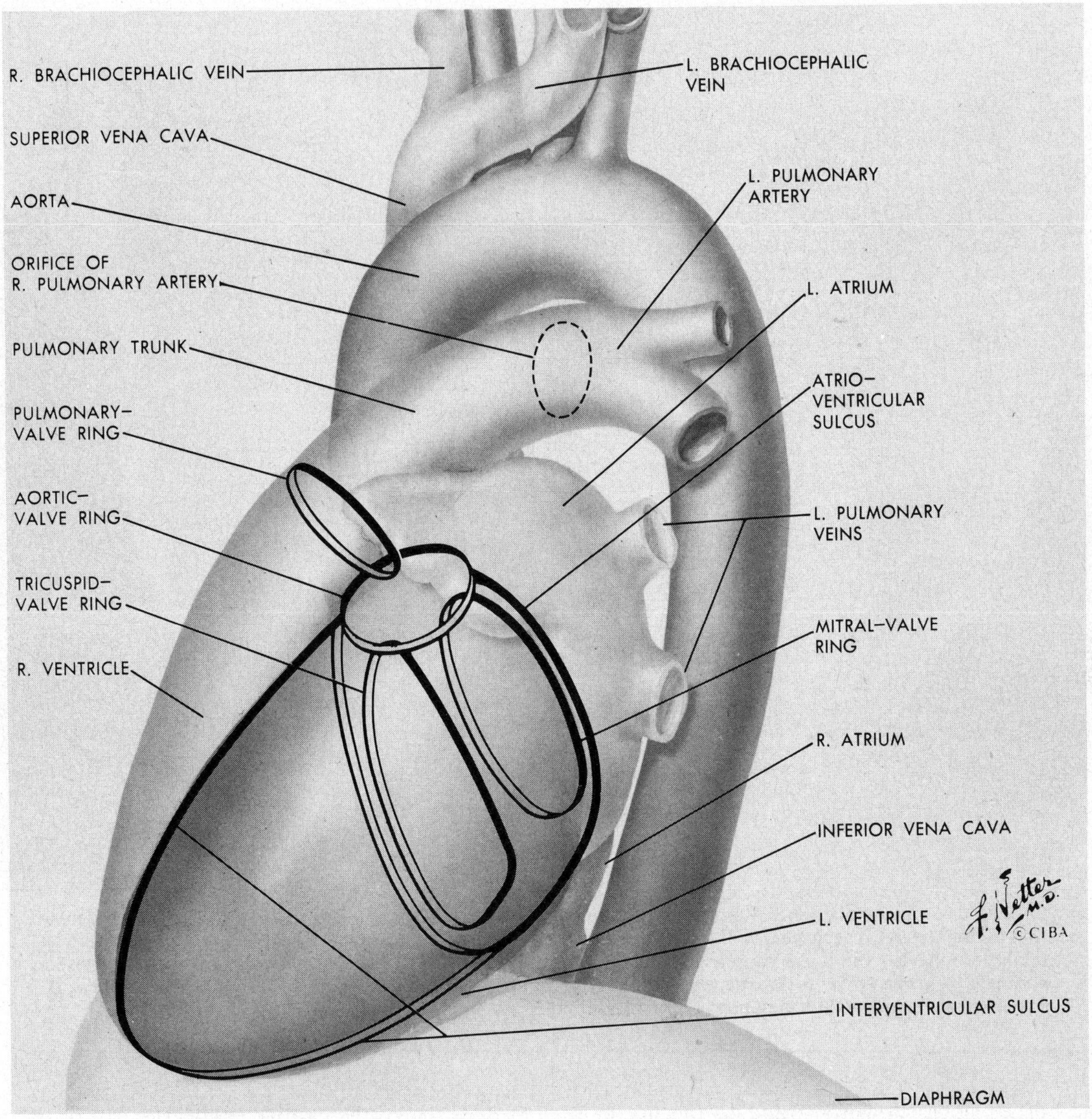

FIGURE 6–5 Lateral projection of the heart. (Reproduced with permission from The CIBA Collection of Medical Illustrations by Frank H. Netter, M.D. Vol. 5, The Heart, edited by F. Y. Yonkman. Copyright 1969, CIBA Pharmaceutical Co., Division of CIBA-GEIGY Corp. All rights reserved.)

eral projection provides a fairly accurate indicator of left ventricular size. The cava can usually be identified as a curvilinear shadow that extends upward and forward from the right diaphragm (see Figure 6–5). The lower part of the cardiac border is formed by the left ventricle and, as it curves forward, it crosses the posterior margin of the caval shadow about 2 cm above the left leaf of the diaphragm. As the left ventricle dilates, the apex of the chamber extends downward, and the point of intersection between the border of the ventricle and the cava moves closer to a diaphragm (Fig. 6–8).[1] However, the accuracy of this sign is considerably diminished if the patient is rotated slightly to either side and the film is not a true lateral projection.[2]

When valvular calcification is identified in the lateral view, fluoroscopy is usually not needed to determine whether the leaflets of the aortic valve or the mitral valve are involved. The two valves can be separated by a line drawn from the origin of the left main bronchus to the anterior costophrenic sulcus. (The bronchus can be recognized because it is projected on end and casts a round, lucent shadow at the lower end of the trachea.) The mitral valve almost always lies below this line, while the aortic valve lies more anteriorly, above the line (Figs. 6–7 and 6–9).[3]

RIGHT ANTERIOR OBLIQUE VIEW (Fig. 6–10). If the patient is properly positioned, the cardiac silhouette will be projected completely to the left of the shadow of the spine. The upper half of the right heart border is formed by the posterolateral wall of the left atrium and its lower half by the back of the right atrium. As in the lateral view, the left atrial contour cannot be satisfactorily delineated unless the esophagus is filled with barium. The ascending aorta forms the relatively straight, upper portion of the left cardiac contour. Beneath this segment,

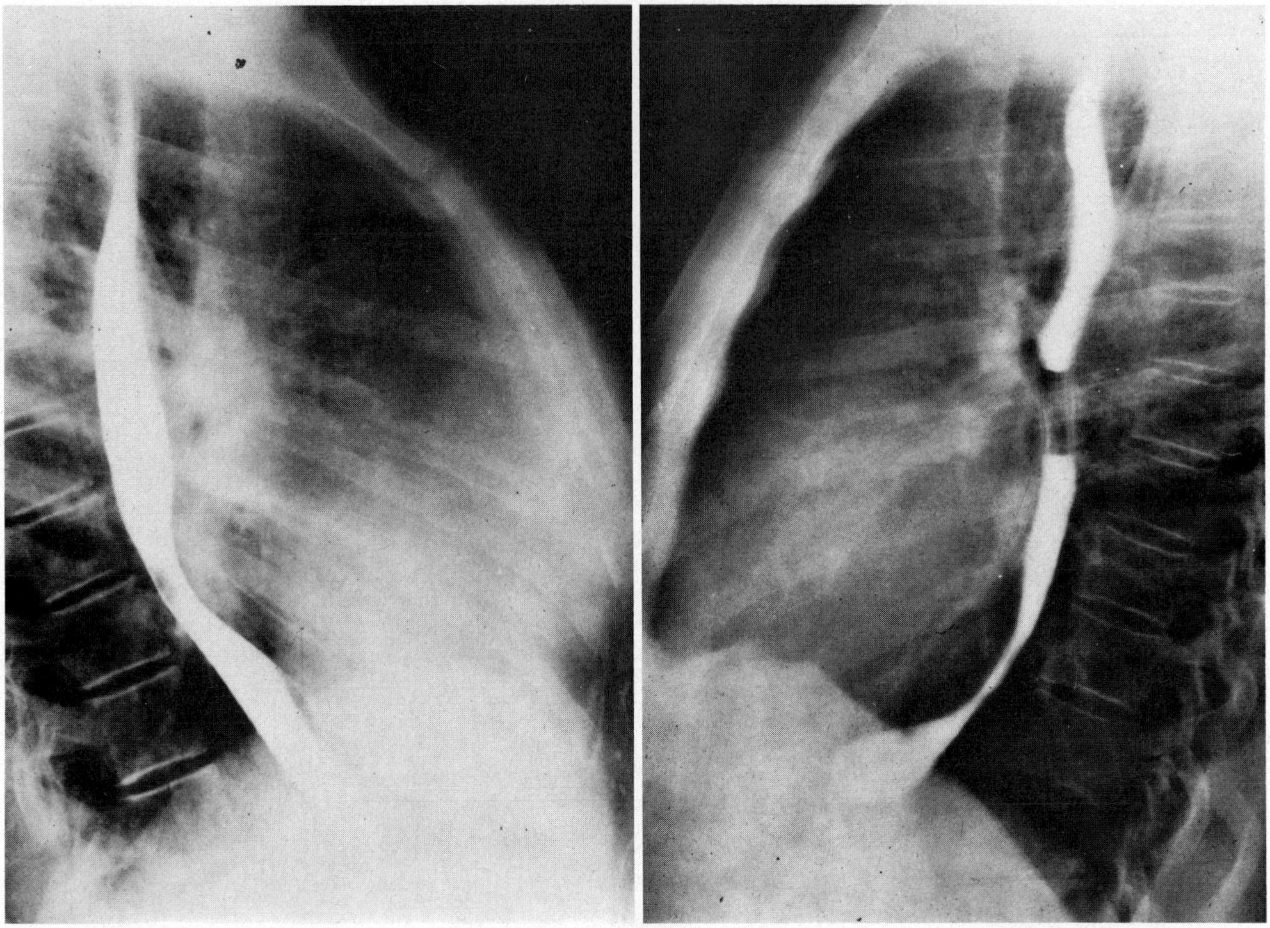

FIGURE 6–6 Indentation of the esophagus by the left cardiac chambers. *A*, Enlarged left atrium. The indentation on the anterior esophageal wall begins just below the level of the carina and involves only the midportion of the esophagus. The lower esophagus is in its normal position and shows no indentation. *B*, Enlarged left ventricle. The dilated ventricle extends posteriorly and impinges on the lowermost portion of the esophagus. The esophageal indentation continues to the diaphragm.

the cardiac border slopes downward and to the left in a shallow curve formed by the margins of the outflow tract of the right ventricle and the main pulmonary artery. The inferior continuation of the curve represents the anterior border of the left ventricle.

The information provided by this view regarding left atrial size is essentially the same as that gained from the lateral projection. When the atrium is large, it indents or displaces the barium-filled esophagus. The lowermost portion of the esophagus will not be affected if the left ventricle is normal in size. When the ventricle is also enlarged, the esophagus is displaced backward in a continuous curve that extends from the carina to the diaphragm.

Dilatation of the outflow tract of the right ventricle and the main pulmonary artery produces a bulge on the left cardiac contour just beneath the straight aortic segment. This is a common finding when there is a sizable left-to-right shunt through an atrial or ventricular septal defect. In mitral valve disease, abnormal prominence of the right ventricular outflow tract usually signifies the presence of pulmonary hypertension (Fig. 6–11).

The right anterior oblique view is the best for detection of mitral valve calcification. The valve is seen within the midportion of the cardiac silhouette, free of the shadow of the spine (Fig. 6–11), and because it is projected tangentially, it exhibits its maximal range of motion between systole and diastole. The valve can be located fluoroscopically because it is aligned with the atrioventricular sulcus in this view. In adults, the sulcus usually contains an accumulation of fat and casts a lucent, vertical, linear shadow that moves from side to side with the heartbeat. If no calcific densities are identified in relation to the sulcus, one can assume that the mitral valve is free of significant calcification. The aortic valve is situated above and slightly to the right of the mitral valve and moves in a vertical direction.

LEFT ANTERIOR OBLIQUE VIEW (Fig. 6–12). This is the only projection of the cardiac series in which the body of the left atrium can be visualized directly. The posterior atrial wall forms the upper third of the left cardiac contour, just beneath the left main bronchus. The lower two-thirds of this contour are formed by the left ventricle. The right border of the cardiac shadow represents mostly right atrium except for a short segment just above the diaphragm, where the right ventricle comes into profile. The arch of the aorta parallels the plane of the film in this view and is projected with a minimum of foreshortening. The

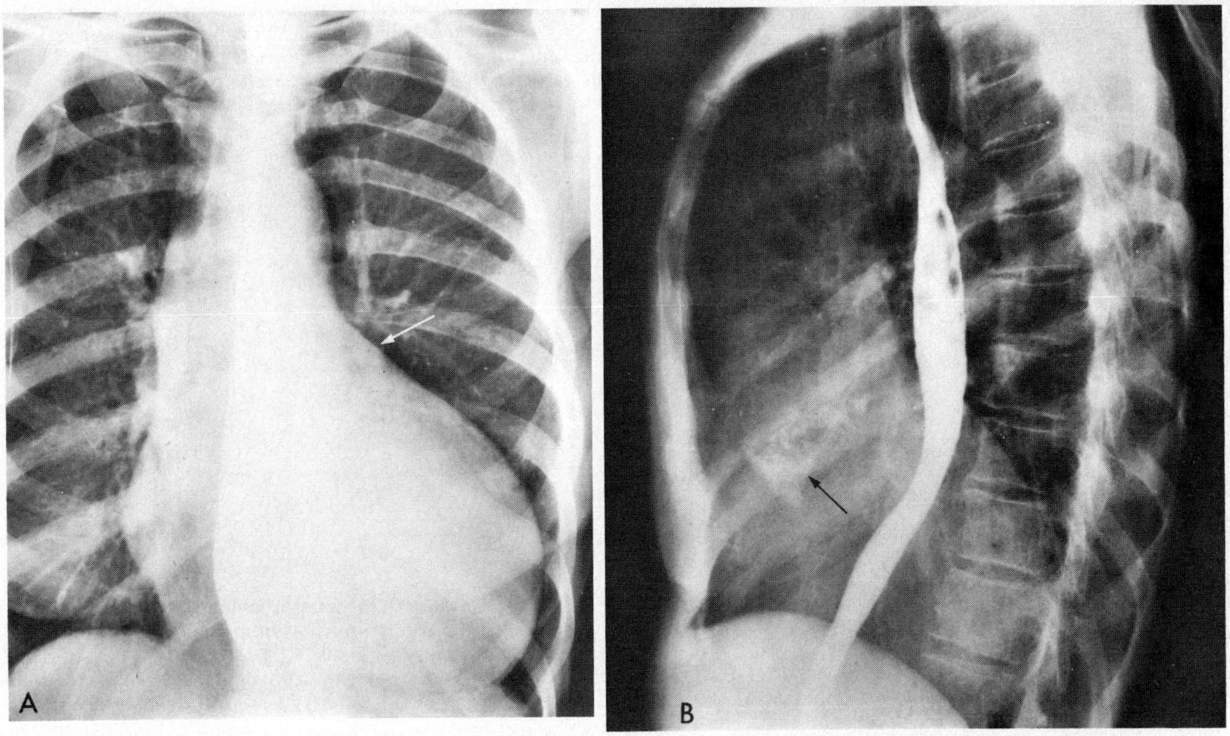

FIGURE 6–7 Dilatation of the left ventricle in aortic valve disease. *A*, Frontal view. The cardiac silhouette is elongated downward and to the left, indicating left ventricular enlargement. There is slight prominence of the left atrial appendage (arrow). The esophagus is displaced medially. *B*, Lateral view. The left ventricle is markedly enlarged and extends posterior to the esophagus. The aortic valve is densely calcified (arrow). The indentation on the anterior wall of the midesophagus is caused by the moderately dilated left atrium. There was no evidence of mitral valve disease.

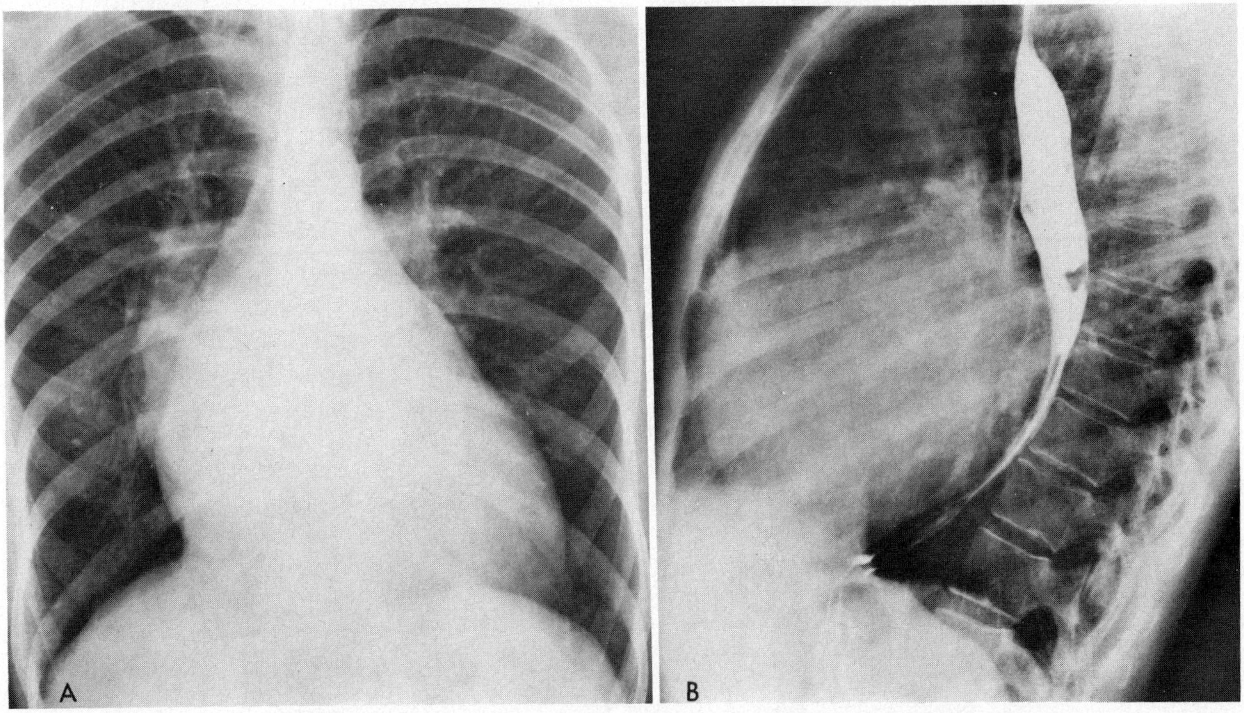

FIGURE 6–8 Enlargement of the left atrium and left ventricle. *A*, Frontal view. The abnormal density of the central portion of the cardiac silhouette and the double contour on the right side indicate enlargement of the left atrium. The bulge of the atrial appendage on the left cardiac border is less prominent than would be expected, considering the size of the atrium, because the widening of the cardiac shadow. The displacement of the apex of the heart downward and to the left is caused by enlargement of the left ventricle. The increased size of the pulmonary vessels in the upper lungs and the narrowed vessels at the bases as well as the Kerley B lines in the costophrenic sulci reflect the presence of pulmonary venous hypertension. *B*, Lateral view. The esophagus is displaced backward in a continuous curve from the carina to the diaphragm. The posterior border of the heart crosses the shadow of the inferior vena cava almost at the level of the diaphragm, confirming the presence of left ventricular enlargement.

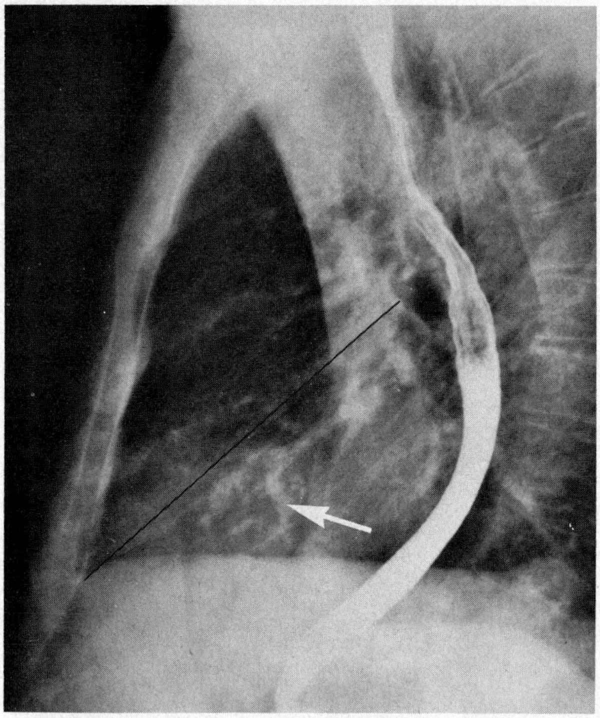

FIGURE 6–9 Mitral valve calcification, lateral view. The valvular calcification (arrow) lies below the line drawn from the left main bronchus to the anterior costophrenic sinus, localizing it to the mitral valve. The aortic valve, in this view, lies more anteriorly, above the line.

FIGURE 6–10 Right anterior oblique projection of the heart. (Reproduced with permission from The CIBA Collection of Medical Illustrations by Frank H. Netter, M.D. Vol. 5, The Heart, edited by F. Y. Yonkman.)

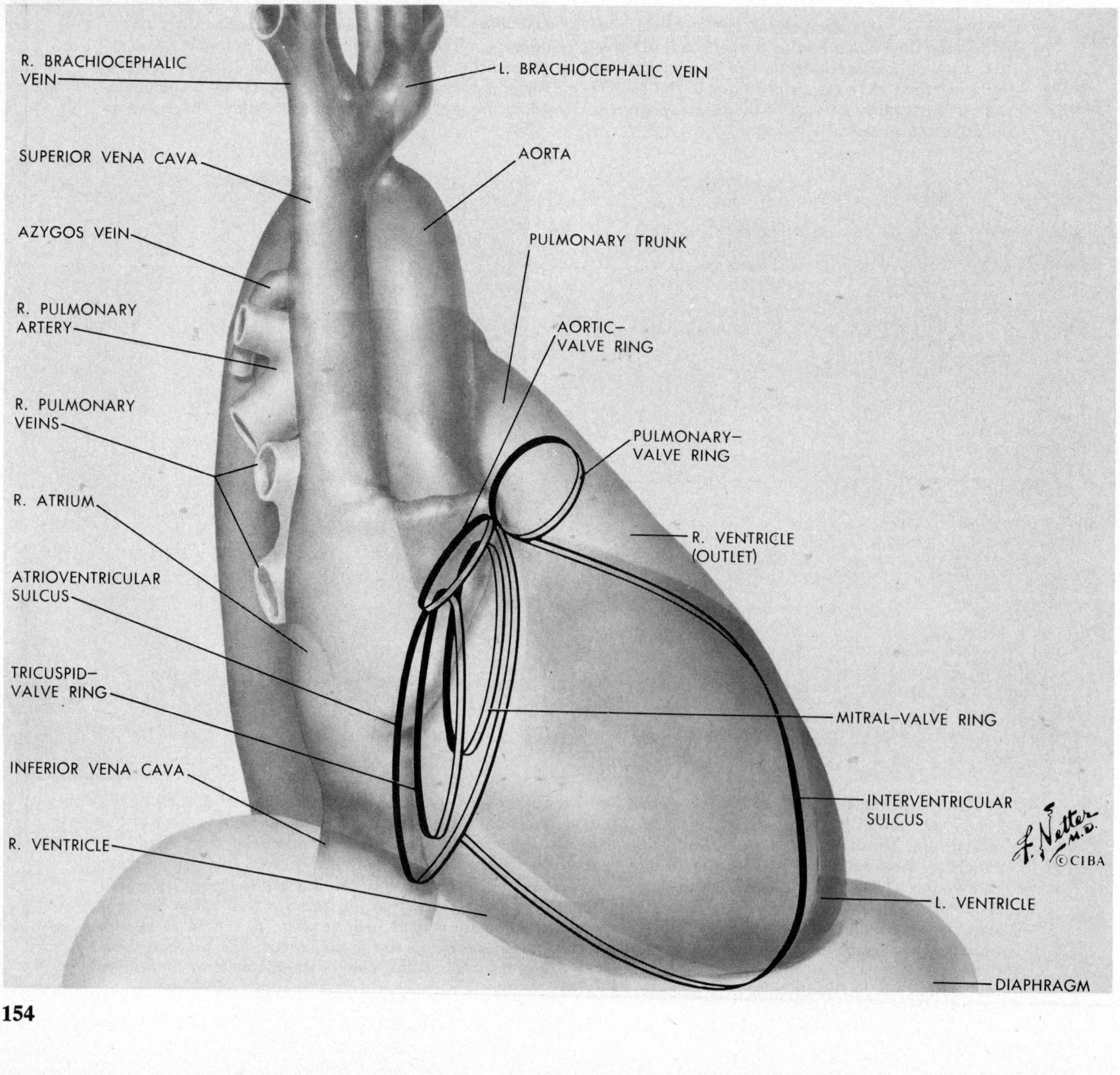

FIGURE 6–11 Mitral valve disease. Right anterior oblique view. The outflow tract of the right ventricle is dilated, indicating elevation of pulmonary artery pressure. The calcified mitral valve (arrow) is clearly visible within the midportion of the cardiac silhouette. The size of the left atrium cannot be evaluated because of esophageal spasm.

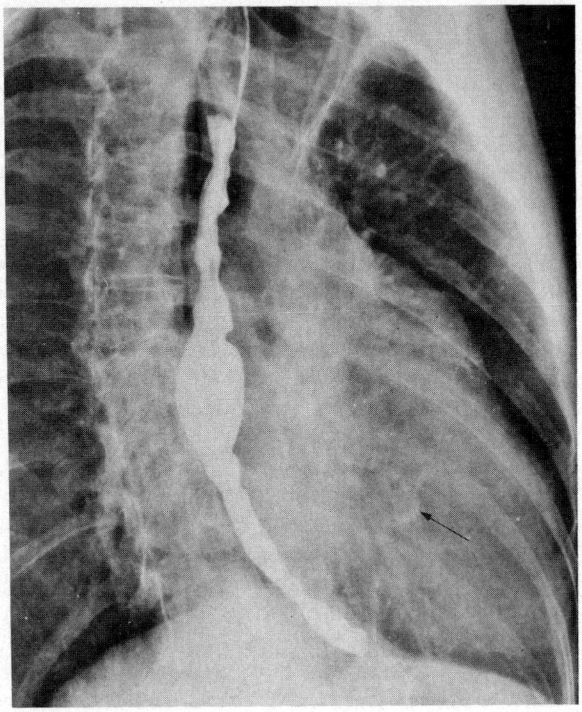

FIGURE 6–12 Left anterior oblique projection of the heart. (Reproduced with permission from The CIBA Collection of Medical Illustrations by Frank H. Netter, M.D. Vol. 5, The Heart, edited, by F. Y. Yonkman. Copyright 1969, CIBA Pharmaceutical Co., Division of CIBA-GEIGY Corp. All rights reserved.)

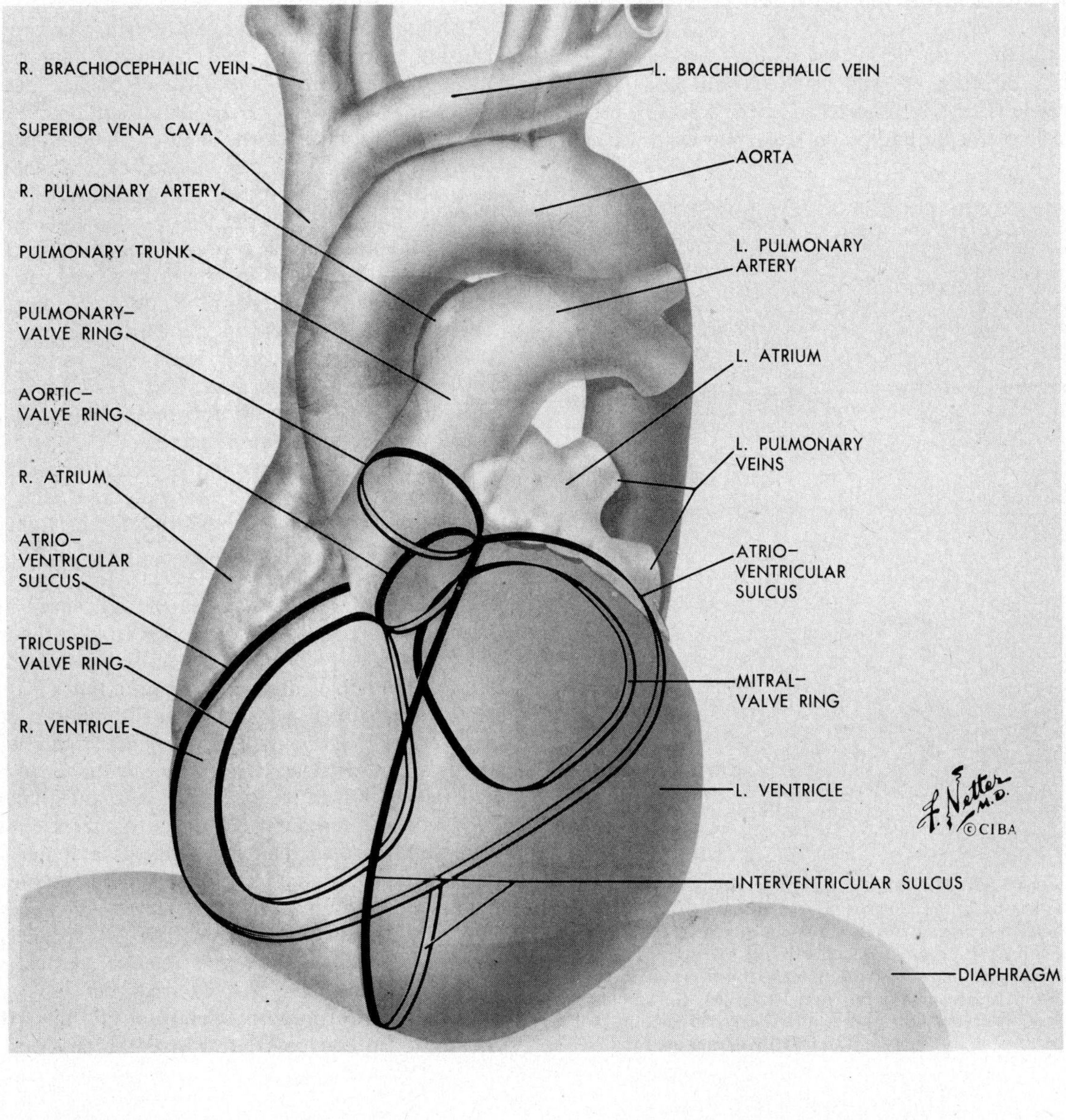

origins of the great vessels are maximally separated. The atrioventricular valves are projected *en face* so that calcification of the mitral valve is more difficult to detect than in the right oblique view. The aortic valve is projected almost tangentially, and calcification of its cusps is easily seen.

Enlargement of the *right atrium* causes widening of the cardiac silhouette to the right and an increase in the curvature of the right cardiac contour (Fig. 6–13). In some instances, it may not be possible to separate the atrial and ventricular components of this border on plain films. This can be resolved by fluoroscopy, because the borders of the chambers move in opposite directions during the cardiac cycle.

Normally, the segment of the left cardiac contour formed by the left atrium is straight or slightly concave. As the chamber increases in size, this border becomes convex (Fig. 6–13) and encroaches on the "aortic window," the clear space beneath the aortic arch. Upward displacement of the left main bronchus is often better seen in this view than in the frontal projection. Because the barium-filled esophagus is often projected over the border of the heart, it may obscure the left atrial contour. The left anterior oblique view, therefore, should be obtained first when filming a cardiac series, before the patient is given barium to swallow.

When the left ventricle dilates, its long axis elongates in a posterior direction as well as downward and laterally. The ventricle is thus foreshortened in the frontal view, and its size can easily be underestimated. However, when the patient is in the left oblique position, the long axis of the ventricle is aligned parallel to the film. For this reason, this view is essential, in addition to the frontal view, for proper evaluation of left ventricular size (Fig. 6–14). Whether the ventricle is elongated (Fig. 6–15) is of considerably greater diagnostic significance than whether the cardiac silhouette is projected clear of the shadow of the spine or not. The latter sign depends to a large extent on the position of the patient.[4] The steeper the oblique angle, the more likely that the shadow of the ventricle—regardless of its size—will not overlap the spine. Even with a standard degree of obliquity, the ventricle that is elongated mainly to the left will tend to clear the spine, whereas the same size ventricle extending more posteriorly will not. In addition, this sign may be falsely positive if the right ventricle is significantly enlarged. An increase in the size of this chamber displaces the left ventricle to the left and posteriorly, and the heart may not clear the shadow of the spine in the left oblique view, even though the left ventricle is normal in size.

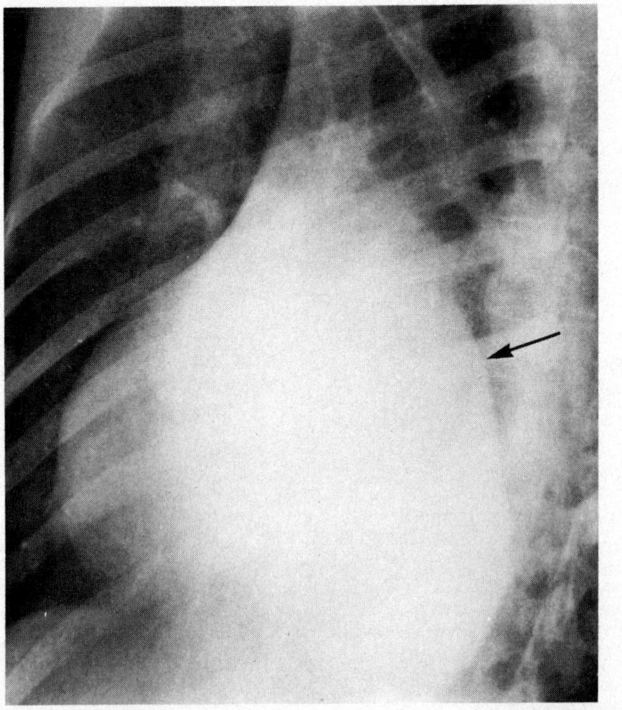

FIGURE 6–13 Left anterior oblique projection showing enlargement of both atria in mitral valve disease. The right side of the cardiac silhouette is enlarged and its curvature increased because of dilatation of the right atrium. The convexity of the upper left cardiac border (arrow) just beneath the left main bronchus indicates that the left atrium is also enlarged. (From Baron, M. G.: Left anterior oblique view for evaluation of left atrial size. Circulation *44*:926, 1971, by permission of the American Heart Association, Inc.)

Heart Size

Although heart disease can certainly be present without causing cardiomegaly, the converse is not true. Enlargement of the heart is indicative of cardiac disease and, at times, may be its first overt manifestation. When a patient is known to have heart disease, changes in cardiac size over a period of time can be used to evaluate the progress of the disease or the results of treatment.

Even though an experienced observer can estimate cardiac size with an acceptable degree of accuracy from the appearance of the cardiac silhouette, a more objective method of measurement is often desirable. A simple measurement of one or more diameters of the cardiac silhouette has little meaning, because normal heart size varies considerably with sex and body habitus. The *cardiothoracic ratio* was designed to compensate for these factors and uses the width of the chest as an indicator of body build. A vertical reference line is drawn on the frontal chest film through the spinous processes of the vertebrae. The sum of the maximum distances from this line to the right and to the left borders of the cardiac silhouette constitutes the transverse cardiac diameter (Fig. 6–16). This value is then divided by the greatest width of the thorax as measured from the inner margins of the ribs to give the cardiothoracic ratio. A value of 0.5 is generally considered to indicate the upper limit of normal heart size, but a figure of 0.6 is preferable, since it will decrease the number of false-positive results.[5,6] Unfortunately, the maximum width of the chest is not a particularly accurate index of body build, and its use introduces a second variable that is independent of the presence or absence of cardiac disease. The transverse cardiac diameter alone is a better measure of heart size if it is compared with standard tables of cardiac diameters in adults of different height and weight.[7]

A more accurate determination of cardiac size can be achieved by calculating the relative cardiac volume.[8,9] Three measurements are required: the long axis of the heart (L) is measured on the frontal film from the break in the right cardiac contour, where the superior vena cava

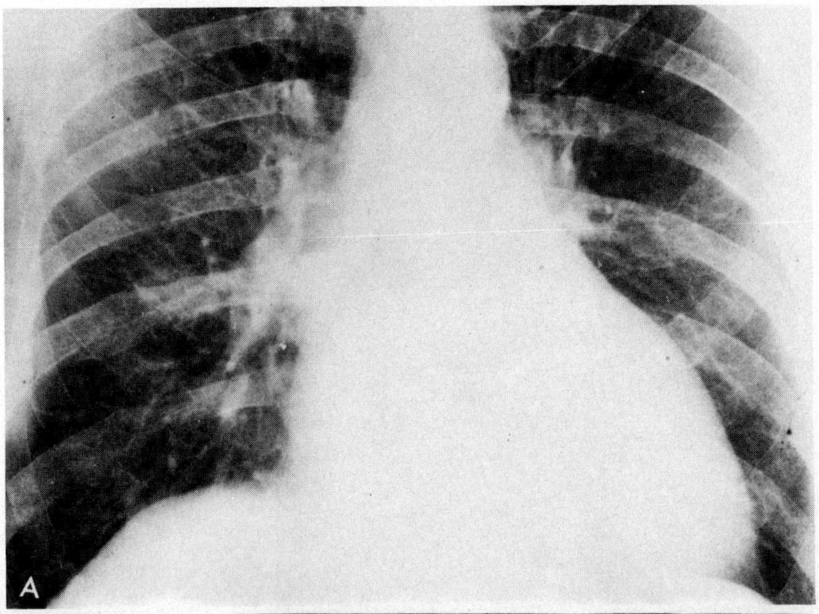

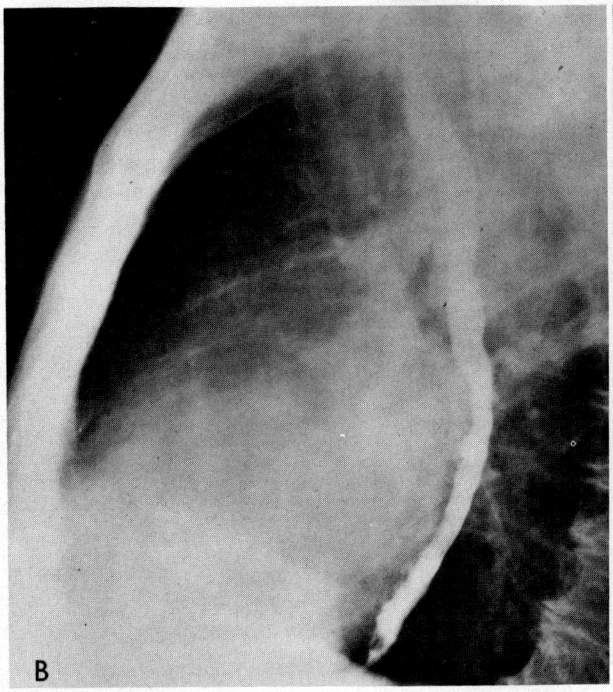

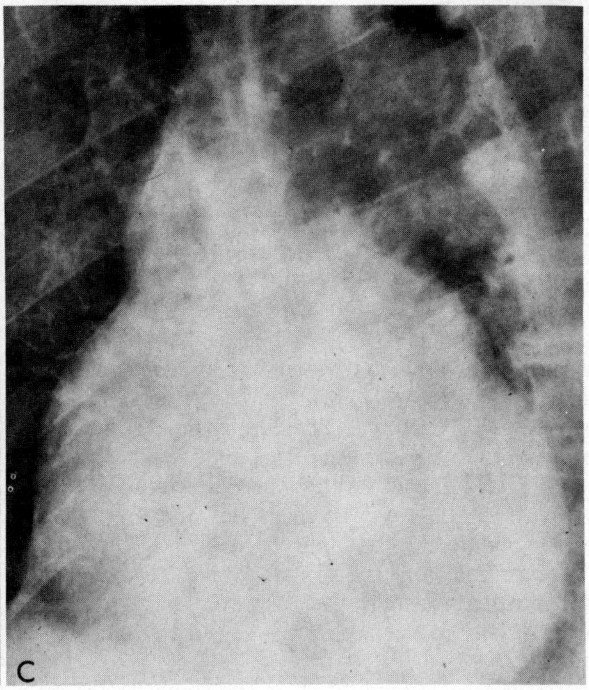

FIGURE 6–14 Left atrial and left ventricular enlargement. *A*, Frontal view. The heart is elongated and has a configuration most suggestive of aortic regurgitation. There is no evidence of left atrial enlargement. *B*, Lateral view. Although the esophagus appears to be displaced backward to some extent, this is difficult to evaluate because it is not well distended. *C*, Left anterior oblique view. The double bulge of the left cardiac contour reflects the considerable increase in size of the left atrium as well as of the left ventricle. Elevation of the left main bronchus is well visualized in this projection. The patient has both aortic and mitral valve disease.

joins the right atrium, to the cardiac apex; the short axis (S) is measured from the right cardiophrenic angle to the junction of the pulmonary artery and left atrial segments on the left heart border; the third dimension (D) represents the greatest anteroposterior diameter of the heart and is measured on the lateral chest film (Fig. 6–17). The final calculation is made from the formula

$$\frac{L \times S \times D \times K}{\text{Body surface area}} = \text{Relative cardiac volume}$$

K is a constant that is related to the distance between the x-ray tube and the film. For the usual 6-foot chest film, K equals 0.42. Figures for body surface area are obtained from the DuBois standards.[10]

A volume of less than 450 cc/m^2 for women and 500 cc/m^2 for men is considered to be normal. Values over 490 cc/m^2 for women and 540 cc/m^2 for men are definitely abnormal. Aside from the inherent mathematical accuracy of this method, it is of particular value because it is not significantly affected by the phase of the cardiac cycle. Even in patients with large stroke volumes and a considerable change in the apparent size of the heart between systole and diastole, the relative cardiac volume varies little because it is determined from the volumes of all four cardiac chambers. When the ventricles contract during systole, the atria become larger as they fill with blood, whereas in diastole the atria decrease in size and the ventricles distend. The measurement has definite prognostic significance in

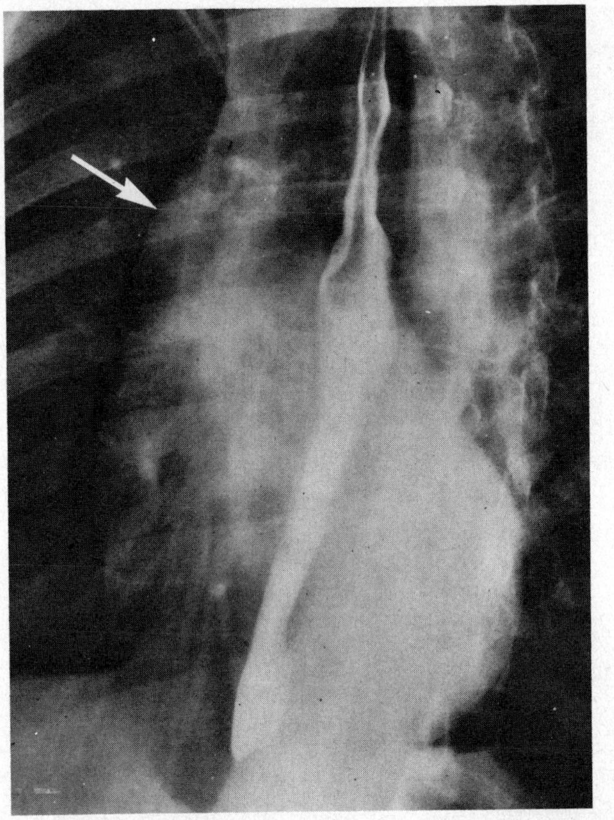

FIGURE 6–15 Left ventricular enlargement, left anterior oblique view. The cardiac silhouette is enlarged downward, to the left, and posteriorly, indicating dilatation of the left ventricle. The ascending aorta is widened (arrow).

ischemic heart disease[11] but not in the presence of aortic regurgitation or mitral valve disease. The measurement will obviously be grossly incorrect if enlargement of the cardiac silhouette is due to a pericardial effusion.

In most instances, calculation of cardiac volume, or even measurement of the transverse cardiac diameter, is too time-consuming to be a routine procedure. A visual estimate of heart size from the frontal film is generally adequate for most clinical purposes. However, several possible pitfalls must be recognized if gross errors are to be avoided.

First, the degree of inspiration is the single factor with the greatest effect on the apparent size of the heart. During a maximal inspiratory effort, a patient should be able to lower his or her diaphragm at least to the level of the tenth rib posteriorly. If the diaphragm is at a higher level, the long axis of the heart lies more horizontally, and its transverse diameter is increased (Fig. 6–18). In addition, because lung volume is decreased, the heart, which does not change in size, occupies a relatively greater portion of the available thoracic space.

Second, because chest films are exposed at random, some are made during diastole and others during systole. In the great majority of patients, the difference in the transverse cardiac diameter between the two phases of the cardiac cycle is relatively small.[12] However, in patients with a slow heart rate and a large stroke volume, such as a trained athlete or a patient with complete atrioventricular block, the change in transverse diameter between systole and diastole may be as much as 2 cm. When two films of such a patient are compared, the differences in heart size can be misinterpreted to indicate an important change in the cardiac status. This error can be avoided by calculation of the relative cardiac volume.

Third, visualization of more of the cardiac apex than is usually seen can cause the heart to appear abnormally large. The heart lies anteriorly and is situated below the highest point of the curve of the diaphragm. In the frontal projection, the cardiac silhouette appears to end at the diaphragm because its lowermost portion is obscured by the shadows of the abdominal viscera. However, when there is a moderate quantity of air in the stomach, the "infradiaphragmatic portion" of the heart may be seen through the gastric air bubble. This causes the cardiac silhouette to appear larger than it really is. Mistakes can be avoided if the area beneath the left diaphragm is simply covered before the size of the heart is assessed (Fig. 6–19).

Fourth, when the anteroposterior diameter of the chest is abnormally narrow because of loss of the thoracic kyphotic curvature, or pectus excavatum, the heart may be compressed between the sternum and the spine and splayed to one or both sides. The transverse cardiac diameter is then abnormally large. The cause of the apparent cardiomegaly is obvious if a lateral film is available. However, the chest deformity can usually be recognized from the appearance of the ribs on the frontal film. The course of the posterior ribs tends to be horizontal or angled upward, while the downward slope of the anterior ends of

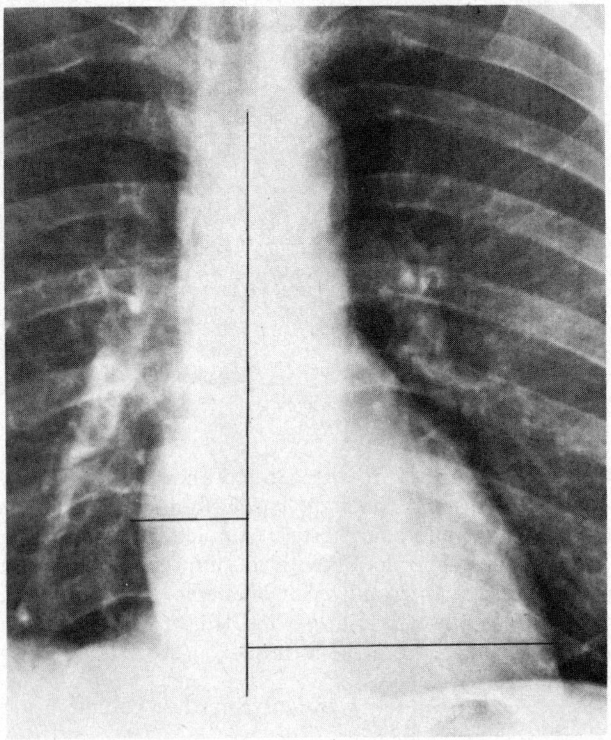

FIGURE 6–16 Measurement of the transverse cardiac diameter. A vertical reference line is first drawn through the spinous processes of the vertebrae. The greatest distances from this line to the right and to the left margins of the cardiac silhouette are then measured. Their sum constitutes the transverse cardiac diameter.

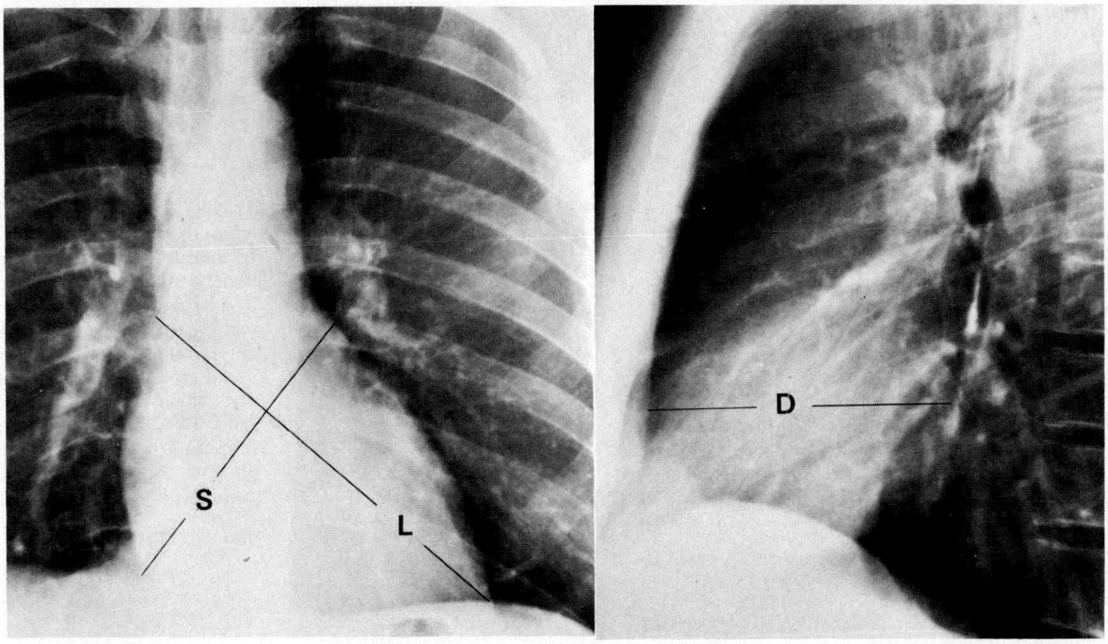

FIGURE 6–17 Measurement of relative cardiac volume. *A*, Frontal projection. The long axis of the heart (L) is measured from the break in the right cardiac contour, where the superior vena cava joins the right atrium, to the apex of the heart. The short diameter (S) extends from the right cardiophrenic angle to the junction of the left atrial and pulmonary artery segments. This line is roughly perpendicular to the long axis. *B*, Lateral view. The widest anteroposterior dimension of the cardiac silhouette constitutes the depth of the heart (D). If the posterior border of the heart cannot be clearly identified, the anterior margin of the barium-filled esophagus can be used as the boundary for this measurement.

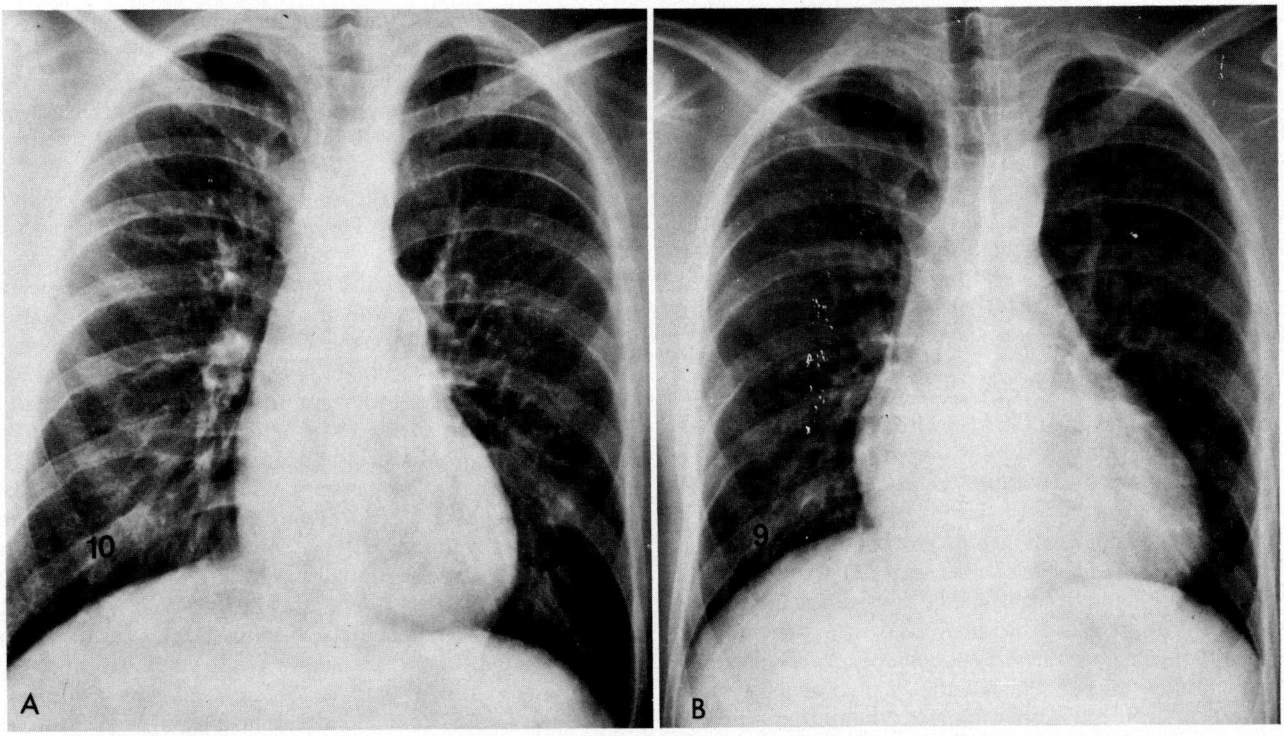

FIGURE 6–18 The effect of respiration on heart size in a patient with coarctation of the aorta. *A*, Deep inspiration. The aortic knob is obscured, and ribs 5 to 9 on the right side and 8 on the left show notching of the undersurface—an appearance pathognomonic of coarctation. The patient has taken a deep inspiration, lowering the diaphragm to the 10th posterior interspace. Although the heart is normal in size, elongation of its long axis indicates some enlargement of the left ventricle. *B*, With a lesser inspiratory effort, the diaphragm is at the level of the 9th posterior interspace. The long axis of the heart is displaced toward the horizontal, increasing the transverse cardiac diameter. The heart appears larger than in *A*.

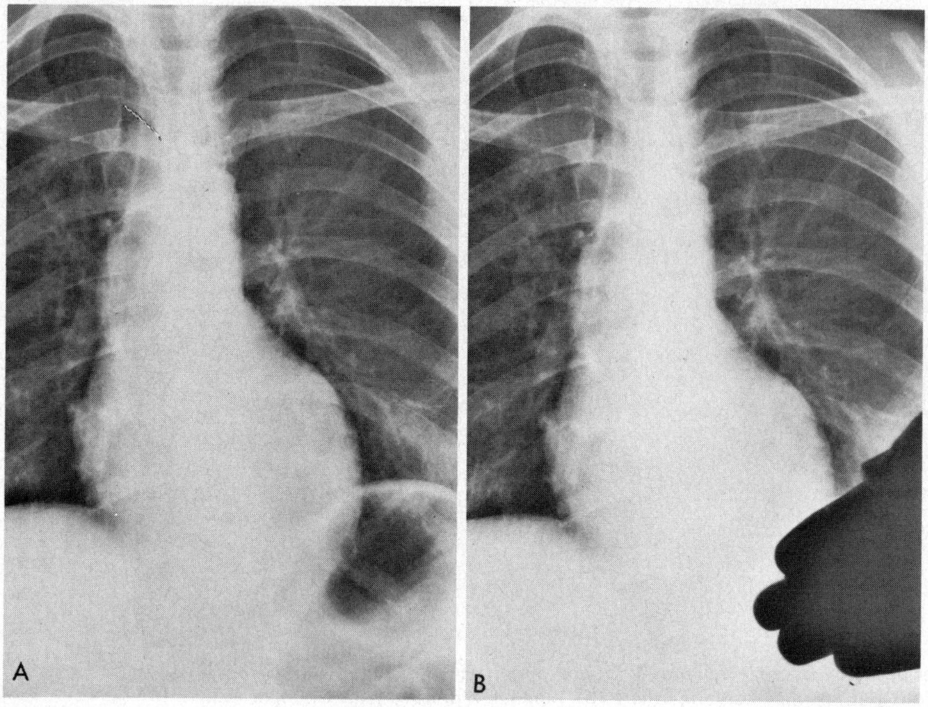

FIGURE 6–19 The "infradiaphragmatic" portion of the cardiac silhouette. *A,* A portion of the apical and diaphragmatic aspects of the heart, usually hidden by the diaphragm and the abdominal organs, is seen through the gastric air bubble. Visualization of this additional area of the heart causes the cardiac shadow to appear enlarged. *B,* Same film. Evaluation of heart size is simplified if the area beneath the diaphragm is covered. The heart is normal.

the ribs is much steeper than normal. In addition, the cardiac silhouette is not as dense as expected for a heart with such a large transverse diameter, and the ribs and vascular markings in the left lower lobe are easily visible through it.

Finally, the size of the cardiac shadow is also determined by the degree to which the heart is magnified on the film. The farther the heart is from the film, or the nearer the x-ray tube to the film, the larger the cardiac silhouette. Most bedside examinations are made with a tube-to-film distance of three feet, with the cassette behind the patient. The shadow of the heart is therefore more magnified and appears larger than on a standard chest film made at a distance of six feet, with the patient facing the cassette. Thus it is extremely difficult to compare the size of the heart on a portable film with that on a standard chest film with any degree of accuracy.

ACQUIRED HEART DISEASE

Coronary Artery Disease (See also Chapter 39)

There is no direct relationship between the appearance of the heart and the presence or severity of coronary artery disease. So long as myocardial function is not significantly impaired, the heart size is normal, even in a patient who may be totally incapacitated by angina. Similarly, if sufficient functioning muscle remains after a myocardial infarction, the heart can retain its normal configuration. On the other hand, the finding of an enlarged heart may at times be the first indication of coronary artery disease.[13,14]

Ischemic heart disease, from a practical standpoint, is a disease of the left ventricle. Enlargement of the heart implies significant impairment of left ventricular function, and the degree of dilatation is roughly related to the degree of limitation of ventricular contractility. Since the size of the heart is an indicator of cardiac decompensation, the chest film is a simple means of following the course of ischemic heart disease.

Deterioration of left ventricular function results in an increase in left ventricular end-diastolic pressure. This, in turn, interferes with left atrial emptying, and the atrium tends to dilate. The appearance of the heart at this stage of left ventricular failure may be similar to that of mitral valve disease (Fig. 6–20). With further progression, the right heart chambers also enlarge, and the cardiac silhouette becomes rounded. The appearance may also resemble that caused by a pericardial effusion; the cardiac pulsations are markedly diminished in both conditions. The two can usually be differentiated by the appearance of the hilar vessels. Cardiac enlargement of this extent is associated with some degree of congestive failure, and the hilar vessels become engorged and unduly prominent. On the other hand, the dilated cardiac silhouette caused by a pericardial effusion tends to obscure the hilar vessels (see Fig. 6–43).[15]

A myocardial infarct cannot be identified on plain films unless it is calcified or forms an aneurysm. In some cases, the abnormal motion of the infarcted segment of the ventricular wall can be noted on fluoroscopic examination, but because the septal and diaphragmatic aspects of the ventricle are not adequately visualized, a large number of infarcts cannot be detected. When calcium is deposited within an infarct, it produces a fine shell that is seen as a dense, curvilinear line when viewed tangentially. However, when projected *en face* or obliquely, the calcific layer is often too thin to cast a recognizable shadow. Both the thinning of the ventricular wall and the calcification, if present, are more easily detected by computed tomography (p. 189).

A calcified infarct is almost always transmural in extent.

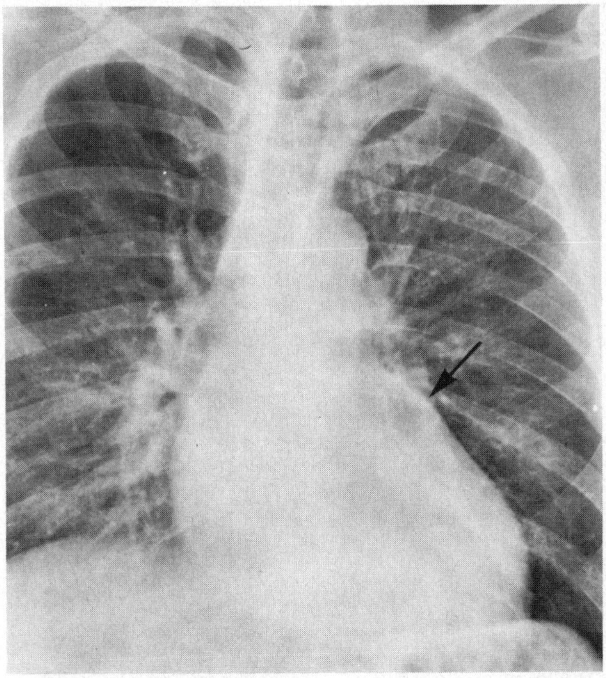

FIGURE 6–20 Mitral configuration in ischemic heart disease. The left ventricle is dilated because of myocardial ischemia. Ventricular end-diastolic pressure is elevated and is the cause of the left atrial dilatation (arrow).

Because the fibrotic scar is thin, the calcific rim lies close to, and parallels, the outer border of the heart (Fig. 6–21). The infarcts visualized in the frontal projection involve the anterolateral wall of the left ventricle or its apex, although on a well-penetrated film it may be possible to detect a calcified infarct of the interventricular septum. Because of its proximity to the outer border of the heart, the calcific rim of an infarct can be confused with calcification of the pericardium. However, calcific deposits on the pericardium are usually coarser and more irregular. In addition, they tend to accumulate over the atrioventricular sulci and the interventricular groove to a greater extent than over the free wall of the left ventricle (Fig. 6–22).

An *aneurysm* that is not calcified can be detected when it projects beyond the normal cardiac contour. Even when the left ventricle is markedly enlarged, the border of the chamber is made up of a single smooth curve. A localized bulge in this curve is presumptive evidence of a ventricular aneurysm (see Figure 6–3*B*). However, some aneurysms project from the cardiac contour only during systole and blend in with the curve of the distended ventricle during diastole. This type of aneurysm may be recognizable by means of fluoroscopy, but as a rule, fluoroscopy is not a very effective method for detection of a ventricular aneurysm. Considerably more than half of all aneurysms will be hidden within the cardiac silhouette and cannot be detected by fluoroscopy.[16] In the occasional case when an aneurysm is so large that it forms most of the left cardiac contour, the appearance of the heart can be almost identical to that of a failing ventricle due to diffuse as opposed to localized myocardial fibrosis (Fig. 6–23). Fluoroscopic examination is useful in this instance to determine the need for angiocardiography. In most cases, an aneurysm of this size will pulsate paradoxically, whereas the pulsations of a dilated, flabby ventricle will be in proper phase, although grossly diminished in amplitude.

Calcific deposits within the coronary arteries are usually thin and their shadows are not very dense. Because of the blurring caused by motion of the heart, they are almost never seen on plain films, and a careful fluoroscopic examination is required for their detection. Most commonly, calcification occurs first in the proximal portions of the coronary arteries near the base of the heart. When the calcification is more extensive, it may be seen more distally in the vessels in the atrioventricular sulci or the interventricular groove. Calcific plaques are too fine to be visible when viewed *en face* and are seen only where they are projected tangentially. Thus, coronary calcification appears as a single, sharp, linear shadow or, if the entire circumference of the vessel is involved, as two parallel linear densities. When the calcified vessel is projected on end, it casts a fine, ring-shaped shadow.

Coronary artery calcification is very common in patients with ischemic heart disease.[17,18] However, it does not always indicate the presence of ischemic heart disease. The significance of calcification of the coronary arteries varies with the age of the patient, the incidence of coronary artery calcification not associated with stenosis increasing with age. It has little importance as an indicator of significant coronary artery narrowing in patients older than 65 or 70.[18,19] On the other hand, there is an extremely high

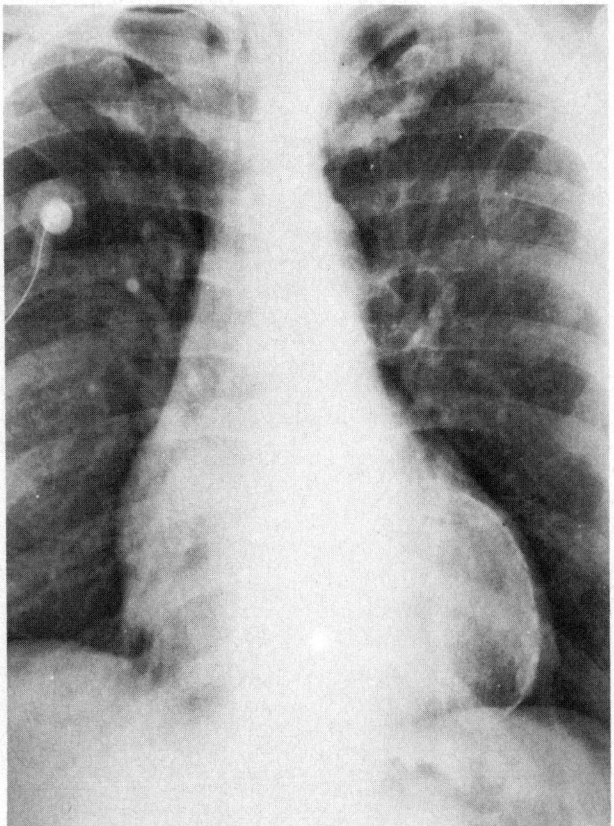

FIGURE 6–21 Calcified myocardial infarct. The rim of calcium paralleling the lateral border of the heart outlines an old infarct of the anterolateral left ventricular wall. Although the calcification extends around to the anterior and posterior surfaces of the ventricle, it is well visualized only where it is projected tangentially.

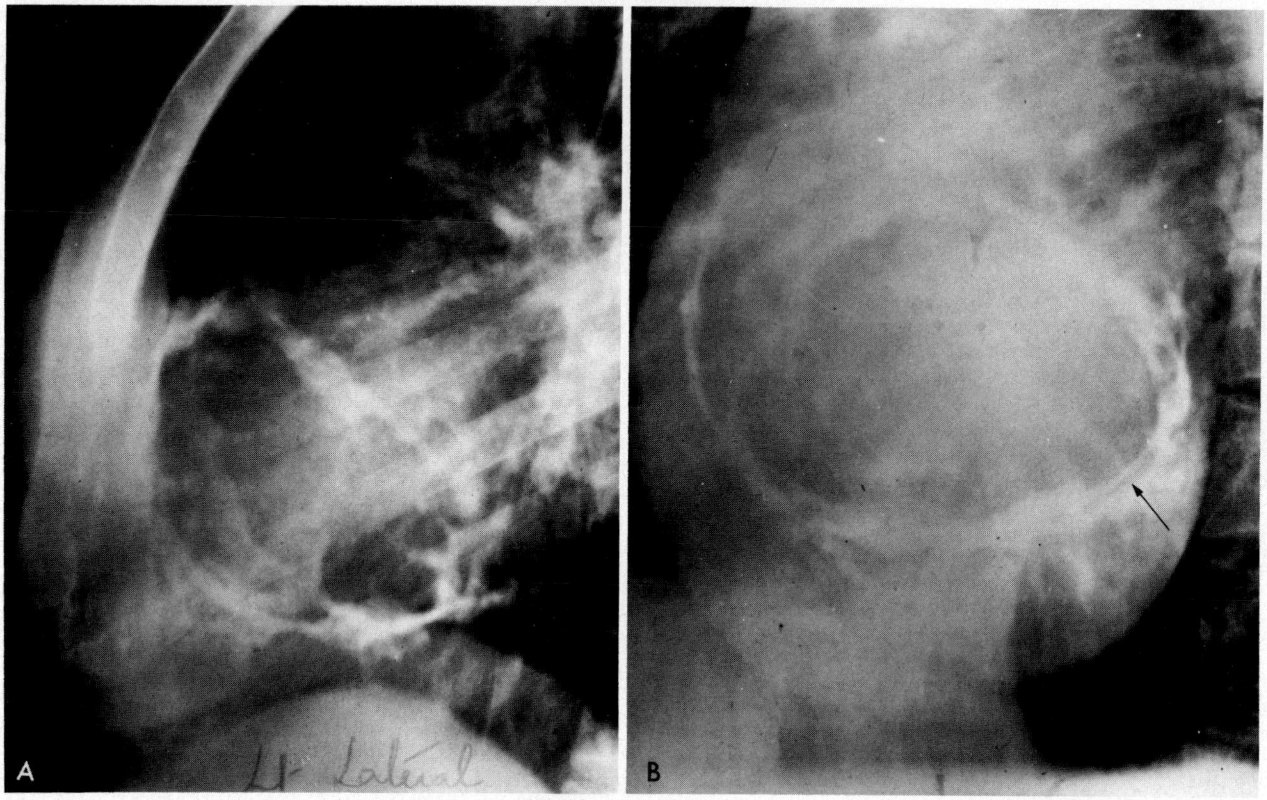

FIGURE 6–22 Pericardial calcification. *A,* Lateral chest film of a young woman showing dense, calcific patches distributed along the course of the atrioventricular sulcus and over the anterior portion of the right ventricle. *B,* Left anterior oblique view. The lucent line within the calcified sulcus (arrow) most likely represents the circumflex branch of the left coronary artery, which is not calcified. (Courtesy of Dr. S. Bharati.)

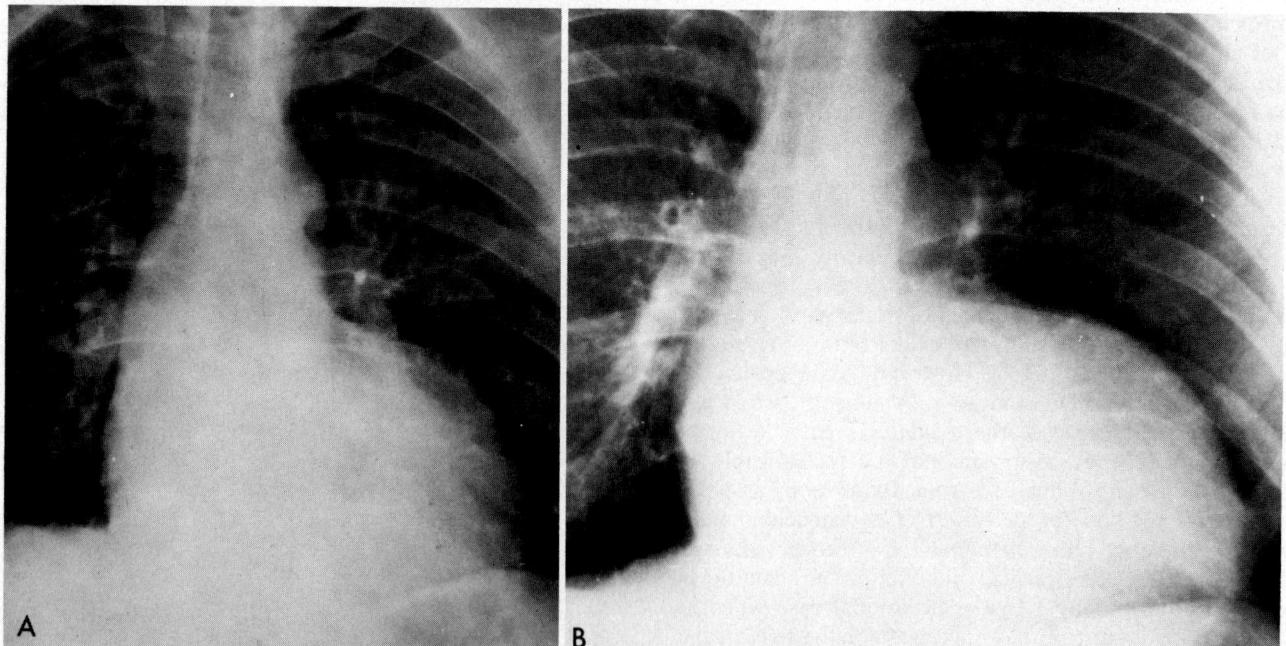

FIGURE 6–23 Left ventricular aneurysm. *A,* The aneurysm is so large that it forms almost the entire lateral profile of the left ventricle. (From Donoso, E., and Gorlin, R. [eds.]: Current Cardiovascular Topics. Vol. 3, Angina Pectoris. New York, Stratton Intercontinental Medical Book Co., 1977.) *B,* An almost identical appearance can be caused by the dilated, failing ventricle that results from diffuse ischemic disease. The two can be distinguished by fluoroscopy, because an aneurysm of this size will show paradoxical pulsations.

correlation between coronary artery calcification and coronary artery disease in patients under the age of 50. Because the search for coronary artery calcification is time-consuming and involves moderate radiation exposure, it is not a suitable screening procedure. There is little point in searching for such calcification in patients who have other evidence of coronary atherosclerosis or who are in the older age group. From a practical standpoint, such a study is best limited to younger patients who have chest pain of unknown etiology.[20]

Mitral Valve Disease (See also Chapter 32)

Disease of the mitral valve, whether it causes stenosis or regurgitation, results in dilatation of the left atrium. When *mitral stenosis* predominates, the heart is usually normal in size, and the left atrium may be the only chamber that is enlarged. There is a poor correlation between the size of the left atrium and the severity of the mitral stenosis, but moderate to marked left atrial enlargement occurs more commonly in patients with atrial fibrillation than in those with normal sinus rhythm.[21,22] In *mitral regurgitation,* diastolic overloading of the left ventricle causes the chamber to enlarge together with the left atrium. In practice, it is difficult to determine which of the two lesions is predominant.

Longstanding, moderate, or severe mitral stenosis is commonly associated with pulmonary arterial hypertension and dilatation of the right ventricle. As a result, the transverse diameter of the heart is widened, and the cardiac apex is displaced to the left. Dilatation of the left ventricle also widens the cardiac silhouette to the left, so that in many cases it is difficult to be sure whether the cardiac enlargement is due to the right ventricle alone or to both ventricles. This is further complicated by the fact that rheumatic heart disease often involves both the aortic and mitral valves. The combination of aortic regurgitation and mitral stenosis can produce a cardiac shape indistinguishable from that associated with mitral regurgitation. Conversely, a marked degree of mitral regurgitation may be present in the absence of significant enlargement of the left ventricle. This is most commonly seen following rupture of a papillary muscle or a chorda tendineae, when regurgitation, although severe, is of recent onset.[23]

Calcification of the mitral valve (Fig. 6–9) is indicative of stenosis (although there may be some accompanying regurgitation). The calcium is usually deposited in clumps on the valve leaflets but may also involve the commissures.[24] Extensive calcification may be visible on chest films, but fluoroscopy is required to detect smaller deposits. Valvular calcification must be distinguished from *calcification of the mitral annulus.* The latter occurs in older patients, particularly women,[25] and as long as the calcification does not extend onto the valve leaflets, it does not signify the presence of mitral valve disease.[26] The calcified annulus appears as a broad, curved shadow that may form a complete ring or, if the entire annulus is not involved, a U-shaped or J-shaped density. The curve of a calcified annulus has a larger diameter than that of a calcified valve, and it tends to appear as one continuous deposit rather than as separate calcific clumps (Fig. 6–24).

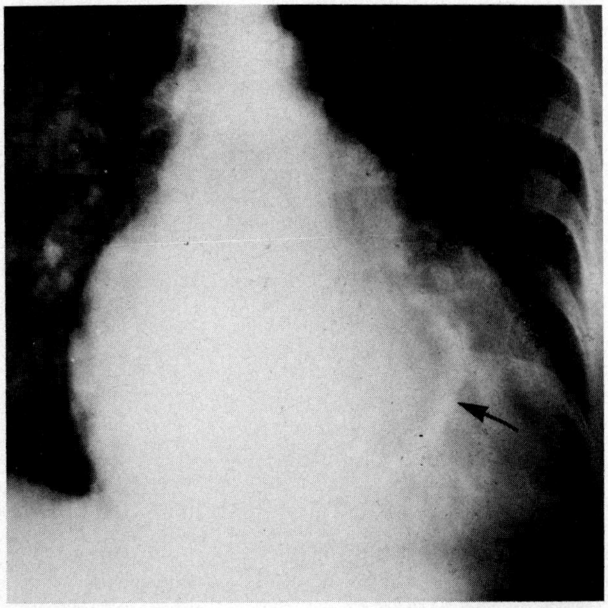

FIGURE 6–24 Calcification of the mitral annulus. The broad, curved density (arrow) in the mitral region represents calcification of the valve annulus. The arc of the calcific shadow is larger than that of the mitral orifice, distinguishing it from calcification of the leaflets, and it is too small for the calcium to be within the atrioventricular sulcus.

Except for its rare occurrence in metabolic calcinosis, calcification of the left atrium signifies mitral stenosis. The calcification may appear as a thin shell completely outlining the atrial wall or as a curvilinear shadow involving only one portion of the atrial circumference. The posterior atrial wall is the area most commonly involved and is best seen in the lateral view, below the carina and just in front of the esophagus (Fig. 6–25). If the atrial appendage is calcified, it presents as a short, arcuate density along the left border of the heart below the pulmonary segment in the frontal view and within the midportion of the cardiac silhouette in the lateral view. In the great majority of cases, a mural thrombus is present when the left atrium is calcified.[27] The calcium is usually deposited within the wall of the atrium but on occasion is present only within the thrombus.[28]

Narrowing of the mitral orifice results in elevation of left atrial and pulmonary venous pressures. Eventually, pulmonary hypertension may result. These changes are associated with a sequence of alterations in the appearance of the lungs and especially of the pulmonary vascular pattern. The resultant pictures are not specific for mitral stenosis but occur with any disease that causes an elevation of left atrial pressure (p. 172). *Pulmonary hemosiderosis* and pulmonary ossifications, however, are rarely encountered with any form of heart disease other than mitral stenosis.

Because of the chronic pulmonary congestion and elevated capillary pressure caused by mitral stenosis, small intraalveolar hemorrhages are common. Hemosiderin from the broken-down red cells is picked up by phagocytes, and clusters of these iron-laden cells form small nodules that can be seen on the chest film.[29,30] Their appearance is almost identical to that seen in idiopathic hemosiderosis or

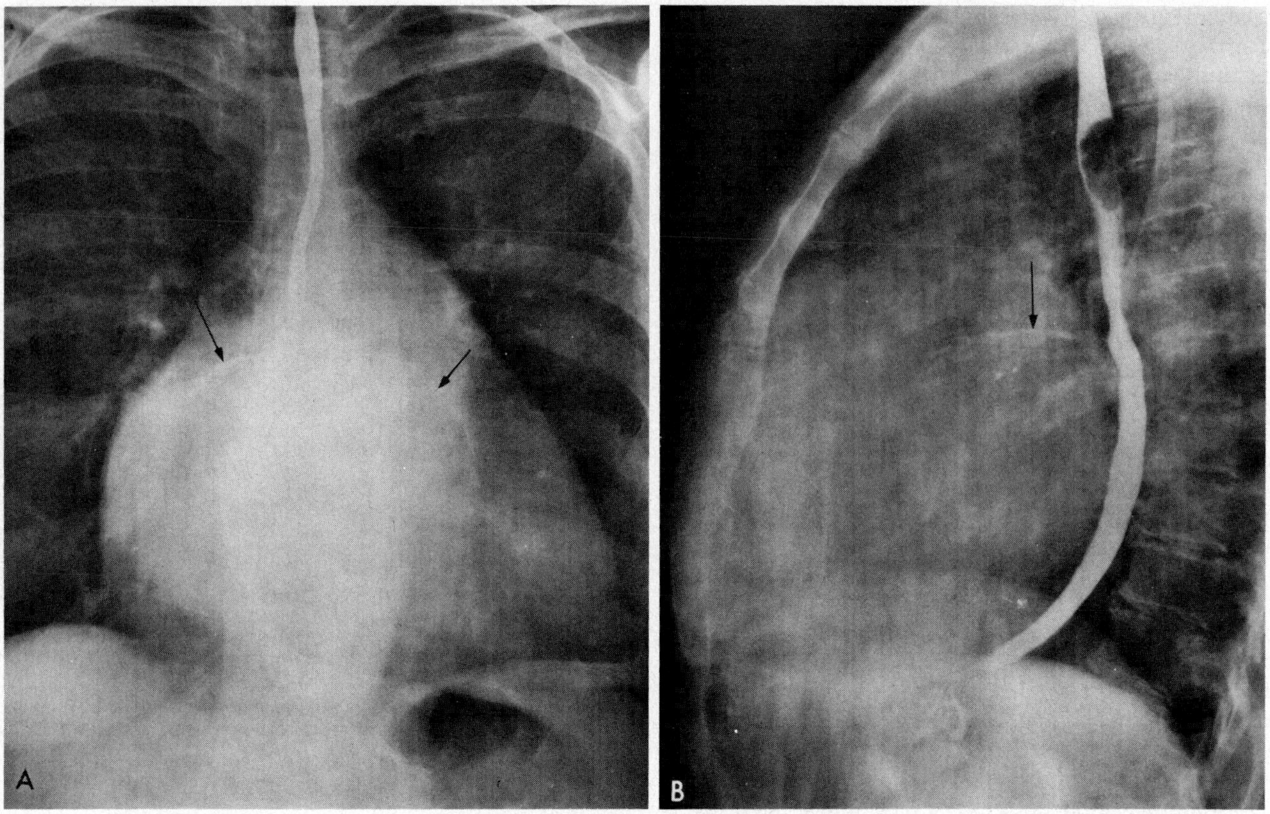

FIGURE 6–25 **Calcification of the left atrium in rheumatic mitral disease. *A,* Frontal view. The left atrium is enlarged, its upper margin outlined by a fine rim of calcium (arrows). The right atrium is dilated, and there is biventricular enlargement. *B,* Lateral view. The calcified superior wall of the atrium is visualized (arrow) just below the level of the carina. The esophagus is displaced backward in a continuous curve that extends to the diaphragm, indicating dilatation of both left atrium and left ventricle.**

in some of the miliary lung diseases (Fig. 6–26*A*). Although in mitral stenosis the nodules are distributed mainly in the mid and lower lung fields, rather than evenly throughout the lungs, the main differential point is the association with a cardiac shadow that has a mitral configuration.

Pulmonary ossifications are probably also the result of intraalveolar hemorrhage. The nodules of bone lie within the alveoli, mostly in the lower portions of the lungs. They are larger and more dense than hemosiderotic nodules and are fewer in number (Fig. 6–26*B*). The nodules vary considerably in size and often have an irregular shape. This, together with their distribution, serves to differentiate them from other calcific nodules in the lungs, such as those caused by histoplasmosis or chickenpox pneumonia.[31] Both pulmonary hemosiderosis and ossifications occur in patients with longstanding mitral disease, often with pulmonary hypertension. However, the two are unrelated, and it is not uncommon for one to be present without the other. The bony nodules are pathognomonic of mitral stenosis but can occur when the valve is partially occluded by a myxoma of the left atrium.[32]

Aortic Valve Disease (See also Chapter 32)

Aortic regurgitation causes elongation and dilatation of the left ventricle. The cardiac apex is displaced downward, to the left, and posteriorly (Fig. 6–4*A*). Often the entire ascending aorta is dilated, and fluoroscopic examination reveals an increase in the amplitude of its pulsations.

Aortic stenosis is more difficult to recognize on chest films. The heart is usually normal in size or only slightly enlarged, even with severe narrowing of the valve. However, the shape of the heart is often abnormal. Concentric hypertrophy of the left ventricle causes an increase in the curvature of the lower left cardiac contour and blunting of the cardiac apex (Fig. 6–27). Elongation of the long ventricular axis occurs occasionally in pure aortic stenosis but is never marked. Significant dilatation of the left ventricle in the absence of aortic regurgitation indicates failure of the myocardium and heralds the end stage of the disease.

Calcification of the aortic valve is common in congenital as well as acquired stenosis.[33,34] Poststenotic dilatation involving the ascending aorta at the junction of its proximal and middle thirds also occurs with both types of aortic stenosis. The poststenotic bulge may protrude from the right side of the mediastinum in the frontal view but is best seen on the left anterior oblique projection.[35] There is no correlation between the degree of poststenotic dilatation and the severity of the stenosis.[36] A similar localized dilatation of the ascending aorta can occur when the stenosis is due to a membranous web in the subvalvular region, but it is not associated with the hypertrophic form of subaortic stenosis.

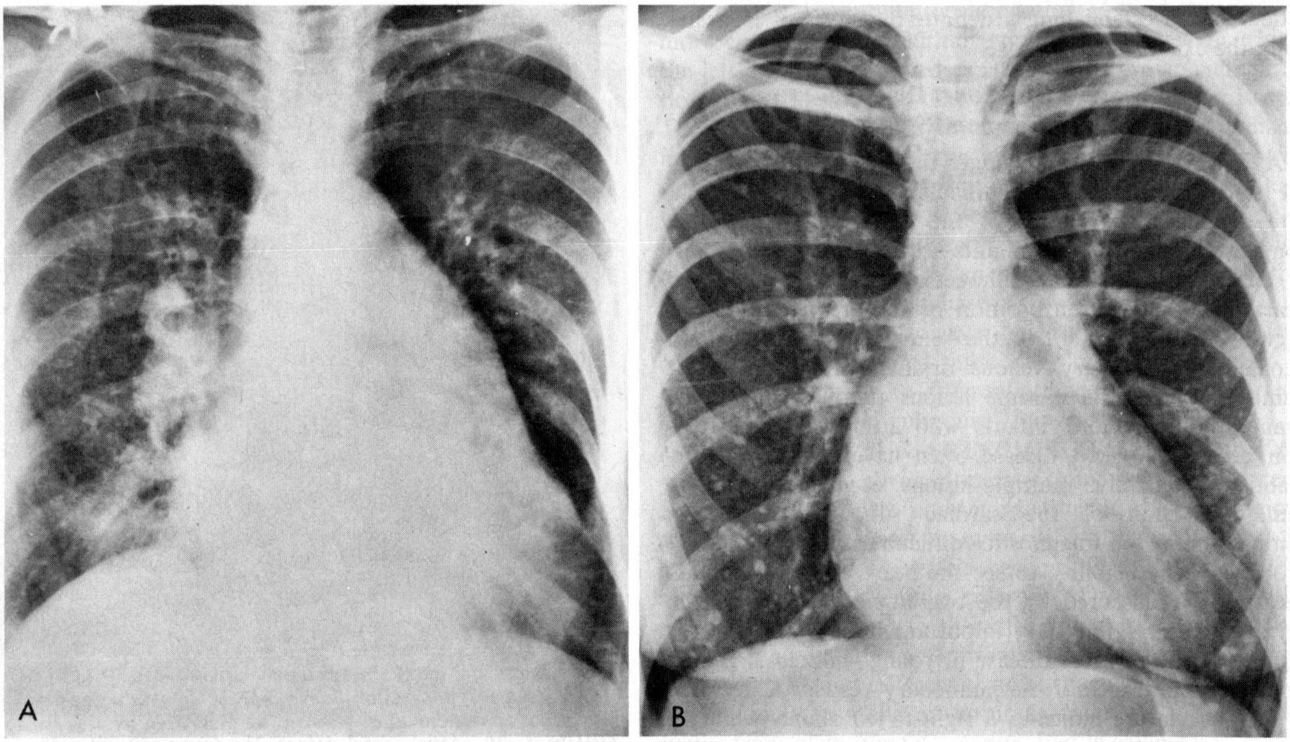

FIGURE 6–26 Lung changes in mitral stenosis. *A*, Pulmonary hemosiderosis. The lower lungs are studded with small nodules of moderate radiodensity. The left atrium and left ventricle are enlarged. Kerley B lines are present in the lateral basal portions of the lungs. *B*, Pulmonary ossifications. Scattered calcific nodules of differing size and shape are present in the lower lungs. They represent foci of organized bone within the alveoli. The left atrium is enlarged, and a double contour can be seen through the right side of the cardiac silhouette. The left atrial appendage is obscured by the dilated left ventricle.

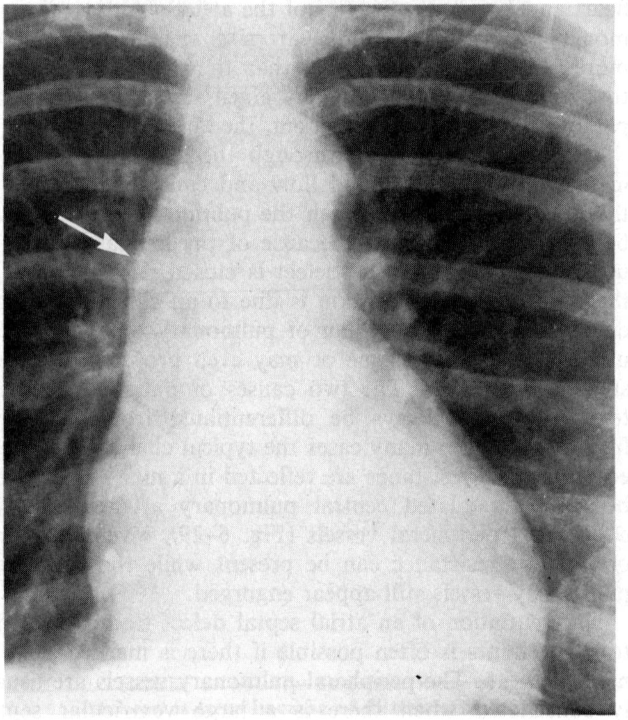

FIGURE 6–27 Aortic stenosis. The transverse diameter of the heart is slightly enlarged, and the curvature of the left cardiac contour is accentuated, suggesting left ventricular hypertrophy. The prominence of the midascending aorta (arrow) is due to poststenotic dilatation. A gradient of 90 mm Hg was measured across the aortic valve.

PRIMARY MYOCARDIAL DISEASE (See also Chapter 41)

The roentgen manifestations depend on whether the main effect of the disease is impairment of myocardial contractility, as in congestive (dilated) cardiomyopathy, or thickening of the ventricular wall, as in restrictive or hypertrophic cardiomyopathy. In either case, the heart may appear normal in the early stages or when the disease is of limited severity. More extensive involvement usually results in cardiac enlargement.

Diminution of ventricular function is reflected in an increase in the size of the ventricles. The cardiac silhouette is enlarged and tends to have a globular shape. The transverse cardiac diameter is widened, the curves of the heart border are accentuated, and cardiac pulsations are diminished. The hilar vessels are often prominent because of elevated left ventricular end-diastolic pressure, and the overall appearance of the heart may be similar to that seen with extensive ischemic disease of the myocardium.

In general, the degree of cardiac dilatation is proportional to the impairment of myocardial function. This relationship does not hold with myocardial hypertrophy. Severe and incapacitating degrees of hypertrophy may be present with only minimal or moderate cardiac enlargement. Most commonly, only the left ventricle is hypertrophied, but both ventricles may be involved. As the wall of the left ventricle thickens, the transverse cardiac diameter increases and the curvature of the left heart border becomes accentuated. This configuration is suggestive of myocardial hypertrophy, but as a rule the chest film is of

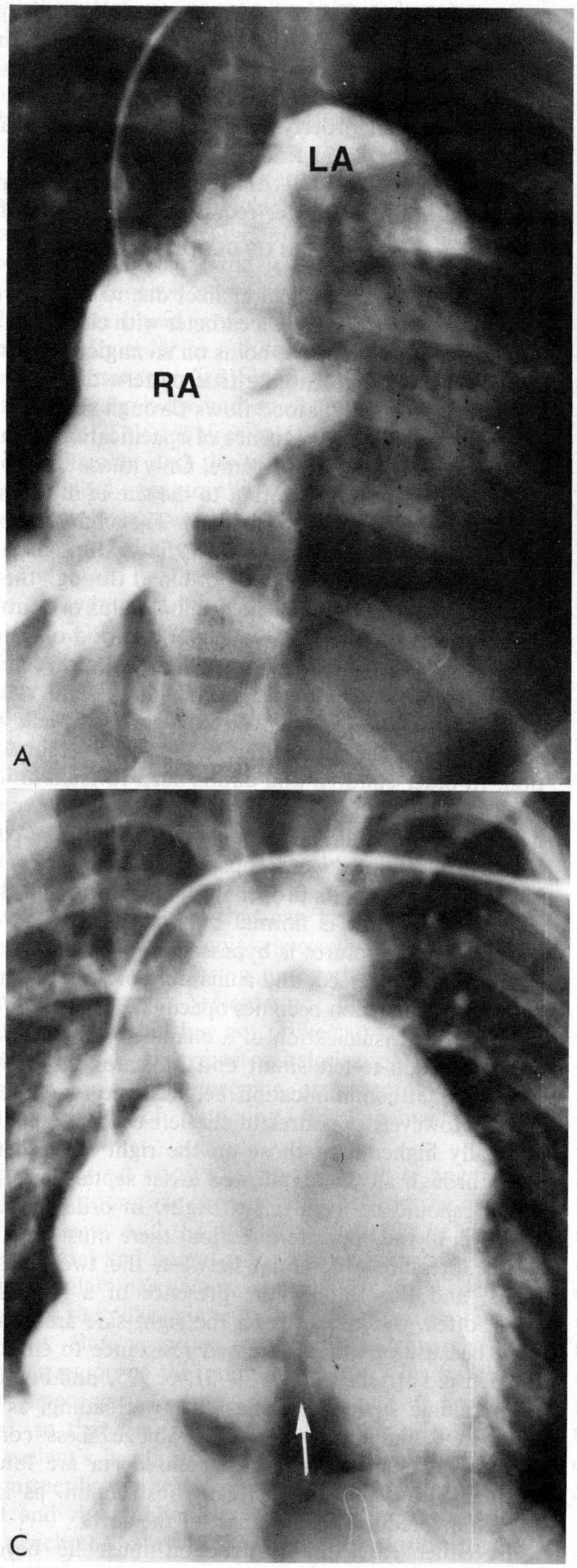

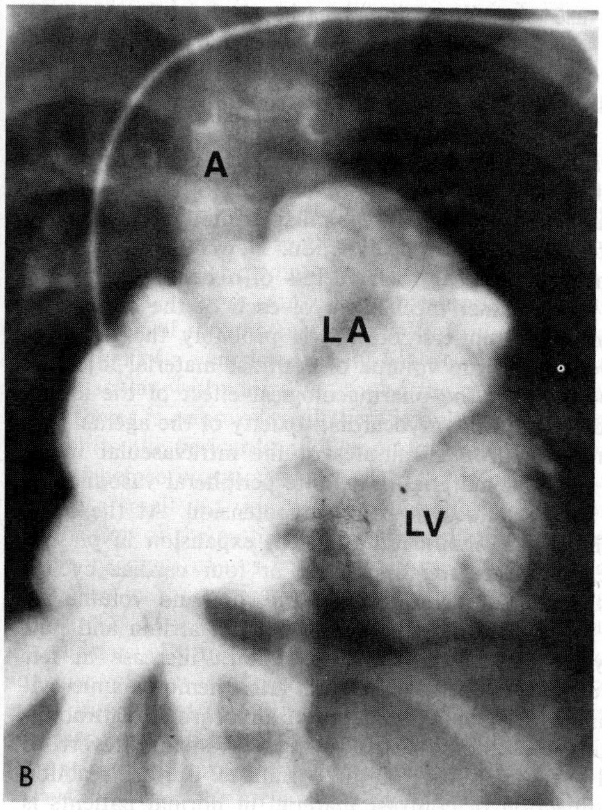

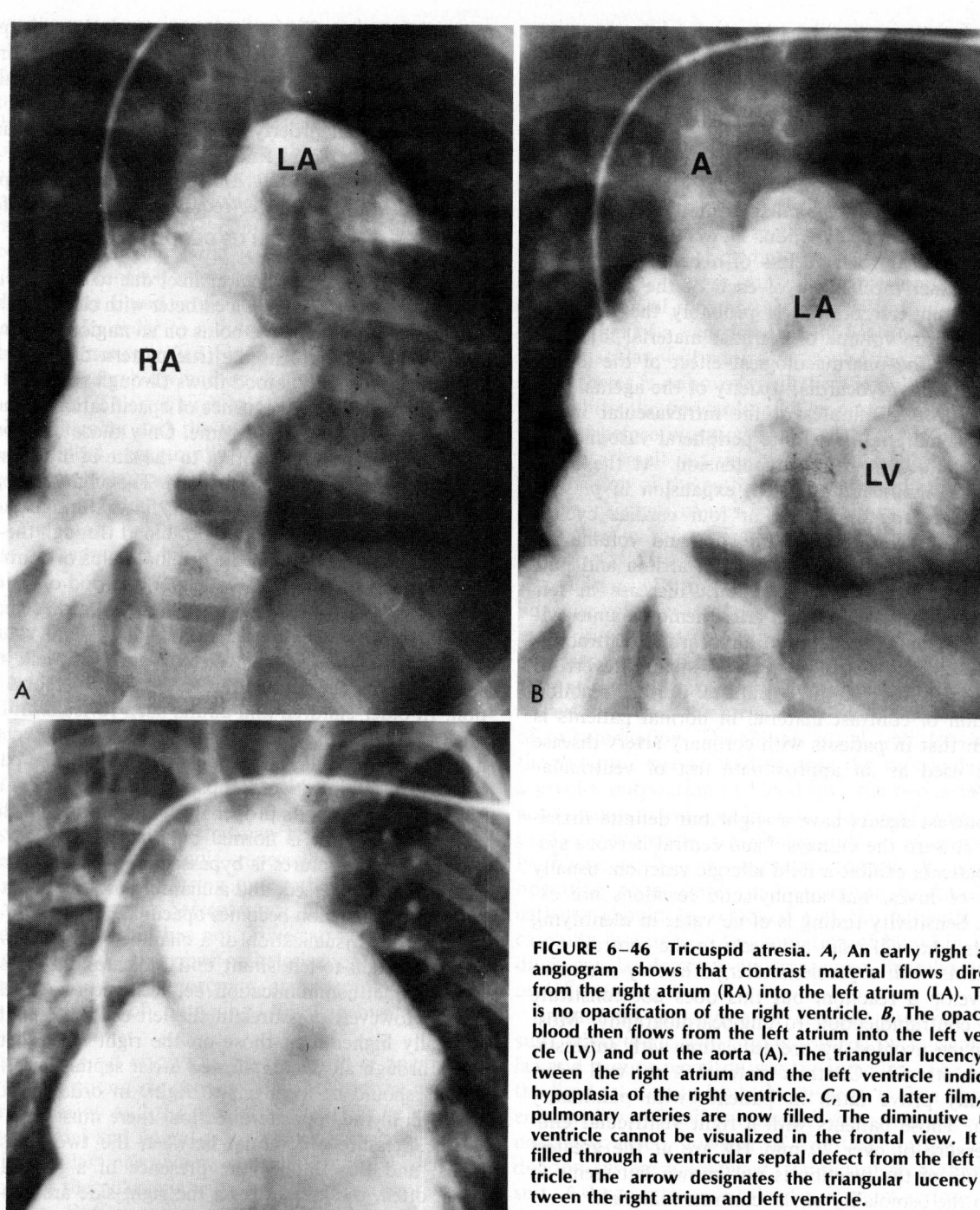

FIGURE 6–46 Tricuspid atresia. *A*, An early right atrial angiogram shows that contrast material flows directly from the right atrium (RA) into the left atrium (LA). There is no opacification of the right ventricle. *B*, The opacified blood then flows from the left atrium into the left ventricle (LV) and out the aorta (A). The triangular lucency between the right atrium and the left ventricle indicates hypoplasia of the right ventricle. *C*, On a later film, the pulmonary arteries are now filled. The diminutive right ventricle cannot be visualized in the frontal view. It was filled through a ventricular septal defect from the left ventricle. The arrow designates the triangular lucency between the right atrium and left ventricle.

result in elevation of the right atrial pressure, it causes an even greater elevation of left atrial pressure, so that the shunt would still be from left to right.

At times, two lesions can be localized from the sequence of opacification of the cardiac chambers. If contrast material injected into the right atrium first opacifies the left atrium, then the left ventricle, and finally the right ventricle, the presumptive diagnosis is tricuspid atresia with a right-to-left shunt through the atrial septum and a left-to-right shunt through a ventricular septal defect (Fig. 6–46).[113,114] More often, the abnormal flow pattern simply indicates the general location of the lesions, and a definitive diagnosis depends upon identification of specific anatomical abnormalities. If the opacified blood flows from the right atrium into the right ventricle as well as into the left atrium, a second injection of contrast material into the right ventricle is usually required in order to study the infundibular region of the right ventricle, the pulmonic valve, and the pulmonary circulation (see Figures 29–36, p. 986, 29–37, p. 987, 29–38, p. 988, and 29–46, p. 992).

Premature visualization of the descending aorta from an injection on the right side of the heart indicates reversed flow through a patent ductus arteriosus. This is most often due to preductal coarctation of the aorta.[115] The ascending aorta and the subclavian and carotid arteries are not visualized because they are filled by antegrade flow of nonopacified blood from the left ventricle. However, if the entire aorta is opacified through the ductus, the pressure in the ascending aorta must be similar to that in the descending aorta, and the possibility of a coarctation is excluded (Fig. 6–47). Usually, this pattern of flow is seen with hypoplasia of the left heart[116,117] but is rarely caused by severe pulmonary hypertension.[118]

Rare exceptions to the rule that two lesions are needed to produce a right-to-left shunt are a pulmonary arteriovenous fistula and anomalous drainage of a systemic vein (such as a persistent left superior vena cava) into the left atrium.[119]

Opacification of a chamber or vessel upstream in relation to the site of injection of the contrast material results from a left-to-right shunt or when a cardiac valve is incompetent. Some retrograde filling of the inferior or superior vena cava from the right atrium or of the pulmonary veins from the left atrium is not abnormal because the orifices of these vessels are not guarded by valves.

Backward visualization of a structure not contiguous to the one in which the contrast material is injected signifies a left-to-right shunt. Accurate localization of the lesion is usually possible when the jet of opacified blood crossing the defect between the two sides of the heart can be identified.[120,121] This usually requires selective injection of contrast material into the chamber from which the shunt arises. If the shunt itself is not visualized, it may be possible to establish the diagnosis by correlating the appearance of the opacified blood on the right side of the heart with the filling of the left-heart structures. For example, if, following a supraaortic injection of contrast material, the pulmonary artery does not become opacified until the proximal descending aorta is filled, a patent ductus is most likely. However, filling of the pulmonary artery when only the ascending aorta is opacified is indicative of an aorticopulmonary window.

In some instances, the defect cannot be localized with certainty without two or more selective angiograms. If the right atrium becomes opacified during the levocardiogram phase of a right ventriculogram, the presence of an atrial septal defect is statistically most likely. However, the shunt could have originated in the left ventricle (atrioventricular septal defect) or in the aorta (ruptured sinus of Valsalva aneurysm). A left ventricular injection, and possibly an aortogram, is required to exclude these lesions. A similar picture can be caused by anomalous drainage of a pulmonary vein into the right atrium. Usually, this need not be excluded, since it will become evident at the time of

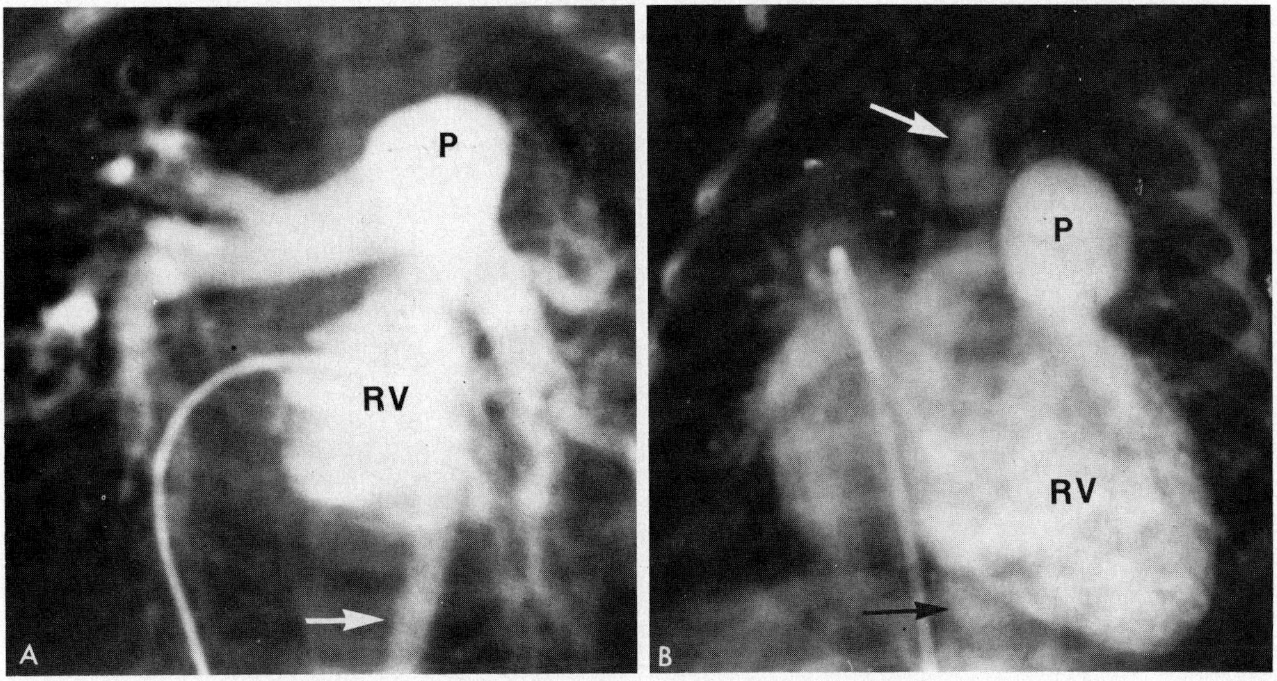

FIGURE 6–47 Patent ductus arteriosus and right-to-left shunt. *A*, Preductal coarctation. Contrast material has been injected selectively into the right ventricle (RV). The descending aorta (arrow) is filled through a patent ductus from the pulmonary artery (P). The ascending aorta and great vessels are not opacified. *B*, Hypoplastic left heart syndrome and interruption of the inferior vena cava. A catheter inserted into the femoral vein reaches the heart by way of the azygos vein, and contrast material is injected selectively into the right ventricle (RV). Both the ascending aorta (white arrow) and the descending aorta (black arrow) are filled from the pulmonary artery (P) by way of a patent ductus arteriosus.

operative repair of the atrial defect. However, if important, the abnormal venous connection can be demonstrated by selective injections into the right and left pulmonary arteries. When there is more than one left-to-right shunt, only the most proximal one that is opacified can be identified with certainty. For example, opacification of the right ventricle from a left ventricular injection indicates the presence of a ventricular septal defect. Forward flow of the opacified blood from the right ventricle rapidly fills the pulmonary artery, and it is usually not possible to recognize the presence of an associated patent ductus arteriosus. A second injection above the aortic valve is needed to evaluate this possibility (Fig. 6–48).

Cardiac Chambers

The size of a cardiac chamber may reflect an abnormal pattern of blood flow and has little diagnostic specificity. Although a chamber may be small because of malseptation, more commonly this is the result of a decreased volume load because of an anomaly that allows blood to bypass the chamber during embryonic life. Thus, tricuspid atresia or pulmonary valve atresia with an intact ventricular septum is associated with a diminutive right ventricle. A small left ventricle is often associated with a double-outlet right ventricle, and when the aortic or mitral valve is atretic, the ventricle may be represented only by an endocardium-lined slit.

When estimating chamber size from the angiogram, it is important to consider the size of the other cardiac chambers, a possible source of distortion. Enlargement of the right ventricle causes posterior displacement of the ventricular septum and the left ventricle. The left ventricle may be rotated medially, so that its lateral projection resembles that normally seen in the left anterior oblique view. The shadow of the ventricle is thus foreshortened, and the chamber, although normal in size, can appear small.

Dilatation of a chamber usually results from a volume overload, as in valvular regurgitation or a shunt, or from a decrease in the functional capacity of the myocardium. The underlying cause of such dilatation can be determined from a properly designed angiographic study. A right-sided angiocardiogram is usually inadequate when the cause of left ventricular enlargement is sought. A selective left ventriculogram is required in order to study contractility of the ventricular wall and to demonstrate regurgitation of the mitral valve. An aortogram is needed to evaluate the competency of the aortic valve and the possibility of

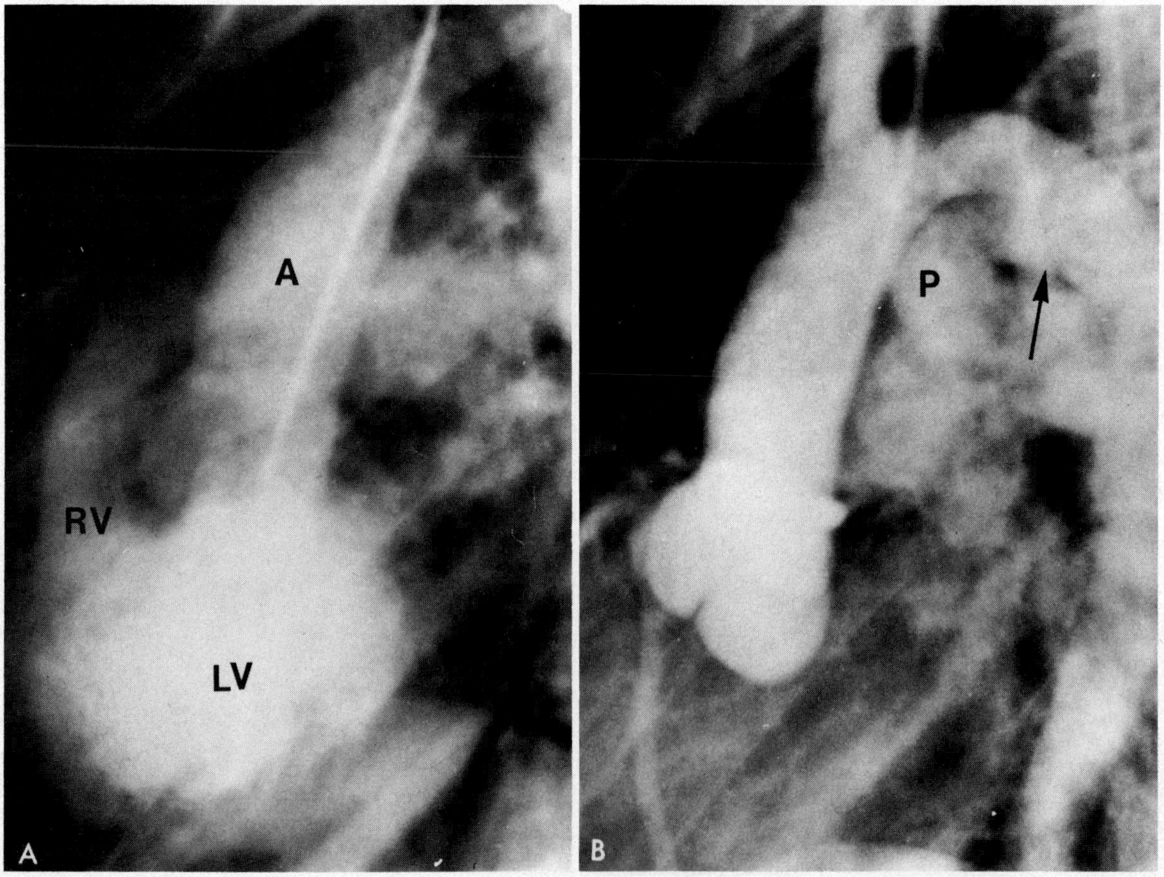

FIGURE 6–48 Multiple left-to-right shunts. *A*, Left ventriculogram, lateral view. Contrast material injected into the left ventricle (LV) flows rapidly across a large ventricular septal defect into the right ventricle (RV). The pulmonary artery is opacified by antegrade flow from the right ventricle. Although the aorta (A) is well opacified, it is not possible to identify a patent ductus arteriosus. *B*, The catheter was withdrawn into the ascending aorta, and a second injection was made. This time the pulmonary artery (P) is opacified by way of a patent ductus arteriosus (arrow). (From Angrissola, A. B., and Puddu, V. [eds.]: Cardiologia D'Oggia. Torino, C. B. Edizion Scientifiche, 1976.)

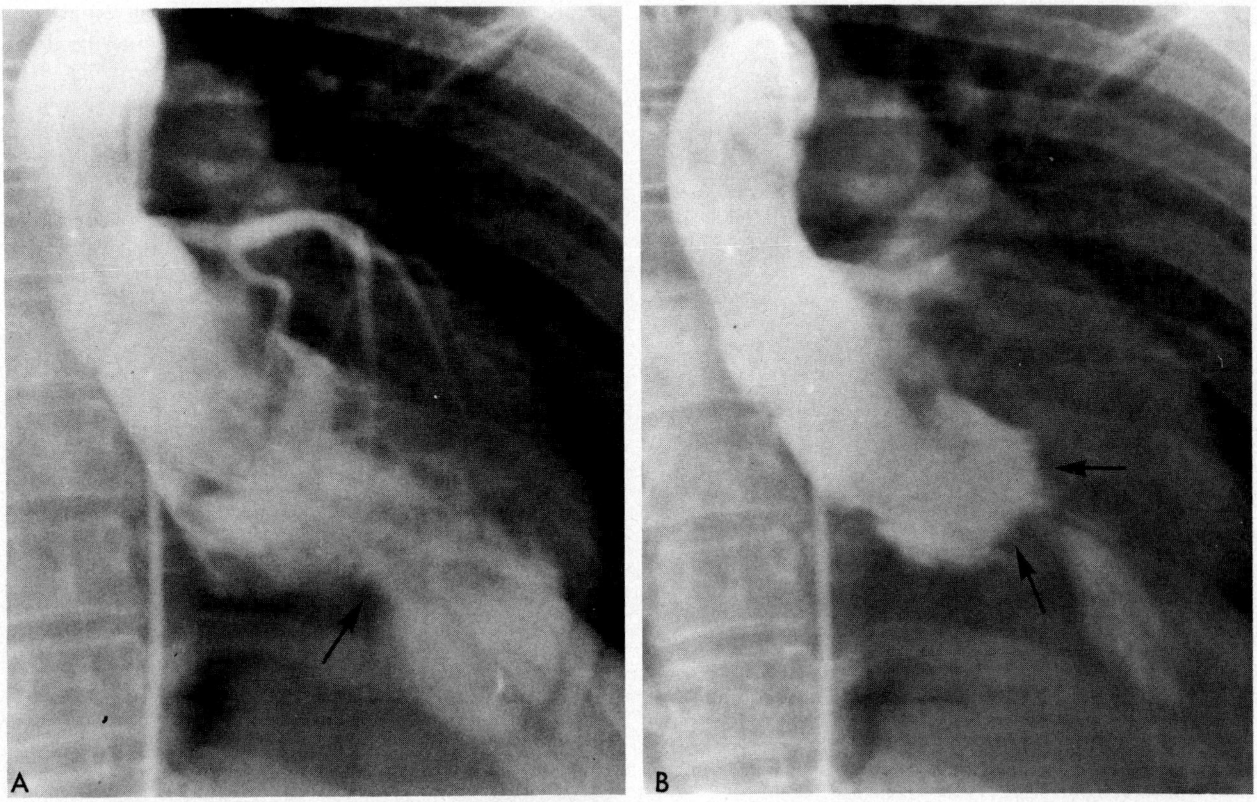

FIGURE 6–49 Left ventriculogram in hypertrophic obstructive cardiomyopathy. *A*, Diastole. The left ventricular wall is abnormally thickened because of muscular hypertrophy. The indentation on the medial aspect of the chamber (arrow) is caused by hypertrophy of the interventricular septum and the medial papillary muscle. *B*, Systole. As the heart contracts, the papillary muscles (arrows) constrict the midbody of the ventricle and sequester the apical region.

an anomalous left coronary artery (see Figure 29–22, p. 972).

Myocardial hypertrophy can be detected on the angiocardiogram. The distance between the edge of an opacified cardiac chamber and the outer border of the heart represents the combined thickness of the cardiac wall and the pericardium. A significant increase in this distance on an angiocardiogram can be due to hypertrophy of the myocardium or a pericardial effusion; however, hypertrophy rarely causes the thickness of the atrial wall to increase by more than a few millimeters. Atrial wall thickness of 8 mm or more is diagnostic of pericardial disease, almost always an effusion.[122]

Filling defects within the opacified atrium that occur early in the angiographic sequence, when contrast material is first injected into the chamber, usually result from incomplete mixing of the contrast material with the incoming nonopaque venous blood. The defects disappear after one or two cardiac cycles. A persistent defect that appears essentially the same from film to film indicates the presence of an intraluminal mass, either a thrombus or a tumor. A local dilution defect, such as that caused by nonopaque blood shunted through an atrial septal defect, can mimic the appearance of a mass. However, these dilution defects are never sharply outlined, and their appearance constantly changes during the cardiac cycle.

Ventricular filling defects are almost always due to hypertrophied musculature. In the right ventricle, the thickened myocardial bands and trabeculae cause scalloped indentations on the margins of the opacified chamber or round filling defects within it. Hypertrophy of the crista supraventricularis and the septal and parietal bands produce a narrowing of the infundibulum. Hypertrophic papillary muscles in the left ventricle are best seen in the frontal projection, since they encroach on the superior and inferior aspects of the ventricular cavity, narrowing the midbody of the chamber (Fig. 6–49). When the interventricular septum hypertrophies, it assumes a fusiform shape and bulges into the adjacent portions of both ventricular cavities.[123,124]

A thin, lucent line stretching across the outflow portion of the left ventricle is usually due to a subaortic membrane. This lesion may be difficult to demonstrate, and multiple views of the opacified ventricle are often required. The subaortic membrane can be delineated without equivocation, if contrast material is injected selectively into the space between the membrane and the aortic valve.[125] A more jagged, V-shaped lucent line seen in the outflow portion of the left ventricle in the frontal view is characteristic of hypertrophic obstructive cardiomyopathy[126] (Fig. 41–13, p. 1417). The linear defect is present only in late systole, when the anterior mitral leaflet swings forward and makes contact with the ventricular septum.

If the minor intrusions of the muscular trabeculae are ignored, the overall shape of the ventricular cavities is regular. Local outpocketings of the lumen are abnormal. On the left side, they usually represent postmyocardial infarction aneurysm (Figure 39–16, p. 1364) or, rarely, a con-

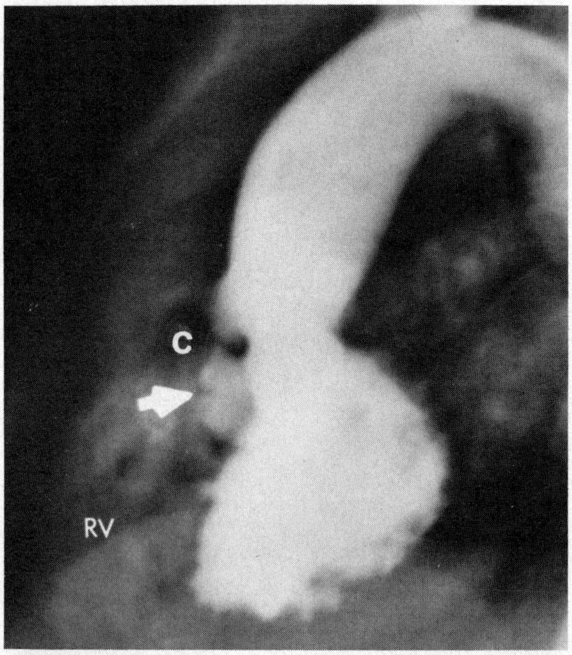

FIGURE 6–50 Aneurysm of the membranous septum. Left ventricular angiocardiogram, lateral view. The scalloped protrusion of the left ventricle (arrow) arises from the region of the membranous septum and extends anteriorly into the right ventricle beneath the crista supraventricularis (C). The right ventricle (RV) is opacified because of a small shunt through a defect in the aneurysm.

genital aneurysm or ventricular diverticulum. As the ventricle contracts, the aneurysm remains unchanged or bulges outward, and the contrast material pools within it. The opacified blood persists in the aneurysm, while it is washed away from the rest of the chamber. Aneurysms of the right ventricle are rare and are usually related to previous surgery.

An aneurysm of the membranous septum communicates with the left ventricular cavity and arises immediately beneath the commissure between the right coronary and noncoronary aortic cusps. The aneurysm usually has a trabeculated contour and extends anteriorly into the outflow tract of the right ventricle (Fig. 6–50). It is likely that most membranous septal aneurysms are misnamed and actually are formed by a portion of the tricuspid valve that has adhered to the margins of a membranous ventricular septal defect.[127,128]

Cineangiocardiography is required for a detailed study of ventricular function. End-diastolic and end-systolic volumes can be calculated from the size of the opacified ventricle in one or two projections and can be used to derive stroke volume, ejection fraction, and other measurements of myocardial performance (Chap. 14). It is also possible to divide the ventricular wall into segments and measure the shortening of each one during systole to disclose abnormalities in regional wall motion that may not be apparent from simple observation of the contracting chamber.[129,130]

Hypercontractility of the musculature is usually associated with hypertrophy and results in abnormal constriction of the ventricular lumen in end systole. In the right ventricle, this is most easily seen in the infundibular region. Normally, this area narrows slightly during systole. However, when the muscular contraction is abnormally forceful, the caliber of the infundibulum may be decreased by 80 per cent or more. Such systolic narrowing of the infundibulum is commonly seen with pulmonic valve stenosis.[131] If the infundibulum distends normally during diastole, the systolic narrowing was caused by hypercontraction of the musculature (Fig. 6–51). However, if the infundibulum is fibrotic, the narrowing is fixed, and it appears essentially the same in systole and diastole.

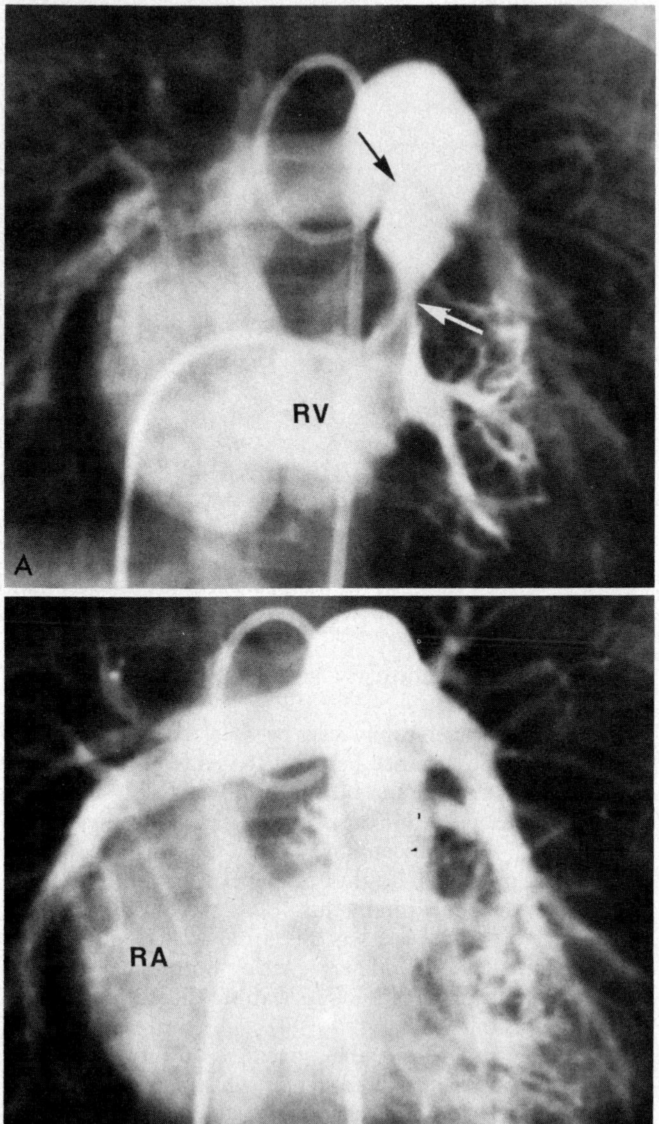

FIGURE 6–51 Pulmonary stenosis with hypercontraction of the infundibulum. *A*, Systole. A catheter has been advanced through the inferior vena cava to the right ventricle (RV). The stenotic pulmonic valve forms a dome (black arrow) bulging away from the ventricle. The infundibulum is markedly narrowed (white arrow). The multiple filling defects within the apical regions of the right ventricle are caused by hypertrophied trabeculae. The second catheter is positioned in the arch of the aorta. *B*, Diastole. The infundibulum appears of normal caliber, indicating that the narrowing was due to muscular contraction and does not represent fixed infundibular stenosis. The right atrium (RA) is opacified because of tricuspid regurgitation. (From Angrissola, A. B., and Puddu, V. [eds.]: Cardiologia D'Oggia. Torino, C. B. Edizion Scientifiche, 1976.)

Hypercontraction of the left ventricle is manifested mainly in the body of the chamber. When there is a diffuse increase in contractility of the ventricular wall, the end-systolic volume of the chamber is decreased, and the cavity of the ventricle, except for its outflow portion, may be completely effaced. This can represent a response to obstruction in the aortic valve or the subaortic region but also occurs without known cause.[132] Eccentric hypertrophy and hypercontractility of the ventricle usually involves the septum and the papillary muscles and produces a pinching of the body of the ventricle that sequesters the apical region from the rest of the chamber (Fig. 6–49).[126,133]

Cardiac Valves

Angiocardiography is probably the best single method for evaluation of the structure of cardiac valves. It is an accurate and sensitive technique for the detection of stenosis of the aortic and pulmonic valves and, to a lesser extent, of the mitral valve. It is not very effective for evaluation of tricuspid stenosis. Regurgitation of all four valves, even of the slightest degree, can be routinely demonstrated.

When the blood on both sides of the valve is opacified, and the valve is viewed tangentially, the cusps normally appear as thin, smooth, curvilinear lucencies. If the valve is projected obliquely or *en face*, the cusps usually cannot be identified. However, because the cusps are sheetlike structures, it is not necessary to visualize both surfaces in order to study their function. For example, on a supravalvular aortogram, the line of demarcation between the opacified blood in the aorta and the radiolucent blood in the ventricle actually represents the aortic surface of the valve cusps. The cusps are more easily seen on this type of examination, and in many instances their motion can be studied in greater detail (Fig. 6–52).

STENOSIS.[134] The cusps of the normal aortic and pulmonic valves are rarely identified during systole because of their rapid motion. Even in the fully opened position, the cusps are not still, since their free margins are unsupported and tend to vibrate in the rapidly flowing arterial stream. However, during diastole, the cusps coapt and support each other so that they are relatively immobile for a considerable part of the cardiac cycle.

When the valve is stenotic, the cusps cannot separate from each other, and they form a membrane with a narrow orifice. During systole, the membrane, stretched taut by the stream of blood ejected from the ventricle, is relatively motionless. A dome-shaped curvilinear lucency, bulging away from the contracting chamber, is the angiographic hallmark of valvular stenosis (Figs. 6–52 and 6–53).[135,136] If the cusps cannot be seen during systole, it may be assumed that the valve is not stenotic. The aortic

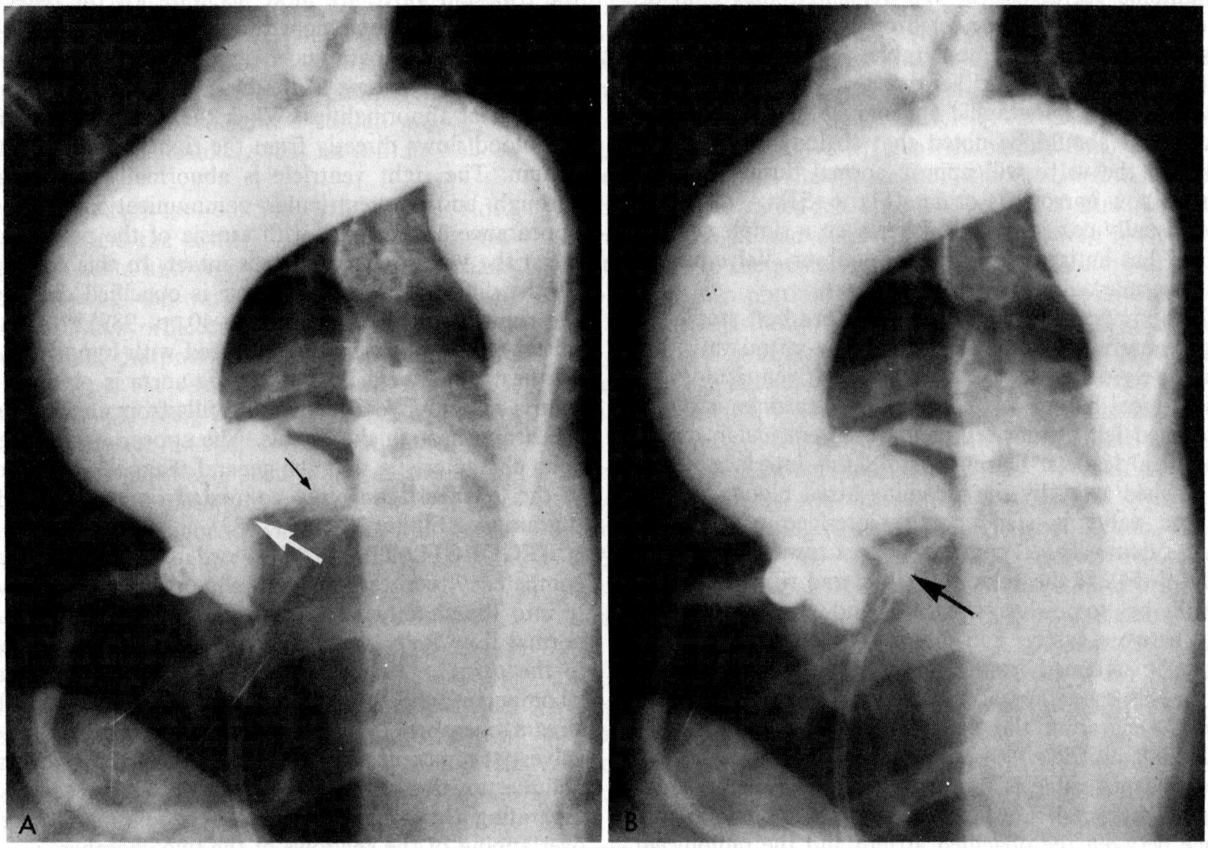

FIGURE 6–52 Aortic stenosis, supravalvular aortogram. *A*, Systole. The aortic valve is rigid and cannot open. The narrow dilution defect (white arrow) represents radiolucent blood ejected from the left ventricle and indicates the diameter of the valve orifice. The irregularity of the left coronary cusp (black arrow) is caused by a vegetation on the valve. There is poststenotic dilatation of the ascending aorta. *B*, Diastole. The valve hardly moves at all, and there is a fine jet of aortic regurgitation (arrow).

with basic electrophysiological properties of the heart; with clinical and laboratory findings; and with anatomical, pathological; and experimental observations.[2] The result has been that electrocardiography can be used, within limits, to identify anatomical, metabolic, ionic, and hemodynamic changes. It is often an independent marker of myocardial disease and occasionally the only indicator of a pathological process.[3–11]

Electrocardiography serves as a gold standard for the diagnosis of arrhythmias. Arrhythmias have been studied by a variety of methods for centuries, but none of the diverse methods has approached the levels of sensitivity and specificity offered by the ECG. Free of the assumptions required for interpreting the electrocardiographic P, QRS, ST, or T waveforms, arrhythmias recorded from the surface of the body, with rare exceptions, accurately reflect intracardiac events. However, even in the area of rhythm analysis, certain limitations must be appreciated. While most arrhythmias are due to disordered impulse formation or conduction (or both) of the specialized tissue, the ECG reflects the electrical behavior of the myocardium and not of the specialized tissue. For simple arrhythmias, this dichotomy poses no problem; however, in complex arrhythmias, when recognition and interpretation of the behavior of specialized tissue is critical, such information must be derived by deductive reasoning. In addition, intracardiac ECG studies have demonstrated that small changes in the speed of conduction, or cycle length, may be a critical determinant of rhythm behavior, but such small changes may not be appreciated in a tracing inscribed with standard direct writing equipment. Furthermore, on rare occasion, arrhythmias induce voltage changes too small to register in the ECG. These limitations, once appreciated as inherent in the ECG, rarely interfere with proper analysis of even the most complex arrhythmias.

The contribution of electrocardiography to the diagnosis and management of patients with heart disease is equaled, if not exceeded, by its impact on clinical and basic electrophysiological research. The clinical ECG continues to stimulate an exchange of ideas between the clinical electrocardiographer and the basic and clinical investigator. Numerous electrophysiological concepts derived through deductive analysis of the ECG have ultimately been confirmed in the laboratory. Similarly, concepts first developed in an animal laboratory have been identified in man by clinical electrocardiographers. As a result of such interaction, electrocardiography, at first a largely empirical body of knowledge, is gradually acquiring firm experimental bases.

As with any other laboratory procedure, the sensitivity and specificity of the ECG and of its individual components are critical determinants of its clinical usefulness. This is far more complex for the ECG than for other laboratory techniques developed for a single purpose, since its multiple waveforms may be identically or differentially influenced by a wide spectrum of physiological, pathophysiological, or anatomical changes. Thus, it may be difficult—if not impossible—to identify a singular cause for an ECG abnormality. Sensitivity and specificity can be enhanced through the examiner's careful formulation of the question the ECG is expected to answer, attention to the intra- and extracellular environment present at the time of the recording, use of proper recording technique, and assessment of serial tracings, all coupled with skillful interpretation of the ECG findings.[12]

THEORETICAL CONSIDERATIONS

Essential to an understanding of the derivation and interpretation of the clinical ECG is information about (1) the physical and electrophysiological events responsible for the electrical potential, recorded as the transmembrane action potential, and the spread of excitation; (2) the role of the volume conductor; and (3) the theoretical basis of the lead systems.

ELECTRICAL BASES AND THEORY (THE DIPOLE, VOLUME CONDUCTOR, MAGNITUDE OF POTENTIAL, AND POLARITY OF THE ELECTRICAL FIELD)

At any moment in time, the cardiac generator can be viewed as a dipole or doublet consisting of a positive and a negative charge separated by a small distance. Since the dipole generates a force that has magnitude and direction, it can be expressed as a vector. By convention the arrowhead of the vector indicates the positive pole. When such a dipole is immersed in a volume conductor, an electrical field is generated.[13,14] In a homogeneous volume conductor, the field is symmetrically distributed. The lines of the electrical field are symmetrical in relation to a line that is perpendicular to and transects the dipole at its midpoint.

At any moment in time, the magnitude of the potential at a given point (P) in the volume conductor can be estimated using the solid-angle concept, or the concept relating the potential to an angle formed by a line drawn from P to the midpoint of the dipole axis and the dipole axis itself (Fig. 7–1).

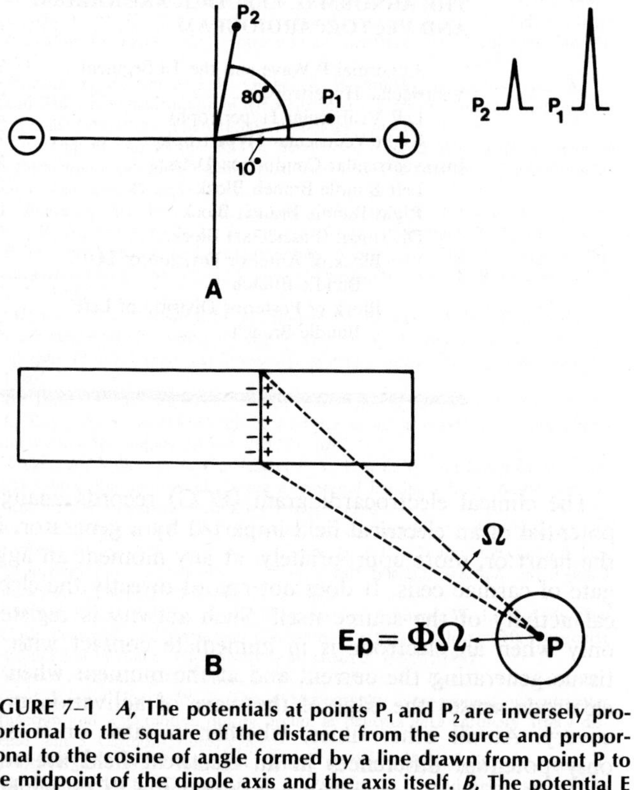

FIGURE 7–1 *A,* The potentials at points P_1 and P_2 are inversely proportional to the square of the distance from the source and proportional to the cosine of angle formed by a line drawn from point P to the midpoint of the dipole axis and the axis itself. *B,* The potential E is proportional to the solid angle Ω and the strength of the charged surface subtending the angle Φ. (Modified from Wolff, L.: Electrocardiography: Fundamentals and Clinical Application. 3rd ed. Philadelphia, W. B. Saunders Co., 1962, p. 15.)

The electrical surface with its boundary projected to P results in a cone and defines the solid angle subtended by the area in question. The segment of a sphere inscribed by a radius of unity drawn about point P, with P as the center of the sphere, and its border delineated by the cone, is proportional to the area of electrical activity. With variables such as tissue resistance and geometry being constant, the voltage at P can be expressed as $Ep = \phi \cdot \Omega$, where ϕ is voltage per unit of the solid angle and Ω is the solid angle.[15,16]

An alternative and perhaps clinically more applicable approach to estimating Ep considers the distance (r) of P from the source, the strength of the source (m), and the cosine of the angle formed by a line drawn from P to the midpoint of the dipole axis and the dipole axis (Θ), with the magnitude of the angle estimated in reference to the positive pole of the dipole. This relationship can be expressed as $Ep = \frac{m \cos \Theta}{\gamma^2}$. According to this formula, when the angle is 90°, the line drawn from P is perpendicular to the dipole axis and the Ep is zero. In the ECG the inscription would be isoelectric or equiphasic. On the other hand, with the angle becoming smaller, the P is closer to the positive pole of the dipole and the voltage becomes greater.[9,15,16]

Assuming that the volume conductor is homogeneous and infinite and has a uniform boundary and that the generator is located in the center of the volume conductor, both approaches for estimation of Ep at P are correct. Such assumptions, however, are not valid in man (see below).

The influence of polarity of the dipole, the distance from the dipole, and the strength of the electrical field on waveform are critical for proper analysis and interpretation of the ECG. These relationships can be studied using a hypothetical experimental dipole or cardiac tissue immersed in a homogeneous volume conductor. An exploring electrode placed in a line with the axis of the dipole and gradually moved from left (negative pole) to right (positive pole) records a negative-positive deflection. A remote electrode, located outside the electrical field, fails to record a potential. However, when the electrode is moved into the negative field, it encounters and records a gradually increasing negativity. As the electrode nears and passes the negative pole of the dipole and finds itself halfway between the two poles, a sharp reversal of polarity is registered (intrinsicoid deflection) and the electrode enters the field of positivity. The positive voltage declines gradually as the electrode moves away from the positive pole. Finally, the electrode moves out of the electrical field and a potential is no longer registered.

A similar sequence of events is registered with the electrode stationary and the electrical field moving relative to the electrode. When the positive field moves toward the electrode, a positive potential is recorded; when the electrode finds itself in the negative field, a negative potential is recorded.

Electrophysiological Bases and Theory

Transmembrane ionic fluxes are responsible for voltage differences between activated and resting tissue. These ionic fluxes are reflected as the transmembrane action potential, the cellular counterpart of the clinical ECG. The ECG counterparts of the TAP phases 0, 1, 2, 3, and 4 are the QRS complex, the ST segment, the T wave, and the isoelectric baseline, respectively (see Chapter 19).

DEPOLARIZATION AND REPOLARIZATION. To progress logically toward an understanding of the ECG, we will review the effect of a muscle strip immersed in a homogeneous volume conductor on the electrical field generated by the muscle strip and on the electrode immersed in the field. A muscle strip, when uniformly positive on the outside, is in a resting or polarized state. Because it exhibits no difference of potential and fails to impart an electrical field, an electrode immersed in the volume conductor registers an isoelectric line. Stimulation of the muscle strip at any given point increases membrane permeability, and positive charges enter the cell. The result is depolarized (relatively negative) muscle in apposition to polarized (relatively positive) muscle, with a potential difference across a boundary. In the surrounding medium the current flows from the positively (source) to the negatively (sink) charged muscle. The moving boundary between the polarized (positive) and the depolarized (negative) muscle can be represented by a dipole or vector. This dipole or vector moves along the muscle fiber from the point of excitation, leaving in its wake tissue that is electrically negative (depolarized) in relation to the still polarized (resting) muscle. When the wave of depolarization reaches the end of the muscle strip, the surface becomes uniformly negative and the strip is now completely depolarized. Since a difference of potential no longer exists, an isoelectric baseline is inscribed. The most intense difference of potential exists at the boundary between depolarized and resting tissue, and the recorded voltage changes reflect the events taking place at this boundary.[13,14]

Restitution of membrane polarity, or *repolarization*, can be viewed as a "wave" of positivity enveloping the cells or tissue. As a result, the outside of the cell is again uniformly positive. Since the boundary moves in the direction of the depolarized, negative muscle, an electrode located at the point of origin of repolarization records a positive potential. An electrode placed at the opposite end records a negative potential. In an isolated preparation of myocardial tissue, the direction of repolarization is the same as that of depolarization but is preceded by the negative pole of the dipole. The repolarization inscribes an area equal to that inscribed by depolarization but of opposite polarity.

EFFECT OF THE BOUNDARY OF DEPOLARIZATION AND REPOLARIZATION ON POLARITY OF THE RECORDED POTENTIAL. Three electrodes placed on a muscle strip will illustrate the effect of a boundary potential, which can be represented as a dipole or vector, on the recording electrode[9] (Fig. 7–2). Electrode A is located at the point of excitation, electrode B at the midpoint of the muscle strip, and electrode C at the end of the muscle strip. Immediately after excitation, electrode A finds itself in the most intensively negative field. As the dipole moves away, the potential becomes less negative, and at the end of depolarization the inscription returns to the baseline. Thus, the electrode at point A inscribes a negative deflection. At the moment of excitation, electrode B is located in the positive field of the dipole. As the dipole moves toward the recording electrode, the latter registers a gradually increasing positivity and records an upright deflection. When the dipole passes the electrode, there is a sudden reversal of polarity, and the electrode finds itself in a strongly negative field. A downward, negative deflection is recorded. With the dipole moving away, the electrode at point B registers a less negative potential, and finally, when the strip is completely depolarized, an isoelectric baseline is recorded. Thus, the electrode at point B registers a positive-negative deflection. Electrode C is located in the positive field throughout the entire process of depolarization. As the dipole approaches the electrode, the field becomes more intensively positive, with the most intense positivity at the moment immediately prior to completion of depolarization. Thus, the electrode at point C records an upright deflection.

SEQUENCE OF ACTIVATION OF THE HEART. For a proper analysis of the ECG, recognition of the se-

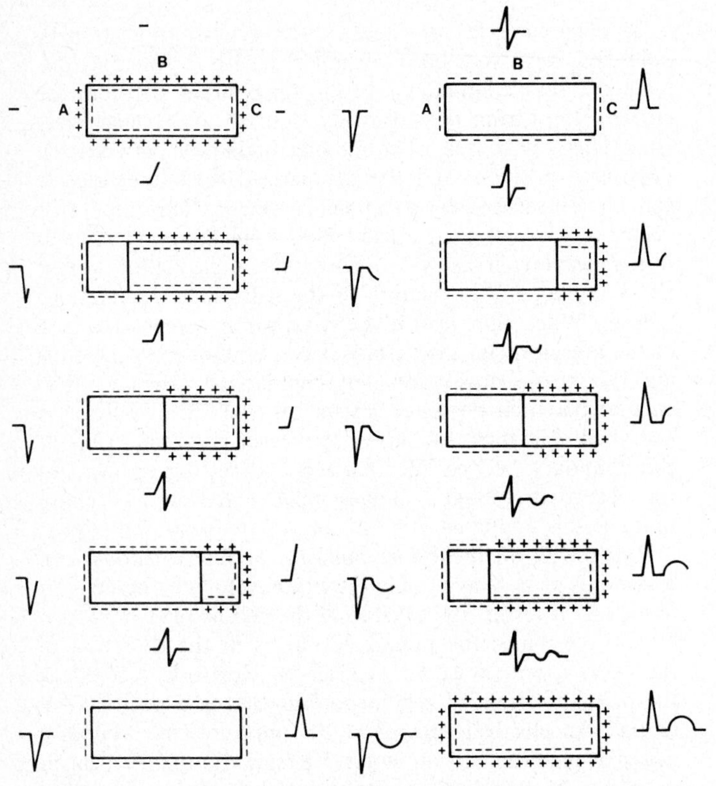

FIGURE 7–2 Potential generated during depolarization (*left vertical sequence of panels*) and repolarization (*right vertical sequence of panels*) recorded with an exploring electrode located at the endocardium (A), epicardium (C), and midway between the two (B). (Modified from Barker, J. M.: The Unipolar Electrocardiogram: A Clinical Interpretation. New York, Appleton-Century-Crofts, Inc., 1952.)

quence of cardiac activation is as important as the understanding of the physical and electrophysiological bases of the cardiac current. The sequence of activation of the heart has been studied in animals, primarily in the dog and in the isolated perfused human heart.[17] The normal impulse originates in the sinoatrial node and traverses the atria in a wavelike front with a velocity of approximately 1000 mm/sec. The wave of atrial activation is described as one resembling a wavefront seen when a pebble is thrown into water. The sinoatrial node is located in the right atrium and initially activates the right atrium in a right and anterior direction, followed by excitation of the left atrium in a left and posterior direction. It has been suggested that preferential internodal pathways connect the sinoatrial node and the atrioventricular (AV) junctional tissue and that these specialized internodal pathways are capable of conducting an impulse in the face of a quiescent atrium.[18] The concept has attracted considerable interest and is the subject of continued investigation.[19]

The impulse arrives at the AV node, where it is delayed, most likely owing to decremental conduction (p. 624).[20] Study of the sequence of ventricular activation in the dog reveals an early (0 to 5 msec) and almost simultaneous activation of the central left side of the septum and the high anterior and apical posterior paraseptal areas of the left ventricle. At 5 to 10 msec after the onset of ventricular activation, the wave of activation envelops left and right ventricular walls and the remainder of the septum; the latter is completely activated at 12 msec. The earliest epicardial breakthrough occurs at the anterior right epicardial surface near the apex, followed by anterior and posterior paraseptal areas of the left ventricle. At 18 msec, activation of the central portion of the two ventricles is complete. Excitation continues along the lateral and basal aspect of the left ventricle, with the basal portion of the septum last to depolarize.[15]

Studies of perfused human heart indicate that its path of activation closely follows that of the canine heart (Fig. 7–3). The results obtained in the resuscitated human heart were validated by comparing the process of activation with that of a perfused and in situ dog heart. The only difference was that the activation proceeded more rapidly in the perfused dog preparation.[17] By means of intracardiac mapping during surgery it has also been shown that epicardial breakthrough occurred in the right ventricle followed by activation of the anterior and inferior left ventricle.[21]

In contrast to the reasonably accurate information regarding the process of activation, knowledge of the sequence of *repolarization* in an intact heart is incomplete and difficult to define. For one thing, the experimental design itself may alter the sequence of repolarization. Simi-

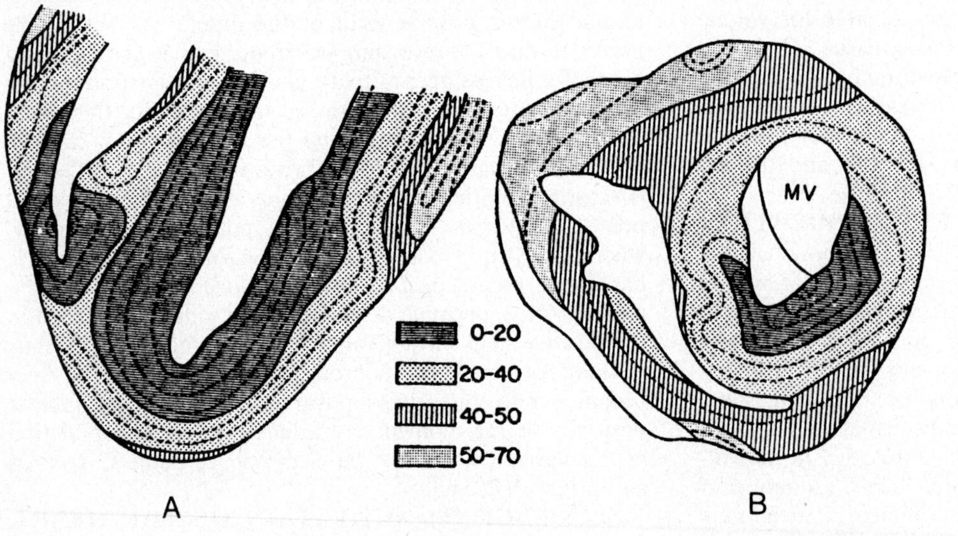

FIGURE 7–3 Sequence of ventricular activation of an isolated human heart. *A* and *B* represent sagittal and coronal sections, respectively. The dotted lines denote 5-msec sequences, while changes in pattern represent 20-msec intervals. (Durrer, D., et al.: Total excitation of the isolated human heart. Circulation *41*:899, 1970, by permission of the American Heart Association, Inc.)

larly, electrodes used to plot the wave of repolarization may induce a current of injury and interfere with the recording of meaningful data. Human studies indicate that atrial repolarization follows approximately the same path as atrial depolarization, with the polarity of repolarization opposite to that of depolarization. Ventricular repolarization proceeds in a direction *opposite* to that of depolarization, and its polarity is therefore the *same* as that of depolarization. The process of repolarization recorded directly from the epicardium indicates that in the intact ventricle repolarization begins at the epicardium—a sequence opposite to that observed in isolated muscle strip. The reason for the in vivo reversal of the order of repolarization is not entirely clear. The presence of a transmural pressure gradient may be an important factor, since it prolongs the duration of the excited state of the endocardium and, consequently, recovery begins at the epicardium.

VENTRICULAR GRADIENT. The concept of ventricular gradient (G), introduced by Wilson, is a method for describing the relationships between depolarization (QRS) and repolarization (T).[22] As stated above, in the isolated muscle strip depolarization and repolarization are equal in duration and follow the same path. The net areas of the QRS complex (AQRS) and the T wave (AT) are equal but of opposite polarity, so that their sum is zero and there is no gradient. In the intact heart, on the other hand, repolarization proceeds from the epicardium to endocardium, in a direction opposite to that of depolarization; the algebraic sum of their respective areas is no longer zero; and a gradient is said to exist. AQRS, AT, and G can be expressed as a vectorial quantity from any two of the three bipolar limb leads of the ECG. AQRS and AT are expressed in the form of vectors and are plotted using the Einthoven triangle or Bayley triaxial reference system. A parallelogram of the AQRS and the AT is constructed, with the resultant diagonal vector being the manifest AQRST vector or gradient (G). The G vector and the mean QRS vector are located in about the same plane. The G forms an angle of approximately 30° with the mean spatial QRS vector.

G is an index of variation in duration of the excited state and thus of the local rate of repolarization. Although it is of theoretical value in the study of T-wave abnormalities, the variations between individuals and in the same individual and the tedious calculations required, especially when small changes may prove important, limit its clinical usefulness. The electrocardiographer intuitively evaluates the ventricular gradient whenever reading the cardiogram.[11]

THEORETICAL BASES OF SURFACE LEADS. At any instant the surface leads reflect projection of the electrical current of the equivalent or "net" dipole expressed as the mean instantaneous spatial vector. Orientation of a lead axis is defined as one that records a maximal voltage when its axis is parallel to that of the axis or vector of the equivalent dipole. The voltage registered in any lead, having magnitude and direction, can be expressed as a vector (lead vector), with the amplitude of deflection in any lead paralleling the magnitude of the vector. Since more than one dipole may exist at any instant, the net potential and consequently the resultant lead vector reflect the contribution of all such dipoles. Furthermore, because dipole vectors may vary in magnitude and direction, the equivalent or "net" dipole is an approximation of these forces and consequently its expression on a lead axis is also an approximation.

THE NORMAL ELECTROCARDIOGRAM AND VECTORCARDIOGRAM

Leads

Bipolar limb leads introduced by Einthoven register the direction, magnitude, and duration of voltage changes in the frontal plane. The three bipolar leads—I, II, and III—record the difference in potential between left arm (LA) and right arm (RA), left leg (LF) and RA, and LF and LA, respectively.

Unipolar limb leads are constructed by connecting all three extremities to a "central terminal" (Fig. 7–4*B*). Although in reality the central terminal registers a small voltage, for practical purposes it is considered to have a zero potential and serves as the *indifferent* or *reference electrode.* The potential differences recorded by the positive terminal, the *exploring electrode,* are dominated by local electrical events. When placed on the right arm, left arm, or left foot, the exploring electrode registers the potential from the respective limb. The letter V identifies a unipolar lead and the letters r, l, and f the respective extremities. If one disconnects the central terminal from the extremity from which the potential is being recorded, the amplitude registered by the respective unipolar limb lead is augmented; such leads are designated as aV_r, aV_l, and aV_f.

Locations of the exploring electrode for the *precordial leads* are as follows: V_1—fourth interspace to the right of the sternum; V_2—fourth interspace to the left of the sternum; V_3—midway between leads V_2 and V_4; V_4—fifth interspace at the midclavicular line; V_5—anterior axillary line at the level of lead V_4; and V_6—midaxillary line at the level of lead V_4[23] (Fig. 7–4*B*).

Of the six precordial leads, it is assumed that leads V_1 and V_2, V_3 and V_4, and V_5 and V_6 face the right side of the septum, the septum itself, and the left side of the septum, respectively, and are referred to as right ventricular, septal or transitional, and left ventricular leads, respectively.

THE NORMAL ELECTROCARDIOGRAM

THE P WAVE

The cardiac impulse originating in the sinoatrial node activates the right and left atria in the general direction

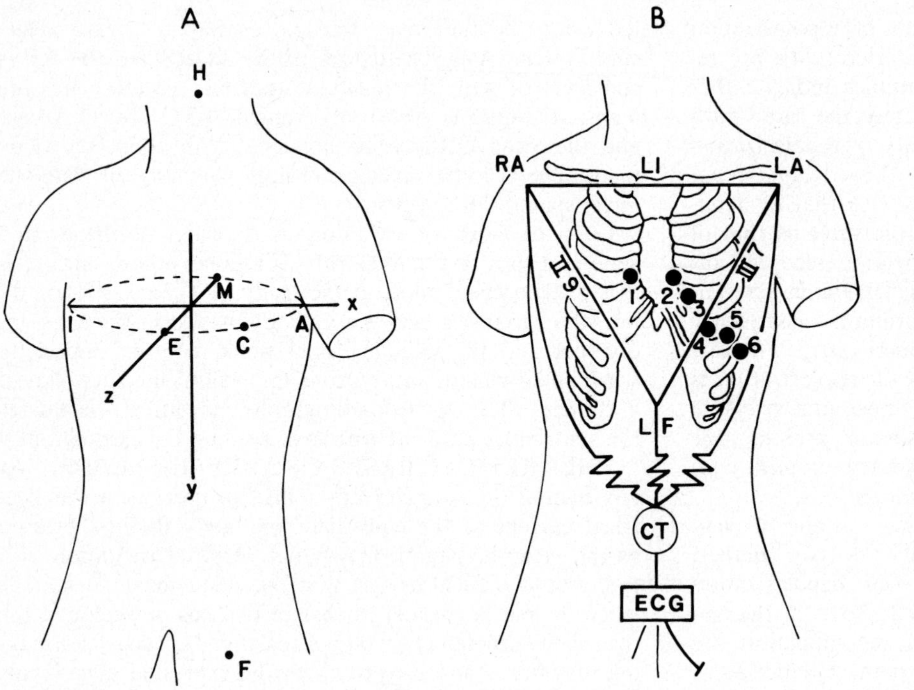

FIGURE 7–4 *A*, Frank electrode system. Five horizontal electrodes are placed at the level where the fifth intercostal space intersects the sternal line. Specific locations include fifth intercostal space and sternum (E), the midaxillary line (A-I), and the vertebral column (M). Electrode C is located halfway between points E and A, while electrodes H and F are on the back of the neck and left lower extremity, respectively. *B*, ECG lead system. Leads I, II, and III are formed by connecting RA-LA, RA-LF, and LA-LF, respectively. The indifferent electrode of the unipolar system is obtained by connecting RA, LA, and LF through 50,000-ohm resistance into a central terminal (CT). (For details about positioning of the exploring unipolar electrode, see p. 199.)

from right to left atrium, inferiorly and posteriorly. Initial activation of the right atrium, an anterior chamber, is directed anteriorly and inferiorly and is followed by activation of the left or posterior atrium, directed to the left, posteriorly, and inferiorly.

The P wave is rounded with a notch corresponding to the separation between right and left atrial activation. Amplitude of the P wave is normally less than 2.5 mm (0.25 mV) with a duration less than 0.12 sec (Table 7–1). The P wave and the *Ta segment*, or atrial repolarization, define atrial electrical systole. The P vector varies from −50° to +60°. In the precordial leads the P wave is positive except in lead V_1, where the P wave may be upright, biphasic, or negative.

The Ta segment is inscribed during the QRS complex and the early part of the ST segment. It is best seen in the

TABLE 7–1

A. P WAVE: HEIGHT AND DURATION IN NORMAL ADULTS

	Lead I	Lead II	Lead III	Lead V_1*
P height (mV)				
Mean	0.49	1.03	0.69	0.40
Range	0.2 to 1.0	0.3 to 2.0	0 to 2.0	0.05 to 0.80
P duration (sec)				
Mean	0.08	0.09	0.07	0.05
Range	0.05 to 0.12	0.05 to 0.12	0.02 to 0.13	0 to 0.08
R-R interval (sec)				
Mean	0.16	0.16	0.16	
Range	0.12 to 0.20	0.12 to 0.20	0.12 to 0.20	

B. AMPLITUDE OF Q, R, S, AND T WAVES ON SCALAR ECG OF 100 NORMAL ADULTS†

	I	II	III	aV_r	aV_l	aV_f	V_1	V_5	V_6
Patients with Q wave	38%	41%	50%	—	38%	40%	0%	60%	75%
Q amplitude									
Mean	0.4	0.6	0.9	—	0.4	0.7	0	0.3	0.3
Range	0 to 1.0	0 to 1.6	0 to 2.3	—	0 to 1.1	0 to 1.7	0	0 to 1.8	0 to 1.8
R amplitude									
Mean	5.6	8.9	4.5	1.3	3.4	6.0	1.9	12.6	10.2
Range	1.0 to 10.0	2.0 to 16.9	1.0 to 12.1	0 to 2.9	0 to 8.2	0 to 13.8	1.0 to 6.0	7.0 to 21.0	5.0 to 18.0
S amplitude									
Mean	2.0	2.1	2.4	7.0	2.6	—	8.0	2.5	1.3
Range	0 to 5.0	0 to 3.7	0 to 6.4	2.2 to 11.8	0 to 5.8	—	3.0 to 13.0	0 to 5.0	0 to 2.0
T amplitude									
Mean	1.9	2.3	1.0	—	0.3	1.7	1.0	3.3	1.0
Range	1.0 to 3.0	1.0 to 4.0	−2.0 to 2.0	—	−1.0 to 2.0	0 to 4.0	−2.0 to 2.0	2.0 to 7.0	1.0 to 4.0

*Twenty-five per cent of the series had a small terminal negative deflection of the P wave in lead V_1.
†Values of Q, R, S and T amplitudes are in millimeters (1 mm = 0.1 mv).
Modified and reproduced from Cooksey, J.D., et al.: Clinical Vectorcardiography and Electrocardiography. 2nd ed. Copyright © 1977 by Year Book Medical Publishers, Inc., Chicago.

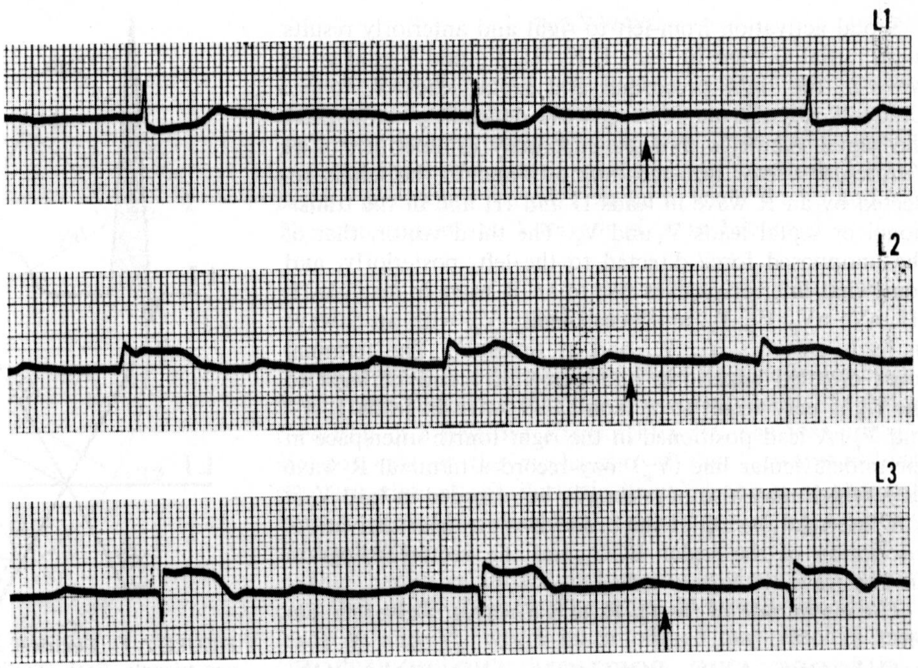

FIGURE 7–5 Atrial infarction. The tracing illustrates sinus rhythm, complete AV block, and an acute inferior myocardial infarction. The Ta segment indicative of atrial infarction is elevated in leads II and III (arrows) and depressed in lead I (arrow).

presence of AV block (Fig. 7–5).[24] Duration of the Ta segment varies from 0.15 to 0.45 sec, and its amplitude is low, reaching 0.08 mV. The magnitude of the Ta is directionally related to the area of the P wave and thus the heart rate. The vector of the Ta is opposite to that of the P vector and is oriented superiorly, to the right, and somewhat posteriorly. Similarly, the P wave and the Ta areas are equal and opposite in direction, and the resultant gradient is zero. In the presence of atrial enlargement, the Ta segment may result in displacement of the ST segment.

THE P-R INTERVAL. The P-R interval includes the intraatrial, AV nodal, and His-Purkinje conduction, and its duration varies from 0.12 to 0.20 or 0.22 sec (Table 7–1). AV conduction is discussed in Chapter 19.

The QRS Complex

Familiarity with the sequence of ventricular activation is a prerequisite for proper analysis of the normal and abnormal QRS complex. As stated above, ventricular activation proceeds more or less symmetrically about the septum and from the endocardium to the epicardium. Consequently, much of its voltage is canceled; in fact, only 10 to 15 per cent of the potential generated by the heart is ultimately recorded on the surface ECG.

The QRS complex can be described by four vectors[11] (Fig. 7–6): (1) initial septal activation from left to right, anteriorly, inferiorly, or superiorly, followed by further septal activation from left to right (0.01 sec); (2) an overlapping wave of excitation involving both ventricles, with the vector directed inferiorly and slightly to the left (0.02 sec); (3) unopposed activation of the apical and central portions of the left ventricle, the thin right ventricular wall having been depolarized, with a resultant vector directed posteriorly, inferiorly, and to the left (0.04 sec); and, finally, (4) activation of the posterior basal portion of the left ventricle and septum, with a vector directed superiorly and posteriorly (0.06 sec).

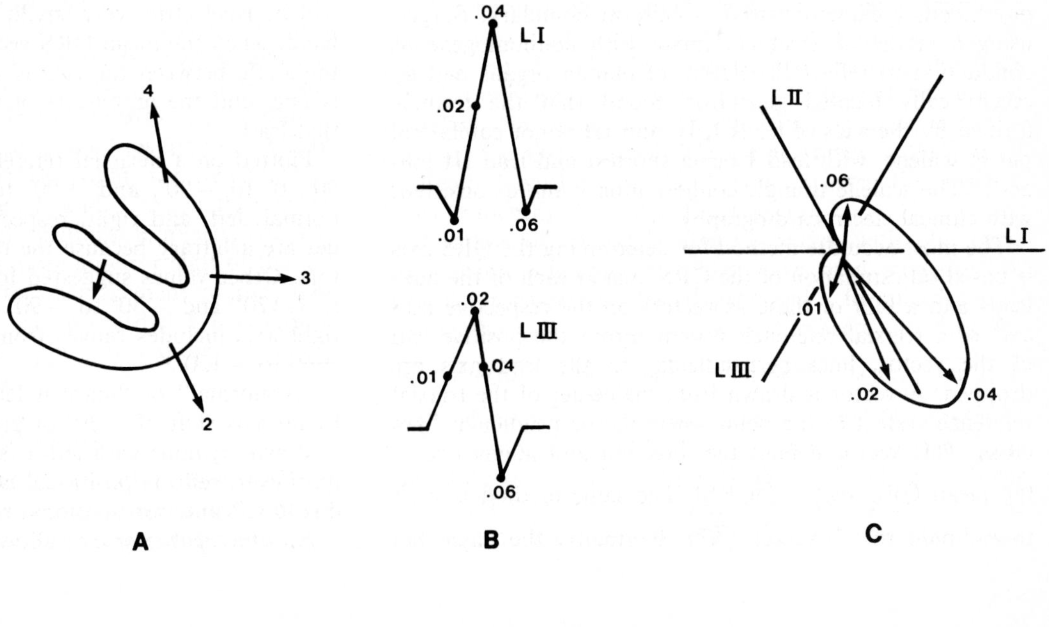

FIGURE 7–6 Correlation between the order of ventricular activation (*A*), scalar ECG (*B*), and vectorcardiogram (*C*). *A*, The sequence of ventricular activation is represented by four instantaneous frontal plane vectors. *B*, The four vectors plotted on leads I and III at the appropriate time during inscription of the QRS. *C*, Using the method of construction of vectors described in Figure 7–7, one can derive each of the four vectors in the frontal plane. A line joining the ends of the vectors results in a frontal plane QRS loop. The same method can be used to derive the orthogonal X, Y, and Z leads from the frontal, transverse, or sagittal planes. (Times given are in seconds.)

low or isoelectric in lead I, and tall—but more importantly, peaked or pointed—in leads II, III, and aV_f (Fig. 7–11*B*). P waves in leads V_{4r}, V_1, and V_2 may be upright and increased in amplitude. A P-wave axis greater than +90° with an isoelectric P wave in lead I is rarely, if ever, a normal finding (Fig. 7–11). In the adult the most common cause of right atrial abnormality is chronic obstructive lung disease. Nonspecificity of P pulmonale is suggested by the presence of the P pulmonale pattern in the absence of right atrial enlargement. Such P waves, termed "pseudo-P pulmonale," have been found in association with a variety of disorders of the left heart, including coronary artery disease with angina pectoris, and less often in the absence of heart disease. It has been suggested that in the presence of left heart disease, "pseudo-P pulmonale" reflects an increase of the left atrial component of the P waves.[58]

Left atrial abnormality is manifest by prolongation of the P wave, shortening or absence of the P-R segment, and a shift of the P vector to the left and posteriorly (Fig. 7–11 *A*). The duration of the P wave is 0.12 sec or longer, the wave is notched, and its axis is shifted to the left. Because

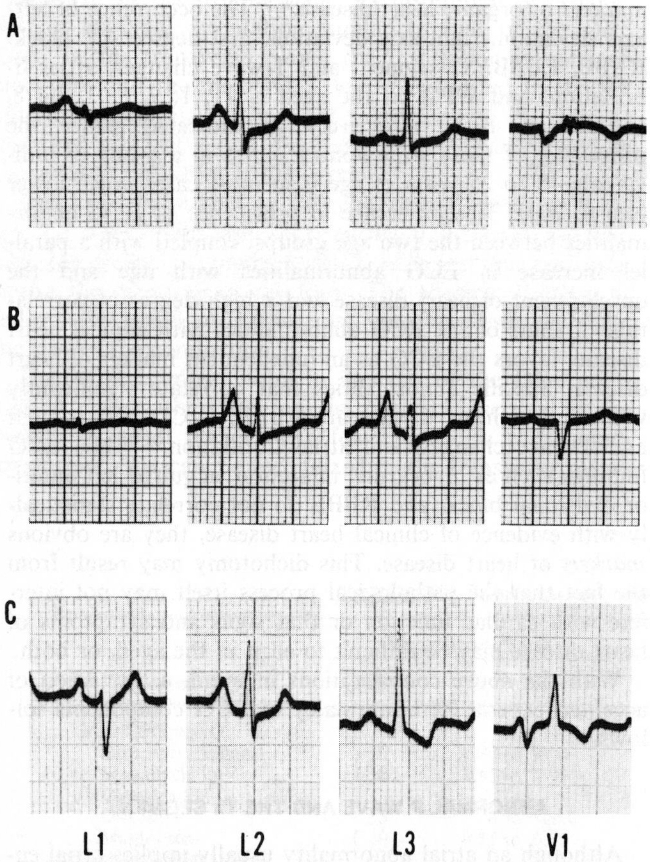

FIGURE 7–11 Atrial hypertrophy, *A*, Recording from a patient with mitral stenosis showing left atrial enlargement characterized by prolonged duration of the P wave, loss of the P-R segment, left-axis deviation of the P wave, and a negative orientation in lead V_1. A common feature not clearly visible in this tracing is notching of the P wave. *B*, Recording from a patient with chronic obstructive lung disease showing right atrial enlargement manifest by right-axis deviation of the P wave and a tall, peaked P wave in leads II and III. *C*, Recording from a patient with mitral stenosis showing biatrial enlargement manifest by a tall P wave in lead II, a notched P wave with left-axis deviation of the terminal component in lead III, and a pronounced large biphasic P wave in lead V_1.

the vector is increased in magnitude and oriented posteriorly, lead V_1 registers a prominent negative P wave. A negative P wave in lead V_1, 0.04 sec in duration and 1 mm in depth, is consistent with left atrial preponderance,[59] the so-called P mitrale. Although this abnormality is common in mitral valve disease, the most frequent cause is left ventricular disease, with the increased left ventricular end-diastolic pressure reflected in the atrium.

In *biatrial* enlargement, both anterior and posterior forces are increased. The abnormality includes a prominent initial part of the P wave coupled with the left axis of the terminal portion of the P wave and a biphasic P wave in leads V_1 and occasionally in V_2 (Fig. 7–11*C*).

In the presence of atrial fibrillation, atrial disease can occasionally be suspected from an analysis of the QRS complex. With severe tricuspid regurgitation, right atrial enlargement displaces the tricuspid valve down and to the left. As a result, lead V_1 (and sometimes V_2), normally subtended by the right ventricle, now reflects the intracavitary (qR) right atrial potential as indicated by QR, qR, or qrS complexes in leads V_1 or V_1 and V_2 followed by a normal progression of R-wave amplitude from leads V_2 or V_3 to V_6 (Fig. 7–12).[10]

Atrial enlargement can also be suspected when coarse, relatively large fibrillatory waves are present, especially in lead V_1. This is in contrast to atrial fibrillation complicating arteriosclerotic and hypertensive heart disease, in which the fibrillatory waves are fine and frequently unidentifiable.

In the VCG, the P loop parallels the changing direction of the maximal P vector.[37,38,60] In the transverse plane, *right atrial enlargement* is recognized when a major portion of the loop is displaced anteriorly. The inscription is counterclockwise. In the right sagittal plane, the loop is inscribed counterclockwise and is displaced anteriorly and inferiorly; the posteriorly located component remains unaltered. In the frontal plane, the loop is narrow and has a vertical orientation.

In the transverse plane, *left atrial enlargement* is inscribed in a counterclockwise direction or in the form of a figure-of-eight. With the exception of an initial component located anteriorly, the loop is shifted posteriorly and to the left. In the right sagittal plane, the loop is located more superiorly than normal and the major portion of the loop is located posteriorly; the inscription is clockwise. In the frontal plane, the loop is shifted to the left.

In *biatrial enlargement*, the horizontal plane loop inscribes both the increased early anterior and the late posterior components of the loop.

Intraatrial conduction abnormalities can result in enlargement of the loop in the absence of dilatation or hypertrophy. The loop displays localized conduction and anatomical abnormalities, the latter in the form of "notches" and "bites."[61]

Alteration of atrial repolarization (Ta), recognized by deviation from the T-P segment, can be either secondary or primary (Figs. 7–5 and 7–13). The usual pathological causes of secondary Ta-segment depression, which may exceed 1 mm (0.1 mV), include atrial dilation, hypertrophy, or intraatrial block. In chronic obstructive lung disease, for example, depression of the Ta segment may be exaggerated and mistaken for ST-segment displacement.

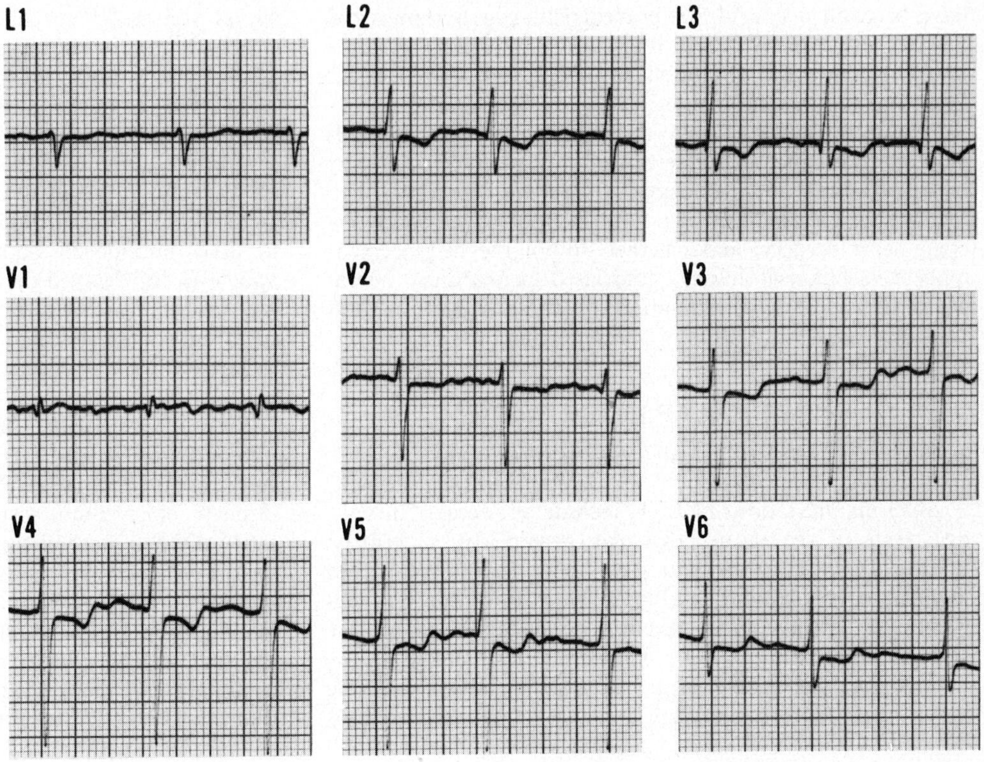

FIGURE 7–12 Rheumatic valvular heart disease with tricuspid regurgitation. The basic rhythm is atrial fibrillation. The right-axis deviation, "squatty" QRS in lead V_1, and clockwise rotation are consistent with mitral valve disease. The QR pattern in V_1 reflects the right atrial intracavitary potential and indicates a regurgitant tricuspid valve.

The usual causes of *primary* Ta-segment changes are pericarditis, atrial infarction, and atrial injury due to penetrating wounds. *Pericarditis* exaggerates the normally negative Ta-segment, and Ta-segment depression is recorded in all leads except aVR, in which it is elevated (Fig. 7–13).[24,62,63] Occasionally, a Ta-segment abnormality may be the only convincing evidence of acute pericarditis.

The incidence of *atrial infarction* in myocardial infarction is variously reported as 1 to 42 per cent.[62,63] Isolated atrial infarction in the absence of ventricular infarction is a most unlikely event. The manifestations of infarction may include elevation of the Ta segment in leads I, II, III, V_5, or V_6 or a depression that may exceed 1.5 mm in precordial leads and 1.0 mm in leads I, II, and III. Reciprocal Ta-segment changes may be present[64] (Fig. 7–5). Attempts to localize the site of atrial infarction electrocardiographically

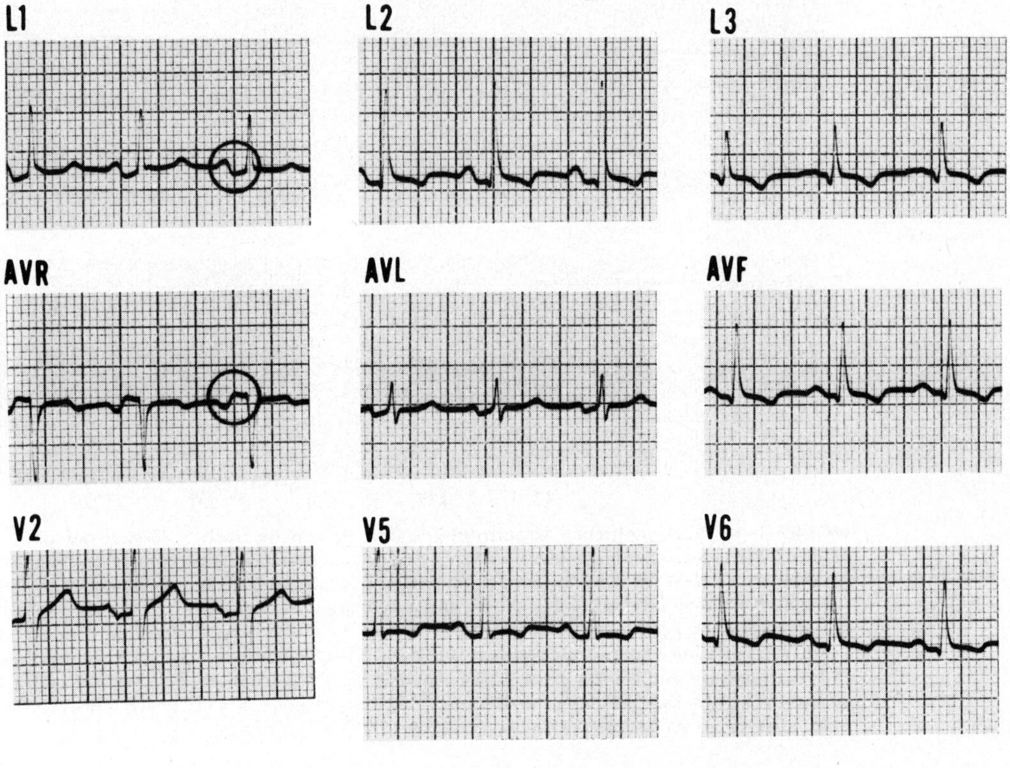

FIGURE 7–13 Acute pericarditis. The tracing shows sinus rhythm with nonspecific ST-segment and T-wave changes. The Ta segment is depressed in leads I, II, V_2, and V_5 and is elevated in lead aV_r. Ta displacement is the only change diagnostic of acute pericarditis.

have been unsuccessful.[65] Supraventricular arrhythmias frequently accompany atrial infarction. The ECG changes that occur in atrial infarction have been reproduced in the experimental animal.[5,66]

Penetrating injury of the atria due to gunshot wounds or perforation in the course of cardiac catheterization may be associated with diagnostic Ta-segment depression. Ta-segment displacement is also frequently observed following open heart surgery, and whether or not the displacement reflects mechanical injury, associated pericarditis, hemopericardium, or a combination of these factors is still unclear.

VENTRICULAR HYPERTROPHY

LEFT VENTRICULAR HYPERTROPHY (LVH)

ECG manifestations of LVH include an increase in voltage; shift of the mean QRS axis posteriorly, superiorly, and to the left; prolongation of depolarization (delayed intrinsicoid deflection); and gradual shift of the ST segment and T wave in a direction opposite to that of the QRS complex (Fig. 7–14). The exact mechanism of the voltage increase is not clear. In addition to the muscle mass, other factors may play a role, such as intracavitary blood volume,[67,68] proximity to the chest wall, conducting properties of intrathoracic organs, location of the heart within the thorax, intraventricular and transmural pressures, and perhaps unopposed inscription of a portion of the QRS complex due to delayed activation.

The left superior and posterior orientation of the mean QRS vector in LVH is most likely related to hypertrophy of the basal portion of the left ventricle with delayed, and at times unopposed, activation. Variables that may be responsible for delayed depolarization include increased muscle mass, decreased Purkinje activation, and localized intraventricular conduction delays. Marked superior orientation is noted in association with left anterior divisional block.

Prolongation of the excited state through the myocardium and prolongation of activation result in a change in the order of repolarization, which proceeds from endocardium to epicardium, resulting in a reversal of T-wave polarity. Of the mechanisms responsible for reversal of repolarization, increased muscle mass without a concomitant increase in the capillary bed—so-called relative coronary insufficiency—may be an important factor. It is also possible that as the muscle mass outgrows the Purkinje fiber mass, more of the activation proceeds through the myocardium, and this can contribute to a change in the T-wave

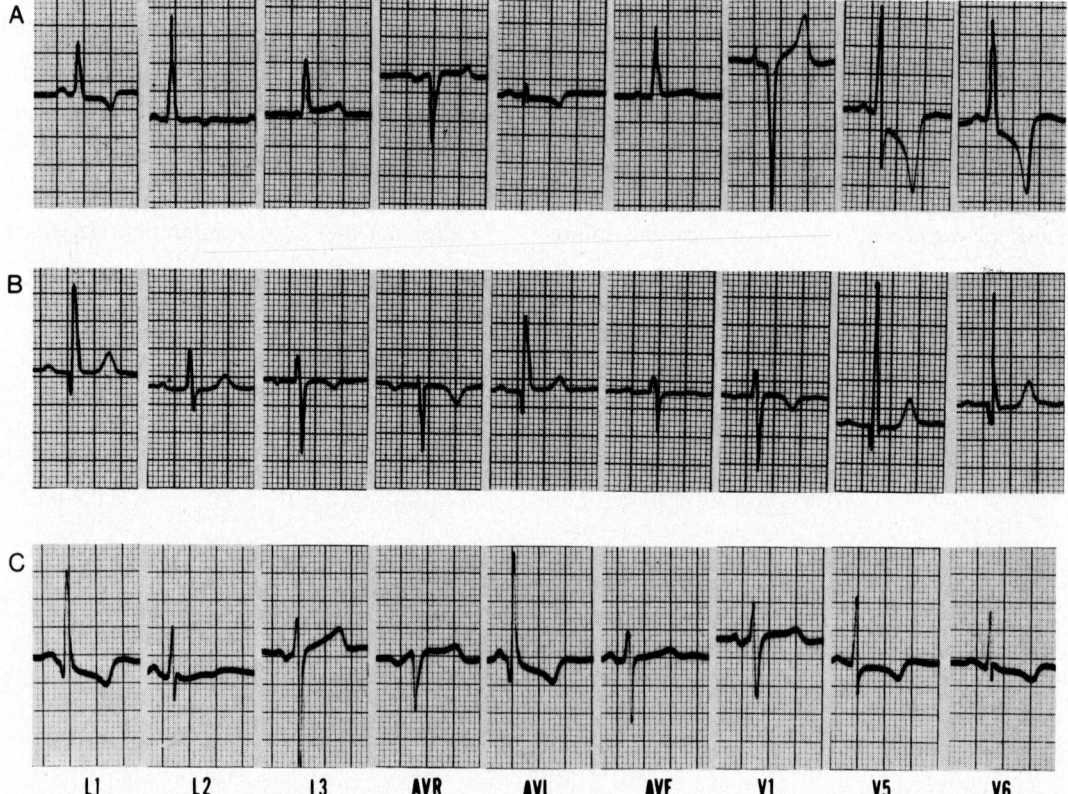

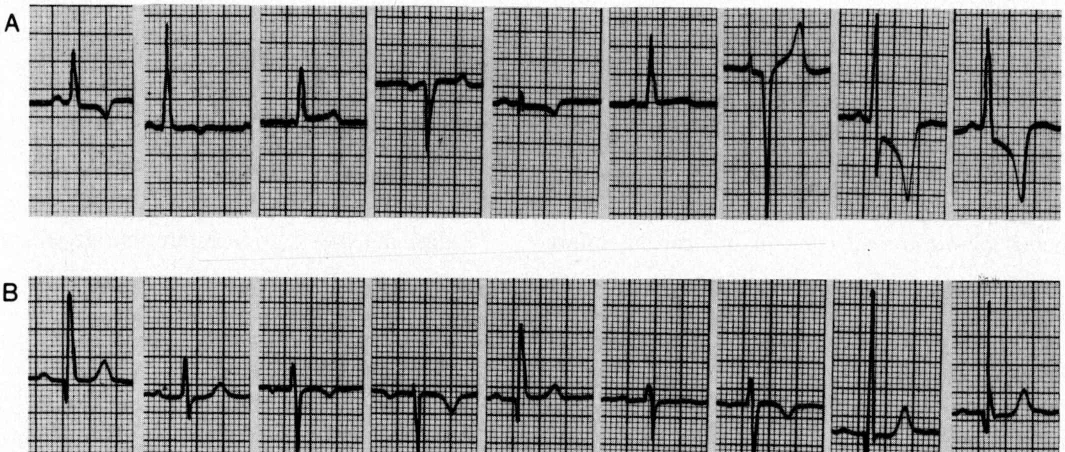

FIGURE 7–14 Left ventricular hypertrophy (LVH). *A*, Tracing from a 23-year-old patient with severe aortic stenosis. The precordial leads were obtained at one-half standard. The voltage and characteristic ST-T changes of LVH are evident. *B*, Tracing from a patient with acute aortic regurgitation due to endocarditis showing a prominent Q wave in leads I, aV_l, and V_5 and a prominent R wave in leads V_5 and V_6. Voltage criteria are consistent with LVH. Prominent Q waves reflect the diastolic overload. *C*, Tracing from a 37-year-old patient with aortic regurgitation demonstrates voltage and ST-T changes consistent with LVH as well as prominent Q waves in leads I and aV_l and a prominent R wave in lead V_1. These changes indicate a diastolic overload component of the LVH. Although prominent septal forces in the presence of LVH nearly always indicate a diastolic overload, absence of such Q waves does not rule out LVH of this type.

vector. ST-segment depression may be due to the onset of repolarization prior to the completion of depolarization.

The mean QRS vector, increased in magnitude and oriented toward the left, posteriorly and superiorly, results in a positive deflection in leads I, II, V_5, and V_6 and a positive or negative deflection in leads III and aV_f. The precordial transitional zone is shifted to the left. Leads V_1 and V_2 record an rS pattern, but in some instances the initial R wave may be absent for reasons that may remain obscure. Lack of the initial R wave may be erroneously interpreted as an anteroseptal myocardial infarction.

QRS voltage criteria for LVH include $R_I + S_{III} \geq 25$ mm, R in $aV_l > 12$ mm, R in $aV_f > 20$ mm, S in $V_1 \geq 24$ mm, R in V_5 or $V_6 > 26$ mm, R in V_5 or V_6 + S in $V_1 >$ 35 mm.[11,69] The following point system for diagnosing LVH has been suggested:[11,70]Amplitude of R or S wave in limb leads $\geq$ 20 mm *or* S_1 in V_1 or $V_2 \geq$ 30 mm *or* R wave in V_5 or $V_6 \geq$ 30 mm = 3 points. ST-segment changes with or without digitalis = 1 or 2 points, respectively. Left atrial enlargement = 3 points. Left-axis deviation −30° or more = 2 points. QRS duration $\geq$ 0.09 sec and intrinsicoid deflection in V_5 and $V_6 \geq$ 0.05 sec = 1 point each. Left ventricular hypertrophy is considered to be likely if the points total 4 and to be present if the total is 5 or more. The diagnosis of LVH is strengthened by a delayed intrinsicoid deflection in lead V_5 or V_6, measuring more than 0.05 sec in the adult. The ST segment and T wave are directed opposite to the QRS complex. Characteristically, the T wave is negative and asymmetrical, its ascending limb being steeper, with occasional terminal positive inscription (Fig. 7–14). The J point and the ST segment are depressed in leads I, aV_l, V_5, and V_6. T-wave inversion is greater in lead V_6 than in V_4. In the presence of a vertical position, the above changes are recorded in leads II, III, and aV_f. Left atrial preponderance is found frequently in LVH.

The shortcomings of the ECG in terms of sensitivity and specificity in the diagnosis of LVH have long been recognized.[71] This is true for both the voltage and the point systems. On the one hand, autopsy data indicate that voltage consistent with LVH can be present in patients without myocardial hypertrophy,[72] while on the other hand, normal ECG values were recorded in about 40 to 50 per cent of patients with LVH, based on echocardiographic findings.[71] This is not surprising, since the ECG reflects an electrical current and only indirectly an anatomical change, and the magnitude of this current is subject to a variety of influences discussed earlier. Furthermore, it is often difficult to differentiate between a delayed intrinsicoid deflection and conduction abnormalities due to focal delays and blocks. Left-axis deviation of less than −30° is of little help in the diagnosis of LVH. Similarly, an axis greater than −30° is often due to intraventricular conduction manifest because of left anterior divisional block and may not be related to LVH. The sensitivity and specificity of the ECG criteria for LVH improve when more than one criterion is applied. An ECG diagnosis of LVH in patients with cardiac disorders that are likely to result in such hypertrophy is secure when the abnormal QRS voltage is accompanied by ST-segment and T-wave changes in the absence of abnormalities that alone may induce these changes.

The concept of *diastolic overload* is found by the author to be clinically useful at times.[73] It may point to such lesions as patent ductus arteriosus, ventricular septal defect, or aortic or mitral valve regurgitation. The ECG pattern is one of LVH but with a prominent Q wave in the leads facing the left side of the septum, namely, I, aV_l, V_5, and V_6, and a reciprocal, prominent R wave in the leads facing the right side of the septum, namely, V_1 and V_2. As a rule, the Q wave is narrow, measuring 0.025 sec or less, and its depth is 2 mm or greater. The concept of systolic or "pressure" overload, characterized by high-amplitude R waves and ST-segment and T-wave changes in the left ventricular leads and present in disorders with an increased resistance to left ventricular outflow, is of limited usefulness (Fig. 7–14).

The VCG changes in LVH are due to an increase in and rotation of the forces further to the left and posteriorly. These events are best reflected in the transverse plane. The VCG loop is increased in magnitude, elongated, inscribed counterclockwise as a rule, and shifted posteriorly. The occasional posterior orientation of the initial part of the loop simulates anteroseptal myocardial infarction. The termination of the loop is anterior, to the right, and superior to the origin of the loop. The loop is therefore open, and this displacement accounts for the ST-segment shift. Secondary T-wave changes shift the T loop to a direction opposite to that of the QRS loop, namely, anteriorly, to the right, and superiorly.[38,74,75]

RIGHT VENTRICULAR HYPERTROPHY (RVH)

In contrast to LVH, RVH is not simply an exaggeration of the normal. For RVH to become manifest, the right ventricular mass must be sufficiently large to overcome the left ventricular forces. For this reason, the specificity of the ECG pattern of RVH is much greater but the sensitivity is relatively low, varying from 25 to 40 per cent depending on the criteria used.[76] While the ECG changes of RVH result largely from the chamber's anatomical dominance, the etiology of the heart disease and associated hemodynamic alterations often contribute to the abnormal ECG pattern. At times, the etiology of the cardiac disorder and the severity of right ventricular pressure can be estimated from an analysis of the ECG.

In RVH the axis shifts to the right, the degree of axis deviation varying with the clinical disorder, and this is accompanied by vertical position and clockwise rotation. Based on the QRS pattern in lead V_1, RVH can generally be separated into three groups, namely, a dominant R wave (R, qR rR, rsR′) (Fig. 7–15), RS (Rs, Rsr′), and rS or rsr′ complex. The different QRS patterns may provide a clue to the degree of elevation in right ventricular pressure. In general a qR complex, a prominent R wave with a slur on the upstroke, or an rsr′ complex (incomplete RBBB) suggest that right ventricular pressure exceeds, is equal to, or is lower than left ventricular pressure, respectively. Examples include severe pulmonary stenosis or primary pulmonary hypertension, tetralogy of Fallot or Eisenmenger complex and atrial septal defect, respectively. In the latter, hypertrophy of the outflow tract of the right ventricle is responsible for the r′ wave.

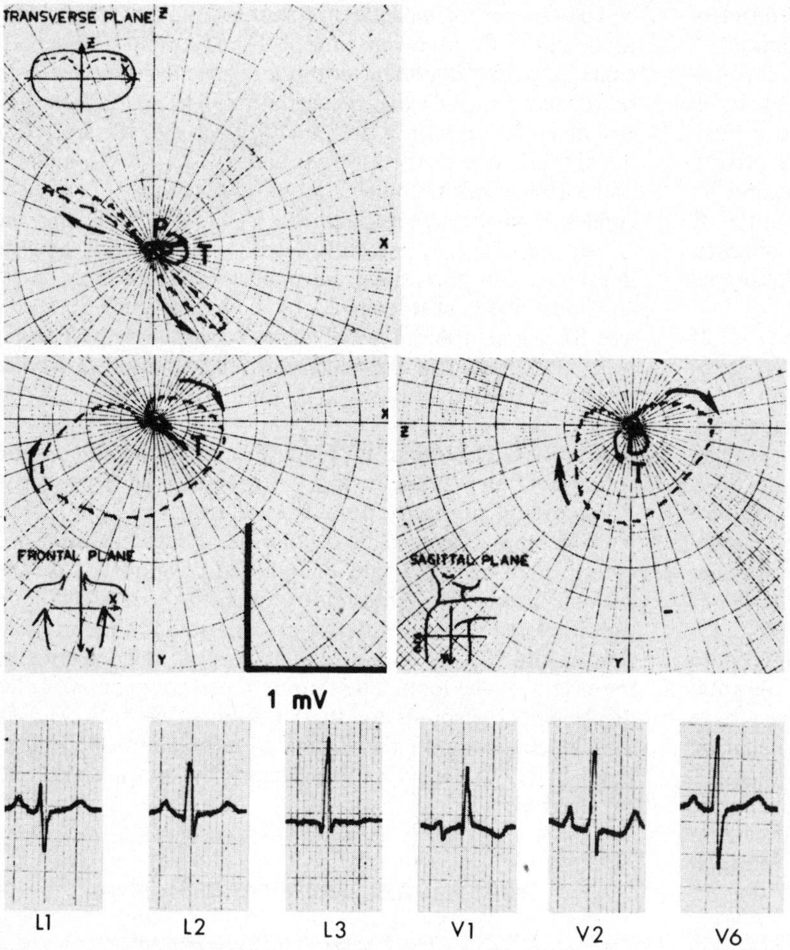

FIGURE 7–15 Right ventricular hypertrophy (RVH). In the transverse plane of the VCG, anterior and rightward displacement of the mid and late portions of the QRS loop with a figure-of-eight inscription can be seen. In the frontal plane, the QRS loop is inscribed clockwise and displaced to the right. In the sagittal plane, the loop is inscribed clockwise and displaced anteriorly. The T-wave loop is inscribed counterclockwise. The time scale is the same for all VCG. The loop is interrupted every 2.5 msec, as indicated by each dot or comma. The ECG illustrates the classic pattern of moderately severe to severe RVH (see text).

In the presence of RVH the delay of ventricular activation results in earlier recovery of the endocardium, and repolarization proceeds from endocardium to epicardium. The ST segment is thereby depressed and the T wave inverted in lead V_1 and occasionally in V_2. Significant ST-segment depression and T-wave inversion is, as a rule, indicative of moderate or severe hypertension.

In the adult with acquired RVH the most commonly encountered ECG changes include right-axis deviation and an R/S ratio $\geq$ 1 in V_1, with an R wave 5 mm or greater. Isolated right-axis deviation in excess of +100° to −90° is considered by some to be indicative of RVH,[77] but this criterion alone is less sensitive. The R/S ratio in lead V_1 alone is not diagnostic of RVH, since it may be recorded in patients with a posterior infarction or occasionally in the absence of heart disease. In the normal subject, an R/S ratio greater than 1 in lead V_1 may also be accompanied by right-axis deviation.

ECG changes due to acute pulmonary embolus with pulmonary hypertension (acute cor pulmonale) and chronic obstructive lung disease often differ from the classic pattern seen in RVH and will be discussed separately.

ACUTE PULMONARY EMBOLUS (ACUTE COR PULMONALE) (see also p. 1578). The most characteristic ECG feature of this disorder is probably the transient nature of the changes (Fig. 7–16). The ECG changes are most likely related to acute pulmonary hypertension with right atrial and ventricular dilatation, hypoxia, and perhaps myocardial ischemia. From time to time, the changes include P pulmonale; right-axis deviation with clockwise rotation; an S1, S2, or S3 pattern; complete or incomplete RBBB; or T-wave inversion in the right precordial and inferior leads. T-wave changes may last a few days, while the axis deviation, clockwise rotation, and RBBB may persist as long as 1 to 3 weeks. The acute atrial dilatation coupled with myocardial ischemia is probably responsible for the frequent atrial arrhythmias. Sensitivity and specificity of the ECG in diagnosis of acute cor pulmonale is relatively low; this test is diagnostic in about 25 per cent of patients. Both transient T-wave alterations and the RBBB, although nonspecific and frequently seen in a variety of chronic cardiac disorders, are of diagnostic value when accompanied by a clinical picture suggestive of acute cor pulmonale.

CHRONIC OBSTRUCTIVE LUNG DISEASE (COLD) AND COR PULMONALE (see also p. 1592). The ECG pattern of COLD and COLD with pulmonary hypertension (cor pulmonale) can be ascribed to a combination of positional changes, increased lung volume, and RVH. ECG changes include right-axis deviation of the P wave, increased amplitude and "peaked" appearance of the P wave in the limb leads, and "peaked" and biphasic morphology wave in lead V_1 (Fig. 7–11, p. 208). A P-wave axis of +90° is highly suggestive of COLD. Because of the large P-wave area, the Ta segment is exaggerated and occasionally interpreted as ST-segment depression. Right-axis deviation and clockwise rotation are characteristic find-

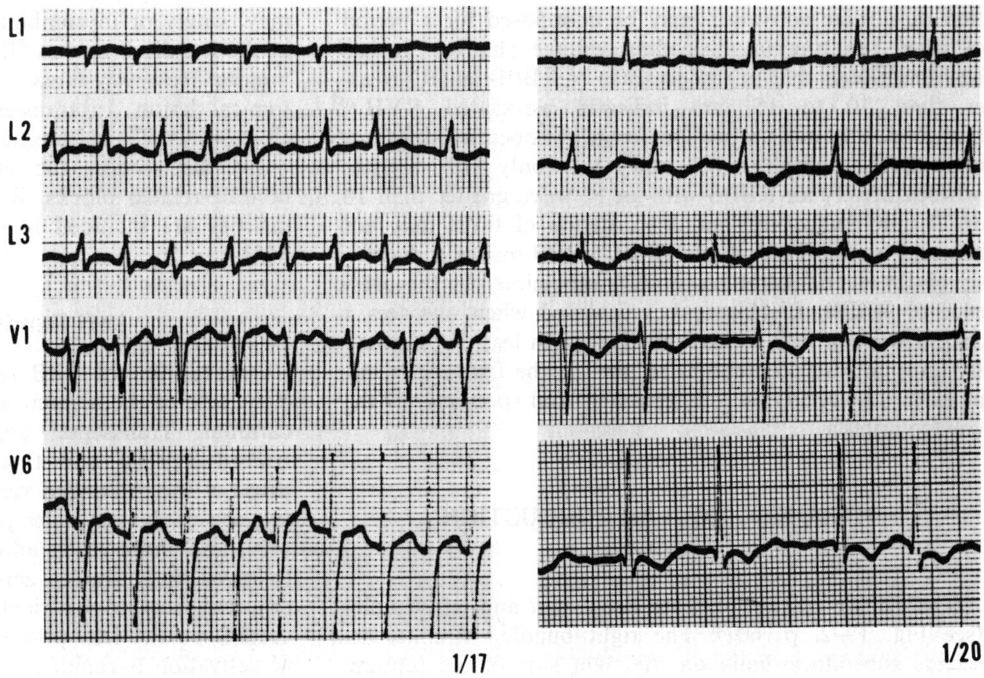

FIGURE 7–16 Acute pulmonary embolus. The basic rhythm is atrial fibrillation. On 1/17 the ventricular rate was about 150 bpm, with the axis shifted to the right and an RS pattern in lead V_6. On 1/20 this rate slowed to about 75 to 100 bpm. The axis and QRS complex in V_6 are both normal.

ings. Occasionally, an S1, S2, S3 pattern may be present. Amplitude of the precordial R wave is reduced in leads V_5 and V_6, often measuring less than 7 mm. When the clockwise rotation is marked, absence of the R wave in precordial leads simulates an anterior myocardial infarction. With progression to pulmonary hypertension and RVH, prominent R waves may appear in leads V_1 and V_2. These changes are probably due to unopposed late activation of the crista terminalis and right ventricular free wall. Right atrial dilatation is probably responsible for the QR pattern in V_1, with the Q wave reflecting right atrial intracavitary potential (as occurs also in tricuspid regurgitation (Fig. 7–12, p. 209). As indicated, the sensitivity of the ECG for cor pulmonale is relatively low, the test being diagnostic in about 25 to 40 per cent of patients with confirmed RVH.[76]

In *biventricular hypertrophy,* the LV forces are dominant and often obscure the RVH.

In RVH, the characteristic VCG changes of the QRS loop are recorded in the transverse plane, with three general patterns recognized (Fig. 7–17). In type A, the loop is inscribed clockwise, occasionally in a figure-of-eight (Fig. 7–15), and is positioned in the right and left anterior quadrants. In type B, the loop is inscribed clockwise, or counterclockwise, is often figure-of-eight, and is located primarily in the left anterior and to a lesser extent in the left and right posterior quadrants. In type C, the loop is inscribed counterclockwise, with 50 per cent of the loop located in posterior left and right quadrants. Of the three, type A usually reflects severe RVH, while type B is most often encountered in patients with atrial septal defect and mitral stenosis. Type C can be recorded with chronic obstructive lung disease.[78,79]

VENTRICULAR HYPERTROPHY IN THE PRESENCE OF CONDUCTION DEFECTS. The diagnosis of ventricular hypertrophy in the presence of BBB is difficult, if not impossible, owing in part to the fact that a por-

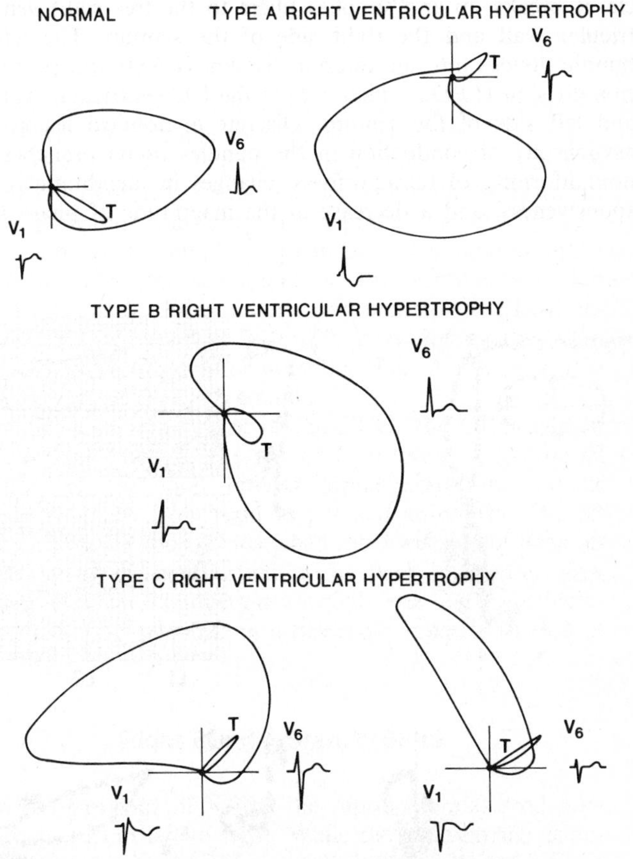

FIGURE 7–17 Diagrammatic representation of the three common, but not exclusive, VCG patterns of right ventricular hypertrophy recorded in the horizontal plane. When compared with the normal, the QRS loops are located in the right and left anterior quadrants in Type A and in the left anterior and to a lesser extent left and right posterior quadrants in Type B; a major portion of the loop is located in the left and right posterior quadrants in Type C. (Modified from Chou, T. C., Helm, R. A., and Kaplan, S.: Clinical Vectorcardiography. 2nd ed. New York, Grune and Stratton, 1974, pp. 87, 99, and 102.)

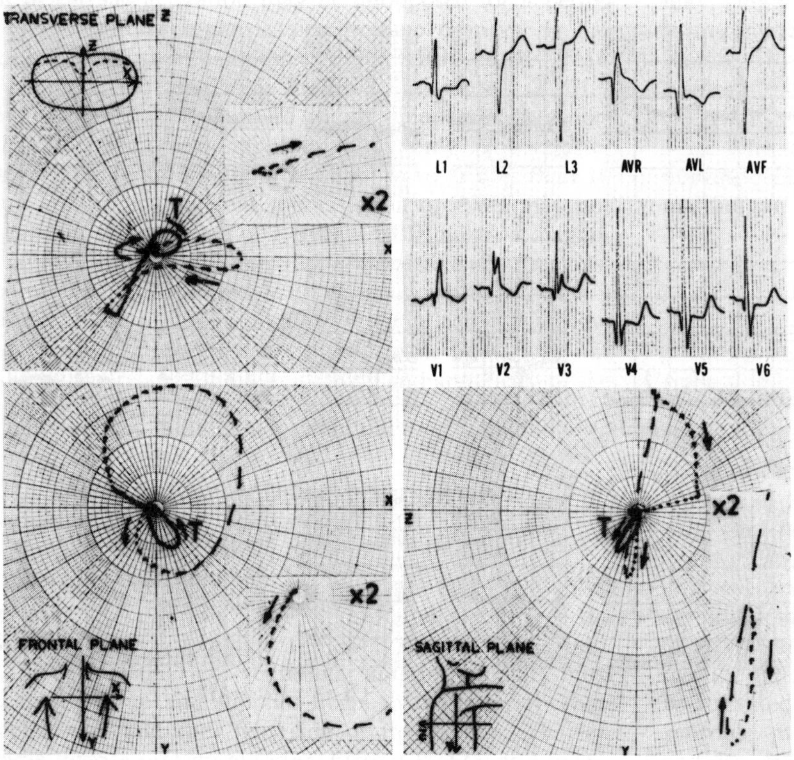

FIGURE 7–20 The ECG illustrates an anterior myocardial infarction, RBBB, and left anterior divisional block (LADB). In the transverse plane, the VCG displays an initial QRS force directed to the right and slightly anteriorly with a clockwise inscription. The decrease in the anteriorly directed initial QRS force is due to the infarction. A delayed terminal QRS loop exhibiting a figure-of-eight inscription is displaced anteriorly. The terminal, anteriorly directed, slowly inscribed part of the loop is due to RBBB. The clockwise-inscribed T-wave loop is oriented in a direction opposite to that of the main QRS force. In the frontal plane, the initial QRS is directed to the right and inferiorly. The loop is inscribed counterclockwise and is displaced superiorly and to the left. The superior and leftward displacement of the loop is due to LADB. The delayed terminal QRS forces are shifted superiorly and to the right. In the sagittal plane, the initial QRS loop is directed inferiorly and slightly anteriorly, with a decrease of the initial anteriorly directed QRS force. The delayed terminal loop is displaced anteriorly and superiorly. The initial portion of the QRS loop is displayed at two times the standard (× 2).

vation of the right ventricle is directed to the right, anteriorly, and either superiorly, inferiorly, or horizontally.

The characteristic ECG changes of RBBB are recorded in lead V_1. The initial normal septal activation inscribes an R wave, followed by an S wave reflecting left ventricular activation and a final R′ wave due to depolarization of the right ventricle from left to right and anteriorly. The depth of the S wave in lead V_1 will vary depending on whether the left ventricular activation generates a more posteriorly or anteriorly oriented vector. In the former, a prominent S wave will separate the R wave from R′ wave, while in the latter, the S wave may be shallow or a slur or, indeed, may be absent. Leads facing the left side of the septum, namely, I, aV_l, V_5, and V_6, record an initial Q wave followed by an R wave of normal duration and a prolonged, relatively shallow S wave. The latter reflects delayed activation of the right ventricle (Figs. 7–20 to 7–22).

The T wave is usually inverted in lead V_1 and occasionally in V_2, while it is upright in the remaining precordial and limb leads.

The characteristic VCG feature is evident in the transverse plane and consists of a slowly inscribed termi-

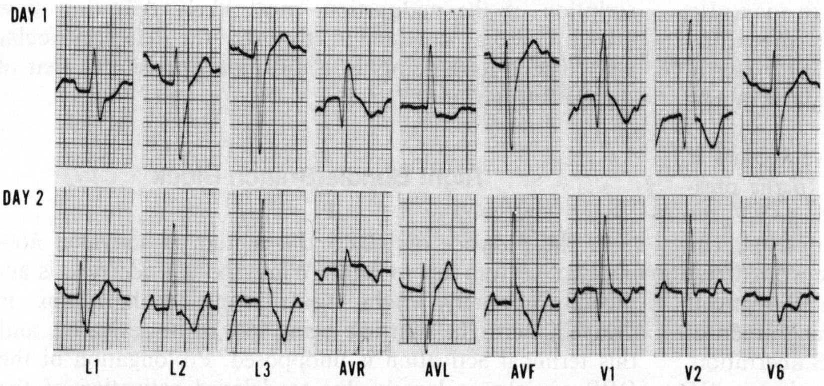

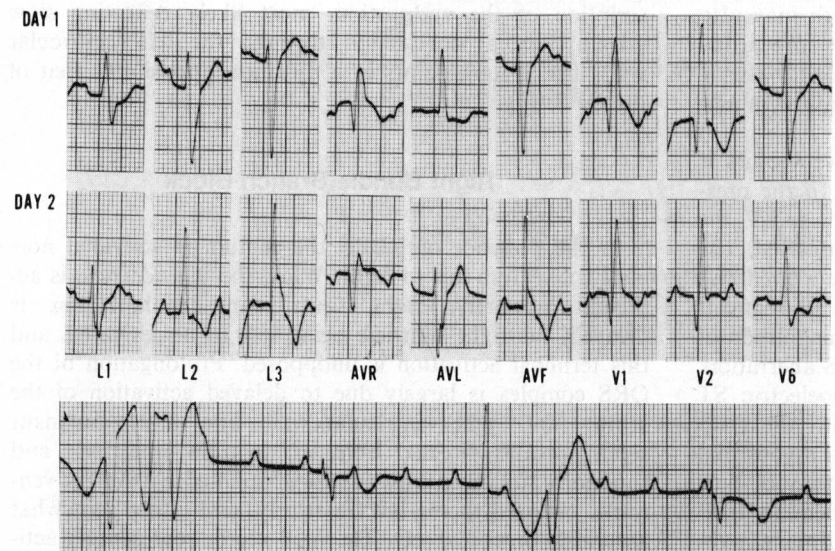

FIGURE 7–21 Acute anterior myocardial infarction complicated by RBBB, LADB, left posterior divisional block (LPDB), and complete AV block. On day 1, the ECG records a sinus rhythm; LADB in leads I, II, and III; RBBB in leads V_1 and V_2; and anterior myocardial infarction manifest by a deep Q wave in leads V_1 and V_2. On day 2, the RBBB and anterior infarction are again noted, but with LPDB recorded in leads I, II, and III. The LPDB is indicated by shift of axis to the right, as estimated on the basis of the initial 0.08 sec of the QRS and the appearance of Q waves and tall R waves in leads II, III, and aV_f. Complete AV block, ventricular premature beats, prolonged Q-T interval, and deeply inverted T waves are recorded in row 3.

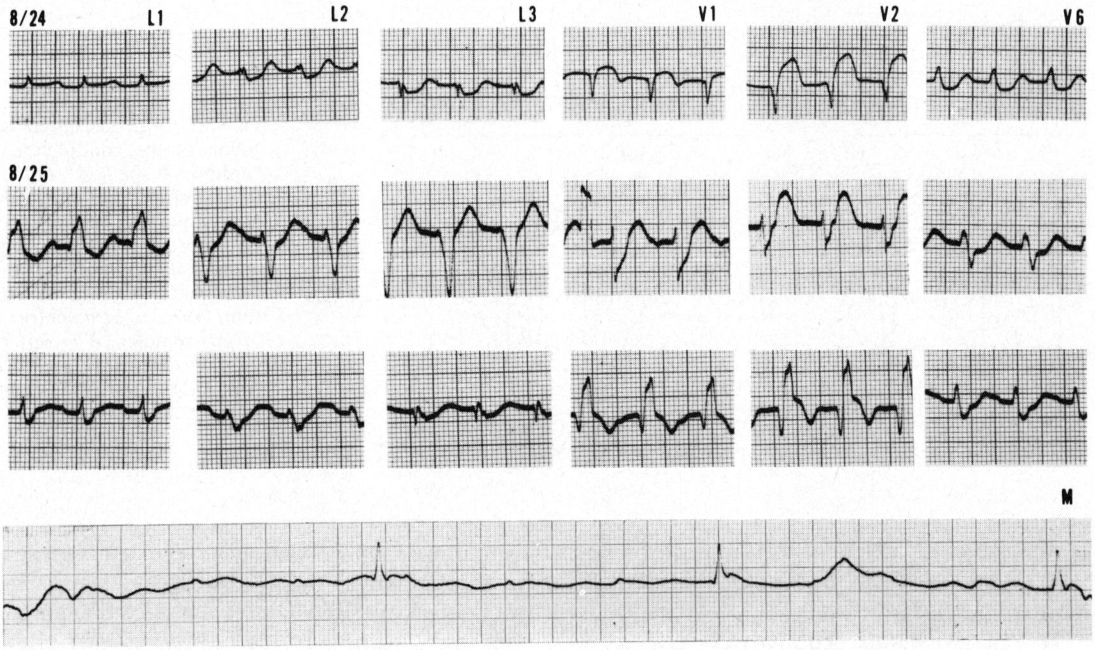

FIGURE 7–22 Acute anterior myocardial infarction complicated by alternating bundle branch block. On 8/24, the acute anterior myocardial infarction is manifest by a QS pattern with elevation of the ST segment in leads V_1 and V_2 and reciprocal ST-segment depression in leads II, III, and V_6. On 8/25, row 2, the pattern is that of LBBB, which obscures the myocardial infarction; in row 3, RBBB and acute anterior myocardial infarction are present. This is followed by complete AV block with an idioventricular rate of about 25 bpm. (M=monitor lead.)

nal appendage directed to the right and anteriorly. The initial septal and left ventricular portion of the loop is normal (Fig. 7–20).[87,88]

Divisional (Fascicular) Blocks

The ventricular conduction system, including the right bundle branch and the two divisions of the left bundle, can be considered for purposes of clinical electrocardiography to consist of three divisions (fascicles) (Fig. 7–23). Some accept the existence of the midseptal "branch" and thus a four-divisional system. However, only patterns consistent with left anterior divisional and left posterior divisional block are recognizable in the ECG. Divisional blocks are, with rare exception, acquired.[33]

According to some investigators, evidence for the existence of anatomically discrete divisions of the left bundle branch is not convincing. However, experimental data tend to support a functional divisional conduction system.[89,90] Furthermore, synchronous endocardial activation at three sites, namely, the anterior right, anterior, and posterior paraseptal areas, is consistent with the concept of existence of functional divisions of the left bundle. This concept is also supported by distinctive and predictable ECG patterns. Thus, from the ECG standpoint, the concept of divisions of the left bundle is a useful one.[91,92]

BLOCK OF ANTERIOR DIVISION OF THE LEFT BUNDLE BRANCH (ANTERIOR FASCICULAR BLOCK). In the presence of left anterior divisional block, the initial septal activation proceeds inferiorly, anteriorly, to the right, and occasionally to the left. This is followed by activation of inferior and apical areas with the vector oriented inferiorly, to the left, and anteriorly. Final activation is that of the anterolateral and posterobasal left ventricular wall, the vector oriented superiorly, posteriorly, and to the left.

The resultant ECG pattern is characteristic (Fig. 7–23). Lead I records a dominant R wave, with or without an initial Q wave. The presence or absence of a Q wave depends on whether the initial septal activation is directed to the right or to the left. Since the initial activation is directed inferiorly, leads II, III, and aV_f inscribe an R wave followed by a deep S wave reflecting activation of the anterolateral and posterobasal segments of the left ventricle. The QRS axis varies from −30° to −90° (Figs. 7–20, 7–21, 7–24, and 7–25).

The precordial transitional zone is frequently displaced to the left. The amplitude of the R wave is diminished, with a prominent S wave in V_5 and V_6 reflecting the superior orientation of the mean left ventricular vector. The S wave is exaggerated when the final order of activation is directed to the right. Because of the inferior orientation of the initial vector, the midprecordial leads may register an initial Q wave. Such patterns could be mistaken for anteroseptal myocardial infarction[93] were it not for the fact that an R wave is recorded when the leads are placed an interspace lower. The T waves are normally upright except in lead aV_r and occasionally in leads aV_l and V_1.

Of the three VCG planes, the frontal is the most useful for visualization of left anterior divisional block (Fig. 7–26). The inscription of the loop is counterclockwise, initially directed to the right and inferiorly, with the major and remaining portion of the loop displaced superiorly. The superior orientation reflects activation of the anterior and lateral left ventricular wall.[38,92–95] Left anterior divisional block is nearly always an acquired abnormality and thus a

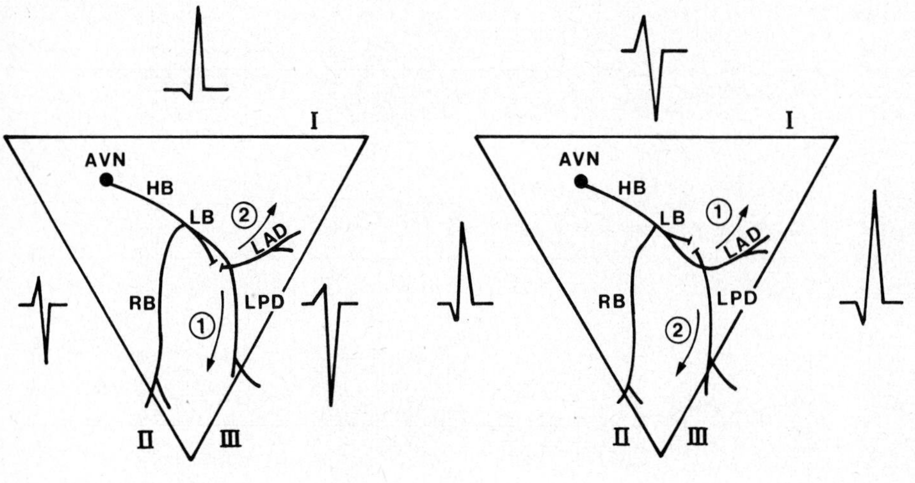

FIGURE 7–23 Diagrammatic representation of the conduction system. Interruption of the LAD (*left*) results in an initial inferior (*1*) followed by a dominant superior (*2*) direction of activation; interruption of the LPD (*right*) results in an initial superior (*1*) followed by a dominant inferior (*2*) direction of activation. AVN = atrioventricular node; HB = His bundle; LB = left bundle; RB = right bundle; LAD = left anterior division; LPD = left posterior division.

marker of organic disease. Often, however, it is present without clinical evidence of heart disease, but the prognosis depends on the underlying disease.

BLOCK OF POSTERIOR DIVISION OF THE LEFT BUNDLE BRANCH (POSTERIOR FASCICULAR BLOCK). Left posterior divisional block is a rare finding and its pattern is nonspecific. It can be recorded in asthenic individuals and patients with emphysema, RVH, and extensive lateral infarction.[91] Diagnosis is secure only if a normal ECG is recorded prior to appearance of the block.

In the presence of left posterior divisional block, activation begins in the midseptal and paraseptal areas, with the vector directed to the left, anteriorly, and superiorly. This is followed by activation of the left ventricular anterior and anterolateral walls, with the vector directed to the left and anteriorly. Final activation is of the inferior and posterior walls with the vector directed inferiorly, posteriorly, and to the right. In the limb leads, the initial superior and left orientation of septal vectors is reflected as an R wave in lead I and a narrow, 0.025-msec Q wave in leads II, III, and aV_f. The R wave in lead I is small and is followed by a deep S wave reflecting the inferior, posterior, and right orientation of the wave of activation (Figs. 7–21 and 7–23). The initial superior force and final inferior force result in a QR complex in leads II, III, and aV_f. The frontal axis varies from about +90° to +120°, or perhaps +80° to +140°. The T wave is usually normal.

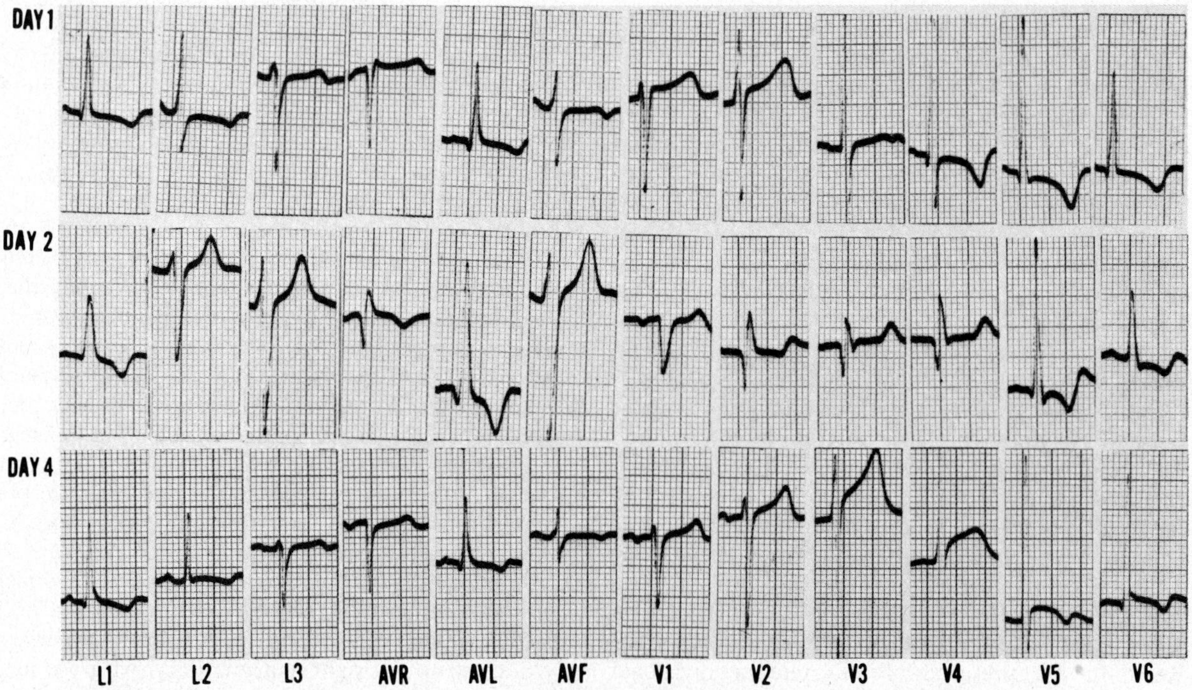

FIGURE 7–24 Transient Q waves and left anterior divisional block (LADB) recorded after aortic valve surgery. On day 1, nonspecific ST-segment and T-wave changes and voltage consistent with LVH are recorded. On day 2, LADB and prolongation of the QRS are accompanied by a Q wave in leads V_1 to V_4. On day 4, the QRS duration is normal, and LADB and Q waves are no longer present.

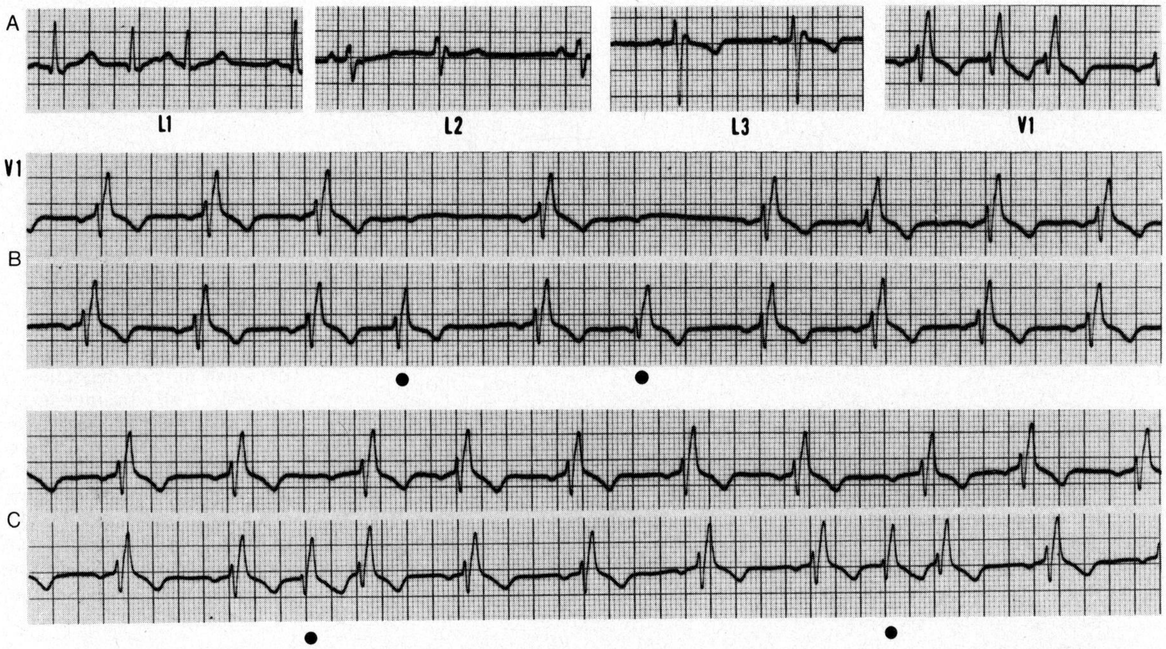

FIGURE 7–25 Concealed junctional discharge manifest as Mobitz (Type II) AV block and intermittent prolongation of the P-R interval. *A*, Normal sinus rhythm interrupted by supraventricular premature complexes, left anterior divisional block, and RBBB. *B*, Mobitz (Type II) AV block due to concealed junctional discharge. The mechanism is supported by the presence of manifest junctional prematures in the second tracing (solid circles). *C*, Isolated, unexpected P-R prolongation (upper tracing) is due to concealed junctional discharge, as suggested by manifest interpolated premature junctional complexes with similar prolongation of the P-R interval in the lower tracing. (Solid circles = manifest junctional impulses.)

In the frontal plane of the VCG, the inscription is clockwise, initially superior and to the left, but with the major portion of the loop located in the right inferior quadrant.[92,96]

RIGHT BUNDLE BRANCH BLOCK AND DIVISIONAL BLOCKS. RBBB with left anterior divisional block is the most common combination of the left divisional and bundle branch blocks. The activation during the first 0.08 sec determines the axis and identifies the left anterior divisional block. The delay of depolarization due to RBBB results in a final activation of the right ventricle to the right and anteriorly (Figs. 7–21 and 7–25).

RBBB with left posterior divisional block is a rare combination. The initial 0.08 sec defines the axis and divisional block while the final delayed activation, oriented to the right and anteriorly, reflects RBBB (Fig. 7–21).

Block of the right bundle and both divisions of the left bundle (trifascicular block) can be entertained in the presence of RBBB with alternating left anterior and posterior divisional blocks. Such patterns are usually associated with Mobitz (type II) AV block. It has been suggested that RBBB with either of these hemiblocks and a prolonged P-R interval may be a manifestation of trifascicular block. Although the prolonged P-R interval may be due to delayed conduction in the remaining division, the delay may also reflect AV nodal delay.[97]

The VCG records the characteristic terminal portion of the RBBB loop in the transverse plane, while the left anterior divisional block[94,98] and left posterior hemiblock[98,99] are best visualized in the frontal plane. The characteristic features of RBBB and left anterior divisional block with and without RBBB are shown in Figures 7–20 and 7–26. An initial inferior with rapid upward displacement of the loop or an initial superior with rapid inferior displacement in the frontal plane is recorded with left anterior or left posterior divisional block, respectively. A terminal and delayed activation to the right and anteriorly in the transverse plane is the characteristic finding in RBBB.

NONSPECIFIC INTRAVENTRICULAR CONDUCTION DEFECT (IVCD). The QRS complex may be abnormally prolonged but without the characteristic pattern of either RBBB or LBBB. Such conduction delays are referred to as "nonspecific" IVCD. These often resemble LBBB or LBBB with an abnormal left-axis deviation, a combination suggesting left anterior hemiblock with peripheral conduction delay. Presence of a normal Q wave supports peripheral delay as the cause of QRS prolongation. Although such a nonspecific prolongation may be due to drugs or electrolyte abnormalities, it is most often due to organic heart disease.

BILATERAL BUNDLE BRANCH BLOCK. This diagnosis can be entertained when alternating RBBB and LBBB are present. Any other combination of conduction delays cannot be differentiated from block in the AV junction. For example, block in both bundles results in complete AV block. Similarly, intermittent delay or block in one bundle and complete block of conduction in the contralateral bundle will manifest either as bundle branch block with a prolonged P-R interval or intermittent AV block. In the presence of BBB, a superimposed AV block due to failure of conduction in the contralateral bundle branch cannot be differentiated from block in the AV junction (Fig. 7–22).[100]

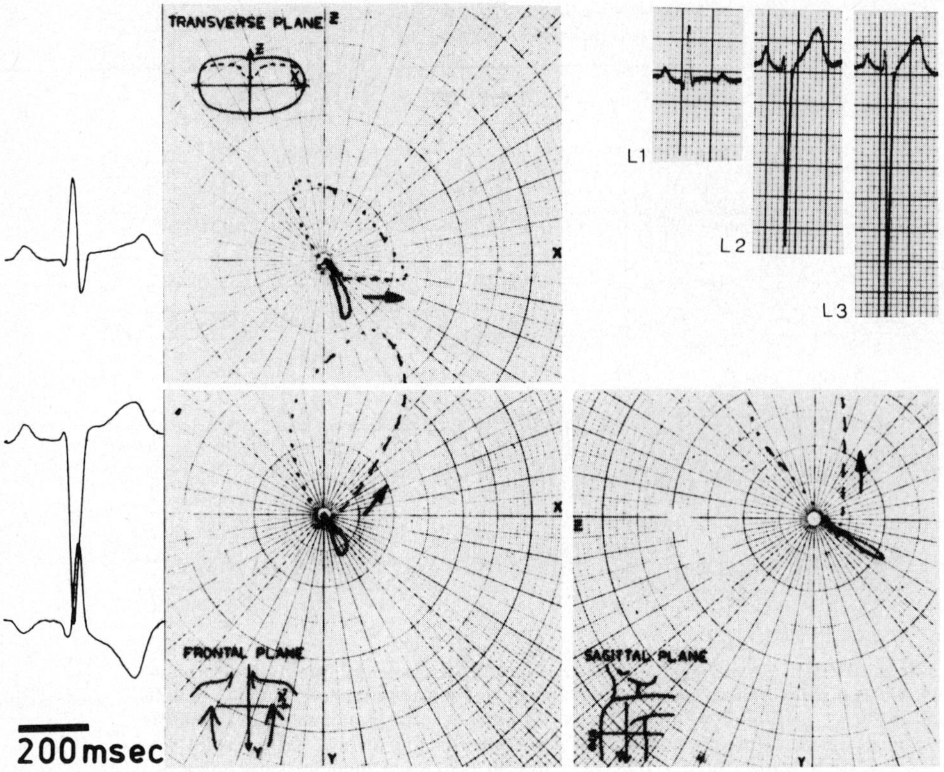

FIGURE 7–26 Left anterior divisional block and left ventricular hypertrophy (LVH). The ECG pattern of qR in lead I and rS in leads II and III indicates presence of left anterior divisional block. The diagnostic VCG features of left anterior divisional block are an initial small inferior deflection with rapid superior and counterclockwise displacement of the loop in the frontal plane, and the major area of the loop located in the left upper quadrant. LVH is suggested on ECG by the ST-T changes in lead I and the QRS voltage in leads II and III. On the VCG, LVH is indicated by posterior displacement of the loop in the horizontal plane.

Wolff-Parkinson-White (WPW) Syndrome

(See also pp. 628 and 712)

WPW, or preexcitation,[101,102] is an electrocardiographic syndrome characterized by a short P-R ($\leq$0.12 sec) interval, prolonged QRS ($\geq$0.12 sec) complex, a slur on the upstroke of the QRS (delta wave), and (as a rule) a normal P-J interval (Figs. 7–27, 7–28). Secondary ST-segment and T-wave changes are nearly always present. Ectopic atrial tachycardia is recorded in about 50 per cent of patients with WPW. The characteristic pattern of WPW can be altered by abnormalities of AV and intraventricular conduction. The prevalence of WPW in the general population is approximately 3 per thousand; the fact that this figure is identical for both the young and the aged supports a congenital origin for WPW.[33]

Although Wilson is credited with the initial report of WPW,[103] it was Cohn who brought the electrocardiograph to America and first described an ECG pattern to become known as WPW. His patient was described in 1913, and suffered from a supraventricular tachycardia.[104] In 1930, this pattern was recognized as a discrete ECG syndrome.[101] Shortly thereafter the bypass concept of WPW was proposed, and this concept has stood the test of time.[105] It is of interest to note that over the years a variety of mechanisms have been proposed to explain the ECG pattern of WPW, including an excitable focus within the ventricle mechanically triggered by contraction of the atrium, accelerated conduction over a segment of the normal AV pathway, and, most recently, AV nodal bypass coupled with conduction through the Mahaim fibers.[106]

In WPW the QRS complex is a fusion between the impulse traversing the bypass and the normal AV junction. The bypass component of the QRS complex, or *delta wave,*

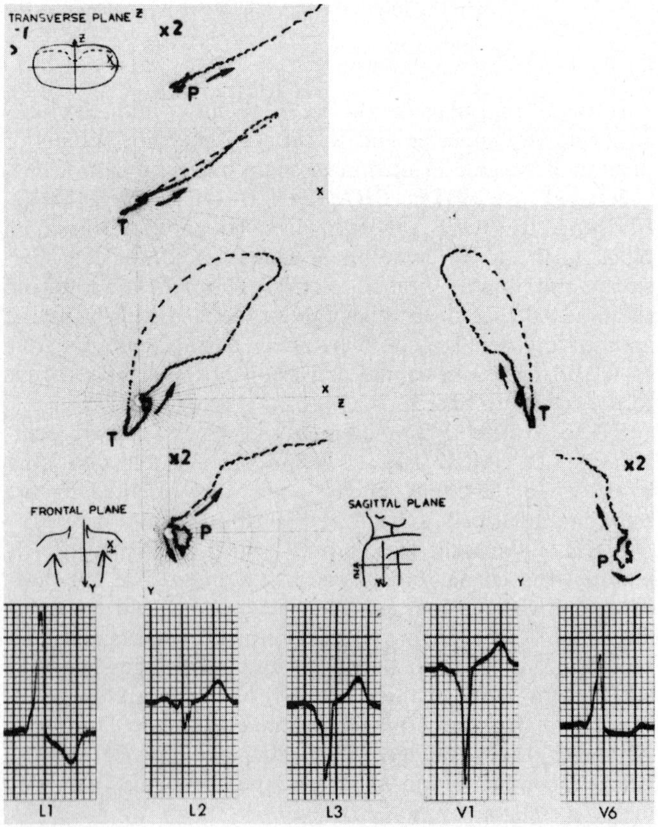

FIGURE 7–27 The ECG illustrates type B Wolff-Parkinson-White syndrome and simulates an inferior myocardial infarction. The VCG displays a delayed initial QRS force, indicated by close spacing of the dots. This initial force is directed to the left, posteriorly, and superiorly. The T-wave loop is oriented in a direction opposite to that of the initial QRS force. The initial portion of the QRS loop is also recorded at twice the standard ($\times$ 2).

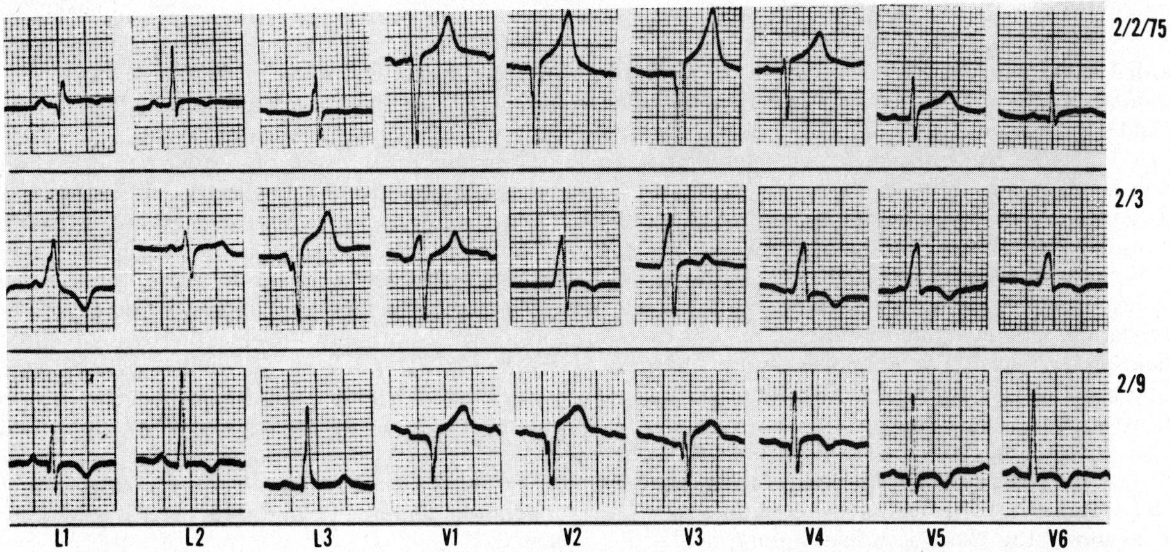

FIGURE 7–28 Anterior myocardial infarction obscured by type A Wolff-Parkinson-White syndrome. On 2/2/75, a Q wave in leads V_1 to V_4 indicates an anterior myocardial infarction. On 2/3, WPW Type A obscures the myocardial infarction. On 2/9, AV conduction is normal, WPW is no longer present, and the anterior myocardial infarction with evolutionary ST-segment and T-wave changes is evident.

varies depending on the size of the ventricular muscle mass activated through the bypass. In some instances, especially in the presence of AV conduction delay, the entire ventricular mass may be activated by the impulse propagated through the bypass, and the entire QRS complex becomes a delta wave.[107]

Traditionally, WPW has been classified into types A and B. *Type A* is characterized by a prominent positive initial QRS deflection in leads V_1 and V_2 (Fig. 7–28) and *type B* by a predominantly negative deflection in leads V_1 and V_2 (Fig. 7–27).[108] In type A, the initial inscription of the QRS complex, the delta wave, reflects early activation of the posterior left ventricle and, in type B, early activation of the anterior superior right ventricle. *Type C WPW*, characterized by a negative delta wave in the left lateral leads, has also been described. Presence of more than one QRS pattern suggests the possibility of multiple bypass tracts. A short P-R interval with a normal QRS complex accompanied by atrial tachycardia (the Lown-Ganong-Levine syndrome) has been suggested as a variant of WPW (p. 713).[109]

First-, second-, and third-degree AV block have been reported with WPW. The mechanisms that could explain the coexistence of WPW and AV block are many, but in any one patient the exact cause is usually unclear.[107] Right and left BBB have been described in association with WPW. In the presence of a BBB, an ipsilateral bypass, by preexciting the ventricle normally activated by the blocked bundle branch, will obscure the BBB.[110] Both supernormal and concealed conduction have been invoked to explain unexpected patterns of behavior of bypass conduction.[111]

WPW often complicates ECG interpretation because it may obscure or simulate a variety of patterns. It may mask (Fig. 7–28) or may simulate myocardial infarction. When the QRS vector is directed toward the left ventricular cavity, the cavity becomes initially positive and a Q wave will not be recorded. A diagnosis of ventricular hypertrophy in the presence of WPW (as in BBB) may be difficult, if not impossible. WPW has been mistaken for RBBB, LBBB, and RVH. Supraventricular arrhythmias with aberration, resulting from conduction through the bypass, have been mistaken for ventricular tachycardia. Aberration due to WPW should be suspected when the ventricular rate is rapid, often approaching 300 bpm, or when the QRS morphology of the bizarre complexes is upright in leads V_1 and V_2 as well as in V_5 and V_6.

The characteristic VCG feature of WPW syndrome is a slowly inscribed initial portion of the loop, the delta wave of the ECG, which is best seen in the horizontal plane.[37,38,112] The delta is defined as that portion of the loop which begins at point E, the resting or isoelectric point of the electronic beam, and ends with resumption of normal conduction speed. The direction of this initial portion of the loop classifies the WPW into type A, B, or C. Normally, the duration of the slow inscription varies from 0.02 to 0.08 sec, depending on how much of the ventricle is activated through the anomalous pathway.

In *type A WPW*, the slow portion of the loop is directed to the left and anteriorly. The remainder of the QRS loop, usually inscribed counterclockwise, maintains the same direction as the delta wave and is located in the left anterior quadrant. In about 20 per cent of cases, the maximal vector of the loop points in the direction of the left posterior quadrant. In the ECG these changes are manifest by an upright QRS complex in leads V_1 and V_6.

Type B WPW is recognized by an initial slow inscription oriented to the left and posteriorly or slightly anteriorly. The major portion of the loop is located in the left posterior quadrant. In the ECG these are reflected as a QS complex in leads V_1 and V_2 and an R wave in leads V_5 and V_6 (Fig. 7–27).

Type C WPW is a rarely encountered variant characterized by a Q wave in leads V_5 and V_6. The slowly inscribed initial portion of the loop is directed anteriorly to the right, with the remainder of the loop inscribed normally.

MYOCARDIAL INFARCTION

Myocardial damage manifest by elevation of the ST segment was first observed in the dog with injection of silver nitrate[113] and shortly thereafter with ligation of a coronary artery.[114] In 1920, the ECG of myocardial infarction was described in man.[115]

The ECG changes of myocardial infarction are those of ischemia, injury, and cellular death and are, within limits, reflected by T-wave changes, ST-segment displacement, and the appearance of Q waves, respectively. Such a clear-cut differentiation, although clinically useful, may be overly simplistic and artificial. For example, T-wave changes may be due to ischemia, injury, or death of muscle. Similarly, a Q wave may be due to impairment of transmembrane ionic fluxes and not necessarily cellular death. However, for the purpose of this discussion, T-wave changes, ST-segment displacement, and appearance of a Q wave are assumed to reflect ischemia, injury, and cell death, respectively.

ISCHEMIA

In the dog, the earliest change following ligation of a coronary artery is the almost immediate appearance of a primary T-wave change. (For a definition of primary and secondary T-wave changes, see page 232.) After 60 to 90 seconds, there is a maximal shift of the ST segment. The T wave is now positive and peaked, and the change is as a rule a primary change.[116–118] In man, unless an ECG is recorded at the moment of occlusion, the initial T wave stage is usually missed. Occasionally, a giant R wave is recorded early during the ischemic episode. This is seen in experimental animals[119,120] and in man.[121,122] Such changes in the QRS could contribute to the T-wave abnormality, and the T-wave alteration would reflect both primary and secondary changes in repolarization.

Normally the process of repolarization proceeds from the epicardium to the endocardium, and an upright T wave is recorded. Ischemia prolongs the regional duration of recovery, with the ischemic area being last to repolarize. If the ischemia is subendocardial, the direction of repolarization remains unchanged and the polarity of the T wave remains upright. In the presence of subepicardial ischemia, the duration of the excited state is longer in the epicardium; the normal order of repolarization is reversed, proceeding from endocardium to epicardium; and an inverted T wave is inscribed. Because of local prolongation of recovery, the late phase of repolarization may be unopposed, and a large and prolonged T wave may be registered.[123]

INJURY

Two concepts based on systolic and diastolic phenomena have been suggested to explain the ST-segment displacement. One postulates local reduction or loss of resting potential, resulting in a *diastolic current of injury.* The second concept assumes an unopposed current flowing from the injured area during the isoelectric ST segment, resulting in a *systolic current of injury.* These systolic and diastolic phenomena cannot be differentiated with the ordinary clinical alternating-current (AC) electrocardiograph but can be recorded experimentally with direct-current (DC) equipment (Fig. 7–29).

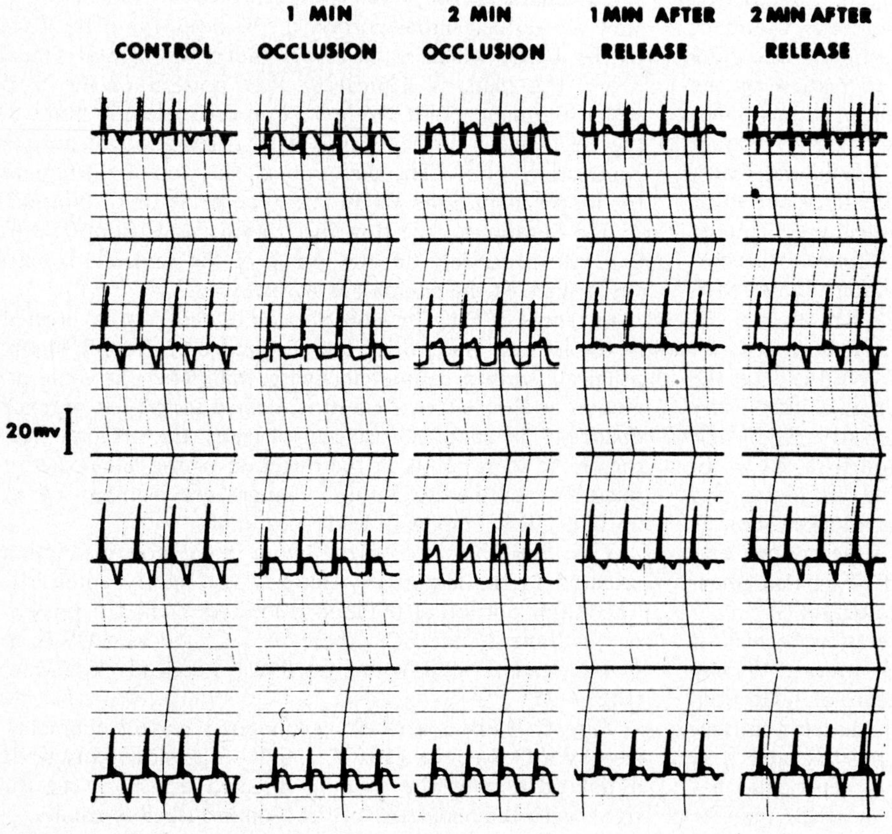

FIGURE 7–29 Simultaneous epicardial electrograms recorded from four sites. The electrodes were distributed randomly in the ischemic area, with some closer to the center of the ischemic area than others. After one minute of occlusion, TQ-segment depression is apparent in all recordings. After two minutes of occlusion, TQ-segment depression has increased. The ST-segment takeoff is slightly elevated or isoelectric in all recordings. The polarity of the T wave is changed from a negative during the control period to positive. These recordings emphasize that major changes in action potential downstroke, shape, and timing can occur without significant alteration of phase 2 and of the action potential. Similarly, T-wave changes can occur without a significant shift of the true ST segment. True TQ-segment depression appears to be the major cause of ST-segment displacement and the true ST-segment shift of lesser magnitude and variable. T waveform is markedly altered with occlusion. (From Vincent, G. M., et al.: Mechanisms of ischemic ST-segment displacement. Circulation *56*:559, 1977, by permission of the American Heart Association, Inc.)

The concept of *diastolic current* proposes that localized injury is associated with a flow of current from the uninjured to the injured area. As a result, the T-Q segment is displaced downward but is automatically shifted to control level by the capacitor-coupled amplifier of the ECG. When the entire heart (including the injured area) is depolarized, the ST segment is elevated with respect to the depressed but rectified (isoelectric) diastolic T-Q segment (Fig. 7–30).

The concept of *systolic current* proposes that during the ST segment, the normal heart is depolarized but the injured area undergoes early repolarization. The result is a current flow from the more positive injured area to a more negative or uninjured area. The result is true elevation of the ST segment. Similarly, if, rather than repolarizing early, the injured area fails to depolarize with the normal myocardium, a current of injury would exist and an elevated ST segment would be recorded (Fig. 7–30). Earlier experimental studies indicate that during injury both systolic and diastolic currents are present,[124] and at times the systolic precedes the diastolic current of injury. A more recent study suggests that the diastolic current predominates while the systolic current plays a lesser role and that the magnitude of the current is modified by the heart rate[125] (Fig. 7–29). As indicated, the clinical ECG does not differentiate between systolic and diastolic currents of injury. Furthermore, unless the onset of the injury is recorded, even a DC coupled ECG would not identify the mechanism of the ST-segment shift.

For reasons outlined earlier, an electrode facing subendocardial injury registers an elevated ST segment, while an epicardial electrode subtended by the normal myocardium registers ST-segment depression. Similarly, an electrode facing epicardial injury registers elevation of the ST segment, while the endocardial electrode inscribes ST-segment depression.

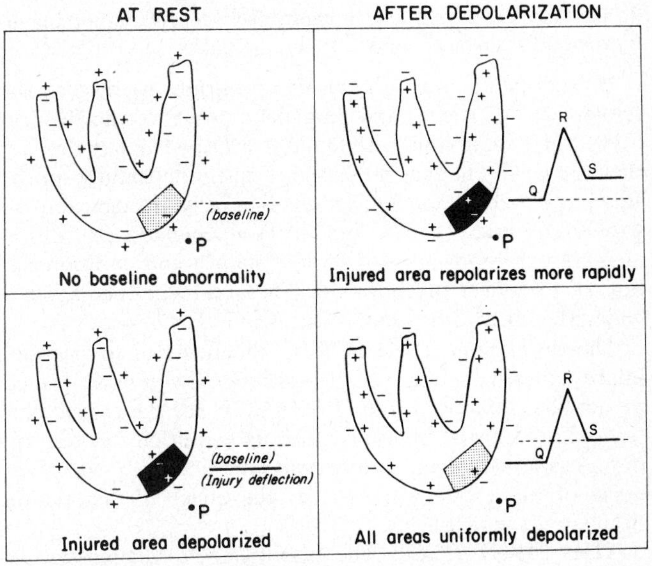

FIGURE 7–30 Systolic (*upper row*) and diastolic (*lower row*) currents of injury. *Upper row,* The ischemic area (shaded) is electrically identical to the nonischemic heart at rest, and there is no shift of the baseline potential. During repolarization, however, the ischemic area (black) has repolarized early and is positive relative to the depolarized heart, the baseline is shifted upward (positive), and the ECG records an elevated ST segment. Similarly, if the ischemic area fails to depolarize with the remainder of the heart, it would be positive relative to the remainder of the heart and a positive ST segment would be recorded. This latter mechanism may also be operative.

Lower row, The ischemic area (black) is depolarized at rest, thus negative relative to the remainder of the heart, and the baseline is shifted down (negative). This shift is not recognizable on ECG. However, with completion of depolarization the injured area is also depolarized; its potential becomes identical to that of the rest of the heart; and the ST segment, although isoelectric, is elevated relative to the depressed baseline, so that an elevated ST segment is registered.

These two mechanisms cannot be differentiated with the ECG, and although both contribute to the current of injury, the systolic is thought to dominate (Fig. 7–29). (From Scher, A. M.: Electrocardiogram. *In* Ruch, I. C., and Patton, H. D. (eds.): Physiology and Biophysics. Philadelphia, W. B. Saunders Co., 1974.)

INFARCTION

Infarction implies necrosis and an electrically inert myocardium. The diagnostic feature of infarction is the *Q wave.* Two concepts have been invoked to explain the appearance of the Q wave. The theory of proximity, the "window" theory, suggests that the electrically inert myocardium allows an electrode to record the intracavitary negativity.[126,127] There is ample evidence, however, to suggest that a Q wave can be recorded in the absence of a transmural infarction.[128] Heterogeneity of electrophysiological changes associated with the dynamic events of ischemia and subsequent healing, with intermingling of fibrous and viable tissue, has been suggested as an explanation.[127,129–131]

According to the vectorial concept, the electrically inert myocardium fails to contribute to the normal electrical forces and the result is a vector that points away from the area of infarction, reflected by a Q wave. Theoretically, the infarction vector represents the force that alters the normal vector. It is equal to but opposite in direction from the vector generated by the infarcted myocardium prior to infarction.[37] If the net vector is directed normally but is reduced in magnitude, a Q wave will not be recorded, but the amplitude of the QRS complex will be reduced, indicating loss of myocardium. However, the specificity of such a change for infarction is low.

DIAGNOSIS OF MYOCARDIAL INFARCTION

(See also p. 1283)

One of the most valuable contributions of the ECG is in the diagnosis of myocardial infarction. Usually it is the first laboratory test performed; the technique is reliable and reproducible, can be applied serially, and when properly interpreted is the cornerstone of the laboratory diagnosis of myocardial infarction. In 1933 Wilson and his associates clearly defined the role of the electrocardiogram in the diagnosis of myocardial infarction (at that time referred to as "coronary occlusion"):

> In general we found the electrocardiogram far more helpful in the diagnosis of coronary occlusion than the physical findings, but of less value than the clinical history. There are many cases in which characteristic electrocardiographic changes are absent, although electrocardiograms that are within normal limits in every respect are relatively rare, especially during the period immediately following the vascular accident. Since the most distinctive of the electrocardiographic signs of infarction occur at this time and are transient, a series of curves taken at frequent intervals

during the first month are far more likely to give important information than a single curve.[132]

It is difficult and perhaps inappropriate to discuss the sensitivity, specificity, and diagnostic power of the ECG in myocardial infarction without first acknowledging the fact that the ECG changes differ significantly depending on the stage and size of the infarction. Similarly, recognition of, and attention to, subtle and atypical changes, realization of the great importance of serial tracings, and an appreciation of the effect of coexisting conduction defects will enhance the diagnostic value of the ECG.

The discussion of the ECG in diagnosis of myocardial infarction will include (a) the earliest change in suspected myocardial infarction, the "first ECG"; (b) the classic pattern of myocardial infarction and its evolution; (c) the minor, subtle, atypical, and nonspecific changes; (d) diagnosis of old infarction; and (e) the effect of conduction defects on the diagnosis.

THE FIRST ECG. The first ECG is "diagnostic" of acute infarction in slightly more than half the patients. This statement should be accepted with the reservation that a single ECG may never be "diagnostic" (see p. 226). However, a pattern of ST-segment displacement, especially with associated Q-wave and T-wave changes, and a clinical history suggestive of ischemic heart disease is highly suggestive—if not diagnostic of acute myocardial infarction. In a study of all patients admitted to an emergency room and subsequently proven to have myocardial infarction, 65 per cent had an initial diagnostic ECG and 20 per cent were said to have a normal tracing.[133] In another study of 198 patients, the ECG recorded on the first day was diagnostic of infarction in 72 per cent of men and 61 per cent of the women. Serial tracing increased the sensitivity to 93 per cent.[134] In a series of 449 patients, the initial ECG was interpreted as diagnostic of myocardial infarction in 229 (51 per cent), probable myocardial infarction in 120 (27 per cent), doubtful in 30 (7 per cent), and no evidence of infarction in 70 (16 per cent). Serial cardiograms increased the accuracy to 83 per cent.[135]

In 150 patients with "slight or subacute infarction" treated at home, a pattern diagnostic of myocardial infarction was seen in 27 patients (18 per cent). Seventy-two patients showed significant but not diagnostic abnormalities. LVH was present in 10 patients and minor, 0.5-mm ST-segment depression and lowering of T waves were present in 24 patients. The ECG was borderline in seven and normal in 10 patients.[136]

CLASSIC PATTERN AND EVOLUTION OF INFARCTION. The sequence of ECG evolution of myocardial infarction in man is, in many respects, similar to that recorded in the experimental animal. If the ECG is inscribed at the onset of myocardial infarction, the characteristic early change—namely, an abnormal T wave—is often recorded. The T wave may be prolonged, increased in magnitude, and either upright or inverted.[122,137] This is followed by ST-segment elevation in leads facing the area of injury, with reciprocal depression in the "opposite leads." The upright T wave may exhibit terminal inversion at a time when the ST segment is still elevated. A Q wave may be present in the first ECG or may not appear for hours or sometimes days. The amplitude of the QRS complex may diminish and may be replaced by a QS pattern.

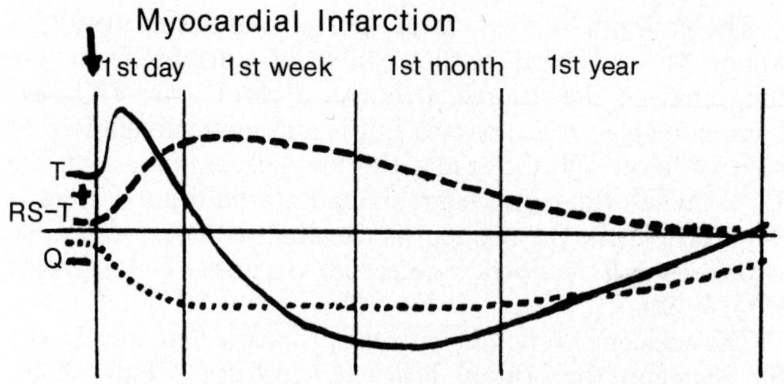

FIGURE 7–31 Evolution of the T wave, ST segment, and Q wave after myocardial infarction. (From Lepeschkin, E.: Modern Electrocardiography. Baltimore, Williams and Wilkins Co., 1951.)

As the ST segment returns to the baseline, symmetrically inverted T waves evolve.[115] The time of appearance and the magnitude of the changes vary from patient to patient.[138,139] Representative time sequences and magnitudes of the T wave, ST segment, and Q wave are illustrated in Figure 7–31.

The classic evolution of acute myocardial infarction is documented in approximately one-half to two-thirds of the patients (Fig. 7–32). In a prospective study of 230 patients, 66 per cent showed diagnostic changes characterized by typical evolution of ST segment and T waves with the appearance of Q waves, while in 34 per cent the infarct was manifest by ST-segment and T-wave changes only (Fig. 7–33).[140]

SUBTLE, ATYPICAL, NONSPECIFIC PATTERNS OF INFARCTION. Atypical features and characteristics of early infarction seen in about 40 to 50 per cent of the first ECG's include a normal ECG; subtle ST-segment and T-wave changes: isolated T-wave abnormality; transient normalization of the ST segment, T wave, or QRS complex (Fig. 7–33); involvement of electrically "silent" areas (Fig. 7–34); or the masking effect of conduction defects (Figs. 7–19, 7–22, and 7–28). Awareness and recognition of the early, nondiagnostic, "atypical" or subtle abnormalities will improve the diagnostic sensitivity of the ECG.

Although ECG changes can be documented within seconds after experimental myocardial infarction,[116] such changes may be delayed in man. A normal initial ECG in a patient with evolving clinical acute myocardial infarction may be due to absence of ischemia at the time of the initial tracing, a delay in evolution of the characteristic pattern, an initially small infarct that produces diagnostic ECG changes only after extension, transient normalization of the ECG in the course of evolution of acute myocardial infarction (Fig. 7–33), or infarction in an electrocardiographically silent area of the myocardium (Fig. 7–34).[135,136]

Evolution of the characteristic ST-segment and T-wave changes coupled with appearance of Q waves is highly specific for acute myocardial infarction. In the first ECG, the sensitivity and specificity of the ST-segment change alone, especially when marked, is high. At times, however, *evolving* changes in the ST segment need to be demonstrated,[136] since conditions such as pericarditis, early repolarization, hyperkalemia, or ventricular aneurysm and Prinzmetal's angina may also manifest ST-segment elevation. Subtle, "minor" ST-segment elevation can be easily overlooked but is a relatively common, isolated early finding.

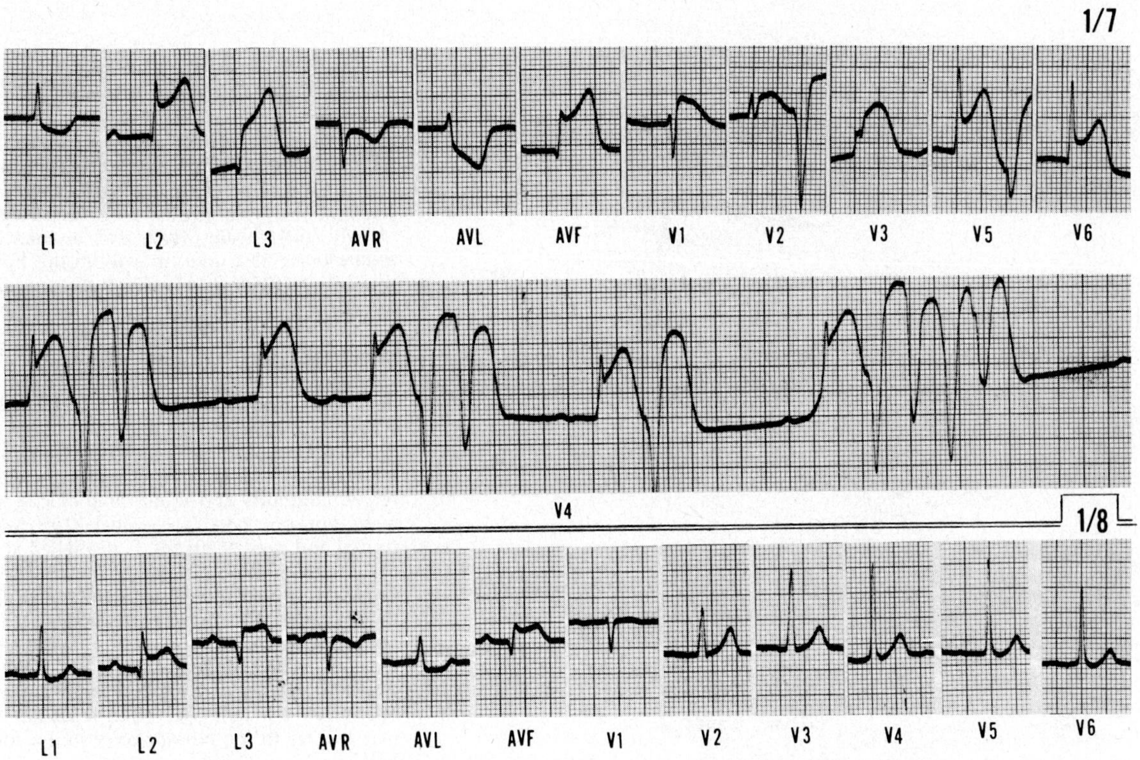

FIGURE 7–32 Acute inferior myocardial infarction and transient extensive anterior injury. Tracing on 1/7 shows elevation of the ST segment in leads II, III, and aV_f. V_1 through V_6 with reciprocal depression of the ST segment in leads I and aV_l. In the second row the acute injury is accompanied by ventricular premature complexes (isolated and couplets) and a short run of ventricular tachycardia. On 1/8, the anterior current of injury is no longer present, and the residual pattern is that of an acute inferior myocardial infarction manifest by a Q wave and ST-segment elevation in leads II, III, and aV_f.

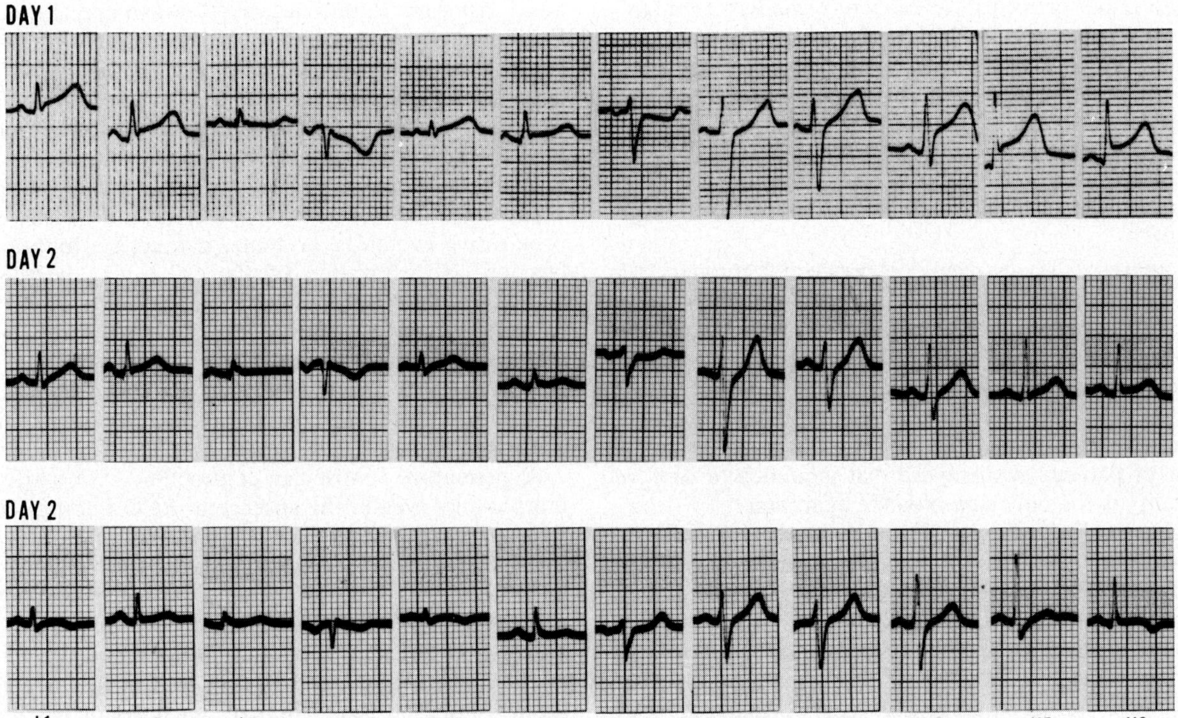

FIGURE 7–33 Normalization of the ECG in the course of evolution of an acute myocardial infarction ultimately manifest by T-wave changes only. Day 1, current of injury in leads I, II, aV_l, V_4, V_5, and V_6. Day 2, row 2, ECG is normal. Day 2, row 3, T waves are inverted in leads I, aV_l, V_5, and V_6. Inversion of the T wave is the only evidence of infarction.

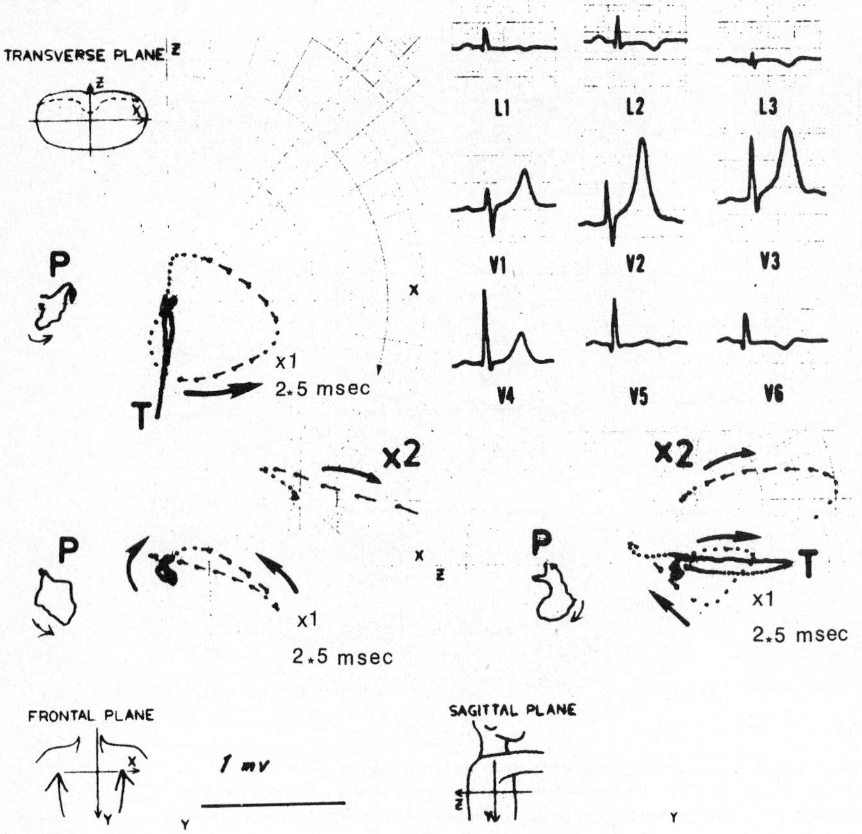

FIGURE 7–34 The ECG illustrates an inferior and posterior infarction. In the transverse plane, the VCG displays anterior displacement of the QRS loop with the anteriorly displaced area about 70 per cent of the entire loop owing to the posterior infarction. The large but narrow T loop is directed anteriorly and to the right and is inscribed counterclockwise at a uniform rate. In the frontal plane, the initial QRS force is directed superiorly and is inscribed clockwise with an inscription of 20 msec located superiorly. The initial leftward QRS magnitude, along the 0 to 180° axis, is 0.25 mV. In the sagittal plane, the initial QRS force is directed superiorly and anteriorly and is inscribed clockwise with a portion displaced superiorly. The entire QRS loop is also shifted anteriorly consistent with a posterior infarction. The large but narrow T-wave loop is directed anteriorly and is inscribed clockwise at an almost uniform rate. The initial QRS force in the frontal and sagittal planes, is displayed at two times the standard (× 2), while the P-wave loop is displayed at four times the standard in each of the three planes. The Q waves in leads II, III, and V_6 and T-wave changes in leads I, II, III, V_5, and V_6 indicate an inferior apical infarction, while the tall R waves in leads V_1, V_2, and V_3 reflect the posterior infarction. The tall T waves in leads V_1, V_2, and V_3 may be due to the inferior or posterior infarction or both.

ST-segment depression may reflect subendocardial ischemia, infarction, or reciprocal changes secondary to infarction at an "opposite" site. It has also been suggested that depression of the ST segment in leads V_1 to V_4 in the presence of an inferior infarction may be due to associated ischemia caused by significant obstruction of the left anterior descending coronary artery.[141] Minor subtle ST-segment depression is a common early finding of acute myocardial infarction and should be viewed with suspicion.[134,142]

Tall, peaked T waves seen in experimental coronary occlusion[116] are occasionally recorded in man and are thought to represent subendocardial ischemia.[122,137] More often, the initial T wave may be isoelectric, negative, or biphasic. This frequently subtle and nonspecific T-wave change is often the earliest recorded sign of infarction and is probably indicative of subepicardial ischemia. In about 20 to 30 per cent of patients with myocardial infarction, a T-wave abnormality is the only sign of acute infarction.

An *abnormal U wave* is a frequent marker of ischemic heart disease. Negative or biphasic U waves have been reported in up to 30 per cent of patients with chronic angina pectoris, either as a persistent finding or as a transient manifestation during an episode of angina. It is most often recorded in leads I, II, and V_4 to V_6. Appearance of a negative U wave during exercise-induced ischemia has been appreciated for some time[31,143,144] and has recently been found to be highly specific for disease of the left anterior descending coronary artery.[145,146] A negative U wave is seen in 10 to 60 per cent of patients with anterior infarction and in up to 30 per cent of patients with inferior infarction.[31] Appearance of a negative U wave may precede other ECG changes of infarction by several hours (Fig. 7–35).[147]

An abnormal QRS complex, ST segment, and T wave may normalize transiently in the course of evolution of acute myocardial infarction (Fig. 7–33). Such normalization, termed the "intermediate phase," may be due to reversible ischemia or injury or conduction defects.[148,149] Frequently, however, it represents a phase during progressive evolution of acute, irreversible myocardial infarction. Normalization of the ECG may be misleading and may suggest regression of the acute process or absence of myocardial infarction. Normalization and subsequent reappearance of ST-segment displacement alone in the presence of other unequivocal ECG signs of infarction may be a manifestation of "reelevation"—a frequent finding in acute infarction.[150]

A premature ventricular contraction with a qR or QR morphology even in the absence of ECG findings of infarction suggests the presence of myocardial infarction.[151] This finding may prove particularly useful when the myocardial infarction is masked, for example, by LBBB or WPW.

OLD INFARCTION (THE Q WAVE). ECG diagnosis of an old infarction is often difficult and frequently impossible without the availability of tracings documenting the acute episode. A definitive diagnosis of old infarction depends on the presence of a pathological Q wave. Only rarely can it be based on T-wave changes alone. While a Q wave may be absent in transmural infarction[152] and present in nontransmural infarction,[130,131,153] in essence, the sensitivity and specificity of the ECG for diagnosis of an old myocardial infarction still depend on the Q wave. The specificity of the Q wave is relatively high; its sensitivity is quite low. Within 6 to 12 months after an acute myocardial infarction, about 30 per cent of the tracings, although abnormal, are no longer diagnostic of infarction.[154] Similarly, by the end of 10 years, or sooner, some 6 to 10 per cent of the cardiograms revert to normal.[155]

In a series of 1184 tracings correlating myocardial infarction with postmortem findings, the specificity and sensitivity of the Q wave were 89 and 61 per cent, respectively, and varied with location of the infarction. Anteriorly located Q waves (leads V_1 to V_4) and inferiorly located Q waves (leads II, III, and aV_f) were falsely positive in 46 per cent, while only 4 per cent of Q waves greater than 0.03 sec present in the lateral leads (V_5 and V_6) or in a combination of anterior and inferior leads with another lead proved to be falsely positive. The sensitivity of the Q wave was lowest for infarction located in the lateral basal portion of the left ventricle.[156] This anatomical area is usually reflected in leads I and aV_l.

In another study, a Q wave of 0.04 sec or more in lead aV_f indicated the presence of coronary artery disease and asynergy of the inferior wall in 94 and 76 per cent of cases, respectively.[157]

MYOCARDIAL INFARCTION AND CONDUCTION DELAYS. Conduction defects may not interfere with, may mask, or may falsely suggest the diagnosis of myocardial infarction. In RBBB, the initial order of activation is normal and thus the pattern of infarction is unaltered (Figs. 7–20 to 7–22). In LBBB the sequence of early activation is altered, with the initial septal vector directed from right to left. As a result the earliest left ventricular intracavitary potential is positive. In keeping with the "window" concept of infarction, a Q wave cannot be registered except when there is extensive septal infarction. Restated in terms of the dipole or vector concept, since the free wall infarct is inscribed during the latter part of the QRS complex after the septal activation is complete, the direction of initial activation expressed as a dipole or vector is unaltered by the infarction, and the infarct is masked (Figs. 7–18, 7–19, and 7–22).

Numerous studies have been designed in an attempt to define diagnostic criteria for myocardial infarction in the presence of LBBB. None of the criteria has proved to be of significant help, and these criteria rarely correlate with autopsy findings.[158,159] In a study of 52 patients with LBBB and autopsy findings of myocardial infarction, the following ECG findings were thought to correlate with myocardial infarction: (1) a Q wave 0.04 sec or greater in leads I, aV_l, V_5, or V_6; (2) rapid serial ST-segment and T-wave changes; (3) acute ST-segment elevation disproportionate to the area of the QRS complex; and (4) a Q wave of any size in lead V_6. Others suggest that a deep S wave in leads

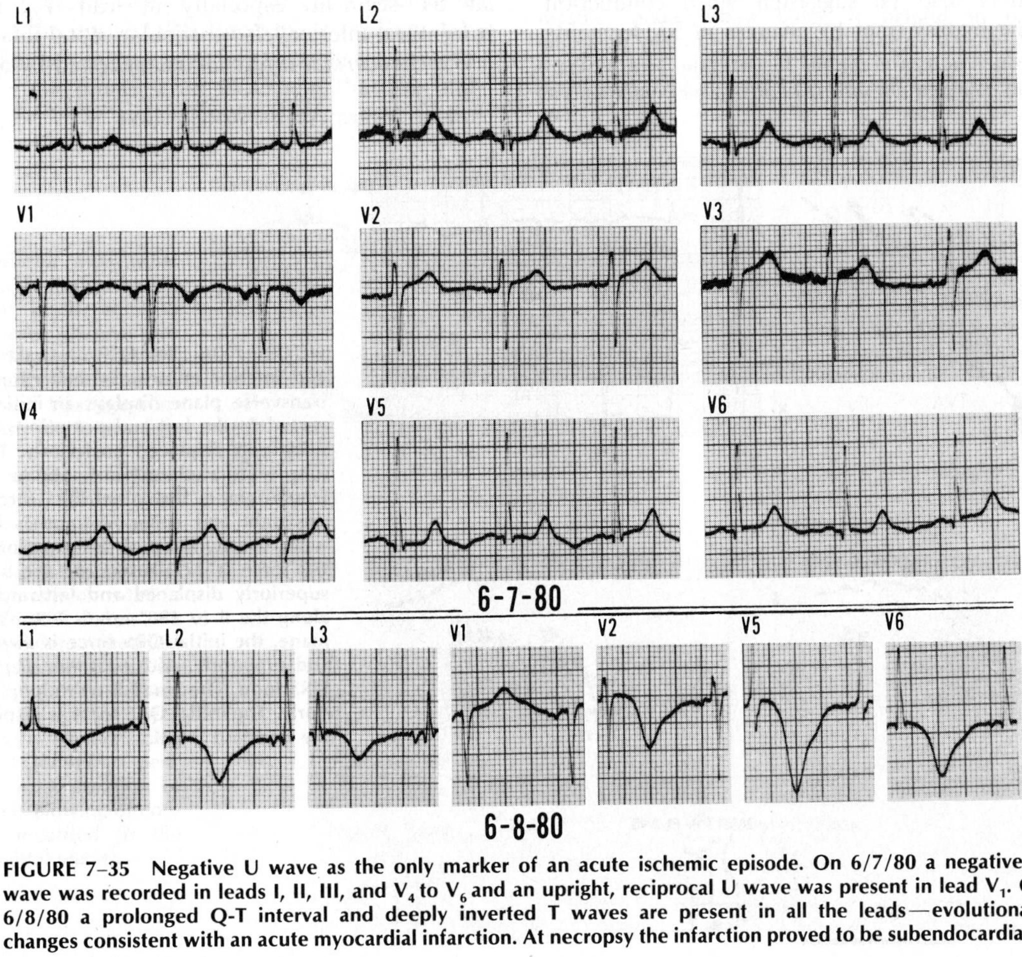

FIGURE 7–35 Negative U wave as the only marker of an acute ischemic episode. On 6/7/80 a negative U wave was recorded in leads I, II, III, and V_4 to V_6 and an upright, reciprocal U wave was present in lead V_1. On 6/8/80 a prolonged Q-T interval and deeply inverted T waves are present in all the leads—evolutionary changes consistent with an acute myocardial infarction. At necropsy the infarction proved to be subendocardial.

infarction. In patients with an inferior or lateral myocardial infarction, an R wave of increased amplitude, 0.04 sec in duration in leads V_1 and V_2, suggests concomitant posterior wall involvement (Fig. 7–34).

Periinfarction block, as originally defined, is a specific conduction abnormality due to myocardial infarction.[178] The ECG changes include a Q wave of 0.04 sec and a QRS complex in the limb leads of 0.10 sec, with a slurred prolonged terminal component facing the site of infarction. Periinfarction block is not synonymous with left anterior divisional block. In our experience periinfarction block may be of help in the diagnosis of old inferior infarction when the characteristic changes are no longer evident. Presence of terminal, somewhat delayed activation facing lead II, III, or aV_f and a terminal negative wave in leads I, V_5, and V_6—signs of periinfarction block—strengthen the diagnosis of myocardial infarction (Figs. 7–37 and 7–38).

THE VCG IN MYOCARDIAL INFARCTION

The appearance of the loop in myocardial infarction depends on the site and size of the infarction. Deviation from normal reflects loss of forces normally generated by the infarcted area and resultant dominance of the noninfarcted myocardium. Anterior myocardial infarction is best visualized in the transverse plane, while an inferior infarction is best displayed in the frontal or sagittal plane.

Anteroseptal myocardial infarction[179] is recognized in the transverse plane by loss of the first 10- to 20-msec forces, with the initial position of the loop oriented posteriorly and to the left. The entire loop is displaced posteriorly with loss of the anterior convexity. In the vast majority of cases, the loop is inscribed in a counterclockwise direction. The initial posterior and left orientation of the loop is reflected in the ECG as a QS complex in leads V_1 to V_4 (Fig. 7–36).

In a *localized anterior infarction,* the transverse loop is similar in appearance to that present in anteroseptal myocardial infarction except for a normally inscribed initial force in a left and anterior direction. This initial inscription is displayed in the ECG as an R wave in lead V_1 and at times in V_2 (Fig. 7–20).

In the transverse plane, an *anterolateral infarction* is inscribed clockwise or as a figure-of-eight. The initial normal part of the loop is followed by posterior and somewhat rightward displacement, reflecting the more extensive loss of left ventricular wall. Loss of the lateral wall may result in an increase in magnitude of the initial left-to-right portion of the loop, reflected in the ECG as a tall R wave inscribed in the right precordial leads.

In an *extensive anterior infarction,* the transverse loop reflects loss of both the septal and free left ventricular walls. The initial normal anteriorly inscribed portion of the loop is lost, and the loop is shifted posteriorly and inscribed clockwise. The ECG shows a loss of R wave, at times, in all precordial leads.

Inferior myocardial infarction is best displayed in the frontal and sagittal planes (Figs. 7–34 and 7–36).[180] In the frontal plane, the loop is most often inscribed in a clockwise direction. The initial portion of the loop is directed superiorly, the superior displacement exceeding 25 to 30 msec. The loop crosses the X axis at 0.30 msec to the left of the point of origin.[180] It has been suggested that when the above diagnostic findings are absent, a shift to the left of the QRS loop combined with clockwise rotation is strongly indicative of an inferior infarction.[181] Occasionally, when the inferior septum is spared, the initial loop may have a normal orientation, that is, to the right and inferiorly. This is followed by clockwise inscription and superior displacement of the remainder of the loop. In such instances the ECG will record a small initial R wave in leads II, III, and aV_f.

In a *posterior myocardial infarction,*[177,182] the initial forces are normal in the transverse plane, but more than half the loop is ultimately displaced anteriorly. In the majority of cases, inscription of the loop is counterclockwise. The anterior displacement of the loop is reflected in the ECG by a prominent R wave in lead V_1 or V_2 that may exceed 0.04 sec in duration (Fig. 7–34).

A summary of VCG criteria for myocardial infarction is presented in Table 7–5.

NONINFARCTION Q WAVES

While the vast majority of abnormal Q waves are due to myocardial infarction, a significant number have other causes, including positional changes, congenital electrophysiological and anatomical abnormalities of the septum, loss of electrical activity without cellular death,[149] replacement of the myocardium by a variety of pathological processes, alteration of the initial vector due to conduction defects or hypertrophy, and other less commonly observed disorders.

Noninfarction Q waves may be transient or permanent.

TABLE 7–5 SUMMARY OF VECTORCARDIOGRAPHIC CRITERIA FOR DIAGNOSIS OF MYOCARDIAL INFARCTION (MI)

Anteroseptal MI (1 and 2)*
1. Initial anterior QRS forces absent
2. 0.02-sec QRS vector directed posteriorly
Localized Anterior MI (1,2, and 3)
1. Initial anterior septal forces present
2. 0.02-sec QRS vector directed posteriorly
3. Voltage criteria for left ventricular hypertrophy absent
Anterolateral MI (1,2, and 3)
1. Initial anterior septal forces normal
2. Initial rightward QRS forces > 0.022 sec
3. Efferent limb of transverse plane QRS loop inscribed clockwise
4. Initial rightward QRS forces > 0.16 mV
5. Maximum frontal plane QRS vector > 40°, QRS loop inscribed counterclockwise
Extensive Anterior MI (1 and 2)
1. Initial anterior QRS forces absent
2. Transverse plane QRS loop inscribed clockwise
Inferior MI (1 or more)
1. Initial superior QRS forces > 0.025 sec
2. Initial superior QRS forces ≥ 0.020 sec, maximum left superior force ≥ 0.25 mV
3. Maximum frontal plane QRS vector < 10°, efferent limb of frontal QRS loop inscribed clockwise
4. Bites in afferent limb of frontal QRS loop
Inferolateral MI (1 and 2)
1. Initial rightward QRS forces > 0.022 sec
2. Initial superior QRS forces > 0.025 sec

*Numbers in parentheses after each type of infarction indicate the minimum requirements for the diagnosis.

From Chou, T.-C., et al.: Clinical Vectorcardiography. 2nd ed. New York, Grune and Stratton, 1974, p. 229.

Transient Q waves have been produced experimentally in animals[153] and observed in patients during anginal attacks.[183,184] Such Q waves have been explained by a transient loss of electrophysiological function, the phenomenon referred to by some as "myocardial concussion."[185] Q waves have been recorded with severe metabolic disturbances accompanying shock or pancreatitis.[186,187] Similarly, transient Q waves have been noted during cardiac surgery and ascribed variously to transient ischemia and hypoxia, spasm, localized metabolic and electrolyte disturbances, and possible hypothermia (Fig. 7–24).[188] Rarely a transient Q wave may result from tachycardia.[189] The author has recorded transient Q waves and ST-segment and T-wave changes due to air embolism of the coronary artery complicating induction of a therapeutic pneumothorax.

The largest group of noninfarction Q waves is that comprising a variety of pathological processes that affect the myocardium,[190] including myocarditis, cardiac amyloidosis, neuromuscular disorders such as progressive muscular dystrophy, myotonia atrophica, Friedreich's ataxia,[191] scleroderma, postpartum myopathy, myocardial replacement by tumor, sarcoidosis, idiopathic cardiomyopathy, and anomalous coronary artery.

Noninfarction Q waves commonly accompany hypertrophic cardiomyopathy[192] and may simulate anterior or inferior myocardial infarction (Fig. 7–39). The exact mechanism of the Q wave in this condition is unclear. Increased septal mass or abnormal depolarization because of anomalous architecture of the septal myocardium, or both, has been proposed as the cause.[193] A recent study suggests that the electrophysiological characteristics of septal muscle may differ from normal. For example, the refractory period of the myocardium responsible for the Q wave exceeds the refractory period of the junctional tissue. This relationship may be altered by tachycardia with disappearance of the Q wave.[194]

A Q wave can be due to COLD with or without cor pulmonale, pulmonary embolism, and pneumothorax. In COLD, findings in the precordial leads frequently simulate anterior myocardial infarction.[195] The mechanism responsible for the QS complex is clockwise rotation and downward displacement of the diaphragm and of the heart. As a result, the electrodes are located superior to the initial vector; when this vector is directed inferiorly, a QS pattern results. By placing the electrode one interspace lower, it is often possible to record an R wave and thus provide strong evidence against myocardial infarction. Occasionally in COLD the Q wave may simulate an inferior myocardial infarction.[196] The positional origin of the anterior or inferior Q waves may be suspected when the Q wave is accompanied by other ECG findings of COLD. However, since both COLD and myocardial infarction frequently coexist, differential diagnosis may at times be difficult or impossible.

Abnormal Q waves, especially in lead III and rarely in lead aV_f, with an S wave in lead I, can be recorded in acute cor pulmonale due to *pulmonary embolism.* Clockwise rotation with superior orientation of the initial vector is most likely reponsible for the Q wave in lead III. A Q wave in lead II is rarely recorded. Occasionally acute pulmonary embolus may simulate anterior myocardial infarction.

Spontaneous pneumothorax, particularly on the left, may result in a pattern simulating anterior myocardial infarction with occasional absence of the R wave in all the precordial leads.[198]

In LBBB the initial forces are directed from right to left and either superiorly or inferiorly. When the inferiorly directed forces dominate, a QS complex may be recorded in the precordial leads, simulating an anterior myocardial infarction.[199,200] If the initial vector is oriented to the left and superiorly, a QS complex may be registered in the inferior leads, suggesting inferior myocardial infarction.[200]

With left anterior divisional block, the transitional zone is shifted to the left, and an initial Q wave may appear in the right precordial leads. Loss of the forces normally contributed by the left anterior division results in a vector directed inferiorly, posteriorly, and to the right. Con-

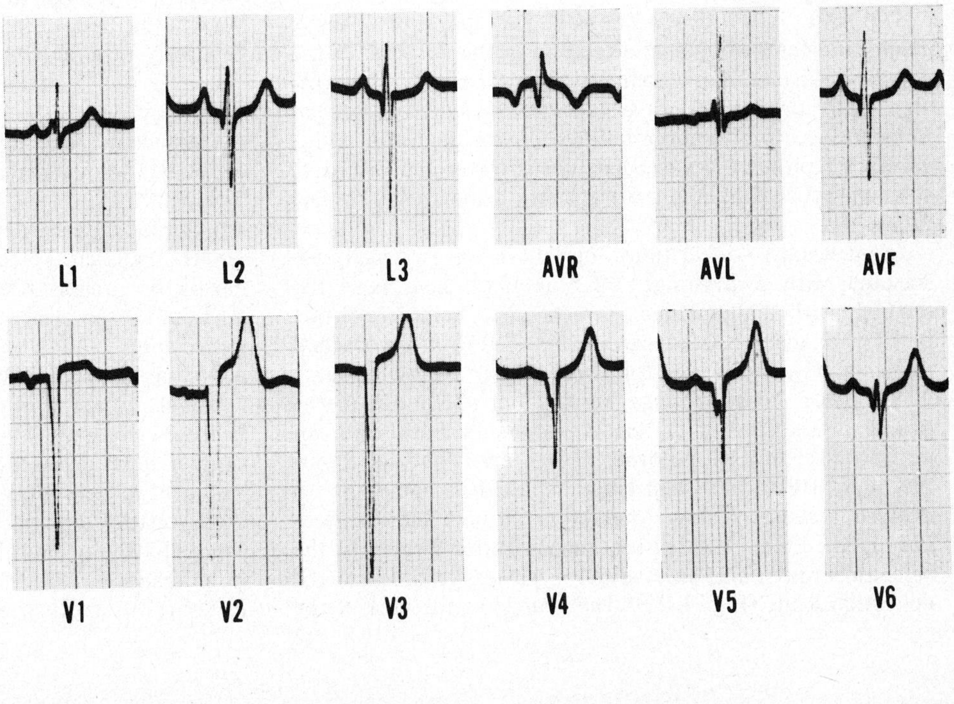

FIGURE 7–39 Noninfarction Q waves due to hypertrophic cardiomyopathy. This tracing recorded in a 16-year-old girl shows left axis deviation and Q waves in leads V_3 to V_6.

sequently, right precordial leads may register a qrS complex suggestive of an anteroseptal infarction. By placing the electrodes one interspace lower, an rS complex can be recorded attesting to the positional nature of the Q wave.[91,93]

Noninfarction Q waves are frequent in WPW (p. 220). WPW type B, with the initial forces directed from right to left, registers a QS complex in the right precordial leads and may be mistaken for anteroseptal or anterior myocardial infarction. Rarely, preexcitation of the left lateral wall, with the vector oriented anteriorly and to the right, simulates lateral infarction.[201] Most often, however, WPW simulates inferior infarction (Fig. 7–27). The Q waves recorded in leads II, III, and aV_f are due to superior orientation of the initial vector and may be seen with either type A or type B WPW.[202]

In LVH, failure to record an R wave in leads V_1 to V_4 may suggest an anteroseptal myocardial infarction.[195] Similarly, reciprocal elevation of the ST segments in these leads may contribute to an erroneous diagnosis of myocardial infarction. The exact mechanism of the initial negative deflection of the QRS is not clear, but it may be related to posterior rotation or inferior orientation of the initial vector.[195,199]

ST-SEGMENT AND T-WAVE CHANGES

ST-SEGMENT ELEVATION. Most of the causes of ST-segment elevation have been discussed in connection with a specific mechanism or etiology. In addition to the three most common organic causes—namely, acute myocardial infarction, pericarditis, and Prinzmetal's angina—ST-segment elevation is occasionally observed in acute cor pulmonale,[203] hypothermia(?), hyperkalemia, cerebrovascular accidents, LVH, LBBB, hypertrophic cardiomyopathy, and invasion of the heart by neoplastic tissue.[204] Elevation of the ST segment may also be an artifact caused by excessive inertia of the stylus of the electrocardiograph. In the normal heart the most common cause of ST-segment elevation is so-called *early repolarization*, a normal variant (see Fig. 7–9*E*, p. 204).

T-WAVE ABNORMALITIES. A *primary T-wave change* indicates a regional alteration in the duration of the depolarized state. Some common clinical conditions associated with primary T-wave changes include myocardial ischemia, electrolyte abnormalities, effects of drugs, and a variety of primary myocardial and extracardiac disorders such as myocarditis and subarachnoid hemorrhage, respectively.

Giant negative or, at times, upright T waves, usually associated with a prolonged Q-T interval have been described with subarachoid hemorrhage, complete heart block with marked bradycardia (Fig. 7–21), in myocardial ischemia (Fig. 7–35), and following cardiac resuscitation.

Secondary T-wave changes result from alterations of the timing or sequencing of depolarization, or both, with an obligatory change of the order of repolarization. For example, in LBBB, left ventricular epicardial activation is delayed because of slow conduction through the ventricular myocardium. As a result, repolarization begins in the subendocardium and an inverted T wave is recorded in the epicardial leads (Fig. 7–22). The change in the area of the QRS complex and T waves is identical but opposite in direction. Occasionally LBBB is associated with an upright T wave in the left ventricular leads, suggesting that in addition to altered activation due to LBBB, regional abnormalities of repolarization contribute to the T-wave morphology.

Intermittent LBBB is an ideal model for evaluating the significance of primary T-wave changes in the presence of LBBB.[161] In a study of 13 patients with primary T-wave changes over the anteroseptal and anterior wall recorded during normal intraventricular conduction, primary T-wave changes were also present after the appearance of LBBB in nine of the 13. On the other hand, two of 14 patients with normal T waves during normal intraventricular conduction exhibited primary ST-segment and T-wave changes with LBBB.[161] Such data suggest that primary T-wave change in the presence of LBBB may be a useful sign of myocardial abnormality. Occasionally, however, normal T waves are recorded during normal intraventricular conduction in patients manifesting primary T waves with LBBB.

Rate-Related T-Wave Changes. Postextrasystolic T-wave change was first described in 1915.[205] Since then, a number of mechanisms have been proposed to explain this observation, including an abnormal pathway of repolarization, prolonged diastolic filling time,[206] and an abrupt change in the cycle length.

Minor T-wave changes may be present following an abrupt cycle change or after an interpolated ventricular premature complex. Each is a physiological phenomenon and in keeping with in vitro studies of normal cardiac tissue. However, more pronounced T-wave alterations suggest a myocardial disorder.[207,208]

T-wave inversion is occasionally noted following supraventricular or ventricular tachycardia. The magnitude of the T-wave inversion varies, and when extreme, it may resemble the T-wave changes seen with cerebrovascular accidents or myocardial ischemia.[209] The exact mechanism of the posttachycardia T wave is obscure.

T Wave Alternans. Isolated T wave alternans, i.e., without a change in either the QRS complex or the P wave, was first noted in the cat papillary muscle.[210] It is relatively rare and its mechanism not clear.[211] Alternans of phases 2 and 3 of the action potential of the T wave has been recorded without any demonstrable change in phase 0, supporting the concept that isolated alternation of repolarization reflected in the T wave is possible. T wave alternans of the type mentioned above is most often present during tachycardia or during a sudden change in cycle length. Isolated T wave alternans, independent of tachycardia or premature systole, is nearly always associated with advanced heart disease or severe electrolyte disturbance (Fig. 7–40)[212] or may follow cardiac resuscitation.

Notched, Bifid T Waves. Notched, bifid T waves are relatively common in the absence of heart disease, especially in the young.[213] They may also be present in congenital organic heart disease, the prolonged Q-T syndrome (Fig. 7–41), central nervous system disorders,[214] and alcoholic cardiomyopathy or following the administration of drugs, especially the phenothiazines.[215] The mechanism of the bifid or notched T wave is unclear. It has been suggested that in some instances it is due to nonuniform repolarization

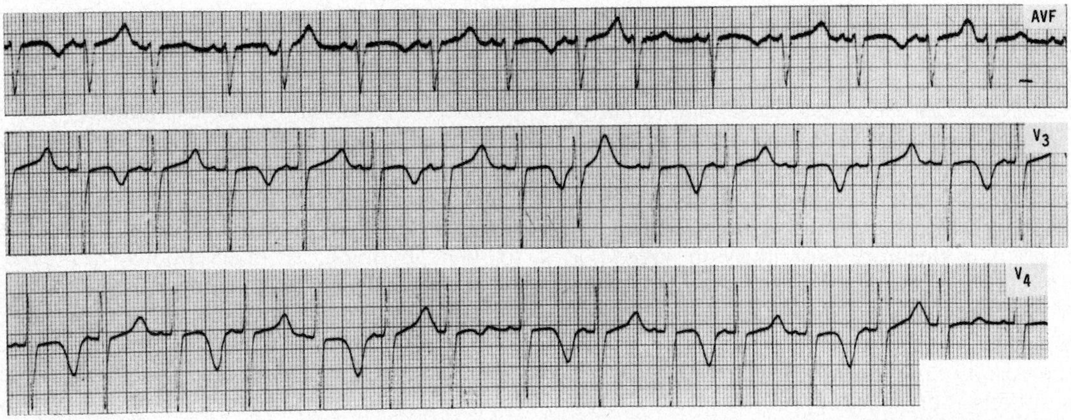

FIGURE 7–40 Isolated alternation of the T wave. The rhythm is sinus with occasional supraventricular premature complexes, probably atrial in origin. The QRS is normal in duration, with alternation of polarity of the T wave.

secondary to differential innervation of the anterior and posterior ventricular walls.[214,216] It has also been proposed that it may reflect regional delay of repolarization secondary to delayed depolarization.

NONSPECIFIC ST-SEGMENT AND T-WAVE CHANGES. Although the ST segment and T wave represent different electrophysiological events and their respective changes may have different clinical connotations, the widespread practice among electrocardiographers is to refer to either one or both as *ST-T changes.* While it is more appropriate to discuss the two separately—and whenever feasible, this will be attempted—it should be recognized that abnormalities of the ST segment and T wave frequently coexist.

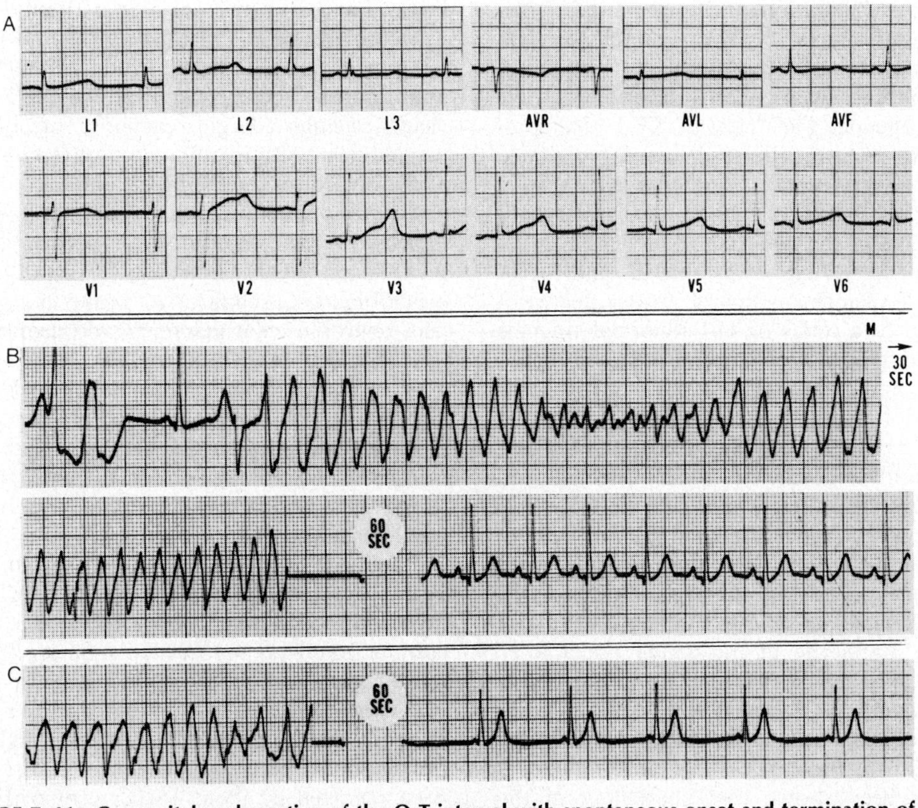

FIGURE 7–41 Congenital prolongation of the Q-T interval with spontaneous onset and termination of ventricular tachycardia and fibrillation. *A,* The rhythm is sinus with a rate of 55 bpm, the Q-T interval measures approximately 0.56 sec, and the T wave is notched. The notched T wave is best seen in leads V_2 to V_4. *B,* The tracing is continuous and illustrates spontaneous onset and termination of a ventricular tachycardia and fibrillation lasting about 90 sec. *C,* Spontaneous termination of an episode of ventricular tachycardia and flutter lasting about 90 msec. Both the Q-T interval and the T-wave morphology normalize after termination of ventricular arrhythmia. In addition to normalization of the Q-T interval and the T wave, the P-R interval is foreshortened. A possible mechanism that could explain the normalization of repolarization and shortening of the P-R interval is an increase in the level of catecholamines in response to the ventricular arrhythmia. The morphology of the T waves in *C* also suggests hyperkalemia.

Nondiagnostic ST-segment and T-wave changes are the most common ECG abnormality and account for about 50 per cent of the abnormal tracings recorded in a general medical hospital.[217] It has been estimated that nondiagnostic T-wave changes comprise 2.4 per cent[217] and 4.5 per cent[218] of all routine cardiograms. An abnormal T wave is extremely common because the wave is highly sensitive to a variety of abnormalities and interventions, and of all the ECG changes it is therefore least likely to suggest a specific diagnosis. This fact has been recognized since 1925, when Wilson first recorded inversion of the T wave following the ingestion of cold water.[219]

Although statistically an abnormal T wave suggests the presence of an abnormal or, more appropriately, an altered state,[220] it is recorded with relative frequency in the absence of any disorder (see Fig. 7–9, p. 204) as a reflection of a physiological event.[221] For these reasons, any T-wave change must be interpreted with extreme caution and must *always* be correlated with all available clinical and laboratory information. Misinterpretation of the significance of a T-wave abnormality is the most common cause of "iatrogenic ECG heart disease." Attempts to identify the etiology of an abnormal ST segment, T wave, or ST-T segment in isolation from clinical and other laboratory findings often fail.

The accepted "classic" ST-T changes, such as those seen with LVH, digitalis administration, and ischemic heart disease, are of relatively low specificity. For example, a negative wave reflecting persistence of a juvenile pattern cannot be differentiated from the symmetrically inverted T wave due to myocardial ischemia. The "classic" ST-T change of LVH may be due to ischemic heart disease or digitalis, while the marked ST-segment depression due to ischemia or subendocardial infarction may be simulated by the administration of digitalis in the presence of moderate or severe disease. When correlated with clinical and other laboratory data, ST-T changes assume a greater degree of diagnostic specificity. In a series of 410 abnormal tracings analyzed without regard to clinical data, 70 per cent could be interpreted only as "nonspecific ST-T change." This number was reduced to 10 per cent when such changes were correlated with available clinical information.[217]

The nonspecific and labile nature of the ST segment and the T wave, especially the latter, should not be unexpected. Repolarization is a much more diverse process than depolarization. Depolarization, i.e., activation, is rapid, with a reasonably uniform potential difference across the boundary of activation and is reflected in the rate of rise of phase 0 and the amplitude of the action potential.[222] Repolarization, displayed as the ST segment and T wave, reflects phases 2 and 3 of the action potential, is considerably longer and is nonuniform, with many simultaneous boundaries and with differing potentials across various boundaries.[223] It has been shown that shortening of the monophasic action potential by as little as 12 to 18 msec will alter the morphology of the T wave, and importantly, the change can be seen with involvement of 10 per cent or less of the myocardial mass. The magnitude of the T-wave changes, unlike that of the QRS complex, is not related to the mass of the myocardium. This condition has been ascribed to cancellation of repolarization voltages and to uneven contributions from the different regions of repolarization to the genesis of the T wave.[224] Such experimental findings explain, at least partially, the nonspecific character of ST-segment and T-wave changes.

Thus, a variety of clinical conditions could alter the ST segment and the T wave.[225] Abnormalities associated with clinically normal hearts were discussed above. Other ST-segment and T-wave changes can be grouped as being due to (1) physiological interventions, (2) pharmacological agents, (3) extracardiac disorders without obvious anatomical abnormality of the heart, (4) myocardial changes due to primary myocardial disease, (5) myocardial disorders secondary to systemic disease, and (6) disorders resulting from coronary artery disease. The last is discussed in connection with myocardial infarction.

Some of the more common *physiological phenomena* responsible for abnormalities of the ST segment and T wave include a change in position and a resultant abnormal ST segment and T wave in leads II, III, and aV_f; effects of cold, hyperventilation, anxiety, food, and especially glucose; and tachycardia and sympathetic and parasympathetic influences. *Pharmacological agents* causing such changes include digitalis, antiarrhythmic drugs, and drugs used in psychophysiological disorders such as phenothiazines, tricyclics, and lithium. In addition to altering the direction of the ST-T segment, drugs may shorten or prolong the Q-T or Q-U interval and may be associated with bifid T waves and often a prominent U wave. *Extracardiac disorders* that alter the ST segment and T wave include, among others, electrolyte abnormalities, cerebrovascular events,[226] shock and hemorrhage, anemia, allergic reactions, infections, endocrine abnormalities (especially hypothyroidism), and acute abdominal disorders. Primary and secondary *diseases of the myocardium* include, among others, congestive cardiomyopathy of unknown etiology, hypertrophic cardiomyopathy, postpartum myocardiopathy, myocarditis, amyloidosis, hemochromatosis, connective tissue abnormalities, sarcoidosis, neuromuscular disorders, and neoplasm.

U-WAVE ABNORMALITY. An abnormal U wave may be increased in amplitude, inverted or prolonged. A negative U wave is documented in about 1 per cent of cardiograms recorded in a general hospital.[227] An exaggerated upright U wave may be due to hypokalemia, a variety of drugs (particularly digitalis), and some of the antiarrhythmic agents (e.g., amiodarone).

The most common causes of a *negative U wave* are hypertension, aortic and mitral valve disease, RVH, and myocardial ischemia (Fig. 7–35). The last was discussed in conjunction with myocardial infarction (p. 226). A negative U wave can occasionally be found in other metabolic or organic diseases. In hypertension, a negative U wave may be the earliest sign of myocardial involvement, appearing long before any change in the T wave, and has been reported in about 16 per cent of ECG's with an upright T wave and 45 per cent with negative T waves. It may revert to normal with control of the hypertension.[31] The majority of patients with aortic regurgitation and about 10 per cent of patients with aortic stenosis manifest a negative U wave. Approximately 5 and 80 per cent of patients with systolic and diastolic overload of the right ventricle, respectively, manifest a negative U wave in leads

II, III, V_1, and V_2.[31] In essence, a negative U wave, even as an isolated finding in an otherwise normal ECG, is strongly indicative of a pathophysiological state.

Q-T INTERVAL ABNORMALITY (see also p. 203). *Shortening of the Q-T interval* may be recorded with hyperkalemia, digitalis, hypercalcemia, and acidosis. *Prolongation of the Q-T interval* may be primary and independent of the QRS, or it may reflect secondary changes of repolarization due to abnormal depolarization, or a combination of the two. Prolongation of the Q-T interval, independent of QRS duration, can be congenital (Fig. 7–41) or acquired.[228,229] Acquired disorders include ischemic heart disease, hypothermia, cardiomyopathy, mitral valve prolapse, complete heart block, a condition following cardiac resuscitation, electrolyte changes, and administration of drugs (p. 243). Q-T interval prolongation is a relatively frequent complication of acquired cerebral lesions, especially subarachnoid hemorrhage, and can also be present during and following neurosurgical procedures.

ELECTRICAL ALTERNANS. This discussion deals only with alternation in amplitude and direction. Alternation of the QRS complex was noted in the experimental animal and man as early as 1908 and 1910, respectively,[230,231] followed by documentation of alternation of the P wave, ST segment, and T wave (Fig. 7–40).

Isolated *alternation of the P wave* is seen frequently in the experimental setting but is rare in man. Most often it accompanies alternation of the QRS complex and occasionally the QRS complex and the T wave. The latter situation is referred to as *total alternans* and suggests pericardial effusion usually due to malignancy and frequently associated with tamponade or impending tamponade.

Although pericardial effusion is the most common cause of alternation of the QRS complex, *QRS alternans* is also seen with myocardial ischemia and myocardial disease due to causes other than ischemia or drugs.[232] Two mechanisms of QRS alternans have been proposed, namely, positional oscillation and aberrancy of intraventricular conduction. The early suggestion that oscillation or alternation of position is the mechanism of alternans of the QRS complex[233] was proved with the advent of echocardiography[234] (see Fig. 5–75, p. 132). The concept of oscillation also explains the fact that P wave alternans is seen predominantly with massive pericardial effusion.

ST segment alternans has been described in dogs after ligation of the coronary artery, in severely ill infants with congenital heart disease, and in patients with Prinzmetal's angina.[232] For a discussion of *T wave alternans,* see page 232. *U wave alternans* is least common. In the few cases described, the difficulty of separating the T wave and U wave as well as differentiation from a bifid T wave makes a definitive diagnosis most difficult.

The mechanism of alternans in severe myocardial disorders but in the absence of pericardial effusion is obscure. It has been ascribed to uneven duration of the excited state or to two alternating foci of impulse formation. However, the fact that alternation of depolarization, activation, and repolarization can be recorded in a single cell suggests that the mechanism is probably related to transmembrane ionic fluxes.[235] Alternans of a human atrial monophasic action potential[236] adds further credence to the primary role of transmembrane ionic events.

THE OSBORNE WAVE. An Osborne wave, seen in hypothermia, is a deflection inscribed between the QRS complex and the beginning of the ST segment (Fig. 7–42).[237] It has been variously suggested that this wave reflects delay of depolarization, a current of injury, or early repolarization.[238] In the left ventricular leads the polarity of the wave is positive and its amplitude is inversely related

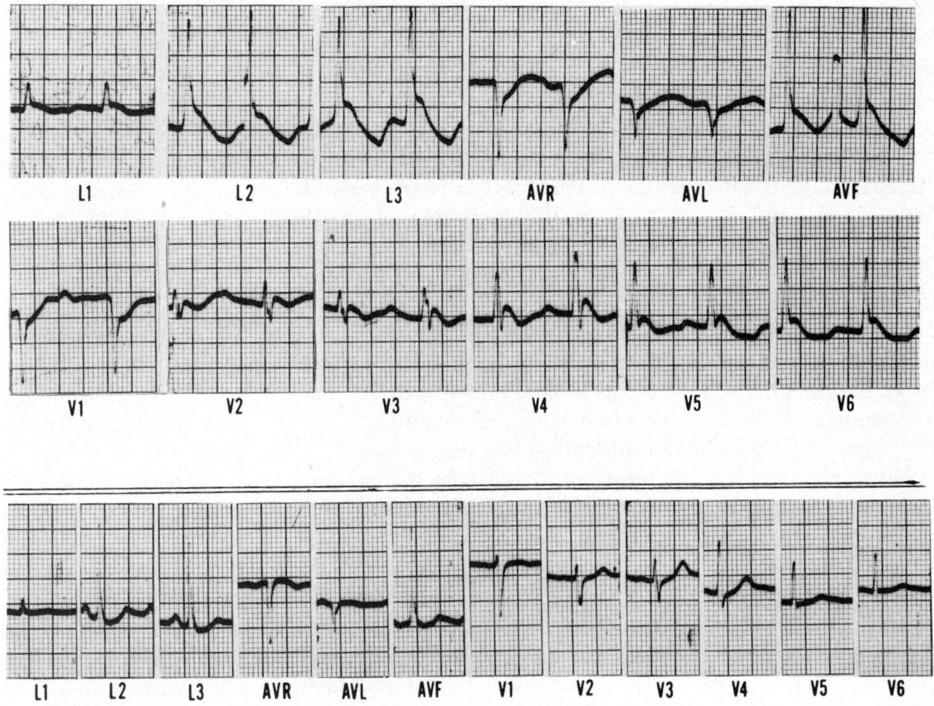

FIGURE 7–42 Osborne wave. *Upper panel,* Recorded during hypothermia, the P-R interval is 0.28 sec; the QRS complex measures 0.10 sec and is followed by a wave (the Osborne wave) that merges with the ST segment; and the T wave is inverted in leads I, II, III, aV_f, V_5, and V_6. It is difficult to separate the Osborne wave from the initial part of the ST segment. *Bottom panel,* Recorded after the temperature returned to normal. The tracing is normal.

to body temperature. The electrophysiological mechanism of the Osborne wave remains unclear.

THE ECG AND ELECTROLYTE ABNORMALITIES

Potassium

HYPERKALEMIA. In experimental hyperkalemia there is a good correlation between plasma K and the surface ECG.[239] The earliest ECG change, at a plasma level of about 5.7 mEq/liter, is a tall, peaked, most often symmetrical T wave with a narrow base and a normal or decreased Q-Tc interval. The QRS complex widens uniformly at a level of 9 to 11 mEq/liter and an occasional acute current of injury resembling myocardial infarction may be present.[240] Reduction in P-wave amplitude, intraatrial conduction delay, and P-R interval prolongation are recorded at a plasma level of about 7.0 mEq/liter. At plasma K levels of about 8.4 mEq/liter or higher, the P wave is no longer recognizable. When the plasma concentration exceeds 12 mEq/liter, either ventricular fibrillation or arrest follows. Sinoatrial node fibers, being more resistant to the depressive action of K than is atrial myocardium, continue to generate impulses that are now delayed in their exit or may fail to propagate because of depressed intraatrial conduction. The result may be Wenckebach (type I) or Mobitz (type II) sinoatrial (SA) block. Junctional escape and junctional rhythm are relatively common in experimental hyperkalemia.[241]

In clinical hyperkalemia, abnormalities of impulse formation and conduction appear at K levels lower than those observed in the experimental animal, and the correlation between plasma K and the ECG is less reliable. A tall, peaked, symmetrical T wave with a narrow base, the so-called "tented" T wave, is the earliest ECG abnormality.[242] The pointed, symmetrical appearance and narrow base of the T wave help to differentiate the effect of hyperkalemia from other causes of tall T waves, often a normal variant. The tented appearance and the narrow base are probably more characteristic of hyperkalemia than is the amplitude of the T wave. T waves suggestive of hyperkalemia are found in about 20 per cent of patients with elevated plasma K levels and are usually best seen in leads II, III, V_2, V_3, and V_4. A decrease in amplitude of the R wave, appearance of a prominent S wave, widening of the QRS complex, depression of the ST segment, and an occasional elevation of the ST segment evolve as plasma K continues to rise and approaches 8 to 9 mEq/liter (Fig. 7–43).[240] A decrease in amplitude and prolongation of the P wave and lengthening of the P-R interval followed by disappearance of the P wave often makes recognition of arrhythmias in hyperkalemia difficult, if not impossible.[243]

With hyperkalemia, depression of intraventricular conduction is characteristically diffuse and fairly uniform and results in prolongation of both the initial and terminal parts of the QRS complex. The resulting pattern may resemble RBBB, LBBB, left anterior or posterior divisional block, or some combination of these. When the ECG resembles RBBB, the initial phase of the QRS complex is prolonged, in contrast to the conventional RBBB, in which only the terminal portion of the QRS complex is delayed.

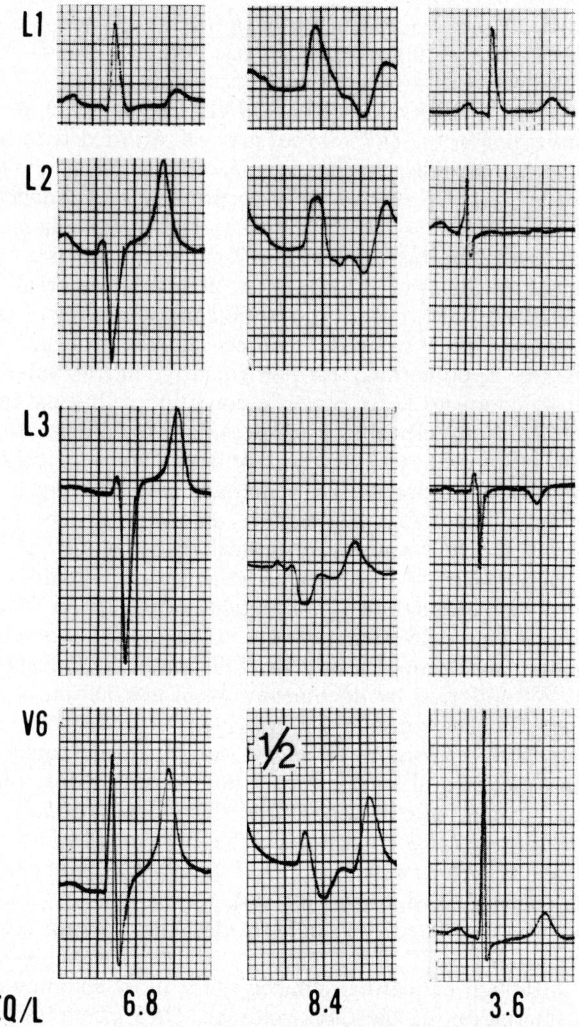

FIGURE 7–43 ECG changes of hyperkalemia. After treatment with potassium (K^+ level = 3.6 mEq/liter), the P-R interval, QRS, and T waves are normal. At a K^+ level of 6.8 mEq/liter the P-R interval and QRS complex are prolonged, with shift of the QRS axis to the left. The T waves are symmetrical, narrow based, and tall—the so-called tented T wave. At a K^+ level of 8.4 mEq/liter, there is further prolongation of the P-R interval, the P wave is difficult to identify, the QRS complex is prolonged to 0.20 sec, and the QRS axis is normal. Prolongation of both initial and terminal portions of the QRS complex, characteristic of K^+-induced intraventricular conduction, is best illustrated in lead V_6. (From Fisch, C.: Electrolytes and the heart. *In* Hurst, J. W. (ed.): The Heart. New York, McGraw-Hill Book Co., 1982, p. 1599.)

Similarly, when the ECG simulates LBBB, an S wave indicates slowing of the terminal portion of the QRS (Fig. 7–43). In conventional LBBB, on the other hand, prolongation involves only the initial component of the QRS complex.

In man, as in animals, SA block (p. 691), either Wenckebach (type I) or Mobitz (type II), passive or accelerated junctional or ventricular escape rhythms may be present. Potassium may normalize physiologically or functionally inverted T waves, but as a rule it has no effect on T-wave inversion due to organic disorders or drugs.[244]

HYPOKALEMIA. Patients treated for diabetic coma have been found to have a prolonged Q-T interval, abnormal T waves, occasionally a depressed ST segment—

changes proved to be due to hypokalemia.[245] There is a reasonable correlation between ECG changes and K concentrations below 2.3 or 3.0 mEq/liter.[246–248] The hypokalemia is characterized by an exaggerated U wave without a significant change in Q-T duration (Fig. 7–44). Depression of the ST segment and its gradual fusion with the U wave, less commonly inversion of the T wave, and an increase in amplitude of the QRS complex may also be present. Prominent U waves with ST-segment and T-wave changes are not specific for hypokalemia, however. Such abnormalities can be the result of digitalis and other drugs, ventricular hypertrophy, and bradycardia.

CALCIUM

The effects of calcium on the ECG were recognized in 1922.[249] In general, the ECG changes due to alteration in Ca levels correlate with the effect of Ca ion on the transmembrane action potential. Changes in duration of phase 2 parallel the altered duration of the ST segment and the Q-T interval.

Hypocalcemia prolongs phase 2, reflected by prolongation of the ST segment and Q-T interval (Fig. 7–45). The Q-aT (Q to the apex of the T wave) and Q-T intervals are prolonged, but the Q-Tc interval rarely exceeds 140 per cent of the normal. If longer, the U wave is likely to be included in the measurement. Hypocalcemia does not affect phase 3 of the action potential or the T wave.[248] Hypocalcemia with hyperkalemia, most often seen in patients with chronic renal disease, results in a prolonged ST segment and a "tented" T wave (Fig. 7–45). Hypocalcemia and hypokalemia exhibit a prolonged ST segment and a prominent terminal wave that includes both T and U waves.[246]

Hypercalcemia shortens phase 2 of the action potential and the ST segment. Occasionally the ST segment is depressed and the Q-T interval shortened (Fig. 7–45).

The correlation between the Q-T interval and serum Ca concentration is unpredictable, largely because the Q-T duration is affected by factors other than calcium levels, such as age, sex, heart rate, myocardial disease, drugs, and other electrolytes. It has been suggested that when one eliminates factors known to alter the Q-T interval, a reasonably good correlation is found between the ECG and calcium levels. This assumption is supported by the fact that Ca levels in pure hypocalcemia induced by EDTA show a reasonably good correlation with the Q-T interval. Of the three intervals—Q-T, Q-oT (Q to the onset of the T wave), and Q-aT—the Q-aT interval can be measured with greatest accuracy and correlates best with the Ca level.[250]

MAGNESIUM

Administration of magnesium may result in a statistically significant shortening of the Q-T interval. As a rule, however, abnormalities of the ST segment due to hypermagnesemia cannot be identified on the ECG because the changes are dominated by calcium.[251] Hypomagnesemia cannot be recognized on the ECG.

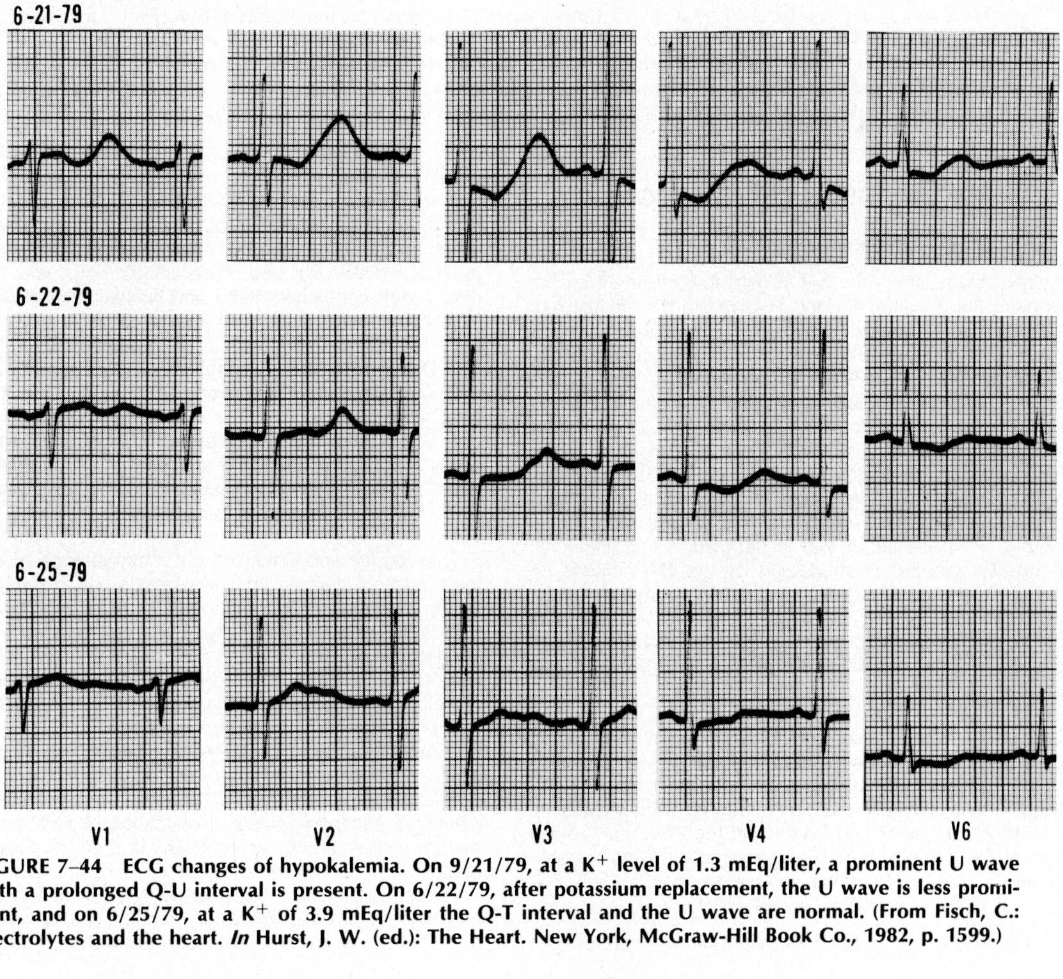

FIGURE 7–44 ECG changes of hypokalemia. On 9/21/79, at a K^+ level of 1.3 mEq/liter, a prominent U wave with a prolonged Q-U interval is present. On 6/22/79, after potassium replacement, the U wave is less prominent, and on 6/25/79, at a K^+ of 3.9 mEq/liter the Q-T interval and the U wave are normal. (From Fisch, C.: Electrolytes and the heart. *In* Hurst, J. W. (ed.): The Heart. New York, McGraw-Hill Book Co., 1982, p. 1599.)

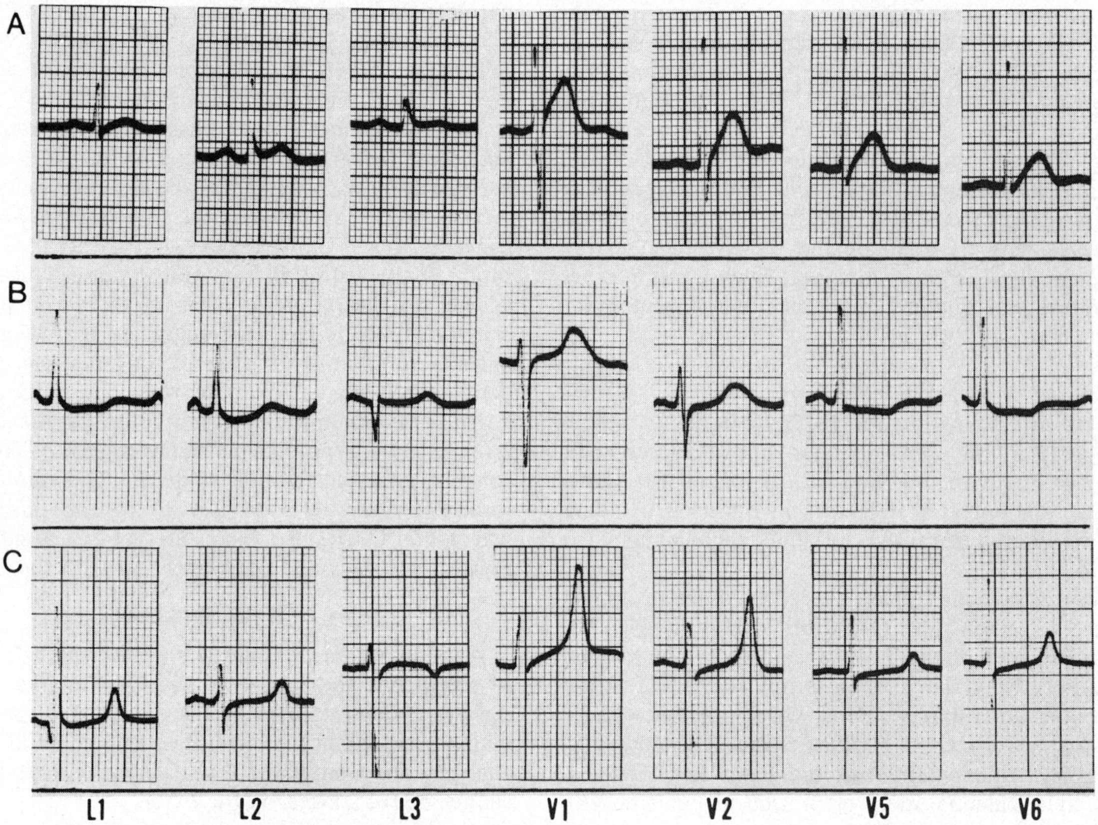

FIGURE 7–45 ECG changes of hypercalcemia, hypocalcemia, and hypocalcemia with hyperkalemia. *A,* Tracing recorded at a Ca^{++} level of 17.0 mg/dl shows short ST segment of hypercalcemia. *B,* At a Ca^{++} level of 5.9 mg/dl the Q-T interval is prolonged characteristic of hypocalcemia. *C,* Tracing recorded at a K^{+} level of 6.2 mEq/liter, Ca^{++} of 5.3 mg/dl, and phosphorus of 12.2 mg/dl. The prolonged Q-T interval and the tented T wave reflect hypocalcemia and hyperkalemia seen in chronic renal disease. (Fisch, C.: Electrolytes and the heart. *In* Hurst, J. W. (ed.): The Heart. New York, McGraw-Hill Book Co., 1982, p. 1599.)

EFFECTS OF DRUGS ON THE ECG

DIGITALIS (See also p. 523)

The cardiac glycosides differ little with regard to their effect on the ECG. Alterations of the ST segment and T wave are the earliest recognizable changes due to digitalis. The T-wave amplitude is lowered, and the ST segment is depressed and shortened, with occasional appearance of a prominent U wave.[252] While the "characteristic" digitalis-induced ST segment is described as sagging, it is often difficult if not impossible to differentiate it from ST-segment depression of other causes. When the ST segment is also shortened, digitalis is the likely cause of the depression. ST-segment displacement due to digitalis may be greatly exaggerated by myocardial disease, tachycardia, and high-amplitude QRS complexes. Rarely, digitalis causes symmetrical inversion of the T wave similar to that in pericarditis and ischemia, but there is usually associated shortening of the Q-T interval. A peaked, "tented" T wave, probably due to concomitant hyperkalemia, can also be present.

Digitalis has no significant effect on depolarization of the atrium or ventricle. Consequently, prolongation of intraatrial and intraventricular conduction is rare.[253]

Classification of Digitalis-Induced Arrhythmias. Digitalis has been known to induce nearly every known arrhythmia, and a comprehensive discussion of the subject is beyond the scope of this review.[254–256] The following general classification, based on the electrophysiological effects of the cardiac glycoside and less so on the ECG morphology or site of origin of the arrhythmia, encompasses most of the digitalis-induced arrhythmias. The classification is enlarged upon in Table 7–6 and is discussed in terms of clinical relevance below.

1. Ectopic rhythms due to enhanced automaticity or reentry or both and, perhaps, to delayed diastolic afterdepolarizations (p. 620) (Fig. 7–46): atrial tachycardia with block (see Fig. 21–13, p. 701), atrial fibrillation and flutter, nonparoxysmal junctional tachycardia, (Fig. 21–19, p. 705), ventricular premature contractions, ventricular tachycardia (Fig. 7–46), ventricular flutter and fibrillation, multiple ectopic rhythms, bidirectional ventricular tachycardia (Fig. 7–47), or accelerated escape.

2. Depression of pacemaker: Sinoatrial node arrest (p. 691).

3. Depression of conduction: SA block, AV block, exit block, or reciprocation.

4. AV dissociation: Suppression of the dominant pacemaker with passive escape of the lower junctional focus or inappropriate acceleration of a subsidiary pacemaker, or, rarely, dissociation within the AV junction (double junctional tachycardia).

Therapeutic and Toxic Effects. Appearance of ectopic rhythms in the course of digitalis administration is nearly always a sign of toxicity. On the other hand, depression of AV conduction may at times be a desirable therapeutic endpoint. Acknowledging that some degree of overlap is unavoidable and that the clinical significance of an arrhythmia may differ depending on the setting, we can divide the effects of digitalis on the ECG into three general groups—therapeutic, excessive and/or toxic, and unequivocally toxic.

Clinically acceptable effects of digitalis include some prolongation of the P-R interval; slowing of the ventricular response in atrial flutter and fibrillation: and in atrial fibrillation, the appearance of isolated AV junctional escape impulses. Conversion of atrial arrhythmias to sinus rhythm, either directly or indirectly, is another desirable effect of the drug.

Excessive or toxic effects, or both, are heralded by the appearance of atrial tachycardia with block, nonparoxysmal junctional tachycardia (Fig. 7–48), AV dissociation, second- and third-degree AV block, SA

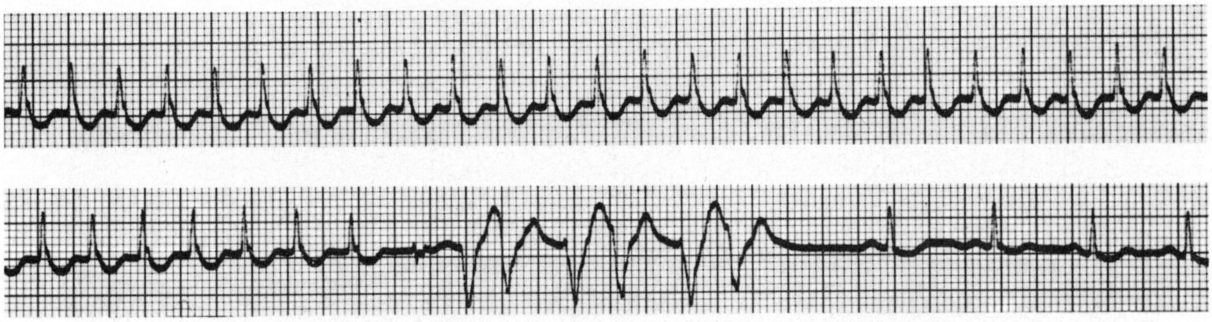

FIGURE 7–46 **Supraventricular tachycardia treated with large doses of digitalis terminating with ventricular tachycardia and 3:2 Wenckebach (type I) exit block. Atrial tachycardia at a rate of 230 bpm is followed by a bigeminal rhythm, with ventricular complexes all of similar morphology. The longer cycles are less than twice the shorter cycle, suggesting a ventricular tachycardia with a 3:2 Wenckebach exit block. The interectopic ventricular cycle length is 0.22 sec. One possible mechanism of the ventricular tachycardia is delayed afterdepolarization, or "triggered" automaticity.**

block, AV junctional rhythm, and reciprocating rhythm. Ventricular arrhythmias due to digitalis are an unequivocal sign of toxicity. This group includes isolated ventricular premature contractions (VPC), ventricular bigeminy, multifocal or multiform VPC, ventricular tachycardia, and "bidirectional" ventricular tachycardia, flutter, and fibrillation.

A *diagnosis of digitalis toxicity* is seldom based on the ECG alone. Pharmacodynamics of the glycoside and extracardiac and cardiac factors that alter tolerance to the drug must be considered.[256] The numerous arrhythmias ascribed to digitalis and summarized in Table 7–6 represent a composite of a number of studies of digitalis toxicity reported over a period of 21 years. The data should be viewed in light of the retrospective nature of the studies and the fact that interpretation and recognition of arrhythmias were subject to changes in our knowledge about electrophysiology and electrocardiography during the interim between studies. For example, atrial tachycardia with block and nonparoxysmal junctional tachycardia were noted in only a small number of early studies but were increasingly recognized as analysis of arrhythmias became more sophisticated. In addition, a serious limitation of any such study is the low specificity of many of the arrhythmias for digitalis toxicity.[257]

The wide spectrum of arrhythmias induced by digitalis and the coexistence of a number of different arrhythmias in the same tracing can be explained by the effects of the interplay of digitalis and myocardial and extracardiac factors on the electrophysiological properties of cardiac tissues. The magnitude of the effect of the drug on specialized tissue, the SA node, specialized atrial tissue, AV junctional tissue, and the Purkinje fibers varies and, in fact, may have an opposite effect on cells with the same functional properties. Furthermore,

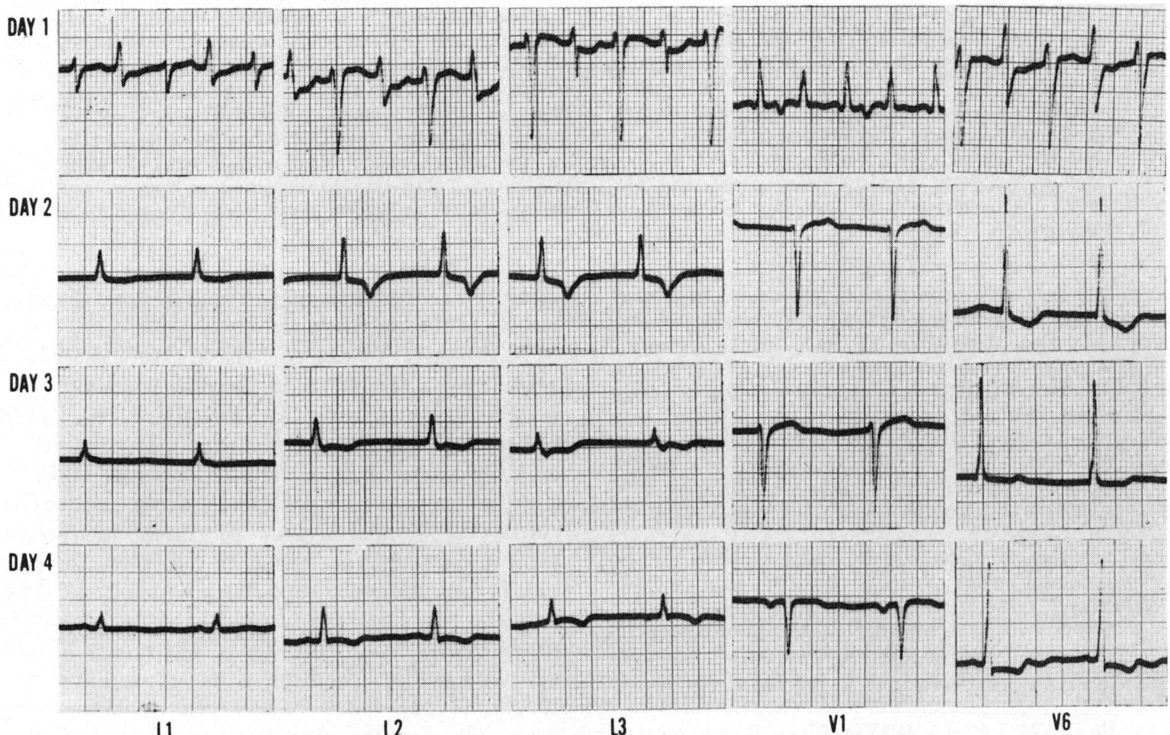

FIGURE 7–47 **Bidirectional ventricular tachycardia and junctional tachycardia due to digitalis. On day 1, the ECG shows bidirectional ventricular tachycardia with alternation of the axis and RBBB. The divisions of the left bundle are the site of the tachycardia. On day 2, the rhythm is junctional at a rate of 83 bpm, with retrograde P waves in leads II and III and an R-P interval of about 0.20 sec. On day 3, the junctional rate is 68 and retrograde P waves follow the R wave by an interval of about 0.08 sec. On day 4, normal sinus rhythm is accompanied by nonspecific T-wave changes in leads II, III, and V_6 and negative U waves in lead V6.**

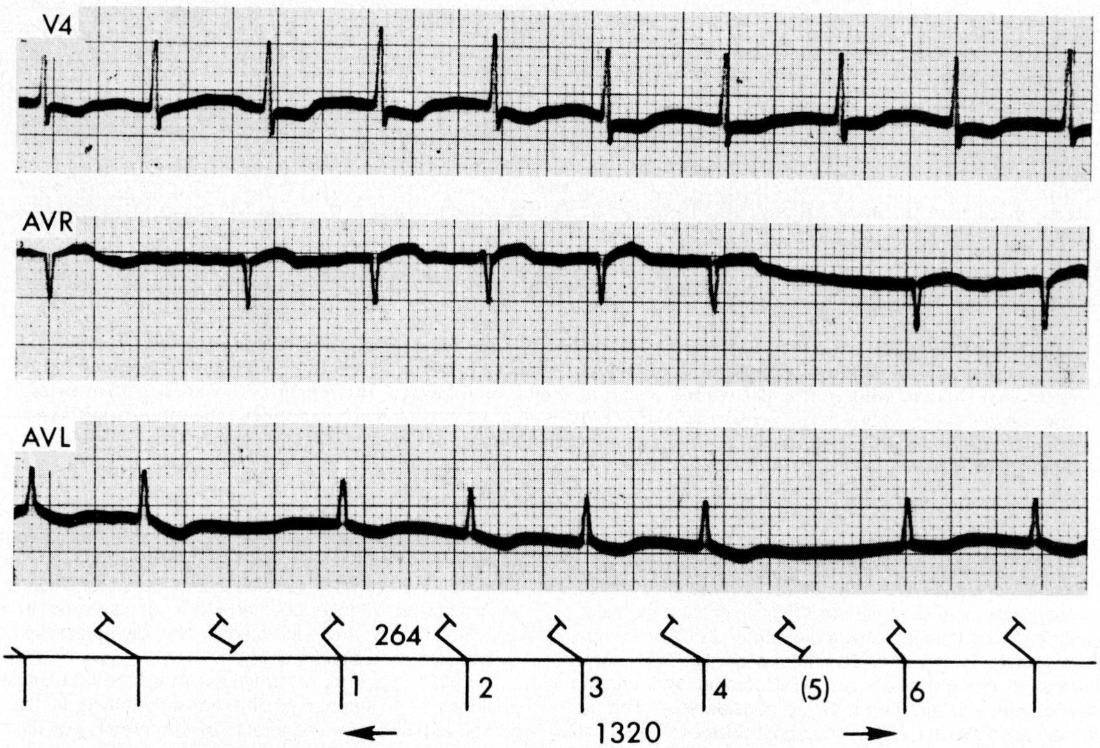

FIGURE 7-48 Atrial fibrillation and nonparoxysmal junctional tachycardia with Wenckebach (type I) exit block due to digitalis intoxication. Lead V_4 illustrates a regular ventricular rhythm at a rate of 107 bpm, characteristic of this arrhythmia. In leads aV_r and aV_l the R-R cycle foreshortens gradually and the long pause is shorter than the length of two of the preceding R-R cycles. This is characteristic of a Wenckebach structure and identifies Wenckebach (type I) exit block from the junctional focus. Although at first glance leads aV_r and aV_l suggest atrial fibrillation, the repetitive Wenckebach structure indicates that there is, in addition, a regular junctional rhythm with a Wenckebach (type I) exit block.

The actual interectopic junctional interval and delay of conduction from the pacemaker to surrounding tissue can be calculated from the ECG with the aid of the Lewis diagram (bottom). The number of *manifest* QRS cycles of the Wenckebach sequence (QRS1 to QRS6) is four. To this number is added one additional pacemaker cycle to take into account the cycle that fails to manifest a QRS(5). The duration of the sequence from QRS1 to QRS6 is 1320 msec. The latter is divided by the five cycles, and the actual interectopic interval of the junctional pacemaker is calculated to be 264 msec. The increased distance between the junctional pacemaker and the manifest QRS is a measure of delay of conduction from the pacemaker to the myocardium. The same method is used to calculate the sinoatrial node (SAN) rate and conduction time to the atrium in the presence of Wenckebach type I exit block. The SAN and P wave are substituted for the junctional pacemaker and QRS, respectively.

the electrocardiographic expression of electrophysiological effects of digitalis is a net result of altered automaticity, refractoriness, excitability, and conduction. Also, digitalis may act directly on the specialized tissue or its action may be mediated through the sympathetic or parasympathetic system or both.[258,259] In addition, the sensitivity of the tissues to digitalis may be altered by factors such as a changing acid-base balance, plasma and intracellular electrolyte levels, oxygen saturation, and mechanical stretch. Similarly, improvement of cardiac function with treatment may alter the variables affecting the electrophysiological properties of the cardiac tissue and consequently the tissue's response to digitalis.

Arrhythmias identical to those due to digitalis toxicity can be caused by heart disease, drugs other than digitalis, and a variety of extracardiac factors.[260]

Selected arrhythmias due to digitalis have been singled out for discussion here because of their frequency and relatively high specificity for digitalis toxicity.

ATRIAL TACHYCARDIA WITH BLOCK (see also p. 701). The cause of this arrhythmia can be ascribed almost equally to severe heart disease and to digitalis toxicity.[260-263] The diagnosis of atrial tachycardia with block may occasionally be difficult. At rapid rates it resembles atrial flutter. The amplitude of the atrial deflections may be low, and only careful attention to lead V_1 may disclose the true nature of the arrhythmia.

NONPAROXYSMAL JUNCTIONAL TACHYCARDIA (see also p. 704). In the proper setting, this arrhythmia is highly specific for digitalis excess or toxicity.[264] Other less common causes of nonparoxysmal junctional tachycardia, namely, acute myocardial infarction, open heart surgery, myocarditis, and general anesthesia, must be ruled out. Nonparoxysmal junctional tachycardia differs from paroxysmal junctional or supraventricular tachycardia. It appears and disappears gradually and, when repetitive, the coupling, or relation of the first ectopic complex, to the dominant impulse varies. The rate is 70 to 130 bpm. AV dissociation resulting from acceleration of the AV junctional pacemaker is recorded in 85 per cent of the cases. The ectopic junctional focus activates both atria and ventricles in the remaining 15 per cent of cases. Rarely, two junctional foci coexist, one controlling the atria and the other the ventricles, resulting in a double junctional tachycardia.[265]

In the absence of exit block, the rhythm in non-

TABLE 7–6 CARDIAC ARRHYTHMIAS DUE TO DIGITALIS (10 STUDIES, 661 PATIENTS)

	No. of Series	No. of Arrhythmias		
Ventricular Arrhythmias		470 (71%)		
Ventricular premature contractions			420	
Bigeminy	9			150
Multifocal	4			121
Not specified	4			79
Other (frequent, unifocal, occasional, etc.)	3			70
Ventricular tachycardia	7		50	
AV Block		194 (29%)		
First-degree	7		87	
Second-degree	10		58	
Wenckebach	3			4
Third-degree	6		37	
Unspecified	2		12	
Atrial Arrhythmias		177 (26%)		
Atrial fibrillation	9		80	
with slow rate	2			21
PAT with block	7		59	
Atrial premature beats	4		27	
Atrial flutter	4		11	
Sinoatrial Node Arrhythmias		85 (13%)		
Sinus tachycardia	3		29	
Sinus bradycardia	4		27	
with nodal escape	1			11
Sinus arrest	2		11	
SA block	3		7	
Wandering pacemaker	3		11	
AV Dissociation	4	65 (9.8%)		
AV Nodal Arryhthmias		47 (7%)		
Nodal tachycardia	4		32	
Nodal rhythm	2		11	
Nodal premature beats	1		4	

From Knoebel, S.B., and Fisch, C.: Recognition and therapy of digitalis toxicity. Progr. Cardiovasc. Dis. *13*:71, 1970.

paroxysmal junctional tachycardia is generally perfectly regular and the diagnosis usually simple. Recognition becomes more difficult in the presence of exit block.[266] A high degree of exit block may suggest a slow junctional rhythm or AV block. If the exit block is Mobitz (type II), with 3:2 exit block, a bigeminal rhythm appears, with longer cycles exact multiples of shorter cycles. If the exit block is Wenckebach (type I), the gradually shortening R-R interval and lack of the expected relationship of the long pause to the shorter cycles (i.e., the pause is not a multiple of the shorter cycle), atrial fibrillation may be suggested (Fig. 7–48). Only a careful search for the Wenckebach structure will reveal the true nature of the arrhythmia. Nonparoxysmal junctional tachycardia with an irregular ventricular response without conforming to the Wenckebach (type I) or Mobitz (type II) structure precludes the diagnosis, and nonparoxysmal junctional tachycardia cannot be differentiated from atrial fibrillation. Occasionally, this arrhythmia is masked and becomes evident with slowing of the dominant rhythm; it may appear as nonparoxysmal junctional tachycardia or as a single accelerated escape impulse.[267]

Differentiation of nonparoxysmal junctional tachycardia with aberrant intraventricular conduction from ventricular tachycardia may be difficult, if not impossible. A rapid heart rate, a bizarre QRS complex, and AV dissociation are common to both arrhythmias. In the presence of WPW, nonparoxysmal junctional tachycardia may be associated with fusion and capture complexes.[107]

VENTRICULAR ARRHYTHMIAS. Ventricular premature contractions (VPC) are the most common manifestation of digitalis toxicity but, at the same time, are the least specific as a sign of glycoside toxicity.[268] None of the morphological features of the QRS complex helps to differentiate VPC due to digitalis from those of other causes. The exception is ventricular bigeminy, with accurate coupling but varying morphology—a criterion that is suggestive of digitalis toxicity.

The problems of recognition associated with digitalis-induced VPC are also applicable to ventricular tachycardia. Ventricular tachycardia with exit block (Fig. 7–46) and bidirectional ventricular tachycardia (Fig. 7–47) strongly suggest digitalis intoxication. A bidirectional tachycardia of supraventricular origin is extremely rare. When the ventricular tachycardia originates in the divisions of the left bundle branch, the QRS complex may be normal in duration,[269] and the diagnosis rests on the presence of ventricular capture and fusion complexes. Studies in animals and man confirm that narrow QRS complex tachycardias may be ventricular in origin.

Digitalis-induced ventricular fibrillation is seldom recorded in man. It is rarely, if ever, the initial manifestation of digitalis toxicity but is usually preceded by other digitalis-induced arrhythmias.

In rare instances, ventricular parasystole is due to digitalis. This is particularly the case when parasystole is accompanied by other arrhythmias known to be due to digitalis intoxication.

The presence of diverse ectopic rhythms, either simultaneously or serially, is strongly suggestive of digitalis toxicity as is the appearance of ectopic rhythms and AV conduction.[253]

AV DISSOCIATION (see also p. 735). AV dissociation appearing in the course of digitalis administration is strongly indicative of digitalis overdosage or intoxication.[270]

AV CONDUCTION DELAY. Depression of AV conduction may be due to a vagal effect of the glycoside and can be reversed with atropine or catecholamines released during normal activities or during exercise. Such depression may also be due to a "direct" extravagal effect of the drug on the cell.[258,259,271]

In contrast to ectopy, depression of conduction may be either a desirable therapeutic effect or a manifestation of digitalis toxicity. The differentiation of the two is a clinical decision. For example, in atrial fibrillation and atrial flutter depression of AV conduction is desirable. In the presence of sinus rhythm, however, AV delay, other than simple prolongation of the P-R interval, is, with rare exception, evidence of digitalis overdose. Although AV block in the presence of sinus rhythm is frequently mentioned as a sign of digitalis intoxication, third-degree AV block is a relatively rare manifestation of glycoside toxicity.

ACCELERATED JUNCTIONAL ESCAPE. This arrhythmia is an interesting manifestation of digitalis intoxication. It is seen in the same clinical conditions as is nonparoxysmal junctional tachycardia and its clinical significance is probably the same in both.[267] Accelerated junctional escape follows the rules set for cardiac arrhythmias induced by delayed afterdepolarization[272] and may be the clinical counterpart of the arrhythmias induced in the Purkinje fiber and the intact animal.

"MASKED" (SUPPRESSED) DIGITALIS TOXICITY. Toxic effects of glycosides, especially enhanced junctional or Purkinje automaticity, may be suppressed by a more rapidly discharging, higher pacemaker. Slowing of the dominant rhythm may unmask the toxic ectopic rhythm, manifesting in the form of a single complex or an ectopic tachycardia. Sinus bradycardia, SA block, AV block, a compensatory pause following a spontaneous ectopic impulse,[267,273] and carotid sinus stimulation may be the mechanisms of slowing of the dominant rhythm and unmasking of toxicity.

The possibility of masked digitalis toxicity should be considered when digitalis is administered to patients with atrial fibrillation in clinical states in which slowing of the ventricular rate by digitalis is difficult or impossible. These include thyrotoxicosis, infection, pulmonary embolism, "high-output" failure, and occasionally intractable and perhaps far advanced heart failure.[257]

Other Drugs

QUINIDINE (see also p. 656). The ECG manifestations of quinidine are secondary to depression of conduction, automaticity, and excitability. At the level of the SA and AV nodes, the effect may be sinus bradycardia, sinus arrest, SA block, P-R interval prolongation, or rarely, a higher degree of AV block. Quinidine prolongs the P wave; slows intraatrial conduction and the rate of atrial flutter and fibrillation; and converts atrial fibrillation to atrial flutter, atrial flutter to fibrillation, and both—ultimately—to sinus rhythm. The combination of a slower flutter rate and acceleration of AV conduction due to the antivagal atropine-like effect of quinidine may result in an atrial flutter with 1:1 AV conduction (Fig. 7–49). Similar-

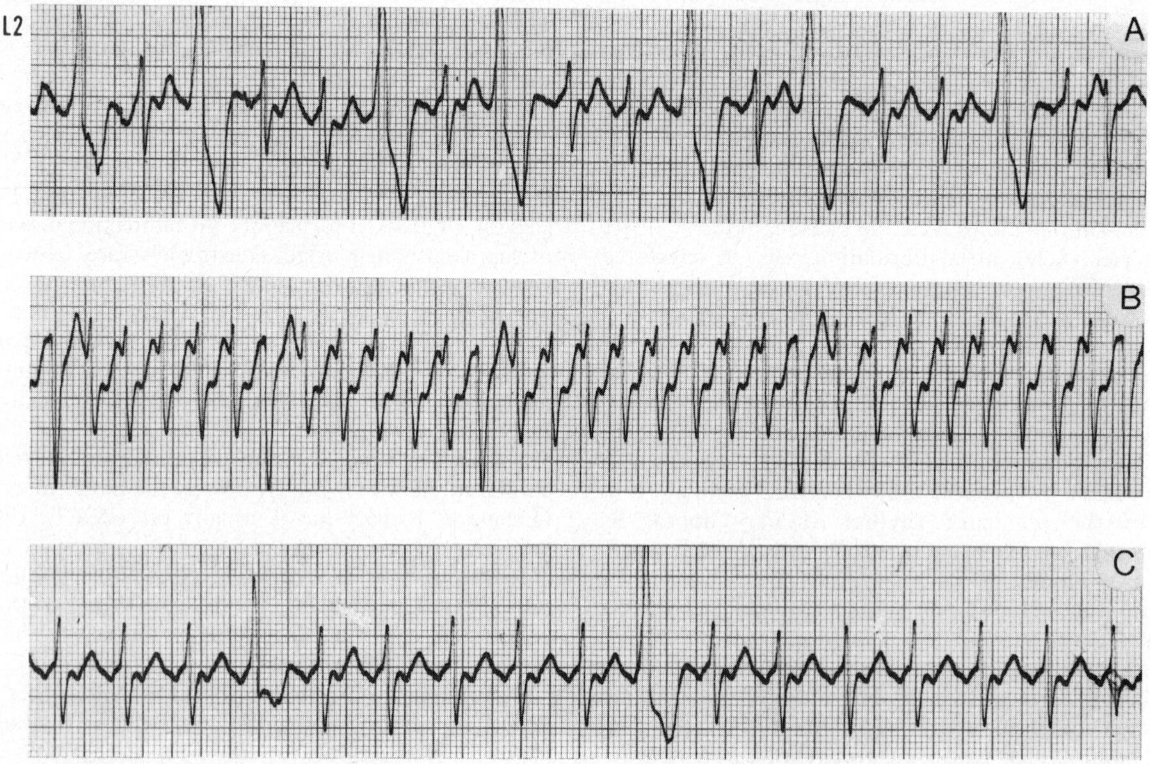

FIGURE 7–49 Acceleration of AV nodal conduction due to a combination of the vagolytic effect of quinidine and slowing of the rate of flutter by the drug. *A,* Atrial flutter with an f-f interval of 0.20 sec, 2:1 AV conduction, and ventricular premature systoles. *B,* Recording after administration of 900 mg of quinidine. The f-f interval is increased to 0.23 sec. Coupled with the vagolytic effect of quinidine on the AV node, this results in 1:1 AV conduction. *C,* Recording after administration of 10 mg of Tensilon shows that 2:1 AV conduction has been reestablished.

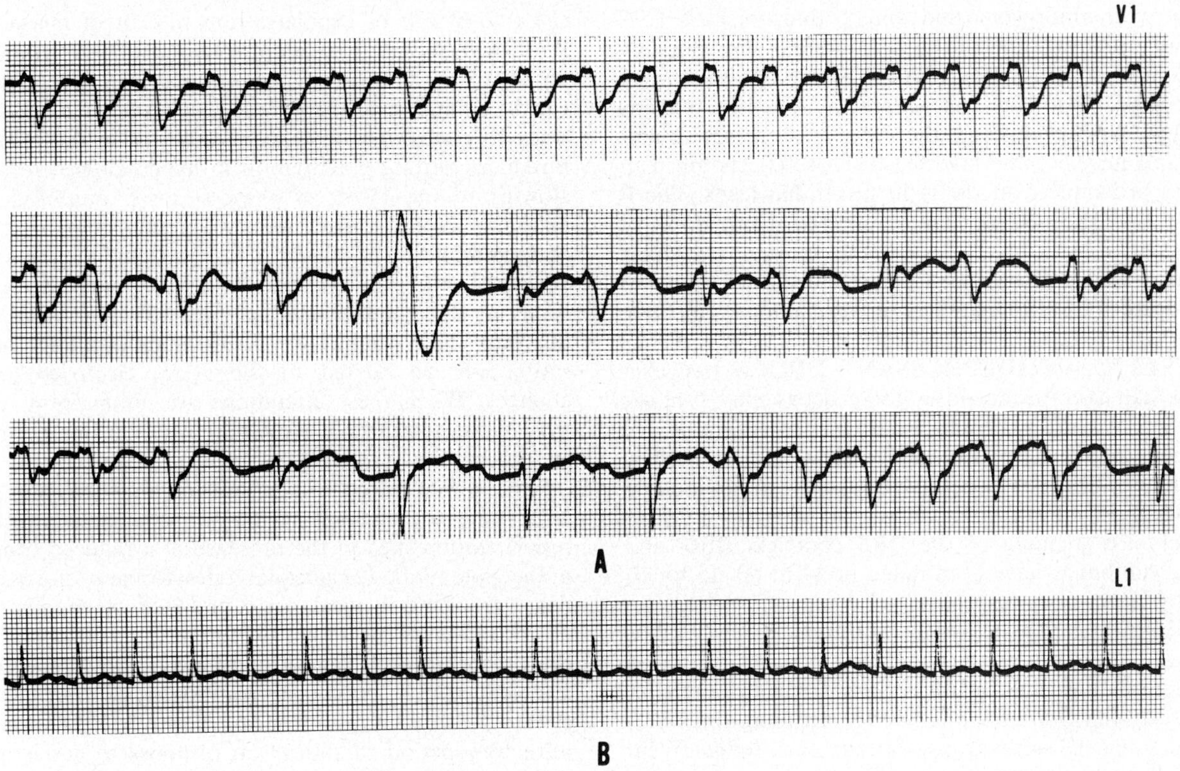

FIGURE 7–50 **Intraventricular aberration due to quinidine and acceleration of the heart rate. In panel *B*, a control tracing, the ECG is normal with a sinus rate of 130 bpm. After administration of quinidine (panel *A*), heart rate is 120 bpm and the QRS widened to 0.20 sec. In row 2, AV conduction changed to a 3:2 Wenckebach (type I) block interrupted by one VPC. P-wave duration is prolonged and the P-R interval measures 0.28 sec. The QRS complex following the longer pause is somewhat narrower, probably owing to a longer period of recovery. In row 3, 1:1 AV conduction is interrupted by 2:1 AV conduction. P waves measure 0.20 sec in duration, the P-R interval is 0.40 sec, and the QRS complexes are foreshortened to 0.16 sec. The intraventricular delay to 0.16 sec is caused by quinidine, while the much wider QRS complexes of 0.20 sec in the presence of 1:1 AV conduction reflect both the effect of quinidine and the accelerated heart rate.**

atrial flutter with 1:1 AV conduction (Fig. 7–49). Similarly, an acceleration of sinus rate and ventricular rate in atrial fibrillation can occur following the administration of quinidine.

At high plasma drug levels, the QRS complex is prolonged, and this usually affects the entire complex (Fig. 7–50).[274] The durations of the T wave and the Q-T interval are also prolonged. Depending on the effect of the drug on the QRS complex, the T-wave change may be secondary, primary, or a combination of the two. An upright T wave may lose amplitude or may become notched or inverted, while an inverted T wave may become more deeply inverted. The ST segment remains isoelectric and the U-wave amplitude is increased.[8] The T-wave changes are indistinguishable from a variety of other abnormal T waves. It has been suggested that the combination of a prolonged QRS complex, an abnormal T wave, and a dominant U wave is fairly specific for quinidine effect. However, similar changes may be seen with other drugs. Digitalis in combination with quinidine causes elongation and depression of the ST segment and a decrease in T wave amplitude. With appearance of a prominent U wave, the pattern is indistinguishable from that of hypopotassemia.[246]

Quinidine toxicity can be dose-dependent or dose-independent. Widening of the QRS complex, AV block, and pronounced bradycardia are usually produced by high levels of quinidine.[274] On the other hand, ventricular arrhythmias including the torsades de pointes variant of ventricular tachycardia and ventricular fibrillation (p. 725) may appear with low plasma levels of quinidine.[275]

PROCAINAMIDE (see also p. 657). The effect of procainamide on the ECG is the same as that of quinidine but quantitatively less pronounced, so that ECG abnormalities are less often encountered. The P wave and P-R intervals may be prolonged, the T wave lower and notched, and the U-wave amplitude increased.[276] As with quinidine, procainamide administered with digitalis results in an ECG pattern indistinguishable from that in hypopotassemia.

DISOPYRAMIDE (see also p. 659). The electrophysiological effects of disopyramide are similar to those of quinidine[277–279] and consist of slowing of the upstroke of phase 0 and prolongation of the transmembrane action potential. In the ECG, depression of conduction is manifest by lengthening of the P-R interval, the P wave, and the QRS complex. The Q-T interval may be prolonged and the T wave lowered and at times notched. Ventricular tachycardia, including torsades de pointes similar to that seen with quinidine, and ventricular fibrillation have been observed with disopyramide.[280]

PHENOTHIAZINES (see also p. 1840). ECG changes due to phenothiazine derivatives reflect the effect of these drugs on ventricular repolarization. Changes are most commonly seen with thioridazine and are less pronounced with chlorpromazine and trifluoperazine[215,281,282] and include prolongation of the Q-T interval and widening and notching of the T wave. The U-wave amplitude may be increased, but the ST segment usually remains unchanged. At higher levels the T wave decreases in amplitude and may become inverted.[283] These effects are usually most pronounced in the right precordial leads. The P wave and the QRS complex are not altered. Large doses of phenothiazines have been observed to induce ventricular arrhythmias and probably are the mechanism of occasional sudden death following ingestion of large amounts of these drugs.

TRICYCLIC ANTIDEPRESSANT DRUGS (see also p. 1838). In therapeutic doses these drugs may prolong the P-R interval, QRS complex, and Q-T interval; alter the ST segment and T wave; and induce atrial and ventricular arrhythmias. Toxic doses of the drugs may, in addition to the above listed effects, result in second- and third-degree AV block. Lengthening of the QRS complex, BBB, and cardiac arrhythmias have been noted in 44 to 50, 15 to 17, and 11 to 17 per cent, respectively.[284]

LITHIUM (see also p. 1841). Lithium affects cardiac repolarization and the sinoatrial node. The most common ECG abnormalities due to lithium are T-wave changes.[285] However, dysfunction of the SA node, including sinus bradycardia, sinoatrial node arrest, or exit block (either Wenckebach [type I] or Mobitz [type II]), is more characteristic of lithium toxicity. Interestingly, the ECG changes occur often at therapeutic levels of the salt. Lithium has no recognizable effects on the P-R interval or the QRS complex. A normal A-H interval with only slight prolongation of the H-V interval has been documented,[286] suggesting a selective action of lithium on the sinoatrial node.

MECHANISMS OF ARRHYTHMIAS DERIVED FROM ECG ANALYSIS

The ECG diagnosis of specific arrhythmias is discussed in Chapter 22, so that only selected mechanisms will be included here. These have been singled out because, in contrast to the arrhythmias discussed in Chapter 22, which can usually be diagnosed clinically, the concepts included in this section can as a rule (1) be inferred only from analysis of the ECG; (2) represent general principles, in that they apply to arrhythmias originating from different sites; (3) are clinically important; and (4) serve as ECG models of basic electrophysiological phenomena.[5,287–290]

ABERRATION

Intraventricular aberration, a term introduced and defined by Lewis, describes a supraventricular impulse with abnormal, bizarre intraventricular conduction (Fig. 7–51).[291] It refers to intraventricular conduction abnormalities related to changing heart rate or other functional alterations in electrophysiological properties, anomalous AV conduction, metabolic and electrolyte abnormalities, and toxic effects of drugs. The term aberration, as used currently, does not include fixed organic conduction defects.

The speed of conduction generally depends on the magnitude of the transmembrane resting potential (phase 4), the rate of rise of depolarization (dV/dt of phase 0), and the amplitude of the action potential. The relation of the dV/dt of phase 0 to the magnitude of the resting potential can be expressed as membrane responsiveness.[292] Excitation prior to completion of repolarization or in the presence of a reduced resting potential, as in hyperkalemia, results in a slowing of the dV/dt of phase 0, lower amplitude of the action potential, and slower conduction. Similarly, a shift of membrane responsiveness to the right, as, for example, with antiarrhythmic drugs such as quinidine, procainamide, or disopyramide, is associated with slowing of conduction.[293] The numerous ECG manifestations of aberration can be related to the above electrophysiological changes. When these alterations are nonuniform, conduction of the specialized tissue may also become nonuniform and aberration results.[294]

More specifically, the mechanisms for aberration include from time to time (1) excitation prior to completion of repolarization (i.e., in the presence of a reduced transmembrane potential), (2) unequal refractoriness of conducting tissue resulting in local delay or block of conduction, (3) prolongation of the action potential due to prolongation of the preceding cycle length and thus voltage-dependent refractoriness, (4) failure of restitution of transmembrane electrolyte concentration during diastole, (5) failure of the refractory period to shorten in response to acceleration of the heart rate, (6) a reduced take-off potential secondary to diastolic depolarization, (7) concealed transseptal conduction with delay or block of bundle branch conduction, (8) diffuse depression of intraventricular conduction including that of specialized as well as myocardial tissue, (9) anomalous ventricular activation due to congenital anatomical abnormalities such as the bundle of Kent and Mahaim and James fibers, and (10) "predestination" of intraventricular conduction secondary to altered intraatrial conduction.[18]

QRS aberration may result when any of the above mechanisms alter conduction in the bundle branches or the divisions of the left bundle branch (or a combination of the two), the Purkinje fibers, or the myocardium. RBBB is the most common form of aberrancy and is frequently associated with left anterior divisional block. Aberrancy due to LBBB is much less common and in our experience nearly always due to heart disease, although the heart disease may not be clinically evident.[295] An abnormality of intraventricular conduction due to diffuse depression of conduction in the Purkinje system and in the myocardium should be suspected when both the initial and terminal portions of the QRS complex are abnormal.

Of the numerous mechanisms and manifestations of aberration, nine will be considered in further detail: (1) premature excitation, (2) the Ashman phenomenon, (3) acceleration-dependent aberrancy, (4) deceleration-dependent aberrancy, (5) concealed conduction, (6) diffuse myocardial depression of conduction, (7) abnormal anatomical pathways, (8) postextrasystolic aberrancy, and (9) electrical (QRS) alternans.

Premature Excitation. Conduction will fail or be delayed if the stimulus falls during the effective or the relative refractory period of recovery.[5] When the impulse falls during the relative refractory period of a single bundle branch, the unilateral delay results in a bundle branch block. The duration of the refractory period may equal that of

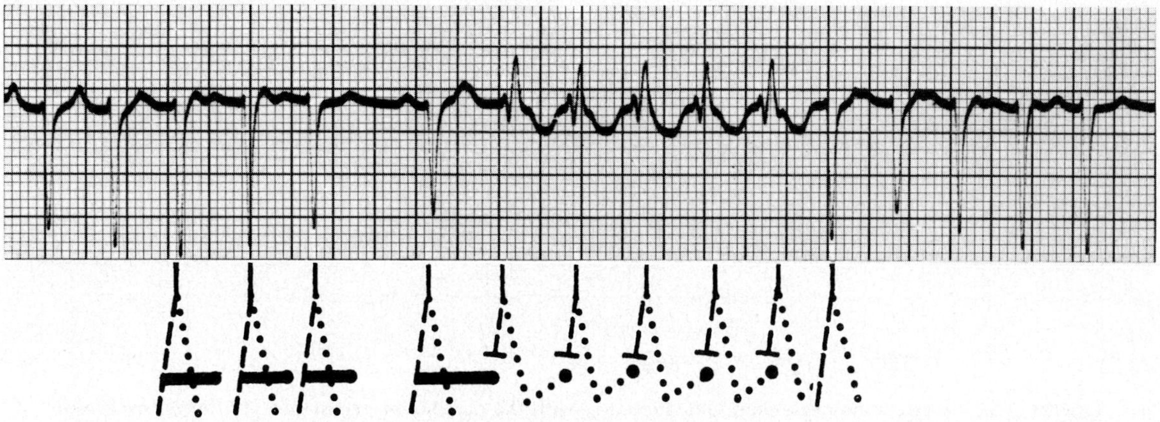

FIGURE 7–51 Atrial tachycardia with Wenckebach (type I) AV block, ventricular aberration due to the Ashman phenomenon, and probably concealed transseptal conduction. The long pause of the atrial tachycardia is followed by five QRS complexes with RBBB morphology. The RBBB of the first QRS reflects the Ashman phenomenon. The aberration is perpetuated by concealed transseptal activation from the left bundle into the right bundle with block of the anterograde conduction of the subsequent sinus impulse in the right bundle. Foreshortening of the R-R cycle, a manifestation of the Wenckebach structure, disturbs the relationship between transseptal and anterograde sinus conduction, and RBB conduction is normalized. In the diagram, the dashes indicate the RBB and the dots the LBB, while the solid bar denotes the refractory period. Following the long pause, the refractory period of the RBB is prolonged and is responsible for the RBBB of the first QRS. The impulse conducted along the LBB is propagated across the septum, engages the RBB, and blocks anterograde conduction of the sinus impulse.

the transmembrane action potential, so-called voltage-dependent refractoriness, or it may exceed it, so-called time-dependent refractoriness. Duration of the refractory period depends to a great extent on the basic heart rate and on the duration of the immediately preceding cycle(s). Normally, the refractory period shortens with acceleration of the heart rate and lengthens with slowing of the heart rate. It is possible, therefore, to maintain fixed coupling of a premature excitation to the dominant impulse but, by prolonging the preceding cycle, to lengthen the refractory period sufficiently to induce aberration.[296]

With all variables affecting conduction being constant, the degree of aberration is largely a function of prematurity of excitation. On rare occasions, however, the opposite may be noted, namely, a shorter R-P interval may be followed by a normal QRS complex while a longer R-P interval will exhibit an abnormal QRS complex (see Gap Phenomenon, p. 252).

The site of conduction depression and thus the morphology of the aberrant QRS complex is determined by the length of the refractory period of the AV node, the bundle of His, and the bundle system itself. Normally, at slow heart rates, the right bundle branch has the longest refractory period, with the left bundle and the AV node somewhat shorter and the bundle of His the shortest. Only at very rapid rates may the duration of the refractory period of the left bundle exceed that of the right bundle.[297]

Effect of Changing Cycle Length on Refractoriness (Ashman Phenomenon). This form of aberrancy, also a function of premature excitation, differs little electrophysiologically from that due to early excitation described above. The difference is that the abnormal conduction is a function of an altered duration of the refractory period rather than of changing prematurity of stimulation. Since the duration of the refractory period is a function of the immediately preceding cycle length, the longer the preceding cycle, the longer the refractory period that follows. Consequently, with a fixed stimulus interval, sudden prolongation of the immediately preceding cycle length may result in aberration. This relationship of aberrancy to changes in the preceding cycle length is known as the Ashman phenomenon.[296] It has been demonstrated that aberrancy so initiated may persist for a number of cycles (Fig. 7–51). With rare exception, aberrancy due to the Ashman phenomenon exhibits the RBBB morphology. The RBBB may be associated with left anterior or rarely with left posterior divisional block.

In the presence of irregular supraventricular rhythms, such as atrial fibrillation, repetitive atrial tachycardia, or atrial tachycardia with Wenckebach (type I) AV block (Fig. 7–51), aberration due to the Ashman phenomenon is suggested by the following: (1) a relatively long cycle immediately preceding the cycle terminated by the aberrant QRS complex, (2) RBBB aberrancy with normal orientation of the initial QRS vector, (3) irregular coupling of the aberrant QRS complex, and (4) lack of a compensatory pause following the aberrant QRS complex.

Acceleration-dependent aberrancy (tachycardia-dependent aberrancy, phase 3 aberrancy). This form of aberration has been recognized since 1913.[298] At certain critical heart rates, impaired intraventricular conduction results in aberrancy (Figs. 7–50 and 7–52). This phenomenon has been described using a variety of terms. The one most commonly used is tachycardia-dependent aberrancy or phase 3 aberrancy; however, neither term is entirely appropriate. Aberration often appears at relatively slow rates, frequently below 75 bpm; similarly, because of the slow rate at which the conduction fails, one would have to postulate an extremely long transmembrane action potential in order to accept excitation during phase 3 as the cause of the impaired conduction. Finally, conduction will also fail with excitation during phase 2 of the action potential. The term *acceleration-dependent aberrancy* appears most appropriate.

The appearance and disappearance of aberration often depends on very small changes in cycle length, a change frequently difficult if not impossible to detect in the ECG. Assuming that a reasonably long recording is available, a comparison of the earliest available cycle length terminated by a normal QRS complex with the cycle length terminated by the first aberrant QRS complex will aid in the diagnosis of acceleration-dependent aberrancy. The difference in the duration of two such cycles is often less than 0.04 sec. The importance of such a minimal foreshortening of the cycle length for this diagnosis can be demonstrated with atrial pacing in which a 10-msec or shorter decrease in cycle length may result in aberrant conduction. In some instances, as in paroxysmal atrial tachycardia, there may be no demonstrable change in cycle length preceding the onset of aberrant conduction. Such aberration is probably a function of the duration of the tachycardia and perhaps due to a failure of restitution of the ionic gradient during diastole (time-dependent refractoriness).[295]

Acceleration-dependent aberrancy differs in a number of respects from the physiological aberrancy observed in a normal heart. Differences include (1) appearance of aberrancy at relatively slow heart rates, (2) predominance of LBBB morphology, (3) independence from the immediately preceding cycle length, (4) occasional appearance with no, or only slight change in cycle length, and (5) association with heart disease.

QRS aberrancy may persist at an R-R interval considerably longer than the interval that initiated the aberrancy (Fig. 7–52). Three mechanisms have been suggested to explain this paradox: (1) concealed

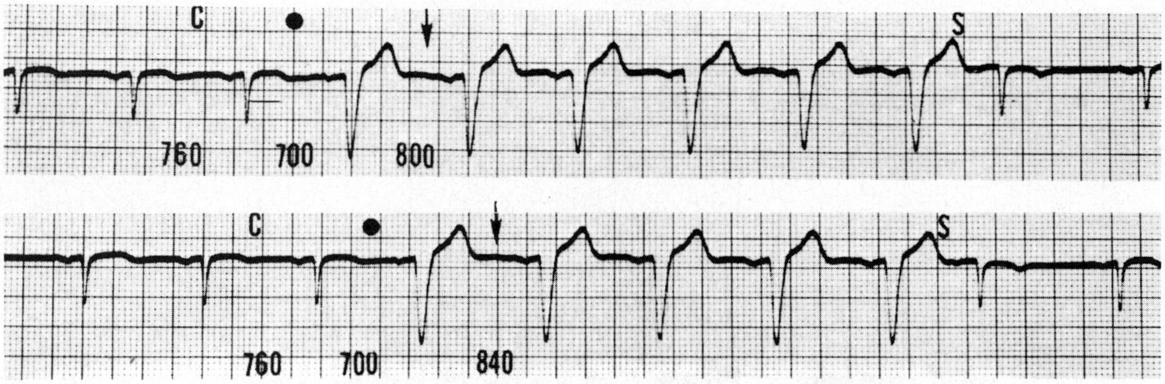

FIGURE 7–52 Acceleration-dependent QRS aberrancy with the paradox of persistence at a longer cycle and normalization at a shorter cycle than that which initiated the aberrancy. LBBB appears at a cycle length of 700 msec and is perpetuated at cycle lengths of 800 and 840 msec; conduction normalizes after a cycle length of 600 msec (S). Perpetuation of LBBB at a cycle length of 800 and 840 msec is probably due to transseptal concealment, similar to that described in Figure 7–51. Unexpected normalization of the QRS (S) following the atrial premature contraction is probably due to equalization of conduction in the two bundles; however, supernormal conduction in the left bundle cannot be excluded. (From Fisch, C., et al.: Rate dependent aberrancy. Circulation *48*:714, 1973, by permission of the American Heart Association, Inc.)

transseptal activation blocking conduction in the contralateral bundle; (2) "fatigue" of the bundle; and (3) concealed transseptal conduction coupled with suppression of conduction due to the increased heart rate, somewhat analogous to suppression of pacemakers by an ectopic tachycardia. A discrepancy of as much as 210 msec between the cycles initiating and terminating the aberration suggests that concealed transseptal conduction may not be the sole factor responsible for the unexpected persistence of aberrancy at the longer cycle lengths. The difference cannot be explained solely on the basis of time consumed by conduction along the contralateral bundle and across the septum.[299] Normal transseptal activation in the human heart is about 60 to 70 msec; in the diseased heart, it may be prolonged to 115 msec.[300] It is likely, therefore, that a combination of mechanisms is operative.

One mechanism that would explain the unexpected delay in normalization of intraventricular conduction is "fatigue."[295] The term "fatigue" is a descriptive one and may reflect failure of restitution of transmembrane ionic gradients and lowering of the transmembrane resting potential and/or a shift of the membrane responsiveness to the right. A different mechanism, namely, concealed conduction, may explain the delayed normalization of bundle branch conduction in patients with atrial fibrillation. Concealed conduction of atrial fibrillatory impulses into the blocked bundle may result in a true bundle-to-bundle interval that is considerably shorter than the manifest QRS interval.

Occasionally, paradoxical normalization of the QRS complex without a change in heart rate—or, in fact, with acceleration of the heart rate—has been documented (Fig. 7–52). Mechanisms that may explain this phenomenon include physiological shortening of the refractory period in response to acceleration of the heart rate, equalization of conduction in the two bundles, conduction during the supernormal period, and the gap phenomenon (p. 252).

Deceleration-dependent aberrancy (bradycardia-dependent aberrancy, phase 4 aberrancy). A prolonged cycle may be terminated by an aberrant QRS and foreshortening of the cycle may normalize the QRS (Fig. 7–53).[103,301] It has been suggested that this form of aberrancy is due to a gradual loss of transmembrane resting potential during a prolonged diastole with excitation from a less negative takeoff potential.[302] Because a small change in resting potential may have a pronounced effect on the rate of rise of phase 0 of the action potential, deceleration aberrancy may be seen with a relatively small prolongation of the cycle length.[303] In order to exclude ventricular escape as the cause for the apparent aberrancy, two or more consecutive aberrant QRS complexes must be recorded and all must be preceded by the same P-R interval. In atrial fibrillation, deceleration-dependent aberrancy cannot be considered because an idioventricular escape rhythm is likely. Similarly, concealed conduction (p. 247) into the bundle with a shorter bundle-to-bundle interval cannot be excluded with certainty. Concealed conduction may also be operative in patients with sinus rhythm and Wenckebach (type I) AV block, with the blocked P wave concealing the bundle and resulting in a short bundle-to-bundle interval and thus in aberrancy of the QRS complex following the Wenckebach pause. In such cases, the bundle-to-bundle interval may be considerably shorter than the manifest QRS cycle and may be even shorter than the QRS cycle during 1:1 AV conduction. Consequently, acceleration-dependent QRS aberrancy, rather than deceleration-dependent QRS aberrancy, may be present. Because both deceleration- and acceleration-dependent aberrancy reflect disordered electrophysiological function, the two often coexist.

Concealed Conduction. Bundle branch conduction may be impaired by concealed penetration of a supraventricular impulse or by transseptal activation from the contralateral bundle (Fig. 7–51). In atrial fibrillation, concealed conduction into a bundle branch can be considered when acceleration-dependent aberrancy persists at a QRS cycle that is longer than a cycle terminated by a normal QRS. Transseptal concealed conduction into a bundle branch from the contralateral bundle should be suspected if aberrancy, once initiated, persists at rates slower than the rate that initiated the aberrancy (Fig. 7–52).

Diffuse Myocardial Depression. Drugs and metabolic and electrolyte disorders are frequent causes of QRS aberrancy (Figs. 7–43 and 7–50). The severity of depression of conduction varies, and the QRS may exhibit RBBB or LBBB, divisional block, or the two combined. As indicated previously, aberrancy can be differentiated from ordinary BBB by the presence of distortion in the initial and terminal components of the QRS complex.

Anomalous AV Conduction. Activation of the ventricle over an abnormal AV pathway results in intraventricular aberration. The pathways of conduction resulting in QRS aberrancy include the Mahaim fibers, the bundle of Kent, and probably a combination of Mahaim and James fibers[18] (see also Fig. 21–26, p. 714).

The Mahaim fibers leave the AV node or the bundle of His and preexcite different areas of the interventricular septum. This mechanism has been invoked to explain aberrant junctional escape complexes when the QRS complex measures less than 0.12 sec. However, similar complexes may originate in the divisions of the left bundle branch, and the two sites of origin cannot be differentiated with certainty.

An AV nodal bypass tract may preferentially activate different parts of the His bundle and result in QRS aberrancy. It has been suggested that a tract bypassing the AV node, as manifested by a short P-R interval, when associated with distal conduction over Mahaim fibers may result in a QRS indistinguishable from WPW. Altered intraatrial conduction or conduction over the internodal pathways with preferential activation of segments of the AV junction, His bundle, or ventricular septum may theoretically result in QRS aberrancy.[18]

Postextrasystolic Aberration. Aberrant intraventricular conduction of a sinus impulse terminating a compensatory pause is rare and

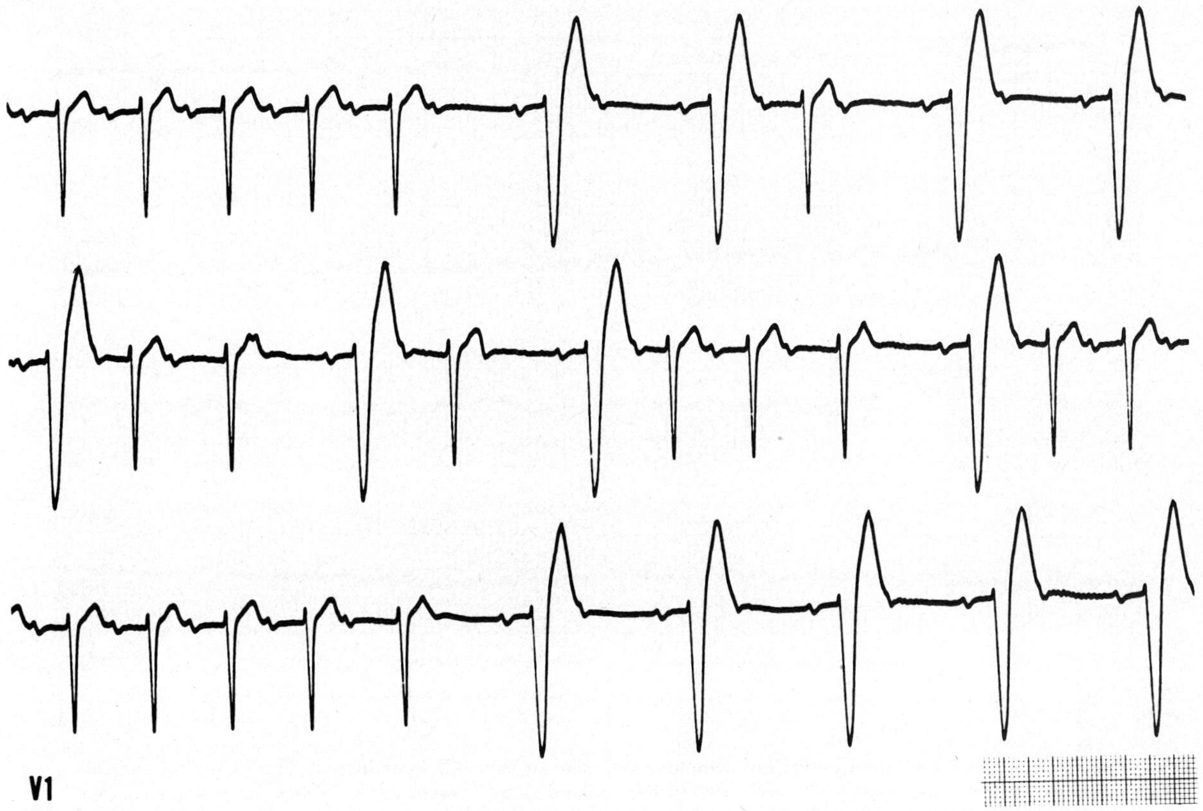

FIGURE 7–53 Deceleration-dependent aberrancy. The basic rhythm is sinus with Wenckebach (type I) AV block. With 1:1 AV conduction, the QRS complexes are normal in duration; with 2:1 AV block or after the longer pause of a Wenckebach sequence, LBBB appears. Slow diastolic depolarization (phase 4 of the transmembrane action potential) during the prolonged cycle is implicated as the cause of the LBBB.

must be differentiated from an aberrant escape complex. The exact mechanism of the postpausal aberrancy is not clear. It may be due to slow diastolic depolarization, unequal recovery of conducting or myocardial tissue, or increased diastolic volume.

Electrical (QRS) Alternans. The exact mechanism of QRS alternans is obscure and may differ from one case to another (p. 132). In supraventricular tachycardia with bidirectional "ventricular" complexes, the alternation is probably a result of alternate conduction over the two divisions of the left bundle with or without accompanying RBBB. In severe myocardial disease or digitalis intoxication, QRS alternans probably reflects nonuniform recovery of the ventricles and the basic mechanism may be related to altered ionic fluxes as suggested by the phenomenon of alternation of the transmembrane action potential. The QRS alternans in cardiac tamponade, as indicated earlier, is due to rotation of the heart.

CONCEALED CONDUCTION

Concealed conduction (CC) is a common manifestation of normal and diseased cardiac tissue, so that an understanding of this concept is prerequisite for analysis of all but the most simple cardiac arrhythmias. To understand CC is to appreciate the fact that the analysis of complex arrhythmias is one of deductive reasoning, since, as stated earlier, the surface ECG reflects electrical activity of myocardial tissue while the genesis of arrhythmias is related to abnormal function of the specialized tissues.

CC was observed and defined by Englemann in the course of studying an isolated heart preparation, some years before Einthoven introduced the electrocardiograph. In 1887, Englemann wrote, "Every effective atrial stimulation, even if it does not elicit a ventricular systole, prolongs the subsequent AV interval."[304] Thirty-eight years later this phenomenon was recorded in the AV node of the dog with the aid of the ECG.[305] Further studies in the intact animal,[299,306] in isolated cardiac cells,[307] and in man using His bundle electrography[308] validated the concept that had been derived by careful deductive analysis of the ECG,[309] i.e., that an incompletely conducted impulse can affect the behavior of subsequent AV conduction.

The concept of CC has been gradually extended to conduction within the sinoatrial node, perinodal tissue, atrium,[310] AV node, ventricular septum, and bundle branches[299] (Fig. 7–54). The concealing impulse may be normal, ectopic, automatic, or reentrant, and its conduction may be antegrade or retrograde.

A number of classifications of CC and its ECG manifestations have been proposed. Consideration of three variables—namely, the site of origin of the impulse which is concealed, the site of concealment, and the ECG manifestation—will define most all forms of CC. Concealed conduction can be grouped according to its effect on impulse formation, conduction, or both. More specifically, the effects include delay of conduction, block of conduction (Fig. 7–25), repetitive concealment, enhancement of conduction, reentrant rhythm, and premature resetting of a pacemaker. ECG manifestations of these six major categories are numerous, and each represents an interesting ECG model of basic electrophysiological phenomena.[290,309,311]

FUSION

A fusion complex, either atrial or ventricular, results from simultaneous activation of the atria or ventricles by impulses originating at two different sites. The resultant fusion complex frequently represents a spectrum of P waves or QRS complexes, their morphology depending on the relative contribution of the two impulses. The timing of the two impulses contributing to the fusion complex must be such that simultaneous excitation of the chambers is possible. For example, in the case of fusion between a sinus and ventricular impulse, the P-R interval must be sufficiently long for the sinus impulse to have reached the ventricle.

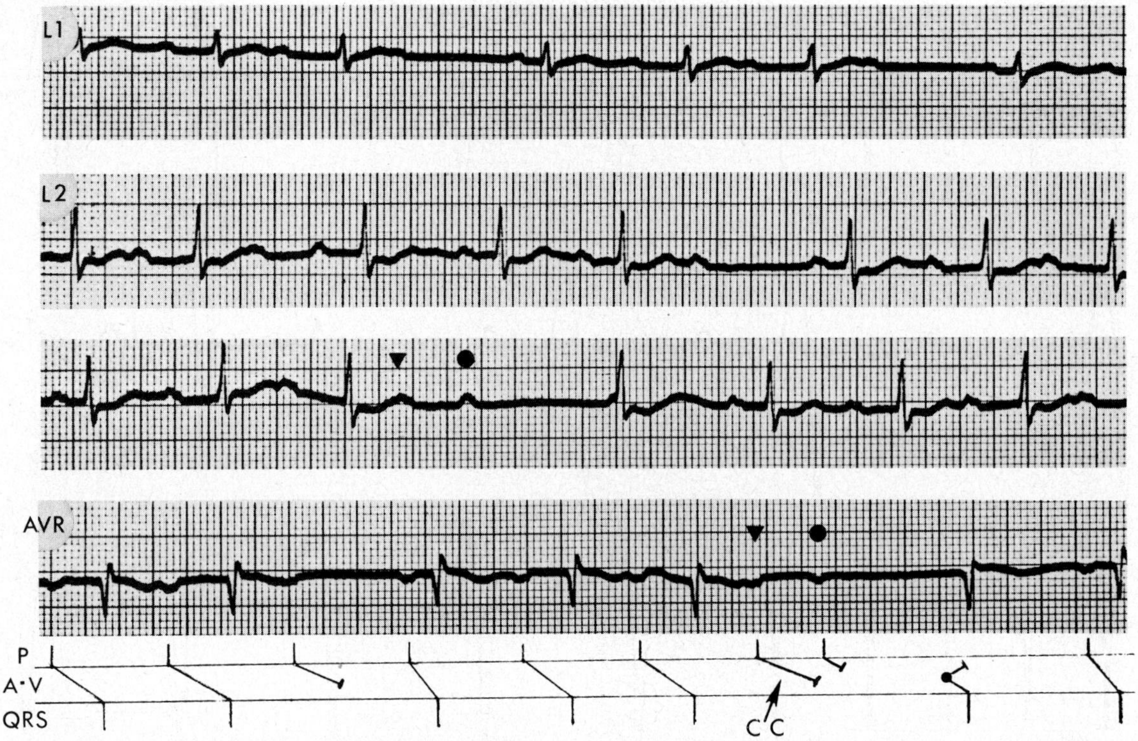

FIGURE 7–54 Block of atrial premature complex (APC) due to concealed conduction. The basic rhythm is sinus with a Wenckebach type I AV block. Two of the blocked sinus P waves of the Wenckebach sequence (▼) are followed by blocked APC (●), in spite of the fact that the APC is sufficiently distant from the preceding QRS (R-P interval) to allow for its conduction. Failure of the APC to conduct results from refractoriness of the AV node secondary to penetration of the preceding blocked sinus P wave (▼) into the AV node (↑CC). The result is unexpected block of the APC. Conduction of the blocked sinus P wave (▼) to the level of the AV node is not recorded in the surface ECG and thus concealed, recognized only by its effect on the subsequent APC, i.e., unexpected block.

Atrial fusions are relatively rare because the unprotected sinoatrial node is discharged by the ectopic impulse, thus eliminating the opportunity for dual excitation of the atria. In addition, because of the low amplitude of the P wave and a frequent lack of morphological detail, atrial fusions may be difficult to recognize. Atrial fusion is usually seen in atrial parasystole or during the interplay of sinoatrial and junctional impulses. Theoretically, it may also result from fusion of two atrial ectopic impulses.

Ventricular fusions are common and clinically important because, with rare exception, their presence confirms the ventricular origin of an arrhythmia. The mechanism of ventricular fusion varies.[312] In AV dissociation, a fusion complex may result from fusion of junctional and ventricular impulses. The ventricular contribution may be that of a single late diastolic VPC, idioventricular rhythm, ventricular parasystole, ventricular tachycardia, or paced ventricular rhythm. Although the supraventricular impulse that fuses with a ventricular complex is usually of sinoatrial origin, it may arise within the atrium or in the AV junction. Rarely a ventricular fusion may be the result of two or more ventricular rhythms.

By definition, a ventricular fusion differs in morphology from the normal, supraventricular QRS complex. However, the aberration may be extremely subtle, and in such instances a careful analysis of the T wave in search of secondary T-wave changes may prove useful. In the presence of BBB, fusion of the supraventricular impulse and an ipsilateral VPC may result in a QRS complex that is normal in appearance.

In WPW, the QRS complex is a fusion, a result of a supraventricular impulse, usually from the sinoatrial node, activating the ventricle through two pathways. The degree of QRS aberrancy depends on a relative contribution of the impulse conducting through the two pathways. Fusion between a supraventricular impulse conducting through an anomalous pathway and an impulse originating in the ventricle or AV junction has also been described.[107]

CAPTURE (See also Fig. 21–48, p. 735)

Capture implies activation of the ventricle by an atrial impulse in the presence of AV dissociation. The timing of the P wave is such that the impulse arrives in the AV junction when the latter is no longer refractory and conduction of the atrial impulse is possible.

In the presence of an idioventricular rhythm, the QRS complex resulting from activation by an atrial impulse (capture) may be normal, aberrant, or a ventricular fusion. The ventricular focus may be discharged and reset by the capture, or it may remain unaffected. If the supraventricular impulse reaches the ventricular pacemaker at the moment it discharges or shortly thereafter, the pacemaker will fail to reset. Similarly, in partial capture, a fusion will fail to discharge the pacemaker. Failure of the early impulse to discharge the pacemaker is due to physiological refractoriness and is an example of *interference*.

In the presence of a dominant junctional rhythm, a concealed penetration, capture of the junctional pacemaker by an atrial impulse will reset and prolong the return cycle length of the junctional focus (see Concealed Conduction p. 247).

PARASYSTOLE (See also p. 622)

Parasystole is most likely an automatic rhythm of an independent and protected focus. The protection is manifest by the inability of an extraneous impulse—be it sinus or ectopic—to alter the rhythmicity of the parasystolic impulse. Parasystolic protection must be demonstrated by activation of the chamber, the site of the parasystolic rhythm, at a time when the extraneous impulse should reset the parasystolic focus yet fails to do so. Functional unidirectional protection of the parasystolic focus, i.e., *entrance block*, is the characteristic feature of parasystole, although the existence of unidirectional protection or block as an absolute prerequisite has been questioned. It has been suggested that the parasystolic rate is more rapid than the manifest rate, and that the slower manifest rate is a manifestation of an exit block.[313] If such is the case, the protection is one of interference between two foci, and a unidirectional block need not be invoked.

Although one of the characteristic features of parasystole is its regularity, spontaneous variations of parasystolic cycle length were recognized as early as 1920.[314] In some instances, the changing rate is probably related to a changing slope of diastolic depolarization of the automatic fibers or to conduction delay from the focus. It has been suggested that a parasystolic rhythm can be altered in a predictable manner by electrotonus generated[315,316] by nonparasystolic impulses. The role of electrotonus in clinical parasystole must await further study.

Parasystole may be continuous or intermittent.[317] Intermittency appears to be due to failure of protection, allowing the extraneous impulse to discharge and to reset the parasystolic pacemaker. In sinus rhythm with intermittent parasystole, for example, the first impulse of each parasystolic sequence exhibits fixed coupling, a relationship which strongly suggests that the parasystolic focus was discharged and reset by the sinus impulse.[318]

Exit block, first described in conjunction with parasystole, explains the occasional failure of a parasystolic impulse to become manifest at a time when the atrium or ventricle is no longer refractory (see p. 251).

Parasystole may originate in the sinoatrial node, atrium, AV junction, and ventricle. Coexistence of an atrial and a ventricular and two or more ventricular parasystolic rhythms has been observed. The ECG manifestations of parasystole include (1) varying coupling of the parasystolic impulse to the dominant impulse; (2) a common denominator of the manifest interectopic intervals, the longer interectopic intervals being multiples of the common denominator, with a variation of 0.04 sec per cycle from the established common denominator acceptable;[288] (3) fusions; and (4) manifestation of the parasystolic impulse whenever the ventricle or the atrium is not in a refractory state.

Atrial parasystole differs from AV nodal or ventricular parasystole in that both the parasystolic and sinus rhythms originate in the same chamber. Because an atrial parasystole discharges the unprotected sinus node and thus is manifest as atrial begeminy, the parasystolic nature of the rhythm is frequently unrecognized. The sinoatrial node is discharged by each parasystolic impulse, and consequently the sinus impulse is entrained to the parasystolic impulse by a fixed interval, i.e., the sinus rate. As a result, a bigeminal relationship exists between the sinoatrial node and the parasystolic rhythms, the sequence being sinus P, parasystolic P–sinus P, parasystolic P. Atrial parasystole is identifiable only when the parasystolic impulse fails to influence the sinus node and the two discharge independently.

An automatic ventricular parasystole discharging rapidly may have to be differentiated from ventricular tachycardia, a nonprotected and most often a reentrant rhythm. Demonstration of protection of the ectopic focus will identify a parasystolic ventricular tachycardia. Protection of a parasystolic focus is present when an extraneous impulse arrives at a moment when the cardiac tissue surrounding the ectopic focus responsible for the tachycardia is no longer refractory but fails to disturb its rhythmicity. This type of protection has to be differentiated from protection due to interference between the tachycardia and the extraneous impulse, the interference due to a physiological refractory state of the surrounding tissue induced by the rapidly discharging ventricular focus. It follows that the parasystolic nature of a tachycardia can be proved only when the rate of the tachycardia is sufficiently slow for the heart, including the pacemaker, to recover its excitability. Clinically the combination of a sufficiently slow rate of the parasystolic tachycardia and presence of an appropriately timed extraneous impulse is rare, so that proof of parasystolic nature of a tachycardia may be difficult. The concept of protection of a pacemaker due to physiological interference is illustrated in Figure 7–55.

Occasionally parasystolic ventricular tachycardia is associated with exit block and a slow manifest heart rate. In such cases the presence of an underlying regular rapid parasystolic focus is suggested when long cycles are multiples of the shortest manifest cycle.

Sinus parasystole has been reported, but such observations are infrequent because the sinus node is rarely protected.[289]

SUPERNORMAL CONDUCTION AND EXCITATION

Supernormal conduction[319] should be differentiated from supernormality of excitability. The latter indicates that a

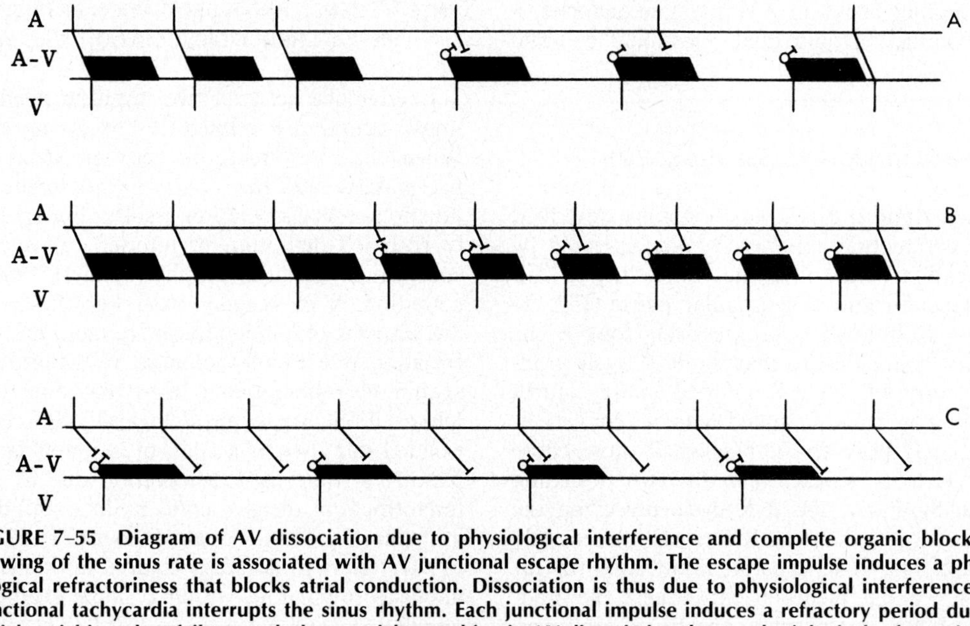

FIGURE 7–55 Diagram of AV dissociation due to physiological interference and complete organic block. A, Slowing of the sinus rate is associated with AV junctional escape rhythm. The escape impulse induces a physiological refractoriness that blocks atrial conduction. Dissociation is thus due to physiological interference. *B*, Junctional tachycardia interrupts the sinus rhythm. Each junctional impulse induces a refractory period during which atrial impulses fail to reach the ventricle, resulting in AV dissociation due to physiological refractoriness. In *A* and *B*, absence of organic block is evident by normal AV conduction when the atrial impulse "clears" the refractory period. Refractoriness also protects the junctional pacemaker from being affected by the atrial impulse. *C*, The ventricular rate is regular and slow and the atrial rate exceeds the ventricular rate, a finding not present in *A* and *B*. Because of the slow rate, AV conduction has ample opportunity to recover and conduct but fails to do so, indicating presence of complete organic AV block. A = atrium, AV = AV nodal (junctional) conduction; V = ventricle; black bar = AV nodal refractory period.

subthreshold stimulus falling within the supernormal period of recovery elicits a propagated response—in other words, its stimulus strength becomes threshold. The phenomenon is commonly seen in the presence of malfunctioning artificial cardiac pacemakers. Pacemaker stimuli that otherwise fail to elicit a propagated response may do so when falling on the downstroke of the T wave, the supernormal period of cardiac recovery, and elicit a propagated ventricular response.

Since supernormality of conduction is a manifestation of depressed tissue and while conduction is slower than normal but more rapid than would be expected under the circumstances, the term *relative supernormality* is more appropriate.[320] Supernormality of conduction has been invoked to explain more rapid AV conduction than expected or conduction when AV block is expected. Similarly, supernormal conduction has been suggested as a mechanism of alternation of the P-R interval with a paradoxical R-P/P-R relationship.

Supernormality of intraventricular conduction is suspected when unexpected normalization of intraventricular conduction occurs at a cycle length shorter than that of the prolonged QRS complexes (Fig. 7–52).[321] In WPW, supernormality of conduction of the anomalous pathway has been reported.[111]

While existence of supernormality of intraventricular conduction is accepted,[322] supernormality of AV conduction is questioned on both experimental and clinical grounds. In a comprehensive review of the subject, a variety of mechanisms have been proposed that could explain paradoxical improvement of conduction without invoking supernormality of conduction. Some of the mechanisms suggested include ventricular fusion, equalization of conduction in both bundles (Fig. 7–52), the gap phenomenon (Fig. 7–55), retrograde excitation of a nonconducting bundle by a PVC, "peeling back" of AV nodal refractories, a vagal effect on conduction, and dual AV nodal conduction.[323]

WENCKEBACH STRUCTURE (See also p. 730)

The Wenckebach (type I) block was originally described as a form of AV conduction abnormality characterized by a gradual prolongation of the P-R interval leading to failure of atrial conduction and a ventricular pause (Fig. 7–50).[324] While the P-R interval is progressively longer, the increment is gradually smaller, so that the R-R cycle gradually shortens. Return of the P-R interval to its control state following the long pause, coupled with the longest P-R interval immediately prior to the blocked P wave, cause the long R-R cycle to be shorter than the two preceding ventricular cycles. Similarly, the R-R cycle preceding the blocked P wave is shorter than the R-R cycle immediately following the pause. This R-R structure is not essential for the diagnosis of AV nodal Wenckebach, because the gradual prolongation of P-R is evident in the ECG. However, Wenckebach block can be a manifestation of conduction of an impulse originating anywhere in the heart, and the delayed conduction, the exit delay per se, may not be evident on the surface ECG. It can be recognized only by the Wenckebach structure of the manifest waves, either P or QRS. Wenckebach block has been described in conjunction with impulses originating in the sinoatrial nodal,[325] ectopic atrial,[326] AV nodal (Fig. 7–48),[254] Purkinje (Fig. 7–46), and perhaps ventricular myocardial foci[327] and impulses generated by artificial pacing.[328]

Wenckebach-type conduction delay has been described in the bundle branches and the divisions of the left bundle.[329] In the former, the block is identified by a sequence of gradual prolongations of bundle branch duration, beginning with a normal QRS complex and ending with a complete BBB.

In the presence of Wenckebach exit from a sinoatrial, AV junctional, or ventricular pacemaker, the true basic interectopic interval of the pacemaker itself is estimated by measuring the interval from the wave initiating the Wenckebach sequence (P-P for exit from sinoatrial pacemaker and R-R for exit from the AV nodal junctional or ventricular pacemaker) to the wave terminating the long pause. This interval is divided by the number of manifest P-P or R-R cycles, adding one in order to account for cycle lost because of the block of an impulse. Having identified and plotted the interectopic intervals, and the manifest P or QRS and by joining the two (Lewis diagram), conduction time from the ectopic focus to the manifest P wave or QRS complex can be estimated. This method is applicable provided that the ectopic rhythm is regular and the exit delay follows the classic Wenckebach pattern. The method of estimating the interectopic interval and conduction time to the surrounding tissue is shown in Figure 7–48.

The precise mechanism responsible for the Wenckebach block is unclear. Decremental conduction, inhomogeneity of the wavefront, concealed reentry, and concealed conduction have all been invoked.

INTERFERENCE AND DISSOCIATION BETWEEN PACEMAKERS (INTERFERENCE DISSOCIATION) (See also p. 735)

Interference between two impulses results from a fortuitous, temporally related discharge of two pacemakers. When the interference is between atrial and ventricular pacemakers and the point of interference is in the AV junction, AV dissociation results (Fig. 7–56). The currently accepted definition of interference is one of failure of conduction because of physiological refractoriness. This definition is in keeping with known electrophysiological mechanisms of conduction or refractoriness or both.[330] Dissociation due to physiological refractoriness (interference) should be differentiated from that due to organic block. Dissociation due to physiological interference may involve isolated impulses or a train of impulses lasting for varying periods of time. AV dissociation due to physiological refractoriness of the AV node is illustrated diagrammatically in Figure 7–55. Although dissociation due to interference usually refers to AV dissociation, interference between two impulses originating within a single chamber and between impulses originating in either cardiac chamber and the AV junction are occasionally encountered.

In the atrium, an early atrial premature complex (APC) reaching the sinoatrial node when the nodal or perinodal tissue is refractory, results in interference between the sinoatrial node and the APC, and an interpolated APC is re-

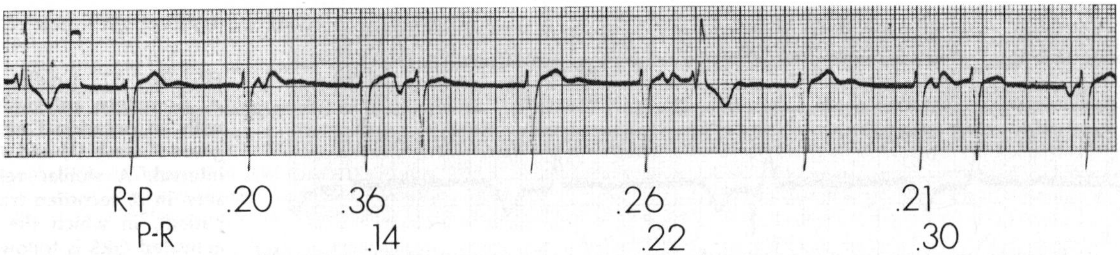

FIGURE 7–56 Gap phenomenon. The tracing shows sinus bradycardia with AV dissociation and occasional ventricular capture. A P wave with an R-P interval of 0.21 sec is followed by a normal QRS, while a P wave with an R-P interval of 0.26 sec results in a QRS complex with RBBB. This paradox is explained by the fact that the P wave that follows the shorter R-P interval is delayed in the AV junction, the P-R interval prolonged to 0.30 sec allowing the RBB to recover. On the other hand, the P wave preceded by a longer R-P interval, measuring 0.26 sec, conducts more rapidly, with a P-R interval of 0.22 sec, and reaches the RBB before it had a chance to recover, so that RBBB results.

corded. Similarly, intraatrial interference is noted when a junctional impulse activates the atrium simultaneously with a sinus impulse. The result is an atrial fusion.

Interference between atrial impulses and a more rapid junctional rhythm due either to inappropriate acceleration of the junctional pacemaker or to slowing of the sinus rate results in AV dissociation.[330–332] Rarely, AV dissociation results from interference between two junctional impulses, a double junctional rhythm.[265] All forms of ventricular rhythm, VPC, ventricular tachycardia, fascicular tachycardia, and accelerated idioventricular rhythm may lead to AV dissociation because of interference between the retrograde ventricular and antegrade conduction of an atrial or junctional impulse. An atrial or junctional impulse may reach the ventricle only to find parts of the ventricle refractory because of activation by an ectopic ventricular impulse, resulting in QRS fusion. Dissociated atrial and junctional foci may synchronize[331] their rates and rhythms and maintain this entrainment for a prolonged period of time. The mechanism of such synchronization is not clear.[333] AV dissociation due to physiological interference may be enhanced by a simultaneous delay of AV conduction. The latter is suggested by failure of P waves to conduct when such conduction would normally be expected. Although both the refractoriness and delayed conduction contribute to the AV dissociation, the relative contribution of each is difficult, if not impossible, to quantitate from the ECG.

VENTRICULOATRIAL AND UNIDIRECTIONAL CONDUCTION

(See also p. 623)

Retrograde conduction in the presence of normal antegrade conduction is a common phenomenon and frequently accompanies VPC[334] and ventricular tachycardia.[335] One-to-one retrograde ventriculoatrial conduction in ventricular tachycardia makes differentiation of supraventricular arrhythmia with aberrancy and ventricular tachycardia from the surface ECG practically impossible.

Unidirectional conduction has been documented experimentally[336,337] and clinically. Retrograde AV conduction in the presence of complete antegrade block is an electrocardiographic example of unidirectional conduction (Fig. 7–57). A number of mechanisms have been proposed to explain this observation,[336] including mechanical stimulation of the atrium by ventricular contraction, stimulation by ventricular contraction of a latent ectopic pacemaker located above the site of AV block, and retrograde conduction along an anomalous or normal AV pathway. Retrograde conduction over a normal AV pathway is the mechanism most widely accepted and supported by clinical and experimental observations. Retrograde conduction with an R-P interval of 0.10 to 0.11 sec may be recorded in the presence of complete anterograde block, supporting the early experimental observation that normal unidirectional conduction can coexist with complete block in an opposite direction. Unidirectional retrograde conduction has been documented following VPC, idioventricular rhythm, and ventricular pacing.[338]

EXIT BLOCK. Exit block is defined as failure of an ectopic impulse to propagate. The most commonly recognized example is sinoatrial exit block (p. 691). Experimental[327,339] and clinical observations suggest that exit block is due largely to delay or failure of impulse propagation and not to abnormal impulse formation. The concept of exit block was first proposed to explain failure of a parasystolic impulse to manifest when the heart was not refractory.[314] It has subsequently been shown to be a property of all spontaneous and artificial pacemaker–induced rhythms.[340,341]

Exit block can manifest the Wenckebach (type I) (Figs. 7–46 and 7–48) or Mobitz (type II) structure. The Wenckebach structure may be identified by the P-P or R-R interval. Type II exit block is suggested by a long pause that is a multiple of the basic cycle length. Even in type II block, however, the long cycle may be slightly shorter than a multiple of the basic cycle length, since conduction from the focus terminating the long cycle may be slightly more rapid than that preceding the exit block. Exit block may fail to conform to either type I or type II block. If the basic P-P or R-R cycles are irregular, a diagnosis of exit block is impossible.

By definition, the diagnosis of exit block can be entertained only when failure of conduction occurs at a time when the surrounding myocardium is not refractory; otherwise, failure of propagation is a manifestation of interference.

ENTRANCE BLOCK. Entrance block is present when an impulse fails to reach and discharge, suppress, or reset a pacemaker. Such an entrance block is, for example, an integral component of parasystole and of some cases inter-

200. Myers, G. B.: QRS-T patterns in multiple precordial leads that may be mistaken for myocardial infarction. III. Bundle branch block. Circulation *2*:60, 1950.
201. Kennedy, R. J., Varriale, P., and Alfenito, J. C.: Textbook of Vectorcardiography. New York, Harper and Row, 1970.
202. Kariv, I.: Wolff-Parkinson-White syndrome simulating myocardial infarction. Am. Heart J. *55*:406, 1958.
203. Spodick, D. H.: Electrocardiographic response to pulmonary embolism. Mechanisms and sources of variability. Am. J. Cardiol. *30*:695, 1972.
204. Harris, T. R., Copeland, G. D., and Brody, D. A.: Progressive injury current with metastatic tumor of the heart. Case report and review of the literature. Am. Heart J. *69*:392, 1965.
205. White, P. D.: Alternation of the pulse: A common clinical condition. Am. J. Med. Sci. *150*:82, 1915.
206. Edmands, R. E., Greenspan, K., and Fisch, C.: Effect of cycle-length alteration upon the configuration of the canine ventricular action potential. Circ. Res. *9*:602, 1966.
207. Scherf, D.: Alterations in the form of the T waves with changes in heart rate. Am. Heart J. *28*:332, 1944.
208. Ashman, R., Ferguson, F. P., and Gremillion, A.: The effect of cycle-length changes upon the form and amplitude of the T deflection of the electrocardiogram. Am. J. Physiol. *143*:453, 1945.
209. Currie, G. M.: Transient inverted T waves after paroxysmal tachycardia. Br. Heart J. *4*:149, 1942.
210. Taussig, H. B.: Electrograms taken from isolated strips of mammalian ventricular cardiac muscle. Bull. Johns Hopkins Hosp. *43*:81, 1928.
211. Fisch, C., Edmands, R. E., and Greenspan, K.: T wave alternans: An association with abrupt rate change. Am. Heart J. *81*:817, 1971.
212. Wellens, H. J. J.: Isolated electrical alternans of the T wave. Chest *62*:319, 1972.
213. Awa, S., Linde, L. M., Oshima, M., Okuni, M., Momma, K., and Nakamura, N.: The significance of late phased dart T wave in the electrocardiogram of children. Am. Heart J. *8*:619, 1970.
214. Millar, K., and Abildskov, J. A.: Notched T waves in young persons with central nervous system lesions. Circulation *37*:597, 1968.
215. Surawicz, B., and Lasseter, K. C.: Effect of drugs on the electrocardiogram. Progr. Cardiovasc. Dis. *13*:26, 1970.
216. Abildskov, J. A.: Central nervous system influence upon electrocardiographic waveforms. *In* Schlant, R. C., and Hurst, J. W. (eds.): Advances in Electrocardiography. New York, Grune and Stratton, 1976.
217. Friedberg, C. K., and Zager, A.: "Nonspecific" ST and T-wave changes. Circulation *23*:655, 1961.
218. Sleeper, J. C., and Orgain, E. S.: Differentiation of benign from pathologic T waves in the electrocardiogram. Am. J. Cardiol. *11*:338, 1963.
219. Wilson, F. N., and Finch, R.: The effect of drinking iced-water upon the form of the T deflection of the electrocardiogram. Heart *10*:275, 1923.
220. Ostrander, L. D., Jr.: The relation of "silent" T wave inversion to cardiovascular disease in an epidemiologic study. Am. J. Cardiol. *25*:325, 1970.
221. Wasserburger, R. H.: The riddle of the labile T wave. Am. J. Cardiol. *2*:179, 1958.
222. Burgess, M. J., and Lux, R. L.: Physiologic basis of the T wave. *In* Schlant, R. C., and Hurst, J. W. (eds.): Advances in Electrocardiography. New York, Grune and Stratton, 1976, pp. 327–337.
223. Abildskov, J. H.: Nonspecificity of ST-T changes. *In* Fisch, C. (ed.): Cardiovascular Clinics, Complex Arrhythmias. Vol. 6. Philadelphia, F. A. Davis Co., 1973, pp. 170–177.
224. Autenrieth, G., Surawicz, B., Kuo, C. S., and Arita, M.: Primary T wave abnormalities caused by uniform and regional shortening of ventricular monophasic action potential in dog. Circulation *51*:668, 1975.
225. Marriott, J. L. H.: Coronary mimicry: Normal variants, and physiologic pharmacologic and pathologic influences that simulate coronary patterns in the electrocardiogram. Ann. Intern. Med. *52*:411, 1960.
226. Abildskov, J. A.: Electrocardiographic wave form and the nervous system (editorial). Circulation *41*:371, 1970.
227. Palmer, J. H.: Isolated U wave negativity. Circulation *7*:205, 1953.
228. Ward, O. C.: New familial cardiac syndrome in children. J. Ir. Med. Assoc. *54*:103, 1964.
229. Abildskov, J. A.: The prolonged QT interval. Ann. Rev. Med. *30*:171, 1979.
230. Hering, H. E.: Experimentalle Studien an Saugetieren uber das Electrocardiogramme. Z. Exp. Pathol. Ther. *7*:363, 1909.
231. Lewis, T.: Notes upon alternation of the heart. Quart. J. Med. *4*:141, 1910.
232. Williams, R. R., Wagner, G. S., and Peter, R. H.: ST-segment alternans in Prinzmetal's angina. A report of two cases. Ann. Intern. Med. *81*:51, 1974.
233. McGregor, M., and Baskind, E.: Electric alternans in pericardial effusion. Circulation *11*:837, 1955.
234. Feigenbaum, H., Zaky, A., and Grabhorn, L. L.: Cardiac motion in patients with pericardial effusion. A study using reflected ultrasound. Circulation *34*:611, 1966.
235. Kleinfeld, M., and Stein, E.: Electrical alternans of components of action potential. Am. Heart J. *75*:528, 1968.
236. Pop, T., and Fleischmann, D.: Alternans in human atrial monophasic action potential. Br. Heart J. *39*:1273, 1977.
237. Osborn, J. J.: Experimental hypothermia. Respiratory and blood pH changes in relation to cardiac function. Am. J. Physiol. *175*:389, 1953.
238. Santos, E. M., and Kittle, C. F.: Electrocardiographic changes in the dog during hypothermia. Am. Heart J. *55*:415, 1958.
239. Winkler, A. W., Hoff, H. E., and Smith, P. K.: Electrocardiographic changes and concentration of potassium in serum following intravenous injection of potassium chloride. Am. J. Physiol. *124*:478, 1948.
240. Levine, H. D., Wanzer, S. H., and Merrill, J. P.: Dialyzable currents of injury in potassium intoxication resembling acute myocardial infarction of pericarditis. Circulation *13*:29, 1956.
241. Fisch, C., Martz, B. L., and Priebe, F. H.: Enhancement of potassium-induced atrioventricular block by toxic doses of digitalis drugs. J. Clin. Invest. *39*:1885, 1960.
242. Levine, H. D., Vasifdar, J. P., Lown, B., and Merrill, J. P.: "Tent-shaped" T waves of normal amplitude in potassium intoxication. Am. Heart J. *43*:437, 1952.
243. Fisch, C.: Electrolytes and the heart. *In* Hurst, J. W. (ed.): The Heart. New York, McGraw-Hill Book Co., 1982, p. 1599.
244. Wasserburger, R. H., and Corliss, R. J.: Value of oral potassium salts in differentiation of functional and organic T wave changes. Am. J. Cardiol. *10*:673, 1962.
245. Bellet, S., and Dyer, W. W.: The electrocardiogram during and after emergence from diabetic coma. Am. Heart J. *13*:72, 1937.
246. Surawicz, B., and Lepeschkin, E.: The electrocardiographic pattern of hypopotassemia with and without hypocalcemia. Circulation *8*:801, 1953.
247. Surawicz, B., Braun, H. A., Crum, W. B., Kemp, R. L., Wagner, S., and Bellet, S.: Quantitative analysis of the electrocardiographic pattern of hypopotassemia. Circulation *16*:750, 1957.
248. Surawicz, B.: Relationship between electrocardiogram and electrolytes. Am. Heart J. *73*:814, 1967.
249. Carter, E. P., and Andrus, E. C.: Q-T interval in human electrocardiogram in absence of cardiac disease. JAMA *78*:1922, 1922.
250. Nierenberg, D. W., and Ransil, B. J.: Q-at$_c$ interval as a clinical indicator of hypercalcemia. Am. J. Cardiol. *44*:243, 1979.
251. Kleeman, C., and Singh, B. N.: Serum electrolytes and the heart. *In* Maxwell, M. H., and Kleeman, C. R. (eds.): Clinical Disorders of Fluid and Electrolyte Metabolism. New York, McGraw-Hill Book Co., 1979, p. 145.
252. Cohn, A. E., Fraser, F. R., and Jamieson, A.: The influence of digitalis on the T wave of the human electrocardiogram. J. Exp. Med. *21*:593, 1915.
253. Fisch, C., Greenspan, K., Knoebel, S. B., and Feigenbaum, H.: Effect of digitalis on conduction of the heart. Progr. Cardiovasc. Dis. *6*:343, 1964.
254. Fisch, C., and Knoebel, S. B.: Recognition and therapy of digitalis toxicity. Progr. Cardiovasc. Dis. *13*:71, 1970.
255. Smith, W. T., and Haber, E.: Digitalis. N. Engl. J. Med. *289*:945, 1010, 1063, and 1125; 1973.
256. Fisch, C., Zipes, D. P., and Noble, R. J.: Digitalis toxicity: Mechanism and recognition. *In* Yu, P., and Goodwin, R. (eds.): Progress in Cardiology. Philadelphia, Lea and Febiger, 1975, pp. 37–70.
257. Surawicz, B., and Mortelmans, S.: Factors affecting individual tolerance to digitalis. *In* Fisch, C., and Surawicz, B. (eds.): Digitalis. New York, Grune and Stratton, 1969.
258. Gold, H., Kwit, N. T., Otto, H., and Fox, T.: On vagal and extravagal factors in cardiac slowing by digitalis in patients with auricular fibrillation. J. Clin. Invest. *18*:429, 1939.
259. Mendéz, C., Aceves, J., and Mendéz, R. J.: The anti-adrenergic action of digitalis on the refractory period of the A-V transmission system. J. Pharmacol. Exp. Ther. *131*:199, 1961.
260. Barker, P. S., Wilson, F. N., Johnston, F. D., and Wishart, S. W.: Auricular paroxysmal tachycardia with auriculoventricular block. Am. Heart J. *25*:765, 1943.
261. Lewis, T.: Paroxysmal tachycardia. Heart *1*:43, 1909.
262. Lown, B., and Levine, H. D.: Atrial Arrhythmias, Digitalis and Potassium. New York, Landsberger Medical Books, 1958.
263. Morgan, W. L., and Breneman, G. M.: Atrial tachycardia with block treated with digitalis. Circulation *25*:787, 1962.
264. Pick, A., and Dominquez, P.: Nonparoxysmal A-V nodal tachycardia. Circulation *16*:1022, 1957.
265. Chevalier, R. B., and Fisch, C.: Dissociation of pacemakers located within the atrioventricular node. Am. J. Cardiol. *5*:654, 1960.
266. Pick, A., Langendorf, R., and Katz, L. N.: A-V nodal tachycardia with block. Circulation *24*:12, 1961.
267. Knoebel, S. B., and Fisch, C.: Accelerated junctional escape. A clinical and electrocardiographic study. Circulation *50*:151, 1974.
268. Friedberg, C. K., and Donoso, E.: Arrhythmias and conduction disturbances due to digitalis. Progr. Cardiovasc. Dis. *2*:408, 1959.
269. Cohen, H. C., Gozo, E. G., Jr., and Pick, A.: Ventricular tachycardia with narrow QRS complexes (left posterior fascicular tachycardia). Circulation *45*:1035, 1972.
270. Jacob, D. R., Donoso, E., and Friedberg, C. K.: A-V dissociation—A relatively frequent arrhythmia. Analysis of 30 cases with detailed discussion of the etiologic significance of digitalis, physiologic mechanisms, and differential diagnosis. Medicine *40*:101, 1961.
271. Hoffman, B. F., and Singer, D. H.: Effects of digitalis on electrical activity of cardiac fibers. Progr. Cardiovasc. Dis. *7*:226, 1964.
272. Rosen, M. R., Fisch, C., Hoffman, B. F., Danilo, P., Jr., Lovelace, D. E., and Knoebel, S. B.: Can accelerated atrioventricular junctional escape rhythms be explained by delayed afterdepolarization? Am. J. Cardiol. *45*:1272, 1980.
273. Castellanos, A., Jr., Lemberg, L., Centurion, M. J., and Berkovits, B. V.: Concealed digitalis-induced arrhythmias unmasked by electrical stimulation of the heart. Am. Heart J. *73*:484, 1967.

274. Gold, H., Otto, H. L., and Satchwell, H.: The use of quinidine in ambulatory patients for the prevention of paroxysms of auricular flutter and fibrillation; with especial reference to dosage and the effects of intraventricular conduction. Am. Heart J. *9*:219, 1933.
275. Selzer, A., and Wray, H. W.: Quinidine syncope: Paroxysmal ventricular fibrillation occurring during treatment of chronic atrial arrhythmias. Circulation *30*:17, 1964.
276. Kayden, H. J., Brodie, B. B., and Steele, J. M.: Procaine amide. A review. Circulation *15*:118, 1957.
277. Kus, T., and Sasyniuk, B.: Electrophysiological action of disopyramide phosphate on canine ventricular muscle and Purkinje fibers. Circ. Res. *37*:844, 1975.
278. Befeler, B., Castellanos, A., Jr., Wells, D. E., Vagueiro, M. C., and Yeh, B. K.: Electrophysiologic effects of the antiarrhythmic agent, disopyramide phosphate. Am. J. Cardiol. *35*:282, 1975.
279. LaBarre, A., Strauss, H. C., Scheinman, M. M., Evans, G. T., Bashore, T., Tiedeman, J. J., and Wallace, A. G.: Electrophysiologic effects of disopyramide phosphate on sinus node function in patients with sinus node dysfunction. Circulation *59*:226, 1979.
280. Wald, R. W., Waxman, M. B., and Colman, J. M.: Torsades de pointes ventricular tachycardia. A complication of disopyramide shared with quinidine. J. Electrocardiol. *14*:301, 1981.
281. Kelly, H. G., Fay, J. E., and Laverty, S. G.: Thioridazine hydrochloride (Mellaril): Its effect on the ECG and a report of two fatalities with ECG abnormalities. Canad. Med. Assoc. J. *89*:546, 1963.
282. Ban, T. A. and St. Jean, A.: The effect of phenothiazines on the electrocardiogram. Canad. Med. Assoc. J. *91*:537, 1964.
283. Wendkos, M. H.: The significance of electrocardiographic changes produced by thioridazine. J. New Drugs *4*:322, 1964.
284. Marshall, J. B., and Forker, A. D.: Cardiovascular effects of tricyclic antidepressant drugs: Therapeutic usage, overdose, and management of complications. Am. Heart J. *103*:401, 1982.
285. Rector, W. G., Jr., Jarzobski, J. A., and Levin, H. S.: Sinus node dysfunction associated with lithium therapy: Report of a case and a review of the literature. Nebr. Med. J. *64*:193, 1979.
286. Wellens, H. J. J., Cats, V. M., and Duren, D. R.: Symptomatic sinus node abnormalities following lithium carbonate therapy. Am. J. Med. *59*:285, 1975.
287. Katz, L. N., and Pick, A.: Clinical Electrocardiography. Philadelphia, Lea and Febiger, 1956.
288. Scherf, D., and Schott, A.: Extrasystoles and Allied Arrhythmias. Chicago, Year Book Medical Publishers, 1973.
289. Schamroth, L.: The Disorders of Cardiac Rhythm. Oxford, Blackwell Scientific Publications, 1979.
290. Pick, A., and Langendorf, R.: Interpretation of Complex Arrhythmias. Philadelphia, Lea and Febiger, 1979.
291. Lewis, T.: Observations upon disorders of the heart's action. Heart *3*:279, 1912.
292. Weidmann, S.: Effect of the cardiac membrane potential on the rapid availability of the sodium carrying system. J. Physiol. *127*:213, 1955.
293. Gettes, L. S.: The electrophysiologic effects of antiarrhythmic drugs. Am. J. Cardiol. *28*:526, 1971.
294. Singer, D. H., and Ten Eick, R. E.: Aberrancy: Electrophysiologic aspects. Am. J. Cardiol. *28*:381, 1971.
295. Fisch, C., Zipes, D. P., and McHenry, P. L.: Rate dependent aberrancy. Circulation *48*:714, 1973.
296. Gouaux, J. L., and Ashman, R.: Auricular fibrillation with aberration simulating ventricular paroxysmal tachycardia. Am. Heart J. *34*:366, 1947.
297. Mendez, C., Gruhzit, C. C., and Moe, G. K.: Influence of cycle length upon refractory period of auricles, ventricles and A-V in the dog. Am. J. Physiol. *184*:287, 1956.
298. Lewis, T.: Certain physical signs of myocardial involvement. Br. Med. J. *1*:484, 1913.
299. Moe, G. K., Mendez, C., and Han, J.: Aberrant A-V impulse propagation in the dog heart: A study of functional bundle branch block. Circ. Res. *16*:261, 1965.
300. Katz, A., and Pick, A.: The transseptal conduction time in the human heart. Circulation *27*:1061, 1963.
301. Dressler, W.: Transient bundle branch block occurring during slowing of the heart beat and following gagging. Am. Heart J. *58*:760, 1959.
302. Singer, D. H., Lazarra, R., and Hoffman, B. F.: Interrelationship between automaticity and conduction in Purkinje fibers. Circ. Res. *21*:537, 1967.
303. Fisch, C., and Miles, W. M.: Deceleration ("bradycardia") dependent left bundle branch block: A spectrum of bundle branch conduction delay. Circulation *65*:1029, 1982.
304. Engelmann, T. W.: Beobachtungen and Versuche am suspendieren Herzen. Pfluegers Arch. *56*:149, 1894.
305. Lewis, T. and Master, A. M.: Observations upon conduction in the mammalian heart. A-V conduction. Heart *12*:209, 1925.
306. Moe, G. K., Abildskov, J. A., and Mendéz, C.: An experimental study of concealed conduction. Am. Heart J. *67*:338, 1964.
307. Hoffman, B. F., Cranefield, P. R., and Stuckey, J. H.: Concealed conduction. Circ. Res. *9*:194, 1961.
308. Rosen, K. M., Rahimtoola, S. H., and Gunnar, R. M.: Pseudo A-V block secondary to premature nonpropagated His bundle depolarization. Documentation by His bundle electrocardiography. Circulation *42*:367, 1970.
309. Langendorf, R.: Newer aspects of concealed conduction of the cardiac impulse. *In* Wellens, H. J. J., Lie, K. I., and Janse, M. J. (eds.): The Conduction System of the Heart: Structure, Function and Clinical Implications. Philadelphia, Lea and Febiger, 1976.
310. Sung, R. J., Myerburg, R. J., and Castellanos, A.: Electrophysiological demonstration of concealed conduction in the human atrium. Circulation *58*:940, 1978.
311. Fisch, C., Zipes, D. P., and McHenry, P. L.: Electrocardiographic manifestations of concealed junctional ectopic impulses. Circulation *53*:217, 1976.
312. Malinow, M. R., and Langendorf, R.: Different mechanisms of fusion beats. Am. Heart J. *62*:320, 1961.
313. Scherf, D., and Bornemann, C.: Parasystole with a rapid ventricular center. Am. Heart J. *62*:320, 1961.
314. Kaufman, R., and Rothberger, C. J.: Beitrage zur Entstehungsweise der extrasystolischer Allorhythmien. Z. ges. exper. Med. *11*:40, 1920.
315. Moe, G. D., Jalife, J., and Mueller, W. J.: Reciprocation between pacemaker sites: Reentrant parasystole? *In* Kulbertus, H. E. (ed.): Reentrant Arrhythmias. Mechanisms and Treatment. Baltimore, Md., University Park Press, 1977, p. 271.
316. Jalife, J., and Moe, G. K.: Effect of electrotonic potentials on pacemaker activity of canine Purkinje fibers in relation to parasystole. Circ. Res. *39*:801, 1976.
317. Fisch, C., and Chevalier, R. B.: Intermittent atrial parasystole. Circulation *22*:1149, 1960.
318. Steffens, T. G.: Intermittent ventricular parasystole due to entrance block failure. Circulation *44*:442, 1971.
319. Adrian, E. D., and Lucas, K.: On the summation of propagated disturbances in the nerve and muscle. J. Physiol. *44*:68, 1912.
320. Adrian, E. D.: The recovery process of excitable tissues. J. Physiol. *54*:1, 1920.
321. Lewis, T., and Master, A. M.: Supernormal recovery phase, illustrated by two clinical cases of heart block. Heart *11*:371, 1924.
322. Mihalick, M. J., and Fisch, C.: Supernormal conduction of the right bundle branch. Chest *57*:395, 1970.
323. Moe, G. K., Childers, R. W., and Merideth, J.: An appraisal of "supernormal" A-V conduction. Circulation *38*:5, 1968.
324. Wenckebach, K. F.: Zur Analyse des unregelmössigen Pulses. II. Uber den regelmössig intermillierenden Pulse. Zschr. Klin. Med. *37*:475, 1899.
325. Schamroth, L., and Dove, E.: The Wenckebach phenomenon in sino-atrial block. Br. Heart J. *28*:350, 1966.
326. Omori, Y.: Repetitive multifocal paroxysmal atrial tachycardia: With cyclic Wenckebach phenomenon under observation for 13 years. Am. Heart J. *82*:527, 1971.
327. Greenspan, K., Anderson, G. J., and Fisch, C.: Electrophysiologic correlate of exit block. Am. J. Cardiol. *28*:197, 1971.
328. Mehta, J., and Khan, A. H.: Pacemaker Wenckebach phenomenon due to antiarrhythmic drug toxicity. Cardiology *61*:189, 1976.
329. Cerqueira-Gomes, M., and Teixeira, A. V.: Wenckebach phenomenon in the posterior division of the left branch. Am. Heart J. *82*:377, 1971.
330. Pick, A.: A-V dissociation. A proposal for comprehensive classification and consistent terminology (editorial). Am. Heart J. *66*:147, 1963.
331. Segers, M., LeQuime, J., and Denolin, H.: Synchronization of auricular and ventricular beats during complete heart block. Am. Heart J. *33*:685, 1947.
332. Fisch, C., and Knoebel, S. B.: Junctional rhythms. Progr. Cardiovasc. Dis. *13*:141, 1970.
333. Levy, M. N., and Edelstein, J.: The mechanism of synchronization in isorhythmic A-V dissociation. II. Clinical studies. Circulation *42*:689, 1970.
334. Kistin, A. D., and Landowne, M.: Retrograde conduction from premature ventricular contractions, a common occurrence in the human heart. Circulation *3*:738, 1951.
335. Kistin, A. D.: Retrograde conduction to the atria in ventricular tachycardia. Circulation *24*:236, 1961.
336. Winternitz, M., and Langendorf, R.: Auriculoventricular block with ventriculoauricular response. Report of six cases and critical review of the literature. Am. Heart J. *27*:301, 1944.
337. Ashman, R., and Hafkesbring, R.: Unidirectional block in heart muscle. Am. J. Physiol. *91*:65, 1929.
338. Castillo, C., and Samet, P.: Retrograde conduction in complete heart block. Br. Heart J. *29*:553, 1967.
339. Anderson, G. J., Greenspan, K., and Fisch, C.: Electrophysiologic studies on Wenckebach structures below the atrioventricular junction. Am. J. Cardiol. *30*:232, 1972.
340. Pick, A., Langendorf, R., and Jedlicka, J.: Exit block. *In* Fisch, C. (ed.): Complex Electrocardiography. Cardiovascular Clinics. Vol. 5. Philadelphia, F. A. Davis Co., 1973, pp. 113–133.
341. Parkinson, J., and Papp, C.: Repetitive paroxysmal tachycardia. Br. Heart J. *9*:241, 1947.
342. Durrer, D.: Electrical aspects of human cardiac activity: A clinical-physiological approach to excitation and stimulation. Cardiovasc. Res. *2*:1, 1968.
343. Gallagher, J. J., Damato, A. N., Caracta, A. R., Varghese, P. J., Josephson, M. E., and Lau, S. H.: Gap in A-V conduction in man: Types I and II. Am. Heart J. *85*:78, 1973.
344. Agha, A. S., Castellanos, A., Jr., Wells, D., Ross, M. D., Befeler, B., and Myerburg, R. J.: Type I, type II and type III gaps in bundle branch conduction. Circulation *47*:325, 1973.

8 EXERCISE STRESS TESTING

by L. Thomas Sheffield, M.D.

EXERCISE TESTING FOR CORONARY ARTERY DISEASE*

Coronary artery disease is a frequent cause of episodic chest discomfort in adults. Unless the description of the episodes (precipitating factors, time course, quality, location, and alleviating factors) is typical of angina pectoris, the physician will usually seek additional information. Diagnosis would be aided if the physician were able to observe the patient during an attack of chest discomfort to determine exactly what degree of stimulus was required to provoke the attack and were able to record an electrocardiogram during the episode. This was the rationale of Goldhammer and Scherf when they introduced exercise stress testing for coronary artery disease in 1933.[1] Their test was individualized to the patient, but Master adapted the electrocardiographic recording to his two-step fitness test and made it a standardized procedure. The two-step test was not very stressful to most subjects, and the notion grew that more vigorous testing might detect disease at an earlier stage.[2] Treadmills and bicycles were found to be better suited for providing patients with strenuous exercise, and with these innovations maximal exercise tests became feasible.[3]

Indications for Noninvasive Exercise Stress Testing. Dynamic exercise testing such as performed on treadmill or bicycle, and hereafter called simply exercise stress testing, has various specific purposes in the diagnosis and treatment of heart disease. It is used to aid in the diagnosis of chest pain in adults, especially when the clinical description is not entirely typical of angina pectoris (Table 8–1). Even when the diagnosis is certain, stress testing is frequently used to determine the approach to therapy, since the results of the test may provide information concerning the risk of complications. Those patients shown to be at high risk should have prompt definitive and often surgical therapy, whereas those with least risk might be best treated more conservatively (Chap. 39). Exercise testing is also useful in evaluating the degree of benefit from vasodilator, beta-blocking, or antiarrhythmic therapy or combinations of these. Among postinfarction patients, it has helped to identify the low-risk subjects who can proceed rapidly toward rehabilitation (Chaps. 38 and 40) and those who should proceed more slowly and perhaps be studied by coronary arteriography because of decreased myocardial reserve, angina, or arrhythmias (pp. 265 and 1293).

Stress testing is generally recommended to minimize the risk among middle-aged persons contemplating a physical fitness program and who are unaccustomed to exercise. Exercise testing has also proved useful in measuring the degree of benefit derived from surgical procedures such as coronary bypass, correction of congenital heart malformations,[4] aortic valve replacement, or iliofemoral bypass. Some controversy attends the use of exercise screening of professionals, such as commercial airline pilots, whose sudden incapacitation could cause great harm to others. This is because the number of false-positive results in asymptomatic individuals is rather high. Those favoring this ap-

TABLE 8–1 INDICATIONS FOR NONINVASIVE EXERCISE STRESS TESTING

To aid in diagnosis of chest pain
To evaluate the prognostic severity of coronary heart disease
To evaluate therapy of known coronary heart disease
To guide rehabilitation following myocardial infarction
To evaluate the benefit of surgical procedures
To provide a safety checkup prior to a fitness program
To screen high-risk professionals
To assess, in part, the risk factor in asymptomatic persons

*The use of radionuclide techniques for the study of the response of the ventricle and of the coronary circulation to exercise is discussed in Chapter 11.

plication argue that the disadvantage of false-positive results is more than offset by the consideration of public safety.

Finally and most controversial is the use of exercise stress testing in the asymptomatic general public. Because the prevalence of coronary artery disease is low in this group, an ischemic type of response in this setting would much more likely be a false-positive than a true one. For that reason the test probably should not be used to seek out unexpected coronary heart disease diagnosis in the asymptomatic public, but it can be used effectively in its proper role as part of a risk factor assessment program in which serum cholesterol, triglyceride, high-density lipoprotein, blood glucose, blood pressure, smoking history, age, and sex are combined with the exercise test in order to give an accurate assessment of an asymptomatic individual's risk of developing coronary heart disease in the future. Considered as a risk factor, the abnormal test result offers an otherwise unavailable opportunity to prevent disease. When positive, it is far more predictive of a coronary event than are the "classical" risk factors (Fig. 8–1).

Controversies Concerning the Application of Stress Testing. Recent issues and concerns in this field have been (1) that the correlation between exercise electrocardiograms and coronary angiograms has been poorer than expected in spite of the good agreement between exercise tests and clinical follow-up[5]; an important reason for this discrepancy has been the wide range of methodological variation among the reported studies[6]; (2) that epidemiological concepts have been introduced to explain why the test cannot be as accurate in screening asymptomatic subjects as it is in adults with chest pain; and (3) that the exercise test has been extended to include heart rate, blood pressure, and endurance observations in addition to the electrocardiogram. These issues are discussed below.

PHYSIOLOGY OF EXERCISE TESTING

CORONARY ARTERIAL RESERVE. The human body incorporates reserve capability in every organ system to permit either performance of function at levels much higher than those required in the resting state or continuation of normal function at moderate levels of performance even though disease processes may have incapacitated a considerable fraction of the total organ function. The heart and blood vessels are no exception, and most measurements of cardiovascular function during the resting state are poor predictors of circulatory performance during vigorous exercise. During exercise, intracardiac shunts that, at rest, are from left to right may reverse and become predominantly right to left. Pulmonary artery pressures and pressure differences across cardiac valves that are unimpressive at rest may become critical during heavy exercise. Left ventricular wall motion in a certain region that is normal at rest may become feeble during vigorous work, simulating an aneurysm. Finally, we have learned that advanced degrees of coronary arterial obstruction may exist without myocardial ischemia, owing to the remarkable physical flow properties of fluids in restricted tubes. Exercise is, at present, the safest and most convenient means of stimulating the myocardium to demand maximal or near maximal blood flow and is the only way of stimulating such a rigorous demand for oxygen delivery that even moderate impairment of coronary blood flow capacity becomes detectable.

CARDIAC OUTPUT INCREASES IN EXERCISE. As an adult exercises maximally, cardiac output may rise from 5 to 25 liters per minute.[7] Vasodilation in the skeletal muscular bed helps permit this increase in flow to take place, but in addition an increase in mean arterial pressure occurs. Pressure increases of 50 per cent are typical, dictating corresponding increases in the contractile force of myocardial fibers, a major determinant of myocardial oxygen consumption. There is typically a slight increase in stroke volume with exercise, although most changes in stroke volume represent adaptation to varying body attitudes, which change the inflow pressure of the returning venous blood.[8] Since adaptation of stroke volume to increasing cardiac output demand is limited, the principal mechanism of increasing cardiac output is that of raising heart rate. With an increasing heart rate, the duration of systolic ejection per beat diminishes. Attainment of normal

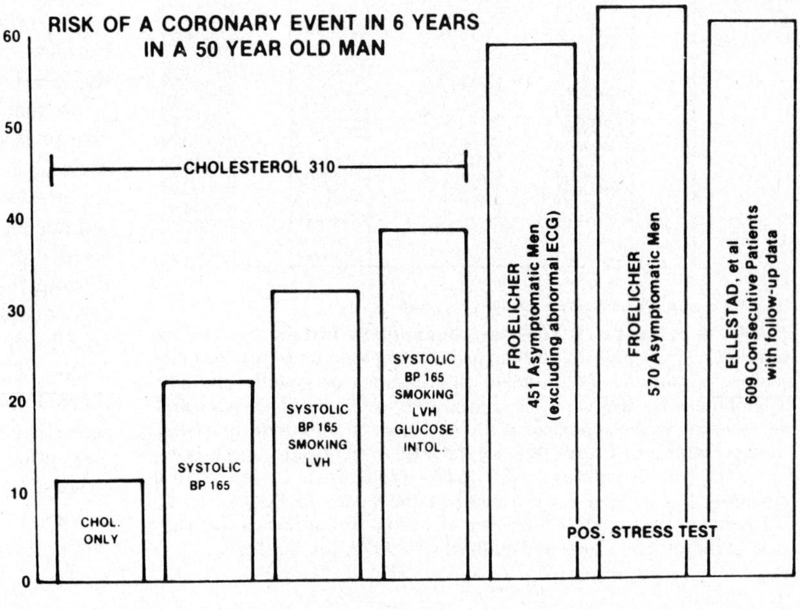

FIGURE 8–1 Graph of the relative capacity to predict coronary events among the various risk factors used in the Framingham Study compared with the stress test. (Reproduced with permission from Ellestad, M. H.: Stress Testing: Principles and Practice. 2nd ed. Philadelphia, F. A. Davis Co., 1980, p. 100.)

systolic emptying in shorter and shorter periods requires increasing the rate of tension development in the myocardial fibers, a valuable adaptive mechanism that parallels increases in contractility but also exacts a price—increasing the oxygen consumption with each contraction.

MYOCARDIAL OXYGEN CONSUMPTION IN EXERCISE. Myocardial oxygen consumption per contraction is determined principally by the tension developed by the myofibrils and the inotropic (contractile) state and is reflected in the rapidity with which tension is generated and shortening occurs[9] (Chap. 36). Both these determinants of myocardial oxygen consumption are greatly increased by exercise, resulting in a net increase in oxygen consumption per contraction during exercise. Myocardial oxygen consumption per minute is a function of heart rate, which increases in proportion to the intensity of exercise; in the normotensive person the increase in heart rate accounts for the greatest increment in coronary blood flow during exercise (Fig. 8–2). Measurements of contractility and heart wall tension are not practical in the intact human; fortunately, there is excellent correlation between myocardial oxygen consumption and the product of heart rate and systolic blood pressure.[10] The rate-pressure product is a reliable index of the myocardial perfusion requirement in patients with coronary artery disease as well as in normal people,[10] and persons with stable angina pectoris tend to experience chest pain at a repeatable rate-pressure product.[11]

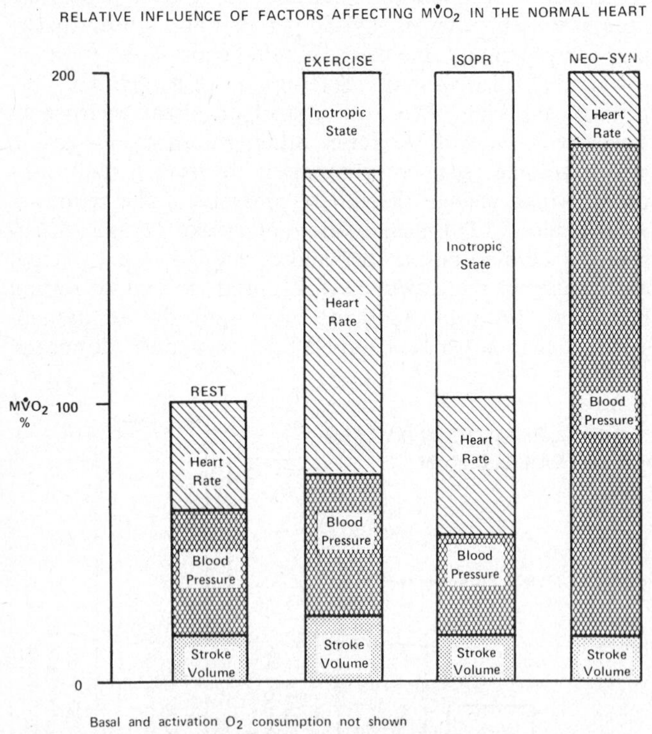

FIGURE 8–2 Myocardial oxygen consumption first in the resting state ($\dot{V}O_{2\,max}$ = 100%) and then as it is increased under various circulatory conditions. The relative contributions of systolic pressure development by the ventricle (blood pressure), the heart rate, and the increase in the inotropic state are shown during mild muscular exercise, infusion of isoproterenol (ISOPR), and infusion of the pressor agent Neo-Synephrine (NEO-SYN). (From Ross, J., Jr.: Factors regulating the oxygen consumption of the heart. *In* Russek, H. I., and Zohman, B. L. (eds.): Changing Concepts in Cardiovascular Disease. Baltimore, Williams and Wilkins Co., 1972, pp. 20–31.)

Because of these changes involved in vigorous exercise, the oxygen consumption per contraction increases from about 1.2×10^{-3} ml/100 gm to about 1.9×10^{-3} ml/100 gm per beat. At normal oxygen content of about 19 ml/dl, and when the fraction of oxygen taken up by the myocardium is essentially unchanged, coronary blood flow must increase from about 60 ml/100 gm at rest to about 240 ml/100 gm during vigorous aerobic exercise.[12] It is apparent that this degree of coronary flow increase may not take place if there is severe or moderately severe obstructive disease of principal coronary arteries, and regions of the heart that are adequately perfused at rest therefore become ischemic during exercise. Exercise stress testing is based on the premise that exercise-induced ischemia may be detected by both subjective and objective means and can be used to make diagnostic inferences.

In view of the high incidence of coronary atherosclerosis as the cause of myocardial ischemia, it is easy to overlook other potential causes. Theoretically, pulmonary insufficiency, by inadequately oxygenating the blood, can cause myocardial ischemia. However, the remarkable vasodilating capability of the normal coronary circulation allows precapillary resistance to drop as a means of compensation. The resulting increase in coronary flow and the high myocardial capacity for oxygen extraction compared with other tissues explain why this is rarely, if ever, a clinical problem.[13] Reduced oxygen transport capacity of the blood, due either to anemia or to carbon monoxide exposure, may occasionally cause myocardial ischemia. More frequently, a marked chronic increase in cardiac loading and secondary hypertrophy of the heart, as in aortic valve stenosis, may result in oxygen requirements that exceed the perfusion capacity of even a normal coronary vasculature. Although none of these conditions is common compared with coronary atherosclerosis, frequently the degree of myocardial hypoperfusion from one of these causes is aggravated by coexisting coronary atherosclerosis.

Although earlier it was thought that maximal exercise might provoke myocardial ischemia in persons with normal coronary arteries,[14] the advent of high-performance exercise testing and angiographic correlation has led to a consensus that the coronary vasculature is not the limiting factor in cardiac performance. In near maximal or maximal exercise, at least as performed in currently employed exercise protocols, myocardial ischemia does not result if the heart and its coronary arteries are normal and if there is no disorder of oxygen transport.[15] However, these exercise protocols employ progressively increasing levels of exercise, so that each level serves as a warm-up period for the level to come. There is some evidence that normal individuals engaging in sprint-type exercise without adequate warm-up may indeed develop myocardial ischemia.[16] If this finding is confirmed, it would suggest that adaptations to vigorous exercise take place in the myocardium and its vessels in the course of vigorous exercise, permitting high levels of coronary blood flow, and without adaptation there may indeed be insufficient myocardial perfusion to serve the heart adequately during bursts of intense exercise. On the other hand, when exercise intensity is increased gradually, not only does the large degree of coronary reserve prevent the development of ischemia when these vessels are normal, but this reserve probably also prevents ischemia when mild or moderate degrees of atherosclerotic obstruction are present. In most studies, correlations of exercise tests with angiograms show that there is a moderately severe or far-advanced degree of coronary atherosclerosis when exertional ischemia is demonstrated.[17–20]

MYOCARDIAL ISCHEMIA DUE TO INSUFFICIENT CORONARY BLOOD FLOW INCREASE. Unfortunately, it is not now known to what extent the coronary blood flow rate appropriate for a given level of myocardial work must be reduced in order to produce evidence of ischemia, measured either by deterioration of some work function or by the electrocardiogram. It is unlikely that a small percentage of reduction, such as 5 per cent below optimal, would be perceptible in the relatively brief exercise tests currently employed.[21,22] On the other hand, tests of longer duration, i.e., 20 or 30 minutes instead of the typical 6 to 9 minutes, would be susceptible to complicating factors such as musculoskeletal conditioning or variations in pulmonary function. In spite of this we do have a basis for roughly estimating the threshold change required to produce ischemia. Patients with uncomplicated angina pectoris undertaking threadmill tests usually make the transition from normal function to ischemia in the course of an increase of one stage in the exercise protocol. Since these stages usually produce an increase in the rate-pressure product of approximately 40 per cent, the threshold for manifestation of detectable ischemia probably lies in this range as well.[23] This phenomenon has definite practical implications with regard to the design of exercise stress protocols, since the incorporation of greater increases in work from one stage to the next would tend to reduce the precision with which one can estimate the ischemic threshold. The importance of accurate estimation of the threshold of ischemia in a given subject is now becoming appreciated and is discussed later in this chapter.

Relationship Between Degree of Coronary Atherosclerosis and Degree of Blood Flow Restriction. With continued refinement of coronary angiography and the widespread availability of coronary revascularization surgery, it is now especially important to know the degree of coronary artery stenosis that corresponds to clinical heart disease as well as the degree of atherosclerosis that is compatible with normal health and therefore unlikely to be responsible for symptoms at present or in the near future. Gould and colleagues studied the degree of reactive hyperemic blood flow that was possible following temporary vascular occlusion with various degrees of external compression of coronary arteries in dogs.[24] They found that in the basal state, over 80 per cent occlusion was necessary before a significant drop in coronary blood flow occurred. Although a measurable reduction in maximal hyperemic flow took place with 40 to 60 per cent occlusion, in order to produce a 50 per cent reduction in hyperemic flow, about 70 per cent occlusion was required. Logan reported similar findings when examining the flow rates possible in diseased coronary arteries removed post mortem and perfused with blood under controlled hydrostatic pressure.[25] In the most common type of stenosis, with the lumen tapering to a minimum diameter and then gradually widening, the degree of dynamic resistance corresponds to the minimum lumen area. On the other hand, if the length of the stenotic segment is increased, the actual resistance will be greater than that predicted by lumen area.[26]

Thus both clinical and laboratory studies confirm the high degree of reserve in normal coronary artery blood flow capacity. They indicate that although degrees of coronary atherosclerosis that obstruct the lumen up to 50 per cent represent a distinct warning, in the sense of indicating the presence of a potentially dangerous atherosclerotic process, such stenosis is unlikely to be responsible for ischemia, even during ordinary exertion. The relative insensitivity of physiological tests such as the exercise test for detecting moderate coronary atherosclerosis makes it all the more important to enhance test sensitivity in any way possible. This requires that the degree of exercise stress be of a very high order, either maximal or nearly so, and that the means of detecting ischemia be enhanced by the use of multiple modes of observation and multiple high-quality electrocardiographic leads.

Interestingly, exercise tests for ischemia, insensitive as they are for predicting exact coronary anatomy, correspond well with follow-up observations of actual coronary heart disease.[27] In a follow-up study of 2700 patients, Ellestad and colleagues found that 1067 normal responders had only a 7 per cent incidence of progression to angina, myocardial infarction, or death in 4 years, whereas 609 patients with abnormal ("positive") responses had a 46 per cent incidence of combined events in the same period.[27] McNeer and colleagues, combining observations of ST segment, exercise endurance, and maximal heart rate from exercise testing of 1472 patients, were able to define 876 patients with chest pain at low risk who had a 7 per cent mortality during 4 years of observation, whereas 134 patients who were classified to be at high risk according to the exercise test demonstrated a 37 per cent mortality during the same interval.[28]

CONSEQUENCES OF MYOCARDIAL ISCHEMIA

Chest Discomfort. Current experience suggests that chest discomfort is not as sensitive an indicator of myocardial ischemia as some of the objective indices used,[29,30] since it occurs only about half as frequently as ST-segment depression.[18,31] However, when angina pectoris does occur during testing, it is a valuable finding and increases the likelihood that significant coronary artery disease is present.

Accurate differentiation of angina pectoris from chest pain of other origin depends upon careful evaluation of the symptom.[32] True angina is a deep visceral discomfort (pp. 5 and 1335). Patients frequently use the terms "pressure," "squeezing sensation," or "a bursting feeling." They may deny that the sensation is actual pain, preferring to call it an unpleasant or disagreeable feeling. Conversely, a sharp, clearly painful sensation is unlikely to be angina pectoris, especially if it is superficial in location. The classic locations of spontaneous angina pectoris—substernal, interscapular, and anterior cervical—are encountered when ischemia is induced by stress testing. Radiation of discomfort to the shoulders, medial aspects of the arms, elbows, and, less commonly, forearms and hands and up the neck into the mandible is also found in stress testing. Nonanginal pain is usually located elsewhere, in the right hemithorax or in the left midclavicular line at the level of the 4th through the 6th interspaces without any central component. The time-intensity course of discomfort helps in its identification. Angina that occurs during diagnostic exercise testing with progressively increasing workload will increase in severity until termination of exercise. "Walk-through angina" may occur with steady mild exercise but is most unlikely during stress testing. Nonanginal chest pain frequently fails to crescendo and may even improve or disappear with continued exercise. Hot, or sometimes cold, discomfort in a bandlike pattern accross the sternum is likely to be an angina-equivalent if the time-intensity characteristic is appropriate. A full description of any chest discomfort and its distinguishing characteristics should be recorded and evaluated as part of every exercise test.

ST-Segment Displacement. Occurrence and disappearance of negative displacement of a flat or downward-sloping ST segment corresponding to the application and termination of exercise stress has been a hallmark of ischemia since introduction of the exercise test (pp. 267 to 269). Positive, or upward, displacement of the ST segment occurs less commonly. Negative ST-segment displacement is probably the result of subendocardial ischemia (p. 222), and ST elevation is probably due to subepicardial or transmural ischemia (p. 223). In both cases the ST-segment phenomenon has a vectorial or directional quality in contrast with the ST-segment elevation of pericarditis, which is found in most leads of the electrocardiogram and is present at rest and usually not altered by exercise. It is well known, but sometimes overlooked, that coronary atherosclerosis is not the only cause of subendocardial ischemia. Poor oxygen delivery by the blood for any reason, coronary arterial spasm (p. 1360), and high left ventricular pressure from any cause may also result in myocardial ischemia and displacement of the ST segment. Nearly all these causes may be readily detected. Unfortunately, displacement of the ST segment sometimes occurs in the absence of any known cause of ischemia and behaves equivocally when certain drugs such as digitalis are present.[33]

Arrhythmias. An additional diagnostic problem is the interpretation of cardiac arrhythmias, particularly ventricular extrasystoles, which occur or increase with exercise. Ischemia is one cause of arrhythmias, yet the nonspecific nature of this finding, if it occurs without any clear evidence of ischemia, has as yet made the presence or absence of exertional arrhythmias almost useless in diagnostic stress testing. It is true that the statistical probability of developing coronary heart disease is some three times greater in otherwise healthy men with exertional ventricular arrhythmias, but how this should affect management of the individual patient is by no means clear.[34] On the other hand, ventricular arrhythmias accompanying ST-segment depression or in the postinfarction patient carry a much more serious prognosis than ST-segment depression occurring alone.[35]

Reduction in Maximal Cardiac Pump Function. In patients without valvular heart disease, myocarditis, or cardiomyopathy, the inability to sustain a normal peak level of cardiac work, as reflected in the heart rate–systolic blood pressure product, suggests significant coronary artery obstruction.[36]Also, patients who develop transient pump failure, as reflected in an actual drop in blood pressure without cessation or reduction of exercise, usually have advanced coronary obstruction.[37] Lastly, inability to continue the progressively increasing exercise of a graded treadmill or bicycle test protocol for a normal time is an important sign of myocardial ischemia when other possible causes have been excluded.[28]

One might think that any measure of the heart's function would therefore deteriorate when myocardial ischemia occurs, either spontaneously or when provoked by exercise stress. This is essentially true when the ischemia is "global," i.e., when the entire left ventricle or a large portion of it becomes ischemic as a result of widespread coronary atherosclerosis. But the issue becomes complex when ischemia is regional and affects primarily a single portion of the left ventricle. In this case, other less affected portions of myocardium may have both the strength and the blood supply to compensate for local deterioration of function, and external measurement of blood pressure and heart rate, the electrocardiogram, or degree of work endurance may not reflect the abnormality. This may occur in the intact myocardium when there is localized stenosis of a minority of the coronary vessels and branches and may also occur in the presence of localized and well-healed infarctions.

TYPES OF EXERCISE TESTS

Exercise tests are used in two distinctly different settings: the noninvasive cardiovascular laboratory in the hospital or physician's office and the cardiac catheterization laboratory. The requirements of these two facilities differ considerably, as can be seen from Table 8–2.

In the *noninvasive laboratory,* generally, the electrocardiographic data assume more importance than in the catheterization laboratory. There is need for higher intensity of exercise, with the aim of detecting maximal coronary reserve. It is necessary to employ a familiar form of exercise in order to secure the greatest possible degree of subject cooperation.

In the *catheterization laboratory,* a major constraint is the necessity of having the subject lie on an x-ray–equipped catheterization table. Surgical draping and other

TABLE 8–2 USES OF EXERCISE TESTING

IN THE NONINVASIVE LABORATORY
- To detect and evaluate ischemia by electrocardiogram and other means
- To evaluate left ventricular performance in exercise by kinetocardiogram or apexcardiogram
- To detect ischemia in exercise by thallium-201 scintigraphy
- To measure left ventricular performance in exercise by gated blood pool scintigraphy
- To evaluate functional capacity as a guide to timing surgical replacement of diseased valves
- To evaluate effects of surgical treatment of congenital heart disease and coronary artery disease
- To measure physical fitness and effects of athletic training in normal individuals and patients with coronary artery disease

IN THE CATHETERIZATION LABORATORY
- To evaluate valve gradients at high flow rates
- To measure shunts and pressures in response to exercise
- To measure left ventricular function in exercise
- To measure coronary blood flow in response to exercise
- To study myocardial metabolism during exercise

practical considerations usually prohibit use of the arms for exercise, leaving leg-pedaling ergometer exercise as the most practical means of stressing the circulation. Circulatory stress is proportional to the mass of exercising muscle, so use of the legs, involving the large hamstring and quadriceps femoris muscle groups, is desirable. On the other hand, maximal gross oxygen consumption and cardiac output in the recumbent position are less than that attainable in the erect position.[38] Although absence of the restraint of gravity on venous return improves venous inflow to the heart and results in larger stroke volumes than in the erect position, high-volume ventilation is less efficient because the diaphragm is more cephalad in the recumbent position. Fortunately most research and diagnostic studies that employ exercise in the catheterization laboratory do not require maximal or near maximal exercise. Measurements made at rest and at two or more progressive levels of exercise allow the construction of a work-response relationship. Whether this involves regulation of coronary blood flow or the hydrodynamic resistance of a valve, useful and usually satisfactory information can be obtained at submaximal exercise levels.

ISOMETRIC EXERCISE. In addition to dynamic exercise, static exercise has received considerable attention recently. In the general population, static exercise has been the subject of books and systems for (usually cosmetic) muscle building and strength improvement. Because of its popularity, investigators have studied the effects of static or isometric exercise on patients with ischemic heart disease.[39,40] The effect of moderate isometric exercise (approximately one-half maximal effort) is to raise the systemic vascular resistance, causing about a one-third increase in mean arterial pressure as well as a moderate (typically 20 per cent) increase in heart rate. Since both these changes contribute to an increase in cardiac work reflected in the rate-pressure product, isometric exercise in the form of a firm, sustained handgrip has been used to provoke either clinical angina pectoris or ventricular dysfunction manifested by a ventricular filling sound or mitral incompetence.[39,41] These occur readily in a patient with a very low anginal threshold, but since the increase in the rate-pressure product caused by this maneuver is only modest, such a clinical test, though useful at the bedside, does not rival a high-performance dynamic exercise test.

RELATIONSHIP OF WORKING MUSCLE MASS TO CIRCULATORY STRESS. The distribution of work among skeletal muscles affects hemodynamic performance. Any specified amount of work is done most efficiently when the largest muscle mass is employed. Thus 300 kpm/min of pedaling work can be performed with the least rise in the rate-pressure product when it is performed by both legs. If performed by a single leg, the rate-pressure product will be higher, and the progressive rise is continued when the work is performed by both arms or a single arm.[38] This relationship also holds true for isometric work. The lowest rate-pressure product is obtained when a weight is carried on the back, and the greatest rise in rate-pressure product occurs when the same weight is carried in one hand.[42]

CHOICE OF EXERCISE MODE. Factors determining the choice of exercise mode are therefore the type of data to be collected, the group of subjects to be studied, the familiarity of the subjects with various exercise devices, and the intensity of exercise intended. When measurement of maximal exercise capacity is intended, possible choices include the motor-driven treadmill and the upright bicycle ergometer.

Treadmill. The motor-driven treadmill permits the highest oxygen consumption rate of any common exercise device, involving as it does both legs, the torso, and both arms. In contrast to electronically controlled bicycle ergometers, treadmills can be calibrated without resort to any special instrumentation. External control of the work rate is attained with a minimum of subject cooperation—either the subject maintains his position on the treadmill without grasping the support rails or he does not. Conversely, the work rate in the step test and with the mechanical bicycle ergometer is controlled entirely by the subject. When the subject becomes tired, adherence to a standard work rate with these devices becomes progressively more difficult. Although the controlled bicycle ergometer maintains work rate by increasing its resistance in proportion to decreasing pedal velocity, this may produce a surprising and threatening aspect to the subject, who may thus discontinue exercise short of the work rate attainable with a more familiar device.

The treadmill provides exercise most familiar to North Americans, and both active and sedentary persons can attain their maximal oxygen consumptions even with untrained legs and knees. The principal disadvantages of the treadmill are that it is expensive, the noisiest of exercise devices, and most demanding of space. Electrocardiographic recordings during treadmill exercise are moderately distorted, owing to both myographic artifact and the bouncing effect of soft tissues with each footstep. Finally, treadmill exercise is not suitable for studies requiring a relatively immobile thorax, such as those involving indwelling vascular catheters or sensitive precordial detectors such as echocardiographs or scintillation cameras.

Bicycle. The upright bicycle excels in providing undistorted electrocardiograms, and it is possible for the subject to maintain the thorax immobile long enough for sensitive precordial measurements, even phonocardiograms, to be recorded during exercise. Intravascular catheters may be kept in place, expired air may be collected easily, and with perseverance both echocardiographic and scintigraphic observations may be made. Mechanical bicycle ergometers cost much less than do electronically regulated ones. All types are quieter than treadmills and require only one-third to one-half the space needed for a treadmill. Their main disadvantages are that they are unfamiliar to many North American adults, a situation which seems now to be improving, and that they depend upon complete subject cooperation in order to maintain a constant work rate in following a specific protocol.

Variable Step. The variable step is the simplest and lowest cost device for attaining maximal exercise in a relatively stationary position.[43] Well suited for athletically trained individuals, it has not proved as acceptable to older or sedentary subjects because of the concentration of stress in the knees and thighs. Step exercise produces the greatest distortion in the electrocardiogram of these three work forms. Because of the vertical motion involved, use of sensitive precordial detectors is impossible, and the employment of intravascular catheters would be least practical with this form of exercise.

TIME COURSE OF EXERCISE INTENSITY. The pattern of exercise intensity should be determined by the purpose of testing and the characteristics of the population to be tested. If the testing is to determine minimal qualification standards for some activity, such as participation in a school sports program or qualification for a certain industrial operation, the test may be limited to a fixed duration of exercise, with the intensity chosen appropriately. The Master two-step test is a popular example of a test of fixed duration with exercise intensity chosen individually for the subject.[29] In a fixed length of time, originally 11/2 minutes and later 3 minutes, a certain number of ascents of a two-step stair are performed, the number being determined by the sex, age, and weight of the subject.

Single-level vs. Multilevel Tests. If the group to be tested is fairly homogeneous in exercise capacity, the exercise test may consist of a single level of exercise suitable for that group. In selecting an exercise test suitable for a wide range of subjects—from sedentary elderly subjects to vigorous younger ones—it is apparent that no single level of exercise would provide suitable stress in each case. For this reason exercise test protocols are dominated by graded or progressive increases in work rate with time. The initial work rate is low enough for the least powerful subject, and the progression continues until work rates suitable for the strongest subject have been reached (Fig. 8–3). In such a progressive test the highest stage completed gives an indication of that subject's functional capacity. The duration of each interval depends upon whether it is intended that the subject reach circulatory steady state in each stage before going on to the next. This requires about 5 or 6 minutes for most subjects. Since exercise tests that last longer than about 20 minutes introduce the possibility of fatigue and internal heat burden, thereby complicating the measurement of functional capacity, the use of stages 6 minutes long would permit only three or four different levels of exercise. A practical compromise involves using stages of 3 minutes' duration, permitting five different exercise intensity levels which may be spaced more closely in terms of work rate and thus may be more precise in measuring maximal functional capacity. The Bruce treadmill protocol is an example of such a test.[44]

Another approach is to employ small increases in work intensity in stages so brief that the rate of work increase is virtually continuous, and the concept of circulatory steady state is set aside entirely.[43] Although such protocols are not well adapted for time-consuming measurements such as oxygen consumption or cardiac output, they can offer a precise measurement of maximal functional capacity. The Balke-Ware test, with stages only 1 minute in duration, is an example of this approach.[45]

An exercise test consisting of individual periods of exercise progressively increasing in intensity and separated by rest periods will permit time-consuming physiological studies during each stage of exercise after steady state has been attained, yet the intervening rest periods will avoid the pitfall of cumulative fatigue from earlier stages. Such tests typically consist of 6-minute exercise periods, 5 to 10 minutes of rest, the next higher exercise level for 6 minutes, and so on, with the progression sometimes carried out over the space of several days.[46] Owing to their precision, such test patterns are favored by work physiologists. On the other hand, because of the protracted nature of such testing, this pattern is not ordinarily well suited for purposes of disease diagnosis.

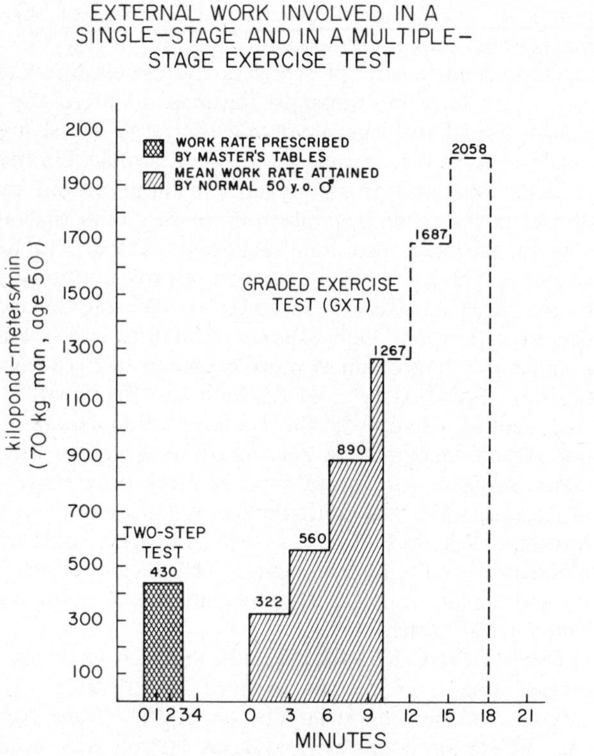

FIGURE 8–3 Rate of energy output in kilopond-meters/minute developed by a 50-year-old, 70-kg man performing a single-stage test (Master two-step); the *rate* of work, i.e., the number of ascents per minute, is the same in the single and double tests. The calculation is as follows:

70 kg (body weight) × 0.46 (height of steps in meters) × 20 (number of ascents) ÷ 1.5 (duration of test in minutes) = 430 (kpm/min). The work rate involved in the GXT (shaded area) is that performed by a normal 50-year-old, 70-kg man who walks 10 minutes on the treadmill while attaining his target heart rate (90% of age-predicted maximal exercise heart rate; see Table 8–3). The external work rate (equivalent rate of climb × body weight) 113 m/min (treadmill speed) × 16% (treadmill grade) × 70 kg (body weight), or 1267 kpm/min. The dotted line outlines the work rates involved in the higher stages for the same body weight. (From Sheffield, L. T., and Roitman, D.: Stress testing methodology. Prog. Cardiovasc. Dis. *19*:33, 1976, by permission of Grune and Stratton.)

Termination of Exercise: Open-ended vs. Closed-ended Tests. Regardless of which exercise protocol is used, exercise should always be terminated upon recognition of any evidence that further exercise may be harmful to the subject. This would include certain arrhythmias and other electrocardiographic changes, a drop in blood pressure, or incoordination of gait. These and other safety considerations will be elaborated later. Tests that are terminated, usually by the subject, before arriving at a scheduled endpoint or before manifesting diagnostic evidence of disease should be termed incomplete or nondiagnostic. For terminating exercise, tests may be considered open-ended or close-ended. In open-ended tests, the duration of the test is determined by the reaction of the subject to exercise, and work is continued until a certain degree of reaction has taken place. Closed-ended tests, generally milder in intensity, are continued for a certain fixed period (for example, the 3-minute double two-step test). Of the open-ended tests, four distinct choices are available for termination of exercise: (1) exercise to a fixed heart rate, such as 150 beats/min[47]; (2) exercise to a variable heart rate, such as 90 per cent of predicted maximal[48]; (3) exercise to symptom-limited maximum tolerance[44]; and (4) exercise to physiologically documented maximal aerobic capacity.[49]

Exercise to a Fixed Heart Rate. Exercise to a fixed heart rate is popular in Europe, especially in Scandinavian countries. It has a physiological basis, since weaker subjects will perform less work in reaching a heart rate of 150 beats/min than will robust subjects who should be stressed harder. Nomograms have been developed that enable one to predict maximal aerobic capacity on the basis of the work level required to attain a heart rate of 150 beats/min.[49] Although such estimates have a variance of 10 to 15 per cent, they provide clinically useful information. The principal disadvantage of this method of testing is that it stresses subjects of different ages unequally. A heart rate of 150 beats/min (or any other chosen value) will be attained at a much smaller fraction of maximal exercise capacity in the younger person than in the older one, for some of whom it may represent a nearly maximal rate. Therefore such a test finds its greatest usefulness in testing groups of persons in approximately the same age range.

Exercise to an Individualized Heart Rate. Exercise to 90 per cent (or some other relatively high percentage) of estimated maximal heart rate has the advantage of avoiding the discomfort of all-out maximal exercise, while retaining test sensitivity by presenting nearly maximal stress to persons of all ages. The highest heart rate anyone can attain during exercise gradually decreases with age. There is a moderate amount of individual variation, one standard deviation of maximal heart rate being ± 10 beats/min.[50,51] Additionally, it has been found that persons actively engaged in athletics have maximal heart rates that are about 7 beats/min lower than physically untrained subjects of the same age.[50] Finally, the regression of maximal heart rate with age differs slightly between the sexes.[51] Thus by taking age, sex, and physical training into account, it is possible to arrive at a target heart rate that is approximately 90 per cent of maximal for that subject.

Post Infarction Exercise Testing. Exercise testing is frequently performed just before the discharge from the hospital of acute myocardial infarction patients, in order to identify those who are at increased risk and thus who may need additional treatment. Such testing can also identify low-risk patients who may safely follow an accelerated convalescence and early return to work. Early testing is indicated when this information can be applied beneficially to the patient's management. Such testing would probably *not* be indicated in the case of the elderly patient, already retired and not intending to resume an active life, especially if the patient was expected to be under regular medical observation after discharge. Predischarge exercise testing is *contraindicated* in the patient with persistent ventricular arrhythmias, any evidence of cardiac failure, or recurrent chest pain.

In the recent postinfarct patient, the modified treadmill stages zero and one-half (or similarly low work levels in other protocols) are employed, and exercise is usually terminated at 70 or 75 per cent of predicted maximal heart rate or at the onset of effort intolerance. Test interpretation is based upon evidence of ischemia and degree of exercise tolerance. The very low-risk category consists of patients able to exercise to the specified heart rate or to the point of normal fatigue and breathlessness without manifesting either ST-segment depression or angina pectoris. Intermediate-risk patients are those demonstrating transient ischemia but normal exercise tolerance; poor-risk patients are those showing evidence of ischemia at a low heart rate or exercise level.

Subjective Maximal Exercise. Subjective maximal exercise testing is easiest to define. The subject simply exercises in a standardized work pattern until unable to continue because of intolerable fatigue, dyspnea, or pain. The high level of circulatory stress provided by maximal exercise makes it possible to demonstrate exertional cardiac ischemia in some cases where lower levels of exercise would have been insufficient to expose it. At any unaccustomed level of exercise there is some slight theoretical danger of precipitating circulatory arrest or myocardial infarction. On the basis of reported instances, however, the frequency of this complication is reassuringly very low.

The subjective nature of the endpoint for this test naturally raises the question of whether all subjects stress themselves to the same degree or whether the more timid ones may tolerate appreciably less fatigue or discomfort than more aggressive subjects. However, proponents of subjective maximal testing report that subjective variability with this test is low.[52] This variability may be reduced by comparing the subject's maximum test heart rate with the predicted target heart rate (Table 8–3). If the attained heart rate is more than 10 beats/min below the target heart rate, if the test is otherwise negative, and if there is no obvious cause of blunted heart rate response, the test may be classified as incomplete and nondiagnostic.

DOCUMENTED MAXIMAL AEROBIC CAPACITY. Exercise to physiologically documented maximal aerobic capacity is a highly valuable investigative tool in work physiology. Typically, interrupted tests of fixed duration are employed with measurement of oxygen uptake at each stage. A level of work will finally be found at which the

TABLE 8–3 GRADED EXERCISE TEST—TARGET HEART RATES

Age (years)	30	35	40	45	50	55	60	65
Predicted maximal heart rate—men	193	191	189	187	184	182	180	178
Target heart rate—men (90% of maximal)	173	172	170	168	166	164	162	160
Predicted maximal heart rate—women	190	185	181	177	172	168	163	159
Target heart rate—women (90% of maximal)	171	167	163	159	155	151	147	143

oxygen uptake reaches a plateau, and the least amount of exercise that clearly demonstrates such a plateau represents maximal aerobic exercise. Any exercise greater than this represents supramaximal or sprint-type exercise, which can be supported only briefly on an anaerobic basis. This type of testing, ideal for studies of normal physiology and the quantitation of training effect, is not well suited for the clinical diagnostic laboratory because of the physical discomfort involved at this level of exercise, the possible hazards, and the large amounts of time involved in interrupted testing.

SPECIFIC EXERCISE TESTS: THE BRUCE, NAUGHTON, AND SHEFFIELD PROTOCOLS. These three tests share the following characteristics: (1) For each subject an appropriate cardiovascular history and examination should be performed prior to the exercise test. (2) The subject should be tested either after an overnight fast or no earlier than 2 hours after a light meal. The patient should be informed of the indications for the test, the details of its procedure, and the potential hazards of testing and should then execute written informed consent. A 12-lead conventional resting electrocardiogram must be recorded and examined for possible exercise contraindications, and the interpretation should be recorded prior to exercise.

During and after exercise, a bipolar CM_5 lead (Naughton test),[53] a CB_5 lead (Bruce test),[54] or Wilson leads V_2 and V_5 and limb lead aV_f (Sheffield test)[48] (Fig. 8–4) should be continuously displayed on an oscilloscope and then recorded on paper at least once per exercise stage and at each minute post exercise. Blood pressure should be measured before exercise, at least once during each exercise stage, and every 2 minutes post exercise until stable.

Exercise is carried out on a motor-driven treadmill according to stages defined in Table 8–4. Exercise is continued by the subject until terminated because of the appearance and progression of symptoms, exhaustion, or the development of ventricular arrhythmia (all tests). Negative tests are classified "incomplete" if the subject did not come within 10 beats/min of target heart rate (Table 8–3); positive tests are valid at any heart rate (Sheffield test).

In the postexercise period, a complete 12-lead electrocardiogram should be recorded immediately and at 2 and 4 minutes post exercise in addition to any other leads. The sitting position is employed because of the discomfort often caused by lying supine and still after near maximal exercise. Brief pulmonary auscultation for rales and wheezes

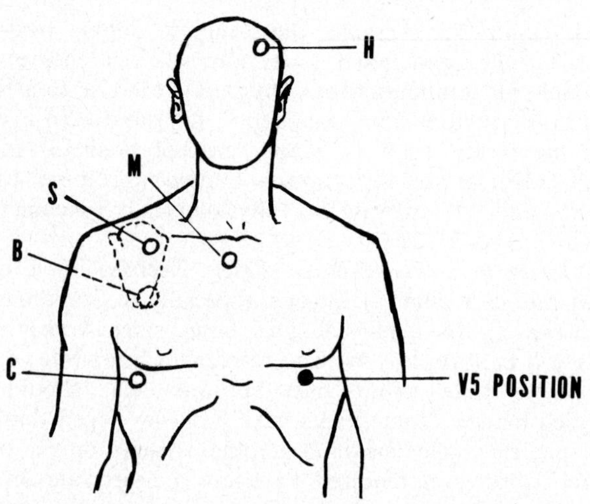

FIGURE 8–4 Locations of electrodes for some commonly used bipolar electrocardiographic leads. These leads are designated "$C(*)_5$," where * is replaced by the letter denoting the negative or reference electrode (e.g., CH_5 indicates that the active electrode is at V_5 and the reference electrode is on the head).

TABLE 8–4 THREE TREADMILL EXERCISE TEST PROTOCOLS

	Stage	Speed (mph)	Elevation (% grade)	Duration (min)	Approximate VO_2/kg/min (ml)
Bruce test	1	1.7	10.0	3	18.0
	2	2.5	12.0	3	25.0
	3	3.4	14.0	3	34.0
	4	4.2	16.0	3	46.0
	5	5.0	18.0	3	55.0
	6	5.5	20.0	3	—
	7	6.0	22.0	3	—
Modified Naughton test	1	2.0	0.0	3	7.0
	2	2.0	3.5	3	10.5
	3	2.0	7.0	3	14.0
	4	2.0	10.5	3	17.5
	5	2.0	14.0	3	21.0
	6	2.0	17.5	3	24.5
	7	3.0	12.5	3	28.0
	8	3.0	15.0	3	31.5
	9	3.0	17.5	3	35.0
	10	3.0	20.0	3	38.5
	11	3.0	22.5	3	42.0
	12	3.4	20.0	3	45.5
	13	3.4	22.0	3	49.0
	14	3.4	24.0	3	52.5
	15	3.4	26.0	3	56.0
Sheffield test* (GXT)	0	1.7	0.0	3	8.0
	½	1.7	5.0	3	12.0
	1	1.7	10.0	3	18.0

*Stages 2 through 7 of the Sheffield test are identical to those of the Bruce test.

is also worthwhile. Cardiac auscultation should be carried out as quickly as possible in order to detect exercise-induced mitral regurgitation or atrial or ventricular gallops. Postexercise observation should continue for 6 minutes or until all exercise-induced abnormalities have disappeared. Exercise testing should be supervised by a physician trained in the procedure, and the exercise laboratory should be equipped and organized for patient safety measures, as described later in this chapter.

EXERCISE ELECTROCARDIOGRAPHY

TYPES OF ST-SEGMENT DISPLACEMENT. When during exercise myocardial perfusion is inadequate to meet increased oxygen requirements, it is the subendocardium that becomes ischemic, since its perfusion is most precarious. As a consequence, a diastolic injury potential characterized by a vector that is opposite in direction to the major QRS vector is produced; hence there is ST-segment depression in leads with dominant R waves. The ST-segment ischemic displacement phenomenon in exercise stress testing, like that produced by angina at rest, is generally of three types.[55–57] The most common type is a displacement beginning at the QRS-ST junction which is downward or negative in polarity and which is followed by an initially upsloping ST segment as it merges into the T wave. As exercise progresses and presumably as ischemia also progresses, the degree of J-point depression increases and the ST segment becomes less and less upsloping. In its most characteristic form the ST segment becomes entirely flat for the first 80 msec of its duration and with further change may actually become negative or downsloping.

As an interpretive criterion, 0.10 mv (1 mm) or more of flat ST-segment displacement in a standard electrocardiographic lead is commonly considered indicative of ischemia. This is a conservative balance between *sensitivity* to detect ischemia and *specificity* to avoid false-positive results. At one time 0.05 mv (0.5 mm) ST displacement was used as a criterion of ischemia, and although the number of patients with obstructive coronary artery disease who were missed was small, the number of normal persons who shared this response was excessive, i.e., there were few false-negatives but many false-positives (high sensitivity, low specificity). Others have required 0.20 mv (2 mm) ST displacement for an ischemic response; this reduces the number of patients with positive tests who do not have ischemic heart disease but misses many patients with documented coronary obstruction; there were few false-positives but many false-negatives (high specificity, low sensitivity).

Other types of electrocardiographic leads (bipolar leads or Frank leads) have sensitivities different from the standard leads, warranting different criteria of ischemia. ST displacement of 0.20 mv (2 mm) is a logical and frequently used criterion for bipolar leads. The corresponding value for Frank leads would lie between 0.05 and 0.10 mv (0.5 to 1 mm) and in practice has not been adequately defined.

When we realize that the spectrum of ischemic ST-segment displacement varies from zero to nearly the amplitude of the QRS in some patients, it is apparent that any criterion we use is arbitrary, dictated partly by the recording format and partly by the desire for an optimal compromise between ability to detect disease and to reject nondisease.

An important feature of this type of response is its prompt improvement as soon as exercise is terminated and remarkably quick disappearance early in the postexercise period (Fig. 8–5, Type I). The brevity of this response makes it almost impossible to detect unless electrocardiographic recording and display are carried out *during* exercise and continued without interruption into the immediate postexercise period.

The second most frequent ST-displacement response begins as in the first example, but instead of immediate improvement with termination of exercise, the response becomes progressively more abnormal for several seconds or minutes following exercise (Fig. 8–5, Type II). In the postexercise period there is additional negative displacement of the flat or downsloping ST, which is frequently, but not always, associated with chest discomfort. In most cases this protracted response shows an evolutionary pattern in the course of returning to normal, developing a downsloping ST segment with upward convexity and merging into an inverted T wave. Usually from 5 to 20 minutes is required for the T wave to become fully upright thereafter and for the ST segment to return fully to its preexercise isoelectric contour. It is thought that the degree of ST-segment shift reflects the severity of myocardial ischemia, whereas the degree of coronary obstruction responsible for ischemia is inversely related to the amount of exercise stress required to provoke ischemia and directly related to the duration of ST-segment depression after exercise, once ischemia is provoked. Thus transient ST

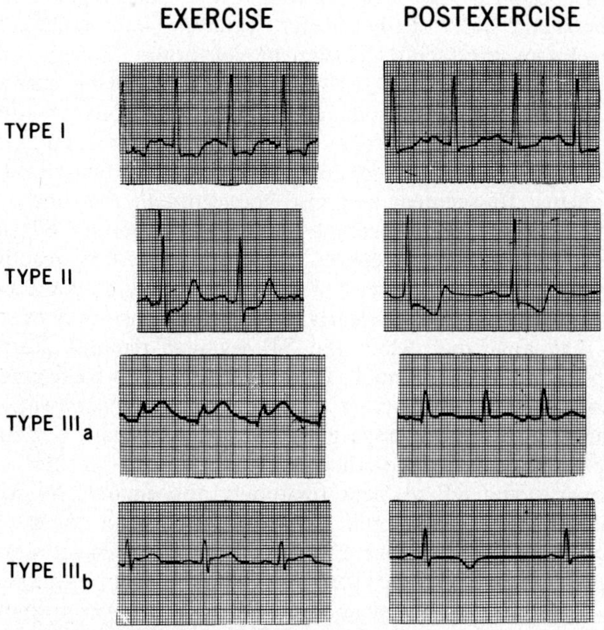

FIGURE 8–5 Types of exertional ST-segment displacement:
- **I:** Transient depression during exercise that has virtually disappeared 1 minute after exercise.
- **II:** Depression during exercise that becomes more pronounced after exercise before belatedly returning to normal.
- **IIIa:** ST elevation characteristic of Prinzmetal's angina.
- **IIIb:** ST elevation of modest degree usually caused by dyskinesis or scarring of the left ventricle.

depression (Type I) occurring only with vigorous exercise would represent minor prognostic abnormality, whereas protracted ST depression (Type II) provoked only by mild exercise would constitute a major prognostic abnormality, such as usually caused by severe multivessel or left main coronary artery disease.

The least common ST-segment response, occurring in only 3 to 5 per cent of most series, consists of ST-segment *elevation* rather than depression. At least two mechanisms can be responsible for ST-segment elevation. Intense, localized transmural ischemia may be produced in Prinzmetal's variant angina by spastic occlusion of a single major coronary vessel. Although episodes of transmural ischemia caused by coronary spasm characteristically occur at rest, there is now substantial evidence that it can be provoked by exercise as well[58] (p. 1242). Similar intense localized ischemia may be provoked by exercise (Fig. 8–5, Type IIIa). This type of response, when severe, usually distorts the QRS complex as well, causing the QRS-T configuration to resemble temporarily a directly recorded monophasic action potential. This response usually goes through a phase of T-wave inversion in the process of disappearing.

A second kind of ST-segment elevation response has been described (Fig. 8–5, Type IIIb). This is most frequently found in the longitudinal leads, reflecting the diaphragmatic surface of the left ventricle. This type of ST-segment elevation does not distort the QRS complex, is not followed by the evolutionary pattern of T-wave inversion in its improvement and disappearance, and has been related to the presence of scarring or dyskinesia due to preexisting disease, rather than to temporary ischemia of otherwise normal myocardium.[59,60] Alternatively, it is possible that during exercise, as a greater quantity of myocardium becomes ischemic and akinetic, the larger noncontractile mass of myocardium behaves like a ventricular aneurysm, producing ST-segment elevation.

Depression of the QRS-ST junction (J) during exercise occurs in normal persons, although usually not more than 0.20 mv (2 mm). When this occurs, an upsloping depression of the ST segment results. Unfortunately, the ischemic ST-segment response goes through this phase in the process of approaching flat or downsloping ST-segment depression. In order to differentiate this reaction from normal, the exercise should, if possible, be continued to a higher level so a clearly ischemic response may evolve in the abnormal while the ST segment remains steeply upsloping in the normal. Thus with respect to ST-segment slope in exercise there are three zones of prognostic significance: a steeply upsloping ST segment (normal), a gently upsloping one (probably abnormal), and a flat or downsloping ST segment (definitely abnormal).[61] As with ST-displacement criteria, any division between zones will be arbitrary, but we have found it useful to consider slopes greater than 1 mv/sec (40 per cent slope when paper speed is 25 mm/sec) normal and those 0 to 1 mv/sec probably abnormal. Another useful rule of thumb is that an upsloping ST segment may be considered abnormal when the degree of depression at 0.06 sec from the J-point is depressed by 1.5 mm or more.[62]

There is renewed interest in R-wave amplitude change as a sign of exertional ischemia.[63,64] The *Brody effect* is an augmentation of the radially directed electrocardiographic signal due to the highly conductive intracavitary blood.[65] Further increase in this blood pool due to ischemic dysfunction might augment the electrocardiographic signal still more. Conversely, animal studies have shown reduction of electrocardiographic signal in response to increase in intraventricular pressure.[66] However, at present there are not enough published data on ischemic QRS-amplitude changes to develop a reliable perspective.[66] Although T-wave changes—specifically T-wave inversions—during exercise are quite uncommon in normal subjects, they are nonspecific and occur not only in patients with coronary artery disease but also in those with hypertension and cardiomyopathy.

Recording Electrocardiographic Effects of Ischemia. As discussed on p. 222, subendocardial ischemia ordinarily produces not ST-segment depression, but rather T-P-QRS elevation.[59,67,68] Since clinical electrocardiographs are not direct-coupled and thus are insensitive to direct-current voltages, it is not possible to distinguish between true depression of one portion of the electrocardiogram, such as the ST segment, and true elevation of every other portion of the electrocardiogram, such as the T-P-Q segment (See Figure 7–29 p. 222). It is only by means of direct-coupled recorders connected to the exposed heart that the true nature of an ST displacement can be established. Although it is helpful to understand the true electrical alteration caused by ischemia, it continues to be impractical (if not impossible) to record and measure *true* shifts in the T-P-Q segment "baseline" by body surface recordings with conventional instruments. *Ischemic ST-segment depression* is a term widely used in this chapter even though it may be technically incorrect or only partially correct.

The Electrode-skin Interface. It has long been recognized by electrocardiographers[69] and electroencephalographers that a nonmetallic electrolyte interface must be interposed between the skin and the metal recording electrode in order to minimize recording artifacts.[70]

In 1959 Shackel described a quick, painless, and effective means of reducing skin impedance for recording purposes.[71] Our adaptation of his method involves the use of a No. 6 spherical dental burr inserted into a variable-speed hobby grinding tool.* When rotating at an intermediate speed and touched lightly to the skin (2 to 5 gm pressure) for 1 second, a pinhead-sized area of cornified epithelium is abraded without pain or bleeding. An exercise electrocardiographic electrode applied over this spot, or alternately over an area prepared by lightly rubbing with fine sandpaper and scrubbing with acetone, will have a contact impedance of 1 to 5 kilohms instead of the 10 to 50 kilohms usually obtained without any kind of dermabrasion.

Silver–silver chloride electrodes are best, but stainless steel electrodes are satisfactory if the active surface is maintained properly. Burnishing the surface with a coarse pencil-shaped typewriter eraser is effective. In either case the metallic electrode should be recessed within a cup-shaped plastic housing filled with electrolyte paste. The more viscous the paste, the more satisfactory the resultant electrocardiograms, and therefore electrolyte cream has not proved satisfactory for this purpose. The electrode is then adhered to the skin with ring-shaped plastic seals which are coated on both sides with adhesive. Recessed, adhesive, disposable exercise electrocardiographic electrodes were developed by Mason and Likar and are now commercially available from numerous sources.[72] The cable that connects the electrodes to the recorder should be shielded, preferably all the way to the electrode, to reduce power-line artifact. The cable should be thin, light, and compliant and should introduce no electrical potential of its own when flexed or agitated. Some exercise electrocardiographic systems contain preamplifier circuits located at the patient end of the cable. This virtually eliminates the problem of power-line artifact while only slightly increasing the bulk of the cable system carried by the subject.

Electrocardiographic Leads for Detection of Ischemia. There is not uniform agreement on the number of electrocardiographic leads required for optimal exercise electrocardiography. Some investigators use only a single bipolar lead, requiring application of only two

*Such as a Dremel Moto-tool, model #380.

or three electrodes, whereas Blackburn et al.,[73] Mason and Likar,[74] and Phibbs and Buckels[75] have shown that some ischemic type of electrocardiographic responses will be missed if only a single lead is recorded. The range of positive yield from a single V_5-like lead has varied from as low as 60 per cent to over 90 per cent of the yield possible when 12 conventional leads are recorded. Blackburn has reported that the positive yield of the 12-lead series can be virtually retained by using the 6 leads V_3 through V_6 and limb leads II and a V_f.[73] Although this appears to be a 50 per cent reduction in the number of leads required, in practice all 4 torso electrodes must be applied in order to record any limb leads or Wilson precordial leads, and therefore to record these 6 leads, 8 electrodes must be applied instead of the 10 electrodes required for all 12 leads. Another practical consideration is that the ready availability of automatic three-channel electrocardiographs makes it easier to record a 12-lead sequence than it would be to select any 6 leads individually. Tubau and coworkers find that a combination of 12 conventional leads and 2 bipolar leads gives greater sensitivity than 1, 2, or 3 leads.[76]

Bipolar electrocardiographic leads were popularized during the era when it was thought that radiotelemetry was necessary to overcome the technical problems of recording the exercise electrocardiogram.[77] The miniature radio transmitters used for this purpose could accept only a bipolar input signal, so this was derived by placing an active electrode over the V_5 position, where the electrocardiographic signal is strongest, and a reference electrode somewhere on the right side of the chest. Various positions for the reference electrode became standardized (Fig. 8–4). On the basis of current evidence the recommended choice of exercise electrocardiographic leads is the conventional 12-lead set using torso (Mason-Likar) locations for limb leads. This procedure is easy to follow using an unmodified automatic three-channel electrocardiographic recorder, and the same leads used during and after exercise may be used for the resting control electrocardiogram.

BIOLOGICAL AND PHARMACOLOGICAL EFFECTS. Ischemic heart disease is one of several causes of ST-segment depression. The subendocardial region is the most distal tissue perfused by the coronary vasculature, and thus perfusion pressure is lowest here. Yet it is this tissue which is subjected to direct ventricular pressure and thus has the greatest intramural force resisting coronary flow. Therefore any disparity between perfusion requirement and supply, short of total arterial occlusion, will affect the subendocardium first and most profoundly and will spread outward with increasingly severe underperfusion.

Pressure Overload. Pressure overload of the left ventricle due to either arterial hypertension or obstruction of ventricular outflow may thus be expected to interfere with subendocardial perfusion, even in the absence of atherosclerosis. Lepeschkin showed that young college students with hypertension may show ST-segment depression with exercise,[78] and it is now generally accepted that ventricular overload may result in a false-positive exercise electrocardiogram.[18]

Another relationship between hypertension and exercise electrocardiography is that diuretics administered as antihypertensive therapy may lower the serum potassium concentration sufficiently to cause equivocal changes in the exercise electrocardiogram. The ability of hypokalemia to confound interpretation of the exercise electrocardiogram has been established,[79] and therefore when conducting an exercise test, one should assure that the potassium concentration is normal or should at least exclude possible causes of hypokalemia.

The mechanism producing the various manifestations of prolapse of the mitral valve (p. 1089) is not understood, be they premature beats, chest discomfort, or ST-segment changes. It is known, however, that these patients develop exertional ST-segment depression in the absence of coronary atherosclerosis.[80]

Abnormal Activation Sequence of Ventricles. Abnormal activation sequence of the ventricles, especially the left, alters repolarization and prohibits interpretation of ST-segment changes.[81] This includes not only left bundle branch block but also the Wolff-Parkinson-White syndrome (a subtle source of false-"positive" reaction if it occurs only during exercise (Fig. 8–6). It has also been claimed that patients with short P-R intervals but no delta waves may have false-positive exercise electrocardiographic responses,[82] but this has not been substantiated. It is generally supposed that left ventricular ischemia may be recognized in the lateral electrocardiographic leads when right bundle branch block is present, though perhaps with somewhat less sensitivity.[83,84]

Digitalis Effect. Digitalis is notorious for its obfuscating effect on the ST segment.[85–87] Even when digitalis effect is not apparent in the resting electrocardiogram, it still may be responsible for exertional ST-segment depression.[78] This effect persists longer than the half-life of the glycoside in the blood would suggest.[85] Therefore a conservative policy would be to discontinue digoxin therapy a week before exercise electrocardiography. If glycoside therapy is necessary for its inotropic effect, one should question seriously whether an exercise test is even indicated. It would be convenient if digitalis caused only a limited degree of ST-segment displacement, e.g., not more than 0.20 mv, for then greater displacement could be attributed to ischemia. Although this is thought to be true in the case of marked ST-segment depression (i.e., ≥0.40 mv), no dependable upper limit of digitalis-caused ST-segment displacement has been defined. On the other hand, digitalis is not accused of causing falsely negative ECG responses. The absence of ST-segment deviation at peak exercise or thereafter may be considered a valid negative response.

Psychoactive Drugs. Tricyclic and other antidepressant drugs are said to cause false-positive and false-negative responses, especially in women.[88] This effect is by no means understood and needs additional study. Women have been said to manifest more false-positive and false-negative exercise electrocardiographic responses than men,[89] but Linhart et al. do not confirm this if drug effects are taken into account.[88] We have found that asymptomatic women show exertional ST depression with the same frequency as do asymptomatic men.[50]

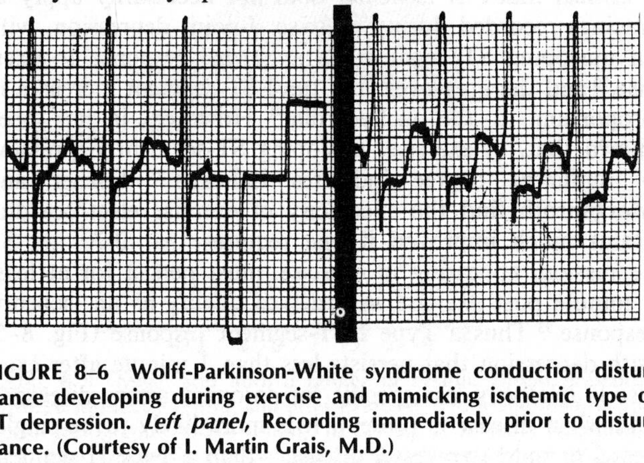

FIGURE 8–6 Wolff-Parkinson-White syndrome conduction disturbance developing during exercise and mimicking ischemic type of ST depression. *Left panel,* Recording immediately prior to disturbance. (Courtesy of I. Martin Grais, M.D.)

ing only a minute or two, the sinus rate increases progressively with each increase in exercise intensity. This is expected, since cardiac output is linearly related to exercise intensity, and heart rate is the principal determinant of cardiac output in exercise. As maximal aerobic exercise capacity is approached, heart rate reaches a plateau just as oxygen consumption does.[107] Maximal exercise heart rate is highest in childhood and becomes lower with age (Fig. 8–10).[50,51] The maximal level of exercise tachycardia is slightly less in trained athletes, averaging 7 beats/min lower than that of sedentary individuals in each age range. This description of normal heart rate response assumes normal sinus rhythm, of course. Abnormal rhythms may cause unpredictable rate responses.

There are two principal abnormal heart rate responses to exercise. First, the heart rate increment per stage of exercise may be lower than normal, and the heart rate may demonstrate a plateau at a distinctly subnormal intensity of work. This may be due to disease of the sinoatrial node and may also be the result of adrenergic blocking agents, such as propranolol. Second, occasionally one also finds a very high heart rate response at low levels of work as a result of either physical deconditioning or marginal circulatory compensation.

The heart rate–systolic blood pressure product—a good, externally derived indicator of myocardial oxygen needs—rises progressively during exercise stress testing, and its peak value serves to characterize the normal cardiovascular performance. Normal individuals usually develop a peak rate-pressure product of 20 to 35 mm Hg × beats/min × 10^{-3}. On the other hand, most patients with overt ischemic heart disease will not be able to generate rate-pressure products exceeding 25 mm Hg × beats/min × 10^{-3}. Although on the average the peak rate-pressure products of normal persons are higher than those of ischemic heart disease patients, there is sufficient overlap in individual cases to prevent this product from being a useful single criterion of disease.[23] As one factor in a multivariate interpretation method, however, it contributes to increased test accuracy.[108]

Systolic time intervals (p. 54) have been advocated by Lewis and colleagues and others for extending the accuracy of the electrocardiogram in exercise stress testing.[109] Since Lance and Spodick have introduced a method of recording systolic time intervals during exercise using procedures unlikely to complicate the stress test unnecessarily, this seems a promising means of extending the diagnostic value of the exercise test.[110] In the absence of sufficient perfusion, the left ventricle responds with less than normal vigor to the adrenergic stimulus of exercise. This results in postexercise prolongation of the left ventricular ejection time index. Additional experience with this method of observation is required in order to gauge the clinical value of systolic time interval measurement.

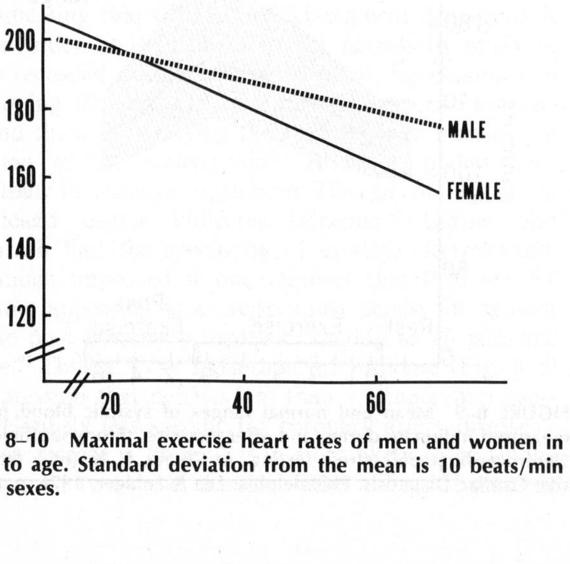

FIGURE 8–10 Maximal exercise heart rates of men and women in relation to age. Standard deviation from the mean is 10 beats/min for both sexes.

MAXIMAL WORK CAPACITY. Maximal work capacity is probably the most important measurement that can be gained from an exercise stress test. On a treadmill exercise protocol calling for increments of about 12 ml of oxygen/kg body weight/minute/3-minute stage, the exercise endurance of adult men is about 11.5 minutes and that of women 7.6 minutes.[50,51] With the bicycle ergometer, average maximal aerobic exercise capacity of men is about 1200 kpm/min.* Average maximal bicycle ergometer capacity for adult women is about 800 kpm/min.[49] The length of time a subject is able to continue exercise by any of the progressive, continuous protocols correlates with the subject's maximal oxygen consumption ($\dot{V}O_{2\ max}$). It is tempting, therefore, to predict $\dot{V}O_{2\ max}$ from treadmill endurance time or to estimate "functional aerobic impairment,"[111] i.e., the difference between the predicted peak $\dot{V}O_2$ and the peak estimated $\dot{V}O_2$ divided by the predicted peak $\dot{V}O_2$. Such estimates should be used with reservation, since the results vary significantly from protocol to protocol and from one test to another on the same protocol.[112,113]

The work capacity of normal sedentary individuals may be increased dramatically with regular training. More than doubling may be attained in young persons, and about a 50 per cent increase is possible in middle-aged individuals. In spite of the wide normal variability of work capacity, the measurement of exercise protocol endurance has great value in the study of patients with chest pain. It has been found that in patients with evidence of ischemia after only 7 minutes of exercise, 5-year prognosis is virtually as good as in patients who show no evidence of ischemia at all, whereas patients demonstrating ischemia after only 3 minutes of exercise or less have four times as high an incidence of disease progression or cardiovascular death.[114]

In view of the great importance of accurately assessing exercise capacity, care should be taken that the subject is acquainted with the exercise device and not intimidated by it. A pretest familiarization visit to the exercise lab is well worthwhile. Exercise should be begun at a sufficiently low level to serve as an unstressful warm-up for later stages. If the treadmill is used, subjects must be coached to walk properly, neither pushing on the front handrail and increasing their work rate ("lawn mower effect") nor partially supporting themselves on the side rails.

When a subject is unable to maintain position on the treadmill without grasping and pulling on the handrails, exercise should be terminated, since work rate drops when the handrails provide assistance. In using the bicycle ergometer, exercise should be terminated as soon as the sub-

*Kilopond-meters per minute = kilogram-weight force × meters per minute.

ject becomes unable to maintain the set pedaling speed. If there are any limitations to maximal exercise capacity other than cardiovascular ones, these should be carefully noted, since psychological, musculoskeletal, or other noncardiovascular limitations do not have the prognostic implications mentioned above.

EFFORT ANGINA. Although numerous kinds of chest discomfort are encountered during exercise testing, the finding of symptoms distinguished clearly as anginal may improve the sensitivity of exercise electrocardiographic testing considerably. Cole and Ellestad report that whereas ST-segment changes alone detect 64 per cent of patients with significant coronary artery disease, when characteristic chest discomfort was also considered a positive finding, the detection rate rose to 85 per cent.[115]

INTERPRETATION OF STRESS TESTS

(See also p. 1340)

Few diseases manifest a wider spectrum of morbidity and length of survival than coronary artery disease. Therefore we need to know not just whether or not a patient has the disease, but also how severely it is likely to affect his future. Exercise stress testing can help determine this, but in order to make the best use of this procedure the dimensions of the test results should be familiar. Terms used in evaluating stress test results are found in Table 8–5.

Figures-of-merit for Evaluating Tests. *Sensitivity* gives an index of the capability of a test to detect abnormality. The value is given as a percentage or decimal fraction. Although one would wish every test to have a sensitivity of 100 per cent, in the medical realm tests with high sensitivity frequently have the disadvantage of yielding some abnormal results erroneously. The sensitivity of near maximal and maximal exercise tests for coronary artery disease is generally between 60 and 70 per cent when only the ST-segment behavior is considered; however, when combined with other exercise test observations, test sensitivity increases to over 90 per cent.[18,115,116]

Specificity indicates the ability of a test to recognize a normal subject. This is a very important characteristic because of the potential harm should diagnosis of a serious disease be applied to a subject in error. Because of this concern, tests are not usually considered for clinical application unless they have high specificity. Specificity of the near maximal exercise electrocardiographic test usually ranges from 90 to 95 per cent.[18,115,116]

Accuracy is the measure of the capability of a test to yield correct results. It gives a general or overall figure-of-merit for a test, since it includes the ability of the test to recognize true-positives as well as true-negatives.

True-positive is the most clinically useful test result because of the avenue it opens for primary or secondary prevention of overt disease. In a predictive sense the true-positive result would identify the individual who, although healthy at present, is destined to manifest angina pectoris, myocardial infarction, or sudden death in the foreseeable future. *False-positive, true-negative,* and *false-negative* results do not require elaboration.

Predictive value indicates the clinical significance of a positive test result. It is the percentage of likelihood that a positive result is true. This term takes into consideration the prevalance of the disease in the population tested. If the prevalence is high, such as the prevalence of coronary atherosclerosis in a population of adults consulting a physician for chest pain, the number of true-positive results will be high and the number of false-positive results will be low, yielding a high predictive value. On the other hand, if the same test is conducted in the population at large in which the prevalence of coronary artery disease is probably between 1 and 2 per cent, the yield of true-positives will be overwhelmed by the large number of false-positives, and the predictive value will be quite low.

Relative risk indicates how a subject's statistical prognosis is changed by virtue of his having undergone a test. Most studies have shown very close agreement on relative risk, finding that persons with abnormal test results have about 13 times greater incidence of coronary disease than those with a negative test result.

When exercise test results are thought of in terms of relative risk instead of clinical diagnosis, justification can be seen for screening selected asymptomatic subjects. Those giving abnormal responses qualify for special attention to reduce risk factors, not to diagnose a disease. Kattus showed the value of this approach in screening 309 asymptomatic executives.[117] Half of those with abnormal responses then participated in a remedial exercise program; all improved their functional capacity, and in one-third electrocardiographic responses converted to normal compared with one-seventh of the nonexercising controls.

Bayes' Theorem (see also Fig. 39–2, p. 1340). In 1763 the English philosopher Thomas Bayes demonstrated the way in which the predictive value of a test is influenced not only by the sensitivity of the test but most especially by the "prior probability" that an individual has the disease tested for (i.e., the prevalence of the disease in

TABLE 8–5 TERMS USEFUL IN EVALUATION OF TEST RESULTS

Sensitivity	=	$\frac{\text{Number of true-positive detections}}{\text{Total number of positives in the group tested}}$
Specificity	=	$\frac{\text{Number of true normals detected}}{\text{Total number of normals in the group tested}}$
Accuracy	=	$\frac{\text{Number of true test results (true-positives + true-negatives)}}{\text{Total number of tests performed}}$
True-positive	=	Abnormal test result in individual who has (or will have) the disease*
False-positive	=	Abnormal test result in one who does not (and will not) have the disease
True-negative	=	Normal test result in one who does not (and will not) have the disease
False-negative	=	Normal test result in one who has (or will have) the disease
Predictive value	=	$\frac{\text{True-positives}}{\text{True-positives + false-positives}}$
Relative risk (risk ratio)	=	$\frac{\text{Disease rate** in persons with a positive test result}}{\text{Disease rate in persons with a negative test result}}$

*Whatever disease the test aims to detect.

**This may be in terms of current prevalence, future incidence, or both and should be specified when the term is used.

the population being tested). This relationship is described by the following formula:

$$P[C/A] = \frac{P[A/C]}{P[A]} = \frac{P[A/C] \cdot P[C]}{P[A/C] \cdot P[C] + P[A_i/C_i] \cdot P[C_i]}$$

where

$P[C/A]$ = probability that a person with a positive test has the disease tested for

C = sensitivity of test

$C_i = 1 -$ specificity of test

A = prevalance of disease

A_i = rarity of disease (complement of A)

Applying this formula to some realistic approximations and assuming that exercise test sensitivity for ischemic heart disease is 80 per cent, that specificity is 90 per cent, and that in a population of North American adults complaining of chest pain the prevalance of ischemic heart disease is 50 per cent, Bayes' theorem would then determine that a patient with a positive exercise test would have an 89 per cent probability of having ischemic heart disease.

If sensitivity = 0.80, specificity = 0.90, and prevalence = 0.50

$$P = \frac{0.50 \times 0.80}{(0.50 \times 0.80) + (0.50 \times 0.10)} = 0.89$$

On the other hand, if the test with unchanged sensitivity and specificity is applied to a group of asymptomatic adults with a disease prevalance of 3 per cent, the probability that an individual with a positive test has ischemic heart disease is only 20 per cent! Of 100 such positive tests, 80 of them would be false-positives.

If sensitivity = 0.80, specificity = 0.90, and prevalence = 0.03

$$P = \frac{0.03 \times 0.80}{(0.03 \times 0.80) + (0.97 \times 0.10)} = 0.20$$

Thus in assessing the meaning of an exercise test result, Bayes' theorem emphasizes the importance of considering the identifiable risk group from which an individual comes.[118] The patient with typical chest pain and positive exercise electrocardiogram, who has an 89 per cent likelihood of having significant coronary artery disease, presents justification for accepting this diagnosis and commencing treatment. However, a patient with atypical chest pain, and thus only about a 20 per cent pretest likelihood of having coronary artery disease, after being tested and found positive will have a 67 per cent probability of coronary disease. That is, there is one chance in three that he does not. In such a case one would like to have additional evidence for the presence of disease before embarking on a potentially dangerous or difficult course of treatment. In the asymptomatic person whose positive test raises his disease probability from 3 to 20 per cent (Fig. 8–1), only moderate preventive measures that would be unlikely to be harmful or burdensome to anyone are justified, although they could be expected to reduce the likelihood of future coronary events.

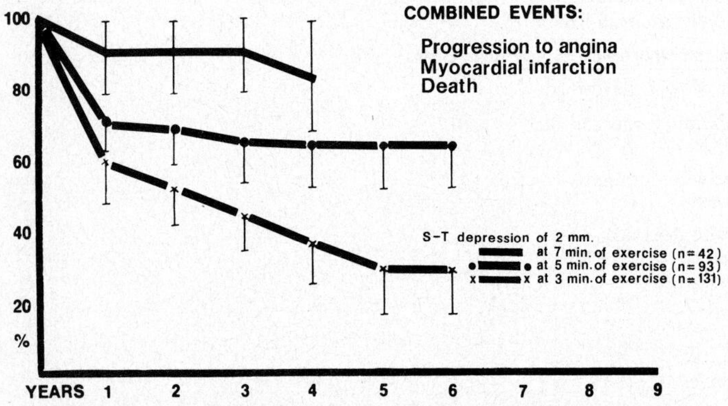

FIGURE 8–11 Continued survival without progression to angina or myocardial infarction with ST depression after 7 minutes (———), 5 minutes (●———●), and 3 minutes (x———x) of exercise. Healthy survival is proportional to exercise capacity. (From Ellestad, M. H.: Stress Testing: Principles and Practice. Philadelphia, F. A. Davis Co., 1975, p. 167.)

PROGNOSTIC SIGNIFICANCE OF EXERCISE TEST RESULTS. The foregoing should have suggested that the exercise test result should be considered as a quantitative risk factor rather than as a simple disease/no disease classification. Persons without clinical evidence of coronary artery disease who manifest ST-segment depression after only mild exercise have a greater than 50 per cent likelihood of progression of coronary heart disease, as reflected in the development of angina or a myocardial infarction, in the succeeding 4 years, those who develop ischemia only after moderate exercise have a less than 50 per cent likelihood of progression, and patients with ischemia only after strenuous exercise have less than 20 per cent likelihood of progression of disease in the next 4 years (Fig. 8–11).[96] The prognostic value of the treadmill test prevails also in survivors of myocardial infarction; 4 years after testing, patients with abnormal treadmill responses had 30 per cent greater progression of coronary disease than did survivors with a normal test response.[96] Limited stress testing 3 weeks after myocardial infarction (p. 1293) identified patients with more than twice the risk of additional coronary events in the next 4 years than those with normal responses.[119]

McNeer and colleagues found that in patients with angiographically significant coronary artery disease, those with exercise-induced ST-segment depression have over three times greater mortality during 4 years of observation than those without.[28] This landmark study utilized the Duke University computerized data bank. Results from 2290 patients were involved. They employed 12-lead electrocardiograms throughout exercise testing and used a conventional criterion of ≥0.10 mv flat or downsloping (or elevated) ST-segment deviation from baseline. The Bruce treadmill stages were used. Negative tests required attainment of ≥85 per cent of predicted maximal heart rate. Follow-ups occurred at 6 months, 1 year, 2 years, 3 years, and 4 years and were 99.5 per cent complete. They also noted the importance of maximum achieved heart rate during testing. Those whose heart rates did not reach 120 beats/min showed less than 75 per cent survival over 4 years, those reaching heart rates of 120 to 159 beats/min showed over 85 per cent survival, and those with exercise heart rates 160 beats/min or greater had 95 per cent survival. By taking into account ST-segment response, exercise duration, and heart rate, it is possible to identify a low-risk group of patients who, even though afflicted with coronary artery disease, may be expected to show over 90 per cent survival in 4 years. On the other hand, it is also possible to identify a high-risk subgroup based on these observations who can expect only 60 per cent survival over the same interval (Fig. 8–12).

Goldschlager and colleagues found that the Type II ST-segment depression (i.e., ST-segment depression which, instead of improving immediately upon cessation of exercise, becomes more pronounced before improvement begins) is useful in predicting severe coronary artery obstruction (Fig. 8–5, Type II).[120] From 86 to 91 per cent of their patients with this finding had advanced two-vessel, three-vessel, or left main coronary disease. Blumenthal and colleagues reported similar findings. The occurrence of a strongly positive exercise stress test had a 57 per cent predictive accuracy for the presence of left main coronary artery disease.[121] The

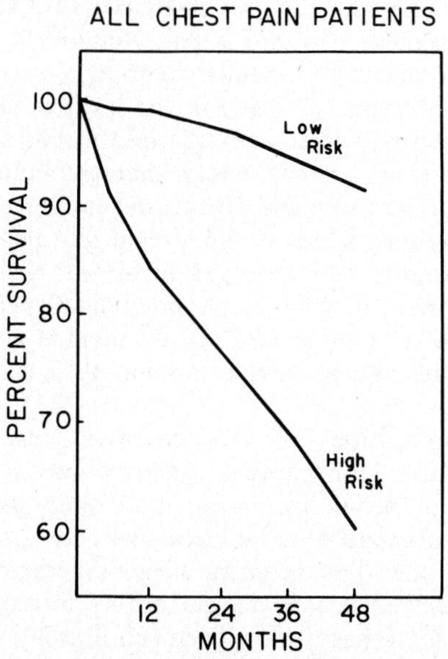

FIGURE 8–12 **Prediction of survival on basis of exercise test. "Low-risk" patients had normal ST-segment, heart rate, and exercise duration responses, whereas "high-risk" patients did not. (From McNeer, J. F., et al.: The role of the exercise test in the evaluation of patients for ischemic heart disease. Circulation *57*:64, 1978, by permission of the American Heart Association, Inc.)**

use of exercise test data makes it possible to separate those patients whose unfavorable risk indicates prompt consideration for coronary arteriography for bypass surgery while also identifying patients who are good candidates for medical, physical, and dietary therapy.[28]

SAFETY OF EXERCISE TESTING

The primary requirements of any elective test are that it be as safe as possible and that the ratio of benefit to risk be favorable. Exercise stress testing enjoys an excellent safety record. Maintenance of a high order of patient safety in testing depends on continual attention to three important factors: contraindications to testing, indications for terminating exercise, and incidence and management of complications.

CONTRAINDICATIONS TO TESTING. It is necessary that the subject considered for exercise stress testing understand the nature of the procedure, the importance of cooperation with the supervising physician, the necessity for reporting all symptoms promptly, and the realization of the very slight but definite risk which the procedure entails in an individual with preexisting cardiovascular disease. Although informed consent may be given verbally to the supervising physician after a discussion of the procedure, use of written and signed informed consent is more likely to avoid omission of important details, will emphasize the importance of the procedure to the subject, and will communicate to the subject the concern which the supervising physician, his coworkers, and his institution have for his well-being.

True contraindications to testing are conditions that are likely to be aggravated by vigorous exercise (Table 8–6). Naturally such a list is headed by unhealed myocardial infarction. Breach of this contraindication has been known to be due to misinterpretation or omission of the resting control 12-lead electrocardiogram. This emphasizes that the supervising physician must be expert in the interpretation of symptoms of coronary heart disease and of resting and exercise electrocardiograms.

Another important contraindication is unstable angina pectoris (p. 1355), variably called preinfarctional angina or intermediate coronary syndrome and defined as "angina pectoris which is newly developed or has definitely become worse in frequency, ease of provocation, and severity (including rest angina) in the last 4 weeks."

Exercise may safely be conducted in the presence of mild to moderate aortic stenosis, with careful attention to blood pressure, the patient's symptoms, and electrocardiogram. Only severe aortic stenosis with palpably prolonged left ventricular ejection time and with clear-cut electrocardiographic left ventricular hypertrophy is a contraindication. The other contraindications are self-explanatory. The AMA Council on Scientific Affairs has recently reported on indications and contraindications for exercise testing, and they are essentially identical with those proposed herein.[122] *Relative* contraindications include known left main coronary disease or the equivalent, severe hypertension, and hypertrophic obstructive cardiomyopathy.

In addition to clinical contraindications, there are conditions which do not compromise safety but which in one way or another limit the usefulness of test results. These include confusing variables such as left ventricular hypertrophy, left bundle branch block, digitalis effect, and others. These were detailed in the preceding section on electrocardiography. When one or more of these conditions are present, one should reconsider whether the expected benefit of the test fully justifies its use.

TERMINATION OF EXERCISE. Termination of exercise has two aspects. Technically, it is determined by whether the test is (1) a subjective maximal one, in which uncomplicated termination is determined by the subject; or (2) a near maximal test, in which an objective endpoint, such as a target heart rate, would be reached and the test then terminated. The aspect of termination most important here is the one of patient safety. In this light items 1 through 11 in Table 8–7 are applicable. These are specific expressions of the general conviction that exercise testing should cease whenever any important sign of work intolerance is recognized or when any condition appears that is more than likely to contribute to morbidity or mortality. Chest pain should convincingly simulate angina pectoris and should be tolerated until it is clear that it is definitely progressing and not stabilizing or regressing in the face of

TABLE 8–6 **CONTRAINDICATIONS TO EXERCISE TESTING**

Myocardial infarction—impending, acute, or healing
Unstable angina pectoris
Acute myocarditis or pericarditis
Known ominous coronary artery disease pattern
Severe aortic stenosis
Congestive heart failure
Severe hypertension
Uncontrolled cardiac arrhythmias
Intracardiac conduction block greater than first-degree
Acute systemic illness
Unwillingness to give informed consent

TABLE 8–7 INDICATIONS FOR TERMINATING GRADED EXERCISE TESTING

1.	Angina-like pain that is progressive during exercise
2.	Excessive degree (≥0.4 mv) of ischemic type of ST-segment depression or elevation during exercise
3.	Ectopic supraventricular tachycardia (regular or irregular)
4.	Ventricular premature beats aggravated by exercise or precipitated by exercise (over 25% of beats)
5.	Electrocardiogram consistent with ventricular tachycardia
6.	*Any* recognized type of intracardiac block precipitated by exercise
7.	Signs of peripheral circulatory insufficiency (pallor, diminished pulse, clammy skin, exhaustion, staggering gait)
8.	Drop in systolic blood pressure during mild or moderate exercise (e.g., below Stage 3 of Bruce test)
9.	Excessive fatigue or dyspnea
10.	Failure of monitoring equipment
11.	Subject wishes to stop exercise

increasing exercise. The "diagnostic degree" of ST-segment depression should be quite pronounced, more than an estimated 2 mm, since ST-segment depression is frequently overestimated during the quick scrutiny possible during exercise, especially when evaluated by means of an oscilloscope.

INCIDENCE OF COMPLICATIONS. The safety of exercise stress testing is well documented. Reports from nine groups, ranging from 500 to 170,000 tests, represent a cumulative experience of about 260,000 tests from about 80 medical centers. The largest single reported experience (170,000 tests) resulted from Rochmis and Blackburn's questionnaire survey of 73 medical centers.[123] They found that 16 deaths were associated with exercise testing and that an additional 40 patients required hospitalization for nonfatal complications such as prolonged chest pain or cardiac arrhythmias. This amounts to a mortality rate of 10 per 100,000 tests and a morbidity rate of 24 per 100,000. Eight of the reports include a total of greater than 90,000 tests, among which there were 13 nonfatal infarctions and 3 deaths.[3,124–130] This yields a mortality rate of 3.3 per 100,000 while maintaining a complication rate comparable to that found in the larger survey.

It is not possible to anticipate and prevent the rare instance when a small coronary arterial plaque—insufficient to provoke detectable ischemia during even maximal exercise—may be the site of subintimal hemorrhage, resulting in dislodgment, occlusion of the vessel, and infarction or death. Such an occurrence is far less likely than the risks patients face every day. The more common risks of exercise testing can be detected by careful, attentive search for contraindications prior to testing; meticulous observation of the patient during exercise with monitoring of the electrocardiogram and the blood pressure as well as the subject's symptoms and appearance; and close attention to the patient after exercise, including auscultation and palpation of the heart and inspection of the cervical veins, skin, and general appearance.

TABLE 8–8 EQUIPMENT AND SUPPLIES FOR MANAGEMENT OF COMPLICATIONS

1.	Direct-current defibrillator with full tube of electrode paste
2.	Assorted airways, ventilation bag, oxygen, and laryngoscope
3.	Intravenous fluid (5% dextrose) with tubing, needles, and assorted syringes
4.	Assorted drugs, including lidocaine, quinidine, disopyramide, procainamide, phenytoin, propranolol, atropine, isoproterenol, norepinephrine, metaraminol, furosemide, digoxin, dopamine

MANAGEMENT OF COMPLICATIONS. Appropriate management of exercise test complications depends primarily on the prior establishment of a protocol to be followed by everyone involved in the testing. This includes knowledge of what persons or services to employ immediately, such as anesthesia/airway therapy, emergency patient transport service, and so on, depending on the local setting. A preselected set of equipment and medications in a specific location and arranged in an established pattern is necessary (see Table 8–8). A previously specified treatment routine is essential and should include arranging for transfer of the patient and admission to a coronary care unit.

Rare complications of exercise stress testing include supraventricular tachycardias, such as paroxysmal atrial tachycardia or atrial fibrillation, and ominous multifocal ventricular premature complexes with excessively close coupling to preceding beats or occurring repetitively. Established ventricular tachycardia occurs infrequently, and in our experience has always been self-limiting upon cessation of exercise except when paroxysmal ventricular tachycardia was a preexisting problem in the patient tested. We have not encountered an episode of primary ventricular fibrillation in the course of approximately 25,000 exercise tests. Other complications include atrioventricular block; vasovagal syncope that has progressed through sinus bradycardia to several seconds of complete cardiac arrest before reverting to completely normal, uncomplicated cardiovascular function; prolonged postexercise angina pectoris; and rare instances of myocardial infarction.

References

1. Goldhammer, S., and Scherf, D.: Elektrokardiographische Untersuchungen bei Kranker mit Angina Pectoris ("ambulatorischer Typus"). Zschr. klin. Med. *122*:134, 1933.
2. Rowell, L. B., Taylor, H. L., Simonson, E., and Carlson, W. S.: The physiologic fallacy of adjusting for body weight in performance of the Master two-step test. Am. Heart J. *70*:461, 1965.
3. Blomqvist, C. G.: Use of exercise testing for diagnostic and functional evaluation of patients with arteriosclerotic heart disease. Circulation *44*:1120, 1971.

3a. Froelicher, V. F.: Exercise testing and training: Clinicial applications. J. Am. Coll., Cardial. *1*:114, 1983.

4. James, F. W., Kaplan, S., Schwartz, D. C., Chou, T., Sandker, M. J., and Naylor, V.: Response to exercise in patients after total surgical correction of tetralogy of Fallot. Circulation *54*:671, 1976.
5. Borer, J. S., Brensike, J. F., Redwood, D. R., Itscoitz, S. B., Passamani, E. R., Stone, N. J., Richardson, J. M., Levy, R. I., and Epstein, S. E.: Limitations of the electrocardiographic response to exercise in predicting coronary-artery disease. N. Engl. J. Med. *293*:367, 1975.
6. Philbrick, J. T., Horwitz, R. I., and Feinstein, A. R.: Methodologic problems of exercise testing for coronary artery disease: Groups, analysis and bias. Am. J. Cardiol. *46*:807, 1980.
7. Epstein, S. E., Beiser, G. D., Stampfer, M., Robinson, B. F., and Braunwald, E.: Characterization of the circulatory response to maximal upright exercise in normal subjects and patients with heart disease. Circulation *35*:1049, 1967.
8. Astrand, P., and Rodahl, K.: Evaluation of physical work capacity on the basis of tests. *In* Textbook of Work Physiology. New York, McGraw-Hill Book Co., 1970, Chapter 11.
9. Braunwald, E., Ross, J., Jr., and Sonnenblick, E. S.: Mechanism of Contraction of the Normal and Failing Heart. 2nd ed. Boston, Little, Brown and Co., 1976, pp. 166–200.
10. Gobel, F. L., Nordstrom, L. A., Nelson, R. R., Jorgensen, C. R., and Wang, Y.: The rate-pressure product as an index of myocardial oxygen consumption during exercise in patients with angina pectoris. Circulation *57*:549, 1978.
11. Robinson, B. F.: Relation of heart rate and systolic blood pressure to the onset of pain in angina pectoris. Circulation *35*:1073, 1967.
12. Cannon, P. J., Weiss, M. B., and Sciacca, R. R.: Myocardial blood flow in coronary artery disease: Studies at rest and during stress with inert gas washout techniques. Prog. Cardiovasc. Dis. *22*:95, 1977.
13. Hillis, L. D., and Braunwald, E.: Myocardial ischemia. N. Engl. J. Med. *296*: 971, 1977.

14. Harrison, T. R., and Reeves, T. J.: Less common and rare causes of ischemic heart disease. *In* Principles and Problems of Ischemic Heart Disease. Chicago, Year Book Medical Publishers, 1968, Chapter 5.
15. Froelicher, V. F., Jr.: Use of the exercise electrocardiogram to identify latent coronary atherosclerotic heart disease. *In* Amsterdam, E. A., Wilmore, J. H., and DeMaria, A. N. (eds.): Exercise in Cardiovascular Health and Disease. New York, Yorke Medical Books, 1977, Chapter 13.
16. Barnard, R. J., MacAlpin, R., Kattus, A. A., and Buckberg, G. D.: Ischemic response to sudden strenuous exercise in healthy men. Circulation *48*:936, 1973.
17. Mason, R. E., Likar, I., Biern, R. O., and Ross, R. S.: Multiple-lead exercise electrocardiography. Experience in 107 normal subjects and 67 patients with angina pectoris, and comparison with coronary cinearteriography in 84 patients. Circulation *36*:517, 1967.
18. Roitman, D., Jones, W. B., and Sheffield, L. T.: Comparison of submaximal exercise ECG test with coronary cineangiocardiogram. Ann. Intern. Med. *72*: 641, 1970.
19. Ascoop, C. A., Simoons, M. L., Egmond, W. E., and Bruschke, A. V. G.: Exercise test, history, and serum lipid levels in patients with chest pain and normal electrocardiogram at rest: Comparison to findings at coronary arteriography. Am. Heart J. *82*:609, 1971.
20. Bartel, A. G., Behar, V. S., Peter, R. H., Orgain, E. S., and Kong, Y.: Graded exercise stress tests in angiographically documented coronary artery disease. Circulation *49*:348, 1974.
21. Wyatt, H. L., Forrester, J. S., Tyberg, J. V., Goldner, S., Logan, S. E., Parmley, W. W., and Swan, H. J. C.: Effect of graded reductions in regional coronary perfusion on regional and total cardiac function. Am. J. Cardiol. *36*: 185, 1975.
22. Waters, D. D., Da Luz, P., Wyatt, H. L., Swan, H. J. C., and Forrester, J. S.: Early changes in regional and global left ventricular function induced by graded reduction in regional coronary perfusion. Am. J. Cardiol. *39*:537, 1977.
23. Sheffield, L. T., and Roitman, D.: Systolic blood pressure, heart rate, and treadmill work at anginal threshold. Chest *63*:327, 1973.
24. Gould, K. L., Hamilton, G. W., Lipscomb, K., Ritchie, J. L., and Kennedy, J. W.: Method for assessing stress-induced regional malperfusion during coronary arteriography. Experimental validation and clinical application. Am. J. Cardiol. *34*:557, 1974.
25. Logan, S. E.: On the fluid mechanics of human coronary artery stenosis. IEEE Trans. Biomed. Eng. *22*:327, 1975.
26. Feldman, R. L., Nichols, W. W., and Pepine, C. J.: What is the coronary hemodynamic significance of the length of a coronary artery obstruction? Clin. Res. *24*:216A, 1976.
27. Ellestad, M. H.: Stress Testing Principles and Practice. Philadelphia, F. A. Davis Co., 1975, p. 175.
28. McNeer, J. F., Margolis, J. R., Lee, K. L., Kisslo, J. A., Peter, R. H., Kong, Y., Behar, V. S., Wallace, A. G., McCants, C. B., and Rosati, R. A.: The role of the exercise test in the evaluation of patients for ischemic heart disease. Circulation *57*:64, 1978.
29. Master, A. M., Friedman, R., and Dack, S.: The electrocardiogram after standard exercise as a functional test of the heart. Am. Heart J. *24*:777, 1942.
30. Ellestad, M. H., Allen, W., Wan, M. C. K., and Kemp, G. L.: Maximal treadmill stress testing for cardiovascular evaluation. Circulation *39*:517, 1969.
31. Weiner, D. A., McCabe, C., Hueter, D., Hood, W. B., Jr., and Ryan, T.: The predictive value of chest pain as an indicator of coronary disease during exercise testing. Circulation *54* (Suppl. II):II-10, 1976.
32. Harrison, T. R., and Reeves, T. J.: Analysis of symptoms. *In* Principles and Problems of Ischemic Heart Disease. Chicago, Year Book Medical Publishers, 1968, Chapter 6.
33. Varnauskas, E.: The ECG and exercise testing. *In* Julian, D. G. (ed.): Angina Pectoris. New York, Churchill Livingstone, 1977, Chapter 7.
34. Koppes, G., McKiernan, T., Bassan, M., and Froelicher, V. F.: Treadmill exercise testing. Part II. Curr. Prob. Cardiol. *7*:1, 1977.
35. Udall, J. A., and Ellestad, M. H.: Predictive implications of ventricular premature contractions associated with treadmill stress testing. Circulation *56*: 985, 1977.
36. Robinson, B. F.: Relation of heart rate and systolic blood pressure to the onset of pain in angina pectoris. Circulation *35*:1073, 1967.
37. Thomson, P. D., and Kelleman, M. H.: Hypotension accompanying the onset of exertional angina. Circulation *52*:28, 1975.
38. Astrand, P., and Saltin, B.: Maximal oxygen uptake and heart rate in various types of muscular activity. J. Appl. Physiol. *16*:977, 1961.
39. Nutter, D. O., Schlant, R. C., and Hurst, J. W.: Isometric exercise and the cardiovascular system. Mod. Concepts Cardiovasc. Dis. *41*:11, 1972.
40. Lowe, D. K., Rothbaum, D. A., McHenry, P. L., Corya, B. C., and Knoebel, S. B.: Myocardial blood flow response to isometric (handgrip) and treadmill exercise in coronary artery disease. Circulation *51*:126, 1975.
41. Helfant, R. H., deVilla, M. A., and Meister, S. G.: Effect of sustained isometric handgrip exercise on left ventricular performance. Circulation *44*:982, 1971.
42. Jackson, D. H., Reeves, T. J., Sheffield, L. T., and Burdeshaw, J.: Isometric effects on treadmill exercise response in healthy young men. Am. J. Cardiol. *31*: 344, 1973.
43. Nagle, F. J., Balke, B., and Naughton, J. P.: Gradational step tests for assessing work capacity. J. Appl. Physiol. *20*:745, 1965.
44. Bruce, R. A., Blackmon, J. R., Jones, J. W., and Strait, G.: Exercising testing in adult normal subjects and cardiac patients. Pediatrics *32*:742, 1963.
45. Balke, B., and Ware, R. W.: An experimental study of "physical fitness" of Air Force Personnel. U.S. Armed Forces Med. J. *10*:675, 1959.
46. Hellerstein, H. K., Hornsten, T. R., Baker, R. A., and Hoppes, W. L.: Cardiac performance during postprandial lipemia and heparin-induced lipolysis. Am. J. Cardiol. *20*:525, 1967.
47. Astrand, P., and Rhyming, I.: A nomogram for calculation of aerobic capacity (physical fitness) from pulse rate during submaximal work. J. Appl. Physiol. *7*: 218, 1954.
48. Sheffield, L. T.: Graded exercise test (GXT) for isochemic heart disease. A submaximal test to a target heart rate. *In* Exercise Testing and Training of Apparently Healthy Individuals: A Handbook for Physicians. American Heart Association Committee on Exercise, 1972, pp. 35-38.
49. Astrand, I.: Aerobic work capacity in men and women with special reference to age. Acta Physiol. Scand. *49* (Suppl. 169):1, 1960.
50. Lester, F. M., Sheffield, L. T., and Reeves, T. J.: Electrocardiographic changes in clinically normal older men following near maximal and maximal exercise. Circulation *36*:5, 1967.
51. Sheffield, L. T., Maloof, J. A., Sawyer, J. A., and Roitman, D.: Maximal heart rate and treadmill performance of healthy women in relation to age. Circulation *57*:79, 1978.
52. Bruce, R. A., Gey, G. O., Cooper, M. N., Fisher, L. D., and Peterson, D. R.: Seattle heart watch: Initial clinical, circulatory and electrocardiographic responses to maximal exercise. Am. J. Cardiol. *33*:459, 1974.
53. Patterson, J. A., Naughton, J., Pietras, R. J., and Gunnar, R. M.: Treadmill exercise in assessment of the functional capacity of patients with cardiac disease. Am. J. Cardiol. *30*:757, 1972.
54. Bruce, R. A., and Hornsten, T. R.: Exercise stress testing in evaluation of patients with ischemic heart disease. Prog. Cardiovasc. Dis. *11*:371, 1969.
55. Feil, H., and Siegel, M. L.: Electrocardiographic changes during attacks of angina pectoris. Am. J. Med. Sci. *175*:255, 1928.
56. Wood, F. C., and Wolferth, C. C.: Angina pectoris. The clinical and electrocardiographic phenomena of the attack and their comparison with the effects of experimental temporary coronary occlusion. Arch. Intern. Med. *47*: 339, 1931.
57. Wilson, F. N., and Johnston, F. D.: The occurrence in angina pectoris of electrocardiographic changes similar in magnitude and kind to those produced by myocardial infarction. Am. Heart J. *22*:64, 1941.
58. Prinzmetal, M., Kennamer, R., Merliss, R., Wada, T., and Bor, N.: Angina pectoris. I. A variant form of angina pectoris. Am. J. Med. *27*:375, 1959.
59. Chahine, R. A., Raizner, A. E., and Ishimori, T.: The clinical significance of exercise-induced ST-segment elevation. Circulation *54*:209, 1976.
60. Fortuin, N. J., and Friesinger, G. C.: Exercise-induced ST segment elevation: Clinical, electrocardiographic and arteriographic studies in twelve patients. Am. J. Med. *49*:459, 1970.
61. Rijneke, R. D., Ascoop, C. A., and Talmon, J. L.: Clinical significance of upsloping ST segments in exercise electrocardiography. Circulation *61*:671, 1980.
62. Ellestad, M. H.: Stress Testing. 2nd ed. Philadelphia, F. A. Davis Co., 1980.
63. Berman, J. L., Wynne, J., and Cohn, P. F.: Multiple-lead QRS changes with exercise testing. Diagnostic value and hemodynamic implications. Circulation *61*:53, 1980.
64. Baron, D. W., Ilsley, C., Sheiban, I., Poole-Wilson, P. A., and Rickards, A. F.: R wave amplitude during exercise. Relation to left ventricular function and coronary artery disease. Br. Heart J. *44*:512, 1980.
65. Brody, D. A.: A theoretical analysis of intracavitary blood mass influence on the heart-lead relationship. Circ. Res. *4*:731, 1956.
66. Lekven, J., Chatterjee, K., Tyberg, J. V., Stowe, D. F., Mathey, D. G., and Parmley, W. W.: Pronounced dependence of ventricular endocardial QRS potentials on ventricular volume. Br. Heart J. *40*:891, 1978.
67. Vincent, G. M., Abildskov, J. A., and Burgess, M. J.: Mechanisms of ischemic ST-segment displacement. Evaluation by direct current recordings. Circulation *56*:559, 1977.
68. Samson, W. E., and Scher, A. M.: Mechanism of S-T segment alteration during acute myocardial injury. Circ. Res. *8*:780, 1960.
69. Einthoven, W.: Weiteres über das Elektrokardiogramm. Arch. ges. Physiol. *122*:517, 1908.
70. Abarquez, R. F., Freiman, A. H., Reichel, F., and LaDue, J. S.: The precordial electrocardiogram during exercise. Circulation *22*:1060, 1960.
71. Shackel, B.: Skin-drilling. A Method of diminishing galvanic skin-potentials. Am. J. Psychol. *72*:114, 1959.
72. Mason, R. E., and Likar, I.: A new system of multiple-lead exercise electrocardiography. Am. Heart J. *71*:196, 1966.
73. Blackburn, H., Katigbak, R., Mitchell, P., and Imbimbo, B.: What electrocardiographic leads to take after exercise? Am. Heart J. *67*:184, 1964.
74. Mason, R. E., and Likar, I.: A new approach to stress tests in the diagnosis of myocardial ischemia. Trans. Am. Clin. Climatol. Assoc. *76*:40, 1964.
75. Phibbs, B. P., and Buckels, L. J.: Comparative yield of ECG leads in multistage stress testing. Am. Heart J. *90*:275, 1975.
76. Tubau, J. F., Chaitman, B. R., Bourassa, M. G., and Waters, D. D.: Detection of multivessel coronary disease after myocardial infarction using exercise stress testing and multiple ECG lead systems. Circulation *61*:44, 1980.
77. Bellet, S., Deliyiannis, S., and Eliakim, M.: The electrocardiogram during exercise as recorded by radioelectrocardiography. Comparison with postexercise electrocardiogram (Master two-step test). Am. J. Cardiol. *8*:385, 1961.
78. Lepeschkin, E., and Surawicz, B.: Characteristics of true-positive and false-

positive results of electrocardiographic Master two-step exercise tests. N. Engl. J. Med. *258*:511, 1958.
79. Riley, C. P., Oberman, A., and Sheffield, L. T.: Electrocardiographic effects of glucose ingestion. Arch. Intern. Med. *130*:703, 1972.
80. Greenspan, M., Iskandrian, A. S., Mintz, G. S., Croll, M. N., Segal, B. L., Kimbiris, D., and Bemis, C. E.: Exercise myocardial scintigraphy with ^{201} thallium. Chest *77*:47, 1980.
81. Whinnery, J. E., Froelicher, V. F., Jr., Stewart, A. J., Longo, M. R., Jr., Triebwasser, J. H., and Lancaster, M. C.: The electrocardiographic response to maximal treadmill exercise of asymptomatic men with left bundle branch block. Am. Heart J. *94*:316, 1977.
82. Astrand, I., Blomqvist, G., and Orinius, E.: ST changes at exercise in patients with short P-R interval. Acta Med. Scand. *185*:205, 1969.
83. Whinnery, J. E., Froelicher, V. F., Jr., Stewart, A. J., Longo, M. R., Jr., and Triebwasser, J. H.: The electrocardiographic response to maximal treadmill exercise of asymptomatic men with right bundle branch block. Chest *71*:335, 1977.
84. Johnson, S., O'Connel, J., Becker, P., Moran, J. F., and Gunnar, R.: The diagnostic accuracy of exercise ECG testing in the presence of complete right bundle branch block. Circulation *52*(Suppl. II):II–48, 1975.
85. Kawai, C., and Hultgren, H. N.: The effect of digitalis upon the exercise electrocardiogram. Am. Heart J. *68*:409, 1964.
86. Liebow, I. M., and Feil, H.: Digitalis and the normal work electrocardiogram. Am. Heart J. *22*:683, 1941.
87. Yu, P. N. G., Lovejoy, F. W., Hulfish, B., Howell, M. M., Joos, H. A., Tenney, S. M., Haroutunian, L. M., and Evans, H. W.: Cardiorespiratory responses and electrocardiographic changes during exercise before and after intravenous digoxin in normal subjects. Am. J. Med. Sci. *224*:146, 1952.
88. Linhart, J. W., Laws, J. G., and Satinsky, J. D.: Maximum treadmill exercise electrocardiography in female patients. Circulation *50*:1173, 1974.
89. Cumming, G. R., Dufresne, C., Kich, L., and Samm, J.: Exercise electrocardiogram patterns in normal women. Br. Heart J. *35*:1055, 1973.
90. Robb, G. P., and Marks, H. H.: Latent coronary artery disease: Determination of its presence and severity by the exercise electrocardiogram. Am. J. Cardiol. *13*:603, 1964.
91. Sheffield, L. T., Holt, J. H., Lester, F. M., Conroy, D. V., and Reeves, T. J.: On-line analysis of the exercise electrocardiogram. Circulation *40*:935, 1969.
92. Kurita, A., Chaitman, B. R., and Bourassa, M. G.: Significance of exercise-induced junctional S-T depression in evaluation of coronary artery disease. Am. J. Cardiol. *40*:492, 1977.
93. Lozner, E. C., and Morganroth, J.: New criteria for evaluating "positive" exercise tests in asymptomatic patients. Am. J. Cardiol. *39*:288, 1977.
94. Blackburn, H., Taylor, H. L., Okamoto, N., Rautaharju, P., Mitchell, P. L., and Kerkhof, A. C.: Standardization of the exercise electrocardiogram. A systematic comparison of chest lead configurations employed for monitoring during exercise. *In* Karvonen, M. J., and Barry, A. J. (eds.): Physical Activity and the Heart. Springfield, Ill., Charles C Thomas, 1967, Chapter 9.
95. Froelicher, V. F., Jr., Wolthius, R., Keiser, N., Stewart, A., Fischer, J., Longo, M. R., Jr., Triebwasser, J. H., and Lancaster, M. C.: A comparison of two bipolar exercise electrocardiographic leads to lead V_5. Chest *70*:611, 1976.
96. Ellestad, M. H., and Wan, M. K. C.: Predictive implications of stress testing. Follow-up of 2700 subjects after maximum treadmill stress testing. Circulation *51*:363, 1975.
97. Weiner, D. A., McCabe, C. H., Fisher, L. D., Chaitman, B. R., and Ryan, T. J.: Similiar rates of false positive and false negative exercise tests in matched males and females (CASS). Circulation *58*(Suppl. II):II–140, 1978.
98. Sheffield, L. T.: The use of the computer in exercise electrocardiography. Prac. Cardiol. *4*:101, 1978.
99. Blomqvist, G.: The Frank lead exercise electrocardiogram. A quantitative study based on averaging technic and digital computer analysis. Acta Med. Scand. *178*(Suppl. 440):5, 1965.
100. McHenry, P. L., Stowe, D. E., and Lancaster, M. C.: Computer quantitation of the the ST segment response during maximal treadmill exercise. Circulation *38*:691, 1968.
101. Simoons, M. L., Boom, H. B. K., and Smallenburg, E.: On-line processing of orthogonal exercise electrocardiogram. Comput. Biomed. Res. *8*:105, 1975.
102. Sheffield, L.T.: The meaning of exercise test findings. *In* Fox, S. M., III (ed.): Coronary Heart Disease. Prevention, Detection, Rehabilitation with Emphasis on Exercise Testing. Denver, Department of Professional Education International Medical Corp., 1974, Chapter 9.
103. Harrison, T. R., and Reeves, T. J.: The exertional electrocardiogram. *In* Principles and Problems of Ischemic Heart Disease. Chicago, Year Book Medical Publishers, 1968, Chapter 25.
104. Wolthuis, R. A., Froelicher, V. F., Jr., Fischer, J., and Triebwasser, J. H.: The response of healthy men to treadmill exercise. Circulation *55*:153, 1977.
105. Morris, S. N., Phillips, J. F., Jordan, J. W., and McHenry, P. L.: Incidence and significance of decreases in systolic blood pressure during graded treadmill exercise testing. Am. J. Cardiol. *41*:221, 1978.
106. Baker, T., Levites, R., and Anderson, G. J.: The significance of hypotension during treadmill exercise testing. Circulation *54*(Suppl. II):II–11, 1976.
107. Andersen, K. L.: The cardiovascular system in exercise. *In* Falls, H. B. (ed.): Exercise Physiology. New York, Academic Press, 1968, Chapter 3.
108. Berman, J. L., Wynne, J., and Cohn, P. F.: Value of a multivariate approach for interpreting treadmill exercise tests in coronary artery disease. Am. J. Cardiol. *41*:375, 1978.
109. Lewis, R. P., Boudoulas, H., Welch, T. G., and Forester, W. F.: Usefulness of systolic time intervals in coronary artery disease. Am. J. Cardiol. *37*:787, 1976.
110. Lance, V. Q., and Spodick, D. H.: Systolic time intervals utilizing ear densitography. Advantages and reliability for stress testing. Am. Heart J. *94*: 62, 1977.
111. Bruce, R. A.: Exercise testing of patients with coronary heart disease. Principles and normal standards for evaluation. Ann. Clin. Res. *3*:323, 1971.
112. Froelicher, V. F., Thompson, A. J., Longo, M. R., Triebwasser, J. H., and Lancaster, M. C.: Value of exercise testing for screening asymptomatic men for latent coronary artery disease. Prog. Cardiovasc. Dis. *18*:265, 1976.
113. Froelicher, V. F., and Lancaster, M. C.: The prediction of maximal oxygen consumption from a continuous exercise treadmill protocol. Am. Heart J. *87*: 445, 1974.
114. Ellestad, M. H.: Stress Testing. Principles and Practice. Philadelphia, F. A. Davis Co., 1975, Chapter 8.
115. Cole, J. P., and Ellestad, M. H.: Significance of chest pain during treadmill exercise: Correlation with coronary events. Am. J. Cardiol. *41*:227, 1978.
116. Aronow, W. S., and Cassidy, J.: Five year follow-up of double Master's test, maximal treadmill stress test, and resting and postexercise apexcardiogram in asymptomatic persons. Circulation *52*:616, 1975.
117. Kattus, A. A., Jorgensen, C. R., Worden, R. E., and Alvaro, A. B.: ST segment depression with near-maximal exercise: Its modification by physical conditioning. Chest *62*:678, 1972.
118. Melin, J. A., Piret, L. J., Vanbutsele, R. J. M., Rousseau, M. F., Cosyns, J., Brasseur, L. A., Beckers, C., and Detry, J. M. R.: Diagnostic value of exercise electrocardiography and thallium myocardial scintigraphy in patients without previous myocardial infarction: A bayesian approach. Circulation *63*:1019, 1981.
119. DeBusk, R. F., Davidson, D. M., Houston, N., and Fitzgerald, J.: Serial ambulatory electrocardiography and treadmill exercise testing after uncomplicated myocardial infarction. Am. J. Cardiol. *45*:547, 1980.
120. Goldschlager, N., Selzer, A., and Cohn, K.: Treadmill stress tests as indicators of presence and severity of coronary artery disease. Ann. Intern. Med. *85*:277, 1976.
121. Blumenthal, D. S., Weiss, J. L., Mellits, E. D., and Gerstenblith, G.: The predictive value of a strongly positive stress test in patients with minimal symptoms. Am. J. Med. *70*:1005, 1981.
122. Council on Scientific Affairs, American Medical Association: Indications and contraindications for exercise testing. J.A.M.A. *246*:1015, 1981.
123. Rochmis, P., and Blackburn, H.: Exercise tests. A survey of procedures, safety and litigation experience in approximately 170,000 tests. J.A.M.A. *217*:1061, 1971.
124. Doyle, J. T., and Kinch, S. H.: The prognosis of an abnormal electrocardiographic stress test. Circulation *41*:545, 1970.
125. Bruce, R. A., Hornsten, T. R., and Blackmon, J. R.: Myocardial infarction after normal responses to maximal exercise. Circulation *38*:552,1968.
126. Jelinek, M. V., and Lown, B.: Exercise stress testing for exposure of cardiac arrhythmia. Prog. Cardiovasc. Dis. *16*:497, 1974.
127. Sheffield, L. T., and Reeves, T. J.: Graded exercise in the diagnosis of angina pectoris. Mod. Conc. Cardiovasc. Dis. *34*:1, 1965.
128. Kattus, A. S., Hanafee, W. N., Lingmise, W. P., Jr., MacAlpin, R. N., and Rivin, A. U.: Diagnosis, medical and surgical management of coronary insufficiency. Ann. Intern. Med. *69*:115, 1968.
129. McHenry, P. L., Morris, S. N., and Jordan, J. W.: Stress testing in coronary heart disease. Heart and Lung *3*:83, 1974.
130. Atterhog, J. H., Jonsson, B., and Samuelsson, R.: Exercise testing: A prospective study of complication rates. Am. Heart J. *98*:572, 1979.

9 CARDIAC CATHETERIZATION

by William H. Barry, M.D., and William Grossman, M.D.

TECHNICAL ASPECTS

Historical Review. According to André Cournand, cardiac catheterization was first performed (and so named) in 1844 by Claude Bernard,[1] who catheterized both the right and the left ventricles of a horse by means of a retrograde approach from the jugular vein and carotid artery. There followed an era of investigation of cardiovascular physiology in animals that resulted in the development of many important techniques and principles—including pressure manometry and the application of the Fick principle for measuring cardiac output—subsequently applied to the study of patients with heart disease.

Although others had previously passed catheters into the great veins, Werner Forssmann is generally credited as the first to pass a catheter into the heart of a living human being.[2] At age 25, he exposed a vein in his own left arm, introduced a ureteral catheter into the venous system, and advanced it under fluoroscopic control into the right atrium. He then walked to the Radiology Department, where the catheter position was documented by a chest x-ray. During the next 2 years, Forssmann continued to perform catheterization studies, including six additional attempts to catheterize himself.

The potential of Forssmann's technique was appreciated by other investigators. In 1930, Klein reported on catheterization of the right ventricle in 11 patients and measurement of cardiac output using the Fick principle.[3] The cardiac outputs were 4.5 and 5.6 liter/min in two patients without heart disease.[1] Except for these and several other studies, application of cardiac catheterization to evaluate the circulation in normal and disease states was limited and fragmentary until the work of Cournand and Richards, who in 1941 began a remarkable series of investigations of right-heart physiology in humans.[4-6] In 1947, Dexter and his colleagues at the Peter Bent Brigham Hospital reported their studies of congenital heart disease and mentioned some observations on "the oxygen saturation and source of pulmonary capillary blood" obtained from a catheter in the pulmonary artery "wedge" position.[7] Subsequent work from Dexter's laboratory[8] and by Lagerlof and Werkö[9] showed that the pressure measured in the pulmonary artery "wedge" position was an accurate estimate of pulmonary venous and left atrial pressure. During this exciting early period, catheterization was used to investigate problems in cardiovascular physiology by McMichael in England,[10] Lenegre in Paris,[11,12] and Cournand, Warren, Stead, Bing, Dexter, Burchell, Wood, and their respective coworkers in this country.[13-22]

Further developments came rapidly. Some of the highlights include the following: Retrograde left-heart catheterization was first introduced by Zimmerman[23] and Limon Lason[24] and their respective coworkers in 1950. The percutaneous technique developed by Seldinger in 1953 was soon applied to cardiac catheterization of both the left and right heart chambers.[25] Transseptal left-heart catheterization was developed[26] and applied clinically by Ross, Braunwald, and Morrow,[27] and it quickly became accepted as a standard technique. Selective coronary arteriography was developed by Sones et al. in 1959[28,29] and was perfected in the ensuing years. In 1970, a practical balloon-tipped flow-guided catheter technique was introduced by Swan, Ganz, and their collaborators, making possible the applicability of catheterization outside the conventional catheterization laboratory.[30] Many other landmark events could be mentioned and the contributions of many individuals could be recognized, but these have been detailed elsewhere.[31]

In this chapter, we discuss current methods of cardiac catheterization, including technical aspects important for optimal use of these methods and accurate interpretation of the data obtained. The development of these techniques and their application to the study of normal and abnormal human cardiac physiology have played a decisive role in improving the diagnosis and treatment of patients with cardiac disease.

Fluoroscopy and Image Intensification. A modern cardiac fluoroscopy unit is a central component of any cardiac catheterization facility. Such a unit[32] consists of three components: an x-ray generating system; an image intensifier; and an image recording system, usually a video camera and monitor and a 35-mm cine camera. The cine camera is used almost exclusively for cardiac angiography.

X-ray Source. An x-ray tube consists of a glass container evacuated of air, containing a cathode, which is the electron source, and an anode, toward which flow the negatively charged electrons emitted from the cathode. The number of electrons flowing from the cathode to the anode per unit of time (current in mA) is largely controlled by the temperature of the cathode. The energy of the electrons is controlled by the potential difference (kv) between the cathode and the anode. When electrons strike the anode, a few pass close to nuclei of the atoms of the anode material and produce "Bremsstrahlung" or "braking radiation" x-ray photons. The radiation spectra thus produced can be filtered (normally with aluminum) to remove lower energy photons that cannot penetrate a human torso but can increase radiation exposure. In operation, the control system for the x-ray tube produces and adjusts the direct-current high voltage (kv), adjusts the x-ray tube current (mA), provides for selection of anode focal spot size, and controls exposure time (pulse width in msec). A small focal spot yields better resolution but produces higher heating, which can shorten the life of the anode.

A portion of the x-ray photons thus produced is allowed to pass upward through an adjustable lead-shielded exit port (cone) and thence through the patient. The interaction of an x-ray photon with body tissue results in attenuation of an x-ray beam, which is influenced by x-ray photon energy. Subject contrast range is determined by minimum and maximum penetration values of the body section and is thus influenced by the energy spectrum of the x-ray photon.

Intensifying Screens. Imaging intensifier screens convert x-ray photons into lower energy photons in the visible light spectrum and amplify the image obtained. The most commonly used input phosphor screen is of the cesium-iodide type, which typically absorbs 50 per cent or more of incident radiation. In this layer, incident x-ray photons are converted into light. In direct contact with the input phosphor is a second layer, the photocathode, which converts the light image into an electron image. The electrons emitted from the photocathode are electrically focused on a smaller output screen, where electrons are absorbed and produce another light image. Input phosphor screens vary from 5 to 12 inches in diameter, and many intensifier systems have two or three interchangeable screens or "tubes" of different sizes that may be selected by the operator when differing degrees of magnification are required. The typical output screen is slightly less than 1 inch in diameter.

Gain in light intensity occurs because of acceleration of electrons between the photocathode and the output screen and because the output screen is smaller in area than is the input screen. Modern image intensifier tubes have a gain of 5000× or more and thus markedly diminish radiation exposure to the patient and operator.

Radiation Hazards. Radiation exposure during cardiac catheterization and angiography ranges from 21 to 39 mrad for the primary operator and from 12 to 20 mrad for the assistant (1 rad = 100 ergs/gm in any tissue).[33] Approximately one-half this exposure occurs during fluoroscopy and one-half during cine operation. On the basis of a recommended maximum dose of 100 mrad/week to the lens of the eye for occupational workers, it is advised that an operator be limited to five procedures per week. Exposure of catheterization personnel should be monitored by means of film badges worn at the collar level. Radiation exposures to patients during cardiac catheterization are significant and range to 28 rad.

The following guidelines help reduce radiation exposure to patients and operators:

1. The smallest x-ray beam possible should be used.
2. Fluoroscopy and cineangiography times should be kept to a minimum.
3. Personnel should remain as far as possible from the patient and should wear lead aprons.
4. Personnel should be shielded during cineangiography if this is practical.

CARDIAC CATHETERIZATION

Catheter Insertion. Of the various approaches to cardiac catheterization, certain ones are of historical interest only (i.e., transbronchial approach, posterior transthoracic left atrial puncture, and suprasternal puncture of the left atrium). The majority of catheterizations performed currently utilize either of two approaches: catheterization by direct exposure of an artery and a vein (including umbilical vessels in neonates) and catheterization by the percutaneous approach (including transseptal catheterization). Each method has its advantages and disadvantages, its adherents and detractors. In reality, the methods are not mutually exclusive but rather complementary, and it is our belief that the physician performing cardiac catheterization should be well versed in both techniques. The methods employed in the authors' laboratories are described below.

Brachial Approach. This approach involves surgical exposure of the brachial artery and basilic vein in the antecubital fossa and insertion of the catheters directly following vessel incision. The percutaneous approach of Seldinger may also be used in adults via the brachial vessels if catheters of small size (No. 5 French) are used.[25] The brachial approach is utilized in patients with obstructive and/or thrombotic arterial disease involving the abdominal aorta, iliac artery, or femoral artery; suspected thrombosis of the femoral vein or inferior vena cava; or coarctation of the aorta. It may also be advantageous in obese patients, in whom the percutaneous femoral technique may be technically quite difficult and in whom bleeding may be hard to control after removal of the catheter.

Procedure. After the brachial artery is localized by means of palpation in the right antecubital fossa, local anesthesia is induced with 5 to 15 ml of 1 to 2 per cent lidocaine, and a single transverse incision is made just proximal to the flexor crease. Tissues are separated by blunt dissection, and a medial vein is isolated and encircled proximally and distally with 3–0 or 4–0 silk. The brachial artery is isolated from adjacent nerves and fascia and is encircled proximally and distally with moistened umbilical tape or silicone Elastomer surgical tape.

Right-heart catheterization is accomplished by means of antegrade passage of an appropriate catheter (e.g., Cournand, Goodale-Lubin, Swan-Ganz) via the basilic or brachial vein to the right atrium, right ventricle, pulmonary artery, and pulmonary capillary "wedge" positions under fluoroscopic guidance. In the wedge position, the catheter occludes the distal pulmonary artery segment, and thus the catheter tip is exposed to only the pulmonary venous pressure. Pressure recorded from the wedge position is accepted as a true wedge pressure only if a characteristic left atrial waveform is exhibited and if completely oxygenated blood (>95 per cent oxygen saturation) can be aspirated from the catheter.[31] Left-heart catheterization is then accomplished by means of retrograde passage of an appropriate catheter (e.g., Eppendorf, Lehman angiographic, Sones, NIH) through a transverse brachial arteriotomy to the ascending aorta and left ventricle.

Systemic administration of heparin (5000 units) at the time of left-heart catheterization and coronary arteriography is indicated to prevent thrombotic complications. In case of difficulty in passing catheters from the brachial artery around the shoulder, an end-hole catheter with a flexible guidewire protruding beyond the tip may be useful. As catheters with or without the aid of guidewires are advanced in the vascular system, their passage should be monitored fluoroscopically; if progress of the catheter is difficult, or if the patient complains of pain, caution should be exercised to avoid dissection or perforation of the vessel wall. Occasionally, spasm of the vessel around the catheter may occur, owing to the relatively small size of vessels in the upper extremities. In this case administration of small amounts of morphine should promptly facilitate catheter manipulation; if not, a catheter of smaller diameter should be used.

Following completion of hemodynamic and angiographic studies, the catheters are withdrawn, and the artery is repaired. In our laboratory, a Fogarty balloon catheter is routinely passed proximally and distally to remove any thrombi that may have formed within the arterial lumen during the catheterization. After proximal and distal flow is deemed adequate, 15 ml of heparinized solution (1500 units in 15 ml of 5 per cent dextrose in water) are infused into the artery proximally and distally through a small polyethylene catheter. The artery is immediately occluded with vascular clamps proximal and distal to the arteriotomy site. A stay suture is placed at each end of the arteriotomy, which is then closed using a continuous stitch of 6–0 Tevdek. It is important not to raise an intimal flap nor to penetrate the posterior intima with the needle. After suturing, first the distal and then the proximal clamp is removed. Minor leaks usually respond to gentle pressure applied directly with a finger over the site of the arteriotomy repair. The radial pulse should be palpable and as strong as it was prior to catheterization. If it is absent or markedly reduced, the artery should be reopened, a Forgarty balloon catheter passed again, and the vessel repaired. If this does not result in return of the pulse, an experienced vascular surgeon should be consulted. The vein may be tied off or repaired directly.

The wound is then flushed with sterile saline and a 1 per cent povidone-iodine solution, and the skin incision is closed with 3–0 to 4–0 nylon, which should be removed within 7 to 10 days. Alternatively, an absorbable material may be used, so that suture removal is unnecessary. Antibiotic ointment (10 per cent povidone-iodine) is applied to the suture line, and the area should be covered with a dressing.

Postcatheterization orders should include the following:

1. Resume all previous medications.
2. Measure blood pressure and pulse and inspect dressing every 15 minutes for 1 hour, every hour for 4 hours, then every 4 hours for 24 hours.
3. Call a house officer or attending physician *and* a member of the catheterization laboratory staff in the event of bleeding, loss of pulse, hypotension, or chest pain.
4. Encourage oral fluid intake of 2 to 3 liters over 6 to 8 hours (if an angiographic contrast agent has been administered).
5. Administer analgesic medication, as needed.

Femoral Approach. Right- and left-heart catheterization via the femoral approach is usually performed from the right groin, although the left groin may be used if necessary. The major landmarks of the femoral area are the anterior superior iliac spine, the pubic tubercle, and the inguinal ligament running between them. The femoral nerve, artery, and vein are located in the femoral triangle below the inguinal ligament. Proceeding from lateral to medial, the relationship of these structures may be remembered with the aid of the mnemonic NAVY (*n*erve, *a*rtery, *v*ein, empt*y* space).

Procedure. The femoral artery is located by means of palpation at a point approximately two fingerbreadths below the inguinal ligament. The skin and subcutaneous tissue over the artery are anesthesized with 10 to 15 ml of 1 per cent lidocaine. The anesthetic must be given carefully and must not be injected directly into a vessel. It is important that percutaneous puncture of the femoral vessels be a correct distance below the inguinal ligament; if it is too high, hemostasis may be impaired, owing to the posterior course of the vessels in the pelvic cavity; if it is too low, the vein may run behind the artery, and the artery may be entered after it bifurcates into the profunda and superficial femoral branches. Although the inguinal crease is usually just below the inguinal ligament, this relationship is not constant, and the use of the inguinal ligament as the primary landmark is therefore advised.

When performing right-heart and left-heart catheterization via the femoral approach, we prefer to enter the femoral vein first. This is accomplished using an 18-gauge Seldinger needle, which consists of a blunt, tapered external cannula with a sharp obturator. After a ¼-inch skin incision has been made at the correct distance below the inguinal ligament and medial to the arterial pulse, the needle and obturator are inserted with a smooth motion at a 45-degree angle. If the patient has discomfort as the needle penetrates the deeper femoral tissues, additional lidocaine can be infiltrated through the needle, after removing the obturator and ascertaining that the needle is extravascular. A small syringe is then attached to the needle, which is slowly withdrawn while continuous gentle aspiration is performed. When the vein is entered, blood is easily aspirated. The syringe is removed without moving the needle, and a Teflon-coated guidewire (preferably a J tip) is inserted into the needle and is advanced into the vein (Fig. 9–1). The guidewire should pass easily, with its course checked fluoroscopically. The needle is then withdrawn over the guide, and a venous sheath of appropriate size with obturator is placed into the vein over the guidewire. The sheath should be inserted with a twisting, forward pressure. The obturator and guidewire are then removed, and the sheath is flushed via a stopcock.

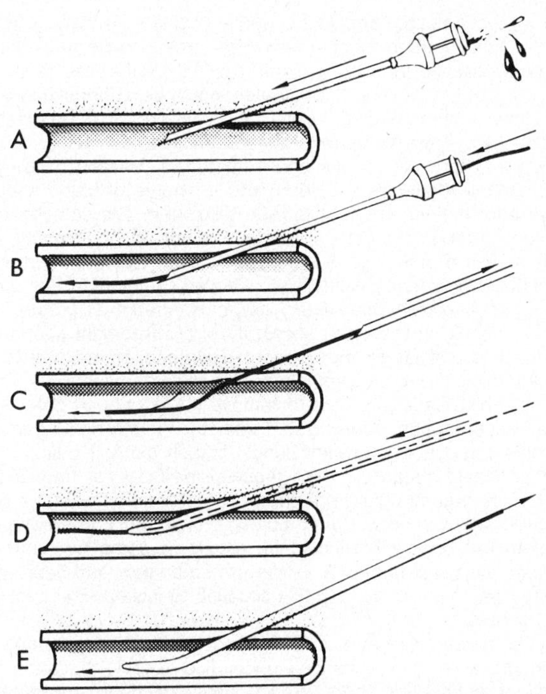

FIGURE 9–1 The Seldinger technique. The Seldinger needle is inserted through the vessel at an angle no steeper than 45 degrees. The needle obturator is withdrawn, and the needle is slowly pulled out until the tip is within the lumen of the vessel (*A*). A flexible tipped guidewire is then inserted into the vessel through the needle (*B*), and the needle is withdrawn (*C*). A catheter (or sheath with obturator) is then inserted into the vessel over the guidewire (*D*). The guidewire is then removed, leaving the catheter (or sheath) in the vessel lumen (*E*). (From Kory, R. C., et al.: A Primer of Cardiac Catheterization. Springfield, Ill. Courtesy of Charles C Thomas, 1965.)

Catheter Insertions. The femoral artery may then be punctured at a 45-degree angle with the Seldinger needle, once a skin incision ¼-inch long and deep has been made directly over the arterial pulse. The obturator is removed, and the needle is slowly withdrawn until the tip enters the artery lumen and a pulsatile flow of arterial blood exits from the needle hub. A Teflon-coated J guidewire is inserted into the needle and advanced into the artery. The guidewire should advance easily, with its position observed on fluoroscopy as it passes into the abdominal aorta. The needle is then withdrawn over the guidewire, and the artery is compressed firmly at the puncture site. A No. 8 French arterial sheath with a proximal hemostasis valve and a side-port extension tube is inserted into the artery over the guidewire. The sheath obturator and guidewire are removed, and the sheath is flushed via the side-arm extension tube, which is connected to a pressure transducer for continuous monitoring of femoral arterial pressure. It is, of course, possible to insert an end-hole catheter into the artery directly over the guidewire without use of a sheath. This would be appropriate if only one arterial catheter were to be used. However, use of the arterial sheath greatly facilitates catheter changes, permits use of a greater variety of catheters, and allows continuous monitoring of femoral artery pressure during left-heart catheterization.[34] With sheaths in the femoral artery vein, and the femoral artery pressure recorded for monitoring purposes, it is possible to proceed to right- and left-heart catheterization.

Right-heart Catheterization. The right-heart catheters used with the femoral approach are the same as those described for the brachial approach (i.e., Cournand, Goodale-Lubin, or Swan-Ganz) (Fig. 9–2). The first two of these catheters have an elbow bend, which facilitates passage from the right ventricle into the pulmonary artery. As the catheter is advanced through the sheath and into the inferior vena cava, its motion should be observed on fluoroscopy. The movement of the catheter should be gentle and the passage effortless; catheter advancement should never be forced. While the right-heart catheter is passed from the groin, it frequently enters the renal or hepatic veins. If this occurs, the catheter should be withdrawn and rotated before it is advanced farther. A guidewire may be used if a tortuous venous system makes catheter passage difficult.

Once the right atrium has been entered, a pressure tracing from this chamber should be recorded, and a sample of blood should be obtained for measurement of oxygen saturation. The catheter is then advanced through the right ventricle and into the pulmonary artery. Blood pressure and oxygen saturation should then be measured in the pulmonary artery. A difference between right atrial (or superior vena caval) and pulmonary artery oxygen saturation of greater than 5 per cent should indicate the possibility of a left-to-right shunt. Occasionally it is difficult to maneuver a Cournand or a Goodale-Lubin catheter from the right ventricle to the pulmonary artery from the groin, in which case it is best to remove the right-heart catheter and use a balloon-tipped, flow-directed catheter for the right-heart study. In addition, in patients with left bundle branch block, a balloon catheter is preferred because of the reduced likelihood of trauma to the right bundle branch during right-heart catheterization with this type of catheter. Catheter-induced right bundle branch block in a patient with complete left bundle branch block results in complete heart block and can cause asystole. A Gorlin or Cournand right-heart pacing catheter may also be used in this situation to initiate emergency pacing, if necessary.

The right-heart catheter is then used to record pulmonary artery wedge pressure; it is advanced under fluoroscopic guidance into a peripheral pulmonary artery branch during a deep inspiration. To record a wedge pressure with a balloon-type catheter, the balloon is inflated while the catheter tip is in a proximal pulmonary artery. The catheter is then advanced until the pressure configuration changes to that of a wedge pressure. Deflation of the balloon at this point should result in reappearance of pulmonary artery pressure. To re-obtain wedge pressure, the balloon is *slowly* inflated while catheter pressure is monitored until the pressure waveform changes to a wedge contour. Overinflation of the balloon, or inflation of the balloon in a distal vessel, carries the risk of pulmonary artery rupture. Also, to reduce the likelihood of pulmonary infarction and/or pulmonary artery rupture, the balloon should not be left inflated for longer than the time required to record pressure and obtain a sample of blood to determine oxygen saturation. Positioning of the Cournand or balloon-tipped catheter during right-heart catheterization may be facilitated by the use of guidewires, but catheters should not be advanced into the wedge position with a guidewire protruding beyond the catheter tip.

Left-heart Catheterization. When using a right femoral artery sheath, this procedure may be performed with a variety of catheters (Fig. 9–2). Closed end-hole catheters (Lehman angiographic, Eppendorf) similar to those used in the direct brachial approach may be introduced through the sheath and advanced into the aorta and left ventricle. However, passage of catheters through the frequently tortuous iliofemoral system is facilitated by the use of end-hole catheters with J guidewires. In our laboratory the most commonly used catheter for this purpose is the "pigtail" catheter, which has multiple side holes and an end hole and can be used for angiography as well as pressure measurement. After introduction of the left-heart catheter, 5000 units of heparin are administered intravenously for anticoagulation.

When preformed catheters are used (pigtail, Judkins, or Amplatz), a J-shaped guidewire is inserted into the catheter prior to introducing the catheter into the sheath. Then, when the catheter tip is within the sheath, the J guide is advanced beyond the tip and into the femoral artery for several centimeters. Under fluoroscopic observation, the catheter is then advanced into the aorta, with the guidewire tip preceding it. Again, the catheter passage should be effortless. When the catheter is in the abdominal aorta, the guidewire is removed, and the catheter and sheath are flushed with heparinized saline. The catheter and sheath should be flushed every 5 minutes after heparin administration and every 2 minutes if heparin is not used.

The catheter is advanced carefully around the aortic arch to avoid inadvertently entering the aortic arch vessels. The pressure just above the aortic valve is recorded along with simultaneous femoral artery pressure via the side arm of the sheath. As will be discussed later, the peak femoral artery pressure is frequently slightly higher than the peak central aortic pressure; however, mean systolic pressures are usually identical. The catheter is then passed across the aortic valve into the left ventricle. If the aortic valve is abnormal, a guidewire may be required to stiffen the catheter to permit crossing of the aortic valve. In aortic stenosis, crossing the valve with a pigtail catheter may not be possible, in which case a right Judkins coronary catheter is usually employed. The valve is traversed with a straight-tip guidewire, and the catheter is then advanced over the wire into the ventricle for pressure measurement. Other catheters, such as the Sones, left Judkins, and Gensini, may be preferable in selected patients. Not more than 15 minutes or so should be expended in attempting to cross an aortic valve with a single type of catheter before trying another.

When the catheter enters the left ventricle, the left ventricular and femoral artery pressures are recorded to evaluate aortic valve function, and the left ventricular and pulmonary artery wedge pressures are recorded to evaluate mitral valve function. Cardiac output is measured, and a right-heart pullback is performed to evaluate the pulmonic and tricuspid valves by recording, in close time sequence, pulmonary artery, right ventricular, and right atrial pressures. If left ventricular angiography is planned, and the aortic valve was not crossed with a pigtail or other catheter suitable for ventricular angiography, an exchange guidewire may be introduced into the left ventricle, the catheter may be removed over the guidewire, and a pigtail catheter may be advanced over the exchange guidewire back into the left ventricle.

Termination of the Procedure. Following completion of the hemodynamic and angiographic studies, the catheters are removed. Preformed arterial catheters should be withdrawn from the artery into the sheath with several centimeters of guidewire protruding from the catheter tip to avoid trauma to the arterial intima. Following administration of protamine to reverse the heparin effect, the arterial and venous sheaths are removed, and the vessels are firmly compressed by hand or a mechanical compressor for 15 to 20 minutes, with control of bleeding during this time. With this technique significant hematoma formation occurs in fewer than 2 per cent of patients. In patients with hypertension, or wide pulse pressure (aortic regurgitation), longer groin compression times may be required to achieve hemostasis.

Postcatheterization orders should include the following:

1. Bed rest until the morning after the procecure, with a sandbag applied to the groin for the first 6 hours.
2. Resume all previous medications.
3. Check vital signs every 15 minutes for 1 hour, every hour for 4 hours, and every 4 hours thereafter for 24 hours.
4. Check right (or left, depending on entry site) groin and pedal pulse at above schedule. Call a house officer or attending physician *and* a member of the catheterization laboratory staff in the event of bleeding, loss of pulse, hypotension, or chest pain.
5. Encourage oral fluid 2 to 3 liters over 6 to 8 hours (if angiographic contrast agent has been administered).

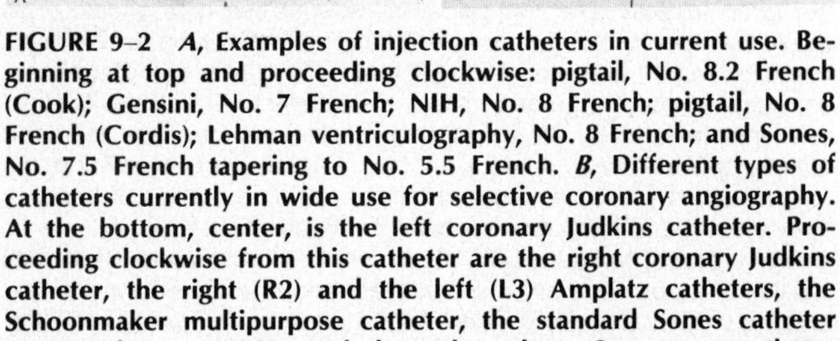

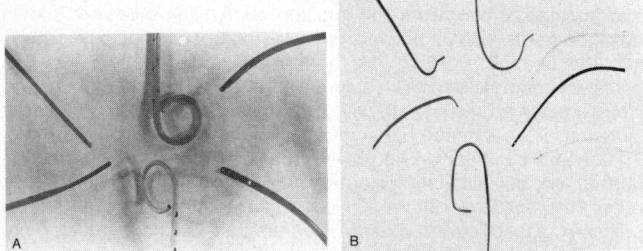

FIGURE 9–2 ***A,*** **Examples of injection catheters in current use. Beginning at top and proceeding clockwise: pigtail, No. 8.2 French (Cook); Gensini, No. 7 French; NIH, No. 8 French; pigtail, No. 8 French (Cordis); Lehman ventriculography, No. 8 French; and Sones, No. 7.5 French tapering to No. 5.5 French.** ***B,*** **Different types of catheters currently in wide use for selective coronary angiography. At the bottom, center, is the left coronary Judkins catheter. Proceeding clockwise from this catheter are the right coronary Judkins catheter, the right (R2) and the left (L3) Amplatz catheters, the Schoonmaker multipurpose catheter, the standard Sones catheter (woven dacron, USCI), and the polyurethane Sones-type catheter (Cordis). (Reproduced with permission from Grossman, W. F.: Cardiac Catheterization and Angiography. 2nd ed. Philadelphia, Lea and Febiger, 1980.)**

6. Administer analgesic medication, as needed. The patient is always seen on rounds by the catheterization team several hours after and the day following catheterization, or more often, if complications develop.

Transseptal Catheterization. When the aortic valve cannot be crossed by the retrograde approach from either the brachial or the femoral artery, and it is essential that the left ventricular pressure be measured, transseptal catheterization of the left ventricle may be performed. In our experience, approximately 5 per cent of severly stenotic valves cannot be crossed in a retrograde manner within a reasonable period of time, and these patients, as well as those with tilting-disc prosthetic aortic valves, are candidates for this procedure. Patients with porcine heterograft valves and ball-cage prosthetic aortic valves can safely undergo retrograde left ventricular catheterization.[35] Transseptal left-heart catheterization is also indicated in patients with suspected mitral valve obstruction in whom a pulmonary artery wedge pressure cannot be measured.

Procedure. Transseptal catheterization is performed in our laboratory using the Teflon 70-cm No. 8 French catheter developed by Brockenbrough and Braunwald.[36] Prior to insertion of the catheter into the right femoral vein, a Brockenbrough needle is inserted into the catheter, with a Bing stylet protruding 1 cm or so beyond the needle tip to prevent penetration of the catheter wall by the needle (Fig. 9–3). The distance (in millimeters) between the catheter butt and the direction indicator on the needle should be measured with the stylet just inside the catheter tip (measurement No. 1), with the needle tip just inside the catheter tip (measurement No. 2), and with the needle tip 1 cm beyond the catheter tip (measurement No. 3). Measurement No. 1 minus measurement No. 2 should equal the distance that the stylet protrudes beyond the needle tip. If the catheter is matched to

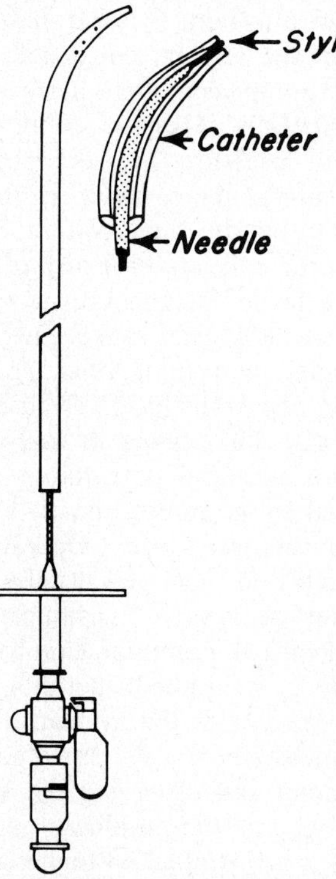

FIGURE 9–3 The Brockenbrough transseptal needle, catheter, and stylet. Use of the stylet prevents inadvertent puncture of the catheter by the needle tip during insertion of the needle into the catheter. The wide flange near the needle hub is pointed on one side to indicate the direction of the needle tip. (From Grossman, W.: Cardiac Catheterization and Angiography. 2nd ed. Philadelphia, Lea and Febiger, 1980.)

the needle, the needle tip should not protrude more than 12 mm beyond the catheter tip when the needle is fully advanced. These measurements are written on a blackboard by a technician for easy reference.

With the patient positioned for a straight frontal projection, the Brockenbrough catheter is advanced to the junction of the right atrium and the superior vena cava by means of a guidewire. The guidewire is removed, the catheter is flushed, and right atrial pressure is recorded. The transseptal needle with its stylet is inserted and then gently advanced through the transseptal catheter under fluoroscopic observation. It is important to allow free rotation of the needle as it is advanced by holding the needle itself (not the direction indicator) between the fingertips. When the tip of the stylet is near the tip of the catheter, the stylet is removed, and the needle is advanced until the needle tip is just within the catheter. The needle is firmly held in this position, with the direction indicator pointing up, to prevent inadvertent extension of the needle tip out of the catheter. The needle is flushed and connected to a pressure transducer, so that a phasic right atrial pressure and a mean pressure can be recorded through the needle and can be verified as similar to that recorded through the catheter prior to insertion of the needle. It is important not to use soft or excessively long lengths of connecting tubing for this purpose, since it is possible to overdamp the pressure recorded through the 21-gauge needle tip.

Puncture of Atrial Septum. After right atrial pressure has been recorded, the direction indicator is rotated clockwise to the 4 o'clock position with fluoroscopic and pressure monitoring. The catheter and needle as a unit are then pulled inferiorly. The catheter will move over the aortic root in a sudden leftward motion; further inferior pull will usually result in a second, smaller leftward motion, as the catheter tip enters the fossa ovalis. Right atrial phasic pressure should be monitored during this time. The catheter and needle (with the needle tip still within the catheter) are then advanced, and the catheter tip will move superiorly, sliding up the interatrial septum. It will usually "hang up" on the lip of the fossa ovalis, at the level of or slightly superior to the plane of the aortic valve. Occasionally, the catheter will pass easily into the left atrium through a patent foramen ovale and will be manifest as leftward motion of the catheter tip and by the appearance of a left atrial phasic waveform. If this occurs, the oxygen saturation of blood aspirated through the needle should be checked and the pressure recorded to document entry into the left atrium. The catheter is then gently advanced 1 or 2 cm over the needle, and the needle is removed. More commonly, the foramen ovale is not patent and must be punctured with the needle tip. This is done during pressure and fluoroscopic monitoring by advancing the needle 1 cm beyond the catheter tip, when the tip is firmly wedged in the fossa ovalis.

After the needle penetrates the interatrial septum, a left atrial pressure waveform (usually a higher mean pressure than in the right atrium) will be evident. Entry into the left atrium should be confirmed by measurement of oxygen saturation. The needle and catheter are then slowly advanced into the left atrium, with the needle position indicator maintained in the 4 o'clock position. Resistance is usually encountered as the catheter tip punctures the septum, and it is important to stabilize the catheter position by holding the catheter in the groin with the left hand while advancing the catheter and needle with the right hand. When the catheter traverses the septum and enters the left atrium (a 1- to 2-cm leftward motion), the needle is withdrawn, the catheter is flushed, left atrial pressure is recorded, and blood is withdrawn for measurement of oxygen saturation through the catheter. Passage of the catheter from the left atrium into the left ventricle is achieved by advancing the catheter tip through the mitral valve. The transseptal catheter may enter a pulmonary vein or left atrial appendage. In this case, the left ventricle may be entered by withdrawing the catheter slowly while rotating it counterclockwise and/or by inserting a coiled-tip occluder to increase the bend in the catheter tip.

It is important to emphasize that transseptal catheterization—as indeed all cardiac catheterization procedures—should be done only by or under the supervision of physicians experienced in the technique. The transseptal needle may perforate the right atrial wall, enter the coronary sinus or the aorta, or perforate the left atrial wall. The small needle tip itself (21-gauge) is not likely to cause a major problem unless an atrial wall is torn; however, passage of the catheter through these structures may result in tamponade and death. Thus, the emphasis placed on pressure monitoring through the needle is important.

Pediatric Cardiac Catheterization. The methods described above are broadly applicable to the cardiac catheterization of children, but *special considerations for the newborn* should be emphasized. In such patients, meticulous attention must be given to maintenance of body temperature by means of heating pads, an infared lamp, or other devices designed for this purpose. In addition, precise attention must be paid to fluid balance, with care being taken to replace exactly the volume of fluid and blood removed, so as to cause neither hypovolemia and hypotension nor hypervolemia with pulmonary edema. In the newborn, the umbilical artery and vein may be used for catheterization for about 72 hours after birth. Of course, catheters should be of small diameters and lengths in procedures involving neonates, infants, and children. The reader is referred to texts and reviews detailing special technical considerations in cardiac catheterization of newborns.[31,37-39]

Catheter Sizes and Construction. In addition to the above-mentioned considerations, it is important that individuals involved in cardiac catheterization understand the sizing of catheters, needles, and guidewires and that they have a knowledge of different methods and materials used in their construction. Cardiac catheters differ in size, length, shape, and material of construction. The last factor determines the friction coefficient, hardness, curve retention, moisture absorption, and autoclavability. In addition, it is clear that different catheter materials have varying degrees of thrombogenicity.[40] Cardiac catheters are usually constructed of woven Dacron, polyethylene, or polyurethane. Some catheter walls are reinforced with stainless steel braids to increase torque control and to enable the catheter to withstand high intraluminal pressures during the injection of angiographic contrast material. In addition, the walls of most cardiac catheters are impregnated with lead or barium salts to render them radiopaque.

The outside diameter (OD) of a catheter is indicated in French units: one French (F) unit = 0.33 mm (0.013 inches). Thus a No. 7 French (7F) catheter has an OD of 2.33 mm. The internal diameter (ID) of a catheter is always, of course, less than the OD, the exact relationship between OD and ID depending on the thickness of the catheter wall. The ID of the catheter determines the thickness of the guidewire that can be passed through the catheter. The guidewire must in turn be small enough to fit through the lumen of the needle used for vessel puncture in percutaneous catheterization techniques. The diameter of the guidewire is usually expressed in inches (0.032, 0.035, 0.038, and so on), whereas needle size is expressed in "gauge," indicating the OD of the needle. An 18-gauge thin-walled needle has an OD of 0.086 inches. The cardiologist beginning to use these techniques must be familiar with these units. In addition, it is wise to check that catheter, guidewire, and needle are all compatible in size and length before the vessel is punctured.

MEASUREMENT OF HEMODYNAMIC PARAMETERS

Pressure Measurement

Theoretical Considerations. Myocardial contractile force is transmitted through the fluid medium of blood as a pressure wave. An important objective of the cardiac catheterization procedure is to assess accurately the forces, and therefore the pressure waves, generated by various cardiac chambers. *A pressure wave may be considered a complex periodic fluctuation in force per unit area,* with one cycle consisting of the time interval from the onset of one wave to the onset of the next. The number of cycles within 1 second is termed the *fundamental frequency* of the waveform. Thus, for a left ventricular pressure waveform at a heart rate of 120 beats/min, the fundamental frequency would be 2 sec^{-1}, or 2 Hz.

Considered as a complex periodic waveform, the pressure wave may be subjected to a type of analysis developed by the French physicist Fourier, whereby any complex waveform may be considered to be the mathematical summation of a series of simple sine waves of differing frequencies and amplitudes.[41-43] The practical consequence of this analysis is that in order to record pressure accurately a system must respond in such a way that output amplitude is directly proportional to input throughout the range of frequencies contained within the pressure wave. If components in a given frequency range are either suppressed or exaggerated by the transducer system, the recorded signal will be a grossly distorted version of the original physiological waveform. For example, the incisura of the aortic pressure wave contains frequencies above 10 cycles/sec; if the pressure measurement system were unable to respond to these, the incisura would be slurred or absent.

The *frequency response* of a pressure measurement system may be defined as the ratio of output amplitude/input amplitude over a range of frequencies of the input or pressure wave. An ideal pressure measurement system would have an output/input ratio of one over an infinite range of input frequencies. In practice this is never the case, and the frequency response characteristics reflect the interaction of the *natural frequency* of the system and the degree of *damping.* If the sensing membrane in the pressure measurement system were shock-excited, in the absence of friction it would oscillate for an indefinite period of time in simple harmonic motion. The frequency of this motion would be the *natural frequency* of the system. The amplitude of the output signal tends to be augmented as the frequency of that signal approaches the natural frequency of the system (Fig. 9–4A). Optimal damping dissipates the energy of the oscillating system gradually, thereby maintaining the nearly flat frequency response curve (constant input/output ratio) as it approaches the region of the pressure measurement system's natural frequency. An extensive literature on the question of what frequency response is desirable and on the testing, construction, and evaluation of different pressure measurement systems is available.[31,44]

Fluid-filled Catheter Systems. With fluid-filled catheters, an external pressure transducer is used to detect changes in pressure at the catheter tip that are transmitted to the transducer by the fluid column in the catheter. A pressure transducer consists basically of a diaphragm that is deformed in a linear fashion by the application of pressure within the physiological range. Deformation of the diaphragm produces a proportional change in electrical resistance within the transducer. By use of a Wheatstone bridge-type circuit, this change in transducer resistance is converted into an electrical potential, which is then amplified and recorded as an analog signal that represents pressure applied to the transducer. Operation of the bridge requires an excitation voltage, usually supplied by the pressure amplifier. A variable resistance control, by means of which the electrical potential can be adjusted to zero when no pressure is applied, permits balancing of the transducer. Calibration of the system is performed by applying known pressures to the transducer by means of a mercury manometer and observing the analog voltage output. The sensitivity of the amplifiers used in pressure recording systems is adjustable, so that a given pressure may be made to correspond to a precise deflection of the recorder.

Because movement of the transducer diaphragm is necessary to produce a voltage output for a given pressure, a certain volume of fluid must move through the catheter-connector tubing system to the transducer to produce a

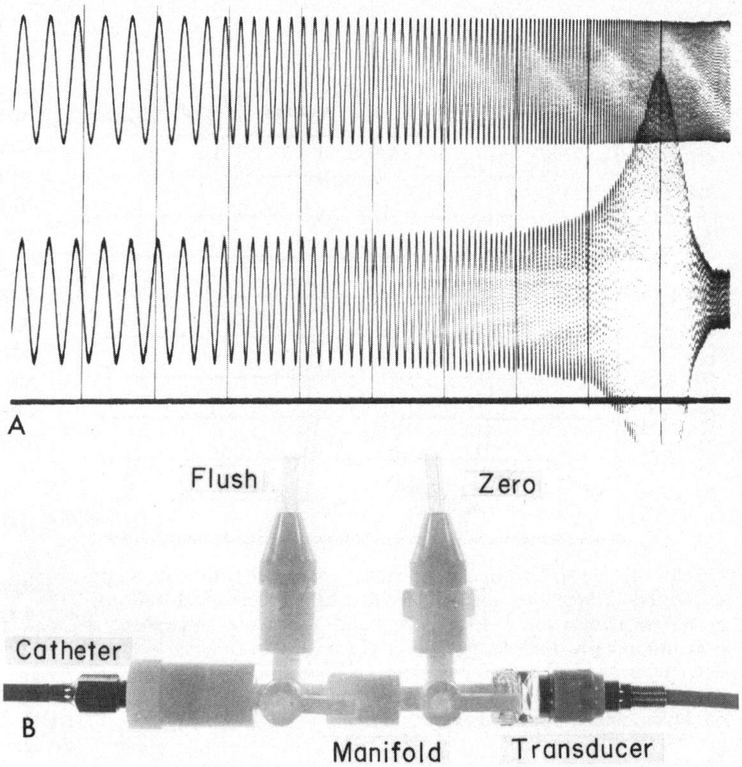

FIGURE 9–4 Recording of phasic pressures with a fluid-filled catheter system.

A, The upper trace shows a "true" phasic pressure of 20 mm Hg (sine wave of increasing frequency) generated within a closed chamber. The lower trace shows the same, pressure recorded with a fluid-filled 110-cm catheter–external transducer system. Note that the pressures are equal in amplitude up to a frequency of about 15 Hz. As the frequency of the pressure sine wave increases above this point, an increase in amplitude occurs owing to resonance in the catheter-transducer system. The "resonant frequency" is about 40 Hz, and above this frequency, the amplitude of the signal falls rapidly. In this case, since the resonant frequency is well above most frequencies contained in the intracardiac pressure waveforms, little distortion of intracardiac pressure by the catheter-transducer recording system will be present. (The vertical lines are 1 sec apart.)

B, The system used to record the pressure in *A.* A small volume-displacement transducer is attached directly to the back end of a two–side-arm manifold. Fluid-filled tubings are attached to the side arms for "zero" pressure reference and catheter flushing, and the front end of the manifold is connected directly to the catheter. Care must be taken during filling of the transducer and manifold to remove all air bubbles, which can markedly lower the resonant frequency of the system.

pressure recording. This tends to cause low-frequency resonance in the system. The resonant frequency of a fluid-filled system should be above the frequencies contained in intracardiac pressure waveforms (see above). For usual clinical purposes, a system with frequency response that is flat to 10 or 12 Hz with a resonant frequency above this level is adequate. This can be achieved most easily by use of small volume-displacement transducers, with imposition of as few stopcocks and connecting tubings as possible between the catheter hub and the transducer. The system used in our cardiac catheterization laboratories is shown in Figure 9–4B.

With an aqueous fluid–filled catheter attached to a transducer, the transducer will indicate zero pressure when the catheter tip is at the same height as the transducer. If the catheter tip is elevated above the transducer, a positive pressure of 1 mm Hg will be indicated for every 1.36 cm of height difference; if the catheter tip is below the transducer level, a negative pressure of the same magnitude will be indicated. These effects are due simply to gravitational force acting on the fluid column in the catheter and the specific gravity of mercury of 13.6. The transducer is therefore positioned at a level approximately the same as that of the heart, usually the midchest. If the transducer is placed at a different height, attaching a second fluid-filled catheter to the transducer and positioning the tip of that catheter at the zero (midchest) level permit proper zeroing of the transducer relative to the catheter tip position within the heart (Fig. 9–4B). It is important to note that pressures measured inside the heart chambers do not necessarily equal the true transmural pressures, because of the normal intrathoracic negative pressure, which ranges between 0 and −8 mm Hg during normal respiration.

Even when a pressure measurement system has a high degree of sensitivity, uniform frequency response, and optimal damping and is properly zeroed and balanced, distortions and inaccuracies in the pressure waveform may occur. Motion of the catheter within the heart and great vessels accelerates the fluid contained within the catheter, and such *catheter whip* artifacts may produce superimposed waves of ± 10 mm Hg. Catheter whip artifacts are particularly common in tracings from the pulmonary arteries and are difficult to avoid.

Manometer-tipped Catheters. In order to minimize artifacts associated with low resonant frequency systems, catheter whip, and excessive damping, many laboratories employ micromanometer-tipped catheters, with which the pressure transducer is actually placed in the cardiac chamber in which pressure is being measured. As is evident in Figure 9–5, there may be a distinct difference in waveform between "true" left ventricular pressure (as recorded using an intracardiac micromanometer) and that recorded through a standard fluid-filled catheter system. Low resonant frequency and inadequate damping of the fluid-filled system in this example resulted in exaggeration of the high-frequency components in the left ventricular pressure rise and fall, with corresponding artifactual overshoot of the pressures in early diastole and early systole. More optimal damping and natural frequency characteristics of the fluid-filled system can minimize these artifacts but cannot eliminate them. In addition, a 30- to 40-msec delay in the pressure waveform occurs with fluid-filled catheter systems, necessitating the use of manometer-tipped catheters in situations in which recording of simultaneous pressure and angiographic volume, echocardiographic, phonocardiographic, or electrocardiographic data is required. The high-frequency response of manometer-tipped catheter transducers (resonant frequency = 25 to 40 kHz) permits their application for the detection and recording of intracardiac sounds.

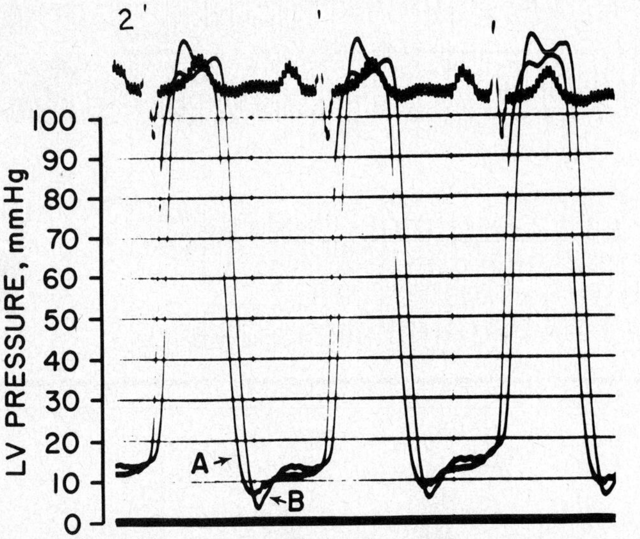

FIGURE 9–5 Left ventricular pressures recorded with a manometer-tipped catheter (*A*) and a fluid-filled catheter–external transducer system with a low resonant frequency (*B*). Note undershoot of pressure in early diastole, overshoot of pressure in early systole, and delay of fluid-filled catheter pressure relative to the "true" pressure. (From Grossman, W.: Cardiac Catheterization and Angiography. 2nd ed. Philadelphia, Lea and Febiger, 1980.)

Most manometer-tipped catheters do not have an endhold and must therefore be inserted via arteriotomy or a vascular sheath. Millar* manufactures a No. 8 French endhole manometer-tipped angiocatheter that can be used with a guidewire. Since the zero level of the manometer-tipped catheter may drift, it is most useful to have a fluid-filled lumen in the catheter by means of which a true zero pressure reference level can be established.

Representative Pressure Tracings. In evaluating pressure tracings, specific phasic and mean pressure values should be measured, the phasic pressure waveform contours noted, and pressures in different chambers compared. Analysis of these data, interpreted in the light of cardiac output and angiographic measurement, permits detection and quantitation of valvular, myocardial, and pericardial abnormalities.

NORMAL PRESSURE WAVEFORMS. An understanding of pressure waveforms, both under normal conditions and in various disease states, is predicated on a thorough comprehension of the events of the cardiac cycle (Fig. 12–25, p. 431). Shown in Figure 9–6 are normal pressure waveforms obtained with fluid-filled catheters.

*Millar Instruments, Inc., P.O. Box 18227, Houston, Texas 77023.

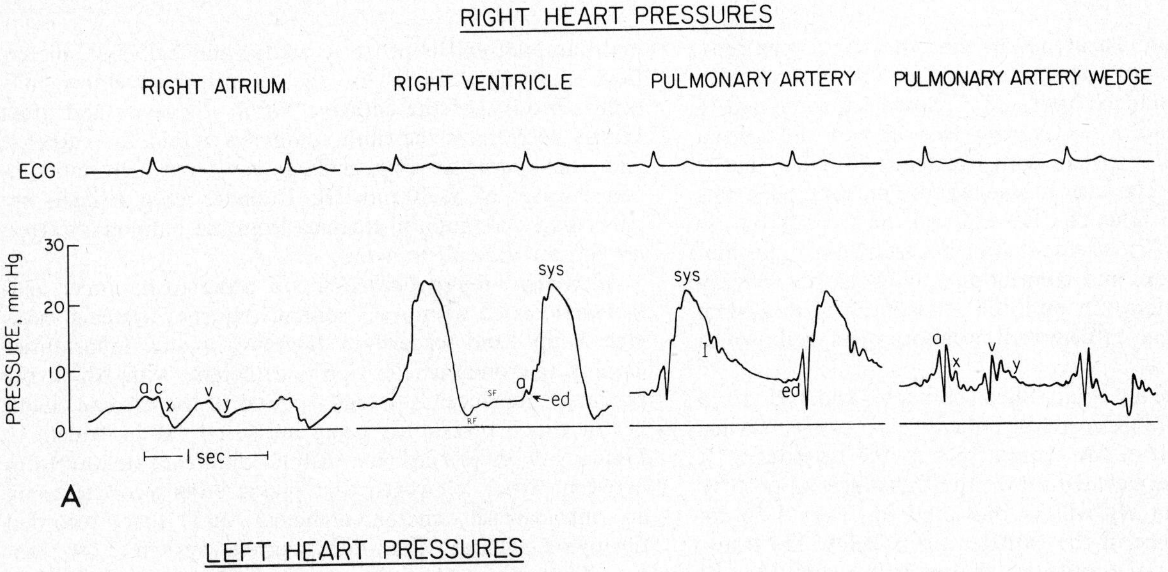

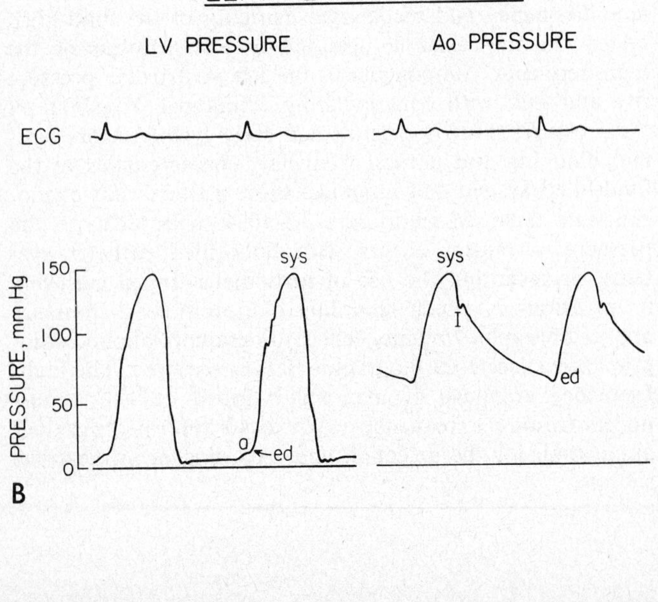

FIGURE 9–6 *A,* Representative normal pressure tracings from the right side of the heart; sys = systolic, ed = end-diastolic. *B,* Representative normal pressures from the left ventricle (LV) and aorta (Ao).

The *right atrial pressure waveform* consists of two major positive deflections—the *a* and *v* waves. The *a* wave is due to atrial systole and follows the P wave of the electrocardiogram. As the pressure declines from the peak of the *a* wave (the *x* decent), a small positive deflection, the *c* wave, occurs concomitant with tricuspid valve closure. After the "*c*" wave, right atrial pressure continues to fall (*x* descent) even though the atrium is filling with blood (the tricuspid valve is closed), owing to atrial relaxation. After full atrial relaxation occurs, at the nadir of the *x* descent, the pressure in the atrium starts to rise as atrial filling continues from peripheral venous return. This rise in the right atrial pressure during right ventricular systole is termed the *v* wave, and it reaches a peak just before the opening of the tricuspid valve. Following opening of the tricuspid valve, the right atrium empties into the right ventricle, and pressure in the atrium falls, constituting the *y* descent. Following the *y* descent, pressure in the atrium is equal to ventricular diastolic pressure and slowly increases as the ventricle fills. Peak *a* and *v* wave pressures are measured, and the mean pressure is obtained electronically. Normal values are shown in Table 9–1.

The *diastolic phase of the right ventricular pressure pulse* consists of an early rapid filling wave, during which approximately 60 per cent of ventricular filling ocurs; a slow filling period, accounting for approximately 25 per cent of ventricular filling; and an atrial systolic wave *(a)*, accounting for approximately 15 per cent of ventricular filling. During diastole, right atrial and right ventricular pressures are nearly equal, because of the low resistance to flow across the tricuspid valve. Two pressures are usually measured: the peak systolic right ventricular pressure and the end-diastolic right ventricular pressure immediately following the *a* wave. The normal range of values for the pressures is shown in Table 9–1.

The *pulmonary artery pressure waveform* contains a systolic pressure owing to flow of blood into the pulmonary artery from the right ventricle. As right ventricular ejection ends, pressure in the pulmonary artery falls, and when right ventricular pressure drops below the pulmonary pressure, the pulmonary valve closes, resulting in the incisura on the pressure waveform. Pressure in the pulmonary artery then falls gradually as blood flows through the pulmonary arteries and veins into the left atrium and ventricle. The nadir of this pressure in late diastole is termed the end-diastolic pulmonary artery pressure. This pressure, the peak systolic pressure, and the mean pulmonary artery pressure are the parameters usually measured. It is not unusual to observe a small (≤ 5 mm Hg) gradient in peak systolic pressure between the right ventricle and the pulmonary artery.

The *pulmonary artery wedge pressure* has a waveform similar to that of the left atrial pressure but is both damped and delayed by transmission through the capillary vessels. A normal wedge pressure should show *a* and *v* waves, which reflect, respectively, left atrial systole and left atrial filling during left ventricular systole (see discussion of right atrial pressure above). However, *c* waves may not be apparent on the wedge pressure tracing. The *x* and *y* descents should be distinct in a wedge pressure tracing if it is not overdamped. The peak *a* and *v* wave pressures are usually measured, as in the mean wedge pressure. In a normal pulmonary circulation of low vascular resistance, the pulmonary artery flow is diminished at end diastole, so that end-diastolic pulmonary artery and mean pulmonary artery wedge pressures are approximately equal. Mean pulmonary artery pressure is always higher than mean wedge pressure. Normal values for pulmonary artery wedge pressure are presented in Table 9–1.

Normal left heart pressure waveforms are shown in Figure 9–6. The *left atrial pressure waveform* was discussed in the description of the pulmonary artery wedge pressure. Unless a transseptal catheterization is performed, pulmonary artery wedge pressure is recorded as an acceptable substitute for the actual left atrial pressure. It is important to recognize that this can be a source of error, unless a properly damped wedge pressure is observed and confirmed by determination of oxygen saturation.

The components of the *left ventricular waveform* are similar to those already described for that of the right ventricle. The pressures in the left ventricle in diastole (as well as systole) are normally higher than those in the right ventricle, owing in part to the greater wall thickness of the left ventricle, which results in greater chamber stiffness.

The *central aortic pressure tracing* consists of a systolic wave, followed by the incisura, which denotes closure of the aortic valve, and then a gradual fall in pressure as the blood flows from the aorta through the peripheral arterial capillary and venous vessels. Pressure is normally measured at peak systole and at end diastole, and the mean pressure is determined electronically.

The *peripheral arterial pressure,* commonly measured

TABLE 9–1 Range of Normal Resting Hemodynamic Values

	a Wave	*v* Wave	Mean	Systolic	End-Diastolic	Mean
Pressures						
Right atrium	2–10	2–10	0–8			
Right ventricle				15–30	0–8	
Pulmonary artery				15–30	3–12	9–16
Pulmonary artery wedge and left atrium	3–15	3–12	1–10			
Left ventricle				100–140	3–12	
Systemic arteries				100–140	60–90	70–105
Oxygen consumption index (ml/min/m²)		110–150				
Arteriovenous oxygen difference (ml/l)		30–50				
Cardiac output index (l/min/m²)		2.5–4.2				
Resistances (dynes-sec-cm^{-5})						
Pulmonary vascular		20–120				
Systemic vascular		770–1500				

probably about 10 per cent.[46,49-52] The Fick oxygen method is most accurate in patients with low cardiac output, in whom the arteriovenous oxygen difference is wide.

Indicator-dilution Method. The Fick method is merely a specific application of the indicator-dilution method, in which O_2 being continuously infused by the lungs is the indicator and is diluted in the pulmonary blood flow. Stewart was the first to use a dye indicator-dilution method to measure cardiac output; he used the continuous infusion technique and reported his first studies in 1897.[53] Numerous indicators have since been successfully employed.[46] Indocyanine green dye has gained the widest acceptance in clinical practice, although recently thermodilution (in which cold saline is the indicator) has become widely used.[54-59] When indocyanine green dye is used, a bolus is rapidly injected into the pulmonary artery, and its appearance and concentration in arterial blood are recorded from a peripheral systemic artery (e.g., brachial, femoral, or radial). A time-concentration curve is thus recorded that exhibits a rapid rise to a peak and then a gradual decline in concentration that is interrupted by a secondary rise due to recirculation of the dye (Fig. 9–10, *top*). The problem of isolating those data that relate only to the first pass of the indicator has been approached by several investigators, but the method originally proposed by Kinsman, Moore, and Hamilton[60] is the one still used most widely today. Kinsman and coworkers showed mathematically that the true "first-pass" curve will be given by plotting the concentration decline on semilogarithmic paper and extrapolating the early linear part of the plot.

The cardiac output (CO) is then calculated as $CO = i/(\bar{c} \times t)$, where i is the quantity of indicator injected, $\bar{c}$ is the average concentration of the indicator during its first pass, and t is the total duration of the curve. The product of $\bar{c}$ and t is easily measured as the area under the first-pass curve, as determined by planimetry. This may be further simplified by the use of any number of available computer methods in which the semilogarithmic replotting, area computation, and cardiac output calculation are all accomplished electronically. More precise methodological details, as well as a discussion of sources of error, can be found elsewhere.[31,46] Most laboratories,[54,61-63] but not all,[57] have found there to be excellent agreement between the indicator-dilution methods and independent methods for measuring cardiac output, particularly when the cardiac output is normal or elevated. The error of the indicator-dilution method is greatest in patients with extremely low outputs, severe mitral or aortic regurgitation, or intracardiac shunts. Therefore it complements the Fick method of cardiac output determination, in which the accuracy is greatest in patients having low cardiac output with wide arteriovenous oxygen differences.

It is important to note that indocyanine green dye can cause interference when oxygen content is determined by spectrophotometric methods. Therefore, if cardiac output is to be determined by both the Fick and the indocyanine green dye indicator-dilution methods *in the same patient,* the former measurement should be done first. Not only does the use of cold saline (thermodilution) as an indicator avoid this problem, but also this technique can be performed repeatedly without buildup of indicator or recirculation problems. For these reasons, the thermo-

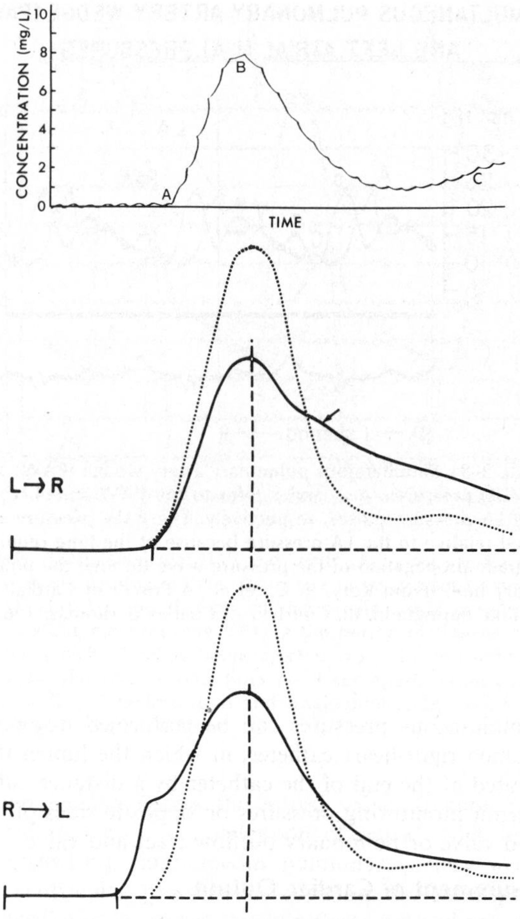

FIGURE 9–10 Time-concentration curves generated by injecting indocyanine green dye into the right heart and sampling in the brachial artery. *Top,* Normal curve showing appearance of the dye in arterial blood (A) and the peak concentration (B), followed by an exponential disappearance and then recirculation of the dye (C). *Center,* The solid line is a schematic drawing of the time-concentration curve in a patient with a left-to-right shunt. There is an early recirculation "bump" (arrow) on the downslope of the curve due to the dye that is shunted from left to right and then reappears in the left circulation. The dotted line represents a normal dye concentration curve. *Bottom,* Time-concentration curve in the presence of a right-to-left shunt, showing early appearance of the dye in the brachial artery. The early appearing dye passes through the shunt and thus does not traverse the pulmonary circulation. The dotted line represents a normal dye concentration curve. (Top panel from Grossman, W.: Cardiac Catheterization and Angiography. 2nd ed. Philadelphia, Lea and Febiger, 1980. Center and lower panels from Kory, R. C., et al.: A Primer of Cardiac Catheterization. Springfield, Ill. Courtesy of Charles C Thomas, 1965.)

dilution method has become the most commonly used indicator-dilution technique for measuring cardiac output.

Angiographic Measurement of Cardiac Output. Measurement of left ventricular end-diastolic and end-systolic volumes by quantitative left ventricular angiography, described on p. 470, permits calculation of left ventricular stroke volume. In the absence of atrial fibrillation or significant mitral or aortic regurgitation, systemic cardiac output may be estimated by multiplying the stroke volume by the heart rate during the angiogram. This method is a less accurate method of measuring cardiac output than either the indicator-dilution or the Fick method.

Regional Blood Flows. The principles discussed above may be applied to measure regional blood flows. Three common examples are intracardiac shunt flow as measured by the Fick principle, coronary sinus flow by thermodilution, and regurgitant valve flow by a combination of angiographic and Fick measurements of cardiac output.

INTRACARDIAC SHUNTS. Detection, localization, and quantification of intracardiac shunts can generally be accomplished with precision at cardiac catheterization. Although intracardiac shunts are usually suspected prior to catheterization, this is not always the case. Therefore, the operator must always be alert to the possibility of an intracardiac shunt and must search for one when unexpected arterial oxygen desaturation is detected or an inappropriately high mixed venous (i.e., pulmonary artery) oxygen saturation is observed.

Detection and Localization of Shunts. In a patient with a *left-to-right shunt* (atrial septal defect, ventricular septal defect, patent ductus arteriosus) pulmonary blood flow is higher than systemic blood flow, and the pulmonary artery oxygen saturation is greater than the true mixed venous blood saturation. The anatomical location of the shunt is determined by obtaining multiple samples for oxygen saturation. In the traditional oximetry run duplicate samples are drawn in rapid succession from the left, right, and main pulmonary arteries[7,64,65]; the outflow tract, body, and inflow area of the right ventricle; the low, mid, and high right atrium; the low and high superior vena cava; and the inferior vena cava at the level of the diaphragm. Oxygen content of blood from these locations normally shows variability due to streaming of up to 20 ml/liter in the right atrium, 10 ml/liter in the right ventricle, and 5 ml/liter in the pulmonary artery.[7,64] Variations above these values generally indicate the entrance of oxygenated blood into the right heart through an abnormal communication. The level of the "oxygen step-up" generally locates the anatomical position of the left-to-right shunt. If, for example, oxygen content of right atrial blood samples is 148, 152, and 156 ml/liter (average 152 ml/liter), that of right ventricular blood samples is 151, 152, and 153 ml/liter (average 152 ml/liter), but that of pulmonary artery blood is 180, 182, and 178 ml/liter (average 180 ml/liter), there is a significant oxygen step-up in the pulmonary artery (+28 ml/liter) indicative of a left-to-right shunt at that level (e.g., patent ductus arteriosus or aortopulmonary window).

One limitation of the oxygen method of detecting intracardiac shunts is its low degree of sensitivity. Small shunts ($\dot{Q}_p/\dot{Q}_s \leq 1.3$) at the level of the pulmonary artery or right ventricle and shunts at the atrial level with $\dot{Q}_p/\dot{Q}_s <$ 1.5 are not consistently detected by this technique alone because of the normal variability in O_2 saturation described above.[65] A more sensitive technique for the detection of small left-to-right intracardiac shunts involves detection of the early appearance of hydrogen in the right heart after inhalation of hydrogen gas using a right-heart hydrogen-sensitive platinum-tipped electrode catheter to measure direct-current voltage changes. In addition, in the presence of a left-to-right shunt, injection of indocyanine green dye into the pulmonary artery with sampling from the femoral artery will demonstrate early recirculation on the downslope of the dye curve.[64,66–68] These techniques are easily performed and can sometimes detect left-to-right shunts too small to be detected by the oxygen step-up method (Fig. 9–10, *center*).

In *right-to-left shunts,* arterial blood is unsaturated, and cyanosis is frequently noted. Clinically, the site of entry of a right-to-left cardiac shunt may be localized by noting which of the left-heart chambers is the first to show desaturation. However, it is usually difficult to enter the pulmonary vein and left atrium in the adult, as discussed previously. Small right-to-left shunts may be detected by injecting indocyanine dye into a vena cava and detecting the early appearance of the dye in arterial blood prior to the primary peak (Fig. 9–10, *bottom*). The site of origin of the shunt can then be localized by injecting dye at a more distal site in the right heart until its early appearance disappears.

It should be remembered that an abnormal catheter position can also be useful in detecting an abnormal communication. This is particularly true for atrial septal defects and for anomalous pulmonary veins emptying into the right atrium. In addition, angiographic methods may be used to detect and localize intracardiac shunts (Chap. 10).

Shunt Quantification. The usefulness of the oximetry run method of shunt detection is enhanced by the fact that the data obtained are also used in quantification of the shunt. When the shunt is unidirectional (e.g., left-to-right), its magnitude is simply calculated as the difference between the pulmonary and systemic blood flows. Pulmonary blood flow ($\dot{Q}_p$) in liters/min is given as:

$$\dot{Q}_p = \frac{O_2 \text{ consumption (ml/min)}}{\underset{\text{(ml/liter)}}{\text{PV } O_2 \text{ content}} - \underset{\text{(ml/liter)}}{\text{PA } O_2 \text{ content}}}$$

where PV and PA refer to pulmonary venous and pulmonary arterial blood, respectively. If a pulmonary vein has not been entered, systemic arterial oxygen content may be used in lieu of PV O_2 content, as long as the systemic arterial oxygen saturation is 95 per cent or more. If systemic oxygen saturation is less than 95 per cent, one must determine whether a right-to-left shunt is present. If such a shunt exists, then a value of PV O_2 content is calculated from the assumption that it is 98 per cent of blood oxygen capacity, and this is used in calculated $\dot{Q}_p$. If arterial desaturation is present but is not due to a right-to-left intracardiac shunt, the observed systemic arterial oxygen content is used to calculate $\dot{Q}_p$.

Systemic blood flow ($\dot{Q}_s$) in liters/min is calculated as

$$\dot{Q}_s = \frac{\dot{Q}_2 \text{ consumption (ml/min)}}{\left[\begin{array}{c}\text{Systemic arterial}\\ O_2 \text{ content (ml/liter)}\end{array}\right] - \left[\begin{array}{c}\text{Mixed venous}\\ O_2 \text{ content (ml/liter)}\end{array}\right]}$$

Mixed venous oxygen content is obtained as the average oxygen content of blood in the chamber immediately upstream in relation to the shunt, as defined by the level of the O_2 step-up in the oximetry run. The formula used to calculate mixed venous oxygen content when the shunt is at the level of the right atrium as in atrial septal defect was derived by Flamm and coworkers.[69] They found that $\dot{Q}_s$ calculated from mixed venous oxygen content derived as

$$\frac{3 \text{ SVC } O_2 \text{ content} + 1 \text{ IVC } O_2 \text{ content}}{4}$$

most closely approximated $\dot{Q}_s$ measured by left ventricular to brachial artery indicator-dilution curves in patients with atrial septal defect.

Calculation of the shunt flow itself is then given as $\dot{Q}_p - \dot{Q}_s$. If the shunt is wholly left-to-right, this value is positive, whereas a negative value is observed in patients with pure right-to-left shunts (e.g., tetralogy of Fallot). When there is *bidirectional shunting*, the more complicated formula at the bottom of the page must be used.[31]

REGURGITANT FLOWS. In aortic or mitral valve regurgitation, left ventricular stroke volume measured angiographically is greater than the forward stroke volume (calculated by dividing the Fick cardiac output by the heart rate), and the difference is the volume of regurgitant blood that leaks across the abnormal valve(s) during each cardiac cycle. Calculation of this regurgitant flow from data obtained during cardiac catheterization can be helpful in evaluating the severity of regurgitant lesions. The regurgitant fraction (RF) is defined as

$$RF = \frac{\begin{bmatrix}\text{Angiographic}\\ \text{stroke volume}\end{bmatrix} - \begin{bmatrix}\text{Fick stroke}\\ \text{volume}\end{bmatrix}}{\text{Angiographic stroke volume}}$$

As a general rule, regurgitant fractions exceeding 30 to 40 per cent are considered hemodynamically important. However, because of potential errors of measurement of both the angiographic and Fick stroke volume, this measurement must be interpreted in light of other hemodynamic, angiographic, and clinical data.

CORONARY SINUS FLOW. Coronary sinus blood flow may be measured during cardiac catheterization by the thermodilution technique.[70] A themodilution catheter is inserted into the coronary sinus via a right antecubital vein. Saline at room temperature is continuously infused, and the temperature of the blood-saline mixture downstream in the coronary sinus is monitored by an external thermistor on the catheter. The temperature of the injected saline is monitored by an internal thermistor near the catheter injection orifice. The relationship is

$$F_B = F_I \times 1.19 \times \left(\frac{T_B - T_I}{T_B - T_M} - 1\right) \text{ml/min}$$

where F_B = coronary sinus blood flow
F_I = flow of room temperature saline injectate (ml/min)
T_B = body temperature (°C)
T_I = injectate temperature (°C)
T_M = temperature of blood-injectate mixture (°C)

F_I must be great enough (usually 40 ml/min) to insure adequate turbulence for blood-injectate mixing in the coronary sinus. This method allows continuous and repeated measurements of coronary sinus blood flow, approximating 95 per cent of coronary arterial flow.[70]

Other techniques may also be used to estimate coronary blood flow.[31] For example, a small amount of the inert gas isotope xenon-133 may be injected selectively into a coronary artery, and the initial washout of radioactivity from the heart can be recorded with a scintillation camera (Chap. 11). The regional myocardial blood flow in the distribution of that coronary artery can be estimated from the rate constant (k) derived from a semilogarithmic plot of the radioactivity washout curve, the partition coefficient of the tracer in myocardial tissue. (λ), and the specific gravity of myocardial tissue (ρ). The formula used is

$$\text{Myocardial blood flow (cm}^3\text{/100 gm tissue} \times \text{min)} = \frac{k\ (\text{min}^{-1})\ \lambda\ 100}{\rho\ (\text{gm/cm}^3)}$$

Inaccuracies in the measurement of coronary blood flow with this method may occur because of recirculation of the isotope, deposition of xenon in myocardial fat, and local inhomogeneity of flow.

Measurement of Vascular Resistance

Theoretical Considerations. Hydraulic resistance (R) is defined by analogy to Ohm's law as the ratio of the mean pressure drop (ΔP) to flow (Q) between two points in a liquid flowing in a tube. The applicability of this simple equation to pulsatile flow in vascular beds is dubious. Nevertheless, vascular resistance calculated in this fashion has become standard practice in hemodynamic laboratories, and the calculated resistances so obtained often yield important clinical information. Poiseuille's studies of laminar steady-state flow in rigid glass tubes showed that

$$Q = \frac{\pi(\Delta P)r^4}{8\eta l}$$

where r = radius of the tube, l = length of the tube, and η = viscosity of the fluid.[43] By rearrangement, it can be seen that resistance (R) is given by

$$R = \frac{\Delta P}{Q} = \frac{8\ \eta l}{\pi r^4}$$

Thus, under the ideal conditions of laminar fluid flow in rigid tubes, resistance is directly proportional to the length of the tube and to the viscosity of the fluid and *inversely proportional to the fourth power of the tube's radius.* It is clear from this that reduction in cross-sectional area of a vessel lumen is the most powerful determinant of resis-

$$L \rightarrow R = \frac{\text{PBF (PA } O_2 \text{ content} - \text{Mixed venous } O_2 \text{ content)}}{\text{(PV* } O_2 \text{ content} - \text{Mixed venous } O_2 \text{ content)}}$$

$$R \rightarrow L = \frac{\text{PBF (PV* } O_2 \text{ content} - \text{BA } O_2 \text{ content) (PV* } O_2 \text{ content} - \text{PA } O_2 \text{ content)}}{\text{(Ba } O_2 \text{ content} - \text{Mixed venous } O_2 \text{ content) (PV* } O_2 \text{ content} - \text{Mixed venous } O_2 \text{ content)}}$$

*If actual PV is not measured, assume 98 per cent blood O_2 capacity in a patient whose pulmonary function is normal or presumed to be so.

tance to flow. It was observed by Reynolds in 1883 that the pressure drop across a length of tubing exeeded that predicted by the Poiseuille equation at a critical flow rate, dependent on the diameter of the tube and the viscosity of the fluid. He defined the Reynold's number (R_e) as being equal to $\frac{\overline{V}D\rho}{\mu}$, where $\overline{V}$= average velocity of flow, D = diameter of the tube, ρ= density of the fluid, and μ = its viscosity.[43] When this number is exceeded, flow becomes turbulent, and the pressure drop exceeds that predicted by the Poiseuille equation, which assumes laminar flows. For blood, $R_e = 2000$, and it appears likely that during normal blood flow in arteries, R_e is not exceeded and that flow remains laminar. However, across severely stenotic valves or in areas of severe luminal arterial narrowing, this may not be the case. This will be considered further in the subsequent discussion of calculation of stenotic valve areas.

Calculations of Vascular Resistance. Vascular resistance for the systemic and pulmonary vascular beds. (SVR and PVR, respectively) is usually calculated as

$$SVR = \frac{80\ (AO_m - RA_m)}{Q_s}$$

and

$$PVR = \frac{80\ (PA_m - LA_m)}{Q_p}$$

where AO_m, RA_m, PA_m, and LA_m are the aortic, right atrial, pulmonary artery, and left atrial mean pressures in mm Hg; Q_s and Q_p are the systemic and pulmonary blood flows in liters/min (which are equal to the cardiac output in the absence of a shunt); and 80 is the factor used to convert resistance from "hybrid" units (mm Hg/liter/min) to metric units (dynes-sec-cm^{-5}). (See also Chap. 25.) These values can be corrected for body size by multiplying (not dividing) them by body surface area—an important factor in evaluating vascular resistance in infants and adolescents.

Cardiac output, usually measured by the Fick or indicator-dilution method, is used in the calculation of blood flow. It is important to appreciate that in the presence of an intracardiac shunt, in which pulmonary and systemic blood flows are not equal, the respective blood flows through each circuit must be measured and used in the calculation of resistance. Often, the mean pulmonary artery wedge pressure is used as an approximation of mean left atrial pressure, since there is ample evidence that these two measurements, when properly obtained, closely approximate each other.[71,72]

The normal value for systemic vascular resistance has been reported to be 1130 $\pm$ 178 dynes-sec-cm^{-5} (mean $\pm$ standard deviation).[73] Thus values for systemic vascular resistance less than 1500 dynes-sec-cm^{-5} are probably normal. The normal pulmonary vascular resistance has been reported as 67 $\pm$ 23 dynes-sec-cm^{-5},[73] and therefore values of pulmonary vascular resistance less than 120 dynes-sec-cm^{-5} are probably normal.

Abnormal increases of systemic and pulmonary vascular resistance may be seen in a variety of conditions (Chaps. 25 and 26). It may be important to determine whether the increased resistance is fixed (i.e., due to chronic anatomical and pathological changes) or functional (i.e., due to increased tone in small muscular arteries and arterioles), since this finding can have important clinical implications. For example, in the systemic bed, major elevations in vascular resistance may lead to a low cardiac output and left ventricular failure, particularly in the presence of mitral regurgitation. Lowering systemic resistance with specific agents (e.g., nitroprusside, hydralazine, prazosin, erythrityl tetranitrate) at the time of cardiac catheterization may yield important information about the potential therapeutic usefulness of such reduction of afterload in chronic therapy (Chap. 16).[74–83] Marked fixed increases in pulmonary vascular resistance in patients with congenital heart disease and abnormal communication between the pulmonary and systemic circuits (e.g., ventricular septal defect, atrial septal defect, patent ductus arteriosus) may contraindicate corrective surgery. Therefore, a demonstration that the increased resistance is not fixed may be of considerable importance in the individual patient. In the catheterization laboratory various agents and manipulations have been utilized to assess the reversibility of high vascular resistance, including oxygen inhalation, infusions of acetylcholine, infusions of tolazoline hydrochloride (Chap. 25), and exercise.[84–93]

Since blood flow is pulsatile, and the vascular beds have nonlinear elastic and capacitative properties, the concept of *vascular impedance* has been employed. Resistance varies continuously with pressure, and blood flow is influenced by many factors, such as inertia, reflected waves, and the phase angle between pulse and flow velocities.[43,94,95] The impedance modulus is calculated to express the spectrum of impedance versus the frequency of a pressure wave.[43]

Stenotic Valves: Calculations of Orifice Area. The evaluation of valvular stenosis in the catheterization laboratory includes a calculation of orifice size based on measurement of the pressure gradient and flow across a valve. The equations used for the aortic and mitral valves were derived and validated by Gorlin.[31,96,97]

The following equations are used when valvular gradients are measured directly:

$$\text{Aortic valve area (cm}^2\text{)} = \frac{F}{44.5\sqrt{\Delta P}}$$

$$\text{Mitral valve area (cm}^2\text{)} = \frac{F}{38.0\sqrt{\Delta P}}$$

where F = flow across the orifice in ml/sec and ΔP = mean pressure gradient in mm Hg across the orifice. A pressure drop across a stenotic valve occurs because of viscous resistance to flow (Poiseuille) and turbulent flow (Reynolds). The empirical constants 44.5 and 38.0 relate these factors to valve area and differ between aortic and mitral valves because of variations in flow pattern.

For specific application to cardiac valves, F is derived as:

$$\text{Flow (F) (ml/sec)} = \frac{\text{Cardiac output (ml/min)}}{\text{DFP (sec/min) or SEP (sec/min)}}$$

The diastolic filling period (DFP) and systolic ejection period (SEP) are derived by measuring the diastolic filling time (mitral valve opening to closure, Fig. 9–8) or systolic ejection time (aortic valve opening to closure, Fig. 9–7) per beat and multiplying by the heart rate.

In a typical patient, cardiac output might be 4300 ml/min, mean transmitral diastolic pressure gradient = 14 mm Hg, diastolic filling time per beat directly measured from the pressure tracings = 0.42 sec/beat, and heart rate = 72 beats/min. Thus, the mitral valve area will be

$$\frac{(4300 \text{ ml/min}) \div (0.42 \text{ sec/beat} \times 72 \text{ beats/min})}{38\sqrt{14 \text{ mm Hg}}} = 1.0 \text{ cm}^2$$

It is important to remember that variations in flow patterns may alter the relationship between orifice area and pressure gradient. In addition, stiff valve leaflets may be more widely opened at high flow velocities (and higher pressure gradients). Therefore, estimation of valve areas, particularly at low flow rates, may be in error and should be considered measurements of functional orifice size. In addition, the presence of valvular regurgitation will result in a falsely low valve area calculation, since the actual valve flow per beat is greater than the flow calculated from the systemic cardiac output. Stenotic valve areas calculated in patients with regurgitation across the stenotic valve should therefore be considered to be the lower limits of the true valve area. In general, errors in estimation of valve flow cause greater inaccuracies in calculations of valve area than do errors in measurement of the pressure gradient across the valve. Nevertheless, hemodynamic measurement of valve area, corrected for body surface area (valve area index), has proved very useful in the clinical management of patients.

Exercise. In many patients with heart disease, hemodynamics may be only slightly disturbed or normal at rest but become markedly abnormal during the stress of exercise. Exercise of a patient during cardiac catheterization (p. 262) can therefore provide very important information regarding the cause of symptoms that are exercise-related. Most commonly, bicycle ergometry in the supine position is used during catheterization; upright bicycle exercise, upper extremity exercise, or straight leg-raising may also be used, if appropriate.

In supine bicycle ergometry, the patient's feet are attached by straps to the pedals of the bicycle ergometer which is attached to the catheterization table or suspended from the ceiling. The workload may be adjusted by varying the speed of and resistance to turning of the pedals. When the subject's feet are upon the pedals, intracardiac pressures normally increase slightly (i.e., by 2 to 4 mm Hg), owing to increased venous return by gravity from the legs and elevation of the diaphragm. As the exercise load is increased, oxygen consumption is increased. Exercise level is frequently expressed as metabolic equivalents of resting O_2 consumption (METS), a level of 2 METS corresponding to a doubling of O_2 consumption and usually achieved at a workload of about 75 kg-meter/min. During exercise, increased O_2 consumption by skeletal muscles is supplied by increased cardiac output and a widened arteriovenous O_2 content difference. When exercise is carried out in the supine position, cardiac output is normally increased mainly by an increase in heart rate, with only slight increases in stroke volume.[98] Patients with cardiac disease may be unable to increase cardiac output normally with exercise because of their inability to maintain stroke volume with increased heart rate and thus will supply most of the increased O_2 required by exercising tissue by means of an increase in the arteriovenous O_2 difference. The "exercise factor" expressed as ΔCO during exercise (ml/min)/ΔO_2 consumption (ml/min) is a measure of this response. It is normally greater than or equal to 6.0, since cardiac output normally increases linearly with increasing O_2 consumption. If the exercise factor is less than 6.0, the increase in cardiac output in response to exercise is impaired.

Changes in intracardiac pressures during exercise are also important. The left ventricular end-diastolic pressure does not normally increase above 16 mm Hg during exercise, but in ischemic, myocardial, and valvular disease it may rise to considerably higher levels. In some patients, exercise may exacerbate mitral or tricuspid regurgitation and usually markedly increases the left atrial–left ventricular pressure gradient in mitral stenosis (Fig. 9–8) (Chap. 32). Thus, an abnormal increase in pressures, an inadequate rise in the cardiac ouput, or both in response to the stress provided by mild to moderate exercise in the supine position can be a very important finding at catheterization (p. 483). In practice, it is important to maintain a given exercise load for at least 3 to 4 minutes before measuring cardiac output and pressures in order to assure a steady state of O_2 consumption and cardiac output. Pressures and the electrocardiogram, as well as the patient's symptoms, should be carefully monitored during exercise to avoid complications.

APPLICATIONS OF CARDIAC CATHETERIZATION

Indications. As with any diagnostic procedure, the decision to perform cardiac catheterization must be based upon a careful balance between the risk of the procedure and the anticipated value of the information obtained. Cardiac catheterization is generally recommended when there is a need to confirm the presence of a clinically suspected condition, define its anatomical and physiological severity, and determine the presence or absence or associated conditions. This need most commonly arises when clinical assessment suggests that the patient may benefit from a *cardiac operation.* Cardiac catheterization is usually coupled with angiographic and/or arteriographic examination and may yield information that will be crucial in defining the need for cardiac operation as well as its risks and anticipated benefit for a given patient.

Although few would disagree that consideration of heart surgery is an adequate reason for performance of catheterization, there are differences of opinion about whether *all* patients being considered for such procedures should undergo preoperative cardiac catheterization.[99,100] In this regard, it should be emphasized that the risks of catheterization are small compared with those of operation in patients in whom (1) an incorrect diagnosis was made, (2) the presence of an unsuspected additional condition prolongs and complicates the planned surgical approach, or (3) the hemodynamic assessment by clinical means was inaccurate. The operating room is not a good place for surprises; preoperative cardiac catheterization can provide the surgical team with a precise and complete road map of the course ahead and thereby permit a carefully reasoned and maximally efficient operative procedure. Futhermore, information obtained by cardiac catheterization may be invaluable in the assessment of the crucial determinants of prognosis, such as left ventricular function and patency of the coronary arteries. For these reasons, we recommend that cardiac catheterization be carried out on almost all adult patients for whom a cardiac operation is contemplated. Of course, it is possible that in time noninvasive techniques may be further perfected and shown to be acceptable substitutes for catheterization data.[101] Following operation, catheterization may be necessary to evaluate the results of operation (graft patency, prosthetic valve function, and so forth).

A second broad indication for performing cardiac catheterization combined with coronary arteriography (Chap. 10) is to clarify the diagnosis in patients with *chest pain of uncertain etiology*, in whom there is confusion regarding the presence of obstructive coronary disease. The data obtained will help relieve the anxiety of the patient and aid the physician in advising the patient concerning the appropriateness of his or her future personal or professional plans. Another example within this category might be the symptomatic patient with a suspected *cardiomyopathy*. Although some may be satisfied with a clinical diagnosis of this condition, the implications of such a diagnosis in terms of therapy and prognosis are so important that cardiac catheterization is usually recommended in such patients in order to rule out potentially correctible conditions (e.g., occult valvular or pericardial disease), even though the likelihood of their presence may appear remote on clinical grounds.

A third important indication for cardiac catheterization is the need to define the response of a patient to *specific pharmacological therapy*. This may be necessary during treatment of an unstable patient (e.g., following acute myocardial infarction) or in an intensive care unit setting, when monitoring of right and left atrial pressures, systemic pressures, and cardiac output is essential to patient management. In addition, the response of patients with chronic heart failure to afterload reduction or to changes in ventricular preload may be most precisely determined by cardiac catheterization. Pharmacological intervention with vasodilators in the treatment of pulmonary hypertension,[102] or with anticoagulation in suspected acute pulmonary embolism (Chap. 46), might well be considered of sufficient potential risk to warrant cardiac catheterization and/or angiography.

Contraindications. If it is important to consider the *indications* for cardiac catheterization in each patient, it is equally important to ascertain whether there are any *contraindications*. Over the past several years, our concept of contraindications has been modified, because patients previously considered too ill for this procedure with serious conditions such as acute myocardial infarction, intractable ventricular tachycardia, and cardiogenic shock have tolerated catheterization and coronary arteriography surprisingly well.[103–105] A long list of relative contraindications must be kept in mind, however, and these include all intercurrent conditions that can be corrected and whose correction would improve the safety of the procedure. Ventricular irritability may greatly increase the risk of left-heart catheterization and can interfere with the interpretation of ventriculography. Hypertension should be controlled prior to and during cardiac catheterization. Other conditions that should be corrected prior to elective cardiac catheterization if at all possible include febrile illness, decompensated left-heart failure, anemia, digitalis toxicity, and electrolyte disturbance. Infective endocarditis and pregnancy are relative though not absolute contraindications to cardiac catheterization.

Anticoagulant therapy is a more controversial contraindication. Some experienced physicians in this field have cautioned against catheterization in patients receiving anticoagulants, particularly when the percutaneous approach is used,[106–108] whereas others suggest that anticoagulation in such patients may be safe or even desirable.[109,110] It is our policy to maintain the prothrombin time less than 18 seconds and to avoid heparin administration for 4 to 6 hours prior to the procedure. If anticoagulant therapy cannot be interrupted, we prefer heparin because it can be easily and immediately reversed by intravenous administration of protamine sulfate should uncontrollable bleeding or cardiac perforation occur in the course of catheterization. If transseptal catheterization is planned, it is mandatory that coagulation be normal.

Design of Catheterization Protocol. Every cardiac catheterization should have a protocol, that is, a carefully reasoned sequential plan designed specifically for the individual patient being studied. Although this protocol may exist only in the mind of the operator, it is our practice to prepare a written protocol and post it prominently in the laboratory so that all personnel are made award of exactly what is planned and thus may be reasonably expected to anticipate the needs of the operator. Certain general principles should be considered in the design of a protocol. First, hemodynamic measurements should precede angiographic studies, so that the physiological state may be as basal as possible at the time of pressure and flow measurements. Second, pressure and blood oxygen saturation should be measured and recorded for each chamber immediately after entry and before passing on to the next chamber. If problems should develop during the later stages of a catheterization procedure (atrial fibrillation or other arrhythmia, pyrogen reaction, hypotension, or reaction to contrast material), the physician will wish that pressures and saturations had been measured initially rather than waiting for the time the catheter is being withdrawn. A third principle is that pressure and cardiac output measurements should be made simultaneously insofar as this is possible. Beyond these general guidelines, the protocol will reflect individual differences from patient to patient. With regard to angiography, it is important to sequence the contrast injections, so that the most important diagnostic study is performed first in a given patient.

Preparation and Premedication of the Patient. The emotional as well as the "medical" preparation of the patient for cardiac catheterization is the responsibility of the operator. It is good practice always to inform the patient and his or her family that there is some risk involved, although unless there are special circumstances they may be reasonably reassured that special problems are unlikely. The discomfort and duration of the procedure should, however, not be understated.

Usually patients scheduled for catheterization are admitted to the hospital 24 to 48 hours prior to the procedure. However, some centers are now performing cardiac catheterization on an outpatient basis for selected stable patients.[111,112] The degree to which this practice will become widely adopted is uncertain at present.

The question of administering prophylactic antibiotics is frequently raised, and some laboratories routinely administer them prior to catheterization,[113] although there are essentially no studies to support their use,[114] and we do not routinely use prophylactic antibiotics in our laboratories.

A wide variety of sedatives has been employed for premedication. We routinely use diazepam (Valium), 5 to 10 mg orally, and diphenhydramine (Benadryl), 25 to 50 mg orally, 1/2 hour prior to starting the procedure. When coronary arteriography is to be part of the procedure, some operators favor the addition of 0.4 mg atropine subcutaneously in order to avoid excessive bradycardia.[115] It is our practice to have the patient fasting (except for oral medications) after midnight. We allow a light breakfast if the patient is not scheduled for catheterization until late in the morning or afternoon.

Prior to catheterization the skin overlying the vessels to be entered (femoral areas or antecubital fossa) should be prepared by shaving and thorough cleansing with iodine or Zephiran chloride solution. This procedure as well as careful sterile technique during the catheterization procedure minimizes the incidence of infection.

Complications of Cardiac Catheterization: Incidence Prevention, and Treatment

There is an extensive literature describing a wide array of complications associated with cardiac catheterization.[107,108,115–144] The incidence of various complications has been reported by the Registry of the Society for Cardiac Angiography.[145] A total of 53,581 patients underwent catheterization and angiography in 66 laboratories over a period of 14 months, beginning in October 1979. There were 75 deaths (0.14 per cent), 40 myocardial infarctions (0.07 per cent), and 35 cerebrovascular accidents (0.07 per cent). The incidence of deaths was greater in patients under 1 year of age (1.75 per cent) and over age 60 (0.25 per cent) than in patients between 1 and 60. In patients undergoing coronary angiography, the mortality ranged from 0.86 per cent in patients with significant left main coronary artery disease to 0 per cent in patients with normal coronary arteries or only minimal coronary disease. Vascular complications occurred in 291 patients (0.57 per cent), the majority (62 per cent) in patients undergoing catheterization via the brachial approach. However, there was no difference between the brachial and femoral techniques in the incidence of serious complications, in contrast to another report.[146]

These data indicate that the incidence of complications of cardiac catheterization as currently practiced is low, although careful attention to detail and meticulous technique are required to achieve this standard of performance.

The problem of *arterial thrombosis* deserves special attention.[113,116–118,122,124,132] Sones has reported 2 to 3 per cent segmental occlusion at the site of arteriotomy.[113] It is generally acknowledged that the incidence of thrombosis is related to the duration of the procedure, the number of catheters used, the presence of underlying arterial disease, and the technique of arterial repair.[31] With regard to the percutaneous femoral approach, local complications include thrombosis, distal embolization, false aneurysm, and delayed hemorrhage.[120,127,128,135,136,142] Serious complications involving the femoral artery are usually related to the presence of preexisting iliofemoral disease, and in such patients it is preferable to avoid a percutaneous femoral approach.

Perforation of the heart or intrathoracic great vessels can occur with any approach but most commonly involves the right ventricular outflow tract and apex.[107] These areas are subject to perforation during right ventricular angiography or pacemaker placement. Perforations of the aorta, iliac artery, subclavian artery, or great veins have all been reported and are generally associated with excessive catheter manipulation. In many such instances, catheter manipulation was continued despite resistance to passage or complaints by the patient of pain related to the catheter passage. Since transseptal left-heart catheterization entails controlled perforation of the interatrial septum, perforation of the heart is its main hazard. Unintentional perforation of the aorta, atrial wall, coronary sinus, or right atrial appendage may occur, leading to cardiac tamponade.

Vagal reactions are common and may be quite serious. They are frequently, but not always, incited by pain in a tense, anxious patient and consist of nausea, hypotension, and bradycardia. In older patients, the entire picture of a vagal reaction may be present without bradycardia. If promptly recognized, vagal reactions usually respond dramatically to cessation of catheter manipulation, intravenous atropine (0.5 to 1.0 mg), and elevation of the legs to increase venous return. If the hypotension and bradycardia persist for any period of time, serious arrhythmias and/or irreversible shock may develop, particularly in patients with ischemic heart disease or aortic stenosis.

Myocardial infarction may complicate cardiac catheterization but rarely occurs unless left ventriculography or coronary arteriography is part of the procedure.[115,122,129–131] Documentation of myocardial infarction, when less than transmural in extent, may be difficult in such patients, since intramuscular injections and soft tissue trauma during the catheterization procedure may lead to increases in serum enzymes (LDH, GOT, and CK) that are often used to diagnose the presence of infarction.[143,144] However, following uncomplicated cardiac catheterization, it was shown that although total CK was increased in nearly all patients, none had elevation of CK-MB activity.[134]

Electrical hazards have been reported in association with cardiac catheterization.[138–141] Currents of only a few microamperes transmitted to a small area of myocardium by the wires of electrode catheters, catheters filled with saline, thermistor catheters, or manometer-tipped catheters may produce ventricular fibrillation. This occurrence is now rare, because of the use of common grounding of all electrical equipment, transformer isolation of electrical equipment from the power line by means of current-limiting devices, and establishment of an equal potential environment.[147]

Contamination of catheters or fluids administered during cardiac catheterization with sterile bacterial products or other foreign substances can result in a *pyrogen reac-*

tion, characterized by rigors followed by temperature elevation. If this occurs during catheterization, catheters and fluids should be set aside for subsequent culture; the reaction itself usually responds to small amounts of morphine sulfate (2 mg) administered intravenously. Pyrogen reactions are best treated by prevention. Careful cleaning and sterilization of catheters are essential in this regard.

Other Procedures Involving Cardiac Catheterization

Cardiac catheterization techniques are now being employed in an increasing number of procedures for purposes other than hemodynamic or angiographic study. In many instances the approaches and catheters used and the indications and complications for these procedures differ, and they will therefore be discussed separately.

INTRACARDIAC ELECTROCARDIOGRAPHY AND PACING. Electrodes mounted on the tips of cardiac catheters can be used to record intracardiac electrical activity and to stimulate the heart at selected sites. This technique is of great value in elucidating the mechanism and treating a variety of arrhythmias, as discussed in Chapters 19, 20, and 21. Both acute and chronic pacing are also carried out, most commonly, through pacing catheters, as described in Chapter 22.

Transvenous Endomyocardial Biopsy. Nonoperative cardiac biopsy was initially developed as a needle biopsy technique similar to needle biopsy of the kidney or liver.[148–150] In 1962, Japanese workers reported a method for transvenous endomyocardial biopsy of the right ventricle[151]; this has subsequently been modified and applied to endomyocardial biopsy of both right and left ventricles by a number of investigators.[152–157] This method is illustrated in Figure 9–11. A No. 9 French venous sheath is placed in the internal jugular vein via a percutaneous approach. The bioptome is inserted into the sheath and advanced to the right atrium and across the tricuspid valve. After positioning of the end of the bioptome against the endocardium of the interventricular septum, by fluoroscopy, the bioptome is opened, gently advanced against the endocardium, and then closed. On withdrawal of the bioptome, a small (1 to 2 mm in diameter) portion of right ventricular myocardium with attached endocardium is obtained. This maneuver is repeated three times, and specimens are processed for light and electron microscopic study. This technique is useful in the diagnoses of hypertrophic and congestive cardiomyopathies (Chap. 41), amyloid and other infiltrative cardiomyopathies (p. 1422), and immunological rejection in cardiac transplant recipients (p. 1445).[152,153,155,158] Serial endomyocardial biopsies have been used to evaluate cardiac toxicity in patients receiving high-dose systemic adriamycin therapy for carcinoma (p. 1690).[159] A particularly promising application of this technique may be in detection of inflammatory myocarditis. In a recent report by Nippoldt et al.[160] of clinicopathological correlates in 100 consecutive patients undergoing right ventricular endomyocardial biopsy at the Mayo Clinic, myocarditis was detected in 15 per cent of patients with unexplained congestive heart failure and in 15 per cent of patients with unexplained dysrhythmia or syncope. In some cases, inflammatory myocarditis and associated congestive heart failure may respond to immunosuppressive drugs.[161] Complications, which have been rare, include cardiac perforation and tamponade, pericarditis, and atrial and ventricular tachyarrhythmias.

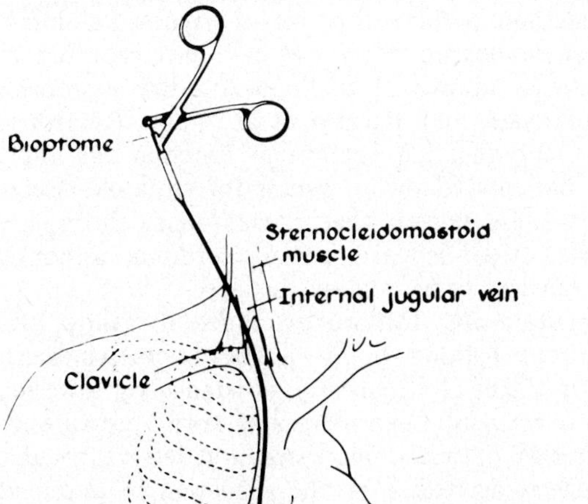

FIGURE 9–11 Endomyocardial biopsy. The biotome is introduced via the right internal jugular vein and is passed across the tricuspid valve into the right ventricle. With the biotome a small segment of right ventricular endocardium is removed from the interventricular septum for microscopic examination. (From Mason, J. W., et al.: Myocardial biopsy. *In* Willerson, J. T., and Sanders, C.A. (eds.): Clinical Cardiology. New York, Grune and Stratton, 1977.)

CORONARY ANGIOPLASTY. Over the past several years, transluminal coronary angioplasty has become an accepted method of treating selected patients with angina pectoris due to atheromatous coronary artery disease (p. 1353). This technique was developed by Grüntzig[162,163] and was an outgrowth of his previous extensive work on transluminal dilation of peripheral arterial stenoses.[162–167] For performance of transluminal dilation of coronary artery stenoses, a small (No. 3 French) dilating catheter is passed down a coronary artery, via a large guiding catheter, placed from the femoral or brachial artery in the coronary artery ostium. Recently, Simpson et al.[168] have developed a dilation catheter that has an independently movable, flexible-tipped guidewire within the dilation catheter, to facilitate passage of the dilation catheter down the appropriate coronary artery branch and crossing of the stenosis (Fig. 9–12). When the stenosis is passed with the dilating catheter, a polyvinyl chloride balloon on the dilating catheter is inflated, compressing and splitting the atheroma (Fig. 9–13).

Results of coronary angioplasty have been encouraging. A report from the Registry of the National Heart, Lung, and Blood Institute[169] indicated that this procedure was successful in 59 per cent of 631 patients, with an average decrease in the degree of stenosis from 83 to 31 per cent. Emergency bypass graft surgery was required in 6 per cent of patients, and the mortality was less than 1 per cent. The majority of patients undergoing the procedure had single-vessel disease (80 per cent), and the success rate appears greatest in lesions of the left anterior descending coronary artery. This technique also appears to be suitable for se-

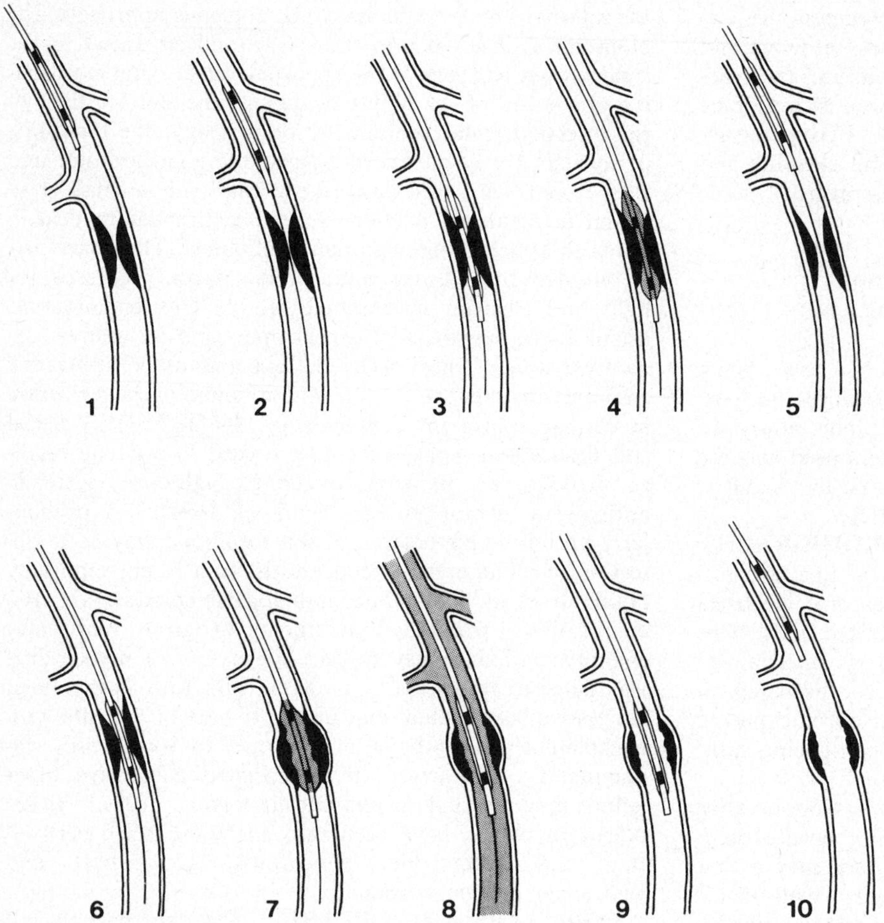

FIGURE 9–12 Schematic diagram of the dilation process: (1) A curved guidewire has been used to direct the balloon catheter away from the most proximal side branch, but it is not suitable for crossing the stenosis. (2) With the dilation catheter maintained beyond the origin of the first branch vessel, the guidewire is withdrawn, straightened, and advanced across the stenosis. (3) The deflated balloon is advanced over the guidewire and into the stenosis. (4) Initial inflation shows a persistent central indentation in the contrast-filled balloon due to incomplete dilation of the stenosis. (5) If myocardial ischemia develops before effective dilation, the guidewire may be advanced as the balloon is withdrawn from the stenosis, permitted reperfusion of the distal vessel. (6) After reperfusion, the balloon is readvanced into the stenosis. (7) Repeated inflation results in elimination of residual balloon deformity. (8) Contrast injection through the guiding catheter demonstrates brisk flow around the deflated balloon. (9) Removal of the guidewire from the dilation catheter permits measurement of the residual transstenotic pressure gradient. (10) Withdrawal of the balloon from the stenosis permits recording of the pullback gradient. (Reproduced with permission from Simpson, J. B. et al.: New catheter system for coronary angioplasty. Am. J. Cardiol. *49*: 1219, 1982.)

lected patients with unstable angina,[170] and improvement in exercise capacity soon after coronary angioplasty has been documented.[161,170,171] This improvement seems to be sustained in approximately 80 per cent of patients for 1 year,[169] whereas 15 to 20 per cent of patients experienced a recurrence of stenosis.

Further improvement in results with continuing development of catheter design and operator experience is to be anticipated, and this technique may eventually be more widely utilized in treating patients with multivessel disease.

Intracoronary Thrombolysis (see also p. 1324). In 1981 Rentrop and colleagues[172] reported on their initial experience with 29 patients with acute myocardial infarction, in whom selective infusion of streptokinase into an obstructed coronary artery was performed. Streptokinase, a plasmin-activating enzyme, was infused directly into the obstructed coronary artery via a standard coronary angiographic catheter at a rate of 2000 units/min, after a bolus of 10,000 to 20,000 units, to an average total dose of 128,000 units. Opening of the occluded vessel occurred within 15 to 90 minutes of initiation of streptokinase infusion in 22 of the 29 patients. An example of the efficacy of intracoronary streptokinase is shown in Figure 9–14. Reports by Ganz[173] and Mathey[174] have confirmed that in 70 to 90 per cent of patients with acute myocardial infarction, recanalization of an occluded artery may be achieved with this technique. Ganz and colleagues[173] have utilized a small selective catheter passed through the coronary angiographic catheter for infusion of a mixture of streptokinase and plasminogen in the immediate vicinity of the coronary thrombosis.

Whether or not reperfusion of coronary arteries with this method reduces the size of myocardial infarction is not yet established. Markis et al.[175] have reported improved myocardial uptake of thallium-201 after coronary artery thrombolysis, and Reduto el al.[176] and Rentrop et al.[177] have found that left ventricular function has improved in some patients following successful streptokinase infusion. These results suggest that intracoronary thrombolysis can indeed salvage jeopardized myocardium, although much work remains to be done in this area.

Percutaneous Intraaortic Balloon Pump Insertion. Intraaortic balloon pump (IABP) counterpulsation provides mechanical circulatory assistance by lowering aortic pressure in systole and increasing aortic pressure in diastole. Cardiac output is increased and left ventricular filling pressure is decreased by the reduction in afterload; myocardial ischemia is alleviated by reduction in oxygen demand while oxygen supply is increased. Therefore, this technique can have a dramatic beneficial effect in patients with cardiogenic shock (p. 1317) and severe, acute myocardial ischemia (p. 1359). It has become a well-accepted method of providing temporary circulatory support for critically ill patients, tiding them over during a stressful procedure, such as cardiac catheterization and angiography, and/or until cardiac surgery can be performed.[178] In

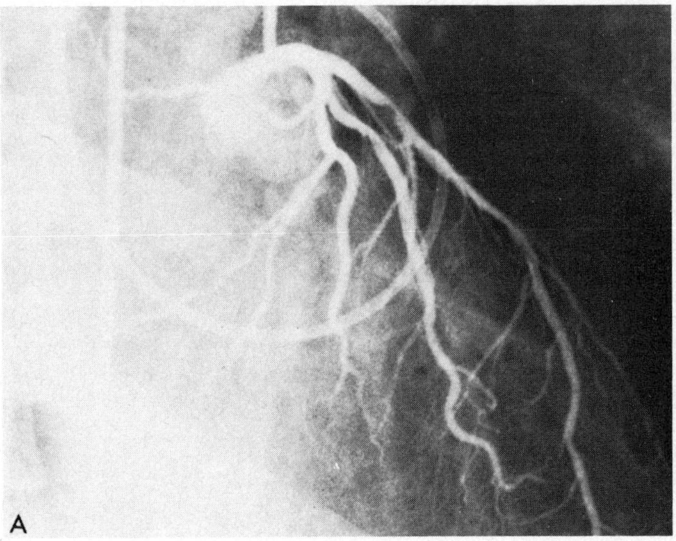

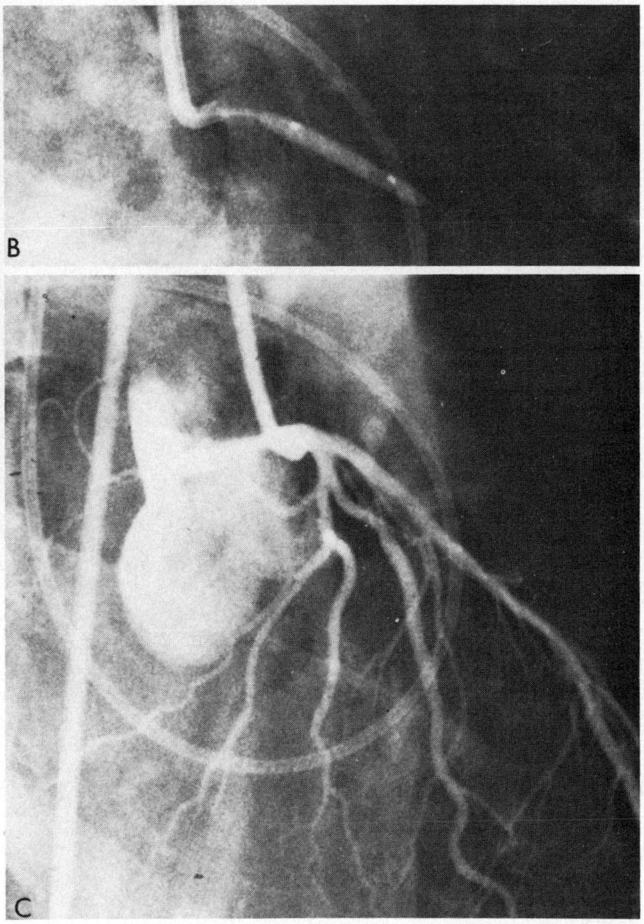

FIGURE 9–13 Balloon dilation of coronary artery. Coronary arteriography cine frames obtained in the right anterior oblique projection before balloon dilation of proximal left anterior descending coronary artery stenosis (*top*), during inflation of the contrast-filled balloon on the dilation catheter, which has been passed across the stenosis over a 0.018-inch guidewire (*middle*), and after balloon dilation of the stenotic region (*bottom*). There is significant relief of stenosis following the dilation procedure. The stenosis was not altered by the intracoronary administration of nitroglycerin. (From Barry, W. H., and Levin, D. unpublished data.)

the past, IABP catheters have been inserted via a direct surgical approach, requiring a cutdown on the femoral artery and surgical repair of the artery after the balloon pump has been removed. With this method, however, the incidence of complications was not inconsiderable. For example, in the series reported by Pace et al.[179] from the Brigham and Women's Hospital, thrombotic or embolic occlusion of the femoral artery occurred in 29 per cent of the patients, and there was a significant incidence of more severe problems, including dissection of the aorta or iliac artery, contributing to an overall mortality associated with the use of the balloon pump of 4.8 per cent.

Because of the widespread applicability of IABP, there has been great interest in developing techniques for percutaneous insertion and removal of the balloon catheter, in hopes of reducing the complication rate. The method that has been developed involves insertion of an IABP catheter through a No. 12 French sheath placed percutaneously in the femoral artery. The catheter is advanced into the central aorta under fluoroscopic control. Passage of the catheter past a tortuous iliac artery is facilitated by use of a 15-inch sheath that allows advancement of the sheath introducer into the abdominal aorta, leading with a guidewire.[180] More recently, an IABP catheter with a central lumen has been developed, and this also allows use of a guidewire during placement of the catheter in the central aorta,[181] as well as monitoring of central aortic pressure during counterpulsation. For removal, the catheter and sheath are withdrawn simultaneously, and the artery is compressed until hemostasis is achieved.

With these methods, successful insertion can be achieved in over 90 per cent of patients. The reported incidence of complications of this technique varies from 0 to 26 per cent[180–183] and is undoubtedly influenced in part by the population of patients in which it is employed. However, the incidence of severe complications, such as aortic or iliac dissection, appears lower with the percutaneous method, especially when the long sheath technique or the central lumen guidewire catheter is employed and fluoroscopy is utilized. The risk of ischemic limb complications remains significant, particularly in persons with atherosclerotic peripheral vascular disease and in women; in these patients the No. 12 French sheath may cause arterial obstruction. Therefore, use of IABP is usually restricted to those patients who are primarily Class IV with refractory myocardial ischemia, congestive heart failure, or cardiogenic shock.

Miscellaneous Therapeutic Procedures. The technique of *balloon atrial septostomy*, developed by Rashkind, has become a standard procedure to improve mixing between systemic and pulmonary circulations in neonates with transposition of the great arteries and in patients with intact atrial septum or inadequate interatrial communication (Chap. 29).[184,185,185a]

There has been extensive experience primarily in Japan and Germany with *nonoperative closure of a patent ductus*

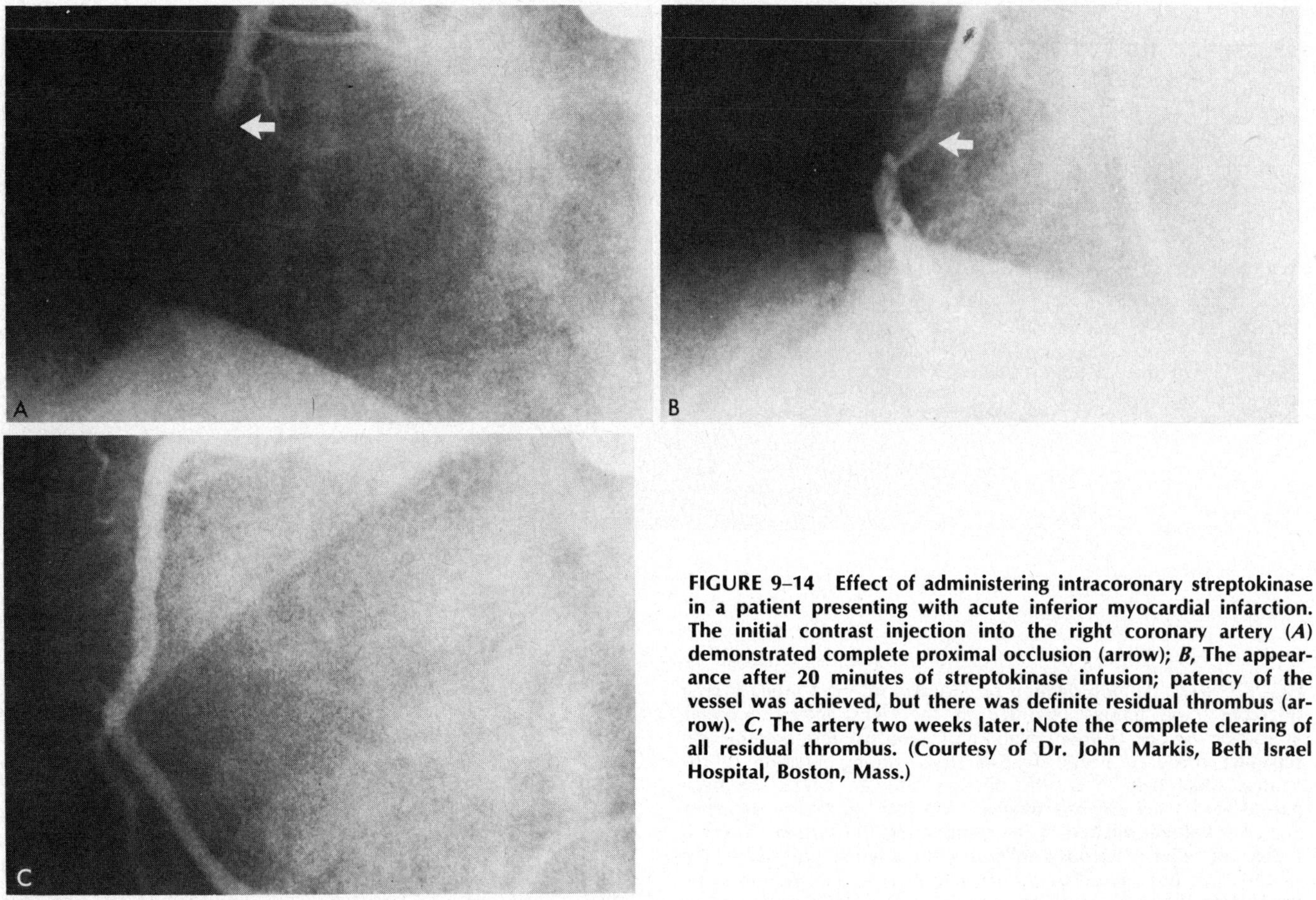

FIGURE 9–14 Effect of administering intracoronary streptokinase in a patient presenting with acute inferior myocardial infarction. The initial contrast injection into the right coronary artery (*A*) demonstrated complete proximal occlusion (arrow); *B*, The appearance after 20 minutes of streptokinase infusion; patency of the vessel was achieved, but there was definite residual thrombus (arrow). *C*, The artery two weeks later. Note the complete clearing of all residual thrombus. (Courtesy of Dr. John Markis, Beth Israel Hospital, Boston, Mass.)

arteriosus (Chap. 30).[185a,186–188] This has been accomplished by insertion of a plug, mounted on the tip of a catheter, into the patent ductus. Extension of this technique to *closure of an atrial septal defect* using a transvenous umbrella technique has bee reported.[185a,189,190]

A technique for *transvenous pulmonary embolectomy* has been devised that utilizes a catheter with a suction-cupped tip.[191,192] This catheter is advanced to the pulmonary artery, and its tip is manipulated by externally controlled, braided wires within its wall until the suction cup makes contact with the embolus. The application of suction by syringe produces adherence of the end of the embolus to the suction cup, and the catheter and suction cup are then withdrawn together with the embolus.

In another interesting therapeutic application of cardiac catheterization, Taylor and colleagues have reported therapeutic *embolization of the pulmonary artery* in pulmonary arteriovenous fistulas.[193]

Special "snare" catheters have been designed to *retrieve from within the heart catheter fragments* introduced iatrogenically.[194,195] Use of these techniques can obviate thoracotomy and cardiotomy.

This is by no means an exhaustive description of all the therapeutic uses of cardiac catheterization but should serve to illustrate how techniques originally developed to perform hemodynamic measurements have evolved into the therapeutic procedures. Thus, it is clear that cardiac catheterization can no longer be considered solely a diagnostic procedure.

References

1. Cournand, A.: Cardiac catheterization. Development of the technique, its contributions to experimental medicine, and its initial application in man. Acta Med. Scand. *579* (Suppl.):1, 1975.
2. Forssmann, W.: Die Sondierung des rechten Herzens. Klin. Wschr. *8*:2085, 1929.
3. Klein, O.: Zur Bestimmung des zirkulatorischen Minutensvolumen nach dem Fickschen Prinzip, Münch. Med. Wschr. *77*:1311, 1930.
4. Cournand, A. F., and Ranges, H. S.: Catheterization of the right auricle in man. Proc. Soc. Exp. Biol. Med. *46*:462, 1941.
5. Richards, D. W.: Cardiac output by the catheterization technique in various clinical conditions. Fed. Proc. *4*:215, 1945.
6. Cournand, A. F., Riley, R. L., Breed, E. S., Baldwin, E. F., and Richards, D. W.: Measurement of cardiac output in man using the technique of catheterization of the right auricle. J. Clin. Invest. *24*:106, 1945.
7. Dexter, L., Haynes, F. W., Burwell, C. S., Eppinger, E. C., Sagerson, R. P., and Evans, J. M.: Studies of congenital heart disease. II. The pressure and oxygen content of blood in the right auricle, right ventricle, and pulmonary artery in control patients, with observations on the oxygen saturation and source of pulmonary "capillary" blood. J. Clin. Invest. *26*:554, 1947.
8. Hellems, H. K., Haynes, F. W., and Dexter, L.: Pulmonary "capillary" pressure in man. J. Appl. Physiol. *2*:24, 1949.
9. Lagerlof, H., and Werkö, L.: Studies on circulation of blood in man. Scand. J. Clin. Lab. Invest. *7*:147, 1949.
10. McMichael, J., and Sharpey-Schafer, E. P.: The action of intravenous digoxin in man. Qt. J. Med. *13*:1123, 1944.
11. Lenegre, J., and Maurice, P.: Premiers recherches sur la pression ventriculaire droite. Bull. Mem. Soc. Med. Hop. Paris *80*:239, 1944.
12. Lenegre, J., and Maurice, P.: La derivation directe intracavitaire des courants electrique de l'oreillette et du ventriculaire droite. Paris Med. *35*:23, 1945.

13. Stead, E. A., Jr., and Warren, J. V.: Cardiac output in man: Analysis of mechanisms varying cardiac output based on recent clinical studies. Arch. Intern. Med. *80*:237, 1947.
14. Stead, E. A., Jr., Warren, J. V., and Brannon, E. S.: Cardiac output in congestive heart failure: Analysis of reasons for lack of close correlation between symptoms of heart failure and resting cardiac output. Am. Heart J. *35*: 529, 1948.
15. Bing, R. J., Hammond, M. M., Handelsman, J. C., Powers, S. R., Spencer, F. C., Eckenhoff, J. E., Goodale, W. T., Italkenschiel, J. H., and Kety, S. S.: Catheterization of coronary sinus and middle cardiac vein in man. Proc. Soc. Exp. Biol. Med. *66*:239, 1947.
16. Bing, R. J., Vandam, L. D., Gregoire, F., Handelsman, J. C., Goodale, W. T., and Echenhoff, J. E.: Measurement of coronary blood flow, oxygen consumption and efficiency of the left ventricle in man. Am. Heart J. *38*:1, 1949.
17. Vandam, L. D., Bing, R. J., and Gray, F. D., Jr.: Physiological studies in congenital heart disease. IV. Measurements of circulation in 5 selected cases. Bull. John Hopkins Hosp. *81*:192, 1947.
18. Bing, R. J., Vandam, L. D., and Gray, F. D., Jr.: Physiological studies in congenital heart disease. I. Procedures. Bull. Johns Hopkins Hosp. *80*:107, 1947.
19. Burchell, H. B.: Cardiac catheterization in diagnosis of various cardiac malformations and diseases. Proc. Mayo Clin. *23*:481, 1948.
20. Wood, E. H., Geraci, J. E., Pollack, A. A., Groom, D., Taylor, B. D., Pender, J. W., and Puch, D. G.: General and special techniques in cardiac catheterization. Proc. Mayo Clin. *23*:494, 1948.
21. Burwell, C. S., and Dexter, L.: Beri-beri heart disease. Trans. Assoc. Am. Physicians *60*:59, 1947.
22. Harvey, R. M., Ferrer, M. I., Cathcart, R. T., Richards, D. W., Jr., and Cournand, A.: Some effects of digoxin upon heart and circulation in man: Digoxin in left ventricular failure. Am. J. Med. *7*:439, 1949.
23. Zimmerman, H. A., Scott, R. W., and Becker, N. D.: Catheterization of the left side of the heart in man. Circulation *1*:357, 1950.
24. Limon Lason, R., and Bouchard, A.: El cateterismo intracardico; cateterization de las cavidades izquierdas en el hombre. Registro simultaneo de presion y electrocardiograma intracavetarios. Arch. Inst. Cardiol. Mexico *21*:271, 1950.
25. Seldinger, S. I.: Catheter replacement of the needle in percutaneous arteriography: A new technique. Acta Radiol. *39*:368, 1953.
26. Ross, J., Jr.: Transseptal left heart catheterization: A new method of left atrial puncture. Ann. Surg. *149*:395, 1959.
27. Ross, J., Jr., Braunwald, E., and Morrow, A. G.: Transseptal left atrial puncture: A new method for the measurement of left atrial pressure in man. Am. J. Cardiol. *3*:653, 1959.
28. Sones, F. M., Jr., Shirey, E. K., Proudfit, W. L., and Westcott, R. N.: Cine coronary arteriography. Circulation *20*:773, 1959.
29. Sones, F. M., Jr., and Shirey, E. K.: Cine coronary arteriography. Mod. Concepts Cardiovasc. Dis. *31*:735, 1962.
30. Swan, H. J. C., Ganz, W., Forrester, J., Marcus, H., Diamond, G., and Chonette, D.: Catheterization of the heart in man with use of a flow directed balloon-tipped catheter. N. Engl. J. Med. *283*:447, 1970.
31. Grossman, W.: Cardiac Catheterization and Angiography. 2nd ed. Philadelphia, Lea and Febiger, 1980.
32. Sprawls, P., Jr.: The Physical Principles of Diagnostic Radiology. Baltimore, University Park Press, 1977, pp. 1–166.
33. Reuter, F. G.: Physician and patient exposure during cardiac catheterization. Circulation *58*:134, 1978.
34. Barry, W. H., Levin, D. C., Green, L. H., Bettman, M. A., Mudge, G. H., Jr., and Phillips, D.: Left heart catheterization and angiography via the percutaneous femoral approach using an arterial sheath. Cathet. Cardiosvasc. Diagn. *5*:401, 1979.
35. Karsh, D. L., Michaelson, S. P., Langon, R. A., Cohen, L. S., and Wolfson, S.: Retrograde left ventricular catheterization in patients with an aortic valve prosthesis. Am. J. Cardiol. *41*:893, 1978.
36. Brockenbrough, E. C., and Braunwald, E.: A new technique for left ventricular angiocardiography and transseptal left heart catheterization. Am. J. Cardiol. *6*: 1062, 1960.
37. Keane, J. F., Freed, M. D., Fellows, K. E., and Fyler, D. C.: Pediatric cardiac angiocardiography using a 4 French catheter. Cathet. Cardiovasc. Diagn. *3*: 313, 1977.
38. Lees, M. H., Bristow, J. D., Way, C., and Brown, M.: Cardiac output by Fick principle in infants and young children. Am. J. Dis. Child. *114*:144, 1967.
39. Jarmakani, J. M.: Cardiac catheterization in heart disease in infants, children, and adolescents. *In* Moss, A. J., Adams, F. H., and Emmanouilides, G. C. (eds.): Heart Disease in Infants and Children. Baltimore, Williams and Wilkins Co., 1977.
40. Nachnani, G. H., Lessin, L. S., Motomiya, T., and Leusen, W. N.: Scanning electron microscopy of thrombogenesis on vascular catheter surfaces. N. Engl. J. Med. *286*:139, 1972.
41. Fry, D. L.: Physiologic recording by modern instruments with particular reference to pressure recording. Physiol. Rev. *40*:753, 1960.
42. Noble, F. W.: Electrical Methods of Blood Pressure Recording. Springfield, Ill., Charles C. Thomas, 1953.
43. McDonald, D. A.: Blood flow in Arteries. 2nd ed. Baltimore, Williams and Wilkins Co., 1974.
44. Wood, E. H., Leusen, I. R., Warner, H. R., and Wright, J. L.: Measurement of pressures in man by cardiac catheters. Circ. Res. *2*:294, 1954.
45. Grossman, W., McLaurin, L. P., and Stefadouros, M. A.: Left ventricular stiffness associated with chronic pressure and volume overloads in man. Circ. Res. *35*:793, 1974.
46. Guyton, A. C., Jones, C. E., and Coleman, T. G.: Circulatory Physiology: Cardiac Output and Its Regulation. 2nd ed. Philadelphia, W. B. Saunders Co., 1973.
47. Fick, A.: Über die Messung des Blutquantums in den Herzventrikeln. Sitz der Physik. Med. Ges. Wurzburg 1870, p. 16.
48. Van Slyke, D. D., and Neill, J. M.: The determination of gases in blood and other solutions by vacuum extraction and manometric measurements. J. Biol. Chem. *8*:654, 1962.
49. Barratt-Boyes, B. G., and Wood, E. H.: The oxygen saturation of blood in the venae cavae, right heart chambers, and pulmonary vessels of healthy subjects. J. Lab. Clin. Med. *50*:93, 1957.
50. Selzer, A., and Sudrann, R. B.: Reliability of the determination of cardiac output in man by means of the Fick principle. Circ. Res. *6*:485, 1958.
51. Thomassen, B.: Cardiac output in normal subjects under standard conditions. The repeatability of measurements by the Fick method. Scand. J. Clin. Lab. Invest. *9*:365, 1957.
52. Visscher, M. B., and Johnson, J. A.: The Fick principle: Analysis of potential errors and its conventional application. J. Appl. Physiol. *5*:635, 1953.
53. Stewart, G. N.: Researches on the circulation time and on the influences which affect it. IV. The output of the heart. J. Physiol. *22*:159, 1897.
54. Hamilton, W. F., Riley, R. L., Attyah, A. M., Cournand, A., Fowell, D. M., Himmelstein, A., Noble, R. P., Remington, J. W., Richards, D. W., Wheeler, N. C., and Witham, A. C.: Comparison of Fick and dye injection methods of measuring cardiac output in man. Am. J. Physiol. *153*:309, 1948.
55. Rahimtoola, S. H., and Swan, H. J. C.: Calculation of cardiac output from indicator dilution curves in the presence of mitral regurgitation. Circulation *31*: 711, 1965.
56. Shepherd, R. L., Higgs, L. M., and Glancy, D. L.: Comparison of left ventricular and pulmonary arterial injection sites in determination of cardiac output by the indicator dilution technique. Chest *62*:175, 1972.
57. Reddy, P. S., Curtiss, E. I., Bell, B., O'Toole, J. D., Salerni, R., Leon, D. F., and Shaver, J. A.: Determinants of variation between Fick and indicator dilution estimates of cardiac output during diagnostic catheterization. Fick vs. dye outputs. J. Lab. Clin. Med. *87*:568, 1976.
58. Branthwaite, M. A., and Bradley, R. D.: Measurement of cardiac output by thermodilution in man. J. Appl. Physiol. *24*:434, 1968.
59. Ganz, W., Donoso, R., Marcus, H. S., Forrester, J. S., and Swan, H. J. C.: A new technique for measurements of cardiac output by thermodilution in man. Am. J. Cardiol. *27*:392, 1971.
60. Kinsman, J. M., Moore, J. W., and Hamilton, W. F.: Studies on the circulation. I. Injection method. Physical and mathematical considerations. Am. J. Physiol. *89*:322, 1929.
61. Moore, J. W., Kinsman, J. M., Hamilton, W. G., and Spurling R. G.: Studies on the circulation. II. Cardiac output determinations; comparison of the injection method with the direct Fick procedure. Am. J. Physiol. *89*:331, 1929.
62. Doyle, J. T., Wilson, J. S., Lepine, C., and Warren, J. V.: An evaluation of the measurement of the cardiac output and of the so-called pulmonary blood volume by the dye-dilution method. J. Lab. Clin. Med. *41*:29, 1953.
63. Eliasch, H., Lagerlof, H., Bucht, H., Ek, J., Eriksson, K., Bergstrom, J., and Werkö, L.: Comparison of the dye dilution and the direct Fick methods for the measurement of cardiac output in man. Scand. J. Lab. Clin. Invest. *7* (Suppl. 20):73, 1955.
64. Dalen, J. E.: Shunt detection and measurement. *In* Grossman, W. (ed.): Cardiac Catheterization and Angiography. Philadelphia, Lea and Febiger, 1974, p. 96.
65. Dexter, L., Haynes, F. W., Burwell, C. S., Springer, E. C., Seibel, R. E., and Evans, J. M.: Studies of congenital heart disease. I. Technique of venous catheterization as a diagnostic procedure. J. Clin. Invest. *26*:547, 1947.
66. Hyman, A. L., Myers, W., Hyatt, K., DeGraff, A. C., Jr., and Quiroy, A. C.: A comparison study of the detection of cardiovascular shunts by oxygen analysis and indicator dilution methods. Ann. Intern. Med. *56*:535, 1962.
67. Swan, H. J. C., and Wood, E. H.: Localization of cardiac defects by dye dilution curves recorded after injection of T-1824 at multiple sites in the heart and great vessels during cardiac catheterization. Proc. Staff Meet. Mayo Clin. *28*: 95, 1953.
68. Castillo, C. A., Kyle, J. C., Gilson, W. E., and Rowe, G. G.: Simulated shunt curves. Am. J. Cardiol. *17*:691, 1966.
69. Flamm, M. D., Cohn, K. E., and Hancock, E. W.: Measurement of systemic cardiac output at rest and exercise in patients with atrial septal defect. Am. J. Cardiol. *23*:258, 1969.
70. Ganz, W., Tamura, K., Marcus, H. S., Donose, R., Yoshida, S., and Swan, H. J. C.: Measurement of coronary sinus blood flow by continuous thermodilution in man. Circulation *44*:181, 1971.
71. Rapaport, E., and Dexter, L.: Pulmonary "capillary" pressure. *In* Methods in Medical Research. Chicago, Year Book Medical Publishers, *7*:85, 1958.
72. Connolly, D. C., Kirklin, J. W., and Wood, E. H.: The relationship between pulmonary artery pressure and left atrial pressure in man. Circ. Res. *2*:434, 1954.
73. Barratt-Boyes, B. G., and Wood, E. H.: Cardiac output and related

measurements and pressure values in the right heart and associated vessels, together with an analysis of the hemodynamic response to the inhalation of high oxygen mixtures in healthy subjects. J. Lab. Clin. Med. *51*:72, 1958.
74. Goldberg, S., Grossman, W., and Mann, J. T.: Vasodilator therapy of heart failure in the setting of valvular heart disease: Determinants of increased cardiac output. Am. J. Med. *65*:161, 1978.
75. Cohn, J. N.: Vasodilator therapy for heart failure. The influence of impedance on left ventricular performance. Circulation *48*:5, 1973.
76. Chatterjee, K.: Vasodilator therapy for heart failure. Ann. Intern. Med. *83*: 421, 1975.
77. Braunwald, E., Welch, G. H., Jr., and Morrow, A. G.: The effects of acutely increased systemic resistance on the left atrial pressure pulse: A method for the clinical detection of mitral insufficiency. J. Clin. Invest. *37*:35, 1958.
78. Grossman, W., Harshaw, C. W., Munro, A. B., Becker, L., and McLaurin, L. P.: Lowered aortic impedance as therapy for severe mitral regurgitation. J. A. M. A. *230*:1101, 1974.
79. Harshaw, C. W., Munro, A. B., McLaurin, L. P., and Grossman, W.: Reduced systemic vascular resistance as therapy for severe mitral regurgitation of valvular origin. Ann. Intern. Med. *83*:312, 1976.
80. Bolen, J. L., and Alderman, E. L.: Hemodynamic consequences of afterload reduction in patients with chronic aortic regurgitation. Circulation *53*:879, 1976.
81. Goodman, D. J., Rossen, R. M., Holloway, E. L., Alderman, E. L., and Harrison, D. C.: Effect of nitroprusside on left ventricular dynamics in mitral regurgitation, Circulation *50*:1025, 1974.
82. Chatterjee, K., Parmley, W. W., Massie, B., Greenberg, B., Werner, J., Klausner, S., and Norman A.: Oral hydralazine therapy for chronic refractory heart failure. Circulation *54*:879, 1976.
83. Miller, R. R., Vismara, L. A., Zelis, R., Amsterdam, E. A., and Mason, D. T.: Clinical use of sodium nitroprusside in chronic ischemic heart disease. Effects on peripheral vascular resistance, venous tone, and on ventricular volume, pump, and mechanical performance. Circulation *51*:328, 1975.
84. Fritts, H. W., Harris, P., Clauss, R. H., Odell, J. E., and Cournand, A.: The effect of acetylcholine on the human pulmonary circulation under normal and hypoxic conditions. J. Clin. Invest. *37*:99, 1958.
85. Wood, P., Besterman, E. M., Towers, M. K., and McIlroy, M. B.: The effect of acetylcholine on pulmonary vascular resistance and left atrial pressure in mitral stenosis. Br. Heart J. *19*:279, 1957.
86. Dresdale, D. T., Michton, R. J., and Schultz, M.: Recent studies in primary pulmonary hypertension including pharmacodynamic observations on pulmonary vascular resistance. Bull. N. Y. Acad. Med. *30*:195, 1954.
87. Rudolph, A. M., Paul, M. H., Sommer, L. S., and Nadas, A. S.: Effects of tolazoline hydrochloride (Priscoline) on circulatory dynamics of patients with pulmonary hypertension. Am. Heart J. *55*:424, 1958.
88. Vogel, J. H. K., Grover, R. F., Jamieson, G., and Blount, S. G., Jr.: Long term physiologic observations in patients with ventricular septal defect and increased pulmonary vascular resistance. Adv. Cardiol. *11*:108, 1974.
89. Grover, R. F., Reeves, T. J., and Blount, S. G., Jr.: Tolazoline hydrochloride (Priscoline): An effective pulmonary vasodilator. Am. Heart J. *61*:5, 1961.
90. Brammel, H. L., Vogel, J. H. K., Pryor, R., and Blount, S. G., Jr.: The Eisenmenger syndrome. Am. J. Cardiol. *28*:679, 1971.
91. Moret, P., Covarrubias, E., Condert, J., and Duchosall, F.: Cardiocirculatory adaptation to chronic hypoxia. Acta Cardiol. (Brux.) *27*:596, 1972.
92. Penazola, D., Sime, F., Banchero, N., Gamboa, R., Cruz, J., and Marticorena, E.: Pulmonary hypertension in healthy men born and living at high altitudes. Am. J. Cardiol. *11*:150, 1963.
93. Vogel, J. H. K., Weaver, W. F., Rose, R. L., Blount, S. G., Jr., and Grover, R. F.: Pulmonary hypertension on exertion in normal men living at 10,150 feet (Leadville, Colorado). Med. Thorac. *19*:461, 1962.
94. Milnor, W. R.: Pulsatile blood flow. N. Engl. J. Med. *287*:27, 1972.
95. Nichols, W. W., Conti, C. R., Walker, W. E., and Milnor, W. R.: Input impedance of the systemic circulation in man. Circ. Res. *40*:421, 1977.
96. Gorlin, R., and Gorlin, G.: Hydraulic formula for calculation of area of stenotic mitral valve, other valves, and central circulatory shunts. Am. Heart J. *41*:1, 1951.
97. Cohen, M. V., and Gorlin, R.: Modified orifice equation for the calculation of mitral valve area. Am. Heart J. *84*:839, 1972.
98. Marshall, R. J., and Shepherd, J. J.: Cardiac function in health and disease. Philadelphia, W. B. Saunders Co., 1968.
99. St. John Sutton, M. G., St. John Sutton, M., Aldershaw, P., Sacchetti, R., Paneth, M., Lennox, S. C., Gibson, R. V., and Gibson, D. G.: Valve replacement without preoperative cardiac catheterization. N. Eng. J. Med. *305*: 1233, 1981.
100. Roberts, W. C.: No cardiac catheterization before cardiac valve replacement—a mistake. Am. Heart J. *103*:930, 1982.
101. Alpert, J. S., Sloss, L. J., Cohn, P. F., and Grossman, W.: The diagnostic accuracy of combined clinical and noninvasive cardiac evaluation: Comparison with findings at cardiac catheterization. Cathet. Cardiovasc. Diagn. *6*:359, 1980.
102. Lupi-Herrera, E., Sandoval, J., Seoane, M., and Bialostozky, D.: The role of hydralazine therapy for pulmonary arterial hypertension of unknown cause. Circulation *65*:648, 1982.
103. Diamond, G., Marcus, H., McHugh, T., Swan, H. J. C., and Forrester, J.: Catheterization of the left ventricle in acutely ill patients. Br. Heart J. *33*:489, 1971.
104. Gold, H. K., Keinbach, R. C., Sanders, C. A., Buckley, M. J., Mundth, E. D., and Austen, W. G.: Intraaortic balloon pumping for ventricular septal defect or mitral regurgitation complicating acute myocardial infarction. Circulation *47*:1191, 1973.
105. Gold, H. K., Leinbach, R. C., Sanders, C. A., Buckley, M. J., Mundth, E. D., and Austen, W. G.: Intraaortic balloon pumping for control of recurrent myocardial ischemia. Circulation *47*:1197, 1973.
106. O'Brien, K. P., Glancy, D. L., and Brandt, P. W. T.: Cardiac catheterization: indications, current techniques, and complications. Ausralast. Radiol. *14*:378, 1970.
107. Braunwald, E., and Swan, H. J. C. (eds.): Cooperative study on cardiac catheterization. Circulation *37* (Suppl. 111):1, 1968.
108. Mortensen, J. D.: Clinical sequelae from arterial needle puncture, cannulation, and incision. Circulation *35*:1118, 1967.
109. Kloster, F. E., Bristow, J. D., and Seaman, A. J.: Cardiac catheterization during anticoagulant therapy. Am. J. Cardiol. *28*:675, 1971.
110. Walker, W. J., Mundall, S. L., Broderick, H. G., Prasad, B., Kin, J., and Ravi, J. M.: Systemic heparinization for femoral percutaneous angiography. N. Engl. J. Med. *288*:826, 1973.
111. Mahrer, P. R., and Eshoo, N.: Outpatient cardiac catheterization and coronary angiography. Cathet. Cardiovasc. Diagn. *7*:355, 1981.
112. Perrigo, E. S., Kuehne, M. L., and Michienzi, F.: Twenty month experience in outpatient cardiac catheterization. Circulation *62*: (Supp. 111):216, 1980.
113. Sones, J. M., Jr.: Cine coronary arteriography. *In* Hurst, J. W., and Logue, R. B. (eds.): The Heart. 2nd ed. New York, McGraw-Hill Book Co., 1970, p. 377.
114. Sande, M. A., Levinson, M. E., Lukas, D. S., and Kaye, D.: Bacteremia associated with cardiac catheterization. N. Engl. J. Med. *281*:1104, 1969.
115. Green, G. S., McKinnon, C. M., Rosch, J., and Judkins, M. P.: Complications of selective percutaneous transfemoral coronary arteriography and their prevention. Circulation *45*:552, 1972.
116. Campion, B. C., Frye, R. L., Pluth, J. R., Fairbairn, J. F., and Davis, G. D.: Arterial complications of retrograde brachial arterial catheterization. Mayo Clin. Proc. *46*:589, 1971.
117. Jeresaty, R. M., and Liss, J. P.: Effects of artery catheterization on arterial pulse and blood pressure in 203 patients. Am. Heart J. *76*:481, 1968.
118. Machleder, H. I., Sweeney, J. P., and Barker, J. F.: Pulseless arm after brachial artery catheterization. Lancet *1*:407, 1972.
119. Bristow, J. D., Seaman, A. J., Kloster, F. E., Herr, R. H., and Griswold, H. E.: Late, heparin-induced bleeding after retrograde arterial catheterization. Circulation *37*:393, 1968.
120. Kloster, F. E., Bristow, J. D., and Griswold, H. E.: Femoral artery occlusion following percutaneous catheterization. Am. Heart J. *79*:175, 1970.
121. Gupta, P. K., and Haft, J. I.: Complete heart block complicating cardiac catheterization. Chest *61*:185, 1972.
122. Chahine, R. A., Herman, M. V., and Gorlin, R.: Complications of coronary arteriography: Comparison of the brachial to the femoral approach. Ann. Intern. Med. *76*:862, 1972.
123. Eshagy, B., Loeb, H. S., Miller, S. E., Scanlon, P. J., Towne, W. D., and Gunnar, R. M.: Mediastinal and retropharyngeal hemorrhage: A complication of cardiac catheterization. J. A. M. A. *226*:427, 1973.
124. Brener, B. J., and Couch, N. P.: Peripheral arterial complications of left heart catheterization and their management, Am. J. Surg. *125*:521, 1973.
125. Hey, E. G., Jr., Dyrda, I., and Joyner, C. R.: Entanglement of a cardiac catheter on a heart valve prosthesis. N. Engl. J. Med. *275*:434, 1966.
126. Goodman, D. J., Rider, A. K., Billingham, M. E., and Schroeder, J. S.: Thromboembolic complications with the indwelling balloon tipped pulmonary arterial catheter. N. Engl. J. Med. *291*:777, 1974.
127. Stanger, P., Heymann, M. A., Tarnoff, H., Hoffman, J. I. E., and Rudolph, A. M.: Complications of cardiac catheterization of neonates, infants and children. Circulation *50*:595, 1974.
128. Murphy, T. O., Piper, C. A., and Anderson, C. L.: Complications of left heart catheterization. Am. Surgeon *37*:472, 1971.
129. Price, H. P., and Takaro, T.: Unusual coronary emboli associated with coronary arteriography. Chest *63*:698, 1973.
130. Walson, W. J., Lee, G. B., and Amplatz, K.: Biplane selective coronary arteriography via percutaneous transfemoral approach. Am. J. Roentgenol. *100* : 332, 1967.
131. Takaro, T., Pifarre, R., and Wuerflein, R. D.: Acute coronary occlusion following coronary arteriography: Mechanisms and surgical relief. Surgery *72*: 1018, 1972.
132. Nicholas, G. G., and DeMuth, W. E.: Long term results of brachial thrombectomy following cardiac catheterization. Ann. Surg. *183*:436, 1976.
133. Smith, W. R., Glauser, F. L., and Jemison, P.: Ruptured chordae of the tricuspid valve: The consequence of flow directed Swan-Ganz catheterization. Chest *70*:790, 1976.
134. Roberts, R., Ludbrook, P. A., Weiss, E. S., and Sobel, B. E.: Serum CPK isoenzymes after cardiac catheterization. Br. Heart J. *37*:1144, 1975.
135. Takahashi, O., Zakheim, R., Park, M. K., Mattioli, L., and Diehl, A. M.: The effects of transfemoral cardiac catheterization on limb blood flow in children. Chest *71*:159, 1977.
136. Rosengart, R., Nelson, R. J., and Emmanoulides, G. C.: Anterior tibial compartment syndrome in a child: An unusual complication of cardiac catheterization. Pediatrics *58*:456, 1967.
137. Dawson, D. M., and Fisher, E. G.: Neurologic complications of cardiac catheterization. Neurology *27*:496, 1977.

138. Bousvaros, G. A., Conway, D., and Hopps, J. A.: An electrical hazard of selective angiocardiography. Can. Med. Assoc. J. *87*:286, 1962.
139. Starmer, C. F., Whalen, R. E., and McIntosh, H. D.: Hazards of electric shock in cardiology. Am. J. Cardiol. *14*:537, 1964.
140. Mody, S. M., and Richings, M.: Ventricular fibrillation resulting from electrocution during cardiac catheterization. Lancet *2*:698, 1962.
141. Starmer, C. F., McIntosh, H. D., and Whalen, R. E.: Electrical hazards and cardiovascular function. N. Engl. J. Med. *284*:181, 1971.
142. Lang, E. K.: A survey of a complications of percutaneous retrograde arteriography, Seldinger technique. Radiology *81*:257, 1963.
143. Adrouny, Z. A., Stephenson, M. J., Straube, K. R., Dotter, C. T., and Griswold, H. E.: Effect of cardiac catheterization and angiocardiography on the serum glutamic oxalozcetic transminase. Circulation *27*:565, 1963.
144. Burckhardt, D., Vera, C. A., LaDue, J. S., and Steinberg, I.: Enzyme activity following angiography. Am. J. Roentgenol. *102*:406, 1968.
145. Kennedy, J. W.: Complications associated with cardiac catheterization and angiography. Cathet. Cardiovasc. Diagn. *8*:5, 1982.
146. Davis, K., Kennedy, J. W., Kemp, H. G., Jr., Judkins, M. P., Gosselin, A. F., and Killip, T.: Complications of coronary arteriography. Circulation *59*:1105, 1979.
147. Shabetai, R., and Adolph, R. J.: Principles of cardiac catheterization *In* Fowler, H. O. (ed.): Cardiac Diagnosis and Treatment. 2nd ed. Hagerstown, Md., Harper and Row, p. 86.
148. Sutton, D. C., and Sutton, G. C.: Needle biopsy of the human ventricular myocardium. Review of 54 consecutive cases. Am. Heart J. *60*:364, 1960.
149. Bulloch, R. T., Murphy, M. L., Pearce, M. B.: Intracardiac needle biopsy of the ventricular septum. Am. J. Cardiol. *16*:227, 1965.
150. Hirose, T., and Bailey, C. P.: New myocardial biopsy needle. Angiology *16*: 288, 1965.
151. Sakakibara, S., and Konno, S.: Endomyocardial biopsy. Jap. Heart J. *3*:537, 1962.
152. Caves, P., Billingham, M. B., Coltart, J., Rider, A., and Stinson, E.: Transvenous endomyocardial biopsy—application of a method for diagnosing heart disease. Postgrad. Med. J. *51*:286, 1975.
153. Hess, O. M., Schneider, J., Turina, M., Heeb, S., Grob, P., and Krayenbuehl, K. P.: Die transvenose Endomyokardbiopsie in der Bewiteilung der kongestivan Kardiomyopathie. Schweiz. Med. Wschr. *109*:293, 1977.
154. Mason, J. W.: Technique for right and left ventricular endomyocardial biopsy. Am. J. Cardiol. *41*:887, 1978.
155. Olsen, E. G. J.: Results of endomyocardial biopsy—histological, histochemical and ultrastructural analysis. Postgrad Med. J. *51*:295, 1975.
156. Peters, T. J., Brooksby, I. A. B., Webb-Peploe, M. M., Wells, G., Jenkins, B. S., and Coltart, D. J.: Enzymic analysis of cardiac biopsy material from patients with valvular heart disease. Lancet *1*:269, 1976.
157. Kawai, C., and Kitaura, Y.: New endomyocardial biopsy catheter for the left ventricle. Am J. Cardiol. *40*:63, 1977.
158. Colucci, W. S., Lorell, B. H., Schoen, F. J., Warhol, M. J., and Grossman, W.: Hypertrophic obstruction due to Fabry's disease, N. Engl. J. Med. *307*:926, 1982.
159. Bristow, M. R., Mason, J. W., Billingham, M. E., and Daniels, J. R.: Doxorubicin cardiomyopathy: Evaluation by phonocardiography, endomyocardial biopsy, and cardiac catherization. Ann. Intern. Med. *88*: 168, 1978
160. Nippoldt, T. B., Edwards, W. D., Holmes, D. R., Relder, G. S., Hartzler, G. O., and Smith, H. C.: Right ventricular endomyocardial biopsy. Clinicopathologic correlates in 100 consecutive patients. Mayo Clin. Proc. *57*: 407, 1982.
161. Mason, J. W., Billingham, M. E., and Ricci, D. R.: Treatment of acute inflammatory myocarditis assisted by endomyocardial biopsy. Am. J. Cardiol. *45*: 1037, 1980.
162. Grüntzig, A. R., Jenning, A., and Siegenthaler, W. E.: Non-operative dilation of coronary artery stenosis. N. Eng. J. Med. *301*:61, 1979.
163. Grüntzig, A.: Transluminal dilatation of coronary artery stenosis. Lancet *1*:263, 1978.
164. Grüntzig, A.: Perkutane Dilatation von Koronarstenosen—Beschreibung eines neuen Kathetersystems. Klin. Wschr. *54*:543, 1976.
165. Grüntzig, A., Schneider, H. J.: Die perkutane dilatation chronischer Koronarstenosen—Experiment und Morphologie. Schweiz. Med. Wschr. *107*: 1588, 1977.
166. Grüntzig, A., Myler, R. K., Hamma, E. S., and Turina, M. I.: Coronary transluminal angioplasty. Circulation *56* (Suppl. 11):316, 1977.
167. Grüntzig, A., and Hepff, H.: Perkuntane Rekanalization chronischer arterieller Verschlusse mitg einen neuen Dilatationkatheter. Deutsch. Med. Wschr. *99*: 2502, 1974.
168. Simpson, J. B., Baim, D. S. Robert, E. W., and Harrison, D. C.: A new catheter system for coronary angioplasty. Am. J. Cardiol. *49*:1216, 1982.
169. Kent, K. M., et al.: Percutaneous transluminal coronary angioplasty: Report from the Registry of the National Heart, Lung, and Blood Institute. Am. J. Cardiol. *49*: 2011, 1982.
170 Williams, D. O., Riley, R. S., Singh, A. K., Gervertz, H., and Most, A. H.: Evaluation of the role of coronary angioplasty in patients with unstable angina pecrotis. Am. Heart J. *102*:1, 1981.
171. Crowley, M. J., Vetorovee, G. W., and Wolfgang, T. C.: Efficacy of percutaneous transluminal coronary angioplasty: Technique, patient selection, laboratory results, limitations, and complications. Am. Heart J. *101*:272, 1981.
172. Rentrop, P., Blanke, H., Karsch, K. R., Daiser, H. Kostering, H, and Leitz, K.: Selective intracoronary thrombolysis in acute myocardial infarction and unstable angina pectoris. Circulation *63*:307, 1981.
173. Ganz, W., Buchburder, N., Marcus, H., Mondkar, A., Maddahi, J., Charuzi, Y., O'Connor, L., Shell, W., Fishbein, M., Kass, R., Miyamoto, A., and Swan, H. J. C.: Intracoronary thrombolysis in evolving myocardial infarction. Am. Heart J. *101*:4, 1981.
174. Mathey, D. G., Kuch, K. H., Tilsner, V., Krebber, H. J., and Bleifeld, W.: Nonsurgical coronary artery recanalization in acute transmural myocardial infarction. Circulation *63*:489–497, 1981.
175. Markis, J. E., Malagold, M., Parker, J. A., Silverman, K. J., Barry, W. H., Als, A. V., Paulin, S., Grossman, W., and Braunwald, E.: Myocardial salvage after intracoronary thrombolysis with streptokinase in acute myocardial infarction. N. Engl. J. Med. *305*:777, 1981.
176. Reduto, L. A., Smalling, R. W., Freund, G. C., and Gould, K. L.: Intracoronary infusion of streptokinase in patients with acute myocardial infarction: Effects of reperfusion on left ventricular performance. Am. J. Cardiol. *48*:403, 1981.
177. Rentrop, P., Blouke, H., and Karsch, K. R.: Effects of non-surgical coronary reperfusion on the left ventricle in human subjects compared with conventional treatment. Am. J. Cardiol. *49*:1, 1982.
178. Levine, F. H., Gold, H. K., Leinbach, R. G., Daggett, W. M., Austen, W. G., and Buckley, M. J.: Management of actute myocardial ischemia with intra-aortic balloon pumping and coronary bypass surgery. Circulation *58*:1, 1978.
179. Pace, P. D., Tilney, N. L., Lesch, M., and Couch, N. P.: Peripheral arterial complications of intra-aortic balloon counterpulsation. Surgery *88*:685, 1977.
180. Vignola, P. A., Swaye, P. S., Gosselin, A. F.: Guidelines for effective and safe intraaortic balloon pump insertion and removal. Am. J. Cardiol. *48*:660, 1981.
181. Leinbach, R. C., Goldstein, J., Gold, H. K., Moses, J. W., Collins, M. B., and Subramanian, V.: Percutaneous wire-guided balloon pumping. Am. J. Cardiol. *49*:1707, 1982.
182. Harvey, J. C., Goldstein, J. E., McCabe, J. C., Hoover, E. L., Gay, W. A., Jr., and Subramanian, V. A.: Complications of percutaneous intraaortic balloon pumping. Circulation *64* (Suppl. 11), 114, 1981.
183. Bregman, D., Nichols, A. B., Weiss, M. B., Powers, E. R., Martin, E. C., and Casarella, W. J.: Percutaneous intraaortic balloon insertion. Am. J. Cardiol. *46*:261, 1980.
184. Rashkind, W. J., and Miller, W. W.: Creation of an atrial septal defect without thoracotomy: A pallative approach to complete transposition of the great vessels. J.A.M.A. *196*:991, 1966.
185. Rashkind, W. J., and Miller, W. W.: Transposition of the great arteries: Results of palliation by balloon atrial septostomy in 31 patients. Circulation *38*:453, 1968.
185a. Rashkind, W. J.: Transcathetler treatment of congenital heart disease, Circulation *67*:711, 1983.
186. Porstmann, W., Wierny, L., and Warnke, H.: Der Verschluss des Ductus Arteriosus Persistens ohne Thorakotomie. Fortschr. Roentgenstr. *109*:133, 1968.
187. Porstmann, W., Wierny, L., Warnke, H., Gertsberger, G., and Romaniuk, P. A.: Catheter closure of patent ductus arteriosus: 62 cases treated without thoractomy. Radiol. Clin. North Am. *9*:203, 1971.
188. Sato, K., Fiyino, M., Kozuka, T., Naito, Y., Kitamura, S., Nakano, S., Ohyama, C., and Kawashima, Y.: Transfemoral plug closure of patent ductus arteriosus: Experience in 61 consecutive cases treated without thoractomy. Circulation *51*:337, 1975.
189. Mills, N. L., and King, T. D.: Nonoperative closure of left to right shunts. J. Thorac. Cardiovasc. Surg. *72*:371, 1976.
190. King, T. D., Thompson, S. L., Steiner, C., and Mills, N. L.: Secundum atrial septal defect. Nonoperative closure during cardiac catheterization. J.A.M.A. *235*:2506, 1976.
191. Scoggins, W. G., and Greenfield, L. J.: Transvenous pulmonary embolectomy for acute massive pulmonary embolism. Chest *71*:213, 1977.
192. Greenfield, L. J., Reif, M., and Guenter, C. A.: Hemodynamic and respiratory response to transvenous pulmonary embolectomy. J. Thorac. Cardiovasc. Surg. *62*:890, 1971.
193. Taylor, B. G., Cockerill, E. M., Manfredi, F., and Klatte, E.: Therapeutic embolization of the pulmonary artery in pulmonary arterio-venous fistula. Ann. J. Med. *64*:360, 1978.
194. Massumi, R. A., and Ross, A. M.: Atraumatic non-surgical techniques for removal of broken catheters from cardiac cavities. N. Engl. J. Med. *277*:195, 1967.
195. Bloomfield, A.: Techniques of non-surgical retrieval of iatrogenic foreign bodies from the heart. Ann. J. Cardiol. *27*:538, 1971.

10 CORONARY ARTERIOGRAPHY

by Goffredo G. Gensini, M.D.

Radner was the first to outline the coronary arteries in living man in 1945.[1] The earliest studies consisted of incidental opacifications of the coronary arteries at the time of retrograde aortography. Later, methods that would permit intentional, satisfactory visualization of the human coronary arteries were tested by many investigators. These methods included random injections, acetylcholine arrest, intrabronchial pressure elevation, occlusion aortography, and differential opacification of the aortic stream. These methods are of historical interest only. Extensive bibliographic references may be found in an earlier work on this subject.[2]

In May, 1959, Sones reported a straightforward approach to achieve opacification of the coronary arteries, i.e., the deliberate, selective catheterization of each vessel with a special catheter, designed by Sones himself.[3,4] He demonstrated that the human coronary arteries can be individually and selectively catheterized with safety, in both health and disease, provided that appropriate instrumentation and methods are used. In this light, all current methods of coronary arteriography may be considered as more or less successful modifications of Sones' original idea. Entire "families" of preshaped catheters have been developed by numerous investigators.[5–9] Generally speaking, these preshaped catheters make possible quick entry into the coronary arteries. In expert hands, both the Judkins' femoral approach[4] and Sones' brachial cutdown method have been shown to provide a high degree of safety and reliability.

TECHNIQUE

REQUISITES FOR SUCCESS. The requisites for successful catheterization of the coronary arteries are few: a properly designed catheter, a first-class imaging system, and an expert hand. A flawless cine camera and good filming techniques are necessary to insure appropriate recording of coronary opacifications. For the safety of the patient, a relatively nontoxic contrast agent, continuous electrocardiographic monitoring, frequent pressure monitoring, and a DC-defibrillator are necessary.

The ingredients for maintenance of efficiency in a cardiovascular laboratory are the quality, experience, and dedication of the personnel. In the author's opinion, selective coronary arteriography should be performed full time by physicians with a solid background in *cardiology.* No amount of elaborate radiological and electronic apparatus can take the place of the trained and experienced operator. On the other hand, in cine coronary arteriography, the appropriate selection and flawless performance of the equipment rank closely in importance to the skill and knowledge of the physician and technical personnel using the equipment.[2]

PATIENT TEACHING AND PREPARATION. The instruction and psychological preparation of the patient scheduled to undergo coronary arteriography should begin as soon as he or she arrives in the hospital. Physicians and nursing personnel caring for patients undergoing cardiovascular diagnostic procedures should be familiar with these tests and should be able to answer intelligently any of the patients' questions. Patients need to feel that the staff is competent and efficient. It is the duty of the cardiovascular team and of all personnel caring for these patients to gain their confidence and dispel doubts and unnecessary fears. The relative benefits and risks of coronary arteriography and what will be expected of the patient and what the patient should expect must be explained beforehand.

In certain x-ray projections, the diaphragm covers the distal portion of the coronary vessels and obscures some important areas of perfusion. During the procedure, therefore, the operator occasionally asks the patient to take a deep breath, hold it, and at the same time avoid bearing down, which would produce a Valsalva effect and elevate the diaphragm.

If signs of bradycardia appear following injection of contrast material into a coronary artery, the patient is instructed to cough. The patient should be told that a strong, immediate cough is expected in response to this directive. Bradycardia is an expected phenomenon in this setting, but if prolonged, it may be followed by extrasystoles and, eventually, ventricular fibrillation. As soon as the operator observes that a patient's heart rate is slowing, the catheter tip should be withdrawn from the coronary ostium, and the patient should be told to cough. Coughing clears the contrast agent from the vessel and acts as a mechanical stimulus to the heart. The instruction to cough should be given only by the physician manipulating the catheter.

I believe that it is desirable for patients to express their feelings about coming to the hospital and the performance of these tests. We encourage them to ask questions, even during the examination. One thing is certain: Patients who are relaxed and confident require less medication and are less likely to experience complications, such as peripheral arterial spasm and nausea, during coronary arteriography.

PREPARATION OF THE PATIENT

Although hospitalization is required for patients whose condition is unstable, and although in many laboratories hospitalization is required for all patients who undergo coronary arteriography, it is the author's practice to carry out coronary arteriography on an outpatient basis in elective, ambulatory cases. We admit such patients to the laboratory on the morning of the examination and discharge them several hours after the procedure, if their condition is stable. In our opinion, the clinical status of the patient and the suspected underlying pathology, rather than the arteriography itself, should dictate the mode of admission and the length of stay in the hospital, that is, which patient should be admitted as an inpatient before the procedure or, having come as an outpatient, should remain in the hospital after the procedure.

The author's facility for outpatient catheterization includes a large room immediately adjacent to the cardiac laboratory. This room is staffed by a nurse and it is furnished with five comfortable Barcaloungers. Privacy, when needed, is achieved using ceiling-mounted curtains that can effectively screen one easy chair from the others. A bed is also provided as a temporary alternative to the easy chair. Upon arrival in the outpatient facility, or upon admission to the hospital, the patient is visited by two members of the cardiovascular laboratory team and given a complete explanation of the procedure before being asked to sign a consent form. The possible risks of coronary arteriography are explained in simple, readily understandable terms. All of this information is also summarized in a booklet that is given to the patient and to his family at the time the appointment for the procedure is arranged.

For a patient with a history of valvular heart disease, ampicillin is ordered or, if he or she is allergic to penicillin, erythromycin. The patient should receive no solid food after midnight on the day of the examination but is encouraged to drink juices and water up to one hour prior to the procedure. One hour before the procedure, an electrocardiogram is recorded. Secobarbital, 100 mg, and diazepam (Valium), 5 mg, are given orally unless congestive heart failure is present, in which case secobarbital is omitted. If a patient takes digitalis daily, he or she should be given this medication before going to the laboratory. We recommend that patients who have been receiving propranolol be instructed to taper the dosage at least three days before any left-heart studies. High doses of propranolol depress myocardial contractility and produce hemodynamic changes that may result in increased left ventricular end-diastolic pressure and decreased ejection fraction.

Before each procedure, cardiovascular technicians specially trained to assist the physician during cardiac catheterization procedures prepare the necessary sterile instruments and pressure gauges. A pressurized drip containing 5000 units of heparin in 500 ml of 5 per cent dextrose and water rather than continuous pressure monitoring is used intraarterially to maintain catheter patency throughout the procedure. (Many laboratories utilize continuous pressure monitoring using a three-stopcock manifold.) Having prepared the pressurized drip, the technicians should make certain that the DC-defibrillator, located in the procedure room, is turned on and available, with paddles already spread with conductive paste for immediate use if necessary.

Upon arrival in the laboratory, the patient reclines on the Cardiodiagnost* unit. Monitoring type electrocardiographic leads† are applied. The technician places surgical drapes on the patient, and the operator performs a cut-down on the right brachial artery under local anesthesia. We never administer general anesthesia, since it adds to the risk, nor do we use prophylactic cardiac pacing or atropine unless they are indicated for reasons independent of the coronary arteriogram and left heart studies. The use of any drug not medically indicated for the treatment of preexisting conditions (except mild sedatives) should be discouraged prior to coronary arteriography. Bradycardia associated with the injection of a contrast agent into a coronary artery is promptly treated by having the patient cough at the appropriate time. In the several thousand procedures we have performed using the Sones' technique, atropine was never used prior to coronary arteriography (unless medically indicated for reasons other than the arteriography), nor was it ever needed during the procedure. Furthermore, published reports[10-12] indicate that atropine may actually be harmful in eurhythmic patients with severe ischemic heart disease in normal sinus rhythm.

THE TRANSBRACHIAL APPROACH (SONES' METHOD)[2-4]

The vessel is isolated by blunt dissection (Fig. 10–1*A*), and a 1-mm vertical incision is made in the vessel with the tip of a No. 11 blade (Fig. 10–1*B*). Bleeding is controlled proximally and distally with umbilical tapes or silicone loops. The Sones catheter, 7, 7½, or 8 French, 80 cm long, is introduced into the distal segment of the brachial artery, and 3 ml of saline solution containing 2500 units of heparin (Panheparin, 5000 units/ml) is injected to prevent clotting from distal arterial stasis during the procedure. The catheter is withdrawn, reintroduced proximally in the same incision (Fig. 10–1*C*), and advanced under fluoroscopic visualization until the tip is at the level of the left ventricle. Baseline pressure measurements, which include left ventricular pressure and dp/dt, are then recorded. While pressures are still being recorded, the catheter is withdrawn from the left ventricle to the ascending aorta to determine if a pressure gradient is present within the left ventricle or between the left ventricle and the aorta.

The Sones catheter is then replaced by a Lehman or Eppendorf thin-walled ventriculography catheter,** 7 or 8 French, 100 cm long, with the tip directed into the left ventricle. An automatic injector delivers 35 ml of contrast material, an agent containing diatrizoate

*Cordis Corporation, Box 370428, Miami, Florida 33137.

†Red Dot monitoring electrodes, 3M Center, Medical Product Division, St. Paul, Minnesota 55101.

**United States Catheter and Instrument Co., a division of C.R. Bard, Inc., Billerica, Massachusetts 01821.

meglumine, 66 per cent, and diatrizoate sodium, 10 per cent (Renografin-76), into the left ventricle. A 35-mm cine camera records the diastolic and systolic phases of the ventricular cycles at a rate of 40 frames each second. Routinely, we take this cine left ventriculogram in the right anterior oblique (RAO) projection. In almost all cases and particularly whenever the presence of a lesion of the interventricular septum is suspected, an additional left ventricular injection is performed and recorded with 30 degrees cranial angulation in a 60-degree left anterior oblique projection.[13]

Whenever contraction abnormalities,[14,15] elevation of left ventricular end-diastolic pressure,[16] or enlargement of the left ventricle is detected, nitroglycerin is injected into the left ventricle in doses of 0.6 mg in 1.5 ml of distilled water. The left ventriculogram is then repeated as soon as the left ventricular end-diastolic pressure has reached its lowest value or 3 minutes later, whichever occurs first.

The ventriculography catheter is then removed, the Sones catheter is reintroduced, and both the right and left coronary arteries are catheterized in both the left anterior oblique and right anterior oblique views. We also routinely take cranial angulation of the left and right coronary artery in anterior oblique views and caudal angulation of the left coronary artery in left anterior oblique views.

The catheter is then removed, and forceful bleeding is allowed to occur for a second or two. The tip of the catheter is reinserted into the distal segment of the brachial artery, and aspiration with a syringe is undertaken until a forceful arterial backflow is obtained. A second dose of 2500 units of heparin is injected into the distal arterial segment, the catheter is removed, and the artery is closed with a 6-0 Polydek* Lock-stitch suture (Fig. 10–1*D*).

*Deknatel, Queens Village, New York.

An inexpensive but highly effective and practical tool that is most helpful for suturing of the vessel is a pair of magnifying goggles.* The skin is sutured with 3-0 silk. A sterile pressure dressing is applied to the wound, and the patient is returned to his or her room. The average laboratory stay per patient is 45 minutes; often, especially in young patients without tortuous brachiocephalic vessels, a procedure may be completed in 30 minutes.

THE PERCUTANEOUS FEMORAL APPROACH (JUDKINS' METHOD)[6]

The percutaneous insertion of a catheter into a peripheral artery was first described by Seldinger in 1953,[26] and this procedure was extensively utilized in Europe in the 1950's. Dotter and Gensini reported on percutaneous transfemoral retrograde catheterization of the left ventricle and systemic arteries of man in 1960; in closing they stated, "In providing a means for direct catheterization of the coronary orifice, it . . . makes possible detailed coronary artery visualization in vivo."[27]

The percutaneous transfemoral approach to coronary arteriography became truly practical when Judkins designed a series of special catheters** made of polyurethane, preformed into curves suitable for the right or left coronary arteries, thereby achieving a "coronary artery–seeking" tip configuration. Each catheter, 100 cm in length, is

*optiVISOR DA-5 (3+), Bowen and Company, Inc., Rockville, Maryland 30852.

**Cordis Corporation, Box 370428, Miami, Florida.

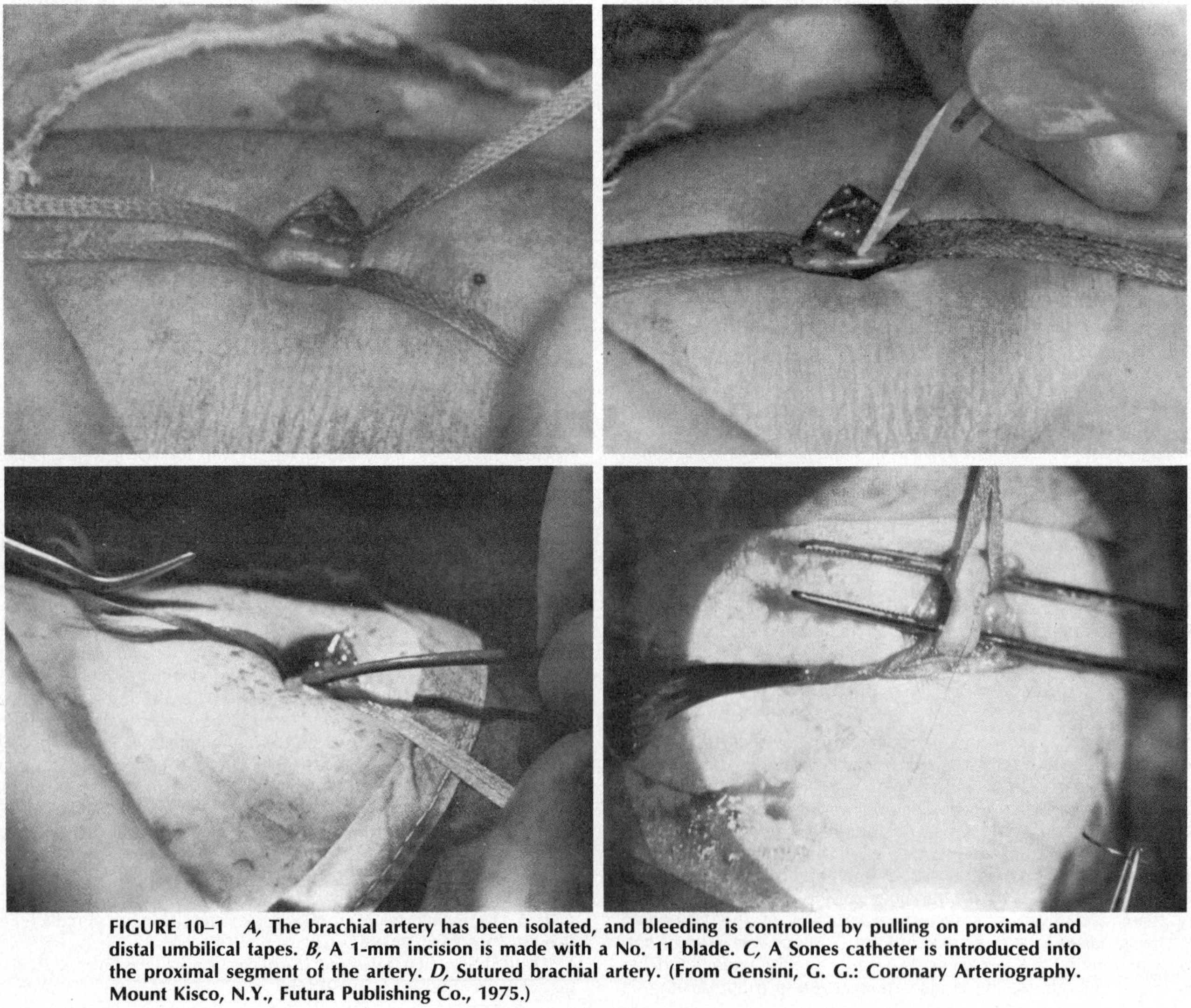

FIGURE 10–1 *A,* The brachial artery has been isolated, and bleeding is controlled by pulling on proximal and distal umbilical tapes. *B,* A 1-mm incision is made with a No. 11 blade. *C,* A Sones catheter is introduced into the proximal segment of the artery. *D,* Sutured brachial artery. (From Gensini, G. G.: Coronary Arteriography. Mount Kisco, N.Y., Futura Publishing Co., 1975.)

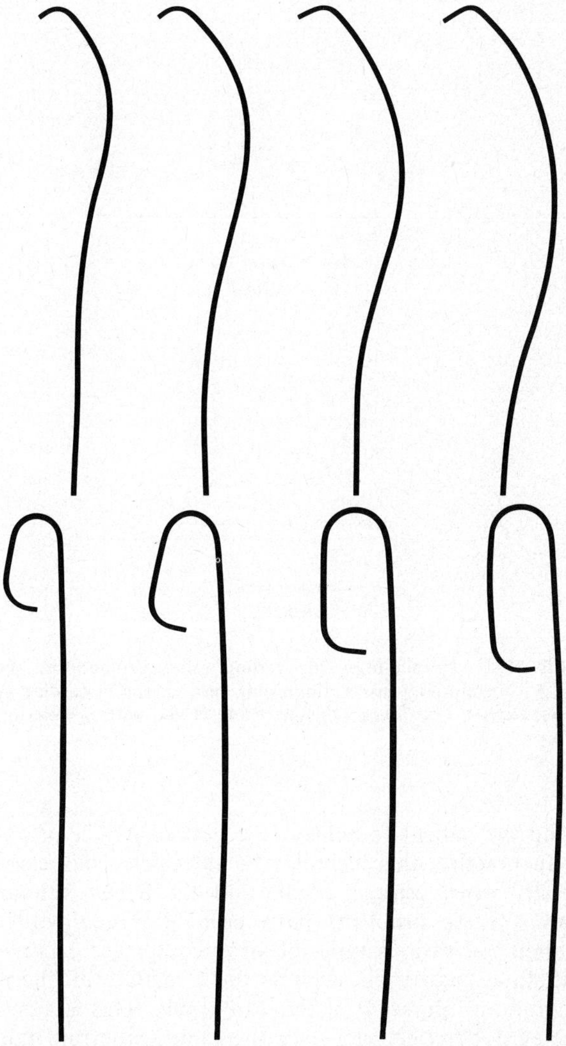

FIGURE 10–2 Judkins' catheters. *Top,* Right coronary tip curves. *Bottom,* Left coronary tip curves. (Courtesy of Cordis Corporation, Miami, Florida.)

now available in sizes 7 or 8 French, with four sizes of the terminal curve. They should be inserted using Teflon-coated guidewires. A catheter introducer may also be utilized in order to avoid damage or kinking of the catheter during its first pass into the artery. The four sizes of the terminal curve are designed to suit different aortic diameters. The appropriate size should be selected according to an assessment made prior to catheterization, based on patient size and the appearance of the aorta on a plain chest x-ray (Fig. 10–2).

From a procedural point of view, the technique of transfemoral coronary arteriography and left ventriculography is simple: The appropriate site of puncture overlying the femoral artery is identified and a small stab wound is made with a No. 11 blade; the opening is enlarged in the direction of the artery with straight, fine forceps. A left ventriculography catheter, either a Gensini*[28] or a pigtail,† is usually introduced first in order to measure the aortic and left ventricular pressures and to perform left ventriculography. With all types of catheters, the soft pliable end of the spring guidewire should protrude for at least an inch to find its way along the aorta and minimize the possibility of vascular trauma. Many investigators use a safety-tip J-shaped wire, so that the possibility of vascular trauma will be further diminished. After left ventriculography is performed, the ventriculography catheter is withdrawn and the left coronary catheter is then introduced. If one observes the protruding wire and/or the catheter entering one of the branches of the aortic arch, the catheter should be drawn back and the guide drawn back into the catheter. The natural curvature present on the catheter can then be used to direct it over the arch and into the ascending aorta. Once in the ascending aorta, the guide is withdrawn and the catheter is advanced while its concavity follows that of the aortic arch (Fig. 10–3*A*). The left-sided catheter naturally seeks the left coronary artery and, therefore, the arteriographer should be very careful in identifying the entrance of the catheter into the left coronary ostium the moment that this takes place. Prior to injecting the contrast agent, the angiographer should be certain that the catheter is not wedged into the left main coronary artery; this can be accomplished by a small test injection of contrast or by monitoring the pressure recorded from the tip of the catheter.

After completion of the visualization of the left coronary artery in multiple views, the left coronary catheter is withdrawn, and the right coronary artery catheter is inserted over the same wire. This catheter is usually manipulated with ease into the ascending aorta by drawing the guidewire back from the tip and advancing the catheter with the angled tip pointed to the inner aspect of the curve of the aortic arch. Once in the root of the aorta, the catheter is rotated so that the tip projects forward and slightly to the right of the patient (Fig. 10–3*B*). This is best accomplished by viewing the patient in the left anterior oblique projection. In this view, one can usually detect whether or not the catheter is approaching the right coronary artery. After the right coronary artery has been successfully visualized, the catheter is withdrawn, and pressure is applied over the inguinal area until adequate hemostasis is achieved. Usually the patient is released from the laboratory with a pressure bandage in place.

After coronary arteriography, the nurse checks the dressing for bleeding and records the patient's blood pressure and right radial pulse rate every 15 minutes for two hours. The pressure bandage is removed 30 minutes after the patient's return to the room, and the wound is re-dressed. The patient rests in bed for two hours and resumes the usual diet.

Later on the same day, the patient is visited by the physician who performed the examination, is told about the results of the procedure, and is advised on the further management of his or her problems.

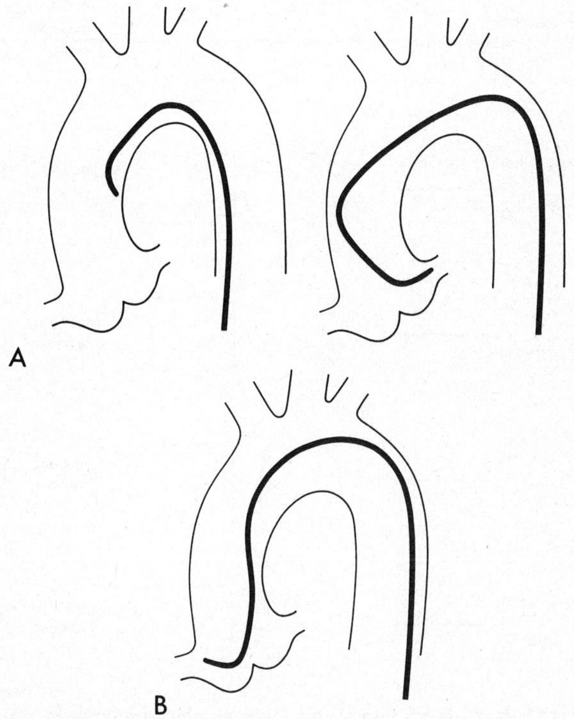

FIGURE 10–3 Judkins' technique of entering the left coronary artery (*A*) and the right coronary artery (*B*).

*United States Catheter and Instrument Co., a division of C. R. Bard, Inc., Billerica, Massachusetts 01821.

†Cordis Corporation, Box 370428, Miami, Florida 33137.

MULTIPLE VIEWS

One of the major problems in interpreting coronary arteriograms has been the considerable overlap and foreshortening of the main left coronary artery, of the proximal branches of the left anterior descending artery, and of the branches of the right coronary artery at the crux. Occasionally, despite the many projections obtained utilizing conventional angulation of the x-ray beam (i.e., perpendicular to the long axis of the patient), doubts may linger as to the integrity of these segments. Consequently, several authors, beginning with Bunnell, Greene, and others in 1973,[17] have described additional views in multiple obliquity, utilizing cranial and caudal angulation of the x-ray beam.[13,17–22,43,47–51]

Throughout this chapter we shall use the terminology proposed by Paulin and illustrated in Figures 10–4 through 10–7.

The most important problem areas are the main left coronary artery and its proximal branches, notably the bifurcation; the initial course of the left anterior descending and circumflex arteries; and the bifurcation between the left anterior descending and its major diagonal branch. In general, whenever there is a reason to question the integrity of these areas, the right anterior oblique projection with caudal angulation is employed. When heart size is normal or almost so, the left anterior oblique with cranial angulation is employed as well; in the presence of cardiomegaly the left anterior oblique projection with caudal angulation is employed.

Cranial angulation is possible with the simple technique of elevating the chest (utilizing a radiolucent wedge) and

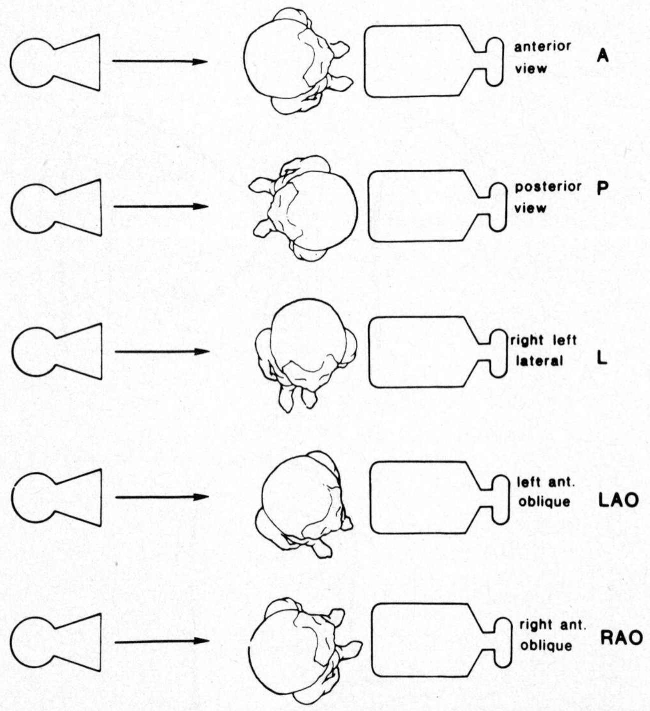

FIGURE 10–4 Terminology for radiographic projections. (From Paulin, S.: Terminology for radiographic projections in cardiac angiography. Cathet. Cardiovasc. Diagn. *7*:341, 1981, with permission.)

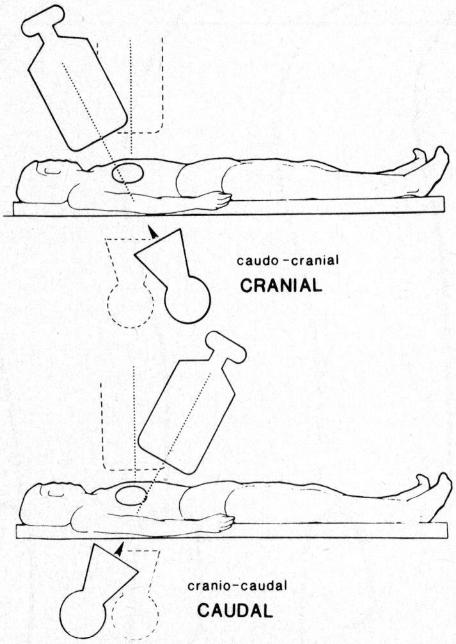

FIGURE 10–5 Terminology for radiographic projections. (From Paulin, S.: Terminology for radiographic projections in cardiac angiography. Cathet. Cardiovasc. Diagn. *7*:341, 1981, with permission.)

rotating the patient to achieve the desired degree of obliquity. In practice, this technique is extremely cumbersome, especially when using a cradle and the Sones technique. However, these problems have been alleviated with the availability of various types of x-ray equipment capable of longitudinal angulation, such as the U or C arm, the parallelogram, or elevation of the x-ray table. This angulation is achieved by either elevating the table (Spectrum table), angling the table and the U arm (Cardiodiagnost*), or angling the x-ray tube and image intensifier (parallelogram, LAD† system).

Like many other technical or procedural refinements, these special views may, at times, be most valuable; however, caution is advised against their overutilization, which could lead to unwarranted prolongation of the study and, consequently, to greater risk for the patient.

COMPLICATIONS

Coronary arteriography is routinely performed in approximately 1000 laboratories of this nation. A report from the National Center for Health Care Technology[29] suggests that nearly 300,000 coronary arteriograms were performed in 1980. In the state of New York alone over 25,000 coronary arteriograms were performed in 1981.[30]

Any diagnostic intervention that is potentially hazardous must be reserved for patients in whom the benefits derived from the procedure outweigh the risks. If the incidence and severity of complications vary from one in-

*North American Philips, United X-Ray Corporation, Fall River, Massachusetts 02723.

†General Electric Medical Division, Westwood, Massachusetts 02090.

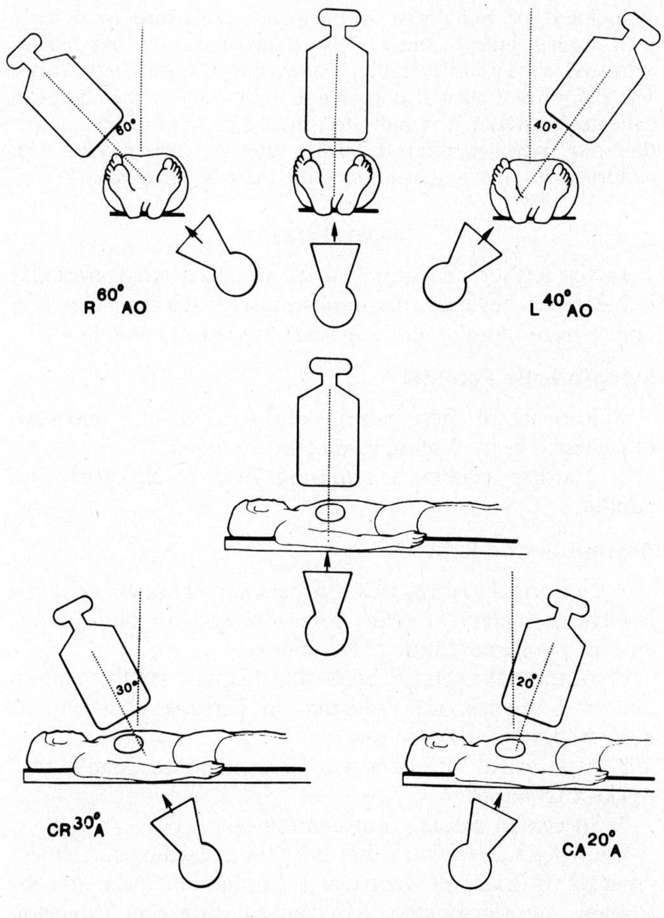

FIGURE 10–6 Terminology for radiographic projections. (From Paulin, S.: Terminology for radiographic projections in cardiac angiography. Cathet. Cardiovasc. Diagn. 7:341, 1981, with permission.)

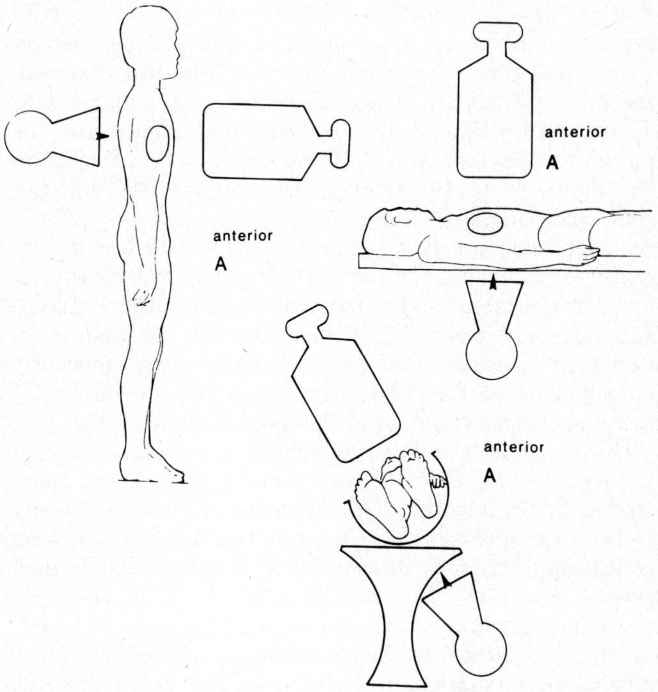

FIGURE 10–7 Terminology for radiographic projections. (From Paulin, S.: Terminology for radiographic projections in cardiac angiography. Cathet. Cardiovasc. Diagn. 7:341, 1981, with permission.)

stitution to another, rules that may be valid in one setting may not apply in another. Earlier nationwide surveys demonstrated that this is indeed the case for coronary arteriography, i.e., that the incidence of serious complications could vary widely. In fact, reports of the mortality of coronary arteriography ranged from 0.05 to 2.37 per cent.[31,32]

The most authoritative and recent reports on mortality and complications related to cardiac catheterization and angiography are those by the Registry Committee of the Society for Cardiac Angiography.[33,34] These reports are based on 53,581 patients studied over a period of 14 months and describe significant complications in 950 patients (1.8 per cent) (Table 10–1). Catheterization-related mortality for the purpose of inclusion in the Society's reports was defined as death that (1) occurred during the procedure, (2) occurred within 24 hours after the procedure and was not attributable to any non–catheterization-related cause, or (3) occurred several days after the procedure but was clearly precipitated by an event occurring during the procedure. An example of the latter is a myocardial infarction occurring during the procedure and resulting in death four days later. There were 75 deaths overall in these 53,581 patients, a mortality rate of 0.14 per cent. However, eight of these deaths occurred among the 457 patients studied under the age of one year (mortality rate in this group = 1.7 per cent). There were 24 deaths in patients between one and 60 years of age, resulting in a mortality rate of 0.07 per cent, and 43 deaths in those over 60 years of age, with a mortality rate of 0.25 per cent. Overall the mortality rate was 0.12 per cent for males and 0.18 per cent for females. Mortality was, as expected, closely related to the patient's functional class.

Patients who were in Class IV had a mortality rate of 0.67 per cent, whereas the mortality rate was 0.02 per cent in Class I and Class II patients. Mortality was also related to the extent of left ventricular dysfunction. In patients with an ejection fraction equal to or better than 50 per cent, the mortality was 0.05 per cent; for those with an ejection fraction of 30 to 49 per cent, the mortality was 0.23 per cent; and for patients with an ejection fraction < 30 per cent, mortality was 0.76 per cent. As anticipated, mortality during or following coronary arteriography was closely related to the extent and severity of coronary artery disease and was highest in the 2,452 patients with left main coronary artery disease—0.86 per cent. There was no mortality among the 11,418 patients who had normal or minimally diseased coronary arteries at the time of angiography.

There was no significant difference in mortality between the patients studied with the brachial technique and those studies by the femoral artery technique. The events leading to the 75 deaths were closely scrutinized and the following conclusions could be drawn: Three of these patients died several days after their catheterization from an unrelated cause and should be excluded from the analysis. Twenty-one patients arrived at the laboratory in extremis and their deaths were expected, irrespective of the catheterization. Most of these patients were either suffering from recent myocardial infarction and cardiogenic shock, or had complex congenital malformations. Thus there were a total of 51 unexpected deaths which were considered to be causally related to the procedure, reducing the mortality rate to 0.10 per cent. In conclusion, according to this authoritative study, catheterization-related mortality occurs mostly in patients with far-advanced cardiac disease. Nearly one third of the unexpected deaths occurred suddenly after a seemingly uneventful procedure. Many of the patients dying unexpectedly had 90 per cent or more obstruction of the left main coronary artery or 90 per cent or more obstruction of all three major vessels.

As shown on Table 10–1, the other major complications were myocardial infarction (0.7 per cent), cerebrovascular accident (0.07 per cent), arrhythmia (0.56 per cent), vascular complications (0.57 per cent), and other unspecified complications (0.41 per cent). An interesting finding concerning indications for and hazards of coronary arteriography is a higher incidence of death within the 24 hours before than within the 24 hours after the tests.[35,36] Fear seems to play a major part in causing death in some of these patients.

The author's belief in the relative safety of properly performed selective coronary arteriography therefore rests on the basis of his experience as well as that of many other institutions where mortality related to the technique is maintained at or below 0.1 per cent. The author shares the opinion expressed by Judkins and Gander[37] that in institutions where the mortality exceeds 0.1 per cent, the entire coronary arteriography program should be reevaluated, and that in those where the rate exceeds 0.3 per cent, these studies should be discontinued.

Sones precisely defined the problem and expressed the sentiment shared by many angiographers[38]:

> The safe performance of consistently superior studies demands a high level of technical competence. At present, it appears that at least two years of special training are required to provide a cardiologist or radiologist with enough experience to perform such studies independently. This responsibility should not be entrusted to enthusiastic but inadequately trained individuals. The risk of mortality attributable to this study in the classes of patients for whom it is indicated should be lower than one per thousand. When significantly higher rates are encountered, inept performance, poor judgment, or both, must be assumed.

TABLE 10–1 MAJOR COMPLICATIONS ASSOCIATED WITH CARDIAC CATHETERIZATION AND ANGIOGRAPHY*

	Number	Per Cent of Total
Death	75	0.14
MI	40	0 .07
CVA	35	0.07
Arrhythmia	287	0.56
Vascular	291	0.57
Other	222	0.41
Total	950	1.82

From Kennedy, W. J., et al.: Complications associated with cardiac catheterization and angiography. Cathet. Cardiovasc. Diagn. 8:8, 1982.

INDICATIONS*

In the author's opinion,[39] when the associated mortality is below 0.1 per cent, the indications for selective cine coronary arteriography and left-heart studies are as follows:

Symptomatic Patients

1. Presence of chest pain in adults in whom a diagnosis of ischemic heart disease cannot be excluded.
2. Cardiac problems requiring open-heart surgery in adults.

Asymptomatic Patients

1. Abnormal resting ECG in persons whose occupations involve the safety of other persons (truck or bus drivers, aircraft pilots, air traffic controllers).
2. Abnormal exercise ECG, or thallium studies consistent with myocardial ischemia, in persons with one or more additional risk factors.
3. Myocardial infarction (studies should be done 4 to 8 weeks afterward).
4. Successful cardiac resuscitation.

Evolving acute myocardial infarction, cardiogenic shock, repeated episodes of ventricular fibrillation, other uncontrollable life-threatening arrhythmias, threat of extension of myocardial infarction, and uncontrollable heart failure such as occurs with septal perforation or papillary muscle rupture are, under certain circumstances, indications for emergency coronary arteriography. It should be understood, however, that these are heroic measures performed in highly specialized centers and that the higher mortality rate associated with these types of patients cannot and should not be confused with or added to the incidence of complications of elective coronary arteriography.

CONTRAINDICATIONS

Coronary arteriography and left-heart studies are usually not performed under the following circumstances:

*Editor's Note: There is considerable variability in currently accepted indications for coronary arteriography. Other discussions of this subject are found in Chapters 38 and 39.

1. If acute myocardial infarction is well established (the patient is asymptomatic) and infarction has been present for longer than 6 hours and for less than 3 weeks.

2. When coronary revascularization must be deferred or is considered to be contraindicated because of other debilitating conditions, including massive obesity.

3. A laboratory incapable of producing films of consistent diagnostic quality or with mortality greater than 3 per 1000 related to arteriography in uncomplicated patients. Such a laboratory should suspend its activity, investigate, identify, and eliminate the causes of its inadequacy.

GOALS OF CORONARY ARTERIOGRAPHY

The primary goal of coronary arteriography is the identification, localization, and assessment of obstructive lesions present within the arteries of the heart. Combined with contrast and hemodynamic studies of the left ventricle, it remains the most important method of defining the presence and severity of coronary atherosclerosis and the adequacy of myocardial function.

An important distinction must be made between arteriography employed in part or entirely for research purposes and that performed strictly for the care of patients. Techniques, methods, and protocols that may be considered acceptable and necessary in selected groups of consenting and informed volunteers for the purpose of conducting needed research studies are not the subject of this chapter, which will deal exclusively with well-established routine techniques of coronary arteriography, utilized in the daily care of patients with known or suspected coronary artery disease. Coronary arteriography is performed for the primary purpose of determining the presence (or the absence), extent, and severity of coronary artery disease and the adequacy of left ventricular function and not specifically for the purpose of determining whether or not a patient is a candidate for coronary bypass surgery.

The knowledge gained through coronary arteriography, left-heart catheterization, and left ventriculography often help in the management of the patient with known or suspected coronary artery disease, regardless of whether or not that particular patient happens to be a possible surgical candidate. To state that coronary arteriography should be performed only to decide on the possibility of coronary bypass surgery would seem to be akin to stating that an electrocardiogram should be performed only to decide whether or not a patient should be admitted to a coronary care unit.

NORMAL CORONARY ARTERY ANATOMY

Strict anatomical descriptions of the coronary arteries are available from standard textbooks of anatomy, and excellent monographs on this subject have been written by James[40] and McAlpine.[41] However, most of the descriptions contained in these works are based on views and perspectives obtained from anatomical specimens. The arteriographer, instead, uses an entirely different set of reference points and is less inclined to emphasize landmarks that are visible on the specimen but which may not be readily recognized on the radiographic image. Since our description is based on selective cine coronary arteriograms and is directed to physicians interested in interpreting them, we shall follow, whenever possible, the point of view of the arteriographer.

DIMENSIONS OF THE CORONARY ARTERIES. Coronary arteriography accurately depicts the origin, distribution, and appearance of the coronary arteries in living intact subjects.[2] *Quantitative* coronary arteriography[23] can actually define the *exact dimensions* of the coronary arteries in living man and their changes during physiological, pharmacological, or surgical interventions. MacAlpin et al. applied this method to calculate the size of human coronary arteries in living patients without coronary artery disease.[42]

On the basis of vessel size, the left coronary artery system is almost always more important than the right coronary artery system in the blood supply to the left ventricle, even in cases classified anatomically as having "right coronary artery preponderance" (see p. 320).

Dimensions of coronary ostia[41] (mm)
Right: $3.7 \pm 1.1 \times 2.4 \pm 0.9$ (Range = 0.5 to 7.0)
Left: $4.7 \pm 1.2 \times 3.2 \pm 1.1$ (Range = 1.0 to 8.5)

THE REGION OF THE CORONARY OSTIA. In the left anterior oblique view, the major axis of the outflow tract of the left ventricle and ascending aorta tips slightly to the left of the observer. Schematically, the outflow tract of the left ventricle and aorta may be regarded as a nearly cylindrical structure with a bulge in the middle, owing to the presence of the aortic sinuses. A line drawn along the *upper* edge of this bulge marks the area of the aortic ring or the plane dividing the aortic sinus from the ascending aorta. A line drawn along the *lower* edge of this bulge divides the floor of the aortic cusps from the outflow tract of the ventricle (the aortoventricular plane).

These landmarks are easily identifiable on an aortogram, and the origin of the two coronary arteries can readily be described in relation to them. Figure 10–8 shows the opacification of the aorta, both in diastole (*A*) and in systole (*B*) in the left anterior oblique view. The plane of the aortic ring and the aortoventricular plane are identified as 1 and 2, respectively. The right sinus of Valsalva (rsv), the left sinus of Valsalva (lsv), and the posterior sinus of Valsalva (psv) are shown in Figure 10–8*A*. In Figure 10–8*B*, R, L, and P identify the semi-open right, left, and posterior cusps, respectively. The origin of the right coronary artery is seen to the left and immediately above the right sinus of Valsalva in *A*. The position of the right coronary artery ostium in relation to the described landmarks may vary. In over 90 per cent of our patients, it was located high in the right sinus of Valsalva, immediately below the level of the ring. Occasionally it was found close to the aortoventricular plane and, in a few cases (1 to 2 per cent), above the ring. The left coronary artery originates from the left sinus of Valsalva. The ostium of the left coronary artery is usually located at the level of the aortic ring, and can often be seen as a small protuberance at this level, directly coinciding with the left edge of the broken line under 1.

A *horizontal section drawn at the level of the aortic valve* shows the relationship of the tip of the catheter as it would approach this valve (Fig. 10–9*A*). In the right anterior oblique view, the noncoronary sinus of Valsalva lies to the left and below the tip of the catheter. The left sinus is above and to the right of it. The right sinus is anterior to

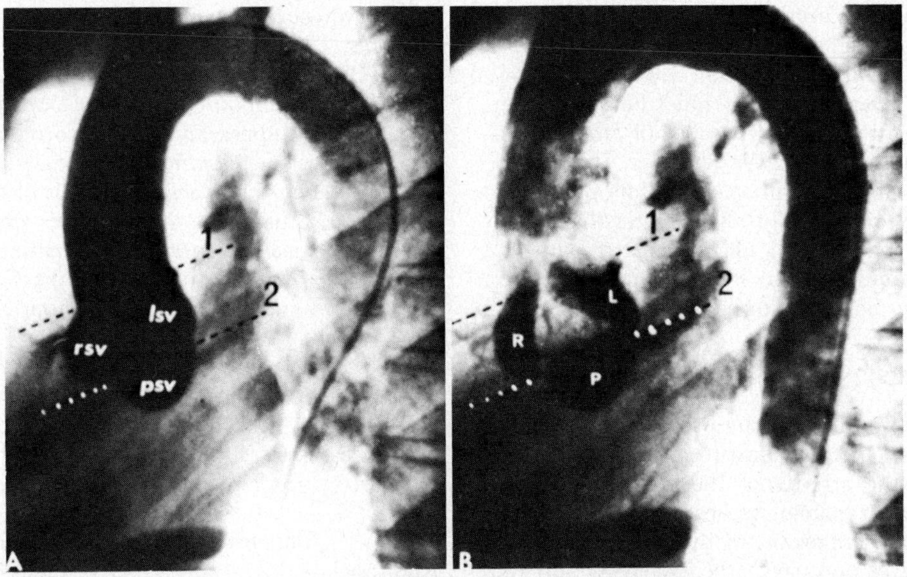

FIGURE 10–8 Left anterior oblique projections showing opacification of the aorta during diastole (*A*) and systole (*B*). See text for explanation. (From Gensini, G. G.: Coronary Arteriography. Mount Kisco, N.Y., Futura Publishing Co., 1975.)

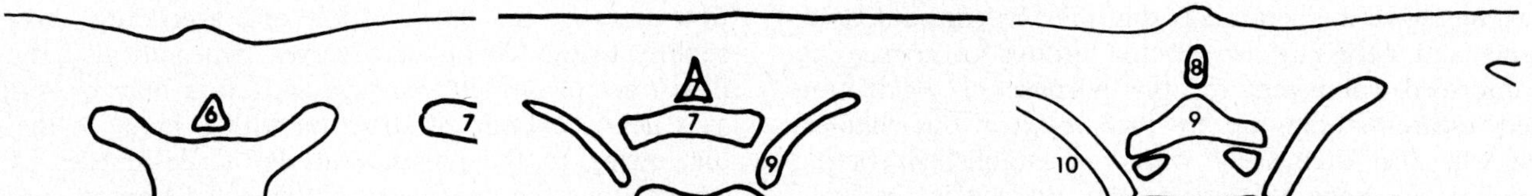

FIGURE 10–9 *A*, Horizontal body section drawn at the level of the aortic valve and seventh thoracic vertebra. *B*, Horizontal body section drawn at the level of the eighth thoracic vertebra. *C*, Horizontal body section drawn at the level of the ninth thoracic vertebra. (From Gensini, G. G.: Coronary Arteriography. Mount Kisco, N.Y., Futura Publishing Co., 1975.)

(3)	Third rib or vertebra	(LA)	Left atrium	(CS)	Coronary sinus
(4)	Fourth rib or vertebra	(SC)	Scapula	(PL)	Posterolateral branch
(5)	Fifth rib or vertebra	(RA)	Right atrium	(LV)	Left ventricle
(6)	Sixth rib or vertebra	(RV)	Right ventricle	(LAD)	Left anterior descending branch
(7)	Seventh rib or vertebra	(psV)	Posterior sinus of Valsalva	(RCA)	Right coronary artery
(8)	Eighth rib or vertebra	(OM)	Obtuse marginal branch	(PD)	Posterior descending branch
(9)	Ninth rib or vertebra	(C)	Circumflex	(AM)	Acute marginal branch
(10)	Tenth rib	(lsV)	Left sinus of Valsalva	(IVC)	Inferior vena cava
(A)	Descending aorta	(D)	Diagonal branch	(rsV)	Right sinus of Valsalva

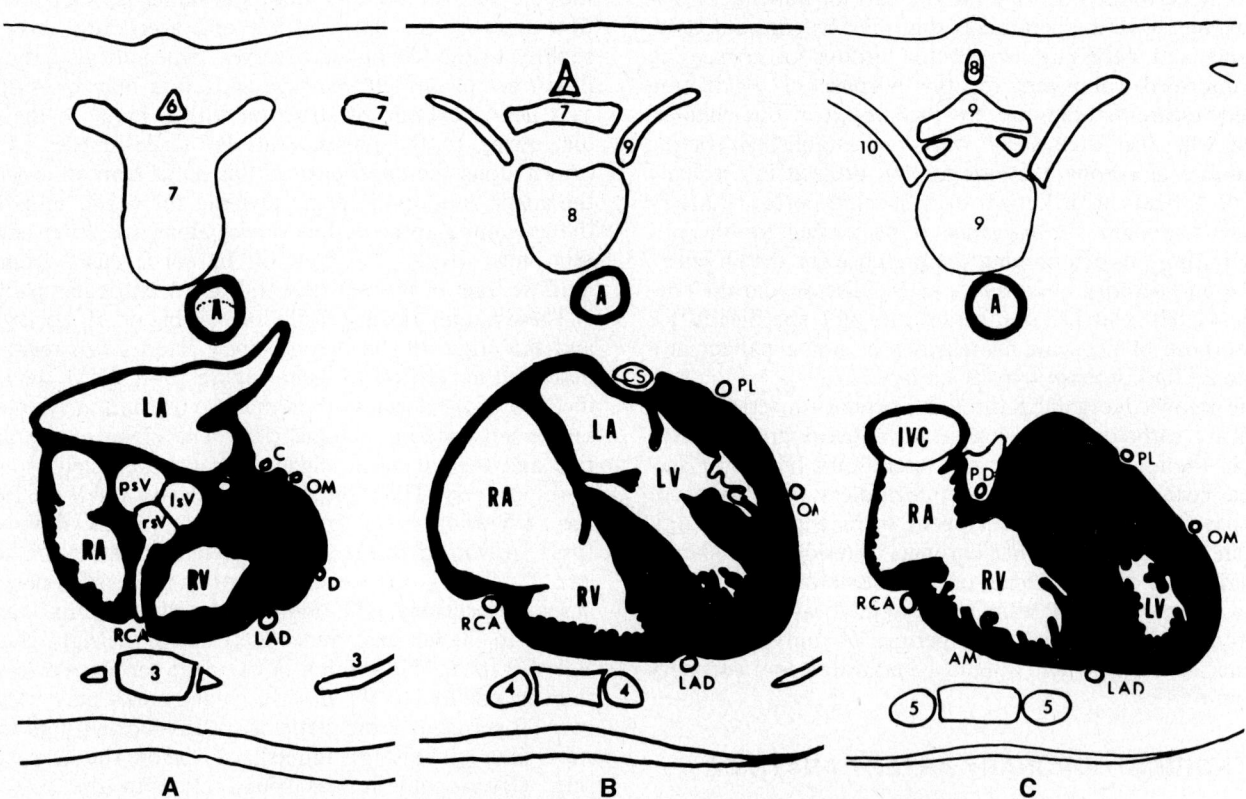

the catheter and is located at a level between the left and the posterior sinuses. The right sinus overlaps the left sinus by two thirds of its area and the posterior sinus by only one third. At this level, the right atrium is to the left of the catheter and the right ventricle is to the right and inferior to it. The left atrium is located posteriorly and to the left. The left ventricle does not yet appear at this level. The right coronary artery is directly anterior to the catheter, whereas the main left coronary artery is above, to the right, and slightly posterior to it. If the patient is positioned for the left anterior oblique projection, the right sinus of Valsalva will appear on the left and the left sinus will be on the right and at a slightly higher level. The noncoronary sinus is posterior and below the other two sinuses. The right atrium will be to the left, whereas the right ventricle will be in front of and to the left of the catheter. The left atrium is on the right and is, in this view, one of the most posterior structures. The coronary arteries will bear the same relationship to the catheter as the one described for their respective sinuses of Valsalva, i.e., the right coronary is to the left and the left coronary to the right of the catheter.

A *horizontal section drawn at the level of the eighth vertebral body* transects all four chambers of the heart (Fig. 10–9*B*). This section is useful to gain an appreciation of the topographical anatomy of the ventricular and atrial septa and the relationship between the major coronary branches, the ventricles, and the atria. In the right anterior oblique view, the main stem of the right coronary artery is anterior and to the left; the left anterior descending branch is anterior and to the right. The obtuse marginal branch is located posteriorly, partially overlapped by the left anterior descending branch. The posterolateral branch of the circumflex is the most posterior one and appears to be located between the right coronary artery and the left anterior descending branch. The posterior descending branch is below this section and thus does not appear at this level. The right atrium and ventricle are the most anterior structures, the atrium on the left and the ventricle on the right. The projection of the edges of the vertebral bodies appears to touch the leftmost border of the right atrium. The descending aorta, which is anterior to and to the side of the spine, is behind the body of the left atrium. The right or anterior atrioventricular groove, along which the right coronary artery runs, overlaps the base of the tricuspid valve. The interventricular and interatrial septa form a wall which, in a 30-degree right anterior oblique projection, is perpendicular to the line of sight of an outside observer looking in. Therefore, the septa are seen together as a curtain that separates the right atrium and ventricle, which are in front of it, and from the left atrium and ventricle, which are behind it. The left or posterior atrioventricular groove and the base of the mitral valve divide the left atrium from the left ventricle. The observer sees the left atrium to the left and the left ventricle to the right.

In the left anterior oblique view, both ventricles are anterior and both atria are posterior to the observer; the right cavities are seen on the left and the left cavities on the right. The major axis of the interventricular septum points directly to the observer when the patient is in a 30-degree left anterior oblique position. When using steeper degrees of obliquity, such as the 45- and 60-degree left anterior oblique views, the anterior aspect of the interventricular septum is slightly to the left of the observer and the posterior aspect tips slightly to the right. The border of the heart shadow, which is to the right of the observer, is the posterolateral wall of the left ventricle. The one on the left is the right anterior atrioventricular groove. The projection of the aorta and of the spine partially overlaps the posterolateral wall of the left ventricle in both the 30- and 45-degree left anterior oblique projection but is distinct from it in the 60-degree left anterior oblique view. The obtuse marginal and posterolateral branches also overlap one another and are superimposed with the edge of the spine and the full width of the descending aorta in shallower left anterior oblique projections (30 and 45 degrees). Therefore, the 60-degree left anterior oblique projection is especially useful to separate these vessels and visualize them apart from the confusing shadows of the vertebral column.

A final *horizontal section drawn at the level of the ninth vertebral body* (Fig. 10–9*C*), has many points in common with the section just described. At this level, however, the left atrium is no longer present and only the apex of the left ventricle appears. A new structure that is visible here is the distal segment of the right coronary artery, which runs directly posterior to the lower segment of the anterior aspect of this artery, so that these two structures appear to be superimposed.

In order to define better the relationship of the coronary arteries to the mass of the heart and to major landmarks of the thorax, it may be useful to utilize an imaginary horizontal projection (Fig. 10–10). In this projection the thorax is transected at the level of the eighth thoracic

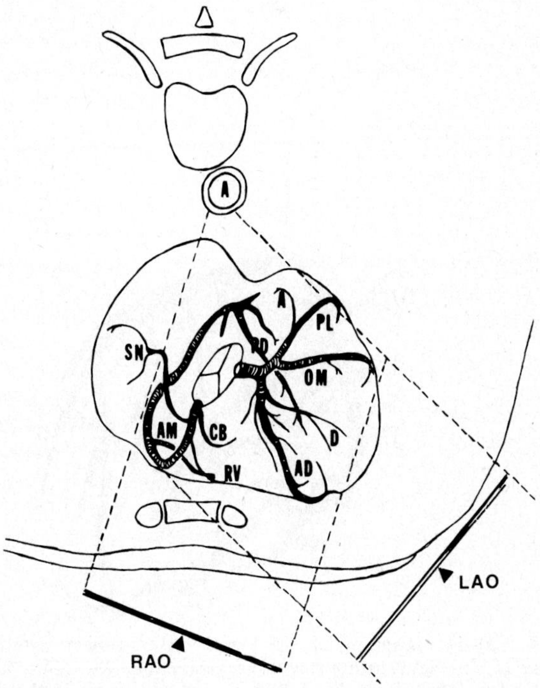

FIGURE 10–10 Horizontal projection of the heart demonstrating the relationship of the coronary arteries to the major landmarks of the thorax. The position of the input screen of the image intensifier over the chest is shown for both the left anterior oblique and the right anterior oblique projections. See text for details. Labels are as described in the legend of Figure 10–11. (From Gensini, G. G.: Coronary Arteriography. Mount Kisco, N.Y., Futura Publishing Co., 1975.)

vertebra, and the coronary arteries are visualized in their entirety, from the sinuses of Valsalva to their terminal branches, as if they were draped over a transparent heart. In this illustration, the input screen of the image intensifier is shown for a 20-degree right anterior oblique and a 45-degree left anterior oblique projection; the outlines of the heart shadow (actually its girth) are drawn as they appear at the level of the eighth vertebral body. The plane of the aortic valve, which is above this section and is steeply inclined from top to bottom, from left to right, and from front to back, appears as an ellipse, owing to its projection on the plane of the section utilized.

In the right anterior oblique projection (Fig. 10–11), the right coronary artery courses along the right atrioventricular groove, at first directed toward the input screen of the image intensifier and then away from it. The considerable foreshortening of the initial and terminal segments of the right coronary artery, which occurs in the right anterior oblique projection, can be adequately appreciated from this illustration. Conversely, these two segments of the right coronary artery are obviously well delineated in the left anterior oblique projection, which instead tends to foreshorten the posterior descending and, to a lesser extent, the right ventricular branches. When visualized in the right anterior oblique projection, the ventricular branches of the right coronary artery are generally directed toward the right border of the screen, whereas the atrial branches (of which only the sinus node branch is illustrated) are directed toward the left border of the screen.

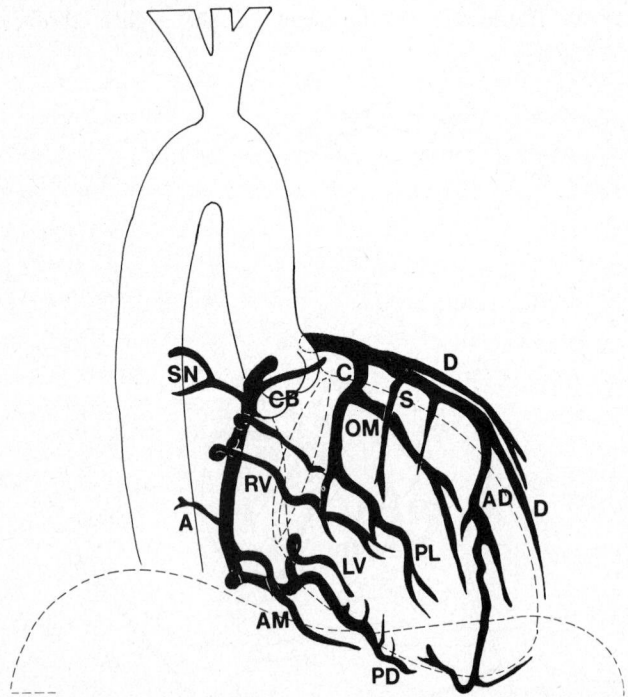

FIGURE 10–11 **Diagram of right and left coronary arteries as viewed in the right anterior oblique projection. The abbreviations shown here and utilized throughout the chapter are as follows: CB = conus branch; SN = sinus node branch; RV = right ventricular branch; AM = acute marginal branch; A = atrial branch; PD = posterior descending branch; LV = left ventricular branch; C or C_x = circumflex; OM = obtuse marginal branch; PL = posterolateral branch; S = septal branch; D = diagonal branch; AD or LAD = left anterior descending branch (preferably LAD). (From Gensini, G. G.: Coronary Arteriography. Mount Kisco, N.Y., Futura Publishing Co., 1975.)**

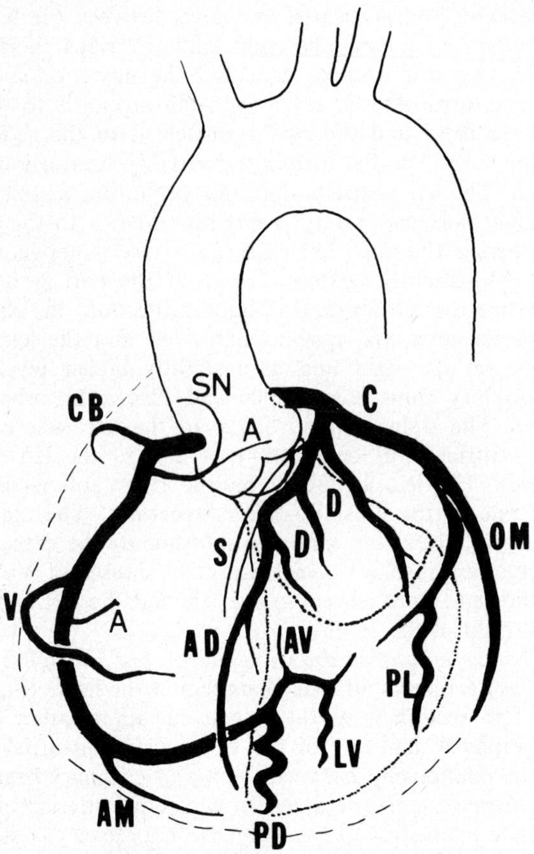

FIGURE 10–12 **Diagram of right and left coronary arteries as viewed in the left anterior oblique projection. (Labels as in Figure 10–11; AV = atrioventricular node branch.) (From Gensini, G. G.: Coronary Arteriography. Mount Kisco, N.Y., Futura Publishing Co., 1975.)**

The main left coronary artery is only moderately inclined in relationship to the plane of the section displayed in this view. The left anterior descending branch and atrioventricular segment of the circumflex, respectively, are directed toward both the right and left anterior oblique projections, and away from the plane of the image intensifier and are thus foreshortened in these views. In order to visualize the left anterior descending artery without foreshortening, the best view is the left lateral projection.

An overview of the entire coronary arterial system and its relationship to the left ventricle and the aorta is demonstrated in the right anterior oblique (RAO) projection in Figure 10–11 and in the left anterior oblique (LAO) projection in Figure 10–12. [The outlines of the left ventricle, the mitral valve, and the diaphragm are shown with dotted or dashed lines.] These illustrations are based on representative coronary arteriograms of healthy individuals and, *when taken as broad outlines,* represent the general appearance and distribution of coronary arteries in the majority of the human population. More as well as less common normal anatomical variations are illustrated and discussed later in the text.

Right Coronary Artery (Table 10–2)

The right coronary artery originates from the right sinus of Valsalva (usually its right half) and is best seen in the left anterior oblique view. In this view, the right coronary

TABLE 10–2 RIGHT CORONARY ARTERY—ANATOMICAL CONSIDERATIONS

Branch of Right Coronary Artery (Abbreviation)	International Anatomical Classification	Percentage of Time From RCA	Other Sites of Origin and Time Present	Area Perfused	Best Angiographic View*	Site of Origin and Route if Comes From RCA	Role in Collateral Blood Supply (Usual)
Right coronary artery (RCA)	Arteria coronaria dextra			RA and part of LA, RV, posterosuperior IV septum, SN, and AV node	$L^{60°}AO$	Right sinus of Valsalva; anteriorly and inferiorly along right AV groove	
Conus branch (CB)	Ramus coni arteriosi	60%	As separate vessel (1 mm from RCA ostium), 40%	Outflow tract, right ventricle	$R^{30°}AO$	Within first 2 cm; runs centrally to left of pulmonic valve	When LAD or RCA is occluded, acts as anastomotic ring of Vieussens
Sinus node (SN(R))	Ramus nodi sinoatrialis dexter	59%	C, 39%; C and RCA, 2%	Right and left atria, sinus node	$R^{30°}AO$	Within first 3 cm (occasionally from mid, rarely from distal portion of RCA); runs cranially, dorsally, and to right base of SVC (opposite direction of CB)	Atrial branches connect with distal portion of RCA or C
Right ventricular (RV)	Ramus ventricularis dexter anterior	100%	Additional RV branches of LAD infrequently seen in angiocardiography	Right ventricle	$R^{30°}AO$	Mid anterior portion of RCA; over anterior surface of right ventricle	Connects with branches of LAD; may connect with more distal RVB or AM
Atrial (A)	Ramus atrialis	100%	None	Right atrium	$R^{30°}AO$	Above or at level of AM directed cranially, posteriorly, and to right	May join branches from SN artery
Acute marginal (AM)	Ramus marginalis dexter	100%	None	Inferior and diaphragmatic surface of RV—occasionally posteroapical IV septum	RAO, LAO $CR^{30°}R^{30°}AO$ $CR^{30°}L^{60°}AO$	At or about acute margin along or close to AM, toward apex	Connects with anterior or posterior descending
AV node (AVN(R))	Ramus nodi atrioventricularis	87.9%	C, 11.9%; RCA and C, 0.2%	AVN, lower portion of IA septum	$CR^{30°}L^{60°}AO$	Originates proximal to or at top of U curve at crux cordis; runs cranially and toward center of heart	May join septal branch of anterior descending
Posterior descending (PD)	Ramus interventricularis	86%	C, 14%; RCA and C, 4%	Posterior and diaphragmatic area of septum	$CR^{30°}L^{60°}AO$ $CR^{30°}L^{30°}AO$	When present, most important terminal branch of RCA; level of crux cordis; posterior IV sulcus	Joins septal and terminal branches of anterior descending
Left ventricular branch (LVB)	Rami posterolaterales dextri (proximales)	80%	C, 20%	Diaphragmatic aspect of LV	$CR^{30°}L^{75°}AO$	Beyond crux cordis, runs centrally in angle formed by left posterior AV groove and posterior IV sulcus; if LV branches are large and numerous, PL branch of C may not be present	Joins branches of C, especially AC and PL branches
Posterolateral (PL)	Rami posterolaterales dextri (distales)	20%	C, 80%	Posterior and diaphragmatic LV wall	$CR^{30°}L^{75°}AO$	Most terminal branch of RCA, when present (See above, LVB)	(See above, LVB)

*The terminology for radiographic projections in cardiac angiography recommended by Paulin[22] has been utilized throughout this chapter. See also Refs. 13, 17–21, 43, 47–51.

Modified from Kelly, A. E., and Gensini, G. G.: Coronary arteriography and left heart studies. Heart Lung *4*:85, 1975.

C = circumflex branch.

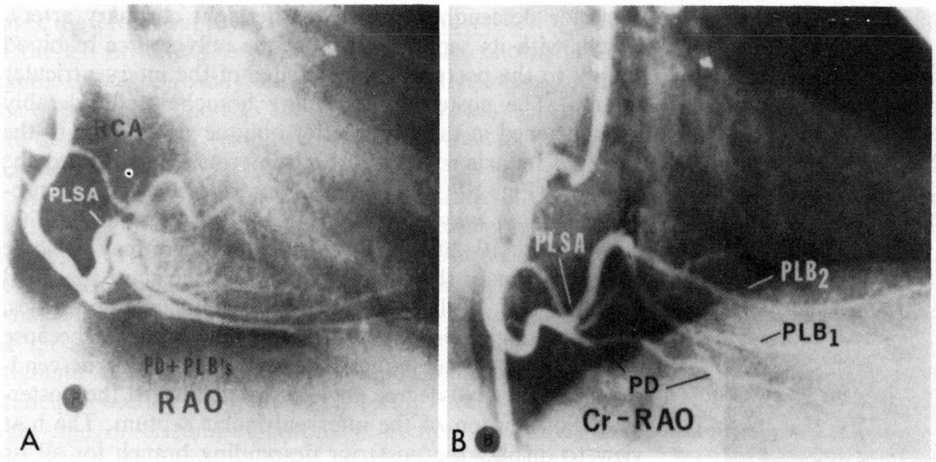

FIGURE 10–21 Selective right coronary arteriogram. *A*, Nonangled right anterior oblique (RAO) view. Note the superimposition of the posterior descending (PD) and posterolateral (PLB's) branches. *B*, Cranial–right anterior oblique (Cr-RAO) view results in a "stair-step" effect of the distal branches. There is separation of the posterior descending branch from the first and second posterolateral branches. Note the improved visualization of the posterolateral segment artery (PLSA). RCA = right coronary artery. (From Elliott, L. P., Green, C. E., Roger, W. J., Mantle, J. A., Papapietro S. E., Hood, W. P., and Russell, R. O.: Advantage of the cranial–right anterior oblique view in diagnosing mid left anterior descending and distal right coronary artery disease. Am. J. Cardiol. *48*:754, 1981.)

times one of these branches originates midway between the acute margin and the posterior interventricular sulcus. In such cases, the posterosuperior portion of the posterior interventricular septum and the AV node are supplied by the most distal posterior descending branch, whereas the posteroinferior portion is supplied by the more proximal posterior descending branch.

In a small percentage of cases (3 per cent), the main stem of the right coronary artery divides even before it reaches the acute margin, runs along the atrioventricular groove, reaches the posterior aspect of the heart, and gives origin to the posterior descending branch. The inferior ramus, on the other hand, runs diagonally along the anterior surface of the right ventricle to the acute margin in order to reach—again, with an oblique path—the posterior aspect of the right ventricle. In such cases, the more proximal ramus of the coronary artery provides the blood supply to the inferior and posterior walls of the right ventricle, whereas the branch running along the posterior atrioventricular groove gives origin to the posterior descending artery.

The most distal branch of the right coronary artery is usually a left atrial branch, which, when present, runs along the posterior-left atrioventricular groove and then curves upward from the crux cordis, superiorly, posteriorly, and away from the right coronary artery. This branch appears to curve upward toward the spine, pointing to the upper right corner of the frame in the left anterior oblique view. The behavior of the terminal portion of the right coronary artery has been the source of a great deal of controversy and misunderstanding. Bianchi,[44] Spalteholz,[45] and Schlesinger,[46] divided the coronary circulation into "right preponderant" and "left preponderant," depending on which artery crossed the crux. When both arteries reached the crux without crossing it, the circulation was considered to be "balanced." Actually, in 84 per cent of our patients the posterior descending is a branch of the right coronary artery and in 70 per cent it runs along the posterior interventricular sulcus up to its mid portion and even farther, toward the direction of the apex. According to these anatomical definitions, the right coronary artery could therefore be considered the preponderant artery in 84 per cent of the population. In reality, as has been demonstrated by many anatomists and as is clearly visible in the majority of coronary arteriograms, the left coronary artery gives rise to the greatest number of ramifications directed toward the thickest part of the left ventricular wall, toward the largest portion of the interventricular septum, toward the largest part of the atria, and toward the smallest portion of the right ventricle. It is therefore evident that the left coronary artery is, by far, the predominant artery in man. The right coronary artery, instead, gives origin to the

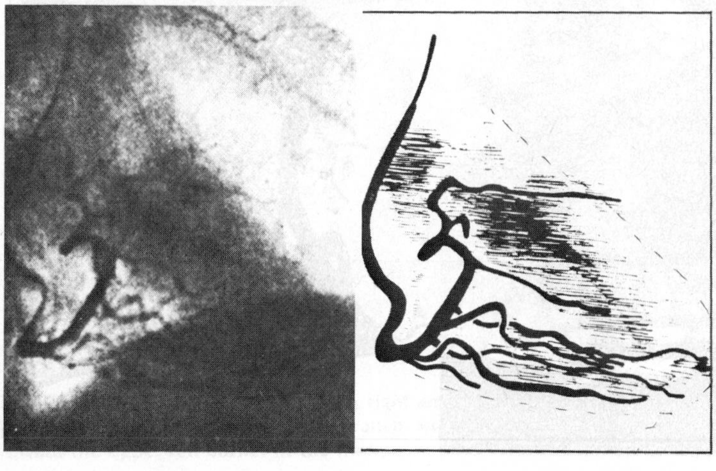

FIGURE 10–22 Definition of the area of the interventricular septum supplied by the posterior descending, obtained by filming past the arterial phase, during the parenchymal phase of the injection. That portion of the interventricular septum supplied by the posterior descending stands out, in the RAO view, as a triangle. (From Gensini, G. G.: Coronary Arteriography. Mount Kisco, N.Y., Futura Publishing Co., 1975.)

branch of the sinus node and to the branch of the AV node in approximately 60 per cent of cases and appears to be more often involved in perfusion of areas of specialized autonomic tissue.

In patients with so-called right preponderant coronary anatomy, the right coronary artery does not terminate with the posterior descending branch, even though this is its most important branch. Instead, the right coronary artery continues beyond the origin of the posterior descending branch and beyond the crux, passing along the diaphragmatic aspect of the left ventricle. In this area it gives off a variable number of posterolateral branches (sometimes referred to as posterior left ventricular branches). These branches can sometimes be quite large, even larger than the posterior descending branch itself. They supply blood to the diaphragmatic aspect of the left ventricle and can be seen best in a 45-degree left anterior oblique projection. In this view, the entire sweep of the right coronary artery resembles a sickle, the blade being formed by the main stem of the right coronary artery and the handle being formed by the posterior descending and posterior left ventricular branches (Fig. 10–13).

From a surgical standpoint, the main question that needs to be resolved is whether or not the right coronary artery gives rise to the posterior descending and, eventually, to important left ventricular branches. Whenever the right coronary artery provides such a branch or branches in patients who are being subjected to coronary artery revascularization, clinically significant obstructions or occlusions of this artery should be bypassed with a graft, placed downstream with respect to the most distal lesion. If the right coronary artery does not give rise to the posterior descending branch, any right-sided lesion is considered surgically insignificant.

Left Coronary Artery (Table 10–3)

The left coronary artery, usually the largest and shortest coronary artery, originates from the left sinus of Valsalva. The ostium of the left coronary artery is usually located at the level of the aortic ring and often can be found immediately above it (Fig. 10–8). Owing to the inclination of the aortic valvular plane over the sagittal, frontal, and horizontal planes, the position of the ostium of the left coronary artery appears to be located at a higher level than the right coronary artery orifice. Often the left coronary ostium appears as much as 1 cm higher than the right. This is true in all the common projections used in coronary arteriography. The axis of the ostium of the left coronary artery is located from 20 to 50 degrees (average = 30 to 40 degrees) posterior to the frontal plane.

Main Stem of the Left Coronary Artery. This vessel is directed anteriorly, to the left, and downward. The path of its axis in the horizontal plane varies from about 30 degrees anteriorly to 20 degrees posteriorly to the frontal plane. This means that the ostium of the left coronary artery is located posterior to the axis of this artery. This anatomical detail is a highly significant arteriographic finding, since it indicates that the catheterization of the main left coronary artery is best approached in a 30-degree right anterior oblique view, but the course of this artery is best outlined by a far shallower view. Owing to its path in the frontal plane, it is not easily identifiable in the left oblique view over 45 degrees, since the artery is then seen almost on end and appears to be greatly foreshortened, being almost perpendicular to the plane of the image intensifier. Because of its position within the chest, the main left coronary artery would be seen best in the anteroposterior view if it were not for the occasional superimposition of the spinal column. An excellent compromise is to film the main left coronary artery in a very shallow (10-degree) right anterior oblique projection, just enough to shift the spine slightly away from this vessel. The main left coronary artery may also be reasonably well visualized in the standard 30-degree right anterior oblique view (Fig. 10–23, *top*) or in a shallow (40- to 45-degree) left anterior oblique view (Fig. 10–23, *bottom*).

Bunnell et al.[17] were the first to introduce the "tilted"[13] or angulated[47–51] views in coronary angiography, primarily

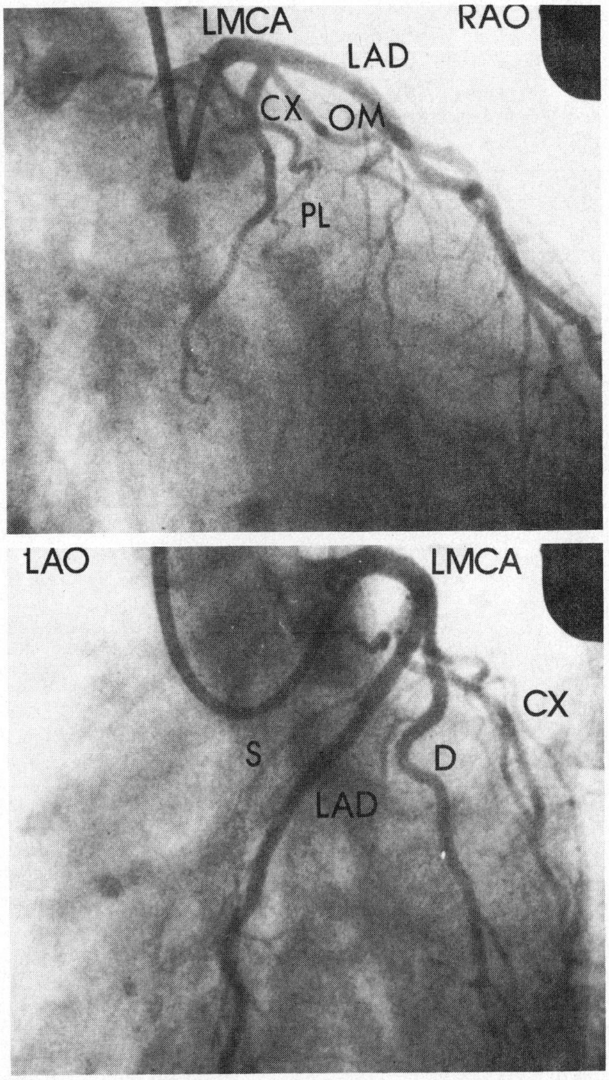

FIGURE 10–23 Left coronary artery. *Top,* Right anterior oblique view. *Bottom,* Left anterior oblique view. (Same patient as in Figures 10–13 and 10–14.) LMCA = left main coronary artery; LAD = left anterior descending artery; CX = circumflex coronary artery; OM = obtuse marginal branch; S = septal branch; D = diagonal branch; PL = posterolateral branch.

TABLE 10–3 LEFT CORONARY ARTERY—ANATOMICAL CONSIDERATIONS

Branch of Left Coronary Artery	Abbreviation	International Anatomical Classification	Number of Vessels	Percentage of Time From LCA
Left main	MLCA	Arteria coronaria sinistra	Absent if C and LAD have separate ostia	
Anterior descending (proximal and mid portion)	LAD	Ramus interventricularis anterior (pars proximalis)	1, rarely 2	98%
First diagonal	1°D	Ramus diagonalis (proximalis)	1	100%
First septal	1°S	Ramus septalis anterior (proximalis)	1	99.8%
Septals (minor)	S	Rami septales anteriores (distales)	Several	100%
Apical portion (interventricular)	IV	Ramus interventricularis anterior (pars distalis)	1	100%
Second diagonal	2°D	Ramus diagonalis (distalis)	1 or 3	100%
Circumflex	C or Cx	Ramus circumflexus	1	97%
Obtuse margin	OM	Ramus marginalis sinister	1 or 2	97%
Sinus node	SN (L)	Ramus nodi sinoatrialis sinister	0 or 1	C, 39%
Atrial circumflex	AC	Ramus atrialis sinister	1	98%
Posterolateral	PL	Rami posterolaterales sinistri	1 or 2	80%
Posterior descending	PD	Ramus interventricularis posterior	1	18%
AV node	AVN (L)	Ramus nodi atrioventricularis	1	11.9%

Modified from Kelly, A. E., and Gensini, G. G.: Coronary arteriography and left heart studies. Heart Lung *4*:85, 1975.

Other Sites of Origin and Time Present	Area Perfused	Best Angiographic View	Site of Origin and Route if Comes From LCA	Role in Collateral Blood Supply (Usual)
2% absent; from RCA, 0.1%	Entire LV, LA except the posterior portion of IV septum and adjacent area when PD is branch of RCA	$CR^{30^\circ}R^{20^\circ}AO$ AP $CR^{30^\circ}L^{45-60^\circ}AO$ $CA^{20^\circ}L^{60^\circ}AO$	LF sinus of Valsalva; runs behind pulmonary artery	None
Left sinus of Valsalva, separate ostium, 2%	Anterior 2/3 of IV septum, anterior portion of LV	$R^{20-30^\circ}AO$ $L^{60^\circ}AO$ $CR^{30^\circ}L^{60^\circ}AO$ $CR^{30^\circ}R^{30^\circ}$ $CA^{20^\circ}R^{30^\circ}AO$	Beneath left auricular appendage and pulmonary artery; runs along IV sulcus	Joins PD through its terminal branches
None	High lateral wall of LV	$CR^{30^\circ}L^{45-60^\circ}AO$	AD; runs in high lateral aspect of LV free wall	Joins lateral branch of C
RCA, 0.2%	Superior and anterior portion of IV septum	(lacks motion) $R^{20^\circ}AO$ $CR^{30^\circ}R^{20-30^\circ}AO$	AD, 90° angle; runs in anterior and superior half of IV septum	Joins posterior septals
None	Inferior and anterior 1/3 of septum	(lacks motion) $CR^{30^\circ}R^{20-30^\circ}AO$	AD, 90° angle; runs in anterior and inferior half of IV septum	Joins posterior septals
	Anterior aspect of apex	$CR^{30^\circ}R^{20-30^\circ}AO$ $L^{60^\circ}AO$	Continuation of AD. Route: Lower IV groove and apex	Joins posterior descending lateral branch of C
	Lower lateral aspect of LV free wall	$L^{60^\circ}AO$ $CR^{30^\circ}L^{45^\circ}AO$	Distal 2/3 of AD. Route: Diagonally along LV free wall	Joins lateral branch of C
RCA, right sinus of Valsalva, 1%; left sinus of Valsalva, separate ostium, 2%	Obtuse margin of heart and its entire posterior wall, post-IV septum when PD is branch of C, left atrium	$R^{30^\circ}AO$ $L^{60^\circ}AO$ $CA^{20^\circ}R^{30^\circ}AO$	Main LCA at level of anterior left AV sulcus beneath left auricular appendage. Route: Along left AV sulcus beneath left auricular appendage and below left pulmonary vein	Joins AD and/or RCA through its terminal branch
RCA, 3%	Obtuse margin of heart and adjacent posterior LV	$R^{30^\circ}AO$ $CA^{20^\circ}R^{30^\circ}AO$	Within first 5 cm C. Route: Laterally and posteriorly along OM of heart	May connect with D, AD, PL, PD
RCA, 59%, RCA and C, 2%	Sinus node, right and left atria	$R^{30^\circ}AO$ $L^{60^\circ}AO$	Initial C, few millimeters beyond origin. Route: Runs cranially, dorsally, to right, to base of SVC	Atrial branches connect with proximal portion of RCA
RCA, 2%	Left atrial wall	$R^{30^\circ}AO$ $L^{60^\circ}AO$	First 4 cm C runs along posterior left AV groove	Joins terminal RCA, terminal C
RCA, 20%	Posterior and diaphragmatic LV wall	$R^{30^\circ}AO$	Terminal C; posterior aspect of left AV groove. Route: Caudally and to left on post-LV	Joins with terminal branches of RCA, with lateral branch of C
RCA, 78%; RCA and C, 4%	Posterior IV septum and diaphragmatic LV	$CR^{30^\circ}R^{30^\circ}AO$ $L^{60^\circ}AO$	Terminal C; to left of crux cordis	Joins septal and terminal branch of C
RCA, 87.9%; RCA and C, 0.2%	AV node, lower portion of IA septum	$L^{60^\circ}AO$	Level of U curve at crux cordis. Route: Runs cranially and to center of heart	Joins septal branch of AD

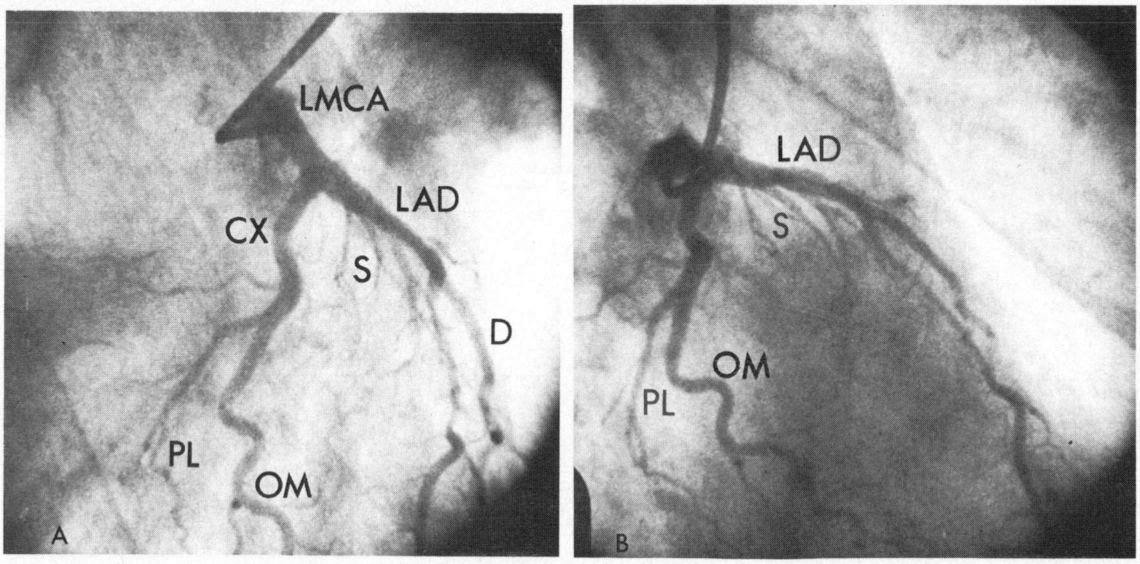

FIGURE 10–24 Left coronary artery. *A,* Hemiaxial left anterior oblique view. Excellent demonstration of main left coronary artery. *B,* Conventional left anterior oblique view. The main left coronary artery is highly foreshortened.

to improve the visualization of the proximal left coronary artery. This most important vessel is particularly well seen $CR^{30°}L^{60°}AO$ and $CR^{30°}R^{30°}AO$ (Fig. 10–24*A*). Occasionally, among patients with horizontal hearts and/or cephalad-directed proximal left coronary artery, a $CA^{30°}L^{60°}AO$ may be quite useful[21,47] (Fig. 10–25*A* and *B*).

The main stem of the left coronary artery is usually the largest of the main trunks, often exceeding 4.5 mm in diameter. It is also one of the shortest among the important vessels of the body. We have observed many left coronary arteries of only 1 or 2 mm in length. Sometimes the main left coronary artery may actually be missing, with the left coronary ostium appearing like a shallow funnel with two separate openings—the left anterior descending and the circumflex. When it is short, visualization of the main left coronary artery may be difficult and could be missed in many frames. In these cases the tip of the catheter appears to be in direct contact with the bifurcation between the left anterior descending and the circumflex branches.

The main left coronary artery divides into its two branches, the anterior descending and the circumflex, while still in the space between the aorta and pulmonary artery. Occasionally, however, its mode of termination may not be a straightforward bifurcation. Indeed, in approximately one fifth of our cases, there were more than two branches. In such patients, in the left anterior oblique view, the branch arching away from the left coronary artery and running in the direction of the crux of the heart is the circumflex branch; the one forming a wide arch and descending vertically toward the apex is the anterior de-

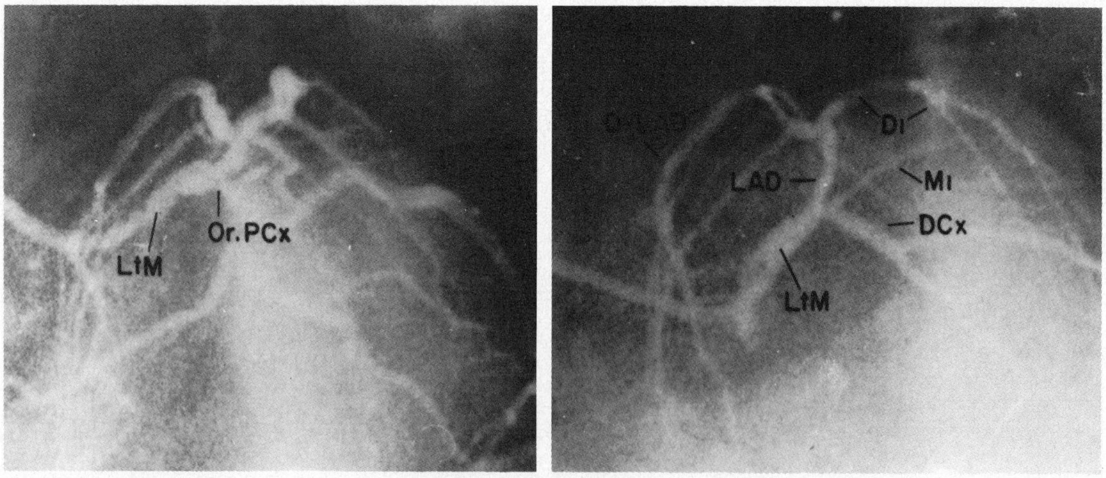

FIGURE 10–25 CA-LAO views in two patients. *Left,* There is severe stenosis of the origin of the proximal circumflex (Or.PCx). This area was unmasked by this view. *Right,* The entire proximal left anterior descending artery (LAD) was narrowed. There is an early-arising first marginal (M^1) which on other views could not be distinguished from a ramus intermedius or first diagonal. The origin of the first diagonal (D^1) is nicely seen. LtM = left main artery; D-LAD=distal left anterior descending artery; DCx=distal circumflex artery. (From Elliot, L. P., Bream, P. R., Soto, B., Russell, R. O., Rogers, W. J., Mantle, J. A., and Hood, W. P.: Significance of caudal left anterior oblique view in analyzing the left main coronary artery and its major branches. Radiology *139*:39, 1981.)

scending branch. The other branches, located between the anterior descending and circumflex and distributing to the free wall of the left ventricle, run in a lateral and caudal direction toward the apex and are named diagonal branches of the left ventricle. The best projection to observe the division of the left main stem into its branches is the $CR^{30°}L^{60°}AO$,[52] but a standard left anterior oblique may be adequate in most cases (Fig. 20–23, *bottom*). In this projection the two principal rami, the circumflex and the anterior descending, run along opposite borders of the cardiac shadow, whereas the diagonal branches occur in the angle subtended by these vessels. When all these branches are particularly evident and tortuous, the ensemble takes on the appearance, in the left oblique projection, of an octopus whose head is represented by the main stem and whose tentacles are represented by the left coronary branches, which seem to wave and contract with each cardiac cycle. In approximately 0.5 per cent of cases, the only artery arising from the left sinus of Valsalva is the anterior descending, since the circumflex is, in those cases, a branch of the right coronary artery.

In patients with high diaphragms, with horizontal hearts, and with horizontal or cephalad-directed left coronary arteries, a "weeping willow" view ($CA^{30°}L^{60°}AO$) may improve the visualization of the division of the left main stem into its branches[47] (Fig. 10–25*A* and *B*).

Left Anterior Descending Coronary Artery. This is the vessel in the human heart with the most constant origin, course, and distribution. Generally, it begins as a continuation of the main left coronary artery, passes to the left of the pulmonic valve, and runs along the anterior interventricular sulcus.

The size, length, and distribution of the left anterior descending are key factors in the balance of the perfusion to the interventricular septum, the lateral wall, and the apex of the left ventricle. Thus, according to D. B. Effler (personal communication), it should be classified arteriographically into Types I, II, and III depending on its length and the amount of myocardium it perfuses. The Type I left anterior descending is a small-caliber vessel that reaches only two thirds of the way from the base of the heart to the apex and that seems to be more prevalent in women. The Type II left anterior descending is a vessel of larger caliber and, by definition, reaches the apex of the left ventricle. The Type III left anterior descending extends from the base of the heart to the apex and around to the diaphragmatic aspect of the left ventricle, where it augments the normal perfusion pattern of the posterior descending artery. Anastomoses with the posterior descending branch are often visualized following occlusion of the right coronary artery.

The left anterior descending coronary artery can be well visualized in all projections. In the right anterior oblique view, it approaches the left border of the cardiac shadow (Fig. 10–11); in the anteroposterior view, it appears as the branch of the left coronary artery that runs caudally, with a more or less vertical course, separating the right from the left ventricle; in the $L^{60°}AO$, left lateral, and $CR^{30°}L^{60°}AO$ views, it is represented by the branch of the left coronary artery that is directed more ventrally than any of the other branches (Fig. 10–23, *bottom*). Sometimes, in both the right anterior oblique and the anteroposterior views, it may be difficult to distinguish the anterior descending from the many left ventricular branches of the circumflex. However, this task can be simplified by observing the film in motion. In so doing, all the anteriorly located vessels (the anterior descending, the septal, and the diagonal branches) appear to move in a direction opposite to the posteriorly located arteries (i.e., the ventricular branches of the circumflex, such as the obtuse and the posterolateral branches). Another cine angiographic feature typical of the left anterior descending (and especially of its septal branches) is their relative lack of motion, when compared to the behavior of the circumflex and of the right coronary artery.

The branches of the left anterior descending artery are, in order of origin, the first diagonal, the first septal, the right ventricular (infrequently demonstrated), the minor septals, the second diagonal, and the apical. From a surgical standpoint, it is helpful to divide the left anterior descending artery into proximal, mid, and apical segments (Fig. 10–26). The most important landmark along the course of this artery is the origin of the major (and usually first) septal branch. That portion of the anterior descending artery located between its origin from the main left coronary artery and the first septal branch is the proximal third. The middle third runs from the origin of the main septal branch to the origin of the second diagonal branch. Distal to that vessel we find the terminal (or apical) segment of the anterior descending, which usually reaches the apex, encircles it, and often runs for a short distance along the posterior interventricular groove (Type III LAD).

In most cases, the first branch of the anterior descending is a rather large vessel that distributes to the free wall of the left ventricle, roughly midway between the anterior interventricular groove and the obtuse margin of the heart. Owing to their diagonal course along the free wall of the left ventricle, this vessel and any other branch of the anterior descending artery with distribution to the same general area of the myocardium are called "diagonals." The first diagonal often originates quite close to the bifurcation of the main left coronary artery and in more than 10 per cent of cases has a separate origin from the main stem, so that the left coronary artery ends in a trifurcation rather than a bifurcation.

The best projections to observe the origin and course of the diagonal branches are the left anterior oblique (Fig. 20–23, *bottom*) and the $CR^{30°}R^{30°}AO$ views (Fig. 10–24*A*). In the right anterior oblique view, the first diagonal is often superimposed on the left anterior descending artery, and it may be quite difficult to separate the two vessels, at least along their more proximal segments. The more distal two thirds of the first diagonal, however, are well visualized in the right anterior oblique view. Here the diagonal appears to run along the border of the left heart shadow roughly parallel to the shadow of the ribs (Figs. 10–20 to 10–23, *top*; Fig. 10–24; and Fig. 10–25*A* and *B*).

Although there may be several small "diagonal" branches, one of these is referred to as the second diagonal branch and serves to separate the apical third of the left anterior descending artery from its middle third. This vessel branches off at an acute angle from the left anterior descending artery and distributes to the lateral portion of the apex.

The septal branches, which vary in number, arise from the left anterior descending artery at about a 90-degree angle. They run along the septum from front to back and in a caudal direction, with distribution to about two thirds of the upper portion of the septum and perfusing almost the entire septum in its inferior third (Figs. 10–24 and 10–25*A* and *B*). The more posterior and superior third of the septum receives its blood supply through the short branches derived from the posterior descending branch. Therefore, in a large percentage of cases, the septum is another important area of anastomosis between the right and left coronary arteries. On the other hand, when the posterior descending branch originates from the circumflex, the left coronary artery is the sole source of blood supply for the entire interventricular septum.

The largest (and usually the first) septal branch is of extreme importance because of its prominent role in supplying blood to the septum and its consistency of origin, course, and distribution. For these reasons, the first septal branch represents a major landmark in the identification and description of the left anterior descending artery, both in health and, especially, in disease. As indicated, its origin serves to separate the first third of the anterior descending artery from its middle third. Any lesions of the anterior descending artery are usually classified in relation to this branch, i.e., as proximal or distal to it. The first septal artery is seen in the right anterior oblique view as that vessel which originates at a clear-cut 90-degree angle from its parent vessel, running vertically toward the diaphragm, in the middle of the heart shadow (Fig. 10–25*A* and *B*). The first septal is seen in an entirely different perspective in the left anterior oblique view, in which it appears to run above the left anterior descending artery, inclining from right to left and from top to bottom, with a course parallel to the left anterior descending artery (Fig. 10–25*C*).

The more cranial septal branches are better demonstrated angiographically than the lower septal branches, since they are of greater length and caliber. Their characteristic branching from the left anterior descending artery and their straight course, lacking the slight tortuosity of the other branches, make them easy to identify (Fig. 10–25*A* and *B*) and, in turn, help to distinguish the anterior descending artery from the large diagonal branches, with which it could be confused in the right anterior oblique view. Another cineangiographic feature, typical of the left anterior descending and septal branches, is their relative lack of motion. This is especially evident when the left coronary artery is viewed against the background of the circumflex in the right anterior oblique view (Fig. 10–25*A* and *B*).

In its course, the left anterior descending artery gives off one or more *branches to the right ventricle.* The highest of these runs toward the conus branch of the right coronary artery, at the level of the pulmonic valve, forming, as a consequence of obstructions or occlusions of either the right coronary or left anterior descending artery, the anastomotic ring of Vieussens[52]; the other branches run obliquely over the right ventricular surface, anastomosing with similar branches of the right coronary artery. These branches are seldom angiographically identifiable in normal subjects; however, they become more readily appreciable in cases of occlusion of the parent vessel, thus acquiring great importance as collateral channels.

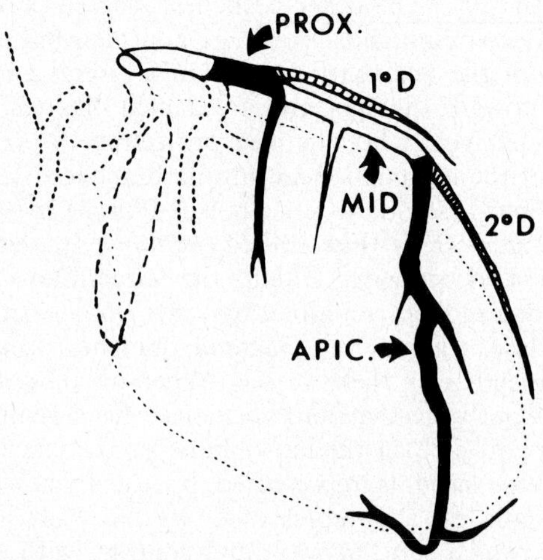

FIGURE 10–26 Diagram of left anterior descending branch in right anterior oblique projection showing its division into proximal, mid, and apical segments. The first and second diagonal branches are also shown. (From Gensini, G. G.: Coronary Arteriography. Mount Kisco, N.Y., Futura Publishing Co., 1975.)

The terminal branches of the Type III left anterior descending artery are the apical branches (Figs. 10–26 to 10–28). They distribute to both the anterior and the diaphragmatic aspects of the apex. Usually at least two branches can be seen (especially in the right anterior oblique view): the recurrent posterior and the recurrent lateral apical branches, the former turning around the apex and supplying its diaphragmatic portion (Figs. 10–26 and 10–27) and the latter supplying the lateral aspect of the apex.

Left Circumflex Artery. This vessel usually departs at a rather sharp angle from the main left coronary artery to run posteriorly along the atrioventricular groove, toward the crux cordis, which, however, it reaches in only 16 per cent of cases. In 84 per cent of cases, the circumflex ends distal to the obtuse margin without reaching the posterior interventricular sulcus. When the circumflex reaches and passes beyond this region, it gives origin to the posterior descending branch (Fig. 10–29); in such cases, the left coronary artery not only is the sole source of blood supply to the entire interventricular septum but also gives origin to the branch supplying the atrioventricular node.

In the anteroposterior and right anterior oblique views, the left circumflex artery usually appears as the vessel first

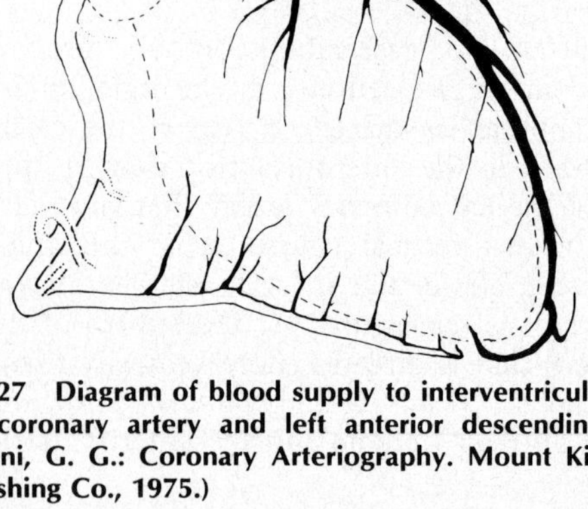

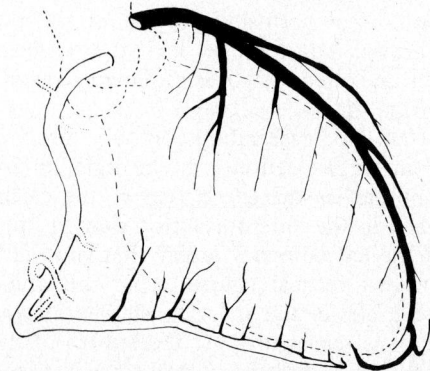

FIGURE 10–27 Diagram of blood supply to interventricular septum from right coronary artery and left anterior descending branch. (From Gensini, G. G.: Coronary Arteriography. Mount Kisco, N.Y., Futura Publishing Co., 1975.)

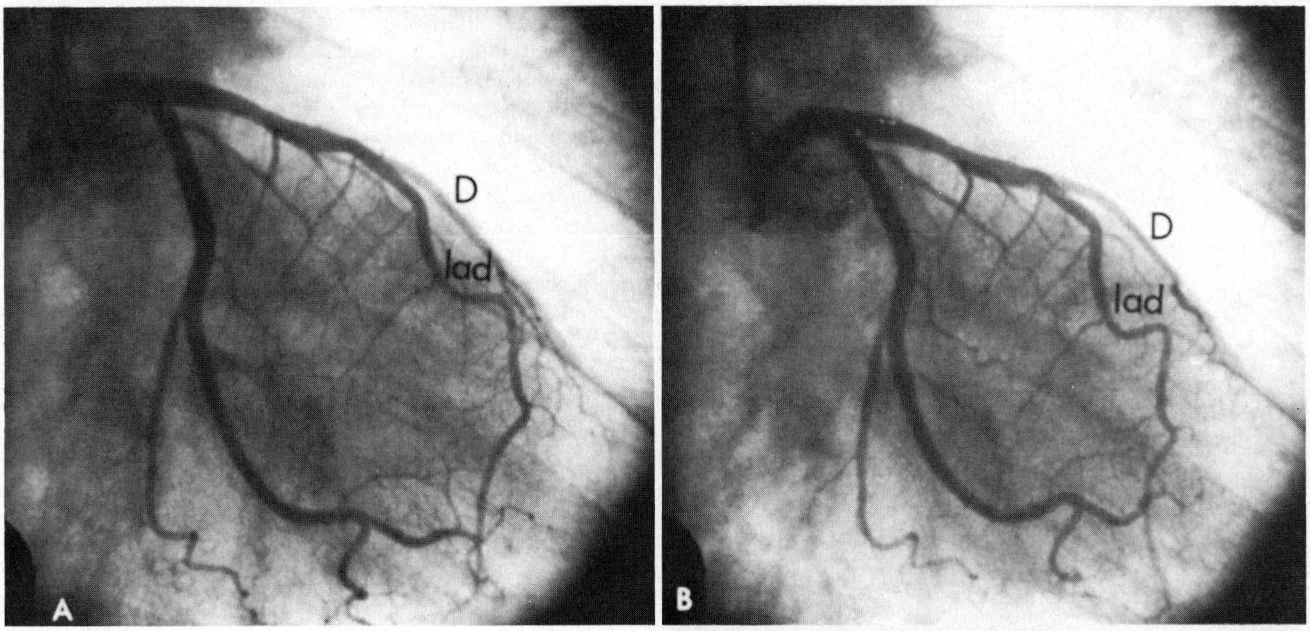

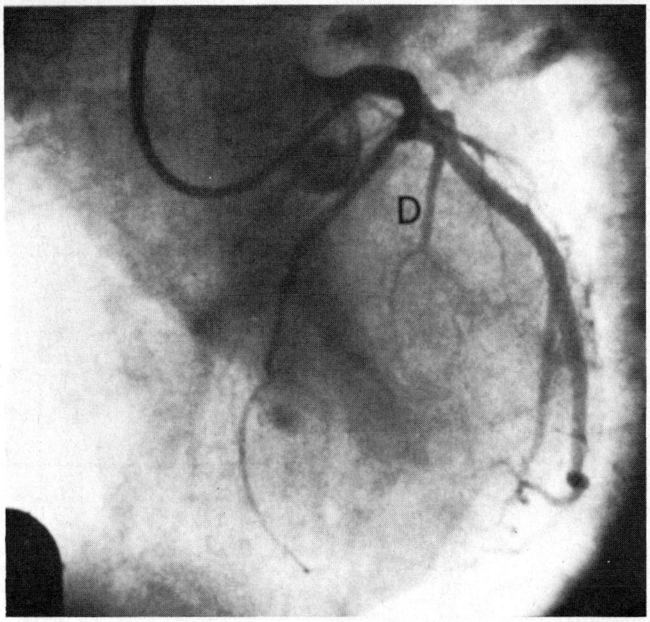

C

FIGURE 10–28 Left coronary artery. Right anterior oblique view in diastole (*A*) and systole (*B*). *C,* Left anterior oblique view. D = diagonal branch; lad = left anterior descending coronary artery.

to depart from the general direction taken by the left coronary artery (Figs. 10–24*B* and 10–28*A* and *B*). It forms a circle directed first caudally and then toward the center of the heart, coursing along the left atrioventricular groove. In the left anterior oblique view (Fig. 10–30), it appears to take the course directly opposite to that of the anterior descending artery, moving caudally and posteriorly toward the vertebral column, occasionally encircling the posterior border of the heart shadow (Figs. 10–23, *top,* and 10–30).

Soon after its origin, the circumflex not infrequently divides into two parallel branches, which are occasionally of nearly equal caliber. The lower, and usually the larger, of the two gives origin to the ventricular branches. The superior one, called the *atrial circumflex,* gives origin to branches for the atrial wall. More commonly, however, the atrial circumflex is a relatively slender branch that runs opposite to the ventricular branches.

In the 41 per cent of cases in which the *sinus node artery* is a branch of the left coronary artery, this vessel usually originates from the initial portion of the circumflex, a few millimeters beyond the origin of the latter. Less frequently, it takes off from the mid portion of the circumflex and rarely from its distal segment.

The largest and most constant branch (or branches) of the circumflex is the *branch* (or branches) *to the obtuse margin.* This vessel (or vessels) arises from the circumflex and runs along the ventricular wall, somewhat posteriorly and in the direction of the apex. Very often one of these branches acquires a special importance and appears as the very large branch which, in the left anterior oblique view, runs along the posterior edge of the left ventricular border (Fig. 10–28*C*). It maintains a path which, in the right anterior oblique view, is slightly inclined in relation to the course of the left anterior descending coronary artery (Fig. 10–28*A* and *B*).

The proximal portions of the obtuse marginal, anterior descending, and diagonal branches may be closely superimposed on one another when the origin of the obtuse

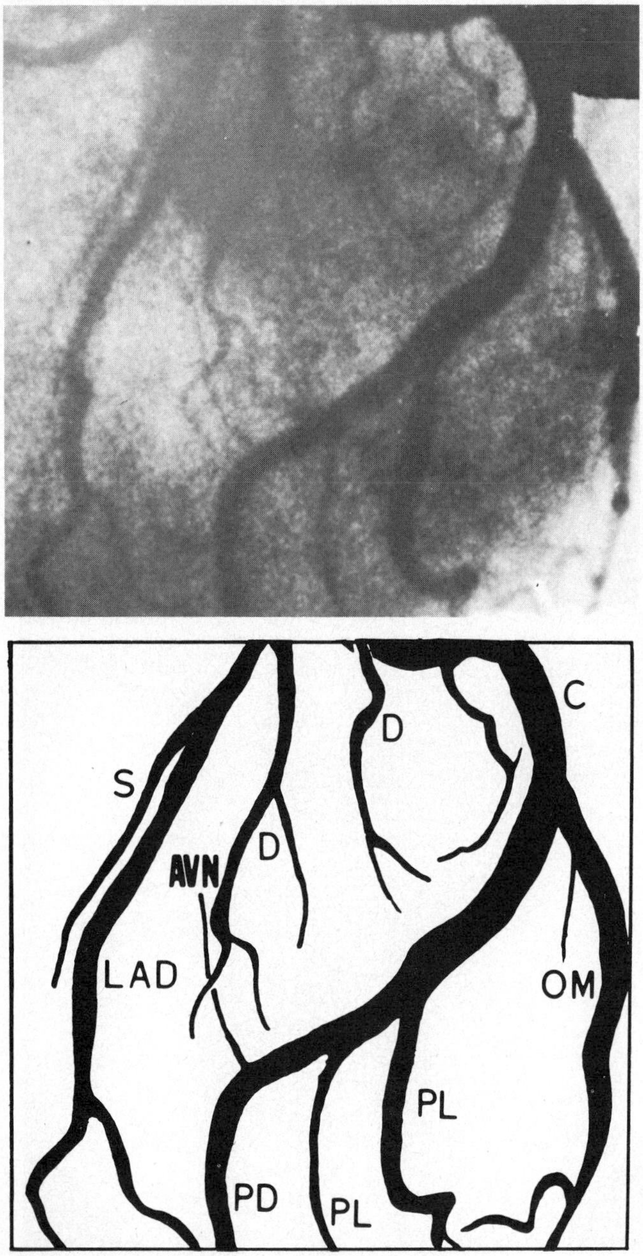

marginal is along the initial segment of the circumflex. This bunching up of several vessels may make it difficult to recognize minor (and sometimes even major) lesions of any one of these branches in either the right or the left anterior oblique view (Figs. 10–23*B* and 10–30). In such cases, the $CA^{20°}R^{30°}AO$ view may be necessary to separate the various branches adequately.

There is considerable variation in the anatomy of the obtuse marginal branches of the left circumflex artery. Anywhere from one to four of these branches may be present, and they vary in size from quite large (as large as the left anterior descending artery) to quite small. They supply the lateral wall of the left ventricle above its diaphragmatic surface. After giving rise to the obtuse marginal branches, the circumflex artery continues along the left atrioventricular groove for a variable distance toward the crux of the heart. Because of its close relationship to the atrioventricular groove (and mitral valve ring), this portion of the circumflex artery moves widely with systole and diastole, i.e., toward the apex in systole and away from it in diastole. This motion is especially evident in the right anterior oblique projection. In over 80 per cent of cases, the circumflex artery does not reach the crux of the heart but terminates along the left atrioventricular groove after giving rise to the obtuse marginal branches. In 14 per cent of cases, the so-called left preponderant coronary anatomy exists (Fig. 10–29). In these patients, the posterior descending and posterolateral branches do not arise from the right coronary artery but instead arise from the left circumflex.

After giving rise to the obtuse marginal branches, the left circumflex artery continues all the way around the left atrioventricular groove. As it passes along this groove and reaches the diaphragm, it gives rise to the posterolateral branches, and when it reaches the crux of the heart, it turns forward to continue along the posterior interventric-

FIGURE 10–29 Left coronary artery, left anterior oblique view. Origin of posterior descending branch (PD) and AV node branch (AVN) from circumflex. (From Gensini, G. G.: Coronary Arteriography. Mount Kisco, N.Y., Futura Publishing Co., 1975.)

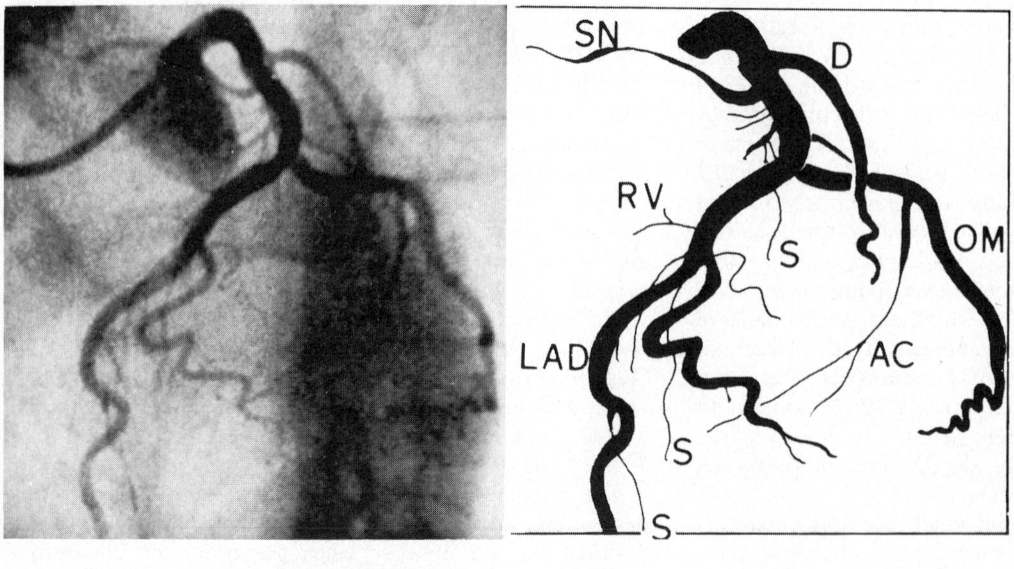

FIGURE 10–30 Left coronary artery, left anterior oblique view. (From Gensini, G. G.: Coronary Arteriography. Mount Kisco, N.Y., Futura Publishing Co., 1975.)

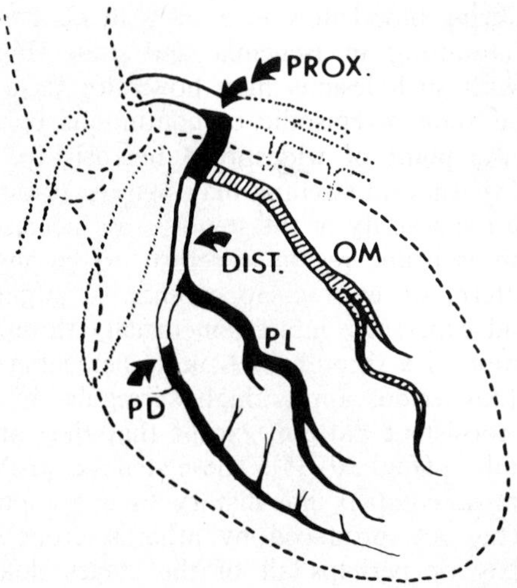

FIGURE 10–31 Diagram of circumflex in right anterior oblique view, showing its division into four segments (or into five segments when the posterior descending is a branch of the circumflex). (From Gensini, G. G.: Coronary Arteriography. Mount Kisco, N.Y., Futura Publishing Co., 1975.)

ular groove as the posterior descending artery. Regardless of its origin—whether it is a branch of the right coronary artery or of the circumflex—the posterior descending coronary artery follows the same course along the posterior interventricular groove and supplies the same portion of the posterior interventricular septum (p. 319). Its origin from the circumflex is best seen in the left anterior oblique view (Fig. 10–29), although it soon becomes foreshortened. For this reason, the best means of observing its middle and distal portions, as well as the posterior septal arteries that issue from it, is by using the right anterior oblique projection. The AV node branch, which originates from the distal segment of the circumflex in 12 per cent of cases, is also well visualized in the left anterior oblique view (Fig. 10–29). It appears as a slender and straight vessel departing from the circumflex at a 90-degree angle in a direction opposite to the posterior descending artery.

From a surgical standpoint, the circumflex is divided into four or five segments (Fig. 10–31).

Tables 10–2 and 10–3 summarize the nomenclature, abbreviations, and course of all the coronary arteries and their major branches.

ANATOMY OF CORONARY ARTERIES IN DISEASE

AGING OF THE CORONARY ARTERIES. Aging of the arterial wall is associated with gradual distention caused by progressive deterioration of the elastic tissue that results in dilatation of the lumen. During the average life span, the cross-sectional area of the arteries increases six or seven times.[53] Degeneration of the elastic fibers in the media may be accompanied by calcification, which can occur without atheroma.[54] Two of these three changes typical of aging, i.e., dilatation of the lumen and calcification of the wall, may occasionally be seen during coronary arteriography in the elderly. This pattern has been noted in a few healthy octogenarians with atypical chest pain or valvular heart disease.

CORONARY ATHEROSCLEROSIS. Coronary atherosclerosis may begin at a relatively young age, i.e., in the twenties or thirties, in patients at high risk and, in the majority of these patients, progresses rapidly[55,56]; on the other hand, if an individual has reached age 50 to 60 with normal coronary arteries, chances are that he or she will remain free of coronary artery disease throughout the entire life span.[55,57]

Postmortem studies have repeatedly demonstrated that the incidence of coronary atherosclerosis peaks at about age 60[58] and declines in the very old, presumably because patients with severe lesions succumb to the disease before they reach an advanced age. Thus, coronary atherosclerosis is not a manifestation of age; on the contrary, longevity and severe coronary atherosclerosis are usually mutually exclusive. However, the changes typical of aging arteries may occasionally coexist with the truly pathological changes of atherosclerosis.[59]

MICROSCOPIC CHANGES

1. *Alterations of the elastic lamina:* There is no obvious arteriographic counterpart of this stage of the atherosclerotic process.

2. *Early deposition of lipid material:* Separation of the elastic fibers and elevation of the surface of the intima occur. These changes appear in the arteriogram as minute nickings and are generally smooth "regular irregularities" (Fig. 10–32).

3. *Fibrous plaques and atheromatous foci:* These fibrolipid plaques may become thick and encroach grossly upon the lumen of the artery, possibly leading to severe obstruction. The lesions are identifiable on the coronary arteriogram as fairly regular reductions in lumen diameter that may, upon serial studies, become progressively more severe in a stepwise fashion (Fig. 10–33).

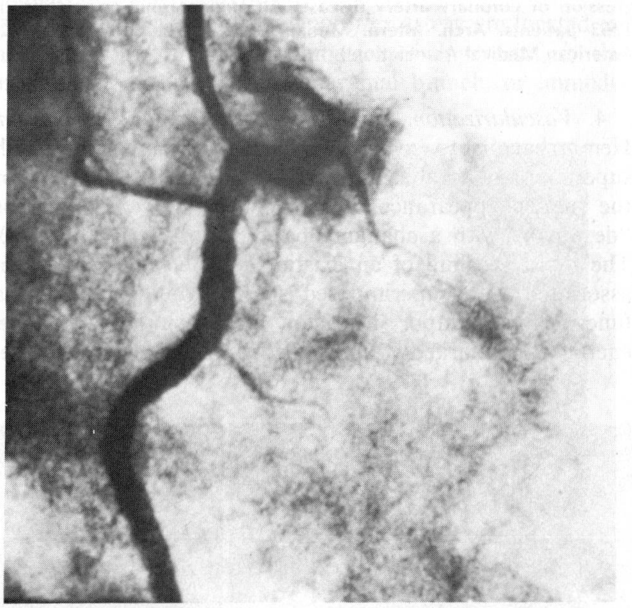

FIGURE 10–32 Right coronary artery, right anterior oblique view. Minute irregularities are observed at several points and resemble minute nickings or scallopings of the wall. (From Gensini, G. G.: Coronary Arteriography. Mount Kisco, N.Y., Futura Publishing Co., 1975.)

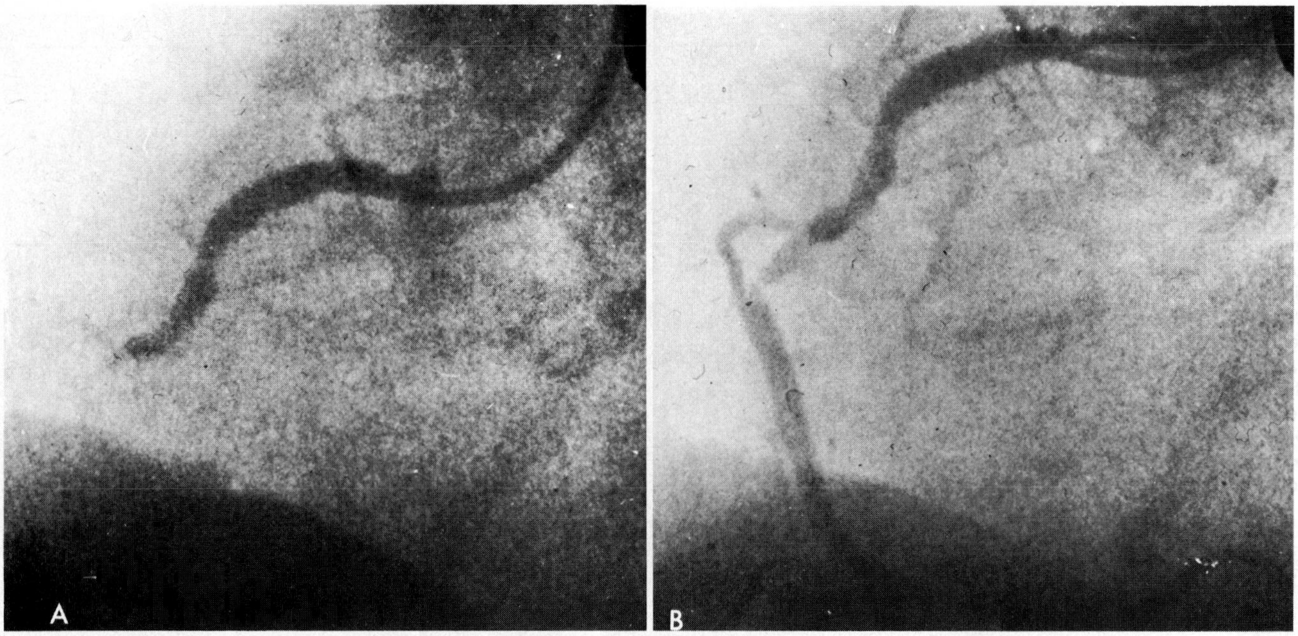

FIGURE 10–43 Right coronary artery, left anterior oblique view, in 49-year-old male. *A,* Apparent total occlusion. No contrast agent progressed beyond the point shown at any time during or after injection. *B,* Five minutes after administration of 5 mg of chewable isosorbide dinitrate (Sorbitrate [Stuart Pharmaceuticals, Division of ICI America, Inc., Wilmington, Delaware]). (From Gensini, G. G.: Coronary Arteriography. Mount Kisco, N.Y., Futura Publishing Co., 1975.)

parenteral nitroglycerin, which should be *injected* into the left ventricle (or intravenously) in doses of 0.4 mg as soon as the ergonovine test is terminated (Fig. 10–44) or at the first sign of an adverse effect such as arrhythmia; reduction in contractility, especially associated with hypotension; a marked rise in left ventricular end-diastolic pressure; coronary artery occlusion; or severe ischemic pain. In refractory spasm nitroglycerin (in boluses of 0.2 mg) may also be injected into the involved coronary artery.

The effect of injection of nitroglycerin is a most rewarding and impressive pharmacodynamic event. Injected as a single 0.4-mg bolus into the left ventricle, it instantly reduces elevated left ventricular end-diastolic pressure, often with simultaneous improvement in the indices of contractility, and it induces moderate reductions in the systolic left ventricular pressure and a minimal increase in the pulse rate.[25] Coronary spasm, if present, promptly disappears; the patient becomes more comfortable, with alleviation of any chest pain or dyspnea; and left ventricular hypokinetic segments begin contracting vigorously.[15]

In over 2500 coronary arteriograms performed we have never observed a serious adverse or deleterious effect arising from administration of nitroglycerin. Most misconceptions and lost therapeutic opportunities appear to have been due to the occasional patient (2 to 3 per cent) who responds with excessive peripheral vasodilatation to the administration of nitroglycerin. This in no way impairs the function of the heart as a pump but warrants prompt treatment with simple elevation of the lower extremities and with intravenous fluids. Theoretically, a pure alpha adrenergic stimulant, such as phenylephrine, should be administered if simple physical measures prove inadequate, but we have never found this to be necessary.

Coronary Occlusion and Thrombolysis

An impressive body of knowledge on the pathophysiology and therapy of myocardial infarction has been accumulated during the last few years, since Rentrop's[74–76] demonstration of the safety and usefulness of coronary arteriography during the acute phases of myocardial infarction. These findings demonstrated that the direct cause of acute myocardial infarction in the majority of patients with symptoms of chest pain and ST-segment elevation is acute intraluminal coronary thrombosis, generally superimposed on an obstructive atherosclerotic lesion.[77,78] Either rupture of the plaque, spasm of the wall or both may precede the final thrombotic occlusion in most patients. Chazov, who first suggested the use of fibrinolytic agents for the treatment of thromboembolism and infarction,[79,80] was also the first to report in 1976[81,82] on the successful intracoronary administration of fibrinolysin in acute myocardial infarction. Mazur[83] earlier had reported on the use of parenteral streptokinase in patients with this condition. Dotter[84] in 1974 described his success with selective intra-arterial perfusion of streptokinase in thrombotic occlusion of peripheral arteries.

The experiences of Rentrop and associates,[74–76] followed by the reports of Ganz et al.,[85] gave the real impetus to this technique, which is now widely applied in many cardiac laboratories including the author's. Recanalization of an occluded coronary artery can be achieved in nearly 80 per cent of patients during the evolving stage of myocardial infarction.[86] However, the quality of the late results appears to be inversely related to the duration of ischemia.[87] It follows that early recognition of the syndrome and prompt catheterization of the affected artery are the key to the

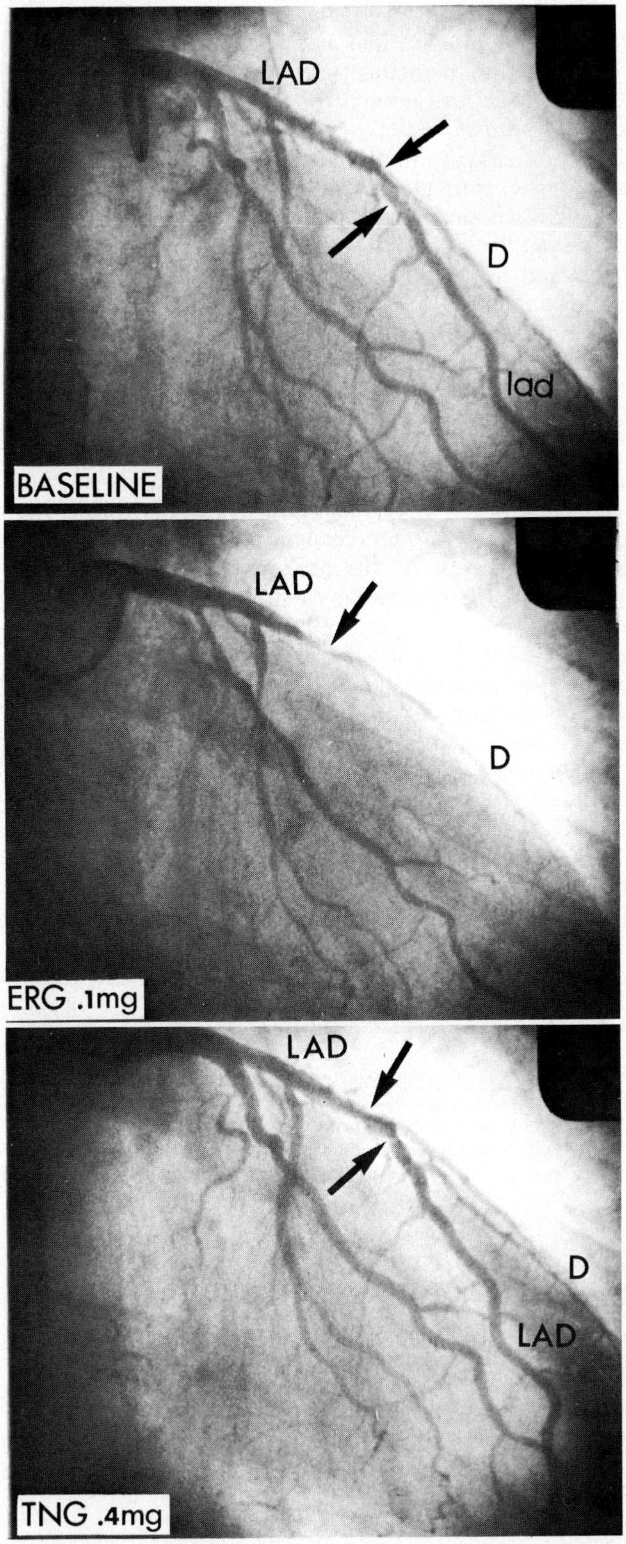

FIGURE 10–44 Left coronary artery, right oblique view. *Top,* Baseline injection. Arrows point to area of 50 to 75 per cent narrowing along left anterior descending branch. *Center,* After administration of 0.1 mg ergonovine in left ventricle. There is complete occlusion of left anterior descending, with total lack of filling of its mid and apical segments. The small *branch* seen is a diagonal branch and not the LAD proper. *Bottom,* Resolution of occluding spasm one minute after injection of 0.4 mg of nitroglycerin into the left ventricle.

successful application of this technique. Our protocol, which has been applied in 100 patients during the last 14 months, is designed with the safety of the patient well in mind and emphasizes simplicity and promptness of action.

PROCEDURE. The St. Joseph's Hospital Emergency Room is usually alerted by the Advance Life Support Unit about the impending arrival of a suspected myocardial infarction patient. As soon as the patient enters the emergency room, he or she is seen by the emergency room physician; if the diagnosis of myocardial infarction is confirmed by the presence of persistent ST-segment elevation, a blood sample for routine and coagulation studies is obtained, an I.V. nitroglycerin drip is started at 30 to 60 μg/min unless severe hypotension (systolic pressure below 80 mm Hg) is present. A lidocaine drip may also be started if frequent extrasystoles are present. If the ST-segment elevation does not disappear within five minutes from the beginning of the administration of nitroglycerin, the cardiovascular laboratory physician and the attending physician are immediately notified, while the patient and/or the family is advised of the availability of the myocardial infarction intervention protocol. If permission is obtained from the patient and the referring physician, the cardiovascular team is summoned and the patient is taken to the cardiovascular laboratory.

A team composed of an experienced cardiac angiographer, two laboratory nurses, and one laboratory technician is available at all times, less than 20 minutes away from the cardiovascular laboratory.

The Sones technique described previously is used; only the Sones catheter is employed for all functions and the left ventriculogram is delayed until the end of the procedure. As soon as the affected artery (or its parent) is entered, an injection of Renografin 76 is made to ascertain the status and level of the occluding lesions. Intracoronary nitroglycerin, 0.4 mg, is given, followed two minutes later by a second opacification of the artery. If the occlusion is persistent, an intracoronary bolus of 10,000 units of streptokinase is given. The streptokinase drip is then begun at 4000 units/min and continued for 30 minutes. Arteriograms are performed at 10, 20, and 30 minutes. A few ventricular premature beats occur at the time of the reopening of the artery. The drip is diminished to 3000 units/min and continued for an additional 30 minutes, again filming every 10 minutes. Generally the infusion is discontinued after 60 minutes.

A left ventriculogram is performed in the RAO view using 25 ml or less of Renografin 76 and the procedure is discontinued. Following the procedure the patient is treated with intravenous heparin (1000 units/hr in patients weighing between 150 and 200 lbs).

IDENTIFICATION AND ASSESSMENT OF JEOPARDIZED MYOCARDIUM

Both an expert and a novice arteriographer can benefit from a *systematic* approach to the analysis of coronary and left ventricular contrast studies. The following are suggested steps for an orderly analysis of a coronary arteriogram and left ventriculogram.

1. *Are the coronary arteries free of atherosclerotic lesions?*

A normal artery has smooth walls, tapers toward the periphery, is free of isolated areas of radiolucency, and possesses all expected important branches unless these originate from another vessel. Nicking and scalloping of an arterial border usually indicate early atherosclerotic changes. With regard to possible anatomical variations, the following three principles should be kept in mind:

a. Coronary artery disease is far more frequent than are unusual anatomical variations.
b. There are thousands of collaterals for any one variant, aberrant, or anomalous vessel.
c. Before an unusual vessel is accepted as a variant, an occlusion or a large collateral channel should be suspected. Conversely, systolic narrowing that disappears during diastole is pathognomonic of "myocardial

bridging" (Fig. 10–45), i.e., the intramyocardial course of an epicardial artery, and should not be confused with a permanent obstruction.

2. *Is the ventricle normal in size, shape, vigor, and symmetry of contraction?*

The normal pattern of left ventricular contraction as seen on cine ventriculography is a uniform, almost concentric inward motion of all points along the inner surface during systolic ejection. This pattern depends on the coordinated and sequential contraction of the myocardial mass, which is intended to produce maximum effective work at minimum cost (myocardial synergy).[88,89]

The normal outline of the human left ventricular cavity, as seen in the right anterior oblique projection during diastole, is that of an ellipsoid, with the tip inclined downward 45 degrees. During systole, the concentric inward motion of the anterior and posterior walls (and to a lesser extent of the apex) squeezes the sides and tips of the ellipsoid toward the center without changing the dimension of the base (mitral valve). At the peak of systolic ejection, the outline of the left ventricular cavity often resembles a pear core or an ice cream cone. When this outline enlarges or loses this characteristic appearance, left ventricular enlargement or asynergy should be suspected (Fig. 10–46).

The distribution of the coronary arteries to the left ventricular myocardium follows a broad outline that allows division of the ventricular mass into a number of segments according to the areas perfused by the major myocardial branches. We have found that division of the left ventricular silhouette into five major segments in the right anterior oblique projection and into two major segments in the left anterior oblique projection is adequate for the description of abnormalities of wall motion (Fig. 10–47). Depending on the degree of motion impairment, each segment can be

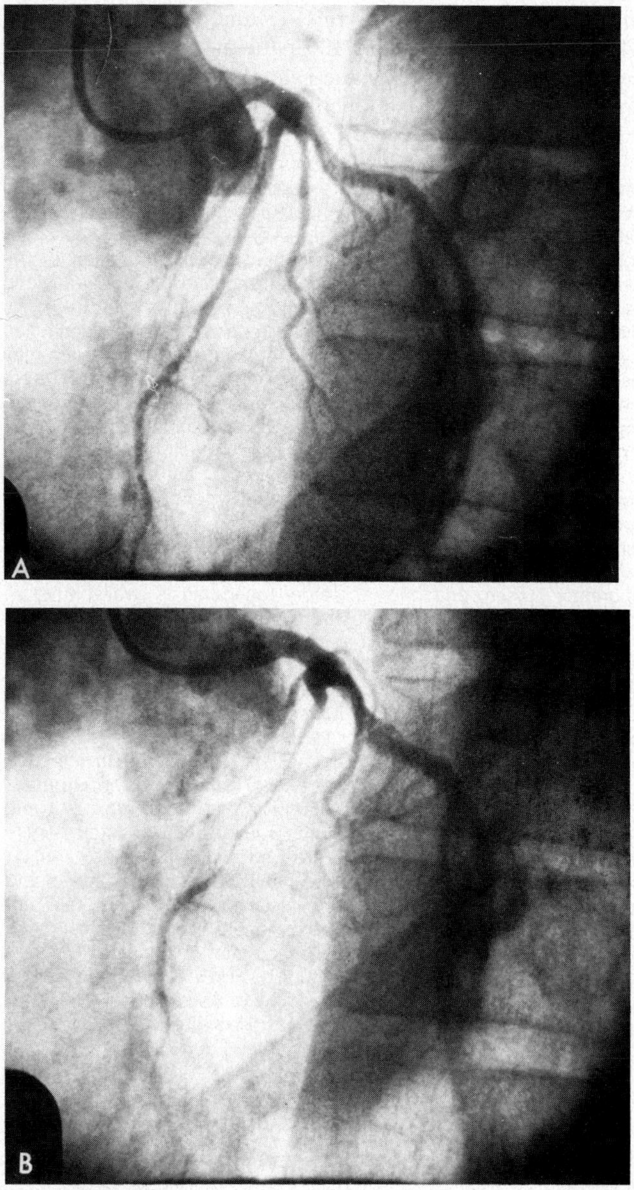

FIGURE 10–45 Left coronary artery, left anterior oblique view. In diastole (*A*) there is slight nicking and scalloping of the left anterior descending coronary artery. During systole (*B*) there is severe systolic narrowing (myocardial bridging) of the left anterior descending coronary artery, which is almost totally obliterated.

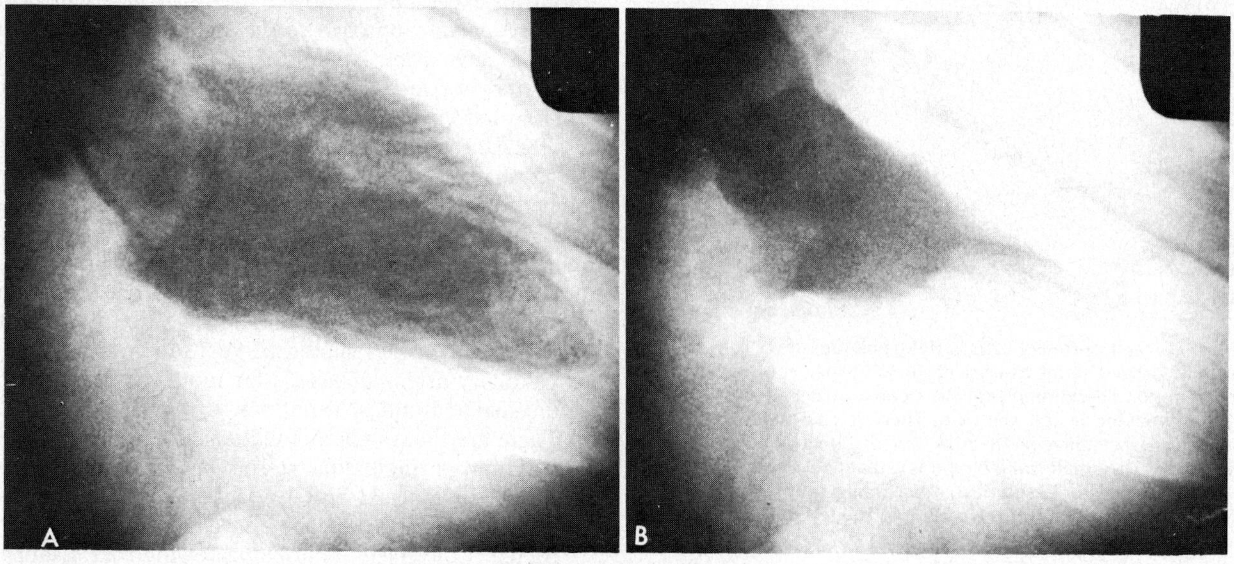

FIGURE 10–46 Normal left ventricle, right anterior oblique view, in diastole (*A*) and systole (*B*).

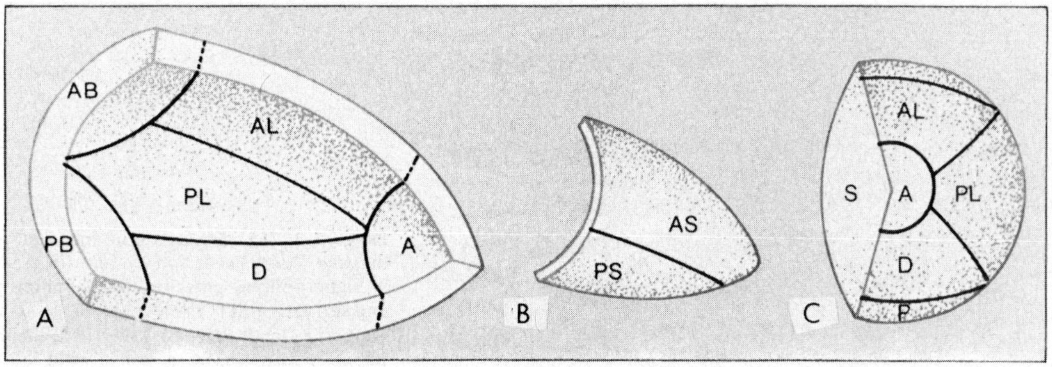

FIGURE 10-47 Schematic division of left ventricular wall, including septum, into seven segments.

A, Shell of free wall of ventricle as seen from front right after removal of interventricular septum. Segments are designated apical (A), anterobasal (AB), anterolateral (AL), diaphragmatic (D), posterobasal (PB), and posterolateral (PL).

B, Shell of interventricular septum as seen in the same projection, with division into portions supplied by anterior septal (AS) and posterior septal (PS) branches.

C, Apical view of left ventricle. S = septum. (From Gensini, G. G.: Coronary arteriography. Role in myocardial revascularization. Postgrad. Med. *63*:121, 1978.)

described as normal, hypokinetic (reduced motion), akinetic (absent motion), dyskinetic (systolic bulging), or aneurysmal (Fig. 10-48).

A useful means of quantifying ventricular performance is the ejection fraction (stroke volume/end-diastolic volume), usually calculated from the right anterior oblique images (Chap. 14). If a ventricle appears not to be enlarged in systole or diastole, if the silhouette conforms with the normal description and exhibits vigorous and symmetrical contraction of all segments, and if the ejection fraction is 55 per cent or greater, the left ventriculogram can be said to be normal. At this point, a patient found to have normal coronary arteries and a normal ventriculogram can be classified as having no evidence of ischemic heart disease caused by obstructive atherosclerosis of the coronary arteries and to have good left ventricular function. He or she should be suitably reassured, and another cause for chest pain should be sought. In our experience, the three most common causes of chest pain or discomfort in patients with normal coronary arteries are reflux esophagitis, cervical arthritis, and psychoneurosis.

3. *If the coronary arteries are not free of disease, is there any lesion that has resulted in a 75 per cent or greater reduction in luminal diameter?*

Experimental studies in animals have shown that stenosis up to 70 or 80 per cent may not impair resting coronary flow, although constrictions of 50 to 60 per cent may cause ischemia during exercise. For this reason, a lesion causing a 75 per cent or greater reduction in luminal diameter (i.e., a reduction to one fourth its original size) is considered capable of producing a perfusion deficit.[90,91] Multiple projections are necessary for accurate assessment of a lesion, because of the possibility of underestimation of slit- or crescent-shaped narrowings.

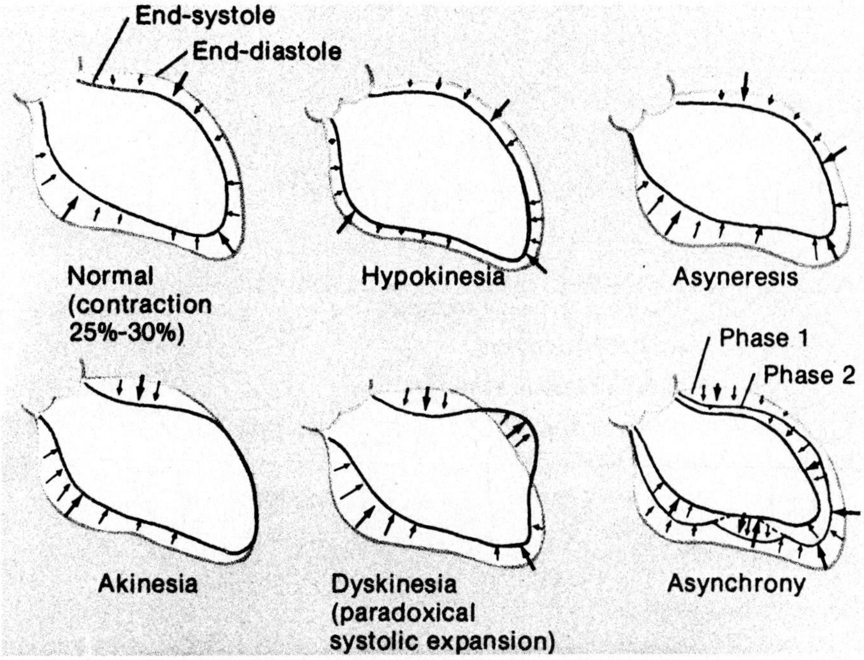

FIGURE 10-48 Localized and generalized abnormalities of cardiac contraction. Arrows represent motion from end-diastole to end-systole. (From Herman, M. V., and Gorlin, R.: Implications of left ventricular asynergy. Am. J. Cardiol. *23*:538, 1969.)

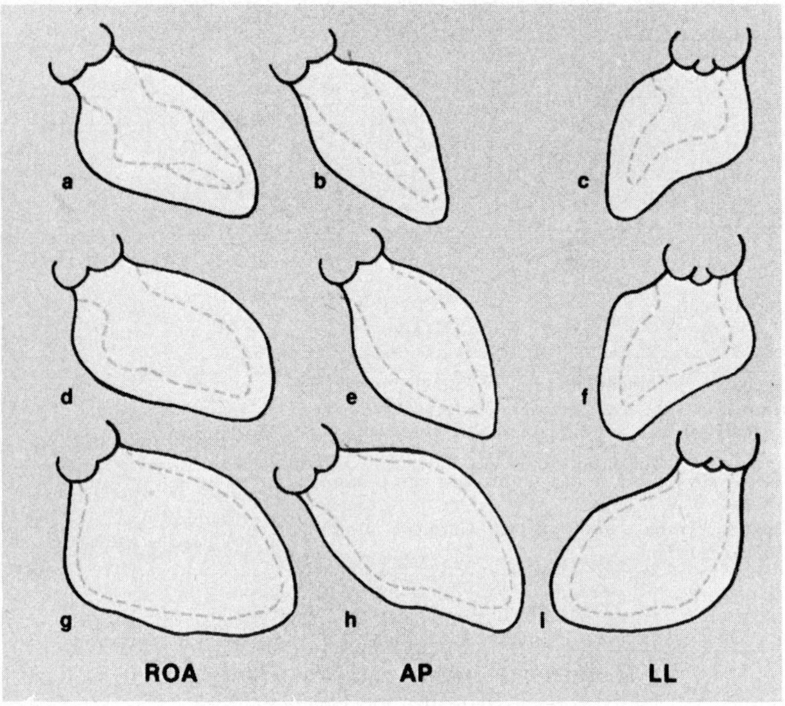

FIGURE 10–49 Diagrams of left ventricular cavity in diastole (solid lines) and systole (dashed lines) as seen in right oblique anterior (ROA), anteroposterior (AP), and left lateral (LL) projections. *a, b,* and *c,* Normal left ventricle (inner dashed lines in *a* denote imprint of papillary muscles). *d, e,* and *f,* Mild left ventricular enlargement, mainly at expense of an increased left ventricular end-systolic volume. *g, h,* and *i,* Severe left ventricular enlargement and hypokinesia. (From Gensini, G. G.: Coronary arteriography. Role in myocardial revascularization. Postgrad. Med. *63*:121, 1978.)

4. *If the ventricle is not normal, describe any abnormalities in terms of alteration of size, vigor, shape, or synergy of contraction.*

Abnormalities observed on the left ventriculogram may involve the entire ventricle or may be localized to a segment. They result in a change of shape and volume or in alterations in the contraction pattern. Additional abnormalities of the left ventriculogram are seen with certain valvular defects, such as mitral regurgitation, mitral stenosis, and aortic stenosis, or with septal perforation.

Table 10–4 summarizes the common abnormalities of the left ventriculogram. Diagrams of a normal ventricle as well as two different degrees of left ventricular enlargement are included in Figure 10–49. Figures 10–50 and 10–51 give additional examples.

5. *Is the luminal narrowing sufficiently proximal to jeopardize a sizable myocardial segment?*

Atherosclerosis is a diffuse process and can be found at all levels along the epicardial course of a coronary artery. Although multiple bypass grafts are now commonplace and are often made to relatively small branches, there is general agreement that a relationship exists between blood flow through the graft (and the size of the anastomosis), on the one hand, and the likelihood of graft patency, on the other. If narrowing involves a small branch or is located at the periphery of a vessel, or if the involved artery

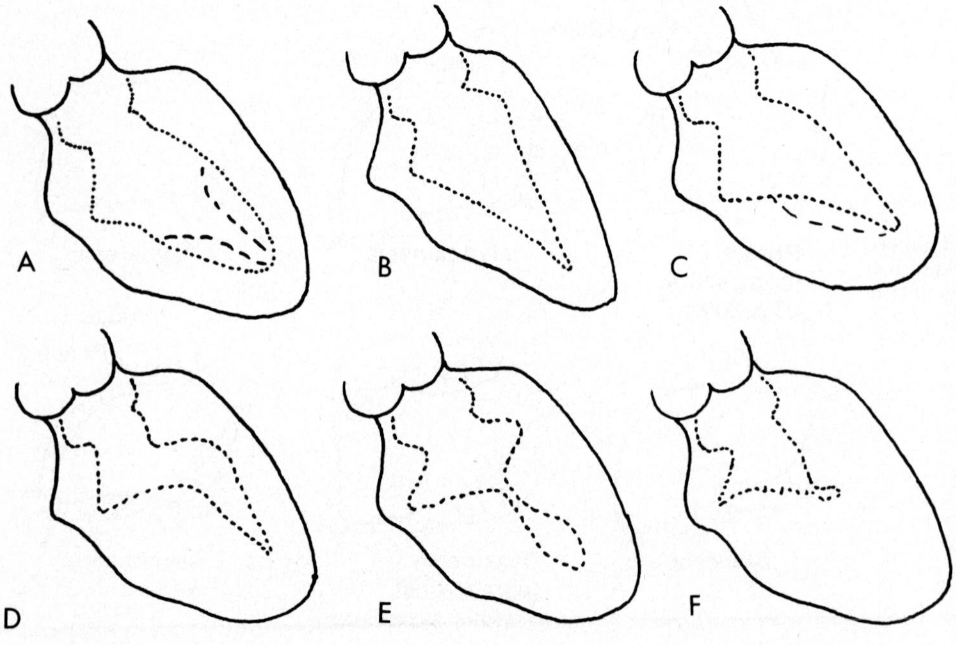

FIGURE 10–50 Diagrammatic representation of the left ventricular cavity in diastole (solid line) and systole (dotted line) as seen in RAO view. *A,* Normal ventricle, with pear-core configuration in systole due to the imprint of the papillary muscles (dashed line). *B,* Normal ventricle, ice cream cone configuration. *C,* Normal ventricle, pointed boot configuration. Only the posterior papillary muscle (dashed line) can be seen faintly. *D,* Ballerina foot configuration due to localized hyperkinesis of the diaphragmatic segment and mild hypokinesis of the anterior segment. *E,* Hourglass configuration due to hypertrophy of the anterior and posterior walls. *F,* Cavity obliteration. (From Gensini, G. G.: Coronary Arteriography. Mount Kisco, N.Y., Futura Publishing Co., 1975.)

TABLE 10–4 THE ABNORMAL LEFT VENTRICULOGRAM

- **Diffuse Abnormalities**
- Abnormalities of volume
  - Enlargement
    - End-systolic
    - End-diastolic
  - Reduction
    - End-diastolic
    - End-systolic (cavity obliteration)
- Abnormalities in rate of volume change
  - Hypokinesia
    - Mild
    - Moderate
    - "Quivering" ventricle
  - Hyperkinesia
    - Mild
    - Moderate
    - Severe
- **Segmental Abnormalities** (Asynergy)
- Decreased function
  - Hypokinesia (asyneresis)
  - Asynchrony
  - Akinesia
  - Dyskinesia
- Increased function
  - Hyperkinesia
  - (Asymmetrical hypertrophy?)
- Segmental early relaxation phenomenon (SERP)
- **Filling Defects**
- **Valvular Involvement**
- Mitral stenosis
- Mitral regurgitation
- Aortic stenosis
- **Septal Perforation** (Acquired Ventricular Septal Defect)

From Gensini, G. G.: Coronary Arteriography. Mount Kisco, N.Y., Futura Publishing Co., 1975.

perfuses a myocardial segment of trivial magnitude, there is little justification for performing or extending surgery for that lesion.

6. *Does the narrowed coronary artery perfuse a viable myocardial segment?*

This is a crucial and often difficult decision to make. Clearly, there is no point in trying to revascularize a scar. Furthermore, reperfusion of a freshly necrotic segment may be undesirable. Many infarctions seen postoperatively may be due to reperfusion of an already necrotic segment rather than to failure of a properly placed graft.[92]

Viability of a myocardial segment is best assessed by the combination of pre- and postintervention ventriculography (p. 1369). If the myocardial segment perfused by an obstructed or occluded artery is either normally contracting or mildly hypokinetic, there should be little doubt as to its viability. Conversely, if it is aneurysmal or clearly dyskinetic, there is no point in considering a bypass to its parent vessel. The difficult part of the decision-making concerns a segment that is severely hypokinetic or akinetic, in which case the segment's behavior must be examined before and after the performance of maneuvers that potentiate contractility. The contractions of the segment should be critically examined during a normally conducted beat and during a postextrasystolic beat (Fig. 10–52) as well as before and after the administration of nitroglycerin (Fig. 10–53).[14,15] If improvement is apparent, the segment may be assumed to be viable and its revascularization is of potential benefit.

7. *Is the distal coronary segment both identifiable (by antegrade flow or through collaterals) and suitable for bypass graft surgery?*

Unless an artery can be positively identified and its course, diameter, branching, and lumen correctly assessed, it should not be chosen as a target for a bypass graft. For example, an arterial segment (distal to an occlusion) that fills incompletely or not at all may be diffusely diseased, may have virtually no lumen, or may be too small for successful anastomosis. If it is the only segment in need of repair, the cardiologist and surgeon would be ill advised in

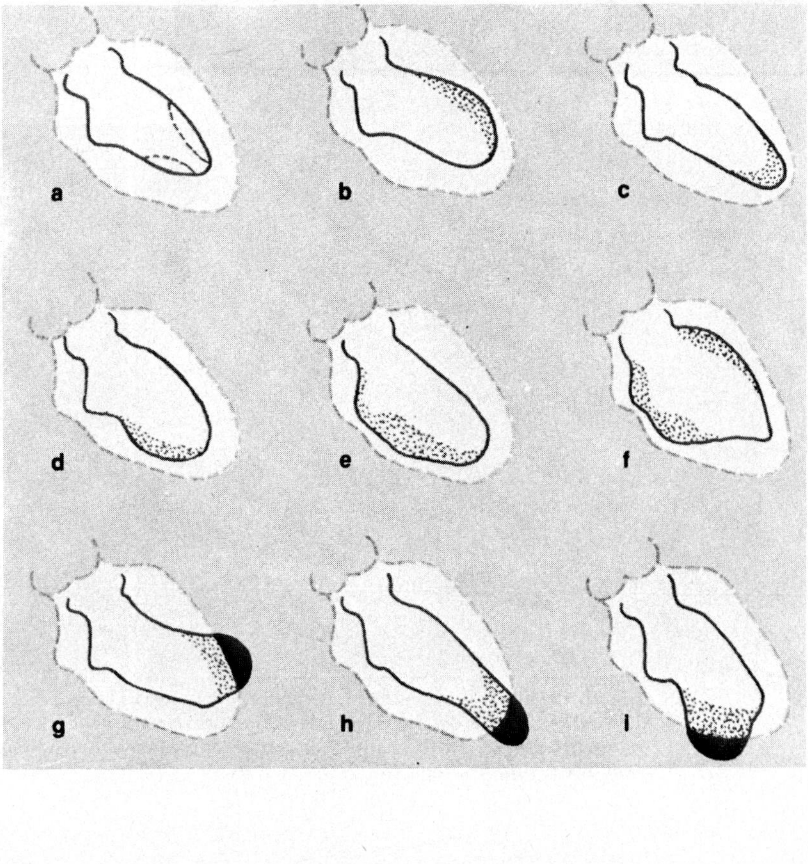

FIGURE 10–51 Selected examples of frequently observed segmental left ventricular contraction abnormalities. Diastole is represented by dashed lines and systole by solid lines; akinetic segments are represented by dotted areas and dyskinetic segments by dotted and black areas; normal end-systolic contour is represented by the white area within the solid line. (Dashed lines within solid line in *a* denote imprint of papillary muscles.) *a,* Normal ventricle. *b,* Anterolateral akinesia. *c,* Apical akinesia. When mild, or simply hypokinetic, pattern is often described as "lazy apex." *d,* Diaphragmatic akinesia, soupspoon configuration. *e,* Posterobasal and diaphragmatic akinesia. *f,* Anterobasal, anterolateral, diaphragmatic, and posterobasal akinesia. *g,* Anterolateral dyskinesia. *h,* Apical dyskinesia. *i,* Diaphragmatic dyskinesia. (From Gensini, G. G.: Coronary arteriography. Role in myocardial revascularization. Postgrad. Med. *63*:121, 1978.)

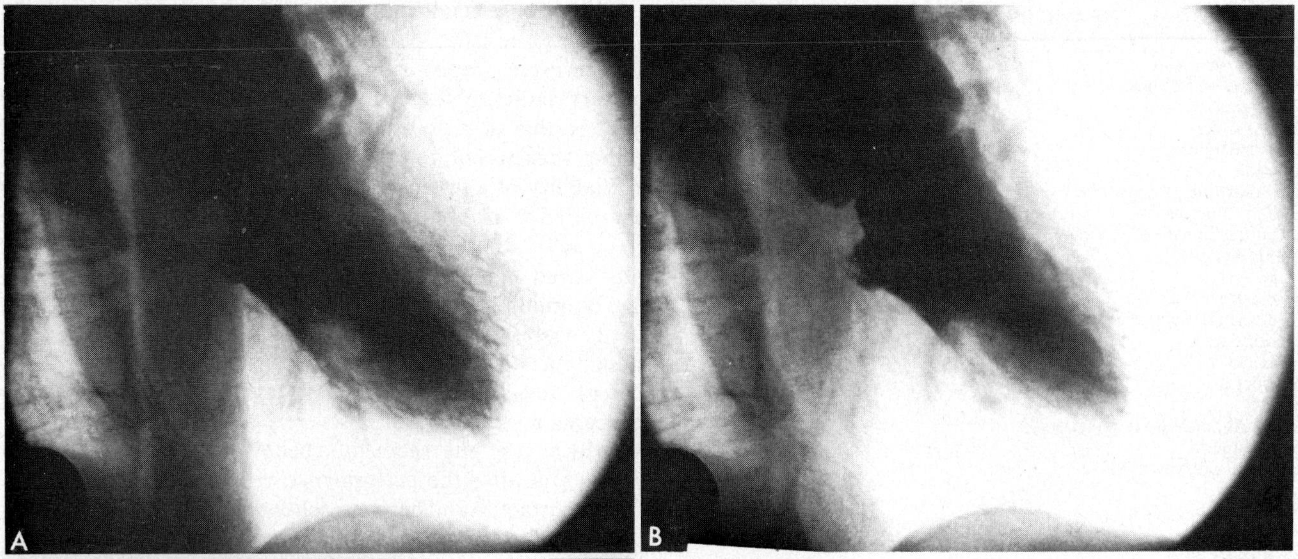

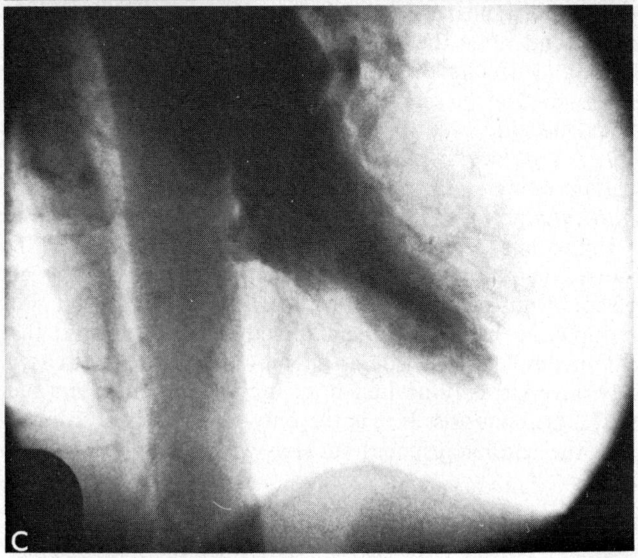

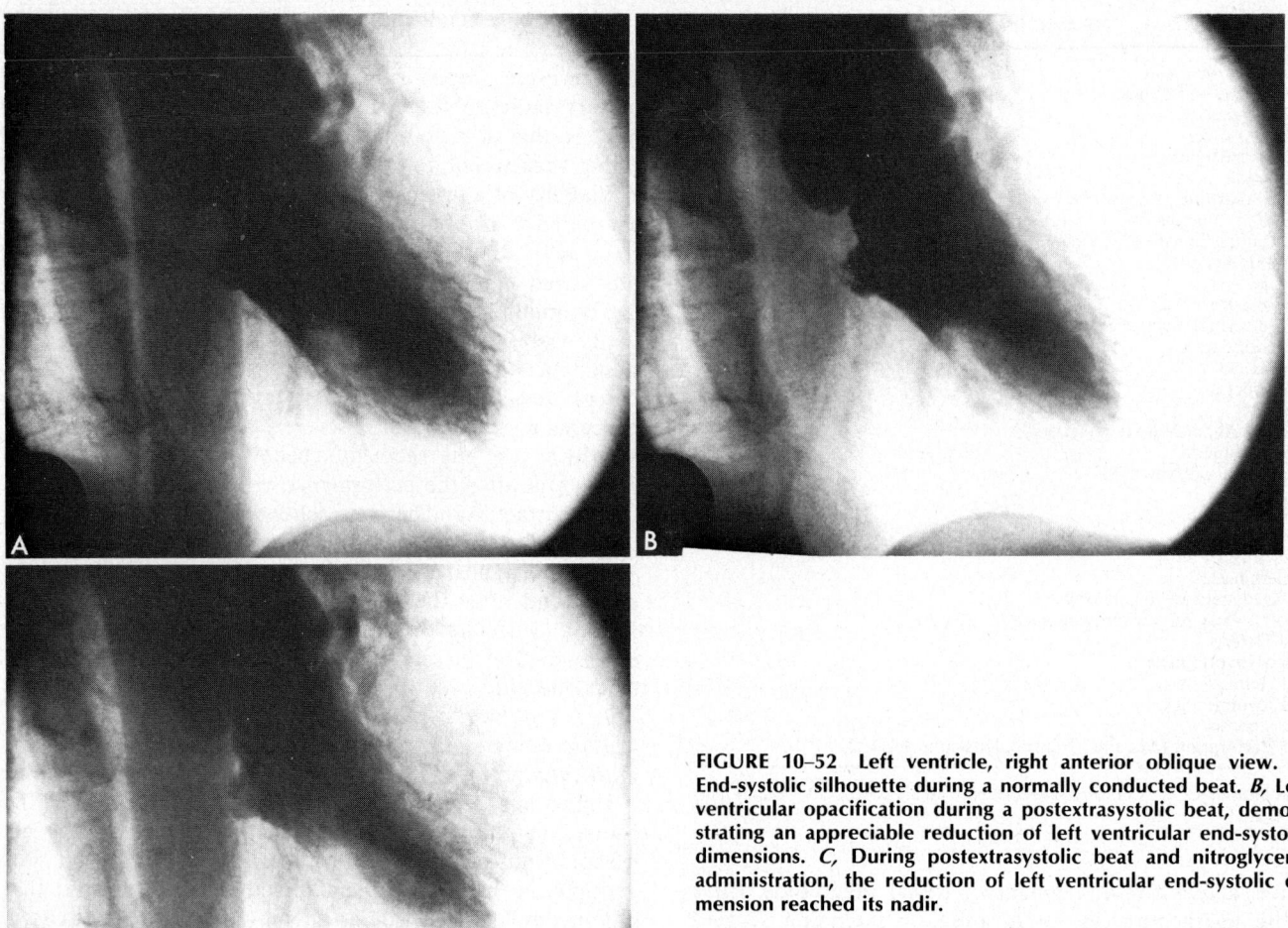

FIGURE 10–52 Left ventricle, right anterior oblique view. *A,* End-systolic silhouette during a normally conducted beat. *B,* Left ventricular opacification during a postextrasystolic beat, demonstrating an appreciable reduction of left ventricular end-systolic dimensions. *C,* During postextrasystolic beat and nitroglycerin administration, the reduction of left ventricular end-systolic dimension reached its nadir.

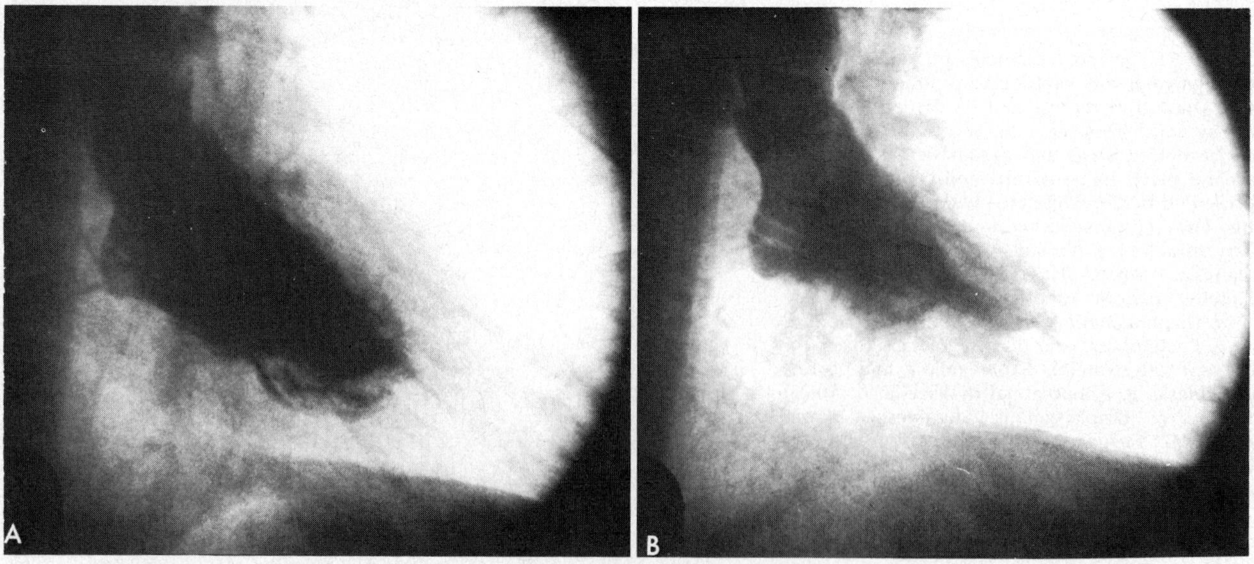

FIGURE 10–53 Left ventricle, end-systolic silhouette, right anterior oblique view. Before (*A*) and after (*B*) administration of 0.4 mg of nitroglycerin in the left ventricle demonstrating a striking improvement of left ventricular synergy, with nearly complete disappearance of diaphragmatic hypokinesis and marked improvement of ejection fraction.

respectively referring and accepting the patient. An exception to this rule is a nonfilling anterior descending coronary artery *in the presence of unimpaired motion of the anterolateral wall.* Should operation be indicated because of the involvement of another artery that could clearly be the target for bypass, exploration of the inadequately identified segment distal to a complete occlusion should be performed in any case in the hope that it might be suitable for a graft. This is frequently the case in occlusions of the left anterior descending artery, when the patency of that segment is maintained by collaterals originating from a conus artery that is inadequately opacified because of its separate ostium in the right sinus of Valsalva.

When the arterial segment beyond a stenosis is adequately opacified, its suitability for a bypass is a function of size, distribution, and the degree of peripheral involvement, as follows:

a. *Size* (diameter of vessel at site of intended anastomosis): A vessel is totally unsuitable if the size is 0.7 mm or less, poor if 0.8 to 1.0 mm, acceptable for internal mammary anastomosis if 1.1 to 1.4 mm, and good for any type of graft if 1.5 mm or larger.
b. *Distribution*: Length of a segment and number of branches beyond the stenosis are expressions of size and importance of the myocardial segment perfused and broadly correlate with flow requirement. Clearly, the larger the segment, the better would be the long-term patency and clinical usefulness of a graft. The necessity of evaluating the distribution pattern of a vessel when considering coronary artery bypass surgery is exemplified by the different size and length of the left anterior descending coronary artery. Classification of this vessel into its three types (see p. 325) is helpful in assessing the prognosis in disease of the left anterior descending artery. Total occlusion of a Type I left anterior descending artery may be associated with little muscle damage, because it perfuses a limited area of the anteroseptal portion of the left ventricle. In contrast, the Type III vessel is usually of a larger caliber and perfuses the anterior two thirds of the interventricular septum, the anteroapical portion of the left ventricle, and even a portion of the diaphragmatic surface of the left ventricle; total occlusion of this vessel may be lethal, and those who do survive usually present with a postinfarction ventricular aneurysm.
c. *Peripheral involvement*: An artery free of disease distal to the intended site of anastomosis is ideal for grafting. Peripheral lesions up to 50 per cent reduction in the lumen may be acceptable, but the expected long-term patency of the graft, or its potential for long-term effectiveness, is diminished.

8. *Is overall myocardial function acceptable for revascularization surgery?*

A few investigators have reported dramatic results with bypass grafts in patients with poor left ventricular function. However, these cases are the exceptions rather than the rule (p. 1368). There is a relatively high surgical mortality among these patients, but in some instances the long-term clinical results have been encouraging.[93]

STRATIFICATION OF CORONARY ARTERY DISEASE: GRADING THE SEVERITY OF OBSTRUCTIVE LESIONS

The universally accepted method of identifying an obstructive lesion on a coronary arteriogram is subjective examination by a trained arteriographer who reviews the film with an experienced but unaided eye. Computer-assisted methods (quantitative angiography)[23] may be utilized for experimental research or for special projects but are still impractical for use on a routine basis.

A grading method that disregards the limitations of the human eye (however well trained it might be) is unrealistic and doomed to failure. The system employed by the author is based on the demonstration that a trained observer can easily distinguish reductions in lumen diameter to one-fourth, one-half, or three-fourths the original size.[2] Obviously it is easy to identify both complete occlusion and lesions that cause almost complete occlusion, classified as "99 per cent" obstructions. Once these fundamental "benchmarks" are established, only one questionable situation remains, i.e., stenosis of 90 per cent, in which the lumen is narrowed by more than three fourths but is not quite reduced to an almost invisible thread (and appears to be about one tenth the size of the original lumen).

A number of approaches and methods for defining the severity of an obstructive lesion have been proposed by various authors. Our classification, adopted by the Ad Hoc Committee on Grading of Coronary Arterial Disease of the American Heart Association, is as follows (Fig. 10–54)[94]:

Normal—Lumen appears perfectly smooth and even; no restriction, indentation, loss of density, or sudden bulging.

25%—Lumen diameter is reduced *by* one fourth its former width.

50%—Lumen diameter is reduced *to* one half its former width.

75%—Lumen diameter is reduced *to* one fourth its former width.

90%—Lumen appears to be reduced to about one tenth its former diameter.

"99%"*—Lumen appears to be almost totally obliterated but some contrast still passes through the obstruction.

Occlusion—Total obstruction of a vessel without any filling of the distal segment from the proximal portion.

The current method of classifying patients with coronary artery disease as having single-, double-, and triple-vessel involvement does not anticipate changes in the natural history of the disease that may occur spontaneously or that could be achieved with a different treatment modality, such as with medical or surgical therapy. The profound difference that exists between 99 per cent obstruction of the proximal left anterior descending artery and 75 per cent obstruction of its apical segment is indisputable, yet both lesions are included in the category of single-vessel disease. Therefore, it is widely recognized that a method that assigns a different severity score depending on the degree of luminal narrowing and the geographical importance of its location would be desirable. A scoring technique which received some recognition was that of Friesinger et al., in which each of the three main coronary trunks was given a score from zero to five, depending on whether the vessel was normal or showed progressively severe changes.[95] Unfortunately, Freisinger's score did not distinguish between proximal and distal lesions or between a lesion of a branch and that of its parent vessel.

*"99%," as used here to describe a degree of luminal narrowing, merely indicates the greatest reduction in lumen diameter detectable with our image intensifier short of vessel separation and is not intended to be mathematically accurate. A simple calculation would show that even when starting with a very large lumen (e.g., 4 mm in diameter), the narrowest segment still identifiable (100 μ) with a cesium iodide image intensifier and 35-mm film would be equivalent to a 97.5 per cent diameter reduction. Thus, "99 per cent" is written in quotes.

Several years ago, recognizing these shortcomings, the author devised a system that takes into consideration the geometrically increasing severity of lesions, the cumulative effects of multiple obstructions, the significance of their locations, the modifying influence of the collaterals, the size and quality of the distal vessel, and the importance of the status of myocardial function.[9] This system requires no additional effort or calculation on the part of the arteriographer, once the location and the severity of each lesion, the presence of collaterals, and the suitability of a graft have been properly scored on a computer card or with the aid of a small keyboard. The fundamental concept forming the basis of this system is the hypothesis that the severity of coronary artery disease must be regarded as a consequence of the functional significance of the vascular narrowing and the extent of the area perfused by the involved vessel or vessels; the presence of an effective coronary collateral circulation may, on the other hand, modify the functional significance of a severe obstruction or occlusion.

The percentage of reduction in lumen diameter (from 0 to 100 per cent) is assigned a degree of severity (called ischemia numerical grade, or ING) from 1 to 32 (Fig. 10–54), each grade being twice as large as the previous one. Using this method, the ING of a "99 per cent" obstruction, for example, is 16 times greater than the one corresponding to a 25 per cent reduction of lumen diameter, a fact in keeping with Poiseuille's law as well as with clinical observation. Just as it is only too obvious that a 90 per cent obstruction is far more severe than a 25 per cent one, it would similarly be illogical to give to 90 per cent stenosis of the main left coronary artery the same "weight" as that assigned to 90 per cent obstruction of the terminal segment of the circumflex coronary artery. Accordingly, the left ventricular myocardium is divided into nine myocardial perfusion areas (MAP's), each receiving its blood supply from a well-defined coronary branch. MAP's are assigned a numerical value of either 0.5 or 1.0, depending on size. Each MAP thus becomes a multiplying factor to be used in the final equation. The value of this multiplying factor and the distribution of the nine MAP's are shown in Figure 10–55. The severity of coronary artery disease equals the MAP multiplied by ING (MAP per ING, or MAPpING). A proximal lesion involves all dependent MAP's. If multiple lesions are present in the same vessel, the ING's are added to a maximum of 32. When collateral circulation (CC) is present, a lower ING is used; in other words, the computer utilizes a formula that takes into consideration the contribution of collateral blood flow to a myocardial perfusion area beyond a severe obstruction or occlusion. This formula proportionally reduces the score of an occlusion or of a severe obstruction according to the quality of reopacification achieved by the collateral channels and the integrity of the distal segment.

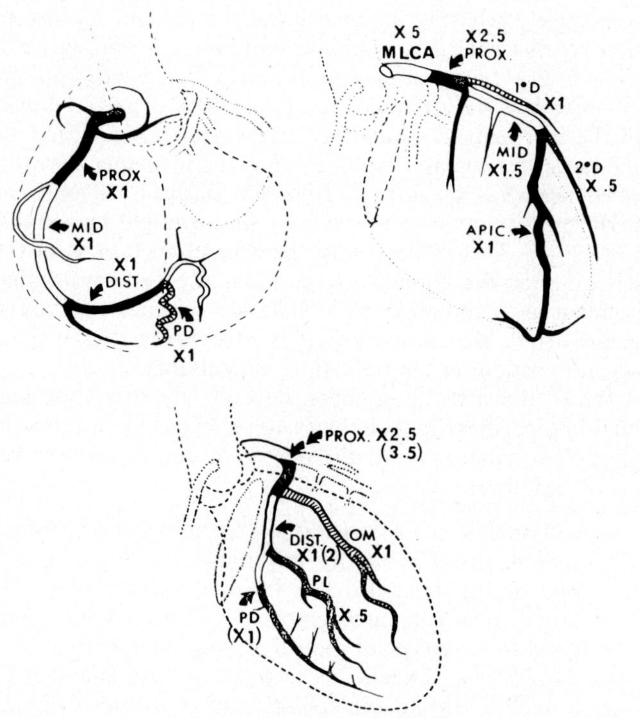

FIGURE 10–55 The principal vascular segments (from left to right) of the right coronary artery, left anterior descending branch, and circumflex. Each segment is followed by a multiplying factor (e.g., X1, X2.5, etc.) to indicate the functional significance of the area supplied by that segment. The numbers shown are based on an "average" coronary circulation but may differ depending on the relative quantities of myocardium perfused by the vessel in question. PROX = proximal segment; MID = midsegment; DIST = distal segment; PD = posterior descending branch; MLCA = main left coronary artery; 1°D = first diagonal; 2°D = second diagonal; APIC = apical; OM = obtuse marginal branch; PL = posterolateral. (From Gensini, G. G.: Coronary Arteriography. Mount Kisco, N.Y., Futura Publishing Co., 1975.)

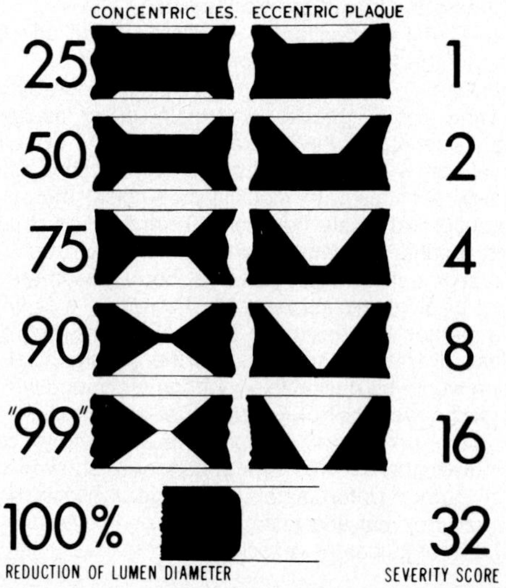

FIGURE 10–54 The roentgenographic appearance of concentric lesions and eccentric plaques resulting in 25, 50, 75, 90, and "99" per cent obstruction as well as complete (100 per cent) occlusion. The column on the right indicates the relative severity of these lesions using a score of 1 for the 25 per cent obstruction and doubling that number as the severity of these obstructions progresses according to the reduction of lumen diameter (left column). (From Gensini, G. G.: Coronary Arteriography. Mount Kisco, N.Y., Futura Publishing Co., 1975.)

After the scores for each segment of the arteries have been calculated, they are added together to produce a severity score per artery; these scores are then added to obtain a total score for the entire coronary system. The final score is obtained by leaving the arterial score unchanged when the ejection fraction (EF) is normal or by adding a progressively larger number (from 20 to 80) for progressively more severe reductions of ejection fraction.[9]

Although this method may not be ideal, it provides more useful information than the simple division of patients into single-, double-, and triple-vessel disease. The advantages of this scoring method are as follows:

1. It provides an accurate stratification of patients according to the functional significance of their disease.[96]
2. It lends itself to computer elaboration, storage, retrieval, and analysis.
3. It provides an opportunity to match patients with similar degrees of coronary artery disease but who are receiving different forms of treatment.
4. It allows for continuous, microprocessor-assisted studies of interobserver and intraobserver variability. Computer hardware and software to elaborate and store this type of information are readily available and are inexpensive.

PITFALLS OF CORONARY ARTERIOGRAPHY

Judkins has properly called attention to "an unheralded complication of coronary arteriography that is frequently overlooked but equal in importance to the most severe . . . the incomplete or nondiagnostic study."[37] Another similarly unheralded "complication" of coronary arteriography is the misinterpretation of the arteriogram,[96a,96b] whether the result of inadequate training, inadequate views, honest mistakes, or limitations of the technique itself.

The following list presents some of the most common problems leading to inappropriate conclusions in the evaluation of coronary arteriograms.

Operator-Related Sources of Error

Iatrogenically Induced Coronary Spasm. The presence of an obstruction immediately distal to the tip of the catheter should suggest the possibility of catheter-induced spasm, especially if the catheter was pushed deeply into a main vessel or became wedged in a small branch vessel. Opacification should be repeated after the vessel in question is not entered for at least 15 minutes and nitroglycerin or isosorbide dinitrate[24,25] has been administered to the patient. In questionable cases, opacification may have to be repeated during an adequate sinus flush injection to exclude the effect of additional catheter manipulation on a potentially hyperactive area of the vessel.

Iatrogenically induced spasm appears more frequently (3 per cent of all cases studied in our laboratory) during catheterization of the right coronary artery, probably because deep penetration by the catheter occurs more easily in this artery. A similar phenomenon involving the main left coronary artery is very rare; we have seen it only once in over 3000 coronary arteriograms.

The following features are typical of iatrogenically induced spasm:

— localization to the initial segment of the right coronary artery, at or within a few millimeters from the catheter
— no apparent hindrance to blood flow
— no association with pain or with ST-segment changes
— tendency to disappear spontaneously within 10 to 20 minutes, provided that the catheter is removed from the coronary artery; spasm may disappear more rapidly with nitroglycerin or isosorbide dinitrate, even though dilatation of the unaffected segment may occur prior to disappearance of the constricting area
— negative ergonovine test

Inadequate Force of Injection. Weak, hesitant injections should be avoided; they provide little information and may lead to misinterpretation. Slow, laminar flow into the injected vessel may result in incomplete mixing and layering[97] of contrast agent and blood. The separation between the two streams may then give the false appearance of luminal narrowing when, in fact, no narrowing exists. If flow into the injected vessel is too rapid, the trickle of contrast agent dripping out of the catheter is quickly swept away with each heart cycle, never *fully* opacifying the vessel under study and occasionally even *failing* to opacify some important branches.

Fixed Number and/or Angle of Projection. The use of fixed anteroposterior and lateral views in coronary arteriography is inappropriate; multiple projections, including hemiaxial views (see p. 308), are necessary to eliminate (or at least minimize) confusion arising because of superimposition, foreshortening, and doubling-up of vessels. During the course of the procedure, the operator should be aware of the specific requirements of the individual set of arteries under study and must vary the number of injections and the angle of obliquity accordingly. Careful attention must be paid to the following segments of vessels: main left coronary artery, initial segment of the left anterior descending artery (Fig. 10–56), the initial segment of the circumflex artery, the first diagonal branch, and the initial segment of the obtuse marginal branch.

Superimposition of The Diaphragm (and Underexposure of the Corresponding Area of Myocardium). This combination results in inadequate visualization of the distal segment and branches of the right coronary artery (and/or of the circumflex) (Fig. 10–57). Severe narrowings may be easily missed, with dire consequences for the patient.

Superselective Catheterization of Branches of Either Left or Right Coronary Artery. In a small number of cases, the main left coronary artery is very short and quickly divides into the anterior descending and the circumflex branches. In a few cases, the main stem is totally missing, and the two arteries originate either from a very short funnel or directly from two separate ostia. These anatomical variations almost invariably lead to the superselective catheterization of either the anterior descending or the circumflex branch. This problem may occur even with main left coronary arteries of normal length. Sometimes the catheter may slip into a secondary branch, such as the obtuse marginal or the diagonal. On the right side, it is possible to enter a conus branch that has a separate ostium or a right ventricular branch, thereby inadvertently preventing opacification of the main stem. Superselective catheterization of branches may be performed intentionally for special reasons, but the unnecessary use of this technique is dangerous for two reasons: first, it may lead to ventricular fibrillation if the amount of contrast agent injected is too large relative to vessel size and flow, and, second, an undetected superselective injection may be mistakenly interpreted as an occlusion of the other branch or branches (Fig. 10–58).

Mistaking a Vein for a Coronary Artery (and Vice Versa).[98] This should be an extremely rare situation. Two conditions, however, may create some confusion: one condition is the forceful injection of the contrast agent through a catheter wedged into a branch (see Superselective Catheterization above), so that the vein draining that segment will be promptly filled; the second condition is encountered when an occluded coronary artery is filled late by collateral circulation, while a normally perfused, adjoining segment is draining the contrast agent in the venous system. In the first situation, a vein may appear to be an artery, whereas in the second, an artery may be mistaken for a vein.

Artifactual Demonstration of Collateral Channels. This is another possible pitfall stemming from forceful injection with the catheter in a wedged position.[97,99]

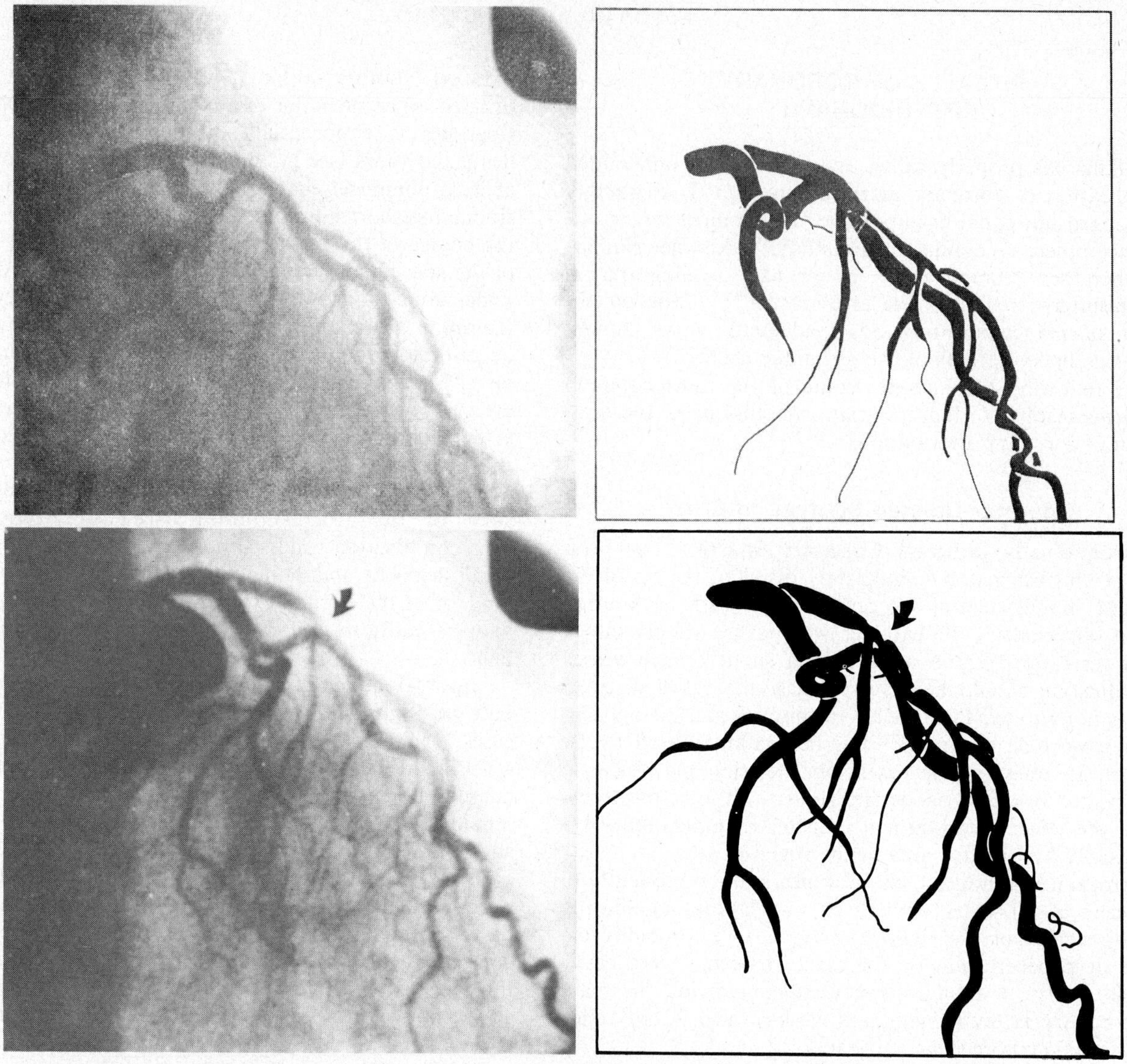

FIGURE 10–56 *Top,* RAO view of left coronary artery shows superimposition of left anterior descending and obtuse marginal branch of circumflex. *Bottom,* Slightly different view uncovers severe narrowing of left anterior descending at level of first septal branch (arrow). (From Gensini, G. G.: Coronary Arteriography. Mount Kisco, N.Y., Futura Publishing Co., 1975.)

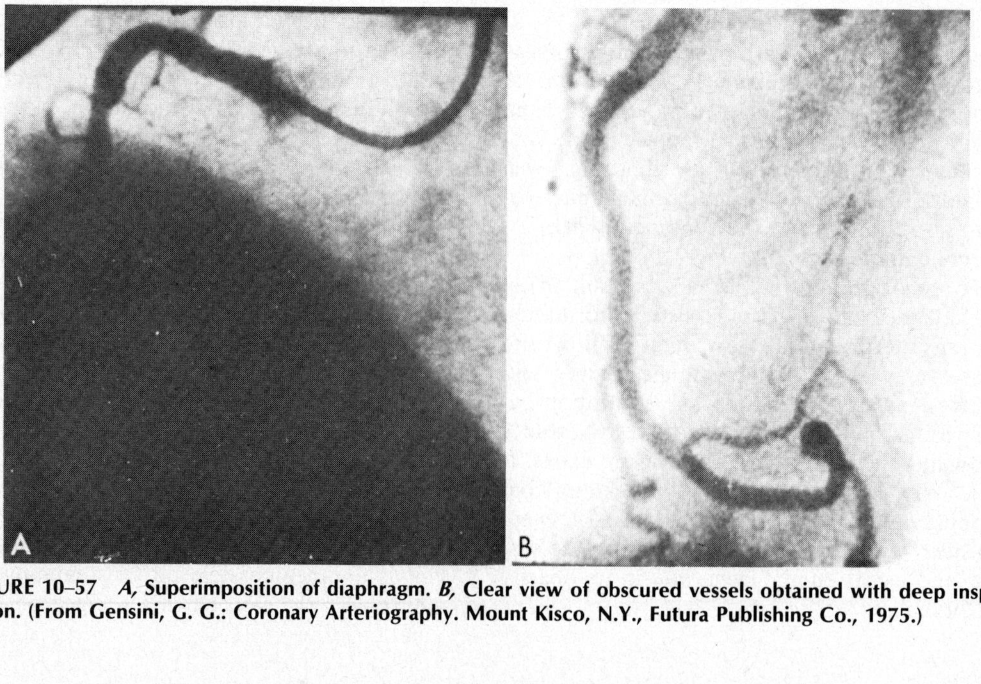

FIGURE 10–57 *A,* Superimposition of diaphragm. *B,* Clear view of obscured vessels obtained with deep inspiration. (From Gensini, G. G.: Coronary Arteriography. Mount Kisco, N.Y., Futura Publishing Co., 1975.)

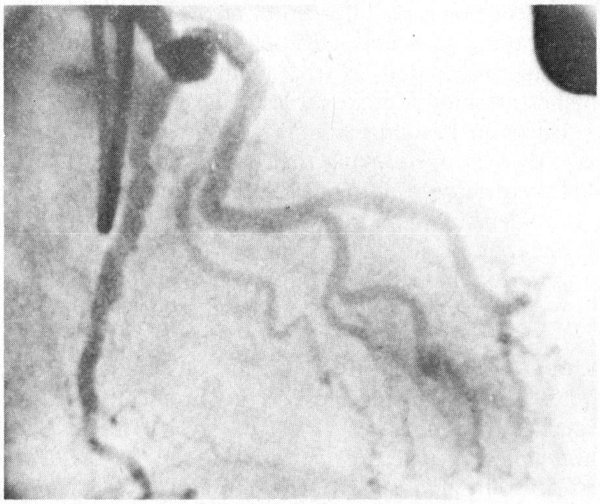

FIGURE 10–58 Left coronary artery, right anterior oblique view. Apparent total occlusion of left anterior descending branch resulting from superselective injection into the circumflex artery. (From Gensini, G. G.: Coronary Arteriography. Mount Kisco, N.Y., Futura Publishing Co., 1975.)

Patient-Related Sources of Error

MYOCARDIAL BRIDGES.[98,100–107] Casual analysis of the arteriogram may lead to the erroneous diagnosis of organic narrowing if the rhythmic changes of the vessel dimensions are overlooked. This error is not likely to occur with cine techniques, especially when the differences between the systolic and the diastolic appearance of the vessel (and therefore the presumed organic lesion) are most pronounced (Fig. 10–45).

Anomalous Origin of a Coronary Artery.[97,102] An anomaly occurring in slightly less than 1 per cent of cases is the origin of the circumflex coronary artery from either the right coronary artery (Fig. 10–59) or the right sinus of Valsalva. Failure to opacify such an anomalous vessel is more likely to occur when there is a separate ostium in the right sinus of Valsalva. However, even when the circumflex is a branch of the right coronary artery, its point of origin is very close to the ostium, and thus slightly deeper penetration of the catheter into the main trunk may lead to failure of visualization (or poor visualization) of the anomalous branch. Overlooking the existence of the right-sided circumflex may then lead to the incorrect diagnosis of occlusion of this artery.

Another relatively common anomaly is the high origin of either the right or the left coronary arteries. In these cases, exploration of the respective sinuses with the catheter will fail to opacify the displaced ostium, since it lies well above the sinuses. Rarer anomalies include (1) origin of the main left coronary artery from either the right sinus of Valsalva or the right coronary artery; (2) origin of the left anterior descending coronary artery from the right sinus of Valsalva; (3) origin of all three coronary arteries from either the right or left sinus of Valsalva via two or three distinct ostia; and (4) a single coronary artery. A variety of anatomical arrangements is possible with the latter anomaly, but the most important clinically is the type in which the left coronary artery originates from either the right sinus of Valsalva or the proximal portion of the right coronary artery and passes between the right ventricular outflow tract and the aorta to reach the left atrioventricular groove. This anomaly may be associated with sudden death.

Unusual Predominance of Right or Left Coronary Artery. Perhaps one of the most common variations is the total preponderance of the left coronary artery. In such cases, the right coronary artery provides only the most proximal atrial and right ventricular branches and sometimes does not even reach the acute margin of the heart. This anatomical variation should not be confused with the results of coronary occlusion.

A slightly more confusing anomaly is the overwhelming predominance of the right coronary artery, extending either over the apex and anterior surface of the left ventricle or over the lateral wall or both. In the first instance, the posterior descending artery continues well beyond its usual area of distribution along the posterior interventricular groove, encircles the apex, and distributes along the inferior third of the anterior interventricular groove. In these cases, an occlusion of the posterior descending artery will affect a much larger area of the interventricular septum

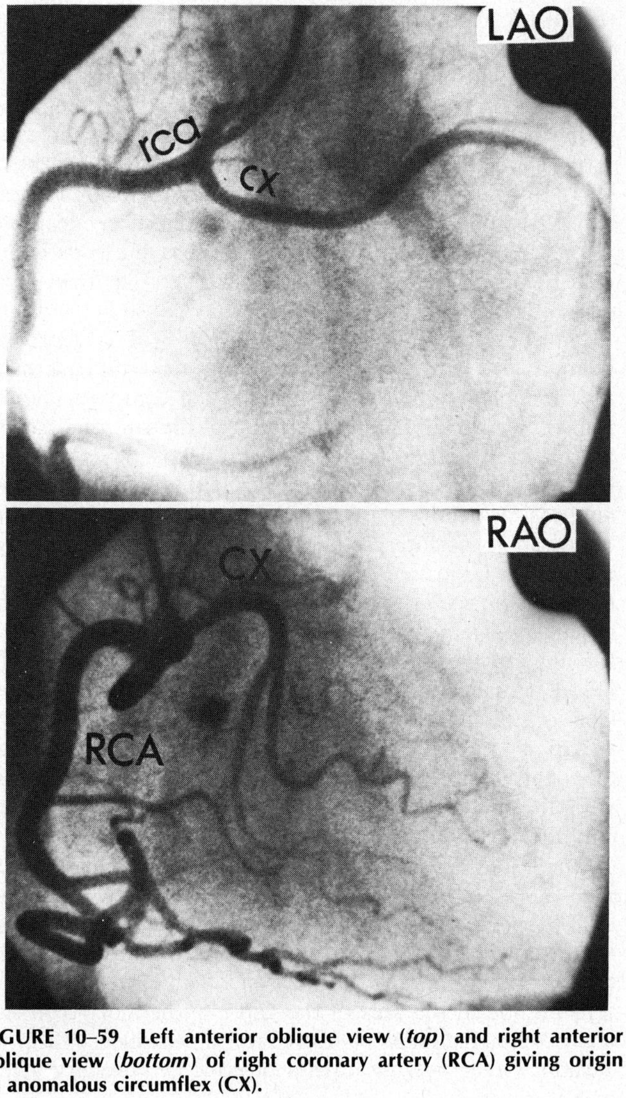

FIGURE 10–59 Left anterior oblique view (*top*) and right anterior oblique view (*bottom*) of right coronary artery (RCA) giving origin to anomalous circumflex (CX).

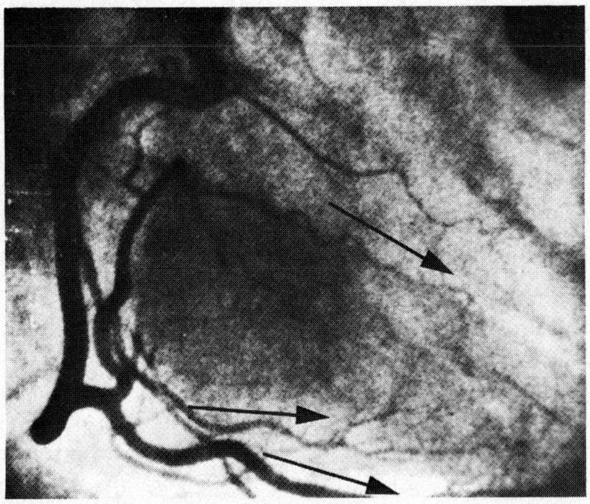

FIGURE 10–60 Right anterior oblique view showing exceptional predominance of right coronary artery sending branches to entire posterolateral and left marginal surface of left ventricle (arrows). (From Gensini, G. G.: Coronary Arteriography. Mount Kisco, N.Y., Futura Publishing Co., 1975.)

and *may* be accompanied by electrocardiographic evidence of diaphragmatic *and* apical infarction or ischemia (and possibly even anterior infarction or ischemia). Misinterpretation of this pattern may conceivably lead to a fruitless search for a possible site for an anterior descending graft, whereas a right-sided graft would be the only one needed. In the second instance, the right coronary artery continues well beyond the left ventricular segments adjoining the posterior interventricular septum and supplies the entire posterolateral and left marginal surface of the left ventricle (Fig. 10–60). Thus, in these patients the left circumflex is expected to be quite small or absent. Absent or incomplete visualization of these branches would be the consequence of a lesion of the right coronary artery rather than of the circumflex branch.

Unrecognized Total "Amputation" of a Coronary Branch. According to Paulin, "the most difficult situation for angiographic assessment is the complete amputation of a coronary branch exactly at the site of its origin and in the absence of any collateral filling of its distal extension. We have seen this occur with regard to the left anterior descending artery: casual scrutiny of the films may lead to misinterpretation, and both a large septal artery and a large side branch to the anterolateral aspect of the left ventricular wall may be confused with it. Do not accept an artery which does not show the typical curve at the apex of the heart as being the left anterior descending before visualization of the corresponding increased extension of the posterior branches indicates the presence of variation."[97] Similar situations may occur with one of the diagonal branches of the left anterior descending artery, with the marginal and posterolateral branches of the circumflex, and with the right or the left ventricular branches of the right coronary artery. Unexplained gaps between their areas of distribution must be critically questioned and repeatedly inspected. Occasionally, minute collateral channels will be identified upon repeated and careful scrutiny; at other times, identification of abnormal segmental wall motion in the area of the gap may be more than adequate "circumstantial" evidence to suspect such a flush occlusion. Other possible causes of error in coronary arteriography include:[109]

1. Absence or early bifurcation of the main left coronary artery, leading to nonvisualization of one of its branches.
2. Superimposition of the main left coronary artery branches masking a proximal lesion.
3. Injection beyond a stenosis of the main left coronary artery, thereby overlooking that lesion.
4. Eccentricity of and/or crescent-shaped stenoses, leading to underestimation of their severity.
5. Separate origin of the conus artery, leading to underestimation of the collateral supply and failure to recognize the distal patency of an occluded left anterior descending artery.
6. Partial recanalization of an occluding thrombus, thereby interpreting as stenosis a chronically or acutely recanalized thrombus.

Anomalies of the coronary arteries can be divided into those affecting myocardial perfusion and those that do not affect perfusion. Among those that affect coronary perfusion are:

1. Coronary artery fistulas. These anomalies, from a coronary artery to any of the four cardiac chambers or the pulmonary artery, may range in size from insignificant to large.
2. Origin of left coronary artery from pulmonary artery.
3. Congenital coronary atresia.
4. Origin of left coronary artery from the right sinus of Valsalva.

Anomalies usually not altering myocardial perfusion include:

1. Origin of the circumflex coronary artery from the right sinus of Valsalva.
2. Origin of the left anterior descending artery from the right sinus of Valsalva (rare).
3. Single coronary artery.
4. Origin of all coronary arteries from one sinus of Valsalva.
5. "Horseshoe coronary artery" with ostia in the left and right sinus of Valsalva.[111]
6. Origin of one or both coronary arteries from above the sinuses of Valsalva.

References

1. Radner, S.: Attempt at roentgenologic visualization of coronary blood vessels in man. Acta Radiol. *26*:497, 1945.
2. Gensini, G. G.: Coronary Arteriography. Mount Kisco, N.Y., Futura Publishing Co., 1975, p. 261.
3. Sones, F. M., Jr.: Acquired heart disease: Symposium on present and future of cineangiocardiography. Am. J. Cardiol. *3*:710, 1959.
4. Sones, F. M., Jr., and Shirey, E. K.: Cine coronary arteriography. Mod. Concepts Cardiovasc. Dis. *31*:735, 1962.
5. Ricketts, H. J., and Abrams, H. L.: Percutaneous selective coronary cine arteriography. J.A.M.A. *181*:620, 1962.
6. Judkins, M. P.: Selective coronary arteriography: A percutaneous transfemoral technic. Radiology *89*:815, 1967.
7. Amplatz, K., Formanek, G., Stanger, P., and Wilson, W.: Mechanics of selective coronary artery catheterization via femoral approach. Radiology *89*: 1040, 1967.
8. Bourassa, M. G., Lesperance, J., and Campeau, L.: Selective coronary arteriography by the percutaneous femoral artery approach. Am. J. Roentgenol. *107*: 377, 1969.
9. Wells, D. E., Befeler, B., Winkler, J. B., Myerburg, R. J., Castellanos, A., and Castillo, C. A.: A simplified method for left heart catheterization including coronary arteriography. Chest *63*:959, 1973.
10. Goldstein, R. E., Karsh, R. B., Smith, E. R., Orland, M., Norman, D., Farnham, G., Redwood, D. R., and Epstein, S. E.: Influence of atropine and of vagally mediated bradycardia on the occurrence of ventricular arrhythmias following acute coronary occlusion in closed-chest dogs. Circulation *47*:1180, 1973.

11 CARDIAC IMAGING

A—Nuclear Cardiology

by B. Leonard Holman, M.D.

GLOSSARY

Absorbed dose The energy absorbed by the patient from the decay of the **radionuclide**; expressed in rads or millirads (1 rad = 100 ergs/g).

Algorithm An explicitly defined process made up of a number of discrete steps or instructions; these instructions are frequently coded into computer languages (computer program, software).

Analog-to-digital conversion (ADC) Conversion of continuous analog signals (voltages) to discrete digital information.

Annihilation photons The two 511-kev **photons** emitted during **positron** decay; these photons are released in opposite directions (180-degree angle between photons).

Background Any radiation coming from an undesired location, including radioactivity emanating from structures surrounding the organ of interest (target organ).

Beta rays Nonpenetrating radiation (electrons) emitted during beta decay; ^{3}H is a **radionuclide** that undergoes beta decay.

Characteristic x-rays Low-energy photons released after electron capture (a type of radioactive decay); thallium-201 is an example of a **radionuclide** that decays by electron capture, and its characteristic x-rays are used for scintigraphic imaging.

Coincidence detection Simultaneous detection of the two **annihilation photons** emitted during positron decay.

Collimator The lens of the imaging system, absorbing photons traveling in inappropriate directions and originating from parts of the body other than the region under investigation; collimators are usually made of lead with holes to allow desired photons to pass through to the **crystal**.

- **(a) Parallel-hole** Collimator with thousands of holes in a lead-absorbing sheet. The holes are parallel to each other and perpendicular to the crystal (straight-bore) or at some other angle to the crystal (for example, at a 30-degree slant). Standard high-sensitivity and high-resolution collimators are types of parallel-hole collimators.
- **(b) High-sensitivity** A collimator designed to achieve high count rates by using large, short holes.
- **(c) High-resolution** A collimator designed to maximize spatial resolution by using small, long holes; as a result, sensitivity is reduced.
- **(d) Pinhole** Single-hole (2 to 8 mm in diameter) collimator in which the magnification and resolution increase with decreas-

ing distance between patient and collimator; allows for high resolution but offers poor sensitivity.

(e) **Converging** A multihole collimator with holes that converge toward the center of the collimator; the field of view is compressed to encompass a small organ on a large crystal; allows for high resolution and high sensitivity.

(f) **Cylindrical (single-bore)** A central hole in a large mass of lead; used only with the scintillation probe.

(g) **Multiple pinhole** A collimator with multiple holes for acquiring tomographic images.

Compton scatter A change in the direction of travel of a photon due to an interaction between the photon and matter (the patient or the crystal); a major cause of loss of spatial resolution; presents most difficulty at lower photon energies.

Count(s) The disintegrations that the detector records. Counts/disintegrations represents the efficiency of the detector.

Count rate The number of counts recorded per unit of time (counts/min).

Crystal (sodium iodide scintillation) A high-density photon absorber that converts the energy of the incident photon to a number of light photons.

Cycle-length window The range of cardiac cycle times (R-R interval times) that will be accepted in a gated radionuclide ventriculogram.

Dead time The time required for the camera-computer system to recover after an interaction between a photon and the crystal; counts will not be recorded during this time ($\sim$5 μsec); the dead time determines the maximum count rate that can be accurately recorded.

Disintegration The radioactive decay of one atom.

Disintegration rate Number of disintegrations per unit of time (disintegrations/sec). The standard units are the curie (2.22×10^{12} disintegrations/min) and the millicurie (1 Ci = 1000 mCi).

Electron volts The unit of energy for the photon; usually expressed in thousands (kev) or millions (Mev) of electron volts (1 Mev = 1.6×10^{-6} erg).

Electronic cursor An electronic device for selecting a **region-of-interest** by manually defining the region on an oscilloscope or video display; light pens and joysticks are examples.

Emission tomography See **Tomography, emission.**

Frames The division of a dynamic study into discrete temporal units; for example, a radionuclide angiocardiogram can be collected at a rate of 20 frames per second.

Functional image, Parametric image An image in which intensity reflects a physiological parameter rather than activity; for example, intensity may be proportional to blood flow or to ejection fraction.

Gamma rays Electromagnetic waves with short wavelengths that originate from nuclear transitions; made up of photons capable of giving up energy in discrete interactions with matter.

Gating (physiological) Acquisition of data only during some physiological event. In cardiovascular applications, acquisition is usually gated to the cardiac cycle. Data may be acquired from the entire cardiac cycle by dividing the R-R interval into frames that represent counts acquired at preset time intervals after the R wave; prospective selection of frame intervals is termed **matrix mode**; retrospective selection is termed **list mode**.

Generator, radionuclide A device (usually an inorganic resin) through which a short-lived nuclide (the daughter) can be eluted (separated) from a long-lived parent (^{99}Mo$\rightarrow$^{99m}Tc, ^{113}Sn$\rightarrow$^{113m}In).

Half-life

(a) **Physical** The time necessary for the activity of a nuclide to decay to one-half its original activity (^{99m}Tc = 6 hours, ^{201}Tl = 73.1 hours).

(b) **Biological** The time necessary for the concentration of the tracer to fall to one-half its original concentration.

Isotope Different nuclides of the same element, having the same proton number but different mass numbers; for example, $^{11}_{6}$C, $^{12}_{6}$C, $^{13}_{6}$C, $^{14}_{6}$C are isotopes of carbon.

kev See **Electron volts.**

List mode **Acquisition of data from a dynamic study** in the form of a sequence of individual scintillation events which can then be re-formatted retrospectively into a variable number of **frames**.

Matrix The two-dimensional array into which positional data from the gamma camera are pigeonholed (32 $\times$ 32, 64 $\times$ 64, 128 $\times$ 128).

Matrix (histogram) mode Acquisition of data from a dynamic study such as a radionuclide angiocardiogram which can be re-formatted into a predefined number of **frames** and framing rate.

Mev See **Electron volts.**

Parametric image See **Functional image.**

Photon A packet of energy associated with electromagnetic radiation (gamma rays, x-rays, or light); the energy units are **electron volts** or kiloelectron volts (kev).

Photopeak The energy of the predominant photons released during decay of the **radionuclide** (^{99m}Tc = 140 kev, ^{201}Tl = 69 to 83 kev).

Pixel A single picture element in a digitized image; one of the **matrix** elements.

Positron A positively charged electron released during positron decay of a nucleus; interacts with an electron, transforming the mass of the electron and the positron into two 511-kev **annihilation photons.**

Pulse-height analyzer An electronic discriminator that selects those pulses arising from photons with energies approximating that of the **photopeak** and rejects pulses due to scattered radiation above and below the **photopeak**; the range of energies that are accepted constitutes the "window" of the analyzer.

Radionuclide An atom or species of atom with an unstable nucleus that will spontaneously decay to a more stable form, emitting radiation in the process; examples include thallium-201 (^{201}Tl), tantalum-178 (^{178}Ta), and technetium-99m (^{99m}Tc, where "Tc" is the abbreviation for the element technetium, "99" is its atomic mass, and "m" indicates the metastable state).

Reformat To rearrange retrospectively the parameters of a study; to convert **list mode** data to **matrix mode** data.

Region-of-interest The **pixels** or matrix elements of a digitized image (or series of images in a dynamic study) that outline a desired structure, organ, or region within the image; may be defined manually with an **electronic cursor.**

Resolution

(a) **Spatial** The ability of the detector to separate adjacent sources of activity.

(b) **Temporal** The maximum combination of framing rate and number of **frames** that can be acquired.

(c) **Energy** The ability of the detector to discriminate between photons of adjacent energies.

Scintigram An image of the distribution of radioactivity obtained with a **scintillation camera** after the internal administration of a **radionuclide.**

Scintigraphy The process of acquiring a **scintigram.**

Scintillation camera

(a) **Single-crystal, Anger-type** An imaging device with a single sodium iodide crystal with a 10- to 15-inch diameter and ¼- to ½-inch thickness; the detector records the spatial distribution of the internally administered radiotracer.

(b) **Multicrystal** An imaging with multiple crystals and a high count rate capability.

Scintillation probe A device that records radioactivity but does not provide positional or spatial information.

Time-activity curve A histogram (in the **matrix mode**) of the change in the count rate as a function of time.

Tomography, emission

(a) **Transaxial** Transverse-section reconstruction of the radionuclide distribution obtained by acquiring images or "slices" (about 1 to 2 cm in thickness) of the head or body; uses **coincidence detection** (positrons) or **single-photon detection** (nuclides such as ^{99m}Tc or ^{201}Tl).

(b) **Limited angle** Images obtained by focusing at varying depths within the organ of interest; the images maintain the same spatial orientation as do conventional images (the two-dimensional image is oriented parallel to the detector); can be obtained with standard **scintillation cameras** and specially designed **collimators.**

Radionuclide methods provide a safe, relatively atraumatic, often quantitative approach to assessing a variety of cardiac functions.[1] Their recent popularity can be attributed to the fact that they can be applied during exercise and other physiological and pharmacological interventions; they can be applied to very ill patients; they can provide a direct measure of cardiac function, myocardial blood flow, and metabolism; and they can provide quantitative landmarks to help evaluate the temporal progress of cardiac disease.

In this chapter, we will describe these methods, discussing first the required instrumentation and then the techniques used to assess cardiac wall motion and hemodynamics, myocardial perfusion, myocardial metabolism, and acute infarction and to detect pulmonary emboli.

INSTRUMENTATION

THE SCINTILLATION (ANGER, GAMMA) CAMERA

The scintillation camera provides a pictorial representation of the distribution of radioactivity. This device consists of a collimator, a position-sensitive detector (a large, flat sodium iodide crystal), and 37 to 91 photomultiplier tubes closely packed against the crystal. When gamma rays interact with the crystal, a portion of the gamma-ray energy is converted to light. The light is then converted into an electrical signal by the photomultiplier tubes. Electronically, the detector then calculates the position of the interaction and the energy of the gamma rays.

The *collimator* is analogous to a lens (Fig. 11–1). It is made from material that readily absorbs gamma rays, usually lead. The gamma rays can reach the crystal only by passing through the holes or channels of the collimator. The most common collimator is the *parallel-hole* collimator. Only gamma rays emitted from the patient in a direction perpendicular to the crystal can enter the detector. The diameter and length of the channels (holes) strongly affect the spatial resolution and sensitivity of the system. *High-resolution* parallel-hole collimators result in high spatial resolution at the expense of sensitivity, while *high-sensitivity* collimators result in an increase in count rate by a factor of two or three over high-resolution collimators but with a loss of resolution of about 25 per cent. A *general-purpose* collimator represents a compromise with regard to both resolution and sensitivity.

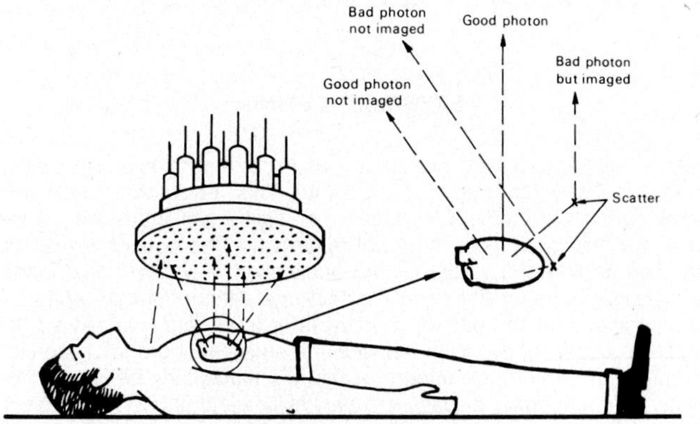

FIGURE 11–1 The multi-channel collimator acts as a lens for photon detection. (From Budinger, T. F., and Rollo, F. D.: Physics and instrumentation. Progr. Cardiovasc. Dis. *20*:19, 1977, by permission of Grune and Stratton, Inc.)

Multiple-hole collimators that diverge toward the patient are sometimes used to increase the field of view of the system (*diverging* collimators). Conversely, holes that converge toward the camera increase sensitivity with a smaller field of view (*converging* collimators). In a *slant-hole* collimator the holes are angled with respect to the detector, and the camera can obtain an oblique view with the detector flat against the chest.

A pinhole collimator can be used to magnify the image. It is considerably less sensitive than a parallel-hole collimator and is therefore used for imaging small organs. A collimator with several pinholes can be used to image an organ from several slightly different angles simultaneously to produce tomographic images.

For nuclear cardiology, a *general-purpose* collimator is used for time-dependent studies such as exercise thallium-201 and gated blood pool imaging. *High-resolution* collimators are generally used for studies obtained at rest. Recently a high-resolution, square-hole collimator has been introduced with increased sensitivity so that it may be used in time-dependent studies, such as during or after exercise. *High-sensitivity* collimators are used when the photon number is limited, as in first-pass radionuclide angiocardiography. *Slant-hole* collimators are used to maximize separation between atria and ventricles and to permit imaging along the long axis of the ventricles. *Seven-pinhole* collimators have been used for limited-angle tomography but offer no significant advantages.

The important performance parameters of the Anger scintillation camera are sensitivity, spatial resolution, field uniformity, energy resolution, and count-rate linearity. *Sensitivity* is defined as the number of recorded counts per gamma ray emitted from a radioactive tracer. The sensitivity of a gamma camera will depend on three principal factors: the gamma ray energy, the thickness of the crystal, and the collimator employed. *Spatial resolution* is a measure of the imaging system's ability to resolve small structural details in an object. One measure of resolution is the camera's response to a line source, expressed as the line spread function. Spatial resolution can be described in terms of the full-width at half-maximum, the width of the line spread function at 50 per cent of the maximum value.

The characteristics of the Anger camera, such as the thickness of the sodium iodide crystal, represent a compromise between sensitivity and spatial resolution. For example, a 12-mm (½ inch-thick) crystal will absorb 98 per cent of the 140 kev photons of technetium-99m and 100 per cent of the 68 to 82 kev photons of thallium-201. A 6-mm (¼ inch-thick) crystal will absorb 84 per cent of the 140 kev photons of technetium-99m and 100 per cent of the 68 to 82 kev photons of thallium-201. The intrinsic resolution of thallium-201 is better with a thinner crystal, although the improvement in resolution drops with distance from the collimator. A ⅜-inch thick crystal is therefore a good compromise if both thallium-201 and technetium-99m are to be imaged with the same camera.

The *standard field of view* of most mobile cameras is 25 cm. Smaller diameters are used on some special-purpose cameras. The diameter should be large enough to encompass the entire heart within the field of view using parallel-hole collimators (20 cm for circular fields of view). Detectors with a large field of view (35 to 50 cm) are useful for pulmonary scintigraphy (see later).

Count-rate linearity refers to a linear increase in the detected count rate as the activity increases. The count-rate loss should be less than 10 per cent of count rates at 50,000 counts per second, but this loss increases rapidly at higher counting rates. Other effects may also be seen at higher counting rates. For example, spurious counts can be recorded due to the coincidence of two low-energy photons. Finally, the uniformity of the camera can change at higher count rates. Recent improvements in camera design based on digital electronics have substantially increased the range of count-rate linearity.

THE MULTICRYSTAL CAMERA

The multicrystal scintillation camera has 294 separate sodium iodide scintillation crystals arranged in a matrix of 14 $\times$ 21 crystals. The crystals are 9.5 mm square and 2.5 mm thick. There are 35 photomultiplier tubes connected to the crystal array. An event is located in a particular crystal through detection of the simultaneous pulse from both a row and a column photomultiplier tube. A digital computer, which is an integral part of the camera, accumulates the image in its memory for display and processing.

The camera has good sensitivity, even at energies above 200 kev, because of its thick crystals. The constant picture element size means that, except for the effects of scattered radiation, image resolution is constant over the full energy range of 50 to 500 kev. The electronics have been designed for very fast processing of scintillation events leading to a short resolving time and a maximum count rate of 400,000 to 500,000 events per second—three to four times faster than the Anger camera. This is an advantage for rapid, dynamic studies, such as first-transit radionuclide angiocardiography.

Disadvantages of the matrix detector are related mainly to the light lost in the complex light guides and the coarse nature of the matrix itself. Approximately 50 per cent of the light from the crystals is lost in the light pipe arrangement. The energy resolution for technetium-99m is therefore about 50 per cent full-width at half-maximum compared to the Anger camera's resolution of 13 per cent. This means that in imaging studies with thick sources at energies from 50 to 200 kev, significant scattered radiation will lead to loss of image contrast. The coarse spatial resolution is determined by the size of the individual crystals (9.5 mm $\times$ 9.5 mm).

THE SINGLE-PROBE DETECTOR

The scintillation probe offers the advantage of portability and enables the measurement of cardiac function in settings where it might be difficult to bring in an Anger scintillation camera (such as the operating room, the recovery room, and the intensive care unit). While cardiac studies performed with the scintillation probe provide reasonably accurate measurements of left ventricular ejection fraction and other measures of global left ventricular function, they do require considerable training to perform and are of limited use in patients with very poor function, when it may be difficult to determine the edge of the ventricle and to determine background.

The standard sodium iodide scintillation probe is 1 to 3 inches in diameter and between 1 and 2 inches in depth. The crystal may be housed in a cylindrical collimator, a parallel-hole collimator similar to the low-resolution/high-efficiency collimators used with scintillation cameras, or a converging collimator. The sodium iodide crystal is used with a high temporal resolution rate meter (10 to 50 msec). Information is acquired after the intravenous injection of an intravascular tracer, such as technetium-99m–labeled red blood cells, and the studies are gated to the patient's electrocardiogram as in the equilibrium radionuclide angiocardiogram (see below). Although the data can be displayed directly on a strip chart recorder, most systems now use a microprocessor for data acquisition and analysis. The time-activity curves are displayed on an oscilloscope, and the processed data are read out through a teleprinter or a console.

More recently, substantially smaller probes have been constructed using *cadmium telluride* crystals. With these smaller systems, it may be possible to monitor patients sequentially over prolonged periods with a probe permanently positioned to the patient's chest. Sequential monitoring may be particularly useful in patients with acute myocardial infarction and other patients in the intensive care setting.

TOMOGRAPHIC IMAGING SYSTEMS

Tomography is used in an attempt to solve one of the major constraints of standard two-dimensional imaging: the overlap of adjacent structures and background on the organ or tissue of interest. Both single-photon and positron-emission tomography are now in use.

Two techniques for performing tomography are *limited-angle* and *transaxial*. The seven-pinhole and rotating slant-hole collimators are examples of limited-angle tomography that are adaptable to standard Anger cameras and single-photon tracers. Because of the limited angle, depth resolution is poor. While the instrumentation is relatively inexpensive, requiring only the purchase of the collimator and reconstruction software, the future of this technique remains uncertain.

Transaxial tomography provides improved depth resolution and is the most promising approach to the quantification of in vivo distribution of radiotracers. *Positron-transaxial tomography* systems are, in fact, being used to quantify regional myocardial metabolism and perfusion (p. 1251). Prototype single-photon transaxial tomographic instruments have been limited either by poor sensitivity (rotating gamma cameras) or poor resolution (ring detector systems). It is anticipated that further improvements in design will overcome these limitations and that tomography may play an increasingly important role by improving the accuracy of current scintigraphic methodologies and by more accurately reflecting the extent of altered myocardial perfusion, wall motion abnormalities, and global ventricular function.

THE COMPUTER

A computer is necessary for nearly all procedures in nuclear cardiology. It may be an integral part of the imaging system or may be separate from the scintillation camera as either a mobile or stationary system. The computer should be adequate for first-pass and equilibrium (gated) radionuclide angiocardiography; this requires high temporal resolution (a minimum of 30 to 40 frames per second) and a matrix capability of at least 64 $\times$ 64 picture elements (pixels). Two basic types of computers are used in nuclear medicine: general-purpose (programmable) and special-purpose (hard-wire) units. The general-purpose systems are more flexible and programs can be developed and changed by the users. Special-purpose systems have fixed programs and are more limited in capability. The size and configuration of the computer system will vary with the types of procedures to be performed and local factors in a given department.

EXERCISE TESTING

An exercise table and bicycle are used for supine exercise testing during radionuclide angiocardiography. This equipment must not move during the study. The patient should be well-stabilized on the table and the table itself must not move while the patient is exercising. The bicycle should permit the application of variable workloads, variable positions for the pedals to facilitate patient comfort, and variable positions for the patient. Some prefer a 45-degree angle for the patient's upper body. With equilibrium angiocardiography, exercise testing in the 45-degree upright position is particularly helpful for patients with pulmonary disease or heart failure and is used routinely in many departments. Equipment for upright exercise should also be available, since this is commonly used for first-pass radionuclide angiocardiography and thallium exercise studies. The most common method for upright exercise with ^{201}Tl-imaging is treadmill ergometry, which is superior to the bicycle because it is more likely to stress the patient maximally.

CARDIAC PERFORMANCE

Cardiac performance is a prime factor in determining appropriate medical and surgical management for patients with coronary heart disease.[2–5] Ventricular ejection fraction and regional wall motion are directly related to clinical prognosis in patients with chronic coronary heart disease[2–4] and after myocardial infarction.[6,7] Although invasive techniques involving left ventricular catheterization and radiocontrast angiography provide reliable measurements of ejection fraction and regional wall motion[8] (p. 473), they have limited application in critically ill patients. Radionuclide techniques are noninvasive, requiring only a peripheral intravenous injection, and thus offer distinct advantages over more conventional, invasive methods. The radionuclide techniques are safe and repeatable and do not induce measurable hemodynamic alterations.[9,10] In addition, cardiac performance can be studied during a variety of physiological or pharmaceutical interventions.

RADIOPHARMACEUTICALS

The primary requirement of a radiopharmaceutical for first-pass radionuclide angiocardiography (p. 356) is that it remain intravascular during its first passage through the right and left heart phases. The secondary requirement is that the physical properties of the radionuclide be satisfactory with respect to the instrumentation being used.

The radionuclide that is used for virtually all phases of radionuclide angiocardiography is technetium-99m. It has a 6-hour half-life, a photon energy of 140 kev, and minimal nonpenetrating radiation, and it effectively labels a large number of pharmaceuticals—a requirement that is particularly important for equilibrium studies. While pertechnetate leaks out rapidly into the extracellular space with an intravascular half-life of approximately one hour, it does remain intravascular during the first intravascular transit. Because the tracer must remain intravascular only during its first transit, technetium-99m pertechnetate can be used for first-pass studies. Since ^{99m}Tc-pertechnetate ($^{99m}TcO_4^-$) is the chemical form of ^{99m}Tc after elution from the ^{99}Mo*→ ^{99m}Tc generator, it is the most readily available and the least expensive of the technetium-99m pharmaceuticals.

The major disadvantage of ^{99m}Tc is its long half-life relative to the duration of the procedure. After intravenous injection, the material persists in the intravascular and extracellular space, precluding serial studies, and only two or three first-pass studies are possible within a 6-hour period. As a result, evaluation in multiple projections or after multiple physiological or pharmacological interventions is not possible.

One approach to increasing the number of serial studies is the use of ^{99m}Tc-sulfur colloid, a radiopharmaceutical extracted by the reticuloendothelial system, thereby radically shortening the biological half-life. The pharmaceutical is extracted primarily by the liver and spleen within several minutes after intravenous injection.[11] The disadvantage of this approach is the relatively high radiation dose to the bone marrow. Approximately 5 per cent of the dose is sequestered by the bone marrow, the most radiosensitive of the body's tissues. ^{99m}Tc-pyrophosphate is an attractive alternative in the coronary care unit. Acute infarct scintigraphy can be performed three hours after the initial first-pass study. Thus, two studies can be performed after the injection of a single radiopharmaceutical. ^{99m}Tc-DTPA (diethylenetriaminepentaacetic acid) has also been suggested for first-pass studies, since clearance of this radiopharmaceutical from the blood is more rapid than that of ^{99m}Tc-pertechnetate, reducing the whole-body radiation dose and, more importantly, shortening the time between sequential studies.[9]

*Mo = molybdenum.

The development of ultrashort-lived nuclides should increase the flexibility of this technique. Gold-195m has a 30-second half-life and an acceptable gamma energy of 262 kev for use with multicrystal cameras and with Anger cameras using medium-energy collimators and adequate shielding.[12] It is obtained from a ^{195}Hg→ ^{195m}Au generator system. Its parent, mercury-195m, has a sufficiently long half-life (41.6 hours) so that each generator will last up to three or four days.

The advantages of gold-195m are that multiple views can be obtained and serial responses to exercise or drug interventions can be studied by repeating the injection at frequent intervals without build-up of significant background activity and with minimal patient radiation dose. Also, because of the reduced patient dose relative to ^{99m}Tc, larger doses can be injected, taking full advantage of the higher count-rate capacities of multicrystal cameras and digital Anger cameras. Limitations of this tracer are that the parent, ^{195m}Hg, may be present as a contaminant in the injected dose; the half-life of the tracer is too short to permit measurement of the parent prior to each injection; high-energy photons result in scattered radiation; and the high cost of the generator will make it practical only in hospitals that carry out a large number of first-pass studies.

Other ultrashort half-life tracers have been introduced, including tantalum-178, with a half-life of 9 minutes,[13] and iridium-191m, with a half-life of 4.9 seconds.[14] Tantalum-178 is used with low-energy imaging systems such as the multiwire proportional camera. Iridium-191m is used for children, in whom the 4.9-second half-life is tolerable. Both tracers are obtained from long-lived parents by elution through generator systems.

The radiopharmaceutical for equilibrium (ECG-gated) studies (p. 360) must remain within the intravascular space throughout the course of the study. If continual monitoring is anticipated, the radiopharmaceutical must remain within the intravascular space for at least one or two half-lives. ^{99m}Tc–human serum albumin (HSA) and ^{99m}Tc-tagged red blood cells (RBCs) have been advocated for this purpose. ^{99m}Tc-HSA is less satisfactory for gated studies because (1) there is proportionately more activity in the liver, since the liver albumin space is larger than the intravascular space; and (2) the blood clearance of ^{99m}Tc-HSA is fairly rapid, precluding prolonged monitoring and repeat studies.

Once the initial equilibration of the tracer has been reached, ^{99m}Tc-RBCs are cleared from the blood very slowly. The red cells can be tagged in vivo by injecting 300 to 400 μg of stannous iron intravenously and injecting ^{99m}Tc-pertechnetate 15 minutes later. Approximately 60 to 80 per cent of the pertechnetate attaches to and labels the red blood cells; the remainder is excreted through the kidneys or labels iodine traps, such as the kidney and stomach. Equilibration is reached after 5 minutes. Since rapid renal clearance is a precondition for optimal studies, this technique is less satisfactory in patients with poor renal clearance and results in high background activity and poor target-to-background ratios. The primary advantage of this technique is the ease with which the red cells can be labeled. Recently, kits have been developed for in vitro labeling of the patient's own red cells. The major advantage of this approach is the high labeling efficiency (greater than or equal to 98 per cent). This technique does take more time than in vivo labeling, but with the newly developed kits, labeling can be performed in 15 to 30 minutes.

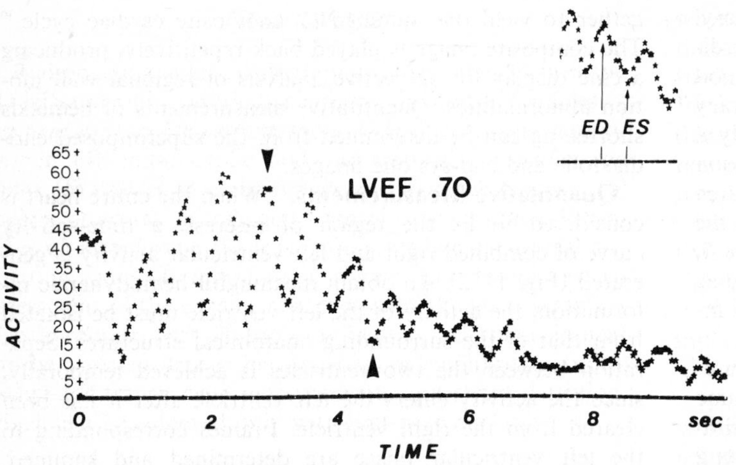

FIGURE 11-3 Time-activity curve from left ventricular region. Each point represents total counts for 40 msec. The highest value (peak) for each cycle corresponds to end-diastole (ED) and the subsequent low value (valley) to end systole (ES). An average left ventricular ejection fraction (LVEF) of 0.70 was calculated for the three cycles between the arrows. (From Ashburn, W. L., et al.: Left ventricular ejection fraction—a review of several radionuclide angiographic approaches using the scintillation camera. Progr. Cardiovasc. Dis. *20*:267, 1978, by permission of Grune and Stratton, Inc.)

count rate minus background:

$$EF = \frac{\text{Diastolic counts} - \text{Systolic counts}}{\text{Diastolic counts} - \text{Background counts}} \quad (6)$$

When multicrystal cameras are used, the counting rate is sufficiently high to allow calculation of the ejection fraction from the maxima and minima of the oscillations on the left ventricular time-activity curve. With single-crystal cameras, the sensitivity, and hence the counting rate, is lower. If only the maximum and minimum counting rates are used for each oscillation, the statistical reliability of the data is compromised.

These techniques for determining ejection fraction have been validated by comparison with values obtained using single-plane and biplane contrast ventriculography. Correlation coefficients ranging from r = 0.94 to r = 0.97 have been reported by a number of groups who have compared the two techniques.[11,15,16]

Left Ventricular Ejection-Phase Indices. A number of ejection-phase performance indices (p. 480) can be measured from the left ventricular time-activity curve. *Left ventricular ejection rate* can be measured from either the equilibrium or the first-pass radionuclide angiocardiogram. A weighted least-squares analysis can be used to fit the ejection phase data (four to nine data points per ejection phase) to a straight line.[11] The slope of this line, representing the change in counts with time, *dC/dT*, is determined and normalized to the average number of counts over the ejection phase ($dC/dT/C_{ave}$). This measurement, unlike the left ventricular ejection fraction, appears to be sensitive to changes in the inotropic state in patients with cardiac disease. The normal value for the normalized left ventricular ejection rate is 3.40 ± 0.17 $dC/dT/C_{ave}$. In patients who have coronary artery disease, this value is 1.22 ± 0.11 $dC/dT/C_{ave}$.

Indices of diastolic function are more sensitive for detecting the effects of myocardial ischemia than are systolic indices such as ejection fraction[31] (p. 1247). These changes in the diastolic properties of the ventricle are seen in acute myocardial ischemia and may be present even at rest in patients with coronary artery disease.[32,33] Both first-pass and equilibrium methods can be used to derive indices of diastolic function (as well as the other phase indices described in this section) from the left ventricular volume curve. The *peak diastolic filling rate* expresses diastolic filling as a fraction of the end-diastolic volume per second. It is calculated from the diastolic portion of the left ventricular volume curve by fitting a third-order polynomial to the first 400 msec of diastole.[34] The point of maximum filling is determined by setting the second derivative of the polynomial to zero. The third-order polynomial is then differentiated to yield the maximum filling rate, which is normalized to the total end-diastolic counts. With this method, the peak diastolic filling rate has been found to be 2.14 ± 0.63 end-diastolic volume/sec in normals and is reduced in about 90 per cent of patients with previous myocardial infarction when they are studied at rest. Patients with coronary artery disease but without previous infarction may also have abnormal filling rates at rest, but the incidence of this abnormality remains controversial (56 to 85 per cent).[34,35]

Right Ventricular Ejection Fraction. Right ventricular performance is difficult to quantitate, since the geometry of the right ventricle is complex, making calculation of the right ventricular ejection fraction by standard geometrical methods extremely difficult. A radionuclide method for this measurement has been developed and is similar in many respects to that for left ventricular ejection fraction.[36] The radiotracer is injected intravenously, through either a large medial antecubital vein or the jugular vein, in a volume of less than 2 ml. The first pass of the radioactive bolus through the central circulation is recorded in the 30-degree right anterior oblique projection. The ejection fraction is measured from the time-activity curve derived from the right ventricular blood pool. A region of interest is assigned to this pool, carefully excluding the right atrium and the pulmonary artery. A second semiannular region of interest is placed outside the right ventricle adjacent to the apical anterior and inferior walls. A high-frequency time-activity curve (25 frames/sec) is generated from both the right ventricular and the background regions of interest. Right ventricular ejection fraction is calculated by dividing the difference in counts between end-diastole and end-systole by the number of counts at end diastole after correcting for background. Three to five beats from the downslope of the right ventricular time-activity curve are used for the calculation.

Background correction of the right ventricular ejection fraction measurement appears necessary only when serial studies are performed, since background activity alters right ventricular ejection fraction by less than 5 per cent.[36]

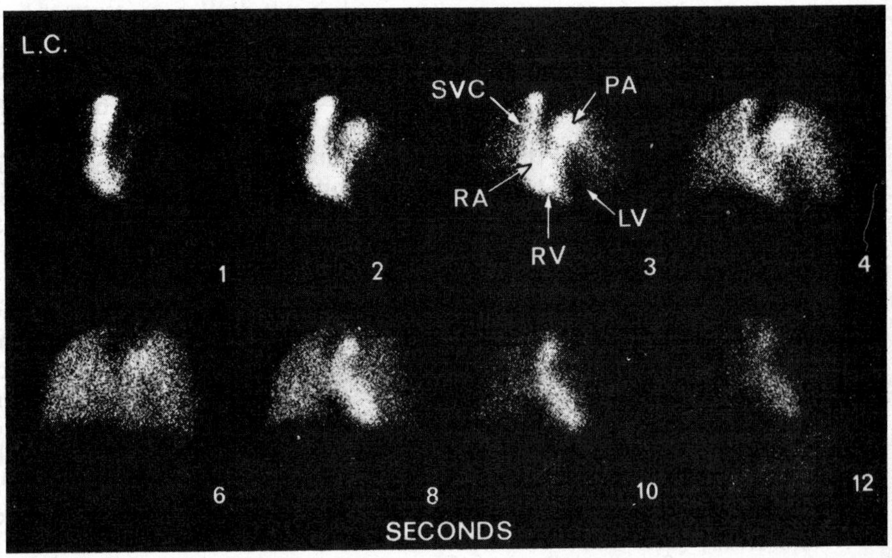

FIGURE 11–4 **First-transit radionuclide angiogram. At one second, the tracer is in the superior vena cava, right atrium, and right ventricle. By three seconds, the radioactivity is entering the lungs through the pulmonary arteries. By eight seconds, the radioactivity has returned to the left side of the heart. The left ventricle and aorta are clearly seen, and the lung background is rapidly diminishing. Numbers represent time of frames in seconds following the injection. (SVC = superior vena cava; RA = right atrium; RV = right ventricle; LV = left ventricle; PA = pulmonary artery.)**

Because the activity is high and the background is low during transit through the right ventricle, single-crystal cameras can be used for this purpose, although multi-crystal cameras provide significantly higher counting rates and therefore improve the statistical reliability of the measurement.[37] Using the first-pass method, investigators have found the mean right ventricular ejection fraction normally to be between 0.52 and 0.57.[36–38]

End-Diastolic Volume. End-diastolic volume can be approximated from a first-pass radionuclide angiocardiogram with high temporal resolution using geometrical techniques. After the time-activity curve has been obtained, those frames representing end-diastolic volume are summed. The left ventricular contour is determined by means of an electronic cursor or an edge-detection algorithm. A grid of known dimensions is then placed between the radioactive source and the detector for size correction, and the volume is determined using the technique of Sandler and Dodge.[39] Since the ventricular edges are not as well defined with first-pass radionuclide angiocardiography as with contrast left ventriculography, and because only one projection is usually obtained, it would not be expected that the resultant measurement would be the most precise, although recent studies have shown a reasonable correlation between the two methods.

SHUNT DETECTION. In normal patients, the lung time-activity curve has a characteristic appearance after intravenous injection of a first-pass tracer. There is an early peak due to the appearance of radiotracer in the lungs. This is followed by rapid clearance as the tracer moves into the systemic circulation. Eventually some recirculation will occur as the tracer returns from the systemic circulation to the right side of the heart and the lungs (Fig. 11–4). In patients with *left-to-right shunts*, tracer passes from the left to the right side of the heart, short-circuiting the systemic circulation and resulting in rapid recirculation to the lungs. On first-pass radionuclide angiocardiography, the three distinct phases (right heart, lungs, and left heart) merge owing to rapid recirculation, and a clear definition of the left ventricle is not possible because of the high level of radioactivity in the lungs (Fig. 11–5).

Several indices have been suggested for quantifying left-

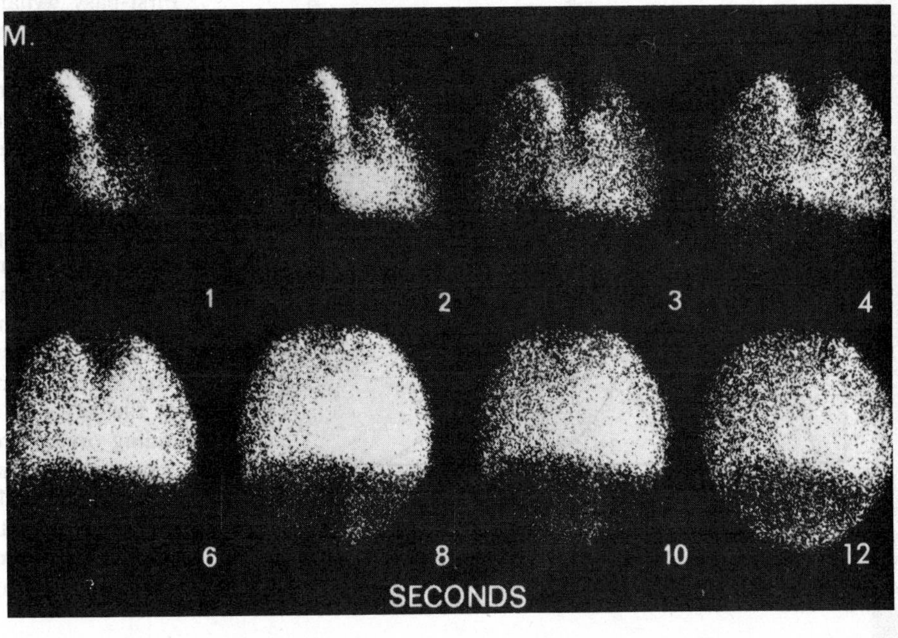

FIGURE 11–5 **Left-to-right shunt at atrial level. Recirculation of radioactivity is seen in the lungs. In addition, radioactivity reappears in the right atrium, right ventricle, and pulmonary artery at 8, 10, and 12 seconds (bottom right). (From Treves, S., et al.: Intracardiac shunts. *In* James, A. E., et al. (eds.): Pediatric Nuclear Medicine. Philadelphia. W. B. Saunders Co., 1974, p. 231.)**

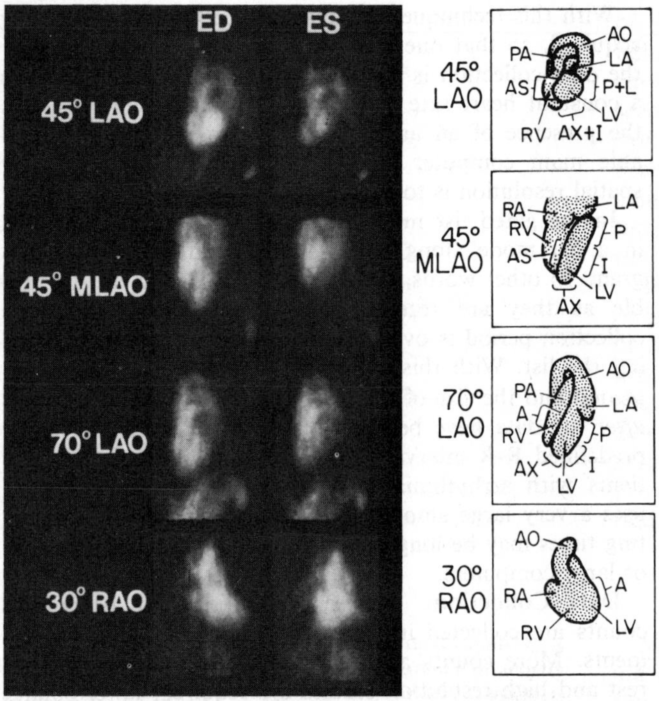

FIGURE 11–9 Normal equilibrium (gated) radionuclide angiocardiogram. LAO = left anterior oblique projection; MLAO = modified left anterior oblique; RAO = right anterior oblique; ED = end diastole; ES = end systole; PA = pulmonary artery; AS = anteroseptal; RV = right ventricle; AX = apex; I = inferior; LV = left ventricle; P = posterior; L = lateral; LA = left atrium; AO = aorta; RA = right atrium.

rived from contrast ventriculography. The left ventricle is divided into anatomical segments, usually the anterior wall (best seen on the 30-degree RAO and 70-degree LAO views), anteroseptum (best seen on the 45-degree LAO or MLAO view), apex (seen on all views), and inferoposterior wall (best seen on the 45-degree MLAO and 70-degree LAO views). Each segment is assigned a score: 3 = normokinesis, 2 = mild hypokinesis, 1 = severe hypokinesis, 0 = akinesis, and −1 = dyskinesis.

Numerical Analysis. Quantitative measurements of global and regional ventricular function can be obtained from the time-activity curves derived from the left and right ventricles and from regions of the ventricles. Since the radiopharmaceutical is uniformly mixed in the blood at equilibrium, a time-activity curve over the ventricles will represent the changes in ventricular volume occurring during the cardiac cycle. However, because activity is distributed throughout the intravascular space, including tissue in front of and behind the heart, accurate background correction is essential.

Wall motion can be assessed by radionuclide methods either from the geometrical approaches used in the standard contrast angiographic method or from analysis of changes in count rate. Background-corrected activity recorded from the region of the left ventricle is directly proportional to this chamber's blood volume. Although the radionuclide method provides limited spatial resolution and edge definition, it does offer an accurate measure of the activity viewed by the detector or a region of the detector. Therefore, assessment of global and regional ventricular function based on changing count rates has two inherent advantages over the geometrical approaches borrowed from contrast angiography: (1) The geometrical approaches assess only that part of the ventricular wall which is tangential to the detector. Techniques based on left ventricular activity assess the three-dimensional space viewed by the corresponding region of the detector, assessing ventricular function regardless of its orientation to the detector. Techniques based on activity do not require assumptions concerning left ventricular shape—a consideration that is particularly important in patients with asynergy, in whom such geometrical assumptions may not be valid. (2) The need to define the margins of the left ventricle during end-systole is eliminated with the count-rate method. During end-systole, the difference between ventricular and background activity may be small and edge resolution particularly poor.

Background Correction. The left ventricular time-activity curve is generated after the left ventricular outline has been defined using a light pen or an electronic cursor and after subtraction of background. As with first-pass probe studies, background correction is critical, since approximately 33 to 50 per cent of the activity emanating from the area of the left ventricle is due to background. The background regions, usually representing areas just lateral and inferior to the heart and including a portion of the interventricular septum, can be defined manually or automatically using predefined computer algorithms.

Several general approaches have been suggested for background correction: (1) fixed ventricular and background regions can be defined from the end-diastolic frame; and (2) a variable left ventricular region, shrinking during systole and expanding during diastole, can be defined. Background regions may be continuous or interrupted and may extend into the septum. Background regions never abut the base of the ventricle. However, each of these approaches can result in accurate measures of ejection fraction if applied carefully and if adequately controlled comparisons are made regularly with measurements derived at cardiac catheterization.

Left Ventricular Ejection Fraction. Once background activity is known with reasonable accuracy, ejection fraction can be determined from changes in count rate rather than from geometrical analysis,[50–53] since changes in left ventricular activity are directly proportional to changes in ventricular blood volume. Ejection fraction is calculated from the formula

$$\mathrm{LVEF} = \frac{\mathrm{EDC} - \mathrm{SC}}{\mathrm{EDC} - \mathrm{BC}} \qquad (8)$$

where LVEF is left ventricular ejection fraction; EDC, or "end-diastolic counts," represents the activity emanating from the region of the left ventricle during the frame corresponding to end diastole; and ESC, or "end-systolic counts," represents left ventricular activity during the end-systolic frame; BC stands for background counts. These two frames can be determined from the time-activity curve and correspond to the maximum and minimum points, respectively. Ejection fraction obtained using this algorithm correlates very well with ejection fractions derived by means of contrast ventriculography ($r = 0.92$).[50]

Ventricular Volume and Cardiac Output. Left ventricular volume can be measured using geometrical or count-rate principles. The count-rate method compares the background-corrected left ventricular activity with the activity in a known volume of the patient's blood.[54] To obtain volumes in milliliters and output in liters/min, attenuation corrections must be introduced.[55] This is the most difficult of the numerical analyses to measure accurately because of the varying attenuation among patients, particularly between men and women, and the careful attention to detail that is required.

Functional Images. It is important for the physician who is accustomed to using contrast ventriculography to keep in mind the differences between contrast and radionuclide studies. The contrast ventriculogram represents volume information relatively poorly because mixing of the contrast is not complete and because there are difficulties with film linearity. However, because it has excellent resolution, it defines the edges of the ventricle well; therefore, volume can be calculated from the two-dimensional silhouette of the ventricle, and edge motion is used to evaluate wall motion. By comparison, the radionuclide angiocardiogram has poor spatial resolution, but the image data are directly proportional to ventricular volume after background correction. For this reason, techniques such as functional imaging have been very useful aids in the interpretation of the radionuclide angiocardiogram. Subjective assessment of the cineangiocardiogram must rely on catching the wall motion abnormality on target, hence the need for multiple views. With function-imaging techniques, we take advantage of the count-rate changes that occur throughout the ventricle and result in intensity changes in the image rather than alterations on the edges of the image.

Functional images are physiological maps. After certain arithmetic operations have been performed on a group of images, the resultant image or images are no longer representative of the basic activity distribution but are representative of some physiological function, such as regional ejection fraction or onset of contraction. In such an image the intensities are proportional to a function rather than to the original activity distributions.

Ejection-Fraction Image. The ejection-fraction image makes use of the proportionality between background-corrected left ventricular count rate and blood volume. By subtracting the end-systolic image from the end-diastolic image, an image of regional stroke volume can be obtained. The stroke-volume image is divided by the background-corrected end-diastolic image to produce an ejection-fraction image, a map of regional ejection fractions throughout the left ventricle.[56]

In the ejection-fraction image, the intensity of each of the matrix areas is directly proportional to the regional ejection fraction. The normal ejection-fraction image is characterized by a peripheral ejection shell comprising matrices with greater than 50 per cent ejection—i.e., a reduction in blood volume of 50 per cent between diastole and systole in any given matrix area within the end-diastolic perimeter of the left ventricle. The width of the normal ejection shell exceeds one-third of the left ventricular transverse diameter throughout its inferoposterior and apical extent. Thinning of the ejection shell corresponds to hypokinesis, and absence of the shell corresponds to akinesis (Fig. 11–10). The accuracy of this technique compares favorably with contrast ventriculography for the detection of ventricular asynergy.[56]

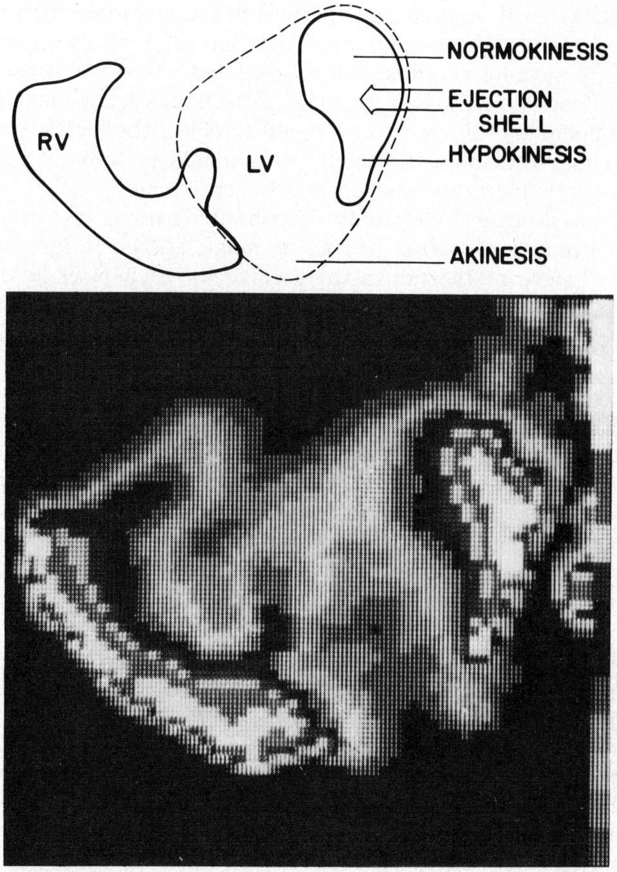

FIGURE 11–10 *A*, Schematic representation of left ventricular ejection shell with thinning (hypokinesis) and fracture (akinesis). *B*, Corresponding ejection fraction image in a patient with a large akinetic segment (apical) and adjacent hypokinesis. (From Maddox, D. E., et al.: The ejection fraction image: A noninvasive index of regional left ventricular wall motion. Am. J. Cardiol. *41*:1230, 1978.)

Paradox Image. If the end-diastolic frame is subtracted from the end-systolic frame, the resultant image will show areas of left ventricular paradox. The presence and extent of paradox in each picture element is determined from the end-diastolic (ED) and end-systolic (ES) counts within that picture element according to the equation

$$\text{Paradox} = \text{ES} - \text{ED} \quad (9)$$

The extent of paradox may be determined in terms of both the number of picture elements (pixels) within the left ventricle demonstrating paradox and the number of counts within those pixels. Both the number of pixels and the number of counts are normalized by dividing the number of pixels demonstrating paradox by the number of picture elements within the entire left ventricle during end diastole and the number of counts within the left ventricle during end diastole, respectively. There is an excellent correlation between this technique and contrast ventriculography for detecting dyskinetic wall motion.[57]

Phase Images. The radionuclide angiocardiogram can be used to assess regional ventricular performance quantitatively at different intervals during the cardiac cycle and to characterize regional asynchrony. For example, the most sensitive components of the cardiac cycle may be during early systole and during relaxation rather than at end systole. Furthermore, delayed regional contraction and early systolic paradox characterize ventricular contraction in zones bordering on previous infarction.[58] Assessment of regional asynchrony is also useful to detect the foci of ventricular activation in patients with altered patterns of contraction due to pacemakers and to arrhythmias.[59]

Phase images pictorially describe the pattern of cardiac contraction. The first Fourier harmonic is used to fit a cosine wave to the time-activity curve for each pixel in the image. This approach therefore assumes that the ventricular volume curve is similar to one cycle or period of a cosine wave. Each pixel in the image is then coded to a color or gray scale to reflect the phase angle or regional phase delay. In normal patients, the onset of contraction is fairly homogeneous throughout the right and left ventricles and begins soon after the R wave. Contraction begins at the base of the interventricular septum and spreads to the body of the septum, the apex, and then laterally throughout the ventricles. In patients with foci of premature ventricular activation, the focus corresponds to the region with an abnormally early onset of ventricular contraction on the phase image.[59]

While phase imaging is imperfect owing to the assumptions necessary in fitting harmonic waves to the ventricular volume curve and to superimposition of normally contracting myocardium on regions of asynchrony, it does provide useful information regarding sequential electrical events from a sequential assessment of mechanical events.

Regional Ejection Fraction. Several methods have been suggested for measuring regional ejection fraction. Basically, one method divides the ventricle into radial sectors while the other divides it into rectangular segments bordering the major and minor axes of the left ventricle.[60,61] Background is subtracted regionally, using areas adjacent to the various regions. Regional ejection fraction is then calculated from the count-rate changes in each segment using Equation 8 (p. 362). Both methods yield similar results. With the rectangular method, normal regional ejection fraction is 0.66 ± 0.13 in the anteroseptum, 0.85 ± 0.12 in the apex, and 0.74 ± 0.16 in the inferoposterior segment.

This method is not as sensitive as functional imaging because normal and abnormal ventricular segments are mixed in the much larger region of interest that must be used for quantification. On the other hand, regional ejection fraction measurements are reproducible and useful in studies that require quantitative measures of wall motion, such as before and during drug therapy.

Right Ventricular Ejection Fraction. Although equilibrium (ECG-gated) radionuclide ventriculography can be used for the sequential assessment of global and regional left ventricular performance, there are anatomical differences between the left and right sides of the heart that make assessment of right ventricular ejection fraction using count-rate techniques and the equilibrium radionuclide angiocardiogram more difficult. The right atrium lies behind the right ventricle to a greater extent than the left atrium overlies the left ventricle. This interference is solved in first-pass radionuclide angiocardiography by imaging in the right anterior oblique projection, thus spatially separating the right atrium from the right ventricle. This cannot be done easily using equilibrium radionuclide ventriculography because the right ventricle is superimposed on the left in that projection. Thus, initial attempts at measuring the ejection fraction by equilibrium methods have necessitated the use of either multiple regions of interest in an effort to define the right ventricular perimeter throughout the cardiac cycle[62] or a background region of interest extending into the right atrium and pulmonary outflow tract.[63]

An alternative method for assessing right ventricular ejection fraction from the equilibrium radionuclide angiocardiogram involves use of the slant-hole collimator, which provides a 30-degree caudal tilt that more effectively separates the right atrium from the right ventricle.[64] A fixed background correction region is defined in the usual manner for measurement of the global left ventricular ejection fraction. The same regions are also used for the right ventricle. Background is then subtracted from each pixel of the end-diastolic and end-systolic frames. The end-diastolic right ventricular perimeter is defined manually from the ejection fraction image and the end-diastolic frame. The ejection fraction image separates the right atrium from the right ventricle since the atrium moves paradoxically in relation to the right ventricle. Time-activity curves are then generated from the right ventricular region of interest to determine the frames corresponding to right ventricular end systole and end diastole.

Right ventricular ejection fraction is then calculated from the formula

$$RVEF = \frac{EDC - ESC}{EDC - BC} \tag{10}$$

where RVEF is right ventricular ejection fraction, EDC represents the counts within the right ventricular region of interest in the frame corresponding to right ventricular end-diastole, ESC represents the counts within the right ventricular region of interest in the right ventricular end-systolic frame, and BC represents the background counts.

With this method, right ventricular ejection fraction in patients without cardiopulmonary disease averages 0.59 ± 0.08 (SD). The correlation between right ventricular ejection fraction measured by both first-pass and equilibrium techniques is excellent.[64]

Valvular Regurgitation. The severity of aortic and mitral regurgitation can be measured from the radionuclide angiocardiogram.[65–67] While first-pass techniques have been described for assessing left-sided regurgitation, the greatest experience has been derived from equilibrium (gated) studies. Radionuclide angiocardiography is performed as described above. Regions of interest are drawn over the left and right ventricles by visual inspection, taking care to include the entire right ventricular or left ventricular area, while excluding as much of the atria, pulmonary artery, and aorta as possible. This is best accomplished with the 30-degree slant-hole collimator and the stroke-volume image for outlining the ventricles. Changes in the counts in each ventricular area between systole and diastole are then determined. Since the same regions of interest are used for both systole and diastole, and since only the absolute change in counts is recorded, background activity is not subtracted. The results are expressed as a ratio of the change in counts in the left ventricular area over the change in counts in the right ventricular area (LV/RV stroke-index ratio).

In patients without aortic or mitral regurgitation, the left-to-right ventricular stroke-index is 1.15 ± 0.15. The ratio is greater than one in normal patients because the right ventricular stroke volume is underestimated owing to overlapping of the right atrium on the right ventricle. In patients with mitral or aortic regurgitation, the ratio is greater than 1.35. There is good agreement between the stroke-volume index and qualitative angiographic estimates of regurgitation.

Some constraints that must be considered when applying this technique are that (1) right-sided regurgitation should not be present, (2) global left ventricular ejection fraction should be greater than 0.30, and (3) there should be good separation of the right atrium from the right ventricle. There is always some overlap of the right atrium on the right ventricle, even with a slant-hole collimator, and this problem may be more severe with significant right atrial enlargement.

Tricuspid regurgitation can be diagnosed and assessed by evaluating the change in liver blood volume during the cardiac cycle.[68] Normally there is no change in liver blood volume; however, with tricuspid regurgitation, liver blood volume increases by 1 per cent or more soon after ventricular end-systole.

EXERCISE

The advantage of radionuclide angiocardiography over other methods for assessing ventricular performance is that it can be performed during physiological stresses and during pharmacological interventions. This is particularly helpful in the evaluation of patients with suspected cardiopulmonary disease because diagnostic and management decisions often cannot be based on resting ventricular performance alone but require additional information about coronary and cardiac reserves.

Exercise is the most frequently applied stress and is particularly useful in evaluating patients suspected of having coronary artery disease[69,70] (p. 366). With equilibrium radionuclide angiocardiography, a resting study is performed with the patient in the same position as will be used later during exercise. This is usually the 45-degree left anterior oblique projection, so that the right and left ventricles can be viewed separately, and with the patient supine or 45 degrees upright. The 45-degree upright position increases the likelihood that the patient will achieve an adequate exercise level but requires an appropriately designed table and camera mount. A high-sensitivity collimator is used because the acquisition time is short. A restraining harness is used to minimize patient motion under the camera during exercise. The imaging table should be secure, with minimal motion. Exercise loads are increased stepwise by 25-watt increments at 3-minute intervals until the patient experiences symptoms of angina, dyspnea, or fatigue of sufficient severity to limit further exercise or until the patient develops hypertension, arrhythmia, or marked ST-segment changes. Electrocardiographic leads are recorded and monitored continuously throughout the study. Multigated blood pool imaging is performed during the final 2 minutes of each exercise period.

This technique requires patient cooperation, since significant movement during the exercise test will substantially reduce spatial resolution and because the patient must maintain his maximal level of exercise for at least two minutes so that adequate counting statistics can be acquired. This may be particularly difficult for many patients who are not accustomed to supine bicycle exercising or who have peripheral vascular disease. As a result, many patients will become fatigued well below their maximum predicted heart rate response.

Exercise radionuclide angiocardiography can also be performed with the first-pass technique. Only resting and peak exercise studies are obtained with ^{99m}Tc tracers; studies can be obtained at each stage of exercise with ^{195m}Au. This method has several advantages in that upright bicycle exercising can be employed. As a result, more patients will achieve maximum levels of stress. The first-pass study also requires that the patient maintain his maximum exercise level for a considerably shorter time than with equilibrium radionuclide angiocardiography and does not require a steady-state heart rate for as long a period as equilibrium imaging.

Other forms of stress, such as isometric hand-grip, atrial pacing, and the cold pressor test, have been suggested as alternative methods, particularly for patients who cannot use the bicycle ergometer.[71,72] With *isometric hand-grip*, an abnormal response in patients with coronary artery disease is based on impaired regional left ventricular performance. The global ejection fraction response alone does not identify patients with coronary artery disease. While some reports have suggested that regional dysfunction occurs in most patients with coronary artery disease,[71] this method is not as sensitive as dynamic exercise.[73] The *cold pressor test* is performed by having the patient place his hand in a bucket of ice water for several minutes. This response to cold results in systemic vasoconstriction mediated through alpha-adrenergic receptors.[74] The increase in the pressure-rate double product may be used to stress patients with coronary disease, resulting in a depression in left ventricular performance.[72] This test appears to be fairly sensitive for the detection of coronary artery disease, provided that the patient is not receiving beta-adrenergic blocker therapy.[74]

Comparison of First-Pass and Equilibrium Angiocardiography

Both the first-pass and equilibrium radionuclide angiocardiogram provide accurate measurement of global left ventricular ejection fraction. Correlation between the two methods is high ($r = 0.87$[75] and $r = 0.89$[9]). Other hemodynamic indices (such as the peak ejection rate) that depend on high temporal resolution of the left ventricular time-activity curve cannot be obtained as accurately from first-pass studies; they require the high counts obtained with gated studies. Regional wall motion can be assessed with either method, although, again, the high counting rate obtained with the gated studies provides superior spatial resolution and improved accuracy, particularly when indices of regional wall motion, such as regional ejection fraction, are measured.

Background is a greater problem with equilibrium studies than with first-pass studies and accounts for as much as half the activity from the left ventricular region-of-interest with the former method. As a result, it may be easier to detect the edges of the left ventricle with first-pass studies despite the lower intrinsic resolution. However, equilibrium studies are superior for patient monitoring and for sequential studies. Imaging can be continued for up to four hours after injection of the radiopharmaceutical, allowing imaging in multiple projections and during physiological or pharmacological interventions. With first-pass studies, a radiopharmaceutical must be administered each time imaging is to be performed. Background activity precludes more than two or three studies during the effective half-life of the tracer, thus limiting the number of sequential studies possible with ^{99m}Tc, for example. On the other hand, physiological or pharmacological interventions with concomitant rapid changes in heart rate may be studied best with the first-pass technique. For both techniques, a steady-state heart rate is necessary, but only five or six heartbeats are required for first-pass studies compared to at least two minutes of heartbeats for the gated studies.

CLINICAL APPLICATIONS

DETECTION AND EVALUATION OF CORONARY ARTERY DISEASE. In patients with coronary artery disease who have not yet sustained an acute myocardial infarction, resting ventricular performance is usually normal because the myocardium is not ischemic. When these patients are stressed, an imbalance between oxygen supply and demand develops, resulting in ischemia. This, in turn, causes a fall in global left ventricular ejection fraction and the development of regional wall motion abnormalities. When radionuclide angiocardiography is applied during exercise in normal patients, left ventricular ejection fraction rises significantly compared to levels at rest, with no left ventricular wall motion abnormalities.[69,70] In patients with coronary artery disease and angina, left ventricular ejection fraction falls during exercise and new regional wall motion abnormalities may develop. The normal increase in ejection fraction with exercise is due primarily to a decrease in end-systolic volume, while the exercise-induced decrease in ejection fraction in patients with angina is due to an increase in end-systolic volume.[75] In patients with coronary artery disease without angina there is usually no change in ejection fraction during exercise, since there is no significant change in end-systolic volume.

The criteria for an abnormal left ventricular ejection fraction response with exercise vary considerably from laboratory to laboratory. Most groups, however, require at least a 5 or 10 per cent increase in ejection fraction to consider the result normal. In normal patients with high resting ejection fractions (>75 per cent), there may be no change in ejection fraction with exercise. In addition to the measurement of global left ventricular function, the cineangiocardiograms obtained at rest and during exercise are evaluated to detect any new wall motion abnormalities. The numerical analyses described previously can also be applied to assess regional and global ventricular performance during exercise.

At first glance, this technique would seem to be particularly accurate for the diagnosis of coronary artery disease. Okada et al. reviewed the literature from 1978 to 1980[76] and found that the sensitivity for detection of regional wall motion abnormalities (the percentage of coronary artery disease patients with this finding) was 73 per cent, while the specificity (the percentage of normal subjects without regional asynergy) was 100 per cent. There was considerable variability in the sensitivity rates from study to study, however, with a range of less than 50 per cent to 100 per cent. It would seem that the sensitivity for detecting wall motion abnormalities should not be high with this method, since only one projection is obtained and the image has poor resolution because of the short acquisition time. The sensitivity of this method for detecting an abnormal left ventricular ejection fraction response in patients with coronary artery disease was 87 per cent with a specificity of 93 per cent.

Other factors will play a major role in determining left ventricular response with exercise. For example, inadequate stress due to peripheral vascular disease or the concurrent administration of beta-adrenergic blocking drugs may result in normal responses in spite of coronary artery disease.[77] It has also been shown that the sensitivity of the test is reduced in women and in men with atypical angina. The ejection fraction response is greater with upright exercise than with supine exercise.[78]

Most important in determining the specificity of the test is the definition of the control population. Exercise response is dependent on the patient's sex, resting ejection fraction, and change in end-diastolic volume.[79–81] Age is a particularly important factor. Most studies have involved control patients who were usually young individuals without cardiopulmonary disease. Patients over the age of 60, however, may demonstrate no increase in ejection fraction with exercise and may in fact demonstrate a decrease in ejection fraction due to aging rather than to coronary artery disease.[80]

In fact, an abnormal ejection fraction response to exercise is expected in any condition in which there is reduced left ventricular reserve, such as volume- or pressure-overload states and states of decreased left ventricular compliance. As a result, abnormal responses have been reported in patients with aortic stenosis,[82] aortic regurgitation,[83] mitral regurgitation,[84] mitral valve prolapse,[85] hypertrophic obstructive cardiomyopathy,[86] chronic obstructive pulmonary disease,[87] beta-thalassemia and chronic iron overload,[88] cystic fibrosis,[89] elderly patients, female patients, and patients receiving propranolol.[90–92]

When interpreting the exercise radionuclide angiocardiogram, it is clear that additional information should be incorporated into the decision-making process. For example, almost three-fourths of patients suspected of having coronary artery disease without a high pretest probability of the disease (i.e., no previous infarction or typical anginal symptoms) can be diagnosed with an 85 per cent certainty by combining the results of exercise radionuclide angiocardiography and clinical variables such as the presence of chest pain and ST-segment changes with exercise.[93] Thus, the radionuclide angiocardiogram is most useful in the noninvasive diagnosis of coronary artery disease when it is coupled with additional clinical information.

In the diagnostic evaluation of patients with suspected coronary artery disease, the exercise electrocardiogram may provide the necessary diagnostic information without resorting to additional noninvasive or invasive methods. If the exercise electrocardiogram is nondiagnostic, an exercise radionuclide study may be useful. At the present time, neither exercise radionuclide angiocardiography nor exercise myocardial perfusion scintigraphy (p. 370) appears clearly to be the procedure of choice. Radionuclide angiocardiography provides higher sensitivity but poorer specificity in patients with valvular heart disease, primary myocardial disease, or severe lung disease. Furthermore, particularly with supine bicycle ergometry, many patients may not achieve an adequate chronotropic response. The exercise radionuclide angiocardiogram does provide more complete information, particularly when imaging is performed at each stage of exercise, which allows cardiac performance to be assessed at various levels of submaximal exercise.

On the other hand, thallium scintigraphy can be performed in multiple projections immediately after exercise and provides a more reliable map of the pattern and location of the regional abnormality. Furthermore, it is more likely that the patient will achieve an adequate exercise response with thallium scintigraphy, since ordinarily the exercise is performed upright and on a treadmill. The choice between the two procedures may depend heavily on the experience of the nuclear cardiology personnel, however.

ACUTE MYOCARDIAL INFARCTION. Ventricular performance is a major factor affecting patient prognosis after acute myocardial infarction. Radionuclide angiocardiography provides information concerning global left ventricular function, the extent and location of regional abnormalities, and the presence and extent of right ventricular involvement. As a result, it provides prognostic information, since the left ventricular ejection fraction is a predictor of early mortality and the development of congestive failure or sudden death.[94,95] In addition, approximately half the patients with inferior infarction will have abnormalities in right ventricular performance.[96–98]

Ventricular function can also be used to assess patient recovery. Global and regional ventricular performance will improve gradually over the first two weeks after infarction but will show a significant improvement by two to four months if uninterrupted by complications such as reinfarction. Additional prognostic information may be gained from submaximal exercise testing of patients prior to discharge from the hospital, since the ventricular response to exercise appears useful in selecting patients at high risk for subsequent complications.[95,99]

VALVULAR HEART DISEASE. Radionuclide angiography provides the only readily available, noninvasive means for quantifying the degree of left-sided valvular regurgitation.[67] While echocardiography offers excellent visualization of valve motion, assesses aortic dilatation, and measures the degree of mitral stenosis, the severity of regurgitation can be estimated only qualitatively, even with Doppler methods.

In addition to its ability to detect and measure left-sided regurgitation, radionuclide angiocardiography may play a role in the management of patients with aortic valve regurgitation. In these patients, the decision to intervene surgically depends on the degree of left ventricular dysfunction (p. 1114). The dysfunction may not be apparent at rest and may show up only during exercise. It has been suggested that by the time symptoms develop in these patients, irreversible myocardial dysfunction has occurred and that functional abnormalities may appear during stress even in the asymptomatic patient.[100,101] As a result, radionuclide assessment of left ventricular function during exercise has been suggested as a means of following patients with aortic regurgitation to determine the optimal time for valve replacement. While this approach appears promising, further validation is required before it can be recommended for routine clinical use.

ASSESSMENT OF VENTRICULAR DYSFUNCTION. Radionuclide angiocardiography is most useful in patients with symptoms suggesting ventricular dysfunction because it can (1) detect ventricular aneurysm, (2) distinguish regional from global dysfunction, (3) evaluate myocardial viability, (4) evaluate right and left ventricular function, and (5) evaluate the effectiveness of therapeutic interventions. It provides a noninvasive method for accurate quantitation of ventricular hemodynamics and regional wall motion in patients too ill to undergo invasive cardiac catheterization. In addition, the technique can be performed sequentially to evaluate the natural history of heart disease and the effectiveness of medical or surgical management.

The technique is comparable in sensitivity to contrast ventriculography in detecting and assessing *aneurysm* and in determining the location and extent of dyskinetic segments and the status of the remaining ventricle. These factors are particularly important in patients with coronary artery disease in whom aneurysmectomy is being considered (p. 1374).[102] As a result, the radionuclide method can be used to screen patients to separate those with diffuse hypokinesis, who are poor candidates for surgery (Fig. 11–11) from those with localized akinesis or aneurysm (Fig.

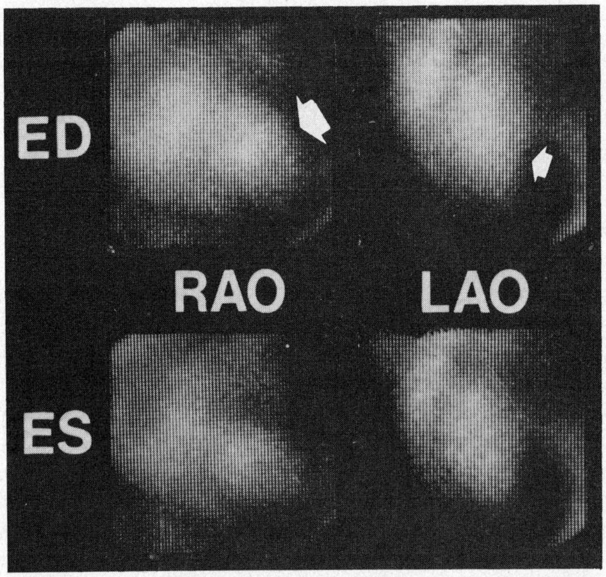

FIGURE 11–11 Equilibrium (gated) radionuclide angiocardiogram of a patient with ischemic cardiomyopathy. There is global asynergy of the markedly enlarged left ventricle (arrows). Note the small difference in size and intensity of left ventricular activity between diastole and systole. The right ventricle is normal in size and performance. ED = end-diastolic frame; ES = end-systolic frame; RAO = 30-degree right anterior oblique projection; LAO = 45-degree modified left anterior oblique projection.

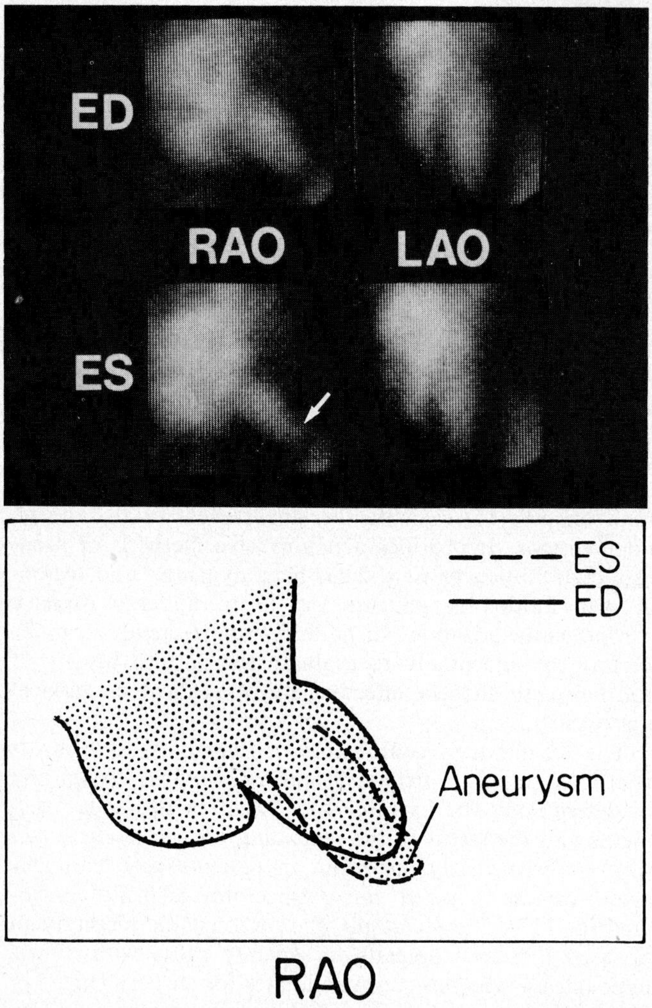

FIGURE 11–12 Equilibrium (gated) radionuclide angiocardiogram of a patient with an apical aneurysm. Note the apical dyskinesis seen best on the RAO projection (arrow). Performance is normal in the other ventricular segments. ED = end-diastolic frame; ES = end-systolic frame; RAO = 30-degree right anterior oblique projection; LAO = 45-degree modified left anterior oblique projection.

11–12), who may then undergo cardiac catheterization prior to surgery.

Regional wall motion abnormalities present at rest may be due to scar from previous myocardial infarction or to reversible ischemia of viable tissue. Since revascularization may improve regional function if the tissue is viable, it is important to *differentiate between reversible ischemia and scar.* Postextrasystolic potentiation and nitroglycerin have been used to help make this distinction, usually at the time of catheterization[103–109] (p. 1369). The exercise radionuclide angiocardiogram can be used to evaluate the change in regional wall motion after exercise.[103,109] In most patients with surgically reversible regional ventricular dysfunction (> 90 per cent), function in that region improves immediately after exercise compared to function at rest. The predictive value of this test is controversial, however, since the number of patients whose regional function does not improve after exercise but does improve after surgery varies from 16[103] to 50 per cent.[109]

Right ventricular function is seriously compromised in patients with *chronic obstructive pulmonary disease* who have pulmonary artery hypertension or pulmonary vasoconstriction (Fig. 11–13). There is a direct relationship between right ventricular dysfunction and prognosis; right ventricular performance is also related to the magnitude of arterial hypoxemia and ventilatory impairment. Abnormal right ventricular function is a warning sign of subsequent cardiopulmonary decompensation.[110] During exercise, the majority of patients with chronic obstructive lung disease will have abnormal right ventricular reserve, as manifested by reduction in the ejection fraction.[111] This response is not necessarily due to intrinsic myocardial dysfunction but is the result of a normal response to elevated pulmonary artery (and right ventricular systolic) pressure during exercise. Left ventricular response in these patients is generally normal.[112]

Radionuclide angiocardiography provides a noninvasive method for *monitoring the acute and chronic effects of drugs* on ventricular performance. A wide variety of drugs has been studied, including inotropic agents such as digitalis and amrinone,[113,114] afterload-reducing agents such as prazosin,[115,116] bronchodilators such as aminophylline,[117] beta-adrenergic blockers such as propranolol,[118] antiarrhythmics such as disopyramide, and slow-channel calcium antagonists such as verapamil or nifedipine.[119] Individual patient response can be studied as well. Ventricular performance can be used as a guide to determine when a particular therapeutic agent has lost its effectiveness and when replacement or combinative therapy may be necessary.

Ventricular performance is an important indicator of cardiotoxicity with drugs, such as doxorubicin, that have a potentially detrimental effect on the heart[120] (p. 1690). By sequentially assessing patients who are receiving these agents, it might be possible to predict when irreversible cardiac failure might develop in an individual patient. As a result, medication can be continued as long as possible and stopped while cardiac failure is still reversible.

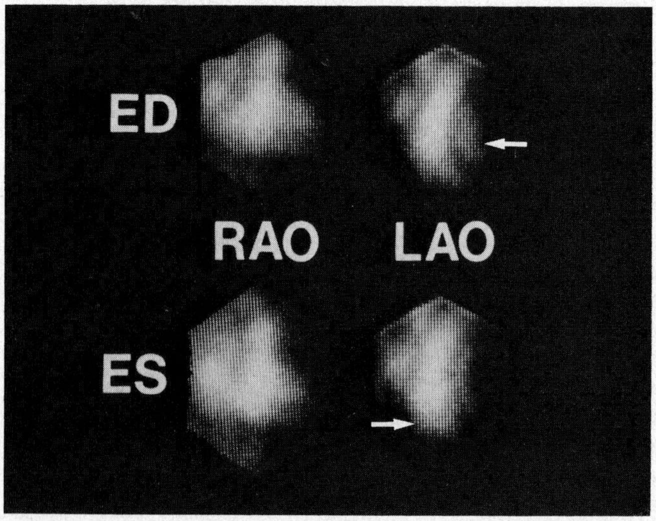

FIGURE 11–13 Equilibrium (gated) radionuclide angiocardiogram of a patient with severe chronic obstructive pulmonary disease and right sided heart failure. Note the dilated, poorly contracting right ventricle (upper arrow) and dilated right atrium. The left ventricle is normal in size and performance (lower arrow). ED = end-diastolic frame; ES = end-systolic frame; RAO = 30-degree right anterior oblique projection; and LAO = 45-degree modified left anterior oblique projection.

MYOCARDIAL PERFUSION SCINTIGRAPHY

The development of newer surgical and medical techniques for the treatment of coronary artery disease has emphasized the need for an objective measure of regional myocardial perfusion. Although the coronary arteriogram can precisely define vessel morphology (Chap. 10), the effect of a coronary artery lesion on tissue perfusion cannot be accurately determined by means of roentgenographic procedures.[121] Furthermore, objective screening procedures are needed to evaluate patients during the early stages of their disease, well before symptoms become severe enough to warrant catheterization. Radionuclide techniques that assess regional myocardial perfusion provide information useful in the detection and evaluation of coronary artery disease and in the assessment of therapies aimed at limiting the degree of ischemia and the extent of tissue necrosis.[122] It is critical to obtain *regional* information, since coronary heart disease is a regional disease with areas of normal myocardium often adjacent to severely diseased tissue. It is also critical to measure perfusion both at rest and during exercise, pacing, or some other stress, since perfusion may be normal at rest even in patients with severe coronary artery disease.

RADIOPHARMACEUTICALS FOR PERFUSION SCINTIGRAPHY

The first radioactive *potassium analogs* available for human use emitted photons that were too energetic for scintillation imaging.[123–125] Potassium-43 was the first of a number of potassium analogs with physical characteristics that were compatible with external imaging techniques.[126] Other potassium analogs have been used for myocardial scintigraphy, including cesium-129,[127] rubidium-81,[128] and thallium-201.[129] While all these radionuclides have limitations because of their long physical half-life, unsatisfactory gamma energies, or limited availability, thallium-201 has emerged clearly as the radiotracer of choice for myocardial perfusion scintigraphy.

Thallium-201 has a physical half-life of 73.1 hours and is a metallic element with properties similar to potassium.[130,131] Its physical characteristics are reasonably well suited for imaging with scintillation camera systems.[132] Characteristic x-rays are emitted in a range from 69 to 83 kev, and these photons are routinely used for external imaging. In addition, gamma emissions of 135 and 167 kev are produced during 10 per cent of the disintegrations. In routine imaging, the pulse height analyzer is centered over the lower energy characteristic x-rays. These low-energy photons result in some loss of spatial resolution because the scattered radiation cannot be separated completely from the primary photopeak. Nevertheless, this energy range does permit imaging with scintillation cameras and enables greater resolution than is obtained with potassium-43, rubidium-81, or cesium-129. Thallium-201 has a number of biological characteristics that make it particularly attractive for perfusion scintigraphy. Clearance of thallium from the blood is almost as rapid as that of potassium or rubidium, and washout from the myocardium is slower. A maximum heart-to-blood ratio is reached within 6 to 8 minutes after injection. *Distribution* of thallium and rubidium is similar throughout the left ventricle, but thallium appears to *concentrate* in myocardial tissue to a somewhat greater degree than potassium or rubidium.[129,132] Extraction of thallium by the myocardium occurs by a cell membrane transport system that can be inhibited by ouabain and is most likely due to activation of the sodium-potassium ATPase system.[133] Thallium appears to bind at two sites on the enzyme system compared to potassium, with one binding site; this may account for the prolonged clearance of thallium from the myocardium.[131]

Technetium-99m is the ideal radionuclide for Anger camera scintigraphy because of its gamma energy of 140 kev, its relatively short physical half-life (6 hours), its low radiation dose to the patient, and its general availability from a long-lived parent via a relatively inexpensive generator system. The development of a ^{99m}Tc myocardial perfusion agent would be quite attractive. A monovalent cation complex has recently been labeled with technetium-99m.[134] In most animal models, myocardial distribution of this tracer is proportional to blood flow. Further study is required to determine whether this tracer or an analog accumulates in the human heart in sufficient concentration to be clinically useful.

When cyclotron-produced positron-emitting potassium analogs and positron imaging devices are used in perfusion scintigraphy, three-dimensional reconstruction of the heart is possible. The very short half-life of these agents also permits multiple studies under various stress states as well as frequent sequential examinations to follow the course of ischemia or infarction. One of these promising tracers is *rubidium-82*, a positron emitter with a 75-second half-life.[135] Aside from the obvious advantage that results from its short half-life, this potassium analog is the daughter of strontium-82, with a 25-day half-life. Since strontium-82/rubidium-82 generator systems have been developed,[136] the parent can be stored for considerable periods of time and eluted whenever rubidium-82 is needed for injection. High-resolution scintiscans have been obtained when coincidence imaging is used with either positron cameras or positron emission–computed tomographic devices.[137] While imaging is not possible with standard Anger scintillation camera systems because of the high gamma energy (511 kev) of rubidium-82, rotating collimators have recently been developed that permit high-resolution scintigraphy after intracoronary injection of the tracer and perhaps even after intravenous injection.[138]

Another positron emitter, *nitrogen-13 ammonium*, has also been used as a marker of myocardial perfusion, and there has been a close correlation between changes in the size of the resultant perfusion defect and the clinical course of patients with acute infarction.[139] Because of the short half-life of this tracer, an on-site cyclotron is necessary for radiotracer production, markedly limiting its availability and capability.

THALLIUM-201 KINETICS

Regional alterations in myocardial perfusion can be measured when myocardial scintigraphy is performed after the intravenous injection of potassium analogs such as thallium-201. This approach is based on the indicator fractionation principle, which postulates that the uptake of these tracers by heart muscle equals the fraction of cardiac output perfusing the myocardium after the intravenous injection of the tracer.[140] Since approximately 5 per cent of the cardiac output supplies the myocardium at rest and since the myocardial extraction of thallium-201 is high, there is sufficient uptake of the tracer by the heart relative to surrounding structures to permit imaging with external detecting systems.

INITIAL DISTRIBUTION. After intravenous injection of thallium-201, the initial distribution of the tracer is equal to the product of regional myocardial blood flow times the extraction fraction, i.e., the percentage of the tracer extracted by the myocardium during a single passage through its circulation. Thus, the degree to which the distribution of thallium-201 reflects myocardial blood flow depends on an unchanging extraction fraction at different flows. However, several factors affect the extraction fraction of thallium-201 in the myocardium. At coronary flow rates while the patient is at rest, the extraction fraction is high, between 85 and 90 per cent. At high flow rates, if the increase in flow is greater than the metabolic needs of the heart, the extraction fraction is reduced, and thallium-201 uptake consequently increases at a lower rate than the increase in coronary blood flow.[141] Another factor that affects the distribution of thallium-201 is the functional integrity of the cell membrane adenosine triphosphatase, which maintains transmembrane electrochemical gradients of sodium and potassium.[142,143,143a] For example, in the presence of severe regional hypoxia with adequate perfusion, the concentration of some potassium analogs is decreased;[144] hypoxia causes a decrease in the extraction fraction of thallium-201 as well.[145] Furthermore, inhibition of either oxidative phosphorylation or glycolytic pathways reduces thallium uptake at the cellular level.[146]

Despite these limitations, regional myocardial uptake of thallium-201 correlates linearly with regional myocardial blood flow from very low flow rates to normal resting levels.[147] At flow rates above the resting level, thallium uptake increases proportionately when the increased flow levels are associated with increases in myocardial oxygen demand[148] and less than proportionately when the increases in flow exceed the metabolic needs of the heart.[141,149,150]

Exercise or other forms of stress are essential to detect coronary stenoses accurately by myocardial perfusion scintigraphy. Regions that are perfused normally at rest but exhibit reduced perfusion during exercise represent ischemic zones, while perfusion defects seen both at rest and during exercise usually represent zones of previous infarction. Abnormal perfusion during stress in patients with transient ischemia is due to a heterogeneous increase in myocardial blood flow. In normal individuals, blood flow increases uniformly throughout the left ventricle during exercise or other forms of stress-simulating interventions. In patients with coronary artery disease, the increase in blood flow to the myocardium distal to a hemodynamically significant arterial stenosis is less than normal and may in fact be absent. There is an inverse relationship between the increase in flow and the percentage of coronary artery stenosis once the lumen is narrowed by approximately 40 to 50 per cent.[151] Thus, the difference between the absolute quantity of radiotracer available for uptake by myocardial cells beyond arterial obstructions and the quantity available in beds supplied by normal coronary arteries is maximal during exercise. Since myocardial thallium clearance is high, the relative differences in regional myocardial blood flow will be reflected in disproportionate concentrations of regional myocardial radioactivity on the scintiscan.[152]

The indicator fractionation principle assumes that the tracer will remain trapped in the organ during the period of observation. This is true for microspheres injected intravenously or intra-arterially, but it is not true for thallium-201, particularly when it is injected during exercise. Redistribution of the tracer begins within 10 minutes after injection.[153] The thallium washout rate has a half-life of 4 hours after intravenous injection.[154] It is prolonged in regions of hypoperfusion[155] and is related to the rate of thallium clearance from the blood.[156]

REDISTRIBUTION. Redistribution of thallium-201 has important implications for patients with coronary artery disease, especially when imaging takes place during exercise. When myocardial perfusion scintigraphy is performed during stress, transiently ischemic myocardium can be detected.[157,158] By taking advantage of the redistribution phenomenon, one can detect exercise-induced ischemia by imaging after the exercise injection of thallium and by repeat delayed imaging when the thallium has partially cleared from the normal myocardium and partially washed into the hypoperfused areas, resulting in the disappearance of the initial perfusion defects.[159] This disappearance with time results in the accumulation of thallium in previously unperfused zones in combination with the washout of the tracers from normal myocardium.[155,160]

Perfusion defects noted on the initial postexercise thallium scintigram may be either reversible or nonreversible. In reversible defects due to transient ischemia associated with viable myocardium, thallium washout is slower in the hypoperfused region compared to normal areas, with concentrations of the tracer in the two regions eventually becoming equal. In nonreversible defects due to acute myocardial infarction or myocardial scar associated with nonviable myocardium, the initial perfusion defects persist with delayed imaging because thallium does not accumulate in the infarcted tissue and there is no washin to these nonviable zones during the redistribution phase; hence, concentrations in the infarcted and normal myocardium do not equalize with time.

The *disadvantage* of this technique is that the time during which the thallium distribution reflects myocardial blood flow is limited, lasting for only a short time after the tracer has cleared from the blood following intravenous injection. Consequently, it is essential that imaging begin very soon after injection and that imaging be performed as rapidly as possible. Furthermore, in the face of transient ischemia, the time it takes for concentrations in the ischemic and normal zones to equalize may vary considerably from patient to patient. While the use of a set time (e.g., 3 to 4 hours after injection) for redistribution imaging will differentiate transient ischemia from infarction in the majority of patients, in others redistribution will occur more slowly and further delayed imaging will be necessary to differentiate the two phenomena.

TECHNIQUE

For exercise myocardial perfusion scintigraphy, thallium-201 is injected at the time of maximal stress during a multistage treadmill test according to the Bruce protocol. The patient should not eat for at least four hours prior to the exercise test so that splanchnic uptake of the tracer is reduced to a minimum. For the detection and evaluation of coronary artery disease, drugs that protect the myocardium, such as beta-adrenergic blockers, should be discontinued for a long enough time before the study to allow the amount of drug in the blood to decrease to less than pharmacologically significant levels. (For propranolol, this would be approximately 48 hours prior to the test.) If the protective effect of the drug is being studied specifically, the dose regimen should be maintained at the levels administered prior to the test.

A 12-lead electrocardiogram is obtained prior to the test, and an intravenous line is inserted for rapid injection of the radiotracer and for emergency use if necessary. Exercise should be graded and the injection made at the time of maximal exercise, which should be maintained for at least 60 to 90 seconds following the injection to allow the tracer to be cleared from the blood. A near maximum exercise level (≥ 85 per cent of predicted maximal heart rate) should be achieved to assess the extent of the disease.[161] It would appear that the heart rate response may be less critical for accurate diagnosis of coronary artery disease, although the incidence of false-negative examinations is high when the patient fails to achieve 70 per cent of the predicted maximal heart rate. Electrocardiographic monitoring should continue throughout the test and during the immediate post-test period. The exercise test should be stopped if hypotension, marked electrocardiographic evidence of ischemia, serious arrhythmias, or significant pain develops.

Imaging may begin 6 to 8 minutes after injection, allowing sufficient time for the thallium to be cleared from the blood but prior to significant redistribution. A camera and collimator with a system spatial resolution of at least 4.5 mm (full-width at half-maximum) for thallium-201 should be used for imaging. Because imaging must be performed as quickly as possible, the low-energy, all-purpose collimator is usually used, although the recently introduced high-resolution parallel square-hole collimator offers better spatial resolution with sensitivity comparable to that of the standard all-purpose collimators. With the latter collimator, care must be taken to keep the amount of the thallium-202 contaminant, with its high-energy emissions, to a minimum at the time of injection. The pulse height analyzer energy window is peaked over the low-energy (69 to 81 kev) thallium-201 photopeak. In cameras with multiple pulse height analyzer energy windows for data collection, the counts resulting from the higher energy gamma rays (135 and 165 kev) should also be collected, substantially increasing camera sensitivity and improving spatial resolution.

Projections obtained during myocardial perfusion scintigraphy include the 30- or 45-degree left anterior oblique, anterior, 70-degree left anterior oblique, and left lateral views. Since the plane of the septum can vary, patient positioning should be tailored to the individual patient and his cardiac anatomy. Care must be taken in interpreting the 70-degree LAO and the left lateral views, particularly when the patient is imaged in the supine position. Increased attenuation of the diaphragm superimposed on the inferior wall of the left ventricle may cause apparent inferior perfusion defects in patients with normal blood flow.[162] Perfusion defects seen only on these views should be confirmed with additional imaging in the 70-degree LAO or left lateral view with the patient lying left side up. At least 300,000 counts are acquired per view; when computer acquisition is used, counts on each view can be collected for a preset time, usually 6 to 10 minutes per view. With a preset time, quantitative comparisons of thallium-201 activity can be made between serial images. These projections are repeated during redistribution imaging 3 to 4 hours after injection. In addition, if perfusion defects persist and the distinction between infarction and transient ischemia is critical, repeat imaging can be performed 24 hours after injection.

Other forms of stress can be employed, including upright and supine bicycle ergometry, hand-grip exercise, and atrial pacing. Treadmill ergometry is preferable, unless patients are physically unable to run. Treadmill testing is the most likely method to force patients to adequate exercise levels and to increase coronary flow sufficiently to permit accurate interpretations of the thallium-201 images.

Pharmacological methods to increase coronary blood flow have a number of compelling advantages, however. Patients can be routinely and reproducibly stressed to a predefined endpoint, and the method can be used in patients who cannot exercise to maximum levels. Perfusion imaging can be performed after the intravenous injection of dipyridamole, a potent coronary vasodilator that produces little if any myocardial ischemia. Initial experience with this method is encouraging; accuracy in detecting coronary artery disease is comparable to that of standard exercise testing,[163–165] with an improvement in image quality. While imaging is probably safer with dipyridamole than with exercise, patients have experienced severe headaches and postural hypotension after administration of this drug. Furthermore, the relationship between increases in flow and thallium activity are probably not linear in the face of a falling extraction fraction due to increasing flow without corresponding increases in metabolic needs.

INTERPRETATION

Most commonly, image interpretation is based on analog images using Polaroid film or x-ray film for hardcopy. In our laboratory, we find Polaroid film using a triple-lens camera (each lens having a different intensity setting) the most satisfactory method for analog-image interpretation, providing a range of photographically contrast-enhanced images and protecting against the pseudodefects that may occur with computer processing (see below).

In the normal scintigram there is uniform distribution of the tracer throughout the left ventricular wall, with a decrease in concentration in the region of the apex in about half the patients (Fig. 11–14).[166] The ventricle has a horseshoe appearance, with its long axis oriented anywhere from horizontal to vertical. Activity tapers near the base of the heart. In the majority of patients, the inferior wall appears thicker than the anterolateral surface. In the central zone, a region of decreased or absent activity is noted and represents the left ventricular cavity. The right ventricular myocardium is not visualized in normal subjects at rest but may be seen as a thin wall extending from the apex

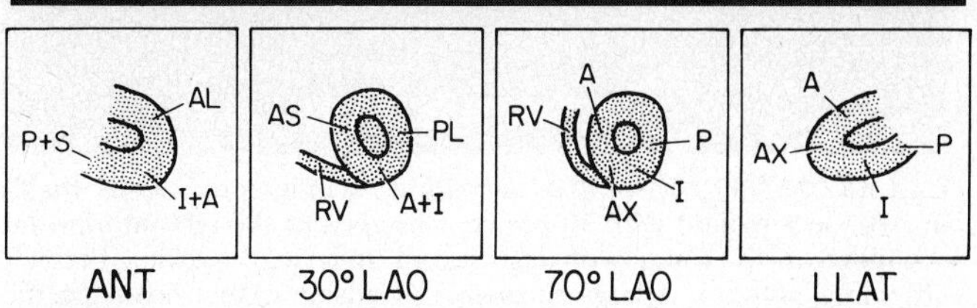

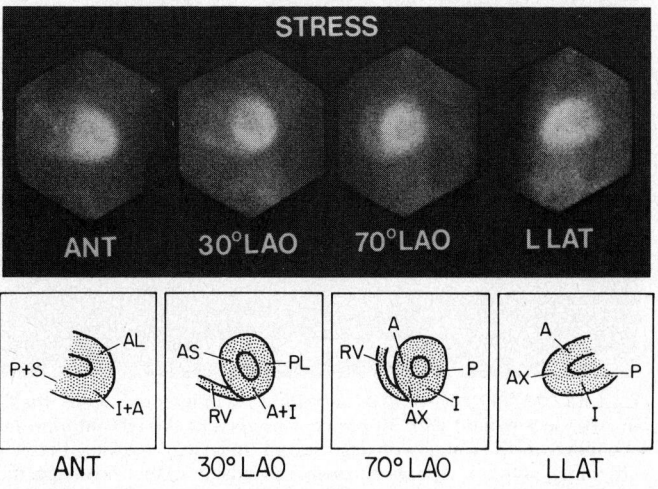

FIGURE 11–14 Normal myocardial perfusion scintigraphy with thallium-201 after stress in four different projections. Notice the uniform uptake of radiotracer throughout the left ventricular wall and the central defect due to the left ventricular cavity. ANT = anterior; 30° LAO = 30-degree left anterior oblique; 70° 70-degree left anterior oblique; LLAT = left lateral; P = posterior; S = septum; AL = anterolateral; I = inferior; A = anterior; PL = posterolateral; AX = apex; RV = right ventricle.

when the injection is made at peak stress during redistribution imaging.

Multiple oblique projections are required, since perfusion defects are seen best on a tangent. In the anterior view, the apical, inferior, and anterolateral walls are well seen. The septum and posterolateral walls are seen best on the 30- to 45-degree LAO views. The anterior free wall, inferior and posterior walls are seen best on the 70-degree LAO and left lateral views. Right ventricular activity is seen when imaging is performed after stress but is less intense than left ventricular activity.[167]

When exercise (stress) and redistribution imaging are performed, it is essential that each of the views obtained during redistribution be acquired in exactly the same position relative to the detector as the corresponding stress image. If proper technique is followed during stress and redistribution imaging, corresponding images can be evaluated for (1) reversible perfusion defects (those that appear on stress imaging but disappear after redistribution and are due to transient ischemia) (Fig. 11–15), (2) nonreversible perfusion defects (abnormalities that persist with equivalent intensity during redistribution imaging and are usually due to scar or infarction) (Fig. 11–16), and (3) normal anatomical variations (such as apical thinning and normally decreased perfusion at the base due to the aortic and mitral valves).

The greatest accuracy is achieved when perfusion defects are seen in the same segment on several views. Stenoses involving the left anterior descending coronary artery result in perfusion defects involving the anterior, septal, and lateral segments. Both the right coronary artery and the left circumflex artery perfuse the inferior and posterior segments; hence, perfusion defects in these segments may be due to stenoses involving either coronary arteries. The apex may be supplied by all three major coronary vessels.

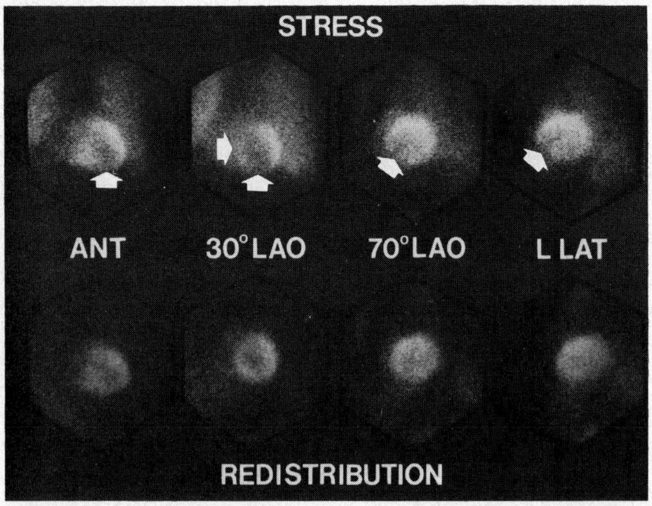

FIGURE 11–15 Myocardial perfusion scintigraphy with thallium-201 in a patient with 90 per cent stenosis of the left anterior descending artery along with less severe stenoses involving the left circumflex system. A large reversible perfusion defect involving the anteroseptal and apical segments of the left ventricle is seen best on the 30-degree LAO immediate postexercise image (arrows). The defect is not present on redistribution imaging four hours later (lower panel) because it is due to transient ischemia. Note the transiently increased lung uptake on the immediate postexercise images (upper panel). (ANT = anterior; 30° LAO = 30-degree left anterior oblique; 70° LAO = 70-degree left anterior oblique; LLAT = left lateral.)

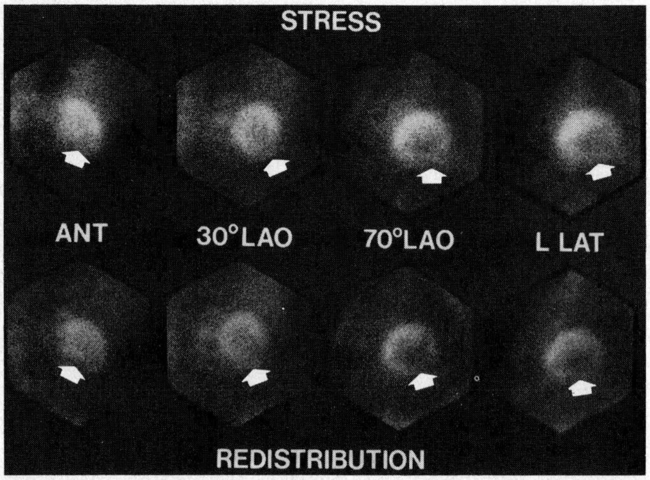

FIGURE 11–16 Myocardium perfusion scintigraphy with thallium-201 in a patient with a previous inferoposterior myocardial infarction. A large nonreversible perfusion defect involving the inferior and posterior segments of the left ventricle is seen best in the 70-degree LAO and LLAT projections. The defect is seen on the immediate poststress images (upper arrows) and involves the same area of the left ventricle on the redistribution images obtained four hours later (lower arrows). The defect is due to nonviable myocardium or to scar tissue. (ANT = anterior; 30° LAO = 30-degree left anterior oblique; 70° LAO = 70-degree left anterior oblique; LLAT = left lateral.)

In addition to interpretation of myocardial thallium-201 activity, attention should also be directed to the size of the cardiac chamber, wall thickness, and pulmonary uptake of thallium-201. An enlarged cardiac chamber may be seen at rest, indicating ventricular dilation. Cardiac chamber enlargement may be seen only during the exercise phase of the study and indicates a transient increase in end-diastolic volume, an index of diminished cardiac reserve in patients with a variety of cardiac diseases including, but not limited to, coronary artery disease. A transient increase in lung activity during exercise results from a transient increase in pulmonary blood volume and is associated with an elevated pulmonary capillary wedge pressure. The increase in pulmonary thallium-201 activity is probably due to an increase in capillary surface area and a resultant increase in tracer extraction. The ratio between lung and heart activity has been quantitated and found to be highly specific but only moderately sensitive for coronary artery disease.[168] More experience is required with this index to determine whether other cardiac or pulmonary diseases result in increased pulmonary blood volume during stress with an attendant increase in thallium activity.

QUANTIFICATION

Visual interpretation of unprocessed thallium-201 myocardial images leads to a significant degree of disagreement among observers and makes sequential assessment of regional myocardial perfusion difficult.[169] Thallium images have a relatively high level of background activity, which interferes with evaluation of the images. Computers are especially useful in thallium imaging because they allow the observer the capability for interactive image processing. It is very helpful in visualizing the subtle differences involved if one can raise the lower and upper thresholds while viewing the images. Overlaying of images is also helpful in comparing initial images with images after redistribution. In addition to simple threshold subtraction, several interpolative methods for background subtraction have been suggested. These take into account the nonuniformity of background that may result in excessive background subtraction.[170,171] Image interpretation should not depend on background-corrected images alone and must take into account the unprocessed image as well.

Quantitative computer analysis of the thallium image has been suggested as a means for standardizing the interpretation of images and eliminating the high degree of subjectivity in visual analysis.[172,173] In general, this technique evaluates the relative concentrations of thallium in the various segments of the left ventricle.[154,171,174–176] Regional activity is assessed quantitatively by breaking up the thallium myocardial image into anatomically defined left ventricular regions. Thallium-201 uptake in these left ventricular segments is considered to be pathologically reduced if count rates are less than 75 to 80 per cent of maximum left ventricular thallium-201 uptake. Thallium-201 distribution may also be analyzed quantitatively as a function of time, measuring the net rate of thallium washin or washout from the myocardium during the redistribution phase of the study.[154]

While initial experience with these quantitative techniques is promising and appears to improve the accuracy with which coronary artery disease can be detected and assessed, more experience is required before these techniques can be routinely applied. In particular, these methods depend heavily on accurate background correction, which is difficult from two-dimensional images; tomographic imaging may be required for accurate background subtraction. Furthermore, excessive contrast enhancement may result in regions of apparently reduced activity called *pseudodefects*, which are produced by a real difference in counts but are caused by statistical considerations, geometry, or inhomogeneous background activity. Accurate background correction is further complicated because thallium-201 uptake is dependent on myocardial perfusion, mass, and metabolism, and these factors determine the ratio of myocardial activity to background activity. In addition, uptake is affected by exercise, dosage and type of cardiac pharmaceuticals, equipment, and the method used for data collection, processing, and display. The accuracy of quantitative techniques is also affected by the low photon energy of thallium-201 with its high attenuation coefficient. The radiation emanating from the posterior wall of the left ventricle is markedly diminished by absorption in blood and body tissues in the anterior view. Overlying breast tissue can produce an artifactual perfusion defect as well.

TOMOGRAPHY

Many of the problems associated with conventional scintigraphy, such as superimposition of one portion of myocardium on another and the heterogeneity of background activities, are overcome by tomography. Both limited-angle and transaxial tomography can be performed using thallium-201.

Limited-angle tomography of the heart can be performed with thallium-201 and a seven-pinhole or a rotating slant-hole collimator.[177] With seven-pinhole tomography, seven two-dimensional images are obtained. The pinholes are at slightly different angles and provide seven different views of the heart. A series of two-dimensional images that focus on various depths within the chest are reconstructed from the original data. The primary advantages of this approach are that commercially available radiopharmaceuticals can be used and currently available instrumentation can be modified to obtain limited-angle tomograms. Depth resolution is poor with limited-angle tomography, and positioning of the patient is technically difficult but critical to obtaining satisfactory results. Furthermore, there does not appear to be a significant difference in accuracy between limited-angle tomography and standard two-dimensional thallium imaging.[178–180]

Transaxial computed tomography can be performed with a rotating scintillation camera system or with a multi-detector system.[181] In the rotating gamma camera system, the detector rotates 180 or 360 degrees around the patient.[182,183] The camera detector makes between 32 and 64 stops; during each of these 20- to 40-second stops, the camera acquires a two-dimensional image. The data from all 32 to 64 images or projections are summed, corrected for attenuation, and reconstructed into a transaxial image. Images of other planes, such as coronal, sagittal, or oblique sections, can be reconstructed from the data as well. Thus, imaging can be performed in planes parallel and perpendicular to the long axis of the left ventricle,[184–188] reducing interpretive errors due to reduced perfusion at the base of the heart in the region of the valve plane.

Myocardial perfusion transaxial tomography has a characteristic appearance in the normal patient (Fig. 11–17). The left ventricle appears horseshoe-shaped at the base heart, with the long axis of the horseshoe oriented between 35 and 45 degrees toward the left anterior oblique. The distribution throughout the septum and anterior and lateral walls is homogeneous. The open end of the horseshoe corresponds anatomically to the region of the aortic valve. Sections obtained at the midventricular plane appear doughnut-shaped, with uniform uptake throughout the doughnut. The central perfusion defect represents the left ventricular cavity. Slices through the apex show a round or oval region of activity with a minimal or absent central defect corresponding to a transverse section through the apical wall caudal to the cardiac chamber. Right ventricular or atrial activity is usually not detected.

In patients with myocardial infarction, regions of markedly reduced perfusion are seen in areas corresponding to the location of the infarct (Fig. 11–18). The extent of the perfusion defect is usually greater on emission tomography than on standard two-dimensional scintigraphy. Similarly, the border between the normally perfused myocardium and perfusion defect is sharper and more clearly defined on tomography, since perfused myocardium is not superimposed on the ischemic tissue as it is with conventional imaging. Tomography also improves the contrast between the myocardium and surrounding structures, such as the lung and liver. In addition to the improved accuracy over conventional two-dimensional imaging, the ability to obtain multiple transaxial slices of the area of the myocar-

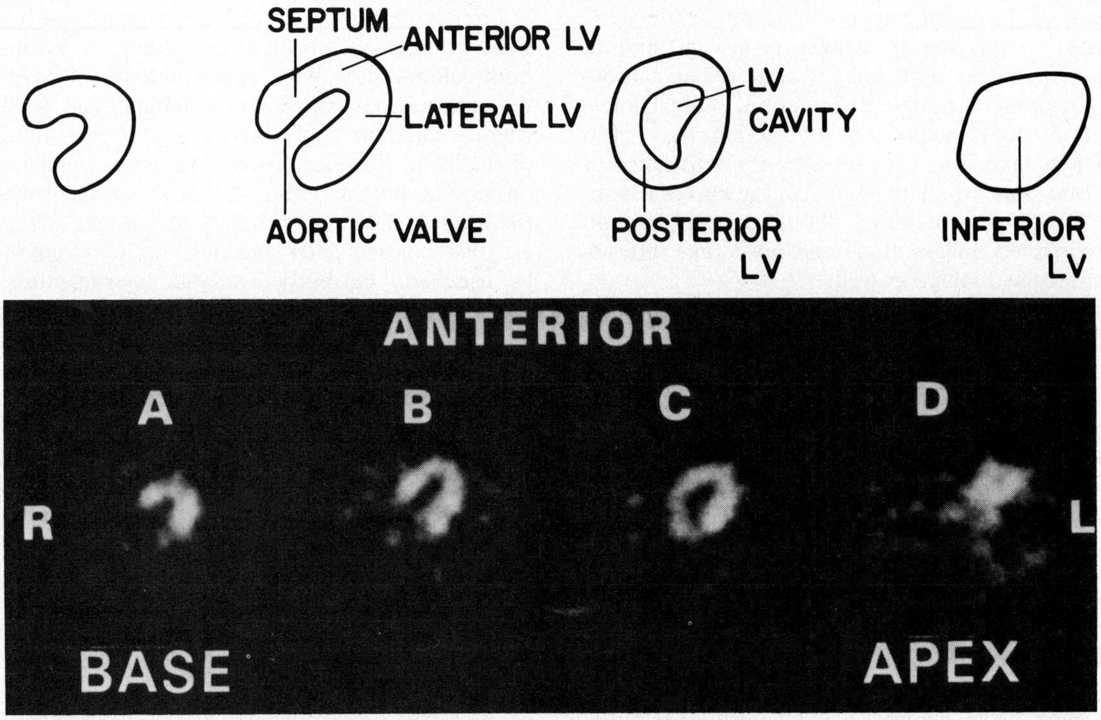

FIGURE 11–17 Normal transaxial myocardial tomograms using thallium-201 in man. The slices are oriented as though the viewer is looking from below with the anterior surface up. Slice A was taken through the base of the left ventricle. The thallium-201 uptake appears horseshoe-shaped owing to the lack of uptake in the region of the valves. Slices obtained more distally through the heart (B and C) show more of a doughnut-shape, with no radioactivity in the region of the left ventricular cavity. At the apex (D), the left ventricular wall is imaged below the cavity, and therefore uptake appears uniform. The right ventricle is not normally seen at rest. (R = right; L = left.) (From Holman, B. L., et al.: Single photon emission computed tomography of the heart in normal subjects and patients with infarction. J. Nucl. Med. *20*:736, 1979.)

dium with the perfusion defect suggests the potential for volumetric quantitation of infarction or ischemia. The ability to quantify the extent of the perfusion defect becomes increasingly important as limitation of infarct size becomes part of the therapeutic strategy in acute myocardial infarction.

CLINICAL APPLICATIONS

DIAGNOSIS OF CORONARY ARTERY DISEASE

The diagnosis of coronary artery disease is the most important application of myocardial perfusion scintigraphy with thallium-201. It is significantly more accurate for the detection of coronary artery disease than the exercise electrocardiogram[189–194] (p. 1341). In a review summarizing the results in over 1800 patients, overall sensitivity for detecting coronary artery disease using thallium-201 was 82 per cent and specificity was 91 per cent. Sensitivity for the exercise electrocardiogram was 60 per cent and specificity was 81 per cent.[76] It has been suggested that temporal and spatial quantitation and tomographic imaging may improve the accuracy of diagnosis somewhat.

Myocardial perfusion scintigraphy with thallium-201 should be used as a complement to exercise electrocardiography. The exercise ECG should be obtained first, prior to perfusion scintigraphy. Thallium-201 scintigraphy should then be carried out when the exercise ECG is nondiagnostic or is abnormal in an asymptomatic patient or when there is a moderate probability of coronary artery disease.[195]

Nondiagnostic electrocardiograms may result when the

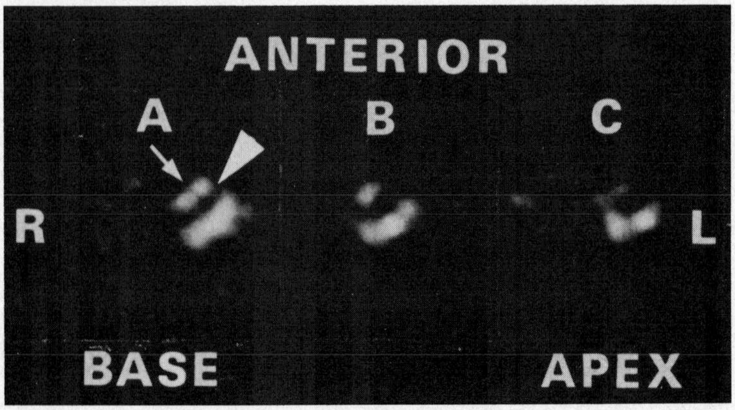

FIGURE 11–18 Transaxial myocardial tomography in a patient with anteroseptal infarct. Note some reduction in perfusion to septum (arrow) and markedly reduced perfusion to anterior wall (arrowhead). (A = slice through base of left ventricle; B = mid-ventricle; C = slice through apex; R = right; L = left.) (From Holman, B. L., et al.: Single photon emission computed tomography of the heart in normal subjects and patients with infarction. J. Nucl. Med. *20*:736, 1979.)

resting electrocardiogram is abnormal but ischemic ST-segment changes cannot be defined. This may occur in patients with left bundle branch block or in those receiving digitalis. In this group of patients, the accuracy of thallium-201 perfusion scintigraphy remains high and is therefore extremely helpful. Another cause for uninterpretable exercise electrocardiograms is failure to achieve 85 per cent of predicted maximal heart rate with no ST-segment changes (p. 1341). In this group of patients, the sensitivity and specificity of thallium-201 imaging are approximately the same as for patients who are able to achieve an adequate heart rate response.[161,196,197] These results suggest that the mechanisms underlying an abnormal stress electrocardiogram and an abnormal myocardial scintigram are different and help to explain why the sensitivities of these tests are additive. When the diagnosis of coronary artery disease is based on both an abnormal stress electrocardiogram and an abnormal thallium-201 test, the diagnostic sensitivity is substantially greater than when either test is used alone. However, it must be remembered that when the two tests are used additively, the diagnostic specificity for coronary artery disease falls substantially.

Patients with *atypical angina pectoris* are reasonable candidates for myocardial perfusion scintigraphy. The likelihood of these patients having coronary artery disease is between 30 and 50 per cent.[198] Perfusion scintigraphy is useful in this group of patients. The accuracy of the exercise electrocardiogram may be too low to affect substantially the likelihood of coronary artery disease, regardless of the outcome of the test (p. 2). The accuracy of myocardial perfusion scintigraphy is higher, so that in patients who are moderately likely to have coronary artery disease, the results of the test can be used to guide medical management. This is not true for patients with *typical angina pectoris*, in whom the likelihood of having the disease is so high prior to diagnostic testing that a normal perfusion test cannot be accepted as strong evidence that the patient does not have coronary artery disease. Similarly, in *asymptomatic* patients, the likelihood of disease is so small prior to testing that this likelihood will change little after the test.[199] Furthermore, if large numbers of asymptomatic patients are studied, a sizable number of false-positive results will occur even when the test's specificity is 90 per cent.

While the test has limited usefulness for asymptomatic patients in general, it is of value in asymptomatic patients with positive stress electrocardiograms. The prevalence of coronary artery disease in this population is approximately 30 per cent.[200] A positive thallium perfusion scintigram raises the likelihood of disease to greater than 80 per cent, while a negative test reduces it to less than 10 per cent.

DIAGNOSING THE EXTENT OF CORONARY ARTERY DISEASE. Thallium-201 perfusion scintigraphy has been most useful in providing the clinician with an objective guide to the severity of a patient's coronary artery disease and the effectiveness of medical therapy. For example, patients with coronary artery disease can be studied while taking propranolol to determine whether they are adequately protected from ischemia at the maximum exercise levels they can achieve while on the drug.

Thallium-201 perfusion scintigraphy has not been particularly useful in determining the number of stenotic coronary arteries nor in identifying which vessels are diseased. The sensitivity is approximately 60 to 80 per cent for identifying obstruction of the left anterior coronary artery, 50 to 60 per cent for the right coronary artery, and 20 to 50 per cent for the left circumflex coronary artery.[201,202] Sensitivity is affected by the severity of the stenosis,[203] with an increasing sensitivity as the degree of stenosis increases. Specific patterns of extensive coronary artery disease that involves either three vessels or the left main coronary artery are helpful when present but are seen in less than half the patients.[204]

The sensitivity for detecting the *extent* of coronary artery disease is directly related to the level of exercise attained.[162] In addition, computer processing (specifically, the measurement of thallium-201 washout at two or three points during the first 6 hours after injection of the tracer) has been suggested to improve the specificity for detecting the number and location of diseased coronary vessels;[205,206] temporal quantitation must be confirmed in other laboratories before it can be applied routinely in clinical practice.

Myocardial perfusion scintigraphy with thallium-201 may be a useful adjunct to coronary angiography for evaluating the *functional significance of coronary stenoses.* The coronary angiogram provides anatomical detail but very little information related to myocardial perfusion. While thallium-201 scintigraphy has been most useful in providing an overall estimate of the functional significance of the disease, it is less useful for defining the functional significance of a borderline coronary artery stenosis. If a perfusion defect is present in the segment supplied by the artery in question, the test result is useful, showing that the lesion is hemodynamically significant. If more severe coronary stenoses in adjacent vessels cause transient ischemia and cessation of the exercise test before the hemodynamically significant stenosis in question causes ischemia, no perfusion defect will appear in that segment.

Perfusion scintigraphy may also be useful as an adjunct to coronary angiography by *differentiating viable from nonviable myocardium.* There is a strong relationship between the degree of redistribution in a region of transient ischemia and the degree of asynergy in that myocardial segment.[207] Furthermore, the better the redistribution, the more likely the segment will contract normally after bypass surgery.[208]

Thallium-201 perfusion scintigraphy has been used to study patients after coronary bypass surgery in whom the question of *graft patency* has arisen. In patients with exercise-induced perfusion defects that become normal after operation, the likelihood of bypass graft patency is high.[209,210] If the segment was normal prior to operation, the postoperative development of transient ischemia indicates that the graft is probably occluded. If perfusion during exercise is normal after operation, the graft is probably patent. If there is no change in perfusion to the segment after surgery, graft patency cannot be predicted accurately.

OTHER CAUSES OF TRANSIENT PERFUSION DEFECTS. Many patients with transient perfusion defects on thallium-201 imaging but considered false-positives in reported studies have coronary stenoses of between 20 and 50 per cent of the vessel diameter.[211] That these patients have a higher incidence of transient ischemia than patients with less severe stenoses may indicate both the difficulty in accurately defining the degree of stenoses using coronary angiography and the possibility that what has traditionally been characterized as subcritical stenoses may result in myocardial hypoperfusion during maximal stress.

Abnormal results may also be seen in patients with *muscular myocardial bridges* without evidence of coronary atherosclerosis[212] and in patients with evidence of *diffuse cardiac disease.*[213] In patients with *aortic stenosis* and normal coronary arteries, exercise-induced subendocardial ischemia[214] or changes in left ventricular wall thickness may develop.[215] This ischemia will result in perfusion defects on thallium-201 imaging. While perfusion defects have been reported in patients with mitral valve prolapse, most studies have not substantiated this observation and have suggested the use of this test for identifying underlying coronary artery disease in patients with prolapse.[216–218]

CORONARY ARTERY SPASM. This may occur in patients without detectable coronary artery stenoses. These patients will have transient perfusion defects on thallium-201 imaging if they are injected during or immediately following spasm.[219–221] Spasm has been demonstrated during exercise in some patients with exertional chest pain and ST-wave elevation who have normal coronary arteries at angiography. Spasm may occur at rest; in this case, perfusion defects are observed even without exercise.

FIXED DEFECTS. *Nonreversible defects,* perfusion defects that are seen both during exercise and at rest, may be due to previous myocardial infarction, hypertrophic obstructive cardiomyopathy,[222] sarcoid heart disease,[223] idiopathic congestive cardiomyopathy,[224] amyloidosis, metastatic disease to the heart, and other infiltrative heart diseases.

Other causes of abnormal tests result from *technical factors.* For example, in patients with negative electrocardiographic exercise tests, the specificity of the test is quite low in women (56 per cent) compared with men (81 per cent) and is due to attenuation of myocardial activity by overlying breast resulting in an apparent perfusion defect in the myocardial segment underlying the breast.[225] As mentioned previously, perfusion defects may appear on the lateral or 70-degree LAO projection in patients studied supine because of attenuation caused by abdominal organs and the diaphragm. Because camera nonuniformity may also result in apparent defects, it is critical to pay close attention to quality control. Probably the single most common cause of apparent perfusion abnormalities is heterogeneous background lung activity, especially when lung activity is high owing to increased pulmonary blood volume. This will result in apparently decreased activity in myocardium that does not overlie the lung and is only partially corrected by interpolative background-correction programs. Emission tomography will alleviate these background problems but may introduce additional problems due to inadequate correction of attenuation.

ACUTE MYOCARDIAL INFARCTION (p. 1288). Perfusion scintigraphy at rest has been used to detect the presence of acute myocardial infarction. Wackers et al. showed defects in 165 of 200 patients (82 per cent).[226] This technique is most sensitive soon after infarction. Thus, 90 of 96 patients had abnormal scintiscans within 24 hours of infarction, while only 75 of 104 had abnormalities after 24 hours. Defects also appear to decrease in size with time, particularly when the initial study is performed within 24 hours of infarction. Since perfusion defects can be seen at rest in some patients with unstable angina and during spasm in patients with Prinzmetal's angina, perfusion scintigraphy cannot always distinguish between these two conditions. The greatest value of this technique lies in obtaining a normal scintigram within 24 hours of suspected infarction, greatly lowering the probability that the patient has sustained acute infarction. In acute infarction the perfusion defect will decrease in size during the first week, while the defect produced by scar tissue will not change in size. Consequently, serial imaging will be necessary to distinguish old from new infarction.

Patients with unstable angina pectoris have abnormal perfusion at the time of chest pain, but they also have abnormal scintigrams after the pain has subsided.[227] Abnormal scintigrams occur more frequently in patients with a complicated course.

Perfusion scintigraphy may provide prognostic information, since it correlates well with estimates of infarct size made by serum creatine kinase curve analysis[228–230] and by pathological studies.[231–233] Initially, the thallium perfusion defect is larger than the acute infarct because of surrounding ischemia, and it may remain larger if the patient has sustained previous infarctions and has myocardial scar in addition to necrosis.

Thallium perfusion scintigraphy may be useful as a prognostic indicator if it is obtained early after the onset of symptoms.[234] Patients with large defects have an extremely high mortality rate compared to patients with smaller defects. To use this test in a predictive way, it is essential that imaging be obtained early or at a predefined time after the onset of symptoms. Since the perfusion defect will shrink with time unless the patient sustains reinfarction or extension of the infarct, it will not be possible to compare the results obtained at variable times after infarction. The predictive value of this test is enhanced when the test is combined with technetium-99m–pyrophosphate scintigraphy (see Infarct-Avid Scintigraphy), particularly with emission computed tomography.

THE RIGHT VENTRICLE. Right ventricular uptake on the resting thallium-201 images correlates with right ventricular overload (Fig. 11–19) and may be seen in either volume overload (atrial septal defect or pulmonic or tricuspid regurgitation) or pressure overload (mitral stenosis, primary pulmonary hypertension, ventricular septal defect, or Eisenmenger's syndrome). There is a direct relationship between the intensity of right ventricular uptake and the hemodynamic measurement of right ventricular work.

THROMBOLYTIC THERAPY. The intracoronary injection of thrombolytic agents such as streptokinase may reduce the extent of irreversible myocardial damage in patients with acute infarction[235,236] (p. 1324). Since a coronary artery catheter is already in place in the vessel, coronary arteriography can be performed to demonstrate the degree to which the vessel has been reopened. In addition, thallium-201 can be injected directly into the coronary artery both before and after thrombolytic therapy to determine the viability of the reperfused myocardium. Only a small amount of thallium (30 to 50 μCi) needs to be injected at each time. The advantage of this approach is that both reperfusion and integrity of the sodium-potassium pump are necessary for thallium accumulation in the cell. Further work is needed to document that the previously ischemic cells that take up thallium-201 will survive.

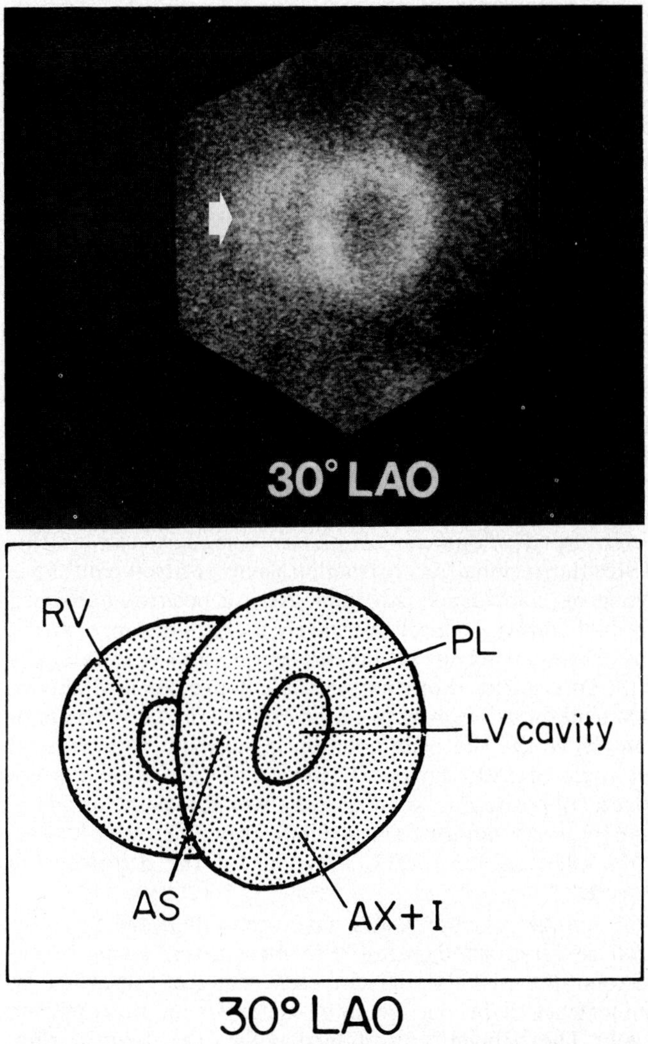

FIGURE 11–19 Myocardial perfusion scintigram in a patient with right ventricular hypertrophy. Note increased thallium-201 uptake in the right ventricle (arrow). 30° LAO = 30-degree left anterior oblique projection; RV = right ventricle; AS = anteroseptal; AX = apex; I = inferior; LV = left ventricular; and PL = posterolateral.

ASSESSMENT OF REGIONAL MYOCARDIAL PERFUSION WITH INVASIVE TECHNIQUES

A number of techniques utilizing radionuclides during or after coronary arteriography have been developed to assess fully the significance of coronary artery lesions. These "invasive" techniques suffer in that they are limited in serial evaluations of patients with coronary artery disease. Nevertheless, they do provide information complementary to that of the coronary arteriogram. Myocardial perfusion may be assessed both in the basal state and following an intervention to determine regional myocardial blood flow distal to coronary artery lesions; thus the hemodynamic significance of the latter may be assessed. It may also be possible to discover those segments of myocardium irreversibly scarred from prior infarction.

Perfusion Scintigraphy with Microparticles. Myocardial perfusion scintigraphy may be performed following intracoronary injection of either macroaggregated albumin[237,238] or radiolabeled microspheres. The primary advantages of this approach are the improved spatial resolution that results from the substantially higher target-to-background ratio and the better physical characteristics of the radiopharmaceutical when it is labeled with ^{99m}Tc. As already mentioned, its major limitations are the need to inject the tracer *directly* into the coronary circulation, usually at the time of coronary angiography, and the impracticality of serial studies.

Myocardial perfusion imaging yields results compatible in most cases to the anatomical lesions found at coronary arteriography[239] and left ventricular angiography. Occasionally, a region of reduced uptake is not associated with abnormal wall motion in the same location. Obstructions of major vessel branches that exceed 70 per cent of the diameter are usually associated with recognizable regional hypoperfusion on the appropriate radionuclide images. This appears to be more marked when there is a relative lack of collateral perfusion, when multiple vessels are involved, and in those cases in which extensive scarring of the myocardium has occurred.

Perfusion scintigraphy with microparticles, performed in the basal state, demonstrates abnormalities in only a portion of patients with significant coronary artery disease.[238] Presumably, in patients with normal scintigrams and coronary obstruction, the latter is not severe enough to limit the flow in the resting state nor is there any scar tissue caused by previous infarction. The finding of abnormal perfusion studies with normal coronary arteriograms may result from several factors. First, since the particles are injected directly into the coronary artery, streaming becomes a potential source of error that may result in artifactual regions of reduced perfusion. Second, other types of cardiac disease may result in increased heterogeneity of blood flow and even of regional scarring. Thus, a perfusion defect on the scintigram may not be specific for coronary artery disease. It is possible, but much less likely, that perfusion defects result from disease not detected arteriographically. Perfusion scintigraphy may also be performed after various types of intervention procedures that include the injection of contrast media.[240] Thus, it may be possible to provide information similar to that obtained with potassium analogs after exercise.

At the present time, it is questionable whether the improvement in spatial resolution obtained with microspheres compensates for the limitations presented by the need for direct injection of the tracer into the coronary arteries and for the difficulty in assessing perfusion during exercise. These problems should be kept in mind, since the difference between spatial resolution obtained with the microsphere technique and that with intravenous myocardial perfusion scintigraphy has been substantially reduced with the introduction of ^{201}Tl.

Intracoronary Rubidium-82. The positron emitter ^{82}Rb can be injected directly into the coronary arteries at the time of coronary angiography.[138] Imaging can be performed with well-shielded Anger cameras using rotating collimators. Because the half-life of the tracer is so short (75 sec), sequential imaging can be performed, with repeat injections made within 5 or 10 minutes of one another. By studying patients at rest and during atrial pacing and by injecting both the left and right coronary arteries, the effectiveness of collateral blood flow can be studied. Because the injection is arterial, catheter streaming remains a problem with this approach. Also, like the microsphere method, it does not permit quantitative measurement of flow.

Inert Gas Washout Method. The inert gas washout method provides a quantitative measure of tissue flow expressed in ml/min/100 gm. The inert gas dissolved in saline is injected directly and rapidly into the coronary artery. Once the tracer has diffused into the tissue, the organ is perfused by tracer-free blood, setting up a concentration gradient between tissue and blood. Since the tracer is not diffusion-limited, the rate at which it diffuses back into the blood depends on the flow rate through the tissue and the solubility partition coefficient between blood and tissue. The more rapid the flow rate, the more rapid the clearance, or washout, from the tissue.

Radiotracers must meet several requirements to be suitable for this technique: (1) they must be freely diffusible into the tissue in which perfusion is to be measured; (2) they cannot be diffusion-limited, since washout of the tracer would then be proportional not only to flow, but also to the time needed for the tracer to diffuse back to the capillary tissue interface; (3) they cannot be metabolized or sequestered in the tissues, since flow measurements depend on the undegraded tracer diffusing freely back into the blood; and (4) if possible, the tracers should not recirculate, since recirculation redistributes a portion of the tracer back into the organ. (If recirculation does occur, corrections must be employed.) The inert gases satisfy these conditions.

For external monitoring, the physical characteristics of the tracer become important. Xenon-133 is the tracer most frequently used. Because the energy of its photon emission is low (81 kev), scattered radiation cannot be easily eliminated from the photopeak by pulse height analysis, and this reduces the spatial resolution of the resultant data. Blood flow measurements are weighted more heavily toward superficial tissue lying closer to the external detector, since the attenuation for 81 kev photons is less than for those from deep structures. Other isotopes of xenon, such as ^{127}Xe, may reduce these problems when they become commercially available. ^{81m}Kr has also been suggested as a tracer to enable quantitation of blood flow.[241] ^{81}Rb is injected into the coronary arteries and serves as an in vivo generator, continually producing ^{81m}Kr (190 kev), which has a 13-second half-life. This technique permits quantitative measurement of transient changes in coronary blood flow following a single injection of ^{81}Rb.

There are advantages to specific flow measurements, particularly in regional perfusion studies. The geometry of the organ is not a factor when external monitoring devices are used, since flow is measured per unit weight. Furthermore, clearance rates are independent of the initial quantity of tracer reaching the tissue (the calculation depends only on the slope of the washout) and are therefore not affected by catheter streaming.

However, the inert gas washout technique has a number of inherent limitations. The relative solubility between lipid and water differs by a factor of 10 for xenon, and the blood:tissue partition coefficient (λ) is difficult to determine accurately. No method is currently available for the in vivo determination of λ. In addition, the washout curve, even the initial portion, may be influenced by cardiac fat, with its high affinity for and correspondingly slow release of xenon, thus underestimating specific flow. Errors result when there is inhomogeneous perfusion in the region in which flow is to be assessed, leading to overestimation of flow because the initial slope reflects predominantly washout of the well-perfused muscle to which the indicator is predominantly distributed. This problem has been overcome to a considerable extent by assessing regional perfusion with scintillation camera systems.

The presence of countercurrent exchange vascular systems may result in underestimation of flow values, since trapping of gas by the system causes its rate of washout to be slower than that predicted from capillary blood flow rates. It has been postulated that in subendocardial regions of heart muscle, some diffusional shunting across arterial or capillary loops may occur.[242,243] The differences in myocardial transit that result from shunting appear to be small and would therefore result in an insignificant error when the inert gas washout method is used to measure transmural flow.

Regional flow measurements present a number of additional problems. Specific flow measurement techniques assume that the perfused tissue is not diffusion-limited.[244] With xenon, the detector is more sensitive to perfusion in the myocardial wall closer to the detector, and studies in multiple projections are therefore desirable. Perfusion gradients across the ventricular wall cannot be detected with this technique. Since the ischemic myocardium will receive little indicator if ischemia occurs in only a part of the tissue included in the xenon clearance curve, the initial part of the washout curve will be determined essentially by the indicator contained in well-perfused zones.

Although the limitations of specific flow techniques must be taken into account, correlation between flow measured directly with electromagnetic flow meters and with the inert gas washout technique has been excellent,[245,246] while regional flow values obtained in the clinic have been quite reproducible and have correlated with the extent of coronary artery disease, particularly during pharmacological or physiological stress.[247]

Global myocardial blood flow has been measured using a scintillation counter as the external detector.[248] Techniques to assess regional myocardial blood flow (RMBF) have been developed recently using the inert gas washout technique with ^{133}Xe and scintillation cameras.[247,249,250] Electronic crystal-splitting techniques or multicrystal cameras allow clearance curves to be monitored from small regions of the myocardium.

Although compartmental analysis can be applied to myocardial washout curves, the initial slope method is the one usually applied. Specific flow is calculated from the equation

$$F/W = \frac{\lambda \cdot k \cdot 100}{\rho} \qquad (11)$$

where F/W is specific flow (ml/min/100 gm), λ is the blood:tissue partition coefficient, k is the slope of the washout curve, and ρ is the specific gravity of myocardium.

The inert gas washout method is most useful in assessing the effect of drugs on coronary blood flow. For example, nitroglycerin has been shown to improve flow preferentially to ischemic regions in some patients with well-developed collaterals.[251] Conversely, nitroprusside has been shown to induce a coronary steal phenomenon in some patients with coronary artery disease.[252]

MYOCARDIAL METABOLISM

Adequate cardiac function requires a sufficient supply of blood to meet the metabolic demands of the myocardium. With conventional radionuclide studies, perfusion of the myocardium and cardiac performance can be assessed. Recently, techniques have been developed to allow measurement of metabolism using the radiotracer method. Direct measurement of the uptake and utilization of fuel substrates may provide a more direct measure of the severity of myocardial ischemia, since ischemia results from a combination of inadequate blood supply and excessive demand for mechanical work. It may also be possible to understand better intrinsic disturbances in myocardial metabolism as might occur in cardiomyopathies and other diseases in which the primary etiology is alteration of biochemical pathways.

Perhaps the greatest impetus to study in this area has been the development of *positron emission tomography.* Three-dimensional reconstruction using positron emitters is based on coincidence detection. After a positron is formed through positron decay, it travels a short distance within the tissue, giving up its kinetic energy, and then interacts with an electron. Both particles are converted into annihilation photons, each with an energy of 511 kev. The photons leave the site of interaction in opposite directions, at an angle of 180 degrees. If two scintillation detectors are placed opposite one another, they will detect the annihilation photons simultaneously (coincidence detection). Scattered photons that reach only one of the detectors are rejected.

A number of approaches have been advocated for positron emission tomography.[253] In most cases, a ring of detectors is used in which each detector operates in coincidence with one or more detectors in the opposite bank. The patient is positioned within the detector ring. After imaging, the data are reconstructed into an image representing the transaxial distribution of the tracer.

Positron emission tomography has a number of advantages: (1) the field of view of the coincidence detectors is highly uniform over a large distance; (2) the coincidence counting rate remains virtually constant, regardless of the position of the radiation source within the absorber; (3) tissue attenuation is less with annihilation photons than with lower energy photon emissions of radionuclides such as technetium-99m and thallium-201; and (4) the short-lived positron-emitting radionuclides such as oxygen-15, nitrogen-13, and carbon-11 offer fundamental advantages in the study of metabolic processes. These last elements are ubiquitous in naturally occurring metabolic processes, and these nuclides are the only isotopes of these elements suitable for imaging. Thus, ^{15}O, ^{13}N, and ^{11}C can be incorporated into radiopharmaceuticals that are true metabolic substrates and consequently can be tailored to the investigation of selected metabolic pathways.[254]

MYOCARDIAL GLUCOSE UPTAKE

Regional myocardial glucose uptake can be measured using ^{18}F 2-fluoro-2-deoxyglucose (FDG).[254a] Fluorine-18 is a positron emitter with a 2-hour half-life. FDG exchanges rapidly across the capillary and cellular membranes in direct proportion to glucose transport. It competes for hexokinase and is phosphorylated to FDG-6-phosphate. Since it is not a substrate for glycolysis, it undergoes no further metabolism and therefore remains in the heart. As a result, the amount of tracer in the heart at the time of equilibrium is directly proportional to the rate of uptake of exogenous glucose.[255,256]

While the initial tissue uptake of the tracer is a function of blood flow and the concentration of tracer in the blood, at the time of equilibrium—approximately 60 to 90 minutes after injection—the tissue activity represents primarily FDG-6-phosphate.[255–258] To measure *exogenous* glucose uptake, positron emission tomography is performed 60 minutes after injection to determine the tissue concentration of the tracer. Arterial glucose and FDG plasma concentrations are also determined, and the information is fit into a three-compartment model consisting of vascular, tissue, and metabolic components.

While this technique is a satisfactory measure of exogenous glucose uptake in man, it measures the glycolytic rate only when all the extracted glucose is used for glycolysis. This occurs only when glycogen stores are depleted, as in ischemia.[259] This technique has a number of technical limitations as well, in that it requires arterial or arterialized blood sampling; a knowledge of the rate constants required for application of the three-compartment model (since these rate constants may change during disease and during ischemia); and correction for washout of the tracer from the myocardium, which occurs late after injection.

When these studies are applied to man, they have provided insights into the biochemical pathways initiated during ischemia. In patients with unstable angina, there is a regional increase in glucose uptake in the ischemic segment despite a decrease in perfusion.[260,261] Even when normal myocardium is metabolizing primarily free fatty acids and hence has low glucose uptake, regions of ischemia may show excessive glucose uptake, indicating the primary reliance on glycolysis for energy in ischemic myocardium.

FATTY ACID METABOLISM

(Also see p. 1250)

Under normal conditions, most of the energy requirements of the heart are met by oxidation of free fatty acids.[260–262] Free fatty acid metabolism has been studied in man using ^{11}C-labeled palmitic acid combined with positron emission tomography.[263,263a] The initial distribution of this tracer in the myocardium is directly proportional to myocardial blood flow.[264] Myocardial clearance depends on the oxygen demand and the availability of alternative substrates. In normal hearts, the slope of the early component of the washout curve corresponds to the rate of oxidation of ^{11}C-palmitic acid.[265–267] Abnormalities in initial clearance may be due to metabolic abnormalities in free fatty acid utilization or to alternative metabolic pathways, as may occur if free fatty acid plasma levels are low and the heart is using primarily glucose and lactic acid.[268] While this method provides a semiquantitative measure of free fatty acid utilization in the heart, accurate measurement is limited by washout of ^{11}C-palmitic acid when oxygen availability is restricted, because of reduced availability of the tracer in regions of markedly reduced flow and because other fatty acids are utilized by the heart.

Positron emission tomography using ^{11}C-palmitate has been used to identify the size and extent of myocardial infarction.[269] In normal subjects tomography shows uniform distribution of the tracer throughout the left ventricle. Tomograms from patients with previous myocardial infarction show diminished accumulation of ^{11}C-palmitate, delineating regions corresponding to the electrocardiographic focus of infarction. (Fig. 36–14, p. 1251)

Since ischemia alters the myocardial metabolism of free fatty acid by decreasing oxidation and increasing conversion to triglycerides, fatty acids labeled with positron-emitting nuclides such as ^{11}C–palmitate may be used to localize zones of transient ischemia. Because of the very short half-life of the tracer, transient changes can be documented by serial injections of the tracer. Thus, regions that are transiently ischemic will show augmented accumulation of the tracer with reperfusion, while zones of infarction will show no change in uptake on sequential studies obtained over a relatively short period of time (up to six hours). It has therefore been suggested that this method may be a useful indicator of cell viability, and since its accumulation is related to blood flow, it may be used as a marker of the severity and extent of tissue infarction.

^{11}C–lactic acid and pyruvic acid may be useful markers for identifying acutely ischemic tissue.[270] Tracer clearance from the myocardium is extremely prolonged in areas of ischemia resulting in zones of increased tracer activity. This method may also prove useful in distinguishing reversible from irreversible ischemia. The underlying metabolic pathways involved in tracer retention are so far unknown.

IODINE-123 FATTY ACIDS. Positron emission tomography will be limited largely to major medical centers and applied largely to research in the foreseeable future. The technology is very expensive, requiring an on-site production facility for most of the short-lived radiopharmaceuticals; even ^{18}F-FDG must be produced nearby. As a result, this method will be used primarily to improve our understanding of the pathophysiology of cardiac disease and may eventually lead to less expensive diagnostic tools, using single photon–emitting radiotracers.

^{123}I-hexadecanoic acid and ^{123}I-heptadecanoic acid have been used for measuring myocardial perfusion and fatty acid metabolism using standard single-photon imaging equipment such as Anger scintillation cameras. These tracers are extracted avidly from the blood and cleared quickly from the myocardial tissue with a half-time of approximately 25 minutes.[271] They are esterified and then undergo beta-oxidation.[272–274] The pattern of uptake and washout in the heart is similar to that for unlabeled free fatty acids.[275,276]

The major limitation of this technique is that the iodide label dissociates rather quickly from the free fatty acid. Subsequent washout of free iodide results in progressively high blood levels of the contaminant. This ^{123}I washout added to the clearance of the free fatty acid makes quantification difficult. Furthermore, the increasing background activity interferes with quantification using two-dimensional imaging or limited-angle tomography. This may explain the discordance in clearance results obtained in ischemic myocardium between ^{11}C-labeled fatty acids and ^{123}I-labeled fatty acids.[277] Corrections have been proposed for this contamination.[278]

^{123}I-labeled fatty acids may also be used to measure myocardial perfusion, since their initial distribution is proportional to blood flow. The rapid washout of the ^{123}I-hexadecanoic and heptadecanoic acids makes high-quality imaging difficult and limits imaging to two-dimensional techniques and to limited-angle tomography. Other fatty acids that are more readily retained by the myocardium are more suitable for this purpose but still suffer because of the low dose of tracer that can be administered to the patient; the high cost of the pharmaceutical; and the high-energy photons associated with the tracer and with its contaminant, ^{124}I, which degrades spatial resolution. As a perfusion agent, the ^{123}I label offers no advantages over thallium-201 and would be clearly inferior to technetium-99m–labeled perfusion agents that localize in the human heart.

INFARCT-AVID MYOCARDIAL SCINTIGRAPHY

In infarct-avid scintigraphy, radiopharmaceuticals are sequestered by acutely infarcted myocardium, resulting in regions of increased myocardial uptake. This procedure has emerged as a useful noninvasive technique to aid in the detection, localization, and quantification of myocardial necrosis. Infarct-avid scintigraphy has potential advantages over other techniques, including serum enzyme tests, electrocardiography, and vectorcardiography, which provide indirect evidence of the presence, size, and location of an infarcted region of the myocardium. These indirect techniques are usually satisfactory for detecting infarction, particularly during its early stages, but may be less useful for measuring the extent of irreversible tissue damage.

RADIOPHARMACEUTICALS

^{99m}Tc-PYROPHOSPHATE

At the present time, ^{99m}Tc-pyrophosphate is the radiotracer of choice for imaging acute myocardial infarction in man.[279–281] Fifty per cent of the injected dose is extracted by bone and the remainder is rapidly excreted through the kidneys in normal subjects. At 90 minutes, less than 5 per cent of the injected dose remains in the blood.

^{99m}Tc-pyrophosphate uptake in acute myocardial infarction depends on a number of factors: (1) regional blood flow, (2) myocardial calcium concentration, (3) irreversible myocardial injury, and (4) time after infarction.

Blood Flow. While the uptake of ^{99m}Tc-pyrophosphate is directly related to the degree of tissue damage, the pharmaceutical must reach the damaged tissue before it can be extracted. Following acute coronary occlusion, increased concentrations of ^{99m}Tc-pyrophosphate are found in regions with only minimally reduced blood flow.[288] In animal studies, tissue concentrations have been found to be about 20 times the concentration in normal myocardium. The highest concentration ratio between damaged and normal myocardium occurs when normal local blood flow is reduced by 20 to 40 per cent. As flow is reduced further, the concentration ratios begin to fall until, in regions of minimal flow (0 to 5 per cent of normal levels), ^{99m}Tc-pyrophosphate concentrations may be normal. Furthermore, there is a greater concentration of the tracer in epicardial than in endocardial segments at the same blood flow.

There are a number of reasons for this flow-dependency.[283] The total extraction of ^{99m}Tc-pyrophosphate can be expressed as a product of the extraction fraction times flow. With marked decreases in blood flow, the amount of ^{99m}Tc-pyrophosphate that is extracted is reduced because the radiopharmaceutical does not reach the tissue. The only way extraction can keep up with marked reductions in flow is if the extraction fraction (i.e., that portion of the radiotracer removed by the tissue during a single transit through the microcirculation) increases proportionately. This does not appear to be the case for ^{99m}Tc-pyrophosphate, and as a result, the total amount of tracer extracted decreases at low flow.

A second reason for reduced tracer uptake at low flow is less direct. The calcium phosphate deposits that appear in the necrotic myocardium soon after infarction may not represent precipitation of intracellular calcium.[284–286] If the deposits are of exogenous origin, their intracellular concentrations will depend on residual blood flow to provide the calcium. Since calcium concentration within the center of the infarct is low and is probably required for binding of the radiotracer, low levels of calcium within the center of the infarct may also account for the decreased concentration of radiotracer in that region in patients with large infarcts.

Myocardial Calcium. This ion probably plays a key role in technetium-99m–pyrophosphate binding in acute infarction. Approximately 50 per cent of the radiopharmaceutical is absorbed by bone in the normal patient. The binding site in bone is probably low-density amorphous calcium phosphate. While binding is possible at both the crystalline and the amorphous calcium phosphate sites, the concentration is twice as high in amorphous calcium phosphate. Furthermore, there is a direct relationship between the number of moles of bone-seeking radiopharmaceutical and the number of moles of calcium.

Irreversibly injured myocardium contains three types of calcium phosphate: amorphous, crystalline, and hydroxyapatite-like deposits. Calcium phosphate deposits are particularly abundant in the periphery of the infarct. Regional ^{99m}Tc-pyrophosphate concentrations parallel the calcium phosphate concentrations with increased radiotracer activities in the periphery of the infarct.[284–289]

The relationship between calcium content and pyrophosphate uptake is not linear, however, probably because the avidity for radiotracer binding depends on the form of the tissue calcium deposit. Much of the calcium in necrotic myocardium is exogenous in origin and results from a complex between the calcium ions and various components of the myocardial cell.[288] Massive calcium accumulation results in precipitation of calcium phosphate deposits. Hydrolysis of amorphous calcium phosphate results in the formation of crystalline hydroxyapatite. While the hydroxyapatite is localized primarily in the mitochondria, the amorphous calcium phosphate deposits are distributed more uniformly throughout the irreversibly damaged cell. Since both the amorphous and hydroxyapatite deposits probably represent binding sites, ^{99m}Tc-pyrophosphate is found in the various cellular fractions, including the mitochondria, the microsomes, and the soluble supernatant fraction.

It has also been suggested that the lack of correlation between calcium and pyrophosphate concentrations may indicate an alternative mechanism for localization, such as binding by polynuclear complexing with denatured macromolecules. In this case, calcium may form a bridge between the denatured protein and the radiotracer.[290] Furthermore, pyrophosphate uptake may be seen in irreversibly damaged myocardium independent of the presence or absence of calcium ion in the perfusate.[291] Thus, there may be binding sites in addition to calcium phosphate deposits within the infarct.

Irreversible Tissue Damage. In man, ^{99m}Tc-pyrophosphate labels acutely necrotic myocardium. The concentration ratio between infarcted and normal myocardium may be as high as 18:1, and the distribution—even in large circumferential infarcts—may be homogeneous throughout the infarct.[292]

In the zone immediately bordering the infarct, the concentration of pyrophosphate is greater than in normal myocardium; however, the increase is less than 50 per cent higher than normal myocardium. Furthermore, this border zone of slightly increased radiotracer concentration extends only a small distance from the necrotic region.

Technetium-99m–pyrophosphate uptake may be increased in patients with unstable angina pectoris, although histopathological examination of several of these patients has indicated multifocal lesions of coagulation necrosis, myocytolysis, and replacement fibrosis.[293] Increased uptake has also been noted in patients with ventricular aneurysm and regions of ventricular dyskinesis. The increase in radiotracer uptake may persist for some time after an acute infarction. In these patients, histopathological examinations have demonstrated myocytolytic degeneration in myocardial foci that have survived initial infarction. Myocytolysis appears to result from more slowly progressive injury compared to coagulation necrosis. This chronic injury occurs in regions of previous myocardial infarction.

Time After Infarction. Uptake of the radiopharmaceutical begins to increase after four hours of permanent coronary artery occlusion.[294] In most patients with transmural myocardial infarction, faint uptake will be seen shortly after this time and will increase in intensity over the next 36 to 48 hours. Intensity will reach a peak by 48 hours and will gradually diminish over the next 5 to 7 days. The time course will vary depending on a number of factors:

1. The larger the infarct, the longer it takes for the intensity of tracer uptake to reach its peak.[295] This is because initial delivery of the radiopharmaceutical is retarded by markedly diminished perfusion, particularly in the center of the infarct. With the development of collateral vessels, more radiopharmaceutical can reach the infarct and the intensity reaches its peak.

2. The intensity will fade more slowly in large transmural infarcts because there may be continuing tissue necrosis well beyond the initial event.

3. There may be extension of the infarct or reinfarction following the initial event. Following this complication, the extent of the radiotracer uptake will increase and the intensity of uptake may also increase.

OTHER INFARCT-AVID TRACERS

The first successful attempt at infarct-avid scintigraphy in man used technetium-99m–tetracycline as the radiotracer.[296,297] Since the optimal time for imaging is 24 hours after injection and liver concentration is high, this tracer has been replaced by the bone-seeking radiotracers. Nevertheless, ^{99m}Tc-tetracycline does more accurately reflect the degree of tissue necrosis, since its myocardial uptake is inversely related to blood flow even at low flow rates.[298]

Other tracers have been suggested, including ^{99m}Tc-glucoheptonate,[299,300] ^{99m}Tc-methylene diphosphonate,[301,302] and ^{99m}Tc-imidodiphosphonate,[303] but these do not appear to have any advantage over ^{99m}Tc-pyrophosphate.

Radiolabeled Antibody Against Cardiac Myosin. Purified radiolabeled antibody against cardiac myosin has also been demonstrated in regions of acute infarction. After intravenous injection of radioiodine-labeled (FAB′)$_2$ fragments of antibodies specific for cardiac myosins, concentration ratios of up to 6:1 between infarcted and normal myocardium may be found in the animal model. There is an inverse relationship between regional myocardial blood flow and uptake of the tracer even in areas of low flow.[304] After intravenous injection, well-defined areas of increased myocardial activity are found by 72 hours after permanent occlusion of a coronary artery in animals. Unfortunately, the concentration of tracer within the infarct is too low to permit external detection of the infarct within the first 24 hours after coronary occlusion unless the tracer is injected directly into the coronary artery.[305] The delay in infarct visualization is the result of prolonged clearance time of the tracer from the blood and slow entry of the tracer into the infarct.

This technique is based on the assumption that these antibodies are highly specific for myocardium and that as capillary and cellular membrane integrity is disrupted by myocardial ischemia, the antibodies attach themselves to the contractile proteins of the myocardium. Initial results demonstrate very slow blood clearance because of the relatively large size of the antibody molecules. When fragments of antimyosin antibody are used, blood clearance is significantly improved without loss of antibody specificity.

The tissue activity of the radiolabeled cardiac myosin antibody fragments is inversely related to blood flow. The radioconcentration is highest in segments of maximal flow reduction and tissue necrosis, unlike ^{99m}Tc-pyrophosphate, which concentrates most in myocardial segments with flow reductions 20 to 40 per cent of normal. Thus, the radiolabeled antibodies are similar to ^{99m}Tc-tetracycline in distribution. The high uptake in low-flow areas results from prolonged intravascular transit, which allows the radiotracer time to reach poorly perfused tissue.

Indium-111–Labeled White Blood Cells. By labeling blood cell components, physiological parameters other than tissue necrosis can be measured. Experimental acute coronary artery thrombosis and experimental infective endocarditis have been detected using indium-111–labeled platelets.[306] Although this technique is promising for evaluating coronary artery bypass graft patency and for assessing the inflammatory component of acute infarction, it is currently limited by the difficulty encountered in routine labeling of platelets.

Indium-111–labeled white blood cells provide an additional tool for visualizing acute myocardial infarctions, particularly for studying their pathophysiology.[307] Migration of polymorphous leukocytes into acutely infarcted myocardium is known to occur, and use of these labeled cells can provide useful information when one is monitoring the inflammatory response in acutely infarcted myocardium as well as the effects of therapeutic intervention.

TECHNIQUE

Patients suspected of having sustained an acute myocardial infarction are usually admitted directly to the coronary care unit. Usually they are at risk for developing either electrophysiological or hemodynamic complications; if so, imaging must be performed at the bedside using a portable scintillation camera. The camera should be a 37-photomultiplier tube, high-resolution instrument used in conjunction with a high-resolution collimator.

Patients who are clinically stable may be brought to the nuclear medicine clinical unit. In this case, the suite used for imaging should contain monitoring equipment, including an electrocardiographic monitor, defibrillator, and emergency drugs. Standard infarct imaging does not require additional equipment. Computer processing has been suggested to subtract uptake by overlying ribs in patients in whom costochondral cartilage uptake obscures the myocardial field. We have found this to be a problem in less than 1 per cent of patients. More sophisticated equipment, such as transaxial tomographic imaging systems with a rotating gamma camera or a multidetector scanning tomograph are necessary for sizing the acute infarction.

For best results, it is essential that the amount of free pertechnetate be kept to an absolute minimum. Poor labeling or rapid breakdown within the vial or syringe will lead to poor clearance of the tracer from the blood pool because of either the presence of free ^{99m}Tc-pertechnetate or excessive labeling of the patient's red blood cells with ^{99m}Tc. Poor clearance will lead to excessive blood pool activity on the scintigrams, resulting in a diffuse myocardial pattern, and may mask underlying focal uptake. Each batch of ^{99m}Tc-pyrophosphate should be tested for labeling efficiency, and free pertechnetate should be less than 1 per cent of the total activity. Once the material is labeled, breakdown will occur with time. It is critical that the radiopharmaceutical be injected shortly after it is prepared.

The specificity of infarct-avid scintigraphy with ^{99m}Tc-pyrophosphate depends on the time intervals between injection and imaging and should be performed at least three hours after the intravenous injection of 10 to 15 mCi of the tracer. When imaging is performed at 90 minutes after injection, there is a high incidence of diffuse blood pool activity, which can lead to a false-positive test for acute infarction. By delaying the imaging time from 90 minutes to three hours, the probability of acute infarction with moderately intense diffuse uptake (greater than or equal to the ribs in intensity) increases from 40 to 75 per cent.[308]

Images are obtained in the anterior, left anterior oblique, and left lateral projections, with at least 400,000 counts collected in each projection. Multiple projections permit accurate localization of the infarct uptake as distinguished from that in overlying bone.

A number of other techniques have also been suggested to improve the specificity of a diffuse pattern. Since the initial distribution of the radiotracer is intravascular, images obtained shortly after injection represent the extent of myocardial blood flow. It may be useful to subtract the initial blood pool image from the final image obtained 3 hours later. If focal myocardial uptake is present, myocardial uptake will involve a smaller area of the myocardium than on the initial blood pool image. Several techniques have been suggested for this purpose, including subjective assessment and computer subtraction.[309,310]

IMAGE INTERPRETATION

THE NORMAL IMAGE. Technetium-99m–pyrophosphate is a bone-seeking radiopharmaceutical. After injection, about half the tracer is extracted by bone and the remainder is excreted through the kidneys. In the normal image, myocardial uptake will be equal to that over the right hemithorax and there will be no identification of a discrete cardiac silhouette (Fig. 11–20). The threshold for abnormal myocardial uptake is controversial, however, and will be described in more detail in the next section. Bone uptake will usually be prominent, with activity in the sternum and anterior ribs seen on all three views. Activity from the thoracolumbar spine will be seen superimposed on the sternum in the anterior view, extending to the left of the sternum on the LAO projection, and forming the border opposite the sternum on the left lateral view. Activity in the scapula may be seen as shine-through on the anterior projection; the inferior tip of the scapula frequently shows disproportionately increased activity compared to

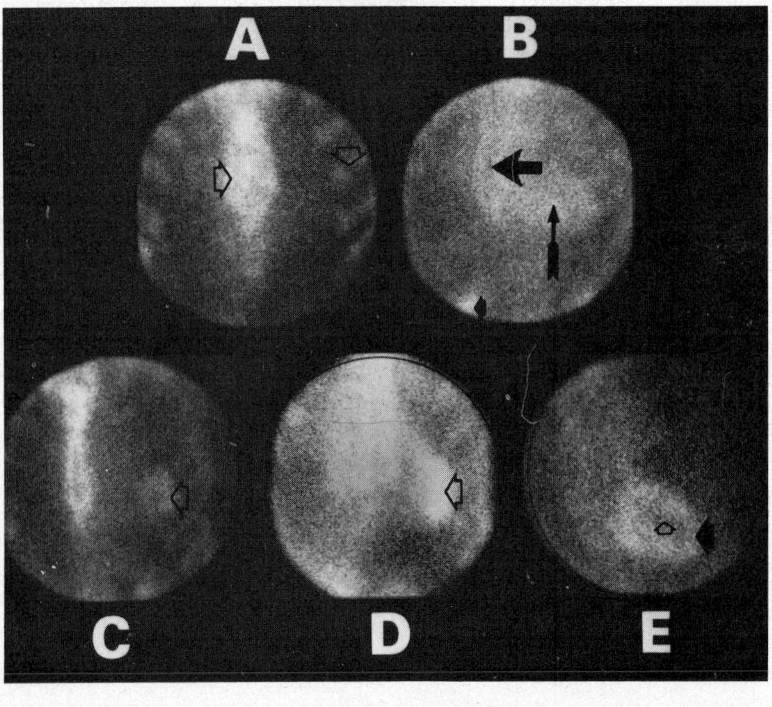

FIGURE 11–20 Scintigraphic classification of myocardial uptake of technetium-99m–pyrophosphate. *A*, Normal (horizontal arrow = sternum; vertical arrow = rib). *B*, Diffuse (upper arrow = sternum; lower arrow = kidney; vertical arrow = myocardial activity). *C*, Focal, less intense than radioactivity in sternum (arrow = focal myocardial activity). *D*, Focal, equal to or greater than radioactivity in sternum (arrow = focal myocardial activity). *E*, Massive (open arrow = central defect due to ventricular cavity; closed arrow = myocardial uptake involving entire left ventricle). (From Holman, B. L., et al.: The prognostic implications of acute myocardial infarct scintigraphy with ^{99m}Tc-pyrophosphate. Circulation *57*:320, 1978, by permission of the American Heart Association, Inc.)

the rest of the bone, and this should not be confused with uptake in the lateral wall of the myocardium.

A number of abdominal structures may be seen on the images. Activity in the renal pelvis may appear as a focal defect and could occasionally be confused with an inferior myocardial infarct, particularly if the kidney lies high in the diaphragm. Activity in the stomach indicates breakdown of the radiopharmaceutical, with free ^{99m}Tc-pertechnetate accumulating in the gastric cells of the antrum. A number of conditions that result in splenic uptake such as infarction, sarcoidosis, tuberculosis, and amyloidosis may be seen occasionally; splenic uptake is usually diffusely distributed throughout the organ and is usually too lateral and posterior to be confused with myocardial uptake. Breast uptake of the radiopharmaceutical has been reported in a wide variety of conditions and may overlie the myocardium, particularly in the anterior projection. Uptake by the breast will be anterior to the sternum and the myocardium on the left lateral projection. Burns to the skin and the underlying chest wall muscle may occur following cardioversion; while superimposition may occur on the anterior view, focal radiotracer uptake will be anterior to the sternum and to the myocardium on the left lateral view. Calcification of the costochondral junctions or the cartilaginous structures of the rib cage may result in focal uptake overlying the myocardial silhouette. While uptake in overlying rib may make interpretation difficult in a small minority of patients, only rarely will rib uptake be confused with myocardial uptake, and again, multiple images in various projections can be used to differentiate the two.

THE ABNORMAL IMAGE. A number of grading systems have been suggested for interpreting the abnormal image. Most systems are based on a grading of 0 to 4+.[281] A grade of 0 means that there is no activity in the heart and indicates a negative myocardial scintigram. A grade of 1+ represents questionable but not definite activity and is also considered to be a negative scintigraphic result. A grade of 2+ indicates definite but faint activity and an abnormal myocardial scintigram, while definite and increased activity within the myocardial image is associated with grades 3+ and 4+. In scintiscans considered to be positive (2+, 3+, and 4+), the area of increased activity (anterior, inferior, lateral, or true posterior) is also described.

Although this classification has proved useful, it suffers from several shortcomings. Grading is highly subjective and prone to interobserver error. Moreover, it does not take into account the difference in accuracy when uptake is focal or diffuse. Several alternative grading systems have been suggested to correct for these limitations.[311] In those that retain the 0 to 4+ grading, the grades are made more objective by differentiating 2+ as activity less than that in the adjacent ribs, 3+ as activity equal to that in adjacent ribs, and 4+ as activity greater than that in adjacent ribs.

A distinction must be made between *diffuse* and *focal* activity. Diffuse uptake will appear as relatively homogeneous radiotracer activity throughout the myocardium, including both ventricles and often the great vessels. Activity frequently extends to the right of the sternum; left ventricular activity does not appear as a photon-deficient area, as would be the case if the activity were primarily in the myocardial walls. In diffuse uptake, activity is most often due to persistent radiotracer in the blood pool resulting from poor renal clearance, as may occur in impaired renal function; a particularly large left ventricular end-diastolic volume, as may occur in congestive heart failure and cardiomyopathies; and red blood cell labeling, as may occur in breakdown of the radiopharmaceutical. The specificity of the diffuse pattern for the diagnosis of acute myocardial infarction is poor.

Because the specificity of the diffuse pattern depends on the time after injection and the intensity of the pattern, we suggest the following grading system when imaging is performed 3 or more hours after injection (Fig. 11–20):

Normal (No identification of the discrete cardiac silhouette): Myocardial uptake that is equal to that over the right hemithorax.

Mild Diffuse (Low probability of acute myocardial infarction): Myocardial uptake exceeding that over the right hemithorax but less intense than that over the ribs and distributed over most or all of the myocardium.

Moderate Diffuse (Indeterminant for the diagnosis of acute infarction): Myocardial uptake equally or more intense than that over the ribs but less intense than that over the sternum.

Focal (High probability of acute infarction): Discrete myocardial uptake.

Massive (High probability of acute myocardial infarction): An increase in myocardial uptake that involves 50 per cent or more of the cardiac silhouette and is equally or more intense than uptake over the sternum. Most often there is a focal central area of decreased activity due either to the left ventricular cavity or to central necrosis.

When myocardial uptake is focal, it can be localized to one or more segments of the myocardial wall from an analysis of the scintigrams obtained in multiple projections. In patients with *anterior myocardial infarcts*, uptake involves much of the left ventricular silhouette on the anterior view; in the left lateral view, the uptake appears as a thin band directly behind the sternum, since the anterior free wall of the left ventricle is being viewed tangentially in this projection (Fig. 11–21). In patients with inferior myocardial infarction, the radiotracer appears curvilinear, usually extending from the lower portion of the sternum laterally toward the ribs on the anterior projection and from the lower portion of the sternum approximately two-thirds of the way toward the vertebrae on the left lateral view. *Inferior infarcts* are always imaged perpendicular to the collimator. The true extent of an inferior infarct can be appreciated only with the aid of single-photon transaxial tomography. *Lateral infarcts* are seen perpendicular to the collimator on the anterior view, usually lying directly under the anterior rib ends and well away from the sternum. Lateral infarcts are seen in their greatest extent on the left lateral or left anterior oblique projections. *Apical infarcts* usually result from uptake in several adjacent walls, usually the inferior and lateral or distal anterior and lateral walls. *Posterior infarction* is usually seen in conjunction with inferior wall uptake and is seen best in the left lateral projection extending superiorly and posteriorly from the inferior wall. Occasionally posterior uptake may be seen in isolation. *Right ventricular uptake* is most often seen in conjunction with inferior left ventricular activity and is appreciated best when there is also uptake in the inferior portion of the left ventricular septum. In this case, the right ventricular activity appears to the right of the septum and inferior wall. The activity may extend horizontally or at various angles from the inferior wall from a horizontal to an almost vertical orientation, depending on the ana-

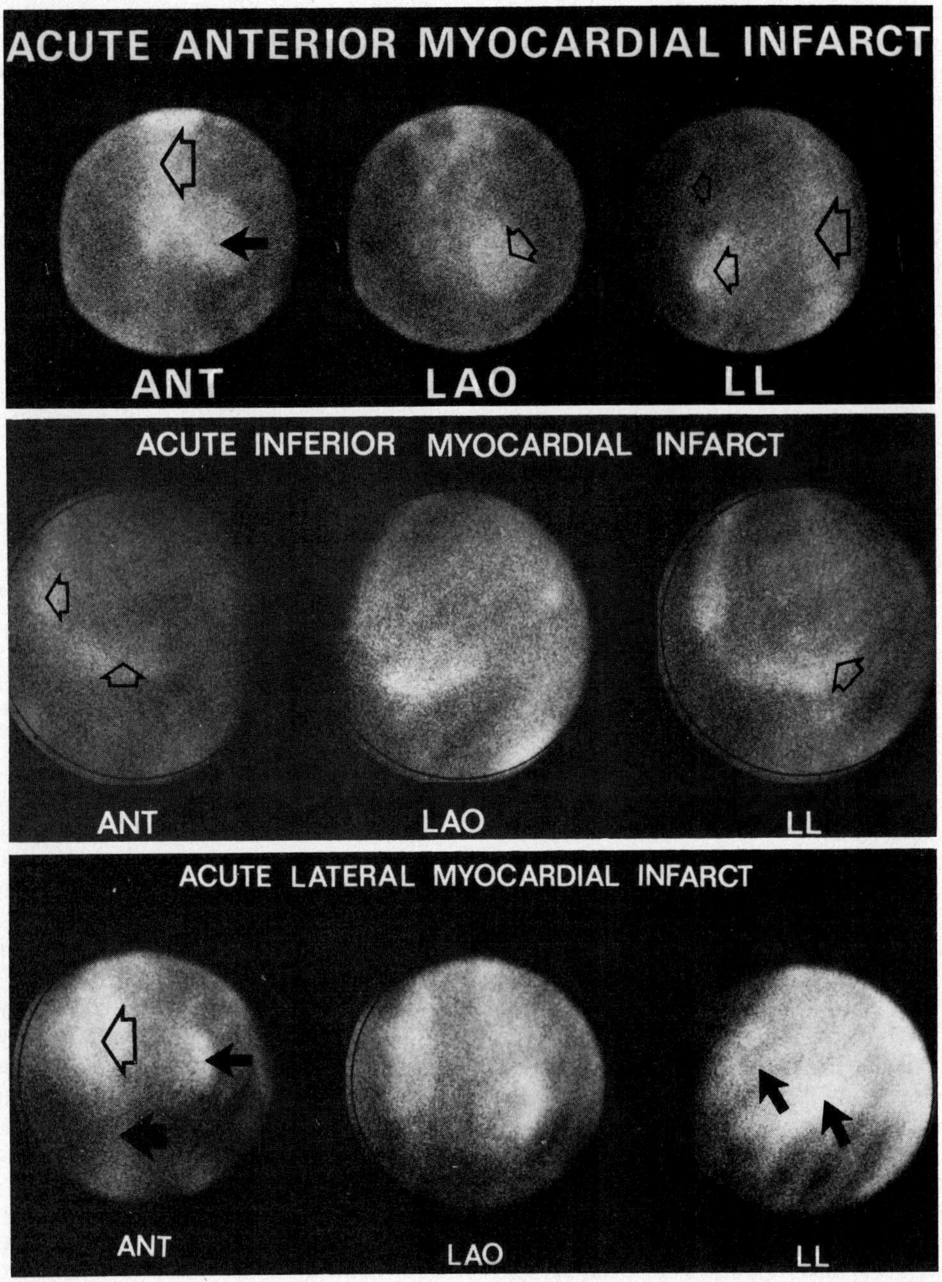

FIGURE 11–21 *A,* Myocardial scintigraphy with ^{99m}Tc-pyrophosphate in patients with acute anterior myocardial infarct. *Anterior*: Open arrow = sternum; arrow = myocardial uptake. *Left anterior oblique*: Arrow = myocardial activity. *Left lateral*: Upper arrow = sternum; lower arrow = myocardial activity; large arrow = vertebrae. *B,* Scintigrams of a patient with acute inferior myocardial infarction. *Anterior*: Upper arrow = sternum; lower arrow = myocardial activity. *Left lateral*: Note posterior wall extension (arrow). *C,* Myocardial scintigraphy in a patient with acute lateral myocardial infarct. *Anterior*: Open arrow = sternum; lower arrow = vertebrae; upper arrow = myocardial activity. *Left lateral*: Upper arrow = ribs; lower arrow = myocardial activity.

tomical position of the right ventricle and of the right ventricular free wall (Fig. 11–22).

In patients with large anteroseptal or anterolateral or circumferential left ventricular infarcts, the pattern of uptake is massive, and in most of these patients, the scintigraphic appearance has been described as a *doughnut pattern* with intense uptake along the borders and relatively diminished intensity in the center. This pattern can be explained in two ways: First, patients presenting with this pattern have large infarcts, and animal data suggest that the central portion of the infarct takes up relatively less radiotracer than do the peripheral zones because of diminished perfusion and decreased radiotracer delivery.[288] Second, even in patients with large myocardial infarcts who present with the doughnut pattern, radiotracer uptake may be uniform throughout the area of tissue necrosis.[292] The explanation for the doughnut pattern in these patients—and perhaps, to some extent, in all patients exhibiting this pattern—is that the intensity in any region is equal to the concentration of the tracer times the weight of the tissue within the field of view. The weight of tissue is considerable in the field of view where the left ventricular wall is being imaged tangentially and where the wall is parallel to the collimator. The weight of tissue is less where the wall is parallel to the detector. Thus, a ^{99m}Tc-pyrophosphate scan in a patient with a large left ventricular infarct has a central photopenic zone similar to the one found in a normal thallium-201 scan.

While most subendocardial and many transmural infarcts will appear normal on infarct-avid scintigraphy after the first week, many transmural infarcts will show persistent accumulation of the radiotracer for considerable periods of time after the initial episode, even when extension or reinfarction has not been documented.[312] In approxi-

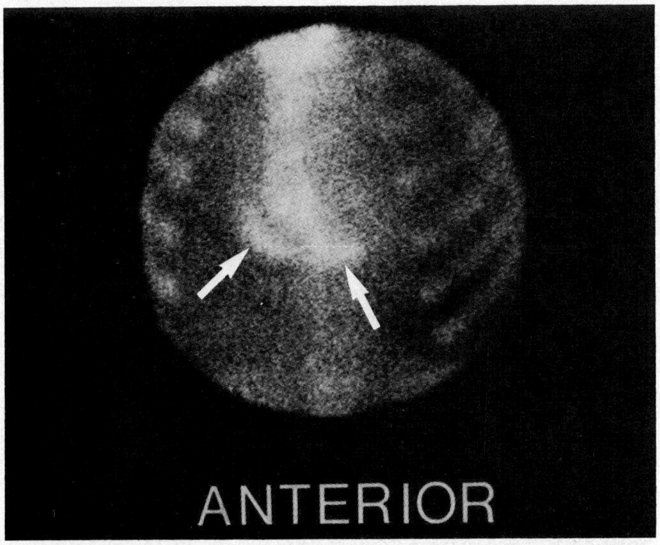

FIGURE 11–22 Infarct-avid scintigraphy with ^{99m}Tc-pyrophosphate in a patient with an acute inferior wall infarct (right arrow) with extensive right ventricular extension (left arrow).

mately 40 per cent of patients with acute myocardial infarction, activity will persist beyond the first several weeks, the intensity of uptake will gradually diminish, and the appearance and the distribution of the radiotracer will appear more diffuse than on the initial scintigrams obtained several days after infarction.

Focal uptake may also be seen in patients with valvular calcifications,[313] repeated high-energy direct-current (DC) cardioversions,[314] ventricular aneurysms,[315] myocardial contusion,[316] and metastatic carcinoma to the heart (Table 11–1). Since myocardial scintigraphy with ^{99m}Tc-pyrophosphate would be a useful technique for examining patients after resuscitation to detect acute infarction, initial case reports and animal studies that reported significant myocardial uptake after DC cardioversion in the absence of ischemic heart disease were discouraging.[314] When patients were studied systematically following cardiopulmonary resuscitation with cardioversion, however, the incidence of pyrophosphate uptake in patients without myocardial infarction was only 13 per cent.[317] With an imaging accuracy of 80 per cent, it would appear that false-positive scintiscans after electrical cardioversion occur infrequently. Similarly, valvular calcification must be extensive, and focal uptake without evidence of infarction is unusual in such patients. Focal uptake in patients with ventricular aneurysms may represent calcification within the aneurysm, or, as in patients with recent infarction, persistent and ongoing cellular necrosis and damage. Pericarditis alone does not result in increased uptake of pyrophosphate.[318] One exception is the hypercalcemic patient with pericardial calcification.[319]

TABLE 11–1 CAUSES OF ^{99m}TC-PYROPHOSPHATE UPTAKE

Focal	Diffuse
Acute myocardial infarction	Acute myocardial infarction† (subendocardial)
Recent myocardial infarction	Unstable angina pectoris†
Breast tumors	Cardiomyopathy†
Left ventricular aneurysms	Left ventricular aneurysms
Rib fractures	Persistent blood pool activity
Skeletal muscle damage	Myocarditis
Cardioversion (secondary to skeletal muscle as well as myocardial damage)*	
Valvular calcification*	
Myocardial contusion	
Skin lesions*	
Calcified costal cartilage	

*Unusual.
†Due to blood pool activity.

Diffuse patterns of increased uptake of ^{99m}Tc-pyrophosphate have been observed in patients with nontransmural acute myocardial infarction, idiopathic cardiomyopathy,[320] unstable angina pectoris,[321] and stable angina pectoris[320,322] and in patients with no apparent heart disease. The high incidence of diffuse uptake in nontransmural infarction and its occurrence in many other conditions suggest that the primary cause for the diffuse pattern is persistent blood pool activity. Most patients with nontransmural infarction have focal necrosis, and even in those patients with global subendocardial infarction, an area of reduced radioactivity corresponding to the left ventricular cavity is rarely seen.[318] This pattern would be observed if the uptake were primarily in the left ventricular wall,[292] but it is seen only in patients with massive transmural infarcts. Persistent blood pool activity is seen when imaging is performed too soon after injection. It occurs in patients with poor renal function, cardiac enlargement, and reduced ejection fraction. Some patients may have persistent blood pool activity without apparent explanation. In these patients, there is probably some dissociation of the ^{99m}Tc from the pyrophosphate, with subsequent binding to either a protein or a red blood cell fraction. Drugs may also cause increased retention of the label within the vascular compartment. This probably accounts for the reports of diffusely abnormal pyrophosphate scans in patients with adriamycin toxicity. Patients who receive this drug have altered tracer kinetics with increased activity outside of the intravascular component when in vivo labeling of red blood cells is performed with ^{99m}Tc-pertechnetate after pyrophosphate injection. Also, blood clearance is delayed when ^{99m}Tc-pyrophosphate is used for myocardial scintigraphy. Other interactions between drugs and radiotracers probably occur as well.

It is possible, however, that processes that affect the myocardium diffusely, resulting in tissue necrosis, may cause diffuse myocardial uptake. One such example has been demonstrated in an animal model of experimental viral myopericarditis. Extensive experience with pyrophosphate imaging in myocarditis in humans has not yet been reported.[323] Similarly, processes that result in extensive calcification within the myocardium may result in diffuse uptake of pyrophosphate. Such a pattern has been reported with amyloidosis.[324]

ASSESSMENT OF THE METHOD

The sensitivity of myocardial scintigraphy with ^{99m}Tc-pyrophosphate for the detection of acute myocardial infarction depends on a number of factors, including the criteria used for interpretation of the images and patient selection. In most large series in which patients were selected either at random or sequentially, the sensitivity of the technique was high. In 24 different series—a total of 1143 patients with documented acute myocardial infarcts—pyrophosphate scans were abnormal in 89 per cent.[308] In a similar group of 19 different series, which included a total of 1482 patients with no evidence of acute infarction, ^{99m}Tc-pyrophosphate scans were normal in 86 per cent.[308] The composite results indicate a false-negative rate of 11 per cent and a false-positive rate of 14 per cent.

These results may be deceiving, however. The low incidence of false-positive results may be attributable to the patient mix, which frequently included a spectrum of chest pain syndromes. The diagnostic problem that is usually faced, however, is in distinguishing unstable angina pectoris from acute infarction. Many patients with unstable angina have abnormal scintiscans. Among 374 patients with a clinical diagnosis of unstable angina pectoris and without clinical evidence of acute infarction, 152 (41 per cent) had positive ^{99m}Tc-pyrophosphate scans.[308]

It has generally been assumed that abnormal scintiscans obtained in patients with unstable angina pectoris represent false-positive results. However, in a small series of patients with unstable angina pectoris or symptomatic ischemic heart disease after myocardial infarction, those patients with abnormal scintigrams were found to have histopathological evidence of multifocal irreversible damage at autopsy.[325] Of those patients with clinical evidence of unstable angina pectoris studied by means of both ^{99m}Tc-pyrophosphate and sequential determination of serum MB-band creatine kinase (MB-CK) activity, total plasma CK and MB-CK activity was elevated in 22 of 36 patients with abnormal images.[326] These studies suggest that, at least in some patients with unstable angina and abnormal scintigrams, underlying tissue necrosis accounts for the uptake of pyrophosphate. Furthermore, patients with abnormal images but without clinical evidence of acute infarction have a poorer prognosis than do those with normal scintigrams (i.e., complication rates of 22 and 5 per cent, respectively).[327]

Another diagnostic problem that is overlooked when composite results are reported is the difference in sensitivity between transmural and nontransmural infarction. Infarct scintigraphy with ^{99m}Tc-pyrophosphate is most sensitive in patients with transmural infarction. However, these patients can usually be diagnosed without the aid of infarct scintigraphy. It is in patients with nontransmural infarction that the diagnosis is frequently in doubt at the time of admission. The diagnosis of nontransmural infarction may be difficult to confirm because the accompanying electrocardiographic changes may be nonspecific. Nontransmural infarction frequently occurs during surgery or in other clinical settings characterized by hemodynamic instability. Furthermore, when patients present with nonspecific ST-segment or T-wave abnormalities several days after a prolonged episode of pain, it may be impossible to establish the diagnosis of acute myocardial infarction using currently available cardiac enzyme techniques.

Although initial reports suggested that myocardial scintigraphy with ^{99m}Tc-pyrophosphate was a very sensitive method for detecting nontransmural myocardial infarction, more recent evidence suggests a substantially lower accuracy.[311] The sensitivity of the technique is high in patients with nontransmural infarction if one is willing to accept a correspondingly low specificity, since approximately 50 per cent of these patients show diffuse uptake that is indistinguishable from that seen in many patients with unstable angina pectoris but without clinical evidence of infarction. When rigid criteria are used and faint diffuse uptake is considered to be a normal finding, the sensitivity for the detection of nontransmural infarction has not been found to be as high as was initially reported. Recent studies report focal uptake in only 40 to 60 per cent of these patients.[326–328]

The incidence of diffuse uptake in patients with nontransmural infarction may be dependent on the spatial resolution of the imaging equipment. Recent studies suggest a lower incidence of diffuse uptake than has been reported previously. Massie et al. found diffuse uptake in only 19 per cent of patients with nontransmural infarction and in 10 per cent of those with stable angina pectoris,[329] whereas Jaffe et al. found focal uptake of pyrophosphate in more than 95 per cent of patients with unstable angina pectoris and elevated MB-CK activity.[326]

The failure of ^{99m}Tc-pyrophosphate scintigraphy to return to normal within one to two weeks in the majority of patients with acute infarction limits the specificity of the technique in patients with recent myocardial infarction and recurrent symptoms. In those patients with infarction and recurrent symptoms, a single study at the time when reinfarction is suspected is of value only if it is negative or intensely positive, since persistently faint or moderately intense uptake may be due to the initial infarct. Sequential scintigraphy is of value if the scintigraphic pattern follows a classic course after the recurrent symptoms. If the intensity of pyrophosphate uptake increases for the first 48 to 72 hours following the development of recurrent symptoms, with a subsequent rapid decrease in intensity, the probability of reinfarction is high. In all other cases, recurrent myocardial infarction cannot be distinguished from recent infarction without a baseline study at the time of initial infarction.

CLINICAL APPLICATIONS

Myocardial scintigraphy with ^{99m}Tc-pyrophosphate is useful in patients with *suspected acute infarction* in whom other clinical and laboratory evidence is nondiagnostic. Thus, scintigraphy is very helpful in patients who present more than 24 hours after the onset of symptoms when very sensitive serum enzyme tests such as MB-band CK may have returned to normal. The probability of acute infarction is high in patients with focal uptake, provided an infarction has not occurred within 6 to 12 months of the acute event. The size and persistence of uptake may provide predictive information as well. Usefulness of the test in the presence of moderately intense diffuse uptake is limited, however. Myocardial scintigraphy can be used to diagnose *right ventricular infarction.* Although an elevation in right ventricular filling pressure may indicate right ventricular involvement, it may also occur in the presence of cor pulmonale. Myocardial scintigraphy with ^{99m}Tc-pyrophosphate provides more direct evidence of acute infarction of the right ventricle.[330]

This technique is also of value in evaluating patients following coronary bypass surgery (Fig. 11–23). The diagnosis of myocardial infarction after cardiac surgery is complicated because chest pain, elevated enzyme levels, and

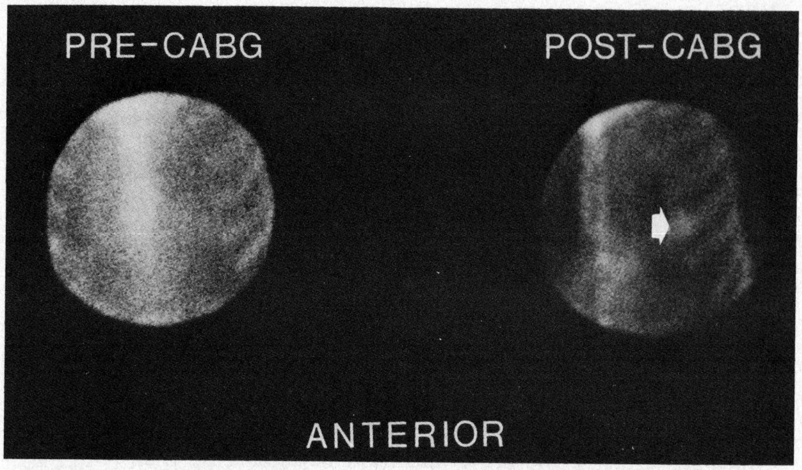

FIGURE 11–23 Infarct-avid scintigraphy with ^{99m}Tc-pyrophosphate in a patient who sustained an intraoperative infarct during coronary artery bypass graft surgery. PRE-CABG = faint diffuse myocardial uptake prior to surgery; POST-CABG = focal apical uptake of the radiotracer (arrow) in the location of the intraoperative infarct.

electrocardiographic changes may result from the operation itself.[331] Infarction occurs in about 10 per cent of these patients, however. ^{99m}Tc-pyrophosphate scintigraphy is accurate in the postoperative patient.[332,333] The importance of preoperative scintigraphy for comparison is controversial. A significant number of patients undergoing bypass surgery will have positive infarct scintigrams preoperatively.[334] In order to interpret postoperative scintigraphy in patients who suffered an infarction within one year prior to the operation, we recommend a baseline study be obtained for comparison.

Extension of an infarction or reinfarction can be determined if a baseline scintigram is available. For example, it has been observed that the abnormalities on infarct scintigraphy may become more prominent in the absence of clinically suspected infarct extension during the first 24 to 48 hours after the onset of symptoms. If serial infarct scintigrams are obtained, certain sequential abnormalities are suggestive of infarct extension. Reinfarction is likely if there is a marked increase in the size of the scintigraphic abnormality observed during the baseline examination, reappearance of an abnormality that has cleared, or appearance of a regional abnormality in an area that was previously normal.

Infarct-avid scintigraphy is useful in patients who develop symptoms suggestive of acute myocardial infarction after heavy exercise. For example, serum creatine kinase activity, including that of the MB isoenzyme fraction, is elevated in marathon runners because of skeletal muscle necrosis. Imaging with ^{99m}Tc-pyrophosphate may be useful to exclude myocardial infarction and to localize the site of tissue necrosis.[335] Similarly, scintigraphic imaging may define the extent of muscle necrosis after electrical injury.

The scintigraphic pattern of myocardial uptake provides clues to the patient's future course, both in the hospital and over the long term.[327] The complication rate, particularly during hospitalization, is directly related to the extent of uptake of pyrophosphate in patients with acute infarction (Fig. 11–24). In fact, in patients with clinical evidence of infarction and small foci of ^{99m}Tc-pyrophosphate myocardial uptake (less than 16 cm^2), complication rates are comparable to those in patients without acute infarction. On the other hand, when the extent of uptake is moderate (16 to 40 cm^2), morbidity is high (67 per cent). When the extent of uptake is considerable (greater than 40 cm^2), mortality is high (87 per cent).

A number of other observations that reflect the extent and intensity of pyrophosphate uptake also have prognostic value. In one study, 67 per cent of patients with a doughnut pattern developed left ventricular failure with infarction.[336] In another series, late complications developed in all patients with the doughnut pattern, compared with 43 per cent of the patients with focal uptake and 12 per cent of those with diffuse uptake.[337] Persistently positive

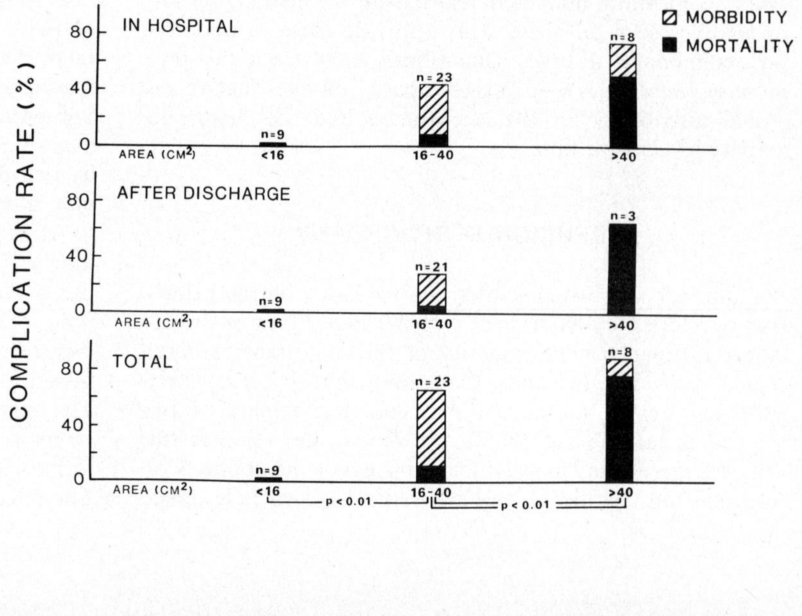

FIGURE 11–24 Complication rates versus area of technetium-99m–pyrophosphate uptake in patients with acute myocardial infarction and patterns C, D, and E. (Single bracket designates complication rate; double bracket designates mortality rate.) (From Holman, B. L., et al.: The prognostic implications of acute myocardial infarct scintigraphy with ^{99m}Tc-pyrophosphate. Circulation *57*:320, 1978, by permission of the American Heart Association, Inc.)

^{99m}Tc-pyrophosphate scintigrams also correlate with mortality and morbidity[295] and with elevated pulmonary artery pressure.[338]

The past decade has seen considerable interest in the concept of infarct size reduction (p. 1318). Since the incidence of pump failure is related directly to the extent of myocardial necrosis, and since at least some of the myocardium at risk may be salvageable during the early hours after infarction, a wide range of therapeutic interventions has been suggested to attempt to limit the size of an infarct. To determine the efficacy of such interventions, accurate quantification of infarct size is necessary. Myocardial scintigraphy with ^{99m}Tc-pyrophosphate allows direct visualization of the necrotic myocardium and may therefore permit accurate estimation of infarct size.

Accurate sizing of the acute infarction be measuring the extent of radiotracer uptake is limited by the geometrical constraints of standard two-dimensional imaging. Single-photon–emission computed tomography provides a three-dimensional map of radionuclide distribution and may yield more accurate assessments of infarct size. Initial studies in an animal model have demonstrated a good correlation between infarct size and measured uptake of ^{99m}Tc-pyrophosphate.[339]

Emission tomography can be performed in humans and provides a three-dimensional map of ^{99m}Tc-pyrophosphate uptake within the heart.[340] In patients with acute anterior infarction, uptake is seen within the anterior wall of the left ventricle, frequently involving the septum (Fig. 11–25). In patients with acute inferior infarction, uptake may occur in the posterior wall of the right ventricle, posterior septum, and posterolateral wall of the left ventricle as well. The advantages of tomography over other methods for infarct sizing is that imaging need be performed only once between 1 and 10 days after infarction. Serum enzyme analysis requires frequent sampling beginning hours after the onset of symptoms. This approach appears to be promising for quantitatively estimating infarct size in humans, especially when coupled with thallium-201 to assess the volume of perfused myocardium.

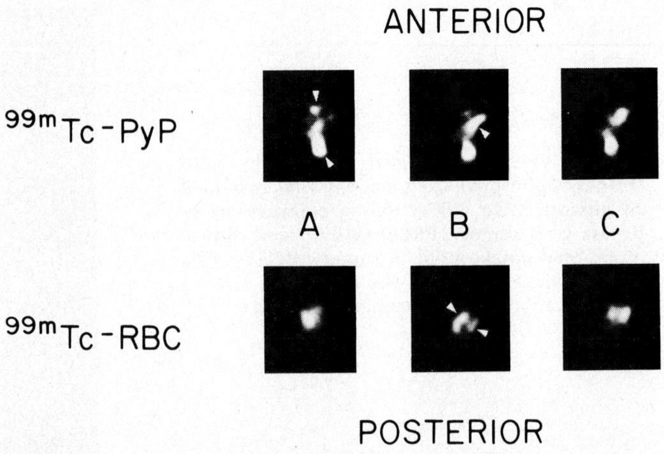

FIGURE 11–25 Transaxial tomograms obtained with technetium-99m pyrophosphate (upper panels) and technetium-99m red blood cells (lower panels) of a patient with an acute anteroseptal infarct. In upper frame A, upper arrow indicates the sternum and lower arrow indicates the spine. In upper frame B, arrow indicates ^{99m}Tc-pyrophosphate uptake in the anterior wall of the left ventricle and the septum. In lower frame B, the upper arrow indicates the right ventricular cavity and the lower arrow indicates the left ventricular cavity. A = transaxial plane corresponding to base of left ventricle; B = midventricle; C = apex.

PULMONARY SCINTIGRAPHY

Pulmonary scintigraphy is a safe, noninvasive method for evaluating regional myocardial perfusion and ventilation. It has been applied most widely in the diagnosis of pulmonary embolism. The radionuclide image provides a map of regional pulmonary perfusion or ventilation. Many abnormalities appear as areas of decreased isotopic uptake on the scan. The presence or absence of these areas, their size and location, and their relationship to anatomical abnormalities seen on chest x-rays provide clues to underlying pulmonary disease. Quantification of regional pulmonary function is also possible based on the relative regional distribution of the radiotracers and the change in activity levels with time.

PERFUSION SCINTIGRAPHY

Pulmonary perfusion scintigraphy is based on the principles developed by Sapirstein: regional blood flow is directly proportional to the quantity of the radiotracer in that region provided (a) that the radiotracer is completely extracted by the tissue, (b) that complete mixing of the tracer has taken place within the blood, and (c) that the radiotracer remains in the tissue and is not metabolized or released from the tissue.[341] When radioactive particles larger in size than the diameter of a pulmonary capillary are injected intravenously, they are mixed in the right side of the heart and are then trapped by the capillary and precapillary vasculature. As a result, the quantity of radioactivity in any region of the lung—and hence the activity emanating from that region—is directly proportional to blood flow to that region.

A number of agents have been used to determine regional pulmonary perfusion by means of the particle-entrapment technique.[342] The first material used clinically was macroaggregated albumin (MAA) labeled with iodine-131. Subsequently, indium-labeled iron hydroxide aggregates came into use and, more recently, technetium-labeled iron hydroxide aggregates, macroaggregated albumin, and human albumin microspheres.

At the present time, either ^{99m}Tc–macroaggregated albumin or ^{99m}Tc–human albumin microspheres are in common use. ^{99m}Tc-microspheres provide a more uniform particle size than other ^{99m}Tc-labeled particles;[343] on the other hand, macroaggregated albumin has been associated with fewer instances of allergic reactions than have the microspheres.[344] The aggregated albumin particles are between 10 and 40 microns in diameter; the albumin microspheres are more uniform in size and are between 20 and 40 microns in diameter. The particles break up slowly after entrapment in the lung;

their biological half-life is approximately 7 hours in normal patients and somewhat longer in patients with pulmonary embolism or parenchymal lung disease. The fragments are then removed from the circulation by the reticuloendothelial system.

Perfusion scintigraphy is a safe procedure with a very low incidence of side effects. It has been estimated that less than 0.1 per cent of the pulmonary capillaries are occluded when 200,000 to 500,000 particles are injected. Iatrogenic impairment of lung function is unlikely, even when the organ is severely compromised by disease, because of the sparsity of occlusion and rich collateral circulation.[345,346] No change is observed in pulmonary diffusing capacity after injection of the radiopharmaceutical,[347] although fatal reactions have been reported to occur after the labeled particles were administered to patients with severe pulmonary hypertension.[348]

Images are obtained, using a standard high-resolution gamma camera, in the right and left lateral, right and left posterior oblique, and anterior and posterior positions. The posterior oblique views have been recently incorporated into the imaging regimen because they provide better delineation of the posterior and lateral basal segments of the lower lobes and eliminate much of the overlapping radioactivity seen from the opposite lung on lateral views.[349] At least 400,000 to 600,000 counts should be obtained in each view. The two lateral views should be imaged for the same time rather than for the same counts; similarly, the two oblique views should be imaged for the same time.

In the normal perfusion lung scintiscan there is uniform distribution of activity throughout the lung, with increasing radioactivity seen from the anterior to the posterior projection if the patient is injected while supine (Fig. 11–26). The margins of the lung's radioactivity are smooth and correspond to the lung outline seen on the chest radiograph. The heart and mediastinal structures produce a midline defect extending to the left, particularly on the anterior view. The heart is usually not seen on the posterior view unless it is enlarged. Occasionally, the aortic notch produces a defect in the midline, particularly when it is tortuous. Diminished perfusion may be seen in the region of an azygos lobe.[350] More subtle changes occur with changes in the position of the diaphragm, particularly if there is central eventration. In patients with diaphragmatic paralysis and those who are very obese, basilar defects in the perfusion scan may cause confusion at times.

Of the pathological conditions that can interfere with regional lung perfusion, the most important are those involving the pulmonary arterial vasculature. These include primary diseases of the pulmonary arteries, either congenital (atresia) or acquired (arteritis); extraluminal compression by interstitial fluid, tumors, lymph nodes, or other mediastinal structures; and intraluminal filling by tumor, fat, air, parasites, amniotic fluid, or blood clots.

Parenchymal diseases (inflammatory, malignant) and extrapulmonic displacement of lung tissue due to pleural effusion or cardiomegaly also compromise regional lung perfusion. Intrapulmonary shunting caused by regional hypoxia diverts blood flow and therefore radioactive particles away from that portion of the lung. Shunts from the bronchial to the pulmonary arteries in bronchiectasis and some bronchogenic carcinomas also keep the particles away from the affected areas.[351] Although clinical attention has focused primarily on the value of pulmonary scintigraphy in detecting thromboembolic disease, it is important to remember that other conditions can interfere with regional perfusion, leading to abnormal scans.

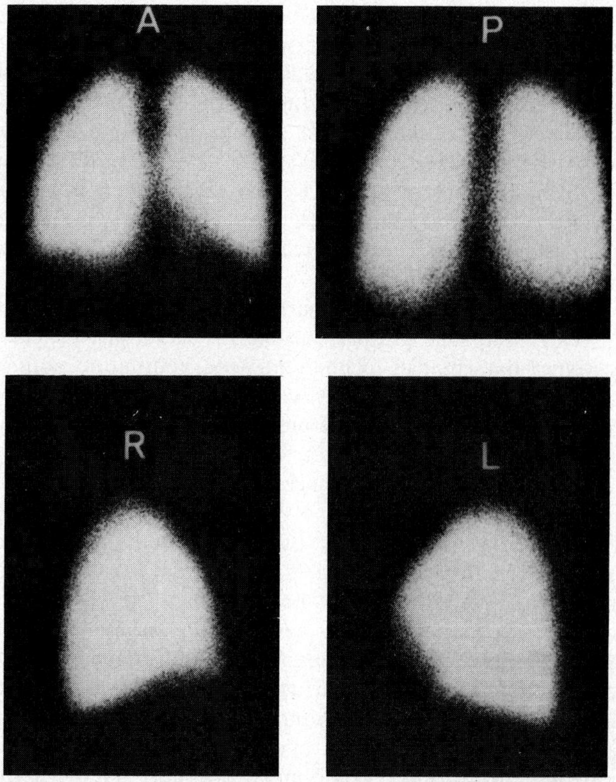

FIGURE 11–26 Normal pulmonary perfusion scintiscan. The distribution of tracer is relatively homogeneous but with a decreasing gradient toward the apex due to decreasing lung volume, an increasing gradient toward the dependent portion of the lung (posterior if injected supine) due to gravitational effects on perfusion, and no radioactivity in the mediastinum. (A = anterior view; P = posterior view; R = right lateral view; L = left lateral view.)

VENTILATION SCINTIGRAPHY

Ventilation scintigraphy is a helpful maneuver in distinguishing between primary perfusion abnormalities and those secondary to regional hypoxia.[352,353] Regional ventilation is usually assessed using the inert gas xenon-133. The maneuver can be performed before perfusion scintigraphy, in which case imaging is performed in the posterior projection. Alternatively, ventilation imaging can be performed after perfusion scintigraphy, in which case the physician has the flexibility to choose the projection to be used for imaging. If ventilation is assessed after perfusion scintigraphy, there is substantial scattered radiation within the xenon-133 energy window due to the higher energy technetium-99m. This interference must be overcome by using higher doses of xenon-133.

Areas of poor ventilation represent deficits in activity on the initial breathholding scintiscan, while regions of relatively increased activity indicate abnormal ventilation during the washout phase. The abnormal retention of xenon during the washout phase is due to air-trapping. The initial breathholding study alone is insufficient because patients with parenchymal disease may have normal ventilation in areas of reduced perfusion on the single-breath image but will trap xenon during the washout phase.[354] When initial breathholding imaging is used alone, without the washout phase of the study, the specificity for detection of pulmonary embolism is only 80 per cent; however, when the additional information obtained from the washout phase of the study is added, the specificity increases to over 90 per cent.

A number of other radiopharmaceuticals have been used for ventilation scintigraphy. Xenon-127 has a photon energy higher than that of technetium-99m. Ventilation scintigraphy can therefore be performed after perfusion imaging with far less interference from technetium-99m. At the present time, xenon-127 is not widely available; it is expensive and requires recycling because of its costs and long half-life.

An alternative approach uses the rubidium-81/krypton-81m generator. The patient inhales krypton-81m during normal respiration.[355,356] Because the primary photopeak of krypton-81m is 190 kev, higher spatial resolution can be obtained than with xenon-133, and imaging can be performed following the perfusion study with little scattered radiation from technetium-99m. The primary disadvantage of this radiotracer—one that will severely limit its implementation in the community hospital—is the short half-life of its parent compound, rubidium-81 (4 hours). Since the physical half-life of this radiotracer is very short (13 seconds), the continual inhalation of krypton-81m results in images that depict the balance between regional ventilation and radioactive decay of the tracer. After about 30 seconds of inhalation, a steady state is reached, and the activity represents the distribution of tidal ventilation.[356] Thus, information contained in a single krypton-81m ventilation scan is only a crude representation of regional ventilation. The short time required for imaging, its simplicity, and the low absorbed radiation dose enable serial high-resolution images of ventilatory flow to be obtained in multiple views. However, because of the short half-life, washout studies cannot be obtained.

PULMONARY EMBOLISM

(See also p. 1586)

The single most important application of pulmonary scintigraphy is in the diagnosis of pulmonary embolism. The clinical manifestations of pulmonary embolism are frequently vague and nonspecific[357] (p. 1586). The most frequent signs and symptoms are tachypnea (92 per cent), dyspnea (81 per cent), pleuritic chest pain (72 per cent), apprehension (59 per cent), cough (54 per cent), and rales (53 per cent). Signs and symptoms more specific for the diagnosis of pulmonary embolism occur much less frequently. For example, hemoptysis is seen in only 34 per cent of patients, cyanosis in 18 per cent, and thrombophlebitis in 33 per cent.

The value of pulmonary scintigraphy in detecting acute pulmonary emboli is based, in part, on its high sensitivity, since a normal lung scan virtually rules out clinically significant pulmonary emboli within the previous 48 hours.[358] Theoretically, microemboli might produce perfusion defects beyond the resolution of present instrumentation, or clots in the central pulmonary artery that only partially occlude the lumen might not affect regional blood flow. Nevertheless, a well-documented case of acute pulmonary embolism with a technically adequate normal perfusion scan obtained within 48 hours of the onset of symptoms has yet to be recorded.

The abnormal scintigram presents more of a problem. Diagnostic information must be garnered from clues derived from the anatomical distribution of the perfusion defects, the relationship between the degree of impairment in regional perfusion and ventilation, and the stability of the perfusion defects over time. In general, acute pulmonary emboli produce sharply delineated polysegmental or lobar defects (Fig. 11–27).[359] These are unlike the anatomically less well-defined defects seen in chronic lung disease. A large proportion of patients with lobar defects have pulmonary embolism, for example.[360,361] On the other hand, subsegmental defects are the predominant perfusion abnormality in only a small fraction of patients with clinically apparent pulmonary embolism. Unilateral absence of perfusion is not pathognomonic of pulmonary embolism; it is also seen in bronchogenic carcinoma, the hyperlucent emphysematous lung, and pulmonary artery atresia.

Most patients with pulmonary emboli have multiple perfusion defects. In one series, for example, only 16 of 104 patients with abnormal lung scintigrams had single perfusion defects.[360] Of these, only three were present in patients with pulmonary embolism. Thus, 93 per cent of patients with pulmonary emboli have multiple perfusion defects. In patients with multiple perfusion defects, 52 per cent of patients with pulmonary embolism have perfusion defects in-

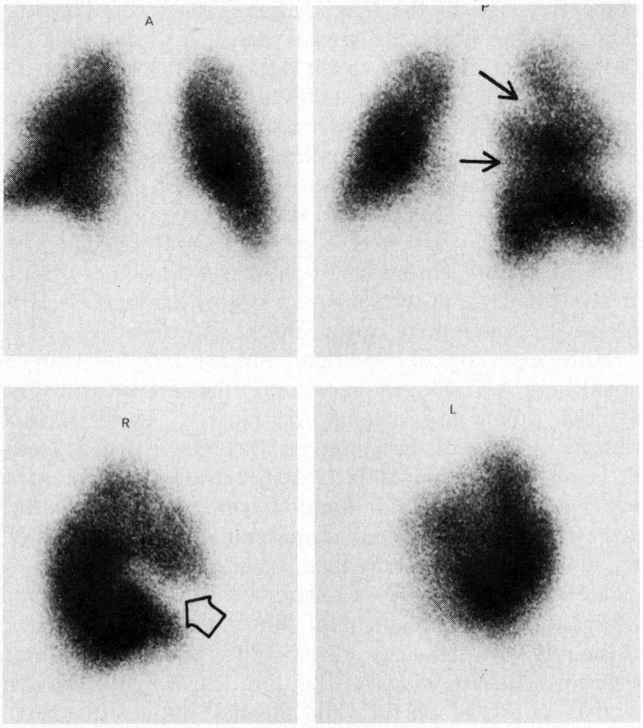

FIGURE 11–27 Perfusion scintiscan demonstrating absent perfusion to a segment of the right middle lobe (open arrow) with additional subsegmental perfusion defects (arrows).

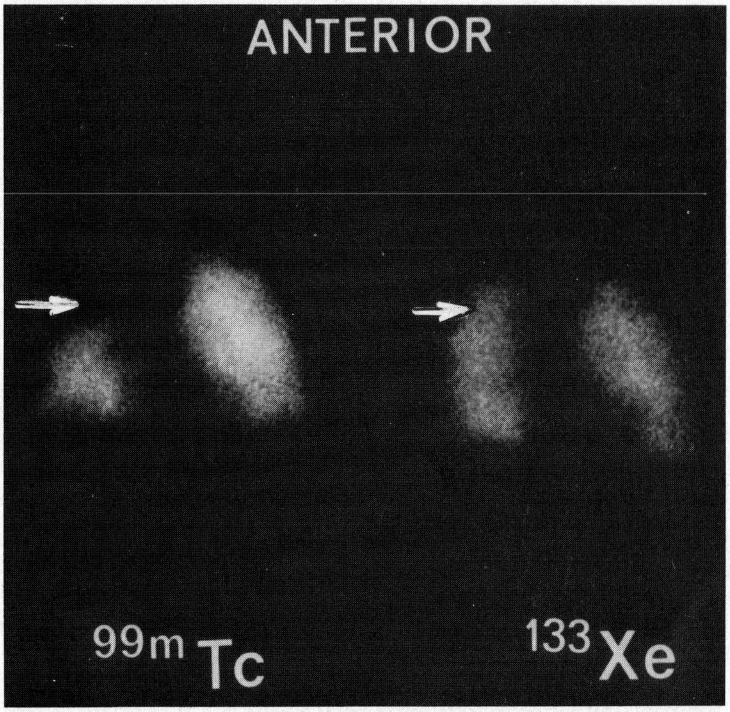

FIGURE 11–28 Perfusion scintiscan demonstrating that perfusion to the right upper lung field is absent (left, arrow). Single-breath ventilation scintiscan demonstrating normal ventilation in this region (right, arrow). Ventilation-perfusion mismatch is consistent with pulmonary embolism.

volving lobar areas. Only 8 per cent of patients without pulmonary emboli had similar findings. Segmental defects occurred with about equal frequency (22 to 33 per cent) in patients with pulmonary embolism and in patients with chronic lung disease. Patients with pulmonary emboli rarely have small subsegmental defects as their largest perfusion defects (2 to 8 per cent).[362] Nevertheless, the pattern of perfusion abnormalities is only a fair discriminator of pulmonary embolism and, if possible, should not constitute the only radiodiagnostic criterion.

Ventilation scintigraphy is a helpful maneuver in distinguishing between primary perfusion abnormalities and those secondary to regional hypoxia.[352–354] In patients with pulmonary emboli, the perfusion abnormality clearly exceeds any abnormality in ventilation (Fig. 11–28). In patients with acute bronchospasm or chronic lung disease, the compromise of regional ventilation usually matches or exceeds that of perfusion. In patients with normal or near-normal chest x-rays, this comparison between perfusion and ventilation is particularly useful in differentiating pulmonary lung disease from pulmonary emboli.

Interpretation becomes more difficult when the chest x-ray is abnormal in the region of the perfusion defect. The pulmonary density seen on the x-ray may represent parenchymal pulmonary disease or may be secondary to pulmonary infarction. Since ventilation will be affected in either case, ventilation scintigraphy is of limited value unless other perfusion defects are present. The size relationship of the perfusion defect and the density on chest x-ray may be helpful, however.[363] If the perfusion defect is small relative to the density on the x-ray, the probability of pulmonary embolism is low (7 per cent). When the perfusion defect is substantially larger than the roentgenographic abnormality, the probability of pulmonary embolism is increased (89 per cent). The perfusion defect must be substantially larger or smaller than the corresponding radiographic abnormalities for these diagnostic criteria to apply. Otherwise, a scintigram with a perfusion defect and accompanying chest x-ray density with no other diagnostic clues is indeterminant for the diagnosis of pulmonary embolism.

Natural evolution of the appearance on perfusion scans after an acute episode is also a useful indicator of pulmonary embolism (Fig. 11–29).[364–366] In general, perfusion scintigraphy returns to normal soon after the embolic event. The rapidity of improvement seems to depend on the patient's age and cardiovascular status and the amount of lung involved. In the absence of heart failure, even major occlusions may revert to normal within weeks. Recurrent embolism is often characterized by the appearance of new regions of involvement as old ones disappear. Frag-

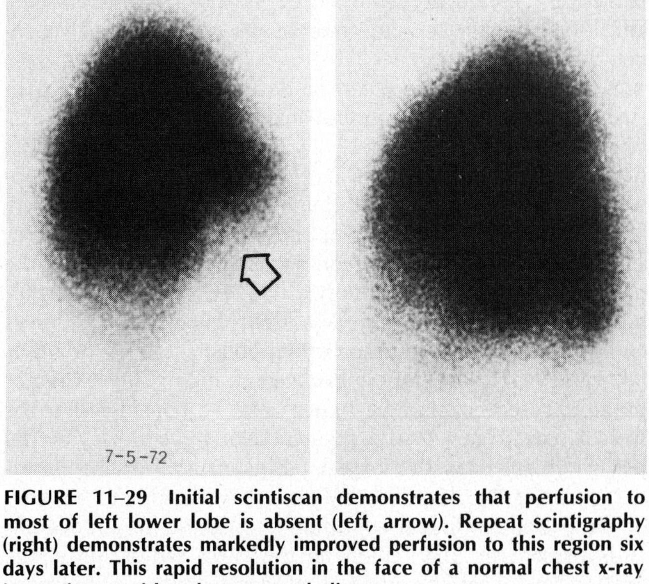

FIGURE 11–29 Initial scintiscan demonstrates that perfusion to most of left lower lobe is absent (left, arrow). Repeat scintigraphy (right) demonstrates markedly improved perfusion to this region six days later. This rapid resolution in the face of a normal chest x-ray is consistent with pulmonary embolism.

TABLE 11–2 THE ROLE OF SCINTIGRAPHY IN PULMONARY EMBOLISM (PE)

Largest Perfusion Defect	X-Ray	Ventilation	Interpretation	Strategy
Normal			No pulmonary embolism within past 48 hours	No pulmonary angiography
Subsegmental		Indicated only if large subsegmental deficit; then interpretation same as segmental or lobar below	Low probability of PE (< 5%)	Pulmonary angiography only if clinical suspicion is high
Segmental or lobar	Normal in region of defect	Perfusion-ventilation match	Low probability of PE	Pulmonary angiography only if clinical suspicion is high
Segmental or lobar	Abnormal density in region of defect	Not indicated	Indeterminate	Pulmonary angiography recommended
Segmental or lobar	Normal in region of defect	Perfusion-ventilation mismatch	High probability of PE (> 90%)	Treat
Segmental or lobar	Normal in region of defect	Cannot be performed	Moderate probability of PE (25% in segmental and 80% in lobar defects)	Pulmonary angiography recommended

mentation of large central thromboemboli can produce new subsegmental defects, however. Because of this natural evolution, it is often difficult to document reembolization in patients already receiving therapy for previous pulmonary emboli.

Conditions other than acute pulmonary embolism can result in ventilation/perfusion mismatches (normal ventilation in regions of decreased or absent perfusion).[367] The ventilation/perfusion mismatch is, after all, evidence only of a vascular rather than a parenchymal etiology. In parenchymal disease, regional hypoxia results in a reflex reduction in decreased pulmonary blood flow to that region. Vascular diseases, such as previous pulmonary embolism, pulmonary artery agenesis or stenosis, vasculitis (polyarteritis nodosa), tuberculosis, pulmonary artery sarcoma, hemangioendotheliomatosis, and pulmonary venoocclusive disease would be expected to result in ventilation/perfusion mismatches. There are sporadic reports of parenchymal lung disease, including emphysema, radiation therapy, intravenous drug abuse, bronchogenic carcinoma, lymphangitic carcinomatosis, and pneumonia that result in ventilation/perfusion mismatch. Despite this extensive differential diagnosis, ventilation/perfusion mismatches and perfusion defects involving large subsegments, segments, and lobes are due to acute pulmonary embolism in over 90 per cent of the cases.

A reasonable strategy can be developed in patients with suspected pulmonary embolism based on the perfusion and ventilation studies (Table 11–2). Patients with normal perfusion scintigrams have not had clinically significant embolism within the previous 48 hours. Pulmonary angiography is not ordinarily indicated in these patients. If the perfusion scintigram contains small subsegmental defects as the predominant perfusion abnormality, the likelihood of pulmonary embolism is low (less than 5 per cent). Unless clinical suspicion of pulmonary embolism is high or other laboratory or radiographic evidence is highly suggestive of pulmonary embolism, the patient can be considered to be free of recent emboli. If a segmental or large subsegmental perfusion defect is the largest perfusion abnormality present, and the ventilation study cannot be performed because of the patient's clinical condition or because an abnormality is present in that region on the chest radiography, the probability of embolization is moderate and a pulmonary arteriogram is necessary for documentation of the disease. While the presence of a lobar defect increases the likelihood of pulmonary embolism, pulmonary angiography is still necessary to document the disease if ventilation scintigraphy cannot be performed or if additional segmental defects do not accompany it. If a large subsegmental or lobar defect is associated with a ventilation/perfusion mismatch, and multiple perfusion defects are present, the likelihood of pulmonary embolism is very high and treatment should be begun immediately. Care must be taken in patients with severe chronic lung disease in which the changes due to pulmonary embolism may be masked by the parenchymal disease. Angiography should be performed in these patients if the perfusion scans are not normal or exhibit only small subsegmental defects.

References

CARDIAC PERFORMANCE

1. Blumgart, H. L., and Weiss, S.: Studies on the velocity of blood flow. II. The velocity of blood flow in normal resting individuals, and a critique of the method used. J. Clin. Invest. *4*:15, 1927.
2. Cohn, P. F., Gorlin, R., Cohn, L. H., and Collins, J. J., Jr.: Left ventricular ejection fraction as a prognostic guide in surgical treatment of coronary and valvular heart disease. Am. J. Cardiol. *34*:136, 1974.
3. Nelson, G. R., Cohn, P. F., and Gorlin, R.: Prognosis in medically treated coronary artery disease: The value of ejection fraction compared with other measurements. Circulation *52*:408, 1975.
4. Feild, B. J., Russell, R. O., Jr., Dowling, J. T., and Rackley, C. E.: Regional left ventricular performance in the year following myocardial infarction. Circulation *46*:679, 1972.
5. Watson, L. E., Dickhaus, D. W., and Martin, R. H.: Left ventricular aneurysm: Preoperative hemodynamics, chamber volume, and results of aneurysmectomy. Circulation *52*:868, 1975.
6. Schelbert, H. R., Henning, H., Ashburn, W. L., Verba, J. W., Karliner, J. S., and O'Rourke, R. A.: Serial measurements of left ventricular ejection fraction by radionuclide angiography early and late after myocardial infarction. Am. J. Cardiol. *38*:407, 1976.
7. Rigo, P., Murray, M., Strauss, H. W., Taylor, D., Kelly, D., Weisfeldt, M., and Pitt, B.: Left ventricular function in acute myocardial infarction evaluated by gated scintigraphy. Circulation *50*:678, 1974.
8. Karliner, J. S., Gault, M. D., Eckberg, D., Mullins, C. B., and Ross, J., Jr.: Mean velocity of fiber shortening: A simplified measure of left ventricular myocardial contractility. Circulation *44*:323, 1971.
9. Ashburn, W. L., Schelbert, H. R., and Verba, J. W.: Left ventricular ejection fraction: A review of several radionuclide angiographic approaches using the scintillation camera. Progr. Cardiovasc. Dis. *20*:267, 1978.
10. Bodenheimer, M. M., Banka, V. S., and Helfant, R. H.: Nuclear cardiology. I. Radionuclide angiographic assessment of left ventricular contraction: Uses, limitations, and future directions. Am. J. Cardiol. *45*:661, 1980.
11. Marshall, R. C., Berger, H. J., Costin, J. C., Freedman, G. S., Wolberg, J., Cohen, L. S., Gottschalk, A., and Zaret, B. L.: Assessment of cardiac performance with quantitative radionuclide angiocardiography. Circulation *56*:820, 1977.

12. Wackers, F. J., Giles, R. W., Hoffer, P. B., Lange, R. C., Berger, H. J., and Zaret, B. L.: Gold-195m, a new generator-produced short-lived radionuclide for sequential assessment of ventricular performance by first pass radionuclide angiocardiography. Am. J. Cardiol. *50*:89, 1982.
13. Holman, B. L., Neirinckx, R. D., Treves, S., and Tow, D. E.: Cardiac imaging with tantalum-178. Radiology *131*:525, 1979.
14. Treves, S., Cheng, C., Samuel, A., Lambrecht, R., Babchyck, B., Zimmerman, R., and Norwood, W.: Iridium-191 angiocardiography for the detection and quantitation of left-to-right shunting. J. Nucl. Med. *21*:1151, 1980.
15. Schelbert, H. R., Verba, J. W., Johnson, A. D., Brock, G. W., Alazraki, N. P., Rose, F. J., and Ashburn, W. L.: Nontraumatic determination of left ventricular ejection fraction by radionuclide angiocardiography. Circulation *51*:902, 1975.
16. Jengo, J. A., Mena, I., Blaufuss, A., and Criley, J. M.: Evaluation of left ventricular function (ejection fraction and segmental wall motion) by single pass radioisotope angiography. Circulation *57*:326, 1978.
17. Parker, J. A., and Treves, S.: Radionuclide detection, localization and quantitation of intracardiac shunts and shunts between the great arteries. Progr. Cardiovasc. Dis. *20*:121, 1977.
18. Lane, S. D., Patton, D. D., Staab, E. V., and Baglan, R. J.: Simple technique for rapid bolus injection. J. Nucl. Med. *13*:118, 1972.
19. Oldendorf, W. H.: Measurement of the mean transit time of cerebral circulation by external detection of an intravenously injected radioisotope. J. Nucl. Med. *3*:382, 1962.
20. Treves, S., Maltz, D. L., and Adlestein, S. J.: Intracardiac shunts. *In* James, A. E., Wagner, H. N., and Cooke, R. E. (eds.): Pediatric Nuclear Medicine. Philadelphia, W. B. Saunders Co., 1974, p. 231.
21. Donato, L.: Basic concepts of radiocardiography. Semin. Nucl. Med. *3*:111, 1973.
22. Ellis, J. H., and Steele, P. P.: Value of combined hemodynamic and radiocardiographic studies in acute respiratory failure. *In* Serafini, A. N., Gilson, A. J., and Smoak, W. M. (eds.): Nuclear Cardiology. New York, Plenum Press, 1977, p. 187.
23. Parker, H., Van Dyke, D., Weber, P., Davies, H., Steele, P., and Sullivan, R.: Evaluation of central circulatory dynamics with the radionuclide angiocardiogram. *In* Wagner, H. (ed.): Diagnostic Nuclear Cardiology. St. Louis, The C. V. Mosby Co., 1974.
24. Pierson, R. N., Jr., and Van Dyke, D. C.: Analysis of left ventricular function. *In* Pierson, R. N., Kriss, J. P., Jones, R. H., and MacIntyre, W. J. (eds.): Quantitative Nuclear Cardiography. New York, John Wiley and Sons, 1975, p. 123.
25. Hamilton, W. F., Moore, J. W., Kinsman, J. M., and Spurling, R. G.: Studies on the circulation. IV. Further analysis of the injection method and of changes in hemodynamics under physiological and pathological conditions. Am. J. Physiol. *99*:534, 1931–32.
26. Razzak, M. A., Botti, R. E., MacIntyre, W. J., and Pritchard, W. H.: Consecutive determination of cardiac output and renal blood flow by external monitoring of radioactive isotopes. J. Nucl. Med. *11*:190, 1970.
27. Thompson, H. K., Starmer, C. E., Whalen, R. E., and McIntosh, H. D.: Indicator transit time considered as a gamma variate. Circ. Res. *14*:502, 1964.
28. Starmer, C. E., and Clark, D. O.: Computer computations of cardiac output using the gamma function. J. Appl. Physiol. *28*:219, 1970.
29. Steadham, R. E., and Blackwell, L. H.: A new method for the determination of the area under a cardiac output curve. I.E.E.E. Trans. Biomed. Engin. *17*: 335, 1970.
30. Kriss, J. P., Enright, L. P., Hayden, W. G., Wexler, L., and Shumway, N. E.: Radioisotope angiocardiography: Wide scope applicability in diagnosis and evaluation of therapy in diseases of the heart and great vessels. Circulation *43*: 792, 1971.
31. Mann, T., Goldberg, S., Mudge, G. H., and Grossman, W.: Factors contributing to altered left ventricular diastolic properties during angina pectoris. Circulation *59*:14, 1979.
32. Hirota, Y.: A clinical study of left ventricular relaxation. Circulation *62*:756, 1980.
33. Ludbrook, P. A., Byrne, J. D., and McKnight, R. C.: Influence of right ventricular hemodynamics on left ventricular diastolic pressure-volume relations in man. Circulation *59*:21, 1979.
34. Polak, J. F., Kemper, A. J., Bianco, J. A., Parisi, A. F., and Tow, D. E.: Resting early peak diastolic filling rate: A sensitive index of myocardial dysfunction in patients with coronary artery disease. J. Nucl. Med. *23*:471, 1982.
35. Bonow, R. O., Bacharach, S. L., Green, M. V., Kent, K. M., Rosing, D. R., Lipson, L. C., Leon, M. B., and Epstein, S. E.: Left ventricular diastolic filling in patients with coronary artery disease (abstr). Circulation *62*:III-77, 1980.
36. Tobinick, E., Schelbert, H. R., Henning, H., LeWinter, M., Taylor, A., Ashburn, W. L., and Karliner, J. S.: Right ventricular ejection fraction in patients with acute anterior and inferior myocardial infarction assessed by radionuclide angiography. Circulation *57*:1078, 1978.
37. Berger, H. J., Matthay, R. A., Marshal, R. A., Gottschalk, A., Cohen, L. S., and Zaret, B. L.: Noninvasive radionuclide technique for right ventricular ejection fraction in man. Circulation *54*(Suppl.):II-109, 1976.
38. Berger, H. J., Matthay, R. A., Loke, J., Marshall, R. C., Gottschalk, A., and Zaret, B. L.: Assessment of cardiac performance with quantitative radionuclide angiocardiography: Right ventricular ejection fraction with reference to findings in chronic obstructive pulmonary disease. Am. J. Cardiol. *51*:897, 1978.
39. Sandler, H., and Dodge, H. T.: Use of single pace cineangiograms for the calculation of left ventricular volume in man. Am. Heart J. *75*:325, 1968.
40. Folse, R., and Braunwald, E.: Pulmonary vascular dilution curves recorded by external detection in the diagnosis of left-to-right shunts. Br. Heart J. *24*:166, 1962.
41. Carter, S. A., Bajec, D. F., Yannicelli, E., and Wood, E. H.: Estimation of left-to-right shunt from arterial dilution curves. J. Lab. Clin. Med. *55*:77, 1960.
42. Alazraki, N. P., Ashburn, W. L., and Hagan, A.: Detection of left-to-right cardiac shunts with the scintillation camera pulmonary dilution curve. J. Nucl. Med. *13*:142, 1972.
43. Maltz, D. L., and Treves, S.: Quantitative radionuclide angiocardiography: Determination of Q_p:Q_s in children. Circulation *47*: 1040, 1973.
44. Greenfield, L. D., and Bennett, L. R.: Detection of intracardiac shunts with radionuclide imaging. Semin. Nucl. Med. *3*:139, 1973.
45. Greenfield, L. D., Vincent, W. R., Graham, L. S., and Bennett, L. R.: Evaluation of intracardiac shunts. CRC Crit. Rev. Clin. Radiol. Nucl. Med. *6*:217, 1975.
46. Braunwald, E., Long, R. T. L., and Morrow, A. G.: Injections of radioactive krypton (Kr^{85}) solution in the detection and localization of cardiac shunts. J. Clin. Invest. *38*:990, 1959.
47. Bosnjakovic, B., Bennett, L., and Vincent, W.: Diagnosis of intracardiac shunts without cardiac catheterization. Circulation *44*:II-144, 1971.
48. Polak, J. F., Podrid, P. J., Lown, B., and Holman, B. L.: Ventricular postextrasystolic potentiation in the dog: A study using list mode radionuclide ventriculography. J. Nucl. Med. (in press).
49. Rabinovitch, M. A., Stewart, J., Chan, W., Dunlap, T. E., Kalff, V., Clare, J., Thrall, J. H., and Pitt, B.: Scintigraphic demonstration of ventriculo-atrial conduction in the ventricular pacemaker syndrome. J. Nucl. Med. *23*:795, 1982.
50. Bacharach, S. L., Green, M. V., Borer, J. S., Hyde, J. E., Farkas, S. P., and Johnson, G. S.: Left-ventricular peak ejection rate, filling rate, and ejection fraction—frame rate requirements at rest and exercise. J. Nucl. Med. *20*:189, 1979.
51. Maddox, D. E., Holman, B. L., Wynne, J., Idoine, J., Parker, J. A., Uren, R., Neill, J. M., and Cohn, P. F.: The ejection fraction image: A noninvasive index of regional left ventricular wall motion. Am. J. Cardiol. *41*:1230, 1978.
52. Parker, J. A., Secker-Walker, R. H., Hill, R. L., Siegel, B. A., and Potchen, E. J.: A new technique for the calculation of left ventricular ejection fraction. J. Nucl. Med. *13*:649, 1972.
53. Secker-Walker, R. H., Resnick, L., Kunz, H., Parker, J. A., Hill, R. L., and Potchen, E. J.: Measurement of left ventricular ejection fraction. J. Nucl. Med. *14*:798, 1973.
54. Slutsky, R., Karliner, J., Ricci, D., Kaiser, R., Pfisterer, M., Gordon, D., Peterson, K., and Ashburn, W.: Left ventricular volumes by gated equilibrium radionuclide angiography: A new method. Circulation *60*:556, 1979.
55. Konstam, M. A., Wynne, J., Holman, B. L., Brown, E. J., Neill, J. M., and Kozlowski, J.: Use of equilibrium (gated) radionuclide ventriculography to quantitate left ventricular output in patients with and without left-sided valvular regurgitation. Circulation *64*:578, 1981.
56. Maddox, D. E., Holman, B. L., Wynne, J., Idoine, J., Parker, J. A., Uren, R., Neill, J. M., and Cohn, P. F.: Ejection fraction image: A noninvasive index of regional left ventricular wall motion. Am. J. Cardiol. *41*:1230, 1978.
57. Holman, B. L., Wynne, J., Idoine, J., Zielonka, J., and Neill, J.: The paradox image: A noninvasive index of regional left ventricular dyskinesis. J. Nucl. Med. *20*:1237, 1979.
58. Holman, B. L., Wynne, J., Idoine, J., and Neill, J.: Disruption in the temporal sequence of regional ventricular contraction. Circulation *61*:1075, 1980.
59. Botvinick, E. H., Frais, M. A., Shosa, D. W., O'Connell, J. W., Pacheco-Alvarez, J. A., Scheinman, M., Hattner, R. S., Morady, F., and Faulkner, D. B.: An accurate means of detecting and characterizing abnormal patterns of ventricular activation by phase image analysis. Am. J. Cardiol. *50*:289, 1982.
60. Pavel, D., Swlryn, S., Lam, W., Byrom, E., Shelkh, A., and Rosen, K.: Ventricular phase analysis of radionuclide gated studies (abstr.). Am. J. Cardiol. *45*:398, 1980.
61. Maddox, D. E., Wynne, J., Uren, R., Parker, J. A., Idoine, J., Siegel, L. C., Neill, J. M., Cohn, P. F., and Holman, B. L.: Regional ejection fraction: A quantitative radionuclide index of regional left ventricular performance. Circulation *59*:1001, 1979.
62. Silber, S., Schwaiger, M., Klein, U., and Rudolph, W.: Quantitative Beurteilung der linksventrikulären Funktion mit der Radionuklid-Ventrikulographie. Herz *5*:146, 1980.
63. Slutsky, R., Hooper, W., Gerber, K., Battler, A., Froelicher, V., Ashburn, W., and Karliner, J.: Assessment of right ventricular function at rest and during exercise in patients with coronary artery disease: A new approach using equilibrium radionuclide angiography. Am. J. Cardiol. *45*:63, 1980.
64. Holman, B. L., Wynne, J., Zielonka, J. S., and Idoine, J.: A simplified technique for measuring right ventricular ejection fraction using the equilibrium radionuclide angiocardiogram and the slant-hole collimator. Radiology *138*: 429, 1981.
65. Rigo, P., Alderson, P. O., Robertson, R. M., Becher, L. C., and Wagner, H. N., Jr.: Measurement of aortic and ventral regurgitation by gated cardiac blood pool scans. Circulation *60*:306, 1979.
66. Nicod, P., Corbett, J. R., Firth, B. G., Dehmer, G. J., Izquierdo, C., Markham, R. V., Jr., Hillis, L. D., Willerson, J. T., and Lewis, S. E.: Radionuclide techniques for valvular regurgitant index: Comparison in patients with normal and depressed ventricular function. J. Nucl. Med. *23*:763, 1982.
67. Alderson, P. O.: Radionuclide quantification of valvular regurgitation. J. Nucl. Med. *23*:851, 1982.
68. Tu'meh, S. S., Tracy, D., Wynne, J., Konstam, M. A., Kozlowski, J. F., Neu-

mann, A. L., and Holman, B. L.: Scintigraphic diagnosis of tricuspid regurgitation. Radiology *145*:463, 1982.
69. Borer, J., Bacharach, S. L., Green, M. V., Kent, K. M., Epstein, S. E., and Johnston, G. S.: Real-time radionuclide cineangiography in the noninvasive evaluation of global and regional left ventricular function at rest and during exercise in patients with coronary-artery disease. N. Engl. J. Med. *296*:839, 1977.
70. Borer, J., Bacharach, S. L., and Green, M. V.: Radionuclide cineangiography in the clinical assessment of patients with coronary and valvular heart diseases. Progr. Nucl. Med. *6*:151, 1980.
71. Bodenheimer, M. M., Banka, V. S., Fooshee, C. M., Gillespie, J. A., and Helfant, R. H.: Detection of coronary heart disease using radionuclide determined regional ejection fraction at rest and during handgrip exercise: Correlation with coronary arteriography. Circulation *58*:640, 1980.
72. Wainwright, R. J., Brennand-Roper, D. A., Cueni, T. A., Sowton, E., Hilson, A. J. W., and Maisey, M. N.: Cold pressor test in detection of coronary heart-disease and cardiomyopathy using technetium-99m gated blood-pool imaging. Lancet *2*:320, 1979.
73. Peter, C. A., and Jones, R. H.: Effects of isometric handgrip and dynamic exercise on left-ventricular function. J. Nucl. Med. *21*:1131, 1980.
74. Wynne, J. W., Borwo, K. M., Holman, B. L., and Mudge, G. H., Jr.: Cold pressor radionuclide ventriculography: Clinical utility. Br. Heart J. (in press).
75. Slutsky, R., Karliner, J., Ricci, D., Schuler, G., Pfisterer, M., Peterson, K., and Ashburn, W.: Response of left ventricular volume to exercise in man assessed by radionuclide equilibrium angiography. Circulation *60*:565, 1979.
76. Okada, R. D., Boucher, C. A., Strauss, H. W., and Pohost, G. M.: Exercise radionuclide imaging approaches to coronary artery disease. Am. J. Cardiol. *46*:1188, 1980.
77. Marshall, R. C., Wisenberg, G., Schelbert, H. R., and Henze, E.: Effect of oral propranolol on rest, exercise and postexercise left ventricular performance in normal subjects and patients with coronary artery disease. Circulation *63*:572, 1981.
78. Poliner, L. R., Dehmer, G. J., Lewis, S. E., Parkey, R. W., Blomqvist, C. G., and Willerson, J. T.: Left ventricular performance in normal subjects: A comparison of the responses to exercise in the upright and supine positions. Circulation *62*:528, 1980.
79. Jones, R. H., McEwan, P., Newman, G. E., Port, S., Rerych, S. K., Scholz, P. M., Upton, M. T., Peter, C. A., Austin, E. H., Leong, K., Gibbons, R. J., Cobb, F. R., Coleman, R. E., and Sabiston, D. C.: Accuracy of diagnosis of coronary artery disease by radionuclide measurements of left ventricular function during rest and exercise. Circulation *64*:586, 1981.
80. Port, S., Cobb, F. R., Coleman, R. E., and Jones, R. H.: Effect of age on the response of the left ventricular ejection fraction to exercise. N. Engl. J. Med. *303*:1133, 1980.
81. Gibbons, R. H., Lee, J. L., Cobb, F. R., Coleman, R. E., and Jones, R. H.: Ejection fraction response to exercise in patients with chest pain, coronary artery disease, and normal coronary arteriograms. Circulation *66*:643, 1982.
82. Borer, J. S., Bacharach, S. L., Green, M. V., Kent, K. M., Rosing, D. R., Seides, S. F., McIntosh, C. L., Conkle, D., Morrow, A. G., and Epstein, S. E.: Left ventricular function in aortic stenosis: Response to exercise and effects of operation (abstr). Am. J. Cardiol. *41*:382, 1978.
83. Borer, J. S., Bacharach, S. L., Green, M. V., Kent, K. M., Henry, W. L., Rosing, D. R., Seides, S. F., Johnston, G. S., and Epstein, S. E.: Exercise-induced left ventricular dysfunction in symptomatic and asymptomatic patients with aortic regurgitation: Assessment with radionuclide cineangiography. Am. J. Cardiol. *42*:351, 1978.
84. Borer, J. S., Gottdiener, J. S., Rosing, D. R., Kent, K. M., Bacharach, S. L., Green, M. V., and Epstein, S. E.: Left ventricular function in mitral regurgitation: Determination during exercise (abstr). Circulation *60*(Suppl.):II-38, 1979.
85. Ahmad, M., Sullivan, T., Haibach, H., Sandock, K., Logan, K., and Holmes, R.: Exercise induced changes in left ventricular function in patients with mitral valve prolapse (abstr). Clin. Res. *27*:146, 1979.
86. Borer, J. S., Bacharach, S. L., Green, M. V., Kent, K. M., Maron, B. J., Rosing, D. R., Seides, S. F., and Epstein, S. E.: Obstructive vs. nonobstructive symmetric septal hypertrophy: Differences in left ventricular function with exercise (abstr). Am. J. Cardiol. *41*:379, 1978.
87. Slutsky, R., Ackerman, W., Hooper, W., Battler, A., Karliner, J., Ashburn, W., and Moser, K.: The response of left ventricular ejection fraction and volume to supine exercise in patients with severe COPD (abstr.). Circulation *60* (Suppl.):II-234, 1979.
88. Leon, M. B., Borer, J. S., Bacharach, S. L., Green, M. V., Benz, E. J., Griffith, P., and Nienhuis, A. W.: Detection of early cardiac dysfunction in patients with severe beta-thalassemia and chronic iron overload. N. Engl. J. Med. *301*: 1143, 1979.
89. Chipps, B. E., Alderson, P. O., Roland, J. M. A., Yang, S., van Aswegen, A., Rosenstein, B. L., and Wagner, H. N.: Ventricular function at rest and during exercise in cystic fibrosis (abstr). J. Nucl. Med. *20*:637, 1979.
90. Port, S., Cobb, F. R., and Jones, R. H.: Effects of propranolol on left ventricular function in normal men (abstr). J. Nucl. Med. *60* (Suppl.):II-91, 1979.
91. Wisenberg, G., Marshal, R., Schelbert, H.,and Rue, C.: The effects of oral propranolol on left ventricular function at rest and during exercise in normal patients and in patients with coronary artery disease as determined by radionuclide angiography (abstr). J. Nucl. Med. it 20:639, 1979.
92. Ehrhardt, J. C., Verani, M. S., and Marcus, M. L.: Exercise isotope ventriculogram: Use in assessing change in left ventricular function (abstr). Circulation *56* (Suppl.):II-141, 1977.
93. Gibbons, R. J., Lee, K. L., Pryor, D., Harrell, F. E., Jr., Coleman, R. E., Cobb, F. R., Rosati, R. A., and Jones, R. H.: The use of radionuclide angiography in the diagnosis of coronary artery disease: A logistic regression analysis. Circulation (*in press*).
94. Nesto, R. W., Cohn, L. H., Collins, J. J., Wynne, J., Holman, L., and Cohn, P. F.: Inotropic contractile reserve: A useful predictor of increased 5 year survival and improved postoperative left ventricular function in patients with coronary artery disease and reduced ejection fraction. Am. J. Cardiol. *50*:39, 1982.
95. Borer, J. S., Rosing, D. R., Miller, R. H., Stark, R. M., Kent, K. M., Bacharach, S. L., Green, M. V., Lake, C. R., Cohen, H., Holmes, D., Donohue, D., Baker, W., and Epstein, S. E.: Natural history of left ventricular function during 1 year after acute myocardial infarction: Comparison with clinical, electrocardiographic and biochemical determinations. Am. J. Cardiol. *46*:1, 1980.
96. Reduto, L. A., Berger, H. J., Gottschalk, A., and Zaret, B. L.: Sequential radionuclide assessment of left and right ventricular performance after acute transmural myocardial infarction. Ann. Intern. Med. *89*:441, 1978.
97. Shah, P. K., Pichler, M., Berman, D. S., Singh, B. N., and Swan, H. J. C.: Left ventricular ejection fraction and first third ejection fraction determined by radionuclide ventriculography in early stages of first transmural myocardial infarction: Relation to short-term prognosis. Am. J. Cardiol. *45*:542, 1980.
98. Rigo, P., Murray, M., Taylor, D. R., Weisfeldt, M. L., Kelley, D. T., Strauss, H. W., and Pitt, B.: Right ventricular dysfunction detected by gated scintigraphy in patients with acute inferior myocardial infarction. Circulation *52*:268, 1975.
99. Pulido, J. I., Doss, J., Twieg, D., Blomqvist, G. C., Faulkner, D., Horn, V., DeBates, D., Tobey, M., Parkey, R. W., and Willerson, J. T.: Submaximal exercise testing after acute myocardial infarction: Myocardial scintigraphic and electrocardiographic observations. Am. J. Cardiol. *42*:19, 1978.
100. Borer, J. S., Bacharach, S. L., Green, M. V., Kent, K. M., Henry, W. L., Rosing, D. R., Seides, S. F., Johnston, G. S., and Epstein, S. E.: Exercise-induced left and right ventricular dysfunction in symptomatic and asymptomatic patients with aortic regurgitation: Assessment with radionuclide cineangiography. Am. J. Cardiol. *42*:351, 1978.
101. Borer, J. S., Rosing, D. R., Kent, K. M., Bacharach, S. L., Green, M. V., McIntosh, C. J., Morrow, A. G., and Epstein, S. E.: Left ventricular function at rest and during exercise after aortic valve replacement in patients with aortic regurgitation. Am. J. Cardiol. *44*:1297, 1979.
102. Watson, L. E., Dickhaus, D. W., and Martin., R. H.: Left ventricular aneurysm. Preoperative hemodynamics, chamber volume, and results of aneurysmectomy. Circulation *52*:868, 1975.
103. Rozanski, A., Berman, D., Gray, R., Diamond, G., Raymond, M., Prause, J., Maddahi, J., Swan, H. J. C., and Matloff, J.: Preoperative prediction of reversible myocardial asynergy by postexercise radionuclide ventriculography. N. Engl. J. Med. *307*:212, 1982.
104. Bodenheimer, M. M., Banka, V. S., Hermann, G. A., Trout, R. G., Pasdar, H., and Helfant, R. H.: Reversible asynergy. Circulation *53*:792, 1976.
105. Chatterjee, K., Swan, H. J. C., Parmley, W. W., Sustaita, H., Marcus, H. S., and Matloff, J.: Influence of direct myocardial revascularization on left ventricular asynergy and function in patients with coronary heart disease: With and without previous myocardial infarction. Circulation *47*:276, 1973.
106. Popio, K. A., Gorlin, R., Bechtel, D., and Levine, J. A.: Postextrasystolic potentiation as a predictor of potential myocardial viability. Am. J. Cardiol. *39*: 944, 1977.
107. Righetti, A., Crawford, M. H., O'Rourke, R. A., Schelbert, H., Daily, P. O., and Ross, J., Jr.: Intraventricular septal motion and left ventricular function after coronary bypass surgery: Evaluation with echocardiography and radionuclide angiography. Am. J. Cardiol. *39*:372, 1977.
108. Helfant, R. H., Pine, R., Meister, S. G., Feldman, M. S., Trout, R. G., and Banka, V. S.: Nitroglycerin to unmask reversible asynergy: Correlation with post coronary bypass surgery. Circulation *50*:108, 1974.
109. DePuey, E. G., Mammen, G. P., Rivas, A. H., Thompson, W. L., Sonnemaker, R. E., Mathur, V., Burdine, J. A., Garcia, E., and Hall, R. J.: Post-exercise potentiation of wall motion to identify myocardial viability. Texas Heart Inst. J. 9:127, 1982.
110. Berger, H. J., Matthay, R. A., Loke, J., Marshall, R. C., Gottschalk, A., and Zaret, B. L.: Assessment of cardiac performance with quantitative radionuclide angiocardiography: Right ventricular ejection fraction with reference to findings in chronic obstructive pulmonary disease. Am. J. Cardiol. *41*:897, 1978.
111. Berger, H. J., and Matthay, R. A.: Noninvasive radiographic assessment of cardiovascular function in acute and chronic respiratory failure. Am. J. Cardiol. *47*:950, 1981.
112. Matthay, R. A., Berger, J. H., Davies, R. A., Loke, J., Mahler, D. A., Gottschalk, A., and Zaret, B. L.: Right and left ventricular exercise performance in chronic obstructive pulmonary disease: Radionuclide assessment. Ann. Intern. Med. *93*:234, 1980.
113. Morrison, J., Coromilas, J., Robbins, M., Ong, L., Eisenberg, S., Stechel, R., Zema, M., Reiser, P., and Scherr, L.: Digitalis and myocardial infarction in man. Circulation *62*:8, 1978.
114. Wynne, J., Malacoff, R. F., Benotti, J. R., Curfman, G. D., Grossman, W., Holman, B. L., Smith, T. W., and Braunwald, E.: Oral amrinone in refractory congestive heart failure. Am. J. Cardiol. *45*:1245, 1980.
115. Goldman, S. A., Johnson, L. L., Escala, E., Cannon, P. J., and Weiss, M. B.: Improved exercise ejection fraction with long-term prazosin therapy in patients with heart failure. Am. J. Med. *68*:36, 1980.

116. Colucci, W. S., Wynne, J., Holman, B. L., and Braunwald, E.: Long-term therapy of heart failure with prazosin: A randomized double blind trial. Am. J. Cardiol. *45*:337, 1980.
117. Matthay, R. A., Berger, H. J., Loke, J., Gottschalk, A., and Zaret, B. L.: Effects of aminophylline upon right and left ventricular performance in chronic obstructive pulmonary disease: Noninvasive assessment by radionuclide angiocardiography. Am. J. Med. *65*:903, 1978.
118. Bonow, R. O., Leon, M. B., Rosing, D. R., Kent, K. M., Lipson, L. C., Bacharach, S. L., Green, M. V., and Epstein, S. E.: Effect of propranolol and verapamil on left ventricular diastolic filling in patients with coronary artery disease (abstr). Circulation *62*:III-85, 1980.
119. Malacoff, R. F., Lorell, B. H., Mudge, G. H., Jr., Holman, B. L., Idoine, J., Bifolck, L., and Cohn, P. F.: Beneficial effects of nifedipine on regional myocardial blood flow in patients with coronary artery disease. Circulation *65*:I-32, 1982.
120. Alexander, J., Dainiak, N., Berger, H. J., Goldman, L., Johnstone, D., Reduto, L., Duffy, T., Schwartz, P., Gottschalk, A., and Zaret, B. L.: Serial assessment of doxorubicin cardiotoxicity with quantitative radionuclide angiocardiography. N. Engl. J. Med. *300*:278, 1979.

MYOCARDIAL SCINTIGRAPHY

121. Abrams, H. L., and Adams, D. F.: The coronary arteriogram. Structural and functional aspects. N. Engl. J. Med. *281*:1276, 1969.
122. Bodenheimer, M. M., Banka, V. S., and Helfant, R. H.: Nuclear cardiology. II. The role of myocardial perfusion imaging using thallium-201 in diagnosis of coronary heart disease. Am. J. Cardiol. *45*:674, 1980.
123. Bennett, K. R., Smith, R. O., Lehan, P. H., and Hellems, H. K.: Correlation of myocardial ^{42}K uptake with coronary arteriography. Radiology *102*:117, 1972.
124. Carr, E. A., Jr., Beierwaltes, W. H., Wegst, A. V., and Bartlett, J. D., Jr.: Myocardial scanning with rubidium-86. J. Nucl. Med. *3*:76, 1962.
125. Carr, E. A., Jr., Walker, B. J., and Bartlett, J., Jr.: The diagnosis of myocardial infarcts by photoscanning after administration of cesium^{131}. J. Clin. Invest. *42*:922, 1963.
126. Hurley, P. J., Cooper, M., Reba, R. C., Poggenburg, K. J., and Wagner, H. N., Jr.: ^{143}KCl: A new radiopharmaceutical for imaging the heart. J. Nucl. Med. *12*:516, 1971.
127. Romhilt, D. W., Adolph, R. J., Sodd, V. C., Levenson, N. I., August, L. S., Nishiyama, H., and Berke, R. A.: Cesium-129 myocardial scintigraphy to detect myocardial infarction. Circulation *48*:1242, 1973.
128. Martin, N. D., Zaret, B. L., McGowan, R. L., Wells, H. P., Jr., and Flamm, M. D.: Rubidium-81: A new myocardial scanning agent. Radiology. *111*:651, 1974.
129. Lebowitz, E., Greene, M. W., Bradley-Moore, P., Atkins, H., Ansari, A., Richards, P., and Belgrave, E.: ^{201}Tl for medical use. J. Nucl. Med. *14*: 421, 1973.
130. Gehring, P. J., and Hammond, P. B.: The interrelationship between thallium and potassium in animals. J. Pharmacol. Exp. Ther. *55*:187, 1967.
131. Britten, J. S., and Blank, M.: Thallium activation of the $(Na^+$-$K^+)$-activated ATPase of rabbit kidney. Biochim. Biophys. Acta *159*:160, 1968.
132. Strauss, H. W., Harrison, K., Langan, J. K., Lebowitz, E., and Pitt, B.: Thallium-201 for myocardial imaging. Relation of thallium-201 to regional myocardial perfusion. Circulation *51*:641, 1975.
133. Zimmer, L., McCall, D., D'Addabbo, L., and Whitney, K.: Kinetics and characteristics of thallium exchange in cultured cells (abstr). Circulation *60* (Suppl.):II-138, 1979.
134. Deutsch, E., Bushong, W., Glavan, K. A., Elder, R. C., Sodd, V. J., Scholz, K. L., Fortman, D. L., and Lukes, S. J.: Heart imaging with cationic complexes of technetium. Science *214*:85, 1981.
135. Budinger, T. F., Yano, Y., and Hoop, B.: A comparison of $^{82}Rb^+$ and $^{13}NH_3$ for myocardial positron scintigraphy. J. Nucl. Med. *16*:429, 1975.
136. Yano, Y., and Anger, H. O.: Visualization of heart and kidneys in animals with ultrashort-lived ^{82}Rb and the positron scintillation camera. J. Nucl. Med. *9*:413, 1968.
137. Vokelman, J., Van Dyke, D., and Yano, Y.: Myocardial scanning with rubidium-82. Stokely Laboratory Reports. Berkeley, CA, University of California Press, 1972, p. 775.
138. Harper, P. V., Ryan, J. W., Al-Sadir, J., Chua, K. G., Resnekov, L., Neirinckx, R., Loberg, M., and the Los Alamos Medical Radioisotope Group: Intracoronary use of rubidium-82. J. Nucl. Med. *23*:P69, 1982.
139. Walsh, W. F., Fill, H. R., and Harper, P. V.: Nitrogen-13–labeled ammonia for myocardial imaging. Semin. Nucl. Med. *7*:59, 1977.
140. Sapirstein, L. A.: Fractionation of the cardiac output of rats with isotopic potassium. Circ. Res. *4*:689, 1956.
141. Weich, H. F., Strauss, H. W., and Pitt, B.: The extraction of Tl-201 by the myocardium. Circulation *56*:188, 1977.
142. Case, R. B.: Ion alterations during myocardial ischemia. Cardiology *56*:245, 1971.
143. Parker, J. O., Chiong, M. A., West, R. O., and Case, R. B.: The effect of ischemia and alterations of heart rate on myocardial potassium balance in man. Circulation *42*:205, 1970.
143a. Goldhaber, S. Z., Newell, J. B., Alpert, N. M., Andrews, E., Pohost, G. M., and Ingwall, J. S.: Effects of ischemic-like insult on myocardial thallium-201 accumulation. Circulation *67*:778, 1983.
144. Levenson, N. I., Adolph, R. J., Romhilt, D. W., Gabel, M., Sodd, V. C., and August, L. S.: Effect of myocardial hypoxia and ischemia on myocardial scintigraphy. Am. J. Cardiol. *35*:251, 1975.
145. Adolph, R., Romhilt, D., Nishiyama, H., Sodd, V., Blue, J., and Gabel, M.: Use of positive and negative imaging agents to visualize myocardial ischemia. Circulation *54*(Suppl.):II-220, 1976.
146. McCall, D., Zimmer, L., D'Addabbo, L., and Whitney, K.: Modification of ^{204}Tl uptake in cultured myocardial cells. Circulation *60*:II-220, 1976.
147. Mueller, T. M., Marcus, M. L., Ehrhardt, J. C., Kerber, R. E., Brown, D. D., and Abboud, F. M.: Limitations of thallium-201 myocardial perfusion scintigrams. Circulation *54*:640, 1976.
148. Nielson, A., Morris, K. G., Murdock, R. H., Bruno, F. P., and Cobb, F. R.: Linear relationship between distribution of thallium-201 and blood flow in ischemic and nonischemic myocardium during exercise. Circulation *60* (Suppl.):II-148, 1979.
149. Strauss, H. W., and Pitt, B.: Noninvasive detection of subcritical coronary arterial narrowings with a coronary vasodilator and myocardial perfusion imaging. Am. J. Cardiol. *39*:403, 1977.
150. Gould, K. L.: Noninvasive assessment of coronary stenoses by myocardial perfusion imaging during pharmacologic coronary vasodilatation. I. Physiological basis and experimental validation. Am. J. Cardiol. *41*:267, 1978.
151. Holman, B. L., Cohn, P. F., Adams, D. F., See, J. R., Roberts, B. H., Idoine, J., and Gorlin, R.: Regional myocardial blood flow during hyperemia induced by contrast agent in patients with coronary artery disease. Am. J. Cardiol. *38*: 416, 1976.
152. Zaret, B. L., Strauss, H. W., Martin, N. D., Wells, H. P., Jr., and Flamm, M. D., Jr.: Noninvasive regional myocardial perfusion with radioactive potassium. Study of patients at rest, with exercise, and during angina pectoris. N. Engl. J. Med. *288*:809, 1973.
153. Schwartz, J. S., Ponto, R., Carlyle, P., Forstrom, L., and Cohn, J. N.: Early distribution of thallium-201 after temporary ischemia. Circulation *57*:332, 1978.
154. Garcia, E., Maddahi, J., Berman, D., and Waxman, A: Space/time quantitation of thallium-201 myocardial scintigraphy. J. Nucl. Med. *22*:309, 1981.
155. Grunwald, A., Watson, D., Holzgrefe, H., Irving, J., and Beller, G. A.: Myocardial thallium-201 kinetics in normal and ischemic myocardium. Circulation *64*:610, 1981.
156. Okada, R., Jacobs, M., Daggett, W., Leppo, J., Strauss, H. W., Newell, J. B., Moore, R., Boucher, C. A., O'Keefe, D., and Pohost, G. M.: Thallium-201 kinetics in nonischemic canine myocardium. Circulation *65*:70, 1982.
157. Berger, H. J., and Zaret, B. L.: Nuclear cardiology. N. Engl. J. Med. *305*:799 and 855, 1981.
158. Jengo, J. A., Freeman, R., Brizendine, M., and Mena, I.: Detection of coronary artery disease: Comparison of exercise stress radionuclide angiocardiography and thallium stress perfusion scanning. Am. J. Cardiol. *45*:535, 1980.
159. Pohost, G. M., Zir, L. M., Moore, R. H., McKusick, K. A., Guiney, T. E., and Beller, G. A.: Differentiation of transiently ischemic from infarcted myocardium by serial imaging after a single dose of thallium-201. Circulation *55*: 294, 1977.
160. Leppo, J., Rosenkrantz, J., Rosenthal, R., Bontemps, R., and Yipintsoi, T.: Quantitative thallium-201 redistribution with a fixed coronary stenosis in dogs. Circulation *63*:632, 1981.
161. McLaughlin, P. R., Martin, R. P., Doherty, P., Daspit, S., Goris, M., Haskell, W., Lewis, S., Kriss, J. P., and Harrison, D. C.: Reproducibility of thallium-201 myocardial imaging. Circulation *55*:497, 1977.
162. Johnstone, D. E., Wackers, F. J., Berger, H. J., Hoffer, P. B., Kelley, M. J., Gottschalk, A., and Zaret, B. L.: Effect of patient positioning on left lateral thallium-201 myocardial images. J. Nucl. Med. *20*:183, 1979.
163. Francisco, D. A., Collins, S. M., Go, R. T., Ehrhardt, J. C., Van Kirk, O. C., and Marcus, M. L.: Tomographic thallium-201 myocardial perfusion scintigrams after maximal coronary artery vasodilation with intravenous dipyridamole. Circulation *66*:370, 1982.
164. Heiss, H. W.: Coronary blood flow at rest and during exercise. *In* Rackman, H., and Hahn, C. H. (eds.): Ventricular Function at Rest and During Exercise. Berlin, Springer-Verlag, 1976, p. 17.
165. Albro, P. C., Gould, K. L., Westcott, R. J., Hamilton, G. W., Ritchie, J. L., and Williams, D. L.: Noninvasive assessment of coronary stenoses by myocardial imaging during pharmacologic coronary vasodilatation. III. Clinical trial. Am. J. Cardiol. *41*:279, 1978.
166. Strauss, H. W., and Pitt, B.: Thallium-201 as a myocardial imaging agent. Semin. Nucl. Med. *7*:49, 1977.
167. Wackers, F. J., Klay, J. W., Laks, H., Schnitzer, J., Zaret, B. L., and Geha, A. S.: Pathophysiological correlations of right ventricular thallium-201 uptake in a canine model. Circulation *64*:1256, 1981.
168. Boucher, C. A., Zir, L. M., Beller, G. A., Okada, R. D., McKusick, K. A., Strauss, H. W., and Pohost, G. M.: Increased lung uptake of thallium-201 during exercise myocardial imaging: Hemodynamic and angiographic implications of patients with coronary artery disease. Am. J. Cardiol. *46*:189, 1980.
169. Okada, R. D., Boucher, C. A., Kirshenbaum, H. D., Kushner, F. G., Strauss, H. W., and Pohost, G. M.: Thallium stress test: Improved diagnostic accuracy for an individual observer using criteria derived from interobserver analysis of variance (abstr). Clin. Res *27*:191, 1979.
170. Goris, M. L., Daspit, S. G., McLaughlin, P., and Kriss, J. P.: Interpolative background subtraction. J. Nucl. Med. *17*:744, 1976.
171. Narahara, K. A., Hamilton, G. W., Williams, D. L., and Gould, K. L.: Myocardial imaging with thallium-201: An experimental model for analysis of the true myocardial and background image components. J. Nucl. Med. *18*:781,1977.

172. Cantez, S., Harper, P. V., Atkins, F., Sbarboro, J., and Karunaratne, H.: Tomography in cardiac imaging. J. Nucl. Med. *18*:642, 1977.
173. Atwood, E., Jensen, D., Froelicher, V., Witztum, K., Gerber, K., Gilpin, E., and Ashburn, W.: Agreement in human interpretation of analog thallium myocardial perfusion images. Circulation *64*:601, 1981.
174. Meade, R. C., Bamrah, V. S., Horgan, J. D., Ruetz, P. P., Kronenwetter, C., and Yeh, E.: Quantitative methods in the evaluation of thallium-201 myocardial perfusion images. J. Nucl. Med. *19*:1175, 1978.
175. Koral, K. F., Rogers, W. L., and Knoll, G. F.: Digital tomographic imaging with time-modulated pseudorandom coded aperture and Anger camera. J. Nucl. Med. *16*:402, 1975.
176. Burow, R. D., Pond, M., Schafer, A. W., and Becker, L.: "Circumferential profiles:" A new method for computer analysis of thallium-201 myocardial perfusion images. J. Nucl. Med. *20*:771, 1979.
177. Vogel, R. A., Kirsh, D. L., LeFree, M. T., Rainwater, O. J., Jensen, D. P., and Steele, P. P.: Thallium-201 myocardial perfusion scintigraphy: Results of standard and multi-pinhole tomographic techniques. Am. J. Cardiol. *43*:787, 1979.
178. Berman, D., Staniloff, H., Freeman, M., Garcia, E., Pantaleo, N., Maddahi, J., Waxman, A., Forrester, J., and Swan, H. J. C.: Thallium-201 stress myocardial scintigraphy: Comparison of multiple pinhole tomography with planar imaging in the assessment of patients undergoing coronary arteriography. Am. J. Cardiol. *45*:481, 1980.
179. Green, A., Alderson, P., Berman, D., Caldwell, J., Thrall, J., and Vogel, R.: A multicenter comparison of standard and 7 pinhole tomographic myocardial perfusion imaging: ROC analysis of qualitative visual interpretation. J. Nucl. Med. *21*:P70, 1980.
180. Berman, D., Garcia, E., Maddahi, J., and Forrester, J.: Quantitative analysis of thallium-201 distribution and washout for comparison of multiple pinhole tomography with planar imaging. Circulation *62*:III-103, 1980.
181. Holman, B. L., Hill, T. C., Wynne, J., Lovett, R. D., Zimmerman, R. E., and Smith, E. M.: Single photon transaxial emission computed tomography of the heart in normal subjects and in patients with infarction. J. Nucl. Med. *20*:736, 1979.
182. Coleman, R. E., Jaszczak, R. J., and Cobb, F. R.: Comparison of 180° and 360° data collection in thallium-201 imaging using single-photon emission computerized tomography (SPECT): Concise communication. J. Nucl. Med. *23*: 655, 1982.
183. Tamaki, N., Muaki, T., Ishii, Y., Fujita, T., Yamamoto, K., Minato, K., Yonekura, Y., Tamaki, S., Kambara, H., Kawai, C., and Torizuka, K.: Comparative study of thallium emission myocardial tomography with 180° and 360° data collection. J. Nucl. Med. *23*:661, 1982.
184. Ritchie, J. L., Olson, D. O., Williams, D. L., Harp, G., Caldwell, J. H., and Hamilton, G. W.: Transaxial computed tomography with ^{201}Tl in patients with prior myocardial infarction (abstr). J. Nucl. Med. *22*:P11, 1981.
185. Coleman, R. E., Cobb, F. R., and Jaszczak, R. J.: Thallium studies using single photon emission computed tomography (SPECT) (abstr). J. Nucl. Med. *22*: P11, 1981.
186. Borello, J. A., Clinthorne, N. H., Rogers, W. L., Thrall, J. H., and Keyes, J. W., Jr.: Oblique-angle tomography: A restructuring algorithm for transaxial tomographic data. J. Nucl. Med. *22*:471, 1981.
187. Besozzi, M. C., Rizi, H. R., Rogers, W. L., Clinthorne, N., Pitt, B., Thrall, J. H., and Keyes, J. W., Jr.: Rotating gamma camera ECT of Tl-201 in the human heart (abstr). J. Nucl. Med. *22*:P11, 1981.
188. Rizzi, R. H., Pasyk, S., Fiedler, V. B., Mori, K. W., Lucchesi, B., Pitt, B., and Keyes, J. W., Jr.: Tl-201 transaxial ECT: In vivo quantification of myocardial ischemia in dogs. J. Nucl. Med. *22*:P11, 1981.
189. Ritchie, J. L., Zaret, B. L., Strauss, H. W., Pitt, B., Berman, D. S., Schelbert, H. R., Ashburn, W. L., Berger, H. J., and Hamilton, G. W.: Myocardial imaging with thallium-201: A multicenter study in patients with angina pectoris or acute myocardial infarction. Am. J. Cardiol. *42*:345, 1978.
190. Verani, M. S., Marcus, M. L., Razzak, M. A., and Ehrhardt, J. C.: Sensitivity and specificity of thallium-201 perfusion scintigrams under exercise in the diagnosis of coronary artery disease. J. Nucl. Med. *19*:773, 1978.
191. Blood, D. K., McCarthy, D. M., Sciacca, R. R., and Cannon, P. J.: Comparison of single-dose and double-dose thallium-201 myocardial perfusion scintigraphy for the detection of coronary artery disease and prior myocardial infarction. Circulation *58*:777, 1978.
192. Ritchie, J. L., Trobaugh, G. B., Hamilton, G. W., Gould, K. L., Narahara, K. A., Murray, J. A., and Williams, D. L.: Myocardial imaging with thallium-201 at rest and during exercise: Comparison with coronary arteriography and resting and stress electrocardiography. Circulation *56*:66, 1977.
193. Botvinick, E. H., Taradash, M. R., Shames, D. M., and Parmley, W. W.: Thallium-201 myocardial perfusion scintigraphy for the clinical clarification of normal, abnormal and equivocal electrocardiographic stress tests. Am. J. Cardiol. *41*:43, 1978.
194. Bailey, I. K., Griffith, L. S. C., Rouleau, J., Strauss, H. W., and Pitt, W.: Thallium-201 myocardial perfusion imaging at rest and during exercise. Comparative sensitivity to electrocardiography in coronary artery disease. Circulation *55*:79, 1977.
195. McCarthy, D. M., Blood, D. K., Sciacca, R. R., and Cannon, P. J.: Single dose myocardial perfusion imaging with thallium-201: Application in patients with nondiagnostic electrocardiographic stress tests. Am. J. Cardiol. *43*:899, 1979.
196. Berger, B. C., Watson, D. D., Taylor, G. T., Craddock, G. B., Martin, R. P., and Beller, G. A.: Sensitivity of quantitative thallium-201 scintigraphy following nondiagnostic exercise stress. Circulation *60*:II-72, 1979.
197. Iskandrian, A. S., and Segal, B. I.: Value of exercise thallium-201 imaging in patients with diagnostic and nondiagnostic exercise electrocardiograms. Am. J. Cardiol. *48*:233, 1981.
198. Diamond, G. A., and Forrester, J. S.: Analysis of probability as an aid in the clinical diagnosis of coronary-artery disease. N. Engl. J. Med. *300*:1350, 1979.
199. Ritchie, J. L.: Myocardial perfusion imaging. Am. J. Cardiol. *49*:1341, 1982.
200. Caralis, D. G., Bailey, I., Kennedy, H. L., and Pitt, B.: Thallium-201 myocardial imaging in evaluation of asymptomatic individuals with ischaemic ST segment depression on exercise electrocardiogram. Br. Heart J. *42*:562, 1979.
201. Rigo, P., Bailey, I. K., Griffith, L. S. C., Pitt, B., Burow, R. D., Wagner, H. N., Jr., and Becker, L. C.: Value and limitations of segmental analysis of stress thallium myocardial imaging for localization of coronary artery disease. Circulation *61*:973, 1980.
202. Lenaers, A.: Thallium-201 myocardial perfusion scintigraphy during rest and exercise. Cardiovasc. Radiol. *2*:195, 1979.
203. Massie, B. M., Botvinick, E. H., and Brundage, B. H.: Correlation of thallium-201 scintigrams with coronary anatomy: Factors affecting region-by-region sensitivity. Am. J. Cardiol. *44*:616, 1979.
204. Dash, H., Massie, B. M., Botvinick, E. H., and Brundage, B. H.: The noninvasive identification of left main and three-vessel coronary artery disease by myocardial stress perfusion scintigraphy and treadmill exercise electrocardiography. Circulation *60*:276, 1979.
205. Beller, G. A., Watson, D. D., Berger, B. C., Martin, R. D., and Taylor, G. J.: Detection of multivessel disease by exercise thallium-201 scintigraphy. Am. J. Cardiol. *45*:482, 1980.
206. Garcia, E., Maddahi, J., Berman, D. S., Waxman, A., and Swan, H. J. C.: A comprehensive model for space-time quantitation of sequential thallium-201 myocardial scintigrams. Circulation *62* (Suppl):II-75, 1980.
207. Bodenheimer, M. M., Banka, V. S., Fooshee, C., Hermann, G. A., and Helfant, R. H.: Relationship between regional myocardial perfusion and the presence, severity and reversibility of asynergy in patients with coronary heart disease. Circulation *58*:789, 1978.
208. Rozanski, A., Berman, D., Gray, R., Levy, R., Raymond, M., Maddahi, J., Pantaleo, N., Waxman, A. D., Swan, H. J. C., and Matloff, G.: Use of thallium-201 redistribution scintigraphy in the preoperative differentiation of reversible and nonreversible myocardial asynergy. Circulation *64*:936, 1981.
209. Greenberg, B. H., Hart, R., Botvinick, E. H., Werner, J. A., Brundage, D. M., Shames, D. M., Chatterjee, K., and Parmley, W. W.: Thallium-201 myocardial perfusion scintigraphy to evaluate patients after coronary bypass surgery. Am. J. Cardiol. *42*:167, 1978.
210. Rehn, T., Griffith, L., Achuff, S., Pond, M., and Becker, L.: Value and limitations of thallium-201 imaging to detect bypass graft patency. Am. J. Cardiol. *43*:434, 1979.
211. Pohost, G. M., Boucher, C. A., Zir, L. M., McKusick, K. A., Beller, G. A., and Strauss, H. W.: The thallium stress test: The quantitative approach revisited. Circulation *60*:II-149, 1979.
212. Ahmad, M., Merry, S. L., and Harbach, H.: Thallium-201 scintigraphic evidence of ischemia in patients with myocardial bridges. Am. J. Cardiol. *45*:482, 1980.
213. Losse, B., Kuhn, H., Kronert, H., Rafflenbeal, D., Fernendegen, L. E., and Loogen, F.: Exercise thallium-201 myocardial perfusion imaging in patients with normal coronary angiogram and ventriculogram. Circulation *60*:II-148, 1979.
214. Bailey, I. K., Come, P. C., Kelly, D. T., Burow, R. D., Griffith, L. S. C., Strauss, H. W., and Pitt, B.: Thallium-201 myocardial perfusion imaging in aortic valve stenosis. Am. J. Cardiol. *40*:889, 1977.
215. Keyes, J. W., Orlandea, N., Heetderks, W. J., Leonard, P. F., and Rogers, W. L.: The humongotron—a scintillation camera transaxial tomograph. J. Nucl. Med. *18*:381, 1977.
216. Gaffney, F. A., Wohl, A. J., Blomqvist, C. G., Parkey, R. W., and Willerson, J. T.: Thallium-201 myocardial perfusion studies in patients with mitral valve prolapse syndrome. Am. J. Med. *64*:21, 1978.
217. Klein, G. J., Kostuk, W. J., Boughner, D. R., and Chamberlain, M. J.: Stress myocardial imaging in mitral leaflet prolapse syndrome. Am. J. Cardiol. *42*: 746, 1978.
218. Massie, B., Botvinick, E. H., Shames, D., Taradash, M., Werner, J., and Schiller, N.: Myocardial perfusion scintigraphy in patients with mitral valve prolapse. Circulation *57*:19, 1978.
219. Maseri, A., Parodi, O., Severi, S., and Pesola, A.: Transient transmural reduction of myocardial blood flow, demonstrated by thallium-201 scintigraphy, as a cause of variant angina. Circulation *54*:280, 1976.
220. Ricci, D. R., Orlick, A. E., Doherty, P. W., Cipriano, P. R., and Harrison, D. C.: Reduction of coronary blood flow during coronary artery spasm occurring spontaneously and after provocation by ergonovine maleate. Circulation *57*: 392, 1978.
221. Waters, D. D., Chaitman, B. R., Dupras, G., Theroux, P., and Mizgala, M. D.: Coronary artery spasm during exercise in patients with variant angina. Circulation *59*:580, 1979.
222. Bulkley, B. H., Rouleau, J., Strauss, W., and Pitt, B.: Idiopathic hypertrophic subaortic stenosis: Detection by thallium-201 myocardial perfusion imaging. N. Engl. J. Med. *293*:1113, 1975.
223. Bulkley, B. H., Rouleau, J. R., Whitaker, J. Q., Strauss, H. W., and Pitt, B.: The use of ^{201}thallium for myocardial perfusion imaging in sarcoid heart disease. Chest *72*:27, 1977.
224. Bulkley, B. H., Hutchins, G. M., Bailey, I., Strauss, H. W., and Pitt, B.: Thallium-201 imaging and gated cardiac blood pool scans in patients with ischemic and idiopathic congestive cardiomyopathy: A clinical and pathologic study. Circulation *55*:753, 1977.

225. Pohost, G. M., Boucher, C. A., Zir, L. M., McKusick, K. A., Beller, G. A., and Strauss, H. W.: The thallium stress test: The qualitative approach revisited. Circulation *60*(Suppl.):II-49, 1979.
226. Wackers, F. J. T., Sokole, E. B., Samson, G., van der Schoot, J. B., Lie, K. I., Liem, K. L., and Wellens, H. J. J.: Value and limitations of thallium-201 scintigraphy in the acute phase of myocardial infarction. N. Engl. J. Med. *295*:1, 1976.
227. Wackers, F. J. T., Lie, K. I., Liem, K. L., Sokole, E. B., Samson, G., van der Schoot, J. B., and Durrer, D.: Thallium-201 scintigraphy in unstable angina pectoris. Circulation *57*:738, 1978.
228. DiCola, V. C., Downing, S. F., Donabedian, R. K., and Zaret, B. L.: Pathophysiological correlates of thallium-201 myocardial uptake in experimental infarction. Cardiovasc. Res. *11*:141, 1977.
229. Henning, H., Schelbert, H. R., Righetti, A., Ashburn, W. L., and O'Rourke, R. A.: Dual myocardial imaging with technetium-99m pyrophosphate and thallium-201 for detecting, localizing and sizing acute myocardial infarction. Am. J. Cardiol. *40*:147, 1977.
230. Mueller, H. S., Fletcher, J. W., and Ayres, S. M.: 201-Thallium image and creatine kinase MB infarct size—evaluation of variable treatment responses (abstr). Circulation *60*:II-163, 1979.
231. Buja, L. M., Parkey, R. W., Stokely, E. M., Bonte, F. J., and Willerson, J. T.: Pathophysiology of technetium-99m stannous pyrophosphate and thallium-201 scintigraphy of acute anterior myocardial infarct in dogs. J. Clin. Invest. *57*: 1508, 1976.
232. Wackers, F. J., Becker, A. E., Samson, G., Sokole, E. B., van der Schoot, J. B., Vet, A. J. T. M., Lie, K. I., Durrer, D., and Wellens, H.: Location and size of acute transmural myocardial infarction estimated from thallium-201 scintiscans: A clinicopathological study. Circulation *56*:72, 1977.
233. Smitherman, T. C., Osborn, R. C., and Narahara, K. A.: Serial myocardial scintigraphy after a single dose of thallium-201 in men after acute myocardial infarction. Am. J. Cardiol. *42*:177, 1978.
234. Silverman, K. J., Becker, L. C., Bulkley, B. H., Burow, R. D., Mellits, E. D., Kallman, C. H. and Weisfeldt, M. L.: Value of early thallium-201 scintrigraphy for predicting mortality in patients with acute myocardial infarction. Circulation *61*:996, 1980.
235. Markis, J. E., Malagold, M., Parker, J. A., Silverman, K. F., Barry, W. H., Als, A. V., Paulin, J. S., Grossman, W., and Braunwald, E.: Myocardial salvage after intracoronary thrombolysis with streptokinase in acute myocardial infarction: Assessment of intracoronary thallium-201. N. Engl. J. Med. *305*: 777, 1981.
236. Maddahi, J., Ganz, W., Ninomiya, K., Hashida, J., Fishbein, M. C., Mondkar, A., Buchbinder, N., Marcus, H., Geft, I., Shah, P. S., Rozanski, A., Swan, H. J. C., and Berman, D. S.: Myocardial salvage by intracoronary thrombolysis in evolving acute myocardial infarction: Evaluation using intracoronary injection of thallium-201. Am. Heart J. *102*:664, 1981.
237. Ashburn, W. L., Braunwald, E., Simon, A. L., Peterson, K. L., and Gault, J. H.: Myocardial perfusion imaging with radioactive-labeled particles injected directly into the coronary circulation of patients with coronary artery disease. Circulation *44*:851, 1971.
238. Jansen, C., Judkins, M. P., Grames, G. M., Gander, M., and Adams, R.: Myocardial perfusion color scintigraphy with MAA. Radiology *109*:369, 1973.
239. MacIntyre, W. J., Cannon, P. J., and Ashburn, W. L.: Measurements of regional myocardial perfusion. *In* Pierson, R. N., Jr., Kriss, J. P., Jones, R. H., and MacIntyre, W. J. (eds.): Quantitative Nuclear Cardiography. New York, John Wiley and Sons, 1975, p. 155.
240. Ritchie, J. L., Hamilton, G. W., Gould, K. L., Allen, D., Kennedy, J. W., and Hammermeister, K. E.: Myocardial imaging with indium-113m–and technetium-99m–macroaggregated albumin: New procedure for identification of stress-induced regional ischemia. Am. J. Cardiol. *35*:380, 1975.
241. Idoine, J. D., Holman, B. L., Jones, A. G., Schneider, R. J., Schroeder, K. L., and Zimmerman, R. E.: Quantification of flow in a dynamic phantom using ^{81}Rb-^{81m}Kr and a sodium iodide detector. J. Nucl. Med. *18*:570, 1977.
242. Yipintsoi, T., Knapp, T. J., and Bassingthwaighte, J. B.: Countercurrent exchange of labelled water in canine myocardium. Fed. Proc. *28*:645, 1969.
243. Yipintsoi, T., and Bassingthwaighte, J. B.: Circulatory transport of iodoantipyrine and water in the isolated dog heart. Circ. Res. *27*:461, 1970.
244. Ter-Pogossian, M. M., Koehler, P. R., and Potchen, E. J.: In vivo autoradiography of xenon-133 distribution in the cystic human kidney. Radiology *91*:358, 1968.
245. Bassingthwaighte, J. B., Strandell, T., and Donald, D. E.: Estimation of coronary blood flow by washout of diffusible indicators. Circ. Res. *23*:259, 1968.
246. Shaw, D. J., Pitt, A., and Friesinger, G. C.: Autoradiographic study of the ^{133}xenon disappearance method for measurement of myocardial blood flow. Cardiovasc. Res. *6*:268, 1972.
247. Cannon, P. J., Weiss, M. B., and Casarella, W. J.: Studies of regional myocardial blood flow: Results in patients with left anterior descending coronary artery disease. Semin. Nucl. Med. *6*:279, 1976.
248. Holman, B. L., Adams, D. F., Jewitt, D., Eldh, P., Idoine, J., Cohn, P. F., Gorlin, R., and Adelstein, S. J.: Measuring regional myocardial blood flow with ^{133}Xe and the Anger camera. Radiology *112*:99, 1974.
249. Cannon, P. J., Dell, R. B., and Dwyer, E. M., Jr.: Measurement of regional myocardial perfusion in man with ^{133}xenon and a scintillation camera. J. Clin. Invest. *51*:964, 1972.
250. Cannon, P. J., Dell, R. B., and Dwyer, E. M., Jr.: Regional myocardial perfusion rates in patients with coronary artery disease. J. Clin. Invest. *51*:978, 1972.
251. Cohn, P. F., Maddox, D., Holman, B. L., Markis, J. E., Adams, D. F., and See, J. R.: Effect of sublingually administered nitroglycerin on regional myocardial blood flow in patients with coronary artery disease. Am. J. Cardiol. *39*: 672, 1977.
252. Mann, T., Cohn, P. F., Holman, B. L., Green, L. H., Markis, J. E., and Philips, D. A.: Effect of nitroprusside on regional myocardial blood flow in coronary artery disease. Results in 25 patients and comparison with nitroglycerin. Circulation *57*:732, 1978.
253. Phelps, M. E., Hoffman, E. J., Huang, S. C., and Kuhl, D. E.: ECAT: A new computerized tomographic imaging system for positron-emitting radiopharmaceuticals. J. Nucl. Med. *19*:635, 1978.
254. Ter-Pogossian, M. M., Klein, M. S., Markham, J., Roberts, R., and Sobel, B. E.: Regional assessment of myocardial metabolic integrity in vivo by positron-emission tomography with ^{11}C-labeled palmitate. Circulation *61*:242, 1980.
254a. Marshall, R. C., Tillisch, J. H., Phelps, M. E., Huang, S-C., Carson, R., Henze, E., and Schelbert, H. R.: Identification and differentiation of resting myocardial ischemia and infarction in man with positron computed tomography, ^{18}F-labeled fluorodeoxyglucose and N-13 ammonia. Circulation *67*:766, 1983.
255. Phelps, M. E., Hoffman, E. J., Selin, C., Huang, S. C., Robinson, G., MacDonald, O., Schelbert, H., and Kuhl, D. E.: Investigation of [^{18}F]2-fluoro-2-deoxyglucose for the measure of myocardial glucose metabolism. J. Nucl. Med. *19*:1311, 1978.
256. Ratib, O., Phelps, M. E., Huang, S. C., Henze, E., Selin, C., and Schelbert, H. R.: Determination of myocardial metabolic rate (MRGlc) by positron computed tomography (PCT) and fluoro-18 deoxyglucose (FDG) (abstr). J. Nucl. Med. *22*:P11, 1981.
257. Huang, S. C., Phelps, M. E., Hoffman, E. J., Sideris, K., Selin, C. J., and Kuhl, D. E.: Noninvasive determination of local cerebral metabolic rate of glucose in man. Am. J. Physiol. *238*:E69, 1980.
258. Phelps, M. E., Huang, S. C., Hoffman, E. J., Selin, C., Sokoloff, L., and Kuhl, D. E.: Tomographic measurement of local cerebral glucose metabolic rate in man with (F-18)2-fluoro-2-deoxy-D-glucose: Validation of method. Ann. Neurol. *6*:371, 1979.
259. Opie, L. H., Owen, P., and Riemersma, R. A.: Relative rates of oxidation of glucose and free fatty acids by ischemic and nonischemic myocardium after coronary ligation in the dog. Eur. J. Clin. Invest. *3*:419, 1973.
260. Neely, J. R., Rovetto, M. J., and Oram, J. F.: Myocardial utilization of carbohydrate and lipids. Progr. Cardiovasc. Dis. *15*:289, 1972.
261. Neely, J. R., and Morgan, H. E.: Relationship between carbohydrates and lipid metabolism and the energy balance of heart muscle. Ann. Rev. Physiol. *36*: 413, 1974.
262. Schelbert, H. R.: The heart. *In* Ell, P. J., and Holman, B. L. (eds.): Computed Emission Tomography. Oxford, Oxford University Press, 1982, p. 91.
263. Henze, E., Perloff, J. K., and Schelbert, H. R.: Alterations of regional myocardial perfusion and metabolism in Duchenne's muscular dystrophy detection by positron computed tomography (abstr). Circulation *64*:IV-279, 1981.
263a. Geltman, E. M., Smith, J. L., Beecher, D., Ludbrook, P. A., Ter-Pogossian, M. M., and Sobel, B. E.: Altered regional myocardial metabolism in congestive cardiomyopathy detected by positron tomography. Am. J. Med. *74*:773, 1983.
264. Schelbert, H. R., Henze, E., Huang, S. C., and Phelps, M. E.: Relationship between myocardial blood flow and uptake and utilization of free fatty acids (abstr). J. Nucl. Med. *22*:P10, 1981.
265. Schön, H., Robinson, G., Barrio, J., Phelps, M., and Schelbert, H.: Extraction and clearance of C-11 palmitate in normal myocardium. Circulation *62*:III-103, 1980.
266. Schön, H. R., Robinson, G., Schelbert, H. R., and Barrio, J. R.: Kinetics of C-11-labeled palmitate in ischemic myocardium (abstr). Am. J. Cardiol. *47*: 414, 1981.
267. Hillis, L. D., and Braunwald, E.: Myocardial ischemia. N. Engl. J. Med. *296*: 971, 1034, and 1093, 1977.
268. Klein, M. S., Goldstein, R. A., Welch, M. J., and Sobel, B. E.: External assessment of myocardial metabolism with [^{11}C]palmitate in rabbit hearts. Am. J. Physiol. *237*:H51, 1979.
269. Goldstein, R. A., Klein, M. S., Welch, M. J., and Sobel, B. E.: External assessment of myocardial metabolism with C-11 palmitate in vivo. J. Nucl. Med. *21*:342, 1980.
270. Goldstein, R. A., Klein, M. S., and Sobel, B. E.: Detection of myocardial ischemia before infarction, based on accumulation of labeled pyruvate. J. Nucl. Med. *21*:1101, 1980.
271. Poe, N. D., Robinson, G. D., Jr., and MacDonald, N. S.: Myocardial extraction of labeled long-chain fatty acid analogs. Proc. Soc. Exp. Biol. Med. *148*: 215, 1975.
272. Reske, S. N., Machulla, H.-J., Biersack, H. J., Lackner, K., Knopp, R., and Winkler, C.: Nicht-invasive Erfassung des regionalen myocardialen Stoffwechsels von J-123-para-Phenylpentadecansaure durch single photon tomography. Nucklearmedizin *19*:258, 1982.
273. Chanusssot, F., and Debry, G.: Incorporation d'acid heptadécanoïque dans les lipides hépatiques du rat Wistar. J. Physiol. (Paris) *76*:831, 1980.
274. Knust, E. J., Kupfernagel, C. H., and Stocklin, G.: Long-chain F-18 fatty acids for the study of regional metabolism in heart and liver: Odd-even effects of metabolism in mice. J. Nucl. Med. *20*:1170, 1979.
275. van der Wall, E. E., Westera, G., den Hollander, W., and Visser, F. C.: External detection of regional myocardial metabolism with radioiodinated hexadecanoic acid in the dog heart. Eur. J. Nucl. Med. *6*:147, 1981.
276. van der Wall, E. E., Heidendal, G. A. K., den Hollander, W., Westera, G., and Roos, J. P.: Metabolic myocardial imaging with I-123 labeled heptadecanoic acid in patients with stable angina pectoris. Eur. J. Nucl. Med. *6*:391, 1981.

11 CARDIAC IMAGING

B—Nuclear Magnetic Resonance Imaging of the Heart

by Adam V. Ratner and Gerald M. Pohost, M.D.

Nuclear magnetic resonance (NMR), a method first applied by chemists to characterize molecular structure, now allows high-resolution tomographic and three-dimensional imaging as well as the acquisition of metabolic information, all without the need for ionizing radiation. Images produced by NMR methods have already shown significant clinical utility, particularly in the assessment of neurological disease.[1] For example, NMR imaging of protons can differentiate gray and white matter, detect demyelination, and define cerebral infarcts and tumors. Images can be generated with spatial resolution approaching that of x-ray computed tomography.

The spectroscopic aspect of NMR promises to provide a means for in vivo assessment of the metabolic function of internal organs. While the exact role that NMR techniques will play in the assessment of cardiac disease is currently not defined, there are many applications in which NMR may provide unique or complementary information when compared to existing diagnostic methods.

GENERAL PRINCIPLES OF NMR

Nucleons (protons and neutrons), the subunits of the atomic nucleus, have an intrinsic spin. Accordingly, certain nuclei (usually with odd numbers of nucleons) have a net nuclear spin. Since the nucleus is charged and a moving charge generates a magnetic field, spinning atomic nuclei possess magnetic fields or *moments* and simulate submicroscopic bar magnets. Such nuclear magnetic moments are required for a nucleus to exhibit NMR. Medically relevant nuclei that exhibit NMR include ^{1}H (proton), ^{13}C, ^{23}Na, and ^{31}P.

In a substance containing magnetic nuclei, the magnetic moments are usually randomly oriented. However, when placed in an external magnetic field, a number of magnetic nuclei align with the field. Most of the nuclei that align are parallel with respect to the field; however, some are antiparallel. The net effect is to generate a macroscopic magnetic moment parallel to the applied magnetic field (Fig. 11–30). The magnitude of the macroscopic magnetic moment is related to the concentration of magnetic nuclei within the sample under investigation.

To detect a magnetic moment it is necessary to displace it from its equilibrium position parallel to the external field. When a magnetic nucleus is rotated away from its original orientation, it will spin or precess about an axis parallel to the extrinsic magnetic field, like a spinning top.

In practice, radiofrequency (RF) pulses are used as the energy source for perturbing the net magnetization of the sample under investigation. The net magnetic moment will be rotated away from the direction of the extrinsic field in proportion to the duration and power of the RF pulse. When the RF pulse is turned off, these nuclei precess at the resonant or Larmor frequency, which is unique for a specific nuclear species at a given magnetic field strength and is determined by the Larmor equation:

Larmor (resonant) frequency = Gyromagnetic ratio (specific for each nucleus) × Magnetic field strength

For example, the resonant frequency of protons in a magnetic field of 0.15 tesla (tesla = unit of magnetic field strength equivalent to 10,000 gauss or 10 kilogauss) is 6.25 MHz, or 6,250,000 cycles/second. For ^{31}P (naturally abundant phosphorus) the resonant frequency would be 2.53 MHz.

The precessing nuclei will release an RF signal at the same unique (Larmor) frequency when they return to their original equilibrium positions. The RF signal released after an RF pulse is known as the free induction decay (FID) and provides the data that are analyzed in both NMR spectroscopy and NMR imaging.

The return of the nuclei to the initial, aligned state is known as relaxation; the time constant describing this process is known as the relaxation time. Actually, two terms mathematically describe the duration of this relaxation process: T1 and T2. T1, the spin-lattice (or longitudinal) relaxation time, describes the time course for the rotated or energized nuclei to return to the initial aligned position and describes

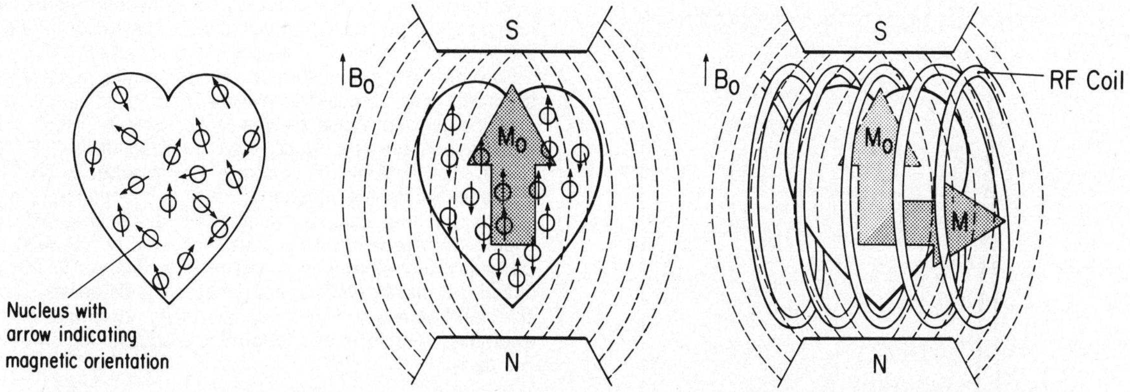

FIGURE 11–30 **Nuclei with randomly oriented moments are depicted within the heart (*left*). When the heart is placed in a magnetic field (B_0), the nuclei align both parallel and antiparallel to the field (*middle*). There is, however, a net moment (M_0) that is aligned in parallel with B_0. When an RF pulse is transmitted at the Larmor frequency of the nuclei, the magnetic moment M_0 is rotated to M, in this case after a 90-degree pulse (*right*).**

the process of energy transfer from the displaced nuclei to the environment. T2, the spin-spin (or transverse) relaxation time, describes the decay of the magnetic field in the transverse plane (perpendicular to the direction of the external field). During the RF pulse, nuclei precess in phase. After the RF pulse, each nucleus continues to experience not only the effects of the external static magnetic field but also the effects of the magnetic properties of neighboring nuclei. Consequently, after a time described by T2, the precession of individual nuclei drifts out of phase, and the net magnetic moment becomes smaller until the nuclei precess randomly and there is no net moment. T2 may never exceed T1 but, in certain instances, may approach it.

NMR SPECTROSCOPY

In 1946, Bloch and Purcell, motivated by theoretical considerations, independently published experimental data demonstrating the existence of NMR.[2,3] Since NMR signals are influenced by the chemical environment, NMR is capable of defining chemical composition. The frequency of a nucleus may be shifted away from the Larmor frequency by interactions of the electrons surrounding the nucleus in question, a so-called chemical shift. After an appropriate RF pulse, the resultant free induction decay signal is converted to a spectrum by using Fourier transformation. The area under each peak on the NMR spectral plot is directly related to the concentration of the chemical constituent containing that nucleus. In principle, NMR spectroscopy may be useful for the detection of many soluble body constituents and, as a result, may be useful over a wide range of medical applications. Using appropriate spectroscopic methods, investigators have studied cardiac metabolism and the effects of various interventions.

Most spectroscopic studies record the RF energy emitted by the sample after numerous bursts of radiofrequency energy. After a single burst, the resulting signal is weak and has considerable noise and by itself is inadequate for spectroscopic analysis. In order to obtain an adequate signal-to-noise ratio, many spectra are summed. Applications of proton, ^{13}C, and ^{31}P NMR spectroscopy to the study of ischemia and myocardial metabolism are summarized below.

Proton (^{1}H) Spectroscopy. Protons (^{1}H) are the most common nuclei in biology. Indeed, they compose approximately 70 per cent of the human body. Since they are so abundant and can emit stronger NMR signals than any other nuclei, protons are used for high-resolution imaging. In addition, since proton relaxation rates can be visualized by NMR imaging methods, proton spectroscopy is being used to define alterations of these proton relaxation parameters in relevant disease states.

Accordingly, Buonanno et al. have used proton spectroscopy to examine the effects of ischemia on T1 and T2 values of cerebral tissue. These investigators produced cerebral ischemia in the gerbil by ligating a carotid artery. Gerbils that were asymptomatic (demonstrated no evidence of hemiparesis) had normal relaxation times in both hemispheres, whereas symptomatic animals had significant increases in T1 and T2 in the hemisphere ipsilateral to the carotid ligation and normal values in the contralateral hemisphere.[4] With regard to myocardium, Williams et al. examined T1 in canine myocardium 30 minutes to 2 hours after coronary ligation. Significant increases in T1 were observed in ischemic myocardium compared with nonischemic myocardium[5] as early as 30 minutes after ligation.

Changes in proton relaxation parameters such as those demonstrated above suggest that, in addition to high-resolution tomography, proton NMR imaging may be useful for characterizing tissue damage during and after an ischemic insult.

^{13}C Spectroscopy. Approximately 1 per cent of natural carbon atoms are stable and the NMR-sensitive ^{13}C and virtually all the rest are ^{12}C. NMR spectroscopy has been applied to biological systems to evaluate metabolic processes using endogenous ^{13}C or ^{13}C-labeled substrates as tracers. Using ^{13}C-labeled precursors, Alger et al. studied glucose and lipid metabolism in various organs in the rat.[6] Bailey et al. studied tricarboxylic acid cycle intermediates in isolated perfused rat hearts.[7] This method has great potential for experimental characterization of metabolic processes and may ultimately be useful for clinical assessment of myocardial metabolism.

^{31}P Spectroscopy. Phosphorus-31, the naturally abundant phosphorus nucleus, is perhaps the most interesting from a biological perspective, since high-energy phosphate metabolism can be directly monitored with NMR techniques. In Figure 11–31, a schematic representation of a ^{31}P spectrum of myocardium, each peak represents a different phosphorus-containing moiety. The area under each peak is related to the relative concentration of each substance. Using ^{31}P spectroscopy in isolated working rat or rabbit hearts, it is possible to monitor the time course and reversibility of changes in high-energy phosphate concentrations with myocardial anoxia, ischemia, and infarction. In addition, the position of the inorganic phosphate peak is related to intracellular pH. Accordingly, changes in intracellular pH can be evaluated using spectroscopic monitoring of the position of the inorganic phosphorous resonance peak. Also, the concentration of magnesium (II) may be measured by examination of the position of the gamma-ATP resonance. When magnesium (II) is bound to ATP, the chemical environment surrounding the gamma phosphorus of ATP changes, altering its resonant frequency. Furthermore, enzyme kinetics and the compartmentalization of metabolites can be studied using a method that "labels" nuclei, enabling specific moieties to be followed even after chemical change. This technique is known as saturation transfer ^{31}P NMR.[8]

Phosphorus-31 spectroscopy has been used to study high-energy phosphate metabolism under normal and pathological conditions. Fossel et al. demonstrated variations in the concentrations of high-energy phosphates during different stages of the cardiac cycle.[9] They found that phosphocreatine and ATP levels were highest and inorganic phosphate levels lowest at end diastole, when aortic pressure was low. Conversely, in systole when aortic pressure was high, high-energy phosphate levels were lowest and inorganic phosphate levels were highest.

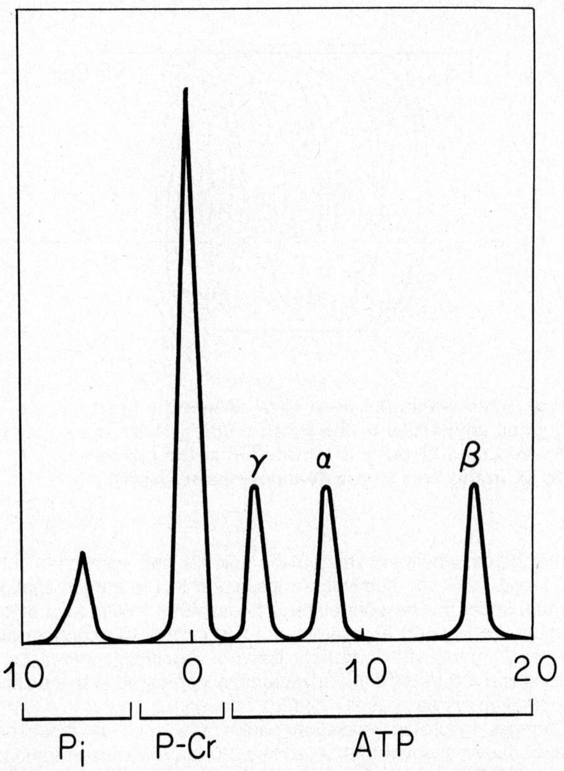

FIGURE 11–31 Schematic diagram of a ^{31}P spectrum of myocardium. Each peak represents a different phosphorus-containing moiety. From left to right are inorganic phosphate (P_i); phosphocreatine (P-Cr); and the gamma, alpha, and beta peaks of ATP. The area under each peak is related to the concentration of each group. The distance between the inorganic phosphate and phosphocreatine peaks is related to the pH. The numbers on the abscissa denote the difference (chemical shift) in the resonant frequency of each peak from the reference peak (phosphocreatine) in parts per million.

The beneficial effects of various interventions have been evaluated using ^{31}P spectroscopy. For example, Pieper et al. demonstrated that the acidosis of ischemic arrest could be significantly reduced with the addition of the beta-adrenergic blocking agent propranolol.[10] Flaherty et al. showed that potassium cardioplegia worked synergistically with hypothermia to preserve myocardial high-energy phosphates during episodes of ischemia.[11] The clinical relevance of these studies is apparent, and techniques are being developed and implemented for clinical application of NMR spectroscopy.

TOPICAL MAGNETIC RESONANCE

By application of specialized methods known as topical magnetic resonance (TMR), NMR spectroscopy can be performed in vivo in one of two ways. One method, the surface coil technique, uses radiofrequency coils placed on the surface of the subject being evaluated to delineate the region of interest. The other technique uses profiling magnetic gradients to designate a small sensitive volume from which spectra are generated. By these means, one may compare the spectra from regions of suspected disease with normal regions, serially follow the course of a disease with or without treatment, and obtain values of pH and metabolite concentrations.

In the *surface coil technique*, a small coil is placed adjacent to the physical region of interest. This technique allows signal acquisition from tissues no deeper than the radius of the coil and is most useful for studying superficial structures in vivo or excised structures. By placing a surface coil over the region of the left anterior descending coronary artery (LAD) on an excised perfused rabbit heart, Nunnally and Bottomley demonstrated that verapamil limited myocardial ischemic damage, as shown by increased high-energy phosphate concentrations after 30 minutes of LAD ligation versus the control.[12]

In the *sensitive volume technique*, a second magnetic field is established electronically that will localize the region of interest without the physical placement of a coil on the sample.[13]

Clinically, using the surface coil technique, a case of McArdle's syndrome was detected in skeletal muscle. In normal skeletal muscle, anaerobic exercise causes lactic acidosis, which shifts the inorganic phosphate resonance peak as observed in ^{31}P TMR spectra. However, in McArdle's syndrome, where lactate is not produced, the inorganic phosphate resonance peak remained fixed, a finding consistent with the absence of acidosis during anaerobic exercise.[14] It should be noted that TMR is not an imaging modality but rather a technique that produces a chemical spectrum similar to that produced in a classic NMR spectrometer. The difference is that the classic spectrometer collects signals from all parts of the sample, whereas TMR allows one to localize a specific region of interest within a sample.

NMR IMAGING

NMR imaging was first performed 10 years ago by Lauterbur using a modified spectrometer.[15] As described earlier, the resonant frequency of a given nucleus is proportional to the magnetic field in which it resides. If two identical nuclei are placed in magnetic fields of different strengths, they will have different resonant frequencies. Different regions of the magnetic field will have different field strengths if a magnetic field gradient is superimposed on the static magnetic field. As a consequence, identical nuclei in different parts of the field will have different resonant frequencies. If the field strength at all parts of the imaging field is known, it is possible to determine the location of nuclei using the emitted radiofrequency.

Most current NMR imaging systems acquire data from one or more planes or from an entire volume at any given time. Volumetric acquisitions allow sampling of an entire anatomical region with selection of the planes of interest to be studied after data collection. This allows retrospective analysis of data and may be particularly useful if the precise location of the suspected disease is unknown.

Intensity in an NMR image depends primarily on several factors, including proton density, T1, T2, and motion. With different pulse sequences, one or more of the above factors may be highlighted. In initial cardiac imaging studies, the NMR imaging group at the Massachusetts General Hospital employed a pulse sequence known as steady-state free precession (SSFP). This pulse sequence generates images related to proton density as well as to both T1 and T2 and is extremely sensitive to motion. The inherent motion sensitivity of this pulse sequence has made it only of historical interest in terms of in vivo cardiac imaging. This pulse sequence is produced by rapidly transmitting pulses while not allowing enough time for either spin-lattice or spin-spin relaxation to be completed.

Saturation recovery (SR) is a pulse sequence that can produce images with both proton density and T1 components. It is produced by employing 90-degree RF pulses interspersed by some time delay, tau (τ). By selecting different tau values, one can control the degree of T1 weighting. In SR images, the longer the time between the two RF pulses, the more complete is relaxation, and there is more proton density weighting and less T1 weighting. The proton density of a given tissue tends to change substantially only late in the course of a pathological process. T1, however, appears to provide additional contrast earlier in the course of certain disease states. When further T1 contrast is desired, an inversion recovery pulse sequence may be used. This pulse sequence is characterized by an initial 180-degree or inversion pulse followed by a 90-degree "read" pulse separated from the inversion pulse by a given tau. After the "read" pulse, a period of time equivalent to at least four to five times the longest T1 present is allowed to pass before the next 180-degree pulse is transmitted, so that complete relaxation can occur. As with saturation recovery, variations in the tau value will lead to changes in tissue contrast.

A spin-echo pulse sequence is used to acquire images with T2 weighting. A spin-echo sequence commences with a 90-degree pulse followed by one or more 180-degree pulses. One such sequence is the Carr-Purcell-Meiboom-Gill (CPMG) pulse sequence, which uses several 180-degree pulses after the 90-degree pulse.

CARDIAC NMR IMAGING

Some of the early images of the heart were of poor quality because the SSFP pulse sequence used was extremely sensitive to motion. Cardiac images obtained by Smith et al. using another ungated approach produced images with substantially better definition of the myocardium.[16] Subsequently, efforts were made to synchronize the RF pulses to the cardiac cycle. This was done by gating to physiologic cardiac parameters such as the arterial pulse or the electrocardiogram. Typically, projections are acquired at the same point in successive cardiac cycles until a complete tomograph is produced (Fig. 11–32). Problems arise in patients with irregular cardiac rhythms; in such patients, image degradation can be expected owing to successive projections being acquired at different points in the cardiac cycle. The ECG tends to provide synchronization that is physiologically superior to hemodynamic parameters, since most changes in cardiac function have a greater effect on the morphology of the arterial pressure wave than on the configuration of the QRS complex. Unfortunately, ECG-gated NMR images can have a high level of noise, since the ECG electrode acts as an antenna and transmits noise into the imaging region.

Myocardial intensity from gated saturation recovery images depends primarily on proton density with some T1 weighting. Because the RF pulses are synchronized with the cardiac cycle, T1 weighting in gated SR images of the heart depends on the heart rate. Gated inversion recovery and CPMG images have not yet been made because of the greater complexity of these pulse sequences. Gated cardiac images in man have been generated by investigators at Case–Western Reserve University Hospital.[17] These images were made using a gated saturation recovery pulse sequence, and they tend to highlight proton density.

Figure 11–33 depicts transverse section cardiac anatomy throughout the cardiac cycle. Anticipated changes in cardiac chamber size are observed during the cardiac cycle. In coronal images at end diastole (Fig. 11–34*A*), the signal intensity of blood in the arteries of the thorax is similar to that found in the surrounding tissue. In systole, as seen in Figure 11–34*B*, motion of the blood causes the signal from within the vessel to diminish. Proton NMR imaging thus differentiates moving blood from the tissue surrounding it. Kaufman, Crooks, and their associates demonstrated the feasibility of making quantitative measurements of flow and flow obstructions in models.[18,19] Thus, in addition to depicting cardiac structures with high resolution, gated proton NMR imaging may provide information concerning vascular flow.

The utility of proton NMR imaging for characterizing myocardium as ischemic or infarcted is now being explored.[19a] As stated earlier, spectroscopic studies showed that a prolonged ischemic insult may affect proton relaxation parameters in both ischemic brain and heart. Buonanno et al. showed that spectroscopically identified differences in T1 and T2 could also be seen in SSFP images of infarcted gerbil cerebral hemispheres.[4] Changes in proton signal strength in myocardium during infarction may result from the formation of edema, lipid accumulation, and fibrosis.

Studies in dogs carried out at the Massachusetts Gener-

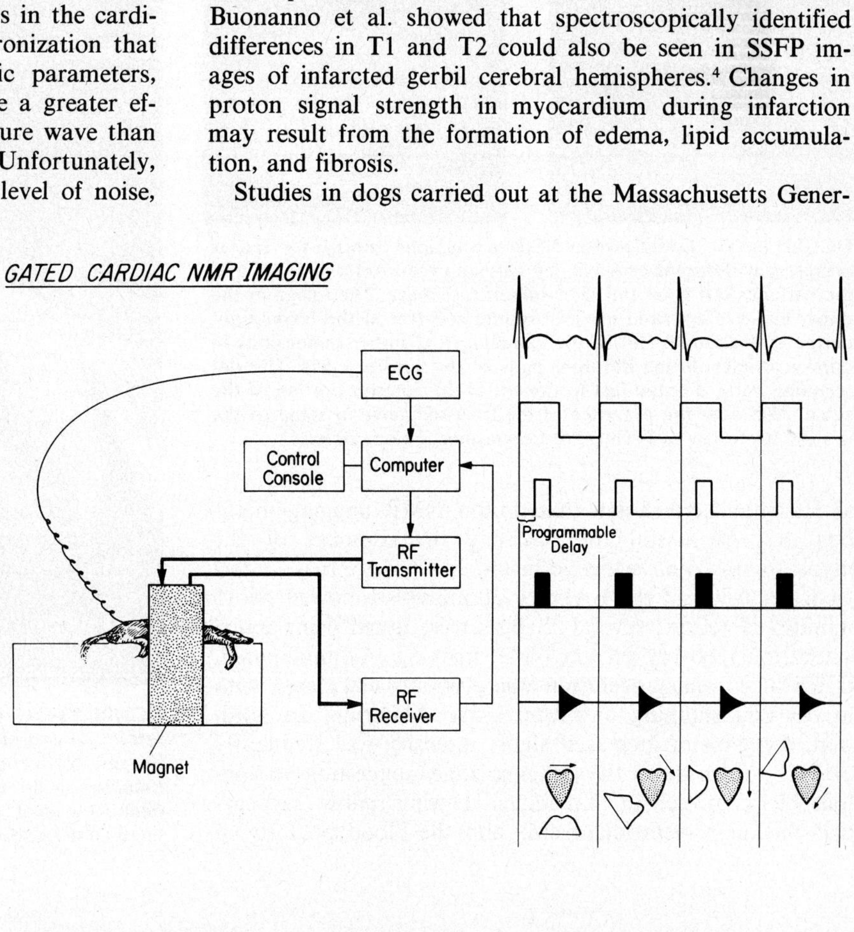

FIGURE 11–32 Schematic diagram of gating technique used in NMR tomographic imaging. A physiologic cardiac parameter such as the R wave of the ECG is converted to a digital signal in order to synchronize NMR imaging pulses with the cardiac cycle. The computer may be programmed to add some delay time to allow signal acquisition from different parts of the cardiac cycle. After the transmitter sends RF pulses into the imaging region, the returned signal (FID) is acquired by the receiver and relayed to the computer for processing of that projection. The system then waits for the next gating pulse to begin acquiring the next projection.

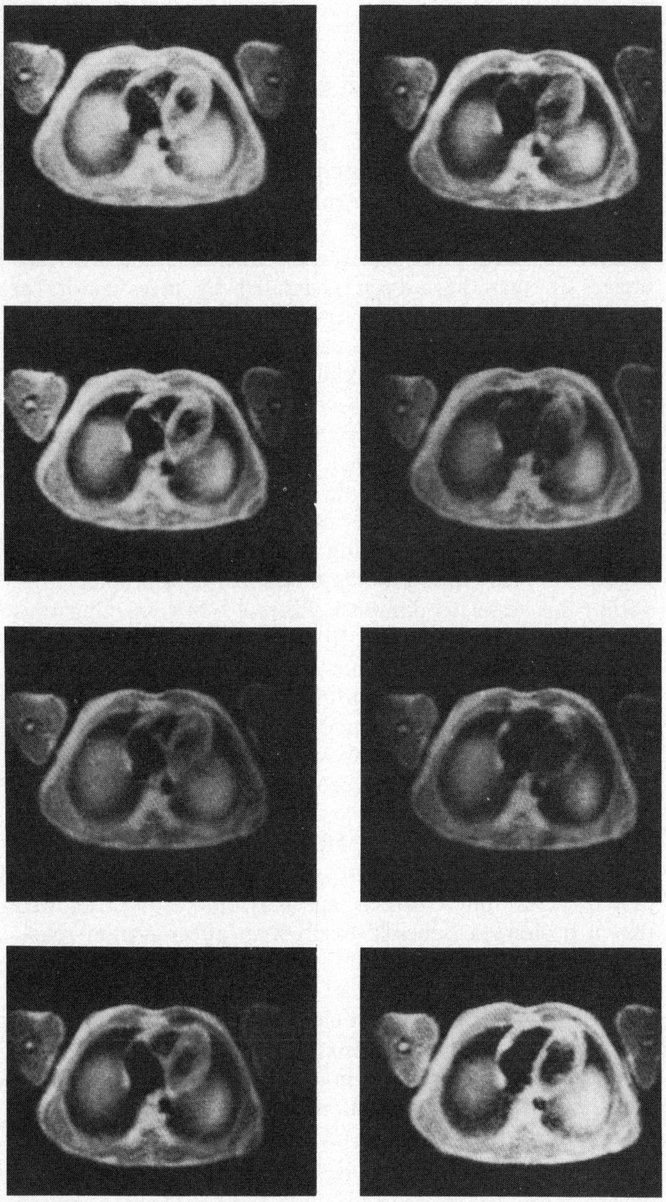

FIGURE 11–33 Gated proton NMR tomographs through the thorax acquired at different times in the cardiac cycle. Anterior is up and the patient's left is on the right side of the image. The image in the upper left was acquired in early systole and that at the lower right during end diastole. Notice the variation in chamber dimensions in both ventricles during different parts of the cardiac cycle. The descending aorta is noted just to the left of the anterior portion of the spine. Also note the presence of the tricuspid valve in some of the images. (Courtesy of Technicare Corporation, Solon, Ohio.)

al Hospital have shown that proton NMR imaging methods may be useful for assessing the response of the myocardium to an ischemic insult. In 16 dogs that underwent occlusion of the LAD for 30 minutes followed by 15 minutes of reflow, several changes were noted using gated saturation recovery proton NMR imaging. As anticipated, transient coronary occlusion was generally associated with myocardial thinning and ventricular dilatation. In addition, a region of increased signal intensity was frequently evident subjacent to the ischemic zone, suggesting anomalous blood motion in that region. During reflow, myocardial thickness, ventricular size, and the blood pool signal tended to revert toward normal. There was no apparent change in the intensity of the myocardial signal in the ischemic zone versus the normal zone. In dogs that underwent 72 hours of occlusion of the LAD without a reflow period, myocardial thinning, ventricular dilatation, and blood stasis also appeared. There were also examples of increased myocardial signal intensity in the ischemic region, which may represent lipid accumulation or asynergy in the necrotic myocardium.[20,21] It appears that cardiac NMR imaging can depict dynamic myocardial responses secondary to ischemia and may also be useful in characterizing the degree of ischemic tissue damage (Fig. 11–35).

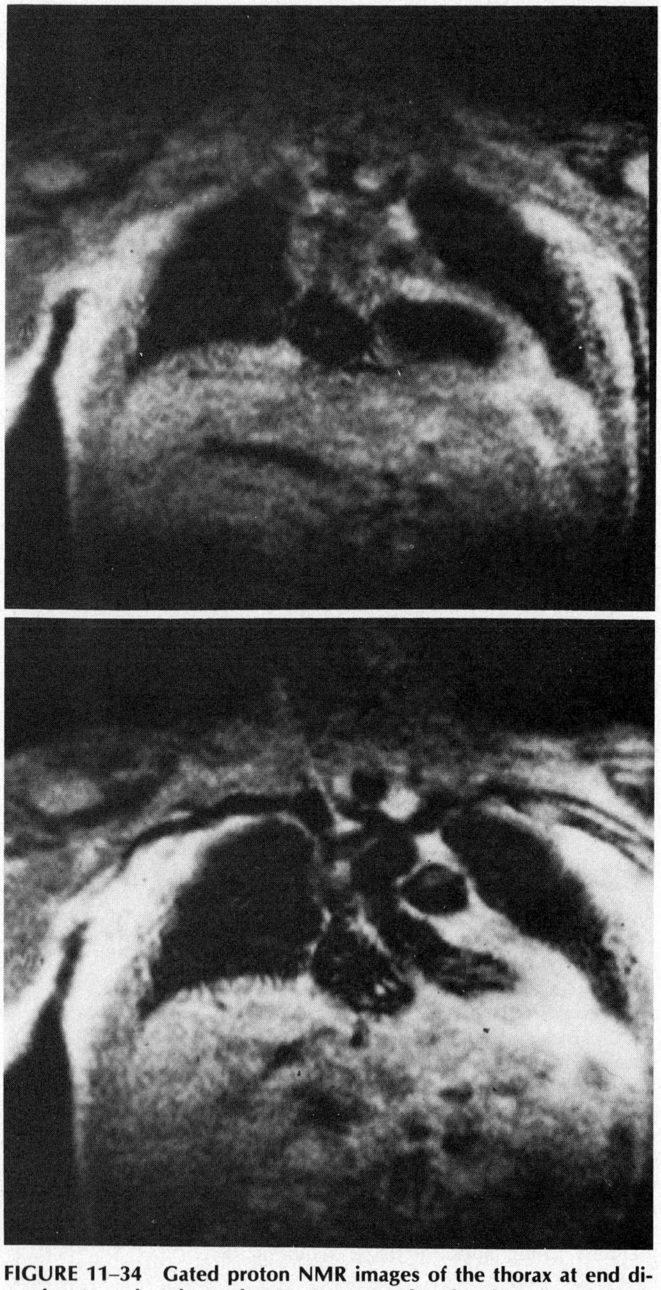

FIGURE 11–34 Gated proton NMR images of the thorax at end diastole (*A*) and end systole (*B*). Compare the chamber sizes in both images. Notice that the aortic outflow tract and its large arterial branches in the thorax, which are not well seen in *A*, are very well delineated in *B*. Motion of the blood is responsible for the heightened contrast. (Courtesy of Technicare Corporation, Solon, Ohio.)

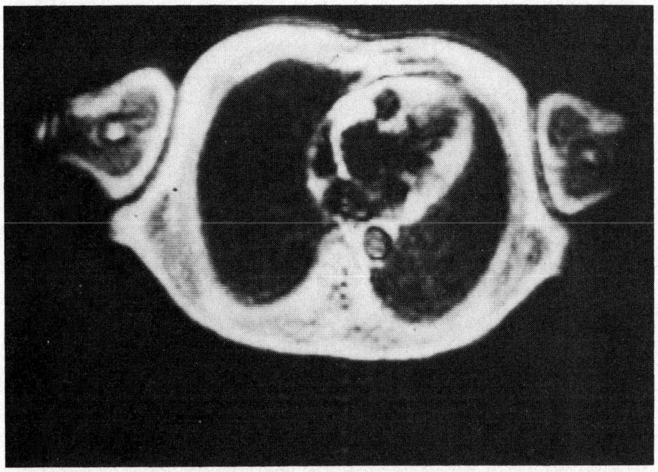

FIGURE 11–35 Gated proton NMR tomograph of a patient with a history of an old infarct. Notice the myocardial thinning and diminished signal intensity at the apex. The patient's left side is at the right side of the image. (Courtesy of Technicare Corporation, Solon, Ohio.)

CONTRAST AGENTS

Paramagnetic substances can modify the relaxation times of NMR-sensitive nuclei and as such may be useful as NMR contrast agents. In general, paramagnetic substances are those with unpaired electrons that can interact with NMR-sensitive nuclei and accelerate both spin-lattice and spin-spin relaxation, significantly shortening T1 and T2. Manganese ion (Mn^{++}) is strongly paramagnetic and has been shown in radionuclide studies to distribute in myocardium in proportion to blood flow.[22] Lauterbur et al. demonstrated spectroscopically that Mn^{++} could be used to label normal myocardium by reducing relaxation times.[23] In canine studies performed at the Massachusetts General Hospital, defects seen in Mn^{++}-enhanced NMR images corresponded closely with triphenyl tetrazolium chloride defects in both 90-minute and 24-hour coronary ligations.[24,25] Unfortunately, free Mn^{++} is a fairly toxic substance, and its clinical utility may therefore be limited.

There are several other paramagnetic substances, including molecular oxygen and stable free radicals, which may be clinically useful and not limited by toxicity. The paramagnetism of molecular oxygen may allow the in vivo assessment of blood oxygen saturation.

FUTURE IMAGING TECHNIQUES

With regard to proton imaging, an approach now being developed by Mansfield has the potential to allow acquisition of an entire tomographic image in less than 100 milliseconds.[26] Tomographic gated cardiac images, as described previously, require several minutes and the acquisition of numerous cardiac cycles. The Mansfield technique, known as "echo planar" imaging, is accomplished by using rapidly switching field gradients and can generate images in a small fraction of the cardiac cycle. Accordingly, the approach does not require gating, since each tomograph represents a single acquisition. Although images produced thus far by this technique have limited spatial resolution, the approach may provide the basis for a future avenue of cardiac NMR imaging.

Another development with potential cardiac applicability was the demonstration by DeLayre et al. that gated ^{23}Na images could be generated from the blood pool of an isolated beating rat heart.[27]

Although ^{31}P accounts for virtually 100 per cent of natural phosphorus, the concentration of phosphorus within most biological samples is very low. This low concentration, combined with the intrinsically lower NMR sensitivity of ^{31}P, contributes to the million-fold difference in the signal strength of phosphorus NMR signals compared to proton signals. While low signal strength may preclude high-resolution imaging of this nucleus, clinically useful low-resolution images may someday be obtained. Phosphorus spectroscopy in vivo is currently possible using TMR as described earlier.

SAFETY CONSIDERATIONS

While both NMR spectroscopic and imaging techniques appear to be safe, there are a few exceptions. Patients with metallic implants (e.g., aneurysm clips) should avoid strong magnetic fields, since the magnetic forces might displace the implant and cause harm. Furthermore, persons with cardiac pacemakers should not come close to an NMR system because of the risk that pacemakers may be reprogrammed or switched into the fixed-rate mode by the magnetic field. Budinger summarizes the potential medical effects and hazards of radiofrequency and magnetic fields and concludes that no biological hazard should be anticipated with NMR imaging systems.[29]

CLINICAL UTILITY OF NMR (Table 11–3)

High-resolution gated proton NMR tomography should permit accurate evaluation of ventricular volumes, myocardial mass, and the relative positions of the cardiac chambers and great vessels. The relaxation times T1 and T2 provide the basis for characterizing myocardial disease in proton NMR imaging, but considerable investigation is still needed to establish the utility of this approach.

The contrast provided by the motion of blood within the vasculature suggests that noninvasive angiography may ultimately be feasible without the need for radiopaque contrast media. In addition, reduced blood motion can be depicted within the cardiac chambers, and consequently, NMR imaging may allow detection of conditions favorable to thrombus formation. Paramagnetic substances provide a basis for myocardial perfusion imaging.

Perhaps the most exciting potential application for cardiac NMR is in the assessment of nuclei other than the proton. Measurement of cardiac high-energy phosphate concentrations and intracellular pH using TMR or imaging approaches may have important ramifications. The ability to assess high-energy phosphates, even with limited spatial resolution, would permit evaluation and monitoring of myocardial health in ischemic or other states.

While echocardiography provides some structural information at a considerably lower cost and during real time,

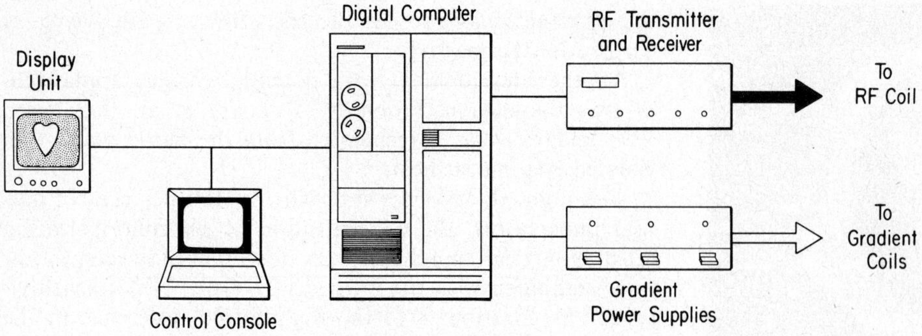

FIGURE 11–36 Schematic diagram of NMR imaging hardware.

proton NMR imaging is not impeded by bone or lung and can provide three-dimensional images as well as the potential for tissue contrast.

The ability to evaluate myocardial perfusion and viability noninvasively is limited to radionuclide approaches using thallium-201 with gamma-camera imaging[30] and positron-emission tomography using radioactive metabolic substrates. Although gamma-camera imaging can be performed at moderate cost, it requires the administration of radiopharmaceuticals with limited shelf-lives and generates reliable tomograms with difficulty. Positron methods are expensive because, for maximum flexibility, a cyclotron is needed to generate the short-lived radiopharmaceuticals. A fundamental problem with all tracer methods is that they require intravenous administration of the substance to be monitored; as a result, distribution is related not only to cell function but also to perfusion. High-energy phosphates, on the other hand, are endogenous, and their concentration directly reflects the state of myocardial health.

Although NMR imaging is at an early stage of development, its proven ability to generate high-resolution, tomographic, and three-dimensional images without the need to employ ionizing radiation will make it a powerful diagnostic tool. In addition, the ability of NMR spectroscopy and TMR to assess metabolic function by analysis of endogenous substrates and metabolic tracers will increase our understanding of cardiac disease and its therapy.

HARDWARE CONSIDERATIONS

NMR techniques are sophisticated and represent the confluence of computer and image-processing technology with radio and magnetic phenomena.

Most NMR imaging systems, whether they utilize resistive or superconducting magnets, employ a system similar to that depicted in Figure 11–36. The central unit, the digital computer, is responsible for image data acquisition and reconstruction. Through peripheral devices such as those shown, the computer can execute the desired RF pulse sequences and make the proper gradient adjustments as well as acquire the resultant NMR signals and reconstruct them into images.

The magnet is central to an NMR system. There are two types of magnets: electromagnets and permanent magnets. Nearly all systems to date have used electromagnets, which can be either resistive

TABLE 11–3 EVALUATION OF NMR IMAGING

Advantages
- High resolution (about 1 mm)
- Intrinsically tomographic or three-dimensional
- Ionizing radiation not employed
- No interference from bone or lung
- Contrast achieved between cardiovascular blood and surrounding structures without contrast media
- Tissue characterization possible

Disadvantages
- Relatively slow speed of image acquisition compared to x-ray and ultrasound methods
- High cost of hardware and site preparation
- Greater impact on cost of medical care
- Potential for changing operating mode of artificial pacemaker
- Potential for displacing metallic implants
- Effects of long-term chronic exposure unknown

Potential Utility
- Proton imaging
  - Noninvasive angiocardiography without contrast media
  - Detection of blood stasis (e.g., in left ventricle associated with myocardial infarction)
  - Characterization of diseased tissue using T1 and T2
  - Noninvasive oximetry
  - Rapid tomography (10 to 100 msec) using "echo-planar" technique
  - Tomographic myocardial perfusion imaging
- Non-proton imaging using ^{13}C, ^{23}Na, and ^{31}P
  - High-energy phosphate metabolism
  - Intracellular pH
  - ^{13}C-labeled substrate metabolism

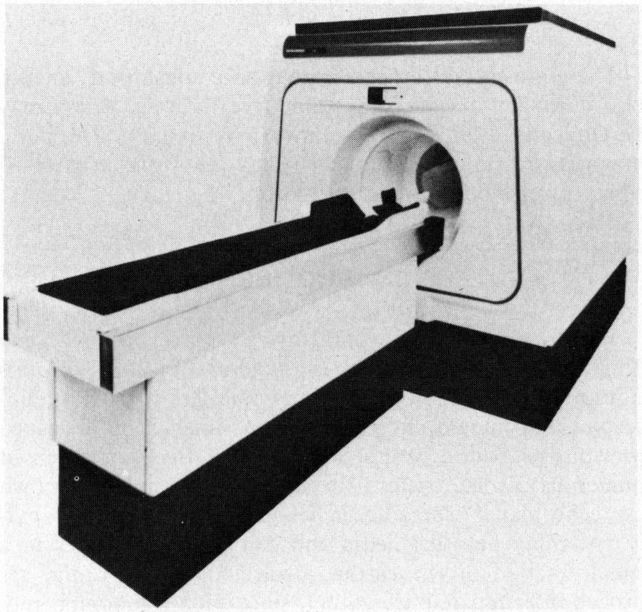

FIGURE 11–37 Photograph of whole-body NMR imaging magnet. (Courtesy of Technicare Corporation, Solon, Ohio.)

or superconducting. Superconducting magnets, although more expensive and considerably more difficult to manufacture, are necessary for work at field strengths above 2.0 to 2.5 kilogauss. Superconducting systems with fields of 3.5 to 5.0 kilogauss are being used for proton work (Fig. 11–37), and 15 kilogauss or higher field systems are used for ^{13}C and ^{31}P TMR. Resistive magnets can produce excellent images and may ultimately allow construction of computed tomography systems at a lower cost than can be produced with radiographic methods.

Resistive magnets consist of conductive copper wrapped around a central core. Such systems consume large amounts of electric current and require magnet power supplies. Superconducting systems consist of niobium alloy wire wrapped around a cylindrical core, which is surrounded by dewars of liquid helium and liquid nitrogen. This wire has an extremely high electrical resistance at room temperature but virtually no electrical resistance at the temperature of the surrounding liquid helium. The liquid nitrogen fills a dewar, which surrounds the liquid helium and serves to reduce the amount of helium boiled off. Both helium and nitrogen require periodic replenishing.

Owing largely to the dewars for the cryogens, superconducting magnets are necessarily larger than resistive magnets. Other considerations when erecting an NMR system include allocation of adequate floor space so that the magnetic field does not interfere with surrounding hospital functions and vice versa. Precautions must be taken to keep the laboratory isolated from large moving metal objects such as elevators because these objects can alter the uniformity of the magnetic field. Care must be taken to keep small ferromagnetic objects away from the NMR system, since the magnetic field can convert such objects into dangerous projectiles. Adequate space must be allocated for the requisite computer, power supplies, control console, and ancillary items crucial for patient safety.

References

1. Bydder, G. M., Steiner, R. E., Young, I. R., et al.: Clinical NMR imaging of the brain: 140 cases. Am. J. Radiol. *139*:215, 1982.
2. Bloch, F.: Nuclear induction. Physiol. Rev. *70*:460, 1946.
3. Purcell, E. M., Torrey, H. C., and Pound, R. V.: Resonance absorption by nuclear magnetic moments in a solid. Physiol. Rev. *69*:37, 1946.
4. Buonanno, F. S., Pykett, I. L., Vielma, J., et al.: Proton NMR imaging of normal and abnormal brain. Experimental and clinical observations. *In* Witcofski, R. L., Karstaedt, N., and Partain, C. L. (eds.): Proceedings of the International Symposium in NMR Imaging. Winston-Salem, N.C., Bowman Gray School of Medicine Press, 1982, pp. 147–157.
5. Williams, E. S., Kaplan, J. I., Thatcher, F., Zimmerman, G., and Knoebel, S. B.: Prolongation of proton spin-lattice relaxation times in regionally ischemic tissue from dog hearts. J. Nucl. Med. *21*:449, 1980.
6. Alger, J. R., Sillerud, L. O., Behar, K. L., Gillies, R. J., and Shulman, R. G.: In vivo carbon-13 nuclear magnetic resonance studies of mammals. Science *214*:660, 1981.
7. Bailey, I. A., Gadian, D. G., Matthews, P. M., Radda, G. K., and Seeley, P. J.: Studies of metabolism in the isolated perfused rat heart using C-13 NMR. FEBS Lett. *123*:315, 1981.
8. Ingwall, J. S.: Phosphorus nuclear magnetic resonance spectroscopy of cardiac and skeletal muscles. Am. J. Physiol. *242*:729, 1982.
9. Fossel, E. T., Morgan, H. E., and Ingwall, J. S.: Measurement of changes in high-energy phosphates in the cardiac cycle using gated P-31 NMR. Proc. Natl. Acad. Sci. *77*:3654, 1980.
10. Pieper, G. M., Todd, G. L., Wu, S. T., Salhany, J. M., Clayton, F. C., and Eliot, R. S.: Attenuation of myocardial acidosis by propranolol during ischemic arrest and reperfusion: Evidence with P-31 nuclear magnetic resonance. Cardiovasc. Res. *14*:646, 1980.
11. Flaherty, J. T., Weisfeldt, M. L., Bulkley, B. H., Gardner, T. J., Gott, V. L., and Jacobus, W. E.: Mechanisms of ischemic myocardial cell damage assessed by phosphorus-31 nuclear magnetic resonance. Circulation *65*:561, 1982.
12. Nunnally, R. L., and Bottomley, P. A.: Assessment of pharmacological treatment of myocardial infarction by phosphorus-31 NMR with surface coils. Science *211*:177, 1981.
13. Ross, B. D., Radda, G. K., Gadian, D. G., Rocker, G., Esiri, M., and Falconer-Smith, J.: Examination of a case of suspected McArdle's syndrome by P-31 NMR. N. Engl. J. Med. *304*:1338, 1981.
14. Gordon, R. E., Hanley, P. E., and Shaw, D.: Topical magnetic resonance. *In* Progress in NMR Spectroscopy, Vol. 15. New York, Pergamon Press, 1982, pp. 1–47.
15. Lauterbur, P. C.: Image formation by induced local interactions: Examples employing nuclear magnetic resonance. Nature *242*:190, 1973.
16. Smith, F. W.: Clinical application of NMR tomographic imaging. *In* Witcofski, R. L., Karstaedt, N., and Partain, C. L. (eds.): Proceedings of the International Symposium in NMR Imaging. Winston-Salem, N.C., Bowman Gray School of Medicine Press, 1982, pp. 125–32.
17. Alfidi, R. J., Haaga, J. R., El-Yousef, S. J., et al.: Preliminary experimental results in humans and animals with a superconducting, whole-body, nuclear magnetic resonance scanner. Radiology *143*:175, 1982.
18. Kaufman, L., Crooks, L. E., Sheldon, P. E., Rowan, W., and Miller, T.: Evaluation of NMR imaging for detection and quantification of obstructions in vessels. Invest. Radiol. *17*:554, 1982.
19. Crooks, L. E., Mills, C. M., Davis, P. L., et al.: Visualization of cerebral and vascular abnormalities by NMR imaging. The effects of imaging parameters on contrast. Radiology *144*:843, 1982.

19a. Ruigrok, T. J. C., van Echteld, C. J. A., Kruijff, B. de, Borst, C., and Meijler, F. L.: Protective effect of nifedipine in myocardial ischemia assessed by phosphorus nuclear magnetic resonance. J. Am. Coll. Cardiol. *1*:666, 1983.

20. Pohost, G. M., Goldman, M. R., Pykett, I. L., et al.: Gated NMR imaging in canine myocardial infarction (Abstract). Circulation *66*: 11-39, 1982.
21. Ratner, A. V., Goldman, M. R., and Pohost, G. M.: Visualization of myocardial ischemic damage using nuclear magnetic resonance imaging (Abstract). Clin. Res., *31*:213a, 1983.
22. Chauncey, D. M., Jr., Schelbert, H. R., Halpern, S. E., Delans, F., McKegney, M. L., Ashburn, W. L., and Hagan, P. L.: Tissue distribution studies with radioactive manganese: A potential agent for myocardial imaging. J. Nucl. Med. *18*:933, 1977.
23. Lauterbur, P. C., Dias, M. H. M., and Rudin, A. M.: Augmentation of tissue water proton spin-lattice relaxation rates by in vivo addition of paramagnetic ions. *In* Dutton, P. L., Leigh, J. S., and Scarpa, A. (eds.): Frontiers of Biological Energetics. New York, Academic Press, p. 752, 1981.
24. Goldman, M. R., Brady, T. J., Pykett, I. L., et al.: Quantification of experimental myocardial infarction using nuclear magnetic resonance imaging and paramagnetic ion contrast enhancement in excised canine hearts. Circulation *66*:1012, 1982.
25. Brady, T. J., Goldman, M. R., Pykett, I. L., Buonanno, F. S., Kistler, J. P., Newhouse, J. H., Burt, C. T., Hinshaw, W. S., and Pohost, G. M.: Proton nuclear magnetic resonance imaging of regionally ischemic canine hearts: Effect of paramagnetic proton signal enhancement. Radiology *144*:343, 1982.
26. Ordidge, R. J., Mansfield, P., Doyle, M., et al.: "Real-time" moving images by NMR. *In* Witcofski, R. L., Karstaedt, N., and Partain, C. L. (eds.): Proceedings of the International Symposium in NMR Imaging. Winston-Salem, N.C., Bowman Gray School of Medicine Press, 1982, pp. 89–92.
27. DeLayre, J. L., Ingwall, J. S., Malloy, C., and Fossel, E. T.: Gated sodium-23 nuclear magnetic resonance images of an isolated perfused working rat heart. Science *212*:935, 1981.
28. New, P. F. J., Rosen, B. R., Brady, T. J., et al.: Potential hazards and artifacts of ferromagnetic and nonferromagnetic surgical and dental materials and devices in NMR imaging. Radiology, *147*:139, 1983.
29. Budinger, T. F.: Thresholds for physiological effects due to RF and magnetic fields used in NMR imaging. IEEE Trans. Nucl. Sci. *NS-26*:2821, 1979.
30. Pohost G. M., and Goldhaber, S. Z.: Nuclear magnetic resonance. *In* Morganroth, J., Parisi, A., and Pohost, G. M. (eds): Noninvasive Cardiac Imaging. Chicago, Year Book Medical Publishers, Inc., 1983, pp. 423–431.

PART II

ABNORMALITIES OF CIRCULATORY FUNCTION

12 CONTRACTION OF THE NORMAL HEART

by Eugene Braunwald, M.D., Edmund H. Sonnenblick, M.D., and John Ross, Jr., M.D.

The function of the heart is to propel unoxygenated blood to the lungs and oxygenated blood to the peripheral tissues in accordance with their metabolic requirements. Heart failure may therefore be defined as the pathophysiological state in which an abnormality of cardiac function is responsible for the failure of the heart to pump blood at a rate commensurate with these requirements. To understand the disturbances in cardiac contraction that characterize heart failure, described in Chapter 13, it is necessary to comprehend the structure and function of the normal cardiac cell and of the normal contractile process, described in this chapter.

STRUCTURE OF THE MYOCARDIAL CELL

MYOCARDIAL CELLS, MYOFIBRILS, AND SARCOMERES. *Ventricular myocardial cells* (fibers) are normally 40 to 100 μ in length and 10 to 20 μ in diameter (Fig. 12–1). Numerous cross-banded strands or bundles, termed *myofibrils,* traverse the length of the fibers and, unlike the case for skeletal muscle, are incompletely separated by clefts of cytoplasm that contain mitochondria and membranous tubules (Fig. 12–1*B*).[1–4]

Myofibrils are composed of longitudinally repeating *sarcomeres* separated by two adjacent dark lines, the Z lines (Fig. 12–1*B* and *C*).[5] Sarcomeres occupy about 50 per cent of the mass of the cardiac cells and are aligned so that the ends of adjacent myofibrils are in register, giving the fiber its striated appearance.[1,2] The length of the sarcomere ranges from 1.6 to 2.2 μ, depending on muscle length. The center of the sarcomere is occupied by a dark band, the A band (the anisotropic or birefringent band that rotates polarized light); the band is composed primarily of myosin and is 1.5 μ in length. The A band is flanked by two lighter bands, termed I (isotropic) bands, which are variable in length depending on the length of the sarcomere. The bands of the sarcomere reflect the disposition of interdigitating myofilaments made up of contractile proteins (Fig. 12–1*C* and 12–3*A*). Thin filaments composed of actin are attached to each Z line and project longitudinally into the middle of the sarcomere, where they interdigitate with an array of thicker filaments composed of myosin molecules.[6] It is the interactions between the thick and thin myofilaments that generate force and shortening of the myocardium.

The *nucleus* is centrally placed within the myocardial cell. *Mitochondria,* which make up about 20 per cent of the

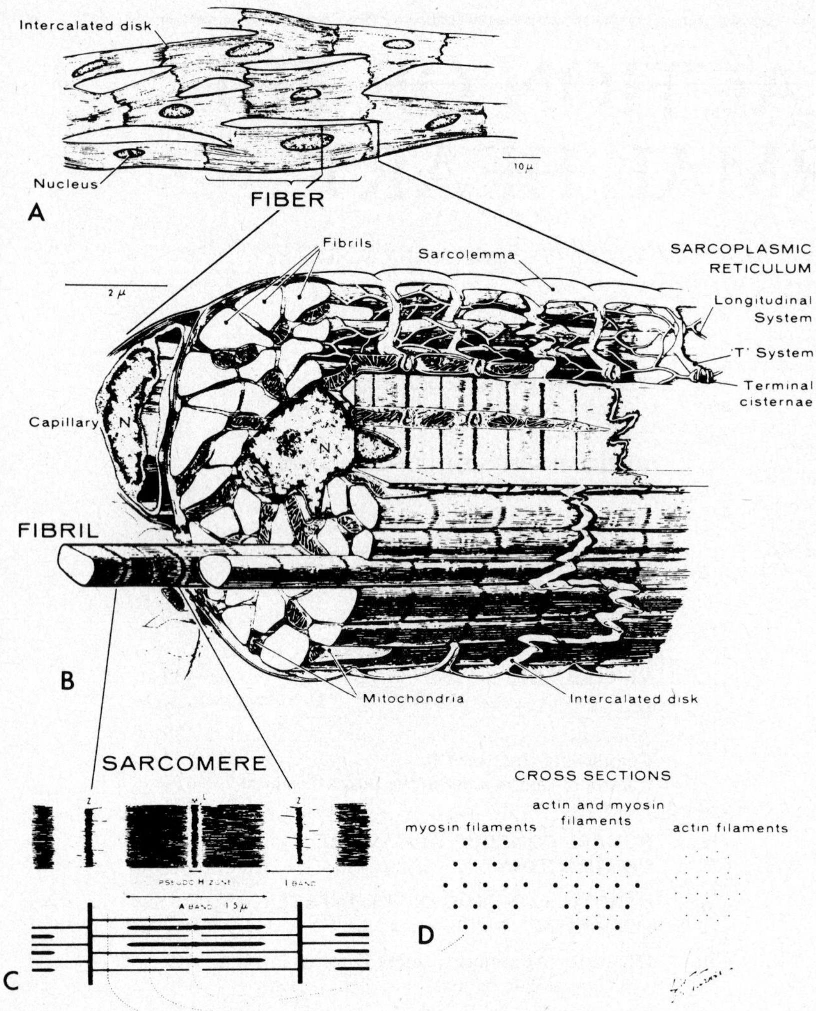

FIGURE 12–1 Schematic diagram of the microscopic structure of heart muscle.

A, Myocardium as seen under the light microscope. Branching of fibers is evident, with each containing a centrally located nucleus. Fibers or cells are connected across intercalated disks.

B, A myocardial cell or fiber reconstructed from electron micrographs, showing the arrangement of multiple parallel fibrils that compose the cell and of serially connected sarcomeres that compose the individual fibril. N = nucleus. The sarcotubular system, which mediates activation, includes the sarcolemma and sarcoplasmic reticulum. An intercalated disk in the center of the reconstruction serves to separate two cells.

C, An individual sarcomere from a myofibril. Diagrammatic representation of the arrangement of myofilaments that make up the sarcomere. Thick filaments, approximately 1.5 microns in length, composed of myosin, are localized to the A band, while thin filaments, 1.0 micron in length, composed primarily of actin, extend from the Z line through the I band into the A band, ending at the edges of the central H zone. The H zone is the central area of the A band where thin filaments are absent. Thick and thin filaments overlap only in the A band.

D, Diagrammatic cross section of the sarcomere showing the specific lattice arrangements of the myofilaments. In the center of the sarcomere (left), only the thick (myosin) filaments arranged in a hexagonal array are seen. In the distal portions of the A band (center), both thick and thin (actin) filaments are found, each thick filament surrounded by six thin filaments. In the I band, only thin filaments are present. (From Braunwald, E., et al.: Mechanisms of Contraction of the Normal and Failing Heart. 2nd ed. Boston, Little, Brown, 1976.)

volume of the cell, are elliptically shaped, approximately 2 to 5 μ by 0.5 μ, and are situated between and in close apposition to the myofibrils as well as just beneath the sarcolemma.[7] Their platelike foldings, or cristae, which contain the enzymes of the tricarboxylic acid cycle, project inward from the surface membrane. The close proximity of the mitochondria, the organelles in which ATP is produced, to the contractile filaments may facilitate the transfer of ATP from its site of production to its site of utilization during the contractile process. *Lysosomes,* membrane-limited vesicles about 0.1 μ in diameter and located near the pole of the nucleus, contain latent hydrolytic enzymes capable of lysing cellular membranes as well as other cellular components.

Myocardial cells that initiate intrinsic activity in the heart, i.e., *pacemaker or automatic cells,* are somewhat smaller than ventricular fibers[8] (p. 605). Those which are specialized for conduction and the spread of excitation, i.e., Purkinje fibers, are very large when compared to contractile fibers; they contain fewer myofibrils and greater quantities of clear cytoplasm, fine intracellular noncontractile filaments, and glycogen in addition to having a rich external investment of capillaries and small nerves.[9]

Myocardial fibers are surrounded by a rich capillary network, and small, nonmyelinated nerves are found lying free in the extracellular space.[3] These nerves have no specific junctions with cardiac cells but do exhibit bulbous ends bearing granules that contain neurotransmitter substances. These substances are *acetylcholine,* located primarily in the atria and in automatic and conduction tissues, and *norepinephrine,* found in these tissues but also in the ventricles; both can be released to act on membrane surface receptors of adjacent cells.

SARCOLEMMA, INTERCALATED DISKS, AND SARCOPLASMIC RETICULUM. A surface membrane, the *sarcolemma,* surrounds the myocardial cells and invaginates the Z lines of the sarcomere.[1,7,7a] It is composed of a thin (7 to 9 nm), bimolecular phospholipid layer, the plasmalemma, which is the site of electrical polarization (Fig. 19–5, p. 609). Just exterior to the plasmalemma is the glycocalyx, i.e., the basement membrane, approximately 50 nm in thickness (Fig. 12–2), which in turn is composed of an inner and an outer coat. The plasmalemma is the major semipermeable membrane between the intracellular cytoplasm and the negatively charged glycocalyx to which Ca^{++} may be bound and which separates the cell from the extracellular matrix. Adjacent myocardial cells are connected end-to-end by a thickened portion of the sarcolemma, termed the *intercalated disk,*[1–3] a segment of which, i.e., the nevus or gap junction, represents a low-resistance pathway to the propagation of electrical activity between cells.[1,8] Myocardial fibers are also interconnected

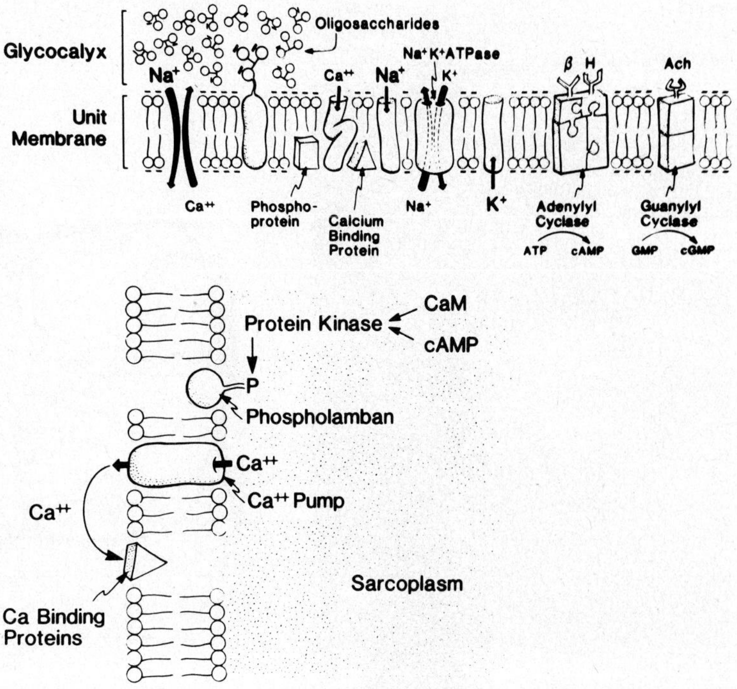

FIGURE 12–2 Schematic of the ultrastructure of the sarcolemma (*top*) and sarcoplasmic reticulum (*bottom*) of ventricular muscle cells. Both membrane systems have a lamina consisting of a sheet of lipids forming the matrix of the membrane and acting as a hydrophobic barrier. The outer surface of the sarcolemma is covered by a negatively charged glycocalyx that appears as a fuzzy layer in electron micrographs. Embedded in the sarcolemma are receptors for hormones and neurotransmitters along with the enzymes that transduce receptor binding to an alteration in intracellular concentrations of cyclic nucleotides. Major proteins in the sarcoplasmic reticulum (SR) are a calcium pump protein; calcium binding proteins that store transported calcium ions; and phospholamban, which, when phosphorylated by cAMP- or calmodulin-dependent protein kinases, alters the calcium pump and induces an increase in the rate of calcium transport into the lumen of the SR. (From Solaro, R. J.: The role of calcium in the contraction of the heart. *In* Flaim, S. F., and Zelis, R. (eds.): Calcium Blockers: Mechanisms of Action and Clinical Applications. Baltimore, Urban and Schwarzenberg, 1982, p. 25.)

by an extensive network of fine microfibrils and microthreads,[10] which play an important role in cell orientation, tissue compliance, and force transmission.

The hydrophobic phospholipid bilayer of the plasmalemma acts as an ionic barrier and maintains higher intracellular than extracellular potassium [K^+] concentrations and lower intracellular than extracellular sodium [Na^+] and calcium [Ca^{++}] concentrations. (Cytoplasmic [Ca^{++}] is of the order of 10^{-7} M; extracellular [Ca^{++}] is 10^{-3} M.) The sarcolemma possesses enzyme systems that utilize ATP for energy in order to maintain these differences in ion concentrations.[11,12] Na^+,K^+-stimulated ATPases (p. 509) are responsible for the active transport of Na^+ and Ca^{++} out of the cardiac cell and for the uptake of K^+. Near the Z lines the sarcolemma contains wide invaginations, *the T system,* which branch, both longitudinally and transversely, through the cell (Fig. 12–3). Closely coupled to but not continuous with the T system is the *sarcoplasmic reticulum* (SR), a complex network of anastomosing, membrane-limited tubular intracellular channels, approximately 300 Å in diameter, which surround each myofibril and play a critical role in excitation of the muscle.[7] Unlike the T system, the SR is not continuous with the extracellular space. Where the SR approaches the T tubules or the sarcolemma, it widens into flattened saclike enlargements (cisternae). At their junction, the SR and T tubules are separated by gaps of 10 to 12 nm. Depolarization of the sarcolemma is channeled through the T system to release Ca^{++} from the SR, which mediates myofibrillar activation (see below). Like the sarcolemma, the SR has a bilayer matrix consisting principally of phospholipids.

CONTRACTILE PROTEINS. The contractile apparatus consists of partially overlapping, rodlike myofilaments that are fixed in length, both at rest and during contraction.[1,13] The thicker filaments, composed of *myosin* molecules, are limited to the A band, are about 100 nm in diameter with tapered ends, and measure 1.5 to 1.6 μ in length.[1,14] They are created by an orderly aggregation of longitudinally stacked molecules of myosin proteins with a molecular weight of approximately 500,000 daltons and are held parallel and in register by centrally located connections at the M line. A rodlike tail, approximately 1300 nm in length, lies along the filament, and a globular bilobed head forms bridgelike outcroppings from the filament that can form a cross bridge which interacts with actin filaments[15] (Fig. 12–4). Myosin exhibits the ability to split ATP, i.e., it acts as an ATPase that is inhibited by Mg^{++} but activated by small amounts of Ca^{++}.[16] When myosin combines with actin, it forms an actomyosin complex that is enzymatically even more active in its ability to split ATP and is stimulated by both Mg^{++} and Ca^{++}. This constitutes the enzyme which is physiologically active in force development. The myosin molecule can be broken down by the proteolytic enzyme trypsin into two fragments, *light meromyosin* and *heavy meromyosin.* The latter contains bilobed globular heads (Fig. 12–4*A*), the site of ATPase activity.

Myosin itself can be separated into three isoenzyme components—V_1, V_2, and V_3—which have a different heavy-chain composition.[17,17a] Only two chemically distinct heavy-chain subunits exist, α and β.[18] V_1 and V_3 comprise αα and ββ while V_2 is a heterodimer, αβ. Myosin ATPase and intrinsic muscle speed (V_{max}) depend on the proportions of these isoenzymes that are present, V_1 being fast and V_3 being slow.[19] As noted on page 449, hypertrophied heart muscle has a lowered V_{max} and a greater amount of V_3.[18]

The thin filament, 1.0 μ in length in ventricular myocardium, is a double alpha-helix that consists of two strands of *actin,* has a molecular weight of 47,000 daltons and a diameter of 55 nm (Fig. 12–5).[20] Actin filaments course from the Z line through the I band and into the A band (Fig. 12–1*C*). The A band is the region of the sarcomere where there is overlapping of thick and thin filaments, while the I band contains only thin filaments. In atrial tissue, thin filament length is more variable.[6]

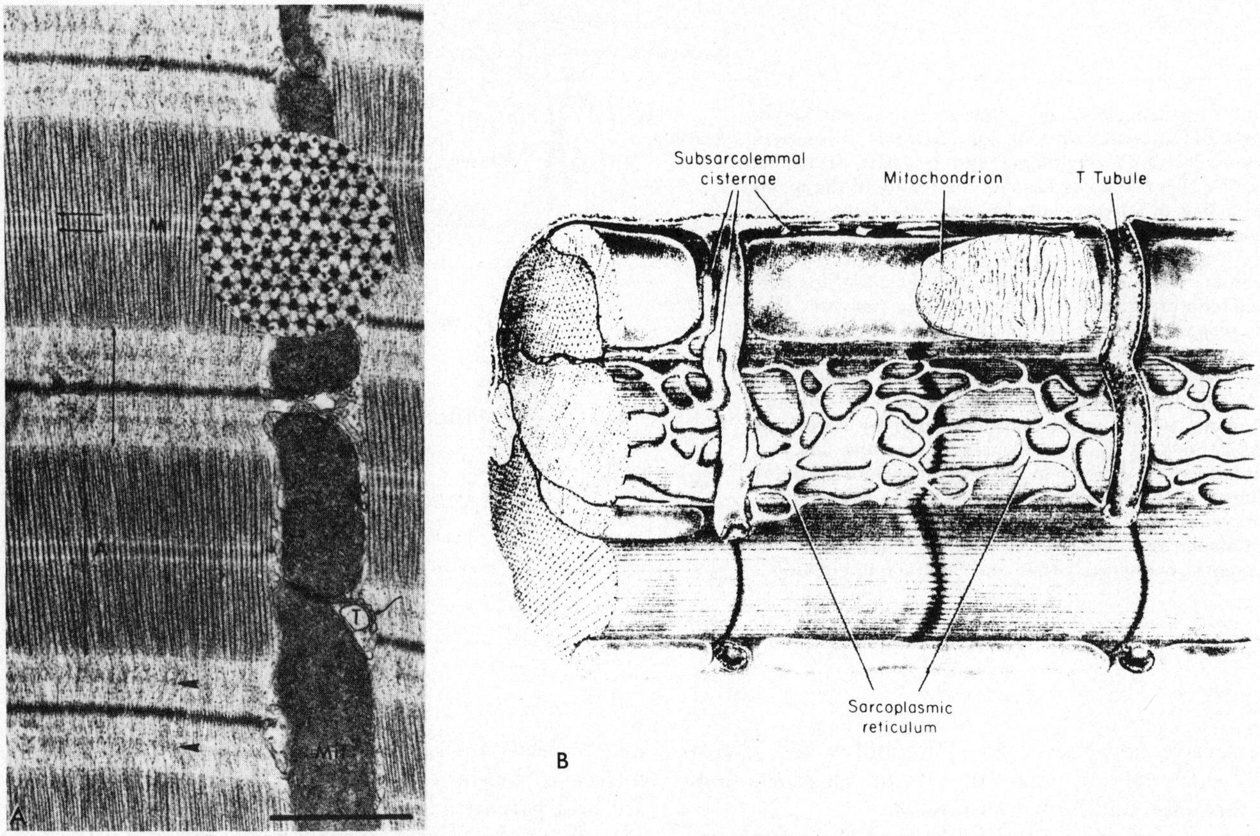

FIGURE 12–3 *A*, Longitudinal section through opossum cardiac muscle; different bands of striated muscle are clearly distinguishable. The A band (A = anisotropic) is composed of thick (myosin) filaments. Between the thick filaments, thin (actin) filaments are visible that slide between the former during contraction. Actin filaments make up the I band (I = isotropic) and are attached to the Z line (Z). Note that in the region of the M line (*inset*) some thin filaments are present equidistant from adjacent filaments. M = M line; arrows = pseudo H or L line; arrowheads = N line; curved arrow = junctional sarcoplasmic reticulum forming interior couplings with transverse tubules (T); Mit = mitochondrion. Bar = 1000 nm. (From Sommer, J. R., and Johnson, E. A.: Ultrastructure of cardiac muscle. *In* Berne, R. M. (ed.): Handbook of Physiology. Section 2, The Cardiovascular System. Vol. I, The Heart. Bethesda, American Physiological Society, 1979, pp. 113–186.)

Inset, Transverse section through region of M line. Note connections between myosin filaments and few actin filaments within the lattice. (From Robinson, T., and Winegrad, S.: Variations of thin filament lengths in heart muscle. Nature *267*:74, 1977.)

B, Schematic of T tubules and sarcoplasmic reticulum of mammalian cardiac muscle. Note how the diffuse tubular network of the sarcoplasmic reticulum forms saccular expansions, the subsarcolemmal cisternae, which are in close apposition to the sarcolemma and T tubules. (From Fawcett, D. W., and McNutt, N. S.: The ultrastructure of the cat myocardium. I. Ventricular papillary muscle. J. Cell Biol. *42*:1, 1969.)

Troponin and *tropomyosin* are regulatory proteins that constitute about 10 per cent of total myofibrillar protein and are associated with the thin filament.[21] Tropomyosin is a rodlike protein, 400 nm in length and 20 to 30 nm in width, with a molecular weight of 70,000 daltons. It comprises two helices, each of which lies slightly off the groove between the actin chains. Tropomyosin forms a continuing strand through the center of the thin filament while the troponin complex is located at intervals of 365 nm. *Troponin* can be separated into three components[22]: (1) troponin C, a "calcium-sensitizing factor" that binds Ca^{++} [23,24]; (2) troponin I, an "inhibitory factor" that inhibits the Mg^{++}-stimulated ATPase of actomyosin; and (3) troponin T, which is necessary for the entire complex to function and serves to allow attachment of the troponin complex to actin and tropomyosin.[24]

In the absence of troponin and tropomyosin, the contractile proteins actin and myosin interact and are fully activated, requiring the presence of only Mg^{++} and ATP to initiate the reaction leading to muscular contraction. When these regulatory proteins are present, however, cross-bridge formation between myosin and actin is inhibited.[21] When Ca^{++} is bound to troponin C, the binding of troponin I to actin is inhibited, which in turn causes a conformational change in tropomyosin, so that the latter, instead of inhibiting, now enhances cross-bridge formation. Ca^{++} may thus be considered to be a "derepressor," since it *inactivates* an *inhibitor* of the reaction between actin and myosin. Inhibition of the interaction between actin and myosin is mediated by the ability of the Ca^{++}-troponin complex to alter the configuration of tropomyosin, which in turn changes the exposure of active sites all along the thin filaments.[21] In relaxed muscle, tropomyosin blocks the active sites of actin that react to form cross bridges with myosin.[25] With cellular depolarization, the myoplasmic [Ca^{++}] rises from 10^{-7} to about 10^{-5} M. Ca^{++} is bound to troponin, and the actin rods are drawn toward the center of the sarcomere.[26] Once such a "stroke" is completed, an

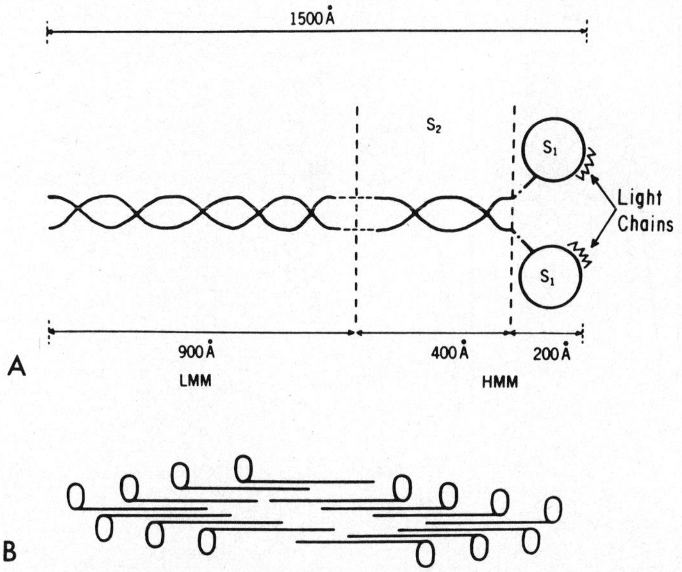

FIGURE 12–4 Structure of the myosin molecule and its aggregation into a thick filament.

***A*, The myosin molecule. The two-stranded portion of the molecule shows a point of cleavage between light meromyosin (LMM) and heavy meromyosin (HMM). Heavy meromyosin can be cleaved into two portions—an S_2 fragment, which is similar to the LMM portion of the molecule, and an S_1 fragment, which contains the ATPase portion of the molecule. Light chains are associated with the S_1 fragment. (From Lowey, S., et al.: Substructure of the myosin molecule. I. Subfragments of myosin by enzymatic degradation. J. Molec. Biol. *42*:1, 1969.)**

***B*, Diagram of the aggregation of myosin filaments into a thick filament. The long portion of the molecule tends to be oriented toward the center of the filament, with the enzymatically active heads of the molecule oriented laterally. Thus, the center of this aggregation will contain no active enzyme sites.**

attached myosin head ejects its ATP hydrolysis products, binds another ATP molecule, and detaches from the actin site. The myosin head then returns to its original orientation and the cycle is repeated, the head attaching to a different actin monomer farther along the thin filament[27] (Fig. 12–6). Thus, shortening of cardiac muscle involves a relative change in position of these two sets of filaments, i.e., actin filaments are displaced by the force-generating process at many cross-bridge sites. If the muscle is not permitted to shorten, i.e., during isometric contraction (in the presence of Ca^{++}), the heavy meromyosin does not undergo a conformational change, the cross bridges between actin and myosin are maintained, and ADP rather than ATP remains bound to myosin.

EXCITATION-CONTRACTION COUPLING: THE ROLE OF CALCIUM

Since the classic experiments of Ringer in 1882, it has been appreciated that cardiac contraction depends on the presence of Ca^{++}.[28] Heart muscle contains 2.5 mmol of Ca^{++} per liter of water, which is several hundred times higher than the concentration required for activation.[20] However, the higher [Ca^{++}] within the relaxed cell is not directly available to initiate contraction but is bound to many structures, including the nucleus, mitochondria, sarcolemma, T system, and particularly the SR. As already indicated, Ca^{++} is required at the contractile sites to trigger the contractile process by repressing troponin, the inhibitor of the actin-myosin interaction. The key event in the initiation of contraction then is the rise in sarcoplasmic [Ca^{++}].[29] The importance of this event had been suspected for many years, but there was no *direct* evidence for it in cardiac muscle until Allen and Blinks succeeded in the difficult task of using the photoprotein aequorin as an intracellular indicator of [Ca^{++}] in cardiac muscle.[30,31]

The Ca^{++} flowing into the cell does not appear to activate the contractile system directly but rather is stored in the membrane sites within the cell, i.e., the T system and the SR (Fig. 12–7). The Ca^{++} that actually activates the contractile system appears to be stored in the cisternae of the SR, which have the capacity to bind Ca^{++} actively and to store it in a bound form within their lumina.[31] A minute amount of Ca^{++}, which enters the cell during the plateau of the action potential but is insufficient to stimulate the contractile apparatus, may be capable of releasing a much larger quantity of Ca^{++} from the SR, allowing activation of the contractile system. This Ca^{++}-mediated release of Ca^{++} has been termed "regenerative" or "calcium-induced" calcium release.[32,33] According to this concept, depolarization of the cell membrane causes release of Ca^{++} from a store, SR_1 (the terminal cisternae of the SR), into the cytoplasm; Ca^{++} binding by troponin molecules results in contractile activity; relaxation is brought about by the active uptake of Ca^{++} into the temporary store, SR_2 (area of the SR adjacent to the contractile proteins), and from there the Ca^{++} eventually returns to SR_1. Thus, in

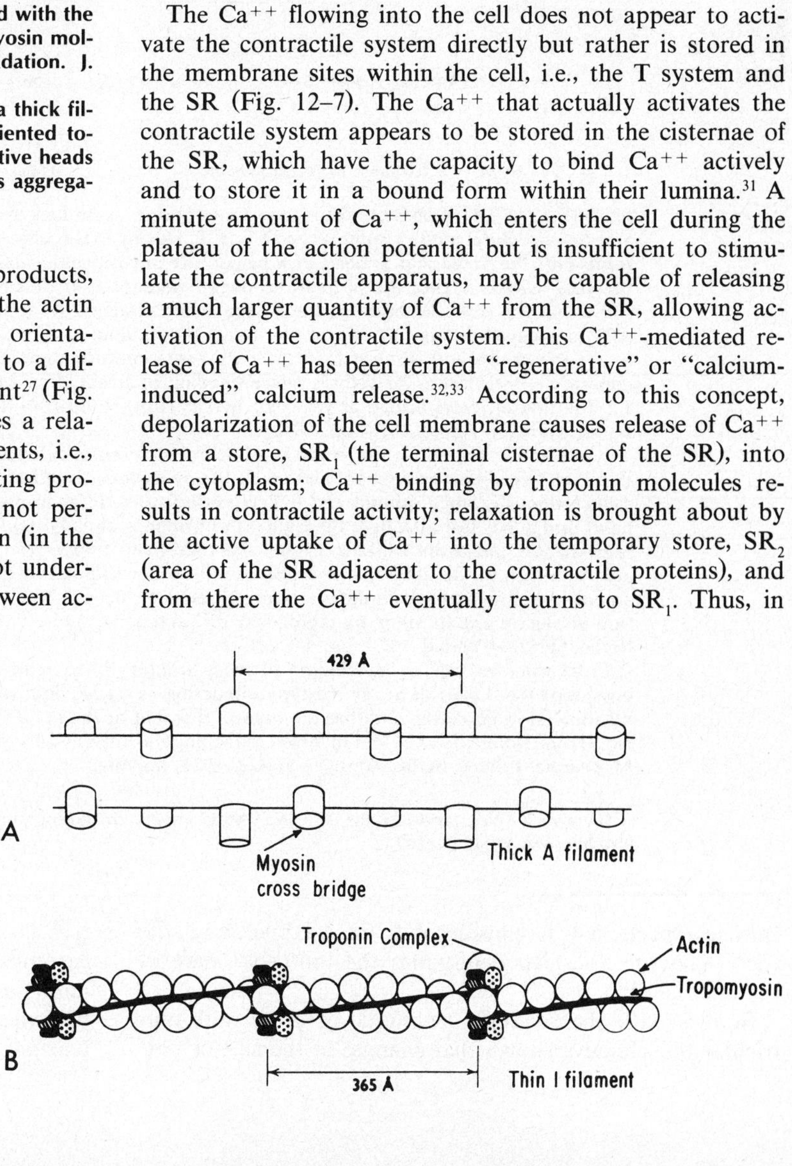

FIGURE 12–5 Structure and relations of the thick (*A*) and thin (*B*) filaments. The active myosin bridges turn progressively as one moves across the filament, with a complete revolution every 429 Å. The thin filament is composed of a double-chained alpha helix of actin molecules. The troponin complex is located at every seventh actin site, while the tropomyosin molecule lies close to the ridge between the two strands of actin. Thus, each strand of seven molecules of actin is associated with one troponin complex and one long molecule of tropomyosin, which extends the length of these seven molecules of actin. (Modified from Perry, S. V.: The control of muscular contraction. Symp. Soc. Exp. Biol. *27*:531, 1973.)

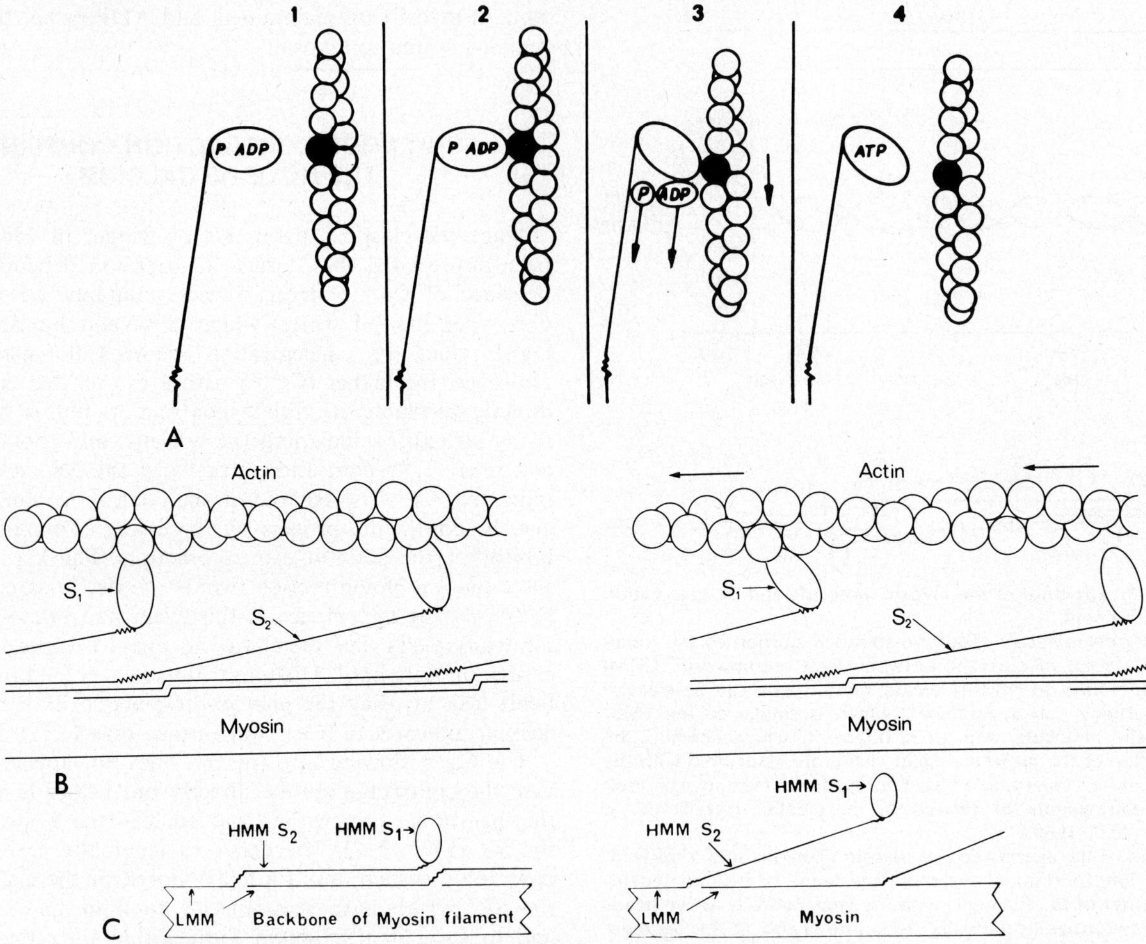

FIGURE 12–6 ***A,*** **A possible four-stage cross-bridge cycle based on the kinetic studies of Lymn and Taylor* and the structural studies summarized by H. E. Huxley.[26] The object on the left in each section of the diagram represents the S_2 tail and S_1 head of a heavy meromyosin molecule, which is joined to the myosin filament at the base of the S_2 rod; the S_1 head (depicted here as a single head) contains ATPase. The actin filament is shown on the right. Rotation of the bridge while attached to actin moves the actin filament along. Probably ADP is released during this part of the cycle. The binding of ATP to the new empty nucleotide binding site releases the bridge and restores it to the right-angle conformation. During this process ATP is hydrolyzed; concomitantly, the affinity for actin is raised, leading to a rebinding and repetition of the cycle. (From Holmes, K. C.: The myosin cross-bridge as revealed by structure studies.** ***In*** **Riecker, G., et al. (eds.): Myocardial Failure. Berlin, Springer-Verlag, 1977, pp. 16–27.)**

B, **An active change in the angle of attachment of cross-bridges (S_1 subunits) to actin filaments could produce relative sliding movements between filaments maintained at constant lateral separation. Bridges can act asynchronously, since subunit and helical periodicities differ in the actin and myosin filaments.** ***Left,*** **The left-hand bridge has just attached; the right-hand bridge is already partly tilted.** ***Right,*** **The left-hand bridge has just reached the end of its working stroke; the right-hand bridge has already detached and will probably not be able to attach to this actin filament again until further sliding brings the helically arranged sites on the actin filament into a favorable orientation. (From Huxley, H. E., and Haselgrove, J. C.: The structural basis of contraction in muscle and its study by rapid x-ray diffraction methods.** ***In*** **Riecker, G., et al. (eds.): Myocardial Failure. Berlin, Springer-Verlag, 1977, pp. 4–15.)**

C, **In order to explain the binding of cross-bridges (S_1) to actin over a range of filament spacings, Huxley[26] envisaged the S_2 part of heavy meromyosin acting as a stiff, light rod with hinges at both ends. The S_1 is thereby allowed to be closer to either the myosin filament or the actin filament, depending on the state of the muscle. (From Holmes, K. C.: The myosin cross-bridge as revealed by structure studies.** ***In*** **Riecker, G., et al. (eds.): Myocardial Failure. Berlin, Springer-Verlag, 1977, pp. 16–27.)**

Lymn, R. W., and Taylor, E. W.: Mechanism of adenosine triphosphate hydrolysis by actomyosin. Biochemisty** ***10**:4617, 1971.**

cardiac muscle, SR_1 is considered to be a labile store, the Ca^{++} content of which determines the inotropic state of the muscle.[33,34]

Studies with the aequorin technique in atrial and ventricular muscle have shown that changes in the rate or pattern of stimulation, in extracellular [Ca^{++}], and in catecholamines all produce a greater increase in cytoplasmic [Ca^{++}].[30] Catecholamines differ from the other inotropic interventions in that they produce a smaller increase in tension production than would be expected from the increase in the cytoplasmic [Ca^{++}], presumably by reducing the sensitivity of the contractile system to Ca^{++}. This decrease in sensitivity results from an increase in the degree of phosphorylation of troponin that is brought about by the cyclic AMP–induced activation of a protein kinase.[31]

As presented in detail on pages 610 to 617, the action potential for cardiac cells is generated by the movement of ions across the cell membrane, which in turn is controlled by variations in membrane permeability and ion concentration gradient in a manner similar to that occurring in nerve cells.[35,35a] The action potential of ventricular myocardium has two components, the spike and the plateau; a large fast inward Na^{+} current passing through "fast Na^{+} channels" is responsible for the early spike, while Ca^{++} influx into the myocardial cell occurs during the plateau phase of the action potential through a separate set of "slow channels" that are permeable primarily to Ca^{++}.[36] The latter are blocked by the organic Ca^{++}-channel blocking agents such as verapamil, nifedipine, diltiazem, and their analogs[37,38,38a] (p. 1350) and by manganese ion, lanthanum ion, and acidosis; additional Ca^{++} channels are recruited by beta-adrenergic stimulation. Total Ca^{++} within the cell is also affected by an exchange of more than $2Na^{+}$ for each Ca^{++} across the sarcolemma, the energy for which is supplied by the Na^{+} gradient generated by the sodium pump.[39] Ca^{++} removal from the cell is enhanced when the Na^{+} gradient is increased, and it is reduced (leading to intracellular Ca^{++} accumulation) when the gradient diminishes. The latter effect may explain the positive inotropic effect of lowering extracellular [Na^{+}] or of inhibiting the Na^{+},K^{+}-stimulated ATPase with digitalis, which elevates intracellular [Na^{+}]; both these interventions alter the transmembrane Na^{+} gradient and elevate intracellular [Ca^{++}] (p. 510).

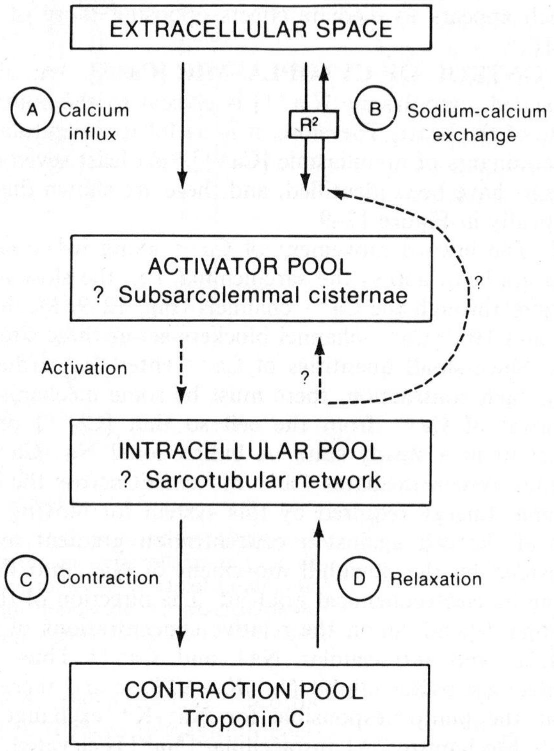

FIGURE 12–7 Calcium fluxes that participate in cardiac excitation-contraction coupling represent movement of calcium between the extracellular space, an activator pool that may be related to the subsarcolemmal cisternae, an intracellular pool that is probably within the sarcoplasmic reticulum, and a contraction pool that represents calcium bound to troponin. Calcium influx (*A*) is a "downhill" flux across the sarcolemma that occurs largely as the electrogenic slow inward current. A sodium-calcium exchange (*B*) can transport calcium in either direction across the sarcolemma but is involved mainly in the "uphill" transport of calcium out of the cell in a nonelectrogenic exchange for sodium, which moves down a concentration gradient into the cell. The intracellular pool that supplies calcium to the sodium-calcium exchange has not been identified but may be related to the sarcoplasmic reticulum. A relatively small calcium flux from the activator pool may trigger the release of a larger amount of calcium from the intracellular pool ("calcium-triggered calcium release") as shown by the arrow labeled "activation." Contraction (*C*) occurs when a large amount of calcium is released from the intracellular pool, most likely when an increase in the calcium permeability of the sarcoplasmic reticulum allows this ion to become available for binding to calcium-binding sites on troponin. Relaxation (*D*) occurs when the ATP-dependent calcium pump of the sarcoplasmic reticulum pumps calcium back into the intracellular membrane system. The resulting fall in cytosolic Ca^{++} concentration causes calcium to become dissociated from its binding site on troponin. (From Katz, A. M.: Physiology of the Heart. New York, Raven Press, 1977.)

As has already been pointed out, the absolute quantity of Ca^{++} that crosses the sarcolemma during the plateau (phase 2) of the action potential, i.e., during the slow inward current, is relatively small and is incapable in and of itself of bringing about full activation of the contractile apparatus. Instead, the major portion of the Ca^{++} used to activate concentration is stored within the cell, largely in the SR, in its subsarcolemmal cisternae (Fig. 12–7), or on the inner surface of the sarcolemma itself.[40] This Ca^{++} diffuses toward the myofibrils and binds to troponin, which, together with tropomyosin but in the absence of Ca^{++}, prevents the interaction between heavy meromyosin and actin. The number of contractile sites activated and therefore the resultant force generated are directly related to the quantity of Ca^{++} present in the vicinity of the myofibrils, which in turn ultimately depends on the influx of Ca^{++} that accompanied the action potential.[41] This influx, in turn, is a function of the extracellular [Ca^{++}], the duration of the action potential,[42] and the number of action potentials per unit time.[34]

Relaxation of cardiac muscle results from a cessation of the inward slow Ca^{++} current coupled with the uptake and storage of Ca^{++} by the SR, in which is embedded a 100,000-dalton membrane-bound protein, phospholamban, which spans the lipid bilayer (Fig. 12–2). This protein, a Ca^{++}-stimulated Mg-ATPase, has a very high affinity for Ca^{++} and is responsible for the active transport of Ca^{++} from the cytoplasm into the lumen of the SR. Thus, during repolarization, the SR in the presence of ATP avidly accumulates myoplasmic Ca^{++} against a concentration gradient, so that intracellular [Ca^{++}] falls to below 10^{-7} M and Ca^{++} detaches from the troponin, resulting in inhibition of the interactions between actin and myosin and hence in relaxation.[42]

INOTROPIC EFFECTS AND CALCIUM KINETICS. There is evidence that (1) the total tension developed, (2) the rate of tension development, and (3) the rate of tension decline during relaxation can be related, respectively, to (1) the quantity of Ca^{++} made available for binding to troponin, (2) the rate of Ca^{++} delivery to troponin, and (3) the rate at which Ca^{++} is removed from

troponin.[43] Many inte
contractile state of h
indeed are caused by
concentrations in hea
frequency relation,[46] i
ing from an increase
postextrasystolic pot
force-frequency relati
such as the cardiac g
amines,[53–55] and xanth
tility—and agents su
Ca^{++}-channel blocke
rhythmic agents, and
Experiments on skinn
erate acidosis causes
released from the SR
for the negative inotr
One proposed mec
amines is shown in F
to act on beta recep
process leads to th
membrane-bound enz
cyclic AMP from A
AMP, in turn, acti
AMP–dependent pro
number of cellular p
by an increase in c
stimulation of the he
protein located near
open state. Such Ca
beta-adrenergic agon
channels." Another
phorylated by cAMI
the rate of Ca^{++} up
evidence that beta-a
tivity of the contrac
of phosphorylation o
protein kinase.[55,58] K
summarized in Figu
beta-receptor stimula
port by the SR, whi
hancement of tensio
of relaxation.
In *summary*, beta-
flux across the sarco
tor-activated) slow

1. Catec
2. Activ
3. Increa
4. Activ
5. Phosp
6. Increa

INCREASED RATE OF

nists in cardiac muscle (and alpha-adrenergic agonists in vascular smooth muscle) increase Ca^{++} influx via the slow inward current, thereby enhancing contractility, frequency and conduction velocity in the heart in the case of $beta_1$ receptors, and the degree of contraction of arterioles in the case of alpha receptors on vascular smooth muscle. Activation of adrenergic receptors does not appear to increase Ca^{++} influx by increasing the size of the Ca^{++} channels or the rates at which their gates open or close but rather appears to recruit an additional number of active channels.[66] It has been proposed that when endogenous adrenergic nervous activity is low or is blocked by an adrenergic-receptor blocker, a certain proportion of the Ca^{++} channels is unable to open in response to a depolarizing stimulus. According to this theory, physiological stimuli or drugs that activate adrenergic receptors elevate cyclic AMP levels in the myocardium, which in turn facilitates transfer of a phosphate in ATP to form a phosphoester bond with one of the proteins in an inactive Ca^{++} channel, permitting the channel to participate in Ca^{++} entry into the cell. As a consequence, adrenergic influences increase Ca^{++} influx across the sarcolemma; the channels acted upon by receptor-mediated events are termed receptor-operated channels (Fig. 12–9, Mechanism 1B).

CALCIUM-CHANNEL BLOCKERS

A number of inorganic cations such as manganese, cobalt, and lanthanum can function as general Ca^{++} antagonists and are effective in blocking a wide variety of Ca^{++}-dependent processes. This nonselectivity of action probably arises from the ability of these cations to substitute for Ca^{++} at a variety of Ca^{++} binding sites. They probably block the function of all Ca^{++} channels or actually enter the cell, where they substitute for Ca^{++} at the intracellular Ca^{++} receptors. Of far more significance to clinical medicine are the organic Ca^{++}-channel blockers. The pioneering work of Fleckenstein[67] revealed that these compounds can produce selective blockade of the slow inward current and produce electromechanical uncoupling in heart muscle.

Since organic Ca^{++}-channel blockers exert their actions at nanomolar concentrations and exhibit stereospecificity, it appears likely that they are recognized by specific structures of the Ca^{++} channel.[37,68–70] However, the diversity of molecular structures of Ca^{++}-channel blockers is consistent with differing modes and sites of action rather than with the tight binding of these drugs to a specific receptor, analogous to the receptor that binds beta-adrenergic blockers.

The action of nifedipine is consistent with the drug actually "plugging" Ca^{++} channels. In contrast, verapamil, and to a lesser extent diltiazem, are "use-dependent," i.e., their Ca^{++}-blocking activities are a function of the frequency of contraction so that they cause an inversion of the myocardium's normal force-frequency relationship, an increase in contraction frequency causing a reduction rather than an augmentation of contraction.[65] This situation is analogous to the better investigated, frequency-dependent inhibition of Na^{+} channels by local anesthetics and Type I antiarrhythmic drugs and suggests that verapamil interacts preferentially with the depolarized, inactivated state of the Ca^{++} channel.

CARDIAC ADRENERGIC RECEPTORS

In 1967 Lands et al. demonstrated that beta-adrenergic receptors could be classified into two types: $beta_1$ receptors, which mediate cardiac stimulation and lipolysis, and $beta_2$ receptors, which mediate relaxation of vascular and bronchial smooth muscle.[71] The effects of catecholamines on the contractile and electrical properties of the heart are mediated predominantly by beta-adrenergic receptors, embedded in the sarcolemma (see Fig. 12–2). As determined by physiologic and radioligand-binding studies, the large majority of myocardial beta receptors are of the $beta_1$ subtype; likewise, the inotropic effects of beta-adrenergic agonists are mediated predominantly, if not exclusively, by $beta_1$ receptors.[71a] However, it has been suggested that chronotropy, i.e., sinoatrial rate, may be mediated by $beta_2$ receptors located in the sinoatrial node.[72] $Beta_1$-adrenergic receptors are located on effector cells in proximity to adrenergic synapses, while $beta_2$ receptors are located at some distance from the synapses.[73] $Beta_1$ receptors appear to respond primarily to neuronally released norepinephrine, whereas $beta_2$ receptors respond preferentially to circulating epinephrine from the adrenal medulla (and to exogenously injected agonists). Also, as in the case of alpha-adrenergic receptors (p. 914), beta-adrenergic receptors located presynaptically on the nerve fiber regulate norepinephrine release. However, as opposed to presynaptic alpha receptors, which have an inhibitory role, stimulation of presynaptic beta receptors stimulates release of norepinephrine.[74] Whereas ventricular receptors are exclusively $beta_1$,[75] approximately 25 per cent of atrial receptors are of the $beta_2$ subtype. Atrial $beta_2$ receptors, presumably located within the sinoatrial node, may mediate the chronotropic effects of catecholamines on the heart.

It appears that catecholamines exert at least some of their effects through myocardial alpha-adrenergic receptors.[75a] As with myocardial beta-adrenergic receptors, stimulation of myocardial alpha receptors augments myocardial contractility.[76,77] The subtype of myocardial alpha-adrenergic receptors is somewhat controversial, although most evidence favors the presence of only $alpha_1$ receptors.[77] A number of observations suggest that the molecular mechanism by which alpha-adrenergic receptors exert a positive inotropic effect is different from that of beta receptors. Whereas stimulation of beta-adrenergic receptors increases intracellular cyclic AMP, which is thought to mediate subsequent events, stimulation of alpha-adrenergic receptors has no effect on cyclic AMP production in myocardium. Also, alpha receptor–mediated effects on inotropy are more sensitive to the extracellular concentration of Ca^{++} or blockade of Ca^{++} influx by Ca-channel blockers than are beta-mediated effects. Based on these observations, it has been suggested that alpha-adrenergic receptors mediate an increase in inotropy almost exclusively by means of an increase in Ca^{++} influx.[78]

MECHANICS OF CARDIAC CONTRACTION

Cardiac contraction can be readily studied in vitro by mounting a mammalian papillary muscle, trabeculae carneae, or strip of atrial myocardium in an oxygenated, physiological salt solution.[79–82] The ends of the muscle are fixed, and the muscle is activated by electrical stimulation. The

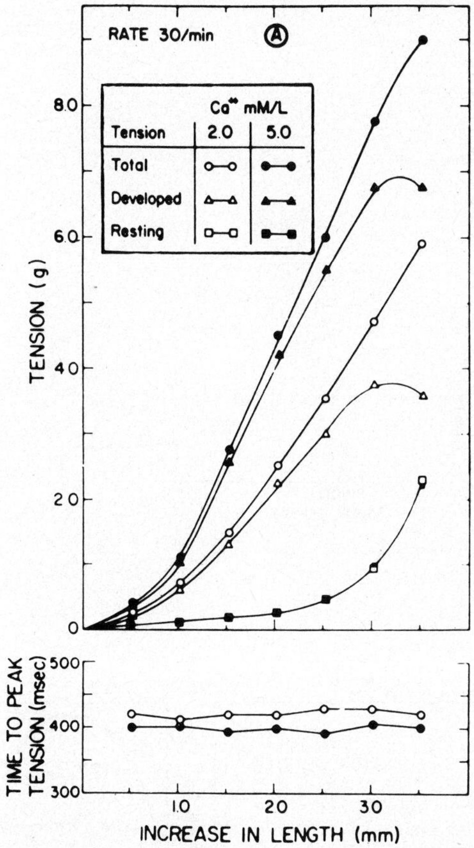

FIGURE 12–11 Effects of increased [Ca^{++}] on the relation between muscle length and tension in an isolated cat papillary muscle. The [Ca^{++}] in the perfusing medium has been increased from 2.0 mM to 5.0 mM. The relation between resting muscle length and tension is not altered. However, the development of tension at any given muscle length is increased at the higher [Ca^{++}] concentration, although L_{max} is not altered. Total tension is the sum of developed and resting tension.

strength of individual isometric cardiac contractions is modified by two major influences: (1) a *change in initial muscle length,* or preload, induced by a change in the passive stretch of the muscle; and (2) a *change in contractility or inotropic state.*[80]

Development of active tension during isometric contraction by the myocardium can be altered by changing initial muscle length, and the relation between these two variables constitutes the length–active tension curve (Fig. 12–11). When a change in contractility is induced by what is termed an *inotropic intervention,* such as the addition of Ca^{++}, digitalis, or norepinephrine to the medium, the peak force developed increases, the rate of force development rises, and the time to reach peak force shortens; these changes in contractile activity occur at a constant preload. Inotropic interventions do not generally alter the relation between the preload (the tension placed on the resting muscle) and the length of the muscle, i.e., the length–resting tension relation, an expression of the resting stiffness of the cardiac muscle.

By adjusting the initial degree of stretch placed on resting muscle, a length of the muscle can be found at which the resultant force development is maximal when the muscle is stimulated to contract isometrically; this length is termed L_{max}. The relation between developed isometric tension (i.e., the increment in tension occurring during contraction) and initial muscle length is termed the *length–active tension relation* (Fig. 12–11). By definition, the length–active tension relation at lengths below L_{max} is termed the *ascending limb* of the curve and the portion above L_{max}, the *descending limb* of the curve. When initial muscle length is altered slightly on either side of L_{max}, active tension is altered substantially; a 10 per cent reduction in muscle length below L_{max} may be responsible for a 30 per cent decrease in actively developed tension.

THE FORCE-VELOCITY RELATION. In order to analyze not only isometric contractions but also the shortening characteristics of the muscle, one end of the muscle is attached to a lever system and its degree of shortening is measured (Fig. 12–12*A*). The preload, a small weight placed on the opposite end of the lever, stretches the passive muscle; a stop is then adjusted above the tip of the lever and any weight added to the lever over and above the preload, termed the *afterload,* may be sensed by the muscle *after* the onset of contraction (Fig. 12–12*B*). The extent and maximum velocity of shortening for each contraction depend on the load (Fig. 12–12*C*), and the inverse relation between the tension (force) developed and the velocity of contraction constitutes the *force-velocity curve* (Fig. 12–12 *D*). When the load is greatest, there is no shortening, i.e., the muscle develops maximal force during isometric contraction (P_0). Conversely, when the load is smallest, the velocity of shortening is greatest. Although the velocity of shortening with zero load cannot be measured directly, since the preload provides for initial length, extrapolation of the curve back to zero load allows approximation of this maximum velocity of unloaded shortening, termed V_{max}.[79–83]

When the *initial muscle length* is altered by increasing the preload, the force-velocity curve is shifted characteristically (Fig. 12–13); the velocity of shortening at any given load is increased as is P_0. However, V_{max} is little altered by a change in initial muscle length. In contrast, when the *contractility* of the papillary muscle is augmented (Fig. 12–14), the rate of tension development is increased, as are the velocity and extent of shortening with a given load.[84] The entire force-velocity curve is shifted upward and to the right with increases in *both* P_0 and V_{max}.[81,82,85]

MUSCLE MODELS

There has been considerable interest in the development of models of muscle contraction, since they provide a method for analyzing contraction of heart muscle[86] as well as some insight into the complexities of ventricular function. Current working models include a *contractile element* (CE), which represents the actively contracting portion of the muscle, arranged in series with a passive elastic component, the *series elastic element* (SE). At rest, CE is considered to be freely extensible, so that resting tension is sustained by another elastic component arranged in parallel, the *parallel elastic component* (PE). Depending on the model chosen, PE spans both CE and SE (Maxwell model) or CE alone (Voight model).

The resting stiffness of cardiac muscle is greater than that of skeletal muscle, but the reasons for this difference are not clear.[87] Myocardial cells are smaller than skeletal muscle cells and therefore possess a relatively greater proportion of stiff sarcolemma per unit weight of tissue; intercellular collagen is also more abundant in heart muscle. The sarcomeres of cardiac muscle resist stretching beyond 2.2 μ, which may also be a factor in the stiffness of PE of heart muscle. An as yet unidentified elastic element, perhaps the protein fibrillin, may reside within the cardiac sarcomeres and be involved in maintaining rigidity.

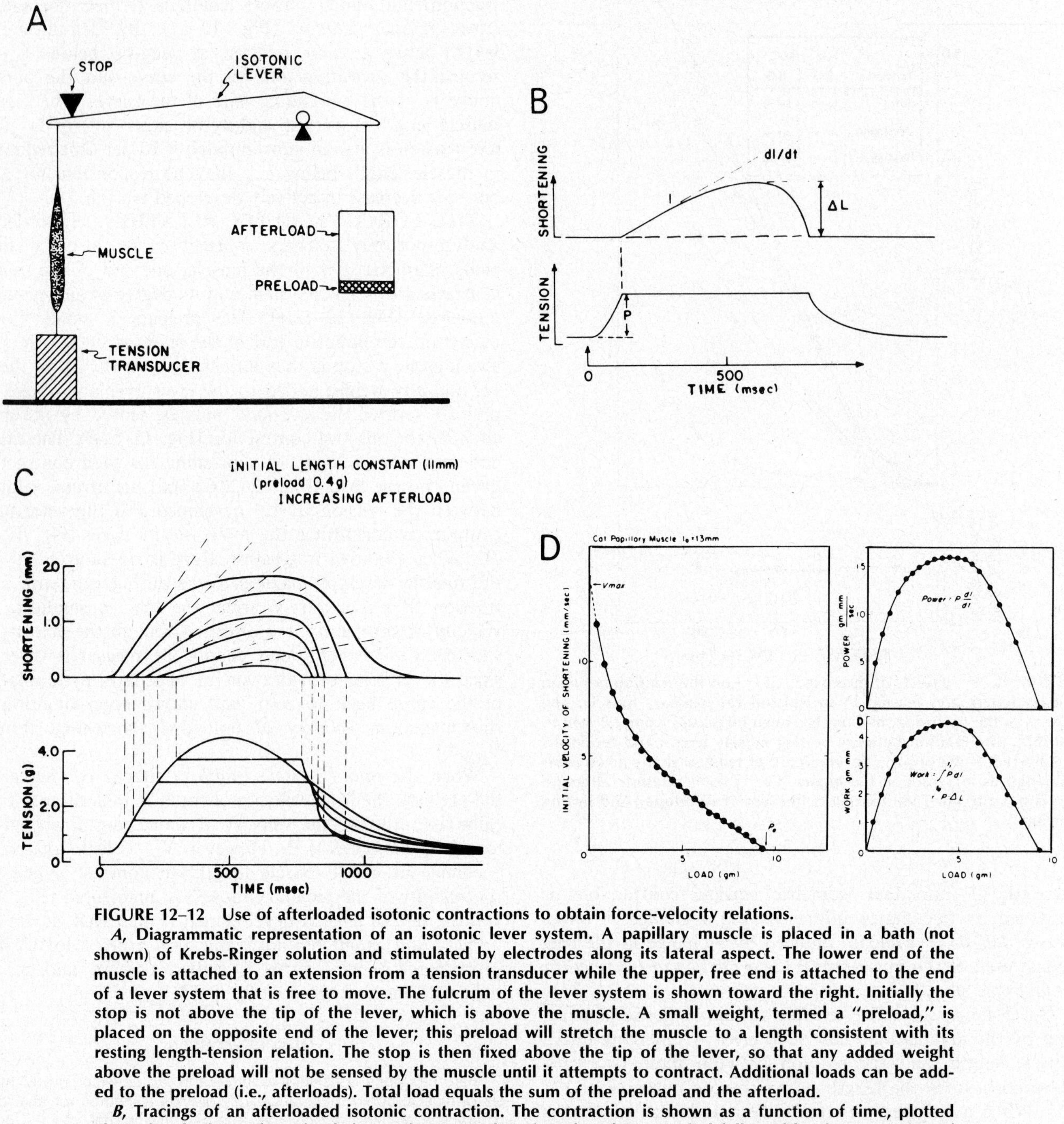

FIGURE 12–12 Use of afterloaded isotonic contractions to obtain force-velocity relations.

A, Diagrammatic representation of an isotonic lever system. A papillary muscle is placed in a bath (not shown) of Krebs-Ringer solution and stimulated by electrodes along its lateral aspect. The lower end of the muscle is attached to an extension from a tension transducer while the upper, free end is attached to the end of a lever system that is free to move. The fulcrum of the lever system is shown toward the right. Initially the stop is not above the tip of the lever, which is above the muscle. A small weight, termed a "preload," is placed on the opposite end of the lever; this preload will stretch the muscle to a length consistent with its resting length-tension relation. The stop is then fixed above the tip of the lever, so that any added weight above the preload will not be sensed by the muscle until it attempts to contract. Additional loads can be added to the preload (i.e., afterloads). Total load equals the sum of the preload and the afterload.

B, Tracings of an afterloaded isotonic contraction. The contraction is shown as a function of time, plotted along the abscissa. After stimulation at time zero, there is a short latent period followed by the generation of isometric force. When the force (P) equals the load, shortening begins, as shown in the upper half of the panel. Maximum velocity is reached shortly after shortening commences, and the tangent to this slope (dl/dt) approximates the maximum velocity of shortening with this particular load. ΔL denotes the extent of shortening. Subsequently the muscle elongates and then relaxes isometrically.

C, Effects of increasing afterloads on the course of tension development and subsequent shortening. Several superimposed contractions are displayed. The muscle develops a force equal to the afterload and thereafter shortens. As the afterload is increased, the velocity of shortening (dashed lines) and the extent of shortening decline.

D, Velocity of shortening plotted as a function of load: the force-velocity relation. As the load is increased, the velocity of shortening decreases. When the load is so high that no external shortening is recorded, velocity is zero, and the force is equivalent to the isometric contraction (P_0). When the curve is extrapolated back to zero load, V_{max} is obtained. Also shown at right are power (*top*) and work (*bottom*) curves as a function of increasing afterloads. Both power and work are zero when the load is zero or with isometric contractions, and both curves peak at an intermediate load. (From Braunwald, E., et al.: Mechanisms of Contraction of the Normal and Failing Heart. 2nd ed. Boston, Little, Brown, 1976.)

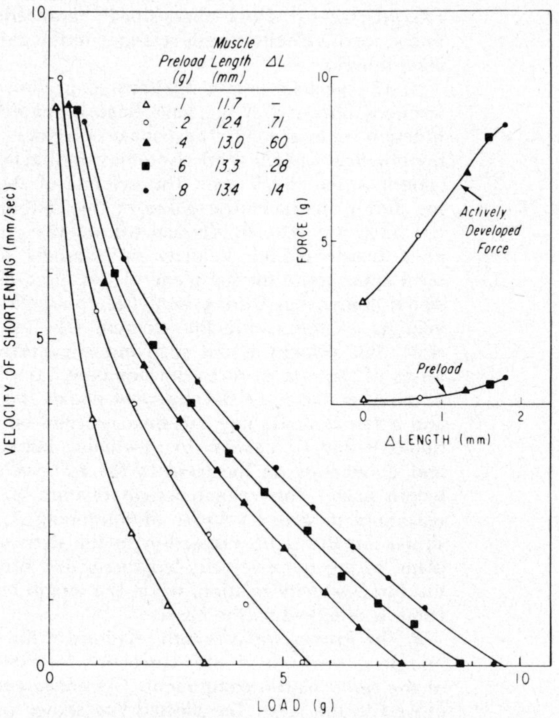

FIGURE 12–13 Relation between peak velocity of afterloaded, isotonic shortening and total load at several initial muscle lengths in a cat papillary muscle. The inset at the right shows the resting and developed active force at these various lengths. When initial muscle length is increased, the actively developed force is augmented, as is the velocity of shortening at any individual load. The maximum velocity of shortening with the preload alone is little altered. Moreover, if these curves were to be extrapolated back to zero load (V_{max}), this value would also show little or no change.

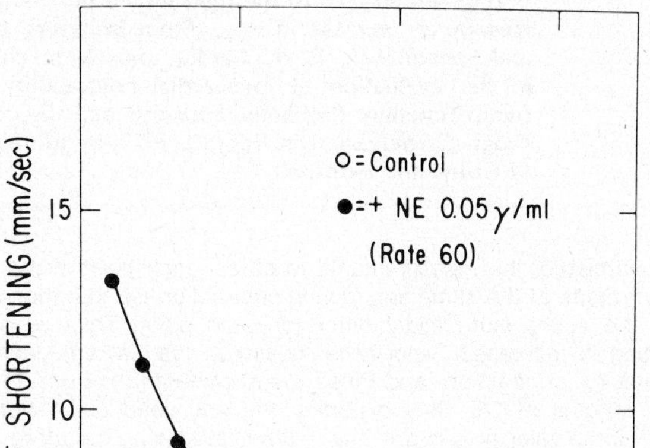

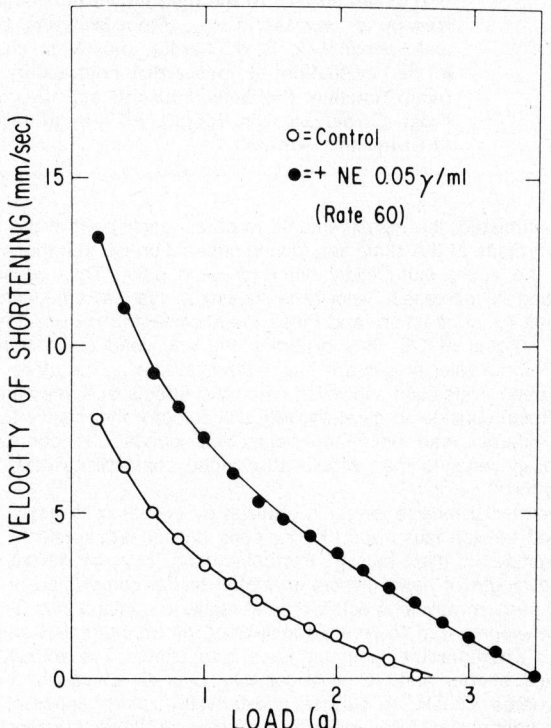

FIGURE 12–14 Effects of the addition of norepinephrine on the force-velocity relation of the cat papillary muscle. Norepinephrine induces an increase in the velocity of shortening at any load, in the maximum force of isometric contraction (P_0), and in the maximum velocity of zero load shortening (V_{max}).

The characteristics of muscular contraction are determined by the time course of activation of CE, its force-generating and shortening properties, and the stiffness of SE. The SE is a "lumped" elasticity, most of it being in elastic connections of the muscle to its points of fixation.

In the simplest model, consisting of only CE and SE, in an *isometric* contraction, with activation of the muscle, the CE shortens, stretching the springlike SE, and the force builds up at the ends of the system in a manner dependent upon the interaction of the shortening properties of the CE and compliance of the SE. On the other hand, in an *afterloaded isotonic* contraction, force is developed as shortening of the CE stretches the SE, until the force equals the load, and the load is then lifted. Muscle shortening occurs with the SE at a fixed length, and the subsequent course of shortening reflects shortening of the CE alone. Viscous elements are identified in the PE of resting heart muscle by the presence of stress relaxation, i.e., a fall in resting tension following a sustained stretch to a long length.

Contraction of muscle depends on its loading. The muscle can be permitted to shorten isotonically with just the preload, i.e., the small load that stretches the resting muscle and sets its initial length. If the ends of the muscle are fixed to prevent shortening, *isometric* force is developed. In the beating heart in vivo, contraction commences isometrically but is followed by shortening against a load, a condition mimicked in the isolated muscle by the *afterloaded isotonic contraction*, in which isometric force develops first and shortening then occurs at a constant force. In such a contraction, force is generated until it equals an imposed load, the *afterload* (Fig. 12–12*B*). The muscle then shortens, bearing the total load (afterload plus preload) until the length–active tension curve is reached. The intensity of the active state then declines; isotonic lengthening, i.e., lengthening at a constant force, occurs first and then the force itself declines. In the intact heart, the load is largely removed during relaxation owing to the closing of the aortic valve. When preload and thus the initial muscle length are increased, both developed force and the extent of afterloaded isotonic shortening are increased. When contractility is stimulated (Fig. 12–11), isometric force development and the extent of afterloaded isotonic muscle and CE shortening are increased. As already pointed out, the *force-velocity relation* obtained from afterloaded isotonic contractions helps to distinguish the two major ways in which cardiac performance is altered[80] (Figs. 12–13 and 12–14).

PROPERTIES OF THE CONTRACTILE ELEMENT

The mechanical activity of the CE reflects the summated contribution of cross bridges between myosin and actin and some form of conformational changes in the heads of the cross bridges, which then generate displacement of the actin filaments (see Fig. 12–6).[88–90] *Active state*, a term adapted from skeletal muscle physiology, has been used to describe the capacity of the CE to shorten in accordance with the force-velocity relation.[85,90,91] It is a mechanical measure of the chemical processes in the CE that generate both force and shortening.

RESTING LENGTH-TENSION RELATIONS

When relaxed heart muscle is stretched progressively, its resting tension increases slightly at first and then rises more markedly (Fig. 12–11). The stiffness of the resting muscle is represented by the slope of the curve relating the change in resting tension (ΔP) to the change in length (ΔL), which is approximately exponential. The resting length-tension relation is not generally altered by interventions that acutely alter the length–active tension curve or the force-velocity-length relation except that ischemia increases the apparent stiffness of the resting muscle (p. 1247), presumably by interfering with relaxation. Marked tachycardia also tends to increase the resting length-tension relation, because relaxation is not complete at the termination of diastole.[92] Aging also causes a significant increase in stiffness; less stress relaxation is exhibited by muscles from old compared to young adult rats, which may account, at least in part, for the age-associated changes in the resting length-tension curve.[93]

FORCE-VELOCITY-LENGTH RELATIONS

The interdependence between force, velocity, and muscle length is demonstrated as a *force-velocity-length diagram.*[94] The projection on the left of each of the panels of Figure 12–15 forms the *force-velocity*

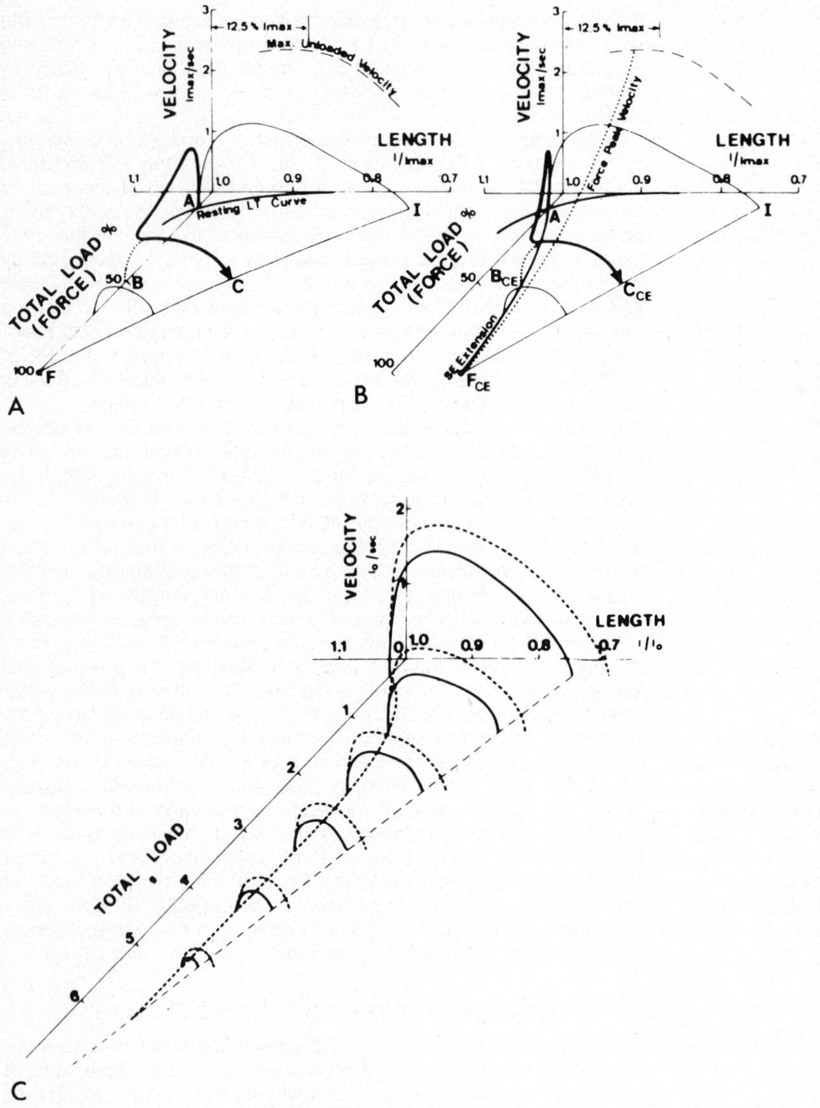

FIGURE 12–15 Three-dimensional representation of the force-velocity-length relations in the cat papillary muscle.

A, The velocity-length relations of isotonic contractions obtained at L_{max} have been replotted as a function of total load. The course of velocity of a hypothetical afterloaded isotonic contraction is superimposed (thick line). The velocity of shortening during the isometric phase of the contractions has been theoretically derived from a two-component muscle model. Velocity rises rapidly to the level appropriate for the plane of this three-dimensional composite. During isometric contraction the velocity of the contractile element falls as force rises. This velocity is not seen but is expressed in terms of the rate of force development, i.e., dP/dt. At point B, the force development equals the load, and external shortening can then proceed between points B and C. Velocity of shortening between B and C depends on the level of the force-velocity-length plane. The velocity-length relation and the maximum unloaded velocity of shortening (V_{max}) is shown on the right. Projection to the right of the plane of the force-velocity-length relation provides the force-velocity relation, while the length-tension curve is reflected on the base.

B, The force-velocity-length relations of the same muscle as shown in *A* after correction for extension of the series elastic component. The entire curve is moved to the right. The dashed line shown on the plane created by the force-velocity-length relation represents the force-velocity curve as obtained from afterloaded contractions.

C, Effect of a positive inotropic intervention (dashed line) on the force-velocity-length relation. The velocity of shortening at any given muscle length is augmented, so that the entire surface relating force-velocity and length is increased, and the extent of shortening is augmented. The projection of this surface to the right would be characterized by an increase in V_{max}. (From Brutsaert, D. L., and Sonnenblick, E. H.: Cardiac muscle mechanics in the evaluation of myocardial contractility and pump function: Problems, concepts and directions. Progr. Cardiovasc. Dis. *16*:337, 1973, by permission of Grune and Stratton.)

relation, the projection to the rear forms the *length-velocity* relation, and the base of this diagram represents the *length-tension* relation. During contraction, the muscle moves in a predictable manner across the surface, describing this relation between force, length, and velocity. With activation, the contractile elements rise onto a hypothetical force-velocity curve, with force increasing and the velocity of the contractile element decreasing until the afterload is reached, after which shortening proceeds across the surface. The force-velocity-length relation is relatively independent of time during a major portion of the shortening phase of contraction.[95] However, late in the course of contraction, shortening diverges from the velocity-length phase planes, indicating that the active state is declining.

Myocardial contractility can be described by the surface of the plane describing the force-velocity-length relation (Fig. 12–15).[94] The full activity of cardiac muscle commences rapidly after stimulation. The surface of the plane describing the force-velocity-length relation is reached rapidly, and its position may be considered to be a definition of the contractile state, since the position of this surface is essentially independent of preload and afterload. The duration of the active state is sufficient to allow shortening to occur to the same end-systolic length, regardless of the initial length if afterload and contractility remain constant.[96] This property of cardiac muscle is crucial to the use of end-systolic cardiac dimensions or volume in the assessment of cardiac contractility (p. 476).[97,98]

While force-velocity curves (Figs. 12–13 and 12–14) appear to provide valid descriptors of the contractile state in a wide variety of circumstances, an important theoretical limitation of such curves must be appreciated; the measurements to obtain each point in the curve are not made at the same time during contraction, so that the intensity of the active state might differ for each point. Thus, when the afterload is increased, velocity is measured later in time after the stimulus for contraction, and these measurements may occur at differing lengths of CE, thus distorting the enscribed curve from the "true" force-velocity curve.[94] The extrapolated V_{max} therefore could have been misleading. However, when the effects of these variables have been considered carefully, with unloading of the muscle to near zero external load once contraction has begun, the conclusions previously reached from simple afterloaded contractions have been supported.[95]

When initial muscle length is reduced by 10 per cent, actively developed tension falls about 30 per cent, but unloaded velocity does not change. In intact muscle, this dependency of force development on the length of heart muscle is related to the compliance of SE.[94] When cardiac muscle is activated and made to contract isometrically, the development of force is accompanied by an internal shortening, so that when maximal isometric force is reached, CE is actually substantially shorter and SE is longer than prior to activation. Indeed, sarcomeres actually do shorten substantially during "apparent" isometric contraction.[99–102] In contrast, isotonic contractions against very small loads do not involve the development of force, stretching of SE, and shortening of CE at the expense of SE; hence, shortening of CE is directly translated into shortening of the muscle, and velocities are measured at longer sarcomere lengths.[99] In studies in which sarcomere dynamics have been measured directly,[100] it appears that only a minor proportion of the SE is associated with the contractile machinery and cross bridges in heart muscle and that the effective SE largely reflects external elastic connections.

LENGTH-DEPENDENT ACTIVATION

In the foregoing discussion of the mechanics of muscular contraction, it has been generally assumed that inotropic interventions and changes in muscle length are independent regulators of myocardial performance. However, evidence is increasing that both inotropic interventions and changes of muscle length may act primarily through mechanisms that involve Ca^{++} activation.[31,103–108] The traditional view that length and inotropic state are independent regulators of myocardial performance was based on the observation that a decline of tension production occurs at short muscle lengths; this would be expected, because tension is lost as a consequence of the double overlap of the thin filaments in the central region of each sarcomere, resulting in interference with normal cross-bridge formation. However, tension production in cardiac muscle falls off much more steeply at muscle lengths below L_{max} than would be expected according to the sliding filament hypothesis.[105]

The inotropic effect of changes in extracellular [Ca^{++}] is dependent on muscle length; the mechanical performance of cardiac muscle is more sensitive to changes in extracellular [Ca^{++}] at longer than at shorter muscle lengths.[31,105,108,109] There is evidence in skeletal muscle too that the affinity of troponin for Ca^{++} is length-dependent,[110] and the same situation may well exist in cardiac muscle. It has been suggested that the same quantity of Ca^{++} released may thus be more actively bound at longer than at shorter sarcomere lengths and that an increase in muscle length (1) does not change or decreases the transsarcolemmal influx of Ca^{++}, (2) increases the release of Ca^{++} triggered by the transsarcolemmal Ca^{++} influx, and/or (3) increases the sensitivity of the myofilaments to Ca^{++}.[31]

Thus, all changes in contractile behavior may result primarily from alterations in the degree of activation of the contractile system, and therefore contractility and muscle length (preload) should not be regarded as totally independent regulators of myocardial performance. While a change in contractility relates to changes in *quantity and rate* of Ca^{++} made available to troponin C, a change in muscle length appears to alter the *sensitivity* of the sarcomere to Ca^{++}. However, the distinct differences in the effects of changes in preload and of contractility on V_{max} (Figs. 12–13 and 12–14), on the duration of the active state, and on the rate of tension development and decline all indicate that, regardless of the similarity in the fundamental molecular mechanism, consideration of preload and contractility as separate determinants of cardiac performance still remains an extremely useful working model.

THE ULTRASTRUCTURAL BASIS OF STARLING'S LAW OF THE HEART

The capacity of the intact ventricle to vary its force of contraction on a beat-to-beat basis as a function of its preload, reflected in the initial (end-diastolic) size, constitutes one of the major principles of cardiac function and is generally referred to as the *Frank-Starling phenomenon,* or *Starling's Law of the Heart.*[111,112] This fundamental property of the heart is based on the myocardial *length–active tension relation,* in which force of contraction and/or extent of shortening depends on initial muscle length,[113] which in turn is dependent on the ultrastructural disposition of thick and thin myofilaments within the sarcomeres.[114] As has already been pointed out (p. 409), the sarcomere is composed of an array of partially overlapping thick and thin filaments. A change in the length of the sarcomeres in striated muscle, whether skeletal or cardiac, creates a predictable change in the extent of overlapping between the two sets of filaments (Fig. 12–16). The critical relation between sarcomere length and isometric tension development was defined for skeletal muscle by A.F. Huxley and associates[114,115] (Fig. 12–17) who found that developed tension was constant with a sarcomere length between 2.0 and 2.2 μ but that when sarcomeres were shortened to less than 2.0 μ, the developed force fell. These changes in force development were explained by the relative position of the two sets of myofilaments within the sarcomere. The thick filaments are about 1.5 μ in length while the thin filaments

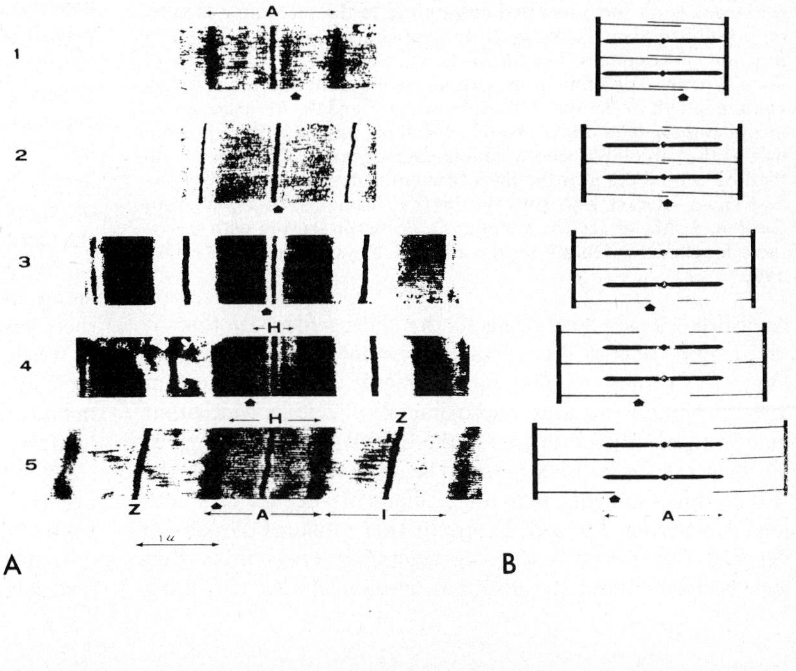

FIGURE 12–16 Relation between changes in sarcomere length and band patterns in skeletal muscle (frog sartorius). *A,* Band patterns as seen with the electron microscope. *B,* Relative disposition of the thick and thin filaments that create these patterns. The arrows in both panels denote the ends of the thin filaments that insert into the Z line to the left. In *A,* (3) represents the sarcomere at the apex of the length-active tension curve, i.e., at L_{max}. In (1) and (2), the sarcomere is shorter, whereas in (4) and (5) it is elongated. Throughout, the A band remains constant in width. The placement of filaments to provide for maximum overlap is shown in *B* (3). In (1), the sarcomere from a greatly shortened muscle is shown; the I band has disappeared, and a secondary dark band has formed at the center of the sarcomere, termed the C contraction band, and is due to the passage of thin filaments through this area. In *A* (4) and (5), an expanding H zone has appeared, owing to the withdrawal of thin filaments of constant length from the A band, as shown diagrammatically in *B* (4) and (5).

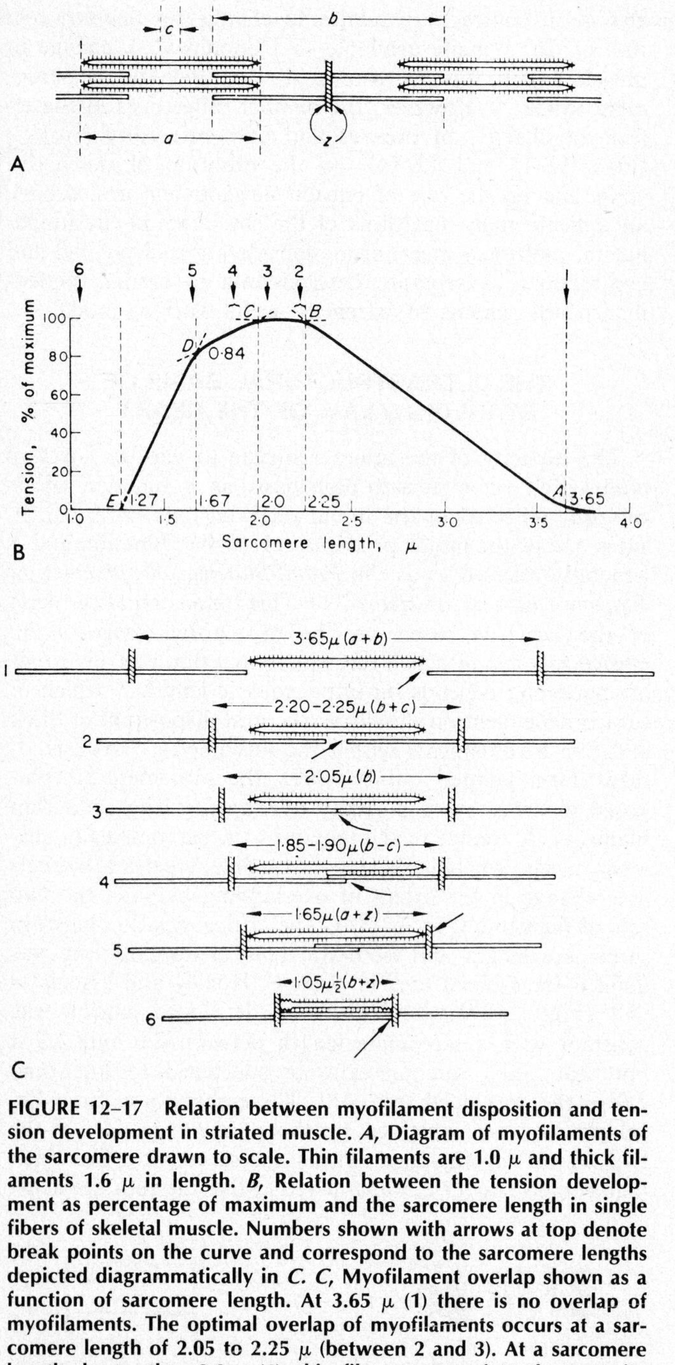

FIGURE 12–17 Relation between myofilament disposition and tension development in striated muscle. *A*, Diagram of myofilaments of the sarcomere drawn to scale. Thin filaments are 1.0 μ and thick filaments 1.6 μ in length. *B*, Relation between the tension development as percentage of maximum and the sarcomere length in single fibers of skeletal muscle. Numbers shown with arrows at top denote break points on the curve and correspond to the sarcomere lengths depicted diagrammatically in *C*. *C*, Myofilament overlap shown as a function of sarcomere length. At 3.65 μ (1) there is no overlap of myofilaments. The optimal overlap of myofilaments occurs at a sarcomere length of 2.05 to 2.25 μ (between 2 and 3). At a sarcomere length shorter than 2.0 μ (4), thin filaments pass into the opposite half of the sarcomere, and a double overlap occurs (5 and 6). Note that the central 0.2 μ of the thick filament is devoid of cross-bridges that could interact with sites on the thin filaments. (Adapted from Gordon, A. M., et al.: The variation in isometric tension with sarcomere length in vertebrate muscle fibers. J. Physiol. (Lond.) *184*:170, 1966.)

measure 1.0 μ.[13] According to the sliding filament theory, the length of both sets remains constant, both at rest and during contraction. The central region of the thick filaments contains an area approximately 0.2 μ in width that is devoid of cross bridges for the formation of force-generating cross links with actin. The optimal overlap of the 1.0 μ thin filaments with thick filaments occurs in sarcomeres between 2.0 and 2.2 μ. In this range of sarcomere lengths, the number of force-generating cross links that can be formed and the resultant developed force are maximal and constant. With sarcomeres longer than 2.2 μ, the fall in developed force may be directly related to the widening H zone and the resultant decrease in overlap between thick and thin filaments, thereby reducing the potential for cross bridge formation. At 3.65 μ, no overlap of filaments remains, and force generation ceases.[115]

When sarcomere lengths are progressively reduced below 2.0 μ, a reduction in tension development also occurs, presumably because (as pointed out earlier [p. 411]) thin filaments of 1.0 μ meet in the center of the sarcomere and bypass one another as sarcomere length is decreased further, resulting in a double overlap of filaments. As noted previously, this may interfere with the formation of cross bridges, may alter the ability of the filaments to bind Ca^{++} for activation, may reduce the sensitivity of the overlapping filaments to Ca^{++},[105] and/or may generate significant internal loads that might impair shortening of the sarcomere. Also, thin filaments may actually be repelled from the opposite half of the A band. All these factors may contribute to the fall in force development with shorter sarcomere lengths.

Although it has been suggested that thin filaments may be pulled by electrostatic forces rather than attaching physically to the thick filaments,[101,116] the concept of cross bridges between thick and thin filaments provides a useful working model that satisfactorily explains most of the observations of a variety of interventions involving cardiac contraction.

RELATION BETWEEN SARCOMERE LENGTH AND THE LENGTH–ACTIVE TENSION CURVE OF HEART MUSCLE

At L_{max}, the length of sarcomeres in mammalian ventricular myocardium averages 2.2 μ[117] (Fig. 12–18). As the resting muscle is shortened to about 85 per cent of L_{max}, sarcomere lengths decrease as a linear function of muscle length.[117,118] With further passive shortening of myocardium, however, little additional passive shortening of sarcomeres occurs, with diastolic sarcomere length remaining at 1.9 μ.

Although the structure of the sarcomere is similar in heart and skeletal muscle, important specialized differences permit cardiac muscle to function on the ascending portion of the length–active tension curve and maintain a length-dependent relation between sarcomere length and force development. First, the stiffness of the passive elastic component of cardiac muscle is such that diastolic sarcomere length is prevented from exceeding 2.3 μ, thus preventing disengagement of the myofilaments (Fig. 12–19). Second, the series elastic component is so compliant that during isometric contraction of cardiac muscle, substantial shortening of the sarcomeres occurs on the steep portion of their length–active tension curve.[119]

When cardiac muscle is stretched beyond L_{max}, resting tension rises to very high levels (Fig. 12–19), while, by definition, actively developed tension falls. However, in contrast to skeletal muscle, sarcomeres in cardiac muscle resist overstretching. With extension of the muscle to 20 per cent beyond L_{max}, sarcomeres elongate only slightly beyond 2.2 μ, but developed tension falls substantially. A decrease in overlap between thick and thin filaments, i.e., disengagement of myofilaments, cannot explain the sub-

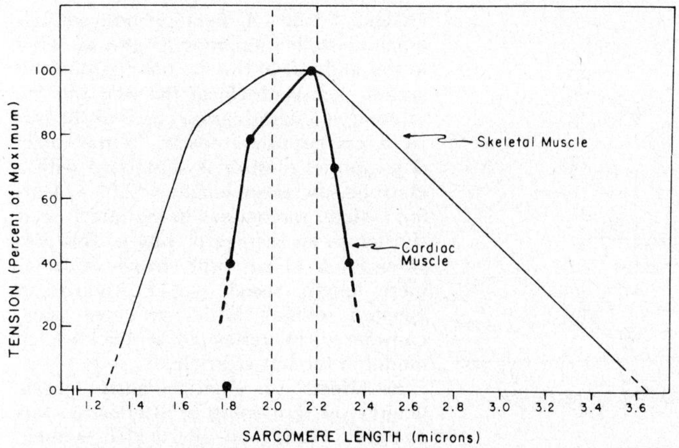

FIGURE 12–18 Relation between tension development and sarcomere length for cardiac muscle. Data were obtained by fixing cat papillary muscles with glutaraldehyde at various diastolic lengths relative to the length-tension curve and determining the average sarcomere length within the tissue using electron microscopic methods. The relation between tension development and sarcomere length obtained with skeletal fibers has been superimposed for comparison. In cardiac muscle, peak tension occurs with a diastolic sarcomere length of 2.2 μ. In skeletal muscle, there is a plateau of developed tension between sarcomere lengths of 2.2 and 2.0 μ, whereas in cardiac muscle this is not the case, and developed tension falls as sarcomere length is decreased below 2.2 μ. Furthermore, the shortest diastolic sarcomere length obtained in cardiac muscle in the absence of activation is 1.8 μ. As the papillary muscle is stretched beyond 2.2 μ, resting tension rises substantially (not shown; see Figure 12–20, p. 426) while actively developed tension falls precipitously. In contrast, in skeletal muscle, actively developed tension falls in a linear fashion between a sarcomere length of 2.2 and 3.6 μ. (From Sonnenblick, E. H., and Skelton, C. L.: Reconsideration of the ultrastructural basis of cardiac length-tension relations. Circ. Res. *35*:517, 1974, by permission of the American Heart Association, Inc.)

stantial decrements in developed force observed under these conditions; cellular damage occurs in cardiac muscle with this degree of overstretching and presumably is responsible, at least in part, for the reduction of tension development.[120]

Figure 12–19 shows the relation between average midwall sarcomere length and filling pressure for the left ventricles of the dog and cat.[121] When the left ventricle is empty, sarcomere length averages 1.9 μ, but as the left ventricle is filled, sarcomere lengths increase, so that at a filling pressure of 12 mm Hg the sarcomere length reaches 2.2 μ. With further ventricular distention, filling pressure rises markedly for small increments in ventricular volume, and only small increases in sarcomere length accompany large increases in intraventricular pressure. The same relation holds for the right ventricle but is scaled to lower filling pressures.[122] The relation between tension developed by the cat papillary muscle over a range of sarcomere lengths has been superimposed on the sarcomere resting length-tension relation in Figure 12–19. The optimal sarcomere length for maximum tension development (i.e., 2.2 μ) corresponds to the upper limits of normal ventricular filling pressure. When diastolic sarcomere length is related simultaneously to ventricular filling pressure and to active tension development, it becomes apparent that the apex of the sarcomere length–active tension curve and the normal upper limit of ventricular filling pressure coincide. Thus, the ventricle normally starts to contract when end-diastolic sarcomere lengths are along the upper half of the ascending portion of the sarcomere length–active tension curve.

In studies of the relation between sarcomere length and ventricular performance in the intact ejecting heart, the canine left ventricle has been fixed in situ during end diastole and end systole.[123,124] Diastolic sarcomere lengths in the midwall of the left ventricle averaged 2.07 μ when filling pressure ranged from 6 to 8 mm Hg.[124] At end systole, when the ventricle had ejected about two-thirds of its end-diastolic volume, the average sarcomere length shortened to 1.8 μ (Fig. 12–20), and when contractility of the ventricle was augmented by postextrasystolic potentiation, maximum systolic emptying was increased substantially and end-systolic sarcomere lengths were 1.6 μ.

Sarcomeres tend to be longest in the midwall of the ventricle and reach a maximal length (2.25 μ) at filling pressures of 10 mm Hg, when subendocardial and subepicardial sarcomeres are shorter.[121] As filling pressure is raised further, sarcomere length increases across the entire wall; this recruitment of shorter sarcomeres from across the wall may constitute one of the principal functional reserves of the Frank-Starling mechanism.[125]

The relative degree of sarcomere shortening cannot be the same across the ventricular wall during ejection; geo-

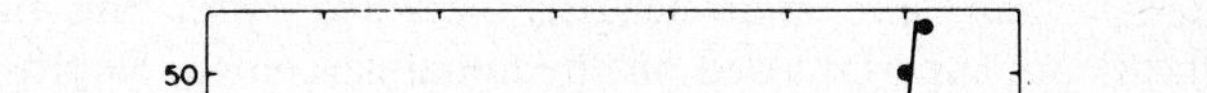

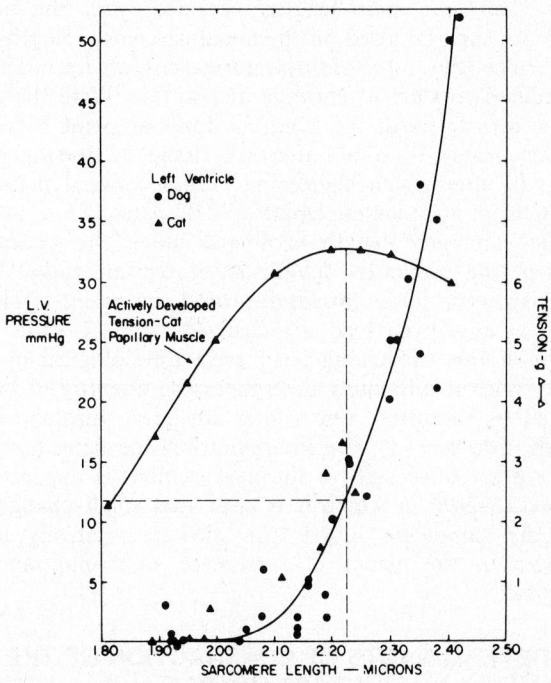

FIGURE 12–19 Relation between left ventricular pressure and average sarcomere length in the midwall of a canine left ventricle. The upper curve represents the relation between tension development and sarcomere length, as obtained from studies of cat papillary muscle. The lower curve relates left ventricular filling pressure to midwall sarcomere length for both dog and cat. At a left ventricular filling pressure of 12 mm Hg, which approximates the upper limit of normal filling pressure in the intact animal, average midwall sarcomere length is about 2.2 μ. This sarcomere length is also associated with the upper limits of the length–active tension curve, as shown by the vertical dashed line. Further increments in filling pressure yield only minor further increments in sarcomere length for very large increments in filling pressure. (From Spotnitz, J. H., et al.: Relation of ultrastructure to function in the intact heart: Sarcomere structure relative to pressure-volume curves of the intact left ventricles of dog and cat. Circ. Res. *18*:49, 1966, by permission of the American Heart Association, Inc.)

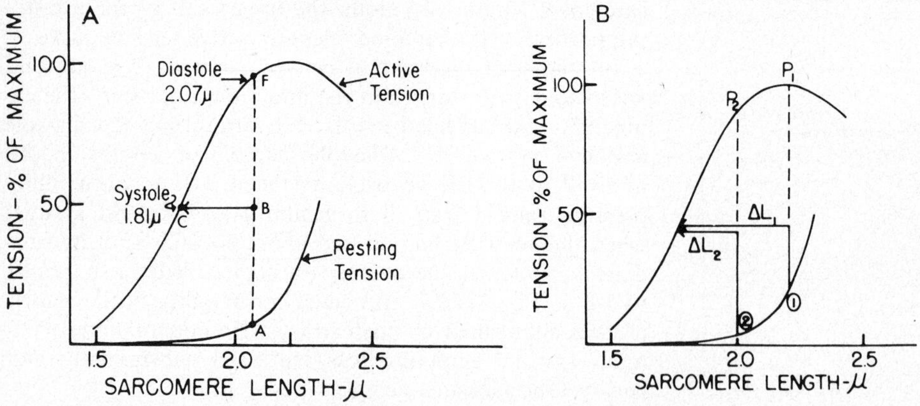

FIGURE 12–20 *A*, **Relation between average diastolic sarcomere lengths as noted in the midwall of the normal diastolic and systolic left ventricle of the dog and the sarcomere length-tension curve of the isolated cat papillary muscle. In the intact dog, normal diastole is associated with a diastolic sarcomere length of 2.07 μ. During systole, sarcomeres in the intact heart shorten to an average of 1.81 μ. This provides for a 13 per cent change in sarcomere length, which would produce an ejection fraction of 55 per cent when considered in terms of a thick-walled model of the left ventricle.**

***B*, Effects of altering initial muscle lengths on shortening of afterloaded sarcomeres. During an afterloaded isotonic contraction (1), the sarcomere begins to shorten from a diastolic length of 2.20 μ (point 1) and to become 1.81 μ (ΔL_1). The isometric force associated with this sarcomere length is noted at P_1. When diastolic sarcomere length is reduced to 2.0 μ (point 2), the sarcomere with the same afterload will shorten to the same point on the length–active tension curve (ΔL_2). This will result in a shortening from 2.00 to 1.81 μ. In this instance the associated isometric force occurs at P_2. Note that despite a minor change in peak developed isometric force, a substantial change in afterloaded isotonic shortening occurs at the same afterload. This would produce a substantial change in the stroke volume when extrapolated to the intact heart; e.g., in a 100-gram canine left ventricle, a change in diastolic sarcomere length from 2.0 to 2.2 μ in the midwall would increase stroke volume from 17 to 42 ml, with end-diastolic volume increasing from 40 to 65 ml. (From Ross, J., Jr., et al.: Architecture of the heart in systole and diastole: Technique of rapid fixation and analysis of left ventricular geometry. Circ. Res. *21*:409, 1967, by permission of the American Heart Association, Inc.)**

metrical considerations dictate that epicardial fibers must shorten relatively less than endocardial fibers. Nevertheless, when sarcomere lengths obtained from the intact heart are superimposed on the initial sarcomere length-tension curve (Fig. 12–20*A*), the normal sarcomere might be considered to start to contract at point A. Were the ends of the muscle fixed, the isometric force at point F would be developed. With an afterload, force is developed to point B, after which shortening occurs between points B and C from a sarcomere length of 2.07 μ to 1.81 μ. As diastolic sarcomere length is altered along the ascending limb of the sarcomere length–active tension curve, both peak isometric force development and the extent of shortening at any given load are changed (Fig. 12–20*B*). The extent of this shortening is of great physiological importance, since it ultimately determines the quantity of blood ejected by the intact ventricle at any given diastolic fiber length. The basis for the Frank-Starling mechanism in the intact heart (discussed in the next section) is apparent in Figure 12–20*B*, in which it is clear that small changes in diastolic sarcomere length can mediate relatively large changes in the extent of sarcomere shortening at any afterload.

DETERMINANTS OF CONTRACTION OF THE INTACT HEART

Although the geometry of the intact ventricle is far more complex than that of papillary muscle, with its parallel, longitudinally disposed fibers, if certain analogies are drawn and assumptions made, it becomes apparent that the basic mechanisms that influence the contraction of isolated cardiac muscle (described above) affect the performance of the whole heart in a similar manner.[94,125–129]

CHANGES IN VENTRICULAR SIZE AND SHAPE

The dimensions of the ventricular cavities, thickness of the ventricular walls, and intrinsic mechanical properties of cardiac tissue are the determinants of passive elasticity or stiffness of the ventricle and therefore of diastolic tension. In this manner they determine the filling of the ventricles, ultimately affecting the length of the sarcomeres at the onset of systole and thereby the contractile events. The shape of the ventricles, the angles of adjacent muscle fibers, and the thickness of the ventricular walls also determine the distribution of active forces within the ventricular myocardium throughout systole and hence affect the extent and speed of muscle shortening. In addition to the changes that occur normally during the cardiac cycle and that are produced by acute physiological stresses, the shape of the ventricle often undergoes major alterations consequent to chronic cardiac disorders, such as valvular abnormalities, or local scarring due to coronary heart disease. The model often applied when one is considering the left ventricle as a thick-walled ellipsoid of revolution, which has practical utility in the calculation of left ventricular volume (p. 471).

The myocardial fibers are arranged in a spiral fashion around the central cavity of the left ventricle. The subendocardial and the subepicardial fibers run largely parallel to the long axis of the cavity, and the midwall fibers are mostly circumferential, i.e., perpendicular to the long axis. All the fibers tend to be perpendicular to the radius of the cavity. During contraction, the myocardial fibers shorten and thicken (Fig. 12–21), and as a consequence the left ventricular cavity decreases circumferentially and longitudinally and the wall thickens. The generation of intraventricular pressure and the displacement of blood from the left ventricular cavity are produced by a combination of fiber shortening and thickening.

During isovolumetric left ventricular contraction, the chordae tendineae become tense, the mitral valve closes, and the ellipsoidal left ventricle becomes more spherical, with slight apex-to-base shortening and a small increase in the minor ventricular diameter. These changes in left ventricular dimensions prior to ejection appear most marked when measured on the external surface of the heart.[130,131] The tendency toward sphericalization and wall thickening

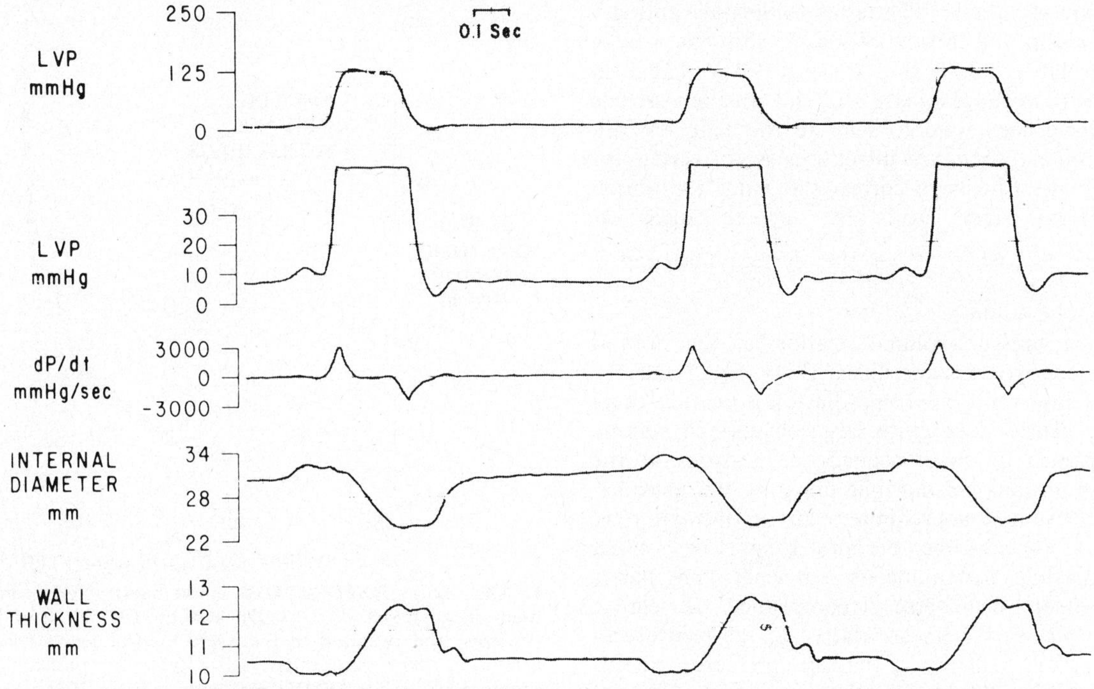

FIGURE 12–21 High-speed tracings obtained in a normal conscious, chronically instrumented dog with sinus arrhythmia. LVP = left ventricular pressure (in the top two tracings, at high and low amplification). dP/dt = the first derivative of left ventricular pressure. The internal diameter of the left ventricle was measured by means of a pair of ultrasonic crystals placed on the endocardium near the minor equator. The wall thickness of the left ventricle was measured by means of a pair of miniature ultrasonic crystals juxtaposed across the free wall near the minor equator. (From Theroux, P., Ross, J., Jr., et al.: Unpublished observations.)

during isovolumetric contraction and toward ellipticalization and wall thinning during isovolumetric relaxation is more pronounced when ventricular size is reduced, as occurs during thoracotomy (i.e., in the absence of a negative intrapleural pressure) or with occlusion of venous inflow into the heart.[132] During ejection, the minor (transverse) axis shortens by only 9 per cent.[132,133] Thus, shortening of the internal minor axis diameter accounts for approximately 85 to 90 per cent of the stroke volume. Measurements of casts of canine left ventricles arrested at end diastole and end systole have provided similar values and in addition have shown that the ratio of the major-to-minor axis changed from an average of 1.49 in diastole to 1.93 in systole.[123]

Similar changes in shape occur in the human left ventricle studied by means of angiography. As the left ventricle empties during systole, the inner surface decreases proportionately more than the external surface, as dictated by the geometry of the heart. Since muscle mass remains constant, an increase in wall thickness must occur; direct measurements of the left ventricular wall in intact animals[133,134] as well as cineangiography in patients[135] have confirmed that left ventricular wall thickness increases by 25 and 35 per cent during systole.

DIASTOLIC PROPERTIES OF THE VENTRICLES

Certain terms are commonly used to describe the mechanical properties of cardiac muscle.[136,137] Since there has been confusion about their meaning, they will be defined explicitly here. *Stress* is the force per unit of cross-sectional area, frequently expressed as gm/cm^2; *strain* is the fractional (or percentage of) change in dimension or size from the unstressed dimension that results from the application of stress; *elasticity* is the property of recovery of a deformed material after removal of the stress; *creep* is the time-dependent strain of tissue maintained at a constant level of stress after a rapid change in stress; *stress relaxation* is the time-dependent reduction of stress when tissue is maintained at a constant level of strain after a rapid change in strain. Like most biological materials, cardiac muscle exhibits a curvilinear relation between passive (diastolic) stress and strain (see Fig. 12–11); this property is responsible for the nonlinear pressure-volume curve (Fig. 12–22) and stress-strain relation of the intact ventricle. *Elastic stiffness* defines the ratio of stress to strain at any defined point of the curve relating these two variables. The *elastic stiffness constant* is the slope of the straight line relating elastic stiffness to the corresponding stress. The term elastic stiffness, sometimes called *volume stiffness* or *chamber stiffness*, has also been used to refer to the stiffness of the ventricular chamber and, by simplification, has been defined as the ratio of the change in pressure (dP) to the change in volume (dV). When the stress-strain relation is analyzed, the term *myocardial stiffness* has been employed to differentiate those effects due to changes in the stiffness properties of each unit of muscle as opposed to those due to increased muscle mass alone, which can affect *chamber stiffness*; thus, in some patients with concentric left ventricular hypertrophy, chamber stiffness is increased and myocardial stiffness is normal, whereas in others, both are elevated.[137] The terms *compliance* and *distensibility* represent the inverse of elastic stiffness, i.e., in referring to isolated muscle it is the ratio of a change in strain relative to a change in stress (d_e/d_s). In the ventricle these terms have been used to refer to the ratio dV/dP. The term *specific compliance* introduces a correction for the initial volume. Efforts to correct this value for ventricles of different sizes have also led to such expressions as $\frac{dV/dP}{V}$, where V in the denominator represents end-diastolic volume.

The diastolic pressure-volume relation of the normal mammalian left ventricle is curvilinear (Figs. 12–22 and 12–23).[138,139] At a low ventricular end-diastolic pressure there is a relatively gentle slope, with large changes in volume being accompanied by small changes in pressure. At the upper limits of normal end-diastolic pressure, the curve becomes steeper[140,141] and approximates an exponential relation, so that as the chamber becomes progressively filled during each diastole, instantaneous ventricular compliance (dV/dP) decreases; the inverse of compliance, i.e., elastic stiffness (dP/dV) bears a linear relation to the pressure in the normal dog left ventricle at diastolic pressures exceeding 3 mm Hg.[142] The slope of the line relating dP/dV to P represents the elastic stiffness constant of the chamber; it is relatively independent of ventricular shape and therefore may be useful for detecting changes in wall stiffness.[135,136] However, caution must be used in drawing conclusions from measuring these variables in one ventricle when the effects of changes in the volume of the other ventricle and the elastic limits of the pericardium cannot be excluded.

Although by definition, and as is apparent from Figures

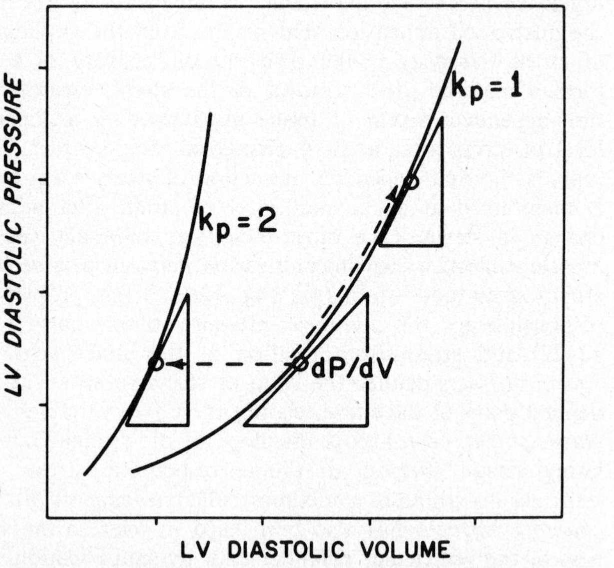

FIGURE 12–22 Diagrammatic representation of left ventricular (LV) diastolic pressure-volume relationships. *Right,* An increase in operative chamber stiffness (dP/dV) occurs in the absence of any change in the modulus of chamber stiffness (K_p). *Left,* An increase in operative chamber stiffness occurs as a result of an increase in the modulus of chamber stiffness (relative to the curve on the right). Because operative chamber stiffness depends on the modulus of stiffness and the level of operative filling pressure, this comparison is made at equivalent levels of pressure. (From Gaasch, W. H., et al.: Left ventricular compliance: Mechanisms and clinical implications. Am. J. Cardiol. *38*:645, 1976.)

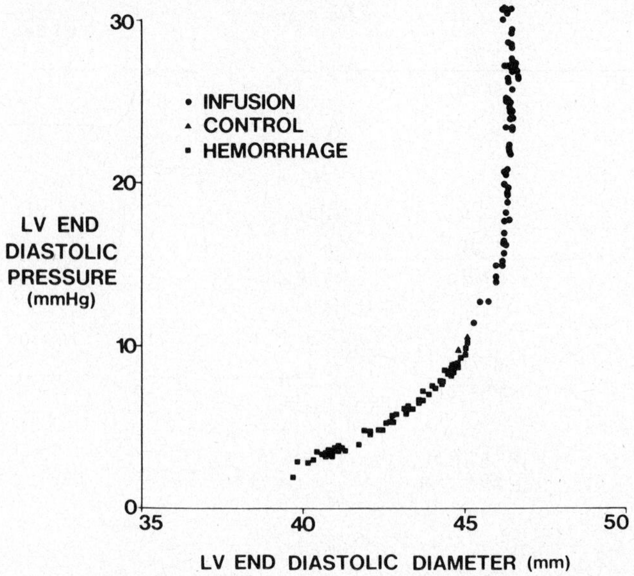

FIGURE 12–23 LVEDP-LVEDD curve constructed from an experiment in an intact dog. LVEDP and LVEDD fell with hemorrhage (squares) and returned to the same control levels (triangles) with reinfusion. With subsequent saline infusion (circles), LVEDP rose considerably, while LVEDD rose only slightly. (From Boettcher, D. H., et al.: Extent of utilization of the Frank-Starling mechanism in conscious dogs. Am. J. Physiol. *234*:H338, 1978.)

12–22 and 12–23, the compliance of the ventricle changes as it fills, an alteration of the compliance of the chamber as a whole can be identified by a change in the shape and position of the curve relating ventricular diastolic volume or dimensions to pressure.[131] As has already been pointed out (p. 421), excluding the incomplete relaxation that occurs in tachycardia and myocardial ischemia, interventions that alter myocardial contractility acutely do not cause significant shifts in the ventricle's diastolic pressure-volume relation. The small changes in the relation reported in some studies may be secondary to effects on time-dependent, inertial, and viscous properties and to the influence of filling of the opposite ventricle (p. 429). Since the diastolic pressure-volume relation is curvilinear, left ventricular diastolic compliance is determined by both the diastolic pressure-volume relation and the level of diastolic pressure at any instant, the so-called operating diastolic pressure (Fig. 12–22).[143] Therefore, ventricular compliance declines, i.e., the chamber elastic stiffness increases as it fills. Increased diastolic filling, as occurs with acute aortic regurgitation, and, conversely, reduced ventricular preload, as occurs after administration of nitroglycerin, result in increased and reduced stiffness, respectively, as the ventricle moves up or down its pressure-volume curve.[143]

Ventricular (chamber) stiffness is a function of muscle stiffness as well as of the thickness and geometry of the ventricle. If the stiffness of cardiac tissue (myocardial stiffness) is increased, as may occur with a fibrous scar or with infiltration of amyloid, but the thickness of the ventricular wall remains normal, ventricular (chamber) stiffness will be increased. An increase in chamber stiffness will also occur if the stiffness of each individual unit of myocardial tissue (myocardial stiffness) is normal but the ventricular wall becomes thicker.

In the intact heart, *stress relaxation* is of significance

only when large increases in ventricular diastolic pressure and volume occur abruptly. For example, there is a small drop in ventricular end-diastolic pressure (about 1 mm Hg) when systolic pressure is suddenly elevated by 70 to 80 per cent in the isovolumetrically contracting left ventricle, which is held at a constant volume. This suggests the presence of viscous elements, but these changes are of relatively minor significance in the intact heart.[144] *Creep*, a time-dependent shift of the left ventricular diastolic pressure-volume relation, has also been documented in the conscious dog after large increases in systolic and diastolic pressures (ventricular diastolic volume being larger at the same levels of diastolic pressure).[145]

The normal *right ventricle is more compliant than the left*, not because of any intrinsic difference in myocardial stiffness but because of its thinner wall.[122] In the isolated, nonbeating normal dog heart, when the left and right ventricles are filled simultaneously to a pressure of 10 mm Hg, the volume of the right ventricle is about 35 per cent greater than that of the left, and the upper limit of normal for right ventricular end-diastolic pressure in man is about one-half (6 mm Hg) that of the left ventricle (12 mm Hg).[140] In man, the end-diastolic volumes of the two ventricles are approximately equal,[146] and therefore the ejection fractions of the two ventricles are normally similar as well.

Ventricular Interdependence. Alterations in the filling of one ventricle can substantially alter the diastolic pressure-volume relation of the opposite chamber.[140] Therefore, when right ventricular volume changes significantly, changes in left ventricular end-diastolic pressure may not be a reliable guide even to directional changes of the diastolic volume of the left ventricle.[147,148] Studies in which the pericardium is intact have shown that not only the diastolic pressure but also the shape of the left ventricle is altered by increased right ventricular filling, which can result in encroachment of the interventricular septum on the left ventricular cavity.[149] Alterations in the right ventricular pressure-volume relation that occur after an alteration in left ventricular loading may not reflect a change in right ventricular myocardial or chamber stiffness but rather may be secondary to changes in the volume of the left ventricle within a pericardial sac that restrains changes in the volume of the entire heart.[150]

ROLE OF THE PERICARDIUM (See also p. 1471)

Experimental data indicate that the normal pericardium has an important effect on the diastolic properties of the ventricles during acute volume overload and therefore could be important during acute heart failure. During acute volume loading in the dog, intrapericardial pressure rises when overall cardiac volume (both right and left heart chambers) is increased beyond the limit of pericardial distensibility, i.e., the pericardium becomes restrictive. This factor may also play a role in the large decreases in left ventricular filling pressures that are observed during nitroprusside vasodilator therapy in human heart failure (p. 1473) when heart size decreases within the pericardial sac, which is no longer restrictive.

Figure 12–24 shows data from a conscious experimental animal instrumented for the measurement of left ventricular segment dimensions and left ventricular end-diastolic pressure; with the pericardium intact, overtransfusion produced a marked shift upward and to the left of the entire diastolic pressure-dimension curve of the left ventricle. Infusion of nitroprusside under these conditions caused a partial shift downward of the entire curve, the degree of the shift being equal to the fall of intrapericardial pressure. Thus, although a portion of the drop in cardiac filling pressure produced by nitroprusside was due to a reduction of cardiac volume, a portion of the fall resulted from the shift of the entire curve due to lowering of the elevated intrapericardial pressure. In contrast, when the pericardium was removed and the same animal was studied several days later, acute volume overloading, followed by the administration of nitroprusside, moved the left ventricle upward and downward on a single diastolic pressure-dimension curve.[151] Further research is needed to establish

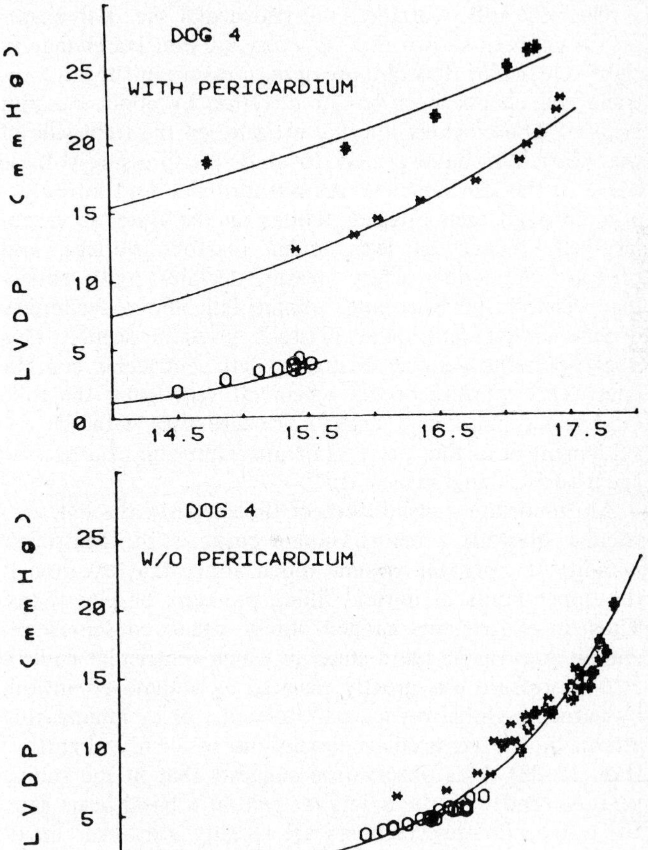

FIGURE 12–24 Relations between the length of a segment of left ventricle and left ventricular diastolic pressure (LVDP) in a conscious dog. Points were obtained during slow cardiac filling (diastasis). *Upper panel,* Relation with the *pericardium intact* before (open symbols) and after intravenous infusion of dextran to produce acute cardiac dilatation (asterisks, upper curve); the middle curve (x's) shows the effect of an intravenous infusion of nitroprusside in the presence of such acute cardiac dilatation. *Lower panel,* the same dog studied *without (W/O) the pericardium* (after its surgical removal). The same interventions, volume loading and nitroprusside, are carried out. The ventricle now appears to be operating on a single diastolic pressure–length relation. (Adapted from Shirato, K., et al.: Alteration of the left ventricular diastolic pressure–segment length relation produced by the pericardium: Effects of cardiac distention and afterload reduction in conscious dogs. Circulation *57*: 1191, 1978. By permission of the American Heart Association, Inc.)

the importance of such effects of the pericardium in human subjects.

While a reduction of left ventricular compliance occurs during angina pectoris (p. 1247), presumably as a consequence of impaired ventricular relaxation, this is not sufficient to account for the marked shifts in the left ventricular pressure-volume relations observed in pacing-induced angina signifying an apparent increase in elastic stiffness, when the pericardium is intact.[152] Furthermore, opposite shifts that suggest *increased* ventricular compliance occur with the administration of nitroglycerin and nitroprusside,[140,141] whereas shifts that suggest *decreased* compliance occur when systemic arterial pressure is raised by angiotensin II. These shifts of the pressure-volume relation may result in part from alterations of extrinsic pressures acting on the left ventricle, which is contained within a relatively stiff container, the pericardial sac. For example, it has been shown that for every 1.0 mm Hg change in right ventricular diastolic pressure, pressure in the left ventricle will change in a similar direction by about 0.5 mm Hg.[149,152] Thus, merely altering pressure on the right side of the heart can be expected to shift the pressure-volume curve of the left ventricle. As nitroprusside and nitroglycerin, through their dilating actions on the systemic vascular bed, reduce left ventricular diastolic volume and pressure, pulmonary artery pressure declines, right ventricular diastolic pressure and volume fall, and a secondary decline in left ventricular diastolic pressure occurs. This does not reflect a true change in left ventricular compliance. The opposite occurs when left ventricular diastolic (and hence pulmonary artery) pressure rises with the development of angina pectoris or upon infusion of a pressor agent such as angiotensin II.[153]

An important consequence of the shape of the left ventricular diastolic pressure-volume curve is the ventricle's inability to augment volume much above that existing at the upper limits of normal filling pressure, despite stress. Thus, in experiments carried out in intact, conscious, reclining dogs in the basal state, in which ventricular end-diastolic pressure was greatly elevated by volume expansion, by inducing global myocardial ischemia, or by augmenting afterload, left ventricular dimensions rose only slightly[154] (Fig. 12–23). This observation suggests that in the supine position, and with the animal at rest, at a basal heart rate, left ventricular muscle fibers are already near their maximal length and that operating from this baseline an increase of preload is *not* an important mechanism responsible for the augmentation of cardiac performance. On the other hand, when ventricular end-diastolic pressure and volume are lowered by hemorrhage, tachycardia, assumption of the upright posture, or opening of the chest, changes in cardiac performance can result from large alterations in ventricular dimensions as a consequence of augmenting blood volume or afterload. Therefore in the resting, reclining, conscious dog, the left ventricle operates near the bend of its pressure-volume curve, end-diastolic dimensions are nearly maximal, and cardiac performance cannot be augmented substantially through an increase in preload; rather, it requires an increase in contractility expressed as more complete systolic emptying from the same end-diastolic volume and an increase in heart rate, to augment cardiac output. Similar considerations apply to patients.[155]

The classic experiments of Starling,[112] Wiggers,[156] Sarnoff,[157] and their coworkers were carried out at unphysiological, high heart rates, with ventricular end-diastolic volumes far from maximal, allowing them to observe a distinct augmentation of ventricular diastolic dimensions with a variety of interventions. However, even in the conscious, intact organism, variations in ventricular performance as a consequence of alterations in preload are not totally unphysiological. They operate on a beat-to-beat basis in maintaining balanced outputs from the two ventricles during normal respiration[157] and allow for an increase in end-diastolic volume during exercise in the upright position, i.e., when baseline volume is not maximal.

PERFORMANCE OF THE INTACT VENTRICLE

The three determinants of performance of isolated cardiac muscle—preload, afterload, and contractility—also affect the performance of the intact ventricle. In addition, heart rate represents a fourth determinant of performance per unit time.

THE CARDIAC CYCLE. The relations between left ventricular pressure, the diameter of the minor equator at the endocardial surface of the left ventricular wall, and the wall thickness in a conscious dog are shown in Figure 12–21, and the events of the cardiac cycle are shown diagrammatically in Figure 12–25. Ventricular end diastole is followed by a brief period of isovolumetric left ventricular contraction, the maximum rate of pressure change (peak dP/dt) occurring just prior to the onset of ejection.[157a] The onset of inward motion of the ventricular wall then commences as blood is ejected into the aorta, and the rate of wall shortening becomes maximal near the middle of ejection. Wall thickness increases during shortening, becoming maximal at the end of ejection. Following isovolumetric relaxation, during which peak negative dP/dt is reached, a rapid increase in the diameter of the ventricle occurs during early diastole, followed by a slow phase of filling in mid-diastole (diastasis); a second, rapid increase in diameter takes place in late diastole, as a consequence of atrial contraction. The time course of changes in ventricular volume closely parallel those shown for ventricular internal diameter during each cardiac cycle. This relation between ventricular pressure and volume can also be plotted as a pressure-volume loop (Fig. 12–26) in a manner analogous to the sarcomere length-pressure (Fig. 12–19) and length-tension (Fig. 12–20) relations. This provides a convenient framework for understanding the responses of individual left ventricular contractions to alterations in preload, afterload, and contractility.

The pressure-volume loop of the left ventricle can be related to the performance of isolated cardiac muscle, in which the active isometric length-tension curve provides the limit of shortening for isotonic contractions. The linear relation between the end-systolic volume and the end-systolic pressure of the left ventricle is analogous to this length-tension relation and has been well defined in the isolated heart preparation[158,159] (Fig. 12–26, upper panel). It has also been studied in conscious animals by infusing a range of doses of a vasoconstrictor (that does not itself

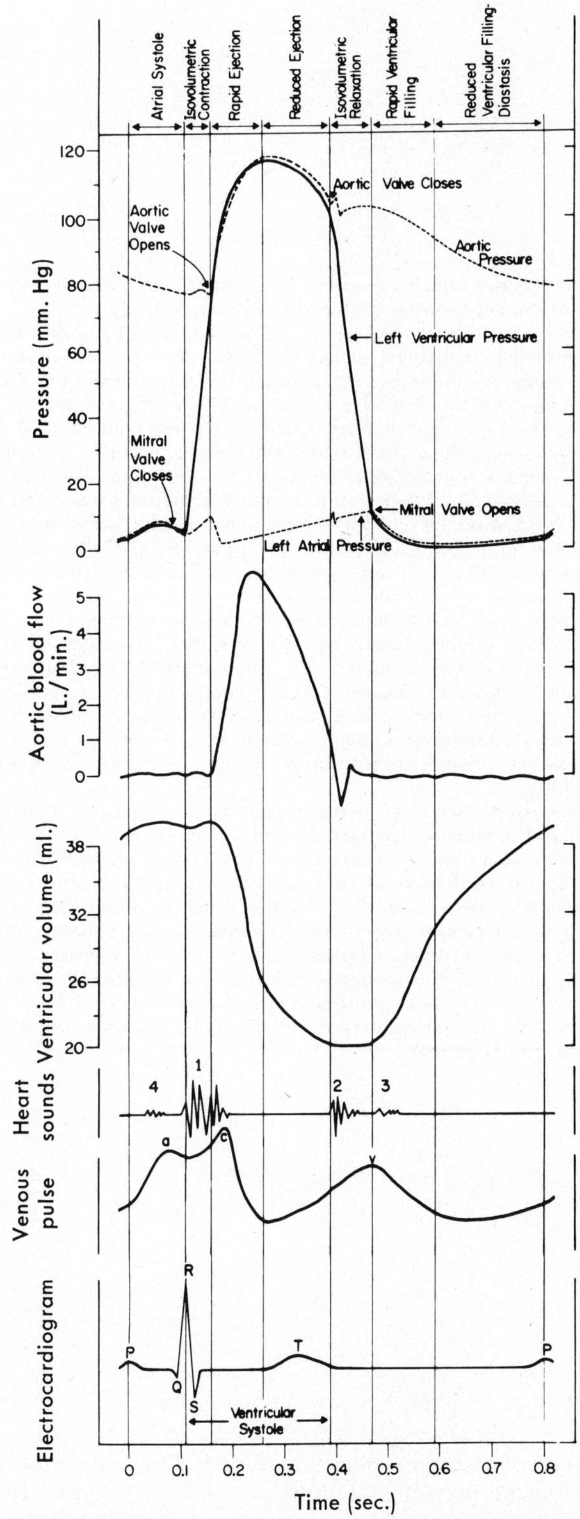

FIGURE 12–25 Events of the cardiac cycle. Left atrial, aortic, and left ventricular pressure pulses are correlated in time with aortic flow, ventricular volume, heart sounds, venous pulse, and electrocardiogram to provide a complete cardiac cycle in the dog. (From Berne, R. M., and Levy, M. N.: Cardiovascular Physiology. 3rd ed. St. Louis, The C. V. Mosby Co., 1977.)

have appreciable inotropic effects, such as the alpha-adrenergic agonist phenylephrine.[160] In man, the end-systolic ventricular volume can be determined by obtaining two or more angiocardiograms during infusion of such a vasoconstrictor, and the end-systolic values are then related to the corresponding ventricular or aortic pressure at the end of ventricular ejection; noninvasive techniques for measuring ventricular dimensions or volume (echocardiography and radionuclide methods) can also be employed. The linear end-systolic pressure-volume relation of the left ventricle has been found to shift downward and to the right in the presence of myocardial disease and to shift upward and to the left (with steepening of its slope) during acute positive inotropic interventions in experimental animals and in man (Fig. 12–26, lower panel).[161]

This relation is of particular importance because it defines the level of inotropic state under acutely changing conditions *independent* of the end-diastolic volume (preload) and the systolic aortic or ventricular pressure (as a measure of afterload). Thus, a given cardiac cycle arrives at end ejection and falls in this linear relation, regardless of the starting point for end-diastolic volume and the level of aortic pressure encountered during ejection, and the entire end-systolic pressure-volume relation is shifted acutely only by a change in inotropic state (Fig. 21–26). However, it should be recognized that under conditions in which there are *chronic* changes in the shape and size of the ventricle or in the thickness of its wall, systolic pressure is not indicative of the level of afterload; under these conditions the end-systolic pressure-volume relation does not define the level of inotropic state, and the wall force must be calculated in order to determine the linear relations between end-systolic volume and end-systolic wall force, which does identify the status of contractility.[162]

In comparing the whole heart to isolated muscle, heart volume and pressure are analogous to muscle length and tension. More complex formulations have also been developed; thus, the average circumferential wall stress (force per unit of cross-sectional area of wall) is related directly to the product of intraventricular pressure and internal radius and inversely to wall thickness. In the simplest versions of Laplace's law for a spherical ventricle, $\sigma = Pa/2h$ and, for an ellipsoidal ventricle, $\sigma = \frac{Pb}{h} \cdot \frac{1-b^2}{2c^2}$ where σ = average circumferential wall stress, P = intraventricular pressure, h = wall thickness; and b and c = the semiminor and semimajor axes at the endocardial surface.[136,158] In the ejecting ventricle, the extent and rate of wall shortening—and thus indirectly the stroke volume—are analogous to the extent and velocity of shortening of isolated muscle. The ventricular pressure during ventricular ejection is closely related to the afterload, although geometrical factors must be considered in order to calculate wall forces in the heart.

In order to clarify these concepts further, the relation between left ventricular systolic pressure and stroke volume was examined in the intact canine ventricle, while ventricular end-diastolic volume was held constant, and the force-velocity relation of the whole ventricle was calculated[163,164] (Fig. 12–27). Aortic pressure was varied independently of ventricular end-diastolic volume by rapid infusion or withdrawal of blood from the aorta during a single diastolic interval while the aortic valve was closed. The next cardiac cycle was then initiated from the same ven-

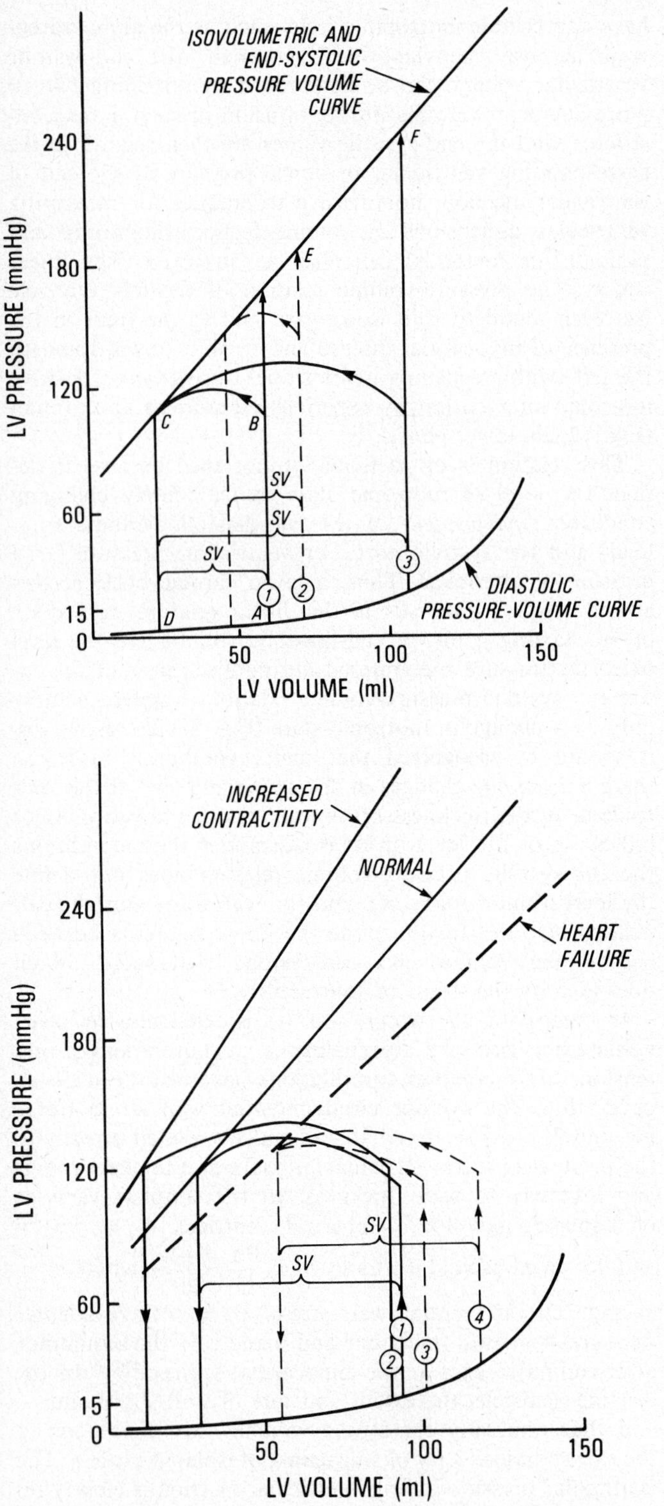

FIGURE 12–26 Effects of several interventions on pressure-volume loops of the left ventricle (LV) shown diagrammatically.

Upper panel, Effects of varying preload and afterload (with level of contractility remaining constant). Contraction 1 commences at end diastole (A) and is isovolumetric (arrow A to B) until the onset of ejection (B); the end of ejection or end-systolic volume (C) is followed by isovolumetric relaxation (C to D), and then filling of the ventricle occurs along the diastolic pressure-volume curve (from D to A). When a contraction originating from the same diastolic volume as contraction 1 is forced to contract isovolumetrically (top arrows), a point on the volume-isovolumetric systolic pressure curve is generated; if beats originating at larger end-diastolic volumes (contractions 2 and 3) are forced to contract isovolumetrically, points E and F are generated on that curve. This active pressure-volume curve provides the limit for the end-systolic volume of ejecting contractions. Ejecting contraction 3 shows that increasing end-diastolic volume causes an increase in stroke volume (SV) when aortic pressure is relatively constant. Ejecting contraction 2 (dashed lines) shows the effect of increasing systolic aortic pressure; when compared with contraction 1, SV is actually less, despite an increased end-diastolic volume, because of the higher level of aortic pressure or afterload.

Lower panel, Effects of increasing contractility (positive inotropic agent) and decreasing contractility (heart failure) on left ventricular pressure-volume loops. Contraction 1 is a normal pressure-volume loop, at a normal level of contractility. Contraction 2 shows that when contractility is increased, a larger stroke volume is generated from a similar or even slightly reduced end-diastolic volume, aortic pressure being relatively constant. In the presence of heart failure, SV may be diminished despite a slightly larger end-diastolic volume at a comparable level of aortic pressure (dashed line, contraction 3); however, SV may be restored if end-diastolic volume is further increased (contraction 4).

tricular end-diastolic volume but could be subjected to a wide range of predetermined pressures, i.e., afterloads. This experimental design mimics that of the isolated muscle contracting under variably afterloaded conditions, when a force-velocity relation is determined from a constant resting muscle length or preload (see Fig. 12–12). The ventricle became shorter auxotonically, i.e., against a *varying* afterload as ventricular wall tension declined when radius fell during ejection, rather than in a manner analogous to the usual papillary muscle preparation, which contracts isotonically, i.e., against a constant afterload. Increases in stroke volume and peak flow rate occurred when aortic pressure was lowered, and the opposite effect was observed when the pressure was elevated. Thus, an inverse relation was observed between myocardial wall stress and the velocity of circumferential fiber shortening (V_{CF}). When aortic pressure was increased to a sufficiently high level during diastole, the ventricle could be forced to contract isovolumetrically. Peak stress (P_0) as well as shortening velocities at all levels of afterload were altered by inotropic influences when ventricular end-diastolic volume was constant. These experiments indicate that the mamma-

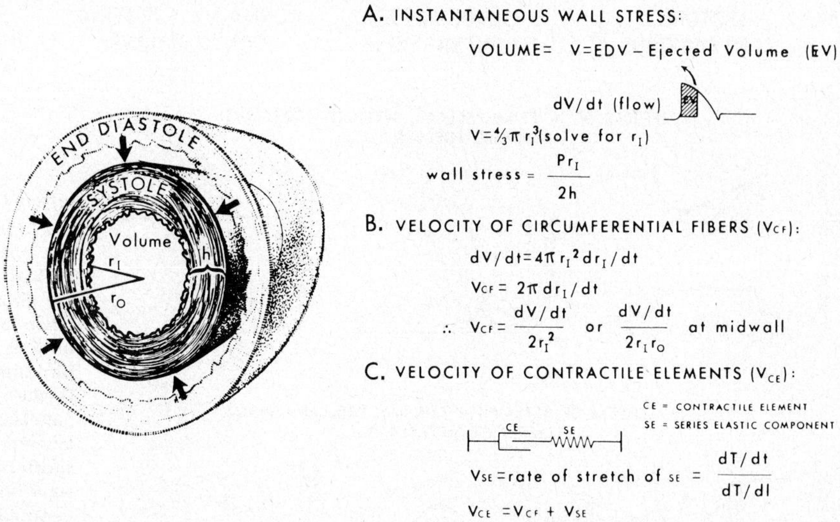

FIGURE 12–27 Diagram of a method of calculating force-velocity relationships in the intact ventricle. The equations assume a spherical model, the transected ventricle being shown at end diastole and during systole, when the instantaneous force-velocity relation is calculated. The wall-thickness (h) has increased from end diastole, and the instantaneous volume (V) can be computed from the aortic flow tracing (shown diagrammatically at the upper right) by subtracting the ejected volume (EV) (the cross-hatched area) from the end-diastolic volume (EDV). The instantaneous mean wall stress can then be calculated by solving the equation under heading *A* for the volume of the sphere to yield the inner radius (r_I). Since the ventricular wall becomes increasingly thick during systole, the velocity of the circumferential fibers (V_{CF}), calculated under heading *B*, employs values of both the inner radius (r_I) and the outer radius (r_O) to arrive at the midwall radius. The first equation under heading *B* represents differentiation of the equation for the volume of the sphere; the second equation represents the rate of shortening of the circumferential fibers (V_{CF}). Under heading *C*, the approach for calculating the velocity of the contractile elements (V_{CE}) is shown; the two-component model for muscle described by A. V. Hill is utilized in which the rate of stretch of the series elastic component (V_{SE}) is directly proportional to the rate of tension development (dT/dt) and is inversely proportional to the stiffness of the series elastic component (dT/dl). V_{CE} is equal to V_{SE} during isovolumetric contraction, whereas during shortening, V_{CE} equals $V_{CF} + V_{SE}$. (From Braunwald, E., et al.: Mechanisms of Contraction of the Normal and Failing Heart. 2nd ed. Boston, Little, Brown, 1976.)

lian ventricle as a whole responds in a manner similar to that of isolated cardiac muscle.

Preload

Starling's Law of the Heart, which states that "the mechanical energy set free on passage from the resting to the contracted state is a function of the length of the muscle fiber, i.e., of the area of chemically active surfaces,"[112] is an expression of the length–active tension curve, reflecting the functional consequences of variations in preload. In the intact heart, ventricular end-diastolic wall stress or tension is analogous to the preload of isolated muscle and ultimately determines the resting length of the sarcomeres (see Fig. 12–19).

The influence of alterations in preload independent of alterations in frequency, afterload, and inotropic state for the isotonically contracting canine left ventricle are shown diagrammatically in Figure 12–28*A*. Increases in preload augment the stroke volume as well as the extent and velocity of wall shortening.[164a] As in isolated muscle, in force-velocity curves obtained in the isotonically contracting heart, the maximum velocity of wall shortening estimated at zero force (V_{max}) does not appear to be altered by changing preload.[163,164] If ejection is prevented and the ventricle contracts isovolumetrically, a direct correlation between preload, as reflected in the end-diastolic volume, and peak left ventricular systolic pressure or calculated wall stress can also be shown (analogous to the length–active tension curve of isolated muscle). These relationships constitute expressions of the Frank-Starling mechanism and provide the basis for ventricular function curves in the normally ejecting heart, which relate ventricular end-diastolic volume or pressure to stroke volume and stroke work.[157] Any of the curves discussed above can, of course, be shifted up or down by positive and negative inotropic influences, respectively (see Fig. 12–26).

ATRIAL CONTRIBUTION TO PRELOAD. Atrial muscle behaves in accord with Starling's law, with increasing stretch resulting in a more forceful contraction.[165] When properly timed, atrial contraction augments ventricular filling and preload. Rapid ventricular filling induced by atrial contraction at the end of diastole abruptly elevates ventricular end-diastolic pressure and volume. This allows a lower mean right or left atrial pressure to exist throughout most of diastole than would be the case if atrial contraction were ineffective (as in atrial fibrillation) or ill-timed (as in nodal rhythm or atrioventricular dissociation).[166] The atrial contribution to ventricular filling is of particular importance in the presence of ventricular hypertrophy and other states of reduced ventricular compliance. In these conditions, the loss of atrial systole reduces ventricular end-diastolic pressure and volume, ultimately impairing myocardial performance.[166a]

DESCENDING LIMB OF STARLING'S CURVE. The question of whether a descending limb of cardiac function exists in the whole left ventricle has been of great interest.[167] In the isovolumetrically contracting isolated canine left ventricle, no reduction of developed wall stress or systolic pressure occurred until the ventricular end-diastolic pressure exceeded 60 mm Hg; when diastolic ventricular pressure was further elevated to 100 mm Hg, developed pressure declined by only 7.5 per cent. At these extremely high end-diastolic pressures, sarcomere lengths averaged 2.27 to 2.30 μ.[168] Based on this and earlier work showing that midwall sarcomere lengths did not exceed 2.27 μ at left ventricular end-diastolic pressures up to 40 mm Hg,[169] may be postulated that the descending limb of ventricular performance, when observed in ejecting heart, is not caused by operation of the heart on a descending limb of the sarcomere length-tension relation,[170] i.e., it is not a consequence of the disengagement of actin and myosin myofilaments. However, a descending limb of curves that relate left ventricular end-diastolic pressure to stroke work was demonstrated in dogs when volume loading was carried out to achieve end-diastolic pressures exceeding 30 mm

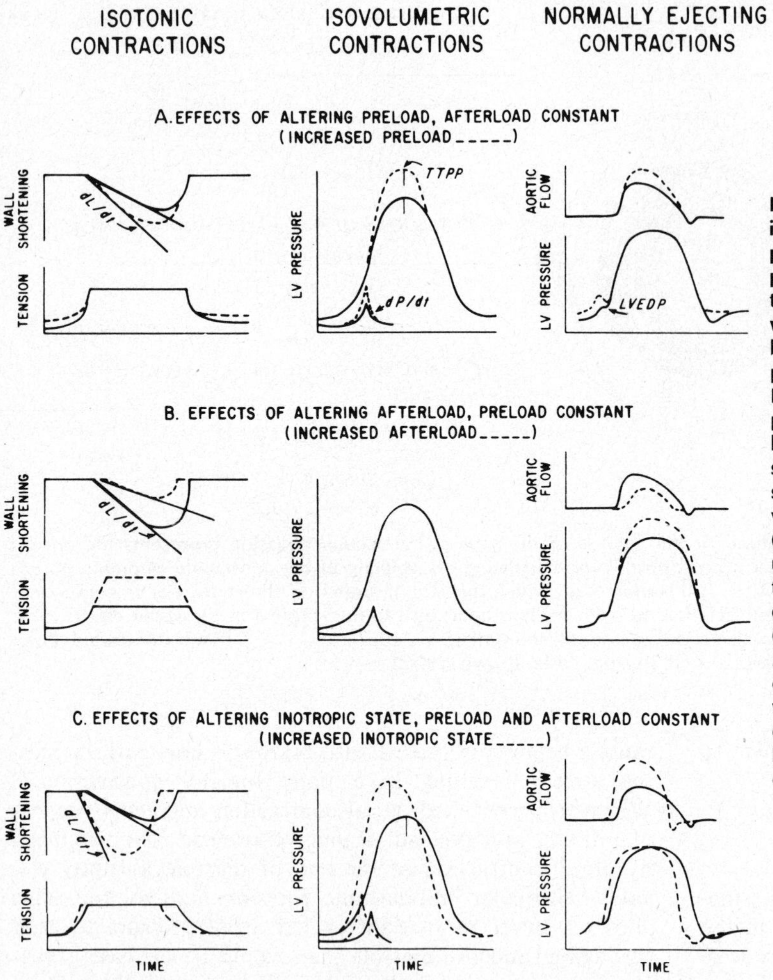

FIGURE 12–28 Effects of changing preload, afterload, and inotropic state on contractions of the whole heart. The upper row of panels (*A*) shows the effects of increasing preload when afterload and contractility are held constant, the middle row (*B*) shows the effects of increasing afterload when preload and contractility are held constant, and the bottom row (*C*) shows the effects of increasing the inotropic state when preload and afterload are held constant. Dashed lines show effects of intervention. Each of the three panels arranged vertically on the left (under the column labeled isotonic contractions) shows the extent of wall shortening, shortening velocity (dL/dt), and tension in superimposed tracings obtained in the isotonic canine left ventricular preparation. The tracings in the middle column (isovolumetric contractions) show isovolumetric left ventricular (LV) pressure tracings, the first derivatives (dP/dt), and time to peak pressure (TTPP). It should be noted that, by definition, an isovolumetric contraction is not afterloaded (since no shortening occurs) and therefore is unchanged in *B*, center panel. The tracings in the right column (normally ejecting contractions) show the effects of these three interventions on superimposed left ventricular contractions ejecting into the aorta, with left ventricular pressure and blood flow in the aortic root being shown. Left ventricular end-diastolic pressure (LVEDP) is also indicated.

Hg, after mean aortic pressure had initially been elevated.[171] Under these circumstances, slight further increases in aortic pressure occurred during the volume loading, which elevated left ventricular filling pressures above 30 mm Hg. It was concluded that the descending limb of function in the ejecting ventricle is only apparent and actually results from reduced myocardial wall shortening due to an increased afterload, when the ventricle is unable to compensate by further increases in sarcomere length. It has also been proposed that the descending limb of function induced in the failing human heart by infusion of a vasopressor agent[172] is due to such an effect of augmented afterload, when preload reserve is absent.[173] The development of mitral regurgitation consequent to ventricular dilatation can also depress forward stroke volume and result in an *apparent* depression of ventricular performance as preload is elevated to very high levels.

In summary, alterations in preload, operating through changes in end-diastolic sarcomere length, serve as an important determinant of the performance of the intact ventricle and provide the basis for the function curves of the intact ventricle. The ability to augment preload provides a functional reserve to the heart in situations of acute stress and operates on a beat-to-beat basis in maintaining balanced outputs of the two ventricles during such normal maneuvers as respiration.[157] The possibility of increasing preload provides a reserve mechanism and allows some augmentation of cardiac performance during severe stresses such as maximum exercise performed in the upright position.[174]

CONTROL OF PRELOAD IN THE INTACT ORGANISM

In the intact organism, preload is determined largely by venous return and total blood volume and its distribution (Fig. 12–29)[175,176] as well as by the activity of the atrium.

Venous Return. In the absence of heart failure in the intact organism, most changes in cardiac output can be accounted for largely by changes in the *return* of blood to the heart, which in turn alters the preload. In the absence of heart failure, simple augmentation of myocardial contractility, as occurs with administration of a cardiac glyco side or institution of sustained postextrasystolic potentiation (paired electrical stimulation), has little effect on cardiac output.[177] In contrast, relatively large changes in output occur during maneuvers that alter venous return, such as lower body positive or negative pressure, positive-pressure respiration, a sudden change in posture, and rapid changes in blood volume.

Conditions that lower peripheral vascular resistance are among the most important of those augmenting venous return and include the opening of arteriovenous fistulas and conditions that mimic the latter, such as patent ductus arteriosus, fever, beriberi, pregnancy, and Paget's disease. (These and other chronic high-output states are discussed in Chapter 24.) A reduction in vascular resistance also occurs during *exercise,* when the arterioles supplying the ex-

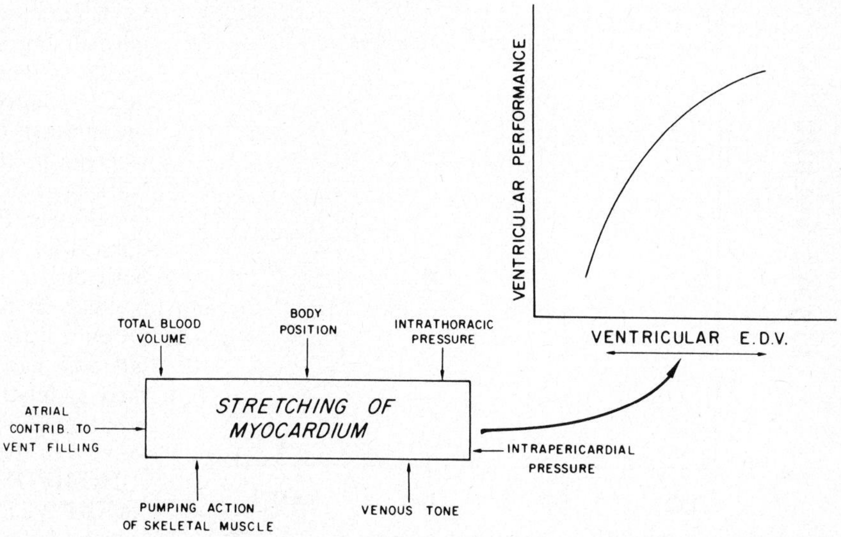

FIGURE 12–29 *Bottom left,* **Major influences that determine the degree of stretching of the myocardium, i.e., the magnitude of end-diastolic volume (E.D.V.).** *Top right,* **Diagram of a Frank-Starling curve, relating ventricular E.D.V. to ventricular performance. (From Braunwald, E., et. al.: Mechanisms of Contraction of the Normal and Failing Heart. 2nd ed. Boston, Little, Brown, 1976.)**

ercising muscle dilate; in severe *anoxia,* when generalized vascular dilation occurs; and in the presence of *anemia,* when blood viscosity and hence resistance to flow in the vascular bed are reduced.

Total Blood Volume. When blood volume is rapidly reduced, cardiac output and particularly stroke volume decline. However, in the intact organism, small (less than 15 per cent of control) or gradual reductions in blood volume can be tolerated with barely perceptible changes in cardiac output, as a consequence of a number of compensatory mechanisms resulting from activation of the adrenergic nervous system.

Distribution of Blood Volume. At any given total blood volume, the ventricular end-diastolic volume is a function of the distribution of blood between the intra- and extrathoracic compartments. The principal determinants of this distribution are as follows.

Body Position. Gravitational forces pool blood in the dependent portions of the body, and assumption of the upright posture therefore increases extrathoracic blood volume at the expense of intrathoracic and ventricular end-diastolic volumes, thereby reducing preload and cardiac output. The effects of negative pressure (suction) applied to the lower extremities and trunk with the subject supine mimic those of assumption of the upright posture, while inflation of a lower-body positive-pressure suit, immersion of the lower extremities and trunk into water, or the absence of gravitational force during space flight increases intrathoracic blood volume and preload.

Intrathoracic Pressure. The negative intrathoracic pressure normally increases thoracic blood volume, improving cardiac filling and augmenting preload and thereby cardiac performance. The intrathoracic pressure becomes most negative during inspiration and approximates atmospheric pressure during expiration. Accordingly, the gradient for venous return (and therefore right ventricular stroke volume) rises during inspiration when the intrathoracic pressure declines. Elevation of mean intrathoracic pressure, as occurs with the application of positive-pressure respiration or the development of pneumothorax, tends to impede total venous return to the heart, diminishes intrathoracic blood volume, and ultimately reduces ventricular performance.[178]

Intrapericardial Pressure. (See also Chapter 43). When pericardial pressure is elevated, as occurs in pericardial effusion, there is interference with cardiac filling, and the resultant reduction in ventricular diastolic volume (preload) reduces ventricular performance. With marked elevations of intrapericardial pressure, cardiac tamponade may occur, which is characterized by marked lowering of stroke volume and arterial pressure with circulatory collapse. Chronic constrictive pericarditis also impedes ventricular filling and thereby lowers stroke volume.[179]

Venous Tone. Smooth muscle in the walls of the veins responds to a variety of neural and humoral stimuli[180]; venoconstriction occurs during exercise, anxiety, deep respiration, or marked hypotension, tending to augment intrathoracic blood volume.[181] A variety of drugs act on venous smooth muscle. Thus, sympathomimetic agents produce venoconstriction,[180] while ganglionic blocking agents and sympatholytic and norepinephrine-depleting drugs or agents such as nitroglycerin that are direct venodilators[182,183] produce extrathoracic pooling and thereby ultimately reduce preload and cardiac output.[184] Extravascular compression of the veins by skeletal muscle plays an important role in augmenting venous return by exercising skeletal muscle.[185]

Atrial Contribution to Ventricular Filling (see p. 433). A vigorous, appropriately timed atrial contraction augments ventricular filling and end-diastolic volume.[165,166]

Afterload

When applied to the intact ventricle, afterload may be defined as the tension, force, or stress (force per unit of cross-sectional area) acting on the fibers in the ventricular wall *after* the onset of shortening, and it is a key determinant of the quantity of blood ejected by the ventricle.[187,188] In the intact heart, abrupt alterations in the impedance to left ventricular ejection cause reciprocal changes in the stroke volume of the left ventricle[159,160,187–189] (Fig. 12–26).

The influence of variations in afterload on the performance of the intact ventricle can be studied using the isotonically contracting heart preparation in which the other two determinants of ventricular performance (preload and contractility) are held constant (Fig. 12–28*B*). Increasing the afterload reduces both stroke volume and the extent

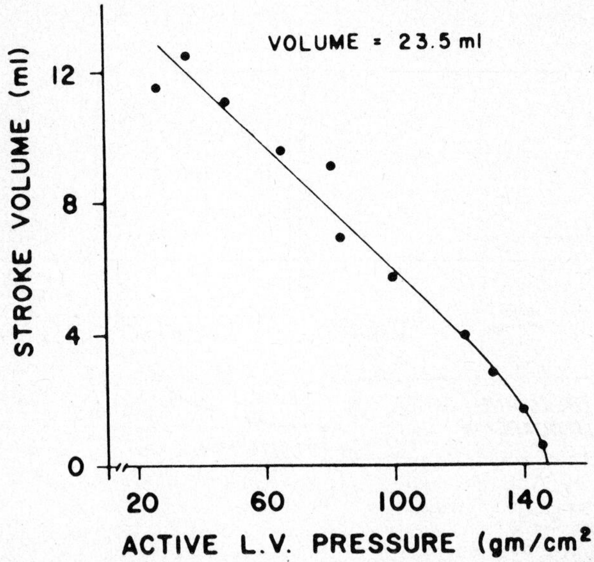

FIGURE 12–30 Relation between left ventricular systolic pressure (active L.V. pressure) and stroke volume in a series of contractions in the isotonically contracting canine left ventricle, in which left ventricular end-diastolic volume was held constant at 23.5 ml. The inverse relation between active pressure and stroke volume is apparent. (From Burns, J. W., et al.: Mechanics of isotonic left ventricular contractions. Am. J. Physiol. *224*:725, 1973.)

and velocity of wall shortening. Curves showing inverse relationships between afterload and stroke volume (Fig. 12–30), extent of wall shortening, and velocity of shortening can be constructed.[163,164,190]

The low impedance to left ventricular ejection (reduction in afterload) produced by mitral regurgitation,[191,192] patent ductus arteriosus, ventricular septal defect, or arteriovenous fistula can increase the extent of shortening and the ejection fraction. In the acutely pressure- and/or volume-overloaded ventricle, when sarcomere length is optimal and there is no preload reserve, any alteration in afterload causes a reciprocal change in stroke volume.[171] It is clear that the more severely depressed the inotropic state of the heart, the greater the influence of a change in afterload on the extent of myocardial fiber shortening. These considerations are relevant to the use of vasodilating agents to augment cardiac output in patients with left ventricular failure (Fig. 16–17, p. 537) and the use of pressor agents in the assessment of left ventricular function (p. 484).

When the ventricle is not operating along the steep portion of its diastolic pressure-volume curve, i.e., when there is still some preload reserve, an elevation of afterload often results in a compensatory elevation of ventricular end-diastolic volume, i.e., a rise in ventricular preload, which enhances myocardial contraction. However, as a consequence of the operation of Laplace's law (p. 431), this compensatory elevation of preload elevates myocardial tension development (afterload) further, and this in turn reduces myocardial fiber shortening. However, geometrical considerations dictate that the relative extent of myocardial fiber shortening required to maintain stroke volume constant is less in the larger ventricle. Hence, stroke volume may remain constant even though myocardial fiber shortening declines. If afterload rises, and if inflow into the ventricle is not restricted and preload can also rise, stroke volume can be maintained. In accord with these considerations, the normal subject responds to a pressor agent by maintaining stroke volume and increasing stroke work while augmenting left ventricular end-diastolic pressure and volume, i.e., the increase in afterload is met by an increase in preload, whereas in the diseased heart stroke volume and stroke work tend to fall because there is little, if any, preload reserve[172] (see Fig. 14–21, p. 485). Thus, the response to increased aortic pressure is dependent in significant measure both on the level of myocardial contractility and on the preload, in that a moderate pressor stress will ordinarily produce little change in stroke volume in the normal heart but will augment stroke volume in heart failure. When there is relative hypovolemia, and preload cannot rise appropriately, an increase in afterload will reduce the stroke volume in the normal heart.

HOMEOMETRIC AUTOREGULATION, OR THE "ANREP EFFECT." A positive inotropic effect has been said to follow abrupt elevation of systolic aortic and left ventricular pressure.[157,193–197] This response was first described by Von Anrep in 1912[198] and has been termed the "Anrep effect," or homeometric autoregulation. This effect occurs during the first minutes after aortic pressure is abruptly elevated, with end-diastolic pressure and circumference then tending to fall as stroke volume and stroke work recover. Force-velocity analyses of the left ventricle in anesthetized dogs suggest that it constitutes a small net positive inotropic effect.[195]

Homeometric autoregulation is most marked in the anesthetized state, and studies in conscious animals show that the initial increases in end-diastolic pressure and dimension are minimal at slow heart rates; however, during tachycardia greater initial increases in end-diastolic pressure and dimensions observed during aortic pressure elevation were followed by a much more marked Anrep effect.[199] These observations, together with the finding that reactive hyperemia in the myocardium occurs if aortic pressure is lower early during the Anrep effect but not after the effect is complete, support the concept that the phenomenon is related to recovery from transient subendocardial ischemia.[199]

CONTROL OF AFTERLOAD IN THE INTACT ORGANISM. In the intact organism, afterload is determined largely by peripheral vascular resistance, the physical characteristics of the arterial tree, and the volume of blood that it contains at the onset of ejection. The critical role played by ventricular afterload in cardiovascular regulation is summarized in Figure 12–31. While increases in both preload and contractility increase myocardial fiber shortening, increases in afterload reduce it; the extent of myocardial fiber shortening and of left ventricular size determines stroke volume. Arterial pressure, in turn, is related to the product of cardiac output and systemic vascular resistance, while afterload is a function of left ventricular size and arterial pressure. For example, when vasoconstriction raises arterial pressure, afterload is also augmented, which, through a negative feedback mechanism, tends to depress myocardial fiber shortening, stroke volume, and cardiac output; the latter, in turn, restores arterial pressure to its previous level.

When left ventricular function is impaired, afterload becomes an increasingly important determinant of cardiac performance. Afterload may rise as a consequence of vasoconstriction resulting from the influence on the arterial bed

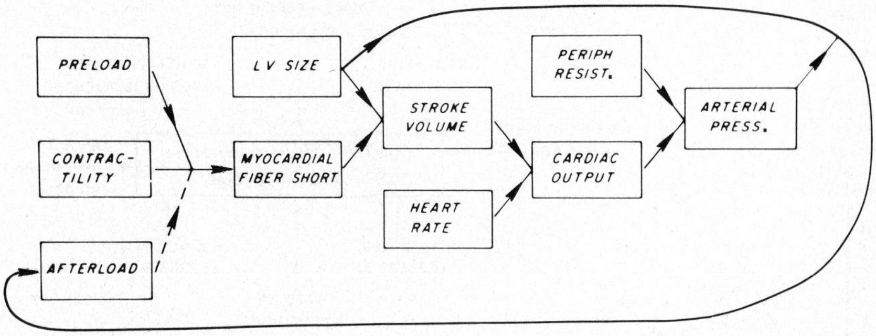

FIGURE 12–31 Schema showing interactions between various components regulating cardiac activity. Solid lines indicate an increasing effect; broken line represents a depressing effect. Note that left ventricular (L.V.) size is a determinant of both stroke volume and afterload. (Reprinted by permission from Braunwald, E.: Regulation of the circulation. N. Engl. J. Med. *290*:1124, 1974.)

of neural, humoral, and structural changes that occur in response to a fall in cardiac output. This increased afterload may reduce cardiac output further; on the other hand, pharmacological reductions of afterload may be beneficial in elevating cardiac output (p. 534).

In summary, when acute changes in arterial pressure occur, the resultant alteration in afterload has an important effect on cardiac performance (Fig. 12–30). An understanding of the effects of changes in afterload is central to an appreciation of the effects of conditions such as systemic or pulmonary arterial hypertension and obstruction to ventricular ejection by valvular disease (aortic and pulmonic stenosis), which increase afterload, and of mitral regurgitation and ventricular septal defect, which reduce it. Adaptation to a chronic increase in afterload by means of wall hypertrophy, in which a gradual increase in wall thickness occurs and tends to return wall stress and wall shortening characteristics toward normal,[200] is discussed in Chapter 13.

Contractility (Inotropic State)

The term "contractility," or "inotropic state," has a different connotation from the term "performance." For practical purposes, it is useful to regard a *change in contractility as an alteration in cardiac performance that is independent of changes resulting from variations in preload or afterload.* When loading conditions remain constant, an improvement in contractility augments cardiac performance (a positive inotropic effect) while a depression in contractility lowers cardiac performance (a negative inotropic effect).

The effects of an increase in contractility induced by a positive inotropic agent such as a catecholamine have been studied in the isotonically contracting heart preparation in which the other determinants of performance (preload, afterload, and contraction frequency) can be held constant.[164,200a] As in isolated muscle, increases in the velocity and extent of wall shortening and increased stroke volume occur while the duration of contraction is shortened (Fig. 12–28*C*). The force-velocity relation is shifted upward, P_0 and V_{max} both increase (Fig. 12–14), and curves relating diastolic volume to active peak isovolumetric pressure are shifted upward (Fig. 12–26). Acute administration of negative inotropic agents produce the opposite effects.[201]

THE INTERVAL-STRENGTH RELATION. In the intact ventricle, as in isolated cardiac muscle, premature depolarization results in a reduced mechanical contraction, the extent of the reduction being directly proportional to the degree of prematurity. However, the ensuing contraction is then more forceful than normal, the degree of augmentation being greater the earlier the extra depolarization is introduced.[49–51] This phenomenon, termed "postextrasystolic potentiation," is clearly *independent* of variations in preload, since it occurs in the isovolumetrically contracting heart in which preload is fixed.[202,203] In the intact organism, when the premature beat is followed by a compensatory pause, the ventricular end-diastolic volume may be augmented, and this increased preload may contribute along with the greater contractility to the enhanced performance that characterizes the postextrasystolic contraction. Postextrasystolic potentiation can be sustained and results in a striking augmentation of myocardial contractility when pairs of stimuli are delivered repetitively to the intact ventricle. In this technique, termed "paired electrical stimulation," the second stimulus is placed immediately after the electrical refractory period and results in only a small secondary contraction.[50,51] It is likely that the additional activation promotes an increased availability of Ca^{++} at the contractile sites. Despite its striking positive inotropic effect, paired electrical stimulation does not increase cardiac output in the nonfailing heart of the intact dog or of human subjects but does have this effect in the presence of experimental heart failure.[204]

Control of Contractility in the Intact Organism

The factors that modify cardiac contractility of the myocardium may be considered to operate by modifying the level of ventricular performance at any given ventricular end-diastolic volume, i.e., the relative position of the entire Frank-Starling curve (Fig. 12–32).

Sympathetic Nerve Activity. The quantity of norepinephrine (NE) released by sympathetic nerve endings in the heart is probably the most important factor regulating myocardial contractility under physiological conditions. Rapid changes in contractility in the intact organism are effected by variations in the impulse traffic in the cardiac adrenergic nerves. Beta-adrenergic receptor blocking agents and NE-depleting drugs interfere with the myocardial response to sympathetic nerve stimuli.

Circulating Catecholamines. When stimulated by nerve impulses, the adrenal medulla releases epinephrine, which is carried by the bloodstream to the myocardium, where it acts upon beta receptors to augment contractility. This mechanism is slower than the response to NE release by cardiac nerves but may be of physiological importance in conditions such as hypovolemia and a variety of chronic stresses, including congestive heart failure.

Interval-Strength Relation. As described above, myo-

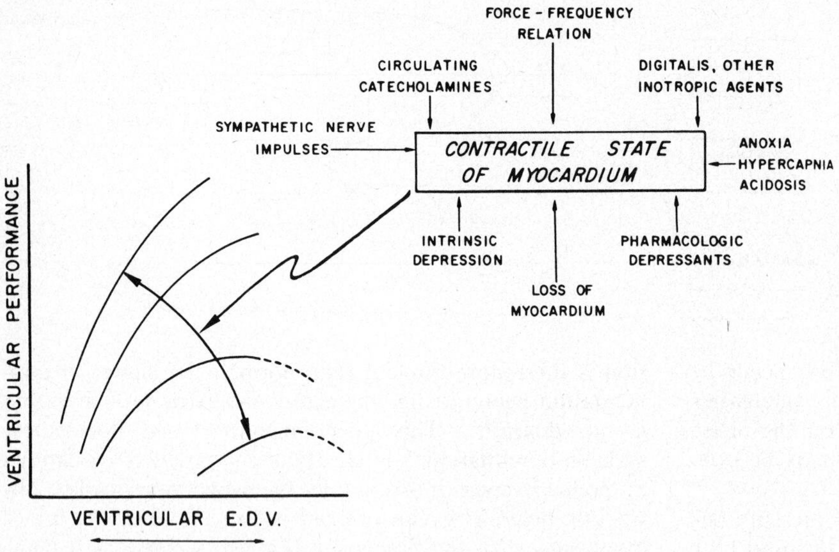

FIGURE 12–32 *Top right,* Diagram showing the major influences that elevate or depress the contractile state of the myocardium. *Bottom left,* Effect of alterations in the contractile state of the myocardium on the level of ventricular performance at any given level of ventricular end-diastolic volume. (From Braunwald, E., et al.: Mechanisms of Contraction of the Normal and Failing Heart. 2nd ed. Boston, Little, Brown, 1976.)

cardial contractility may be influenced profoundly by the rate and rhythm of cardiac contraction. For example, a ventricular extrasystole augments contractility, although to a decreasing extent, for several cardiac cycles. A simple increase in frequency in the physiological range also augments cardiac contractility, but this effect is more prominent in isolated heart muscle or in the intact heart with depressed function than it is in the normal heart of the intact organism.

Exogenous Inotropic Agents. The cardiac glycosides, sympathomimetic agents, Ca^{++}, caffeine, theophylline, amrinone, and their derivatives (see Chap. 16) all augment cardiac contractility.

Physiological and Pharmacological Depressants. These include anoxia,[205] ischemia (Chap. 36),[206] acidosis,[207] and local anesthetics (Chap. 20), barbiturates, and most general anesthetics.

Loss of Contractile Mass. When a portion of the ventricle becomes necrotic, as occurs in ischemic heart disease, the overall performance of the ventricle at any given end-diastolic volume is reduced, even though the contractility of the remaining myocardium may be normal (Chap. 37).

Intrinsic Myocardial Depression. Although, as indicated in Chapter 13, the fundamental mechanism responsible for depression of myocardial contractility in heart failure still remains to be elucidated, it is now apparent that the contractile state of each unit of myocardium is depressed in this condition.

Heart Rate

Accelerating the frequency of contraction generally does not induce a shift of the ventricular function curve, i.e., the relation between ventricular end-diastolic pressure and stroke work, in the open-chest anesthetized dog; however, it does increase stroke power (rate of performance of stroke work) at any given level of filling pressure,[157,208] a finding consistent with improvement of myocardial contractility and with observations on the effects of increases in the frequency of contraction in isolated cardiac muscle. Pacing-induced increases in contraction frequency, unaccompanied by sympathetic stimulation of the ventricle, also increase the calculated V_{max} and elevate the force-velocity relation of the ventricle in the anesthetized open-chest dog.[47]

The positive inotropic effect resulting from an increase in the frequency of contraction is more prominent in the anesthetized animal, in the depressed heart, and in isolated cardiac muscle than in the normal heart of the intact, conscious dog.[48] In the last situation, venous return to the heart is reflexly and metabolically stabilized, so that artificially varying heart rate between about 60 and 160 beats/minute has little effect on cardiac output, despite the above-mentioned modest changes in contractility that accompany changes in heart rate.[208,208a] However, if the diastolic volume of the heart is maintained, by increasing venous return as heart rate is increased, an elevation of frequency will augment cardiac output, and during exercise, tachycardia normally plays the major role in increasing cardiac output. However, since an increased heart rate augments the total fraction of each cardiac cycle occupied by systole, the corresponding reduction in the duration of diastole at very rapid rates can interfere with ventricular filling, ultimately limiting the rise in cardiac output associated with tachycardia.

Since, at a constant stroke volume, cardiac output is a linear function of heart rate, the ability to alter the latter is a critically important mechanism in the adjustment of cardiac output.[208b] The importance of heart rate in the maintenance of cardiac output is reflected in the inability of patients or experimental animals with fixed heart rates to elevate cardiac output appropriately, even when myocardial function is entirely normal. Under normal circumstances, heart rate is determined largely by the slope of phase 4 (spontaneous depolarization) of the sinoatrial node (p. 616); the intrinsic rhythmicity may be altered by a variety of influences, such as temperature and metabolism, rising with fever and thyrotoxicosis and falling with hypothermia and hypothyroidism. The two neurotransmitters released by autonomic nerves innervating the sinoatrial node play a critical role in the control of heart rate; acetylcholine slows while NE accelerates the slope of diastolic depolarization.

NEURAL CONTROL OF CARDIAC CONTRACTION

The autonomic nervous system is of critical importance in the moment-to-moment regulation of heart rate and contractility and of the capacitance and resistance of the vascular bed, thereby controlling cardiac output, blood flow distribution, and arterial pressure. Neural regulation is capable of producing considerable changes in cardiocirculatory function within seconds, before more slowly acting mechanisms, such as those mediated by the metabolic stimuli, circulating catecholamines, and the renin-angiotensin system, exert any effect.

ANATOMICAL CONSIDERATIONS. Sympathetic and parasympathetic preganglionic cells represent the final common pathways of neural impulses to the cardiovascular system. These cells receive both excitatory and inhibitory impulses from all levels of the central nervous system but most importantly from the cardiovascular center in the medulla and from spinal neurons. The medullary cardiovascular centers, operating independently of higher structures, are capable of regulating cardiac contractility and rate, arterial pressure, and even blood flow distribution, but under normal conditions their activity is regulated by influences from higher centers, notably the cerebral cortex, especially its cingulate gyrus, the hypothalamus, and the reticular substance in the pons and the mesencephalon. The impulse traffic from the vasomotor center is heightened by wakefulness, pain, mental and muscular effort, or emotional stress. Tonic activity in the medullary cardiovascular-excitatory center is constantly inhibited by impulses from the cardiovascular mechanoreceptors (both the high-pressure receptors in the carotid sinuses, aorta, and left ventricle and the low-pressure receptors in the atria, pulmonary vascular bed, and ventricles), but the medullary centers also receive input from chemoreceptors in skeletal muscle, skin, the viscera, and the special senses.

The cell bodies of the sympathetic preganglionic neurons lie in the intermediolateral horns of the spinal cord; most of their axons leave the spinal cord through the anterior roots of the thoracic and first two lumbar spinal nerves, synapse with postganglionic neurons in the chains of ganglia on each side of the spinal cord or in the peripheral sympathetic ganglia, and then traverse peripheral sympathetic nerves or spinal nerves to the heart and blood vessels. Some preganglionic sympathetic nerve fibers pass directly through the sympathetic chains, through the splanchnic nerves, and into the adrenal medulla where they synapse with secretory cells, which are analogous to postganglionic neurons. Catecholamines (predominantly epinephrine) may be released thereby from the adrenal medulla into the bloodstream at times when sympathetic efferent activity involving other organs is heightened. These two means of sympathetic stimulation (neural and humoral) supplement each other, the former acting rapidly but often briefly and the latter acting slowly but in a more sustained fashion.

While considerable overlap of autonomic innervation exists within most portions of the heart, certain regions receive their major supply from restricted sources. The sympathetic nerves originating from the right stellate ganglion are distributed primarily to the sinoatrial node and the right atrium, while the left ventrolateral cardiac nerve provides the primary supply to the posterolateral surfaces of the left atrium and ventricle; the central representation of these nerves may allow selective and rapid regulation of cardiac function. Contractility of both the epicardial and endocardial surfaces of the left ventricle can be independently altered, and it is now clear that certain nerves preferentially supply nodal tissues while others innervate contractile tissues.[209] The sympathetic nerve endings in the atria and ventricles are interposed between muscle bundles. The terminal innervation of the heart is a plexiform structure, the so-called *perimuscular* or *perimysial plexus,* which extends around the muscle cells in close apposition to, but without penetrating, the myocardial cells. The cardiac muscle cells and innervating fibers might be considered to be analogous to a neuromuscular unit in skeletal muscle. When the rate of liberation of the neurotransmitter exceeds the capacity of the enclosed units to utilize or metabolize it, it may overflow into vascular channels.[210,211]

The NE present in the heart is synthesized and then stored in the sympathetic nerve fibers rather than in the myocardial cells per se. Chemical sympathectomy with 6-hydroxydopamine, cardiac denervation, and treatment with catecholamine-depleting drugs such as reserpine all result in a striking reduction in NE content of the heart as well as in the disappearance of histochemical fluorescence. Sympathetic nerve endings contain neurosecretory granules ranging in size from 400 to 700 nm, and the depolarization of the neurons triggers the release of NE from these vesicles and thence from the adrenergic neuron.

The effects of released NE are terminated by three mechanisms (Fig. 12–33): (1) reuptake into the adrenergic neuron by means of an energy-dependent pump; once inside the neuron, much of the transmitter is again taken up into the neurosecretory granules and is available for subsequent re-release; (2) escape of NE into the circulation is metabolized by catechol-O-methyl transferase (COMT) to normetanephrine, some of which is further converted into vanillylmandelic acid (VMA) via the action of monoamine oxidase (MAO); and finally (3) conversion of NE intraneuronally to 3,4-dihydroxymandelic acid by MAO and then to VMA by COMT. The heart and other organs exhibit supersensitivity to NE after surgical denervation or the administration of cocaine. Both these interventions block the neuronal uptake of NE, thus making a larger quantity of neurotransmitter available for binding to the receptor sites.

The peripheral effects mediated by NE and epinephrine have been classified as alpha or beta. An important effect of NE is to cause vasoconstriction, an action on postsynaptic $alpha_1$ receptors on vascular smooth muscle. However, NE also acts on receptors on the neuron terminal itself. These *presynaptic* alpha receptors (termed $alpha_2$ receptors) serve as feedback inhibitors of the release of NE from the neuron terminal and reduce the release of neurotransmitter. The mechanisms by which NE acts upon cardiac beta and alpha receptors is discussed on page 418.

As we have seen, NE, the natural transmitter for sympathetic neurons, has both alpha and beta receptor–stimulating properties. When NE is given systemically, the alpha vasoconstrictor action predominates, and the elevation of arterial pressure results in reflex bradycardia and an increase in stroke volume and coronary blood flow but no change in cardiac output. *Epinephrine,* synthesized only

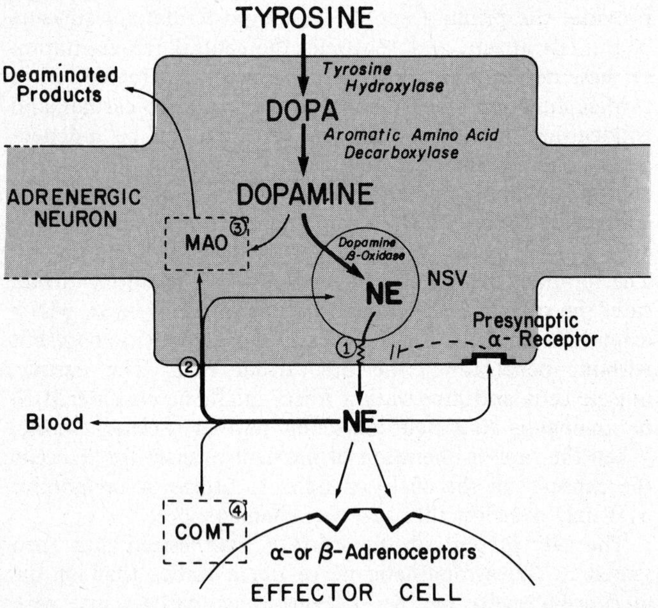

FIGURE 12–33 Synthesis, storage, secretion, and disposition of the adrenergic neurotransmitter norepinephrine (NE). A varicosity of the adrenergic neuron is depicted diagrammatically. Multiple varicosities occur at intervals along the terminal segments of peripheral adrenergic neurons and are juxtaposed to effector sites within target organs. Tyrosine is transported into the adrenergic neuron to provide substrate for the synthesis of NE. The rate-limiting enzyme is tyrosine hydroxylase, and the final enzyme, dopamine β-oxidase, is located within the neurosecretory vesicle (NSV).

1, Depolarization of the neuron leads to release of NE by a calcium-dependent process of "excitation-secretion coupling." in which the neurosecretory vesicle fuses with the neuronal membrane and by exocytosis discharges its soluble contents, including NE and dopamine β-oxidase.

2, Much of the NE released into the synaptic cleft between the neuron and the effector cell is removed from this area by a specialized membrane transport system, known as the NE pump, which transports NE back into the neuron against a concentration gradient. This transport system is relatively unspecific and is responsible for the uptake of a number of ring-substituted amines such as tyramine, ephedrine, and guanethidine. It is competitively inhibited by the tricyclic antidepressants. Released NE may act on adrenoreceptors, "spill" into the bloodstream, or be metabolized extraneuronally (see *4*).

3, The major pathway for intraneuronal bioinactivation of NE (and dopamine) is via monoamine oxidase (MAO).

4, Extraneuronally, a major pathway of NE metabolism is via catechol-O-methyl transferase (COMT), to which NE is exposed at some effector cells and in remote organs such as the liver. (From Oates, J. A., and Shand, D. G.: Clinical pharmacology of the autonomic nervous system. *In* Isselbacher, K. J., et al. (eds.): Harrison's Principles of Internal Medicine. 9th ed. New York, McGraw-Hill Book Co., 1980, p. 390.)

in the adrenal medulla, also has combined alpha and beta actions, but its beta effects are more striking than those of NE, especially in low doses; therefore, it produces tachycardia and an elevation of cardiac output. *Dopamine* (p. 542) is the third naturally occurring catecholamine that subserves a transmitter function in the central nervous system. When infused, it has both alpha and beta effects and in addition acts on what appear to be specific dopamine receptors. At low doses (1 to 5 μg/kg/min, administered intravenously), it dilates mesenteric and renal vessels, producing increased renal blood flow and sodium excretion by its action on dopamine receptors. At slightly higher doses (5 to 10 μg/kg/min), beta stimulation increases cardiac output with relatively little tachycardia. At even higher doses (> 10 μg/kg), tachycardia and alpha stimulation occur. *Isoproterenol* is a synthetic compound with pure beta-agonist activity, causing a reduction in peripheral vascular resistance with an increase in heart rate and contractility and thus an increase in cardiac output.

CARDIAC CONTROL IN THE INTACT ORGANISM (Fig. 12–34)

In the normal state, interference with one or even more of the above-mentioned mechanisms that affect cardiac performance may not influence the cardiac output. For example, a moderate reduction of blood volume or loss of the atrial contribution to ventricular contraction can ordinarily be sustained without a reduction of cardiac output in the resting state. Presumably, other factors such as an increase in adrenergic nerve impulse traffic, which augments contractility, and venoconstriction, which increases ventricular filling, can compensate for this depression.[212] Mechanisms are also available to prevent unnecessary elevation of cardiac output. For example, in normal subjects, expansion of blood volume, a simple increase in heart rate induced by atropine or pacing, or augmentation of myocardial contractility by means of cardiac glycosides does not increase cardiac output[213,214]; the latter reduces the frequency of adrenergic nerve impulses to the heart, thereby tending to oppose the direct inotropic effect.[215] More importantly, since the normal heart is capable of expelling all the blood returned to it under most physiological conditions, cardiac output is ordinarily a function of venous return, not of the level of contractility.[177] The latter does not limit the volume of blood ejected by the heart in the normal subject except perhaps under the most severe stress, and therefore stimulation of myocardial contractility alone would not be expected to elevate cardiac output in a normal subject at rest or during mild activity unless there is a simultaneous reduction in peripheral arterial resistance (as occurs with isoproterenol administration).[216] In the presence of congestive heart failure, on the other hand, cardiac output is usually limited by the contractile state of the myocardium, and a positive inotropic influence raises cardiac output.[204]

Circulatory Adjustment During Exercise

Peripheral Circulatory Responses. As important as the heart may be in mediating the body's response to exercise, alterations in the peripheral circulation are of at least equal significance. Indeed, the elevation of cardiac output achieved in the resting state through infusion of a maximal dose of isoproterenol, which greatly augments cardiac rate and contractility, does not approach the level commonly observed during exercise. Changes in the peripheral circulation act in concert to augment the capacity of the vascular bed to return blood to the heart.[217] Perhaps the most important of these is the vasodilation that takes place in the blood vessels supplying the exercising muscles. The marked reduction in systemic vascular resistance acts in a

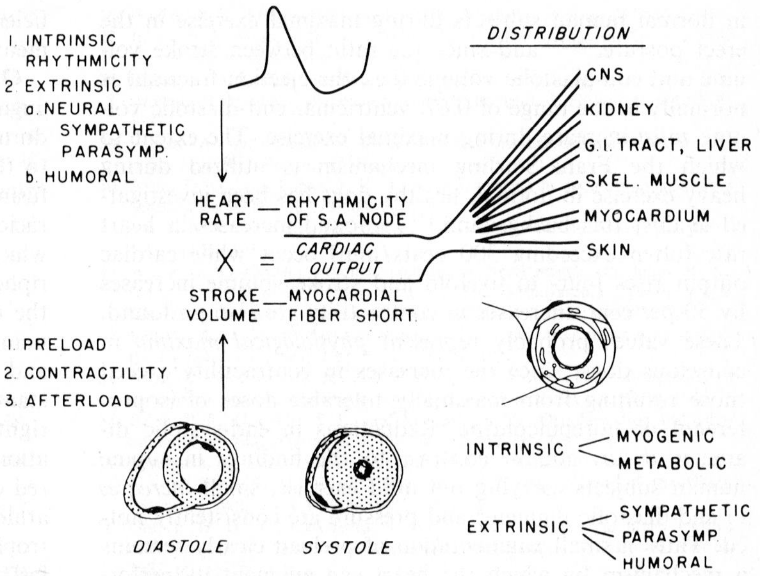

FIGURE 12–34 Schema of factors affecting systemic circulation. In the center, cardiac output is shown with its two determinants, heart rate and stroke volume; the former is a function of the automaticity of the sinoatrial (S.A.) node, while the latter is dependent on the extent of myocardial fiber shortening. The principal determinants of heart rate and stroke volume are listed at the extreme left. Distribution of cardiac output through various vascular beds is shown at the upper right (CNS = central nervous system). The two principal influences (intrinsic and extrinsic) on the lumen of the peripheral resistance vessels and their major determinants are shown at the lower right. (Reprinted by permission from Braunwald, E.: Regulation of the circulation. N. Engl. J. Med. *290*:1124, 1974.)

manner analogous to the opening of multiple arteriovenous fistulas and greatly reduces the resistance to the return of blood ejected from the left ventricle back to the right atrium. Vascular dilatation also tends to reduce afterload and thereby facilitates left ventricular emptying. However, despite profound vasodilation in the metabolizing muscles during exercise, arterial pressure tends to rise, primarily as a consequence of the elevation of cardiac output but also as a result of vasoconstriction, which occurs in many vascular beds other than in the heart and the exercising limbs.[218] Other factors that facilitate venous return during exercise include the rhythmic tensing of the skeletal muscles, not only of the exercising limbs but of the abdomen and thorax as well, which compresses the veins and displaces blood centrally.[217]

Ventricular Volumes and Dimension. The cardiac response to exercise is complex and involves the interaction of changes in heart rate, contractility, preload, and afterload. In man, the elevation of cardiac output that occurs during mild exercise in the supine position results almost exclusively from an increase in heart rate, with stroke volume showing little change.[219] In contrast, in individuals at rest in the erect position, stroke volume is less than in the supine position but increases markedly during strenuous exertion; these increases in stroke volume contribute substantially to the elevation of cardiac output. Indeed, during maximal treadmill exercise, stroke volume increases to approximately twice the levels present at rest in the upright position.[220,221]

The effects of *light* muscular exercise in the supine position on ventricular dimensions have been studied in patients by determining the distances between roentgenopaque markers sewn onto the epicardium.[222] End-diastolic dimensions in both ventricles decreased slightly[223,224] while myocardial contractility rose, as attested to by a shift of the force-velocity relation.[224] Maximal exercise in the dog[174] or strenuous exercise in semirecumbent[225] or upright[226] humans results in an increase in end-diastolic dimensions.

Heart Rate. The ability to alter heart rate is an extremely important mechanism for the adjustment of cardiac output during exercise. Indeed, changes in heart rate normally account in large measure for changes in cardiac output. The increase in cardiac output that occurs in man during light to moderate exercise in the supine position is accompanied by a parallel augmentation of heart rate, while, as just noted, the stroke volume remains essentially unchanged. When heart rate fails to rise normally, as in patients with heart block, the maximal cardiac output that can be achieved during exercise is reduced.

The Adrenergic Nervous System. The effects of adrenergic blockade have been studied in an effort to elucidate the role of adrenergic nervous activity in the cardiovascular response to exercise. Beta blockade reduces the endurance for maximal activity, cardiac output, mean arterial pressure, left ventricular minute work, and maximal oxygen uptake and increases the arteriovenous oxygen difference and central venous pressure in normal human subjects during maximal exercise in the upright position.[220] This intervention has no significant effect on ventricular dimensions recorded at rest in the supine position, indicating that there is little tonic adrenergic support under these circumstances. However, after beta blockade, little augmentation of the contractile state was observed during exercise; despite some elevations of heart rate, ventricular end-diastolic dimensions do not decrease during exercise, as is the case in the unblocked state.[224]

The Frank-Starling Mechanism. The finding that with light exercise, performed in the supine position, ventricular end-diastolic dimensions decline has been used to support the view that the Frank-Starling mechanism is *not* involved in the cardiac response to exercise.[225,226] In the intact subject the increase in end-diastolic volume that occurs during light exercise may not be evident because of the opposing effects of the tachycardia per se and the increased sympathetic activity normally occurring during exercise, both of which contribute to the reduction of end-diastolic dimensions; indeed, in the presence of beta blockade, exercise no longer reduces end-diastolic size. This conclusion is consonant with studies on denervated dogs[227] in which exercise results in small but significant increases in ventricular end-diastolic dimensions as well as stroke volume.

There is considerable evidence that the *intensity* of exercise also conditions the cardiac response to this stimulus. Indeed, since, as already noted, stroke volume may double

coplasmic reticulum after coronary artery occlusion for 60 and 90 minutes. Circ. Res. *20*:439, 1967.
117. Varley, K. G., and Dhalla, N. S.: Excitation-contraction coupling in heart: XII. Subcellular calcium transport in isoproterenol-induced myocardial necrosis. Exp. Mol. Pathol. *19*:94, 1973.
118. Kim, N. D., and Harrison, C. E.: $^{45}Ca^{2+}$ accumulation by mitochondria and sarcoplasmic reticulum in chronic potassium depletion cardiomyopathy. *In* Dhalla, N. S., and Rona, G. (eds.): Myocardial Biology. Vol. 4. Baltimore, University Park Press, 1972, pp. 551–562.
119. Lindenmayer, G. E., Sordahl, L. A., Harigaya, S., Allen, J. C., Besch, H. R., Jr., and Schwartz, A.: Some biochemical studies on subcellular systems isolated from fresh recipient human cardiac tissue obtained during transplantation. Am. J. Cardiol. *27*:277, 1971.
120. Khatter, J. C., and Prasad, K.: Myocardial sarcolemmal ATPase in dogs with induced mitral insufficiency. Cardiovasc. Res. *10*:637, 1976.
121. Prasad, K., Khatter, J. C., and Bharadwaj, B.: Intra- and extracellular electrolytes and sarcolemmal ATPase in the failing heart due to pressure overload in dogs. Cardiovasc. Res. *13*:95, 1979.
122. Braunwald, E., and Ross, J., Jr.: Control of Cardiac Performance. *In* Berne, R. M. (ed.): Handbook of Physiology. Section 2, The Cardiovascular System, Vol. 1, The Heart. Bethesda, American Physiological Society, 1979, pp. 533–580.
123. Chidsey, C. A., Harrison, D. C., and Braunwald, E.: Augmentation of plasma norepinephrine response to exercise in patients with congestive heart failure. N. Engl. J. Med. *267*:650, 1962.
124. Goldstein, D. S.: Plasma norepinephrine as an indicator of sympathetic neural activity in clinical cardiology. Am. J. Cardiol. *48*:1147, 1981.
125. Maurer, W., Ablasser, A., Tschada, R., Hausen, M., Saggau, W., and Kubler, W.: Myocardial catecholamine metabolism in patients with chronic aortic regurgitation. Circulation *66*(Suppl. 1):139, 1982.
125a. Malliani, A., and Pagani, M.: The role of the sympathetic nervous system in congestive heart failure. Eur. Heart J. *4*(Suppl. A):49, 1983.
126. Chidsey, C. A., Braunwald, E., and Morrow, A. G.: Catecholamine excretion and cardiac stores of norepinephrine in congestive heart failure. Am. J. Med. *39*:442, 1965.
127. Thomas, J. A., and Marks, B. H.: Plasma norepinephrine in congestive heart failure. Am. J. Cardiol. *41*:233, 1978.
128. Cody, R. J., Franklin, K. W., Kluger, J., and Laragh, J. H.: Sympathetic responsiveness and plasma norepinephrine during therapy of chronic congestive heart failure with captopril. Am. J. Med. *72*:791, 1982.
129. Levine, T. B., Francis, G. S., Goldsmith, S. R., Siomon, A. B., and Cohn, J. N.: Activity of the sympathetic nervous system and renin-angiotensin system assessed by plasma hormone levels and their relation to hemodynamic abnormalities in congestive heart failure. Am. J. Cardiol. *49*:1659, 1982.
130. Kluger, J., Cody, R. J., and Laragh, J. H.: The contributions of sympathetic tone and the renin-angiotensin system to severe chronic congestive heart failure: Response to specific inhibitors (prazosin and captopril). Am. J. Cardiol. *49*:1667, 1982.
130a. Turini, G. A., Waeber, B., and Brunner, H. R.: The renin-angiotensin system in refractory heart failure: Clinical, hemodynamic and hormonal effects of captopril and enalapril. Eur. Heart J. *4*(Suppl. A):189, 1983.
131. Colucci, W. S., Alexander, R. W., Williams, G. H., Rude, R. E., Holman, B. L., Konstam, M. A., Wynne, J., Mudge, G. H., Jr., and Braunwald, E.: Decreased lymphocyte beta-adrenergic-receptor density in patients with heart failure and tolerance to the beta-adrenergic agonist pirbuterol. N. Engl. J. Med. *305*:185, 1981.
132. Chidsey, C. A., Kaiser, G. A., Sonnenblick, E. H., Spann, J. F., Jr., and Braunwald, E.: Cardiac norepinephrine stores in experimental heart failure in dogs. J. Clin. Invest. *43*:2386, 1964.
133. Coulson, R. L., Yazdanfar, S., Rubio, E., Bove, A. A., Lemole, G. M., and Spann, J. F.: Recuperative potential of cardiac muscle following relief of pressure overload hypertrophy and right ventricular failure in the cat. Circ. Res. *40*:41, 1977.
134. Bristow, M. R., Ginsburg, R., Minobe, W., Cubicciotti, R. S., Sageman, W. S., Lurie, K., Billingham, M. E., Harrison, D. C., and Stinson, E. B.: Decreased catecholamine sensitivity and beta-adrenergic-receptor density in failing human hearts. N. Engl. J. Med. *307*:205, 1982.
135. Spann, J. F., Jr., Sonnenblick, E. H., Cooper, T., Chidsey, C. A., Willman, V. L., and Braunwald, E.: Cardiac norepinephrine stores and the contractile state of heart muscle. Circ. Res. *19*:317, 1966.
136. Spann, J. F., Jr., Chidsey, C. A., Pool, P. E., and Braunwald, E.: Mechanism of norepinephrine depletion in experimental heart failure produced by aortic constriction in guinea pig. Circ. Res. *17*:312, 1965.
137. Sole, M. J., Lo, C., Laird, O., Sonnenblick, E. H., and Wurtman, R. J.: Norepinephrine turnover in the heart and spleen of the cardiomyopathic Syrian hamster. Circ. Res. *37*:855, 1975.
138. Sole, M. J.: Alterations in sympathetic and parasympathetic neurotransmitter activity. *In* Braunwald, E., Mock, M. B., and Watson, J. (eds.): Congestive Heart Failure: Current Research and Clinical Applications. New York, Grune and Stratton, 1982, p. 101.
139. Pool, P. E., Covell, J. W., Levitt, M., Gibb, J., and Braunwald, E.: Reduction of cardiac tyrosine hydroxylase activity in experimental congestive heart failure. Its role in depletion of cardiac norepinephrine stores. Circ. Res. *20*:349, 1967.
140. Sole, M. J., Kamble, A. B., and Hussain, M. N.: A possible change in the rate-limiting step for cardiac norepinephrine synthesis in the cardiomyopathic Syrian hamster. Circ. Res. *41*:814, 1977.
141. Rutenberg, H. L., and Spann, J. F., Jr.: Alterations in cardiac sympathetic neurotransmitter activity in congestive heart failure. Am. J. Cardiol. *32*:472, 1973.
142. Mathes, P., Cowan, C., and Gudbjarnarson, S.: Storage and metabolism of norepinephrine after experimental myocardial infarction. Am. J. Physiol. *220*:27, 1971.
143. Covell, J. W., Chidsey, C. A., and Braunwald, E.: Reduction of the cardiac response to postganglionic sympathetic nerve stimulation in experimental heart failure. Circ. Res. *19*:51, 1966.
144. Gaffney, T. E., and Braunwald, E.: Importance of the adrenergic nervous system in the support of circulatory function in patients with congestive heart failure. Am. J. Med. *34*:320, 1963.
145. Epstein, S. E., and Braunwald, E.: The effect of beta-adrenergic blockade on patterns of urinary sodium excretion: Studies in normal subjects and in patients with heart disease. Ann. Intern. Med. *75*:20, 1966.
146. Vogel, J. H. K., and Chidsey, C. A.: Cardiac adrenergic activity in experimental heart failure assessed with beta-receptor blockade. Am. J. Cardiol. *24*:198, 1969.
147. Goldstein, R. E., Beiser, G. D., Stampfer, M., and Epstein, S. E.: Impairment of autonomically mediated heart rate control in patients with cardiac dysfunction. Circ. Res. *36*:571, 1975.
148. Higgins, C. B., Vatner, S. F., Eckberg, D. L., and Braunwald, E.: Alterations in the baroreceptor reflex in conscious dogs with heart failure. J. Clin. Invest. *51*:715, 1972.
149. White, C. W.: Reversibility of abnormal arterial baroreflex control of heart rate in heart failure. Am. J. Physiol. *241*(Heart Circ. Physiol. 10):H778, 1981.
150. Cohn, J. N., Taylor, N., Vrobel, T., and Moskowitz, R.: Contrasting effect of vasodilators on heart rate and plasma catecholamines in patients with hypertension and heart failure. Clin. Res. *26*(Abstr.):547A, 1978.
151. Mark, A. L., Mayer, H. E., Schmid, P. G., Heistad, D. D., and Abboud, F. M.: Adrenergic control of the peripheral circulation in cardiomyopathic hamsters with heart failure. Circ. Res. *33*:74, 1973.
152. Eckberg, D. L., Drabinsky, M., and Braunwald, E.: Defective cardiac parasympathetic control in patients with heart disease. N. Engl. J. Med. *285*:877, 1971.
153. Roskoski, R., Jr., Schmid, P. G., Mayer, H. E., and Abboud, F. M.: In vitro acetylcholine biosynthesis in normal and failing guinea pig hearts. Circ. Res. *36*:547, 1975.
154. Schmid, P. G., Lund, D. D., and Roskoski, R., Jr.: Efferent autonomic dysfunction in heart failure. *In* Abboud, F. M., Fozzard, H. A., Gilmore, J. P., and Reis, D. J. (eds.): Disturbances in Neurogenic Control of the Circulation. Bethesda, Md., American Physiological Society, 1981, p. 138.
155. Amorim, D. S., Heer, K., Jenner, D., Richardson, P., Dargie, H. J., Brown, M., Olsen, E. G. J., and Goodwin, J. F.: Is there autonomic impairment in congestive (dilated) cardiomyopathy? Lancet *1*:525, 1981.
156. Gauer, O. H., and Henry, J. P.: Neurohumoral control of plasma volume. *In* Guyton, A. C., and Cowley, A. W. (eds.): International Review of Physiology. Cardiovascular Physiology II. Baltimore, University Park Press, 1976, pp. 145–190.
157. Nonidez, J. F.: Identification of the receptor areas in the venae cavae and pulmonary veins which initiate reflex cardiac acceleration (Bainbridge's reflex). Am. J. Anat. *61*:203, 1937.
158. Thoren, P., and Ricksten, S.-E.: Cardiac C-fiber endings in cardiovascular control under normal and pathophysiological conditions. *In* Abboud, F. M., Fozzard, H. A., Gilmore, J. P., and Reis, D. J. (eds.): Disturbances in Neurogenic Control of the Circulation. Bethesda, Md., American Physiological Society, 1981, p. 17.
159. Abboud, F. M., Thames, M. C., and Mark, A. L.: Role of cardiac afferent nerves in regulation of circulation during coronary occlusion and heart failure. *In* Abboud, F. M., Fozzard, H. A., Gilmore, J. P., and Reis, D. J. (eds.): Disturbances in Neurogenic Control of the Circulation. Bethesda, Md., American Physiological Society, 1981, p. 65.
160. Belleau, L., Mion, H., Simard, S., Granger, P., Bertranou, E., Nowacynski, W., Boucher, R., and Genest, J.: Studies on the mechanism of experimental congestive heart failure in dogs. Can. J. Physiol. Pharmacol. *48*:450, 1970.
161. Zehr, J. E., Hawe, A., Tsakiris, A. G., Rastelli, G. C., McGoon, D. C., and Segar, W. E.: ADH levels following nonhypotensive hemorrhage in dogs with chronic mitral stenosis. Am. J. Physiol. *221*:312, 1971.
162. Greenberg, T. T., Richmond, W. H., Stocking, R. A., Gupta, P. D., Meehan, J. P., and Henry, J. P.: Impaired atrial receptor responses in dogs with heart failure due to tricuspid insufficiency and pulmonary artery stenosis. Circ. Res. *32*:424, 1973.
163. Zucker, I. H., Earle, A. M., and Gilmore, J. P.: The mechanism of adaptation of left atrial stretch receptors in dogs with chronic congestive heart failure. J. Clin. Invest. *60*:323, 1977.
164. Zucker, I. H., Earle, A. M., and Gilmore, J. P.: Changes in the sensitivity of left atrial receptors following reversal of heart failure. Am. J. Physiol. *237*:H555, 1979.
165. Riegger, G. A. J., Liebau, G., and Kocksiek, K.: Antidiuretic hormone in congestive heart failure. Am. J. Med. *72*:49, 1982.
166. Weber, K. T., and Janicki, J. S.: The heart as a muscle-pump system and the concept of heart failure. Am. Heart J. *98*:371, 1979.

14 ASSESSMENT OF CARDIAC FUNCTION

by Eugene Braunwald, M.D.

THEORETICAL CONSIDERATIONS

Assessment of cardiac function is a challenging and critically important task in the evaluation of patients with real or suspected heart disease. Since the heart's prime function is to deliver sufficient oxygenated blood to meet the metabolic requirements of the tissues, it is understandable that measurement of cardiac output has become a time-honored method for assessing cardiac performance and that therapeutic interventions in patients with heart disease are frequently evaluated in terms of their effects on cardiac output. Determination of cardiac output does indeed provide a useful measure of the pumping ability of the heart; however, we have seen from the discussion in Chapter 12 that cardiac output is dependent on two other influences in addition to contractility—preload and afterload.* Therefore, measurement of cardiac output alone is of limited value in the characterization of cardiac function.[1]

At any level of contractility, the extent of myocardial fiber shortening, and therefore the stroke volume, varies directly with the preload and inversely with the afterload.[2] When the latter is progressively raised, an increasing proportion of the muscle's contractile energy is expended in the generation of tension and a correspondingly smaller fraction in myocardial fiber shortening (Fig. 12–12, p. 420). For example, when aortic impedance† is progressively raised while ventricular end-diastolic volume is held constant, stroke volume declines until a level of impedance is reached at which the maximum force-generating capacity of the myocardium is exceeded, and ventricular ejection ceases, i.e., the contraction becomes isovolumetric. Conversely, when the aortic impedance falls (afterload is reduced), stroke volume rises. From these considerations, it is clear that when changes in afterload occur, reciprocal changes in cardiac output take place that need not reflect changes in myocardial contractility (Fig. 12–30, p. 436). For example, an increase in cardiac output in a patient with heart failure following relief of severe aortic stenosis or the successful treatment of hypertension may be due to reduction in afterload or an improvement in contractility or both. Similarly, the elevated cardiac output associated with severe anemia (low blood viscosity), fever (arteriolar dilatation), or patent ductus arteriosus (arteriovenous fistula) may be explained in part or entirely by a reduction in aortic impedance, which reduces afterload (Fig. 12–26, p. 432, and Fig. 24–1, p. 808); again, an augmentation of contractility such as occurs with stimulation of cardiac sympathetic nerves need not necessarily be invoked.

The effects of simple alterations of preload on cardiac output are even more widely appreciated. Thus, the depression of cardiac output that occurs with hypovolemia (e.g., hemorrhagic shock), displacement of blood from the thorax (e.g., positive-pressure ventilation), or cardiac compression (e.g., pericardial tamponade) may be explained solely by a reduction of preload (Fig. 12–28, p. 434, and Fig. 12–29, p. 435), and the elevation of cardiac output that occurs in some patients with polycythemia vera or acute glomerulonephritis does not reflect an augmentation of contractility but rather a higher preload resulting from the hypervolemia (p. 820).

When myocardial contractility is normal, cardiac output is dependent more upon peripheral factors and their influence on ventricular preload and afterload than on the exact level of myocardial contractility. For example, both

*Heart rate, the fourth determinant of cardiac performance (p. 438), is so easily measurable that it will not be considered further, although it is recognized that changes in heart rate per se affect myocardial contractility.

†Aortic impedance is defined as the sum of the external factors that oppose ventricular ejection. It is the ratio of pressure to flow in the aorta and is determined by the physical properties of blood and the vascular wall; it includes the viscosity and density of blood, the diameter of the aorta and the viscoelasticity of the aortic wall, and the reflected pressure and flow waves generated in distal parts of the arterial tree; aortic impedance is generally expressed as the sum of a series of sinusoidal functions of pressure and flow waves ("harmonics") superimposed on the mean pressure and flow.[3]

digitalis glycosides and paired electrical stimulation exert powerful inotropic influences yet do not raise cardiac output in normal human subjects or experimental animals. By contrast, in the presence of myocardial failure these stimuli significantly elevate cardiac output.[4]

The relation between a chain and its links may be a useful, though obviously oversimplified, analogy for explaining the relation between cardiac output and myocardial contractility; the total weight that the chain can support will increase only if its weakest link is strengthened. Thus, in a patient with heart failure and a depressed myocardium, stimulation of contractility, which may be thought of as strengthening the weakest link in the chain of factors controlling cardiac output, will elevate cardiac output. On the other hand, when one or both of the other links of the chain (i.e., preload and/or afterload) are limiting, it is not surprising that strengthening a link that is not weakest (i.e., improving myocardial contractility) does not improve cardiac output.

From the foregoing discussion, and as is evident from Figure 12–31 (p. 437), cardiac output can be lowered by reduction of contractility and preload, and by elevation of afterload—operating singly or in combination—and it is not possible to deduce from the measurement of a reduced cardiac output that contractility is depressed. Conversely, cardiac output may be normal when depression of contractility is accompanied by an augmented preload or a reduced afterload or both. Therefore, assessment of cardiac performance should include—but must not be limited to—measurement of cardiac output, i.e., it should also provide an analysis both of contractility and of the heart's loading conditions.

It is often desirable in the clinical care of patients with heart disease to ascertain the basal level of myocardial contractility and in other instances to determine the effects of therapeutic interventions, such as a drug or an operation, on contractility. In isolated cardiac muscle or in the isolated heart, the individual influence of each of the three major determinants of cardiac performance (preload, afterload, and contractility) can be analyzed by maintaining two of these three variables constant and determining the effects of changing the third on muscle or cardiac performance. However, it is far more difficult to make analogous measurements in patients with heart disease in whom preload or afterload, or both, may be abnormal and cannot be controlled or held constant. For example, it is often desirable to ascertain in a patient with valvular heart disease, ventricular hypertrophy, and symptoms of heart failure whether it is the abnormality in loading produced by the valvular lesion or a depression of myocardial contractility (or a combination of these two factors) that is responsible for the clinical manifestations. Similarly, it is frequently necessary to study the effects on myocardial contractility of a pharmacological agent that may also act on the arterial and venous beds and therefore may change preload and afterload. Such considerations have led to the search for methods of evaluating ventricular function that go beyond simple analysis of the pumping function of the ventricle and that are directed toward quantification of contractility. Although a number of indices of contractility have been proposed and investigated empirically, conclusions drawn about them have involved an element of circular reasoning, since, unfortunately, there is no *absolute* hemodynamic or mechanical measure of this property of the myocardium with which these indices can be compared.

The Frank-Starling Mechanism

The earliest efforts to separate loading conditions from contractility in assessing ventricular performance utilized the Frank-Starling relation, i.e., the relation between ventricular filling pressure or end-diastolic volume, on the one hand, and ventricular mechanical activity, as expressed in the pressure generated, the volume output, or the product of these two variables (i.e., stroke work), on the other. It was shown in the heart-lung preparation that the stroke volume is a function both of diastolic fiber length (i.e., of preload) and of contractility. The failing heart was found to deliver a smaller than normal stroke volume from a normal or elevated end-diastolic volume.[5] Later, Sarnoff and his collaborators examined ventricular stroke work over a range of mean atrial or ventricular end-diastolic pressures and termed the resulting relation "the ventricular function curve."[6] A family of such curves reflects a spectrum of contractile states, and the position of a given curve provides a description of ventricular contractility (Fig. 12–32, p. 438). Movement along a single curve (Fig. 12–29, p. 435) represents the operation of the "Frank-Starling principle," where stroke work or volume varies directly with changes in preload. By contrast, upward or

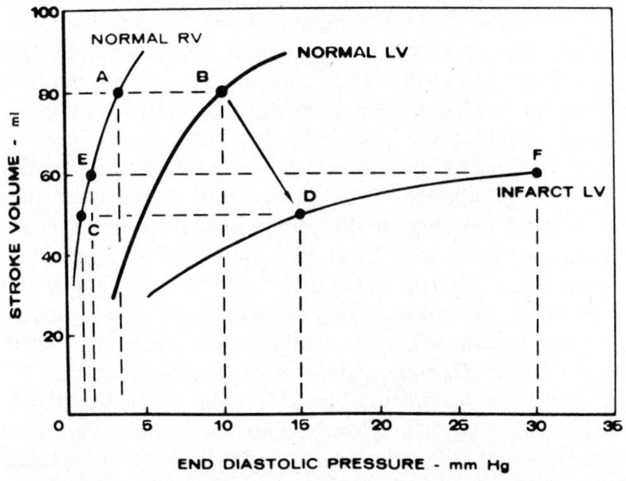

FIGURE 14–1 Schematic right ventricular (RV) and left ventricular (LV) function curves before and after left ventricular infarction. The normal RV function curve is to the left of the normal LV function curve, since, at any stroke volume, RV end-diastolic pressure is less than LV end-diastolic pressure. However, since the two ventricles have the same average stroke volume in a steady state, they operate on the same horizontal line. Under normal circumstances, the right ventricle would be at point A and the left ventricle at point B, both with a stroke volume of 80 ml. Following infarction, which predominantly affects the left ventricle, the LV curve is shifted down and to the right (point D), although the RV curve may not be initially affected. Stroke volume decreases to 50 ml, and the function of the right ventricle moves to point C. A volume load at this point might increase stroke volume to 60 ml, and the function of the right ventricle would move to point E, whereas that of the left ventricle would move to point F. At this high filling pressure, the patient might well go into pulmonary edema. (From Parmley, W. W.: Hemodynamic monitoring in acute ischemic disease. *In* Fishman, A. P. [ed.]: Heart Failure. New York, McGraw-Hill Book Co., 1978, p. 113.)

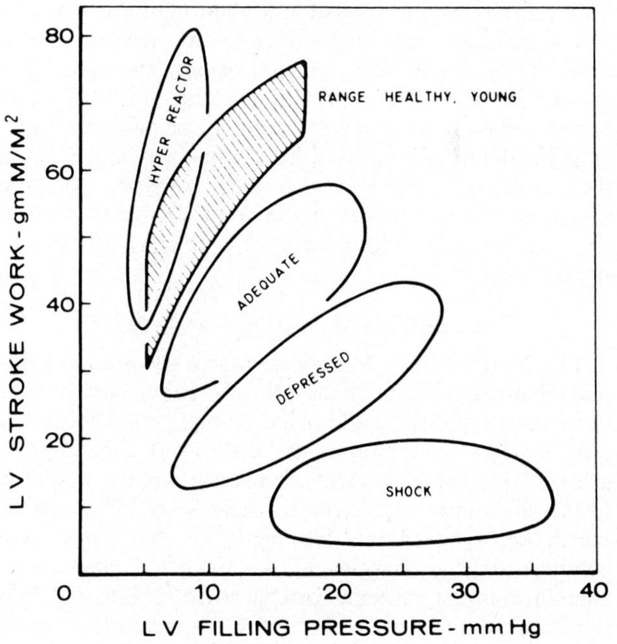

FIGURE 14–2 Hemodynamic consequences of myocardial infarction expressed as varying levels of left ventricular function. The cross-hatched area represents the range of left ventricular (LV) function in healthy, young individuals. Following acute myocardial infarction, there is wide variability in the hemodynamic response. Some patients with small infarcts and increased sympathetic tone may be in the normal or supernormal range. As the size of the infarct increases, however, function is progressively shifted down and to the right, so that all patients with cardiogenic shock fall in the lower right-hand group. (From Parmley, W. W.: Hemodynamic monitoring in acute ischemic disease. *In* Fishman, A. P. [ed.]: Heart Failure. New York, McGraw-Hill Book Co., 1978, p. 114.)

downward displacement of the *entire* curve (Fig. 12–32, p. 438) represents a positive or negative inotropic effect, i.e., an augmentation or depression of contractility, respectively (Figs. 14–1 and 14–2). In experimental animal preparations, ventricular function curves are usually recorded at a constant mean arterial pressure,[4] since the level of stroke work is pressure-dependent, just as the work of isolated muscle is afterload-dependent (Fig. 12–12, p. 420). Thus, at any level of contractility, stroke work is influenced also by the afterload, being low when outflow pressure is very low, increasing to a maximal level as pressure is raised, and again declining to zero when the afterload is so high as to prevent ventricular ejection (i.e., when ventricular contraction is isovolumetric and stroke volume is zero).[7] It should be recognized that even when outflow pressure is held constant, the standard ventricular function curve (Fig. 12–29, p. 435) represents a complex interaction of preload and afterload, since as preload is augmented and heart size increases, according to Laplace's law (p. 431), afterload rises at a constant aortic pressure.

ASSESSING CARDIAC PERFORMANCE BASED ON PRESSURES, FLOWS, VOLUMES, AND DIMENSIONS

Despite the theoretical limitations alluded to above, the simplest, most straightforward approaches for assessing resting levels of contractility and their changes are still based on measurements of intravascular and intracardiac pressures, stroke volume (or cardiac output), and ventricular volume and/or dimensions.

CARDIAC INDEX. The normal range for the cardiac index in the basal (resting) state and the supine position is wide—between 2.5 and 4.2 liters/min/square meter—making this variable a very *insensitive* assessment of cardiac function; it can be within normal limits, decline by almost 40 per cent as a consequence of myocardial failure, and still remain within these limits. Therefore, when the cardiac index falls below normal, it usually represents a gross disturbance in *circulatory,* though not necessarily *cardiac,* performance (p. 447), and such a degree of impairment is usually readily detectable clinically. Despite these limitations, measurement of cardiac index in the basal state is of value, since it provides an assessment of the heart's most critical function, i.e., the delivery of blood to the metabolizing tissues.

A measurement that detects milder degrees of cardiac impairment with greater sensitivity than does the measurement of cardiac output in the basal state is the level of cardiac output in response to the stress of exercise. Most commonly, the effect of exercise on cardiac output is determined in the cardiac catheterization laboratory as the patient pedals a stationary bicycle in the supine position, and both oxygen consumption and cardiac output are measured at rest and during exercise (p. 294). The increase in cardiac output is a function not only of the heart's pumping capacity but also of the severity of exercise, which can be expressed by the patient's total oxygen consumption. The increase in cardiac output normally exceeds 6 ml/min for each ml increase in oxygen consumption per minute.

INTRACARDIAC PRESSURES. The accuracy of the assessment of cardiac performance can be increased by adding a measurement of ventricular filling pressure* to that of cardiac (or stroke) index. In the basal state, when the ventricular end-diastolic pressure is abnormally elevated *and* cardiac performance (expressed as cardiac [or stroke] index or work) is depressed, myocardial contractility is *probably* impaired. However, elevation of ventricular filling pressure does not necessarily indicate an elevation of end-diastolic volume, since ventricular compliance may be reduced (Fig. 12–22, p. 428). Such a reduction of compliance may be caused, for example, by pericardial disease, by restrictive endocardial or myocardial disease, by cardiac hypertrophy, or by myocardial ischemia; it can elevate the ventricular filling pressure while end-diastolic volume remains normal.

Despite the problems mentioned above, the combination of ventricular end-diastolic pressure and cardiac output or work is often helpful (Figs. 14–1 and 14–2). For example,

*Ventricular filling pressure refers to ventricular end-diastolic pressure, or an index thereof; in the absence of disease of the atrioventricular valve, this is reflected in the mean atrial or, preferably, the mean diastolic atrial pressure or the atrial pressure at the *z* point, i.e., at the time of onset of ventricular contraction. In the case of the left ventricle, the mean pulmonary capillary wedge pressure or, in the case of the right ventricle, the central venous pressure provides a reasonably accurate approximation of ventricular end-diastolic pressure, except when there is a tall *a* wave in the ventricular pressure pulse, in which case the end-diastolic ventricular pressure exceeds the mean atrial pressure, or when there is a tall *v* wave, in which case the mean atrial pressure exceeds the end-diastolic ventricular pressure.

the finding of the combination of a normal cardiac index (>2.5 $l/min/m^2$) and ventricular filling pressure (<12 mm Hg) is a more accurate indicator of normal contractility than is either measurement alone. However, a further obvious limitation of this combination of measurements emerges when cardiac output (or work) is depressed while filling pressure is within the normal range (6 to 12 mm Hg) or low (<6 mm Hg); such findings could reflect a depression of contractility and/or a reduction of preload in the presence of normal contractility.

One approach to overcome the problems described above is to measure cardiac performance (cardiac or stroke index or work) both in the basal state and after preload has been raised by increasing intravascular volume. Normally, an elevation of preload is accompanied by a clear-cut increase in cardiac output. In addition, the effects of an intervention on the slope of the relation between filling pressure and cardiac work can be evaluated. For example, as shown in Figure 14–3, in a patient recovering from myocardial infarction, cessation of the infusion of glucose-insulin-potassium depressed the ventricular function curve.[8]

From the foregoing consideration of the importance of ventricular compliance, measurement of ventricular end-diastolic volume obviously is superior to that of filling pressure in the assessment of left ventricular preload (end-diastolic fiber stretch). Angiographic techniques, described below, provide the most widely accepted means for measuring ventricular cavity volumes as well as wall thickness and thereby allow calculation of the extent and velocity of

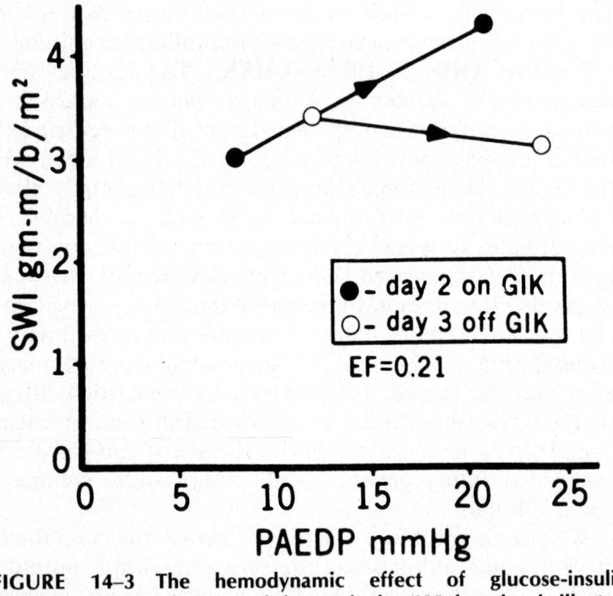

FIGURE 14–3 The hemodynamic effect of glucose-insulin-potassium (GIK) solution on left ventricular (LV) function is illustrated by the slope of the ventricular function curve in a patient with acute myocardial infarction. After the patient had been on the GIK solution for 2 days, the slope of the function curve was steeper than on day 3, 24 hours after the GIK solution had been discontinued. These changes indicate the positive inotropic effect of the metabolic solution on the viable and/or marginally ischemic myocardium surrounding the infarction site. Ventricular function is expressed as the relation between pulmonary artery end-diastolic pressure (PAEDP), reflecting left ventricular filling pressure and left ventricular stroke work index (SWI). (Reproduced with permission from Rackley, C. E., Russell, R. O., Jr., Rogers, W. J., et al.: Clinical experience with glucose-insulin-potassium therapy in acute myocardial infarction. Am. Heart J. *102*:1038, 1981.)

wall shortening and of regional abnormalities of wall motion and, when combined with pressure measurements, estimation of ventricular compliance and the forces acting within the wall that oppose shortening. Such calculations permit left ventricular performance to be analyzed in terms used for describing isolated heart muscle (Chap. 12); when the results are expressed in units corrected for muscle length or circumferences of the ventricle, comparisons can be made between individuals with widely differing heart sizes.

Quantitative Angiocardiography

TECHNIQUES. Measurements of the volumes of cardiac chambers can be made utilizing either large, cut films or cineangiograms (single plane or biplane).[9] Cineangiography, which is emerging as the method of choice, provides a larger number of sequential observations per unit of time (30 to 60 frames per second), whereas the large, cut films, which are exposed less frequently (6 to 12 per second), produce sharper margins of the opacified chambers. Although contrast material can be injected into the pulmonary artery and left atrium, the left ventricle is outlined more clearly by means of direct injection into its cavity; therefore, this latter mode is used in most patients, except in those with severe aortic regurgitation, in whom the contrast material may be injected into the aorta, with the resultant reflux outlining the left ventricular cavity. Digital subtraction augiography utilizing peripheral vein injections may also be employed.[9a,9b]

Unless the effects of premature contractions and of the resultant postextrasystolic potentiation are to be examined specifically,[10] ventricular irritability should be avoided during injection by assuring that the tip of the catheter is not in contact with the myocardium and that a multiholed catheter is used to diminish the impact of the jet of contrast agent striking the endocardium. If premature contractions are induced, the results are subject to serious misinterpretation, since the premature contraction itself and the first and second postpremature beats may result in marked changes in cardiac function. However, since the contrast material is usually injected within 2 to 3 seconds and filming is carried out within 5 to 8 seconds, one to two cycles are usually available for analysis even if a single premature contraction occurs at the beginning of the injection. Injection of the contrast agent does not begin to produce hemodynamic changes (except for premature beats) until approximately the sixth beat post injection.[11] Moreover, the hyperosmolarity produced by the contrast agent increases the blood volume, which begins to raise preload and heart rate within 30 seconds of the injection, an effect which may persist for as long as 2 hours. Accordingly, when multiple observations in a comparable state are desired, it is essential to monitor hemodynamics to assure that they have returned to control levels before the angiogram is repeated. Ordinarily, the exposure of each pair of angiographic films or cineangiographic frames is recorded on a multichannel recorder and related to a simultaneously recorded electrocardiogram and to intracardiac pressure.

In calculating ventricular volume or, for that matter, ventricular dimension, from radiographs, it is essential to take into account and apply appropriate correction factors for magnification as well as for distortion resulting from nonparallel x-ray beams.[12–14] In order to apply these correction factors, care must be exercised to determine the tube-to-patient and tube-to-film distances with great accuracy. With cine technique, correction is best accomplished by filming a calibrated grid at the position of the ventricle.[15]

NONINVASIVE METHODS FOR ASSESSING CARDIAC PERFORMANCE

Cardiac catheterization and quantitative angiography are the standard tools for evaluating the function and contractility of the heart, but these invasive procedures are not free of risk or discomfort, and they are not suitable for multiple application in the same patient. Therefore, as has already been pointed out, there has been a continuing search for reliable noninvasive methods of assessing cardiac performance. Such methods are particularly needed in detecting serial changes in cardiac function with time and in evaluating both acute and chronic effects of drug therapy and cardiac operations. Discussed elsewhere are the three principal noninvasive methods for assessing cardiac performance: systolic time intervals (p. 55), M-mode and cross-sectional echocardiography[15a] (p. 102), and radionuclide angiography (p. 357). The last two techniques are alternatives to contrast angiography for measurement of ventricular volume and/or dimensions, and both allow the noninvasive estimation of ejection phase indices. Afterload can be estimated from systemic arterial pressure and ventricular wall thickness in patients other than those with aortic stenosis; wall thickness can be determined by echocardiography.

Mean velocity of circumferential fiber shortening (V_{CF}) can be simply determined from echocardiographic measurements of end-diastolic and end-systolic dimensions. Since the ventricle is approximately circular at its minor axis, the circumference is equal to $\pi \cdot D$. Mean V_{CF} is therefore the difference between end-diastolic and end-systolic circumference (in centimeters) divided by the product of the duration of ejection (in seconds) and the end-diastolic circumference (in centimeters). Values of V_{CF} obtained by echocardiography compare closely with those determined from cineangiograms.[16]

Prolongation of the preejection period (PEP) and shortening of the left ventricular ejection time (LVET) reflect reduced left ventricular dP/dt and stroke volume, respectively, and there is an empirical inverse correlation between the ratio PEP/LVET (which is elevated in left ventricular dysfunction) and ejection fraction (EF).[17]

LEFT VENTRICULAR VOLUME. The area-length method developed by Dodge is still the most useful for calculating left ventricular volume[12,18] (Fig. 14–4). The longest length of the ventricular chamber, i.e., from the apex to the root of the aortic valve, is measured directly, and the diameter of the ventricle is calculated from the formula $D = 4A/\pi L$, where D = calculated diameter in centimeters; L = length in centimeters; and A = area of left ventricular cavity in square centimeters determined by planimetry. Ordinarily this calculation is made for films exposed in both anteroposterior (AP) and lateral projections. The shape of the left ventricle usually resembles a prolate ellipsoid, with one major and two minor diameters.[12,19,20] With this assumption, left ventricular volume is calculated from the formula

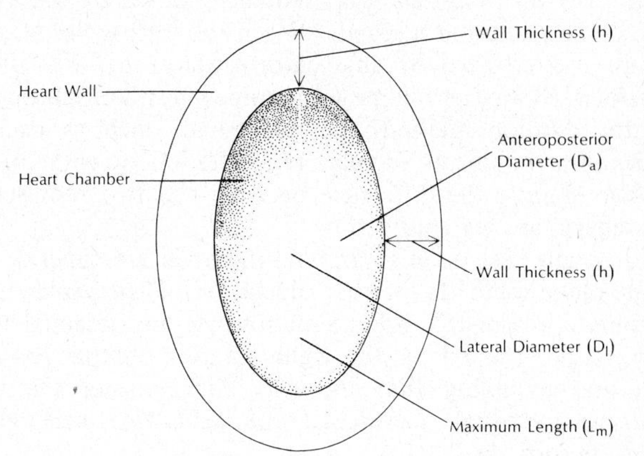

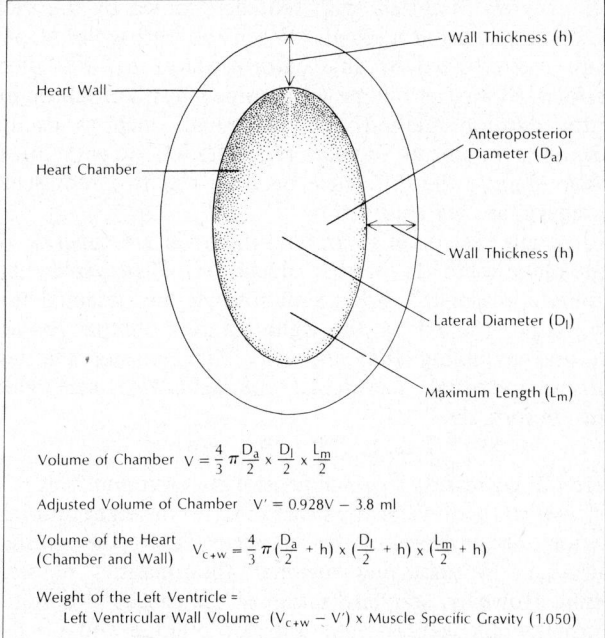

Volume of Chamber $V = \frac{4}{3}\pi \frac{D_a}{2} \times \frac{D_l}{2} \times \frac{L_m}{2}$

Adjusted Volume of Chamber $V' = 0.928V - 3.8$ ml

Volume of the Heart (Chamber and Wall) $V_{C+W} = \frac{4}{3}\pi (\frac{D_a}{2} + h) \times (\frac{D_l}{2} + h) \times (\frac{L_m}{2} + h)$

Weight of the Left Ventricle =
Left Ventricular Wall Volume $(V_{C+W} - V') \times$ Muscle Specific Gravity (1.050)

FIGURE 14–4 Diagram illustrating the approach used to calculate left ventricular volume by means of quantitative angiocardiography. Margins of the projected image of the left ventricular chamber are traced, and maximum length is measured in the anteroposterior and lateral views. Minor axes are derived from the planimetered areas of the chamber in both views; all dimensions are corrected to allow for distortion due to nonparallel x-rays. Left ventricular volumes are calculated using the formula for the volume of an ellipsoid, since (with regression-equation adjustment) this has given results that tally closely with directly measured ventricular volume. To determine left ventricular mass, volume of the ventricular chamber is subtracted from volume of chamber plus wall; multiplying wall volume by the specific gravity of cardiac muscle converts volume to heart weight or mass. (From Dodge, H. T.: Hemodynamic aspects of cardiac failure. *In* Braunwald, E. [ed.]: The Myocardium: Failure and Infarction. New York, HP Publishing Co., 1974, p. 70.)

$$V = 4/3\pi\,(L/2) \cdot (D_{AP}/2) \cdot (D_{lat}/2)$$

where V = volume in milliliters; L = longest length in centimeters in the AP or lateral projection; and D_{AP} and D_{lat} = the diameters (minor axes) in centimeters calculated from the AP and lateral projection angiocardiograms, respectively. These diameters, in turn, are calculated from the formula for the area of an ellipse (A) as follows:

$$D = \frac{4A}{\pi L}$$

A, the area of the opacified ventricle, can be conveniently determined by a hand or electronic planimeter and an X-Y platter.[15] *Actual* ventricular volume is determined from the calculated volume using the aforementioned correction factors and a regression formula that takes into account the volume occupied by the papillary muscles and chordae tendineae within the ventricular chamber (see adjusted volume, Fig. 14–4). Studies based on human autopsy specimens as well as on models and casts thereof have proved the accuracy of this approach.[9]

Left ventricular stroke volume is calculated as the difference between end-systolic and end-diastolic volumes. An important validation of the angiographic method for measuring ventricular volume has been provided by the observation that the stroke volume, calculated by angiocardiography, correlates closely with that determined by the Fick or indicator dilution method.[21] When the ventricular stroke volume (determined by angiocardiography) and the effective forward stroke volume (determined by the Fick or indicator dilution method) are not equal, such as occurs with aortic or mitral valvular regurgitation or with intracardiac shunts, the difference between the two represents the regurgitant (or shunt) flow.

Although biplane angiographic methods are superior to single-plane methods for the calculation of left ventricular volume, a reasonable approximation can be obtained utilizing either the AP or the right anterior oblique projection and assuming that the two diameters of the left ventricle are equal. Ventricular volume is then calculated from the formula

$$V = L \cdot D^2 \cdot CF^3 \cdot \pi/6$$

where CF represents a one-dimensional correction factor.[9]

In patients with ischemic heart disease, the right and left anterior oblique views of the left ventricle are the optimal projections for assessing regional abnormalities of wall motion. However, standardization of the degree of obliquity, usually 30 degrees right anterior oblique and 60 degrees left anterior oblique, is required for application of any particular correction factor in the calculation of ventricular volume. A close correlation has been found between left ventricular volume determined in the right anterior oblique view and true cardiac volume; however, the overestimation of true volume is greater than that using the biplane oblique volume method, and appropriate corrections must be made.[22]

Just as the prolate ellipsoid provides a frame of reference for the shape of the left ventricle, the right ventricle is shaped like a pyramid with a triangular base, and the formula for deriving the volume of this geometrical figure should be employed in the calculation of right ventricular volume.[23] The atria resemble ellipsoids, and their volumes can be determined using the area-length method.[24]

LEFT VENTRICULAR MASS. This value can also be determined by angiocardiography. Wall thickness, as visualized and measured along the free lateral wall of the left ventricle just below the equator during diastole (best measured on the AP or RAO angiogram), is added to the major and minor semiaxes to compute the volume of the chamber plus wall. This volume minus the chamber volume equals wall volume. The product of wall volume and the specific gravity of heart muscle (1.050) equals left ventricular mass.[25] Thus, left ventricular mass (M) in grams can be calculated from the formula

$$M = ([4/3 \cdot \pi \frac{(L + 2h)}{2} \cdot \frac{(D_{AP} + 2h)}{2} \cdot \frac{(D_{lat} + 2h)}{2}] - V) \cdot (1.050)$$

where h = left ventricular wall thickness in centimeters; 1.050 = specific gravity of heart muscle; D_{AP} and D_{lat} are the ventricular diameters in centimeters in the AP and lateral views, respectively; and V = left ventricular volume in cubic centimeters. A major assumption made with this method and one that undoubtedly introduces some inaccuracy is that left ventricular wall thickness is uniform around the entire left ventricular cavity. However, this method has been validated by postmortem studies comparing actual and calculated left ventricular weights.[15]

LEFT VENTRICULAR FORCES. The *forces* acting within the ventricular wall can be calculated from knowledge of the dimensions of the left ventricular cavity, wall thickness, and pressure.[26] *Tension* (force/cm), which, according to Laplace's law, is a product of the intraventricular pressure and radius (p. 431), may be defined as the force acting on a hypothetical slit in the ventricular wall that would tend to pull its edges apart. *Wall stress* is the force or tension (in dynes) per unit of cross-sectional area of the ventricular wall (in square centimeters). From a clinical viewpoint, the most useful calculation is *circumferential wall stress,* which is the largest force generated and supported within the ventricular wall at the equator

$$CWS = \frac{(P \cdot b)}{h} (1 - b^2/2a^2 - h/2b + h^2/8a^2)$$

where CWS = circumferential wall stress in dynes/square centimeters × 10^3; P = left ventricular pressure in dynes/square centimeters; and a and b are the major and minor semiaxes (i.e., half the longest lengths), respectively, in centimeters and h = left ventricular wall thickness in centimeters.[27]

Simultaneous recording of a biplane angiogram and intraventricular pressure pulse (recorded preferably with a high-fidelity micromanometer to avoid the artifacts inherent in the usual catheter–external manometer systems) allows calculation of *left ventricular tension* and *stress* throughout the cardiac cycle. Another method of analyzing the instantaneous force-velocity-length relations of the left ventricle consists of recording left ventricular pressure simultaneously with left ventricular diameter across the minor axis of the left ventricle recorded by means of an M-mode echocardiogram[27a]* (Fig. 5–16, p. 98). This combination of measurements provides all the data necessary to calculate ventricular circumferential fiber shortening, at either the endocardium or the midwall, and midwall circumferential stress, using minor modifications of the equations presented above.[28]

Ventricular *preload* may be expressed as end-diastolic wall stress and *afterload* as peak or mean systolic wall stress. During ejection, as the left ventricular cavity decreases in size and wall thickness increases, systolic wall stress (and tension) declines rapidly even though pressure is maintained (Fig. 14–5). *Left ventricular power* can be calculated as the product of intracavitary pressure and the rate of change of ventricular volume. Simultaneously recorded ventricular volumes and pressures during diastole allow the calculation of *left ventricular chamber and muscle compliance*[29] (Fig. 12–22, p. 428).

VENTRICULAR WALL MOTION. Quantitative angiography also permits study of ventricular wall motion. The most gross focal abnormalities of the extent of contraction can be appreciated by visual inspection of cineventriculograms. Segments of abnormal ventricular contraction can be localized by superimposing end-diastolic and

*However, use of M-mode echocardiography is based on the assumption of uniform wall motion; this assumption can be made with reasonable assurance in conditions that affect left ventricular function uniformly, such as dilated cardiomyopathy, or aortic regurgitation, but is not warranted in conditions that produce localized or regional dysfunction, such as coronary artery disease.

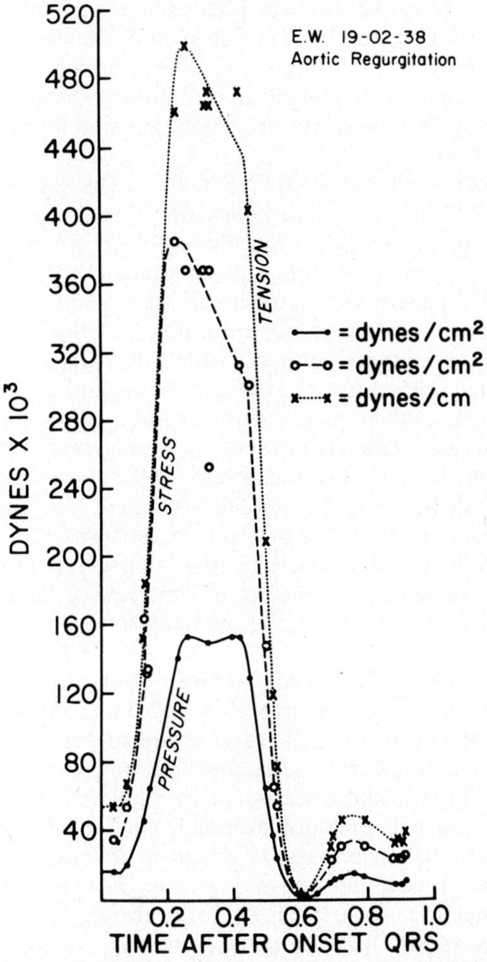

FIGURE 14–5 Sequential changes in left ventricular tension, stress, and pressure are illustrated throughout the cardiac cycle in a patient with aortic regurgitation. Note that tension, but particularly stress, declines during ejection (i.e., while the left ventricular volume decreases), although left ventricular pressure is maintained. (From Rackley, C. E.: Quantitative evaluation of left ventricular function by radiographic techniques. Circulation *54*:862, 1976, by permission of the American Heart Association, Inc.)

end-systolic outlines of the left ventricular cavity and tracing both the central x-ray beam and the cavity silhouette on paper or by using a computer (Fig. 10–48, p. 339).[30] *Akinesis* is present when a portion of each of the two silhouettes shares a common line; *dyskinesis* is present when the end-systolic silhouette extends outside the end-diastolic silhouette. The abnormally contracting segments (both akinetic and dyskinetic) are expressed as percentages of the total end-diastolic circumference (Fig. 14–6). *Hypokinesis* (focal decreases in the extent of contraction) as well as *asynchrony* (abnormalities of timing of contraction) are less severe disturbances of contraction. High filming rates, with analysis of wall motion from multiple cine frames, and the use of computer techniques to assist in data reduction and analysis are necessary for the detection of these more subtle abnormalities.[31] By use of such techniques, it is apparent that focal hypokinesis that cannot readily be detected by visual inspection of cineangiograms is a common disturbance and that abnormalities of timing of segmental wall motion are nearly as common as abnormalities of the extent of contraction. Focal hypokinesis is often associated with hyperkinesis of other wall regions, presumably as a compensatory mechanism.[25,31] Two-dimensional echocardiography[32,33] (p. 102) and radionuclide angiography (p. 357) have provided useful approaches for assessing wall motion noninvasively.

Applications

VENTRICULAR VOLUME. The normal left ventricular end-diastolic volume averages 70 ± 20 (SD) ml/square meter.[15,25] When ventricular end-diastolic volume is clearly elevated (i.e., >108 ml/square meter, or >2 SD's above the normal average) and *total* stroke volume and/or cardiac index and work are either reduced or within normal limits, while heart rate and afterload are normal, cardiac contractility is depressed.

EJECTION FRACTION. The ratio of stroke volume to end-diastolic volume, the ejection fraction (EF), is a

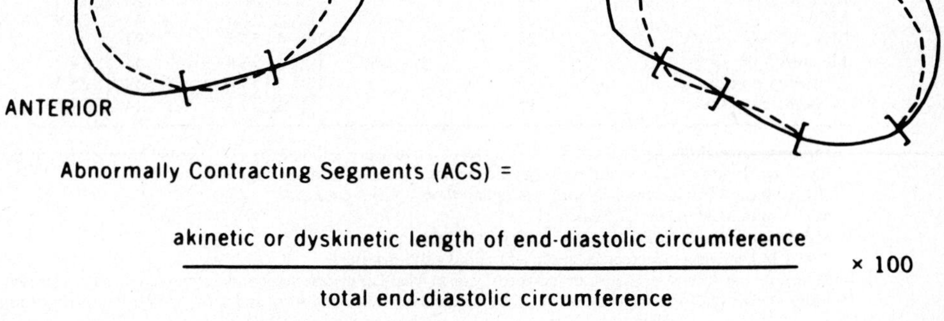

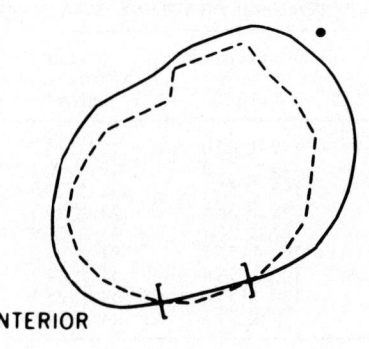

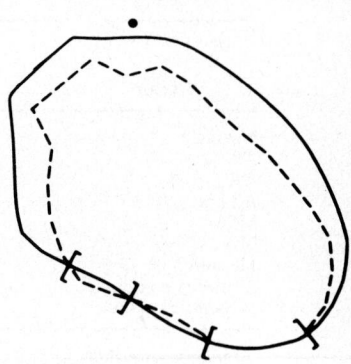

$$\text{Abnormally Contracting Segments (ACS)} = \frac{\text{akinetic or dyskinetic length of end-diastolic circumference}}{\text{total end-diastolic circumference}} \times 100$$

FIGURE 14–6 Systolic (dashed) and diastolic (solid) lateral and anteroposterior (AP) angiocardiograms are superimposed with a central lead marker as a reference point. The abnormally contracting segments are enclosed by brackets on the diastolic silhouette. (From Rackley, C. E.: Quantitative evaluation of left ventricular function by radiographic techniques. Circulation *54*:862, 1976, by permission of the American Heart Association, Inc.)

global index of the extent of ventricular fiber shortening and has been considered, on the basis of a number of empirical studies, to provide one of the most useful measures of left ventricular pump function. EF averages 0.67 ± 0.08 (SD) in normal subjects[15,25] and ranges from 0.45 to 0.70 in experimental animals, depending on the heart rate, the method used to measure cardiac volume, and whether the animal is anesthetized or awake.[34] EF is closely related to and can be predicted accurately from the percentage of shortening during systole of left ventricular minor axis dimension, and this provides the basis for assessing ejection fraction by echocardiography (p. 103).[35,36] Most commonly, the diameter perpendicular to the midpoint of the long axis is used, and its fractional shortening (FS) is calculated as follows

$$FS = \frac{\text{(Left ventricular) end-diastolic dimension} - \text{End-systolic dimension}}{\text{End-diastolic dimension}}$$

and is expressed as a percentage.

In addition to myocardial contractility, both preload and afterload affect EF, FS, and the mean velocity of circumferential fiber shortening (V_{CF}). The last-named, expressed in circumferences per second, is calculated as the quotient of circumferential fiber shortening during ejection (in circumferences) and ejection time (in seconds). The lower limit of normal for mean V_{CF} is 1.1 circumferences per second.[37] Studies in conscious or lightly sedated baboons[38] and conscious human subjects[39] have shown that moderate changes in preload have little effect on mean or maximum velocity of fiber shortening. However, when end-diastolic volume (preload) is acutely reduced or aortic pressure (afterload) is acutely elevated or both, the so-called *ejection phase indices of ventricular performance* (i.e., EF, FS, and mean and peak V_{CF}) all decline (Fig. 12–28, p. 434). Conversely, the ejection phase indices may be normal in conditions in which afterload is reduced, such as mitral regurgitation, even when contractility is depressed (p. 1079). These findings suggest that *changes* in EF, FS, and V_{CF}, like changes in stroke volume, do not simply reflect variations in contractility. However, as will be pointed out below, the ejection phase indices are often useful for determining the level of contractility in the basal state in the presence of chronic heart disease, in which the influence of changes in preload and afterload tends to be corrected for by compensatory dilatation and hypertrophy[40] (Table 14–1).

VENTRICULAR DIMENSIONS. The extent and velocity of ventricular wall shortening during ejection have been employed to determine the effects of a variety of interventions on contractility using implanted ultrasonic dimension gauges in conscious dogs and primates[35] and by cineradiographic recording of the motion of radiopaque markers sutured to the epicardium at the time of cardiac operations in patients.[41] Mean and peak V_{CF} can be used to evaluate acute inotropic interventions provided that afterload remains constant or almost so.[42] V_{CF} probably shows little change fortuitously during acute elevations in preload alone had afterload remained constant.[35,36,43,44] The mean and peak V_{CF} incorporate the important element of the velocity of myocardial fiber shortening and appear to be more sensitive measures of contractility than EF and FS, which simply reflect the pumping function of the ventricle.

LEFT VENTRICULAR MASS. Left ventricular wall thickness normally averages 10.9 ± 2.0 mm (SD)[15] and left ventricular mass 92 ± 16 gm/square meter body surface area.[9,24] Chronic cardiac dilatation secondary to valvular or primary myocardial disease increases left ventricular mass, as does chronic pressure overload. Characteristically, hypertrophy due to pressure overload is characterized by an increased muscle mass resulting from an augmentation of wall thickness with, at first, little change in ventricular chamber volume (concentric hypertrophy); in contrast, hypertrophy due to volume overload of myocardial disease is characterized by an increased muscle mass resulting from ventricular dilatation, with a slight increase in wall thickness (eccentric hypertrophy [Fig. 13–7, p. 452). There is often a correlation between stroke work of the left ventricle and left ventricular mass in chronic valvular heart disease, but no such relation exists in primary myocardial disease[24] (Table 14–1).

TABLE 14–1 LEFT VENTRICULAR VOLUME DATA IN PATIENTS

Group	Number of Patients	End-diastolic volume (ml/m^2)	Stroke Volume (ml/m^2)	Mass (gm/m^2)	Ejection Fraction
Normal*	–	70 ± 20.0	45 ± 13.0	92 ± 16.0	0.67 ± 0.08
AS	14	84 ± 22.9	44 ± 10.1	172 ± 32.7	0.56 ± 0.17
AR	22	193 ± 55.4	92 ± 30.9	223 ± 73.0	0.56 ± 0.13
AS and AR	13	138 ± 36.5	75 ± 19.1	231 ± 56.9	0.53 ± 0.10
MS	37	83 ± 21.2	43 ± 11.9	98 ± 24.1	0.57 ± 0.14
MR	29	160 ± 53.1	87 ± 21.3	166 ± 49.9	0.47 ± 0.10
MS and MR	29	106 ± 34.4	58 ± 14.7	119 ± 27.8	0.57 ± 0.12
A and M combined	45	130 ± 55.8	69 ± 25.5	156 ± 55.9	0.55 ± 0.12
Myocardial disease	15	199 ± 75.7	44 ± 14.5	145 ± 27.6	0.25 ± 0.09

*Normal values from Kennedy, J. W., et al.: Quantitative angiocardiography. The normal left ventricle in man. Circulation *34*:272, 1966.
AS = aortic valve stenosis with peak systolic pressure gradient > 30 mm Hg.
AR = aortic valve insufficiency with regurgitant flow > 30 ml per beat.
MS = mitral valve area < 1.5 sq cm.
MR = mitral valve regurgitant flow > 20 ml per beat.
A and M combined = combined aortic and mitral valve disease.
Myocardial disease = primary cardiomyopathy or myocardial disease secondary to coronary atherosclerosis.
From Dodge, H. T., and Baxley, W. A.: Left ventricular volume and mass and their significance in heart disease. Am. J. Cardiol. *23*:528, 1969.

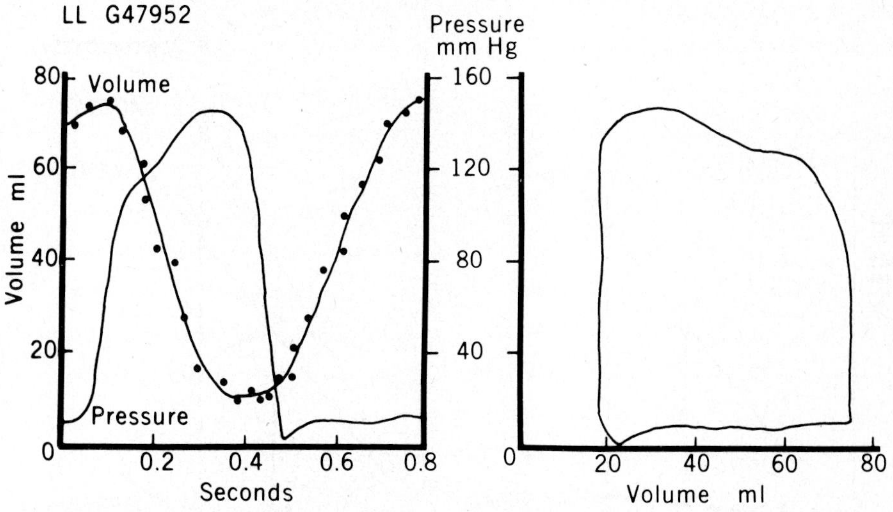

FIGURE 14–7 Volume and pressure changes obtained from a patient with a normal left ventricle are displayed on the left, timed with respect to onset of the QRS complex in the electrocardiogram. On the right, pressure and volume are related to construct a pressure-volume loop. (From Grossman, W. [ed.]: Cardiac Catheterization and Angiography. 2nd ed. Philadelphia, Lea and Febiger, 1980.)

THE PRESSURE-VOLUME LOOP. When ventricular pressure and volume are related to each other over an entire cardiac cycle, a pressure-volume loop can be constructed (Fig. 14–7). The timing of valve opening and closing can be indicated on such a loop; the height and width of the loop are determined by the systolic pressure and stroke volume, respectively.[25] The area subtended by the systolic portion of the curve provides a measure of stroke work performed by the left ventricle during systole, whereas the area subtended by the diastolic limb provides a measure of diastolic work performed *on* the left ventricle in distending it during diastole. Net work is the difference between the two. Diastolic work may be thought of as the energy supplied to the ventricle required for "priming the pump." In the absence of valvular regurgitation, diastolic work is largely generated by the left atrium and right ventricle, and its elevation is the physiological basis, at least in part, for the right ventricular failure observed in patients with left ventricular failure and secondary pulmonary hypertension.[25] With left ventricular failure and a rise in left ventricular diastolic pressure, there is an increase in diastolic work relative to systolic work and thus a decrease in net work. Characteristic changes in the left ventricular pressure-volume loops occur in various disease states (Fig. 14–8 and Table 14–1).

VENTRICULAR END-SYSTOLIC PRESSURE-VOLUME RELATIONS. The extent of myocardial fiber shortening reflects the interaction of preload, afterload, and contractility. As afterload increases, the extent of systolic fiber shortening declines (Fig. 12–30, p. 436, and Fig. 24–3, p. 808) resulting in progressively greater end-systolic fiber lengths[45–48] (Fig. 12–26, p. 432). Thus, end-systolic fiber length is a direct function of afterload (Fig. 14–9). Myocardial contractility can be evaluated by making use of this fundamental property of heart muscle and focusing attention on the relation of the residual volume, i.e., the volume of blood remaining in the ventricle at the end of systole, and the ventricular pressure at that instant. At any level of contractility the end-systolic volume to which a ventricle contracts is a linearly increasing function of end-systolic ventricular pressure. End-systolic volume varies inversely and end-systolic pressures vary directly with contractility (Fig. 14–9). There is little difference between the end-systolic pressure-volume relation in isovolumetric and ejecting contractions. Indeed, the virtual identity of isometric and

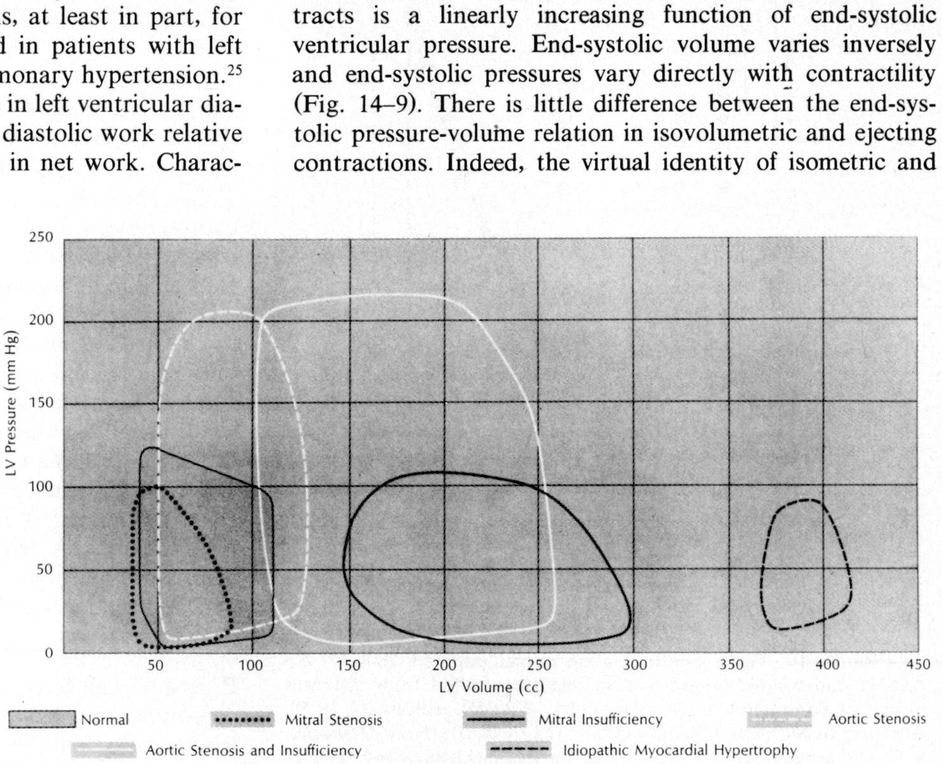

FIGURE 14–8 Left ventricular pressure-volume curves from patients with different varieties of heart disease. The height of each curve is determined by systolic pressure and the width by stroke volume. The two smallest curves—one from a patient with mitral stenosis, the other from a patient with primary cardiomyopathy—indicate similar stroke volumes; however, in the latter, the dilated left ventricle is functioning at an inappropriately large volume, and the ejection fraction is low. The curve in mitral insufficiency demonstrates volume overload by the large excursion along the volume axis and the absence of an isovolumetric contraction period. The shape of the curve in aortic stenosis shows the effect of pressure overload. In aortic stenosis and insufficiency the curve demonstrates the influence of pressure and volume overload, with the large area subtended by the curve. (From Dodge, H. T.: Hemodynamic aspects of cardiac failure. *In* Braunwald, E. [ed.]: The Myocardium: Failure and Infarction. New York, HP Publishing Co., 1974, p. 70.)

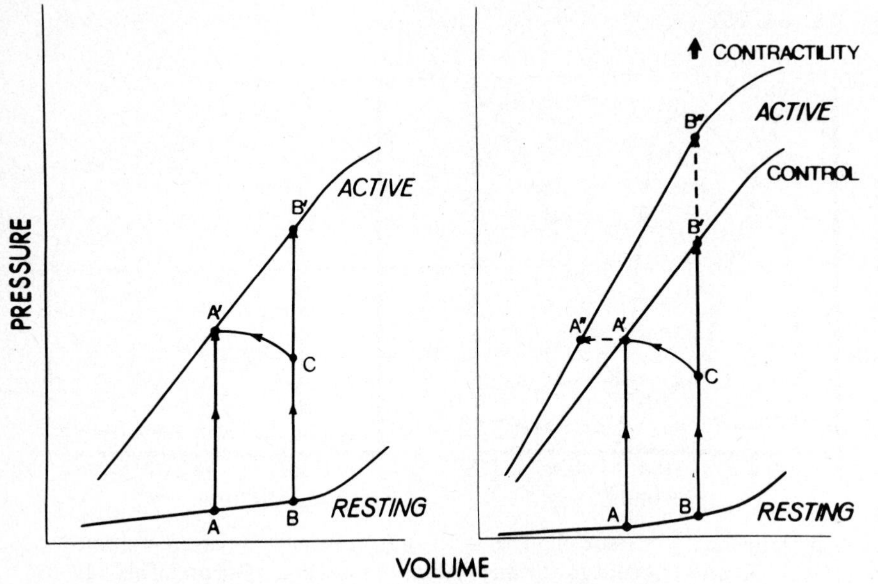

FIGURE 14–9 Schematic representation of the theoretical relationship of ventricular preload, afterload, and contractility for isovolumetric and ejecting beats. *Left,* Isovolumetric (A → A′, B → B′) and ejecting (B → C → A′) pathways illustrate the identity of isovolumetric and ejecting end-systolic pressure-volume relations. *Right,* The effect of increased myocardial contractility is to produce a higher pressure in isovolumetric beats (B′ → B″) and a smaller end-systolic volume in ejecting beats (B → C → A′ → A″). Note that end-systolic volume at the higher contractile state (A″) is independent of end-diastolic volume or preload, in that it is the final volume for ejecting beats originating from both the higher (B → C → A′ → A″) and lower (A → A′ → A″) preloads. (From Grossman, W., Braunwald, E., Mann, T., McLaurin, L. P., and Green, L. H.: Contractile state of the left ventricle in man as evaluated from end-systolic pressure-volume relations. Circulation *56*:845, 1977, by permission of the American Heart Association, Inc.)

isotonic length-tension curves has been demonstrated in isolated cat papillary muscle[49,50] (Fig. 14–10) and in the intact heart[51–55] (Fig. 14–11). Figure 14–11*B* shows the pressure-volume diagrams from a left ventricle connected to a pump system, which allowed the ventricle to eject the fluid at any desired afterload.[54] The large dots, which represent the peak pressures that this ventricle reached in isovolumetric contractions, lie very close to the solid lines, which connect the end-systolic pressure-volume relations of ejecting beats. Figure 14–11*C* shows pressure-volume

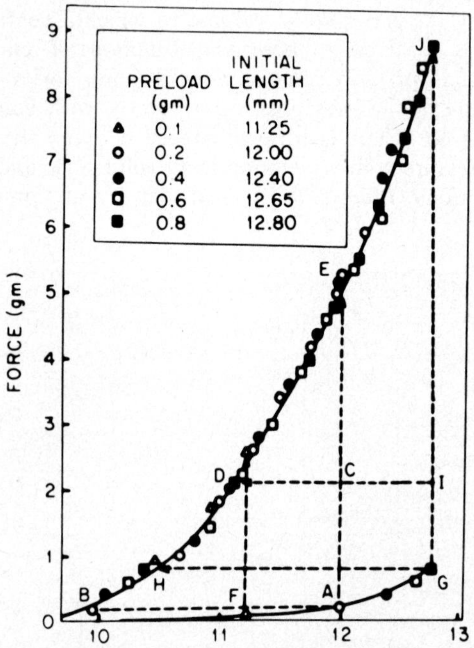

FIGURE 14–10 Force-length relation in cat papillary muscle. No distinct end-systolic length-tension relation resulted from different modes of contraction, such as isometric (F to D), isotonic (A to B), and afterloaded isotonic contractions (G to I to D). (From Downing, S. E., and Sonnenblick, E. H.: Cardiac muscle mechanics and ventricular performance. Force and time parameters. Am. J. Physiol. *207*: 705, 1964.)

loops from a left ventricle that ejected blood from different end-diastolic volumes but at identical systolic pressures. The end-systolic pressure-volume relations are identical. When the ventricle contracted at different afterloads,[51,52] the left ventricular end-systolic pressure-volume relations again formed a straight line. Figure 14–11*D* shows the effects of decreasing venous return; there was a progressive reduction in end-diastolic and end-systolic diameters as well as left ventricular wall stress. However, the stress-diameter relation remained constant.[56]

The end-systolic pressure-volume relationship for both isovolumetric and ejecting contractions can be expressed as

$$P_{es} = E_{es}(V_{es} - V_d)$$

where P_{es} and V_{es} are end-systolic pressure and end-systolic volume, respectively; E_{es} is the slope of the line relating these two variables (the solid lines in Figure 14–11); and V_d is the intercept of this line on the volume axis (Fig. 14–11*C*). Thus, E_{es} is a numerical expression of myocardial contractility; a higher value indicates a steeper slope and a smaller end-systolic volume, i.e., more complete systolic emptying at any given end-systolic pressure.

There appear to be a number of theoretical advantages to the use of end-systolic pressure–volume relations as an approach to the assessment of myocardial contractility.[56a] First, since afterload is already incorporated into the calculation of E_{es}, the observed changes assess contractility directly rather than the mixture of changes in contractility and afterload that affect the ejection phase indices;[57] and second, since E_{es} is independent of preload,[51,55] difficulties with the ejection phase indices that are affected by end-diastolic volume[58] are obviated.[56] E_{es} can be measured by rearranging the equation as follows:

$$E_{es} = P_{es}/(V_{es} - V_d)$$

P_{es} and V_{es} can be measured relatively easily in patients; the determination of V_d requires measurement of P_{es} and V_{es} from contractions at a constant contractility but at different afterloads. P_{es} and V_{es} can be measured at two pressures by either raising resistance with phenylephrine or lowering

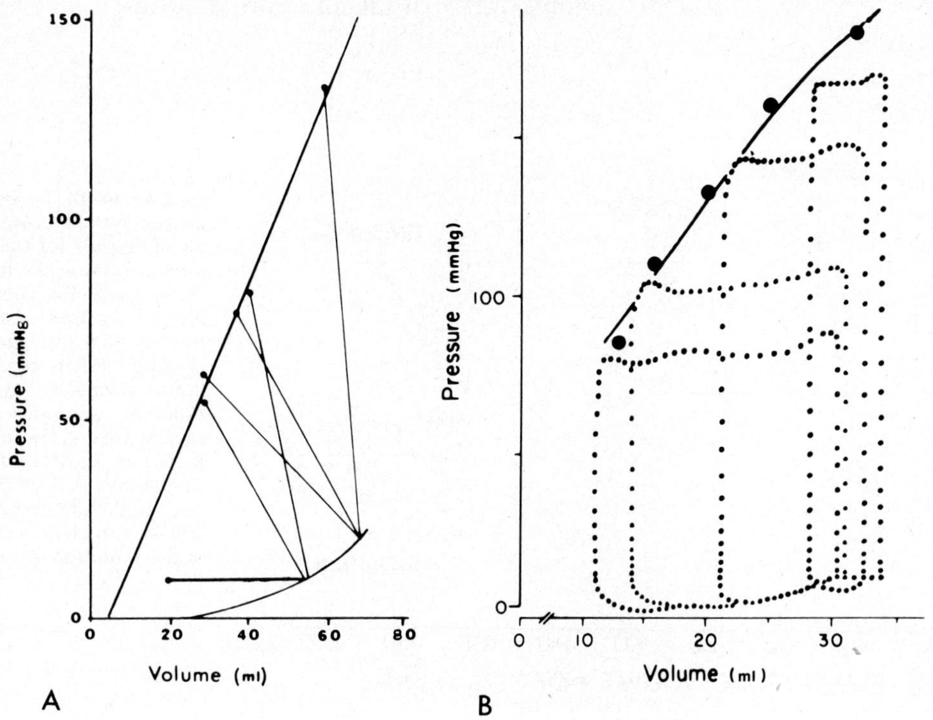

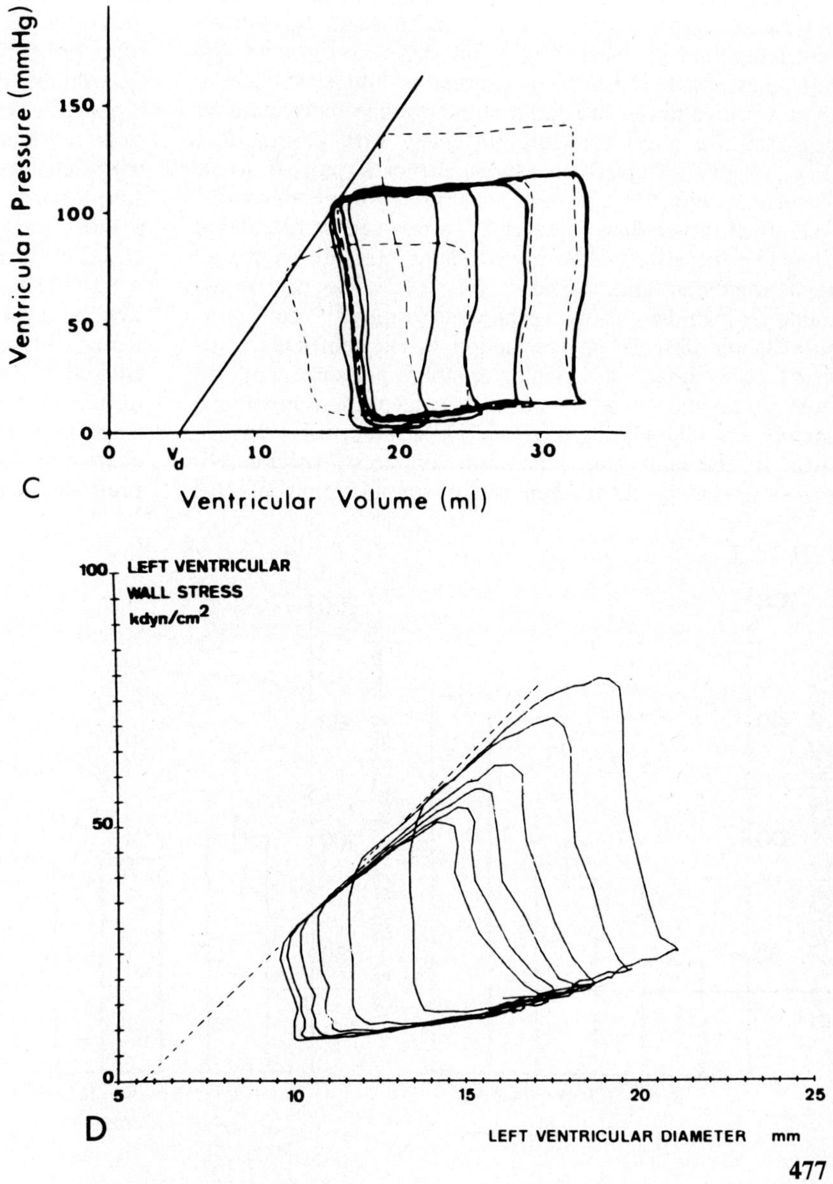

FIGURE 14–11 Pressure-volume (P-V) diagrams in canine ventricles. *A*, P-V diagram obtained in an isolated left ventricle that was filled with air and connected to an air chamber. The ventricle compressed air during systole. (From Monroe, R. G., and French, G. N.: Left ventricular pressure-volume relationships and myocardial oxygen consumption in the isolated heart. Circ. Res. *9*:362, 1961, by permission of the American Heart Association, Inc.). *B*, P-V diagram obtained in an isolated left ventricle that ejected liquid against a hydraulic servo-controlled loading system. The large dots near the solid line represent the peak isovolumetric pressures at various volumes.) (From Weber, K. T., et al.: Left ventricular force-length relations of isovolumic and ejecting beats. Am. J. Physiol. *231*:337, 1976.) *C*, P-V diagram obtained in a left ventricle ejecting blood. Volume was measured by a cardiometer while venting the right ventricles. (From Sagawa, K.: The ventricular pressure-volume diagram revisited. Circ. Res. *43*:677, 1978, by permission of the American Heart Association, Inc.) *D*, Beat-to-beat changes in left ventricular stress-diameter loop during a decrease in venous return in an open-chest dog. The dotted line corresponds to the end-systolic–stress end-systolic diameter line. The stress-diameter relations are linear during most of the ejection. The slope of this linear phase is much less affected by the maneuver than is the end-systolic diameter. (Reproduced with permission from Pouleur, H., Rousseau, M. F., van Eyll, C., van Mechelen, H., Brasseur, L. A., and Charlier, A. A.: Assessment of left ventricular contractility from late systolic stress-volume relations. Circulation *65*:1204, 1982, by permission of the American Heart Association, Inc.)

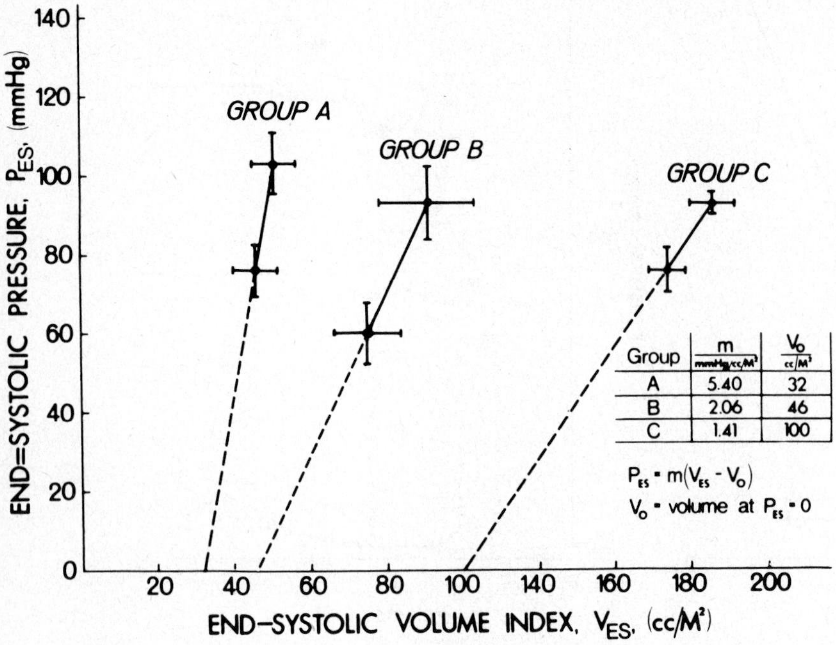

FIGURE 14–12 Average values for left ventricular end-systolic volume and pressure at two levels of systolic load are plotted for subjects with normal contractile function (group A, ejection fraction $\geq$ 0.60), intermediate function (group B, ejection fraction = 0.41 to 0.59), and poor contractile function (group C, ejection fraction $\leq$ 0.40). Points represent average values, and brackets indicate standard errors of the means. Volumes are index for body surface area in square meters. (From Grossman, W., Braunwald, E., Mann, T., McLaurin, L. P., and Green, L. H.: Contractile state of the left ventricle in man as evaluated from end-systolic pressure-volume relations. Circulation *56*:845, 1977, by permission of the American Heart Association, Inc.)

it with nitroglycerin (Fig. 14–12). The method can be further simplified by measuring V_{es} at the operating end-systolic pressure, if the latter is normal or almost so. Under these circumstances the end-systolic volume (corrected for body surface area) correlates inversely with contractility (Fig. 14–13). Although measurements of P_{es} appear to be useful clinically,[59,60] it is more accurate to use end-systolic wall *stress* rather than pressure;[60–63] stress can be calculated from considerations of intraventricular pressure and from cavity diameter and thickness (p. 472).[61] The use of M-mode or two-dimensional echocardiography,[61,63] cuff pressure (in the absence of obstruction to left ventricular outflow) to estimate ventricular systolic pressure, and an indirect carotid pulse to aid in the determination of end systole are all helpful in providing a noninvasive assessment of the end-systolic pressure (or stress)–volume (dimension) index. A further useful simplification of this index can be derived by determining the ratio of peak systolic pressure/end-systolic volume, the former parameter determined by sphygmomanometry and the latter by radionuclide ventriculography.[64–66,66a,66b] Normally, this ratio rises markedly during exercise but fails to do so in patients with left ventricular dysfunction. The end-systolic pressure/volume ratio at rest and during exercise appears to be a more sensitive index than the ejection fraction (at rest and during exercise) in identifying ventricular dysfunction.

The left ventricular end-systolic pressure–volume relation is of particular value in assessing contractility in patients with mitral regurgitation, in whom this is otherwise particularly difficult.[60] Since isovolumetric systole is absent in mitral regurgitation, isovolumetric indices cannot be employed. The reduced afterload and augmented preload characteristic of mitral regurgitation complicate the interpretation of the ejection phase indices as well. The relation

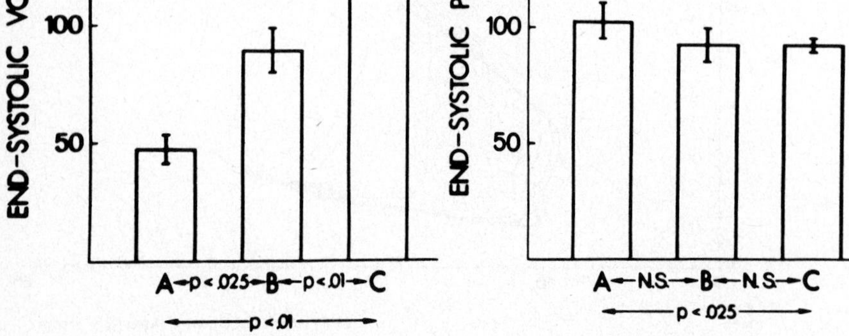

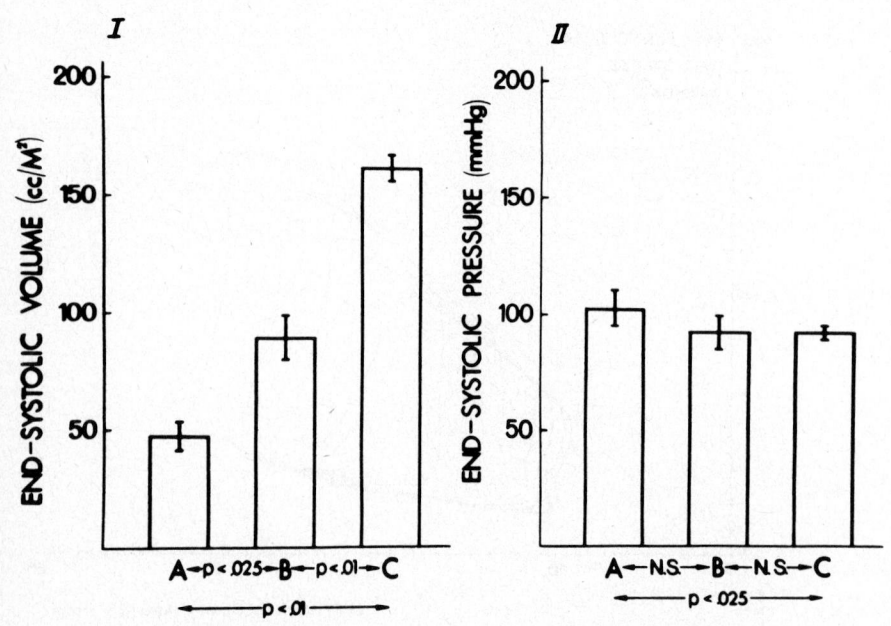

FIGURE 14–13 Values for end-systolic volume and pressure in groups A, B, and C (defined in legend to Figure 14–12). Resting end-systolic volume closely reflects overall left ventricular contractile performance, as indicated by the clear separation of groups A, B, and C. Bars represent mean values, and brackets indicate standard errors of the means. (From Grossman, W., Braunwald, E., Mann, T., McLaurin, L. P., and Green, L. H.: Contractile state of the left ventricle in man as evaluated from end-systolic pressure-volume relations. Circulation *56*:845, 1977, by permission of the American Heart Association, Inc.)

between arterial pressure and wall stress, determined by echocardiography, has been used to classify patients with hypertension into those with normal or impaired left ventricular function.[65] The left ventricular stress-dimension relation, determined noninvasively, has also been found helpful in identifying positive inotropic interventions.[63]

WALL MOTION ABNORMALITIES. The mildest disturbance of ventricular performance in ischemic heart disease consists of focal abnormality of contraction in the presence only of a reduction in diastolic distensibility but with a normal end-diastolic volume and EF.[67] A slightly more severe disturbance consists of a normal EF at rest, but a failure to rise during exercise. This is followed by a reduced EF and an elevated filling pressure in the presence of a normal end-diastolic volume at rest. The elevated filling pressure reflects reduced compliance of the scarred ventricle rather than systolic failure. Similar abnormalities may occur with acute ischemia and may be induced by stress through atrial pacing or by exercise. When abnormal wall motion involves more than approximately one-sixth of the endocardial surface, the ventricular end-diastolic volume at rest rises. Cardiac output declines with abnormal contraction involving more than approximately one-fourth of the endocardial surface.[67]

VENTRICULAR dP/dt. Since *changes* in the maximum rate of rise of ventricular pressure (peak dP/dt) are known to be highly sensitive to acute *changes* in contractility[68,69] (Fig. 14–14), measurement of ventricular dP/dt may be employed along with ventricular end-diastolic volume and filling pressure in the assessment of *directional changes* in contractility with an intervention. Peak dP/dt cannot be reliably measured with the catheter-manometer systems ordinarily used during cardiac catheterization, unless special precautions are taken to prevent artifacts and the frequency response of the system is carefully determined.[70] High-fidelity catheter-tip micromanometers should be employed, but even with these, artifacts due to flicking catheter motion during the cardiac cycle must be assiduously avoided.

Peak dP/dt is largely independent of changes in afterload, provided it occurs *before* aortic valve opening.[44,71] Studies carried out in both dogs[72] and human patients[44] have shown that peak dP/dt is little altered by steady-state alterations in aortic pressure, and although it appears to be much more markedly affected by changes in contractility than by alterations in preload, the latter influence cannot be disregarded; therefore, even when contractility is constant, a large change in preload can cause a modest alteration in dP/dt in the same direction. Another difficulty with peak dP/dt is that it cannot be corrected for changes in muscle mass produced by ventricular hypertrophy. Although peak dP/dt, in general, correlates with the basal level of contractility, it is not as useful for assessing this property of cardiac function as are the ejection phase indices (see below).

ASSESSING CARDIAC PERFORMANCE BASED ON FORCE-VELOCITY-LENGTH CONCEPTS

In the final analysis, irrespective of theoretical considerations, any index that is proposed for assessing ventricular function must be reproducible in the same individual under constant conditions and must be capable of differentiating patients with normal cardiac function from those with reduced cardiac function.[73] The principles of myocardial muscle mechanics, outlined in Chapter 12, have provided a framework for analysis for two classes of indices: one group based on events during isovolumetric contraction and a second group based on events during ejection. These indices are employed for two purposes: (1) determining absolute levels of contractility, i.e., whether the basal level of contractility is normal or not; and (2) determining directional changes of contractility, i.e., whether any given intervention exerts a positive or negative inotropic effect.

Isovolumetric Phase Indices. V_{max}, the maximum velocity of shortening of the unloaded contractile elements (CE), theoretically provides a measure of myocardial contractility independent of preload or afterload. Controversy continues to surround calculation of CE V_{max}, both in isolated muscle and, even more so, in the intact heart, in which case the calculation must be based on many assumptions.[74] Despite these difficulties, however, observations in the intact left ventricle (p. 435) indicate that its V_{max}, determined by extrapolation of the force-velocity relation derived from multiple variably afterloaded beats, is, like the V_{max} of isolated cardiac muscle, not significantly al-

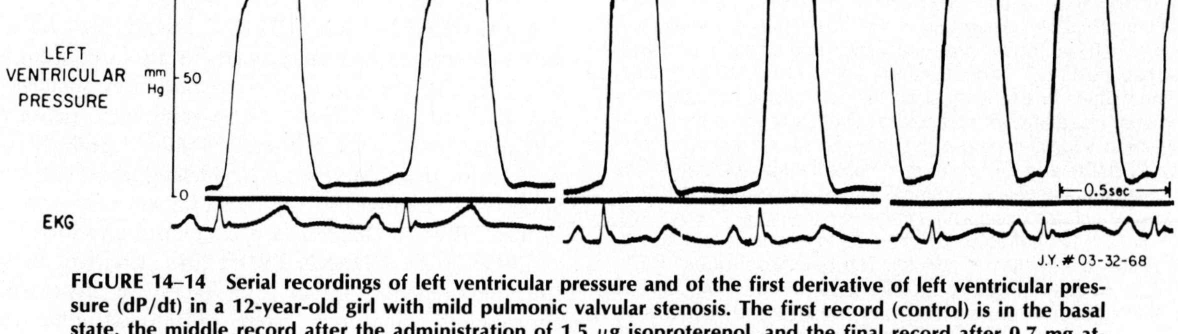

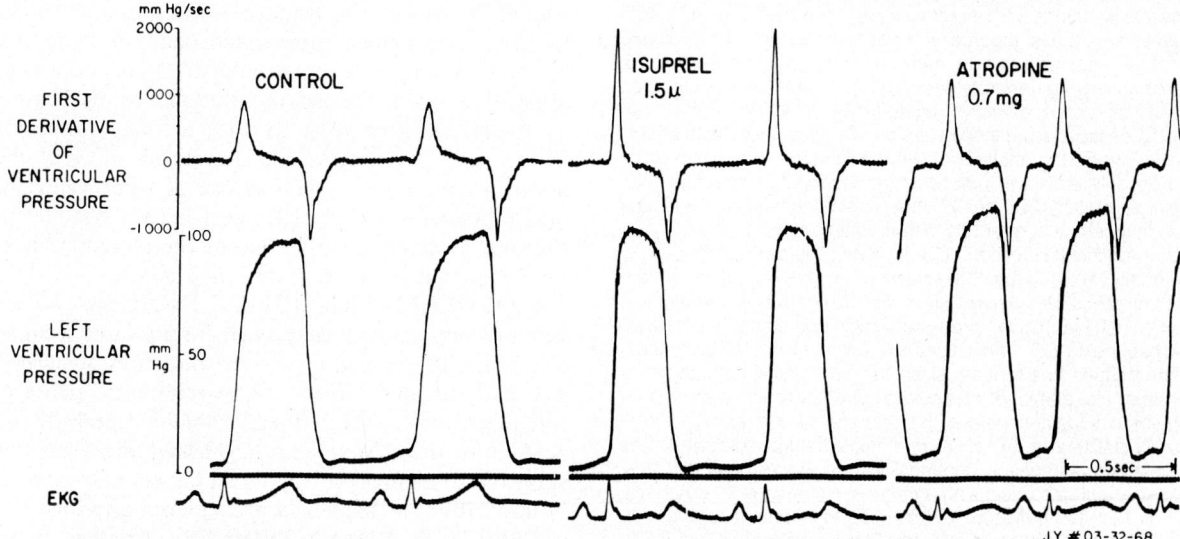

FIGURE 14–14 Serial recordings of left ventricular pressure and of the first derivative of left ventricular pressure (dP/dt) in a 12-year-old girl with mild pulmonic valvular stenosis. The first record (control) is in the basal state, the middle record after the administration of 1.5 μg isoproterenol, and the final record after 0.7 mg atropine. (From Gleason, W. L., and Braunwald, E.: Studies on the first derivative of the ventricular pressure pulse in man. J. Clin. Invest. *41*:80, 1962.)

tered by alterations of preload within the physiological range but is markedly sensitive to inotropic stimuli.[75]

CE velocity in the intact heart has been estimated assuming a muscle model in which CE and SE (series elastic element) are in series (p. 419). At any instant the velocity of SE extension (V_{SE}), and hence of V_{CE}, is directly proportional to the rate of force development (dF/dt) and is inversely related to the stiffness of SE.[76] When ejection of the canine ventricle is prevented experimentally and the calculated V_{CE} is plotted against the corresponding wall stress, an inverse relation between V_{CE} and stress is described.[77] V_{max} has been estimated from isovolumetric contractions by extrapolation of the V_{CE} stress relation to zero stress; maximum isovolumetric wall stress (P_0) can also be calculated. Such force-velocity curves obtained from the intact dog ventricle during inotropic interventions[77] exhibit changes resembling those calculated in a similar manner, albeit with fewer assumptions, from isometric twitches as well as from variably afterloaded contractions in isolated cardiac muscle.

It is obviously impractical in patients to determine V_{max} either in variably afterloaded or completely isovolumetric beats. However, a mathematical derivation of CE V_{max} can be obtained in the normally ejecting heart, using only the isovolumetric phase of contraction and employing one of the so-called isovolumetric phase indices described below. In one approach that has been applied clinically,[78] V_{CE} is calculated as dP/dt/KP (where K is an assumed stiffness constant for the series elastic element) and is plotted against instantaneous wall stress (calculated from intraventricular pressure, volume, and wall thickness) during the isovolumetric phase of left ventricular systole, and the curve is then extrapolated to zero stress to obtain V_{max}. However, if it is further assumed that contraction of the myocardium during isovolumetric contraction is truly isometric, then pressure and wall stress are linearly related to one another, and no calculation of wall stress is required to determine V_{max};[79] calculated V_{CE} is simply plotted against the instantaneous intraventricular pressure and extrapolated to zero pressure. This index of V_{max} is relatively independent of acute changes in preload at low left ventricular end-diastolic pressures[80] but declines at end-diastolic pressures exceeding 10 mm Hg.[81]

Determination of V_{max} in the intact heart, as described above, requires a number of assumptions concerning the characteristics of the SE and PE (parallel elastic elements) and the type of muscle model that exists in the intact heart,[73] little information is available about how chronic heart disease alters these characteristics.[74] Furthermore, the validity of the assumption that isovolumetric contraction is truly isometric has been questioned.[82] Since this estimate of V_{max} declines as left ventricular end-diastolic pressure rises,[37] it will underestimate contractility when ventricular compliance is reduced, as occurs in ventricular hypertrophy. In addition, this index of V_{max} may be maintained in the presence of acute ischemia despite depression of pump performance, presumably because it reflects the behavior of normal muscle in series with nonfunctioning segments of myocardium. In addition to these theoretical objections, errors in calculating V_{max} can arise from artifacts in measuring dP/dt from inadequate catheter-manometer systems; from whipping motion of the catheter; and from the presence of mitral regurgitation, which prevents even brief periods of isovolumetric contraction. Despite these limitations, when data derived from analysis of the isovolumetric phase are considered to be only *empirical indices of the inotropic state* rather than *true measures of behavior of CE*, they can be useful for detecting *changes* in myocardial contractility with an intervention.

Some of the difficulties cited above involving the calculation of V_{max} can be partially avoided by the selection of certain points on the curve relating dP/dt/DP, where DP is the developed left ventricular pressure (i.e., left ventricular pressure minus end-diastolic pressure) to the corresponding DP. These measures tend to be relatively independent of changes in afterload, since they are usually computed at a DP of 40 mm Hg, a level of pressure generation which in most clinical circumstances occurs before the opening of the aortic valve.[83] The ratio dP/dt/DP at a DP of 40 mm Hg, although somewhat less sensitive to acute changes in contractility than simple peak dP/dt, is nonetheless useful for assessing *directional* changes in contractility,[42,44,83,84] since it is unaffected by changes in afterload and is relatively insensitive to changes in preload. The peak level of dP/dt/TP, termed "V_{pm}" (where TP refers to total pressure development), is also relatively independent of both preload and afterload but sensitive to changes in the inotropic state,[85,86] and it has been advocated as an index of the contractility in the basal state, as discussed further below.

Ejection Phase Indices. The most commonly used ejection phase indices include ejection fraction (EF), peak and mean fractional shortening (FS) of ventricular myocardium, and peak and mean velocity of circumferential fiber shortening.[73] Contractility can be evaluated using high-fidelity catheter-tip manometers and cineangiography[87] or a catheter-tip velocity flow meter in the ascending aorta[88] to determine the instantaneous relation between wall stress or tension and midwall or endocardial shortening velocity throughout ejection. Ejection phase indices can also be obtained noninvasively by echocardiography.[61,64] V_{CF} at peak wall stress has been chosen for many calculations, since at that instant the rate of change in wall force (and therefore the rate of change in the length of SE) is zero, and V_{CF} equals V_{CE}.

DETERMINATION OF DIRECTIONAL CHANGES IN CONTRACTILITY

At constant levels of ventricular filling pressure, end-diastolic volume or dimensions (as evidence of constant ventricular preload); aortic or left ventricular systolic pressure (as evidence of constant afterload); and a variety of measures of left ventricular performance, such as the ejection phase indices (EF, peak and mean FS, and V_{CF}) as well as stroke volume, stroke work, stroke power, and peak left ventricular dP/dt (see below), all vary as functions of myocardial contractility. Thus, acute enhancement or depression of contractility may be assumed to occur if any of these indices of mechanical performance increases while filling pressure or end-diastolic volume and aortic pressure remain unchanged or vary in a manner that affects performance in a direction *opposite* to the change in contractility.[58,89] For example, at a similar aortic pressure, the finding of a reduction of stroke volume or dP/dt while ventricular filling pressure or end-diastolic volume remains constant or rises reflects a depression of contractility.

Although the absolute levels of ventricular filling pressure do not correlate with end-diastolic volume in chronic heart disease[25,90] (Fig. 14–8), acute *changes* in ventricular filling pressure are *directionally* similar to changes in end-diastolic volume (except in the presence of myocardial ischemia or marked tachycardia [p. 428]). Therefore, a *change* in ventricular filling pressure can be related to a *change* in one of the hemodynamic measures of left ventricular performance enumerated above in order to assess *directional* changes of contractility.[58,89] This approach is not applicable when preload or afterload or both are altered by the intervention so as to cause a change in performance in the same direction as the presumed effect of the alteration in contractility, such as occurs when ventricular filling pressure rises or left ventricular systolic pressure declines or both occur as one of the aforementioned indices of ventricular performance increases.

ISOVOLUMETRIC PHASE INDICES. In assessing acute *changes* in contractility, there does not seem to be an advantage in the use of derived measures such as "V_{max}," which is calculated from the isovolumetric phase pressure tracings, over the more directly obtained peak $dP/dt/DP_{40}$, since both these isovolumetric phase indices are highly responsive to changes in the inotropic state and are relatively insensitive to changes in preload and afterload.[42]

EJECTION PHASE INDICES. Changes in the relation between the velocity or extent of myocardial wall shortening (measured from cineangiographic frames,[91] echocardiograms, or a catheter-tip velocity meter[88]) and the simultaneous ventricular wall stress at any given length

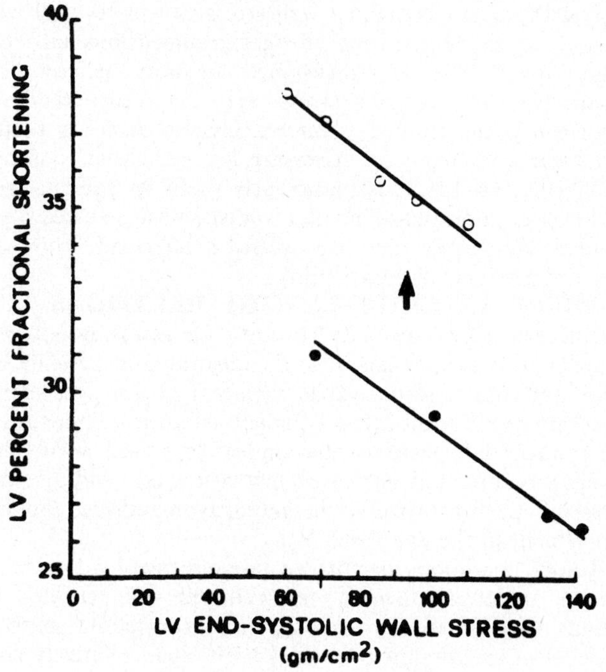

FIGURE 14–15 Comparison of the LV end-systolic wall stress-shortening lines joining points at different afterloads for control (closed circles) and increased (open circles) contractile states produced by dobutamine in a representative subject. With the dobutamine infusion, the percentage of ΔD is higher for any level of end-systolic wall stress. (Reproduced with permission from Borow, K. M., Green, L. H., Grossman, W., and Braunwald, E.: Left ventricular end-systolic stress-shortening and stress-length relations in humans. Am. J. Cardiol. *50*:1301, 1982.)

reflect acute changes in contractility. For instance, an augmentation of instantaneous velocity of minor axis shortening (V_{CF}) at any given ventricular length and wall stress signifies an improvement of contractility. The relation between end-systolic meridional wall stress and of left ventricular fractional shortening provides a sensitive index by which an inotropic intervention can be assessed[63] (Fig. 14–15).

DETERMINATION OF CONTRACTILITY IN THE BASAL STATE

ISOVOLUMETRIC PHASE INDICES. As already stated, these isovolumetric phase indices—$dP/dt/DP_{40}$, peak dP/dt, V_{pm}, and V_{max}—are usually of little value in assessing *basal levels* of contractility and in *comparing* contractility in different patients or in any given patient at different times.[73] Empirically, it has been observed that of these several indices, V_{pm}—i.e., the physiological maximum observed velocity of myocardial shortening, calculated as the maximum dP/dt/P—is superior to the others in separating *groups* of patients with normal and depressed contractility, but even this index is unreliable in classifying individual patients.[92] Although the average values of normal subjects and of patients with left ventricular dysfunction differ significantly, there is sufficient overlap so that any given patient cannot be reliably assessed by V_{pm} or any other isovolumetric phase index.

EJECTION PHASE INDICES. In contrast to the above-mentioned limitations of the isovolumetric phase indices, the ejection phase indices—EF, FS, and mean and peak V_{CF} as well as the rate of left ventricular wall thickening during systole[93]—and the closely related mean systolic ejection rate can be employed to define basal contractility (Fig. 14–16) despite their sensitivity to variations in loading. Acute elevations of afterload cause an inverse change in ejection phase indices; however, these indices are less sensitive to changes in preload. In experimental animals, both FS and V_{CF} remain normal when measured at various time intervals following a chronic volume overload despite progressive cardiac dilatation, unless acute cardiac failure occurs.[95] Therefore compensation of the heart by chronic dilatation and hypertrophy for a chronic volume overload does *not* preclude the usefulness of ejection phase indices for assessing the basal level of contractility. Ejection phase indices may also be useful in assessing basal levels of contractility in the chronically pressure-overloaded heart that

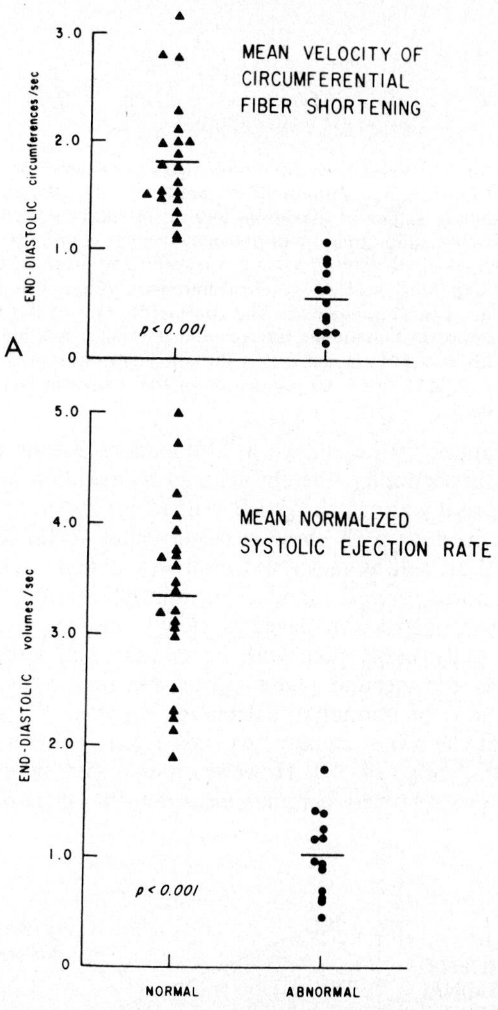

FIGURE 14–16 *A*, Mean velocity of circumferential fiber shortening (mean V_{CF}) plotted in circumferences per second (corrected for end-diastolic circumference). *B*, Mean systolic ejection rate (corrected for end-diastolic volume). Triangles represent patients with normal ventricular function; circles represent patients with clearly abnormal ventricular function as determined from other criteria. In addition to significant separation between the two groups, there is little overlap among individual patients. The superiority of these two ejection phase indices in separating these two groups of patients compared with the isovolumetric phase indices is evident. (From Peterson, K. L., et al.: Comparison of isovolumic and ejection phase indices of myocardial performance in man. Circulation *49*:1088, 1974, by permission of the American Heart Association, Inc.)

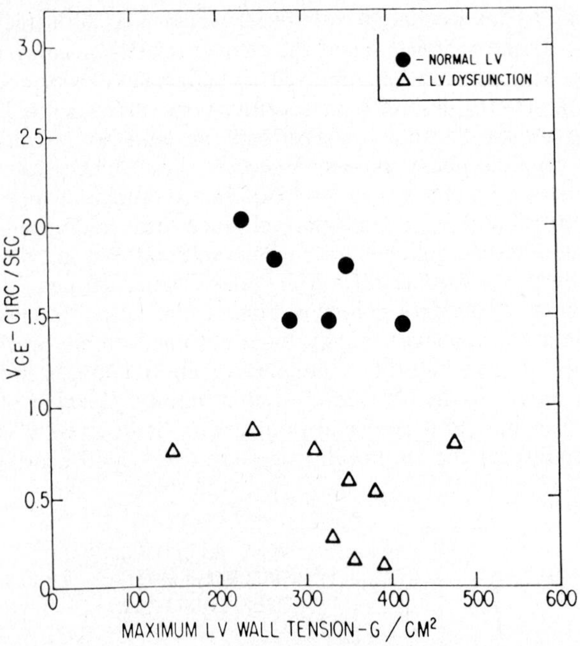

FIGURE 14–17 Velocity of circumferential fiber shortening at maximal wall tension (V_{CE}, contractile element velocity) plotted against corresponding values of maximum tension in subjects with normal left ventricles (solid circles) and patients with left ventricular disease (open triangles) are plotted against corresponding levels of left ventricular wall tension. Circ = circumferences. (From Gault, J. H., Ross, J., Jr., and Braunwald, E.: The contractile state of the left ventricle in man: Instantaneous tension-velocity-length relations in patients with and without disease of the left ventricular myocardium. Circ. Res. *22*:451, 1968, by permission of the American Heart Association, Inc.)

has adapted to the change in afterload by means of concentric hypertrophy, thereby tending to maintain afterload or restore it to normal. As left ventricular hypertrophy develops, in dogs with chronic experimental aortic constriction, FS as well as mean and peak V_{CF} at first decline but then return to and stabilize at normal levels.[96] Indeed, when the obstruction develops slowly and compensatory hypertrophy keeps pace with it, so that wall stress does not rise, the ejection phase indices remain normal.[97] The lower limit of normal of calculated V_{CE} (i.e., V_{CF} at peak stress at the minor equator) exceeds 1.4 circumferences per second[87,98] (Fig. 14–17). However, it may not be essential to use this relatively complex measurement, since V_{CE} (i.e., V_{CF} at the time of maximal wall stress) correlates well with mean V_{CF}, calculated from changes in dimensions and ejection time.[94] The aforementioned relation between left ventricular end-systolic stress and per cent fractional shortening, determined noninvasively,[63] provides a useful, practical framework for assessing left ventricular contractility (Fig. 14–18). It is particularly useful in patients with reduced ejection phase indexes to distinguish reduced myocardial shortening due to excessive afterload from depressed myocardial contractility.

FORCE-VELOCITY-LENGTH RELATIONS. The usefulness of force-velocity concepts for assessing left ventricular contractility has been demonstrated in patients before and after aortic valve replacement for free *aortic regurgitation.*[98] Although all patients studied demonstrated an improved forward cardiac index, increased aortic diastolic pressure, and decreased left ventricular end-diastolic pressure postoperatively, the majority manifested no improvement in the depressed V_{CF}.

Under conditions of chronic pressure overload, such as occurs in *aortic stenosis,* the ventricle compensates by means of hypertrophy, adding more contractile units in parallel in an attempt to maintain afterload relatively constant. It has been pointed out that if hypertrophy is inadequate or fails to keep pace with an increasingly severe pressure overload, wall stress rises, and in keeping with the inverse force-velocity relation of cardiac muscle, there are reciprocal obligatory declines in the various ejection phase indices.[26,97] Therefore, for these indices to provide an index of contractility, they must be related to wall stress. In some patients with pressure overload, wall stress is elevated, and contractility, as reflected in the fiber shortening–wall stress relation, is normal despite absolute depressions of the ejection phase indices. A true depression of contractility is present when these indices of shortening are lowered even when the existing level of afterload is taken into account (Fig. 13–9, p. 453). These observations illustrate the usefulness of characterizing myocardial function by utilizing force-velocity concepts.[99]

Studies in experimental animals have demonstrated that acute *mitral regurgitation* is associated with a marked reduction in intramyocardial wall tension (i.e., afterload) but enhanced ventricular emptying and increased EF, FS, and V_{CF}.[100,101] In patients with severe mitral regurgitation in the clinically compensated state, these ejection phase indices

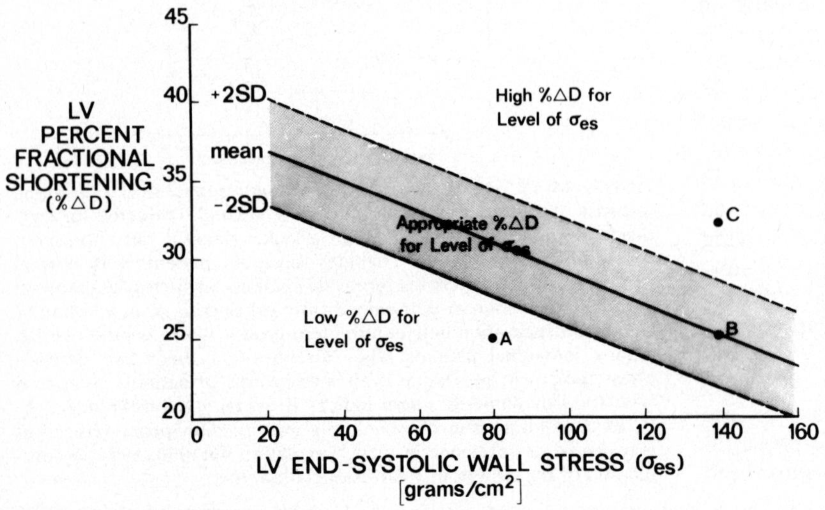

FIGURE 14–18 Diagram of the LV end-systolic wall stress (σ_{es}-shortening percentage of ΔD) relation. This relation may be useful in distinguishing depressed myocardial shortening due to excessive afterload (point B) from an intrinsic contractile abnormality (point A). Hypercontractile states would be characterized by a higher than predicted percentage of ΔD for any σ_{es} (point C versus point B). (Reproduced with permission from Borow, K. M., Green, L. H., Grossman, W., and Braunwald, E.: Left ventricular end-systolic stress-shortening and stress-length relations in humans. Am. J. Cardiol. *50*:1301, 1982.)

are also elevated. Although left ventricular fiber shortening and ejection phase indices may be normal[102] in patients with chronic mitral regurgitation in heart failure, it is impaired in patients with left ventricular failure due to cardiomyopathy, aortic stenosis, and chronic aortic regurgitation. A likely explanation for this difference between mitral regurgitation and these other causes of left heart failure is that in mitral regurgitation there is a low-impedance systolic leak into the left atrium, which reduces left ventricular afterload, increases myocardial fiber shortening, and reduces end-systolic volume.[100,102,103]

Thus, in chronic severe mitral regurgitation, myocardial contraction is affected by two opposing influences: the tendency of a low-impedance leak to increase myocardial shortening and of impaired myocardial function secondary to prolonged volume overload to reduce it. The important implication of this observation is that values for ejection phase indices in the normal range in patients with severe mitral regurgitation often represent impaired myocardial function and moderately reduced values are usually indicative of much more severe myocardial impairment than are similar values recorded in patients with cardiomyopathy, aortic stenosis, or chronic aortic regurgitation. Many patients with chronic mitral regurgitation, marked left ventricular dilatation, low-normal ejection fraction, and eccentric cardiac hypertrophy manifest progressive worsening of myocardial shortening and lack of regression of hypertrophy after mitral valve replacement presumably as a consequence of the increase in left ventricular afterload with abolition of the regurgitant leak.[104]

Patients with *cardiomyopathy* without clearly abnormal hemodynamic function, i.e., without volume or pressure overload, can be distinguished from normal subjects by the presence of depressed ejection phase indices and lower levels of V_{CE}.[91,92]

In conclusion, the ejection phase indices are more useful than the isovolumetric phase indices for the evaluation of basal levels of contractility. However, unlike the isovolumetric phase indices, the ejection phase indices are exquisitely sensitive to afterload.[44,105]

When a ventricle is stressed by a hemodynamic overload, at first it utilizes all its compensatory mechanisms to maintain normal mechanical performance, and the ejection phase indices are maintained within normal limits. However, when the Frank-Starling mechanism, the development of hypertrophy, and endogenous adrenergic stimulation are all maximally utilized and contractility becomes impaired, an abnormally elevated afterload results in reduced myocardial performance, as reflected in depressed ejection phase indices, a mechanical expression of depressions of contractility, which may occur despite maintenance of a normal cardiac output at rest.[105] With further depressions of contractility, these indices decline more, ultimately resulting in a reduction in stroke volume, a rise in ventricular filling pressure, and the clinical manifestations of heart failure (described in Chap. 15).

ASSESSMENT OF THE VENTRICULAR RESPONSE TO STRESS

A number of approaches have been used to detect mild to moderate left ventricular dysfunction, when the basal values for left ventricular performance—including the filling pressure, cardiac index, and ventricular stroke and minute work—ejection fraction, and other ejection indices are all within the normal range. In many such patients the cardiovascular response to stress is nonetheless subnormal. The stresses most commonly employed are isotonic exercise, isometric exercise, pacing, and increased afterload.

As pointed out earlier (p. 294), during *dynamic exercise* in the supine posture, the cardiac output normally rises by more than 6 ml/min for each milliliter of increase in oxygen consumption/min;[106] stroke volume and ejection fraction usually rise, and left ventricular end-diastolic pressure at rest is less than 12 mm Hg and rises slightly, remains unchanged, or decreases slightly. With impairment of left ventricular function, however, the left ventricular end-diastolic pressure rises by more than 3 mm Hg, usually to exceed 12 mm Hg, and stroke volume and ejection fraction either remain constant or decline.[107–109] There are various intermediate degrees of impairment between the normal response and that of the failing left ventricle to the stress of isotonic exercise[108,109a] (Figs. 14–19 and 14–20*A*). When dynamic exercise is carried out in the erect position, end-diastolic volume may rise in normal subjects,[110] and both end-diastolic and end-systolic volumes rise markedly in patients with impaired left ventricular function (Fig. 14–20*B*). It is important to recognize that the response to exercise is altered by age and physical training. In elderly normal subjects (> 65 years) during upright exercise, ejection fraction declines rather than increases,[111] as it does in normal young subjects. It is possible that stiffening of the arterial system with age results in a greater afterload during exercise and thereby reduces the ejection fraction.[112] Although both untrained and trained healthy young subjects experienced increased ejection fraction during supine exercise, untrained subjects tended to have an increase in end-dia-

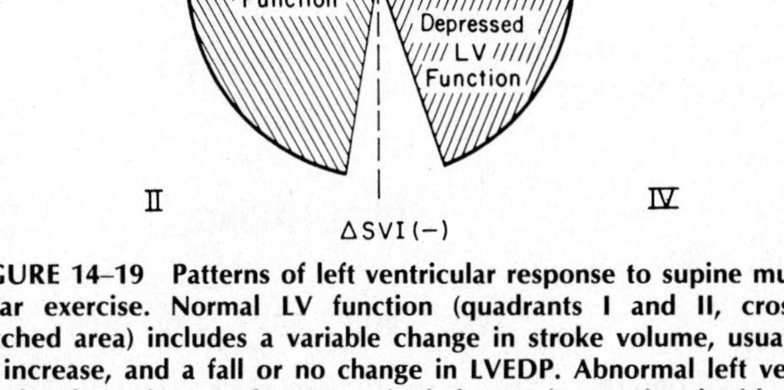

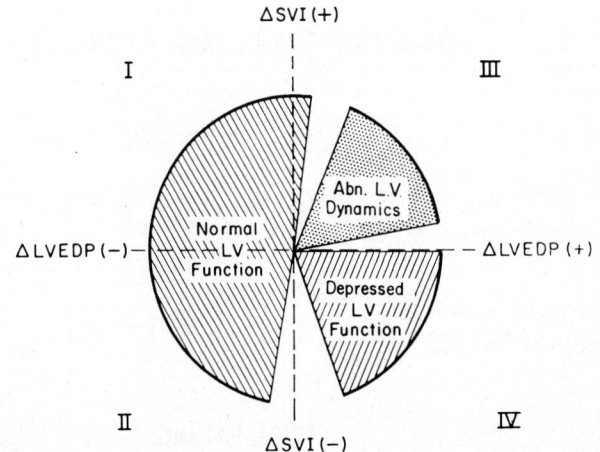

FIGURE 14–19 Patterns of left ventricular response to supine muscular exercise. Normal LV function (quadrants I and II, cross-hatched area) includes a variable change in stroke volume, usually an increase, and a fall or no change in LVEDP. Abnormal left ventricular dynamics (quadrant III, stippled area) is associated with an increase in stroke volume index (SVI) and an increase in LVEDP. Depressed LV function (quadrant IV, cross-hatched area) is characterized by no change or a fall in SVI and an increase in LVEDP. The areas between the shaded sectors include responses that cannot be definitively classified. (From Ross, J., Jr., and Braunwald, E.: Left ventricular performance during muscular exercise in patients with and without cardiac dysfunction. Circulation *34*:597, 1966, by permission of the American Heart Association, Inc.)

stolic volume, whereas trained subjects showed decreased end-systolic volume.[113] Obviously, these variations must be kept in mind in interpreting the results of patients with suspected heart disease.

Isometric exercise, usually sustained handgrip,[114] has the advantage over isotonic exercise in that it requires minimal movement of the patient and therefore allows simultaneous measurements, such as phonocardiograms and echocardiograms.[115] It is a simple, convenient test of left ventricular function.[116] The centrally mediated increase in heart rate, arterial pressure, and cardiac output appears to be designed to maintain flow in the compressed vascular bed of skeletal muscle.[117] The normal left ventricle responds to the stress of isometric exercise with little change or a decline in filling pressure and end-diastolic volume, but with an increase in stroke work. In contrast, the ventricle whose function is impaired displays an increase in filling pressure and end-diastolic volume, but little change or an actual fall in stroke work[118,119] (Fig. 14–20*B*).

The response of stroke volume, stroke work, and ventricular end-diastolic pressure before and during an *increase in left ventricular afterload* induced by the infusion of a pressor agent such as angiotensin is another useful method of evaluating the left ventricle under stress.[120] Whereas the normal left ventricle responds to this stress with little change or even an increase in stroke volume, an increase in stroke work, and a small rise in filling pressure and end-diastolic volume, when left ventricular contractility is impaired, filling pressure rises markedly, but stroke volume falls, whereas stroke work either remains constant or declines (Fig. 14–21).

With *atrial pacing* in normal subjects, cardiac output and arterial pressure remain constant and stroke volume varies inversely with heart rate;[121] both end-diastolic and end-systolic volumes decline, whereas ejection fraction shows little change. In patients with ischemic heart disease, atrial pacing may cause ischemia with an elevation of left ventricular end-diastolic pressure if the tachycardia produces ischemia (Fig. 14–20*D*).[108]

The left ventricular responses to these various forms of stress are useful not only in detecting the impairment of myocardial functional reserve but also in expressing the se-

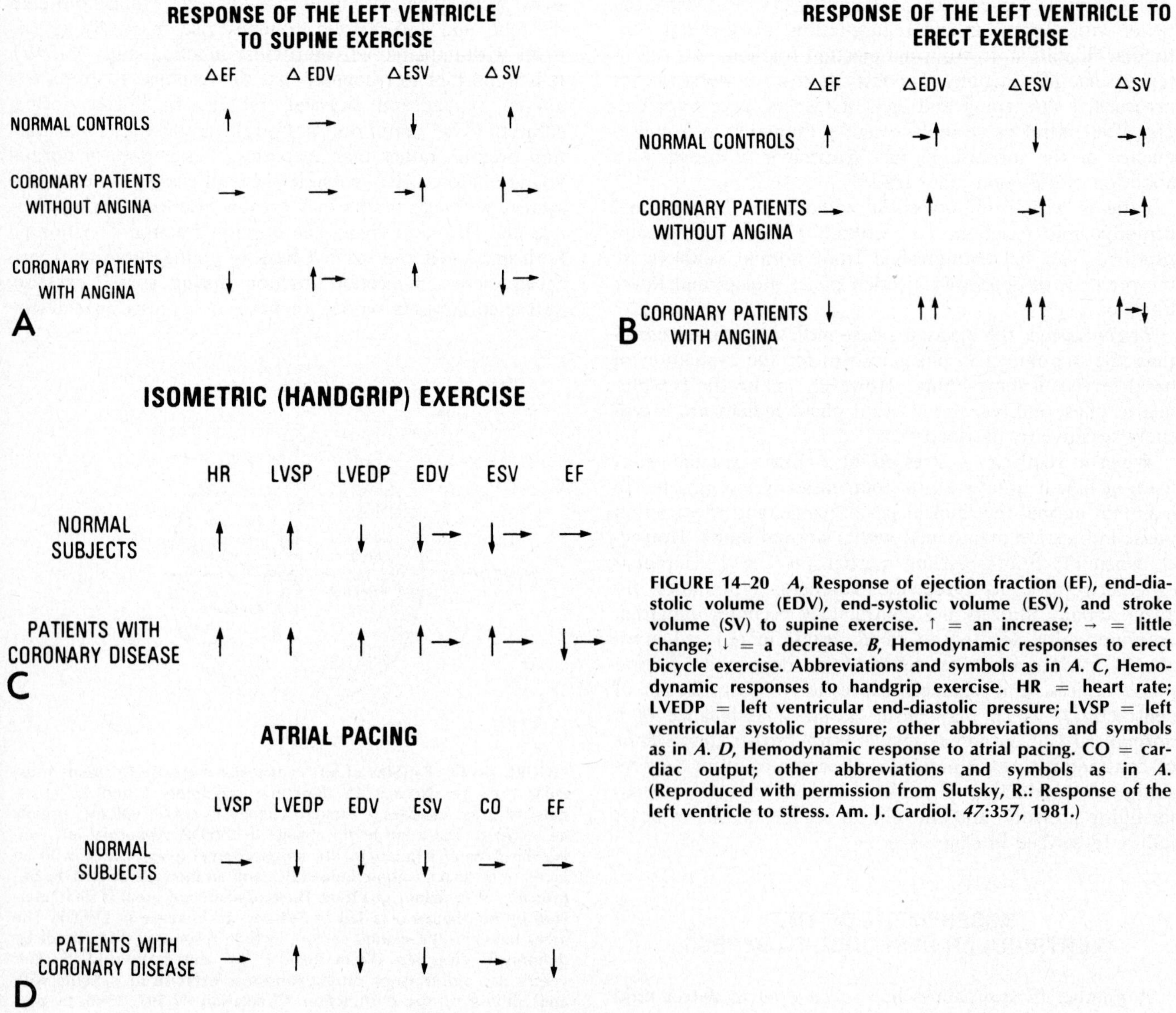

FIGURE 14–20 *A*, Response of ejection fraction (EF), end-diastolic volume (EDV), end-systolic volume (ESV), and stroke volume (SV) to supine exercise. ↑ = an increase; → = little change; ↓ = a decrease. *B*, Hemodynamic responses to erect bicycle exercise. Abbreviations and symbols as in *A*. *C*, Hemodynamic responses to handgrip exercise. HR = heart rate; LVEDP = left ventricular end-diastolic pressure; LVSP = left ventricular systolic pressure; other abbreviations and symbols as in *A*. *D*, Hemodynamic response to atrial pacing. CO = cardiac output; other abbreviations and symbols as in *A*. (Reproduced with permission from Slutsky, R.: Response of the left ventricle to stress. Am. J. Cardiol. *47*:357, 1981.)

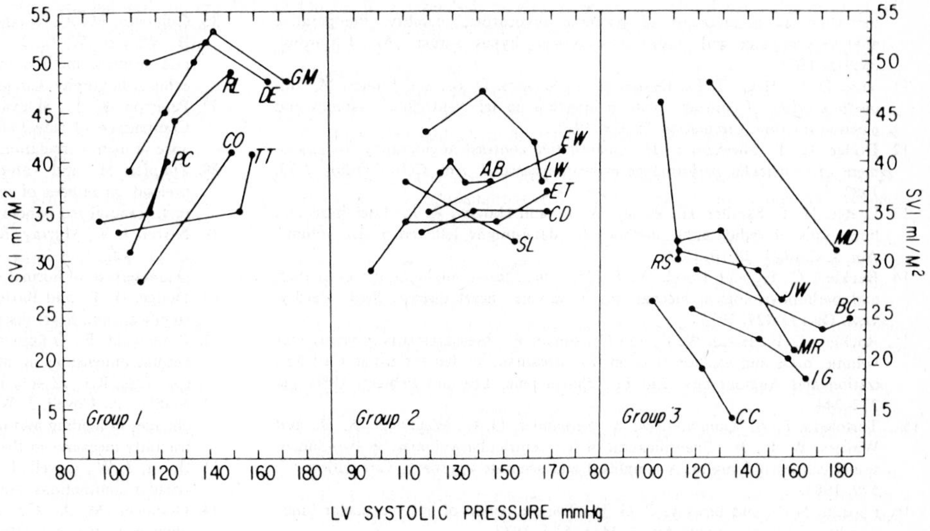

FIGURE 14–21 Relations between elevations of left ventricular (LV) systolic pressure and the stroke volume index (SVI) induced by angiotensin infusion in a group of patients with normal left ventricular function (Group 1), minor left ventricular dysfunction (Group 2), and cardiac dilatation and severe left ventricular dysfunction (Group 3). In each group, substantial and comparable increases in left ventricular end-diastolic pressure also occurred. (From Ross, J., Jr., and Braunwald, E.: A study of left ventricular function in humans by increasing resistance to ventricular ejection with angiotensin. Circulation *29*:739, 1964, by permission of the American Heart Association, Inc.)

verity of this impairment quantitatively and for studying the effects of interventions such as drugs on the diseased heart faced with an increased load. Considerable effort is now under way to apply such stresses in a standardized manner by employing noninvasive techniques to evaluate the effects on ventricular performance.

CONCLUSIONS

The isovolumetric phase indices are most useful for measuring *acute directional changes* in contractility. Left ventricular $dP/dt/DP_{40}$ is relatively simple to obtain and has the advantage over maximum dP/dt in that it is relatively independent of the time and level of arterial pressure at the instant of aortic valve opening; it is insensitive to changes in afterload but increases slightly with large changes in preload. Although V_{max}, calculated using developed pressure, is not preload- or afterload-dependent, its determination is beset by many serious theoretical problems, and it appears to have little advantage over V_{pm}, i.e., the maximum dP/dt/P or $dP/dt/DP_{40}$.

Stroke volume and stroke work are useful for detecting acute changes in contractility if they can be related to directional changes in ventricular end-diastolic volume or filling pressure or if they can be determined at various levels of ventricular filling pressure. The ejection phase indices (ejection fraction, fractional shortening of the ventricular circumference or a ventricular dimension, and the mean and peak velocities of circumferential fiber shortening) are responsive to acute changes in contractility and are relatively insensitive to acute changes in preload, but they are markedly influenced by acute alterations in afterload, so that they cannot be used to assess variations in contractility when acute changes in aortic pressure occur. However, the end-systolic pressure-volume (or stress-dimension) relation can be used to assess changes in contractility even when afterload varies, and this relation is preload-independent as well.

A number of invasive and noninvasive approaches appear useful for separating *groups of patients* with normal left ventricular function from those with abnormal function. Of the isovolumetric phase indices, V_{pm} and V_{max} based on total pressure appear to be the most reliable, although considerable overlap exists between individuals in normal and abnormal groups.

Ejection phase indices are capable of detecting depressed contractility in the basal state in individual patients and are clearly preferable to the isovolumetric phase indices for this purpose. End-systolic pressure-volume, stress-dimension, and stress-shortening relations provide a particularly useful approach to assessing basal levels of contractility in individual patients.

Determination of the effect of an acute stress, such as isotonic or isometric exercise, or of pressure overloading by pharmacological means on stroke volume, stroke work, filling pressure, or ejection phase indices may be useful in detecting reductions of myocardial reserve when no abnormality is apparent in the basal state. Noninvasive techniques may be used for assessing left ventricular ejection phase indices and are particularly useful in serial assessments of cardiac performance in individual patients.

References

1. Braunwald, E.: On the difference between the heart's output and its contractile state (Editorial). Circulation *43*:171, 1971.
2. Ross, J., Jr.: Cardiac function and myocardial contractility: A perspective. J. Am. Coll. Cardiol. *1*:52, 1983.
3. Nichols, W. W., Conti, C. R., Walker, W. E., and Milnor, W. R.: Input impedance of the systemic circulation in man. Circ. Res. *40*:451, 1977.
4. Frommer, P. L., Robinson, B. F., and Braunwald, E.: Paired electrical stimulation. A comparison of the effects on performance of the failing and nonfailing heart. Am. J. Cardiol. *18*:738, 1966.
5. Starling, E. H.: Linacre Lecture on the Law of the Heart (1915). London, Longmans, 1918.
6. Sarnoff, S. J., and Mitchell, J. H.: Control of function of heart. *In* Hamilton, W. F., and Dow, P. (eds.): Handbook of Physiology. Section 2. Circulation, Vol. 1. Washington, D.C., American Physiological Society, 1962, pp. 489–532.
7. Suga, H., Sagawa, K., and Demer, L.: Determinants of instantaneous pressure in canine left ventricle: Time and volume specification. Circ. Res. *46*:256, 1980.
8. Rackley, C. E., Russell, R. O., Rogers, W. J., Mantle, J. A., McDaniel, H. G., and Papapietro, S. E.: Clinical experience with glucose-insulin-potassium therapy in acute myocardial infarction. Am. Heart J. *102*:1038, 1981.
9. Rackley, C. E.: Quantitative evaluation of left ventricular function by radiographic techniques. Circulation *54*:862, 1976.

9a. Tobis, J., Nalcioglu, O., Johnston, W. D., Seibert, A., Iseri, L. T., Roeck, W., and Henry, W. L.: Digital aniography in assessment of ventricular function and wall motion during pacing in patients with coronary artery disease. Am. J. Cardiol. *51*:668, 1983.

9b. Kronenberg, M. W., Price, R. R., Smith, C. W., Robertson, R. M., Perry, J. M., Pickens, D. R., Domanski, M. J., Partain, C. L., and Friesinger, G. C.: Evaluation of left ventricular performance using digital subtraction angiography. Am. J. Cardiol. *51*:837, 1983.

10. Popio, K. A., Gorlin, R., Bechtel, D., and Levine, J. A.: Postextrasystolic po-

15 CLINICAL MANIFESTATIONS OF HEART FAILURE

by Eugene Braunwald, M.D.

It is impossible thoughtfully to survey, in the light of early experience, the field of medical work covering diseases of the heart without realizing the central problem to be failure of the heart to accomplish its work in lesser or greater degree. . . . The very essence of cardiovascular practice is recognition of early heart failure and discrimination between different grades of failure. . . . When a patient seeks advice and heart disease is suspected, or is known to be present, two questions are of chief importance. Firstly, has the heart the capacity to do the work demanded of it when the body is at rest? Secondly, what is the condition of the heart's reserve? These questions can be correctly answered in almost all cases by simple interrogations and by bedside signs.

In this, the opening paragraph of his classic text *Diseases of the Heart,* published in 1933, Sir Thomas Lewis identified the diagnosis and assessment of heart failure as the cardinal problem in clinical cardiology.[1] Now, a half century later, the situation has changed little, in that a principal complication of virtually all forms of heart disease is heart failure, defined as the pathophysiological state in which an abnormality of cardiac function is responsible for the failure of the heart to pump blood at a rate commensurate with the requirements of the metabolizing tissues (p. 447). Included in this definition is a wide spectrum of clinical-physiological states, ranging from the rapid impairment of pumping function, occurring when a massive myocardial infarction or tachy- or bradyarrhythmia develops suddenly, to the gradual impairment of myocardial function, observed only during stress and occurring in a patient whose heart sustains a pressure or volume overload for a prolonged period.[2]

The clinical manifestations of heart failure vary enormously and depend on a variety of factors, including the age of the patient, the extent and rate of development of the impairment of cardiac performance, the etiology of the heart disease, the precipitating causes of heart failure, and the specific chambers involved in the disease process.[3]

FORMS OF HEART FAILURE

Forward vs. Backward Heart Failure

The clinical manifestations of heart failure arise as a consequence of inadequate cardiac output and/or damming up of blood behind one or both ventricles. These two principal mechanisms are the basis of the so-called forward and backward pressure theories of heart failure. The *backward failure hypothesis,* first proposed in 1832 by James Hope, indicates that when the ventricle fails to discharge its contents, blood accumulates and pressure rises in the atrium and the venous system emptying into it.[4] There is substantial physiological evidence in favor of this theory. As discussed on page 475, the inability of cardiac muscle to shorten against a load alters the relationship between ventricular end-systolic pressure and volume, so that residual volume rises. The following sequence of adaptations then occurs that at first tends to maintain normal cardiac output: (1) Ventricular end-diastolic volume and pressure increase; (2) the volume and pressure rise in the atrium behind the failing ventricle; (3) the atrium contracts more vigorously (a manifestation of Starling's Law of the Atrium);[5] (4) the pressure rises in the venous bed behind (upstream to) the failing ventricle; (5) the capillary pressure upstream to the failing ventricle rises; (6) transudation of fluid from the capillary bed into the interstitial space (pulmonary or systemic) rises; and (7) extracellular fluid volume increases. Many of the symptoms characteristic of heart failure result from this sequence of events and the subsequent increase in fluid in the interstitial spaces of the lungs, liver, subcutaneous tissues, and serous cavities.

Cardiac output in the basal state is a relatively *insensitive* index of cardiac function. (p. 469). In many patients a portion of or, indeed, the entire sequence of events outlined above may be well established while cardiac output *at rest* is still within normal limits. Indeed, the backward pressure theory of heart failure reflects one of the principal compensatory mechanisms in heart failure, i.e., the operation of Starling's Law of the Heart,[6] in which distention of the ventricle helps to maintain cardiac output. The failing ventricle operates on an ascending, albeit depressed and flattened, function curve[7] (Figure 13–17, p. 463), and the augmented ventricular end-diastolic volume and pressure characteristic of heart failure must be regarded as aiding in the maintenance of cardiac output. When this compensatory mechanism is interfered with (e.g., by means of dietary sodium restriction and treatment with diuretics), there may be clinical improvement due to loss of extracellular fluid volume, with its accompanying reduction in tissue congestion, but at the same time cardiac output may decline,[8] and the symptoms secondary to a reduction of cardiac output may actually intensify. Thus, although many of the clinical manifestations of heart failure are secondary to excessive retention of fluid, the elevation of preload constitutes an important compensatory mechanism.

Hope's backward pressure theory of cardiac failure incorporates the concept that the cardiac chambers may fail independently and that an imbalance in performance of the ventricles may result. If one considers, for simplicity, the development of left ventricular failure consequent to aortic stenosis or of right ventricular failure secondary to pulmonic stenosis, the initial clinical manifestations of each relate primarily to the damming up of blood behind the affected ventricle. An important extension of the backward failure theory is the sequential development of right ventricular failure as a consequence of left ventricular failure (Fig. 15–1). According to this concept, the elevation of left ventricular diastolic, left atrial, and pulmonary venous pressures results in backward transmission of pressure and leads to pulmonary hypertension, which ultimately causes right ventricular failure. Often, pulmonary vasoconstriction plays a part in this form of pulmonary hypertension as well (p. 828).

Eighty years after publication of Hope's work, Mackenzie proposed the *forward failure hypothesis*, which relates clinical manifestations of heart failure to inadequate delivery of blood into the arterial system.[9] According to this hypothesis, the principal clinical manifestations of heart failure are due to reduced cardiac output, which results in diminished perfusion of vital organs, including the brain, leading to mental confusion; skeletal muscles, leading to weakness; and kidneys, leading to sodium and water retention through a series of complex mechanisms (Chap. 52). This renal effect, in turn, augments extracellular fluid volume and ultimately leads to symptoms due to congestion of organs and tissues. The heart then fails "as a whole," since there can be no imbalance between the output of the two ventricles in the steady state.

Although these two seemingly opposing views concerning the pathogenesis of heart failure led to lively controversy during the first half of this century, it no longer seems fruitful to make a rigid distinction between backward and forward heart failure, since both mechanisms operate in the majority of patients with *chronic* heart failure. Exceptions may occur, however, and some patients, particularly those with *acute* decompensation, develop relatively pure forms of forward or backward failure. An example of relatively pure forward failure occurs in the patient with acute right ventricular failure secondary to massive pulmonary embolism in whom shock—perhaps even death—due to inadequate cardiac output may ensue within minutes or hours. Although right ventricular diastolic pressure and volume and right atrial and systemic venous pressure all rise markedly, the patient may succumb before sufficient extracellular fluid has accumulated to produce symptoms of systemic venous congestion. This presentation may be contrasted with that of the patient who develops chronic cor pulmonale as a result of multiple pulmonary emboli and gradually rising pressures in the pulmonary artery, right side of the heart, and systemic venous bed. Cardiac

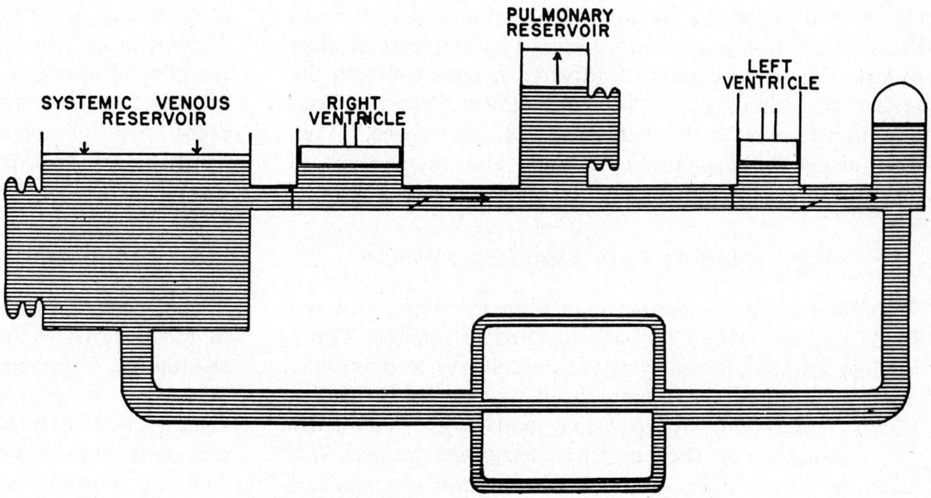

FIGURE 15–1 Diagram of the circulation explaining the etiology of pulmonary congestion. Since the capacity of the systemic venous reservoir is much larger than that of the pulmonary venous reservoir, transfer of small quantities of blood from the systemic circulation would produce a relatively large increase in pulmonary vascular volume and pressure. A slight imbalance in output between the right and left ventricles could produce significant pulmonary congestion. A sustained increase in left ventricular filling pressure could produce chronic pulmonary congestion without appreciable increase in total blood volume. (From Rushmer, R. F.: Cardiac compensation, hypertrophy and myopathy and congestive heart failure. *In* Rushmer, R. F. [ed.]: Cardiovascular Dynamics. Philadelphia, W. B. Saunders Co., 1976, p. 532.)

output and perfusion of the renal bed may be normal, at least in the resting state, but abnormal retention of extracellular fluid volume, with congestive hepatomegaly, ankle edema, and ascites, may occur. Such a patient manifests relatively pure backward failure.

Similar considerations apply to disorders affecting the left ventricle. For instance, a massive myocardial infarction may result in either (1) forward failure with a marked reduction of left ventricular output and cardiogenic shock (p. 591) and clinical manifestations secondary to impaired perfusion (hypotension, mental confusion, oliguria, and so on) or (2) backward failure with a transient inequality of output between the two ventricles, resulting in acute pulmonary edema. More commonly, patients with large myocardial infarctions develop a combination of forward and backward failure, with symptoms resulting from both inadequate cardiac output and pulmonary congestion. Early in the course of acute myocardial infarction, patients might succumb to these forms of heart failure long before renal retention of salt and water can occur. However, if the patient survives the acute insult, expansion of the extracellular fluid volume and manifestations resulting therefrom usually occur.

The relative importance of forward and backward failure in the genesis of clinical manifestations of heart failure also depends on the specific anatomical abnormality. For instance, in conditions involving interference with filling of the right side of the heart, i.e., tricuspid stenosis or constrictive pericarditis, systemic venous pressure is markedly elevated; one can readily appreciate how this leads to systemic venous congestion, capillary transudation, hepatomegaly, edema, and ascites, i.e., to backward heart failure. Patients with chronic left ventricular failure secondary to coronary artery disease or hypertension may exhibit marked accumulation of sodium and water in the systemic venous bed with no or only minimal elevation of systemic venous pressure. In these patients, accumulation of fluid is largely due to impairment of renal perfusion, i.e., forward heart failure accompanied by excessive renal tubular sodium reabsorption.

There is general agreement that fluid retention in heart failure (Figure 52–3, p. 175) is due in part to reduction in glomerular filtration rate and in part to activation of the renin-angiotensin-aldosterone system.[10] Reduced cardiac output is associated with a lowered glomerular filtration rate and an increased elaboration of renin, which, through the activation of angiotensin, results in the release of aldosterone. The combination of impaired hepatic function due to hepatic venous congestion and reduced hepatic blood flow interferes with the metabolism of aldosterone,[11,12] further raising its plasma concentration and augmenting the retention of sodium and water.

Right-sided vs. Left-sided Heart Failure

Implicit in the backward failure theory is the idea that fluid localizes behind the specific cardiac chamber that is initially affected. Thus, symptoms secondary to pulmonary congestion initially predominate in patients with left ventricular infarction, hypertension, and aortic and mitral valve disease, i.e., they manifest *left heart failure.* With time, however, fluid accumulation becomes generalized, and ankle edema, congestive hepatomegaly, ascites, and pleural effusion occur, i.e., the patients later exhibit *right heart failure* as well. Less commonly, prolonged right ventricular failure with massive accumulation of extracellular fluid may be associated with dyspnea, particularly when the patient is in the supine position and when large pleural effusions are present.

Although a disturbance of contractile function initially takes place in the ventricle subjected to the abnormal burden, with the passage of time the other ventricle undergoes changes as well. For example, the depletion of norepinephrine that occurs in experimental animals subjected to ventricular pressure overload is not confined to the stressed ventricle, but also involves the opposite ventricle[13,14] (Figure 13–12, p. 459). Similarly, alterations in the activity of actomyosin ATPase have been observed in both ventricles of animals in which the hemodynamic burden was placed on only one.[15] These findings are not suprising when one considers that both ventricles share a common wall—the interventricular septum—and that the muscle bundles constituting the ventricles are continuous. Thus, specific lesions that place an abnormal load on only one ventricle may eventually be responsible for failure of the heart as a whole.

Acute vs. Chronic Heart Failure

As has already been pointed out, the clinical manifestations of heart failure depend importantly on how rapidly the syndrome develops and specifically on whether sufficient time has elapsed for compensatory mechanisms to become operative and for fluid to accumulate in the interstitial space. For example, when a previously normal person suddenly develops a serious anatomical or functional abnormality of the heart (such as massive myocardial infarction, heart block with a very slow ventricular rate [<40/min], a tachyarrhythmia with a very rapid rate [>180/min], rupture of a valve secondary to infective endocarditis, or occlusion of a large segment of the pulmonary vascular bed by a pulmonary embolus), either a marked, sudden reduction in cardiac output with symptoms due to inadequate organ perfusion and/or acute congestion of the venous bed behind the affected ventricle will occur. If the same anatomical abnormality develops gradually, a host of compensatory mechanisms, especially cardiac hypertrophy, will allow the patient to adjust to and tolerate not only the anatomical abnormality but also a reduction in cardiac output, with less difficulty. Frequently, the clinical manifestations of chronic heart failure are suppressed by treatment. Under these circumstances, an acute event such as an infection, an arrhythmia, or discontinuation of therapy may precipitate manifestations of acute heart failure.

Low-output vs. High-output Heart Failure

Low cardiac output characterizes heart failure occurring in most forms of heart disease, i.e., congenital, valvular, rheumatic, hypertensive, coronary, and cardiomyopathic. A variety of high-output states, including thyrotoxicosis, arteriovenous fistula, beriberi, Paget's disease of bone, anemia, and pregnancy (described in detail in Chap. 24), lead to heart failure as well. Low-output heart failure is characterized by clinical evidence of impairment of the peripheral circulation, with peripheral vasoconstriction and cold, pale, and sometimes cyanotic extremities; in late stages, as the stroke volume declines, the pulse pressure narrows. In contrast, in high-output heart failure the extremities are usually warm and flushed, and the pulse pressure is widened or at least normal. The ability of the heart to deliver the quantity of oxygen required by the metabolizing tissues is reflected in the arterial–mixed venous oxygen difference, which is abnormally widened (i.e., > 5.0 ml/dl in the basal state) in patients with low-output heart failure but is normal or even reduced in high-output states, owing to elevation of the mixed venous oxygen saturation by the admixture of blood that has been shunted away from metabolizing tissues. However, the arterial–mixed venous oxygen difference still exceeds the level that existed *prior* to the development of heart failure, and cardiac output, though frequently elevated in absolute terms, is lower than it had been before the development of heart failure.

Heart Failure in the Neonate and Infant

Heart failure in the neonate or infant has a different clinical expression from that in the older child or adult[16] (Table 29–4, p. 948). Feeding difficulties, failure to gain weight and grow, tachypnea, and excessive diaphoresis are manifestations of heart failure occurring in the first year of life. Obstruction of the airways due to enlargement of the left atrium and main pulmonary artery may result in either emphysematous expansion of the left lung or, in more severe cases, atelectasis. Excessive sweating and repeated pulmonary infections are common features of heart failure in infants. Tachypnea accompanies a reduction in tidal volume, which is secondary to the presence of interstitial pulmonary edema. Respiratory distress is manifested by flaring of the alae nasi, grunting, and retraction of the ribs, features rarely seen in adults. Peripheral perfusion is poor, with cool limbs and delayed capillary filling. Hepatomegaly is a common manifestation of both left and right heart failure in infants, as is a paradoxical pulse secondary to wide variations in ventricular filling as a consequence of marked swings in intrapulmonary pressure. Peripheral edema, ascites, and pulsus alternans occur far less frequently in infants than in older children or adults with heart failure. On the other hand, facial edema, an uncommon finding in adults, is more common than peripheral edema in infants.

Because of the short neck of infants, distention of the jugular veins is difficult to detect. However, prominence of the veins on the back of the hand is a valuable sign of systemic venous congestion. Although most neonates and infants with cardiac failure have heart disease that is obvious on clinical examination, it is sometimes difficult to distinguish respiratory distress arising from cardiac disease from that associated with primary pulmonary disorders. Specifically, heart failure may be confused with bronchiolitis, asthma, or pneumonia. The presence of cyanosis and heart murmurs on physical examination and of cardiomegaly and pulmonary congestion on radiological examination are helpful though not decisive signs in the differential diagnosis.

CAUSES OF HEART FAILURE

It is useful to divide the causes of heart failure into three separate categories: (1) *underlying causes*, comprising the structural abnormalities—congenital or acquired—that affect the peripheral and coronary vessels, pericardium, myocardium, or cardiac valves and lead to the increased hemodynamic burden or myocardial or coronary insufficiency responsible for heart failure; (2) *fundamental causes*, comprising the biochemical and physiological mechanisms through which either an increased hemodynamic burden or a reduction in oxygen delivery to the myocardium results in impairment of myocardial contraction (Chap. 13); and (3) *precipitating causes*, comprising the specific causes or incidents that precipitate heart failure in approximately 50 per cent of episodes of clinical heart failure.[17]

It is helpful to recognize both the underlying and the precipitating causes of heart failure. Appropriate management of the underlying heart disease (e.g., surgical correction of a congenital heart defect or of an acquired valvular abnormality or pharmacological management of hypertension) may prevent the development or recurrence of heart failure. Similarly, treatment of the precipitating cause will usually rapidly terminate an episode of heart failure and may be life-saving.

Overt heart failure may, of course, also be precipitated if there is progression of the underlying heart disease. A previously stable, compensated patient may develop heart failure that is apparent clinically for the first time when the intrinsic process has advanced to a critical point, such as with progressive obliteration of the pulmonary vascular bed in a patient with cor pulmonale or further narrowing of a stenotic aortic valve. Alternatively, decompensation may occur as a result of failure or exhaustion of the compensatory mechanisms but without any change in the volume load on the heart.

Precipitating Causes of Heart Failure

Inappropriate Reduction of Therapy. Perhaps the most common cause of decompensation in a previously compensated patient with heart failure is inappropriate relaxation in the intensity of treatment—be it dietary sodium restriction, reduced physical activity, a drug regimen, or, most commonly, a combination of these measures. Many patients with serious underlying heart disease, regardless of whether they previously experienced heart failure, may be relatively asymptomatic for as long as they carefully adhere to their treatment regimen. However, without proper instruction, the patient who has become asymptomatic may incorrectly assume that his underlying condition has been cured and may voluntarily diminish the intensity of therapy, precipitating a bout of congestive heart failure. Perhaps the most serious example of this situation is the patient who adjusts his digitalis dosage on the basis of symptoms, discontinuing the drug when there are no symptoms of heart failure but taking three, four, or even more times the maintenance dose when symptoms of heart failure are present. Obviously, this practice can lead to wide variations in digitalis levels, exacerbation of heart failure, and digitalis intoxication.

Dietary excesses of sodium, incurred particularly on vacations or holidays or during an illness of the spouse responsible for preparing the patient's meals, are related frequent causes of sudden cardiac decompensation.

Arrhythmias (see also Chap. 21). Cardiac arrhythmias are far more common in patients with underlying structural heart disease than in normal subjects and commonly precipitate or intensify heart failure. Arrhythmias impair cardiac function through several mechanisms. (1) *Tachyarrhythmias* reduce the time available for ventricular filling, When there is already an impairment of ventricular filling, as in mitral stenosis or ventricular hypertrophy, tachycardia will raise left atrial pressure and reduce cardiac output further. In addition, tachyarrhythmias increase myocardial oxygen demands and, in a patient with obstructive coronary artery disease, may induce or intensify myocardial ischemia, which, in turn, impairs both cardiac relaxation and systolic function, thereby raising left atrial pressure further and causing symptoms secondary to pulmonary congestion. (2) *Marked bradycardia* in a patient with underlying heart disease usually depresses cardiac output, since stroke volume may already be maximal and cannot rise further to maintain cardiac output. (3) *Dissociation between atrial and ventricular contraction,* which occurs in many arrhythmias, results in loss of the atrial booster pump mechanism, which impairs ventricular filling, lowers cardiac output, and raises atrial pressure.[18] This loss is particularly deleterious in patients with impaired ventricular filling due to concentric cardiac hypertrophy, e.g., in systemic hypertension, aortic stenosis, and hypertrophic obstructive cardiomyopathy. (4) *Abnormal intraventricular conduction,* which occurs in many arrhythmias such as ventricular tachycardia, impairs myocardial performance because of loss of the normal synchronicity of ventricular contraction.

Systemic Infection. Although patients with congestive heart failure are particularly susceptible to pulmonary infections, *any* infection may precipitate cardiac failure. The mechanisms include increased total metabolism as a consequence of fever, discomfort, and cough, which increase the hemodynamic burden on the heart; the accompanying sinus tachycardia, secondary to fever and discomfort, plays an additional adverse role.

Pulmonary Embolism. Patients with congestive heart failure, particularly when confined to bed, are at high risk of developing pulmonary emboli, which may increase the hemodynamic burden on the right ventricle by elevating right ventricular systolic pressure further and may cause fever, tachypnea, and tachycardia, the deleterious effects of which have already been discussed.

Physical, Environmental, and Emotional Excesses. Intense, prolonged exertion or severe fatigue, such as may result from prolonged travel or emotional crises, and a severe climatic change, such as to a hot, humid environment, are relatively common precipitants of cardiac decompensation.

Cardiac Infection and Inflammation. Myocarditis due to a recurrence of acute rheumatic fever (p. 1646) or to infective endocarditis (p. 1152) or as a consequence of a variety of allergic inflammatory or infectious processes (including viral myocarditis) (p. 1432) may impair myocardial function directly and exacerbate existing heart disease. The anemia and tachycardia that accompany these processes are also deleterious. In patients with infective endocarditis, additional valvular damage may also precipitate cardiac decompensation.

High-Output States. As indicated in Chapter 24, anemia, thyrotoxicosis, or pregnancy and other high-output states by themselves rarely, if ever, produce heart failure; however, the development of these conditions in the presence of underlying heart disease often precipitates heart failure. In these states the requirements of the peripheral tissues for oxygen can be satisfied only by an increase in cardiac output. Although the normal heart is capable of augmenting its output, this may not be true of the diseased heart. Thus, acute heart failure may be precipitated in patients with underlying heart disease who develop one of the hyperkinetic circulatory states.

Development of an Unrelated Illness. Heart failure may be precipitated in patients with compensated heart disease when an unrelated illness develops. For example, renal failure may further impair the ability of patients with heart failure to excrete sodium and thus may intensify the accumulation of fluid. Similarly, blood transfusion or the administration of sodium-containing fluid in the postoperative state may result in sudden heart failure in patients with underlying heart disease. Prostatic obstruction in the elderly male, parenchymal liver disease, and administration of corticosteroids or estrogens with sodium-retaining properties may also precipitate heart failure in patients with underlying heart disease.

Administration of a Cardiac Depressant or Salt-Retaining Drug. A variety of drugs depress cardiac function; these include alcohol, beta-adrenergic blocking agents, disopyramide (p. 659), and antineoplastic drugs such as adriamycin and cyclophosphamide (p. 1690). Others, such as estrogens, androgens, glucocorticoids, and nonsteroidal antiinflammatory agents, may cause salt and water retention. Any of these drugs, when administered to a patient with heart disease, can precipitate or aggravate heart failure.

Development of a Second Form of Heart Disease. Patients with one form of heart disease often remain compensated until they develop a second form of heart disease. For example, a patient with chronic hypertension and left ventricular hypertrophy but without left ventricular failure may be asymptomatic until a myocardial infarction develops (which may be silent) and precipitates sudden heart failure.

It is essential to make a careful and systematic search for one or more of these precipitating causes in all patients with congestive heart failure, since lack of recognition or treatment or both may be responsible for otherwise refractory heart failure. In most instances these precipitating causes can be treated effectively, after which appropriate measures should be instituted to avoid any recurrence. When a precipitating cause of heart failure can be identified, it generally signifies a better prognosis than when a similar degree of heart failure is due simply to progression of the underlying cardiac disease.

SYMPTOMS OF HEART FAILURE

Respiratory Distress

Breathlessness, a cardinal manifestation of left ventricular failure, may present with progressively increasing severity as (1) exertional dyspnea, (2) orthopnea, (3) paroxysmal nocturnal dyspnea, (4) dyspnea at rest, and (5) acute pulmonary edema.

Dyspnea (see also p. 1789). The principal difference between exertional dyspnea in normal subjects and in cardiac patients is the degree of activity necessary to induce the symptom. Indeed, at first, exertional dyspnea may simply represent an aggravation of the breathlessness that occurs in normal subjects during activity. Patients usually report that a specific task which they were able to carry out without difficulty for many years, e.g., climbing three flights of stairs, evokes more breathlessness than previously or requires them to stop briefly midway or both. As left ventricular failure advances, the intensity of exercise resulting in breathlessness declines progressively. Engorged pulmonary vessels and interstitial pulmonary edema reduce the compliance of the lungs and increase airway resistance, which increases the work of the respiratory muscles required for ventilation. However, there is no close correlation between subjective exercise capacity and objective left ventricular performance at rest in patients with heart failure.[19]

Orthopnea. This symptom may be defined as dyspnea that develops in the recumbent position and is relieved by sitting or standing. In the recumbent position there is reduced pooling of fluid in the lower extremities and abdomen; movement of fluid from the dependent parts into the circulation causes displacement of blood from the extrathoracic to the thoracic compartment.[20] The failing left ventricle, operating on the flat portion of its depressed Starling curve (see Figure 13–17, p. 463), cannot accept and pump out the extra volume of blood delivered to it by the competent right ventricle, and pulmonary venous and capillary pressures rise further.

The patient with orthopnea generally elevates his head on several pillows to prevent nocturnal breathlessness and the development of paroxysmal nocturnal dyspnea (see below); in fact, the severity of orthopnea is conveniently estimated from the number of pillows required. Patients frequently awaken short of breath if the head has slipped off the pillows and they then often seek and find relief by sitting in front of an open window. In advanced left ventricular failure, orthopnea may be so severe that the patient cannot lie down at all and must spend the entire night in the sitting position. Often such patients are observed sitting at the side of the bed, slumped over a night table or bedside stand.

A nonproductive *cough* in patients with heart failure is often a "dyspnea equivalent." It may be caused by pulmonary congestion, occurs under the same circumstances as dyspnea (i.e., during exertion or recumbency), and is relieved by treatment of heart failure.

Paroxysmal Nocturnal Dyspnea. These attacks may be considered exaggerations of orthopnea. They usually occur at night, and the patient awakens with a feeling of extreme suffocation, sits bolt upright, and gasps for breath. Bronchospasm, which may be caused by congestion of the bronchial mucosa and which increases ventilatory difficulty and the work of breathing, is a common complicating factor of paroxysmal nocturnal dyspnea. The commonly associated wheezing is responsible for the alternate name of this condition, *cardiac asthma.* In contrast to orthopnea, which may be relieved by sitting upright at the side of the bed with the legs dependent, attacks of paroxysmal nocturnal dyspnea generally persist even in this position. The reason for the common occurrence of these episodes at night is not clear, but it seems likely that the combination of (1) reduced adrenergic drive to the left ventricle during sleep, (2) elevation of thoracic blood volume during recumbency, and (3) normal nocturnal depression of the respiratory center, plays a major role. Attacks of paroxysmal dyspnea rarely occur during the daytime and are provoked by effort or excitement.

Pulmonary Edema. The most severe form of breathlessness, pulmonary edema, is associated with a number of unique pathophysiological and clinical features and is described in Chapter 17.

MECHANISMS OF DYSPNEA. Increased awareness of respiration or difficulty in breathing is associated with pulmonary capillary hypertension and results from an elevation of left atrial or left ventricular filling pressure. Patients with left ventricular failure typically exhibit a restrictive ventilatory defect, characterized by a reduction of vital capacity as a consequence of the replacement of the air in the lungs with blood or interstitial fluid or both. Consequently, the lungs become stiffer, air trapping occurs because of earlier than normal closure of dependent airways,[21] and the work of breathing is increased because higher intrapleural pressures are required to distend the stiff lungs.[22] Tidal volume is reduced, and respiratory frequency rises in a compensatory fashion (Fig. 15–2). En-

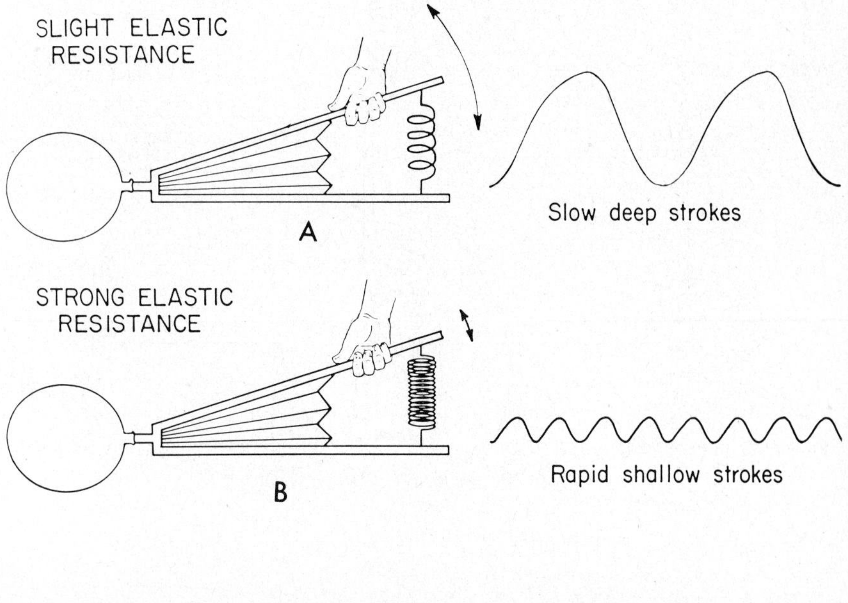

FIGURE 15–2 Mechanism for tachypnea in heart failure. To pump equal volumes of air per unit time against strong elastic resistance, a spring-loaded bellows should be operated with short rapid strokes to achieve greatest efficiency and reduce the total work. Congested lungs tend to resist normal inspiratory distention, so that rapid shallow breathing tends to reduce the work of breathing, particularly when respiratory minute volume must be increased, as during exertion. This suggests that the breathing pattern observed in patients with congestive heart failure may actually minimize the excess work of breathing imposed by the rigidity of the lungs. (From Rushmer, R. F.: Cardiac compensation, hypertrophy and myopathy and congestive heart failure. *In* Rushmer, R. F. [ed.]: Cardiovascular Dynamics. Philadelphia, W. B. Saunders Co., 1976, p. 532.)

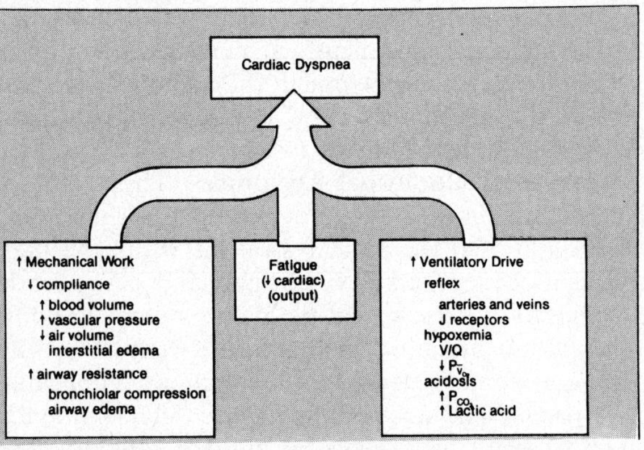

FIGURE 15–3 Factors that induce an increase in mechanical work of ventilation and ventilatory drive in states of pulmonary venous hypertension resulting from increased left heart filling pressure. The simultaneous occurrence of these factors and muscular fatigue converge to produce the sensation of dyspnea. (Reproduced with permission from Turino, G. M.: Origins of cardiac dyspnea. Primary Cardiol. *7*:76, 1981.)

gorgement of blood vessels may reduce the caliber of the peripheral airways, increasing the airway resistance. In addition, there are alterations in the distribution of ventilation and perfusion (p. 1783), resulting in widened alveolar-arterial differences for oxygen, hypoxemia, and an increased ratio of dead space to tidal volume. Whatever abnormalities in mechanics and gas exchange function of the lung exist at rest are aggravated during exercise when pulmonary venous and capillary pressures rise further. Transudation of fluid from the intravascular to the extravascular space results in greater stiffening of the lungs, an augmentation in the work of breathing, and increased resistance to air flow.[23] There is an increased ventilatory drive, as a consequence of the stimulation of stretch receptors in the pulmonary vessels and interstitium, as well as a result of hypoxemia and metabolic acidosis. The increased work of breathing, combined with a low cardiac output and resulting impaired perfusion of the respiratory muscles, causes fatigue[24] and ultimately the sensation of dyspnea[25] (Fig. 15–3).

Thus, dyspnea (during exertion or at rest) and orthopnea are clinical expressions of pulmonary venous and capillary congestion. Paroxysmal nocturnal dyspnea reflects the presence of *interstitial* edema, whereas pulmonary edema, in which there is transudation and expectoration of blood-tinged fluid (Chap. 17), is a manifestation of *alveolar* edema. The precise mechanism (or mechanisms) responsible for the respiratory distress of heart failure have not been definitively elucidated,[26] but a number of factors may be in operation (Figs. 15–3 and 15–4). It is well known that dyspnea occurs whenever the work of respiration is excessive. Increased force generation is required for the respiratory muscles to move a given volume of air if the compliance of the lungs is reduced or the resistance to air flow is increased; both these changes occur in left heart failure. Although patients are more likely to become dyspneic when the work of respiration is augmented, this increased work does not account for the perceptual difference between a deep breath with a normal mechanical load and a normal-sized breath with an increased mechanical load. The amount of work may be the same with both breaths, but the normal breath with the increased load will be associated with discomfort. A more appealing theory of the mechanism of dyspnea involves the inappropriateness of length to tension in the respiratory muscles. It has been proposed that discomfort arises when there is misalignment of the nerve spindles, which sense tension, in relation to muscle length. This misalignment could lead to the sensation of getting an insufficient breath for the tension generated by the respiratory muscles.[27]

DIFFERENTIATION BETWEEN CARDIAC AND PULMONARY DYSPNEA (see also Chap. 54). In most patients with dyspnea, there is obvious clinical evidence of disease of either the heart or the lungs, but in some the differentiation between cardiac and pulmonary dyspnea may be difficult. The dyspnea of chronic obstructive lung disease tends to develop more gradually than that of heart disease; exceptions, of course, occur in patients with *ob-*

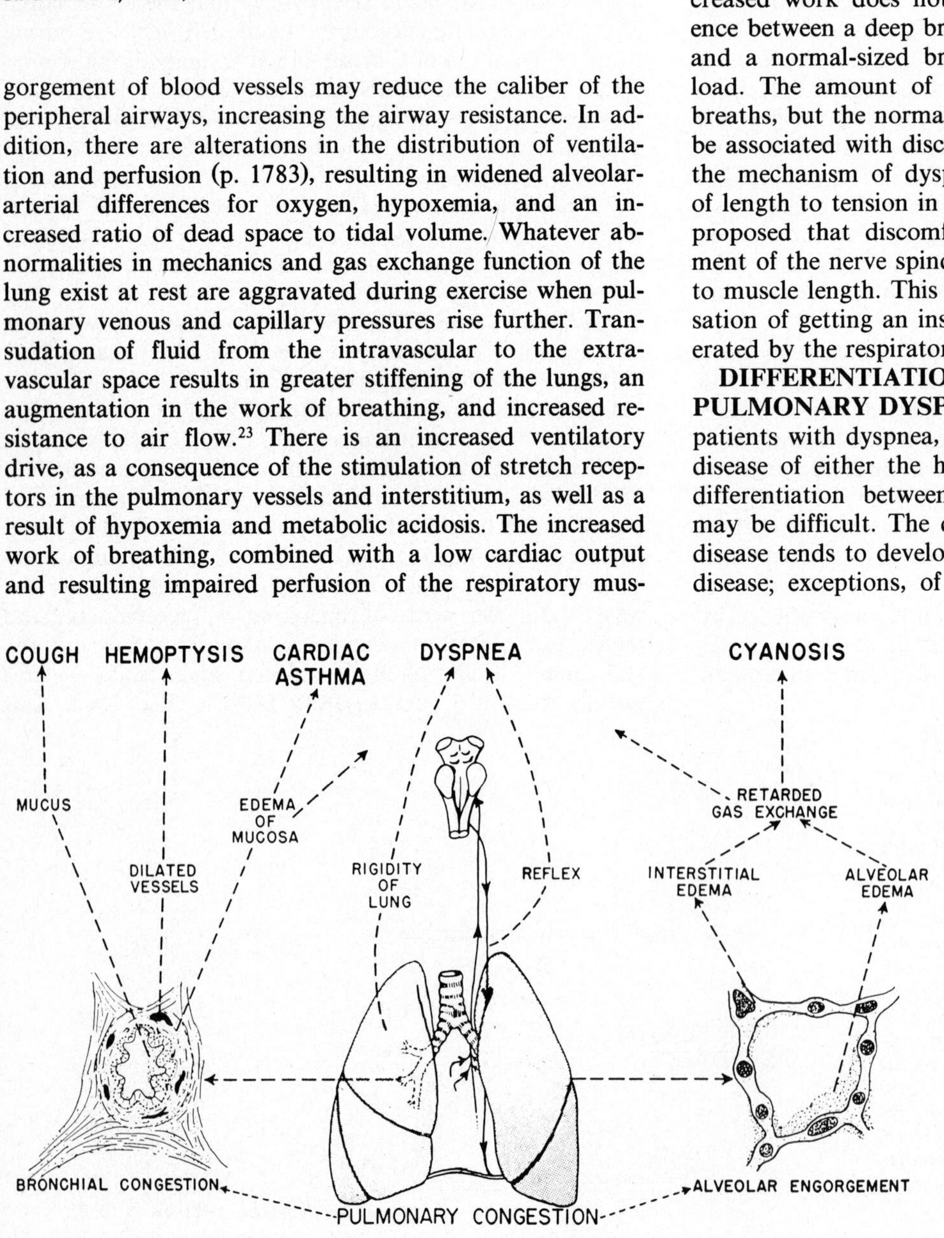

FIGURE 15–4 Etiology of respiratory symptoms from pulmonary congestion. Since most bronchial capillaries drain by way of the pulmonary veins, congestion develops simultaneously in alveolar and bronchial vascular networks. Bronchial congestion tends to stimulate production of mucus, leading to a productive cough. The distended bronchial capillaries may rupture, causing the patient to cough up blood-tinged sputum (hemoptysis). Edema of the bronchial mucosa increases resistance to air flow, producing respiratory distress similar to asthma. Dyspnea results primarily from reflexes initiated by vascular distention but may be supplemented by increased rigidity of the lungs and by impaired gas exchange resulting from interstitial edema and the accumulation of fluid in alveolar sacs. (From Rushmer, R. F.: Cardiac compensation, hypertrophy and myopathy and congestive heart failure. *In* Rushmer, R. F. [ed.]: Cardiovascular Dynamics. Philadelphia, W. B. Saunders Co., 1976, p. 532).

structive lung disease who experience an episode of infectious bronchitis, pneumonia or pneumothorax or an exacerbation of asthma. Like patients with cardiac dyspnea, patients with chronic obstructive lung disease may also waken at night with dyspnea, but this is usually associated with sputum production; the dyspnea is relieved after the patient rids himself of secretions by coughing rather than specifically by sitting up.

Acute cardiac asthma (paroxysmal nocturnal dyspnea with prominent wheezing) usually occurs in patients who have obvious clinical evidence of heart disease and may be further differentiated from acute bronchial asthma by the presence of diaphoresis, more bubbly airway sounds, and the more common occurrence of cyanosis. The difficulty in distinguishing between cardiac and pulmonary dyspnea may be compounded by the coexistence of diseases involving both organ systems. Thus, patients with a history of chronic bronchitis or asthma who develop left ventricular failure tend to develop particularly severe bronchoconstriction and wheezing in association with bouts of paroxysmal nocturnal dyspnea and pulmonary edema.

Pulmonary function testing should be carried out in patients in whom the etiology of dyspnea is unclear despite detailed clinical evaluation. The results may be helpful in determining whether dyspnea is produced by heart disease, lung disease, a combination of the two, or anxiety. In addition to the usual clinical means of assessing patients for heart disease (Chaps. 1 and 2), the arm-to-tongue circulation time may be useful, since in patients with cardiac dyspnea, this value usually exceeds the upper limit of normal (16 seconds) by 4 seconds or more (unless high-output heart failure is present).

The major alterations in pulmonary function tests in congestive heart failure are reductions of vital capacity, total lung capacity, pulmonary diffusion capacity at rest and particularly during exercise, and pulmonary compliance; resistance to air flow is moderately increased. Often there is hyperventilation at rest and during exercise, an increase in dead space, and some abnormalities of ventilation-perfusion relations with slight reductions in arterial pCO_2 and pO_2.

Rarely, it may be difficult to differentiate between cardiac dyspnea, dyspnea based on *malingering,* and dyspnea due to an *anxiety neurosis.* Careful observation for the appearance of effortless or irregular respiration during exercise testing often helps to identify the patient in whom dyspnea is related to these two noncardiac causes. Patients whose anxiety neurosis focuses on the heart may fear the presence of (nonexistent) heart disease and may exhibit sighing respiration and difficulty in taking a deep breath as well as dyspnea at rest. Their breathing pattern is not rapid and shallow, as in cardiac dyspnea. In some patients, a "therapeutic test" is helpful, and amelioration of dyspnea accompanied by a weight loss exceeding 2 kg induced by administration of a diuretic supports a cardiac origin for the dyspnea. Conversely, failure of these measures to achieve weight reduction in excess of 2 kg and to diminish dyspnea weighs heavily against a cardiac origin.

Other Symptoms

Fatigue and Weakness. Although these symptoms, often accompanied by a feeling of heaviness in the limbs, are generally related to poor perfusion of the skeletal muscles in patients with a lowered cardiac output, they may also be caused by sodium depletion, hypovolemia or both, as a consequence of excessive treatment with diuretics and restriction of dietary sodium.

Urinary Symptoms. *Nocturia* occurs relatively early in the course of heart failure. Urine formation is suppressed during the day when the patient is upright and active; this is due, at least in part, to a redistribution of blood flow away from the kidneys during activity[28] (see Figure 13–16, p. 462). When the patient rests in the recumbent position at night, the deficit in cardiac output in relation to oxygen demands is reduced, renal vasoconstriction diminishes, and urine formation increases. This diurnal pattern of urine flow characteristic of heart failure contrasts sharply with that existing in renal failure, in which urine formation occurs at a reasonably constant rate, both day and night. *Oliguria* is a sign of late cardiac failure and is related to the suppression of urine formation as a consequence of severely reduced cardiac output.

Cerebral Symptoms. Confusion, impairment of memory, anxiety, headache, insomnia, bad dreams or nightmares, and rarely psychosis with disorientation, delirium, and even hallucinations may occur in elderly patients with advanced heart failure, particularly in those with accompanying cerebral arteriosclerosis.

Symptoms of Predominant Right Heart Failure. Breathlessness, the cardinal manifestation of left ventricular failure, is uncommon in isolated right ventricular failure because pulmonary congestion is usually absent. Indeed, when a patient with mitral stenosis or left ventricular failure develops right ventricular failure, the more severe forms of dyspnea (i.e., paroxysmal nocturnal dyspnea and episodic pulmonary edema) tend to diminish in frequency and intensity, because the inability of the right ventricle to augment its output prevents the temporary imbalance between blood flow into and out of the pulmonary vascular bed. On the other hand, when cardiac output becomes markedly reduced in patients with terminal right heart failure, as may occur in the terminal phases of primary pulmonary hypertension and of pulmonary thromboembolic disease, severe dyspnea (air hunger) may occur, presumably as a consequence of the reduced cardiac output, poor perfusion of respiratory muscle, hypoxemia, and metabolic acidosis. In addition, dyspnea may be a prominent symptom in some patients with right ventricular failure and anasarca, hydrothorax, and ascites as a consequence of lung compression; these patients may even have orthopnea.

As in patients with predominant left ventricular failure, fatigue, a sense of heaviness of the limbs, and anorexia may be troubling symptoms in patients with predominant right heart failure. In patients with severe obstruction of right ventricular outflow of any cause and right ventricular failure, right ventricular stroke volume cannot be augmented, and dizziness and syncope may occur on exertion, just as in patients with aortic stenosis.

Congestive hepatomegaly may produce pain in the right upper quadrant or epigastrium, generally described as a dull ache or heaviness. This discomfort, which is caused by stretching of the hepatic capsule, may be severe when the liver enlarges rapidly, as in acute right heart failure. In contrast, chronic hepatic enlargement is generally painless. Other gastrointestinal symptoms, including anorexia, nausea, a sense of fullness after meals, and constipation, occur owing to congestion of the liver and gastrointestinal tract. In severe, preterminal heart failure, inadequate bowel perfusion can cause abdominal pain, distention, and bloody stools. Nausea, anorexia, and emesis may also be due to cardiac drugs, particularly digitalis (p. 525) and quinidine (p. 656).

FUNCTIONAL CLASSIFICATION. A classification of patients with heart disease based on the relation between symptoms and the amount of effort required to provoke them has been developed by the New York Heart Association.[29] Although there are obvious limitations to assigning numerical values to subjective findings, this classification is extremely useful in comparing groups of patients as well as the same patient at different times.

Class I—*No limitation:* Ordinary physical activity does not cause undue fatigue, dyspnea, or palpitation.

Class II—*Slight limitation of physical activity:* Such patients are comfortable at rest. Ordinary physical activity results in fatigue, palpitation, dyspnea, or angina.

Class III—*Marked limitation of physical activity:* Although patients are comfortable at rest, less than ordinary activity will lead to symptoms.

Class IV—*Inability to carry on any physical activity without discomfort:* Symptoms of congestive failure are present even at rest. With any physical activity, increased discomfort is experienced.

As discussed on page 13, the accuracy and reproducibility of this classification are limited. To overcome these limitations, Goldman et al. have developed a useful classification based on the estimated metabolic cost of various activities (Table 1–2, p. 13).[30]

PHYSICAL FINDINGS

General Appearance. Patients with mild or moderate heart failure appear to be in no distress after a few minutes of rest. However, they may be obviously dyspneic during and immediately after activity, such as coming to the physician's office or undressing. Patients with left ventricular failure may become uncomfortable if asked to lie flat for more than a few minutes. Those with severe heart failure appear anxious and may exhibit signs of air hunger. Patients with heart failure of recent onset appear acutely ill but are usually well nourished, whereas those with chronic cardiac failure often appear malnourished and wasted. Chronic, marked elevation of systemic venous pressure may produce exophthalmos and severe tricuspid regurgitation and may lead to visible systolic pulsation of the eyes.[31]

Reduced Stroke Volume. In mild or moderately severe heart failure, stroke volume is normal at rest; in severe heart failure, it is reduced, and this reduction is reflected in a diminished pulse pressure and dusky discoloration of the skin. With very severe failure, particularly if cardiac output drops acutely, systolic arterial pressure may be reduced. The pulse may be rapid, weak, and thready.

Adrenergic Activity. Increased activity of the adrenergic nervous system is a principal compensatory mechanism for support of the circulation in the presence of reduced cardiac output (p. 458). It is responsible for a number of physical signs, including peripheral vasoconstriction, which is manifested as pallor and coldness of the extremities and cyanosis of the digits. There may be diaphoresis with tachycardia, loss of normal sinus arrhythmia, and obvious distention of the peripheral veins secondary to venoconstriction. Diastolic arterial pressure may even be slightly elevated.

Pulmonary Rales. Moist rales that result from the transudation of fluid into the alveoli are heard over the lung bases and are often accompanied by some dullness to percussion. They are characteristic of congestive heart failure of at least moderate severity. (In acute pulmonary edema, coarse, bubbling rales and wheezes are heard over both lung fields and are accompanied by the expectoration of frothy, blood-tinged sputum [p. 570].) With congestion of the bronchial mucosa, excessive bronchial secretions or bronchospasm or both may give rise to rhonchi and wheezes. Rales are usually bilateral, but if unilateral they usually occur on the right side. When rales are audible *only* over the left lung in a patient with heart failure, they may signify the presence of pulmonary embolism to that lung.

Systemic Venous Hypertension (see also pp. 20 to 21). This can be detected more readily by inspection of the jugular veins, which provides a useful index of right atrial pressure. The upper limit of normal of the jugular venous pressure is approximately 4 cm above the sternal angle. When tricuspid regurgitation is present, the *v* wave and *y* descent are most prominent; however, with impedance to right ventricular filling (tricuspid stenosis) or right ventricular emptying (pulmonary hypertension, pulmonic stenosis), the *a* wave is most prominent. Normally, the jugular venous pressure declines on exertion, but in patients with heart failure it rises. Rarely, venous pressure may be so high that the peripheral veins on the dorsum of the hands or in the temporal region are dilated.

Congestive Hepatomegaly. The liver often enlarges *before* overt edema develops, and it may remain so even after other symptoms of right-sided heart failure have disappeared. Inspection of the abdomen may reveal epigastric fullness and, on percussion, dullness in the right upper quadrant. If hepatomegaly has occurred rapidly and relatively recently, the liver is usually tender owing to stretching of its capsule. In long-standing heart failure this tenderness disappears, even though the liver remains enlarged.

In patients with tricuspid regurgitation, the prominent right atrial *v* wave may be transmitted to the liver, which pulsates during systole (Fig. 15–5). A prominent presystolic pulsation in the liver due to an enlarged right atrial *a* wave can occur in tricuspid stenosis, constrictive pericarditis, restrictive cardiomyopathy, pulmonary hypertension, and pulmonic stenosis. In patients with mild right heart failure, the jugular venous pressure may be normal at rest but rises to abnormal levels with compression of the abdomen, a sign known as the *abdominojugular reflux.* In order to elicit this sign, the periumbilical region should be compressed firmly, gradually, and continuously for 1 minute while the veins of the neck are observed. The patient should be advised to avoid straining or holding his breath. A positive test, i.e., expansion of the jugular veins during and immediately after compression, usually reflects the combination of a congested abdomen (particularly the liver) and inability of the right side of the heart to accept or

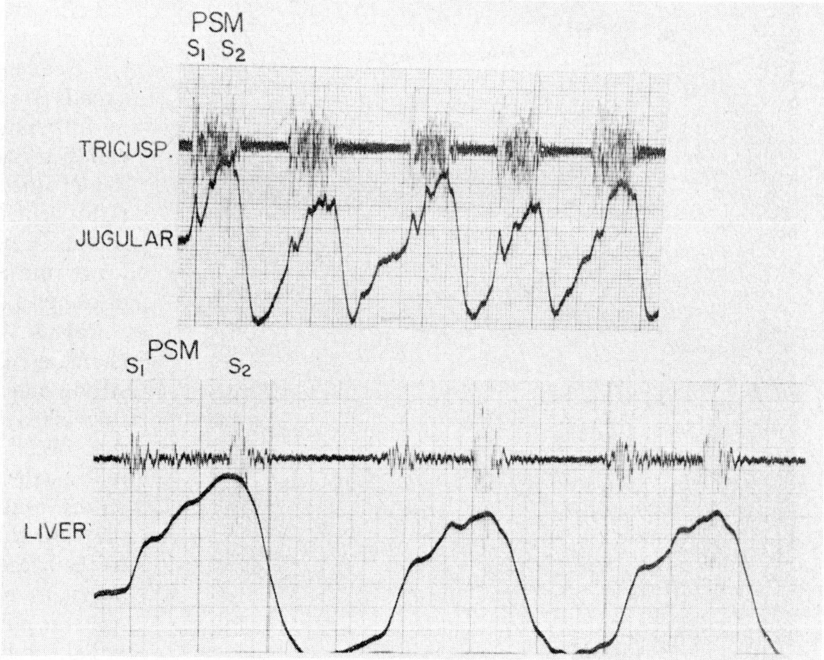

FIGURE 15–5 Jugular venous and hepatic pulse tracings and phonocardiogram from a 42-year-old woman with mitral stenosis and marked tricuspid regurgitation. A pansystolic murmur (PSM) was heard in the tricuspid area. Atrial fibrillation was present. The phonocardiogram shows the pansystolic murmur in the tricuspid region. Graphs of the jugular vein and liver show "ventricularization" of the systolic pulse wave. The rise of the regurgitant venous and liver pulses is synchronous with the first sound. Paper speed at the top tracing is 25 mm/sec, in the bottom tracing 75 mm/sec. (From Dressler, W.: Pulsations of the cervical veins and liver. *In* Dressler, W. [ed.]: Clinical Aids in Cardiac Diagnosis. New York, Grune and Stratton, 1970, p. 190, by permission of Grune and Stratton.)

eject this transiently increased venous return. Thus, a positive abdominojugular reflux is helpful in differentiating hepatic enlargement due to heart failure from that due to other conditions.

Edema. Although a cardinal manifestation of congestive heart failure, edema does not correlate well with the level of systemic venous pressure. As already noted, in patients with chronic left ventricular failure and a low cardiac output, extracellular fluid volume may be sufficiently expanded to produce edema in the presence of normal or only minimal elevations of systemic venous pressure. A substantial gain of extracellular fluid volume, a minimum of 5 liters in adults, must usually take place before peripheral edema is manifested. Therefore, edema may develop over a number of days and may not be present initially in patients with acute heart failure and marked systemic venous hypertension.

Edema is usually symmetrical and generally occurs first in the dependent portions of the body, where the systemic venous pressure rises to its highest levels. Accordingly, cardiac edema in ambulatory patients is usually first noted in the feet or ankles at the end of the day and generally resolves after a night's rest. In bedridden patients it is most commonly found over the sacrum. Facial edema seldom appears in adults but, as mentioned earlier, may occur in infants and young children. Late in the course of heart failure, edema may become massive and generalized (anasarca); it can involve the upper extremities, the thoracic and abdominal walls, and particularly the genital area. Rarely, when edema is severe and develops suddenly, it may cause rupture of the skin and extravasation of fluid. Long-standing edema results in pigmentation, reddening, and induration of the skin of the lower extremities, usually the dorsum of the feet and the pretibial areas. In patients with hemiplegia, edema is usually more marked on the paralyzed side.

Hydrothorax. Since the pleural veins drain into both the systemic and the pulmonary venous beds, hydrothorax is observed most commonly in patients with hypertension involving both venous systems, but it may also occur when there is marked elevation of pressure in either venous bed. An increase in capillary permeability probably also plays a role in the pathogenesis of cardiac hydrothorax, since the protein content of the pleural fluid is usually significantly greater (2 to 3 gm/dl) than that found in edema fluid (0.5 gm/dl). Hydrothorax is usually bilateral, but when unilateral it is usually confined to the right side of the chest and is caused most commonly by severe systemic venous hypertension, as occurs in tricuspid stenosis or constrictive pericarditis. Conversely, if the hydrothorax is limited to the left side, it is most commonly secondary to pulmonary venous hypertension (e.g., mitral stenosis). When hydrothorax develops, dyspnea usually becomes intensified owing to a further reduction in vital capacity. Although the excess fluid in hydrothorax is usually resorbed as the condition of the heart improves, interlobar effusions sometimes persist.

Ascites. This complication occurs in patients with increased pressure in the hepatic veins and in the veins draining the peritoneum (Fig. 15–6). Ascites usually reflects long-standing systemic venous hypertension, and in patients with organic tricuspid valve disease and chronic constrictive pericarditis, it may be more prominent than subcutaneous edema. As in the case of hydrothorax, there is increased capillary permeability because the protein content is similar to that of hepatic lymph, i.e., four to six times that of edema fluid. Protein-losing enteropathy may occur in patients with visceral congestion,[32] and the resultant reduced plasma oncotic pressure may lower the threshold for the development of ascites.

CARDIAC FINDINGS

Cardiomegaly. This finding is nonspecific and occurs in the majority of patients with chronic heart failure. Notable exceptions are heart failure due to chronic constrictive pericarditis, restrictive cardiomyopathy, and a variety

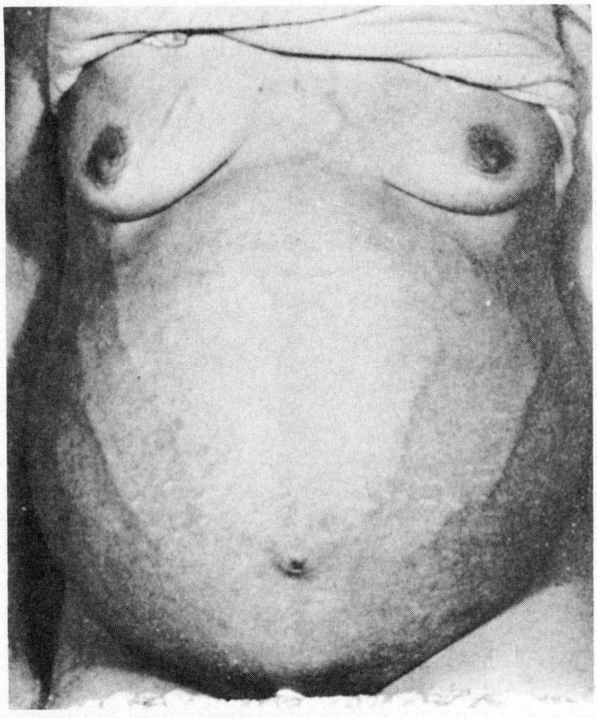

FIGURE 15–6 Gross ascites due to congestive heart failure. The everted umbilicus, distended abdominal veins, and striae are typical. (From Oram, S.: Heart failure. *In* Oram, S. [ed.]: Clinical Heart Disease. 2nd ed. London, William Heinemann Medical Books, Ltd., 1981, p. 666.)

of acute insults such as acute myocardial infarction, the sudden development of arrhythmias, or rupture of a valve or chordae tendineae; in such circumstances heart failure may occur before the heart has had a chance to enlarge.

Gallop Sounds. Protodiastolic sounds, generally emanating from the left ventricle (but occasionally from the right) and occurring 0.13 to 0.16 second after the second heart sound, are common findings in healthy children and young adults. Such physiological sounds are rarely audible in healthy persons after the age of 40 years but occur in patients of all ages with heart failure and are referred to as protodiastolic, or S_3, gallops. Thus, in older adults, they generally signify the presence of heart failure (p. 50). Protodiastolic gallops are caused by the sharp deceleration of ventricular inflow that occurs immediately after the early filling phase, perhaps accompanied by simultaneous closure of the atrioventricular valve; a reduction in ventricular distensibility, i.e., the ventricle operating on the steep portion of its diastolic pressure-volume curve (see Figure 12–23, p. 428), may contribute to their genesis. In patients with mitral or tricuspid regurgitation or left-to-right shunts, torrential flow into the ventricle in early diastole contributes to the generation of an S_3 (p. 50), but under these conditions this sound is not to be interpreted as signifying the presence of heart failure. In heart failure the atrioventricular pressure gradient during early filling may be high as a consequence of elevated atrial pressure, and the distensibility of the ventricle may be altered, resulting in a protodiastolic gallop. Thus, a protodiastolic gallop sound is an excellent sign of heart failure when other causes, such as a physiological S_3 occurring in a healthy child or young adult, constrictive pericarditis, mitral and tricuspid regurgitation, or a left-to-right shunt, can be excluded.

Left ventricular gallop sounds are best heard at the apex with the patient in the left lateral recumbent position and are frequently palpable, whereas right ventricular gallop sounds are best heard at the left sternal edge in the fourth or fifth interspace with the patient supine. Protodiastolic gallop sounds originating from the left ventricle tend to be louder *after* inspiration, whereas those originating from the right ventricle are best heard *during* inspiration. Gallop sounds are more readily audible in the presence of a rapid heart rate and may sometimes be elicited by a brief bout of exercise.

Pulsus Alternans (see also p. 25). This condition is characterized by a regular rhythm with alternation of strong and weak contractions (Fig. 15–7). It should be distinguished from the alternation of strong and weak beats that occurs in pulsus bigeminus, in which the weak beat follows the strong beat by a shorter time interval than the strong beat follows the weak, whereas in pulsus alternans they are equally spaced or the weak beat is slightly closer to the succeeding than to the preceding beat. Severe pulsus alternans may be detected either by palpation of the peripheral pulses (the femoral more readily than the brachial, radial, or carotid) or by sphygmomanometry. As the cuff is slowly deflated, only alternate beats are audible for a variable number of millimeters of Hg below the systolic level, depending on the severity of the alternans, and then all beats are heard. Occasionally, the weak beat is so small that the aortic valve is not opened, and this results in an apparent halving of the pulse rate, a condition referred to as *total alternans.* Pulsus alternans may be accompanied by alternation in the intensity of the heart sounds and of existing heart murmurs. With total alternans there is a first heart sound for each contraction, but the second heart sound may be absent, with the weak contractions owing to failure of the semilunar valves to open.

Pulsus alternans occurs most commonly in heart failure secondary to increased resistance to left ventricular ejection, as occurs in systemic hypertension and aortic stenosis, as well as in coronary atherosclerosis and cardiomyopathy. It is frequently associated with a ventricular protodiastolic gallop sound (S_3), usually signifies advanced myocardial disease, and often disappears with treatment of heart failure. Rarely, it may also occur in normal persons during tachycardia or following a single premature beat. In patients with heart failure, pulsus alternans can often be elicited by reduction in systemic venous return, as occurs with assumption of the erect posture or application of venous tourniquets, and it is reduced by an increase in venous return, as in recumbency or with exercise. In patients with heart disease, it tends to be present during tachycardia and is often initiated by a premature beat (Fig. 15–7).

Pulsus alternans is attributed to an alternation in the stroke volume ejected by the left ventricle[33] and ultimately to a deletion in the number of contracting cells in every other cycle due to incomplete recovery. Alternans is almost always concordant in the two sides of the circulation, i.e., the strong and weak beats occur simultaneously in the two ventricles. Rarely, pulsus alternans is accompanied by electrical alternans; however, the latter condition is usually not due to mechanical alternans but rather to alternating position of the heart within the fluid-filled pericardial sac (Figure 5–75, p. 132).

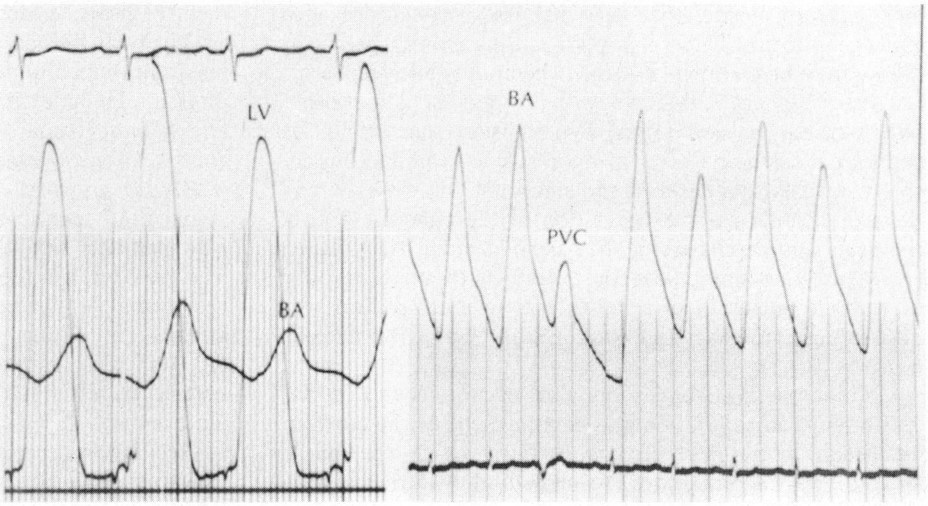

FIGURE 15–7 Pulsus alternans: *Left,* A classic strong-weak-strong-weak pattern in both brachial and left ventricular pulse pressures in tracings from a patient with aortic stenosis. *Right,* Premature ventricular contraction precipitates pulsus alternans, facilitating detection of this sign of left ventricular failure. (From Perloff, J. K.: The clinical manifestations of cardiac failure in adults. Hosp. Pract. *5*:43, 1970; and Braunwald, E. [ed.]: The Myocardium: Failure and Infarction. New York, HP Publishing Co., 1974, p. 93.)

Accentuation of P_2. With the development of left ventricular failure, pulmonary artery pressure rises, and P_2 becomes accentuated—often louder than A_2—and more widely transmitted. As the patient improves, P_2 becomes softer.

Systolic murmurs are common in heart failure owing to the relative mitral or tricuspid regurgitation that may occur secondary to ventricular dilatation. Often these murmurs diminish or disappear when compensation is restored.

Fever. A low-grade temperature ($<38°C$), which results from cutaneous vasoconstriction and therefore impairment of heat loss, may occur in severe heart failure; fever usually subsides when compensation is restored. Greater elevations of temperature often signify the presence of an infection, pulmonary infarction, or infective endocarditis.

Cardiac Cachexia. Long-standing, severe congestive heart failure, particularly of the right ventricle, may lead to anorexia, owing to hepatic and intestinal congestion and sometimes to digitalis intoxication. Occasionally, there is impaired intestinal absorption of fat[34] and rarely protein-losing enteropathy.[32] Patients with heart failure may also exhibit an increase in total metabolism, secondary to (1) an augmentation of myocardial oxygen consumption, as occurs in patients with aortic stenosis and hypertension; (2) excessive work of breathing; and (3) low-grade fever. The combination of a reduced caloric intake and increased caloric expenditure may lead to marked weight loss and, in severe cases, to cardiac cachexia.[35] In some patients the cachexia may be severe enough to suggest the presence of disseminated malignant disease.

Cheyne-Stokes Respiration. This condition, also known as periodic or cyclic respiration, is characterized by the combination of depression in the sensitivity of the respiratory center to carbon dioxide and left ventricular failure.[36,37] During the apneic phase, arterial pO_2 falls and pCO_2 rises; this combination excites the depressed respiratory center, resulting in hyperventilation and subsequently hypocapnia, followed by another period of apnea. The principal cause of Cheyne-Stokes respiration is a cerebral lesion such as cerebral arteriosclerosis, stroke, or head injury. These causes are often exaggerated by sleep, barbiturates, and narcotics, all of which further depress the sensitivity of the respiratory center. Left ventricular failure, which prolongs the circulation time from the lung to the brain, results in a sluggish response of the system and is responsible for the oscillations between apnea and hyperpnea and prevents return to a steady state of ventilation and blood gases. Occasionally, the patient with heart failure awakens at night with dyspnea precipitated by periodic (Cheyne-Stokes) respiration; this form of nocturnal dyspnea is not considered as ominous as classic paroxysmal nocturnal dyspnea.[38]

PATHOLOGICAL FINDINGS

Lungs. The lungs are enlarged, firm, dark, and filled with bloody fluid. When pulmonary congestion has been long-standing, they are brown with deposition of hemosiderin and usually do not seep edema fluid. On microscopic examination, the capillaries are engorged and there is thickening of the alveolar septa as well as extravasation of large mononuclear cells containing red blood cells or hemosiderin granules or both.[39] Often the pulmonary vessels show medial hypertrophy and intimal hyperplasia (p. 831).

Liver. In acute right heart failure, the liver is enlarged, firm, and filled with fluid. On microscopic examination, the central hepatic veins and sinusoids are dilated. With long-standing right heart failure, the liver returns to normal size, subsequently atrophies, and becomes "nutmeg" in appearance as a consequence of the dark red areas of central venous congestion and the lighter, fatty area in the periphery of the lobule. Cardiac cirrhosis is characterized by central lobular necrosis and atrophy as well as extensive fibrous retraction;[40] sometimes there is sclerosis of the hepatic veins. Since cardiac cirrhosis develops as a function of the level of hepatic venous pressure and the duration of its elevation, it is not surprising that it occurs most commonly in patients with chronic constrictive pericarditis and organic tricuspid valve disease who often have prolonged elevation of systemic venous pressure. In patients with left ventricular failure, central hepatic necrosis without evidence of passive congestion may be present.[41] Liver biopsies in patients with acute heart failure exhibiting fulminant hepatic failure showed replacement of hepatocytes by red blood cells.[42] Presumably, the hypoxia caused by hypoperfusion produces hepatocyte necrosis;[43] erythrocytes may then enter the space of Disse between damaged endothelial cells. These changes resulting from acute heart failure may be transient if there is hemodynamic recovery.

Other Viscera. Patients with chronic hepatic venous hypertension develop portal hypertension that results in congestive splenomegaly. On microscopic examination, the spleen reveals dilatation of the sinusoids and fibrosis, and there is chronic passive congestion of the pancreas and of the veins and capillaries of the gastrointestinal tract. Rarely, intense mesenteric vasoconstriction without thrombotic or embolic occlusion of a mesenteric artery may lead to a hemorrhagic, nonbacterial enterocolitis,[44] with hemorrhagic necrosis.

Chronic venous congestion also occurs in the kidney and brain, with dilatation and engorgement of the capillaries. Small infarcts are frequently observed in the spleen and kidneys of patients with long-standing atrial fibrillation.

LABORATORY FINDINGS

Proteinuria and a high urine specific gravity are common findings in heart failure. Blood urea nitrogen and creatinine levels are often moderately elevated secondary to reductions in renal blood flow and glomerular filtration rate[10] (p. 1750). The erythrocyte sedimentation rate is usually quite low secondary to impaired fibrinogen synthesis and resultant decreased fibrinogen concentrations.

SERUM ELECTROLYTES. Serum electrolyte values are generally normal in patients with heart failure prior to treatment. However, in severe heart failure, prolonged, rigid sodium restriction, coupled with intensive diuretic therapy as well as the inability to excrete water, may lead to hyponatremia (p. 1750). The hyponatremia is dilutional and occurs despite an expansion of extracellular fluid volume and an increase in total body sodium. It may be accompanied by, and presumably is caused in part by, elevated concentrations of circulating vasopressin.[45] Serum potassium levels are usually normal, although the prolonged administration of kaliuretic diuretics, such as the thiazides or loop diuretics, may result in hypokalemia (p. 531). Hyperkalemia may occur in patients with very severe heart failure who show marked reductions in glomerular filtration rate and inadequate delivery of sodium to the distal tubular sodium-potassium exchange sites, particularly if these patients are also receiving potassium-retaining diuretics (p. 1752).

Congestive hepatomegaly and cardiac cirrhosis are often associated with impaired hepatic function, characterized by abnormal values of serum glutamic oxaloacetic transaminase (SGOT) and other liver enzymes.[46,47] Hyperbilirubinemia, secondary to an increase in both the directly and the indirectly reacting bilirubins, is common, and in severe cases of acute (right or left) ventricular failure, frank jaundice may occur. Acute hepatic venous congestion can result in severe jaundice with a bilirubin level as high as 15 to 20 mg/dl, elevation of SGOT to more than 10 times the upper limit of normal, and elevation of the serum alkaline phosphatase level, as well as prolongation of the prothrombin time. Both the clinical and the laboratory pictures may resemble viral hepatitis, but the impairment of hepatic function is rapidly ameliorated by successful treatment of heart failure. In patients with long-standing cardiac cirrhosis, albumin synthesis may be impaired, with resultant hypoalbuminemia, intensifying the accumulation of fluid. Hepatic hypoglycemia, fulminant hepatic failure, and hepatic coma are rare, late, and sometimes terminal complications of cardiac cirrhosis.[48–51]

Venous pressure can be conveniently measured with a spinal fluid manometer while the patient is in the recumbent position and the arm is abducted from the thorax. The baseline for the measurement should be 5 cm below the sternal angle, i.e., the estimated position of the right atrium. The venous pressure is often elevated (i.e., > 12 cm H_2O) at rest, but in mild or borderline cases it may be normal at rest but rises with hepatic compression or during exercise.

Circulation time can be measured by rapid intravenous injection of 3 to 5 ml of 20 per cent dehydrocholic acid (Decholin), with a bitter taste designating the endpoint. The normal range in adults is 9 to 16 seconds. Circulation time varies directly with the volume of blood in which the indicator is diluted and inversely with the velocity of blood flow. Therefore, pulmonary and/or systemic venous congestion, as well as reduced cardiac output, causes prolongation. Because of the high velocity of blood flow, circulation time tends to be normal or even shortened in patients with high-output heart failure. Although circulation time is not a particularly sensitive test for heart failure, it may be useful in differentiating between pulmonary or cardiac dyspnea and between low- and high-output cardiac failure.

THE VALSALVA MANEUVER. This maneuver—forced expiration against a closed glottis—is helpful in the diagnosis of heart failure.[52] The standard test consists of asking the patient to blow against an aneroid manometer and to maintain a pressure of 40 mm Hg for 30 seconds. The Valsalva maneuver raises intrathoracic pressure, venous return to the heart diminishes, stroke volume falls, and venous pressure rises. Arterial pressure tracings normally show four distinct phases (Fig. 15–8): (1) an initial rise in arterial pressure, which represents transmission to the periphery of the increased intrathoracic pressure; (2) with continuation of the strain and the accompanying reduction of venous return, reductions in systolic, diastolic, and pulse pressures accompanied by a reflex increase in heart rate; (3) on release of the strain, a sudden drop of arterial pressure equivalent to the fall in intrathoracic pressure; and (4) an overshoot of arterial pressure to above control levels, with a wide pulse pressure and bradycardia due to the combination of the inrush into the heart of blood that had been dammed up in the venous bed and reflex vasoconstriction and tachycardia secondary to the low perfusion pressure of the carotid and baroreceptors during phase 3.

In heart failure[52] (Fig. 15–9), phases 1 and 3 are normal, i.e., there is normal transmission of the elevated intrathoracic pressure into the arterial tree during phase 1 and sudden loss of this with the release of the strain during phase 3. However, since the heart operates on the flat portion of its Starling curve (see Figure 13–17, p. 463), the impedance of venous return during phase 2 does not affect stroke volume. Therefore the baroreceptor reflex is not activated, and there is no overshoot upon release of the

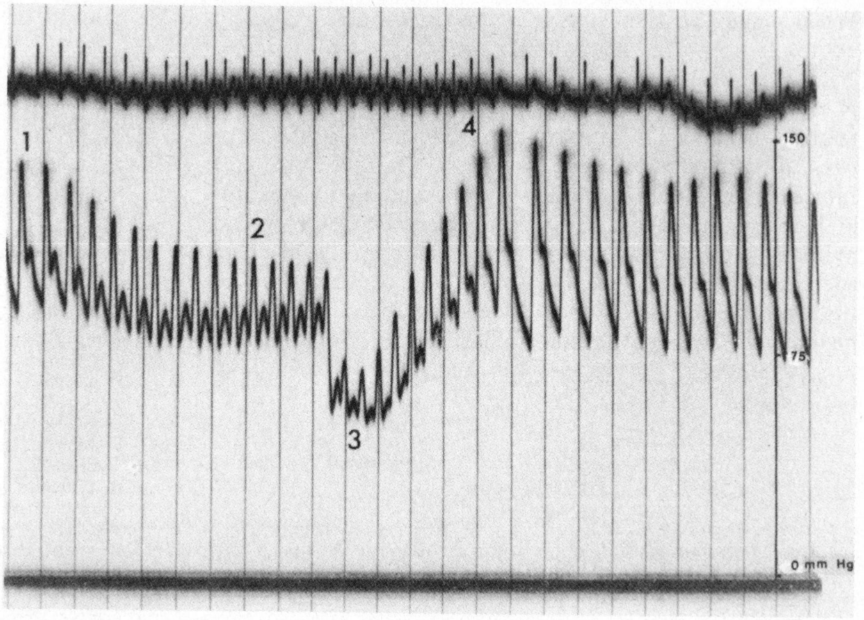

FIGURE 15–8 Normal response to Valsalva maneuver. Intraarterial pressure tracing. The four phases (see text) are denoted. (From Oram, S.: Further bedside examination. *In* Oram, S. [ed.]: Clinical Heart Disease. 2nd ed. London, William Heinemann Medical Books, Ltd., 1981, p. 668.)

strain. This results in a "square-wave" appearance of the tracing. Although the Valsalva maneuver can be recorded most accurately through an indwelling needle, careful palpation of the pulse in normal individuals allows detection of phases 2 and 4 and their absence, in particular, slowing of the pulse in phase 4 in heart failure.[53]

The Chest Roentgenogram

(See also Chap. 6)

Two principal features of the chest roentgenogram are useful in the patient with congestive heart failure.

The *size and shape of the cardiac silhouette* provide important information concerning the precise nature of the underlying heart disease. Both the cardiothoracic ratio (see Figure 6–16, p. 158) and the heart volume determined on the plain film (see Figure 6–17, p. 159) are relatively specific but insensitive indicators of increased left ventricular end-diastolic volume and reduced ejection fraction.

In the presence of normal pulmonary capillary and venous pressure in the erect position, the lung bases are better perfused than the apices, and the vessels supplying the lower lobes are significantly larger than are those supplying the upper lobes. With elevation of left atrial, pulmonary venous, and capillary pressures, interstitial and perivascular edema develops and is most prominent at the lung bases because hydrostatic pressure is greater there.[54] The resultant compression of pulmonary vessels in the lower lobes causes equalization in size of the vessels to the apices and bases when pulmonary capillary pressure is slightly elevated, i.e., approximately 13 to 17 mm Hg.[55,56] With greater pressure elevation (approximately 18 to 23 mm Hg), actual pulmonary vascular redistribution occurs, i.e., further constriction of vessels leading to the lower lobes and dilatation of vessels leading to the upper lobes.

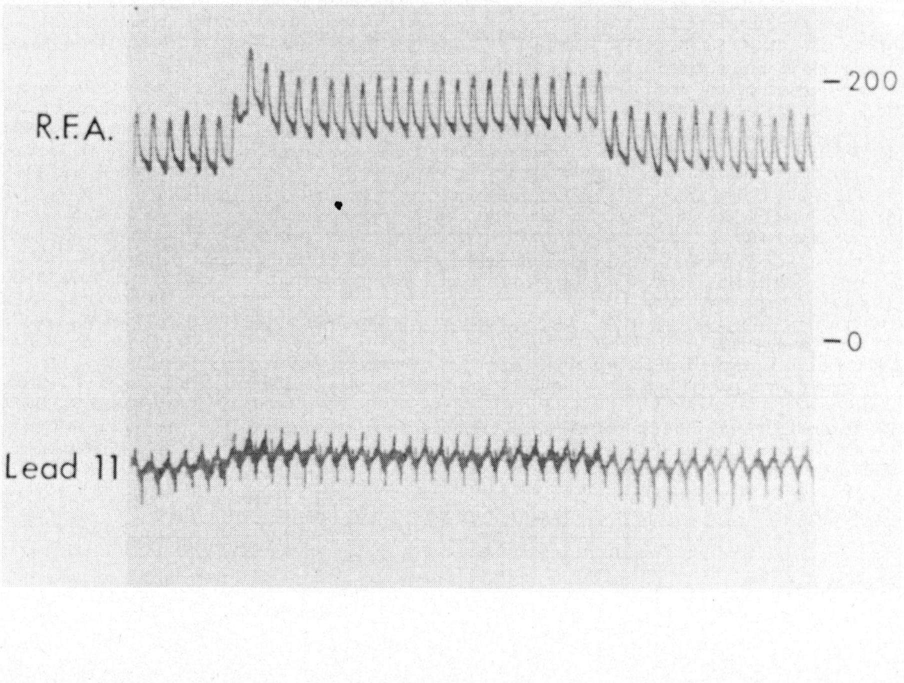

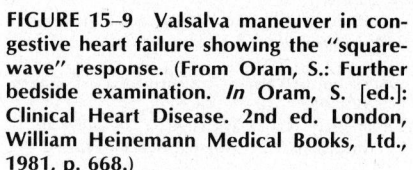

FIGURE 15–9 Valsalva maneuver in congestive heart failure showing the "square-wave" response. (From Oram, S.: Further bedside examination. *In* Oram, S. [ed.]: Clinical Heart Disease. 2nd ed. London, William Heinemann Medical Books, Ltd., 1981, p. 668.)

When pulmonary capillary pressures exceed approximately 20 to 25 mm Hg, interstitial pulmonary edema occurs. This may be of several varieties: (1) *septal,* producing Kerley's lines (i.e., sharp, linear densities of interlobular interstitial edema); (2) *perivascular,* producing loss of sharpness of the central and peripheral vessels; and (3) *subpleural,* producing spindle-shaped accumulations of fluid between the lung and adjacent pleural surface. When pulmonary capillary pressure exceeds 25 mm Hg, alveolar edema, with a cloudlike appearance and concentration of the fluid around the hili in a "butterfly pattern," and large pleural effusions may occur.[56] With elevation of systemic venous pressure, the azygos vein and superior vena cava may enlarge.[57]

References

1. Lewis, T.: Diseases of the Heart. New York, The Macmillan Co., 1933, p. 1.
2. Braunwald, E., Mock, M. B., and Watson, J. (eds.): Congestive Heart Failure. Current Research and Clinical Applications, New York, Grune and Stratton, 1982, 384 pp.
3. O'Brien, C. P.: Approaches to heart failure. *In* Brandenburg, R. O. (ed.): Office cardiology. Cardiovasc. Clin. *10*:33, 1980.
4. Hope, J. A.: Treatise on the Diseases of the Heart and Great Vessels. London, Williams-Kidd, 1832.
5. Williams, J. F., Jr., Sonnenblick, E. H., and Braunwald, E.: Determinants of atrial contractile force in intact heart. Am. J. Physiol. *209*:1061, 1965.
6. Starling, E. H.: Linacre Lecture on the Law of the Heart (1915). London, Longmans, 1918.
7. Ross, J., Jr., and Braunwald, E.: Studies on Starling's law of the heart. IX. The effects of impeding venous return on performance of the normal and failing human left ventricle. Circulation *30*:719, 1964.
8. Stampfer, M., Epstein, S. E., Beiser, G. D., and Braunwald, E.: Hemodynamic effects of diuresis at rest and during intense upright exercise in patients with impaired cardiac function. Circulation *37*:900, 1968.
9. Mackenzie, J.: Disease of the Heart. 3rd ed. London, Oxford University Press, 1913.
10. Hricik, D. E., and Kassirer, J. P.: Azotemia in cardiac failure. J. Cardiovasc. Med. (In press.)
11. Davis, J. O.: The mechanism of salt and water retention in cardiac failure. In Braunwald, E. (ed.): The Myocardium: Failure and Infarction. New York, HP Publishing Co., 1974, pp. 80–92.
12. Tan, S. Y., and Mulrow, P. J.: Aldosterone in hypertension and edema. *In* Bondy, P. K., and Rosenberg, L. E. (eds.): Metabolic Control and Disease. 8th ed. Philadelphia, W. B. Saunders Co., 1980, p. 1516.
13. Spann, J. F., Chidsey, C. A., Pool, P. E., and Braunwald, E.: Mechanism of norepinephrine depletion in experimental heart failure produced by aortic constriction in the guinea pig. Circ. Res. *17*:312, 1965.
14. Chidsey, C. A., Kaiser, G. A., Sonnenblick, E. H., Spann, J. F., and Braunwald, E.: Cardiac norepinephrine stores in experimental heart failure in the dog. J. Clin. Invest. *43*:2386, 1964.
15. Chandler, B. M., Sonnenblick, E. H., Spann, J. F., and Pool, P. E.: Association of depressed myofibrillar adenosinetriphosphate and reduced contractility in experimental heart failure. Circ. Res. *21*:717, 1967.
16. Artman, M., and Graham, T. P., Jr.: Congestive heart failure in infancy: Recognition and management. Am. Heart J. *103*:1040, 1982.
17. Sodeman, W. A., and Burch, G. E.: The precipitating causes of congestive heart failure. Am. Heart J. *15*:22, 1938.
18. Braunwald, E., and Frahm, C. J.: Studies on Starling's law of the heart. IV. Observations on the hemodynamic functions of the left atrium in man. Circulation *24*:633, 1961.
19. Franciosa, J. A., Park, M., and Levine, T. B.: Lack of correlation between exercise capacity and indexes of resting left ventricular performance in heart failure. Am. J. Cardiol. *47*:33, 1981.
20. Perera, G. A., and Berliner, R. W.: The relation of postural hemodilution to paroxysmal dyspnea. J. Clin. Invest. *22*:25, 1943.
21. Collins, J. V., Clark, T. J. H., and Brown, D. J.: Airway function in healthy subjects and in patients with left heart disease. Clin. Sci. Molec. Med. *49*:217, 1975.
22. Marshall, R., McIroy, M. B., and Christie, R. V.: The work of breathing in mitral stenosis. Clin. Sci. *17*:667, 1958.
23. Fishman, A. P. (ed.): Pulmonary Diseases and Disorders. New York, McGraw-Hill Book Co., 1980, pp. 44–67.
24. Macklem, P. T.: Respiratory muscles: The vital pump. Chest *78*:753, 1980.
25. Turino, G. M.: Origins of cardiac dyspnea. Primary Cardiol. *7*:76, 1981.
26. Fishman, A. P., and Ledlie, J. F.: Dyspnea. Bull. Eur. Physiopathol. Resp. *15*: 789, 1979.
27. Campbell, E. J. M., Agostoni, E., and Newsom Davis, J.: The Respiratory Muscles: Mechanisms and Neural Control. 2nd ed. Philadelphia, W. B. Saunders Co., 1970.
28. Higgins, C. B., Vatner, S. F., Franklin, D., and Braunwald, E.: Effects of experimentally produced heart failure on the peripheral vascular response to severe exercise in conscious dogs. Circ. Res. *31*:186, 1972.
29. Criteria Committee, New York Heart Association, Inc.: Diseases of the Heart and Blood Vessels. Nomenclature and Criteria for Diagnosis. 6th ed. Boston, Little, Brown and Co., 1964, p. 114.
30. Goldman, L., Hashimoto, B., Cook, E. F., and Loscalzo, A.: Comparative reproducibility and validity of symptoms for assessing cardiovascular functional class. Advantages of a new specific activity scale. Circulation *64*:1227, 1981.
31. Earnest, D. L., and Hurst, J. W.: Exophthalmos, stare and increase in intraocular pressure and systolic propulsion of the eyeballs due to congestive heart failure. Am. J. Cardiol. *26*:351, 1970.
32. Strober, W., Cohen, L. S., Waldmann, T. A., and Braunwald, E.: Tricuspid regurgitation: A newly recognized cause of protein-losing enteropathy, lymphocytopenia and immunologic deficiency. Am. J. Med. *44*:842, 1968.
33. Gleason, W. L., and Braunwald, E.: Studies on Starling's law of the heart. VI. Relationships between left ventricular end-diastolic volume and stroke volume in man with observations on the mechanism of pulsus alternans. Circulation *25*: 841, 1962.
34. Berkowitz, D., Croll, M. N., and Likoff, W.: Malabsorption as a complication of congestive heart failure. Am. J. Cardiol. *11*:43, 1963.
35. Pittman, J. G., and Cohen, P.: The pathogenesis of cardiac cachexia. N. Engl. J. Med. *27*:403, 1964.
36. Brown, H. W., and Plum, F.: The neurological basis of Cheyne-Stokes respiration. Am. J. Med. *30*:849, 1940.
37. Lange, R. L., and Hecht, H. H.: The mechanism of Cheyne-Stokes respiration. J. Clin. Invest. *41*:42, 1962.
38. Rees, P. J., and Clark, T. J. H.: Paroxysmal nocturnal dyspnoea and periodic respiration. Lancet *2*:1315, 1979.
39. Friedman-Mor, Z., Chalon, J., Turndorf, H., and Orkin, L. R.: Cardiac index and incidence of heart failure cells. Arch. Pathol. Lab. Med. *102*:418, 1978.
40. Moschcowitz, E.: The morphology and pathogenesis of cardiac fibrosis of the liver. Ann. Intern. Med. *36*:933, 1952.
41. Cohen, J. A., and Kaplan, M. M.: Left-sided heart failure presenting as hepatitis. Gastroenterology *74*:583, 1978.
42. Kanel, G. C., Ucci, A. A., Kaplan, M. M., and Wolfe, H. J.: A distinctive perivenular hepatic lesion associated with heart failure. Am. J. Clin. Pathol. *73*: 235, 1980.
43. Nouel, O., Henrion, J., Bernuau, J., DeGott, C., Rueff, B., and Benhamou, J.-P.: Fulminant hepatic failure due to transient circulatory failure in patients with chronic heart disease. Dig. Dis. Sci. *25*:49, 1980.
44. Wilson, R., and Qualheim, R. E.: A form of acute hemorrhagic enterocolitis afflicting chronically ill individuals. Gastroenterology *27*:431, 1954.
45. Szatalowicz, V. L., Arnold, P. E., Chaimovitz, C., Bichet, D., Beri, T., and Schrier, R. W.: Radioimmunoassay of plasma arginine vasopressin in hyponatremic patients with congestive heart failure. N. Engl. J. Med. *305*:263, 1981.
46. West, M., Pilz, C. G., and Zimmerman, H. J.: Serum enzymes in disease: III. Significance of abnormal serum enzyme levels in cardiac failure. Am. J. Med. Sci. *241*:350, 1960.
47. Kaplan, M. M.: Liver dysfunction secondary to congestive heart failure. Practical Cardiol. *6*:39, 1980.
48. Kaymakcalan, H., Dourdourekas, D., Szanto, P. B., and Steigmann, F.: Congestive heart failure as cause of fulminant hepatic failure. Am. J. Med. *65*:384, 1978.
49. Dunn, G. D., Hayes, P., Breen, K. J., and Schenker, S.: The liver in congestive heart failure. A review. Am. J. Med. Sci. *265*:174, 1973.
50. Benzing, G., III, Schubert, W., Hug, G., and Kaplan, S.: Simultaneous hypoglycemia and acute congestive heart failure. Circulation *40*:209, 1969.
51. Kisloff, B., and Schaffer, G.: Fulminant hepatic failure secondary to congestive heart failure. Am. J. Dig. Dis. *21*:895, 1976.
52. Gorlin, R., Knowles, J. H., and Storey, C. F.: The Valsalva maneuver as a test of cardiac function. Pathologic physiology and clinical significance. Am. J. Med. *22*:197, 1957.
53. Elisberg, E. I.: Heart rate response to the Valsalva maneuver as a test of circulatory integrity. J.A.M.A. *186*:200, 1963.
54. Jefferson, K., and Rees, S.: Pulmonary venous hypertension. *In* Jefferson, K., and Rees, S. (eds.): Clinical Cardiac Radiology. London, Butterworth and Co., 1973, pp. 84–94.
55. Levin, D. C., Hessel, S. J., Mann, T., Swensson, R. G., Grossman, W., Baumstark, A., and Abrams, H. L.: Estimation of pulmonary capillary wedge pressure from chest radiographs. Radiology (in press).
56. Spindola-Franco, H.: Plain film diagnosis of congestive heart failure. J. Med. Soc. N.J. *75*:783, 1978.
57. Daves, M. L.: Cardiac Roentgenology. Chicago, Year Book Medical Publishers, 1981, pp. 78–86.

16 THE MANAGEMENT OF HEART FAILURE

by Thomas W. Smith, M.D., and Eugene Braunwald, M.D.

INTRODUCTION

Three general approaches are employed in the treatment of heart failure:

1. *Removal of the Underlying Cause.* This—the most desirable approach—involves surgical correction of structural abnormalities responsible for heart failure, such as congenital malformations and acquired valvular lesions, or medical treatment of conditions such as infective endocarditis or hypertension.

2. *Removal of the Precipitating Cause.* The recognition, prompt treatment, and, whenever possible, prevention of the specific causes or incidents that produce or exacerbate heart failure, such as infections, arrhythmias, and pulmonary emboli (p. 491), are critical to successful management of heart failure.

3. *Control of the Congestive Heart Failure State.* This approach, the subject of this chapter, may be divided into three categories (Table 16–1):

a. *Improvement of the heart's pumping performance,* which consists of efforts to restore the contractility of the failing heart toward normal.

b. *Reduction of the heart's workload,* which involves reduction of the demands placed on the heart to generate pressure and/or to pump blood.

c. *Control of excessive salt and water retention,* i.e., control of the expansion of extracellular fluid volume, which is the principal cause of many manifestations of heart failure, such as dyspnea and edema.

In each of these last three categories, a number of therapeutic measures are available. As outlined in Table 16–2, numbers 2 (digitalis) and 6 (other inotropic agents) contribute to the direct improvement of the heart's pumping performance; numbers 1 (restriction of physical activity) and 5 (vasodilators) involve reducing the heart's workload; while numbers 3 (restriction of sodium intake), 4 (diuretics), and 7 (physical removal of excess fluid) involve control of excessive salt and water retention.

TABLE 16–1 CONTROL OF CONGESTIVE HEART FAILURE

1. *Improvement of Pumping Performance*
   (A) Digitalis glycoside
   (B) Sympathomimetic agents
   (C) Other positive inotropic agents
   (D) Pacemaker
2. *Reduction of Workload*
   (A) Physical and emotional rest
   (B) Treatment of obesity
   (C) Vasodilator therapy
   (D) Assisted circulation
3. *Control of Excessive Salt and Water Retention*
   (A) Low-sodium diet
   (B) Diuretics
   (C) Mechanical removal of fluid
      (1) Thoracentesis
      (2) Paracentesis
      (3) Dialysis
      (4) Phlebotomy

TABLE 16–2 OUTLINE OF TREATMENT OF CHRONIC CONGESTIVE HEART FAILURE*

1. *Restriction of Physical Activity*
   (A) Discontinue exhausting sports and heavy labor
   (B) Discontinue full-time work or equivalent activity, introduce rest periods during the day
   (C) Confine to house
   (D) Confine to bed-chair
2. *Digitalis Glycoside*
   (A) Usual maintenance dose
   (B) Maximally tolerable dose
3. *Restriction of Sodium Intake*
   (A) Eliminate saltshaker at table (Na = 1.6 to 2.8 gm)
   (B) Eliminate salt in cooking and at table (Na = 1.2 to 1.8 gm)
   (C) Institute A and B above plus low-sodium diet (Na = 0.2 to 1.0 gm)
4. *Diuretics*
   (A) Moderate diuretics (thiazide†)
   (B) "Loop" diuretic (ethacrynic acid or furosemide)
   (C) "Loop" diuretic plus distal tubular (potassium-sparing) diuretic
   (D) "Loop" diuretic plus thiazide and distal tubular diuretic
5. *Vasodilators*
   (A) Hydralazine plus isosorbide dinitrate combination or prazosin
   (B) Captopril
   (C) Intravenous nitroprusside
6. *Other Inotropic Agents* (dopamine, dobutamine)
7. *Special Measures* (thoracentesis, paracentesis, dialysis, assisted circulation, cardiac transplantation)

*Numbers and letters correspond to Figure 16–1.
†Thiazide or a diuretic of approximately equal potency, such as metolazone.

THERAPEUTIC STRATEGY IN THE TREATMENT OF HEART FAILURE

CHRONIC HEART FAILURE. A condition as variable as congestive heart failure cannot be treated according to a simple formula. Intelligent management depends on an appreciation of the nature of the underlying condition and the rapidity of its progression; the presence of associated illnesses; the patient's age, occupation, personality, life style, family setting, and ability and motivation to cooperate with treatment; and, importantly, the response to therapeutic measures.[1] With the recognition that wide differences exist among individual patients, Figure 16–1 is presented as a general guide to the therapy of adult patients with chronic congestive heart failure in whom the underlying disease is not amenable to further treatment and in whom precipitating causes have been eliminated to the maximum extent possible. The course of heart failure is rarely smoothly progressive; rather, it is usually punctuated by a series of abrupt downward steps due to acute decompensation, generally as a consequence of one of the precipitating causes of heart failure described on p. 492. When the precipitating cause has been removed and treatment has been intensified, the patient's previous condition is often restored. In other patients there are long periods—many months or even years—when the course is stable without any discernible deterioration.

Ordinarily, treatment of heart failure is not begun until the first symptoms of diminished cardiac reserve occur, i.e., until the patient enters New York Heart Association Class II. The general strategy is to utilize, first, relatively simple means, such as administration of digitalis glycosides or diuretics, mild restriction of physical activity, and reduction of sodium dietary intake. If symptoms and signs of heart failure persist despite these measures, progressively stricter and more aggressive measures must be employed. As has been pointed out elsewhere (p. 493), the earliest symptoms of heart failure usually appear during heavy exertion. When symptoms of dyspnea on exertion or orthopnea are due to ischemia-induced impairment of ventricular diastolic relaxation rather than to diminished systolic contraction, specific measures to reduce myocardial ischemia are in order (see Chapter 40). When it has become clear that these symptoms are indeed related to impaired cardiovascular reserve, two forms of treatment are begun simultaneously: discontinuation of intense physical exertion, i.e., heavy labor and competitive or exhausting sports (1A*); and improvement of the pumping performance of the heart with a usual maintenance dose of a digitalis glycoside (2A*). Obese patients should be encouraged to lose weight, and systemic hypertension, if present, must be treated vigorously. Most patients initially respond to these relatively simple measures, but if symptoms secondary to extracellular fluid accumulation again appear, dietary sodium intake should be restricted. This may consist merely of eliminating the saltshaker at the table (3A*). If heart failure persists or advances despite these measures, an oral diuretic such as a thiazide or an agent of similar potency should be administered (4A*).

When, despite the measures outlined above, a patient is symptomatic upon ordinary exertion such as nondemanding work, shopping, cleaning the home, i.e., when de-

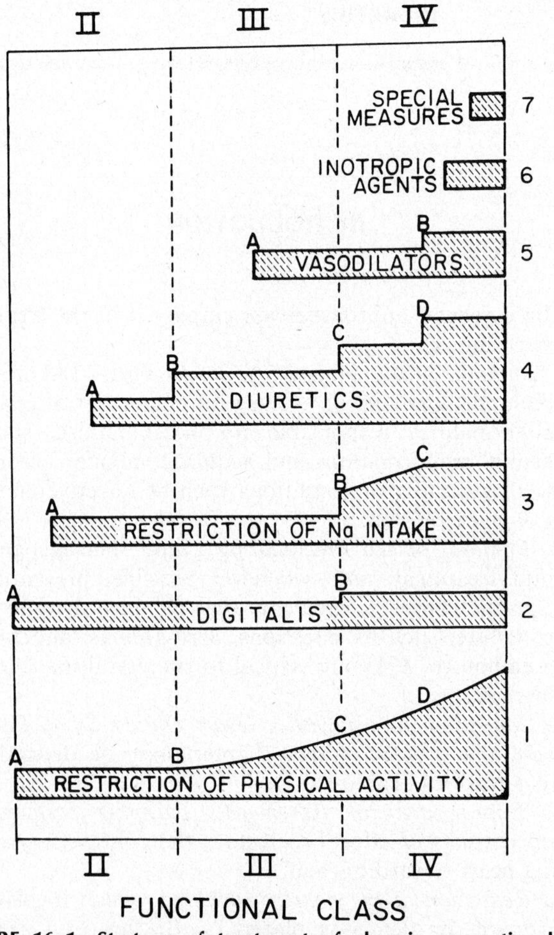

FIGURE 16–1 Strategy of treatment of chronic congestive heart failure in the adult. Various modes of therapy and the intensity of their application at various stages of the patient's course are plotted. For further explanation, see Table 16–2.

terioration into functional Class III (p. 496) has occurred, certain of the measures already taken should be intensified. Full-time work or its equivalent is reduced, the patient is advised to take one or two rest periods during the day (1B*), and a more powerful diuretic—furosemide or ethacrynic acid—is substituted for the thiazide (4B*). When a patient becomes a "late Class III" and is increasingly symptomatic upon ordinary activity, vasodilators may be given (5A*). In some clinical circumstances (e.g., mitral regurgitation), vasodilators may be of particular value and should be considered earlier in the clinical course.

In patients who are symptomatic at rest or with minimal activity, i.e., functional Class IV, confinement to the home is necessary (1C*), and the dose of the cardiac glycoside is cautiously raised to achieve the maximum level consistent with an adequate margin of safety (2B*). All salt is eliminated at the table and in cooking (3B*), and a potassium-sparing diuretic that acts on the distal tubule, such as spironolactone or triamterene, is added to the "loop" diuretic (4C*). If further deterioration occurs, hospitalization is usually required. Other inotropic agents such as a sympathomimetic amine (6*) are administered, physical activity is drastically curtailed (1D*), a low-sodium (200 mg) diet is instituted (3C*), the number and/or dose of diuretics is increased (4D*), intravenous vasodilators may be administered (5B*), and the application of special measures (7*) such as the physical removal of fluid (thoracentesis, paracentesis, or dialysis) or, under special circumstances, the application of assisted circulation or cardiac transplantation may be considered.

To reemphasize the importance of individualizing the treatment of heart failure, a few explanations of this therapeutic strategy are in order.

1. It appears more logical to commence therapy by improving cardiac contractility with a cardiac glycoside and to reduce or eliminate those activities that usually precipitate symptoms of cardiac failure (i.e., to diminish the discrepancy between the heart's ability to pump blood and the requirements of the metabolizing tissues [Fig. 16–2]) as opposed to commencing therapy with diuretics, which treat a complication of heart failure (i.e., the abnormal retention of sodium and water). Nevertheless, certain subsets of patients, such as those with mild symptoms and signs of failure whose physical activity is limited by age or other infirmity, may be treated initially with thiazide diuretics with a more favorable risk-benefit ratio. Also, certain patients with an unusual propensity to develop overt digitalis toxicity may be more appropriately treated initially with a diuretic.

2. Restriction of physical activity is carried out in a manner so as to disturb the patient's life style as little as possible (p. 506).

3. Similarly, restriction of sodium intake need be only mild initially and consist of eliminating the saltshaker at the table, unless heart failure is severe. The availability of potent diuretics allows the patient to eat a nutritious and palatable diet for the major portion of the course of the disease.

4. There is considerable debate about when in the course of heart failure vasodilator treatment should be initiated. It has been proposed that the treatment of heart failure can begin with these drugs rather than with digitalis or diuretics. While the efficacy of this mode of therapy is unquestioned, many patients do not derive long-term benefit (or cannot tolerate side effects) from the chronic oral use of vasodilators (p. 541). Furthermore, in the absence of pulmonary congestion, vasodilators produce little if any rise in cardiac output and may cause a dangerous fall in arterial pressure. Accordingly, it is recommended that vasodilator therapy be begun when the patient has become symptomatic upon mild activity despite optimal use of digitalis and loop diuretics. It is appropriate to use these agents *before* rigid dietary sodium restriction, multiple diuretics, or intravenous inotropic agents are employed.

Since there are many exceptions to this general thera-

*These number and letter designations refer to both Figure 16–1 and Table 16–2.

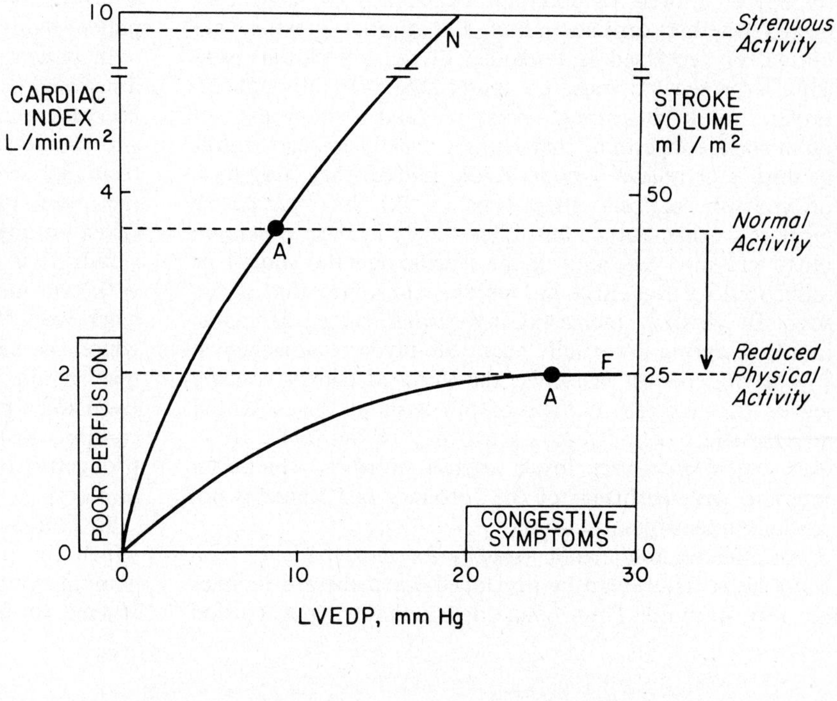

FIGURE 16–2 Diagram demonstrating the relationship between left ventricular end-diastolic pressure (LVEDP) and cardiac index (left ordinate) or stroke volume (right ordinate) in a normal (N) and a failing (F) heart. The upper limit of normal of LVEDP (12 mm Hg) and lower limit of normal of CI (2.2 liters/min/m²) are shown, as are the values associated with congestive symptoms (LVEDP > 20 mm Hg) and with impaired perfusion (< 2.2 liters/min/m²). A and A′ represent the operating points at rest of a hypothetical patient with heart failure and of a normal person, respectively. Reduction of physical activity allows the failing heart to meet the demands of the metabolizing tissues. A positive inotropic agent displaces the curve from F toward N.

peutic strategy, a few examples are provided to demonstrate how it may be modified in specific circumstances:

1. If a patient's livelihood is dependent on physical labor and transfer to a more sedentary occupation cannot be readily accomplished, moderate restriction of sodium intake and diuretics can be begun along with digitalis, and marked restriction of physical activity can be deferred, often for a number of years. Also, the administration of digitalis (with or without ancillary use of verapamil or a beta-adrenergic blocking agent), by controlling ventricular rate in a patient with atrial fibrillation and limitation of functional activity, may restore the patient to near-normal cardiac reserve, and restriction of physical activity can be avoided.

2. Occasional patients with left ventricular failure exhibit symptoms of paroxysmal nocturnal dyspnea that are particularly troublesome, yet they are able to engage in almost normal physical activity during the day. In such patients the paroxysmal nocturnal dyspnea can often be prevented by the administration in the evening of a long-acting venodilator such as nitroglycerin ointment or other transdermal preparation, or by the intensification of diuretic therapy, and they can be maintained in functional Class II.

3. Some patients cannot tolerate vasodilators. They become severely hypotensive, develop an adverse reaction to one of the drugs after prolonged use (e.g., the lupus-like syndrome due to hydralazine), or are unwilling (or unable) to take multiple medications several times a day. Such patients may fare better with more rigid restriction of dietary sodium at an early stage of the disease, and the vasodilator can be held in reserve until later.

4. Occasional patients are particularly prone to accumulate fluid in serous cavities, in which case thoracentesis and/or paracentesis may rapidly relieve dyspnea and need not be reserved until a more advanced phase of the illness.

ACUTE HEART FAILURE (see also p. 571). Treatment of patients with acute congestive cardiac failure usually involves a choice among diuretics, vasodilators, and inotropic agents. In selecting from these three modes of therapy it is well to ascertain by clinical or laboratory means whether cardiac output and arterial pressure are normal or depressed and whether or not myocardial ischemia is present. It must be appreciated that although *diuretics* diminish filling pressure and symptoms of pulmonary congestion, they do not usually increase cardiac output or relieve hypoperfusion; indeed, they may have precisely the opposite effect (Fig. 16–12). *Inotropic agents* increase cardiac output but differ widely in their effects on blood pressure. Selection of the specific agent(s) should be influenced by the effect on vascular resistance that is desired. By virtue of increasing myocardial oxygen demands, inotropic agents potentially aggravate myocardial ischemia. In the presence of ischemia, therefore, afterload-reducing agents that increase cardiac output without this potential adverse effect of inotropic agents may be desirable. However, *vasodilators* may lower arterial pressure, which can interfere with perfusion of the coronary bed, thereby potentially intensifying ischemia.

An effective therapeutic strategy for most patients with acute heart failure can be developed when these principles are kept in mind. Thus, congestion without hypoperfusion should be treated with diuretics. If blood pressure is elevated or normal, vasodilators are indicated if heart failure is severe. The combination of congestion and hypoperfusion should be treated with a vasodilator and diuretic as long as arterial pressure is not depressed, and with positive inotropic agents when blood pressure is depressed.

In transient acute heart failure (e.g., that following acute cardiopulmonary bypass), the most effective therapy may consist of a short period of additional inotropic support with infusion of a sympathomimetic agent, or of reduction of the cardiac workload by applying intraaortic balloon counterpulsation.

General Measures

REST. Reduced physical activity is critical in the care of patients with heart failure throughout their entire course (Fig. 16–1). The intensity of the restriction should depend, of course, on the severity of the heart failure. Until relatively recently it was common practice to reduce markedly the physical activity of patients with enlarged hearts in functional Class II; as a consequence, these patients led unnecessarily restricted lives for many years. Now, the usual recommendation is to tailor the degree of physical activity depending on the symptoms in patients with impaired cardiac reserve. For example, if dyspnea occurs only while a patient is loading cartons into a truck or climbing four flights of stairs, he or she should be advised to make every effort to discontinue these particular activities. If it is essential for them to be continued, they should be carried out more slowly and should be interrupted by rest periods. Competitive or exhausting sports should be discontinued. As is the case in patients with angina pectoris (p. 1346), regular physical activity to a level which does not regularly produce symptoms is desirable in patients with congestive heart failure. Often relatively minor adjustments in activity will allow a patient with mild heart failure to remain gainfully employed or a homemaker to continue routine tasks. Insofar as recreation is concerned, again, minor adjustments, such as the use of a golf cart, may allow the patient many hours of pleasurable activity.

In patients with more severe heart failure, i.e., those in functional Class III, the problem of continued employment becomes more difficult. Such patients are usually unable, and should not be encouraged, to work full-time, even at a relatively sedentary job. This should not mean, however, that total unemployment is necessary or even desirable. Often an adjustment of the work schedule is feasible, e.g., a reduction of the working day from 8 to 5 or 6 hours, with two mandatory one-hour rest periods, or a four-day work week, with a day in the middle of the week during which the patient remains at home to rest. Evening activities should be curtailed but need not be discontinued. Even some patients who are in functional Class IV and are confined to the home are able to lead more satisfying and productive lives by working for two or three hours a day at a desk.

In contrast to the situation in chronic heart failure, in which the patient is urged to remain active short of becoming symptomatic, *physical activity should be rigidly restricted in the presence of acute cardiac decompensation.*

Under these circumstances it is almost always desirable to hospitalize the patient, since this will facilitate work-up and the search for a precipitating cause and will allow adjustment of medication and institution of additional therapeutic measures while the patient is under observation. Hospitalization also facilitates more rigid restriction of sodium intake than is usually possible at home and allows more rigorous control of the restriction of physical activity. Although physical rest plays a crucial role in the treatment of heart failure, complete physical rest does not mean complete rest in bed. Indeed, patients are usually more comfortable and the venous return (and therefore the cardiac preload) is lower when the patient is sitting rather than supine. Also, patients should not be forced to use the bedpan, and trips to the bathroom can usually be allowed. On the other hand, too much relaxation of the rules restricting physical activity can obviate the value of physical rest. For examples, frequent walks to another room on the hospital floor to visit with family or friends, watch television, eat, or use the telephone may nullify the potential benefit of rest.

The hazards of phlebothrombosis and pulmonary embolization should be recognized, and deep-breathing exercises, leg exercises, and elastic stockings are advisable. The use of anticoagulants (minidose heparin, p. 1588) should be considered in patients with heart failure with or without a previous history of thromboembolic disease.

Emotional and mental rest are as important as physical rest. Hospitalization is often beneficial because it removes the patient from a situation that is anxiety-provoking. Since emotional stress can retard convalescence from an episode of acute congestive heart failure, visitors and incoming telephone calls should be limited. The physician should serve as a thoughtful, sympathetic listener with whom the patient can discuss a variety of problems. In particular, the patient must be given a realistic appraisal of the prognosis, and it must be emphasized that if a precipitating cause of heart failure can be identified, acute cardiac decompensation does not signify a hopeless outlook. It is important that the patient sleep well each night, and the use of flurazepam, 15 to 30 mg, as a hypnotic may be advisable. Diazepam, 2 to 5 mg twice a day, may be helpful as well in patients with marked anxiety.

There is no formula for deciding on the duration of rigid restriction of physical activity for patients with acute cardiac decompensation. It should depend principally on the patient's response to the overall treatment program. As a general rule, it is advisable to maintain the patient at rest as long as *more* than a trace of ankle edema or a few moist rales at the lung bases persist. At this point the patient can usually be discharged to continue convalescence at home or in a nursing home. Although the restriction of physical activity can be relaxed at this point, it should continue in a modified form for two to four weeks, depending on the rigidity of the patient's convalescence.

DIET. Before effective oral diuretics were available, diet played a more important role in the control of salt and water retention than it does today. It is now possible to recommend only modest restriction of sodium intake in most patients with heart failure, with intensification of the diuretic regimen to prevent accumulation of extracellular fluid. Nonetheless, restriction of sodium intake remains one of the cornerstones of the treatment of congestive heart failure. The normal daily sodium content of the unrestricted American diet ranges from 3.0 to 6.0 gm; simple elimination of the saltshaker at the table and a few common foods such as pretzels, popcorn, salted nuts, potato chips, candy bars, smoked and salt-cured meats (including ham, bacon, and sausage), delicatessen meats, herring, and condiments such as olives and pickles will reduce this to approximately half (1.5 to 3.0 gm). Potassium chloride (salt substitute) may be used in place of ordinary table salt. There is no need to eliminate the salt in cooking and to make the diet unpalatable unless fluid retention occurs despite intensive use of diuretics. Indeed, the monotony and unpalatability of a low-sodium diet has caused unnecessary hardship to patients and their families and has often interfered with adequate nutrition.

Reduction of sodium intake to between 1.2 and 1.5 gm/day can be achieved by simply eliminating all salt from cooking and from the table. If it is necessary to reduce the sodium intake to 0.2 gm daily in patients with Class IV congestive heart failure, many common foods must be eliminated. Spices and herbs should be used to flavor the food in place of sodium chloride, and as wide a variety of foods as possible should be employed to diminish the monotony. A variety of books and pamphlets are available to aid in the preparation of salt-poor diets. It must be recognized that while the elimination of dietary salt may be necessary in patients with severe heart failure, this can result in a marked reduction of caloric intake, leading to malnutrition and even cardiac cachexia (p. 499).

Opinion concerning *water intake* in heart failure has varied widely in the past. At one time rigid restriction of water intake was advised; then it became clear that the total extracellular fluid volume was primarily dependent on the body sodium content. For some years it was thought that excessive water intake (exceeding 3 liters/day) would increase the elimination of salt, i.e., it would "flush out" sodium. There is no evidence in favor of this concept, and therefore it is advisable simply to leave the water intake to the patient's own desire. However, in far-advanced congestive heart failure the ability to excrete a free-water load may be impaired, with resulting dilutional hyponatremia (p. 1750). Only under these circumstances is it desirable to restrict water intake so that the serum sodium concentration does not fall below approximately 130 mEq/liter. Modest reductions of serum sodium (i.e., to 130 to 142 mEq/liter) do not usually require specific therapy.

OXYGEN. The use of oxygen in patients with pulmonary edema and with acute myocardial infarction is discussed elsewhere (pp. 571 and 1303). Oxygen inhalation, most conveniently by means of nasal prongs at 4 to 6 liters/min, should be employed in patients with other forms of congestive heart failure if the arterial oxygen saturation falls below 90 per cent. Oxygen therapy is particularly useful in patients with heart failure precipitated by pulmonary infection or pulmonary infarction. Many patients consider the inhalation of oxygen a sign of terminal illness, and it is important to explain to them that in most instances its use is temporary.

PHYSICAL REMOVAL OF FLUID. Ordinarily, mechanical removal of fluid from the pleural and abdominal cavities is unnecessary in patients with congestive heart

ministration of daily maintenance doses of digitoxin without a loading dose will result in gradual digitalization, with the 4- to 6-day half-life of the drug resulting in establishment of the final steady-state plateau after 3 to 4 weeks.

DESLANOSIDE (CEDILANID-D). This agent is structurally identical to digoxin except for the presence of an additional terminal glucose residue. This alteration results in poor gastrointestinal absorption, and thus the drug is recommended only for parenteral use. Its half-life is essentially identical to that of digoxin. Although its onset of action is somewhat more rapid, it probably enjoys no substantial advantages over parenteral use of digoxin unless rapidity of effect is an overriding consideration; however, if this is the case, ouabain may be preferable.

OUABAIN AND ACETYLSTROPHANTHIDIN. *Ouabain* is the most polar and rapidly acting of the cardiac glycosides currently available for routine clinical use. Like the other cardiac glycosides, its excretion from the body follows first-order pharmacokinetics, with a fixed proportion of the residual drug in the body being excreted each day. For ouabain, the plasma half-life in normal subjects is about 21 hours—similar to the half-life of positive inotropic effect and of ventricular rate slowing in patients with atrial fibrillation.[140] The quantity of ouabain in the body, and also the risk of toxicity, in a patient placed on a regular maintenance dosage schedule without a loading dose will continue to rise for four to five half-lives (4 to 5 days) until a plateau is reached. Impairment of renal function will prolong the half-life of ouabain and also the period during which accumulation will continue.

Although ouabain is predominantly excreted unchanged via the renal route, its gastrointestinal excretion is substantial after intravenous administration in both dog and man.[141] The drug appears to enter the gastrointestinal tract by pathways other than the biliary tract. In normal human subjects, urinary excretion accounted for an average of only 47 per cent of the intravenous dose. Ouabain is poorly absorbed from the gastrointestinal tract and is not available for oral use.

Acetylstrophanthidin, a rapidly acting synthetic C-3 acetyl ester of the aglycone strophanthidin, has been used in both experimental and clinical investigations but is available for clinical use only on an investigative basis. In human subjects, the principal exponential decline of plasma acetylstrophanthidin commences 10 to 30 minutes after intravenous infusion, and the mean half-life in plasma is 2.3 hours, in keeping with the known short duration of clinical effect. Urinary excretion averages only 22 per cent of the intravenous dose.[142]

Detailed reviews of cardiac glycoside pharmacokinetics and metabolism are available.[61,143]

BIOAVAILABILITY

Three decades ago, Gold and his colleagues evaluated the relative efficacy of cardiac glycosides given by oral and parenteral routes. The ventricular rate of patients in atrial fibrillation was used as a quantitative indicator of digitalis effect.[116] Oral digoxin was found to be about two thirds as effective in slowing the ventricular rate as an equivalent intravenous dose,[118] whereas digitoxin was almost equally effective when given by either route.[116] Thus, the bioavailability of digoxin as determined by this clinical bioassay was about 67 per cent, whereas that of digitoxin was nearly 100 per cent.

A number of subsequent studies have documented incomplete absorption of digoxin from the gastrointestinal tract.[144,145] Individual patient variation, circumstances of drug administration, and characteristics of the pharmaceutical preparation ingested are all known to affect digoxin bioavailability.[146] Patients with malabsorption syndromes may absorb digoxin poorly and erratically.[147] However, patients with maldigestion due to pancreatic insufficiency, despite comparable degrees of steatorrhea, appear to absorb the drug more normally. Administration of digoxin after meals is likely to decrease peak serum levels achieved, but total absorption is not affected to any noteworthy degree. Absorption of digoxin tends to be enhanced by drugs that decrease gastrointestinal motility and to be reduced by drugs that increase motility, particularly if the preparations have limited bioavailability. In addition, nonabsorbed substances, such as cholestyramine, colestipol, kaolin and pectin (Kaopectate), and nonabsorbable antacids, when taken concurrently can interfere with gastrointestinal absorption of digoxin; neomycin has also been shown to interfere with digoxin absorption. Because of previously documented variations in the bioavailability of commercially available digoxin preparations, bioavailability specifications provided by the FDA and USP are currently in effect.[148–150]

Biological availability uniformly approaching 100 per cent probably cannot be achieved with any oral digoxin preparation, but a recently marketed encapsulated gel preparation is reported to have 90 to 100 per cent bioavailability. After intravenous administration of digoxin, 6-day urinary recovery by radioimmunoassay averaged 76 per cent of the administered dose. Intramuscular digoxin caused severe pain at the injection site, and bioavailability was only 83 per cent that of intravenous digoxin. Digoxin elixir was significantly more bioavailable (65 per cent of intravenous) than the tablet form studied (55 per cent of intravenous).[149]

Since the studies of Gold et al., oral absorption of digitoxin has generally been considered to be virtually 100 per cent, and no recent studies have cast doubt on that estimate. As with digoxin, binding to nonabsorbable substances such as cholestyramine can interfere with initial absorption.[138] Patients receiving such anion-exchange resins in addition to a cardiac glycoside should be instructed to ingest the cardiac glycoside two hours before the resin to minimize this effect.

CLINICAL USE OF DIGITALIS

A sound working knowledge of the pharmacokinetics of the commonly used cardiac glycosides is essential to the optimal use of these drugs. Computer programs and nomograms[151,152] can provide initial approximations of optimal dose, but further dosage adjustments based on close clinical observation of the patient are often required. In many cases the variability in serum digoxin concentrations among different patients remains unexplained even after adjustments for dose, body size, and renal function have been made and measurement of digoxin concentrations and their use for feedback dosage adjustments have been suggested.[153]

The clinical use of cardiac glycosides is complicated by the absence of a readily measurable therapeutic objective (except in certain atrial arrhythmias), the lack of reliable means to predict individual cardiac responses, and the difficulty in defining proximity to toxicity. The acetylstrophanthidin tolerance test has been used investigatively[154,155] but carries potential risk and is not generally available for clinical use. Other experimental approaches employ electrical pulses to assess the degree of digitalization, on the basis of the observation that cardioversion may elicit rhythm disturbances in digitalized patients.[156]

CONGESTIVE HEART FAILURE. Cardiac glycosides are of potential value in most patients with symptoms and signs of *congestive heart failure* due to ischemic, valvular, hypertensive, or congenital heart disease, dilated cardiomyopathies, and cor pulmonale. Improvement of depressed myocardial contractility increases cardiac output, promotes diuresis, and reduces the filling pressure of the failing ventricle(s), with consequent reduction of pulmonary vascular congestion and central venous pressure.

As previously noted, digitalis is of no demonstrable benefit in isolated *mitral stenosis* with normal sinus rhythm unless right ventricular failure has supervened. Similarly, little benefit may result in patients with *pericardial tamponade* or *constrictive pericarditis* except when there is invasion of the myocardium in the latter. Hypertrophic obstructive cardiomyopathy represents another process in which digitalis is often of little value and may actually be deleterious because it can increase left ventricular outflow obstruction by augmenting the contractility of the hypertrophic outflow-tract segment. It is our impression that patients with left ventricular hypertrophy and well-preserved left ventricular ejection fractions, even in the presence of symptoms related to elevated filling pressures, benefit little from digitalis. In the later stages of hypertrophic cardiomyopathy, in which ventricular dilation and congestive problems may predominate over obstructive ones, cardiac glycosides may be beneficial. Patients who develop congestive heart failure in response to a specific precipitating stress (p. 491) may benefit from temporary use of digitalis but will not necessarily require long-term maintenance digitalization. The risk:benefit ratio must be reassessed with any change in clinical status and will often be found to favor discontinuation of digitalis when an acute stress such as infection, anemia, or thyrotoxicosis is no longer present.[62]

Digitalis glycosides may improve symptoms of angina pectoris when it coexists with cardiomegaly and congestive heart failure. As discussed subsequently, however, an increase in angina may occur unless the tendency toward increased oxygen consumption is offset by decreased ventricular size and wall tension.

Prophylactic digitalization of the patient with diminished cardiac reserve about to undergo a major stress such as surgery remains controversial (p. 1821). In the absence of obvious cardiomegaly or other evidence of overt congestive heart failure, most clinicians prefer to withhold digitalis until a specific indication arises. Prophylactic digitalization has been recommended for patients undergoing aortocoronary bypass surgery on the basis of a significant reduction in supraventricular arrhythmias.[157] Evidence of a difference in ultimate outcome between digitalized and nondigitalized patients was not documented, however, and another study of 140 consecutive patients undergoing myocardial revascularization showed a *higher* incidence of supraventricular tachyarrhythmias in patients receiving prophylactic digitalis.[158]

The availability of reliable pervenous catheter endocardial pacing techniques has helped to resolve the problem of digitalis use in patients with marginal atrioventricular conduction or established atrioventricular block. One can now carry out pacemaker implantation at minimal risk even in severely ill patients and then give digitalis without fear of aggravating conduction problems.

Arrhythmias (See also Chapter 22). Digitalis is of potential use in the management of four types of supraventricular tachyarrhythmias.

1. *Paroxysmal superventricular tachycardia* (p. 702), whether of atrial or atrioventricular junctional origin, usually responds to digitalization when simpler measures such as carotid sinus pressure alone have failed. Many clinicians now prefer to use verapamil as the drug of first choice in this clinical setting (p. 665). When digitalis is used, carotid sinus pressure should be repeated during the course of digitalization, since the combination of partial digitalization and carotid sinus pressure will often succeed when neither measure alone suffices. Maintenance digitalization usually abolishes or reduces the frequency of recurrent attacks. Use of digitalis in the setting of paroxysmal supraventricular tachycardia demands that digitalis intoxication be excluded as a cause of the arrhythmia.

2. *Atrial fibrillation* with a rapid ventricular response is one of the most common indications for the use of digitalis. Both vagal and direct mechanisms result in increased blockade of impulses arriving at the atrioventricular junction, with slowing of the ventricular rate. Conversion to normal sinus rhythm may occur in the course of digitalization. Addition of beta-adrenergic blocking agents or verapamil[159] may be useful in circumstances in which the ventricular rate is difficult to control without the emergence of toxic symptoms (e.g., untreated thyrotoxicosis) and congestive heart failure is absent or minimal.

3. *Atrial flutter*, usually accompanied by 2:1 atrioventricular block in untreated cases, can often be managed with digitalis in doses sufficient to produce a degree of atrioventricular blockade that results in a ventricular rate in the range of 70 to 100/min. This effect may require doses considerably in excess of the usual range. As in atrial fibrillation, when the arrhythmia is poorly tolerated by the patient, it is often advisable to attempt direct-current cardioversion before administration of doses of digitalis that would render the procedure hazardous.

4. *Wolff-Parkinson-White syndrome* tachyarrhythmias (p. 712) may be terminated or prevented by digitalis in cases in which preferential effects on conduction or refractoriness in the normal or anomalous conduction pathways result in interruption of the reentrant circus movement. Other antiarrhythmic drugs may be more effective in other cases. Sellers et al. concluded on the basis of detailed electrophysiological studies of responses to digoxin in 21 patients that no a priori prediction about the effect of digitalis on the antegrade conduction of accessory pathways can be made, suggesting that formal electrophysiological studies are indicated in many of these patients to predict their response to maintenance digoxin therapy.[160] Potential hazards of digitalis use in patients with the Wolff-Parkinson-White syndrome and episodes of atrial fibrillation are discussed on page 718.

DOSAGE SCHEDULES

Specific recommendations for digoxin dosage have been developed on the basis of the pharmacokinetic principles previously discussed. Usually there is no reason to use a loading dose far in excess of what the steady-state body content will be with the usual maintenance dose. A patient with entirely normal renal function who excretes 37 per cent of the digoxin in his body each day will, on a maintenance dose of 0.25 or 0.50 mg/day, have a steady-state total body content of about 0.67 or 1.35 mg, respectively. If a reasonable estimate of 75 per cent absorption of the tablet form of digoxin is made, estimates for the loading dose become 0.5 and 1.0 mg, respectively, for maintenance doses of 0.25 and 0.50 mg/day. This amount can be given over a period of a day or so in several increments, or the same level of digitalization can be achieved over a period of about a week in a patient with normal renal function by administration of the daily maintenance dose without any loading dose. The latter procedure is often preferable in outpatient practice. It must be remembered, however, that severe renal impairment will prolong the half-life of digoxin to a maximum of about 4.4 days and hence extend the period required to reach a steady-state plateau to a maximum of about 3 weeks. Lean body mass should be considered in selection of both loading and maintenance digoxin doses. In adult patients with cardiac disease, initial intravenous loading doses of about 0.50 to 0.75 mg/45 kg (100 lb) of body weight, given in increments, are unlikely to cause toxicity and can be supplemented by further increments if indicated by the clinical course.

The maintenance digoxin dose required to replace daily losses will vary from about 37 per cent of the total body content in patients with normal renal function to nonrenal losses averaging about 14 per cent in patients who are essentially anephric. Between the extremes of normal renal function and no renal function, digoxin excretion is linearly related to glomerular filtration rate or creatinine clearance (C_{Cr}). A reasonable approximation of daily percentage of loss of digoxin is as follows[161]:

$$14 + \frac{C_{Cr} \text{ in ml/min}}{5}$$

Since accurate creatinine clearance values will often not be immediately available, one can use the following estimate based on a stable serum creatinine in mg/100 ml, abbreviated as c:

$$C_{Cr} \text{ (men)} = \frac{100}{c} - 12$$

and

$$C_{Cr} \text{ (women)} = \frac{80}{c} - 7$$

These expressions can be combined so that

$$\% \text{ daily loss (men)} = 11.6 + \frac{20}{c}$$

and

$$\% \text{ daily loss (women)} = 12.6 + \frac{16}{c}$$

The daily maintenance digoxin dose is intended to replace daily losses after an appropriate loading dose, so that the above value for daily percentage of loss multiplied by the loading dose that produced a satisfactory therapeutic response gives a reasonable initial approximation of the proper daily maintenance dose. Jelliffe and Brooker have developed a useful nomogram for digoxin therapy that takes into account body weight and renal function and provides guidelines for determining both loading and maintenance doses.[152]

The recommended oral loading dose of digoxin, based on *lean body weight* and administered in the form of digoxin elixir, is 25 to 35 μg/kg for full-term infants; 35 to 60 μg/kg for infants from 1 to 24 months; 30 to 40 μg/kg for ages 2 to 5 years; 20 to 35 μg/kg for 5 to 10 years; and 10 to 15 μg/kg for children over 10 years. For premature infants a loading dose of 20 to 30 μg/kg is recommended. Daily maintenance doses *for patients with normal renal function* are estimated as 20 to 30 per cent of the oral loading dose for premature infants and as 25 to 35 per cent of the oral loading dose for full-term infants through children 10 years of age and older. Parenteral (intravenous) loading and maintenance dose recommendations are approximately 75 per cent of the oral dosages.[162]

For digitoxin, half-lives usually range within 20 per cent of a mean value of 4.8 days, and relatively little variation in the body pool would be expected among individual patients receiving a given maintenance dose of the drug. The average steady-state digitoxin pool in a patient receiving 0.1 mg/day is about 0.8 mg, and as with digoxin, there is usually no reason to give a loading dose substantially in excess of the expected steady-state body pool achieved with usual maintenance doses. A loading dose of about 0.010 to 0.012 mg/kg allows compensation for variations in body size. Gradual digitalization without a loading dose is feasible with digitoxin, but because four to five half-lives are required to reach the steady-state plateau, this will take 3 to 4 weeks.

Estimates of loading and maintenance doses based on the above considerations are average values intended only as initial approximations and in no way diminish the need for further adjustments based on frequent and careful observation of the patient.

THERAPEUTIC ENDPOINTS

In addressing the difficult problem of defining the elusive state of optimal digitalization, one might begin by stating that it is not necessarily the largest dose that can be tolerated without emergence of overt toxicity. The toxic:therapeutic ratio for cardiac glycosides is small at best, and the availability of other measures of treating heart failure, particularly potent oral diuretics and vasodilators, usually obviates balancing therapy at the edge of toxicity. Electrocardiographic ST-segment and T-wave changes of "digitalis effect" are, unfortunately, limited indicators of the state of digitalization. The perils of depending on slowing of sinus tachycardia to gauge the adequacy of digitalis dosage are well known.

In patients with atrial flutter or fibrillation, control of the ventricular response provides a relatively straightforward endpoint. Failure of atropine or exercise to increase the ventricular response has been used as an additional indicator of "full digitalization" in such patients, but overly vigorous pursuit of this goal may result in unduly slow resting heart rates or other evidence of impending or overt toxicity.

When congestive heart failure is the indication for use of digitalis, it is helpful to remember that positive inotropy is a graded response that is appreciable at doses well short of "maximally tolerated doses." As already stated, available data suggest that further inotropic benefit may not occur clinically beyond serum digoxin levels in the 1.0 to 2.0

TABLE 16–5 FACTORS INFLUENCING INDIVIDUAL SENSITIVITY TO DIGITALIS

- Type and severity of underlying cardiac disease
- Serum electrolyte derangements
  - Hypokalemia or hyperkalemia
  - Hypomagnesemia
  - Hypercalcemia
  - Hyponatremia
- Acid-base imbalance
- Concomitant drug administration
  - Anesthetics
  - Catecholamines and sympathomimetics
  - Antiarrhythmic agents
- Thyroid status
- Renal function
- Autonomic nervous system tone
- Respiratory disease

ng/ml range.[62] Carotid sinus massage can provide useful bedside clues to impending digitalis excess. Rhythm disorders such as second-degree atrioventricular block, accelerated atrioventricular junctional rhythm, and ventricular premature beats or bigeminy may emerge in response to carotid sinus stimulation before they occur spontaneously.[163]

INDIVIDUAL SENSITIVITY TO DIGITALIS. It is considerably easier to calculate theoretical body pools of cardiac glycosides than to decide, at the bedside, when optimal digitalization has been achieved in an individual patient. A number of factors influencing individual sensitivity to cardiac glycosides are listed in Table 16–5. Changes in absorption or bioavailability increase the probability of suboptimal digitalization because of fluctuations that can occur on a supposedly fixed dosage regimen. Such changes are reflected by changes in serum glycoside concentrations, however, and do not represent an actual change in sensitivity to the drug's effects. Quite distinct from the clinical problem of variable bioavailability is the enhanced sensitivity to lower serum concentrations of cardiac glycosides noted in up to 10 to 15 per cent of patients.

ELECTROLYTE AND ACID-BASE DISTURBANCES. Disturbances of potassium homeostasis clearly influence the action of digitalis.[61,164] Myocardial concentrations of digoxin tend to decrease with increasing serum potassium concentration. Furthermore, hypokalemia has a primary arrhythmogenic effect, both decreasing the effective refractory period of Purkinje cells and shortening the coupling interval for ventricular premature beats.[165] Depression of atrioventricular nodal conduction can occur with both digitalis excess and either very low or extremely high levels of serum K^+.[166,167] Diuretic therapy, insulin administration or carbohydrate loading, renal disease, and acid-base disturbances must all be borne in mind as potential causes of clinically significant alterations in potassium homeostasis, which can, in turn, affect importantly the response to cardiac glycoside.

Disturbances in serum levels of other electrolytes may also influence myocardial sensitivity to digitalis, although less profoundly than K^+ concentration. Administration of Mg^{++} salts suppresses digitalis-induced arrthythmias and hypomagnesemia appears to predispose to digitalis toxicity.[168] There is some evidence that the digitalis-induced K^+ efflux from the myocardium is reduced by Mg^{++} salts.[169] Magnesium depletion may become clinically important with the chronic administration of diuretic agents[170] and with gastrointestinal disease, diabetes mellitus, or poor nutritional states. Moreover, in patients with congestive heart failure, significant depletion of total body Mg^{++} stores may occur owing to prolonged secondary aldosteronism. The frequency and clinical importance of Mg^{++} depletion in digitalis therapy remain unresolved.[171,172]

Elevated serum Ca^{++} levels increase ventricular automaticity, and this effect is at least additive to and perhaps synergistic with the effects of digitalis. In one early study, ventricular ectopic activity occurred at lower doses of ouabain in hypercalcemic patients.[173] Furthermore, patients with digitalis intoxication have been reported to respond successfully to calcium-chelating agents.[174] The clinician should be alert for the possibility of enhanced digitalis sensitivity when treating hypercalcemic patients or when administering calcium parenterally to digitalized patients.

The interactions of digitalis with acid-base disturbances are complex. Perturbations in potassium homeostasis that follow shifts in hydrogen ion concentration obviously will affect myocardial binding of cardiac glycosides and the development of digitalis-related arrhythmias, as will primary changes in serum K^+ concentration. Similarly, acid-base status will influence the serum levels of ionized Ca^{++}, with attendant effects on automaticity. Whether alkalosis itself, independent of these changes, increases sensitivity to digitalis is controversial.[175,176] Acidosis independent of changes in $[K^+]$ does not appear to enhance sensitivity to the arrthythmogenic effects of digitalis[177] and may even render the myocardium more resistant to digitalis intoxication.[178]

DRUG INTERACTIONS. Concomitant drug administration may interact with the effects of digitalis through several mechanisms. As noted above, certain drugs such as cholestyramine and neomycin may decrease oral absorption of digoxin, thereby altering the serum and myocardial levels ultimately achieved. In addition, nonabsorbable antacids and Kaopectate may have a similar effect in some patients.

Drugs that affect metabolism or excretion of various digitalis preparations will influence toxicity through variations in the levels of serum and myocardial digitalis achieved rather than through altered sensitivity to the action of the glycosides themselves. Quinidine reduces both the renal and nonrenal elimination of digoxin and also appears to decrease the apparent volume of distribution of this glycoside.[179] The net result is an increase in serum digoxin concentration that averages two-fold in patients in whom conventional doses of quinidine are added to a maintenance digoxin regimen[179]; unfortunately, individual responses to quinidine may vary substantially and close surveillance of clinical status (and, if possible, serum digoxin concentration) is needed to reduce the risk of precipitating overt digoxin toxicity. Preliminary studies of a possible interaction between digitoxin and quinidine have yielded conflicting results, and this issue remains unsettled.[61] Procainamide and disopyramide do not appear to alter serum digoxin levels, but verapamil does increase serum digoxin concentration by decreasing volume of distribution and clearance of digoxin.[180,181] Other calcium channel blocking agents, including nifedipine and tiapamil, can also increase serum digoxin levels,[182,183] and both short- and long-term amiodarone administration has been found to increase steady-state serum digoxin concentration.[184,185] Other newly introduced drugs will require close surveillance for interactions with cardiac glycosides.

Diuretic agents potentially enhance the occurrence of digitalis toxicity both by decreasing glomerular filtration rate and through a variety of electrolyte disturbances, including hypokalemia, hypomagnesemia, and (for thiazide diuretics) hypercalcemia. By counteracting the cardiac toxic manifestations of digitalis excess, concurrent administration of some antiarrhythmic agents may create the impression of a relative resistance to digitalis toxicity.

Several anesthetic agents are arrhythmogenic, and experimental studies suggest that this effect may be synergistic with digitalis enhancement of ventricular automaticity in the case of cyclopropane[186] and succinylcholine.[187] The profound systemic effects of general anesthesia introduce many variables that could affect digitalis sensitivity, thus greatly complicating the detailed assessment of individual anesthetic agents. The interrelationships between catecholamines and sympathomimetic drugs and cardiac glycosides are intriguing but incompletely characterized. Several experimental studies have demonstrated that catecholamine-induced increases in ventricular automaticity add to the arrhythmogenic effects of digitalis[188]; however, detailed clinical correlation has not been forthcoming. It is reasonable for the clinician to assume that sympathomimetic agents increase the likelihood of enhanced automaticity of ectopic pacemakers in patients receiving digitalis.

TYPE AND SEVERITY OF UNDERLYING HEART DISEASE

The effects of digitalis on the heart are modified by the type and severity of the underlying heart disease.[189] This is dramatically demonstrated in otherwise healthy subjects who ingest massive doses of digitalis. Toxicity in such situations is frequently manifested by progressively diminished atrioventricular conduction or by sinoatrial exit block, rather than by enhanced automaticity and ventricular ectopic activity as seen in patients with underlying heart disease.[190,191] In many patients with ischemic, myocardial, or valvular heart disease the effects of digitalis are superimposed on an electrophysiologically unstable condition with preexisting abnormalities of impulse formation and conduction. The more severe and advanced the heart disease, the more likely the occurrence of focal ischemia, myocardial fibrosis, and ventricular dilatation with stretching of Purkinje fibers and resultant tendency toward increased automaticity. The clinical observation that digitalis toxicity is particularly common in patients with amyloidosis involving the heart may be accounted for, at least in part, by digoxin binding by amyloid fibrils.[192]

DIGITALIS AND ISCHEMIC HEART DISEASE. The use of digitalis in patients with ischemic heart disease deserves special attention. In experiments employing an isolated canine cardiac preparation, it was shown that acetylstrophanthidin administration increased myocardial oxygen consumption in the normal heart, whereas consumption was decreased in the failing heart.[193] The increase in oxygen consumption in the normal heart can be explained by the increased velocity of contraction and increased wall tension. In the failing heart, decreased oxygen consumption can be explained by a decrease in left ventricular end-diastolic pressure, resulting in a reduction in end-diastolic volume and consequently, on the basis of the Laplace relation, a decline in intramyocardial tension.

Changes in oxygen consumption are always the net result of two opposing effects of digitalis: a potential reduction in wall tension and an increase in contractility. Thus, in the failing heart the net result depends on the balance of these effects, and either a diminution of oxygen consumption or no change may be observed. In the nonfailing heart, oxygen consumption increases with digitalis administration.[194] These considerations are of clinical importance when a decision must be made about whether to use digitalis in patients with coronary disease. Angina pectoris has been observed to improve after digitalization in patients with heart failure but occasionally to worsen in those who are well compensated. An objective study of the effect of ouabain on the response of the left ventricle in patients with angina pectoris showed that the depressed myocardial performance noted on exercise was improved by digitalization in the majority of patients studied.[195] Despite these beneficial effects on left ventricular performance, however, there was no consistent alteration in exercise tolerance or the pressure-rate product at which angina occurred. Other studies have demonstrated an increased cardiac output on exercise after digitalization, suggesting that the reduction in myocardial oxygen consumption that followed digitalis-induced improvement in left ventricular function probably masked any increase caused by its positive inotropic action.[196] No deterioration of myocardial metabolism with acute ouabain administration was found in patients with chronic coronary artery disease either at rest[197] or with pacing-induced myocardial ischemia.[198] Improved myocardial perfusion judged by means of thallium-201 scans was found in response to maintenance doses of digoxin in patients with coronary artery disease and left ventricular dysfunction.[199] The combination of propranolol and digoxin in patients with angina pectoris appears to be advantageous in the subgroup with angina pectoris and abnormal ventricular function or large hearts.[200]

There are still many unanswered questions concerning the role of digitalis therapy after acute myocardial infarction. There is little to be gained from administration of the drug to patients who have uncomplicated infarction without cardiomegaly (p. 1315).[201] There is limited clinical documentation of its value in cardiogenic shock, a syndrome in which no pharmacological agent has been demonstrated to be highly effective. Indeed, rapid digitalization may occasionally be harmful, owing to the vasoconstrictor properties of the drug.[202] Small increases in cardiac index and stroke work as well as a reduction in left ventricular end-diastolic pressure have been observed after digitalization in patients with left ventricular failure following myocardial infarction.[203] Although ouabain did not alter cardiac output in another series of patients with acute myocardial infarction,[204] it caused significant improvement in other indices of left ventricular performance, such as end-diastolic pressure and stroke work. Similar benefits were noted in patients convalescing from myocardial infarction.[205]

The issue of increased susceptibility to the toxic effects of digitalis in recent or acute myocardial infarction remains controversial. In animal models, the dose of digitalis required to reach a toxic endpoint clearly is reduced after experimentally induced myocardial infarction.[206,207] However, in a study of patients with acute myocardial infarction, 89 per cent tolerated a full dose of acetylstrophanthidin, suggesting no significant enhancement of sensitivity to the drug.[155] In patients with acute myocardial infarction treated with intravenous digoxin using a double-blind randomized protocol, no difference in incidence of rhythm disturbances was found between digoxin-treated and control patients.[208] There appears to be no convincing evidence for an increased incidence of arrhythmias complicating digitalization in patients with acute infarction when serum levels do not exceed the conventional therapeutic range.[209]

The clearest indication for digitalis after acute myocardial infarction is in the treatment of atrial fibrillation with a rapid ventricular rate. Electrical cardioversion may be preferred in the treatment of other supraventricular tachyarrhythmias.[210]

Evidence based on a retrospective analysis by Moss et al.[211] suggests that mortality within the first 4 months after myocardial infarction may be increased in a high-risk subset of patients with congestive heart failure and ventricular arrhythmias, but this finding has not yet been confirmed by prospective studies, and, indeed, has been contested.[211a]

In summary, current evidence indicates that digitalis has no well-defined role in the management of acute myocardial infarction without congestive heart failure or supraventricular tachyarrhythmias. Judicious patient selection and management of drug doses will minimize the potentially deleterious effects of digitalis in acute myocardial infarction.

ADVANCED AGE. Advanced age per se has been considered by some to be a risk factor in the development of digitalis toxicity because of an enhanced sensitivity to the drug.[212,213] However, diminished glomerular filtration rate with age will alone lead to prolonged half-life of digoxin and thus to increased serum levels and an increased probability of toxicity on a given dosage regimen. Advanced age is frequently associated with other factors that increase the likelihood of digitalis intoxication, including more severe heart disease; impairment of pulmonary, renal, and neurological function; and an increased number of concurrent medications.

RENAL FAILURE (See also page 1759). Renal failure, particularly in patients requiring hemodialysis, is a disease state in which factors influencing digitalis absorption and elimination and rapid shifts of electrolytes profoundly affect the response to digitalis. The marked diminution of glomerular filtration rate with renal failure prolongs the half-life of digoxin and thus increases serum digoxin levels. Toxicity from this predictable response can be avoided by careful and frequent adjustments of dosage to correlate with the level of renal function present. Less predictably, dialysis can cause at least a transient decrease in serum potassium that will increase the tendency toward digitalis-induced arrhythmias. Depending on the magnesium content of the dialysate and the use of magnesium-containing antacids by the patient, there may be significant aberrations of serum magnesium levels in patients on dialysis.[172] Some evidence suggests that increased serum levels of digoxin may reflect a decreased volume of distribution, so that relatively higher levels may be needed to achieve a certain effect.[214] The clinician is well advised to use the minimum drug dosage that produces the desired clinical effect in this condition noted for its extreme fluctuations in fluid and electrolyte balance.

THYROID DISEASE. It is well known that thyroid disease alters digitalis pharmacokinetics. In hypothyroid patients the serum digoxin half-life is consistently prolonged, while in those with hyperthyroidism serum digoxin levels tend to be decreased.[215] Since some studies have not documented significant changes in metabolism or serum half-life of digoxin in hyperthyroid patients,[216] it has been suggested that an increased distribution space for digoxin may exist. This hypothesis is of interest in light of experimental findings indicating higher levels of Na^+,K^+-ATPase activity in the myocardium[217] and other tissues of hyperthyroid animals.[218] In any event the apparent resistance or sensitivity to digitalis in thyroid disease is dependent, at least in part, on changes in the pharmacokinetics of digoxin. Changes in the response of the heart to a given serum level of drug probably also occur (for example, the difficulty in controlling the ventricular response in patients with thyrotoxicosis and atrial fibrillation), but these changes have not been well defined either in the experimental laboratory or in the clinical setting. As discussed previously, autonomic neural influences on the effect of digitalis on the heart have long been appreciated. Such changes in autonomic tone may to some extent explain the apparent resistance to digitalis effect seen in thyrotoxicosis.

PULMONARY DISEASE. There has been considerable interest in the use of digitalis in patients with pulmonary disease.[219] A number of authors have noted that ventricular ectopic activity consistent with digitalis toxicity frequently occurs in patients with respiratory disease who are receiving digitalis.[220–222] Such reports are difficult to interpret, however, because respiratory failure and hypoxemia frequently provoke arrhythmias indistinguishable from those associated with digitalis excess.[223,224] A population of 931 patients admitted consecutively to a medical service and studied prospectively demonstrated an increased incidence of rhythm disturbances consistent with digitalis toxicity among patients with acute or chronic lung disease.[225]

When excessive sensitivity to digitalis in patients with pulmonary disease was investigated utilizing acetylstrophanthidin tolerance testing, it was observed that of 18 patients with chronic lung disease who did not receive digitalis previously, six demonstrated increased sensitivity, all of whom had cor pulmonale and hypercapnia and five of whom were hypoxemic.[226] These findings are corroborated by the relatively frequent discordance between serum digoxin levels and tolerance to acetylstrophanthidin in patients with pulmonary disease.[227] In a group of patients with severe respiratory failure, 18 had rhythm disturbances consistent with digitalis toxicity at a time when serum digoxin levels were within a range not usually associated with toxicity.[228] Only the presence of more severe hypoxemia distinguished these patients from those with pulmonary disease who appeared toxic only at higher serum concentrations.

Therefore the evidence is highly suggestive that pulmonary disease predisposes to the development of digitalis intoxication at relatively low serum concentrations. It would appear that hypoxemia is an important factor associated with this enhanced sensitivity to digitalis. However, the degree of hypoxemia may be merely an index of the severity of the respiratory failure and its associated physiological derangements rather than a factor that by itself is causally related to digitalis sensitivity. Although not adequately subdivided into acute or chronic respiratory illnesses, the available epidemiological data suggest that patients with stable chronic lung disease are at increased risk of developing digitalis intoxication. Particularly as a result of diuretic therapy, these patients are subject to derangements in potassium homeostasis and the development of metabolic alkalosis—both predisposing to digitalis toxicity. What role exogenous catecholamines and the sympathomimetic agents commonly used in the therapy of chronic airway disease may have in the development of digitalis-related arrhythmias is not known. No published studies have shown convincing enhancement of ventricular ectopic activity in patients receiving catecholamines by inhalation in either the presence or the absence of digitalis.

From the data available, then, it is reasonable for the clinician to assume that patients with a variety of pulmonary diseases may be sensitive to the arrhythmogenic effects of digitalis at relatively low serum concentrations.

SERUM OR PLASMA CONCENTRATIONS OF DIGITALIS GLYCOSIDES

It has long been apparent clinically that alterations in cardiac rhythm as well as extracardiac manifestations of digitalis action, such as gastrointestinal and central nervous system symptoms, are dose-related.[229] It has now been demonstrated convincingly in a number of studies that plasma digitalis concentrations are also correlated with the amount of drug administered.[189] One would therefore expect that a correlation would exist between plasma digitalis concentration and the symptoms and signs of toxicity. In both animal and human studies, after attainment of equilibrium, a relatively constant ratio of plasma to myocardial digoxin concentration has been observed,[230,231] although not all the digoxin present in myocardium is bound to specific receptors relevant to the pharmacological action of the drug. As discussed earlier, the available evidence that digitalis glycosides act on receptors similar or identical to Na^+,K^+-ATPase and hence in close proximity to the cell surface suggests that digitalis concentration at these receptor sites would be influenced readily by the concentration in plasma. Animal experiments have confirmed the expected relation between plasma digoxin concentrations and electrophysiological effects on the heart.[232]

The availability of methods for measuring serum or plasma digitalis concentrations* in the clinical laboratory has led to extensive studies concerning the relation between serum levels and manifestations of toxicity in man.[61] Methods practically applicable to evaluation of patient serum samples are based on physicochemical separation, inhibition of Na^+,K^+-ATPase or its transmembrane cation transport function, or competitive protein binding employing either a specific antibody or a preparation containing Na^+,K^+-ATPase. Available methods are discussed in detail elsewhere.[233]

RADIOIMMUNOASSAY. Most published clinical studies have employed specific antibody as the binding protein in a competitive binding assay. This procedure is readily adaptable to the clinical laboratory. Small volumes of serum or plasma may be used directly, without prior extraction, necessitating a minimal number of manipulations. Appropriately selected antisera have exceptionally high degrees of affinity and specificity for the cardiac glycoside of interest, allowing the measurement of subnanogram amounts.[234] However, as with other radioimmunoassays, these are subject to certain pitfalls that may cause erroneous results if careful attention is not paid to selection of antisera, assurance of purity of standards and tracers, and appropriate counting techniques.[235]

Further details of available techniques for measurement of circulating cardiac glycoside concentrations are provided in reviews of this subject.[61,233,234] With the proliferation of commercial kits for measuring cardiac glycoside concentrations, it is particularly important for the clinician and clinical investigator to be certain that the values reported by the laboratory are accurate. Moreover, uncertainty can be introduced if sufficient time has not elapsed since the last previous dose to allow full equilibration of the drug between intravascular and peripheral compartments. In practice, a safe time for sampling of serum or plasma is 6 hours or more after the last dose of the cardiac glycoside.

CLINICAL CORRELATIONS. Although several techniques have been used to measure the concentrations of digoxin and digitoxin, there is substantial agreement regarding these values in patients receiving usual maintenance doses of these drugs.[61] Mean serum or plasma digoxin concentrations in groups of patients without evidence of toxicity average about 1.4 ng/ml. As would be expected, increasing digoxin doses or decreasing renal function is correlated with higher mean serum levels. Mean serum digoxin concentrations tend to be two to three times higher in patients with clinical evidence of digoxin toxicity, and the difference in mean levels is statistically significant in the vast majority of studies.[61] It must be emphasized that overlap of levels between groups with and without evidence of toxicity has been observed in most series and tends to be more pronounced in prospective, blind studies than in retrospective studies.[225] Despite this overlap, use of serum digoxin concentration measurements to guide therapy has been associated with a reduction in the incidence of digitalis toxicity.[236]

Analogous data correlating serum digitoxin concentrations with clinical state[61] indicate that although levels average about 10-fold higher than those of digoxin because of digitoxin binding to serum proteins, patients with clinical evidence of toxicity again have mean levels about two times higher than those without evidence of a toxic response. As in the case of digoxin, substantial overlap in levels occurs among groups of patients with and without evidence of toxicity despite the statistically significant differences in mean serum concentrations.

Although cardiac digitalis toxicity is accompanied by relatively well-defined relations between rhythm disturbance and serum glycoside concentration, it is more difficult to correlate therapeutic effects with serum levels in

*Serum and plasma digoxin, digitoxin, and ouabain concentrations are equivalent and will hereafter be referred to as serum concentrations.

man. A correlation has been reported between plasma digoxin levels and slowing of previously rapid ventricular rates in patients with atrial fibrillation.[237] Another measure of the degree of digitalization is the cumulative dose of acetylstrophanthidin required to reach a toxic endpoint.[227] Substantial variation in acetylstrophanthidin sensitivity was demonstrated among individual patients at any given serum digoxin level, indicating a continuing need to correlate serum digoxin concentration with other, independent methods of assessing myocardial sensitivity to cardiac glycosides.

The multifactorial determinants of digitalis intoxication and the overlap in serum digitalis concentrations between toxic and nontoxic states preclude the use of these levels as a sole guide to digitalis dosage. A Bayesian approach (page 273) to the use of serum digoxin levels in clinical decision making is logical and theoretically attractive.[238] Serum levels considered within a particular clinical context together with other available information can be a valuable aid to therapeutic decision-making. Suspected manifestations of digitalis intoxication in the absence of an adequate history, fluctuating renal function, presence of overt or suspected malabsorption, and use of preparations of uncertain bioavailability are among the circumstances in which knowledge of the serum level is most helpful. More generally, it is our opinion that measurement of serum cardiac glycoside concentrations is indicated whenever an unanticipated response to these drugs (either suspected toxicity or absence of an expected therapeutic effect) is encountered.

DIGITALIS TOXICITY

Toxic manifestations of digitalis persist as one of the most prevalent adverse drug reactions encountered in clinical practice.[61,239,240] The true incidence is difficult to determine accurately but at present is probably in the range of 5 to 15 per cent in hospitalized patients receiving these drugs. The variability in available estimates relates to differing definitions of digitalis intoxication, the retrospective nature of many studies, and differences in the groups under study. In a prospective investigation, 931 consecutive admissions to a single medical facility were studied. Of these, 15 per cent of patients had taken digitoxin, digoxin, or digitalis leaf up to 48 hours or less before admission. Digitalis intoxication was diagnosed electrocardiographically by the presence of typical disturbances of impulse formation and conduction that disappeared when the drug was withheld. Of the digitalized patients, 23 per cent fulfilled criteria for definite digitalis toxicity and another 6 per cent were judged to be possibly toxic. Other prospective studies have reported a comparable incidence of toxicity.[61] There is some evidence that increased understanding of pharmacokinetics and the use of serum level data to guide therapy have reduced this alarming incidence,[236] but constant vigilance on the part of the physician is required.

Mechanisms of Digitalis Intoxication (See also p. 238)

The major manifestations of digitalis intoxication include gastrointestinal and central nervous system symptoms and disturbances of cardiac rhythm. Anorexia, nausea, and vomiting are probably mediated by chemoreceptors located in the area postrema of the medulla rather than by a direct irritant effect of the drug on the gastrointestinal tract.[241] The precise mechanism underlying this and other central nervous system effects remains unclear, but several studies have demonstrated the presence of digoxin in the cerebrospinal fluid of patients treated with this drug.[242,243] Therefore, the drug clearly penetrates the blood-brain barrier in appreciable amounts and may, in addition, exert effects in regions that lack a normal blood-brain barrier, such as the area postrema of the medulla.[82,244]

The genesis of cardiac arrhythmias depends, at least in part, on the effect of the drug on the electrical activity of cardiac cells. Digitalis-induced disturbances of impulse formation and conduction are conventionally explained in terms of alterations in refractory period, impulse transmission, and automaticity of cardiac tissues, although alterations in sympathetic activity and changes in vagal tone may also be of considerable importance in some situations, as discussed previously. Interesting data have been obtained from experiments in which isolated canine Purkinje fibers were perfused with the blood of intact donor dogs and ouabain-induced changes in the donor dog's electrocardiogram were correlated with changes in the Purkinje fiber transmembrane potential[245,246] (Fig. 16–6). At the time of onset of early ouabain toxicity in the donor dog, defined as junctional or ventricular premature contractions or junctional tachycardia, Purkinje fiber recordings showed decreases in action-potential amplitude, resting membrane potential, maximum velocity of the upstroke of the action potential, action-potential duration, and plateau phase. Slowing of conduction was also apparent, often varying in extent from cycle to cycle. With further progression of toxicity to ventricular tachycardia in the donor dog, changes in transmembrane potential became still more marked, as shown in Figure 16–6.

In additional experiments, increased automaticity was found to occur at the time of early toxicity at plasma potassium concentrations below 4 mEq/liter. Increased automaticity was more frequent when Purkinje fibers had been stretched and in the presence of hypokalemia, which correlates well with clinical observations of increased frequency of digitalis toxicity in the dilated failing heart as well as in the presence of hypokalemia. Additional evidence bearing on the particular sensitivity of Purkinje fibers to the toxic electrophysiologic effects of digitalis comes from studies showing greater effects of acute and chronic digoxin administration on monovalent cation transport in Purkinje fibers compared with adjacent working myocardium.[37]

Regarding the cellular mechanism of digitalis toxicity, until recently most investigators favored a sequence in which digitalis-induced inhibition of Na^+ and K^+ transport caused increased intracellular $[Na^+]$, decreased intracellular $[K^+]$, and gradual depolarization. This in turn

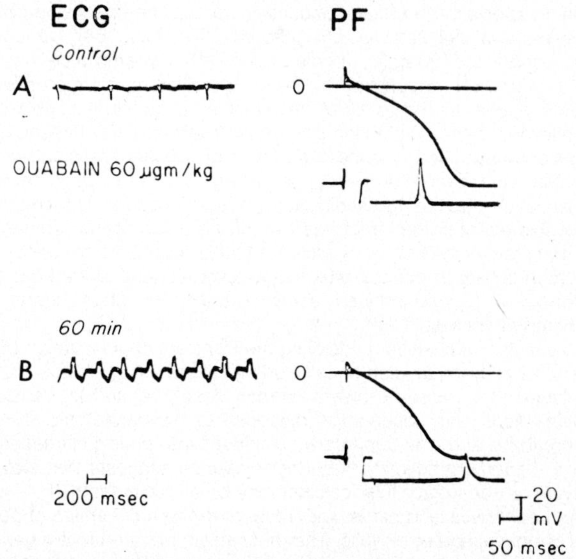

FIGURE 16–6 Effects of ouabain on the electrocardiogram (ECG) of an intact donor dog and on the Purkinje fiber (PF) action potential of an isolated preparation perfused with blood from the donor dog. Sinus rhythm (panel A) is succeeded by ventricular tachycardia (panel B) 60 minutes after administration of a toxic dose of ouabain. At the onset of ventricular tachycardia, the Purkinje fiber action potential shows significant loss of amplitude, duration, and maximum velocity of the phase 0 upstroke. The lower trace in each PF panel shows the first derivative of voltage with respect to time during phase 0. (From Rosen, M. R., et al.: Correlation between effects of ouabain on the canine electrocardiogram and transmembrane potentials of isolated Purkinje fibers. Circulation *47*:65, 1973, by permission of the American Heart Association, Inc.)

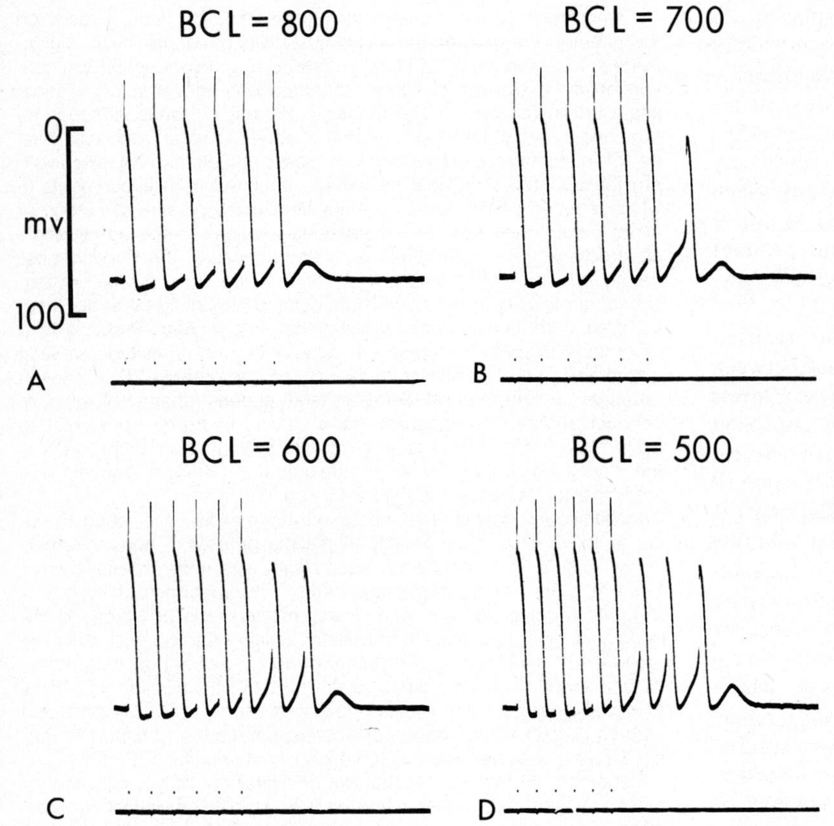

FIGURE 16–7 Sequential development (*A* to *D*) of a train of spontaneous beats due to transient depolarizations (also called oscillatory afterpotentials) in a canine Purkinje fiber exposed to acetylstrophanthidin and then driven at varying basic cycle lengths (BCL), indicated in milliseconds at the top of each panel. (From Ferrier, G. R., et al.: A cellular mechanism for the generation of ventricular arrhythmias by acetylstrophanthidin. Circ. Res. *32*:600, 1973, by permission of the American Heart Association, Inc.)

led to increased automaticity, conduction disturbances, and finally inexcitability. Recent experimental evidence suggests that cardiac glycosides promote a hitherto unrecognized mechanism of spontaneous activity in specialized cardiac conducting tissue. The underlying cellular event is a depolarizing afterpotential that has been variously called "enhanced diastolic depolarization,"[247] "low-amplitude potential,"[248] "transient depolarization,"[249] or "oscillatory afterpotentials" (p. 620), shown in Figure 16–7. In panel A, a transient depolarization follows a train of six action potentials. It falls short of threshold in this instance but can influence conduction of subsequent impulses.[250] With increased driving frequency, as shown in panel B, the transient depolarization reaches threshold, and excitation occurs. The counterpart of this event in the intact heart would be a ventricular premature beat. Panels C and D show multiple repetitive responses to further increases in driving frequency, which may be analogous to the beat dependence of digitalis-induced ectopic activity in intact hearts of experimental animals.[251,252]

The cellular mechanism underlying the transient depolarization phenomenon has been studied in calf Purkinje fibers using voltage-clamp techniques.[253] A transient inward current closely related to transient depolarizations was observed in response to the cardiotonic steroid strophanthidin and was temporally coincident with phasic increases in tension ("aftercontraction").[254] Further evidence suggests that elevated levels of free intracellular calcium may be a crucial factor,[254,255] just as has been discussed earlier with respect to the mechanism of positive inotropic action of digitalis. The mechanism involved in the generation of digitalis-induced transient depolarizations clearly differs both from that underlying normal phase 4 spontaneous depolarization and from the slow inward current.[256]

Potential or overt toxic effects of digitalis on cardiac electrophysiology will now be briefly summarized:

SINUS NODE AND ATRIUM

Digitalis-induced slowing of the sinus rate in patients without congestive heart failure is usually minor in degree and is largely mediated by vagal effects on the sinoatrial node. Patients with transplanted, denervated hearts do not respond to conventional doses of digoxin with any change in sinus rate.[257] As far as direct effects of digitalis are concerned, the atrium seems more sensitive than the sinus node. Experimentally, at higher doses, there is a depression in sinus node automaticity.[258,259] A combination of vagal and direct effects on the sinus node probably contributes to sinus bradycardia as well as to occasional cases of sinoatrial arrest or exit block seen in digitalis intoxication. This bradycardia predisposes to the emergence of junctional ventricular escape rhythms.

Digitalis, even in therapeutic doses, can impair sinoatrial conduction. Although usually well tolerated in patients with sick sinus syndrome, occasionally sinus node dysfunction is precipitated by digoxin, even in doses not usually associated with toxicity. Digitalis shortens the refractory period of the atrial myocardium in experimental studies, but has relatively minor and variable effects in the human heart.[61]

ATRIOVENTRICULAR NODE

The effective refractory period of the atrioventricular node is prolonged by digitalis. As with the sinus node, this longer period is in part related to increased vagal activity and in part to direct action on nodal fibers, although the vagal effect appears to predominate in subjects without intrinsic diseases of the cardiac conduction system.[190] Decreased amplitude and upstroke velocity of the action potential from the node itself and from nodal-His fibers have been recorded by means of microelectrode studies of isolated tissues in response to cardiac glycosides.[260]

The therapeutic effect of digitalis in slowing ventricular response in atrial flutter or fibrillation depends in part on the entry of concealed atrial impulses into the atrioventricular node, with failure to reach the His-Purkinje system by virtue of decremental conduction within the node (p. 624). When atrioventricular block of second or third degree occurs as a result of digitalis intoxication, however, the principal mechanism is failure of propagation within the atrioventricular node.[260]

HIS-PURKINJE SYSTEM

Digitalis-induced increases in the automaticity of the His-Purkinje system may come about because of enhanced spontaneous diastolic (phase 4) depolarization or the more recently described transient depolarization mechanism discussed above and elsewhere.[61] The appearance of new pacemakers is manifest clinically by premature junctional or ventricular beats or by accelerated junctional or ventricular rhythms. The nonuniform effect of digitalis on ventricular and Purkinje fibers and simultaneous enhancement of automaticity, depression of conduction velocity, and local block may also predispose to arrhythmias based on reentry mechanisms that may progress to ventricular tachycardia and fibrillation.[61]

Clinical Manifestations

Gastrointestinal Symptoms. Anorexia is often an early manifestation of digitalis intoxication.[225] Nausea and vomiting follow as clear consequences of digitalis overdose and result from central nervous system mechanisms.[241] It may be difficult, in clinical situations, to attribute these symptoms to digitalis, since they may also be caused by cardiac failure or by associated illnesses.

Neurological Symptoms. These include headache, fatigue, malaise, neuralgic pain, disorientation, confusion, delirium, and seizures. Visual symptoms are not infrequent and include scotomas, flickering, halos, and changes in color perception.[261] As with gastrointestinal symptoms, it is often difficult to determine whether neurological symptoms are a consequence of digitalis excess, associated fluid and electrolyte disturbances, or associated illnesses.

Cardiac Toxicity (see also pages 238 to 242). Cardiac toxicity manifested by arrhythmias can take the form of essentially every known rhythm disturbance.[61] Common arrhythmias include atrioventricular junctional escape rhythms, ventricular bigeminy or trigeminy, nonparoxysmal atrioventricular junctional tachycardia, unifocal or multifocal ectopic ventricular beats, and ventricular tachycardia. Atrioventricular junctional exit block, paroxysmal atrial tachycardia with atrioventricular block, sinus arrest, and Mobitz type I (Wenckebach) second-degree atrioventricular block also occur. This list should not be considered exhaustive. There are no unequivocal electrocardiographic features that distinguish digitalis-toxic rhythm disturbances from rhythms due to intrinsic cardiac disease, although rhythms combining features of increased automaticity of ectopic pacemakers with impaired conduction, such as paroxysmal atrial tachycardia with atrioventricular dissociation and an accelerated atrioventricular junctional pacemaker, strongly suggest digitalis toxicity. However, even rhythms such as atrial tachycardia with AV block, considered typical of digitalis toxicity, are frequently due to underlying heart disease rather than to digitalis excess.[262] The difficulty in determining whether or not ventricular ectopic activity is due to digitalis excess is exemplified by a study in which 142 patients with this rhythm disturbance, most of whom were on maintenance digoxin doses, were given incremental doses of the rapidly acting agent acetylstrophanthidin to determine their response.[263] Frequency of ventricular premature beats decreased in 46 per cent of patients, remained unchanged in 26 per cent, and increased in 28 per cent in response to the additional doses of digitalis. The cause of an arrhythmia may at times be clarified (but not defined with complete certainty) by demonstration of a reversion to normal rhythm when the drug is withheld. Clinical and electrocardiographic findings associated with digitalis toxicity have been reviewed extensively.[61,264–266]

Other Manifestations. Allergic skin lesions are rare but have been reported.[267] Gynecomastia is occasionally induced in men,[268] and sexual dysfunction has been reported.[269]

Massive Cardiac Glycoside Overdose

Digitalis overdose, either suicidal or accidental, is occasionally encountered as a life-threatening problem.[190,191,270] Patients without underlying heart disease tend to tolerate large doses, with serum digoxin concentrations ranging as high as 10 to 15 ng/ml.[190]

The principal manifestations in patients without intrinsic heart disease are most often sinus bradycardia; atrioventricular block of first, second, or third degree; or sinoatrial exit block. Atropine alone is often successful in reversing these manifestations but is not invariably effective.[61,190] Ventricular pacing with a pervenous endocardial catheter electrode is usually successful, although ventricular standstill unresponsive to pacing has been reported.[190]

Patients with preexisting heart disease tend to be more difficult to manage, in that ectopic ventricular arrhythmias are frequently the initial manifestation of digitalis intoxication.[190] Phenytoin, lidocaine, procainamide, and potassium have been used in treatment.[61] Direct-current cardioversion may also be required for refractory, life-threatening supraventricular or ventricular tachycardia or for ventricular fibrillation, despite the known hazards of this therapeutic modality in patients with digitalis toxicity. Not infrequently, the ventricular arrhythmias in this group lead to a fatal outcome despite the most vigorous therapeutic efforts.

Refractory hyperkalemia can occur at extremely high digoxin doses and serum concentrations.[190,191,271] Greater elevations of serum K^+ concentration were associated with worsening prognosis in a large series of patients after massive doses, usually of digitoxin.[272] It is likely that elevation of serum potassium is a consequence of inhibition of Na^+,K^+-ATPase throughout the body, with consequent impairment of monovalent cation transport across cell membranes.

The half-time for digoxin clearance from plasma is shortened when levels are very high.[190,273] This effect may be related to an altered ratio between plasma and tissue concentrations, allowing a relatively large quantity of the drug to be presented to the kidney for excretion.

Treatment of Digitalis Intoxication

The key to successful treatment is early recognition that an arrhythmia is related to digitalis intoxication. The more common manifestations—including occasional ectopic beats, marked first-degree atrioventricular block, or atrial fibrillation with a slow ventricular response—require only temporary withdrawal of the drug, electrocardiographic monitoring (if indicated) until the arrhythmia has disappeared, and subsequent adjustment of the dosage schedule to prevent recurrence. Rhythm disturbances that impair cardiac output because of too rapid or too slow ventricular rates, or those that portend ventricular fibrillation, require more active intervention. Ventricular tachycardia due to digitalis intoxication demands immediate vigorous treatment. Sinus bradycardia, sinoatrial arrest, and atrioventricular block of second or third degree are sometimes treated effectively with atropine, as previously indicated. Occasionally, electrical pacing will be required. It has been recommended that nonparoxysmal atrioventricular junctional rhythms with rates greater than 90 or with exit block be treated actively.[274] Atrioventricular junctional escape rhythms may simply be monitored if the rate is satisfactory.

Phenytoin and Lidocaine (see also pages 653 and 661). Phenytoin and lidocaine are useful drugs in the treatment of ectopic arrhythmias due to digitalis toxicity.[61] They have little adverse effect on sinoatrial rate, atrial conduction, atrioventricular conduction, or conduction in the

His-Purkinje system.[275–277] Indeed, phenytoin may improve sinoatrial block and atrioventricular conduction under some circumstances.[277,278] A recommended regimen for phenytoin is 100 mg administered by slow intravenous infusion every 5 minutes until onset of toxicity or control of the arrhythmia, followed by an oral maintenance dose of 400 to 600 mg/day if control of the arrhythmia is achieved. Lidocaine is given intravenously in 100-mg bolus doses every 3 to 5 minutes, followed by the continuous infusion of 15 to 50 μg/kg of body weight/min as required to maintain control of the rhythm disturbances.

Potassium. Therapy with potassium is recommended for ectopic tachyarrhythmias when hypokalemia is present but must be used with caution in other circumstances because of the risks associated with hyperkalemia.[61] Particular care is necessary when conduction disturbances are present, since elevations of plasma potassium concentration may impair atrioventricular conduction.[279]

Propranolol. Propranolol has been useful in the treatment of some digitalis-toxic arrhythmias. Because of its antiadrenergic effects, it causes a decrease in automaticity, whereas by virtue of its direct myocardial effects, it shortens the refractory period of atrial muscle, ventricular muscle, and Purkinje fibers; slows the rate of depolarization; and slows conduction velocity.[280] Potential undesirable effects include depression of atrioventricular conduction and of sinoatrial and atrioventricular junctional pacemakers, with asystole or marked bradycardia, and depression of myocardial contractility with hemodynamic deterioration.

Quinidine and Procainamide (see also pages 656 and 657). Quinidine and procainamide carry a risk of cardiac toxicity, such as depression of the sinoatrial node and of atrioventricular and His-Purkinje conduction, as well as the potential for eliciting ventricular arrhythmias. They are also capable of depressing myocardial contractility. Quinidine may actually intensify digitalis intoxication by raising serum level, as discussed on p. 519. Other agents are usually preferable for use in digitalis intoxication.[274]

Direct-Current Countershock (see also page 669). Whereas countershock is generally inadvisable in the presence of digitalis intoxication because of the severe arrhythmias that may ensue, it must occasionally be used when all other methods have failed in the face of a life-threatening rhythm disturbance. The risk is decreased when lower energy levels are employed.[61,281] In contrast to the increased risk reported in the presence of overt digitalis toxicity, cardioversion appears to be a benign procedure in patients without digitalis-induced rhythm disturbances.[282]

Steroid-Binding Resins. As previously noted (p. 514), digitoxin undergoes some enterohepatic circulation, and agents that bind the drug within the gastrointestinal lumen should shorten its half-life. Cholestyramine induced a reduction in serum half-life of chloroform-extractable activity from 6.0 to 4.5 days after tritiated digitoxin administration in man,[138] and colestipol appears to have a similar effect.[283] These effects may provide a means of reducing the duration of digitoxin toxicity but are probably not of sufficient magnitude or rapidity to be of great importance in the management of severe, life-threatening toxicity. Although digoxin has only a minimal enterohepatic circulation,[144] cholestyramine tends to interfere with its initial absorption from the gastrointestinal tract.[284]

Reversal of Toxicity by Specific Antibody. The use of cardiac glycoside–specific antibodies and their Fab fragments for treatment of advanced digitalis intoxication has been studied in considerable detail.[285–287] A possible mechanism for the reversal of both inotropic and arrhythmogenic effects of cardiac glycosides was suggested in experiments demonstrating that high-affinity cardiac glycoside–specific antibodies are able to reverse established glycoside-induced inhibition of myocardial Na^+,K^+-ATPase[288] and monovalent cation active transport.[289]

Fab fragments provide advantages over purified intact antibodies as potential therapeutic agents. Each intact IgG antibody molecule of molecular weight 150,000 is cleaved by the proteolytic enzyme papain into an Fc fragment and two Fab fragments, each of which contains a specific binding site and has a molecular weight of 50,000. This smaller molecular species has a greater rate and volume of distribution after intravenous infusion and reverses experimentally induced digoxin-toxic arrhythmias more rapidly than does intact antibody.[287] The smaller size of the Fab molecule also allows it to pass through the mammalian glomerulus, unlike intact IgG. Fab fragments are excreted to an appreciable extent in the urine, but intact IgG is not.[290] Whereas injection of intact antibody markedly prolongs the plasma half-life of digoxin (although it is largely antibody-bound), digoxin bound to Fab fragments is excreted much more rapidly.[291] Rapid reversal of otherwise lethal experimentally induced digitoxin toxicity with specific antibodies and Fab fragments has been demonstrated,[292] together with substantial acceleration by Fab of the renal excretion of digitoxin. This rapid renal excretion of Fab fragments may be of importance in reducing the immunogenicity of the foreign protein.[293]

A series of 26 patients with life-threatening digoxin or digitoxin toxicity has been treated with purified digoxin-specific Fab fragments.[191] All these patients had advanced cardiac rhythm disturbances and in 9 cases hyperkalemia was present as well, owing, in the majority, to ingestion of very large digitalis doses accidentally or with suicidal intent. All patients treated had an initial favorable response to intravenously administered Fab. Four patients eventually died as a result of cerebral or myocardial damage from prolonged low output states prior to Fab administration; available Fab supplies were insufficient to provide adequate treatment in a fifth case. In the remaining 21 patients, cardiac arrhythmias and hyperkalemia were reversed rapidly with full recovery.[191] Efforts are underway to make this therapeutic modality more widely available.

DIURETICS

A diuretic is a drug that increases urinary excretion of salt and water. Certain agents *indirectly* increase urine production by enhancing renal blood flow and the rate of glomerular filtration. Examples of such agents are digitalis, which effects a diuresis indirectly by enhancing cardiac output, and dopamine, which not only increases cardiac output but also acts directly on the renal vasculature; the diuretic action of albumin and dextran is through expansion of plasma volume. Most diuretics, however, act *directly* on the kidney to inhibit solute and water absorption, thereby increasing urine volume. While it is generally assumed that diuretics exert their favorable clinical effects by promoting excretion of excess salt and water and reducing abnormally elevated preload, there is evidence that furosemide administration can produce a diuresis accompanied by improved performance of the failing left ventricle and reduced afterload without alteration of the left ventricular diastolic dimension as an index of preload.[294]

Nonreabsorbable solutes such as mannitol are freely filtered at the glomerulus. Since their osmotic effects inhibit water reabsorption, thereby causing a diuresis, such substances are termed osmotic diuretics.[295] Many pharmacological agents interfere with active ion transport, resulting in increased urine flow secondary to the enhanced excretion of ions and the water they osmotically obligate (Fig. 16–8). The precise cellular sites of action of most diuretics are not known. They may interfere with any of the three steps in the sequence of sodium reabsorption: (1) the entry of the solute into the cell, (2) the generation and utilization of energy for sodium transport, and (3) the transfer of sodium from the cell to peritubular blood through the antiluminal membrane.[296,297] *Water diuresis* may be induced by agents such as demeclocycline or lithium that block the cellular action of vasopressin, which normally allows the reabsorption of water along the distal nephron and collecting system.

SITES AND MECHANISMS OF ACTION OF DIURETIC AGENTS (See Figures 16–9 and 16–10 and Table 16–6)

PROXIMAL TUBULE

Since 50 to 75 per cent of filtered sodium and water is reabsorbed by the proximal tubule, substances that inhibit transport in this segment of the nephron would be expected to be potent diuretic agents.[298] Although no available diuretic completely prevents proximal tubular sodium reabsorption, the carbonic anhydrase inhibitors such as acetazolamide act primarily by inhibiting proximal reabsorption. It has been shown under experimental conditions that thiazide diuretics,[299,300] metolazone, and furosemide[301] possess mild carbonic anhydrase inhibitory activity, but this action does not appear to be clinically important. Acetazolamide is actively absorbed and concentrated within cells of the proximal tubule and causes diuresis by inhibiting the formation of hydrogen ions needed to reabsorb filtered sodium bicarbonate. The demands of electroneutrality require that sodium and, to a lesser extent, potassium be retained in the tubular lumen to offset the accumulating negative charge from unreabsorbed bicarbonate anion, causing a sodium, potassium, and bicarbonate diuresis. The effectiveness of carbonic anhydrase inhibitors is proportional to the filtered load of bicarbonate. It follows that their efficacy is impaired by metabolic acidosis and enhanced by metabolic alkalosis.[302] Moreover, because these agents induce loss of $NaHCO_3$, they induce metabolic acidosis, which progressively limits their effectiveness.

A significant fraction of proximal sodium and chloride reabsorption is passive, being dependent on the generation of a favorable chloride gradient between tubular fluid and plasma. The active reabsorption of

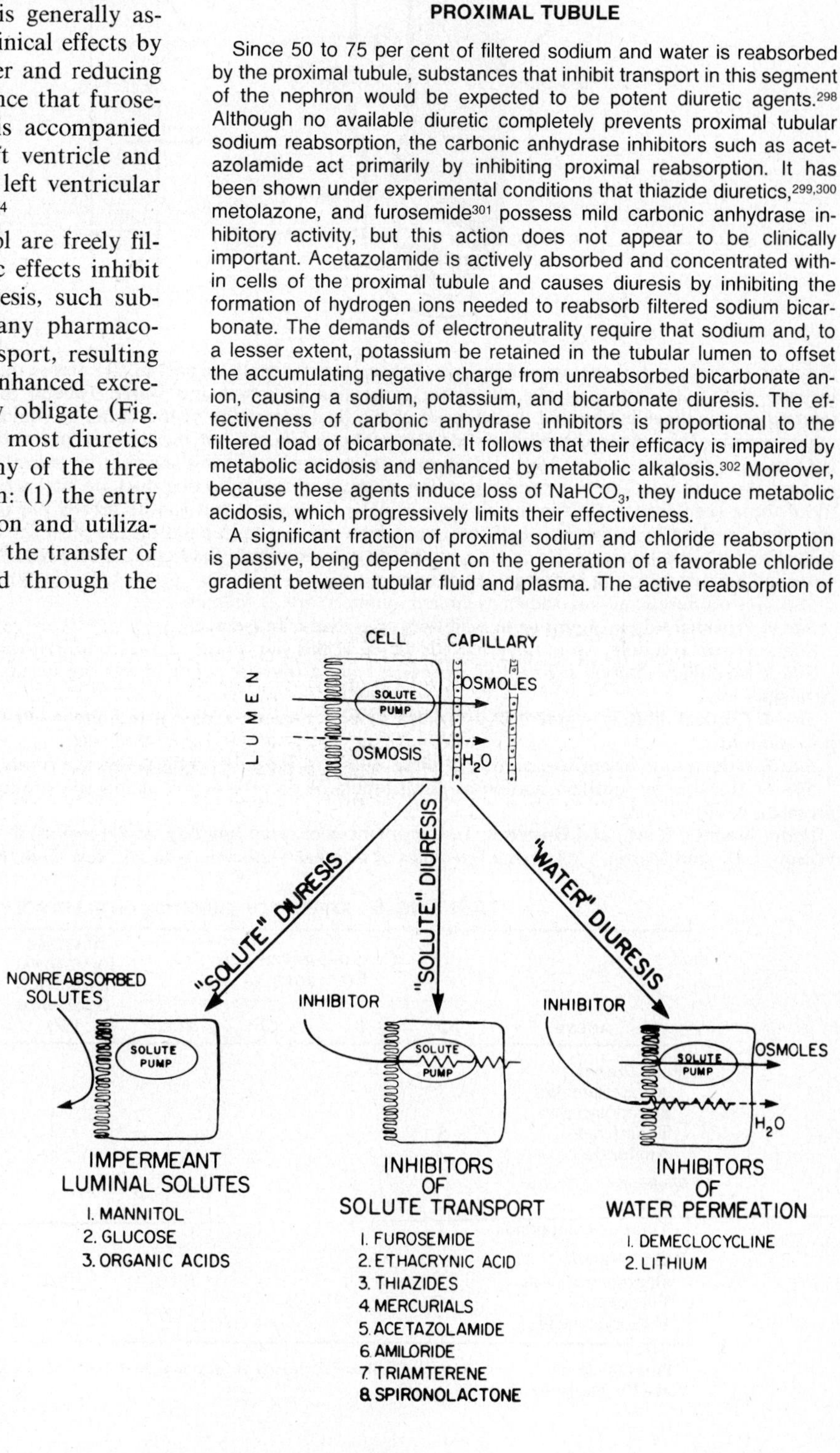

FIGURE 16–8 General mechanisms of diuresis. Glomerular filtrate is absorbed in renal tubules by the active transport of solute (osmoles) and the passive transport of water (osmosis). Two types of diuresis can occur due to interference with tubular absorption: (1) "Solute" diuresis follows the glomerular filtration of nonreabsorbable solute or in consequence of the inhibition of solute pumps. (2) "Water" diuresis is seen when the osmotic permeability to water is decreased selectively. (From Grantham, J. J., and Chonko, A. M.: The physiological basis and clinical use of diuretics. *In* Brenner, B. M., and Stein, J. H. (eds.): Sodium and Water Homeostasis. Vol. I. New York, Churchill Livingstone, 1978, p. 179.)

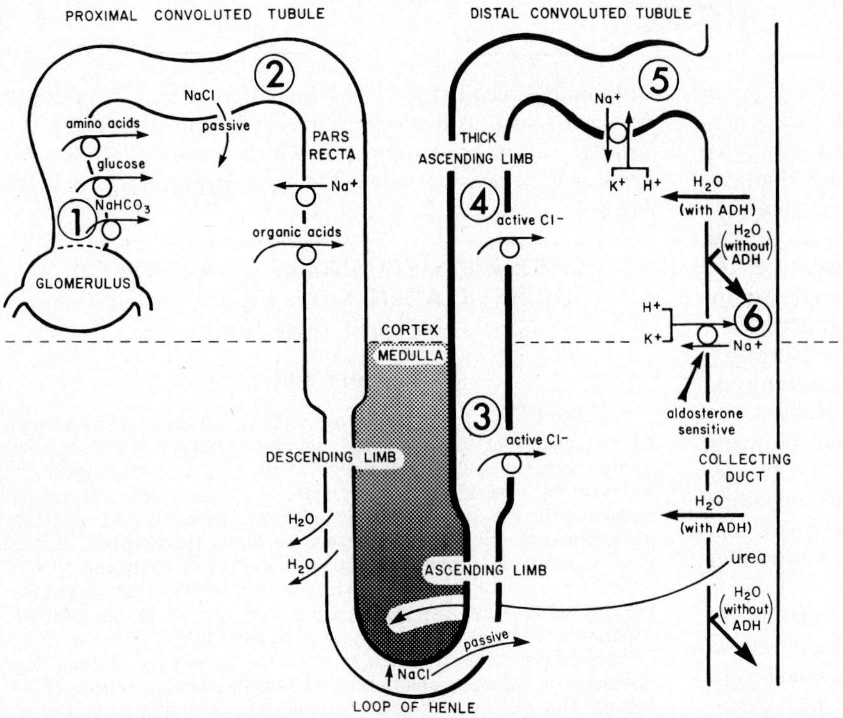

FIGURE 16–9 Transport functions of the various anatomical segments of the mammalian nephron. Fluid reabsorption across the proximal tubule is isosmotic and accounts for approximately two-thirds of the reabsorption of filtered Na^+ and H_2O. $NaHCO_3$ is reabsorbed by a nonelectrogenic mechanism, most likely via H^+ secretion. The active transport of these solutes results in transepithelial concentration and effective osmotic pressure gradients promoting H_2O flow across the proximal tubule into the peritubular capillaries. The rise in tubular fluid Cl^- concentration is a consequence of the decreased luminal HCO_3^- concentration and becomes an important force for the outward passive transport of Cl^- down its concentration gradient. The pars recta of the proximal tubule is capable of active electrogenic transport of Na^+. Normally, approximately one-third of the glomerular filtrate enters the descending limb of Henle's loop. Because the thin descending limb is incapable of active outward NaCl transport and is characterized by low permeability to Na^+ but high H_2O permeability, H_2O is extracted passively as the fluid approaches the end of Henle's loop. Hypertonic fluid with a greater NaCl concentration but lower urea concentration than the surrounding medullary interstitium thus enters the thin ascending limb of Henle. This segment differs from the descending limb in that it is largely impermeable to H_2O and urea but highly permeable to NaCl. These characteristics allow for passive diffusion of NaCl out of the ascending limb. Active electrogenic transport of Cl^- across the water-impermeable thick ascending limb of Henle, with Na^+ following passively, allows for separation of solute and water. Tubular fluid therefore becomes dilute, and the medullary interstitium becomes hypertonic. Irrespective of the final osmolality of the urine, the fluid that enters the distal convoluted tubule is always hypo-osmotic. This segment exhibits active Na^+ reabsorption. All but the terminal portion of the distal convoluted tubule is impermeable to H_2O, even in the presence of ADH. Aldosterone exerts its effect in this segment by enhancing Na^+ reabsorption, which is variably coupled to K^+ and H^+ secretion. The cortical and papillary portions of the collecting duct are sites where ADH exerts its principal effect. The permeability of these segments to H_2O in the absence of ADH is very low but can be greatly enhanced in the presence of ADH. These segments are also characterized by active Na^+ reabsorption, which appears to depend on the presence of mineralocorticoids. In the absence of ADH, the collecting tubule is impermeable to H_2O, so that hypotonic tubule fluid courses through it. However, in the presence of ADH, water is avidly absorbed here, resulting in hypertonic final urine.

The sites of diuretic action, shown as circled numbers, are as follows:

Site 1: Proximal tubule. Sensitive to inhibitors of carbonic anhydrase.

Site 2: Proximal tubule. An osmotic diuretic acting at this site results in *increased* free-water production and *increased* potassium loss.

Site 3: Medullary diluting segment of ascending limb. A diuretic acting at this site results in *decreased* free-water production and *increased* potassium loss.

Site 4: Cortical diluting segment of ascending limb. A diuretic acting at this site results in *decreased* free-water production and *increased* potassium loss.

Site 5: Aldosterone-insensitive portion of distal tubule. A diuretic acting at this site produces *decreased* potassium loss.

Site 6: Aldosterone-sensitive portion of distal tubule. A diuretic acting at this site produces *decreased* potassium loss but acts only in the presence of aldosterone.

(From Brenner, B. M., and Hostetter, T.: Disturbances of renal function. *In* Petersdorf, R. G., Adams, R. D., Braunwald, E., Isselbacher, K. J., Wilson, J. D., and Martin, J. M. (eds.): Principles of Internal Medicine. 10th ed. New York, McGraw-Hill Book Co., 1983, p. 1602.)

TABLE 16–6 EFFECTS OF DIURETICS ON ELECTROLYTE EXCRETION

	Changes in Urinary Electrolytes				Maximal Fractional Excretion of Sodium	Inhibitory Factors		Site(s) of Action (see Figure 16–19 for Site Numbers)
Agent	*Na^+*	*K^+*	*Cl^-*	*HCO_3^-*	(%)	*Acidosis*	*Alkalosis*	
Weak Diuretics								
Acetazolamide	↑	↑	↓	↑	~4	+		1
Spironolactone	↑	↓	↑	↑	~2			6
Triamterene	↑	↓	↑	↑	~2			5
Amiloride	↑	↓	↑	↑	~2			5
Moderately Effective Diuretics								
Thiazide compounds	↑	↑	↑	↑	~8			4
Potent Diuretics								
Organomercurials	↑	↑	↑		~20		+	3,4
Furosemide	↑	↑	↑		~23			3,4
Ethacrynic acid	↑	↑	↑		~23			3,4?,5,6

From Brater, D. C., and Thier, S. O.: Renal disorders. *In* Melmon, K. L., and Morrelli, H. F. (eds.): Clinical Pharmacology. New York, The Macmillan Co., 1978, p. 349.

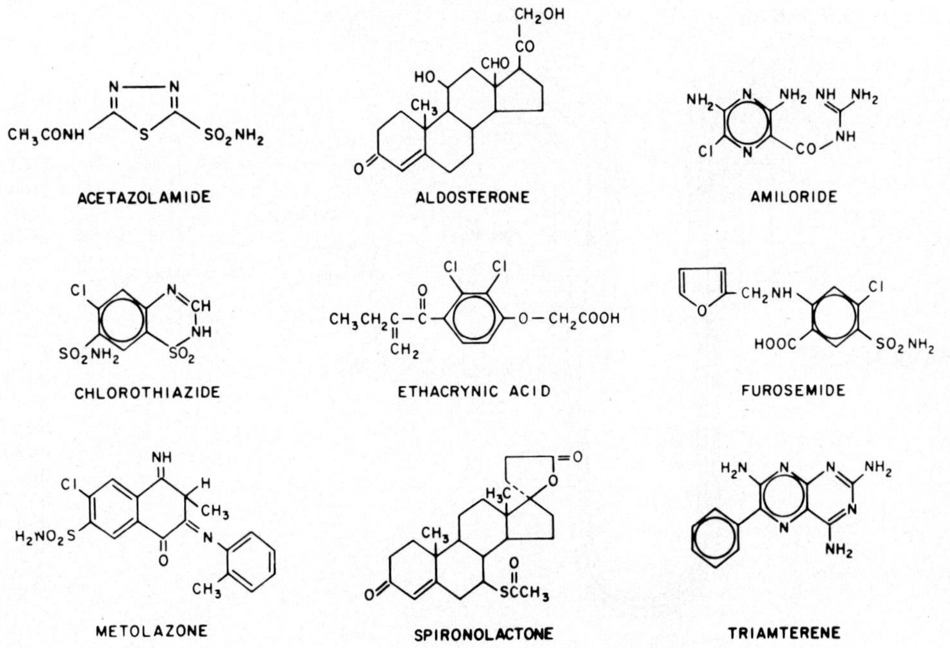

FIGURE 16–10 Structures of diuretics.

sodium bicarbonate and water increases this luminal concentration of chloride, thereby creating a favorable chemical gradient for the passive movement of chloride into the peritubular blood. The positive luminal charge engendered by loss of chloride enables sodium to move passively down its electrochemical gradient into the blood. Water passively follows NaCl along its osmotic gradient.[303] Reduction of proximal tubular bicarbonate reabsorption by inhibition of carbonic anhydrase will therefore appreciably decrease sodium and chloride transport. However, the increased delivery of sodium chloride to the distal tubule merely results in enhanced reabsorption there, and as a consequence, carbonic anhydrase inhibition may produce little diuresis. However, when distal reabsorption is interfered with by another diuretic, such as ethacrynic acid or chlorothiazide, acetazolamide's inhibition of proximal reabsorption is unmasked.[302] In some patients who develop normokalemic hypochloremic alkalosis as a consequence of treatment with furosemide and spironolactone, inhibitors of proximal tubular reabsorption may be effective.[304]

LOOP OF HENLE

The thin and thick portions of the ascending limb of Henle's loop are impermeable to water but permeable to solute (Fig. 16–9). Sodium chloride *passively* exits from the thin segment, whereas *active* chloride transport, accompanied passively by sodium, accounts for loss of solute from the thick ascending segment.[305,306] Loss of luminal solute but retention of water renders luminal fluid dilute and interstitial tissue concentrated. In the distal tubule and early cortical collecting duct, water moves out of the lumen, down its osmotic gradient, but the relative impermeability of these segments to urea causes the luminal urea concentration to increase. In the late medullary collecting duct, urea moves passively into the interstitium where it accumulates and exerts a major osmotic effect on the water-permeable but sodium chloride–impermeable descending limb. Water leaves this segment—in response to a high concentration of urea in the interstitium—causing the remaining sodium chloride concentration to increase progressively. The luminal solute concentration is increased above that of the interstitium, allowing sodium chloride to exit *passively* from the thin ascending limb.

Diuretics such as *furosemide, ethacrynic acid,* and the *organic mercurials,* which act, in part, by inhibiting chloride transport in the ascending limb, enhance the excretion not only of that solute but also of water, by removing the gradient for passive water movement from the descending limb of Henle's loop and the medullary collecting duct into the renal interstitium. The mechanism by which these diuretics inhibit chloride reabsorption in the ascending limb has not been elucidated, although considerable evidence supports the view that they block the entry of chloride into the cell at the luminal membrane (Fig. 16–11). It has also been proposed that chloride transport in the ascending limb is in some way dependent on Na^+,K^+ATPase activity and that this inhibition of ATPase activity[307] plays a role in the diuretic effects of furosemide, ethacrynic acid, and the mercurials. Indeed, furosemide has been shown to inhibit selectively Na^+,K^+-ATPase in the loop of Henle,[308] but the relationship between this inhibition and its diuretic effects is still debated.[296,297] Some studies have suggested that the diuretic effect of ethacrynic acid may, at least in part, be related to its inhibition of prostaglandin degradation.[309] Both furosemide and ethacrynic acid inhibit adenylate cyclase[310] and prostaglandin dehydrogenase[311] and increase the urinary excretion of prostaglandin E_2.[309] Since indomethacin, aspirin, and presumably other prostaglandin synthetase inhibitors can blunt the natriuretic effect of furosemide,[312,313] the possibility that local prostaglandins may be involved in mediating the action of furosemide in the tubule must be considered. This change in sodium excretion may be caused by inhibition of the increased renal blood flow usually associated with furosemide administration. Another possibility is that indomethacin reduces the renal clearance of furosemide.

There is agreement that the loop diuretics, furosemide and ethacrynic acid, exert their effects on the luminal membrane and therefore must be secreted from peritubular capillaries into the proximal tubular fluid.[314–319] At least in the case of furosemide, the efficiency of this transport system is one determinant of the magnitude of the diuresis; the time-course of furosemide excretion is another. Progressive reabsorption of diuretic-free glomerular filtrate causes relatively high concentrations of the drug to be presented to the ascending limb of Henle's loop, where furosemide, ethacrynic acid, and mercurials exert their direct tubular effects. The observation that probenecid (an inhibi-

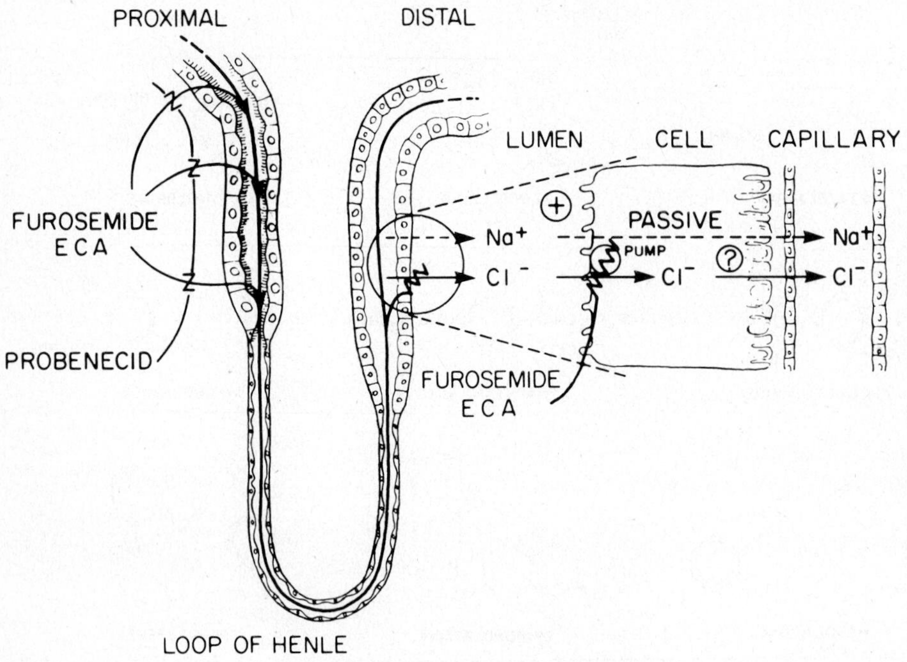

FIGURE 16–11 The mechanism of action of "loop" diuretics. Furosemide and ethacrynic acid (ECA) are actively secreted into the urine in the proximal tubule by a process that is inhibited by probenecid. Ethacrynic acid is modified to the cysteine adduct, the active form of the drug in the urine. These diuretics interfere with chloride transport at the luminal membrane of the ascending limb to decrease net solute absorption. Consequently, the drugs interfere with the formation of dilute urine and the concentration of interstitial solutes by a single inhibitory action. (From Grantham, J. J., and Chonko, A. M.: The physiological basis and clinical use of diuretics. *In* Brenner, B. M., and Stein, J. H. (eds.): Sodium and Water Homeostasis. Vol 1. New York, Churchill Livingstone, 1978, p. 178.)

tor of aryl acid transport) in the proximal tubule blocks the diuresis caused by furosemide supports this sequence of events.[320]

THE DISTAL NEPHRON

Thiazides act in the distal convoluted tubule,[300] perhaps by reducing the permeability of the luminal membrane to both sodium and chloride. However, they also enhance the excretion of potassium both by increasing its delivery to the distal tubule and by enhancing its secretion along this segment.[321] The molecular basis of the diuretic effect of the thiazides is still unknown.

Sodium chloride absorption and sodium-potassium exchange in the distal convoluted tubule, cortical collecting tubules, and perhaps the papillary collecting ducts are modulated by aldosterone. *Spironolactone* inhibits sodium reabsorption and potassium secretion indirectly by binding both to cytosolic and to nuclear protein receptors of aldosterone, displacing the hormone, and thereby preventing its effect.[322] Thus, it is a true competitive inhibitor of aldosterone, and its diuretic and antikaliuretic effects are dependent upon the presence of this hormone. Two other diuretics, *triamterene* and *amiloride*, also inhibit both the distal reabsorption of sodium and the secretion of potassium. However, these agents differ from spironolactone in that they are effective even in the absence of aldosterone. It has been proposed that they reduce the sodium permeability of the luminal surface of the tubular cell membrane, thus lowering the sodium available for transport across the antiluminal membrane[323]; this effect, in turn, is thought to interfere with potassium secretion.[324] In addition to their effects on distal sodium and potassium transport (perhaps secondary to potassium retention[325]), triamterene,[323] amiloride,[323] and spironolactone[326] are all capable of inhibiting urinary hydrogen ion secretion. There is evidence that furosemide and ethacrynic acid, in addition to their primary effect on the thick segment of the ascending limb of the loop of Henle, also act on the *collecting tubules* by inhibiting the action of vasopressin.[327,328]

PRINCIPLES OF DIURETIC ACTION

Diuretics stimulate regulatory processes that tend to counter their renal effects. Diuresis-induced plasma volume contraction, acting through a series of complex physical and hormonal signals, enhances tubular avidity for sodium, thereby tending to neutralize the diuretic effect. As a consequence, the efficacy of any diuretic in an intact system is much less than would be predicted from its action in an isolated preparation. Also, when a diuretic is given repeatedly, its activity diminishes as a result of progressively increased fractional reabsorption of sodium in the portion of the nephron unaffected by the diuretic. In this manner, salt balance is reestablished, albeit at a lower total body sodium than before diuretic administration. Hypovolemia may enhance sodium reabsorption by suppression of the postulated natriuretic hormone[329] and by activation of the renin-angiotensin system, which stimulates release of aldosterone. Other mediators, such as catecholamines and prostaglandins, may also affect the "tubuloglomerular feedback" system, which accounts for increased proximal tubular reabsorption of sodium in response to hypovolemia.

Since renal blood flow usually falls to a greater extent than does glomerular filtration during hypovolemia, a greater fraction of blood delivered to the kidney is filtered. Removal of a greater amount of protein-free fluid at the glomerulus causes the albumin concentration of postglomerular and peritubular blood to increase, and this increased oncotic pressure enhances the proximal reabsorption of sodium. Diuretics acting on the more distal nephron become progressively less effective as the glomerular filtration rate falls and increased reabsorption of sodium occurs in the proximal tubule. Therefore, drugs that act at different sites, such as furosemide and acetazolamide, tend to have additive diuretic effects. The combination of furosemide and metolazone has been reported to be effective in some patients with refractory edema,[330] and Wollam et al. have reported a successful diuretic response to combined hydrochlorothiazide and furosemide therapy in patients with renal insufficiency (serum creatinine range 1.3 to 4.9 mg/dl) who had a poor response to either drug alone.[331] We have found this combination to be effective in patients with refractory congestive heart failure without intrinsic renal disease. Also, intermittent courses of acetazolamide may induce diuresis in patients with refractory heart failure who have developed normokalemic hypochloremic alkalosis as a result of treatment with furosemide and spironolactone.[304] In addition, diuretics that act at the same site via different mechanisms, such as spironolactone and triamterene, may be additive. The action of one diuretic may counteract an undesirable effect of a second agent. Thus, spironolactone may reduce the potassium loss caused by thiazides without interfering with their diuretic action. It should be recognized that some degree of salt restriction is essential if negative sodium balance is to be achieved with potent but short-acting diuretics such as furosemide, because sodium lost after diuretic administration will otherwise be regained by renal conservation throughout the remainder of the day.[332]

RENAL BLOOD FLOW AND GLOMERULAR FILTRATION RATE. The acute administration of either furosemide or ethacrynic acid causes a significant increase in renal blood flow and reduction of renal vascular resistance.[333] Since both these agents also cause an increase in renal renin release, and since the renin-angiotensin system mediates vasoconstriction, some other prominent vasodilatory influence (perhaps enhanced synthesis of prostaglandin E[309,311]) must override this effect. In contrast, thiazides and acetazolamide diminish renal blood flow.[309,334] If as a consequence of diuretic administration plasma volume decreases and the left ventricular function curve moves to the left, (Figure 16–12), cardiac output, renal blood flow, and glomerular filtration rate will all decline, reducing the effectiveness of additional diuretic administration.

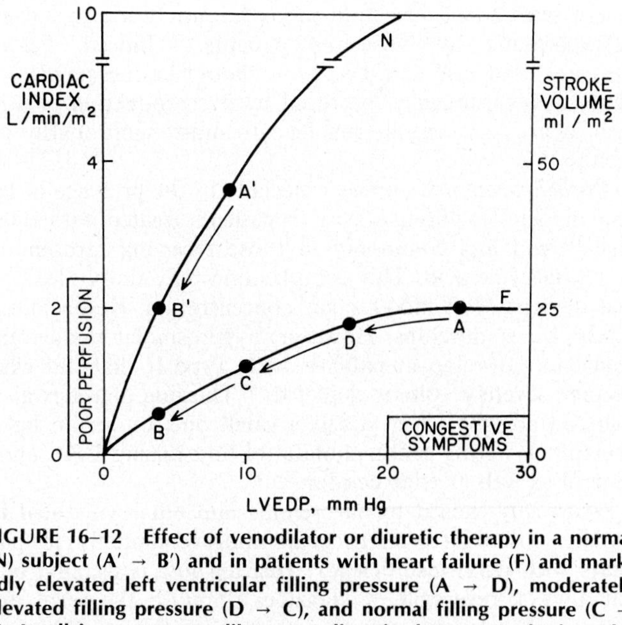

FIGURE 16–12 Effect of venodilator or diuretic therapy in a normal (N) subject (A′ → B′) and in patients with heart failure (F) and markedly elevated left ventricular filling pressure (A → D), moderately elevated filling pressure (D → C), and normal filling pressure (C → B). In all instances venodilators or diuretic therapy results in a decline in filling pressure; except in the patient with marked elevation of filling pressure, cardiac output declines.

Some diuretics reduce the glomerular filtration rate, related in part to lowered extracellular fluid volume and consequent lowering of cardiac output. In the case of furosemide, there is an initial rise in glomerular filtration rate, and, as extracellular fluid volume is reduced, renal blood flow and glomerular filtration rate fall. In contrast, ethacrynic acid may cause a fall in filtration rate despite concurrent replacement of fluid losses.[335] Since these diuretics increase peripheral venous compliance and reduce venous return[336–338]—actions independent of their renal effects—it is possible that renal blood flow and filtration rate may fall despite maintenance of extracellular fluid volume. The thiazides, mercurials, and carbonic anhydrase inhibitors also cause a decrease in glomerular filtration rate when diuretic losses are replaced. There is evidence that these effects may be secondary to an intrarenal feedback mechanism that couples distal salt delivery with filtration rate in individual nephrons.[339–341]

POTASSIUM EXCRETION. Urinary potassium excretion is dependent, in part, on the rate of volume flow past the distal convoluted and cortical collecting tubules. Therefore, acetazolamide, furosemide, ethacrynic acid, the thiazides, and osmotic diuretics such as mannitol tend to enhance urinary potassium loss.[342] In addition, activation of the renin-angiotensin-aldosterone system, which occurs in heart failure and also as a result of the contraction of the extracellular fluid volume induced by diuresis, further increases potassium secretion in the distal nephron. The aldosterone component of potassium-wasting becomes blunted, since hypokalemia decreases the adrenal secretion of aldosterone.[343] Also, contraction of the extracellular fluid compartment enhances the proximal reabsorption of glomerular filtrate, thereby reducing flow into the distal nephron and thus inhibiting further excretion of potassium. Thus, enhanced potassium excretion is usually not sustained if the extracellular fluid volume has been markedly contracted.[344] Indeed, urinary potassium loss and resultant potassium depletion are most pronounced in patients receiving diuretics with large sodium chloride and water intake.[345] Metabolic alkalosis is also a potent stimulus to distal potassium secretion and further loss of potassium into the urine.[346] Under these circumstances, supplemental intake of potassium chloride and administration of spironolactone or triamterene may be necessary.

COMPLICATIONS OF DIURETIC THERAPY

(See Table 16–7)

The increased distal delivery of sodium and water during diuretic therapy enhances secretion of potassium and hydrogen ions. *Potassium depletion,* in turn, further enhances hydrogen ion secretion and increases ammonia production through stimulation of renal glutaminase activity. The consequent reduction of hydrogen ion concentration produces a *metabolic alkalosis.* With contraction of the extracellular fluid volume and loss of sodium chloride ("contraction alkalosis"), there is increased reabsorption of sodium bicarbonate, maintaining the *metabolic alkalosis.*[347,348] Contraction alkalosis will usually respond to reduction of the dose of diuretic and reexpansion of the extracellular fluid volume[347] as well as to potassium

TABLE 16–7 COMPLICATIONS OF DIURETIC TREATMENT

Diuretic	Hyper-uricemia	Hypo-kalemia	Hyper-kalemia	Acidosis	Alkalosis	Other
Osmotic	−	+	−	−	+ (Contraction)	Hyper- or hypoosmolality
Acid-forming salts	−	+	−	+	−	
Organomercurials	−	+	+ (Rare, acute)	−	+	Tubular necrosis, hypersensitivity reactions
Acetazolamide	?	+	−	+	−	Urinary tract calculi, hepatic coma
Thiazides	+	+	−	−	+	Cutaneous vasculitis, agranulocytosis, thrombocytopenia, anemia, pancreatitis, glucose intolerance, hepatic coma
Ethacrynic acid	+	+	−	−	+	Hyper- and hypoglycemia, gastrointestinal bleeding, deafness, hepatic coma
Furosemide	+	+	−	−	+	Glucose intolerance, deafness, hepatic coma
Spironolactone	−	−	+	−	−	Gynecomastia
Triamterene	−	−	+	+	−	Azotemia, muscle cramps
Amiloride	−	−	+	+	−	Azotemia

From Brater, D. C., and Thier, S. O.: Renal disorders. *In* Melmon, K. L., and Morrelli, H. F. (eds.): Clinical Pharmacology. New York, The Macmillan Co., 1978, p. 349.

supplementation.[348] Diuretic-induced potassium depletion clearly predisposes some patients without overt cardiac disease to high-grade ventricular arrhythmias,[349] and this tendency is an even greater potential problem in patients with known cardiac disease. It must also be remembered, however, that *hyperkalemia* is also a serious risk in patients receiving potassium-sparing diuretics, especially in the elderly, in those with impaired renal function, and in those with diabetes mellitus.[350] Beta-adrenergic blocking agents will tend to accentuate any tendency to hyperkalemia in all of these states. These agents act, in part, by reducing renin release as well as by diminishing the extrarenal capacity for potassium uptake.[351]

Metabolic acidosis may occur as a complication of treatment with acetazolamide, which causes a sodium bicarbonate diuresis by reducing its proximal reabsorption. Spironolactone, by antagonizing aldosterone, may also limit the ability to excrete hydrogen ions, resulting in a hyperchloremic metabolic acidosis.[326]

Hyponatremia, an important complication of diuretic therapy, results from an imbalance between water ingestion and renal diluting capacity. Furosemide, ethacrynic acid, and thiazides inhibit free water generation and cause excretion of relatively concentrated urine. When water intake is increased, hyponatremia may occur.[352] In addition, stimuli for the secretion of antidiuretic hormone (ADH), including volume contraction,[353] morphine, pain, and mechanical ventilation, may be present in these patients. Since total body sodium is usually normal or increased in patients with heart failure receiving diuretics, restriction of water intake below external and insensible loss (usually $\leq$ 1000 ml/day) will increase the serum sodium concentration. Temporary interruption of diuretic therapy and, if possible, improvement of cardiac function with inotropic agents or treatment of a precipitating cause of heart failure are useful measures.

Hyperuricemia is a common complication of chronic diuretic therapy with thiazides, furosemide, and ethacrynic acid. Furosemide and ethacrynic acid compete with uric acid for secretion by the proximal organic acid transport system. This competition plus enhanced proximal and distal reabsorption of uric acid (caused by diuretic-induced contraction of the extracellular fluid volume) combine to elevate sodium uric acid. Most patients tolerate hyperuricemia well and require no specific treatment.[354] Sustained plasma urate concentrations up to 10 mg/100 ml appear to have no deleterious effect on renal function. Occasionally clinical gout develops, particularly in patients with a previous history of gout or hyperuricemia. Levels higher than 10 mg/100 ml may warrant the use of allopurinol.[355] It appears unlikely that moderate hyperuricemia (men $<$ 13 mg/dl; women $<$ 10 mg/dl) exerts a deleterious effect on renal function.[356] At higher levels or in patients with a history of gout, allopurinol can be used with diuretics.[355] There seem to be few indications for uricosuric agents in asymptomatic hyperuricemic patients.[357] Indeed, before they are used uric acid excretion should be measured, because if hyperuricemia is caused by overproduction of uric acid, a uricosuric agent can lead to urate nephropathy or stones.

Carbohydrate intolerance, especially in the presence of latent diabetes mellitus, occurs in patients treated with thiazides[358] and less commonly in those receiving furosemide and ethacrynic acid. This complication may simply lead to loss of control of blood sugar concentration. Ketoacidosis rarely if ever develops. However, hyperosmolar nonketotic coma may develop in patients with Type II diabetes who become severely volume depleted.[354] Thiazide diuretics also exert an adverse effect, albeit a small one, on serum lipoproteins, lowering HDL cholesterol and raising LDL cholesterol as well as triglycerides.[359,360]

Ototoxicity caused by furosemide and ethacrynic acid is usually dose-related and occurs most commonly in patients with renal insufficiency. Hearing loss is usually, but not always, reversible.[298] Thiazides diminish the renal excretion of calcium, and *hypercalcemia* is an occasional complication of their use. It occurs, in particular, in patients with hyperparathyroidism.

Endocrine disorders, particularly gynecomastia, impotence, diminished libido, and irregular menses, may result from chronic administration of spironolactone, which appears to antagonize androgen activity.[361]

INDIVIDUAL DIURETICS (See Table 16–8 and Figure 16–10)

THIAZIDES. The thiazides can induce a maximal increase in sodium excretion to 3 to 6 per cent of the filtered load, placing them in the "moderately potent" category. Their major natriuretic activity occurs as a result of their ability to block sodium reabsorption at the cortical diluting site in the late ascending limb of the loop of Henle and the early distal convoluted tubule (see Fig. 16–9). Thiazides cause the excretion of equivalent quantities of sodium and chloride. Although the diuretic response to thiazides is not affected by alkalosis or acidosis, their administration may lead to metabolic alkalosis. These agents have achieved preeminence in the treatment of mild to moderate congestive heart failure because of their relative safety and their record of side effects that are usually managed easily.

The thiazides are relatively ineffective in patients with glomerular filtration rates below 30 ml/min,[362] which may account for their lack of effectiveness in the therapy of severe congestive heart failure, in which renal blood flow is markedly reduced. The dosages and durations of action of various thiazides are shown in Table 16–8.

METOLAZONE. This is a quinethazone derivative, the site of action and the potency of which are similar to those of chlorothiazide.[363,364] However, unlike the thiazides,[365] metolazone in usual doses does not generally reduce renal blood flow or glomerular filtration rate[363,366]—a fact of importance in patients whose renal hemodynamics are already compromised. Thus, unlike the thiazides, metolazone may be effective in patients with markedly reduced renal function.[366] Metolazone has a duration of action of 24 to 48 hours,[363] much longer than that of most of the thiazides. Both the thiazides and metolazone are weak carbonic anhydrase inhibitors and therefore exert a mild inhibitory effect on proximal tubular sodium reabsorption.[363,364,367]

ETHACRYNIC ACID AND FUROSEMIDE. Although ethacrynic acid and furosemide are quite dissimilar structurally, they are similar in their functional characteristics (Figs. 16–10 and 16–11). Both drugs are powerful diuretics capable of increasing the fractional sodium excretion to more than 20 per cent of the filtered load for short periods.

The maximal single oral or intravenous dose of furosemide or ethacrynic acid ranges from 200 to 250 mg. Higher doses are given to patients with acute or chronic renal failure and occasionally effect an increased urine volume. In some patients with heart failure large doses of either of these loop diuretics given orally may yield a poor response, while a much smaller intravenous dose may be effective. Both drugs have a rapid onset and short duration of action and inhibit active chloride reabsorption in the ascending limb of the loop of Henle. Their diuretic effect may also be due to some extent to reversal of the shunting of blood from cortical to juxtamedullary nephrons, which is common in heart failure. These agents can cause hypovolemia, potassium depletion, and alkalosis secondary to loss of potassium and hydrogen ions. Like the thiazides, their activity is not affected by alkalosis or acidosis. Furosemide also exerts a weak effect on the proximal tubule as a carbonic anhydrase inhibitor. These drugs are equipotent, and there is little reason to choose between them except for patients who are allergic to sulfa drugs, in which case ethacrynic acid should be employed. Gastrointestinal distress and ototoxicity occur more commonly with ethacrynic acid than with furosemide.

SPIRONOLACTONE, TRIAMTERENE, AND AMILORIDE. These three diuretics are relatively weak and rarely are used as the sole diuretic agent. Rather, they are usually added to thiazides or "loop" diuretics, where they exert an additive diuretic effect and, in addition, antagonize the kaliuretic actions of the most potent diuretics. Since triamterene and amiloride act directly on distal tubular cells to diminish potassium secretion, they are capable of antikaliuretic effects independent of the presence or absence of aldosterone.[368] Triamterene and amiloride act more

TABLE 16–8 CHARACTERISTICS OF DIURETICS

Generic Name	Brand Name	How Supplied	Usual Dosage	Onset of Effect	Peak Effect	Duration
Acetazolamide	Diamox	250-mg tablet	250 to 375 mg/day	1 hr	2 to 4 hr	8 hr
Chlorothiazide	Diuril	500-mg tablet	500 to 1000 mg/day	1 hr	4 hr	6 to 12 hr
Hydrochlorothiazide	HydroDiuril	50-mg tablet	50 to 100 mg/day	2 hr	4 hr	12 hr or more
Trichlormethiazide	Metahydrin, Naqua	4-mg tablet	4 to 8 mg/day	2 hr	6 hr	24 hr
Chlorthalidone	Hygroton (generic)	100-mg tablet	100 mg/day	2 hr	6 hr	24 hr or more
Meralluride	Mercuhydrin	10-ml vial	0.50 to 2.00 ml IM 3 times/week	2 hr	6 to 9 hr	12 to 24 hr
Mercaptomerin	Thiomerin	10-ml vial	0.25 to 2.00 ml IM 3 times/week	2 hr	6 to 9 hr	12 to 24 hr
Metolazone	Zaroxolyn	2.5-, 5-, and 10-mg tablets	5 to 10 mg/day	1 hr	2 to 4 hr	24 to 48 hr
Triamterene	Dyrenium	100-mg capsule	100 to 300 mg/day	2 hr	6 to 8 hr	12 to 16 hr
Spironolactone	Aldactone	25-mg tablet	25 mg 4 times/day	Gradual onset	1 to 2 days after initiation of therapy	2 to 3 days after cessation of therapy
Furosemide	Lasix	40-mg tablet	40 to 120 mg/day	Oral, 1 hr; IV, 5 min	Oral, 1 to 2 hr; IV, 30 min	Oral, 6 hr; IV, 2 hr
Ethacrynic acid	Edecrin	50-mg tablet	50 to 100 mg/day	Oral, 30 min; IV, 15 min	Oral 2 hr; IV, 45 min	Oral, 6 to 8 hr; IV, 3 hr

Adapted from Frazier, H. S., and Yager, H.: The clinical use of diuretics; renal regulation of salt and water balance. N. Engl. J. Med. *288*:248, 1973.

rapidly than does spironolactone—within hours versus two to three days—but unlike the aldosterone antagonists, they may produce azotemia. It must be recognized that all three drugs inhibit the exchange of potassium not only for sodium but also for hydrogen and may induce metabolic acidosis as well as hyperkalemia. Amiloride may cause anorexia, nausea, and vomiting.[367] Unlike triamterene it does not cause renal calculi; unlike spironolactone, it does not cause gynecomastia. Potassium-sparing diuretics should be used with caution in patients with renal failure, diabetes, or advanced age.

Mercurial Diuretics. While quite effective when administered parenterally, these agents are ineffective when given orally. They are rarely used because more effective, less toxic drugs, such as furosemide and ethacrynic acid, are available and can be given orally. Mercurials inhibit the reabsorption of sodium in the thick portion of the ascending limb of the loop of Henle and in the distal convoluted tubule. Potassium secretion tends to be reduced, so that urinary losses of this electrolyte are less prominent than after doses of thiazides, ethacrynic acid, or furosemide, which produce comparable losses of sodium. Metabolic alkalosis, however, is a frequent sequela of diuresis with mercurials. Sudden death, presumably from cardiac arrhythmia, is a rare complication of intravenous administration. Renal failure, nephrotic syndrome, and hemorrhagic colitis may occur with chronic therapy, particularly in patients with renal insufficiency, and probably represent a form of heavy-metal poisoning.[369]

VASODILATORS

GENERAL CONSIDERATIONS

Cardiac function can be profoundly affected by alterations in the resistance and capacitance of the peripheral vascular bed. Thus, it has been appreciated for many years that both in animals with experimentally induced mitral regurgitation[370,371] and in patients with this valvular lesion[372] the volume of regurgitant flow varies directly, and the forward stroke volume varies inversely, with afterload. The response of the left ventricle to an augmentation of afterload induced by the infusion of a pressor agent is a direct function of myocardial contractility (see Figure 14–21, p. 485); when contractility is normal, elevating afterload leads to a marked increase in stroke work, with little elevation of ventricular end-diastolic volume of pressure and little decline in stroke volume. In patients with impaired contractility, however, as afterload is increased, stroke volume falls, and left ventricular end-diastolic pressure and volume rise, often sharply.[373] Arterial counterpulsation, a mechanical technique that reduces left ventricular afterload (p. 593), appears to have been the first deliberate clinical use of afterload reduction in the treatment of left ventricular failure,[374] although effective treatment of hypertension has undoubtedly achieved this goal in many instances since the introduction of antihypertensive drugs.

Majid et al. took an important step forward when they infused the alpha-adrenergic blocking agent phentolamine into normotensive patients with persistent left ventricular dysfunction after myocardial infarction and demonstrated that the induced fall in systemic vascular resistance was accompanied by considerable elevation of cardiac output and reduction of pulmonary artery pressure.[375] Since that report, vasodilators have appropriately achieved wide use in the treatment of heart failure.[376–379]

With few exceptions, vasodilators do not exert a direct effect on the heart, but their ability to relax vascular smooth muscle, directly or indirectly, can result in profound improvement in both the clinical and hemodynamic state of the patient. By dilating arterioles and/or veins, these agents have the capacity to alter profoundly the loading conditions on the heart and thereby to modify cardiac performance. *Arteriolar dilatation* results in a reduction in afterload and may augment cardiac output, while venodilatation produces a reduction in preload, lowers ventricular filling pressure, and thereby may diminish symptoms of pulmonary congestion. However, like all other drugs useful in the management of congestive heart failure, vasodilator agents must be used with caution and a thorough understanding of their mechanism of action, since their inappropriate administration can result in deterioration rather than improvement of the patient's circulatory status.

Venodilators result in a redistribution of the blood volume. Since the capacity of the venous bed (also referred to as the "capacitance bed") is large, a relatively small reduction in venous tone can result in the pooling of substantial quantities of blood in this bed and its redistribution from the pulmonary to the systemic circuit.[380] Patients with heart failure often exhibit intense and inappropriate venoconstriction,[381] thus augmenting pulmonary blood volume and contributing to pulmonary congestion. The hemodynamic effects of a pure venodilator resemble those of a diuretic (Fig. 16–12) and result in a shift to the left on the left ventricular function curve. In a normal subject this reduction in preload can result in an undesirable decline of cardiac output (A′ → B′). However, it is not sufficiently appreciated that in a patient with heart failure but normal filling pressure, venodilatation (or further diuresis) may also result in a decline in cardiac performance (C → B). Only in the patient with heart failure and an elevated filling pressure can venodilatation (or diuresis) reduce filling pressure and thereby produce relief of symptoms of pulmonary congestion without depressing cardiac output (A → D). Many patients with heart failure present with a moderate elevation of filling pressure (D); in them the cardiac output response will be intermediate between that observed in patients with marked elevation (A) and those without elevation (C) of filling pressure; i.e., they will experience some clinical improvement resulting from reduction of the moderately elevated pulmonary capillary pressure but at the expense of some reduction in cardiac output (D → C). Fundamental aspects of the effects of afterload reduction on myocardial energetics have been reviewed by Ford,[382] and Packer and LeJemtel have reviewed the conceptual framework for vasodilator therapy in heart failure.[383]

CHOICE OF VASODILATOR. From a theoretical point of view, therefore, one would expect the administration of a pure venodilator to be (1) *desirable* in patients whose principal clinical manifestation of heart failure is

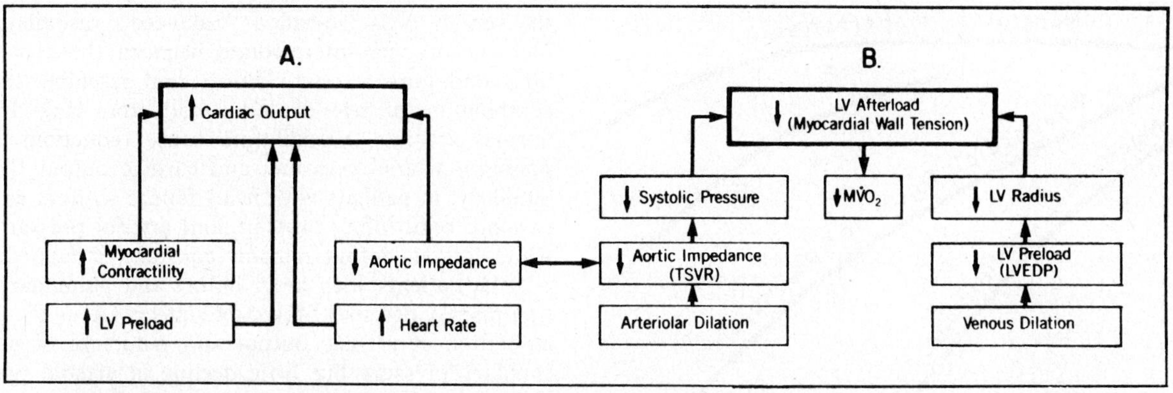

FIGURE 16–13 *A,* **Representation of four principal determinants of cardiac output (CO).** *B,* **Representation of two major determinants of left ventricular (LV) afterload. TSVR indicates total systemic vascular resistance. LVEDP = left ventricular end-diastolic pressure; MVO_2 = myocardial oxygen requirements. Arteriolar dilation raises CO (reduces fatigue), decreases LV afterload, and diminishes MVO_2 (antianginal effect). Venous dilation decreases LVEDP (reduces dyspnea), decreases LV afterload, and diminishes MVO_2 (anti-ischemic effect). Combined arteriolar and venous dilation raises CO, decreases LVEDP, diminishes LV afterload, and reduces MVO_2. (Reproduced with permission from Mason, D. T., Awan, N. A., Joye, J. A., Lee, G., DeMaria, A. N., and Amstersdam, E. A.: Treatment of acute and chronic congestive heart failure by vasodilator-afterload reduction. Arch. Intern. Med.** ***140*****:1577, 1980.)**

pulmonary congestion secondary to elevated left ventricular filling pressure rather than to a lowered cardiac output and resultant poor perfusion, (2) *contraindicated* in patients in whom the preload or filling pressure has already been restored to normal by means of diuretic therapy and/or dietary sodium restriction, and (3) *useful in combination with arteriolar dilators* in patients whose clinical manifestations of failure are related to both reduction of perfusion and pulmonary congestion.[384]

Arteriolar dilators act as *afterload reducing agents.* As shown in Figures 16–13 and 16–14, as well as in Figures 12–28 (p. 434) and 12–30 (p. 436), at any level of preload and myocardial contractility, the extent of myocardial fiber shortening (and therefore stroke volume) is inversely related to the afterload. As discussed elsewhere (p. 435), afterload is related to the instantaneous wall stress in the muscle fibers of the ventricle. Therefore, it is also closely related to the aortic impedance, i.e., the instantaneous relationship between pressure and flow in the aorta during ejection. Impedance, in turn, is closely related to systemic vascular resistance, i.e., the average relationship between pressure and flow. Just as the effects of venodilatation and the resultant reduction of ventricular preload are dependent on the filling pressure (Fig. 16–12), so are the effects of afterload dependent on myocardial contractility. Figures 16–14 and 16–15 display the effects of afterload reduction on ventricular fiber shortening in normal and failing hearts. In the normal heart (Fig. 16–14) a reduction of afterload (from B to C) results in only a minor augmentation of myocardial fiber shortening (B → F to C → G). In contrast, an identical reduction in afterload results in a substantial augmentation of myocardial fiber shortening in the failing heart (B → D to C → E). In the intact heart, as outlined in Figure 16–15, the consequences of increased afterload thus are substantially greater in the presence of heart failure than when normal contractile function is present.

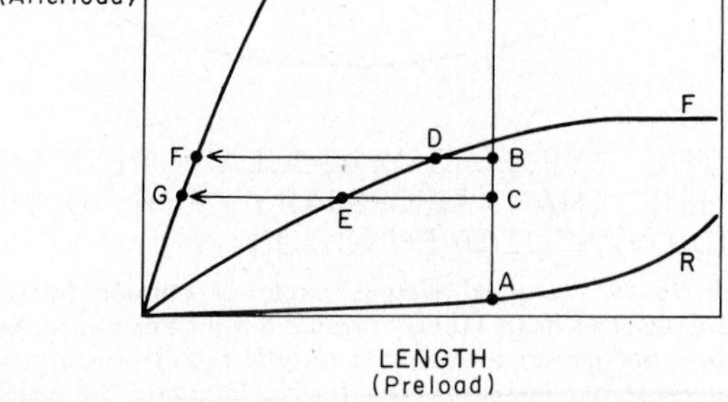

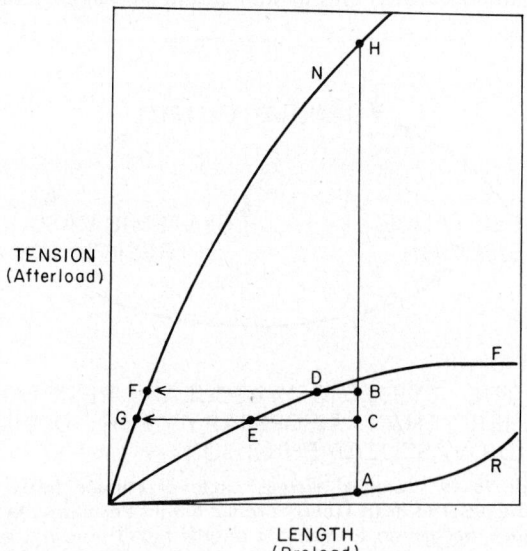

FIGURE 16–14 Length-tension relations in normal (N) and failing (F) heart muscle. R = length-resting tension curve for both normal and failing heart muscle. The effects of reducing afterloads from B to C on shortening are contrasted. In the normal muscle, shortening increases only slightly (from B → F to C → G). In failing muscle, there is substantial enhancement of shortening (B → D to C → E). H represents isometric tension development by normal muscle.

In patients with congestive heart failure the arterial vascular bed (just like the venous bed) is often inappropriately constricted. (Fig. 16–16).[381] The vasoconstriction is related to that observed in other conditions such as hypovolemic shock, in which there is a reduction of cardiac output, and it represents a fundamental response of the organism, the survival value of which is to maintain the perfusion pressure of vital organs, such as the brain and the heart, at the expense of less immediately essential vascular beds, such as the skin, gut, and kidney. While this maintenance of perfusion pressure may be a desirable evolutionary development insofar as hypovolemic shock is concerned, it plays a deleterious role in patients with congestive heart failure. (Presumably there is little evolutionary selective advantage to the survival of individuals with heart failure.) At least four mechanisms appear to be involved in the inappropriate elevation of systemic vascular

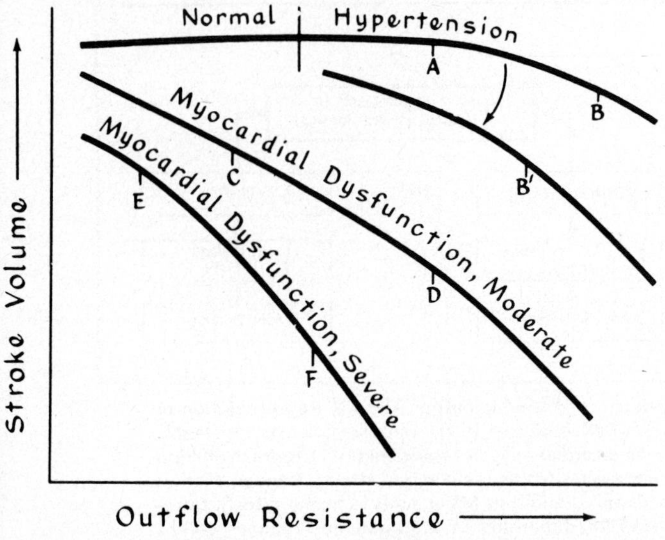

FIGURE 16–15 Relation of left ventricular stroke volume to systemic outflow resistance in normal and diseased hearts. A family of curves may be described, depending on the severity of the myocardial disease. If cardiac function is normal, a rise in resistance results in hypertension, since cardiac output remains fairly constant. Heart failure in a hypertensive patient could be shown by a move to either point B, a high resistance with normal function, or point B′, which represents a shift to a slightly depressed ventricular function curve. When myocardial dysfunction is more severe, as shown by the lower two curves, blood pressure is no longer directly determined by resistance, since stroke volume and resistance are inversely related. Consequently, arterial pressure may be similar at points E and F despite marked differences in cardiac output and resistance. It is also apparent that a reduction in outflow resistance will not affect significantly the stroke volume of the normal ventricle. However, it can produce a marked increase in the stroke volume of the failing ventricle (F → E). (Reproduced with permission from Cohn, J. N., and Franciosa, J. A.: Vasodilator therapy of cardiac failure. N. Engl. J. Med. *297*:27, 1977.)

resistance, arterial pressure, and therefore ventricular afterload in patients with congestive heart failure: (1) increased sympathetic vasoconstrictor tone; (2) elevated concentrations of circulating catecholamines; (3) elaboration of renin, with resultant increase in the potent vasoconstrictor angiotensin II; and (4) increased thickness of arteriolar walls, presumably related to extracellular fluid accumulation in the blood vessels themselves.[385,386]

Arteriolar dilators (afterload-reducing agents) are capable of augmenting stroke volume (and cardiac output) in patients with heart failure (Fig. 16–17, A → H) and in this manner reduce symptoms caused by poor perfusion. The reduction in vascular resistance induced by the vasodilator will be offset by the large increase in cardiac output, and arterial pressure may decline only slightly or not at all. In normal subjects the reduction of systemic vascular resistance induced by afterload-reducing agents is associated with no or only small increases in cardiac output (A′ → H′), and their administration may result in a marked reduction of arterial pressure accompanied by a reflex tachycardia. In patients with depressed contractility and normal preload, arterial dilatation may produce a small augmentation of cardiac output (C → H″), but in contrast to the situation existing in patients with an elevated preload, arterial pressure may decline to dangerously low levels.

A number of vasodilators act on both the arterial and the venous beds (so-called "balanced" vasodilators), and their actions are intermediate between those of pure venous and pure arterial dilators and resemble those of a combination of arterial and venodilators (Fig. 16–17). In normal subjects, vasodilators cause reductions in filling pressure, arterial pressure, and cardiac output (A′ → P′). Similarly, in patients with heart failure without an elevated preload, both filling pressure and arterial pressure decline, while cardiac output remains constant or falls slightly (C → P″). Patients with heart failure and pulmonary congestion display decisively favorable effects (A → P), with augmentation of cardiac output and reduction of pulmonary capillary pressure but little decline in arterial pressure or elevation of heart rate.

From these considerations, it is apparent that patients with depressed myocardial contractility *and* an elevated preload are likely to benefit significantly from vasodilator therapy, with an increase in cardiac output resulting chiefly from arterial dilators, a reduction in pulmonary congestion resulting from venodilators, and a combination of effects resulting from "balanced" dilators. Patients with heart disease but with normal or almost normal hemodynamics (cardiac output and filling pressure) are unlikely to benefit from the use of vasodilators; indeed, they are likely to experience a reduction of cardiac output and/or arterial pressure. In patients with heart disease, impaired myocardial contractility, and normal preload (often achieved by means of vigorous diuretic therapy), the effects of vasodilator therapy are more difficult to predict; venodilators usually decrease left ventricular performance; arteriolar dilators or balanced dilators may achieve a modest increase in cardiac output, but often at the expense of perfusion pressure. It therefore becomes evident that (in the absence of mitral regurgitation) vasodilator therapy is not desirable in the earliest stages of heart failure but is more appropriate when the use of other measures is inadequate to maintain cardiac output and filling pressure at or near normal.

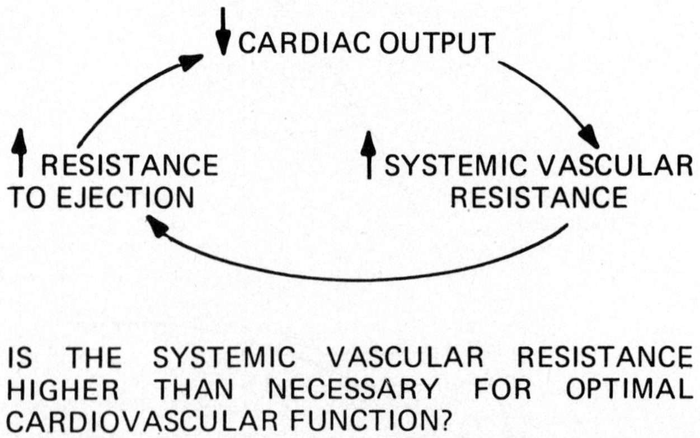

FIGURE 16–16 Potential vicious circle of chronic heart failure. With the onset of heart failure, cardiac output decreases. As a compensatory mechanism to maintain arterial blood pressure, systemic vascular resistance increases. This further increases the resistance or impedance to ejection of the left ventricle, which will result in a further reduction in cardiac output. The patient will spiral down this cycle until a new steady-state relation is reached in which cardiac output may be lower and systemic vascular resistance higher than is really optimal for the benefit of the patient. (From Parmley, W. W., and Chatterjee, K.: Vasodilator therapy. Curr. Probl. Cardiol. Vol. 2, No. 12, 1978, p. 15.)

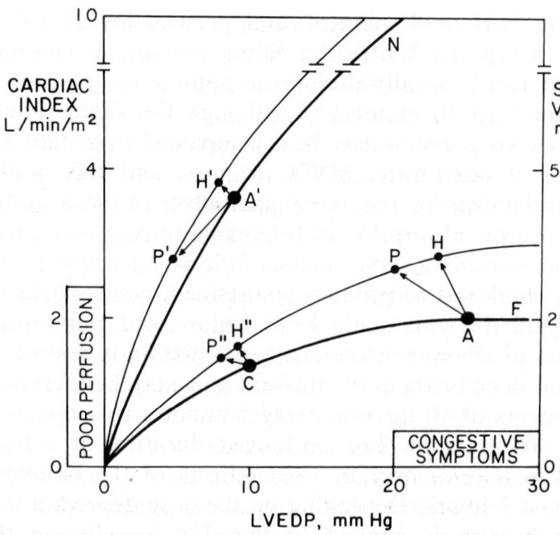

FIGURE 16–17 Effects of various vasodilators on the relationship between left ventricular end-diastolic pressure (LVEDP) and cardiac index or stroke volume in normal (N) and failing (F) hearts. H represents hydralazine or any other pure arterial dilator. It produces only a minimal increase in cardiac index in the normal subject (A' → H') or in the patient with heart failure with normal LVEDP (C → H"). In contrast, it elevates output in the patient with heart failure and elevated LVEDP (A → H). P represents a balanced vasodilator, such as sodium nitroprusside or prazosin. It reduces filling pressure in all patients, elevates cardiac output in patients with heart failure and elevated LVEDP (A → P), lowers cardiac output in normal subjects (A' → P'), and has little effect on cardiac output in heart failure patients with normal filling pressures (C → P").

Although the classification of vasodilators as predominant arterial or venodilators or as "balanced" vasodilators has proved to be useful in understanding their action and in the rational selection of a particular agent for a specific patient, the intimate interactions between cardiac preload and afterload that exist in the intact circulation must be considered. Since afterload, i.e., myocardial systolic wall tension, is a function not only of intraventricular pressure but also of ventricular volume, it may be readily appreciated that a venodilator that reduces preload will also lower afterload by reducing ventricular volume without altering systemic vascular resistance. Conversely, an arterial dilator that diminishes arterial pressure and thereby enhances stroke volume and ventricular emptying, i.e., reduces ventricular volume in both systole and diastole, will also reduce preload. The lower filling pressure will result in greater reduction of systolic wall tension (afterload) than of arterial pressure.

Since wall tension is a principal determinant of myocardial oxygen consumption ($M\dot{V}O_2$) and since both arteriolar and venodilators reduce wall tension in patients with heart failure, vasodilators reduce $M\dot{V}O_2$ while increasing cardiac output. These actions of vasodilators compare favorably with those of (1) positive inotropic agents, which (like vasodilators) augment cardiac output but either increase $M\dot{V}O_2$ or maintain it at a constant level; or (2) beta-adrenergic blocking agents, which (like vasodilators) reduce $M\dot{V}O_2$ but depress cardiac performance.

MONITORING. The use of vasodilators in the treatment of acute myocardial infarction is discussed in detail elsewhere (p. 1314). When these agents are used in patients with coronary artery disease, it is important to bear in mind that reductions in coronary perfusion pressure in the face of critical coronary obstruction can further impair blood flow through narrowed, though not occluded, coronary arteries, or through collaterals. Therefore, vasodilator therapy must be employed cautiously in patients with coronary artery disease, particularly those with acute myocardial infarction or other acute ischemia syndromes, to avoid the intensification of ischemia. Arterial pressure should be monitored carefully during vasodilator therapy in patients with known or suspected coronary artery disease. In view of the importance of ventricular filling pressure as a determinant of the response to vasodilators (Figs. 16–12 and 16–17), the monitoring of pulmonary artery or pulmonary capillary wedge pressure by means of a Swan-Ganz catheter is extremely helpful in regulating the dose of vasodilators during intravenous therapy. Since, in addition to the reduction in pulmonary wedge pressure, the elevation of cardiac output is an important endpoint, it is desirable to make serial measurements of cardiac output in acutely ill patients receiving intravenous vasodilators. In patients without ischemic heart disease, monitoring of intraarterial pressure during *intravenous* vasodilator therapy may be desirable but is not essential as long as pressure is measured indirectly at frequent intervals. Invasive monitoring is obviously not practical or necessary for patients treated for prolonged periods with agents administered orally, sublingually, or in ointment form. However, it is highly desirable to make frequent measurements of arterial pressure in the supine and upright positions when therapy is initiated or the dosage is being adjusted.

VASODILATOR AGENTS

SODIUM NITROPRUSSIDE. Probably the most widely used vasodilator in the treatment of *acute* congestive heart failure, sodium nitroprusside is ultrashort-acting and must be given intravenously. It acts directly to relax vascular smooth muscle in both arterioles and veins. For many years sodium nitroprusside has been employed successfully to treat hypertensive crisis (p. 923) but was introduced for the treatment of congestive heart failure only as recently as 1972.[387–390] Since sodium nitroprusside is a balanced (arteriolar and venous) dilator, its hemodynamic action in the presence of severe impairment of left ventricular function is both to increase cardiac output and to diminish pulmonary congestion (Fig. 16–17). The initial infusion rate in adults is usually about 10 μg/min and is increased by increments of 5 to 10 μg/min every 5 minutes until the desired effect is achieved or hypotension or other side effects limit further dose increments. The maximum dose in adults is 500 μg/min.

The most important hazardous effect is hypotension, which is actually an extension of its therapeutic action and is reversed within 10 minutes after discontinuation of the drug. If this waiting period would pose a danger, hypotension can be treated more rapidly by infusion of a vasoconstrictor such as phenylephrine or norepinephrine, a combination vasoconstrictor–positive inotropic agent. Nitroprusside releases hydrocyanic acid, which theoretically could lead to cyanide poisoning.[391] However, this is an extremely uncommon complication, since hydrocyanic acid is converted to thiocyanate in the presence of thiosulfate. Thiocyanate is excreted by the kidney, and in the presence

tion by vasodilator drugs of neurohumoral forces that promote peripheral vasoconstriction and tachycardia[448] and sodium retention.[449] Franciosa has reviewed the clinical status of long-term vasodilator therapy in the chronic heart failure setting.[434]

The contribution of vasodilator therapy to the support of the circulation may be difficult to assess in patients with severe heart failure who are already receiving oral vasodilator therapy. If clinical circumstances dictate, hospitalization may be advisable, and the effects of raising the dose of vasodilator may be assessed. Occasionally it is desirable to substitute or add a course of therapy with intravenous sodium nitroprusside and/or a sympathomimetic amine (p. 546).

SYMPATHOMIMETIC AMINES

Catecholamines and other sympathomimetic amines (Fig. 16–21) exert potent inotropic effects by interacting with myocardial (beta$_1$) adrenergic receptors. For many years attempts were made to utilize these properties in the treatment of heart failure, but these efforts were largely unsuccessful because of the other effects of these agents (Tables 16–9 and 16–10). Thus, isoproterenol, and to a lesser extent epinephrine, causes tachycardia and hypotension by stimulating beta$_1$-adrenergic receptors in the sinoatrial node and beta$_2$ receptors in the systemic vascular bed. Norepinephrine, on the other hand, by stimulating alpha-adrenergic receptors, causes vasoconstriction and hypertension. Two agents introduced relatively recently, dopamine and dobutamine, produce less tachycardia and fewer peripheral vascular effects and are used frequently in the treatment of acute heart failure.

DOPAMINE

This endogenous catecholamine, the immediate precursor of norepinephrine (Fig. 12–33, p. 440), stimulates myocardial contractility by acting directly on beta$_1$-adrenergic

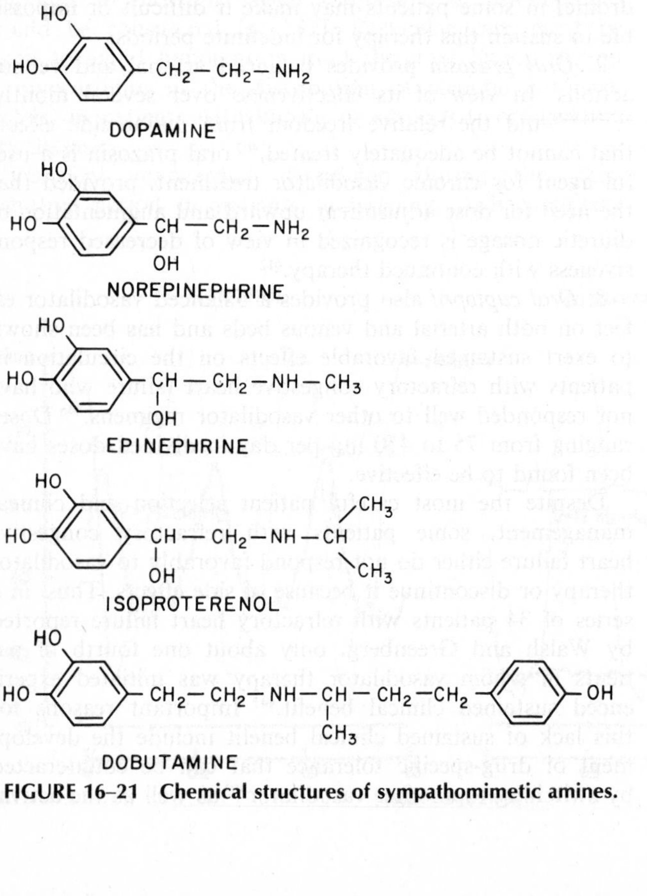

FIGURE 16–21 Chemical structures of sympathomimetic amines.

TABLE 16–9 SOME RECEPTOR ACTIONS OF CATECHOLAMINES

Adrenergic Receptor	Site	Action
Beta$_1$	Myocardium	Increase atrial and ventricular contractility
	Sinoatrial node	Increase heart rate
	Atrioventricular conduction system	Enhance atrioventricular conduction
Beta$_2$	Arterioles	Vasodilation
	Lungs	Bronchodilation
Alpha	Peripheral arterioles	Vasoconstriction

TABLE 16–10 ADRENERGIC RECEPTOR ACTIVITY OF SYMPATHOMIMETIC AMINES

	Alpha Peripheral	Beta$_1$ Cardiac	Beta$_2$ Peripheral
Norepinephrine	++++	++++	0
Epinephrine	++++	++++	++
Dopamine*	++++	++++	++
Isoproterenol	0	++++	++++
Dobutamine	+	++++	++
Methoxamine	++++	0	0

*Causes renal and mesenteric dilatation by stimulating dopaminergic receptors.
Both tables from Sonnenblick, E. H., et al.: Dobutamine: A new synthetic cardioactive sympathetic amine. N. Engl. J. Med. *300*:18, 1979.

receptors in the myocardium and indirectly by releasing norepinephrine from sympathetic nerve terminals, which in turn also stimulates beta$_1$ receptors[450] (Tables 16–9 and 16–10). All *cardiac* effects of dopamine are antagonized by beta-adrenergic blockers.[450] However, there is considerable evidence that the vasodilation mediated by dopamine is secondary to activation of specific dopaminergic receptors.[451,452] Dopamine-induced vasodilation, which is not blocked by propranolol and therefore is not related to activation of beta$_2$ receptors, occurs in the renal, mesenteric, coronary, and cerebral vascular beds.[450] This vasodilation is not due to release of acetylcholine,[450,453] histamine,[450] or prostaglandins.[454] However, dopaminergic vasodilation is antagonized by phenothiazines, such as chlorpromazine, and butyrophenone compounds, such as haloperidol.[455] Dopamine also causes vasodilation of dog hind limb vasculature that can be prevented by section of the nerves innervating these vessels,[456] and it has been suggested that this response is due to a ganglionic blocking action of this amine[457] or to inhibition of transmission in the postganglionic sympathetic nerve.[458] Dopamine-induced diuresis is common in patients with heart failure and is secondary to a combination of inotropic and renal vasodilator effects[450]; studies in both dog[459] and man[460] have demonstrated that dopamine preferentially dilates vessels in the renal cortex.

When larger doses of dopamine are administered, the dilation is reversed, and dopamine causes constriction of arteries and veins in all vascular beds.[450] Although the vasoconstriction has been attributed to action of the drug on alpha-adrenergic receptors,[450,461] the doses of the alpha-receptor blockers phentolamine and phenoxybenzamine required to prevent the dopamine-induced vasoconstriction are higher than those required to antagonize the vasoconstriction caused by other alpha-adrenergic agonists. Dopamine-induced contractions of isolated canine vessels can be attenuated by concentrations of the serotonin-blocking agent cyproheptadine that do not antagonize the actions of norepinephrine. These findings suggest that dopamine may cause contraction of vascular smooth muscle, in part, by action on serotonin- or tryptamine-sensitive receptors.[456]

Because dopamine in small and large doses acts on receptors that mediate opposing effects in animal experiments, it is not surprising that the effects of this drug on vascular resistance and arterial pressure are dose-dependent in patients as well. With infusion rates of 2 to 5 μg/kg/min, cardiac contractility, cardiac output, and renal blood flow increase, with little change in heart rate and either a reduction or no change in total peripheral resistance.[462] With higher infusion rates (5 to 10 μg/kg/min), arterial pressure, peripheral resistance, and heart rate increase[463] and renal blood flow may decline.

Like other sympathomimetic amines that increase cardiac contractility, dopamine increases coronary blood flow[450,464] secondary to the increase in myocardial oxygen consumption that results from increased cardiac work.[465] Direct coronary vasodilation through action on dopaminergic receptors is a secondary mechanism involved in the increase in coronary flow.[466] However, as is the case in other vascular beds, large doses of dopamine may increase coronary artery resistance by direct action on receptors mediating constriction.[450] Ultimately, the effects of dopamine, like those of other catecholamines, depend on myocardial oxygen utilization and coronary blood flow, which in turn are affected by the sum total of its several actions. Augmented heart rate, contractility, and arterial pressure will increase oxygen utilization, whereas reduced peripheral resistance and heart size will decrease oxygen utilization. Stimulation of dopaminergic receptors increases coronary blood flow, while stimulation of alpha-adrenergic receptors decreases it.

In early investigations, Goldberg et al. found that in patients with heart failure, dopamine increased sodium excretion and cardiac output[467,468]; infusion rates of 2.1 to 5.8 μg/kg/min increased cardiac index (+26 per cent) without significant change in heart rate or total body oxygen consumption. Peripheral resistance was reduced, and pulmonary resistance, when elevated, also fell. Left ventricular dP/dt increased by 58 per cent, glomerular filtration rate by 38 per cent, renal plasma flow by 79 per cent, and sodium excretion by an average of 48 per cent.[468] Thus, in patients with congestive heart failure, dopamine exerts important beneficial hemodynamic and renal effects. However, care must be taken to adjust the infusion rate carefully to prevent excessive positive inotropic effect, tachycardia, and increased peripheral resistance.

In normotensive patients with otherwise refractory heart failure, infusions are begun at low rates (0.5 to 1.0 μg/kg/min) and are gradually increased until urine flow is augmented or until increments in diastolic pressure and heart rate are observed. The infusion rate should then be decreased or the infusion discontinued. In patients with cardiogenic shock, both the vasoconstrictor and the more intense inotropic effects of higher doses may be desirable (pp. 595 and 1317).

USE IN CARDIAC SURGERY

Dopamine has become widely used for the treatment of acute heart failure during and after cardiac surgery. In a comparison of the effects of three catecholamines in 22 patients with low cardiac output states following surgery, dopamine increased cardiac index by 1.10 liters/min/m^2, mean arterial blood pressure by 7 mm Hg, heart rate by 19 beats/min, and urine flow by 75 ml/hr. In contrast, norepinephrine increased cardiac index by much less (only 0.20 liter/min/m^2) and mean arterial pressure by much more (23 mm Hg), while heart rate rose by 9 beats/min and urine flow *decreased* by 8 ml/hr. Isoproterenol resembled dopamine by increasing cardiac index by 0.95 liter/min/m^2 but caused a more severe tachycardia, increasing heart rate by 28 beats/min. Urine flow increased by 28 ml/hr, while mean arterial pressure decreased by 7 mm Hg. These observations demonstrate the superiority of dopamine over previously used sympathomimetic agents in this clinical setting.[469] Sometimes the use of sympathomimetic amines permits the discontinuation of cardiopulmonary bypass in patients who cannot be weaned from the pump. Here also dopamine appears to be superior to isoproterenol.[451] Combined use of intraaortic balloon counterpulsation with dopamine and nitroprusside has been reported to be effective in patients with low cardiac output and elevated systemic vascular resistance following cardiopulmonary bypass.[470]

DOBUTAMINE

Dobutamine is a synthetic cardioactive sympathomimetic amine that stimulates beta$_1$-, beta$_2$-, and alpha-adrenergic receptors.[471–474] Radioligand binding studies suggest that beta$_1$ activity predominates over beta$_2$, and that alpha$_1$ predominates over alpha$_2$ activity of this drug.[475] Under some circumstances, dobutamine has been shown to exert alpha-adrenergic antagonist activity in vascular tissue.[476] At equivalent cardiac contractile force responses, dobutamine exerts a much weaker beta$_2$-adrenergic action than does isoproterenol and a much weaker alpha-adrenergic action than does either norepinephrine or dopamine. Injections of dobutamine into the femoral vascular bed cause slight vasoconstriction at low doses and a biphasic vasoconstrictor-vasodilator response at higher doses; phenoxybenzamine blocks the vasoconstrictor component and propranolol blocks the vasodilator component.[451]

In contrast to dopamine, which increases renal blood flow in all dose ranges, dobutamine does not alter renal blood flow but does cause a redistribution of cardiac output in favor of the coronary and skeletal muscle beds over the mesenteric and renal vascular beds.[477,477a] Gillespie and colleagues administered dobutamine to patients with acute myocardial infarction and found that the drug improved hemodynamic parameters without provoking undesirable effects and without increasing the extent of myocardial injury.[478] Favorable hemodynamic effects sustained for weeks to a few months in patients with congestive cardiomyopathy treated for two or three days with intravenous dobutamine have been reported.[479,479a] Improvement in cardiac index (mean increase 54 per cent) and stroke work index (mean increase 65 per cent) has also been reported in response to dobutamine infusion in patients with chronic heart failure associated with ischemic heart disease, with infrequent precipitation of overt myocardial ischemia.[480]

Adverse Effects of Dopamine and Dobutamine. Cardiac arrhythmias constitute the most serious adverse effect of sympathomimetic amines. The electrophysiological properties of dopamine and dobutamine resemble those of other sympathomimetic amines[450,481,482] and consist of an acceleration of the spontaneous depolarization of sino-atrial cells, thereby increasing heart rate, accelerating diastolic depolarization and facilitating activation of latent pacemaker cells, shortening the refractory period of atrial and ventricular muscle, and speeding atrioventricular conduction. Ventricular arrhythmias have been observed with the use of both drugs.[450,483–485] Since ventricular arrhythmias are more prone to develop with increased peripheral resistance during halothane anesthesia, dobutamine is less likely to cause such arrhythmias than are vasoconstricting doses of dopamine.[486] In patients with coronary artery disease, both dobutamine and dopamine may precipitate angina pectoris.[450,483,487]

In patients with preexisting vascular disease, dopamine may cause gangrene of the digits.[488,489] Tissue necrosis similar to that produced by norepinephrine can also occur if an infusion of dopamine extravasates into tissue; this can be prevented by infiltrating the area promptly with 5 to 10 mg of phentolamine diluted in saline. Dopamine differs from the other catecholamines in that it causes nausea and vomiting in some patients, an effect more commonly observed with high doses.[450,460] Since the cardiovascular effects of dopamine (in contrast to dobutamine) are potentiated by prior therapy with monoamine oxidase inhibitors,[450] the dose of dopamine in such patients should be reduced to approximately 10 per cent of the usual dose.

Comparisons Between Dopamine and Dobutamine.[489a,489b] There has been considerable interest in comparing the effects of dobutamine and dopamine in patients with severe congestive heart failure. In one study dobutamine raised cardiac index while lowering left ventricular end-diastolic pressure and leaving mean aortic pressure unchanged.[490] Dopamine also improved cardiac index but at the expense of a greater increase in heart rate than occurred with dobutamine. Dopamine was ineffective in lowering left ventricular end-diastolic pressure but increased mean aortic pressure. Because dobutamine has little effect on two major determinants of myocardial oxygen consumption, i.e., heart rate and aortic pressure, and reduces a third, i.e., ventricular filling pressure—a determinant of ventricular size, it may be superior to dopamine in patients with low-output syndrome associated with ischemic heart disease. In these patients, heart rate and arterial pressure rise and end-diastolic pressure remains constant.[490]

In another study comparing the acute hemodynamic effects of dobutamine and dopamine in patients with chronic low-output cardiac failure, it was observed that at dosages adjusted to achieve similar increments in cardiac output, dobutamine reduced left ventricular filling pressure from an average of 25 to 17 mm Hg, while dopamine increased it to 30 mm Hg.[491] This response to dopamine was probably the result of its vasoconstrictor actions and illustrates the potential advantages of using a more cardioselective agent such as dobutamine when the desired goal of therapy is to improve ventricular function by direct inotropic stimulation.

In a comparison between the two sympathomimetic amines in patients with severe heart failure, dobutamine in doses up to 10 μg/kg/min progressively increased cardiac output while decreasing systemic and pulmonary vascular resistance and filling pressure, without a significant effect on heart rate and ventricular irritability. In contrast, dopamine at doses above 4 μg/kg/min increased not only cardiac output but also filling pressure and ventricular ectopic activity; at doses greater than 6 μg/kg/min, dopamine increased heart rate and systemic and pulmonary resistance. Infusion rates above 4 μg/kg/min had little additional effect on cardiac output, presumably because of the increase in systemic vascular resistance.[492]

The heart rate–systolic blood pressure product, an index related to myocardial oxygen demands, increases with both agents but more so with dopamine than with dobutamine. Furthermore, at any increase in the heart rate–systolic pressure product, the increase in cardiac output with dobutamine is nearly twice as great as with dopamine. With prolonged infusions of optimal doses of both agents (dopamine 3.7 to 4.0 μg/kg/min and dobutamine 7.3 to 7.7 μg/kg/min), only dobutamine *maintained* the elevations in stroke volume, cardiac output, urinary sodium excretion, urine flow rate, and creatinine clearance.[492]

Thus, the hemodynamic effects are adverse in *normotensive* patients with advanced heart failure, i.e., left ventricular filling pressures rise, with agents such as norepinephrine or dopamine in large doses, which cause vasoconstriction, but often respond well to vasodilator therapy, to dobutamine, or to a combination of a vasodilator and dopamine or dobutamine. Since the inotropic effects of dopamine are in part mediated by release of endogenous cardiac catecholamines, which may be depleted in patients with chronic heart failure (p. 459), low doses of this drug may be insufficient to achieve the desired inotropic effect of an increase in cardiac output, while larger doses may produce unwanted vasoconstriction.

Although dopamine can improve renal and mesenteric perfusion by selective nonbeta-adrenergic vasodilation (and this unique property of dopamine is not shared by dobutamine[472]), this beneficial effect on regional perfusion is often reversed when dopamine is given in the large doses sometimes required to achieve a sufficient inotropic effect. It is possible, however, to use dopamine in low doses (1.2 to 2.5 μg/kg/min) to provide selective vasodilation in mesenteric and renal vascular beds and combine it with dobutamine, or with a vasodilator, to achieve optimal hemodynamic improvement (p. 547). In patients

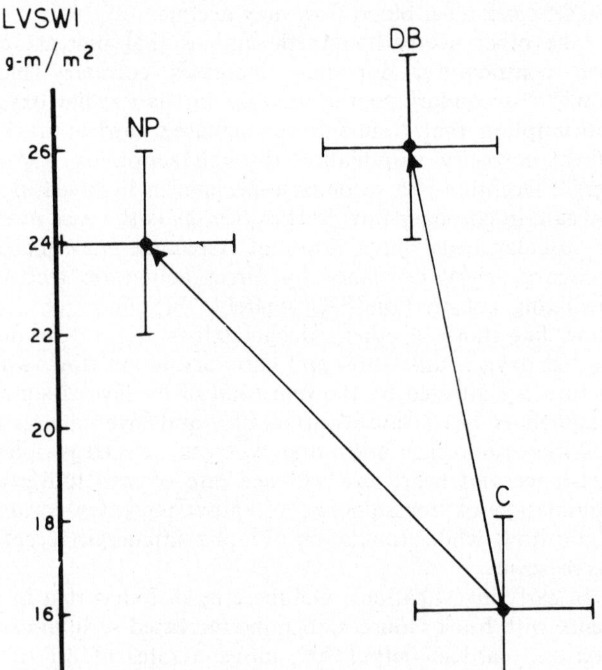

FIGURE 16–22 Left ventricular stroke work index (LVSWI) is plotted on the vertical axis, and left ventricular filling pressure (LVFP) is plotted on the horizontal axis. C = control; NP = nitroprusside; DB = dobutamine. The plots move upward and to the left during infusion of both agents, suggesting improved ventricular performance. Data are from 19 patients in chronic low-output (Class III or IV) congestive heart failure despite use of digitalis and diuretics. (From Berkowitz, C., et al.: Comparative responses to dobutamine and nitroprusside in patients with chronic low output cardiac failure. Circulation *56*:918, 1977, by permission of the American Heart Association, Inc.)

with frank hypotension, dopamine, with its greater vasoconstrictor properties, may be superior to dobutamine.

In a comparison between sodium nitroprusside and dobutamine, it was found that both drugs reduced systemic vascular resistance.[493] The reduction produced by dobutamine results primarily from withdrawal of compensatory vasoconstriction, as a consequence of elevation of cardiac output,[494] the direct peripheral vasodilator effect of dobutamine playing only a minor role.[495,496] On the other hand, sodium nitroprusside infusion reduces systemic vascular resistance more than does dobutamine, suggesting that dobutamine might be preferable to nitroprusside for augmenting cardiac output in borderline hypotensive patients or in patients with preexisting vascular disease, particularly those with coronary artery disease, in whom blood flow to vital organs may be largely dependent upon arterial pressure. Nitroprusside, however, is more effective than dobutamine in lowering elevated filling pressure (Fig. 16–22). Dobutamine consistently increases heart rate, albeit only moderately, in patients with heart failure,[482,483,491,497,498] whereas sodium nitroprusside, which lacks direct chronotrophic activity, has a variable effect on heart rate in patients with heart failure.[499] When increases in heart rate do occur during nitroprusside infusion, they probably result from compensatory reflexes[500] secondary to excessive hypotension.[501,502] Therefore, nitroprusside is preferable to dobutamine for emergency treatment of patients who require rapid reduction of pulmonary venous pressure.

ORALLY ACTIVE SYMPATHOMIMETIC AMINES

Several orally active beta-adrenergic agonists have undergone clinical study recently, although none of these newer agents is available for routine clinical use in the United States at this time.

Pirbuterol has been found to have favorable hemodynamic effects in patients with refractory congestive heart failure that may derive from both vasodilator and positive inotropic actions.[446] Awan and colleagues have documented improved cardiac output with lowered ventricular filling pressures in patients with chronic severe congestive heart failure[503] and found responses to an oral dose of pirbuterol similar to those observed with intravenous dopamine.[504] Dawson et al. also observed improved pump performance of the heart in patients with chronic heart failure in response to oral pirbuterol,[505] and Rude and colleagues observed substantial acute hemodynamic improvement in patients with chronic congestive heart failure, with no evident increased requirement for coronary blood flow or myocardial oxygen delivery.[506] No provocation of myocardial ischemia was noted in six patients with coronary artery disease and chronic congestive heart failure refractory to digitalis and diuretics. Of concern, however, is the finding of Colucci et al. that tolerance to the favorable hemodynamic effects of pirbuterol developed over a one-month period of chronic administration of the drug. This was accompanied by decreased numbers of beta-adrenergic receptors on lymphocytes of these patients, suggesting a possible mechanism for reduced responsiveness after long-term therapy with pirbuterol.[507]

Prenalterol is an orally active $beta_1$ selective adrenergic agonist with positive inotropic effects that has undergone recent clinical testing. At appropriate doses, positive inotropic effects have been observed with little increase in heart rate,[508–512,512a] but increased ventricular ectopic activity has also been observed in some patients.[509]

Other beta-adrenergic agonists originally introduced as bronchodilators, including *terbutaline*[513] and *salbutamol*,[514] have also been found to exert favorable hemodynamic effects owing to vasodilator and/or positive inotropic properties.

AMRINONE

Appreciable clinical experience has accumulated with amrinone, an orally active drug still in investigational status at this writing with both vasodilator and positive inotropic properties initially thought to act through a mechanism separate from those of the cardiac glycosides or sympathomimetic amines.[515] Recent evidence suggests, however, that amrinone acts as a phosphodiesterase inhibitor, thus increasing intracellular cyclic AMP levels.[516,517,517a] Since the initial report of Benotti et al.,[518] several studies have documented substantial increases in cardiac output and left ventricular ejection fraction together with lowered ventricular filling pressures in patients with severe congestive heart failure.[519–521]

Favorable hemodynamic effects were not associated with adverse effects on myocardial oxygen consumption or coronary blood flow requirements in patients with congestive heart failure due to coronary artery disease.[522] Improved exercise capacity has also been documented in selected patients with heart failure in response to amrinone given acutely[523,524] and chronically.[523,525] A combination of amrinone and hydralazine produced greater hemodynamic benefit than either agent alone.[526] Side effects, including dose-related thrombocytopenia, have been relatively frequent in clinical testing and require further study. Recently, milrinone, a congener of amrinone, has been found to have about 15 times the potency of the parent compound and far fewer side effects.[526a,526b] Although it appears to be an effective drug in the treatment of refractory heart failure, its ultimate clinical role remains to be determined.

REFRACTORY AND INTRACTABLE HEART FAILURE

Heart failure is considered to be *refractory* when it persists or the patient's condition deteriorates despite intensive therapy. It is defined as *intractable* when it is resistant to all known therapeutic measures. The first step in treating a patient in refractory failure is to exclude any underlying disease that might be reversible. Thus, both the nature and hemodynamic consequences of the underlying illness should be reassessed, and surgical treatment should be considered or reconsidered; often cardiac catheterization and angiography should be carried out or repeated at this time. For example, resection of a large ventricular aneurysm might have been deferred as long as the patient responded to medical treatment for heart failure because of the potentially high surgical risk, but reconsideration might be in order when such a response wanes. Similar considerations may apply to patients with known multivessel coronary artery disease or advanced valvular heart disease and poor left ventricular function. Other forms of heart disease that may lead to refractory heart failure and that are treatable surgically but are not readily recognized on clinical examination include cardiac tumors (Chap. 42), endomyocardial fibrosis (p. 1427), and constrictive pericarditis without calcification. Such conditions should at least be considered and, if possible, excluded assuming that the heart failure state is refractory.

In the absence of any correctable underlying heart disease, one must next consider whether some precipitating cause has not been properly identified and treated. A number of possibilities should come to mind:

1. Could the patient be "cheating" on the restricted sodium diet?

2. Is the patient not complying with the medication schedule prescribed, despite protestations to the contrary?

3. Has excessive diuresis occurred, and are lethargy and weakness due not to refractory heart failure but rather to a low cardiac output state secondary to an inadequate preload?

4. Could digitalis intoxication be present? Digitalis toxicity can occur despite a serum glycoside level in the usual therapeutic range and can cause fatigue, lethargy, and anorexia that may mimic refractory heart failure.

5. Has the patient been receiving optimal doses of cardiac glycosides? A glycoside level in the usual therapeutic range does not necessarily mean that the patient has been receiving the optimal dose of the glycoside. A greater inotropic effect may sometimes be provided by the addition of a very small dose of digitalis (0.125 mg digoxin daily or every other day) above the maintenance dose without precipitating signs or symptoms of toxicity.

6. Has an electrolyte imbalance, such as hypokalemic alkalosis or hyponatremia, developed as a consequence of excessive diuresis and severe restriction of sodium intake?

7. Could the patient be suffering from unrecognized pulmonary embolism (p. 1578)? This condition is often silent and manifests itself only by slight tachycardia, anxiety, tachypnea, and intensification of heart failure. Densities on the chest roentgenogram may make it difficult or impossible to interpret lung scans, and a pulmonary angiogram may be required to establish the diagnosis. Although this procedure is not without risk, a positive result may lead to treatment such as anticoagulants and/or vena caval interruption that could prevent further emboli and prove to be life-saving.

8. Could pulmonary infection be present? Pneumonitis may be difficult to recognize in patients with chronic congestive heart failure who often have a chronic low-grade fever as well as increased interstitial markings on chest roentgenogram and pulmonary rales on clinical examination. Is the suspicion of pulmonary infection high enough to warrant sputum culture and consideration of a course of antibiotics?

9. Could hyperthyroidism or infective endocarditis be present? Thyrotoxicosis (often apathetic in the elderly) and infective endocarditis in the presence of heart failure may not present with typical clinical manifestations, but their presence can lead to refractory heart failure. Should tests including an assessment of thyroid function and multiple blood cultures be obtained?

10. Could the diagnosis of refractory heart failure be incorrect, and could the patient with established heart disease be suffering from an unrelated illness, such as an occult neoplasm, viral hepatitis, or hepatic cirrhosis?

11. Could alcohol be playing a role? Alcohol is a potent myocardial depressant. In addition to producing cardiomyopathy (p. 1406), it can contribute to the heart failure state when it is not the primary cause of heart failure but is superimposed on some other form of heart disease.

12. Does the patient have inappropriate bradycardia due to sinus node dysfunction or atrioventricular block that could be corrected by means of a pacemaker?

13. Is the patient receiving any medications with salt-retaining (e.g., corticosteroids, estrogens, non-steroidal antiinflammatory drugs) or negative inotropic (e.g., disopyramide,[527] beta-adrenergic blocking agents, verapamil[528]) effects?

14. Is vasodilator therapy causing an increased tendency to salt and fluid retention?

15. Can *any* aspect of therapy be intensified without producing untoward effects?

These and related questions can usually be answered only if the patient is hospitalized; if *every* aspect of the diagnosis, including underlying and precipitating causes of heart failure, is carefully assessed; and if *every* aspect of therapy is meticulously reconsidered. If the patient has been placed at rest and has received optimal doses of cardiac glycosides and diuretics, and if electrolyte imbalance has been corrected and large volumes of fluid in the serous cavities not mobilized by diuretics have been removed mechanically, then the patient should receive a course of intravenous therapy with a vasodilator, a sympathomimetic agent, or both for 4 to 7 days. Individual use of vasodilators or of sympathomimetic amines has been discussed previously (pp. 534 and 542). In addition, combinations of nitroprusside or nitroglycerin[502] and dobutamine or dopamine have been remarkably effective. The *combined administration* of a sympathomimetic amine and vasodilator may be of benefit in patients with severe heart failure in whom the use of one of these agents alone is insufficient. Thus, in one series of patients with severe chronic congestive heart failure, nitroprusside alone reduced left ventricular end-diastolic pressure from 25 to 14 mm Hg and increased cardiac index from 2.4 to 3.0 liters/min/m^2. Dopamine alone caused a greater elevation of cardiac index, to 3.4 liters/min/m^2, but did not reduce end-diastolic pressure. Simultaneous infusion of the two agents resulted in favorable alterations in *both* hemodynamic variables: left ventricular end-diastolic pressure declined to 16 mm Hg and cardiac index rose to 3.5 liters/min/m^2.[529]

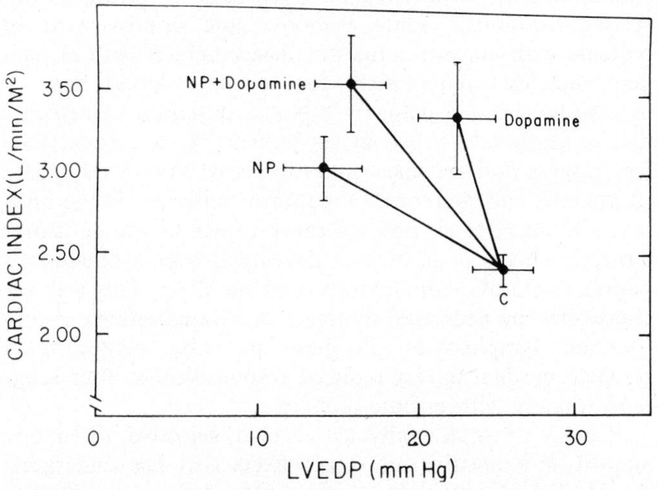

FIGURE 16–23 Effect of nitroprusside (NP), dopamine, and the combination of NP and dopamine on left ventricular end-diastolic pressure and cardiac index. Data are from 9 patients with chronic congestive heart failure (Class III) despite use of digitalis and diuretics; digitalis was discontinued 72 hours before this study. (From Miller, R. R., et al.: Combined dopamine and nitroprusside therapy in congestive heart failure. Circulation *55*:881, 1977, by permission of the American Heart Association, Inc.)

Thus, the combination of dopamine and nitroprusside provides the principal beneficial actions of both drugs in patients with heart failure. The combination raises cardiac output considerably while markedly reducing elevated filling pressure (Fig. 16–23). Combined use of digoxin with nitroprusside has also been shown to be more effective than nitroprusside alone in heart failure complicating acute myocardial infarction.[530] Such treatment can, of course, be carried out only in the hospital, with careful monitoring of filling pressure, cardiac output, and arterial pressure. If it is successful and the patient can be weaned from the intravenous therapy, larger doses of oral vasodilators and experimental drugs such as oral sympathomimetics or amrinone (or its congener, milrinone, p. 545) may provide sustained benefit.

Heart failure can properly be termed intractable if it persists despite the application of all the measures cited above. Then, the possibilities of cardiac transplantation and assisted circulation may be considered in selected instances.

OTHER MEASURES

Cardiac Transplantation

This procedure was first performed in humans in 1967.[531,532] Despite its technical feasibility, the high mortality rates resulting from graft rejection led to its abandonment in most institutions. As of May 1, 1983, a total of 263 transplants had been carried out at Stanford University Medical Center, where experience with cardiac transplantation has been most extensive. One hundred and seven of these patients are current survivors, and the longest living recipient underwent transplantation 13.3 years ago. Currently the one-year survival rate after cardiac transplantation at Stanford is 82 per cent, which is comparable to the results obtained with cadaver kidney programs.[533,534] Recent improved results reflect the potency and effectiveness of the immunosuppressive agent, Cyclosporin A.[534a]

Potential recipients of cardiac transplants must have advanced heart disease, should be in Class IV with intractable heart failure (as defined above, on p. 545), and should have a poor prognosis for one-year survival. Candidates should be stable psychologically and should have a history of compliance with medical therapy. Since younger patients have better survival rates, 50 years is the usual upper age limit for potential recipients. Contraindications to cardiac transplantation include severe pulmonary hypertension, parenchymal pulmonary disease, recent pulmonary infarction, donor-specific cytotoxic antibodies, active infection, diabetes mellitus requiring insulin, and other diseases considered likely to limit survival or rehabilitation. Over half the recipients at Stanford Medical Center have had coronary artery disease, while the remainder have had idiopathic, viral, or rheumatic cardiomyopathies. Thus, the ideal recipient has been a young person who is dying of end-stage cardiac disease and who is otherwise vigorous, emotionally stable, and willing to risk a complex procedure and course for the chance of functional improvement. Combined transplantation of the heart and lungs has been employed successfully in the treatment of irreversible, severe pulmonary hypertension.[535]

The majority of heart donors have sustained irreversible cerebral damage due to trauma or intracranial hemorrhage. However, donor supply remains critical, and the experience at Stanford has been that an appreciable number (approximately one third) of recipients awaiting transplant die before a suitable donor heart becomes available. The success of using hearts removed from donors and transported under conditions of hypothermic ischemia for up to 3 hours has broadened the sources of donor supply.[536] It is likely that continuous hypothermic perfusion with an oxygenated hyperosmolar solution will extend the duration of possible storage to 24 hours.[537] Other than choosing a heart from a donor less than 35 years of age of appropriate weight, ABO type, and absence of a positive lymphocyte cross match, no prospective histocompatibility typing has been used for cardiac transplantation. The results of HLA typing have been disappointing in predicting long-term survival.

After placing the recipient on cardiopulmonary bypass, the heart is removed, leaving the posterior walls of the atria with their venous connections in place.[532] The donor atria are sutured to the corresponding structures of the in situ residual atria of the recipient, and the great vessels are anastomosed last. Alternatively, in *heterotopic heart transplantation*, the recipient's heart is left in situ, and the donor heart is placed in parallel, with anastomoses between the two right atria, pulmonary arteries, left atria, and aortae. The stated advantage of this technique is that should acute donor heart failure occur, chances for the patient's survival are improved by his own heart; retransplantation is possible if the donor heart becomes nonfunctional because of rejection or any other reason.[538] Immunosuppression has been accomplished with high-dose prednisone and azathioprine and antithymocyte globulin, the dosage being adjusted according to the patient's course. More recently, the combination of cyclosporin-A, a fungal metabolite which is a cyclic oligopeptide, and low-dose prednisone has proved to be a promising immunosuppressive regimen.[539]

In the absence of rejection, the transplanted heart, which of course is denervated and lacks autonomic neural control, has the capacity to maintain a normal resting cardiac output. During exercise, stroke volume rises first, after which increased levels of circulating catecholamines cause tachycardia. As a consequence of this near-normal circulatory response, the transplanted heart has allowed functional rehabilitation in 90 per cent of the long-term survivors in the Stanford program.[540,541]

Transplant recipients are monitored in order to detect a fall in electrocardiographic QRS voltage (reflecting myocardial edema), atrial arrhythmias, and an S_3 gallop as early manifestations of the rejection process. These changes can be confirmed by histopathological examination of tissue obtained by percutaneous transvenous (internal jugular) biopsy of the right ventricular endomyocardium (p. 297).[542] Acute rejection can be treated successfully in more than 90 per cent of patients by high-dose boluses of methylprednisolone and antithymocyte globulin. Infections complicating intense immunosuppression are still the major hazard to survival. Continued medical surveillance is required at 2- to 4-week intervals. In the late postoperative course the threat of rejection continues, but its likelihood is considerably less than it is earlier in the course. However, accelerated coronary atherosclerosis, presumably due to rejection-induced injury to the coronary arterial intima, develops in the transplanted heart of a small number of patients. As in kidney transplant programs involving chronic immunosuppression, malignant neoplasms, usually of the lymphoreticular type, have been observed in a few recipients.

Patients who survive for three months have a better than 75 per cent two-year survival rate. Patients younger than 40 years and those who have had previous cardiac surgery associated with blood transfusions exhibit even better survival. Subsequent attrition is approximately 5 per cent per year and reflects the continuing hazards threatening immunosuppressed patients.[543] Despite advances in distant heart procurement procedures,[536] it is likely that the supply of donor hearts will continue to be a limiting factor in the number of cardiac transplants performed.

MECHANICAL CIRCULATORY SUPPORT

INTRAAORTIC BALLOON COUNTERPULSATION. This method of partial circulatory support is described on page 1317 and is illustrated in Figure 18–10 (p. 593). The phased inflation during diastole of a balloon inserted into the descending aorta through the femoral artery generally increases cardiac output by 10 to 20 per cent and elevates arterial diastolic pressure while reducing arterial systolic pressure.[544–546] A major application of this technique has been in patients with acute left ventricular failure secondary to acute myocardial infarction (cardiogenic shock), but it has also been utilized to support the circulation in patients with acute ischemic syndromes who are undergoing cardiac catheterization, angiocardiography, and coronary arteriography.[549] Of increasing importance is the use of intraaortic balloon counterpulsation during the perioperative period in patients undergoing cardiac surgery and developing acute heart failure. Usually this method of therapy is applied for 24 to 48 hours, after which an attempt is made to wean the patient from the support provided by the balloon. In some instances, counterpulsation has been continued for as long as two weeks.

The principal advantage of the technique is its relative simplicity and low risk. Ease of insertion of the device has been improved by the introduction of percutaneous methods not requiring surgical cutdown (p. 298). The major disadvantage is that it offers only modest circulatory support (elevation of cardiac index up to 0.8 liter/min/m^2) and cannot sustain life in extremely severe heart failure or in the presence of chaotic cardiac rhythms.

TEMPORARY LEFT VENTRICULAR ASSISTANCE. For patients who cannot be resuscitated or sustained by pharmacologic therapy and intraaortic balloon assistance, a more effective means of circulatory support is required. In patients in whom recovery of left ventricular function is anticipated and where removal of the pump is expected, several groups have developed left ventricular assist devices consisting of a pump with afferent and efferent conduits attached to the left ventricular apex and ascending thoracic aorta, respectively[550–552,552a,552b] (Fig. 16–24). The inflow and outflow conduits each contain a xenograft (porcine) valve to provide unidirectional flow. The pneumatic power source and control circuit are extracorporeal, and the pump itself rests on the anterior chest wall. Pumping is accomplished by the introduction of carbon dioxide under pressure into the space between the flexible bladder and rigid housing. Stroke volumes of 85 ml and rates of 100 beats/min can be achieved.

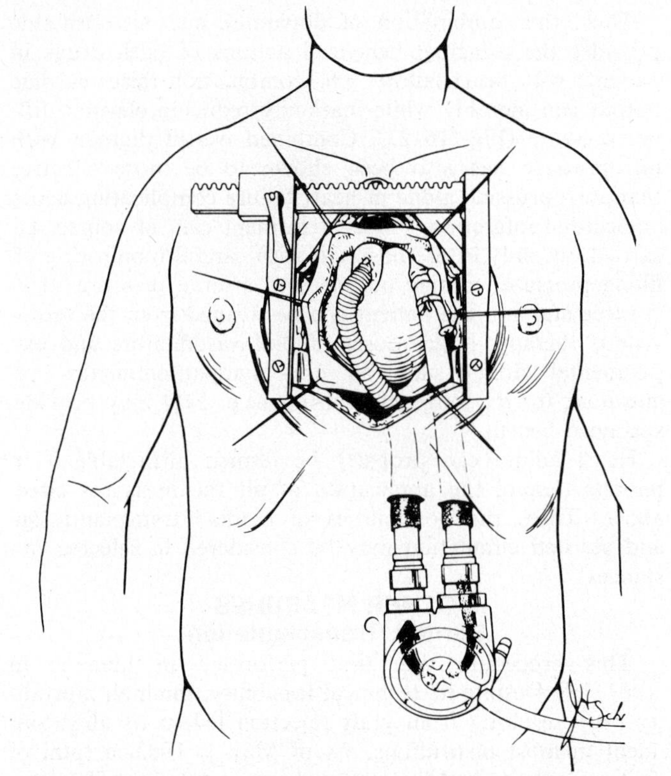

FIGURE 16–24 Pneumatically powered ventricular-assist pump as employed after cardiac operation but before chest closure. Blood is removed from the left atrium and pumped into the ascending aorta. (Reproduced with permission from Pierce, W. S., et al.: Ventricular-assist pumping in patients with cardiogenic shock after cardiac operations. N. Engl. J. Med. *305*:1606, 1981.)

Clinical trials are currently underway in patients who have had corrective cardiac surgery and in whom (1) pump oxygenator dependence develops in spite of intensive treatment with conventional measures, including intraaortic balloon counterpulsation, and (2) refractory cardiogenic shock occurs within 72 hours of the operation. In addition, it is being tested in patients with terminal heart failure secondary to acute (presumably viral) myocarditis and in patients with acute myocardial infarction and refractory cardiogenic shock.

When the left ventricular assist device is first applied to the patient, it handles almost the total left-heart output, while the patient's left ventricle performs little work. If, as a result of this "rest" period for 48 to 72 hours, the myocardium recovers, the left ventricle may be allowed to resume pumping a gradually increasing fraction of systemic blood flow, and attempts to wean the patient from the assist device are undertaken. Temporary reductions in the output of the mechanical device are made, and if adequate cardiac output and arterial pressures are maintained without a marked increase in left atrial pressure, withdrawal of mechanical support can be planned. Severe right-heart failure leads to inadequate left-heart filling, and the low preload precludes adequate inflow into the left ventricular assist device. Inotropic support of the right heart with catecholamines is therefore frequently necessary.

Norman, Cooley, and colleagues have developed an intracorporeal (abdominal) left ventricular assist device that is undergoing clinical testing,[553] and Rose et al. have reported clinical experiences in 16 patients with perioperative myocardial infarction and shock who could not be weaned from cardiopulmonary bypass despite use of inotropic agents and the intraaortic balloon pump and were treated with partial left heart (left atrium–aorta) bypass; eight patients survived.[554]

There is increasing evidence that approximately 25 per cent of patients whose hearts cannot sustain life despite pharmacologic therapy and intraaortic balloon counterpulsation can be maintained alive, survive discontinuation of left ventricular assistance, and leave the hospital. Obviously, long-term survival from this temporary period of support can be attained only if the cardiac insult is reversible.

PERMANENT LEFT VENTRICULAR ASSISTANCE. Patients whose left ventricles have sustained permanent damage and in whom recovery of function sufficient to support the circulation is not anticipated would be candidates for permanent left ventricular assistance. Potential candidates are patients with end-stage left ventricular disease, resulting from ischemic or other cardiomyopathies, patients with left ventricular infarction and shock, and postoperative patients with intractable left ventricular failure who are dependent on and cannot be weaned from temporary left ventricular assistance. These permanent devices, currently undergoing refinement and chronic testing in animals, are similar to those described above for temporary left ventricular assistance, except that the pump which fills from the left atrium or left ventricle and ejects blood into the aorta is implanted into the thorax or abdominal cavity. The energy source for these pumps is external and either an air tube or a wire passes through the skin. The native heart remains in situ, and survival requires continued function of the right ventricle. Such devices have functioned in calves for several months,[555,556] but at the time of this writing they have not been employed successfully for prolonged periods in human patients.

THE TOTAL ARTIFICIAL HEART. Also known as the biventricular replacement device, the *total* artificial heart involves the use of two mechanical pumps that replace the natural ventricles and support both the systemic and pulmonary circulations. With such a device the natural heart is excised. The contemplated use of the total artificial heart is in patients who could not otherwise survive and in whom the natural heart is permanently useless or even a threat to life, such as patients with large left ventricular infarctions and with rupture of the left ventricle or an irreparable ventricular septal defect or patients in whom catastrophic injury to the heart occurs during operation.

Since the first report describing the implantation of an artificial heart in an experimental animal in 1958, progress has been made, albeit gradually, toward the goal of developing a practical, totally implanted device that will support the circulation and allow a comfortable existence.[557] When successful clinical cardiac transplantation was first accomplished, the concept that a mechanical heart would become a useful therapeutic device was in doubt. However,

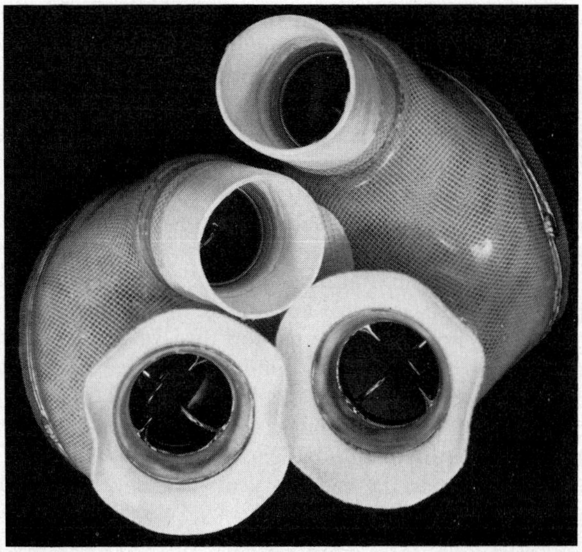

FIGURE 16–26 Utah total artificial heart. (Reproduced with permission from DeVries, W. C.: The total artificial heart. In Sabiston, D. C., Jr., and Spencer, F. C. (Eds.): Surgery of the Chest, 4th Ed. Philadelphia, W. B. Saunders Company, 1983.)

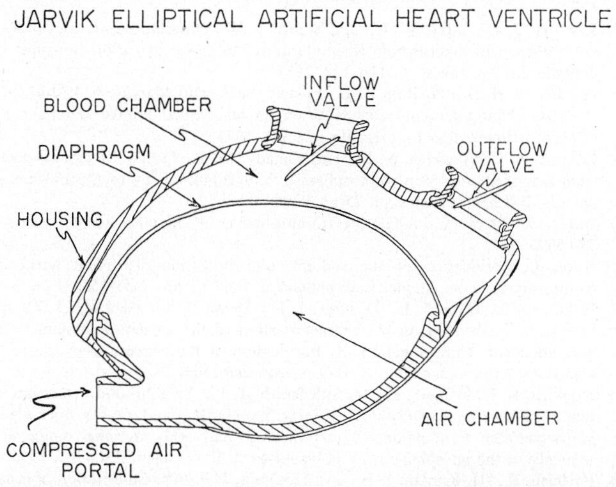

FIGURE 16–25 Cutaway of pneumatic ventricle. (Reproduced with permission from DeVries, W. C.: The total artificial heart. In Sabiston, D. C., Jr., and Spencer, F. C. (Eds.): Surgery of the Chest, 4th Ed. Philadelphia, W. B. Saunders Company, 1983.)

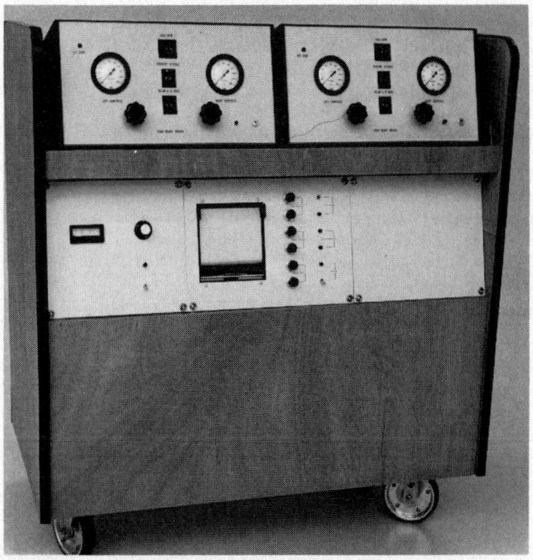

FIGURE 16–27 Utah heart drive system. (Reproduced with permission from DeVries, W. C.: The total artificial heart. In Sabiston, D. C., Jr., and Spencer, F. C. (Eds.): Surgery of the Chest, 4th Ed. Philadelphia, W. B. Saunders Company, 1983.)

the serious problems faced in obtaining donor hearts and in coordinating donor heart availability and recipient need have forced a reevaluation of transplantation as the ultimate solution to intractable heart failure.

A variety of devices is now being tested in experimental animals. A promising artificial heart recently developed[557a] consists of an electronic control system and two smooth-surfaced, sac-type pumps made of segmental polyurethane (Fig. 16–25 and 16–26). Two pneumatic power units (Fig. 16–27) pulse air intermittently to move the diaphragm, thereby moving blood into and out of the blood chamber (Fig. 16–25). Four pyrolitic carbon disc valves assure the unidirectional blood flow. A similar device[556,558] totally assumed the function of the heart for as long as six months in calves, which ate well and gained weight, and for more than three months in one patient, Dr. Barney Clark. The control system has the capability of balancing the output automatically during exercise. Bulky, electrically driven air-powered units (Fig. 16–27) positioned alongside the recipient power the artificial ventricles through air tubes. Current research centers on the development of pumps powered by implanted compact electrical motors.[556,558,559] At this time it appears that the problems inherent in the development of a totally implanted heart capable of permanent support of the circulation, although they have not been solved, are not insurmountable.

References

Digitalis Glycosides

1. Opie, L. H.: Principles of therapy for congestive heart failure. Europ. Heart J. *4*(Suppl. A):199, 1983.
2. Withering, W.: An account of the foxglove and some of its medical uses, with practical remarks on dropsy, and other diseases. *In* Willis, F. A., and Keys, T. E. (eds.): Classics of Cardiology. New York, Henry Schuman, Inc., 1941, p. 231.
2a. Marshall, P. G.: Steroids: Cardiotonic glycosides and aglycons: Toad poisons. *In* Coffey, S. (ed.): Rodd's Chemistry of Carbon Compounds. 2nd ed. Vol. 2D, Steroids. Amsterdam, Elsevier Publishing Co., 1970, p. 360.
3. Hoffman, B. F., and Bigger, J. T., Jr.: Digitalis and allied cardiac glycosides. *In* Gilman, A. G., Goodman, L. S., and Gilman, A. (eds.): The Pharmacological Basis of Therapeutics. 2nd ed. New York, Macmillan Publishing Company, Inc., 1980.
4. Lee, K. S., and Klaus, W.: The subcellular basis for the mechanism of inotropic action of cardiac glycosides. Pharmacol. Rev. *23*:193, 1971.
5. Schwartz, A., Lindenmayer, G. E., and Allen, J. C.: The sodium-potassium adenosine triphosphatase: Pharmacological, physiological and biochemical aspects. Pharmacol. Rev. *27*:1, 1975.
6. Akera, T., and Brody, T. M.: The role of Na^+,K^+-ATPase in the inotropic action of digitalis. Pharmacol. Rev. *29*:187, 1977.
7. Smith, T. W., and Barry, W. H.: Monovalent cation transport and mechanisms of digitalis-induced inotropy. Yale Symposium, 1982, in press.
8. Moran, N. C.: The effects of cardiac glycosides on mechanical properties of heart muscle. *In* Marks, B. H., and Weissler, A. M. (eds.): Basic and Clinical Pharmacology of Digitalis. Springfield, Ill., Charles C Thomas, 1972, p. 94.
9. Koch-Weser, J., and Blinks, J. R.: Analysis of the relation of the positive inotropic action of cardiac glycosides to the frequency of contraction of heart muscle. J. Pharmacol. Exp. Ther. *136*:305, 1962.
10. Farah, A. E.: The effects of the ionic milieu on the response of cardiac muscle to cardiac glycosides. *In* Fisch, C., and Surawicz, B. (eds.): Digitalis. New York, Grune and Stratton, 1969, p. 55.
11. Spann, J. F., Jr., Sonnenblick, E. H., Cooper, T., Chidsey, C. A., Willman, V. L., and Braunwald, E.: Studies on digitalis. XIV. Influence of cardiac norepinephrine stores on the response of isolated heart muscle to digitalis. Circ. Res. *19*:326, 1966.
12. Koch-Weser, J.: Beta-receptor blockade and myocardial effects of cardiac glycosides. Circ. Res. *28*:109, 1971.
13. Entman, M. L., Cook, J. W., Jr., and Bressler, R.: The influence of ouabain and alpha angelica lactone on calcium metabolism of dog cardiac microsomes. J. Clin. Invest. *48*:229, 1969.
14. Katz, A. M.: Contractile proteins of the heart. Physiol. Rev. *50*:63, 1970.
15. Coleman, H. N.: Role of acetylstrophanthidin in augmenting myocardial oxygen consumption. Circ. Res. *21*:487, 1967.
16. Weingart, R., Kass, R. S., and Tsien, R. W.: Is digitalis inotropy associated with enhanced slow inward calcium current? Nature *273*:389, 1978.
17. Lederer, W. J., and Eisner, D. A.: The effects of sodium pump activity on the slow inward current in sheep cardiac Purkinje fibers. Proc. Roy. Soc., Series B.
18. Marban, E., and Tsien, R. W.: Enhancement of cardiac calcium current during digitalis inotropy: Positive feedback regulation by intracellular calcium? J. Physiol. (London) *329*:589, 1982.
19. Fabiato, A., and Fabiato, F.: Activation of skinned cardiac cells. Subcellular effects of cardioactive drugs. Eur. J. Cardiol. *1*:145–155, 1973.
20. Bailey, L. E., and Harvey, S. C.: Effect of ouabain on cardiac ^{45}Ca kinetics measured by indicator dilution. Am. J. Physiol. *216*:123, 1969.
21. Langer, G. A., and Serena, S. D.: Effects of strophanthidin upon contraction and ionic exchange in rabbit ventricular myocardium: Relation to control of active state. J. Molec. Cell. Cardiol. *1*:65, 1970.
22. Biedert, S., Barry, W. H., and Smith, T. W.: Inotropic effects and changes in sodium and calcium contents associated with inhibition of monovalent cation active transport by ouabain in cultured myocardial cells. J. Gen. Physiol. *74*:479, 1979.
22a. Morgan, J. P., and Blinks, J. R.: Intracellular Ca^{++} transients in the cat papillary muscle. Can. J. Physiol. Pharmacol. *60*:524, 1982.
23. Schatzmann, H. J.: Herzglykoside als Hemmstoffe für den activen Kalium- and Natriumtransport durch die Erythrocytenmembran. Helv. Physiol. Pharmacol. Acta *11*:346, 1953.
24. Skou, J. C.: Enzymatic basis for active transport of Na^+ and K^+ across cell membrane. Physiol. Rev. *43*:596, 1965.
25. Repke, K., Est, M., and Portius, H. F.: Über die Ursache der Speciesunterschiede in der Digitalisempfindlichkeit. Biochem. Pharmacol. *14*:1785, 1965.
26. Schwartz, A., Matsui, H., and Laughter, A. H.: Tritiated digoxin binding to Na^+, K^+-activated adenosine-triphosphatase: Possible allosteric site. Science *160*:323, 1968.
27. Flasch, H., and Heinz, N.: Correlation between inhibition of NaK-membrane-ATPase and positive inotropic activity of cardenolides in isolated papillary muscles of guinea pig. Naunyn Schmiedebergs Arch. Pharmakol. *304*:37–44, 1978.
28. Allen, J. C., and Schwartz, A.: A possible biochemical explanation for the sensitivity of the rat to cardiac glycosides. J. Pharmacol. Exp. Ther. *168*:42, 1969.
29. Akera, T., Baskin, S. I., Tobin, T., and Brody, T. M.: Ouabain: Temporal relationship between the inotropic effect and the in vitro binding to, and dissociation from, (Na^+,K^+)-activated ATPase. Naunyn Schmiedebergs Arch. Pharmakol. *277*:151, 1973.
30. Ku, D., Akera, T., Pew, C. L., and Brody, T. M.: Cardiac glycosides: Correlation among Na^+,K^+-ATPase, sodium pump and contractility in the guinea pig heart. Naunyn Schmiedebergs Arch. Pharmakol. *285*:185, 1974.
31. Akera, T., Olgaard, M. K., Temma, K., and Brody, T. M.: Development of the positive inotropic action of ouabain: Effects of transmembrane sodium movement. J. Pharmacol. Exp. Ther. *203*:675, 1977.
32. Wasserman, O., and Holland, W. C.: Effects of tetrodotoxin and ouabain on atrial contractions. Pharmacol. Res. Commun. *1*:236, 1969.
33. Barry, W. H., Liechty, L., Beaudoin, D., and Smith, T. W.: Comparison of effects of a low extracellular potassium concentration and cardiac glycoside on contractility, monovalent cation transport and Na-Ca exchange in cultured ventricular cells. Trans. Assoc. Amer. Phys. *95*:12, 1982.
34. Eisner, D. A., and Lederer, W. J.: The role of the sodium pump in the effects of potassium-depleted solutions on mammalian cardiac muscle. J. Physiol. (London) *294*:279–301, 1979.
35. Akera, T., Larsen, F. S., and Brody, T. M.: Correlation of cardiac sodium- and potassium-activated adenosine triphosphatase activity with ouabain-induced inotropic stimulation. J. Pharmacol. Exp. Ther. *173*:145, 1970.
36. Hougen, T. J., and Smith, T. W.: Inhibition of myocardial monovalent cation active transport by subtoxic doses of ouabain in the dog. Circ. Res. *42*:856, 1978.
37. Somberg, J. C., Barry, W. H., and Smith, T. W.: Differing sensitivities of Purkinje fibers and myocardium to inhibition of monovalent cation transport by digitalis. J. Clin. Invest. *67*:116–123, 1981.
38. Prindle, K. H., Jr., Skelton, C. L., Epstein, S. E., and Marcus, F. I.: Influence of extracellular potassium concentration on myocardial uptake and inotropic effect of tritiated digoxin. Circ. Res. *28*:337, 1971.
39. Bonting, S. L., Hawkins, N. M., and Canady, M. R.: Studies of sodium-potassium activated adenosine triphosphatase. VII. Inhibition by erythrophleum alkaloids. Biochem. Pharmacol. *13*:13, 1964.
40. Akera, T.: Membrane adenosine triphosphatase: A digitalis receptor? Science *198*:569, 1977.
41. Kyte, J.: Purification of the sodium- and potassium-dependent adenosine triphosphatase from canine renal medulla. J. Biol. Chem. *246*:4157, 1971.
42. Hokin, L. E., Dahl, J. L., Deupree, J. D., Dixon, J. F., Hackney, J. F., and Perdue, J. F.: Studies on the characterization of the sodium-potassium transport adenosine triphosphatase. X. Purification of the enzyme from the rectal gland of a *Squalus acanthias*. J. Biol. Chem. *248*:2593, 1973.
43. Hopkins, B. E., Wagner, H., Jr., and Smith, T. W.: Sodium- and potassium-activated adenosine triphosphatase of the nasal salt gland of the duck (*Anas platyrhynchos*): Purification, characterization, and NH_2^-terminal amino acid sequence of the phosphorylating polypeptide. J. Biol. Chem. *251*:4365, 1976.
44. Forbush, B., III, Kaplan, J. H., and Hoffman, J. F.: Characterization of a new photoaffinity derivative of ouabain: Labelling of the large polypeptide and of a proteolipid component of the Na,K-ATPase. Biochemistry *17*:3667, 1978.
45. Kyte, J.: The titration of the cardiac glycoside binding site of the (Na^{++} K^+)-adenosine triphosphatase. J. Biol. Chem. *247*:7634, 1972.

46. Pitts, B. J. R., and Schwartz, A.: Improved purification and partial characterization of (Na+,K+)-ATPase from cardiac muscle. Biochim. Biophys. Acta *401*:184, 1975.
47. Calhoun, J. A., and Harrison, T. R.: Studies in congestive heart failure. IX. The effect of digitalis on the potassium content of the cardiac muscle of dogs. J. Clin. Invest. *10*:139, 1931.
48. Ellis, D.: The effects of external cations and ouabain on the intracellular sodium activity of sheep heart Purkinje fibers. J. Physiol. (London) *273*:211, 1977.
49. Lee, C. O., Kang, D. H., Sokol, J. H., and Lee, K. S.: Relation between intracellular Na ion activity and tension of sheep cardiac Purkinje fibers exposed to dihydro-ouabain. Biophys. J. *29*:315, 1980.
50. Cohen, C. J., Fozzard, H. A., and Shen, S-S.:Increase in intracellular sodium ion activity during stimulation in mammalian cardiac muscle. Circ. Res. *50*:651, 1982.
51. Langer, G. A.: Relationship between myocardial contractility and the effects of digitalis on ionic exchange. Fed. Proc. *36*:2231, 1977.
52. Baker, P. F., Blaustein, M. P., Hodgkin, A. L., and Steinhardt, R. A.: The influence of calcium on sodium efflux in squid axons. J. Physiol. (London) *200*:431, 1969.
53. Glitsch, H. G., Reuter, H., and Scholz, H.: The effect of the internal sodium concentration on calcium fluxes in isolated guinea pig auricles. J. Physiol. (London) *209*:25–43, 1970.
54. Akera, T., Bennett, R. T., Olgaard, M. K., and Brody, T. M.: Cardiac (Na+ + K+)-adenosine triphosphatase inhibition by ouabain and myocardial sodium: A computer simulation. J. Pharmacol. Exp. Ther. *199*:287, 1976.
55. Gervais, A., Lane, L. K., Anner, B. M., Lindenmayer, G. E., and Schwartz, A.: A possible molecular mechanism of the action of digitalis: Ouabain action on calcium binding to sites associated with a purified sodium-potassium-activated adenosine triphosphatase. Circ. Res. *40*:8, 1977.
56. Lüllman, H., and Peters, T.: Action of cardiac glycosides on the excitation-contraction coupling in heart muscle. Progr. Pharmacol. *2*:1, 1979.
57. Schon, R., Schonfeld, W., Menke, K.-H., and Repke, K. R. H.: Mechanism and role of Na+/Ca++ competition in (NaK)-ATPase. Acta Biol. Med. Germ. *29*:643, 1972.
58. Okita, G. T.: Dissociation of Na+,K+-ATPase inhibition from digitalis inotropy. Fed. Proc. *36*:2275, 1977.
59. Schwartz, A.: Brief reviews: Is the cell membrane Na+,K+-ATPase enzyme system the pharmacological receptor of digitalis? Circ. Res. *39*:2, 1976.
60. Noble, D.: Mechanism of action of therapeutic levels of cardiac glycosides. Cardiovasc. Res. *14*:495–514, 1980.
61. Smith, T. W., Antman, E. M., Friedman, P. L., Blatt, C. M., and Marsh, J. D.: Digitalis glycosides: Mechanisms and manifestations of toxicity. Progr. Cardiovasc. Dis. In Press.
62. Smith, T. W., and Barry, W. H.: The role of NaK-ATPase as a cardiac glycoside receptor. *In* Haft, J., and Karliner, J. (eds.): Textbook on Cardiac Receptors. In Press.
63. Goldman, R. H., Deutscher, R. N., Schweizer, E., and Harrison, D. C.: Effect of a pharmacologic dose of digoxin on inotropy in hyper- and normokalemic dogs. Am. J. Physiol. *223*:1438, 1972.
64. Seller, R. H.: The role of magnesium in digitalis toxicity. Am. Heart J. *82*:511, 1971.
65. Hoffman, J. F.: The red cell membrane and the transport of sodium and potassium. Am. J. Med. *41*:666, 1966.
66. Perrone, J. R., and Blostein, R.: Asymmetric interaction of inside-out and right-side–out erythrocyte membrane vesicles with ouabain. Biochim. Biophys. Acta *291*:680, 1973.
67. Caldwell, P. C., and Keynes, R. D.: The effect of ouabain on the efflux of sodium from a squid axon. J. Physiol. (London) *148*:8P, 1959.
68. Smith, T. W., Wagner, H., Jr., Markis, J. E., and Young, M.: Studies on the localization of the cardiac receptor. J. Clin. Invest. *51*:1777, 1972.
69. Smith, T. W., Wagner, H., Jr., and Young, M.: Cardiac glycoside interaction with solubilized myocardial sodium- and potassium-dependent adenosine triphosphatase. Molec. Pharmacol. *10*:626, 1974.
70. Rosen, M. R., Wit, A. L., and Hoffman, B. F.: Electrophysiology and pharmacology of cardiac arrhythmias. IV. Cardiac antiarrhythmic and toxic effects of digitalis. Am. Heart J. *89*:391, 1975.
71. Dhingra, R. C., Amat-Y-Leon, F., Wyndham, C., Wu, D., Denes, P., and Rosen, K. M.: The electrophysiological effects of ouabain on sinus node and atrium in man. J. Clin. Invest. *56*:555, 1975.
72. Goodman, D. J., Rossen, R. M., Ingham, R., Rider, A. K., and Harrison, D. C.: Sinus node function in the denervated human heart: Effects of digitalis. Br. Heart J. *37*:612, 1975.
73. Goodman, D. J., Rossen, R. M., Cannom, D. S., Rider, A. K., and Harrison, D. C.: Effect of digoxin on atrioventricular conduction: Studies in patients with and without cardiac autonomic innervation. Circulation *51*:251, 1975.
74. Kim, Y. I., Noble, R. J., and Zipes, D. P.: Dissociation of the inotropic effect of digitalis from its effect on atrioventricular conduction. Am. J. Cardiol. *36*:459, 1975.
75. Hordof, A. J., Spotnitz, A., Mary-Rabine, L., Edie, R., and Rosen, M. R.: The cellular electrophysiologic effects of digitalis on human atrial fibers. Circulation *56*:223, 1978.
76. Przybyla, A. C., Paulay, K. L., Stein, E., and Damato, A. N.: Effects of digoxin on atrioventricular conduction patterns in man. Am. J. Cardiol. *33*:344, 1974.
77. Rosen, M. R., Hordof, A. J., Hodess, A. B., Verosky, M., and Vulliemoz, Ouabain-induced changes in electrophysiologic properties of neonatal, young and adult canine cardiac Purkinje fibers. J. Pharmacol. Exp. Ther. *194*:255, 1975.
78. Rogers, M. C., Willerson, J. T., Goldblatt, A., and Smith, T. W.: Serum digoxin concentrations in the human fetus, neonate, and infant. N. Engl. J. Med. *287*:1010, 1972.
79. Weingart, R.: Influence of cardiac glycosides on electrophysiologic processes. *In* Greeff, K. (ed.): Cardiac Glycosides. Vol. 56, Part I, Handbook of Experimental Pharmacology. Berlin, Springer-Verlag, 1981.
79a.Gillis, R. A., and Quest, J. A.: The role of the nervous system in the cardiovascular effects of digitalis. Pharmacol. Rev. *31*:19–97, 1979.
80. Pace, C. B., and Gillis, R. A.: Neuroexcitatory effects of digoxin in the cat. J. Pharmacol. Exp. Ther. *199*:583, 1976.
81. Gillis, R. A., Raines, A., Sohn, Y. J., Levitt, B., and Standaert, F. G.: Neuroexcitatory effects of digitalis and their role in the development of cardiac arrhythmias. J. Pharmacol. Exp. Ther. *183*:154, 1972.
81a.Levitt, B., Cagin, N. A., Somberg, J., Bounous, H., Mittag, T., and Raines, A.: Alteration of the effects and distribution of ouabain by spinal cord transection in the cat. J. Pharmacol. Exp. Ther. *185*:24, 1973.
82. Somberg, J. C., and Smith, T. W.: Localization of the neurally mediated arrhythmogenic properties of digitalis. Science *204*:321, 1979.
83. Somberg, J. C., Risler, T., and Smith, T. W.: Neural factors in digitalis toxicity: Protective effect of C-1 spinal cord transection. Am. J. Physiol. *235*:H531–536, 1978.
84. Mudge, G. H., Jr., Lloyd, B. L., Greenblatt, D. J., and Smith, T. W.: Inotropic and toxic effects of a polar cardiac glycoside derivative in the dog. Circ. Res. *43*:847, 1978.
85. Smith, T. W.: The future of inotropic drugs in clinical practice. Eur. Heart J. *3*: 149, 1982.
86. Wiggers, C. J., and Stimson, B.: Studies on cardiodynamic action of drugs. III. The mechanism of cardiac stimulation by digitalis and g-strophanthin. J. Pharmacol. Exp. Ther. *30*:251, 1927.
87. Cattell, M., and Gold, H.: The influence of digitalis glycosides on the force of contraction of mammalian cardiac muscle. J. Pharmacol. Exp. Ther. *62*:116, 1938.
88. Braunwald, E., Bloodwell, R. D., Goldberg, L. I., and Morrow, A. G.: Studies on digitalis. IV. Observations in man on the effects of digitalis preparations on the contractility of the non-failing heart and on total vascular resistance. J. Clin. Invest. *40*:52, 1961.
89. Cotten, M. deV., and Stopp, P. E.: Action of digitalis on the nonfailing heart of the dog. Am. J. Physiol. *192*:114, 1958.
90. Spann, J. F., Jr., Buccino, R. A., Sonnenblick, E. H., and Braunwald, E.: Contractile state of cardiac muscle obtained from cats with experimentally produced ventricular hypertrophy and heart failure. Circ. Res. *21*:341, 1967.
91. Burwell, C. S., Neighbors, DeW., and Regen, E. M.: The effect of digitalis upon the output of the heart in normal man. J. Clin. Invest. *5*:125, 1927.
92. Harvey, R. M., Ferrer, M. I., Cathcart, R. T., and Alexander, J. K.: Some effects of digoxin on the heart and circulation in man: Digoxin in enlarged hearts not in clinical congestive failure. Circulation *4*:366, 1951.
93. Sonnenblick, E. H., Williams, J. F., Jr., Glick, G., Mason, D. T., and Braunwald, E.: Studies on digitalis. XV. Effects of cardiac glycosides on myocardial force-velocity relations in the nonfailing human heart. Circulation *34*:532, 1966.
94. Smith, T. W.: Medical treatment of advanced congestive heart failure: Digitalis and diuretics. *In* Braunwald, E., Moch, M. B., and Watson, J. T. (eds.): Congestive Heart Failure. New York, Grune and Stratton, Inc., 1982, pp. 261–278.
95. Arnold, S. B., Byrd, R. C., Meister, W., Melmon, K., Cheitlin, M. D., Bristow, J. D., Parmley, W. W., and Chatterjee, K.: Long-term digitalis therapy improves left ventricular function in heart failure. N. Engl. J. Med. *303*:1443–1448, 1980.
96. Lee, D. C.-S., Johnson, R. A., Bingham, J. B., Leahy, M., Dinsmore, R. E., Goroll, A. H., Newell, J. B., Strauss, H. W., and Haber, E.: Heart failure in outpatients. A randomized trial of digoxin versus placebo. N. Engl. J. Med. *306*:699–705, 1982.
97. Murray, R. G., Tweddel, A. C., Martin, W., Pearson, D., Hutton, I., and Lawrie, T. D. V.: Evaluation of digitalis in cardiac failure. Br. Med. J. *284*:1526–1528, 1982.
98. Fleg, J. L., Gottlieb, S. H., and Lakatta, E. G.: Is digoxin really important in treatment of compensated heart failure? Am. J. Med. *73*:244–250, 1982.
99. Williams, F. J., Jr., Klocke, F. J., and Braunwald, E.: Studies on digitalis. XIII. A comparison of the effects of potassium on the inotropic and arrhythmia-producing actions of ouabain. J. Clin. Invest. *45*:346, 1965.
100. Klein, M., Nejad, N. S., Lown, B., Hagemeijer, F., and Barr, I.: Correlation of the electrical and mechanical changes in the dog heart during progressive digitalization. Circ. Res. *29*:635, 1971.
101. Beiser, G. D., Epstein, S. E., Stampfer, M., Robinson, B., and Braunwald, E.: Studies on digitalis. XVII. Effects of ouabain on the hemodynamic response to exercise in patients with mitral stenosis in normal sinus rhythm. N. Engl. J. Med. *278*:131, 1968.
102. Mason, D. T., Zelis, R., and Amsterdam, E. A.: Unified concept of the mechanism of action of digitalis: Influence of ventricular function and cardiac disease on hemodynamic response to fundamental contractile effect. *In* Marks, B. H., and Weissler, A. M. (eds.): Basic and Clinical Pharmacology of Digitalis. Springfield, Ill., Charles C Thomas, 1972, p. 206.
103. Ross, J., Jr., Waldhausen, J. A., and Braunwald, E.: Studies on digitalis. I. Direct effects on peripheral vascular resistance. J. Clin. Invest. *39*:930, 1960.
104. Goldman, M. R., Wold, S. W., Rulten, D. L., and Powell, W. J., Jr.: Effect of

ouabain on total vascular capacity in the dog. J. Clin. Invest. *69*:175–184, 1982.
105. Mason, D. T., and Braunwald, E.: Studies on digitalis. X. Effects of ouabain on forearm vascular resistance and venous tone in normal subjects and in patients in heart failure. J. Clin. Invest. *43*:532, 1964.
106. Stark, J. J., Sanders, C. A., and Powell, W. J., Jr.: Neurally mediated and direct effects of acetylstrophanthidin on canine skeletal muscle vascular resistance. Circ. Res. *30*:274, 1972.
107. Garan, H., Smith, T. W., and Powell, W. J., Jr.: The central nervous system as a site of action for the coronary vasoconstrictor effect of digoxin. J. Clin. Invest. *54*:1365, 1974.
108. Sagar, K. B., Hanson, E. C., and Powell, W. J.: Neurogenic coronary vasoconstrictor effects of digitalis during acute global ischemia in dogs. J. Clin. Invest. *60*:1248, 1977.
109. Kumar, R., Yankopoulos, N. A., and Abelmann, W. H.: Ouabain-induced hypertension in a patient with decompensated hypertensive heart disease. Chest *63*:105, 1973.
110. Cohn, J. N., Tristani, F. E., and Khatri, I. M.: Cardiac and peripheral vascular effects of digitalis in clinical shock. Am. Heart J. *78*:318, 1969.
111. Shanbour, L. L., and Jacobson, E. D.: Digitalis and the mesenteric circulation. Am. J. Dig. Dis. *17*:826, 1972.
112. DeMots, H., Rahimtoola, S. H., McAnulty, J. H., and Porter, G. A.: Effects of ouabain on coronary and systemic vascular resistance and myocardial oxygen consumption in patients without heart failure. Am. J. Cardiol. *41*:88, 1978.
113. Zelis, R., and Mason, D. T.: Compensatory mechanisms in congestive heart failure: The role of the peripheral resistance vessels. N. Engl. J. Med. *282*:962, 1970.
114. Strickler, J. C., and Kessler, R. H.: Direct renal action of some digitalis steroids. J. Clin. Invest. *40*:311, 1961.
115. Torretti, J., Hendler, E., and Weinstein, E.: Functional significance of Na-K-ATPase in the kidney: Effects of ouabain inhibition. Am. J. Physiol. *222*:1398, 1972.
116. Gold, H., Cattell, M., Modell, W., Kwit, N. T., Kramer, M. L., and Zahm, W.: Clinical studies on digitoxin (Digitaline Nativelle): With further observations on its use in the single average full dose method of digitalization. J. Pharmacol. Exp. Ther. *82*:187, 1944.
117. Gold, H., Modell, W., Kwit, N. T., Shane, S. J., Dayrit, C., Kramer, M. L., Zahm, W., and Otto, H. L.: Comparison of ouabain with strophanthidin-3-acetate by intravenous injection in man. J. Pharmacol. Exp. Ther. *94*:39, 1948.
118. Gold, H., Cattell, M., Greiner, T., Hanlon, L. W., Kwit, N. T., Modell, W., Cotlove, E., Benton, J., and Otto, H. L.: Clinical pharmacology of digoxin. J. Pharmacol. Exp. Ther. *109*:45, 1953.
119. Cardiac Glycosides. Part II: Pharmacokinetics and Clinical Pharmacology. *In* Greeff, K. (ed.): Handbook of Experimental Pharmacology, Vol. 56. Berlin, Springer-Verlag, 1981.
120. Smith, T. W.: Drug therapy: Digitalis glycosides. N. Engl. J. Med. *288*:719, 1973.
121. Peters, V., Falk, L. C., and Kalman, S. M.: Digoxin metabolism in patients. Arch. Intern. Med. *138*:1074–1076, 1978.
122. Lindenbaum, J., Tse-Eng, D., Butler, V. P., Jr., and Rund, D. G.: Urinary excretion of reduced metabolites of digoxin. Am. J. Med. *71*:67–74, 1981.
122a. Lindenbaum, J., Rund, D. G., and Butler, V. P., Jr.: Inactivation of digoxin by the gut flora: reversal by antibiotic therapy. N. Engl. J. Med. *305*:789, 1981.
123. Halkin, H., Sheiner, L. B., Peck, C. C., and Melmon, K. L.: Determinants of the renal clearance of digoxin. Clin. Pharmacol. Ther. *385*:394, 1975.
124. Linday, L. A., Engle, M. A., and Reidenberg, M. M.: Maturation and renal digoxin clearance. Clin. Pharmacol. Ther. *30*:735–738, 1981.
125. Marcus, F. L., Burkhalter, L., Cuccia, C., Pavlovich, J., and Kapadia, G. G.: Administration of tritiated digoxin with and without a loading dose: A metabolic study. Circulation *34*:865, 1966.
126. Ackerman, G. L., Doherty, J. E., and Flanigan, W. J.: Peritoneal dialysis and hemodialysis of tritiated digoxin. Ann. Intern. Med. *67*:718, 1967.
127. Coltart, D. J., Chamberlain, D. A., Howard, M. R., Kettlewell, M. G., Mercer, J. L., and Smith, T. W.: The effect of cardiopulmonary bypass on plasma digoxin concentrations. Br. Heart J. *33*:334, 1971.
128. Coltart, D. J., Watson, D., and Howard, M. R.: Effect of exchange transfusions on plasma digoxin levels. Arch. Dis. Child. *47*:814, 1972.
129. Ewy, G. A., Groves, B. M., Ball, M. F., Nimmol, L., Jackson, B., and Marcus, F.: Digoxin-metabolism in obesity. Circulation *44*:810, 1971.
130. Cogan, J. J., Humphreys, M. H., Carlson, C. J., Benowitz, N. L., and Rapaport, E.: Acute vasodilator therapy increases renal clearance of digoxin in patients with congestive heart failure. Circulation *64*:973, 1981.
131. Dungan, W. T., Doherty, J. E., Harvey, C., Char, F., and Dalrymple, G. V.: Tritiated digoxin. XVIII. Studies in infants and children. Circulation *46*:983, 1972.
132. O'Malley, K., Coleman, E. N., Doig, W. B., and Stevenson, I. H.: Plasma digoxin levels in infants. Arch. Dis. Child. *48*:55, 1973.
133. Leahey, E. B., Jr., Reiffel, J. A., Drusin, R. E., Heissenbuttel, R. H., Lovejoy, W. P., and Bigger, J. T., Jr.: Interaction between quinidine and digoxin. J.A.M.A. *240*:533, 1978.
134. Lukas, D. S., and DeMartino, A. G.: Binding of digitoxin and some related cardenolides to human plasma proteins. J. Clin. Invest. *48*:1041, 1969.
135. Storstein, L.: Studies on digitalis. I. Renal excretion of digitoxin and its cardioactive metabolites. Clin. Pharmacol. Ther. *16*:14, 1974.
136. Storstein, L.: Studies on digitalis. II. The influence of impaired renal function on the renal excretion of digitoxin and its cardioactive metabolites. Clin. Pharmacol. Ther. *16*:25, 1974.
137. Okita, G. T.: Distribution, disposition and excretion of digitalis glycosides. *In* Fisch, C., and Surawicz, B. (eds.): Digitalis. New York, Grune and Stratton, 1969, p. 13.
138. Caldwell, J. H., Bush, C. A., and Greenberger, N. J.: Interruption of the enterohepatic circulation of digitoxin by cholestyramine. II. Effect on metabolic disposition of tritium-labeled digitoxin and cardiac systolic intervals in man. J. Clin. Invest. *50*:2638, 1971.
139. Solomon, H. M., and Abrams, W. B.: Interactions between digitoxin and other drugs in man. Am. Heart J. *83*:277, 1972.
140. Selden, R., and Smith, T. W.: Ouabain pharmacokinetics in dog and man: Determination by radioimmunoassay. Circulation *45*:1176, 1972.
141. Selden, R., Margolies, M. N., and Smith, T. W.: Renal and gastrointestinal excretion of ouabain in dog and man. J. Pharmacol. Exp. Ther. *188*:615, 1974.
142. Selden, R., Klein, M. D., and Smith, T. W.: Plasma concentration and urinary excretion kinetics of acetylstrophanthidin. Circulation *47*:744, 1973.
143. Cardiac Glycosides. Part II: Pharmacokinetics and Clinical Pharmacology. *In* Greeff, K. (ed.): Handbook of Experimental Pharmacology, Volume 56. Berlin, Springer-Verlag, 1981.
144. Doherty, J. E., Flanigan, W. J., Murphy, M. L., Bulloch, R. T., Dalrymple, G. V., Beard, O. W., and Perkins, W. H.: Tritiated digoxin. XIV. Enterohepatic circulation, absorption and excretion studies in human volunteers. Circulation *42*:867, 1970.
145. Beermann, B., Hellstrom, K., and Rosen, A.: The absorption of orally administered (12α-^{3}H) digoxin in man. Clin. Sci. *43*:507, 1972.
146. Greenblatt, D. J., Smith, T. W., and Koch-Weser, J.: Bioavailability of drugs: The digoxin dilemma. Clin. Pharmacokinet. *1*:36–51, 1976.
147. Heizer, W. D., Smith, T. W., and Goldfinger, S. E.: Absorption of digoxin in patients with malabsorption syndromes. N. Engl. J. Med. *285*:257, 1971.
148. Lindenbaum, J., Mellow, M. H., Blackstone, M. O., and Butler, V. P.: Variation in biologic availability of digoxin from four preparations. N. Engl. J. Med. *285*:1344, 1971.
149. Greenblatt, D. J., Smith, T. W., and Koch-Weser, J.: Bioavailability of drugs: The digoxin dilemma. Clin. Pharmacokinet. *1*:36, 1976.
150. Harter, J. G., Skelly, J. P., and Steers, A. W.: Digoxin—The regulatory viewpoint. Circulation *49*:395, 1974.
151. Jelliffe, R. W., Buell, J., and Kalaba, R.: Reduction of digitalis toxicity by computer-assisted glycoside dosage regimens. Ann. Intern. Med. *77*:891, 1972.
152. Jelliffe, R. W., and Brooker, G.: A nomogram for digoxin therapy. Am. J. Med. *57*:63, 1974.
153. Peck, C. C., Sheiner, L. B., Martin, C. M., Combs, D. L., and Melmon, K. L.: Computer-assisted digoxin therapy. N. Engl. J. Med. *289*:441, 1973.
154. Lown, B., Hagemeijer, F., Barr, I., and Klein, M.: Digitalis intoxication: Clinical and experimental assessment of the degree of digitalization. *In* Marks, B. H., and Weissler, A. M. (eds.): Basic and Clinical Pharmacology of Digitalis. Springfield, Ill., Charles C Thomas, 1972, p. 299.
155. Lown, B., Klein, M. D., Barr, I., Hagemeijer, F., Kosowsky, B. D., and Garrison, H.: Sensitivity to digitalis drugs in acute myocardial infarction. Am. J. Cardiol. *30*:388, 1972.
156. Kleiger, R., and Lown, B.: Cardioversion and digitalis. II. Clinical studies. Circulation *33*:878, 1966.
157. Johnson, L. W., Dickstein, R. A., Freuhan, C. T., Kane, P., Potts, J. L., Smulyan, H., Webb, W. R., and Eich, R. H.: Prophylactic digitalization for coronary artery bypass surgery. Circulation *53*:819, 1976.
158. Tyras, D. H., Stothert, J. C., Jr., Kaiser, G. C., Barner, H. B., Codd, J. E., and Willman, V. L.: Supraventricular tachyarrhythmias after myocardial revascularization: A randomized trial of prophylactic digitalization. J. Thorac. Cardiovasc. Surg. *77*:310, 1979.
159. Schwartz, J. B., Keefe, D., Kates, R. E., Kirsten, E., and Harrison, D. C.: Acute and chronic pharmacodynamic interaction of verapamil and digoxin in atrial fibrillation. Circulation *65*:1162–1170, 1982.
160. Sellers, T. D., Bashore, T. M., and Gallagher, J. J.: Digitalis in pre-excitation syndrome—Analysis during atrial fibrillation. Circulation *56*:260, 1977.
161. Jelliffe, R. W.: Factors to consider in planning digoxin therapy. J. Chron. Dis. *24*:407, 1971.
162. Package Insert—Lanoxin Brand of Digoxin. Burroughs Wellcome Company, March, 1981.
163. Lown, B., and Levine, S. A.: The carotid sinus: Clinical value of its stimulation. Circulation *23*:766, 1961.
164. Sampson, J. J., Albertson, E. C., and Kondo, B.: The effect on man of potassium administration in relation to digitalis glycosides with special reference to blood serum potassium, the electrocardiogram and ectopic beats. Am. Heart J. *26*:164, 1943.
165. Fisch, C.: Relation of electrolyte disturbances to cardiac arrhythmias. Circulation *47*:408, 1973.
166. Davidson, S., and Surawicz, B.: Ectopic beats and atrioventricular conduction disturbances. Arch. Intern. Med. *120*:280, 1967.
167. Fisch, C., Martz, B. C., and Priebe, F. H.: Enhancement of potassium-induced atrioventricular block by toxic doses of digitalis drugs. J. Clin. Invest. *39*:1885, 1960.
168. Ghani, M. F., and Smith, J. R.: The effectiveness of magnesium chloride in the treatment of ventricular tachyarrhythmias due to digitalis intoxication. Am. Heart J. *88*:621, 1974.

169. Neff, M. S., Mendelssohn, S., Kim, K. E., Banach, S., Swartz, C., and Seller, R. H.: Magnesium sulfate in digitalis toxicity. Am. J. Cardiol. *29*:377, 1972.
170. Editorial: Calcium, magnesium, and diuretics. Br. Med. J. *1*:170, 1975.
171. Holt, D. W., and Goulding, R.: Magnesium depletion and digoxin toxicity. Br. Med. J. *1*:627, 1975.
172. Beller, G. A., Hood, W. B., Jr., Smith, T. W., Abelmann, W. H., and Wacker, W. E. C.: Correlation of serum magnesium levels and cardiac digitalis intoxication. Am. J. Cardiol. *33*:225, 1974.
173. Gold, H., and Edwards, D. J.: The effects of ouabain on the heart in the presence of hypercalcemia. Am. Heart J. *3*:45, 1927.
174. Surawicz, B.: Use of the chelating agent, EDTA, in digitalis intoxication and cardiac arrhythmias. Progr. Cardiovasc. Dis. *2*:432, 1959.
175. Warren, M. C., Gianelly, R. E., Cutler, S. L., and Harrison, D. C.: Digitalis toxicity. II. The effect of metabolic alkalosis. Am. Heart J. *75*:358, 1968.
176. Galmarini, D., Campdonico, J. F., and Wenk, R. D.: Effect of alkalosis on ouabain toxicity in the dog. J. Pharmacol. Exp. Ther. *186*:199, 1973.
177. Williams, J. F., Jr., Boyd, D. C., and Border, J. F.: Effects of acute hypoxia and hypercapnic acidosis on the development of acetylstrophanthidin induced arrhythmias. J. Clin. Invest. *47*:1885, 1968.
178. Tisi, G. M., and Moser, K. M.: Effect of acute changes in pO_2, pCO_2, and pH on digitalis toxicity. Circulation *36*:11, 1967.
179. Bigger, J. T.: The quinidine-digoxin interaction. Int. J. Cardiol. *1*:109–116, 1981.
180. Pedersen, K. E., Dorph-Pedersen, A., Hvidt, S., Klitgaard, N. A., and Nielsen-Kudsk, F.: Digoxin-verapamil interaction. Clin. Pharmacol. Ther. *30*:311–316, 1981.
181. Klein, H. O., Lang, R., Weiss, E., Segni, E. D., Libhaber, C., Guerrero, J., and Kaplinsky, E.: The influence of verapamil on serum digoxin concentration. Circulation *65*:998–1003, 1982.
182. Belz, G. G., Aust, P. E., and Munkes, R.: Digoxin plasma concentrations and nifedipine. Lancet *1*:844–845, 1981.
183. Lessem, J., and Bellinetto, A.: Interaction between digoxin and calcium antagonists. Am. J. Cardiol. *49*:1025, 1982.
184. Moysey, J. O., Jaggarao, N. S. V., Grundy, E. N., and Chamberlain, D. A.: Amiodarone increases plasma digoxin concentrations. Br. Med. J. *282*:272–273, 1981.
185. Nademanee, K., Kannan, R., Hendrickson, J., Burnam, M., Kay, I., and Singh, B.: Amiodarone-digoxin interaction during treatment of resistant cardiac arrhythmias. Am. J. Cardiol. *49*:1026, 1982.
186. Morrow, D. H., and Townley, N. T.: Anesthesia and digitalis toxicity: An experimental study. Anesth. Analg. *43*:510, 1964.
187. Dowdy, E. G., and Fabian, L. W.: Ventricular arrhythmias induced by succinylcholine in digitalized patients. Anesth. Analg. *42*:501, 1963.
188. Becker, D. J., Nankin, P. M., Bennett, L. D., Kimball, S. G., Sternberg, M. S., and Wasserman, F.: Effect of isoproterenol in digitalis cardiotoxicity. Am. J. Cardiol. *10*:242, 1962.
189. Smith, T. W.: Contribution of quantitative assay technics to the understanding of the clinical pharmacology of digitalis. Circulation *46*:188, 1972.
190. Smith, T. W., and Willerson, J. T.: Suicidal and accidental digoxin ingestion: Report of five cases with serum digoxin level correlations. Circulation *44*:29, 1971.
191. Smith, T. W., Butler, V. P., Jr., Haber, E., Fozzard, H., Marcus, F. I., Bremner, W. F., Schulman, I. C., and Phillips, A.: Treatment of life-threatening digitalis intoxication with digoxin-specific Fab fragments: Experience in 26 cases. N. Engl. J. Med. *307*:1357, 1982.
192. Rubinow, A., Skinner, M., and Cohen, A. S.: Digoxin sensitivity in amyloid cardiomyopathy. Circulation *63*:1285–1288, 1981.
193. Covell, J. W., Braunwald, E., Ross, J., Jr., and Sonnenblick, E. H.: Studies on digitalis. XVI. Effects on myocardial oxygen consumption. J. Clin. Invest. *45*:1535, 1966.
194. Sonnenblick, E. H., Ross, J., Jr., and Braunwald, E.: Oxygen consumption of the heart: Newer concepts of its multifactorial determination. Am. J. Cardiol. *22*:328, 1968.
195. Glancy, D. L., Higgs, L. M., O'Brien, K. P., and Epstein, S. E.: Effects of ouabain on the left ventricular response to exercise in patients with angina pectoris. Circulation *43*:45, 1971.
196. Sharma, B., Majid, P. A., Meeran, M. K., Whitaker, W., and Taylor, S. H.: Clinical, electrocardiographic and haemodynamic effects of digitalis (ouabain) in angina pectoris. Br. Heart J. *34*:631, 1972.
197. DeMots, H., Rahimtoola, S. H., Kremkau, E. L., Bennett, W., and Mahler, D.: Effects of ouabain on myocardial oxygen supply and demand in patients with chronic coronary artery disease: A hemodynamic, volumetric, and metabolic study in patients without heart failure. J. Clin. Invest. *58*:312, 1976.
198. Loeb, H. S., Streitmatter, N., Braunstein, D., Jacobs, W. R., Croke, R. P., and Gunnar, R. M.: Lack of ouabain effect on pacing-induced myocardial ischemia in patients with coronary artery disease. Am. J. Cardiol. *43*:995, 1979.
199. Vogel, R., Kirch, D., LeFree, M., Frischknecht, J., and Steele, P.: Effects of digitalis on resting and isometric exercise myocardial perfusion in patients with coronary artery disease and left ventricular dysfunction. Circulation *56*:355, 1977.
200. Crawford, M. H., LeWinter, M. M., O'Rourke, R. A., Karliner, J. S., and Ross, J.: Combined propranolol and digoxin therapy in angina pectoris. Ann. Intern. Med. *83*:449, 1975.
201. Karliner, J. S., and Braunwald, E.: Present status of digitalis treatment of acute myocardial infarction. Circulation *45*:891, 1972.
202. Cohn, J. N., Tristani, F. E., and Khatri, I. M.: Cardiac and peripheral vascular effects of digitalis in clinical cardiogenic shock. Am. Heart J. *78*:318, 1969.
203. Ratshin, R. A., Rackley, C. E., and Russell, R. O., Jr.: Hemodynamic evaluation of left ventricular function in shock complicating myocardial infarction. Circulation *45*:127, 1972.
204. Rahimtoola, S. H., Sinno, M. Z., Chuquimia, R., Loeb, H. S., Rosen, K. M., and Gunnar, R. M.: Effects of ouabain on impaired left ventricular function in acute myocardial infarction. N. Engl. J. Med. *287*:527, 1972.
205. Rahimtoola, S. H., DiGilio, M. M., Sinno, M. Z., Loeb, H. S., Rosen K. M., and Gunnar, R. M.: Effects of ouabain on impaired left ventricular function during convalescence after acute myocardial infarction. Circulation *44*:866, 1971.
206. Morris, J. J., Jr., Taft, C. V., Whalen, R. E., and McIntosh, H. D.: Digitalis and experimental myocardial infarction. Am. Heart J. *77*:342, 1969.
207. Kumar, R., Hood, W. B., Jr., Joison, J., Gilmour, D. P., Norman, J. C., and Abelmann, W. H.: Experimental myocardial infarction. VI. Efficacy and toxicity of digitalis in acute and healing phase in intact conscious dogs. J. Clin. Invest. *49*:358, 1970.
208. Reičansky, I., Conradson, T. B., Holmberg, S., Rydén, L., Waldenström, A., and Wennerblom, B.: The effect of intravenous digoxin on the occurrence of ventricular tachyarrhythmias in acute myocardial infarction in man. Am. Heart J. *91*:705, 1976.
209. Rahimtoola, S. H., and Gunnar, R. M.: Digitalis in acute myocardial infarction: Help or hazard? Ann. Intern. Med. *82*:234, 1975.
210. Selzer, A.: The use of digitalis in acute myocardial infarction. Progr. Cardiovasc. Dis. *10*:518, 1968.
211. Moss, A. J., Davis, H. T., Conard, D. L., DeCamilla, J. J., and Odoroff, C. L.: Digitalis-associated cardiac mortality after myocardial infarction. Circulation *64*:1150, 1981.
211a. Ryan, T. J., Bailey, K. R., McCabe, C. H., Luk, S., Fisher, L. D., Mock, M. B., and Killip, T.: The effects of digitalis on survival in high-risk patients with coronary artery disease. The coronary artery surgery study (CASS). Circulation *67*:735, 1983.
212. Dall, J. L.: Digitalis intoxication in the elderly. Lancet *1*:194, 1965.
213. Hermann, G. R.: Digitoxicity in the aged. Geriatrics *21*:109, 1966.
214. Szefler, S. J., and Jusko, W. J.: Decreased volume of distribution of digoxin in a patient with renal failure. Res. Commun. Chem. Pathol. Pharmacol. *6*:1095, 1973.
215. Croxson, M. S., and Ibbertson, H. K.: Serum digoxin in patients with thyroid disease. Br. Med. J. *3*:566, 1975.
216. Doherty, J. E., and Perkins, W. H.: Digoxin metabolism in hypo- and hyperthyroidism: Studies with tritiated digoxin in thyroid disease. Ann. Intern. Med. *64*:489, 1966.
217. Curfman, G. D., Crowley, T. J., and Smith, T. W.: Thyroid-induced alterations in myocardial sodium- and potassium-activated adenosine triphosphatase, monovalent cation active transport, and cardiac glycoside binding. J. Clin. Invest. *59*:586, 1977.
218. Ismail-Beigi, F., and Edelman, I. S.: The mechanism of the calorigenic action of thyroid hormone: Stimulation of $Na^+ + K^+$-activated adenosine-triphosphatase. J. Gen. Physiol. *57*:710, 1971.
219. Green, L. H., and Smith, T. W.: The use of digitalis in patients with pulmonary disease. Ann. Intern. Med. *87*:459, 1977.
220. Hargreave, F. D.: Digitalis and cor pulmonale. Br. Med. J. *2*:943, 1965.
221. Carazza, L. J., and Pastor, B. H.: Cardiac arrhythmias in chronic cor pulmonale. N. Engl. J. Med. *259*:862, 1958.
222. Rodensky, P. L., and Wasserman, F.: Observations on digitalis intoxication. Arch. Intern. Med. *108*:171, 1961.
223. Hudson, L. D., Kurt, T. L., Petty, T. L., and Genton, E.: Arrhythmias associated with acute respiratory failure in patients with chronic airway obstruction. Chest *63*:661, 1973.
224. Thomas, A. J., and Valabhji, P.: Arrhythmia and tachycardia in pulmonary heart disease. Br. Heart J. *31*:491, 1969.
225. Beller, G. A., Smith, T. W., Abelmann, W. H., Haber, E., and Hood, W. B., Jr.: Digitalis intoxication: Prospective clinical study with serum level correlations. N. Engl. J. Med. *284*:989, 1971.
226. Baum, G. L., Dick, M. M., Schotz, S., and Gumpel, R. C.: Digitalis toxicity in chronic cor pulmonale. South. Med. J. *49*:1037, 1956.
227. Klein, M. D., Lown, B., Barr, I., Hagemeijer, F., Garrison, H., and Axelrod, P.: Comparison of serum digoxin level measurement with acetyl strophanthidin tolerance testing. Circulation *49*:1053, 1974.
228. Harrison, D. C., Robinson, M. D., and Kleiger, R. E.: Role of hypoxia in digitalis toxicity. Am. J. Med. Sci. *256*:352, 1968.
229. Lely, A. H., and van Enter, C. H. J.: Non-cardiac symptoms of digitalis intoxication. Am. Heart J. *83*:149, 1972.
230. Doherty, J. E., and Perkins, W. H.: Tissue concentration and turnover of tritiated digoxin in dogs. Am. J. Cardiol. *17*:47, 1966.
231. Doherty, J. E., Perkins, W. H., and Flanigan, W. J.: The distribution and concentration of tritiated digoxin in human tissues. Ann. Intern. Med. *66*:116, 1967.
232. Barr, I., Smith, T. W., Klein, M. D., Hagemeijer, F., and Lown, B.: Correlation of the electrophysiologic action of digoxin with serum digoxin concentration. J. Pharmacol. Exp. Ther. *180*:710, 1972.
233. Smith, T. W., and Curfman, G. D.: Radioimmunoassay of cardiac glycosides. *In* Strauss, W., and Pitt, B. (eds.): Cardiovascular Nuclear Medicine. 2nd ed. St. Louis, C. V. Mosby Co., 1979, p. 394.

234. Smith, T. W., and Haber, E.: The current status of cardiac glycoside assay techniques. *In* Yu, P. N., and Goodwin, J. F. (eds.): Progress in Cardiology. Philadelphia, Lea and Febiger, 1973, p. 49.
235. Smith, T. W., and Haber, E.: Clinical value of the radioimmunoassay of the digitalis glycosides. Pharmacol. Rev. *25*:219, 1973.
236. Duhme, D. W., Greenblatt, D. J., and Koch-Weser, J.: Reduction of digoxin toxicity associated with measurement of serum levels. Ann. Intern. Med. *80*:516, 1974.
237. Chamberlain, D. A., White, R. J., Howard, M. R., and Smith, T. W.: Plasma digoxin concentrations in patients with atrial fibrillation. Br. Med. J. *3*:429, 1970.
238. Eraker, S. A., and Sasse, L.: The serum digoxin test and digoxin toxicity: A Bayesian approach to decision-making. Circulation *64*:409–420, 1981.
239. Hurwitz, N., and Wade, O. L.: Intensive hospital monitoring of adverse reactions to drugs. Br. Med. J. *1*:531, 1969.
240. Ogilvie, R. I., and Ruedy, J.: Adverse drug reactions during hospitalization. Canad. Med. Assoc. J. *97*:1450, 1967.
241. Borison, H. L., and Wang, S. C.: Physiology and pharmacology of vomiting. Pharmacol. Rev. *5*:193, 1953.
242. Gayes, J. M., Greenblatt, D. J., Lloyd, B. L., Harmatz, J. S., and Smith, T. W.: Cerebrospinal fluid digoxin concentrations in humans. J. Clin. Pharmacol. *18*:16, 1978.
243. Allonen, H., Andersson, K.-E., Iisalo, E., Kanto, J., Strömblad, L. G., and Wettrell, G.: Passage of digoxin into cerebrospinal fluid in man. Acta Pharmacol. Toxicol. *41*:193, 1977.
244. Somberg, J. C., Kuhlman, J. E., and Smith, T. W.: Localization of the neurally mediated coronary vasoconstrictor properties of digitalis in the cat. Circ. Res. *49*:226–233, 1981.
245. Rosen, M. R., Gelband, H., and Hoffman, B. F.: Correlation between effects of ouabain on the canine electrocardiogram and transmembrane potentials of isolated Purkinje fibers. Circulation *47*:65, 1973.
246. Rosen, M. R., and Gelband, H.: Effect of ouabain on canine Purkinje fibers in situ or perfused with blood. J. Pharmacol. Exp. Ther. *186*:366, 1973.
247. Davis, L. D.: Effect of changes in cycle length on diastolic depolarization produced by ouabain in canine Purkinje fibers. Circ. Res. *32*:206, 1973.
248. Rosen, M. R., Gelband, H., Merker, C., and Hoffman, B. F.: Mechanisms of digitalis toxicity. Effects of ouabain on phase 4 of canine Purkinje fiber transmembrane potentials. Circulation *47*:681, 1973.
249. Ferrier, G. R., Saunders, J. H., and Mendez, C.: A cellular mechanism of the generation of ventricular arrhythmias by acetylstrophanthidin. Circ. Res. *32*:600, 1973.
250. Saunders, J. H., Ferrier, G. R., and Moe, G. K.: Conduction block associated with transient depolarizations induced by acetylstrophanthidin in isolated canine Purkinje fibers. Circ. Res. *32*:610, 1973.
251. Zipes, D. P., Arbel, E., Knope, R. F., and Moe, G. K.: Accelerated cardiac escape rhythms caused by ouabain intoxication. Am. J. Cardiol. *33*:248, 1973.
252. Ferrier, G. R.: Digitalis arrhythmias: Role of oscillatory afterpotentials. Progr. Cardiovasc. Dis. *19*:459, 1977.
253. Lederer, W. J., and Tsien, R. W.: Transient inward current underlying arrhythmogenic effects of cardiotonic steroids in Purkinje fibers. J. Physiol. (London) *263*:73, 1976.
254. Kass, R. S., Lederer, W. J., Tsien, R. W., and Weingart, R.: Role of calcium ions in transient inward currents and aftercontractions induced by strophanthidin in cardiac Purkinje fibers. J. Physiol. (London) *281*:187, 1978.
255. Tsien, R. W., Weingart, R., Lederer, W. J., and Kass, R. S.: On the inotropic and arrhythmogenic effects of digitalis. *In* Riecker, G., Weber, A., and Goodwin, J. (eds.): Myocardial Failure. New York, Springer-Verlag, 1977, p. 331.
256. Kass, R. S., Tsien, R. W., and Weingart, R.: Ionic basis of transient inward current induced by strophanthidin in cardiac Purkinje fibers. J. Physiol. (London) *281*:209, 1978.
257. Goodman, D. J., Rossen, R. M., Ingham, R., Rider, A. K., and Harrison, D. C.: Sinus node function in the denervated human heart. Effect of digitalis. Br. Heart J. *37*:612–618, 1975.
258. Hoffman, B. F., and Singer, D. H.: Effects of digitalis on electrical activity of cardiac fibers. Progr. Cardiovasc. Dis. *7*:226, 1964.
259. James, T. N., and Nadeau, R. A.: The chronotropic effect of digitalis studied by direct perfusion of the sinus node. J. Pharmacol. *139*:42, 1960.
260. Watanabe, Y., and Dreifus, L. S.: Interactions of lanatoside C and potassium on atrioventricular conduction in rabbits. Circ. Res. *27*:931, 1970.
261. Lely, A., and van Enter, C.: Large-scale digitoxin intoxication. Br. Med. J. *3*:737, 1970.
262. Storstein, O., and Rasmussen, K.: Digitalis and atrial tachycardia with block. Br. Heart J. *36*:171, 1974.
263. Lown, B., Graboys, T. B., Podrid, P. J., Cohen, B. H., Stockman, M. B., and Gaughan, C. E.: Effect of a digitalis drug on ventricular premature beats. N. Engl. J. Med. *296*:301, 1977.
264. Chung, E. K.: Principles of Cardiac Arrhythmias. Baltimore, Williams and Wilkins, 1971.
265. Fisch, C., Zipes, D. P., and Noble, R. J.: Digitalis toxicity: Mechanism and recognition. *In* Yu, P. N., and Goodwin, J. F. (eds.): Progress in Cardiology. Vol. 4. Philadelphia, Lea and Febiger, 1975, p. 35.
266. Wellens, H. J. J.: The electrocardiogram in digitalis intoxication. *In* Yu, P. N., and Goodwin, J. F. (eds.): Progress in Cardiology. Vol. 5. Philadelphia, Lea and Febiger, 1976, p. 271.
267. Brauner, G. J., and Greene, M. H.: Digitalis allergy: Digoxin-induced vasculitis. Cutis *10*:441, 1972.
268. LeWinn, E. B.: Gynecomastia during digitalis therapy: Report of eight additional cases with liver-function studies. N. Engl. J. Med. *248*:316, 1953.
269. Neri, A., Aygen, M., Zuckerman, A., and Bahary, C.: Subject of assessment of sexual dysfunction of patients on long-term administration of digoxin. Arch. Sexual Behav. 9:343–347, 1980.
270. Bismuth, C., Motte, G., Conso, F., Chauvin, M., and Gaultier, M.: Acute digitoxin intoxication treated by intracardiac pacemaker: Experience in sixty-eight patients. Clin. Toxicol. *10*:443, 1977.
271. Citrin, D., Stevenson, I. H., and O'Malley, K.: Massive digoxin overdose: Observations on hyperkalaemia and plasma digoxin levels. Scott. Med. J. *17*:275, 1972.
272. Gaultier, M., Fournier, E., Efthymiou, M. L., Frejaville, J. P., Jouannot, P., and Dentan, M.: Intoxication digitalique aiguë (70 observations). Bull. Soc. Med. Hop. Paris *119*:247, 1968.
273. Hobson, J. D., and Zettner, A.: Digoxin serum half-life following suicidal digoxin poisoning. J.A.M.A. *223*:147, 1973.
274. Bigger, J. T., Jr., and Strauss, H. C.: Digitalis toxicity: Drug interactions promoting toxicity and the management of toxicity. Semin. Drug Treat. *2*:147, 1972.
275. Bigger, J. T., Jr., and Mandel, W. J.: Effect of lidocaine on the electrophysiological properties of ventricular muscle and Purkinje fibers. J. Clin. Invest. *49*:63, 1970.
276. Bigger, J. T., Jr., Bassett, A. L., and Hoffman, B. F.: Electrophysiological effects of diphenylhydantoin on canine Purkinje fibers. Circ. Res. *22*:221, 1968.
277. Strauss, H. C., Bigger, J. T., Jr., Bassett, A. L., and Hoffman, B. F.: Actions of diphenylhydantoin on the electrical properties of isolated rabbit and canine atria. Circ. Res. *23*:463, 1968.
278. Helfant, R. H., Scherlag, B. J., and Damato, A. N.: The electrophysiological properties of diphenylhydantoin sodium as compared to procaine amide in the normal and digitalis-intoxicated heart. Circulation *36*:108, 1967.
279. Fisch, C., Knoebel, S. B., Feigenbaum, H., and Greenspan, K.: Potassium and the monophasic action potential, electrocardiogram, conduction and arrhythmias. Progr. Cardiovasc. Dis. *8*:387, 1966.
280. Davis, L. D., and Temte, J. V.: Effects of propranolol on the transmembrane potentials of ventricular muscle and Purkinje fibers of the dog. Circ. Res. *22*:661, 1968.
281. Lown, B., Kleiger, R., and Williams, J.: Cardioversion and digitalis drugs: Changed threshold to electric shock in digitalized animals. Circ. Res. *17*:519, 1965.
282. Ditchey, R. V., and Karliner, J. S.: Safety of electrical cardioversion in patients without digitalis toxicity. Ann. Intern. Med. *95*:676–679, 1981.
283. Bazzano, G., and Bazzano, G. S.: Digitalis intoxication: Treatment with a new steroid-binding resin. J.A.M.A. *220*:828, 1972.
284. Goldfinger, S. E., Heizer, W. D., and Smith, T. W.: Absorption of digoxin in patients with malabsorption syndrome. *In* Storstein, O. (ed.): International Symposium on Digitalis. Oslo, Gyldendal Norsk Forlag, 1973, p. 224.
285. Smith, T. W., Butler, V. P., Jr., and Haber, E.: Cardiac glycoside-specific antibodies in the treatment of digitalis intoxication. *In* Haber, E., and Krause, R. M. (eds.): Antibodies in Human Diagnosis and Therapy. New York, Raven Press, 1977.
286. Butler, V. P., Jr., Smith, T. W., Schmidt, D. H., and Haber; E.: Immunological reversal of the effects of digoxin. Fed. Proc. *36*:2235, 1977.
287. Lloyd, B. L., and Smith, T. W.: Contrasting rates of reversal of digoxin toxicity by digoxin-specific IgG and Fab fragments. Circulation *58*:280, 1978.
288. Smith, T. W.: Ouabain-specific antibodies: Immunochemical properties and reversal of Na^+, K^+-activated adenosine triphosphatase inhibition. J. Clin. Invest. *51*:1583, 1972.
289. Hougen, T. J., Lloyd, B. L., and Smith, T. W.: Effects of inotropic and arrhythmogenic digoxin doses and of digoxin-specific antibody on myocardial monovalent cation transport in the dog. Circ. Res. *44*:23, 1979.
290. Waldmann, T. A., and Strober, W.: Metabolism of immunoglobulins. Progr. Allergy *13*:1, 1969.
291. Butler, V. P., Jr., Schmidt, D. H., Smith, T. W., Haber, E., Raynor, B. D., and McMartini, P.: Effects of sheep digoxin-specific antibodies and their Fab fragments on digoxin pharmacokinetics in dogs. J. Clin. Invest. *59*:345, 1977.
292. Ochs, H. R., and Smith, T. W.: Reversal of advanced digitoxin toxicity and modification of pharmacokinetics by specific antibodies and Fab fragments. J. Clin. Invest. *60*:1303, 1977.
293. Smith, T. W., Lloyd, B. L., Spicer, N., and Haber, E.: Immunogenicity and kinetics of distribution and elimination of sheep digoxin-specific IgG and Fab fragments in the rabbit and baboon. Clin. Exp. Immunol. *36*:384, 1979.

Diuretics

294. Wilson, J. R., Reichek, N., Dunkman, W. B., and Goldberg, S.: Effect of diuresis on the performance of the failing left ventricle in man. Am. J. Med. *70*:234, 1981.
295. Gennari, F. J., and Kassirer, J. P.: Osmotic diuresis. N. Engl. J. Med. *291*:714, 1974.
296. Grantham, J. J., and Chonko, A. M.: The physiologic basis and clinical use of diuretics. *In* Brenner, B. M., and Stein, J. H. (eds.): Contemporary Issues in Nephrology: Sodium and Water Homeostasis. Vol. 1. New York, Churchill Livingstone, 1978, p. 178.

297. Warnock, D. G., and Eveloff, J.: NaCl entry mechanism in the luminal membrane of the renal tubule. Am. J. Physiol. *242*:F561–F574, 1982.
298. Reineck, H. J., and Stein, J. H.: Mechanisms of action and clinical uses of diuretics. *In* Brenner, B. M., and Rector, F. C. (eds.): The Kidney. 2nd ed. Philadelphia, W. B. Saunders Co., 1981.
299. Beyer, K., and Baer, J.: Physiologic basis for the action of newer diuretic agents. Pharmacol. Rev. *13*:517, 1961.
300. Kunau, R. T., Weller, D. R., and Webb, H. L.: Clarification of the site of action of chlorothiazide in the rat nephron. J. Clin. Invest. *56*:401, 1975.
301. Stein, J. H., Wilson, C. B., and Kirkendall, W. M.: Differences in the acute effects of furosemide and ethacrynic acid in man. J. Lab. Clin. Med. *71*:654, 1968.
302. Chou, S., Porush, J. G., Slater, P. A., Flombaum, C. D., Shafi, T., and Fein, P. A.: Effects of acetazolamide on proximal tubule Cl, Na, HCO_3 transport in normal and acidotic dogs during distal blockade. J. Clin. Invest. *60*:162, 1977.
303. Rector, F. C., Martinez-Maldonado, M., Brunner, F. P., and Seldin, D. W.: Evidence of passive reabsorption of sodium chloride in the proximal tubule of rat kidney. J. Clin. Invest. *45*:1060, 1966.
304. Khan, M. I.: Treatment of refractory congestive heart failure and normokalemic hypochloremic alkalosis with acetazolamide and spironolactone. Can. Med. Assoc. J. *123*:883, 1980.
305. Burg, M. B., and Green, N.: Function of the thick ascending limb of Henle's loop. Am. J. Physiol. *224*:659, 1973.
306. Rocha, A. S., and Kokko, J. P.: Sodium chloride and water transport in the medullary thick ascending limb of Henle: Evidence for active chloride transport. J. Clin. Invest. *52*:612, 1973.
307. Burg, M., and Stoner, L.: Renal tubular chloride transport and mode of action of some diuretics. Ann. Rev. Physiol. *38*:37, 1976.
308. Schmidt, U., and Dubach, U. C.: The behavior of Na-K activated adenosine triphosphate in various structures in the rat nephron after furosemide application. Nephron *7*:447, 1970.
309. Patak, R., Rosenblatt, S., Fadem, S., Lifschitz, M. D., and Stein, J. H.: Diuretic induced changes in renal blood flow and prostaglandin E excretion in the dog. Am. J. Physiol. *236*:F494, 1979.
310. Ebel, H.: Effects of diuretics on renal Na-K ATPase and adenyl cyclase. Naunyn Schmiedebergs Arch. Pharmakol. *281*:301, 1974.
311. Abe, K., Yasuima, M., Cheiba, L., Irokawa, N., Ipo, P., and Yoshinaga, K.: Effect of furosemide on urinary excretion prostaglandin E in normal volunteers and patients with essential hypertension. Prostaglandins *14*:513, 1977.
312. Patak, R. V., Mookerjee, B. K., Bentzel, C. J., Hysert, P. E., Babej, M., and Lee, J. B.: Antagonism of the effects of furosemide by indomethacin in normal and hypertensive man. Prostaglandins *10*:649, 1975.
313. Bailie, M. D., Barbour, J. A., and Hook, J. B.: Effects of indomethacin on furosemide-induced changes in renal blood flow. Proc. Soc. Exp. Biol. Med. *148*:1173, 1975.
314. Bowman, R. H.: Renal secretion of [^{35}S] furosemide and its depression by albumin binding. Am. J. Physiol. *229*:93, 1975.
315. Burg, M. B.: The mechanism of action of diuretics in renal tubules. *In* Wesson, L. G., and Fanelli, G. M. (eds.): Recent Advances in Renal Physiology and Pharmacology. Baltimore, University Park Press, 1974, pp. 99–109.
316. Charnock, J. S., and Almeida, A. F.: Ethacrynic acid accumulation by renal tissue. Biochem. Pharmacol. *21*:647, 1972.
317. Mitch, W. E., and Wilcox, C. S.: Disorders of body fluids, sodium and potassium in chronic renal failure. Am. J. Med. *72*:536, 1982.
318. Essig, A.: Competitive inhibition of renal transport of *p*-aminohippurate by analogues of chlorothiazide. Am. J. Physiol. *201*:303, 1961.
319. Hirsch, G. H., Pakuts, A. P., and Bayne, A. J.: Furosemide accumulation by renal tissue. Biochem. Pharmacol. *24*:1943, 1975.
320. Hook, J. B., and Williamson, H. E.: Influence of probenecid and alterations in acid base balance on the saluretic activity of furosemide. J. Pharmacol. Exp. Ther. *149*:404, 1965.
321. Costanzo, L. S., and Windhager, E. E.: Calcium and sodium transport by the distal convoluted tubule of the rat. Am. J. Physiol. *4*:F492, 1978.
322. Edelman, I., and Fimognari, G.: On the biochemical mechanisms of action of aldosterone. Recent Prog. Hormone Res. *24*:1, 1968.
323. Crabbe, J.: A hypothesis concerning the mode of action of amiloride and triamterene. Arch. Int. Pharmacodyn. Ther. *173*:474, 1968.
324. Stoner, L. C., Burg, M. B., and Orloff, J.: Ion transport in cortical collecting tubule; effect of amiloride. Am. J. Physiol. *227*:453, 1974.
325. Tannen, R. L.: Relationship of renal ammonia production and potassium homeostasis. Kidney Int. *11*:453, 1977.
326. Manuel, M. A., Beirne, G. J., Wagnild, J. P., and Weiner, M. W.: An effect of spironolactone on urinary acidification in normal man. Arch. Intern. Med. *134*:472, 1974.
327. Abramow, M.: Effects of ethacrynic acid on the isolated collecting tubule. J. Clin. Invest. *53*:796, 1974.
328. Hantman, D., Rossier, B., Zohlman, R., and Schrier, R.: Rapid correction of hyponatremia in the syndrome of inappropriate secretion of antidiuretic hormone: An alternative treatment to hypertonic saline. Ann. Intern. Med. *78*:870, 1973.
329. deWardener, H. E.: Natriuretic hormone. Clin. Sci. Molec. Med. *53*:1, 1977.
330. Epstein, M., Lepp, B. A., Hoffman, D. S., and Levinson, R.: Potentiation of furosemide by metolazone in refractory edema. Current Therap. Res. *21*:656, 1977.
331. Wollam, G. L., Tarazi, R. C., Bravo, E. L., and Dristan, H. P.: Diuretic potency of combined hydrochlorothiazide and furosemide therapy in patients with azotemia. Am. J. Med. *72*:929, 1982.
332. Wilcox, C. S., Mitch, W. E., Kelly, R. A., Skorecki, K., Meyer, T., Friedman, P., and Souney, P.: Effect of salt intake on sodium homeostasis during furosemide administration. Kidney Int. *21*:160, 1982.
333. Stein, J. H., Lameire, N. H., and Earley, L. E.: Renal hemodynamic factors in the regulation of sodium excretion. *In* Andriole, T. E., Hoffman, J. F., and Fanestil, D. D. (eds.): Physiology of Membrane Disorders. New York, Plenum Press, 1978, p. 739.
334. Mathisen, O., Raeder, M., Sejersted, O. M., and Kiil, F.: Effect of acetazolamide on glomerulo-tubular balance and renal metabolic rate. Scand. J. Clin. Lab. Invest. *36*:617, 1976.
335. Clapp, J. R., Nottebohm, G. A., and Robinson, R. R.: Proximal site of action of ethacrynic acid. Importance of filtration rate. Am. J. Physiol. *220*:1355, 1971.
336. Ogilvie, R. I., and Ruedy, J.: Hemodynamic effects of ethacrynic acid in anephric dogs. J. Pharmacol. Exp. Ther. *176*:389, 1971.
337. Ogilvie, R. I., and Schlieper, E.: Comparative effects of ethacrynic acid, furosemide and diazoxide in the perfused dog hindlimb. Canad. J. Physiol. Pharmacol. *49*:1038, 1971.
338. Dikshit, K., Vyden, J. D., Forrester, J. S., and Swan, H. J. C.: Renal and extrarenal hemodynamic effects of furosemide in congestive heart failure after acute myocardial infarction. N. Engl. J. Med. *288*:1087, 1973.
339. Wright, F. S.: Intrarenal regulation of glomerular filtration rate. N. Engl. J. Med. *291*:135, 1974.
340. Wright, F. S., and Schnermann, J.: Interference with feedback control of glomerular filtration rate by furosemide, triflocin and cyanide. J. Clin. Invest. *53*:1695, 1974.
341. Seely, J. F., and Dirks, J. H.: Editorial: Site of action of diuretic drugs. Kidney Int. *11*:1, 1977.
342. Giebisch, G.: Effects of diuretics on renal transport of potassium. *In* Martinez-Maldonado, M. (ed.): Methods in Pharmacology. Vol. 4A. Renal Pharmacology. New York, Plenum Press, 1976, pp. 121–164.
343. Sealey, J. E., and Laragh, J. H.: A proposed cybernetic system for sodium and potassium homeostasis: Coordination of aldosterone and intrarenal physical factors. Kidney Int. *6*:281, 1974.
344. Davidson, C., McLachlan, M. S. F., Burkinshaw, L., and Morgan, D. B.: Effect of long-term diuretic treatment on body potassium in heart disease. Lancet *2*:1044, 1976.
345. Venkata, C., Ram, S., Garrett, B. N., and Kaplan, M.: Moderate sodium restriction and various diuretics in the treatment of hypertension. Arch. Intern. Med. *141*:1015, 1981.
346. Seldin, D. W., and Rector, F. C., Jr.: The generation and maintenance of metabolic alkalosis. Kidney Int. *1*:306, 1972.
347. Editorial: Hypokalemia and diuretics—Analysis of publications. Br. Med. J. *1*:905, 1980.
348. Garella, S., Chazan, J. A., and Cohen, J. J.: Saline-resistant metabolic alkalosis or "chloride-wasting nephropathy." Ann. Intern. Med. *73*:31, 1970.
349. Holland, O. B., Nixon, J. V., and Kuknert, L.: Diuretic-induced ventricular ectopic activity. Am. J. Med. *70*:762, 1981.
350. Kelly, R. A., Wilcox, C. S., and Mitch, W. E.: Diuretics: An update. J. Cardiovasc. Med. *7*:1153, 1982.
351. Rosa, R. M., Silva, P., Young, J. B., Landsberg, L., Brown, R. S., Rowe, J. W., and Epstein, F. N.: Adrenergic modulation of extrarenal potassium disposal. N. Engl. J. Med. *302*:431, 1980.
352. Kennedy, R. M., and Earley, L. E.: Profound hyponatremia resulting from thiazide induced decrease in urinary diluting capacity in a patient with primary polydipsia. N. Engl. J. Med. *282*:1185, 1970.
353. Verney, E. V.: Croonian Lecture: The anti-diuretic hormone and the factors which determine its release. Proc. Roy. Soc. Lond. (Series B) *135*:25, 1947.
354. Davies, D. L., and Wilson, G. M.: Diuretics: Mechanism of action and clinical application. Drugs *9*:178, 1975.
355. Berger, L., and Yü, T.: Renal function in gout. IV. An analysis of 524 gouty subjects including long-term follow-up studies. Am. J. Med. *59*:605, 1975.
356. Fessel, W. J.: Renal outcomes of gout and hyperuricemia. Am. J. Med. *67*:74, 1979.
357. Johnson, M. W., and Mitch, W. E.: The risks of asymptomatic hyperuricaemia and the use of uricosuric diuretics. Drugs *21*:220, 1981.
358. Glodner, M. G., Zarowitz, H., and Akgun, F.: Hyperglycemia and glucosuria due to thiazide derivatives administered in diabetes mellitus. N. Engl. J. Med. *262*:403, 1960.
359. Helgsland, A., Huermann, I., Holme, I., and Leren, P.: Serum triglycerides and serum uric acid in untreated and thiazide-treated patients with mild hypertension. Am. J. Med. *64*:34, 1978.
360. Bauer, J. H., Brooks, C. S., Weinstein, I., Wilcox, H. H., Heimberg, M., Burch, R. N., and Barkley, R.: Effects of diuretic and propranolol on plasma lipoprotein lipids. Clin. Pharmacol. Therap. *30*:35, 1981.
361. Loreaux, L., Menard, R., Taylor, A., Patpita, J. C., and Santen, R.: Spironolactone and endocrine dysfunction. Ann. Intern. Med. *85*:630, 1976.
362. Reubi, F. C.: The action and use of diuretics in renal disease. *In* Friedberg, C. K. (ed.): Heart, Kidney and Electrolytes. New York, Grune and Stratton, 1962, p. 169.
363. Steinmuller, S. R., and Puschett, J. B.: Effects of metolazone in man: Comparison with chlorothiazide. Kidney Int. *1*:169, 1972.
364. Fernandez, P. C., and Puschett, J. B.: Proximal tubular actions of metolazone and chlorothiazide. Am. J. Physiol. *225*:954, 1973.

365. Heinemann, H. O., Demartini, E. E., and Laragh, J. H.: The mode of action and use of chlorothiazide on renal excretion of electrolytes and free water. Am. J. Med. *26*:853, 1959.
366. Craswell, P. W., Ezzat, E., Kopstein, J., Varghese, Z., and Moorhead, J. F.: Use of metolazone, a new diuretic, in patients with renal disease. Nephron *12*:63, 1973.
367. Multicenter Diuretic Cooperative Study Group. Arch. Intern. Med. *141*:482, 1982.
368. Crosley, A. P., Jr., Ronquillo, L. M., Strickland, W. H., and Alexander, F.: Triamterene, a new natriuretic agent: Preliminary observations in man. Ann. Intern. Med. *56*:241, 1962.
369. Frazier, H. S., and Yager, H.: The clinical use of diuretics. N. Engl. J. Med. *288*:246 and 455, 1973.

Vasodilators

370. Wiggers, C. J., and Feely, H.: The cardiodynamics of mitral insufficiency. Heart *9*:141, 1921–22.
371. Braunwald, E., Welch, G. H., Jr., and Sarnoff, S. J.: Hemodynamic effects of quantitatively varied experimental mitral regurgitation. Circ. Res. *5*:539, 1957.
372. Braunwald, E., Welch, G. H., Jr., and Morrow, A. G.: The effects of acutely increased systemic resistance on the left atrial pressure pulse: A method for the clinical detection of mitral insufficiency. J. Clin. Invest. *37*:35, 1958.
373. Ross, J., Jr., and Braunwald, E.: The study of left ventricular function in man by increasing resistance to ventricular ejection with angiotensin. Circulation *29*:739, 1964.
374. Clauss, R. H., Birtwell, W. C., Albertel, G. A., Lunzer, S., Taylor, W. J., Fosberg, A. M., and Harkin, D. E.: Assisted circulation. I. The arterial counterpulsator. J. Thorac. Cardiovasc. Surg. *41*:447, 1961.
375. Majid, P. A., Sharma, B., and Taylor, S. H.: Phentolamine for vasodilator treatment of severe heart failure. Lancet *2*:719, 1971.
376. Massie, B. M., Chatterjee, K., and Parmley, W. W.: Vasodilator therapy for acute and chronic heart failure. *In* Yu, P. N., and Goodwin, J. F. (eds.): Progress in Cardiology. Vol. 8. Philadelphia, Lea and Febiger, 1979.
377. Mason, D. T. (ed.): Symposium on vasodilator and inotropic therapy of heart failure. Am. J. Med. *65*:101, 1978.
378. Cohn, J. N., and Franciosa, J. A.: Vasodilator therapy of cardiac failure. N. Engl. J. Med. *297*:27 and 254, 1977.
379. Cohn, J. N.: Vasodilators: Rationale, application, and future prospects. *In* Braunwald, E., Mock, M. B., and Watson, J. (eds.): Congestive Heart Failure: Current Research and Clinical Applications. New York, Grune and Stratton, 1982, p. 279.
380. Braunwald, E., Ross, J., Jr., Kahler, R. L., Gaffney, T. E., Goldblatt, A., and Mason, D. T.: Reflex control of the systemic venous bed: Effects on venous tone of vasoactive drugs and of baroreceptor and chemoreceptor stimulation. Circ. Res. *12*:539, 1963.
381. Zelis, R., and Flaim, S. F.: Alterations in vasomotor tone in congestive heart failure. Prog. Cardiovasc. Dis. *24*:437–459, 1982.
382. Ford, L. E.: Effect of afterload reduction on myocardial energetics. Circ. Res. *46*:161–166, 1980.
383. Packer, M., and LeJemtel, T. H.: Physiologic and pharmacologic determinants of vasodilator response: A conceptual framework for rational drug therapy for chronic heart failure. Prog. Cardiovasc. Dis. *24*:275–292, 1982.
384. Miller, R. M., Fennell, W. H., Young, J. B., Palomo, A. R., and Quinones, M. A.: Differential systemic arterial and venous actions and consequent cardiac effects of vasodilator drugs. Prog. Cardiovasc. Dis. *24*:353–374, 1982.
385. Zelis, R., Mason, D. T., and Braunwald, E.: A comparison of the effects of vasodilator stimuli on peripheral resistance vessels in normal subjects and in patients with congestive heart failure. J. Clin. Invest. *47*:960, 1968.
386. Zelis, R., Lee, G., and Mason, D. T.: Influence of experimental edema on metabolically determined blood flow. Circ. Res. *34*:482, 1974.
387. Franciosa, J. A., Guiha, N. M., Limas, C. J., Rodriguera, E., and Cohn, J. N.: Improved left ventricular function during nitroprusside infusion in acute myocardial infarction. Lancet *1*:650, 1972.
388. Pepine, C. J., Nichols, W. W., Curry, R. C., Jr., and Conti, C. R.: Aortic input impedance during nitroprusside infusion. A reconsideration of afterload reduction and beneficial action. J. Clin. Invest. *64*:643, 1979.
389. Pouleur, H., Covell, J. W., and Ross, J., Jr.: Effects of nitroprusside on venous return and central blood volume in the absence and presence of acute heart failure. Circulation *61*:328, 1980.
390. Cogan, J. J., Humphreys, M. H., Carlson, C. J., and Rapaport, E.: Renal effects of nitroprusside and hydralazine in patients with congestive heart failure. Circulation *61*:316, 1980.
391. Davies, D. W., Kadar, D., Steward, D. J., and Munro, I. R.: A sudden death associated with the use of sodium nitroprusside for induction of hypotension during anesthesia. Canad. Anaesth. Soc. J. *22*:547, 1975.
392. Miller, R. R., Vismara, L. A., Williams, D. O., Amsterdam, E. A., and Mason, D. T.: Pharmacological mechanisms for left ventricular unloading in clinical congestive heart failure: Differential effects of nitroprusside, phentolamine, and nitroglycerin on cardiac function and peripheral circulation. Circ. Res. *39*:127, 1976.
393. Taylor, S. H., Sutherland, G. R., MacKenzie, M. B., Staunton, H. P., and Donald, K. W.: The circulatory effects of intravenous phentolamine in man. Circulation *31*:741, 1955.
394. Stern, M. A., Gohlke, H. K., Loeb, H. S., Croke, R. P., and Gunnar, R. M.: Hemodynamic effects of intravenous phentolamine in low output cardiac failure. Dose-response relationships. Circulation *58*:157, 1978.
395. Henning, R. J., Shubin, H., and Weil, M. H.: Afterload reduction with phentolamine in patients with acute pulmonary edema. Am. J. Med. *63*:568, 1977.
396. Warren, S. E., and Francis, G. S.: Nitroglycerin and nitrate esters. Am. J. Med. *65*:53, 1978.
397. Williams, D. O., Amsterdam, E. A., and Mason, D. T.: Hemodynamic effects of nitroglycerin in acute myocardial infarction. Decrease in ventricular preload at the expense of cardiac output. Circulation *51*:421, 1975.
398. Flaherty, J. T., Reid, P. R., Kelly, D. T., Taylor, D. R., Weisfeldt, M. L., and Pitt, B.: Intravenous nitroglycerin in acute myocardial infarction. Circulation *51*:132, 1975.
399. Franciosa, J. A., and Cohn, J. N.: Sustained hemodynamic effects without tolerance during long-term isosorbide dinitrate treatment of chronic left ventricular failure. Am. J. Cardiol. *45*:648, 1980.
399a. Leier, C. V., Huss, P., Magorien, R. D., and Unverferth, D. V.: Improved exercise capacity and differing arterial and venous tolerance during chronic isosorbide dinitrate therapy for congestive heart failure. Circulation *67*:817, 1983.
400. Pierpont, G. L., Brown, D. C., Franciosa, J. A., and Cohn, J. N.: Effect of hydralazine on renal failure in patients with congestive heart failure. Circulation *61*:323, 1980.
401. Packer, M., Meller, J., Medina, N., Gorlin, R., and Herman, M. V.: Dose requirements of hydralazine in patients with severe chronic congestive heart failure. Am. J. Cardiol. *45*:655, 1980.
402. Packer, M., Meller, J., Medina, N., Gorlin, R., and Herman, M. V.: Importance of left ventricular chamber size in determining the response to hydralazine in severe chronic heart failure. N. Engl. J. Med. *303*:250–255, 1980.
403. Packer, M., Meller, J., Medina, N., Yushak, M., and Gorlin, R.: Hemodynamic characterization of tolerance to long-term hydralazine therapy in severe chronic heart failure. N. Engl. J. Med. *306*:57–62, 1982.
404. Massie, B., Ports, T., Chatterjee, K., Parmley, W., Ostland, J., O'Young, J., and Haughom, F.: Long-term vasodilator therapy for heart failure: Clinical response and its relationship to hemodynamic measurements. Circulation *63*:269–278, 1981.
405. Franciosa, J. A., Weber, K. T., Levine, T. B., Kinasewitz, G. T., Janicki, J. S., West, J., Henis, M. M., and Cohn, J. N.: Hydralazine in the long-term treatment of chronic heart failure: Lack of difference from placebo. Am. Heart J. *104*:587–594, 1982.
406. Franciosa, J. A., and Cohn, J. N.: Effects of minoxidil on hemodynamics in patients with congestive heart failure. Circulation *63*:652–657, 1981.
407. Colucci, W. S.: Alpha-adrenergic receptor blockade with prazosin: Consideration of hypertension, heart failure, and potential new applications. Ann. Intern. Med. *97*:67–77, 1982.
408. Lowenstein, J., and Steele, J., Jr.: Prazosin. Am. Heart J. *95*:262, 1978.
409. Awan, N. A., Miller, R. R., and Mason, D. T.: Comparison of effects of nitroprusside and prazosin on left ventricular function and the peripheral circulation in chronic refractory congestive heart failure. Circulation *57*:152, 1978.
410. Mehta, J., Iacona, M., Feldman, R. L., Pepine, C. J., and Conti, C. R.: Comparative hemodynamic effects of intravenous nitroprusside and oral prazosin in refractory heart failure. Am. J. Cardiol. *41*:925, 1978.
411. Packer, M., Meller, J., Gorlin, R., and Herman, H. V.: Hemodynamic and clinical tachyphylaxis to prazosin-mediated afterload reduction in severe congestive heart failure. Circulation *59*:531, 1979.
412. Colucci, W. S., Wynne, J., Holman, B. L., and Braunwald, E.: Chronic therapy of heart failure with prazosin: A randomized double-blind trial. Am. J. Cardiol. *45*:337–344, 1980.
413. Goldman, S. A., Johnson, L. L., Escala, E., Cannon, P. J., and Weiss, M. D.: Improved exercise ejection fraction with long-term prazosin therapy in patients with heart failure. Am. J. Med. *68*:36–42, 1980.
413a. Rutishauser, W.: A review of the long-term effects of prazosin and hydralazine in chronic congestive heart failure. Europ. Heart J. *4*(Suppl. A):149, 1983.
414. Awan, N. A., Miller, R. R., Miller, M. P., Specht, K., Vera, Z., and Mason, D. T.: Clinical pharmacology and therapeutic application of prazosin in acute and chronic refractory congestive heart failure. Balanced systemic venous and arterial dilation improving pulmonary congestion and cardiac output. Am. J. Med. *65*:146, 1978.
415. Dzau, V. J., Colucci, W. S., Hollenberg, N. K., and Williams, G. H.: Relation of the renin-angiotensin-aldosterone system to clinical state in congestive heart failure. Circulation *63*:645–651, 1981.
416. Levine, E., Franciosa, J. A., and Cohn, J. N.: Acute and long-term response to an oral converting enzyme inhibitor, captopril, in congestive heart failure. Circulation *62*:35–41, 1980.
417. Dzau, V. J., Colucci, W. S., Williams, G. H., Curfman, G., Meggs, L., and Hollenberg, N. K.: Sustained effectiveness of converting-enzyme inhibition in patients with severe congestive heart failure. N. Engl. J. Med. *302*:1373–1379, 1980.
418. Ader, R., Chatterjee, K., Ports, T., Brundage, B., Hiramatsu, B., and Parmley, W.: Immediate and sustained hemodynamic and clinical improvement in chronic heart failure by an oral angiotensin-converting enzyme inhibitor. Circulation *61*:931–937, 1980.
419. Dzau, V. J.: Angiotensin-converting enzyme inhibition in the treatment of hypertension and congestive heart failure. *In* Isselbacher, K. J., et al. (eds.):

with severe congestive heart fa
62:28–34, 1980.
523. Weber, K. T., Andrews, V., J
Amrinone and exercise perforn
J. Cardiol. *48*:164–169, 1981.
524. Siskind, S. J., Sonnenblick, E.
H.: Acute substantial benefit
hemodynamics and metabolisr
64:966–973, 1981.
525. Maskin, C. S., Forman, R., K
T. H.: Long-term amrinone th
J. Med. *72*:113–118, 1982.
526. Siegel, L. A., Keung, E., Sisk
Efstathakis, D., Sonnenblick,
amrinone-hydralazine combina
pacity in patients with severe
1981.
526a. McDowell, A., Baim, D., Che
man, W.: Hemodynamic effect
tients with refractory heart fail
526b. Maskin, C. S., Sinoway, L., C
T. H.: Sustained hemodynamic
WIN 47203, in patients with
1065, 1983.
527. Podrid, P. J., Schoenberger, A
by oral disopyramide. N. Engl.
528. Chew, C. Y. C., Hecht, H. S.,
N.: Influence of severity of ver
to intravenously administered
Cardiol. *47*:917–922, 1981.
529. Miller, R. R., Awan, N. A., Jo
sterdam, E. A., and Mason,
therapy in congestive heart fail
530. Raabe, D. S., Jr.: Combined t
failure complicating acute myo

Other Measures

531. Barnard, C. N.: The operation.
532. Stinson, E. B., Dong, E., Jr., Il
plantation in man. III. Surgical
533. Schroeder, J. S.: Current statu
241:2069, 1979.
534. Watson, D. C., Reitz, B. A., E
Stinson, E. B., and Shumway,
tation. Surgery *86*:56, 1979.
534a. Hess, M. L. Hastillo, A., Tho
Status of cardiac transplantati
Am. Coll. Cardiol. *1*:721, 1983
535. Reitz, B. A., Wallmork, J. L.,
Oyer, P. E., Stinson, E. B., an
N. Engl. J. Med. *306*:557, 1982
536. Billingham, M. E., Baumgartne
M. A., Raney, A. A., Oyer, P.
tant heart procurement for hu
11–19, 1980.
537. Wiscomb, W., Cooper, D. K. C
N.: Orthotopic transplantation
ervation by continuous hy
hyperosmolar solution. J. Thora
538. Losiman, J. G., and Barnard, C
id alternative to orthotopic tran
tages. J. Surg. Res. *32*:297, 1982
539. Oyer, P. E., Jamieson, S. W., a
end-stage congestive heart failu
son, J. (eds.): Congestive Heart
pp. 317–328.
540. Hunt, S. A., Rider, A. K., Stins
rison, D. C., and Shumway, N

Updates of Internal Medicine, IV. New York, McGraw-Hill, 1982, pp. 137–146.

419a. Cody, R. J., Covit, A. B., Schaer, G. L., and Laragh, J. H.: Evaluation of a long-acting converting enzyme inhibitor (Enalapril) for the treatment of chronic congestive heart failure. J. Am. Coll. Cardiol. *1*:1154, 1983.

420. Fouad, F. M., Ceimo, J. M. K., Tarazi, R. C., and Bravo, E. L.: Contrasts and similarities of acute hemodynamic responses to specific antagonism of angiotensin II ([Sar^1, Thr^8] A II) and to inhibition of converting enzyme (Captopril). Circulation *61*:163, 1980.

421. Vrobel, T., and Cohn, J. N.: Comparative hemodynamic effects of converting enzyme inhibitor and sodium nitroprusside in severe heart failure. Am. J. Cardiol. *45*:331, 1980.

422. Swartz, S. L., Williams, G. H., Hollenberg, N. K., Crantz, F. R., Moore, T. J., Levine, L., Sasahara, A. A., and Dluhy, R. G.: Endocrine profile in the long-term phase of converting-enzyme inhibition. Clin. Pharmacol. Ther. *28*:499, 1980.

423. Lijnen, P., Fagard, R., Staessen, J., VerSchueren, L. J., and Amery, A.: Role of various vasodepressor systems in the acute hypotensive effect of captopril in man. Eur. J. Clin. Pharmacol. *20*:1, 1981.

424. Levine, T. B., Franciosa, J. A., and Cohn, J. N.: Acute and long-term responses to an oral converting-enzyme inhibitor, captopril, in congestive heart failure. Circulation *62*:35, 1980.

425. Gavras, H., Faxon, D. P., Berkoben, J., Brunner, H. R., and Ryan, T. J.: Angiotensin converting enzyme inhibition in patients with congestive heart failure. Circulation *58*:770, 1978.

426. Curtiss, C., Cohn, J. N., Vrobel, T., and Franciosa, J. A.: Role of the renin-angiotensin system in the systemic vasoconstriction of chronic congestive heart failure. Circulation *58*:763, 1978.

427. Creager, M. A., Halperin, J. L., Bernard, D. B., Faxon, D. P., Melidossian, C. D., Gavras, H., and Ryan, T. J.: Acute regional circulatory and renal hemodynamic effects of converting-enzyme inhibition in patients with congestive heart failure. Circulation *64*:483, 1981.

428. Maslowski, A. H., Ikram, H., Nicholls, M. G., and Espiner, E. A.: Haemodynamic, hormonal and electrolyte responses to captopril in resistant heart failure. Lancet *1*:71, 1981.

429. Davis, R., Ribner, H. S., Keung, E., LeJemtel, T. H., and Sonnenblick, E. H.: Treatment of chronic congestive heart failure with captopril, an oral inhibitor of angiotensin-converting enzyme. N. Engl. J. Med. *301*:177, 1979.

429a. Kramer, B. L., Massie, B. M., and Topic, N.: Controlled trial of captopril in chronic heart failure: A rest and exercise hemodynamic study. Circulation *67*:807, 1983.

429b. Awan, N. A., Amsterdam, E. A., Hermanovich, J., Bommer, W. J., Needham, K. E., and Mason, D. T.: Long-term hemodynamic and clinical efficacy of captopril therapy in ambulatory management of severe chronic congestive heart failure. Am. Heart J. *103*:474, 1982.

430. Faxon, D. P., Creager, M. A., Halperin, J. L., Gavras, H., Coffman, J. D., and Ryan, T. J.: Central and peripheral hemodynamic effects of angiotensin inhibition in patients with refractory congestive heart failure. Circulation *61*:925, 1980.

431. Pierpont, G. L., Hale, K. A., Franciosa, J. A., and Cohn, J. N.: Relationship between pulmonary vascular and hypoxemic effects of vasodilators in left ventricular failure. Circulation *56*(Suppl. III):III–163, 1977 (abstract).

432. Collste, P., Haglund, K., Lundgren, G., Magnusson, G., and Ostman, J.: Reversible renal failure during treatment with captopril. Br. Med. J. *2*:612–613, 1979.

433. Case, D. B., Atlas, S. A., Mouradian, J. A., Fishman, R. A., Sherman, R. L., and Laragh, J. H.: Proteinuria during long-term captopril therapy. J.A.M.A. *244*:346–349, 1980.

434. Franciosa, J. A.: Effectiveness of long-term vasodilator administration in the treatment of chronic left ventricular failure. Prog. Cardiovasc. Dis. *24*:319–330, 1982.

435. DiSegni, E., Kaplinsky, E., Klein, H. O., and Levy, M.: Treatment of ruptured interventricular septum with afterload reduction. Arch. Intern. Med. *138*:1427, 1978.

436. Greenberg, B. H., Massie, B. M., Brundage, B. H., Botvinick, E. H., Parmley, W. W., and Chatterjee, K.: Beneficial effects of hydralazine in severe mitral regurgitation. Circulation *58*:273, 1978.

437. Greenberg, B. H., DeMots, H., Murphy, E., and Rahimtoola, S.: Beneficial effects of hydralazine on rest and exercise hemodynamics in patients with chronic severe aortic insufficiency. Circulation *62*:49–55, 1980.

437a. Fioretti, P., Benussi, B., Scardi, S., Klugmann, S., Brower, R. W., and Camerini, F.: Afterload reduction with nifedipine in aortic insufficiency. Am. J. Cardiol. *49*:1728–1732, 1982.

438. Rubin, L. J., and Peter, R. H.: Hemodynamics at rest and during exercise after oral hydralazine in patients with cor pulmonale. Am. J. Cardiol. *47*:116–122, 1981.

439. Colucci, W. S., Holman, L., Wynne, J., Carabello, B., Malacoff, R., Grossman, W., and Braunwald, E.: Improved right ventricular function and reduced pulmonary vascular resistance during prazosin therapy of congestive heart failure. Am. J. Med. *71*:75–80, 1981.

440. Weber, K. T., Kinasewitz, G. T., West, J. S., Janicki, J. S., Reichek, N., and Fishman, A. P.: Long-term vasodilator therapy with trimazosin in chronic cardiac failure. N. Engl. J. Med. *303*:242, 1980.

440a. Lemke, R., Trompler, A., Kaltenbach, M., and Bussmann, W. D.: Wirkung von Prazosin bei der therapierefraktären chronischen Herzinsuffizienz. Dtsch. Med. Wschr. *104*:1769, 1979.

441. Franciosa, J. A., and Cohn, J. N.: Immediate effects of hydralazine isosorbide dinitrate combination on exercise capacity and exercise hemodynamics in patients with left ventricular failure. Circulation *59*:1085, 1979.

442. Pierpont, G. L., Cohn, J. N., and Franciosa, J. A.: Combined oral hydralazine-nitrate therapy in left ventricular failure. Hemodynamic equivalency to sodium nitroprusside. Chest *73*:8, 1978.

443. Massie, B., Kramer, B., and Haughom, F.: Postural hypotension and tachycardia during hydralazine-isosorbide dinitrate therapy for chronic heart failure. Circulation *63*:658–644, 1981.

444. Aronow, W. S., Lurie, M., Turbow, M., Whittaker, K., VanCamp, S., and Hughes, D.: Effects of prazosin vs. placebo on chronic left ventricular heart failure. Circulation *59*:344, 1979.

445. Aronow, W. S., and Danahy, D. T.: Efficacy of trimazosin and prazosin therapy on cardiac and exercise performance in outpatients with chronic congestive heart failure. Am. J. Med. *65*:155, 1978.

446. Sharma, B., Hoback, J., Francis, G. S., Hodges, M., Asinger, R. W., Cohn, J. N., and Taylor, C. R.: Pirbuterol: A new oral sympathomimetic amine for the treatment of congestive heart failure. Am. Heart J. *102*(Part 2):533–541, 1981.

447. Walsh, W. F., and Greenberg, B. H.: Results of long-term vasodilator therapy in patients with refractory congestive heart failure. Circulation *64*:499–505, 1981.

448. Packer, M., Meller, J., Medina, N., Yushak, M., and Gorlin, R.: Determinants of drug response in severe chronic heart failure. I. Activation of vasoconstrictor forces during vasodilator therapy. Circulation *64*:505–514, 1981.

449. Colucci, W. S., Williams, G. H., Alexander, R. W., and Braunwald, E.: Mechanisms and implications of vasodilator tolerance in the treatment of congestive heart failure. Am. J. Med. *71*:89–99, 1981.

Sympathomimetic Amines

450. Goldberg, L. I.: Cardiovascular and renal actions of dopamine: Potential clinical applications. Pharmacol. Rev *24*:1, 1972.

451. Goldberg, L. I., Hsieh, Y.-Y., and Resnekov, L.: Newer catecholamines for treatment of heart failure and shock: An update on dopamine and a first look at dobutamine. Progr. Cardiovasc. Dis. *19*:327, 1977.

452. Goldberg, L. I.: The dopamine vascular receptor: New areas for biochemical pharmacologists. Biochem. Pharmacol. *24*:651, 1975.

453. Toda, N., Hojo, M., Sakae, K., and Usui, H.: Comparison of the relaxing effect of dopamine with that of adenosine, isoproterenol and acetylcholine in isolated canine coronary arteries. Blood Vessels *12*:290, 1975.

454. Dressler, W. E., Rossi, G. V., and Orzechowski, R. F.: Evidence that renal vasodilation by dopamine in dogs does not involve release of prostaglandin. J. Pharm. Pharmacol. *27*:203, 1975.

455. Yeh, B. K., McNay, J. L., and Goldberg, L. I.: Attenuation of dopamine renal and mesenteric vasodilation by haloperidol: Evidence for a specific receptor. J. Pharmacol. Exp. Ther. *168*:303, 1969.

456. Gilbert, J. C., and Goldberg, L. I.: Characterization by cyproheptadine of the dopamine-induced contraction in canine isolated arteries. J. Pharmacol. Exp. Ther. *193*:435, 1975.

457. Willems, L. J., and Bogaert, M. G.: Dopamine-induced neurogenic vasodilation in isolated perfused muscle preparation of the dog. Naunyn Schmiedebergs Arch. Pharmakol. *286*:413, 1975.

458. Enero, M. A., and Langer, S. Z.: Inhibition of dopamine of ^{3}H-noradrenaline release elicited by nerve stimulation of the isolated cat's nictitating membrane. Naunyn Schmiedebergs Arch. Pharmakol. *289*:179, 1975.

459. Hardaker, W. T., Jr., and Wechsler, A. S.: Redistribution of renal intracortical blood flow during dopamine infusion in dogs. Circ. Res. *33*:437, 1973.

460. Hollenberg, N. K., Adams, D. F., Mendell, P., Abrams, H. L., and Merrill, J. P.: Renal vascular responses to dopamine. Haemodynamics and angiographic observations in normal man. Clin. Sci. Molec. Med. *45*:733, 1973.

461. Goldberg, L. I., and Toda, N.: Dopamine-induced relaxation of isolated canine renal, mesenteric and femoral arteries contracted with prostaglandin-$F_{2\alpha}$. Circ. Res. *36*(Suppl. I):I-97, 1975.

462. Goldberg, L. I.: Dopamine: Clinical uses of an endogenous catecholamine. N. Engl. J. Med. *291*:707, 1974.

463. Allwood, M. J., and Ginsburg, J.: Peripheral vascular and other effects of dopamine infusion in man. Clin. Sci. *27*:271, 1964.

464. Vincenti, F., and Goldberg, L. I.: Combined use of dopamine and prostaglandin A_1 in patients with acute renal failure and hepatorenal syndrome. Prostaglandins *15*:463, 1978.

465. Brooks, H. L., Stein, P. D., Matson, J. L., and Hyland, J. W.: Dopamine-induced alterations in coronary hemodynamics in dogs. Circ. Res. *24*:699, 1969.

466. Toda, N., and Goldberg, L. I.: Effects of dopamine on isolated canine coronary arteries. Cardiovasc. Res. *9*:384, 1975.

467. Goldberg, L. I., McDonald, R. H., Jr., and Zimmerman, A. M.: Sodium diuresis produced by dopamine in patients with congestive heart failure. N. Engl. J. Med. *269*:1060, 1963.

468. Rosenblum, R., Tai, A. R., and Lawson, D.: Dopamine in man: Cardiorenal hemodynamics in normotensive patients with heart disease. J. Pharmacol. Exp. Ther. *183*:256, 1972.

469. Marino, R. J., Romagnoli, A., and Keats, A. S.: Selective venoconstriction by

dopamine in comparison with isoprc
43:570, 1975.
470. Sturm, J. T., Guhrman, T. M., Stc
Norman, J. C.: Combined use of dc
junction with intra-aortic balloon p
omy low-output syndrome. J. Thora
471. Tuttle, R. R., and Mills, J.: Dopami
selectively increase cardiac contractil
472. Vatner, S. F., Higgins, C. B., and B
coronary circulation and left ventric
Res. 34:812, 1974.
473. Sonnenblick, E. H., Frishman, W.
new synthetic cardioactive sympathe
474. Fuchs, R. M., Rutlen, D. L., and F
systemic capacity in the dog. Circ. R
475. Williams, R. S., and Bishop, T.: Sele
tor subtypes: *In vitro* analysis by rac
1711, 1981.
476. Fleisch, J. H., and Spaethe, S. M.: V
lated perfused rat mesenteric vascu
vascular pharmacology of dobutamir
477. Robie, N. W., and Goldberg, L. I.:
dynamic effects of dopamine and dol
477a. Magorien, R. D., Unverferth, D.
Dobutamine and hydralazine: Comp
vasodilation on coronary blood fl
chemic congestive heart failure. J. A
478. Gillespie, J. A., Ambos, H. D., S
dobutamine in patients with acute
39:588, 1977.
479. Unverferth, D. V., Magorien, R. D.,
benefit of dobutamine in patients wi
J. 100:622–630, 1980.
479a. Applefeld, M. M., Newman, K. A.,
S., Reed, W. P., and Linberg,
dobutamine infusion in the manage
Cardiol. 51:455, 1983.
480. Bendersky, R., Chatterjee, K., Parn
T. A.: Dobutamine in chronic ischer
ular function and coronary hemodyn
481. Aronson, R. S., and Gelles, J. M.:
sheep cardiac Purkinje fibers. J. Pha
482. Loeb, H. S., Sinno, M. Z., Saudye,
Electrophysiologic properties of dob
483. Loeb, H. S., Khan, M., Klodnycky,
Gunnar, R. M.: Haemodynamic ef
2:29, 1975.
484. Tinker, J. H., Tarhan, S., White, R
Dobutamine for inotropic support
bypass. Anesthesiology 44:281, 1976
485. Lipp, H., Falicov, R. E., Resnekov,
on depressed myocardial function
closed-chest dog. Am. Heart J. 84:2(
486. Holloway, G. A., Jr., and Frederick
nist. Anesth. Analg. 53:616, 1974.
487. Pozen, R. G., DiBianco, R., Katz
Fletcher, R. D.: Myocardial m
dobutamine in heart failure complic
63:1279–1285, 1981.
488. Alexander, C. S., Sako, Y., and M
the use of dopamine. N. Engl. J. Me
489. Greene, S. I., and Smith, J. W.:
294:114, 1976.
490. Stoner, J. D., Bolen, J. L., and Ha
and dopamine in treatment of severe
491. Loeb, H. S., Bredakis, J., and Gunn
dopamine for augmentation of cardi
put cardiac failure. Circulation 55:37
492. Leier, C. V., Heban, P. T., Huss, P.
tive systemic and regional hemodyn
in patients with cardiomyopathic he
493. Berkowitz, C., McKeever, L., Crok
Gunnar, R. M.: Comparative resp
patients with chronic low output car
494. Mason, D. T., and Braunwald, E.:
on forearm vascular resistance and
tients in heart failure. J. Clin. Invest
495. Robie, N. W., Nutter, D. O., Mooc
of adrenergic receptor activity of c
1974.
496. Vatner, S. F., McRitchie, R. J., and
left ventricular performance, coron
output in conscious dogs. J. Clin. In
497. Akhtar, N., Mikulic, E., Cohn, J. N
fect of dobutamine in patients wi
36:202, 1975.

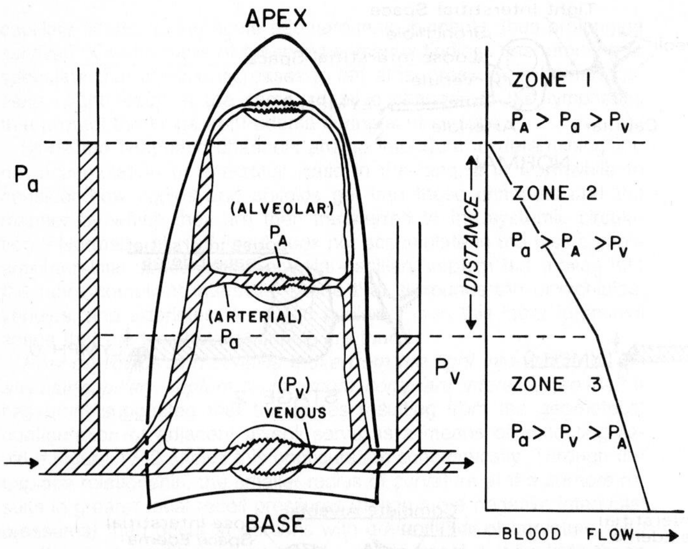

FIGURE 17–4 Schematic representation of the gravity-dependent, apex-to-base distribution of pulmonary blood flow in an upright lung according to West.[30] Pulmonary artery pressure (P_a) and pulmonary venous pressure (P_V) increase on a hydrostatic basis as the base is approached. Alveolar pressure (P_A) is constant with vertical distance. (The three zones are described at length in the text.)

confirmed that apical capillaries are bloodless.[31] On the other hand, gamma-emitting isotope studies in normal humans indicate that, although blood flow is strikingly diminished at the apex, no *true* Zone 1 (with total absence of flow) exists.[32]

In Zone 2, arterial pressure exceeds alveolar pressure, which in turn exceeds venous pressure. Here, each vessel is similar to a collapsible tube in a pressure chamber, and an analogy has been drawn between these vessels and a Starling resistor. An interesting property of the Starling resistor is as follows: When chamber pressure (analogous to alveolar pressure) exceeds the downstream pressure (analogous to venous pressure), the pressure drop for flow is not equal to the difference between upstream (arterial) and downstream (venous) pressures but rather to the difference between upstream (arterial) and chamber (alveolar) pressures. It is in this zone that large increases in flow occur per unit of distance of descent down the lung. These are due to large increases in perfusing pressures with no change in alveolar pressures.

In Zone 3, venous pressure exceeds alveolar pressure, resulting in distention of collapsible capillaries. Mean intravascular pressures are greatest in this zone; hence, with elevations of venus pressure or with disruption of alveolar-capillary membranes, edema formation is both more rapid and greatest here. It is only in this zone that the usual calculation of pulmonary vascular resistance holds true, and it is the only zone in which a valid pulmonary capillary wedge pressure measurement can be obtained. Increases in blood flow with increasing distance from the apex are more gradual in this zone because increases in pulmonary arterial pressures are offset by identical increases in venous pressures. The basis for the increase in flow with distance is the greater mean distending intravascular pressure with greater distention of the vessels as the base is approached.

Thus, in normal, erect humans, perfusion is greater in the basilar lung regions than in the more apical ones. Deviation from this gravity-dependent pattern has been called *vascular redistribution.* There are several ways to view the phenomenon of redistribution. Any encroachment of Zone 1 upon Zone 2 secondary to increased pulmonary venous pressure is, in a sense, redistribution, since regional blood flow is distributed differently after such a change. In like manner, greater relative perfusion of Zone 2 with increases in pulmonary artery pressure distributes more blood to the apex. However, true redistribution is generally considered to be a relative reduction in perfusion of the bases with a relative increase in apical perfusion. This phenomenon is most likely due to compression of the lumina of basilar vessels secondary to the greater and more rapid formation of edema at the lung bases and the tendency for extravascular liquid formed elsewhere to gravitate toward the bases.[5] In addition, pulmonary arteriolar constriction secondary to alveolar hypoxia, which may also contribute to this redistribution, is more prominent at the lung bases.[33] Several experimental studies either imply[34] or demonstrate[35] that vascular redistribution occurs only *after* the acute onset of alveolar edema. If this were the case in human disease, as it seems likely to be, redistribution should be no more subtle a finding than auscultatory abnormalities.

The situation with *chronic* elevations of left atrial pressure, as in mitral stenosis or chronic congestive heart failure, should be contrasted with that of acute pulmonary edema. Clinical experience with such chronic conditions suggests that redistribution of flow does occur with minimal or no evidence of interstitial edema and in the absence of alveolar edema. Because of the pathological changes found in such lungs at postmortem examination,[36] i.e., interstitial fibrosis of basilar lung regions and narrowing of basilar arteries and arterioles by lesions that often occur with pulmonary hypertension, it is more likely that redistribution is secondary to such changes.

CLASSIFICATION OF PULMONARY EDEMA

The two most common forms of pulmonary edema are those initiated by an imbalance of Starling forces and those initiated by disruption of one or more components of the alveolar-capillary membrane (Table 17–1).[37,37a] Less often, lymphatic insufficiency can be involved as a predisposing, if not initiating, factor in the genesis of edema. Although the initiating or primary mechanism may be clearly identifiable, multiple factors come into play during the development of edema, and irrespective of the initiating event, the stage of alveolar flooding is characterized most often by disruption of the alveolar-capillary membrane.

IMBALANCE OF STARLING FORCES. *Increased pulmonary capillary pressure* is a straightforward initiating event, whether due to mitral stenosis, left ventricular failure, or pulmonary venoocclusive disease.[38] Although pulmonary capillary wedge pressures must be abnormally high to increase the flow of interstitial liquid, at a time when edema is clearly present, these pressures may not correlate with the severity of pulmonary edema.[39] In fact, pulmonary capillary wedge pressures may have returned to normal at a time when there is still considerable pulmonary edema, since the rate of removal of both interstitial and alveolar edema appears to be relatively slow.[38] Other

TABLE 17–1 CLASSIFICATION OF PULMONARY EDEMA BASED UPON INITIATING MECHANISM

- I. Imbalance of Starling Forces
  - A. Increased pulmonary capillary pressure
    1. Increased pulmonary venous pressure without left ventricular failure (e.g., mitral stenosis)
    2. Increased pulmonary venous pressure secondary to left ventricular failure
    3. Increased pulmonary capillary pressure secondary to increased pulmonary arterial pressure (so-called overperfusion pulmonary edema)*
  - B. Decreased plasma oncotic pressure
    1. Hypoalbuminemia secondary to renal, hepatic, protein-losing enteropathic, or dermatological disease or nutritional causes**
  - C. Increased negativity of interstitial pressure
    1. Rapid removal of pneumothorax with large applied negative pressures (unilateral)
    2. Large negative pleural pressures due to acute airway obstruction along with increased end-expiratory volumes (asthma)*
  - D. Increased interstitial oncotic pressure
    1. No known clinical or experimental example
- II. Altered Alveolar-capillary Membrane Permeability (Adult Respiratory Distress Syndrome)
  - A. Infectious pneumonia—bacterial, viral, parasitic
  - B. Inhaled toxins (e.g., phosgene, ozone, chlorine, Teflon fumes, nitrogen dioxide, smoke)
  - C. Circulating foreign substances (e.g., snake venom, bacterial endotoxins, alloxan†, alpha-naphthyl thiourea†)
  - D. Aspiration of acidic gastric contents
  - E. Acute radiation pneumonitis
  - F. Endogenous vasoactive substances (e.g., histamine, kinins*)
  - G. Disseminated intravascular coagulation
  - H. Immunological—hypersensitivity pneumonitis, drugs (nitrofurantoin), leukoagglutinins
  - I. Shock lung in association with nonthoracic trauma
  - J. Acute hemorrhagic pancreatitis
- III. Lymphatic Insufficiency
  - A. Post lung transplant
  - B. Lymphangitic carcinomatosis
  - C. Fibrosing lymphangitis (e.g., silicosis)
- IV. Unknown or Incompletely Understood
  - A. High-altitude pulmonary edema
  - B. Neurogenic pulmonary edema
  - C. Narcotic overdose
  - D. Pulmonary embolism
  - E. Eclampsia
  - F. Post cardioversion
  - G. Post anesthesia
  - H. Post cardiopulmonary bypass

*Not certain to exist as a clinical entity.
**Not certain that this, as a single factor, leads to clinical pulmonary edema.
†Predominantly an experimental technique.

factors obscure the relationship between the severity of edema and measured pulmonary capillary pressures in addition to slower rates of removal after edema has collected. The rate of increase in lung liquid at any given elevation of capillary pressure is related to the functional capacity of lymphatics,[40,41] which may vary from patient to patient, and to variations in interstitial oncotic and hydrostatic pressures.[38]

The question of increased capillary pressures secondary to increased pulmonary artery pressure due to overperfusion is difficult to place in a clinical context.[41a] Indeed, experimental resection of well over half the pulmonary capillary bed has been shown to produce pulmonary edema.[42] The most relevant clinical observation has been the description of pulmonary edema in one lung or lobe following the creation of an end-to-end shunt from a systemic artery to a single pulmonary artery for the treatment of cyanotic congenital heart disease.[43] The question might be raised of why pulmonary edema does not occur with severe pulmonary hypertension (e.g., primary pulmonary hypertension). The obvious answer is that the arteriolar bed is severely narrowed in the latter instance, and thus capillaries are not exposed to the increased pressure, whereas in the former instance, the arteriolar bed is not narrowed, and increased pressures are found in the pulmonary capillaries.

Hypoalbuminemia is well known to produce dependent systemic edema without elevations of systemic venous pressures. In contrast, pulmonary edema does *not* develop with hypoalbuminemia alone. Hypoalbuminemia may alter the fluid conductivity of the interstitial gel so that liquid moves more easily between capillaries and lymphatics to add to the lymphatic safety factor.[44] Thus, there must be, in addition to hypoalbuminemia, some elevations of pulmonary capillary pressure, albeit only small increases are necessary before pulmonary edema ensues. Indeed, in such patients, only moderate fluid overload can precipitate overt pulmonary edema in the absence of left ventricular failure.

Increased negativity of interstitial pressure due to rapid removal of pleural air for relief of a relatively complete pneumothorax may be associated with pulmonary edema. Usually, the pneumothorax has been present for several hours to days, allowing time for alterations in surfactant, so that large negative pressures are necessary to open collapsed alveoli.[45,46] In this instance the edema is unilateral and is most often only a radiographic finding with few clinical findings.

Large negative pleural pressures thought to approximate interstitial pressures have been shown experimentally to increase the rate of edema formation in dogs.[47] Stalcup and Mellins have shown that the degree of negativity of the mean intrapleural pressure in asthma correlates with the severity of an attack and have speculated that there might be associated pulmonary edema, although it is radiographically inapparent owing to the hyperinflation of the lung in this condition.[10] This interesting hypothesis should be tested, since asthma is a common condition that is often treated with large volumes of intravenous fluids. Animal experiments involving inspiratory loading and increased lung volume as a means of increasing pleural pressure swings have demonstrated increases in left atrial transmural pressures along with diminution in left ventricular end-diastolic dimensions and decreases in cardiac output.[48–50] Thus, it is possible that diminution of left ventricular diastolic filling and an elevation of left atrial pressures accompany such large negative intrapleural pressures.

There is no known clinical or experimental example of pulmonary edema initiated by *increased interstitial oncotic pressure.* However, after the appearance of increased concentrations of macromolecules in the liquid of the interstitium or in alveoli, extravascular oncotic forces undoubtedly serve to intensify and perpetuate the process of edema formation.

PRIMARY ALVEOLAR-CAPILLARY MEMBRANE DAMAGE. Many diverse medical and surgical conditions are associated with pulmonary edema that appears to be due not to primary alteration in Starling forces but rather to damage of the alveolar-capillary membrane. These conditions include acute pulmonary infections and pulmonary effects of gram-negative septicemia and nonthoracic trauma as well as any condition associated with disseminated intravascular coagulation.[51–53] Despite the diversity of underlying causes, once diffuse alveolar-capillary injury has occurred, the pathophysiological and clinical sequence of events is quite similar in most patients. Because of the resemblance of the clinical picture to that seen with respiratory distress of the neonate, these conditions have been referred to as the *adult respiratory distress syndrome* (ARDS).[54] This similarity includes the superimposition of secondary factors, either occurring spontaneously or induced by therapeutic interventions, that serve to perpetuate or worsen the clinical course. An example of a spontaneously occurring secondary factor is the appearance of left ventricular failure with elevation of pulmonary capillary pressure during the course of the illness; a frequent consequence of therapeutic intervention is fluid overload of the patient due to the administration of excessive volumes of intravenous fluids.

Direct evidence for increased capillary permeability has come mainly from experimental studies in which pulmonary edema has been produced by endotoxin infusion;[55] hemorrhagic shock;[56,57] infusion of oleic acid;[58] and inhalation of high concentrations of oxygen[59] or toxic gases, such as phosgene,[60] ozone,[61] and nitrogen dioxide.[62] Reliable clinical data are far more difficult to obtain, since (1) macromolecules in alveolar liquid may be diluted by tracheobronchial secretion, resulting in an underestimation of the extent of the alveolar-capillary leak, and (2) such macromolecules, secondary to previously elevated capillary pressures, can be present at a time when intravascular pressures have returned to normal levels, hence leading to the erroneous conclusion that alveolar-capillary membrane damage was the primary event. Nonetheless, clinical studies of ARDS with normal pulmonary capillary wedge pressures have been reported and have shown either an elevation of protein in the liquid aspirated from the tracheobronchial tree[63,64] or appearance in this liquid of foreign macromolecules injected intravenously.[65] Thus, it is probable, though not yet proved, that increased permeability of the alveolar-capillary membrane is an initiating event in most of the cases designated as ARDS.

There are many similarities between ARDS from diverse etiologies and the respiratory distress syndrome seen in infants, which is due only to immaturity of the surfactant system. Although surfactant deficiency cannot be assigned a *primary* role in the pathogenesis of ARDS, there are many data to support the idea that changes in the properties of surfactant are added to the initial impairment and serve to perpetuate pulmonary dysfunction. Impairment of surfactant has been shown to occur with cardiogenic pulmonary edema,[66] exposure to various plasma constituents,[67] and high concentrations of oxygen[68] and in association with systemic hypotension.[69] Closely related to the pulmonary edema in the ARDS is that which is commonly associated with all forms of shock—the so-called "shock lung." The theories of pathogenesis of shock lung are shown in Table 17–2. (For further discussion of ARDS and shock lung, see p. 583.)

TABLE 17–2 THEORIES OF PATHOGENESIS OF SHOCK LUNG

I Hemodynamic
- A. Backward theory—pulmonary venular constriction (?centrally mediated; ?cerebral hypoxia)
- B. Forward theory—pulmonary hypertension. See IV, Microemboli (below)

II. Circulating humoral agent(s)
- A. Soluble factor(s) released from extrapulmonary cells injures vascular endothelium

III. Cellular agent(s)
- A. Locally released in lung injures vascular endothelium

IV. Microemboli—altered permeability arises from diffuse microembolization of lung
- A. Subtheories: why emboli form
  - 1. Exogenous from transfusions
  - 2. Increased rate of formation (platelet, leukocyte, or erythrocyte aggregates)
  - 3. Decreased breakdown (altered fibrinolysis)
  - 4. Decreased removal by reticuloendothelial system (liver)
    - a. Humoral—deficient opsonin
    - b. Decreased hepatic phagocytosis
- B. Mechanism of injury
  - 1. Hemodynamic (forward theory—severe, unevenly distributed pulmonary arterial hypertension transmitted to pulmonary capillaries, leading to shear stress and mechanical injury)
  - 2. Chemical (endothelium is injured by clot products: platelet, leukocyte, or erythrocyte aggregates)

From Robin, E. D.: Permeability pulmonary edema, *In* Fishman, A. P., and Renkin, E. M. (eds.): Pulmonary Edema. Bethesda, American Physiological Society, 1979, p. 217.

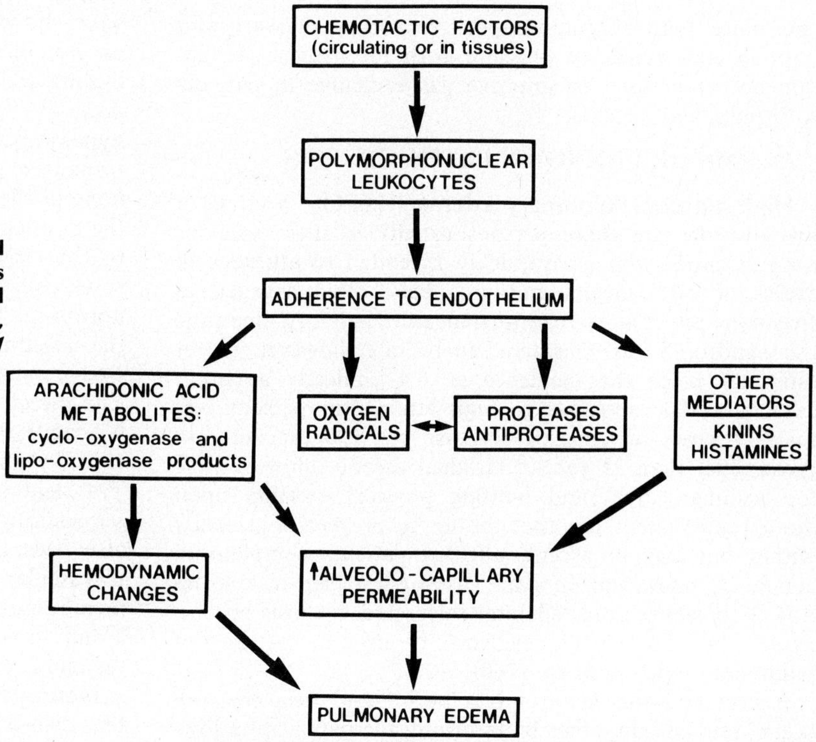

FIGURE 17–5 Flow chart showing the proposed mechanisms for chemotaxin and leukocyte interactions to produce alveolar-capillary membrane damage and pulmonary edema. (After Repine, J. E., Bowman, C. M., and Tate, R. M.: Neutrophils and lung edema. Chest *81* (Suppl.): 5, 1982.)

Recent experimental data strongly imply either a causal or a major and necessary role for interaction of polymorphonuclear leukocytes in the blood and circulating or cellular chemotactic macromolecules for the initiation, perpetuation, or amplification of lung injury leading to ARDS. The precise sequence of events is not truly settled but comprises some combination of items II, III, IVA, and B in Table 17–2. Figure 17–5 gives the elements of the potential role of leukocytes and chemotactic agents.[70] Chemotaxins in the circulating blood (e.g., the fifth component of complement, C5a) or from alveolar macrophages can recruit polymorphonuclear leukocytes, cause them to adhere to the pulmonary capillary endothelium, and activate them to produce several toxic substances that alter alveolar-capillary membrane permeability or cause circulatory changes or both. Because of the location of the polymorphonuclear leukocytes, their peripheral depletion and pulmonary vascular sequestration in many forms of acute lung injury, and their ability, when activated, to produce arachidonic acid metabolites (by both cyclo- and lipo-oxygenase pathways), oxygen radicals, proteases, and other mediators that alter permeability and influence vasomotoricity, the hypothesis is an appealing one.

Since these chemotaxins can arrive from distal sources in the body to inflict injury or can be derived from the alveolar macrophages of the alveolar side, systemic events such as gram-negative septicemia, distal events such as pancreatitis, and local pulmonary events such as inhalational injury can all be accommodated by this hypothesis.[71,72] Moreover, since the leukocyte aggregates often include platelets, the thrombocytopenic and consumptive coagulopathic states often accompanying ARDS can be explained. Recent clinical studies appear to support this hypothesis.[71] Bronchoalveolar lavage liquid from patients with ARDS has shown a predominance of neutrophils, leukocytic elastase, and partially inactivated alpha$_1$ antitrypsin.[73,74] Further, there is a strong correlation between neutrophil-aggregating activity in the plasma and the subsequent development of ARDS in clinical conditions that are often associated with this syndrome.[75] To date, no observations are available to refute this hypothesis, yet the many potential and complex interactions await elucidation before preventive or therapeutic measures can be devised and translated into clinical practice for the avoidance or arrest of lung injury.

LYMPHATIC DYSFUNCTION. Abnormalities in pulmonary lymphatics can produce abnormalities of liquid transport in the lung. However, the question remains whether such alterations alone ever account for pulmonary edema. Experimental studies have been in direct conflict on this point.[40,76] From the clinical standpoint, however, there are clear examples to suggest the importance of pulmonary lymphatics. In silicosis, with the invariably associated obliterative lymphangitis, only moderate elevations of left atrial pressures result in impressive pulmonary edema.[41] Similar observations have been made following lung transplantation with complete disruption of lymphatics[13] and in association with obstruction of lymphatics due to lymphangitic carcinomatosis.[77]

There are experimental studies showing that lymphatic dysfunction can be present *without structural abnormalities.* For example, Hall and colleagues have shown that the normal rhythmic contractions of pulmonary lymphatic vessels in sheep disappear when the animals are anesthetized.[78] Cessation of lymphatic pumping would be expected to result in a net gain of interstitial liquid, and this may leave a clinical counterpart of pulmonary edema following anesthesia or sedative drug overdose. Impairment of lymphatic flow with a net gain of lung liquid content has also been shown to occur in sheep given continuous positive airway pressure.[79] The clinical occurrence or importance of this finding has yet to be established, but the question is a significant one, since both continuous positive airway pressure and positive end-expiratory pressure with mechanical ventilation are often used to improve gas exchange in patients with pulmonary edema.

FORMS OF UNKNOWN PATHOGENESIS

High-altitude Pulmonary Edema (HAPE). Victims of this disorder are those persons usually in their teens or early twenties who have quickly ascended to altitudes in excess of 2700 meters and who have often engaged in strenuous physical exercise at that altitude.[80,81] At one time this syndrome was considered to be rare; however, recent estimates place the incidence at 6.4 clinically apparent cases per 100 exposures to high altitude in persons less than 21 years of age and 0.4 case per 100 exposures in those older than 21 years.[82] Gradual ascent, allowing time for acclimatization, and limiting physical exertion upon more rapid ascent are thought to be preventive. Usually within one day of ascent, affected patients complain of cough, dyspnea, and, in some cases, chest pain in association with tachycardia, bilateral rales, and cyanosis accompanied by radiographic evidence of discrete patches of pulmonary infiltrate (Fig. 17–6).

Reversal of this syndrome is both rapid (less than 48 hours) and certain either by returning the patient to a lower altitude or by administering a high inspiratory concentration of oxygen. Sleeping below 8000 ft, gradual acclimatization, and avoidance of heavy exertion for the first 2 or 3 days at high altitude appear to be preventive. Although formerly thought to occur only in persons from low altitudes who ascend quickly for mountaineering or skiing,[83,84] it has recently been documented to occur among natives of high-altitude regions upon their return from altitudes below 2200 meters.[85] No single mechanism satisfactorily explains the pathogenesis of HAPE, yet several possible mechanisms have been proposed. Although most have shown pulmonary arterial hypertension, the pulmonary capillary wedge pressures have been near normal,[86] a finding which has led to the suggestion that direct disruption of the walls of small arteries proximal to the hypoxically constructed arterioles in patients with hyperresponsive pulmonary vessels may be responsible.[87] Clearly, none of the catheterization data have been obtained during the development of, nor at the peak of, pulmonary edema, so that transitory elevations of pulmonary capillary pressures could have been present and could have returned to normal at the time of measurement. However, in view of the existing data showing normal pulmonary capillary wedge pressures, other mechanisms have been proposed. The direct effect of alveolar hypoxia on increasing alveolar-capillary membrane permeability was initially considered,[88] yet more recent studies do not support that idea.[89] Transient intravascular coagulation secondary to hypoxic sequestration of platelets in the pulmonary circulation has also been implicated;[90] however, it is possible that the intravascular coagulation is secondary to alveolar-capillary membrane disruption rather than a cause. At this point, it is fair to state that the pathogenesis is unknown,[91] but the response to simple treatment is dramatic.

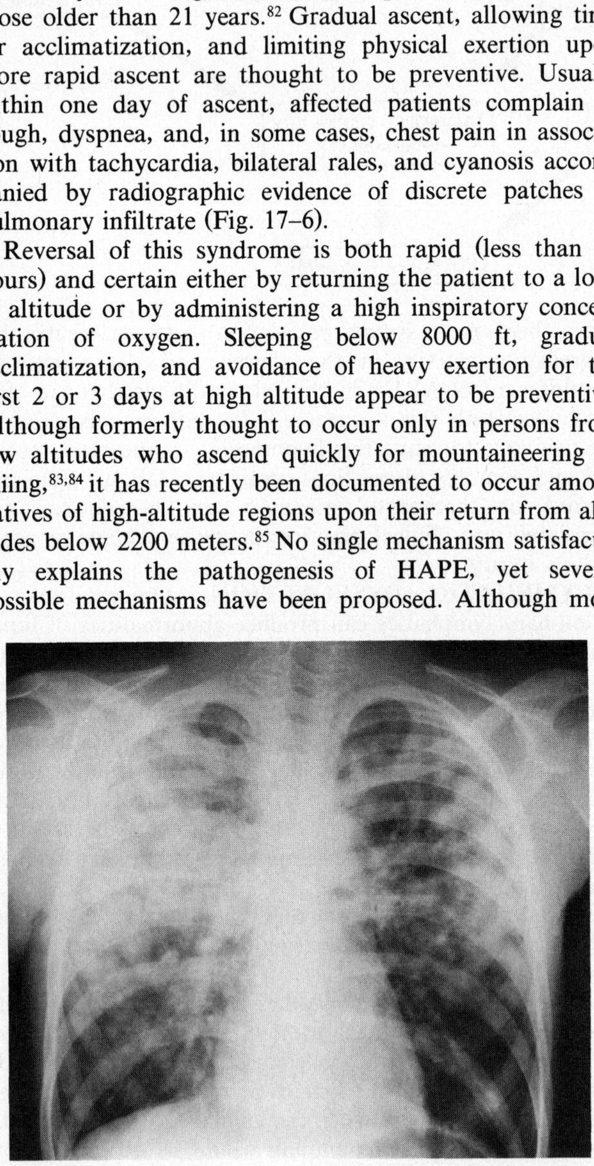

FIGURE 17–6 Chest x-ray of a 10-year-old boy in whom pulmonary edema developed on his return to his home at an elevation of 3100 meters after a visit to low altitude. Note patchy infiltrates scattered throughout both lung fields. Normal heart size indicates absence of left heart failure. (From Grover, R. F., et al.: High-altitude pulmonary edema. *In* Fishman, A. P., and Renkin, E. M. (eds.): Pulmonary Edema. Bethesda, American Physiological Society, 1979, p. 229.)

Neurogenic Pulmonary Edema. Central nervous system disorders ranging from head trauma to grand mal seizures can be associated with acute pulmonary edema (without detectable left ventricular disease). An early experimental model for this syndrome, consisting of fibrin injections into the fourth ventricle of dogs,[92] has been used to show that sympathectomy completely prevented the accumulation of lung liquid.[93] Indeed, observation that a variety of sympatholytic drugs serve to prevent neurogenic pulmonary edema makes it likely that the sympathetic nervous system plays a key role. Although not completely supported by direct measurements, the current idea is that sympathetic overactivity produces shifts of blood volume from the systemic to the pulmonary circulation, with secondary elevations of left atrial and pulmonary capillary pressures.[94] Thus, it would appear that an imbalance of Starling forces is the basis for this form of pulmonary edema, although capillary pressure quickly returns to normal after the acute and transitory sympathetic discharge. An unusually timely set of observations made on a patient with a pulmonary arterial catheter who experienced a grand mal seizure lent support to this idea. Wray and Nicotra observed transitory and severe elevations of pulmonary capillary wedge pressure in this patient during and immediately following the seizure.[95] Pulmonary edema diagnosed by both radiographic and clinical criteria was clearly present after wedge pressures had returned to normal levels. It should be emphasized that although sympatholytics prevent neurogenic pulmonary edema, they appear to have no place in the *treatment* of this syndrome, since pulmonary capillary pressures have returned to near normal when the syndrome is diagnosed.

The idea of a transitory sympathetic neural discharge of sufficient magnitude to account for high-pressure pulmonary edema as the basis for the neurogenic variety has not gone without challenge. Hakim et al. have presented data showing modest increases in pulmonary endothelial permeability without elevation of pressures produced by stellate ganglion stimulation in dogs,[96] and Simon and coworkers have demonstrated neurally mediated elevations in permeability during status epilepticus in anesthetized and paralyzed sheep, also without elevations of pulmonary capillary pressures.[97] Both of these observations, though demonstrating only a modest effect, suggest that neural mechanisms can alter membrane permeability. However, whether these changes are of sufficient magnitude to produce pulmonary edema is open to question. Nonetheless, in viewing the available data, we think the hemodynamic hypothesis to be the most appealing.

Narcotic Overdose Pulmonary Edema. Acute pulmonary edema is a well-recognized sequence of heroin overdose.[98] Because of the illicit traffic in this drug given by the intravenous route, the syndrome was initially thought to be due to injected impurities rather than to the heroin itself. However, since oral methadone or dextropropoxyphene can also be associated with pulmonary edema,[99,100] the syndrome cannot be attributed to injected impurities.

The well-known respiratory depressant effects of opiates lead to severe hypoxemia and hypercapnia with respiratory acidosis, which may account for the cerebral edema seen in many of these patients.[101] Cerebral edema, along with opiate-induced hypothalamic dysfunction,[102] raises the possibility of a neurogenic mechanism. Transient impairment of lymphatic pumping capacity may be a contributory factor.[78] The fact that edema fluid contains protein concentrations nearly identical to those found in plasma[103] and that pulmonary capillary wedge pressures, when measured, are normal[104] would appear to argue for an alveolar-capillary membrane leak as the initiating cause. In animal experiments, histamine has been shown to be released in the lung after both heroin and morphine administration.[105] Thus, it is possible that the well-known effects of histamine on vascular permeability might play a role in this syndrome. However, there is not sufficient experimental or clinical evidence in support of such a role. As with several other pulmonary edema syndromes of uncertain etiology that develop quickly, the possibility must be considered that transitory pulmonary capillary pressure elevations account for the edema and that the reported normal measurements were made during the phase of resolution.

Pulmonary Embolism. Acute pulmonary edema in association with either a massive embolus or multiple smaller emboli has been well described and most often attributed to concomitant left ventricular dysfunction due to a combination of hypoxemia and encroachment of the interventricular septum on the left ventricular cavity. Although this sequence is quite likely to be applicable in the case of massive embolism, whether it applies equally well to instances of multiple small emboli or microemboli is open to question. There are data to suggest, in the latter instance, that an increase in permeability of the alveolar-capillary membrane occurs.[52] Figure 17–7 outlines a hypothesis that implicates both clotting factors and formed elements in the pathogenesis of a pulmonary capillary leak due to microembolism.[106] Thrombin generated by the clotting process and in association with the embolus causes aggregation of platelets, complement activation, and leukostasis. It is proposed that the sequence then follows that outlined in Figure 17–5. Experimental support for this notion comes from the blunting of the capillary leak process following defibrinogenation[107] or leukocyte depletion.[108]

Eclampsia. Acute pulmonary edema frequently complicates eclampsia.[109] Multiple factors such as cerebral dysfunction with massive sympathetic discharge, left ventricular dysfunction secondary to acute systemic hypertension, hypervolemia, hypoalbuminemia (secondary to renal losses), and disseminated intravascular coagulation probably play a role in the pathogenesis.

Post Cardioversion. Although pulmonary edema has been documented to occur following cardioversion,[110] the mechanism is poorly understood. Ineffective left atrial function immediately following cardioversion has been suggested as a contributing factor, yet left ventricular dysfunction and neurogenic mechanisms are also possible.

Post Anesthesia. In previously healthy subjects, pulmonary edema has been found in the early postanesthesia period without a clear relationship to fluid overload or any subsequent evidence of left ventricular disease.[111] The basis for this disorder is unknown, but it is tempting to invoke some role for temporary lymphatic dysfunction under anesthesia, as previously shown in sheep.[78]

Post Cardiopulmonary Bypass. Although all patients who undergo cardiopulmonary bypass obviously have significant heart disease, the development of edema has been associated with normal left atrial pressures.[112,113] Alterations of surfactant due to prolonged collapse of the lung during the procedure, with subsequent need to apply high negative intrapleural pressures for reexpansion, and release of toxic substances have been suggested as mechanisms. The matter is not settled, but the syndrome is fortunately rare.

CARDIOGENIC PULMONARY EDEMA

CLINICAL MANIFESTATIONS. It would be satisfying to relate signs, symptoms, radiographic changes, and measurable dysfunction to all three stages of pulmonary edema. Unfortunately, in its earliest stage—i.e., increased lymph flow without net gain of interstitial liquid—there is currently no reliable way to detect pulmonary edema clinically or to quantitate it. If the process is initiated by an in-

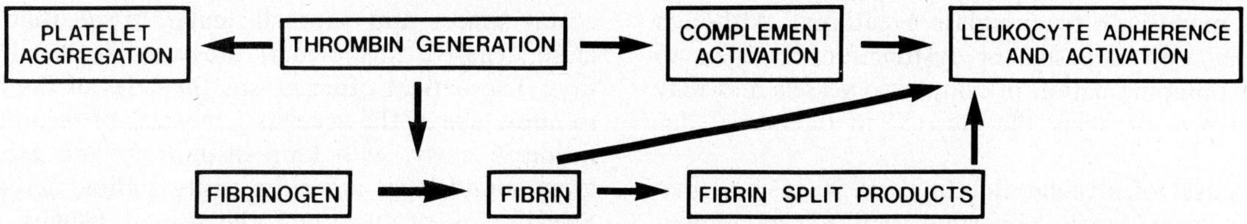

FIGURE 17–7 Flow chart showing the proposed mechanism for microembolic generation of increased permeability through the route shown in Figure 17–5. (After Malik, A. B., Tahamont, M. V., Minnear, F. L., Johnson, A., and Kaplan, J. E.: Lung fluid and protein exchange after pulmonary vascular thrombosis. Chest *81*:5, 1982.)

crease in left atrial or pulmonary venous pressures, prominent pulmonary veins with secondary prominence of pulmonary arteries would be an expected radiographic finding. Although earlier studies were able to relate vascular dimensions to intravascular pressures, those measurements were made only under conditions of *chronic* pressure elevations;[114] therefore, the findings might not apply to acute changes. Nonetheless, it is likely, given the pressure-diameter characteristics of both pulmonary veins and pulmonary arteries, that acute changes could be easily detectable radiographically, especially if serial films were available. Concerning measurable dysfunction, Hogg and coworkers were able to demonstrate in animal studies an increase in resistance of peripheral airways during pulmonary venous hypertension and to show that this finding could be attributed to competition for space between vessels and airways within the bronchovascular sheaths, with consequent compression of small airways.[115] There is some indirect evidence that the same phenomenon may be seen in human disease in which there is increased pulmonary blood volume.[116] Compromise of the lumina of small airways, predominantly in the more dependent portions of the lung, would be expected to increase both the alveolar-to-arterial difference for oxygen and the wasted ventilation ratio and to lead to a measurable increase in closing volume (Chap. 54). Since such mild changes in other settings rarely lead to symptoms, it is doubtful that any symptoms, except for exertional dyspnea, would accompany these abnormalities in Stage 1 edema. In like manner, physical findings in the lungs would be scarce except for mild inspiratory rales due to opening of closed airways.

Interstitial (or Stage 2) edema presents similar problems, in that correlative studies are scarce or nonexistent. Radiographic changes have been attributed to the increase in liquid in the loose interstitial space contiguous with the perivascular tissue of larger vessels and containing venules and arterioles. These changes (p. 173) are a loss of the normally sharp radiographic definition of pulmonary vascular markings, haziness and loss of demarcation of hilar shadows, and thickening of interlobular septa (Kerley B lines). Competition for space between vessels, airways, and increased liquid within the loose interstitial space produces greater compromise of small airway lumina than does Stage 1 edema. Thus, greater hypoxemia, more wasted ventilation, and more impressive elevations of closing volume occur. Indeed, in the setting of acute myocardial infarction, the degree of hypoxemia correlates with the degree of elevation of the pulmonary capillary wedge pressure.[117] *Tachypnea* is a frequent finding with interstitial edema and has been attributed to stimulation by the edema of interstitial J-type receptors or to stretch receptors in the interstitium rather than to hypoxemia, which is rarely of sufficient magnitude to stimulate breathing.[7] Although the tachypnea itself is a sign of dysfunction, it serves to augment the pumping action of lymphatic vessels and may serve to minimize or delay the increase in interstitial liquid.

With the onset of alveolar flooding, or Stage 3 edema, gas exchange is extremely abnormal, with severe hypoxemia and hypocapnia. Alveolar flooding can proceed to such a degree that many large airways are filled with blood-tinged foam that can be expectorated. Although hypocapnia is the rule, it has been well documented that hypercapnia with acute respiratory acidemia can occur in more severe cases.[118] It is in such instances that morphine, with its well-known respiratory depressant effects, should be used with caution.

As indicated above, pulmonary edema developing during acute myocardial infarction most often is thought to be due to pulmonary capillary hypertension, yet recent experimental data in dogs with acute ligation of coronary arteries indicate another possible contributory mechanism. Richeson et al. showed that edema developing after coronary artery ligation occurred when pulmonary capillary pressures were normal and that the increases in lung water were blocked when animals were pretreated with indomethacin.[119] This finding suggests that inhibition of cyclooxygenase or cyclic nucleotide phosphodiesterase reduced pulmonary edema secondary to increased permeability of the alveolar-capillary membrane. Whether and to what extent these findings will apply to the human illness must await further study. Occasionally, patients with acute myocardial infarction and pulmonary edema present with normal pulmonary capillary wedge pressures.[120] It is possible that delay in radiographing clearance after a fall in pulmonary venous pressure is responsible, but it is also possible that in some patients an increase in permeability of the alveolar-capillary membrane secondary to low cardiac output, i.e., a form of "cardiogenic shock" lung, causes the pulmonary edema.

DIAGNOSIS. Acute cardiogenic pulmonary edema is the most dramatic symptom of left heart failure. Impaired left ventricular function, mitral stenosis, or whatever cause of elevated left atrial and pulmonary capillary pressures leading to cardiogenic pulmonary edema interferes with oxygen transfer in the lungs and, in turn, depresses arterial oxygen tension. At the same time the sensation of suffocation intensifies the patient's fright, elevates heart rate, and further restricts ventricular filling. The increased discomfort and work of breathing place an additional load on the heart, and cardiac function becomes further depressed by the hypoxia. If this vicious cycle is not interrupted, it may rapidly lead to death.

Acute cardiogenic pulmonary edema differs from orthopnea and paroxysmal nocturnal dyspnea in the more rapid development of extreme pulmonary capillary hypertension. Acute pulmonary edema is a terrifying experience for both patient and bystander; usually extreme breathlessness develops suddenly, and the patient becomes extremely anxious, coughs, and expectorates pink, frothy liquid, causing him to feel as if he is literally drowning. The patient usually sits bolt upright, exhibits air hunger, and may thrash about. The respiratory rate is elevated, the alae nasi are dilated, and there is inspiratory retraction of the intercostal spaces and supraclavicular fossae that reflects the large negative intrapleural pressures required for inspiration. The patient often grasps the sides of the bed in order to allow use of the accessory muscles of respiration. Respiration is noisy, with loud inspiratory and expiratory gurgling sounds that are often easily audible across the room. Sweating is profuse, and the skin is usually cold, ashen, and cyanotic, reflecting low cardiac output and increased sympathetic drive.

On auscultation the lungs are noisy, with rhonchi,

wheezes, and moist and fine crepitant rales that appear at first over the lung bases but then extend upward to the apices as the condition worsens. Cardiac auscultation may be difficult because of the respiratory sounds, but a third heart sound and an accentuated pulmonic component of the second heart sound are frequently present.

The patient may suffer from intense precordial pain if the pulmonary edema is secondary to acute myocardial infarction. Unless cardiogenic shock is present, arterial pressure is usually elevated above the patient's normal level as a result of excitement and sympathetic vasoconstriction. Because of the presence of systemic hypertension, it may be inappropriately suspected that the pulmonary edema is due to hypertensive heart disease. However, it should be noted that this condition is now quite rare, and if arterial pressure is elevated, examination of the fundi will usually indicate whether or not hypertensive heart disease is actually present (p. 17). Obviously, if the attack is not terminated, arterial pressure declines preterminally.

It may be difficult to differentiate severe bronchial asthma from acute pulmonary edema, since both conditions may be associated with extreme dyspnea, pulsus paradoxicus, demands for an upright posture, and diffuse wheezes that interfere with cardiac auscultation. In bronchial asthma, there is most often a history of previous similar episodes, and the patient is frequently aware of the diagnosis. During the acute attack, the asthmatic patient does not usually sweat profusely, and arterial hypoxemia, though present, is not usually of sufficient magnitude to produce cyanosis. In addition, the chest is hyperexpanded and hyperresonant, and use of accessory muscles is prominent. The wheezes are more high-pitched and musical than in pulmonary edema, and other adventitious sounds such as rhonchi and rales are less prominent in asthma. The patient with acute pulmonary edema most often perspires profusely and is frequently cyanotic owing to desaturation of arterial blood *and* decreased cutaneous blood flow. The chest is often dull to percussion, there is no hyperexpansion, accessory muscle use is less prominent than in asthma, and moist, bubbly rales and rhonchi are heard in addition to wheezes. The radiological changes in pulmonary edema are discussed on page 174 and illustrated in Figures 6–38 through 6–42, pages 173 to 175.

Measurement of pulmonary artery wedge pressure by means of a Swan-Ganz catheter may be critical to the differentiation between pulmonary edema secondary to an imbalance of Starling forces, i.e., cardiogenic pulmonary edema, and that secondary to alterations of the alveolar-capillary membrane. Specifically, a pulmonary capillary wedge or pulmonary artery diastolic pressure exceeding 25 mm Hg in a patient without previous pulmonary capillary pressure elevation (or exceeding 30 mm Hg in a patient with chronic pulmonary capillary pressure elevation) and with the clinical features of pulmonary edema strongly suggests that the edema is cardiogenic in origin.

Following effective treatment of the pulmonary edema, the patient is often rapidly restored to the condition that existed before the attack, although he usually feels exhausted; between attacks of pulmonary edema there may be few symptoms or signs of heart failure.

TREATMENT. In the treatment of acute pulmonary edema, a physician cannot usually work alone, since multiple simultaneous maneuvers are required. Therefore, if logistics and time permit, the patient should be transferred to an intensive care unit, and cardiac rhythm should be monitored. However, it is important to emphasize that transfer of the patient and institution of monitoring *must not delay initial therapy*, which must often be begun in the house or ambulance. While initial treatment is under way, it is frequently advisable to place an arterial catheter to record intraarterial pressure and obtain frequent samples for arterial blood gas measurements. If possible, a Swan-Ganz catheter should be inserted, so that pulmonary arterial diastolic and capillary wedge pressures can be measured and monitored.

The strategy of treatment of cardiogenic pulmonary edema is threefold: (1) a series of nonspecific measures are applied; (2) the precipitating factor is identified, if possible, and treated; and (3) attention is directed to the underlying condition, which is then corrected, if possible.

Nonspecific Measures

1. *Inhalation of oxygen-enriched inspired gas*, often with the aid of mechanical ventilation, is useful, as discussed below (p. 574).

2. The patient should be placed in the *sitting position*. Often this is not necessary, because the patient recognizes that distress is increased when he lies down and that he is more comfortable sitting up. However, it is often helpful to seat the patient at the side of the bed or in a chair in order to lower the feet and thereby further diminish venous return.

3. *Morphine sulfate* remains an extremely valuable drug in the treatment of cardiogenic pulmonary edema. By its narcotic action it diminishes the patient's distress, reduces the work of breathing, and, perhaps most importantly, diminishes the sympathetically induced venous and arteriolar constriction. Thus, even though morphine is not a direct vasodilator, in the setting of acute pulmonary edema it results in arteriolar and especially in venous dilation.[121]

Three to 5 mg of morphine sulfate may be injected intravenously over a 3-minute period, while the patient is observed for both its beneficial action (i.e., relief of pulmonary edema) and its principal adverse effect (i.e., respiratory depression). This dose may usually be repeated two or three times at 15-minute intervals, if necessary. When the situation is somewhat less urgent, 8 to 15 mg of morphine sulfate may be injected subcutaneously or intramuscularly, and this dose can be repeated every 3 to 4 hours. Morphine antagonists should be readily available whenever morphine is administered. Morphine should be avoided if acute pulmonary edema is associated with intracranial bleeding; disturbed consciousness; bronchial asthma; chronic pulmonary disease; or reduced ventilation, as reflected in an elevated arterial P_{CO_2}.

4. *Reduction of preload* can be accomplished by applying rotating tourniquets of wide, soft rubber tubing or blood pressure cuffs to the extremities. These should be placed several inches below the groin and shoulders, and the cuffs should be inflated to approximately 10 mm Hg below diastolic pressure, thus permitting arterial inflow to the limbs but restricting venous outflow. Only three of the four extremities should be compressed at one time, and every 15 to 20 minutes one of the tourniquets should be released and rotated to the free extremity.

Hg) without hypercapnia, oxygen enrichment of the inspired gas may suffice and can be given by nasal prongs, Venturi masks, or reservoir bag masks, depending upon the degree of oxygen enrichment required to elevate the PaO_2 sufficiently. If arterial oxygen tensions cannot be maintained at or near 60 mm Hg despite 100 per cent oxygen at 20 liters per minute, or if there is progressive hypercapnia, intubation and institution of mechanical ventilation are usually necessary.

In the instance of progressive hypoxemia without hypercapnia, the role of mechanical ventilation is not to increase alveolar ventilation but to increase mean lung volume during the respiratory cycle, which in turn opens more alveoli for gas exchange. If hypoxemia is not corrected by mechanical ventilation or if toxic doses of oxygen are necessary for prolonged periods, further improvements in arterial oxygenation at the same inspired oxygen concentration or equivalent levels of arterial oxygenation at lower concentrations of oxygen can be achieved by increasing end-expiratory lung volumes by the addition of positive end-expiratory pressure (PEEP).[129] Since maintenance of oxygenation is absolutely necessary for survival, reports that mechanical ventilation with positive end-expiratory pressure actually increases the liquid content of the lung[79] may unsettle the physician who must utilize these techniques but will make him or her aware that this form of treatment should be discontinued as soon as possible.

Two complications of mechanical ventilation with positive end-expiratory pressure deserve special mention. The first is that high intrathoracic pressures and increasing lung volumes serve to impede venous return and increase the afterload to the right ventricle, with attendant decreases in cardiac output.[48] In the case of cardiogenic pulmonary edema, the impedance of venous return may provide some benefit with decreases in central pressures but no decline in cardiac output. However, in other forms of pulmonary edema, a fall in cardiac output may be detrimental to the oxygen transport system. A fall in blood pressure or urine output or both may be the only indication that a severe diminution in cardiac output has occurred unless cardiac output is monitored during this form of therapy. The predominant basis for the decrease in cardiac output is increased intrathoracic pressure, which directly impedes venous return.[48,49] An additional contribution may come from greater pulmonary vascular resistance due to increased lung volume.[48] The result of increased right ventricular afterload is a displacement of the interventricular septum, which impedes left ventricular diastolic filling.[50,130,131,132] It is also likely that direct compression of the left ventricle by the inflated lung also restricts diastolic filling.[133,134] The second complication of mechanical ventilation, barotrauma (pneumomediastinum, pneumothorax, and subcutaneous emphysema), requires appropriate decompressive therapy.[135]

When it is not possible to maintain oxygenation utilizing the above techniques, extracorporeal membrane oxygenators have been tried with the hope that life could be maintained during critical periods while reparative processes in the heart or lung or both are taking place. However, a National Heart, Lung, and Blood Institute trial designed to evaluate this heroic and costly form of life support has not been shown to improve the clinical outcome.

When hypercapnia with respiratory acidosis is present, mechanical ventilatory support may be necessary for improving alveolar ventilation in addition to improving oxygenation. If hypercapnia has resulted from excessively vigorous use of morphine, antagonist drugs might avert the need for mechanical ventilation.

In any situation in which cardiac output is diminished and arterial oxygenation is impaired, there may be insufficient oxygen delivered for aerobic metabolic demands; hence anaerobic metabolism with excessive production of lactic acid results in metabolic acidemia. Clearly, the primary aim is to improve both cardiac output and arterial oxygenation; however, sodium bicarbonate may be given intravenously as a temporary measure while more basic

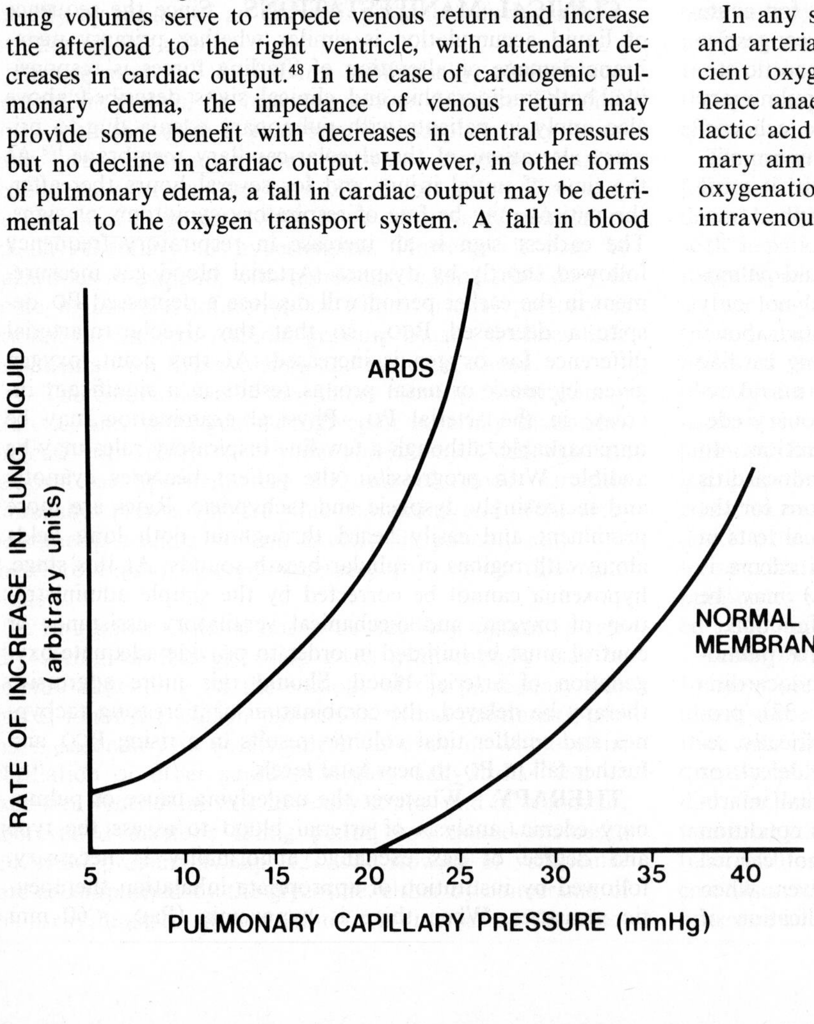

FIGURE 17–8 Schematic representation of the deleterious effects of acceptably normal capillary pressures in combination with pulmonary capillary leak. (Based upon the data of Prewitt, R. M., McCarthy, J., and Wood, L. D. H.: Treatment of acute low pressure pulmonary edema in dogs: Relative effects of hydrostatic and oncotic pressure, nitroprusside, and positive end-expiratory pressure. J. Clin. Invest. *67*:409, 1981.)

therapeutic measures are undertaken. Occasionally, when large quantities of sodium bicarbonate are required, there is a danger of sodium overload.

Measures aimed against increased capillary permeability in ARDS are frustratingly nonspecific and have not been shown to alter the time course or outcome of the illness. A possible exception is the use of specific antibiotic therapy directed against a causative or complicating bacterial infection. Adrenal glucocorticosteroid therapy leads the list of nonspecific measures that have yet to be of proven benefit.[38] In cases of pulmonary edema related to or complicated by disseminated intravascular coagulation, low molecular weight dextran and heparin have been used without any clear evidence of an effect on the severity of the lung lesion.[38]

An obvious and not often emphasized principle is to maintain pulmonary capillary pressures at the lowest possible levels (i.e., compatible with maintaining cardiac and urinary outputs and blood pressure) when there is increased permeability. Prewitt et al. have shown, using a dog model of oleic acid–induced pulmonary edema, that the rate of formation of pulmonary edema is cut to less than half when pulmonary capillary wedge pressures are decreased from 12 to 6 mm Hg.[136] The principle is schematized in Figure 17–8.

Since both increases in pulmonary capillary pressure and primary alveolar-capillary damage result in interstitial edema and alveolar flooding with liquid-containing erythrocytes and macromolecules, indicating severe membrane disruption, it is difficult to evolve a rationale for the use of intravenous colloids such as albumin or high molecular weight dextrans. In fact, large molecular weight compounds administered intravenously have been shown to appear rapidly in alveolar liquid.[65] Furthermore, there is experimental evidence that the administration of colloid to dogs with experimental lung injury actually *slows* the resolution of ultrastructural changes in the interstitium.[137] Since there is no firm clinical evidence that treatment with protein-containing solutions results in more rapid recovery from acute pulmonary edema,[135] and since there are strong intuitive reasons and some experimental data to suggest detrimental results, the use of albumin and other colloids should generally be avoided. There are, however, two situations in which albumin can be reasonably considered. First, if there is hypoalbuminemia, administration of albumin in addition to interventions designed to lower pulmonary capillary pressures seems rational. Second, the suggestion has been made that albumin might hasten the rate of resolution of pulmonary edema once alveolar-capillary membrane integrity has been reestablished.[138]

References

1. Laennec, R. T. H.: Traité de l'Auscultation Médiate. Vol. 2. Paris, Brosson and Chaude, 1819, p. 9.
2. Visscher, M. B., Haddy, F. J., and Stephens, G.: The physiology and pharmacology of lung edema. Pharmacol. Rev. *8*:389, 1956.
3. Drinker, C. K.: Pulmonary Edema and Inflammation. Cambridge, Harvard University Press, 1945.
4. Guyton, A. C., and Lindsey, A. W.: Effect of elevated left atrial pressure and decreased plasma protein concentration on the development of pulmonary edema. Circ. Res. *7*:649, 1959.
5. Staub, N. C.: Pulmonary edema. Physiol. Rev. *54*:678, 1974.
6. Yu, P. N.; Pulmonary edema. Circulation *63*:724, 1981.
7. Szidon, J. P., Pietra, G. G., and Fishman, A. P.: The alveolar-capillary membrane and pulmonary edema. N. Engl. J. Med. *286*:1200, 1972.
8. Guyton, A. C., Parker, J. C., Taylor, A. E., Jackson, T. E., and Moffatt, D. S.: Forces governing water movement in the lung. *In* Fishman, A. P., and Renkin, E. M. (eds.): Pulmonary Edema. Bethesda, American Physiological Society, 1979, p. 70.
9. Lai-Fook, S. J.: Perivascular interstitial fluid pressure measured by micropipettes in isolated dog lung. J. Appl. Physiol. *52*:9, 1982.
10. Stalcup, S. A., and Mellins, R. B.: Mechanical forces producing pulmonary edema in acute asthma. N. Engl. J. Med. *297*:592, 1977.
11. Parker, J. C., Parker, R. E., Granger, D. N., and Taylor, A. E.: Vascular permeability and transvascular fluid and protein transport in the dog lung. Circ. Res. *48*:549, 1981.
12. Staub, N. C.: Pulmonary edema due to increased microvascular permeability to fluid and protein. Circ. Res. *43*:143, 1978.
13. Ersalan, S., Turner, M. D., and Hardy, J. D.: Lymphatic regeneration following lung reimplantation in dogs. Surgery *56*:970, 1964.
14. Sampson, J. J., Leeds, S. E., Uhley, H. N., and Friedman, M.: The lymphatic system and pulmonary disease. *In* Mayerson, H. S. (ed.): Lymph and the Lymphatic System. Springfield, Ill., Charles C Thomas, 1968, p. 200.
15. Carlson, R. W., Schaeffer, R. C., Jr., Michaels, S. G., and Weil, M. H.: Pulmonary edema fluid. Circulation *60*:1161, 1979.
16. Bruderman, I., Somers, K., Hamilton, W. K., Tooley, W. H., and Butler, J.: Effect of surface tension on circulation in the excised lungs of dogs. J. Appl. Physiol. *19*:707, 1964.
17. Yoffey, J. M., and Courtice, F. C.: Lymphatics, Lymph and the Lymphomeyloid Complex. London, Academic Press, 1970.
18. Rusznyak, J., Földi, M., and Szabo, G.: Lymphatics and Lymph Circulation: Physiology and Pathology. 2nd ed. Oxford, Pergamon Press, 1967.
19. Hammersen, F.: Ultrastructure and functions of capillaries and lymphatics. Arch. Physiol. *336* (Suppl.):S43, 1972.
20. Casley-Smith, J. R.: The role of the endothelial intercellular junctions in the functioning of the initial lymphatics. Angiologica *9*:106, 1972.
21. Hall, J. G., Morris, B., and Wooley, G.: Intrinsic rhythmic propulsion of lymph in the unanesthetized sheep. J. Physiol. *180*:336, 1965.
22. Lambert, R. K., and Gremels, H.: On the factors concerned in the production of pulmonary edema. J. Physiol. (London) *61*:98, 1926.
23. Rush, S., Abildskov, J. A., and McFee, R.: Resistivity of body tissues at low frequencies. Circ. Res. *12*:40, 1963.
24. Vanselow, K., and Heuck, F.: Theoretische Untersuchungen über eine Messmethode zur quantitativen Bestimmung des Wasser-Luft-Verhältnisses des Lungengewebes. Fortschr. Röntgenstr. *100*:441, 1964.
25. Ahluwalia, B. D., Brownell, G. L., Hales, C. A., and Kazemi, H.: An index of pulmonary edema measured with emission computed tomography. J. Comput. Assist. Tomogr. *5*:690, 1981.
26. Chinard, F. P.: Estimation of extravascular lung water by indicator-dilution techniques. Circ. Res. *37*:137, 1975.
26a. Sibbald, W. J., Warshawski, F. J., Short, A. K., Harris, J., Lefcoe, M. S., and Holliday, R. L.: Clinical studies of measuring extravascular lung water by the thermal dye technique in critically ill patients. Chest *83*:725, 1983.
27. Fishman, A. P.: Pulmonary edema. *In* Fishman, A. P. (ed.): Pulmonary Diseases and Disorders. New York, McGraw-Hill Book Co., 1980, p. 733.
28. Staub, N. C., Nagano, H., and Pearce, M. L.: Pulmonary edema in dogs, especially the sequence of fluid accumulation in lungs. J. Appl. Physiol. *22*:227, 1967.
29. Agostoni, E.: Mechanics of the pleural space. Physiol. Rev. *52*:57, 1972.
30. West, J. B.: Ventilation Blood Flow and Gas Exchange. Oxford, Blackwell Scientific Publications, 1970.
31. Glazier, J. B., Hughes, J. M. B., Maloney, J. E., and West, J. B.: Measurements of capillary dimensions and blood volume in rapidly frozen lung. J. Appl. Physiol. *26*:65, 1969.
32. Dollery, C. T., Heimberg, P., and Hugh-Jones, P.: Relationships between blood flow and clearance rate of radioactive carbon dioxide and oxygen in normal and oedematous lungs. J. Physiol. (London) *162*:93, 1962.
33. Dawson, A.: Regional pulmonary blood flow in sitting and supine man during and after acute hypoxia. J. Clin. Invest. *48*:301, 1969.
34. Ritchie, B. C., Schauberger, G., and Staub, N. C.: Inadequacy of perivascular edema hypothesis to account for distribution of pulmonary blood flow in lung edema. Circ. Res. *24*:807, 1969.
35. Muir, A. L., Hogg, J. C., Naimark, A., Hall, D. L., and Chernecki, W.: Effect of alveolar liquid on distribution of blood flow in dog lungs. J. Appl. Physiol. *39*:885, 1975.
36. Parker, F., Jr., and Weiss, S.: The nature and significance of the structural changes in the lungs in mitral stenosis. Am. J. Pathol. *12*:573, 1936.
37. Ayres, S. M.: Mechanisms and consequences of pulmonary edema: Cardiac lung, shock lung, and principles of ventilatory therapy in adult respiratory distress syndrome. Am. Heart J. *103*:97, 1982.
37a. Sprung, C. L., Rackow, E. C., Fein, I. A., Jacob, A. I., and Isikoff, S. K.: The spectrum of pulmonary edema: Differentiation of cardiogenic, intermediate, and noncardiogenic forms of pulmonary edema. Ann. Rev. Respir. Dis. *124*:718, 1981.
38. Robin, E. D., Cross, C. E., and Zelis, R.: Pulmonary edema. N. Engl. J. Med. *288*:239 and 292, 1973.
39. Pietra, G. G., Szidon, J. P., Leventhal, M. M., and Fishman, A. P.: Hemoglobin as a tracer in hemodynamic pulmonary edema. Science *166*:1643, 1969.

40. Földi, M.: Diseases of Lymphatics and Lymph Circulation. Springfield, Ill., Charles C Thomas, 1969.
41. Cross, C. E., Shaver, J. A., Wilson, R. J., and Robin, E. D.: Mitral stenosis and pulmonary fibrosis: Special reference to pulmonary edema and lung lymphatic function. Arch. Intern. Med. *125*:248, 1970.
41a. Landolt, C. C., Matthay, M. A., Albertine, K. H., Roos, P. J., Wiener-Kronish, J. P., and Staub, N. C.: Overperfusion, hypoxia, and increased pressure cause only hydrostatic pulmonary edema in anesthetized sheep. Circ. Res. *52*:335, 1983.
42. Hultgren, H. N., and Grover, R. F.: Circulatory adaptation to high altitude. Annu. Rev. Med. *19*:119, 1968.
43. Albers, W. H., and Nadas, A. S.: Unilateral chronic pulmonary edema and pleural effusion after systemic-pulmonary arterial shunts for cyanotic congenital heart disease. Am. J. Cardiol. *19*:861, 1967.
44. Kramer, G. C., Harms, B.A., Gunther, R. A., Renkin, E. M., and Demling, R. H.: The effects of hypoproteinemia on blood-to-lymph fluid transport in sheep lung. Circ. Res. *49*:1173, 1981.
45. Ziskind, M. M., Weil, H., and George, R. A.: Acute pulmonary edema following the treatment of spontaneous pneumothorax with excessive negative intrapleural pressure. Am. Rev. Respir. Dis. *92*:632, 1965.
46. Trapnell, D. H., and Thurston, J. G. B.: Unilateral pulmonary oedema after pleural aspiraton. Lancet *1*:1367, 1970.
47. Mellins, R. B., Levine, O. R., Skalak, R., and Fishman, A. P.: Interstitial pressure in the lungs. Circ. Res. *24*:197, 1969.
48. Scharf, S. M., Caldini P., and Ingram, R. H., Jr.: Cardiovascular effects of increasing airway pressure. Am. J. Physiol. *1*:35, 1977.
49. Scharf, S. M., Brown, R., Saunders, N. A., Green, L. H., and Ingram, R. H., Jr.: Changes in left ventricular size and configuration with positive end-expiratory pressure. Circ. Res. *44*:672, 1979.
50. Scharf, S. M., and Brown, R.: Influence of the right ventricle on canine left ventricular function with PEEP. J. Aopl. Physiol. *52*:254, 1982.
51. Malik, A. B., and Staub, N. C. (eds.): Mechanisms of Lung Microvascular Injury. New York, New York Academy of Sciences, 1982.
52. Staub, N. C.: Pulmonary edema due to increased microvascular permeability. Ann. Rev. Med. *32*:291, 1981.
53. Carlson, R. W., Schaeffer, R. C., Jr., Puri, V. K., Brennan, A. P., and Weil, M. H.: Hypovolemia and permeability pulmonary edema associated with anaphylaxis. Crit. Care Med. *9*:883, 1981.
54. Ashbaugh, D. G., Bigelow, D. B., Petty, T. L., and Levine, B. E.: Acute respiratory distress in adults. Lancet *2*:319, 1967.
55. Snell, J. D., Jr., and Ramsey, L. H.: Pulmonary edema as a result of endotoxemia. Am. J. Physiol. *217*:170, 1969.
56. Ratliff, N. B., Wilson, J. W., Horckel, D. B., and Martin, A. M., Jr.: The lung in hemorrhagic shock. II. Observations on alveolar and vascular ultrastructure. Am. J. Pathol. *58*:353, 1970.
57. Moss, G. S., Das Gupta, T. K., Newson, B., and Nyhus, L. M.: Morphologic changes in the primate lung after hemorrhagic shock. Surg. Gynecol. Obstet. *134*:3, 1972.
58. Parker, F. B., Jr., Wax, S. D., Kusajima, K., and Webb, W. R.: Hemodynamic and pathological findings in experimental fat embolism. Arch. Surg. *108*:70, 1974.
59. Kapanci, Y., Weibel, E. R., Kaplan, H. P., and Robinson, P. V. M.: Pathogenesis and reversibility of the pulmonary lesions of oxygen toxicity in monkey. II. Ultrastructural and morphometric studies. Lab. Invest. *20*:101, 1969.
60. Cameron, G. R., and Courtice, F. C.: The production and removal of oedema fluid in the lungs after exposure to carbonyl chloride (phosgene). J. Physiol. (London) *105*:175, 1946.
61. Bils, R. F.: Ultrastructural alterations of alveolar tissue of mice. III. Ozone. Arch. Environ. Health *20*:468, 1970.
62. Sherwin, R. P., and Richters, V.: Lung capillary permeability: nitrogen dioxide exposure and leakage of tritiated serum. Arch. Intern. Med. *128*:61, 1971.
63. Gelb, A. F., and Klein, E.: Hemodynamic and alveolar protein studies in noncardiac pulmonary edema. Am. Rev. Respir. Dis. *114*:831, 1976.
64. Sprung, C. L., Rackow, E. C., Fein, I. A., Jacob, A. I., and Isikoff, S. K.: The spectrum of pulmonary edema: differentiation of cardiogenic, intermediate, and noncardiogenic forms of pulmonary edema. Am. Rev. Respir. Dis. *124*:718, 1981.
65. Robin, E. D., Carey, L. C., Grenvik, A., Glauser, F., and Gaudio, R.: Capillary leak syndrome with pulmonary edema. Arch. Intern. Med. *130*:66, 1972.
66. Pattle, R. E.: Properties, function, and origin of the alveolar lining layer. Nature (London) *175*:1125, 1955.
67. Said, S. I., Avery, M. E., Davis, R. K., Banjaree, C. M., and El-Gohar, M.: Pulmonary surface activity in induced pulmonary edema. J. Clin. Invest. *44*: 458, 1965.
68. Miller, W. W., Waldhausen, J. A., and Rashkind, W. J.: Comparison of oxygen poisoning of the lung in cyanotic and acyanotic dogs. N. Engl. J. Med. *282*:943, 1970.
69. Henry, J. N.: The effect of shock on pulmonary alveolar surfactant. Its role in refractory respiratory insufficiency of the critically ill or severely injured patient. J. Trauma *8*:756, 1968.
70. Repine, J. E., Bowman, C. M., and Tate, R. M.: Neutrophils and lung edema. Chest *81*(Suppl.):5, 1982.
71. Rinaldo, J. E., and Rogers, R. M.: Adult respiratory-distress syndrome: Changing concepts of lung injury and repair. N. Engl. J. Med. *306*:900, 1982.
72. Brigham, K. L., Loyd, J. E., Newman, J. H., Snapper, J. R., Ogletree, M. L., and English, D. K.: Granulocytes in acute lung vascular injury in unanesthetized sheep. Chest *81* (Suppl.):5, 1982.
73. Lee, C. T., Fein, A. M., Lippman, M., Holtzman, H., Kimbel, P., and Weinbaum, G.: Elastolytic activity in pulmonary lavage fluid from patients with adult respiratory distress syndrome. N. Engl. J. Med. *304*:192, 1981.
74. Cohen, A. B., and Cochrane, C. G.: Studies on the pathogenesis of the adult respiratory distress syndrome. J. Clin. Invest. *69*:543, 1982.
75. Hammerschmidt, D. E., Weaver, L. J., Hudson, L. D., Craddock, P. R., and Jacob, H. S.: Association of complement activation and elevated plasma-C5a with adult respiratory distress syndrome: Pathophysiological relevance and possible prognostic value. Lancet *1*:947, 1980.
76. Magno, M., and Szidon, J. P.: Hemodynamic pulmonary edema in dogs with acute and chronic lymphatic ligation. Am. J. Physiol. *231*:1777, 1976.
77. Trapnell, D. H.: Radiological appearances of lymphangitis carcinomatosa of the lung. Thorax *19*:251, 1964.
78. Hall, J. G., Morris, B., and Wooley, G.: Intrinsic rhythmic propulsion of lymph in the unanesthetized sheep. J. Physiol. (London) *180*:336, 1965.
79. Permutt, S.: Mechanical influences on water accumulation in the lungs. *In* Fishman, A. P., and Renkin, E. M. (eds.): Pulmonary Edema. Bethesda, American Physiological Society, 1979, p. 175.
80. Sutton, J. R., and Lassen, N.: Pathophysiology of acute mountain sickness and high altitude pulmonary oedema. An hypothesis. Bull. Eur. Physiopathol. Respir. *15*:1045, 1979.
81. Lockhart, A., and Saiag, B.: Altitude and the human pulmonary circulation. Clin. Sci. *60*:599, 1981.
82. Hultgren, H. N.: High altitude pulmonary edema. Adv. Cardiol. *5*:24, 1970.
83. Hultgren, H. N., Spickard, W. B., Hellriegel, K., and Houston, C. S.: High altitude pulmonary edema. Medicine (Baltimore) *40*:289, 1961.
84. Fred, H. L., Schmidt, A. M., Bates, T., and Hecht, H. H.: Acute pulmonary edema of altitude: Clinical and physiologic observations. Circulation *25*:929, 1962.
85. Scoggin, C. H., Myers, T. M., Reeves, J. T., and Grover, R. F.: High altitude pulmonary edema in the children and young adults of Leadville, Colorado. N. Engl. J. Med. *297*:1269, 1977.
86. Hultgren, H. N., Lopez, C. E., Lundberg, E., and Miller, H.: Physiologic studies of pulmonary edema at high altitude. Circulation *29*:393, 1964.
87. Whayne, T. F., Jr., and Severinghaus, J. W.: Experimental hypoxic pulmonary edema in the rat. J. Appl. Physiol. *25*:279, 1968.
88. Warren, M. F., and Drinker, C. K.: The flow of lymph from the lungs of the dog. Am. J. Physiol. *136*:207, 1942.
89. Goodale, R. L., Goetzman, B., and Visscher, M. B.: Hypoxia and iodoacetic acid and alveolo-capillary membrane permeability to albumin. Am. J. Physiol. *219*:1226, 1970.
90. Gray, G. W., Bryan, A. C., Freedman, M. H., Houston, C. S., Lewis, W. F., McFadden, D. M., and Newell, G.: Effect of altitude exposure on platelets. J. Appl. Physiol. *39*:648, 1975.
91. Grover, R. F., Hyers, R. M., McCurty, I. F., and Reeves, J. T.: High-altitude pulmonary edema. *In* Fishman, A. P., and Renkin, E. M. (eds.): Pulmonary Edema. Bethesda, American Physiological Society, 1979, p. 229.
92. Cameron, G. R., and De, S. N.: Experimental pulmonary oedema of nervous origin. J. Pathol. Bacteriol. *61*:375, 1949.
93. Sarnoff, S. J., and Sarnoff, L. C.: Neurohemodynamics of pulmonary edema. II. The role of sympathetic pathways in the elevation of pulmonary and systemic vascular pressures following the intracisternal injection of fibrin. Circulation *6*:51, 1952.
94. Theodore, J., and Robin, E. D.: Speculations on neurogenic pulmonary edema (NPE). Am. Rev. Respir. Dis. *113*:405, 1976.
95. Wray, N. P., and Nicotra, M. B.: Pathogenesis of neurogenic pulmonary edema. Am. Rev. Respir. Dis. *118*:783, 1978.
96. Hakim, T. S., van der Zee, H., and Malik, A. B.: Effects of sympathetic nerve stimulation on lung fluid and protein exchange. J. Appl. Physiol. *47*:1025, 1979.
97. Simon, R. P., Bayne, L. L., Tranbaugh, R. F., and Lewis, F. R.: Elevated pulmonary lymph flow and protein content during status epilepticus in sheep. J. Appl. Physiol. *52*:91, 1982.
98. Steinberg, A. D., and Karliner, J. S.: The clinical spectrum of heroin pulmonary edema. Arch. Intern. Med. *122*:122, 1968.
99. Fraser, D. W.: Methadone overdose: Illicit use of pharmaceutically prepared narcotics. J.A.M.A. *217*:1387, 1971.
100. Bogartz, L. J., and Miller, W. C.: Pulmonary edema associated with propoxyphene intoxication. J.A.M.A. *215*:259, 1971.
101. Richter, R. W., Baden, M. N., and Pearson, J.: Cerebral edema seen in many "sudden death" heroin victims. J.A.M.A. *212*:967, 1970.
102. Jaffe, J. H.: Narcotic analgesics. *In* Goodman, L. S., and Gilman, A. (eds.): The Pharmacological Basis of Therapeutics. 4th ed. New York, Macmillan, 1970, p. 237.
103. Katz, S., Aberman, A., Frand, U. I., Stein, I. M., and Fulop, M.: Heroin pulmonary edema: Evidence for increased pulmonary capillary permeability. Am. Rev. Respir. Dis. *106*:472, 1972.
104. Gopinathan, K., Saroja, D., Spears, J. R., Gelb, A., and Emmanuel, G. E.: Hemodynamic studies in heroin induced acute pulmonary edema. Circulation *42* (Suppl. 3):44, 1970.
105. Brashear, R. E., Kelly, M. T., and White, A. C.: Elevated plasma histamine after heroin and morphine. J. Lab. Clin. Med. *83*:451, 1974.
106. Malik, A. B., Tahamont, M. V., Minnear, F. L., Johnson, A., and Kaplan, J.

E.: Lung fluid and protein exchange after pulmonary vascular thrombosis. Chest *81*:5, 1982.
107. Johnson, A., and Malik, A. B.: Effect of defibrinogenation on lung water accumulation after pulmonary microembolism in dogs. J. Appl. Physiol. *49*:841, 1980.
108. Flick, M. R., Perel, A., and Staub, N. C.: Leukocytes are required for increased lung microvascular permeability after microembolization in sheep. Circ. Res. *48*:344, 1981.
109. Rovinsky, J. J., and Guttmacher, A. F.: Medical, Surgical, and Gynecologic Complications of Pregnancy. 2nd ed. Baltimore, Williams and Wilkins Co., 1965.
110. Resnekow, L., and McDonald, L.: Complications in 220 patients with cardiac dysrhythmias treated by phased direct current shock and indications for electroconversion. Br. Heart J. *29*:926, 1967.
111. Cooperman, L. H., and Price, H. L.: Pulmonary edema in the operative and postoperative period: A review of 40 cases. Ann. Surg. *172*:883, 1970.
112. Rittenhouse, E. A., and Merendino, K. A.: Acute pulmonary edema in the absence of left ventricular failure. Circulation *40*:823, 1969.
113. Culliford, A. T., Thomas, S., and Spencer, F. C.: Fulminating noncardiogenic pulmonary edema: A newly recognized hazard during cardiac operations. J. Thorac. Cardiovasc. Surg. *80*:868, 1980.
114. Teichmann, V., Jezek, V., and Herles, F.: Relevance of width of right descending branch of pulmonary artery as a radiological sign of pulmonary hypertension. Thorax *25*:91, 1970.
115. Hogg, J. C., Agarawal, J. B., Gardiner, A. J. S., Palmer, W. H., and Macklem, P. T.: Distribution of airway resistance with developing pulmonary edema in dogs. J. Appl. Physiol. *32*:20, 1972.
116. DeTroyer, A., Yernault, J., and Englert, M.: Mechanics of breathing in patients with atrial septal defect. Am. Rev. Respir. Dis. *115*:413, 1977.
117. Fillmore, S. J., Giumaraes, A. C., Scheidt, S. S., and Killip, T.: Blood gas changes and pulmonary hemodynamics following acute myocardial infarction. Circulation *45*:583, 1972.
118. Aberman, A., and Fulop, M.: The metabolic and respiratory acidosis of acute pulmonary edema. Ann. Intern. Med. *76*:173, 1972.
119. Richeson, J. F., Paulshock, C., and Yu, P. N.: Non-hydrostatic pulmonary edema after coronary artery ligation in dogs. Circ. Res. *50*:301, 1982.
120. Timmis, A. D., Fowler, M. B., Burwood, R. J., Gishen, P., Vincent, R., and Chamberlain, D. A.: Pulmonary oedema without critical increase in left atrial pressure in acute myocardial infarction. Br. Med. J. *283*:636, 1981.
121. Vismara, L. A., Leaman, D. M., and Zelis, R.: The effects of morphine on venous tone in patients with acute pulmonary edema. Circulation *54*:335, 1976.
122. Iff, H. W., and Flenley, D. C.: Blood-gas exchange after furosemide in acute pulmonary edema. Lancet *1*:616, 1971.
123. Scheinman, M., Brown, M., and Rapaport, E.: Hemodynamic effects of ethacrynic acid in patients with refractory acute left ventricular failure. Am. J. Med. *50*:291, 1971.
124. Dikshit, K., Vyden, J. K., Forrester, J. S., Chatterjee, K., Prakash, R., and Swan, H. J. C.: Renal and extrarenal hemodynamic effects of furosemide in congestive heart failure after acute myocardial infarction. N. Engl. J. Med. *288*: 1087, 1973.
125. Wilson, J. R., Reichek, N., Dunkman, W. B., and Goldberg, S.: Effect of diuresis on the performance of the failing left ventricle in man. Am. J. Med. *70*: 234, 1981.
126. Mitenko, P. A., and Ogilvie, R. I.: Rational intravenous doses of theophylline. N. Engl. J. Med. *289*:600, 1973.
127. Tai, E., and Read, J.: Response of blood gas tensions to aminophylline and isoprenaline in patients with asthma. Thorax *22*:543, 1967.
128. Hildner, F. J.: Pulmonary edema associated with low left ventricular filling pressures. Am. J. Cardiol. *44*:1410, 1979.
129. Rizk, N. W., and Murray, J. F. : PEEP and pulmonary edema. Am. J. Med. *72*:381, 1982.
130. Cassidy, S. S., and Mitchell, J. H.: Effects of positive pressure breathing on right and left ventricular preload and afterload. Fed. Proc. *40*:2178, 1981.
131. Jardin, F., Farcot, J.-C., Boisante, L., Curien, N., Margairaz, A., and Bourdarias, J.-P.: Influence of positive end-expiratory pressure on left ventricular performance. N. Engl. J. Med. *304*:387, 1981.
132. Lorell, B. H., Palacios, I., Daggett, W. M., Jacobs, M. L., Fowler, B. N., and Newell, J. B.: Right ventricular distension and left ventricular compliance. Am. J. Physiol. *240*:H87, 1981.
133. Wead, W. B., and Norton, J. F.: Effects of intrapleural pressure changes on canine left ventricular function. J. Appl. Physiol. *50*:1027, 1981.
134. Fewell, J. E., Abendschein, D. R., Carlson, C. J., Rapaport, E., and Murray, J. F.: Continuous positive-pressure ventilation does not alter ventricular pressure-volume relationship. Am. J. Physiol. *240*:H821, 1981.
135. Pontoppidan, H., Wilson, R. S., Rie, M. A., and Schneider, R. C.: Respiratory intensive care. Anesthesiology *47*:96, 1977.
136. Prewitt, R. M., McCarthy, J., and Wood, L. D. H.: Treatment of acute low pressure pulmonary edema in dogs: Relative effects of hydrostatic and oncotic pressure, nitroprusside, and positive end-expiratory pressure. J. Clin. Invest. *67*: 409, 1981.
137. Lowe, R. J., and Moss, G. S.: Pulmonary failure after trauma. Surg. Annu. *8*: 63, 1976.
138. Tullis, J. L.: Albumin. I. Background and use. J.A.M.A. *237*:355 and 460, 1977.

18 CARDIAC AND NONCARDIAC FORMS OF ACUTE CIRCULATORY FAILURE (SHOCK)

by Burton E. Sobel, M.D.

Viewed quite simply, the systemic circulation comprises a pump (the left ventricle) in series with a compliant system of conduits (the arteries) that direct blood to the resistance vessels (the arterioles), which in turn lead to a network of vessels in which exchange of gas and metabolites occurs (the capillary bed) and then to a capacitance system (the venous bed) that returns the blood to the right atrium. *Circulatory failure* occurs when transport of blood through this circuit is not sufficient to provide oxygen and nutrients to vital organs or to remove accumulating metabolites at rates commensurate with metabolic requirements. *Transient* circulatory failure, occurring, for example, as a consequence of brief asystole, is frequently manifested by syncope, discussed in Chapter 28. Circulatory failure that results from depression of cardiac function and gives rise to maldistribution of the vascular volume with accumulation of blood in the systemic and/or pulmonary venous beds is termed *congestive heart failure* and is discussed in Chapters 13 and 15. Acute severe circulatory failure, regardless of etiology, has been termed *shock.* Cardiac function may be normal, at least initially, in many forms of circulatory failure, such as those that occur when the vascular volume is inadequate or when vascular tone is impaired.

The common denominator of shock, regardless of its etiology, is *reduction of blood flow to vital organs* due to reduction of total cardiac output or maldistribution of flow or both. Although specific entities give rise to shock with disparate clinical and hemodynamic characteristics, shock is often associated with profound arterial hypotension, restlessness and impaired cerebration, diminished urine output, and tachypnea. Depression of the central nervous system with somnolence is typically observed, and in late stages, coma ensues.

Laboratory findings may differ depending on the specific etiology, and the stage at which the patient is being studied, but profound derangements are generally evident. Hemodilution occurs in hemorrhagic shock when sufficient time has elapsed to permit the transfer of interstitial fluid into the vascular space, but hemoconcentration is characteristic of shock due to dehydration or loss of vascular volume accompanying conditions such as burns or acute pancreatitis. Hyperglycemia resulting from diminished pancreatic perfusion and from the effects of epinephrine on glycogenolysis is common. Accumulation of H^+ and lactate in hypoperfused organs and consequently in the blood contributes to systemic acidosis along with accumulation of other anions because of impaired renal excretion. Tests of renal and liver function are abnormal, arteriovenous oxygen differences are typically elevated when cardiac output is reduced, and pH and the chest roentgenogram may exhibit infiltration and edema associated with "shock lung." When the shock state is associated with infection with gram-negative organisms, there may be increased cardiac output early in the course and a reduced arteriovenous oxygen difference due to arteriovenous shunting. Respiratory alkalosis with a depressed pCO_2 is frequently superimposed on the metabolic acidosis, since the respiratory system is driven by acidemia and by reflex responses to altered fluid in the lung. Disseminated intravascular coagulation with severe thrombocytopenia sometimes occurs. Increased blood viscosity and aggregation of erythrocytes may aggravate hypoperfusion of the microcirculation.[1–7]

ETIOLOGY AND PROGNOSIS

Although the clinical syndrome of shock results from multiple pathophysiological mechanisms, it is convenient to characterize shock in terms of the primary etiology (Table 18–1). Even such a simple classification, which divides the etiology of shock into four categories—cardiogenic, obstructive, oligemic, and distributive—emphasizes the diversity of etiologies leading to shock, and within a single category of shock, the dominant physiological derangements change as a function of time and therapy. Thus, we are faced with a complex array of syndromes with varying hemodynamic characteristics. In addition, elements of more than one etiology are frequently present simultaneously in an individual patient. However, as already stated, *the common denominator of all forms and etiologies of shock is impaired perfusion of and oxygen delivery to vital organs.*

Although prolonged shock from any cause is incompatible with survival, prompt and appropriate intervention can reverse most forms of shock rapidly. A wide variety of responses to treatment can be expected. At one end of the spectrum is the young, otherwise healthy person who experiences acute, massive hemorrhage and for whom adequate blood replacement is provided promptly. If bleeding can be controlled quickly and the complications of transfusion can be avoided, survival, restitution of normal hemodynamics, and no permanent sequelae can be anticipated. At the other end of the spectrum is the elderly patient with multisystem disease and cardiogenic shock due to acute myocardial infarction; this condition is associated with an extremely high mortality (75 to 90 per cent) despite therapy.[6–8] Survival in conditions such as endotoxin shock ranges from 40 to 80 per cent[9–11] and appears to be dependent upon factors such as the age and sex of the patient, the duration of shock prior to specific therapy, the specific infecting organisms, appropriate selection of antibiotic therapy, hepatic function, and the status of the immune system. In all forms of shock, survival is inversely related to the duration of hypoperfusion and is improved by therapy aimed at correcting both the cause, such as myocardi-

TABLE 18–1 ETIOLOGIES OF SHOCK

Cardiogenic

1. Secondary to arrhythmias
   a. Bradyarrhythmias
   b. Tachyarrhythmias
2. Secondary to cardiac mechanical factors
   a. Regurgitant lesions
      (1) Acute mitral or aortic regurgitation
      (2) Rupture of interventricular septum
      (3) Massive left ventricular aneurysm
   b. Obstructive lesions
      (1) Left ventricular outflow tract obstruction, e.g., congenital or acquired valvular aortic stenosis and hypertrophic obstructive cardiomyopathy
      (2) Left ventricular inflow tract obstruction, e.g., mitral stenosis, left atrial myxoma, atrial thrombus
3. Myopathic
   a. Impairment of left ventricular contractility, as in acute myocardial infarction or congestive cardiomyopathy
   b. Impairment of right ventricular contractility due to right ventricular infarction
   c. Impairment of left ventricular relaxation or compliance as in restrictive or hypertrophic cardiomyopathy

Obstructive (due to factors extrinsic to cardiac values and myocardium)

1. Pericardial tamponade
2. Coarctation of aorta
3. Pulmonary embolism
4. Primary pulmonary hypertension

Oligemic

1. Hemorrhage
2. Fluid depletion or sequestration due to vomiting, diarrhea, dehydration, diabetes mellitus, diabetes insipidus, adrenal cortical failure, peritonitis, pancreatitis, burns, ascites, villous adenoma, or pheochromocytoma

Distributive

1. Septicemic
   a. Endotoxic
   b. Secondary to specific infection, such as dengue fever
2. Metabolic or toxic
   a. Renal failure
   b. Hepatic failure
   c. Severe acidosis or alkalosis
   d. Drug overdose
   e. Heavy metal intoxication
   f. Toxic shock syndrome (possibly due to a staphylococcal exotoxin)
   g. Malignant hyperthermia
3. Endocrinologic
   a. Uncontrolled diabetes mellitus with ketoacidosis or hyperosmolar coma
   b. Adrenal cortical failure
   c. Hypothyroidism
   d. Hyper- or hypoparathyroidism
   e. Diabetes insipidus
   f. Hypoglycemia secondary to excess exogenous insulin or a beta-cell tumor
4. Microcirculatory impairment due to altered blood viscosity
   a. Polycythemia vera
   b. Hyperviscosity syndromes, including multiple myeloma, macroglobulinemia, and cryoglobulinemia
   c. Sickle cell anemia
   d. Fat emboli
5. Neurogenic
   a. Cerebral
   b. Spinal
   c. Dysautonomic
6. Anaphylactic

al failure or septicemia, and the manifestations, such as hypoxemia and acidemia.

STAGES OF SHOCK

Oligemic shock has been divided into reversible and irreversible stages. This type of shock reflects decreased tissue perfusion due to diminished effective blood volume and is manifested by systemic hypotension and tachycardia. It is almost always reversible early in its course. Thus, patients suffering from simple hemorrhage and exhibiting profound hypotension when first seen respond dramatically to prompt replacement of blood and may show no sequelae of the insult after several days. Early in the evolution of such a process, compensatory mechanisms are called into play in part as a response to declining systemic arterial and right-sided filling pressures and to acidosis. Compensation usually fails if blood volume depletion exceeds 20 per cent, at which time systemic manifestations of shock, including hypotension and tachycardia, appear and are accompanied by progressive manifestations of injury to vital organs.[12] Although integrated reflex and neurohumoral control of the peripheral circulation may protect the patient during the early stages of shock, it may also mask the underlying disorder unless there is reason for a high index of suspicion. Accordingly, the nature of such compensation merits special consideration.

When systemic arterial pressure falls, decreased afferent activity emanates from baroreceptors in the carotid and aortic arteries.[13] Under physiological conditions, increased afferent activity in the baroreceptors inhibits sympathoadrenal efferent activity and vasoconstrictor tone and augments parasympathetic efferent activity to the heart via the vagi. In hypotension, this inhibition of the sympathoadrenal system is withdrawn, and vagal efferent activity is enhanced. Reflex vasoconstriction, tachycardia, and augmented cardiac output result, reflecting the increases in rate and contractility.[14]

Reflex responses are also modulated by afferent impulses originating in the atrial and ventricular myocardium.[15,16] Vagal afferent fibers from the heart and coronary vascular bed may be stimulated by metabolites accumulating locally or by changes in stretch or pressure.[17–20] Chemical, pharmacological, or electrical stimulation of selected afferents in the left ventricle elicits bradycardia as well as arterial and venous dilation,[17] possibly contributing to the syncope and exacerbation of hypotension associated with some forms of cardiogenic shock. Stimulation of other ventricular afferents gives rise to reflex tachycardia, increased contractility, and sympathetic vasoconstrictor impulses to the kidneys.

Stretch receptors in the atria and in the cavae (involved in the Bainbridge reflex) influence the flow of sympathetic impulses to the heart and kidneys as well as the secretion of antidiuretic hormone (ADH) (p. 462). Thus, shock in which left atrial pressure is elevated, i.e., cardiogenic shock, may be accompanied by renal vasodilatation, decreased circulating ADH, and a relative preservation of normal urine output, in contrast to shock in which left atrial pressure is low, which may be accompanied by profound renal vasoconstriction, high ADH levels, and therefore oliguria out of proportion to the reduction of renal perfusion. Secretion of both ADH and aldosterone is influenced by reflexes involving stretch receptors in the right atrium (p. 462). Thus, decreased stretch augments efferent renal sympathetic activity, increases renin secretion and consequently angiotensin II concentration, and ultimately increases aldosterone secretion, which tends to limit excretion of sodium and water and thereby maintains blood volume.

In concert, the reflex response to hypotension resulting from oligemia is compensatory, since the decline in perfusion pressure of vital organs is limited by vasoconstriction, tachycardia, and augmented cardiac contractility. However, redistribution of blood flow occurs as well. In many forms of shock, cutaneous, skeletal muscle, renal, and splanchnic perfusion decrease primarily because of vasoconstriction mediated by the rich alpha-adrenergic innervation of the arterioles supplying these organs.[21]

Reflex responses to oligemia also result in characteristic humoral changes. Plasma renin activity increases as a consequence of sympathetic stimulation of the juxtaglomerular apparatus as well as the direct response of the kidney to reduced glomerular filtration. Elevated circulating angiotensin II contributes to maintenance of systemic vascular resistance along with the markedly increased circulating catecholamines released from the adrenal medulla and nerve endings. Elaboration of aldosterone released in response to angiotensin II, and of ADH released in response to reflex stimulation mediated by a reduction of atrial pressure, potentiates maintenance of vascular volume and systemic arterial pressure. Vasoactive prostaglandins, catabolized by the lung under physiological conditions, may accumulate. Together, these substances affect hemodynamics not only by influencing vascular volume and tone but also by modulating central and peripheral adrenergic activity.[22–27]

When oligemia is so severe that compensatory mechanisms cannot maintain adequate pressure for perfusion of vital organs, or when the metabolic derangements overpower compensatory mechanisms, decompensation occurs, manifested by a marked decline in systemic arterial pressure, diminished cardiac output, and the biochemical changes of ischemia and hypoxia in vital organs (Fig. 18–1). Anaerobic glycolysis compensates for diminished oxygen delivery and leads to the production of lactate and its elaboration from skeletal muscle, liver, and other organs into the circulation, resulting in progressive lactic acidosis. Diminished hepatic metabolism of circulating lactate, coupled with decreased renal excretion, potentiates the acidosis. Impaired pulmonary function causes hypoxemia, and the ensuing ventilatory response, mediated reflexly by chemoreceptor stimulation, leads to hypocapnia. Hyperglycemia in response to catecholamine stimulation of glycogenolysis, coupled with inhibition of insulin release, is a typical finding until glycogen stores are depleted, at which point hypoglycemia may supervene. Despite the lipolytic actions of catecholamines, the concentration of circulating free fatty acids may fall, possibly because of limited perfusion of adipose tissue. In endotoxic shock, hypertriglyceridemia may be prominent, possibly because of depressed lipoprotein lipase activity in adipose tissue and the myocardium.[28]

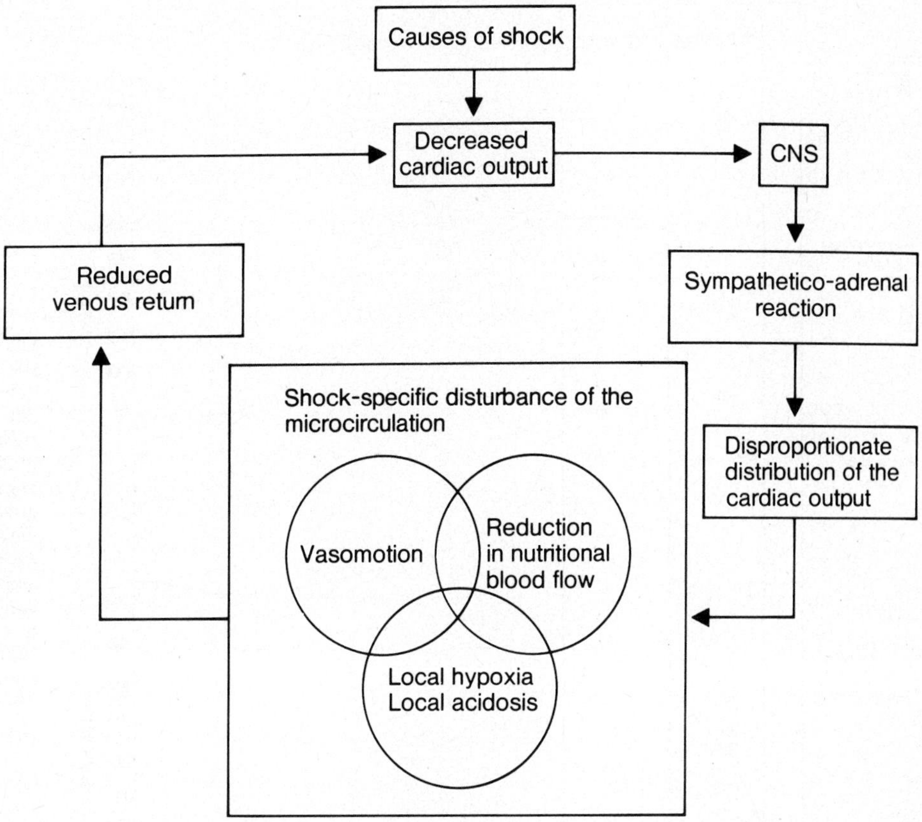

FIGURE 18–1 Diagram depicting the vicious circle typically manifested in shock associated with a low cardiac output. Regardless of etiology, impairment of vasomotor tone mediated by manifestations of tissue hypoxia including local acidosis contributes to reduced venous return and consequent further diminution of cardiac output with progressive reduction of effective vascular volume and perfusion of vital organs, including the heart itself. An analogous picture evolves even when the shock state is initially associated with a high cardiac output, such as in cases of distributive shock due to sepsis. Under these conditions, reduction of effective vascular volume ultimately compromises cardiac output progressively. (From Messmer, K.: Pathophysiological aspects and problems of shock. Triangle, *13*:85, 1974.)

Circulating levels of lysosomal hydrolases increase not only because of liberation of these enzymes from damaged ischemic cells, primarily in splanchnic organs, but also because of impaired function of the reticuloendothelial system—an important site of enzyme removal under physiological conditions.[29–32]

COMPENSATED AND DECOMPENSATED SHOCK

In animals subjected to hemorrhage, a phenomenon referred to as "taking up" can be demonstrated. When blood pressure is reduced profoundly by bleeding, but this blood is reinfused within one to two hours, restoration of circulatory integrity can be anticipated. However, if the interval of hypotension is prolonged, reinfusion of blood is not associated with a corresponding augmentation of arterial pressure. Thus, vasodilatation within some elements of the vascular bed leads to pooling of blood, and augmentation of blood volume fails to increase the "effective" vascular volume, i.e., the blood that actually perfuses metabolizing tissues.[33]

It has been difficult to delineate the mechanisms involved in the *irreversibility* of shock in humans because of generalizations derived from experimental animal models, in which the responsible factors may be quite different. For example, in dogs subjected to hemorrhage, irreversibility appears to be related to associated endotoxemia and its sequelae. Loss of the intestinal epithelium's barrier function to bacteria and bacterial products is the putative factor.[34] However, irreversible shock occurs in germ-free animals,[35] and evidence to corroborate an endotoxic mechanism in oligemic shock in man has been lacking.

Irreversibility of shock has also been attributed to the effects of numerous humoral agents, many of which seem to be released from cells subjected to ischemia (Fig. 18–2), including histamine,[36] serotonin, kinins, lactate, hydrogen ions, proteases, catecholamines, prostaglandins, angiotensin II, and lysosomal enzymes.[22–27,37–39] A decline in plasma histaminase activity may account, in part, for the increased concentrations of circulating histamine.[39] Physiological decompensation may be mediated in part by late inhibition of adrenergic vascular control due to inhibitory actions of prostaglandins on the peripheral adrenergic nervous system.[40] Thus, inhibitors of prostaglandin synthesis help to maintain vascular tone in animal preparations subjected to shock.

Marked and sustained increases in the blood levels of vasopressin and angiotensin II accompany hemorrhagic shock.[23,41–43] Both of these hormones are powerful constrictors of the mesenteric vascular bed and may contribute to ischemia of the gut and liver, potentially contributing to irreversibility. Administration of a nonapeptide that blocks conversion of angiotensin I to angiotensin II (the physiologically active moiety) precluded the development of intense vasoconstriction and increased the survival of dogs subjected to hemorrhage. In addition, administration of the angiotensin-converting inhibitor to dogs with experimentally induced diabetes insipidus maintained peripheral vascular conductance and cardiac output in the face of hemorrhage. Accordingly, prevention of intense mesenteric vasoconstriction mediated by angiotensin II and ADH ap-

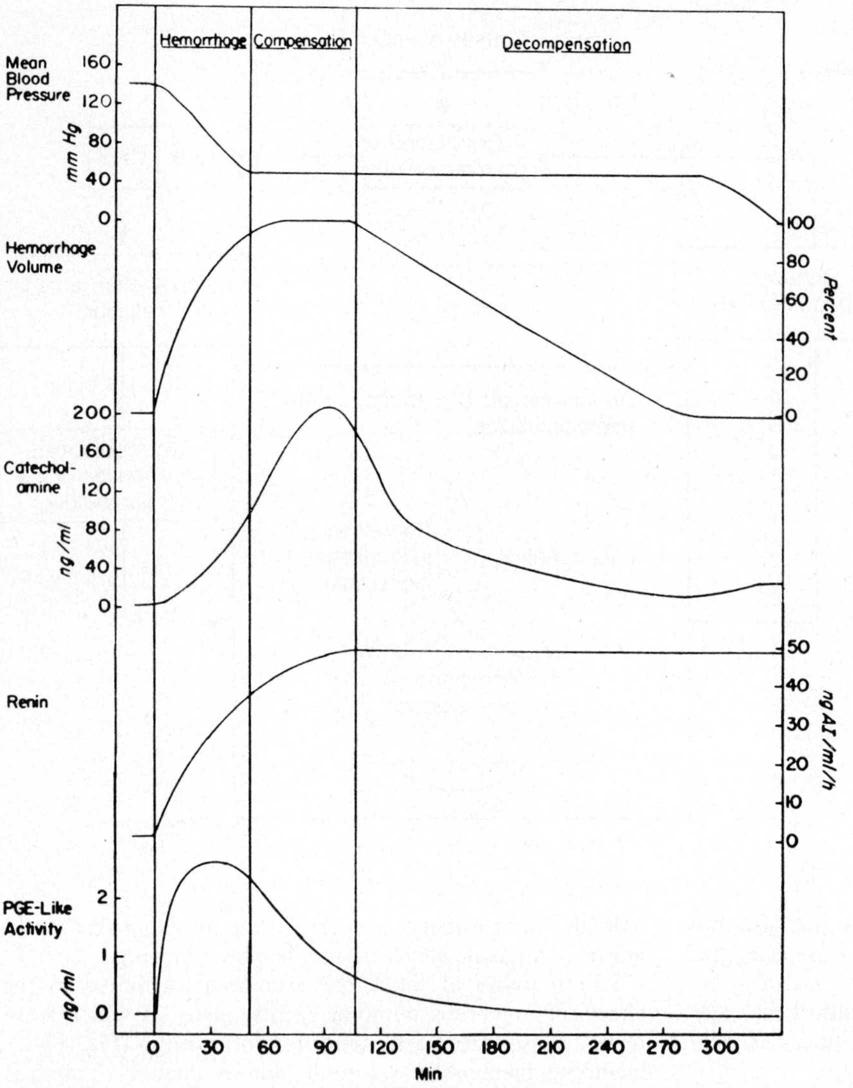

FIGURE 18–2 Diagrammatic representation of the characteristic temporal profile of plasma catecholamines, renin, and prostaglandin E (PGE)–like activity in dogs subjected to hemorrhage sufficient to induce a decline of mean arterial blood pressure to approximately 50 mm Hg. Decompensation (manifested by the need for progressive infusion of blood to maintain the same mean arterial pressure) was characterized by an associated decline in levels of plasma catecholamines and PGE-like activity but a persistent elevation of plasma renin activity. (From Jakschik, B. A., et al.: Profile of circulating vasoactive substances in hemorrhagic shock and their pharmacologic manipulation. J. Clin. Invest. *54*:842, 1974.)

pears to be protective in the canine model of hemorrhagic shock.

Several observations also suggest that shock is mediated in part by endorphins released from the pituitary gland,[44] since opiate antagonists such as naloxone maintain hemodynamics and prolong survival in experimental animals subjected to hemorrhagic shock.[45,46] Thromboxanes have also been implicated because of the elevated levels which occur, the prevalence of disseminated intravascular coagulation, and the protective effects of thromboxane synthetase inhibitors in endotoxic shock in animals.[47,48] Prostacyclin (PGI_2), a physiological antagonist of thromboxane A_2, may reverse lethal endotoxemia under some circumstances,[49] and both PGI_2 and PGI_2-analogs are undergoing clinical trials for evaluation of treatment of shock.

Ischemia due to hypoperfusion is responsible for profound organ damage in shock. Mucosal lesions in the small intestine occur in patients as well as in experimental animals in shock.[50] Ultrastructural alterations in pancreatic tissue from patients in shock are more likely due to the direct effects of ischemia than to injury mediated by activation of lysosomal enzymes.[51] Damage to the renal tubules with back-diffusion of glomerular filtrate as well as redistribution of renal blood flow contributes to oliguria.[52,53] The resting transmembrane potential of skeletal muscle declines in hemorrhagic shock, a finding indicative of impaired membrane transport function secondary to ischemia.[54]

Disseminated intravascular coagulation, induced by thromboplastic substances released into the circulation,[4] may also play an important role in potentiating regional ischemia by impairing flow through the microcirculation. This may be accentuated by arteriolar and venular constriction, even though perfusion pressure is maintained.

It appears likely that irreversible shock results from destruction of cells in vital organs due to the combined effects of ischemia and of noxious circulating and local metabolites. The onset of irreversible shock in animals correlates with accumulated oxygen debt exceeding 120 ml/kg of body weight.[55]

ROLE OF THE HEART IN IRREVERSIBLE SHOCK. Prolonged shock, regardless of its etiology, leads to impairment of cardiac function (Fig. 18–3). Adequate ventricular function is dependent on aerobic metabolism of the myocardium, which like any other organ, is dependent on an adequate oxygen supply. In experimental animals in which the oxygen delivered to the heart can be manipulated by changes in the hemoglobin content of the blood, impaired ventricular performance in association with hemorrhagic shock has been directly related to oxy-

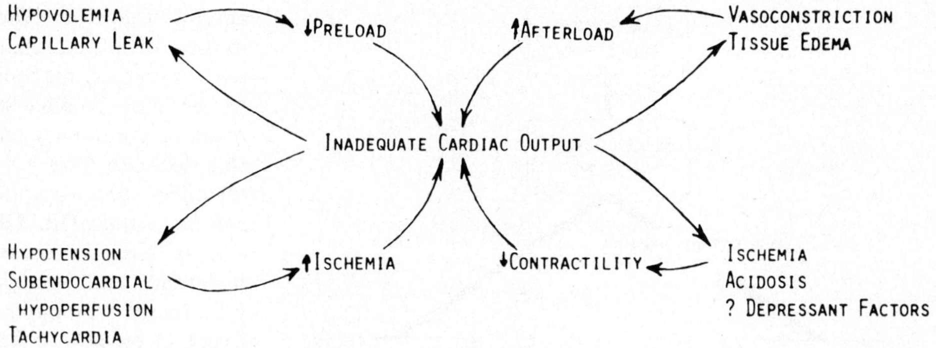

FIGURE 18–3 The interaction of factors that compromise cardiac output in noncardiac shock syndromes. The inadequate preload, consequent to hypovolemia, capillary damage, or failure of vascular autoregulation, initiates a series of responses that further compromises cardiac output and tissue perfusion, ultimately leading to microcirculatory failure. (Reproduced with permission from Shine, K. I.: Aspects of the management of shock. Ann. Intern. Med. *93*:723, 1980.)

gen availability.[56–58] Depletion of cellular ATP may lead to irreversible myocardial injury through several mechanisms, including failure to maintain cation transport, with consequent cell swelling, or activation of lytic enzymes capable of degrading cell membranes.

Although contributing factors such as metabolic acidosis, loss of sympathetic stimulation to the heart,[59] circulating myocardial depressant factors,[60] and limited substrate availability[61] may all play a role in the impairment of myocardial contractility in shock, irreversibility of shock from any cause may depend in part on deterioration of cardiac function.[62,63] Preservation of myocardial function may be afforded by calcium antagonists such as verapamil, which exert favorable hemodynamic and metabolic effects and prolong survival in dogs subjected to hemorrhagic shock.[64] Since the coronary vascular bed can be constricted by alpha-adrenergic stimulation[65] (p. 1242), with resultant diminution of myocardial oxygen availability, the massive adrenergic stimulation that accompanies shock may contribute to the limitation of myocardial oxygen availability, which impairs cardiac performance and leads in turn to irreversibility.

EFFECTS OF SHOCK ON TARGET ORGANS

It is convenient to consider the pathophysiology of shock in terms of the initiating cause(s), the effects of the shock state on target organs, and the vicious circles that contribute to perpetuation and progression of the syndrome. Before considering specific categories of shock classified according to initiating cause (Table 18–1), the effects on target organs are discussed.

THE LUNG (See also page 566)

Pulmonary failure is one of the most important potentially lethal complications of shock. (Prior to the use of dialysis, renal failure predominated in this regard.) Indeed, among patients with noncardiogenic shock, pulmonary failure is the most common cause of death, affecting an estimated 150,000 patients annually with a case fatality rate exceeding 50 per cent.[66] Atelectasis and infection are contributing but probably not primary factors. The syndrome, now frequently referred to as the adult respiratory distress syndrome (ARDS), shock lung, post-transfusion lung, or stiff lung, cannot be explained in simple terms. Distressingly often, ARDS follows shock, regardless of its etiology, within 24 to 72 hours,[67] although most frequently it follows massive hemorrhage or trauma. Interstitial and alveolar pulmonary edema are the hallmarks of ARDS. Pathogenetic factors include (1) increased permeability of the alveolar-capillary membrane; (2) increased capillary hydrostatic pressure; (3) decreased plasma oncotic pressure; (4) interference with function of the pulmonary lymphatics, especially by depressant drugs or anesthetics; (5) deficient production of surfactant (Fig. 18–4);[68] (6) loss of alveolar type I cells, and their replacement with type II cells; (7) capillary obliteration; and, as a late event, (8) extensive fibrosis.[66] In addition to shock, exposure of the lung to high concentrations of inspired oxygen or other toxins causes similar injury to the alveolar-capillary membrane.[69]

The initial phase of ARDS may occur when cardiac output is still depressed or has already been restored after having been depressed. Interstitial edema accompanied by hypocapnia is an important initial finding. Factors responsible for this early accumulation of fluid in the lungs include (1) an increase in the permeability of the pulmonary capillaries to plasma proteins secondary to the effects of ischemia on the lung, with platelet aggregation, oxygen toxicity, and deleterious humoral stimuli playing contributory roles;[70] (2) a lowering of plasma oncotic pressure, sometimes potentiated by the administration of excessive volumes of crystalloid solutions; and (3) an elevated pulmonary capillary pressure. In addition, complement-mediated aggregation of neutrophils, associated with release of proteases and potentially responsive to administration of corticosteroids, contributes to pulmonary capillary stasis and endothelial injury.[66,71] Once protein has extravasated into the pulmonary interstitial or alveolar space, its oncotic pressure may enhance further accumulation of fluid.

ARDS is characterized by tachypnea and diffuse, bilateral inspiratory rales in association with severe hypoxemia and radiographic opacification of both lung fields.[72–77] Pulmonary compliance and functional residual capacity are both reduced, and ventilation-perfusion ratios are altered markedly, causing venous admixture and, as the process becomes more advanced, intrapulmonary right-to-left shunting, a condition in which the depressed arterial pO_2 is not responsive to ventilation with 100 per cent O_2. Although ischemia of the alveolar-capillary membrane alone does not appear to give rise to ARDS, the pathophysiology does appear to reflect increased membrane permeability

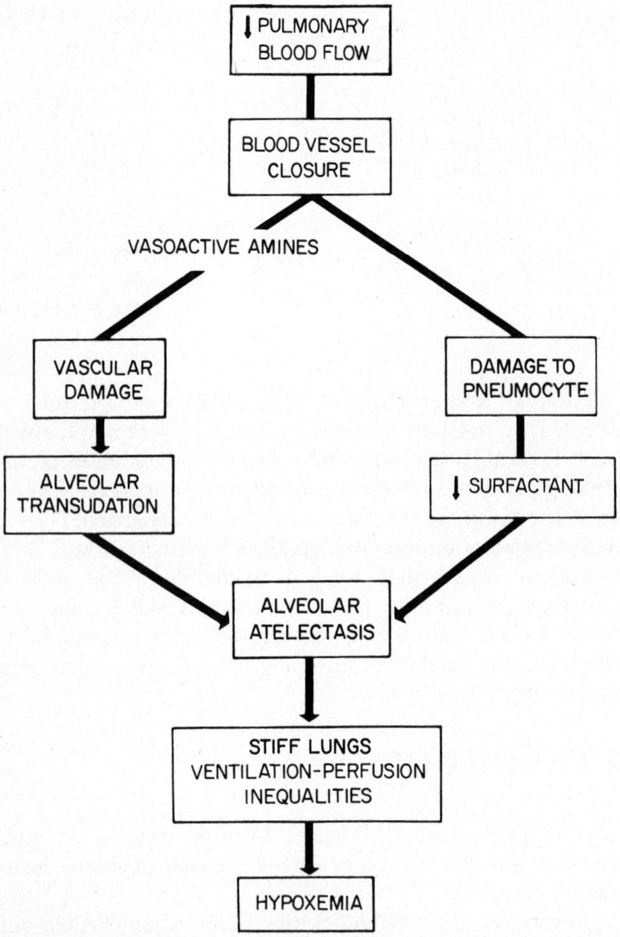

FIGURE 18–4 Pathways involved in the genesis of adult respiratory distress syndrome (ARDS) accompanying shock. (From Kones, R. J.: Cardiogenic Shock. New York, Futura Publishing Co., 1974.)

as well as augmented filtration due to altered pulmonary hemodynamics.[78] Exposure of the lung to bacterial insults occurring concomitantly with shock of another etiology potentiates pulmonary failure,[79] as does excessive administration of intravenous crystalloid solutions.[80,81] Impaired function of the reticuloendothelial system, reflecting, in part, deficiency of fibronectin, a serum opsonin, results in reduced clearance not only of bacterial components in septic shock but also of fibrin and fibrinogen degradation products and injured platelets—all of which contribute to formation of pulmonary edema.[82] This phenomenon has given rise to trials of the administration of fibronectin to patients with shock of diverse etiologies, including the toxic shock syndrome.[83–85] The possible role of neural stimulation in causing damage to the alveolar-capillary membrane has been suggested by studies in which unilateral pulmonary denervation conferred protection on the denervated lung in experimental animals subjected to hemorrhagic shock.[86–88] Impaired integrity of the alveolar-capillary membrane may be a consequence of the same circulating metabolites as those potentially contributing to irreversible injury in other organs.

Since solutions containing albumin or other colloids can extravasate into the lung when the integrity of the alveolar-capillary membrane has been compromised,[89] excessive administration of such fluids to patients with ARDS may actually exacerbate the syndrome. On the other hand, diminution of intravascular colloid osmotic pressure correlates with increased mortality in patients with shock (Fig. 18–5), perhaps because it is a critical factor in the development of pulmonary edema.[90,91] The mechanisms underlying this decrease have not been totally elucidated, but in some instances inappropriate administration of colloid-free fluid can be implicated. Other factors underlying the progression of ARDS include perivenular leakage, potentiated by histamine and bradykinin[92] with increased filtration and pulmonary lymphatic flow early in shock; inadequate delivery of oxygen to fulfill the high oxygen requirements of Type II alveolar cells, which are responsible for synthesis of surfactant; sequestration of platelets and polymorphonuclear leukocytes[93] with liberation of proteases; immunological factors; pulmonary vasoconstrictor effects of acidosis;[94] and consequences of decreased ventilation-perfusion ratios induced by atelectasis and edema. The suggestion that impaired production of pulmonary surfactant may underlie or contribute to ARDS is based on analysis of bronchoalveolar lavage fluid,[95] and the potential importance of pulmonary venoconstriction in the genesis of the syndrome has been demonstrated in experiments on sheep. Altered pulmonary vasoreactivity contributing to edema formation may be mediated by increased synthesis of vasodilatory prostaglandins in arteries and of thromboxane-like vasoconstrictor compounds in veins; these vasoactive substances may act directly on pulmonary vascular tissue or may alter vascular responsiveness to neurohumoral agents such as norepinephrine and serotonin.[96]

TREATMENT OF ARDS (see also p. 573). Since ARDS potentiates the severity of shock and may be lethal even if circulatory failure is corrected, aggressive therapy is required. Tracheal intubation is often necessary to prevent or treat hypoxemia and permit control of pulmonary secretions. The concentration of inhaled oxygen (FIO_2) should not be elevated above the level needed to maintain arterial pO_2 within the range of 60 to 90 mm Hg and should not

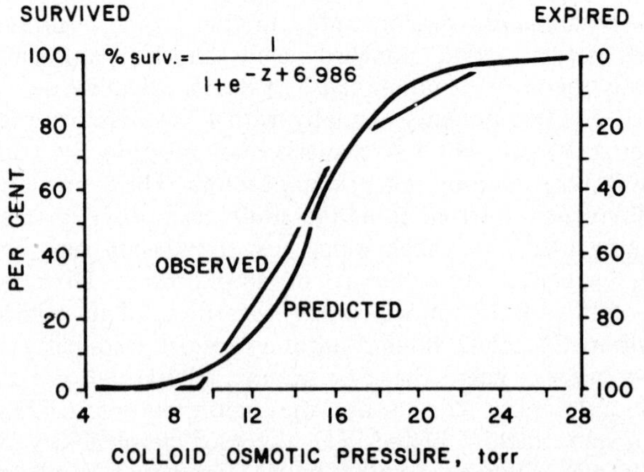

FIGURE 18–5 The relationship between survival and plasma colloid osmotic pressure among 99 patients with shock due to diverse etiologies. The mean survival time for patients who expired was 5.4 days. Based on the lowest value for colloid osmotic pressure obtained in serial determination, correct classification (survival versus mortality) was obtained with the use of the equation shown in the inset in 79 per cent of cases. (From Morissette, M., et al.: Reduction in colloid osmotic pressure associated with fatal progression of cardiopulmonary failure. Crit. Care Med. *3*:115, 1975.)

exceed 0.60. Positive end-expiratory pressure (PEEP) or continuous positive airway pressure (CPAP) may diminish intrapulmonary right-to-left shunting by recruiting previous closed alveolar units and should be employed when an FIO_2 of 0.60 fails to maintain an arterial pO_2 of 60 mm Hg.[97] The use of PEEP or CPAP in patients with ARDS may not decrease cardiac output, particularly when left ventricular end-diastolic pressure exceeds 15 mm Hg. A paradoxical increase in cardiac output may, in fact, occur because of the salutary effects of improved oxygenation of the blood on a failing left ventricle.

Maintenance of normal levels of vascular volume is desirable; colloid should not be administered in excess, and crystalloids should be administered only in volumes that replace losses. In fact, augmentation of pulmonary blood flow per se, by expansion of blood volume or administration of dopamine or isoproterenol, may accentuate venous admixture due to further mismatch of ventilation and perfusion.[98] Intravascular colloid osmotic pressure can be stabilized by the judicious intravenous administration of loop diuretics, furosemide or ethacrynic acid; the use of albumin is fraught with difficulty because of the rapidity with which it leaves the circulation and enters the pulmonary interstitium and alveoli.

Vigorous treatment of sepsis is necessary, and supportive measures designed to stabilize cardiac rhythm and function are helpful. Glucocorticoids may modify the course of the syndrome favorably, particularly when they are administered soon after the onset of the insult.[100–103] Potential benefit may also accrue from inhibition of complement-mediated neutrophil aggregation and proteolysis and an increase in lung vascular permeability.[66] Although cyclooxygenase inhibitors, anticoagulants, and fibronectin have not yet been proven helpful, they and agents that elevate serum antiprotease acitivity, such as Danazol, are being evaluated intensively.[104] When shock is treated successfully and the underlying initiating cause is removed, abnormalities of pulmonary function or sequelae of ARDS sometimes persist.[105] The value of antifibrotic agents such as penicillamine or analogs of proline has not yet been established but is under investigation.

THE HEART

CARDIAC METABOLISM IN SHOCK. Under physiological conditions, the heart derives its energy almost exclusively from oxidative processes in mitochondria (Chap. 36). Oxidation of fatty acids and pyruvate predominates, but when the supply of these preferred substrates or of oxygen is limited, aerobic glycolysis is unable to meet the heart's metabolic needs. Net glycogenolysis does not occur in well-oxygenated myocardium, even in the face of maximal adrenergic stimulation.[106] However, myocardial anoxia or ischemia leads to rapid depletion of glycogen stores mediated by the phosphorylase reaction (Fig. 18–6). Under anaerobic conditions, myocardial viability appears to depend, in part, on glycolysis, since supplementation of perfusates with glucose improves ventricular performance[107] and maintains the biochemical integrity of anoxic tissue.[108] Nevertheless, the ability of anaerobic metabolism alone to maintain high-energy phosphate stores is limited, and myo-

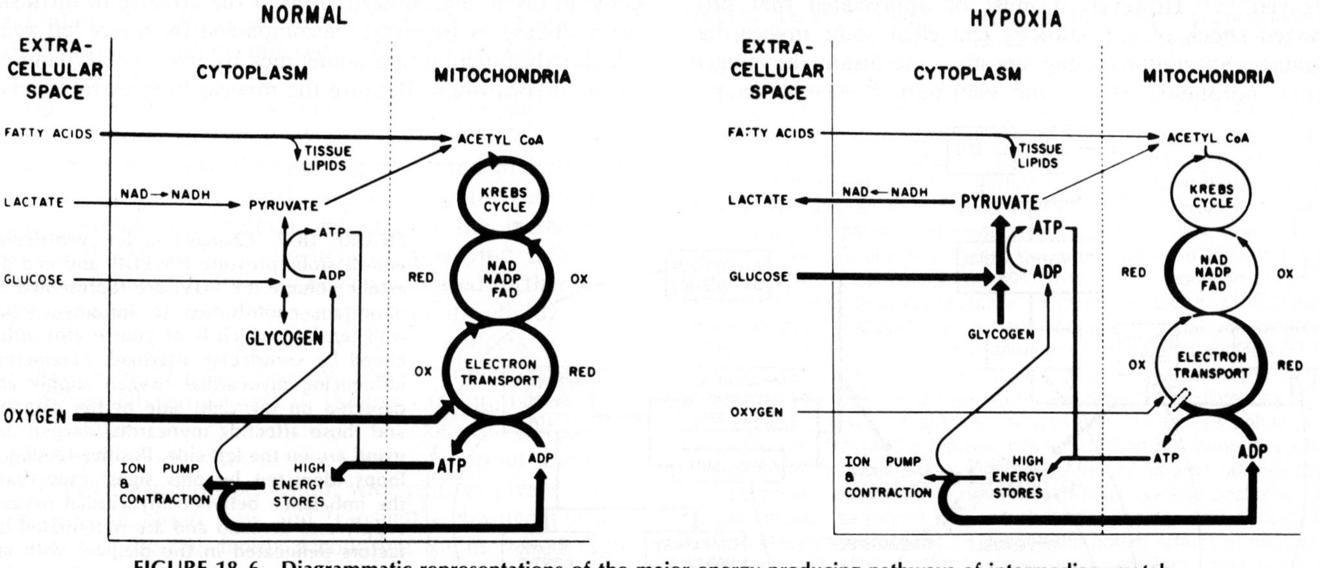

FIGURE 18–6 Diagrammatic representations of the major energy-producing pathways of intermediary metabolism in normal (left) and hypoxic (right) myocardium. Under physiological conditions, energy production depends on oxidation of fatty acids and carbohydrates, with a final common pathway being oxidation of acetyl-CoA via the tricarboxylic acid cycle (the Krebs cycle) with associated electron transport through intermediates such as reduced (RED) and sequentially oxidized (OX) pyridine nucleotides (NAD and NADP) and flavoprotein (FAD) intermediates and a final electron-acceptor role for oxygen, which is converted to water. The concomitant production of ATP permits the cell to maintain vital functions and provide chemical energy in a form suitable for mediating contraction of myofibrillar proteins. Under conditions of tissue hypoxia, such as those accompanying shock, oxidation of acetyl-CoA is inhibited because of the lack of a terminal electron acceptor (oxygen). Thus, formation of ATP depends virtually exclusively on anaerobic glycolysis, which cannot proceed beyond formation of lactate and which gives rise to a much smaller amount of ATP per mole of glucose metabolized than is the case when oxidative metabolism is present. (From Kones, R. J.: Cardiogenic Shock. New York, Futura Publishing Co., 1974.)

magnitude of hemodynamic impairment appears to be directly related to the amount of myocardium involved, with shock likely when the cumulative volume of infarcted tissue constitutes 40 per cent or more of the left ventricle. It is not yet clear whether the specific location of involved ventricular myocardium (i.e., anterior wall, diaphragmatic wall, apex, septum, etc.) is a significant determinant of the presence or absence of shock, unless specialized regions such as the conduction system or valvular supporting apparatus are involved.[204]

CLINICAL FEATURES. Cardiogenic shock accompanies myocardial infarction in 10 to 15 per cent of patients who survive sufficiently long to reach the hospital.[8,167,176,177] The primary defect is severe impairment of left ventricular contractile function with resultant circulatory failure. The patient is generally restless and confused but may be stuporous, with cool, moist skin reflecting reflex sympathetic reduction of cutaneous perfusion and stimulation of diaphoresis. Core temperature may be reduced, peripheral pulses are generally rapid and thready, arterial pressure is reduced, and pulse pressure is narrow. Early in the course, pressure may not be reduced despite profound impairment of perfusion of vital organs. Diminished urine output is characteristic, and persistent or recurrent chest pain is common.

Disturbances of cardiac rhythm of almost any type, including sinus tachycardia, ventricular tachyarrhythmias and premature complexes, sinus bradycardia, atrioventricular block, and supraventricular tachycardias, are common. In the absence of hypovolemia, the clinical features of acute pulmonary edema may be present (chap. 17) with bronchospasm, suffocating dyspnea, copious pulmonary secretions, and profound cyanosis. Rapid shallow respirations are typical, but Cheyne-Stokes respiration may supervene, especially when patients are treated aggressively with narcotics or when there is concomitant cerebrovascular disease. If right ventricular failure occurs, either consequent to pulmonary hypertension, secondary to left ventricular failure or primarily as a result of right ventricular infarction, systemic venous distention may be evident rather than the virtual absence of visible peripheral veins due to venoconstriction.

Cardiac signs include diminished intensity of heart sounds, reflecting greatly reduced contractility, the other auscultatory manifestations of acute myocardial infarction, pericarditis, papillary muscle dysfunction, or left or right ventricular failure. Cardiomegaly is common, but if there is concomitant hypovolemia, as may result from excessive prolonged diaphoresis, vomiting, or prior treatment with diuretics, the heart may not be enlarged. Laboratory findings include those associated with myocardial infarction, congestive heart failure, and shock. Thus, metabolic (often lactic) acidosis, hypocapnia and hypoxemia, hypo- or hyperkalemia and azotemia, markedly elevated activity of plasma enzymes, leukocytosis, and numerous nonspecific laboratory manifestations of massive neurohumoral stimulation and progressive organ injury are prevalent.

HEMODYNAMICS. Because impaired myocardial contractility secondary to loss of contractile mass is the primary defect responsible for the syndrome of cardiogenic shock secondary to acute myocardial infarction, cardiac output is invariably low, even when ventricular filling pressure is increased by intravenous administration of colloid. The elevation of left ventricular filling pressure[167,168] is usually in excess of that expected from the only modest increase in left ventricular end-diastolic volume because of reduction in left ventricular compliance.[179,180] In the presence of associated hypovolemia, left ventricular preload may not be adequate despite normal or even modestly elevated left ventricular end-diastolic pressure because of diminished ventricular compliance, and it may be necessary to augment ventricular filling pressure substantially above normal with the use of intravenous infusion of colloid to improve cardiac output, by taking maximum advantage of the Frank-Starling mechanism.[167,180,181]

The presence of reduced cardiac output, associated with systemic hypotension, in the face of an elevated left ventricular filling pressure, is the hallmark of cardiogenic shock. Since left ventricular filling pressure is often estimated from pulmonary artery occlusive pressure (an index of left atrial pressure), mitral regurgitation or impairment of left ventricular filling by mitral stenosis, thrombus, or tumor must be excluded to establish that the left ventricular diastolic pressure is truly elevated. The low cardiac output is associated with depressions of stroke volume, left ventricular work and isovolumetric and ejection phase indices of contractility. The elevation of pulmonary artery resistance and pressure, augmented by hypoxemia and acidosis, contribute to the development of right ventricular failure.[182]

On the other hand, right ventricular failure may also result from right ventricular infarction in the absence of marked elevation of pulmonary artery pressure. Regardless of its cause, right ventricular failure is accompanied by elevation of right atrial and central venous pressures; right ventricular failure may be complicated by tricuspid regurgitation, due either to dilatation of the tricuspid annulus or to ischemia or infarction of right ventricular papillary muscles. In the absence of right ventricular failure and despite profound cardiogenic shock, central venous pressure may be normal or only slightly elevated, and accordingly, monitoring of this parameter may be a misleading guide to therapy (Fig. 18–8).

The neurohumoral response to severe left ventricular failure usually includes an elevated systemic vascular resistance, although not all patients with cardiogenic shock exhibit peripheral vasoconstriction.[183–185] Thus, the typical hemodynamic picture of cardiogenic shock includes systolic arterial pressure less than 80 mm Hg, diastolic pressure less than 50 mm Hg, mean arterial pressure less than 60 mm Hg, mean central venous pressure greater than 9 mm Hg; pulmonary artery occlusive pressure greater than 18 mm Hg; heart rate greater than 95 beats/min; cardiac index less than 1.8 $l/min/m^2$; and total peripheral resistance greater than 2000 dyne-sec-cm^{-5}.

Pulmonary complications of cardiogenic shock are common because the same factors that affect the lung in shock of any etiology exist in this condition (p. 583) but are intensified by the pulmonary venous hypertension characteristic of cardiogenic shock. Impairment of pulmonary function exaggerates arterial hypoxemia, thereby exacerbating the functional deterioration of the heart (p. 438). The increased work of breathing in cardiogenic shock diverts an inappropriate fraction of the cardiac output to the respiratory muscles, further impairing perfusion of other beds (Fig. 54–10, p. 1789).

A variety of pharmacological agents commonly used in the treatment of patients with acute myocardial infarction exert negative inotropic effects, particularly antiarrhythmic, beta-adrenergic blocking, and central nervous system depressant agents, and the use of these drugs may contribute to the impairment of cardiac output. Tolerance of ischemic myocardium to cardiac glycosides is decreased,[186] and the vasoconstrictor actions of these compounds may influence the coronary bed itself.[187] Occult hypovolemia or unrecognized vasovagal reactions superimposed on the underlying cardiogenic process may intensify the shock and limit the efficacy of therapy directed against the primary disorder.

MANAGEMENT

(See also Chapter 38, pp. 1316 to 1318)

Primary Therapy. When cardiogenic shock is due to a mechanical defect, such as rupture of the interventricular septum, acute mitral regurgitation due to papillary muscle rupture or dysfunction, or ventricular aneurysm, primary therapy consists of surgical correction of the lesion. Unfortunately, emergency surgery is plagued by technical difficulties related to repair of tissue undergoing active necrosis, and results have been somewhat disappointing. If systemic hemodynamics can be stabilized by means of medical management or appropriate use of intraaortic balloon counterpulsation (IABP) for one week or longer, surgical results are generally more favorable.[169,188,189] In present practice, the balloon is inserted percutaneously or via an arterial cutdown into the thoracic aorta via the femoral artery. Phased pulsations synchronized with the electrocardiogram are utilized to commence inflation at the time of closure of the aortic valve and to initiate deflation just prior to the onset of systole. The augmented coronary perfusion pressure during diastole facilitates coronary blood flow, since coronary vascular resistance is minimal during this portion of the cardiac cycle (Fig. 18–10). Since the balloon is deflated throughout systole, the left ventricle ejects against a lower impedance. Hemodynamic changes generally include a 10 to 20 per cent increase in cardiac output, a reduction in systolic and increase in diastolic arterial pressure with little change in mean pressure, a diminution of heart rate, and an increase in urine output.[190–196]

Serious complications of IABP are infrequent but include damage to or perforation of the aortic wall, ischemia distal to the site of insertion of the balloon in the femoral artery, thrombocytopenia hemolysis, renal emboli, and mechanical failures such as rupture of the balloon.[197] Although left ventricular rupture has been observed in as many as 7 per cent of patients,[196] this phenomenon appears to be a manifestation of the underlying extensive transmural infarction rather than a complication of IABP itself. Use of echocardiography to evaluate the dimensions of the aorta and location and function of the balloon may help to minimize some of these complications.[198] Contraindications to IABP include aortic regurgitation and aortic aneurysm; tachyarrhythmias or irregular rhythms are relative contraindications and must be controlled for effective functioning of the device.

Unfortunately, IABP often fails to stabilize the hemodynamic status of patients with cardiogenic shock secondary to mechanical lesions, such as ventricular septal defect or mitral regurgitation, long enough to defer surgical intervention for even a few days.[190] Under these circumstances, surgery should not be deferred. In cases of emergency surgery for mechanical causes of cardiogenic shock, patient

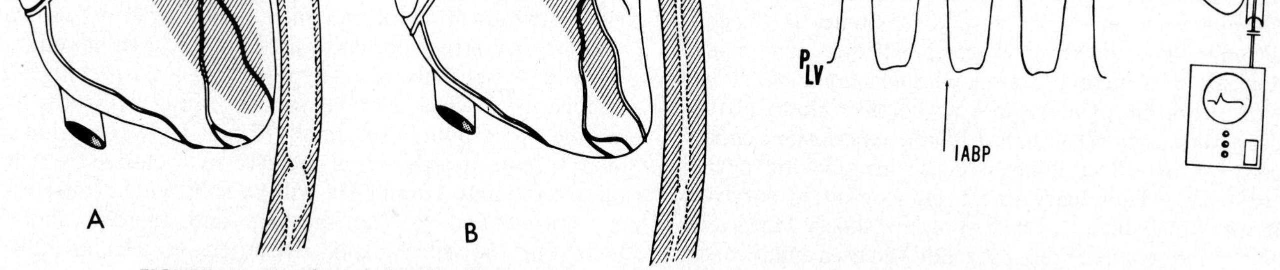

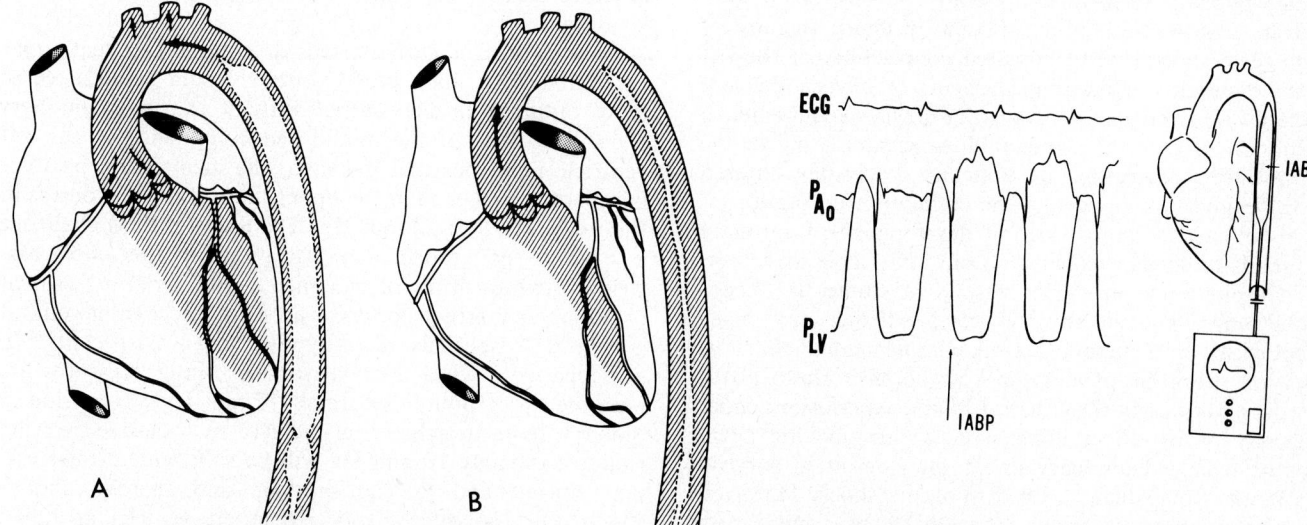

FIGURE 18–10 The relationship between the cardiac cycle and balloon inflation when intraaortic balloon counterpulsation is being utilized. During diastole (panel A) the balloon is inflated, augmenting the prevailing pressure in the proximal aorta and hence coronary arterial perfusion pressure. During systole (panel B) the left ventricular chamber dimension decreases with antegrade ejection of blood into the proximal aorta. During this portion of the cardiac cycle the balloon is deflated, facilitating ejection of blood into the periphery where systemic arterial resistance vessels are dilated maximally because of the preceding inhibition of perfusion by the inflated balloon during diastole. As shown in the inset on the right, utilization of intraaortic balloon counterpulsation (IABP) results in augmentation of diastolic arterial blood pressure (P_{A_0}) with a modest reduction in systolic left ventricular pressure (P_{LV}). (From Bolooki, H.: Clinical Application of Intra-aortic Balloon Pump. New York, Futura Publishing Co., 1977.)

survival may exceed 40 per cent,[191–193] far better than the almost uniformly dismal outlook for such patients without surgical intervention.[190,194] Even in patients whose hemodynamic status is stabilized by IABP, surgical treatment should be undertaken promptly to avoid the development of complications such as renal failure, ARDS, or infection. IABP, while useful as a "holding maneuver," does not constitute adequate therapy. In patients with cardiogenic shock and mechanical lesions, surgery may be deferred in the rare instance when weaning from IABP is possible within 12 to 24 hours and if hemodynamic stability is then maintained without the mechanical support. IABP also permits additional diagnostic studies, such as coronary angiography and ventriculography, to be performed with considerable safety in patients with cardiogenic shock.[195–200] Although survival is better in patients operated upon relatively late, i.e., more than two weeks after the development of the mechanical lesion, this may be related to patient selection; patients who are more gravely ill simply do not survive that long.

Results in patients with cardiogenic shock without mechanical lesions demonstrate conclusively that hemodynamic improvement can be achieved with IABP. Unfortunately, the large majority of such patients soon become balloon-dependent. However, IABP does permit support of the circulation, so that patients can be studied intensively in relative safety, and in some cases it makes possible detection and then surgical correction of mechanical lesions that would otherwise have been impossible.[200,201] Another mechanical approach employed recently to support the circulation in patients with cardiogenic shock is ventricular-assist pumping. This modality is particularly promising for patients undergoing open heart surgical procedures who develop post–cardiac surgery cardiogenic shock and who cannot otherwise be weaned successfully from cardiopulmonary bypass[202] (Fig. 16–24, p. 548).

From a theoretical point of view, primary therapy of cardiogenic shock due to impaired contractility of the left ventricle should include improvement of oxygen delivery to the heart; reduction of myocardial oxygen requirements; facilitation of removal of metabolites accumulating in the myocardium; protection of ischemic, reversibly injured myocardium; and support of the circulation during an interval sufficiently long to permit development of coronary collaterals to sustain jeopardized but still viable myocardium. Despite some promising results in studies in experimental animals, it is not yet clear whether any pharmacological or metabolic regimen implemented after the onset of shock in patients will accomplish these goals. However, very early (less than 4 hours) reperfusion, either surgically or by direct infusion of a thrombolytic agent into the occluded coronary artery, may result in survival of a number of patients with cardiogenic shock. However, the appropriate comparisons have not yet been made with appropriate control groups. Other than the above-mentioned anecdotal reports, the mortality associated with cardiogenic shock approaches 100 per cent when criteria for the diagnosis are rigorous.[6,8,203,204]

Secondary Therapy. Despite the lack of proof that pharmacological protection of ischemic myocardium, untilizing approaches considered in detail in Chapter 38, will reduce mortality associated with cardiogenic shock, it is sensible to predicate therapy in part on approaches designed to preserve jeopardized myocardium. General support for the patient with cardiogenic shock is vital. Relief of pain with adequate doses of morphine may reduce unrecognized vasovagal contributions to circulatory impairment, diminish profuse diaphoresis and the associated fluid loss that can complicate management, and reduce adrenergic stimulation of the heart, thereby diminishing tachyarrhythmias and potentially harmful excess metabolic requirements.

Rarely, cardiogenic shock may be complicated by a significant component of excess vagal tone, usually manifested by sinus bradycardia and other bradyarrhythmias accompanying the profound hypotension and common during the earliest phases of myocardial infarction. Atropine may be particularly helpful in reversing hemodynamic abnormalities under these circumstances.[205] Other general measures are helpful, including reduction of fever, treatment of nausea and vomiting, administration of oxygen and ventilatory assistance if hypoxemia persists, prompt treatment of arrhythmias, treatment of bronchospasm with aminophylline, and correction of electrolyte and acid-base abnormalities.

The principles underlying the medical management of cardiogenic shock include (1) maximization of ventricular performance by adjustment of left ventricular filling pressure to provide an optimal preload; (2) modification of peripheral vascular resistance to optimize impedance to left ventricular ejection; (3) stimulation of contractility, qualified by the proviso that augmentation of oxygen requirements in jeopardized ischemic tissue may be deleterious; (4) vigorous treatment of brady- and tachyarrhythmias; (5) maintenance of the physiological sequential relationship between atrial and ventricular contraction to facilitate atrial transport and the maintenance of ventricular filling pressure; and (6) control of heart rate to facilitate ventricular filling.

Since preload is an important determinant of ventricular performance (p. 433), blood volume should be adjusted so as to optimize cardiac output without causing pulmonary edema. Because of the diminished compliance of the left ventricle in myocardial ischemia, the ideal filling pressure is generally higher than the upper limit of normal and is in the range of 18 to 22 mm Hg. The use of a fluid challenge by means of graded administration of low molecular weight dextran in 50-ml increments with serial assessment of pulmonary artery occlusive pressure and cardiac output is helpful,[180] especially when hypovolemia is suspected.[167] In some patients whose left ventricular filling pressures are near the upper limits of normal (12 mm Hg), expansion of blood volume to achieve an increase in occlusive pressure to approximately 20 mm Hg will be sufficient to raise cardiac output and arterial pressure and thereby abolish shock. On the other hand, when left ventricular filling pressure exceeds 20 mm Hg and/or when pulmonary edema is present, diuresis with intravenous furosemide or ethacrynic acid should be carried out. Furosemide may reduce pulmonary capillary pressure well before it induces diuresis because of its effects on reducing venous capacitance[243] and ventricular afterload[206] (p. 527). Not only will this maneuver diminish pulmonary edema, but since it reduces ventricular dimensions, it also lowers left ventricular wall tension, a principal determinant of myocardial oxygen consumption.

If systolic arterial blood pressure remains depressed, signs of poor peripheral perfusion do not resolve, and total peripheral resistance and left ventricular filling pressure remain markedly elevated, increasing cardiac output by stimulating myocardial contractility with agents such as dopamine or dobutamine may be helpful. *Dopamine* (p. 542) may improve cardiac output by increasing contractility.[206a] At low doses (less than 2 to 5 μg/kg/min), its vasodilatory effect on the renal and other vascular beds may modestly augment renal perfusion and decrease total peripheral resistance. At doses of 5 to 8 μg/kg/min, its positive inotropic effects on beta-1 receptors in the myocardium becomes dominant and at doses in excess of 8 μg/kg/min, it exerts a vasoconstrictor effect by stimulating alpha-adrenergic receptors. Despite its relatively modest positive chronotropic effect, infusion of dopamine must be titrated carefully to avoid precipitating ventricular arrhythmias or severe peripheral vasoconstriction, which occurs at high doses (greater than 20 μg/kg/min). Cardiac output and renal blood flow may be enhanced by the combined use of an alpha-adrenergic blocking agent such as phentolamine to counteract the vasoconstriction induced by dopamine alone.[207] Despite the absence of definitive effects on long-term survival, dopamine, alone or in combination with prazosin (an alpha-adrenergic receptor antagonist) or salbutamol (a $beta_2$-agonist, currently investigational in the United States), has improved hemodynamics and short-term survival.[209–212]

Dobutamine, another catecholamine congener, acts on $beta_1$-, $beta_2$-, and alpha-adrenergic receptors, although its $beta_2$-agonist and alpha- actions are markedly less than those of isoproterenol or norepinephrine, respectively. Its potential advantage compared to dopamine is its consistent *reduction* of systemic vascular resistance.[213] Isoproterenol has also been used to treat cardiogenic shock because of its positive inotropic effects. However, tachycardia, arrhythmia, increased myocardial oxygen requirements, excessive peripheral vasodilatation, and precipitous declines in systemic arterial pressure are major disadvantages. Its use should probably be discontinued or, at most, reserved for rare circumstances in which peripheral vasoconstriction is extreme and accompanied by bradycardia.

It is tempting, on theoretical grounds and on the basis of studies in patients without shock,[214] to utilize vasodilator agents to diminish impedance to left ventricular ejection and to reduce myocardial oxygen requirements. However, therapy with vasodilators alone or even in combination with other agents such as salbutamol[215] or modalities such as intraaortic balloon counterpulsation in patients with cardiogenic shock is potentially hazardous and has not yet proven to be helpful. Peripheral perfusion may increase in some organ beds, and under some circumstances so may cardiac output, but the decline of peripheral resistance in a setting of profound systemic hypotension may decrease systemic diastolic perfusion pressure and hence coronary perfusion pressure. Since left ventricular filling pressure usually must be maintained in the range of 20 mm Hg to optimize cardiac output, any further decline in systemic arterial diastolic pressure produced by a vasodilator will not be offset by a decrease in diastolic tension within the ventricular wall, and hence the net driving pressure supporting coronary perfusion diminishes, potentially exacerbating myocardial ischemia.

For many years alpha-adrenergic agonists provided the sole pharmacological approach to the treatment of cardiogenic shock. Use of these drugs was predicated on the concept (now recognized to be overly simplistic) that peripheral vascular resistance and arterial pressure should be augmented. Such a view neglects the primacy of the need for enhancement of *perfusion* rather than of arterial *pressure*. Agonists with both alpha- and beta-receptor actions, such as norepinephrine, then became the mainstay of treatment, because their combined effects on the heart and peripheral vascular resistance may raise arterial pressure when the circulatory system is responsive to no other drug. Metaraminol, by virtue of its direct alpha-agonistic and indirect beta-agonistic properties, mediated by local catecholamine release, has also been utilized widely. However, it has now become clear that these agents not only fail to improve overall mortality associated with cardiogenic shock but may actually exert substantial deleterious effects on the heart.[177] Although some increase in cardiac output and systemic arterial pressure can be achieved with agents such as norepinephrine, the lowest effective doses necessary should be used to avoid additional damage to the heart secondary to greater ischemia and afterload.[220]

In addition to beta-adrenergic agonists, other agents with positive inotropic effects—particularly digitalis glycosides—have been utilized. Although the beneficial effects of digitalis on ventricular performance in congestive heart failure are unequivocal (p. 513), and the net effects of digitalis on ischemic myocardium are protective in the presence of heart failure,[217] the relative inefficacy of digitalis in the setting of cardiogenic shock may be explained on both theoretical and empirical grounds. Tolerance to the drug under these circumstances is diminished, and its propensity to produce arrhythmia is accentuated.[186,218] The peripheral and coronary vasoconstrictor actions of intravenous glycosides may be deleterious in that they elevate arterial pressure (afterload) and reduce coronary blood flow. Alterations in pH and electrolyte status reduce the toxic/therapeutic ratio. Perhaps most important, the primary defect in cardiogenic shock is impaired cardiac contractility due to limited coronary perfusion and therefore impaired delivery of oxygen and substrate, so that the efficacy of glycosides for improving cardiac function may be severely limited. Uncontrolled or recurrent supraventricular tachyarrhythmias unresponsive to vagotonic maneuvers are the principal indication for use of parenteral digitalis glycosides in patients with cardiogenic shock. Digitalis may exert some beneficial effect on ventricular performance in cardiogenic shock even when these specific indications are absent, but a favorable effect on the overall course of the syndrome is unproven. Accordingly, doses should be modest to avoid inducing serious toxic effects when major benefits cannot be anticipated.

SHOCK DUE TO LEFT VENTRICULAR OUTFLOW TRACT OBSTRUCTION

Profound reduction of left ventricular output causing cardiogenic shock may be due to anatomical obstruction of the aortic outflow tract at the supra-, infra-, or aortic valvular levels. Lesions include supravalvular aortic stenosis (Chaps. 29 and 30), congential or acquired valvular aortic stenosis (Chap. 32), or hypertrophic obstructive cardiomyopathy (Chap. 41). Any of these lesions, when sufficiently severe, may produce chronic heart failure, but if this is not treated surgically, cardiac output may continue to decline to levels that ultimately result in cardiogenic shock. At this juncture, surgical correction, while long overdue, may still be the only life-saving therapy. It is important to be aware that left ventricular outflow obstruction due to hypertrophic obstructive cardiomyopathy may be exacerbated by agents with positive inotropic effects, particularly beta-adrenergic agonists. Thus, these drugs may exaggerate the hemodynamic disturbance and should be avoided (p. 1418). Similarly, agents such as nitrates, which cause venous pooling of blood and hence diminished ventricular volume, may intensify the obstruction associated with hypertrophic cardiomyopathy and contribute to hemodynamic deterioration. Administration of calcium antagonists such as verapamil in doses of 80 to 120 mg orally at 6-hour intervals may improve ventricular performance by diminishing systolic dynamic obstruction, increasing diastolic compliance, or both[229] (p. 1420). Vasodilator agents are contraindicated in patients with shock due to obstruction to left ventricular outflow.[264]

OTHER TYPES OF OBSTRUCTIVE SHOCK. A variety of other conditions can impair outflow from the heart and cause systemic hypoperfusion and hypotension. One category comprises lesions affecting left ventricular inflow, including critical, far-advanced mitral stenosis (p. 1064); "ball-valve" thrombus that occludes flow through the mitral valve; and left atrial myxoma, which can produce the same hemodynamic abnormalities. Although ball-valve thrombi and myxomas generally give rise to intermittent circulatory insufficiency with syncope, transitory pulmonary venous hypertension, and/or postural hypotension, propagation of the thrombus with persistent occlusion of the atrioventricular orifice or persistent occlusion due to myxoma can also lead to shock (Chap. 42).

Pericardial tamponade is a prime example of obstructive shock and is discussed on page 1480.

HEMORRHAGIC SHOCK

PRIMARY THERAPY. Rapid loss of 30 per cent or more of the blood volume generally produces oligemic shock. Although this form of shock is accompanied by hemodilution, reexpansion of the plasma volume evolves slowly, with effects on the hematocrit often not evident for 3 to 6 hours. Additional blood loss must be halted as soon as hemodynamics have been stabilized by rapid repletion of vascular volume, preferably with type-specific whole blood or washed red blood cells and frozen plasma, but if necessary with colloid and crystalloid solutions. If volume repletion is initiated after more than a short interval following the onset of shock, administration of blood substantially in excess of the amount lost may be required.[12] When more than 2 liters is required, fresh blood is desirable to avoid thrombocytopenia and dilution of clotting factors. Although crystalloids such as normal saline or Ringer's lactate solution can be utilized initially, adequate amounts of colloid to maintain vascular volume should be included. Despite its availability, plasma is not necessarily the colloid of choice because of the risk of hepatitis. Albumin is useful, but the half-life of intravenously administered purified albumin is short. Dextran may interfere with coagulation or with blood-typing because of nonspecific agglutination of red cells and may induce a hypersensitivity reaction. Plasma expanders such as hydroxyethyl starch may not have these disadvantages.[221]

SECONDARY THERAPY. The hemodynamic picture that accompanies hemorrhagic shock is dominated by the direct consequences of a diminished blood volume (decreased cardiac output and systemic arterial pressure) and the sympathoadrenal response manifested by tachycardia, cutaneous vasoconstriction, venoconstriction, and redistribution of organ blood flow in relation to regional sympathetic tone. Capillary filtration may be enhanced because of the increased venous tone, and accordingly alpha-adrenergic blockade may be useful in association with expansion of vascular volume.[222] However, adequate and prompt repletion of vascular volume is usually sufficient without this adjunct.

If the hemodynamic derangements induced by hemorrhagic shock are not corrected promptly, impaired cardiac function may result and may subsequently contribute to the reduced cardiac output apparently on the basis of damage sustained as a consequence of myocardial ischemia[58,223] (Fig. 18–3). Although administration of large quantities of bank blood might depress cardiac contractility by chelating free calcium in the plasma with citrate, other manifestations of hypocalcemia, such as tetany, are usually evident first. Nevertheless, in rare circumstances, administration of intravenous calcium may be helpful when hypocalcemia is suggested by prolongation of the Q-T interval on the electrocardiogram or is documented by measurement of plasma ionized calcium.[224]

The use of glucocorticoids has been advocated for the treatment of shock of virtually all etiologies, including hemorrhagic shock.[225–228] Their use has been recommended because of their (1) potential direct stimulation of cardiac function;[229] (2) inhibition of vasoconstrictor actions of catecholamines and vasopressin; (3) restoration of phagocytic function of the reticuloendothelial system;[227] (4) diminution of platelet aggregation; (5) reduction of postganglionic sympathetic nerve transmission;[230] (6) stabilization of lysosomal membranes;[231] (7) blockade of alpha-adrenergic receptors or direct vasodilation;[232,233] (8) protection of the lung and prevention of ARDS;[234] and (9) favorable effects on the oxygen affinity of hemoglobin with enhanced oxygen delivery to the tissues.[235] However, their clinical efficacy in shock, with the exception of shock due to adrenocortical failure and possibly septic shock, has not been established.

When arterial pressure cannot be restored promptly by restitution of intravascular volume, it may be necessary to support the circulation with the use of vasoactive drugs. The previous reliance on norepinephrine, indirectly acting sympathomimetics such as metaraminol, and alpha-adrenergic agonists has been modified by favorable experience with other agents such as dopamine (2 to 5 $\mu g/kg/min$), a drug with positive inotropic effects and dopaminergic vasodilatory effects on mesenteric, renal, and cerebral vessels. As already noted, at higher doses dopamine may produce vasoconstriction. Its combined actions of increasing cardiac output and maintaining perfusion of vital organs have made it a valuable agent in the treatment of oligemic shock.[236–238]

Pure alpha- or beta-adrenergic agonists should not be used routinely for the treatment of oligemic shock, since nutritive flow may not be enhanced even though arterial pressure or cardiac output may be increased. Similar limitations apply to alpha-adrenergic receptor blocking agents to reduce vasoconstriction, since the potential advantages of vasodilatation are frequently outweighed by a decline in systemic pressure from already low levels, with consequent further compromise of perfusion of the heart and other vital organs.

Nonhemorrhagic Oligemic Shock

Reduction of effective vascular volume may result from sequestration of fluid in a "third space" in disorders such as hemorrhagic pancreatitis, burns, surgical wounds, or trauma to skeletal muscle; in the abdominal cavity with ascites; or in the intestinal lumen with obstructive or adynamic ileus. Excessive filtration of plasma sometimes accompanies pheochromocytoma with manifestations of postural hypotension and occasionally shock due to the combined effects of diminished plasma volume and rarely myocarditis, apparently induced by catecholamines (p. 1734).[239,240] The more commonly manifested vasoconstrictor effects of the circulating catecholamines released by the tumor may be masked by the profound diminution of blood volume with or without accompanying cardiac dysfunction.

Oligemic shock may also occur in association with: (1) salt-wasting nephritis; (2) protracted fluid loss from the gastrointestinal tract due to vomiting or diarrhea, cholera, or gastroenteritis in infancy;[241–243] (3) uncontrolled diabetes mellitus; (4) diabetes insipidus; (5) sodium depletion accompanying adrenocortical failure; (6) excessive diuresis induced pharmacologically; (7) or any other condition in which components of the vascular volume are sequestered or lost. The hemodynamic hallmark is hypotension, generally accompanied by arteriolar vasoconstriction and tachycardia. Systemic venous pressure is reduced, and oliguria is usually prominent. Because of the loss of plasma volume and retention of red cells, hemoconcentration is a prominent feature.

Primary therapy of nonhemorrhagic, oligemic shock consists of rapid replacement of lost fluid. Shock accompanying pheochromocytoma necessitates infusion of plasma, albumin, or another plasma expander and crystalloid solution. In the absence of unrecognized complicating factors (such as marked sodium loss and impaired vascular tone in the case of an Addisonian crisis, or impaired cardiac function accompanying profound myxedema), early oligemic shock responds promptly to adequate repletion of plasma volume, as long as additional fluid losses are controlled and the initiating cause is corrected.

Acute renal failure often accompanies intravascular hemolysis, particularly when the latter is associated with severe or persistent hypotension, despite the lack of demonstrable nephrotoxic effects of pure hemoglobin. Its etiology appears to depend in part upon deleterious effects of other, not yet delineated constituents of the red cell stroma. Administration of mannitol may be helpful in preventing or minimizing irreversible renal damage.[244] When a diuretic phase follows early renal failure associated with rhabdomyolysis, hypercalcemia may occur, presumably from remobilization of calcium previously deposited in damaged muscle,[245] as well as transient secondary hyperparathyroidism. Unrecognized or inadequately treated electrolyte abnormalities, including alterations in plasma ionized calcium, may be responsible for the occurrence of severe arrhythmias and even sudden death.

DISTRIBUTIVE SHOCK

Shock due to sepsis, neurological disturbances, anaphylaxis, and metabolic, toxic, or endocrine depression of vasomotor tone share the common features of inappropriate vasodilatation, causing maldistribution of vascular volume, reduction of systemic arterial pressure, and impaired perfusion of vital organs.[246] Calculated total peripheral vascular resistance is generally markedly decreased and arterial pressure is reduced, but cardiac output may be normal, increased, or reduced. Cutaneous vasodilatation is often present, and the patient exhibits so-called warm shock.

SEPTIC SHOCK (Table 18–2)

In septic shock severe infection leads to circulatory collapse.[246–249] The clinical picture frequently includes chills, rigors, and fever as high as 106°F (41°C). Cerebral function is frequently impaired, venous pressure is markedly reduced, and oliguria is prominent. When the cutaneous bed is dilated, the patient is often alert, the skin is warm and dry, and cardiac output is frequently increased, even though perfusion of many tissues is reduced. While vasodilatation often predominates early in the pyrogenic phase, later in the course profound vasoconstriction occurs, peripheral resistance rises, and cardiac output declines; at this stage the prognosis is ominous.[250]

The most common offending agents are gram-negative enteric bacilli, although other bacterial organisms, including gram-positive cocci, gram-negative diplococci, and clostridia, as well as nonbacterial organisms, including viruses, rickettsia, and fungi, may be responsible.[251] Compromise of a host by immunosuppressive drugs, antimetabolite therapy, or prolonged administration of glucocorticoids may predispose to the condition. "Warm shock" is particularly prominent when the initiating bacteremia is due to gram-negative enteric bacteria, presumably because of the effects of endotoxin. A substantial fraction of the blood volume pools in the venous bed, with consequent reduction of effective circulating volume. Metabolic acidosis, elevation of plasma lactate, low arteriovenous oxygen content, differences due to arteriovenous shunting, fever, and leukopenia followed by leukocytosis are typical.

Endotoxins, i.e., large macromolecular lipopolysaccharide complexes derived from the cell walls of a variety of gram-negative bacilli, produce shock when injected intravenously into experimental animals, resulting in pathophysiological disturbances that resemble septic shock in man (Fig. 18–11). Hepatic and splanchnic venoconstriction limits venous return to the heart, contributing to the decline in cardiac output and to systemic arterial hypotension. Endothelial damage, aggregation of cellular blood elements leading to thrombocytopenia and leukopenia, and stasis and microthrombi in the microcirculation contribute to impaired perfusion of vital organs.

Because endotoxin can activate the coagulation, fibrinolytic, complement, and kallikrein systems, both hyper- and hypocoagulability may occur. Activation of complement and the production of kinins appear to contribute to enhanced vascular permeability; bradykinin may contribute to the decline in systemic arterial resistance and to bradycardia. Prostaglandins are also involved, since inhibition of prostaglandin synthesis favorably modifies the hemodynamic response to the insult.[252]

Since endotoxin can activate hepatic glycogenolysis, the initial hyperglycemia—characteristic of all forms of shock because of the effect of glucocorticoids and catecholamines—may be accentuated. A secondary hypoglycemia is common when carbohydrate reserves have been depleted.[253] The disturbances of carbohydrate metabolism

TABLE 18–2 PATHOPHYSIOLOGIC SEQUELAE OF ENDOTOXEMIA

Activation of Hageman factor
Hypotension (kinin system)
Disseminated intravascular coagulation
Changes in peripheral blood levels (granulocytes and lymphocytes)
Activation of fibrinolytic pathways
Activation of classic and alternative pathways of complement
Release of vasoactive and coagulation-promoting substances from platelets
Endothelial damage
Release of effector substances from neutrophils and mononuclear cells

Reproduced with permission from Shine, K. I., Kuhn, M., Young, L. S., and Tillisch, J. H.: Aspects of the management of shock. Ann. Intern. Med. *93*:723, 1980.

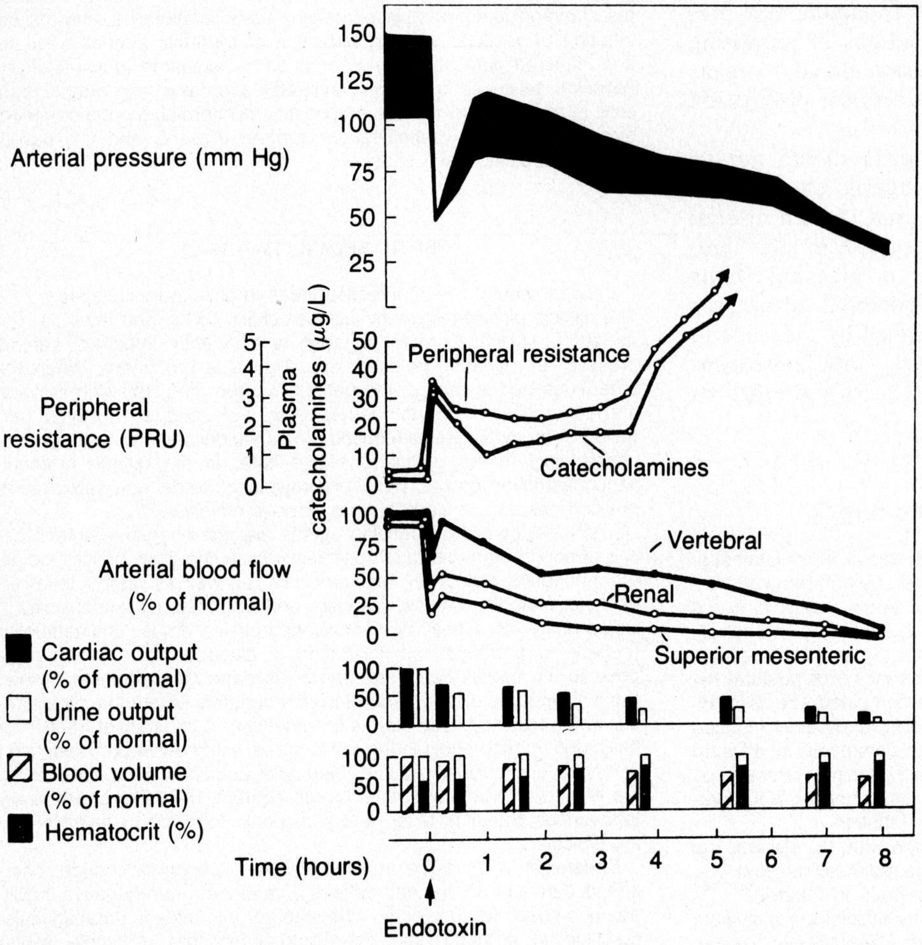

FIGURE 18–11 Characteristic hemodynamic changes induced experimentally in dogs subjected to endotoxic shock. Early in the evolution of shock, peripheral vascular resistance is inappropriately low with respect to arterial blood pressure despite the elevation of plasma catecholamines. Late in the evolution of the condition, peripheral vascular resistance increases markedly but systemic arterial blood pressure continues to decline. Progressive hemoconcentration accompanies the diminution of vascular volume. Both reflect effusion of plasma into the interstitial fluid space, further compromising cardiac output, systemic arterial pressure, and urine output. (From Niazi, Z., et al.: Use of monitoring to improve survival in shock. Geriatrics *30*:93, 1975.)

include hypoinsulinemia, mediated in part by alpha-adrenergic inhibition of insulin secretion.[253,254]

Primary Therapy. Primary therapy of septic shock includes administration of antibiotics once specimens of blood, urine, sputum, cerebrospinal fluid, and, when present, wound exudates have been obtained for culture and sensitivity tests. Initial selection of antibiotic therapy must frequently be made on an empirical basis, depending on the probable source of infection and organism involved. An aminoglycoside should be administered for suspected enteric organisms, with carbenicillin when *Pseudomonas* is suspected; penicillinase-resistant penicillins or cephalosporins are often the agents of choice when the probability of infection with a gram-positive organism is higher. Suspected *Bacteroides fragilis* infection should be treated with clindamycin.

Secondary Therapy. Large volumes of fluid and plasma expanders are needed to sustain effective vascular volume and maintain normal plasma oncotic pressure. The hemodynamic response to intermittent fluid challenges, analogous to that utilized in patients with cardiogenic shock (p. 1317), can be employed to assess the adequacy of vascular volume. If systemic hypotension persists, agents such as dopamine may be useful. Alpha-adrenergic agonists should not be utilized, since they may further compromise perfusion of vital organs in the face of vasoconstriction.

The possible benefit of corticosteroids in the treatment of septic shock remains controversial. Doses utilized have been as much as 50- to 100-fold greater than those required for replacement therapy in patients with adrenocortical failure. Dexamethasone (40 mg intravenously followed by 20 mg at 4-hour intervals) has been employed to increase cardiac output and decrease peripheral arterial resistance, improve oxygenation, and decrease metabolic acidosis.[255] Gastrointestinal bleeding may be a relative contraindication to treatment with these agents.

The efficacy of other suggested measures, such as glucose-insulin-potassium,[256] antihistamines to antagonize vasodilatation mediated by histamine release,[257] and inhibitors of prostaglandin synthesis,[258] has not yet been established. When disseminated intravascular coagulation has been documented, heparin should be administered,[259] although controlled studies have not demonstrated improved survival. When there is widespread fibrinolysis, the use of agents such as epsilon-aminocaproic acid may be justified.[259]

NEUROGENIC SHOCK

Central nervous system disease, including cerebrovascular disorders, marked or rapid elevations of cerebrospinal fluid pressure from any cause, hypertensive encephalopathy, hemorrhage into the basal ganglia or into the cerebellum; vascular or traumatic injury to the spinal cord; deep general or spinal anethesia; or toxic depression of the nervous system by heat stroke, dehydration, drug overdose, or other metabolic insults may result in shock mediated in part by profound disturbance of autonomic nervous system function. Often vasodilatation, vagotonia, and suppression of sympathetic support of vascular tone with shock accompanied by bradycardia are prominent. Primary therapy consists of treatment of the underlying disturbance. Supportive therapy, primarily vigorous administration of colloid and crystalloid solutions, is similar to that utilized in the *distributive shock* of other etiologies, such as sepsis.[246,260–262] Infusion of agents with positive inotropic effects, such as dopamine, or alpha-adrenergic agonists such as methoxamine and phenylephrine may be useful, but only as a temporizing measure, until expansion of blood volume can be achieved. With the exception of neurogenic shock related to visceral pain, which may respond dramatically to analgesics, the outcome of neuropathic shock is generally grave.

SHOCK DUE TO METABOLIC, TOXIC, OR ENDOCRINE FACTORS

Drug abuse or suicide attempts with agents such as barbiturates, phenothiazines, glutethemide, diazepam, and other central nervous system depressants may give rise to shock, as may hepatic and renal failure, uncontrolled diabetes mellitus, anoxia, hypercarbia, and respiratory and metabolic acidosis (including lactic ketoacidosis), hyperosmolality,[263] alkalosis,[264] dehydration, and hypoglycemia.[263] Excessive transfusions with banked blood and chelation of calcium without adequate replacement, or injudicious administration of vasodilators or diuretics, may cause shock in patients whose circulation is already compromised. Heavy metal intoxication, often complicated by vomiting and diarrhea, intoxication with carbon monoxide, ingestion of ethylene glycol with resultant metabolic acidosis, and toxicity from venoms may all impair maintenance of vascular tone, with consequent development of shock.

Addisonian crisis, whether due to (1) disease intrinsic to the adrenal cortex (sometimes manifest only with surgical or traumatic stress); (2) hemorrhagic infarction of the adrenal glands precipitated by meningococcal infection; or (3) hemorrhage into the adrenals associated with excessive anticoagulation, may cause shock not only because of failure of sodium retention secondary to mineralocorticoid deficiency, but also because of diminished cardiac contractility and impaired vascular tone.[265–267] Pressor reactivity to catecholamines is reduced by adrenalectomy in experimental animals and can be restored by the administration of adrenocorticoid hormones.[265] Shock due to adrenocortical failure responds initially to the administration of large volumes of saline, and the accompanying hypoglycemia responds to hypertonic glucose. However, the administration of mineralocorticoids and glucocorticoids is necessary as well.

Circulatory collapse with mortality exceeding 50 per cent may accompany other serious endocrine disturbances, including myxedema (p. 1729) and hyperparathyroidism.[263] Myxedema leads to depressed myocardial contractility, myocardial injury, and hypovolemia (p. 1730). It should be suspected when shock is accompanied by hypothermia, an inappropriately slow heart rate, low voltage on the electrocardiogram, soft heart sounds, an inactive precordium, ascites or other serous effusions, and the stigmata of myxedema, such as thickened, dry skin. Circulatory collapse is an end-stage manifestation of profound thyroid deficiency and may be due in part to the loss of the permissive role of thyroid hormone in the maintenance of receptors to adrenergic agonists.[268,269]

The success of therapy of these forms of shock is dependent on the recognition of the etiology, on the prompt implementation of primary treatment directed against the specific impairment, and on appropriate attention to accompanying alterations in blood volume and electrolyte balance.

ANAPHYLACTIC SHOCK

Anaphylactic shock is a disorder that generally occurs precipitously in response either to exposure to an antigen in the natural environment or as a result of drug administration. In sensitized individuals, the antigen interacts with an IgE-specific antibody on mast cells and other cell surfaces. Mediators liberated from sensitized mast cells (Fig. 18–12) include histamine and leukotrienes. Other substances that are involved include prostaglandins, thromboxane A_2, kinins, chemotactic factors, and catecholamines. Tissue mast cells and basophils in the peripheral blood are important sources of these mediators.[270–272]

Life-threatening anaphylaxis occurs within minutes after exposure to the antigen and is manifested by marked respiratory distress and bronchospasm, plasma volume depletion with hemoconcentration, circulatory collapse, decreased cardiac output, increased peripheral resistance, and frequently urticaria. Supraventricular and ventricular tachyarrhythmias are common. Milder forms of anaphylactic shock present with partial airway obstruction, hives, tachycardia, and mild hyper- or hypotension.

The diagnosis of anaphylactic shock is usually based on the history and knowledge of the setting in which the episode occurs, as well as recognition of the unique combination of bronchospasm and cardiovascular collapse often accompanied by cutaneous manifestations. However, in some cases, the diagnosis is confounded when vascular collapse occurs without antecedent respiratory compromise.[274]

Primary Therapy. Primary therapy includes immediate vigorous efforts to eliminate or reduce exposure to antigen, e.g., by placing a tourniquet above an injection site when the episode occurs after administration of heterologous protein or a pharmacological agent; by using epinephrine (0.1 mg intravenously and 0.4 mg subcutaneously) both to support the circulation and to enhance intracellular cyclic AMP levels, thereby inhibiting release of mediators; or by further augmenting intracellular cyclic AMP levels with the use of a phosphodiesterase inhibitor such as aminophylline (500 mg intravenously over 10 to 20 minutes). Administration of antihistamines such as diphenhydramine hydrochloride (50 to 100 mg intravenously over an interval of several minutes) may be helpful but is rarely definitive. Glucocorticoids may reduce the likelihood of protracted anaphylaxis but are of little help in treating the acute episode. Epinephrine remains the mainstay of primary therapy. Intramuscular injections are advantageous when cutaneous vasoconstriction is prominent.

Secondary Therapy. Systemic arterial pressure should be maintained with infusion of large volumes of crystalloid solutions and oxygenation by mechanical support of respiration.[272,274] Since loss of plasma volume is a major consequence of anaphylactic shock, the efficacy of vasoconstrictor agents such as norepinephrine is questionable. Ventilation must be supported immediately with oxygen delivered through an endotracheal tube, since laryngeal edema may occur rapidly. Because of the possibility of recurrent anaphylaxis, it is essential to observe the patient for at least several hours after the circulatory and respiratory status have been restored to normal. The patient must be instructed to avoid subsequent exposure to the offending antigen and provided with such ancillary devices as bracelets describing his or her susceptibility to an allergic reaction.

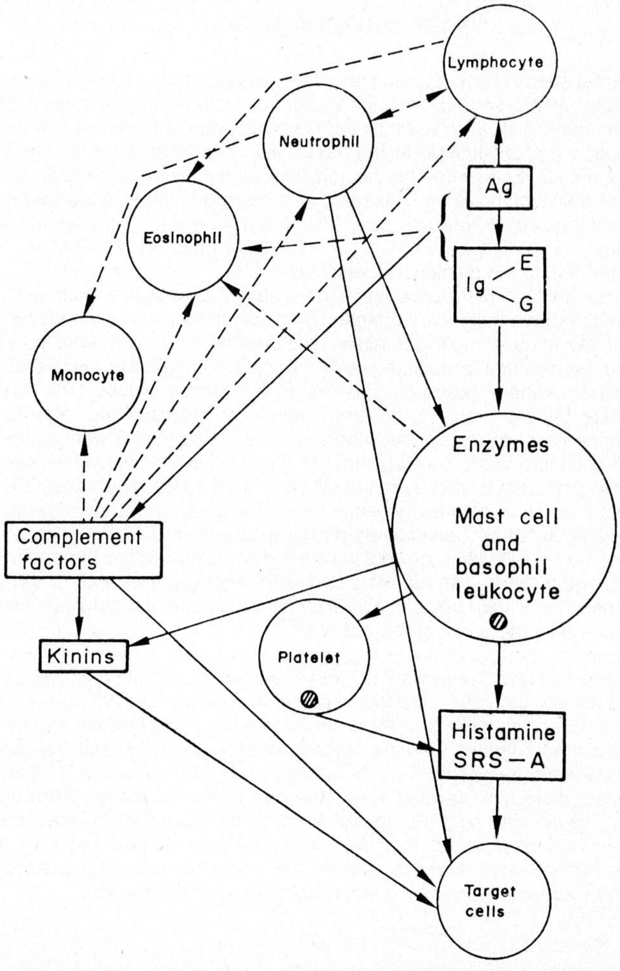

FIGURE 18–12 Interaction of antigen (Ag) with immunoglobulins (Ig), particularly of the E and G classes, influences a variety of cells, including mast cells and lymphocytes, to release mediators that either directly affect target cells in the lung and other organs or induce liberation of other mediators from platelets and other cells that, in turn, impinge on target cells. (From Austen, K. F., and Becker, E. L. (eds.): Biochemistry of the Acute Allergic Reactions—Second International Symposium. London, Blackwell Scientific Publications, 1971.)

PULMONARY EMBOLISM (See also Chapter 46)

Antecedent shock is common when massive pulmonary embolism causes death. On the other hand, except for transitory increases of pulmonary arterial pressure, marked derangements of circulatory function are uncommon in the vast majority of patients with pulmonary emboli. Even when the hemodynamic concomitants of the immediate insult of massive pulmonary embolism are marked, persistent circulatory insufficiency is rare. The improvement in hemodynamics reflects primarily two mechanisms—fibrinolysis and distal migration of emboli within the pulmonary vasculature.[275]

The primary hemodynamic manifestations of massive pulmonary emboli include pulmonary arterial hypertension; right ventricular failure with elevation of right ventricular end-diastolic and right atrial pressure, sometimes associated with tricuspid regurgitation; increased systemic venous pressure; and diminished cardiac output. Left ventricular filling pressure is generally normal or reduced, and total peripheral vascular resistance is increased. Supraventricular arrhythmias are common, but if the magnitude of the insult is so severe that systemic perfusion is impaired, arrhythmias of all types may occur. Despite massive pulmonary embolism, death is uncommon when anticoagulation is implemented promptly to prevent further embolization. Partial resolution of obstruction due to emboli within the pulmonary vasculature can be detected with angiographic and isotopic techniques within days[276] and may be complete as early as two weeks after the onset of the episode.[275]

Primary therapy of shock associated with massive pulmonary embolism includes prevention of further embolization with anticoagulation or an umbrella inserted into the inferior vena cava, relief of dynamic factors adding to the obstruction such as hypoxemia and the associated pulmonary arterial vasoconstrictor response, and the use of systemic fibrinolytic therapy (urokinase or streptokinase).[276] Secondary therapy is directed toward supporting the circulation with cardiac glycosides and vigorously treating the arrhythmias that are commonly associated. Pulmonary embolectomy is indicated only if the patient is in extremis despite the above-mentioned measures, combined with the use of isotropic agents such as dopamine.

SHOCK DUE TO MISCELLANEOUS CAUSES

Shock may occur in relatively unusual conditions such as *malignant* hyperthermia, a hereditary disorder in which profound hyperpyrexia, marked elevations of plasma creatine kinase activity, and circulatory collapse occur in response to anesthesia or other stresses.[277–279] In this disorder, refractory shock may follow triggering events unless the diagnosis is suspected and appropriate precautions are taken to avoid use of agents likely to precipitate the syndrome. The shock appears to be due to profound augmentations in anaerobic metabolism resulting from compensatory responses to an intrinsic defect in calcium binding by the sarcoplasmic reticulum.[278,280] Dantrolene sodium in doses of 1 to 10 mg/kg intravenously appears to be effective in blunting the abnormal metabolic activity and aborting the syndrome.[280] Once circulatory failure has occurred, the outlook is poor despite supportive therapy.

Cyclic episodes of shock have been observed in syndromes such a *periodic edema, angioneurotic edema* associated with hereditary deficiency of an inhibitor of the complement system, *periodic fever*, and *hyperglobulinemias*.[281,282] Effective management of these disorders is directed toward the primary derangement and prevention of shock.

References

1. Shine, K. I., Kuhn, M., Young, L. S., and Tillisch, J. H.; Aspects of the management of shock. Ann. Intern. Med. *93*:723, 1980.
2. Eldridge, F. L.: Relationship between lactate turnover rate and blood concentration in hemorrhagic shock. J. Appl. Physiol. *37*:321, 1974.
3. Messmer, K., and Sunder-Plassmann, L.: Microcirculatory and rheologic changes in shock. *In* Shoemaker, W. C., and Taveres, B. L. (eds.): Current Topics in Critical Care Medicine. Basel, S. Karger, 1976, p. 16.
4. Hardaway, R. M., Dixon, R. S., Foster, E. F., Karabin, B. L., Schifres, F. D., and Meyers, T.: The effect of hemorrhagic shock on disseminated intravascular coagulation. Ann. Surg. *184*:43, 1976.
5. Kantrowitz, A., Krakauer, J. S., Butner, A. M., Freed, P. S., Jaron, D., Rosenbaum, A., and Goodman, P. M.: Phase-shift balloon pumping in cardiogenic shock. Progr. Cardiovasc. Dis. *12*:293, 1969.
6. Scheidt, S., Arscheim, R., and Killip, T., III: Shock after acute myocardial infarction. Am. J. Cardiol. *26*:556, 1970.
7. Gunnar R. M., Cruz, A., Boswell, J., Co, B. S., Pietras, R. J., and Tobin, J. R., Jr.: Myocardial infarction with shock: Hemodynamic studies and results of therapy. Circulation *33*:753, 1966.
8. Cohn, J. N., and Franciosa, J. A.: Pathophysiology of shock in acute myocardial infarction. *In* Yu, P. N., and Goodwin, J. F. (eds.): Progress in Cardiology. Philadelphia, Lea and Febiger, 1973, p. 207.
9. Lees, N. W.: The diagnosis and treatment of endotoxin shock. Anaesthesia *31*: 897, 1976.
10. Hassen, A.: Gram-negative bacteremic shock. Med. Clin. North Am. *57*:1403, 1973.
11. McArdle, C. S., MacDonald, J. A. E., and Ledingham, I. M.: A three year retrospective analysis of septic shock in a general hospital. Scott. Med. J. *20*:79, 1975.
12. Pardy, B. J., and Dudley, H. A. F.: Sequential patterns of haemodynamic and metabolic changes in experimental hypovolaemic shock. I. Responses to acute haemorrhage. Br. J. Surg. *66*:84, 1979.
13. Bronk, D. W., and Stella, G.: Afferent impulses in the carotid sinus nerve: I. The relation of the discharge from single end organs to arterial blood pressure. J. Cell. Physiol. *1*:113, 1932.
14. Abboud, F. M., Heistad, D. D., Mark, A. L., and Schmid, P. D.: Reflex control of the peripheral circulation. Progr. Cardiovasc. Dis. *17*:371, 1976.
15. Paintal, A. S.: Cardiovascular receptors. *In* Neil, E. (ed.): Enteroceptors. Berlin, Springer-Verlag, 1972, p. 1.
16. Oberg, B., and Thoren, P.: Increased activity in left ventricular receptors during hemorrhage or occlusion of caval veins in the cat—A possible cause of the vaso-vagal reaction. Acta Physiol. Scand. *85*:164, 1972.
17. Mark, A. L., Abboud, F. M., Schmid, P. G., and Heistad, D. D.: Reflex vascular responses to left ventricular outflow obstruction and activation of ventricular baroreceptors in dogs. J. Clin. Invest. *52*:1147, 1973.
18. Jarisch, A., and Zotterman, Y.: Depressor reflexes from the heart. Acta Physiol. Scand. *16*:31, 1948.
19. Davies, G. S., and Comroe, J. H.: Chemoreflexes from the heart and lungs. Physiol. Rev. *34*:167, 1954.
20. Linden, R. J.: Function of cardiac receptors. Circulation *48*:463, 1973.
21. Green, H. D., and Kepchar, J. H.: Control of peripheral resistance in major systemic vascular beds. Physiol. Rev. *39*:617, 1959.
22. Jakschik, B. A., Marshall, G. R., Kourik, J. L., and Needleman, P.: Profile of circulating vasoactive substances in hemorrhagic shock and their pharmacologic manipulation. J. Clin. Invest. *54*:842, 1974.
23. Hall, R. C., and Hodge, R. L.: Changes in catecholamine and angiotensin levels in the cat and dog during hemorrhage. Am. J. Physiol. *221*:1305, 1971.
24. Scornik, O. A., and Paladini, A. C.: Angiotensin blood levels in hemorrhagic hypotension and other related conditions. Am. J. Physiol. *206*:553, 1964.
25. Hollenberg, N. K., Waters, J. R., Toews, M. R., Davies, R. O., and Nickerson, M.: Nature of cardiovascular decompensation during hemorrhagic hypotension. Am. J. Physiol. *219*:1476, 1970.
26. Starke, K., Werner, U., Hellerforth, R., and Schumann, H. J.: Influence of peptides on the output of noradrenaline in isolated rabbit hearts. Eur. J. Pharmacol. *9*:136, 1970.
27. Collier, J. G., Herman, A. G., and Vane, J. R.: Appearance of prostaglandins in the renal venous blood of dogs in response to acute systemic hypotension produced by bleeding or endotoxin. J. Physiol. *230*:19, 1973.
28. Bagby, G. J., and Spitzer, J. A.: Lipoprotein lipase activity in rat heart and adipose tissue during endotoxin shock. Am. J. Physiol. *238*:H325, 1980.
29. Tung, S. H., Bettice, J., Wang, B. C., and Brown, E. G., Jr.: Intracellular and extracellular acid-base changes in hemorrhagic shock. Respir. Physiol. *26*:229, 1976.
30. Daniel, A. M., Pierce, C. H., MacLean, L. E., and Shizgal, H. M.: Lactate metabolism in the dog during shock from hemorrhage, cardiac tamponade or endotoxin. Surg. Gynec. Obstet. *143*:581, 1976.
31. Arfman, R. C., Loegering, D. J., and Smith, J. J.: Changes in plasma levels of lysosomal and nonlysosomal enzymes during hemorrhagic hypotension. Proc. Soc. Exp. Biol. Med. *149*:1029, 1975.
32. Roberts, R., and Sobel, B. E.: The inactivation and clearance of enzymes. *In* Hearse, D. J., and DeLeiris, J. (eds.): Enzymes in Cardiology: Diagnosis and Research. Chichester, England, John Wiley and Sons, Ltd., 1979.
33. Wiggers, C. J.: The present status of the shock problem. Physiol. Rev. *22*:74, 1942.
34. Fine, J.: Septic shock. J.A.M.A. *188*:127, 1964.
35. McNulty, W. P., Jr., and Linares, R.: Hemorrhagic shock of germfree rats. Am. J. Physiol. *198*:141, 1960.
36. Krause, S. M., and Hess, M. L.: Diphenhydramine protection of the failing myocardium during gram-negative endotoxemia. Circ. Shock *6*:75, 1979.
37. Rocha e Silva, M., Jr.: Participation of the kinin-system in different kinds of shock. *In* Bertelli, A., and Back, N. (eds.): Shock: Biochemical, Pharmacological, and Clinical Aspects. New York, Plenum Press, 1970, p. 135.
38. Lefer, A. M.: Blood-borne humoral factors in the pathophysiology of circulatory shock. Circ. Res. *32*:129, 1973.
39. Rai, V., Pandey, S. K., Singh, R. H., and Udupa, K. N.: Systemic histamine and histaminase changes during haemorrhagic shock. Indian J. Exp. Biol. *14*: 187, 1976.

40. Bond, R. F., Bond, C. H., Peissner, L. C., and Manning, E. S.: Prostaglandin modulation of adrenergic vascular control during hemorrhagic shock. Am. J. Physiol. *241*:H85, 1981.
41. Errington, M. L., and Rocha e Silva, M., Jr.: Vasopressin clearance and secretion during haemorrhage in normal dogs and in dogs with experimental diabetes insipidus. J. Physiol. *227*:395, 1972.
42. Regoli, D., and Vane, J. R.: The continuous estimation of angiotensin formed in the circulation of the dog. J. Physiol. *183*:513, 1966.
43. Errington, M. L., and Rocha e Silva, M., Jr.: On the role of vasopressin and angiotensin in the development of irreversible haemorrhagic shock. J. Physiol. *242*:119, 1974.
44. Holaday, J. W., O'Hara, M., and Faden, A. I.: Hypophysectomy alters cardiorespiratory variables: Central effects of pituitary endorphins in shock. Am. J. Physiol. *241*:H479, 1981.
45. Curtis, M. T., and Lefer, A. M.: Protective actions of naloxone in hemorrhagic shock. Am. J. Physiol. *239*:H416, 1980.
46. Holaday, J. W., and Faden, A. I.: Naloxone reversal of endotoxin hypotension suggests role of endorphins in shock. Nature *275*:450, 1978.
47. Cook, J. A., Wise, W. C., and Halushka, P. V.: Elevated thromboxane levels in the rat during endotoxic shock. J. Clin. Invest. *65*:227, 1980.
48. Wise, W. C., Cook, J. A., Halushka, P. V., and Knapp, D. R.: Protective effects of thromboxane synthetase inhibitors in rats in endotoxic shock. Circ. Res. *46*:854, 1980.
49. Krausz, M. M., Utsunomiya, T., Feuertein, G., Wolfe, J. H. N., Shepro, D., and Hechtman, H. B.: Prostacyclin reversal of lethal endotoxemia in dogs. J. Clin. Invest. *67*:1118, 1981.
50. Haglund, U., Hulten, L., Ahren, C., and Lundgren, O.: Mucosal lesions in the human small intestine in shock. Gut *16*:979, 1975.
51. Jones, R. T., Garcia, J. H., Mergner, W. J., Pendergrass, R. E., Valigorsky, J. M., and Trump, B. F.: Effects of shock on the pancreatic acinar cell. Arch. Pathol. *99*:634, 1975.
52. Passmore, J. C., Leffler, C. W., and Neiberger, R. E.: A critical analysis of renal blood flow distribution during hemorrhage in dogs. Circ. Shock *5*:327, 1978.
53. Dunnill, M. D., and Jerrome, D. W.: Renal tubular necrosis due to shock: Light-and-electron-microscope observation. J. Pathol. *118*:109, 1976.
54. Arango, A., Illner, H., and Shires, G. T.: Role of ischemia in the induction of changes in cell membrane during hemorrhagic shock. J. Surg. Res. *20*:473, 1976.
55. Guyton, A. C.: Circulatory Physiology. Philadelphia, W. B. Saunders Co., 1973.
56. Wiggers, C. H., and Werle, J. M.: Cardiac and peripheral resistance factors as determinants of circulatory failure in hemorrhagic shock. Am. J. Physiol. *136*: 421, 1942.
57. Jones, C. E., Smith, E. E., DuPont, E., and Williams, R. D.: Demonstration of nonperfused myocardium in late hemorrhagic shock. Circ. Shock *5*:97, 1978.
58. Lee, J. C., and Downing, S. E.: Myocardial oxygen availability and cardiac failure in hemorrhagic shock. Am. Heart J. *92*:201, 1976.
59. Siegel, H. W., and Downing, W. E.: Reduction of left ventricular contractility during acute hemorrhagic shock. Am. J. Physiol. *218*:772, 1980.
60. Lefer, A. M.: Myocardial depressant factor and circulatory shock. Klin. Wochenschr. *52*:358, 1974.
61. Kashyap, M. L., Tay, J. S. L., Sothy, S. P., and Morrison, J. A.: Role of adipose tissue in free fatty acid metabolism in hemorrhagic hypotension and shock. Metabolism *24*:855, 1975.
62. Guntheroth, W. G., Jacky, J. P., Kawabori, I., Stevenson, J. G., and Moreno, A. H.: Left ventricular performance in endotoxin shock in dogs. Am. J. Physiol. *242*:H172, 1982.
63. Parker, J. L., and Adams, H. R.: Contractile dysfunction of atrial myocardium from endotoxin-shocked guinea pigs. Am. J. Physiol. *240*:H954, 1981.
64. Hackel, D. B., Mikat, E. M., Reimer, K., and Whalen, G.: Effects of verapamil on heart and circulation in hemorrhagic shock in dogs. Am. J. Physiol. *241*:H12, 1981.
65. Feigl, E. O.: Control of myocardial oxygen tension by sympathetic coronary vasoconstriction in the dog. Circ. Res. *37*:88, 1975.
66. Rinaldo, J. E., and Rogers, R. M.: Adult respiratory-distress syndrome: Changing concepts of lung injury and repair. N. Engl. J. Med. *306*:900, 1982.
67. Weil, M. H., Carlson, R., Schaeffer, R., Jr., and Shubin, H.: Acute respiratory failure associated with shock. Antibiot. Chemother. *21*:106, 1976.
68. Hopewell, P. H., and Murray, J. F.: The adult respiratory distress syndrome. *In* Creger, W. P., Coggins, C. H., and Hancock, E. W. (eds.): Annual Review of Medicine: Selected Topics in Clinic Sciences. Vol. 27. Palo Alto, Calif., Annual Reviews, Inc., 1976, p. 343.
69. Katzenstein, A., Bloor, C. M., and Leibow, A. S.: Diffuse alevolar damage—the role of oxygen, shock, and related factors. Am. J. Pathol. *85*:210, 1976.
70. Gump, F. E., Mashima, R., Jorgensen, S., and Kinney, J. M.: Simultaneous use of three indicators to evaluate pulmonary capillary damage in man. Surgery *70*:262, 1971.
71. Hammerschmidt, D. E., White, J. G., and Craddock, P. R.: Corticosteroids inhibit complement-induced granulocyte aggregation: A possible mechanism for their efficacy in shock states. J. Clin. Invest. *63*:798, 1979.
72. Robin, E. D., Carey, L. C., Grenvik, A., Glauser, F., and Gaudio, R.: Capillary leak syndrome with pulmonary edema. Arch. Intern. Med. *130*:66, 1972.
73. Ratliff, N. B., Young, W. G., Jr., Hackel, D. B., Mikat, E., and Wilson, J. W.: Pulmonary injury secondary to extracorporeal circulation. J. Thorac. Cardiovasc. Surg. *65*:425, 1973.
74. Petty, T. L., and Ashbaugh, D. G.: The adult respiratory distress syndrome: Clinical features, factors influencing prognosis and principles of management. Chest *60*:233, 1971.
75. Joffe, N., and Simon, M.: Pulmonary oxygen toxicity in the adult. Radiology *92*:460, 1969.
76. Burford, T. H., and Burback, B.: Traumatic wet lung: Observations on certain physiologic fundamentals of thoracic trauma. J. Thorac. Surg. *14*:415, 1945.
77. Senior, R. M., Wessler, S., and Avioli, L. V.: Pulmonary oxygen toxicity. J.A.M.A. *127*:1373, 1971.
78. Tiefenbrun, J., Dikman, S., and Shoemaker, W. C.: The correlation of sequential changes in the distribution of pulmonary blood flow in hemorrhagic shock with the histopathologic anatomy. Surgery *78*:618, 1975.
79. Esrig, B. C., and Fulton, R. L.: Sepsis, resuscitated hemorrhagic shock and "shock lung": An experimental correlation. Ann. Surg. *182*:218, 1975.
80. Gaisford, W. D., Pandley, N., and Jensen, C. G.: Pulmonary changes in treated hemorrhagic shock: II. Ringer's lactate solution versus colloid infusion. Am. J. Surg. *124*:738, 1972.
81. Jenkins, M. T., Jones, R. F., Wilson, B., and Moyer, C. A.: Congestive atelectasis—a complication of the intravenous infusion of fluids. Ann. Surg. *132*: 327, 1950.
82. Dillon, B. C., and Saba, T. M.: Fibronectin deficiency and intestinal transvascular fluid balance during bacteremia. Am. J. Physiol. *242*:H557, 1982.
83. McKenna, U. G., Meadows, J. A., III, Brewer, N. S., Wilson, W. R., and Perrault, J.: Toxic shock syndrome, a newly recognized disease entity: Report of 11 cases. Mayo Clin. Proc. *55*:663, 1980.
84. Blumenstock, F. A., Saba, T. M., Weber, P., and Lafin, R.: Biochemical and immunological characterization of human opsonic a_2SB glycoprotein: Its identity with cold-insoluble globulin. J. Biol. Chem. *253*:4287, 1978.
85. Saba, T. M., and Jaffe, E.: Plasma fibronectin (opsonic glycoprotein): Its synthesis by vascular endothelial cells and role in cardiopulmonary integrity after trauma as related to reticuloendothelial function. Am. J. Med. *68*:577, 1980.
86. Moss, G., and Stein, A. A.: The centrineurogenic etiology of the respiratory distress syndrome: Protection by unilateral chronic pulmonary denervation in hemorrhagic shock. J. Trauma *16*:361, 1976.
87. Lopes, O. U., Pontieri, V., Rocha e Silva, M., Jr., and Velasco, I. T.: Hyperosmotic NaCl and severe hemorrhagic shock: Role of the innervated lung. Am. J. Physiol. *241*:H883, 1981.
88. Valesco, I. T., Pontieri, V., Rocha e Silva, M., Jr., and Lopes, O. U.: Hyperosmotic NaCl and severe hemorrhagic shock. Am. J. Physiol. *239*:H664, 1980.
89. Holcroft, J. W., and Trunkey, D. D.: Pulmonary extravasation of albumin during and after hemorrhagic shock in baboons. J. Surg. Res. *18*:91, 1975.
90. Moss, G., and Stein, A. A.: The respiratory distress syndrome: Hypoalbuminemia as a predisposing factor. Crit. Care Med. *4*(Abstract):95, 1976.
91. Morissette, M., Weil, M. H., and Shubin, H.: Reduction in colloid osmotic pressure associated with fatal progression of cardiopulmonary failure. Crit. Care Med. *3*:115, 1975.
92. Attar, S. M. A., Tingey, H. B., McLaughlin, J. S., and Cowley, R. A.: Bradykinin in human shock. Surg. Forum *18*:46, 1967.
93. Hallett, J. W., Jr., Sneiderman, C. A., and Wilson, J. W.: Pulmonary effects of arterial infusion of filtered blood in experimental hemorrhagic shock. Surg. Gynecol. Obstet. *138*:517, 1974.
94. Shubrooks, S. J., Jr., Schneider, B., Dubin, H., and Turino, G. M.: Acidosis and pulmonary hemodynamic in hemorrhagic shock. Am. J. Physiol. *225*:225, 1973.
95. Petty, T. L., Reiss, O. K., Paul, G. W., Silvers, G. W., and Elkins, N. D.: Characteristics of pulmonary surfactant in adult respiratory distress syndrome associated with trauma and shock. Am. Rev. Respir. Dis. *115*:531, 1977.
96. Greenberg, S., McGowan, C., and Glenn, T. M.: Pulmonary vascular smooth muscle function in porcine splanchnic arterial occlusion shock. Am. J. Physiol. *241*:H34, 1981.
97. Demling, R. H., Selinger, S. L., Bland, R. D., and Staub, N. C.: Effect of acute hemorrhagic shock on pulmonary microvascular fluid filtration and protein permeability in sheep. Surgery *77*:512, 1975.
98. Jardin, F., Eveleigh, M. C., Gurdjian, F., Delille, F., and Margairaz, A.: Venous admixture in human septic shock: Comparative effects of blood volume expansion, dopamine infusion and isoproterenol infusion on mismatching of ventilation and pulmonary blood flow in peritonitis. Circulation *60*:155, 1979.
99. Woolverton, W. C., Brigham, K. L., and Staub, N. C.: Effect of continuous positive airway pressure breathing on pulmonary fluid filtration and content in sheep. Physiologist *16*:490, 1973.
100. James, P. M., Jr.: Treatment of shock lungs. Am. Surg. *41*:451, 1975.
101. Harken, A. H., Brennan, M. F., Smith, B., and Barsamian, E. M.: The hemodynamic response to positive end-expiratory ventilation in hypovolemic patients. Surgery *76*:786, 1974.
102. Chinard, F. P., Enns, T., and Nolan, M. D.: Permeability characteristics of alveolar-capillary barrier. Trans. Assoc. Am. Phys. *75*:253, 1962.
103. Staub, N. C.: Pathogenesis of pulmonary edema. Am. Rev. Respir. Dis. *109*: 358, 1974.
104. Gadek, J. E., Fulmer, J. D., Gelfand, J. A., Frank, M. M., Petty, T. L., and Crystal, R. G.: Danazol-induced augmentation of serum α_1-antitrypsin levels in individuals with marked deficiency of this antiprotease. J. Clin. Invest. *66*: 82, 1980.
105. Simpson, D. L., Goodman, M., Spector, S. L., and Petty, T. L.: Long-term follow-up and bronchial reactivity testing in survivors of the adult respiratory distress syndrome. Am. Rev. Respir. Dis. *117*:449, 1978.

106. Sobel, B. E., and Mayer, S. E.: Cyclic adenosine monophosphate and cardiac contractility. Circ. Res. *32*:407, 1973.
107. Weissler, A. M., Kruger, F. A., Baba, N., Scarpelli, D. G., Leighton, R. F., and Gallimore, J. K.: Role of anaerobic metabolism in the preservation of functional capacity and structure of anoxic myocardium. J. Clin. Invest. *47*: 403, 1968.
108. Henry, P. D., Sobel, B. E., and Braunwald, E.: Protection of hypoxic guinea pig hearts with glucose and insulin. Am. J. Physiol. *226*:309, 1974.
109. Clark, A. J., Gaddie, R., and Stewart, C. P.: The anaerobic activity of the isolated frog's heart. J. Physiol. *75*:321, 1932.
110. Kubler, W., and Spieckermann, P. G.: Regulation of glycolysis in the ischemic and the anoxic myocardium. J. Mol. Cell. Cardiol. *1*:351, 1970.
111. Brachfeld, N., Ohtaka, Y., Klein, I., and Kawade, M.: Substrate perference and metabolic activity of the aerobic and the hypoxic turtle heart. Circ. Res. *31*:453, 1972.
112. Huckabee, W. E.: Relationships of pyruvate and lactate during anaerobic metabolism. I. Effects of infusion of pyruvate or glucose and of hyperventilation. J. Clin. Invest. *37*:244, 1958.
113. Mueller, H., Ayres, S. M., Gregory, J. J., Giannelli, S., Jr., and Grace, W. J.: Hemodynamics, coronary blood flow, and myocardial metabolism in coronary shock; response to l-norepinephrine and isoproterenol. J. Clin. Invest. *49*: 1885, 1970.
114. Whalen, D. A., Jr., Hamilton, D. C., Ganote, C. E., and Jennings, R. B.: Effect of a transient period of ischemia on myocardial cells. I. Effects on cell volume regulation. Am. J. Pathol. *74*:381, 1974.
115. Remme, W. J., de Jong, J. W., and Verdouw, P. D.: Effects of pacing-induced myocardial ischemia on hypoxanthine efflux from the human heart. Am. J. Cardiol. *40*:55, 1977.
116. de Jong, J. W., and Goldstein, S.: Changes in coronary venous inosine concentration and myocardial wall thickening during regional ischemia in the pig. Circ. Res. *35*:111, 1974.
117. Sobel, B. W.: Salient biochemical features in ischemic myocardium. Circ. Res. *35*(Suppl.):III-173, 1974.
118. Agress, C. M., Jacobs, H. I., Glasner, H. F., Lederer, M. A., Clark, W. G., Wroblewski, F., Karmen, A., and LaDue, J. S.: Serum transaminase levels in experimental myocardial infarction. Circulation *11*:711, 1955.
119. Nachlas, M. D., Friedman, M. D., and Cohen, S. P.: A method for the quantitation of myocardial infarcts and the relation of serum enzyme levels to infarct size. Surgery *55*:700, 1964.
120. Kjekshus, J. K., and Sobel, B. E.: Depressed myocardial creatine phosphokinase activity following experimental myocardial infarction in rabbit. Circ. Res. *27*:403, 1970.
121. Shell, W. E., Kjekshus, J. K., and Sobel, B. E.: Quantitative assessment of the extent of myocardial infarction in the conscious dog by means of analysis of serial changes in serum creatine phosphokinase activity. J. Clin. Invest. *50*: 2614, 1971.
122. Weissmann, G., Hoffstein, S., Gennaro, D., and Fox, A. C.: Lysosomes in ischemic myocardium with observations on the effects of methylprednisolone. *In* Lefer, A. M., Kelliher, G. J., and Rovetto, M. J. (eds.): Pathophysiology and Therapeutics of Myocardial Ischemia. New York, Spectrum Publications, Inc., 1977, p. 367.
123. Harnarayan, C., Bennett, M. A., Pentecost, B. L., and Brewer, D. B.: Quantitative study of infarcted myocardium in cardiogenic shock. Br. Heart J. *32*: 728, 1970.
124. Page, D. L., Caulfield, J. B., Kastor, J. A., DeSanctis, R. W., and Sanders, C. A.: Myocardial changes associated with cardiogenic shock. N. Engl. J. Med. *285*:133, 1971.
125. Tennant, R., and Wiggers, C. J.: The effect of coronary occlusion on myocardial contraction. Am. J. Physiol. *112*:351, 1935.
126. Gutovitz, A. L., Sobel, B. E., and Roberts, R.: Progressive nature of myocardial injury in selected patients with cardiogenic shock. Am. J. Cardiol. *41*:469, 1978.
127. Steenberger, C., Deleeuw, G., Rich, T., and Williamson, J. R.: Effects of acidosis and ischemia on contractility and intracellular pH of rat heart. Circ. Res. *41*:469, 1978.
128. Braunwald, E., and Kloner, R. A.: The stunned myocardium: Prolonged, postischemic ventricular dysfunction. Circulation *66*:1146, 1982.
129. da Luz, P. L., Weil, M. H., and Shubin, H.: Current concepts on mechanisms and treatment of cardiogenic shock. Am. Heart J. *92*:103, 1976.
130. Borda, L., Schuchleib, R., and Henry, P. D.: Effects of potassium on isolated canine coronary arteries: Modulation of adrenergic responsiveness and release of norepinephrine. Circ. Res. *41*:778, 1977.
131. Carlson, E. L., Selinger, S. L., Utley, J., and Hoffman, J. I. E.: Intramyocardial distribution of blood flow in hemorrhagic shock in anesthetized dogs. Am. J. Physiol. *230*:41, 1976.
132. Lloyd, B. L., and Taylor, R. R.: Augmentation of myocardial digoxin concentration in hemorrhagic shock. Circulation *51*:718, 1975.
133. Peterson, D. F., and Brown, A. M.: Pressor reflexes produced by stimulation of afferent fibers in the cardiac sympathetic nerves of the cat. Circ. Res. *28*: 605, 1971.
134. Malliani, A., Peterson, D. F., Bishop, V. S., and Brown, A. M.: Spinal sympathetic cardiocardiac reflexes. Circ. Res. *30*:158, 1972.
135. Bradfonbrener, M., and Geller, H. M.: Effect of dibenamine on renal blood flow in hemorrhagic shock. Am. J. Physiol. *171*:482, 1952.
136. Stein, J. H., Lifschitz, M. D., and Barnes, L. D.: Current concepts on the pathophysiology of acute renal failure. Am. J. Physiol. *234*:F171, 1978.
137. Levinsky, N. G.: Pathophysiology of acute renal failure. N. Engl. J. Med. *296*: 1453, 1977.
138. Van Den Berg, C. J., and Pineda, A. A.: Plasma exchange in the treatment of acute renal failure due to low molecular-weight dextran. Mayo Clin. Proc. *55*: 387, 1980.
139. Hollenberg, N. K., Adams, D. F., Oken, D. E., Abrams, H. L., and Merrill, J. P.: Acute renal failure due to nephrotoxins: Renal hemodynamic and angiographic studies in man. N. Engl. J. Med. *282*:1329, 1970.
140. Vatner, S. F.: Effects of hemorrhage on regional blood flow distribution in dogs and primates. J. Clin. Invest. *54*:225, 1974.
141. Fink, G. D., Chapnick, B. M., Goldberg, M. R., Paustian, P. W., and Kadowitz, P. J.: Influence of prostaglandin E_2, indomethacin, and reserpine on renal vascular responses to nerve stimulation, pressor and depressor hormones. Circ. Res. *41*:172, 1977.
142. Reubi, F. C., and Vorburger, C.: Renal hemodynamics and physiopathology of acute renal failure and shock in man. *In* Giovannetti, S., Bonomini, V., and D'Amico, G. (eds.): Advances in Nephrology: Physiology, Hypertension, Renal Diseases, Renal Failure, Dialysis and Transplantation. Sixth International Congress of Nephrology. Basel, S. Karger, 1975, p. 554.
143. Lucas, C. E., Rector, F. E., Werner, M., and Rosenberg, I. K.: Altered renal homeostasis with acute sepsis: Clinical significance. Arch. Surg. *106*:444, 1973.
144. Gorfinkel, H. J., Szidon, J. P., Hirsch, L. H., and Fishman, A. P.: Renal performance in experimental cardiogenic shock. Am. J. Physiol. *222*:1260, 1972.
145. Kreisberg, J. I., Bulger, R. E., Trump, B. F., and Nagle, R. B.: Effects of transient hypotension on the structure and function of rat kidney. Virchows Arch. (Cell. Pathol.) *22*:121, 1976.
146. Levinsky, N. G., Davidson, D. G., and Berliner, R. W.: Effects of reduced glomerular filtration on urine concentration in the presence of antidiuretic hormone. J. Clin. Invest. *38*:730, 1959.
147. Shier, M. R., Bradley, V. E., Ledgerwood, A. M., Rosenberg, I. K., and Lucas, C. E.: Renal function and the postresuscitative hypertension syndrome. Surg. Forum *26*:56, 1975.
148. Carlson, R. P., and Lefer, A. M.: Hepatic cell integrity in hypodynamic states. Am. J. Physiol. *231*:1408, 1976.
149. Loegering, D. J.: Humoral factor depletion and reticuloendothelial depression during hemorrhagic shock. Am. J. Physiol. *232*:H283, 1977.
150. Kaplan, J. E., and Saba, T. M.: Humoral deficiency and reticuloendothelial depression after traumatic shock. Am. J. Physiol. *230*:7, 1976.
151. Loegering, D. J., and Saba, T. M.: Hepatic Kupffer cell dysfunction during hemorrhagic shock. Circ. Shock *3*:107, 1975.
152. Saba, T. M.: Reticuloendothelial systemic host defense after surgery and traumatic shock. Circ. Shock *2*:91, 1975.
153. Williams, L. F., Jr.: Vascular insufficiency of the intestines. Gastroenterology *61*:757, 1971.
154. Okuda, M., and Fukui, T.: Myocardial depressant factor—A peptide: Its significance in cardiogenic shock. Jap. Circ. J. *38*:497, 1974.
155. Lundgren, O., Haglund, U., Isaksson, O., and Abe, T.: Effects on myocardial contractility of blood-borne material released from the feline small intestine in simulated shock. Circ. Res. *38*:307, 1976.
156. Meagher, D. M., Piermattei, D. L., and Swan, H.: Platelet aggregation during progressive hemorrhagic shock in pigs: Possible effects on reperfusion syndrome. J. Thorac. Cardiovasc. Surg. *62*:822, 1971.
157. Bridenbaugh, G. A., and Lefer, A. M.: Influence of humoral shock factors in in vitro aggregation of dog platelets. Thromb. Res. *8*:599, 1976.
158. Lecompte, F., II, Aberkane, H., Azoulay, E., Muffat-Joly, M., and Pocidalo, J. J.: Blood affinity for oxygen in experimental hemorrhagic shock with metabolic acidosis. Pfluegers Arch. *359*:147, 1975.
159. Agostoni, A., Lotto, A., Stabilini, R., Bernasconi, C., Gerli, G., Gattinoni, L., Iapickino, G., and Salvade, P.: Hemoglobin oxygen affinity in patients with low-output heart failure and cardiogenic shock after acute myocardial infarction. Eur. J. Cardiol. *3*:53, 1975.
160. Kostuk, W. J., Suwa, K., Bernstein, E. F., and Sobel, B. E.: Altered hemoglobin oxygen affinity in patients with acute myocardial infarction. Am. J. Cardiol. *31*:295, 1973.
161. Lambertson, C. J., Semple, S. J. G., Smyth, M. G., and Gelfand, R.: H^+ and pCO_2 as chemical factors in respiratory and cerebral circulatory control. J. Appl. Physiol. *16*:473, 1961.
162. Harper, A. M.: Autoregulation of cerebral blood flow: Influence of the arterial blood pressure on the blood flow through the cerebral cortex. J. Neurol. Neurosurg. Psychiatry *29*:398, 1966.
163. Kariman, K., Hempel, F. G., Jobsis, F. F., Burnes, S. R., and Saltzman, H. A.: In vivo comparison of cerebral tissue PO_2 and cytochrome aa_3 reduction-oxidation state in cats during hemorrhagic shock. J. Clin. Invest. *68*:21, 1981.
164. Siesjo, B. J., and Zwetnow, N. N.: The effect of hypovolemic hypotension on extra- and intracellular acid-base parameters and energy metabolites in the rat brain. Physiol. Scand. *79*:114, 1970.
165. Baek, S.-M., Makabali, G. G., Bryan-Brown, C. W., Kusek, J. M., and Shoemaker, W. C.: Inadequacy of high central venous pressure as a guide to volume therapy. Surg. Forum *24*:14, 1973.
166. Niazi, A., Beckman, C., Shatney, C., and Lillehei, R. C.: Use of monitoring to improve survival in shock. Geriatrics *30*:93, 1975.
167. Rackley, C. E., Russell, R. O., Jr., Mantle, J. A., and Moraski, R. E.: Cardiogenic shock: Recognition and management. Cardiovasc. Clin. *7*:251, 1975.

168. Forrester, J. S., Diamond, G., Chatterjee, K., and Swan, H. J. C.: Medical therapy of acute myocardial infarction by application of hemodynamic subsets (Parts I and II). N. Engl. J. Med. *295*:1356, 1976.
169. Loisance, D. Y., Cachera, J. P., Poulain, H., Aubry, P. H., Juvin, A. M., and Galey, J. J.: Ventricular septal defect after acute myocardial infarction: Early repair. J. Thorac. Cardiovasc. Surg. *80*:61, 1980.
170. Cohn, J. N., Guiha, N. H., Broder, M. I., and Limas, C. J.: Right ventricular infarction. Am. J. Cardiol. *33*:209, 1974.
171. Strauss, H. D., Sobel, B. E., and Roberts, R.: The influence of occult right ventricular infarction on enzymatically estimated infarct size, hemodynamics and prognosis. Circulation *62*:503, 1980.
172. Gewirtz, H., Gold, H. K., Fallon, J. T., Pasternak, R. C., and Leinbach, R. C.: Role of right ventricular infarction in cardiogenic shock associated with inferior myocardial infarction. Br. Heart J. *42*:719, 1979.
173. Lorell, B., Leinbach, R. C., Pohost, G. M., Gold, H. K., Dinsmore, R. E., Hutter, A. M., Jr., Pastore, J. O., and DeSanctis, R. W.: Right ventricular infarction: Clinical diagnosis and differentiation from cardiac tamponade and pericardial constriction. Am. J. Cardiol. *43*:465, 1979.
174. Iqbal, M. A., and Liebson, P. R.: Counterpulsation and dobutamine: Their use in treatment of cardiogenic shock due to right ventricular infarct. Arch. Intern. Med. *141*:247, 1981.
175. Rackley, C. E., Russel, R. O., Mantle, J. A., Rogers, W. J., Papapietro, S. A., and Schwartz, K. M.: Right ventricular infarction and function. Am. Heart J. *101*:215, 1981.
176. Wackers, F. J., Lie, K. I., Becker, A. E., Durrer, D., and Wellens, H. J. J.: Coronary artery disease in patients dying from cardiogenic shock or congestive heart failure in the setting of acute myocardial infarction. Br. Heart J. *38*:906, 1976.
177. Amsterdam, E. A., DeMaria, A. N., Hughes, J. L., Hurley, E. J., Lurie, A. J., Williams, D. O., Miller, R. R., and Mason, D. T.: Myocardial infarction shock: Mechanisms and management. *In* Mason, D. T. (ed.): Congestive Heart Failure: Mechanisms, Evaluations and Treatment. New York, Dun-Donnelly, 1976, p. 365.
178. Bleifeld, W., Hanrather, P., Mathey, D., and Merx, W.: Acute myocardial infarction. V. Left and right ventricular haemodynamics in cardiogenic shock. Br. Heart J. *36*:822, 1974.
179. Diamond, G., and Forrest, J. S.: Effect of coronary artery disease and acute myocardial infarction on left ventricular compliance in man. Circulation *45*:11, 1972.
180. Russell, R. O., Jr., Rackley, C. E., Pombo, J., Hunt, D., Potanin, C., and Dodge, H. T.: Effects of increasing left ventricular filling pressure in patients with acute myocardial infarction. J. Clin. Invest. *49*:1539, 1970.
181. Cohn, J. N., Luria, M. H., Daddario, R. C., and Tristani, F. E.: Studies in clinical shock and hypotension. V. Hemodynamic effects of dextran. Circulation *35*:316, 1967.
182. Ferrer, M. I.: Disturbances in the circulation in patients with cor pulmonale. Bull. NY Acad. Med. *41*:942, 1965.
183. Kezdi, P., Misra, S. N., Kordenat, R. D., Spickler, J. W., and Stanley, E. L.: The role of vagal afferents in acute myocardial infarction. Am. J. Cardiol. *26*: 642, 1970.
184. Costanin, L.: Extracardiac factors contributing to hypotension during coronary occlusion. Am. J. Cardiol. *11*:205, 1963.
185. Brown, A. M.: Excitation of afferent cardiac sympathetic nerve fibres during myocardial ischaemia. J. Physiol. *190*:35, 1967.
186. Kumar, R., Hood, W. B., Jr., Joison, J., Gilmour, D. P., Norman, J. C., and Abelmann, W. H.: Experimental myocardial infarction. VI. Efficacy and toxicity of digitalis in acute and healing phase in intact conscious dogs. J. Clin. Invest. *49*:358, 1980.
187. Sagar, K. B., Hanson, E. C., and Powell, W. J., Jr.: Neurogenic coronary vasoconstrictor effects of digitalis during acute global ischemia in dogs. J. Clin. Invest. *60*:1248, 1977.
188. Buckley, M. J., Mundth, E. D., Daggett, W. M., DeSanctis, R. M., Sanders, C. A., and Austen, W. G.: Surgical therapy for early complications of myocardial infarction. Surgery *70*:814, 1971.
189. Guiliani, E. R., Danielson, G. K., Pluth, J. R., Odyniec, N. A., and Wallace, R. B.: Postinfarction ventricular septal rupture: Surgical considerations and results. Circulation *49*:455, 1974.
190. Bardet, J., Masquet, C., Kahn, C., Gourgon, R., Bourdarias, J., Mathivat, A., and Bouvrian, Y.: Clinical and hemodynamic results of intraaortic balloon counterpulsation and surgery for cardiogenic shock. Am. Heart J. *93*:280, 1977.
191. Miller, M. G., Weintraub, R. M., Hedley-Whyte, J., and Restall, D. S.: Surgery for cardiogenic shock. Lancet *2*:1342, 1974.
192. Kantrowitz, A., Krakauer, J. S., Rosenbaum, A., Butner, A. M., Freed, P. S., and Jaron, D.: Phase-shift balloon pumping in medically refractory cardiogenic shock: Results in 27 patients. Arch. Surg. *99*:739, 1969.
193. Snow, N., Lucas, A. E., and Richardson, J. D.: Intra-aortic balloon counterpulsation for cardiogenic shock from cardiac contusion. J. Trauma *22*: 426, 1982.
194. Mundth, E. D., Buckley, M. J., Daggatt, W. M., McEnany, M. T., Leinbach, R. C., Gold, H. K., and Austen, W. B.: Intra-aortic balloon pump assistance and early surgery in cardiogenic shock. Adv. Cardiol. *15*:159, 1975.
195. Leinbach, R. C., Dinsmore, R. E., Mundth, E. D., Buckley, M. J., Dunkman, W. B., Austen, W. B., and Sanders, C. A.: Selective coronary and left ventricular cineangiography during intraaortic balloon pumping for cardiogenic shock. Circulation *45*:845, 1972.
196. Scheidt, S., Wilner, G., Mueller, H., Summers, D., Lesch, M., Wolff, G., Krakauer, J., Rubenfire, M., Felming, P., Noon, G., Oldham, N., Killip, T., and Kantrowitz, A.: Intra-aortic balloon counterpulsation in cardiogenic shock: Report of a co-operative clinical trial. N. Engl. J. Med. *288*:979, 1973.
197. Isner, J. M., Cohen, S. J., Viruari, R., Lawrikson, W., and Roberts, W. C.: Complications of the intra-aortic balloon counterpulsation device: Clinical and morphologic observations in 45 necropsy patients. Am. J. Cardiol. *45*:250, 1980.
198. Weir, J., Yacoub, M., and Pridies, R. B.: Echocardiography of the intraaortic balloon. Br. Heart J. *37*:1045, 1975.
199. Bergmann, S. R., Lerch, R. A., Fox, K. A. A., Ludbrook, P. A., Welch, M. J., Ter-Pogossian, M. M., and Sobel, B. E.: The temporal dependence of beneficial effects of coronary thrombolysis characterized by positron tomography. Am. J. Med., *73*:573, 1982.
200. DeWood, M. A., Notske, R. N., Hensley, G. R., Shields, J. P., O'Grady, W. P., Spores, J., Goldman, M., and Ganji, J. H.: Intraaortic balloon counterpulsation with and without reperfusion for myocardial infarction shock. Circulation *61*:1105, 1980.
201. Lamberi, J. J., Jr., Cohn, L. H., Lesch, M., and Collins, J. J., Jr.: Intraaortic balloon counterpulsation: Indications and long-term results in postoperative left ventricular power failure. Arch. Surg. *109*:766, 1974.
202. Pierce, W. S., Parr, G. V. S., Myers, J. L., Pae, W. D., Jr., Bull, A. P., and Waldhausen, J. A.: Ventricular-assist pumping in patients with cardiogenic shock after cardiac operations. N. Engl. J. Med. *305*:1606, 1981.
203. Swan, H. J. C., Forrester, J. S., Danzig, R., and Allen, H. N.: Power failure in acute myocardial infarction. Progr. Cardiovasc. Dis. *12*:568, 1970.
204. Mundth, E. D., Buckley, M. J., Leinbach, R. C., Gold, H. K., Daggett, W. M., and Austen, W. G.: Surgical intervention for the complication of acute myocardial ischemia. Ann. Surg. *178*:379, 1973.
205. Warren, J. V., and Lewis, R. P.: Beneficial effects of atropine in the prehospital phase of coronary care. Am. J. Cardiol. *37*:68, 1976.
206. Dikshit, K., Vden, J. K., Forrester, J. S., Chatterjee, K., Prakash, R., and Swan, H. J. C.: Renal and extrarenal hemodynamic effects of furosemide in congestive heart failure after acute myocardial infarction. N. Engl. J. Med. *288*: 1087, 1973.
206a. Richard, C., Ricome, J. L., Rimailho, A., Bottineau, G., and Auzepy, P.: Combined hemodynamic effects of dopamine and dobutamine in cardiogenic shock. Circulation *67*:620, 1983.
207. MacCannell, K. L., McNay, J. L., Meyer, M. B., and Goldberg, L. I.: Dopamine in the treatment of hypotension and shock. N. Engl. J. Med. *275*:1389, 1966.
208. Goldberg, L. I., Hsieh, Y., and Resnekov, L.: Newer catecholamines for treatment of heart failure and shock: An update on dopamine and a first look at dobutamine. Prog. Cardiovasc. Dis. *19*:327, 1977.
209. Holzer, J., Karline, J. S., O'Rourke, R. A., Pitt, W., and Ross, J., Jr.: Effectiveness of dopamine in patients with cardiogenic shock. Am. J. Cardiol. *32*: 79, 1973.
210. Goldberg, L. I., Talley, R. C., and McNay, J. L.: The potential role of dopamine in the treatment of shock. Progr. Cardiovasc. Dis. *12*:40, 1969.
211. Oliver, L. E., Horowitz, J. D., Dynon, M. K., Jarrott, B., Brennan, J. B., Gobel, A. M., and Louis, W. J.: Use of dopamine and prazosin combined in the treatment of cardiogenic shock. Med. J. Aust. (Special Supplement, July) *26*:42, 1980.
212. Timmis, A. D., Fowler, M. B., and Chamberlain, D. A.: Comparison of haemodynamic responses to dopamine and salbutamol in severe cardiogenic shock complicating acute myocardial infarction. Br. Med. J. *282*:7, 1981.
213. Tuttle, R. R., and Mills, J.: Development of a new catecholamine to selectively increase cardiac contractility. Circ. Res. *36*:185, 1975.
214. Shell, W. E., and Sobel, B. E.: Protection of jeopardized ischemic myocardium by reduction of ventricular afterload. N. Engl. J. Med. *291*:481, 1974.
215. Fowler, M. B., Timmis, A. D., and Chamberlain, D. A.: Synergistic effects of a combined salbutamol-nitroprusside regimen in acute myocardial infarction and severe left ventricular failure. Br. Med. J. *16*:435, 1980.
216. Diamond, G., Forrester, J., Danzig, R., Parmley, W. W., and Swan, H. J. C.: Haemodynamic effects of glucagon during acute myocardial infarction with left ventricular failure in man. Br. Heart J. *33*:290, 1971.
217. Watanabe, T., Covell, J. W., Maroko, P. R., Braunwald, E., and Ross, J., Jr.: The effects of increased arterial pressure and positive inotropic agents on the severity of myocardial ischemia in the acutely depressed heart. Am. J. Cardiol. *30*:371, 1972.
218. Williams, J. R., Jr., Boyd, D. L., and Border, J. F.: Effect of acute hypoxia and hypercapnia acidosis on the development of acetylstrophanthidin-induced arrhythmias. J. Clin. Invest. *47*:1885, 1968.
219. Rosing, D. R., Kent, K. M., Maron, B. J., and Epstein, S. E.: Verapamil therapy: A new approach to the pharmacologic treatment of hypertrophic cardiomyopathy. II. Effects on exercise capacity and symptomatic status. Circulation *60*:1208, 1979.
220. Johnson, A. M.: Aortic stenosis, sudden death, and the left ventricular baroceptors. Br. Heart J. *33*:1, 1971.
221. Smith, J. A. R., Norman, J. N., Smith, A., and Smith, G.: Comparison of dextran 70 and hydroxyethyl starch in volume replacement. Br. J. Surg. *62*:666, 1975.

222. Nickerson, M.: Sympathetic blockade in therapy of shock. Am. J. Cardiol. 12: 619, 1963.
223. MacDonald, J. A. E., Milligan, G. F., Mellon, A., and Ledingham, I. M.: Ventricular function in experimental hemorrhagic shock. Surg. Gynecol. Obstet. 140:572, 1975.
224. Drop, L. J., and Laver, M. B.: Low plasma ionized calcium and response to calcium therapy in critically ill man. Anesthesiology 43:300, 1975.
225. Vargish, T., Turner, C. S., Bagwell, C. E., and James, P. M., Jr.: Dose-response relationships in steroid therapy for hemorrhagic shock. Rev. Surg. 33: 363, 1976.
226. Weil, M. H., and Whigham, H.: Corticosteroids for reversal of hemorrhagic shock in rats. Am. J. Physiol. 209:815, 1965.
227. Altura, B. M., and Altura, B. T.: Peripheral vascular actions of glucocorticoids and their relationship to protection in circulatory shock. J. Pharmacol. Exp. Ther. 190:300, 1974.
228. Schumer, W., and Nyhus, L. M.: Corticocosteroid effect on biochemical parameters of human oligemic shock. Arch. Surg. 100:405, 1970.
229. Vargish, T., Shircliff, A., and James, P. M.: Effect of steroids on cardiac function. Am. Surg. 40:688, 1974.
230. Motsay, G. J., Romero, L. H., and Lillehei, R. C.: Use of corticosteroids in the treatment of shock. Int. Surg. 59:593, 1974.
231. Tanaka, K., and Iizuka, Y.: Suppression of enzyme release from isolated rat liver lysosomes by non-steroidal anti-inflammatory drug. Biochem. Pharmacol. 17:2023, 1968.
232. Lillehei, R. C., and MacLean, L. D.: Physiological approach to successful treatment of endotoxin shock in the experimental animal. Arch. Surg. 78:116, 1959.
233. Dietzman, R. H., and Lillehei, R. C.: The treatment of cardiogenic shock. V. The use of corticosteroids in the treatment of cardiogenic shock. Am. Heart J. 75:274, 1968.
234. Sladen, A.: Methylprednisolone: Pharmacologic doses in shock lung syndrome. J. Thorac. Cardiovasc. Surg. 71:800, 1976.
235. Bryan-Brown, C. W.: Tissue blood flow and oxygen transport in critically ill patients. Crit. Care Med. 3:103, 1975.
236. Reid, P. R., and Thompson, W. L.: The clinical use of dopamine in the treatment of shock. Johns Hopkins Med. J. 137:276, 1975.
237. Dopamine for treatment of shock. The Medical Letter, Vol. 17, 1975.
238. Nagakawa, B., Goldberg, L., McCartney, J., and Matsumoto, T.: The effect of dopamine on renal microcirculation in hemorrhagic shock in dogs. Surg. Gynecol. Obstet. 142:871, 1976.
239. Engelman, K., Watts, R. W. E., Klinenberg, J. R., Sjoerdsma, A., and Seegmiller, J. E.: Clinical, physiological and biochemical studies of a patient with xanthinuria and pheochromocytoma. Am. J. Med. 38:839, 1964.
240. Sjoerdsma, A., Engelman, K., Waldman, T. A., Cooperman, L. H., and Hammond, W. G.: Pheochromocytoma: Current concepts of diagnosis and treatment. Ann. Intern. Med. 65:1302, 1966.
241. Arthurson, G.: Burn shock. Triangle 13:105, 1974.
242. Facey, F. L., Weil, M. H., and Rosoff, L.: Mechanism and treatment of shock associated with acute pancreatitis. Am. J. Surg. 111:374, 1966.
243. Weil, M. H., and Shubin, H.: Critical Care Medicine: Current Principles and Practices. Hagerstown, MD, Harper & Row, 1976.
244. Rowland, L. P., and Penn, A. S.: Myoglobinuria. Med. Clin. North Am. 56: 1233, 1972.
245. de Torrente, A., Berl, T., Cohn, P. D., Kawamoto, E., Hertz, P., and Schrier, R. W.: Hypercalcemia of acute renal failure: Clinical significance and pathogenesis. Am. J. Med. 61:119, 1976.
246. Weil, M. H., and Shubin, H.: Proposed reclassification of shock states with special reference to distributive defects. *In* Hinshaw, L. B., and Cox, B. G. (eds.): The Fundamental Mechanisms of Shock. New York, Plenum Press, 1972, p. 13.
247. Wright, C. J., McLean, A. P. H., and MacLean, L. D.: Regional capillary blood flow and oxygen uptake in severe sepsis. Surg. Gynecol. Obstet. 132: 637, 1971.
248. Hinshaw, L. B.: Role of the heart in the pathogenesis of endotoxin shock: A review of the clinical findings and observations on animal species. J. Surg. Res. 17:134, 1974.
249. Lansing, A. M.: Septic shock. J. Canad. Med. Assoc. 89:583, 1963.
250. Metabolic and cardiac alterations in shock and trauma. Circ. Shock 1 (Suppl.):1, 1979.
251. Weil, M. H., Shubin, H., and Nishijima, H.: Gram-negative shock: Definition, diagnosis and mechanisms. Antibiot. Chemother. 21:178, 1976.
252. Fletcher, J. R., Ramwell, P. W., and Herman, C. M.: Postaglandins and the hemodynamic course of endotoxin shock. J. Surg. Res. 20:589, 1976.
253. McClure, J. J.: Endotoxic shock. Vet. Clin. North Am. 6:193, 1976.
254. Cryer, P. E., Herman, C. M., and Sode, J.: Carbohydrate metabolism in the baboon subjected to gram-negative (*Escherichia coli*) septicemia. II. Depressed insulin secretion with glucose intolerance and sensitivity to exogenous insulin. Curr. Top. Surg. Res. 3:117, 1971.
255. Shatney, C. H., Dietzman, R. H., and Lillehei, R. C.: The effects of corticosteroids on systemic oxygenation and pulmonary shunting in septic shock: *In* Shoemaker, W. C., and Tavares, B. M. (eds.): Current Topics in Critical Care Medicine. Basel, S. Karger, 1974, p. 92.
256. Weisul, J. P., O'Donnell, T. F., Jr., Stone, M. A., and Clowes, G. H. A., Jr.: Myocardial performance in clinical septic shock: Effects of isoproterenol and glucose potassium insulin. J. Surg. Res. 18:357, 1975.
257. Lowry, P., Blanco, T., and Santiago-Delpin, E. A.: Histamine and sympathetic blockage in septic shock. Am. J. Surg. 43:12, 1977.
258. Fletcher, J. R., Herman, C. M., and Ramwell, P. W.: Improved survival in endotoxemia with aspirin and indomethacin pretreatment. Surg. Forum 27:11, 1976.
259. Bergentz, S. E.: Septic shock and disturbances in coagulation. Triangle 13:129, 1974.
260. Shubin, H., and Weil, M. H.: Shock associated with barbiturate intoxication. J.A.M.A. 215:263, 1971.
261. Schwartzman, R. J.: Cerebrovascular disorders causing coma or shock: CVAs and hypertensive crisis. *In* Findeiss, J. C. (ed.): Emergency Management of the Critical Patient. New York, Stratton Intercontinental Publ. Co., 1975, p. 175.
262. Fauci, A. S., Wolff, S. M., and Johnson, J. S.: Effect of cyclophosphamide upon the immune response in Wegener's granulomatosis. New Engl. J. Med. 285:1493, 1971.
263. Taylor, A. L.: Metabolic disorders causing coma and shock. *In* Findeiss, J. C. (ed.): Emergency Management of the Critical Patient. New York, Stratton Intercontinental Publ. Co., 1975, p. 175.
264. Griggs, D. M., Jr.: Cardiac output and peripheral resistance influenced by acidosis and alkalosis. *In* Oaks, W. W., and Moyer, J. H. (eds.): Pre- and Postoperative Management of the Cardiopulmonary Patient. New York, Grune and Stratton, 1970, p. 227.
265. Nahas, G. G., Brunson, J. G., King, W. M., and Cavert, H. M.: Functional and morphologic changes in heart-lung preparations following administration of adrenal hormones. Am. J. Pathol. 34:717, 1958.
266. Grollman, A. P., and Gamble, J. L., Jr.: Metabolic alkalosis, a specific effect of adrenocortical hormones. Am. J. Physiol. 196:135, 1959.
267. Sambhi, M. P., Weil, M. H., and Udhoji, V. N.: Pressor responses to norepinephrine in humans before and after corticosteroids. Am. J. Physiol. 203:961, 1962.
268. Lefkowitz, R. J., Limbird, L. E., Mukherjee, C., and Caron, M. G.: The β-adrenergic receptor and adenylate cyclase. Biochem. Biophys. Acta 457:1, 1976.
269. Fregly, M. H., Resch, G. E., Nelson, E. L., Jr., Field, F. P., and Tyler, P. E.: Effect of hypothyroidism on responsiveness to β-adrenergic stimulation. Can. J. Physiol. Pharmacol. 54:200, 1976.
270. Piper, P. J.: Anaphylaxis and the release of active substances in the lung. Pharmacol. Ther. [B]3:75, 1977.
271. Wasserman, S. I., and Austen, K. F.: Arylsulfatase B of human lung: Isolation, characterization, and interaction with slow-reacting substance of anaphylaxis. J. Clin. Invest. 57:738, 1976.
272. Lockey, R. F., and Bukantz, S. C.: Allergic emergencies. Med. Clin. North Am. 58:147, 1974.
273. Ellis, E. F., and Henney, C. S.: Adverse reactions following administration of human gamma globulin. J. Allergy Clin. Immunol. 43:45, 1969.
274. Austen, K. F.: Systemic anaphylaxis in the human being. N. Engl. J. Med. 291: 661, 1974.
275. Dalen, J. E., and Alpert, J. S.: Natural history of pulmonary embolism. Progr. Cardiovasc. Dis. 17:259, 1975.
276. The Urokinase Pulmonary Embolism Trial. Circulation 47(Suppl. II):1, 1973.
277. Britt, B. A.: Malignant hyperthermia: A pharmacogenetic disease of skeletal and cardiac muscle. N. Engl. J. Med. 290:1140, 1974.
278. Denborough, M. A., Forster, J. F. A., Hudson, M. C., Carter, N. G., and Zapf, P.: Biochemical changes in malignant hyperpyrexia. Lancet 1:1137, 1970.
279. Harriman, D. G. F., Sumner, D. W., and Ellis, F. R.: Malignant hyperpyrexia myopathy. Q. J. Med. 42:639, 1973.
280. Dantrolene for malignant hyperthermia during anesthesia. Med. Lett. Drugs Ther. 22:61, 1980.
281. Moulds, R. F. W., and Denborough, M. A.: Biochemical basis of malignant hyperpyrexia. Br. Med. J. 2:241, 1974.
282. Larcan, A., Laprevote, M. C., and Lambert, H.: Cyclical shock with hyperglobulinemia. Bibl. Anat. 13:343, 1975.

19 GENESIS OF CARDIAC ARRHYTHMIAS: ELECTROPHYSIOLOGICAL CONSIDERATIONS

by Douglas P. Zipes, M.D.

ANATOMY OF THE CARDIAC CONDUCTION SYSTEM

Sinus Node. In man, the sinus node[1] is a spindle-shaped structure composed of a fibrous tissue matrix with closely packed cells. It is 10 to 20 mm long, 2 to 3 mm wide, and thick, tending to narrow caudally toward the inferior vena cava. It lies less than 1 mm from the epicardial surface, laterally in the right atrial sulcus terminalis, at the junction of the superior vena cava and right atrium[2,3] (Fig. 19–1). Supplying the sinus node is a prominent artery branching from the right (55 to 60 per cent of the time) or the left circumflex (40 to 45 per cent) coronary artery.[4] The artery may approach the node from a clockwise or counterclockwise direction around the superior vena caval–right atrial junction.[3] The relationship of the artery to the node is thought to be constant, provoking concepts of a physiological interrelation between pulsation, arterial diameter, and sinus discharge rate in a feedback control system.[5] However, more recent evidence suggests an inconsistent relationship between the artery and node and has thrown the postulated servomechanism[5] into question.[3]

Cellular Structure. Cell types in the sinus node include nodal cells, transitional cells, and atrial muscle cells. *Nodal cells* are small (5 to 10 μm), ovoid, primitive-appearing cells with cytoplasm that contains relatively few organelles and myofibrils. Although nuclei are of normal size, nodal cells contain fewer mitochondria compared to contractile cells. The mitochondria are distributed randomly and are variable in size and shape.[6] No transverse tubular system exists. Nodal cells stain poorly, have a pale appearance on light and electron microscopy, and are grouped in elongated clusters located centrally in the sinus node.[6] Although contact between nodal cells was thought to occur mainly by opposing cell membranes—a factor possibly related to the slow conduction within the sinus node—more recent studies suggest the presence of nexus connections.[7] Nodal cells are thought to be the source of normal impulse formation in the sinus node.[7–9]

Transitional cells, or T cells, are elongated cells intermediate in size and complexity between nodal cells and atrial muscle cells. These plentiful cells have large numbers of myofibrils and are heterogeneous in structure, with some T cells more organized and complex than others. T cells near nodal cells have simple intercellular connections, while more fully developed intercalated discs exist between T cells and atrial myocardium. Since nodal cells make contact only with each other or T cells, the latter may provide the only functional pathway for distribution of the sinus impulse formed in the nodal cells to

several parts of the atria, the coronary sinus, atrioventricular valves, portions of the AV junction, and the His-Purkinje system. Ordinarily kept from reaching the level of threshold potential by the more rapidly firing sinus node, ectopic pacemaker activity at one of these latent sites can become manifest when sinus nodal discharge rate slows or block occurs at some level between the sinus node and the ectopic pacemaker site, permitting *escape* of the latent pacemaker at the latter's normal discharge rate. A clinical ECG correlate would be sinus bradycardia to a rate of 45 bpm that permits an AV junctional escape complex to occur at a rate of 50 bpm.

Alternatively, the discharge rate of the latent pacemaker can speed up inappropriately and usurp control of the cardiac rhythm from the sinus node that had been discharging at a normal rate. A clinical example would be interruption of normal sinus rhythm at a rate of 70 bpm by a premature ventricular complex or a burst of ventricular tachycardia. It is important to remember that such disorders of impulse formation can be due to a speeding or slowing of a *normal* pacemaker mechanism (e.g., phase 4 diastolic depolarization that is ionically normal for the sinus node or for an ectopic site such as a Purkinje fiber but occurs inappropriately fast or slow) or due to an ionically *abnormal* pacemaker mechanism. The patient with persistent sinus tachycardia at rest or sinus bradycardia during exertion exhibits inappropriate sinus nodal discharge rates, but the ionic mechanisms responsible for sinus nodal discharge may still be normal. Conversely, when a patient experiences ventricular tachycardia during an acute myocardial infarction, abnormal ionic mechanisms are probably operative to generate this tachycardia. Although pacemaker activity is generally not found in ordinary working myocardium, myocardial ischemia can conceivably bestow abnormal pacemaker properties on cells such as ventricular muscle fibers, permitting them to depolarize automatically. Based on the rate response to catecholamine administration of isolated fibers exhibiting normal phase 4 diastolic depolarization and on in vivo studies during stellate ganglion stimulation, it is likely that rates much in excess of 200 bpm are not due to enhanced normal automaticity.[12,79,131]

Mechanisms responsible for *normal* automaticity were described earlier (p. 616). *Abnormal* automaticity may arise from cells that have reduced maximum diastolic potentials, often in the range of −50 to −60 mV. This type of abnormal automaticity has been found in Purkinje fibers removed from dogs subjected to myocardial infarction,[126] in rat myocardium damaged by epinephrine (Fig. 19–16),[132] in human atrial samples,[133,134] and in ventricular myocardial specimens from patients undergoing aneurysmectomy and endocardial resection for recurrent ventricular tachyarrhythmias.[99,100] It can be produced in normal muscle[135] or Purkinje fibers[136] by appropriate interventions such as current passage that reduces diastolic potential (Fig. 19–17). Automatic discharge rate speeds up with progressive depolarization, while hyperpolarizing pulses slow the spontaneous firing. Other interventions, such as barium administration,[137] produce automaticity during which action potentials are similar to those produced by current passage. It is possible that partial depolarization and failure to reach normal maximal diastolic potential can induce automatic discharge in most if not all cardiac fibers.[131] The responsible ionic mechanisms (which are probably not the same in all the examples) are not clear, but in some preparations they may relate to reduction in an outward K current or impaired Na-K active transport.[113] In other instances, this type of abnormal automatic activity may be due to I_{si} because slow and not fast channel blockers suppress it.[99,101,135,136] Although this type of spontaneous automatic activity has been found in human atrial[133] and ventricular[99-101] fibers, its relation to the genesis of clinical arrhythmias has not been established.

Oscillatory activity may develop in cells both before and after full repolarization (Fig. 19–16). Oscillations with a variety of contours have been observed[100] and may represent another cause of automatic activity; however, their relation to clinical arrhythmias as well as their ionic causes and distinction from other types of depolarizations (see below) remain to be worked out.

TRIGGERED ACTIVITY. This newly recognized form of impulse formation has been observed in several types of fibers. Its demonstration requires a more precise consideration of the term "automaticity." Triggered activi

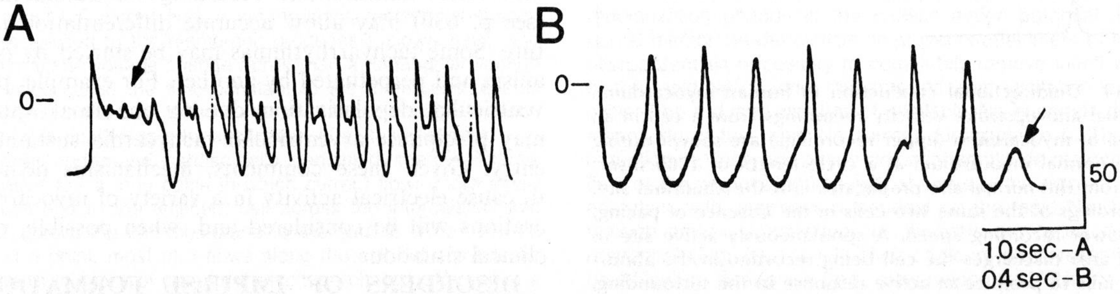

FIGURE 19–16 Triggered sustained rhythmic activity (see Fig. 19–18) recorded in rat myocardium damaged by epinephrine given 24 hours previously. *A,* Triggered activity arises from early afterdepolarizations (arrow) that occur during the plateau of the cardiac action potential. These oscillations arise from relatively low membrane potentials (< −60 mV). *B,* Spontaneous activity in the terminal phase of a triggered burst of activity is demonstrated and exhibits delayed afterdepolarizations. The delayed afterdepolarizations occur after complete repolarization, and subsequent action potentials triggered by this mechanism arise from membrane potentials of −60 to −80 mV. When a delayed afterdepolarization fails to reach threshold (end of recording, arrow), spontaneous activity ceases. (Modified from Gilmour, R. F., Jr., and Zipes, D. P.: Electrophysiological characteristics of rodent myocardium damaged by adrenaline. Cardiovasc. Res. *14*:582, 1980.)

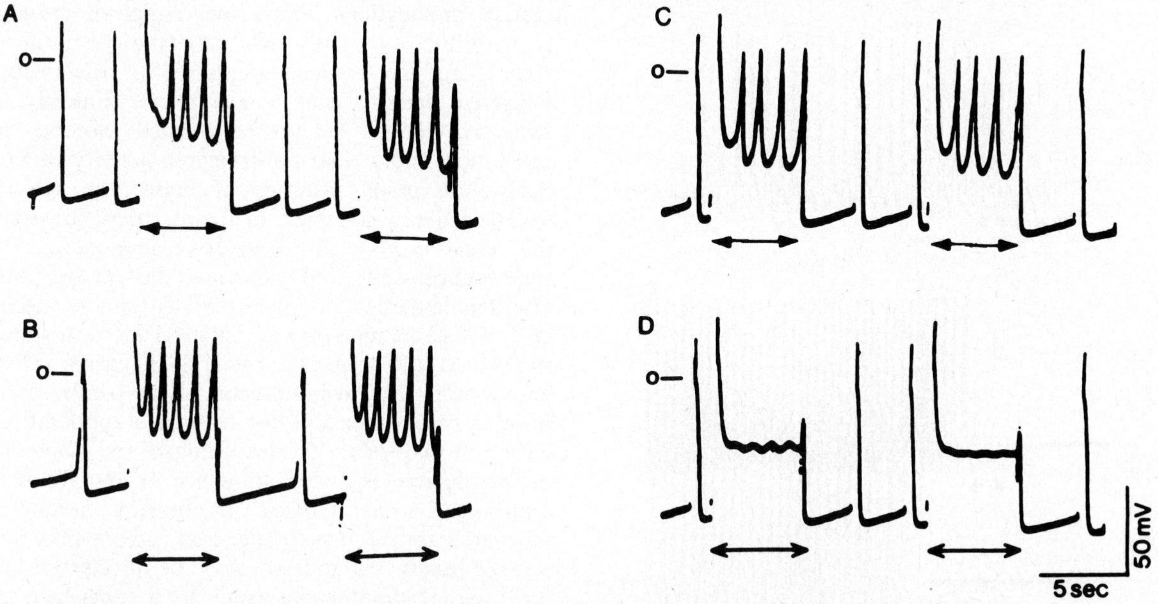

FIGURE 19–17 Abnormal automaticity during depolarization in canine Purkinje fiber. Depolarizing current pulses were delivered (across a single sucrose gap) at various times, as indicated by the intervals between arrowheads. Depolarization reduced membrane potential from −85 to −50 mV and initiated more rapid automaticity. While the fiber was at the more negative resting potential it also spontaneously discharged. Lidocaine (3 mg/L) and verapamil (3×10^{-6} M) exerted differential effects on automaticity initiated at high and low levels of transmembrane potential. *A,* Control. *B,* During superfusion with lidocaine. Lidocaine slowed the spontaneous discharge rate and reduced the amplitude of action potentials arising from the high (more negative) levels of membrane potential but did not alter action potentials or spontaneous rate at the low (less negative) level of membrane potential. *C,* Return to control after 30 minutes of washout. *D,* During superfusion with verapamil. Verapamil suppressed automaticity at the low (less negative) level of membrane potential without altering the spontaneous discharge rate at the high level of membrane potential. (From Elharrar, V., and Zipes, D. P.: Voltage modulation of automaticity in cardiac Purkinje fibers. *In* Zipes, D. P., et al. (eds.): The Slow Inward Current and Cardiac Arrhythmias. The Hague, Martinus Nijhoff, 1980, p. 357.)

ty is pacemaker activity that results *consequent to* a preceding impulse or series of impulses, without which electrical quiescence occurs (Fig. 19–18). Technically, that is not an automatic self-generating mechanism. *Automaticity* is the property of a fiber to initiate an impulse *spontaneously,* without need for prior stimulation, so that electrical quiescence does not occur. *Triggered activity* is initiated by impulses variously called low-amplitude potentials, transient depolarizations, or oscillatory afterpotentials.[138] These depolarizations may occur before or after full repolarization of the fiber (Figs. 19–16 and 19–18) and are best termed *early or late afterdepolarizations,* respectively.[139] They may arise from cells exhibiting high or low diastolic membrane potentials. Afterdepolarizations that reach threshold potential may trigger another afterdepolarization and thus self-perpetuate. Early afterdepolarizations may be precipitated by abrupt reduction in $[K]_o$, by high concentrations of catecholamines, and by some antiarrhythmic drugs[131] and may also be found in myocardium damaged by catecholamines[132] or in myocardium removed from patients who have ventricular arrhythmias.[100,101]

Delayed afterdepolarizations and triggered activity have been demonstrated in Purkinje fibers,[138,140] specialized atrial fibers[141] and ventricular muscle fibers[138] exposed to digitalis preparations and in normal Purkinje fibers exposed to Na-free superfusates.[142] When fibers in the rabbit,[143] canine,[144] simian,[145] and human[146] mitral valves and in the canine tricuspid valve[147] and coronary sinus[148] are superfused with norepinephrine, they exhibit the capacity for sustained triggered rhythmic activity. In general, the fibers exhibit delayed afterhyperpolarizations (i.e., membrane potential following depolarization transiently becomes more negative than the resting potential), followed by delayed afterdepolarizations capable of reaching threshold and triggering sustained rhythmic activity. Action potentials of the mitral valve possess less negative resting membrane potentials and slower upstrokes than do action potentials in the coronary sinus and more clearly resemble slow-response action potentials. Verapamil suppresses the triggered activity in these preparations and it is possible that the slow inward current plays a role in their genesis. The membrane potential of the fibers, however—particularly those in the coronary sinus—is not sufficiently depressed to inactivate the fast response completely or to activate the slow response. Similar triggered activity not requiring norepinephrine for initiation has been recorded in the rabbit atrial pectinate muscle.[149] Triggered activity due to delayed afterdepolarizations has also been noted in diseased human atrial[150] and ventricular[100,101] fibers studied in vitro. In vivo, atrial and ventricular arrhythmias apparently due to triggered activity have been reported in the dog[151] and possibly in humans.[152–154] However, as indicated earlier, it is very difficult to be certain that a particular mechanism is operative in vivo, given our present state of knowledge. It is tempting to ascribe certain clinical arrhythmias to triggered activity, such as some atrial tachycardias that might originate in the coronary sinus, those arrhythmias in patients who have mitral valve prolapse, or those arrhyth-

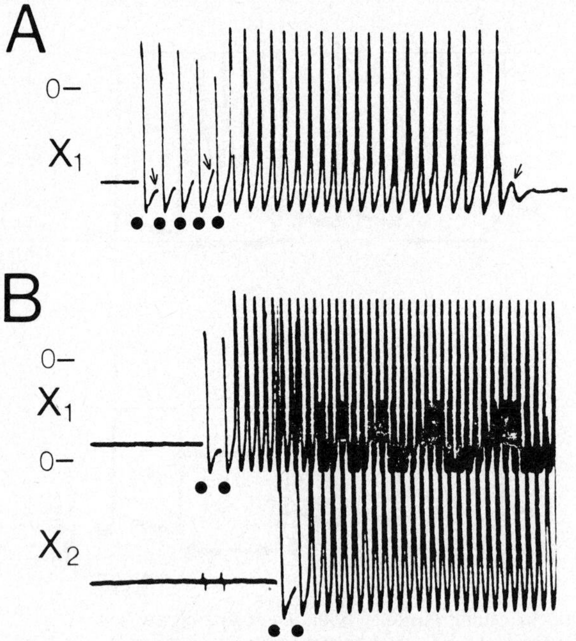

FIGURE 19–18 Triggered sustained rhythmic activity in diseased human ventricle. *A,* Spontaneous activity triggered by a series of driven action potentials (indicated by the dots) at a recording site X1. Note the gradual increase in the size of the afterdepolarizations (arrows) until the afterdepolarization reaches threshold and maintains sustained rhythmic activity after cessation of pacing. The sustained rhythmic activity finally terminates when the last afterdepolarization fails to reach threshold (arrow). *B,* Initiation of triggered activity by intracellular current injection (indicated by dots beneath the respective action potential recordings) at sites X1 and X2, which lie along the same trabeculum. Although sites X1 and X2 were only about 4 mm apart, triggered sustained rhythmic activity from one site did not propagate to the other site, indicating complete dissociation between these two sites. For current pulses, cycle length = 2000 msec; pulse duration = 10 msec; pulse intensity = 200 na. Vertical calibration: 50 mV. Horizontal calibration: 10 sec. (From Gilmour, R. F., Jr., et al.: Cellular electrophysiological abnormalities of diseased human ventricular myocardium. Am. J. Cardiol. *51*:137, 1983.)

mias precipitated by digitalis, but this approach is purely speculative at present.[155]

The ionic mechanism(s) responsible for delayed afterdepolarizations is not clear and may be varied. Because catecholamines and increases in $[Ca]_o$ enhance while verapamil suppresses activity of delayed afterdepolarizations, I_{si} is assumed to play a role. However, the negative level of resting membrane potential at which delayed depolarizations occur as well as the fact that tetrodotoxin[156,157] and antiarrhythmic agents at concentrations that affect only the fast current[158] depress or eliminate delayed afterdepolarizations caused by digitalis suggests that an inward Na current may play a role. Voltage clamp studies indicate that Na carries the inward current,[159,160] leading to the explanation that digitalis, by impairing the Na,K-ATPase exchange system, causes an increase in $[Na]_i$ which, in exchange for $[Ca]_o$, increases $[Ca]_i$. The latter in turn alters membrane conductance to a Na current that generates the afterdepolarization. Recent evidence indicates that electrogenic Na extrusion significantly influences the termination of triggered activity in the canine coronary sinus.[161]

Several features of triggered activity may have important clinical implications. First, since triggered activity appears to be induced so easily in a variety of fibers in vitro, and since suggestive evidence supports its occurrence in vivo, triggered activity may cause some clinically occurring tachyarrhythmias yet to be defined. Second, pacing at rates more rapid than the triggered activity rate (overdrive pacing) in many instances increases the amplitude and shortens the cycle length of the afterdepolarization following cessation of pacing (overdrive acceleration)[138,162] rather than suppressing and delaying the escape rate of the afterdepolarization, as in normal automatic mechanisms[113] (Fig. 19–12). Premature stimulation exerts a similar effect; the shorter the premature interval, the larger the amplitude and shorter the escape interval of the triggered event. The mechanisms responsible for overdrive acceleration are not clear but may relate to steepening of the slope of diastolic depolarization and the influence of Na/K electrogenic pumping.[161] The clinical implication might be that tachyarrhythmias due to triggered activity may not be suppressed easily or, indeed, may be precipitated by rapid rates, either spontaneous (such as a sinus tachycardia) or pacing-induced. Finally, because a single premature stimulus can both initiate and terminate triggered activity, differentiation from reentry (see below) becomes quite difficult.[152,155]

Rhythms due to automaticity may be slow atrial, junctional and ventricular escape rhythms, certain types of atrial tachycardias (such as those produced by digitalis), accelerated junctional (nonparoxysmal junctional tachycardia), and idioventricular rhythms and parasystole (see Ch. 21).

PARASYSTOLE. Electrophysiological concepts about *parasystole* have been drastically revised in the last several years.[163–165] Classically, parasystole has been considered similar to a fixed-rate, asynchronously discharging pacemaker: its timing is not altered by the dominant rhythm, it produces depolarization when the myocardium is excitable, and the intervals between discharges are multiples of a basic interval. Complete *entrance block,* constant or intermittent,[166] insulates and protects the parasystolic focus from surrounding electrical events and accounts for such activity. Occasionally, the focus may exhibit *exit block,* during which it may fail to depolarize excitable myocardium.[167] Data from recent experiments indicate that, in fact, the dominant cardiac rhythm may modulate parasystolic discharge to speed up or slow down its rate. Experimental simulations of parasystole (using a sucrose gap technique, in which a segment of block is created in a fiber by superfusing it with a solution that prevents active impulse propagation in a localized area) demonstrate that the discharge rate of an isolated, "protected" focus can be modulated by electrotonic interactions with the dominant rhythm across an area of depressed excitability. Brief subthreshold depolarizations induced during the first half of the cardiac cycle of a spontaneously discharging pacemaker will delay the subsequent discharge, while similar depolarizations induced in the second half of the cardiac cycle will accelerate it (Figs. 19–19 and 19–20).[168] Complex interactions of complete silence, concealed or manifest bigeminy, trigeminy, quadrigeminy, and periods of more complex group beating may occur owing to the entraining effects of the dominant rhythm on the ectopic focus. Similar exam-

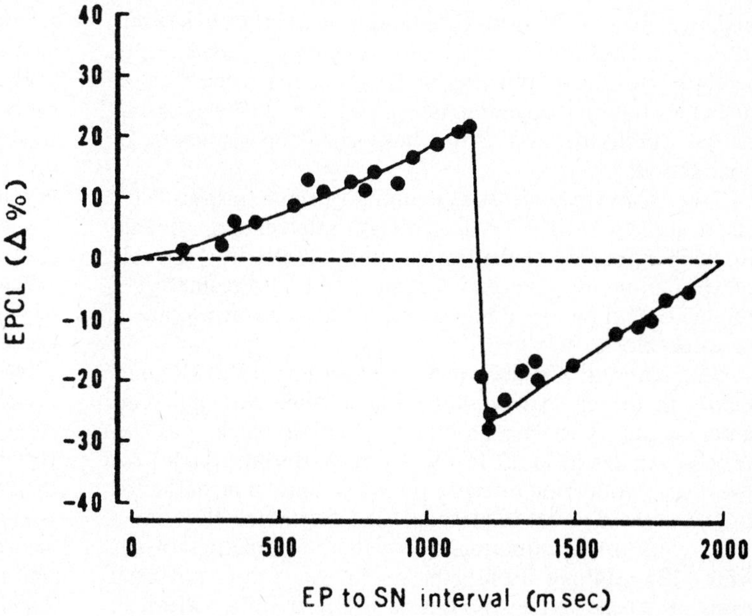

FIGURE 19–19 Phase response curve of a Purkinje fiber pacemaker mounted in a sucrose gap preparation. The x axis (EP to SN interval) represents the time after a spontaneous discharge of the pacemaker (EP) at which stimulated responses (SN) were evoked in the segment of fiber beyond the gap. The y axis (EPCL) represents the prolongation (first half) or abbreviation (second half) of the pacemaker cycle as a function of that time. EPCL = ectopic pacemaker cycle length; EP to SN interval = time after ectopic pacemaker discharge (EP) at which an evoked response (SN) was generated to simulate a ventricular response of sinus nodal (SN) origin. Intrinsic cycle length of EP, in the absence of electrotonic influence, was about 2000 msec. Abrupt phase reversal occurred at about 58 per cent of the intrinsic cycle length. These data indicate that stimulation early in the spontaneous cycle of a "parasystolic" pacemaker (EP) by a beat of sinus origin (SN) (left portion of curve) *delays* the next spontaneous discharge of EP, while stimulation late in the spontaneous cycle (right portion of the cycle) shortens the time to the next response of EP (see Figure 19–20). (From Jalife, M. J., and Moe, G. K.: A biologic model of parasystole. Am. J. Cardiol. *43*:761, 1979.)

ples have been noted in human ventricular tissue (Fig. 19–20).[101] Exactly how these observations will alter the "rules" established to diagnose parasystole electrocardiographically is still being established. However, there appear to be clinical examples[169] to support these experimental observations.

DISORDERS OF IMPULSE CONDUCTION. Conduction delay and block can result in bradyarrhythmias or tachyarrhythmias, the former when the propagating impulse blocks and is followed by asystole or a slow escape rhythm, and the latter when the delay and block produce reentrant excitation (see below). Various factors, involving both active and passive membrane properties,[78,79,170] determine the conduction velocity of an impulse and whether or not conduction is successful. Among these factors are the stimulating efficacy of the propagating impulse, which is related to the amplitude and rate of rise of phase 0,[171] and the excitability of the tissue into which the impulse conducts.[116,172] Over a range of take-off potentials (i.e., membrane potential at the time of excitation) that are more positive than −70 mV, action potential amplitude and rate of rise of phase 0 play prominent roles,[171] while at take-off potentials between −70 and −110 mV, conduction velocity appears to vary more directly with the level of excitability.[116,172] The explanation for this difference is as follows: At take-off potentials close to but more negative than −70 mV, the take-off potential, being closer to threshold, requires less current than a more polarized cell to reduce membrane potential to threshold potential and produce a regenerative response—i.e., the excitability threshold is reduced. Conduction improves even if action potential amplitude and $\dot{V}max$ are lowered. At take-off potentials less

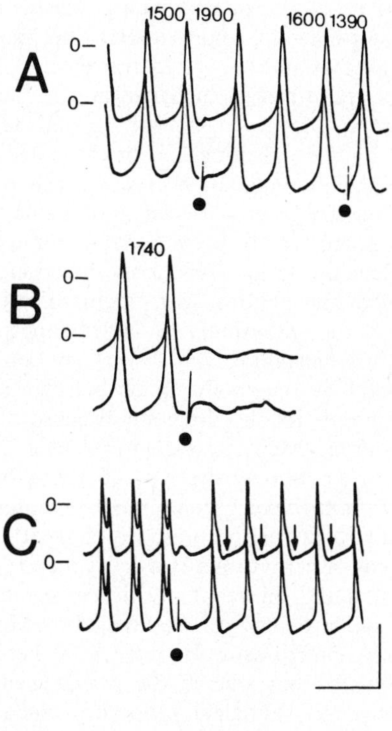

FIGURE 19–20 Modulation of pacemaker activity by subthreshold current pulses in diseased human ventricle. *A,* Two recording sites along the same trabeculum in a spontaneously active preparation. Current pulses (indicated by the dots) of 30 msec duration were injected through the lower microelectrode at various times. The interval between the spontaneous action potentials is given in milliseconds above each cycle. Injection of a subthreshold current pulse through the lower microelectrode relatively early in the spontaneous cycle (about 680 msec after initiation of the rapid portion of the preceding action potential upstroke) produced a subthreshold depolarization in the upper recording and delayed the next spontaneous discharge by 400 msec to 1900 msec. This response would fall in the first half of the curve indicated in Figure 19–19. A current pulse of the same intensity and duration delivered later in the spontaneous cycle (950 msec after the preceding upstroke) accelerated the next discharge by 210 msec to 1390 msec, relative to the previous two action potentials. The response to this current injection falls in the second half of the graph depicted in Figure 19–19.

B, A stimulus at a precise interval in the cardiac cycle (called the singular point [in this example, 930 msec after the preceding action potential upstroke]) abolished pacemaker activity.

C, A single subthreshold pulse (dot) can also alter the contour of the subsequent spontaneous action potentials and convert biphasic action potentials to action potentials with a single active component followed by delayed afterdepolarizations (arrows). Vertical calibration: 50 mV. Horizontal calibration: 2 sec in *A* and *B* and 4 sec in *C.* (From Gilmour, R. F., Jr., et al.: Cellular electrophysiological abnormalities of diseased human ventricular myocardium. Am. J. Cardiol. *51*:137, 1983.)

negative than −70 mV, threshold potential may become more positive (moves "away" from resting membrane potential). This factor plus Na inactivation that occurs at reduced membrane potential (see p. 613) makes action potential amplitude and V̇max important determinants of conduction.

Other features such as alterations in refractoriness,[173–175] electrotonic effects,[176,177] the role of intercellular connections,[178] uniformity of the propagating wavefront,[179] the role of the autonomic nervous system,[59] and the geometry of the tissue[180] may all influence conduction, to accelerate it or cause block.[174,181]

Decremental Conduction. This term is used commonly in the clinical literature but is often misapplied to describe any Wenckebach-like conduction block, i.e., responses similar to block in the AV node during which progressive conduction delay precedes the nonconducted impulse (see Ch. 21). Correctly used, decremental conduction refers to the situation in which the properties of the fiber change along its length so that the action potential loses its efficacy as a stimulus to excite the fiber ahead of it.[37,72,182,183] Thus, the stimulating efficacy of the propagating action potential diminishes progressively, possibly as a result of its decreasing amplitude and V̇max. Whether or not decremental conduction, as defined above, accounts for Wenckebach AV block is not yet resolved.

Electrical activity during each normal cardiac cycle begins in the sinus node and continues until the entire heart has been activated. Each cell, interconnected electrically, becomes activated in turn and the cardiac impulse dies out when all fibers have been discharged and are completely refractory. During this absolute refractory period, the cardiac impulse has "no place to go" and must be extinguished. If, however, a group of fibers not activated because of unidirectional block during the initial wave of depolarization recovers excitability in time to be discharged before the impulse dies out, they may serve as a link to reexcite areas that were just discharged and have now recovered from the initial depolarization. Such a process is given various names, all meaning approximately the same thing: reentry, reentrant excitation, circus movement, reciprocal or echo beat, or reciprocating tachycardia.

McWilliam,[184] Mayer,[185] Mines,[186,187] and Garrey,[188] experimenting on the pulsating bell of the medusa, the jellyfish, turtle, and mammalian hearts, worked out the basic concepts of reentry over a 20-year period early in this century. Mines noted that to prove reentry, three features had to be established: (1) an area of unidirectional block, (2) recirculation of the impulse to its point of origin, and (3) elimination of the arrhythmia by cutting the pathway. He warned against mistaking for reentry an automatic beat that originated at one point in the circuit and traveled around the circuit in one direction because of block near its site of origin. Many investigators have continued to study these concepts over the past 70 years, but the models they have used have become more complex, making it more difficult to prove the presence of reentry. Often, the diagnosis that an arrhythmia is due to reentry is made far too liberally, based on scanty evidence and certainly not adhering to the basic criteria established by Mines.

The primary prerequisite for reentry is the development of unidirectional block due to the presence of tissue with disparate electrophysiological properties. Such asymmetrical depression of conduction occurs commonly in experimental preparations, even those having the simple, relatively uniform geometry of an isolated Purkinje fiber.[177,189] Fibers participating in the reentrant pathway may be contiguous, such as adjacent AV nodal cells or Purkinje fibers, or they may be anatomically separated, such as the AV node and an accessory pathway (see p. 714). Because the two (or more) pathways have different properties—e.g., a refractory period longer in one pathway than the other, decreased excitability in one pathway, ineffectiveness of the wavefront to activate all fibers, or other reasons—the impulse (1) blocks in one pathway (site *x* in Fig. 19–21*A*; site A in Fig. 19–21*B*) and (2) propagates slowly in the adjacent pathway (arrow from *x* to *y* in Fig. 19–21*A*; serpentine arrow, D to C, Fig. 19–21*B*). If conduction in this alternative route is sufficiently depressed, the slowly propagating impulse excites tissue beyond the blocked pathway (hatched and stippled areas in Fig. 19–21*A* and *B*) and returns in a reversed direction along the pathway initially blocked (*y* to *x* in Fig. 19–21*A*; B to A in Fig. 19–21*B*) to (3) reexcite tissue proximal to the site of block (*x* to 1 in Fig. 19–21*A*; A to D in Fig. 19–21*B*). For reentry of this type to occur, the time for conduction within the depressed but unblocked area and for excitation of the distal segments must exceed the refractory period of the initially blocked pathway (*x* in Fig. 19–21*A*; A in Fig. 19–21*B*) and the tissue proximal to the site of block (A in Fig. 19–21*A*; D in Fig. 19–21*B*). Stated another way, continuous reentry requires that the anatomical length of the circuit traveled equal or exceed the reentrant wavelength. The latter is equal to mean conduction velocity of the impulse multiplied by the longest refractory period of the elements in the circuit. Conditions that depress conduction velocity or abbreviate the refractory period will promote the development of reentry, while prolonging refractoriness and speeding conduction velocity will hinder its development. For example, if conduction velocity (0.30 M/sec) and refractoriness (350 msec) for ventricular muscle were normal, a pathway of 105 mm (0.30 M/sec ×0.35 sec) would be necessary for reentry to occur. However, under certain conditions, conduction velocity in ventricular muscle and Purkinje fibers can be very slow (0.03 M/sec),[190] and if refractoriness is not greatly prolonged (600 msec), a pathway of only 18 mm (0.03 M/sec × 0.60 sec) may be necessary. Such reasoning may have clinical implications. For example, it has been reported recently that some antiarrhythmic agents converted nonsustained ventricular tachycardia to sustained ventricular arrhythmias, possibly because the drugs greatly slowed conduction velocity with little effect on ventricular refractoriness.[191] Prior to drug therapy in these patients, when nonsustained ventricular tachycardia occurred, the reentrant impulse may have traveled too fast for the anatomical and physiological length of the circuit and may have encroached on refractory tissue, consequently causing the tachycardia to terminate.[192] Drugs that prolong conduction with little effect on refractoriness may allow sufficient time for full repolarization of the elements in the reentrant pathway and perpetuation of the ventricular tachycardia.

Reflection.[79,193,194] This can be considered as a special subclass of reentry. As in reentry, an area of conduction delay is required and the total time for the impulse to leave and return to its site of origin must exceed the refractory period of the proximal segment. Reflection differs from reentry in that the impulse does not require a circuit, as diagrammed in Figure 19–21*A* and *B*, but appears to travel along the *same* pathway in both directions. The impulse travels in one direction and meets an area of impaired conduction where active transmission pauses (Fig. 19–21*C*). Electrotonically (see p. 618), the impulse spans the zone of impairment, activates the distal segment, and returns electrotonically across the zone of impaired conduction to reexcite the proximal segment. A single reflection could cause a coupled premature complex, while continued reflection back and forth across an inexcitable zone could cause a tachycardia. Recent data[193] suggest that reflection and parasystole (or reentry) are part of a continuous spectrum, without a critical boundary to separate them.

Reentry is probably the cause of many tachyarrhythmias, including various kinds of supraventricular and ventricular tachycardias, flutter, and fibrillation. It is important to remember, however, that circa 1900, investigators were able to demonstrate reentry by using simple preparations. In more complex preparations, such as large pieces of tissue in vitro or the intact heart, it becomes much more difficult to prove that reentry exists. It is very hard technically to record from sufficient sites to meet Mines' criteria. Initiation or termination of tachycardia by pacing stimuli, the demonstration of electrical activity bridging diastole, fixed coupling, and a variety of other clinically used techniques,

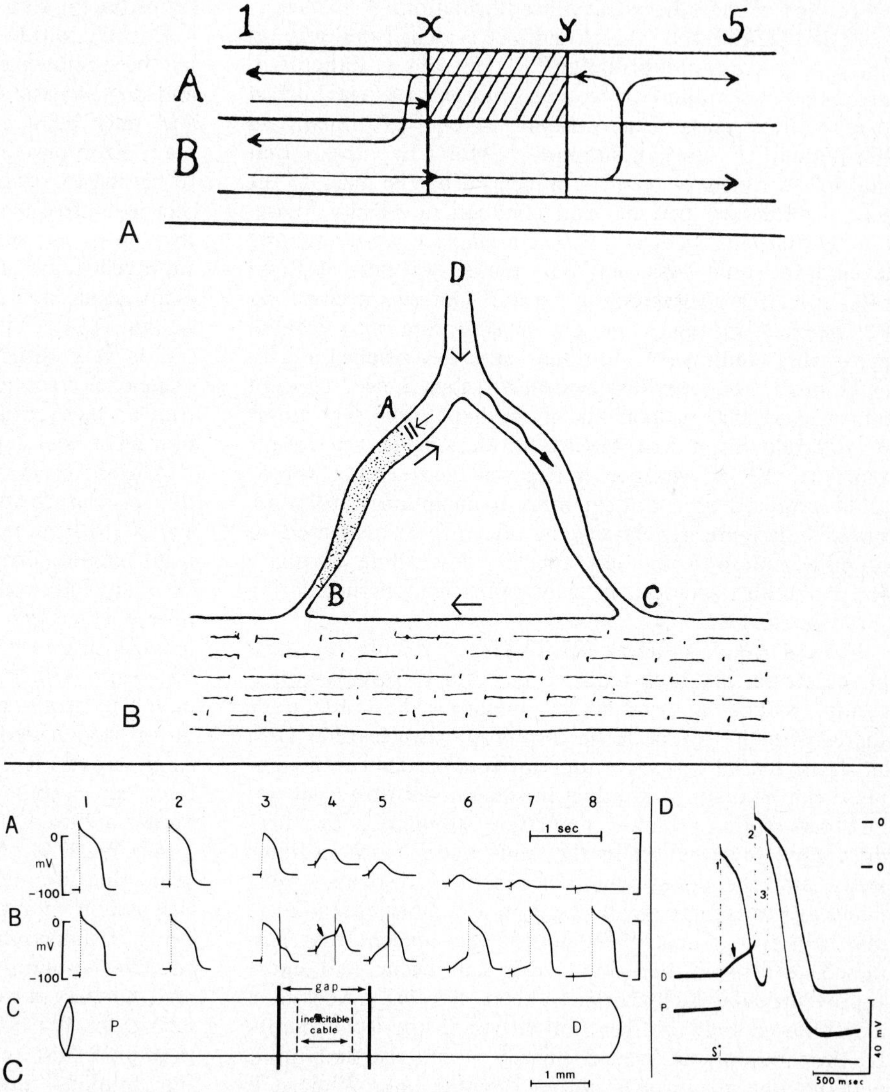

FIGURE 19–21 Diagrams of reentry published by Schmitt and Erlanger in 1928.

A, Reentry is depicted as occurring in contiguous pathways, based on observations that these pathways can undergo functional longitudinal dissociation. Initial propagation begins at site 1 but is able to reach site 5 only in pathway B (lower arrow). Pathway A exhibits unidirectional block (from left to right) at site *x* in the cross-hatched area. The impulse can then reenter pathway A from pathway B and travel from *y* to *x*, reexciting tissue proximal to the site of block. Such concepts of reentry can be applied to any site in the heart.

B, A Purkinje fiber (D) divides into two pathways (B and C), both of which join ventricular muscle (stippled area). It is assumed that the original impulse travels down D, blocks in its anterograde direction at site A (arrow followed by double bar), but continues slowly down C (serpentine arrow) to excite ventricular muscle. The impulse then reenters the Purkinje twig at B and retrogradely excites A and D. If the impulse continues to propagate through D to the ventricular myocardium and elicits ventricular depolarization, a reentrant ventricular extrasystole results. Continued reentry of this type would produce ventricular tachycardia.

C, Reflection. Top panel, schematic representation of electrotonic transmission across an area of inexcitability in a Purkinje fiber. The central compartment (gap) of the tissue bath contains a solution that prevents active conduction in the central segment (inexcitable cable) of the Purkinje fiber. Action potentials from various locations along the Purkinje fiber are presented in panel A when transmission across the inexcitable area is unsuccessful and in panel B when transmission is successful. In panel A, the regenerative impulse encountering the region of block decays along the length of the blocked segment. In panel B, the slowly rising electrotonic potential (arrow) resulting from the activity in the proximal tissue brings the distal segment to threshold and thus restores, after a delay, active propagation via electrotonic transmission. The amplitude of the electrotonic potential emerging from the distal end of the inexcitable cable must be sufficiently large to bring that membrane to the threshold if transmission is to succeed.

When the delay in transmission across the gap is sufficiently long, electrotonic transmission in the reverse direction over the same blocked segment can reexcite the proximal segment and generate a repetitive response, which, under these experimental conditions, is termed *reflection.* This is illustrated in panel D. The two traces were recorded from the two active segments on the proximal (P) and distal (D) sides of the inexcitable gap. The bottom trace is the stimulus marker (S). Stimulation of the proximal segment (1) was transmitted to the distal segment (2) following a slowly developing electrotonic depolarization (arrow) that reached the threshold of the tissue beyond the inexcitable gap after the delay of 300 msec. Electrotonic transmission in the reverse direction induced a closely coupled (404 msec), reflected response (3) in the proximal segment after expiration, of its refractory period. Thus, to-and-fro electrotonic transmission across an inexcitable segment of tissue occurs over the *same pathway* and must be differentiated conceptually from a micro-reentrant circuit that uses *different pathways* in each direction. (From Antzelevitch, C., and Moe, G. K.: Electrotonically-mediated delayed conduction and reentry in relation to "slow responses" in mammalian ventricular conducting tissue. Circ. Res. *49*:1129, 1981. By permission of the American Heart Association, Inc.)

while consistent with reentry, do not constitute proof of its existence.

ATRIAL FLUTTER (p. 697). Lewis[195] considered that atrial flutter was due to a circus movement, but his evidence was not very convincing. Subsequent experiments by Rosenblueth and Garcia Ramos[196] provided more substantial evidence by showing that a well-placed cut interrupted atrial flutter initiated by rapid stimulation in dogs in which intercaval blockade had been produced. These data plus mapping studies[197,198] in animals and mapping and stimulation studies in man[199,200] provide some evidence to suggest that many forms of atrial flutter are due to reentry. Patients may also have dissimilar atrial rhythms in which all or part of one atrium exhibits atrial flutter while all or part of the other atrium has fibrillation.[201]

FIBRILLATION. Much indirect evidence supports reentry as a cause of fibrillation,[202,203] but this is difficult to prove beyond question. Several studies have established that a critical mass of myocardium is required to maintain fibrillation,[204,205] lending support to Moe's hypothesis that multiple wavelets of reentry, influenced by the mass of the tissue, refractory periods, and conduction velocity, maintain fibrillation.[206] Lewis felt that a single wave circulating around the vena cava sent out smaller wavelets at rapid rates to activate surrounding tissue.[207] Garrey's decisive experiments,[188] in which he cut myocardium into smaller pieces that continued to fibrillate until they reached a critically small size, provided evidence against Lewis' concept and also against proponents of the hypothesis that single or multiple firing foci caused fibrillation. In the canine ventricle, the left ventricular free wall and septum appear to be required as a critical mass to maintain fibrillation, since, if they are depolarized by injecting a small amount of potassium into the left anterior descending coronary and circumflex arteries, the right ventricle stops fibrillating spontaneously.[205]

SINUS AND ATRIAL REENTRY. Reentry in parts of the atrium has been reported to occur in several experimental models as well as in humans. The sinus node shares with the AV node electrophysiological features such as the potential for *dissociation of conduction*, i.e., an impulse can be made to conduct in some nodal fibers but not in others.[208] For example, premature stimulation can produce slow propagation in the sinus node, block in some areas, and the development of repetitive responses most likely due to reentry. Evidence from a number of studies in man[209,210] and animals[208,211] support the concept that sustained reentry in the sinus node can occur and cause supraventricular tachycardia (p. 694). Recently, Allessie et al.[211] showed that the reentrant circuit in the isolated rabbit preparation was located entirely within the sinus node and that the atrium was not an essential link. While it is possible that the sinus node responds to premature stimulation with an increase in its discharge rate, under some circumstances as a form of triggered sustained rhythmic activity or overdrive acceleration, and that supraventricular tachycardias thought to be caused by sinus nodal reentry are actually due to triggered activity, experimental evidence does not support these conclusions. The sinus node ordinarily manifests overdrive suppression after a period of rapid pacing,[212] a characteristic that may separate it from automaticity due to other slow-response models. An increase in sinus nodal discharge rate may occur transiently at times following rapid pacing, possibly owing to adrenergic stimulation or vagal withdrawal in response to the pacing-induced rate increase. Premature stimulation of the sinus node may shorten or lengthen the return cycle, depending on the coupling interval of the premature beat, which determines whether the sinus node is reset or is influenced electrotonically[213–215] or if a pacemaker shift occurs. Often, the atrial event does not reflect the true response to premature stimulation of the sinus nodal pacemaker cells. However, triggered sustained rhythmic activity in the sinus node as a cause of persistent supraventricular tachycardia does not seem likely, and the weight of evidence suggests that reentry in the sinus node is responsible for this rhythm disturbance.

Reentry within the atrium, unrelated to the sinus node, has been shown experimentally to occur in the rabbit[216,217] and dog atrium,[218] with or without an anatomical obstacle, and may be a cause of supraventricular tachycardia in man. Examples of supraventricular tachycardia purported to be due to atrial reentry have been cited,[209,220,221] but their relative infrequency in the published literature suggests that this is not a commonly recognized cause of supraventricular tachycardia in man. Distinguishing atrial tachycardia due to automaticity from atrial tachycardia sustained by reentry over very small areas, i.e., micro-reentry, is very difficult, and therefore conclusions regarding clinical electrophysiological mechanisms of this supraventricular tachycardia based on currently available information must be accepted cautiously.

Allessie et al.[216] have shown in isolated rabbit atrium that premature stimulation elicited a reentrant circuit (6 to 8 mm) with radial propagation to the periphery. The reentrant circuit propagated around a functionally inactive core and followed a course along fibers that had a shorter refractory period, blocking in one direction in fibers with a longer refractory period. An anatomical obstacle was not necessary. The refractory period and conduction velocity in the reentrant pathway determined its length. This type of reentry, called the "leading circuit concept,"[217] has a small reentrant circuit, making it difficult to distinguish from an automatic focus unless minute mapping techniques are used.

AV NODAL REENTRY. It has been known for 75 years that stimulation of the ventricle could propagate to the atrium and then back to the ventricles,[222] sometimes being sustained to cause a reciprocating rhythm.[186,187] Although the bundle of fibers described by Kent was considered to play a role in this circus movement[186,187,223] even before the Wolff-Parkinson-White syndrome was described in man, Scherf and Shookhoff[224] ascribed the mechanism to "longitudinal functional dissociation" in the AV junction. They produced (and first used the term) "return ventricular extrasystoles" in dogs by giving quinine to delay AV nodal conduction and suggested that some fibers of the AV conduction system had shorter refractory periods and were able to conduct in one direction while conduction in other fibers with longer refractory periods was blocked. The impulse was then able to reexcite the previously refractory fibers. For a return ventricular extrasystole to occur, the R-P interval (i.e., between the onset of the QRS and the retrograde P wave) must lengthen to a critical ex-

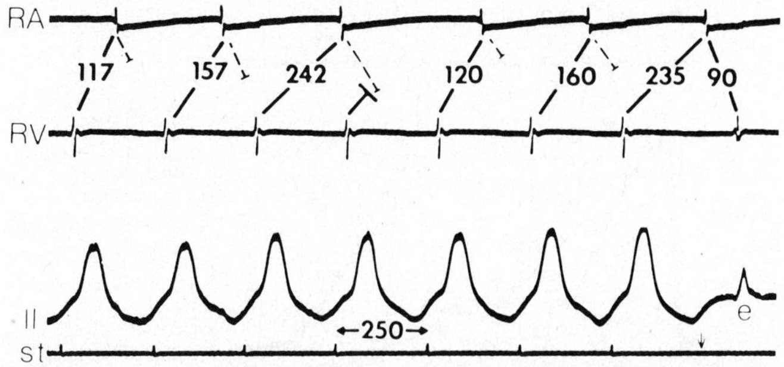

FIGURE 19–22 Return ventricular extrasystoles associated with retrograde Wenckebach conduction. A stable 4:3 retrograde Wenckebach conduction was established in a dog by rapid right ventricular pacing (left half of the figure, first four stimuli). When the eighth ventricular stimulus in the series was omitted (right half of the figure at arrow), the retrograde atrial impulse returned to the ventricle to produce a ventricular echo. Such an event can be explained by the effects of concealed reentry (see p. 247). Solid lines indicate manifest conduction and interrupted lines indicate concealed conduction. Numbers in milliseconds represent ventriculoatrial conduction time. Electrograms recorded from the epicardial surface of the right atrium (RA), right ventricle (RV), and standard lead II. St = stimulus; e = ventricular echo. (From Zipes, D. P., et al.: Some examples of Wenckebach periodicity in cardiac tissues, with an appraisal of mechanisms. *In* Rosenbaum, M. B. (ed.): Cardiac Arrhythmias. The Hague, Martinus Nijhoff [in press].)

tent, and conduction cannot block in the AV junction before the impulse reaches the site of reentry[225] (Fig. 19–22).

In canine and some human studies, the R-P interval is inversely proportional to the P-R interval,[225] i.e., the longer it takes the ventricular impulse to reach the atrium, the less time it takes the return impulse to reach the ventricle. This reciprocal relationship may result if some part of the pathway is common to both anterograde and retrograde conduction. Therefore, a longer ventriculoatrial conduction time permits a longer recovery period for the common pathway and a faster conduction time anterogradely. A short ventriculoatrial conduction time may be followed by a long atrioventricular conduction time. The final common pathway is most likely the mid and distal regions of the AV node.[125] Return extrasystoles, or echoes, can be elicited in the opposite direction as well, in contrast to the conclusions of Rosenblueth.[226] These atrial echoes have characteristics similar to ventricular echoes.[227,228]

In many patients, the ventriculoatrial conduction time may remain relatively fixed in spite of changes in the premature interval (p. 703). Longitudinal dissociation in the AV node, where reentry most likely occurs, remains a plausible mechanism. In fact, Mendez et al.[229] demonstrated that an impulse traveling from ventricle to atrium, if timed properly, did not prevent another impulse traveling simultaneously from atrium to ventricle from reaching the His bundle. For this to occur, the impulses traveling in opposite directions must be conducting in different AV nodal pathways.

Microelectrode studies on isolated rabbit AV nodal preparations provide further evidence to support these concepts of longitudinal AV nodal dissociation and reentry.[179] Cells in the upper portion of the AV node can be dissociated during propagation of premature stimuli, so that one group of cells, called alpha, can discharge in response to a premature stimulus at a time when another group of cells, called beta, fails to discharge.[125,230] The impulse can then propagate to the mid and lower portions of the AV node and turn around (without needing to activate the His bundle) to reexcite the beta group of cells and produce an atrial echo (Fig. 19–23). Experiments by Janse et al.[231] using multiple simultaneous microelectrode recordings, and by Wit et al.,[232] who created episodes of sustained AV nodal tachycardia in isolated rabbit atria, largely confirmed these observations. Although these studies provide the most conclusive animal experimental evidence supporting the presence of AV nodal reentry, they do not prove it unequivocally. In such a complex preparation, all the "rules" established by Mines cannot be met, and the evidence does not exclude, for example, the possibility of a triggered impulse responsible for the returning wavefront.

Mines postulated that reentry within AV nodal connections might be responsible for some clinically occurring arrhythmias, while several other investigators suggested similar concepts based on electrocardiograms recorded in patients.[233–236] The argument by Lewis[237] that rapid atrial conduction time should produce supraventricular tachycardia rates faster than those observed was countered by Barker, who suggested that a circus movement involving the sinus or AV nodes could explain the slower rates. Kistin, using esophageal leads,[238] offered the possibility that two or more AV nodal pathways accounted for reciprocal rhythms.

One of the first studies employing premature electrical stimulation to initiate and terminate a paroxysmal supraventricular tachycardia in situ was performed in a dog.[239] Subsequent investigations in man support the concept[240,241] that reentry, initiated by a critical degree of AV nodal conduction delay,[242,243] can be localized to the AV node, possibly occurring over functionally distinct dual AV nodal pathways.[244] The premature atrial response can block anterogradely in one AV nodal pathway that conducts more rapidly (fast pathway, or beta pathway in Figure 19–23) but has a longer refractory period than a second pathway (slow pathway, or alpha pathway in (Figure 19–23). The premature atrial response travels to the ventricle over the slow (alpha) pathway and back to the atrium over the fast (beta) pathway.[198,245] Less commonly, the premature atrial response can block in the slow pathway and travel in the fast pathway anterogradely, using the slow pathway retrogradely.[246] Conceivably, some patients may have three or more pathways.[245]

In patients who have dual AV nodal physiology, both pathways exhibit electrophysiological responses in the anterograde direction characteristic of AV nodal fibers. However, in some patients, the electrophysiological features of the retrogradely conducting pathway differ greatly from those of the anterogradely conducting pathway, in response not only to atrial or ventricular pacing but also to various drugs.[221,245,247–249] Thus, it is not clear whether the retrogradely conducting pathway is extranodal, is intranodal but insulated from the rest of the AV node, or includes only a small amount of AV nodal tissue.

It is also not settled whether the retrogradely conducting pathway is distinct from the fast and slow anterogradely conducting pathways, which appear to be composed of AV nodal fibers. The geometry and direction of conduction,[250] effects of summation,[251] autonomic tone,[252] as well as the electrophysiological characteristics of the fi-

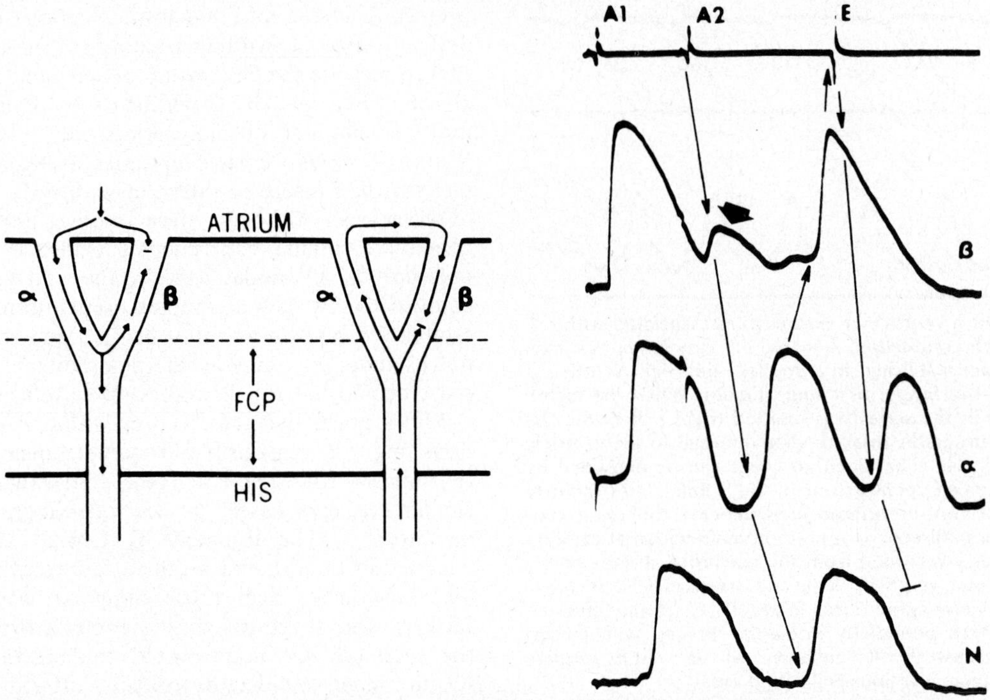

FIGURE19–23 Atrial echoes. *Left,* Schematic representation of intranodal dissociation responsible for an atrial echo. A premature atrial response fails to penetrate the beta pathway, which exhibits unidirectional block but propagates anterogradely through the alpha pathway. Once the final common pathway (FCP) is engaged, the impulse may return to the atrium via the now recovered beta pathway to produce an atrial echo. The neighboring diagram illustrates the pattern of propagation during generation of a ventricular echo. A premature response in the His bundle traverses the final common pathway, encounters a refractory beta pathway (unidirectional block), reaches the atrium over the alpha pathway, and returns through a now recovered beta pathway to produce a ventricular echo. Such events can explain the findings in Figure 19–22.

Right, Actual recordings from the atrium (top tracing), cells impaled in the beta region (second tracing), alpha region (third tracing), and N portion of the AV node (bottom tracing) in an isolated rabbit preparation. The basic response to A_1 activated both alpha and beta pathways and the N cell (first tier of action potentials). The premature atrial response, A_2, caused only a local response in the beta cell (heavy arrow), was delayed in transmission to the alpha cell, and was further delayed in propagation to the N cell. Following the alpha response, a retrograde spontaneous response occurred in the beta cell and propagated to the atrium (E). This atrial response represents an atrial echo. The echo returned to stimulate the alpha cell but was not propagated to the N cell. (From Mendez, C., and Moe, G. K.: Demonstrations of a dual AV nodal conduction system in the isolated rabbit heart. Circ. Res. *19*:378, 1966. By permission of the American Heart Association, Inc.)

bers, all may influence conduction and the response to drugs. A drug such as procainamide may effect retrograde but not anterograde AV nodal conduction in patients with presumably normal AV nodes.[253] It is likely that the anatomical as well as the electrophysiological features of AV nodal pathways may not be the same in all patients who have AV nodal reentrant supraventricular tachycardia. Recent evidence suggests that, in some patients who appear to have AV nodal reentrant supraventricular tachycardia, the retrogradely conducting pathway may exhibit electrophysiological properties consistent with AV nodal tissue but is located in an extranodal site, since it gives rise to an abnormal sequence of retrograde atrial activation.[254] The anatomical basis for such observations may be an eccentric AV node or an accessory pathway with AV nodal characteristics.

The necessary role of atrial participation in the reentrant circuit is still debated. Mendez et al.[229] demonstrated the need for the atrium in generating ventricular echoes caused by AV nodal reentrant activity in dogs, and such a circuit is implicit in their diagram in Figure 19–23. Studies in animals[227] and patients[174,255–257] have challenged the interpretations of Mendez et al. and have suggested that ventricular echoes due to AV nodal reentry can occur *without* activation of the atrium. Figure 19–24 is an example of apparent dissociation of the atrium with uninterrupted continuation of the supraventricular tachycardia, leading to the conclusion that the atrium may *not* be a necessary part of the reentrant circuit in humans (see Chap. 21). However, since rhythms in the atria may become dissimilar,[201] a portion of the atrium may control, or participate in, the cardiac rhythm without recognition of this fact from observation of a scalar ECG or, indeed, from recordings within the right atrium or coronary sinus.[258] Therefore, data refuting the role of the atrium as a necessary link in the reentrant pathway must be obtained from studies in which both atria are carefully mapped for the presence of localized atrial activity, particularly near the upper AV node.[231,232,259]

PREEXCITATION SYNDROME (See also p. 712). The accumulated anatomical and electrophysiological data support a reentrant mechanism to explain tachycardias related to an accessory pathway more than they support that mechanism for any other kind of tachycardia.[260–263] In fact, Mines[187] and deBoer[223] both attempted to explain the mechanism of paroxysmal tachycardia by reentry over the bundle described by Kent[264,265] even before the preexcitation syndrome was ever described in man.

Electrophysiological studies have demonstrated that, in

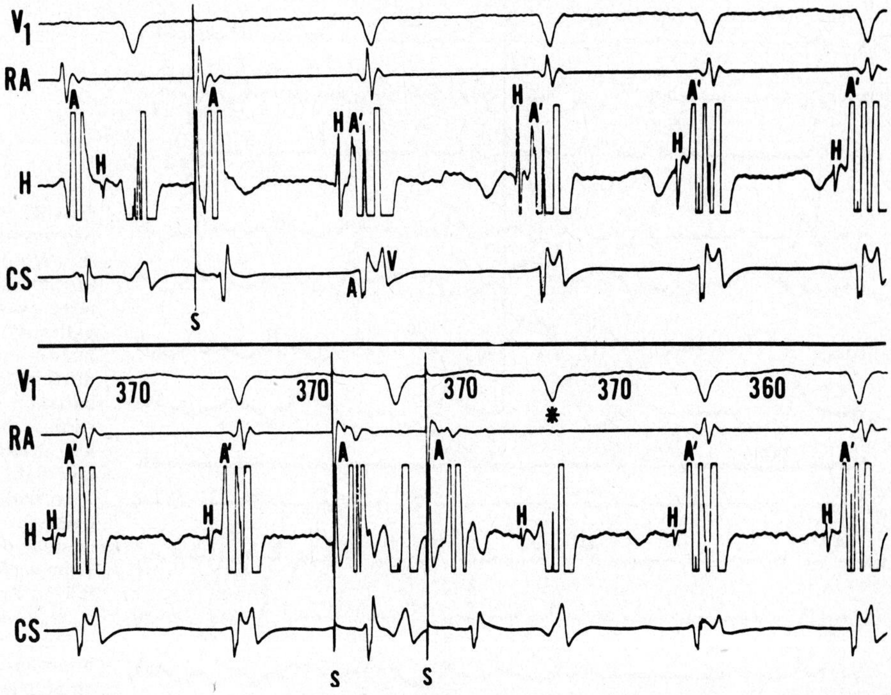

FIGURE 19–24 Dissociation of atria from ventricles without interrupting AV nodal reentrant supraventricular tachycardia. During sinus rhythm, a single premature atrial complex (S, *top panel*) was conducted with AV nodal delay (prolonged A-H interval) and initiated an AV nodal reentrant supraventricular tachycardia. Note that retrograde atrial activation (A′) occurred prior to onset of the QRS complex. Two premature atrial stimuli (S-S, *bottom panel*) captured the atria on both occasions without altering the regular cycle length of the AV nodal reentrant supraventricular tachycardia. Note that the QRS complex marked by an asterisk has no accompanying atrial complex, suggesting that atrial participation in the reentrant circuit was not required. V_1 = scalar lead; RA = right atrial electrogram; H = His bundle electrogram; CS = coronary sinus electrogram.

most patients who have reciprocating tachycardia associated with the Wolff-Parkinson-White syndrome, the accessory pathway conducts more rapidly than does the normal AV node but takes a longer time to recover excitability, i.e., the anterograde refractory period of the accessory pathway exceeds that of the AV node.[261,266] Consequently, a premature atrial complex that occurs sufficiently early blocks anterogradely in the accessory pathway and continues to the ventricle over the normal AV node and His bundle. After the ventricles have been excited, the impulse is able to enter the accessory pathway retrogradely and return to the atrium. A continuous conduction loop of this kind establishes the circuit for the tachycardia. Although exceptions occur, the usual activation wave during such a reciprocating tachycardia in a patient with an accessory pathway occurs in this fashion: anterogradely over the normal AV node–His-Purkinje system and retrogradely over the accessory pathway, resulting in a normal QRS complex (Fig. 19–25). Because the circuit requires both atria and ventricles, the term "supraventricular tachycardia" may not be precisely correct. The term "reciprocating tachycardia" or "circus movement tachycardia" has been substituted. Use of the latter terms assumes that the mechanism of the tachycardia is one of reentry. In some patients, the accessory pathway may be capable only of retrograde conduction,[262,267,268] but the circuit and mechanism of tachycardia remain the same. Less commonly, the accessory pathway may conduct only anterogradely.[262,269]

In addition to the response of the reciprocating tachycardia to premature stimulation, one of the strongest lines of evidence supporting a reentrant mechanism is that interruption of the presumed reentrant loop at widely separated points (i.e., by surgically cutting the normal AV node–His bundle pathway *or* the accessory pathway) eliminates the ability to develop supraventricular tachycardia.

Other pathways may constitute the circuit for reciprocating tachycardias in patients who have some form of the Wolff-Parkinson-White syndrome. Conduction may proceed anterogradely over the accessory pathway and retrogradely over the AV node–His bundle, so-called "antidromic tachycardia." Two accessory pathways may form the circuit. In the Lown-Ganong-Levine syndrome (short P-R interval and normal QRS complex),[270] conduction over a James fiber[271] that connects atrium to the distal portion of the AV node and His bundle may play a role, although the presence of this entity as a distinct syndrome is unsettled[31] (see p. 713).

For some patients, electrophysiological findings may be consistent with communications between the AV node and the ventricle (nodoventricular) or the His-bundle–bundle branches and the ventricle (fasciculoventricular).[272] Tachycardia in patients with nodoventricular fibers may be due to reentry using these fibers as the anterograde pathway and the His-Purkinje fibers and a portion of the AV node retrogradely. No direct relationship may exist between fasciculoventricular fibers and tachycardia. Thus, the accessory pathway concept suggested by Holzmann and Scherf[273] and Wolferth and Wood[274] can be expanded to encompass a variety of syndromes.

VENTRICULAR REENTRY (See also pp. 721 to 728). Reentry in the ventricle as a cause of sustained ventricular arrhythmias was suggested by the work of Mines.[186,187] Later, Schmitt and Erlanger[183] produced probable functional longitudinal dissociation with undirectional block in strips of turtle ventricle exposed unequally to different depressant agents. This resulted in repetitive excitation, likely due to reentry, reflection, or both, and they suggested that the event could occur in a peripheral Purkinje fiber bundle. Their diagram (Fig. 19–21*A* and *B*) has been reproduced many times. Wenckebach and Winterberg[275] raised similar possibilities. A strong objection to this explanation[276] was that the impulse conducted too quickly in cardiac tissue for a pathway to be of reasonable length to support reentry. Studies by Cranefield[189,277] and Wit[190,278] dispelled these doubts by demonstrating that high [K] could depress conduction velocity in peripheral Purkinje

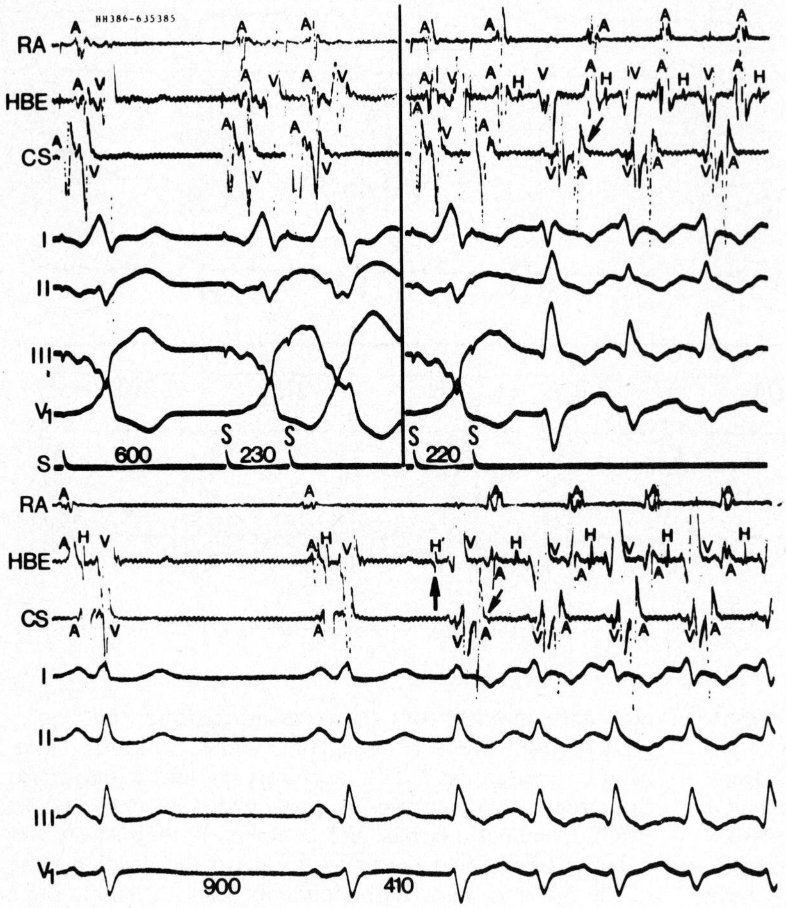

FIGURE 19–25 Spontaneous and induced initiation of paroxysmal reciprocating tachycardia in a patient with the Wolff-Parkinson-White syndrome. *Top left,* Premature left atrial stimulation (S-S) at a cycle length of 230 msec was followed by conduction over the accessory pathway to the ventricle. *Top right,* Shortening the premature interval (S-S) to 220 msec was followed by conduction to the ventricle over the normal pathway and initiation of reciprocating tachycardia, during which the earliest retrograde atrial activation was recorded in the left atrium (CS lead, arrow) followed by activity in the low right atrial (HBE) and high right atrial (RA) leads. This finding is consistent with a left-sided accessory pathway. *Bottom recording,* Premature depolarization in or near the His bundle (H′, upright arrow) initiated the same tachycardia spontaneously. The QRS complex following the H′ is totally normal because the impulse originates distal to the atrial insertion of the accessory pathway and therefore conducts over the normal AV node–His bundle pathway to the ventricle. Retrograde atrial activation (arrow) occurs over the left-sided accessory pathway as in the top right panel.

twigs to 0.01 to 0.10 M/sec and permit reentry, probably due to the slow response, to occur in loops of Purkinje fibers (Fig. 19–26). Spontaneous activity in unbranched fibers could also be elicited in these studies and in others using a sucrose gap technique (Fig. 19–21*C*). The latter studies clearly showed reflection as a cause of repetitive excitation.

Sasyniuk and Mendez[279] demonstrated repetitive firing in papillary muscle–false tendon preparations in which a premature stimulus delivered to a Purkinje fiber blocked at some Purkinje-muscle junctions, conducted through others, and propagated back to its site of origin. Reentry was facilitated in this preparation because the duration of the action potential and refractoriness shortened in the fibers proximal to the site of initial block, allowing early recovery and reexcitation. Related events may occur in damaged fibers.[280] Whether such reentry takes place in the heart in situ is not known; however, reentry has been demonstrated to occur over the bundle branches in the in situ dog heart[281–283] (Fig. 19–27) and probably in man as well.[262,284] The occurrence of bundle branch reentry explains several interesting electrocardiographic phenomena, to be discussed later (p. 727). Bundle branch reentry does not appear to be a common cause of sustained ventricular tachycardia in the dog or in man.[152,285,286,286a] More likely, reentry in ventricular muscle, with or without contribution from specialized tissue, is responsible for many ventricular tachycardias.

Reentry in ventricular muscle is difficult to prove by Mines' criteria because the large muscle mass makes complete mapping of the reentrant loop and interruption of the pathway difficult. Fontaine et al.[287] have shown that an appropriately placed ventriculotomy incision could interrupt sustained ventricular tachycardia in man. In general, experimental studies provide only supportive evidence of reentry.[288] Ischemia, both acute and chronic, has been a favorite model to investigate because it generates fragmented, delayed activation that may be conducive to the generation of reentrant excitation.[289,290] However, even the demonstration of continuous electrical activity spanning diastole that is linked temporally and perhaps causally to the generation of sustained ventricular arrhythmia[286,291,292] constitutes only circumstantial proof. For example, such continuous electrical activity could be produced by oscillatory pacemaker activity (Figs. 19–16 and 19–17) conducting with delay to the surrounding myocardium and could be unrelated to reentry. We have already indicated that initiation and termination of a sustained tachycardia is not proof of reentry, since triggered activity can respond in a similar fashion. Several recent animal studies using an extensive array of extracellular electrodes[293–296] have provided important information concerning the sequence of activation during ventricular tachyarrhythmias, strongly suggesting in some of the studies that reentry is the responsible mechanism. Even though more data meeting Mines' postulates are required to exclude completely other mechanisms responsible for ventricular tachycardia, current information suggests that a great many ventricular tachycardias occurring in man are due to reentrant excitation.

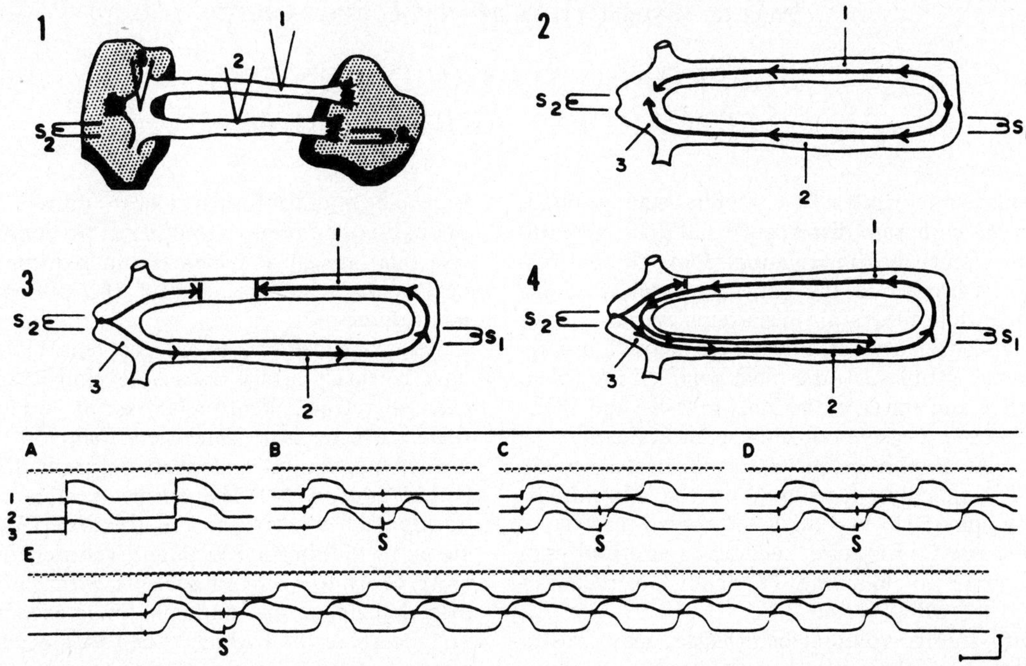

FIGURE 19–26 Sustained circus-movement "ventricular tachycardia" in an isolated preparation from a calf heart. Format of top half of figure: *Panel 1,* Schematic of preparation; stimulating electrodes at S_1 and S_2, recording microelectrodes at 1, 2, and 3; muscle = shaded area; Purkinje fibers = clear strips. *Panel 2,* Conduction of S_1 corresponding to panel B below. *Panel 3,* Conduction of S_2 corresponding to panel C below. *Panel 4,* Conduction of S_2 corresponding to panel D and E below. *Panel A,* Recordings obtained in normal Tyrode's solution. *Panels B to E,* Recordings obtained after exposure to high $[K]_o$ and epinephrine. S = premature stimulus at site 2. In panels B to E the basic drive (S_1) was applied at site 1, followed by a premature stimulus (S_2) applied at site 3. During the basic drive (S_1), activation appears almost simultaneously at sites 1 and 2 but with delay at site 3 (panel 2, above). Application of premature stimulus at S_2 in panel B causes excitation to travel from site 3 to site 2, but it does not reach site 1. Premature stimulus in panel C causes excitation to travel from site 3 to 2 and then to 1 (panel 3, above). In panel D, S_2 results in a sequence similar to that in panel C, which then continues back to site 3 and site 2 (panel 4, above). In panel E, premature stimulation results in several full circuits of this reentrant loop. Calibrations: Vertical = 100 mV; time marks are at 100-msec intervals. (From Wit, A. L., et al.: Slow conduction and reentry in the ventricular conducting system. II. Single and sustained circus movement in networks of canine and bovine Purkinje fibers. Circ. Res. *30*:11, 1972. By permission of the American Heart Association, Inc.)

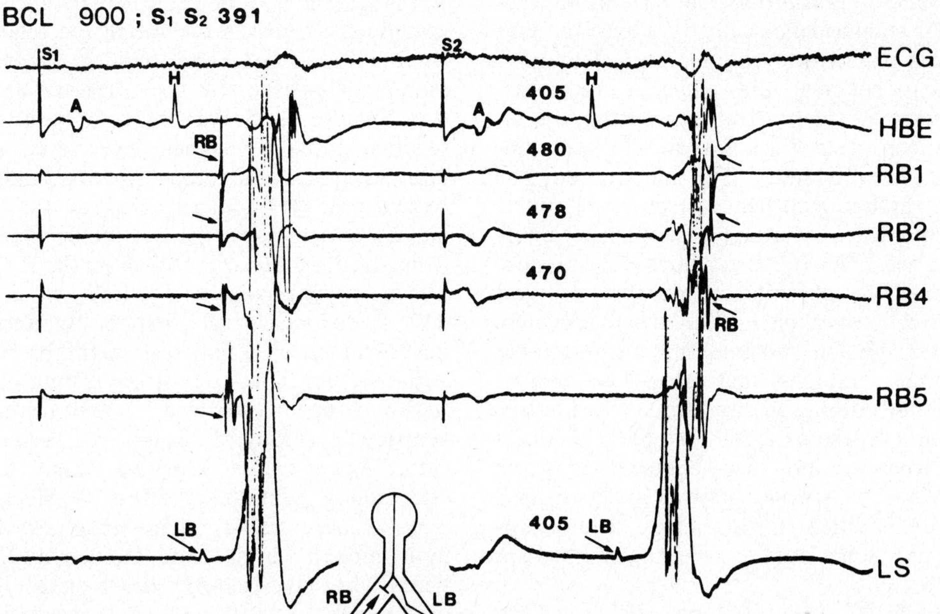

FIGURE 19–27 Reentry in the bundle branches of the dog heart. Recordings have been made with an electrode in the His bundle area (HBE), a multipolar plaque electrode sewn on the right bundle branch portraying activation from base to apex direction in electrograms RB_1 to RB_5 and from the left bundle branch (LB) in the left septal lead (LS). During the last basic cycle, S_1 applied to the atrium causes conduction to proceed from the His bundle through the left and right bundle branches to the ventricle. Note orderly progression of conduction from RB_1 to RB_5. At a premature right atrial interval of 391 msec, conduction is blocked distal to His, travels to the ventricle over the left bundle branch without any delay between left bundle branch deflections, and then activates the right bundle branch retrogradely from RB_4 to RB_2 to RB_1. Retrograde right bundle branch deflection in RB_5 cannot be seen. *Insert* shows activation sequence in bundle branches following S_2. (From Glassman, R. D., and Zipes, D. P.: Site of anterograde and retrograde functional right bundle branch block in the intact canine heart. Circulation *64*:1277, 1981. By permission of the American Heart Association, Inc.)

APPROACH TO THE DIAGNOSIS OF CARDIAC ARRHYTHMIAS

It is important to remember that the physician evaluates a *patient* who has a rhythm disturbance and does not evaluate a rhythm disturbance in isolation. Some rhythm disturbances are hazardous to the patient regardless of the clinical setting, while others are hazardous *because* of the clinical setting. Evaluation of the patient should usually progress from the simplest to the most complex test, from the least invasive and safest to the most invasive and risky, and from the least expensive out-of-hospital evaluations to those that require hospitalization and sophisticated, costly procedures. Occasionally, depending on the clinical circumstances, the physician may wish to proceed directly to a high-risk, expensive procedure, such as an electrophysiological study, prior to obtaining a 24-hour electrocardiographic (ECG) recording.

Patients with cardiac rhythm disturbances may present with a variety of complaints, but commonly symptoms such as palpitations, syncope, presyncope, or congestive heart failure cause them to seek a physician. Their awareness of regular or irregular cardiac rhythm varies greatly. Some patients may perceive slight variations in their heart rhythm with uncommon accuracy, while others are oblivious even to sustained episodes of ventricular tachycardia; still others complain of palpitations when they actually have regular sinus rhythm. The following tests can be used to evaluate patients who have cardiac arrhythmias.

TRANSTELEPHONIC ELECTROCARDIOGRAPHIC TRANSMISSION. Transmitters that send an electrocardiographic signal transtelephonically to a receiver unit may be used to transmit electrocardiographic information.[297] Such an instrument converts the patient's electrocardiogram to an audiotone, which, when transmitted to a recorder-receiver, is converted back to an electrocardiographic signal for interpretation. This device may be indicated when the rhythm disturbance is sufficiently infrequent that continuous ECG recording is impractical. Some recorders can store the ECG signal for later transmission. The arrhythmia must be of sufficient duration (several minutes) to permit the recording for the actual transmission or for later transmission and must not be associated with syncope or other symptoms that prevent the patient from transmitting or recording. A disadvantage to this approach is that it relies on the patient's perception of a cardiac rhythm disturbance, and many patients may be unaware of significant or serious bradyarrhythmias and tachyarrhythmias. In addition, the technique requires access to a receiver and some sort of receiving mechanism available 24 hours a day.

EXERCISE TESTING (See also pp. 257 to 278). About one-third of normal subjects develop ventricular ectopy in response to exercise testing. Ectopy is more likely to occur at faster heart rates, usually in the form of occasional, premature ventricular complexes (PVCs) of constant morphology,[298–304] or even pairs of PVCs, and is not reproducible from one stress test to the next.[298,300–302] Although multiform PVCs and ventricular tachycardia usually do not develop in normal patients, they can occur and therefore their presence does not establish the existence of ischemic or other forms of heart disease. Supraventricular premature complexes are often more common during exercise than at rest and increase in frequency with age; their occurrence does not suggest the presence of structural heart disease.[298]

Approximately 50 to 60 per cent[301–305] of patients who have coronary artery disease develop PVCs in response to exercise testing. Ventricular ectopy appears in these patients at lower heart rates (less than 130 bpm) than in the normal population and often occurs in the early recovery period as well.[306,307] The ectopy is more reproducible[301–304] during each stress test, and frequent PVCs (greater than 10/min), multiform PVCs, and ventricular tachycardia are more likely to occur in patients with coronary artery disease than in normal patients. Since exercise may suppress or exacerbate the frequency of PVCs occurring at rest, alteration in PVC frequency does not appear to be a helpful prognostic indicator.[305] The frequency of sudden cardiac death is increased in patients with coronary artery disease who develop ventricular ectopy at heart rates less than 130 bpm with exercise[301,302] and in whom the ectopy is associated with ST-segment changes, presumably as a manifestation of the relationship between ventricular ectopy and ischemia.[308]

Patients who have symptoms consistent with an arrhythmia induced by exercise (syncope, sustained palpitation, and the like) should be considered for stress testing. Stress testing may be indicated to uncover more complex grades of ectopy, to determine the relationship of the arrhythmia to activity, and to aid in choosing antiarrhythmic therapy. However, the test must be interpreted with caution because of the variability in results obtained in consecutive tests.[300,301] When two tests are performed 45 minutes apart, less ectopy is consistently recorded on the second test.[309] Hence, a decrease in the frequency of PVCs on the post-therapy test cannot be taken as absolute evidence of drug efficacy. However, the inability to reproduce sustained ventricular tachycardia on a second test, after it was produced at the first, or the absence of a deleterious effect on a second test might be helpful in assessing antiarrhythmic therapy. Stress testing appears to be more sensitive than a standard 12-lead resting ECG to detect ventricular ectopy.[300,304] However, prolonged ambulatory recording is more sensitive than exercise testing in establishing ventricular ectopy.[310] Since either technique may uncover serious arrhythmias which the other technique misses,[311] both examinations may be indicated for patients who have ischemic heart disease in whom frequent or complex ventricular ectopy is suspected.

LONG-TERM ELECTROCARDIOGRAPHIC RECORDING. Prolonged ECG recording (Holter monitoring, ambulatory monitoring) in patients engaged in normal daily activity permits quantitation of arrhythmia frequency and complexity, correlation with patient's symptoms, and evaluation of the effect of antiarrhythmic therapy on the arrhythmia.[310,312–316] In addition, such recording can document alterations in QRS, ST, and T contours, depending on the recorder used.[317] It is useful in detecting arrhythmias in symptomatic patients, correlating the ECG with symptoms, detecting pacemaker malfunction, and assessing the response to drug therapy.[317a]

Significant rhythm disturbances are fairly uncommon in healthy young persons. However, sinus bradycardia with heart rates of 35 to 40 bpm, sinus arrhythmia with pauses of even 2 seconds, Wenckebach second-degree AV block (often during sleep), a wandering atrial pacemaker, junctional escape complexes, and infrequent premature atrial complexes (PACs) and PVCs are not necessarily abnormal.[318,319,319a] Frequent ectopic complexes and complex atrial and ventricular rhythm disturbances are rarely recorded, however, and type II second-degree AV conduction disturbances are not recorded in normal patients. Elderly patients may have a greater prevalence of arrhythmias,[320] some of which may be responsible for neurological symptoms.[321,322]

A majority of patients who have ischemic heart disease, particularly those recovering from acute infarction, exhibit PVCs when monitored for periods of 6 to 24 hours. Although the presence of simple PVCs in some[323,324] but not all[325] studies appears to be of little therapeutic or prognostic significance, the following characteristics of ventricular ectopy have been reported to be associated with a worse prognosis in patients with ischemic heart disease: (1) frequent PVCs,[326–329] (2) multiform PVCs,[328–330] (3) early coupling intervals (R-on-T phenomenon),[323–330] (4) pairs of PVCs,[330] (5) bigeminy,[327,330] and (6) ventricular tachycardia.[331,332] Complexity may be related to the frequency of PVCs, and long-term recordings beyond 24 hours increases their detection.[316] There is no universal agreement as to the significance of each of these characteristics, but it is generally conceded that more complex forms of ventricular ectopy imply an increased risk of sudden cardiac death.[333–335b] Whether the ventricular ectopy is related causally to the subsequent sudden death or is only a marker identifying the patient at increased risk is unknown, but it is thought to be an independent risk factor. The frequency and complexity of ventricular rhythm disturbances recorded late in the hospital course or after hospitalization may bear no relation to those recorded during the acute phase.[336] In fact, the frequency of PVCs progressively increases over the first several weeks and months after hospitalization.[337] Serious ventricular ectopy correlates closely with the degree of impaired left ventricular function[336,338] and persistent ST-segment elevation[329] and with the extent of obstructive coronary vascular disease.[336]

Long-term ECG recording has often exposed potentially serious supraventricular tachyarrhythmias or frequent and complex ventricular ectopy in patients with hypertrophic cardiomyopathy[339,340] (p. 1415) and mitral valve prolapse[341–344] (p. 1091). Ventricular tachycardia or fibrillation does not necessarily result in patients who have complex ventricular rhythm disturbances, and sudden cardiac death has occurred in patients who have no documented arrhythmia on prolonged recordings.[345]

In patients who have otherwise unexplained syncope (Fig. 19–28) or transient vague cerebrovascular symptoms, potentially treatable rhythm disturbances are sometimes found on long-term ECG recordings to be the cause.[321,322,346,347] Such recordings may permit one to correlate symptoms with arrhythmias in several situations, including sinus node dysfunction,[348,349] the bradycardia-tachycardia syndrome,[350] and the Wolff-Parkinson-White syndrome.[351] For symptomatic patients with conduction disturbances, such as right bundle branch block and left axis deviation, invasive electrophysiological (His bundle) studies may be useful (p. 634). However, if these studies are nonrevealing particularly in patients with normal resting electrocardiograms, the diagnosis can be obtained by long-term ECG recording (Fig. 19–29). Long-term ECG recording may also be useful for documenting pacemaker malfunction[352] (p. 764).

In normal subjects and in patients with serious rhythm disturbances, the cardiac rhythm may vary markedly from one recording period to the next. To prove the efficacy of antiarrhythmic therapy, it is essential to demonstrate that the frequency of the abnormal rhythm disturbance is reduced more by the agent than by chance alone. Spontaneous reductions in the frequency of PVCs of up to 90 per cent have been demonstrated to occur between two recording periods.[314,353] Therefore, an antiarrhythmic agent must reduce the frequency of premature ventricular complexes by about 75 to 85 per cent, and the frequency of complex ventricular complexes 70 per cent, from one 24-hour recording period to another in order to be considered effective.[354]

Interpretative accuracy of long-term tape recordings varies with the system used. When technicians interpret the tape without semiautomated computer systems, an excellent qualitative analysis may be provided, i.e., detection of PVCs, ventricular tachycardia, asystolic intervals, and so forth, but not a quantitative account of the actual number of each event. With semiautomated interpreting systems, the error rate is 5 to 10 per cent of ectopic complexes. Recently developed fully automated computers reportedly miscount or misinterpret less than 3 per cent of ectopic complexes.[355,356] The clinical utility of such accuracy is questionable, since it is not clear that it really matters

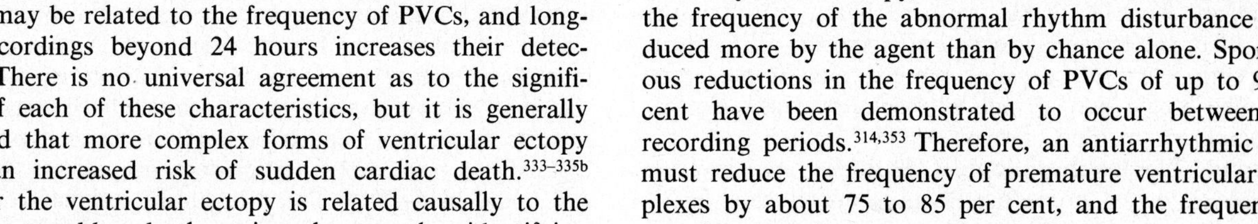

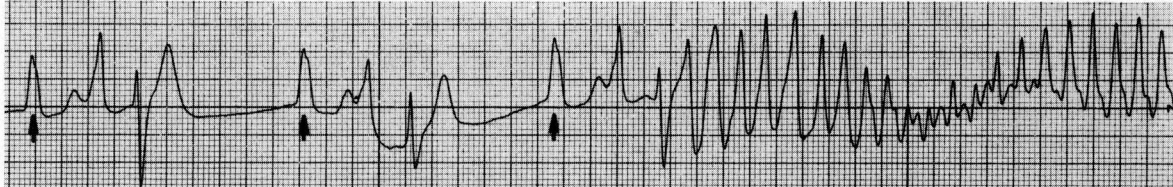

FIGURE 19–28 Onset of ventricular tachycardia–ventricular fibrillation during long-term ECG recording. This 41-year-old female presented with several episodes of presyncope. Bundle branch block and premature ventricular complexes were seen on 12-lead ECG. An electrophysiological study was totally normal (except for the presence of bundle branch block), and neither AV heart block nor ventricular tachyarrhythmias were initiated. After six weeks of *continuous* ECG recording, the patient had another syncopal spell, during which the ECG shown here was obtained. Arrows indicate sinus-initiated beats conducting with a left bundle branch block pattern. The patient could not be resuscitated.

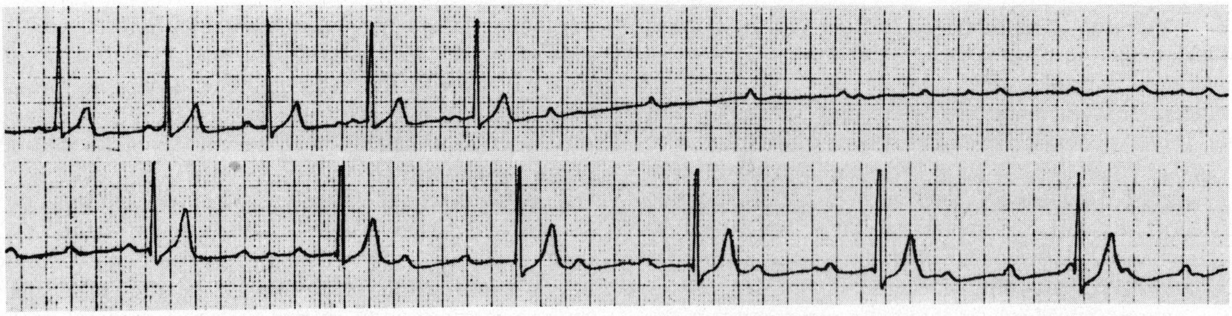

FIGURE 19–29 Paroxysmal complete atrioventricular block in a 25-year-old man with recurrent syncope for seven years. All studies, including an electrophysiological study, were totally normal. Long-term ECG recordings demonstrated intermittent complete AV block of unknown etiology. (From Zipes, D. P., and Noble, R. J.: Assessment of electrical abnormalities. *In* Hurst, J. W. (ed.): The Heart. 5th ed. New York, McGraw-Hill Book Co., 1982, pp. 333–357.)

whether a patient demonstrates 97 or 100 PVCs over a 24-hour period. All systems can potentially record more information than the physician knows how to assimilate. So long as the system detects ectopy, ventricular tachycardia, or asystolic intervals and semiquantitates those abnormalities, the physician probably receives all the clinical information that is needed. Though some physicians and regulatory agencies request information on the actual number of PVCs, until it is clearly demonstrated that reducing the number of PVCs improves prognosis, the necessity for such PVC quantitation is uncertain.

A variety of other recording devices exist that automatically record samples of the cardiac rhythm through the day or that are triggered to record a specific ECG event that occurs at a rate exceeding preset limits. Some record other physiologic signals such as respiratory rate, electroencephalogram, or blood pressure.

Invasive Electrophysiological Studies. An invasive electrophysiological procedure involves introducing multipolar catheter electrodes into the venous and/or arterial system, positioning the electrodes at various intracardiac sites to record electrical activity from portions of the atria or ventricles or from the region of the His bundle, and stimulating the atria or ventricles electrically. Such studies are performed diagnostically to provide information on the type of rhythm disturbance and insight into its electrophysiological mechanism. The procedure is used therapeutically to terminate a tachycardia by electrical stimulation as well as to evaluate effects of therapy by determining whether a particular intervention prevents electrical induction of a tachycardia.[357] Finally, these tests have been used prognostically to identify patients at risk for sudden cardiac death.[358,359] The study may be helpful in patients who have AV block, intraventricular conduction disturbance, sinus node dysfunction, tachycardia, and unexplained syncope or palpitations. It is important to remember that a negative test result—that is, not finding a particular abnormality—does not necessarily mean the patient may not experience the problem at another time. Thus, false-negative results are common with certain rhythm disturbances. A false-positive result, i.e., induction of a nonclinical arrhythmia, may be less common, depending on the stimulation protocol used, although accurate figures must be established for certain arrhythmias, like ventricular tachycardia. Several factors may explain the disparity between test results and spontaneous clinical occurrences, including altered autonomic tone in a supine patient undergoing study, therapeutic lidocaine serum concentrations resulting from local infiltration to introduce the catheters,[360] changing anatomy after the study, and the fact that the test employs an artificial "trigger" (electrical stimulation) to induce the arrhythmia.[152]

AV BLOCK (See also pp. 730, 733, and 735). In patients with AV block, the site of block usually dictates the clinical course of the patient and whether or not a pacemaker is needed.[361,362] Generally, the site of AV block can be determined from an analysis of the scalar ECG. When the site of block cannot be determined from such an analysis, and when knowing the site of block is imperative for patient management, an invasive electrophysiological study is indicated. Candidates include patients who have second-degree AV block and bundle branch block, fixed 2:1 AV block, and syncope and AV block. Patients with block in the His-Purkinje system more commonly become symptomatic because of periods of bradycardia or asystole and require pacemaker implantation than do patients who have AV nodal block.[363–366] The mechanism responsible for the block, such as concealed His extrasystoles[367,368b] (Fig. 19–30), can sometimes be determined from such a study and can also influence the therapeutic course (p. 710).

INTRAVENTRICULAR CONDUCTION DISTURBANCE. For patients with an intraventricular conduction disturbance, an electrophysiological study provides information on the duration of the H-V interval, which can be prolonged with a normal P-R interval or normal with a prolonged P-R interval. A prolonged H-V interval is associated with a greater likelihood of developing trifascicular block, having organic disease, and higher mortality.[369] Some data suggest that finding very long H-V intervals (> 80 to 90 msec) identifies patients at significant risk of developing AV block. During the study, atrial pacing is used to uncover abnormal His-Purkinje conduction.[365,370] In addition to stressing the His-Purkinje system by pacing the atria at fast rates and short premature intervals, drug infusion, such as with procainamide or ajmaline, sometimes exposes abnormal His-Purkinje conduction.[371,372] Ajmaline may cause arrhythmias and should be used cautiously.[373]

An electrophysiological study is indicated only if the patient has symptoms that appear to be related to a bradyarrhythmia (syncope or presyncope) and when no other cause for syncope is found. For many of these patients, ventricular *tachyarrhythmias* rather than AV block may be the cause of their symptoms.[369] In patients who develop bundle branch block associated with acute anteroseptal myocardial infarction, finding a prolonged H-V in-

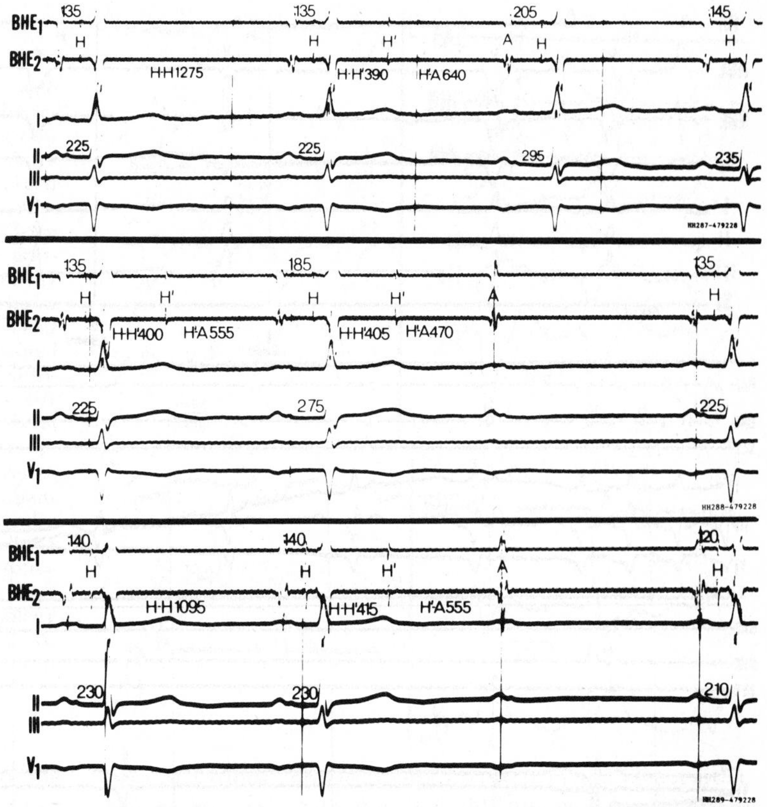

FIGURE 19–30 Concealed discharge from the bundle of His mimicking first-degree (top), type I (middle), and type II (bottom) second-degree AV block. Numbers are in milliseconds. Time lines are one second. (Magnification differs in the three panels.) Numbers in the bipolar His electrogram (BHE_1) indicate A-H intervals; the H-V interval is constant. Numbers in lead II indicate the P-R interval. H-H = interval between His responses in normal conducted cycles. H-H′ = interval between the last normal His discharge and the premature His discharge. H′-A = interval between the premature His depolarization and the next normal sinus-initiated atrial discharge. H′ invaded the AV node and lengthened the A-H interval or produced AV nodal block of the next atrial depolarization. (From Bonner, A. J., and Zipes, D. P.: Lidocaine and His bundle extrasystoles. His bundle discharge conducted normally, conducted with functional right or left bundle branch block or blocked entirely (concealed). Arch. Intern. Med. *136*:700, 1976.)

terval may help identify those who are at greater risk of developing complete AV block or ventricular tachyarrhythmias and of dying.[374,375] Patients who develop bifascicular block and transient high-grade AV block during acute myocardial infarction may not require electrophysiological study, since pacemaker therapy is often recommended on the basis of their clinical course alone[375–377] (see pp. 744 and 756).

SINUS NODAL DYSFUNCTION. The demonstration of slow sinus rates, sinus exit block, or sinus pauses temporally related to symptoms strongly suggests a causal relationship and may obviate further diagnostic studies. Carotid sinus pressure that results in complete cardiac asystole with associated symptoms may expose the patient with a hypersensitive carotid sinus reflex[378] (p. 692). Carotid sinus massage must be done cautiously.[379] Neurohumoral agents or stress testing[380] may be employed to evaluate effects of autonomic tone on sinus nodal function. Atropine,[381,382] isoproterenol,[383] propranolol,[384] and combined atropine and propranolol to produce pharmacological denervation[381,385,386] have been used to identify the patient with sinus node dysfunction due to abnormal autonomic tone. Invasive electrophysiological studies to evaluate sinus node function include assessment of sinus node automaticity and sinoatrial conduction time. Electrophysiological studies should be considered in patients who have symptoms attributable to bradycardia or asystole, such as presyncope or syncope, and for whom noninvasive approaches have provided no explanation for the symptoms.

Overdrive suppression appears to be one of the more useful and sensitive tests to evaluate sinus node function.[212,387–389] The interval between the last paced high right atrial response and the first spontaneous (sinus) high right atrial response after termination of pacing is measured to determine the *sinus node recovery time.* Since spontaneous sinus cycle length influences sinus node recovery time, the *corrected sinus node recovery time* may be used, calculated by subtracting the spontaneous sinus node cycle length (prior to pacing) from the sinus recovery time (Fig. 19–31). Normal values are generally less than 525 msec.[388,389] Prolonged sinus node recovery time has been found in 35 to 93 per cent of patients suspected of having sinus node dysfunction.[198,349,390] The wide range in these values probably depends on whether the patient population includes many who have ECG evidence only of sinus bradycardia.[198,349,391] Such patients often have normal corrected sinus node recovery times. After cessation of pacing, the first return sinus cycle may be normal and may be followed by secondary pauses (Fig. 19–31). Secondary pauses appear to be more common in patients whose sinus node dysfunction is caused by sinoatrial exit block. It is important to evaluate AV nodal and His-Purkinje function in patients with sinus node dysfunction, since many also exhibit impaired AV conduction.[392]

Sinoatrial conduction time can be estimated, based on the assumptions that (1) conduction times into and out of the sinus node are equal, (2) no depression of sinus node automaticity occurs, and (3) the pacemaker site does not shift following premature stimulation. Since these assumptions cannot be applied to all patients, determining sinus node conduction time is less useful than determining corrected sinus node recovery time when sinus node function in human beings is evaluated.[392a]

Marked sinus arrhythmia invalidates the calculation of sinoatrial conduction time; to eliminate its effects, brief periods of atrial pacing at rates just faster than the sinus rate have been used instead of testing during sinus rhythm.[393] The accuracy of this test is comparable to that achieved when testing during sinus rhythm.[393] Generally, measurement of sinoatrial conduction time is an insensitive indicator of sinus node dysfunction, since the time is prolonged in less than half the patients with clinical findings of sinus

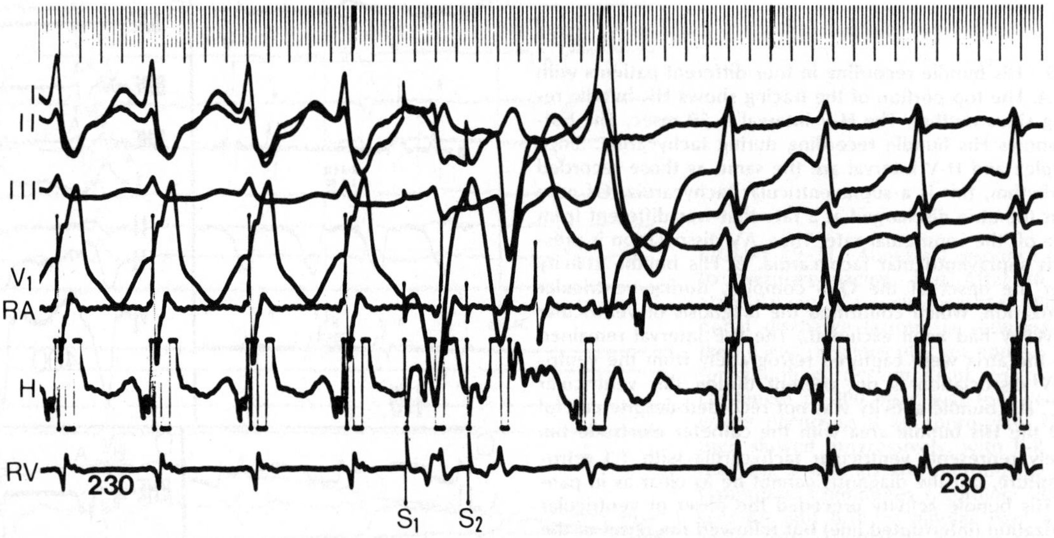

FIGURE 19–34 A wide QRS tachycardia was initiated in this patient. Despite numerous changes in catheters and in catheter positions, an adequate His bundle electrogram could not be recorded, and the diagnosis of ventricular tachycardia could not be excluded. Premature ventricular stimulation (S_1-S_2) normalized the QRS complex at an identical cycle length as the wide QRS tachycardia. Premature right ventricular stimulation thus eliminated the functional right bundle branch block and established the diagnosis of supraventricular tachycardia with aberrancy. (From Zipes, D. P., and Noble, R. J.: Assessment of electrical abnormalities. *In* Hurst, J. W. (ed.): The Heart, 5th ed. New York, McGraw-Hill Book Co., 1982, pp. 333–357.)

gical approaches are developed that may preferentially affect one or the other mechanism.

An electrophysiological study should be considered in patients who have symptomatic, recurrent, or drug-resistant tachyarrhythmias or tachyarrhythmias occurring too infrequently to permit adequate diagnostic or therapeutic assessment. Such inclusion criteria apply to patients who have supraventricular tachyarrhythmias (e.g., reciprocating tachycardia, atrial flutter, or fibrillation with a very rapid ventricular response [often, though not always associated with the Wolff-Parkinson-White syndrome]) and to patients who have symptomatic ventricular tachyarrhythmias. The studies appear useful to guide diagnosis and therapy in patients resuscitated from out-of-hospital sudden death associated with ventricular tachyarrhythmias.[404]

Electrophysiological testing may help identify patients at risk for the subsequent development of ventricular tachycardia or sudden death, not by eliciting a spontaneous premature ventricular complex, called a repetitive ventricular response following a single premature ventricular stimulus delivered during sinus rhythm or atrial pacing[359,405–409] as was originally suggested,[358] but by inducing ventricular tachycardia in susceptible patients.[410,410a]

PATIENTS WITH UNEXPLAINED PALPITATIONS OR SYNCOPE. The three common arrhythmic causes of syncope or palpitations include sinus node dysfunction, tachyarrhythmias, and AV block. Of the three, tachyarrhythmias are probably most reliably initiated in the electrophysiology laboratory, followed by sinus node abnormalities and then His-Purkinje block. The electrophysiological study may fail to explain the patient's symptoms if the arrhythmia cannot be induced or if an abnormal rhythm is induced and the patient remains asymptomatic. However, induction of an arrhythmia that replicates the patient's symptoms may explain the cause of the palpitations or syncope. Patients considered for a study are those whose recurrent syncopal spells remain undiagnosed despite complete general and neurological evaluation, repeated 24-hour ECG recordings, stress testing, and other noninvasive cardiac tests. The presence of palpitations alone is *not* an indication for an electrophysiological study. However, an electrophysiological study may be useful if the patient complains of symptoms such as angina, shortness of breath, or lightheadedness during the palpitations; if there is evidence that the palpitations may represent a significant rhythm disturbance, and if noninvasive studies fail to reveal a cause of the palpitations.

Sensitivity and Specificity. Some understanding of the sensitivity and specificity of the results obtained from electrophysiological testing is required to decide which patients might benefit from such a study. Invasive electrophysiological studies provide important information when a particular abnormality can be demonstrated. Electrophysiological testing initiates paroxysmal supraventricular tachycardia due to Wolff-Parkinson-White syndrome or AV node reentry in over 90 per cent of patients who have spontaneously occurring tachycardias. The ability to precipitate ventricular tachycardia in patients who have spontaneous episodes varies with the etiology of the heart disease and nature of the ventricular tachycardia. During right ventricular pacing, ventricular tachycardia can be induced most often in patients who have ischemic heart disease and sustained ventricular tachycardia and least often in those with heart disease unrelated to ischemia and nonsustained ventricular tachycardia[411] (Fig. 19–28).

More aggressive pacing techniques (e.g., using three premature stimuli), administration of drugs (e.g., isoproterenol), or left ventricular pacing[412] may increase the success rate of ventricular tachycardia induction. The increased sensitivity of the test is paralleled by a decreased specificity because of the induction of nonclinical ventricular tachyarrhythmias. Initiation of sustained supraventricular[219] or ventricular[402,413] tachyarrhythmia during an electrophysiological study provides important information that the induced tachyarrhythmia *may* be clinically significant and responsible for the patient's symptoms. Induction of *sustained* supraventricular or ventricular tachycardia (not pleomorphic ventricular tachycardia progressing to ventricular fibrillation) during an electrophysiological study in patients who are not subject to the spontaneous development of the tachycardia appears to be uncommon, although *appropriate control groups, particularly for ventricular tachycardia, have not yet been reported.* The frequency of induction of ventricular tachycardia in patients who have no history of ventricular tachycardia but have heart disease comparable to those that do have a history of ventricular tachycardia is *not known* and needs to be established using the same stimulation protocols employed to induce ventricular tachyarrhythmias in patients with a history of ventricular tachycardia.[117] Generally, abnormalities such as sustained tachycardia, prolonged pauses following overdrive right atrial pacing, or type II AV block cannot be induced in patients who do not or may not experience these abnormalities spontaneously. In these examples, electrophysiological studies may have a high level of specificity.

Failure to initiate an arrhythmia does not exclude it as a possible cause of the patient's symptoms because of false-negative responses, as mentioned earlier. This caveat is particularly applicable to patients with sinus node dysfunction. Initiation of an abnormally long pause following overdrive pacing, for example, is uncommon in patients without abnormal sinus node function. However, as many as 50 per cent of patients with sinus bradycardia and 20 per cent of those with sinus pauses or sinus exit block may respond normally to overdrive pacing.[198,349,391] His-Purkinje block of a spontaneous or electrically-induced premature atrial complex may occur in normal patients, particularly when the basic cycle length is long and AV nodal propagation is fairly rapid (Fig. 19–35). However, development of block in the His-Purkinje system during sinus rhythm, at atrial-paced rates less than 130 to 150 bpm,[365] at premature intervals (H_1-H_2) longer than about 450 msec,[370] indicates abnormal refractoriness and/or conduction in the His-Purkinje system. However, this is often difficult to produce.

The yield from electrophysiological studies in patients who have syncope appears to vary with the population studied. In one report, such testing revealed a possible cause of the syncope in 68 per cent of 25 patients, most of whom had abnormal ECGs and forms of organic heart disease.[414] In a second study,[415] electrophysiological testing was useful in only 12 per cent of 34 patients who had a normal ECG and no evidence of organic heart disease. Thus, patient selection may influence the usefulness of such testing in patients with unexplained syncope. In these latter situations the sensitivity of the test is low.

Cognizance of the sensitivity and specificity of electrophysiological study for each rhythm disturbance is important, since the risks of these studies, although small (about 2 per cent), far exceed the risks associated with noninvasive tests used to assess electrical abnormalities.[416] Morbidity is the same as that for any cardiac catheterization procedure (p. 296) and includes any vascular complications such as bleeding, thrombosis, thrombophlebitis, pulmonary embolus, inadvertent puncture of the femoral artery, development of arteriovenous fistula, and cardiac perforation. If the left ventricle is mapped or stimulated, morbidity increases, with possible problems associated

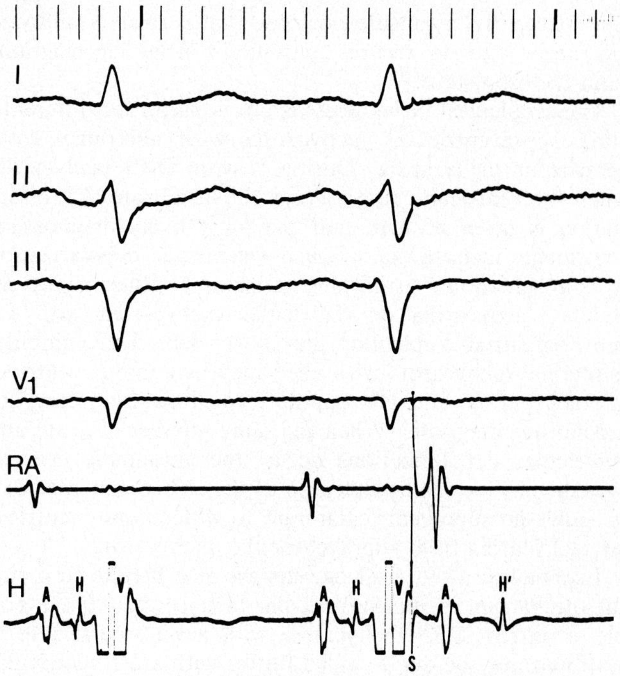

FIGURE 19–35 Premature atrial complex blocking distal to the His bundle recording site. The first two beats are of sinus origin at a cycle length of 670 msec. A premature right atrial stimulus prolongs the A-H interval from 80 msec during sinus rhythm to 150 msec. The premature His response (H′) occurs at an H-H′ interval of 370 msec, and the impulse blocks distal to the His bundle recording site. I, II, III, and V_1 = scalar leads; RA = right atrial lead; H = His bundle lead; A = atrial deflection; H′ = His bundle deflection; V = ventricular depolarization; S = premature right atrial stimulus. (Dark time lines = 50 msec.)

with an arterial puncture and left heart catheterization. If the subclavian approach is used, pneumothorax or arterial puncture may occur. Since precipitation of AV block or a tachyarrhythmia is often a desirable goal of the study, symptoms from such rhythm disturbances may result, compounding the morbidity. Mortality from the study should be near zero, although this depends on how ill the patient may be. In patients with significant myocardial dysfunction, it may be possible to precipitate a ventricular tachyarrhythmia that cannot be terminated by direct-current cardioversion or that results in cerebral, renal, or cardiac ischemia or infarction before termination.

Finally, the procedures are time-consuming[417] and expensive and require sophisticated equipment and personnel trained in catheterization techniques, cardiopulmonary resuscitation, and clinical cardiac electrophysiology. The cost of a three-day hospitalization plus electrophysiological study may exceed the cost of 20 to 25 long-term (24-hour) ECG recordings.

ESOPHAGEAL ELECTROCARDIOGRAPHY. Esophageal electrocardiography is a useful noninvasive technique to diagnose arrhythmias.[200,418,419] The esophagus is adjacent to the posterior atria, and an electrode inserted into the esophagus can record atrial potentials. Bipolar recording appears superior to unipolar recording.[200,420,421] In addition, atrial and occasionally ventricular pacing can be performed via a catheter electrode inserted into the esophagus, and initiation and termination of tachycardias can be accomplished.[422] In adults, optimum atrial recordings are obtained when the distal electrode on the esophageal lead is positioned approximately 40 cm from the patient's nares.[419] Recently, a capsule electrode that is easily swallowed has been used to record continuous atrial electrograms from the esophagus.[418]

The esophageal atrial electrogram is useful for differentiating supraventricular tachycardia with aberrancy from ventricular tachycardia. During a wide QRS tachycardia when the ventricular rate exceeds the atrial rate, AV dissociation is often present, and the most likely diagnosis is ventricular tachycardia. If each ventricular depolarization is coupled to an atrial depolarization, either supraventricular tachycardia or ventricular tachycardia with 1:1 ventriculoatrial conduction may be present. Uncommonly, junctional tachycardia with aberrancy may mimic ventricular tachycardia, and His bundle recordings are needed for a definitive diagnosis. When the same number of atrial and ventricular depolarizations occur, the autonomic nervous system may be manipulated to evoke AV nodal block or to slow the supraventricular rate to differentiate ventricular tachycardia from supraventricular tachycardia.

Esophageal atrial electrograms are also helpful to define the mechanism of supraventricular tachycardias. For example, a narrow QRS tachycardia with a ventricular rate of 150 bpm may be due to atrial flutter with a 2:1 ventricular response, confirmed by finding an atrial rate of 300 bpm. If atrial and ventricular depolarization occur simultaneously during paroxysmal supraventricular tachycardia, reentry utilizing an accessory AV pathway (Wolff-Parkinson-White) can be excluded, and AV nodal reentry is the most likely mechanism for the tachycardia (p. 707).

BODY SURFACE MAPPING. Isopotential body surface maps are used to provide a complete picture of the effects of the currents from the heart on the body surface.[423] The potential distributions are represented by contour lines of equal potential, and each distribution is displayed instant-by-instant throughout activation or recovery, or both.

Body surface maps have been used for preliminary clinical application in the following areas:[423] localizing and sizing myocardial infarction,[424–426] detecting areas of ischemia (especially those apparent only with exercise), localizing ectopic foci[427] or accessory pathways,[428] and differentiating aberrant supraventricular conduction from ventricular origin.

DIRECT CARDIAC MAPPING: RECORDING POTENTIALS DIRECTLY FROM THE HEART. Cardiac mapping is a method whereby potentials recorded directly from the heart are spatially depicted as a function of time in an integrated manner. The location of recording electrodes (epicardial, intramural, or endocardial) and the recording mode used (unipolar versus bipolar) as well as the method of display (isopotential versus isochrone maps) depend upon the problem under consideration.

Direct cardiac mapping via catheter electrodes or at the time of cardiac surgery can be used to localize accessory pathways associated with the Wolff-Parkinson-White syndrome,[429,430] to delineate the anatomical course of the His bundle during open-heart surgery to avoid injury during procedures to correct congenital heart defects.[431] and to identify the site of rhythm disturbances in patients with supraventricular and ventricular tachyarrhythmias refractory to medical therapy; it has also fostered surgical approaches for extirpation of the latter[287,401,403,432] (p. 672). Areas of myocardial ischemia or infarction can be identified to revascularize or to define margins for surgical resection in the treatment of ischemic heart disease.[433,434] These approaches are discussed in greater detail under the individual arrhythmias in Chapter 21.

SIGNAL-AVERAGING TECHNIQUES. Signal averaging is a method that improves signal-to-noise ratio when signals occur recurrently and the noise is random, i.e., not synchronous with the signal. In conjunction with other methods of noise reduction, signal averaging can detect cardiac signals of a few microvolts. With this method, potentials generated by the sinus and AV nodes,[435] His-bundle, and bundle branches are detectable at the body surface.[436–438] The duration of the His-Purkinje waveform corresponds to the H-V interval recorded by the catheter technique. A new development permits high amplification, "on-line" His bundle recordings from the skin surface.[436] Signal averaging has also been applied to improve resolution of potentials that are detectable by standard recording techniques. Examples of such application include recording fetal electrocardiograms[439] as well as recording P waves and ST waves during exercise.[440]

Detecting late ventricular activation in patients with intraventricular conduction delay and ventricular tachycardias may become clinically useful.[441] Delayed activation potentials may serve as a portent of serious ventricular arrhythmias,[442,443] a guide to antiarrhythmic therapy, a diagnostic aid in detecting heart disease, or a means of differentiating between reentrant and automatic ectopic beats. It is likely that signal averaging and other techniques of signal conditioning will become increasingly important in the next several years.

References

1. Keith, A., and Flack, M. W.: The form and nature of the muscular connections between the primary divisions of the vertebrate heart. J. Anat. Physiol. *41*:172, 1907.
2. James, T. N.: Anatomy of the conduction system of the heart. *In* Hurst, J. W. (ed.): The Heart. New York, McGraw-Hill Book Co., 1982.
3. Anderson, R. H., and Becker, A. E.: Gross anatomy and microscopy of the conducting system. *In* Mandel, W. J. (ed.): Cardiac Arrhythmias, Their Mechanisms, Diagnosis and Management. Philadelphia, J. B. Lippincott, 1980.
4. James, T. N.: Anatomy of the Coronary Arteries. New York, Harper and Row, 1961.
5. James, T. N.: The sinus node as a servomechanism. Circ. Res. *32*:307, 1973.
6. James, T. N., Sherf, L., Fine, G., and Morales, A. R.: Comparative ultrastructure of the sinus node in man and dog. Circulation *34*:139, 1966.
7. Masson-Pevet, M., Bleeker, W. K., and Gas, D.: The plasma membrane of leading pacemaker cells in the rabbit sinus node: A qualitative and quantitative ultrastructural analysis. Circ. Res. *45*:621, 1979.
8. Trautwein, W., and Uchizono, K.: Electron microscopic and electrophysiologic study of the pacemaker in the sino-atrial node of the rabbit heart. Z. Zellforsch. Mikrosk. Anat. *61*:96, 1963.
9. Bleeker, W. K., Mackaay, A. J., Masson-Pevet, M., Bouman, L. N., and Becker, A. E.: Functional and morphological organization of the rabbit sinus node. Circ. Res. *46*(1):11, 1980.
10. Becker, A. E., Bouman, L. N., Janse, M. J., and Anderson, R. H.: Functional anatomy of the cardiac conduction system, Harrison, D. C. (ed.): Cardiac Arrhythmias: A Decade of Progress. Boston, G. K. Hall, 1981, p. 3.
11. Levy, M. N., and Martin, P. J.: Neural control of the heart. *In* Berne, R. M., et al. (eds.): Handbook of Physiology. Section 2, The Cardiovascular System. Vol. I, The Heart. Bethesda, Md., American Physiological Society, 1979, p. 581.
12. Randall, W. C.: Sympathetic control of the heart. *In* Randall, W. C. (ed.): Neural Regulation of the Heart. New York, Oxford University Press, 1977.
13. Zipes, D. P., Mihalick, M. J., and Robbins, G. T.: Effects of selective vagal and stellate ganglion stimulation on atrial refractoriness. Cardiovasc. Res. *8*:647, 1974.
14. Prystowsky, E. N., Naccarelli, G. V., Jackman, W. M., Rinkenberger, R. L., Heger, J. J., and Zipes, D. P.: Enhanced vagal tone produced by neck collar suction shortens atrial refractoriness in man. Am. J. Cardiol. *47*:496, 1981.

15. Takahashi, N., and Zipes, D. P.,: Pre- and postsynaptic modulation of adrenergic effects on canine sinus nodal automaticity and AV nodal conduction by vagal stimulation. Clin. Res. *30*:485A, 1982.
16. James, T. N.: The connecting pathways between the sinus node and the AV node and between the right and left atrium in the human heart. Circulation *53*: 609, 1963.
17. Hogan, P. M., and Davis, L. D.: Electrophysiological characteristics of canine atrial plateau fibers. Circ. Res. *28*:62, 1971.
18. Sherf, L., and James, T. N.: Fine structure of cells and their histologic organization within internodal pathways of the heart: clinical and electrocardiographic implications. Am. J. Cardiol. *44*:345, 1979.
19. Roberts, D. E., Hersch, L. T., and Scher, A. M.: Influence of cardiac fiber orientation on wavefront voltage, conduction velocity, and tissue resistivity in the dog. Circ. Res. *44*:701, 1979.
20. Scher, A. M., and Spach, M. S.: Cardiac depolarization and repolarization and the electrocardiogram. *In* Berne, R. M., et al. (eds.): Handbook of Physiology, The Cardiovascular System. Bethesda, Md., American Physiological Society, 1979, p. 357.
21. Vassalle, M., and Hoffman, B. F.: The spread of sinus activation during potassium administration. Circ. Res. *17*:285, 1965.
22. Waldo, A. L., Bush, H. L., Jr., Gelband, H., Zorn, G. L., Vitikainen, K. J., and Hoffman, B. F.: Effects on the canine P wave of discrete lesions in the specialized atrial tracts. Circ. Res. *29*:452, 1971.
23. Spach, M. S., Lieberman, M., Scott, J. G., Barr, R. C., Johnson, E. A., and Kootsey, J. M.: Excitation sequences of the atrial septum and the AV node in isolated hearts of the dog and rabbit. Circ. Res. *29*:156, 1971.
24. Janse, M. J., and Anderson, R. H.: Specialized internodal atrial pathways—Fact or fiction? Eur. J. Cardiol. *2*:117, 1974.
25. Hoffman, B. F.: Fine structure of internodal pathways. Am. J. Cardiol. *44*:385, 1979.
26. Wagner, M. L., Lazzara, R., Weiss, R. M., and Hoffman, B. F.: Specialized conducting fibers in the interatrial band. Circ. Res. *18*:502, 1966.
27. Childers, R. W., Merideth, J., and Moe, G. K.: Supernormality in Bachmann's bundle: An *in vitro* and *in vivo* study in the dog. Circ. Res. *22*:363, 1968.
28. Becker, A. E., and Anderson, R. H.: Morphology of the human atrioventricular junctional area. *In* Wellens, H. J. J., et al. (eds.): The Conduction System of the Heart. Philadelphia, Lea and Febiger, 1976, p. 263.
29. Hecht, H. H., Kossmann, C. E., Childers, R. W., Langendorf, R., Ler, M., Rosen, K. M., Pruitt, R. D., Truex, R. L., Uhley, H. N., and Watt, T. B.: Atrioventricular and intraventricular conduction. Revised nomenclature and concepts. Am. J. Cardiol. *31*:232, 1973.
30. James, T. N.: Morphology of the human atrioventricular node, with remarks pertinent to its electrophysiology. Am. Heart J. *62*:652, 1961.
31. Jackman, W. M., Prystowsky, E. N., Naccarelli, G. B., Heger, J. J., and Zipes, D. P.: Enhanced AV nodal conduction: Prevalence and anatomic substrate. Circulation *67*:441, 1983.
32. Kulbertus, H. E., and Demoulin, J. C.: Pathological basis of concept of left hemiblock. *In* Wellens, H. J. J., et al. (eds.): Conduction System of the Heart. Philadelphia, Lea and Febiger, 1976, p. 287.
33. Massing, G. K., and James, T. N.: Anatomic configuration of the His bundle and bundle branches in the human heart. Circulation *53*:609, 1976.
34. Rosenbaum, M. B., Elizari, M. V., and Lazzari, J. O.: The Hemiblocks. Oldsmar, Fla., Tampa Tracings, 1970.
35. Gilmour, R. F., Jr., and Zipes, D. P.: Different electrophysiological responses of canine endocardium and epicardium to combined hyperkalemia, hypoxia and acidosis. Circ. Res. *46*:814, 1980.
36. Janse, M. J., van Capelle, F. J. L., Anderson, R. H., Toubone, P., and Billette, J.: Electrophysiology and structure of the atrioventricular node of the isolated rabbit heart. *In* Wellens, H. J. J., et al. (eds.): The Conduction System of the Heart. Philadelphia, Lea and Febiger, 1976, p. 296.
37. Paes de Carvalho, A., and de Almeida, D. F.: Spread of activity through the atrioventricular node. Circ. Res. *8*:801, 1960.
38. Anderson, R. H., Janse, M. J., van Capelle, F. J. L., Billette, J., Becker, A. E., and Durrer, D.: A combined morphological and electrophysiological study of the atrioventricular node of the rabbit heart. Circ. Res. *35*:909, 1974.
39. Weidmann, S.: The diffusion of radiopotassium across intercalated disks of mammalian cardiac muscle. J. Physiol. *187*:323, 1966.
40. James, T. N., and Spence, C. A.: Distribution of cholinesterase within the sinus node and AV node in the human heart. Anat. Rec. *155*:151, 1966.
41. Thaemert, J. C.: Atrioventricular node innervation in ultrastructural three dimensions. Am. J. Anat. *128*:239, 1970.
42. Wallace, A. G., and Sarnoff, S. J.: Effects of cardiac sympathetic nerve stimulation on conduction in the heart. Circ. Res. *14*:86, 1964.
43. Yanowitz, F., Preston, J. B., and Abildskov, J. A.: Functional distribution of right and left stellate innervation to the ventricles: Production of neurogenic electrocardiographic changes by unilateral alteration of sympathetic tone. Circ. Res. *18*:416, 1966.
44. Randall, W. C., and Armour, J. A.: Gross and microscopic anatomy of the cardiac innervation. *In* Randall, W. C. (ed.): Neural Regulation of the Heart. New York, Oxford University Press, 1977, p. 13.
45. Kralios, F. A., Martin, L., Burgess, M. J., and Millar, K.: Local ventricular repolarization changes due to sympathetic nerve branch stimulation. Am. J. Physiol. *228*:1621, 1975.
46. Martins, J. B., and Zipes, D. P.: Epicardial phenol interrupts refractory period responses to sympathetic but not vagal stimulation in canine left ventricular epicardium and endocardium. Circ. Res. *47*:33, 1980.
47. Mueller, T. M., Barber, M. J., David, B., and Zipes, D. P.: Phenol topically applied to left ventricular epicardium interrupts sympathetic but not vagal afferents. Clin. Res. *30*:208A, 1982.
48. Martins, J. B., and Zipes, D. P.: Effects of sympathetic and vagal nerves on recovery properties of the endocardium and epicardium of the canine left ventricle. Circ. Res. *46*:100, 1980.
49. Han, J., and Moe, G. K.: Nonuniform recovery of excitability in ventricular muscle. Circ. Res. *14*:44, 1964.
50. Angelakos, E. T., King, M. P., and Millard, R. W.: Regional distribution of catecholamines in hearts of various species. Ann. NY Acad. Sci. *156*:219, 1969.
51. Dahlstrom, A., Fuxe, K., Mya-tu, M., and Zellerstrom, B. E. M.: Observations on adrenergic innervation of the dog heart. Am. J. Physiol. *209*:689, 1965.
52. Kent, K. M., Epstein, S. E., Cooper, T., and Jacobowitz, D. M.: Cholinergic innervation of the canine and human ventricular conducting system: Anatomic and electrophysiologic correlations. Circulation *50*:948, 1974.
53. Schmidt, P. G., Grief, B. J., Lund, D. D., and Roskowski, R., Jr.: Regional choline acetyltransferase activity in the guinea pig heart. Circ. Res. *42*:657, 1978.
54. Brown, O. M.: Cat heart acetylcholine, structural proof and distribution. Am. J. Physiol. *231*:781, 1966.
55. Fields, J. Z., Roeske, W. R., Morkin, E., and Yamamura, H. I.: Cardiac muscarinic cholinergic receptors. J. Biol. Chem. *253*:3251, 1978.
56. Levy, M. N.: Sympathetic-parasympathetic interactions in the heart. Circ. Res. *29*:437, 1971.
57. Ruffy, R., Lovelace, D. E., Knoebel, S. B., and Zipes, D. P.: Influence of secobarbital and alphachloralose and of vagal and sympathetic interruption on left ventricular activation following acute coronary artery ligation in the dog. Circ. Res. *48*:884, 1981.
58. Prystowsky, E. N., Jackman, W. M., Rinkenberger, R. L., Heger, J. J., and Zipes, D. P.: Effect of autonomic blockade on ventricular refractoriness and atrioventricular conduction in humans: Evidence supporting a direct cholinergic action on ventricular muscle refractoriness. Circ. Res. *49*:511, 1981.
59. Zipes, D. P., Martins, J. B., Ruffy, R., Prystowsky, E. N., Elharrar, V., and Gilmour, R. F., Jr.: Roles of autonomic innervation in the genesis of ventricular arrhythmias. *In* Abboud, F. M., et al. (eds.): Disturbances in Neurogenic Control of the Circulation. Bethesda, Md., American Physiological Society, 1981, pp. 225–250.
60. Thames, M. D., Klopfenstein, H. S., Abboud, F. M., Mark, A. L., and Walker, J. L.: Preferential distribution of inhibitory cardiac receptors with vagal afferents to the inferoposterior wall of the left ventricle activated during coronary occlusion in the dog. Circ. Res. *43*:512, 1978.
61. Katz, A. M., Messineo, F. C., and Herbette, L.: Ion channels in membranes. Circulation *65*(Suppl. 1):2, 1982.
62. Hille, B.: Ionic channels in nerve membranes. Progr. Biophys. Mol. Biol. *21*:1, 1970.
63. Langer, G. A., and Brady, A. J.: The Mammalian Myocardium. New York, John Wiley, 1974.
64. Fozzard, H. A.: Cardiac muscle: Excitability and passive electrical properties. Progr. Cardiovasc. Dis. *19*:343, 1977.
65. Sperelakis, N.: Origin of the cardiac resting potential. *In* Berne, R. M., et al. (eds.): Handbook of Physiology, The Cardiovascular System. Bethesda, Md., American Physiological Society, 1979, p. 187.
66. McNutt, N. S.: Ultrastructure of intercellular junctions in adult and developing cardiac muscle. Am. J. Cardiol. *25*:169, 1970.
67. Lowenstein, W. R., Kanno, U., and Socolar, S. J.: The cell-to-cell channel. Fed. Proc. *37*:2645, 1978.
68. Carmeliet, E., and Vereecke, J.: Electrogenesis of the action potential and automaticity. *In* Berne, R. M., et al. (eds.): Handbook of Physiology. Bethesda, Md., American Physiological Society, 1979, p. 269.
69. Electrophysiology of the heart. *In* Berne, R. M., et al. (eds.): Handbook of Physiology. Bethesda, Md., American Physiological Society, 1979, pp. 187–428.
70. Page, E.: The electrical potential difference across the cell membrane of heart muscle. Circulation *26*:582, 1962.
71. Thomas, R. C.: Electrogenic sodium pump in nerve and muscle cells. Physiol. Rev. *52*:563, 1972.
72. Hoffman, B. F., and Cranefield, P. F.: Electrophysiology of the Heart. New York, McGraw-Hill Book Co., 1960.
73. Vassalle, M.: Cardiac automaticity and its control. *In* Levy, M. N., and Vassalle, M. (eds.): Excitation and Neural Control of the Heart. Bethesda, Md., American Physiological Society, 1982.
74. Goldman, D. E.: Potential, impedance and rectification in membranes. J. Gen. Physiol. *27*:27, 1943.
75. Baker, P. F., Blaustein, M. P., Hodgkin, A. L., and Skinhardt, L. A.: Influence of calcium on sodium efflux in squid axons. J. Physiol. (Lond.) *200*:431, 1969.
76. Reuter, H., and Seitz, N.: Dependence of calcium efflux from cardiac muscle on temperature and external ion composition. J. Physiol. (Lond.) *195*:451, 1968.
77. Weidmann, S.: The effect of the cardiac membrane potential on the rapid availability of the sodium carrying system. J. Physiol. (Lond.) *127*:213, 1955.
78. Hodgkin, A. L., and Huxley, A. F.: Quantitative description of membrane current and its application to conduction and excitation in nerve. J. Physiol. *117*:500, 1952.
79. Cranefield, P. F.: The Conduction of the Cardiac Impulse, Mt. Kisco, N.Y., Futura Publ. Co., 1975.

80. Zipes, D. P., Bailey, J. C., and Elharrar, V.: The Slow Inward Current and Cardiac Arrythmias. The Hague, Martinus Nijhoff, 1980.
81. Reuter, H., and Scholtz, H.: A study of the ion selectivity and the kinetic properties of the calcium dependent slow inward current in mammalian muscle. J. Physiol. (Lond.) *264*:17, 1977.
82. Akiyama, T., and Fozzard, H. A.: Ca and Na selectivity of the active membrane of rabbit AV nodal cells. Am. J. Physiol. *236*(1):C1, 1979
83. Mary-Rabine, L., Hoffman, B. F., and Rosen, M. R.: Participation of slow inward current in the Purkinje fiber action potential overshoot. Am. J. Physiol. *237*:H204, 1979.
84. Coraboeuf, E.: Voltage clamp studies of the slow inward current. *In* Zipes, D. P., et al. (eds.): The Slow Inward Current and Cardiac Arrhythmias. The Hague, Martinus Nijhoff, 1980. p. 25.
85. Carmeliet, E.: The slow inward current: Nonvoltage clamp studies. *In* Zipes, D. P., et al. (eds.): The Slow Inward Current and Cardiac Arrhythmias. The Hague, Martinus Nijhoff, 1980, p. 97.
86. Gilmour, R. F., Jr., and Zipes, D. P.: Basic electrophysiology of the slow inward current. *In* Antman, E., and Stone, P. H.: Calcium Blocking Agents in the Treatment of Cardiovascular Disorders. Futura Publ. Co., Mt. Kisco, N.Y. (in press).
87. Niedergerke, R., and Orkand, R. K.: The dual effect of calcium on the action potential of the frog's heart. J. Physiol. (Lond.) *184*:291, 1966.
88. Reuter, H.: Properties of two inward membrane currents in the heart. Ann. Rev. Physiol. *41*:413, 1979.
89. Hauswirth, O., and Singh, B. N.: Ionic mechanisms in heart muscle in relation to the genesis and the pharmacological control of cardiac arrhythmias. Pharmacol. Rev. *30*:5, 1979.
90. Watanabe, A. M., Lindemann, J. P., Jones, L. R., Besch, H. R., Jr., and Bailey, J. C.: Biochemical mechanisms mediating neural control of the heart. *In* Abboud, F. M., Fozzard, H. A., Gilmore, J. P., and Leis, D. J. (eds.): Disturbances in neurogenic control of the circulation. Bethesda, Md., American Physiological Society, 1981.
91. Watanabe, A. M., Jones, L. R., Manalan, A. S., and Besch, H. R., Jr.: Cardiac autonomic receptors: Recent concepts from radiolabeled ligand binding studies. Circ. Res. *50*:161, 1982.
92. Giles, W., and Noble, S. J.: Changes in membrane current in bullfrog atrium produced by acetylcholine. J. Physiol. (Lond.) *261*:103, 1976.
93. Zipes, D. P., and Mendez, C.: Action of manganese ions and tetrodotoxin on atrioventricular nodal transmembrane potentials in isolated rabbit hearts. Circ. Res. *32*:447, 1973.
94. Irisawa, H., and Yanagihara, K.: The slow inward current of the rabbit sinoatrial nodal cells. *In* Zipes, D. P., et al. (eds.): The Slow Inward Current and Cardiac Arrhythmias. The Hague, Martinus Nijhoff, 1980, p. 265.
95. Merideth, J., Mendez, C., Mueller, W. J., and Moe, G. K.: Electrical excitability of atrioventricular nodal cells. Circ. Res. *23*:69, 1968.
96. Zipes, D. P., Besch, H. R., and Watanabe, A. M.: Role of the slow current in cardiac electrophysiology (editorial). Circulation *51*:761, 1975.
97. Nishimura, M., Kokubun, S., Noma, A., Irisawa, H., and Watanabe, Y.: Membrane current systems in the rabbit atrioventricular node. The first voltage clamp study (abstract). Am. J. Cardiol. *47*:429, 1981.
98. Gilmour, R. F., Jr., and Zipes, D. P.: Electrophysiological response of vascularized hamster cardiac transplants to ischemia. Circ. Res. *50*:599, 1982.
99. Spear, J. F., Horowitz, L. N., and Moore, E. N.: The slow response in human ventricle. Zipes, D. P., et al. (eds.): The Slow Inward Current and Cardiac Arrhythmias. The Hague, Martinus Nijhoff, 1980, p. 309.
100. Singer, D. H., Baumgarten, C. M., and Ten Eick, R. E.: Cellular electrophysiology of ventricular and other dysrhythmias: Studies on diseased and ischemic heart. Progr. Cardiovasc. Dis. *24*:97, 1981.
101. Gilmour, R. F., Jr., Heger, J. J., Prystowsky, E. N., and Zipes, D. P.: Cellular electrophysiological abnormalities of diseased human ventricular myocardium. Am. J. Cardiol. (still in press).
102. Kenyon, J. L., and Gibbons, W. R.: Effects of low-chloride solutions on action potentials of sheep cardiac Purkinje fibers. J. Gen. Physiol. *70*:635, 1977.
103. Isenberg, G., and Trautwein, W.: Outward current and electrogenic sodium pump in Purkinje fibers. *In* Fleckenstein, A., and Dhalla, N. S. (eds.): Recent Advances in Studies on Cardiac Structure and Metabolism. Vol. 5. Baltimore, University Park Press, 1975, p. 43.
104. Coraboeuf, E., Deroubaix, E., and Coulombe, A.: Effect of tetrodotoxin on action potentials of the conducting system in the dog. Am. J. Physiol. *236*:H561, 1979.
105. DiFrancesco, D.: A new interpretation of the pacemaker current in calf Purkinje fibers. J. Physiol. (Lond.) *314*:359, 1981.
106. Carmeliet, E., and Saikawa, T.: Shortening of the action potential and reduction of pacemaker activity by lidocaine, quinidine, and procainamide in sheep cardiac Purkinje fibers. An effect on Na or K currents? Circ. Res. *50*:257, 1982.
107. DeMello, W. C.: Some aspects of the interrelationship between ions and electrical activity in specialized tissue of the heart. *In* Paes de Carvalho, A., et al. (eds.): The Specialized Tissues of the Heart. Amsterdam, Elsevier Publ. Co., 1961.
108. Brown, H. F.: Electrophysiology of the sinoatrial node. Physiol. Rev. *62*:505, 1982.
109. Wit, A. L., and Cranefield, P. F.: Effect of verapamil on the sinoatrial and atrioventricular nodes of the rabbit and the mechanism by which it arrests reentrant atrioventricular nodal tachycardia. Circ. Res. *35*:413, 1974.
110. Zipes, D. P., and Fischer, J. C.: Effects of agents which inhibit the slow channel on sinus node automaticity and atrioventricular conduction in the dog. Circ. Res. *34*:184, 1974.
111. Tse, W. W.: Evidence of presence of automatic fibers in the canine atrioventricular node. Am. J. Physiol. *225*:716, 1973.
112. Wit, A. L., and Cranefield, P. F.: Mechanisms of impulse initiation in the atrioventricular junction and the effects of acetylstrophanthidin. Am. J. Cardiol. *49*:921, 1982.
113. Vassalle, M.: Electrogenic suppression of automaticity in sheep and dog Purkinje fibers. Circ. Res. *27*:361, 1970.
113a. Gaskell, W. H.: On the innervation of the heart with special reference to the heart of the tortoise. J. Physiol. *4*:43, 1884.
114. Zipes, D. P., Wallace, A. G., Sealy, W. C., and Floyd, W. L.: Artificial atrial and ventricular pacing in the treatment of arrhythmias. Ann. Intern. Med. *70*:885, 1969.
115. Boineau, J., Schuessler, R. B., Wylds, A. C., Miller, C. B., and Autry, L. A.: Response of atrial pacemaker complex to pharmacologic infusion and cardiac nerve stimulation. Circulation *64*(Suppl. IV):327, 1981.
116. Peon, J., Ferrier, G. R., and Moe, G. K.: The relationship of excitability to conduction velocity in canine Purkinje tissue. Circ. Res. *43*:125, 1978.
117. Zipes, D. P.: New approaches to antiarrhythmic therapy. New Engl. J. Med. *304*:475, 1981.
118. Gadsby, D. C., and Wit, A. L.: Normal and abnormal electrophysiology of cardiac cells. *In* Mandel, W. J. (ed.): Cardiac Arrhythmias. Philadelphia, J. B. Lippincott, 1980, p. 55.
119. Jennings, R. B., Ganote, C. E., and Reimer, K. A.: Ischemic tissue injury. Am. J. Pathol. *81*:179, 1975.
120. Hill, J. L., and Gettes, L. S.: Effect of acute coronary artery occlusion on local myocardial extracellular K^+ activity in swine. Circulation *61*:768, 1980.
121. Rovetto, M. J.: Energy metabolism in the ischemic heart. Tex. Rep. Biol. Med. *39*:397, 1979.
122. Corr, P. B., and Sobel, B. E.: The importance of metabolites in the genesis of ventricular dysrhythmia induced by ischemia. II. Biochemical factors. Mod. Conc. Cardiovasc. Dis. *48*:49, 1979.
123. Wit, A. L., Rosen, M. R., and Hoffman, B. F.: Electrophysiology and pharmacology of cardiac arrhythmias. II. Relation of normal and abnormal electrical activity of cardiac fibers to the genesis of arrhythmias. b. Reentry. Sec. II. Am. Heart J. *88*:798, 1974.
124. Sasyniuk, B. I., and Mendez, C.: A mechanism for reentry in canine ventricular tissue. Circ. Res. *28*:3, 1971.
125. Mendez, C., and Moe, G. K.: Some characteristics of transmembrane potentials of AV nodal cells during propagation of premature beats. Circ. Res. *19*:993, 1966.
126. Friedman, P. L., Stewart, J. R., and Wit, A. L.: Spontaneous and induced cardiac arrhythmias in subendocardial Purkinje fibers surviving extensive myocardial infarction in dogs. Circ. Res. *22*:612, 1973.
127. Myerburg, R. J., Gelband, H., Nilsson, K., Sung, R. J., Thurer, R. J., Morales, A. R., and Bassett, A. L.: Long-term electrophysiological abnormalities resulting from experimental myocardial infarction in cats. Circ. Res. *41*:73, 1977.
128. Barber, M. J., Mueller, T. M., and Zipes, D. P.: Transmural myocardial infarction produces sympathectomy in noninfarcted myocardium apical to the infarct. Am. J. Cardiol. *49*:888, 1982.
129. Elharrar, V., and Zipes, D. P.: Cardiac electrophysiologic alterations during myocardial ischemia. Am. J. Physiol. *233*:H329, 1977.
130. Zipes, D. P., Watanabe, A. W., and Besch, H. R.: Clinical electrophysiology and electrocardiography. *In* Willerson, J. T., and Sanders, C. A. (eds.): The Science and Practice of Clinical Medicine: Clinical Cardiology. New York, Grune and Stratton, 1977, p. 235.
131. Hoffman, B. F., and Rosen, M. R.: Cellular mechanisms for cardiac arrhythmias. Circ. Res. *49*:1, 1981.
132. Gilmour, R. F., Jr., and Zipes, D. P.: Electrophysiological characteristics of rodent myocardium damaged by adrenaline. Cardiovasc. Res. *14*:582, 1980.
133. Rosen, M. R., and Hordof, A. J.: The slow response in human atrium. *In* Zipes, D. P., et al. (eds.): The Slow Inward Current and Cardiac Arrhythmias. The Hague, Martinus Nijhoff, 1980, p. 295.
134. Ten Eick, R. E., and Singer, D. H.: Electrophysiological properties of diseased human atrium. I. Low diastolic potential and altered cellular response to potassium. Circ. Res. *44*:545, 1979.
135. Surawicz, B.: Depolarization-induced automaticity in atrial and ventricular myocardial fibers. *In* Zipes, D. P., et al. (eds.): The Slow Inward Current and Cardiac Arrhythmias. The Hague, Martinus Nijhoff, 1980, p. 375.
136. Elharrar, V., and Zipes, D. P.: Voltage modulation of automaticity in cardiac Purkinje fibers. *In* Zipes, D. P., et al. (eds.): The Slow Inward Current and Cardiac Arrhythmias. The Hague, Martinus Nijhoff, 1980, p. 357.
137. Foster, P. R., Elharrar, V., and Zipes, D. P.: Accelerated ventricular escapes induced in the intact dog by barium, strontium and calcium. J. Pharmacol. Exp. Ther. *200*:373, 1977.
138. Ferrier, G. R.: Digitalis arrhythmias: Role of oscillatory afterpotentials. Progr. Cardiovasc. Dis. *19*:459, 1977.
139. Cranefield, P. F.: Action potentials, afterpotentials and arrhythmias. Circ. Res. *41*:415, 1977.
140. Rosen, M. R., Merker, C., Gelband, H., and Hoffman, B. F.: Mechanisms of digitalis toxicity: Effects of ouabain on phase 4 of canine Purkinje fiber transmembrane potentials. Circulation *47*:681, 1973.
141. Hashimoto, K., and Moe, G. K.: Transient depolarizations induced by acetylstrophanthidin in specialized tissue of dog atrium and ventricle. Circ. Res. *32*:618, 1973.
142. Cranefield, P. F., and Aronson, R. S.: Initiation of sustained rhythmic activity

by single propagated action potentials in canine Purkinje fibers exposed to sodium-free solution or to ouabain. Circ. Res. *34*:477, 1974.
143. Makarycheu, V. A., Kosharskaya, I. L., and Ulyninsky, L. S.: Automatic activity of the pacemaker cells of the atrioventricular valves in the rabbit heart. Bull. Exp. Biol. Med. *81*:646, 1976.
144. Wit, A. L, Fenoglio, J. J., Wagner, B. M., and Bassett, A. L.: Electrophysiological properties of cardiac muscle in the anterior mitral valve leaflet and the adjacent atrium in the dog: Possible implications for the genesis of atrial dysrhythmias. Circ. Res. *32*:771, 1973.
145. Wit, A. L., and Cranefield, P. F.: Triggered activity in cardiac muscle fibers of the simian mitral valve. Circ. Res. *38*:85, 1976.
146. Wit, A. L., Fenoglio, J. J., Hordof, A. J., and Reemtsma, K.: Ultrastructure and transmembrane potentials of cardiac muscle in the human anterior mitral valve leaflet. Circulation *59*:1284, 1979.
147. Bassett, A. L., Fenoglio, J. J., Jr., Wit, A. L., Myerburg, R. J., and Gelband, J.: Electrophysiological and ultrastructural characteristics of canine tricuspid valve. Am. J. Physiol. *230*:1366, 1976.
148. Wit, A. L., and Cranefield, P. F.: Triggered and automatic activity in the canine coronary sinus. Circ. Res. *41*:435, 1977.
149. Saito, T., Otosuro, M., and Matsubara, T.: Electrophysiologic studies on the mechanism of electrically-induced sustained rhythmic activity in the rabbit right atrium. Circ. Res. *42*:199, 1978.
150. Mary-Rabine, L., Hordof, A. J., Danilo, P., Jr., Malm, J. R., and Rosen, M. R.: Mechanisms for impulse initiation in isolated human atrial fibers. Circ. Res. *47*:267, 1980.
151. Zipes, D. P., Arbel, E., Knope, R. F., and Moe, G. K.: Accelerated cardiac escape rhythms caused by ouabain intoxication. Am. J. Cardiol. *33*:248, 1974.
152. Zipes, D. P., Foster, P. R., Troup, P. J., and Pedersen, D. H.: Atrial induction of ventricular tachycardia: Reentry or triggered automaticity. Am. J. Cardiol. *44*:1, 1979.
153. Rosen, M. R., Fisch, C., Hoffman, B. F., Danilo, P., Jr., Lovelace, D. E., and Knoebel, S. B.: Can accelerated atrioventricular junctional escape rhythms be explained by delayed afterdepolarizations? Am. J. Cardiol. *45*:1272, 1980.
154. Wellens, H. J. J., Brugada, P., Vanagt, E. J. D. M., Ross, D. L., and Bär, F. W. H. M.: New studies with triggered automaticity. *In* Harrison, D. C. (ed.): Cardiac Arrhythmias: A Decade of Progress. Boston, G. K. Hall, 1981, p. 601.
155. Zipes, D. P.: A defense of triggered automaticity (symposium). *In* Harrison, D. C. (ed.): Cardiac Arrhythmias: A Decade of Progress. Boston, G. K. Hall, 1981.
156. Rosen, M. R., and Danilo, P.: Effects of tetrodotoxin, lidocaine, verapamil and AHR-2666 on ouabain-induced delayed afterdepolarizations in canine Purkinje fibers. Circ. Res. *46*:117, 1980.
157. Tsien, R. W., and Carpenter, D. O.: Ionic mechanisms of pacemaker activity in cardiac Purkinje fibers. Fed. Proc. *37*:2127, 1978.
158. Elharrar, V., Bailey, J. C., Lathrop, D. A., and Zipes, D. P.: Effects of aprindine HCl on slow channel action potentials and transient depolarizations in canine Purkinje fibers. J. Pharmacol. Exp. Ther. *205*:410, 1978.
159. Vassalle, M., and Mugelli, A.: An oscillatory current in sheep cardiac Purkinje fibers. Circ. Res. *48*:618, 1981.
160. Kass, R., Tsien, R., and Weingert, R.: Ionic basis of transient inward current induced by strophanthidin in cardiac Purkinje fibers. J. Physiol. (Lond.) *281*:209, 1978.
161. Wit, A. L., Cranefield, P. F., and Gadsby, D. C.: Electrogenic sodium extrusion can stop triggered activity in the canine coronary sinus. Circ. Res. *49*:1029, 1981.
162. Vassalle, M., Cummins, M., Castro, C., and Stuckey, J. H.: The relationship between overdrive suppression and overdrive excitation in ventricular pacemakers in dogs. Cir. Res. *38*:367, 1976.
163. Jalife, J., Antzelevitch, C., and Moe, G. K.: Models of parasystole and reflection. *In* Rosenbaum, M. B. (ed.): Cardiac Arrhythmias. The Hague, Martinus Nijhoff, 1982.
164. Antzelevitch, C., Moe, G. K., and Jalife, J.: Electrotonic modulation of pacemaker activity. Further biological and mathematical observations in the behavior of modulated parasystole. Circulation *66*:1225, 1982.
165. Moe, G. K., Jalife, J., Mueller, W. J., and Moe, B.: A mathematical model of parasystole and its application to clinical arrhythmias. Circulation *56*:968, 1977.
166. Cohen, H., Langendorf, R., and Pick, A.: Intermittent parasystole: Mechanism of protection. Circulation *48*:761, 1973.
167. Nau, G. J., Aldariz, A. E., Aconzo, R. S., Chiale, P. A., Elizari, M. V., and Rosenbaum, M. B.: Concealed ventricular parasystole uncovered in the form of ventricular escapes of variable coupling. Circulation *64*:199, 1981.
168. Jalife, J., and Antzelevitch, C.: Phase resetting and annihilation of pacemaker activity in cardiac tissue. Science *206*:695, 1979.
169. Nau, G. T., Aldariz, A. E., Aconzo, R. S., Halpern, S., Davidenko, J. M., Elizari, M. V., and Rosenbaum, M. B.: Modulation of parasystolic activity by non-parasystolic beats. Circulation *66*:462, 1982.
170. Hunter, P. J., McNaughton, P. A., Noble, D.: Analytical models of propagation in excitable cells. Progr. Biophys. Mol. Biol. *30*:99, 1975.
171. Singer, D. H., Lazzara, R., and Hoffman, B. F.: Interrelationships between automaticity and conduction in Purkinje fibers. Circ. Res. *21*:537, 1967.
172. Dominguez, G., and Fozzard, H.: Influence of extracellular K^+ concentration on cable properties and excitability of sheep cardiac Purkinje fibers. Circ. Res. *26*:565, 1970.
173. Simson, M. B., Spear, J. F., and Moore, E. N.: The relationship between atrioventricular nodal refractoriness and the functional refractory period in the dog. Circ. Res. *44*:121, 1979.
174. Pick, A., and Langendorf, R.: Interpretation of Complex Arrhythmias. Philadelphia, Lea and Febiger, 1979, p. 127.
175. Zipes, D. P., and Noble, R. J.: Assessment of electrical abnormalities. *In* Hurst, J. W. (ed.): The Heart. 5th ed. New York, McGraw-Hill Book Co., 1982, p. 333.
176. Ferrier, G. R., and Rosenthal, J. E.: Automaticity and entrance block induced by focal depolarization of mammalian ventricular tissues. Circ. Res. *47*:238, 1980.
177. Antzelevitch, C., and Moe, G. K.: Electrotonically-mediated delayed conduction and reentry in relation to "slow responses" in mammalian ventricular conducting tissue. Circ. Res. *49*:1129, 1981.
178. Lieberman, M., Kootsey, J. M., and Johnson, E. A.: Low conduction in cardiac muscle. A biophysical model. Biophys. J. *13*:37, 1973.
179. Watanabe, Y., and Dreifus, L. S.: Inhomogeneous conduction in the AV node: A model for reentry. Am. Heart J. *70*:505, 1965.
180. de la Fuente, D., Sasyniuk, B., and Moe, G. K.: Conduction through a narrow isthmus in isolated canine atrial tissue. A model of the WPW syndrome. Circulation *44*:803, 1971.
181. Zipes, D. P.: Second degree atrioventricular block. Circulation *60*:465, 1979.
182. Erlanger, J.: Further studies on the physiology of heart block: The effects of extrasystoles upon the dog's heart and upon strips of terrapin's ventricle in the various stages of block. Am. J. Physiol. *16*:160, 1906.
183. Schmitt, F. O., and Erlanger, J.: Directional differences in the conduction of the impulse through heart muscle and their possible relation to extrasystolic and fibrillatory contractions. Am. J. Physiol. *87*:326, 1929.
184. McWilliam, J. A.: Fibrillar contraction of the heart. J. Physiol. (Lond.) *8*:296, 1897.
185. Mayer, A. G.: Rhythmical pulsation in scyphomedusae. Publ. No. 47 of Carnegie Institution of Washington, 1906.
186. Mines, G. R.: On dynamic equilibrium in the heart. J. Physiol. (Lond.) *46*:349, 1913.
187. Mines, G. R.: On circulating excitations in heart muscles and their possible relation to tachycardia and fibrillation. Trans. Roy. Soc. Canad. (Sec. IV) *8*:43, 1914.
188. Garrey, W. E.: The nature of fibrillary contraction of the heart. Its relation to tissue mass and form. Am. J. Physiol. *33*:397, 1914.
189. Cranefield, P. F., Klein, H. O., and Hoffman, B. F.: Conduction of the cardiac impulse. I. Delay, block and one-way block in depressed Purkinje fibers. Circ. Res. *28*:199, 1971.
190. Wit, A. L., Cranefield, P. F., and Hoffman, B. F.: Slow conduction and reentry in the ventricular conducting system. II. Single and sustained circus movement in networks of canine and bovine Purkinje fibers. Circ. Res. *30*:11, 1972.
191. Rinkenberger, R. L., Prystowsky, E. N., Jackman, W. M., Heger, J. J., and Zipes, D. P.: Conversion of nonsustained ventricular tachycardia to sustained ventricular tachycardia during drug therapy as determined by serial electrophysiology studies. Am. Heart J. *103*:177, 1982.
192. Prystowsky, E. N., Heger, J. J., Jackman, W. M., Naccarelli, G. V., and Zipes, D. P.: Incessant supraventricular tachycardia following myocardial infarction. Am. Heart J. *103*:426, 1982.
193. Antzelevitch, C., Jalife, J., and Moe, G. K.: Frequency-dependent alterations of conduction in Purkinje fibers. A model of phase 4 facilitation and block. *In* Rosenbaum, M. B. (ed.): Cardiac Arrhythmias. The Hague, Martinus Nijhoff, 1982.
194. Antzelevitch, C., Jalife, J., and Moe, G. K.: Characteristics of reflection as a mechanism of reentrant arrhythmias and its relationship to parasystole. Circulation *61*:182, 1980
195. Lewis, T.: Observations upon flutter and fibrillation. Part IV. Impure flutter; theory of circus movement. Heart *7*:293, 1920.
196. Rosenblueth, A., and Garcia Ramos, J.: Studies on atrial flutter and fibrillation. II. The influence of artificial obstacles on experimental auricular flutter. Am. Heart J. *33*:677, 1947.
197. Boineau, J. P., Mooney, C. R., Hudson, R. D., Hughes, D. G., Erdin, R. A., Jr., and Wilds, A. C.: Observations on reentrant excitation pathways and the refractory period distributions in spontaneous and experimental atrial flutter in the dog. *In* Kulbertus, H. E. (ed.): Reentrant Arrhythmias. Baltimore, University Park Press, 1977, pp. 72–98.
198. Pastelin, G., Mendez, R., and Moe, G. K.: Participation of atrial specialized conduction pathways in atrial flutter. Circ. Res. *42*:386, 1978.
199. Josephson, M. E., and Seides, S. F.: Clinical Cardiac Electrophysiology. Philadelphia, Lea and Febiger, 1979, p. 68.
200. Waldo, A. L., MacLean, W. H., Karp, R. B., Kouchoukos, N. T., and James, T. N.: Entrainment and interruption of atrial flutter with atrial pacing. Studies in man following open heart surgery. Circulation *56*:737, 1977.
201. Zipes, D. P., and DeJoseph, R. L.: Dissimilar atrial rhythms in man and dog. Am. J. Cardiol. *32*:618, 1973.
202. Schecter, D. C.: Flashbacks: Ventricular fibrillation. Part I. PACE *2*:490, 1979.
203. Schecter, D. C.: Flashbacks: Ventricular fibrillation. Part II. PACE *2*:648, 1979.
204. Porter, W. T.: On the results of ligation of the coronary arteries. J. Physiol. (Lond.) *15*:121, 1894.
205. Zipes, D. P., Fischer, J., King, R. M., Nicoll, A., and Jolly, W. W.: Termination of ventricular fibrillation in dogs by depolarizing a critical amount of myocardium. Am. J. Cardiol. *36*:37, 1975.
206. Moe, G. K., and Abildskov, J. A.: Atrial fibrillation as a self-sustaining arrhythmia independent of focal discharge. Am. Heart J. *58*:59, 1969.

207 Moe, G. K.: On the multiple wavelet hypothesis of atrial fibrillation. Arch. Intern. Pharmacodyn. *140*:183, 1962.
208. Han, J., Malozzi, A. M., and Moe, G. K.: Sinoatrial reciprocation in the isolated rabbit heart. Circ. Res. *22*:355, 1968.
209. Wu, D., Amat-y-Leon, F., Denes, P., Dhingra, R. C., Pietras, R. J., and Rosen, K. M.: Demonstration of sustained sinus and atrial reentry as a mechanism of paroxysmal supraventricular tachycardia. Circulation *51*:234, 1975.
210. Weisfogel, G. M., Batsford, W. P., Paulay, K. L., Josephson, M. E., Ogunkelu, J. B., Akhtar, M., Seides, S. F., and Damato, A. N.: Sinus node reentrant tachycardia in man. Am. Heart J. *90*:295, 1975.
211. Allessie, M. A., and Bonke, F. I. M.: Direct demonstration of sinus nodal reentry in the rabbit heart. Circ. Res. *44*:557, 1979.
212. Mandel, W. J., Hayakawa, H., Danzing, R., and Marcus, H. S.: Evaluation of sinoatrial node function in man by overdrive suppression. Circulation *44*:59, 1971.
213. Klein, H. O., Singer, D. H., and Hoffman, B. F.: Effects of atrial premature systoles on the sinus rhythm in the rabbit. Circ. Res. *32*:480, 1973.
214. Prystowsky, E. N., Grant, A. O., Wallace, A. G., and Strauss, H. C.: An analysis of the effects of acetylcholine on conduction and refractoriness in the rabbit sinus node and atrium. Circ. Res. *44*:112, 1979.
215. Steinbeck, G., Allessie, M. A., Bonke, F. I. M., and Lammers, W. J. E. P.: Sinus node response to premature atrial stimulation in the rabbit studied with multiple microelectrode impalement. Circ. Res. *43*:695, 1978.
216. Allessie, M. A., Bonke, F. I. M., and Schopman, F. J. G.: Circus movement in rabbit and atrial muscle as a mechanism of tachycardia. II. The role of nonuniform excitability in the occurrence of unidirectional block, as studied with multiple microelectrodes. Circ. Res. *39*:168, 1976.
217. Allessie, M. A., Bonke, F. I. M., and Schopman, F. J. G.: Circus movement in rabbit atrial muscle as a mechanism of tachycardia. III. The "leading circle" concept: A new model of circus movement in cardiac tissue without the involvement of an anatomical obstacle. Circ. Res. *41*:9, 1977.
218. Boineau, J. P., Schuessler, R. B., Mooney, C. R., Miller, C. B., Wylds, A. C., Hudson, R. D., Borremans, J. M., and Brockus, C. W.: Natural and evoked atrial flutter due to circus movement in dogs. Am. J. Cardiol. *45*:1167, 1980.
219. Coumel, P., and Barold, S. S.: Mechanisms of supraventricular tachycardia. *In* Narula, O. (ed.): His Bundle Electrocardiography and Clinical Electrophysiology. Philadelphia, F. A. Davis Co., 1975, p. 203.
220. Coumel, P., Flammang, D., Attuel, P., and Leckercq, J. F.: Sustained intra-atrial reentrant tachycardia. Electrophysiologic study of 20 cases. Clin. Cardiol. *2*:176, 1979.
221. Wu, D., Denes, P., Amat-y-Leon, F., Dhingra, R., Wyndham, C. R. C., Bauernfeind, R., Latif, P., and Rosen, K. M.: Clinical electrocardiographic and electrophysiologic observations in patients with paroxysmal supraventricular tachycardia. Am. J. Cardiol. *41*:1045, 1978.
222. Hering, H. E.: Ueber die Automatie des Saugethierherzens. Arch. ges. Physiol. *116*:143, 1907.
223. deBoer, S.: Fortgesetzte Untersuchung über Kammerflimmern. Arch. ges. Physiol. *188*:67, 1921.
224. Scherf, D., and Shookoff, C.: Experimentelle Untersuchungen über die "Umkehr-Extrasystole" (reciprocating beat). Wien. Arch. inn. Med. *12*:501, 1926.
225. Scherf, D., and Shookhoff, C.: An experimental study of reciprocating rhythm. Arch. Intern. Med. *67*:372, 1941.
226. Rosenblueth, A., and Rubio, R.: La influencia de la frecuencia de estimulacion sobre los tiempos de propagacion auriculoventricular y ventriculo-auricular. Arch. Inst. Cardiol. (Mexico) *25*:535, 1955.
227. Mignone, R. J., and Wallace, A. G.: Ventricular echoes: Evidence for dissociation of conduction and reentry within the AV node. Circ. Res. *19*:638, 1966.
228. Moe, G. K., and Mendez, C.: Physiological basis of reciprocal rhythm. Progr. Cardiovasc. Dis. *8*:461, 1966.
229. Mendez, C., Han, J., Garcia de Jalon, P. D., and Moe, G. K.: Some characteristics of ventricular echoes. Circ. Res. *16*:562, 1965.
230. Mendez, C., and Moe, G. K.: Demonstration of dual AV conduction system in the isolated rabbit heart. Circ. Res. *19*:378, 1966.
231. Janse, M. J., Van Capelle, F. J. L., Freud, G. E., and Durrer, D.: Circus movement within the AV node as a basis for supraventricular tachycardia as shown by multiple microelectrode recording in the isolated rabbit heart. Circ. Res. *28*:403, 1971.
232. Wit, A. L., Goldreyer, B. N., and Damato, A. N.: An in vitro model of paroxysmal supraventricular tachycardia. Circulation *43*:862, 1971.
233. White, P. D.: A study of atrioventricular rhythm following auricular flutter. Arch. Intern. Med. *16*:517, 1915.
234. Drury, A. N.: Paroxysmal tachycardia of AV nodal origin, exhibiting retrograde heart block and reciprocal rhythm. Heart *11*:405, 1924.
235. Gallavardin, L., and Veil, P.: Deux cas de nouveaux tachycardie en salves chez de jeunes sujets. Arch. Med. Coeur *20*:1, 1927.
236. Scherf, D., and Cohen, J.: The Atrioventricular Node and Selected Cardiac Arrhythmias. New York, Grune and Stratton, 1964, p. 226.
237. Lewis, T.: Mechanism and Graphic Registration of the Heart Beat. London, Shaw and Son, 1925, p. 396.
238. Kistin, A. D.: Atrial reciprocal rhythm. Circulation *32*:687, 1965.
239. Moe, G. K., Cohen, W., and Vick, R. L.: Experimentally induced paroxysmal AV nodal tachycardia in the dog. Am. Heart J. *65*:87, 1963.
240. Schulienburg, R. N., and Durrer, D.: Atrial echo beats in the human heart elicited by induced atrial premature beats. Circulation *37*:680, 1968.
241. Hunt, N. C., Cobb, F. R., Waxman, M. B., Zeft, H. J., Peter, R. H., and Morris, J. J., Jr.: Conversion of supraventricular tachycardias with atrial stimulation. Evidence for reentry mechanism. Circulation *38*:1060, 1968.
242. Bigger, J. T., and Goldreyer, B. N.: The mechanism of supraventricular tachycardia. Circulation *42*:673, 1970.
243. Goldreyer, B. N., and Damato, A. N.: Essential role of atrioventricular conduction delay in the initiation of paroxysmal supraventricular tachycardia. Circulation *43*:679, 1971.
244. Denes, P., Wu, D., Dhingra, R. C., Chuquimia, R., and Rosen, K. M.: Demonstration of dual AV nodal pathways in patients with paroxysmal supraventricular tachycardia. Circulation *48*:549, 1973.
245. Wu, D.: Dual atrioventricular nodal pathways: A reappraisal. PACE *5*:72, 1982.
246. Wu, D., Denes, P., Amat-y-Leon, F., Wyndham, C. R. C., Dhingra, R., and Rosen, K. M.: An unusual variety of atrioventricular nodal reentry due to retrograde dual atrioventricular nodal pathways. Circulation *56*:50, 1977.
247. Spurrell, R. A. J., Krikler, D. M., and Sowton, E.: Effects of verapamil on electrophysiological properties of anomalous atrioventricular connection in Wolff-Parkinson-White syndrome. Brit. Heart J. *36*:256, 1974.
248. Wellens, H. J. J., Tan, S. L., Bar, F. W. H., Duren, D. R., Lie, K. I., and Dohmen, H. M.: Effects of verapamil studied by programmed electrical stimulation of the heart in patients with paroxysmal reentrant supraventricular tachycardia. Brit. Heart J. *39*:1058, 1977.
249. Rinkenberger, R. L., Prystowsky, E. N., Heger, J. J., Troup, P. J., Jackman, W. M., and Zipes, D. P.: Effects of intravenous and chronic oral verapamil administration in patients with supraventricular tachyarrhythmias. Circulation *62*:996, 1980.
250. Janse, M. J.: Influence of the direction of the atrial wavefront on AV nodal transmission in isolated hearts and rabbits. Circ. Res. *25*:439, 1969.
251. Zipes, D. P., Mendez, C., and Moe, G. K.: Evidence for summation and voltage dependency in rabbit atrioventricular nodal fibers. Circ. Res. *32*:170, 1973.
252. Rahilly, G. T., Zipes, D. P., Naccarelli, G. V., Jackman, W. M., Heger, J. J., and Prystowsky, E. N.: Autonomic blockade in patients with normal and abnormal atrioventricular nodal function. Am. J. Cardiol. *49*:898, 1982.
253. Shenasa, M., Gilbert, C. J., Schmidt, D. H., and Akhtar, M.: Procainamide and retrograde atrioventricular nodal conduction in man. Circulation *65*:355, 1982.
254. Denes, P., Kehoe, R., and Rosen, R. M.: Multiple reentrant tachycardias due to retrograde conduction of dual atrioventricular bundles with atrioventricular nodal-like properties. Am. J. Cardiol. *44*:162, 1973.
255. Langendorf, R., and Pick, A.: Manifestations of concealed reentry in the atrioventricular junction. Eur. J. Cardiol. *1*:11, 1973.
256. Josephson, M. E., and Kastor, J. A.: Paroxysmal supraventricular tachycardia. Is the atrium a necessary link? Circulation *54*:430, 1976.
257. Ko, P. T., Naccarelli, G. V., Gulamhusein, S., Prystowsky, E. N., Zipes, D. P., and Klein, G. J.: Atrioventricular dissociation during paroxysmal junctional tachycardia. PACE *4*:670, 1981.
258. Zipes, D. P., Gaum, W. E., Genetos, B. C., Glassman, R. D., Noble, R. J., and Fisch, C.: Atrial tachycardia without P waves masquerading as an AV junctional tachycardia. Circulation *55*:253, 1977.
259. Schulienburg, R. M., Durrer, D.: Further observations on the ventricular echo phenomenon elicited in the human heart. Is the atrium part of the echo pathway? Circulation *45*:629, 1972.
260. Wolff, L., Parkinson, J., and White, P. D.: Bundle branch block with short P-R interval in healthy young people prone to paroxysmal tachycardia. Am. Heart J. *5*:685, 1950.
261. Durrer, D., Schoo, L., Schulienburg, R. M., and Wellens, H. J. J.: The role of premature beats in the initiation and the termination of supraventricular tachycardia in the Wolff-Parkinson-White syndrome. Circulation *36*:644, 1967.
262. Zipes, D. P., DeJoseph, R. L., and Rothbaum, D. A.: Unusual properties of accessory pathways. Circulation *49*:1200, 1974.
263. Gallagher, J. J., Pritchett, E. L. C., Sealy, W. C., Casell, J., and Wallace, A. G.: The pre-excitation syndromes. Progr. Cardiovasc. Dis. *20*:285, 1978.
264. Kent, A. F. S.: Researches on the structure and function of the mammalian heart. J. Physiol. *14*:233, 1893.
265. Kent, A. F. S.: Observations on the auriculo-ventricular junction of the mammalian heart. Quart. J. Exp. Physiol. *7*:193, 1913.
266. Wellens, H. J. J.: The electrophysiologic properties of the accessory pathway in the Wolff-Parkinson-White syndrome. *In* Wellens, H. J. J., et al. (eds.): The Conduction System of the Heart. Philadelphia, Lea and Febiger, 1976.
267. Coumel, P., and Attuel, P.: Reciprocating tachycardia in overt and latent preexcitation. Influence of functional bundle branch block on the rate of the tachycardia. Eur. J. Cardiol. *1*:423, 1974.
268. Barold, S. S., Coumel, P.: Mechanisms of atrioventricular junctional tachycardia. Role of reentry and concealed accessory bypass tracts. Am. J. Cardiol. *39*:97, 1977.
269. Hammill, S. C., Pritchett, E. L. C., Klein, G. J., Smith, W. M., and Gallagher, J. J.: Accessory atrioventricular pathways that conduct only in the antegrade direction. Circulation *62*:1335, 1980.
270. Lown, B., Ganong, W. F., and Levine, S. A.: The syndrome of short PR interval, normal QRS complex and paroxysmal rapid heart action. Circulation *5*:693, 1952.
271. James, T. N.: The Wolff-Parkinson-White syndrome: Evolving concepts of its pathogenesis. Progr. Cardiovasc. Dis. *13*:159, 1970.
272. Gallagher, J. J., Smith, W. M., Kasell, J. H., Benson, D. W., Jr., Sterba, R., and Grant, A. O.: Role of Mahaim fibers in cardiac arrhythmias in man. Circulation *64*:176, 1981.

273. Holzmann, M., and Scherf, D.: Über Elektrokardiogramme mit verkürzter Vorhof-Kammer-Distanz und positiven P-Zacken. Klin. Med. *121*:404, 1932.
274. Wolferth, C. C., and Wood, F. C.: Mechanisms of production of short PR intervals and prolonged QRS complexes in patients with presumably undamaged hearts: Hypothesis of accessory pathway of auriculoventricular conduction (bundle of Kent). Am. Heart J. *8*:297, 1933.
275. Wenckebach, K. F., and Winterberg, H.: Die Unregelmässige Herztätigkeit. Leipzig, Engelmann, 1927.
276. Scherf, D., and Schott, A. Extrasystoles and Allied Arrhythmias. New York, Grune and Stratton, 1953.
277. Cranefield, P. F., and Hoffman, B. F.: Conduction of the cardiac impulse. II. Summation and inhibition. Circ. Res. *28*:220, 1971.
278. Wit, A. L., Hoffman, B. F., and Cranefield, P. F.: Slow conduction and reentry in the ventricular conducting system. I. Return extrasystole in canine Purkinje fibers. Circ. Res. *30*:1, 1972.
279. Sasyniuk, B. I., and Mendez, C.: A mechanism for reentry in canine ventricular tissue. Circ. Res. *28*:3, 1973.
280. Friedman, P. L., Stewart, J. R., Fenoglio, J. J., Jr., and Wit, A. L.: Survival of subendocardial Purkinje fibers after extensive myocardial infarction in dogs. In vitro and in vivo correlations. Circ. Res. *33*:597, 1973.
281. Moe, G. K., Mendez, C., and Han, J.: Aberrant AV impulse propagation in the dog heart: A study of functional bundle branch block. Circ. Res. *16*:261, 1965.
282. Zipes, D. P.: Reentry in the ventricles. *In* Recent Advances in Ventricular Conduction. Advances in Cardiology. Vol. 14. Basel, Karger, 1975, p. 51.
283. Glassman, R. D., and Zipes, D. P.: Site of antegrade and retrograde functional right bundle branch block in the intact canine heart. Circulation *64*:1277, 1981.
284. Akhtar, M., Gilbert, C., Wolf, F. G., and Schmidt, D. H.: Reentry within the His-Purkinje system. Elucidation of reentrant circuit using right bundle branch and His bundle recordings. Circulation *58*:295, 1978.
285. Spurrell, R. A. J., Sowton, E., and Deuchar, D. C.: Ventricular tachycardia in 4 patients evaluated by programmed electrical stimulation of the heart and treated in two patients by surgical division of anterior radiation of left bundle branch. Br. Heart J. *35*:1014, 1973.
286. Josephson, M. E., Horowitz, L. N., Farshidi, A., and Kastor, J. A.: Recurrent sustained ventricular tachycardia. I. Mechanisms. Circulation *57*:431, 1978.
286a. Lloyd, E. A., Zipes, D. P., Heger, J. J., and Prystowsky, E. N.: Sustained ventricular tachycardia due to bundle branch re-entry. Am. Heart J. *104*:1095, 1982.
287. Fontaine, G., Guiraudon, G., Frank, R., Fillette, F., Cabrol, C., and Grosgogeat, Y.: Surgical management of ventricular tachycardia unrelated to myocardial ischemia or infarction. Am. J. Cardiol. *49*:397, 1982.
288. Wallace, A. G., Mignone, R. J.: Physiologic evidence concerning the reentry hypothesis for ectopic beats. Am. Heart J. *72*:60, 1966.
289. Scherlag, B. J., Helfant, R. H., Haft, J. I., and Damato, A. N.: Electrophysiology underlying ventricular arrhythmias due to coronary ligation. Am. J. Physiol. *219*:1665, 1970.
290. Boineau, J. P., and Cox, J. L.: Slow ventricular activation in acute myocardial infarction. A source of reentrant premature ventricular contractions. Circulation *48*:703, 1973.
291. El-Sherif, N., Hope, R. R., Scherlag, B. J., and Lazzara, R.: Reentrant ventricular arrhythmias in the late myocardial infarction period. I. Conduction characteristics in the infarction zone. Circulation *55*:686, 1977.
292. El-Sherif, N., Hope, R. R., Scherlag, B. J., and Lazzara, R.: Reentrant ventricular arrhythmias in the late myocardial infarction period. II. Patterns of initiation and termination of reentry. Circulation *55*:702, 1977.
293. El-Sherif, N., Smith, R. A., and Evans, K.: Canine ventricular arrhythmias in the late myocardial infarction period. 8. Epicardial mapping of reentrant circuits. Circ. Res. *49*:255, 1981.
294. Wit, A. L., Allessie, M. A., Bonke, F. I. M., Lammers, W., Smeets, J., and Fenoglio, J. J., Jr.: Electrophysiologic mapping to determine the mechanism of experimental ventricular tachycardia initiated by premature impulses. Experimental approaches and initial results demonstrating reentrant excitation. Am. J. Cardiol. *49*:166, 1982.
295. Ideker, R. E., Klein, G. J., Harrison, L., Smith, W. M., Kasell, J., Reimer, K. A., Wallace, A. G., and Gallagher, J. J.: The transition to ventricular fibrillation induced by reperfusion after acute ischemia in the dog: A period of organized epicardial activation. Circulation *63*:1371, 1981.
296. Janse, M. J., van Capelle, F. J. L., Morsink, H., Kleber, A. G., Wilms-Schopman, F., Cardinal, R., d'Aloncourt, C. N., and Durrer, D.: Flow of "injury" current and patterns of excitation during early ventricular arrhythmias in acute regional myocardial ischemia in isolated porcine and canine hearts. Evidence for two different arrhythmogenic mechanisms. Circ. Res. *47*:151, 1980.
297. Furman, S., Parker, B., and Escher, D. J. W.: Transtelephonic pacemaker clinic. J. Thorac. Cardiovasc. Surg. *61*:287, 1971.
298. McHenry, P. L., Fisch, C., Jordan, J. W., and Corya, B. R.: Cardiac arrhythmias observed during maximal treadmill exercise testing in clinically normal men. Am. J. Cardiol. *29*:331, 1972.
299. Blackburn, H., Taylor, H., Hamrell, B., Buskirk, E., Nicholas, W. C., and Thorsen, R. D.: Premature ventricular complexes induced by stress testing. Am. J. Cardiol. *31*:441, 1973.
300. Faris, J. V., McHenry, P. L., Jordan, J. W., and Morris, S. N.: Prevalence and reproducibility of exercise-induced ventricular arrhythmias during maximal exercise testing in normal men. Am. J. Cardiol. *37*:617, 1976.
301. McHenry, P. L., Morris, S. N., Kavalier, M., and Jordan, J. W.: Comparative study of exercise-induced ventricular arrhythmias in normal subjects and patients with documented coronary artery disease. Am. J. Cardiol. *37*:609, 1976.
302. Morris, S. N., and McHenry, P. L.: Cardiac arrhythmias during exercise testing and exercise conditioning. Cardiovasc. Clin. *9*:57, 1978.
303. McHenry, P. L., Morris, S. N., and Kavalier, M.: Exercise-induced arrhythmias—Recognition, classification, and clinical significance. Cardiovasc. Clin. *6*: 245, 1974.
304. Goldschlager, N., Cohn, K., and Goldschlager, A.: Exercise-related ventricular arrhythmias. Mod. Conc. Cardiovasc. Dis. *48*:67, 1979.
305. Goldschlager, N., Cake, D., and Cohn, K.: Exercise-induced ventricular arrhythmias in patients with coronary artery disease. Their relation to angiographic findings. Am. J. Cardiol. *31*:434, 1973.
306. Goldschlager, N., Selzer, A., and Cohn, K.: Treadmill stress tests as indicators of presence and severity of coronary artery disease. Ann. Intern. Med. *85*:277, 1976.
307. Irving, J. B., and Bruce, R. A.: Exertional hypotension and post exertional ventricular fibrillation in stress testing. Am. J. Cardiol. *39*:849, 1977.
308. Helfant, R. H., Pine, R., Kabde, V., and Banka, V. S.: Exercise-related ventricular premature complexes in coronary heart disease. Ann. Intern. Med. *80*:589, 1974.
309. Sheps, D. S., Ernst, J. C., Briese, F. R., Lopez, L. V., Conde, C. A., Castellanos, A., and Myerburg, R. J.: Decreased frequency of exercise-induced ventricular ectopic activity in the second of two consecutive treadmill tests. Circulation *55*:891, 1977.
310. Kennedy, H. L.: Comparison of ambulatory electrocardiography and exercise testing. Am. J. Cardiol. *47*:1359, 1981.
311. Crawford, M., O'Rourke, R. A., Ramakrishna, N., Henning, H., and Ross, J., Jr.: Comparative effectiveness of exercise testing and continuous monitoring for detecting arrhythmias in patients with previous myocardial infarction. Circulation *50*:301, 1974.
312. Holter, N. J.: New method for heart studies: Continuous electrocardiography of active subjects over long periods is now practical. Science *134*:1214, 1961.
313. Kennedy, H. L.: Ambulatory Electrocardiography and Holter Recording Technology. Philadelphia, Lea and Febiger, 1981.
314. Harrison, D. C., Fitzgerald, J. W., and Winkle, R. A.: Ambulatory electrocardiography for diagnosis and treatment of cardiac arrhythmias. N. Engl. J. Med. *294*:373, 1976.
315. Wenger, N. K., Mock, M. B., and Ringquist, I.: Ambulatory Electrocardiographic Recording. Chicago, Year Book Medical Publishers, 1981.
316. Winkle, R. A.: Recent status of ambulatory electrocardiography. Am. Heart J. *102*:757, 1981.
317. Foucachet, Y., Rosier, S. P., Planeix, T., Boisante, L., Delescaut, M. F., Bardet, J., Bourdaris, J. P.: Valeur de l'enregistrenment l'electrocardiographique continue par la methode de Holter pour le diagnostic et al surveillance de l'ischemie myocardique. Arch. Mal Coeur, *74*:427, 1981.
317a. Smith, M. S., and Pritchett, E. L. C.: Electrocardiographic monitoring in ambulatory patients with cardiac arrhythmias. Cardiol. Clin. (in press).
318. Barrett, P. A., Peter, C. T., Swan, H. J., Singh, B. N., and Mandel, W. J.: The frequency and prognostic significance of electrocardiographic abnormalities in clinically normal individuals. Progr. Cardiovasc. Dis. *23*:299, 1981.
319. Sobotka, P. A., Mayer, J. H., Bauernfeind, R. A., Kanakis, C., Jr., and Rosen, K. M.: Arrhythmias documented by 24 hour continuous ambulatory electrocardiographic monitoring in young women without apparent heart disease. Am. Heart J. *101*:753, 1981.
319a. Scott, O., Williams, G. J., and Fiddler, G. I.: Results of 24 hour ambulatory monitoring of electrocardiogram in 131 healthy boys aged 10 to 13 years. Brit. Heart J. *44*:304, 1980.
320. Olec, M. D., Smith, N., McNeill, G. P., and Wright, D. S.: Dysrhythmias in apparently healthy subjects. Age-Aging *8*:173, 1979.
321. Abdon, N. J.: Frequency and distribution of long-term ECG recorded cardiac arrhythmias in an elderly population. With special reference to neurological symptoms. Acta Med. Scand. *209*:175, 1981.
322. Mikolich, J. R., Jacobs, W. C., and Fletcher, G. F.: Cardiac arrhythmias in patients with acute cerebrovascular accidents. JAMA *246*:1314, 1981.
323. Lown, B., and Wolf, M.: Approaches to sudden death from coronary heart disease. Circulation *44*:130, 1971.
324. Kennedy, H. L., Chandra, V., Sayther, K. L., and Caralis, D. G.: Effectiveness of increasing hours of continuous ambulatory electrocardiography in detecting maximal ventricular ectopy. Am. J. Cardiol. *42*:925, 1978.
325. Rabkin, S. W., Mathewson, F. A., and Tate, R. B.: Relationship of ventricular ectopy in men without apparent heart disease. Am. Heart J. *101*:135, 1981.
326. Kotler, M. N., Tabatznik, M., Mower, M. M., and Tominagra, S.: Prognostic significance of ventricular ectopic beats with respect to sudden death in the late postinfarction period. Circulation *47*:959, 1973.
327. Moss, A. J., DeCamilla, J., Engstrom, F., Hoffman, W., Odoroff, C., and Davis, H.: The post-hospital phase of myocardial infarction: Identification of patients with increased mortality risk. Circulation *49*:460, 1974.
328. Moss, A. J., DeCamilla, J., Mietlowski, W., Greene, W. A., Goldstein, S., and Locksley, R.: Prognostic grading and significance of ventricular premature beats after recovery from myocardial infarction. Circulation *51*:204, 1975.
329. Vismara, L. A., Amsterdam, E. A., and Mason, D. T.: Relation of ventricular arrhythmias in the late hospital phase of acute myocardial infarction to sudden death after hospital discharge. Am. J. Med. *59*:6, 1975.
330. Ruberman, W., Weinblatt, E., Goldberg, J. D., Frank, C. W., and Shapiro, S.: Ventricular premature beats and mortality after myocardial infarction. N. Engl. J. Med. *297*:750, 1977.
331. Anderson, K. P., DeCamilla, J., and Moss, A. J.: Clinical significance of ven-

tricular tachycardia (3 beats or longer) detected during ambulatory monitoring after myocardial infarction. Circulation *57*:890, 1978.
332. Bigger, J. T., Jr., Weld, F. M., and Rolnitzky, L. M.: Prevalence characteristics and significance of ventricular tachycardia (three or more complexes) detected with ambulatory electrocardiographic recording in the late hospital phase of acute myocardial infarction. Am. J. Cardiol. *48*:815, 1981.
333. Rozanski, J. J., Castellanos, A., and Myerburg, R. J.: Ventricular ecotopy and sudden death. Cardiovasc. Clin. *11*:127, 1980.
334. Ruberman, W., Weinblatt, E., Frank, C. W., Goldberg, J. D., and Shapiro, S.: Repeated one hour of electrocardiograph monitoring of survivors of myocardial infarction at 6 month intervals: Arrhythmia detection and relation to prognosis. Am. J. Cardiol. *47*:1197, 1981.
335. Ruberman, W., Weinblatt, E., Goldberg, J. D., Frank, C. W., Chaudhary, B. S., and Shapiro, S.: Ventricular premature complexes and sudden death after myocardial infarction. Circulation *64*:297, 1981.
335a. Weaver, W. D., Cobb, L. A., and Hallstrom, A. P.: Ambulatory arrhythimias in resuscitated victims of cardiac arrest. Circulation *66*:212, 1982.
335b. Nikolic, G., Bishop, R. L., and Singh, J. B.: Sudden death recorded during Holter monitoring. Circulation *66*:218, 1982.
336. Vismara, L. A., Vera, Z., Forester, J. M., Amsterdam, E. A., and Mason, D. T.: Identification of sudden death risk factors in acute and chronic coronary artery disease. Am. J. Cardiol. *39*:821, 1977.
337. Fitzgerald, J. W., and DeBusk, R. F.: Early post-infarction ambulatory monitoring and exercise testing in detection of arrhythmias. Am. J. Cardiol. *35*:136, 1975.
338. Schulze, R. A., Jr., Strauss, H. W., and Pitt, B.: Sudden death in the year following myocardial infarction. Am. J. Cardiol. *62*:192, 1977.
339. Maron, B. J., Savage, D. D., Wolfson, J. K., and Epstein, S. E.: Prognostic significance of 24 hour ambulatory electrocardiographic monitoring in patients with hypertrophic cardiomyopathy: A prospective study. Am. J. Cardiol. *48*:252, 1981.
340. McKenna, W. J., England, D., Doi, Y. L., Deanfield, J. E., Oakley, C., and Goodwin, J. F.: Arrhythmia in hypertrophic cardiomyopathy. I. Influence on prognosis. Brit. Heart J. *46*:168, 1981.
341. Leichtman, D., Nelson, R., Gobel, F. L., Alexander, C. A., and Cohn, J. N.: Bradycardia with mitral valve prolapse. Ann. Intern. Med. *85*:453, 1976.
342. Winkle, R. A., Lopes, M. G., Popp, R. L., and Hancock, E. W.: Life-threatening arrhythmias in the mitral valve prolapse syndrome. Am. J. Med. *60*:961, 1976.
343. LeClercq, J. F., Malergue, M. C., Milosevic, D., Rosengarten, M. D., Attuel, P., and Coumel, P.: Ventricular arrhythmias and mitral valve prolapse. A study of 35 cases. Arch. Mal Coeur *73*:276, 1980.
344. Greenspon, A. J., and Schaal, S. F.: AV node dysfunction in the mitral valve prolapse syndrome. PACE *3*:60, 1980.
345. Shappell, S. D., Marshall, C. E., Brown, R. E., and Bruce, T. A.: Sudden death and the familial occurrence of midsystolic click, late systolic murmur syndrome. Circulation *48*:1128, 1973.
346. Lipski, J., Cohen, L., Espinoza, J., Motro, M., Dack, S., and Donoso, E.: Value of Holter monitoring in assessing cardiac arrhythmias in symptomatic patients. Am. J. Cardiol. *37*:102, 1976.
347. Tzivoni, D., and Stern, S.: Pacemaker implantation based on ambulatory ECG monitoring in patients with cerebral symptoms. Chest *67*:274, 1975.
348. Bigger, J. T., Jr., and Reiffel, J. A.: Sick sinus syndrome. Ann. Rev. Med. *30*:91, 1979.
349. Prystowsky, E. N.: The sick sinus syndrome—Diagnosis and treatment. *In* Donoso, F. (ed.): Advances and Controversies in Cardiology. New York, Grune and Stratton, 1981, p. 93.
350. Crook, B. R. M., Cashman, P. M. M., Stott, F. D., and Raftery, E. B.: Tape monitoring of the electrocardiogram in ambulant patients with sinoatrial disease. Brit. Heart J. *35*:1009, 1973.
351. Hindman, M. C., Last, J. H., and Rosen, K. M.: Wolff-Parkinson-White syndrome observed by portable monitoring. Ann. Intern. Med. *79*:654, 1973.
352. Bleifer, S. B., Bleifer, D. J., Hansmann, D. R., Sheppard, J. J., and Karpman, H. I.: Diagnosis of occult arrhythmias by Holter electrocardiography. Progr. Cardiovasc. Dis. *16*:569, 1974.
353. Winkle, R. A.: Antiarrhythmic drug effect mimicked by spontaneous variability of ventricular ectopy. Circulation *57*:1116, 1978.
354. Morganroth, J., Michelson, E., Horowitz, L. N., Josephson, M. E., Pearlman, A. S., and Dunkman, W. B.: Limitations of routine long-term ambulatory electrocardiographic monitoring to assess ventricular ectopy frequency. Circulation *58*:408, 1978.
355. Michelson, E. L., Morganroth, J.: How to use Holter monitoring to your patient's best advantage. J. Cardiovasc. Med. *5*:119, 1980.
356. Knoebel, S. B., Lovelace, D. E., Rasmussen, S., and Wash, S. E.: Computer detection of premature ventricular complexes: A modified approach. Am. J. Cardiol. *38*:440, 1976.
357. Fisher, J. D.: Role of electrophysiologic testing in the diagnosis and treatment of patients with known and suspected bradycardias and tachycardias. Progr. Cardiovasc. Dis. *24*:25, 1981.
358. Greene, L. H., Reid, P. R., and Schaeffer, A. H.: The repetitive ventricular response in man: A predictor of sudden death. New Engl. J. Med. *299*:729, 1978.
359. Naccarelli, G. V., Prystowsky, E. N., Jackman, W. M., Heger, J. J., Rinkenberger, R. L., and Zipes, D. P.: Repetitive ventricular response. Prevalence and prognostic significance. Brit. Heart J. *46*:152, 1981.
360. Nattel, S., Rinkenberger, R. L., Lehrman, L. L., and Zipes, D. P.: Therapeutic blood lidocaine concentration after local anesthesia for cardiac electrophysiologic studies. New Engl. J. Med. *301*:418, 1979.
361. Dreifus, L. S.: Clinical judgment is sufficient for the management of conduction defects. Cardiovasc. Clin. *8*:195, 1977.
362. Wu, D., and Rosen, K. M.: Clinical judgment is not sufficient for the management of conduction defects. Indications for diagnostic electrophysiologic studies. Cardiovasc. Clin. *8*:203, 1977.
363. Langendorf, R., and Pick, A.: Atrioventricular block, type II (Mobitz). Its nature and clinical significance. Circulation *38*:819, 1968.
364. Dhingra, R. C., Denes, P., Wu, D., Chuquimia, R., and Rosen, K. M.: The significance of second-degree atrioventricular block and bundle branch block. Observations regarding site and type of block. Circulation *49*:638, 1978.
365. Dhingra, R. C., Wyndham, C., Bauernfeind, R., Swiryn, S., Deedwania, P. C., Smith, T., Denes, P., and Rosen, K. M.: Significance of block distal to the His bundle induced by atrial pacing in patients with chronic bifascicular block. Circulation *60*:1455, 1979.
366. Strasberg, B., Amat-y-Leon, F., Dhingra, R. C., Palileo, E., Swiryn, S., Bauernfeind, R., Wyndham, C., and Rosen, K. M.: Natural history of chronic second degree atrioventricular nodal block. Circulation *63*:1043, 1981.
367. Bonner, A. J., and Zipes, D. P.: Lidocaine and His-bundle extrasystole. His-bundle discharge conducted normally, conducted with functional right or left bundle branch block or blocked entirely (concealed). Arch. Intern. Med. *136*:700, 1976.
368. Fisch, C., Zipes, D. P., and McHenry, P. L.: Electrocardiographic manifestations of concealed junctional ectopic impulses. Circulation *53*:217, 1976.
368a. Langendorf, R., and Mehlman, J. S.: Block (non-conducted) AV nodal premature systoles imitating first and second degree AV block. Am. Heart J. *34*:500, 1947.
368b. Rosen, K. M., Rahimtoola, S. H., and Gunnor, R. M.: Pseudo AV block secondary to non-premature non-propagated His-bundle depolarizations: Documentation by His-bundle electrocardiography, Circulation *42*:367, 1970.
369. Dhingra, R. C., Palileo, E., Strasberg, B., Swiryn, S., Bauernfeind, R. A., Wyndham, C. R., and Rosen, K. M.: Significance of the HV interval in 517 patients with chronic bifascicular block. Circulation *64*:1265, 1981.
370. Damato, A. N., Varghese, P. J., Caracta, A. R., Akhtar, M., and Lau, S. H.: Functional 2:1 block within the His-Purkinje system: Simulation of type II second degree AV block. Circulation *47*:534, 1973.
371. Puech, P., Grolleau, R., and Guimond, L.: Incidence of different types of AV block and their localization by His bundle recordings. *In* Wellens, H. J. J., et al. (eds.): The Conduction System of the Heart. Philadelphia, Lea and Febiger, 1976, p. 467.
372. McKenna, W. J., Rowland, E., Davies, J., and Krikler, D. M.: Failure to predict development of atrioventricular block with electrophysiological testing supplemented by ajmaline. PACE *3*:666, 1980.
373. Wellens, H. J. J., Bar, F. W., and Vanagt, E. J.: Death after ajmaline administration (letters to editor). Am. J. Cardiol. *45*:905, 1980.
374. Lie, K. I., Wellens, H. J. J., Schuilenburg, R. M., Becker, A. E., and Durrer, D.: Factors influencing prognosis of bundle branch block complicating acute anteroseptal infarction. The value of His-bundle recordings. Circulation *50*:935, 1974.
375. Fisch, G. R., Zipes, D. P., and Fisch, C.: Bundle branch block and sudden death. Progr. Cardiovasc. Dis. *23*:187, 1980.
376. Hindman, M. C., Wagner, G. S., JaRo, M., Atkins, J. M., Scheinman, M. M., DeSanctis, R., Hutter, A. H., Jr., Yeatman, L., Rubenfire, M., Pujura, C., Rubin, M., and Morris, J. J.: The clinical significance of bundle branch block complicating acute myocardial infarction. I. Clinical characteristics, determinants of mortality and one-year followup. Circulation *58*:679, 1978.
377. Hindman, M. C., Wagner, G. S., JaRo, M., Atkins, J. M., Scheinman, M. M., DeSanctis, R., Hutter, A. H., Jr., Yeatman, L., Rubenfire, M., Pujura, C., Rubin, M., and J. J.: The clinical significance of bundle branch block complicating acute myocardial infarction. II. Indications for temporary and permanent pacemaker insertion. Circulation *58*:789, 1978.
378. Solti, F., Szabo, Z., Czako, E., Bodor, E., and Renyi-Vamos, F., Jr.: Adams-Stokes attacks associated with cartoid sinus syncope. Pathogenesis and therapy of the carotid sinus syncope. Kardiologie *69*:656, 1980.
379. Beal, M. F., Park, T. S., and Fisher, C. M.: Cerebral atheromatous embolism following carotid sinus pressure. Arch. Neurol. *38*:310, 1981.
380. Holden, W., McAnulty, J. H., and Rahimtoola, S. H.: Characterization of heart rate response to exercise in the sick sinus syndrome. Brit. Heart J. *40*:923, 1978.
381. Jordan, J. A., Yamaguchi, I., and Mandel, W. J.: Studies on the mechanisms of sinus node dysfunction in a sick sinus syndrome. Circulation *57*:217, 1978.
382. Eckberg, D. L., Drabinsky, M., and Braunwald, E.: Defective cardiac parasympathetic control in patients with heart disease. New Engl. J. Med. *285*:877, 1971.
383. Cleaveland, C. R., Rangno, R. E., and Shand, D. G.: A standardized isoproterenol sensitivity test: The effects of sinus arrhythmia, atropine and propranolol. Arch. Intern. Med. *130*:147, 1972.
384. Stern, S., and Eisenberg, S.: The effect of propranolol (Inderal) on the electrocardiogram of normal subjects. Am. Heart J. *77*:192, 1969.
385. Kang, P. S., Gomes, J. A., Kelen, G., and El-Sherif, N.: Role of autonomic regulatory mechanism in sinoatrial conduction and sinus nodal automaticity in sick sinus syndrome. Circulation *64*:832, 1981.
386. Desae, J. M., Scheinman, M. M., Strauss, H. C., Massie, B., and O'Young, J.: Electrophysiologic effects of combined autonomic blockade in patients with sinus node disease. Circulation *63*:953, 1981.
387. Strauss, H. C., Bigger, J. T., Sardoff, A. C., and Giardina, E. G.: Electrophysiologic evaluation of sinus node function in patients with sinus node dysfunction. Circulation *53*:763, 1976.

388. Breidthardt, G., Seipel, L., and Loogen, F.: Sinus node recovery time and calculated sinoatrial conduction time in normal subjects and patients with sinus node dysfunction. Circulation *56*:43, 1977.
389. Steinbeck, G., and Luderitz, B.: Comparative study of sinoatrial conduction time and sinus node recovery time. Brit. Heart J. *37*:956, 1975.
390. Bigger, J. T., Jr., Cramer, M., and Reid, S.: Ability of Holter electrocardiographic recording and atrial stimulation to detect sinus node dysfunction in symptomatic and asymptomatic patients with sinus bradycardia. Am. J. Cardiol. *40*:189, 1977.
391. Rosen, K. M., Loeb, H. S., Sinno, M. Z., Rahimtoola, S. H., and Gunnar, R.: Cardiac conduction in patients with symptomatic sinus node disease. Circulation *43*:836, 1971.
392. Narula, O. S.: Atrioventricular conduction disturbances in patients with sinus bradycardia. Circulation *44*:1096, 1971.
392a. Kerr, C. R., Grant, A. O., Wenger, T. L., and Strauss, H. C.: Sinus node dysfunction. Cardiol. Clin. (still in press).
393. Narula, D. S., Shanto, N., Vasquez, M., Towne, W. D., and Linhart, J. W.: A new measurement of sino-atrial conduction time. Circulation *58*:706, 1978.
394. Hariman, R. J., Krongrad, E., Boxer, R. A., Weiss, M. B., Steeg, C. N., and Hoffman, B. N.: Method for recording electrical activity of the sinoatrial node and automatic atrial foci during cardiac catheterization in human subject. Am. J. Cardiol. *45*:775, 1980.
395. Wellens, J. H. H., Bär, F. W. H. M., and Lie, K. I.: The value of the electrocardiogram in the differential diagnosis of a tachycardia with a widened QRS complex. Am. J. Med. *64*:27, 1978.
396. Wellens, H. J. J., and Durrer, D.: Supraventricular tachycardia with left aberrant conduction due to retrograde invasion into the left bundle branch. Circulation *38*:474, 1968.
397. Wu, D., Amat-y-Leon, F., Simpson, R. J., Jr., Latif, P., Wyndham, C. R. C., Denes, P., and Rosen, K. M.: Electrophysiologic studies with multiple drugs in patients with atrioventricular reentrant tachycardia utilizing an extranodal pathway. Circulation *56*:727, 1977.
398. Mason, J. W., and Winkle, R. A.: Electrode-catheter arrhythmia induction in the selection and assessment of antiarrhythmia drug therapy for recurrent ventricular tachycardia. Circulation *58*:971, 1978.
399. Horowitz, L. N., Spielman, S. R., Greenspan, A. M., and Josephson, M. E.: Role of programmed stimulation in assessing vulnerability to ventricular arrhythmias. Am. Heart J. *103*:604, 1982.
400. Heger, J. J., Prystowsky, E. N., Jackman, W. M., Naccarelli, G. V., and Zipes, D. P.: Comparison between results obtained from electrophysiologic testing, exercise testing and ambulatory ECG recording. *In* Wenger, N. K., et al. (eds.): Ambulatory Electrocardiographic Recording. Chicago, Year Book Medical Publishers, 1981, p. 379.
401. Gallagher, J. J., Kasell, J. H., Cox, J. L., Smith, W. M., Ideker, R. E., and Smith, W. M.: Techniques of intraoperative electrophysiologic mapping. Am. J. Cardiol. *49*:221, 1982.
402. Josephson, M. E., Kastor, J. A., and Horowitz, L. N.: Electrophysiologic management of recurrent ventricular tachycardia in acute and chronic ischemic heart disease. Cardiovasc. Clin. *11*:35, 1980.
403. Boineau, J. P., and Cox, J. L.: Rationale for a direct surgical approach to control ventricular arrhythmias. Relation of specific intraoperative techniques to mechanism and location of arrhythmic circuit. Am. J. Cardiol. *49*:381, 1982.
404. Ruskin, J. N., DiMarco, J. P., and Garan, H.: Out-of-hospital cardiac arrest: Electrophysiologic observations and selection of long-term antiarrhythmic therapy. N. Engl. J. Med. *303*:607, 1980.
405. Mason, J. W.: Repetitive beating after single ventricular extrastimuli: Incidence and prognostic significance in patients with recurrent ventricular tachycardia. Am. J. Cardiol. *45*:1126, 1980.
406. Farshidi, A., Michelson, E. L., Greenspan, A. M., Spielman, S. R., Horowitz, L. N., and Josephson, M. E.: Repetitive responses to ventricular extrastimuli: Incidence, mechanism and significance. Am. Heart J. *100*:59, 1980.
407. Ruskin, J. N., DiMarco, J. P., and Garan, H.: Repetitive responses to single ventricular stimuli in patients with serious ventricular arrhythmias: Incidence and clinical significance. Circulation *63*:767, 1981.
408. Akhtar, M.: The clinical significance of the repetitive ventricular response (editorial). Circulation *63*:773, 1981.
409. Gomes, J. A., Kang, P. S., Khan, R., Kelen, G., and El-Sherif, N.: Repetitive ventricular response: Its incidence, inducibility, reproducibility, mechanism and significance. Brit. Heart J. *46*:159, 1981.
410. Richards, D. A., Cody, D. V., Denniss, A. R., Russell, P. A.,Uther, J. B., and Young, A. A.: Ventricular electrical instability during the first year following myocardial infarction (abstract). Am. J. Cardiol. *49*:929, 1982.
410a. Hamer, A., Vohra, J., Hunt, D., and Sloman, G.: Prediction of sudden death by electrophysiologic studies in high risk patients surviving acute myocardial infarction. Am. J. Cardiol. *50*:223, 1982.
411. Naccarelli, G. V., Prystowsky, E. N., Jackman, W. M., Heger, J. J., Rahilly, G. T., and Zipes, D. P.: Role of electrophysiologic testing in managing patients who have ventricular tachycardia unrelated to coronary artery disease. Am. J. Cardiol. *50*:165, 1982.
412. Robertson, J. F., Cain, M. E., Horowitz, L. N., Spielman, S. R., Greenspan, A. M., Waxman, H. L., and Josephson, M. E.: Anatomic and electrophysiologic correlates of ventricular tachycardia requiring left ventricular stimulation. Am. J. Cardiol. *48*:263, 1981.
413. Vandepol, C. J., Farshidi, A., Spielman, S. R., Greenspan, A. M., Horowitz, L. N., and Josephson, M. E.: Incidence and clinical significance of induced ventricular tachycardia. Am. J. Cardiol. *45*:725, 1980.
414. DiMarco, J., Garan, H., and Ruskin, J.: Efficacy of quinidine in the treatment of ventricular arrhythmias: The role of electrophysiologic testing. Circulation *64*(Suppl. 4):38, 1981.
415. Gulamhusein, S., Naccarelli, G. V., Ko, P. T., Prystowsky, E. N., Zipes, D. P., Barnett, H. J. M., Heger, J. J., and Klein, G. J.: Value and limitations of the clinical electrophysiologic study in the assessment of patients with unexplained syncope. Am. J. Med. *73*:700, 1982.
416. DiMarco, J. P., Garan, H., and Ruskin, J. N.: Morbidity associated with electrophysiologic procedures. Am. J. Cardiol. *49*:959, 1982.
417. Ross, D. L., Farre, J., Bär, F. W. H. M., Vanagt, E. J., Vassen, W. R. M., Wiener, I., and Wellens, H. J. J.: Comprehensive clinical and electrophysiologic studies in the investigation of documented or suspected tachycardia. Circulation *61*:1010, 1980.
418. Jenkins, J. M., Wu, D., and Arzbacher, R. C.: Computer diagnosis of supraventricular and ventricular arrhythmias. A new esophageal technique. Circulation *60*:977, 1979.
419. Prystowsky, E. N., Pritchett, E. L. C., and Gallagher, J. J.: Origin of the atrial electrogram recorded from the esophagus. Circulation *61*:1017, 1980.
420. Barold, S. S.: Filtered bipolar esophageal electrocardiography. Am. Heart J. *83*:431, 1972.
421. Hammill, S. C., and Pritchett, E. L.: Simplified esophageal electrocardiography using bipolar recording leads. Ann. Intern. Med. *95*:14, 1981.
422. Gallagher, J. J., Smith, W. M., Kerr, C. R., Kasell, J., Cook, L., Reiter, M., Sterba, R., and Harte, M.: Esophageal pacing: A diagnostic and therapeutic tool. Circulation *65*:336, 1982.
423. Spach, M. S., and Barr, R. C.: Physiological correlation and clinical application of isopotential surface maps. *In* Hoffman, I. (ed.): Vectorcardiography 2: Proceedings of Tenth International Symposium on Vectorcardiography. Amsterdam, North-Holland Publ. Co., 1971.
424. Flowers, N. C., Horan, L. B., Sohi, G. S., Hand, R. C., and Johnson, T. C.: New evidence for inferoposterior myocardial infarction on surface potential maps. Am. J. Cardiol. *38*:576, 1976.
425. Holt, H. J., Jr., Barnard, A. C. L., and Kramer, J. O.: Body surface potentials in ventricular hypertrophy: Analysis using a multiple dipole model of the heart. *In* Alper, T. (ed.): Cardiac Hypertrophy. New York, Academic Press, 1971, p. 611.
426. Mirvis, V. M.: Body surface distributions of repolarization potentials after acute myocardial infarction. II. Relationship between isopotential mapping and ST segment potential summation methods. Circulation *63*:623, 1981.
427. Eifler, W. J., Macchi, E., Ritsema van Eck, H. J., Horacek, B. M., and Rautaharju, P. M.: Mechanism of generation of body surface electrocardiographic P waves in normal middle and lower sinus rhythms. Circ. Res. *48*:168, 1981.
428. Benson, D. W., Jr., Sterba, R., Gallagher, J. J., Walston, A., and Spach, M. S.: Localization of the site of preexcitation with body surface maps in patients with Wolff-Parkinson-White syndrome. Circulation *65*:1259, 1982.
429. Durrer, D., and Roos, J. P.: Epicardial excitation of the ventricles in a patient with Wolff-Parkinson-White syndrome (type B). Circulation *35*:15, 1967.
430. Boineau, J. P., Moore, E. N., and Sealy, W. C.: Epicardial mapping in Wolff-Parkinson-White syndrome. Arch. Intern. Med. *135*:422, 1975.
431. Waldo, A. L., and James, T. N.: The cardiac conduction system: Electrophysiological studies during open heart surgery. Arch. Intern. Med. *135*:411, 1975.
432. Josephson, M. E., Horowitz, L. N., Spielman, S. R., Waxman, H. L., and Greenspan, A. M.: Role of catheter mapping in the preoperative evaluation of ventricular tachycardia. Am. J. Cardiol. *49*:207, 1982.
433. Kaiser, G. A., Waldo, A. L., and Bowman, F. O.: The use of ventricular electrograms in operation for coronary artery disease and its complications. Ann. Thorac. Surg. *10*:153, 1970.
434. Fontaine, G., Frank, R., and Bonnet, M.: Methode d'etude experimentale et clinique des syndromes de Wolff Parkinson White et d'ischemie myocardique par cartographie de la depolarisation ventriculaire epicardique. Coeur Med. Interne *12*:105, 1973.
435. Hombach, V., Braun, V., Hopp, H. W., Gil-Sanchez, D., Scholl, H., Behrenbeck, D. W., Pauchert, M., and Hilger, H. H.: The applicability of the signal-averaging technique in clinical cardiology. Clin. Cardiol. *5*:107, 1982.
436. Flowers, N. C., Shvartsman, V., Kennelly, B. M., Sohi, G. S., and Horan, L. G.: Surface recording of His-Purkinje activity on an every-beat basis without digital averaging. Circulation *63*:948, 1981.
437. Hishimoto, Y., and Toshitami, S.: Noninvasive recording of His-bundle potential in man: Simplified method. Brit. Heart J. *37*:635, 1975.
438. Berbari, E. J., Scherlag, B. J., and El-Sherif, N.: The His-Purkinje electrocardiogram in man: An initial assessment of its uses and limitations. Circulation *54*:219, 1976.
439. Hon, E. H., and Lee, S. T.: Noise reduction in fetal electrocardiography. Am. J. Obstet. Gynecol. *87*:1086, 1963.
440. Brody, D. A., Arzbacher, R. C., Woosley, M. D., and Sato, T.: The normal atrial electrocardiogram: Morphologic and quantitative variability in bipolar extremity leads. Am. Heart J. *74*:4, 1967.
441. Rozanski, J. J., Mortara, D., Myerburg, R. J., and Castellanos, A.: Body surface detection of delayed depolarizations in patients with recurrent ventricular tachycardia and left ventricular aneurysm. Circulation *63*:1172, 1981.
442. Simson, M. B.: Use of signals in the terminal QRS complex to identify patients with ventricular tachycardia after myocardial infarction. Circulation *64*:235, 1981.
443. Simson, M. B.: Clinical application of signal averaging. Cardiol. Clin. *1*:109, 1983.

20 MANAGEMENT OF CARDIAC ARRHYTHMIAS

Pharmacological, Electrical, and Surgical Techniques

by Douglas P. Zipes, M.D.

PHARMACOLOGICAL THERAPY

PRINCIPLES OF CLINICAL PHARMACOKINETICS

Pharmacological treatment of a patient with a cardiac arrhythmia has as its primary objectives to reach an effective and well-tolerated serum drug concentration as rapidly as possible and to maintain this concentration for as long as required without producing adverse effects. In many[1] but not all[2] situations nor with all drugs,[3] serum concentration after equilibration strongly correlates with the antiarrhythmic effect of the drug. Therapeutic serum concentrations for most antiarrhythmic agents are listed in Table 20–1 and are based on concentrations of drugs that exert therapeutic effects without adverse effects in a majority of patients. However, the therapeutic concentration for any individual patient is the amount of drug required *for that patient* to suppress or terminate the cardiac arrhythmia without producing adverse effects. For a specific patient, one must consider the response both of the patient and of the arrhythmia to the drug, and the actual serum concentration of the drug is often of secondary importance. In some patients measured serum concentrations can be useful to establish concentrations needed for prophylaxis, to judge the sensitivity or resistance of the arrhythmia to the drug, and to evaluate symptoms that suggest drug toxicity. Serum concentrations can also be used to determine the effects of changing physiological states on drug concentrations, establish drug compliance or abuse, search for drug interactions, and establish the importance of physiologically active metabolites of the parent compound. Active metabolites may be suspected when the clinical effect of the drug outlasts the therapeutic serum concentration of the drug.

Normally, because antiarrhythmic agents have a narrow toxic-therapeutic relationship, important complications of therapy may result from amounts of drug that only slightly exceed the amount necessary to produce beneficial effects; lesser concentrations are often subtherapeutic. It is obvious that careful dosing with these agents is essential to maintain adequate but nontoxic amounts of drug in the body, a task facilitated by understanding drug pharmacokinetics, which consists of a quantitative assessment of drug absorption, distribution, metabolism, and excretion. Alterations in the rate of any of these processes may account for significant intra- and interpatient variations in serum concentrations.[4,5] In addition, changes in the functional status of any of the organs involved, primarily the liver and kidneys, may significantly alter dose requirements in a given patient.

Absorption. Drug absorption from the intestinal tract occurs for most drugs with a half-time of absorption in the range of 20 to 30 minutes. Completeness of absorption may vary between 50 and over 90 per cent, depending on the drug, with most absorption occurring in the small intestine. Different preparations of the same drug, e.g., digoxin or phenytoin, may undergo different rates of absorption in the same patient because the tablet preparations have different dissolution rates. Thus, two brands of drug may not result in the same serum concentration.[5] Large amounts of some orally administered drugs, such as propranolol or verapamil, are transformed to inactive metabolites in the liver before they reach the systemic circulation—the so-called first-pass hepatic effect. For such an agent, much more drug must be administered orally than intravenously to achieve the same physiological effect.

Disease states and other factors can alter the rate and completeness of drug absorption. For example, heart failure can cause mucosal edema of the gut and impair the absorption of orally administered drugs, as can decreased intestinal blood flow. Malabsorption syndromes, concomitant use of other drugs, or changes in gut motility caused by diarrheal states or the use of cathartics may alter absorption. Since most antiarrhythmic agents are basic compounds, they are ionized and poorly absorbed at normal gastric pH, and some drugs may decompose at gastric pH. Conditions that delay gastric emptying increase the absorption lag phase between ingestion of these drugs and their arrival in the small intestine, where most absorption takes place, and therefore may decrease absorption. In patients with severe hypotension, shock, or cardiac arrest, impaired tissue perfusion prevents reliable absorption of intramuscularly administered agents; so that these patients should receive all medications by the intravenous (IV) route.

The rate of drug absorption, determined by the time required to achieve maximum serum concentration, and the fraction of drug absorbed influence the drug's *bioavailability*, which is a measure of the amount of drug that reaches the systemic circulation intact. Bioavailability of a drug includes factors such as lack of pill dissolution, metabolism by gut mucosa, hepatic metabolism and binding, and absorption. It is a most important property of the drug. Absorption is thus only one component affecting bioavailability. The fraction of an orally administered drug reaching the systemic circulation intact, or *systemic availability*, can be calculated (assuming equal clearances for IV and oral forms of drug) by comparing the area under the plasma concentration curve achieved with oral and intravenous administrations from the following relationship: systemic availability equals the area under the plasma concentration curve following oral administration/the area under the plasma concentration curve following IV administration times 100 (assuming equal IV and oral doses).

Drug Distribution. Most antiarrhythmic drugs in the therapeutic range are eliminated according to first-order kinetics, which means that the amount of drug eliminated per unit time is directly proportional to the amount (or concentration) of drug in the body. More drug in the body results in more drug excreted by the kidneys or metabolized by the liver, so that the *fraction* of drug eliminated per unit of time remains constant regardless of the amount of drug in the body. For example, one-half the drug may be eliminated in 6 hours whether the total amount of drug in the body is 4 gm or 10 gm, resulting in elimination of 2 gm in the first example and of 5 gm in the second. As a consequence, the elimination half-life, or time required to eliminate half the body load (or to halve the plasma concentration) of such a drug is constant and independent of the total body load. The following discussion will assume first-order kinetics unless otherwise stated.

Generally two models, a *one-compartment open model* and a *two-compartment open model*, are used with relative accuracy to describe and predict serum concentrations at a given time for a variety of dose regimens. Even though these models are oversimplified representations of drug disposition, they provide guidelines for choosing loading doses and maintenance dose schedules for a given patient. In the one-compartment open model, drugs are considered to enter and to be eliminated from a single homogeneous unit that represents the entire body. Drugs entering the compartment are considered to be distributed immediately throughout the compartment, making the concentration of the drug equal to the amount of drug in the compartment divided by the volume of the compartment. The latter equals the amount of the drug in the compartment divided by the drug concentration.

In reality, a one-compartment open model is not entirely appropriate because a certain amount of time is needed to distribute the drug throughout the volume of the compartment. However, the one-compartment model predicts plasma concentration as a function of time and dose, if distribution is significantly faster than the rate of administration or of excretion, which is the case for many antiarrhythmic drugs.

If the rate of drug administration is rapid in relation to drug distribution (e.g., intravenous administration), a two-compartment open model more accurately predicts drug concentrations (Fig. 20–1). In this model the drug enters the system by the central compartment and can leave the system only by distribution into a peripheral compartment or elimination from the central compartment. The central compartment, in dynamic equilibrium with the more slowly equilibrating peripheral compartment, is assumed to consist of the blood volume and extracellular fluid of highly perfused tissues such as heart, lungs, kidneys, and liver, while the peripheral compartment, acting as a reservoir, consists of less well perfused tissue such as muscle, skin, and adipose tissue. The first-order rate constants $K_{1\rightarrow 2}$ and $K_{2\rightarrow 1}$ determine the rate of transfer of drug between the central and peripheral compartments or vice versa, with K_e representing the overall elimination rate constant. K_e relates the sum of all methods of irreversible drug elimination from the central compartment to the concentration of drug in that compartment (Fig. 20–1). For antiarrhythmic drugs, the peripheral compartment is generally larger than the central compartment. The concepts of distribution volumes and drug movement are more complex in the two-compartment open model than in the one-compartment open model.[6,7] The two-compartment model may behave similarly to the one-compartment model when drugs are infused slowly or given orally and K_1 approximates K_2, but pronounced differences exist when injections are given rapidly.

Following administration of drugs for which the kinetics are described by a two-compartment model, the curve of plasma drug concentration demonstrates two distinct phases: an early phase (alpha, or distribution phase), characterized by rapidly falling plasma drug concentrations due to distribution between the central compartment and the peripheral compartment, and a second phase (beta, or elimination phase) of slower decline in plasma drug concentration, representing primarily elimination of drugs from the central compartment (Fig. 20–2). *Alpha* is often referred to as the *rate constant for distribution* and *beta* as the *rate constant for elimination.* During the latter beta phase, when the drug is in distribution equilibrium, serum concentrations correlate with the pharmacological effects of the drug. The distribution for quinidine is shown in Figure 20–3.

Several important concepts need to be considered. The extent of extravascular distribution of a drug is obtained by measuring the apparent *volume of distribution*, which is the hypothetical volume into which a dose of drug would have to be diluted to give the observed plasma concentration. It is determined by the dose administered divided by the plasma concentration at time 0. It equals the sum of A and B on the logarithmic plasma concentration axis obtained by extrapolating the alpha and beta phases back to 0 time (Fig. 20–2).[4] A large volume of distribution indicates a wide distribution and extensive tissue uptake of the drug and often exceeds by several times the amount of total body water. The large volume of distribution for most antiarrhythmic agents indicates that they are present in higher concentrations in some tissues than in the plasma. The volume of distribution is dependent on the relative serum and tissue binding characteristics of the drug and may be constricted in some patients, such as those with renal failure, during which a change in serum protein or tissue binding may occur. Quinidine decreases the volume of distribution of digoxin, probably as a result of a decrease in tissue binding of digoxin.

Drug Metabolism and Excretion. Approximately 97 per cent of the dose of any drug is removed from the body in a time equal to five half-lives.[8] *Serum elimination half-life* is defined as the time interval for 50 per cent of the drug present in the body at the beginning of the interval to be eliminated. After one half-life, 50 per cent of the drug remains in the body (assuming no further drug is administered), after two half-lives 25 per cent remains, after three half-lives 12.5 per cent remains, and so forth. Half-life is determined from the relationship $t_{1/2} = 0.693/\text{beta}$ for a two-compartment model (Fig. 20–2). Since changes in drug distribution influence elimination half-life, the equation can be rewritten as $t_{1/2} = 0.693 \times$ volume of distribution/total body clearance.

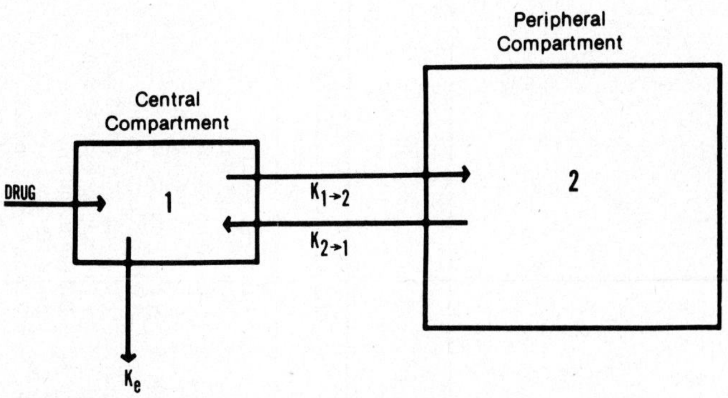

FIGURE 20–1 Two-compartment open model. A smaller central compartment into which drug is administered and from which it is eliminated (K_e) connects in dynamic equilibrium with a larger peripheral compartment.

TABLE 20–1 DOSAGE AND THERAPEUTIC SERUM CONCENTRATIONS FOR ANTIARRHYTHMIC AGENTS

Drug	Usual Dose Ranges: Intravenous (mg) Loading	Intravenous (mg) Maintenance	Oral (mg) Loading	Oral (mg) Maintenance	Time to Peak Plasma Concentration (Oral)	Effective Serum or Plasma Concentration (μg/ml)	Elimination Half-Life After Oral Dose (hr)	Bioavailability (%)	Major Route of Elimination
Lidocaine	1 to 3 mg/kg at 20 to 50 mg/min	1 to 4 mg/min	N/A	N/A	N/A	1 to 5	1 to 2	N/A	Liver
Quinidine	6 to 10 mg/kg at 0.3 to 0.5 mg/kg/min		600 to 1000	300 to 600 q6h	1.5 to 3.0	3 to 6	5 to 9	60 to 80	Liver
Procainamide	6 to 13 mg/kg at 0.2 to 0.5 mg/kg/min	2 to 6 mg/min	500 to 1000	350 to 1000 q3–6h	1	4 to 10	3 to 5	70 to 85	Kidneys
Disopyramide	1 to 2 mg/kg over 15 min* 1 to 2 mg/kg over 45 min	1 mg/kg/hr*	300 to 400	100 to 400 q6–8h	1 to 2	2 to 5	8 to 9	80 to 90	Kidneys
Phenytoin	100 mg q5min for ≤ 1000 mg		1000	100 to 400 q12–24h	8 to 12	10 to 20	18 to 36	50 to 70	Liver
Propranolol	0.25 to 0.5 mg, q5min for ≤ 0.15 to 0.20 mg/kg			10 to 200 q6–8h	2 to 4	0.04 to 0.90	3 to 6	20 to 50	Liver
Bretylium	5 to 10 mg/kg at 1 to 2 mg/kg/min	½ to 2 mg/min	N/A	4 mg/kg/day*		0.5 to 1.5	8 to 14	25	Kidneys
Verapamil	10 mg over 1 to 2 min	0.005 mg/kg/min		80 to 120 q6–8h	1 to 2	0.10 to 0.15	3 to 8	10 to 35	Liver
Amiodarone*	5 to 10 mg/kg		800 to 1200 qid for 1 to 4 weeks	200 to 800 qid	4	1 to 5	30 to 50 days		Liver
Aprindine*	200 mg at 2 mg/min 100 mg at 2 mg/min 30 min later 100 mg at 2 mg/min 6 hr later		100 q6h day 1 75 q6h day 2 50 q6h day 3	25 to 50 q6–12h	2	1 to 2	20 to 30	80 to 90	Liver
Encainide*	0.6 to 0.9 mg/kg		N/A	25 to 75 q6–8h	1 to 2	0.5 to 1.0	3 to 4	40	Liver
Mexiletine*	500 mg	0.5 to 1.0 gm/24 hr	400 to 600	200 to 300 q6–8h	2 to 4	1 to 2		90	Liver
Tocainide*	750 mg		400 to 600	400 to 800 q8–12h	1 to 2	6 to 12	10 to 17	90	Liver
Ethmozine*			300	100 to 400 q8h		0.1			
Flecainide*	2 mg/kg			100 to 300 q12h	1.5 to 3.0	0.2 to 0.8	14 to 20	95	Liver
Lorcainide*	1 to 2 mg/kg			100 q8h		0.3 to 1.0	6 to 20	50	Liver
Propafenone*	1 to 2 mg/kg		600 to 900	150 to 300 q8–12h	1 to 3	2	3 to 4	50 to 75	Liver
Bethanidine*	5 to 20 mg/kg		20 to 30 mg/kg	5 to 10 mg/kg q8h	1 to 4		14	60 to 90	Kidneys
Cibenzoline*	1.0 to 1.2 mg/kg			65 to 81.25 q6h	1 to 2	0.2 to 0.6	7 to 20	100	Kidneys

* Investigational.
Results presented may vary according to doses, disease state, and IV or oral administration.

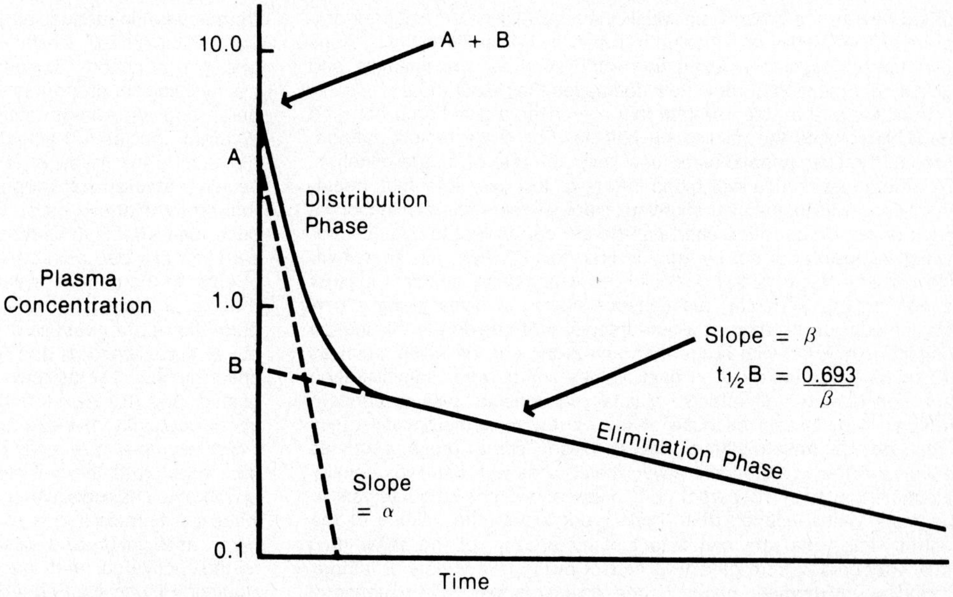

FIGURE 20–2 Schematic diagram of the semilogarithmic plot of drug plasma concentration as a function of time following rapid intravenous injection, according to the principles outlined for a two-compartment open model. (From Gibaldi, M., and Perrier, D.: Drugs and the pharmaceutical sciences. *In* Pharmacokinetics, Vol. I. New York, Marcel Dekker, 1975.)

Drug clearance is analogous to the concept of renal clearance and is the volume of blood totally cleared of drug in unit time. It is the sum of the clearances for each process by which the drug is eliminated and can be calculated from the relationship: clearance = dose of the drug/area under the plasma concentration time curve (AUC). Expressed differently, clearance equals volume of distribution × beta, or volume of distribution × 0.693/half-life. A larger volume of distribution increases the elimination half-life at a given clearance. The larger volume of distribution of antiarrhythmic drugs accounts for the relatively long half-life despite their large clearance rates. Quinidine prolongs digitoxin's half-life by decreasing total body clearance.[5] Clearance of drugs with high extraction ratios strongly depends on

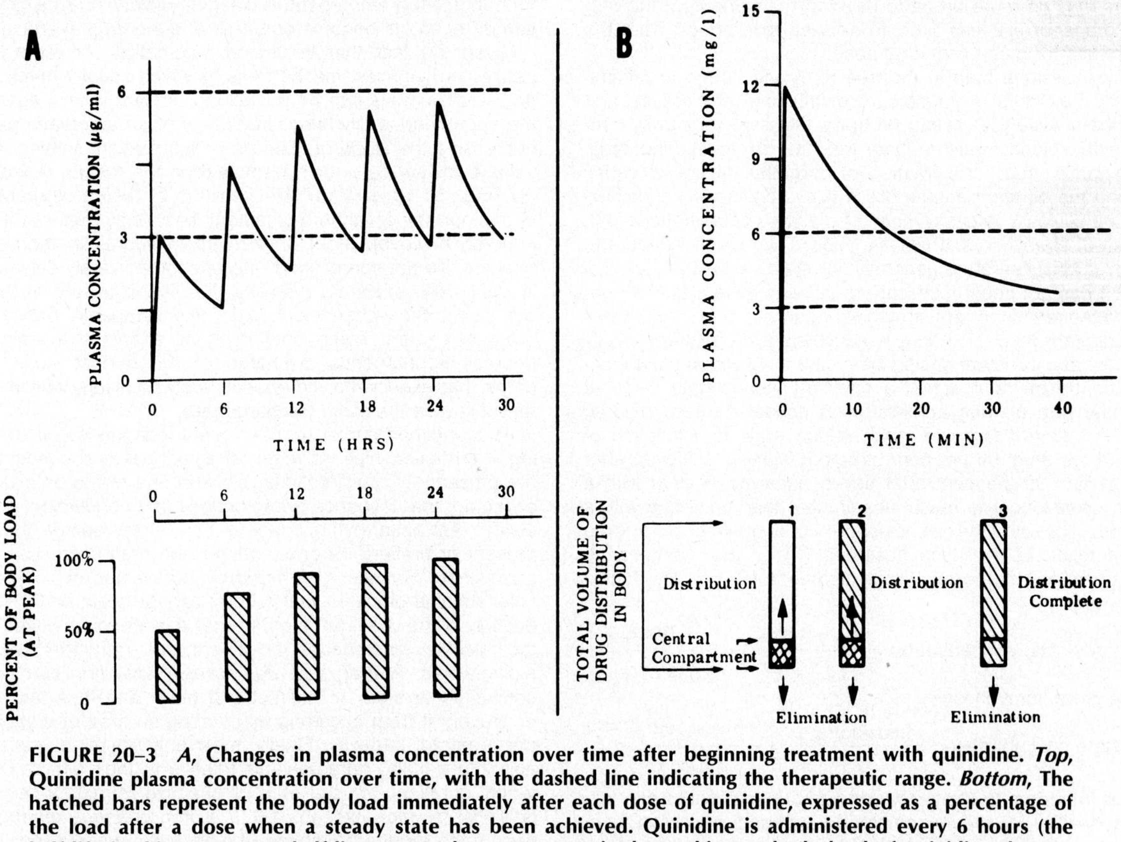

FIGURE 20–3 *A,* Changes in plasma concentration over time after beginning treatment with quinidine. *Top,* Quinidine plasma concentration over time, with the dashed line indicating the therapeutic range. *Bottom,* The hatched bars represent the body load immediately after each dose of quinidine, expressed as a percentage of the load after a dose when a steady state has been achieved. Quinidine is administered every 6 hours (the half-life in this case). Four half-lives, or 24 hours, are required to achieve a body load of quinidine that exceeds 90 per cent of the load at steady state. *B, top,* Plasma concentrations produced by administering a full intravenous loading dose of quinidine as a bolus, with the therapeutic range shown by a dashed line. *Bottom,* The numbered vertical boxes indicate the volume of distribution of quinidine. Just after the drug is given, it is dissolved only in the small central compartment, as in box 1, and very high peak concentrations are achieved (in the toxic range). The drug then distributes throughout the rest of the body. Distribution has a half-life of about 8 minutes and is complete by 30 minutes (box 3). Quinidine concentration is now in the therapeutic range, and further decreases in plasma concentration are due solely to drug elimination. (From Nattel, S., and Zipes, D.P.: Clinical pharmacology of old and new antiarrhythmic drugs. Cardiovasc. Clin. *11*:221, 1980.)

blood flow to the organ from which they are eliminated, such as propranolol, verapamil, or lidocaine in the liver. For antiarrhythmic drugs that have a high renal extraction ratio, such as procainamide and quinidine, reduction of renal flow decreases their clearance.

Function of the organ system that eliminates a given drug from the body determines the elimination half-life. For drugs rapidly metabolized in the liver, hepatic blood flow limits the rate of drug elimination. Disorders that reduce liver blood flow (e.g., low cardiac output, hepatic disease with portacaval shunting) markedly slow the elimination of such drugs. Drugs with a short half-life are convenient to use by intravenous infusion but not by chronic oral dosing, since the short half-life requires frequent oral doses to maintain a fairly constant plasma concentration. Generally, maintenance dosing involves giving a certain amount of the drug at a time interval that equals the elimination half-life. However, with drugs that have very long half-lives, such as 12 hours, this may result in peak values shortly after administration and consequent side effects.[4] Maintaining constant plasma concentrations is necessary because of the narrow toxic-therapeutic ratios exhibited by antiarrhythmic agents. Also, some drugs such as encainide (see p. 667) have active metabolites with half-lives considerably longer than the parent compound, allowing dosing intervals to be more widely spaced than those predicted by the half-life of the parent drug. The rate and extent of metabolism of the same drug may vary greatly from patient to patient owing to a variety of factors, including environment, genetics, age, disease states, and influence of other drugs given concomitantly. A genetically controlled acetyltransferase enzyme system influences the metabolism of some drugs, making about half the American population "rapid" and half "slow acetylators." Rapid acetylators metabolize a greater proportion of a drug dose than do slow acetylators, who may require less drug to achieve any desired serum level or pharmacological effect. Also, rapid acetylators may be more prone to develop reactions from the metabolites of drugs[5] or are less likely to develop side effects from the parent compound for a constant drug dose.

Drugs exist in plasma both in the free form and bound to plasma proteins. Only free drug is capable of distributing into tissues and exerting a pharmacological action. Virtually all assays for drug concentration in the blood measure *both* free and protein-bound drug. For antiarrhythmic drugs, the fraction of drug that is bound varies greatly among the different agents but is fairly constant for individual drugs over the clinically relevant range of plasma concentrations with the exception of phenytoin and disopyramide. Total serum concentrations of a given drug therefore generally correlate well with its clinical effects, and it has not been necessary to develop assays to measure free drug concentrations for antiarrhythmic agents.

When a constant dose of a drug is administered repeatedly (orally or parenterally) at a constant dosing interval, accumulation occurs until drug concentration approaches a constant steady-state level, at which time the rate of drug administration equals the rate of drug elimination. The time it takes to reach steady state is a function of the half-life of the drug; 94 per cent of steady state is achieved after four half-lives and 99 per cent after seven half-lives. A drug with a long half-life takes longer to reach steady state than does one with a short half-life. The average steady-state concentration of a drug equals the fraction of the dose absorbed (F) × the maintenance dose ($dose_m$) divided by the total body clearance (Cl_s) × the dosing interval (τ):

$$\text{Average steady state concentration} = \frac{F \times dose_m}{CL_s \times \tau} = \frac{F \times dose_m\, t_{1/2}}{0.693 \times V_d\, \tau}$$

If the drug is given intravenously,[5]

$$\text{Steady state concentration} = \frac{\text{Infusion rate}}{Cl_s} = \frac{\text{Infusion rate } t_{1/2}}{0.693\ V_d}$$

Finally, it is important to stress that drug pharmacokinetics may differ in normal healthy volunteers compared to patients who have a variety of illnesses. Therefore, information derived from patients as well as normal subjects must be considered when one is planning dosing regimens.

GENERAL CONSIDERATIONS REGARDING ANTIARRHYTHMIC DRUGS

Segregating drugs into various classes, although useful conceptually, will not be emphasized in this chapter.[9] Such classifications* suffer from several inadequacies: (1) all drugs assigned to a single group do not exhibit entirely similar actions, and some drugs exert more than one type of action; (2) classifications are based primarily on the electrophysiological properties exerted by the drugs on normal Purkinje fibers, and the drugs may exert different effects on muscle, on different species, on acutely or chronically damaged tissue, or when the electrolyte milieu is abnormal; in vitro studies on healthy fibers usually establish the properties of antiarrhythmic agents rather than their antiarrhythmic properties;[10] (3) many antiarrhythmic agents produce their effects in vivo not by direct electrophysiological actions on cardiac cells but indirectly by metabolic or anti-ischemic actions, by effects on the central or peripheral autonomic nervous system, by improving circulatory hemodynamics, or by active metabolites; (4) some drugs do not fit neatly into one class, leading to formulation of a variety of classifications; and (5) insights into the mechanisms by which antiarrhythmic agents may affect ion transfer are only recently being gained, and this new knowledge will undoubtedly influence concepts about how antiarrhythmic agents function.

For example, a recently proposed model suggests that antiarrhythmic drugs cross the cell membrane and interact with receptors in the membrane channels when the latter are in the rested, activated, or inactivated states and that each of these interactions is characterized by an association and dissociation rate constant. Transitions among rested, activated, and inactivated states are governed by standard Hodgkin-Huxley–type equations. When the drug is bound (associated) to the channel, the latter cannot conduct, even in the activated state.[11] Some drugs exert greater inhibitory effects at more rapid rates of stimulation, a characteristic called "use-dependence." It is possible that this use-dependence results from preferential interaction of the antiarrhythmic drug with either the open or the inactive channel and little interaction with the resting channels of the unstimulated cell. With increased time spent in diastole (slower rate), a greater proportion of receptors become drug-free and the drug exerts less effect.

Given the fact that enhanced automaticity or reentry can cause cardiac arrhythmias, mechanisms by which antiarrhythmic agents suppress arrhythmias can be postulated. Antiarrhythmic agents can slow the spontaneous discharge frequency of an automatic pacemaker by depressing the slope of diastolic depolarization, shifting the threshold voltage toward zero, or hyperpolarizing the resting membrane potential (Fig. 19–13, p. 618). Mechanisms by which different drugs suppress normal or abnormal automaticity may not be the same. In general, however, most antiarrhythmic agents in therapeutic doses depress the automatic firing rate of spontaneously discharging ectopic sites while minimally affecting the discharge rate of the normal sinus node. Slow-channel blockers like verapamil, beta blockers like propranolol, and some antiarrhythmic agents like amiodarone also depress spontaneous discharge of the normal sinus node, while drugs that exert vagolytic effects, such as disopyramide or quinidine, may increase the sinus discharge rate.

As mentioned earlier (p. 624), reentry depends critically on the timing interrelationships between refractoriness and conduction velocity, the presence of unidirectional block in one of the pathways, and other factors that influence refractoriness and conduction, such as excitability. An antiarrhythmic agent can stop reentry that is already present or prevent it from starting if the drug improves *or* depresses conduction. For example, *improved conduction* can (1) eliminate the unidirectional block so that reentry cannot begin or (2) facilitate conduction in the reentrant loop so that the returning wavefront reenters too quickly, encroaches on fibers still refractory, and becomes extinguished. A drug that *depresses conduction* can transform the unidirectional block to bidirectional block and thus terminate reentry or prevent it from occurring by creating an area of complete block in the reentrant pathway. Finally, most antiarrhythmic agents share the ability to prolong refractoriness relative to their effects on action potential duration, i.e., the ratio of effective refractory period to action potential duration exceeds 1.0. If a drug *prolongs refractoriness* of fibers in the reentrant pathway, the pathway may not recover excitabili-

*Classification of antiarrhythmic drugs:

Class I—Drugs that reduce $\dot{V}$max: Lidocaine, quinidine, procainamide, disopyramide, aprindine, encainide, mexiletine, tocainide, ethmozine, flecainide, lorcainide, propafenone, cibenzoline.

Class II—Drugs that inhibit sympathetic activity: Propranolol.

Class III—Drugs that prolong action potential duration: Amiodarone, bethanidine, bretylium, sotalol.

Class IV—Drugs that block the slow inward current: Verapamil.

ty in time to be depolarized by the reentering impulse, and the reentrant propagation ceases. Conversely, a drug that slows conduction without producing block or lengthening refractoriness significantly may promote reentry.

When one is discussing any of the properties of a drug, it is important that the situation and/or model from which conclusions are drawn be defined with care. Electrophysiological, hemodynamic, autonomic, pharmacokinetic, and adverse effects all may differ in normal subjects compared to patients, in normal tissue compared to abnormal tissue, in muscle compared to specialized fibers, and in different species.

LIDOCAINE

Electrophysiological Actions (Tables 20–2 and 20–3). Lidocaine does not affect normal sinus nodal automaticity[12] but does depress both normal[13] and some abnormal forms of automaticity in Purkinje fibers in vitro. External environment significantly influences the effects of lidocaine. At $[K]_o \leq 4.5$ mM/liter, therapeutic concentrations of lidocaine exert little effect on $\dot{V}max$ of phase 0 in normal cardiac Purkinje fibers, while at $[K]_o > 6.0$ mM/liter, therapeutic concentrations of lidocaine reduce $\dot{V}max$ at any level of membrane potential.[14] In the presence of acidosis, lidocaine significantly reduces canine cardiac Purkinje fiber resting membrane potential, action potential amplitude, and $\dot{V}max$ and increases conduction time, at the same concentrations that exert minimal effects when the pH is normal.[15] Therapeutic concentrations of lidocaine depress activity in abnormal ventricular muscle fibers that have survived experimental myocardial infarction.[16–18] The infarct area exhibits elevated $[K]_o$ and reduced pH, and in this environment, lidocaine exaggerates the action potential changes and quickens the time course produced by ischemia, possibly converting areas of unidirectional block into bidirectional block and preventing development of ventricular fibrillation by preventing fragmentation of organized large wavefronts into heterogeneous wavelets.[19] Lidocaine may be arrhythmogenic if it depresses conduction but not to the point of bidirectional block.[12,20] For example, it may create an area of unidirectional block and another area of conduction delay (see p. 623) and promote reentry.

Lidocaine does *not* affect slow-channel–dependent action potentials. In fact, its depressant effect on ischemic potentials and depressed fast responses supports the notion that these ischemic potentials are depressed fast responses rather than slow responses.[19,21] Lidocaine significantly reduces the action potential duration and the effective refractory period of Purkinje fibers and ventricular muscle[13] but not of ordinary or specialized atrial fibers.[12,22] The decrease in action potential duration in Purkinje fibers, thought to relate in large part to an increase in potassium conductance (gk_1), enhancing potassium's loss from the cell, appears to be due to blocking of tetrodotoxin-sensitive sodium channels, decreasing entry of sodium into the cell.[23] In some in vitro preparations, lidocaine can improve conduction by hyperpolarizing tissues depolarized as a result of stretch or low external potassium concentration.[24]

In vivo, lidocaine has a minimal effect on automaticity or conduction except in unusual circumstances. Patients with preexisting sinus nodal dysfunction,[7] abnormal His-Purkinje conduction,[25] or junctional escape rhythms during ischemia[26] may develop depressed automaticity or conduction. This drug may shorten His-Purkinje refractoriness in man.[27] Part of its effects may be to inhibit cardiac sympathetic nerve activity.[28,29]

Hemodynamic Effects. Clinically significant adverse hemodynamic effects are rarely noted unless left ventricular function is severely impaired.

Pharmacokinetics (Table 20–1). Lidocaine is used only parenterally because oral administration results in extensive first-pass hepatic metabolism and unpredictable, low plasma levels with excessive metabolites that may produce toxicity. Hepatic metabolism of lidocaine depends greatly on hepatic blood flow, so that clearance of this drug almost equals (and can be approximated by) measurements of this flow.[30] Severe hepatic disease or reduced hepatic blood flow, as in heart failure or shock, can mark-

TABLE 20–2 IN VIVO ELECTROPHYSIOLOGICAL CHARACTERISTICS

	Electrocardiographic Intervals						Electrophysiological Intervals				
Drug	*Sinus Rate*	*P-R*	*QRS*	*Q-T*	*A-H*	*H-V*	*ERP AVN*	*ERP HPS*	*ERP A*	*ERP V*	*ERP AP*
Lidocaine	0	0	0	0	0↓	0↑	0↓	0↑	0	0	0
Quinidine	0↑	↓0↑	↑	↑	↓0↑	0↑	↓0↑	0↑	↑	↑	↑
Procainamide	0	0↑	↑	↑	0↑	0↑	0↑	0↑	↑	↑	↑
Disopyramide	0↑	0	0↑	0↑	0	0↑	0↓	↑	↑	↑	↑
Phenytoin	0	0	0	0↓	0↓	0	0↓	↓	0	0	0
Propranolol	↓	0↑	0	0↓	0↑	0	↑	0	0	0	0
Bretylium	0↓	0↑	0	0↑							0
Verapamil	0↓	↑	0	0	↑	0	↑	0	0	0	0
Amiodarone	↓	0↑	0	↑	↑	0	↑	↑↑	↑	↑	↑
Aprindine	↓	↑	↑	0↑	↑	↑	↑	↑	↑	↑	↑
Encainide	0	↑	↑	↑	↑	↑	↑	↑	↑	↑	↑
Mexiletine	0	0	0	0	0↑	0↑	0↑	0↑	0	0	0
Tocainide	0↓	0	0	0↓	0↑	0	↓	0	0↓	0↓	0
Ethmozine	0↓	0↑	0↑	0					↑	↑	
Flecainide		↑	↑	↑	↑	↑	↑		↑	↑	↑
Lorcainide		0↑	↑	↑	0	↑	0		0	0	↑
Propafenone	0↓	↑	↑	0↑	↑	↑	0↑		0↑	↑	↑
Bethanidine	0↓	0	0	0↑							0
Cibenzoline	↑	↑	↑	0↑	0	↑	0		0	↑	

Results presented may vary according to tissue type, experimental conditions, and drug concentration. ↑ = increase; ↓ = decrease; 0 = no change; 0↑ or 0↓ = slight inconsistent increase or decrease. A = atrium; AVN = AV node; HPS = His-Purkinje system; V = ventricle; AP = accessory pathway (WPW); ERP = effective refractory period—longest S_1-S_2 interval at which S_2 fails to produce a response.

TABLE 20–3 IN VITRO ELECTROPHYSIOLOGICAL CHARACTERISTICS

Drug	APA	APD	dV/dt	MDP	ERP	Conduction Velocity	Sinus Nodal Automaticity	PF Normal Phase 4	Membrane Responsiveness	ET	VFT	Contractility	Slow Inward Current	Autonomic Nervous System	Local Anesthetic Effect
Lidocaine	0↓	↓	0↓	0	↓	0↓	0	↓	0↓	0↑	↑	0	0	0	Yes
Quinidine	↓	↑	↓	0	↑	↓	0	↓	↓	↑	↑	0	0	Antivagal alpha blocker	Yes
Procainamide	↓	↑	↓	0	↑	↓	0	↓	↓	↑	↑	0	0	Slight antivagal	Yes
Disopyramide	↓	↑	↓	0	↑	↓	↑0↓	↓	↓	↑	↑	↓	0	Central: antivagal, antisympathetic	Yes
Phenytoin	0	↓	↑0↓	0	↓	0	0	↓	0↑	0			0	0	No
Propranolol	0↓	0↓	0↓	0	↓	0	↓	↓	0↑	0	0↑	↓	0	Antisympathetic	Yes
Bretylium	0	↑	0	0	↑	0	0↓	0	0	0	↑	0↑	0	Antisympathetic	Yes
Verapamil	0	↓	0	0	0	0	↓	↓	0	0	0	↓	Inhibit	? Block alpha receptors	Yes
Amiodarone	0	↑	0↓	0	↑	↓	↓	↓	↓			↓	0↓	Antisympathetic	No
Aprindine	↓	↓	↓	0	↓	↓	0↓	↓	↓	↑	↑	↓	0↓	0	Yes
Encainide	↓	↓	↓	0	↑	↓	0	↓	↓	↑			0	0	Yes
Mexiletine	0	↓	↓	0	↓	↓	0	↓	↓	↑	↑	↓	0	0	Yes
Tocainide	0	↓	0↓	0	↓	↓	0	↓	↓	↑	↑	0	0	0	Yes
Ethmozine	↓	↓	↓	0	↓	↓	0	0	↓	↑	0		0	0	No
Flecainide	↓	↑	↓	0	↑	↓	0	↓	↓				0	0	Yes
Lorcainide	↓	↑	↓	0	↑	↓	0	↓	↓				0		Yes
Propafenone	↓		↓	0		↓	↓		↓	↑	↑	↓	May inhibit	0	Yes
Bethanidine	0	↑	0	0	↑	0		0	0	0	↑		0	Antisympathetic	Yes
Cibenzoline	↓	↑	↓	0	↑	↓	0	↓	↓	↑		↓	0	Slight antivagal	Yes

Key: APA = action potential amplitude; APD = action potential duration; dV/dt = rate of rise of action potential; MDP = maximum diastolic potential; ERP = effective refractory period; PF = Purkinje fibers; ET = excitability threshold; VFT = ventricular fibrillation threshold.

edly decrease the rate of lidocaine metabolism. Prolonged infusion can reduce lidocaine clearance. Its elimination half-life averages about 1 to 2 hours in normal subjects, more than 4 hours in patients after relatively uncomplicated myocardial infarction, more than 10 hours in patients after myocardial infarction complicated by cardiac failure, and even longer in the presence of cardiogenic shock.[31] Maintenance doses should be reduced by one-third to one-half for patients with low cardiac output.

Dosage and Administration (Table 20–1). Although lidocaine may be given intramuscularly, the intravenous route is most commonly used (Fig. 20–4). Intramuscular lidocaine is given in doses of 4 to 5 mg/kg (250 to 350 mg), resulting in effective serum levels at about 15 minutes and lasting for about 90 minutes.[32] Intravenously, lidocaine is given as an initial bolus of 1 to 2 mg/kg body weight at a rate of approximately 20 to 50 mg/min, with a second injection of one-half the initial dose 20 to 40 minutes later.[7] Patients treated with an initial bolus followed by a maintenance infusion may experience transient subtherapeutic plasma concentrations at 30 to 120 minutes after initiation of therapy.[33] A second bolus of about 0.5 mg/kg without increasing the maintenance infusion rate reestablishes therapeutic serum concentrations. If recurrence of arrhythmia appears after a steady state has been achieved (e.g., six to ten hours after starting therapy), a similar bolus should be given and the maintenance infusion rate increased. Increasing the maintenance infusion rate only without an additional bolus results in a very slow increase is plasma lidocaine concentrations, reaching a new plateau in over six hours (four elimination half-lives), and is therefore not recommended.

If the initial bolus of lidocaine is ineffective, up to two more boluses of 1 mg/kg may be administered at 5-minute intervals. Patients who require more than one bolus to achieve a therapeutic effect have arrhythmias that respond only to higher lidocaine plasma concentrations, and a greater maintenance dose may be necessary to sustain these higher concentrations. Patients requiring only a single initial bolus of lidocaine should probably receive a maintenance infusion of 30 μg/kg/min, while those requiring two or three boluses may need infusions at 40 to 50 μg/kg/min.[33] Loading doses may also be administered by rapid infusion and a constant-rate intravenous infusion may be used to maintain an effective concentration. Maintenance infusion rates in the range of 1 to 4 mg/min produce steady-state plasma levels of 1 to 5 μg/ml in patients with uncomplicated myocardial infarction, but these rates must be reduced during heart failure or shock because of concomitant reduced hepatic blood flow.[7]

Clinical Indications. Lidocaine is a very useful antiarrhythmic agent because it demonstrates great efficacy against ventricular arrhythmias of diverse etiology, the ability to achieve effective plasma concentrations rapidly,

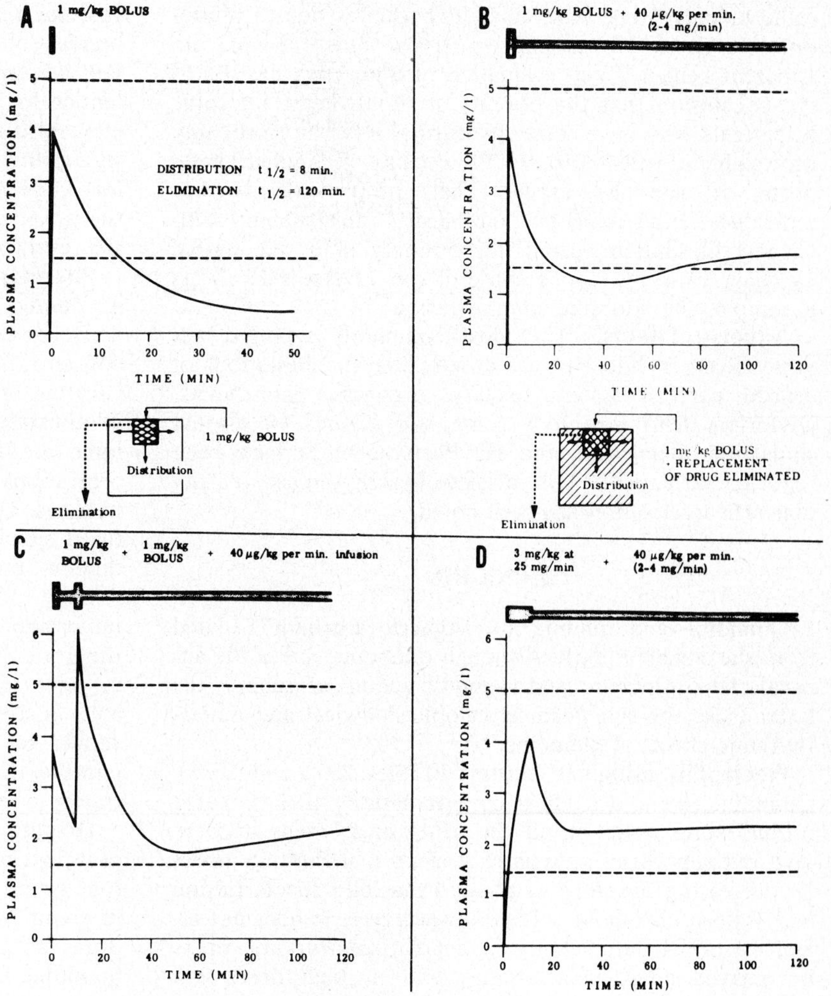

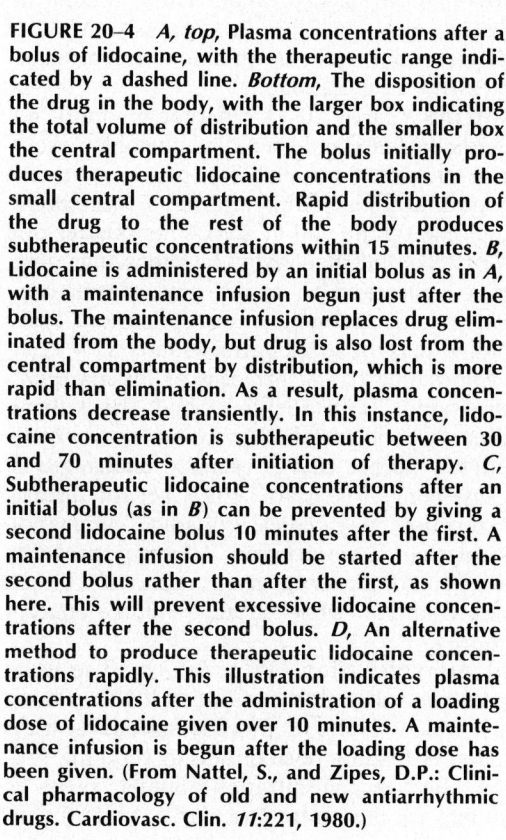

FIGURE 20–4 *A, top,* Plasma concentrations after a bolus of lidocaine, with the therapeutic range indicated by a dashed line. *Bottom,* The disposition of the drug in the body, with the larger box indicating the total volume of distribution and the smaller box the central compartment. The bolus initially produces therapeutic lidocaine concentrations in the small central compartment. Rapid distribution of the drug to the rest of the body produces subtherapeutic concentrations within 15 minutes. *B,* Lidocaine is administered by an initial bolus as in *A,* with a maintenance infusion begun just after the bolus. The maintenance infusion replaces drug eliminated from the body, but drug is also lost from the central compartment by distribution, which is more rapid than elimination. As a result, plasma concentrations decrease transiently. In this instance, lidocaine concentration is subtherapeutic between 30 and 70 minutes after initiation of therapy. *C,* Subtherapeutic lidocaine concentrations after an initial bolus (as in *B*) can be prevented by giving a second lidocaine bolus 10 minutes after the first. A maintenance infusion should be started after the second bolus rather than after the first, as shown here. This will prevent excessive lidocaine concentrations after the second bolus. *D,* An alternative method to produce therapeutic lidocaine concentrations rapidly. This illustration indicates plasma concentrations after the administration of a loading dose of lidocaine given over 10 minutes. A maintenance infusion is begun after the loading dose has been given. (From Nattel, S., and Zipes, D.P.: Clinical pharmacology of old and new antiarrhythmic drugs. Cardiovasc. Clin. *11*:221, 1980.)

and a fairly wide toxic-to-therapeutic ratio with a low incidence of hemodynamic complications and other side effects. However, its first-pass hepatic effect precludes oral administration, and it is generally ineffective against supraventricular arrhythmias. Although lidocaine has been reported to decrease the ventricular response in patients with atrial fibrillation and Wolff-Parkinson-White syndrome,[34] a recent study demonstrates that when the effective refractory period of the accessory pathway is relatively short, lidocaine generally has no significant effect and may even accelerate the ventricular response during atrial fibrillation.[35]

Lidocaine is used primarily for patients with acute myocardial infarction or recurrent ventricular tachyarrhythmias. In patients resuscitated from out-of-hospital ventricular fibrillation and studied in a randomized, blinded trial,[36] lidocaine was comparable to bretylium in preventing recurrent episodes of ventricular tachyarrhythmia. In patients less than 70 years old who were admitted within six hours of onset of symptoms associated with acute myocardial infarction, lidocaine prophylaxis reduced episodes of ventricular fibrillation compared to results in an untreated control group (p. 1309). However, treated patients had a 15 per cent incidence of lidocaine toxicity, which was greater in older patients, and hospital mortality did not differ between treated and control groups, since in all instancesof lidocaine toxicity, which was greater in older37 Other studies have not shown a protective effect of lidocaine in preventing ventricular arrhythmias due to infarction,[38] and of 15 randomized trials, most showed no apparent benefit.[39] Yet, evaluation of these data has led to the conclusion that the benefits of prophylactic lidocaine in patients who have acute myocardial infarction probably outweigh the risks[39,40] (p. 1309). Because of conflicting reports, it can be argued that prophylaxis is not indicated for all patients,[7] since death from primary ventricular fibrillation occurs uncommonly in a well-staffed coronary care unit and because of the adverse side effects accompanying lidocaine administration.

Adverse Effects. The most commonly reported adverse effects of lidocaine are dose-related manifestations of central nervous system toxicity: dizziness, paresthesias, confusion, delirium, stupor, coma, and seizures. Occasional sinus node depression and His-Purkinje block have been reported. In patients with atrial tachyarrhythmias, ventricular rate acceleration has been noted.

QUINIDINE

Quinidine and quinine are isomeric alkaloids isolated from the cinchona bark. Although quinidine shares the antimalarial, antipyretic, and vagolytic actions of quinine, the latter lacks the significant electrophysiological and antiarrhythmic effects of quinidine.[41]

Electrophysiological Actions (Tables 20–2 and 20–3). Quinidine exerts little effect on automaticity of the isolated normal sinus node[7] or on the denervated[42] sinus node in vivo but suppresses automaticity in normal Purkinje fibers by decreasing the slope of phase 4 diastolic depolarization and shifting threshold voltage toward zero. It does not affect abnormal automaticity in depolarized Purkinje fibers or delayed afterdepolarizations, and in high doses can cause abnormal automatic discharge in Purkinje fibers.[7] Because of its significant anticholinergic effect[42,43] and reflex sympathetic stimulation resulting from alpha-adrenergic blockade that causes peripheral vasodilation, quinidine may increase sinus nodal discharge rate and may improve AV nodal conduction in the innervated heart in vivo. In patients with the sick sinus syndrome, quinidine can depress sinus nodal automaticity greatly.[7] Direct myocardial effects may prolong AV nodal and His-Purkinje conduction times.[42] Quinidine prolongs duration of action potential of atrial and ventricular muscle and Purkinje fibers slightly (quinine shortens it[41]), while markedly prolonging the effective refractory period without significantly changing resting membrane potential.[44] Action potential amplitude, overshoot, and $\dot{V}$max of phase 0 are reduced. Because of its vagolytic actions, produced through muscarinic blockade,[43] quinidine can shorten Purkinje fiber action potential when the latter has been prolonged by vagal inhibition of beta-adrenergic receptor stimulation.[45] Quinidine appears to bind to inactive sodium channels and unbind from resting channels in a voltage-dependent fashion. This observation helps explain quinidine's greater depressant effects at faster heart rates (when the cells spend a greater percentage of the cardiac cycle in an active state), so-called use-dependence,[46] and predicts that potentially greater toxic effects of quinidine may occur at faster heart rates.

Hemodynamic Effects. Quinidine decreases peripheral vascular resistance and may cause significant hypotension because of its alpha-adrenergic blocking effects. Concomitant administration of vasodilators may exaggerate the potential for hypotension. In some patients, quinidine can increase cardiac output, possibly by reducing afterload. No significant direct myocardial depressant action occurs unless large doses are given rapidly, intravenously. Most of the adverse effects of intravenous quinidine are probably the result of excessive vasodilation.

Pharmacokinetics (Table 20–1). Although orally administered quinidine sulfate and quinidine gluconate exhibit similar degrees of systemic availability, plasma quinidine concentrations peak at about 90 minutes after oral administration of quinidine sulfate and at 3 to 4 hours after oral administration of quinidine gluconate.[7] Intramuscular quinidine produces a higher and an earlier peak plasma concentration[8] but results in incomplete absorption and tissue necrosis. Quinidine may be given intravenously if it is infused slowly. Approximately 80 per cent of plasma quinidine is protein-bound. Both the liver and the kidneys remove quinidine, hepatic metabolism being more important. Approximately 20 per cent is excreted unchanged in the urine.[8] Because congestive heart failure, hepatic disease, or poor renal function may reduce quinidine elimination and increase plasma concentration, dosage probably should be reduced and the drug given cautiously to patients with these disorders while serum quinidine concentration is monitored.

Dosage and Administration (Table 20–1). The usual oral dose of quinidine sulfate for an adult is 300 to 600 mg four times daily, which results in a steady state level within about 24 hours. A loading dose of 600 to 1000 mg produces an earlier effective concentration.[7] Similar doses of quinidine gluconate are used intramuscularly, while the intravenous dose of quinidine gluconate is 6 to 10 mg/kg given at a rate of 0.3 to 0.5 mg/kg/min as blood pressure and ECG parameters are checked frequently.[47] Anticonvulsant drugs may shorten quinidine's half-life and reduce quinidine serum concentration for a given dose.

Clinical Indications. Quinidine is a versatile antiarrhythmic agent, useful for treating both supraventricular and ventricular premature complexes and sustained tachyarrhythmias. It may prevent spontaneous recurrences of AV nodal reentrant paroxysmal supraventricular tachycardia and inhibit tachycardia induced by programmed electrical stimulation by prolonging atrial and ventricular refractoriness and depressing conduction in the retrograde fast pathway.[48] In patients with the Wolff-Parkinson-White syndrome,[49] quinidine prolongs the effective refractory period of the accessory pathway and, by so doing, may prevent reciprocating tachycardias and slow the ventricular response owing to conduction over the accessory pathway during atrial flutter or atrial fibrillation in this disorder. Quinidine and other antiarrhythmic agents may also prevent recurrences of tachycardia by suppressing the "trigger," i.e., the premature atrial or ventricular complex that initiates a sustained tachycardia.

Quinidine successfully terminates atrial flutter or atrial fibrillation in about 10 to 20 per cent of patients, with higher success rates if the arrhythmia is of more recent onset and if the atria are not enlarged. Incremental dosing with quinidine at 2-hour intervals is no longer indicated to terminate atrial flutter or fibrillation. Prior to administering quinidine to these patients, the ventricular response should be slowed sufficiently with digitalis, propranolol, or verapamil, since quinidine-induced slowing of the atrial flutter rate—e.g., from 300 to the range of 200 bpm—plus its vagolytic effect on AV nodal conduction may convert a 2:1 atrioventricular response (two atrial impulses for each QRS complex) to a 1:1 atrioventricular response, with an *increase* in the ventricular rate. Prior to elective cardioversion of patients with atrial fibrillation, quinidine should probably be given for one to two days, since this regimen restores sinus rhythm in some patients, thus obviating DC cardioversion, and helps maintain sinus rhythm once it is achieved.[50] In most patients, quinidine should probably be administered as long as sinus rhythm continues.

Quinidine has prevented sudden death in patients resuscitated because of out-of-hospital cardiac arrest,[51] particularly those who maintained adequate plasma drug levels.[52] In one series, quinidine provided effective long-term control of ventricular tachycardia and ventricular fibrillation in about one-third of patients evaluated by electrophysiological study.[53] The patient population studied probably has a bearing on quinidine's efficacy and may reduce this success rate to less than one-third.

Adverse Effects. The most common adverse effects of chronic oral quinidine therapy are gastrointestinal, including nausea, vomiting, diarrhea, abdominal pain, and anorexia. Central nervous system toxicity includes tinnitus, hearing loss, visual disturbances, confusion, delirium, and psychosis. Cinchonism is the term usually applied to these side effects. Allergic reactions may be manifest as rash, fever, immune-mediated thrombocytopenia, hemolytic anemia, and rarely anaphylaxis. Thrombocytopenia is due to the presence of antibodies to quinidine-platelet complexes, causing platelets to agglutinate and lyse. In patients receiving oral anticoagulants, quinidine may cause bleeding.[54] Side effects may preclude long-term administration of quinidine in 30 to 40 per cent of patients.

A prominent electrocardiographic feature of quinidine toxicity is slowing of cardiac conduction, sometimes to the point of block. This may become manifest as prolongation of the QRS duration and Q-T interval or SA or AV nodal conduction disturbances. Quinidine-induced cardiac toxicity may be treated with molar sodium lactate.

Quinidine may produce syncope in 0.5 to 2.0 per cent of patients, most often the result of a self-terminating episode of a polymorphic ventricular tachyarrhythmia,[55,56] commonly of a specific variety called *torsades de pointes*[57] (see pp. 725 and 727). Quinidine prolongs the Q-T interval in most patients, whether or not ventricular arrhythmias occur, but significant Q-T prolongation (Q-T interval of 500 to 600 msec) is a general characteristic of quinidine syncope. Many of these patients were also receiving digitalis. Apparently syncope is not related to plasma concentrations of quinidine or duration of therapy.[55] Recently, a diastolic wave following the T wave has been described in patients who experience ventricular arrhythmias while receiving quinidine; however, the significance of this finding needs to be established.[58] Therapy for quinidine syncope requires immediate discontinuation of the drug and avoidance of other drugs that have similar pharmacological effects, such as disopyramide (see p. 659). In spite of the observations regarding "use-dependence," atrial or ventricular pacing may be used to suppress the ventricular tachyarrhythmia and may act by shortening refractoriness at faster rates. For some patients, drugs that do not prolong the Q-T interval, such as lidocaine or phenytoin, may be tried. When pacing is not available, isoproterenol may be given *with caution.*

Drugs that induce hepatic enzyme production, such as phenobarbital or phenytoin, may shorten the duration of quinidine's action by increasing its rate of elimination. Quinidine may elevate serum digoxin[59] and digitoxin[5] concentrations by decreasing total body clearance of digitoxin and by decreasing the clearance, volume of distribution, and affinity of tissue receptors for digoxin[60] (see p. 519).

PROCAINAMIDE

In 1936, Mautz demonstrated that direct application of procaine to the myocardium elevated the threshold of ventricular muscle to electrical stimulation.[61] However, procaine's therapeutic value as an antiarrhythmic agent was limited by its short duration of action and prominent central nervous system effects. A systematic study of procaine congeners and metabolites led to the development of procainamide,[62] which differs from procaine in that it replaces the ester linkage with an amide structure and has a longer duration of action, is effective when given orally, and exhibits increased cardiac effects with decreased central nervous system effects.

Electrophysiological Actions (Tables 20–2 and 20–3). The cardiac actions of procainamide on automaticity, conduction, excitability, and membrane responsiveness resemble those of quinidine and result in depression of excitability in atrium and ventricle, slowing of conduction, and prolongation of the effective refractory period. Like quinidine, procainamide usually prolongs the effective refractory period (ERP) more than it prolongs the action potential duration (APD).[63] When the ERP duration/APD exceeds 1.0, the earliest premature impulse that can be initiated during repolarization arises when the cell has returned to its most negative potential. Premature responses induced at this potential are more likely to have greater $\dot{V}max$ and amplitude, presumably establishing better conduction (see p. 618). Thus the antiarrhythmic agent prevents early responses, arising from less negative resting potentials, that might conduct slowly or block, thereby potentiating the development of arrhythmias. A drug that decreases the ratio of ERP duration/APD may allow earlier premature responses to occur at a time when the membrane potential is more positive. Compared to disopyramide and quinidine, procainamide exerts the least anticholinergic effects[43] but does produce more local anesthetic effects than quinidine. It does not affect normal sinus nodal automaticity.

In vitro studies on cat myocardium subjected to acute and chronic myocardial infarction reveal that procainamide decreases differences in refractoriness between tissue types by prolonging action potential duration and refractoriness most markedly in acutely ischemic cells with the shortest action potential duration and refractoriness and least in chronically injured cells with the longest action potential duration and refractoriness; the drug produced intermediate changes in normal cells.[64] In dogs subjected to a previous myocardial infarction, procainamide in vivo decreases excitability and prolongs refractoriness of abnormal myocardium, preventing reinitiation of sustained ventricular tachyarrhythmias in about half the dogs studied and markedly increasing the cycle length of arrhythmias that were still inducible.[65]

The electrophysiological effects of *N*-acetylprocainamide (NAPA), procainamide's major metabolite, differ from those of the parent compound. NAPA (10 to 40 mg/liter) does not suppress the rate of phase 4 diastolic depolarization of Purkinje fibers and does not alter resting membrane potential, action potential amplitude, or $\dot{V}max$ of phase 0 of the action potential of Purkinje fibers or ventricular muscle. However, NAPA prolongs the action potential duration of ventricular muscle and Purkinje fibers in a dose-dependent manner. Toxic doses produce early afterdepolarizations and triggered activity. NAPA given to dogs (50 to 100 mg/kg intravenously) produces single instances as well as salvos of ventricular extrasystoles that at times degenerate to ventricular fibrillation. Doses up to 100 mg/kg intravenously exert slight antiarrhythmic effects in dogs subjected to myocardial infarction 24 hours previously.[66] Procainamide appears to exert greater electrophysiological effects than NAPA.[67]

Hemodynamic Effects. Procainamide may depress myocardial contractility in high doses. It does not produce alpha blockade but may result in peripheral vasodilation via a mild ganglionic blocking action that impairs cardiovascular reflexes.[7]

Pharmacokinetics (Table 20–1). Following intramuscular administration, peak plasma concentrations occur in 15 to 60 minutes, while oral administration produces peak plasma concentration in about one hour. Absorption may be reduced in the first week after myocardial infarction. Approximately 80 per cent of oral procainamide is bioavailable, with 20 per cent bound to serum proteins. The overall elimination half-life for procainamide is three to five hours, with the majority of the drug eliminated unchanged in the urine and 10 to 30 per cent eliminated by hepatic metabolism.[5] A prolonged-release form of procainamide given every 6 hours provides steady-state plasma levels of the drug equivalent to an equal total daily dose of short-acting procainamide given every 3 hours.[68]

The drug is acetylated to NAPA, which is excreted almost exclusively by the kidneys. As renal function decreases and in patients with heart failure, procainamide levels—and particularly NAPA levels—increase and, because of the risk of serious cardiotoxicity, need to be carefully monitored in such situations. NAPA has an elimination half-life of 7 to 8 hours but exceeds 10 hours if high doses are used.[69] Small amounts of procainamide are present in patients receiving NAPA because of deacetylation.[70]

Dosage and Administration (Table 20–1). Procainamide may be given by the oral, intravenous, or intramuscular route to achieve serum concentrations that produce an antiarrhythmic effect in the range of 4 to 10 μg/ml. Occasionally plasma concentrations exceeding 10 μg/ml have been required,[71,72] but the probability of adverse effects may increase with higher plasma concentrations.[73] Several intravenous regimens have been used to administer procainamide. Twenty-five to 50 mg can be given over a one-minute period and then repeated every five minutes until the arrhythmia is controlled, hypotension results, or the QRS complex is prolonged more than 50 per cent. Rather large doses of 6 to 13 mg/kg at a maximum infusion rate of 0.5 mg/kg/min have been used.[47] Another method employs 50 mg/min with the same endpoints.[72] A constant-rate intravenous infusion of procainamide can be given at a dose of 2 to 6 mg/min.[7] The upper limits regarding total dose are flexible and range between 1000 and 2000 mg, depending upon the patient's response.

Oral administration of procainamide requires a 3- or 4-hour dosing interval at a total daily dose of 2 to 6 gm, with a steady state reached within one day. When a loading dose is used, it should be twice the maintenance dose. Frequent dosing is required because of the short elimination half-life in normal subjects. For the prolonged-release form of procainamide, dosing is at 6-hour intervals.[68] A longer half-life may be seen in some cardiac patients, allowing longer intervals between drug administration, but this needs to be documented for the individual patient. Procainamide is well absorbed after intramuscular injection, with virtually 100 per cent of the dose bioavailable.[7]

It has been suggested recently that the plasma concentration of procainamide required to suppress premature ventricular complexes (PVC) in patients who have acute myocardial infarction may be less than the plasma concentration required to prevent spontaneous episodes of symptomatic sustained ventricular tachycardia. Procainamide, 9 μg/ml, suppressed spontaneous episodes of ventricular tachycardia but decreased PVC frequency by only 36 per cent, whereas the mean concentration required to suppress 85 per cent of PVCs was 15 μg/ml. This study raises interesting questions regarding differences in antiarrhythmic thresholds as influenced by the nature of the heart disease as well as by the arrhythmia.[74]

Clinical Indications. Procainamide is used to treat both supraventricular and ventricular arrhythmias and has a spectrum of application comparable to that of quinidine. Although both drugs have similar electrophysiological actions, either drug may effectively suppress a supraventricular or ventricular arrhythmia that is refractory to the other drug.

Procainamide may be used to convert atrial fibrillation of recent onset to sinus rhythm.[75] As with quinidine, prior treatment with digitalis, propranolol, or verapamil is recommended to prevent acceleration of the ventricular response following procainamide therapy. In patients with paroxysmal supraventricular tachycardia, procainamide may inhibit the induction of sustained AV nodal reentrant tachycardia as a result of selective depression of retrograde AV nodal conduction in the fast pathway. In a small number of patients, apparent vagolytic effects of procainamide potentiated the induction of sustained tachycardia.[76] Recently it has been shown that procainamide almost uniformly depresses retrograde AV nodal conduction in patients who do not have tachycardias due to AV nodal reentry or accessory pathways. Therefore, this effect in patients who do have tachycardias cannot be interpreted to indicate the response of a specific tissue type.[77] Procainamide may block conduction in the accessory pathway of patients with the Wolff-Parkinson-White syndrome and has been used intravenously to identify those patients who have a short anterograde effective refractory period of the accessory pathway[78] (p. 712).

Procainamide has been only partially effective in preventing the induction of ventricular tachycardia by programmed stimulation during electrophysiological studies in patients with a history of ventricular tachycardia or ventricular fibrillation. High doses, 500 to 1000 mg orally every 4 hours, resulting in a plasma concentration of up to 13.5 μg/ml may be necessary to suppress ventricular tachycardia in some patients.[71] Most consistently, procainamide slows the rate of the induced ventricular tachycardia.[79] Recently it has been suggested that the response to programmed electrical stimulation of patients receiving procainamide could predict their response to other conventional agents. Failure to induce sustained ventricular tachycardia while patients received procainamide predicted noninducibility while they received other conventional agents. Conversely, the induction of sustained ventricular tachycardia while patients received procainamide predicted the inducibility of ventricular tachycardia when they received other conventional agents and suggested that alternative treatments with investigational drugs, surgery, or electrical therapy be considered. This interesting study requires confirmation.[80] Procainamide may facilitate the induction of ventricular tachycardia, an effect shared by many other antiarrhythmic agents.[81] It can also induce a polymorphic ventricular tachycardia associated with Q-T interval prolongation.[82] NAPA appears to be a less effective antiarrhythmic agent than procainamide, and the antiarrhythmic response to procainamide does not predict the response to NAPA.

Adverse Effects. Multiple adverse noncardiac effects have been reported with procainamide administration and include skin rashes, myalgias, digital vasculitis, and Raynaud's phenomenon. Gastrointestinal side effects are less frequent than with quinidine, and adverse central nervous system side effects are less frequent than with lidocaine. Procainamide may cause giddiness, psychosis, hallucinations, and depression. Toxic concentrations of procainamide can diminish myocardial performance and promote hypotension. A variety of conduction disturbances or ventricular tachyarrhythmias may occur similar to those produced by quinidine, including prolonged Q-T syndrome and polymorphous ventricular tachycardia.[82] However, ventricular tachyarrhythmias do not appear to occur as frequently following procainamide therapy as they do following treatment with quinidine. In the absence of sinus node disease, procainamide does not adversely affect sinus node function. In patients with sinus dysfunction, procainamide tends to prolong corrected sinus node recovery time and may worsen symptoms in some patients who have the bradycardia-tachycardia syndrome.[83] Fever and agranulocytosis may be due to hypersensitivity reactions, and white blood cell and differential blood counts should be performed at regular intervals. Procainamide does not increase the serum digoxin concentration.[7]

Arthralgia, fever, pleuropericarditis, hepatomegaly, and hemorrhagic pericardial effusion with tamponade have been described in a systemic lupus erythematosus (SLE)–like syndrome[84] (p. 1660). The syndrome may occur more frequently and earlier in patients who are "slow acetylators" of procainamide, although this is not entirely clear. The aromatic amino group on procainamide appears important for induction of SLE syndrome, since acetylating this amino group to form NAPA appears to block the SLE-inducing effect.[85] Procainamide-induced SLE syndrome differs from naturally occurring lupus syndrome by sparing the brain and kidney, uncommonly producing hematological complications, and not producing false-positive serological tests for syphilis. Patients who develop drug-induced SLE have antibodies against single-stranded DNA, while those who have naturally occurring SLE develop antibodies against double-stranded DNA. Almost all patients with drug-induced SLE have antibodies to histones, while only one-third of patients with naturally occurring SLE develop antihistone antibodies. Sixty to 70 per cent of patients who receive procainamide develop antinuclear antibodies, with clinical symptoms in 20 to 30 per cent, but this is reversible when procainamide is stopped. When symptoms occur, SLE cell preparations are often positive. Positive serological tests are not necessarily a reason to discontinue drug therapy, but the development of symptoms or a positive anti-DNA antibody is, except for patients whose life-threatening arrhythmia is controlled only by procainamide. Steroid administration in those patients may eliminate the symptoms.[7]

DISOPYRAMIDE

Disopyramide has been approved in the United States for oral but not intravenous adminstration to treat ventricular arrhythmias. Generally, it exerts efficacy comparable to that of quinidine and procainamide against a similar spectrum of arrhythmias but has important side effects including cardiovascular depression, generation of ventricular arrhythmias, and bothersome anticholinergic properties.

Electrophysiological Actions (Tables 20–2 and 20–3). Similar to the in vitro effects of quinidine and procainamide, disopyramide decreases the slope of phase 4 diastolic depolarization in Purkinje fibers. It produces a rate-dependent depression of $\dot{V}$max of phase 0, prolongs the effective refractory period more than it prolongs the action potential duration,[86] and lengthens conduction time in normal and depolarized Purkinje fibers.[87] Similar to the effects of procainamide in an experimental infarct model studied in vitro,[64] disopyramide reduces the differences in action potential duration between normal and infarcted tissue by lengthening the action potential of normal cells more than it lengthens the action potential of cells from infarcted regions of the heart.[88]

Stereochemical properties influence the effects of disopyramide. Racemic (clinically used) and (+) disopyramide prolong canine Purkinje fiber action potential, while (−) disopyramide shortens it. The (+) isomer exerts approximately three times more vagolytic effects than does the (−) isomer. If Purkinje fibers are treated with isoproterenol (to shorten action potential duration) and then acetylcholine (to antagonize the catecholamine effect and lengthen action potential duration), the vagolytic action of disopyramide eliminates the cholinergic antagonism of beta stimulation, and the action potential shortens.[43] By a similar vagolytic mechanism, disopyramide is capable of speeding up the sinus nodal discharge rate and shortening AV nodal conduction time and refractoriness when the nodes are restrained by cholinergic influences, either in vitro or in vivo.[86,89] Atropine tends to nullify or even reverse this effect. Disopyramide exerts greater anticholinergic effects than quinidine and does not appear to affect alpha- or beta-adrenergic receptors.

Although not a slow-channel blocker, disopyramide can slow the sinus nodal discharge rate by a direct action when given in high concentration[90] and can significantly depress sinus nodal activity in patients with sinus node dysfunction.[91] Atrial and ventricular refractory periods increase. Disopyramide's effect on AV nodal conduction and refractoriness in vivo is not consistent.[89,92,93] AV block may occur occasionally,[94] and since disopyramide can prolong His-Purkinje conduction time, it is possible that infra-His block may result. However, His-Purkinje block did not occur in 22 patients who had bundle branch block and were given disopyramide intravenously.[93] Disopyramide may be administered safely to patients who have first degree or Type I second degree AV block and narrow QRS complexes.[94a] Disopyramide increases the conduction time and effective refractory period of the accessory pathway in Wolff-Parkinson-White syndrome.[95]

Hemodynamic Effects. Maximum hemodynamic effects in patients with left ventricular dysfunction occur immediately after intravenous administration of 2 mg/kg disopyramide and consist of reductions in systemic blood pressure, cardiac index, and stroke index. Right atrial pressure and total peripheral resistance increase. Profound hemodynamic deterioration developed in two of nine patients in this study.[96] Patients who have abnormal ventricular function tolerate the negative inotropic effects of disopyramide quite poorly, and in these patients the drug should be used with extreme caution or not at all.

Pharmacokinetics (Table 20–1). Disopyramide is 80 to 90 per cent absorbed, with a mean elimination half-life of 8 to 9 hours in healthy volunteers but almost 10 hours in patients with heart failure. Total body clearance and volume of distribution decreases in these patients, and mean serum concentration is higher than reported in normal subjects.[97] Renal insufficiency prolongs the elimination time. Thus, in patients who have renal, hepatic, or cardiac insufficiency, loading and maintenance doses need to be reduced. One study of patients who had ventricular arrhythmias showed an elimination half-life of 18 to 19 hours.[98] Peak blood levels after oral administration are seen in 1 to 2 hours, and bioavailability exceeds 80 per cent. The fraction of disopyramide bound to serum protein varies inversely with the total plasma concentration of the drug but may be more stable (30 to 40 per cent) at clinically relevant concentrations of 3 μg/ml.[7,92] About half an oral dose is recovered unchanged in the urine, with about 30 per cent as the mono N-dealkylated metabolite. The metabolites appear to exert less effect than the parent compound.

Dosage and Administration (Table 20–1). Doses are generally 100 to 200 mg orally every six hours with a range of 400 to 1200 mg/day. The intravenous (investigational) dose is 1 to 2 mg/kg as an initial bolus given over 5 to 10 minutes, which may be followed by an infusion of 1 mg/kg/hour.[95]

Clinical Indications. The usefulness of disopyramide in treating multiple categories of atrial and ventricular arrhythmias is still incompletely resolved. Disopyramide appears comparable to quinidine in reducing the frequency of premature ventricular complexes and initial data suggest that it effectively prevents recurrence of ventricular tachycardia in selected patients.[93,99] Its role in preventing arrhythmias and reducing mortality in patients after acute myocardial infarction has not been established[100] and may not be as potent as orally administered aprindine.[101] Disopyramide has been combined safely and effectively with mexiletine to treat patients who had recurrent ventricular tachycardia and/or ventricular fibrillation and were evaluated during electrophysiological study.[102]

Disopyramide terminates attacks of acute paroxysmal supraventricular tachycardia and decreases the frequency of recurrences.[103] It helps prevent recurrence of atrial fibrillation after successful cardioversion as effectively as quinidine[93] and may terminate atrial flutter. In treating patients with atrial fibrillation, and particularly atrial flutter, the ventricular rate must be controlled prior to administering disopyramide, or the atrial rate may decrease sufficiently, aided by the vagolytic effects of disopyramide, to create 1:1 conduction during atrial flutter.[104] Disopyramide prolongs the anterograde and retrograde refractory period of the accessory pathway in patients with the Wolff-Parkinson-White syndrome[95] and may prevent reciprocating tachycardias or slow the ventricular rate during atrial flutter or atrial fibrillation.

Adverse Effects. Three categories of adverse effects are seen following disopyramide administration. The most common adverse effect relates to the drug's potent parasympatholytic properties and includes urinary hesitancy or retention, constipation, blurred vision, closed-angle glaucoma, and dry mouth. Second, disopyramide may produce ventricular tachyarrhythmias that are commonly associated with Q-T prolongation and the ventricular tachycardia called torsades de pointes.[57,93,105,106] Some patients may have "cross sensitivity" to both quinidine and disopyramide and develop torsades de pointes while receiving either drug. When drug-induced torsades de pointes occur, agents that prolong the Q-T interval should be used with great caution. Finally, disopyramide may reduce contractility of the normal ventricle but the depression of ventricular function is much more pronounced in patients with preexisting ventricular failure.[107] Occasionally, cardiovascular collapse can result.[108]

Disopyramide does not appear to alter digitalis metabolism. However, phenytoin may decrease plasma concentration of disopyramide by altering its metabolism.[109]

PHENYTOIN (DIPHENYLHYDANTOIN)

Phenytoin was employed originally to treat seizure disorders and was noted subsequently to abolish ventricular tachycardia in dogs after coronary artery ligation. Although it has been used for many years, phenytoin's value as an antiarrhythmic agent remains limited.

Electrophysiological Actions (Tables 20–2 and 20–3). Therapeutic concentrations of phenytoin do not alter the discharge rate of rabbit sinus nodal tissue but may depress normal automaticity in cardiac Purkinje fibers in vitro[7] or spontaneous ventricular rate in vivo by presumably increasing potassium conductance (the I_{K_1} channel). Phenytoin is very effective in abolishing abnormal automaticity caused by digitalis-induced delayed afterdepolarizations in cardiac Purkinje fibers[110,111] and in suppressing certain digitalis-induced arrhythmias in man.[112] Similar to lidocaine, phenytoin abbreviates Purkinje fiber action potential duration more than it shortens the effective refractory period, thus increasing the ratio of effective refractory period to action potential duration.[7] Phenytoin can cause depolarized cells to repolarize by increasing potassium conductance and, in so doing, may increase the $\dot{V}$max of phase 0 in Purkinje fibers,[113] particularly when these are depressed by digitalis. The rate of rise of action potentials initiated early in the relative refractory period is increased, as is membrane responsiveness, possibly reducing the chance for impaired conduction and block.[63] Phenytoin may slow conduction at high potassium concentrations. Sinus discharge rate and AV conduction in man are minimally affected by phenytoin.

Some of phenytoin's antiarrhythmic effects may be neurally mediated, since phenytoin may reduce the increase in impulse traffic in cardiac sympathetic nerves caused by ouabain toxicity.[114] Injected into the central nervous system, phenytoin protects against digitalis-induced ventricular arrhythmias.[115] The drug may also modulate vagal efferent activity centrally. It has no peripheral cholinergic or beta-adrenergic blocking actions.

Phenytoin exerts minimal *hemodynamic effects.*

Pharmacokinetics (Table 20–1). The pharmacokinetics of phenytoin are less than ideal. Absorption following oral administration is incomplete and delayed and varies with the brand of drug, and plasma concentrations reach their peak 8 to 12 hours later. Ninety per cent of the drug is protein-bound.[8] Phenytoin has limited solubility at physiologic pH, and intramuscular administration is associated with pain, muscle necrosis, sterile abscesses, and variable absorption. Therapeutic serum concentrations of phenytoin (10 to 20 μg/ml) are similar for treating both cardiac arrhythmias and epilepsy. Lower concentrations may suppress certain digitalis-induced arrhythmias or other arrhythmias when decreased plasma protein binding occurs (as in uremia), since a larger fraction of drug is free and pharmacologically active.

Over 90 per cent of a dose is hydroxylated in the liver to presumably inactive compounds. Some families have a genetically determined inability to hydroxylate phenytoin, while others have a higher than usual capability for hydroxylation.[8] Elimination half-time is about 24 hours and may be slowed in the presence of liver disease or when phenytoin is administered concomitantly with drugs such as phenylbutazone, dicumarol, isoniazid, chloramphenicol, and phenothiazines that compete with phenytoin for hepatic enzymes.[113] Because of the large number of medications that may increase or decrease phenytoin levels during chronic therapy, phenytoin plasma concentration should be determined frequently when changes are made in other medications. In some patients, maintenance dose regimens of phenytoin are difficult to predict because the enzyme system that metabolizes phenytoin becomes saturated at plasma concentrations within the therapeutic range. The half-life then increases with increasing phenytoin load, particularly as plasma concentrations approach the therapeutic range. Above the saturation point, phenytoin elimination follows zero-order kinetics, so that only a fixed amount of drug is eliminated per unit time. These concentration-dependent kinetics for elimination can cause unexpected toxicity, since disproportionately large changes in plasma concentration may follow dose increases.[7]

Dosage and Administration (Table 20–1). To achieve therapeutic plasma concentrations rapidly, 100 mg of phenytoin should be administered intravenously every 5 minutes until the arrhythmia is controlled, adverse side effects result, or about 1 gm has been given. Generally, 700 to 1000 mg will control the arrhythmia. A large vein should be used to avoid pain and development of phlebitis produced by the severely alkalotic (pH 11.0) vehicle in which phenytoin is dissolved.[7] Orally, phenytoin is given as a loading dose of approximately 1000 mg the first day, 500 mg on the second and third days, and 400 mg daily thereafter. All maintenance doses can be given once or twice daily, depending on the brand, because of the long half-life of elimination.

Clinical Indications. Phenytoin has been used successfully to treat atrial and ventricular arrhythmias caused by digitalis toxicity but is much less effective in treating ventricular arrhythmias in patients with ischemic heart disease[7,116] or with atrial arrhythmias not due to digitalis toxicity.[113] The drug has been somewhat more successful in treating ventricular arrhythmias associated with general anesthesia and cardiac surgery.

Adverse Effects. The most common manifestations of phenytoin toxicity are central nervous system effects of nystagmus, ataxia, drowsiness, stupor, and coma. Progression of such symptoms can be correlated with increases in plasma drug concentration. Neurological signs, such as nystagmus on lateral gaze, develop at plasma drug levels of about 20 μg/ml.[7] Nausea, epigastric pain, and anorexia are also relatively common effects of phenytoin. Long-term administration may result in hyperglycemia, hypocalcemia, skin rashes, megaloblastic anemia, gingival hypertrophy, lymph node hyperplasia (a syndrome resembling malignant lymphoma), peripheral neuropathy, and drug-induced systemic lupus erythematosus.[8]

PROPRANOLOL

(See also p. 1349)

Although six beta-adrenergic receptor blocking drugs have been approved for use in the United States (Table 39–5, p. 1350), only propranolol and timolol have been approved to treat arrhythmias or to prevent sudden death after myocardial infarction. It is generally considered that no beta blocker offers distinct advantages over the others and that, when titrated to the proper dose, all can be used effectively to treat cardiac arrhythmias, hypertension, or other disorders.[117] However, differences in pharmacokinetic or pharmacodynamic properties that confer safety, reduce adverse effects, or affect dosing intervals or drug interactions influence the choice of agent.

Beta receptors can be separated into those that affect predominately the heart ($beta_1$) or the bronchi and blood vessels ($beta_2$).[118] In low doses, selective beta blockers can block $beta_1$ receptors more than they block $beta_2$ receptors and might be preferable for treating patients with pulmonary or peripheral vascular diseases. In high doses, the selective $beta_1$ blockers also block $beta_2$ receptors.

Some beta blockers exert intrinsic sympathomimetic activity, i.e., they slightly activate the beta receptor. These drugs appear to be as efficacious as beta blockers without intrinsic sympathomimetic actions and may cause less slowing of heart rate at rest and less prolongation of AV nodal conduction time.[117] Recently, they have been shown to induce less depression of left ventricular function than beta blockers without intrinsic sympathomimetic activity.[119]

The following discussion will concentrate on the use of propranolol as an antiarrhythmic agent.

Electrophysiological Actions. Beta blockers may exert an electrophysiological action by competitively inhibiting catecholamine binding at beta adrenoreceptor sites, an effect almost entirely due to the (−) levorotatory stereoisomer,[117] or by their quinidine-like or direct membrane-stabilizing action. The latter is a local anesthetic effect that depresses I_{Na} and membrane responsiveness in cardiac Purkinje fibers,[120] occurs at concentrations generally 10 times that necessary to produce beta blockade, and most likely plays an insignificant antiarrhythmic role. At low, beta-blocking concentrations, propranolol slows spontaneous automaticity in the sinus node or in Purkinje fibers that are being stimulated by adrenergic tone. In the absence of adrenergic tone, only high concentrations of propranolol slow normal automaticity in Purkinje fibers, probably by a direct membrane action.[121,122] In low concentrations that cause beta-receptor blockade but no local anesthetic effects, beta-blocking drugs do not alter the normal resting membrane potential, maximum diastolic potential, amplitude, $\dot{V}max$, repolarization, or refractoriness of atrial, Purkinje, or ventricular muscle cells[121,122] when these tissues are not being superfused with catecholamines. However, in the presence of isoproterenol, a pure beta-receptor stimulator, beta blockers reverse isoproterenol's accelerating effects on repolarization; in the presence of norepinephrine, beta blockade permits unopposed alpha-adrenergic stimulation to prolong action potential duration in Purkinje fibers.

If values for these action potential parameters were abnormally low to start and were increased by catecholamines, such as a slow response generated in a high-potassium, catecholamine environment, beta-receptor blockade might depress conduction by removing the catecholamine stimulatory effect. At higher concentrations exceeding 3 $\mu g/ml$, propranolol depresses $\dot{V}max$, action potential amplitude, membrane responsiveness, and conduction in normal atrial, ventricular, and Purkinje fibers[121,122] without altering resting membrane potential. These effects probably result from depression of sodium conductance. The direct effect of propranolol shortens the action potential duration of Purkinje fibers and, to a lesser extent, of atrial and ventricular muscle fibers.[121,122] Long-term administration of propranolol may lengthen action potential duration. Similar to the effects of lidocaine, acceleration of repolarization of Purkinje fibers is most marked in areas of the ventricular conduction system in which the action potential duration is greatest. The reduction in refractory period is not as great as the reduction in action potential duration (effective refractory period duration/action potential duration > 1.0). At least one beta blocker, sotalol, markedly increases the time course of repolarization in Purkinje fibers and ventricular muscle.

Propranolol slows the sinus discharge rate in humans by 10 to 20 per cent, while severe bradycardia occasionally results if the heart is particularly dependent on sympathetic tone or if sinus node dysfunction is present. The slowing is probably due to beta blockade because D-propranolol does not significantly slow the sinus discharge rate in doses comparable to the racemic mixture. The P-R interval lengthens, as does AV nodal conduction time and refractoriness (if the heart rate is maintained constant), but refractoriness and conduction in the His-Purkinje system remain unchanged even after high doses of propranolol.[123] Therefore, therapeutic doses of propranolol in humans do not exert a direct depressant or "quinidine-like" action but influence cardiac electrophysiology via a beta-blocking action. Beta blockers do not affect conduction in ventricular muscle, as evidenced by their lack of effect on the QRS complex, and they insignificantly prolong the right ventricular effective refractory period[124] and uncorrected Q-T interval.[125,126]

Several observations suggest that the beta-blocking action of propranolol is responsible for its antiarrhythmic effects. The dextrorotatory stereoisomer of beta blockers retains the direct membrane action without beta-blocking properties[127] and does not prevent arrhythmias provoked by catecholamine administration. Also, 1/50th to 1/100th of the plasma concentration necessary to achieve membrane depressant effects on $\dot{V}max$ and overshoot in isolated cardiac muscle possesses antiarrhythmic effects. Thus, beta blockade without direct membrane action prevents many arrhythmias that result from activation of the autonomic nervous system. However, beta blockers with direct membrane action appear necessary to suppress certain experimental arrhythmias, such as those that occur in the dog one to two days after coronary artery ligation or those due to some types of digitalis toxicity.[121,122] In man, the direct membrane effects of beta blockers do not appear necessary for clinical antiarrhythmic actions, and the antiarrhythmic spectrum of clinical effectiveness of beta blockers without direct membrane effects seems to be the same as that of beta blockers with direct membrane effects, including arrhythmias resulting from digitalis intoxication and myocardial infarction. The possible importance of direct membrane effect of some of these drugs cannot be discounted totally because beta blockers with direct membrane actions may affect transmembrane potentials of diseased cardiac fibers at much lower concentrations than are needed to affect normal fibers directly. In addition, the role of important metabolites of propranolol and other beta blockers that may exert electrophysiological actions is not clearly established.

Hemodynamic Effects. Propranolol exerts negative inotropic effects on cardiac contractility and may precipitate or worsen heart failure. By blocking beta receptors, this drug may cause peripheral vasoconstriction.

Pharmacokinetics (Table 20–1). Although various types of beta blockers exert similar pharmacological effects, their pharmacokinetics differ substantially.[117] Propranolol is almost 100 per cent absorbed, but the effects of first-pass hepatic metabolism reduce bioavailability to about 30 per cent and produce significant interpatient variability of plasma concentration for a given dose. Reduction in hepatic blood flow, as in patients with heart failure, decreases the hepatic extraction of propranolol, and in these patients propranolol may further decrease its own elimination rate by reducing cardiac output and hepatic blood flow.[128] Beta blockers eliminated by the kidney tend to have longer half-lives and exhibit less interpatient variability of drug concentration than do those beta blockers metabolized by the liver.

Dosage and Administration (Table 20–1). The appropriate dose of propranolol is best determined by a measure of the patient's physiological response, such as changes in resting heart rate or in the prevention of exercise-induced tachycardia, since wide individual differences exist between the observed physiological effect and plasma concentration. For example, intravenous dosing is best achieved by titrating the dose to a clinical effect, beginning with 0.25 to 0.50 mg and administering doses every five minutes until either a desired effect or toxicity is produced or a total of 0.15 to 0.20 mg/kg has been given. Orally, propranolol is given in four divided doses, usually ranging from 40 to 160 mg a day to more than 1 gram a day. Generally, if one agent in adequate doses proves to be ineffective, other beta blockers will be ineffective also.

Clinical Indications. As an antiarrhythmic agent, propranolol is used most commonly to treat supraventricular tachyarrhythmias. Its effectiveness and mechanism of action vary depending on the arrhythmia. Propranolol may be employed to decrease the rate of persistent sinus tachycardia that results from excessive sympathetic stimulation. Arrhythmias associated with thyrotoxicosis, pheochromocytoma, and anesthesia with cyclopropane or halothane or arrhythmias largely due to excessive cardiac adrenergic stimulation, such as those initiated by exercise or emotion, often respond to propranolol therapy. Beta-blocking drugs usually do not convert chronic atrial flutter or atrial fibrillation to normal sinus rhythm but may be successful if the arrhythmia is of recent onset. The rate of the atrial flutter generally is not changed, but the ventricular response during atrial flutter and atrial fibrillation decreases because beta blockade prolongs AV nodal conduction time and refractoriness. For reentrant supraventricular tachycardias using the AV node as one of the reentrant pathways, such as AV nodal reentrant tachycardia and reciprocating tachycardias in Wolff-Parkinson-White syndrome, or for sinus reentrant tachycardia, propranolol may terminate the tachycardia and be used prophylactically to prevent a recurrence. Combining propranolol with digitalis, quinidine, or a variety of other agents—some of which are investigational—may be effective when propranolol as a single agent fails.

Several other groups of arrhythmias respond particularly well to beta blockade. These include digitalis-induced arrhythmias such as atrial tachycardia, nonparoxysmal AV junctional tachycardia, premature ventricular complexes, or ventricular tachycardia. Part of the effects of propranolol against arrhythmias induced by digitalis results from its action on the central nervous system. If a significant degree of AV block is present during a digitalis-induced arrhythmia, lidocaine or phenytoin may be preferable to propranolol. Propranolol may also be useful to treat ventricular arrhythmias associated with the prolonged Q-T interval syndrome[129] and with mitral valve prolapse.[130] For patients with ischemic heart disease, propranolol generally has not prevented episodes of chronic recurrent ventricular tachycardia that occur in the absence of acute ischemia. However, several clinical trials have demonstrated a reduction in the incidence of overall death and sudden cardiac death after myocardial infarction in patients treated chronically with a variety of beta blockers. The mechanism of this reduction in mortality is not entirely clear and may relate to reduction in the extent of ischemic damage, an antiarrhythmic effect, or both. Survival benefits seem most striking in the first one to two years after myocardial infarction.[131–136, 136a]

Adverse Effects. Adverse cardiovascular effects from propranolol include unacceptable hypotension, bradycardia, or congestive heart failure. The bradycardia may be due to sinus bradycardia or AV block. Uncommonly, propranolol may precipitate left ventricular failure in the absence of previous failure. Sudden withdrawal of propranolol in patients with angina pectoris can precipitate worsening of angina, cardiac arrhythmias, and acute myocardial infarction,[137] possibly owing to heightened sensitivity to beta agonists caused by previous beta blockade. Heightened sensitivity may begin several days after cessation of propranolol therapy and may last five or six days.[138] Other adverse effects of propranolol include worsening of asthma or chronic obstructive pulmonary disease, intermittent claudication, Raynaud's phenomenon, mental depression, increased risk of hypoglycemia among insulin-dependent diabetic patients, easy fatigability, disturbingly vivid dreams or insomnia, and impaired sexual function.

BRETYLIUM TOSYLATE

Bretylium was introduced as an antihypertensive agent in 1959, and its antiarrhythmic potential was recognized several years later.

Electrophysiological Actions (Tables 20–2 and 20–3). Bretylium is selectively concentrated in sympathetic ganglia and their postganglionic adrenergic nerve terminals. After initially *causing* norepinephrine release, bretylium *prevents* norepinephrine release from sympathetic nerve terminals, without depressing pre- or postganglionic sympathetic nerve conduction, impairing conduction across sympathetic ganglia, depleting the adrenergic neuron of norepinephrine, or decreasing the responsiveness of adrenergic receptors.[7] During chronic bretylium treatment, the beta-adrenergic responses to circulating catecholamines are increased. The initial release of catecholamines results in several transient electrophysiological responses such as an increase in the discharge rates of the isolated perfused sinus node and of in vitro Purkinje fibers, often making quiescent fibers automatic. Bretylium initially increases conduction velocity and excitability and decreases refractoriness in the rabbit atrium,[139] and partially depolarized fibers may hyperpolarize. Pretreatment with reserpine or propranolol will prevent these early changes. Initial catecholamine release may aggravate some arrhythmias, such as those caused by digitalis excess[139] or myocardial infarction. Prolonged drug administration lengthens the duration of the action potential and refractoriness of atrial and ventricular muscle and Purkinje fibers.[7,140] The ratio of effective refractory period to action potential duration does not change, nor do membrane responsiveness and conduction velocity. Bretylium exerts little effect on diastolic excitability but increases ventricular fibrillation thresholds significantly.[141] Other adrenergic neuronal blocking agents, such as guanethidine, do not elevate the ventricular fibrillation threshold, while ordinary quaternary ammonium analogs that are not adrenergic neuron blockers can elevate this threshold.[7] Thus, although the chemical sympathectomy-like state may be antiarrhythmic, other factors may be important as well. Recent data obtained from studies of subendocardial Purkinje fibers from infarcted canine hearts indicate that bretylium lengthens the action potential duration most in cells located in proximal areas of the specialized conducting system of normal myocardium and least in cells located within the infarct in which the action potential duration was already lengthened.[142] Perhaps the reduced disparity between action potential duration and refractory period between regions of normal and infarcted myocardium may account for some of the antifibrillatory effects of bretylium in myocardial ischemia. Procainamide[64] and disopyramide[88] exert similar effects. When bretylium was given to conscious dogs subjected to premature electrical stimulation three to six days after myocardial infarction, the drug appeared to prevent the onset of ventricular tachycardia.[143] Bretylium has no effect on vagal reflexes and does not alter the responsiveness of cholinergic receptors in the heart.[7]

Hemodynamic Effects. Bretylium does not depress myocardial contractility, even at high doses.[7] After an initial increase in blood pressure, the drug may cause significant hypotension by blocking the efferent limb of the baroreceptor reflex. Hypotension results most commonly when patients are sitting or standing but may also occur in the supine position in seriously ill patients. Bretylium reduces the extent of the vasoconstriction and tachycardia reflexes during standing. We have noted (unpublished) that orthostatic hypotension may persist for several days after the drug has been discontinued.

Pharmacokinetics (Table 20–1). Bretylium is effective orally as well as parenterally, but it is absorbed poorly and erratically from the gastrointestinal tract. Bioavailability may be less than 50 per cent and elimination almost exclusively by renal excretion without significant metabolism or active metabolites recognized. Elimination half-life is 5 to 10 hours but with fairly wide variability. A recent study of the pharmacokinetics of intravenous and oral bretylium in 12 patients who were survivors of ventricular tachycardia or ventricular fibrillation revealed an elimination half-life of 13.5 hours following single intravenous dosing, which was similar to previous results in normal subjects. Renal clearance accounted for virtually all elimination. Onset of action after intravenous administration occurs within several minutes, but full antiarrhythmic effects may not be seen for 30 minutes to 2 hours. Doses should be reduced in patients with renal insufficiency.[144]

Dosage and Administration (Table 20–1). Bretylium is approved for parenteral administration only and can be given intravenously in doses of 5 to 10 mg/kg body weight diluted in 50 to 100 ml of 5 per cent dextrose in water and administered slowly over 10 to 20 minutes.[145] This dose can be repeated in 1 to 2 hours if the arrhythmia persists. The total daily dose should probably not exceed 30 mg/kg. A similar initial dose, but undiluted, can be given intramuscularly. The maintenance intravenous dose is 0.5 to 2.0 mg/min. Intramuscular injection during cardiopulmonary resuscitation from cardiac arrest and in shock states should be avoided because of unreliable absorption during reduced tissue perfusion. In this situation, bretylium should be given intravenously.

Clinical Indications. Bretylium is currently recommended for use in patients who are in an intensive care setting and who have life-threatening recurrent ventricular tachyarrhythmias that have not responded to lidocaine, quinidine, procainamide, or disopyramide. Bretylium has been remarkably effective in treating some of these patients with drug-resistant tachyarrhythmias.[145,146] In a recent study, bretylium was compared with lidocaine as the initial drug therapy in 46 victims of out-of-hospital ventricular fibrillation in a randomized, blinded trial. No instance of chemical defibrillation was observed with either drug in this study, and bretylium afforded neither significant advantage nor disadvantage compared with lidocaine in the initial management of ventricular fibrillation.[36] However, it can be argued that bretylium was not allowed sufficient time to be effective in this study.

Adverse Effects. Hypotension, most prominently orthostatic but also supine, appears to be the most significant side effect and can be prevented with tricyclic drugs such as protriptyline. Transient hypertension, increased sinus rate, and worsening of arrhythmias,[144] often those due to digitalis excess,[139] may follow initial drug administration and may be due to initial release of catecholamines. Bretylium should be used cautiously or not at all in patients who have a relatively fixed cardiac output, such as those with severe aortic stenosis. Vasodilators or diuretics may enhance these hypotensive effects. Nausea and vomiting may occur following parenteral administration. Parotid pain primarily during meals commonly occurs after 2 to 4 months of oral therapy and is associated with increased salivation without parotid swelling or inflammation.

VERAPAMIL

Verapamil, a synthetic papaverine derivative, was first introduced in 1962 as a smooth muscle relaxant that produced peripheral and coronary vasodilation in animals and man.[92,147] Representing a new class of drugs called "calcium antagonists,"[148–150] oral and intravenous forms of verapamil have recently been approved for clinical use. Oral nifedipine has also been approved for clinical use, but since it exhibits minimal electrophysiological effects at clinically used doses, it will not be discussed here (see p. 1351). Diltiazem has electrophysiological actions similar to verapamil[151,152] but at the time of this writing is approved for use only in the treatment of angina in the United States.

Electrophysiological Actions (Tables 20–2 and 20–3). By blocking the slow inward current (see p. 615) verapamil exhibits electrophysiological effects different from those of other antiarrhythmic agents. In concentrations comparable to those achieved clinically, verapamil, in vitro, does not affect the action potential amplitude, $\dot{V}$max of phase 0, or resting membrane voltage in cells that have fast-response characteristics (atrial and ventricular muscle, the His-Purkinje system). The plateau height of the action potential may be reduced, muscle action potential slightly shortened, and total Purkinje fiber action potential slightly prolonged.[149,153–155] However, in fast-channel cells rendered abnormal by disease, these concentrations of verapamil may suppress electrical activity in atrial[156] or ventricular[157,158] muscle fibers that have reduced resting potentials, suggesting that activity in these cells depends on transmembrane ionic flux through the slow channel. Similarly, verapamil suppresses slow responses elicited by a variety of experimental methods.[148,149] Verapamil also suppresses triggered sustained rhythmic activity and early and late afterdepolarizations (see p. 620). Verapamil and other slow-channel blockers in concentrations that do not affect action potentials of fast-channel dependent cells suppress activity in the normal sinus and AV nodes.[159–165] Verapamil depresses the slope of diastolic depolarization in sinus nodal cells, $\dot{V}$max of phase 0, maximum diastolic potential, and action potential amplitude in the sinus and AV nodal cells and prolongs conduction time and the effective and functional refractory periods of the AV node. The blocking effects of verapamil are more apparent at faster rates of stimulation (use-dependency).

It is important to remember, however, that verapamil does exert some local anesthetic activity[9] because the dextrorotatory stereoisomer of the clinically used racemic mixture exerts slight blocking effects on the fast sodium current. The levorotatory stereoisomer blocks the slow inward current carried by calcium, as well as other ions, traveling through the slow channel. Verapamil does not modify calcium uptake, binding, or exchange by cardiac microsomes nor does it affect calcium-activated ATPase.[166] Verapamil does not block beta receptors, but recent data suggest that it may block alpha receptors. Verapamil may also exert other effects that indirectly alter cardiac electrophysiology, such as decreasing platelet adhesiveness or reducing the extent of myocardial ischemia.[167]

In vivo, both in experimental animals and man, verapamil prolongs conduction time through the AV node (the A-H interval) without affecting the P-A, H-V, or QRS intervals and lengthens the functional and effective refractory periods of the AV node.[168] Spontaneous sinus rate may decrease slightly, an event only partially reversed by atropine. More commonly, the sinus rate does not change significantly in vivo because verapamil causes peripheral vasodilation, transient hypotension, and reflex sympathetic stimulation that mitigates any direct slowing effect verapamil may exert on the sinus node. If verapamil is given to a patient who is also receiving a beta blocker, the sinus nodal discharge rate may slow because reflex sympathetic stimulation is blocked.[169] Verapamil does not exert a direct effect on atrial or ventricular refractoriness or on antegrade or retrograde properties of accessory pathways.[170–172] However, reflex sympathetic stimulation may affect the electrophysiological properties of these fibers and, for example, increase the ventricular response during atrial fibrillation in patients with the Wolff-Parkinson-White syndrome.[171,173] Reflex sympathetic stimulation does not eliminate the direct effects of verapamil on AV nodal properties.

Hemodynamic Effects. Since verapamil interferes with excitation-contraction coupling, it inhibits vascular smooth muscle contraction and causes marked vasodilation in coronary and other peripheral vascular beds.[92] Propranolol does not block the vasodilation produced by verapamil. Reflex sympathetic effects may reduce in vivo the marked negative inotropic action of verapamil on isolated cardiac muscle, but direct myocardial depressant effects of verapamil may predominate when the drug is given in high doses. In patients with well-preserved left ventricular function, combined therapy with propranolol and verapamil appears to be well tolerated,[174] but beta blockade can accentuate the hemodynamic depressant effects produced by oral verapamil.[175] Patients who have reduced left ventricular function may not tolerate the combined blockade of beta receptors and of slow channels and the combined use of verapamil and propranolol in these patients must be undertaken cautiously or not at all. Verapamil decreases myocardial demand for oxygen while decreasing coronary vascular resistance[166] and reduces the extent of ischemic damage in experimental preparations.[176,177] Such changes may be antiarrhythmic.[177,178]

Peak alterations in hemodynamic variables occur 3 to 5 minutes after completion of the verapamil injection, the major effects being dissipated within 10 minutes.[92] Mean arterial pressure decreases and left ventricular end-diastolic pressure increases; systemic resistance decreases and left ventricular dP/dt max decreases. Heart rate, cardiac index, left ventricular minute work, and mean pulmonary artery pressure do not change significantly. Thus, afterload reduction produced by verapamil significantly minimizes its negative inotropic action so that cardiac index may not be reduced. In addition, when verapamil slows the ventricular rate in a patient with a tachycardia, cardiac slowing may also improve hemodynamics. Nevertheless, caution should be exercised when giving verapamil to patients with severe myocardial depression or those receiving beta blockers or disopyramide, because hemodynamic deterioration may progress in some patients.

Pharmacokinetics (Table 20–1). Following single oral doses of verapamil, measurable effects on AV nodal conduction time occur in 30 minutes and last for as long as six hours.[179] After intravenous administration, the onset of action on AV nodal conduction occurs within 1 to 2 minutes. Changes in the A-H interval are still detectable after six hours[180] and correlate with the plasma concentration of verapamil.[181] Effective plasma concentrations necessary to terminate supraventricular tachycardia are in the range 125 ng/ml following doses of 0.075 mg/kg to 0.150 mg/kg.[182] After oral administration absorption is almost complete, but an overall bioavailability of 10 to 35 per cent suggests substantial first-pass metabolism in the liver. The elimination half-life of verapamil is 3 to 8 hours, with up to 70 per cent of the drug excreted by the kidneys. In patients with atrial fibrillation, an intravenous bolus of 15 mg results in an elimination half-life of 8 hours for verapamil and 10.5 hours for norverapamil, a major metabolite that may contribute to verapamil's electrophysiological actions.[183] Serum protein binding is approximately 90 per cent.[184]

Dosage and Administration (Table 20–1). The most commonly used intravenous dose is 10 mg infused over 1 to 2 minutes while cardiac rhythm and blood pressure are monitored. A second injection of equal dose may be given 30 minutes later. The initial effect achieved with the first bolus injection, such as slowing of the ventricular response during atrial fibrillation, may be maintained by a continuous infusion of the drug at a rate of 0.005 mg/kg/min. The oral dose is 80 to 120 mg, given three or four times a day.[171]

Clinical Indications. Intravenous verapamil is the treatment of choice for terminating sustained paroxysmal supraventricular tachycardia that does not terminate following simple vagal maneuvers. Verapamil should definitely be tried prior to attempting termination by digitalis administration, pacing, electrical direct-current cardioversion, or acute blood pressure elevation with vasopressors. This recommendation applies to sinus nodal reentry or to any supraventricular tachycardia, such as AV nodal reentry or reciprocating tachycardias associated with the Wolff-Parkinson-White syndrome, when one of the reentrant pathways is the AV node. Verapamil terminates more than 80 per cent of episodes of paroxysmal supraventricular tachycardias within several minutes.[171,182,185] In patients with AV nodal reentry, the most common mechanism of termination appears to be block in the anterograde or slowly conducting pathway, with block less often in the fast pathway conducting retrogradely.[171,182] In patients who experience reciprocating tachycardias during the Wolff-Parkinson-White syndrome, block terminating the tachycardia almost exclusively occurs in the AV node, not in the accessory pathway.[171]

Verapamil decreases the ventricular response over the AV node in the presence of atrial fibrillation or atrial flutter,[186,187] converting a small number of episodes to sinus rhythm, particularly if the atrial flutter or fibrillation is of recent onset. Some patients who exhibit atrial flutter may develop atrial fibrillation following verapamil administration. Quinidine appears to be more effective than verapamil in establishing and maintaining sinus rhythm in patients with chronic atrial fibrillation.[50] As noted earlier, in patients with atrial fibrillation associated with the Wolff-Parkinson-White syndrome, verapamil may accelerate the ventricular response, and therefore the drug is relatively contraindicated in that situation.[171,173] Less information is available regarding the efficacy of verapamil in treating other types of supraventricular tachycardia. Verapamil may terminate supraventricular tachycardia due to sinus nodal reentry and occasionally may terminate ectopic atrial tachycardias.

Orally, verapamil may prevent the recurrence of AV nodal reentrant and reciprocating tachycardias associated with the Wolff-Parkinson-White syndrome as well as help maintain a decreased ventricular response during atrial flutter or atrial fibrillation.[188] In this regard, the effectiveness of verapamil appears to be enhanced when given concomitantly with digitalis.[171] Verapamil generally has not been effective in treating patients who have recurrent ventricular tachyarrhythmias.[189] However, data from animal models suggest that verapamil may be useful in reducing or preventing ventricular arrhythmias due to acute myocardial ischemia,[177,178] and conceivably, this agent may be useful to help prevent sudden death after acute myocardial infarction.[167]

Adverse Effects. Verapamil must be used cautiously in patients with significant hemodynamic impairment or in those receiving beta blockers, as previously noted. Hypotension, bradycardia, AV block, and asystole are more likely to occur when the drug is given to patients who are already receiving beta blocking agents. Verapamil should also be used with caution in patients with sinus nodal abnormalities, since marked depression of sinus nodal function or asystole may result in some of these patients.[190] Isoproterenol, calcium, glucagon infusion, or atropine (which may be only partially effective) and temporary pacing may be necessary to counteract some of the adverse effects of verapamil. Isoproterenol may be more effective for treating bradyarrhythmias and calcium for treating hemodynamic dysfunction. Contraindications to the use of verapamil include the presence of advanced heart failure, second- or third-degree AV block without a pacemaker in place, significant sinus node dysfunction, cardiogenic shock, or other hypotensive states. While the drug probably should not be used in patients with manifest heart failure, if the latter is due to a supraventricular tachyarrhythmia, verapamil may restore sinus rhythm or significantly decrease the ventricular rate, leading to hemodynamic improvement. Finally, it is important to note that verapamil may decrease the excretion of digoxin by about 30 per cent. Hepatotoxicity may occur on occasion.

NEW ANTIARRHYTHMIC AGENTS
(Tables 20–1 to 20–3)

In the last several years, many new antiarrhythmic agents have been developed and are now undergoing clinical testing in the United States and other countries. The following discussion will serve as a brief review of selected investigational drugs.

Amiodarone. Amiodarone is a benzofuran derivative that was introduced more than 15 years ago as a smooth muscle relaxant and coronary vasodilator to treat patients with angina. Subsequently, its antiarrhythmic actions were noted.[92,191,192] Amiodarone prolongs action potential duration and refractoriness in atrial and ventricular muscle and Purkinje fibers,[92,191] decreases the slope of diastolic depolarization of sinus nodal activity, and minimally decreases $\dot{V}max$ of phase 0 and resting membrane potential of Purkinje fibers.[192] In vivo, amiodarone suppresses arrhythmias induced experimentally by a variety of means. It slows spontaneous sinus nodal discharge rate in anesthetized dogs even after pretreatment with propranolol and atropine. In patients, it prolongs the Q-T interval and often produces sinus bradycardia. Right atrial monophasic action potentials are prolonged[193] as is the effective refractory period of atrial and ventricular muscle, accessory pathways, and the AV node following oral administration. Amiodarone given intravenously does not prolong the refractory period of atrial or ventricular muscle. P-R interval and AV nodal conduction time lengthen but the QRS complex does not.[194–196] Amiodarone apparently exerts a moderate antiadrenergic effect that is still incompletely characterized.[92]

When administered intravenously in doses of 2.5 to 10 mg/kg, amiodarone decreases heart rate, systemic vascular resistance, left ventricular contractile force, and left ventricular dP/dt. However, left ventricular output increases.[92] Peak plasma concentrations occur approximately 4 hours after a single oral dose, with an elimination half-life of approximately 5 hours. The onset of action is 5 to 10 minutes after intravenous administration. Steady-state plasma concentrations are reached 2 to 4 weeks after oral therapy is begun, producing therapeutic plasma concentrations ranging from 1 to 3 μg/ml. Suppression of cardiac arrhythmias may require therapy for 10 to 14 days or longer, although some patients respond sooner. Estimated elimination half-life after achieving steady state ranges between 30 and 50 days and amiodarone's antiarrhythmic action may last several weeks after cessation of drug therapy. Thus, based on preliminary data, the drug is cleared rapidly after single doses but slowly after chronic dosing, and it can still be found in the serum one year after cessation of oral therapy.[197] The intravenous dose is 5 to 10 mg/kg and the oral maintenance dose ranges between 200 and 800 mg daily. Higher loading doses have been recommended. To minimize side effects, the maintenance dose should be reduced to the lowest effective amount.

Amiodarone exhibits a broad spectrum of antiarrhythmic efficacy and suppresses a variety of supraventricular and ventricular tachyarrhythmias in adults as well as in children.[195,198–200] Although drug-resistant ventricular tachyarrhythmias can be suppressed, it is of interest that the response of the patient to premature ventricular stimulation during electrophysiological study does not appear to predict the clinical outcome.[195,201] Ventricular tachycardia can still be induced with premature stimulation in many patients who are taking the drug who do not develop a spontaneous recurrence. Even though amiodarone prolongs the Q-T interval, it may suppress arrhythmias in patients with the long Q-T syndrome.[202] Amiodarone may prevent recurrence of AV nodal reentry, reciprocating tachycardias associated with the Wolff-Parkinson-White syndrome, recurrent atrial flutter, and atrial fibrillation.[191]

Adverse effects include corneal microdeposits, bluish skin discoloration, neuromuscular disturbances (particularly at higher doses), elevation (often transient) of hepatic enzymes, hyper- or hypothyroidism, pulmonary alveolitis, and fibrosis.[195,203] Cardiovascular toxicity is minimal, although marked sinus bradycardia requiring pacemaker implantation may occur on occasion.[195] Amiodarone may elevate digitalis levels and may increase the anticoagulant effects of warfarin drugs.

Aprindine. Aprindine exerts prominent local anesthetic effects. In isolated cardiac preparations, aprindine shortens the duration of the action potential more than it shortens the effective refractory period of Purkinje fibers. In cardiac muscle fibers, action potential duration is slightly reduced while the effective refractory period is lengthened.[204–206] $\dot{V}max$ of phase 0 is depressed (more so at rapid rates) at higher extracellular potassium concentrations and to a greater degree than exerted by comparable amounts of lidocaine. Spontaneous phase 4 diastolic depolarization in Purkinje fibers is also depressed or abolished. Aprindine reduces digitalis-induced increases in potassium permeability and suppresses transient depolarizations caused by acetylstrophanthidin in canine Purkinje fibers.[204,207] At slightly elevated concentrations, aprindine depresses slow-channel–dependent membrane oscillations and both the fast and slow inward currents.[206] In intact dogs, aprindine injected into the sinus nodal artery decreases the spontaneous sinus rate; injected into the AV nodal artery, it prolongs the functional refractory period and conduction time of the AV node.[208] Aprindine slows conduction in all cardiac tissues and prolongs the refractory period of the ventricle. It exacerbates ischemia-induced conduction delay and increases the incidence of ventricular arrhythmias induced by acute coronary artery occlusion in dogs[209] when given prior to the occlusion, probably because of increased concentration in the ischemic zone.[2] Therapeutic doses mildly depress myocardial function, slightly decreasing systolic and mean aortic blood pressure during exercise, myocardial contractility, and peak left ventricular dP/dt. Aprindine is well absorbed, has high systemic bioavailability, and is 85 to 95 per cent protein-bound.

Approximately 95 per cent of the hydroxylated metabolites undergo glucuronidation in the liver. Sixty-five per cent of aprindine and its metabolites are found in the urine, with the remaining 35 per cent in the feces. Elimination half-life ranges between 20 and 30 hours. In patients treated chronically with aprindine, the N-desethyl metabolite is present in small amounts in the plasma and exerts some antiarrhythmic actions. Clinically, the full antiarrhythmic effect of aprindine may not occur for several days, even when the drug is administered initially in a loading dose.[147,210] Aprindine is given orally in loading doses of 100 mg every six hours for the first day, 75 mg every six hours the second day, and 50 mg every six hours the third day. The dose is then adjusted, with most patients requiring and tolerating 100 to 150 mg/day, which produces a mean plasma concentration of 1 to 2 μg/ml. Intravenous doses are similar.[211] Response to intravenous aprindine during electrophysiological study in patients who had recurrent ventricular arrhythmias appears to predict the subsequent response to the oral dose.[212]

Aprindine is effective in patients who have both supraventricular and ventricular tachyarrhythmias. Since it prolongs conduction time and refractoriness in the AV node and prolongs the refractory period of the accessory pathway in patients with the Wolff-Parkinson-White syndrome, it may be used to suppress arrhythmias in patients with AV nodal reentry and to produce block in the accessory pathway.[213] Aprindine also suppresses drug-resistant recurrent ventricular tachyarrhythmias[211] and may be useful in patients whose ventricular arrhythmias are associated with mitral valve prolapse[214] or due to digitalis. The toxic-therapeutic ratio for aprindine is narrow, and side effects are common, particularly during the initial loading period and adjustment of the maintenance dose. These side effects, related to the dose and serum concentration of aprindine, include most commonly a tremor of the hand and fingers. As the serum concentration increases, dizziness, intention tremor, ataxia, nervousness, hallucinations, diplopia, memory impairment, or seizures may occur. Neurological side effects are minimal or absent at serum aprindine concentrations less than 1 μg/ml. Cholestatic jaundice and agranulocytosis have been reported to occur generally between the fourth and sixteenth week of aprindine therapy. The estimated incidence of agranulocytosis is approximately 1 per cent, and the condition is reversible if the drug is discontinued in time. Aprindine may cause Q-T prolongation and polymorphous ventricular tachycardia.[215] A derivative, moxaprindine, has undergone preliminary clinical testing, and initial results are encouraging.[216,217]

Encainide. Encainide is a new antiarrhythmic agent that decreases phase 4 diastolic depolarization in Purkinje fibers and decreases action potential duration, $\dot{V}max$ of phase 0, and propagation velocity in atrial, ventricular, and Purkinje fibers without altering resting membrane potential. It does not affect the slow response in vitro. Encainide has several active metabolites, one of which is more potent than the parent compound.[218] In patients, oral encainide prolongs atrial, ventricular, and accessory pathway refractory periods; A-H and H-V intervals; and P-R, QRS, and Q-T intervals.[219] Active metabolites may contribute to its antiarrhythmic efficacy,[219,220] and variation in the conversion of encainide to its active metabolites may be a source of interpatient differences in drug response.[221] Encainide does not alter myocardial contractility or ejection indices in patients with relatively normal ventricular function; in those with markedly reduced ventricular function, as evidenced by elevated left ventricular end-diastolic pressures and reduced cardiac output, encainide further decreases cardiac output slightly.[222]

Encainide exhibits a wide range of bioavailability and a relatively short half-life of 3 to 4 hours. However, the existence of one or more active metabolites permits a long interval between dosing during which the concentration of encainide metabolites exceeds that of the parent compound and is probably responsible for the delayed return (13 hours) of arrhythmias following drug withdrawal.[223] The drug is useful in treating some patients who have supraventricular tachycardias associated with AV nodal reentry or Wolff-Parkinson-White syndrome.[219,224] Encainide suppresses premature ventricular complexes,[225,226] is effective in about 25 to 30 per cent of patients with chronic recurrent ventricular tachyarrhythmias refractory to conventional agents,[227,228] and has a wide therapeutic-to-toxic ratio.[223] Encainide is generally administered orally four times daily in doses of 100 to 300 mg/day. Dose changes should not be made more frequently than every 48 hours. Adverse effects include dizziness, diplopia, vertigo, paresthesia, leg cramps, and a metallic taste in the mouth. Most significant is its potential to cause or exacerbate serious ventricular tachyarrhythmias in approximately 10 per cent of patients treated. Commonly, a polymorphous ventricular tachycardia ensues and may result in hemodynamic collapse. Often, this is not associated with marked Q-T prolongation and may not terminate spontaneously.[229,230]

Mexiletine. Mexiletine, a local anesthetic with anticonvulsant properties, is similar to lidocaine in many of its electrophysiological actions. In vitro, mexiletine shortens the duration of action potential and refractory period, depresses $\dot{V}max$ of phase 0, and depresses automaticity of Purkinje fibers but not of the normal sinus node.[92,231] It may result in severe bradycardia and abnormal sinus nodal recovery time in patients with sinus node disease and may depress His-Purkinje conduction in some patients. The effects of mexiletine on sinus and AV nodal properties appear to be variable,[227] possibly because mexiletine may produce different results when tested on abnormal tissue, as may lidocaine. Mexiletine does not appear to affect the refractory period of human atrial and ventricular muscle.

Mexiletine has been reported to be rapidly and almost completely absorbed after oral ingestion by volunteers, with peak plasma concentrations attained in 2 to 4 hours. Elimination half-life in healthy subjects is approximately 10 hours and in patients after myocardial infarction, 17 hours.[92] Therapeutic plasma levels of 1 to 2 μg/ml are maintained by oral doses of 200 to 300 mg every six to eight hours. Absorption is delayed and incomplete in patients who have myocardial infarction and in patients receiving narcotic or analgesic agents that retard gastric emptying.[232] Bioavailability of orally administered mexiletine is approximately 90 per cent, and about 70 per cent of the drug is protein-bound. The apparent volume of distribution is large, reflecting extensive tissue uptake. Normally, mexiletine is eliminated metabolically by the liver, with less than 10 per cent excreted unchanged in the urine. Renal clearance of mexiletine decreases as urinary pH increases.

Several European studies have shown mexiletine to be an effective antiarrhythmic agent for both acute and chronic ventricular arrhythmias.[233,234] Experience in the United States has yielded mixed results. Data from one study of patients who had recurrent ventricular arrhythmias resistant to conventional drugs revealed that only 4 of 19 demonstrated sufficient tolerance of the drug and antiarrhythmic efficacy to continue long-term therapy.[235] However, other studies[236,237] have had more encouraging results, and it seems clear that mexiletine can be effective in some patients with recurrent ventricular tachyarrhythmias. The combinations of mexiletine and amiodarone[238] and mexiletine and disopyramide[102] have been reported to be particularly efficacious. Thirty to 40 per cent of patients may require a change in dose or discontinuation of mexiletine therapy as a result of adverse effects,[239] including tremor, dysarthria, dizziness, paresthesia, diplopia, nystagmus, mental confusion, anxiety, nausea, vomiting, and dyspepsia. Cardiovascular side effects are most often seen after intravenous dosing and include hypotension, bradycardia, and exacerbation of arrhythmia.[240] Adverse effects of mexiletine appear to be dose-related and toxic effects occur at plasma concentrations only slightly higher than therapeutic levels. Therefore, effective use of this antiarrhythmic drug requires careful titration of dose and monitoring of plasma concentration.

Tocainide. Tocainide, a primary amine analog of lidocaine that is effective orally, exerts electrophysiological effects very similar to those of lidocaine.[241] In patients with compensated left ventricular dysfunction, intravenous infusion of tocainide moderately decreases mean arterial pressure and slightly increases pulmonary and systemic vascular resistance and left ventricular end-diastolic pressure without altering heart rate, cardiac index, or left ventricular dP/dt.[242] Bioavailability of tocainide is almost 100 per cent, with virtually no hepatic first-pass effect, which is significantly different from lidocaine. The drug is rapidly and completely absorbed, yielding peak plasma concentrations 1 to 1.5 hours after oral ingestion. Oral regimens of 400 to 600 mg every eight hours produce therapeutic plasma concentrations of 6 to 12 μg/ml. Elimination half-life is approximately 14 hours.

Although tocainide effectively reduces the frequency of premature ventricular complexes,[243,244] it has been less effective in preventing chronic recurrent ventricular tachycardia–ventricular fibrillation in some[227,242,245] but not all[246,247] studies. It did not reduce the incidence of ventricular fibrillation or symptomatic ventricular tachycardia in a double-blind controlled study of 112 patients after myocardial infarction.[248] Response to lidocaine therapy may help predict an individual's response to tocainide. If lidocaine fails to suppress the ventricular arrhythmia, tocainide has about a 15 per cent chance of being effective. If lidocaine suppresses the ventricular arrhythmia, tocainide has about a 60 per cent chance of being effective.[242,247] Adverse effects are dose-related, similar to those produced by lidocaine, and include nausea, vomiting, anorexia, tremulousness, memory impairment, skin rash, sweating, paresthesia, diplopia, dizziness, anxiety, and tinnitus. Occasionally, tocainide may produce pulmonary fibrosis or induce or aggravate ventricular arrhythmias.[247,249]

Ethmozine. Ethmozine is a phenothiazine derivative that decreases $\dot{V}max$ of phase 0, action potential amplitude, and action potential duration in canine Purkinje fibers and decreases the force of Purkinje fiber contraction.[250] Injected into the sinus or AV nodal arteries of dogs, ethmozine does not alter sinus discharge rate or AV nodal conduction at therapeutic concentrations[251] and produces minimal electrophysiological changes in patients.[252] It is well absorbed and extensively metabolized, but little is known about the potential activity of its metabolites. Ethmozine suppresses premature atrial and ventricular arrhythmias but the data from controlled studies are too preliminary at present to draw meaningful conclusions.[253] However, it appears to be well tolerated and offers promise as a new antiarrhythmic agent.

Flecainide. Flecainide exerts electrophysiological effects similar to those of quinidine and procainamide and exhibits a wide spectrum of antiarrhythmic effectiveness. The drug has an elimination half-life of about 20 hours and effectively suppresses premature ventricular complexes[254] and nonsustained episodes of ventricular tachycardia.[255] The effective dose is approximately 200 mg every 12 hours, producing therapeutic plasma concentrations of about 600 ng/ml.[254,255] Side effects in early studies have been minimal and include mild and transient neurological reactions such as blurred vision, lightheadedness, and headache. No significant adverse hemodynamic effects have been noted.[254] Flecainide prolongs conduction time in all cardiac fibers, so that intraatrial, AV nodal, His-Purkinje, and intraventricular conduction times lengthen. High-degree AV block may develop in patients with preexisting bundle branch block.[256] P-R, QRS, and Q-Tc intervals increase at increasing doses, in parallel with antiarrhythmic efficacy.[255] Q-T prolongation and ventricular tachycardia have been reported.[257]

Lorcainide. Lorcainide is an acetanilide derivative with local anesthetic effects that decreases $\dot{V}max$ of phase 0 and conduction velocity and slightly prolongs the effective refractory period of Purkinje fibers. It does not affect the slow response and prolongs conduction time in the atria, His-Purkinje system, and ventricles. Elimination half-life ranges in different studies between 5 and 12 hours.[258,259] Important first-pass hepatic effects that reduce bioavailability occur with single 100-mg doses, but bioavailability increases after higher and multiple doses.[258] Lorcainide appears effective against ventricular arrhythmias.[259,260] Insomnia is an important side effect that is effectively treated with diazepam and gradually disappears after continued dosing.

Propafenone. Propafenone appears to be a fairly well tolerated antiarrhythmic agent that prolongs sinus nodal recovery time and lengthens the effective refractory period of the atrium, AV node, ventricle, and accessory pathways.[261] Intraatrial, AV nodal, and His-Purkinje conduction times are prolonged. Elimination half-life is approximately 4 hours, with protein binding exceeding 90 per cent. Preliminary data indicate that this drug is effective against ventricular arrhythmias.[262]

Bethanidine. Bethanidine is a closely related chemical analog of bretylium with similar pharmacological and antifibrillatory actions on the ventricle. Unlike bretylium, bethanidine is rapidly and effectively absorbed after oral administration. Preliminary data demonstrate important antiarrhythmic efficacy.[263]

Other antiarrhythmic agents, such as clofilium,[264] meobentine, cibenzoline, sotalol, and antidepressant drugs such as imipramine and nortriptyline[265] are currently undergoing evaluation.

ELECTRICAL THERAPY OF CARDIAC ARRHYTHMIAS

DIRECT CURRENT CARDIOVERSION

The successful application of external cardioversion[266,267] culminated the research begun in 1899[268] and carried out subsequently by many investigators. Electrical cardioversion offers obvious advantages over drug therapy.[269] Under conditions optimal for close supervision and monitoring, a precisely regulated "dose" of electricity can restore sinus rhythm immediately and safely. The distinction between supraventricular and ventricular tachyarrhythmias—crucial to the proper medical management of arrhythmias—becomes less significant, and the time-consuming titration of drugs with potential side effects is abolished.

MECHANISMS. Electrical cardioversion appears to terminate most effectively those tachycardias presumed to be due to reentry, including atrial flutter and atrial fibrillation, AV nodal reentry, reciprocating tachycardias associated with Wolff-Parkinson-White syndrome, most forms of ventricular tachycardia, ventricular flutter, and ventricular fibrillation. The electric shock, by depolarizing all excitable myocardium, interrupts reentrant circuits, discharges foci, and establishes electrical homogeneity that terminates reentry. A shock that does not end the tachycardia may fail to depolarize critical areas involved in the maintenance of the tachycardia. A tachycardia that terminates and then restarts may be reinitiated by factors provoking the tachycardia in the first place. For example, a tachycardia can be considered according to conditions that initiate it and those that maintain it. A premature depolarization due to enhanced automaticity may initiate a tachycardia that is then maintained by reentrant excitation. Thus, a cardioversion shock may terminate the reentry but not affect the premature systole. The latter may restart the tachycardia after a short period of sinus rhythm. If the precipitating factors are no longer present, interrupting the tachyarrhythmia for only the brief time produced by the shock may prevent its return for long duration even though the anatomical and electrophysiological substrates required for the tachycardia are still present.

Tachycardias thought to be due to disorders of impulse formation (automaticity) include parasystole, some forms of atrial tachycardias with or without AV block, nonparoxysmal AV junctional tachycardia and accelerated idioventricular rhythms. An attempt to cardiovert these tachycardias electrically in most instances is not indicated for several reasons. First, the ventricular rate generally is not very fast and the patient is hemodynamically stable. The tachycardia may terminate spontaneously or with drug therapy. Second, digitalis toxicity may be a cause, in which case electrical countershock would be contraindicated. Third, if these arrhythmias are due to enhanced automaticity, the precipitating and maintaining mechanisms may be the same, i.e., accelerated phase 4 diastolic depolarization. Thus, an electric shock might only "reset" the pacemaker cycle, with the tachycardia continuing after the shock. It is possible that the shock can terminate tachycardias due to enhanced automaticity or triggered activity, but this notion is conjectural at present.

TECHNIQUE. After the procedure has been explained to the patient, a careful physical examination, including palpation of all pulses, should be performed prior to elective cardioversion. A 12-lead electrocardiogram is obtained before and after cardioversion as well as a rhythm strip during the electroshock. The patient should be "metabolically balanced," i.e., blood gases, pH, and electrolytes should be normal with no drug toxicity present. The patient should fast for 6 to 8 hours prior to the shock, if possible. Because patients receiving digitalis without clinical evidence of digitalis toxicity appear to be at low risk for serious postcardioversion ventricular arrhythmias, even when serum digoxin levels are modestly elevated,[270] it does not seem necessary to withhold digitalis for several days prior to elective cardioversion. Maintenance quinidine administration 1 to 2 days before electrical cardioversion of patients with atrial fibrillation may revert 10 to 15 per cent to sinus rhythm and help prevent recurrence of atrial fibrillation once sinus rhythm is restored.

Paddle placement, paddle size, and maximum delivered energy from the external cardioverter have been the subject of some recent controversy.[271–274] A paddle with a 12-cm diameter delivers maximum intracardiac current in dogs. Since the size and configuration of the dog's thorax differ considerably from those of man, the results in dogs may not be applicable to humans. Although 13-cm diameter paddles may not be too large for adult human hearts and should deliver increased intracardiac current,[275] the benefits of a larger paddle size have not been proved for man.[276] The amount of current reaching the heart significantly influences the effectiveness of the shock.[277] For example, an amount of current needed to depolarize a critical mass of excitable myocardial cells appears necessary to terminate fibrillation.[278] Doubling the amount of current that reaches the heart requires a fourfold increase in transthoracic energy.[277] However, it is generally agreed that defibrillators delivering larger energies than those currently commercially available probably are not necessary, even for very large patients,[279] particularly if paddles with large diameters are used. Larger paddles also distribute the intracardiac current over a wider area and may reduce shock-induced myocardial necrosis.

Paddles must be placed in firm contact with the chest wall[273] and are generally positioned in the left infrascapular region (on which the patient lies) and over the upper sternum at the third interspace (Fig. 20–5). A second position is one paddle to the right of the sternum at the level of the first or second rib and the other in the left midclavicular line at the fourth or fifth intercostal space. The effectiveness of these two positions appears fairly comparable.[273]

A synchronized shock, i.e., one delivered during the QRS complex, is used for all cardioversions except for very rapid ventricular tachyarrhythmias, such as ventricular flutter or fibrillation. Because myocardial damage increases directly with increases in applied energy, the minimum effective energy should be used. Therefore, shocks are "titrated" when the clinical situation permits. Except for atrial fibrillation, shocks in the range of 25 to 50 joules successfully terminate most nondigitalis-induced supraventricular tachycardias and should be tried initially. If unsuccessful, a second shock of higher energy may be delivered. The starting level to terminate atrial fibrillation

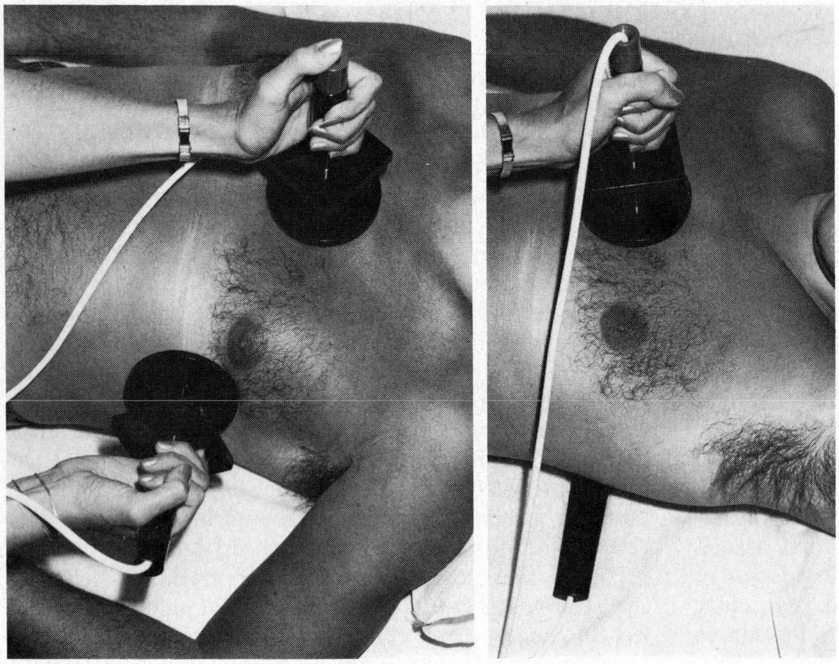

FIGURE 20–5 Paddle position for cardioversion. *Top,* The patient is lying on a flat posterior paddle centered at the tip of the left scapula; the anterior paddle is positioned just below the sternomanubrial joint. *Bottom,* The anterior paddle is in the same position, while the second paddle is placed over the cardiac apex.

should probably be 50 to 100 joules. For patients with stable ventricular tachycardia, starting levels in the range of 25 to 50 joules may be employed. If there is some urgency to terminate the tachyarrhythmia, one can begin with higher energies. To terminate ventricular fibrillation, 200 to 400 joules are used.

During elective cardioversion, a short-acting barbiturate, such as methohexital in intravenous doses of 25 to 75 mg, or an amnesic, such as diazepam given in incremental intravenous doses of 2.5 to 5 mg at 30-second intervals, may be used. A physician skilled in airway management should be in attendance (preferably an anesthetist, if possible), an intravenous route should be established, and all equipment necessary for emergency resuscitation should be immediately accessible. Before cardioversion, 100 per cent oxygen may be administered for 5 to 15 minutes and is continued throughout the procedure. Manual ventilation of the patient may be necessary to avoid hypoxia during periods of deepest sleep.

INDICATIONS. Before considering electrical cardioversion, the likelihood of establishing and maintaining sinus rhythm using electrical countershock should be weighed against the risks of other forms of therapy. As a rule, any tachycardia that produces complications such as hypotension, congestive heart failure, or angina and does not respond promptly to medical management should be terminated electrically. In almost all instances, the patient's hemodynamic status improves after cardioversion. An occasional patient may develop hypotension, reduced cardiac output, or congestive heart failure following the shock. The reasons for this are not entirely clear but may relate to complications of the cardioversion, such as embolic events, myocardial depression resulting from the anesthetic agent, hypoxia, or lack of restoration of left atrial contraction despite return of electrical atrial systole.[280] Direct-current countershock should not be used in patients with digitalis-induced tachyarrhythmias because electrical cardioversion in that situation may precipitate life-threatening ventricular tachyarrhythmias.

Favorable candidates for electrical cardioversion of atrial fibrillation include those patients who (1) have symptomatic atrial fibrillation and derive significant hemodynamic benefits from sinus rhythm; (2) have embolic episodes; (3) continue to have atrial fibrillation after the precipitating cause has been removed, e.g., following treatment of thyrotoxicosis, pericarditis or myocarditis, myocardial infarction, pneumonia, or pulmonary embolism or after corrective cardiac surgery; (4) have idiopathic atrial fibrillation of less than 12 months' duration; and (5) have a rapid ventricular rate that is difficult to slow. The success rate is high for maintaining sinus rhythm after electrical cardioversion of atrial fibrillation in patients with atria of normal size and in whom atrial fibrillation has been present for less than a year.

Unfavorable candidates for electrical cardioversion of atrial fibrillation include (1) patients with digitalis toxicity, (2) asymptomatic elderly patients who have a well-controlled ventricular rate without therapy, (3) patients with sinus node dysfunction and various unstable supraventricular tachyarrhythmias or bradyarrhythmias (often the bradycardia-tachycardia syndrome) who finally develop and maintain atrial fibrillation (which in essence represents a "cure" of the sick sinus syndrome), (4) those who derive little or no benefit from normal sinus rhythm and promptly revert to atrial fibrillation after cardioversion despite drug therapy, (5) those who have a large left atrium and atrial fibrillation of long standing, (6) those who have infrequent episodes of atrial fibrillation that revert spontaneously to sinus rhythm, (7) those in whom mechanical atrial systole does not accompany the return of electrical atrial systole, (8) those who have atrial fibrillation and advanced heart block, (9) those for whom cardiac surgery is planned in the near future, and (10) those who cannot tolerate antiarrhythmic drugs. Atrial fibrillation is likely to recur after cardioversion in patients who have significant chronic obstructive lung disease, congestive heart failure, or mitral valve disease, particularly mitral insufficiency.

In patients with atrial flutter, slowing the ventricular

rate by administering digitalis or terminating the flutter with quinidine may be difficult, so that electrical cardioversion appears to be the initial treatment of choice. For the patient with a supraventricular tachycardia, electrical cardioversion may be employed when maneuvers to enhance vagal tone or simple medical management have failed to terminate the tachycardia and the clinical setting indicates that fairly prompt restoration of sinus rhythm is desirable because of hemodynamic decompensation or electrophysiological consequences of the tachycardia (e.g., very rapid ventricular rates during atrial fibrillation in a patient with Wolff-Parkinson-White syndrome may progress to ventricular fibrillation). Similarly for patients with ventricular tachycardia, the hemodynamic and electrophysiological consequences of the arrhythmias—e.g., the adequacy of hemodynamic compensation during ventricular tachycardia or the possibility of ventricular tachycardia progressing to ventricular fibrillation—determine the need and urgency for direct current-cardioversion (p. 669). Electrical countershock is the initial treatment of choice for ventricular flutter or ventricular fibrillation.

If, after the first shock, reversion to sinus rhythm does not occur, a higher energy level should be tried. When transient ventricular arrhythmias result after an unsuccessful shock, a bolus of lidocaine may be given prior to delivering a shock at the next energy level. If sinus rhythm returns only transiently and is promptly supplanted by the tachycardia, a repeat shock may be tried, depending on the tachyarrhythmia being treated and its consequences. Administration of an antiarrhythmic agent intravenously may be useful prior to delivering the next cardioversion shock. After cardioversion, the patient should be monitored at least until full consciousness has been restored and preferably for several hours thereafter.

RESULTS. Cardioversion restores sinus rhythm in 70 to over 95 per cent of patients, depending upon the type of tachyarrhythmia.[268] But, as an example, less than one-third to one-half the patients with chronic atrial fibrillation remain in sinus rhythm after 12 months. Thus, maintenance of sinus rhythm once established is the difficult problem, not the immediate termination of the tachycardia, and depends on the particular arrhythmia, the presence of underlying heart disease, and the adequacy of antiarrhythmic drug therapy.

COMPLICATIONS. Arrhythmias after cardioversion may be produced by the clinical conditions that caused the initial tachycardia or the effects of the electrical discharge. Arrhythmias induced by the shock generally are caused by inadequate synchronization, with the shock occurring during the ST segment or T wave. It is important to remember that, occasionally, a properly synchronized shock may produce ventricular fibrillation (Fig. 20–6).[276] Post-shock arrhythmias usually are transient and do not require therapy. A variety of delayed tachyarrhythmias have been described, sometimes associated with quinidine or digitalis therapy, but their nature is not clear. In some instances, post-shock arrhythmias may be related to the significant autonomic discharge of thoracic parasympathetic and sympathetic nerve terminals produced by the transthoracic shock.[281,282] Generally these autonomic imbalances are tran-

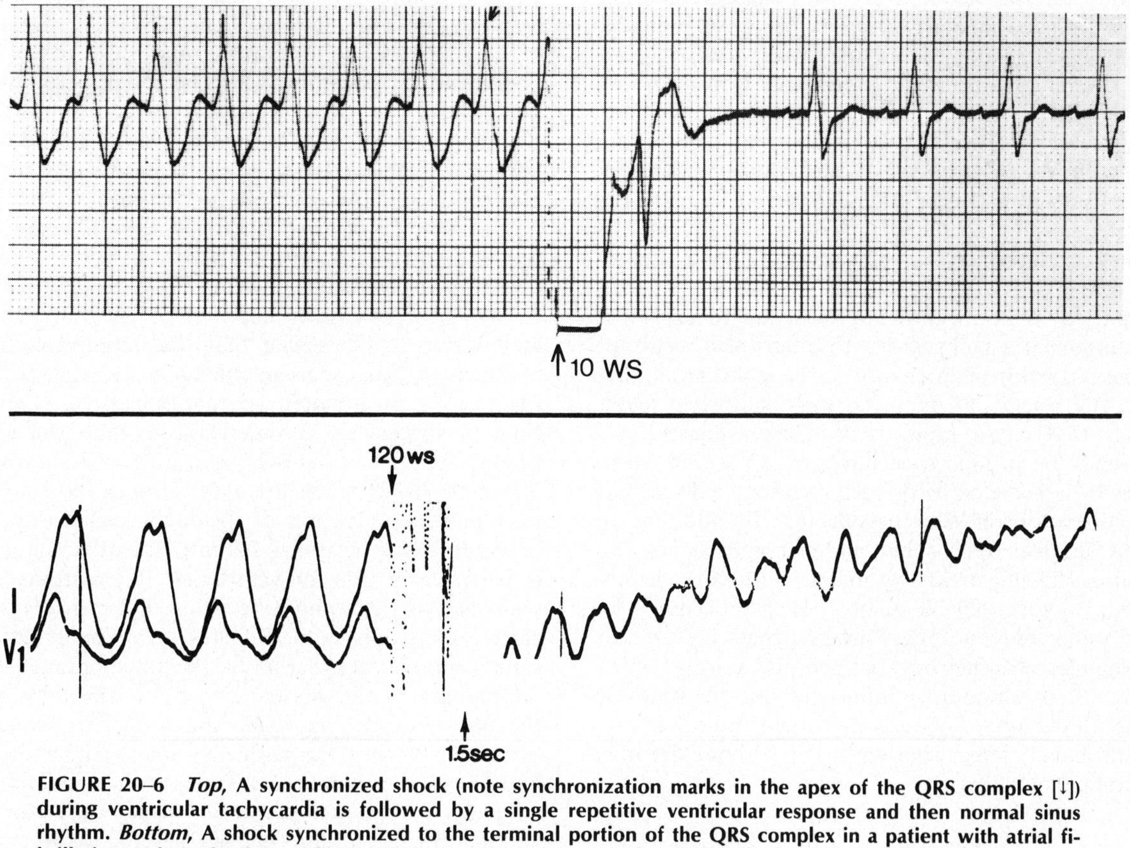

FIGURE 20–6 *Top,* A synchronized shock (note synchronization marks in the apex of the QRS complex [↓]) during ventricular tachycardia is followed by a single repetitive ventricular response and then normal sinus rhythm. *Bottom,* A shock synchronized to the terminal portion of the QRS complex in a patient with atrial fibrillation and conduction to the ventricle over an accessory pathway (WPW syndrome) results in ventricular fibrillation that was promptly terminated by a 400-msec shock. Recording was lost for 1.5 sec (↑) owing to baseline drift after the shock.

sient and do not require therapy. Embolic episodes are reported to occur in 1 to 3 per cent of the patients converted to sinus rhythm.[283,284] Prior anticoagulation for 1 to 2 weeks should be considered for patients who have no contraindication to such therapy and who are at high risk for emboli, such as those with mitral stenosis and atrial fibrillation of recent onset, a history of recent or recurrent emboli, a prosthetic mitral valve, enlarged hearts (including left atrial enlargement), or congestive heart failure.[283,284] Anticoagulation with warfarin for several weeks afterward is recommended. However, it must be emphasized that few controlled studies to support this approach have been published.

Although direct-current shock has been demonstrated in animals to cause cardiac injury,[285] studies in man indicate that elevations of myocardial enzymes after cardioversion are not common.[286] ST-segment elevation may occur with elective direct-current cardioversion, although cardiac enzymes and myocardial scintigraphy may be unremarkable.[287]

New Developments. Ultrasound cardioversion,[288] synchronized transvenous cardioversion by a catheter electrode,[289,290,290a] and defibrillation with implantable devices (see p. 729)[291–293] have all been developed recently. Several of these techniques have undergone clinical testing and offer great promise. Cardioversion of ventricular tachycardia can also be achieved by a chest thump.[294] Its mechanism of termination probably relates to a mechanically induced premature atrial or ventricular complex that interrupts a tachycardia. The thump cannot be timed very well and is probably only effective when delivered during a nonrefractory part of the cardiac cycle. Care must therefore be taken, because the thump can alter a ventricular tachycardia[295] and possibly induce ventricular flutter or fibrillation.[296]

PACEMAKER CONTROL OF CARDIAC ARRHYTHMIAS

Pacing for bradyarrhythmias is well established. More recently, pacing has been shown to terminate effectively a variety of supraventricular tachyarrhythmias. Its use for treating ventricular tachyarrhythmias is limited by its potential for exacerbating the rhythm disturbance (see Chap. 21).

SURGICAL THERAPY OF TACHYARRHYTHMIAS

Use of cardiac surgery to treat patients with recurrent symptomatic tachyarrhythmias has increased in frequency as knowledge about mechanisms of tachycardia and pathways involved in the maintenance of a tachycardia has been gained and new operative approaches have been developed. At present, patient selection remains relatively restricted to severely symptomatic individuals who have had recurrent arrhythmia despite adequate drug therapy. Conceivably, in some instances, such as recurrent tachycardia associated with Wolff-Parkinson-White syndrome, surgery might be considered early for a young person to spare the patient a lifetime of drug therapy, assuming that morbidity, mortality, and chances for surgical cure were acceptable.

The objectives of a surgical approach are to excise or isolate the origin of a tachycardia, to interrupt a reentrant pathway necessary for maintenance of the tachycardia, and to induce AV block in patients with supraventricular tachycardias that cause rapid ventricular responses. AV block also may be produced to interrupt a requisite reentrant pathway associated with reciprocating tachycardias in the Wolff-Parkinson-White syndrome. In addition to these direct surgical approaches, indirect approaches can be useful in selected patients by improving cardiac hemodynamics and myocardial blood flow. Such procedures include aneurysmectomy, coronary artery bypass grafting, or relief of valvular insufficiency or stenosis. Cardiac sympathectomy alters autonomic influences on the ventricle and has been effective in occasional patients who have recurrent ventricular tachycardia with[129] or without the long Q-T syndrome.[297–301]

SUPRAVENTRICULAR TACHYCARDIAS

At the present time, there are primarily three groups of patients who have symptomatic, drug-resistant, recurrent supraventricular tachycardias and are candidates for surgery: (1) those in whom the origin of the tachycardia is confined to a relatively localized area in the atrium; (2) those who have uncontrollably rapid ventricular rates during a supraventricular tachycardia and in whom creation of AV block is desirable; and (3) those with the preexcitation syndrome or one of its variants. Other groups, such as those with AV nodal reentrant tachycardia, may also be candidates in the future owing to the relative ease of creating AV block by means of a new catheter electrode technique.[302,303] Surgery is *not* indicated for eliminating episodes of atrial flutter or atrial fibrillation.

Preoperative assessment of these surgical candidates involves an electrophysiological study to determine whether the tachycardia can be initiated by programmed electrical stimulation to be certain that the initiated tachycardia is identical to that occurring clinically and that the tachycardia can be precipitated so that it can be studied at the time of surgery. It is important to map the tachycardia preoperatively (see below) because general anesthesia, cooling of the heart when the chest is open, and other factors may prevent induction of the tachycardia at surgery and preclude the opportunity for intraoperative mapping. (This is particularly true for ventricular tachycardias.) Also, for tachycardias that cannot be induced electrically, the preoperative electrophysiological study can be performed at a time when the tachycardia has begun spontaneously.

Mapping in the present context is the term applied to the procedure during which the activation sequence—i.e., the origin of and the pathways followed by the electrical impulse as it depolarizes the heart—is determined. Preoperatively, mapping is performed using catheters that bear at their tip electrodes that are several millimeters to one centimeter apart. For a supraventricular tachycardia, the catheter is positioned at various endocardial right atrial sites, around the margin of the tricuspid ring, and along the length of the coronary sinus to obtain recordings of left atrial activity at the region of the AV ring and, at times, through a probe-patent foramen ovale or by a trans-septal puncture to map left atrial endocardium. Local activation times recorded with the electrodes at the catheter tip are determined from the rapid component of unipolar electrode recordings or the first peak of the rapid inflection of bipolar recordings. The activation time along with the anatomical position of the electrode establish the site of the earliest area of activation and the subsequent activation sequence.

In patients with the Wolff-Parkinson-White syndrome, mapping can be performed to define both atrial and ventricular insertions of the accessory pathway. The *ventricular insertion* can be determined by locating the earliest site of ventricular activation when the ventricle is depolarized over the accessory pathway during stable sinus rhythm, during atrial pacing from a site near the accessory pathway, or during stable reciprocating tachycardia characterized by anterograde conduction over the accessory pathway and retrograde conduction over the normal pathway. Ventricular mapping of this type is very difficult to do with a catheter electrode and is best done at the time of surgery. Finding the shortest interval between the stimulus applied to various atrial sites and the delta wave of the QRS complex may be helpful, based on the assumption that the shortest interval results when the atrial pacing stimulus is delivered at a site closest to the accessory pathway. The *atrial insertion* of the accessory pathway is determined by locating the earliest site of atrial activation when the atrium is depolarized over the accessory pathway during ventricular pacing or during reciprocating tachycardia characterized by anterograde conduction over the normal pathway and retrograde conduction over the accessory pathway. Atrial mapping during tachycardia is preferable to be certain that the retrograde atrial activation is due solely to conduction over the accessory pathway and is not a fusion P wave. In some patients with multiple accessory pathways, the retrograde P wave may be a fusion of activation from two or more accessory pathways, and one must search carefully for the presence of multiple accessory pathways.[304] Accurate maps obtained in this fashion can localize the atrial and ventricular insertions of the accessory pathway to be opposite each other across the AV groove. Mapping is repeated at the time of operation.[305,306] In patients who have free-wall AV connections, the earliest epicardial activation of the ventricle occurs before or simultaneously with the onset of the delta wave, while in patients with septal connections, the area of earliest epicardial activation of the ventricle occurs after the onset of the surface delta wave.

Various surgical approaches have evolved during which an incision is made at the presumed insertion site of the accessory pathway and the dissection is extended for at least 1 cm on each side of this area. Accessory pathways can be buried in fat pads, can be positioned at the endocardium or epicardium, and may insert in the ventricular septum or free wall of either ventricle. Exceptionally careful dissection is required when the accessory pathway is in a paraseptal location to avoid damaging the AV node or His bundle. After the accessory pathway has been severed, an attempt is made to reinitiate the tachycardia and another map is obtained to be certain that the operation was successful and that no other accessory pathways exist. Since the first report of successful surgical interruption of an accessory pathway in a patient with the Wolff-Parkinson-White syndrome[307] significant experience has been gained that permits a direct approach to achieve interruption. In addition to cutting the connection, cryosurgery, which involves freezing a portion of the myocardium to interrupt conduction, has been used successfully in some patients.[308] Mortality from the operation is less than 1 to 2 per cent and the success rate for interrupting the AV connection and eliminating the tachycardia exceeds 90 per cent.[309]

Relatively little experience has been acquired with regard to the surgical treatment of supraventricular tachycardias due to abnormalities other than an accessory AV pathway.[310] When the atrial tachycardia is localized to a portion of the atrium, surgical excision of a focal area, such as in the atrial appendage, has effectively removed the tachycardia.[311,312] Of interest, microelectrode studies on the excised tissue in one patient revealed an inducible rhythm localized to a small area of the atrial endocardium, consistent with triggered activity.[311] Electrocautery[313] and cryosurgery[312] have eliminated tachycardia in several patients. In one patient, an encircling incision that contained the earliest point of activation during tachycardia excluded a portion of the left atrium and both pulmonary veins from the remainder of the left atrium[314] and isolated the tachycardia.

Interrupting the AV node–His bundle junction by suture, electrocauterization, incision of the septal portion of the right atrium, and cryothermic ablation have been used in patients with atrial tachycardias with rapid ventricular responses that cannot be slowed by means of drug therapy. Cryothermic ablation appears to represent a preferable technique[315,316] and also has been used to ablate an AV junctional tachycardia arising in the region of the His bundle.[312] Recently, a new technique has been devised to ablate the His bundle by delivering direct-current shocks through a catheter electrode positioned in the His bundle area. In effect, this approach cauterizes the area of His bundle to produce AV block and obviates cardiac surgery.[302,303] It offers a promising, minimally invasive approach to producing AV block and could conceivably be adapted to eliminate sites of ectopic arrhythmia formation or accessory pathways in other parts of the heart.

VENTRICULAR TACHYCARDIA

Surgical therapy for patients with recurrent, drug-resistant, symptomatic ventricular tachycardias is influenced by whether or not patients have ischemic heart disease.

ISCHEMIC HEART DISEASE. In almost all patients who have ventricular tachycardia associated with ischemic heart disease, the arrhythmia, regardless of its configuration on the surface ECG, arises in the left ventricle or on the left ventricular side of the interventricular septum.[317] The contour of the ventricular tachycardia may change either spontaneously or after premature stimulation from a right bundle branch block to a left bundle branch block pattern without a change in the earliest activation site, suggesting that the left ventricular site of origin remains the same, often near a left ventricular aneurysm, but its exit pathway is altered.[318]

Indirect surgical approaches, including cardiac thoracic sympathectomy, coronary artery bypass grafting, and ventricular aneurysm or infarct resection (without mapping) with or without bypass grafting, have been successful in about 60 per cent of reported cases.[319] Better patient selection would probably improve the success rate. For example, coronary artery bypass grafting limited to patients who experience ventricular tachycardia during documented exercise-induced ischemia can prevent recurrence of ventricular tachycardia in almost 100 per cent of patients.[320] However, the number of patients in this group is relatively small compared to the number of patients who have recurrent ventricular tachycardia unrelated to exercise but associated with ischemic heart disease, old myocardial infarction, and scarring. In these latter patients, three types of surgical procedures have been used: isolation, resection, and ablation.

The *encircling endocardial ventriculotomy*[321] involves a transmural ventriculotomy placed perpendicularly or obliquely,[322] relative to the endocardial wall to isolate areas of endocardial fibrosis that are recognized visually. The incision, sparing the epicardium and overlying coronary vessels, is then repaired. When the septum is involved, the ventriculotomy is approximately 1 cm in depth. The rationale for this procedure is to separate arrhythmogenic areas into small islands that become anatomically and electrophysiologically isolated. However, recent animal data suggest that cardiac blood flow to the isolated myocardium may be reduced, adversely affecting myocardial function.[319]

The rationale for the second approach, *endocardial resection,* is based in part on animal data indicating that arrhythmias in dogs subjected to myocardial infarction arise in the subendocardial borders between normal and infarcted tissue.[323] Endocardial resection involves peeling off a layer of endocardium, generally in the rim of an aneurysm, that has been demonstrated by means of mapping procedures to be the site of earliest activation recorded during the ventricular tachycardia (Fig. 20–7). This resection procedure may cause less disruption to the left ventricular wall than does the encircling endocardial ventriculotomy. Tachycardias arising from the papillary muscles cannot be approached in this fashion,[324] and the papillary muscle may need to be resected if the tachycardia arises in that area. Overall operative mortality for encircling ventriculotomy is slightly higher (13 per cent) than for endocardial resection (7 per cent), and the success rate with endocardial resection is somewhat higher compared to that of encircling endocardial ventriculotomy.[322] However, the number of patients treated with both procedures is still fairly small. Ablative procedures involving ventriculotomy and cryosurgery are mentioned below.

Electrophysiological mapping to find the site of earliest

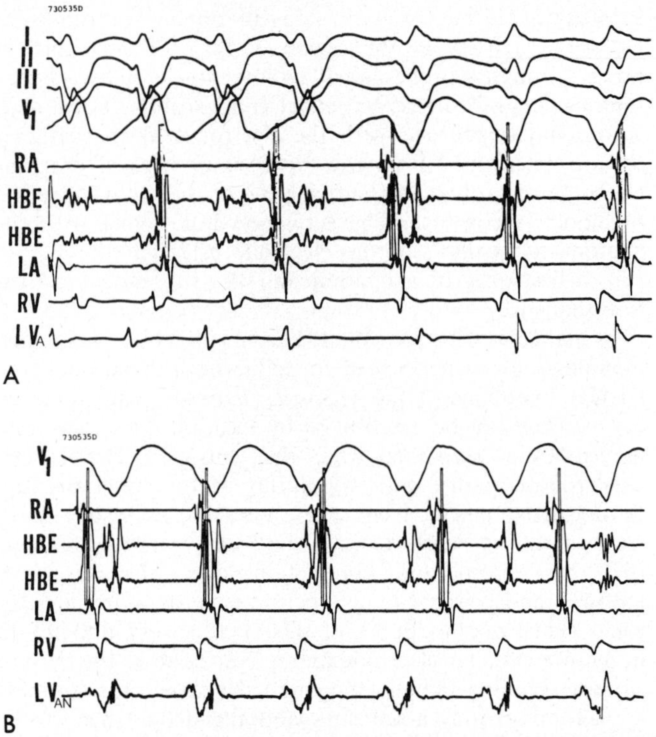

FIGURE 20–8 Spontaneous alteration in QRS contour during ventricular tachycardia. Premature right ventricular stimulation initiated a sustained ventricular tachycardia that initially exhibited a left bundle branch block contour (not shown). The QRS contour during the tachycardia spontaneously changed from left bundle branch block (LBBB) contour to right bundle branch block (RBBB) contour and back again (*A*). Note that ventricular activation recorded from the left ventricular apex during the RBBB contour tachycardia preceded right ventricular activation (*left*), but that left ventricular activation occurred after right ventricular activation during the LBBB contour tachycardia (*right*). Interpretation of these recordings might suggest that the tachycardia changed its site of origin from the left ventricle during the RBBB contour tachycardia to the right ventricle during the LBBB contour tachycardia. However, repositioning the catheter in the left ventricle to an area near the patient's ventricular aneurysm revealed that even during the LBBB contour tachycardia, an early site of activation in the left ventricle could be located, suggesting that the site of origin remained in the left ventricle and that the impulse simply exited in a different fashion to produce a change in the QRS complex[318] (*B*). I, II, III, and V_1 = scalar leads; RA = right atrial electrogram; HBE = His bundle electrogram; LA = left atrial electrogram via the coronary sinus; RV = right ventricular apical electrogram; LVA = left ventricular apical electrogram; LVAN = left ventricular electrogram near aneurysm.

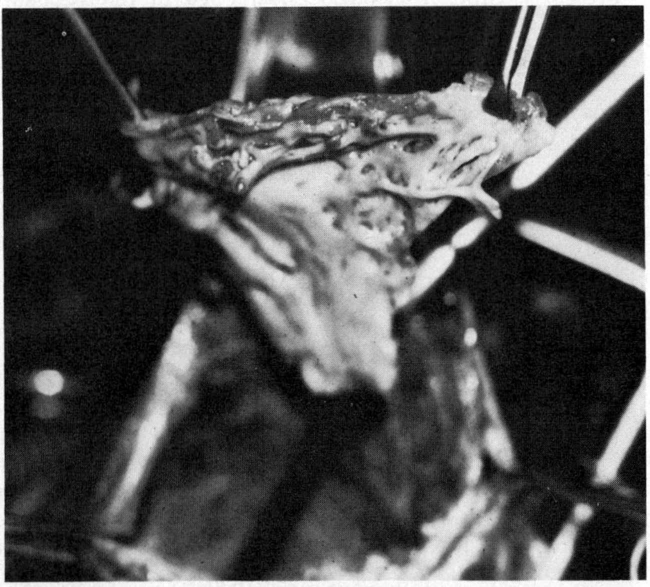

FIGURE 20–7 Endocardial resection. A piece of endocardium resected from the left ventricle in a patient with drug-resistant recurrent ventricular tachycardia. (Surgery was performed by John W. Brown, M.D.)

recorded activation during the ventricular tachycardia is generally used to pinpoint the area to be resected. To obtain a map preoperatively, catheters are positioned at multiple right and left ventricular sites and fluoroscopy directed in several planes establishes their anatomical position. Stable catheter positions are generally at the right ventricular apex, in the His bundle area, and often in the coronary sinus to provide reference electrograms and anatomical reference points to the septum (catheter at the right ventricular apex) and the posterobasal portion of the heart (coronary sinus catheter)[317,325] (Fig. 20–8). Tachycardias that are too rapid, short in duration, or pleomorphic cannot be accurately mapped. In such situations, administering a drug such as procainamide may slow the ventricular tachycardia and transform a nonsustained pleomorphic ventricular tachycardia into a sustained ventricular tachycardia of uniform contour that can be mapped.

Ventricular mapping is also performed at the time of surgery[306] using a handheld electrode moved from site to site. The activation time recorded by this electrode and its anatomical position are compared to the activation time recorded by stationary or reference electrodes fixed at particular positions on the right and left ventricles. The sequence of activation during ventricular tachycardia can then be plotted and the area of earliest activation determined (Figs. 20–9 and 20–10). Using a handheld probe, the ventricular tachycardia must be stable and of uniform configuration, generally for several hundred cycles. Recording from multiple sites simultaneously, coupled with on-line computer techniques that instantaneously provide an activation map cycle-by-cycle, reduces the time necessary to generate an activation sequence map and will greatly speed and simplify intraoperative mapping. *Cryothermal mapping and ablation* has also been used to confirm the site of origin of a ventricular arrhythmia and then to destroy it. A cryoprobe is cooled to 0°C and its influence on the arrhythmia is noted. If it terminates the tachycardia, the temperature is reduced to −60°C and the area frozen.[326]

Several points are worthy of emphasis. Recording electrical activity in damaged tissue may produce broad, low-amplitude electrograms that may originate from the tissue being sampled or from more distant sites; their onset is difficult to measure accurately. Timing of propagation may be distorted because of changing conduction velocities as the wavefront enters specialized conducting tissue, large muscle bundles, or damaged tissue. During ventricular tachycardia, the origin of the arrhythmia is generally ascribed to electrical activity recorded 25 to 50 msec in advance of the QRS complex. However, that is an arbitrary value, and it is quite clear that such activity may be late following the preceding cycle or early in advance of the next cycle. In addition, when such activity is recorded well after termination of the QRS complex, it becomes difficult to determine with certainty whether the deflections represent depolarization or repolarization. Potentials recorded *prior* to the onset of the surface QRS complex suggest that the origin of the tachycardia is nearby. When the earliest

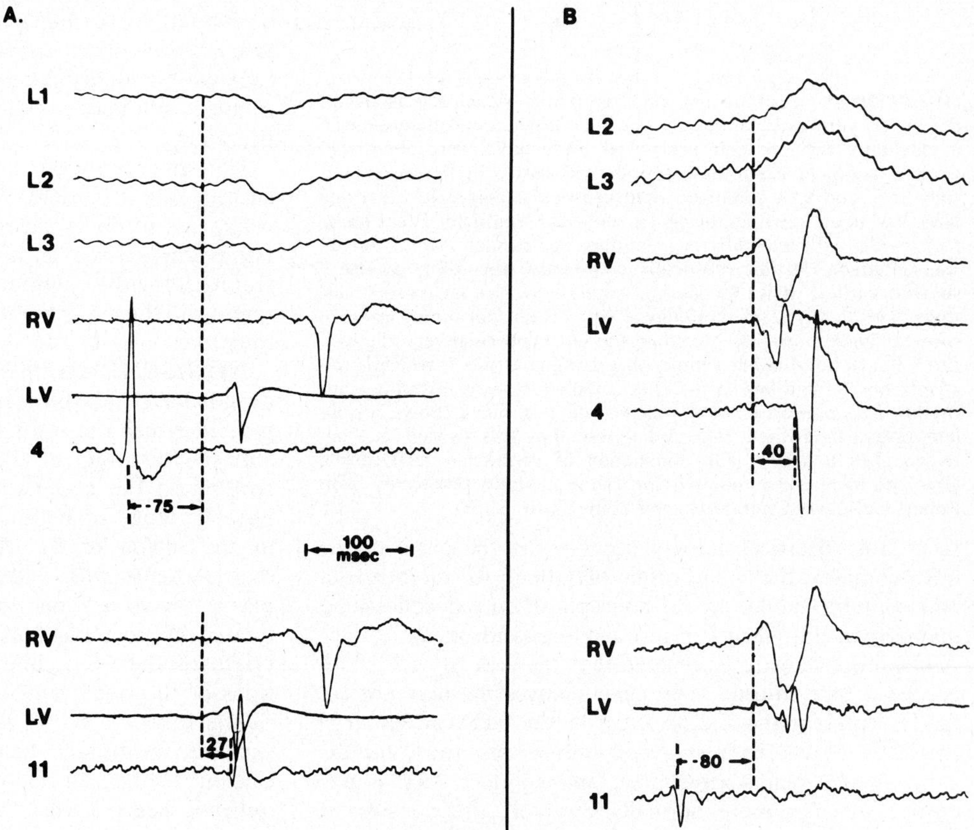

FIGURE 20–9 Intraoperative mapping for ventricular tachycardia. *A*, One beat of a ventricular tachycardia, as displayed in leads I, II, and III, is shown. Stationary reference electrodes have been sewn on the right ventricular (RV) and left ventricular (LV) epicardium. A handheld exploring electrode reveals that the earliest site of ventricular activation is recorded at site 4, 75 msec in advance of the QRS complex (dotted line). Site 11 (shown below) was activated 27 msec after onset of the QRS complex. Site 4 was resected and the ventricular tachycardia could no longer be initiated. *B*, Postoperatively the patient once again developed ventricular tachycardia but with a different contour (leads II and III). Surgery was repeated and mapping now illustrates that electrical activity was recorded first at site 11, 80 msec in advance of the QRS complex, while activity at site 4 occurred 40 msec after the onset of the QRS complex. Site 11 was resected, and this second form of ventricular tachycardia could no longer be initiated. The patient was discharged without antiarrhythmic drug therapy, with no recurrence of ventricular tachycardia during a follow-up period of one year. (Mapping was performed with the help of John W. Brown, M.D., Eric N. Prystowsky, M.D., and James J. Heger, M.D.)

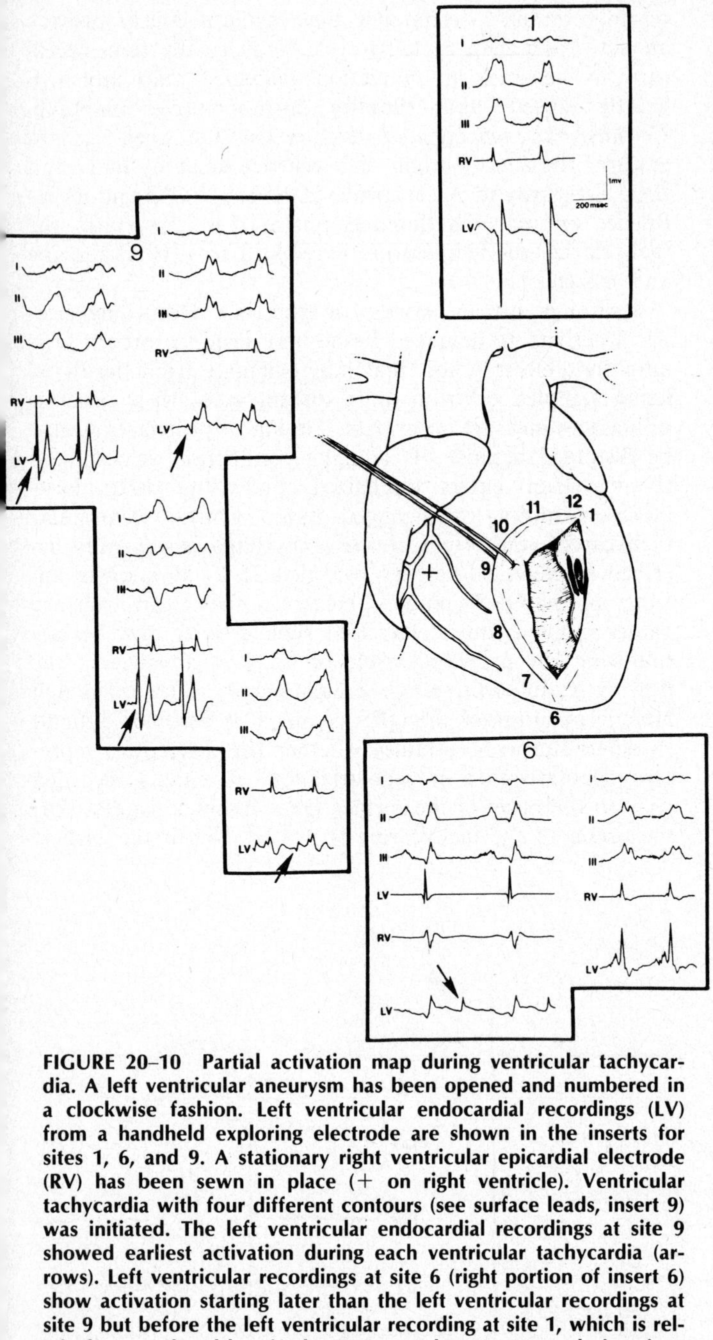

FIGURE 20–10 Partial activation map during ventricular tachycardia. A left ventricular aneurysm has been opened and numbered in a clockwise fashion. Left ventricular endocardial recordings (LV) from a handheld exploring electrode are shown in the inserts for sites 1, 6, and 9. A stationary right ventricular epicardial electrode (RV) has been sewn in place (+ on right ventricle). Ventricular tachycardia with four different contours (see surface leads, insert 9) was initiated. The left ventricular endocardial recordings at site 9 showed earliest activation during each ventricular tachycardia (arrows). Left ventricular recordings at site 6 (right portion of insert 6) show activation starting later than the left ventricular recordings at site 9 but before the left ventricular recording at site 1, which is relatively normal and late in the QRS complex. However, during sinus rhythm (left portion of insert 6), recording at site 6 shows a split, late potential (arrow). Endocardial resection was carried out between sites 6 and 9 with elimination of ventricular tachycardia. (Tracings have been redrawn for clarity.) (Study performed with Robert L. Rinkenberger, M.D., and Robert Kiny, M.D.)

recordable electrical activity occurs *after* the onset of the QRS complex, the site of origin may be in the interventricular septum (similar to the concepts discussed concerning mapping in the Wolff-Parkinson-White syndrome).

It is important to emphasize that the area of earliest recorded activity during ventricular tachycardia may not actually represent the site of origin of the tachycardia, since the latter may originate several centimeters away, for example in a small scarred area, and conduct very slowly until it reaches more normally excitable tissue where it generates a recordable extracellular complex. However, this area of early activation is probably closely related to the origin of the tachycardia and, based on our present state of knowledge and results from surgery, warrants surgical intervention at that site. Finding an area of "continuous electrical activity"[327] does not necessarily mean that reentry is present or that this is the origin of the tachycardia, since similar activity can be produced by automatically discharging foci; by recording slowly propagating, overlapping, or fragmented wavefronts from several areas;[328,329] or by recording repolarization activity. However, it is likely that the origin of the tachycardia is close by. Of interest is that the site of epicardial breakthrough may be distant from the earliest area of recordable endocardial activity,[317,325,325a] further emphasizing the need for endocardial mapping.

Mapping during sinus rhythm allows one to detect abnormal areas evidenced by delayed activation, fragmentation, abnormal Q waves, delayed potentials, and potentials with decreased voltage and very slow conduction.[325] This technique may also be useful to demonstrate that areas of early activation during ventricular tachycardia represent late activation during sinus rhythm.[319] Whether such abnormal electrograms during sinus rhythm can be used to identify patients prone to tachycardia or whether such areas should be resected is not clear.[330] Delayed epicardial potentials recorded during sinus ryhthm may not adequately localize the origin of the tachycardia in patients with ventricular tachycardia and ischemic heart disease.[325a]

Pace-mapping[331,332] involves stimulation of various ventricular sites to initiate a QRS contour that duplicates the QRS contour of the ventricular tachycardia, thus establishing the apparent site of origin of the arrhythmia. This technique is limited by several methodological problems and by the possibility that conduction arising from the same site of origin may change and produce a QRS contour with a totally different shape[318] and that stimulating a different site may produce QRS complexes of a similar appearance.

It is not clear whether mapping improves the surgical success rate in patients with ischemic heart disease[333–335] as it appears to do in patients with nonischemic heart disease (see below). However, myocardial resection guided by electrophysiological mapping may reduce the amount of tissue removed, thus helping to preserve myocardial contractile function.

NONISCHEMIC HEART DISEASE. In patients who do not have ischemic heart disease, tachycardias can originate in either the right or the left ventricle, and the type and site of origin of the ventricular tachycardia vary according to the underlying heart disease. In patients who have tetralogy of Fallot, ventricular tachycardia may arise in the region of the right ventricular infundibulectomy scar. Patients with arrhythmogenic right ventricular dysplasia[336] have a right ventricular tachycardia and can be treated by a simple ventriculotomy at the apparent site of origin of the ventricular tachycardia or by isolating portions of the right ventricular free wall from the remainder of the heart.[319,322,337,338] Mapping during sinus rhythm and sustained ventricular tachycardia has been successful in localizing ventricular tachycardia in some patients without ischemic heart disease.[338] The overall surgical success rate and low mortality for this group of patients are promising but still need improvement.[319,337,338] Similarly, mapping may help localize the origin of the ventricular tachycardia in some patients with cardiomyopathies.[326]

Patients who have prolonged Q-T or Q-U syndrome are thought to have arrhythmias due to preponderant left stellate sympathetic tone, and accordingly, left stellate ganglionectomy has been useful therapeutically.[129,339] In some patients with mitral valve prolapse and associated ventricular tachycardia, valve replacement may eliminate the tachycardia.[319]

Acknowledgment

For critical review of Chapters 19 and 20, the author thanks Charles Antzelevitch, Ph.D., Anton Becker, M.D., Robert F. Gilmour, Ph.D., James J. Heger, M.D., Eric N. Prystowsky, M.D., Roger Winkle, M.D., Kevin Browne, M.D., Donald Chilson, M.D., Richard Hauer, M.D., and Elwyn Lloyd, M.D. Unflagging secretarial help was provided by Lee Northcutt and Shirley Myers.

References

1. Giardina, E. G. V., and Bigger, J. T., Jr.: Procainamide against reentrant ventricular arrhythmias: Lengthening RV intervals of coupled ventricular premature depolarization as an insight into the mechanism of action of procainamide. Circulation *48*:959, 1973.
2. Nattel, S., Pederson, D. H., and Zipes, D. P.: Alterations in regional myocardial distribution and arrhythmogenic effects of aprindine produced by coronary artery occlusion in the dog. Cardiovasc. Res. *15*:80, 1981.
3. Heger, J. J., Prystowsky, E. N., and Zipes, D. P.: Clinical choice of antiarrhythmic drugs. *In* Josephson, M. E. (ed.): Ventricular Tachycardia—Mechanisms and Management. Mt. Kisco, N.Y., Futura Publishing Co., 1982.
4. Shanks, R. G., and Harrison, D. W.: Pharmacokinetic Principles in Cardiac Arrhythmias: A Decade of Progress. Boston, G. K. Hall, 1981, p. 91.
5. Fenster, P. E., and Perrier, D.: Applications of pharmacokinetic principles to cardiovascular drugs. Mod. Conc. Cardiovasc. Dis. *51*:91, 1982.
6. Goldstein, A., Arono, W. L., and Kalman, S. M.: Principles of Drug Action. New York, Harper and Row, 1968.
7. Bigger, J. T., Jr.: Management of arrhythmias. *In* Braunwald, E. (ed.): Heart Disease: A Textbook of Cardiovascular Medicine. Philadelphia, W. B. Saunders Co., 1980, p. 717.
8. Harrison, D. C., Meffin, P. J., and Winkle, R. A.: Clinical pharmacokinetics of antiarrhythmic drugs. Progr. Cardiovasc. Dis. *20*:217, 1977.
9. Singh, B. N., and Vaughn Williams, E. M.: A fourth class of antidysrhythmic action? Effects of verapamil on ouabain toxicity, on atrial and ventricular intracellular potentials and on other features of cardiac function. Cardiovasc. Res. *6*:109, 1972.
10. DuPuis, B. A., and Vincent, A. C.: Experimental arrhythmia models. Critical study of correlations with arrhythmias observed in clinical practice. Arch. Mal. Coeur *74*:17, 1978.
11. Hondeghem, L., and Katzung, B. G.: Test of a model of antiarrhythmic drug action. Effects of quinidine and lidocaine on myocardial conduction. Circulation *61*:1217, 1980.
12. Mandel, W. J., and Bigger, T. J., Jr.: Electrophysiological effects of lidocaine on isolated canine and rabbit atrial tissue. J. Pharmacol. Exp. Ther. *178*:81, 1971.
13. Bigger, J. T., Jr., and Mandel, W. J.: Effect of lidocaine on the electrophysiological properties of ventricular muscle and Purkinje fibers. J. Clin. Invest. *49*:63, 1970.
14. Singh, B. N., and Vaughn Williams, E. M.: Effect of altering potassium concentration on the action of lidocaine and diphenylhydantoin on rabbit atrial and ventricular muscle. Circ. Res. *29*:286, 1971.
15. Nattel, S., Elharrar, V., Zipes, D. P., and Bailey, J. C.: The pH dependent electrophysiological effects of quinidine and lidocaine on canine cardiac Purkinje fibers. Circ. Res. *48*:55, 1981.
16. Kupersmith, J., Antman, E. M., and Hoffman, B. F.: In vivo electrophysiological effects of lidocaine in canine acute myocardial infarction. Circulation *36*:84, 1975.
17. Kupersmith, J.: Electrophysiological and antiarrhythmic effects of lidocaine in canine acute myocardial ischemia. Am. Heart J. *97*:360, 1979.
18. El-Sherif, N., Scherlag, B. J., Lazzara, R., and Hope, R. R.: Reentrant ventricular arrhythmias in the late myocardial infarction period. 4. Mechanism of action of lidocaine. Circulation *56*:395, 1977.
19. Cardinal, R., Janse, M. J., vanEeden, I., Werner, G., d'Alnoncourt, C. N., and Durrer, D.: The effects of lidocaine on intracellular and extracellular potentials, activation, and ventricular arrhythmias during acute regional ischemia in the isolated porcine heart. Circ. Res. *49*:792, 1981.
20. Patterson, E., Gibson, J. K., and Lucchesi, B. R.: Electrophysiologic actions of lidocaine in a canine model of chronic myocardial ischemic injury. Arrhythmogenic actions of lidocaine. Circulation *64*(Suppl. IV):123, 1981.
21. Gilmour, R. F., Jr., and Zipes, D. P.: Electrophysiological response of vascularized hamster cardiac transplants to ischemia. Circ. Res. *50*:599, 1982.
22. Rosen, M. R., Merker, C., and Pippenger, C. E.: The effects of lidocaine on the canine ECG and electrophysiologic properties of Purkinje fibers. An effect on steady state sodium currents? Am. Heart J. *91*:191, 1976.
23. Colatsky, I.: Mechanisms of action of lidocaine and quinidine on action potential duration in rabbit cardiac Purkinje fibers. Circ. Res. *50*:17, 1982.
24. Arnsdorf, M. F., and Bigger, J. T., Jr.: Effect of lidocaine hydrochloride on membrane conductance in mammalian cardiac Purkinje fibers. J. Clin. Invest. *51*:2252, 1972.
25. Badui, E., Gracia-Rubi, D., and Estanol, B.: Inadvertent massive lidocaine overdose causing temporary complete heart block in myocardial infarction. Am. Heart J. *102*:801, 1981.
26. Kuo, C. S., and Reddy, C. P.: Effect of lidocaine on escape rate in patients with complete atrioventricular block. B. Proximal His bundle block. Am. J. Cardiol. *47*:1315, 1981.
27. Ruskin, J. N., Akhtar, M., Damato, A. N., and Foster, J. R.: The effect of lidocaine on reentry within the His-Purkinje system in man. Circulation *62*:388, 1980.
28. Miller, B. D., Mark, A. L., and Thames, M. D.: Inhibition of cardiac sympathetic nerve activity with intravenous administration of lidocaine. Circulation *64*(Suppl. IV):288, 1981.
29. Gilmour, R. F., Jr., Maesaka, J. F., Morrical, D. G., and Zipes, D. P.: Tetrodotoxin exacerbates ischemia-induced electrogram changes in the dog. Circulation *64*(Suppl. IV):192, 1981.
30. Neis, A. S., Shand, D. G., and Wilkinson, G. R.: Altered hepatic blood flow and drug disposition. Clin. Pharmacokinetics *1*:135, 1976.
31. Prescott, L. F., Adjepon-Yamoah, K. K., and Talbot, R. G.: Impaired lidocaine metabolism in patients with myocardial infarction and cardiac failure. Br. Med. J. *2*:939, 1976.
32. Lie, K. I., Leim, K. L., Louridtz, W. J., Janse, M. J., Willebrands, A. F., and Durrer, D.: Efficacy of lidocaine preventing primary ventricular fibrillation within one hour after a 300 mg intramuscular injection. A double-blind randomized study of 300 hospitalized patients with acute myocardial infarction. Am. J. Cardiol. *43*:486, 1978.
33. Nattel, S., and Zipes, D. P.: Clinical pharmacology of old and new antiarrhythmic drugs. Cardiovasc. Res. *11*:221, 1980.
34. Josephson, M. E., Kitchen, J. G., III, and Kastor, J. A.: Lidocaine and Wolff-Parkinson-White syndrome with atrial flutter. Ann. Intern. Med. *84*:44, 1976.
35. Akhtar, M., Gilbert, C. J., and Shenasa, M.: Effect of lidocaine on atrioventricular response via the accessory pathway in patients with Wolff-Parkinson-White syndrome. Circulation *63*:435, 1981.
36. Haynes, R. E., Chinn, T. L., Copass, M. K., and Cobb, L. A.: Comparison of bretylium tosylate and lidocaine in management of out-of-hospital ventricular fibrillation: A randomized clinical trial. Am. J. Cardiol. *48*:353, 1981.
37. Lie, K. I., Wellens, H. J., VanCapelle, F. J., and Durrer, D.: Lidocaine in the prevention of primary ventricular fibrillation. A double-blind randomized study of 212 consecutive patients. N. Engl. J. Med. *291*:132, 1974.
38. Pentecost, B. L., deGiovanni, J. V., Lamb, P., Cadigan, P. J., Evemy, K. L., and Flint, E. J.: Reappraisal of lignocaine therapy in management of myocardial infarction. Br. Heart J. *45*:42, 1981.
39. DeSilva, R. A., Hennekens, C. H., Lown, B., and Casscells, W.: Lignocaine prophylaxis an acute myocardial infarction: An evaluation of randomized trials. Lancet *2*:855, 1981.
40. Harrison, D. C.: Should lidocaine be administered routinely to all patients after acute myocardial infarction? Circulation *58*:581, 1978.
41. Mirro, M. J., Watanabe, A. M., and Bailey, J. C.: Electrophysiologic effects of the optical isomers of disopyramide and quinidine in the dog: Dependence on stereochemistry. Circ. Res. *48*:867, 1981.
42. Mason, J. W., Winkle, R. A., Rider, A. K., Stinson, E. E., and Harrison, D. C.: The electrophysiologic effects of quinidine in the transplanted human heart. J. Clin. Invest. *59*:481, 1977.
43. Mirro, M. J., Manalan, A. S., Bailey, J. C., and Watanabe, A. M.: Anticholinergic effects of disopyramide and quinidine on guinea pig myocardium: Mediation by direct muscarinic receptor blockade. Circ. Res. *47*:855, 1980.
44. Hoffman, B. F., Rosen, M. R., and Wit, A. L.: Electrophysiology and pharmacology of cardiac arrhythmias. VII: Cardiac effects of quinidine and procainamide. Am. Heart J. *89*:804, 1975.
45. Mirro, M. J., Watanabe, A. M., and Bailey, J. C.: Electrophysiological effects of disopyramide and quinidine on guinea pig atria and canine cardiac Purkinje fibers: Dependence on underlying cholinergic tone. Circ. Res. *46*:660, 1980.
46. Weld, F. M., Coromilas, J., Rothman, J. N., and Bigger, J. T., Jr.: Mechanisms of quinidine-induced depression of maximum upstroke velocity in bovine cardiac Purkinje fibers. Circ. Res. *50*:369, 1982.
47. Mason, J. W., and Winkle, R. A.: Electrode-catheter arrhythmia induction in the selection and assessment of antiarrhythmic drug therapy for recurrent ventricular tachycardia. Circulation *58*:971, 1978.
48. Wu, D., Hung, J. S., Kuo, C. T., Hsu, K. S., and Shieh, W. B.: Effects of quinidine on atrioventricular nodal reentrant paroxysmal tachycardia. Circulation *64*:823, 1981.
49. Wellens, H. J. J., and Durrer, D.: Effect of procainamide, quinidine and ajmaline in the Wolff-Parkinson-White syndrome. Circulation *50*:114, 1974.
50. Rasmussen, K., Wang, H., and Fausa, D.: Comparative efficiency of quinidine

and verapamil in the maintenance of sinus rhythm after DC conversion of atrial fibrillation. A controlled clinical trial. Acta Med. Scand. *645*(Suppl.):23, 1981.

51. Ruskin, J. N., DiMarco, J. P., and Garan, H.: Out-of-hospital cardiac arrest: Electrophysiologic observations and selection of long-term antiarrhythmic therapy. N. Engl. J. Med. *303*:607, 1980.
52. Myerburg, R. J., Conde, C. A., Sheps, D. S., Appel, R. A., Kiem, I., Sung, R. J., and Castellanos, A.: Antiarrhythmic drug therapy in survivors of pre-hospital cardiac arrest: Comparison of effects on chronic ventricular arrhythmias and recurrent cardiac arrest. Circulation *59*:855, 1979.
53. DiMarco, J. P., Garan, H., and Ruskin, J. N.: Efficacy of quinidine in the treatment of ventricular arrhythmias: The role of electrophysiologic testing. Circulation *64*(Suppl. IV):38, 1981.
54. Cohen, I. S., Jick, H., and Cohen, S. I.: Adverse reactions to quinidine in hospitalized patients: Findings based on data from the Boston Collaborative Drug Surveillance Program. Progr. Cardiovasc. Dis. *20*:151, 1977.
55. Selzer, A., and Wray, H. W.: Quinidine syncope: Paroxysmal ventricular fibrillation occurring during treatment of chronic atrial arrhythmias. Circulation *30*:17, 1964.
56. Denes, P., Gabster, A., and Huang, S. K.: Clinical electrocardiographic and followup observations in patients having ventricular fibrillation during Holter monitoring. Role of quinidine therapy. Am. J. Cardiol. *48*:9, 1981.
57. Smith, W. M., and Gallagher, J. J.: "Les torsades de pointes": An unusual ventricular arrhythmia. Ann. Intern. Med. *93*:578, 1980.
58. Ejvinsson, G., and Orinius, E.: Prodromal ventricular premature beats preceded by a diastolic wave. Acta Med. Scand. *208*:445, 1980.
59. Schenck-Gustafsson, K., Jogestrand, T., Nordlander R., and Dahlquis, T. R.: Effect of quinidine on digoxin concentration skeletal muscle and serum in patients with atrial fibrillation. Evidence for reduced binding of digoxin in muscle. N. Engl. J. Med. *305*:209, 1981.
60. Ball, W. J., Jr., Tse-Eng, D., Wallick, E. T., Bilezikian, J. P., Schwartz, A., and Butler, V. P., Jr.: Effect of quinidine on the digoxin receptor in vitro. J. Clin. Invest. *68*:1065, 1981.
61. Mautz, F. R.: Reduction of cardiac irritability by epicardial and systemic administration of drugs as a protection in cardiac surgery. J. Thorac. Surg. *5*:612, 1936.
62. Mark, L. C., Kayden, H. J., Steele, J. M., Cooper, J. R., Berlin, I., Rovenstein, E. A., and Brodie, B. B.: The physiological disposition and cardiac effects of procainamide. J. Pharmacol. Exp. Ther. *102*:5, 1951.
63. Moe, G. K., and Abildskov, J. A.: Antiarrhythmic drugs. *In* Goodman, L. S., and Gilman, A. (eds.): The Pharmacological Basis of Therapeutics. New York, MacMillan, 1975, p. 694.
64. Myerburg, R. J., Bassett, A. L., Epstein, K., Gaide, M. S., Kozlovskis, P., Wong, S. S., Castellanos, A., and Gelband, H.: Electrophysiological effects of procainamide in acute and healed experimental ischemic injury of cat myocardium. Circ. Res. *50*:386, 1982.
65. Michelson, E. L., Spear, J. F., and Moore, E. N.: Effects of procainamide on strength interval relations in normal and chronically infarcted canine myocardium. Am. J. Cardiol. *47*:1223, 1981.
66. Dangman, K. H., and Hoffman, B. F.: In vivo and in vitro antiarrhythmic and arrhythmogenic effects of N-acetylprocainamide. J. Pharmacol. Exp. Ther. *217*:851, 1981.
67. Jaillon, P., and Winkle, R. A.: Electrophysiologic comparative study of procainamide and N-acetylprocainamide in anesthetized dogs: Concentration response relationships. Circulation *60*:1385, 1979.
68. Giardina, E. G., Fenster, P., Paul, E., Bigger, J. T., Jr., Mayersohn, M., Perrier, D., and Marcus, F. I.: Efficacy, plasma concentrations and adverse effects of a new sustained release procainamide preparation. Am. J. Cardiol. *46*: 855, 1980.
69. Roden, D. M., Reele, S. B., Higgins, S. B., Wilkinson, G. R., Smith, R. F., Oates, J. A., and Woosley, R. L.: Antiarrhythmic efficacy, pharmacokinetics and safety of N-acetylprocainamide in human subjects: Comparison with procainamide. Am. J. Cardiol. *46*:463, 1980.
70. Kluger, J., Leech, S., Reidenberg, M. M., Lloyd, V., and Drayer, D. E.: Long-term antiarrhythmic therapy with acetylprocainamide. Am. J. Cardiol. *48*:1124, 1981.
71. Greenspan, A. M., Horowitz, L. N., Spielman, S. R., and Josephson, M. E.: Large dose procainamide therapy for ventricular tachycardia. Am. J. Cardiol. *46*:453, 1980.
72. Horowitz, L. N., Josephson, M. E., Farshidi, A., Spielman, S. R., Michelson, E. L., and Greenspan, A. M.: Recurrent sustained ventricular tachycardia. 3. Role of the electrophysiologic study in selection of antiarrhythmic regimens. Circulation *58*:986, 1978.
73. Boccardo, D., Pitchon, R., and Wiener, I.: Adverse reactions and efficacy of high dose procainamide therapy in resistant tachyarrhythmias. Am. Heart J. *102*:797, 1981.
74. Myerburg, R. J., Kessler, K. M., Kiem, I., Pefkaros, K. C., Conde, C. A., Cooper, D., Castellanos, A.: Relationship between plasma levels of procainamide, suppression of premature ventricular complexes and prevention of recurrent ventricular tachycardia. Circulation *64*:280, 1981.
75. Halpern, S. W., Ellrodt, G., Singh, B. N., and Mandel, W. J.: Efficacy of intravenous procainamide infusion in converting atrial fibrillation to sinus rhythm. Relation to left atrial size. Br. Heart J. *44*:589, 1980.
76. Wu, D., Denes, P., Amat-y-Leon, F., Dhingra, R., Wyndham, C. R. C., Bauernfeind, R., Latif, P., and Rosen, K. M.: Clinical electrocardiographic and electrophysiologic observations in patients with paroxysmal supraventricular tachycardia. Am. J. Cardiol. *41*:1045, 1978.
77. Shenasa, M., Gilbert, C. J., Schmidt, D. H., and Akhtar, M.: Procainamide and retrograde atrioventricular nodal conduction in man. Circulation *65*:355, 1982.
78. Wellens, H. J. J., Braat, S., Brugada, P., Gorgels, A. P. M., and Bar, F. W.: Use of procainamide in patients with the Wolff-Parkinson-White syndrome to disclose a short refractory period of the accessory pathway. Am. J. Cardiol. *50*:1087, 1982.
79. Engel, T. R., Meister, S. G., and Luck, J. C.: Modification of ventricular tachycardia by procainamide in patients with coronary artery disease. Am. J. Cardiol. *46*:1033, 1980.
80. Waxman, H. L., Sadowski, L. M., and Josephson, M. E.: Response to procainamide during electrophysiologic study for sustained ventricular tachycardia predicts response to other drugs. Circulation *64*(Suppl. IV):87, 1981.
81. Prystowsky, E. N., Heger, J. J., Jackman, W. M., Naccarelli, G. V., and Zipes, D. P.: Incessant supraventricualr tachycardia following myocardial infarction. Am. Heart J. *103*:426, 1982.
82. Strasberg, B., Sclarovsky, S., Erdberg, A., Duffy, C. E., Lan, W., Swiryn, S., Agmon, J., and Rosen, K. M.: Procainamide-induced polymorphous ventricular tachycardia. Am. J. Cardiol. *47*:1309, 1981.
83. Goldberg, D., Reiffel, J. A., Davis, J. C., Gang, E., Livelli, F., and Bigger, J. T., Jr.: Electrophysiologic effects of procainamide on sinus node function in patients with and without sinus node disease. Am. Heart J. *103*:75, 1982.
84. Ladd, A. T.: Procainamide-induced lupus erythematosus. N. Engl. J. Med. *267*:1357, 1962.
85. Kluger, J., Drayer, D. E., Reidenberg, M. M., and Lahita, R.: Acetylprocainamide therapy in patients with previous procainamide induced lupus syndrome. Ann. Intern. Med. *95*:18, 1981.
86. Danilo, F., Jr., and Rosen, M. R.: Cardiac effects of disopyramide. Am. Heart J. *92*:532, 1976.
87. Frame, L. H., and Hoffman, B. F.: Disopyramide's effects are enhanced by fast pacing rates in depolarized tissue. Circulation *64*(Suppl. IV):272, 1981.
88. Sasyniuk, B. I., and Kus, T.: Cellular electrophysiologic changes induced by disopyramide phosphate in normal and infarcted hearts. J. Int. Med. *4*:20, 1976.
89. Birkhead, J. S., and Vaughan Williams, E. M.: Dual effect of disopyramide on atrial and atrioventricular conduction and refractory periods. Br. Heart J. *39*:657, 1977.
90. Katoh, T., Karagueuzian, H., Jordan, J., and Mandel, W.: The cellular electrophysiologic mechanism of the dual actions of disopyramide on rabbit sinus node function. Circulation *66*:1216, 1982.
91. LaBarre, A., Strauss, H. C., Scheinman, M. M., Evans, G. T., Bashore, T., Tiedeman, J. S., and Wallace, A. G.: Electrophysiologic effects of disopyramide phosphate on sinus node function in patients with sinus node dysfunction. Circulation *59*:226, 1979.
92. Singh, B. N., Collett, J. T., and Chew, C. Y. C.: New perspectives in the pharmacologic therapy of cardiac arrhythmias. Progr. Cardiovasc. Dis. *22*:243, 1980.
93. Morady, F., Scheinman, M. M., and Desai, J.: Disopyramide. Ann. Intern. Med. *96*:337, 1982.
94. Timins, B. I., Gutman, J. A., and Haft, J. I.: Disopyramide-induced heart block. Chest *79*:477, 1981.

94a. Wilkinson, P. R., Desai, J., Hollister, J., Gonzalez, R., Abbott, J. A., and Scheinman, M. M.: Electrophysiologic effects of disopyramide in patients with atrioventricular nodal dysfunction. Circulation *66*:1211, 1982.

95. Kerr, C. R., Prystowsky, E. N., Smith, W. M., Cook, L., and Gallagher, J. J.: Electrophysiological effects of disopyramide phosphate in patients with Wolff-Parkinson-White syndrome. Circulation *65*:869, 1982.
96. Leach, A. J., Brown, J. E., and Armstrong, P. W.: Cardiac depression by intravenous disopyramide in patients with left ventricular dysfunction. Am. J. Med. *68*:839, 1980.
97. Landmark, K., Bredesen, J. E., Thaulow, E., Simonsen, S., and Amlie, J. P.: Pharmacokinetics of disopyramide in patients with imminent to moderate cardiac failure. Eur. J. Clin. Pharmacol. *19*:187, 1981.
98. Hulting, J., and Rosenhamer, G.: Hemodynamic and electrocardiographic effects of disopyramide in patients with ventricular arrhythmia. Acta Med. Scand. *199*:41, 1976.
99. Heel, R. C., Brogden, R. N., Speight, T. M., and Avery, G. S.: Disopyramide: A review of its pharmacological properties and therapeutic use in treating cardiac arrhythmias. Drugs *15*:331, 1978.
100. Wilcox, R. G., Rowley, J. M., Hampton, J. R., Mitchell, J. R., Roland, J. M., and Banks, D. C.: Randomised placebo-controlled trial comparing oxprenolol with disopyramide phosphate in immediate treatment of suspected myocardial infarction. Lancet *2*:765, 1980.
101. Pouleur, H., Chaudron, J. M., and Reyns, P.: Effects of disopyramide and aprindine on arrhythmias after acute myocardial infarction. Eur. J. Cardiol. *5*:397, 1977.
102. Breithardt, G., Seipel, L., and Abendroth, R. R.: Comparison of the antiarrhythmic efficacy of disopyramide and mexiletine against stimulus induced ventricular tachycardia. J. Cardiovasc. Pharmacol. *3*:1026, 1981.
103. Swiryn, S., Bauernfeind, R. A., Wyndham, C. R. C., Dhingra, R. C., Palileo, E., Strasberg, B., and Rosen, K. M.: Effects of oral disopyramide phosphate on induction of paroxysmal supraventricular tachycardia. Circulation *64*:169, 1981.
104. Robertson, C. E., and Miller, H. C.: Extreme tachycardia complicating the use of disopyramide in atrial flutter. Br. Heart J. *44*:602, 1980.
105. Dhurandhar, R. W., Nademanee, K., and Goldman, A. M.: Ventricular tachy-

cardia flutter associated with disopyramide therapy: A report of three cases. Heart and Lung 7:783, 1978.

106. Tzivoni, D., Keren, A., Stern, S., and Gottlieb, S.: Disopyramide-induced torsades de pointes. Arch. Intern. Med. 141:946, 1981.
107. Podrid, P. J., Schoeneberger, A., and Lown, B.: Congestive heart failure caused by disopyramide. N. Engl. J. Med. 302:614, 1980.
108. Desai, J. M., Scheinman, M. M., Hirschfeld, D., Gonzalez, R., and Peters, R. W.: Cardiovascular collapse associated with disopyramide therapy. Chest 79:545, 1981.
109. Matos, J. A., Fisher, J. D., and Kim, S. G.: Disopyramide-phenytoin interaction. Circulation 64(Suppl. IV):264, 1981.
110. Ferrier, G. R.: Digitalis arrhythmias: Role of oscillatory afterpotentials. Progr. Cardiovasc. Dis. 19:459, 1977.
111. Rosen, M. R., Danilo, P., Jr., Alonso, M. B., and Pippenger, C. E.: Effects of therapeutic concentrations of diphenylhydantoin on transmembrane potentials of normal and depressed Purkinje fibers. J. Pharmacol. Exp. Ther. 197:594, 1976.
112. Fisch, C., Zipes, D. P., and Noble, R. J.: Digitalis toxicity: Mechanism and recognition. Yu, P., and Goodwin, R. (eds.): Progress in Cardiology 4:37, 1975.
113. Wit, A. L., Rosen, M. R., and Hoffman, B. F.: Electrophysiology and pharmacology of cardiac arrhythmias. VIII. Cardiac effects of diphenylhydantoin. Am. Heart J. 90:397, 1975.
114. Gillis, R. A., McClellan, J. R., Sauer, T. S., and Standaert, F. G.: Depression of cardiac sympathetic nerve activity by diphenylhydantoin. J. Pharmacol. Exp. Ther. 179:599, 1971.
115. Garan, H., Ruskin, J. N., and Powell, W. J., Jr.: Centrally mediated effect of phenytoin on digoxin-induced ventricular arrhythmias. Am. J. Physiol. 241: H67, 1981.
116. Peter, T., Ross, D., Duffield, A., Luxton, M., Harper, R., Hunt, D., and Slowman, G.: Effect on survival after myocardial infarction of long-term treatment with phenytoin. Br. Heart J. 40:1356, 1978.
117. Koch-Weser, J., and Frishman, W. H.: Beta-adrenoreceptor antagonists: New drugs and new indications. N. Engl. J. Med. 305:500, 1981.
118. Lands, A. M., Arnold, A., McAuliff, P., Luduena, F. P., and Brown, T. G., Jr.: Differentiation of receptor systems activated by sympathomimetic amines. Nature 214:597, 1967.
119. Taylor, S. H., Silke, B., and Lee, P. S.: Intravenous beta blockade in coronary heart disease. N. Engl. J. Med. 306:631, 1982.
120. Davis, L. D., and Temte, J. V.: Effects of propranolol on the transmembrane potentials of ventricular muscle and Purkinje fibers of the dog. Circ. Res. 22:661, 1968.
121. Wit, A. L., Hoffman, B. F., and Rosen, M. R.: Electrophysiology and pharmacology of cardiac arrhythmias. IX. Cardiac electrophysiologic effects of beta adrenergic receptor stimulation and blockade (Part B). Am. Heart J. 90:665, 1975.
122. Wit, A. L., Hoffman, B. F., and Rosen, M. R.: Electrophysiology and pharmacology of cardiac arrhythmias. IX. Cardiac electrophysiologic effects of beta adrenergic receptor stimulation and blockade (Part C). Am. Heart J. 90:795, 1975.
123. Josephson, M. E., and Seides, S. F.: Clinical Cardiac Electrophysiology. Philadelphia, Lea and Febiger, 1979, p. 68.
124. Prystowsky, E. N., Jackman, W. M., Rinkenberger, R. L., Heger, J. J., and Zipes, D. P.: Effect of autonomic blockade on ventricular refractoriness and atrioventricular conduction in humans: Evidence supporting a direct cholinergic action on ventricular muscle refractoriness. Circ. Res. 49:511, 1981.
125. Ahnve, S., and Vallin, H.: Influence of heart rate and inhibition of autonomic tone on the QT interval. Circulation 65:435, 1982.
126. Browne, K. F., Zipes, D. P., Heger, J. J., and Prystowsky, E. N.: The influence of the autonomic nervous system on the QT interval. Am. J. Cardiol. 49:898, 1982.
127. Alexander, R. W., Williams, L. T., and Lefkowitz, R. T.: Identification of cardiac beta adrenergic receptors by (−) [3H] alprenol binding. Proc. Natl. Acad. Sci. (USA) 72:1564, 1975.
128. Nies, A. S., and Shand, D. G.: Clinical pharmacology of propranolol. Circulation 52:6, 1975.
129. Moss, A. J., and Schwartz, P. J.: Delayed repolarization (QT or QTU prolongation) and malignant ventricular arrhythmias. Mod. Conc. Cardiovasc. Dis. 51:85, 1982.
130. Barlow, J. B., and Pocock, W. A.: Mitral valve prolapse, the specific billowing mitral valve leaflet syndrome, or an insignificant non-ejection systolic click. Am. Heart J. 97:227, 1979.
131. Multicentre International Study: Improvement in prognosis of myocardial infarction by long-term beta-adrenoceptor blockade using practolol: A multicentre international study. Br. Med. J. 3:735, 1977.
132. Ahlmark, G., and Saetre, H.: Long-term treatment with beta blockers after myocardial infarction. Eur. J. Pharmacol. 10:77, 1976.
133. Wilhelmsen, C., Wilhelmsen, L., and Vedin, J. A.: Reduction of sudden death after myocardial infarction by treatment with alprenolol. Lancet 2:1157, 1974.
134. Beta Blocker Heart Attack Study Group: The beta blocker heart attack trial. J.A.M.A. 246:2073, 1981.
135. Hjalmarson, A.: Effect on mortality of metoprolol in acute myocardial infarction: A double-blind randomized trial. Lancet 2:823, 1981.
136. The Norwegian Multicentre Study Group: Timolol-induced reduction in mortality and reinfarction in patients surviving acute myocardial infarction. N. Engl. J. Med. 304:801, 1981.
136a. Gundersen, T., Abrahamsen, A. M., Kjekshus, J., and Rønnevik, P. K. for the Norwegian Multicenter Study Group: Timolol-related reduction in mortality and reinfarction in patients ages 65-75 years surviving acute myocardial infarction. Circulation 66:1179, 1982.
137. Miller, R. R., Olson, H. G., Amsterdam, E. A. L., and Mason, D. T.: Propranolol withdrawal rebound phenomenon. N. Engl. J. Med. 293:416, 1975.
138. Nattel, S., Rango, R. E., and Vanloon, G.: Mechanism of propranolol withdrawal phenomenon. Circulation 59:1158, 1979.
139. Gillis, R. A., Clancy, M. M., and Anderson, R. J.: The deleterious effects of bretylium in cats with digitalis-induced ventricular tachycardia. Circulation 47:976, 1973.
140. Waxman, M. B., and Wallace, A. G.: Electrophysiologic effects of bretylium tosylate on the heart. J. Pharmacol. Exp. Ther. 183:264, 1972.
141. Bacaner, M. B.: Bretylium tosylate for suppression of induced ventricular fibrillation. Am. J. Cardiol. 17:528, 1966.
142. Cardinal, R., Sasyniuk, D. I., Electrophysiological effects of bretylium tosylate in subendocardial Purkinje fibers from infarcted canine hearts. J. Pharmacol. Exp. Ther. 204:159, 1978.
143. Patterson, E., Gibson, J. K., and Lucchesi, B. R.: Prevention of chronic canine ventricular tachyarrhythmias with bretylium tosylate. Circulation 64:1045, 1981.
144. Anderson, J. L., Patterson, E., Wagner, J. G., Johnson, T. A., Lucchesi, B. R., and Pitt, B.: Clinical pharmacokinetics of intravenous and oral bretylium tosylate in survivors of ventricular tachycardia or fibrillation: Clinical application of a new assay for bretylium. J. Cardiovasc. Pharmacol. 3:485, 1981.
145. Holder, D. A., Sniderman, A. D., Fraser, G., and Fallen, E. L.: Experience with bretylium tosylate by a hospital cardiac arrest team. Circulation 55:541, 1977.
146. Cohen, H. C., Gozo, E. G., Jr., Langendorf, R., Kaplan, B. M., Chan, A., Pick, A., and Glick, G.: Response of resistant ventricular tachycardia to bretylium: Relation to site of ectopic focus and location of myocardial disease. Circulation 47:331, 1973.
147. Zipes, D. P., and Troup, P. J.: New antiarrhythmic agents. Am. J. Cardiol. 41:1005, 1978.
148. Cranefield, P. F.: The Conduction of the Cardiac Impulse. Mt. Kisco, N.Y., Futura Publishing Co., 1975.
149. Zipes, D. P., Bailey, J. C., and Elharrar, V.: The Slow Inward Current and Cardiac Arrhythmias. The Hague, Martinus Nijhoff, 1980.
150. Antman, E. M., Stone, P. H., Mueller, J. E., and Braunwald, E.: Calcium channel blocking agents in the treatment of cardiovascular disorders. Ann. Intern. Med. 93:875, 1980.
151. Henry, P. D.: Comparative pharmacology of calcium antagonists: Nifedipine, verapamil, and diltiazem: Am. J. Cardiol. 46:1047, 1980.
152. Lathrop, D. A., Valle-Aguilera, J. R., Millard, R. W., Gaum, W. E., Hannon, D. W., Francis, P. D., Nakaya, H., and Schwartz, A.: Comparative electrophysiologic and coronary hemodynamic effects of diltiazem, nisoldipine and verapamil on myocardial tissue. Am. J. Cardiol. 49:613, 1982.
153. Gilmour, R. F., and Zipes, D. P.: Basic electrophysiology of the slow inward current. *In* Antman, E. M., and Stone, P. H.: Cardiac Arrhythmias. Mt. Kisco, N. Y., Futura Publishing Co. (*in press*).
154. Cranefield, P. F., Aaronson, R. S., and Wit, A. L.: Effect of verapamil on the normal action potential and on a calcium dependent slow response of canine cardiac Purkinje fibers. Circ. Res. 34:204, 1974.
155. Rosen, M. R., Wit, A. L., and Hoffman, B. F.: Electrophysiology and pharmacology of cardiac arrhythmias. VI. Cardiac effects of verapamil. Am. Heart J. 89:665, 1975.
156. Hordof, A. J., Edie, R., Malm, J. R., Hoffman, B. F., and Rosen, M. R.: Electrophysiologic properties and response to pharmacologic agents of fibers from diseased human atria. Circulation 54:774, 1976.
157. Spear, J. F., Horowitz, L. N., and Moore, E. N.: The slow response in human ventricle. *In* Zipes, D. P., Bailey, J. C., and Elharrar, V. (eds.): The Slow Inward Current and Cardiac Arrhythmias. The Hague, Martinus Nijhoff, 1980, p. 309.
158. Gilmour, R. F., Jr., Heger, J. J., Prystowsky, E. N., and Zipes, D. P.: Cellular electrophysiological abnormalities of diseased human ventricular myocardium. Am. J. Cardiol. (*in press*).
159. Zipes, D. P., and Mendez, C.: Action of manganese ions and tetrodotoxin on atrioventricular nodal transmembrane potentials in isolated rabbit hearts. Circ. Res. 32:447, 1973.
160. Zipes, D. P., and Fischer, J. C.: Effects of agents which inhibit the slow channel on sinus node automaticity and atrioventricular conduction in the dog. Circ. Res. 34:184, 1974.
161. Yamagishi, S.: Effects of tetrodotoxin on the pacemaker action potential of the sinus node. Proc. Jap. Acad. Sci. 42:1194, 1966.
162. Lenfant, J., Mironneau, J., and Gargouil, Y. M.: Analyse de l'activité electrique spontanée de centre de l'automatisme cardiaque de lapin par les inhibiteurs de permeabilités membranaires. CR Acad. Sci. [D] Paris 266:901, 1968.
163. Rougier, O., Vassort, G., and Garnier, D.: Existence and role of the slow inward current during the frog atrial action potential. Pfluegers Arch. 308:91, 1969.
164. Wit, A. L., and Cranefield, P. F.: Effect of verapamil on the sinoatrial and atrioventricular nodes of the rabbit and the mechanism by which it arrests reentrant atrioventricular nodal tachycardia. Circ. Res. 35:413, 1974.
165. Okada, T.: Effect of verapamil on electrical activities of SA node, ventricular muscle and Purkinje fibers in isolated rabbit hearts. Jap. Circ. J. 40:329, 1976.
166. Naylor, W. G., and Szeto, J.: Effect of verapamil on contractility, oxygen utili-

zation, and calcium exchange ability in mammalian heart muscle. Cardiovasc. Res. *6*:120, 1972.
167. Zipes, D. P., and Gilmour, R. F.: Calcium antagonists and their potential role in the prevention of sudden coronary death. Ann. NY Acad. Sci. *382*:258, 1982.
168. Wellens, H. J. J., Tan, S. L., Bär, F. W. H., Duren, D. R., Lie, K. I., and Dohmen, H. M.: Effects of verapamil studied by programmed electrical stimulation of the heart in patients with paroxysmal reentrant supraventricular tachycardia. Br. Heart J. *39*:1058, 1977.
169. Breidthardt, G., Seipel, L., and Wiebringhaus, E.: Dual effect of verapamil on sinus node function in man. *In* Bonke, F.I.M. (ed.): The Sinus Node. The Hague, Martinus Nijhoff, 1978, p. 129.
170. Spurrell, R. A. J., Krikler, D. M., and Sowton, E.: Effects of verapamil on electrophysiological properties of anomalous atrioventricular connection in Wolff-Parkinson-White syndrome. Br. Heart J. *36*:256, 1974.
171. Rinkenberger, R. L., Prystowsky, E. N., Heger, J. J., Troup, P. J., Jackman, W. M., and Zipes, D. P.: Effects of intravenous and chronic oral verapamil administration in patients with supraventricular tachyarrhythmias. Circulation *62*:996, 1980.
172. Matsuyama, E., Konishi, T., Okazaki, H., Matsuda, H., Kawai, C.: Effects of verapamil on accessory pathway properties and induction of circus movement tachycardia in patients with the Wolff-Parkinson-White syndrome. J. Cardiovasc. Pharmacol. *3*:11, 1981.
173. Gulamhusein, S., Ko, P., Carruthers, S. G., and Klein, G. J.: Acceleration of the ventricular response during atrial fibrillation in the Wolff-Parkinson-White syndrome after verapamil. Circulation *65*:348, 1982.
174. Kieval, J., Kirsten, E. B., Kessler, K. M., Mallon, S. M., and Myerburg, R. J.: The effects of intravenous verapamil on hemodynamic status of patients with coronary artery disease receiving propranolol. Circulation *65*:653, 1982.
175. Packer, M., Mellen, J., Medina, N., Yushak, M., Smith, H., Holt, J., Guerrero, J., Todd, G. D., McAllister, R. G., and Gorlin, R.: Hemodynamic consequences of combined beta-adrenergic and slow calcium channel blockade in man. Circulation *65*:660, 1982.
176. Reimer, K. A., Lowe, J. E., and Jennings, R. B.: The effects of calcium antagonist verapamil on necrosis following temporary coronary artery occlusion in dogs. Circulation *55*:581, 1977.
177. Clusin, W. T., Bristow, M. R., Baim, D. S., Schroeder, J. S., Jaillon, P., Brett, P., and Harrison, D. C.: The effects of diltiazem and reduced serum ionized calcium on ischemic ventricular fibrillation in the dog. Circ. Res. *50*:518, 1982.
178. Elharrar V., Goum, W. E., and Zipes, D. P.: Effects of various drugs on antiarrhythmias during acute myocardial ischemia. Am. J. Cardiol. *37*:134, 1976.
179. Krikler, D. M.: Verapamil in cardiology. Eur. J. Cardiol. *2*:3, 1974.
180. Puech, P.: Dissection de la Conduction Sinoventriculaire pour l'Etude du Verapamil Injectable. Montpellier, Centre Hospitalier, 1972.
181. Mangiardi, L. M., Hariman, R. J., McAllister, R. G., Bhargava, V., Surawicz, B., and Shabetai, R.: Electrophysiologic and hemodynamic effects of verapamil. Circulation *57*:366, 1978.
182. Sung, R. J., Elser, B., and McAllister, R. G., Jr.: Intravenous verapamil for termination of reentrant supraventricular tachycardias. Intracardiac studies correlated with plasma verapamil concentrations. Ann. Intern. Med. *93*:682, 1980.
183. Kates, R. E., Keefe, D. L., Schwartz, J., Harapats, S., Kirsten, E. B., and Harrison, D. C.: Verapamil disposition kinetics in chronic atrial fibrillation. Clin. Pharmacol. Ther. *30*:44, 1981.
184. Schomerus, M., Spiegelhalder, B., and Steiren, B.: Physiological disposition of verapamil in man. Cardiovasc. Res. *10*:605, 1976.
185. Hamer, A., Peter, T., Platt, M., and Mandel, W. J.: Effects of verapamil on supraventricular tachycardia in patients with overt and concealed Wolff-Parkinson-White syndrome. Am. Heart J. *101*:600, 1981.
186. Schamroth, L.: Immediate effects of intravenous verapamil on atrial fibrillation. Cardiovasc. Res. *5*:419, 1971.
187. Waxman, H. L., Myerburg, R. J., Appel, R., and Sung, R. J.: Verapamil for control of ventricular rate in paroxysmal supraventricular tachycardia and atrial fibrillation or flutter: A double-blind randomized cross-over study. Ann. Intern. Med. *94*:1, 1981.
188. Schwartz, J. B., Keefe, D., Kates, R. E., Kirsten E., and Harrison, D. C.: Acute and chronic pharmacodynamic interaction of verapamil and digoxin in atrial fibrillation. Circulation *65*:1163, 1982.
189. Wellens, H. J. J., Farre, J., and Bär, F. W.: The role of the slow inward current in the genesis of ventricular tachycardias in man. *In* Zipes, D. P., Bailey, J., and Elharrar, V. (eds.): The Slow Inward Current and Cardiac Arrhythmias. The Hague, Martinus Nijhoff, 1980, p. 507.
190. Benaim, M. E.: Asystole after verapamil. Br. Med. J. *2*:169, 1972.
191. Rosenbaum, M. B., Chiale, P. A., Ryba, D., and Elizari, M.: Control of tachyarrhythmias associated with Wolff-Parkinson-White syndrome by amiodarone hydrochloride. Am. J. Cardiol. *34*:215, 1974.
192. Rosenbaum, M. B., Chiale, P. A., Halpern, M. S., Nau, G. J., Przybylski, J., Levi, R. J., Lazzari, J. O., and Elizari, M. V.: Clinical efficacy of amiodarone as an antiarrhythmic agent. Am. J. Cardiol. *38*:934, 1976.
193. Olsson, S. B., Brorson, L., and Varnauskas, E.: Antiarrhythmic action in man. Observations from monophasic action potential recordings in amiodarone treatment. Br. Heart J. *35*:1255, 1973.
194. Wellens, H. J. J., Lie, K. I., Bär, F. W., Wesdorf, J. C., Dohmen, H. J., Duren, D. R., and Durrer, D.: Effect of amiodarone in the Wolff-Parkinson-White syndrome. Am. J. Cardiol. *38*:189, 1976.
195. Heger, J. J., Prystowsky, E. N., Jackman, W. M., Naccarelli, G. V., Warfel, K. A., Rinkenberger, R. L., and Zipes, D. P.: Amiodarone: Clinical efficacy and electrophysiology during long-term therapy for recurrent ventricular tachycardia. N. Engl. J. Med. *305*:539, 1981.
196. Nademanee, K., Hendrickson, J. A., Cannom, D. S., Goldreyer, B. N., and Singh, B. N.: Control of refractory life-threatening ventricular tachyarrhythmias by amiodarone. Am. Heart J. *101*:759, 1981.
197. Haffajee, C., Lesko, L., Kanada, A., and Alpert, J. S.: Clinical pharmacokinetics of amiodarone. Circulation *64*(Suppl. IV):263, 1981.
198. Podrid, P. J., and Lown, B.: Amiodarone therapy and symptomatic sustained refractory atrial and ventricular tachyarrhythmias. Am. Heart J. *101*:374, 1981.
199. Marcus, F. T., Fontaine, G. H., Frank, R., and Grosgogeat, Y.: Clinical pharmacology and therapeutic applications of the antiarrhythmic agent, amiodarone. Am. Heart J. *101*:480, 1981.
200. Coumel, P., and Fidelle, J.: Amiodarone in the treatment of cardiac arrhythmias in children: 135 cases. Am. Heart J. *100*:1063, 1980.
201. Hamer, A. W., Finerman, W. B., Jr., Peter, T., and Mandel, W. J.: Disparity between clinical and electrophysiologic effects of amiodarone in the treatment of recurrent ventricular tachyarrhythmias. Am. Heart J. *102*:992, 1981.
202. Bashour, T., Jokhadar, M., and Cheng, T. O.: Effective management of the long QT syndrome with amiodarone. Chest *79*:704, 1981.
203. Sobel, S. M., and Rakita, L.: Pneumonitis and pulmonary fibrosis associated with amiodarone treatment: A possible complication of a new antiarrhythmic drug. Circulation *65*:819, 1982.
204. Elharrar, V., Bailey, J. C., Lathrop, D. A., and Zipes, D. P.: Effects of aprindine HCl on slow channel action potentials and transient depolarizations in canine Purkinje fibers. J. Pharmacol. Exp. Ther. *205*:410, 1978.
205. Carmeliet, E., and Verdonck, F.: Effects of aprindine and lidocaine on transmembrane potentials and radioactive K-efflux in different cardiac tissues. Acta Cardiol. Suppl. *18*:73, 1974.
206. Gilmour, R. F., Chikharev, V. N., Jurevichus, J. A., Zacharov, S. I., Zipes, D. P., and Rozenshtraukh, L. V.: Effect of aprindine on transmembrane currents and contractile force in frog atria. J. Pharmacol. Exp. Ther. *217*:390, 1981.
207. Foster, P. R., King, R. M., Nicoll, A. D., and Zipes, D. P.: Suppression of ouabain-induced ventricular arrhythmias with aprindine HCl. A comparison with other antiarrhythmic agents. Circulation *53*:315, 1976.
208. Zipes, D. P., Elharrar, V., Gilmour, R. F., Heger, J. J., and Prystowsky, E. N.: Studies with aprindine. Am. Heart J. *100*:1055, 1980.
209. Elharrar, V., Gaum, W. E., and Zipes, D. P.: Effect of drugs on conduction delay and the incidence of ventricular arrhythmias induced by acute coronary occlusion in dogs. Am. J. Cardiol. *39*:544, 1977.
210. Van Durme, J. P., Rousseau, M., and Mbuyamba, P.: Treatment of chronic ventricular dysrhythmias with a new drug aprindine (AC1802). Acta Cardiol. (Brux) (Suppl.) *18*:335, 1974.
211. Fasola, A. F., Noble, R. J., and Zipes, D. P.: Treatment of recurrent tachycardia and fibrillation with aprindine. Am. J. Cardiol. *39*:903, 1977.
212. Strassberg, B., Palileo, E., Prechel, D., Bauernfeind, R., Swiryn, S., Wyndham, C. R., Dhingra, R. C., Kehoe, R., and Rosen, K. M.: Ventricular tachycardia: Prediction of response to oral aprindine with intravenous aprindine. Am. J. Cardiol. *47*:676, 1981.
213. Zipes, D. P., Gaum, W. E., Foster, P. R., Rosen, K. M., Wu, D., Amat-y-Leon, F., and Noble, R. J.: Aprindine for treatment of supraventricular tachycardias with particular application to WPW syndrome. Am. J. Cardiol. *40*:586, 1977.
214. Troup, P. J., and Zipes, D. P.: Aprindine treatment of recurrent ventricular tachycardia in patients with mitral valve prolapse. Am. Heart J. *97*:322, 1979.
215. Scagliotti, D., Strasberg, B., Hai, H., Kehoe, R., and Rosen, K. M.: Aprindine-induced polymorphous ventricular tachycardia. Am. J. Cardiol. *49*:1297, 1982.
216. Waleffe, A., Guillaume, D., Mary-Rabine, L., and Kulbertus, H.: The efficacy of intravenous moxaprindine on ventricular ectopic activity. Acta Cardiol. (Brux.) *35*:257, 1980.
217. Staessen, J., Kesteloot, H.: Moxaprindine in the acute treatment of ventricular arrhythmias in patients with cardiovascular disease. Eur. J. Clin. Pharmacol. *19*:167, 1981.
218. Elharrar, V., and Zipes, D. P.: Effects of encainide metabolites (MJ14030 and MJ19444) on canine cardiac Purkinje and ventricular fibers. J. Pharmacol. Exp. Ther. *220*:440, 1982.
219. Jackman, W. M., Zipes, D. P., Naccarelli, G. V., Rinkenberger, R. L., Heger, J. J., and Prystowsky, R. H.: Electrophysiology of oral encainide. Am. J. Cardiol. *49*:1270, 1982.
220. Winkle, R. A., Peters, F., Kates, R. E., and Harrison, D. C.: The contribution of encainide metabolites to its long-term antiarrhythmic efficacy. Circulation *64*(Suppl. IV):264, 1981.
221. Carey, E. L., Duff, H. J., Roden, D. M., Primm, R. K., Oates, J. A., and Woosley, R. L.: Relative electrocardiographic and antiarrhythmic effects of encainide and its metabolites in man. Circulation *64*(Suppl. IV):264, 1981.
222. Harrison, D. C., Winkle, R. A., Sami, M., and Mason, J. W.: Encainide: A new and potent antiarrhythmic agent. *In* Harrison, D. C. (eds.): Cardiac Arrhythmias: A Decade of Progress. Boston, G. K. Hall, 1981, p. 315.
223. Winkle, R. A., Peters, F., Kates, R. E., Tucker, C., and Harrison, D. C.: Clinical pharmacology and antiarrhythmic efficacy of encainide in patients with chronic ventricular arrhythmias. Circulation *64*:290, 1981.
224. Prystowsky, E. N., Klein, G., Rinkenberger, R. L., Heger, J. J., Nacarelli, G. V., and Zipes, D. P.: Clinical efficacy and electrophysiologic effects of encainide in patients with Wolff-Parkinson-White syndrome. Circulation (*in press*).

225. Roden, D. M., Reele, S. B., Higgins, S. B., Mayol, R. F., Gammans, R. E., Oates, J. A., and Woosley, R. L.: Total suppression of ventricular arrhythmias by encainide. N. Engl. J. Med. *302*:877, 1980.
226. Sami, M., Harrison, D. C., Kraemer, H., Houston, N., Shimasaki, C., and DeBusk, R. F.: Antiarrhythmic efficacy of encainide and quinidine: Validation of a model for drug assessment. Am. J. Cardiol. *48*:147, 1981.
227. Heger, J. J., Prystowsky, E. N., and Zipes, D. P.: Clinical choice of antiarrhythmic drugs. *In* Josephson, M. E. (ed.): Ventricular Tachycardia—Mechanisms and Management. Mt. Kisko, N.Y., Futura Publishing Co., 1982.
228. Mason, J. W., and Peters, F. A.: Antiarrhythmic efficacy of encainide in patients with refractory recurrent ventricular tachycardia. Circulation *63*:670, 1981.
229. Rinkenberger, R. L., Prystowsky, E. N., Jackman, W. M., Heger, J. J., and Zipes, D. P.: Conversion of nonsustained ventricular tachycardia to sustained ventricular tachycardia during drug therapy as determined by serial electrophysiology studies. Am. Heart J. *103*:177, 1982.
230. Winkle, R. A., Mason, J. W., Griffin, J. C., and Ross, D.: Malignant ventricular tachyarrhythmias associated with use of encainide. Am. Heart J. *102*:857, 1981.
231. Yamaguchi, I., Singh, B. N., and Mandel, W. J.: Electrophysiological action of mexiletine on isolated rabbit atria and canine ventricular muscle and Purkinje fibers. Cardiovasc. Res. *13*:288, 1979.
232. Prescott, L. F., Pottage, A., and Clements, J. A.: Absorption, distribution and elimination of mexiletine. Postgrad. Med. J. *53*(Supp. I):50, 1977.
233. Campbell, N. P. S., Pantridge, J. F., and Adjey, A. A. J.: Mexiletine and the management of ventricular dysrhythmias. Eur. J. Cardiol. *6*:245, 1977.
234. Talbot, R. G., Julian, D. G., and Prescott, L. F.: Long-term treatment of ventricular arrhythmias with oral mexiletine. Am. Heart J. *91*:58, 1976.
235. Heger, J. J., Nattel, S., Rinkenberger, R. L., and Zipes, D. P.: Mexiletine therapy in 15 patients with a drug-resistant ventricular tachycardia. Am. J. Cardiol. *45*:627, 1980.
236. Podrid, P. J., and Lown, B.: Mexiletine for ventricular arrhythmias. Am. J. Cardiol. *47*:895, 1981.
237. DiMarco, J. P., Garan, H., and Ruskin, J. N.: Mexiletine for refractory ventricular arrhythmias: Results using serial electrophysiologic testing. Am. J. Cardiol. *47*:131, 1981.
238. Waleffe, A., Mary-Rabine, L., Legrand, V., Demoulin, J. C., and Kulbertus, H. E.: Combined mexiletine and amiodarone treatment of refractory recurrent ventricular tachycardia. Am. Heart J. *100*:788, 1980.
239. Campbell, N. P. S., Pantridge, J. F., and Adgey, A. A. J.: Long-term oral antiarrhythmic therapy with mexiletine. Br. Heart J. *40*:796, 1978.
240. Cocco, G., Strozzi, C., Chu, D., and Pansini, R.: Torsades de pointes as a manifestation of mexiletine toxicity. Am. Heart J. *100*:878, 1980.
241. Horowitz, L. N., Josephson, M. E., and Farshidi, A.: Human electropharmacology of tocainide, a lidocaine congener. Am. J. Cardiol. *42*:276, 1978.
242. Winkle, R. A., Meffin, P. J., and Harrison, D. C.: Long-term tocainide therapy for ventricular arrhythmias. Circulation *57*:1008, 1978.
243. Michael, R. A., Neffin, P. J., Fitzgerald, J. W., and Harrison, D. C.: Clinical efficacy and pharmacokinetics of a new orally effective antiarrhythmic, tocainide. Circulation *54*:884, 1976.
244. Woosley, R. L., McDivitt, D. G., Nies, A. S., Smith, R. F., Wilkinson, G. R., and Oates, J. A.: Suppression of ventricular ectopic depolarizations by tocainide. Circulation *56*:980, 1977.
245. Roden, D. M., Reele, S. B., Higgins, S. B., Carr, R. K., Smith, R. F., Oates, J. A., and Woosley, R. L.: Tocainide therapy for refractory ventricular arrhythmias. Am. Heart J. *100*:15, 1980.
246. Young, M. D., Hadidian, Z., Horn, H. R., Johnson, J. L., and Vassalo, H. G.: Treatment of ventricular arrhythmias with oral tocainide. Am. Heart J. *100*:1041, 1980.
247. Podrid, P., and Lown, B.: Tocainide for refractory symptomatic ventricular arrhythmias. Am. J. Cardiol. *49*:1279, 1982.
248. Ryden, L., Arnman, K., Conradson, T. B., Hofvendahl, S., Mortenson, A., and Smedgard, P.: Prophylaxis of ventricular tachyarrhythmias with intravenous and oral tocainide in patients with and recovering from acute myocardial infarction. Am. Heart J. *100*:1006, 1980.
249. Engler, R. L., and LeWinter, M.: Tocainide-induced ventricular fibrillation. Am. Heart J. *101*:494, 1981.
250. Danilo, P., Langen, W. B., Rosen, M. R., and Hoffman, B. F.: Effects of the phenothiazine analog, EN 313, on ventricular arrhythmias in the dog. Eur. J. Pharmacol. *45*:127, 1977.
251. Ruffy, R., Rozenshtraukh, L. V., Elharrar, V., and Zipes, D. P.: Electrophysiologic effects of ethmozin on canine myocardium. Cardiovasc. Res. *13*:354, 1979.
252. Morganroth, J., Michelson, E. L., Kitchen, J. G., and Dreifus, L. S.: Ethmozin: Electrophysiologic effects in man. Circulation *64*(Suppl. IV):263, 1981.
253. Podrid, P. J., Lyakishev, A., Lown, B., and Mazur, N.: Ethmozin: A new antiarrhythmic drug for suppressing ventricular premature complexes. Circulation *61*:450, 1980.
254. Anderson, J. L., Stewart, J. R., Perry, B. A., vanHamersveld, D. D., Johnson, T. A., Conard, G. J., Chang, S. F., Kvam, D. C., and Pitt, B.: Oral flecainide acetate for the treatment of ventricular arrhythmias. N. Engl. J. Med. *305*:473, 1981.
255. Duff, H. J., Roden, D. M., Naffucci, R. J., Vesper, B. S., Conard, G. J., Higgins, S. B., Oates, J. A., Smith, R. F., and Woosley, R. L.: Suppression of resistant ventricular arrhythmias by twice daily dosing with flecainide. Am. J. Cardiol. *48*:1133, 1981.
256. Hodges, M., Haugland, J. M., Granrud, G., Conard, G. J., Asinger, R. W., Mikell, F. L., and Krejei, J.: Suppression of ventricular ectopic depolarization by flecainide acetate, a new antiarrhythmic agent. Circulation *65*:879, 1982.
257. Lui, H. K., Lee, G., Dietrich, P., Low, R. I., and Mason, D. T.: Flecainide-induced QT prolongation and ventricular tachycardia. Am. Heart J. *103*:567, 1982.
258. Ronfeld, R. A.: Pharmacokinetics of new antiarrhythmic drugs in cardiac arrhythmias. Harrison, D. C. (ed.): A Decade of Progress. Boston, G. K. Hall, 1981, p. 135.
259. Somani, P.: Pharmacokinetics of lorcainide, a new antiarrhythmic drug, in patients with cardiac rhythm disorders. Am. J. Cardiol. *48*:157, 1981.
260. Somberg, J. C., Willens, S. H., Camilleri, W., Maguire, W., and Miura, D. S.: Effect of lorcainide on suppressing ventricular tachycardia induced by programed stimulation. Circulation *64*(Suppl. IV):37, 1981.
261. Waleffe, A., Mary-Rabine, L., de Rijbel, R., Soyeur, D., Legrand, V., and Kulbertus, H. E.: Electrophysiological effects of propafenone studied with programmed electrical stimulation of the heart in patients with recurrent paroxysmal supraventricular tachycardia. Eur. Heart J. *2*:345, 1981.
262. Chilson, D. A., Zipes, D. P., Heger, J. J., Browne, F. F., Lloyd, E. A., and Prystowsky, E. N.: Clinical and electrophysiological effeccts of propafenone, a new drug for treating ventricular tachycardia. Clin. Res. *30*:706, 1982.
263. Bacaner, M. B., Hoey, M. F., and Macres, M. G.: Suppression of ventricular fibrillation and positive inotropic action of bethanidine sulfate, a chemical analog of bretylium tosylate that is well absorbed orally. Am. J. Cardiol. *49*:45, 1982.
264. Greene, H. L., Werner, J. A., Gross, B. W., Kime, G. M., Trobaugh, G. B., and Cobb, L. A.: Selective prolongation of cardiac refractory times in man by clofilium, a new antiarrhythmic agent. Circulation *64*(Suppl. IV): 137, 1981.
265. Giardina, E. V., Bigger, J. T., Jr., and Johnson, L. L.: The effect of imipramine and nortriptyline on ventricular premature depolarizations and left ventricular function. Circulation *64*(Suppl. IV):316, 1981.
266. Zoll, P. M., Linenthal, A. J., Gibson, W., Paul, M. H., and Norman, L. R.: Termination of ventricular fibrillation in man by externally applied electric countershock. N. Engl. J. Med. *254*: 727, 1956.
267. Lown, B., Amarasingham, R., and Newman, J.: New method for terminating cardiac arrhythmias. J.A.M.A. *182*:548, 1962.
268. Lown, B.: Electrical reversion of cardiac arrhythmias. Br. Heart J. *29*:469, 1967.
269. Zipes, D. P.: The clinical application of cardioversion. Cardiovasc. Clin. *2*:239, 1970.
270. Ditchey, R. V., and Karliner, J. S.: Safety of electrical cardioversion in patients without digitalis toxicity. Ann. Intern. Med. *95*:676, 1981.
271. Adgey, A. A. J., Patton, J. N., Campbell, N. P. S., and Webb, S. W.: Ventricular defibrillation: Appropriate energy levels. Circulation *60*:219, 1979.
272. Tacker, W. A., Jr., and Ewy, G. A.: Emergency defibrillation dose: Recommendations and rationale. Circulation *60*:223, 1979.
273. Kerber, R. E., and Sarnat, W.: Factors influencing the success of ventricular defibrillation in man. Circulation *60*:226, 1979.
274. Gascho, J. A., Crampton, R. S., Cherwek, M. L., Sipes, J. N., Hunter, F. P., and O'Brien, W. M.: Determinants of ventricular defibrillation in adults. Circulation *60*:231, 1979.
275. Ewy, G. A.: Effectiveness of direct current defibrillation. Role of paddle electrode size. Am. Heart J. *93*:674, 1977.
276. Kerber, R. E., Jensen, S. R., Grayzel, J., Kennedy, J., and Hoyt, R.: Elective cardioversion: Influence of paddle electrode location and size on success rate and energy requirements. N. Engl. J. Med. *305*:658, 1981.
277. Hoyt, R., Grayzel, J., and Kerber, R. E.: Determinants of intracardiac current in defibrillation. Experimental studies in dogs. Circulation *64*:818, 1981.
278. Zipes, D. P., Fischer, J., King, R. M., Nicoll, A.deB., and Jolly, W. W.: Termination of ventricular fibrillation in dogs by depolarizing a critical amount of myocardium. Am. J. Cardiol. *36*:37, 1975.
279. Lown, B., Crampton, R. S., DeSilva, R. A., and Gascho, J.: The energy for ventricular defibrillation—too little or too much? N. Engl. J. Med. *298*:1252, 1978.
280. Mitchell, J. H., and Shapiro, W.: Atrial function and the hemodynamic consequences of atrial fibrillation in man. Am. J. Cardiol. *23*:556, 1969.
281. Cobb, F. R., Wallace, A. G., and Wagner, G. S.: Cardiac inotropic and coronary vascular responses to countershock: Evidence for excitation of intracardiac nerves. Circ. Res. *23*:731, 1968.
282. Ten Eick, R. E., White, S. R., Ross, S. M., and Hoffman, B. F.: Postcountershock arrhythmia in untreated and digitalized dogs. Circ. Res. *21*:375, 1967.
283. Resenkov, L., and McDonald, L.: Complications in 220 patients with cardiac dysrhythmias treated by phased direct current shock and indications for electroconversion. Br. Heart J. *29*:926, 1967.
284. Bjerkelund, C. J., and Orning, O. M.: The efficacy of anticoagulant therapy in preventing embolism related to DC electrical conversion of atrial fibrillation. Am. J. Cardiol. *23*:208, 1969.
285. DiCola, V. C., Freedman, G. S., Downing, S. E., and Zaret, B. L.: Myocardial uptake of technetium-99m stannous pyrophosphate following direct current transthoracic countershock. Circulation *54*:980, 1976.
286. Reiffel, J. A., Gambino, S. R., McCarthy, D. M., and Leahey, E. B., Jr.: Direct current cardioversion: Effect on creatine kinase lactic dehydrogenase and myocardial isoenzymes. J.A.M.A. *239*:122, 1978.
287. Chun, P. K., Davia, J. E., and Donohue, D. J.: ST segment elevation with elective DC cardioversion. Circulation *63*:220, 1981.
288. Smailys, A., Dulevicius, Z., Muckus, K., and Dauska, K.: Investigation of the possibilities of cardiac defibrillation by ultrasound. Resuscitation *9*:233, 1981.

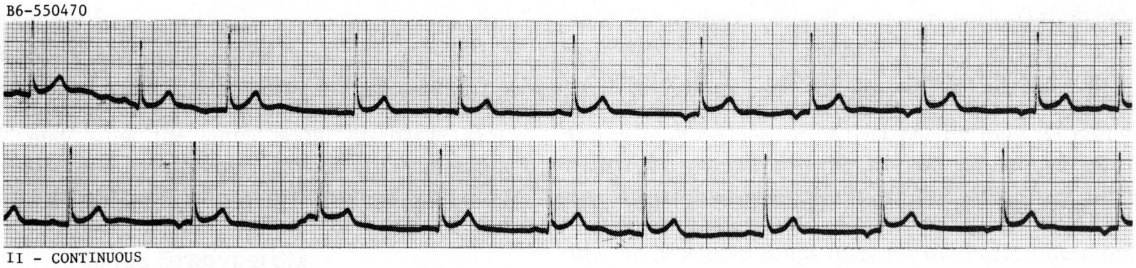

FIGURE 21–5 Wandering atrial pacemaker. As the heart rate slows, the P waves become inverted and then gradually revert toward normal when the heart rate speeds up again. The P-R interval shortens to 0.14 sec with the inverted P wave and is 0.16 sec with the upright P wave. This phasic variation in cycle length with varying P-wave contour suggests a shift in pacemaker site and is characteristic of wandering atrial pacemaker.

may produce type II SA exit block. SA exit block is usually transient. It may be of no clinical importance except to prompt a search for the underlying cause. Occasionally, syncope may result if the SA block is prolonged and unaccompanied by an escape rhythm.

Therapy for patients who have symptomatic SA exit block is as outlined for sinus bradycardia.

Wandering Pacemaker (Fig. 21–5)

This variant of sinus arrhythmia, involves the passive transfer of the dominant pacemaker focus from the sinus node to latent pacemakers that have the next highest degree of automaticity located in other atrial sites or in AV junctional tissue. Thus, only one pacemaker at a time controls the rhythm, in sharp contrast to AV dissociation (p. 735). As with other forms of sinus arrhythmia, the change occurs in a gradual fashion over the duration of several beats. The ECG displays a cyclical increase in R-R interval; a P-R interval that gradually shortens and may become less than 120 msec; and a change in the P-wave contour, which becomes negative in lead I or II (depending on the site of discharge) or is lost within the QRS complex. Generally, these changes occur in reverse as the pacemaker shifts back to the sinus node. Rarely the rate may remain unchanged during these P-wave transitions.

Wandering pacemaker is a normal phenomenon that often occurs in the very young or old and particularly in athletes, presumably because of augmented vagal tone. Persistence of an AV junctional rhythm for long periods of time, however, may indicate underlying heart disease. *Treatment* is usually not indicated but, if necessary, is the same as that for sinus bradycardia (see above).

Hypersensitive Carotid Sinus Syndrome (Fig. 21–6) (See also p. 932)

Electrocardiographic Recognition. This condition is most frequently characterized by cessation of atrial activity due to sinus arrest or SA exit block and ventricular asystole. AV block is observed less frequently, probably in part because the absence of atrial activity due to sinus arrest precludes the manifestations of AV block. However, if an atrial pacemaker maintained an atrial rhythm (Fig. 22–23, p. 768) during the episodes, a higher prevalence of AV block probably would be noted. In symptomatic patients, AV junctional or ventricular escapes generally do not occur or are present at very slow rates, suggesting that heightened vagal tone can suppress subsidiary pacemakers located in the ventricles as well as supraventricular structures.

Clinical Features. Two types of hypersensitive carotid sinus responses are noted. *Cardioinhibitory* carotid sinus hypersensitivity is defined as ventricular asystole exceeding 3 seconds during carotid sinus stimulation, although it should be emphasized that normal limits have not been carefully established. Asystole exceeding 3 seconds during carotid sinus massage may occur in some normal subjects. *Vasodepressor* carotid sinus hypersensitivity is defined as a decrease in systolic blood pressure of 50 mm Hg or more without associated cardiac slowing or a decrease in systolic blood pressure exceeding 30 mm Hg when the patient's symptoms are reproduced.[21]

Hyperactive carotid sinus reflex is common in older patients, but most are asymptomatic. Even if they complain of syncope or presyncope, the hyperactive reflex elicited with carotid sinus massage may not necessarily be responsible for these symptoms.[22] Direct pressure or extension on the carotid sinus such as head turning, neck tension, and tight collars may reproduce syncope in these patients. However, it must be remembered that such procedures may be a source of syncope by reducing blood flow through the vertebral arteries also.

Because intrinsic sinus nodal dysfunction is generally not the major cause for asystole after carotid sinus stimulation in this syndrome,[23] patients with hypersensitive carotid sinus syndrome may be distinguished from those with sick sinus syndrome (p. 693).[21] Hypersensitive carotid sinus reflex is most commonly associated with coronary artery disease.[24] The mechanism responsible for hypersensitive carotid sinus reflex is not known, but possibilities include a high level of resting vagal tone, hyperrespon-

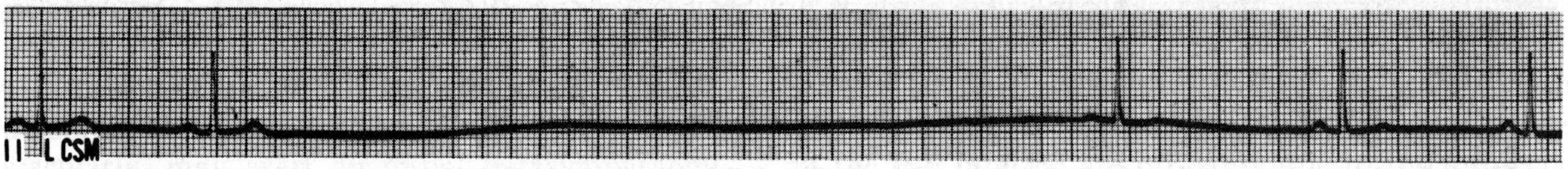

FIGURE 21–6 Hypersensitive carotid sinus syndrome. Gentle left carotid sinus massage (LCSM) produced a prolonged period of asystole. Lead II.

siveness to acetylcholine, excessive release of acetylcholine, and inadequate cholinesterase activity to metabolize the acetylcholine released. Carotid sinus receptors, autonomic centers of the brain stem, and the afferent limb of the reflex have all been incriminated.[21]

TREATMENT. Atropine abolishes cardioinhibitory carotid sinus hypersensitivity. However, the majority of symptomatic patients require pacemaker implantation. It must be stressed that because AV block may occur during the periods of hypersensitive carotid reflex, some form of *ventricular* pacing, with or without atrial pacing, is generally required. Atropine does not prevent the decrease in systemic blood pressure in the vasodepressor form of carotid sinus hypersensitivity, which may result from inhibition of sympathetic vasoconstrictor nerves and possibly activation of cholinergic sympathetic vasodilator fibers. Combinations of vasodepressor and cardioinhibitory types may occur, and vasodepression[25] may account for continued syncope after pacemaker implantation in some patients. Patients who have a hyperactive carotid sinus reflex that does not cause symptoms require no treatment.[22] Drugs such as digitalis, alpha-methyldopa, clonidine,[26] or propranolol may enhance the response to carotid sinus massage and be responsible for symptoms in some patients. Severe vasodepressor or mixed vasodepressor and cardioinhibitory responses may require treatment with either radiation therapy or surgical denervation of the carotid sinus.

Sick Sinus Syndrome

This term[27,28] is applied to a syndrome encompassing a number of sinus nodal abnormalities that include (1) persistent spontaneous sinus bradycardia not caused by drugs, and inappropriate for the physiological circumstance, (2) apparent sinus arrest or exit block, (3) combinations of SA and AV conduction disturbances, or (4) alternation of paroxysms of rapid regular or irregular atrial tachyarrhythmias and periods of slow atrial and ventricular rates (bradycardia-tachycardia syndrome,[29,30] Fig. 21–7). More than one of these conditions can be recorded in the same patient on different occasions, and often their mechanisms can be shown to be causally interrelated and combined with an abnormal state of AV conduction or automaticity.[29,31]

More than one pathophysiological mechanism can produce the clinical manifestations of sick sinus syndrome. The spontaneous clinical arrhythmia and the response to electrophysiological testing (see Chapter 19) depend on the underlying mechanism of sinus nodal dysfunction.[32] Patients who have sinus node disease may be categorized as having intrinsic sinus node disease unrelated to autonomic abnormalities[33,34] or combinations of intrinsic and autonomic abnormalities. Symptomatic patients with sinus pauses and/or SA exit block frequently show abnormal responses on electrophysiological testing and can have a relatively high incidence of life-threatening arrhythmias.[35] In one study of 128 patients diagnosed as having sinus node dysfunction, 33 had sinus bradycardia, 37 had SA block or arrest, and 58 had the bradycardia-tachycardia syndrome. Additional heart disease, predominantly ischemic, was found in 56 per cent. During a followup of about 3 years, nine possible or proven systemic embolic events occurred.[36] In children, sinus node dysfunction most commonly occurs in those with congenital or acquired heart disease, particularly following corrective cardiac surgery. However, it may occur in the absence of other cardiac abnormalities.[37,38] Type I, type II, and complete SA exit block apparently can occur in healthy young boys.[16] Also, excessive training apparently can heighten vagal tone and produce syncope related to sinus bradycardia or AV conduction abnormalities in otherwise normal individuals.[39] The course of the disease is frequently intermittent and unpredictable, influenced by the severity of the underlying heart disease.[39a]

The anatomical basis of sick sinus syndrome may involve total or subtotal destruction of the sinus node, areas of nodal-atrial discontinuity, inflammatory or degenerative changes of the nerves and ganglia surrounding the node, and pathological changes in the atrial wall. Fibrosis and fatty infiltration occur, and the sclerodegenerative processes generally are not limited to the sinus node but involve the AV node or the bundle of His and its branches or distal subdivisions.[40–42] In a study of 111 patients, the amount of nodal cells remaining in the sinus node was found to be inversely proportional to the age of the patient. Chronic SA block was associated with extensive lesions of the approaches to the AV node or of the AV node itself, and the bradycardia-tachycardia syndrome was associated with lesions of the sinus node and atrial muscle. Fibrosis was the main feature of the sinus node lesion.[43]

TREATMENT. For patients with sick sinus syndrome, treatment depends on the basic rhythm problem but generally involves permanent pacemaker implantation when symptoms are manifest (see Chapter 22). Pacing for the bradycardia combined with drug therapy to treat the tachycardia is required in those who fit the bradycardia-tachycardia subset. In these patients, drug therapy without pacing may aggravate the bradycardia. Although some

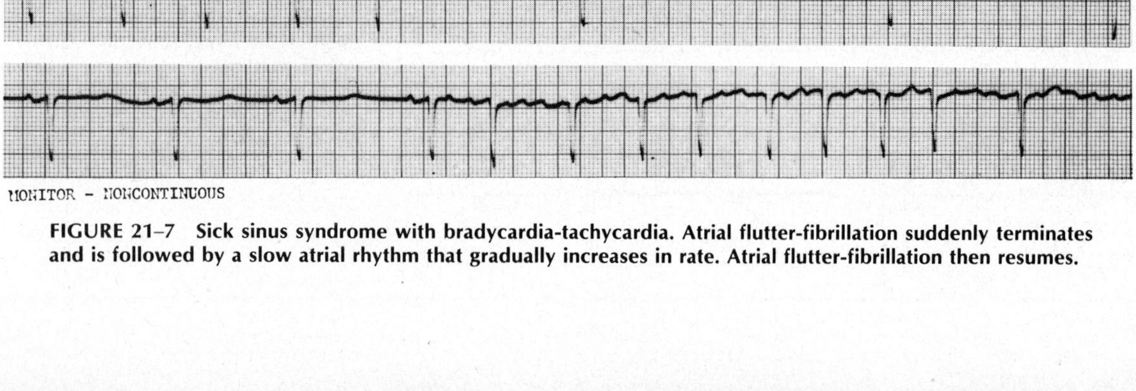

FIGURE 21–7 Sick sinus syndrome with bradycardia-tachycardia. Atrial flutter-fibrillation suddenly terminates and is followed by a slow atrial rhythm that gradually increases in rate. Atrial flutter-fibrillation then resumes.

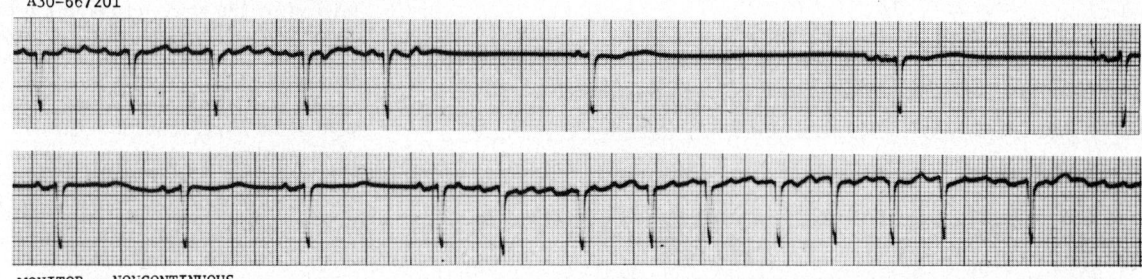

controversy exists about using digitalis, it should be noted that digitalis in therapeutic doses may depress intrinsic sinus nodal function in patients with normal as well as abnormal sinus nodal function. These effects of digitalis are independent of its vagal and antiadrenergic effects, and the drug should be used cautiously in patients with sick sinus syndrome without a pacemaker.[44] Prolonged sinoatrial conduction time in the absence of symptoms is not an indication for prophylactic pacing.[45] Therapy is directed toward control of symptoms.

Sinus Nodal Reentry

(Fig. 21–8) (See also p. 622)

The rate of sinus nodal reentrant tachycardia varies from 80 to 200 beats/min but is generally slower than the other forms of supraventricular tachycardia, with an average rate of 130 to 140 beats/min. Electrocardiographically, P waves are identical or very similar to the sinus P wave morphologically; the P-R interval is related to the tachycardia rate, but generally the R-P interval is long, with a shorter P-R interval (Fig. 21–9*D*). AV block may occur without affecting the tachycardia, and vagal maneuvers may slow and then abruptly terminate the tachycardia. Electrophysiologically, the tachycardia may be initiated and terminated by premature atrial and, uncommonly, premature ventricular stimulation (Fig. 21–8). Initiation of sinus nodal reentry does not depend on a critical degree of intraatrial or AV nodal conduction delay and the atrial activation sequence is the same as during sinus rhythm. AV nodal Wenckebach block during the tachycardia is common.[46–50] The development of bundle branch block does not affect the cycle length or P-R interval during tachycardia. Prolongation of AV nodal conduction time or development of AV nodal block may occur prior to termination of the tachycardia but does not affect the sinus nodal reentry.

Sinus nodal reentry may account for 5 to 10 per cent of cases of supraventricular tachycardia. It occurs in all age groups without sex predilection. Patients may be slightly older and have a higher incidence of heart disease than do patients with supraventricular tachycardia due to other mechanisms. Many may not seek medical attention because the relatively slow rate of the tachycardia does not result in serious symptoms. On the other hand, sinus nodal reentry may be responsible for apparent "anxiety-related sinus tachycardia" in some patients. Drugs such as propranolol, verapamil, and digitalis may be effective in terminating and preventing recurrences of sinus node reentrant tachycardia.[51]

ATRIAL RHYTHM DISTURBANCES

Premature complexes are one of the most common causes of an irregular pulse. They may originate from any area in the heart, most frequently from the ventricles, less often from the atria and from the AV junctional area, and rarely from the sinus node. Although premature complexes arise in normal hearts, they are more often associated with organic heart disease and increase in frequency with age.

Premature Atrial Complexes

Electrocardiographic Recognition (Fig. 21–10). The electrocardiographic diagnosis of premature atrial complexes is indicated by a premature P wave with a P-R interval exceeding 120 msec (except in WPW syndrome when the P-R interval may be less than 120 msec). Although the contour of the premature P wave may resemble the normal sinus P wave, it generally differs. Variations in the basic sinus rate at times may make the diagnosis of prematurity difficult, but differences in the contour of the P waves are usually apparent and indicate a different focus

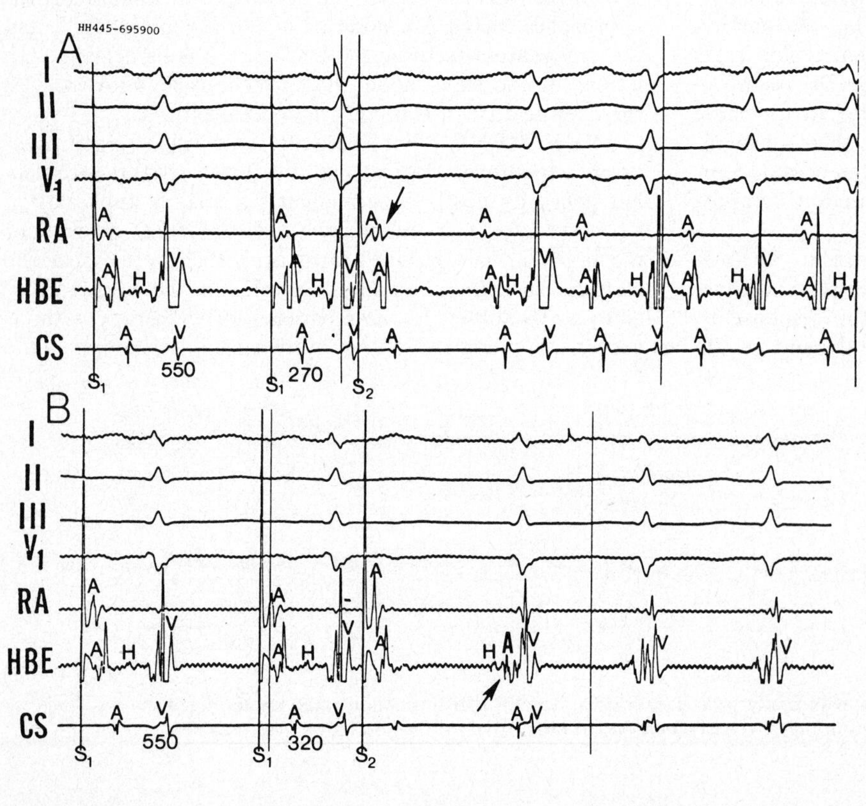

FIGURE 21–8 *A, Sinoatrial nodal reentry.* Premature stimulation of the high right atrium at an S_1-S_2 interval of 270 msec initiates an atrial tachycardia with an activation sequence similar to that occurring during high right atrial pacing. The premature P wave blocks proximal (arrow) to the His bundle but the tachycardia is still initiated. *B, AV nodal reentry.* Premature stimulation of the high right atrium at an S_1-S_2 interval of 320 msec results in a prolonged A-H interval and initiation of *AV nodal reentry.* Retrograde low right atrial activation recorded in the HBE lead occurs before ventricular activation and is followed by left atrial (CS) and high right atrial activation (arrow). This is in sharp contrast to *A*, in which the atrial activation sequence begins in the high right atrium, then the low right atrium (HBE), and then finally the left atrium (CS).

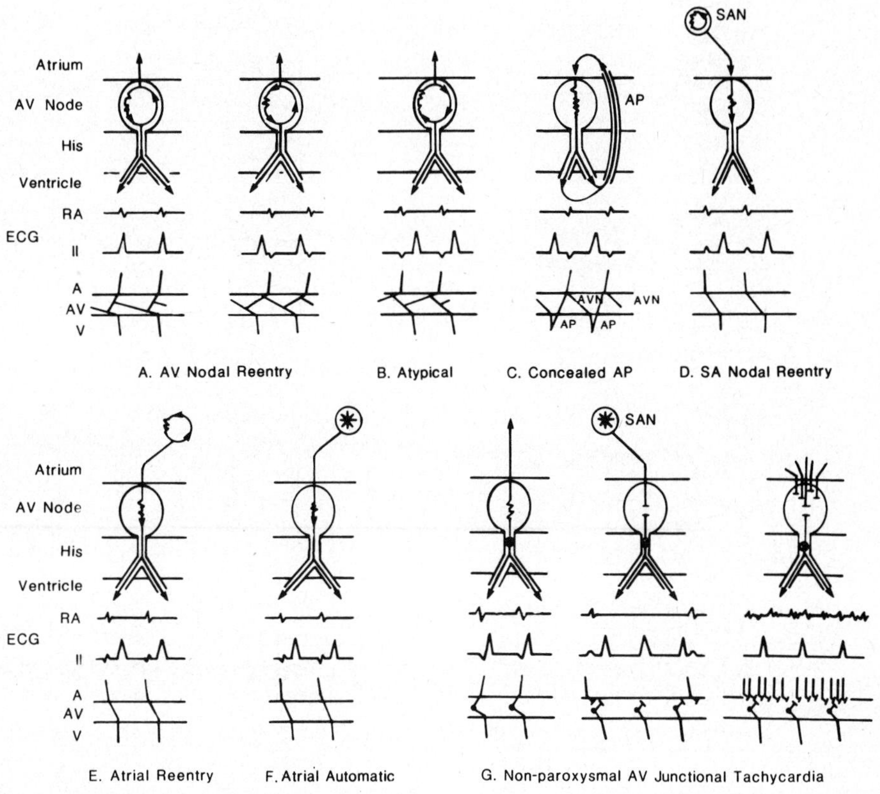

FIGURE 21–9 Diagrammatic representation of various tachycardias. In the top portion of each example, a schematic of the presumed anatomical pathways is drawn; in the bottom half, the ECG presentation and the explanatory ladder diagram are depicted. *A*, AV nodal reentry. In the left example, reentrant excitation is drawn confined to the AV node, with retrograde atrial activity occurring simultaneously with ventricular activity owing to anterograde conduction over the slow AV nodal pathway and retrograde conduction over the fast AV nodal pathway. In the right example, atrial activity occurs slightly later than ventricular activity, owing to retrograde conduction delay. *B*, Atypical AV nodal reentry due to anterograde conduction over a fast AV nodal pathway and retrograde conduction over a slow AV nodal pathway. *C*, Concealed accessory pathway. Reciprocating tachycardia is due to anterograde conduction over the AV node and retrograde conduction over the accessory pathway. Retrograde P waves occur after the QRS complex. *D*, Sinus nodal reentry. The tachycardia is due to reentry within the sinus node, which then conducts to the rest of the heart. *E*, Atrial reentry. Tachycardia is due to reentry within the atrium, which then conducts to the rest of the heart. *F*, Automatic atrial tachycardia. Tachycardia is due to automatic discharge in the atrium, which then conducts to the rest of the heart; it is difficult to distinguish from atrial reentry. *G*, Nonparoxysmal AV junctional tachycardia. Various presentations of this tachycardia are depicted with retrograde atrial capture, AV dissociation with the sinus node in control of the atria, and AV dissociation with atrial fibrillation.

of origin. When a premature atrial complex occurs early in diastole, conduction may not be completely normal. The AV junction may still be refractory from the preceding beat and prevent propagation of the impulse (blocked or nonconducted premature atrial complex, Fig. 21–10*A*) or cause conduction to be slowed (premature atrial complex with a prolonged P-R interval). As a general rule, the R-P interval is inversely related to the P-R interval: thus, a short R-P interval produced by an early premature atrial complex occurring close to the preceding QRS complex is followed by a long P-R interval. When premature atrial complexes occur early in the cardiac cycle, the premature P waves may be difficult to discern because they are superimposed on T waves. Careful examination of tracings from several leads may be necessary before the premature atrial complex can be recognized as a slight deformity of the T wave. Often such premature atrial complexes may block before reaching the ventricle and may be misinterpreted as a sinus pulse or sinus exit block (Fig. 21–10*A*).

The length of the pause following any premature complex or series of premature complexes is determined by the interaction of several factors. If the premature atrial complex occurs when the sinus node and perinodal tissue are not refractory, the impulse may conduct into the sinus node, discharge it prematurely, and cause the next sinus cycle to begin from that time. The interval between the two normal P waves flanking a premature atrial complex that has reset the timing of the basic sinus rhythm is less than twice the normal P-P interval and the pause after the premature atrial complex is said to be "noncompensatory." Referring to Figure 21–10*E*, reset (noncompensatory pause) occurs when A_1-A_2 interval + A_2-A_3 interval < two times the A_1-A_1 interval, and A_2-A_3 interval > A_1-A_1 interval. The interval between the premature atrial complex (A_2) and the following sinus-initiated P wave (A_3) exceeds one sinus cycle but is less than "fully compensatory" (see below), because the A_2-A_3 interval is lengthened by the time it takes the ectopic atrial impulse to conduct to the sinus node and depolarize it and then for the sinus impulse to return to the atrium. These factors lengthen the return cycle, i.e., the interval between the premature atrial complex (A_2) and the following sinus-initiated P wave (A_3) (Fig. 21–10*E*). Premature discharge of the sinus node by an early premature atrial complex may temporarily depress sinus nodal automatic activity, causing the sinus node to beat more slowly initially[52] (Fig. 21–10*D*). Often when this happens, the interval between the A_3 and the next sinus initiated P wave exceeds the A_1-A_1 interval.

Less commonly, the premature atrial complex may encounter a refractory sinus node or perinodal tissue, in which case the timing of the basic sinus rhythm is not altered, since the sinus node is not reset by the premature atrial complex and the interval between the two normal, sinus-initiated P waves flanking the premature atrial complex is twice the normal P-P interval. The interval following this premature atrial discharge is said to be a "full compensatory pause," i.e., of sufficient duration so that the P-P interval bounding the premature atrial complex is twice the normal P-P interval. However, sinus arrhythmia may lengthen or shorten this pause. Rarely, an *interpolated*

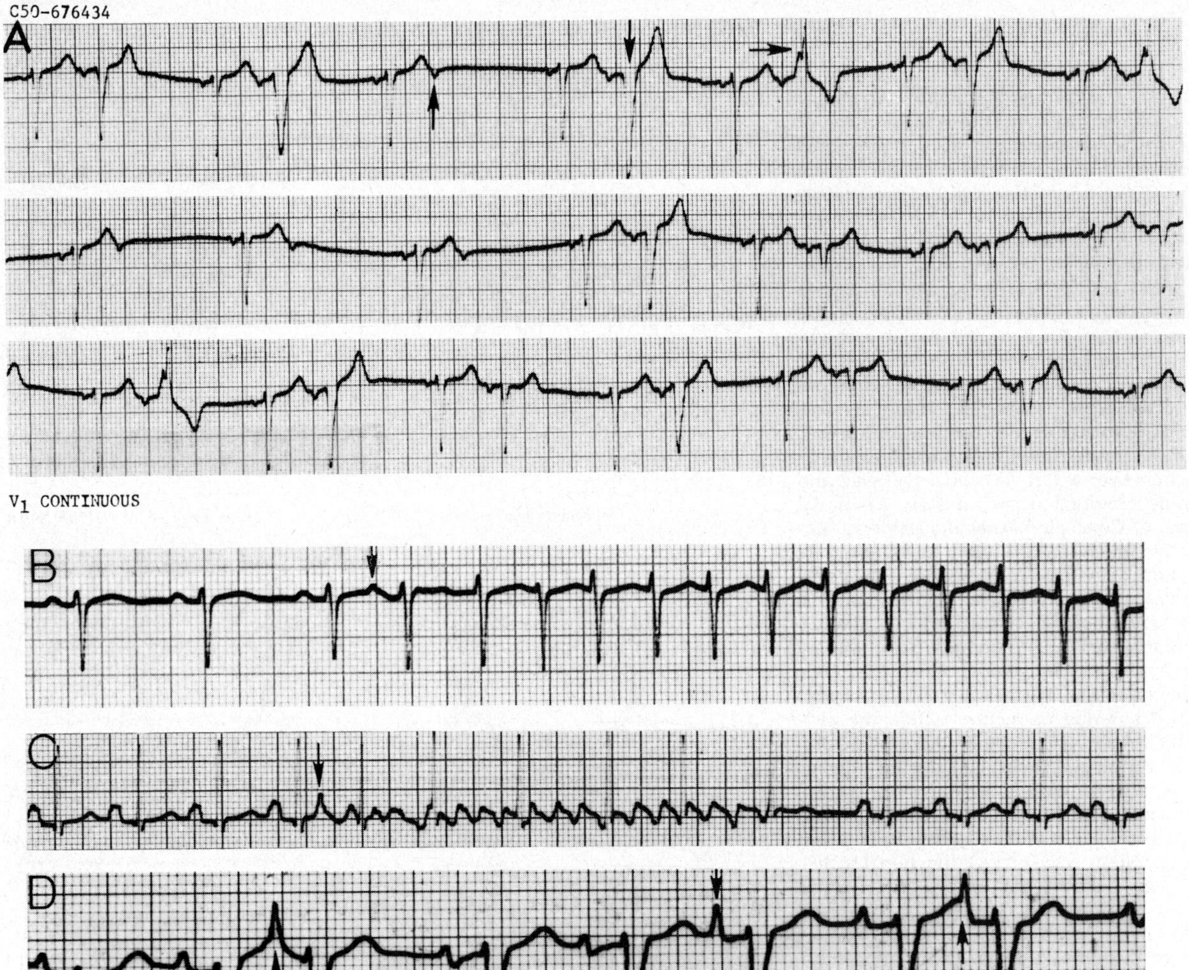

FIGURE 21–10 *A,* **Premature atrial complexes that block entirely or conduct with functional right or functional left bundle branch block. Depending on preceding cycle length and coupling interval of the premature atrial complex, the latter blocks entirely in the AV node (↑) or conducts with functional left bundle branch block (↓) or functional right bundle branch block (→).**

B, **Premature atrial complex (↓) initiates a supraventricular tachycardia probably due to AV nodal reentry.**

C **and** ***D,*** **A premature atrial complex (↓) initiating a short run of atrial flutter (*C*) and a premature atrial complex (↑) depressing the return of the next sinus nodal discharge (*D*). A slightly later premature atrial complex (↓) does not depress sinus nodal automaticity. Panels B=D monitor leads.**

E, **Diagrammatic example of effects of a premature atrial complex. Sinus interval ($A_1 - A_1$) equals X. Third P wave represents premature atrial complex (A_2) that reaches and discharges SA node, causing the next sinus cycle to begin at that time. Therefore, the P′–P (A_2–A_3) equals X+2Y msec, assuming no depression of SA nodal automaticity. (Modified from Zipes, D. P., and Fisch, C.: Premature atrial contraction. Arch. Intern. Med.** ***128*****: 453, 1971.)**

premature atrial complex may occur. In this case, the pause after the premature atrial complex is very short and the interval bounded by the normal sinus-initiated P waves on each side of the premature atrial complex is only slightly longer than or equals one normal P-P cycle length. The interpolated premature atrial complex fails to affect the sinus nodal pacemaker, and the sinus impulse following the premature atrial complex is conducted to the ventricles, often with a slightly lengthened P-R interval. An interpolated premature complex of any type represents the only type of premature systole that does not actually replace the normally conducted beat. Premature atrial complexes may originate in the sinus node and are identified by premature P waves that have a contour identical to the normal sinus P wave. The cycle after the premature sinus complex equals or is slightly shorter than the basic sinus cycle. Premature sinus complexes are not commonly recognized.[53]

On occasion, when the AV node has had sufficient time to repolarize and conduct without delay, the supraventricular QRS complex initiated by the premature atrial complex may be aberrant in configuration because the His-Purkinje system or ventricular muscle has *not* completely repolarized and conducts with functional delay or block (Fig. 21–10*A*). It is important to remember that the refractory period of cardiac fibers is related directly to heart rate. (In the adult, AV nodal effective refractory period prolongs at shorter cycle lengths.) A slow heart rate (long cycle length) produces a longer refractory period than a faster heart rate. Because of this, a premature atrial complex that follows a long R-R interval (long refractory period) may result in functional bundle branch block (aberrant ventricular conduction, p. 214). Since the right bundle branch has a longer refractory period than the left bundle branch, aberration with a right bundle branch block pattern occurs more commonly than aberration with a left bundle branch block pattern. At shorter cycles, the refractory period of the left bundle branch exceeds that of the right bundle branch[155] and a left bundle branch block pattern may be more likely to occur.

Clinical Features. Premature atrial complexes may occur in a variety of situations, for example, during infection, inflammation, or myocardial ischemia, or they may be provoked by a variety of medications, by tension states, or by tobacco, alcohol, or caffeine. Premature atrial complexes may precipitate or presage the occurrence of sustained supraventricular (Fig. 21–10*B* and *C*) and rarely ventricular tachyarrhythmias.[54–59]

Treatment. Premature atrial complexes generally do not require therapy. In symptomatic patients or when the premature atrial complexes precipitate tachycardias, treatment with digitalis, propranolol, or verapamil may be tried. If these drugs are unsuccessful trials with quinidine, procainamide, or disopyramide should be instituted.

Atrial Flutter (Fig. 21–11) (See also p. 626)

Electrocardiographic Recognition. The atrial rate during atrial flutter is usually 250 to 350 beats/min, although drugs such as quinidine, procainamide, or disopyramide may reduce the rate to the range of 200 beats/min. If this occurs, the ventricles may respond in a 1:1 fashion to the slower atrial rate.[60] Ordinarily the flutter rate is in the range of 300 beats/min, and in untreated patients, the ventricular rate is half the atrial rate, i.e., 150 beats/min (Fig. 21–11*A*). A significantly slower ventricular rate (in the absence of drugs) suggests abnormal AV conduction. In children, in patients with the preexcitation syndrome (p. 712), occasionally in patients with hyperthyroidism, or in those whose AV nodes conduct rapidly,[61,62] atrial flutter may conduct to the ventricle in a 1:1 fashion, producing a ventricular rate of 300 beats/min.

The ECG reveals identically recurring regular sawtooth flutter waves (Figs. 21–10*C* and 21–11*B*) and evidence of continual electrical activity (lack of an isoelectric interval between flutter waves), often best visualized in leads II, III, aVf, or V_1. The flutter waves are commonly inverted (negative) in these leads and less often are upright (positive). If the AV conduction ratio remains constant, the ventricular rhythm will be regular; if the ratio of conducted beats varies (usually the result of a Wenckebach AV block), the ventricular rhythm will be irregular. Alternation between 2:1 and 4:1 AV conduction often occurs and may be due to two levels of block—2:1 high in the AV node and 3:2 lower down.[63,64] The irregular ventricular response frequently has the structure that results from Wenckebach periodicity. Recurrent alternation of short and long ventricular intervals may be due to concealed conduction (p. 247).[65] Conduction may also be influenced by various degrees of penetration into the AV junction by the flutter impulses, which then affect conduction of subsequent impulses. The ratio of flutter waves to conducted ventricular complexes most often is an even number (e.g., 2:1, 4:1, and so on).[27] Impure flutter (flutter-fibrillation or "flitter"), occurring at a rate faster then pure flutter, shows variability in the contour and spacing of the flutter waves and in some instances may represent dissimilar atrial rhythms, i.e., fibrillation in one atrium and a slower, more regular rhythm resembling atrial flutter in the opposite atrium.[4,66,67] Prolonged atrial conduction time has been found to be a major predisposing factor for the development of atrial flutter.[68]

Clinical Features. Atrial flutter is less common than is atrial fibrillation. Paroxysmal atrial flutter may occur in patients without organic heart disease, while chronic (persistent) atrial flutter is usually associated with underlying heart disease such as rheumatic or ischemic heart disease or cardiomyopathy. It may occur as a result of atrial dilation from septal defects, pulmonary emboli, mitral or tricuspid valve stenosis or regurgitation, or chronic ventricular failure. Toxic and metabolic conditions that affect the heart, such as thyrotoxicosis, alcoholism, or pericarditis, may cause atrial flutter. Occasionally, it may be congenital.[69] Atrial flutter tends to be unstable, reverting to sinus rhythm or degenerating into atrial fibrillation. Uncommonly, the atria may continue to flutter for months or years. In atrial flutter the atria contract, which may, in part, account for less systemic emboli than during atrial fibrillation.

Atrial flutter usually responds to carotid sinus massage with a decrease in ventricular rate in stepwise multiples, returning in a reverse manner to the former ventricular rate at the termination of carotid massage. Very rarely sinus rhythm follows carotid sinus massage. Exercise, by enhancing sympathetic or lessening parasympathetic tone, may reduce the AV conduction delay and produce a doubling of the ventricular rate.

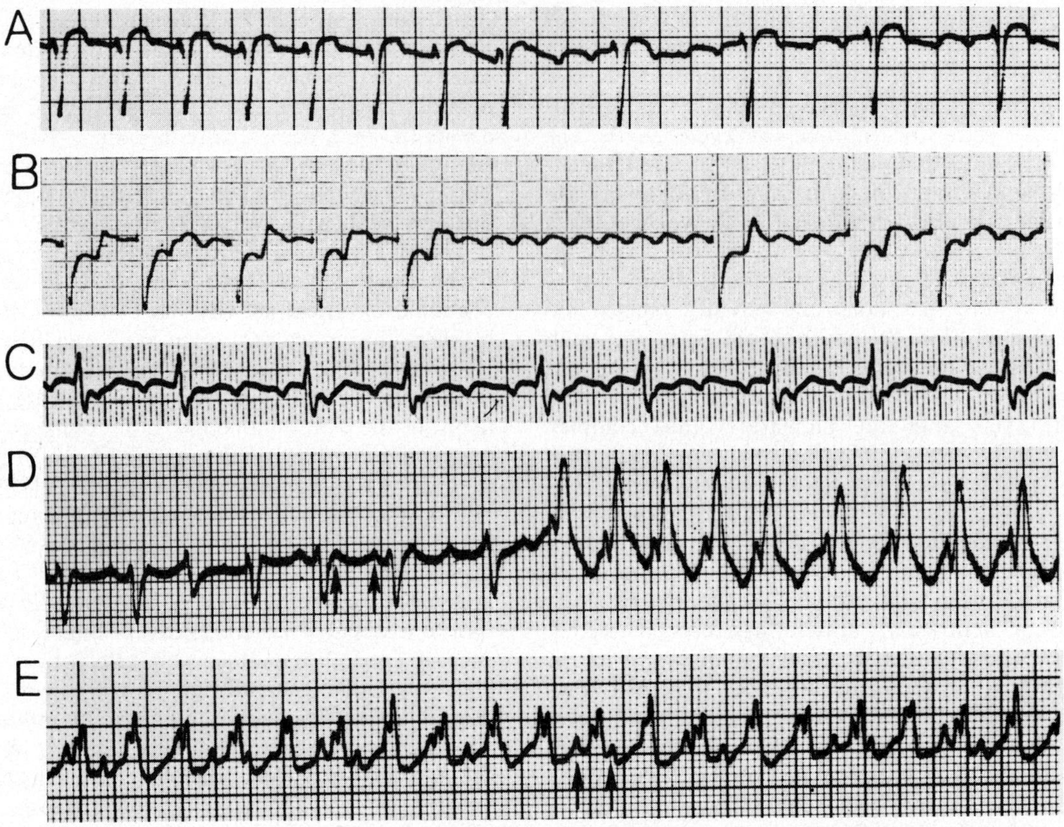

FIGURE 21–11 Various manifestations of atrial flutter. *A*, Atrial flutter at a rate of 300 beats/min conducts to ventricles with 2:1 block. In the midportion of the tracing, carotid sinus massage converts the block to 4:1 and the ventricular rate slows to 75 beats/min. *B*, Carotid sinus massage produces a transient period of AV block clearly revealing the flutter waves. *C*, Quinidine has slowed the atrial flutter rate to approximately 188 beats/min. The block is variable. *D*, Wide QRS complexes with an RSR′ configuration in V_1 begin after a short cycle that follows a long cycle in the midportion of the ECG strip. This represents functional right bundle branch block. *E*, the QRS complexes are 0.12 sec in duration and have a regular interval at a rate of 200 beats/min. Atrial activity is also regular at a rate of 300 beats/min and independent from the ventricular activity. Thus, atrial flutter is present with a probable ventricular tachycardia, an example of complete AV dissociation. Flutter waves are indicated by the arrows. Monitor leads in *A*, *B*, *C*, and *E*.

Physical examination may reveal rapid flutter waves in the jugular venous pulse. If the relationship of flutter waves to conducted QRS complexes remains constant, the first heart sound will have a constant intensity. Occasionally, sounds caused by atrial contraction may be auscultated.

Treatment. Synchronous direct-current (DC) cardioversion (p. 669) is commonly the initial treatment of choice for atrial flutter, since cardioversion promptly and effectively restores sinus rhythm, often requiring relatively low energies (< 50 joules). If the electrical shock results in atrial fibrillation, a second shock at a higher energy level may be used to restore sinus rhythm or, depending on the clinical circumstances, the atrial fibrillation may be left untreated. The latter will usually revert to atrial flutter or sinus rhythm. If the patient cannot successfully be electrically cardioverted or if electrical cardioversion is contraindicated—for example, after administering large amounts of digitalis—*rapid atrial pacing* can effectively terminate atrial flutter in many patients, producing atrial fibrillation with a slowing of the ventricular rate and concomitant clinical improvement or sinus rhythm.[70–72] Termination of atrial flutter by atrial pacing may be associated with entrainment, whereby at critical rates of overdrive atrial pacing the flutter morphology changes but the flutter does not terminate.[70] Using such pacing techniques, two types of atrial flutter have been recognized. Both types have uniform beat-to-beat atrial cycle length, morphology, polarity, and amplitude of right atrial electrograms, but one type, slower than the other, is influenced by rapid atrial pacing from the high right atrium while the other is not.[73]

Verapamil (p. 665), given as an initial bolus of 5 to 10 mg IV, followed by a constant infusion at a rate of 5 μg/kg/min to slow the ventricular response, may be tried.[74] Verapamil may restore sinus rhythm in patients with atrial flutter of recent onset but less commonly terminates chronic atrial flutter.

If the flutter cannot be electrically cardioverted or terminated by pacing or by verapamil, or if it recurs at frequent intervals, a *short-acting digitalis preparation* (such as digoxin or deslanoside) can be given. The dose of digitalis necessary to slow the ventricular response varies and at times may result in toxic levels because it is often difficult to slow the ventricular rate during atrial flutter. Frequently, atrial fibrillation develops after digitalis administration and may revert to normal sinus rhythm on withdrawal of digitalis; occasionally, normal sinus rhythm may occur without intervening atrial fibrillation. *Propranolol* (p. 662) effectively diminishes the ventricular response to atrial flutter and may be used together with digitalis in patients whose ventricular rate is not decreased after digitalis. Propranolol does not appear to affect the atrial rate during atrial flutter.

If the atrial flutter persists, *quinidine sulfate* (p. 656), 200 to 400 mg orally every six hours, can be used to restore sinus rhythm. Large doses of quinidine given every 2 hours to terminate atrial flutter or atrial fibrillation prior to the development of DC cardioversion are no longer warranted. If atrial flutter persists after digitalis and quinidine, disopyramide or procainamide administration can be tried empirically. If conversion occurs, the patient is given maintanence doses of digitalis and quinidine, disopyramide, or procainamide. Sometimes treatment of the underlying disorder, such as thyrotoxicosis, is necessary to effect conversion to sinus rhythm. In certain instances atrial flutter may continue, and if the ventricular rate can be controlled with digitalis, conversion may not be indicated. Quinidine maintenance therapy should be discontinued if flutter remains.

It is important to reemphasize that quinidine, procainamide, and disopyramide should *not* be used unless the ventricular rate during atrial flutter has been slowed with digitalis, verapamil, or propranolol. Because of the vagolytic action of quinidine, procainamide, and disopyramide (see Chap. 20) and also their direct effect to slow the atrial rate, AV conduction may be facilitated sufficiently to result in a 1:1 ventricular response to the atrial flutter.[60]

Prevention of recurrent atrial flutter is often difficult to achieve but should be approached as outlined for the prevention of paroxysmal supraventricular tachycardia due to AV nodal reentry (p. 709). If recurrences cannot be prevented, therapy is directed toward controlling the ventricular rate when the flutter does recur, with digitalis alone or combined with propranolol or with oral verapamil.*

Atrial Fibrillation (Fig. 21–12) (See also p. 626)

Electrocardiographic Recognition. This arrhythmia is characterized by totally disorganized atrial depolarizations without effective atrial contraction. Electrical activity of the atrium may be detected electrocardiographically as small irregular baseline undulations of variable amplitude and morphology, called F waves, at a rate of 350 to 600 beats/min. At times, small, fine, rapid F waves may occur and are detectable only by right atrial leads, intracavitary, or esophageal electrodes. The ventricular response is grossly irregular ("irregularly irregular") and, in the untreated patient with normal AV conduction, is usually between 100 and 160 beats/min. Atrial fibrillation should be suspected when the ECG shows supraventricular complexes at an irregular rhythm and no obvious P waves. The recognizable F waves probably do not represent total atrial activity but depict only the larger vectors generated by the multiple wavelets of depolarization that occur at any given moment.

Each recorded F wave is not conducted through the AV junction so that a rapid ventricular response comparable to the atrial rate does not occur. Many atrial impulses are canceled, owing to a collision of wavefronts, or are blocked, owing to the varying penetration of many atrial impulses into the AV junction without reaching the ventricles (i.e., concealed conduction [see p. 247]). Such variable penetration affects the conduction of subsequent impulses by delaying or blocking their passage in the AV junction and accounts for the irregular ventricular rhythm during atrial fibrillation. When the ventricular rate is very rapid or very slow, it may appear to be more regular. Even though the conversion of atrial fibrillation to atrial flutter is accompanied by slowing of the atrial rate because of less concealed conduction, an increase in the ventricular response may result, since more atrial impulses are transmitted to the ventricle. Also, it is easier to slow the ventricular rate with drugs during atrial fibrillation than during atrial flutter because the increased concealed conduction makes it easier to produce AV block. A pause in the ventricular rhythm after a premature ventricular complex results from concealed retrograde conduction (p. 247) of the ventricular beat into the AV junction, thus preventing conduction of a number of subsequent atrial impulses.[75] During atrial fibrillation with conduction solely through the AV node, a significant correlation exists between the shortest and mean R-R intervals and the AV nodal functional refractory period, as well as with the shortest ventricular cycle length during atrial pacing that results in 1:1 AV conduction.[61,76]

Clinical Features. Atrial fibrillation may be chronic or intermittent; the former is almost always associated with underlying heart disease, while the latter may occur in apparently normal hearts. Underlying heart disease is more

*At the time of this writing, the use of oral verapamil for this purpose is still investigational, although intravenous verapamil has been approved by the FDA to treat supraventricular tachycardias.

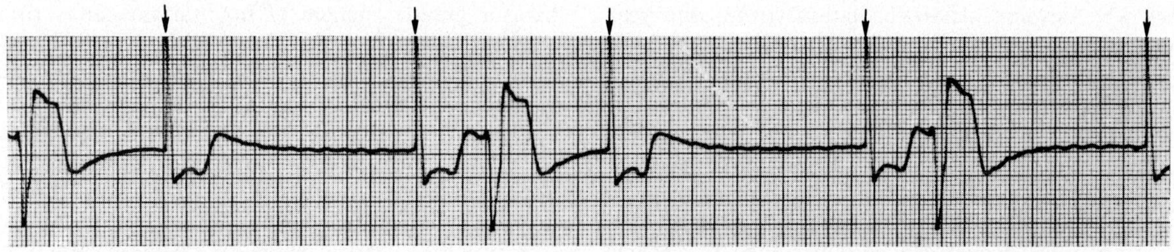

FIGURE 21–12 Atrial fibrillation with a high degree of AV block. Arrows indicate the normally conducted QRS complexes that occur at a very slow rate owing to AV block in the absence of drugs. When the R-R cycle is long, a premature ventricular complex follows, which conforms to the "rule of bigeminy"[27] and indicates that long ventricular cycles tend to be followed by premature ventricular complexes. Monitor lead.

frequent in patients with atrial flutter than in those with atrial fibrillation. The arrhythmia commonly results in patients who have rheumatic heart disease, especially with mitral valve involvement, cardiomyopathy, hypertensive heart disease, pulmonary emboli, pericarditis, and coronary heart disease. Occult or manifest thyrotoxicosis should always be considered in a patient with atrial fibrillation of recent onset.[77] The presence of cardiac failure and rheumatic heart disease are risk factors for the development of atrial fibrillation. Hypertensive cardiovascular disease is the most common antecedent disease, largely because of its frequency in the general population. The development of chronic atrial fibrillation is associated with a doubling of overall mortality and of mortality from cardiovascular disease.[78] Intermittent episodes of atrial fibrillation may recur in some patients only once or twice and in others more frequently. The duration of a single paroxysm may range from less than 24 hours to several weeks. Atrial fibrillation may become permanent in 25 per cent of these patients observed for more than one year.[79]

Mortality is unchanged in patients who have paroxysmal atrial fibrillation with no other identified cardiovascular impairment. However, paroxysmal atrial fibrillation with associated mitral stenosis or coronary disease has been found to be associated with significantly increased mortality. Chronic atrial fibrillation with or without other impairment entails a much higher mortality risk than does paroxysmal atrial fibrillation and is highest in patients with mitral stenosis.[80] Occasionally, patients with long-standing atrial fibrillation may develop spontaneous reversion to sinus rhythm. In the majority of these patients the ECG shows first-degree AV block (see p. 730) after return to sinus rhythm and low-amplitude P waves. Left atrial contraction may not occur in some patients with mitral valve disease, possibly owing to loss of atrial muscle.[81]

Patients with chronic atrial fibrillation are at greatly increased risk of *embolic stroke.* In the absence of rheumatic heart disease, chronic atrial fibrillation is associated with more than a fivefold increase in the incidence of stroke and a seventeenfold increase in patients with rheumatic heart disease. The occurrence of stroke increases directly with the duration of atrial fibrillation.[82] In an autopsy study of patients with atrial fibrillation, embolism was noted in 35 to 40 per cent of patients with mitral valve disease or ischemic heart disease, in 17 per cent of those with other types of heart disease, and in only 7 per cent of a control group of patients with ischemic heart disease without atrial fibrillation. These findings suggest a high risk of embolism from atrial fibrillation of any origin but particularly from that caused by mitral and ischemic heart disease.[83]

Patients who develop atrial fibrillation within one year after acute myocardial infarction are generally older, have a more severe infarction, have higher total mortality at 3 and 12 months after infarction, and have a greater frequency of ventricular tachyarrhythmias and right bundle branch block than do patients who do not develop atrial fibrillation.[84] The presence of atrial fibrillation appears to be related to the type of underlying heart disease, as well as to left atrial size,[85] which can be determined by cardiac echocardiography but not by the amplitude of the F waves on the ECG.[86] The left atrial diameter measured by echocardiography is smaller in patients with paroxysmal atrial fibrillation that terminates spontaneously compared to that in patients who require DC cardioversion or who have persistent atrial fibrillation.[87] Atrial fibrillation in children is rare and is an indication for a thorough clinical investigation.[88]

The presence or absence of symptoms as a result of atrial fibrillation is determined by multiple factors, the most important of which is cardiac status. The rapid ventricular rate and loss of atrial contraction detrimentally affect cardiac output. Physical findings in patients exhibiting atrial fibrillation include a slight variation in the intensity of the first heart sound, absence of *a* waves in the jugular venous pulse, and an irregularly irregular ventricular rhythm. Often with fast ventricular rates a significant pulse deficit appears, during which the apical rate is faster than the rate palpated at the wrist because each contraction is not sufficiently strong to open the aortic valve or to transmit an arterial pressure wave through the peripheral artery. If the rhythm becomes regular in patients with atrial fibrillation, conversion to one of the following rhythms should be suspected: sinus rhythm, atrial tachycardia, atrial flutter with a constant ratio of conducted beats, or development of junctional or ventricular tachycardia.

Treatment. When one is treating the patient with atrial fibrillation for the first time, it is important to search for a precipitating cause, such as thyrotoxicosis, mitral stenosis, pulmonary emboli, or pericarditis, and to treat it appropriately, if found. The patient's clinical status determines initial therapy, the objectives being to slow the ventricular rate and to restore atrial systole. If the sudden onset of atrial fibrillation with a rapid ventricular rate results in acute cardiovascular decompensation, electrical cardioversion is the treatment of choice. In the absence of decompensation, the patient may be treated with digitalis to maintain a resting apical rate of 60 to 80 beats/min that does not exceed 100 beats/min after slight exercise. The speed, route, dosage, and type of digitalis preparation administered are determined by the status of the patient. The combined use of digitalis and a beta or calcium-entry blocker[74,89] may be useful in slowing the ventricular rate. Quinidine, given with digitalis, is often necessary to convert to sinus rhythm. The use of large doses of quinidine to produce reversion to normal sinus rhythm is no longer indicated. Prior to electrical cardioversion, maintenance doses of quinidine sulfate in the range of 1.2 to 2.4 grams/day should be administered for a few days. During this time normal sinus rhythm will resume in 10 to 15 per cent of patients. DC cardioversion establishes normal sinus rhythm in over 90 per cent of patients, but sinus rhythm remains for 12 months in only 30 to 50 per cent. Patients with atrial fibrillation of less than 12 months' duration have a greater chance of maintaining sinus rhythm after cardioversion than do those without left atrial enlargement.[90,90a] The role of anticoagulation prior to cardioversion is somewhat controversial because of imperfect studies. Most investigators feel that anticoagulation prior to drug or electrical cardioversion is indicated in patients with a high risk of emboli, i.e., those with mitral stenosis, atrial fibrillation of recent onset, recent or recurrent emboli, a prosthetic mitral valve, or cardiomegaly. Some recommend two weeks of anticoagulation prior to elective cardioversion of atrial fibrillation present for more than about one week, if no contraindications to anticoagulation exist, and continuing anticoagulation for two additional weeks.[90a]

The incidence of embolization during conversion to normal sinus rhythm is 1 to 2 per cent.[91–93] In one noncontrolled study, 454 electrical conversions in 348 patients who had atrial fibrillation, atrial flutter, or atrial tachycardia of long duration resulted in two embolic events in 186 patients who had received anticoagulant therapy over the long term and 11 embolic events in 162 patients who did not receive anticoagulant therapy.[93] Disopyramide or procainamide[94] may be tried in place of quinidine. Serial electrophysiological testing can be used to select appropriate drugs to prevent recurrence of atrial fibrillation in some patients.[95] Rapid atrial pacing will *not* terminate atrial fibrillation.

Many elderly patients tolerate atrial fibrillation well without therapy because the ventricular rate is slow as a result of concomitant AV nodal disease. These patients often have associated sick sinus syndrome, and the development of atrial fibrillation represents a cure of sorts. Such patients may demonstrate serious supraventricular and ventricular arrhythmias or asystole after cardioversion, so that the likelihood of establishing and maintaining sinus rhythm should be weighed against the risks of cardioversion or other forms of therapy.

Atrial Tachycardia With Block (Fig. 21–13)

Electrocardiographic Recognition. In atrial tachycardia, sometimes called atrial tachycardia with block or paroxysmal atrial tachycardia with block (PAT with block), the atrial rate is generally 150 to 200 beats/min. When the tachycardia is due to digitalis excess, the atrial rate may increase gradually as the digitalis is continued (a similar response may occur in nonparoxysmal AV junctional tachycardia) and may be associated with gradual prolongation of the P-R interval. If the atrial rate is not excessive and AV conduction is not significantly depressed by the digitalis, each P wave may conduct to the ventricles. As the atrial rate increases and AV conduction becomes impaired, Wenckebach (Mobitz type I) second-degree AV block may ensue, hence the term atrial tachycardia with block. Frequently, other manifestations of digitalis excess, such as premature ventricular complexes, are present. In nearly half the cases of atrial tachycardia with block, the atrial rate is irregular. Characteristic isoelectric intervals between P waves, in contrast to atrial flutter, are usually present in all leads. However, at rapid atrial rates the distinction between atrial tachycardia with block and atrial flutter may be difficult.

The term "paroxysmal" is used to indicate a tachycardia of sudden onset that changes from sinus rhythm to a tachycardia in one beat—for example, a premature atrial complex precipitating a paroxysmal supraventricular tachycardia (Fig. 21–10*B*). In contrast, the term "nonparoxysmal" refers to a tachycardia that has a gradual onset and termination, similar to the warm-up phenomenon characteristic of automaticity (p. 620). Nonparoxysmal AV junctional tachycardia is such a tachycardia. Because the atrial tachycardia described above appears to be a "nonparoxysmal" variety, the term "paroxysmal atrial tachycardia with block" would be inappropriate.

Clinical Features. Atrial tachycardia with block occurs most commonly in patients with significant organic heart disease, such as coronary artery disease, with or without myocardial infarction, cor pulmonale, or digitalis intoxication. Digitalis toxicity accounts for 50 to 75 per cent of cases of atrial tachycardia with block. Potassium depletion may precipitate the arrhythmia in patients taking digitalis. The signs, symptoms, and prognosis are usually related to underlying cardiovascular status. Because this arrhythmia occurs primarily in patients suffering from serious heart disease, clinical deterioration may result from the arrhythmia.

Physical findings include a variable rhythm and intensity of the first heart sound, owing to the varying AV block and P-R interval. An excessive number of *a* waves may be seen in the jugular venous pulse. Carotid sinus massage increases the degree of AV block by slowing the ventricular rate in a stepwise fashion, as in atrial flutter. It should be performed cautiously in patients who have digitalis toxicity.

Treatment. Atrial tachycardia with block in a patient not receiving digitalis is treated in a manner similar to other atrial tachyarrhythmias. Depending on the clinical situation, digitalis may be administered to slow the ventricular rate and then if atrial tachycardia with block remains, quinidine, disopyramide, or procainamide may be added. If atrial tachycardia with block appears in a patient receiving digitalis, digitalis should initially be assumed to be respon-

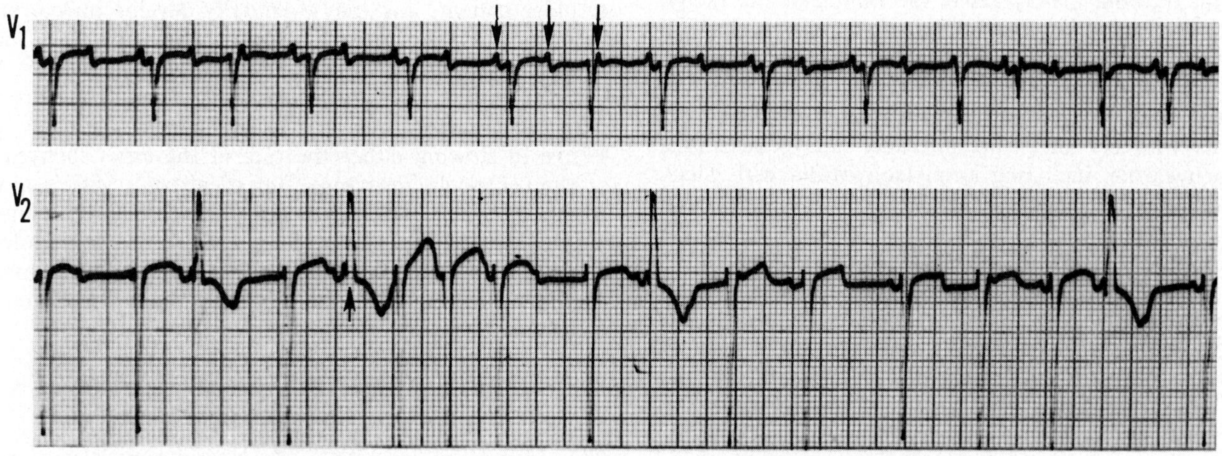

FIGURE 21–13 Atrial tachycardia with varying degrees of AV nodal Wenckebach block. A 3:2 Wenckebach grouping is indicated by the arrows. In V_2, functional right bundle branch block occurs when a short cycle follows a long cycle (arrow).

sible for the arrhythmia. Therapy includes cessation of digitalis and administration of potassium chloride orally or intravenously if serum [K^+] is not abnormally elevated, or drugs such as lidocaine, propranolol, or phenytoin while cardiac rhythm is monitored. Often, the ventricular response is not excessively fast and simply withholding digitalis is all that is necessary.

Two types of atrial tachycardias have been distinguished electrophysiologically: automatic and reentrant atrial tachycardia. While it is likely that one or both of these atrial tachycardias is responsible for atrial tachycardia with block, described above, the relationship, if any, is not clear at present, and these two tachycardias will be discussed separately.

Automatic Atrial Tachycardia
(Fig. 21–9*F*)

Electrocardiographic Features. Automatic atrial tachycardia is characterized electrocardiographically by a supraventricular tachycardia that generally accelerates after its initiation, with heart rates less than 200 beats/min. The P wave differs from the sinus P wave, the P-R interval is influenced directly by the tachycardia rate, and AV block may exist without affecting the tachycardia. Vagal maneuvers generally do not terminate the tachycardia, even though they may produce AV nodal block. Thus, pharmacological or physiological maneuvers that selectively produce AV block do not affect the automatic focus nor does the development of bundle branch block alter the P-R or R-P interval unless it is associated with prolongation of the H-V interval.

Electrophysiologically, initiation of tachycardia with premature atrial stimulation is generally not possible but is independent of intraatrial or AV nodal conduction delay when it occurs. The atrial activation sequence usually differs from a sinus-initiated P wave, and the A-H interval is related to the tachycardia rate. The rate may gradually accelerate after initiation. The first P wave of the tachycardia is the same as the subsequent P waves of the tachycardia in contrast to most forms of reentrant supraventricular tachycardias, in which the initial and subsequent P waves differ.[96–98] Usually the tachycardia cannot be terminated by pacing; the introduction of premature atrial complexes during tachycardia merely resets the timing of the tachycardia. It is very difficult to differentiate this mechanism from micro-reentry, using the leading circle concept of Allessi (see pp. 622 and 626).

Clinical Features. Many supraventricular tachycardias associated with AV block are probably due to automatic atrial tachycardia, including atrial tachycardia with block due to digitalis intoxication (Fig. 21–13). Automatic atrial tachycardia occurs in all age groups; is thought to be due to enhanced automaticity; and is seen in a setting of myocardial infarction, chronic lung disease (especially with acute infection), acute alcohol ingestion, and a variety of metabolic derangements. Digitalis appears to be a particularly important precipitating agent. Differentiation from other tachycardias such as sinus nodal reentry (if the P waves of the automatic atrial tachycardia resemble the sinus-initiated P waves), atrial reentry (particularly if caused by micro-reentry), and some other mechanisms may be difficult. In view of the experimental findings of triggered activity from a variety of atrial fibers, including human mitral valve (see p. 620), it is possible that such activity also occurs in man. However, many automatic atrial tachycardias are not suppressed by verapamil.[99]

Therapy is as discussed under atrial tachycardia with block (p. 701).

Atrial Tachycardia due to Reentry
(Fig. 21–9*E*) (See also p. 626)

Electrocardiographic Recognition. This arrhythmia presents electrocardiographically with a P wave that has a contour different from the sinus P wave, a P-R interval influenced directly by the tachycardia rate, and the ability to develop AV block without interrupting the tachycardia. Electrophysiologically, initiation of the tachycardia occurs with premature stimulation during the atrial relative refractory period, resulting in a critical degree of intraatrial conduction delay, an atrial activation sequence different from that which occurs during sinus rhythm, and an AV nodal conduction time related to the tachycardia rate. Vagal maneuvers generally do not terminate the tachycardia and may produce AV block.[49,100–102]

Clinical Features. The relative infrequency of published reports suggests that atrial reentry is not a commonly recognized cause of supraventricular tachycardia. In a recent report of a group of 20 patients with sustained tachycardia due to intraatrial reentry,[101] the average rate of the tachycardia was 130 beats/min and was started by an atrial extrastimulus, progressively accelerating atrial pacing or an atrial escape beat. In all cases, premature stimulation terminated the tachycardia. Spontaneous termination could be either sudden, with progressive slowing, or alternating long-short cycle lengths.

Chaotic Atrial Tachycardia (Fig. 21–14)

Chaotic (sometimes called multifocal) atrial tachycardia is characterized by atrial rates between 100 and 130 beats/min, with marked variation in P-wave morphology and totally irregular P-P intervals.[103] Generally at least three P-wave contours are noted, with most P waves conducted to the ventricles.[104] This tachycardia occurs commonly in patients with pulmonary disease and in diabetics or older patients and may eventually develop into atrial fibrillation. Digitalis appears to be an unusual cause. Chaotic atrial tachycardia can occur in childhood.[105]

Treatment. Therapy is primarily directed toward the underlying disease. Antiarrhythmic agents are often ineffective in slowing either the rate of the atrial tachycardia or the ventricular response. Empirical trials with standard drugs, with care being taken not to exacerbate the underlying disease (e.g., using verapamil instead of propranolol in patients with bronchospastic pulmonary disease) or to produce drug toxicity, may be warranted in symptomatic patients.

AV JUNCTIONAL RHYTHM DISTURBANCES

AV Junctional Escape Beats

Automatic fibers that are prevented from initiating depolarization by a pacemaker such as the sinus node pos-

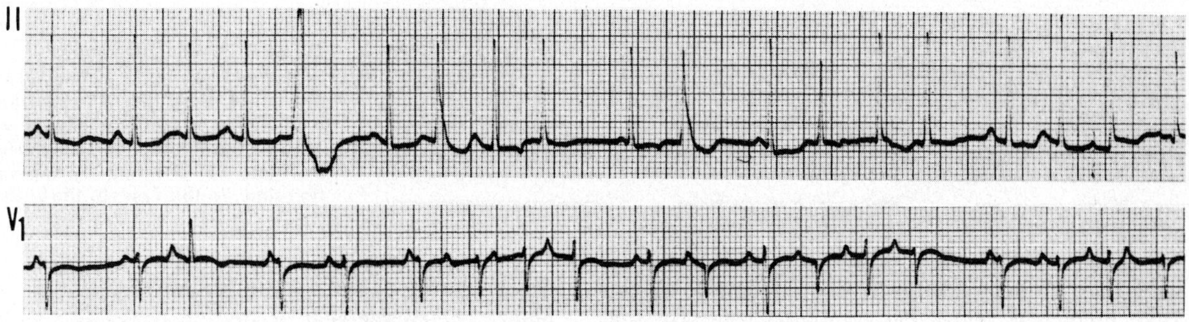

FIGURE 21–14 Chaotic multifocal atrial tachycardia. Premature atrial complexes occur at varying cycle lengths and with differing contours.

sessing a more rapid rate of firing are called *latent pacemakers.* Such latent pacemakers are found in some parts of the atrium, in the AV node–His bundle area, in the right and left bundle branches, and in the Purkinje system. Under usual conditions automatic fibers are *not* found in atrial or ventricular myocardium. It is possible that the N region of the AV node may be automatic, at least in some species.[106,107] A latent pacemaker can become the dominant pacemaker by default or usurpation, that is, by passive or active mechanisms. A decrease in the number of impulses arriving at a latent pacemaker site, the result of slowing of the sinus node or interruption of the propagation of the normal impulse anywhere along its course, allows the latent pacemaker to escape and initiate depolarization passively, by default. An increase in the discharge rate of a latent pacemaker can capture pacemaker control actively, by usurpation. As will be seen, the implication of the two different mechanisms of ectopic impulse formation is important from a therapeutic standpoint.

Electrocardiographic Recognition. An AV junctional escape beat occurs when the rate of impulse formation of the primary pacemaker, generally the sinus node, becomes less than that of the AV junctional region, or when impulses from the primary pacemaker do not penetrate to the region of the escape focus and allow the AV junctional focus to reach threshold and discharge. The interval from the last normally conducted beat to the AV junctional escape beat is a measure of the initial discharge rate of the AV junctional focus and generally corresponds to a rate of 35 to 60 beats/min (Fig. 21–2*B*). Although an AV junctional escape rhythm is usually fairly regular, intervals between subsequent escape beats after the initial escape beat may gradually shorten as the rate of discharge of the escape focus increases, the so-called *rhythm of development* or *warm-up phenomenon.*

The electrocardiogram displays pauses longer than the normal P-P interval, interrupted by a QRS complex of supraventricular configuration with absent, retrograde, fusion, or sinus P waves that do not conduct to the ventricle. If P waves precede the QRS, they have a P-R interval generally less than 0.12 sec. The exact site of impulse formation (i.e., AN, N, or NH regions; low atrium; or His bundle) is not known and may differ from patient to patient and be influenced by the cause of the arrhythmia.

Treatment, if any, lies in increasing the discharge rate of the higher pacemakers and improving AV conduction and may require pacing. Frequently, no treatment is necessary.

Premature AV Junctional Complexes

(Figs. 21–15 to 21–17)

Premature AV junctional complexes are characterized by an impulse that arises prematurely in the AV junction (the exact site—i.e., AN, N, or NH regions; low atrium; or His bundle—is not known and may vary from patient to patient) and that attempts conduction in anterograde and retrograde directions. If unimpeded in its course, the impulse discharges the atrium to produce a premature retrograde P wave and a premature QRS complex with a supraventricular contour. The retrograde P wave may occur before, during, or after the QRS complex (Fig. 21–15). Alterations in conduction time may influence the P-R or R-P relationships without a change in the site of origin of the impulse (Fig. 21–16). Premature AV junctional

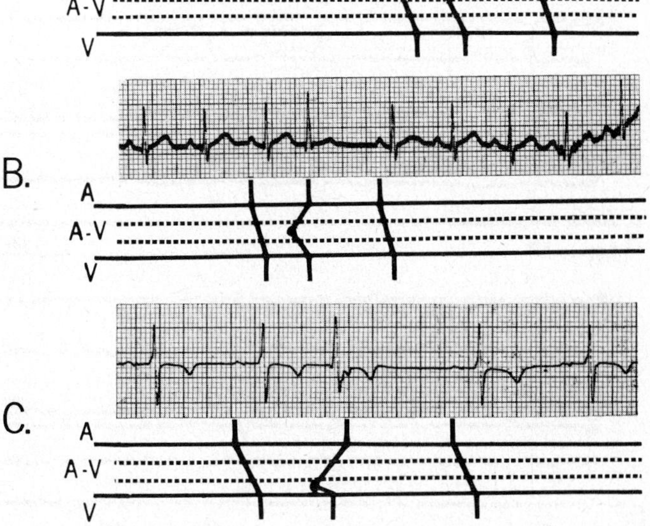

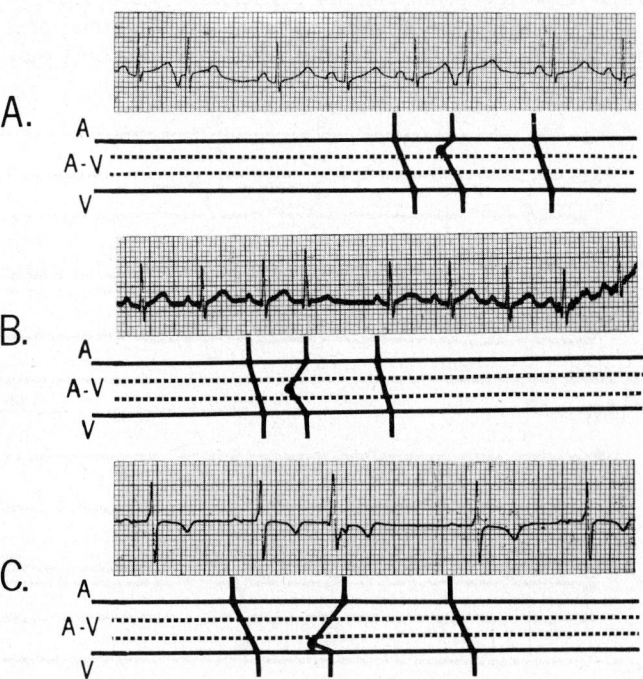

FIGURE 21–15 Premature AV junctional complexes. *A,* The premature AV junctional complex is preceded by a P wave. *B,* The atrial activity associated with this complex cannot be seen but may occur in the terminal portion of the QRS complex. *C,* A retrograde P wave follows the premature AV junctional complex. The ladder diagram indicates the position of the retrograde P wave in relation to the QRS complex by assuming (without adequate basis, see Fig. 21–16) that the premature AV junctional complex arises from upper, mid, and lower regions of the AV node.

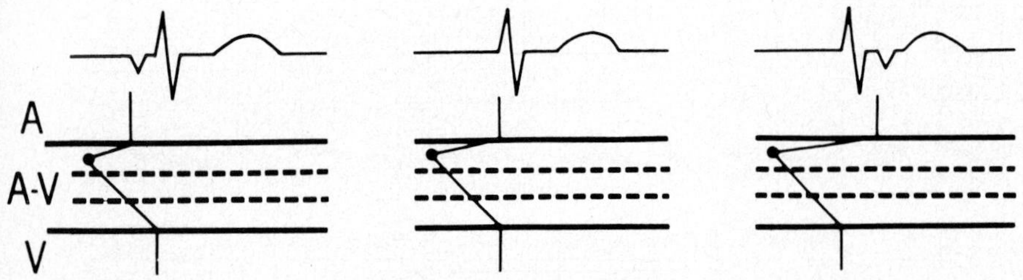

FIGURE 21–16 Diagrammatic representation of premature AV junctional complexes, indicating that the AV junctional focus maintaining a constant site of origin may achieve the P and QRS relationships shown in Figure 21–15 simply by varying conduction time, in this case, to the atrium.

complexes that conduct aberrantly are difficult to distinguish from premature ventricular complexes using the scalar ECG (Fig. 21–17).

Treatment of premature AV junctional complexes is generally not necessary. However, since they may arise distal to the AV node, they may occur early in the cardiac cycle and can initiate a ventricular tachyarrhythmia in some instances. Under these circumstances therapy may be approached as for premature ventricular complexes (see p. 719).

AV Junctional Rhythm (Fig. 21–18)

If the AV junctional escape beats continue for a period of time, the rhythm is called an AV junctional rhythm. Since the inherent rate of the AV junctional tissue is 35 to 60 beats/min, the AV junctional tissue can assume the role of the dominant pacemaker at this rate only by passive default of the sinus pacemaker. The ECG displays a normally conducted QRS complex, which may conduct retrogradely to the atrium or may occur independently of atrial discharge, producing AV dissociation (see p. 735).

An AV junctional escape rhythm may be a normal phenomenon in response to the effects of vagal tone or it may occur during pathological sinus bradycardia or heart block. The escape beat or rhythm serves as a safety mechanism to prevent the occurrence of ventricular asystole. *Physical findings* vary depending on the P-QRS relationship. Large *a* waves in the jugular venous pulse and a loud, soft, or changing intensity of the first heart sound may be present if atrial contraction occurs when the tricuspid valve is shut.

Therapy is discussed under AV junctional escape beats (see above).

Nonparoxysmal AV Junctional Tachycardia (Figs. 21–19 and 21–20)

Electrocardiographic Recognition. To usurp dominant pacemaker status, the AV junctional tissue must exhibit enhanced discharge rate such as during nonparoxysmal AV junctional tachycardia. Nonparoxysmal AV junctional tachycardia is usually of gradual onset and termination, hence the modifier "nonparoxysmal." On occasion, nonparoxysmal AV junctional tachycardia may become manifest abruptly because of slowing of the dominant pacemaker that may then allow sudden capture and control of the rhythm by the AV junctional focus.[108] The

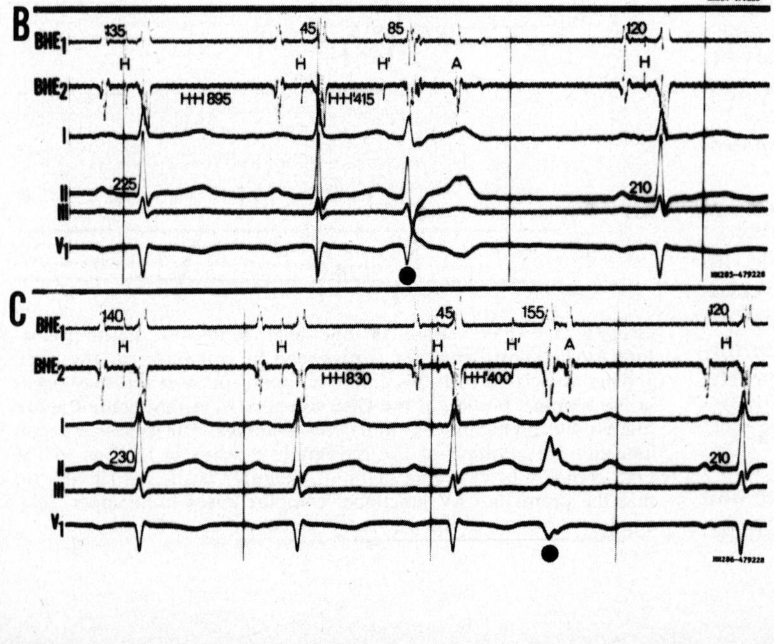

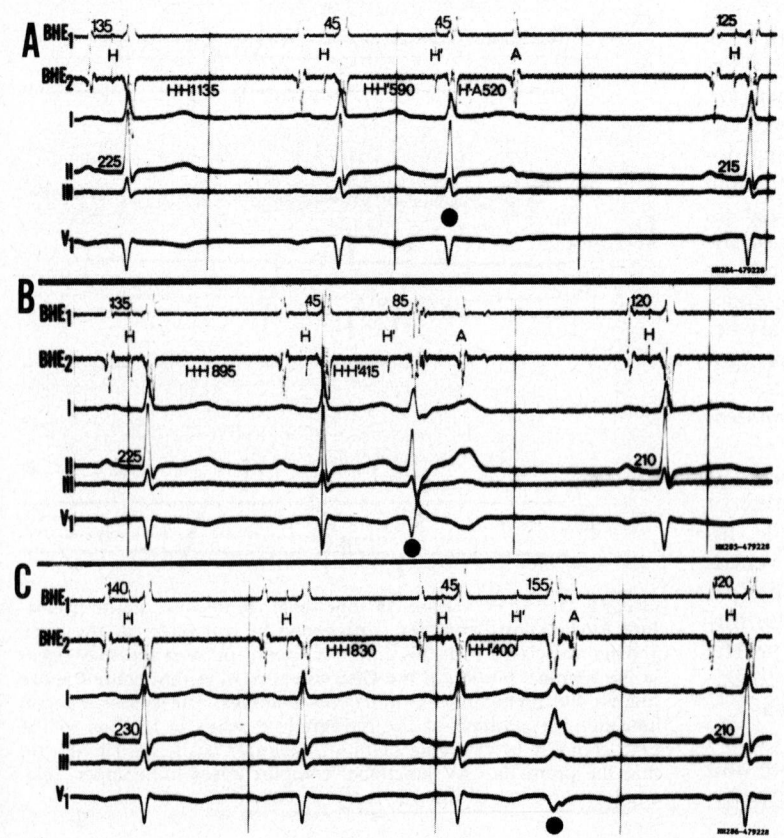

FIGURE 21–17 Premature AV junctional complexes arising in or near the bundle of His (H′) conduct normally (*A*) or with functional right (*B*) and functional left (*C*) bundle branch block. The filled circles indicate the premature junctional complex. Anterograde conduction of the premature junctional (H′) discharges depends on the coupling interval between the last normal His discharge (H) and (H-H′) interval and the spontaneous cycle length (H-H) that preceded H′. When H′ follows a shorter preceding cycle length and occurs at longer coupling intervals, a normal QRS complex results. As the preceding H-H cycle lengthens or as the H-H′ interval shortens, a zone of functional right bundle branch block occurs, followed by a zone of functional left bundle branch block. Not shown are premature His discharges that fail to conduct entirely (see Fig. 19–30, p. 635). Numbers in milliseconds. Time lines=1 sec in each panel. (Magnification is not the same in all three panels.) (From Bonner, A. J., and Zipes, D. P.: Lidocaine and His bundle extrasystoles. His bundle discharge conducted normally, conducted with functional right or left bundle branch block, or blocked entirely (concealed). Arch. Intern. Med. *136*: 700, 1976.)

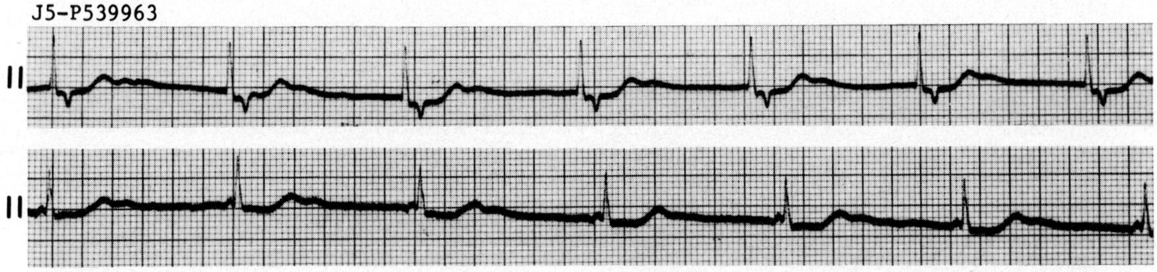

FIGURE 21–18 AV junctional rhythm. *Top,* AV junctional discharge occurs fairly regularly at a rate of approximately 50 beats/min. Retrograde atrial activity follows each junctional discharge. *Bottom,* Recording made on a different day in the same patient; the AV junctional rate is slightly more variable, and retrograde P waves precede the onset of the QRS complex. The positive terminal portion of the P wave gives the appearance of AV dissociation, which was not present.

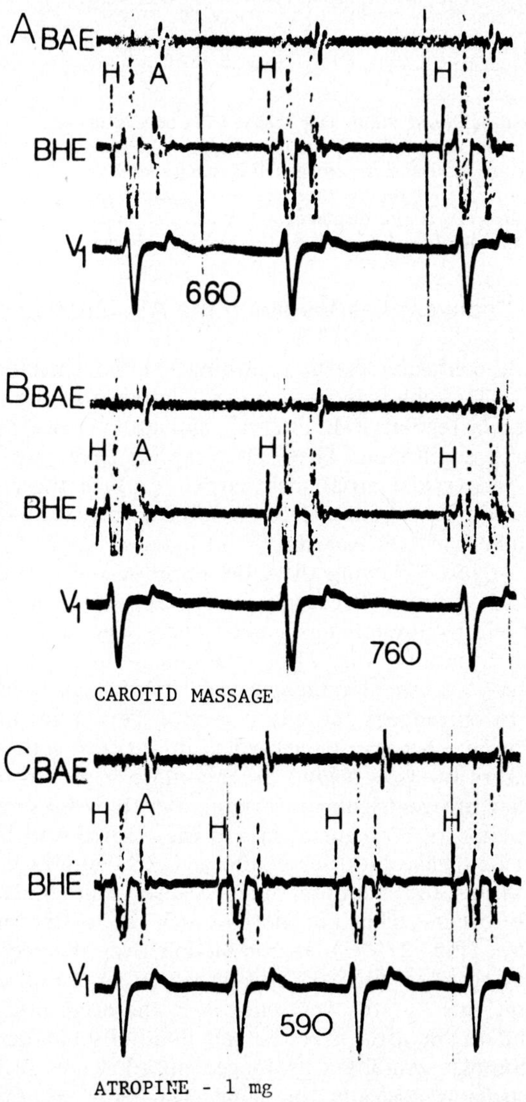

FIGURE 21–19 Nonparoxysmal AV junctional tachycardia. *A,* Control; *B,* response to carotid sinus massage; *C,* response to atropine, 1 mg intravenously. Note that His bundle depolarization is the earliest recordable electrical activity in each cycle. The atria are depolarized retrogradely (low right atrial activity recorded in BHE precedes high right atrial activity recorded in BAE). Note also that carotid sinus massage slows the junctional discharge rate while atropine speeds it up. From these tracings alone one could not distinguish the rhythm from some other types of supraventricular tachycardias. However, onset and termination of this tachycardia was typical of nonparoxysmal AV junctional tachycardia.

rate of discharge is commonly between 70 and 130 beats/min. Although accepted terminology confers the label of tachycardia to rates exceeding 100 beats/min, this term—although not entirely correct—has generally been accepted, since rates exceeding 60 beats/min represent in effect a tachycardia for the AV junctional tissue.[109,110]

Nonparoxysmal AV junctional tachycardia is recognized by a QRS of supraventricular configuration at a fairly regular rate of 70 to 130 beats/min. Enhanced vagal tone may slow while vagolytic agents may speed up the discharge rate. Although retrograde activation of the atria may occur, the atria commonly are controlled by an independent sinus, atrial, or on occasion a second AV junctional focus resulting in AV dissociation (Fig. 21–9*G*). The electrocardiographic diagnosis may be complicated by the presence of entrance and exit blocks at the AV junctional tissue level and incomplete forms of AV dissociation.

The cause of this arrhythmia probably is *accelerated automatic discharge* in or near the His bundle. It is possible that nonparoxysmal AV junctional tachycardia originates in atrial fibers without recognition of the latter's role from analysis of the scalar ECG or on intracardiac electrograms, unless a careful search is made.[111] Wenckebach periods may occur (Fig. 7–48, p. 240), but the presence of exit block has not yet been demonstrated by His bundle recording in humans, and the block may be in the AV node with the origin of the nonparoxysmal AV junctional tachycardia proximal to the site of the His bundle recording.[111,112] Accelerated junctional escape beats that have shorter escape intervals when following premature atrial complexes has raised the possibility of *overdrive acceleration* (p. 620) in these fibers.[113]

Clinical Features. Nonparoxysmal AV junctional tachycardia occurs most commonly in patients with underlying heart disease, such as inferior infarction, myocarditis (often the result of acute rheumatic fever), or after open-heart surgery.[114,115] Probably the most important cause is excessive digitalis, which may also produce the ECG manifestations of varying degrees of exit block (usually Wenckebach type) from the accelerated AV junctional focus. Nonparoxysmal AV junctional tachycardia can occur in otherwise healthy individuals without symptoms (Fig. 21–20) or can be a serious and difficult to control tachycardia,[116] occasionally chronic and longlasting.[117]

The clinical features vary depending on the rate of the arrhythmia and the underlying etiology and severity of heart disease. As in most arrhythmias, the physical signs are determined by the relationship of the P wave to the

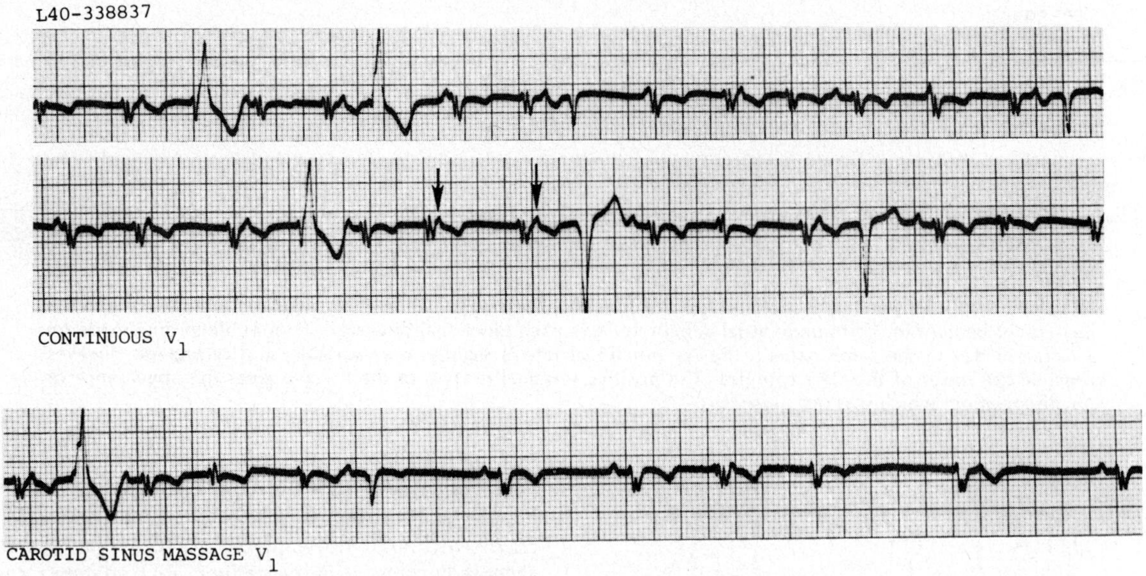

FIGURE 21–20 Nonparoxysmal AV junctional tachycardia in a healthy young adult. This tachycardia occurs at a fairly regular interval ("W-shaped" complexes) and is interrupted intermittently with atrial captures that produce functional right and left bundle branch block. Two P waves are indicated by arrows. The junctional discharge rate is approximately 120 beats/min (cycle length=500 msec) and the rhythm irregular, sometimes shortened by atrial captures or delayed by concealed conduction that resets and displaces the junctional focus (see Chap. 7). In the bottom strip, carotid sinus massage slows the junctional as well as the sinus discharge rate.

QRS complex and the rate of atrial and ventricular discharge. The first heart sound may therefore be constant or varying, and cannon *a* waves may or may not occur in the jugular venous pulse.

The ventricular rhythm may be regular or irregular, often in a constant fashion. It is especially important to recognize slowing and regularization of the ventricular rhythm in a patient with atrial fibrillation as being a possible early sign of *digitalis intoxication* (p. 239). Initially, during atrial fibrillation, the regular ventricular rhythm may result from an AV junctional escape rhythm because the depressed AV conduction caused by digitalis blocks the passage of impulses from the fibrillating atria (Fig. 21–9*G*). As digitalis administration is continued, the ventricular rate may then speed because of increased discharge of the AV junctional pacemaker but may still be regular. Further digitalis administration may produce a rate that is slow and irregular because of varying degrees of AV junctional exit block. The rhythm may be misdiagnosed as resumption of conduction from the fibrillating atria. The rate then may increase further because of development of a ventricular tachycardia.

Therapy is directed toward the underlying etiological factor and functional support of the cardiovascular system. If the rhythm is regular, the cardiovascular status is compromised, and the patient is not taking digitalis, digitalis administration should be considered. Cardioversion may be tried if necessary; theoretically, however, if the nonparoxysmal AV junctional tachycardia is due to enhanced automaticity, cardioversion may be ineffective. If the patient tolerates the arrhythmia well, careful monitoring and attention to the underlying heart disease is usually all that is required. The arrhythmia usually will abate spontaneously. If digitalis toxicity is the cause, the drug must be stopped and potassium, lidocaine, phenytoin, or propranolol administered.

Tachycardias Involving the AV Junction

Much confusion exists regarding the nomenclature of tachycardias characterized by a supraventricular QRS complex, a regular R-R interval, and no evidence of ventricular preexcitation. These tachycardias have often been called paroxysmal atrial tachycardia (PAT) if the P wave occurred in front of the QRS complex or paroxysmal nodal or junctional tachycardia (PJT) if the P wave occurred within or just following the QRS complex and exhibited a retrograde contour. Because it is now apparent that a variety of electrophysiological mechanisms can account for these tachycardias (Fig. 21–9), the nonspecific term paroxysmal supraventricular tachycardia (PSVT) has been proposed to encompass the entire group. This term may be inappropriate because tachycardias in patients with accessory pathways (see below) are no more supraventricular than they are ventricular in origin, since they may require participation of both the atria and the ventricles in the reentrant pathway, and they exhibit a QRS complex of normal contour and duration only because anterograde conduction occurs over the normal AV node–His bundle pathways (Fig. 21–9*C*). If conduction over the reentrant pathway reverses direction and travels in an "antidromic" direction—i.e., to the ventricles over the accessory pathway and to the atria over the AV node–His bundle—the QRS complex exhibits a prolonged duration, although the tachycardia is basically the same. The term *reciprocating tachycardia* has been offered as a substitute for paroxysmal supraventricular tachycardia, but use of such a term presumes the mechanism of the tachycardia to be reentrant (which is probably the case for many supraventricular tachycardias). Reciprocating tachycardia is probably the mechanism of many ventricular tachycardias as well. Thus, no universally acceptable nomenclature exists for these tachycardias. In this chapter, descriptive titles, although

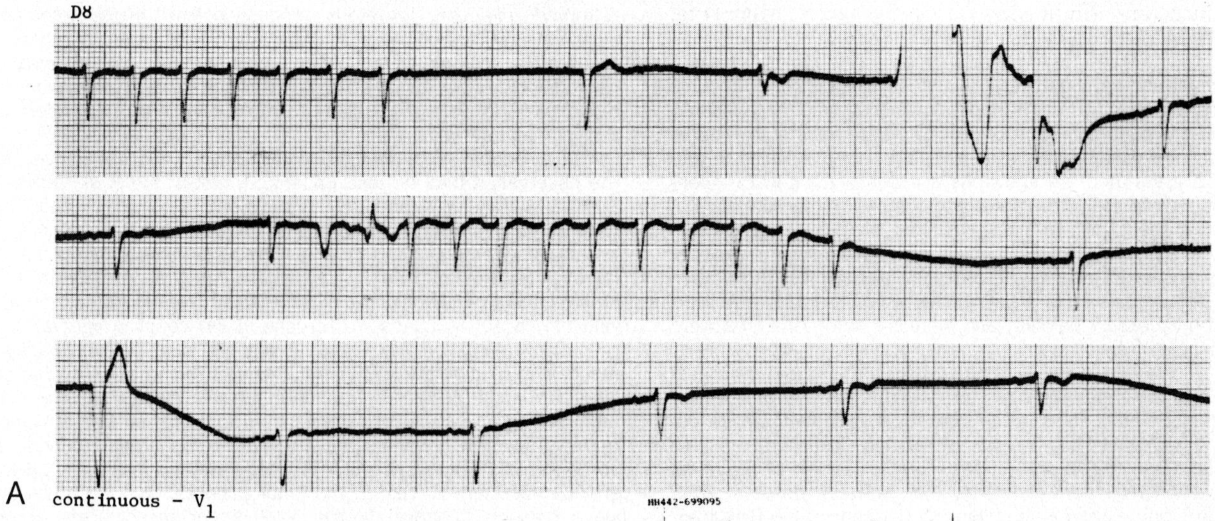

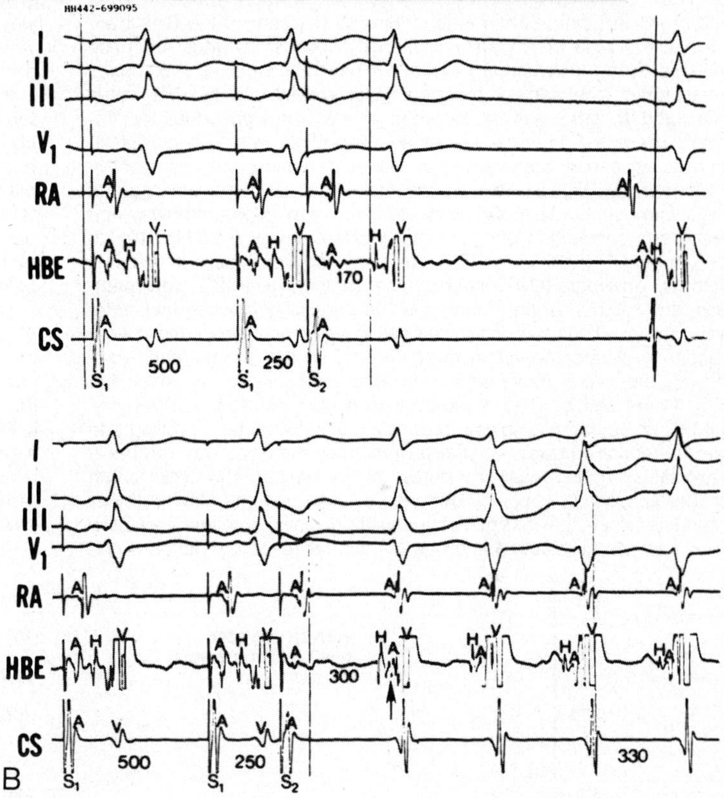

FIGURE 21–21 *A,* Sudden termination of paroxysmal supraventricular tachycardia, probably AV nodal reentry. Tachycardia abruptly terminates in the top recording following a short period of carotid sinus massage. Several escape beats occur followed by another short run or paroxysmal supraventricular tachycardia, which again terminates abruptly. A sinus bradycardia ensues and gradually speeds up. Suppression of sinus nodal activity following termination of a tachycardia is common and is a manifestation of overdrive suppression. *B,* Initiation of AV nodal reentrant tachycardia in a patient with dual atrioventricular nodal pathways. Upper and lower panels show the last two paced beats of a train of stimuli delivered to the coronary sinus at a pacing cycle length of 500 msec. The results of premature atrial stimulation at an S_1–S_2 interval of 250 msec on two occasions are shown. In the *upper panel,* S_2 was conducted to the ventricle with an AH interval of 170 msec and then was followed by a sinus beat. In the *lower panel,* S_2 was conducted with an AH interval of 300 msec and initiated AV nodal reentry. Note that the retrograde atrial activity occurs (arrow) prior to the onset of ventricular septal depolarization and is superimposed on the QRS complex. Retrograde atrial activity begins first in the low right atrium (HBE lead) and then progresses to the high right atrium (RA) and coronary sinus (CS) recordings.

cumbersome, will be used for the sake of clarity. In addition, the mechanism of reentry will be assumed operative when the weight of evidence supports its presence even though unequivocal proof is lacking (see p. 623).

Atrioventricular (AV) Nodal Reentrant Tachycardia

Electrocardiographic Recognition. Reentrant tachycardia in the AV node is characterized by a tachycardia with a QRS complex of supraventricular origin, with sudden onset and termination generally at rates between 150 and 250 beats/min (commonly 180 to 200 beats/min in adults), and with a regular rhythm. Uncommonly, the rate may be as low as 110 beats/min and occasionally, especially in children, may exceed 250. Unless functional aberrant ventricular conduction or a previous conduction defect exists, the QRS complex is normal in contour and duration. AV nodal reentry recorded at the onset begins abruptly, usually following a premature atrial complex that conducts with a prolonged P-R interval (see Figs. 21–9*A* and 21–10*B* and Fig. 19–24, p. 629). The abrupt termination is sometimes followed by a brief period of asystole or bradycardia (Fig. 21–21*A*). The R-R interval may shorten over the course of the first few beats at the onset or lengthen over the course of the last few beats preceding termination of the tachycardia. Variation in cycle length is usually caused by variation in AV nodal conduction time. Carotid sinus massage may slow the tachycardia slightly prior to its termination or, if termination does not occur, may produce only slight slowing of the tachycardia (Fig. 21–21*A*).

Electrophysiological Features. An atrial complex that conducts with a critical prolongation of AV nodal conduction time[118–120] generally precipitates AV nodal reentry (Fig. 21–21*B*). Several AV nodal pathways can be diagrammed to explain this tachycardia. In Figure 19–22 (p. 627), the atria are shown as a necessary link in the reentrant pathway, while in Figure 21–9*A* and *B* (p. 695), the atria are not incorporated in the circuit. In most examples, the retrograde P wave occurs at the onset of the QRS complex, clearly excluding the possibility of an accessory pathway. If an accessory pathway in the ventricle were part of the circuit, the ventricles would have to be activated before the accessory pathway and therefore before the atria were depolarized (see Preexcitation Syndrome, p. 712). In approximately 30 per cent of instances, atrial activation begins at the end of, or just after, the QRS complex, giving rise to a discrete P wave on the surface ECG (Fig. 21–9*B*), while in the majority of patients P waves are not seen, since they are buried within the inscription of the QRS complex (Fig. 21–9*A*). In the most common variety of AV nodal reentrant tachycardia, the V-A interval (i.e., between onset of QRS and onset of atrial activity) is less than 50 per cent of the R-R interval and the ratio of A-V to V-A interval exceeds 1.0. Most of these patients during tachycardia have a V-A minimum value of ≤ 61 msec measured to the earliest recorded atrial activity and of ≤ 95 msec measured to atrial activity recorded in the high right atrial electrogram. These V-A intervals are longer in patients with tachycardia related to accessory pathways[121] as well as in some other forms of AV nodal reentry (Fig. 21–9*B*). In the majority of patients, anterograde conduction occurs to the ventricle over the slow (alpha) pathway and retrograde conduction over the fast (beta) pathway (see Fig. 19–23, p. 628, and Fig. 21–9*A* and *B*). An atrial complex blocks in the fast pathway anterogradely, travels to the ventricle over the slow pathway, and returns to the atrium over the previously blocked fast pathway. The proximal and distal final pathways for this circus movement appear to be located within the AV node, so that, as currently conceived, the circus movement is located totally within the AV node (Fig. 21–9*A* and *B*). The reentrant loop is slow AV nodal pathway → final distal common pathway (probably distal AV node) → retrograde fast AV nodal pathway → final proximal common pathway (probably proximal AV node, possibly a portion of low atrium). The cycle length of the tachycardia generally depends on how well the slow pathway conducts, since the fast pathway usually exhibits excellent capability for retrograde conduction and has the shorter refractory period in the retrograde direction. Therefore, conduction times in the anterograde slow pathway are a major determinant of the cycle length of the tachycardia. In one study, patients with shorter A-H intervals appeared more likely to have AV nodal reentrant tachycardia because these patients were more likely to have excellent retrogradely conducting fast pathways.[122]

The evidence supporting the dual pathway concept derives from the observation that in these patients, a plot of the A_1-A_2 versus the A_2-H_2 or A_1-A_2 versus the H_1-H_2 intervals shows a discontinuous curve (Fig. 21–22). The explanation is that, at a critical A_1-A_2 interval, the impulse suddenly blocks in the fast pathway and conducts with delay over the slow pathway, with sudden prolongation of the A_2-H_2 (or H_1-H_2) interval. Generally, the A-H interval increases at least 50 msec with only a 10- to 20-msec decrease in the coupling interval of the premature atrial complex. Less commonly, dual pathways may be manifested by different P-R or A-H intervals during sinus rhythm or at identical paced rates or by a sudden jump in the A-H interval during atrial pacing at a constant cycle length. Some patients with AV nodal reentry may not have discontinuous refractory period curves, and some patients who do not have AV nodal reentry may exhibit discontinuous refractory curves. In the latter patients, dual AV nodal pathways may be a benign finding.[123,129] Similar mechanisms of tachycardia can occur in children.[124] Triple AV nodal pathways may be demonstrated in occasional patients.[125]

In less than 5 to 10 per cent of patients with AV nodal reentry, anterograde conduction proceeds over the fast pathway and retrograde conduction over the slow pathway (termed the unusual form of AV nodal reentry), causing atrial activation to begin *after* the QRS complex and producing a long V-A interval and a relatively short A-V interval (generally A-V/V-A < 0.75, Fig. 21–9*B*).[100,102,126–132] Finally, it is possible to have tachycardias that use either the antegrade slow or fast pathways and a retrograde concealed accessory pathway (see below).[133,134]

The ventricles and apparently the atria are not needed to maintain AV nodal reentry in man, and spontaneous AV block has been noted on occasion, particularly at the onset of the arrhythmia. Such block can take place in the AV node distal to the reentry circuit between the AV node and bundle of His, within the bundle of His, or distal to it. Rarely the block may be located between the reentry circuit in the AV node and the atrium.[135,135a] Most commonly when block appears, it is below the bundle of His. Termination of the tachycardia generally results from block in the anterogradely conducting slow pathway ("weak link"), so that a retrograde atrial response is not followed by a His or ventricular response.

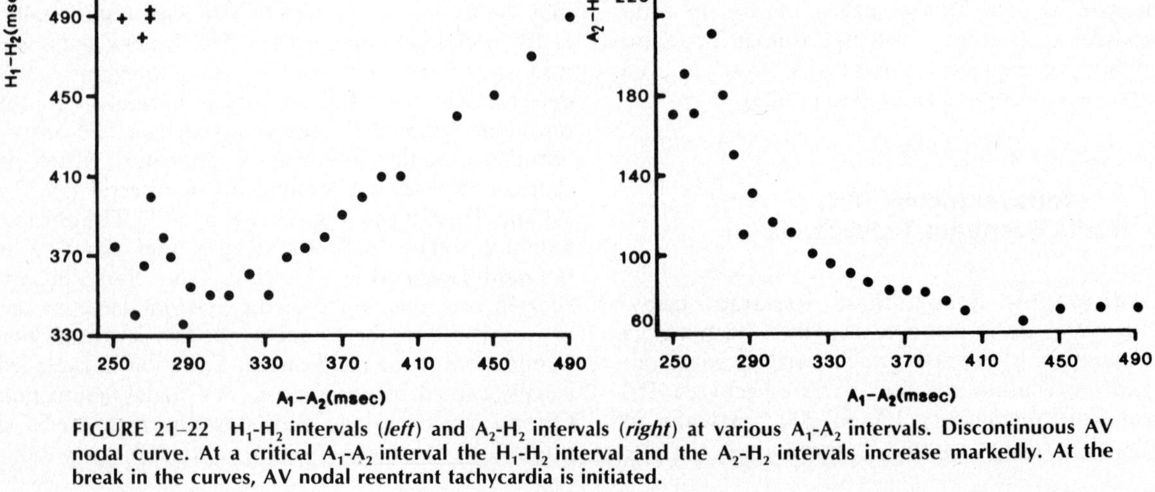

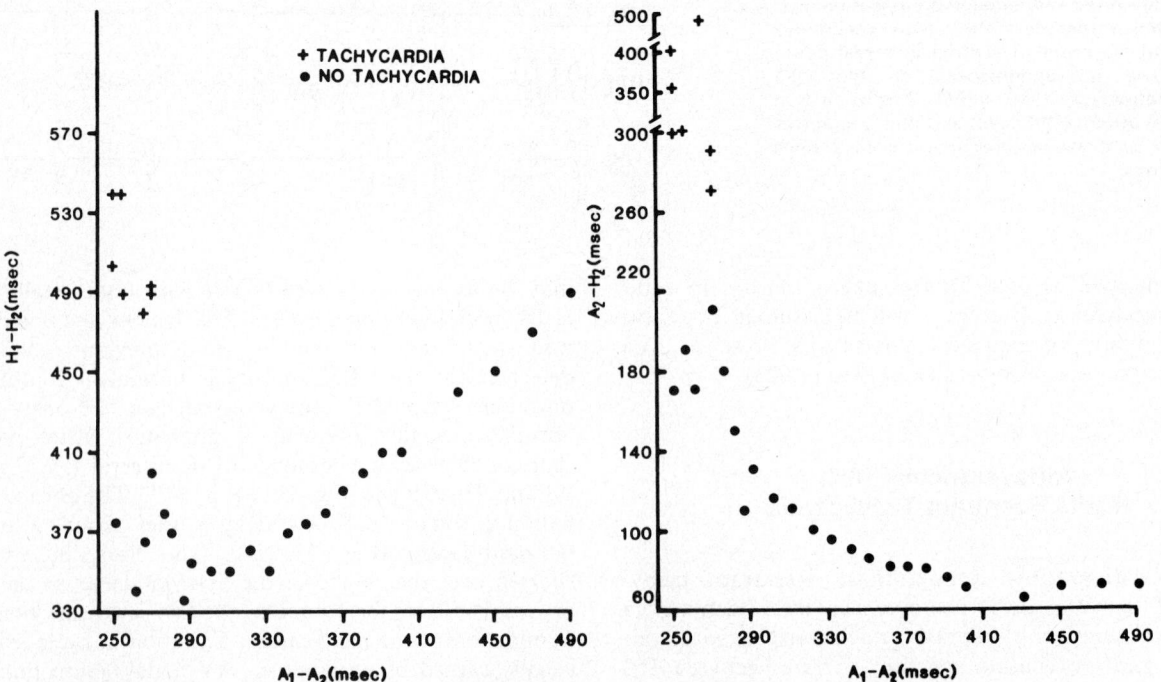

FIGURE 21–22 H_1-H_2 intervals (*left*) and A_2-H_2 intervals (*right*) at various A_1-A_2 intervals. Discontinuous AV nodal curve. At a critical A_1-A_2 interval the H_1-H_2 interval and the A_2-H_2 intervals increase markedly. At the break in the curves, AV nodal reentrant tachycardia is initiated.

The sequence of retrograde atrial activation is normal during AV nodal reentrant supraventricular tachycardia. This means that the earliest site of atrial activation during retrograde conduction over the fast pathway is recorded in the His bundle electrogram followed by electrograms recorded from the os of the coronary sinus and then spreading to depolarize the rest of the right and left atria. During retrograde conduction over the slow pathway in the atypical type of AV nodal reentry, atrial activation recorded in the proximal coronary sinus may precede atrial activation recorded in the low right atrium, suggesting that the slow and fast pathways may enter the atria at slightly different positions.[136] Functional bundle branch block during AV nodal reentrant tachycardia does not modify the tachycardia significantly.

Clinical Features. AV nodal reentry commonly occurs in patients who have no organic heart disease. Symptoms frequently accompany the tachycardia and range from feelings of palpitations, nervousness, and anxiety to angina, heart failure, syncope, or shock, depending on the duration and rate of the tachycardia and the presence of organic heart disease. Tachycardia may cause syncope because of the rapid ventricular rate, reduced cardiac output, and cerebral circulation, or because of asystole when the tachycardia terminates, owing to tachycardia-induced depression of sinus node automaticity (Fig. 21–21). The prognosis for patients without heart disease is usually good.

Hemodynamic consequences of supraventricular tachyarrhythmias in patients with normal ventricular function are due primarily to a marked decrease in left ventricular end-diastolic and stroke volumes with an increase in ejection rate and cardiac output without a significant change in ejection fraction as heart rate is increased and the atrial contribution to ventricular filling is lost.[10] Heart disease or tachycardia may reduce the ejection fraction.[137] Initial hypotension during tachycardia evokes a sympathetic response that increases blood pressure and in turn causes a rise in vagal tone that may terminate the tachycardia.[138]

Treatment. Treatment of the acute attack depends on the underlying heart disease, how well the tachycardia is tolerated, and the natural history of previous attacks in the individual patient. For some patients, rest, reassurance, and sedation may be all that are required to abort an attack. Vagal maneuvers, including carotid sinus massage, Valsalva and Mueller maneuvers, and gagging, serve as the first line of therapy. These maneuvers may slightly slow the tachycardia rate, which then may speed up to the original rate following cessation of the attempt, or they may terminate the tachycardia. Vagal maneuvers should be tried *again* after each pharmacological approach.

Verapamil[99,139–141] (see p. 665), 5 to 10 mg IV, terminates AV nodal reentry successfully in about 2 minutes in over 90 per cent of instances. This drug, or one of the other calcium-entry blockers, such as diltiazem,[142] has become the treatment of choice should simple vagal maneuvers fail. At the time of this writing diltiazem is still an investigational drug for treating arrhythmias.

Cholinergic drugs, particularly edrophonium chloride (Tensilon), a short-acting cholinesterase inhibitor, may terminate AV nodal reentry when administered initially at a trial dose of 3 to 5 mg IV and, if unsuccessful, repeated at a dose of 10 mg IV. Its action is rapid in onset and short in duration, with minimal side effects. Edrophonium should be used cautiously or not at all in patients who are hypotensive or who have lung disease, especially a history of asthma. Treating arrhythmias is not an FDA-approved indication for use of edrophonium.

If these initial approaches are unsuccessful, *intravenous digitalis* administration may be attempted using one of the following short-acting digitalis preparations: ouabain, 0.25 to 0.5 mg IV, followed by 0.1 mg every 30 to 60 minutes, if needed, keeping the total dose less than 1.0 mg within a 24-hour period or 0.01 mg/kg as a single dose over 10 to 15 minutes; digoxin, 0.5 to 1.0 mg IV given over 10 to 15 min, followed by 0.25 mg every 2 to 4 hours, with a total dose less than 1.5 mg within any 24-hour period; or deslanoside, 0.8 mg IV, followed by 0.4 mg every 2 to 4 hours, restricting the total dose to less than 2.0 mg within a 24-hour period. *Oral digitalis* administration to terminate an acute attack is generally not indicated. Vagal maneuvers, previously ineffective, may terminate the tachycardia following digitalis administration and therefore should be repeated.

Propranolol given intravenously at a rate of 0.5 to 1.0 mg/min for a total dose of 0.5 to 3.0 mg may be tried if digitalis administration is unsuccessful. Higher doses may be used in some patients (see Chap. 20). Propranolol must be used cautiously, if at all, in patients with heart failure, chronic lung disease, or a history of asthma because its beta-adrenergic receptor blocking action depresses myocardial contractility and may produce bronchospasm.

Prior to administering digitalis or propranolol, it is advisable to reassess the clinical status of the patient and consider whether DC cardioversion may be advisable. DC shock, administered to patients who have received excessive amounts of digitalis, may be dangerous and may result in serious post-shock ventricular arrhythmias (p. 671). Particularly if signs or symptoms of cardiac decompensation occur, DC electrical shock should be considered early. DC shock, synchronized to the QRS complex to avoid precipitating ventricular fibrillation, successfully terminates AV nodal reentry with energies in the range of 10 to 50 watt-seconds; higher energies may be required in some instances (pp. 626 and 669).

In the event that digitalis has been given in large doses and DC shock is contraindicated, *atrial or ventricular pacing* may restore sinus rhythm. In some instances, esophageal pacing may be useful (p. 756).

Procainamide, quinidine, or disopyramide may be required to terminate AV nodal reentry in some patients. Unless contraindicated, DC cardioversion generally should be employed prior to using these agents, which are more often administered to prevent recurrences. These three drugs selectively depress conduction in the retrograde fast pathway.[143] Disopyramide may at times depress conduction in the slow pathway antegradely.[144] Cardiac glycosides and beta and calcium-entry blockers selectively depress antegrade slow pathway conduction but occasionally may depress conduction in the retrograde fast pathway.

Pressor drugs may terminate AV nodal reentry by inducing reflex vagal stimulation mediated by baroreceptors in the carotid sinus and aorta when the systolic blood pressure is acutely elevated to levels of about 180 mm Hg. One of the following drugs, diluted in 5 to 10 ml of 5 per cent dextrose and water, may be given over 1 to 3 minutes: phenylephrine (Neo-Synephrine), 0.5 to 1.0 mg; methoxamine (Vasoxyl), 3 to 5 mg; or metaraminol (Aramine), 0.5 to 2.0 mg. Pressor drugs should be used cautiously or not at all in the elderly and in patients who have organic heart disease, significant hypertension, hyperthyroidism, or acute myocardial infarction. Today, this potentially dangerous and almost always uncomfortable procedure is rarely needed unless the patient is also hypotensive.

Prevention of recurrences is often more difficult than terminating the acute episode. Initially, one must decide whether the frequency and severity of the attacks warrant long-term drug prophylaxis. If the attacks of paroxysmal tachycardia are infrequent, well tolerated, and either terminate spontaneously or are easily terminated by the patient, no prophylactic therapy may be necessary. If the attacks are sufficiently frequent to necessitate therapy, the patient may be treated with drugs empirically or based on serial electrophysiological testing. Because drug responses are variable, serial electrophysiological testing of multiple drugs appears reasonable in some patients with poorly tolerated tachycardias that recur only sporadically (p. 634).[145]

If empirical testing is desirable, the following choices are recommended: Digitalis is generally the initial drug of choice. It has the advantages of being well- tolerated and requiring administration only once daily. The clinical situation determines the speed of digitalization. Using digoxin, rapid oral digitalization can be accomplished in 24 to 36 hours with an initial dose of 1.0 to 1.5 mg, followed by 0.25 to 0.5 mg every 6 hours for a total dose of 2.0 to 3.0 mg. A less rapid oral regimen digitalizes in 2 to 3 days with an initial dose of 0.75 to 1.0 mg, followed by 0.25 to 0.50 mg every 12 hours for a total dose of 2.0 to 3.0 mg. Alternatively, digoxin administered as a maintenance dose of 0.125 to 0.500 mg achieves digitalization in about one week. Digitoxin, which has a longer duration of action, may be used instead of digoxin. Oral digitalization with digitoxin may be accomplished in 24 to 36 hours with an initial dose of 0.5 to 0.8 mg, followed by 0.2 mg every 6 to 8 hours until a total dose of 1.2 mg is reached. A slower approach involves administering 0.2 mg three times daily for 2 to 3 days. Complete digitalization can also be accomplished in about one month by simply giving a daily maintenance dose of 0.05 to 0.20 mg.

If digitalis alone is unsuccessful, one can then add verapamil, 80 to 120 mg every 6 or 8 hours, quinidine sulfate, 300 to 500 mg every 6 hours, or propranolol, 10 to 40 mg every 6 hours. Procainamide or disopyramide can be used instead of quinidine. In some patients, concomitant administration of digitalis, propranolol, and quinidine or procainamide or disopyramide may be necessary.

For many patients, pacemaker implantation provides acceptable treatment (p. 756). Competitive atrial pacing promptly terminates AV nodal reentry, restoring sinus rhythm immediately or sometimes after a transient episode of atrial flutter or atrial fibrillation, and avoids the necessity of daily drug administration with potential side effects.

Reentry Over a Retrograde Conducting (Concealed) Accessory Pathway

Electrocardiographic Recognition. The presence of an accessory pathway that conducts unidirectionally from the ventricle to the atrium but not in the reverse direction is not apparent in the scalar ECG during sinus rhythm because the ventricle is not preexcited. Therefore, the ECG manifestations of the Wolff-Parkinson-White (WPW) syndrome (see p. 712) are absent and the accessory pathway is said to be "concealed."[146-151] However, since the mechanism responsible for most tachycardias in patients who have the WPW syndrome is probably macro-reentry caused by anterograde conduction over the AV node–His bundle pathway and retrograde conduction over an accessory pathway, the latter, even if it only conducts retrogradely, can still participate in the reentrant circuit. Electrocardiographically, a tachycardia due to this mechanism may be *suspected* when the QRS complex is normal and the retrograde P wave occurs *after* completion of the QRS complex, in the ST segment or early T wave (Fig. 21–9*C*).

This relationship between P wave and QRS complex results because the ventricle must be activated before the propagating impulse can enter the accessory pathway and excite the atria retrogradely. Therefore, the retrograde P wave must follow ventricular excitation in contrast to AV nodal reentry, in which the atria can be excited during ventricular activation (Fig. 21–9*A*). Also, the contour of the retrograde P wave may differ from the usual retrograde P wave, since the atria may be activated eccentrically, i.e., in a manner other than the normal retrograde activation sequence, starting at the low right atrial septum as in AV nodal reentry. This occurs because the concealed accessory pathway in most instances is left-sided, i.e., inserts into the left atrium, making the left atrium the first site of retrograde atrial activation and causing the retrograde P wave to be negative in lead I (Fig. 21–23).[152] Finally, since the tachycardia circuit involves the ventricles, if functional bundle branch block occurs in the same ventricle in which the accessory pathway is located, the cycle length of the tachycardia is prolonged.[147] This important change ensues because the bundle branch block lengthens the reentrant circuit (see Preexcitation Syndrome, p. 712). For example, the normal activation sequence for a reciprocating tachycardia circuit with a left-sided accessory pathway without functional bundle branch block progresses from atrium → AV node–His bundle → right and left ventricles → accessory pathway → atrium. However, during functional left bundle branch block, for example, the tachycardia circuit travels from atrium → AV node–His bundle → right ventricle → septum → left ventricle → accessory pathway → atrium. The additional time required for the impulse to travel from the right to the left ventricle before reaching the accessory pathway and atrium lengthens the V-A interval, which lengthens the cycle length of the tachycardia by an equal amount, assuming no other changes in conduction times occur within the circuit. Thus, lengthening of the tachycardia cycle length by more than 35 msec during ipsilateral functional bundle branch block is diagnostic of a free wall accessory pathway if the lengthening can be shown to be due to V-A prolongation only and not to prolongation of the H-V interval (which may develop with the appearance of bundle branch block). In an occasional patient, the increase in cycle length due to prolongation of VA conduction may be nullified by a simultaneous decrease in the P-R (A-H) interval.[153,153a] Patients with septal accessory pathways have VA prolongation of 25 msec or less with functional right or left bundle branch block.[153a] Functional bundle branch block, particularly functional left bundle branch block, during tachycardia occurs much more commonly in patients who have an accessory pathway than in those with AV nodal reentry, probably because in the latter, slow pathway anterograde conduction allows for longer recovery time of the His-Purkinje system, while in tachycardias associated with accessory pathways, anterograde conduction over the AV node may be more rapid.[154] Functional left bundle branch block may occur more commonly during rapid tachycardias, possibly because the refractory period of the right bundle branch appears to be shorter than the left bundle branch at short cycle lengths.[155] Functional bundle branch block in the ventricle contralateral to the accessory pathway does not lengthen the tachycardia cycle if the H-V interval does not lengthen.

An exception to these observations must be noted. If the patient has a septal accessory pathway (see Preexcitation Syndrome, p. 712), retrograde atrial activation will be normal and the cycle length of the tachycardia may not change appreciably with the development of functional bundle branch block. Invasive electrophysiological confirmation may be necessary (see below).

Vagal maneuvers, by acting predominantly on the AV node, produce a response similar to AV nodal reentry, and the tachycardia may transiently slow or transiently slow and then terminate. General-

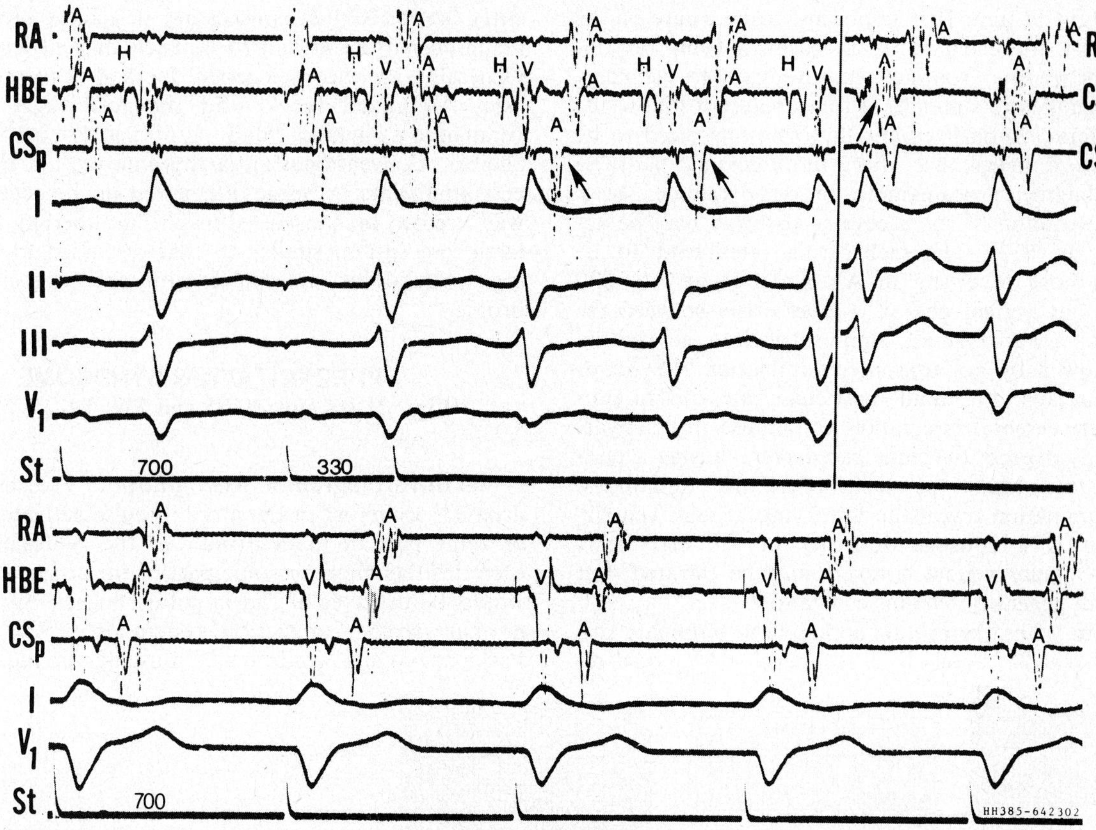

FIGURE 21–23 Retrograde "concealed" accessory pathway and initiation of reciprocating tachycardia in a patient with a left-sided accessory pathway that conducts retrogradely only. The last two stimuli in a train of eight at a cycle length of 700 msec are displayed in the top panel. Premature right atrial stimulation at an interval of 330 msec initiates a reciprocating tachycardia. After the premature stimulus, the A-H interval lengthens slightly and retrograde atrial activity occurs *following* termination of the QRS complex (arrows), beginning first in the CS_p (proximal coronary sinus) electrogram and proceeding to the low right atrial (HBE) and high right atrial (RA) electrograms. Insert at top right indicates that left atrial activity during tachycardia is recorded first in the distal coronary sinus (CS_d) electrogram (arrow) consistent with a left lateral accessory pathway. Catheter electrode that is recording CS is at lateral heart border. No evidence of anterograde conduction over an accessory pathway occurred at any cycle length during pacing of the right or left atrium. Right ventricular pacing at a constant cycle length of 700 msec (bottom) initiated the same sequence of retrograde atrial activation seen during the reciprocating tachycardia, thus confirming the presence of retrograde atrial activity over a "concealed" left lateral accessory pathway. (From Zipes, D. P., et al.: Aprindine for treatment of supraventricular tachycardias. Am. J. Cardiol. *40*:586, 1977.)

ly, termination occurs in the anterograde direction, so that the last retrograde P wave fails to conduct to the ventricle.

Electrophysiological features. Electrophysiological criteria supporting the diagnosis of tachycardia involving reentry over a concealed accessory pathway include the fact that initiation of tachycardia depends on a critical degree of atrioventricular delay (necessary to allow time for the accessory pathway to recover excitability), but the delay can be in the AV node or His-Purkinje system, i.e., a critical degree of A-H delay is not necessary. Occasionally, a tachycardia may start with little or no measurable lengthening of AV nodal or His-Purkinje conduction time.[156] The AV nodal refractory period curve is smooth, in contrast to the discontinuous curve found in many patients with AV nodal reentry. Dual AV nodal pathways occasionally may be noted as a concomitant but unrelated finding.

Accessory pathways can be diagnosed by demonstrating that during ventricular pacing premature ventricular stimulation activates the atria prior to retrograde depolarization of the His bundle, indicating that the impulse reached the atria before it depolarized the His bundle and must have traveled a different pathway to do so. Also, if the ventricles can be stimulated prematurely during tachycardia at a time when the His bundle is refractory, and the impulse still conducts to the atrium, this indicates that retrograde propagation traveled to the atrium over a pathway other than the bundle of His.[146] If the premature ventricular complex depolarizes the atria at the same coupling interval at which the premature ventricular complex occurred, one assumes that the stimulation site (i.e., ventricle) is within the reentrant circuit without intervening His-Purkinje or AV nodal tissue that might increase the V-A and therefore A-A intervals. In addition, if a premature ventricular complex delivered at a time when the His bundle is refractory terminates the tachycardia, an accessory pathway is most likely present.[146,157]

The V-A interval (conduction over the accessory pathway) generally is constant over a wide range of ventricular paced rates and coupling intervals of premature ventricular complexes as well as during the tachycardia in the absence of aberration. Similar short V-A intervals may be observed in patients during AV nodal reentry, but if the VA conduction time or R-P interval is the same during tachycardia *and* ventricular pacing at comparable rates, an accessory pathway is almost certainly present (Fig. 21–23). The V-A interval is usually less than 50 per cent of the R-R interval.[147] The tachycardia can be easily initiated following premature ventricular stimulation that conducts retrogradely in the accessory pathway but blocks in the AV node or His bundle.[157] Atria and ventricles are required components of the macroreentrant circuit, and therefore continuation of the tachycardia in the presence of AV or VA block excludes an accessory atrioventricular pathway as part of the reentrant circuit.

Clinical Features. The prevalance of concealed accessory pathways is estimated to account for at least 30 per cent of patients with apparent supraventricular tachycardia referred for electrophysiological evaluation. The great majority of these accessory pathways are located between left ventricle and left atrium, uncommonly between right ventricle and right atrium. It is important to be aware of the possibility of a concealed accessory pathway being responsible for apparently "routine" supraventricular tachycardia, since therapeutic response at times may not follow the usual guidelines. Antiarrhythmic targeting may need to be directed toward drugs that affect the accessory pathway such as quinidine, procainamide, or disopyramide. Also, surgical interruption of the accessory pathway may be accomplished (p. 672). The tachycardia rates tend to be faster than those occurring in AV nodal reentry (≥ 200 beats/min), but a great deal of overlap exists between the two groups.[158] Paroxysmal supraventricular tachycardia may be followed by polyuria after termination.[159] Syncope may occur because the rapid ventricular rate fails to provide adequate cerebral circulation or because the tachyarrhythmia may depress the sinus pacemaker, causing a period of asystole when the tachyarrhythmia terminates. Physical examination reveals an unvarying, regular ventricular rhythm with constant intensity of the first heart sound. The jugular venous pressure may be elevated, but the waveform generally remains constant.[160]

Treatment. The therapeutic approach to terminate this form of tachycardia acutely is as outlined for AV nodal reentry (see p. 709). It is necessary to achieve block of a single impulse from atrium to ventricle or ventricle to atrium. Generally, the most successful method is to produce transient AV nodal block, and therefore vagal maneuvers, verapamil, digitalis, and propranolol are acceptable choices. Conventional antiarrhythmic agents that prolong activation time or refractory period in the accessory pathway need to be considered as chronic therapy for prophylactic prevention, similar to that discussed for reciprocating tachycardias associated with the preexcitation syndrome.

W20-147489

PREEXCITATION SYNDROME

(Figs. 21–24 and 21–25 and Fig. 19–25, p. 630)

Electrocardiographic Recognition. Preexcitation syndrome[161] occurs when the atrial impulse activates the whole or some part of the ventricle, or the ventricular impulse activates the whole or some part of the atrium, earlier than would be expected if the impulse traveled by way of the normal specific conduction system only.[162] In the Wolff-Parkinson-White syndrome,[163] muscular connections com-

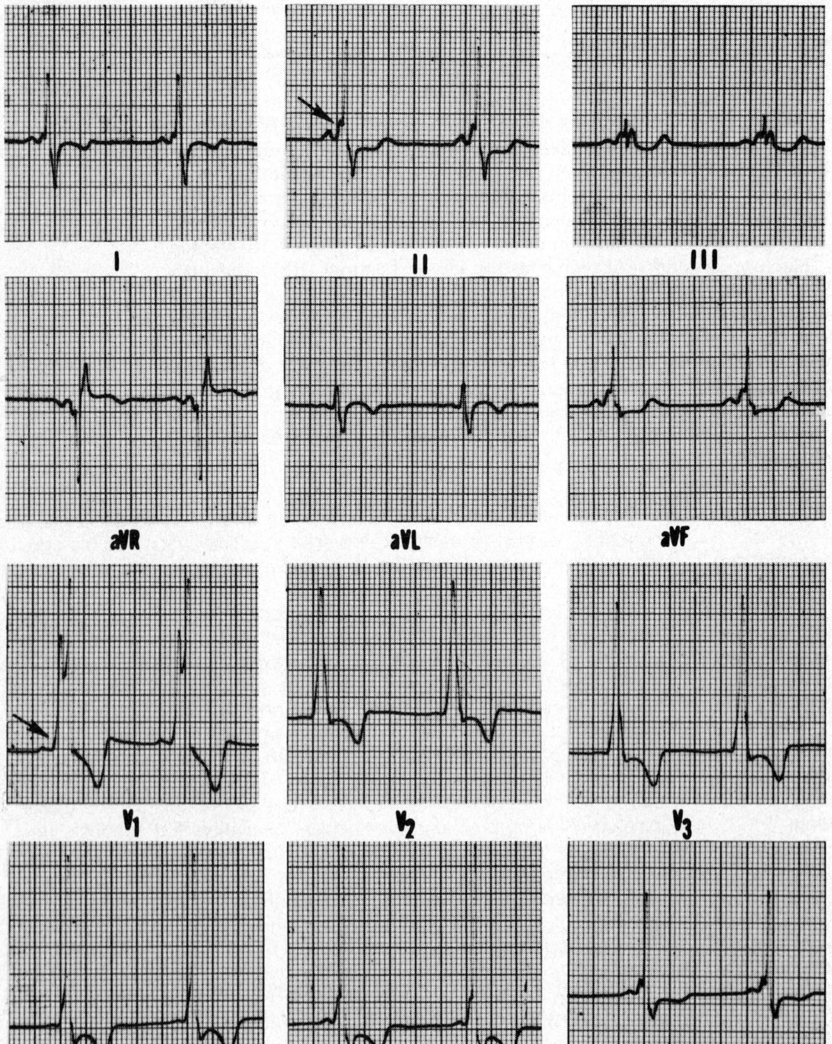

FIGURE 21–24 Wolff-Parkinson-White syndrome due to an accessory pathway, probably located in the left anterior (area 9 in Fig. 21–28) or anterior paraseptal (area 10) position. The delta wave and short P-R intervals can be clearly seen (arrows). The duration of the QRS complex exceeds 120 msec and secondary T-wave changes are present. (From Zipes, D. P., et al.: Preexcitation syndrome. Cardiovasc. Clin. *6*:210, 1974.)

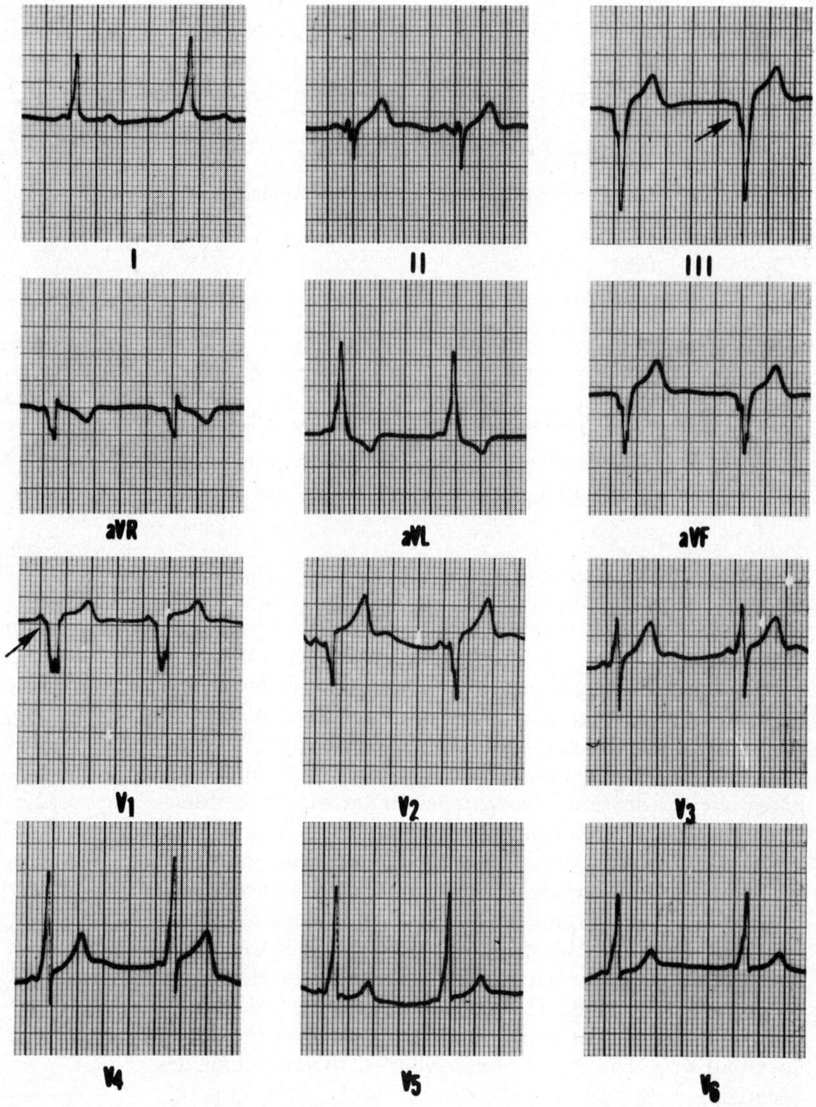

FIGURE 21–25 Wolff-Parkinson-White syndrome probably due to a right lateral accessory pathway (area 3 in Fig. 21–28). The delta wave is indicated by an arrow. (From Zipes, D. P., et al.: Preexcitation syndrome. Cardiovasc. Clin. *6*:210, 1974.)

posed of working myocardial fibers exist outside the specialized conducting tissue, in the presence or absence of a well-developed fibrous annulus, and connect atrium and ventricle.[164] They are named *accessory atrioventricular pathways* or connections, commonly called *Kent bundles*,[165,166] and are responsible for the most common variety of preexcitation. Three basic features typify the ECG abnormalities (Figs. 21–24 and 21–25) of patients with the usual form of WPW syndrome caused by an AV connection: (1) P-R interval less than 120 msec during sinus rhythm; (2) QRS complex duration exceeding 120 msec with a slurred, slowly rising onset of the QRS in some leads (delta wave) and usually a normal terminal QRS portion: and (3) secondary ST-T wave changes that are generally directed opposite to the major delta and QRS vectors.

The term *Wolff-Parkinson-White* (WPW) *syndrome* is applied when the patient has symptoms, generally due to tachyarrhythmias. The most common tachycardia is characterized by a normal QRS, by ventricular rates of 150 to 250 beats/min (generally faster than AV nodal reentry), and by sudden onset and termination, behaving in most respects like the tachycardia described for conduction utilizing a concealed pathway (p. 710). The major difference between the two syndromes is the capacity for anterograde conduction over the accessory pathway during atrial flutter or atrial fibrillation (see below).

A variety of other anatomical substrates exist that provide the basis for different ECG manifestations of several variations of the preexcitation syndrome[167] (Fig. 21–26). Fibers from atrium to His bundle bypassing the physiological delay of the AV node are called atriohisian tracts (Fig. 21–26*B*) and are associated with a short P-R interval and a normal QRS complex. Although demonstrated anatomically[168] (see below), the electrophysiological significance of these tracts in the genesis of tachycardias remains to be established. Indeed, evidence does not support the presence of a specific Lown-Ganong-Levine (LGL) syndrome[169] comprising a short P-R interval, normal QRS complex, and tachycardias related to an atriohisian bypass tract.[170] The short P-R intervals reported in many patients probably represent one end of the spectrum of normal AV conduction.[61] Two varieties of Mahaim fibers[171] include those passing from the AV node to the ventricle, called nodoventricular fibers (Fig. 21–26*C*), and those arising in

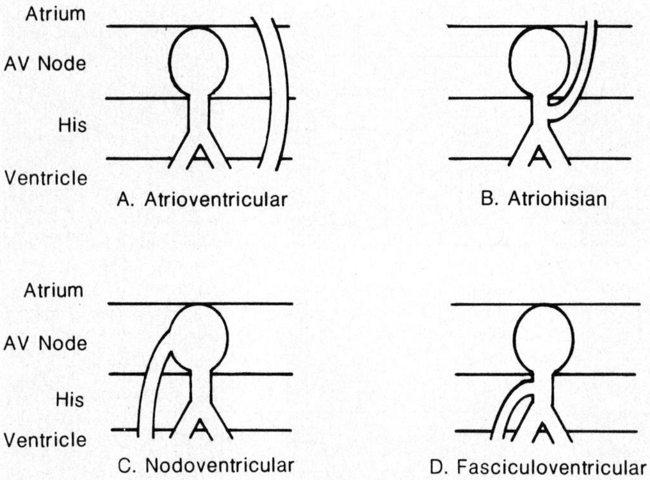

FIGURE 21–26 Schematic representation of accessory pathways.

the His bundle or bundle branches and inserting in the ventricular myocardium, called fasciculoventricular fibers (Fig. 21–26*D*). For nodoventricular connections, the P-R interval may be normal or short, and the QRS complex is a fusion beat. Fasciculoventricular connections create a normal P-R interval and a fixed, anomalous QRS complex.[172]

Electrophysiological Features (See also pp. 634 and 711). If the Kent bundle accessory pathway is capable of antegrade conduction, two parallel routes of AV conduction are possible, one subject to physiologic delay over the AV node and the other passing directly without delay from atrium to ventricle. This produces the typical QRS complex that is a fusion beat due to depolarization of the ventricle in part by the wavefront traveling over the accessory pathway and in part by the wavefront traveling over the normal AV node–His bundle route. The delta wave represents ventricular activation from input over the accessory pathway. The extent of contribution to ventricular depolarization by the wavefront over each route depends upon their relative activation times. If AV nodal conduction delay occurs, for example, because of a rapid atrial pacing rate or premature atrial complex, more of the ventricle becomes activated over the accessory pathway, and the QRS complex becomes more anomalous in contour. Total activation of the ventricle over the accessory pathway can occur if the AV nodal delay is sufficiently long. In contrast, if the accessory pathway is relatively far from the sinus node, for example, a left lateral accessory pathway, or if AV nodal conduction time is relatively short, more of the ventricle may be activated by conduction over the normal pathway (Fig. 21–27). The normal fusion beat during sinus rhythm has a short H-V interval, or His bundle activation actually begins after the onset of ventricular depolarization, because part of the atrial impulse bypasses the AV node and activates the ventricle early, at a time when the atrial impulse traveling the normal route just reaches the His bundle. This finding of a short or negative H-V interval occurs only during conduction over an accessory pathway or from retrograde His activation during a ventricular tachycardia.

Pacing the atrium at rapid rates, at premature intervals, or from a site close to the atrial insertion of the Kent bundle accentuates the anomalous activation of the ventricles and shortens the H-V interval even more (His activation may become buried in the ventricular electrogram, Fig. 21–27). The position of the accessory pathway can be determined by a careful analysis of the spatial direction of the delta wave in the 12-lead ECG in maximally preexcited beats[173] (Fig. 21–28) as well as by body surface maps. T-wave abnormalities can occur after disappearance of preexcitation with orientation of the T wave according to the site of preexcitation.[174] In patients who have an atriohisian tract, theoretically the QRS complex would remain normal and the short A-H interval fixed or show little increase during atrial pacing at more rapid rates. Rapid atrial pacing in patients who have

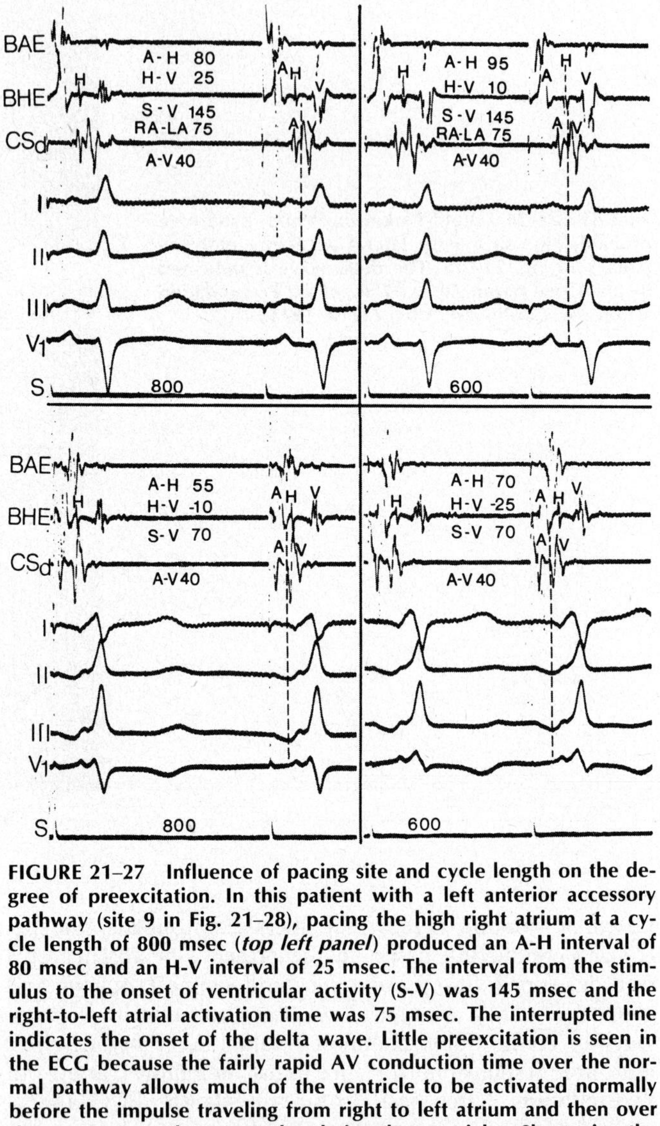

FIGURE 21–27 Influence of pacing site and cycle length on the degree of preexcitation. In this patient with a left anterior accessory pathway (site 9 in Fig. 21–28), pacing the high right atrium at a cycle length of 800 msec (*top left panel*) produced an A-H interval of 80 msec and an H-V interval of 25 msec. The interval from the stimulus to the onset of ventricular activity (S-V) was 145 msec and the right-to-left atrial activation time was 75 msec. The interrupted line indicates the onset of the delta wave. Little preexcitation is seen in the ECG because the fairly rapid AV conduction time over the normal pathway allows much of the ventricle to be activated normally before the impulse traveling from right to left atrium and then over the accessory pathway can depolarize the ventricles. Shortening the pacing cycle length to 600 msec (*top right panel*) without changing the pacing site lengthened the A-H interval by 15 msec and shortened the H-V interval by 10 msec. The other intervals remained the same and the QRS complex changed very slightly. In the *bottom left panel*, the coronary sinus is paced at a cycle length of 800 msec. Even though the A-H interval shortens to 55 msec because of coronary sinus pacing, the S-V shortens to 70 msec, His bundle activation follows the onset of ventricular depolarization by 10 msec, and the QRS complex becomes more aberrant. By pacing at a site near the atrial insertion of the accessory pathway, conduction rapidly reaches the ventricle over the accessory pathway to activate more of the ventricle than when pacing the right atrium at the same cycle length. In the *bottom right panel*, shortening the pacing cycle length to 600 msec lengthens the A-H interval 15 msec, and His bundle activation begins 25 msec after the onset of QRS complex. The S-V and A-V intervals remain unchanged and the QRS complex becomes even more aberrant.

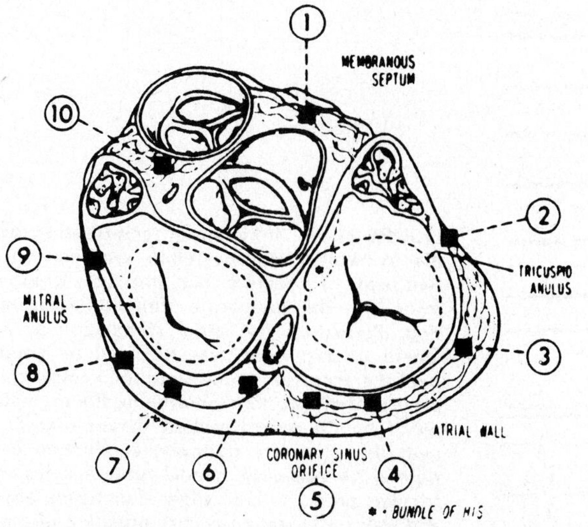

1 RIGHT ANTERIOR PARASEPTAL
2 RIGHT ANTERIOR
3 RIGHT LATERAL
4 RIGHT POSTERIOR
5 RIGHT PARASEPTAL
6 LEFT POSTERIOR PARASEPTAL
7 LEFT POSTERIOR
8 LEFT LATERAL
9 LEFT ANTERIOR
10 LEFT ANTERIOR PARASEPTAL

DELTA WAVE POLARITY

	I	II	III	AVR	AVL	AVF	V1	V2	V3	V4	V5	V6
①	+	+	+(±)	-	±(+)	+	±	±	+(±)	+	+	+
②	+	+	-(±)	-	+(±)	±(-)	±	+(±)	+(±)	+	+	+
③	+	±(-)	-	-	+	-(±)	±	±	±	+	+	+
④	+	-	-	-	+	-	±(+)	±	+	+	+	+
⑤	+	-	-	-(+)	+	-	±	+	+	+	+	+
⑥	+	-	-	-	+	-	+	+	+	+	+	+
⑦	+	-	-	±(+)	+	-	+	+	+	+	+	-(±)
⑧	-(±)	±	±	±(+)	-(±)	±	+	+	+	+	-(±)	-(±)
⑨	-(±)	+	+	-	-(±)	+	+	+	+	+	+	+
⑩	+	+	+(±)	-	±	+	±(+)	+	+	+	+	+

± = Initial 40 msec delta wave isoelectric
+ = Initial 40 msec delta wave positive
- = Initial 40 msec delta wave negative

FIGURE 21–28 In this schematic representation (*top*), sites of the potential position of the accessory pathway are indicated by filled boxes numbered 1 through 10. The delta wave polarity in the 12-lead ECG for each of the 10 sites is depicted in the table at the bottom. (From Gallagher, J. J., et al.: The preexcitation syndromes. Progr. Cardiovasc. Dis. *20*:285, 1978.)

nodoventricular connections shortens the H-V interval and widens the QRS complex but, in contrast to patients who have an atrioventricular connection, (Fig. 21–27) the A-V interval also lengthens. In patients who have fasciculoventricular connections, the H-V interval and QRS complex remain unchanged during rapid atrial pacing.

It is important to remember that, even though the Kent bundle conducts more rapidly than does the AV node (conduction velocity is faster in the accessory pathway), the Kent bundle usually has a longer refractory period during long cycle lengths (e.g., sinus rhythm)—i.e., it takes longer for the accessory pathway to recover excitability than it does for the AV node. Consequently, a premature atrial complex can occur sufficiently early to block anterogradely in the accessory pathway and conduct to the ventricle only over the normal AV node–His bundle (Fig. 21–29). The resultant H-V interval and the QRS complex become normal. Such an event may initiate the most common type of reciprocating tachycardia, which is characterized by anterograde conduction over the normal pathway and retrograde conduction over the accessory pathway (orthodromic)[173,175] (Figs. 21–29 and 21–30). The accessory pathway, blocking in an anterograde direction, recovers excitability in time to be activated following the QRS complex, in a retrograde direction, completing the reentrant loop. Much less commonly, patients can have tachycardias called antidromic tachycardias during which anterograde conduction occurs over the accessory pathway and retrograde conduction over the AV node. The resultant QRS complex is abnormal owing to total ventricular activation over the accessory pathway (Fig. 21–30*C*). In both tachycardias the accessory pathway is an obligatory part of the reentrant circuit.

Rarely, patients may have multiple accessory pathways that maintain the reentrant loop anterogradely over one accessory pathway and retrogradely over the other.[176] Patients who have nodoventricular fibers have tachycardias with a left bundle branch block morphology assumed to be due to a macro-reentrant circuit using the nodoventricular fiber anterogradely and the His-Purkinje system with a portion of the AV node retrogradely[172,177] (Fig. 21–30*F*). This circuit still remains to be established definitively, and it is possible that the nodoventricular pathway is a bystander without participation in the reentrant circuit. No direct relationship between fasciculoventricular fibers and observed arrhythmias has been found.[172] Anatomical-electrophysiological correlative evidence supports the presence and functional significance of nodoventricular fibers.[178]

An incessant form of supraventricular tachycardia has been recognized[179] that generally occurs with a long R-P interval that exceeds the P-R interval (Fig. 21–31) and may be due to an accessory pathway that conducts very slowly, with electrophysiological properties similar to those of the AV node. Tachycardia is maintained by anterograde AV nodal conduction and retrograde conduction over the accessory pathway[180–182] (Fig. 21–30*D*). The long anterograde conduction times over the accessory pathway may prevent ECG manifestations of accessory pathway conduction during sinus rhythm. The QRS is prolonged during sinus rhythm only when conduction times through the AV node–His bundle exceed those in the accessory pathway.[183] Patients can have recurrent, sustained wide QRS tachycardia due to anterograde conduction through the accessory pathway and retrograde conduction over the AV node. Most of these mechanisms found in adults also occur in children.[184]

When retrograde atrial activation during tachycardia occurs over an accessory pathway that connects the left atrium to the left ventricle, the earliest retrograde activity is recorded from a left atrial electrode usually positioned in the coronary sinus (Fig. 21–29). When retrograde atrial activation during tachycardia occurs over an accessory pathway that connects the right ventricle to the right atrium, the earliest retrograde atrial activity generally is recorded from a lateral right atrial electrode. Participation of a septal accessory pathway creates earliest retrograde atrial activation in the low right atrium situated near the septum. These mapping techniques with catheter electrodes and at the time of surgery (pp. 640 and 672) provide the most accurate assessment of the position of the accessory pathway, which can be anywhere in the AV groove except where the ventricles are contiguous (Fig. 21–28). However, it may be difficult to distinguish AV nodal reentry from participation of a septal accessory connection using the retrograde sequence of atrial activation because activation sequences during both tachycardias are similar. Other approaches to demonstrate retrograde atrial activation over the accessory pathway must be tried and can be accomplished by inducing premature ventricular complexes during tachycardia to determine whether retrograde atrial preexcitation can occur at a time when the His bundle is refractory. Since ventriculoatrial conduction cannot occur over the normal conduction system because the His bundle is refractory, an accessory pathway must be present for the atria to become preexcited and must be participating in the tachycardia circuit. No patient with a reciprocating tachycardia due to an accessory AV pathway has a V-A interval less than 70 msec measured from the onset of ventricular depolarization to the onset of the earliest atrial activity recorded on an esophageal lead or less than 95 msec when measured to the high right atrium. In contrast, in the majority of patients with reentry in the AV node, intervals from the onset of ventricular activity to the earliest onset of atrial activity recorded in the esophageal lead are less than 70 msec[185] (see p. 708).

The rhythm of reciprocating tachycardias using an accessory pathway may spontaneously change into atrial flutter or fibrillation.[186] Spontaneous termination of reciprocating tachycardia is common and multiple mechanisms may be involved, with block in the accessory pathway, AV node, or His-Purkinje system.[187]

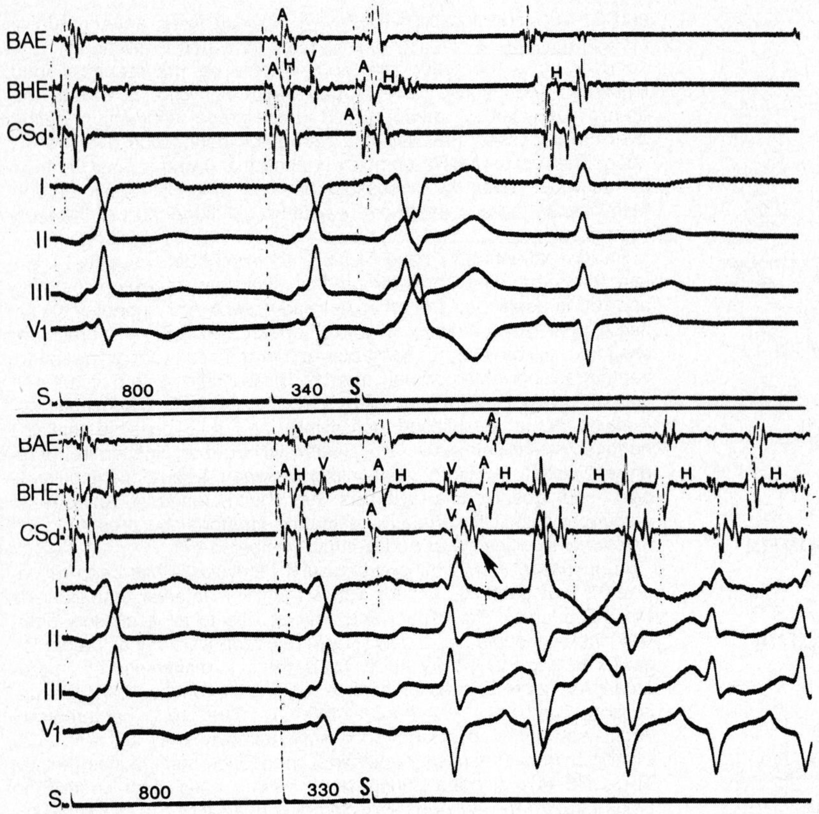

FIGURE 21–29 **Initiation of reciprocating tachycardia in Wolff-Parkinson-White syndrome. The last two beats of a regular train at a cycle length of 800 msec and the premature stimulus (S) are shown. *Top,* Premature left atrial stimulation at a cycle length of 340 msec was followed by conduction over the accessory pathway to the ventricle and full preexcitation. *Bottom,* Shortening the premature interval by 10 msec resulted in anterograde block over the accessory pathway, conduction over the normal AV node–His bundle route and loss of ventricular preexcitation (slight functional aberration and H-V prolongation occur). Initiation of a reciprocating tachycardia follows. Note that during reciprocating tachycardia, atrial activation is recorded earliest in the coronary sinus lead, followed by low and high right atrial activation, and is consistent with a left-sided accessory pathway (arrow).**

Patients may have other types of tachycardia during which the accessory pathway is an "innocent bystander," i.e., uninvolved in the mechanism responsible for the tachycardia. For example, in patients with atrial flutter or atrial fibrillation, the accessory pathway is not a requisite part of the mechanism responsible for tachycardia, and the latter occurs in the atrium unrelated to the accessory pathway (Fig. 21–30*E*). Propagation to the ventricle during atrial flutter or atrial fibrillation therefore can occur over the normal AV node–His bundle or accessory pathway. Patients who have paroxysmal atrial fibrillation almost always have inducible reciprocating tachycardias as well.[188] Atrial fibrillation presents a potentially serious risk because of the possibility for very rapid conduction over the accessory pathway. At more rapid rates, the refractory period of the accessory pathway may shorten significantly and permit an extremely rapid ventricular response during atrial flutter or atrial fibrillation (Fig. 21–32) that may lead to ventricular fibrillation.[189–191] The rapid ventricular response probably exceeds the ability of the ventricle to follow in an organized fashion, resulting in fragmented disorganized ventricular activation

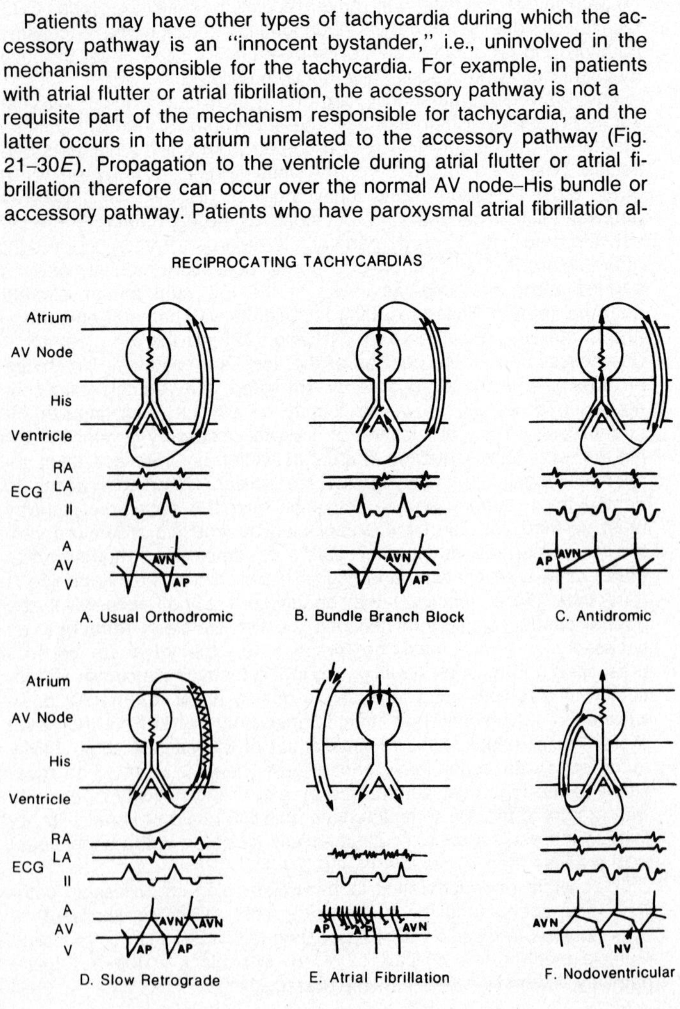

FIGURE 21–30 **Schematic diagram of tachycardias associated with accessory pathways. Format as in Figure 21–9. *A,* Orthodromic tachycardia with anterograde conduction over the AV node–His bundle route and retrograde conduction over the accessory pathway (left-sided for this example as depicted by LA activation preceding RA activation). *B,* Orthodromic tachycardia and ipsilateral functional bundle branch block. *C,* Antidromic tachycardia with anterograde conduction over the accessory pathway and retrograde conduction over the AV node–His bundle. *D,* Orthodromic tachycardia with a slowly conducting accessory pathway. *E,* Atrial fibrillation with the accessory pathway as a bystander. *F,* Anterograde conduction over a portion of the AV node and a nodoventricular pathway and retrograde conduction over the AV node.**

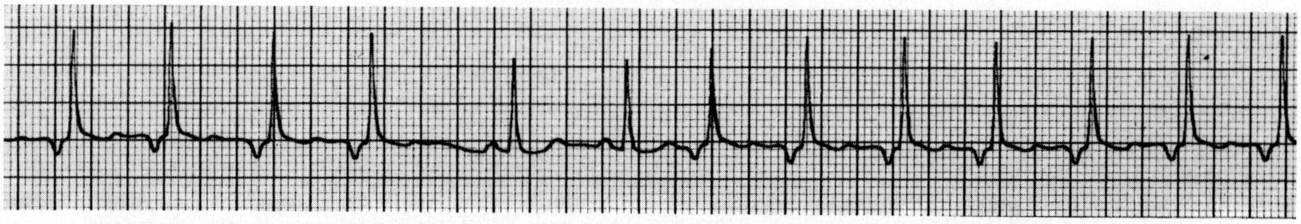

FIGURE 21–31 Scalar ECG appearance of incessant tachycardia due to anterograde conduction over the AV node–His bundle and retrograde conduction over a slowly conducting accessory pathway. Lead II.

and hypotension, and leads to ventricular fibrillation. Alternatively, supraventricular discharge bypassing AV nodal delay may activate the ventricle during the vulnerable period of the antecedent T wave and precipitate ventricular fibrillation.[192] Patients who have had ventricular fibrillation have ventricular cycle lengths during atrial fibrillation in the range of 200 msec or less.[189]

Finally, it is important to remember that patients with preexcitation syndrome may have other causes of tachycardia such as AV nodal reentry,[146] sometimes with dual AV nodal curves,[193] sinus nodal reentry, or even ventricular tachycardia unrelated to the accessory pathway. Accessory pathways may conduct only anterogradely as well as only retrogradely (p. 710).[146,194] If the pathway conducts only anterogradely, it cannot participate in the usual form of reciprocating tachycardia (Fig. 21–30*A*). It can, however, participate in antidromic tachycardia (Fig. 21–30*C*) as well as conduct to the ventricle during atrial flutter or atrial fibrillation (Fig. 21–30*E*). Some data suggest that the accessory pathway demonstrates automatic activity,[27,195] which could conceivably be responsible for some instances of tachycardia.

Clinical Features. The reported incidence of preexcitation syndrome depends in large measure on the population studied, varying from 0.1 to 3.0 per thousand in apparently healthy subjects, with an average of about 1.5 per thousand. The incidence of the electrocardiographic pattern of Wolff-Parkinson-White conduction in 22,500 healthy aviation personnel was 0.25 per cent with a prevalence of documented tachyarrhythmias of 1.8 per cent. However, in a group of referred patients the prevalence of tachyarrhythmias was 20 per cent.[196] It occurs in all age groups, from the newborn to the elderly, in identical twins, and more often in males (60 to 70 per cent of cases). The majority of adults with preexcitation syndrome have normal hearts,[197] although a variety of acquired and congenital cardiac defects have been reported, including Ebstein's anomaly,[198,199] mitral valve prolapse, and cardiomyopathies. Patients with Ebstein's anomaly (p. 996) often have multiple accessory pathways, right-sided either in the posterior septum or posterolateral wall, with preexcitation localized to the atrialized ventricle. They often have reciprocating tachycardia with a long V-A interval and a right bundle branch block morphology.[199]

Four to 80 per cent of patients with preexcitation syndrome experience recurrent tachyarrhythmias, depending on the patient population, with 80 per cent of these patients having a reciprocating tachycardia, 15 to 30 per cent with atrial fibrillation, and 5 per cent with atrial flutter. Ventricular tachycardia occurs uncommonly. The anomalous complexes may mask or mimic myocardial infarction (p. 230), bundle branch block, or ventricular hypertrophy, and the presence of the preexcitation syndrome may call attention to an associated cardiac defect. Sinus node dysfunction has been reported to be more frequent in patients with the preexcitation syndrome.[200] The prognosis is excel-

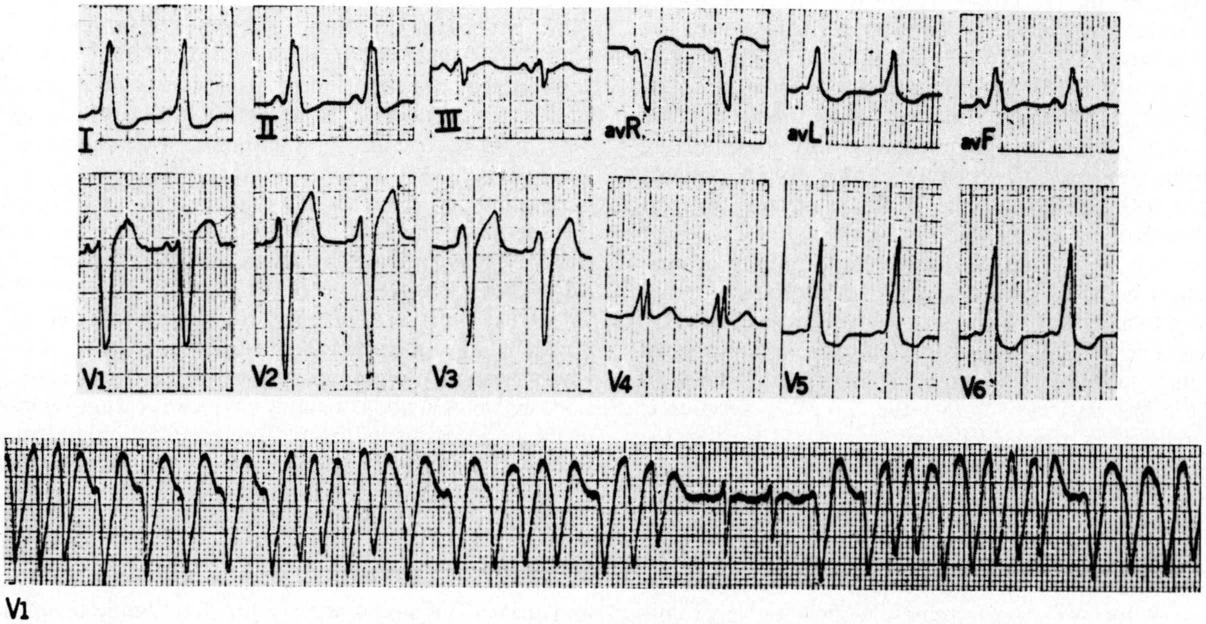

FIGURE 21–32 Preexcitation syndrome is apparent in the 12-lead ECG and may represent a right lateral accessory pathway. During atrial fibrillation the ventricular rate is extremely rapid, at times approaching 350 beats/min. The gross irregularity of the cycle lengths, wide QRS complexes interspersed with normal QRS complexes, and very rapid rate should suggest the diagnosis of atrial fibrillation and an atrioventricular bypass tract.

lent in patients without tachycardia or an associated cardiac anomaly. In patients with recurrent tachycardia the prognosis is good in most, but sudden death occurs rarely, especially when the ventricular rate during tachycardia such as atrial fibillation is rapid or associated congenital defects are present.

It is very likely that acquisition of an accessory pathway occurs congenitally, although its manifestations may present in later years and appear to be "acquired."[156] Some children and adults may lose their tendency to develop tachyarrhythmias as they grow older,[201] possibly owing to fibrotic or other changes at the site of the accessory pathway insertion.[202] The presence or absence of tachycardia associated with the preexcitation syndrome may depend on small changes in activation times in the reentrant loop.

Treatment. Patients with ventricular preexcitation may have no or only occasional tachyarrhythmias unassociated with significant symptoms. These patients do not require electrophysiological evaluation or therapy. However, if a patient has frequent episodes of tachyarrhythmias and/or the arrhythmias cause significant symptoms, therapy should be instituted. Those who suffer significant hemodynamic consequences from the tachycardia should be considered for electrophysiological study (p. 634).

Drugs that increase the refractory period of the accessory pathway or AV node, slow conduction, or cause block in one of the reentry pathways may suppress the reciprocating tachycardia. Verapamil, propranolol, and digitalis prolong conduction time and refractoriness in the AV node. Verapamil[99] and propranolol do not directly affect conduction in the accessory pathway, while digitalis has had variable effects.[203,204] Recently studied, intravenous ouabain had no significant effect on either anterograde or retrograde anomalous pathway refractoriness and did not interfere with the induction of tachycardia in most patients.[205] Because digitalis has been reported to shorten refractoriness in the accessory pathway[204] and speed the ventricular response in some patients with atrial fibrillation,[203] it is advisable *not* to use digitalis as a single drug in patients with the WPW syndrome who have or may develop atrial flutter or atrial fibrillation. Since many patients may develop atrial fibrillation during the reciprocating tachycardia, this caveat probably applies to *all* patients who have tachycardia and the WPW syndrome. Rather, drugs that prolong the refractory period in the accessory pathway such as quinidine, disopyramide, and procainamide should be used. Lidocaine does not prolong refractoriness of the accessory pathway in patients whose effective refractory period ≤ 300 msec.[206] Verapamil[99,207] and lidocaine[206] may increase the ventricular rate during atrial fibrillation in patients with the WPW syndrome. Isoproterenol may expose WPW syndrome and shorten the refractory period of the accessory pathway.[208]

Termination of the acute episode of reciprocating tachycardia, suspected electrocardiographically by a normal QRS complex, regular R-R intervals, a rate of about 200 beats/min, and a P wave in the ST segment, should be approached as for AV nodal reentry. Following vagal maneuvers, verapamil or a similar calcium-entry blocker or edrophonium should be considered as the initial treatment of choice. For atrial flutter or fibrillation, the latter suspected by an anomalous QRS complex and grossly irregular R-R intervals (Fig. 21–32), drugs that prolong refractoriness in the accessory pathway often coupled with drugs that prolong AV nodal refractoriness (e.g., quinidine and propranolol) must be used. In some patients, particularly with a very rapid ventricular response, electrical cardioversion should be the *initial* treatment of choice.

For long-term therapy to *prevent a recurrence,* it is not always possible to predict which drugs may be most effective for an individual patient. Some drugs actually can increase the frequency of episodes of reciprocating tachycardia by prolonging anterograde and not retrograde refractory periods of the accessory pathway, thereby making it easier for a premature atrial complex to block anterogradely in the accessory pathway. Administration of two drugs, such as quinidine and propranolol or procainamide and verapamil, to decrease conduction capabilities in both limbs of the reentrant circuit may be beneficial. Depending on the clinical situation, empirical drug trials or serial electrophysiological drug testing may be employed to determine optimal drug therapy for patients with reciprocating tachycardia. For patients who have atrial fibrillation with a rapid ventricular response, induction of atrial fibrillation while the patient is receiving therapy is essential to be certain that the ventricular rate is controlled.

Although drugs suppress or modify tachycardia in most patients, an occasional patient may require *surgical ablation* of the accessory pathway (p. 672). Surgical division of the accessory pathway is advisable for patients with frequent symptomatic arrhythmias that are not fully controlled by drugs or with rapid AV conduction over the accessory pathway during atrial flutter or fibrillation and in whom significant slowing of the ventricular response during tachycardia cannot be obtained by drug therapy. Patients who have accessory pathways with very short refractory periods may be poor candidates for drug therapy, since the refractory periods may be prolonged insignificantly in response to the standard agents.[209] *Pacing therapy* may be useful in this syndrome as in many other supraventricular tachyarrhythmias (p. 756), with the exception that precipitation of atrial flutter or atrial fibrillation in a patient with an accessory pathway may result in very rapid ventricular rates and clinical deterioration.[210]

In *summary,* electrocardiographic clues are often present that permit differential diagnosis of the various supraventricular tachycardias.[211] P waves during tachycardia identical to sinus P waves and occurring with a long R-P interval and a short P-R interval are most likely due to sinus nodal reentry. Retrograde (inverted in II, III, and aV_f) P waves generally represent reentry involving the AV junction, either AV nodal reentry or reciprocating tachycardia using an accessory pathway. Tachycardia without manifest P waves is probably due to AV nodal reentry (P waves buried in QRS), while a tachycardia with an R-P interval exceeding 60 to 70 msec may be due to an accessory pathway. AV dissociation or AV block during tachycardia excludes the presence of a functioning accessory pathway and makes AV nodal reentry unlikely. Some tachycardias, such as sinus and AV nodal reentry, can occur either simultaneously or at different times in the same patient[99,212] (Fig. 21–8, p. 694). Tachycardia due to intra-His reentry has been described, although the clinical importance of this entity is not established.

VENTRICULAR RHYTHM DISTURBANCES

Premature Ventricular Complexes

Electrocardiographic Recognition. A premature ventricular complex is characterized by the premature occurrence of a QRS complex that is bizarre in shape and has a duration usually more prolonged than the dominant QRS complex, generally exceeding 120 msec. The T wave is commonly large and opposite in direction to the major deflection of the QRS. The QRS complex is not preceded by a premature P wave but may be preceded by a sinus P wave occurring at its expected time. The diagnosis of premature ventricular complex can never be made with unequivocal certainty from the scalar electrocardiogram, since a supraventricular beat or rhythm may mimic the manifestations of ventricular arrhythmia (Figs. 21–17 and 21–33). Retrograde transmission to the atria from the premature ventricular complex occurs fairly frequently but is often obscured by the distorted QRS complex and T wave. If the retrograde impulse discharges and resets the sinus node prematurely, it produces a pause that is not fully compensatory. More commonly, the sinus node and atria are not discharged prematurely by the retrograde impulse, since interference of impulses frequently occurs at the AV junction (see p. 735), establishing a collision between the anterograde impulse conducted from the sinus node and the retrograde impulse conducted from the premature ventricular complex. Therefore, a fully compensatory pause usually follows a premature ventricular complex: the R-R interval produced by the two sinus-initiated QRS complexes on either side of the premature complex equals twice the normally conducted R-R interval. The premature ventricular complex may not produce any pause and may therefore be interpolated (Fig. 21–33), or it may produce a postponed compensatory pause when an interpolated premature complex causes P-R prolongation of the first post-extrasystolic beat to such a degree that the P wave of the second post-extrasystolic beat occurs at a very short R-P interval and is therefore blocked.[213]

Interference within the ventricle may result in *ventricular fusion beats* (see p. 721), which may on occasion be narrower than the dominant beat. For example, a right bundle branch block pattern of a premature ventricular complex arising in the left ventricle of a patient with left bundle branch block may fuse with the dominant left bundle branch block pattern to produce a normally shaped QRS complex. This might also occur when the ventricle with a bundle branch block pattern is paced artificially, producing a narrow ventricular fusion beat between the paced and the sinus-conducted beats. Narrow premature ventricular complexes also have been explained as originating at a point equidistant from each ventricle in the ventricular septum and by arising high in the fascicular system.[214] Whether a compensatory or noncompensatory pause, retrograde atrial excitation, or an interpolated complex, fusion complex or echo beat (p. 627) occurs (Fig. 21–33), it is merely a function of how the AV junction conducts and the timing of the events taking place.

The term *bigeminy* refers to pairs of complexes and indicates a normal and premature complex; *trigeminy* indicates a premature complex following two normal beats; a premature complex following three normal beats is called

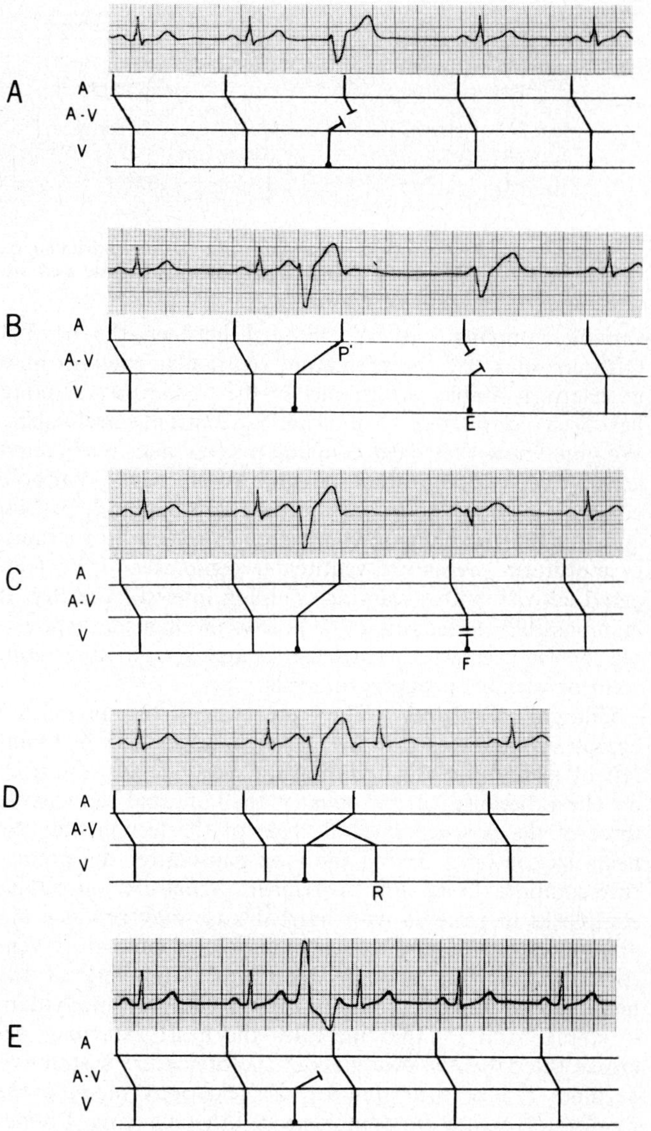

FIGURE 21–33 **Premature ventricular complexes. *A* to *D* were recorded in the same patient. *A*, A late premature ventricular complex results in a compensatory pause. *B*, A slower sinus rate and a slightly earlier premature complex result in retrograde atrial excitation (P′). The sinus node is reset, producing a noncompensatory pause. Before the sinus-initiated P wave that follows the retrograde P wave can conduct to the ventricle, a ventricular escape occurs (E). *C*, Events are similar to those in *B* except that a ventricular fusion beat (F) results following the premature ventricular complex owing to a slightly faster sinus rate. *D*, The impulse propagating retrogradely to the atrium reverses its direction after a delay and returns to reexcite the ventricles (R) to produce a ventricular echo. *E*, An interpolated premature ventricular complex is followed by a slightly prolonged P-R interval of the sinus-initiated beat. Lead II.**

quadrigeminy, and so on. Two successive premature ventricular complexes are termed a pair or a couplet, while three successive premature ventricular complexes are called a triplet. Arbitrarily, three or more successive premature ventricular complexes are termed ventricular tachycardia. Premature ventricular complexes may have different contours and often are called multifocal (Fig. 21–34). More properly they should be called "multiform," "polymorphic," or "pleomorphic," since it is not known whether multiple foci are discharging or whether conduction of the impulse originating from one site is merely changing.

Premature ventricular complexes may exhibit fixed or

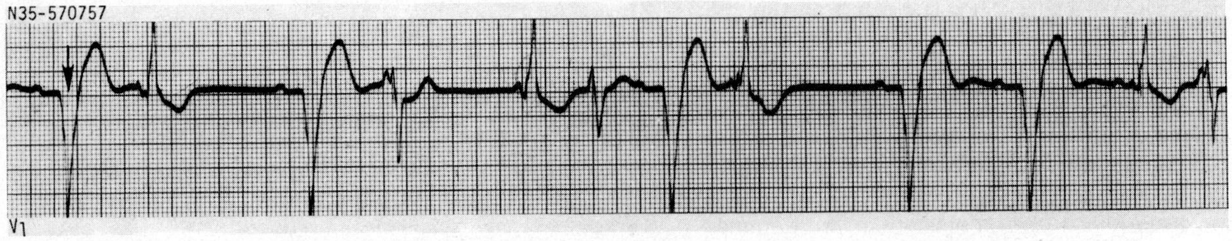

FIGURE 21–34 Multiform premature ventricular complexes. The normally conducted QRS complexes exhibit a left bundle branch block contour (arrow) and are followed by premature ventricular complexes with three different morphologies.

variable coupling, i.e., the interval between the normal QRS complex and the premature ventricular complex may be relatively stable or variable. In the past, fixed coupling has been considered to indicate a reentrant mechanism. We now know that fixed coupling may be due to triggered activity (p. 620) or other possible mechanisms. Variable coupling may be due to parasystole (see Chapter 7, p. 248, and p. 622), to changing conduction in a reentrant circuit, to multiform premature ventricular complexes, or to triggered activity with a varying coupling interval. Usually, it is impossible to determine the precise mechanism responsible for the premature ventricular complex with either constant or variable coupling intervals.

Clinical Features. The prevalence of premature complexes increases with age. Their presence may be manifest by symptoms of palpitations or discomfort in the neck or chest because of the greater than normal contractile force of the post-extrasystolic beat or the feeling that the heart has stopped during the long pause after the premature complex. Long runs of frequent premature ventricular complexes in patients with heart disease may produce angina or hypotension. Frequent interpolated premature ventricular complexes actually represent a doubling of the heart rate and may compromise the patient's hemodynamic status. Activity that increases the heart rate may decrease the patient's awareness of the premature systoles or at times reduce their number. Exercise may increase the number of premature complexes in other patients. Premature systoles may be quite uncomfortable in patients who have aortic regurgitation because of the large stroke volume.

Premature ventricular complexes occur in association with a variety of stimuli and can be produced by direct mechanical, electrical, and chemical stimulation of the myocardium. Often they are seen during infection, in ischemic or inflamed myocardium, or during anesthesia or surgery. They may be provoked by a variety of medications, by tension states, and by excessive use of tobacco, caffeine, or alcohol. Both central and peripheral autonomic stimulation have profound effects on heart rate, which may produce or suppress premature complexes.[215]

Physical examination reveals the presence of a premature beat followed by a pause that is longer than normal. A fully compensatory pause may be distinguished from one that is not fully compensatory, since the former does not change the timing of the basic rhythm. The premature beat is often accompanied by a decrease in intensity of the heart sounds, often with just the first heart sound being heard, which may be sharp and snapping. The relationship of atrial to ventricular systole determines the presence of normal *a* waves or giant *a* waves in the jugular venous pulse, and the length of the P-R interval determines the intensity of the first heart sound. The second heart sound may be abnormally split.

The importance of premature ventricular complexes varies depending on the clinical setting. In the absence of underlying heart disease, the presence of premature ventricular complexes usually has no significance regarding longevity or limitation of activity, and antiarrhythmic drugs are not indicated; the patient should be reassured if he or she is symptomatic. An exception may be middle-aged men, because premature ventricular systoles and complex ventricular arrhythmias occurring in apparently healthy middle-aged men are associated with the presence of coronary heart disease and with a greater risk of subsequent death from coronary heart disease.[216–219] However, it has not been demonstrated that premature ventricular systoles or complex ventricular arrhythmias play a *precipitating* role in the genesis of sudden death in these patients, and the arrhythmias may simply be a marker of heart disease (p. 633). It has not been shown convincingly that antiarrhythmic therapy given to suppress the premature ventricular systoles or complex ventricular arrhythmias reduces the incidence of sudden death in such apparently healthy men. The presence of premature ventricular complexes are thought to reflect an increased risk of cardiac death in patients with hypertrophic cardiomyopathy and mitral valve prolapse. A strong association exists between myocardial infarction size and frequency of premature ventricular complexes found while patients were in the coronary care unit[220] and between poor left ventricular function and frequency of premature ventricular complexes during recovery.[221] In patients suffering from acute myocardial infarction, it has been commonly held that so-called "warning arrhythmias," such as premature ventricular complexes occurring close to the preceding T wave, greater than five or six per minute, bigeminal, multiform, or occurring in salvoes of two, three, or more, may presage or precipitate the occurrence of ventricular tachycardia or fibrillation. However, about half the patients who develop ventricular fibrillation have no "warning arrhythmias" and half who do have "warning arrhythmias" do not develop ventricular fibrillation[222] (p. 728).

Treatment. Extremes of heart rate, both fast and slow, may provoke the development of premature ventricular complexes. Premature ventricular complexes accompanying slow ventricular rates caused by sinus bradycardia or AV block may be abolished by increasing the basic rate with atropine or isoproterenol or by pacing. Conversely, in some patients with sinus tachycardia, slowing the heart rate may eradicate premature ventricular complexes. In the hospitalized patient, lidocaine given intravenously (p. 653) is generally the initial treatment of choice to suppress premature ventricular complexes. Lidocaine can be given intramuscularly in some instances. If maximum dosages of lidocaine are unsuccessful, then procainamide intravenously may be tried. Quinidine may be given intravenously slowly and cautiously. The use of disopyramide intravenously is still investigational. Propranolol or phenytoin may be tried if the other drugs have been unsuccessful. For long-term oral maintenance, quinidine, disopyramide, or procainamide is used, as for the prevention of ventricular tachycardia (p. 723).

Ventricular Tachycardia

Ventricular tachycardia arises in the specialized conduction system distal to the bifurcation of the His bundle, in ventricular muscle, or in combinations of both tissue types. The mechanisms include disorders of impulse formation and conduction (p. 619). The electrocardiographic diagnosis of ventricular tachycardia is suggested when a series of three or more bizarrely shaped premature ventricular complexes occur that exceed 120 msec, with the ST-T vector pointing opposite to the major QRS deflection. The R-R interval may be exceedingly regular or may vary. Atrial activity may be independent of ventricular activity (AV dissociation, p. 735), or the atria may be depolarized by the ventricles retrogradely (VA association). As will be discussed, depending on the particular type of ventricular tachycardia, the rate ranges from 70 to 250 beats/min, and the onset may be paroxysmal (sudden) or nonparoxysmal. QRS contours during the ventricular tachycardia may be unchanging (uniform) or may vary in a random fashion (multiform, polymorphic, or pleomorphic), vary in a more or less repetitive manner (torsades de pointes), vary in alternate complexes (bidirectional ventricular tachycardia), or vary in a stable but changing contour (i.e., right bundle branch contour changing to left bundle branch contour (see Fig. 20–8*A*, p. 674). Ventricular tachycardia may be sustained, defined arbitrarily as lasting longer than 30 seconds or requiring termination because of hemodynamic collapse, or nonsustained when it stops spontaneously in less than 30 seconds.[223,224]

The electrocardiographic distinction between supraventricular tachycardia with aberration and ventricular tachycardia may be extremely difficult at times, since features of

TABLE 21–2 MAJOR FEATURES IN THE DIFFERENTIAL DIAGNOSIS OF WIDE QRS BEATS OR TACHYCARDIA

Supports SVT	Supports VT
Slowing or termination by ↑ vagal tone	Fusion beats
Onset with premature P wave	Capture beats
RP interval $\leq$ 100 msec	AV dissociation
P and QRS rate and rhythm linked to suggest ventricular activation depends on atrial discharge, e.g., 2:1 AV block	P and QRS rate and rhythm linked to suggest atrial activation depends on ventricular discharge, e.g., 2:1 VA block
RSR′ V_1	
Long-short cycle sequence	"Compensatory" pause
	Left axis deviation QRS duration > 140 msec specific QRS contours (see text)

SVT = supraventricular tachycardia;
VT = ventricular tachycardia.

both arrhythmias overlap and under certain circumstances a supraventricular tachycardia can mimic all the criteria established for ventricular tachycardia. Ventricular complexes with bizarre or prolonged configuration indicate only that conduction through the ventricle is abnormal, and they can occur in supraventricular rhythms characterized by preexisting bundle branch block, aberrant conduction during incomplete recovery of repolarization, conduction over accessory pathways, and several other conditions (see p. 244). They do not necessarily indicate the origin of impulse formation or the reason for the abnormal conduction. Conversely, ectopic beats originating in the ventricle uncommonly can have a fairly normal duration and shape.

During the course of a tachycardia characterized by widespread, bizarre QRS complexes, the presence of *fusion beats* and *capture beats* provides maximum support for the diagnosis of ventricular tachycardia (Table 21–2). Fusion beats indicate activation of the ventricle from two different foci, implying that one of the foci had a ventricular origin. Capture of the ventricle by the supraventricular rhythm with a normal configuration of the captured QRS complex at an interval shorter than the tachycardia in question indicates that the impulse has a supraventricular origin (Fig. 21–35). Atrioventricular dissociation (p. 735) has long

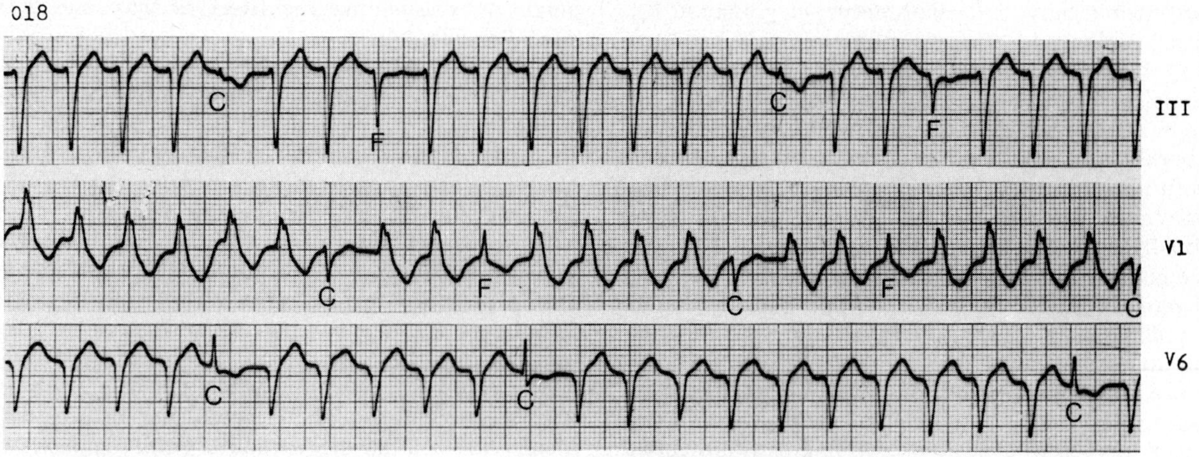

FIGURE 21–35 Fusions and capture beats during a probable ventricular tachycardia. The QRS complex is prolonged, and the R-R interval is regular except for occasional capture beats (C) that have a normal contour and are slightly premature. Complexes intermediate in contour represent fusion beats (F). Thus, even though atrial activity is not clearly apparent, it is likely that AV dissociation is present during a ventricular tachycardia and produces intermittent capture and fusion beats.

been considered a hallmark of ventricular tachycardia. However, retrograde VA conduction to the atria from ventricular beats occurs in a large percentage of patients, and therefore ventricular tachycardia may not exhibit AV dissociation.[225] Atrioventricular dissociation can occur uncommonly during supraventricular tachycardias (see Fig. 19–32*A*, p. 637). Even if a P wave appears to be related to each QRS complex it is at times difficult to determine whether the P wave is conducted anterogradely to the next QRS complex (i.e., supraventricular tachycardia with aber rancy) or retrogradely from the preceding QRS complex (i.e., a ventricular tachycardia). As a general rule, however, AV dissociation during a wide QRS tachycardia is strong presumptive evidence that the tachycardia is of ventricular origin.

Because of the overlapping features of ventricular and supraventricular tachycardias, and because differentiating clues may not be present on a given tracing, it appears best to ascribe a certain probability to the diagnosis that may weigh in favor of its ventricular or supraventricular origin. Some electrocardiographic features characterizing supraventricular arrhythmia with aberrancy include (1) consistent onset of the tachycardia with a premature P wave, (2) a very short R-P interval (≤ 0.1 sec) often requiring an esophageal recording to visualize the P waves, (3) a QRS configuration the same as that which occurs from known supraventricular conduction at similar rates, (4) P and QRS rate and rhythm linked to suggest that ventricular activation depends on atrial discharge (e.g., A-V Wenckebach block), and (5) slowing or termination of the tachycardia by vagal maneuvers.

Analysis of specific QRS contours also may be helpful. For example, QRS contours suggesting a ventricular tachycardia include left-axis deviation in the frontal plane and a QRS duration exceeding 140 msec with a QRS of normal duration during sinus rhythm. During ventricular tachycardia with right bundle branch block appearance, (1) the QRS complex is monophasic or biphasic in V_1 with an initial deflection different from sinus-initiated QRS complex, (2) the amplitude of the R wave in V_1 exceeds the R′, and (3) small R and large S wave or a QS pattern in V_6 may be present. With a ventricular tachycardia having a left bundle branch block contour, (1) the axis may be rightward with negative deflections deeper in V_1 than in V_6, (2) a broad prolonged (> 40 msec) R wave in V_1, and (3) a small Q, large R wave or QS pattern in V_6 may exist. A QRS complex that is similar in V_1 through V_6, either all negative or all positive, favors a ventricular origin as does the presence of 2:1 ventriculoatrial block. Supraventricular beats with aberration often have a triphasic pattern in V_1, an initial vector of the abnormal complex similar to that of the normally conducted beats, and a wide QRS complex that terminates a short cycle length which follows a long cycle (long-short cycle sequence). During atrial fibrillation fixed coupling, short coupling intervals, a long pause after the abnormal beat, and runs of bigeminy rather than a consecutive series of abnormal complexes, all favor ventricular origin of the premature complex rather than supraventricular origin with aberration.[226,227] A grossly irregular, wide QRS tachycardia with ventricular rates faster than 200 beats/min should raise the question of atrial fibrillation with conduction over an accessory pathway (see p. 712 and Fig. 21–32).[226,227] Exceptions exist to all the criteria enumerated above, especially in patients who have preexisting conduction disturbances or preexcitation syndrome; when in doubt, one must rely on sound clinical judgment, considering the ECG as only one of several helpful ancillary tests.

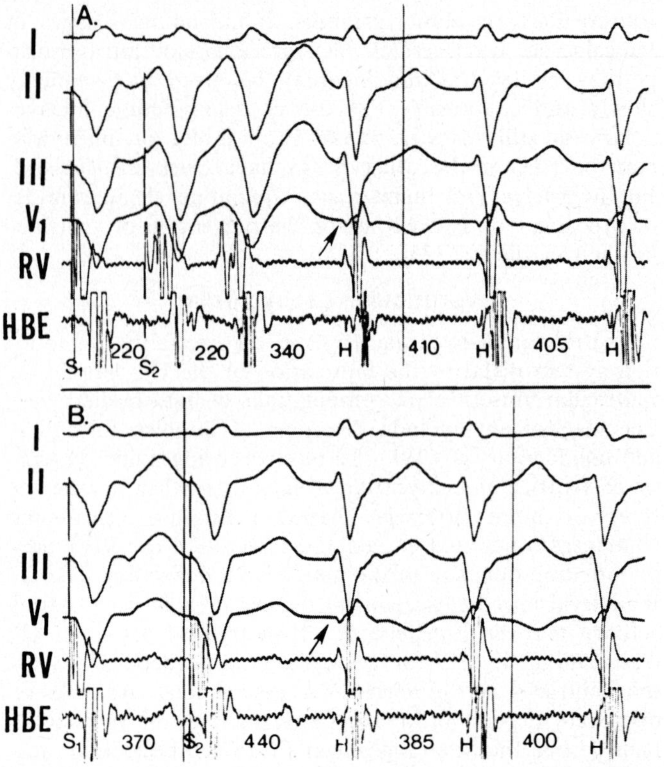

FIGURE 21–36 Precipitation and termination of sustained ventricular tachycardia by premature ventricular stimulation. *A*, The last paced beat (S_1) of a train at a basic cycle length of 550 msec is displayed. Premature ventricular stimulation at an S_1-S_2 interval of 220 msec is followed by a repetitive ventricular response, probably bundle branch reentry (a possible retrograde His depolarization is unlabeled) and then initiation of ventricular tachycardia (arrow). Note that His activation follows the onset of the QRS complex during the ventricular tachycardia. The latter exhibits right bundle branch block and left-axis deviation. *B*, Premature ventricular stimulation at an S_1-S_2 interval of 370 msec initiates the same ventricular tachycardia without a bundle branch reentrant response. (From Zipes, D. P., et al.: Atrial induction of ventricular tachycardia: Reentry versus triggered automaticity. Am. J. Cardiol. *44*:1, 1979.)

ELECTROPHYSIOLOGICAL FEATURES. Electrophysiologically, ventricular tachycardia can be distinguished by a short or negative H-V interval (i.e., H begins after the onset of ventricular depolarization) because of retrograde activation from the ventricles (see Fig. 19–32, p. 637, and Fig. 21–36). His bundle deflections dissociated from ventricular activation are diagnostic of ventricular tachycardia,[228] with rare exception.[229] His bundle deflections usually are not apparent because they are obscured by simultaneous ventricular septal depolarization or because of inadequate catheter position. The latter must be determined during supraventricular rhythm before the onset or after the termination of the ventricular tachycardia. Ventricular tachycardia may produce QRS complexes of narrow duration and of short H-V interval, most likely when the site of origin is close to the His bundle in the fascicles.[230]

Successful electrical induction of ventricular tachycardia

by premature stimulation of the ventricle (Fig. 21–36)[228,231] depends strongly on the characteristics of the ventricular tachycardia and the anatomic substrate. Sustained ventricular tachycardia and ventricular tachycardia due to coronary artery disease are induced with greater success than are nonsustained ventricular tachycardia and ventricular tachycardia due to noncoronary-related causes.[223] In general, it is more difficult to induce ventricular tachycardia with late premature stimuli compared to early premature stimuli, during sinus rhythm compared to ventricular pacing, and with one premature stimulus compared to two or three. The specificity of ventricular tachycardia induction using more than two premature ventricular stimuli has yet to be established, and preliminary data suggest that nonsustained pleomorphic ventricular tachycardia can be induced in patients who have no history of ventricular tachycardia.[232,233] Occasionally, ventricular tachycardia can be initiated only from the left ventricle[228] or from specific sites in the right ventricle.[234] No clinical, anatomical, electrocardiographic, or electrophysiological features are useful to predict whether left ventricular programmed stimulation will be required to induce ventricular tachycardia in patients.[235] Drugs such as isoproterenol,[236] various antiarrhythmic agents,[237] and alcohol[238] can facilitate the induction of ventricular tachycardia.

The capability of terminating ventricular tachycardia by pacing depends significantly on the rate of the ventricular tachycardia. Slower ventricular tachycardias are more easily terminated and with fewer stimuli than are more rapid ventricular tachycardias. An increasing number of stimuli are required to terminate more rapid ventricular tachycardias, which increases the risks of pacing-induced acceleration of the ventricular tachycardia.[239,240] Following premature stimulation during ventricular tachycardia, a pause may result but the tachycardia continues, suggesting that the origin of the tachycardia is relatively protected.[54,241] Ventricular tachycardia can also be induced and terminated during atrial pacing (see Fig. 19–33, p. 637).[54,59]

With the advent of acceptable surgical techniques to treat some forms of ventricular tachycardia it has become important to localize its origin. The 12-lead electrocardiogram may give misleading information regarding the origin of sustained ventricular tachycardia[242] and extensive endocardial and epicardial mapping studies are generally necessary (see Chapter 19). *Radionuclide phase mapping* of ventricular tachycardia is feasible and appears to provide data consistent with the known electrophysiology of ventricular tachycardia.[243]

CLINICAL FEATURES. Symptoms occurring during ventricular tachycardia depend on the ventricular rate, duration of tachycardia, the presence and extent of the underlying heart disease, and peripheral vascular disease. The location of impulse formation and therefore the way in which the depolarization wave spreads across the myocardium may also be important in some instances of delicate hemodynamic compensation. Physical findings depend in part on the P to QRS relationship. If atrial activity is dissociated from the ventricular contractions, the findings of AV dissociation (p. 735) will be present. If the atria are captured retrogradely, regularly occurring cannon *a* waves appear when atrial and ventricular contractions occur simultaneously and the signs of AV dissociation are absent.

In the author's series of 516 patients treated for symptomatic recurrent ventricular tachycardia, 284 patients have had ischemic heart disease, 74 cardiomyopathy (both congestive and hypertrophic), 75 primary electrical disease, 45 mitral valve prolapse, 20 valvular heart disease, and 18 miscellaneous causes. Primary electrical disease includes patients with ventricular tachycardia and no evidence of structural heart disease. The nature of ischemic heart disease may take various forms including patients with and without a past history of myocardial infarction, angina, congestive heart failure, or left ventricular aneurysm. Coronary artery spasm with normal coronary arteries may cause transient myocardial ischemia with severe ventricular arrhythmias in some patients.[244] In patients resuscitated from sudden cardiac death (Chap. 23) the majority (75 per cent) have severe coronary artery disease and ventricular tachyarrhythmias can be induced by premature ventricular stimulation in approximately 75 per cent.[245,246] When ventricular tachycardia occurs in the ambulatory patient, it is uncommonly induced by R-on-T premature ventricular complexes.[247] Even short runs of ventricular tachycardia consisting of three or four complexes can be important. When detected in the late hospital phase of acute myocardial infarction, ventricular tachycardia identifies a group of patients with a 38 per cent one-year mortality rate compared to 11.6 per cent in a group without tachycardia.[248] Sustained recurrent ventricular tachycardia can also occur in children with or without associated cardiovascular disease.[249,250] In some patients an acute emotional disturbance may be related temporally to the onset of life-threatening ventricular arrhythmias. However, the causal role played by the emotional stress needs to be established.[251]

Termination of a tachycardia by triggering vagal reflexes is considered diagnostic of supraventricular tachycardias. However, ventricular tachycardia uncommonly can be stopped in a similar manner.[1,2] Valsalva may terminate ventricular tachycardia most likely related to an abrupt reduction in cardiac dimension.[252]

TREATMENT. The most important question is deciding which patients should be treated.[252a] The relative risks of symptoms or sudden death for each type of ventricular tachycardia determine the course of therapy. Generally, patients who have sustained ventricular tachycardia with or without structural heart disease and those who have nonsustained ventricular tachycardia with structural heart disease are treated. Patients who have nonsustained ventricular tachycardia without structural heart disease but are symptomatic should be treated while those who are asymptomatic and otherwise healthy may not need therapy but should be followed closely.

Ventricular tachycardia that does not cause hemodynamic decompensation can be treated medically to achieve acute termination by administering lidocaine IV according to the doses indicated on page 657. If lidocaine abolishes the ventricular tachycardia, a continuous IV infusion can be given. If maximum doses of lidocaine are unsuccessful, procainamide or bretylium can be administered IV and, if successful, given as an IV infusion. Although quinidine can be used intravenously, great caution is needed.

If the arrhythmia does not respond to medical therapy, electrical direct-current (DC) cardioversion can be employed. Ventricular tachycardia that precipitates hypotension, shock, angina, or congestive heart failure or symptoms of cerebral hypoperfusion should be treated *promptly* with DC cardioversion (p. 669). Very low energies may terminate ventricular tachycardia, beginning with a synchronized shock of 10 to 50 watt-seconds. Digitalis-induced ventricular tachycardia is best treated pharmacologically. After reversion of the arrhythmia to a normal rhythm, it is essential to institute measures to prevent a recurrence.

Striking the patient's chest, sometimes called "thumpversion," may terminate ventricular tachycardia by mechanically inducing a premature ventricular complex that presumably interrupts the reentrant pathway necessary to support the ventricular tachycardia.[253] Stimulation at the time of the vulnerable period during ventricular tachycardia may accelerate the ventricular tachycardia or possibly provoke ventricular fibrillation.[254]

In patients with recurrent ventricular tachycardia, a pacing catheter can be inserted into the right ventricle and single, double, or multiple stimuli can be introduced competitively to terminate the ventricular tachycardia. This procedure incurs the risk of accelerating the ventricular tachycardia to ventricular flutter or ventricular fibrillation.[240] A new catheter electrode has been developed recently through which synchronized cardioversion can be performed (see Fig. 22–13, p. 759).

Intermittent ventricular tachycardia, interrupted by several supraventricular beats, is generally best treated pharmacologically with lidocaine, quinidine, bretylium, procainamide, or disopyramide. Propranolol or rarely phenytoin may be useful. If these drugs fail, a wide range of investigational antiarrhythmic drugs are available (see Chap. 20).

A search for reversible conditions contributing to the initiation and maintenance of ventricular tachyarrhythmias should be made and the conditions corrected if possible. For example, ventricular arrhythmia related to hypotension or hypokalemia at times may be terminated by vasopressors or potassium, respectively. Slow ventricular rates that are caused by sinus bradycardia or AV block may permit the occurrence of premature ventricular complexes and ventricular tachyarrhythmias that can be corrected by administering atropine, by temporary isoproterenol administration, or by transvenous pacing. (Fig. 22–11, p. 757).

Prevention of recurrences is generally more difficult than is terminating the acute episode. Initial preventive drug therapy for recurrent ventricular arrhythmias in the ambulatory patient should involve quinidine, procainamide, or disopyramide. Propranolol or phenytoin may be tried next, but they are often unsuccessful unless the ventricular tachycardia is related to ischemia, catecholamine stimulation, or digitalis toxicity. Investigational drugs such as amiodarone (p. 666) may be required. Different thresholds for arrhythmic suppression may exist. For example, the serum concentration of procainamide necessary to suppress spontaneous ventricular tachycardia may be lower than the concentration necessary to achieve a significant suppression of premature ventricular complexes.[255] Combinations of drugs with different mechanisms of action may be successful when single drugs fail and allow one to use low doses of both agents rather than high or toxic doses of one drug. Most of the combinations represent empirical trials, but we generally attempt to combine drugs to which the patient has exhibited a partial therapeutic response. A trial of ventricular or atrial pacing, combined with antiarrhythmic agents if necessary, may be tested; if successful, permanent pacing may be instituted (p. 756). Generally, unless the ventricular tachycardia is initiated by significant bradycardia, such as ventricular rates less than 40 due to complete AV block, attempts at rapid "overdrive" pacing are ineffective over the long term.

Surgery may be used to treat ventricular tachycardia in selected patients. A ventriculotomy in patients who have ventricular tachycardia related to right ventricular dysplasia, encircling endocardial ventriculotomy, or endocardial resection directed by electrophysiological mapping techniques in patients who have ventricular tachycardia related to coronary disease may eliminate recurrences or may make previously ineffective drug regimens efficacious. Coronary bypass surgery alone, without electrophysiological mapping and myocardial resection, in patients who do not have ventricular tachycardia definitely associated with ischemia—e.g., ventricular tachycardia induced by stress testing—has not been very successful (p. 672).

Evaluating the effectiveness of therapy in patients with widely spaced episodes of ventricular tachycardia is a difficult problem because there exists no adequate end point to judge therapy until the patient has another spontaneous recurrence. Because of this, aggressive approaches using programmed electrical stimulation have been used, as described on pages 636 to 638.[256,257]

Specific Types of Ventricular Tachycardia

A variety of fairly specific types of ventricular tachycardia have been identified, related either to a constellation of distinctive electrocardiographic and electrophysiological features or to a specific set of clinical events. While our understanding of electrophysiological mechanisms responsible for clinically occurring ventricular tachycardias is still naïve, being able to identify different kinds of ventricular tachycardias is the first step toward understanding their mechanisms.

Accelerated Idioventricular Rhythm

Electrocardiographic Recognition. The ventricular rate, commonly between 60 and 110 beats/min, usually hovers within 10 beats of the sinus rate, so that control of the cardiac rhythm may be passed back and forth between these two competing pacemaker sites. Consequently, fusion beats often occur at the onset and termination of the arrhythmia as the pacemakers vie for control of ventricular depolarization (Fig. 21–37). Because of the slow rate, capture beats are common. The onset of this arrhythmia is generally gradual (nonparoxysmal) and occurs when the rate of the ventricular tachycardia exceeds the sinus rate because of sinus slowing or SA or AV block. The ectopic mechanism may also begin after a premature ventricular complex, or the ectopic ventricular focus may simply accelerate sufficiently to overtake the sinus rhythm. The slow rate and nonparoxysmal onset avoid the problems initiated by excitation during the vulnerable period and, conse-

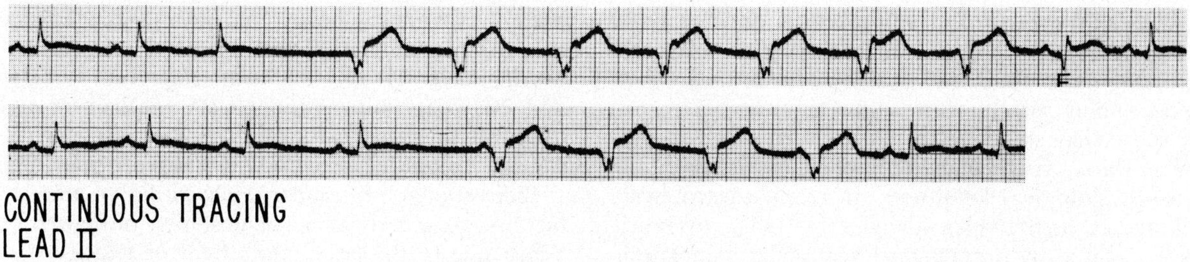

FIGURE 21–37 **Accelerated idioventricular rhythm.** ***Top,*** **A premature atrial complex delays the next sinus initiated P wave and allows escape of an accelerated idioventricular rhythm at a rate of about 70 beats/min. The accelerated idioventricular rhythm is again suppressed when the sinus node resumes control of the cardiac rhythm at the end of the tracing. The next to last QRS complex is a fusion beat (F).** ***Bottom,*** **Progressive sinus bradycardia allows the escape of the accelerated idioventricular rhythm.**

quently, precipitation of more rapid ventricular arrhythmias is rarely seen. Termination of the rhythm generally occurs gradually as the dominant sinus rhythm accelerates or as the ectopic ventricular rhythm decelerates. The ventricular rhythm may be regular or irregular and occasionally may show sudden doubling, suggesting the presence of exit block. Many characteristics suggest enhanced automaticity as the responsible mechanism.

The arrhythmia occurs as a rule in patients who have heart disease, e.g., those with acute myocardial infarction or with digitalis toxicity. It is transient and intermittent, with episodes lasting a few seconds to a minute, and does not appear to affect seriously the course or prognosis of the patient.

Treatment. Suppressive therapy is rarely necessary because the ventricular rate is generally less than 100 beats/min. The following conditions exist during which therapy may be considered: (1) when AV dissociation results in loss of sequential AV contraction and with it the hemodynamic benefits of atrial contribution to ventricular filling; (2) when accelerated idioventricular rhythm occurs together with a more rapid ventricular tachycardia; (3) when accelerated idioventricular rhythm begins with a premature ventricular complex that has a short coupling interval, which causes discharge in the vulnerable period of the preceding T wave; (4) when the ventricular rate is too rapid and produces symptoms; and (5) if ventricular fibrillation develops as a result of the accelerated idioventricular rhythm. This last event appears to be fairly rare.[258] Therapy, when indicated, should be with IV lidocaine, followed by quinidine, bretylium, procainamide, or disopyramide. Often simply increasing the sinus rate with atropine or atrial pacing suppresses the accelerated idioventricular rhythm.[259–261]

Torsades De Pointes

Electrocardiographic Recognition. The term "torsades de pointes" refers to a ventricular tachycardia characterized by QRS complexes of changing amplitude that appear to twist around the isoelectric line and occur at rates of 200 to 250/min (Fig. 21–38*A*). Originally described in the setting of bradycardia due to complete heart block, torsades de pointes connotes a *syndrome*, not simply an ECG description of the QRS complex of the tachycardia.[262,263] Prolonged ventricular repolarization with Q-T intervals exceeding 500 msec occurs as part of the syndrome. The U wave may also become prominent, but its role in this syndrome and in the long Q-T syndrome is not clear. Premature ventricular complexes may discharge during the termination of the T wave, precipitating successive runs of ventricular tachycardia during which the peaks of the QRS complexes appear successively on one side and then on the other of the isoelectric baseline, giving the typical twisting appearance with continuous and progressive

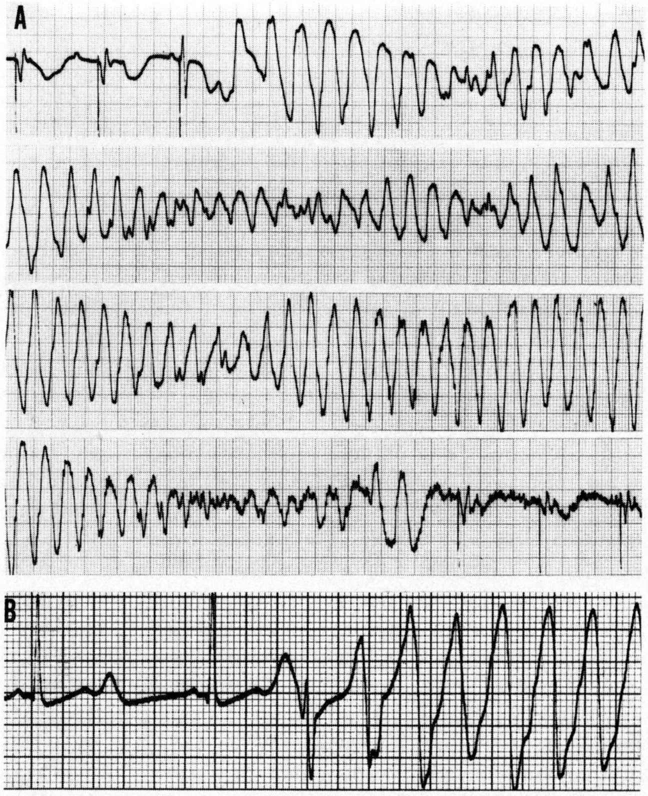

FIGURE 21–38 **Torsades de pointes** ***A,*** **continuous recording monitor lead. A demand ventricular pacemaker (VVI) had been implanted because of type II second-degree AV block. After treatment with amiodarone for recurrent ventricular tachycardia, the Q-T interval became prolonged (about 640 msec during paced beats), and the patient developed episodes of torsades de pointes. In this recording, the tachycardia spontaneously terminates and a paced ventricular rhythm is restored. Motion artifact is noted at the end of the recording as the patient lost consciousness.** ***B,*** **Tracing from a young boy with a congenital long Q-T syndrome. The Q-TU interval in the sinus beats is at least 600 msec. Note TU wave alternans in the first and second complexes. A late premature complex occurring in the downslope of the TU wave initiates an episode of ventricular tachycardia.**

changes in QRS contour and amplitude. The tachycardia may terminate with progressive prolongation of cycle lengths and larger and more distinctly formed QRS complexes, ending with a return to the basal rhythm, a period of ventricular standstill, or a new attack of torsades de pointes. Rarely ventricular fibrillation supervenes.[263]

Electrophysiological Features. In recent electrophysiological studies, arrhythmias similar to torsades depointes have been induced by programmed ventricular stimulation in patients who did not have this ventricular tachycardia spontaneously and in whom the Q-T interval of the sinus beats was normal or only slightly prolonged.[264,265] This pleomorphic ventricular tachycardia occurred without the other distinctive features characteristic of the full syndrome of torsades de pointes. The ventricular tachycardia that occurs spontaneously in the *syndrome* is often difficult to initiate by premature stimulation in patients who have it spontaneously.[266] Electrophysiological mechanisms responsible for torsades de pointes are not well understood and may be due to intraventricular reentry. This explanation appears more probable than the original hypothesis, suggesting the presence of an arrhythmia with two variable opposing foci, although data from one animal study support the latter theory.[267]

Clinical Features. Although many predisposing factors have been cited, the most common are severe bradycardia, potassium depletion, or drugs such as quinidine or disopyramide.[268,269] An imbalance between right and left sympathetic innervations may be important in some patients (see The Long Q-T Syndrome, p. 727).[270] When attacks are prolonged, syncope may result.

Management of ventricular tachycardia with a polymorphic pattern depends on whether or not it occurs in the setting of a prolonged Q-T interval. For this practical reason and because the mechanism of the tachycardia may differ depending on whether or not a long Q-T interval is present, it is important to restrict the definition of torsades de pointes to the typical morphology in the setting of a long Q-T and/or a polymorphic U wave[263] in the basal complexes. In all patients with torsades de pointes, administration of antiarrhythmic agents such as quinidine, disopyramide, and procainamide tends to increase the abnormal Q-T interval and worsen the arrhythmia. Temporary ventricular or atrial pacing should be instituted.[263,271,272] Pacing rapidly suppresses the ventricular tachycardia, which often does not recur even after cessation of pacing. Isoproterenol can be tried until pacing is instituted. The cause of the long Q-T should be determined and corrected if possible. When the Q-T interval is normal, polymorphic ventricular tachycardia *resembling* torsades de pointes is diagnosed, and standard antiarrhythmic drugs may be given. In borderline cases, the clinical context may help determine whether treatment should be initiated with antiarrhythmic drugs. In doubtful cases when the Q-T interval is at upper limits of normal, treatment with pacing is preferable.

Bidirectional Ventricular Tachycardia

This is an uncommon ventricular tachycardia characterized by QRS complexes with a right bundle branch block pattern, alternating polarity in the frontal plane from −60 to −90 degrees to +120 to +130 degrees and a regular rhythm (Fig. 21–39). The ventricular rate is between 140 and 200 beats/min. Although the mechanism and site of origin of this tachycardia has remained somewhat controversial,[273] recent evidence supports a ventricular origin.[274–276]

Bidirectional ventricular tachycardia occurs commonly but not exclusively as a manifestation of digitalis excess.[274] When due to the latter, the extent of toxicity is often advanced, with a poor prognosis. Bidirectional ventricular tachycardia occurs typically in older patients and in those with severe myocardial disease but has been noted in an otherwise asymptomatic 18-year-old with mild hyperkalemic periodic paralysis.[275]

Drugs useful to treat digitalis toxicity such as lidocaine, potassium, phenytoin, and propranolol should be considered if excessive digitalis administration is suspected. Otherwise, the usual therapeutic approach to ventricular tachycardia is recommended (p. 723).

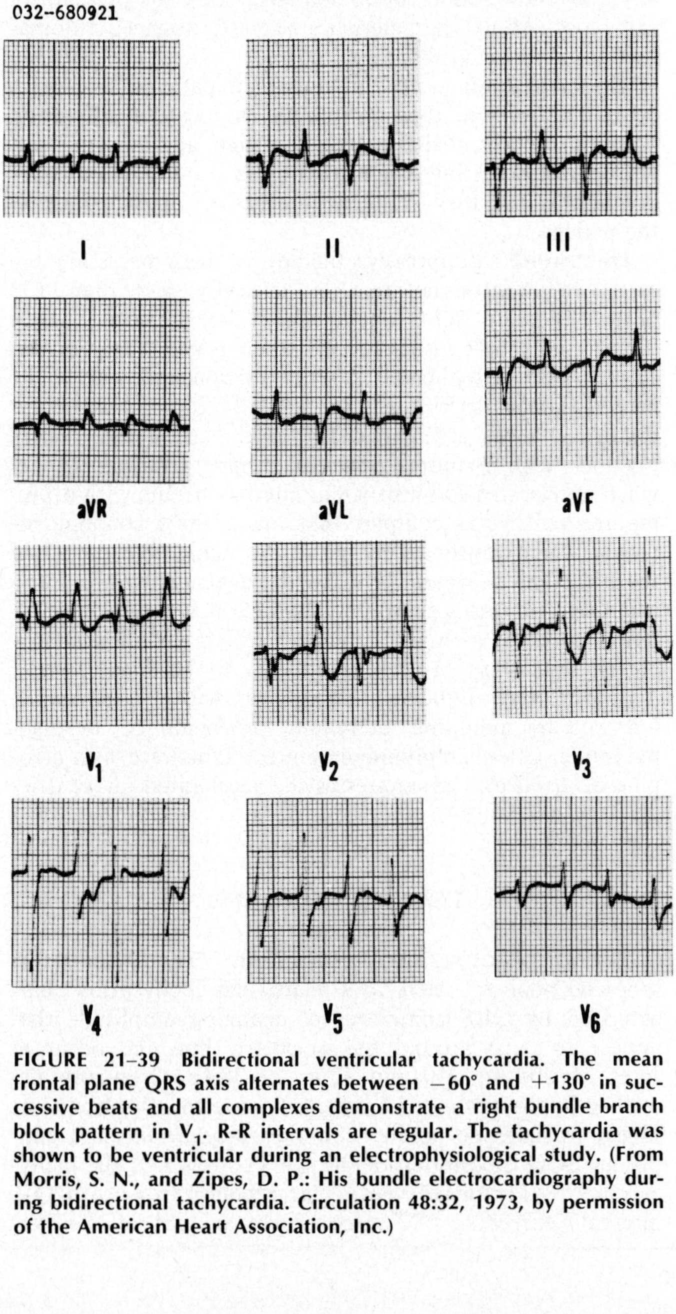

FIGURE 21–39 Bidirectional ventricular tachycardia. The mean frontal plane QRS axis alternates between −60° and +130° in successive beats and all complexes demonstrate a right bundle branch block pattern in V_1. R-R intervals are regular. The tachycardia was shown to be ventricular during an electrophysiological study. (From Morris, S. N., and Zipes, D. P.: His bundle electrocardiography during bidirectional tachycardia. Circulation 48:32, 1973, by permission of the American Heart Association, Inc.)

Repetitive Monomorphic Ventricular Tachycardia

Repetitive monomorphic ventricular tachycardia is defined as three or more consecutive premature ventricular complexes with only brief periods of intervening sinus complexes. Ventricular complexes generally occur in groups of 3 to 15, but occasionally the ventricular tachycardia may be almost continuous. All ventricular complexes have a uniform QRS morphology and interectopic, sinus-conducted complexes have a normal QRS without intraventricular conduction delay or pathologic Q waves (Fig. 21–40). Cycle lengths of the ventricular tachycardia are fairly regular, and the rate ranges between 100 and 150 beats/min, occasionally becoming as rapid as 250 beats/min. Episodes of ventricular tachycardia tend to cluster around certain time periods in an individual patient. Late cycle and variably coupled premature ventricular complexes are common. The tachycardia is difficult to induce with premature ventricular stimulation even though patients may have multiple episodes of spontaneous ventricular tachycardia during the study. Electrophysiological parameters are normal. Abnormal automaticity may be responsible for the tachycardia.[277,277a]

Repetitive monomorphic ventricular tachycardia is often associated with no or minimal structural heart disease and young age and in this setting appears to have an excellent prognosis.[277–281] Arrhythmia-related deaths are reported infrequently.[282] The arrhythmia may disappear with time, perhaps accounting for its reduced prevalence in older populations. The exact prevalence of the tachycardia is difficult to assess, since often it produces no symptoms and may be identified only during routine examination. Of the last 250 patients referred to our hospital for evaluation of ventricular tachycardia, 18 (7 per cent) had this arrhythmia.

When repetitive monomorphic ventricular tachycardia occurs in patients who have normal, sinus-conducted QRS complexes and trivial or no structural heart disease, the ventricular tachycardia appears to be benign and the prognosis favorable. Therapy, as outlined on p. 723, is reserved for patients who are symptomatic from palpitations or have very rapid rates of the ventricular tachycardia.

Bundle Branch Reentrant Tachycardia. Ventricular tachycardia due to bundle branch reentry is characterized by a QRS morphology determined by the circuit established over the bundle branches. Retrograde conduction over the left bundle branch system and anterograde conduction over the right bundle branch will create a QRS complex with a left bundle branch block contour. The frontal plane axis may be about +30 degrees. Electrophysiologically, bundle branch reentrant complexes occur only after a critical S_2-H_2 or S_3-H_3 delay. The H-V interval of the bundle branch reentrant complex equals or exceeds the H-V interval of the spontaneous normally conducted QRS complex.[283,283a]

Although bundle branch reentry has been clearly demonstrated to occur in animals (Fig. 19–27, p. 631) and probably occurs in humans as well, sustained ventricular tachycardia due to bundle branch reentry is a rare event. The long refractory period and rapid conduction velocity of the His-Purkinje system probably prevent sustained circuits of bundle branch reentry from occurring and therefore make it an uncommon mechanism of ventricular tachycardia in man.[283,283a,284]

The therapeutic approach is as for other ventricular tachycardias. Conceivably, creation of bundle branch block might eliminate the tachycardia.

Long Q-T Syndrome (Fig. 21–38*B*)

Electrocardiographic Recognition. The upper limit for the duration of the normal Q-T interval *corrected* for heart rate (Q-Tc) is 0.44 sec. However, it is possible that the formulas used to correct for heart rate, derived from normal subjects not receiving drugs, are not applicable to patients with abnormal repolarization syndromes or after drugs such as quinidine are administered or after myocardial infarction.[285] Nevertheless, delayed repolarization has been defined as a Q-Tc exceeding 0.44 sec or when the Q-TU pattern appears abnormal in configuration. The nature of the U-wave abnormality and its relationship to the long Q-T syndrome are not clear. Notched bifid and sinusoidal T waves may occur.[286]

Clinical Features. Repolarization abnormalities can be divided into two groups: (1) primary or idiopathic, which is a congenital, often familial disorder (p. 1626) that is sometimes,[58] but not always,[287,288] associated with deafness, and (2) an acquired group caused by various drugs like quinidine,[289,290] disopyramide,[291] phenothiazines, or tricyclic antidepressants; metabolic abnormalities such as hypokalemia; the results of the liquid protein diet[292,293]; central nervous system lesions[294]; autonomic nervous system dysfunction[295]; coronary artery disease with myocardial infarction[295–298]; cardiac ganglionitis[299]; and mitral valve prolapse.[300] The autonomic dysfunction may result from a preponderance of left sympathetic tone.[301–304] Probucol, a

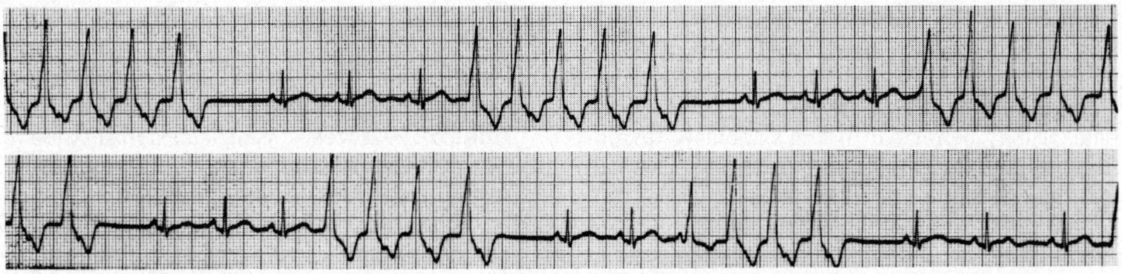

FIGURE 21–40 Repetitive monomorphic ventricular tachycardia. Short episodes of a monomorphic ventricular tachycardia at a rate of 120 to 130 beats/min repeatedly interrupt the normal sinus rhythm. The sinus-initiated QRS complexes are normal in contour with a normal ST segment and T wave.

lipid-lowering agent, has been shown to produce Q-T prolongation and ventricular arrhythmias in dogs and monkeys but not in man.[305]

Symptomatic patients with long Q-T syndrome develop ventricular tachycardias that in many instances are due to torsades de pointes (p. 725). Since sudden death may occur in this group of patients, it is obvious that, in some, the ventricular arrhythmia becomes sustained and probably results in ventricular fibrillation. Patients with congenital long Q-T syndrome who are at increased risk for sudden death include those who have family members who died suddenly at an early age and those who have experienced syncope. Electrocardiograms should be obtained for all family members when the propositus presents with symptoms. Patients should undergo prolonged ECG recording, with various stresses designed to evoke ventricular arrhythmias, such as auditory stimuli,[306] psychological stress,[307] cold pressor stimulation, and exercise. Recently, it has been suggested that the Valsalva maneuver lengthens the Q-T interval and causes T wave alternans and ventricular tachycardia in patients who have prolonged Q-T syndromes with ventricular tachycardia.[308] Catecholamines may be infused in some patients, but this challenge must be performed cautiously, with resuscitative equipment close at hand. Stellate ganglion stimulation and blockade may be useful[304] to provoke or abolish arrhythmias. Premature ventricular stimulation generally does not induce arrhythmias in this syndrome.

Treatment. For patients who have the idiopathic long Q-T syndrome but do not have syncope, complex ventricular arrhythmias, or a family history of sudden cardiac death, no therapy is recommended. In asymptomatic patients with complex ventricular arrhythmias or a family history of premature sudden cardiac death, beta blockers at maximally tolerated doses are recommended. In patients with syncope, beta blockers at maximally tolerated doses, at times combined with phenytoin and phenobarbital, are suggested. For patients who continue to have syncope despite triple drug therapy, left-sided cervicothoracic sympathetic ganglionectomy that interrupts the stellate ganglion and the first three or four thoracic ganglia has been proposed.[286,302]

ARRHYTHMOGENIC RIGHT VENTRICULAR DYSPLASIA

In this infrequently recognized disorder, patients present with ventricular tachycardia that has a left bundle branch block contour, often with right-axis deviation, with T waves inverted over the right precordial leads. Supraventricular arrhythmias may also occur.[309] Premature ventricular stimulation can initiate sustained ventricular tachycardia.

Arrhythmogenic right ventricular dysplasia is a cardiomyopathy with hypokinetic areas involving the wall of the right ventricle. It may be related to Uhl's anomaly (parchment-thin right ventricular wall) in some patients and can be an important cause of ventricular arrhythmias in children and young adults with an apparently normal heart as well as in older patients.[310] Right heart failure or asymptomatic right ventricular enlargement may be present with normal pulmonary vasculature. Males predominate and all patients show an abnormal right ventricle by echo or right ventricular angiography.[309] ECG during sinus rhythm exhibits complete or incomplete right bundle branch block. Although the conventional pharmacological approaches to therapy may be appropriate, surgical manipulations have been successful in some of these patients[309,311–313] (p. 672).

TETRALOGY OF FALLOT

Chronic serious ventricular arrhythmias may occur in patients some years after repair of tetralogy of Fallot. In one series, almost half of 72 patients had serious ventricular arrhythmias within five years after repair, and four patients had experienced cardiac arrest.[314] Sustained ventricular tachycardia after repair may be caused by reentry at the site of previous operation in the right ventricular outflow tract[315] and may be cured by resection of this area.[316]

CATECHOLAMINE-SENSITIVE VENTRICULAR TACHYCARDIA

Some patients may have ventricular tachycardia due to a sensitivity to the effects of catecholamine stimulation.[317] Stress or exercise may exacerbate these ventricular arrhythmias, which can be suppressed with beta blocker therapy.[318]

Ventricular Flutter and Ventricular Fibrillation

Electrocardiographic Recognition. These arrhythmias represent severe derangements of the heart beat that usually terminate fatally within 3 to 5 minutes unless corrective measures are undertaken promptly. Ventricular flutter presents as a sine wave in appearance: regular large oscillations occurring at a rate of 150 to 300/min (usually about 200) (Fig. 21–41*A*). The distinction between rapid ventricular tachycardia and ventricular flutter may be difficult and is usually of academic interest only. Ventricular fibrillation is recognized by the presence of irregular undulations of varying contour and amplitude (Fig. 21–41*B*). Distinct QRS complexes, ST segments, and T waves are absent.

In an animal model of ischemia, ventricular fibrillation begins as an organized rhythm, with activation occurring in an orderly, rapidly repeating sequence at the border of the ischemic reperfused region. Activation then passes through the nonischemic portion of the ventricles as a single organized wavefront to the opposite side of the heart, with the time between successive activation fronts decreasing. However, the time for each activation front to traverse the ventricles increases, resulting in overlapping cycles in which a new activation front arises before the previous front terminates. This produces totally disorganized electrical activity on the scalar ECG at a time when epicardial electrical activity is still fairly organized.[319]

Clinical Features. Ventricular fibrillation occurs in a variety of clinical situations, most commonly associated with coronary artery disease and as a terminal event. It may occur during antiarrhythmic drug administration, hypoxia, ischemia, atrial fibrillation and very rapid ventricular rates in the preexcitation syndrome, after electric shock administered during cardioversion (Fig. 20–6) or accidentally by improperly grounded equipment, and uncom-

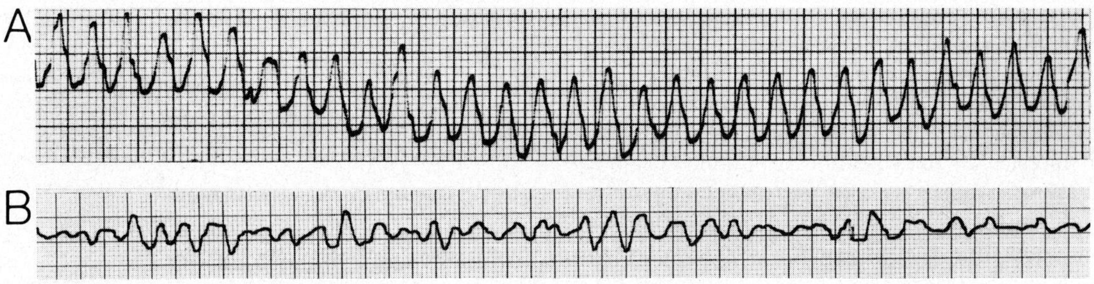

FIGURE 21–41 Ventricular flutter and ventricular fibrillation. ***A,*** **The sine wave appearance of the complexes occurring at a rate of 300 beats/min is characteristic of ventricular flutter.** ***B,*** **The irregular undulating baseline typifies ventricular fibrillation.**

monly during competitive cardiac pacing at slow rates (see Chapter 22). Ventricular flutter or ventricular fibrillation results in faintness, followed by loss of consciousness, seizures, and apnea and eventually, if the rhythm continues untreated, death. The blood pressure is unobtainable and heart sounds are usually absent. The atria may continue to beat as an independent rhythm for a time or in response to impulses from the fibrillating ventricles. Eventually, electrical activity of the heart is completely absent.

In patients resuscitated from out-of-hospital cardiac arrest, all but a few have ventricular fibrillation. A nonarrhythmic cause of sudden cardiac death occurs in only a very small number of patients who have acute myocardial infarction.[320] Although 75 per cent of patients resuscitated from sudden cardiac death have significant coronary artery disease, only 20 to 30 per cent evolve acute myocardial infarction. Those who do not evolve a myocardial infarction have a recurrence rate for ventricular fibrillation of approximately 22 per cent in one year and 40 per cent in two years[321] (p. 793). Patients who have ventricular fibrillation and acute myocardial infarction have a recurrence rate at one year of 2 per cent.

The time from warning arrhythmias to development of ventricular fibrillation is short in many patients. In one series, an R-on-T premature ventricular complex occurred in 33 of 48 patients who developed ventricular fibrillation outside the hospital and, along with an increase in heart rate prior to the onset of ventricular fibrillation, appeared to be the most important initiating factor.[322] Another group at high risk for the development of ventricular fibrillation are patients who suffer an anteroseptal myocardial infarction complicated by right or left bundle branch block.[323]

Treatment (See also pp. 672 and 756). Immediate nonsynchronized DC electrical shock using 200 to 400 joules is mandatory treatment for ventricular fibrillation and for ventricular flutter that has caused loss of consciousness. Cardiopulmonary resuscitation is employed only until defibrillation equipment is readied. Time should not be wasted with cardiopulmonary resuscitation if electrical defibrillation can be done promptly. If the circulation is markedly inadequate despite return to sinus rhythm, closed-chest massage with artificial ventilation as needed should be instituted. The use of anesthesia during electric shock is obviously dictated by the patient's condition and is generally not required. After reversion of the arrhythmia to a normal rhythm, it is essential to monitor the rhythm continuously and to institute measures to prevent a recurrence.

Metabolic acidosis quickly follows cardiovascular collapse, and sodium bicarbonate, 1 to 3 ampoules containing 44 mEq of sodium bicarbonate per ampoule, may be needed initially. Additional ampoules judged by results of frequent blood gas and pH determinations may be given every 5 to 8 minutes until adequate cardiorespiratory function is achieved. If the arrhythmia is terminated within 30 to 60 seconds, significant acidosis does not occur. Also, in this short period of time, artificial ventilation by means of a tightly fitting rubber face mask and an Ambu bag is quite satisfactory and eliminates the delay attending intubation by inexperienced personnel. If such a mask and bag are not available, mouth-to-mouth or mouth-to-nose resuscitation is indicated. It is important to reemphasize that there should be no delay in instituting electrical shock. If the patient is not monitored and it cannot be established whether asystole or ventricular fibrillation caused the cardiovascular collapse, the electric shock should be administered *without* wasting precious seconds attempting to obtain an electrocardiogram. The DC shock may cause the asystolic heart to begin discharging as well as terminate ventricular fibrillation, if the latter is present.

A search for conditions contributing to the initiation of ventricular flutter or fibrillation should be made and the conditions corrected, if possible. A ventricular arrhythmia related to hypotension may at times be terminated by the use of vasopressors. Slow ventricular rates that are due to sinus bradycardia or AV block may permit the occurrence of premature ventricular complexes and ventricular tachyarrhythmias that can be effectively treated by speeding the heart rate. Initial medical approaches to prevent a recurrence of ventricular fibrillation include intravenous administration of lidocaine, bretylium, procainamide, quinidine, or disopyramide. Usually, when ventricular fibrillation occurs, it is irreversible and lethal unless countermeasures are instituted immediately.

HEART BLOCK

Heart block is a disturbance of impulse conduction that may be permanent or transient, owing to anatomical or functional impairment. It must be distinquished from *interference,* a normal phenomenon which is a disturbance of impulse conduction caused by physiological refractoriness due to inexcitability from a preceding impulse. Either interference or block may occur at any site where impulses are conducted, but they are recognized most commonly between the sinus node and atrium (SA block), between the atria and ventricles (AV block), within the atria (intra-atrial block), or within the ventricles (intraventricular block). During AV block, the block may occur in the AV node, His bundle, or bundle branches.[324,325] In some instances of bundle branch block, for example, the impulse may only be delayed and not completely blocked in the bundle branch, yet the resulting QRS complex may be indistinguishable from a QRS complex generated by complete bundle branch block.

The conduction disturbance is classified by severity in three categories. During *first-degree heart block,* conduction time is prolonged but all impulses are conducted. *Second-degree heart block* occurs in two forms: Mobitz type I (Wenckebach) and type II. Type I heart block is characterized by a progressive lengthening of the conduction time until an impulse is not conducted. Type II heart block denotes occasional or repetitive sudden block of conduction of an impulse without prior measurable lengthening of conduction time. When no impulses are conducted, *complete or third-degree block is present.* The degree of block may depend in part on the direction of impulse propagation. For unknown reasons, normal retrograde conduction can occur in the presence of advanced anterograde AV block, for example (see Fig. 7–57, p. 252).[326] The reverse can also occur.

Certain features of type I second-degree block deserve special emphasis because when actual conduction times are not apparent in the electrocardiogram, for example, during SA, junctional, or ventricular exit block (see pp. 251 and 691), type I conduction disturbance may be difficult to recognize. During type I block, the increment in conduction time is greatest in the second beat of the Wenckebach group, and the absolute *increase* in conduction time *decreases* progressively over subsequent beats. These two features serve to establish the characteristics of classic Wenckebach group beating: (1) the interval between successive beats progressively decreases, although the conduction time increases (but by a decreasing function); (2) the duration of the pause produced by the nonconducted impulse is less than twice the interval preceding the blocked impulse (which is usually the shortest interval); and (3) the cycle following the nonconducted beat (beginning the Wenckebach group) is longer than the cycle preceding the blocked impulse. Although much emphasis has been placed on this characteristic grouping of cycles, primarily to be able to diagnose Wenckebach exit block, this typical grouping occurs in less than 50 per cent of patients who have type I Wenckebach AV nodal block.

Differences in cycle-length patterns may result from changes in pacemaker rate (e.g., sinus arrhythmia), in neurogenic control of conduction, and changes in the increment of conduction delay. For example, if the P-R increment in the last cycle increases, the R-R cycle of the last conducted beat may lengthen rather than shorten. In addition, since the last conducted beat is often at a critical state of conduction, it may become blocked, producing a 5:3 or 3:1 conduction ratio instead of a 5:4 or 3:2 ratio. During a 3:2 Wenckebach structure, the cycle following the nonconducted beat will be the same as the cycle preceding the nonconducted beat. Finally, *concealed or manifest reentry* (pp. 247 and 250) may alter the P-R interval during Wenckebach block.[327] As the cardiac cycle length is decreased, the AV nodal effective refractory period normally lengthens in adults and the AV nodal functional refractory period shortens slightly.[328,329] In Wenckebach cycles, a progressive increase in AV nodal effective refractory period results.[330]

Atrioventricular (AV) Block

AV block exists when the atrial impulse is conducted with delay or is not conducted at all to the ventricle at a time when the AV junction is not physiologically refractory.

FIRST-DEGREE AV BLOCK. During first-degree AV block, every atrial impulse conducts to the ventricles, producing a regular ventricular rate, but the P-R interval exceeds 0.20 sec in the adult. P-R intervals as long as 1.0

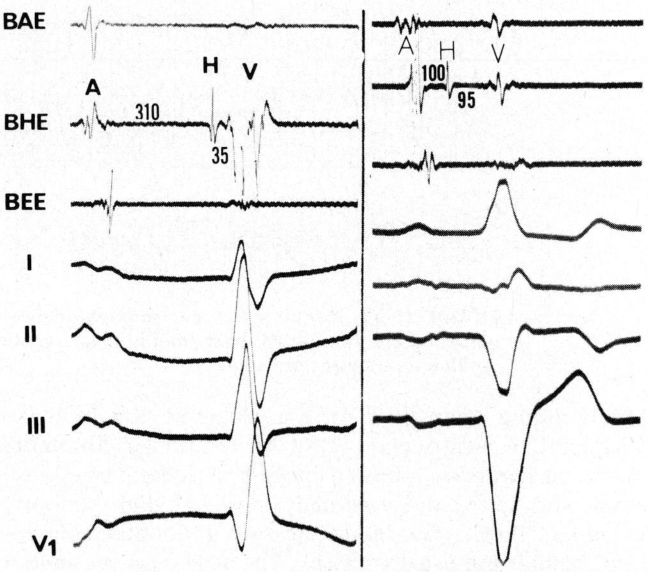

FIGURE 21–42 First-degree AV block. One complex during sinus rhythm is shown. The P-R interval in the left panel measured 370 msec (P-A=25 msec; A-H=310 msec; H-V=35 msec) during a right bundle branch block. Conduction delay in the AV node causes the first-degree AV block. In the panel on the right, the P-R interval is 230 msec (P-A=35 msec; A-H=100 msec; H-V=95 msec) during a left bundle branch block. The conduction delay in the His-Purkinje system causes the first-degree AV block.

sec have been noted and at times may be longer than the P-P interval, a phenomenon known as "skipped" P waves. (Fig. 7–35, p. 227). Clinically important P-R interval prolongation may result from conduction delay in the AV node (A-H interval), in the His-Purkinje system (H-V interval), or at both sites. Equally delayed conduction over both bundle branches uncommonly may produce P-R prolongation without significant QRS complex aberration (Fig. 21–29). Occasionally, intraatrial conduction delay may result in P-R prolongation. If the QRS complex in the scalar ECG is normal in contour and duration, the AV delay almost always resides in the AV node, rarely within the His bundle itself. If the QRS complex shows a bundle branch block pattern, conduction delay may be within the AV node and/or His-Purkinje system (Fig. 21–42). In this latter instance, His bundle electrocardiography is necessary to localize the site of conduction delay. Acceleration of the atrial rate or enhancement of vagal tone by carotid massage may cause first-degree AV nodal block to progress to type I second-degree AV block. Conversely, type I second-

TABLE 21–3 SITE OF SECOND-DEGREE ATRIOVENTRICULAR BLOCK

Type of Block	Normal QRS	BBB
Type I	AVN> > > >HPS	AVN>HPS
Type II	HPS>AVN	HPS> > > >AVN
1:1 → 2:1: fixed 2:1 or greater	HPS=AVN	HPS> >AVN

Except for the location of type I AV block with a normal QRS and type II AV block with a bundle branch block, quantitative data regarding the other sites of block are not available and these statements must be regarded as the author's impressions.

Abbreviations: AVN = atrioventricular node; HPS = His-Purkinje system; BBB = bundle branch block. Arrows > indicate relative frequency of second-degree AV block at different sites, with one arrow meaning slightly more frequent, and four arrows meaning far more frequent.

From Zipes, D. P.: Second-degree atrioventricular block. Circulation *60*:465, 1965, by permission of the American Heart Association, Inc.

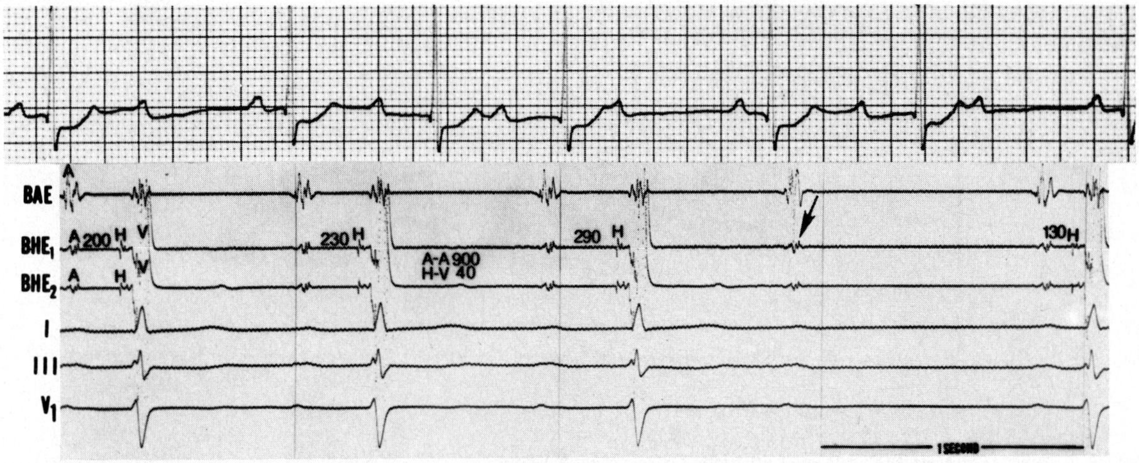

FIGURE 21–43 Type I (Wenckebach) second-degree AV block. In the top strip from a lead II scalar ECG recording, the P-R interval progressively lengthens, and the R-R intervals progressively shorten, culminating in a blocked P wave. The duration of the pause produced by the blocked P wave is less than twice the shortest P-P interval. In the electrophysiological recording shown below, progressive AV nodal conduction delay increases until one P wave (arrow) blocks proximal to the His bundle. The cycle then begins again with marked shortening of the A-H interval to 130 msec. (The first P wave in the electrophysiological recording is not the first P wave of the Wenckebach cycle. Hence, the A-H interval exceeds 130 msec.)

degree AV nodal block may revert to first-degree block with deceleration of the sinus rate.

SECOND-DEGREE AV BLOCK (Table 21–3). Atrial impulses not conducted to the ventricle at a time when physiologic interference is not involved constitutes second-degree AV block. The nonconducted P wave may be intermittent or frequent, at regular or irregular intervals, and may be preceded by fixed or lengthening P-R intervals. A distinguishing feature is that conducted P waves relate to the QRS complex with recurring P-R intervals, i.e., the association of P with QRS is not random. Wenckebach and Hay, by analyzing the *a-c* and *v* waves in the jugular venous pulse, described two types of second-degree AV block. After the introduction of the electrocardiograph, Mobitz classified them as type I and type II.[331] Electrocardiographically, typical type I second-degree AV block is characterized by progressive P-R prolongation culminating in a nonconducted P wave (Fig. 21–43), while in type II second-degree AV block, the P-R interval remains constant prior to the blocked P wave (Fig. 21–44). In both instances the AV block is intermittent and generally repetitive and may block several P waves in a row. Often, the eponyms Mobitz type I and Mobitz type II are applied to the two types of block, while the term "Wenckebach block" refers to type I block only.

Although it has been suggested that type I and type II AV block may be different manifestations of the same electrophysiological mechanism, differing only quantitatively in the size of the increments,[332] clinically separating second-degree AV block into type I and type II serves a useful function and, in most instances, the differentiation can be made easily and reliably from the surface ECG. Type II AV block often antedates the development of Adams-Stokes syncope and complete AV block, while type I AV block with a normal QRS complex is generally more benign and does not progress to more advanced forms of AV conduction disturbance.[333–335]

In the patient with an acute myocardial infarction, type I AV block usually accompanies inferior infarction, is transient, and does not require temporary pacing, whereas type II AV block results in the setting of an acute anterior myocardial infarction, may require temporary or permanent pacing, and is associated with a high rate of mortality, generally due to pump failure[333,336] (p. 1287). A high degree of AV block can occur in patients with acute inferior myocardial infarction and is associated with more myocardial damage and a higher mortality rate compared to those without AV block.[337]

While type I conduction disturbance is ubiquitous and may occur in any tissue in the *in situ* heart, as well as *in vitro,* the site of block for the usual forms of second-degree AV block can be judged with sufficient reliability from the surface ECG to permit clinical decisions without requiring invasive electrophysiological studies in most instances (Table 21–2). Type I AV block with a normal QRS complex almost always takes place at the level of the AV node, proximal to the His bundle.[338] An exception is the uncommon patient with type I intrahisian block.[339] Type II AV block, particularly when it occurs in association with a bundle branch block, is localized to the His-Purkinje system.[338–340] Type I AV block in a patient with a bundle branch block may represent block in the AV node or in the His-Purkinje system.[331,334] Type II AV block in a patient with a normal QRS complex may be due to intrahisian AV block, but the block is likely to be type I AV nodal block, which exhibits small increments in AV conduction time.[341]

The above generalizations encompass the vast majority of patients who present with second-degree AV block. However, certain caveats must be heeded to avoid misdiagnosis because of subtle ECG changes or exceptions:

1. Two:one AV block may be a form of type I or type II AV block (Fig. 21–45). If the QRS complex is normal, the block is more likely to be type I, located in the AV node, and one should search for a transition of the 2:1 block to 3:2 block, during which the P-R interval lengthens in the second cardiac cycle. If a bundle branch block is present, the block may be located either in the AV node or in the His-Purkinje system.
2. AV block may occur simultaneously at two or more levels and may render the distinction between types I and II difficult.

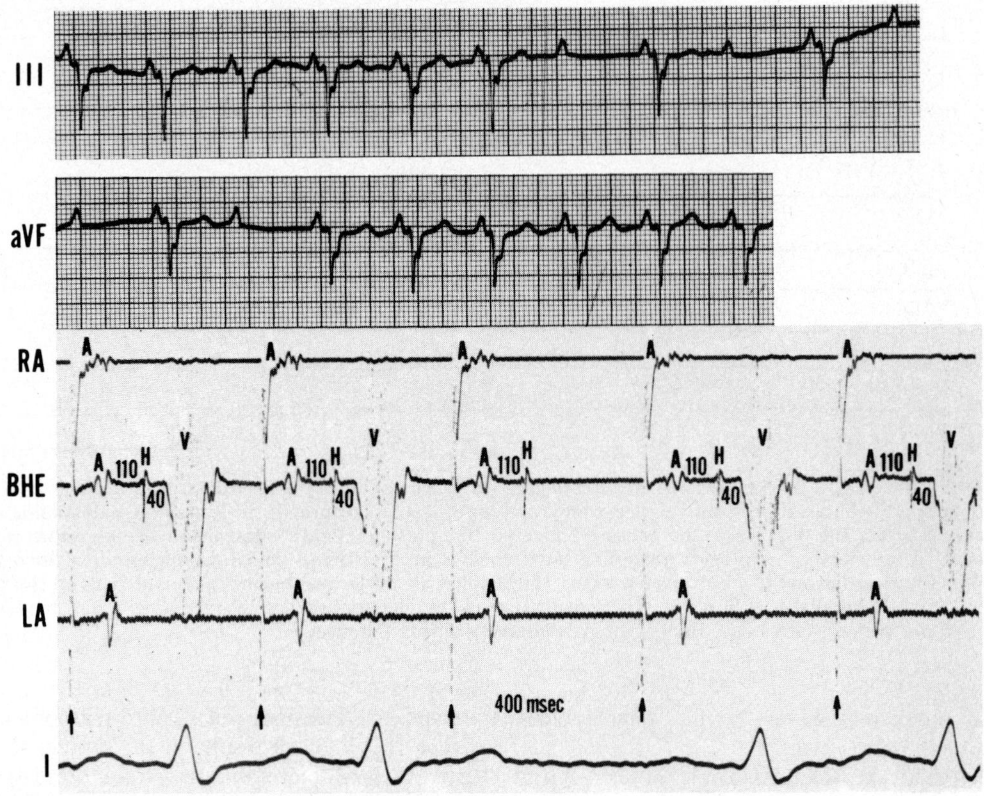

FIGURE 21–44 **Type II second-degree AV block.** ***Top,*** **The surface electrocardiogram illustrates type II AV block in a patient with right bundle branch block and left anterior hemiblock.** ***Bottom,*** **During right atrial pacing at a basic cycle length of 400 msec (pacing spikes indicated by small upright arrows), the A-H and H-V intervals remain constant. Sudden failure of conduction occurs distal to the His bundle recording site following the third P wave.**

3. If the atrial rate varies, it may alter conduction times and cause type I AV block to simulate type II or change type II AV block into type I. For example, if the shortest atrial cycle length that just achieved 1:1 AV nodal conduction at a constant P-R interval is decreased by as little as 10 or 20 msec, the P wave of the shortened cycle may block at the level of the AV node without an apparent increase in the antecedent P-R interval.[342] Apparent type II AV block in the His-Purkinje system may be converted to type I in the His-Purkinje system in some patients by increasing the atrial rate.[331]

4. Concealed premature His depolarizations may create electrocardiographic patterns that simulate type I or type II AV block[343,344] (see Fig. 19–30, p. 635, and Figs. 7–51 and 7–52, pp. 245 and 246).

5. Abrupt, transient alterations in autonomic tone may cause sudden block of one or more P waves without altering the P-R interval of the conducted P wave before or after block.[345] Thus, apparent type II AV block would be produced at the AV node. In the absence of atrial pacing, a burst of vagal tone probably lengthens the P-P interval as well as producing AV block.[346]

6. The response of the AV block to autonomic changes, either spontaneous or induced, to distinguish type I from type II AV block may be misleading. Although vagal stimulation generally increases and vagolytic agents decrease the extent of type I AV block,[347,348] such conclusions are based on the assumption that the intervention acts primarily on the AV node and fail to consider rate changes. For example, atropine may minimally improve conduction in the AV node and markedly increase the heart rate, resulting in an increase in AV conduction time and the degree of AV block as a result of the faster atrial rate. Conversely, if an increase in vagal tone minimally prolongs AV conduction time but greatly slows the heart rate, the net effect on type I AV block may be to improve conduction. In general, however, carotid sinus massage improves and atropine worsens AV conduction in patients with His-Purkinje block, while the opposite results are to be expected in patients who have AV nodal block. These two interventions may help differentiate the site of block without invasive study.[349]

7. During type I AV block with high ratios of conducted beats, the increment in P-R interval may be quite small and simulate type II AV block if only the last few P-R intervals prior to the blocked P wave are measured. By comparing the P-R interval of the first beat in the long Wenckebach cycle with that of the beats immediately preceding the blocked P wave, the increment in AV conduction becomes readily apparent.[350]

8. The classic AV Wenckebach structure depends on a stable atrial rate and a maximal increment in AV conduction time for the second P-R interval of the Wenckebach cycle, with a progressive decrease in subsequent beats. Unstable or unusual alterations in the increment or atrial rate, often seen with long Wenckebach cycles, result in atypical forms of type I AV block in which the last R-R interval may lengthen and are common.[351,352]

9. Finally, it is important to remember that the P-R interval in the scalar ECG is made up of conduction through the atrium, the AV node, and the His-Purkinje system. An increment in HV conduction, for example, can be masked in the scalar ECG by a reduction in the A-H interval, and the resulting P-R interval will not reflect the entire increment in His-Purkinje conduction time.[331] Very long P-R intervals (>200 msec) are more likely to result from AV nodal conduction delay (and block), with or without concomitant His-Purkinje conduction delay.

First-degree and type I second-degree AV block can occur in normal healthy children,[353] and Wenckebach AV block may be a normal phenomenon in well-trained athletes, probably related to an increase in resting vagal tone.[354,355] Occasionally, progressive worsening of the Wenckebach AV conduction disorder may result.[356] In patients who have chronic second-degree AV nodal block (proximal to the His bundle) without organic heart disease, the course is relatively benign, while in those who have organ-

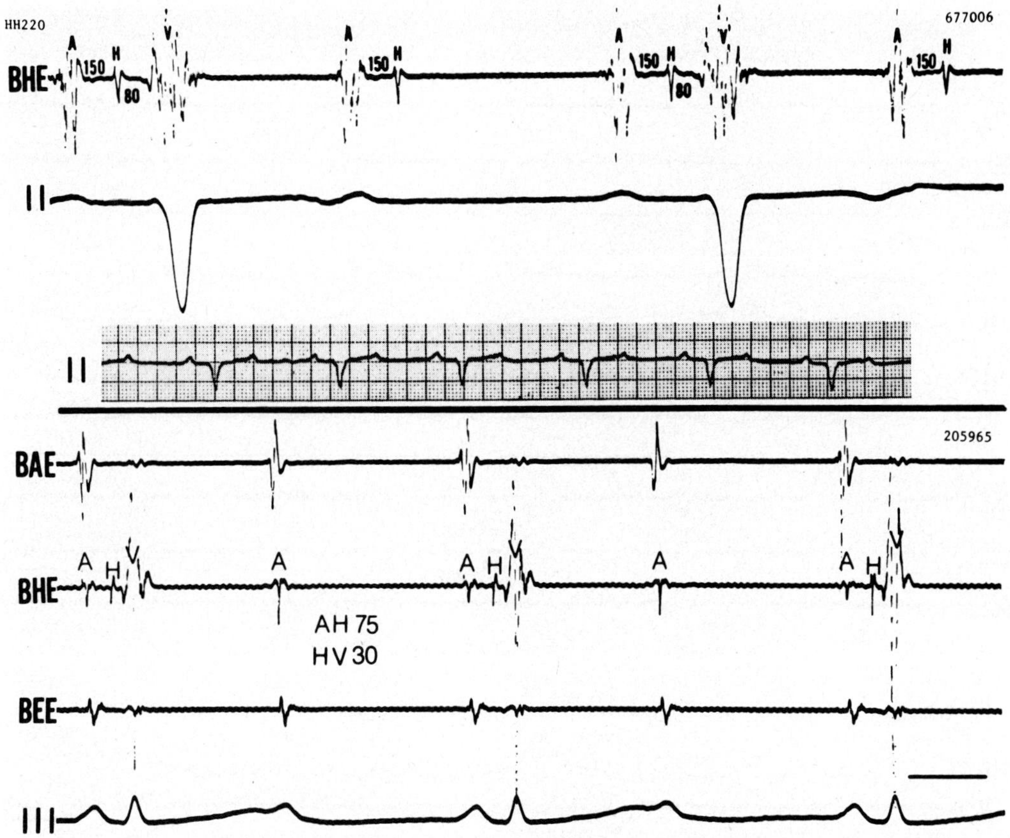

FIGURE 21–45 2:1 AV block proximal and distal to the His bundle deflection in two different patients. *Top,* 2:1 AV block seen in the scalar ECG occurs distal to the His bundle recording site in a patient with right bundle branch block and left anterior hemiblock. The A-H interval (150 msec) and H-V interval (80 msec) are both prolonged. *Bottom,* 2:1 AV block occurs proximal to the bundle of His in a patient with a normal QRS complex. The A-H interval (75 msec) and the H-V interval (30 msec) remain constant and normal.

ic heart disease the prognosis is poor and related to underlying heart disease.[357]

Complete AV Block

Electrocardiographic Recognition. Complete AV block occurs when no atrial activity conducts to the ventricles and therefore the atria and ventricles are controlled by independent pacemakers. Thus, complete AV block is one type of complete AV dissociation (see p. 735). The atrial pacemaker may be sinus or ectopic (tachycardia, flutter, or fibrillation) or may result from an AV junctional focus occurring above the block with retrograde atrial conduction. The ventricular focus is usually located just below the region of block, which may be above or below the His bundle bifurcation. Sites of ventricular pacemaker activity that are in, or closer to, the His bundle appear to be more stable and may produce a faster rate than those located more distally in the ventricular conduction system. The ventricular rate in complete heart block is less than 40 beats/min but may be faster in congenital complete AV block. The ventricular rhythm, usually regular, may vary owing to premature ventricular complexes, a shift in the pacemaker site, an irregularly discharging pacemaker focus, or autonomic influences.

Clinical Features. Complete AV block may result from block at the level of the AV node (usually congenital) (Fig. 21–46), within the bundle of His, or distal to it in the Purkinje system (usually acquired) (Fig. 21–47). The first two types of block generally exhibit normal QRS complexes and rates of 40 to 60 beats/min because the escape focus that controls the ventricle arises in or near the His bundle. In complete AV nodal block, the P wave is not followed by a His deflection, but each ventricular complex is preceded by a His deflection (Fig. 21–46). His bundle electrocardiography may be useful to differentiate AV nodal from intrahisian block, since the latter may carry a more serious prognosis than the former. Intrahisian block is recognized infrequently without invasive studies. In patients with AV nodal block atropine usually speeds both the atrial and the ventricular rate. Isometric exercise may reduce the extent of AV nodal block.[358] Acquired complete AV block occurs most commonly distal to the bundle of His owing to trifascicular conduction disturbance. Each P wave is followed by a His deflection, and the ventricular escape complexes are not preceded by a His deflection (Fig. 21–47). The QRS complex is abnormal and the ventricular rate is usually less than 40 beats/min.

Unusual forms such as paroxysmal AV block[359,360] or AV block following a period of rapid ventricular rate may occur.[361] Paroxysmal AV block in some instances may be due to hyperresponsiveness of the AV node to vagotonic reflexes.[362] Surgery, electrolyte disturbances, endocarditis, tumors, Chagas' disease, rheumatoid nodules, calcific aortic stenosis, myxedema, polymyositis,[363] infiltrative processes (such as amyloid, sarcoid, or scleroderma), and an

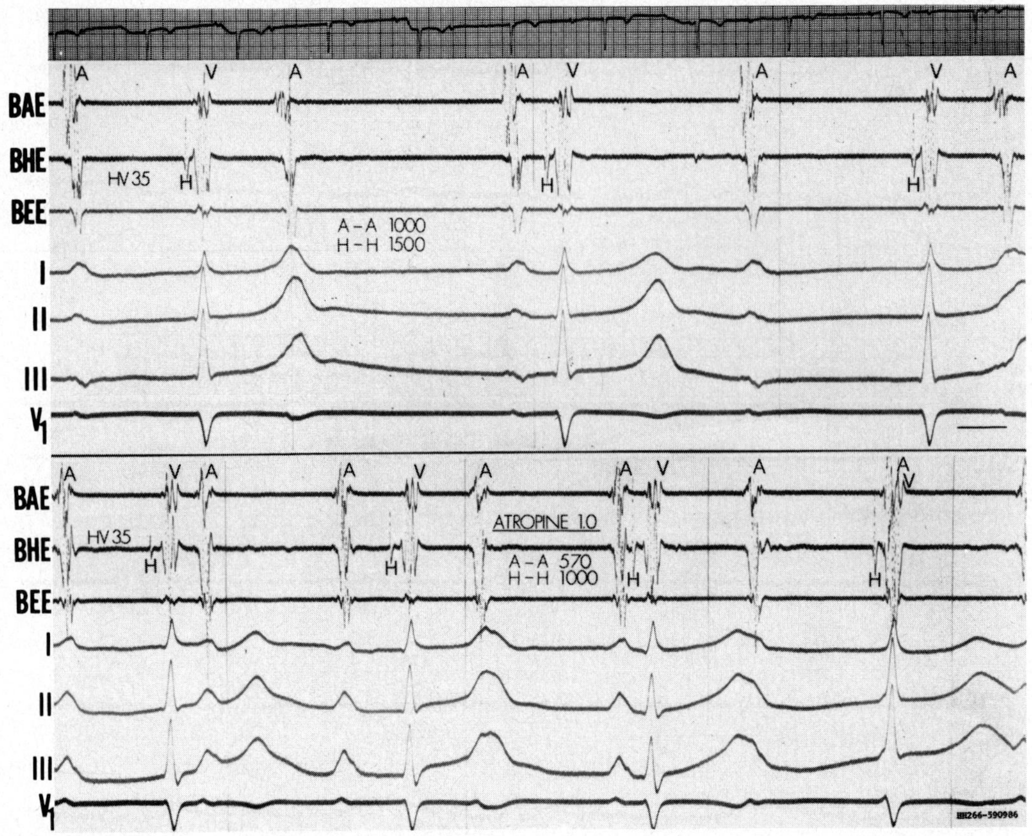

FIGURE 21–46 Congenital complete AV block in a young adult at the level of the AV node. The V_1 surface tracing (*top*) illustrates complete AV block with a normal QRS complex. The top panel of the His bundle recording demonstrates the site of block to be proximal to the His bundle depolarization, at the level of the AV node. The H-V interval is normal (35 msec). The atrial cycles (1000 msec) are completely dissociated from the ventricular cycles (1500 msec). In the bottom panel, after atropine administration (1 mg IV), both the atrial and ventricular rates speed up (A-A interval=570 msec; H-H interval=1000 msec), but complete AV block remains.

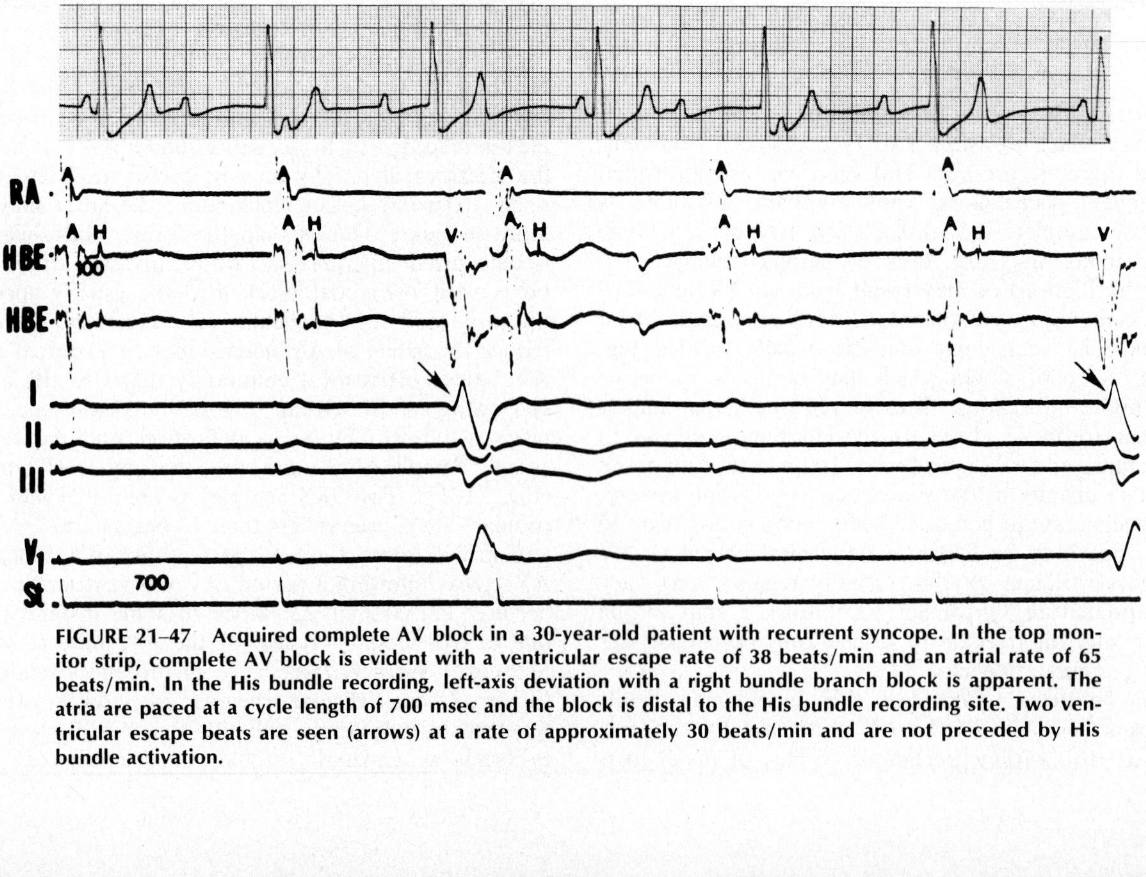

FIGURE 21–47 Acquired complete AV block in a 30-year-old patient with recurrent syncope. In the top monitor strip, complete AV block is evident with a ventricular escape rate of 38 beats/min and an atrial rate of 65 beats/min. In the His bundle recording, left-axis deviation with a right bundle branch block is apparent. The atria are paced at a cycle length of 700 msec and the block is distal to the His bundle recording site. Two ventricular escape beats are seen (arrows) at a rate of approximately 30 beats/min and are not preceded by His bundle activation.

almost endless assortment of common and unusual conditions may produce AV block. In the adult, drug toxicity, coronary disease,[364] and degenerative processes appear to be the most common causes of AV heart block. The degenerative process produces partial or complete anatomical or electrical disruption within the AV nodal region, the AV bundle, or both bundle branches.[365–367]

In children, the most common cause of AV block is congenital (p. 1014). Under such circumstances the AV block may be an isolated finding or associated with other lesions. Children are most often asymptomatic[368]; however, some may develop symptoms that require pacemaker implantation.[369] Mortality from congenital AV block is highest in the neonatal period, is much lower during childhood and adolescence, and increases slowly later in life. Stokes-Adams attacks may occur in patients with congenital heart block at any age. It is difficult to predict the prognosis in the individual patient.[370] A persistent heart rate at rest of 50 beats/min or less correlates with the incidence of syncope, and extreme bradycardia may contribute to the prevalence of Adams-Stokes attacks in children with congenital complete AV block.[371] The site of block may not separate symptomatic children who have congenital or surgically induced complete heart block from those without symptoms. Prolonged recovery times of escape foci following rapid pacing (see discussion of sinus node recovery time, p. 635) and the occurrence of paroxysmal tachycardias may be predisposing factors to the development of symptoms.[372]

Many of the signs of AV block are demonstrated at the bedside. First-degree AV block may be recognized by a long *a-c* wave interval in the jugular venous pulse and by diminished intensity of the first heart sound as the P-R interval lengthens. In type I second-degree AV block, the heart rate may increase imperceptibly with gradually diminished intensity of the first heart sound, widening of the *a-c* interval terminated by a pause, and an *a* wave not followed by a *v* wave. Intermittent ventricular pauses and *a* waves in the neck not followed by *v* waves characterize type II AV block. The first heart sound maintains a constant intensity. In complete AV block, the findings are the same as those in AV dissociation (see below).

Significant clinical manifestations of first- and second-degree AV block are uncommon and usually consist of palpitations or feelings of the heart "missing a beat." Complete AV block may be accompanied by signs and symptoms of reduced cardiac output, syncope or presyncope, angina, or palpitations due to ventricular tachyarrhythmias.

Treatment. As discussed in detail in Chapter 22, drugs cannot be relied on to increase the heart rate for more than several hours to several days in patients with symptomatic heart block without producing significant side effects. Therefore, temporary or permanent pacemaker insertion is indicated in patients with symptomatic bradyarrhythmias.[373,374] For short-term therapy when the block is likely to be evanescent but still requires treatment or until adequate pacing therapy can be established, vagolytic agents such as atropine are useful for patients who have AV nodal disturbances, while catecholamines such as isoproterenol may be used transiently to treat patients who have heart block at any site (see treatment for Sinus Bradycardia, above). Isoproterenol should be used with extreme caution or not at all in patients who have acute myocardial infarction.

ATRIOVENTRICULAR (AV) DISSOCIATION

(See also pp. 249 and 250)

As the term indicates, dissociated or independent beating of atria and ventricles defines AV dissociation. Pick,[375] proposing a comprehensive classification and consistent terminology, emphasized that AV dissociation is never a *primary* disturbance of rhythm but is a "symptom" of an underlying rhythm disturbance produced by one of three causes or a combination of causes (Fig. 21–48), that pre-

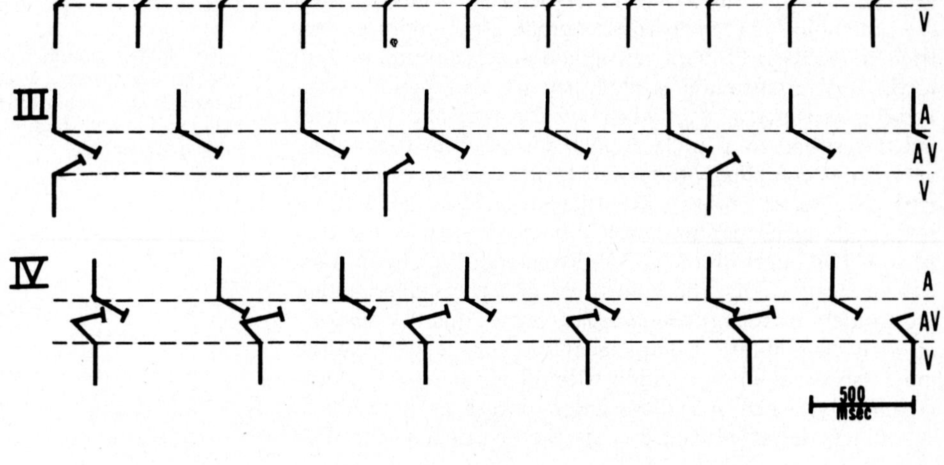

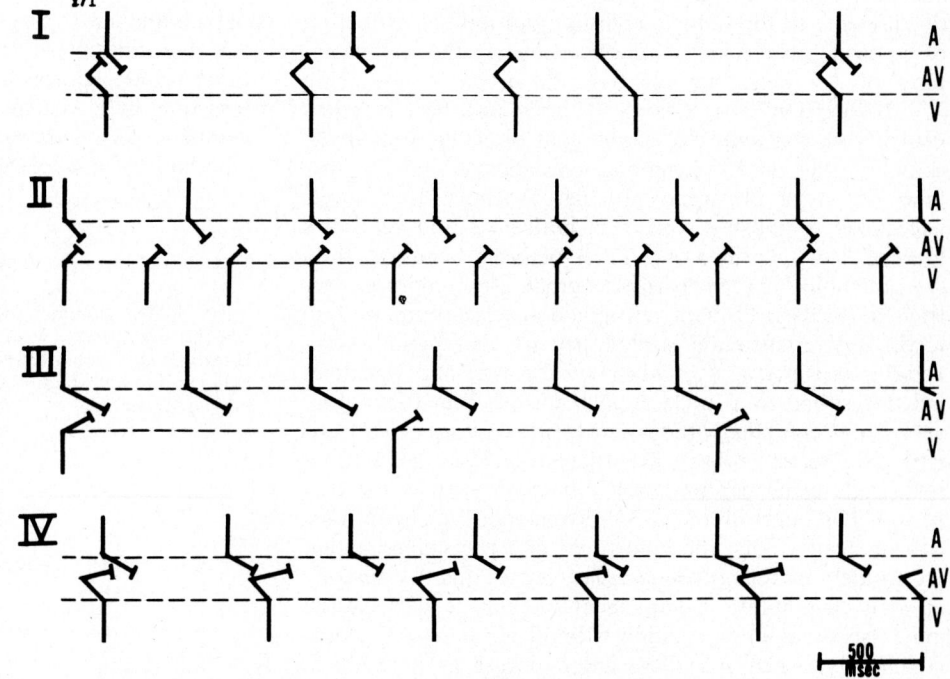

FIGURE 21–48 Diagrammatic illustration of the causes of AV dissociation. A sinus bradycardia that allows the escape of an AV junctional rhythm which does not capture the atria retrogradely illustrates cause I (top panel). Intermittent sinus captures occur (third P wave) to produce incomplete AV dissociation (see Fig. 21–2*B*, p. 689). For cause II, a ventricular tachycardia without retrograde atrial capture produces complete AV dissociation (see Fig. 21–20, p. 706 and 21–35, p. 721). As the third cause, complete AV block with a ventricular escape rhythm is diagrammed (see Figs. 21–46 and 21–47, p. 734). The combination of causes II and III is shown in panel IV, representing a nonparoxysmal AV junctional tachycardia and some degree of AV block.

vent the normal transmission of impulses from atrium to ventricle, as follows:

1. Slowing of the dominant pacemaker of the heart (usually the sinus node), which allows escape of a subsidiary or latent pacemaker. AV dissociation by *default* of the primary pacemaker to a subsidiary one in this manner is often a normal phenomenon. It may occur during sinus arrhythmia or sinus bradycardia, permitting an independent AV junctional rhythm to arise (see Fig. 21–2, p. 689).

2. Acceleration of a latent pacemaker that *usurps* control of the ventricles. Abnormally enhanced discharge rate of a usually slower subsidiary pacemaker is pathological and commonly occurs during nonparoxysmal AV junctional tachycardia or ventricular tachycardia without retrograde atrial capture (see Figs. 21–20 and 21–35, pp. 706 and 721).

3. Block, generally at the AV junction, that prevents impulses formed at a normal rate in a dominant pacemaker from reaching the ventricles and allows the ventricles to beat under the control of a subsidiary pacemaker. Junctional or ventricular escape rhythm during AV block, without retrograde atrial capture, are common examples in which block gives rise to AV dissociation. It is important to remember that complete AV block is *not* synonymous with complete AV dissociation: patients who have complete AV block have complete AV dissociation, but patients who have complete AV dissociation may or may not have complete AV block (Figs. 21–46 and 21–47).

4. A combination of causes may exist, for example, when digitalis excess results in the production of a nonparoxysmal AV junctional tachycardia associated with SA or AV block.[109]

With this classification in mind, it is important to emphasize that the term "AV dissociation" is *not* a diagnosis and is analogous to the terms "jaundice" or "fever." One must state that "AV dissociation is present *due to* . . ." and then give the cause. The accelerated rate of a slower, normally subsidiary pacemaker or the slowed rate of a faster, normally dominant pacemaker that prevents conduction due to physiologic collision and mutual extinction of opposing wavefronts (interference), or the manifestations of AV block are the basic disturbances producing AV dissociation. The atria in all these cases beat independently from the ventricles, under control of the sinus node, ectopic atrial, or AV junctional pacemakers, and may exhibit any type of supraventricular rhythms. If a single pacemaker establishes control of both atria and ventricles for one beat (capture) or a series of beats (sinus rhythm, AV junctional rhythm with retrograde atrial capture, ventricular tachycardia with retrograde atrial capture, and so forth), AV dissociation is abolished for that period. Conversely, as stated above, whenever the atria and ventricles fail to respond to a single impulse for one beat (premature ventricular complex without retrograde capture of the atrium) or a series of beats (ventricular tachycardia without retrograde atrial capture), AV dissociation exists for that period. The interruption of AV dissociation by one or a series of beats under the control of one pacemaker, either antegradely or retrogradely, indicates that the AV dissociation is incomplete. Complete or incomplete dissociation may also occur in association with all forms of AV block. Commonly, when AV dissociation occurs as a result of AV block the atrial rate exceeds the ventricular rate. For example, a subsidiary pacemaker with a rate of 40 beats/min may escape in the presence of a 2:1 AV block when the atrial rate is 78. If the AV block is bidirectional, AV dissociation results.

ELECTROCARDIOGRAPHIC AND CLINICAL FEATURES. The electrocardiogram demonstrates the independence of P waves and QRS complexes. The P-wave morphology depends on the rhythm controlling the atria (sinus, atrial tachycardia, junctional, flutter, or fibrillation). During complete AV dissociation both the QRS complex and the P waves appear regularly spaced without a fixed temporal relationship to each other. When the dissociation is incomplete, a QRS complex of supraventricular contour occurs early and is preceded by a P wave at a P-R interval exceeding 0.12 seconds and within a conductable range. This indicates ventricular capture by the supraventricular focus. Similarly, a premature P wave with a retrograde morphology and a conductable R-P interval may indicate retrograde atrial capture by the subsidiary focus.

The physical findings include a variable intensity of the first heart sound as the P-R interval changes, atrial sounds, and *a* waves in the jugular venous pulse lacking a consistent relationship to ventricular contraction. Intermittent large (cannon) *a* waves may be seen in the jugular venous pulse when atrial and ventricular contraction occur simultaneously. The second heart sound may split normally or paradoxically, depending on the manner of ventricular activation. A premature beat representing a ventricular capture may interrupt a regular heart rhythm. When the ventricular rate exceeds the atrial rate, a cyclic increase in intensity of the first heart sound is produced as the P-R interval shortens, climaxed by a very loud sound (bruit de canon). This intense sound is followed by a sudden reduction in intensity of the first heart sound and the appearance of giant *a* waves as the P-R interval shortens and P waves "march through" the cardiac cycle.

TREATMENT. Treatment is directed toward the underlying heart disease and precipitating cause. The individual components *producing the AV dissociation*—not the AV dissociation per se—determine the specific type of antiarrhythmic approaches. Therapy ranges from pacemaker insertion in a patient who has AV dissociation due to complete AV block to lidocaine administration in a patient who has AV dissociation due to a ventricular tachycardia.

Acknowledgments

The author gratefully acknowledges the thoughtful comments of Eric N. Prystowsky, M.D., and James J. Heger, M.D.; also Kevin Brown, M.D., Donald Chilson, M.D., Elwyn Lloyd, M.D., William Miles, M.D., and Brian Skale, M.D. Lee Northcutt and Shirley Myers provided secretarial help.

References

1. Waxman, M. B., and Wald, R.: Termination of ventricular tachycardia by an increase in cardiac vagal drive. Circulation *56*:385, 1977.
2. Hess, D. S., Hanlon, T., Scheinman, M., Budge, R., and Desai, J.: Termination of ventricular tachycardia by carotid sinus massage. Circulation *65*:627, 1982.
3. Beal, M. F., Park, T. S., and Fisher, C. M.: Cerebral atheromatous embolism following carotid sinus pressure. Arch. Neurol. *38*:310, 1981.

4. Zipes, D. P., and DeJoseph, R. L.: Dissimilar atrial rhythms in man and dog. Am. J. Cardiol. *32*:618, 1973.
5. Jenkins, J. M., Wu, D., and Arzbacher, R. C.: Computer diagnosis of supraventricular and ventricular arrhythmias. A new esophageal technique. Circulation *60*:977, 1979.
6. Prystowsky, E. N., Pritchett, E. L. C., and Gallagher, J. J.: Origin of the atrial electrogram recorded from the esophagus. Circulation *61*:1017, 1980.
7. Barold, S. S.: Filtered bipolar esophageal electrocardiography. Am. Heart J. *83*: 431, 1972.
8. Hammill, S. C., and Pritchett, E. L.: Simplified esophageal electrocardiography using bipolar recording leads. Ann. Intern. Med. *95*:14, 1981.
9. Gallagher, J. J., Smith, W. M., Kerr, C. R., Kasell, J., Cook, L., Reiter, M., Sterba, R., and Harte, M.: Esophageal pacing: A diagnostic and therapeutic tool. Circulation *65*:336, 1982.
10. Hung, J., Kelly, D. T., Hutton, B. F., Uther, J. B., and Baird, D. K.: Influence of heart rate and atrial transport on left ventricular volume and function: Relation to hemodynamic changes produced by supraventricular arrhythmia. Am. J. Cardiol. *48*:632, 1981.
11. Levy, M. N., and Martin, P. J.: Neural control of the heart. *In* Berne, R. M., et al. (eds.): Handbook of Physiology, The Cardiovascular System. Vol. I. Bethesda, Md., American Physiological Society, 1979, p. 581.
12. Jalife, J., and Moe, G. K.: Phasic effects of vagal stimulation on pacemaker activity of the isolated sinus node of the young cat. Circ. Res. *45*:595, 1979.
13. Sheffield, L. T., Holt, J. H., and Reeves, T. J.: Exercise graded by heart rate in electrocardiographic testing for angina pectoris. Circulation *32*:622, 1965.
14. Bauernfeind, R. A., Amat-y-Leon, F., Dhingra, R. C., Kehoe, R., Wyndham, C., and Rosen, K. M.: Chronic nonparoxysmal sinus tachycardia in otherwise healthy persons. Ann. Intern. Med. *91*:702, 1979.
15. Brodsky, M., Wu, D., Denes, P., Kanakis, C., and Rosen, K. M.: Arrhythmias documented by 24-hour continuous electrocardiographic monitoring in 50 male medical students without apparent heart disease. Am. J. Cardiol. *39*:390, 1977.
16. Scott, O., Williams, G. J., and Fiddler, G. I.: Results of 24-hour ambulatory monitoring of electrocardiogram in 131 healthy boys age 10 to 13 years. Br. Heart J. *44*:304, 1980.
17. Adgey, A. A. J., Geddes, J. S., Mulholland, H. C., Keegan, D. A. J., and Pantridge, J. F.: Incidence, significance and management of early bradyarrhythmia complicating acute myocardial infarction. Lancet *2*:1097, 1968.
18. Norris, R. M., Mercer, C. J., and Yeates, S. E.: Sinus rate in acute myocardial infarction. Br. Heart J. *34*:901, 1972.
19. Goldberg, S., Greenspon, A. J., Urban, P. L., Muza, B., Berger, B., Walinsky, P., Maroko, P. R.: Reperfusion arrhythmia: A marker of restoration of antegrade flow during intracoronary thrombolysis for acute myocardial infarction. Am. Heart J. *105*:26, 1983.
20. Weiss, A. T., Rod, J. L., Gotsman, M. S., and Lewis, B. S.: Hydralazine in the management of symptomatic sinus bradycardia. Eur. J. Cardiol. *12*:261, 1981.
21. Walter, P. F., Crawley, I. S., and Dorney, E. R.: Carotid sinus hypersensitivity and syncope. Am. J. Cardiol. *42*:396, 1978.
22. Merx, W., Effert, S., Hanrath, P., Pop, T., Rehder, W., and Schweizer, P.: Hyperactive carotid sinus reflex. Dtsch. Med. Wnschr. *106*:135, 1981.
23. Davies, A. B., Stephens, M. R., and Davies, A. G.: Carotid sinus hypersensitivity in patients presenting with syncope. Br. Heart J. *42*:583, 1979.
24. Brown, K. A., Maloney, J. D., Smith, C. H., Hartzler, G. O., and Ilstup, D. M.: Carotid sinus reflex in patients undergoing coronary angiography: Relationship of degree and location of coronary artery disease in response to carotid sinus massage. Circulation *62*:697, 1980.
25. Wenger, T. L., Dohrmann, M. L., Strauss, H. C., Conley, M. J., Wechsler, A. S., and Wagner, G. S.: Hypersensitive carotid sinus syndrome manifested as cough syncope. PACE *3*:332, 1980.
26. Thorman, J., Neuss, H., Schlepper, M., and Mitrovic, V.: Effects of clonidine on sinus node function in man. Chest *80*:201, 1981.
27. Pick, A., and Langendorf, R.: Interpretation of Complex Arrhythmias. Philadelphia, Lea and Febiger, 1979, p. 127.
28. Lown, B.: Electrical reversion of cardiac arrhythmias. Br. Heart J. *29*:469, 1967.
29. Zipes, D. P., Wallace, A. G., Sealy, W. C., and Floyd, W. L.: Artificial atrial and ventricular pacing in the treatment of arrhythmias. Ann. Intern. Med. *70*: 885, 1969.
30. Short, D. S.: The syndrome of alternating bradycardia and tachycardia. Br. Heart J. *16*:208, 1954.
31. Narula, O. S.: Atrioventricular conduction disturbances in patients with sinus bradycardia. Circulation *44*:1096, 1971.
32. Jordan, J. A., Yamaguchi, I., and Mandel, W. J.: Studies on the mechanisms of sinus node dysfunction in a sick sinus syndrome. Circulation *57*:217, 1978.
33. Kang, P. S., Gomes, J. A., Kelen, G., and El-Sherif, N.: Role of autonomic regulatory mechanism in sinoatrial conduction and sinus nodal automaticity in sick sinus syndrome. Circulation *64*:832, 1981.
34. Desae, J. M., Scheinman, M. M., Strauss, H. C., Massie, B., and O'Young, J.: Electrophysiologic effects of combined autonomic blockade in patients with sinus node disease. Circulation *63*:953, 1981.
35. Scheinmann, M. M., Strauss, H. C., Abbott, J. A., Evans, G. T., Peters, R. W., Benditt, D. G., and Wallace, A. G.: Electrophysiologic testing in patients with sinus pauses and/or sinoatrial exit block. Eur. J. Cardiol. *8*:51, 1978.
36. Simonsen, E., Nielsen, J. S., and Nielsen, B. L.: Sinus node dysfunction in 128 patients. A retrospective study with followup. Acta Med. Scand. *208*:343, 1980.
37. Yabek, S. M., Swensson, R. E., and Jarmakani, J. M.: Electrocardiographic recognition of sinus node dysfunction in children and young adults. Circulation *56*:235, 1977.
38. Mackintosh, A. F.: Sinoatrial disease in young people. Br. Heart J. *45*:62, 1981.
39. Rasmussen, V., Haunso, S., and Skagen, K.: Cerebral attacks due to excessive vagal tone in heavily trained persons. A clinical and electrophysiologic study. Acta Med. Scand. *204*:401, 1978.
39a. Kerr, C. R., Gant, A. O., Wenger, T. L., and Strauss, H. C.: Sinus node dysfunction. Cardiol. Clin. (*in press*).
40. Rosen, K. M., Loeb, H. S., Sinno, M. Z., Rahimtoola, S. H., and Gunnar, R.: Cardiac conduction in patients with symptomatic sinus node disease. Circulation *43*:836, 1971.
41. DeMoulin, J. C., and Kulbertus, H. E.: Histopathological correlates of sinoatrial disease. Br. Heart J. *40*:1384, 1978.
42. Bharati, S., Nordenberg, A., Bauernfeind, R., Varghese, J. P., Carvalho, A. G., Rosen, K. M., and Lev, M.: The anatomic substrate for the sick sinus syndrome in adolescents. Am. J. Cardiol. *46*:163, 1980.
43. Thery, C., Gosselin, B., Lekieffre, J., and Warembourg, H.: Pathology of the sinoatrial node. Correlation with electrocardiographic findings in 111 patients. Am. Heart J. *93*:735, 1977.
44. Gomes, J. A., Kang, P. S., and El-Sherif, N.: Effects of digitalis on the human sick sinus node after pharmacologic autonomic blockade. Am. J. Cardiol. *48*: 783, 1981.
45. Dhingra, R. C., Amat-y-Leon, F., Wyndham, C., Deedwania, P. C., Wu, D., Denes, P., and Rosen, K. M.: Clinical significance of prolonged sinoatrial conduction time. Circulation *55*:8, 1977.
46. Paulay, K. L., Varghese, P. J., and Damato, A. N.: Atrial rhythms in response to an early atrial premature depolarization in man. Am. Heart J. *85*:323, 1973.
47. Curry, P. V. L., Evans, T. R., and Krikler, D. M.: Paroxysmal reciprocating sinus tachycardia. Eur. J. Cardiol. *6*:199, 1977.
48. Narula, O. S.: Sinus node reentry. A mechanism for supraventricular tachycardia. Circulation *50*:1114, 1974.
49. Wu, D., Amat-y-Leon, F., Denes, P., Dhingra, R. C., Pietras, R. J., and Rosen, K. M.: Demonstration of sustained sinus and atrial reentry as a mechanism of paroxysmal supraventricular tachycardia. Circulation *51*:234, 1975.
50. Weisfogel, G. M., Batsford, W. P., Paulay, K. L., Josephson, M. E., Ogunkelu, J. B., Akhtar, M., Seides, S. F., and Damato, A. N.: Sinus node reentrant tachycardia in man. Am. Heart J. *90*:295, 1975.
51. Fauchier, J. P., Latour, F., Neel, C., Charbonnier, B., and Brochier, M.: Paroxysmal sinoatrial tachycardia. Arch. Mal Coeur *73*:165, 1980.
52. Pick, A., Langendorf, R., and Katz, L. N.: Depression of cardiac pacemakers by premature impulses. Am. Heart J. *41*:49, 1951.
53. Langendorf, R., and Mintz, S. S.: Premature systoles originating in the sinoauricular node. Br. Heart J. *8*:178, 1946.
54. Zipes, D. P., Foster, P. R., Troup, P. J., and Pedersen, D. H.: Atrial induction of ventricular tachycardia: Reentry or triggered automaticity. Am. J. Cardiol. *44*:1, 1979.
55. El-Sherif, N., Myerburg, R. J., Scherlag, B. J., Befeler, B., Aranda, J. M., Castellanos, A., Jr., and Lazzara, R.: Electrocardiographic antecedents of primary ventricular fibrillation. Br. Heart J. *38*:415, 1976.
56. Myerburg, R. J., Sung, R. J., Gerstenblith, G., Mallon, S. M., Castellanos, A., Jr., and Lazzara, R.: Ventricular ectopic activity after premature atrial beats in acute myocardial infarction. Br. Heart J. *39*:1033, 1977.
57. Sakamoto, T., Yamada, T., and Hiejima, K.: Ventricular fibrillation induced by conducted sinus or supraventricular beat. Circulation *48*:438, 1973.
58. Jervell, A., and Lange-Nielsen, F.: Congenital deaf-mutism, functional heart disease with prolongation of the QT interval and sudden death. Am. Heart J. *54*:59, 1957.
59. Wellens, H. J. J., Bär, F. W., Farre, J., Ross, D. L., Wiener, I., and Vanagt, E. J.: Initiation and termination of ventricular tachycardia by supraventricular stimuli. Am. J. Cardiol. *46*:576, 1980.
60. Robertson, C. E., and Miller, H. C.: Extreme tachycardia complicating the use of disopyramide in atrial flutter. Br. Heart J. *44*:602, 1980.
61. Jackman, W. M., Prystowsky, E. N., Naccarelli, G. V., Heger, J. J., and Zipes, D. P.: Reevaluation of enhanced AV nodal conduction: Evidence to suggest a continuum of normal nodal physiology. Circulation *67*:441, 1983.
62. Moleiro, F., Mendoza, I. J., Medina-Ravell, V., Castellanos, A., and Myerburg, R. J.: One to one atrioventricular conduction during atrial pacing at rates of 300/min in absence of Wolff-Parkinson-White syndrome. Am. J. Cardiol. *48*:789, 1981.
63. Besoain-Santander, M., Pick, A., and Langendorf, R.: AV conduction in auricular flutter. Circulation *2*:604, 1950.
64. Ashman, R., and Hull, H.: Essentials of Electrocardiography. New York, Macmillan Co., 1947, p. 203.
65. Langendorf, R.: Concealed AV conduction: The effect of blocked impulses on the formation and conduction of subsequent impulses. Am. Heart J. *35*:542, 1948.
66. Suarez, L. D., Kretz, A., Alvarez, J. A., Martinez, J. A., and Perosio, A. M.: Dissimilar atrial rhythms. A patient with triple right atrial rhythm. Am. Heart J. *100*:678, 1980.
67. Gomes, J. A., Kang, P. S., Matheson, M., Gough, W. B., Jr., and El-Sherif, N.: Coexistence of sick sinus rhythm and atrial flutter-fibrillation. Circulation *63*:80, 1981.
68. Simpson, R. J., Foster, J. R., and Gettes, L. S.: Atrial excitability and conduction in patients with interatrial conduction defects. Am. J. Cardiol. *50*:1331, 1982.

69. Anderson, K. J., Simmons, S. C., and Hallidie-Smith, K. A.: Fetal cardiac arrhythmia: Antepartum diagnosis of a case of congenital atrial flutter. Arch. Dis. Child. *56*:472, 1981.
70. Waldo, A. L., MacLean, W. H., Karp, R. B., Kouchoukos, N. T., and James, T. N.: Entrainment and interruption of atrial flutter with atrial pacing. Studies in man following open heart surgery. Circulation *56*:737, 1977.
71. Camm, J., Ward, D., and Spurrell, R.: Response of atrial flutter to overdrive atrial pacing and intravenous disopyramide phosphate, singly and in combination. Br. Heart J. *44*:240, 1980.
72. Zipes, D. P.: The contribution of artificial pacemaking to understanding the pathogenesis of arrhythmias. Am. J. Cardiol. *28*:211, 1971.
73. Wells, J. L., MacLean, W. A. H., James, T. N., and Waldo, A. L.: Characterization of atrial flutter. Studies in man after open heart surgery using fixed atrial electrodes. Circulation *60*:665, 1979.
74. Waxman, H. L., Myerburg, R. J., Appel, R., and Sung, R. J.: Verapamil for control of ventricular rate in paroxysmal supraventricular tachycardia and atrial fibrillation or flutter: A double-blind randomized cross-over study. Ann. Intern. Med. *94*:1, 1981.
75. Pritchett, E. L., Smith, W. M., Klein, G. J., Hammill, S. C., and Gallagher, J. J.: The "compensatory pause" of atrial fibrillation. Circulation *62*:1021, 1980.
76. Rowland, E., Curry, P., Fox, K., and Krikler, E. R.: Relation between atrioventricular pathways and ventricular response during atrial fibrillation and flutter. Br. Heart J. *45*:83, 1981.
77. Forfar, J. C., Miller, H. C., and Toft, A. D.: Occult thyrotoxicosis: A correctable cause of "idiopathic" atrial fibrillation. Am. J. Cardiol. *44*:9, 1979.
78. Kannel, W. B., Abbott, R. D., Savage, D. D., and McNamara, P. M.: Epidemiologic features of chronic atrial fibrillation: The Framingham study. N. Engl. J. Med. *306*:1018, 1982.
79. Takahashi, N., Seki, A., Imataka, K., and Fujii, J.: Clinical features of paroxysmal atrial fibrillation: An observation of 94 patients. Japn. Heart J. *22*:143, 1981.
80. Gajewski, J., and Singer, R. B.: Mortality in an insured population with atrial fibrillation. J.A.M.A. *245*:1540, 1981.
81. Olsson, S. B., Orndahl, G., Ernestrom, S., Eskielson, J., Persson, S., Grennert, M. L., and Johanson, B. W.: Spontaneous reversion from longlasting atrial fibrillation to sinus rhythm. Acta Med. Scand. *207*:5, 1980.
82. Wolf, P. A., Dawber, P. R., Thomas, H. E., Jr., and Kannel, W. B.: Epidemiologic assessment of chronic atrial fibrillation and risk of stroke: The Framingham study. Neurology *28*:973, 1978.
83. Hinton, R. C., Kistler, J. P., Fallon, J. T., Friedlich, A. L., and Fisher, C. M.: Influence of etiology of atrial fibrillation on incidence of systemic embolism. Am. J. Cardiol. *40*:509, 1977.
84. Hunt, D., Sloman, G., and Penington, C.: Effects of atrial fibrillation on prognosis of acute myocardial infarction. Br. Heart J. *40*:303, 1978.
85. Watson, D. C., Henry, W. L., Epstein, S. E., and Morrow, A. G.: Effects of operation on left atrial size and the occurrence of atrial fibrillation in patients with hypertrophic subaortic stenosis. Circulation *55*:178, 1977.
86. Morganroth, J., Horowitz, L. N., Josephson, M. E., and Kastor, J. A.: Relationship of atrial fibrillatory wave amplitude to left atrial size and etiology of heart disease. An old generalization reexamined. Am. Heart J. *97*:184, 1979.
87. Ewy, G. A., Ulfers, L., Hager, W. D., Rosenfeld, A. R., Roeske, W. R., and Goldman, S.: Response of atrial fibrillation to therapy: Role of etiology and left atrial diameter. J. Electrocardiol. *13*:119, 1980.
88. Radford, D. J., and Izukawa, T.: Atrial fibrillation in children. Pediatrics *59*:250, 1977.
89. Stern, E. H., Pitchon, R., King, B. D., Guerrero, J., Schneider, R. R., and Wiener, I.: Clinical use of oral verapamil in chronic and paroxysmal atrial fibrillation. Chest *81*:308, 1982.
90. Hansen, J. F., Anderson, E. D., Olesen, K. H., Steiness, E., Lyngborg, K., Anderson, J. D., Efsen, F., Henningsen, P., and Wennevold, A.: DC cardioversion of atrial fibrillation after mitral valve operation. An analysis of long-term results. Scand. J. Thorac. Cardiovasc. Surg. *13*:267, 1979.
90a. Mancini, G. B. J., and Goldberger, A. L.: Cardioversion of atrial fibrillation: Consideration of embolization, anticoagulation, prophylactic pacemaker and long term success. Am. Heart J. *104*:617, 1982.
91. Lown, B.: Electrical reversion of cardiac arrhythmias. Br. Heart J. *29*:469, 1967.
92. Resenkov, L., and McDonald, L.: Complications in 220 patients with cardiac dysrhythmias treated by phased direct current shock and indications for electroconversion. Br. Heart J. *29*:926, 1967.
93. Bjerkelund, C. J., and Orning, O. M.: The efficacy of anticoagulant therapy in preventing embolism related to DC electrical conversion of atrial fibrillation. Am. J. Cardiol. *23*:208, 1969.
94. Halpern, S. W., Ellrodt, G., Singh, B. N., and Mandel, W. J.: Efficacy of intravenous procainamide infusion in converting atrial fibrillation to sinus rhythm. Relation to left atrial size. Br. Heart J. *44*:589, 1980.
95. Bauernfeind, R. A., Swiryn, S. P., Strasberg, B., Palileo, E., Scagliotti, D., and Rosen, K. M.: Electrophysiologic drug testing in prophylaxis of sporadic paroxysmal atrial fibrillation: Technique application and efficacy in severely symptomatic preexcitation patients. Am. Heart J. *103*:941, 1982.
96. Goldreyer, B. N., Gallagher, J. J., and Damato, A. N.: The electrophysiologic demonstration of atrial ectopic tachycardia in man. Am. Heart J. *85*:205, 1973.
97. Scheinmann, M. M., Basu, D., and Hollenberg, M.: Electrophysiologic studies in patients with persistent atrial tachycardia. Circulation *50*:266, 1974.
98. Gillette, P. C., and Garson, A., Jr.: Electrophysiologic and pharmacologic characteristics of automatic ectopic atrial tachycardia. Circulation *56*:571, 1977.
99. Rinkenberger, R. L., Prystowsky, E. N., Heger, J. J., Troup, P. J., Jackman, W. M., and Zipes, D. P.: Effects of intravenous and chronic oral verapamil administration in patients with supraventricular tachyarrhythmias. Circulation *62*:996, 1980.
100. Coumel, P., and Barold, S. S.: Mechanisms of supraventricular tachycardia. *In* His Bundle Electrocardiography and Clinical Electrophysiology. Narula, O. S. (ed.): Philadelphia, F. A. Davis Co., 1975, p. 203.
101. Coumel, P., Flammang, D., Attuel, P., and Leclercq, J. F.: Sustained intraatrial reentrant tachycardia. Electrophysiologic study of 20 cases. Clin. Cardiol. *2*:176, 1979.
102. Wu, D., Denes, P., Amat-y-Leon, F., Dhingra, R., Wyndham, C. R. C., Bauernfeind, R., Latif, P., and Rosen, K. M.: Clinical electrocardiographic and electrophysiologic observations in patients with paroxysmal supraventricular tachycardia. Am. J. Cardiol. *41*:1045, 1978.
103. Schine, K. I., Kastor, J. A., and Yurchak, E. M.: Multifocal atrial tachycardia. Clinical and electrocardiographic features in 32 patients. N. Engl. J. Med. *279*:344, 1968.
104. Lipson, M. J., and Naimi, S.: Multifocal atrial tachycardia (chaotic atrial tachycardia). Circulation *42*:397, 1970.
105. Bisset, G. S., Siegel, S. F., Gaum, W. E., and Kaplan, S.: Chaotic atrial tachycardia in childhood. Am. Heart J. *101*:268, 1981.
106. Tse, W. W.: Evidence of presence of automatic fibers in the canine atrioventricular node. Am. J. Physiol. *225*:716, 1973.
107. Wit, A. L., and Cranefield, P. F.: Mechanisms of impulse initiation in the atrioventricular junction and the effects of acetylstrophanthidin. Am. J. Cardiol. *49*:921, 1982.
108. Scherf, D., and Cohen, J.: The Atrioventricular Node and Selected Cardiac Arrhythmias. New York, Grune and Stratton, 1964, p. 226.
109. Pick, A., and Dominguez, P.: Nonparoxysmal AV nodal tachycardias. Circulation *16*:1022, 1957.
110. Kastor, J. A., and Yurchak, P. M.: Recognition of digitalis intoxication in the presence of atrial fibrillation. Ann. Intern. Med. *67*:105, 1967.
111. Zipes, D. P., Gaum, W. E., Genetos, B. C., Glassman, R. D., Noble, R. J., and Fisch, C.: Atrial tachycardia without P wave masquerading as an AV junctional tachycardia. Circulation *55*:253, 1977.
112. Castellanos, A., Sung, R. J., and Myerburg, R. J.: His bundle electrocardiography in digitalis-induced atrioventricular junctional Wenckebach periods with irregular HH intervals. Am. J. Cardiol. *43*:653, 1979.
113. Rosen, M. R., Fisch, C., Hoffman, B. F., Danilo, P., Jr., Lovelace, D. E., and Knoebel, S. B.: Can accelerated atrioventricular junctional escape rhythms be explained by delayed afterdepolarizations? Am. J. Cardiol. *45*:1272, 1980.
114. Zipes, D. P., and Fisch, C.: Atrioventricular dissociation. Arch. Intern. Med. *132*:130, 1973.
115. Rosen, K. M.: Junctional tachycardia. Mechanisms, diagnosis, differential diagnosis and management. Circulation *47*:654, 1973.
116. Gordon, A., and Gillette, P. C.: Junctional ectopic tachycardia in children: Electrocardiography, electrophysiology and pharmacologic response. Am. J. Cardiol. *44*:98, 1979.
117. Palileo, E. V., Bauernfeind, R. A., Swiryn, S. P., Wyndham, C. R., and Rosen, K. M.: Chronic nonparoxysmal junctional tachycardia. Chest *80*:106, 1981.
117a. Heddle, B., Brugada, P., Bär, F., and Wellens, H. J. J.: Cycle length change after initiation of reentrant tachycardia. Circulation *66* (Suppl. II): 269, 1982.
118. Bigger, J. T., and Goldreyer, B. N.: The mechanism of supraventricular tachycardia. Circulation *42*:673, 1970.
119. Goldreyer, B. N., and Bigger, J. T.: Site of reentry and paroxysmal supraventricular tachycardia in man. Circulation *43*:15, 1971.
120. Goldreyer, B. N., and Damato, A. N.: Essential role of atrioventricular conduction delay in the initiation of paroxysmal supraventricular tachycardia. Circulation *43*:679, 1971.
121. Benditt, D. G., Pritchett, E. L., Smith, W. M., and Gallagher, J. J.: Ventriculoatrial intervals: Diagnostic use in paroxysmal supraventricular tachycardia. Ann. Intern. Med. *91*:161, 1979.
122. Bauernfeind, R. A., Swiryn, S., Strasberg, B., Palileo, E., Wyndham, C., Duffy, C., and Rosen, K. M.: Analysis of anterograde and retrograde fast pathway properties in patients with dual atrioventricular nodal pathways. Observations regarding the pathophysiology of the Lown-Ganong-Levine syndrome. Am. J. Cardiol. *49*:283, 1982.
123. Casta, A., Wolff, G. S., Mehta, A. V., Tamer, D., Garcia, O. L., Pickoff, A. S., Ferrer, P. L., Sung, R. H., and Gelband, H.: Dual atrioventricular nodal pathways: A benign finding in arrhythmia-free children with heart disease. Am. J. Cardiol. *46*:1013, 1980.
124. Garson, A., Jr., and Gillette, P. C.: Electrophysiologic studies of supraventricular tachycardia in children. I. Clinical-electrophysiologic correlations. Am. Heart J. *102*:233, 1981.
125. Swiryn, S., Bauernfeind, R. A., Palileo, E., Strasberg, B., Duffy, C. E., and Rosen, K. M.: Electrophysiologic study demonstrating triple antegrade AV nodal pathways in patients with spontaneous and/or induced supraventricular tachycardia. Am. Heart J. *103*:168, 1982.
126. Brugada, P., Bär, F. W., Vanagt, E. J., Friedman, P. L., and Wellens, H. J. J.: Observations in patients showing AV junctional echoes with a shorter PR than RP interval. Am. J. Cardiol. *48*:611, 1981.

127. Akhtar, M., Damato, A. N., Ruskin, J. N., Batsford, W. T., Reddy, C. P., Ticzon, A. R., Dhatt, M. S., Gomes, J. A. C., and Calon, A. H.: Antegrade and retrograde conduction characteristics in three patterns of paroxysmal atrioventricular junctional reentrant tachycardia. Am. Heart J. *95*:22, 1978.
128. Coumel, P.: Functional reciprocating tachycardias. The permanent and paroxysmal forms of AV nodal reciprocating tachycardias. J. Electrocardiol. *8*:79, 1975.
129. Denes, P., Wu, D., Dhingra, R., Amat-y-Leon, F., Wyndham, C., and Rosen, K. M.: Dual atrioventricular nodal pathways: A common electrophysiological response. Br. Heart J. *37*:1069, 1975.
130. Denes, P., Wu, D., Dhingra, R. C., Chuquimia, R., and Rosen, K. M.: Demonstration of dual AV nodal pathways in patients with paroxysmal supraventricular tachycardia. Circulation *48*:549, 1973.
131. Wu, D.: Dual atrioventricular nodal pathways: A reappraisal. PACE *5*:72, 1982.
132. Wu, D., Denes, P., Amat-y-Leon, F., Wyndham, C. R. C., Dhingra, R., and Rosen, K. M.: An unusual variety of atrioventricular nodal reentry due to retrograde dual atrioventricular nodal pathways. Circulation *56*:50, 1977.
133. Amat-y-Leon, F., Wyndham, C. R., Wu, D., Denes, P., Dhingra, R. C., and Rosen, K. M.: Participation of fast and slow AV nodal pathways in tachycardias complicating the Wolff-Parkinson-White syndrome. Circulation *55*:663, 1977.
134. Rosen, K. M., Bauernfeind, R. A., Swiryn, S., Strasberg, B., and Palileo, E. V.: Dual AV nodal pathways and AV nodal reentrant paroxysmal tachycardia. Am. Heart J. *101*:691, 1981.
135. Wellens, H. J. J., Westorp, J. C., Duren, D. R., and Lie, K. I.: Second degree block during reciprocal atrioventricular nodal tachycardia. Circulation *53*:595, 1976.
135a. Ko, P. T., Naccarelli, G. V., Gulamhusein, S., Prystowsky, E. N., Zipes, D. P., and Klein, G. J.: Atrioventricular dissociation during paroxysmal junctional tachycardia. PACE *4*:670, 1981.
136. Sung, B. J., Waxman, H. L., Saksena, S., and Juma, Z.: Sequence of retrograde atrial activation in patients with dual atrioventricular nodal pathways. Circulation *64*:1059, 1981.
137. Swiryn, S., Pavel, D., Byrom, E., Wyndham, C., Pietras, R., Bauernfeind, R., and Rosen, K. M.: Assessment of left ventricular function by radionuclide angiography during induced supraventricular tachycardia. Am. J. Cardiol. *47*: 555, 1981.
138. Waxman, M. B., Sharma, A. B., Cameron, D. A., Huerta, F., and Wald, R. W.: Reflex mechanisms responsible for early spontaneous termination of paroxysmal supraventricular tachycardia. Am. J. Cardiol. *49*:259, 1982.
139. Sung, R. J., Elser, B., and McAllister, R. G., Jr.: Intravenous verapamil for termination of reentrant supraventricular tachycardias: Intracardiac studies correlated with plasma verapamil concentrations. Ann. Intern. Med. *93*:682, 1980.
140. Krikler, D. M.: Verapamil in cardiology. Eur. J. Cardiol. *2*:3, 1974.
141. Waxman, H. L., Myerburg, R. J., Appel, R., and Sung, R. J.: Verapamil for control of ventricular rate in paroxysmal supraventricular tachycardia and atrial fibrillation or flutter: A double-blind randomized cross-over study. Ann. Intern. Med. *94*:1, 1981.
142. Betriu, A., Chaitman, B. R., Bourassa, M. G., Brévers, G., Scholl, J., Bruneau, P., Gagne, P., and Chabot, M.: Beneficial effect of intravenous diltiazen in the acute management of paroxysmal supraventricular tachyarrhythmias. Circulation *67*:88, 1983.
143. Wu, D., Hung, J. S., Kuo, C. T., Hsu, K. S., and Shieh, W. B.: Effects of quinidine on atrioventricular nodal reentrant paroxysmal tachycardia. Circulation *64*:823, 1981.
144. Swiryn, S., Bauernfeind, R. A., Wyndham, C. R. C., Dhingra, R. C., Palileo, E., Strasberg, B., and Rosen, K. M.: Effects of oral disopyramide phosphate on induction of paroxysmal supraventricular tachycardia. Circulation *64*:169, 1981.
145. Bauernfeind, R. A., Wyndham, C. R., Dhingra, R. C., Swiryn, S. P., Palileo, E., Strasberg, B., and Rosen, K. M.: Serial electrophysiologic testing of multiple drugs in patients with atrioventricular nodal reentrant paroxysmal tachycardia. Circulation *62*:1341, 1980.
146. Zipes, D. P., DeJoseph, R. L., and Rothbaum, D. A.: Unusual properties of accessory pathways. Circulation *49*:1200, 1974.
147. Coumel, P., and Attuel, P.: Reciprocating tachycardia in overt and latent preexcitation. Influence of functional bundle branch block on the rate of the tachycardia. Eur. J. Cardiol. *1*:423, 1974.
148. Neuss, H., Schlepper, M., and Thormann, J.: Analysis of reentry mechanisms in the three patients with concealed Wolff-Parkinson-White syndrome. Circulation *51*:75, 1975.
149. Spurrell, R. A. J., Krikler, D. M., and Sowton, E.: Concealed bypasses of the atrioventricular node in patients with paroxysmal supraventricular tachycardia revealed by intracardiac electrical stimulation and verapamil. Am. J. Cardiol. *33*:590, 1974.
150. Slama, R., Coumel, P., and Bouvrain, Y.: Les syndromes de Wolff-Parkinson-White de type A inapparents ou latents en rythme sinusal. Arch. Mal Coeur *66*:639, 1973.
151. Barold, S. S., and Coumel, P.: Mechanisms of atrioventricular junctional tachycardia. Role of reentry and concealed accessory bypass tracts. Am. J. Cardiol. *39*:97, 1977.
152. Puech, P., Grolleau, R., and Cinca, J.: Reciprocating tachycardia using a latent left-sided accessory pathway. Diagnostic approach by conventional ECG. *In* Kulbertus, H. E. (ed.): Reentrant Arrhythmias. Baltimore, University Park Press, 1977. p. 117.
153. Pritchett, E. L. C., Tonkin, A. M., Dugan, F. A., Wallace, A. G., and Gallagher, J. J.: Ventriculoatrial conduction time during reciprocating tachycardia with intermittent bundle branch block in Wolff-Parkinson-White syndrome. Br. Heart J. *38*:1058, 1976.
153a. Kerr, C. R., Gallagher, J. J. and German, L. D.: Changes in ventriculoatrial intervals with bundle branch block aberration during reciprocating tachycardia in patients with accessory atrioventricular pathways. Circulation *66*:196, 1982.
154. Prystowsky, E. N., Pritchett, E. L. C., Smith, W. M., Wallace, A. G., Sealy, W. C., and Gallagher, J. J.: Electrophysiologic assessment of the atrioventricular conduction system after surgical correction of ventricular preexcitation. Circulation *59*:789, 1979.
155. Chilson, D. A., Zipes, D. P., Heger, J. J., Browne, K. F., Lloyd, E. A., and Prystowsky, E. N.: Functional bundle branch block in man: Evidence of longer refractoriness of left than right bundle branch at faster heart rates. Clin. Res. *30*:705A, 1982.
156. Prystowsky, E. N., Heger, J. J., Jackman, W. M., Naccarelli, G. V., and Zipes, D. P.: Postmyocardial infarction incessant supraventricular tachycardia due to concealed accessory pathway. Am. Heart J. *103*:426, 1982.
157. Akhtar, M., Shenasa, M., and Schmidt, D. H.: Role of retrograde His-Purkinje block in the initiation of supraventricular tachycardia by ventricular premature stimulation in the Wolff-Parkinson-White syndrome. J. Clin. Invest. *67*: 1047, 1981.
158. Farshidi, A., Josephson, M. E., and Horowitz, L. N.: Electrophysiologic characteristics of concealed bypass tracts: Clinical and electrocardiographic correlates. Am. J. Cardiol. *41*:1052, 1978.
159. Wood, P.: Polyuria in paroxysmal tachycardia and paroxysmal atrial flutter and fibrillation. Br. Heart J. *25*:273, 1963.
160. Harvey, W. P., and Ronan, J. A., Jr.: Bedside diagnosis of arrhythmias. Progr. Cardiovasc. Dis. *8*:419, 1966.
161. Oehnell, R. F.: Preexcitation, a cardiac abnormality. Acta Med. Scand. *152* (Suppl.):78, 1944.
162. Durrer, D., Schuilenburg, R. M., and Wellens, H. J. J.: Preexcitation revisited. Am. J. Cardiol. *25*:690, 1970.
163. Wolff, L., Parkinson, J., and White, P. D.: Bundle branch block with short P-R interval in healthy young people prone to paroxysmal tachycardia. Am. Heart J. *5*:685, 1950.
164. Becker, A. H., and Anderson, R. H.: The Wolff-Parkinson-White syndrome and its anatomical substrates. Anat. Rec. *201*:169, 1981.
165. Kent, A. F. S.: Researches on the structure and function of the mammalian heart. J. Physiol. *14*:233, 1893.
166. Kent, A. F. S.: Observations on the auriculo-ventricular junction of the mammalian heart. Quart. J. Exp. Physiol. *7*:193, 1913.
167. Anderson, R. H., Becker, A. E., Brechenmacher, C., Davies, M. J., and Rossi, L.: Ventricular preexcitation nomenclature for its substrates. Eur. J. Cardiol. *3*: 27, 1975.
168. Brechenmacher, C.: Atrio-His bundle tracts. Br. Heart J. *37*:853, 1975.
169. Lown, B., Ganong, W. F., and Levine, S. A.: The syndrome of short PR interval, normal QRS complex and paroxysmal rapid heart action. Circulation *5*: 693, 1952.
170. Bauernfeind, R. A., Ayres, B. F., Wyndham, C. C., Dhingra, R. C., Swiryn, S. P., Strasberg, B., and Rosen, K. M.: Cycle length in atrioventricular nodal reentrant paroxysmal tachycardia with observations on Lown-Ganong-Levine syndrome. Am. J. Cardiol. *45*:1148, 1980.
171. Mahaim, I.: Kent's fibers and the AV paraspecific conduction through the upper connections of the bundle of His-Tawara. Am. Heart J. *33*:651, 1947.
172. Gallagher, J. J., Smith, W. M., Kasell, J. H., Benson, D. W., Jr., Sterba, R., and Grant, A. O.: Role of Mahaim fibers in cardiac arrhythmias in man. Circulation *64*:176, 1981.
173. Gallagher, J. J., Pritchett, E. L. C., Sealy, W. C., Casell, J., and Wallace, A. G.: The pre-excitation syndromes. Progr. Cardiovasc. Dis. *20*:285, 1978.
174. Nicolai, P., Medevdowsky, J. L., Delaahe, M., Barnay, C., Blache, E., and Pisapia, A.: Wolff-Parkinson-White syndrome: T wave abnormalities during normal pathway conduction. J. Electrocardiol. *14*:295, 1981.
175. Durrer, D., Schoo, L., Schuilenberg, R. M., and Wellens, H. J. J.: The role of premature beats in the initiation and the termination of supraventricular tachycardia in the Wolff-Parkinson-White syndrome. Circulation *36*:644, 1967.
176. Cinca, J., Valle, V., Gutierrez, L., Figueras, J., and Rius, J.: Reciprocating tachycardia using bilateral anomalous pathways: Electrophysiologic and clinical implications. Circulation *62*:657, 1980.
177. Ko, P. T., Naccarelli, G. V., Gulamhusein, S., Prystowsky, E. N., Zipes, D. P., and Klein, G. J.: Atrioventricular dissociation during paroxysmal junctional tachycardia. PACE *4*:670, 1981.
178. Motté, G., Brechenmacher, C., Davy, J. M., and Belhassen, B.: Association of nodoventricular and atrioventricular fibers with the origin of reciprocating tachycardia. Electrophysiological and anomal pathological anatomopathological aspect. Arch. Mal Coeur *73*:737, 1980.
179. Coumel, P., Attuel, P., and Mugica, J.: Junctional reciprocating tachycardias. *In* Kulbertus, H. C. (ed.): Reentrant Arrhythmias. Baltimore, University Park Press, 1977.
180. Gallagher, J. J., and Sealy, W. C.: The permanent form of junctional reciprocating tachycardia. Further elucidation of the underlying mechanism. Eur. J. Cardiol. *8*:413, 1978.

181. Wellens, H. J. J.: Observations in patients showing AV junctional echoes with a shorter PR than RP interval. Distinction between intranodal reentry or reentry using an accessory pathway with a long conduction time. Am. J. Cardiol. *48*:611, 1981.
182. Touboul, P., Atallah, G., and Kirkorian, G.: Role of accessory atrioventricular pathways in the genesis of permanent junctional tachycardia. Arch. Mal Coeur *73*:1131, 1980.
183. Gillette, P. C., Garson, A., Cooley, D. A., and McNamara, D. G.: Prolonged and decremental antegrade conduction properties in right anterior accessory connections: Wide QRS antidromic tachycardia of left bundle branch block pattern without Wolff-Parkinson-White configuration in sinus rhythm. Am. Heart J. *103*:166, 1982.
184. Gillette, P. C., Garson, A., Jr., and Kugler, J. D.: Wolff-Parkinson-White syndrome in children: Electrophysiologic and pharmacologic characteristics. Circulation *60*:1487, 1979.
185. Gallagher, J. J., Smith, W. M., Kasell, J., Smith, W. M., Grant, A. O., and Benson, D. W.: Use of the esophageal lead in the diagnosis of mechanisms of reciprocating supraventricular tachycardia. PACE *3*:440, 1980.
186. Sung, R. J., Castellanos, A., Mallon, S. M., Bloom, M. G., Gelband, H., and Myerburg, R. J.: Mechanisms of spontaneous alternation between reciprocating tachycardia and atrial flutter-fibrillation in the Wolff-Parkinson-White syndrome. Circulation *56*:409, 1977.
187. Ross, D. L., Farre, J., Bär, F. W., Vanagt, E. J., Brugada, T., Wiener, I., and Wellens, H. J. J.: Spontaneous termination of circus movement tachycardia using an atrioventricular accessory pathway: Incidence, site of block and mechanisms. Circulation *63*:1129, 1981.
188. Bauernfeind, R. A., Wyndham, C. R., Swiryn, S. P., Palileo, E. V., Strasberg, B., Lam, W., Westveer, D., and Rosen, K. M.: Paroxysmal atrial fibrillation in the Wolff-Parkinson-White syndrome. Am. J. Cardiol. *47*:562, 1981.
189. Klein, G. H., Bashore, T. M., Seller, T. B., Pritchett, E. L. C., and Gallagher, J. J.: Ventricular fibrillation in the Wolff-Parkinson-White syndrome. N. Engl. J. Med. *301*:1080, 1979.
190. Dreifus, L. S., Haiat, R., Watanabe, Y., Arriaga, J., and Reitman, N.: Ventricular fibrillation: A possible mechanism of sudden death in patients with Wolff-Parkinson-White syndrome. Circulation *43*:520, 1971.
191. Boineau, J. P., and Moore, E. N.: Evidence for propagation of activation across an accessory atrioventricular connection in types A and B preexcitation. Circulation *41*:375, 1970.
192. Campbell, R. W., Smith, R. A., Gallagher, J. J., Pritchett, E. L., and Wallace, A. G.: Atrial fibrillation in the preexcitation syndrome. Am. J. Cardiol. *40*: 514, 1977.
193. Pritchett, E. L., Prystowsky, E. N., Benditt, D. G., and Gallagher, J. J.: "Dual atrioventricular nodal pathways" in patients with Wolff-Parkinson-White syndrome. Br. Heart J. *43*:7, 1980.
194. Hammil, S. C., Pritchett, E. L., Klein, G. J., Smith, W. M., and Gallagher, J. J.: Accessory atrioventricular pathways that conduct only in the antegrade direction. Circulation *62*:1335, 1980.
195. Bosc, E., Grolleau, R., Puech, P., Latour, H., and Souchon, H.: Automatic activity of the preexcitation pathways. Arch. Mal Coeur *72*:359, 1979.
196. Davidoff, R., Schamroth, C. L., and Myerberg, D. P.: The Wolff-Parkinson-White pattern in healthy air crew. Aviat. Space Environ. Med. *52*:554, 1981.
197. Newman, D. J., Donoso, E., and Friedberg, C. K.: Arrhythmias in the Wolff-Parkinson-White syndrome. Progr. Cardiovasc. Dis. *9*:147, 1966.
198. Bharati, S., Rosen, K., Steinfield, L., Miller, R. A., and Lev, M.: The anatomic substrate for preexcitation in corrected transposition. Circulation *62*:831, 1980.
199. Smith, W. M., Gallagher, J. J., Kerr, C. R., Sealy, W. C., Kasell, J. H., Benson, D. W., Jr., Reiter, M. J., Sterba, R., and Grant, A. O.: The electrophysiologic basis and management of symptomatic recurrent tachycardia in patients with Ebstein's anomaly of the tricuspid valve. Am. J. Cardiol. *49*:1223, 1982.
200. Hindman, M. C., Last, J. H., and Rosen, K. M.: Wolff-Parkinson-White syndrome observed by portable monitoring. Ann. Intern. Med. *79*:654, 1973.
201. Wolff, G. S., Han, J., and Curran, J.: Wolff-Parkinson-White syndrome in the neonate. Am. J. Cardiol. *41*:559, 1978.
202. Klein, G. J., Hackel, D. B., and Gallagher, J. J.: Anatomic substrate of impaired antegrade conduction over an accessory atrioventricular pathway in the Wolff-Parkinson-White syndrome. Circulation *61*:1249, 1980.
203. Sellers, T. D., Bashore, T. M., and Gallagher, J. J.: Digitalis in the preexcitation syndrome: Analysis during atrial fibrillation. Circulation *56*:260, 1977.
204. Wellens, H. J. J., and Durrer, D.: Effect of digitalis on atrioventricular conduction and circus movement tachycardias in patients with Wolff-Parkinson-White syndrome. Circulation *47*:1229, 1973.
205. Dhingra, R. C., Palileo, E. V., Strasberg, B., Swiryn, S., Bauernfeind, R., Wyndham, C., and Rosen, K. M.: Electrophysiologic effects of ouabain in patients with preexcitation and circus movement tachycardia. Am. J. Cardiol. *47*: 139, 1981.
206. Akhtar, M., Gilbert, C. J., and Shenasa, M.: Effect of lidocaine on atrioventricular response via the accessory pathway in patients with Wolff-Parkinson-White syndrome. Circulation *63*:435, 1981.
207. Gulamhusein, S., Ko, P., Carruthers, S. G., and Klein, G. J.: Acceleration of the ventricular response during atrial fibrillation in the Wolff-Parkinson-White syndrome after verapamil. Circulation *65*:348, 1982.
208. Przybylski, J., Chiale, P. A., Halpern, M. S., Nau, G. J., Elizari, M. V., and Rosenbaum, M. B.: Unmasking of ventricular preexcitation by vagal stimulation or isoproterenol administration. Circulation *61*:1030, 1980.
209. Wellens, H. J. J., Bär, F. W., Dassen, W. R., Brugada, P., Vanagt, E. J., and Farre, J.: Effect of drugs in the Wolff-Parkinson-White syndrome. Importance of initial length of effective refractory period of the accessory pathway. Am. J. Cardiol. *46*:665, 1980.
210. Zipes, D. P., Rothbaum, D. A., and DeJoseph, R. L.: Preexcitation syndrome. Cardiovasc. Clin. *1*:210, 1974.
211. Josephson, M. E.: Paroxysmal supraventricular tachycardia: An electrophysiologic approach. Am. J. Cardiol. *41*:1123, 1978.
212. Paulay, K. L., Ruskin, J. N., and Damato, A. N.: Sinus and atrioventricular nodal reentrant tachycardia in the same patient. Am. J. Cardiol. *36*:810, 1975.
213. Langendorf, R.: Ventricular premature systoles with postponed compensatory pause. Am. Heart J. *46*:401, 1953.
214. Castillo, C., Castellanos, A., Jr., Agha, A. S., and Myerberg, R.: Significance of His bundle recordings with short H-V intervals. Chest *60*:142, 1971.
215. Winkle, R. A.: The relationship between ventricular ectopic beat frequency and heart rate. Circulation *66*:439, 1982.
216. Hinkle, L. E., Carver, S. T., and Stevens, M.: The frequency of asymptomatic disturbances of cardiac rhythm and conduction in middle-aged men. Am. J. Cardiol. *24*:629, 1969.
217. Chiang, B. N., Perlman, L. V., Ostrander, L. D., and Epstein, F. H.: Relationship of premature systoles to coronary heart disease and sudden death in the Tecumseh epidemiologic study. Ann. Intern. Med. *70*:1159, 1969.
218. Moss, A. J., DeCamilla, J., Davis, H., and Bayer, L.: The early post-hospital phase of myocardial infarction: Prognostic stratification. Circulation *54*:58, 1976.
219. Ruberman, W., Weinblatt, E., Goldberg, J. D., Frank, C. W., and Shapiro, S.: Ventricular premature beats and mortality after myocardial infarction. N. Engl. J. Med. *297*:750, 1977.
220. Ambos, H. D., Roberts, R., Oliver, G. C., Cox, J. R., Jr., and Sobel, B. E.: Infarct size: A determinant of persistence of severe ventricular dysrhythmia. Am. J. Cardiol. *37*:116, 1976.
221. Schulze, R. A., Jr., Strauss, H. W., and Pitt, B.: Sudden death in the year following myocardial infarction: Relation to ventricular premature contractions in the late hospital phase and ventricular ejection fraction. Am. J. Med. *62*:192, 1977.
222. Lie, K. I., Wellens, H. J. J., and Durrer, D.: Characteristics and predictability of binary ventricular fibrillation. Eur. J. Cardiol. *1*:379, 1974.
223. Naccarelli, G. V., Prystowsky, E. N., Jackman, W. M., Heger, J. J., Rahilly, G. T., and Zipes, D. P.: Role of electrophysiologic testing in managing patients who have ventricular tachycardia unrelated to coronary artery disease. Am. J. Cardiol. *50*:165, 1982.
224. Rinkenberger, R. L., Prystowsky, E. N., Jackman, W. M., Heger, J. J., and Zipes, D. P.: Conversion of nonsustained ventricular tachycardia to sustained ventricular tachycardia during drug therapy as determined by serial electrophysiology studies. Am. Heart J. *103*:177, 1982.
225. Kisten, A. D.: Retrograde conduction to the atria in ventricular tachycardia. Circulation *24*:236, 1961.
226. Wellens, J. H. H., Bär, F. W. H. M., and Lie, K. I.: The value of the electrocardiogram in the differential diagnosis of a tachycardia with a widened QRS complex. Am. J. Med. *64*:27, 1978.
227. Sandler, I. A., and Marriott, H.: The differential morphology of anomalous ventricular complexes of RBBB type in lead V_1. Ventricular ectopy versus aberration. Circulation *31*:551, 1965.
228. Josephson, M. E., Horowitz, L. N., Farshidi, A., and Kastor, J. A.: Recurrent sustained ventricular tachycardia. I. Mechanisms. Circulation *57*:431, 1978.
229. Morady, F., Scheinman, M. M., Gonzalez, R., and Hess, E.: His-ventricular dissociation in a patient with reciprocating tachycardia and a nodoventricular bypass tract. Circulation *64*:839, 1981.
230. Cohen, H. C., Gozo, E. G., Jr., and Pick, A.: Ventricular tachycardia with narrow QRS complexes (left posterior fascicular tachycardia). Circulation *45*: 1035, 1972.
231. Wellens, H. J. J.: Value and limitations of programmed electrical stimulation of the heart in the study and treatment of tachycardia. Circulation *57*:845, 1978.
232. Gomes, J. A., Kang, P. S., Khan, R., Kelen, G., and El-Sherif, N.: Repetitive ventricular response: Its incidence, inducibility, reproducibility, mechanism and significance. Br. Heart J. *46*:159, 1981.
233. Brugada, P., Heddle, B., and Wellens, H. J. J.: Results of a ventricular stimulation protocol using a maximum of four premature stimuli in patients without documented or suspected ventricular arrhythmias. Circulation *66*(Suppl. II): 79, 1982.
234. Prystowsky, E. N., Naccarelli, G. V., Rahilly, G. T., Jr., Heger, J. J., and Zipes, D. P.: Electrophysiologic and anatomic characteristics associated with ventricular tachycardia induced at the right ventricular outflow tract but not at the apex. Am. J. Cardiol. *49*:959, 1982.
235. Robertson, J. F., Cain, M. E., Horowitz, L. N., Spielman, S. R., Greenspan, A. M., Waxman, H. L., and Josephson, M. E.: Anatomic and electrophysiologic correlates of ventricular tachycardia requiring left ventricular stimulation. Am. J. Cardiol. *48*:263, 1981.
236. Reddy, C. P., and Gettes, E. S.: Use of isoproterenol as an aid to electric induction of chronic recurrent ventricular tachycardia. Am. J. Cardiol. *44*:705, 1979.

237. Rinkenberger, R. L., Prystowsky, E. N., Jackman, W. M., Heger, J. J., and Zipes, D. P.: Conversion of nonsustained ventricular tachycardia to sustained ventricular tachycardia during drug therapy as determined by serial electrophysiology studies. Am. Heart J. *103*:177, 1982.
238. Greenspon, A. J., Stang, J. M., Lewis, R. P., and Schaal, S. F.: Provocation of ventricular tachycardia after consumption of alcohol. N. Engl. J. Med. *301*: 104, 1979.
239. Wellens, H. J. J., Lie, K. I., and Durrer, D.: Further observations on ventricular tachycardia as studied by electrical stimulation of the heart: Chronic recurrent ventricular tachycardia and ventricular tachycardia during acute myocardial infarction. Circulation *49*:647, 1974.
240. Naccarelli, G. V., Zipes, D. P., Rahilly, G. T., Heger, J. J., and Prystowsky, E. N.: Influence of tachycardia cycle length and antiarrhythmic drugs on pacing termination and acceleration of ventricular tachycardia. Am. Heart J. *105*: 1, 1983.
241. Josephson, M. E., Horowitz, L. N., Farshidi, A., Spielman, S. R., Michaelson, E. L., and Greenspan, A. M.: Sustained ventricular tachycardia: Evidence for protected localized reentry. Am. J. Cardiol. *42*:416, 1978.
242. Josephson, M. E., Horowitz, L. N., Waxman, H. L., Cain, M. E., Spielman, S. R., Greenspan, A. M., Marchlinski, F. E., and Ezri, M. D.: Sustained ventricular tachycardia: Role of the 12-lead electrocardiogram in localizing site of origin. Circulation *64*:257, 1981.
243. Swiryn, S., Pavel, T., Byrom, M. E., Bauernfeind, R. A., Strasberg, B., Palileo, E., Lam, W., Wyndham, C. R., and Rosen, K. M.: Sequential regional phase mapping of radionuclide gated biventriculograms in patients with sustained ventricular tachycardia: Close correlation with electrophysiologic characteristics. Am. Heart J. *103*:319, 1982.
244. Hess, O. M., Graf, C., Frey, R., Dettli, R., and Siegenthaler, W.: Coronary artery spasm with normal coronary arteries as the cause of recurrent ventricular fibrillation. Schweiz. Med. Wnschr. *111*:755, 1981.
245. Ruskin, J. N., DiMarco, J. P., and Garan, H.: Out-of-hospital cardiac arrest: Electrophysiologic observations and selection of long-term antiarrhythmic therapy. N. Engl. J. Med. *303*:607, 1980.
246. Josephson, M. E., Horowitz, L. N., Spielman, S. R., and Greenspan, A. M.: Electrophysiologic and hemodynamic studies in patients resuscitated from cardiac arrest. Am. J. Cardiol. *46*:948, 1980.
247. Winkle, R. A., Derrington, D. C., and Schroeder, J. S.: Characteristics of ventricular tachycardia in ambulatory patients. Am. J. Cardiol. *39*:487, 1977.
248. Bigger, J. T., Jr., Weld, F. M., and Rolnitzky, L. M.: Prevalence characteristics and significance of ventricular tachycardia (three or more complexes) detected with ambulatory electrocardiographic recording in the late hospital phase of acute myocardial infarction. Am. J. Cardiol. *48*:815, 1981.
249. Pedersen, D. H., Zipes, D. P., Foster, P. R., and Troup, P. J.: Ventricular tachycardia and ventricular fibrillation in a young population. Circulation *60*: 988, 1979.
250. Vetter, V. L., Josephson, M. E., and Horowitz, L. N.: Idiopathic recurrent sustained ventricular tachycardia in children and adolescents. Am. J. Cardiol. *47*:315, 1981.
251. Reisch, P., DeSilva, R. A., Lown, B., and Murawski, B. J.: Acute psychological disturbance preceding life-threatening ventricular arrhythmias. J.A.M.A. *246*:233, 1981.
252. Waxman, M. B., Wald, R. W., Finley, J. P., Bonnet, J. F., Downar, E., and Sharma, A. B.: Valsalva termination of ventricular tachycardia. Circulation *62*: 843, 1980.
252a. Vlay, S. C., and Reid, P. R.: Ventricular ectopy: Etiology, evaluation and therapy. Am. J. Med. *73*:899, 1982.
253. Pennington, J. E., Taylor, J., and Brown, B.: Chest thump for reverting ventricular tachycardia. N. Engl. J. Med. *283*:1192, 1970.
254. Sclarovsky, S., Kracoff, O., Arditi, A., Strasberg, B., Zafrir, N., Lewin, R. F., and Agmon, J.: Ventricular tachycardia. "Pleomorphism" induced by chest thump. Chest *81*:97, 1982.
255. Myerburg, R. J., Kessler, K. M., Kiem, I., Pefkaros, K. C., Conde, C. A., Cooper, D., and Castellanos, A.: Relationship between plasma levels of procainamide, suppression of premature ventricular complexes and prevention of recurrent ventricular tachycardia. Circulation *64*:280, 1981.
256. Horowitz, L. N., Spielman, S. R., Greenspan, A. M., and Josephson, M. E.: Role of programmed stimulation in assessing vulnerability to ventricular arrhythmias. Am. Heart J. *103*:604, 1982.
257. Josephson, M. E., Kastor, J. A., and Horowitz, L. N.: Electrophysiologic management of recurrent ventricular tachycardia in acute and chronic ischemic heart disease. Cardiovasc. Clin. *11*:35, 1980.
258. Zipes, D. P., and Fisch, C.: Accelerated ventricular rhythm. Arch. Intern. Med. *129*:650, 1972.
259. Rothfeld, E. L., Zucker, I. R., Parsonnet, V., and Alinsonorin, C. A.: Idioventricular rhythm in acute myocardial infarction. Circulation *37*:203, 1968.
260. DeSoyza, N., Bissett, J. K., Kane, J. J., Murphy, M. L., and Doherty, J. E.: Association of accelerated idioventricular rhythm and paroxysmal ventricular tachycardia in acute myocardial infarction. Am. J. Cardiol. *34*:667, 1974.
261. Lichstein, E., Riebas-Meneclier, C., Guptka, P. K., and Chadda, K. D.: Incidence and description of accelerated idioventricular rhythm complicating acute myocardial infarction. Am. J. Med. *58*:192, 1975.
262. Dessertenne, F.: Considerations sur l'electrocardiogramme de la fibrillation ventriculaire. Arch. Mal Coeur *57*:1421, 1964.
263. Fontaine, G., Frank, R., and Grosgogeat, Y.: Torsades de pointes: Definition and management. Mod. Conc. Cardiovasc. Dis. *51*:103, 1982.
264. Krikler, D. M., and Curry, P. V. L.: Torsades de pointes, an atypical ventricular tachycardia. Br. Heart J. *38*:117, 1976.
265. Horowitz, L. N., Greenspan, A. M., Spielman, S. R., and Josephson, M. E.: Torsades de pointes: Electrophysiologic studies in patients without transient pharmacologic or metabolic abnormalities. Circulation *63*:1120, 1981.
266. Wellens, H. J. J., and Lie, K. I.: Ventricular tachycardia: The value of programmed electrical stimulation. *In* Krikler, D., and Goodwin, J. F. (eds.): Cardiac Arrhythmias. London, Saunders, 1975.
267. Baroy, J. H., Ungerleider, R. M., Smith, W. M., and Ideker, R. E.: A mechanism of torsades de pointes in a canine model. Circulation *67*:52, 1983.
268. Smith, W. M., and Gallagher, J. J.: "Les torsades de pointes": An unusual ventricular arrhythmia. Ann. Intern. Med. *93*:578, 1980.
269. Keren, A., Tzivoni, D., Gavish, D., Levi, J., Gottleib, S., Benhorin, J., and Stern, S.: Etiology warning signs and therapy of torsades de pointes—a study of ten patients. Circulation *64*:1167, 1981.
270. Schwartz, P. J., Periti, M., and Malliani, A.: The long Q-T syndrome. Am. Heart J. *89*:378, 1975.
271. Khan, M. M., Logan, K. R., McComb, J. M., and Adgey, A. A.: Management of recurrent ventricular tachyarrhythmias associated with QT prolongation. Am. J. Cardiol. *47*:1301, 1981.
272. Kastor, J. A., Horowitz, L. N., Harken, A. H., and Josephson, M. E.: Clinical electrophysiology of ventricular tachycardia. N. Engl. J. Med. *304*:1004, 1981.
273. Rosenbaum, M. B., Elizari, M. V., and Lazzari, L. D.: The mechanism of bidirectional tachycardia. Am. Heart J. *78*:4, 1979.
274. Morris, S. N., and Zipes, D. P.: His bundle electrocardiography during bidirectional tachycardia. Circulation *48*:32, 1973.
275. Kastor, J. A., and Goldreyer, B. N.: Ventricular origin of bidirectional tachycardia: Case report of a patient not toxic from digitalis. Circulation *48*:897, 1973.
276. Cohen, S. I., Deisseroth, A., and Hecht, H. S.: Infra-His bundle origin of bidirectional tachycardia. Circulation *47*:1260, 1973.
277. Rahilly, G. T., Prystowsky, E. N., Zipes, D. P., Naccarelli, G. V., Jackman, W. M., and Heger, J. J.: Clinical and electrophysiologic findings in patients with otherwise normal electrocardiograms. Am. J. Cardiol. *50*:459, 1982.
277a. Coumel, P., Leclercq, J. F., Attuel, P., Rosengarten, M., Milosevic, D., Slama, P., and Sourrain, Y.: Tachycardies ventriculaires in salves. Etude electrophysiologique et therapeutique Arch. Mal Coeur *73*:153, 1980.
278. Froment, R., Gallavardin, L., and Cahen, P.: Paroxysmal ventricular tachycardia: A clinical classification. Br. Heart J. *15*:172, 1953.
279. Gallavardin, L., and Veil, P.: Deux nouveaux cas d'extrasystolie-ventriculaire avec salves tachycardiques. Arch. Mal Coeur *22*:738, 1929.
280. Parkinson, J., and Papp, C.: Repetitive paroxysmal tachycardia. Br. Heart J. *9*: 241, 1947.
281. Lesch, M., Lewis, E., Humphries, J. O., and Ross, R.: Paroxysmal ventricular tachycardia in the absence of organic heart disease. Ann. Intern. Med. *66*:950, 1967.
282. Steffens, T. G., Pierce, P. L., and Zegerius, R. J.: Multiple ventricular premature beats in 5 adolescents. Eur. J. Cardiol. *8*:177, 1978.
283. Lloyd, E. A., Zipes, D. P., Heger, J. J., and Prystowsky, E. N.: Sustained ventricular tachycardia due to bundle branch reentry. Am. Heart J. *104*:1095, 1982.
283a. Welch, W. J., Strasberg, B., Coelho, A., and Rosen, K. M.: Sustained macroreentrant ventricular tachycardia. Am. Heart J. *104*:166, 1982.
284. Reddy, C. P., and Slack, J. D.: Recurrent ventricular tachycardia: Report of a case with His bundle branch reentry as the mechanism. Eur. J. Cardiol. *11*:23, 1980.
285. Browne, K. F., Zipes, D. P., Heger, J. J., and Prystowsky, E. N.: The influence of the autonomic nervous system on the QT interval. Am. J. Cardiol. *49*: 898, 1982.
286. Moss, A. J., and Schwartz, P. J.: Delayed repolarization (QT or QTU prolongation) and malignant ventricular arrhythmias. Mod. Conc. Cardiovasc. Dis. *51*:85, 1982.
287. Romano, C., Gemme, G., and Pongiglione, R.: Aritmie cardiache rare dell'eta pediatrica. II. Accessi sincopali per fibrillazione ventricolare parossistica. La Clinic. Paed. *45*:656, 1963.
288. Ward, O. C.: New familial cardiac syndrome in children. J. Irish Med. Assoc. *54*:103, 1964.
289. Selzer, A., and Wray, H. W.: Quinidine syncope: Paroxysmal ventricular fibrillation occurring during treatment of chronic atrial arrhythmias. Circulation *30*: 17, 1964.
290. Reynolds, E. W., and Vander Ark, C. R.: Quinidine syncope and delayed repolarization syndromes. Mod. Conc. Cardiovasc. Dis. *55*:117, 1976.
291. Tzivoni, D., Keren, A., Stern, S., and Gottlieb, S.: Disopyramide-induced torsades de pointes. Arch. Intern. Med. *141*:946, 1981.
292. Singh, B. N., Gaardner, T. D., Kanegae, T., Goldstein, M., Montgomerie, J. Z., and Mills, H.: Liquid protein diets and torsades de pointes. J.A.M.A. *240*: 115, 1978.
293. Siegel, R. J., Cabeen, W. R., Jr., and Roberts, W. C.: Prolonged QT interval–ventricular tachycardia syndrome from massive rapid weight loss utilizing the liquid protein modified fast diet. Sudden death with sinus node ganglionitis and neuritis. Am. Heart J. *102*:121, 1981.
294. Burch, G. E., Myers, R., and Abildskov, J. A.: New electrocardiographic pattern observed in cerebrovascular accidents. Circulation *9*:719, 1954.
295. Schwartz, P. J., and Wolf, S.: QT interval prolongation as predictor of sudden death in patients with myocardial infarction. Circulation *57*:1074, 1978.

296. Ahnve, S., Lundman, T., and Shoaleh-var, M.: The relationship between QT interval and ventricular arrhythmias in acute myocardial infarction. Acta Med. Scand. *204*:17, 1978.
297. Taylor, G. J., Crampton, R. S., Gibson, R. S., Stebbins, P. T., Waldman, M. T., and Beller, G. A.: Prolonged QT interval at onset of acute myocardial infarction in predicting early phase ventricular tachycardia. Am. Heart J. *102*:16, 1981.
298. Haynes, R. E., Hallstrom, A. P., and Cobb, L. A.: Repolarization abnormalities in survivors of out-of-hospital ventricular fibrillation. Circulation *57*:654, 1978.
299. James, T. N., Zipes, D. P., Finegan, R. E., Eisele, J. W., and Carter, J. E.: Cardiac ganglionitis associated with sudden unexpected death. Ann. Intern. Med. *91*:727, 1979.
300. Bekheit, S., and Ali, A.: QT interval in idiopathic prolapsed mitral valve. Am. J. Cardiol. *41*:374, 1978.
301. Yanowitz, F., Preston, J. B., and Abildskov, J. A.: Functional distribution of right and left stellate innervation to the ventricles: Production of neurogenic electrocardiographic changes by unilateral alteration of sympathetic tone. Cir. Res. *18*:416, 1966.
302. Moss, A. J., and McDonald, J.: Unilateral cervicothoracic sympathetic ganglionectomy for the treatment of long QT syndrome. N. Engl. J. Med. *285*:903, 1971.
303. Schwartz, P. J.: The long QT syndrome. *In* Kulbertus, H. E., and Wellens, H. J. J. (eds.): Sudden Death. The Hague, Martinus Nijhoff, 1980, pp. 358–378.
304. Crampton, R.: Preeminence of left stellate ganglion in the long QT syndrome. Circulation *59*:769, 1979.
305. Zipes, D. P., Martins, J. B., Ruffy, R., Prystowsky, E. N., Elharrar, V., and Gilmour, R. F., Jr.: Roles of autonomic innervation in the genesis of ventricular arrhythmias. *In* Abboud, F. M., et al. (eds.): Disturbances in Neurogenic Control of the Circulation. Bethesda, Md., American Physiological Society, 1981, pp. 225–250.
306. Wellens, H. J. J., Vermeulen, A., and Durrer, D.: Ventricular fibrillation occurring on arousal from sleep by auditory stimuli. Circulation *46*:661, 1972.
307. Lown, B., Temte, J. V., Reich, P., Gaughan, C., Regestein, Q., and Hai, H.: The basis for recurring ventricular fibrillation in the absence of coronary heart disease and its management. N. Engl. J. Med. *294*:623, 1976.
308. Mitsutake, A., Takeshita, A., Kuroiwa, A., and Nakamura, M.: Usefulness of the Valsalva maneuver in management of the long QT syndrome. Circulation *63*:1029, 1981.
309. Marcus, F. I., Fontaine, G. H., Guiraudon, G., Frank, R., Laurenceau, J. L., Malergue, C., and Grosgogeat, Y.: Right ventricular dysplasia: A report of 24 adult cases. Circulation *65*:384, 1982.
310. Dungan, W. T., Garson, A., Jr., and Gillette, P. C.: Arrhythmogenic right ventricular dysplasia. A cause of ventricular tachycardia in children with apparently normal hearts. Am. Heart J. *102*:745, 1981.
311. Guiraudon, G. M., Klein, G. J., Gulamhusein, S. S., Painvin, G. A., DelCampo, C., Gonzales, J. C., and Ko, P. T.: Total disconnection of the right ventricular free wall: Surgical treatment of right ventricular tachycardia associated with right ventricular dysplasia. Ann. Thorac. Surg. (*in press*).
312. Fontaine, G., Guiraudon, G., Frank, R., Fillette, F., Cabrol, C., and Grosgogeat, Y.: Surgical management of ventricular tachycardia unrelated to myocardial ischemia or infarction. Am. J. Cardiol. *49*:397, 1982.
313. Klein, G. J., and Guiraudon, G. M.: Surgical therapy of cardiac arrhythmias. *In* Zipes, D. P. (ed.): Cardiology Clinics. Philadelphia, W. B. Saunders Co., 1983, *in press*.
314. Kavey, R. E., Blackman, M. S., and Sondheimer, H. M.: Incidence and severity of chronic ventricular dysrhythmias after repair of tetralogy of Fallot. Am. Heart J. *103*:342, 1982.
315. Horowitz, L. N., Vetter, V. L., Harken, A. H., and Josephson, M. E.: Electrophysiologic characteristics of sustained ventricular tachycardia occurring after repair of tetralogy of Fallot. Am. J. Cardiol. *46*:446, 1980.
316. Harken, A. H., Horowitz, L. N., and Josephson, M. E.: Surgical correction of recurrent sustained ventricular tachycardia on complete repair of tetralogy of Fallot. J. Thorac. Cardiovasc. Surg. *80*:779, 1980.
317. Coumel, P., Fidelle, J., Lucet, V., Attuel, P., and Bouvrain, Y.: Catecholamine induced severe ventricular arrhythmias with Adams-Stokes syndrome in children: Report of four cases. Br. Heart J. *40*(Suppl.):37, 1978.
318. Coumel, P., Rosengarten, M. D., Leclercq, J. F., and Attuel, P.: Role of sympathetic nervous system in nonischemic ventricular arrhythmias. Br. Heart J. *47*:137, 1982.
319. Ideker, R. E., Klein, G. J., Harrison, L., Smith, W. M., Kasell, J., Reimer, K. A., Wallace, A. G., and Gallagher, J. J.: The transition to ventricular fibrillation induced by reperfusion after acute ischemia in the dog: A period of organized epicardial activation. Circulation *63*:1371, 1981.
320. Raizes, G., Wagner, G. S., and Hackel, D. B.: Instantaneous nonarrhythmic cardiac death in acute myocardial infarction. Am. J. Cardiol. *39*:1, 1977.
321. Cobb, L. A., Werner, J. A., and Trobaugh, G. B.: Sudden cardiac death. I. A decade's experience with out-of-hospital resuscitation. Mod. Conc. Cardiovasc. Dis. *49*:31, 1980.
322. Adgey, A. A., Devlin, J. E., Webb, S. W., and Mulholland, H. C.: Initiation of ventricular fibrillation outside hospital in patients with acute ischemic heart disease. Br. Heart J. *47*:55, 1982.
323. Lie, K. I., Liem, K. L., Schuilenburg, R. M., David, G. K., and Durrer, D.: Early identification of patients developing late in-hospital ventricular fibrillation after discharge from the coronary care unit: A 5½ year retrospective and prospective study of 1,897 patients. Am. J. Cardiol. *41*:674, 1978.
324. Watanabe, Y., and Dreifus, L. S.: Atrioventricular block. Basic concepts. *In* Mandel, W. J., (ed.): Cardiac Arrhythmias. Philadelphia, J. B. Lippincott Co., 1980, p. 406.
325. Narula, O., and Shantha, N.: Atrioventricular block: Clinical concepts and His bundle electrocardiography. *In* Mandel, W. J. (ed.): Cardiac Arrhythmias. Philadelphia, J. B. Lippincott Co., 1980, p. 437.
326. Winternitz, M., and Langendorf, R.: Auriculo-ventricular block with ventriculoauricular response. Am. Heart J. *27*:301, 1944.
327. Damato, A. N., Varghese, P. J., Lau, S. H., Gallagher, J. J., and Bobb, G. A.: Manifest and concealed reentry: A mechanism of AV nodal Wenckebach phenomenon. Circ. Res. *30*:283, 1972.
328. Denes, P., Wu, D., Dhingra, R., Pietras, R., and Rosen, K. M.: The effects of cycle length on cardiac refractory periods in man. Circulation *49*:32, 1974.
329. Wiener, I., Kunkes, S., Rubin, D., Kupersmith, J., Packer, M., Pitchon, R., and Schweitzer, P.: Effects of sudden change in cycle length on human atrial, atrioventricular, nodal and ventricular refractory periods. Circulation *64*:245, 1981.
330. Simson, M. B., Spear, J. F., and Moore, E. N.: Electrophysiologic studies on atrioventricular nodal Wenckebach cycles. Am. J. Cardiol. *41*:244, 1978.
331. Zipes, D. P.: Second degree atrioventricular block. Circulation *60*:465, 1979.
332. El-Sherif, N., Scherlag, D. J., and Lazzara, R.: Pathophysiology of second degree atrioventricular block: A unified hypothesis. Am. J. Cardiol. *35*:421, 1975.
333. Langendorf, R., and Pick, A.: Atrioventricular block, type II (Mobitz). Its nature and clinical significance. Circulation *38*:819, 1968.
334. Dhingra, R. C., Denes, P., Wu, D., Chuquimia, R., and Rosen, K. M.: The significance of second-degree atrioventricular block and bundle branch block. Observations regarding site and type of block. Circulation *49*:638, 1978.
335. Donoso, E., Adler, L. N., and Friedberg, C. K.: Unusual forms of second degree atrioventricular block, including Mobitz type II block, associated with the Morgagni-Adams-Stokes syndrome. Am. Heart J. *67*:150, 1964.
336. Rosen, K. M., Loeb, H. S., Chuquimia, R., Sinno, M. Z., Rahimtoola, S. H., and Gunnar, R. M.: Site of heart block in acute myocardial infarction. Circulation *42*:925, 1970.
337. Tans, A. C., Lie, K. I., and Durrer, D.: Clinical setting and prognostic significance of high degree atrioventricular block in acute inferior myocardial infarction: A study of 144 patients. Am. Heart J. *99*:4, 1980.
338. Damato, A. N., Lau, S. H., Helfant, R. H., Stein, E., Patton, R. D., Scherlag, B. J., and Berkowitz, W. D.: A study of heart block in man using His bundle recordings. Circulation *39*:297, 1969.
339. Narula, O. S., and Samet, P.: Wenckebach and Mobitz type II AV block due to block within the His bundle and bundle branches. Circulation *41*:947, 1970.
340. Schuilenburg, R. M., and Durrer, D.: Observations on atrioventricular conduction in patients with bilateral bundle branch block. Circulation *41*:967, 1970.
341. Rosen, K. M., Loeb, H. S., Gunnar, R. M., and Rahimtoola, S. H.: Mobitz type II block without bundle branch block. Circulation *44*:1111, 1971.
342. Spear, J. F., and Moore, E. N.: Electrophysiologic studies on Mobitz type II second degree heart block. Circulation *44*:1087, 1971.
343. Langendorf, R., and Mehlman, J. S.: Block (non-conducted) AV nodal premature systoles imitating first and second degree AV block. Am. Heart J. *34*:500, 1947.
344. Rosen, K. M., Rahimtoola, S. H., and Gunnar, R . M.: Pseudo AV block secondary to nonpremature nonpropagated His-bundle depolarizations: Documentation by His bundle electrocardiography. Circulation *42*:367, 1970.
345. Spear, J. F., and Moore, E. N.: Influence of brief vagal and stellate nerve stimulation on pacemaker activity and conduction within the atrioventricular conduction system of the dog. Circ. Res. *32*:27, 1973.
346. Massie, B., Scheinman, M. M., Peters, R., Desai, J., Hirschfield, D., and O'Young, J.: Clinical and electrophysiologic findings in patients with paroxysmal slowing of the sinus rate and apparent Mobitz type II atrioventricular block. Circulation *58*:305, 1978.
347. Wenckebach, K. F., and Winterberg, H.: Die Unregelmässige Herztätigkeit. Leipzig, Engelmann, 1927.
348. Gilchrist, A. R.: Clinical aspects of high-grade heart block. Scott. Med. J. *3*: 53, 1958.
349. Mangiardi, L. M., Bonamini, R., Conte, M., Gaita, F., Orzan, F., Presbitero, P., and Brusca, A.: Bedside evaluation of atrioventricular block with narrow QRS complexes: Usefulness of carotid sinus massage and atropine administration. Am. J. Cardiol. *49*:1136, 1982.
350. El-Sherif, N., Aranda, J., Befeler, B., and Lazzara, R.: Atypical Wenckebach periodicity simulating Mobitz II AV block. Br. Heart J. *40*:1376, 1978.
351. Simson, M. B., Spear, J. F., and Moore, E. N.: Electrophysiologic studies on atrioventricular nodal Wenckebach cycles. Am. J. Cardiol. *41*:244, 1978.
352. Denes, P., Levy, L., Pick, A., and Rosen, K. M.: The incidence of typical and atypical AV Wenckebach periodicity. Am. Heart J. *89*:26, 1975.
353. Southall, D. P., Johnston, F., Shinebourne, E. A., and Johnston, P. G.: 24-hour electrocardiograph study of heart rate and rhythm patterns in population of healthy children. Br. Heart J. *45*:281, 1981.
354. Zeppilli, P., Fenici, R., Sassara, M., Pirrami, M. M., and Caselli, G.: Wenckebach second degree AV block in top ranking athletes: An old problem revisited. Am. Heart J. *100*:281, 1980.
355. Vitasalo, M. T., Kala, R., and Eisalo, A.: Ambulatory electrocardiographic recording in endurance athletes. Br. Heart J. *47*:213, 1982.

356. Young, D., Eisenberg, R., Fish, B., and Fisher, J. D.: Wenckebach atrioventricular block (Mobitz I) in children and adolescents. Am. J. Cardiol. *40*:393, 1977.
357. Strasberg, B., Amat-y-Leon, F., Dhingra, R. C., Palileo, E., Swiryn, S., Bauernfeind, R., Wyndham, C., and Rosen, K. M.: Natural history of chronic second degree atrioventricular nodal block. Circulation *63*:1043, 1981.
358. Ferrari, I., Bonazzi, O., Gardumi, M., Gregorini, L., Perondi, R., and Mancia, G.: Modulation of atrioventricular conduction by isometric exercises in human subjects. Circ. Res. *49*:265, 1981.
359. Coumel, P., Fabiato, A., Wayneberger, M., Motte, G., Slama, R., and Bouvrain, Y.: Bradycardia-dependent atrioventricular block. J. Electrocardiol. *4*:168, 1971.
360. Rosenbaum, M. B., Elizari, M. V., Levi, R. J., and Nau, G. J.: Paroxysmal atrioventricular block related to hypotension and spontaneous diastolic depolarization. Chest *63*:678, 1973.
361. Wald, R. W., and Waxman, M. B.: Depression of distal AV conduction following ventricular pacing. PACE *4*:84, 1981.
362. Strasberg, B., Lam, W., Swiryn, S., Bauernfeind, R., Scagliotti, D., Palileo, E., and Rosen, K. M.: Symptomatic spontaneous paroxysmal AV nodal block to localized hyperresponsiveness of the AV node to vagotonic reflexes. Am. Heart J. *103*:795, 1982.
363. Kehoe, R. F., Bauernfeind, R., Tommaso, C., Wyndham, C., and Rosen, K. M.: Cardiac conduction defects in polymyositis: Electrophysiological studies in four patients. Ann. Intern. Med. *94*:41, 1981.
364. Ginks, W., Sutton, R., Siddons, H., and Leatham, A.: Unsuspected coronary artery disease as a cause of chronic atrioventricular block in middle age. Br. Heart J. *44*:699, 1980.
365. Ohkawa, S., Sugiura, M., Itoh, Y., Kitano, K., Hiraoka, K., Ueda, J., and Murakama, M.: Electrophysiologic and histologic correlates in chronic complete atrioventricular block. Circulation *64*:215, 1981.
366. Lev, M.: The pathology of complete atrioventricular block. Progr. Cardiovasc. Dis. *6*:317, 1964.
367. Lenegre, J.: Bilateral bundle branch block. Cardiologia *48*:134, 1966.
368. Ayres, C. R., Boineau, J. P., and Spach, M. S.: Congenital complete heart block in children. Am. Heart J. *72*:381, 1966.
369. Besley, D. C., McWilliams, G. J., Moodie, D. S., and Castle, L. W.: Long-term followup of young adults following permanent pacemaker placement for complete heart block. Am. Heart J. *103*:332, 1982.
370. Esscher, E.: Congenital complete heart block. Acta Pediat. Scand. *70*:131, 1981.
371. Karpawich, P. P., Gillette, P. C., Garson, A., Jr., Hesslein, P. S., Porter, C. B., and McNamara, D. G.: Congenital complete atrioventricular block: Clinical and electrophysiologic predictors of need for pacemaker insertion. Am. J. Cardiol. *48*:109, 1981.
372. Benson, D. W., Jr., Spach, M. S., Edwards, S. B., Sterba, R., Serwer, G. A., Armstrong, B. E., and Anderson, P. A.: Heart block in children. Evaluation of subsidiary ventricular pacemaker recovery times and ECG tape recordings. Pediat. Cardiol. *2*:39, 1982.
373. Mond, H. G.: The bradyarrhythmias: Current indications for permanent pacing (Part I). PACE *4*:432, 1981.
374. Mond, H. G.: The bradyarrhythmias: Current indications for permanent pacing (Part II). PACE *4*:538, 1981.
375. Pick, A.: AV dissociation: A proposal for a comprehensive classification and consistent terminology. Am. Heart J. *66*:147, 1963.

22 CARDIAC PACEMAKERS

by Douglas P. Zipes, M.D., and Edwin G. Duffin, Ph.D.

The artificial cardiac pacemaker is an electronic device that delivers electrical stimuli to the heart to treat bradycardias and tachycardias. Essential elements include a power source, usually a battery, which supplies energy for the stimuli and circuitry; an electronic circuit to regulate the timing and characteristics of the stimuli; and a lead composed of electrodes on a catheter or wire to connect the battery and circuit to the heart. The electrode is the uninsulated portion of the lead in contact with the body. At first, pacemakers were external units that provided temporary pacing by delivering stimuli to the skin[1] or to the heart through a lead, with the electronics and power source remaining outside the body. For many clinical situations, temporary pacemakers are still needed. The first totally implantable devices were reported in the late 1950s.[2,3] Today, an estimated one million patients worldwide have implanted pacemakers (500,000 in the United States). Advances in technology have been applied rapidly to pacemaker systems, and pacemakers themselves have changed dramatically from the 250-gram, asynchronous devices of the early 1960s. Present-day systems provide noninvasively programmable single- and dual-chamber pacemakers, which weigh typically 40 to 50 grams, last an estimated six to ten years, and are highly reliable.

INDICATIONS FOR PACING

Pacemakers are employed to treat patients who have symptomatic bradycardias and tachycardias. (The use of pacing as a diagnostic tool is discussed in Chapter 20.) The nature of the arrhythmia and how likely it will persist or recur determine whether pacing, either temporary or permanent, is indicated (Table 22-1). As a general rule, drugs do not successfully and reliably speed up the heart rate or improve atrioventricular (AV) conduction for longer than several hours to several days in patients who have symptomatic bradycardias, without producing intolerable side effects. Therefore, regardless of the arrhythmia causing the bradycardia (e.g., sinus bradycardia or AV block), pacing may be indicated in such cases. In addition, pacing may be used both to terminate and to prevent a recurrence of some forms of tachycardia. The type of tachycardia and clinical setting determine whether pacing should be employed. Most often, other therapeutic approaches, particularly drugs and electrical cardioversion, are tried before pacing is instituted. The choice between temporary and permanent pacing is based on whether the rhythm disturbance is likely to be transient or permanent.

TEMPORARY PACING FOR BRADYCARDIAS. Temporary pacing is indicated in a variety of circumstances in which a symptomatic bradycardia is present or is likely to occur, such as after cardiac surgery,[4] during right heart catheterization in patients with preexisting left bundle branch block, during administration of some drugs that might inappropriately slow the heart rate, and prior to implanting a permanent pacemaker in patients with symptomatic bradycardia. Temporary pacing may also be useful in some patients who have symptoms of heart failure associated with reduced cardiac output secondary to a slow rate (Table 22–1).

Temporary Pacing During Acute Myocardial Infarction (See also p. 1306). The role of temporary pacing during acute myocardial infarction (MI) in patients who develop *AV conduction disturbances* is controversial because the risk-to-benefit ratio is unclear. For untreated patients who develop AV block in this situation the mortality rate is not well established, often because reported studies are spuriously influenced by forms of AV block that do not require pacing. For example, patients who develop an inferior wall MI may have first-degree or type I second-degree AV block combined with an accelerated AV junctional rhythm, giving rise to complete AV dissociation (p. 735). These patients are commonly misclassified as having complete AV block. Since the second-degree AV block and junctional rhythm are usually transient and do not require therapy,[5] this group is considered erroneously to have recovered from complete AV block, a classification that favorably biases the results regarding the natural history of complete AV block during acute MI. Furthermore, causes of death not directly related to the conduction disturbance, such as ventricular fibrillation, may lead to sudden death of these patients.[6] Such a death may be reported incorrectly as being due to complete heart block. However, it seems fairly clear, that the extent of myocardial involvement and resultant degree of heart failure are the most important prognostic factors in patients who develop AV conduction disturbances during acute MI.[7,8]

P-R interval prolongation during acute MI has been reported to be associated with an increased incidence of progression to high-degree AV block.[6,7,9,10] Although P-R prolongation often occurs in patients in whom high-degree AV block follows, the significance of this finding in any given patient is obscure. In the setting of bundle branch block, it may reflect block at the AV nodal level, combined AV nodal and His-Purkinje system conduction delay, or His-Purkinje delay alone. Abrupt complete heart block frequently occurs without demonstrable prior P-R prolongation. Therefore, although P-R interval prolongation and the development of high-degree AV block may be related statistically, they may not be causally related. For example, P-R interval delay may be due to preexistent AV nodal disturbance, while sudden complete heart block may be due to an acute His-Purkinje block. Thus, first-degree AV block that develops before or during acute MI as an isolated finding is not an indication for temporary pacing.

Type I second-degree AV block (p. 731) most commonly occurs during acute *inferior* MI, presumably owing to transient ischemia or increased vagal tone in the region of the AV node, while *type II second-degree AV block* (p. 731) commonly occurs during acute *anterior* MI, resulting from a large infarction that includes the interventricular septum.[11–13] Type I second-degree AV block generally is transient, blocks in the AV node, is not associated with symptoms, and does not require pacing. On the other hand, type II second-degree AV block is most commonly due to block in the His-Purkinje system, occurs in the setting of a bundle branch block, may progress to complete AV block, and requires temporary pacing.[14,15] Whether or not pacing is attempted, type II AV block is associated with a high mortality because of the concomitant large MI.[16]

Patients who develop first-degree or type I second-degree AV block with a normal QRS complex and only axis deviation generally do not require prophylactic pacing. Uncommonly, acute inferior MI results in a bradycardia that does require pacing. This may be a sinus bradycardia, or second-degree or complete AV block that is not transient and does not respond satisfactorily to atropine.[10]

Available data on the significance of *H-V interval prolongation* as an indicator of progression to high-degree AV block in acute MI have led to controversial conclusions. Most patients studied who progress to complete heart block do demonstrate H-V interval prolongation during acute MI.[6] However, this finding does not necessarily imply that complete heart block is imminent, particularly if the H-V interval prolongation preceded the onset of acute MI—a fact not always known. Thus, the clinical usefulness of recording the H-V interval to predict subsequent development of complete AV block as well as survival during acute MI is still not settled.[7]

Development of *complete AV block* should be considered in the same manner as type II second-degree AV block. As mentioned earlier, it is important not to confuse the diagnosis of complete AV dissociation with complete AV block (see Chapter 21). Mortality is influenced in large measure by the severity of the underlying heart disease. However, patients who develop type II second-degree or complete AV block without pulmonary edema or shock still have a higher mortality rate than patients who do not have advanced AV block, with many deaths due to the abrupt development of AV block.[16] Therefore, temporary pacing is clearly indicated in this group of patients.

Temporary pacing is warranted in patients who develop *bifascicular block* (defined as alternating right and left bundle branch block), right bundle branch block with left axis deviation, right bundle branch block with right axis deviation, and perhaps left bundle branch block with P-R interval prolongation when they appear to be at increased risk of developing high-degree AV block.[7,10,15,16] Left bundle branch block with P-R prolongation is included in this group, because while these findings may represent bifascicular block in association with AV nodal disease, the majority of these patients have a prolonged H-V interval and probably trifascicular disease.

The role of prophylactic pacing in the setting of acute anterior MI with new right bundle branch block and a normal axis or with new left bundle branch block and a normal P-R interval is more controversial; however, some evidence of decreased morbidity associated with pacing seems to justify its use in patients who do not have heart failure, provided that the complication rate of inserting a temporary pacing catheter is low.[7] It would appear that *preexisting, stable* right bundle branch block or left bundle branch block with or without axis deviation is *not* an indication for prophylactic pacing, whether the block is present in a patient who has an acute infarction or in other situations, such as in patients undergoing surgery. While the development of bifascicular block is associated with a higher incidence of progression to advanced AV block, the mortality among patients who develop new bundle branch block and acute MI is similar to that among patients who had bundle branch block prior to the infarction.[17,19]

In summary, prophylactic temporary pacing appears warranted in patients who have an acute MI and who develop type II second- or third-degree AV block or bifascicular block of recent onset.[7] Bundle branch block complicating acute MI identifies the individual at significant risk of developing congestive heart failure, with mortality often secondary to myocardial failure or refractory ventricular arrhythmias. The presence of high-degree AV block per se appears to increase mortality in patients without pump failure, and immediate survival may be enhanced by prophylactic pacing in patients at high risk for developing abrupt complete heart block complicating acute

TABLE 22–1 PACING INDICATIONS

	Definitely Indicated	Probably Indicated	Probably Not Indicated	Definitely Not Indicated
Complete AV Block				
Congenital (AV nodal)				
Asymptomatic				X
Symptomatic	T,P			
Acquired (His-Purkinje)				
Asymptomatic		T,P		
Symptomatic	T,P			
Surgical (persistent)				
Asymptomatic	T	P		
Symptomatic	T,P			
Second-degree AV Block				
Type I (AV nodal)				
Asymptomatic				X
Symptomatic	T,P			
Type II (His-Purkinje)				
Asymptomatic		T,P		
Symptomatic	T,P			
First-degree AV Block				
AV Nodal				
Asymptomatic				X
Symptomatic			X	
His-Purkinje				
Asymptomatic				X
Symptomatic			X	
Bundle Branch Block				
Asymptomatic				X
Symptomatic				
Normal H-V		P‡		
Prolonged H-V	P			
Distal His block at paced atrial rates < 130/min	P			
LBBB during right heart catheterization	T			
Acute Myocardial Infarction				
Newly acquired bifascicular BBB	T			
Preexisting BBB				X
Newly acquired BBB plus transient complete AV block	T	P		
Second-degree AV block				
Type I (asymptomatic)				X
Type II	T	P		
Complete AV block	T	P		
Atrial Fibrillation with Slow Ventricular Response				
Asymptomatic				*X*
Symptomatic	*T,P*			
Sick Sinus Syndrome				
Asymptomatic			X	
Symptomatic	T,P			
Hypersensitive Carotid Sinus Syndrome				
Asymptomatic			X	
Symptomatic	T,P			
Bradycardia-Tachycardia Syndrome				
Asymptomatic			X	
Symptomatic	T,P			
Bradycardia-Miscellaneous				
Asymptomatic			X	
Symptomatic	T,P			
Tachycardia Prevention$^{\Delta}$				
Associated with bradycardia	T,P			
Associated with long Q-T, torsades de pointes	T	P		
Not associated with bradycardia, long Q-T, torsades de pointes (after drug failure)		T	P**	

TABLE 22–1 PACING INDICATIONS (*Continued*)

	Definitely Indicated	Probably Indicated	Probably Not Indicated	Definitely Not Indicated
Tachycardia Termination (after drug failure) **Δ				
Atrial flutter	T,P			
Atrial fibrillation				X
AV nodal reentry	T,P			
Reciprocating tachycardia in WPW syndrome	T,PΠ			
Ventricular tachycardia	Tss	Pss		

T = Temporary pacing; P = permanent pacing; X = pacing not indicated
BBB = Bundle branch block; LBBB = left bundle branch block
HV = Measure of His-Purkinje conduction time
Δ = Site and rate of stimulation may influence success
Π = Atrial fibrillation with a rapid ventricular response may be a complication
** = Prove efficacy with temporary pacing
ss = May accelerate VT
‡ = No other cause found for symptoms

MI but who do not manifest evidence of heart failure. The assumption that prophylactic pacing improves the survival of patients who have bundle branch block and significant heart failure complicating acute MI remains speculative. Finally, patients who develop symptomatic bradycardia of any type that responds poorly to drug therapy should be considered as candidates for pacing.

TEMPORARY PACING FOR TACHYCARDIAS (See also p. 672 and Chapter 21). Temporary pacing may be useful to *terminate* a variety of tachycardias, including atrial flutter (p. 697), reciprocating tachycardias involving the sinus or AV node or an accessory pathway (p. 707), and some sustained ventricular tachycardias (p. 724). Isolated examples of other tachycardias terminated by pacing have been reported. Pacing does *not* terminate atrial or ventricular fibrillation. It is used generally when drug therapy has been ineffective and/or electrical cardioversion is contraindicated (suspicion of digitalis toxicity, for example), when cardioversion is required repeatedly owing to frequent recurrence of the tachycardia, or when a pacing catheter is already in place.[20]

Pacing can *prevent* several types of tachycardias, such as those associated with significant bradycardias like complete AV block or with a prolonged Q-T interval that result in torsades de pointes[21,22] (see Fig. 21–38, p. 725). Patients who have the bradycardia-tachycardia syndrome may require pacing after termination of the tachycardia to prevent the bradycardia (p. 693). Use of rapid pacing rates may suppress premature beats and prevent some tachycardias from recurring. Paired or coupled atrial pacing may reduce the venticular rate if the premature atrial complex blocks in the AV junction; paired or coupled ventricular stimulation may reduce the effective ventricular rate if the premature ventricular complex results in electrical without mechanical systole. However, such premature stimulation risks precipitation of fibrillation. Finally, temporary atrial pacing has been used as a stress test in patients suspected of having coronary artery disease.[23]

PERMANENT PACING FOR BRADYCARDIAS. As with temporary pacing, permanent pacing is indicated in patients who have *symptomatic bradycardia*, regardless of the nature of the arrhythmia, as long as the bradycardia is likely to be permanent or recurrent; i.e., it is not associated with a transient condition such as acute MI or drug toxicity. The most common indication for permanent pacing—responsible for 50 percent of all implants—is fixed or intermittent complete third-degree AV block,[24] with sclerotic degeneration of the AV conducting system being the primary etiology. An additional 26 percent of pacemaker implants are to treat patients who have the sick sinus syndrome,[24] manifest as sinus arrest or block, severe sinus bradycardia, or alternating periods of bradycardia and supraventricular tachycardia (brady-tachy syndrome, see p. 693). In these patients, drugs used to treat the tachycardia may aggravate the bradycardia, requiring permanent pacing for the latter. Patients symptomatic from sinus bradycardia or AV block caused by hypersensitive carotid sinus syndrome[25] or slow ventricular rates during chronic atrial fibrillation[26] are also candidates for pacemakers. Sometimes asystole or bradycardia occurs only at the termination of a tachycardia and may be responsible for the patient's symptoms.

Major questions arise when one is considering prophylactic permanent pacing. There is general—although not complete—agreement that permanent pacing is indicated in *asymptomatic* patients who have acquired complete AV block or well-documented, type II second-degree AV block, since their natural history appears to progress to the point of symptoms. Although patients with documented transient high-degree AV block are at a substantial risk of sudden death, one could argue against permanently pacing a sedentary elderly individual who has complete AV block but has been completely asymptomatic.

The prognosis for patients who have *chronic bundle branch block* depends to a large extent on the presence and etiology as well as the severity of the associated heart disease. In most patients, the terminal event is usually one of heart failure or the complications of coronary artery disease. In the absence of clinically detectable heart disease, the long-term prognosis for this group of patients is good without pacing. Ventricular arrhythmias occur more often in patients who have chronic bundle branch block than in the normal population, but the mechanism of sudden death in any given patient is speculative. Most patients who die suddenly, especially those who have coronary artery disease, probably develop ventricular fibrillation. No clinical variable (such as age, syncope, angina, or shortness of breath), physical finding (such as an S_3 gallop, cardiomegaly, or heart failure), or electrocardiographic finding (such as right bundle branch block with left axis deviation, right bundle branch block with right axis devation, or P-R interval prolongation) is useful in predicting progression to complete heart block. All the above variables occur frequently in patients who have bundle branch block, yet the progression to complete heart block is relatively infrequent.

A recent study indicates that more patients who have chronic bifascicular block with a prolonged H-V interval develop AV block than do patients who have a normal H-V interval (0.6 vs. 4.5 per cent), but the risk of developing trifascicular block is still small, and routine permanent pacing is not warranted in patients with chronic bifascicular block with a prolonged H-V interval.[27] Development of His-Purkinje block during atrial pacing at rates less than 130 ppm appears to be a possible marker for development of complete heart block.[28] However, the opposite—namely a normal H-V interval—does not exclude progression to complete heart block. Data for patients with unexplained recurrent syncope or presyncope and bundle branch block suggest that permanent pacing is reasonable therapy only after an effort has been made to exclude noncardiac and other cardiac causes for the symptoms. Some observers believe that documentation of bradyarrhythmia or measurement of the H-V interval is essential prior to institution of pacing in these patients.

Finally, several studies indicate that permanent prophylactic pacing reduces sudden death in survivors of acute MI complicated by bundle branch block and transient high-degree AV block. However, the number of patients studied is small and the data are not conclusive.[10,16]

PERMANENT PACING FOR TACHYCARDIAS. Preventing tachycardia has become an important therapeutic application of pacing, for which several approaches are available. Tachycardias that occur only in the setting of bradycardias can be prevented by pacing at normal rates. In general, pacing at accelerated rates to prevent recurrences of tachycardias in patients who otherwise have normal heart rates and rhythms is not successful over the long term. Therefore, except for bradycardia-related tachycardia, the most successful application of antitachycardia pacing in this area is to *terminate* tachycardias after they start[4,29–31] rather than to *prevent* their occurrence.[29,32–34]

PACEMAKER MODALITIES

Pacemakers perform basically two functions: they all stimulate the heart, and most can sense impulses as well, i.e., they are equipped with amplifiers that register or recognize (sense) a spontaneous cardiac electrical event and then use that information to modulate the timing of the electrical stimulus delivered (pace). These two functions can be carried out in the atrium or ventricle, or in both chambers.[35,36] Sensing and stimulation are accomplished with electrode pairs directly contacting the myocardium (a bipolar system) or with one electrode located at the heart and a second electrode, usually the pacemaker case, located remotely (a unipolar system).

Because pacemakers operate in a variety of complex combinations, a letter code—originally three positions[37] and now five[38]—has been devised as a shorthand notation to identify the different types of pacemakers (Table 22–2). Symbols placed in the first two positions indicate the chambers in which the pacemaker paces (first position) and in which it senses (second position). "A" or "V" indicates that the device paces or senses the atrium or the ventricle; "D" indicates that it paces or senses in both chambers. "S" indicates a single-chamber unit designed to be suitable for either atrial or ventricular pacing, depending on how its parameters are programed. The third position signifies in what manner the pacemaker responds to spontaneous electrical activity. "O" indicates that the pacemaker does not sense spontaneous electrical activity and therefore discharges at a fixed rate and is not influenced by cardiac events. "I" indicates that the pacemaker is inhibited from delivering a stimulus for a certain period of time in response to sensed electrical activity; i.e.,

TABLE 22–2 FIVE-POSITION PACEMAKER CODE

I. Chamber Paced	II. Chamber Sensed	III. Mode of Response	IV. Programmability	V. Tachyarrhythmia Functions*
V = Ventricle	V = Ventricle	I = Inhibited	P = Programmable rate and/or output	B = Burst
A = Atrium	A = Atrium	T = Triggered	M = Multiprogrammable	N = Normal rate competition
D = Atrium and ventricle	D = Atrium and ventricle	D = Atrial triggered and ventricular inhibited	O = None	S = Scanning
	O = None	R = Reverse		E = Externally activated
S = single chamber	S = single chamber	O = None		O = None

This table provides a "shorthand" description of pacemaker operation. Symbols placed in the first two positions indicate chambers in which the pacemaker functions; a symbol in the third position, the mode of operation of the pacemaker; in the fourth position, its programmable characteristics; and in the fifth position, its antitachycardia features. For example, if the pacing lead were inserted into the ventricle and the pulse generator were a ventricular demand inhibited unit, the chamber paced would be ventricle and the first letter in the five position code would be "V." The chamber sensed would be ventricle and, therefore, the second letter in the five-position code would also be "V." The mode of response of the pacemaker would be to inhibit a pacing spike when spontaneous electrical activity were sensed and, therefore, "I" would be in the third position. If only the rate and/or output of the pulse generator could be programed externally, "P" would be in the fourth position. If the pacemaker were used to treat tachycardias, the tachyarrhythmia function would be indicated in the fifth position. Pulse generators that pace or sense in both atrium and ventricle are indicated by the designation "D," meaning dual. If the pacemaker does not have a function in one of the classifications, "O" is used. Finally, some pacemakers have a "reverse" function in that they discharge when the rate becomes too fast (and are thus used to terminate tachycardias). These pacemakers are indicated by the letter "R" in the third position. The different types of tachyarrhythmia functions are discussed in the chapter. Recently, the letter "C" has been suggested for the fourth position to indicate a "communicating" function, i.e., telemetry, with programmable features assumed.

An "S" may be used as a manufacturer's designation to label multiprogrammable single-chamber pacemakers adaptable for either atrial or ventricular use.

* The fourth and fifth positions are optional, as is a comma separating the third and fourth positions.

its discharge cycle is "reset" by the spontaneous event. "T" indicates that a stimulus is discharged in response to sensed activity, while "D" in the third position indicates that the pacemaker responds to sensed atrial activity by delivering a stimulus to the ventricle; i.e., it acts as an artificial AV node but responds to sensed ventricular activity by inhibiting its ventricular stimulus (it is reset). "R" indicates the response mode of a special type of pacemaker used to treat patients who have certain kinds of tachycardias. It discharges stimuli when the sensed heart rate *exceeds* a preset value and is quiescent at normal heart rates. Thus, it functions in reverse relative to most pacemakers, which are usually quiescent when the heart rate exceeds a particular value and discharge when the patient's rate falls below that preset value.

The fourth and fifth positions have been newly added. Position four indicates whether and to what extent pacemaker function can be reversibly changed noninvasively ("programed"). "P" indicates that only the rate and/or output can be altered, while "M" designates that other functions—such as sensitivity, duration of amplifier refractoriness, and so forth—can also be programed. Recently, a "C" has been added to indicate a "communicating" feature, i.e., telemetry, with programmable functions assumed to be present. The fifth position is reserved for pacemakers used to treat tachycardias. Stimuli may be delivered as a burst, "B" (a short train of generally rapid sequential stimuli); at a normal rate, "N," in fixed-rate competition with the tachycardia; or at various intervals that automatically scan the cardiac cycle, "S," in an effort to find the appropriate premature interval that will successfully terminate the tachycardia.

TABLE 22–3 SENSING AND PACING CAPABILITIES OF AVAILABLE PACING MODALITIES

		Senses		Paces	
Pacemaker Type	ICHD Code	*Atrium*	*Ventricle*	*Atrium*	*Ventricle*
Atrial asynchronous	AOO			X	
Ventricular asynchronous	VOO				X
Atrial demand	AAI, AAT	X		X	
Ventricular demand	VVI, VVT		X		X
Atrial synchronous	VAT	X			X
Atrial synchronous ventricular inhibited	VDD	X	X		X
AV sequential	DVI		X	X	X
Optimal sequential	DDD	X	X	X	X

The most commonly implanted pacemaker today is the demand ventricular pacemaker. It paces the ventricle (V), senses ventricular activity (V), and is inhibited from discharging (I) by sensed ventricular events—hence, the VVI pacemaker. If its rate and output only were programmable (P) and it delivered a burst of stimuli (B) in response to a tachycardia, it would be designated VVIPB.

Each of the pacing modalities has different functional capabilities (Table 22–3) and therefore specific indications and contraindications, which will be reviewed (Table 22–4).

TABLE 22–4 INDICATIONS AND CONTRAINDICATIONS FOR AVAILABLE PACING MODES

Mode	Indications	Contraindications	Advantages	Disadvantages
AOO	• Obsolete			
VOO	• Obsolete			
AAI, AAT	• SSS with normal AV conduction	• Atrial inexcitability • High atrial threshold • Abnormal AV conduction	• Simplest system providing properly timed sequential AV contraction; requires only one lead	• Ventricle not paced should AV block develop
VVI, VVT	• SSS without retrograde AV conduction • SSS with no hemodynamic benefit of atrial pacing • Chronic atrial fibrillation or flutter with AV block and a slow ventricular rate	• Hemodynamic insufficiency due to loss of AV synchrony ("pacemaker syndrome")	• Historical inertia • Relative simplicity	• Does not provide AV synchronous contraction • Rate does not change in response to external demands
VAT, VDD	• Normal sinus node function with impaired AV conduction	• Inappropriate atrial tachycardia or bradycardia • Retrograde atrial activation following ventricular stimulation or PVCs	• Maintains atrial transport and normal sinus control of ventricular rate when atrial rate is within tracking limits of pacemaker	• Does not maintain synchronous contractions during atrial bradycardia, since it does not pace the atria • Requires two leads
DVI	• Atrial bradyarrhythmias with or without impaired AV conduction	• Extended periods of atrial fibrillation/flutter	• Maintains sequential AV contraction during sinus bradycardia	• Does not alter rate in response to physiological demands • Does not maintain AV synchronous contractions during periods of normal sinus rhythm and AV block • Competitive atrial pacing during normal sinus rhythm • Requires two leads
DDD	• Atrial bradyarrhythmias with or without impaired AV conduction • Normal sinus node function with impaired AV conduction	• Retrograde atrial activation following ventricular stimulation or PVCs • Extended periods of atrial fibrillation/flutter • Frequent atrial tachycardias	• Maintains sequential AV contraction and sinus control of ventricular rate during normal sinus rhythm and during sinus bradycardia	• Requires two leads

SSS = Sick sinus syndrome

ATRIAL ASYNCHRONOUS

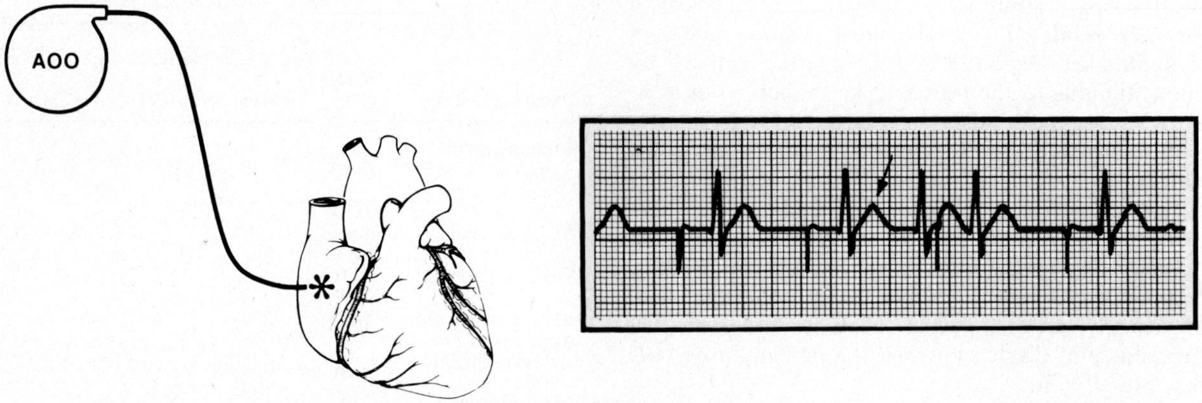

FUNCTION: PACES ATRIUM

FIGURE 22–1 Atrial asynchronous pacemaker (AOO). *Left,* Schematic diagram of heart with an asynchronous atrial pacemaker connected to the right atrium. Asterisk at atrial lead termination indicates that the device stimulates in the atrium. Letters labeling the pacemaker conform to the first three positions of the pacemaker code, as indicated in Table 22–2. *Right,* Representative ECG produced by atrial asynchronous pacing. The first, second, fourth, and fifth ventricular complexes are normally conducted following atrial paced complexes. The third ventricular complex was normally conducted following a spontaneous atrial depolarization (arrow). Pacemaker timing was not reset by this spontaneous atrial event because the pacemaker has no sensing capability.

ATRIAL AND VENTRICULAR ASYNCHRONOUS PACEMAKERS (AOO, VOO). The original pacemakers simply stimulated the myocardium at a constant rate independent of the underlying cardiac rhythm; used for pacing only, these pacemakers could not sense any spontaneous activity. Placed in the atrium, the pacemaker is called an asynchronous atrial pacemaker (AOO) (Fig. 22–1); in the ventricle, it is a ventricular asynchronous pacemaker (VOO) (Fig. 22–2). Asynchronous pacemakers are rarely used today.

ATRIAL AND VENTRICULAR DEMAND PACEMAKERS (AAI, AAT, VVI, VVT). In the early 1970s, sensing circuits were added to pacemakers so that they stimulated only on demand when they could sense no appropriate underlying spontaneous rhythm. This sensing function prevented both competitive pacing and the attendant risk of inducing ventricular fibrillation. *Demand pacemakers* may operate in inhibited (I) and triggered (T) modes. Inhibited devices withhold the stimulus and reset their timing upon sensing spontaneous cardiac activity. *Triggered devices* are designed to deliver a stimulus immediately upon sensing spontaneous depolarization, into the absolute refractory period of the tissue, and simultaneously to reset their timing. Both types deliver a stimulus at the end of their timing cycle (pacemaker escape interval) if no spontaneous cardiac activity is detected (Figs. 22–3

VENTRICULAR ASYNCHRONOUS

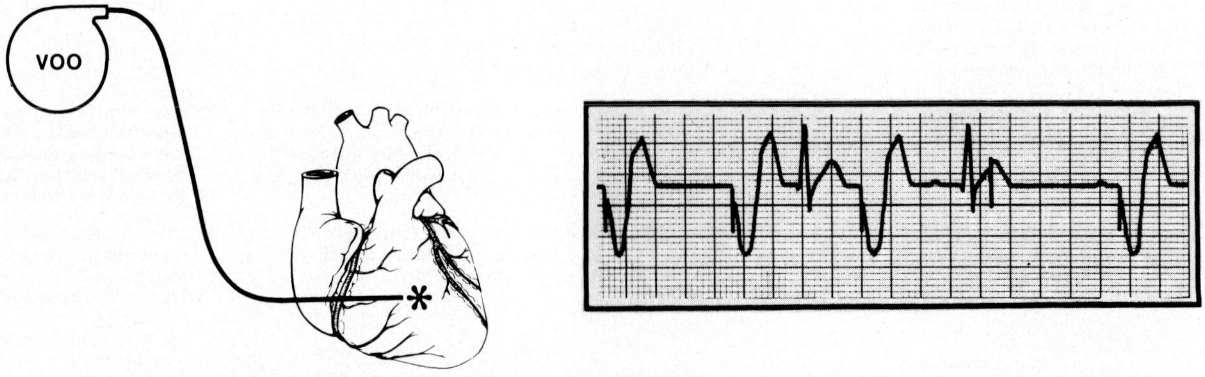

FUNCTION: PACES VENTRICLE

FIGURE 22–2 Ventricular asynchronous pacemaker (VOO). *Left,* Schematic diagram showing a VOO pacemaker connected to the right ventricle, with an asterisk at the lead termination to indicate that the pacemaker stimulates in the ventricle. *Right,* Representative ECG produced by ventricular asynchronous pacing. The first, second, fourth, and sixth ventricular complexes are produced by ventricular pacing. The third and fifth complexes result from conduction of normal sinus atrial activity and do not alter the pacemaker timing, since this device has no sensing capability. The stimulus in the T wave of the next-to-last QRS complex is ineffective because it occurs during the ventricular refractory period.

ATRIAL DEMAND

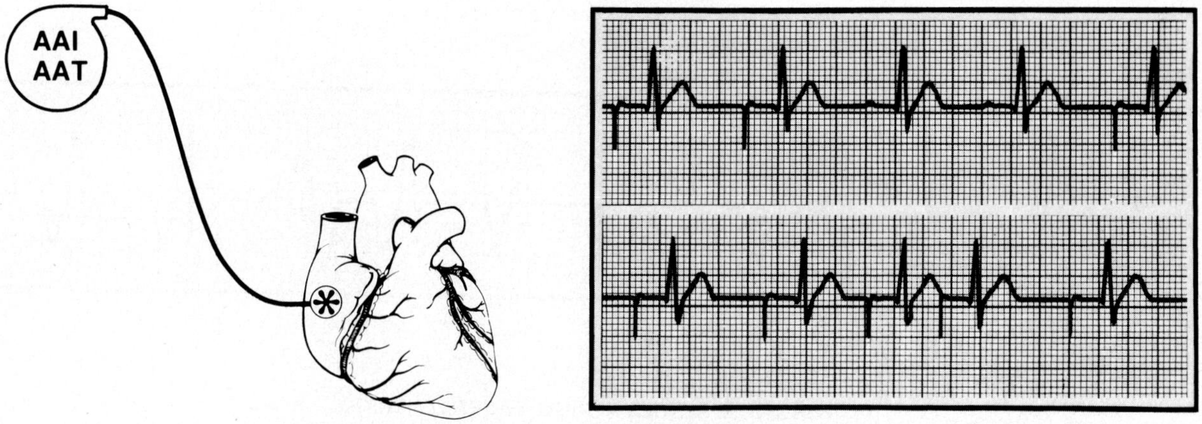

FUNCTION: PACES, SENSES ATRIUM

FIGURE 22–3 Atrial demand pacemakers (AAI, AAT). *Left,* Schematic diagram showing an atrial demand pacemaker connected to the right atrium. The lead termination is marked with a circle to indicate that the pacemaker senses atrial cardiac activity and an asterisk to indicate that the pacemaker stimulates in the atrium. *Right,* Representative ECGs produced by atrial inhibited (AAI, upper tracing) and atrial triggered (ATT, lower tracing) pacing. In the upper tracing, the first, second, and fifth atrial complexes are pacemaker-induced; the third and fouth atrial complexes are spontaneous and reset the pacemaker timing while inhibiting delivery of the stimulus. In the lower tracing, the first, second, and fifth atrial complexes are pacemaker-induced; the third and fourth atrial complexes are spontaneous and reset the pacemaker timing while triggering delivery of the stimulus into refractory atrial tissue. Note that the stimulus is delivered *after* the onset of the third and fourth P waves but initiates the other P waves.

and 22–4). The sensing circuits of these pacemakers are turned off for a period of time following delivery of a stimulus or sensing of spontaneous activity to avoid recognition of inappropriate signals such as T waves. This time interval is called the *pacemaker refractory period.*

The triggered mode was proposed to address concerns that unipolar inhibited devices might allow a patient to become asystolic if extracardiac signals were sensed (e.g, pectoral muscle potentials, electrical signals from radio transmitters or power lines) and were erroneously interpreted to be cardiac signals and thus inhibited pacemaker output. Modern circuitry has reduced the likelihood

VENTRICULAR DEMAND

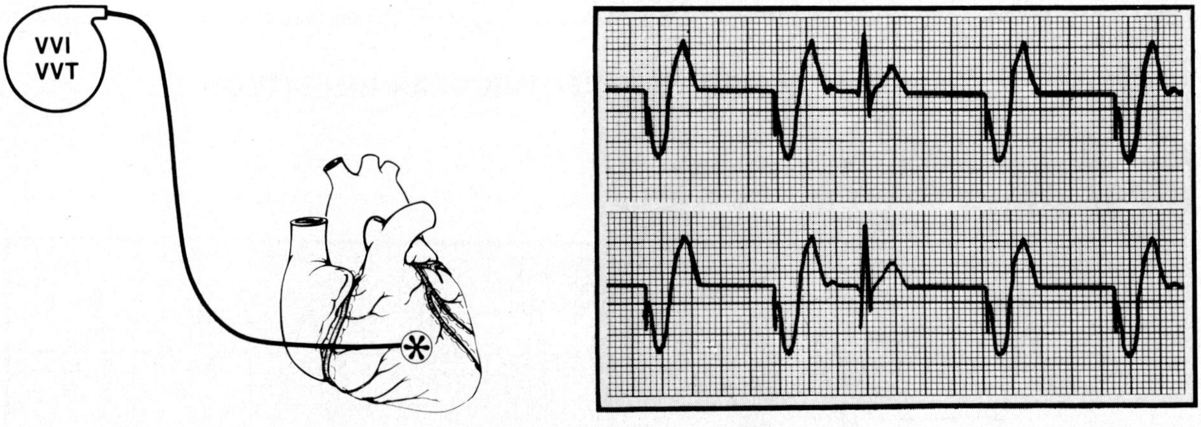

FUNCTION: PACES, SENSES VENTRICLE

FIGURE 22–4 Ventricular demand pacemakers (VVI, VVT). *Left,* Schematic diagram showing a ventricular demand pacemaker connected to the right ventricle, with a circle and an asterisk at the lead termination to indicate that the pacemaker senses ventricular cardiac activity and stimulates in the ventricle. *Right,* Representative ECGs produced by ventricular inhibited (VVI, upper tracing) and ventricular triggered (VVT, lower tracing) pacing. In the upper tracing, the first, second, fourth, and fifth ventricular complexes are pacemaker-induced; the third ventricular complex results from normally conducted sinus activity. This ventricular complex resets the pacemaker timing and inhibits delivery of the ventricular stimulus. In the lower tracing, the first, second, fourth, and fifth ventricular complexes are pacemaker-induced; the third ventricular complex is the result of normally conducted sinus activity. This ventricular complex resets the pacemaker timing and triggers delivery of the stimulus into the refractory ventricular tissue. Note that the stimulus is delivered *after* the onset of the third QRS complex but initiates the other QRS complexes.

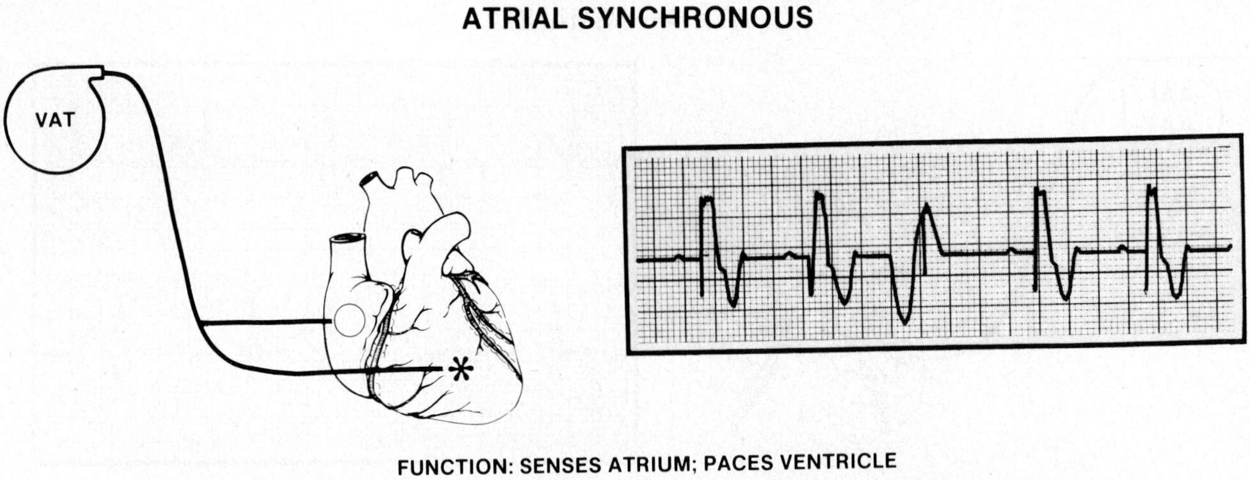

FIGURE 22–5 Atrial synchronous pacemaker (VAT). *Left,* Schematic diagram showing a VAT pacemaker with leads connected to the right atrium and ventricle. The circle at the atrial lead termination indicates that the pacemaker senses atrial activity and the asterisk at the ventricular lead termination indicates that the pacemaker stimulates in the ventricle. *Right,* Representative ECG produced by atrial synchronous ventricular pacing. The first, second, fourth, and fifth ventricular complexes are stimulated by the pacemaker in response to pacemaker sensing of the spontaneous atrial activity. The third ventricular complex is a PVC that occurs simultaneously with a sinus-initiated atrial event. Since the pacemaker does not sense ventricular activity, it is triggered by the P wave (obscured by the PVC) and delivers a ventricular stimulus into the ST segment of the PVC.

of such occurrences. The disadvantages of stimulating when not really necessary, such as distorting the ECG waveform and draining more power from the pacemaker, have resulted in relatively little use of the triggered mode. However, the triggered mode can be valuable in terminating some tachycardias. For example, since the implanted unit senses electrical activity, it can be triggered to pace the heart in response to a series of stimuli delivered to the patient's chest wall from an external source. Also, triggered units are helpful diagnostically to be certain when or if the pacemaker sensed a spontaneous event, since in essence it "marks" that event by delivering a stimulus. Triggered function, therefore, is generally available in modern programmable pacemakers as an option for either permanent or temporary (diagnostic) purposes.

ATRIAL SYNCHRONOUS VENTRICULAR PACEMAKERS (VAT, VDD). To approximate normal cardiac function more closely, sophisticated dual-chamber (atrium and ventricle) "physiologic" pacemakers were developed. The *atrial synchronous ventricular pacemaker* (VAT) (Fig. 22–5) was designed for use in patients with normal sinus node function but impaired AV conduction.[39] This device senses atrial activity by means of an electrode in the atrium and, after a suitable delay, paces the ventricles; it does not pace the atrium. This method of atrial sensing and ventricular pacing preserves the atrial contribution to ven-

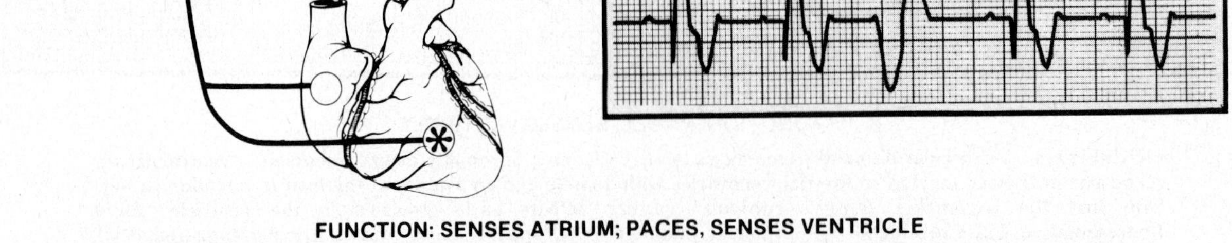

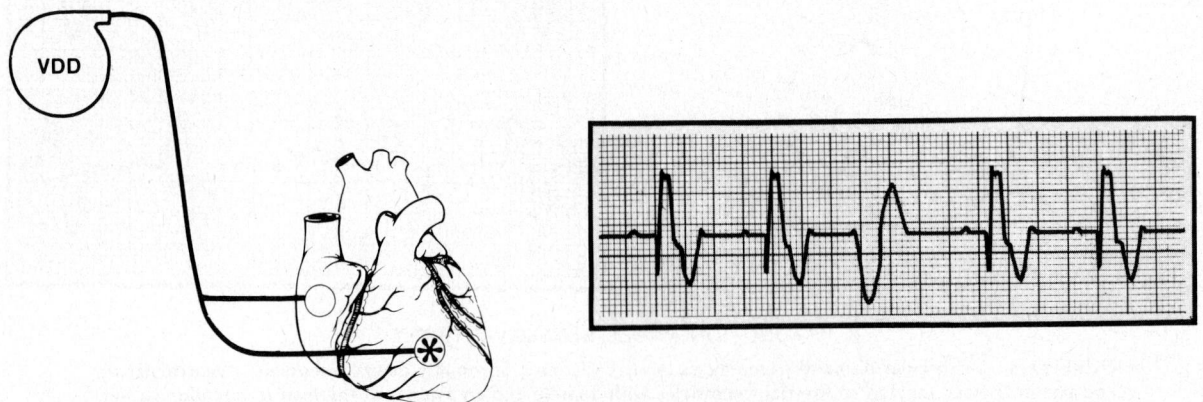

FIGURE 22–6 Atrial synchronous ventricular inhibited pacemaker (VDD). *Left,* Schematic diagram showing a VDD pacemaker with leads connected to the right atrium and ventricle. The circle at the atrial lead termination indicates that the pacemaker senses atrial activity and the circle and asterisk at the ventricular lead termination indicate that the pacemaker senses spontaneous ventricular activity and stimulates in the ventricle. *Right,* Representative ECG produced by VDD pacing. This recording is identical to the VAT pacemaker ECG shown in Figure 22–5 except that the PVC is sensed by the ventricular amplifier and prevents the pacemaker from synchronizing to the sinus P wave (obscured by the PVC) and pacing into the ST segment of the PVC.

tricular filling and maintains sinus control over the ventricular rate. Thus, exercise that stimulates acceleration of the sinus rate concomitantly increases the paced ventricular rate. Rate limitation is one design feature of this pacemaker, so that during atrial bradycardia the unit paces as an asynchronous ventricular pacemaker at a predetermined back-up rate. During atrial tachycardia the pacemaker paces no faster than its upper rate limit, yielding an AV response to sensed atrial activity that is 2:1, or similar to type I second-degree AV block. The VAT device has been refined by the addition of a ventricular sense amplifier, resulting in a new type of pacemaker called the *atrial synchronous ventricular inhibited pacemaker*[40] (VDD) (Fig. 22–6). Addition of the ventricular sense amplifier is important because it provides a demand mode for back-up pacing during bradycardia. It also prevents the atrial amplifier from triggering a ventricular stimulus in the event that a premature ventricular complex (PVC) produces a strong enough signal to be detected at the atrial electrode. To prevent such undesirable triggering, the system is designed to ensure that ventricular amplifer sensing takes precedence. Finally, ventricular sensing prevents competitive pacing when a PVC occurs during the A-V interval while the device is tracking normal sinus activity.

Like the VAT pacemaker, the VDD pacemaker still does not pace the atrium, but it does sense and pace the ventricle. During sinus bradycardia, VAT and VDD pacemakers function in the VOO and VVI modes, respectively, and therefore, under such circumstances, do not maintain sequential AV contraction. Contraindications to VDD pacing include the presence of atrial tachycardias and bradycardias and the occurrence of retrograde conduction to the atria with a long V-A interval during ventricular pacing or PVCs. Such retrograde activation will be sensed by a VDD pacemaker, triggering a ventricular stimulus and initiating a pacemaker-induced tachycardia.

AV SEQUENTIAL PACEMAKERS (DVI). For patients with abnormal sinus node function (sinus bradycardia, sinus arrest, and so forth) as well as impaired AV conduction, the atrial contribution to ventricular filling can be preserved by means of an AV sequential pacemaker[41] (DVI) (Fig. 22–7). This pacemaker senses only ventricular activity but is capable of stimulating both the atrium and the ventricle. Following ventricular sensed or paced events, this device monitors the ventricular electrogram. If ventricular activity is not detected within a prescribed pacemaker escape interval, the device stimulates the atrium. The pacemaker then waits long enough to allow passage of a normal AV interval and, if no ventricular activity occurs, paces in the ventricle. Some AV sequential pacemakers are of the committed type, i.e., they do not wait for normal AV conduction to occur but, instead, always deliver a stimulus to the ventricles following delivery of an atrial stimulus.[42,43] Sensed spontaneous ventricular activity inhibits the ventricular stimulus and resets all pacemaker timing. If the ventricular rate is sufficiently rapid, atrial stimuli from the pacemaker are also inhibited. It is important to reemphasize that the DVI pacemaker does *not* sense spontaneous atrial activity and therefore cannot alter the paced rate in response to physiologic needs.

OPTIMAL SEQUENTIAL PACEMAKERS (DDD). The optimal sequential pacemaker[44] (DDD) combines features of the AAI, VDD, and DVI pacemakers by functioning as an atrial demand pacemaker (AAI) during normally conducted sinus bradycardia, as an atrial synchronous pacemaker (VDD) during normal sinus rates that block or conduct with delay to the ventricle, and as an AV sequential pacemaker (DVI) during sinus bradycardia character-

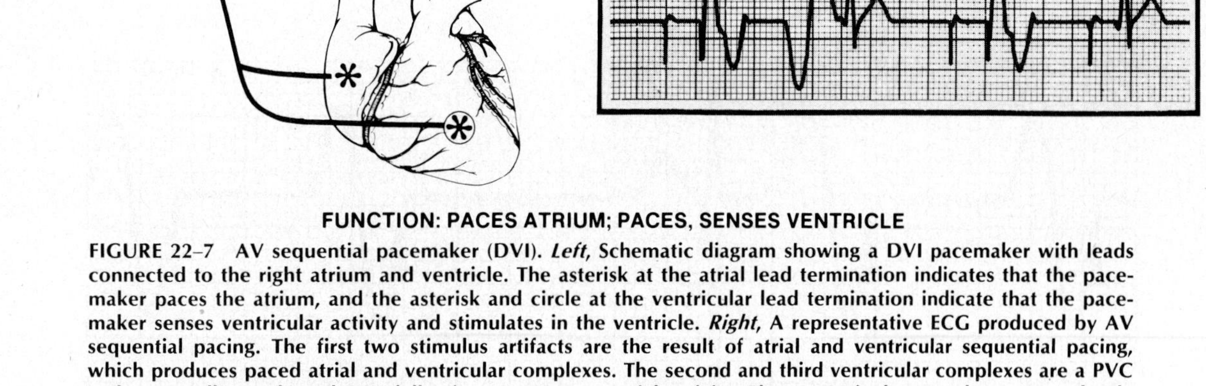

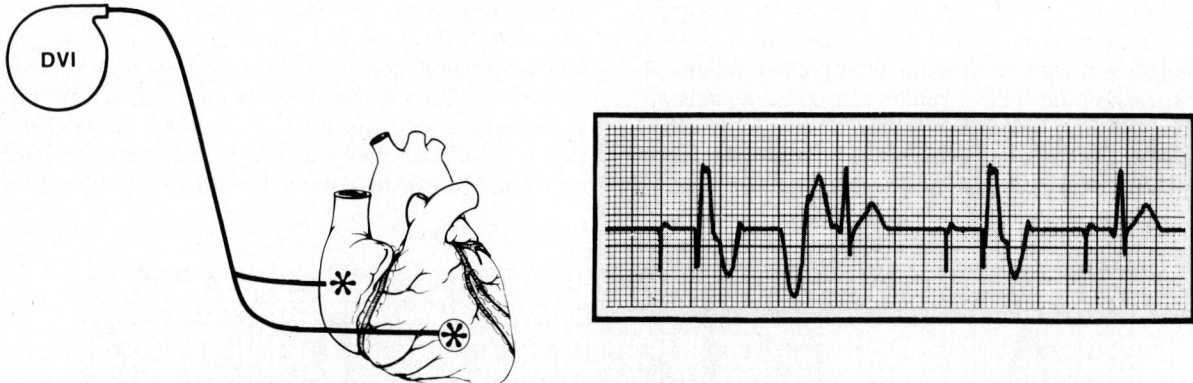

FIGURE 22–7 AV sequential pacemaker (DVI). *Left,* Schematic diagram showing a DVI pacemaker with leads connected to the right atrium and ventricle. The asterisk at the atrial lead termination indicates that the pacemaker paces the atrium, and the asterisk and circle at the ventricular lead termination indicate that the pacemaker senses ventricular activity and stimulates in the ventricle. *Right,* A representative ECG produced by AV sequential pacing. The first two stimulus artifacts are the result of atrial and ventricular sequential pacing, which produces paced atrial and ventricular complexes. The second and third ventricular complexes are a PVC and a normally conducted QRS following spontaneous atrial activity. These ventricular complexes (sensed only by the ventricular amplifier) inhibit both the atrial and ventricular stimuli. The third and fourth stimulus artifacts are again atrial and ventricular sequential pacing, occurring because no additional spontaneous ventricular activity took place within the pacemaker's escape interval. The final stimulus artifact, an atrial stimulus, produced an atrial complex that conducted normally to the ventricles. This conducted ventricular activity inhibited the ventricular stimulus and reset all pacemaker timing.

OPTIMAL SEQUENTIAL

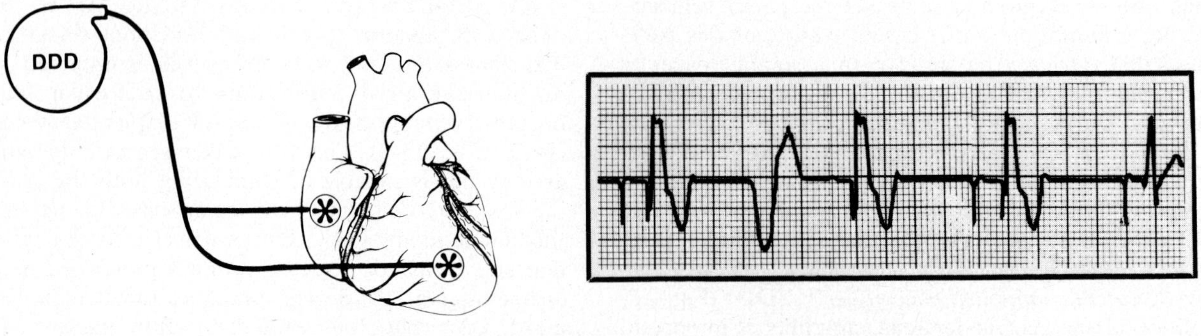

FUNCTION: PACES, SENSES ATRIUM; PACES, SENSES VENTRICLE

FIGURE 22–8 Optimal sequential pacemaker (DDD). *Left,* Schematic diagram of a DDD pacemaker with leads connected to the right atrium and ventricle. Asterisks and circles at the atrial and ventricular lead terminations indicate that the pacemaker paces and senses in both atrium and ventricle. *Right,* A representative ECG produced by DDD pacing. The first and fourth cardiac cycles, each preceded by two stimulus artifacts, are produced by atrial and ventricular sequential stimulation. The second QRS complex is a PVC, which resets all pacemaker timing and inhibits pacing. The third QRS complex is the result of ventricular pacing triggered by the pacemaker's sensing of the preceding sinus atrial event. The fifth QRS complex is the normally conducted result of atrial pacing.

ized by blocked or prolonged AV conduction. During normally conducted sinus impulses, the pacemaker is totally inhibited (Fig. 22–8). Thus, this pacemaker most closely approaches the normal electrophysiology of the heart in order to preserve the optimal hemodynamic relationships between atrial and ventricular contraction.

Current contraindications to its use are (1) the presence of atrial tachycardias that are inappropriate for governing ventricular rate (since the DDD pacemaker senses the atrial rate and paces the ventricle accordingly), and (2) as with the VDD units, retrograde conduction to the atrium with a long V-A conduction time following paced ventricular beats (the retrograde atrial response is sensed, triggers a paced ventricular beat, and thus creates an iatrogenic pacemaker-induced tachycardia). Ultimately, the latter will be eliminated as a contraindication as improved designs allow atrial tracking devices to handle retrograde signals appropriately. Except for these circumstances, in which a DVI pacemaker might be preferred, the DDD pacemaker can be substituted for all existing pacemakers.

HYSTERESIS. Pacemakers with hysteresis are designed to operate as follows: the pacemaker escape interval (interval between the last sensed spontaneous activity and the first paced beat) exceeds the interval between subsequent consecutive pacing cycles, so that normal sinus rhythm can be maintained over a wide range of rates (pacemaker-inhibited) while ensuring an adequate pacing rate when needed. This type of operation is displayed in Figure 22–9.

It is important to recognize the different rate capabilities offered by different pacemakers. AAI, AAT, VVI, VVT, and DVI pacemakers have a fixed rate that can be changed by reprograming the pacemaker. The AAI and AAT pacemakers (assuming normal AV conduction) ensure that both atrial and ventricular rates do not drop below a minimal constant value while the VVI and VVT devices maintain a minimal constant ventricular rate. The DVI pacemaker behaves like the AAI pacemaker except that it also paces the ventricle to maintain the ventricular rate equal to the atrial rate. The VDD pacemaker "tracks"

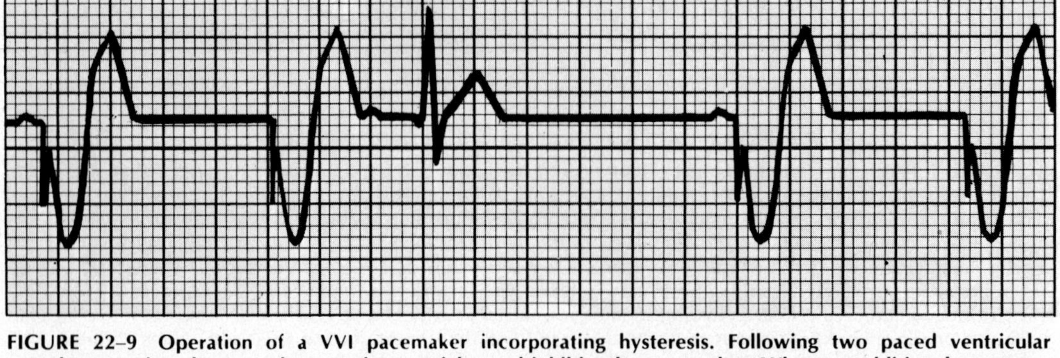

FIGURE 22–9 Operation of a VVI pacemaker incorporating hysteresis. Following two paced ventricular complexes, a sinus beat conducts to the ventricles and inhibits the pacemaker. When no additional spontaneous ventricular activity occurs, the pacemaker "escapes" at an interval of 1200 msec, with subsequent pacing intervals of 857 msec. Thus, the escape interval of the pacemaker exceeds the pacing interval, thereby allowing the patient to remain in a normally conducted rhythm for as much time as possible.

the atrial rate between the lower escape interval of the pacemaker, at which it functions at a constant rate in the VVI mode, and an upper rate limit at which the pacemaker creates second-degree AV block to maintain a fairly constant ventricular rate. The DDD pacemaker functions as a VDD pacemaker through the normal and fast rates but maintains a constant rate for atria and ventricles in the lower range by functioning in the AAI or DVI mode. Naturally, each of these pacemakers can be inhibited by changes in the spontaneous rhythm that alters the heart rate.

HEMODYNAMIC CONSEQUENCES OF SEQUENTIAL AV CONTRACTION

Ventricular (VVI) pacing provides symptomatic improvement for the vast majority of patients who have sick sinus syndrome or impaired AV conduction by establishing a basal ventricular rate that ensures adequate cardiac output. Increasing evidence suggests that some patients are not well served by ventricular pacing,[45–49] either because this pacing mode does not restore sufficient cardiac function to meet the demands of normal daily activity, or because the unnatural cardiac activation sequence associated with VVI pacing interferes with effective cardiac pumping. During ventricular pacing, atrial contractions may be absent, dissociated from ventricular activity, or improperly coupled to ventricular events by retrograde conduction. Inappropriately timed atrial systole effectively eliminates the booster pump action of the atrium present during normal sinus rhythm and impairs valve function.[50]

A consistent ventriculoatrial activation sequence may be associated with even greater hemodynamic compromise than is random AV dissociation because of significant decreases in systemic and left ventricular blood pressure and cardiac output, with concomitant increases in right atrial, ventricular, and pulmonary pressures.[51] In some patients, congestive heart failure may result.[46] Numerous acute studies have shown gains in cardiac output that vary from 2% to 67% after substitution of AV sequential[52–55] or atrial synchronous ventricular pacing[56] for ventricular pacing. Maintenance of hemodynamic gains chronically has been shown in more recent studies in which ventricular demand and atrial synchronous ventricular pacing were compared using measurements obtained by invasive means from exercising patients.[57,58] Patients were first paced for three-month intervals in either the VDD or the VVI mode and were then switched to the other mode. Invasive hemodynamic studies at rest and during exercise after each three-month interval revealed that during the heaviest workload, VDD pacing increased cardiac output 3.8 liters/min (mean) compared to VVI pacing despite a substantial compensatory increase in stroke volume that occurred with VVI pacing. Arteriovenous oxygen concentration differences during the heaviest workload and arterial lactate levels were lower during VDD pacing. Mean working capacity increased 23% and was statistically the same in patients both below and above 65 years of age. A progressive decrease in long-term performance with VVI pacing was evidenced by decreased work capacity, increased heart size, and increased pulmonary artery pressure, while the significant gains seen with VDD pacing were maintained chronically.

Thus, it seems clear that appropriately timed atrial systole has an important influence on cardiac performance. One question remains unresolved: whether dual-chamber devices should be considered for all patients or only for selected groups, such as those whose cardiovascular function is impaired and those who require significant increases in cardiac output (e.g., youngsters or athletically active people).

MODE SELECTION

Selection of an appropriate pacemaker modality for a given patient can be rather complex, requiring knowledge of the electrophysiological performance of the sinus node, AV conduction pathways and hemodynamic status. When available, these data can be used with the algorithm illustrated in Figure 22–10 to select the most suitable type(s) of device. We begin by considering whether sinus node function is normal or abnormal. If it is normal (right branch, Fig. 22–10) and the patient does not suffer angina at elevated rates, an atrial tracking pacemaker (VDD, DDD) may be appropriate, provided that the patient does not have prolonged retrograde conduction time to the atrium following ventricular paced beats. Such retrograde conduction would produce a pacemaker-mediated tachycardia if combined with an atrial tracking device. If there is retrograde conduction, or if there is need to control the upper pacing rate either to limit it in order to prevent angina or to ensure AV synchrony via atrial overdrive, an AV sequential (DVI) pacemaker would be selected. If sinus node function is abnormal (left branch, Fig. 22–10), with frequent periods of atrial fibrillation or flutter, a ventricular demand pacemaker (VVI, VVT) would be chosen. If atrial flutter or fibrillation is not present and AV conduction is normal, an atrial demand pacemaker (AAI, AAT) can be implanted unless the patient has *hypersensitive carotid sinus syndrome.* An atrial pacemaker is inappropriate therapy for patients with this syndrome, since AV conduction is frequently blocked by the excessive vagal tone (although this response is often veiled by concomitant sinus arrest). In patients with hypersensitive carotid sinus syndrome, a DVI pacemaker is the preferred type. If the predominant atrial rhythm is normal with infrequent or brief episodes of atrial bradyarrhythmia, it is likely that an atrial tracking pacemaker (VDD, DDD) may be suitable. The considerations cited above (potential for angina, retrograde conduction) should be reviewed before proceeding with selection of a tracking pacemaker. Finally, if sinus function

TABLE 22–5 CONCISE SUMMARY OF INDICATIONS FOR AVAILABLE PACING MODES

	Atrial Rhythm		
AV Conduction	*Normal*	*Bradycardia*	*Bradycardia-Tachycardia*
Normal	O	AAI	AAI
AV block without prolonged retrograde conduction time	VDD,DDD	DDD,DVI	DVI,VVI
AV block with prolonged retrograde conduction time	DVI	DVI	DVI

O = No pacemaker indicated

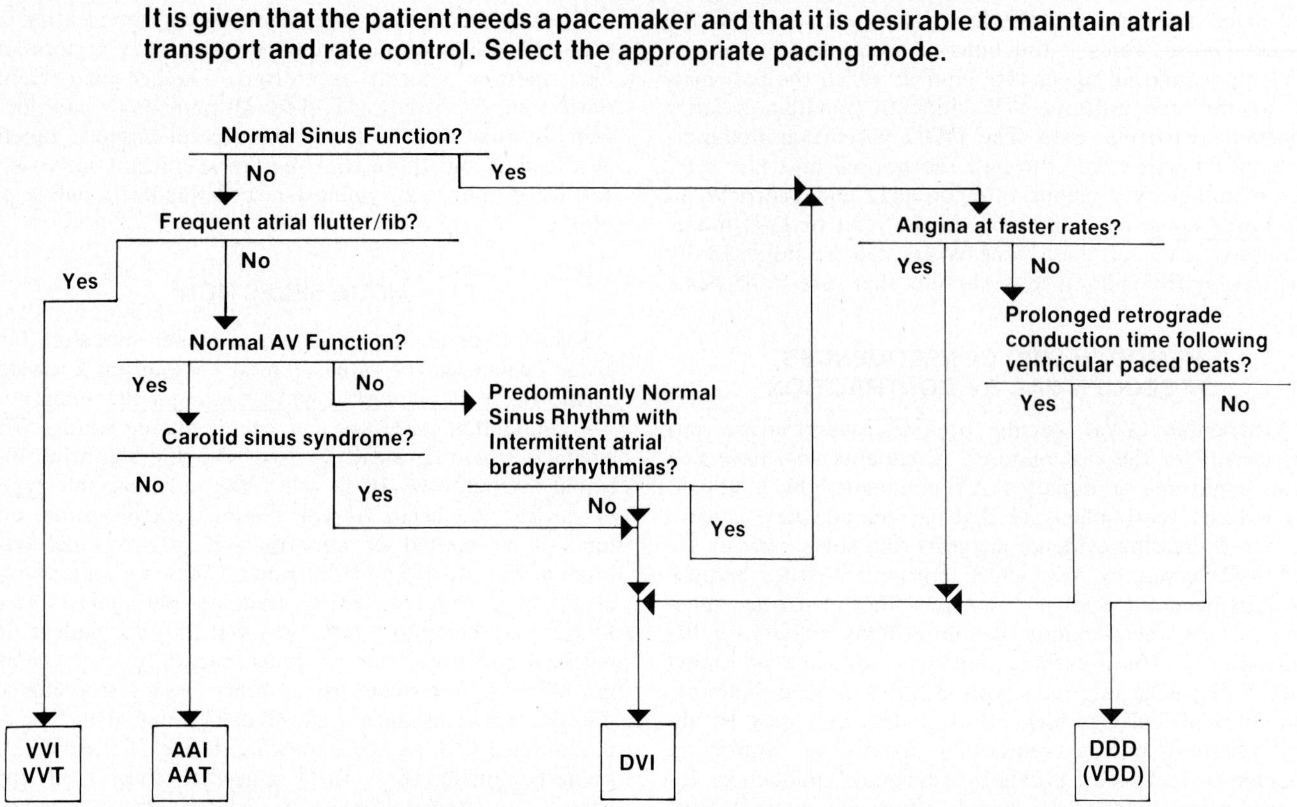

FIGURE 22-10 A flow chart providing an algorithm for selection of an appropriate pacemaker modality. This decision tree is described in detail in the text.

and AV conduction are both abnormal, atrial flutter or fibrillation is infrequent or absent, and the patient has extended periods of bradycardia, a DVI pacemaker should be selected.

A concise summary of the resultant pacemaker mode selection produced by the algorithm of Figure 22-10 is presented in Table 22-5.

PACING FOR TACHYCARDIAS[20,29,59–61]

Pacing to treat patients with tachycardias can be divided into four categories: (1) the need to maintain a normal rate when a required antiarrhythmic regimen produces bradycardia, (2) slowing the ventricular rate, (3) prevention of recurrence of tachycardia, and (4) termination of tachycardia already present.[29]

In the first category, drugs such as digitalis, propranolol, clonidine, and amiodarone (see Chapter 21) may result in symptomatic bradycardias that require some form of pacing to maintain normal heart rates. Similarly, His-bundle ablation to interrupt AV conduction in a patient with drug-refractory supraventricular tachycardia with a rapid ventricular rate results in a bradycardia (due to the AV block) that requires pacing.[62,63] Classically, VVI pacemakers have been used for this purpose, although dual-chamber devices may be more desirable under specific circumstances in which the patient may be capable of achieving sustained periods of AV synchrony.

An infrequently used alternative approach to patients with uncontrollable supraventricular tachycardia is the use of rapid atrial stimulation, which may initiate atrial fibrillation and/or AV block and thus reduce ventricular rate.[64,65] Coupled atrial pacing has also been used to reduce ventricular rate in drug-resistant atrial tachycardia.[66] These approaches reduce the ventricular rate if atrial impulses block in the AV junction. Paired or coupled ventricular pacing for supraventricular or ventricular tachycardias reduces the *effective* ventricular rate by producing an electrical but not a mechanical response. The required closely coupled premature venticular stimulation may produce ventricular fibrillation.

Pacing successfully prevents recurrence of tachycardia only in selected circumstances. In 1960 Linenthal and Zoll demonstrated that ventricular pacing at slightly elevated but generally normal rates usually eliminated ventricular tachyarrhythmias in patients with advanced AV block and slow heart rates punctuated by bouts of ventricular tachycardias.[67] The occurrence of ventricular tachyarrhythmias in association with bradycardia may be related in part to a greater disparity between action potential duration and refractory period at slow heart rates (p. 619). This temporal dispersion of recovery of excitability may be accentuated by a premature extrasystole, causing inhomogeneous areas of conduction delay and block that may lead to reentry. Pacing at faster rates in the absence of ischemia may improve the synchrony of recovery and alleviate the ventricular arrhythmias (Fig. 22-11).

It is important to note that accelerating the heart rate in the presence of ischemia may increase the degree of conduction delay occurring in the ischemic area and increase the temporal dispersion of refractoriness. These changes may result in ventricular tachycardia and ventricular fibrillation.[68] When one is pacing patients who have had a myocardial infarction, care should be taken to find an optimal heart rate that will alleviate the arrhythmias but will not exacerbate the ischemia or provoke new arrhythmias.

In some cases simply improving the patient's hemodynamic status[32] or restoring normal AV synchrony by means of an appropriate standard pacemaker[33,69] will prevent the development of tachycardia. In others, pacing at moderately elevated rates suppresses ectopy and the recurrence of tachycardias. This effect must be well documented before a permanent pacemaker is implanted, because permanent pacing often fails to prevent recurrence of tachycardia over the long term. Also, the site of pacing—atrial or ventricular—may make a difference in efficacy. Short-term, temporary rapid pacing may effectively suppress ventricular tachycardias associated with torsades de pointes and Q-T prolongation. The mechanism by which this pacing mode is successful in some instances may relate to the phenomenon of overdrive suppression (p. 620). In patients who have accessory pathways, an atrial synchronous or DDD pacemaker with a suitably short A-V interval may preclude development of a reciprocating tachycardia while preserving normal sinus control of ventricular rate.[70]

Selected drug-resistant tachycardias, not amenable to surgical therapy, can sometimes be terminated by a pacemaker designed to produce an appropriate sequence of electrical stimuli. Some of the pacemakers are activated by the *patient* when he perceives the presence of a tachyarrhythmia,[31,71–73] while others automatically discharge when the *pacemaker* senses that a tachycardia is present.[74,75] Various cadences of stimuli can be delivered, including short bursts at high rates (Fig. 22-12), stimuli that scan the cardiac cycle and automatically change rate[76] or shift the timing of one or more premature stimuli,[77] and coupled or paired stimuli. A "dual-demand" pacemaker automatically delivers stimuli at a fixed but relatively slow (e.g., 70 bpm) rate when it senses the presence of a bradycardia (e.g., rates less than 70 bpm) or tachycardia (e.g., rates greater than 150 bpm).[78] The tachycardia is terminated when an appropriately timed stimulus occurs during a particular part of the tachycardia cycle; this is called "underdrive termination." Dual-chamber (DVI) pacemakers can be made to operate in the dual-demand mode and pace with short A-V intervals for patients who have accessory pathways.[79,80] Unique custom-built devices with characteristics tailored for specific patients can also be applied.

Although a tachycardia that could be terminated by pacing stimuli was previously believed to be due to reentry, we now know this is not necessarily so, in view of the phenomenon of triggered activity, discussed on p. 620. Nevertheless, assuming reentry to be the mechanism sustaining a tachycardia, we can consider certain principles of

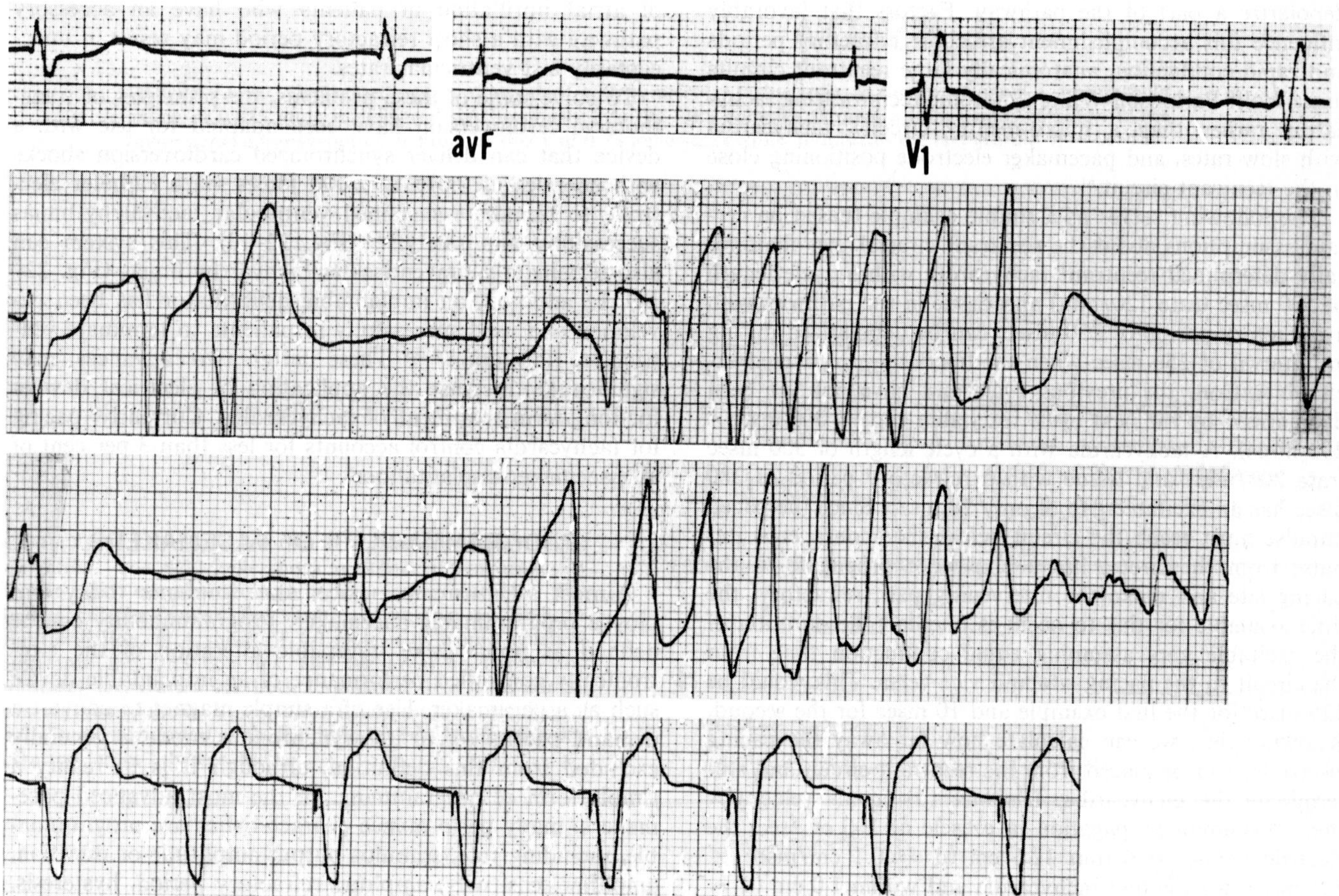

FIGURE 22–11 Electrocardiogram showing runs of ventricular tachycardia consequent to an inadequate ventricular escape rate in a patient with chronic atrial fibrillation and complete AV block (upper panels). Ventricular pacing at a rate of 85 ppm abolished the ventricular arrhythmia (lower panel).

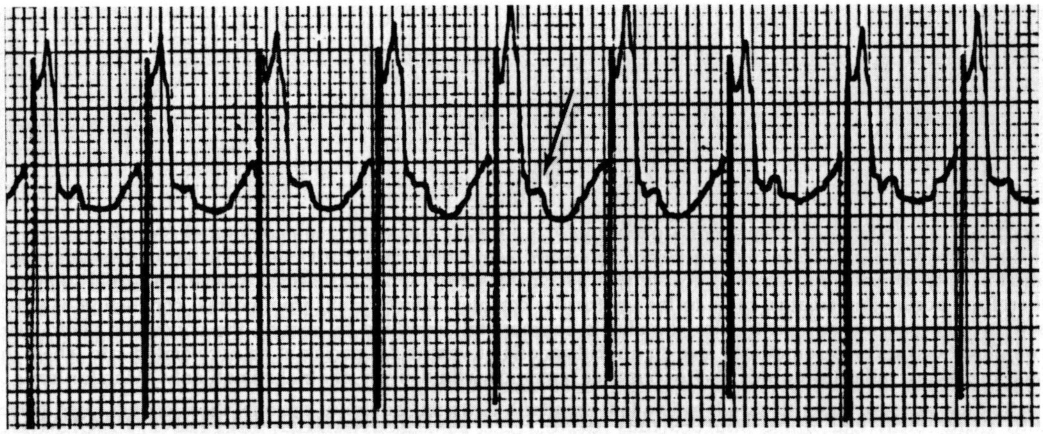

FIGURE 22–22 Electrocardiogram of a patient with a DDD pacemaker demonstrating pacemaker-induced tachycardia due to retrograde atrial activation. Each ventricular stimulus produces a retrograde P wave, which in turn triggers the pacemaker to produce yet another ventricular stimulus. This process usually repeats at a rate equal to the pacemaker's maximum tracking rate, which in this example is 135 ppm. Retrograde P wave indicated by arrow. (Lead I.)

in this example (failure to sense and failure to pace), it is highly probable—although not absolutely certain—that there is a common cause. The most likely etiologies are as follows:

Lack of Capture:
Lead dislodgment, perforation.
Lead wire fracture.
Lead insulation failure.
Pulse generator failure.
Inappropriate programming of output energy.
High threshold.
Misread ECG ("loss of capture" seen only when stimulus occurs during cardiac refractory period).

Lack of Sensing:
Lead dislodgment, perforation.
Lead wire fracture.
Lead insulation failure.
Pulse generator failure.
Inappropriate programming of amplifier sensitivity or refractory period.
Inadequate electrogram amplitude (due to infarct, electrolyte disturbance, myocardial disease).
Electromagnetic interference induced reversion to asynchronous mode.
Stuck reed switch.
Misread ECG (fusion beats).

Analysis should begin by comparing a recent 12-lead ECG to a baseline tracing that predates occurrence of the problem. The current tracing should be carefully reviewed to exclude misinterpretation of fusion beats as sensing failure or of pacing stimuli occurring during the cardiac refractory period as lack of capture. Reversion to the asynchronous mode due to electromagnetic interference usually can be eliminated as a cause of nonsensing if a 12-lead ECG shows no signs of electrical interference. Comparing the current and baseline ECGs establishes the presence or absence of lead position changes, including perforation, as evidenced by shifts in the vectors of the paced QRS complexes and pacing artifacts. It is important to remember that digital ECG systems with low sampling rates can-

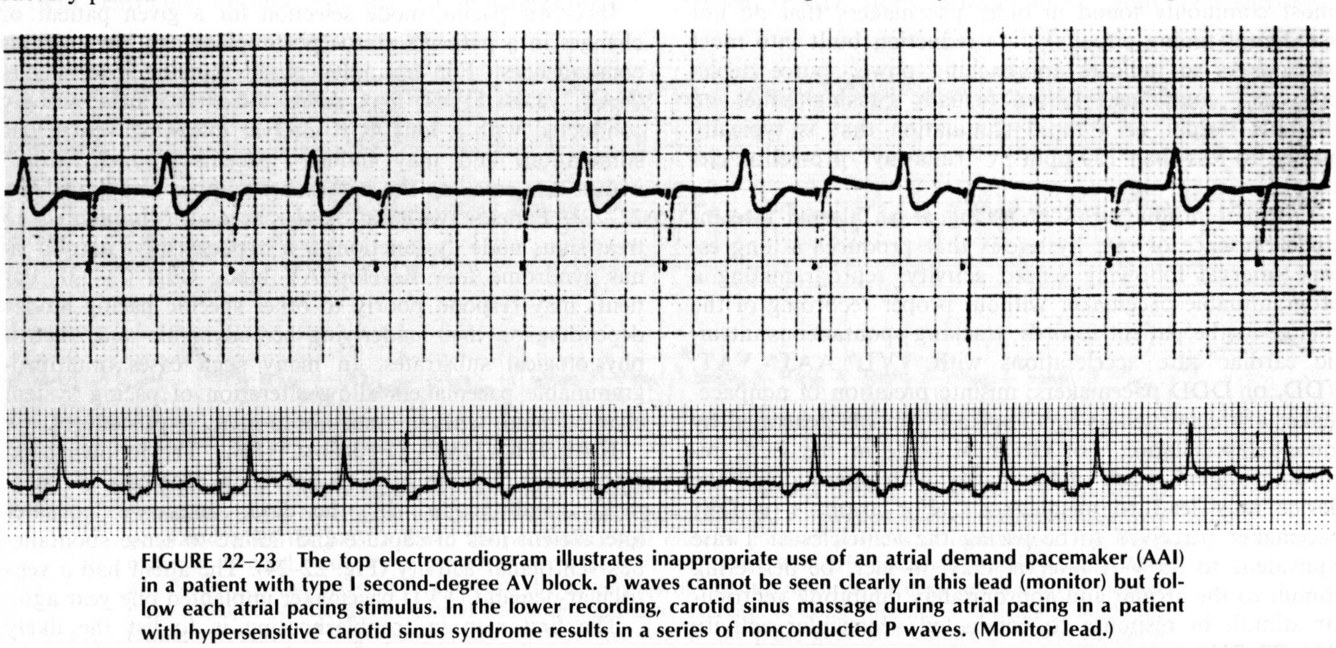

FIGURE 22–23 The top electrocardiogram illustrates inappropriate use of an atrial demand pacemaker (AAI) in a patient with type I second-degree AV block. P waves cannot be seen clearly in this lead (monitor) but follow each atrial pacing stimulus. In the lower recording, carotid sinus massage during atrial pacing in a patient with hypersensitive carotid sinus syndrome results in a series of nonconducted P waves. (Monitor lead.)

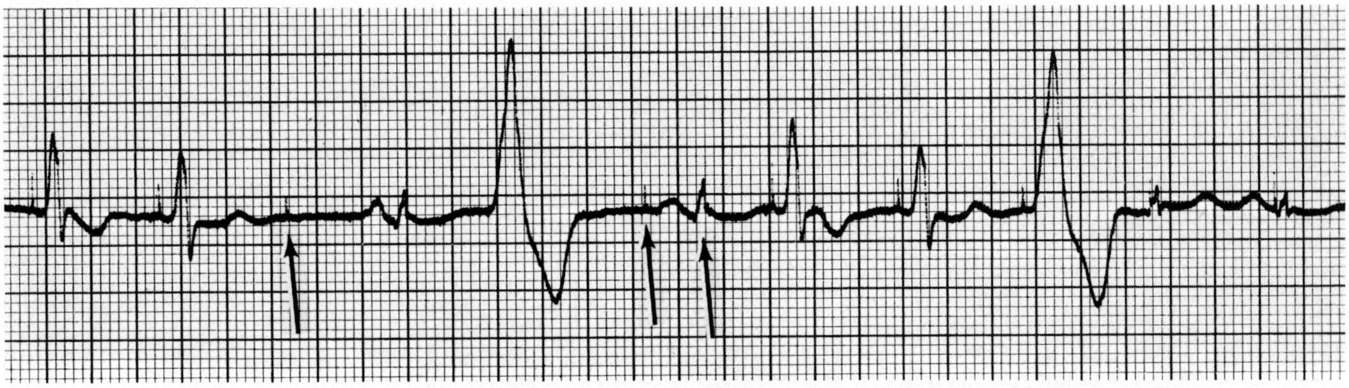

FIGURE 22–24 Failure of a VVI pacemaker. Note that pacing stimuli occasionally fail to elicit a paced QRS complex (first and second arrows), and the pacemaker occasionally fails to sense spontaneous ventricular activity (third arrow) even though it occurs after completion of the ventricular amplifier's refractory period. (Monitor lead.)

not be used to determine the vector of the pacemaker stimulus reliably. An x-ray or fluoroscopy is used to help diagnose lead dislodgment. Insulation defects in the lead result in vector changes in the pacing artifact, but not in the paced QRS complex.

Applying a magnet results in pacing without sensing. In most pacemakers, magnet application alters the pacing rate (sometimes by only a few milliseconds) to confirm that the reed switch is functioning and to eliminate the possibility of nonsensing due to a jammed reed switch.

Inappropriate programming can be evaluated by reprogramming the amplifier sensitivity and refractory period to restore sensing and to increase the stimulus intensity to restore capture. If such reprogramming failed to resolve the problem, or if the parameter settings required are not within normally accepted values, inappropriate programming can be excluded.

Wire fracture can produce nonsensing and lack of capture, but it is generally accompanied by random resetting of the escape interval as the broken wire ends touch intermittently. An x-ray pinpoints some but not all fractures. In this example (Fig. 22–24) the regularity of the escape intervals probably eliminates wire fractures as the cause of the problem.

At this point, noninvasive procedures have been explored to evaluate most potential causes for the reported malfunctions. Threshold elevation, inadequate electrogram characteristics, and pulse generator failure all require invasive evaluation, although some noninvasive determinations can be obtained if the patient has a sophisticated multiprogrammable pulse generator. Some of these devices can telemeter the intracardiac electrogram, facilitating evaluation of sensing problems. They also allow the user to obtain noninvasive threshold measurements. Nevertheless, correction of sensing and pacing failures due to any of these causes will require invasive procedures.

In the example cited, ECG evidence, shown in Figure 22–25, is most consistent with a lead dislodgment. Note the axis shift in the pacemaker-stimulus artifact and in the paced QRS complexes. Lead displacement is the most common cause of sensing and capture failures.

To extend the troubleshooting process to dual-chamber systems, the electrocardiograms of Figure 22–26 are analyzed. These records are taken from a patient who has a bipolar noncommitted atrioventricular sequential pacemaker (DVI), which was programed to an A-V interval of 150 msec. The patient's electrocardiogram exhibited variable A-V intervals up to 200 msec. (Fig. 22–26, upper panel) with no evidence of ventricular pacing. If the pacing system were functioning normally, no A-V interval would exceed the programed 150 msec. Potential causes for failure to pace include broken lead, defective pacemaker/lead connection, "cross talk" between atrial and ventricular channels of dual-chamber pacemakers, component failure, battery depletion, or oversensing. Oversensing could be due to sensing of P or T waves, myopotentials, electromagnetic interference, lead polarization after potentials, and cross talk (sensing of the atrial stimulus by the ventricular amplifier of a dual-chamber device) as well as detection of make-break potentials created by intermittent contact of broken electrode wires or loose connections at the pulse generator (Fig. 22–20).

As shown in the lower tracing of Figure 22–26, placement of the magnet over the pulse generator restored normal AV sequential pacing. This strongly suggests a problem due to oversensing. Myopotential inhibition can be excluded, since the generator is bipolar (muscle inhibition of bipolar generators is exceedingly rare) and because the atrial stimuli continue to occur without prolonged pauses. Electromagnetic interference is also eliminated because the generator is bipolar and there is no evidence of interference in the ECG. T-wave sensing is not a possible cause because the T waves occur after the point in the pacemaker timing cycle when a ventricular stimulus should have been generated. A loose connection is eliminated by manipulating the generator in the pocket while recording the ECG. Lead fractures are relatively uncommon, there was no evidence of pacing failure with the magnet in place, and x-ray examination showed no evidence of conductor failure. Measurement of the A-V intervals in the upper panel of Figure 22–26 reveals that the third, fifth, seventh, and ninth atrial stimuli were timed from the preceding QRS complexes (the V-A interval for this pacemaker is programed to 600 msec). The remaining stimuli were timed from their preceding occurrence rather than from the preceding QRS complexes. Thus, it is fairly evident that this pacemaker is being affected by "cross-talk" between its atrial and ventricular channels. Each atrial stimulus is sensed by the ventricular amplifier that inhibits delivery of a ventricular stimulus. When the spontaneous

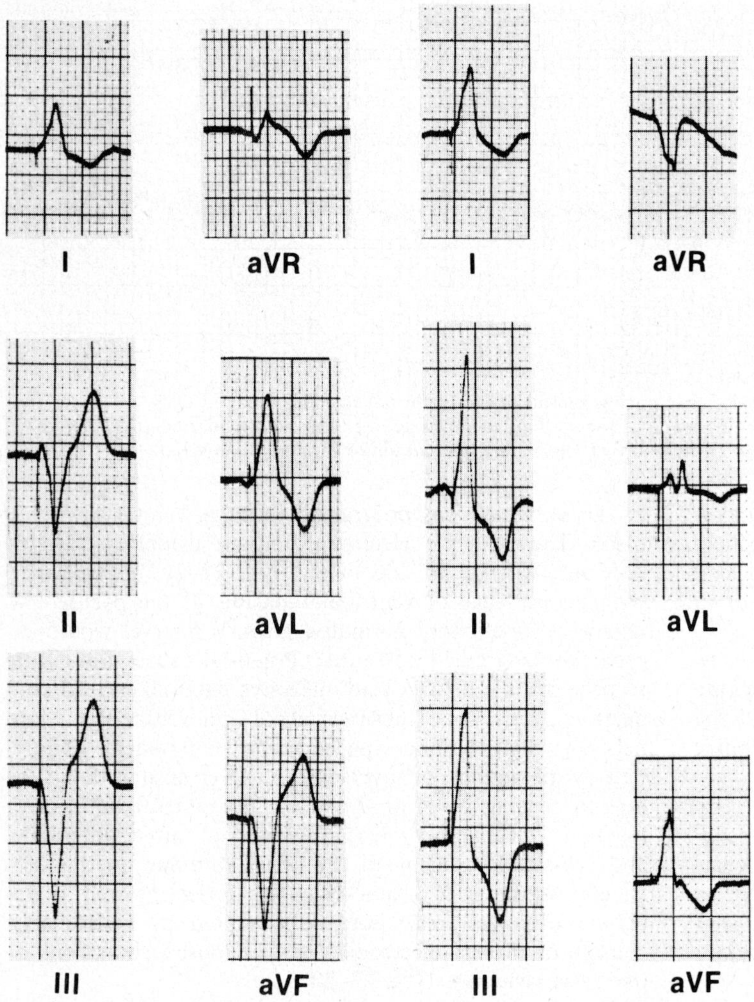

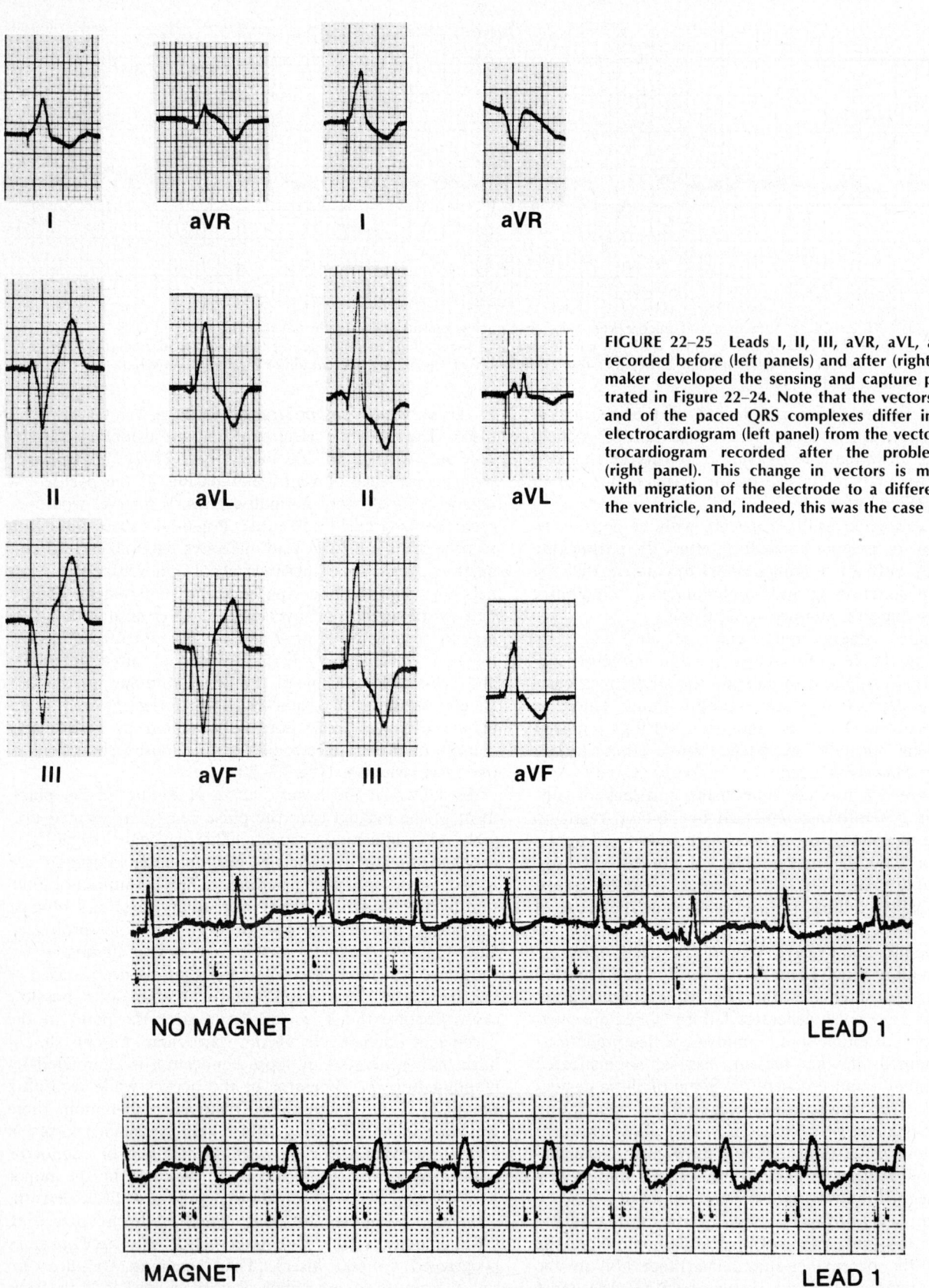

FIGURE 22–25 Leads I, II, III, aVR, aVL, and aVF were recorded before (left panels) and after (right panels) pacemaker developed the sensing and capture problems illustrated in Figure 22–24. Note that the vectors of the spikes and of the paced QRS complexes differ in the baseline electrocardiogram (left panel) from the vectors in the electrocardiogram recorded after the problem developed (right panel). This change in vectors is most consistent with migration of the electrode to a different position in the ventricle, and, indeed, this was the case here.

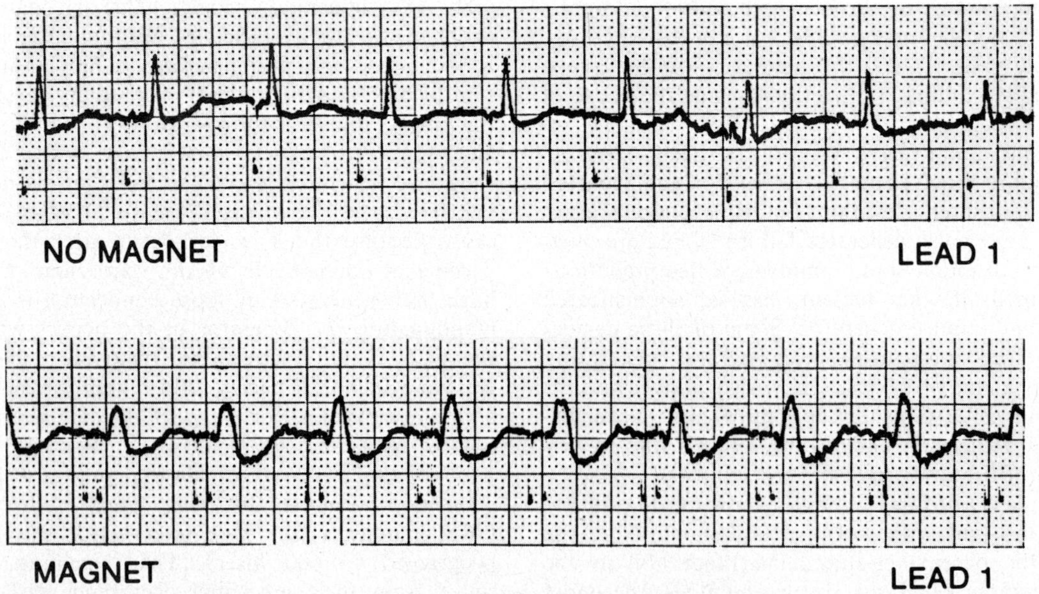

FIGURE 22–26 Electrocardiogram of a patient with a bipolar noncommitted AV sequential (DVI) pacemaker programed to a V-A interval of 600 msec and an A-V interval of 150 msec. The upper tracing, recorded without a magnet over the generator, shows A-V intervals as long as 200 msec with no evidence of ventricular pacing. Placement of a magnet over the generator converts it to asynchronous pacing and restores the ventricular pacing function (lower panel). This is an example of "cross talk," a malfunction in which the ventricular stimulus is inhibited by inappropriate ventricular sensing of the atrial stimulus. In this case the cause was current leakage from damaged insulation on the atrial lead. (Lead I.)

QRS complex occurs sufficiently late after the atrial stimulus so that the QRS falls outside the ventricular amplifier refractory period (200 msec), the pacemaker timing is reset for a second time by the ventricular complex. Consequently, the atrial pacing rate is variable and the A-V interval is not controlled by the pacemaker. The patient's ventricular escape rhythm maintains the cardiac rhythm.

After the pacemaker pocket was opened it was found that a 4.5-volt pacing stimulus delivered to the atrial lead reset the ventricular amplifier, thus confirming the diagnosis. Lead impedance measurements indicated a defect in the atrial lead insulation, which was found at the curvature on its J portion after removal of the lead. The insulation break allowed leakage currents from the atrial stimulus to create sufficient voltage at the ventricular lead to inhibit ventricular output. Replacement of the atrial lead corrected the problem.

These two examples are chosen to illustrate that pacing problems cover the range from being fairly simple to quite complex. Very sophisticated knowledge is required to deal with selection, implantation, and management of modern, multiprogrammable dual-chamber pacing devices.

PATIENT CONCERNS

A pacemaker can extend the patient's longevity and may greatly improve his quality of life. Yet the patient's psychological needs must be considered as well if therapy is to provide maximal benefit. The patient should understand why he has a pacemaker, how it works (in simple terms), and what it will and will not do for him (many patients think that a pacemaker cures or makes the heart stronger). He should be told what, if any, lifestyle restrictions must be observed. If this is not explained, patients may become excessively apprehensive to the point of even avoiding bathing lest they "short-circuit" their pacemakers. The patient will be greatly concerned about his dependency on the pacemaker, the risks of its failing, the anticipated longevity of the system, and the severity of the replacement procedure. If these issues are addressed with clear concise answers in lay terms, the patient with a pacemaker can fully enjoy the extension and better quality of life that this device makes possible.

Acknowledgment

The authors thank Serge Barold, M.D., for critical comments.

References

1. Zoll, P.: Resuscitation of the heart in ventricular standstill by external electric stimulation. N. Engl. J. Med. *247*:768, 1952.
2. Elmquist, R., and Senning, A.: An implantable pacemaker for the heart. Proc. 2nd Int. Conf. Med. Elec. Eng., London, Iliffe and Sons, Ltd. 1959.
3. Zoll, P., and Linenthal, A.: Long-term electrical pacemakers for Stokes-Adams disease. Circulation *22*:341, 1960.
4. Waldo, A., Wells, J., Cooper, T., and MacLean, W.: Temporary cardiac pacing: Applications and techniques in the treatment of cardiac arrhythmias. Prog. Cardiovasc. Dis. *23*(6):451, 1981.
5. Lev, M., Kinare, S., and Pick, A.: The pathogenesis of atrioventricular block in coronary artery disease. Circulation *42*:409, 1970.
6. Lie, K., Wellens, H., Schulienburg, R., Becker, A., and Durrer, D.: The factors influencing prognosis of bundle branch block complicating acute anteroseptal infarction. The value of His-bundle recordings. Circulation *50*:935, 1974.
7. Fisch, G., Zipes, D., and Fisch, C.: Bundle branch block and sudden death. Prog. Cardiovasc. Dis. *23*:187, 1980.
8. Nimitz, A., Shubrooks, S., Hutter, A., and DeSanctis, R.: The significance of bundle branch block during acute myocardial infarction. Am. Heart J. *90*:439, 1975.
9. Atkins, J., Leshin, S., Blomqvist, G., et al.: Ventricular conduction blocks and sudden death in acute myocardial infarction. N. Engl. J. Med. *288*:281, 1973.
10. Hindman, M. C., Wagner, G. S., JaRo, M., Atkins, J., DeSanctis, R., Hutter, A., Morris, J., Rubenfire, M., Scheinman, M., and Yeatman, L.: The clinical significance of bundle branch block complicating acute myocardial infarction. II. Indications for temporary and permanent pacemaker therapy. Circulation *58*:689, 1978.
11. Langendorf, R., and Pick, A.: Atrioventricular block type II (Mobitz)—Its nature and clinical significance. Circulation *38*:819, 1968.
12. McNally, E., and Benchimol, A.: Medical and physiological considerations in the use of artificial cardiac pacing. Part 1. Am. Heart J. *75*:380, 1968.
13. Zipes, D.: Second degree atrioventricular block. Circulation *60*:465, 1979.
14. Dhingra, R., Denes, P., Wu, D., Chuquimia, R., and Rosen, K.: The significance of second degree atrioventricular block and bundle branch block. Observations regarding site and type of block. Circulation *49*:638, 1974.
15. Rosen, K., Lobe, M., Chuquimia, R., Sinno, M., Rahimtoola, S., and Gunnar, R.: Site of heart block in acute myocardial infarction. Circulation *42*:925, 1970.
16. Hindman, M., Wagner, G., JaRo, M., Atkins, J., Scheinman, M., DeSanctis, R., Hutter, H., Yeatman, L., Rubenfire, M., Pujura, C., Rubin, M., and Mars, J.: The clinical significance of bundle branch block complicating acute myocardial infarction. I. Clinical characteristics, hospital mortality, and one year follow-up. Circulation *58*:679, 1978.
17. Gann, D., Balachandran, P., El-Sherif, N., and Samet, P.: Prognostic significance of chronic versus acute bundle branch block in acute myocardial infarction. Chest *67*:298, 1975.
18. Godman, M., Lassers, B., and Julian, D.: Complete bundle branch block complicating acute myocardial infarction. N. Engl. J. Med. *282*:237, 1970.
19. Gould, L., Venkataraman, K., Mohammad, N., and Gomprecht, R.: Prognosis of right bundle branch block in acute myocardial infarction. J.A.M.A. *219*:502, 1972.
20. Batchelder, J., and Zipes, D. P.: Treatment of tachyarrhythmias by pacing. Arch. Intern. Med. *135*:1115, 1975.
21. Keren, A., Tzivoni, D., Gavish, D., Levi, J., Gottlieb, S., BenHorin, J., and Stern, S.: Etiology, warning signs and therapy of Torsade de Pointes. Circulation *64*:1167, 1981.
22. Smith, W., and Gallagher, J.: "Les Torsade de Pointes": An unusual ventricular arrhythmia. Ann. Intern. Med. *93*:578, 1980.
23. Robson, R. H., Pridie, R., and Fluck, D. C.: Evaluation of rapid atrial pacing in diagnosis of coronary artery disease. Br. Heart J. *38*:986, 1976.
24. Goldman, B. S., and Parsonnet, V.: World survey on cardiac pacing. PACE *2*(5):W1, 1979.
25. Sutton, R., Perrins, J., and Citron, P.: Physiological cardiac pacing. PACE *3*:207, 1980.
26. Furman, S.: Cardiac pacing and pacemakers. I. Indications for pacing bradyarrhythmias. Am. Heart J. *93*(4):523, 1977-B.
27. Dhingra, R., Palileo, E., Strasberg, B., Swiryn, S., Bauernfeind, R., Wyndham, C., and Rosen, K.: Significance of the HV interval in 517 patients with chronic bifascicular block. Circulation *64*:1265, 1981.
28. Dhingra, R., Wyndham, C., Bauernfeind, R., Swiryns, S., Deedwania, P., Smith, T., Senes, P., and Rosen, K.: Significance of block distal to the His bundle induced by atrial pacing in patients with chronic bifascicular block. Circulation *60*:1455, 1979.
29. Citron, P., and Duffin, E.: Implantable pacemakers for management of tachyarrhythmias. Herz *4*(3):269, 1979.
30. Cooper, T., MacLean, W., and Waldo, A.: Overdrive pacing for supraventricular tachycardia: A review of theoretical implications and therapeutic techniques. PACE *1*(2):196, 1978.
31. Kahn, A., Morris, J., and Citron, P.: Patient-initiated rapid atrial pacing to manage supraventricular tachycardia. Am. J. Cardiol. *38*:200, 1976.
32. Hyman, A.: Permanent programmable pacemakers in the management of recurrent tachycardias. PACE *2*(1):28, 1979.
33. Khan, M., Logan, K., McComb, J., and Adgey, A.: Management of recurrent ventricular tachyarrhythmias associated with QT prolongation. Am. J. Cardiol. *47*(6):1301, 1981.
34. Leclercq, J., Rosengarten, M., Delcourt, P., Attuel, P., Coumel, P., and Slama, R.: Prevention of intraatrial reentry by chronic atrial pacing. PACE *3*:163, 1980.
35. Harthorne, J.: Indications for pacemaker insertion: Types and modes of pacing. Prog. Cardiovasc. Dis. *23*(6):393, 1981.
36. Sutton, R., and Citron, P.: Electrophysiological and hemodynamic basis for application of new pacemaker technology in sick sinus syndrome and atrioventricular block. Br. Heart J. *41*:600, 1979.
37. Parsonnet, V., Furman, S., and Smyth, N. P. D.: Implantable cardiac pacemakers: Status report and resource guideline. Circulation *50*:A21, 1974.
38. Parsonnet, V., Furman, S., and Smyth, N. P. D.: A revised code for pacemaker identification. PACE *4*(4):400, 1981-B.
39. Nathan, D., Center, S., and Wu, C.: An implantable synchronous pacemaker for the long-term correction of complete heart block. Am. J. Cardiol. *11*:362, 1963.

40. Kruse, I., Ryden, L., and Duffin, E.: Clinical evaluation of atrial synchronous ventricular inhibited pacemakers. PACE *3*:641, 1980.
41. Berkovits, B., Castellanos, A., and Lemberg, L.: Bifocal demand pacing. Circulation *39*:44, 1969.
42. Barold, S., Falkoff, M., Ong, L., and Heinle, R.: Committed and uncommitted AV sequential DVI pulse generators. Arrhythmias and electrocardiographic manifestations of normal function. Stimucoeur 9:353, 1981.
43. Barold, S., Falkoff, M., Ong, L., and Heinle, R.: Characterization of pacemaker arrhythmias due to normally functioning AV demand (DVI) pulse generators. PACE *3*(6):712, 1980.
44. Funke, H. D.: Three years' experience in optimized sequential cardiac pacing. Stimucoeur *9*(1):26, 1981.
45. Alicandri, C., Fouad, F., Tarazi, R., Castle, L., and Morant, V.: Three cases of hypotension and syncope with ventricular pacing: Possible role of atrial reflexes. Am. J. Cardiol. *42*:137, 1978.
46. Davidson, D., Braak, C., Preston, T., and Judge, R.: Permanent ventricular pacing: Effect on long-term survival, congestive heart failure, and subsequent myocardial infarction and stroke. Ann. Intern. Med. *77*:345, 1972.
47. Gamal, M., and Van Gelder, L.: Chronic ventricular pacing with ventriculoatrial conduction versus atrial pacing in three patients with symptomatic sinus bradycardia. PACE *4*:100, 1981.
48. Miller, M., Fox, S., Jenkins, R., Schwartz, J., and Toonder, F.: Pacemaker syndrome: A noninvasive means to its diagnosis and treatment. PACE *4*:503, 1981.
49. Patel, A., Yap, V., and Thomsen, J.: Adverse effects of right ventricular pacing in a patient with aortic stenosis. Chest *72*:103, 1977.
50. Samet, P., Bernstein, W., and Levine, S.: Significance of the atrial contribution to ventricular filling. Am. J. Cardiol. *15*:195, 1965-B.
51. Ogawa, S., Dreifus, L., Shenoy, P., Brockman, S., and Berkovits, B.: Hemodynamic consequences of atrioventricular and ventriculoatrial pacing. PACE *1*:8, 1978.
52. Chamberlain, D., Leinbach, R., Vassaux, C., Kastor, J., DeSanctis, R., and Sanders, C.: Sequential atrioventricular pacing in heart block complicating acute myocardial infarction. N. Engl. J. Med. *282*:577, 1970.
53. Hartzler, G., Maloney, J., and Curtis, J., and Barnhorst, D.: Hemodynamic benefits of atrioventricular sequential pacing after cardiac surgery. Am. J. Cardiol. *40*:232, 1977.
54. Samet, P., Castillo, C., and Bernstein, W.: Hemodynamic consequences of sequential atrioventricular pacing. Am. J. Cardiol. *21*:207, 1968.
55. Samet, P., Castillo, C., and Bernstein, W.: Hemodynamic sequelae of atrial, ventricular, and sequential atrioventricular pacing in cardiac patients. Am. Heart J. *72*:725, 1966.
56. Karlof, I.: Hemodynamic effect of atrial triggered versus fixed rate pacing at rest and during exercise in complete heart block. Acta Med. Scand. *197*:195, 1975.
57. Kruse, I., Arnman, K., Conradson, T., and Ryden, L.: A comparison of acute and long-term hemodynamic effects of ventricular inhibited and atrial synchronous ventricular inhibited pacing. Circulation *65*:846, 1982.
58. Kruse, I., and Ryden, L.: A comparison of physical work capacity and systolic time intervals with ventricular inhibited and atrial synchronous ventricular inhibited pacing. Br. Heart J. *46*:129, 1981.
59. Haft, J.: Treatment of arrhythmias by intracardiac electrical stimulation. Prog. Cardiovasc. Dis. *16*(6):539, 1974.
60. Wellens, H., Bar, F., Gorgels, A., and Muncharaz, J.: Electrical management of arrhythmias with emphasis on the tachycardias. Am. J. Cardiol. *41*:1025, 1978-A.
61. Wellens, H.: Value and limitations of programmed electrical stimulation of the heart in the study and treatment of tachycardias. Circulation *57*:845, 1978-B.
62. Gallagher, J., Svenson, R., Kasell, J., German, L., Bardy, G., Broughton, A., and Critelli, G.: Catheter technique for closed-chest ablation of the atrioventricular conduction system: A therapeutic alternative for the treatment of refractory supraventricular tachycardia. N. Engl. J. Med. *306*:194, 1982.
63. Giannelli, S., Ayres, S. M., Gomprecht, R. F., Conklin, E. F., and Kennedy, R. J.: Therapeutic surgical division of the human conduction system. J.A.M.A. *199*:123, 1967.
64. Davidson, R., Wallace, A., Sealy, W., and Gordon, M.: Electrically induced atrial tachycardia with block; a therapeutic application of permanent radio frequency atrial pacing. Circulation *44*:1014, 1971.
65. Preston, T., Haynes, R., Gavin, W., and Hessel, E.: Permanent rapid atrial pacing to control supraventricular tachycardia. PACE *2*:331, 1979.
66. Arbel, E., Cohen, H., Langendorf, R., and Glick, G.: Successful treatment of drug-resistant atrial tachycardia and intractable congestive heart failure with permanent coupled atrial pacing. Am. J. Cardiol. *41*:336, 1978.
67. Zoll, P. M., Linenthal, A. J., and Zarsky, L. R.: Ventricular fibrillation: Treatment and prevention by external electric currents. N. Engl. J. Med. *262*:105, 1960.
68. Zipes, D., and Knoebel, S.: Rapid rate-dependent ventricular ectopy. Adverse responses to atropine induced rate increase. Chest *62*:255, 1972.
69. Levy, S., Gerard, R., Jausseran, J., Boyer, C., Clementy, J., Baudet, E., and Bricaud, H.: Long-term results of permanent atrioventricular sequential demand pacing. PACE *2*:175, 1979.
70. Leclercq, J. F., Attuel, P., and Coumel, P.: Les stimulateurs cardiaques destines à traiter les tachycardies paroxystiques. Stimucoeur *7*(1):8, 1979.
71. Hartzler, G., Holmes, D., and Osborn, M.: Patient-activated transvenous cardiac stimulation for the treatment of supraventricular and ventricular tachycardia. Am. J. Cardiol. *47*:903, 1981.
72. Hartzler, G.: Treatment of recurrent ventricular tachycardia by patient-activated radio frequency ventricular stimulation. Mayo Clin. Proc. *54*:75, 1979.
73. Ruskin, J., Garan, H., Poulin, F., and Harthorne, J.: Permanent radiofrequency ventricular pacing for management of drug-resistant ventricular tachycardia. Am. J. Cardiol. *46*:317, 1980.
74. Griffin, J., Mason, J., and Calfee, R.: Clinical use of an implantable automatic tachycardia-terminating pacemaker. Am. Heart J. *100*:1093, 1980.
75. Neumann, G., Funke, H. D., Bakels, N., Kirchoff, P. G., and Schaede, A.: A new atrial demand pacemaker for the management of supraventricular tachycardias. Proc. VIth World Symp. Cardiac Pacing, 27-7, 1979.
76. Mandel, W. J., Laks, M. M., Yamaguchi, I., Fields, J., and Berkovits, B.: Recurrent reciprocating tachycardias in the Wolff-Parkinson-White syndrome. Chest *69*:769, 1976.
77. Camm, A., Nathan, A., Hellestrand, K., Ward, D., and Spurrell, R.: The clinical evaluation of tachycardia termination by utilizing autodecremental atrial pacing. PACE *4*(3):A-84, 1981.
78. Curry, P., Rowland, E., and Krikler, D.: Dual-demand pacing for refractory atrioventricular reentry tachycardia. PACE *2*(2):137, 1979.
79. Castellanos, A., Waxman, M., Maleiro, F., Berkovits, B., and Sung, R.: Preliminary studies with an implantable multimodal AV pacemaker for reciprocating atrioventricular tachycardias. PACE *3*:257, 1980.
80. Maloney, J., Medina-Ravell, V., Pieretti, O., Portillo, B., Maduro, C., Castellanos, A., and Berkovits, B.: Follow-up assessment of dual-demand, dual-chamber DVI-DVO pacing for automatic conversion, control, and prevention of refractory paroxysmal supraventricular tachycardia. PACE *4*(3):A-57, 1981.
81. Jackman, W. M., and Zipes, D. P.: Low energy synchronous cardioversion of ventricular tachycardia using a catheter electrode in a canine model of subacute myocardial infarction. Circulation *66*:187, 1982.
82. Zipes, D., Jackman, W., Heger, J., Chilson, D., Browne, K., Nacarelli, G., Rahilly, G., and Prystowsky, E.: Clinical transvenous cardioversion of recurrent life-threatening ventricular tachyarrhythmias: Low energy synchronized cardioversion of ventricular tachycardia and termination of ventricular fibrillation in patients using a catheter electrode. Am. Heart J., *103*:789, 1982.
83. Zipes, D., Prystowsky, E., Browne, K., Chilson, D., and Heger, J.: Additional observations on transvenous cardioversion of recurrent ventricular tachycardia. Am. Heart J., *104*:163, 1982.
84. Mirowski, M., Reid, P. R., Watkins, L., Weisfeldt, M. L., and Mower, M. M.: Clinical treatment of life-threatening ventricular tachyarrhythmias with the automatic implantable defibrillator. Am. Heart J. *102*:265, 1981.
85. Mirowski, M., Reid, P. R., Mower, M. M., Watkins, L., Gott, V., Schauble, J., Langer, A., Heilman, M., Kolenik, S., Fischell, R., and Weisfeldt, M.: Termination of malignant ventricular arrhythmias with an implanted automatic defibrillator in human beings. N. Engl. J. Med. *303*(6):322, 1980.
86. Furman, S., and Pannizzo, F.: Output programmability and reduction of secondary intervention after pacemaker implantation. J. Thorac. Cardiovasc. Surg. *81*(5):713, 1981-A.
87. Hayes, D. L., Maloney, J. D., Merideth, J., Holmes, D. R., Gersh, B., Broadbent, J. C., Osborn, M. J., and Fetter, J.: Initial and early follow-up assessment of the clinical efficacy of a multiparameter-programmable pulse generator. PACE *4*(4):417, 1981.
88. Parsonnet, V., and Rodgers, T.: The present status of programmable pacemakers. Prog. Cardiovasc. Dis. *23*(6):401, 1981-C.
89. Parsonnet, V.: Cardiac pacing and pacemakers. VII. Power sources for implantable pacemakers. Part 1. Am. Heart J. *94*(4):517, 1977.
90. Owens, B.: The role of solid electrolytes in lithium pacemaker batteries. Solid State Ionics *3*:273, 1981-B.
91. Bilitch, M., Hauser, R. G., Goldman, B.S., Furman, S., and Parsonnet, V.: Performance of cardiac pacemaker pulse generators. PACE *5*(1):139, 1982.
92. Hurzeler, P., Morse, D., Leach, C., Sands, B.S., Milton, J., Pennock, R., and Zinberg, A.: Longevity comparisons among lithium anode power cells for cardiac pacemakers. PACE *3*:555, 1980.
93. Owens, B., Brennen, K., and Kim, J.: Lithium pacemaker reliability. Stimucoeur 9:371, 1981-A.
94. Greatbatch, W.: Metal electrodes in bioengineering. CRC Crit. Rev. Bioeng. *5*(1):1, 1981.
95. Smyth, N. P. D.: Techniques of implantation: Atrial and ventricular, thoracotomy and transvenous. Prog. Cardiovasc. Dis. *23*(6):435, 1981.
96. DeCaprio, V., Hurzeler, P., and Furman, S.: A comparison of unipolar and bipolar electrograms for cardiac pacemaker sensing. Circulation *56*:750, 1977.
97. Littleford, P., Parsonnet, V., and Spector, S.: Method for the rapid and atraumatic insertion of permanent endocardial pacemaker electrodes through the subclavian vein. Am. J. Cardiol. *43*:980, 1979.
98. Parsonnet, V.: Routine implantation of permanent transvenous pacemaker electrodes in both chambers. A technique whose time has come. PACE *4*(1):109, 1981-A.
99. Parsonnet, V., Werres, R., Atherley, T., and Littleford, P.: Transvenous insertion of double sets of permanent electrodes. J.A.M.A. *243*:62, 1980.
100. Bisping, H., Kreuzer, J., Birkenheier, H.: Three years' clinical experience with a new endocardial screw-in lead with introduction protection for use in the atrium and ventricle. PACE *3*(4):424, 1980.
101. El Gamal, M., vanGelder, B.: Preliminary experience with the helifix electrode for transvenous atrial implantation. PACE *2*(4):444, 1979.
102. Furman, S., Pannizzo, F., and Campo, I.: Comparison of active and passive adhering leads for endocardial pacing. II. PACE *4*(1):78, 1981-B.

103. Furman, S., Pannizzo, F., and Campo, I.: Comparison of active and passive adhering leads for endocardial pacing. PACE *2*(4):417, 1979.
104. Messenger, J., Castellanet, M., Ellestadt, M., Greensberg, P., Wilson, W., and Stephenson, N.: New permanent endocardial atrial J lead: Implantation techniques and clinical performance. PACE *4*(3):A-59, 1981.
105. Mond, H., and Sloman, G.: Small tined ventricular pacemaker leads—reduction of lead complications. PACE *4*(3):A-60, 1981.
106. Smyth, N. P. D., Citron, P., Keshishian, J. M., Garcia, J. M., and Kelly, L. C.: Permanent pervenous atrial sensing and pacing with a new J shaped lead. J. Thorac. Cardiovasc. Surg. *72*:565, 1976.
107. deFeyter, P., Majid, P., Hoitsma, H., Stroes, W., and Roos, J.: Permanent cardiac pacing with sutureless myocardial electrodes: Experience in first one hundred patients. PACE *3*(2):144, 1980.
108. Zoll, P., Zoll, R., and Belgard, A.: External noninvasive electric stimulation of the heart. Crit. Care Med. *9*(5):393, 1981.
109. Furman, S., Hurzeler, P., and Mehra, R.: Cardiac pacing and pacemakers. IV. Threshold of cardiac stimulation. Am. Heart J. *94*(1):115, 1977-E.
110. Furman, S., Hurzeler, P., and DeCaprio, V.: Cardiac pacing and pacemakers. III. Sensing the cardiac electrogram. Am. Heart J. *93*(6):794, 1977-D.
111. Furman, S.: Cardiac pacing and pacemakers. VIII. The pacemaker follow-up clinic. Am. Heart J. *94*(6):795, 1977-C.
112. MacGregor, D., Correy, H., Noble, E., Smardon, S., Wilson, G., Goldman, B., and Wigle, E.: Computer assisted reporting system for the follow-up of patients with cardiac pacemakers. PACE *3*(5):568, 1980.
113. Zipes, D. P.: Pacing 1980. PACE *4*(2):182, 1981.
114. Cook, A. M., and Webster, J. G.: Therapeutic Medical Devices. Englewood Cliffs, N.J., Prentice Hall, Inc., 1981.
115. Furman, S.: Cardiac pacing and pacemakers. VI. Analysis of pacemaker malfunction. Am. Heart J. *94*(3):378, 1977-A.
116. Kaul, J., Macfarlane, P., Thomson, R., and Bain, W.: An analysis of electrocardiographic, radiographic, and vector cardiographic findings in patients with implanted cardiac pacemakers. Am. Heart J. *99*:686, 1980.
117. Williams, D., and Thomas, D.: Muscle potentials simulating pacemaker malfunction. Br. Heart J. *38*:1096, 1976.

23 CARDIOVASCULAR COLLAPSE AND SUDDEN CARDIAC DEATH

by Bernard Lown, M.D.

HISTORICAL BACKGROUND

The problem of sudden cardiac death has been recognized since the dawn of recorded history, yet it now looms as a major problem in contemporary cardiology. In the industrially developed world, its sheer magnitude is compelling, constituting 15 to 20 per cent of all natural fatalities. In the United States, as many as 450,000 persons succumb to this condition annually. About 60 to 65 per cent of the more than 700,000 deaths from coronary heart disease every year are sudden and occur outside the hospital while the victim is attending to normal, routine activities. Although multiple causes of this phenomenon have been identified, in the majority of cases the essential pathophysiological factors relate to myocardial ischemia—the consequence of coronary atherosclerosis.

Until the advent of the coronary care unit (CCU) for treating acute myocardial infarction in the early 1960's, a sense of futility prevailed in dealing with the problem of sudden cardiac death. Its occurrence was unpredictable—the seemingly healthy subject was afflicted outside the hospital—and the pathological findings almost invariably implicated far-advanced coronary atherosclerosis. Therefore it was not illogical to deem it a stage in the inexorable advance of coronary disease, thereby generating an attitude of inevitability, irreversibility, and helplessness. However, the growth of experience in the CCU made clear that sudden death, which was most likely to occur at the inception of a myocardial ischemic episode, was reversible and could be prevented (Chap. 37).[1] An outgrowth of the CCU was the initiation of mobile coronary units to expedite treatment of the victim of myocardial infarction within the community.[2-7] These developments, as well as the widespread popularization of cardiopulmonary resuscitation techniques among nonmedical personnel, have shed new light on the syndrome of sudden cardiac death and have demonstrated decisively that this problem can be contained.

DEFINITION OF SUDDEN DEATH

The term *sudden death* is subject to wide-ranging interpretations, depending on whether it is employed by the epidemiologist, the pathologist, the clinician, the medical examiner, or the nonmedical public.[8] Customarily, the medical designation encompasses only death from natural causes and therefore excludes homicide, accidents, poisoning, or suicide. An essential element of the definition is its unanticipated occurrence. Differences in the definition of sudden death relate to the meaning imparted to "sudden" in the temporal sense. The problem is frequently compounded by the fact that the death may not have been witnessed. Death may be instantaneous or may be a process of intermediate duration, not exceeding 24 hours. Thus there are three essential elements: (1) a natural process, (2) an unexpected occurrence, and (3) a rapid development.

Sudden death can thus be defined as an unexpected, nontraumatic, non–self-inflicted fatality in patients with or without preexisting disease who die within 1 hour of the onset of the terminal event. In the case of unwitnessed death, the victim has been seen to be well within the preceding 24 hours.

DIFFERENTIAL DIAGNOSIS OF CARDIOVASCULAR COLLAPSE

Sudden cardiovascular collapse does not invariably denote a cardiac catastrophe leading to death. Most often it is a benign condition in which a quick recovery can be expected without therapeutic intervention. However, when the collapse is due to inadequate cardiac output, dire consequences ensue. Since cerebral metabolism is aerobic and depends on an uninterrupted blood supply, more than 4 minutes of asystole result in brain damage. Moreover, as little as 2 minutes of elapsed time of cardiac arrest affect the ease and outcome of resuscitation attempts, a fact probably related to the rapid development of acidosis in the hypoxic heart.[9] Prompt action is therefore mandatory, but before appropriate action is initiated, it is exigent to distinguish between simple syncope and cardiovascular collapse. A brief examination of the differential diagnosis of cardiovascular collapse is therefore in order; yet even a list as seemingly comprehensive as that shown in Table 23–1 is hardly exhaustive. As is frequently the case with clinical classifications such as this one, diverse mechanisms preclude physiological logic in developing the schematization. Necessarily more than one mechanism is involved in any of the conditions listed.

Syncope, also discussed in Chapter 28, is an abrupt, transient loss of consciousness which is the consequence of impaired cerebral metabolism due to deprivation of essential substrates such as oxygen and glucose. Four levels of possible derangements may contribute to the cerebral abnormality[10]: (1) diminution or interruption of the cerebral circulation; (2) inadequacy of cardiac output; (3) compromise of systemic blood pressure; and (4) insufficiency of oxygen and/or energy substrates in the blood delivered to the brain. In each of the clinical conditions listed in Table 23–1, various combinations of these four factors are implicated. For example, when there is loss of consciousness due to rapid tachyarrhythmia, all four factors are involved. The rapid heart action is associated with a low cardiac output that necessarily leads to reduced blood pressure, impaired cerebral circulation, and diminished oxygen tension in the blood.

The physician encountering a patient in *cardiovascular collapse* must determine whether the problem (1) relates to a self-terminating functional derangement or (2) is the result of an organic condition. The former circumstance is benign and ephemeral and resolves with time; the latter is serious and major, jeopardizes survival, and requires prompt and precisely defined measures. Up to 30 per cent of apparently healthy adults will report having experienced at least a single syncopal attack.[11] A second consideration is whether the cause is cardiac or noncardiac. Although cardiac causes are implicated in the vast majority of instances of cardiovascular collapse, the most common basis for loss of consciousness is *vasodepressor syncope.* When observed at its onset, vasodepressor syncope is preceded by symptoms of autonomic hyperactivity, including marked pallor and profuse sweating; during the collapse itself, a pulse is generally present, though faint. In contrast, *cardiac arrest* is characterized by deepening cyanosis of rapid onset, absence of heart sounds, and a lack of detectable pulses in the major vessels. These findings are sufficient to diagnose cardiac arrest.

TABLE 23–1 DIFFERENTIAL DIAGNOSIS OF CARDIOVASCULAR COLLAPSE

I. *Cardiovascular Factors*
  A. Arrhythmias
    1. Tachyarrhythmias
      a. Ventricular
      b. Supraventricular, including junctional
    2. Bradyarrhythmias
      a. Sinus node failure
      b. AV nodal disease
      c. His-Purkinje conduction impairment and Adams-Stokes syndrome
    3. Asystole
  B. Low-output states
    1. Acute myocardial infarction
      a. Congestive heart failure
      b. Cardiogenic shock
    2. Cardiomyopathy
    3. Acquired valvular stenosis
      a. Aortic stenosis
      b. Mitral stenosis
      c. Tricuspid stenosis
    4. Pericardial tamponade
    5. Hypovolemia
      a. Diuretic drugs
      b. Vasodilator drugs
    6. Postural hypotension
  C. Rupture of the heart (intracardiac or extracardiac)
  D. Aortic dissection
  E. Miscellaneous cardiac conditions
    1. Coronary embolism
    2. Cardiac tumors
    3. Subacute bacterial endocarditis
    4. Primary pulmonary hypotension
II. *Respiratory Factors*
  A. Pulmonary embolism
  B. Sudden infant death syndrome
  C. Pneumonitis
  D. Bronchial asthma
  E. "Café coronary"
  F. Asphyxia
  G. Exposure to volatile hydrocarbons ("sniffing death")
  H. Tussive syncope
  I. Pickwickian syndrome
III. *Central Nervous System Factors*
  A. Vasodepressor syncope (common faint)
  B. Carotid sinus sensitivity
  C. Stroke
    1. Cerebrovascular hemorrhage
    2. Thrombosis or embolism
  D. Pulseless disease (Takayasu's disease)
  E. Epilepsy
  F. Post micturition
  G. Infection (meningitis and encephalomyelitis)
  H. Psychologically initiated syncope
    1. Hyperventilation syndrome
    2. Hysteria
IV. *Metabolic Factors*
  A. Hypoxia
  B. Hypoglycemia
  C. Adrenal insufficiency
  D. Hypercalcemia
V. *Miscellaneous Conditions*
  A. Drugs
  B. Alcoholism
  C. Cirrhosis of the liver
  D. Hemorrhage
  E. Allergic reactions
  F. Trauma (air and fat embolism)
  G. Poisoning
  H. Electrical shock
  I. Stings and bites
  J. Overwhelming sepsis

It is essential to consider briefly the important noncardiac conditions associated with cardiovascular collapse and to differentiate them from sudden cardiac death.

PULMONARY DISEASE

Although a multiplicity of pulmonary conditions may be associated with cardiovascular collapse, only those that present problems in the differential diagnosis of sudden cardiac death, as defined earlier, will be briefly considered.

Pulmonary Embolism (See also Chap. 46). Though extremely common, pulmonary embolism is frequently an elusive diagnostic entity. When it occurs in the absence of pulmonary infarction, the classic triad indicative of pulmonary embolism with infarction, i.e., hemoptysis, pleuritic chest pain, and dyspnea, is present in only a minority of patients. Pulmonary embolism should be suspected when there is dyspnea of sudden onset in an elderly patient with congestive heart failure or in patients who have undergone recent surgical procedures, especially orthopedic, or who have been immobilized for whatever reason. The possibility of pulmonary embolism should also be entertained in cases in which young women taking oral contraceptives experience unexplained dyspnea. When embolism is massive, obstructing at least two main pulmonary arteries as identified by angiographic studies, sudden unexplained dyspnea is the most characteristic initial symptom. There is often little else in the history, physical examination, or chest roentgenogram to lend credence to the diagnosis.

Tachypnea and tachycardia were the most commonly observed signs, occurring in 88 per cent and 63 per cent of patients, respectively.[12] Unexpected cardiovascular collapse and death in presumably normal subjects as a result of pulmonary embolism is most unusual.

Syncope may be the initial manifestation of pulmonary embolism.[13] Of 132 patients with angiographically documented pulmonary embolism, 14 per cent[14] experienced syncope, and in two-thirds of these patients, syncope was the initial symptom which caused them to seek medical attention. There were no differences between the group with syncope and that without with regard to age, associated heart disease, or the presence of congestive heart failure. However, the majority of the patients were women exhibiting severe hypotension, which was observed in 76 per cent of the patients with syncope. By contrast, only 12 per cent of the 115 patients with pulmonary embolism who did not have syncope exhibited hypotension. Nearly all the patients with syncope had evidence of right ventricular failure, were strikingly hypoxemic, and demonstrated obstruction of more than 50 per cent of the pulmonary circulation. Pulmonary infarction was uncommon among them. Some electrocardiographic evidence of acute cor pulmonale (new S_I-Q_{III}-T_{III} pattern) or new incomplete right bundle branch block was present in 60 per cent of the patients with syncope as opposed to only 12 per cent of those without syncope.

The problem of diagnosis is less difficult when syncope is caused by pulmonary embolism in the hospitalized patient. Considering the possibility of pulmonary embolism in the differential diagnosis of syncope is not an academic exercise, for the majority of patients survive when appropriately treated with heparin.[15] Rarely, pulmonary embolism, when massive, may cause electromechanical dissociation, as shown in Figure 23–1, and little else may be present to indicate the correct diagnosis. Acute rhythm disorders secondary to transient increases in pulmonary arterial pressure may also result from pulmonary arteriolar constriction. Such arterial narrowing may be secondary to the release of vasoactive substances following embolization of small pulmonary arteries in which direct mechanical factors cannot be responsible for the cardiac collapse.

Sudden Infant Death Syndrome (SIDS). Crib death is the leading cause of fatality in the first year of life and occurs with a frequency of 1 to 3 per 1000 live births. It has been estimated to claim 8,000 to 10,000 infants annually. It is defined as the sudden infant death syndrome (SIDS) and is diagnosed after autopsy by the exclusion of inherently lethal pathologic findings.[16] Death occurs during quiet sleep in infants between 1 and 6 months of age. There is significant association of SIDS with winter months, lower socioeconomic class, and a history of prematurity.[17] Eighty per cent of the affected infants, however, are not premature. An upper respiratory infection may have been recognized for a day or more.

The paucity of autopsy findings in SIDS has suggested a cardiac arrhythmia as the underlying mechanism. The abnormalities implicated have included progressive bradycardia cured by selective thoracic vagotomy[18] and ventricular fibrillation.[19,20] Schwartz has suggested that asymmetrical sympathetic innervation of the heart is the basis for the long Q-T syndrome and that this results from congenital underdevelopment of the right stellate ganglion.[20] He proposed that there may be a similar asymmetrical condition during maturation of the normal infant; the stress of hypoxia may then stimulate the left stellate ganglion and favor ventricular fibrillation.

A number of observations argue *against* the preeminence of a cardiac factor in SIDS. Among infants the age of frequent arrhythmias is the first month of life and does not correspond with the age of vulnerability to SIDS, which spares the first month and peaks during the third or fourth month.[16] A careful study of electrocardiograms of families of SIDS victims has failed to corroborate the presence of Q-T prolongation as reported by Maron et al.[19] When 108 first-degree relatives of 26 patients with SIDS were compared with 99 subjects from 22 control families, there were no demonstrable differences in Q-T interval duration.[21] The postresuscitation electrocardiograms of 21 aborted SIDS infants showed *no* prolongation of the Q-T interval.[22] Furthermore, in postmortem studies of SIDS the oxygen tension in the left heart has been found to be consistently low, suggesting that the heart beat continued *after* respiration ceased.[23] In a separate autopsy study, Beckwith found a high percentage of completely unclotted blood in SIDS, thought to be due to continued perfusion of tissues under profoundly hypoxic conditions with attendant release of fibrinolysins.[24]

It seems likely that the majority of crib deaths are not related to arrhythmia or a primary cardiac factor. A more probable explanation is that the condition is due to apnea, with a defect in regulation of alveolar ventilation.[25] Postmortem histological findings in many victims of SIDS indicate a history of chronic hypoxemia. These include pulmonary arteriolar hypertrophy, retention of brown fat, prolonged extramedullary hematopoiesis, hypertrophy of carotid bodies, and an enlarged right ventricle.[26] No doubt some infant fatalities are related to a cardiac mechanism, but these constitute a minority, perhaps accounting for less than 10 per cent of all such deaths.

Café Coronary. This condition is often confused with sudden death from coronary disease, since it typically afflicts the middle-aged man with dentures who is partaking of a hearty meal. An incidence of 0.66 per 100,000 population has remained constant over the past two decades.[27] Invariably, alcoholic beverages have been imbibed. While talking heatedly, he will take a large morsel of beef which will stick in the oropharynx and cause tracheal obstruction. The patient rapidly becomes blue, clutching at the throat and upper chest in desperate attempts at ventilation; the futile struggle merely augments the cyanosis. These symptoms are frequently misinterpreted as being due to a heart attack. Rather than maneuvers to dislodge the impacted bolus, futile attempts at chest pressure and mouth-to-mouth ventilation prove to be of no avail, and the patient succumbs unnecessarily from asphyxiation.

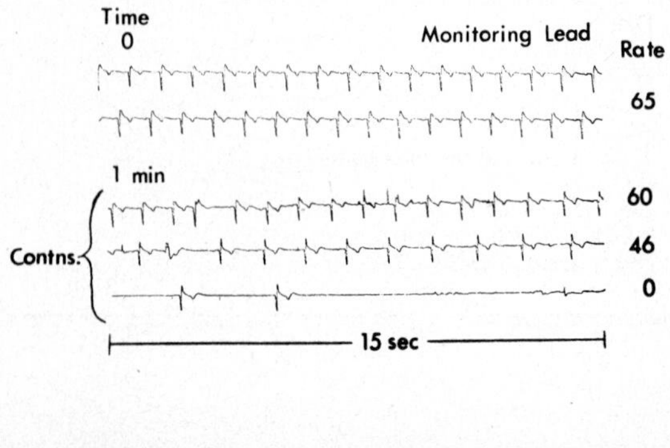

FIGURE 23–1 Electrocardiogram of patient with coronary artery disease and congestive heart failure. During trendscription, loss of blood pressure, pulse, consciousness, and pupil dilation occurred. One minute later cardiac rhythm was still regular, but within the ensuing 60 seconds, bradycardia became marked, terminating in asystole. Resuscitation was unavailing. On postmortem examination, massive embolism was found to have obstructed the main pulmonary artery. Pulse was lost at the inception of this recording, at a time when the electrocardiographic tracing was unaltered.

Volatile Hydrocarbon Inhalation. More and more ecological hazards are emerging as new products with uncertain effects on the cardiovascular system become available. An epidemic of 110 sudden deaths has been described among American youngsters, primarily on the West Coast and predominantly in white males ages 11 to 23, which resulted from sniffing airplane glue or hairsprays.[28] Severe cardiac arrhythmias intensified by hypercapnia and stress of activity are presumed to have caused the almost instantaneous fatality. Generally, after inhaling these toxic substances, the subjects will start running and will suddenly drop dead. The volatile hydrocarbons most frequently involved in deaths caused by aerosol sniffing are trichlorofluoromethane, dichlorodifluoromethane, and cryofluorane. It has long been known that the release of catecholamines that accompanies exercise and exertion potentiates the cardiac effects of volatile hydrocarbons.

CENTRAL NERVOUS SYSTEM FACTORS (see also Chap. 28)

Vasodepressor Syncope. The most common form of syncope is ascribable to a vasodepressor syndrome with vagal activation. It is primarily related to peripheral arteriolar vasodilatation with or without attendant bradycardia. Unfortunately, such collapse mimics a cardiac arrest, and the inexperienced bystander may institute cardiopulmonary resuscitation, resulting in serious visceral injury as well as rib fractures.

Carotid Sinus Syndrome. Although Weiss and Baker first emphasized that a hypersensitive carotid sinus may be responsible for syncopal episodes, appreciation of this possibility probably antedates its more recent description.[29] The Greeks may have been aware that compression of the carotid artery affected cerebral function, for the term "carotid" derives from *karos*, a Greek word meaning "heavy sleep." The earliest medical report is that of Parry in 1799, who noted that pressure on the bifurcation of the common carotid artery produced dizziness and slowing of the heart.[30] The episode, whether occurring spontaneously or induced deliberately, depends upon marked slowing of the heart rate, reduction in arterial pressure, or both.

Syncopal attacks due to carotid sinus sensitivity can be distinguished from seizures of other etiology in that they occur predominantly while the patient is standing, their onset is rapid and duration short, the postictal sensorium is clear, and they can be reproduced by means of brief carotid sinus massage.

Attacks may be precipitated by any factor that exerts direct pressure or tension on the carotid sinus. When carotid sinus sensitivity exists, it can usually be elicited on both sides, albeit to unequal degrees. This syndrome is due to sensitization not of the efferent outflow of the vagus as it enters the heart muscle but rather of the afferent nerve endings within the carotid sinus itself. It must be borne in mind that the carotid sinus in some individuals is quite sensitive, even to the extent that massage will precipitate loss of consciousness, and yet no spontaneous symptoms have ever occurred. Sensitization to carotid sinus stimulation is afforded by digitalis drugs, aging, and coronary artery disease; thus, carotid sinus syndrome represents merely an accentuation of the normal baroreflex.

Stroke. It is generally believed that stroke accounts for 10 to 20 per cent of sudden deaths.[31–33] Much of the literature on this subject derives from reports of medical examiners in metropolitan areas. These data are somewhat limited in value in that the types of cases reported include many that are medically unattended; significant numbers are also missed because they do not fall under the purview of the medical examiner. Furthermore, many patients who survive long enough will die in the hospital.

A recent prospective study conducted in a defined population is relevant to the problem of sudden death in victims of cerebrovascular accidents.[34] Among 993 new cases of strokes of all types occurring in residents of Rochester, Minnesota, during a 15-year period there were 255 deaths due to a first stroke. Fifty-two patients (30 women and 22 men) died within 24 hours, and in each case, this was the first clinically apparent stroke. The median age was 65 years, and the median time from onset to death was 10 hours. Only three deaths were virtually instantaneous, and all were due to subarachnoid hemorrhage. Most of these sudden deaths, unlike in the case of cardiac death, occurred *after* the patient had reached a hospital. All but 10 of the patients survived to reach the hospital, and in all but a few of the cases the nature of the illness was known before death occurred.

Epilepsy. Unexpected sudden death unrelated to status epilepticus has been described in epileptics in the absence of accident or concomitant natural disease. Lancisi, who wrote the first treatise on sudden death in Rome in 1707, already mentioned such a termination in victims who had a history of "fits."[35] In a careful study of eight fatal episodes by Hirsch and Martin, patients ranged from 6 to 30 years of age, and death occurred suddenly without manifestations of a motor seizure except for a brief tonic phase.[36] No satisfactory anatomical cause of death was established at autopsy in any case. Death has been ascribed to a pathophysiological mechanism in which seizure discharge in the brain stem leads to acute disruption of cardiac or respiratory function or both.

DRUGS. Only a fraction of the possible associated factors implicated in sudden cardiovascular collapse are listed in Table 23–1. Of these the most important etiological factor relates to the use or abuse of drugs.

A few key drugs of cardiovascular significance will be considered here. The most important group of agents includes the digitalis glycosides, quinidine, and psychotropic drugs.

Digitalis Glycosides (see also p. 523). It is well appreciated that these drugs can cause a profusion of diverse arrhythmias. There is veritably no abnormal cardiac mechanism that has not been reported at one time or another to have been precipitated by an excess of digitalis or by sensitization of glycoside action by potassium deficit.[37] An unusual recent epidemic of digitalis intoxication provided the first opportunity for studying the epidemiology of digitalis overdosage in a community.[38] Because of an error in manufacture, a large number of patients mistakenly received 0.20 mg of digitoxin and 0.05 mg of digoxin instead of 0.25 mg of digoxin. One hundred and seventy-nine patients were studied, 125 of whom had taken the faulty tablets for more than 3 weeks. There were six sudden deaths. Extreme fatigue and major disturbances in vision were observed in 95 per cent of the patients. A sense of "deadly tiredness or miserable feeling," a diminution in muscular strength, and difficulty in walking were common prodromes to the occurrence of major arrhythmias. Psychic disturbances such as bad dreams, restlessness, nervousness, agitation, listlessness, drowsiness, and fainting as well as pseudohallucination and delirium were noted in 65 per cent of the patients. Of the visual disturbances, most had hazy vision and had difficulty reading. Nearly all patients experienced a disturbance in red-green color perception.[38] Death that results from excessive digitalis is invariably due to ventricular fibrillation rather than to complete heart block.

Quinidine (see also p. 656). Almost since the introduction of quinidine, reports have appeared of syncopal episodes and sudden death during the course of treatment. Quinidine-induced syncope is heralded by few or no prodromes. Ventricular fibrillation is invariably demonstrated as the cause (Fig. 23–2). Attacks are characteristically sudden, are seldom preceded by warning symptoms, and consist of an abrupt loss of consciousness with cessation of respiration and involuntary muscle contractions. Occasionally grand mal seizures occur, in which case there is usually rapid and complete but possibly transient recovery. Syncopal attacks usually occur within 1 to 3 hours after the last dose of quinidine and are generally not observed with high doses of the drug. In most cases, the syncope occurs while the patient is receiving maintenance doses of quinidine. Blood levels at the time of the episode have invariably been within a low therapeutic range.[39] A majority of patients do not have prolongation of the Q-T interval,

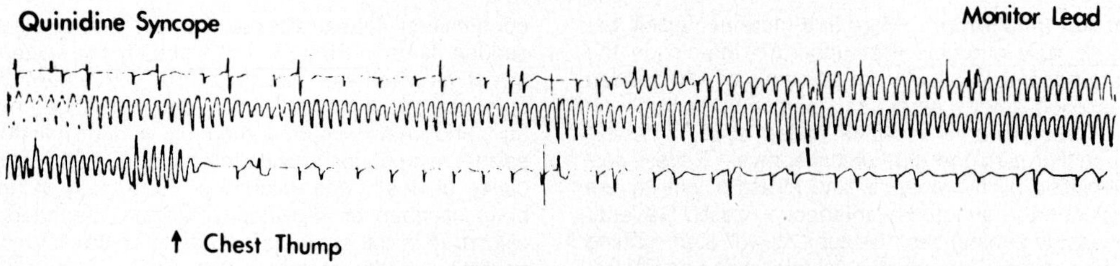

FIGURE 23–2 Within 48 hours following cardioversion for atrial fibrillation, the patient began to experience ventricular bigeminy while receiving 1.2 gm of quinidine in divided doses daily. Ventricular fibrillation ensued and was terminated by means of a chest thump. Numerous such bouts recurred over the next 3 hours. Blood quinidine level was 2.8 μcg/ml.

though hypokalemia may be an important predisposing factor. Nonsustained ventricular fibrillation is the basis for the syncope. Generally, these patients have also been receiving digitalis drugs. It may be that in the presence of hypokalemia, digitalis evokes ventricular ectopic activity, and quinidine, by lengthening the refractory period in the conduction system, promotes reentrant arrhythmias.

Phenothiazines and Tricyclic Antidepressants (see also pp. 1838 and 1891). With introduction of the phenothiazines and tricyclic antidepressant drugs, sudden death had been ascribed to these psychotropic agents. However, in Massachusetts more than a century ago, Dr. Luther Bell reported sudden death in schizophrenic patients in whom autopsy revealed no adequate explanation.[40] This has been referred to as "Bell's mania," "lethal catatonia," or "exhaustion death." Thus, although sudden, unexplained death in the mentally ill is a phenomenon that has been described for over a century, in the past two decades it has been largely attributed to phenothiazines. Whether the so-called phenothiazine deaths are due to the drug itself or to the syndrome of "lethal catatonia" or whether they merely reflect the increasing recognition of the widespread occurrence of sudden death in the community is not certain.[41]

There appears to be an increased risk of sudden death in cardiac patients receiving amitriptyline. In a hospital-based drug information survey, Coull and coworkers have investigated unexpected death in patients diagnosed as having disease and who were receiving this drug.[42] Of 53 patients with cardiac disease, 6 died suddenly after receiving the drug compared with none of 53 control patients matched for sex and age, diagnosis, and length of stay in the hospital. This high frequency of unexpected death was not found in patients receiving imipramine nor in patients receiving amitriptyline who did not have cardiac disease.

SUDDEN CARDIAC DEATH

The prevailing point of view is that sudden cardiac death in the United States is most frequently due to coronary heart disease. Scars of prior myocardial infarction are common, and coronary atherosclerosis is extensive. The problem resides not in the hospital but within the community. The prospective pooled epidemiological studies in Framingham and Albany have confirmed that sudden, unexpected death observed to occur within 1 hour of collapse is the initial and terminal expression of coronary heart disease in over half of the decedents.[43]

SOME EPIDEMIOLOGICAL CONSIDERATIONS. Among patients with ischemic heart disease, the incidence of sudden death increases with age. Indeed, when all known risk factors are combined, age continues to be a potent predictor of a coronary event. This is particularly true among individuals with high-risk coronary profiles.[44] The incidence of sudden death from ischemic heart disease in the age range of 50 to 60 has been estimated to be approximately 2.0 per thousand per year for white men, 1.3 for black men, 1.1 for black women, and 0.5 for white women.[43,45,46] In these retrospective studies of sudden death, up to half the decedents have had known heart disease, they are predominantly male, and risk of sudden death increases with age, hypertension, heavy cigarette smoking, and diabetes mellitus. It is therefore pertinent to examine whether there exists a particular risk-factor profile predisposing to sudden cardiac death.

Role of Coronary Risk Factors. In the pooled prospective study cited above, the question of whether certain characteristics define a coronary population more susceptible to sudden death was carefully examined.[43,47] The population studied involved 4120 men ages 45 to 74. With 1 hour serving as the cutoff point to define sudden death, 109 coronary deaths were adjudged sudden and 125 nonsudden. The classic risk factors (Chap. 35) evaluated were hypercholesterolemia, hypertension, and smoking. No combination of risk factors permitted identification of patients destined to die suddenly. In some population subsets, however, the presence of certain risk factors isolated enhanced susceptibility to sudden death according to sex or race. For example, there was a high prevalence (55 per cent) of hypertension among black women who died suddenly, white women who were heavy smokers had a fourfold higher risk of sudden death, and a higher risk was also noted for divorced and single women, regardless of race.[48]

There are no persuasive data to show that correcting hyperlipidemia will protect against sudden death; however, lowering of blood pressure may exert a beneficial effect, and there is a suggestion that cessation of smoking may be salutary. Wilhelmson et al. have shown that among patients who stopped smoking after suffering myocardial infarction, the risk of sudden death appeared to be reduced in the succeeding 2 years.[49] From the point of view of the clinician who might wish to institute prophylactic measures, the risk factors at present identified define enhanced susceptibility to coronary heart disease, but no combination of currently recognized risk factors uniquely selects out a subset of the population prone to sudden cardiac death. It must be emphasized, however, that death, though often unexpected, is not entirely unpredictable, since three-fourths of those dying suddenly have been recognized previously as having hypertension, heart disease, or diabetes mellitus.[50]

Prodromes to Sudden Cardiac Death. In the second and third decades of this century when myocardial infarction was first recognized as a distinctive syndrome, pioneers such as Herrick[51] and Levine[52] were already aware of the presence in some patients of a symptomatic phase antedating the acute attack. The incidence of such symptoms was not appreciated until Feil[53] and Sampson and Eliaser[54] reported the presence of premonitory pains in the period prior to hospitalization in patients with myocardial infarction. Since the advent of the coronary care unit in the late 1960's, it has been found that two-thirds of the patients experiencing myocardial infarction develop prodromal symptoms in the period prior to infarction.[55,56] (See also Chapter 37.)

Pain is the most common premonitory symptom and has been noted in 70 to 100 per cent of the patients having prodromes. Other symptoms were much less common and include weakness, dyspnea, fatigue, nausea, nervousness, palpitation, and depression. The problem is more complex when one attempts to assess the occurrence of prodromes among victims of sudden cardiac death, because in this case, the only knowledgeable witness is not available to provide testimony. However, the fact that many patients who present with myocardial infarction have experienced worsening angina has suggested that sudden cardiac death might also be preceded by such warnings which, if heeded, could permit institution of prophylactic measures.[50,57]

It is therefore pertinent to examine prospective studies that have focused on prodromes in the hope of identifying patients susceptible to myocardial infarction and sudden death. In a defined population of 25,000 men between the ages of 35 and 69 living in Edinburgh, Scotland, complete information on all acute heart attacks was obtained from general practitioners.[58] During a 6-month period, 87 patients died suddenly within 1 hour of the onset of symptoms and 104 patients sustained myocardial infarction. Only 10 (12 per cent) of those who died suddenly had recently consulted their doctor because of new or worsening anginal pain compared with the 34 (33 per cent) who subsequently sustained infarction. A further point of interest was that of the 87 patients who died suddenly, 40 (46 per cent) had seen a doctor within the preceding 4 weeks. However, of these, only 10 patients had referred to symptoms of angina pectoris; the majority saw their physicians for a variety of reasons unrelated to the heart. This study was then extended to a period of 2½ years involving 251 patients with unstable angina referred by general practitioners from their communities.[59] Of those patients enrolled during this period, only 10 per cent progressed to definite myocardial infarction; an additional 2 per cent had a possible myocardial infarction; and 3 per cent died suddenly. It is therefore evident that only a small proportion of sudden cardiac deaths in the community could be identified by means of a change in or new occurrence of cardiac symptoms.

From these facts a number of epidemiologists have concluded that the risk factors for sudden death are identical to those factors predisposing to coronary artery atherosclerosis, with similar therapeutic and prophylactic implications.[60] The long-held view that sudden cardiac death is the consequence of acute myocardial infarction has been the basis for its use as a model in the experimental laboratory; however, since an acute myocardial lesion is not necessarily the basis for sudden cardiac death, and it is possible that a wrong model has been selected, an entirely different set of risk factors may require investigation.

PATHOLOGY OF SUDDEN CARDIAC DEATH. In the large majority of patients with sudden cardiac death, severe occlusive atherosclerotic disease of major epicardial coronary vessels is present.[61,62] In nearly two-thirds of cases, three vessels showed more than 75 per cent luminal stenosis.[63] The particular arteries involved in victims of sudden cardiac death were the left anterior descending (96 per cent), right coronary (79 per cent), left circumflex (66 per cent), and left main coronary (34 per cent) arteries. The vascular obstruction was generally found in both proximal and distal segments of epicardial arteries.[64–66] Surprisingly, left main coronary artery involvement is rare. Davies[65] found this lesion in only 4 of 194 victims of sudden cardiac death (2 per cent), whereas Baroldi et al.[62] noted it in 10 of 208 cases (5 per cent).

Acute coronary arterial events such as thrombosis of the diseased vessel, hemorrhage into a plaque, or rupture of a plaque have been sought as possible explanations for sudden death. Such vascular lesions are, in fact, observed in only a minority of cases.[62] The incidence of acute occlusive thrombosis is related to the length of survival. Fewer than one-third of patients will exhibit such a lesion when survival is 1 hour.[67,68] However, in nearly 90 per cent of patients dying from acute transmural myocardial infarction, fresh thrombotic lesions will be evident in one or more coronary arteries when death is long delayed, leading to the observation that thrombosis may be the *consequence* rather than the *cause* of myocardial infarction.[65,68] (See also Chap. 37 for a discussion of this subject.)

Abnormalities of intramyocardial arteries are rarely the principal vascular lesion in sudden cardiac death and virtually never exist apart from significant involvement of the epicardial vessels.[62,63,69] Coronary microembolism may play a role in the pathologic conditions of a small percentage of patients dying suddenly and may be of platelet, thrombotic, or atheromatous origin.[70] Platelet aggregates have been found in small coronary vessels in a majority of cases of sudden cardiac death studied by Haerem[70] but not by Lie and Titus[69] or by Davies.[65] Pertinent in this context is the observation of Folts and coworkers that cyclic reductions in flow to zero occurred when the lumen of a canine coronary artery was obstructed by 60 to 80 per cent.[71] Periodic cessation of flow was due to platelet aggregates, and this process was prevented by aspirin administration. It may well be that by the time ventricular fibrillation supervenes, the provocative platelet nidus has disaggregated, thereby explaining its absence on postmortem study. Specific lesions in the vessels of the sinoatrial or atrioventricular nodes are, as a rule, absent.[62] Lie and Titus found discrete infarctions or hemorrhage in the atrioventricular junction or peripheral bundle branches in only 2 of 49 victims of sudden cardiac death.

Selective myocardial necrosis, characterized by widely scattered myofibrillar degeneration, is found in about 80 per cent of cases of sudden cardiac death.[61] Changes typical of myocardial infarction are unusual. Cardiomegaly of moderate degrees is observed in about one-half to two-thirds of cases.[62,69]

Thus, it can be concluded that sudden cardiac death does not exhibit a *distinctive* constellation of pathomorphological lesions. Advanced degrees of coronary atherosclerosis and its myocardial consequences are the rule, and the spectrum of lesions extends from the minor and trivial to the most severe. Acute thrombosis is noted in about 10 per cent of cases and recent myocardial infarction in about 5 per cent.[61,62] That the underlying cardiac disease is not the exclusive variable is indicated by the fact that when subjects afflicted with cardiac arrest are promptly resuscitated, they survive for prolonged periods and frequently without significant limitations due to the underlying heart disease.

Pertinent new data relating to coronary pathology and myocardial impairment are now being derived from angiographic and hemodynamic studies of patients resuscitated from imminent sudden cardiac death. Weaver and coworkers have examined coronary anatomy and left ventricular function in 64 patients with ischemic heart disease who were successfully resuscitated after out-of-hospital ventricular fibrillation.[72] The majority (72 per cent) had a previous history of cardiovascular disease, and in the remaining 28 per cent ventricular fibrillation was the first indication of the presence of a cardiac problem. In 60 of the 64 patients the diameter of at least one major coronary artery was reduced 70 per cent or more. Severe stenosis of two coronary arteries was observed in 28 per cent, and 33 per cent had triple-vessel disease. Distribution of coronary lesions showed nearly equal involvement of the left anterior descending, circumflex, and right coronary arteries. The left main coronary artery showed moderate stenosis in only four patients and severe narrowing in only one. In 20 patients (30 per cent) more than half the left ventricular wall circumference contracted abnormally, and only 19 patients (30 per cent) were free of left ventricular contraction abnormalities. Mitral regurgitation was present in nine patients and was judged to be moderate in four and mild in five. Of these 64 resuscitated patients, 14 subsequently died suddenly or had recurrent episodes of ventricular fibrillation and showed more extensive abnormalities of the coronary artery and myocardium.

The studies of Cobb and coworkers, however, lend support to the view that while coronary artery disease is extensive, myocardial infarction is not usual.[73] Thus, only 57 of 305 patients resuscitated from ventricular fibrillation showed sequential electrocardiographic changes consistent with acute transmural infarction (Fig. 23–3). Even this low incidence of 20 per cent may be an excessive figure with regard to the precipitation of sudden cardiac death by acute myocardial infarction. It is possible that in patients with extensive coronary vascular disease, cessation of myocardial perfusion during ventricular fibrillation as well as the attendant stresses of cardiopulmonary resuscitation is the cause of infarction.

CLINICAL BACKGROUNDS FOR NONISCHEMIC SUDDEN CARDIAC DEATH. Although coronary heart disease plays a preeminent role and accounts for over 75 per cent of sudden cardiac deaths, other cardiac conditions are implicated in about 20 per cent. Table 23–2 lists a number of these conditions, but is not intended to be exhaustive. Those conditions in which there is particular interest will now be considered briefly.

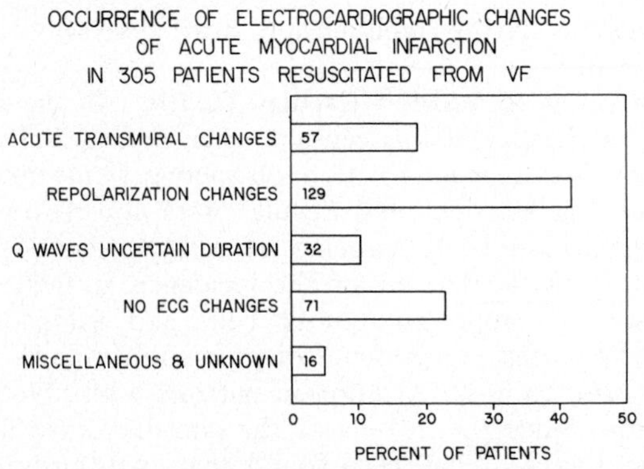

FIGURE 23–3 This tabulation of electrocardiographic changes of acute myocardial infarction after resuscitation from ventricular fibrillation derives from the Seattle experience. (From Cobb, L. A., et al.: Clinical predictors and characteristics of the sudden cardiac syndrome. *In* Proceedings of the First U.S.–U.S.S.R. Symposium on Sudden Death, Yalta, October 3–5, 1977. U.S. Department of Health, Education, and Welfare, Public Health Service, National Institutes of Health, D.H.E.W. Publication No. NIH78-1470, 1978.)

Mitral Valve Prolapse Syndrome (see also p. 1089). The wide clinical application of echocardiography has emphasized the prevalence of abnormal mitral valve motion syndromes. Arrhythmias associated with this syndrome include ventricular premature beats, ventricular tachycardia, paroxysmal atrial tachycardia, and atrial fibrillation.[74–78] In the majority of patients, the ventricular premature beats decrease during sleep.[79]

Despite the ubiquity of ventricular arrhythmias among patients with prolapse of the mitral valve, sudden cardiac death is uncommon.[80,81] When it does occur, sudden death has been presumed to be due to ventricular fibrillation. A composite clinical profile emerges: a woman in her thirties or forties, with significant prolapse of the mitral valve, advanced grades of ventricular ectopic activity, and a history

TABLE 23–2 CAUSES OF SUDDEN CARDIAC DEATH IN ABSENCE OF CORONARY ARTERY DISEASE

- I. *Congenital Heart Disease*
  - A. Structural anomalies
  - B. Electrical derangements due to
    1. Sinoatrial disease
    2. Atrioventricular nodal disease
    3. Accessory bypass tracts
    4. Hereditary Q-T prolongation syndromes
       - a. Jervell and Lange-Nielsen syndrome
       - b. Romano-Ward syndrome
- II. *Acquired Heart Disease*
  - A. Acute pericardial tamponade
  - B. Myocardial disease
    1. Obstructive and nonobstructive cardiomyopathy
    2. Myocarditis
    3. Infiltrative disease (e.g., amyloid, sarcoid, hemochromatosis, scleroderma, and so on)
    4. Primary degeneration of conduction system
    5. Metastatic malignant disease
    6. Cardiac tumors (e.g., atrial myxomas)
  - C. Valvular disease
    1. Subacute bacterial endocarditis
    2. Mitral valve prolapse syndrome
    3. Aortic stenosis
    4. Displacement of valve prosthesis
  - D. Coronary embolism
  - E. Cardiac rupture and dissection
- III. *Apparently Normal Heart*

of syncopal or presyncopal attacks. Rarely, bradycardia and asystole are demonstrated to be the mechanisms for syncope.[82] Among patients with prolapse of the mitral valve and syncope, as in syncope of any etiology, there is need to define the causative mechanism precisely before launching into a prophylactic program against recurrent cardiovascular collapse.

Hereditary Q-T Prolongation Syndromes (see also pp. 727 and 1626). Two syndromes have been related to hereditary prolongation of the Q-T interval. These are characterized by a family history of syncopal episodes and sudden death due to paroxysmal ventricular arrhythmias. When associated with autosomal recessive inheritance and congenital deafness, it has been designated the *Jervell and Lange-Nielsen syndrome.*[83] When the pattern of inheritance is autosomal dominant and no deafness is present, it has been termed the *Romano-Ward syndrome.*[84,85] Asymmetrical activation of the peripheral sympathetic nervous system had been suggested as the factor possibly responsible for the Q-T prolongation.[86,87] This may result in a reduction in neural activity of the right cardiac sympathetic nerves and/or enhanced activity of the left. Schwartz and colleagues have recently called attention to multiple reports of low resting heart rates in affected individuals and to failure of exercise to increase the rate appropriately.[87] Stimulation of the left stellate ganglion prolongs the Q-T interval, reduces the threshold for ventricular fibrillation, and enhances ventricular excitability.[88] Changes in the Q-T interval and T wave analogous to those found in the hereditary Q-T interval prolongation syndromes have been produced in experimental animals by means of right stellate ganglion section and left stellate ganglion stimulation.[89,90] Indeed, unilateral cervicothoracic sympathetic ganglionectomy has been reported to eliminate recurrent malignant arrhythmias.[91] However, some investigators have failed to demonstrate clearcut sympathetic imbalance to account for the Q-T prolongation.[92] The Q-T interval reflects the duration of myocardial electrical refractoriness. When this interval is prolonged, disparity in recovery of excitability is increased in myocardial fibers. Thus, an impulse discharged prematurely is more likely to encounter varying degrees of recovery and will traverse an erratic path favoring reentrant depolarization and self-sustaining electrical activity.

Preexcitation Syndromes (see also pp. 628 and 712). Accelerated conduction from atrium to ventricle, usually engaging accessory pathways that either bridge the atrioventricular groove or merely bypass atrioventricular junction nodal tissue, is usually a benign congenital disorder. Disabling arrhythmias afflict only a minority of these patients. Sudden death, however, has been reported in the Wolff-Parkinson-White syndrome.[93,94] Two mechanisms are believed to be implicated in the precipitation of ventricular fibrillation. The first involves the development of an early premature atrial depolarization which traverses the bypass tract and captures the ventricle during its vulnerable period. The second mechanism is due to ultrarapid tachycardia as a consequence of atrial fibrillation and the antegrade conduction of the impulse down the anomalous pathway. The rapid ventricular rate may cause inadequate coronary artery flow and lead to ischemia, cardiac hypoxia, and ventricular fibrillation. At times digitalis glycosides may shorten the refractory period in the anomalous pathway and thus, in the presence of atrial fibrillation, paradoxically accelerate the ventricular response. In the presence of rates of 300 beats/min or more, ventricular ischemia ensues and fibrillation may be precipitated. Among 25 patients with Wolff-Parkinson-White syndrome who experienced ventricular fibrillation, in all the mechanism was atrial fibrillation with rapid ventricular response from antegrade conduction over the accessory pathway.[94]

Left Ventricular Outflow Tract Obstruction, Obstructive and Nonobstructive Cardiomyopathy, and Aortic Valvular Stenosis (see also Chaps. 30, 32, and 41). The association of aortic stenosis with sudden cardiac death has been appreciated in children as well as in adults of all ages, including patients with bicuspid valves irrespective of etiology (i.e., of congenital, rheumatic, or calcific origin).[95–97] Syncope and sudden death have also been reported to have occurred in patients with subvalvular stenosis. The predisposing factors for syncope and sudden death in patients with aortic valvular stenosis include (1) a large left ventricle, (2) a high systolic gradient across the aortic valve with a markedly reduced valve area, and (3) replacement of myocardium by fibrosis. In a hemodynamic study of 29 patients with aortic stenosis, near syncope was found to be associated with a fall in cardiac output, without significant arrhythmias.[96] Sudden death is also a problem among long-term survivors of aortic valve replacement. Sixteen such patients were distinguished from a control group of 52 survivors by the occurrence of ventricular arrhythmias (44 per cent vs. 10 per cent, $p < 0.05$) and the greater incidence of congestive heart failure (62 per cent vs. 8 per cent, $p < 0.05$).[98] Late sudden death has also been reported after surgical repair of *coarctation of the aorta.* Among 343 such patients followed for an average of 12 years, there were 38 late fatalities, of which 16 were sudden and unexpected, an incidence of 47 per cent.[99] The incidence of sudden death was much higher in patients operated on after puberty than in children and may relate to the duration of the hypertensive stress on the aorta, since rupture of an aortic aneurysm is not uncommon.

Sudden death is observed not uncommonly in various forms of hypertrophic obstructive cardiomyopathy. It has been estimated that this condition accounts for 1 in every 200 sudden deaths, occurring most often in those under age 30.[100] The comprehensive studies of this syndrome by Frank and Braunwald showed that among 126 patients for whom the natural history of their disease was fully described, 10 died as a consequence of their disease, and 6 of these deaths were sudden and unexpected.[101]

Chronic Bifascicular Block (see also page 219). It has been presumed that sudden death in patients with chronic bifascicular block is due to progression to complete heart block, and therefore the insertion of a pacemaker has been deemed the proper prophylactic measure. However, current studies indicate that the incidence of spontaneous progression to complete heart block is relatively low.[102,103] There is, on the other hand, a high incidence of sudden cardiac death in patients with bifascicular block. Among 277 patients with bifascicular block, 60 had complete left bundle branch block, 196 had complete right bundle branch block with left anterior fascicular block, and 21 had complete right bundle branch block with left posterior fascicular block. Sixty-eight of these patients died (24.5 per cent), 30 of whom died suddenly during a mean follow-up of 555 $\pm$ 24 days. There was a significantly higher incidence of left bundle branch block, a significantly lower incidence of right bundle branch block, and a greater prevalence of ventricular premature beats in those who died suddenly. Electrophysiological studies showed no significant differences in the atrial-His (A-H) and His-ventricular (HV) intervals between the groups who died and those who survived. Ten of the deaths were instantaneous and were not preceded by any symptoms. In four cases in which death was documented electrocardiographically, ventricular fibrillation was the terminal event. These investigators believe that ventricular fibrillation rather than progression to complete heart block constitutes the basis for sudden cardiac death among patients with advanced degrees of intraventricular conduction impairment.[102,103]

Subjects with Normal Hearts. Any review of the literature concerning sudden cardiac death reveals a small percentage of individuals in whom, after the most careful pathomorphological search, no explanation is found for the unexpected fatality[104,105]; this is a more common finding among the young. In 18 patients who experienced recurrent ventricular fibrillation or ventricular tachycardia, 6 had no demonstrable cardiac abnormalities by extensive noninvasive and invasive studies.[106] As the practice of out-of-hospital resuscitation becomes more widespread and effective, increasing numbers of individuals with few demonstrable structural cardiovascular abnormalities will probably be found. It is conceivable that the lethal derangements in rhythm in these individuals are due to neurochemical as well as electrophysiological malfunction that cannot be identified with the use of present techniques. It has been suggested that ventricular fibrillation triggered by higher neural activity accounts for these sudden fatalities.[107,108] However, in a group of 29 highly conditioned athletes who died suddenly, Maron et al.[109] found structural cardiovascular abnormalities in 28. The most common cause of death, which was overlooked during life, was hypertrophic cardiomyopathy, which was present in 14 athletes. An additional rare cause of unheralded sudden death in previously healthy persons has been attributed to intramural bridging of the left anterior descending coronary artery.[110] In each of three subjects, death occurred during strenuous exercise.

Miscellaneous Causes. The list of unusual causes of sudden death is extensive and variegated. These causes alter with the fashion of the times. With popularization of liquid protein diets for rapid weight reduction, there have been numerous healthy people, especially young women, who have suddenly died. Isner et al.[111] reported on 17 such patients who were free of cardiovascular disease prior to dieting. All but one were severely obese women. In an average of 5 months of rigorous caloric restrictions, they lost 35 per cent of their predicted body weight. Electrocardiograms made during dieting were available in 10 patients; 9 of these showed Q-T interval prolongations and all 10 exhibited paroxysmal ventricular tachycardia. A detailed prospective study of the effects of a liquid protein diet was conducted by Lantigua et al.[112] in six grossly obese subjects. In three of the six, life-threatening arrhythmias were documented by means of 24-hour Holter monitoring. These developed within 4 weeks of initiating the reducing diet. The arrhythmias were unrelated to changes in body potassium balance. Prolongation of the Q-T interval present in many of these patients predisposes to malignant ventricular arrhythmias. But the basis for the Q-T alteration remains obscure and is not accounted for by hypokalemia, hypocalcemia, or hypomagnesemia. Unkown deficiencies of proteins, trace elements, and micronutrients may be the critical factor; on the other hand, starvation induces pathological alteration in the hypothalamic-pituitary axis, which may account for both the Q-T interval changes and the arrhythmia.[183]

SUDDEN CARDIAC DEATH RELATED TO ISCHEMIC HEART DISEASE. The overwhelming majority of sudden deaths are related to impaired coronary perfusion of the myocardium in patients with extensive atherosclerotic vascular disease. When sudden cardiac death develops as a consequence of myocardial infarction, prodromal symptoms are usually present and frequently lead to hospitalization. In the absence of myocardial infarction, death is frequently instantaneous. Sudden cardiac death therefore may be considered in these two circumstances and may occur either in the hospital or in the community.

Death in the Hospital. In hospitalized patients with acute myocardial infarction, sudden cardiac death is due to one of three mechanisms: (1) ventricular fibrillation; (2) bradyarrhythmia, including complete heart block; or (3) electromechanical dissociation. The tendency for ventricular fibrillation to occur, both in experimental animals following coronary artery ligation and in humans, is strikingly enhanced at the very inception of an acute ischemic episode. In humans, it has been estimated that ventricular fibrillation is 25 times more frequent during the initial 4 hours after the onset of symptoms than in the following 24 hours.[113] If resuscitation is promptly effected, the fact that ventricular fibrillation had occurred may not in itself alter the prognosis of patients with myocardial infarction. Indeed, life expectancy is essentially the same as in those patients with comparable infarcts who had not experienced ventricular fibrillation.[114,115]

Bradyarrhythmias with hypotension and asystole or complete heart block are responsible for a small percentage of cases of sudden cardiac death in patients with acute myocardial infarction. These disorders are more common when the transmural lesion is in an inferior position than when it is located elsewhere. Indeed, 61 per cent of patients with inferior infarction exhibit such disorders within 1 hour after onset of symptoms.[3,114]

A small group of patients with acute myocardial infarction who die suddenly present a most unusual sequence of events:[1] There is loss of consciousness, pulse, and blood pressure; heart sounds are inaudible; respiration is gasping; and yet the electrocardiographic pattern is seemingly unaltered. Rapidly the rate of ventricular depolarization decreases; P waves flatten and then disappear; and the QRS widens progressively until it becomes broad and deformed, eventuating in a completely asystolic straight line. Resuscitation and cardiac pacing are unavailing. This stage has been termed electromechanical dissociation.[1,115] Possible explanations include cardiac rupture, reflex sympathetic inhibition, and massive extension of infarction.

A small number of sudden deaths due to arrhythmia occur among patients convalescing from acute myocardial infarction after discharge from the coronary care unit.[116,117] Post CCU in-hospital sudden cardiac death has been reported to afflict 3 to 20 per cent of patients who succumb during the hospitalization.[118] Certain clinical features during this convalescence period help identify those at increased risk for in-hospital sudden cardiac death and include the following:

1. Persistent sinus tachycardia.
2. Anterior location of transmural infarct.
3. High incidence of complex ventricular arrhythmias at the onset of acute infarction.
4. Development of recent fascicular or bundle branch block.
5. High prevalence of arrhythmias associated with pump failure, such as atrial tachycardia, atrial flutter, and atrial fibrillation.
6. Presence of significant left ventricular failure.

There is no correlation between the occurrence of ventricular arrhythmia at the onset of myocardial infarction and the prevalence of ectopic activity during later in-hospital convalescence.[119] By contrast, occurrence of significant ventricular arrhythmias in the late hospital phase following recovery from acute myocardial infarction is associated with an increased incidence of sudden cardiac death during the 7 months after hospitalization.[118] This association is especially striking in those patients who, in addition to having an arrhythmia, had a reduced left ventricular ejection fraction.[118]

Death Outside the Hospital. The advent of coronary care units and their success in resuscitating patients with ventricular fibrillation have led to the development of mobile life support units to help alleviate the problem of sudden cardiac death occurring outside the hospital setting. Especially instructive has been the broadly based, ongoing community effort in Seattle, Washington.[6,72,73,120,121] During a 6-year period, over 400 patients with ventricular fibrillation have been resuscitated before admission to the hospital and were ultimately discharged as long-term survivors. An important aspect of this program is the extensive system of public education in cardiopulmonary resuscitation. In approximately 35 per cent of cases of cardiac arrest, resuscitation is initiated by 1 of the 125,000 citizens who have completed a specialized training program. In those instances in which resuscitation was initiated by bystanders, the frequency of long-term survival doubled in comparison with those in which resuscitation was delayed until the arrival of specialized emergency teams.

Cobb and coworkers made the important observation that there is a very high rate of recurrence of ventricular fibrillation among survivors of cardiopulmonary resuscitation.[73,120,121] The mortality rate at 1 year was 26 per cent; at 2 years it was 36 per cent. Among the 305 patients successfully resuscitated who had ischemic heart disease, there were 112 deaths, of which 86 (77 per cent) were due to repeated episodes of ventricular fibrillation or sudden cardiac death. Interestingly, when ventricular fibrillation had resulted from acute myocardial infarction, the mortality at 1 year was only 4 per cent and at 2 years 11 per cent. These figures are consistent with the experience in coronary care units already discussed, i.e., that ventricular fibrillation at the inception of an ischemic coronary attack may not adversely affect prognosis.[114,115]

At present two syndromes of sudden cardiac death can be distinguished (Table 23–3).[122] A minority of patients experience myocardial infarction with prodromes of chest pain during the preceding several weeks, and death is delayed during this terminal episode. In the majority of those dying suddenly (about 80 per cent) primary electrical failure occurs, prodromes are absent, the predisposition to recurrent ventricular fibrillation following successful resuscitation continues, and death is usually instantaneous. The precipitating factors in this latter group remain to be defined. Exercise and undue exertion are unusual provocative factors; indeed, nearly 75 per cent of all sudden deaths occur at home and 8 to 12 per cent at work.[32,123] In fewer than 5 per cent of the victims, sudden cardiac death has been preceded by diverse strenuous physical exertion. Although the incidence of sudden cardiac death increases with age, there is a suggestion that death outside the hospital is more likely to occur in the young.

The underlying mechanism in the majority of those who die suddenly and who have been monitored is ventricular fibrillation. The mechanism of this arrhythmia is considered on p. 626.

APPROACHES TO CONTAINING THE PROBLEM OF SUDDEN CARDIAC DEATH

There are essentially two approaches now being considered for containing the problem of sudden cardiac death. The first is a community-wide program of cardiopulmonary resuscitation. The major limitations of this approach relate first to the fact that the patient is reached only *after* the event and even a trivial delay in the initiation of cardiopulmonary support or minor errors in technique can often spell failure. In the second place, even the most successful outcome provides no assurance against recurrence, and the victim may not be fortunate enough to have a witness to his cardiac arrest.

The second approach is identification of the patient susceptible to ventricular fibrillation *before* the event and initiation of a prophylactic antiarrhythmic program. How is the patient predisposed to sudden cardiac death to be recognized? An essential hypothesis has been that certain types of ventricular premature beats (VPB's) in patients with ischemic heart disease are indicators of enhanced risk.[124–127]

VPB's AS RISK INDICATORS. Increasingly, medical attention is being directed to ventricular ectopic activity, an interest which derives from experience in the coronary care unit.[1] The hypothesis relating VPB's to electrical instability of the heart and to a predisposition to ventricular fibrillation led to a corollary formulation that suppression of ventricular extrasystoles in patients with ischemic heart disease may protect against sudden cardiac death.[124–127] These hypotheses derive from experience with acute myocardial infarction. However, it does not necessarily follow that the presence of VPB's is a risk indicator for

TABLE 23–3 SUDDEN CARDIAC DEATH SYNDROMES

Characteristic Findings	Myocardial Infarction	Electrical Failure
Prodromes	Present	Absent
Duration of final episode	Minutes to hours	Seconds
Pathological findings		
Thrombotic or atheromatous coronary artery occlusion	Frequently present	Absent
Acute myocardial infarction	Present	Absent
Post resuscitation (changes of myocardial infarction)		
ECG	Present	Absent
Enzymes	Sequential	Absent
Monitoring (VPB's)	Present	Advanced grades
Recurrence of ventricular fibrillation (1-year follow-up)	Low (<5%)	High (=30%)

instantaneous death in the absence of an overt myocardial ischemic event. Obviously this question is of critical importance and must be answered.

Prevalence of VPB's. A routine electrocardiogram recorded in healthy men, which provides about 45 seconds of monitoring information, generally detects few, if any, VPB's. Thus, among 67,375 asymptomatic men in the military services, Hiss and coworkers noted a prevalence rate of ectopic beats of only 0.6 per cent.[128] Complex forms of VPB's were even more unusual. Heart rate did not correlate with the presence of arrhythmia.

The advent of monitoring technology has permitted surveillance of ambulatory subjects while they are engaged in usual activities. Brodsky and coworkers examined 50 normal male medical students who ranged in age from 23 to 27 years.[129] All were free of the stigmata of cardiovascular disease. The subjects participated in routine daily activities. Fifty-six per cent had one or more atrial premature beats, and 50 per cent exhibited one or more VPB's. However, the frequency of ectopic beats per hour was low, and only one subject had more than 50 VPB's during the 24-hour monitoring period. Multiform VPB's were noted in six, and early ectopic beats interrupting the T wave were observed in three. In one subject an episode of ventricular tachycardia consisting of five consecutive cycles at a rate of 136 beats/min occurred during sleep. These observations lend support to the view that the mere presence of VPB's does not necessarily imply a diseased heart and, furthermore, that frequent or complex forms of ventricular ectopic beats are unusual in young, healthy adult males.

Individuals without demonstrable heart disease as determined by current techniques may, however, exhibit multiform and repetitive ventricular ectopic arrhythmias without suffering adverse effects and without experiencing a dire prognosis. Thus, Kennedy and Underhill studied 25 asymptomatic and apparently healthy subjects who exhibited such multiple ventricular arrhythmias.[130] In 18, no cardiac abnormalities were discovered by means of cardiac catheterization and coronary angiography. In seven, mild heart derangements, if any, were suspected. The arrhythmias had been known to be present for an average of 6 years (range 1 to 30 years). In 19 of the 24 patients VPB's were predominantly of right ventricular origin, and in 21 of 23 they disappeared during maximal exercise testing. Antiarrhythmic drug regimens were generally ineffective.

Hinkle and coworkers monitored for 6 hours 811 employed men ranging in age from 35 to 65 years.[131] Of these, 325 were judged to be at high risk for coronary heart disease. Occurrence of VPB's was found to be a function of age. The frequency of multiform VPB's correlated with VPB prevalence, whereas early VPB's interrupting the T waves were found in 5.5 per cent and were associated with multiformity. All men having greater than 10 VPB's per 1000 beats exhibited coronary heart disease, hypertension, or chronic lung disease.[132] Eighty-eight per cent of 184 patients with ischemic heart disease who were monitored for 24 hours exhibited VPB's.[133] As might be anticipated, the occurrence of VPB's in a population with ischemic heart disease is directly related to the duration of monitoring (Table 23–4).

Patterns of VPB's. The ubiquity of VPB's among patients with coronary heart disease would make their mere presence an unlikely risk indicator for sudden cardiac death. It may well be that risk resides in some specific attribute of the VPB, such as the degree of prematurity, QRS complex morphology, site of origin, or repetitive pattern.

Degree of Prematurity. Even before the era of the coronary care unit, Smirk and Palmer suggested that extrasystoles which interrupt T waves, the so-called "R-on-T phenomenon," predispose to sudden death.[134] It has long been appreciated that the presence of a prolonged Q-T interval, which places the vulnerable period later in the cardiac cycle, is associated with sudden fatality. Han and Goel have emphasized that ventricular fibrillation is more readily induced by early VPB's in the presence of clinical or electrocardiographic evidence of myocardial infarction, bradycardia, Q-T prolongation, and increased T-wave duration.[135] Experimental studies indicate that very early

TABLE 23–4 EXTENT OF EXPOSURE OF VPB'S IN PATIENTS WITH CORONARY HEART DISEASE AND DURATION OF MONITORING

	Patients with VPB's (%)	Duration of Monitoring (min)
ECG recording	10 to 14	≃ 1
Trendscription	40	30
Sedentary monitoring	50	60
Exercise testing	56	15 to 20
Ambulatory monitoring	85 to 88	24 hours

VPB's which interrupt the T wave occur during the ventricular vulnerable period. This period of enhanced susceptibility to fibrillation may be approximated by the ratio between the onset of the QRS complex of the VPB (QR′) as related to the QRS of the preceding normal cycle and the Q-T interval. Thus, when the QR′/QT ratio is less than 1.0, the VPB is likely to depolarize the heart during the vulnerable period with a high risk of ventricular fibrillation.[1,136] In dogs with acute myocardial infarcts, Epstein and associates demonstrated that ventricular fibrillation occurred only in those animals exhibiting ectopic beats within 0.43 sec of the preceding QRS complex, though not in all of them.[137] In contrast, ventricular ectopy beyond 0.43 sec was never associated with fibrillation.

The significance of the R-on-T phenomenon has been questioned.[138] When local bipolar electrocardiograms were recorded in the acutely infarcted heart, isolated areas of fractionation and increased duration of refractoriness with delayed epicardial activation were noted. These sustained areas of excitation apparently functioned as a source for reentrant ectopic beats.[139–141] In fact, in the presence of ischemia, the duration of the vulnerable period cannot be defined precisely from the Q-T interval of the surface electrocardiogram. Williams and coworkers observed that spontaneous tachyarrhythmias, as well as the ectopic mechanism induced by paced beats, were almost invariably initiated by pulses with long coupling intervals.[142] Ventricular tachycardia always followed the ectopic beat with the greatest fractionation and delay recorded in the electrogram of the ischemic zone.

Some clinical studies indicate that the onset of ventricular tachycardia or repetitive ventricular activity does not require an early ectopic beat. Thus, DeSoyza and coworkers found that the mean coupling interval of ectopic beats initiating ventricular tachycardia in patients with acute myocardial infarction was not different from that of isolated ectopic beats in the same patient.[143] In fact, only 12 per cent of episodes of ventricular tachycardia were initiated by VPB's with T-wave interruptions. In these same patients 16 per cent of such early VPB's were not followed by repetitive activity. On the other hand, Rothfeld and colleagues found that in patients with acute myocardial infarction, 25 per cent of the paroxysms of ventricular tachycardia were initiated by VPB's with T-wave interruption; furthermore, they emphasize that these episodes were more resistant to lidocaine and more often degenerated into fibrillation.[144] Wellens and colleagues, employing programmed stimulation of the myocardium, scanned the entire period of diastole, including the Q-T interval.[145] They were unable to induce ventricular tachyarrhythmias in patients with acute myocardial infarction who had had ventricular tachycardia. El-Sherif and associates found that the R-on-T phenomenon initiated 10 of 20 episodes of primary ventricular fibrillation.[146] However, 200 of 430 patients with acute myocardial infarction exhibited such early VPB's without developing repetitive ventricular arrhythmias.

It is of course possible that the pathophysiology of ventricular tachycardia is different from that of ventricular fibrillation. Furthermore, it has already been emphasized that out-of-hospital sudden cardiac death is, in a majority of instances, unrelated to acute myocardial infarction. Early VPB's interrupting T waves probably have prognostic significance for sudden death. Thus, Ruberman and associates have found an increased mortality among coronary heart disease patients who exhibit the R-on-T phenomenon.[147] Similarly, Oliver et al., who monitored patients in the late hospital phase and early post-hospital period after recovery from myocardial infarction, found evidence suggesting that R-on-T is associated with augmented risk for sudden cardiac death.[148] Indeed, they maintain that this is the single most reliable VPB characteristic for identifying those individuals predisposed to sudden death. Campbell and coworkers,[149] in a comprehensive study of this issue, examined the continuously recorded electrocardiographic recording of 1787 patients admitted to a coronary care unit within 12 hours of acute myocardial infarction. Of 17 patients with primary ventricular fibrillation, the arrhythmia was initiated by R-on-T VPB complex in 16 (QR′/QT $\leq$ 0.85), whereas only 4 of 265 of ventricular tachycardia episodes were so initiated.

Morphology of the QRS Complex. It has been suggested that the QRS complex of the VPB widens with age and with the severity of heart disease.[150] Soloff studied 411 patients and categorized VPB's into classic forms (i.e., those having smooth depolarization and smooth, oppositely directed repolarization) and bizarre forms (i.e., those having variable deformities of the QRS complex and T wave).[151] Of the 169 with classic morphologic findings, 71 (42 per cent) had no heart disease; by contrast, only 18 (7 per cent) of the 242 with bizarre forms were free of cardiac illness. To date no data have been presented ascribing prognostic implications for sudden cardiac death to differing QRS configurations of the VPB.

Site of Origin. Hiss and coworkers observed in normal individuals a 3:1 ratio of VPB's originating in the right ventricle (left bundle branch block pattern) compared with those originating in the left ventricle (right bundle branch block pattern).[128] Manning et al. noted that the majority of VPB's in patients with ischemic heart disease originated in the left ventricle.[152] Rosenbaum has asserted that VPB's in normal individuals possess a characteristic morphology, since they nearly always arise in the area approximating the anterior papillary muscle of the right ventricle.[153] Our experience does not support such a differentiation between VPB's in relation to the presence or absence of heart disease. Brodsky and coworkers also found both morphologic types among normal medical students.[129]

Repetitive Activity. As early as 1929, Esler and White pointed out that VPB's in bigeminal patterns or in pairs, especially when multiform or bidirectional, were evidence of serious heart disease.[154] Such forms are unusual in the young and in those with normal hearts. Thus, Hiss et al. observed only 3 subjects with multiform VPB's among 952 exhibiting ectopic activity, and only 6 had brief repetitive salvos.[128] Bigger et al.[155] have reported that occurrence of even a single episode of ventricular tachycardia of three or more beats during 24-hour monitoring inordinately increases late mortality in patients surviving acute myocardial infarction. In 50 patients exhibiting this finding, overall 1-year mortality was 38.0 per cent compared with 11.6 per cent in a control group without tachycardia ($p < 0.001$). Multiple logistic regression analysis showed the presence

TABLE 23–5 A GRADING SYSTEM FOR VPB'S

		VPB Characteristics
Grade	0	No ventricular beats
	1A	Occasional, isolated VPB's (less than 30/hr) less than 1/min
	1B	Occasional, isolated VPB's (less than 30/hr) more than 1/min
	2	Frequent VPB's (more than 30/hr)
	3	Multiform VPB's
	4A	Repetitive VPB's couplets
	4B	Repetitive VPB's salvos
	5	Early VPB's (i.e., abutting or interrupting the T wave)

This grading system is applied to a 24-hour monitoring period and indicates the number of hours within that period during which a patient has VPB's of a particular grade, expressed as superscripts in the resulting "equation." Subscripts indicate particular aspects of the VPB's of a given grade. For example, in the equation below, the subscript for grade 2 indicates the approximate total number of grade 2 VPB's over the 24-hour period; for grade 3 it denotes the number of different forms observed in any single hour; for grade 4B the two subscripts indicate the largest number of paroxysms of tachycardia in a single hour and the maximum number of successive cycles, respectively; for grade 5 the subscript represents the largest number of early ectopic beats in any single hour. A complete translation of this particular equation is as follows:

$$0^{3} \quad 1A^{0} \quad 1B^{4} \quad 2^{6}_{760} \quad 3^{6}_{2} \quad 4A^{2}_{3} \quad 4B^{2}_{4\text{–}7} \quad 5^{1}_{3}$$

Grade	0	Occurred during 3 hours
	1A	No infrequent VPB's
	1B	Infrequent VPB's but more than 1/min observed during 4 hours
	2	Occurred during 6 hours (with a total of 760 VPB's)
	3	Occurred during 6 hours; exhibited two forms
	4A	Occurred during 2 hours; greatest frequency in any single hour was 3
	4B	Occurred during 2 hours; there were 4 paroxysms, and the longest duration was 7 cycles
	5	An early VPB observed 3 times during a single hour in the 24-hour monitoring session

of paroxysms of tachycardia to be an independent predictor of high risk.

Our experimental findings have indicated that repetitive ectopic cycles reduce the threshold for ventricular fibrillation in the vulnerable period. The triggering of fibrillation is enhanced when salvos of ectopic beats tend to accelerate with progressive abbreviation in cycle length.[156,157] Therefore, evidence to date suggests that it is not the mere presence of VPB's but their type, frequency, and repetitive form that have prognostic implications for sudden cardiac death.

Grading of VPB's. The mere presence of simple VPB's in 1 hour of monitoring has little prognostic significance.[158] The fact that VPB's are noted in 85 per cent of patients with ischemic heart disease argues that if VPB's are risk predictors for sudden cardiac death, this property inheres not in their mere occurrence but rather in some specific attributes. These considerations impelled us to devise a grading system based on clinical experience, intuition, and common sense (Table 23–5).[126] Implicit in this categorization of VPB's is the fact that some grades carry a higher risk for sudden cardiac death.

Support for the VPB hypothesis has been provided in two large epidemiological studies.[147,158,159] The Coronary Drug Project Study was a long-term, randomized, double-blind trial to evaluate the safety of drugs that lower lipid levels in an attempt to prolong the life of survivors of one or more documented myocardial infarctions.[159] Eligible men were between the ages of 30 and 65 years at the time of enrollment, had survived their most recent infarction for at least 3 months, and were free of cardiac manifestations of their disease. Of the 8342 recruited survivors of infarction, one-third (2789) were randomly assigned to a placebo-treated group. Complete, edited baseline data for all measured variables were available from 2035 men who had composed the cohort that was subsequently followed up for 3 years. Among these, the resting baseline electrocardiogram in 235 men (11.5 per cent) showed one or more VPB's. During the follow-up period, there were 256 deaths. These were twice as frequent among those with any VPB's (21.7 per cent) compared with those with none (11.4 per cent). Excess, long-term risk of death, including sudden death, was associated with frequent VPB's, with couplets and runs (grade 4), and possibly with early-cycle VPB's. The excess risk associated with these grades of VPB's was independent of 28 other variables related to baseline electrocardiographic and clinical characteristics.

The second investigation involved 1739 men with prior myocardial infarctions selected from the New York Health Insurance Plan study of 120,000 men, ages 35 to 74 years.[147,158] These patients were monitored for 1 hour while sedentary. The average follow-up was 24.4 months. Sudden cardiac death was defined as occurring within minutes of a patient's usual state of health and in the absence of symptoms or findings, suggesting acute myocardial infarction. Analysis of survival data that take account of other important prognostic variables established that the presence of complex VPB's (e.g., R-on-T, runs of two or more, multiform or bigeminal VPB's) in the monitoring hour was asso-

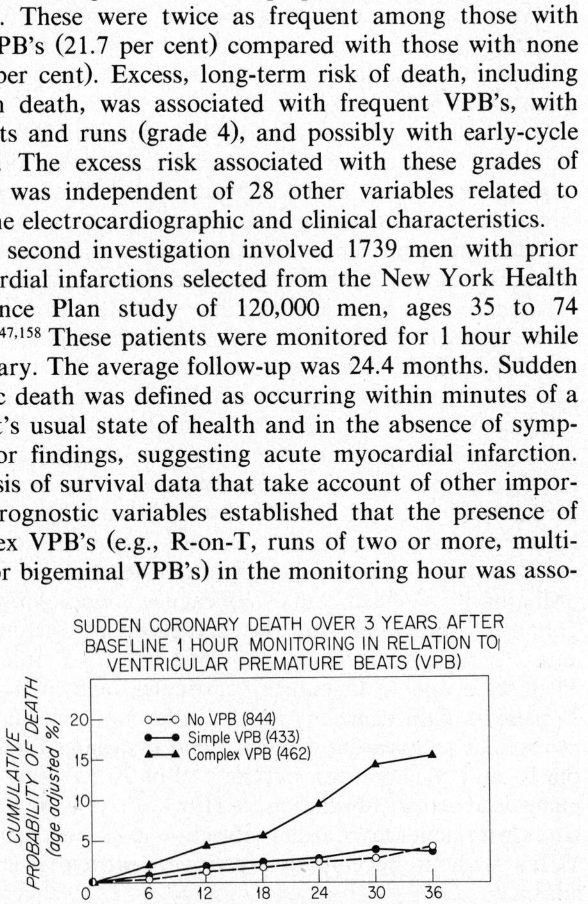

FIGURE 23–4 The mere presence of VPB's, even when they are frequent, does not increase the risk for sudden cardiac death. However, complex forms are associated with a more than threefold increase in mortality. (From Ruberman, W., et al.: Ventricular premature beats and mortality after myocardial infarction. N. Engl. J. Med. *279*:750, 1977.)

ciated with a risk of sudden cardiac death that was three times greater than that observed in men free of complex VPB's (Fig. 23–4).

VPB's and Severity of Heart Disease. It may be argued that advanced grades of VPB's carry adverse prognostic implications, because they reflect the severity of the underlying ischemic heart disease.[160] CCU studies have already indicated a correlation between infarct size, as estimated by creatinine phosphokinase and isoenzymes, and the frequency and grade of ventricular arrhythmias.[161] Epidemiological studies have related the prevalence of VPB's to the extent of myocardial damage. A number of clinical studies have shown an association between the degree of ventricular functional impairment and the occurrence of advanced grades of VPB's.[162–164]

Calvert et al. monitored the electrocardiograms of 124 patients for 24 hours prior to catheterization and coronary angiography.[165] VPB's were demonstrated in 83 per cent. Patients exhibiting only one-vessel disease did not differ from normal persons in the frequency or grade of VPB's; however, those with multivessel disease had a significantly higher incidence of VPB's of advanced grade. Similarly, the presence of elevated left ventricular end-diastolic pressure of asynergy was associated with increased ventricular ectopy. Persistence of VPB's of advanced grade, namely, their recurrence over 3 or more hours, was found only in the presence of multivessel involvement.[165] Among 15 patients with both asynergy and significantly elevated left ventricular end-diastolic pressures (> 19 mm Hg), paroxysms of ventricular tachycardia were noted in 40 per cent and coupled beats in 67 per cent compared with 6 and 12 per cent, respectively, in the 34 patients without these hemodynamic abnormalities ($p < 0.005$).

Similar findings have been reported by Schulze and coworkers, who monitored a small number of patients subjected to cardiac catheterization during the late hospital phase following recovery from acute myocardial infarction.[163,164] Patients with complicated arrhythmias (multiform, coupled, or ventricular premature beats with T-wave interruption or ventricular tachycardia) had a greater number of proximally obstructed major coronary arteries and more extensive atherosclerotic disease than those who demonstrated infrequent or no ectopic activity. Equally persuasive are the studies of Cobb and coworkers.[73] Coronary arteriography and left ventriculography were performed in 64 patients with ischemic heart disease who had been successfully resuscitated from ventricular fibrillation. The majority had extensive abnormalities in left ventricular contraction and stenotic lesions involving two or more vessels. Advanced pathological impairment in coronary flow as well as in asynergy of left ventricular wall motion was the most ominous finding predictive of recurrent ventricular fibrillation.[72]

On the basis of these data, it may be argued that prognostic implications do not reside in the VPB but rather in the extent of cardiac disease, for the grade of ectopic activity is largely an expression of the severity of the ischemic process. A corollary inference may be adduced regarding the futility of attempting to control ventricular arrhythmia when the ultimate outcome is determined by the extent of the heart disease. A recent study by Schulze et al. counters such a conclusion.[118] Although advanced grades of VPB's were limited to those patients with ejection fractions of

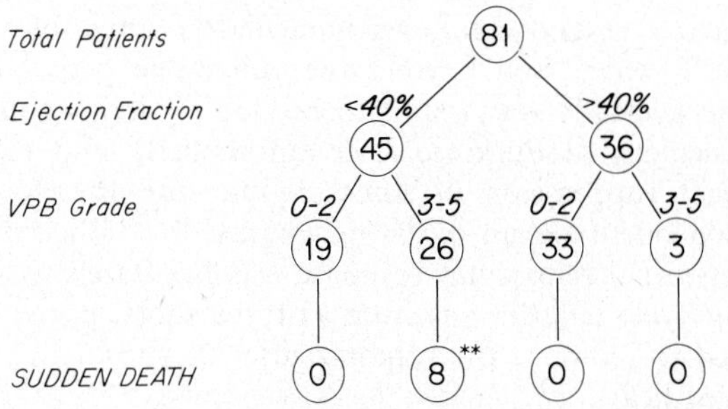

FIGURE 23–5 Among 81 patients who recovered from acute myocardial infarction, 45 had reduced ejection fraction, and those who died suddenly were only a subset of patients with VPB's of grades 3 to 5. (From Schultze, R. A., et al.: Sudden death in the year following myocardial infarction. Am. J. Med. *62*:192, 1977.)

** $p < 0.02$.

less than 40 per cent, sudden, out-of-hospital death was encountered only in those with advanced grades of ectopic beats (Fig. 23–5). Thus, among 45 patients with impaired ejection, 19 did not have significant grades of VPB's, and in a 7-month follow-up period none died. By contrast, among 26 patients with similar hemodynamic deficit but with advanced grades of VPB's, 8 died suddenly ($p < 0.02$). It may well be that extensive cardiac disease predisposes to advanced grades of oft-recurring ventricular arrhythmia, but the presence of these ectopic beats increases the chances of sequential VPB's discharging during the vulnerable period and thereby precipitating ventricular fibrillation.

DIRECT EXPOSURE OF CARDIAC ELECTRICAL INSTABILITY. Reliance on VPB's as an indicator of electrical instability presents a number of limitations. First, it is an elusive target—sporadic and random in occurrence. Second, advanced grades of VPB's have a reproducibility of only about 40 per cent.[165] Third, VPB's may represent the wrong target. In any one individual there is no certainty that the presence of VPB's is synonymous with an electrically unstable myocardium. Although we aim at ventricular ectopic activity, the target is actually ventricular fibrillation. It may well be that in a particular patient the two are disparate electrophysiological phenomena. Fourth, there is no certainty that controlling VPB's will prevent sudden cardiac death. Finally, exposing the presence of VPB's is time-consuming and costly. Direct measurements of electrical instability are therefore necessary, and the following are a number of electrophysiological approaches that are now being applied clinically with increasing frequency.

Repetitive Ventricular Ectopic Activity. Massive electrical currents delivered outside the vulnerable period of the cardiac cycle fail to provoke arrhythmias other than standstill. Even during the vulnerable period, impulses of as much as 50,000 microjoules, which greatly exceed threshold, are required to elicit repetitive activity. This is seven orders of magnitude above the threshold for inducing a single propagated response in diastole, for which as little as 1 microjoule may suffice. We have found in animal experiments that the cardiac glycosides predispose the heart to repetitive ventricular response with threshold energies, i.e., energies just sufficient to induce a single depolarization in diastole.[166–168] This has been designated as the repetitive ventricular response (RVR) phenomenon. The most sensitive part of the cardiac cycle for the repetitive ventricular response follows immediately after inscription of the T wave, well beyond the vulnerable period of the cardiac cycle. It was found to be due to digitalis-induced enhancement of Purkinje fiber automaticity and required transient suppression of sinus rhythm and therefore was not dependent on an initiating impulse.[167,168] Elicitation of the repetitive ventricular response was facilitated by abbreviating cycle length[168]; as little as three short, paced cycles sufficed to reinduce the response after its subsidence in the unpaced heart.

The unmasking of enhanced Purkinje fiber automaticity following digitalization has been employed by Jenzer and coworkers to assess the presence of electrical instability in the ischemic myocardium.[169] Following acute coronary occlusion and the development of myocardial ischemia, a single stimulus delivered early in diastole elicited the repetitive ventricular ectopic activity. Green and coworkers have demonstrated that in patients this phenomenon can be used to expose the presence of electrical instability.[170] They studied 50 patients with recurrent and refractory symptomatic ventricular tachycardia, 18 of whom had been resuscitated from cardiac arrest, and an additional 12 normal patients referred for various chest pain syndromes. Forty-four of the 50 patients with recurrent ventricular tachycardia demonstrated the repetitive ventricular response, whereas such a response was observed in none of the 12 normal patients ($p < 0.001$). During the ensuing year of follow-up, symptomatic ventricular tachycardia or sudden cardiac death occurred in 73 per cent with the repetitive ventricular response compared with only 14 per cent who did not show the response ($p < 0.001$). A "Lown Class 4B and 5A" arrhythmia on Holter monitoring prior to hospital discharge was more frequent among patients with subsequent sudden cardiac death or ventricular tachycardia[170] compared with those free of these arrhythmias ($p < 0.02$).

Repetitive Extrasystole. A different approach to exposing the presence of electrical instability is the use of sequential pulsing during the vulnerable period. It has been postulated that electrical instability is present when a stimulus of just threshold intensity induces repetitive electrical activity when discharged during the ventricular vulnerable period.[171] In animals with coronary artery occlusion, salvos of extrasystoles precede the emergence of ventricular fibrillation.[156,157] By altering the intensity and timing of the third pulse in a sequence of triple pulsing, one can probe for changes in cardiac electrical stability. This technique has been designated sequential R-on-T pulsing.[157,172]

To study alterations in electrical stability in the presence of acute myocardial infarction, an animal model was employed in which a 10-minute period of coronary artery occlusion was followed by abrupt release.[157] Two minutes after abrupt, closed-chest occlusion of the left anterior descending coronary artery in dogs, sequential R-on-T pulsing demonstrates a striking drop in the threshold for ventricular fibrillation[157] and a lengthening in duration of the vulnerable period (Fig. 23–6). Thus, whereas the control threshold for ventricular fibrillation averaged 56 mA, with occlusion it fell to 1.6 mA, returned to control levels, and immediately upon release was reduced to 3.6 mA. During both occlusion and release, there was a material lengthening in the duration of the vulnerable period as well. The time course of these changes in cardiac vulnera-

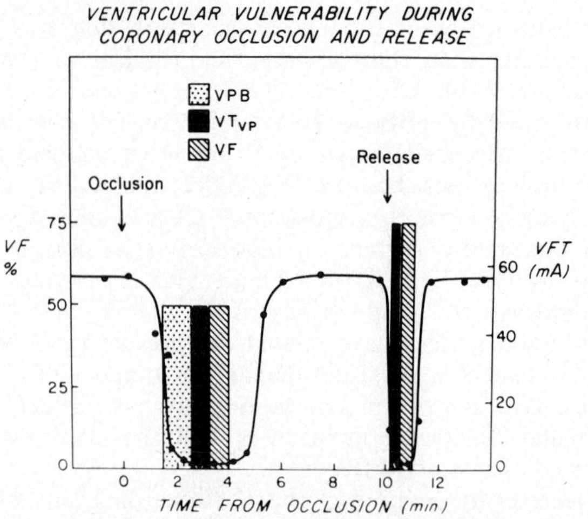

FIGURE 23–6 Measurement of ventricular fibrillation threshold (VFT) (i.e., ventricular vulnerability) during 10-minute coronary artery occlusion and release. The threshold is strikingly reduced within 2 minutes of occlusion, only to rebound within 5 minutes. A sharp drop then recurs with reperfusion. The time course of vulnerability is analogous to the emergence and recession of ventricular arrhythmia.

bility paralleled the emergence and recession of arrhythmias and the altered susceptibility to ventricular fibrillation after coronary artery occlusion and release. If the coronary occlusion was maintained beyond the point of spontaneous arrhythmias, sequential pulsing elicited ventricular fibrillation with pulses within the physiological range of intensity. Unlike the repetitive ventricular response phenomenon, in which an extrasystole occurs after a pause following the stimulus, in repetitive extrasystole the response is early. Thus, at a time when the animal appeared fully recovered and free of ventricular ectopic activity, a tendency toward repetitive electrical activity could still be demonstrated. The objective of this technique is not to induce tachyarrhythmia but to elicit repetitive ventricular ectopic activity.

Electrical Stimulation. Durrer et al.[173] and Coumel et al.[174] in 1967 independently reported on the use of programmed electrical stimulation of the heart for provoking and terminating supraventricular tachyarrhythmias in patients afflicted with these disorders. One or more extrastimuli are delivered to the endocardium at various sites and at variable pacing rates. Stimulation close to the pathway with the longest refractory period facilitates induction of the tachycardia. Arrhythmias can be reproducibly initiated as well as terminated (p. 634).

The recent development of electrophysiological *mapping techniques* for determining the site of origin of the potentially lethal ventricular tachyarrhythmias has promoted insight into the mechanism of ventricular fibrillation in humans and has provided methods for medical as well as surgical management.[175–180] Ventricular tachyarrhythmias could be induced by programmed electrical stimulation in 40 of 59 patients who had been resuscitated from out-of-hospital cardiac arrest.[181] In 23 patients the arrhythmia was sustained ventricular tachycardia, in 10 the mechanism was *torsades de pointes* (p. 725), and in 7 it was ventricular fibrillation. In the 19 patients with noninducible arrhythmia, 9 had coronary artery disease (48 per cent), compared with 34 of 40 (85 per cent) in whom an arrhythmia could be provoked. This initiation of arrhythmia was dependent upon the emergence of fragmented systolic and diastolic electrical activity.[182]

These invasive procedures, though proving invaluable in facilitating the management of refractory ventricular tachyarrhythmias, are unlikely to prove practicable in the detection of patients predisposed to sudden death among those who are free of malignant arrhythmias, who constitute the overwhelming majority of the victims of sudden death.

TRANSIENT RISK FACTORS FOR VENTRICULAR FIBRILLATION. If electrical instability is an abnormal electrophysiological condition of prolonged duration, a pertinent question relates to the possible trigger factors that provoke ventricular fibrillation at the particular time when it does occur. Since no structural lesions have been shown to precipitate the catastrophic arrhythmia, one must turn to transient functional inputs to the heart sufficient to derange its electrophysiological properties. Among the transient risk factors that should be considered are those originating in higher nervous centers.

It has long been appreciated that stimulation of the brain can provoke a variety of arrhythmias and can lower the ventricular vulnerable threshold. In the animal with acute myocardial ischemia, such central nervous system stimulation suffices to provoke ventricular fibrillation.[108,183] Vagal neural traffic or adrenal catecholamines are not the conduits for this brain-heart linkage nor are accompanying increases in heart rate or blood pressure prerequisites for the changes in cardiac excitability.

Sympathetic Neural Activity. Electrical instability of the heart can also be induced by stimulating the stellate ganglia, way stations of sympathetic neural traffic from brain to heart.[183] R-on-T pulsing of the right ventricle with twice threshold currents does not provoke ventricular fibrillation unless either the right or the left stellate ganglion is stimulated simultaneously.[184] Control of heart rate by pacing and prevention of the rise in blood pressure by controlled exsanguination do not decrease the incidence of ventricular fibrillation during R-on-T pulsing and peripheral sympathetic stimulation. When efferent fibers to the stellate ganglion are sectioned or when the animal is pretreated with reserpine, these changes in cardiac vulnerability are prevented.

Quantitative as well as qualitative differences between the right and left stellate ganglia have been defined.[185–187] The left ganglion exerts its influence predominantly on the posterior ventricular surface, whereas the right ganglion affects mainly the anterior ventricular wall.[89] Left stellate stimulation produces exclusively inotropic effects, whereas right stellate stimulation results in both chronotropic and inotropic changes.[188] Brown has shown that there is a surge of sympathetic discharge during the onset of acute myocardial infarction.[189] Malliani and colleagues have recorded increased firing from sympathetic preganglionic fibers at the level of the third thoracic vertebra during acute myocardial ischemia.[190] If sympathetic neural discharge is a factor in determining the heart's vulnerability to ventricular fibrillation, pharmacologic adrenergic ablation should protect the acutely ischemic heart from arrhythmias. In closed-chest dogs, pretreatment with propranolol prevents the reduction in threshold for ventricular fibrillation attendant to occlusion of the left anterior descending coronary artery.[191] However, beta-adrenergic blockade does not prevent the lowering in threshold that follows coronary reperfusion. These findings indicate that activation of the sympathetic nervous system is largely responsible for the enhanced predisposition to fibrillation during the early period of coronary artery occlusion but is not a factor in the genesis of arrhythmia immediately upon reestablishment of flow.

It has also been demonstrated that reflex lessening of sympathetic activity decreases cardiac vulnerability.[192] Since acute increases in blood pressure reduce cardiac sympathetic tone, pharmacologic and mechanical measures were employed to induce hypertension and determine neural effects on the heart. Injection of the alpha-adrenergic–stimulating drug phenylephrine or constriction of the thoracic aorta, which resulted in a rise of blood pressure, increased the threshold for ventricular fibrillation.[192] Cervical vagotomy did not prevent the protection from acute hypertension, but carotid denervation did. A protective effect resulting from an increase in blood pressure was also demonstrated in dogs during acute myocardial ischemia.[193] These findings indicate that reflex diminution of sympathetic tone such as that evoked by elevations in arterial blood pressure may decrease the susceptibility to ventricular fibrillation in animals subjected to coronary artery occlusion. Blood pressure manipulation during reperfusion, however, produces no changes in vulnerability.

Vagal Nerve Activity. A prevailing attitude among physiologists and clinicians until recently has been that vagus innervation is limited to supraventricular structures with only negligible, if any, effects on the ventricles. Persuasive evidence has now been amassed demonstrating parasympathetic influences on both inotropic and chronotropic properties of the ventricular myocardium.[194] There is also anatomical evidence indicating a rich cholinergic network juxtaposed to ventricular conduction tissue; this indicates that vagal nerve activity might modify ventricular excitability as well.[195,196] These recent findings are in accord with an observation made more than a century ago. In 1859 Einbrodt, a Russian investigator working in Karl Ludwig's laboratory, found that vagal stimulation raised the threshold for ventricular fibrillation in open-chest dogs.[197] Kent and coworkers[195] and Myers et al.[198] confirmed and extended this observation. They showed that stimulation of the vagus increases the threshold of the vulnerable period in normal as well as in ischemic dogs. When, instead of open-chest dogs, intact animals were studied by Kolman and colleagues, no salutary effect could be attributed to the vagus.[199] Under conditions of reduced sympathetic discharge, intense vagal stimulation had only slight effects on ventricular vulnerability. However, when sympathetic activity was augmented by thoracotomy or by direct stimulation of cardiac sympathetic fibers, a definite antifibrillatory vagal effect was demonstrated. Similar findings were observed when ventricular excitability was the object of investigation.[200]

The effect of the vagus nerve in opposing vulnerability changes induced by sympathetic neural discharge applies equally to neurohumoral adrenergic release.[201] Vagal stimulation restores the fibrillation threshold, which is reduced by norepinephrine administration, but the restoration is only to the control level. The action of the vagus nerve on cardiac vulnerability is related to its muscarinic properties and can be abolished by atropine.[202] The principal locus of vagal projection in the ventricle is the His-Purkinje system, which is also richly endowed with sympathetic neuroeffector terminals.[196] This provides the anatomical substrate for sympathetic-parasympathetic interactions on ventricular excitability. There is also evidence of such interactions at the molecular level.[203–205]

Psychological Factors. A crucial question is whether behavioral and psychological variables can alter cardiac vulnerability and thereby predispose to ventricular fibrillation. Until recently no such experimental data were available.

It has long been appreciated that when the intensity of electrical discharge during the vulnerable period is increased progressively, repetitive extrasystoles frequently precede the emergence of ventricular fibrillation (Fig. 23–7).[206] In order for the threshold for repetitive extrasystoles to be used as a marker for fibrillation, it was necessary to demonstrate (1) a constant quantitative relationship between the current for repetitive extrasystole and the current for ventricular fibrillation, namely, a fixed coincidence of the two indices within the cardiac cycle; and (2) a constant relationship under diverse experimental conditions, especially those involving neural intervention. Experimental observations suggested that repetitive extrasystole and ventricular fibrillation share a common electrophysiological basis and that the threshold for repetitive extrasystoles *can* be used as a reliable endpoint for assessing susceptibility to fibrillation.[207] The psychological paradigm consisted of exposing the animal to two environments, one of which was stressful. The latter consisted of a Pavlovian sling in which the dog received a single 5-joule transthoracic shock at the end of each experimental period on 3 successive days.[208] In the sling, the dogs were restless, salivated excessively, exhibited somatic tremor, and had a mean heart rate of 136 beats/min. In the cage, the stimulus current for repetitive extrasystoles averaged 43 mA, whereas in the sling, the mean threshold was markedly reduced to 14 mA ($p < 0.001$). These findings indicate that psychological stress can profoundly lower the cardiac threshold for ventricular fibrillation. That this reduction was mediated by

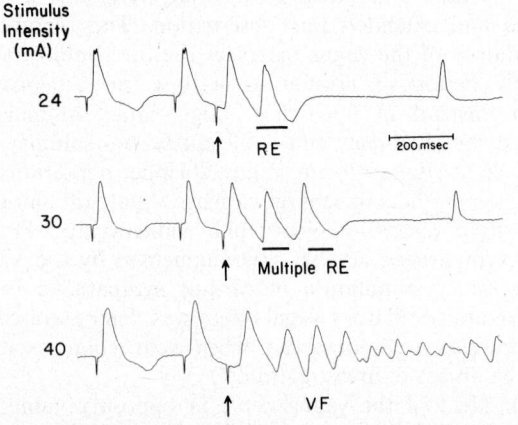

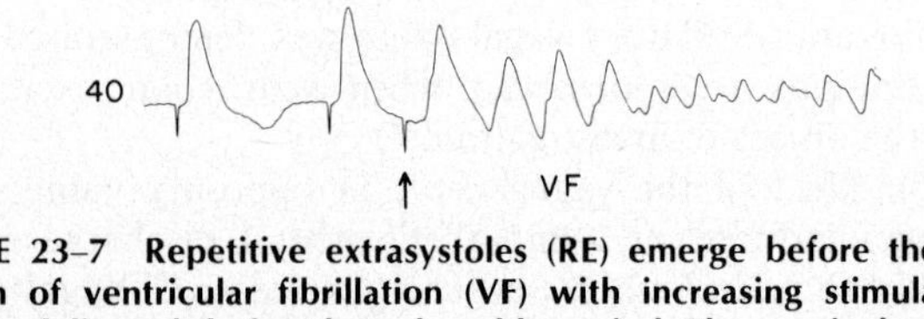

FIGURE 23–7 Repetitive extrasystoles (RE) emerge before the induction of ventricular fibrillation (VF) with increasing stimulating currents delivered during the vulnerable period. Thus, a single stimulus at currents less than 24 milliamperes (mA) elicits but a single response. However, with higher currents, dual and multiple repetitive extrasystoles emerge, and finally, with 40 mA, ventricular fibrillation is provoked.

sympathetic neural activity is further supported by the fact that the cardiospecific, beta-adrenergic–blocking drug tolamolol hydrochloride completely eliminated the stress-induced alteration in cardiac vulnerability.[209]

Psychological stress can also provoke spontaneous arrhythmias in animals with coronary artery occlusion. When animals conditioned in both cage and sling environments later underwent coronary artery ligation, they consistently developed arrhythmias, including ventricular tachycardia and R-on-T extrasystoles,[210] when returned to the sling environment. The arrhythmias promptly disappeared once the animals were returned to the nonaversive cage.

Animal experiments thus demonstrate that different environmental stresses may alter the vulnerability of the heart to ventricular fibrillation. In animals with acute coronary occlusion, psychological stress is a sufficient factor for provoking malignant arrhythmias. Although these effects are mediated by neurophysiological inputs to the heart, remaining to be defined are the precise neural pathways and neurochemical processes that integrate psychological activity and determine the specific neural traffic within the sympathetic nervous system that alters cardiac electrical stability.

Neurochemical Studies. If central neural traffic traversing the sympathetic nervous system modulates cardiac predisposition to arrhythmias, it is reasonable to surmise that neural outflow may be affected centrally. It has indeed been found that intravenous administration of the biochemical precursor of serotonin, either L-tryptophan or 5-hydroxy-L-tryptophan, inhibits sympathetic neural outflow.[211–213] Pretreatment with the decarboxylase inhibitor carbidopa, which circulates peripherally without crossing the blood-brain barrier, tends to restrict the formation of serotonin to the central nervous system. Because the serotonin thus formed would rapidly oxidize, the systemic monoamine oxidase inhibitor phenelzine is given to protect central serotonin from degradation. This results in accumulation of serotonin within the central nervous system but not in the periphery. When dogs are given the serotonin precursor L-tryptophan or 5-hydroxy-L-tryptophan in conjunction with the monoamine oxidase inhibitor phenelzine and the selective peripheral L–amino acid decarboxylase inhibitor carbidopa, ventricular vulnerability is markedly elevated.[214] These findings, though preliminary, nonetheless suggest that we are at the threshold of an era of neurochemical discoveries promising profound insights concerning brain-heart interactions.

Psychological Stress and Sudden Cardiac Death. It is widely believed that emotions can profoundly alter cardiac function and may predispose to sudden cardiac death. Engel has provided a compendium of anecdotal reports gleaned from the daily press relating the occurrence of sudden death to intense emotions such as grief, fear, frustration, rage, joy, and so forth.[215] Wellens and coworkers have described a 14-year-old girl who experienced syncopal attacks on being awakened from sleep by auditory stimuli.[216] Hemodynamic and electrophysiological studies failed to identify structural cardiac abnormalities, and the coronary angiogram was also normal. During these episodes, the electrocardiogram registered prolongation of the Q-T interval followed by ventricular ectopic activity and spontaneously terminating attacks of ventricular fibrillation. Objective evidence from clinical studies has shown that emotional stress occasioned by public speaking,[217] automobile driving,[218] and spectator sports[219] results in significant ST-segment and T-wave alterations and in increases of ventricular ectopic beats and of serum catecholamines. These changes can be suppressed by beta-adrenergic blockade.[217,218] Sleep, during which sympathetic tone is reduced, usually causes diminution in VPB's. In 45 patients who had VPB's while awake during 24-hour monitoring, 78 per cent exhibited a reduction in both frequency and grade of ectopic activity during sleep.[220]

Although it can be documented in humans that stress increases both sympathetic neural traffic and ventricular ectopy, the possibility of a direct relationship between psychological factors and sudden cardiac death is subject to considerable speculation and does not lend itself to precise documentation.[221] Epidemiological studies indicate an increased prevalence of sudden death during bereavement[222] and following significant life changes (p. 1834).[223] In the first 6 months after loss of a spouse, the death rate among 4486 widows and widowers, 55 years of age or older, increased 40 per cent above the expected rate for a married population matched for age.[222] Rahe and coworkers retrospectively interviewed the families of 226 victims of sudden cardiac death in Helsinki, Finland, and noted that significant life changes such as divorce, grief, and altered work patterns had occurred during the 6 months preceding death compared with status in the same interval 1 year earlier (see Table 57–2, p. 1834).[223] Among patients recovering from acute myocardial infarction, one risk factor for sudden cardiac death proved to be ward rounds.[224] A fivefold greater incidence of sudden death occurred during medical daily ward rounds than would have been anticipated had these deaths been random. The physician-in-chief's rounds, held only once weekly, accounted for half the sudden fatalities. Increasing experience with patients resuscitated from non–infarct-related, out-of-hospital sudden cardiac death is proving instructive with regard to the possible role of psychological factors. In one such patient, a 39-year-old man who had twice experienced ventricular fibrillation, extensive studies, including coronary angiography, showed no evidence of cardiovascular disease.[107] However, data were amassed indicating a role for higher nervous activity in the genesis of the ventricular arrhythmia. These included the psychiatric make-up of the patient, the emotional stress attending the first cardiac arrest, the provocation of advanced grades of VPB's and ventricular tachycardia during ward rounds, the prevalence of arrhythmia during the rapid eye movement (REM) stage of sleep when he had violent dreams, the occurrence of the second episode of ventricular fibrillation during a similar period of sleep, and finally the observations that meditation and cardioselective beta-adrenergic–blocking drugs decreased the ventricular arrhythmia.

The studies cited above sanction the view that higher nervous activity may constitute a transient risk factor for sudden cardiac death. So far, a major role can be ascribed to the sympathetic limb of the autonomic nervous system; the cardiac mechanism involves reduction in the vulnerable period threshold for ventricular fibrillation. In patients with ischemic heart disease and electrical instability, such neural traffic primarily engaging the adrenergic system may suffice to provoke lethal ventricular arrhythmias.

ALTERNATIVE HYPOTHESES FOR THE MECHANISM OF SUDDEN CARDIAC DEATH. So far, the major thrust of the discussion has related sudden cardiac death to the occurrence of cardiac arrhythmias triggered by transient risk factors and predisposed to by electrical instability. In the experimental animal, ventricular fibrillation can be induced by two different mechanisms, namely, obstruction of coronary flow and its release, with resulting reperfusion. The latter is unrelated to neural factors and is the more likely to provoke ventricular fibrillation.[157,191] Occlusion for as brief an interval as 4 to 6 minutes activates those factors responsible for inducing ventricular fibrillation on release. It may well be that transient interference with coronary flow is critical for the genesis of ventricular fibrillation. In this context it is possible that platelet aggregates and coronary vasospasm may transiently infringe on coronary blood flow. These two mechanisms therefore deserve consideration.

Platelet Function. Hughes and Tonks were the first to demonstrate that microemboli of platelet aggregates can lodge in the microcirculation of the rabbit heart and cause multiple myocardial necrotic lesions.[225,226] Later, Jorgensen et al. conducted studies in swine in which the direct coronary infusion of adenosine diphosphate (ADP) caused rapid onset of transient circulatory collapse accompanied by electrocardiographic changes of myocardial ischemia; in some animals ventricular fibrillation developed.[227] At the time of these cardiac effects the concentration of platelets in coronary venous blood was reduced to 70 to 75 per cent of the pre-ADP infusion values. These effects abated within 10 minutes. Numerous platelet aggregates were noted in the coronary microcirculation of animals sacrificed during the height of this phenomenon. When these swine were made thrombocytopenic by administering ^{32}P, ADP infusion was unaccompanied by myocardial changes. Folts and coworkers demonstrated a cyclic disappearance of coronary flow in vessels that had been narrowed externally.[71] During these cycles of myocardial ischemia, ventricular arrhythmia emerged. Platelet aggregates were identified in the partially obstructed arteries. This phenomenon of cyclic reduction in coronary flow was prevented by pretreatment with aspirin. Haerem found platelet aggregates in the intramyocardial vessels of patients dying suddenly of coronary artery disease, but these lesions were absent in those that died from other causes.[70]

In addition to their capacity for mechanical obstruction by aggregation, platelets release humoral factors that may contribute to impairment of blood flow. It has been established that the vasoactive amines, released by thrombin from the platelets coating the emboli, contribute to the magnitude of the vascular response in pulmonary embolism.[228,229] The platelet humoral factors are responsible for vascular and airway constriction and contribute to the mortality rate caused by such embolisms.[230,231] As early as 1953, Comroe and coworkers suggested that serotonin (5-hydroxytryptophan) might be the responsible agent for the reflex and direct cardiopulmonary changes associated with pulmonary embolism.[232] Zervas et al. have also shown that pretreatment with reserpine prevented vasospasm in animals subjected to experimental subarachnoid hemorrhage.[233] The protective effect was related to marked reduction in blood serotonin. The feeding of kanamycin to monkeys inhibited cerebrovascular vasospasm.[234] The effect was again associated with and seemingly related to a marked reduction of blood serotonin concentration.

Additional evidence that platelets may be implicated in the mechanism of sudden cardiac death was provided by Ellis and coworkers, who found that when human platelets are aggregated by thrombin, material is released that causes strips of tissue cut from the porcine coronary artery to contract.[235] Peak contraction occurred within 1 minute and dissipated within 4 to 8 minutes. Indomethacin, which inhibits prostaglandin synthesis, prevented the shortening of the coronary artery strip, suggesting that the contractile substance was a prostaglandin. These investigators adduced evidence that thromboxane A_2, one of the principal biologically active prostaglandins released from aggregated platelets, was the contractile factor.[235]

Pertinent to the platelet hypothesis in relation to sudden cardiac death is the fact that infusion of catecholamines such as norepinephrine induces subendocardial necrosis, which is associated with platelet aggregates in the myocardial microcirculation.[236,237] Stress itself may initiate such platelet aggregation in the coronary circulation. Total vascular occlusion occurred in rats subjected to such stressful stimuli as heat or electric shock.[238] The cardiac lesions produced by stress are similar to those observed following catecholamine administration and have also been reported in patients dying from pheochromocytoma.[239] Barr and coworkers have noted an association between thrombocythemia and the occurrence of ventricular arrhythmias.[240] The patient, a young woman with angiographically normal coronary arterial vessels, experienced recurring episodes of Prinzmetal's variant angina pectoris and episodes of nocturnal ventricular tachycardia. The only abnormality was a blood platelet count of 1,000,000/mm^3. Symptoms as well as arrhythmia abated after the initiation of salicylate therapy.

The following hypothesis appears to be supported by substantial evidence: Given a myocardium with electrical instability due to extensive coronary atherosclerosis, psychophysiological stress or enhanced neural sympathetic tone favors formation of platelet aggregates in regions of plaques and turbulent flow; there follows release of biogenic amines and prostaglandins, which induce spasm of large vessels, leading to major coronary artery obstruction as well as to impaired flow in tributaries. Ventricular fibrillation is triggered on platelet disaggregation and the abrupt onset of reperfusion.

Coronary Arterial Spasm (see also p. 1360). The reality of coronary arterial spasm is better appreciated since the description by Prinzmetal et al. of a variant form of angina pectoris.[241] The absence of significant coronary atherosclerosis among a number of patients with this syndrome has been widely reported.[242–244] The role of vasospasm was first conclusively demonstrated by Dhurandhar et al.[245] and by Oliva et al.[246] and has been amply confirmed.[247–250] Especially persuasive are the observations of Maseri and coworkers, who have found that coronary vasospasm is not only limited to variant angina but also is an initiating event in myocardial infarction.[248,249] The concept of vascular spasm in the coronary circulation has profound implications. The investigations of Mudge and coworkers are especially relevant.[251] They measured coronary vascular resistance before and during the initial portion of a cold pressor test in patients with normal and with diseased coronary arteries. Although coronary resistance did not change in the former group, it rose in those with ischemic heart disease. The alpha-adrenergic–blocking drug phentolamine abolished reflex coronary vasoconstriction in several patients who experienced angina pectoris. In patients with Prinzmetal's angina, coronary arterial spasm can also be induced by ergot alkaloids[252,253] as well as by the vagotonic agent methacholine.[254,255]

Relevant to the problem of sudden cardiac death is the fact that Prinzmetal's angina is associated with a ubiquity of VPB's, which may be of advanced grade. It is well appreciated that the current of injury as well as coronary spasm may occur without the patient feeling any discomfort, and one may therefore surmise that in the electrically unstable heart, diverse neural traffic to the heart may provoke coronary vascular spasm, which enhances myocardial ischemia and triggers arrhythmia, which in turn may culminate in ventricular fibrillation at the onset of impaired flow or upon reperfusion. There may also be platelet aggregates and release of diverse biogenic amines, prostaglandins as well as bradykinins, which participate in varying degrees and contribute to the final denouement.

CLINICAL APPROACHES TO SUDDEN CARDIAC DEATH

Patients with Acute Myocardial Infarction. Among those dying suddenly, a major problem is delay in seeking medical attention (Chap. 57).[256] Patients' denial of the gravity of their condition or misinterpretation of symptoms is a significant reason for delayed hospitalization.[7,257–259] Curiously, patients with previous myocardial infarction or with preexisting angina pectoris delay the longest in seeking help.[258] In the pre-hospital phase of myocardial infarction, the most important component of patient delay relates to self-treatment and seeking advice from family, friends, and neighbors.[259] Arrival at the hospital is invariably delayed well beyond the critical first hour, when about 60 per cent of all sudden cardiac deaths occur. Clearly, part of the problem is lack of education on the part of both the medical profession and the lay public about the need for expeditious hospitalization with the advent of symptoms that suggest a heart attack. However, one cannot be overly optimistic that education alone, no matter how intensive, will overcome entrenched habit and fear. Experience with physicians who have heart attacks is sadly instructive; they frequently procrastinate longer than laymen. Certainly this is not due to ignorance of the consequences.

The physician can, however, shorten delay by advising patients with ischemic heart disease to proceed immediately to an appropriate health care facility if there is an abrupt onset of chest pain or if preexisting angina changes in quality or duration. The patient should be instructed to contact an emergency ambulance service directly and bypass calling a physician if symptoms are disabling. When the physician is in the presence of a patient having an acute coronary episode, the first therapeutic objective is to allay anxiety and to assuage pain. The former requires a reassuring demeanor and encouragement; the latter is readily controlled by parenteral morphine. The next objective is to protect against fatal arrhythmia. Monitoring is not required for the initiation of appropriate measures. Even if the heart rate is regular on auscultation or even if an electrocardiographic monitor shows an absence of VPB's, an unheralded outburst of ventricular fibrillation is not precluded.[146,260] The administration of a bolus of 75 mg of lidocaine intravenously followed by 300 mg intramuscularly will prevent malignant ventricular arrhythmia in a large majority of patients. Double-blind studies have demonstrated the protective effect of lidocaine at the very inception of a coronary ischemic event.[261,262] If symptomatic bradycardia is present and heart rates are less than 50 per minute, the judicious use of small doses of atropine may prove salutary. Self-administration of either of these drugs by the patient places an unwarranted burden on the victim. The precise guidelines for the proper use of these medications require medical appraisal and sound clinical judgment.

Patients with Primary Electrical Failure. This syndrome usually lacks prodromes, and death is frequently instantaneous. When time does elapse, the patient may find symptoms difficult to interpret properly and is unlikely to summon help. When help is summoned, it may be too late. As already noted, there are essentially two distinct strategies: (1) reach the patient at the inception of the terminal event and provide emergency cardiopulmonary resuscitative care; and (2) identify the potential victim and initiate prophylactic measures against fatal arrhythmia.

Emergency Care. Current medical efforts for coping with sudden death place major reliance upon cardiopulmonary resuscitation, the intent being to reach the patient expeditiously at the very onset of the potentially lethal attack in order to terminate the ventricular fibrillation and stabilize the heart rhythm. Community-based ambulance services are beginning to incorporate the expertise and facilities found in the coronary care unit and are now gaining popularity. The essential concepts and guidelines for resuscitation were enunciated during the first National Conference on Standards for Cardiopulmonary Resuscitation and Emergency Cardiac Care, held in May, 1973.[263] Two essential strategies were defined and have been recently updated:[264,264a] basic life support and advanced life support.

Emergency first aid procedures, consisting of the recognition of airway obstruction and of respiratory and cardiac arrest and the proper application of cardiopulmonary resuscitation (CPR), constitute the elements of *basic life support.* CPR involves opening and maintaining a patent airway, providing artificial ventilation by means of rescue breathing, and maintaining artificial circulation by means of external cardiac compression. Paramount among the goals of CPR is to restore a cardiac mechanism as expeditiously as possible. The interval between the onset of cardiac arrest and the restoration of a normal cardiac rhythm will determine the success of defibrillation, the capacity to maintain an effective rhythm, the extent of neurologic damage as well as the achievement of long-term survival. Therefore the objectives in cardiac resuscitation are the prompt delivery of oxygenated blood to vital organs by means of cardiac massage and the reestablishment of a heartbeat by means of defibrillation. The priority given to these two procedures depends upon the conditions under which cardiac arrest occurs. Thus, if the arrest is witnessed and a defibrillator is close at hand, one aims first to restore a cardiac mechanism. If, however, the event is unwitnessed, or the area is not equipped with a defibrillator, routine cardiopulmonary efforts are initiated and defibrillation is deferred.

Advanced life support includes, in addition to the basic life support outlined above, a number of adjunctive procedures, including intravenous fluid and drug administration, cardiac defibrillation, stabilization of blood pressure, rhythm monitoring, control of arrhythmias, and postresuscitation care.

CARDIOPULMONARY RESUSCITATION (CPR)

THUMPVERSION At the very inception of ventricular fibrillation, there is frequently observed an ultrarapid regular rhythm designated as ventricular tachycardia of the vulnerable period—$VT_{(vp)}$.[136] This mechanism is believed to result from a self-sustained reentrant wavefront of depolarization circulating around the perimeter of an infarct or of an ischemic area. This view is supported by the observation that one or more threshold pulses delivered directly to the endocardium may terminate this arrhythmia. $VT_{(vp)}$ can also be abolished by one hundredth of the energy required to defibrillate the heart transthoracically. This fact is of profound clinical significance, since such low energies can be delivered to the heart by means of a chest thump.[265] If thumping of the lower sternum is delayed, even momentarily, ventricular fibrillation emerges and is resistant to this maneuver. Effectiveness of the chest thump is due to transduction of the mechanical input to an electrical pulse, i.e., an extrasystole, which depolarizes part of the pathway traversed by the abnormal reentrant excitation.[266] This technique is especially valuable in the patient who is being monitored and when the arrest has been witnessed.

In utilizing the precordial thump, the following guidelines must be observed:

1. One should deliver a sharp, quick blow to the midportion of the sternum, hitting with the lower, fleshy portion of the fist from a distance of 8 to 12 inches above the chest.
2. It must be administered during the first minute after onset of the cardiac arrest.
3. If there is no cardiac response on repeating the chest thump, basic life support must not be further delayed.

Artificial Ventilation. An important factor in successful resuscitation is the immediate establishment of a patent airway (Fig. 23–8). This requires examination of the mouth to assure that no obstruction is present, such as loosely fitting dentures, vomitus, or any other foreign body. The most common cause of airway obstruction in the unconscious person is the tongue, which recedes to the posterior pharyngeal wall. Patency of the airway is assured by tilting the victim's head backward as far as possible. This simple maneuver may suffice for the resumption of spontaneous respiration. With the victim lying on his back, his neck fully extended, so that the base of the tongue no longer obstructs the upper end of the trachea, the rescuer

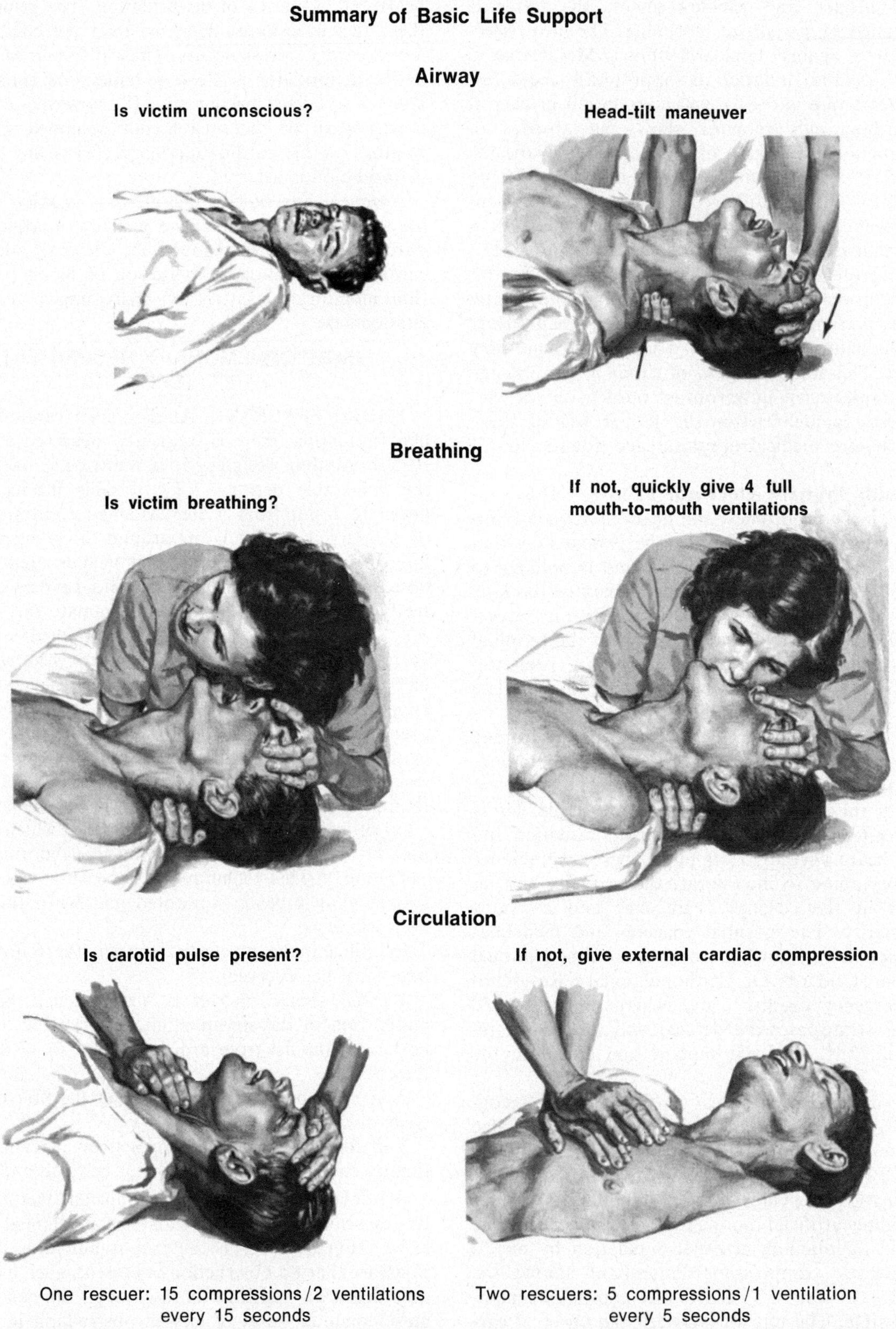
Summary of Basic Life Support
Airway
Is victim unconscious?
Head-tilt maneuver
Breathing
Is victim breathing?
If not, quickly give 4 full mouth-to-mouth ventilations
Circulation
Is carotid pulse present?
If not, give external cardiac compression
One rescuer: 15 compressions/2 ventilations every 15 seconds
Two rescuers: 5 compressions/1 ventilation every 5 seconds

FIGURE 23–8 Emergency maneuvers in a patient with cardiac or cardiorespiratory arrest. (© Copyright 1974 CIBA Pharmaceutical Company, Division of CIBA-GEIGY Corporation. Reprinted with permission from Clinical Symposia, illustrated by Frank H. Netter, M.D. All rights reserved.)

accomplishes the head tilt maneuver by placing one hand beneath the victim's neck and the other hand on the forehead and then lifting the neck while pressing the head backward. The head must be maintained in this position throughout resuscitation. Thereupon, mouth-to-mouth or mouth-to-nose breathing is initiated. A plastic airway can be used if available. With one hand behind the victim's neck, holding the victim's head in a position of maximum backward tilt, the rescuer pinches the victim's nostrils together with the thumb and index finger of the other hand, opens his mouth widely, takes a deep breath, places his mouth over the victim's mouth to create a tight seal, and exhales completely.

This is a simple and effective means of delivering oxygenated air by untrained personnel. The cycle should be repeated every 5 seconds for as long as respiratory inadequacy persists. By observing the rise and fall of the chest and by noting the escape of air during exhalation as well as the resistance encountered during inspiration as the victim's lungs expand, the rescuer can determine whether ventilation is adequate. Often much valuable time is wasted by medical or paramedical personnel in attempting to insert an endotracheal tube as the initial measure in management of cardiac arrest. In the majority of instances, endotracheal intubation is not required. Mouth-to-nose ventilation is preferred and is recommended when it is impossible to open the victim's mouth, when there is injury to the mouth, or when it is difficult to achieve a tight seal.

Artificial Circulation. Cardiac arrest is recognized by the absence of a pulse in the large arteries of an unconscious victim who is not breathing. Having rapidly ventilated the subject four times, one instantly checks for a carotid pulse. While maintaining the head tilt with one hand on the forehead, the rescuer now initiates external cardiac compression, which consists of rhythmic application of pressure to the lower half of the sternum but not over the xiphoid process. External cardiac compression is always accompanied by artificial ventilation. This method is relatively simple and can be used successfully by personnel who have had only a minimum of training. It involves compression of the heart between sternum and spine; lateral cardiac motion is limited by the pericardium. The patient must be in a horizontal position on a hard surface, preferably the floor, if one is indoors. Elevation of lower extremities while the rest of the body remains horizontal may promote venous return and augment artificial circulation during external cardiac compression. The pressure required must be of a magnitude to depress the lower sternum by a minimum of 3 to 5 cm. The long axis of the heel of one's hand is placed parallel to and over the long axis of the lower half of the sternum, and the heel of the other hand is placed on the dorsum of the first. If applied too high, the massage will prove ineffective and may cause multiple rib fractures. The arms are kept straight at the elbow to allow pressure to be applied almost vertically. The shoulders of the resuscitator should be directly above the victim's sternum, so that compression can be carried out by forceful movements of the back and shoulders with elbows fully extended rather than by flexion and extension of the arm at the elbow. Compressions must be regular, uninterrupted, and carried out at a frequency of 60 per minute; relaxation should be abrupt and equal to compression in duration. A ratio of 5:1 is maintained between ventilation and cardiac compression.

Cardiopulmonary resuscitation is best accomplished by two rescuers, one on either side of the patient, who can then switch positions when necessary without any significant interruption of the 5:1 rhythm. If the rescuer is alone, 18 compressions should be applied, and the lungs should be ventilated two times, and this cycle should be continued until help arrives. To attain proficiency one must practice these resuscitative maneuvers using mannequins and under the direction of skilled instructors.

The effectiveness of CPR has been ascribed to compression of the arrested heart between the sternum and the vertebral column. However, early observations indicated that similar intrathoracic arterial and venous pressure levels prevailed during chest compression.[267] Weisfeldt and associates[268] have questioned whether the pumping action of the heart during CPR is a critical factor in maintaining blood flow. They have noted that the effectiveness of CPR correlates with the rise of intrathoracic pressure; for example, in patients with flail chest, no arterial blood pressure is generated until paradoxical thoracic expansion is prevented by binding the chest. Furthermore, by transiently preventing expiration or by maintaining pressure on the AMBU bag in intubated patients, arterial pressure is increased with the greater intrathoracic pressure. In extensive studies, these workers[268] failed to find a pressure gradient across the heart during chest compression. However, they did observe an extrathoracic arteriovenous gradient. Flow occurs because of a rise in intrathoracic pressure, which generates an extrathoracic arteriovenous gradient. These observations are in accord with the demonstration by Criley et al.[269] that continuous coughing can maintain consciousness in the arrested patient.

ADVANCED LIFE SUPPORT. Advanced life support does not imply abandoning cardiopulmonary resuscitation but rather supplementing it with more definitive measures as additional resources and personnel reach the scene. It entails the use of supplemental oxygen as soon as it becomes available. Exhaled air ventilation delivers generally about 16 to 17 per cent oxygen to the victim. This may produce an alveolar oxygen tension of 80 torr. However, because of the low cardiac output associated with external cardiac compression, the presence of intrapulmonary shunting, and ventilation-perfusion abnormalities, marked discrepancies will occur between alveolar and arterial oxygen tension, and hypoxemia will invariably be present. Monitoring for arrhythmia defines the cardiac mechanism and permits the institution of defibrillation. However, blind defibrillation is preferred if time is to be wasted in gaining an adequate electrocardiographic signal.

Defibrillation. The electrode paddles to be applied to the chest as well as the chest areas involved must be adequately covered with electrode paste in order to lower electrical impedance. One electrode is placed in the right 2nd intercostal space rather than over the sternum. The other electrode is either placed in the midaxillary line in the 5th interspace or, if a flat paddle is available, positioned posteriorly at the angle of the left scapula. An energy setting of 400 wsec suffices to revert all patients with primary ventricular fibrillation. With currently used defibrillators, the energy delivered at such a setting is generally about 320 wsec. Recommendations have been made that the energy output of defibrillators currently in use be increased above this limit.[270,271] These suggestions are based on experimental studies in animals and have presumed that the energy of defibrillation is largely a function of body weight. It has been stated that a maximal setting of 400 wsec is inadequate for defibrillating 35 per cent or more of patients who weigh in excess of 50 kg.[271] However, clinical experience is at variance with these opinions. Indeed, Pantridge et al.[272] and Crampton[273] have maintained the contrary, namely, that the maximum energies currently employed for defibrillation are excessive. A single 200-wsec shock reverted 73 of 82 (89 per cent) patients with ventricular fibrillation; a second discharge at the same setting restored sinus rhythm in an additional 7 per cent, resulting in a total success rate of 96 per cent.[272] There was no correlation between ease of reversion and body weight. In one recent clinical experience a man weighing 190 kg (418 lb) was successfully resuscitated with a single 400-wsec shock after a prolonged episode of ventricular fibrillation.[274]

Kerber and Sarnat[275] found no difference in body weight in patients successfully defibrillated compared with those in whom the procedure failed. Nor was there a difference of energy per body weight in the two groups. Patients who were defibrillated were less acidotic and were younger in age.

The question of the energy to be employed is not a minor issue, since electrical discharge can prove injurious even when delivered transthoracically, and these injuries are directly related to the energy content of the shock.[276] Such myocardial injury may prevent successful resuscitation. It needs to be emphasized that when a single discharge fails to revert, repeating the discharge at the same energy level will frequently prove successful. This is due to the fact that the initial discharge lowers skin impedance and thus more current is being delivered with the second discharge.

Intravenous Medications. Once ventilation and cardiac massage are being well sustained, an intravenous route must be established. If circulation is not restored, sodium bicarbonate, 1 mEq/kg, should be injected to combat metabolic acidosis and is repeated after 10 minutes. Once an effective rhythm is restored, further drug administration is governed by arterial blood gas and pH measurements. Epinephrine is an essential drug that proves of great value at times. Although this catecholamine theoretically predisposes to ventricular fibrillation, in practice it has been shown to enhance defibrillation, especially when fine-wave arrhythmia prevails. If, after defibrillation, an ineffectual contraction is restored, the ensuing myocardial hypoxia predisposes to recurrence of the arrhythmia. Since epinephrine increases myocardial contractility and elevates perfusion pressure, it not only lowers the threshold for defibrillation but may also prevent electromechanical dissociation. A dose of 0.5 ml of a 1/1000 solution diluted to 10 ml should be administered intravenously every 5 minutes during the resuscitation effort. When an intravenous route cannot be established, intracardiac administration of this drug may be essential.

When reversion results in profound bradycardia and there is resumption of fibrillation, the intravenous administration of 0.5 mg of atropine may prove salutary. Such a bolus can be repeated in 5 minutes to accelerate the heart rate above 60 per minute. Another essential drug to be used early in resuscitation is lidocaine. This drug raises the fibrillation threshold and has minimal deleterious effects on myocardial contractility, systemic arterial pressure, and venous return. It also diminishes or entirely eliminates advanced grades of VPB's and may thereby reduce recurrence of tachyarrhythmias. Lidocaine is to be given as a 75-mg bolus intravenously, repeated in 2 minutes, and then followed by a continuous infusion of 2 to 3 mg/min but not exceeding 4 mg/min. Bretylium tosylate, an adrenergic-blocking agent, raises the threshold for ventricular fibrillation in experimental animals and may cause spontaneous defibrillation in humans. In a randomized blind trial comparing bretylium with lidocaine in 146 victims of out-of-hospital ventricular fibrillation, no advantage or disadvantage was noted for either drug.[276a]

Two other drugs may be useful. If the resuscitated patient experiences chest pain, *morphine sulfate* will both relieve pain and assuage anxiety. It is especially valuable when pulmonary edema attends the onset of acute myocardial infarction, which was the cause of the cardiac arrest. The intravenous administration of 5 to 8 mg generally suffices. At times it may be necessary to use *calcium chloride*, which increases myocardial contractility, prolongs systole, and enhances ventricular automaticity. Again, this should be used when defibrillation has been repeated several times or when the heart cannot be defibrillated because of fine, rapid oscillations of the fibrillatory wave pattern. The usual recommended dose of calcium chloride is 2.5 ml to 5 ml of a 10 per cent solution providing 3.4 to 6.8 mEq of calcium. When calcium gluconate is infused, the dose is 10 ml of a 10 per cent solution providing 4.8 mEq of calcium.

The initial management of cardiac arrest is crucial. One frequently encounters a patient with a badly damaged brain who lingers as a tragic reminder of belated, inadequate, or improper CPR. Unfortunately during such emergencies there are no adequate records kept to provide insight into precisely what went wrong. In many hospitals cardiac arrest teams do not exist, and the responsibility for CPR devolves on those in the immediate vicinity of the victim. The multitude of bystanders tend to impede the resuscitative effort, which is neither well coordinated nor well directed, thereby jeopardizing survival.

MANAGEMENT OF THE PATIENT AT RISK FOR SUDDEN CARDIAC DEATH

Basically three approaches are available for preventing sudden cardiac death: (1) mass prophylaxis with antiarrhythmic drugs, (2) implanted defibrillators, or (3) individualized antiarrhythmic therapy.

MASS PROPHYLAXIS. The most logical approach is to initiate a prophylactic program with some effective antiarrhythmic measure for those deemed to be at risk for sudden cardiac death. The target population is large, including not only patients with overt manifestations of ischemic heart disease but also those having high-risk profiles for coronary disease. The latter population represents two-thirds of the victims. Currently available antiarrhythmic measures are not suitable for wide prophylactic use, because of the potential of serious adverse reactions. The following calculation makes clear the poor trade-off in employing antiarrhythmic drugs. Patients who have recovered from acute myocardial infarction constitute a high-risk group for sudden cardiac death. In such a group, one may anticipate an annual mortality of 4 per cent, with a 3 per cent incidence of sudden cardiac death. Assuming the availability of an antiarrhythmic drug that would reduce mortality by 30 per cent, sudden death could be prevented in 1 patient per 100 survivors of myocardial infarction per year. However, 99 patients would be burdened with the inconvenience of taking daily medications, at significant psychological and economic costs. Furthermore current antiarrhythmic drugs generally induce toxic reactions in about 30 per cent of recipients. Thus, although one patient might be saved, 30 others certainly might suffer adverse reactions. Until safe and highly effective measures are found, employment of prophylactic antiarrhythmic drugs requires precise identification of the potential victim.

SURVIVORS OF OUT-OF-HOSPITAL CARDIAC ARREST. Ample experience has now been gained with out-of-hospital cardiac arrest to permit definition of the decisive variables determining survival. Eisenberg et al.[277] have shown that survival relates to four factors: (1) whether cardiac arrest was witnessed, (2) the cardiac rhythm at the time of arrest, (3) whether or not CPR was initiated by lay bystanders, and (4) speed in arrival time of paramedic unit. In 611 patients with out-of-hospital cardiac arrest, these variables were predictive of outcome (Table 23–6). Among 22 patients with favorable findings on all four predictive factors, 15, or 70 per cent, were discharged alive. This contrasts with only 1 survivor among 97 patients with all four unfavorable findings. Myerburg et al.[278] have also ascribed critical importance to the cardiac arrest rhythm. Among 352 consecutive victims of out-of-hospital cardiac arrest, of 24 patients presenting with ventricular tachycardia, 16, or 67 per cent, were ultimately discharged alive. When the arrhythmia was ventricular fibrillation, 55, or 23 per cent, recovered. However, when a bradyarrhythmia was the initial mechanism, of 108 such patients only 9 were resuscitated and none survived. Another helpful predictor is the heart rate immediately after defibrillation. Only 5 per cent survived when the rate was less than 60 beats/min, and 17 per cent when it ranged from 60 to 100 beats/min; of these 43 per cent were long-term survivors.[278]

TABLE 23–6 OUTCOME AMONG 611 PATIENTS WITH OUT-OF-HOSPITAL CARDIAC ARREST

Event Witnessed	Number of Patients	Discharged Alive (%)
+	380	28*
–	231	3
Arrythmia of Cardiac Arrest		
VT or VF	389	28*
Asystole	222	3
Bystander-Initiated CPR		
+	168	32*
–	443	14
Response Time (min)		
<4.0	39	56
4.0–8.0	139	35
>8.0	186	17

*p <0.01.
From Eisenberg, M., et al.: The ACLS score: Predicting survival from out-of-hospital cardiac arrest. J.A.M.A. *246*:50, 1981.

Improvement in results of resuscitation following out-of-hospital cardiac arrest has been progressive. In the period from 1971 to 1973, overall survival was 14 per cent, whereas from 1973 to 1978, it had increased to 23 per cent.[278] At present, the hospital discharge rate from out-of-hospital ventricular fibrillation is up to 30 per cent.[279] However, long-range survival has been poor. In a prospective follow-up of 276 resuscitated patients who were discharged alive from the hospital, the probability of remaining alive at 4 years was only 49 per cent, compared with 80 per cent of a normal population adjusted for age and sex and 66 per cent for a population of patients discharged after myocardial infarction.[280] But even those surviving are not spared major neurologic and intellectual impairments. In a prospective study of 63 survivors, seizure activity was observed in 30 per cent.[281] Most commonly, it began within 12 hours, usually occurring either as partial seizures or as myoclonic activity and rarely as a tonic-clonic type of "shivering." A good prognosis for survival and sound neurologic outcome was related to the presence, at the time of admission to hospital, of pupillary responses to light, oculocephalic reflexes, purposeful responses to pain, and spontaneous respiration.

Promise of reducing the inordinate toll of sudden death is being provided by the beta-adrenergic–blocking drugs that result in a low incidence of adverse reactions. Numerous studies have reported favorable results in long-term treatment of patients with ischemic heart disease, and these have been recently reviewed.[282] The most persuasive report is the Norwegian Multicenter Study with timolol in patients surviving acute myocardial infarction.[283] The number of sudden deaths was reduced by about 50 per cent among 1884 randomized to either placebo or timolol groups and followed an average of 17 months.

IMPLANTATION OF DEFIBRILLATORS. For the patient who is greatly threatened by the possibility of recurring ventricular fibrillation, Mirowski et al.[284,285] have suggested the intriguing approach of implanting in the chest a standby automatic defibrillator system. Such a completely implanted defibrillator unit can reverse ventricular fibrillation in dogs. Compared with transthoracic delivery of the shock, intracardiac defibrillation requires only a fraction of the energy. Though this method is fraught with technical difficulties, on first examination it is impressive in its seeming logic. However, difficult problems remain to be surmounted, such as sensing the onset of ventricular fibrillation, prevention of electrical injury, and absence of methods for determining operational readiness and efficacy of an implanted unit.[286] It is our view that placing an electronic device in the chest does not appear to be the answer to the problem of sudden cardiac death. For the immediate future, the potential victim will need to be identified and protected by an individualized antiarrhythmic program.

SELECTION OF PATIENTS FOR ANTIARRHYTHMIC TREATMENT. At present, antiarrhythmic drugs are to be employed largely for those individuals identified as being at high risk for sudden cardiac death. The following constitute the essential subgroups of patients for whom therapy is indicated:

1. Patients who previously experienced primary ventricular fibrillation without associated evidence of acute myo-

cardial infarction. These patients are at highest risk of sudden cardiac death; nearly one-third will succumb within a year of their initial resuscitation.

2. Patients with ischemic heart disease who on monitoring or exercise stress testing exhibit ventricular tachycardia of more than three successive cycles and with rates in excess of 180 beats/min. The risk of sudden cardiac death is greater if the arrhythmia is ventricular tachycardia of the vulnerable period, or $VT_{(vp)}$, or if the salvos consist of accelerating cycles.

3. Patients within the first 6 months after recovery from acute myocardial infarction who have angina pectoris of recent onset or who demonstrate grade 4 or 5 VPB's.

4. Patients who are being subjected to profound psychological stress or are in a state of bereavement because of loss of spouse and have developed grade 4 or 5 VPB's for the first time.

5. Patients with prolonged Q-T intervals who have experienced unexplained syncope and have VPB's of grade 2 or higher.

6. Young women with prolapse of the mitral valve who on monitoring show episodic Q-T interval prolongation and VPB's. Treatment is even more essential if they have experienced syncope or if there is a history of sudden death among close family members.

7. Patients in whom exercise stress induces both ST-segment depression ≥ 2 mm and grade 4 and 5 VPB's either at peak exercise or immediately upon recovery.

8. Patients who develop ventricular ectopic activity when they experience angina pectoris.

9. Patients who are severely disabled because of frequent VPB's.

Patients are generally unaware that they are experiencing VPB's. Often the physician's well-meaning but misguided concern over the presence of cardiac irregularities cues the patient to the abnormal pulse and provokes undue anxiety and psychological disquiet, which may then stimulate further arrhythmia. The mere appearance of VPB's does not portend a dire prognosis and should not be a cause for alarm. The vast majority of individuals with VPB's require little more than reassurance from the physician about the benign nature of this condition. Treatment of sporadic VPB's is directed only at the symptomatic individual in whom simple conservative measures fail to allay anxiety. In these patients, continued and oft-repeated reassurance, instruction in relaxation techniques, encouragement of adequate participation in recreation, initiation of an aerobic exercise program, discontinuation of caffeine-containing beverages and of cigarette smoking, and the judicious use of minor doses of beta-adrenergic–blocking agents (propranolol, 10 to 20 mg three to four times daily; metoprolol, 50 mg twice daily; or atenolol, 25 mg once daily) will suffice for allaying symptoms. In many cases the use of medications may be tailored to the patient's individual problem, e.g., if arrhythmia occurs primarily with exercise, solely at night, or only during periods of intense turmoil, then the beta-blocking agent or some other drug is administered only during or in anticipation of these specific situations.

STRATEGY OF MANAGEMENT. Physicians increasingly encounter patients who either have been resuscitated from ventricular fibrillation or experience oft-recurring bouts of ventricular tachycardia which result in either syncope or profound hemodynamic compromise leading to rapid deterioration of cardiac function. These groups of rhythm disorders have been labeled *malignant ventricular arrhythmias.*[105] To date, there is a paucity of clinical guidelines for managing these patients. Therapeutic measures have been empirical and haphazard. Our experience over the past decade with patients who have had malignant ventricular arrhythmias suggests the following elements for a successful management program.[105,287]

1. Thorough evaluation of the cardiac as well as the human problem is required. There is need to focus attention on the psychological stresses that not infrequently predispose to or cause the arrhythmia.[107] Although the physician may be unable to alter the complex social and psychological milieu, merely the expression of interest and sympathy is profoundly therapeutic.

2. In order to define the prevalence and type of ventricular arrhythmia, 24-hour monitoring as well as exercise stress testing is required.

3. Acute drug testing employing programmed trendscription (i.e., a compressed recording of heart rhythm [p. 799] is a prerequisite for the expeditious screening of drugs for efficacy as well as for appropriate dosage. It also indicates which drug or drugs may aggravate rather than lessen arrhythmia.

4. If advanced grades of VPB's are infrequent or nonreproducible, as is true in 15 per cent of patients with malignant arrhythmias, repetitive ventricular response (RVR) testing is employed to assess drug efficacy.

5. An antiarrhythmic drug should be tried for 48 to 72 hours at each selected dosage. Exercise testing and 24-hour monitoring must be conducted with every dose level.

6. The therapeutic objective is to suppress grades 4 and 5 ventricular arrhythmias. This goal may not be readily achieved; a reduction in frequency of these grades may be the only option. However, if rapid ventricular tachyarrhythmias are provoked during exercise, drugs must be manipulated until the rhythm disturbances are completely suggested. If extrastimulus testing is employed, the endpoint is abolition of nonsustained ventricular tachycardia consisting of three or more cycles.

7. The use of drug combinations is indicated in all instances of ventricular fibrillation. A "fail-safe" system of drug protection, namely, the employment of two or more agents that have proved effective is mandated by the risk of recurrence. In other disorders physicians may have an opportunity to remedy therapeutic error, but this is infrequently the case with ventricular fibrillation.

8. The digitalis glycosides may contribute to suppression of ventricular arrhythmia. The benefit of digitalis drugs is best judged by the use of acetylstrophanthidin.[288]

9. Psychological stress testing may expose advanced grades of ventricular ectopy and may thereby provide useful insights into the factors contributing to the genesis of arrhythmia. This type of provocation also defines the adequacy of a selected antiarrhythmic program.

10. Psychiatric support for the patient and the use of relaxation techniques such as meditation facilitate management of the so-called intractable ventricular arrhythmias.

11. Accurate and meticulous record keeping, as already emphasized by Winkle et al., is mandatory.[289] Daily tabula-

tion of data, including precise time of drug administration, dosage, trendscription findings, and monitoring and exercise results as well as any untoward reactions, is essential to the development of an effective drug program.

Our experience indicates that the majority of patients with recurrent malignant ventricular arrhythmias can be protected by a combination of medical measures.

Ambulatory 24-Hour Electrocardiographic Monitoring. The most effective method for recognizing rarely occurring arrhythmic events is to monitor a patient equipped with a portable recorder for 24 hours while the individual is performing usual daily activities. As already indicated, nearly 90 per cent of patients with ischemic heart disease will demonstrate VPB's and 41 per cent will exhibit repetitive ectopic beats of grade 4 as their maximal grade during at least 1 monitoring hour. It should be emphasized that advanced grades are nonpersistent, sporadic, and relatively rare events. Thus, among 100 men with ischemic heart disease (mean age 57), grade 4 arrhythmia was present in 40 patients during at least 1 hour, but only half these patients demonstrated this grade of VPB's during 2 monitored hours and only 7 (17.5 per cent) exhibited this grade during 12 of the 24 hours.[133] There is an additional problem of reproducibility in successive monitoring sessions.

Monitoring for VPB's by means of 24-hour recordings presents additional problems. It is costly, it is difficult to correlate occurrence of arrhythmia precisely with life events, and there is a variable time lag between monitoring tape interpretation and transmittal of data to the physician. Furthermore, interpretation of the record must rely on sample selection by a third party, the technician reading the tapes, who is generally unfamiliar with the clinical problem. Nonetheless, this technique remains for the present the foundation for defining the patient at risk for sudden cardiac death as well as assessing the therapeutic efficacy of various drug regimens.

Trendscription. This method provides an immediate print-out that permits the physician to examine all the data and then interpret these within the context of clinical circumstances.[290] It fills the gap between the limited arrhythmia information provided by the recording of a routine electrocardiogram and the veritable deluge of output derived from 24-hour monitoring (Fig. 23–9). Thirty minutes of information is presented in a compressed form, recorded on a rotating drum. This method of data condensation is coupled with statistical time sampling and instantaneously provides the physician with significant trends of ectopic activity by means of a print-out that can be easily visualized and readily interpreted. Its greatest value is its use in judging the efficacy and safety of antiarrhythmic drugs.[291]

Exercise Stress Testing to Expose VPB's. In the experimental animal as well as in humans, the frequency of ventricular ectopic beats increases as a function of the presence and extent of myocardial ischemia. Exercise burdens the myocardium with accelerated heart rate, rise in blood pressure, preloading of the ventricle, enhanced sympathetic nervous activity, augmented catecholamine excretion, and, in patients with restricted coronary flow, tissue hypoxia and acidosis. Jelinek and Lown have demonstrated that maximal exercise stress is an effective method for exposing ventricular premature beats in patients with ischemic heart disease.[292] These VPB's are observed primarily during the peak of exercise and in the immediate postexercise recovery period. Whereas normal subjects may develop arrhythmia with exercise, advanced grades of VPB's are more common in those subjects with ischemic heart disease. Indeed, several studies have correlated the occurrence and grade of ectopic activity with the severity of angiographically demonstrated coronary artery disease and with the extent of abnormalities in the motion of the left ventricular wall.[293–295] In some patients with severe ischemic heart disease and recurrent ventricular fibrillation, 24-hour monitoring does not expose the presence of high grades of VPB's, which are demonstrated only with exercise.

Psychological Stress Testing. As with exercise testing, the objective of psychological stress testing has been to devise a method that will reproducibly precipitate ventricular arrhythmias. The basis for this method derives from clinical observations as well as earlier cited investigations. The fact that a 24-hour monitoring period consistently shows a greater frequency of advanced grades of VPB's compared with maximal exercise stress argues for a psychological rather than a hemodynamic trigger for the ectopic beats. At no time during such a 24-hour monitoring period does the patient achieve peak heart rates as high as those that occur during the exercise stress. To date, we have been only episodically successful in precipitating VPB's in about 25 per cent of patients by means of psychological stress. This is a promising but as yet unexplored area.[296]

Problems in Managing Patients with Malignant Ventricular Arrhythmias. The mainstay of prevention of sudden cardiac death consists of the use of antiarrhythmic drugs to subdue advanced grades of VPB's or electrophysi-

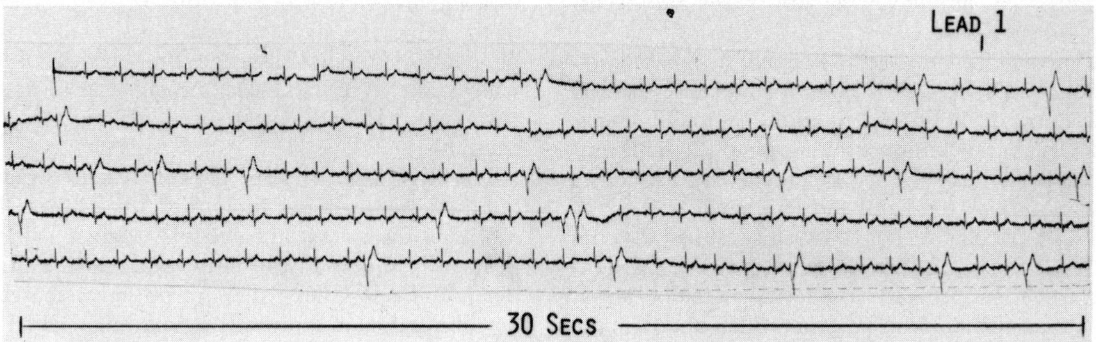

FIGURE 23–9 Part of a trendscription, presenting half the width of the usual record, which inscribes an entire minute of information in a single line. The ease of recognizing VPB's is evident.

ologically provoked ventricular repetitive activity. However, merely administering an antiarrhythmic drug in the hope of preventing fatality is an exercise in futility. Schaffer and Cobb found that 73 per cent of 64 patients who had recurrent ventricular fibrillation were receiving antiarrhythmic therapy at the time of sudden death.[120]

Therapy must be individualized. When an antiarrhythmic drug fails to prevent a recurrence, there is no certainty about whether an improper drug had been chosen or whether an incorrect dose had been administered. Generally, when an antiarrhythmic agent is used, the physician gauges therapeutic efficacy by abatement of symptoms or prevention of recurrence of sustained and demonstrable arrhythmia. When a disordered mechanism of the heartbeat is devoid of symptoms, repeated Holter monitoring sessions are required to determine whether a drug is of value. When ectopic beats are infrequent and sporadic, there is no certainty—even with longer or more frequent periods of monitoring—that the selected drug is effective. Clearly, new techniques are needed to determine drug effectiveness as well as proper dosage for the individual patient with VPB's.

We have therefore attempted to streamline drug therapy by introducing the method of *acute drug testing*.[291] The essential principle is based on the conception that the effectiveness of most antiarrhythmic drugs is related to the establishment of a so-called significant therapeutic blood concentration (see Chap. 20). This can be achieved rapidly by administering a single large oral dose. The purpose of acute drug testing is thus to establish therapeutic blood levels during a brief period of time in order to define during the course of drug action its effects on arrhythmia and to observe immediately whether any possible toxic complication ensues. Since only a single dose is used, drug effects are short-lived and any risk to the patient is of brief duration. After performing a series of such tests with different drugs, one can establish within a relatively short period of time which drugs are optimally effective in any given patient. This is referred to as "phase-one" study.

Quinidine is generally the first drug tested. This is followed by procainamide, diphosphopyramide, and propranolol. The doses employed are 600 mg for quinidine, 1.5 gm for procainamide, 300 mg for diphosphopyramide, and 80 mg for propranolol. These are administered as single oral doses. Then a number of newer drugs, such as mexiletine, tocainide, aprindine, ethmozine, encainide, lorcainide, propafonone, and amiodarone, are tested. Whether further study of any particular agent is undertaken is determined by its efficacy as well as by the occurrence of any untoward effects.

Once the most effective drug is defined, a "phase-two" study is initiated. The patient is given maintenance therapy with the selected drug for a period of 48 to 72 hours. Drug efficacy is then determined by means of 24-hour ambulatory monitoring as well as maximum exercise stress testing on a motorized treadmill and in a small percentage by repetitive ventricular response (RVR) testing. Psychological stress testing is also employed to provoke arrhythmia and thereby to provide additional certainty about adequacy of a particular drug program. Such a systematic approach removes much of the guesswork in antiarrhythmic management and permits tailoring of the drug to the particular response of the individual patient.

Use of Digitalis Glycosides. It has been shown that acetylstrophanthidin may reduce or abolish VPB's.[288] Testing with this drug therefore identifies those patients who may profit from glycoside administration.[297] The reduction of ventricular premature beats by acetylstrophanthidin is not due to the positive inotropic effect of this drug. Only 15 of 65 patients in whom acetylstrophanthidin reduced or abolished ventricular arrhythmia were in cardiac decompensation at the time the test was performed. An alternative explanation relates the salutary effect on VPB's to the vagotonic action of the cardiac glycosides.[298,299] It has long been appreciated that digitalis increases carotid sinus sensitivity and thereby augments vagal action.[299] Evidence was presented earlier indicating that the vagus nerve has a profound indirect effect on cardiac excitability by opposing heightened adrenergic tone. Relevant are the findings that parasympathetic maneuvers such as carotid sinus massage [298] or administration of agents with vagotonic actions[300–302] decrease the frequency of VPB's or abolish ventricular tachycardia. The findings related to acetylstrophanthidin have been replicated in some patients by maintenance digitalis therapy. Our experience indicates, however, that glycosides are *adjunctive* but cannot serve as the sole therapeutic agent against malignant ventricular arrhythmias.

Psychiatric Support and Relaxation Techniques. The patient who has experienced ventricular fibrillation or who is threatened with sudden cardiac death is subjected to inordinate emotional tension. In many instances the anxiety is of such enormity that it can be controlled by the patient only by a demeanor of quietude and complete insouciance. These feelings are blanketed by profound depression manifested in somatic and psychological symptoms at times completely unrelated to the heart. Insomnia and impotence are frequent problems. Loss of concentration and seeming indifference to current events or earlier ambitions are part of the psychological state. Unless the physician addresses the emotional dimension boldly and judiciously with sympathy and understanding, there is little likelihood of successfully managing the patient with an arrhythmia. A therapeutic objective is to promote confidence and incorrigible optimism about the future.

Patients are also encouraged to meditate for brief periods each day in order to foster inner relaxation. The practice is noncultic, and no mantra is employed. Psychological equanimity is also promoted by an aerobic exercise program adapted to the particular experience, aptitudes, and predilections of the individual patient. Again, fetishism and overindulgence are discouraged. Open discussion of the subject of sudden death and the fact that it now can be controlled helps assuage the burden of uncertainty, which, like a veritable Damoclean sword, haunts the patient who has once experienced malignant ventricular arrhythmia.

Effectiveness of the Therapeutic Program. A key question is whether diminution of advanced grades of VPB's affords any protection against sudden cardiac death. This question can be resolved most expeditiously by determining whether patients who have recurrent ventricular fibrillation are protected from this lethal arrhythmia when VPB's are suppressed. We examined this question in 114 consecutive patients referred for management of intractable malignant ventricular arrhythmias.[303] Of this group 72 per cent had experienced primary ventricular fibrillation, and the remainder had symptomatic recurrent ventricular tachycardia associated either with syncope or with hemodynamic compromise. Seventy-three patients (64 per cent) had coronary heart disease, 24 (21 per cent) had miscellaneous forms of heart disease, and 17 (14.9 per cent) were free of demonstrable cardiac disease; the average age was 53 years. Of the 114 patients, 88 (77 per cent) were controlled, as evidenced by elimination of grades 4B and 5 VPB's on both 24-hour Holter monitoring as well as during maximum symptom-limited treadmill exercise stress testing. Twenty-six patients were not controlled. Among the group deemed to have been controlled, only 4 experienced sudden cardiac death over an average follow-up of 21.5 months. However, 13 of the 26 not controlled died suddenly after an average follow-up of 155 months.

The evidence presented indicates that in patients with ischemic heart disease the occurrence of VPB's is associated with an increased risk of sudden cardiac death. Such risk is further enhanced when the VPB's are of advanced grade. Although abolition of arrhythmia appears to reduce susceptibility to ventricular fibrillation, it is not clear whether protection results from reduction in VPB's or as a consequence of changes in the fibrillation threshold quite apart from the ectopic suppressive action. The above-mentioned experience suggests that a majority of patients having recurrent malignant arrhythmias can be protected by medical measures. This subset of patients, however, represents but a small minority of those at risk from sudden death. Newer methods are needed for identifying the large groups that are threatened. A noninvasive screening test for electrical instability of the myocardium must now be developed.

VALUE OF CARDIAC OPERATIONS FOR CONTROL OF MALIGNANT ARRHYTHMIAS

(See also Chap. 20)

Coronary artery bypass grafting and ventricular aneurysmectomy have been the surgical procedures most commonly employed for managing drug-resistant, oft-recurrent ventricular tachyarrhythmias. Successful suppression of arrhythmia by such blind approaches is achieved in fewer than 30 per cent of patients.[304] Although the majority of patients with these arrhythmias do have multivessel coronary artery disease as well as ventricular aneurysms, electrophysiological mapping techniques (p. 640) have demonstrated that the sites of origin of the reentrant mechanisms are at or near the subendocardium at the border of infarction and/or aneurysm.[176,177,180–182] These areas are generally not resected during standard aneurysmectomy. The fact that these arrhythmias often have a precisely localizable anatomical basis invites resection of the nidus for the arrhythmia. The most extensive experience with intraoperative mapping has been reported by Josephson and coworkers.[305] Endocardial resection was carried out in 60 patients with recurrent ventricular tachyarrhythmias; 52 had concomitant aneurysmectomies, whereas 40 received in addition an average of 1.6 grafts per patient. There were 5 operative deaths. Of the remaining 55, in 42 ventricular tachycardia was not inducible, and they were discharged without medication. In 13 patients, arrhythmias could be induced during electrophysiological testing. In a follow-up period of 2 to 41 months, there have been 9 late deaths among the 55 patients surviving operation. At follow-up of 40 months, the predicted actuarial survival curve on patients who had endocardial resection is 62 per cent. In the absence of a medically treated control group, the significance of these results remains uncertain.

With the advent of new and more effective antiarrhythmic drugs, there will be less need to resort to complex and costly operative procedures. In the above-cited study of Josephson et al.,[305] only 10 patients had received experimental drugs. In any case surgery cannot be the strategy of care for the multitudes who are predisposed to sudden cardiac death.[306]

CONCLUDING COMMENTS

Sudden cardiac death continues to exact an inordinate toll in premature and preventable fatalities. In the brief decade since this phenomenon has received increased medical attention, there have been a number of substantial advances. The mechanism has been decisively identified as being due to ventricular fibrillation. Acute anatomical lesions have been shown to be absent. Fatality has been proved to be due to an electrical accident. Resuscitation has been often accomplished, and long survival has been assured for many. Community CPR programs have evolved which have resulted in many lives being saved. VPB's have been established as indicators of increased susceptibility to sudden cardiac death, and advanced grades of ectopic beats have been shown to be largely implicated. Increasingly, patients at risk are being identified. Methodological approaches have been developed which permit tailoring of antiarrhythmic drugs to individual needs. Newer and more effective antiarrhythmic drugs are becoming available to the clinician. Electrophysiological techniques have emerged that permit identification of the precise site of initiation of the reentrant mechanism. The role of higher nervous factors in the genesis of ventricular arrhythmias and ventricular fibrillation has been demonstrated. Finally, the long-prevalent attitude of pessimism and futility is being replaced by a sense of challenge and opportunity. One can be hopeful that it will not require the passage of still another decade before this problem will be largely controlled.

References

1. Lown, B., Fakhro, A. M., Hood, W. B., Jr., and Thorn, G. W.: The coronary care unit: New perspectives and directions. J.A.M.A. *199*:188, 1967.
2. Pantridge, J. F., and Geddes, J. S.: A mobile intensive care unit in the management of myocardial infarction. Lancet *2*:271, 1967.
3. Pantridge, J. F., and Adgey, A. A. J.: Prehospital coronary care: The mobile coronary care unit. Am. J. Cardiol. *24*:666, 1969.
4. Nagel, E. L., Hirschman, J. C., Nussenfeld, S. R., Rankin, D., and Lunbland, E.: Telemetry-medical command in coronary and other mobile emergency care systems. J.A.M.A. *214*:332, 1970.
5. Grace, W. J.: The mobile coronary care unit and the intermediate coronary care unit in the total systems approach to coronary care. Chest *58*:363, 1970.
6. Cobb, L. A., Conn, R. D., Samson, W. E., and Philbin, J. E.: Prehospital coronary care: The role of rapid response mobile intensive coronary care system. Circulation *43*:II-139, 1971.
7. Liberthson, R. R., Nagel, E. L., Hirschman, J. C., and Nussenfeld, S. R.: Prehospital ventricular defibrillation. Prognosis and followup course. N. Engl. J. Med. *291*:317, 1974.
8. Paul, O., and Schatz, M.: On sudden death. Circulation *43*:7, 1971.
9. Chazan, J. A., Stevson, R., and Kurland, G. S.: The acidoses of cardiac arrest. N. Engl. J. Med. *278*:360, 1968.
10. Noble, J. R.: The patient with syncope. J.A.M.A. *237*:1372, 1977.
11. Murdoch, B. D.: Loss of consciousness in healthy South African men: Incidence, causes and relationship to EEG abnormality. S. Afr. Med. J. *57*:771, 1980.
12. Wenger, N. K., Stein, P. D., and Willis, P. W.: Massive acute pulmonary embolism: The deceivingly nonspecific manifestations. J.A.M.A. *220*:843, 1972.
13. Levine, S. A.: Clinical Heart Disease. Philadelphia, W. B. Saunders Co., 1958, p. 297.
14. Thames, M. D., Alpert, J. S., and Dalen, J. E.: Syncope in patients with pulmonary embolism. J.A.M.A. *238*:2509, 1977.
15. Alpert, J. S., Smith, R., Carlson, C. J., Ockéne, I. S., Dexter, L., and Dalen, J.

E.: Mortality in patients treated for pulmonary embolism. J.A.M.A. *236*:1477, 1976.
16. Gutheroth, W. G.: Sudden infant death syndrome (crib death). Am. Heart J. *93*:784, 1977.
17. Valdes-Dapena, M. A.: Sudden unexpected death in infancy. A review of the world literatures. 1954–1966. Pediatrics *39*:123, 1967.
18. Coryllos, E.: Vagal dysfunction and sudden infant death syndrome: One possible cause and its management. N. Y. State J. Med. *82*:731, 1982.
19. Maron, B. J., Clark, C. E., Goldstern, R. E., and Epstein, S. E.: Potential role of Q-T interval prolongation in sudden infant death syndrome. Circulation *54*: 423, 1976.
20. Schwartz, P. J.: Cardiac sympathetic innervation and the sudden infant death syndrome. Am. J. Med. *60*:167, 1976.
21. Kukolich, M. K., Telsey, A., Ott, J., and Motulsky, A. G.: Sudden infant death syndrome: Normal QT interval on ECG relatives. Pediatrics *60*:51, 1977.
22. Kelly, D. H. R., Shannon, D. C., and Liberthson, R. R.: The role of the QT interval in the sudden infant death syndrome. Circulation *55*:633, 1977.
23. Patrick, J. R.: Cardiac or respiratory death. *In* Bergman, A. B., Beckwith, J. B., and Ray, C. J. (eds.): Sudden Infant Death Syndrome. Seattle, University of Washington Press, 1970, p. 130.
24. Beckwith, J. B.: Observations on the pathological anatomy of sudden infant death syndrome. *In* Bergman, A. B., Beckwith, J. B., and Ray, C. J. (eds.): Sudden Infant Death Syndrome. Seattle, University of Washington Press, 1970, pp. 83–132.
25. Shannon, D. C., Kelly, D. H., and O'Connell, K.: Abnormal regulation of ventilation in infants at risk for sudden infant death syndrome. N. Engl. J. Med. *297*:747, 1977.
26. Naeye, R. L.: Pulmonary arterial abnormalities and the sudden infant death syndrome. N. Engl. J. Med. *289*:1167, 1973.
27. Mittleman, R. E., and Wetli, C. V.: The fatal cafe coronary: Foreign-body airway obstruction. J.A.M.A. *247*:1285, 1982.
28. Bass, M.: Sudden sniffing death. J.A.M.A. *212*:2075, 1970.
29. Weiss, S., and Baker, J. P.: The carotid sinus reflex in health and disease. Its role in the causation of fainting and convulsions. Medicine *12*:297, 1933.
30. Parry, C. H.: An inquiry into symptoms and causes of syncope anginosa, commonly called angina pectoris. Bath, England, Cruttwell, 1799.
31. Burch, G. E., and DePasquale, N. P.: Sudden, unexpected, natural death. Am. J. Med. Sci. *249*:86, 1965.
32. Kuller, L.: Sudden and unexpected nontraumatic deaths in adults: A review of epidemiologic and clinical studies. J. Chron. Dis. *19*:1165, 1966.
33. Spain, D. M., Brades, V. A., and Mohr, C.: Coronary atherosclerosis as a cause of unexpected and unexplained death: An autopsy study from 1949–1959. J.A.M.A. *174*:384, 1960.
34. Phillips, L. H., Whisnant, J. P., and Reagan, T. J.: Sudden death from stroke. Stroke *8*:392, 1977.
35. Lancisi, G. M.: De Subitaneis Mortibus. Rome, Buagnai, 1707. Translated by P. D. White and A. V. Boursy. New York, St. John's University Press, 1971.
36. Hirsch, C. S., and Martin, D. L.: Unexpected death in young epileptics. Neurology *21*:682, 1971.
37. Lown, B., and Levine, S. A.: Current Advances in Digitalis Therapy. Boston, Little, Brown and Co., 1954.
38. Lely, A. H., and Van Enter, H. J.: Large scale digitoxin intoxication. Br. Med. J. *2*:734, 1970.
39. Selzer, A., and Wray, H. W.: Quinidine syncope: Paroxysmal ventricular fibrillation occurring during treatment of chronic atrial arrhythmias. Circulation *30*: 17, 1964.
40. Bell, L. V.: On a form of disease resembling mania and fever. Am. J. Insanity *6*:97, 1849.
41. Peele, R., and Von Loetzen, I. S.: Phenothiazine deaths: A critical review. Am. J. Psychiatry *130*:306, 1973.
42. Coull, D. C., Crooks, J., Dingwall-Fordyce, I., Scott, A. M., and Weir, R. D.: Amitriptyline and cardiac disease: Risk of sudden death identified by monitoring system. Lancet *2*:590, 1970.
43. Kannel, W. B., Doyle, J. T., McNamara, P. M., Quickenton, P., and Gordon, T.: Precursors of sudden coronary death. Factors related to incidence of sudden death. Circulation *51*:608, 1975.
44. Kannel, W. B., and Thomas, H., Jr.: Sudden coronary death: The Framingham Study. Ann. N. Y. Acad. Sci. *382*:3, 1982.
45. Weinblatt, E., Shapiro, S., Frank, C., and Sager, R.: Prognosis of men after the first myocardial infarction. Am. J. Pub. Health *58*:1329, 1968.
46. Kuller, L. H., Lilienfeld, A., and Fisher, R.: An epidemiologic study of sudden and unexpected deaths in adults. Medicine *48*:341, 1968.
47. Doyle, J. T., Kannel, W. B., McNamara, R. M., Quickenton, P., and Gordon, T.: Factors related to the suddenness of death from coronary disease: Combined Albany-Framingham Studies. Am. J. Cardiol. *37*:1073, 1976.
48. Kuller, L. H., Perper, J., and Cooper, M.: Demographic characteristics and trends in arteriosclerotic heart disease mortality: Sudden death and myocardial infarction. Circulation *52*:III–1, 1975.
49. Wilhelmson, C., Vedin, J. A., Elmfeldt, E., Tibblin, G., and Wilhelmsen, L.: Smoking and myocardial infarction. Lancet *1*:415, 1975.
50. Kuller, L. H., Cooper, M., and Perper, J.: Epidemiology of sudden death. Arch. Intern. Med. *129*:714, 1972.
51. Herrick, J. B.: Clinical features of sudden obstruction of the coronary arteries. J.A.M.A. *59*:2015, 1912.
52. Levine, S. A.: Coronary thrombosis: Its various clinical features. Medicine *8*: 245, 1929.
53. Feil, H.: Preliminary pain in coronary thrombosis. Am. J. Med. Sci. *193*:42, 1937.
54. Sampson, J. J., and Eliaser, M.: The diagnosis of impending acute coronary artery occlusion. Am. Heart J. *13*:675, 1937.
55. Solomon, H. A., Edwards, A. L., and Killip, T.: Prodromata in acute myocardial infarction. Circulation *40*:463, 1969.
56. Stowers, M., and Short, D.: Warning symptoms before major myocardial infarction. Br. Heart J. *32*:833, 1970.
57. Feinleib, M., Simon, A. B., Gillum, R. F., and Margolis, J. R.: Prodromal symptoms—signs of sudden death. Circulation *52*:III–155, 1975.
58. Fulton, M., Lutz, W., Donald, K. W., Kirby, B. J., Duncan, B., Morrison, S. L., Kerr, F., Julian, D. G., and Oliver, M. F.: Natural history of unstable angina. Lancet *1*:860, 1972.
59. Duncan, B., Fulton, M., Morrison, S. L., Lutz, W., Donald, K. W., Kerr, F., Kirby, B. J., Julian, D. G., and Oliver, M. F.: New and worsening angina. Br. Med. J. *1*:981, 1976.
60. Doyle, J. T.: Profile of risk of sudden death in apparently healthy people. Circulation *52*:III–176, 1975.
61. Reichenback, D. D., Moss, N. S., and Meyer, E.: Pathology of the heart in sudden cardiac death. Am. J. Cardiol. *39*:865, 1977.
62. Baroldi, G., Falzi, G., and Mariani, F.: Sudden coronary death: A postmortem study in 208 selected cases compared to 97 "control" cases. Am. Heart J. *98*: 20, 1979.
63. Titus, J. L., Oxman, H. A., Connolly, D. C., and Nobrega, F. T.: Sudden unexpected death as the initial manifestation of coronary heart disease. Clinical and pathologic observations. Singapore Med. *14*:291, 1973.
64. Roberts, W. C.: Coronary arteries in fatal acute myocardial infarction. Circulation *45*:215, 1972.
65. Davies, J. M.: Pathological view of sudden cardiac death. Br. Heart J. *45*:88, 1981.
66. Roberts, W. C., and Jones, A. A.: Quantification of coronary arterial narrowing at necropsy in sudden coronary death: Analysis of 31 patients and comparison with 25 control subjects. Am. J. Cardiol. *44*:39, 1979.
67. Schwartz, C., and Gerrity, R. G.: Anatomical pathology of sudden unexpected cardiac death. Circulation *52*:III–18, 1975.
68. Spain, D. M., and Brades, V. A.: Sudden death from coronary heart disease. Chest *58*:107, 1970.
69. Lie, J. T., and Titus, J. L.: Pathology of the myocardium and the conduction system in sudden coronary death. Circulation *52*:III–41, 1975.
70. Haerem, J. W.: Platelet aggregates in intramyocardial vessels of patients dying suddenly and unexpectedly of coronary artery disease. Atherosclerosis *15*:199, 1972.
71. Folts, J. D., Crowell, E. R., and Rowe, G. G.: Platelet aggregation in partially obstructed vessels and its elimination with aspirin. Circulation *54*:365, 1976.
72. Weaver, D. W., Lorch, G. S., Alvarez, H. A., and Cobb, L. A.: Angiographic findings and prognostic indicators. Circulation *54*:895, 1976.
73. Cobb, L. A., Hallstrom, A. P., Weaver, D. W., Copass, M. K., and Haynes, R. E.: Clinical predictors and characteristics of the sudden cardiac death syndrome. *In* Proceedings of the First U.S.–U.S.S.R. Symposium on Sudden Death, Yalta, October 3–5, 1977. U.S. Department of Health, Education, and Welfare, Public Health Service, National Institutes of Health, D.H.E.W. Publication No. NIH 78–1470, 1978.
74. Criley, J. M., Lewis, K. B., Humphries, J. O., and Ross, R.: Prolapse of the mitral valve: Clinical and cine-angiographic findings. Br. Heart J. *28*:488, 1966.
75. Hancock, E. W., and Cohn, K.: The syndrome associated with midsystolic click and late systolic murmur. Am. J. Med. *41*:183, 1966.
76. Shell, W. E., Walton, J. A., Clifford, M. E., and Willis, P. W.: The familial occurrence of the syndrome of mid-late systolic click and late systolic murmur. Circulation *39*:327, 1969.
77. Stannard, M., Sloman, J. G., Hare, W. S. C., and Goble, A. J.: Prolapse of the posterior leaflet of the mitral valve: A clinical, familial and cineangiographic study. Br. Med. J. *3*:71, 1967.
78. DeMaria, A. N., Amsterdam, E. A., Vismara, L. A., Markson, W., Broochini, R., and Mason, D. T.: The variable spectrum of rhythm disturbances in the mitral valve prolapse syndrome (abstract). Circulation *50*:III–222, 1974.
79. Winkle, R. A., Lopes, M. G., Fitzgerald, J. W., Goodman, D. J., Schroeder, J. S., and Harrison, D. C.: Arrhythmias in patients with mitral valve prolapse. Circulation *52*:73, 1975.
80. Jeresaty, R. M.: Sudden death in the mitral valve prolapse-click syndrome. Am. J. Cardiol. *37*:317, 1976.
81. Allen, H., Harris, A., and Leatham, A.: Significance and prognosis of an isolated late systolic murmur: a nine to 22 year follow up. Br. Heart J. *36*:525, 1974.
82. Leichtman, D., Nelson, R., Gobel, F. L., Alexander, C. S., and Cohn, J. N.: Bradycardia with mitral valve prolapse: A potential mechanism of sudden death. Ann. Intern. Med. *85*:453, 1976.
83. Jervell, A., and Lange-Nielsen, F: Congenital deaf mutism, functional heart disease with prolongation of Q-T interval and sudden death. Am. Heart J. *54*: 59, 1957.
84. Romano, C., Gemme, G., and Pongiglione, R.: Aritmie cardiache rare dell'eta pediatrica. La Clinic Paed. *45*:656, 1963.
85. Ward, O. C.: A new familial cardiac syndrome in children. J. Irish Med. Assoc. *54*:103, 1964.

86. Vincent, G. M., Abildskov, J. A., and Burgess, M. J.: Q-T internal syndromes. Progr. Cardiovasc. Dis. *16*:527, 1974.
87. Schwartz, P. J., Periti, M., and Malliani, A.: The long QT syndrome. Am. Heart J. *89*:378, 1975.
88. Han, J., and Moe, G. K.: Nonuniform recovery of excitability in ventricular muscle. Circ. Res. *14*:44, 1964.
89. Yanowitz, F., Preston, J. B., and Abildskov, J. A.: Functional distribution of right and left stellate innervation to the ventricles: Production of neurogenic electrocardiographic changes by unilateral alteration of sympathetic tone. Circ. Res. *18*:416, 1966.
90. Schwartz, P. J., and Malliani, A.: Electrical alternation of the T wave: Clinical and experimental evidence of its relationship with the sympathetic nervous system and the long Q-T syndrome. Am. Heart J. *89*:45, 1975.
91. Moss, A., and McDonald, J.: Unilateral cervicothoracic sympathetic ganglionectomy for the treatment of long Q-T interval syndrome. N. Engl. J. Med. *285*:903, 1971.
92. Curtiss, E. I., Heibel, R. H., and Shaver, J. A.: Autonomic maneuvers in hereditary Q-T interval prolongation (Romano-Ward syndrome). Am. Heart J. *95*:420, 1978.
93. Dreifus, L. S., Haiat, R., Watanabe, Y., Arriaga, J., and Reitman, N.: Ventricular fibrillation. A possible mechanism of sudden death in patients with Wolff-Parkinson-White syndrome. Circulation *43*:520, 1971.
94. Klein, G. J., Bashere, T. M., Sellers, T. D., Pritchett, E. L. C., Smith, W. M., and Gallagher, J. J.: Ventricular fibrillation in the Wolff-Parkinson-White syndrome. N. Engl. J. Med. *301*:1080, 1979.
95. Braunwald, E., Goldblatt, A., Aygen, M., Rockoff, S. D., and Morrow, A. G.: Congenital aortic stenosis: Clinical and hemodynamic findings in 100 patients. Circulation *27*:426, 1963.
96. Flann, M. D., Braniff, B. A., Kimball, R., and Hancock, E. W.: Mechanism of effort syncope in aortic stenosis. Circulation *26*:II–109, 1967.
97. Schwartz, L. S., Goldfischer, J., Sprague, G. J., and Schwartz, S. P.: Syncope and sudden death in aortic stenosis. Am. J. Cardiol. *23*:647, 1969.
98. Santinga, J. T., Marvin, M., Kirsh, M. D., Flora, J. D., and Brymer, J. F.: Factors relating to late sudden death in patients having aortic valve replacement. Ann. Thorac. Surg. *29*:249, 1980.
99. Forfang, K., Rostad, H., Sörland, S., and Levorstad, K.: Late sudden death after surgical correction of coarctation of the aorta. Acta Med. Scand. *206*:375, 1979.
100. Editorial: A cause of sudden death. Br. Med. J. *1*:129, 1971.
101. Frank, S., and Braunwald, E.: Idiopathic hypertrophic subaortic stenosis: clinical analysis of 126 patients with emphasis on the natural history. Circulation *37*:759, 1968.
102. Dhingra, R. C., Denes, P., Wu, D., Wyndham, C. R., Amat-y-Leon, F., Towne, W. D., and Rosen, K. M.: Prospective observations in patients with chronic bundle branch block and marked H-V prolongation. Circulation *53*: 600, 1976.
103. Denes, P., Dhingra, R. C., Wu, D., Wyndham, C. R., Amat-y-Leon, F., and Rosen, K. M.: Sudden death in patients with chronic bifascicular block. Arch. Intern. Med. *137*:1005, 1977.
104. Moritz, A. R., and Zamcheck, N.: Sudden and unexpected deaths of young soldiers: Disease responsible for such deaths during World War II. Arch. Pathol. *42*:459, 1946.
105. Lown, B., and Graboys, T. B.: Management of patients with malignant ventricular arrhythmias. Am. J. Cardiol. *39*:910, 1977.
106. Pederson, D. H., Zipes, D. P., Foster, P. R., and Troup, P. J.: Ventricular tachycardia and ventricular fibrillation in a young population. Circulation *60*: 988, 1979.
107. Lown, B., Temte, J. V., Reich, P., Gaughan, C., Regestein, Q., and Hai, H.: Basis for recurring ventricular fibrillation in the absence of coronary heart disease and its management. N. Engl. J. Med. *294*:623, 1976.
108. Lown, B., and Verrier, R. L.: Neural activity and ventricular fibrillation. N. Engl. J. Med. *294*:1165, 1976.
109. Maron, B. J., Roberts, W. C., McAlister, H. A., Rosing, D. R., and Epstein, S. E.: Sudden death in young athletes. Circulation *62*:218, 1980.
110. Morales, A. R., Romanell, R., and Boucek, R. J.: The mural left anterior descending coronary artery, strenuous exercise and sudden death. Circulation *62*: 230, 1980.
111. Isner, J. M., Sours, H. E., Paris, A. L., Ferman, V. J., and Roberts, W. C.: Sudden, unexpected death in avid dieters using the liquid protein fast diet: Observation in 17 patients and role of the prolonged QT interval. Circulation *60*: 1401, 1979.
112. Lantigua, R. A., Amatruda, J. M., Biddle, T. L., Forbes, G. B., and Lockwood, D. H.: Cardiac arrhythmias associated with a liquid protein diet for the treatment of obesity. N. Engl. J. Med. *303*:735, 1980.
113. Lawrie, D. M., Higgins, M. R., Godman, M. J., Oliver, M. F., Julian, D. G., and Donald, K. W.: Ventricular fibrillation complicating acute myocardial infarction. Lancet *2*:523, 1968.
114. Geddes, J. S., Adgey, A. A. J., and Pantridge, J. F.: Prognosis after recovery from ventricular fibrillation complicating ischemic heart disease. Lancet *2*:273, 1967.
115. Lown, B., Klein, M. D., and Hershberg, P. I.: Coronary and precoronary care. Am. J. Med. *46*:705, 1969.
116. Thompson, P., and Sloaman, G.: Sudden death in hospital after discharge from coronary care unit. Br. Med. J. *2*:136, 1971.
117. Graboys, T. B.: In-hospital sudden death after coronary care unit discharge. Arch. Intern. Med. *135*:512, 1975.
118. Schultze, R. A., Strauss, H. W., and Pitt, B.: Sudden death in the year following myocardial infarction. Am. J. Med. *62*:192, 1977.
119. Vismara, L. A., DeMaria, A. N., Hughes, J. L., Mason, D. T., and Amsterdam, E. A.: Evaluation of arrhythmias in the late hospital phase of acute myocardial infarction compared to coronary care unit ectopy. Br. Med. J. *37*: 598, 1975.
120. Schaffer, W. A., and Cobb, L. A.: Recurrent ventricular fibrillation and modes of death in survivors of out-of-hospital ventricular fibrillation. N. Engl. J. Med. *293*:260, 1975.
121. Cobb, L. A., Baum, R. S., Alvarez, H., and Schaffer, W. A.: Resuscitation from out of hospital ventricular fibrillation: 4 years follow-up. Circulation *52*: III–223, 1975.
122. Lown, B., and Graboys, T. B.: Sudden death: An ancient problem newly perceived. Cardiovasc. Med. *2*:219, 1977.
123. Wikland, B.: Death from arteriosclerotic heart disease outside hospitals. Acta Med. Scand. *184*:129, 1968.
124. Lown, B., and Ruberman, W.: The concept of precoronary care. Mod. Concepts Cardiovasc. Dis. *39*:97, 1970.
125. Lown, B.: Sudden death from coronary artery disease. *In* Waldenstrom, J., Larson, T., and Ljungestedt, N. (eds.): Early Phases of Coronary Heart Disease: The Possibility of Prediction (Skandia International Symposia). Stockholm, Nordiska Bokhandelns Forlag, 1973, pp. 255–277.
126. Lown, B., Vassaux, C., Hood, W. B., Jr., Fakhro, A. M., Kaplinsky, E., and Roberge, G.: Unresolved problems in coronary care. Am. J. Cardiol. *20*: 494, 1967.
127. Lown, B., and Wolf, M.: Approaches to sudden death from coronary heart disease. Circulation *44*:130, 1971.
128. Hiss, R., Averill, K., and Lamb, L.: EKG findings in 67,375 asymptomatic subjects. Am. J. Cardiol. *6*:96, 1960.
129. Brodsky, M., Wu, D., Denes, P., Kanakis, C., and Rosen, K. M.: Arrhythmias documented by 24 hour continuous electrocardiographic monitoring in 50 male medical students without apparent heart disease. Am. J. Cardiol. *39*:390, 1977.
130. Kennedy, J., and Underhill, S. J.: Frequent or complex ventricular ectopy in apparently healthy subjects: A clinical study of 25 cases. Am. J. Cardiol. *38*: 141, 1976.
131. Hinkle, L. E., Jr., Carver, S. T., and Argyros, D. C.: The prognostic significance of ventricular premature beats in healthy people and in people with coronary heart disease. Acta Cardiol. *18* (Suppl.):5, 1974.
132. Hinkle, L. E., Jr., Carver, S. T., and Stevens, M.: Frequency of asymptomatic disturbances of cardiac rhythm and conduction in middle-aged men: Study of 301 active American men with 6 hour monitoring. Am. J. Cardiol. *24*:629, 1969.
133. Lown, B. Calvert, A. F., Armington, R., and Ryan, M.: Monitoring for serious arrhythmias and high risk of sudden death. Circulation *52*:189, 1975.
134. Smirk, F. H., and Palmer, D. G.: A myocardial syndrome: With particular reference to the occurrence of sudden death and of premature systoles interrupting antecedent T-waves. Am. J. Cardiol. *6*:620, 1960.
135. Han, J., and Goel, B.: Electrophysiologic precursors of ventricular arrhythmia. Arch. Intern. Med. *129*:749, 1972.
136. Wolff, G. A., Veith, F., and Lown, B.: A vulnerable period for ventricular tachycardia following myocardial infarction. Cardiovasc. Res. *2*:111, 1968.
137. Epstein, S. E., Beiser, G. D., Rosing, D. R., Talano, J. V., and Karsh, R. B.: Experimental acute myocardial infarction. Characterization and treatment of the malignant premature ventricular contractions. Circulation *47*:446, 1973.
138. Engel, R. T., Meister, S. G., and Frankl, W. S.: The "R on T" phenomenon: an update and critical review. Ann. Intern. Med. *88*:221, 1978.
139. Scherlag, B. J., El-Sherif, N., Hope, R., and Lazzara, R.: Characterization and localization of ventricular arrhythmias resulting from myocardial ischemia and infarction. Circ. Res. *35*:372, 1974.
140. Waldo, A. L., and Kaiser, G. A.: A study of ventricular arrhythmias associated with acute myocardial infarction in the canine heart. Circulation *47*:1222, 1973.
141. Boineaux, J. P., and Cox, J. T.: Slow ventricular activation in acute myocardial infraction: A source of re-entrant premature ventricular contractions. Circulation *48*:702, 1973.
142. Williams, D. O., Scherlag, B. J., Hope, R. R., El-Sherif, N., and Lazzara, R.: The pathophysiology of malignant ventricular arrhythmias during acute myocardial ischemia. Circulation *50*:1163, 1974.
143. DeSoyza, N., Bissett, J. K., Kane, J. J., Murphy, M. L., and Doherty, J. E.: Ectopic ventricular prematurity and its relationship to ventricular tachycardia in acute myocardial infarction in man. Circulation *50*:529, 1974.
144. Rothfeld, E. L., Parsonnet, J., McGorman, W., and Linden, S.: Harbingers of paroxysmal ventricular tachycardia in acute myocardial infarction. Chest *71*: 142, 1977.
145. Wellens, H. J. J., Durrer, D. R., and Lie, K. I.: Observations on mechanisms of ventricular tachycardia in man. Circulation *54*:237, 1976.
146. El-Sherif, N., Myerburg, R. J., Scherlag, B. J., Befeler, R., Aranda, J. M., Castellanos, A., and Lazzara, R.: Electrocardiographic antecedents of primary ventricular fibrillation. Value of R on T phenomenon in myocardial infarction. Br. Heart J. *38*:415, 1976.
147. Ruberman, W., Weinblatt, E., Goldberg, J. D., Frank, C. W., Chaudhary, B. S., and Shapiro, S.: Ventricular premature complexes and sudden death after myocardial infarction. Circulation *64*:297, 1981.
148. Oliver, G. C.: Ventricular arrhythmias in coronary artery disease and their relationship to sudden death. *in* Proceedings of the First U.S.–U.S.S.R. Sympo-

sium on Sudden Death, Yalta, October 3–5, 1977. U. S. Department of Health, Education, and Welfare, Public Health Service, National Institutes of Health, D.H.E.W. Publication No. NIH 78–1470, 1978.

149. Campbell, R. W. F., Murray, A., and Julian, D. G.: Ventricular arrhythmias in the first 12 hours of acute myocardial infarction: Natural history study. Br. Heart J. *46*:351, 1981.
150. Huppert, B., and Berliner, K.: The intraventricular conduction time of ventricular premature systoles. Cardiologica *27*:87, 1955.
151. Soloff, L.: Ventricular premature beat—diagnostic of myocardial disease. Am. J. Med. Sci. *242*:289, 1969.
152. Manning, G., Ahuja, A., and Gutierrea, M. R.: Electrocardiographic differentiation between ventricular premature beats from subjects with normal and diseased hearts. Cardiologia *23*:462, 1968.
153. Rosenbaum, M.: Classification of ventricular extrasystoles according to form. J. Electrocardiol. *2*:289, 1969.
154. Estler, J., and White, P. D.: Clinical significance of ventricular premature beats with reference to heart rate. Arch. Intern. Med. *43*:606, 1929.
155. Bigger, T. J., Weld, F. M., Rolnitzky, M. L.: Prevalence, characteristics and significance of ventricular tachycardia (three or more complexes) detected with ambulatory electrocardiographic recording in the late hospital phase of acute myocardial infarction. Am. J. Cardiol. *48*:815, 1981.
156. Thompson, P., and Lown, B.: Sequential R/T pacing to expose electrical instability in the ischemic ventricle. Clin. Res. *20* (Abstr.):401, 1972.
157. Axelrod, P. J., Verrier, R. L., and Lown, B.: Vulnerability to ventricular fibrillation during acute coronary arterial occlusion and release. Am. J. Cardiol. *36*: 776, 1976.
158. Ruberman, W., Weinblatt, E., Goldberg, J. D., Frank, C. W., and Shapiro, S.: Ventricular premature beats and mortality after myocardial infarction. N. Engl. J. Med. *279*:750, 1977.
159. The Coronary Drug Project Research Group: Prognostic importance of premature beats following myocardial infarction. Experience in the Coronary Drug Project. J.A.M.A. *223*:1116, 1973.
160. Moss, A. J., Davis, H. T., DeCamilla, J., and Bayer, L. W.: Ventricular ectopic beats and their relation to sudden and nonsudden cardiac death after myocardial infarction. Circulation *60*:998, 1979.
161. Roberts, R., and Sobel, B.: Relationship between infarct size and ventricular arrhythmia. Br. Heart J. *37*:1169, 1975.
162. Sharma, S. D., Ballantyne, F., and Goldstein, S.: The relationship of ventricular asynergy in coronary artery disease to ventricular premature beats. Chest *66*:358, 1974.
163. Schulze, R. A., Jr., Rouleau, J., Rigo, P., Bowers, S., Strass, H. W., and Pitt, B.: Ventricular arrhythmias in late hospital phase of acute myocardial infarction; relation to left ventricular function detected by gated cardiac blood pool scanning. Circulation *52*:1006, 1975.
164. Schulze, R. A., Jr., Humphries, J. O., Griffith, L. S. C., Ducci, H., Achuff, S., Baird, M. G., Mellits, E. D., and Pitt, B.: Left ventricular and coronary angiographic anatomy: Relationship to ventricular irritability in the late hospital phase of acute myocardial infarction. Circulation *55*:839, 1977.
165. Calvert, A., Lown, B., and Gorlin, R.: Ventricular premature beats and anatomically defined coronary heart disease. Am. J. Cardiol. *39*:627, 1977.
166. Lown, B., Cannon, R. L., III, and Ross, M. A.: Electrical stimulation and digitalis drugs. Repetitive response in diastole. Proc. Soc. Exp. Biol. Med. *126*: 698, 1967.
167. Lown, B., and Cannon, R. L., III: Electrical stimulation to estimate the degree of digitalization: Experimental studies. Am. J. Cardiol. *22*:251, 1968.
168. Hagemeijer, F., and Lown, B.: Effect of heart reate on electrically induced repetitive ventricular responses in the digitalized dog. Circ. Res. *27*:333, 1970.
169. Jenzer, H., Lohrbauer, L., and Lown, B.: Response to single threshold stimuli following acute myocardial infarction. Proc. Soc. Exp. Biol. Med. *141*:606, 1972.
170. Green, L. H., Reid, P. R., and Schaeffer, A. H.: The repetitive ventricular response in man: an index of ventricular electrical instability. Am. J. Cardiol. *41* (Abstr.):400, 1978.
171. Lown, B.: New concepts and approaches to sudden cardiac death. Schweiz. Med. Wschr. *106*:1522, 1976.
172. Lown, B., Verrier, R. L., and Blatt, C. M.: Precordial mechanical stimulation for exposing electrical instability of the heart. Am. J. Cardiol. *42*:425, 1978.
173. Durrer, D., Schoo, L., Schuilenburg, R. M., and Wellens, H. J. J.: The role of premature beats in the initiation and termination of supraventricular tachycardia in Wolff-Parkinson-White syndrome. Circulation *36*:644, 1967.
174. Coumel, P. H., Cabrol, C., Fabiato, A., Gourgon, R., and Slama, R.: Tachycardia permanente par rhythme reciproque. Arch. Mal Coeur *60*:1830, 1967.
175. Wellens, H. J. J.: Value and limitations of programmed electrical stimulation of the heart in the study and treatment of tachycardias. Circulation *57*:845, 1978.
176. Josephson, M. E., Horowitz, L. N., Farshidi, A., and Kastor, J. A.: Recurrent sustained ventricular tachycardia: Mechanism. Circulation *57*:431, 1978.
177. Horowitz, L. N., Josephson, M. E., and Kastor, A. J.: Intracardiac electrophysiologic studies as method for the optimization of drug therapy in chronic ventricular arrhythmias. Prog. Cardiovasc. Dis. *23*:81, 1980.
178. Fontaine, G., Guiraudon, G., Frank, R., Gerbaux, A., Cousteau, J. P., Varillon, A., Gay, J., Cabral, C., and Focquet, J.: La cartographie épicardique et le traitement chirurgical par simple ventriculotomie de certaines tachycardies ventriculaires rebelles par réentrée. Arch. Mal Coeur *68*:113, 1975.
179. Ruskin, J. N., DiMarco, J. P., and Garan, H.: Out-of-hospital cardiac arrest. N. Engl. J. Med. *303*:607, 1980.
180. Horowitz, L. N., Josephson, M. E., Kastor, J. A., and Harken, A. H.: Ventricular resection guided by epicardial and endocardial mapping for treatment of recurrent ventricular tachycardia. N. Engl. J. Med. *302*:589, 1980.
181. Horowitz, L. N., Spielman, S. R., Greenspan, A. M., and Josephson, M. E.: Mechanism in the genesis of recurrent ventricular tachyarrhythmias as revealed by clinical electrophysiologic studies. Ann. N. Y. Acad. Med. *382*:116, 1982.
182. Josephson, M. E., Horowitz, L. N., and Farshidi, A.: Continuous local electrical activity: A mechanism of recurrent ventricular tachycardia. Circulation *57*: 659, 1978.
183. Lown, B., Verrier, R. L., and Rabinowitz, S. H.: Neural psychologic mechanisms and the problem of sudden cardiac death. Am. J. Cardiol. *39*:890, 1977.
184. Verrier, R. L., Thompson, P., and Lown, B.: Ventricular vulnerability during sympathetic stimulation: role of heart rate and blood pressure. Cardiovasc. Res. *8*:602, 1974.
185. Schwartz, P. J., Verrier, R., and Lown, B.: Effect of stellectomy and vagotomy on ventricular refractoriness in dogs. Circ. Res. *40*:536, 1977.
186. Schwartz, P. J., Snebold, N. G., and Brown, A. M.: Effects of unilateral cardiac sympathetic denervation on the ventricular fibrillation threshold. Am. J. Cardiol. *37*:1036, 1976.
187. Schwartz, P. J., Stone, H. L., and Brown, A. M.: Effects of unilateral stellate ganglion blockade on the arrhythmias associated with coronary occlusion. Am. Heart J. *92*:589, 1976.
188. Randall, W. C., and Rohse, W. G.: The augmentor action of the sympathetic cardiac nerves. Circ. Res. *4*:470, 1956.
189. Brown, A. M.: Excitation of afferent cardiac sympathetic nerve fibers during myocardial ischaemia. J. Physiol. (Lond.) *190*:703, 1969.
190. Malliani, A., Schwartz, P. J., and Zanchetti, A.: A sympathetic reflex elicited by experimental coronary occlusion. Am. J. Physiol. *217*:703, 1969.
191. Corbalan, R., Verrier, R. L., and Lown, B.: Differing mechanisms for ventricular vulnerability during coronary artery occlusion and release. Am. Heart J. *92*: 223, 1976.
192. Verrier, R., Calvert, A., Lown, B., and Axelrod, P.: Effect of acute blood pressure elevation on the ventricular fibrillation threshold. Am. J. Physiol. *226*:893, 1974.
193. Blatt, C. M., Verrier, R. L., and Lown, B.: Acute blood pressure elevation and ventricular fibrillation threshold during coronary artery occlusion and reperfusion in the dog. Am. J. Cardiol. *39*:523, 1977.
194. Higgins, C. B., Vatner, S. F., and Braunwald, E.: Parasympathetic control of the heart. Pharmacol. Rev. *25*:119, 1973.
195. Kent, K. M., Smith, E. R., Redwood, D. R., and Epstein, S. E.: Electrical stability of the acutely ischemic myocardium: Influences of heart rate and vagal stimulation. Circulation *47*:291, 1973.
196. Kent, K. M., Epstein, S. E., Cooper, T., and Jacobowitz, D. M.: Cholinergic innervation of the canine and human ventricular conducting system: anatomic and electrophysiologic correlations. Circulation *50*:948, 1974.
197. Einbrodt, E.: Über Herzreizung und ihr Verhältnis zum Blutdruck. Vienna, Akademie der Wissenschaften Sitzungsberichte *38*:345, 1859.
198. Myers, R. W., Pearlman, A. S., Hyman, R. M., Goldstein, R. A., Kent, K. M., Goldstein, R. E., and Epstein, S. E.: Beneficial effects of vagal stimulation and bradycardia during experimental acute myocardial ischemia. Circulation *49*:943, 1974.
199. Kolman, B. S., Verrier, R. L., and Lown, B.: The effect of vagus nerve stimulation upon vulnerability of the canine ventricle: Role of sympathetic-parasympathetic interactions. Circulation *52*:578, 1975.
200. Kolman, B. S., Verrier, R. L., and Lown, B.: The effect of vagus nerve stimulation upon excitability of the canine ventricle: Role of sympathetic-parasympathetic interactions. Am. J. Cardiol. *37*:1041, 1975.
201. Verrier, R. L., Rabinowitz, S. H., and Lown, B.: Vagal and adrenergic interactions and ventricular electrical stability. Clin. Res. *23*:212A, 1975.
202. Rabinowitz, S. H., Verrier, R. L., and Lown, B.: Muscarinic effects of vagosympathetic trunk stimulation on the repetitive extrasystole threshold. Circulation *53*:622, 1976.
203. Murad, F., Chi, Y. M., and Rall, T. W.: Adenylcyclase. III. The effect of catecholamines and choline esters on the formation of adenosine-3′,5′-phosphate by preparations from cardiac muscle and liver. J. Biol. Chem. *237*:1233, 1962.
204. LaRaia, P. J., and Sonnenblick, E. H.: Autonomic control of cardiac C-AMP. Circ. Res. *28*:377, 1971.
205. Watanabe, A. M., and Besch, H. R., Jr.: Interaction between cyclic adenosine monophosphate and cyclic guanosine monophosphate in guinea pig ventricular myocardium. Circ. Res. *37*:309, 1975.
206. Wiggers, C. J., and Wegria, R.: Ventricular fibrillation due to single, localized induction and condenser shocks applied during the vulnerable phase of ventricular systole. Am. J. Physiol. *128*:520, 1940.
207. Matta, R. J., Verrier, R. L., and Lown, B.: The repetitive extrasystole as an index of vulnerability to ventricular fibrillation. Am. J. Physiol. *230*:1469, 1976.
208. Lown, B., Verrier, R. L., and Corbalan, R.: Psychologic stress and threshold for repetitive ventricular response. Science *182*:834, 1973.
209. Matta, R. J., Lawler, J. E., and Lown, B.: Ventricular electrical instability in the conscious dog: Effects of psychologic stress and beta adrenergic blockade. Am. J. Cardiol. *38*:594, 1976.
210. Corbalan, R., Verrier, R., and Lown, B.: Psychologic stress and ventricular arrhythmias during myocardial infarction in the conscious dog. Am. J. Cardiol. *34*:692, 1974.
211. Antonaccio, M. J., and Robson, R. D.: Cardiovascular effects of 5-hydroxytryptophan in anesthetized dogs. J. Pharm. Pharmacol. *25*:495, 1973.

212. Antonaccio, M. J., and Robson, R. D.: Centrally mediated cardiovascular effects of 5-hydroxytryptophan in MAO-inhibited dogs: modification by autonomic antagonists. Arch. Int. Pharmacodyn. Ther. *231*:200, 1975.
213. Baum, T., and Shropshire, A. T.: Inhibition of efferent sympathetic nerve activity by 5-hydroxytryptophan and centrally administered 5-hydroxytryptamine. Neuropharmacology *142*:227, 1975.
214. Rabinowitz, S. H., and Lown, B.: Central neurochemical factors related to serotonin metabolism and cardiac ventricular vulnerability for repetitive electrical activity. Am. J. Cardiol. *41*:516, 1978.
215. Engel, G. L.: Sudden and rapid death during psychologic stress. Folk lore or folk wisdom? Ann. Intern. Med. *74*:771, 1971.
216. Wellens, J. J. H., Vermuelen, A., and Durrer, D.: Ventricular fibrillation occurring on arousal from sleep by auditory stimuli. Circulation *46*:661, 1972.
217. Taggart, P., Carruthers, M., and Somerville, W.: Electrocardiograms, plasma catecholamines and lipids, and their modification by oxyprenolol, when speaking before an audience. Lancet *2*:341, 1973.
218. Taggart, P., Gibbons, D., and Somerville, W.: Some effects of motor-car driving on the normal and abnormal heart. Br. Med. J. *4*:130, 1969.
219. Rose, K. D.: The post-coronary patient as a spectator sportsman, *In* Eliot, R. S. (ed.): Stress and the Heart. New York, Futura Publishing Co., 1974, p. 207.
220. Lown, B., Tykocinski, M., Garfein, A., and Brooks, P.: Sleep and ventricular premature beats. Circulation *48*:691, 1973.
221. Lown, B., DeSilva, R. A., Reich, P., and Murawski, B. J.: Psychophysiologic factors in sudden cardiac death. Am. J. Psychiatry *137*:1325, 1980.
222. Parkes, C. M., Benjamin, B., and Fitzgerald, R.: Broken heart: Statistical study of increased mortality among widowers. Br. Med. J. *1*:740, 1969.
223. Rahe, R. H., Bennett, L., Romo, M., Siltanen, P., and White, R. J.: Subjects' recent life changes and coronary heart disease in Finland. Am. J. Psychiatry *130*:1222, 1973.
224. Jarvinen, K. A. J.: Can ward rounds be a danger to patients with myocardial infarction? Br. Med. J. *1*:318, 1955.
225. Hughes, A., and Tonks, R. S.: Experimental embolic carditis. J. Pathol. Bacteriol. *72*:497, 1956.
226. Hughes, A., and Tonks, R. S.: The role of microemboli in the production of carditis in hypersensitivity experiments. J. Pathol. Bacteriol. *77*:207, 1959.
227. Jorgensen, L., Roswell, H. C., Hovig, T., Glynn, M. F., and Mustard, J. F.: Adenosine diphosphate–induced platelet aggregation and myocardial infarction in swine. Lab. Invest. *17*:616, 1967.
228. Halmagyi, D., Starzechi, B., and Horner, G.: Humoral transmission of cardiorespiratory changes in experimental lung embolism. Circ. Res. *14*:546, 1964.
229. Thomas, D., Gurewich, V., and Ashford, T.: Platelet adherence to thromboemboli in relation to the pathogenesis and treatment of pulmonary embolism. N. Engl. J. Med. *274*:953, 1966.
230. Gurewich, V., Thomas, D., Stem, M., and Wessler, S.: Bronchoconstriction in the presence of pulmonary embolism. Circulation *27*:339, 1963.
231. Smith, G., and Smith, A.: The role of serotonin in experimental pulmonary embolism. Surg. Gynecol. Obstet. *101*:691, 1955.
232. Comroe, J., VanLingen, B., Stroud, B., and Roncoroni, A.: Reflex and direct cardiopulmonary effects of 5-OH-tryptamine (serotonin). Am. J. Physiol. *173*: 379, 1953.
233. Zervas, N. T., Kuwayama, A., Rosoff, C. B., and Salzman, E. W.: Modification by inhibition of platelet function. Arch. Neurol. *28*:400, 1973.
234. Zervas, N. T., Hori, H., and Rosoff, C. B.: Experimental inhibition of serotonin by antibiotic: prevention of cerebral vasospasm. J. Neurosurg. *41*:259, 1974.
235. Ellis, E. L., Oelz, O., Roberts, L. J., II, Payne, N. A., Sweetman, B. J., Nies, A. S., and Oates, J. A.: Coronary arterial smooth muscle contraction by a substance released from platelets: Evidence that it is thromboxane A2. Science *193*: 1135, 1976.
236. Hoak, J. C., Warner, E. D., and Connor, W. E.: New concepts of levarterenol-induced acute myocardial necrosis. Arch. Pathol. *87*:332, 1969.
237. Haft, J. I., Krantz, P. D., Albert, F. J., and Fani, K.: Intravascular platelet aggregation in the heart by norepinephrine. Microscopic studies. Circulation *46*: 698, 1972.
238. Haft, J. I., and Fani, K.: Stress and the induction of intravascular platelet aggregation in the heart. Circulation *48*:164, 1973.
239. VanVliet, P. D., Burchell, H. B., and Titus, J. L.: Focal myocarditis associated with pheochromocytoma. N. Engl. J. Med. *274*:1102, 1966.
240. Barr, I., Cohen, P., Berken, A., and Lown, B.: Thrombocythemia and myocardial ischemia with normal coronary angiogram. Arch. Intern. Med. *134*:528, 1974.
241. Prinzmetal, M., Ekmekci, A., Kennamer, R., Kwoczynski, J. K., Shubin, H., and Toyoshima, H.: Variant form of angina pectoris: Previously undelineated syndrome. J.A.M.A. *174*:1794, 1960.
242. Whiting, R. B., Klein, M. D., VanderVeer, J., and Lown, B.: Variant angina pectoris. N. Engl. J. Med. *282*:709, 1970.
243. MacAlpin, R. N., Kattus, A. A., and Alvaro, A. B.: Angina pectoris at rest with preservative of exercise capacity: Prinzmetal's variant angina. Circulation *47*:946, 1973.
244. Endo, M., Kanda, L., Hosoda, S., Hayashi, H., Kirosawa, K., and Konno, S.: Prinzmetal's variant form of angina pectoris: re-evaluation of mechanism. Circulation *52*:33, 1975.
245. Dhurandhar, R. W., Watt, D. L., Silver, M. D., Trimble, A. S., and Adelman, A. S.: Prinzmetal's variant form of angina with arteriographic evidence of coronary arterial spasm. Am. J. Cardiol. *30*:902, 1972.
246. Oliva, P. B., Potts, D. E., and Pluss, R. G.: Coronary arterial spasm in Prinzmetal's angina: Documentation by coronary arteriography. N. Engl. J. Med. *288*:745, 1973.
247. Cheng, T. O., Bashour, T., Kelsar, G. A., Weiss, L., and Bacos, J.: Variant angina of Prinzmetal with normal coronary arteriograms. A variant of the variant. Circulation *47*:476, 1973.
248. Maseri, A., L'Abbate, A., Baroldi, G., Chierchia, S., Marzilli, M., Ballestra, A. M., Severi, S., Parodi, O., Biagini, A., Distante, A., and Pesola, P.: Coronary vasospasm as a possible cause of myocardial infarction: A conclusion derived from the study of "preinfarction" angina. N. Engl. J. Med. *299*:1271, 1978.
249. Maseri, A., Severi, S., and Marzullo, P.: Role of coronary arterial spasm in sudden coronary ischemic death. Ann. N. Y. Acad. Sci. *382*:204, 1982.
250. Hillis, D., and Braunwald, E.: Coronary arterial spasm. N. Engl. J. Med. *299*: 695, 1978.
251. Mudge, F. H., Jr., Grossman, W., Mills, R. M., Jr., Lesch, M., and Braunwald, E.: Reflex increase in coronary vascular resistance in patients with ischemic heart disease. N. Engl. J. Med. *295*:1333, 1976.
252. Clark, D. A., Quint, R. A., Bolen, J., and Schroeder, J. S.: The angiographic demonstration of coronary artery spasm in patients with suspected variant angina: Method and therapeutic implications. Am. J. Cardiol. *35*(Abstr.):127, 1975.
253. Huepler, F., Proudfit, W., Siegel, W., Shirey, E., Razavi, M., and Sones, M. F.: The ergonovine maleate test for the diagnosis of coronary artery spasm. Circulation *52* (Abstr.):II–11, 1975.
254. Yasue, H., Touyama, M., and Shimamoto, M.: Role of autonomic nervous system in the pathogenesis of Prinzmetal's variant form of angina. Circulation *50*: 534, 1974.
255. Athanasopoulos, C., and Maroutsos, C.: Prinzmetal's angina. Br. Heart J. *39*: 911, 1977.
256. Hackett, T., and Cassem, N.: Factors contributing to delay in responding to the signs and symptoms of acute myocardial infarction. Am. J. Cardiol. *24*: 651, 1969.
257. Whipple, G.: Physician-induced treatment delays in the pre-CCU period. *In* Proceedings of the National Conference on Standards for CPR and Emergency Cardiac Care, 1975, p. 139.
258. Goldstein, S., Moss, A. J., and Greene, W.: Sudden death in acute myocardial infarction. Arch. Intern. Med. *129*:720, 1972.
259. Gillum, R., Feinleib, M., Margolis, J. R., Fabsitz, R. R., and Brasch, R. C.: Delay in the hospital phase of acute myocardial infarction. Arch. Intern. Med. *136*:649, 1976.
260. Lie, K. I., Wellens, H. J., Downar, E., and Durrer, D.: Observations on patients with primary ventricular fibrillation complicating acute myocardial infarction. Circulation *52*:755, 1975.
261. Lie, K. I., Wellens, H. J., VanCapelle, F. J., and Durrer, D.: Lidocaine in the prevention of primary ventricular fibrillation. N. Engl. J. Med. *291*:1324, 1974.
262. Valentine, P. A., Frew, J. L., Mashford, M. L., and Sloman, J. G.: Lidocaine in the prevention of sudden death in the pre-hospital phase of acute infarction: A double-blind study. N. Engl. J. Med. *291*:1327, 1974.
263. American Heart Association and National Resuscitation Council: Standards for cardiopulmonary resuscitation (CPR) and emergency cardiac care (ECC). J.A.M.A. *277*:836, 1974.
264. Standards and guidelines for cardiopulmonary resuscitation (CPR) and emergency cardiac care (ECC). J.A.M.A. *244*:453, 1980.
264a. Silverberg, R. A., and Weil, M. M.: Changing concepts in cardiac resuscitation. McIntosh, M. D. (ed.): Baylor College of Medicine, Cardiology Series, Vol. 5, No. 2, 1982, 27 pp.
265. Pennington, J. E., Taylor, J., and Lown, B.: Chest thump for reverting ventricular tachycardia. N. Engl. J. Med. *283*:1192, 1970.
266. Lown, B., and Taylor, J.: "Thump-version." N. Engl. J. Med. *283*:1223, 1970.
267. Weale, F. E., and Rothwell-Jackson, R. L.: The efficiency of cardiac massage. Lancet *1*:990, 1982.
268. Weisfeldt, M. I., Chandra, N., Tsitlik, J. E., and Rudikoff, M.: New attempts to improve blood flow during CPR. *In* Schluger, J., and Lyon, F. E. (eds.): CPR and Emergency Cardiac Care. New York, EM Books, 1980, p. 29.
269. Criley, J. M., Blaufuss, A. N., and Kissel, G. L.: Cough-induced cardiac resuscitation. J.A.M.A. *236*:1246, 1976.
270. Geddes, L. A., Tacker, W. A., Rosborough, J. P., Moore, A. G., and Geddes, P.: Electrical dose for ventricular defibrillation of large and small animals using precordial electrodes. J. Clin. Invest. *53*:310, 1974.
271. Tacker, W. A., Galioto, F., Guitiani, E., Geddes, L. A., and McNamara, D.: Energy dosage for human defibrillation. N. Engl. J. Med. *290*:214, 1974.
272. Pantridge, J. F., Adgey, A. A. J., and Geddes, J. S.: The Acute Coronary Attack. New York, Grune and Stratton, 1975, pp. 66–78.
273. Crampton, R. S.: Low-energy ventricular defibrillation and miniature defibrillators. J.A.M.A. *235*:2284, 1976.
274. DeSilva, R. A., and Lown, B.: Energy requirements for defibrillation of a markedly overweight patient. Circulation *57*:827, 1978.
275. Kerber, R. E., and Sarnat, W.: Factors influencing the success of ventricular defibrillation in man. Circulation *60*:226, 1979.
276. Lown, B., Crampton, R. S., and DeSilva, R. A.: The energy for ventricular fibrillation defibrillation—Too little or too much? N. Engl. J. Med. *298*:1252, 1978.
276a. Haynes, R. E., Chin, T. L., Copass, M. K., and Cobb, L. A.: Comparison of bretylium tosylate and lidocaine in management of out of hospital ventricular fibrillation: A randomized clinical trial. Am. J. Cardiol. *48*:353, 1981.

277. Eisenberg, M., Hallstrom, A., and Bergner, L.: The ACLS score: Predicting survival from out-of-hospital cardiac arrest. J.A.M.A. *246*:50, 1981.
278. Myerburg, R. J., Kessler, K. M., Zaman, L., Conde, C. A., and Castellanos, A.: Survivors of prehospital cardiac arrest. J.A.M.A. *247*:1485, 1982.
279. Cobb, L. A., Werner, J. A., and Trobough, G. B.: Sudden cardiac death. I. A decade's experience with out-of-hospital resuscitation. Mod. Concepts Cardiovasc. Dis. *49*:31, 1980.
280. Eisenberg, M., Hallstrom, A., and Bergner, L.: Long-term survival after out-of-hospital cardiac arrest. N. Engl. J. Med. *306*:1340, 1982.
281. Snyder, B. D., Hauser, W. A., Loewenson, R. B., Leppik, I. E., Ramirez-Lassepas, M., and Gummit, R. J.: Neurologic prognosis after cardiopulmonary arrest. III. Seizure activity. Neurology *30*:1292, 1980.
282. Hjalmarsen, A.: Beta blocking agents, current status in the prevention of sudden coronary death. Ann. N. Y. Acad. Sci. *382*:805, 1982.
283. Norwegian Multicenter Study Group: Timolol-induced reduction in mortality and reinfarction in patients surviving acute myocardial infarction. N. Engl. J. Med. *304*:801, 1981.
284. Mirowski, M., Mower, M., Staewen, W. S., Tabatznik, B., and Mendeloff, A. I.: Standby autonomic defibrillator: An approach to prevention of sudden coronary death. Arch. Intern. Med. *126*:158, 1970.
285. Mirowski, M., Mower, M. M., Reid, P. P., and Watkins, L., Jr.: Implantable automatic defibrillators—Their potential in prevention of sudden coronary death. Ann. N.Y. Acad. Sci. *382*:371, 1982.
286. Lown, B., and Axelrod, P.: Implanted stand-by defibrillators. Circulation *46*: 637, 1972.
287. Lown, B., Podrid, P. J., DeSilva, R. A., and Graboys, T. B.: Sudden cardiac death—Management of the patient at risk. Curr. Prob. Cardiol. *4*:1, 1980.
288. Lown, B., Graboys, T. B., Podrid, P. J., Cohen, B. H., Stockman, M. B., and Gaughan, C. E.: Effect of a digitalis drug on ventricular premature beats (VPB's). N. Engl. J. Med. *296*:301, 1977.
289. Winkle, R. A., Alderman, E. L., Fitzgerald, J. W., and Harrison, D. C.: Treatment of recurrent symptomatic ventricular tachycardia. Ann. Intern. Med. *85*: 1, 1976.
290. Lown, B., Matta, R. J., and Besser, H. W.: Programmed "Trendscription:" A new approach to electrocardiographic monitoring. J.A.M.A. *232*:39, 1975.
291. Gaughan, C. E., Lown, B., Lanigan, J., Voukydis, P., and Besser, H. W.: Acute oral testing for determining antiarrhythmic drug efficacy. I. Quinidine. Am. J. Cardiol. *38*:677, 1976.
292. Jelinek, M. V., and Lown, B.: Exercise stress testing for exposure of cardiac arrhythmias. Prog. Cardiovasc. Dis. *16*:497, 1974.
293. Zaret, B. L., and Conti, C. R., Jr.: Exercise-induced ventricular irritability: hemodynamic and angiographic correlations. Am. J. Cardiol. *29*:298, 1972.
294. Helfant, R. H., Pine, R., Kalde, V., and Banka, V.: Exercise related ventricular premature complexes in coronary heart disease: Correlation with ischemia and angiographic severity. Ann. Intern. Med. *80*:589, 1974.
295. Goldschlager, N., and Selzer, A.: Treadmill test as an indicator of presence and severity of coronary artery disease. Ann. Intern. Med. *85*:277, 1976.
296. Lown, B., and DeSilva, R. A.: Roles of psychologic stress and autonomic nervous system changes in provocation of ventricular premature beats. Am. J. Cardiol. *41*:979, 1978.
297. Lown, B., Klein, M. D., Barr, I., Hagemeijer, F., Kosowsky, B. D., and Garrison, H.: Sensitivity to digitalis drugs in acute myocardial infarction. Am. J. Cardiol. *30*:388, 1972.
298. Lown, B., and Levine, S. A.: The carotid sinus: Clinical value of its stimulation. Circulation *23*:776, 1961.
299. Nichol, A. D., and Strauss, H.: The effects of digitalis, urginin, congestive cardiac failure and atropine on the hyperactive carotid sinus. Am. Heart J. *25*: 746, 1943.
300. Nalhauson, M. H.: Action of acetylbetamethylcholine on ventricular rhythm induced by adrenalin. Proc. Soc. Exp. Biol. Med. *32*:1297, 1943.
301. Waxman, M. B., Downar, E., Berman, N. D., and Felderhof, D. H.: Phenylephrine (neosynephrine) terminated ventricular tachycardia. Circulation *50*: 656, 1974.
302. Weiss, T., Lattin, G. M., and Engelman, K.: Vagally mediated suppression of premature ventricular contractions in man. Am. Heart J. *89*:700, 1975.
303. Lown, B., and Graboys, T. B.: Ventricular premature beats and sudden cardiac death. *In* McIntosh, H. (ed.): Baylor Coll. Med. Card. Series *3*:4, 1980.
304. Harken, A. H., Horowitz, R. M., and Josephson, M. E.: Comparison of standard aneurysmectomy with directed endocardial resection for treatment of recurrent sustained ventricular tachycardia. J. Thorac. Cardiovasc. Surg. *80*: 527, 1980.
305. Josephson, M. E., Horowitz, L. N., and Harken, A. H.: Surgery for recurrent sustained ventricular tachycardia associated with coronary artery disease: The role of subendocardial resection. Ann. N. Y. Acad. Sci. *382*:381, 1982.
306. Lown, B.: Sudden cardiac death: The major challenge confronting contemporary cardiology. Am. J. Cardiol. *43*:313, 1979.

24 HIGH–CARDIAC OUTPUT STATES

by *William Grossman, M.D., and Eugene Braunwald, M.D.*

METABOLIC DETERMINANTS OF CARDIAC OUTPUT

Discussion of high–cardiac output states should begin with a definition of normal cardiac output and a brief review of the factors that determine cardiac output. The quantity of blood delivered to the systemic circulation per unit of time is termed the *cardiac output,* generally expressed in liters per min. For a normal adult weighing 70 kg, resting cardiac output is approximately 6.25 liters/min.[1] Since the total volume of blood contained in the vascular system is approximately 75 ml/kg body weight in normal subjects,[2] or 5.2 liters in a 70-kg man, it is apparent that the total blood volume is moved around the circulation in a little less than 1 minute. Transient but substantial increases in cardiac output normally occur in response to changing metabolic demands, such as with exercise. However, a sustained increase in cardiac output—the subject of this chapter—is distinctly abnormal and contributes significantly to the symptoms and clinical presentation of several disease states.

The blood pumped by the heart delivers oxygen and a variety of substrates to the metabolizing tissues and removes carbon dioxide and other products of metabolism. In addition, blood transfers the heat generated by metabolic activity from the internal organs to the cutaneous bed, where it is dissipated. Derangement of any of the homeostatic mechanisms by which these functions are regulated can result in sustained deviations of the cardiac output (either increases or decreases) from its normal value.

Oxygen Requirements of the Tissues

The average normal adult consumes 130 ml/sq meter of oxygen each minute, delivered by the blood to metabolically active tissues. If arterial blood normally contains 19 ml O_2/dl (95 per cent saturation if oxygen carrying capacity equals 20 ml O_2/dl), and if cardiac output equals 3.25 liters/min/sq meter, then by Fick's principle (p. 289) the mixed venous blood returning from metabolically active tissue will have an oxygen content of approximately 15 ml/dl, i.e., an oxygen saturation of 75 per cent. The arteriovenous oxygen difference of 4 ml/dl represents the average normal extraction of oxygen by the body's tissues in the basal state. This average extraction represents a heterogeneity of metabolic activities, with skin, kidney, and skeletal muscle extracting relatively little oxygen in the basal state, whereas the heart extracts approximately 12 ml O_2/dl at rest.

As tissue metabolism increases, the arteriovenous oxygen difference rises and is limited at constant flow by a factor termed the *extraction reserve.* The normal extraction reserve for oxygen is 3, which means that given the augmented metabolic demand, the tissues can extract three times the normal quantity of oxygen, i.e., 3×4 ml O_2/dl $= 12$ ml O_2/dl.[3] Thus, if arterial saturation remains constant at 95 per cent, full utilization of the extraction reserve results in a mixed venous oxygen content of 7 ml/dl ($19 - 12$ ml/dl), or 35 per cent saturation, which corresponds to the pulmonary arterial oxygen saturation found in normal subjects studied at maximal exercise.

It is of interest that this value of 3 for the extraction reserve of oxygen predicts that in progressive cardiac decompensation, in order to meet the basal oxygen requirements of the body, oxygen extraction will increase until the arteriovenous oxygen difference has tripled, i.e., until the limit of extraction reserve has been reached and cardiac output has fallen to one-third its normal value. Further reduction of cardiac output results in systemic hypoxia, anaerobic metabolism, metabolic acidosis, and eventually circulatory collapse. It has been observed repeatedly that a persistent fall in resting cardiac output to below one-third of normal resting values is incompatible with life. However, long before the cardiac output has declined to this low level, the heart will be unable to meet the augmented requirements of the metabolizing tissues during activity or in resting patients with a hyperkinetic state, such as pregnancy or hyperthyroidism.

Under basal or near-basal conditions in the intact subject, most changes in cardiac output can be accounted for by changes in the capacity of the peripheral vascular bed to return blood to the heart, which, in turn, causes alterations in the preload. Conditions that lower peripheral vascular resistance are among the most important factors augmenting the venous return and therefore elevating cardiac output. These include anemia, arteriovenous fistulas, beriberi, thyrotoxicosis, pregnancy, and Paget's disease. A reduction in vascular resistance also occurs in (1) muscular exercise, in which dilatation occurs in the arterioles supplying the exercising muscles; (2) fever, in which there is reduced vascular resistance as a consequence of dilated cutaneous vessels; and (3) severe anoxia, in which generalized vascular dilatation also often occurs. These reductions in vascular resistance increase cardiac output not only by lowering ventricular afterload but also by reducing the impedance to venous return, thus tending to increase ventricular preload.

Guyton has properly emphasized the significance of venous return in the regulation of cardiac output.[3] He has pointed out that the ratio of blood volume to capacitance of the systemic circulation determines the level of peripheral venous pressure and that this ratio is a prime determinant of the venous pressure gradient (i.e., the pressure difference between the small veins and the right atrium), which is closely related to the force that returns blood to the heart. According to this formulation, an augmentation of blood volume or reduction of venous capacitance will raise this gradient, augment venous return, and, in the presence of normal cardiac function, increase cardiac output.

As pointed out in Chapters 13 and 14, cardiac output depends upon the interactions of intrinsic myocardial contractility with the prevailing conditions of myocardial loading. Figure 24–1 describes this interaction in terms of the resting and active left ventricular pressure-volume relationships. According to this formulation,[4-6] ACDE represents the control cardiac cycle (Fig. 24–1). End-diastolic pressure and volume are indicated by point A, isovolumetric contraction by line ABC, ejection by line CD, isovolumetric relaxation by line DE, and diastolic filling by segment EA. This type of construction is based on the concept that at constant contractility, ventricular pressure and volume at end systole (point D) always return to the active pressure-volume relationship (upper curve) (Fig. 12–26, p. 432). When left ventricular afterload is decreased, as occurs with the reduction of systemic vascular resistance and blood viscosity (characteristic of most of the conditions discussed in this chapter[7]), the resultant cardiac cycle is denoted by ABFG, which has a considerably larger stroke volume (SV_Y) than the control stroke volume for cycle ABCDE (SV_X). If left ventricular preload now rises, as occurs with an arteriovenous fistula and many of the other conditions to be discussed, the resultant cardiac cycle would be denoted by HIFG, with stroke volume SV_Z rising further still. Thus, the reduction of afterload and increase in preload act in concert to augment stroke volume, in some instances quite strikingly. With no change in heart rate or preload, this lowering of afterload will be translated into an increase in cardiac output.

Increases in contractility, not illustrated in Figure 24–1, would cause the active pressure-volume relationship curve to shift upward and to the left, so that at any given preload and afterload left ventricular ejection would proceed to a smaller end-systolic volume, thereby delivering a larger stroke volume. Since the minute cardiac output is the product of stroke volume and heart rate, the latter is also an important determinant of the cardiac output.

Left ventricular afterload is influenced by a number of variables, including the tone of the systemic arterioles, elasticity of the aorta and large arteries, viscosity of the blood, presence of aortic stenosis, and size and thickness of the left ventricle (Chap. 14). Left ventricular preload is a function of the condition of the mitral valve, compliance of the left ventricle, blood volume, venous tone, and vigor and timing of left atrial contraction. Most importantly, it

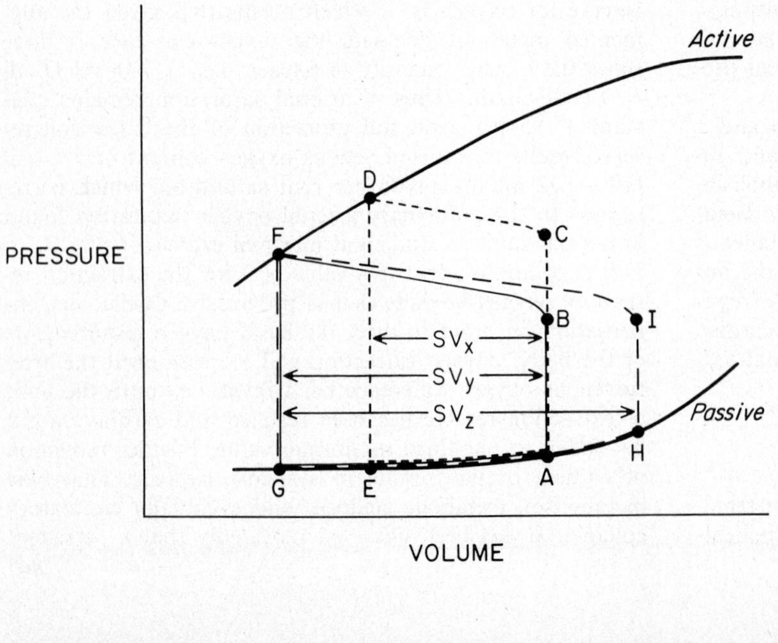

FIGURE 24–1 Influence of alterations in preload and afterload on left ventricular stroke volume. Reduction in afterloads leads to augmentation of stroke volume if preload is held constant, whereas augmentation of preload increases stroke volume if afterload is constant. In most conditions associated with a high-cardiac output state, both afterload reduction and preload augmentation are present. The control cardiac cycle is inscribed by points ABCDE; pure afterload reduction leads to cycle ABFG; a cycle demonstrating both afterload reduction and preload augmentation is indicated by HIFG. SV_X represents the stroke volume of the control cycle, SV_Y the augmented stroke volume effected by afterload reduction alone, and SV_Z the stroke volume with combined afterload reduction and preload augmentation, as might be seen with an arteriovenous fistula.

is a function of the venous return to the left atrium; this in turn is determined by the pressure gradient responsible for the return of blood from the systemic veins to the right atrium and, of course, by the function of the right side of the heart as well as pulmonary vascular resistance. When the latter two parameters are normal, the venous return pressure gradient becomes the principal determinant of left ventricular preload.

Heat Dissipation and Conservation

Body temperature and its regulation are important determinants of cardiac output. Hypothermia lowers cardiac output and hyperthermia raises it in an exponential relationship.[8,9] Temperature elevation raises cardiac output by means of two distinct mechanisms: (1) Cellular metabolism, and therefore oxygen consumption, and the production of vasodilator metabolites are a function of body temperature. With increased oxygen consumption and production of vasodilator metabolites, cardiac output rises as a consequence of reduced afterload and increased venous return, as described above. (2) Cutaneous blood flow is the principal means available to the body for temperature regulation. When total body metabolism is augmented or body temperature rises or both, marked increases in cutaneous blood flow to dissipate heat may be sufficient to increase total cardiac output substantially. The importance of this mechanism is evident in patients with the common forms of low-output congestive heart failure who are unable to increase cardiac output, cannot augment cutaneous blood flow, and therefore exhibit considerable difficulty with heat dissipation.

Substantial increases in cardiac output normally occur in response to increased environmental heat and humidity. Burch and associates have reported that in the humid tropical summer weather of New Orleans, measurements of cardiac output were 57 per cent greater than in an air-conditioned ward.[8,9] Since oxygen consumption was higher in the hot, humid environment, it was not possible to determine whether the increased output was simply a response to increased metabolic demand. However, the arterial–mixed venous oxygen difference either remained unchanged or fell, suggesting that the rise in cardiac output exceeded the oxygen requirement and reflected the body's attempt to increase the effectiveness of heat dissipation. Systemic arteriolar resistance falls in a hot and humid environment,[8] presumably reflecting dilatation of the cutaneous bed, and the resultant reduction in ventricular afterload and augmentation of venous return may be an important mechanism in mediating cardiac output.

CARDIAC RESPONSE TO INCREASES IN OUTPUT LOAD

Just as the normal cardiovascular system can increase its activity to meet the augmented peripheral demands imposed by muscular exertion, the normal heart can tolerate the higher demands imposed by hypermetabolic states (e.g., fever, pregnancy, and hyperthyroidism) and hyperkinetic, nonhypermetabolic conditions (e.g., anemia, arteriovenous fistula, and beriberi) in which reduction of afterload and augmentation of venous return and preload lead to increased flow load. Relying on dilatation and hypertrophy as its principal compensatory mechanisms, the heart can maintain normal tissue oxygenation for many years. On the other hand, when imposed on a heart whose function is intrinsically impaired, these increased demands cannot be met, and the physiological and clinical manifestations of heart failure appear.

Obviously there are exceptions to these basic principles. Extreme anemia (hematocrit < 15 per cent); the combination of severe anemia (hematocrit $= 15$ to 20 per cent) and arteriovenous fistula, as occurs in patients with renal failure with placement of an external shunt for hemodialysis (p. 1756); and the rapid development of severe hyperthyroidism (e.g., thyroid storm) or a large arteriovenous fistula (e.g., aortocaval) may overwhelm even a normal heart and result in heart failure.

Adaptation of the heart to an abnormal burden depends not only on the baseline state of myocardial function when the additional burden is imposed and on the magnitude of the burden, but also on the *rate* at which the new burden is added. Thus, severe anemia, thyrotoxicosis, and an arteriovenous fistula are far more likely to lead to cardiac decompensation when they develop suddenly rather than slowly. For this reason, conditions such as Paget's disease or Albright's syndrome, in which volume overload develops slowly, rarely, if ever, cause heart failure.

HIGH-OUTPUT HEART FAILURE. Cardiac output that was markedly elevated before the development of heart failure tends to remain high afterward, a condition termed *high-output heart failure.* The mechanisms responsible for the development of heart failure in these patients are complex and depend on the underlying disease process. In most of these conditions the heart is called upon to pump an abnormally large volume, and the effect on the myocardium is similar to that which occurs with regurgitant valvular lesions (Chap. 32). In addition, as discussed below, thyrotoxicosis and beriberi may impair myocardial metabolism directly, and severe anemia may interfere with myocardial function by producing myocardial hypoxia.

Clinically, it is sometimes difficult to distinguish between low-output and high-output heart failure. The normal range of cardiac output in the basal state is wide (2.6 to 4.0 liters/min/sq meter), and in many patients with so-called low-output heart failure, the cardiac output *at rest* may actually be within normal limits. On the other hand, in patients with high-output failure, cardiac output may not be excessive but rather is close to the upper limit of normal, particularly when heart failure is severe. Regardless of the absolute level of output, however, cardiac failure may be said to be present when the characteristic clinical manifestations are accompanied by a depression of the curve relating ventricular end-diastolic volume to cardiac performance or by a depression in the end-systolic or active ventricular pressure-volume relation (Figure 14–11, p. 477).

In the usual forms of low-output heart failure, the characteristically inadequate delivery of oxygen to the metabolizing tissues is reflected in an abnormally widened arterial–mixed venous oxygen difference (Chap. 14). In mild cases, this abnormality may become evident only during the stress of increased activity. In patients with high-output heart failure, the arterial–mixed venous oxygen difference is usually normal or may even be abnormally low, as in arteriovenous fistula, because the mixed venous oxygen saturation is raised by the admixture of blood that has been shunted away from some of the metabolizing tissues. In such cases delivery of oxygen to these tissues is reduced, despite the low arterial–mixed venous oxygen difference. When heart failure occurs in patients with high cardiac output, the arterial–mixed venous oxygen difference still exceeds the level that existed after the level of cardiac output rose but *prior* to the development of heart failure, and therefore the cardiac output, although high in the normal range or elevated, is nonetheless lower than it was before heart failure developed.

CONDITIONS ASSOCIATED WITH SUSTAINED INCREASES IN CARDIAC OUTPUT

Anemia

Physiological Mechanisms. Anemia is most commonly responsible for a sustained increase in cardiac output, which occurs consistently when the hematocrit falls below 25 per cent.[10] When the anemia is associated with a condition that produces a marked rise in blood viscosity (which increases afterload), such as multiple myeloma or macroglobulinemia, cardiac output may fail to rise even in the absence of heart disease. Studies by Richardson and Guyton have supported a role for the lowered viscosity of blood in the high cardiac output of anemia.[7] In addition, Murray and Escobar found that when exchange transfusions were carried out in dogs with methemoglobinemia using blood in which viscosity was unaltered, cardiac output remained unchanged.[11] However, when a reduction of oxygen carrying capacity similar to that in methemoglobinemia was produced by an exchange transfusion with low-viscosity dextran, cardiac output rose. Fowler and Holmes produced acute anemia in dogs by exchange transfusion with low molecular weight (70,000 daltons) or high molecular weight (500,000 daltons) dextran.[12] The former produced a 93 per cent increase in cardiac output and the latter only a 43 per cent increase. Since the severity of the anemia was the same in both groups (hematocrit = 18 per cent), they concluded that the difference in cardiac output probably reflected the substantial differences in viscosity. Since an increase in cardiac output still occurred in the dogs with normal blood viscosity who received high molecular weight dextran, it is clear that lowered viscosity, although important, cannot be the sole cause of increased cardiac output. The reduced left ventricular afterload in anemia results from a reduction not only in blood viscosity but in systemic arteriolar tone as well. The mechanism responsible for the latter change is unclear, but local tissue hypoxia, lactic acidemia, and the accumulation of vasodilator metabolites such as adenosine and possibly of bradykinin may all play a role.

To investigate the adjustment of the peripheral circulation to severe anemia, Vatner et al. induced anemia in conscious dogs by progressive phlebotomy and volume replacement over a period of 2 to 4 weeks.[13] At a hematocrit of 22 per cent, heart rate was elevated and resistance to flow in the coronary and iliac beds was strikingly reduced, whereas resistance in the mesenteric and renal beds remained essentially constant. In the presence of more severe anemia (hematocrit = 14 per cent), resistance in the mesenteric and renal beds also declined. On exercise, both coronary and iliac blood flow rose further, but, in contrast to nonanemic dogs, in which mesenteric and renal flow remained constant during exercise, both the mesenteric and the renal blood flow fell markedly (Fig. 24–2). Thus in resting, conscious dogs, reduction in visceral flow is *not* a feature of the cardiovascular response to severe anemia, although some redistribution of blood flow does occur; however, the added stress of exercise during severe anemia results in substantial reductions in flow in at least the mesenteric and renal vascular beds.

There is evidence that the autonomic nervous system plays a key role in the circulatory adaptation to anemia. The responses to severe isovolemic anemia in intact dogs were compared with those in dogs subjected to chronic cardiac denervation. The elevation of cardiac output was significantly greater in the intact animals than in the denervated ones. In intact dogs, the increase in cardiac output stemmed predominantly from a rise in heart rate, whereas elevations in stroke volume played a less important role. In contrast, in the cardiac denervated dogs, the increase in cardiac output tended to be the result of an augmented stroke volume.[14] In this connection the finding of Liang and Huckabee that tissue hypoxia can lead to an autonomic reflex response resulting in reduced arteriolar resistance is of considerable interest.[15] Thus, it may be concluded that an intact autonomic nervous system is necessary for mediation of the normal circulatory response to acutely induced anemia.

Duke and Abelmann studied 24 patients with chronic

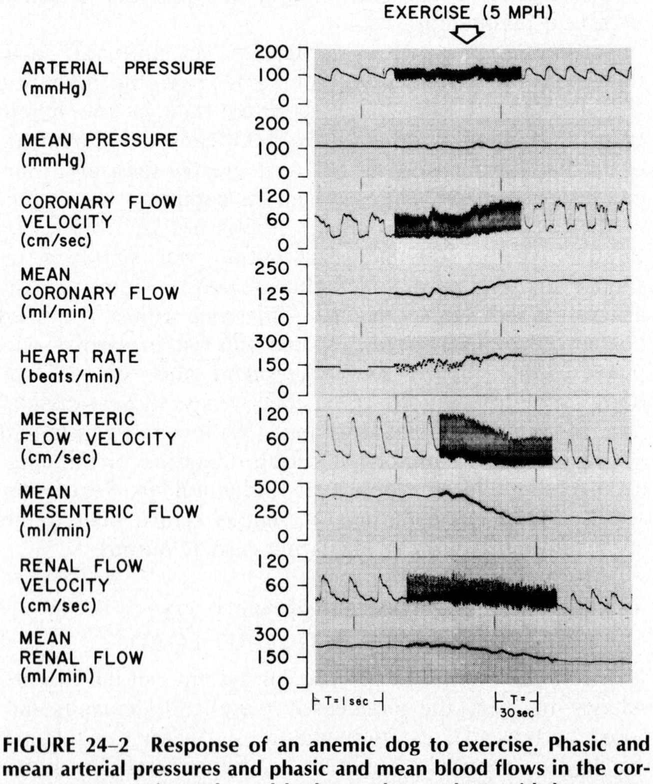

FIGURE 24–2 Response of an anemic dog to exercise. Phasic and mean arterial pressures and phasic and mean blood flows in the coronary, mesenteric, and renal beds are shown along with heart rate. In each case regional flow was initially recorded simultaneously with arterial pressure. (From Vatner, S. F., et al.: Regional circulatory adjustments to moderate and severe chronic anemia in conscious dogs at rest and during exercise. Circ. Res. *30*:731, 1972, by permission of the American Heart Association, Inc.)

anemia (iron deficiency or megaloblastic) and found that with corrective treatment, the cardiac index fell to normal (from 4.7 to 3.4 liters/min/sq meter), heart rate decreased (from 83 to 70 beats/min), and systemic vascular resistance rose (from 1017 to 1526 dynes-sec-cm^{-5}).[16] These changes could be reproduced acutely while the subjects were still anemic by infusion of methoxamine or assumption of the upright posture, suggesting that a combination of vasodilatation and a redistribution of blood volume might be responsible for mediating the hyperkinetic circulatory response to chronic anemia.

Clinical Findings. The consequences of anemia depend to an important extent on its rate of development. When it occurs rapidly, as in hemorrhage, blood volume is not maintained, and the picture of hypovolemic shock predominates (Chap. 18). If anemia develops more slowly, so that blood volume is maintained, cardiac output rises—predominantly as a result of tachycardia—with little change in stroke volume. In chronic severe anemia, heart rate is usually normal or only minimally elevated, and cardiac output is therefore elevated principally as a consequence of augmented stroke volume; the latter is associated with cardiac dilatation and hypertrophy. Not only is the cardiac output elevated at rest, but the augmentation of output during exercise tends to be excessive, often exceeding 1000 ml/100 ml increase in oxygen consumption per minute (normal = 550 to 800 ml).[17] This excessive response is sometimes seen in patients with only mild anemia (hematocrit = 30 per cent) who have normal resting cardiac outputs.[18] Since cardiac output is elevated while pulmonary artery pressure is normal, calculated pulmonary vascular resistance (like calculated systemic vascular resistance) is often reduced, and this variable declines further during exercise.[19] Left ventricular end-diastolic pressure remains within normal limits even in severe anemia, unless heart failure supervenes.[20]

The effect of *acute* anemia on cardiac function was studied by Case et al., who found that in normal dogs left ventricular function became depressed when the hematocrit was reduced below 24 per cent.[21] However, the otherwise normal human heart can tolerate moderately severe anemia (hematocrit = 20 to 25 per cent) for many years without showing any impairment of function; when heart failure occurs in patients with this degree of anemia, *it usually signifies the presence of underlying heart disease that had been compensated until the burden of an augmented cardiac output was added.* Similar considerations apply to the development of angina pectoris and other manifestations of myocardial ischemia. However, two important exceptions should be noted: (1) patients with severe anemia (hematocrit ≤ 15 per cent), in whom clinical evidence of impaired cardiac function can exist even in the absence of apparent underlying heart disease; and (2) patients with sickle cell anemia (p. 1678), who do *not* exhibit a reduction of viscosity and therefore lose this hemodynamic benefit imparted by other forms of anemia. Also, in these patients small thrombi characteristically develop in the pulmonary and coronary vessels, thereby impairing both systemic and cardiac oxygenation and leading to pulmonary hypertension, cor pulmonale, and perhaps even myocardial fibrosis secondary to ischemia. In addition, there may be arterial oxygen unsaturation secondary to pulmonary venous-arterial shunting. These patients exhibit hyperventilation, an increased alveolar-arterial oxygen tension gradient, abnormal ventilation of the dead space during exercise, and a disturbance of pulmonary perfusion with venous-arterial shunting. The most likely basis for these changes is the sickling phenomenon within the pulmonary vascular bed.[22] Arterial hypoxemia, produced by the pulmonary shunt, probably accounts for some of the exercise hyperpnea, partly by increasing chemoreceptor drive and by augmenting lactic acidemia.[23]

History. Chronic anemia produces surprisingly few symptoms, which may consist of easy fatigability, mild exertional dyspnea, and occasionally palpitations and cardiac awareness (Chap. 49). If heart failure or angina pectoris is present, it is likely that the high cardiac output is superimposed on some specific cardiac abnormality, such as valvular stenosis or regurgitation, or coronary artery obstruction. Patients with sickle cell anemia and hemoglobin sickle cell (SC) disease may complain of chest pain and unexplained dyspnea due to in situ pulmonary thrombosis and infarction.[22]

Physical Examination. The anemic patient generally has a pale "pasty" appearance; in black, brown, or tanned persons in whom examination of the skin color is of little help, a finding of paleness of the conjunctivae, mucous membranes, and palmar creases is helpful. Arterial pulses are bounding, "pistol shot" sounds can be heard over the femoral arteries (Duroziez's sign), and subungual capillary pulsations (Quincke's pulse) are present as in patients with aortic regurgitation. A medium-pitched, midsystolic murmur along the left sternal border, generally Grade 1/6 to 3/6 in intensity (rarely accompanied by a thrill), is common. Heart sounds are accentuated, and the pulmonic component of the second heart sound may be particularly prominent in patients with sickle cell anemia and pulmonary hypertension; in these patients a right ventricular lift can usually be palpated. Elevation of cardiac output and the physical findings characteristic of anemia are present in patients with sickle cell anemia and hemoglobin SC disease at *higher* hemoglobin levels than in patients with other forms of anemia.[20] A mid-diastolic flow murmur secondary to augmented blood flow across the mitral value orifice, holosystolic murmurs resulting from tricuspid and mitral regurgitation secondary to ventricular dilatation, and, rarely, diastolic murmurs resulting from aortic and pulmonic value incompetence secondary to dilatation of these vessels may be heard. Occasionally, a third heart sound is audible at the cardiac apex. Jugular venous distention is uncommon, and although peripheral edema and hepatomegaly are occasionally present, they may be due not only to heart failure but also to accompanying abnormalities such as hypoproteinemia and nutritional deficiency.

Laboratory findings in patients with severe anemia usually include mild or moderate cardiomegaly on chest roentgenogram. The electrocardiogram usually does not show any specific changes but may show T-wave inversions in lateral precordial leads. The echocardiogram generally shows a modest and symmetrical increase in size of all chambers, with large systolic excursions of the septal and posterior left ventricular walls and a normal ejection fraction. Hematological and blood chemical findings reflect the specific type of anemia present.

Treatment. Treatment of heart failure associated with severe anemia should be specific for the anemia (e.g., iron, folate, vitamin B_{12}, and so forth). When congestive heart failure is present, diuretics and cardiac glycosides are advisable, although some clinicians feel that the latter drugs are not helpful in this condition. It is our opinion that since most patients with heart failure and anemia have significant underlying heart disease, the administration of glycosides is desirable, because these drugs augment the depressed contractility on which the anemia is superimposed.

When both heart failure and anemia are severe, treatment must be carried out on an urgent basis and presents a difficult challenge. On the one hand, correction of the anemia is desirable to reduce the heart's workload; on the other hand, a too rapid expansion of the blood volume could intensify the manifestations of heart failure. The diagnostic steps for determining the etiology of the anemia should be taken immediately (e.g., blood withdrawn for serum iron, folate, and vitamin B_{12} measurements). *Packed red blood cells* should then be transfused slowly (250 to 500 ml/24 hr), preceded or accompanied by vigorous diuretic therapy (e.g., furosemide, 20 to 40 mg IV immediately followed by 40 mg orally every 8 hours), and the patient should be observed *closely* for the development or exacerbation of dyspnea and pulmonary rales, so that the transfusion can be discontinued immediately to avoid precipitating pulmonary edema. Vasodilator therapy is rarely helpful, since impedance to left ventricular emptying is already markedly reduced in most cases.

Hyperthyroidism (See also p. 1727)

Physiological Mechanisms. Substantial increases in cardiac output commonly occur in hyperthyroidism, and cardiac indexes of 5 to 7 liters/min/sq meter are common,[24–26] generally resulting from both increased stroke volume and increased heart rate. At least four mechanisms appear to contribute to this high-output state:

1. Augmented metabolic rate that causes vasodilation as seen with muscular exercise. It has been well documented that systemic vascular resistance is decreased in hyperthyroidism.[24–26]
2. Increased heat production consequent to the augmented metabolism characteristic of hyperthyroidism results in elevation of cardiac output owing to cutaneous dilatation. This latter mechanism is particularly important in patients with thyroid storm in whom hyperthermia—with temperatures occasionally as high as 106°F (41°C)—is associated with an intense cardiac drive to maintain an elevated cardiac output,[27,28] occasionally resulting in high-output failure and circulatory collapse.
3. Thyroid hormone has a direct, stimulating effect on myocardial contractility,[29–32] which augments stroke volume at any preload and afterload. This effect has been clearly documented in animal experiments[29,31,33] as well as in humans[30,32] and may involve a fundamental alteration in myocardial contractile proteins, such as increased activity of myosin ATPase.[33–36]
4. There is still an undefined relationship between the hyperthyroid state and the sympathoadrenal system, characterized by suppression of the manifestations of the hyperthyroid state by administration of antiadrenergic agents. The tachycardia, widened pulse pressure, and shortened circulation time all return toward normal with beta-receptor blockade,[24–26,30] indicating that adrenergic influences play a role in maintaining the high-output state in hyperthyroid patients. However, it should be noted that the tachycardia of thyrotoxicosis is due not only to the *direct* effects of thyroid hormone and adrenergic influences on the sinoatrial node but also to a reduction in the cholinergic restraint. This does not appear to result from decreased responsiveness of the end organ or impaired release of the cholinergic nerve transmitter but rather from a reduction in cholinergic discharge in the thyrotoxic state, which may result from an abnormality in central or afferent mechanisms.[37] Beta-adrenergic stimulation potentiates certain biochemical changes induced at the cell membrane level by triiodothyronine.[38]

Clinical Findings. Symptoms may include nervousness, personality disorder, heat intolerance, or weight loss with increased appetite and fatigue. Palpitations are common, and atrial fibrillation is occasionally the presenting manifestation. Symptoms of congestive heart failure are rare and, as discussed below, suggest underlying cardiac disease of a different nature.

The principal *physical findings* of hyperthyroidism include tremor; widened palpebral fissures with resultant "stare"; lid lag; exophthalmos; warm, moist, smooth skin; and hyperactive deep tendon reflexes. Cardiovascular examination often reveals tachycardia, a widened pulse pressure, and brisk carotid and peripheral arterial pulsations. The cardiac apex is hyperkinetic on palpation. The first heart sound is loud, and third and fourth sounds are occasionally present. A midsystolic murmur along the left sternal border, secondary to increased flow, is common; occasionally this murmur has an unusual scratchy component (the so-called Means-Lerman scratch) thought to be due to the rubbing together of normal pleural and pericardial surfaces as a consequence of hyperkinetic heart action. Rarely, systolic murmurs of mitral and tricuspid regurgitation, presumably secondary to papillary muscle dysfunction, may occur in thyrotoxicosis and disappear with the establishment of the euthyroid state.

Laboratory findings are those of hyperthyroidism and include elevated levels of thyroxine or triiodothyronine, mild normochromic normocytic anemia, occasional relative lymphocytosis, low serum cholesterol levels, and occasional elevation of serum alkaline phosphatase.

The *chest roentgenogram* is usually normal, although the echocardiogram may show increased left ventricular wall thickness and chamber dimensions and a normal or increased ejection fraction and velocity of shortening.[32] Systolic time intervals may show a low value for the ratio of the preejection period to left ventricular ejection time (PEP/LVET ratio), consistent with increased myocardial contractility (Chap. 3).

The *electrocardiogram* shows widespread but nonspecific ST-segment elevation and upward coving, with terminal T-wave inversion in about one-fourth of patients and shortening of the Q-T interval.[39] ST-segment depression is uncommon in the absence of coronary artery disease. Varying degrees of atrioventricular block,[40] presumably owing to inflammatory changes in the atrioventricular node induced by hyperthyroidism, are occasional manifestations. Atrial fibrillation may occur and is often associated with an unusually rapid ventricular response (i.e., 170 to 220 beats/min) as a consequence of the markedly shortened refractory period of the atrioventricular conduction system. There is relative resistance to slowing of the ventricular rate with digitalis.[41] Spontaneous reversion to sinus rhythm is common.

Treatment. Management of the cardiovascular manifestations of hyperthyroidism depends primarily on treatment of the endocrine abnormality, as outlined in Chapter 51. However, the elevated heart rate, systolic pressure, pulse pressure, and cardiac output, palpitations, and other manifestations of cardiac hyperactivity, as well as tremor, lid lag, hyperreflexia, and widened palpebral fissures can be reduced by administering antiadrenergic agents.[42] The rapid ventricular rate of atrial fibrillation responds particularly well to intravenous propranolol, which may be administered in 1-mg increments every 5 minutes until the ventricular rate is controlled; sometimes sinus rhythm is restored. *Thyroid storm* with hyperpyrexia, marked tachycardia, and pulmonary edema also responds to propranolol, 1 to 2 mg administered intravenously as above, together with sodium iodide (to prevent further release of stored thyroid hormones), and diuretics, adrenal glucocorticoids, cooling blankets, aspirin, and intravenous fluids.[43] Oral propranolol in divided doses ranging from 160 to 400 mg/day (or equivalent doses of another beta blocker [p. 1349]) is also usually effective in controlling many of the cardiovascular manifestations of hyperthyroidism described above. It must be appreciated, however, that despite the salutary effects of beta-blocking agents, they are only adjunctive measures and do not affect the underlying disease process. Indeed, they do not reduce the elevated metabolic rate.

THYROTOXIC HEART DISEASE. As in many other high-output states, the hyperkinetic state of hyperthyroidism does not usually lead to heart failure or angina pectoris in the absence of underlying cardiac or coronary artery disease; the normal heart appears capable of tolerating the burden imposed by hyperthyroidism simply by means of dilatation and hypertrophy. A rare exception is the development of heart failure in patients with neonatal thyrotoxicosis without underlying heart disease.[44] However, when the elevated flow load of hyperthyroidism is superimposed on a reduced cardiovascular reserve (i.e., asymptomatic or only mildly symptomatic heart disease), congestive heart failure is likely to ensue. Similarly, in a patient with obstructive coronary artery disease who is asymptomatic or who has only mild evidence of ischemia in the euthyroid state, the demand for increased coronary blood flow with hyperthyroidism frequently leads to an exacerbation of angina.

Beta-adrenergic blockade may be both helpful and harmful in patients with thyrotoxic heart disease and *heart failure.* Although it may be beneficial by lowering the ventricular rate, particularly by prolonging the refractory period of the atrioventricular conduction system in patients with atrial fibrillation, it may also diminish myocardial contractility by blocking the adrenergic support of the heart. Therefore it must be administered cautiously to the patient with thyrotoxic heart disease and heart failure and only after treatment with glycosides, with the patient at rest and under careful observation. The initial dose should be small (e.g., propranolol, 0.5 mg IV or 10 mg orally), and the patient should be observed after the administration to assure that heart failure is not intensified. Propranolol is particularly useful in the management of angina pectoris associated with hyperthyroidism, and in this condition larger doses are usually well tolerated.

The association of thyrotoxicosis and anginal pain has been demonstrated in the presence of normal coronary vessels on arteriography.[45] These patients showed ischemia in that pacing resulted in lactate production. The possibility of thyrotoxicosis should therefore be considered in the differential diagnosis of patients having anginal pain and normal coronary arteriograms (Chap. 39).

It is particularly important to recognize so-called *apathetic hyperthyroidism,* a condition in which the usual clinical manifestations of hyperthyroidism (i.e., palpitations, tachycardia, and moist skin) are not present. In these patients the first clinical signs of thyrotoxicosis may be unexplained heart failure, an exacerbation of angina pectoris, or unexplained atrial fibrillation, usually but not always with a rapid ventricular rate. Hence it is important to consider the diagnosis of hyperthyroidism in all patients, particularly those over the age of 55 years, who present in this fashion.

Systemic Arteriovenous Fistulas

Systemic arteriovenous fistulas may be congenital or acquired; the latter are either post-traumatic or iatrogenic. Increased cardiac output associated with such fistulas depends on the size of the communication and the magnitude of the resultant reduction in systemic vascular resistance. An increased right atrial pressure does not seem to be necessary to maintain the high-output state, although plasma volume is generally increased.

An experimental model of chronic high-output heart failure due to an arteriovenous fistula has been developed in the rat.[46] At 2 months after creation of an aortocaval fistula, cardiac output and left ventricular end-diastolic pressure were increased, and there was significant biventricular hypertrophy. Blood flow to the splanchnic bed was decreased, but flow to the heart, brain, and kidneys was preserved. Many other physiological characteristics in this model resemble findings in the clinical situation.

The *physical findings* depend in part on the underlying disease and the location of the shunt. In general, a widened pulse pressure, brisk carotid and peripheral arterial pulsations, and mild tachycardia are present. *Branham's sign* (also called Nicaladoni-Branham's sign), which consists of slowing of the heart following manual compression of the fistula,[47,48] is present in the majority of cases; this maneuver also raises arterial and lowers venous pressure. The tachycardia associated with arteriovenous fistula has been studied in an experimental preparation,[49] and the results suggest the operation of a cardioaccelerator reflex with both afferent and efferent pathways in the vagus nerves.

The skin overlying the fistula is warmer than normal, and a "machinery" murmur and thrill are usually present over the lesion. Third and fourth heart sounds are commonly heard, as well as a precordial midsystolic murmur. The electrocardiographic changes of left ventricular hypertrophy are often seen. Rarely, the fistula may become infected, leading to bacterial endarteritis.

CONGENITAL ARTERIOVENOUS FISTULAS. Congenital arteriovenous fistulas result from arrest of the normal embryonic development of the vascular system and are structurally similar to embryonic capillary networks. They range from barely noticeable strawberry birthmarks to enormous clusters of engorged vascular channels that may deform an entire extremity. Most frequently, the vessels of the lower extremities are involved (i.e., femoral, iliac, and popliteal), and the resultant clinical manifestations vary enormously.[50] When fistulas are large, patients generally complain of disfigurement as well as of swelling and pain in the limb (Table 24–1). Left heart failure occurs, particularly in patients with larger lesions that involve the pelvis as well as the extremities.[51,52] Physical examination shows hemangiomatous changes associated with venous distention, deformity, and increased limb length. The fistulous connection may involve any vascular bed, including the internal mammary artery–pulmonary artery connection. Angiography is useful in confirming the diagnosis and in determining the physical extent of the anomaly.

Surgical excision is the ideal treatment, but in many instances the lesions are not sufficiently localized to permit this. The results of ligation and excision have been unsatisfactory in the majority of cases, since the congenital arteriovenous communications are usually not confined to a single anatomical segment or to a circumscribed anatomical region. Complete cure of these lesions is possible in only a few instances. Embolization of Gelfoam pellets delivered through a catheter has been reported to obliterate multiple systemic arteriovenous fistulas and thereby diminish high-output heart failure.[53]

Hereditary hemorrhagic telangiectasia (Osler-Weber-Rendu disease) may be associated with arteriovenous fistulas, particularly in the lungs and liver; the latter condition can produce a hyperkinetic circulation as well as hepatomegaly with abdominal bruits. Because of the presence of oxygenated blood in the inferior vena cava and right atrium, this condition may be misdiagnosed as atrial septal defect.[54]

The congenital arteriovenous communication resulting from *hemangioendothelioma of the liver* is commonly associated with marked increases in cardiac output, sometimes as high as 10.5 liters/min/sq meter, and congestive heart failure.[55,56] These lesions, which are extremely difficult to treat surgically, may be quite large, increase in size with time, and lead to heart failure even in infancy. They are often associated with sizable cutaneous hemangiomas, which should alert the clinician to the possibility of their presence. Hepatic hemangioendotheliomas have been reported to respond to prednisone in the newborn[55] or to hepatic artery ligation.[56]

TABLE 24–1 CONGENITAL ARTERIOVENOUS ANOMALIES

Common Complaints	
Disfigurement	20%
Swelling	19%
Pain	15%
Other (pulsation, ulceration, increased length of limb)	20%
Physical Signs	
Hemangioma, varices, bruit, or swelling, alone or in combination	100%
Color changes	
Erythema	40%
Cyanosis	12%

Adapted from Szilagyi, D. E., et al.: Congenital arteriovenous anomalies of the limbs. Arch. Surg. *111*:423, 1976. Copyright 1976, American Medical Association.

ACQUIRED ARTERIOVENOUS FISTULAS. Naturally acquired arteriovenous fistulas occur most frequently following injuries such as gunshot wounds and may involve any part of the body, most frequently the thigh.[57] Blood flow in the affected limb distal to the fistula diminishes after the creation of the fistula but then returns to normal and often increases with the passage of time. The affected limb is usually larger than its opposite member, and the overlying skin is warmer; cellulitis, venostasis, edema, and dermatitis with pigmentation frequently occur, in part as a consequence of chronically elevated venous pressure. Surgical repair or excision is generally advisable in fistulas that develop following gunshot wounds or trauma. An arteriovenous fistula may be produced by inadvertent damage to blood vessels during an operation, most frequently in nephrectomy, laminectomy, or cholecystectomy.

A rare form of acquired arteriovenous fistula results from spontaneous rupture of an aortic aneurysm into the inferior vena cava. This usually produces an enormous arteriovenous shunt and rapidly progressive left ventricular failure. On physical examination a pulsating mass can be readily palpated superficially in the abdomen, and a continuous bruit is audible.

Massive fistulas may be associated with Wilms' tumor of the kidney, and these have, on rare occasions, caused high-output cardiac failure in children.[58]

Several reports have appeared describing high-output congestive heart failure resulting from the arteriovenous shunts surgically constructed for vascular access in patients on chronic hemodialysis.[59–62] Cardiac outputs as high as 10 liters/min/sq meter, which decrease substantially during temporary occlusion of the shunt, have been found in such patients. These values undoubtedly also reflect the chronic anemia present in many of these patients, but it is clear that it is the added hemodynamic burden imposed by the shunt that precipitates heart failure in patients who had previously tolerated chronic anemia without apparent impairment of cardiac function. It is usually possible to revise or band the fistula to reduce it to the appropriate size for dialysis without compromising cardiac function (Fig. 24–3).[61]

As is the case with other hyperkinetic lesions, the rapidity of the onset of the load and its size, as well as the presence and severity of the underlying heart disease, determines whether or not heart failure will develop.

Beriberi Heart Disease

Pathogenesis and Clinical Considerations. This condition is due to severe thiamine deficiency persisting for at least 3 months. Clinical beriberi is found most frequently in the Far East, although even in that part of the world it is far less prevalent now than in the past. It occurs predominantly in those individuals whose staple diet consists of polished rice, which is deficient in thiamine but high in carbohydrates. The presence of thiamine in the enriched flour used in white bread has virtually eradicated this disease in the United States and Western Europe, where beriberi is found most commonly in diet faddists and

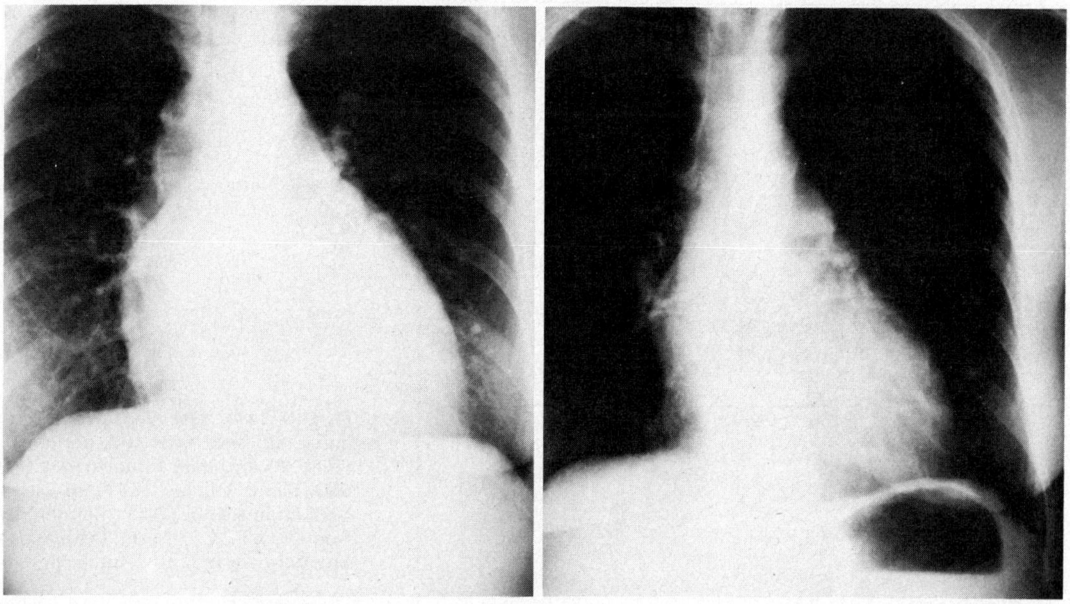

FIGURE 24–3 *Left,* Chest roentgenogram demonstrating cardiomegaly and pulmonary vascular congestion in patient with high-output cardiac failure attributable to end-to-side cephalic vein–radial artery fistula in wrist. *Right,* One month after banding of vein, cardiomegaly has decreased and pulmonary vascular congestion has improved. (From Anderson, C. B., et al.: Cardiac failure and upper extremity arteriovenous dialysis fistulas. Arch. Intern. Med. *136*:292, 1976. Copyright 1976, American Medical Association.)

alcoholics; like polished rice, alcohol is low in vitamin B_1 but has a high carbohydrate content. In the West, alcoholics become thiamine-deficient not only because of a low intake of the vitamin but also because they eat "junk" foods or drink large quantities of beer, with their high carbohydrate content and therefore their great demand for thiamine. A reappearance of beriberi heart disease has been reported in Japan, mainly in teenagers, and has been attributed to the recent tendency for teenagers to ingest excessive amounts of sweet carbonated drinks, instant noodles, and polished rice.[62a] Most cases presented in the summer months and were believed to be precipitated by strenuous physical exercise with a resultant sudden increase in thiamine requirements. All of the patients presented with edema ("wet beriberi") with general malaise and fatigue. Neurological manifestations were uncommon. Hemodynamic findings in those studied before and after treatment with thiamine are presented in Figure 24–4. Since their original description by Wenckebach,[63,64] the hemodynamic abnormalities associated with beriberi heart disease have gained considerable attention.[65–68] The elevation of cardiac output is presumably secondary to the reduced systemic vascular resistance, and it is suspected that the latter is caused by lesions of the sympathetic nuclei.

The role of thiamine diphosphate as a coenzyme is well established. In mammals, thiamine diphosphate is required for a variety of reactions that have in common the cleavage of carbon-carbon bonds—the oxidative decarboxylation of alpha-keto acids (pyruvate and alpha-ketoglutarate) and keto analogs of leucine, isoleucine, and valine and the transketolase reaction in the pentose phosphate pathway. Thiamine triphosphate is important in the binding of thiamine diphosphate to its various apoenzymes. The entire spectrum of changes in thiamine deficiency can be explained by the inhibition of these key enzymatic reactions and, in some instances, by the accumulation of proximal metabolites.

Physical findings in most cases presenting in Western countries are those of the high-output state and usually of severe generalized malnutrition and vitamin deficiency. Evidence of peripheral neuropathy with sensory and motor deficits is common (so-called dry beriberi), as is the presence of nutritional cirrhosis characterized by paresthesias of the extremities, decreased or absent knee and ankle jerks, painful glossitis, the anemia of combined iron and folate deficiency, and hyperkeratinized skin lesions. However, the recent cases in Japanese teenagers[62a] were not characterized by other signs of vitamin or nutritional deficiency, and it is possible that similar cases (wet beriberi above) may present in Western teenagers indulging in similar dietary fads.

Beriberi heart disease[69–71] is characterized by evidence of biventricular failure, sinus rhythm, and marked edema (so-called wet beriberi). There is arteriolar vasodilatation, and the cutaneous vessels may be dilated, or in later cases with congestive heart failure, they may be constricted. Therefore, the absence of warm hands does not discount the diagnosis of beriberi. A third heart sound and an apical systolic murmur are heard almost invariably, and there is a wide pulse pressure characteristic of the hyperkinetic state.

The electrocardiogram characteristically exhibits low voltage of the QRS, prolongation of the Q-T interval, and low voltage or inversion of T waves. The chest roentgenogram usually shows biventricular enlargement, pulmonary congestion, and pleural effusions. In alcoholics with beriberi heart disease, the left ventricular ejection fraction and peak left ventricular dP/dt are usually reduced.[69] The role played by alcoholic cardiomyopathy (p. 1406) in this hemodynamic picture is not clear. The cardiac output falls, and the peripheral resistance rises acutely when thiamine is administered in the catheterization laboratory.[69]

Laboratory diagnosis can be made by demonstration of increased serum pyruvate and lactate levels in the presence

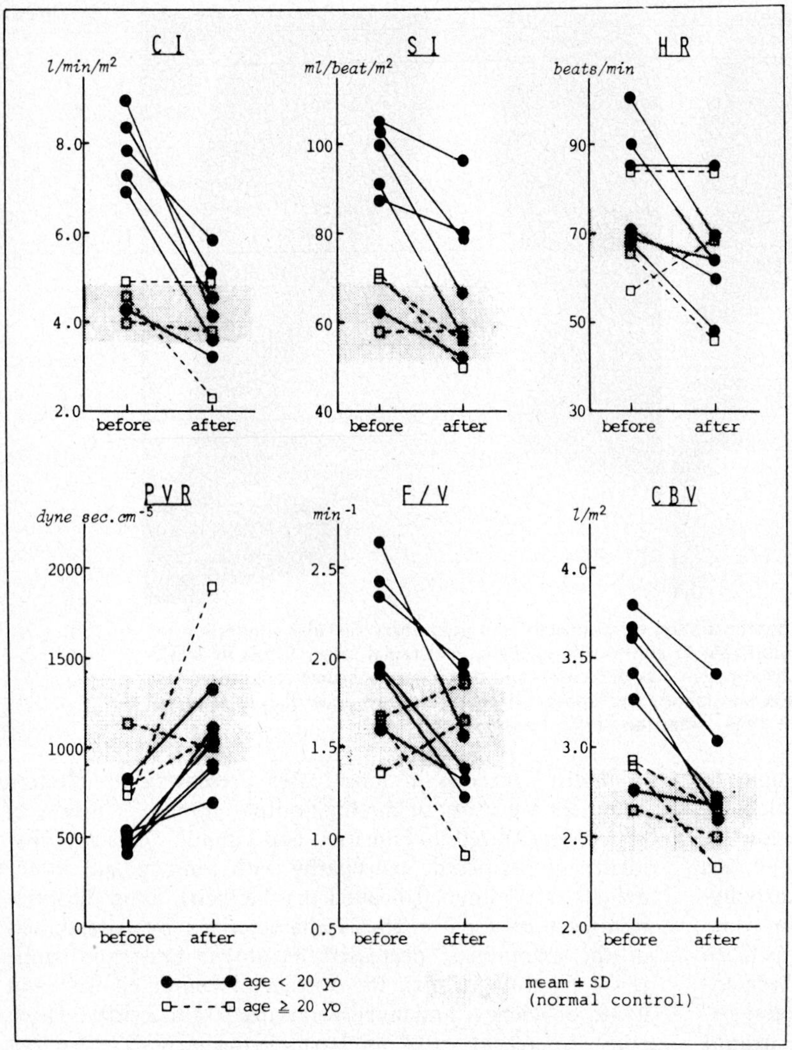

FIGURE 24–4 Changes in cardiac index (CI), stroke index (SI), heart rate (HR), peripheral vascular resistance (PVR), blood turnover rate (F/V), and circulatory blood volume (CBV) in patients treated for beriberi in Kyoto, Japan. (Reprinted with permission from Kawai, C., et al.: Reappearance of beriberi heart disease in Japan. Am. J. Med. *69*:383, 1980.)

of a low transketolase level.[72] Thiamine concentration may be determined in biological fluids,[73–75] and the blood thiamine level furnishes an index of thiamine availability, whereas transketolase activity indicates the ability to convert thiamine into metabolically active forms. The most reliable test of thiamine deficiency is the augmentation of whole blood or erythrocyte transketolase (ETK) activity with treatment (the absolute levels being of little aid). Thiamine functions as a coenzyme for transketolase in the pentose phosphate pathway of glucose metabolism. An increase of circulating ETK activity with treatment or when thiamine diphosphate is added to the patient's blood in vitro (the so-called TPP [thiamine pyrophospate] effect) is helpful in the diagnosis. In the in vitro test, the normal TPP effect is a 0 to 14 per cent increase of ETK activity; a 15 to 24 per cent increase is a borderline response, and a 25 per cent or more increase is evidence of clinical thiamine deficiency.[76] Leukocyte transketolase activity may prove to be a more sensitive index of the thiamine deficiency than the erythrocyte activity.

At *postmortem examination* the heart usually shows simple dilation without other changes. On microscopic examination, there is sometimes edema and hydropic degeneration of the muscle fibers. Nonspecific but abnormal histological and electron microscopic changes have been found in cardiac biopsy specimens.

Heart failure may develop explosively in beriberi, and some patients succumb to the illness within 48 hours of the onset of symptoms. So-called "Shoshin" beriberi, seen most frequently in the Orient, is a fulminating form of the disease[77] characterized by hypotension, tachycardia, and lactic acidosis; if left untreated, the patients die in pulmonary edema. Thus, since the course of the disease may advance rapidly, treatment must be begun immediately once the diagnosis has been established. In the Western world this fulminant form of the disease is quite uncommon.

Treatment. Akbarian and coworkers have reported careful hemodynamic studies which suggest that vasomotor depression or paralysis may be responsible for the depressed vascular resistance.[68] They studied four patients in whom ethanol excess was responsible for the thiamine deficiency. All had increased heart rate and cardiac output (averaging 6 liters/min/sq meter) and reduced arterial–mixed venous oxygen difference and systemic vascular resistance. Right and left ventricular filling pressure and blood volume were also elevated. In one patient intravenous thiamine led to a decrease in cardiac output (from 8.0 to 3.9 liters/min) and an elevation of systemic vascular resistance (from 969 to 1863 dynes-sec-cm^{-5}). Since ouabain then led to substantial improvement, the investigators concluded that the thiamine had converted high-output failure to low-output failure. In other studies, they found that the low systemic vascular resistance did not respond to methoxamine infusion until after correction of the thiamine deficiency.

Patients with beriberi heart disease fail to respond adequately to digitalis and diuretics alone. However, improvement after the administration of thiamine (up to 100 mg IV followed by 25 mg per day orally for 1 to 2 weeks) may be dramatic. Marked diuresis, decrease in heart rate and size, and clearing of pulmonary congestion may occur within 12 to 48 hours.[68,78] However, the acute reversal of the vasodilatation induced by correction of the deficiency may cause the unprepared left ventricle to go into low-output failure. Therefore, patients should receive a glycoside and diuretic therapy along with thiamine.

Latent beriberi deficiency may occur in conditions such as alcoholic cardiomyopathy and in other forms of refractory congestive heart failure. The possibility of thiamine deficiency should be considered in many patients with heart failure of obscure origin. It should be pointed out that the development of thiamine deficiency has been reported in patients receiving prolonged treatment with furosemide.[78a] Thus, patients with heart failure from other etiologies could develop superimposed beriberi heart disease unless adequate thiamine intake is maintained.

Paget's Disease

Pathogenesis. Paget's disease of bone is an asymmetrical process characterized by extremely rapid bone formation and resorption of the involved areas. Histologically, this excessive formation and resorption of bone is mediated by osteoblasts and is followed by replacement of normal marrow by vascular fibrous connective tissue, increases in the vascularity of the diseased bones, and an increase in the size of the vessels originating from the periosteal plexus with an augmentation of periosteal vascularity. Increased blood flow occurs through extremities involved by Paget's disease and may be as high as nine times the normal level.[79,80] Because of the increased vascularity of bone affected by Paget's disease, it has been assumed that this high flow occurred through the involved bone.[79,81,82] However, studies with radioactive technetium-labeled microspheres injected into the femoral arteries of patients with Paget's disease have shown no evidence of arteriovenous shunting.[83] Instead, it appears that the additional blood flow through an affected, resting limb passes through the *cutaneous tissue* overlying the involved bone, possibly secondary to local heat production resulting from the increased metabolic activity of affected bone.[80]

Clinical Findings. These are a function of the extent of the disease and the specific bones involved. Involvement of at least one-third of the skeleton by Paget's disease in an active stage, accompanied by a high alkaline phosphatase level, is necessary before a clinically significant augmentation of cardiac output is observed. The physical findings are those of Paget's disease of bone with swelling or deformity of one or more long bones, enlargement of the skull, facial pain, headache, backache or pain, and an elevated blood alkaline phosphatase level. The cardiovascular findings are not distinguishable from those in other conditions with high-output states. In addition, metastatic calcifications are characteristic. If they involve the heart, they may lead to sclerosis and calcification of the valve rings, with extension into the interventricular septum, and may produce abnormalities of atrioventricular or interventricular conduction.

Treatment. Treatment is generally unsatisfactory, although the long-term use of salmon calcitonin may be beneficial; however, the reported effects of such treatment on the high-output state are mixed.[82,84] Recently oral etidronate disodium has been introduced. This diphosphonate is similar in structure to pyrophosphate, which modifies the crystal growth of calcium hydroxyapatite by adsorption onto the crystal surface, where it inhibits either crystal resorption or crystal growth. There is suppression of rapid turnover of bone, as reflected in bone scans, as well as reduction of urinary hydroxyproline and serum alkaline phosphatase. Etidronate disodium provides symptomatic relief, including reduced bone pain, in many patients. In two-thirds of patients the elevated cardiac output returns to normal within 3 months.[85]

Cytotoxic drugs, including actinomycin D and mithramycin, have also been found to be useful in lowering the elevated cardiac output in Paget's disease, but these potent agents have serious toxic side effects.

Fibrous Dysplasia (Albright's Syndrome)

This condition, in which there is proliferation of fibrous tissue in bone, may also be associated with an elevated cardiac output.[86-89] Fibrous dysplasia has the appearance typical of fibromas, in which are embedded areas of coarse fiber bone with wide osteoid seams, prominent cement lines, and many thin-walled sinusoids; it has been postulated that these sinusoids act as multiple minute arteriovenous fistulas, leading to deformity and fractures. There is abnormal cutaneous pigmentation (i.e., dark brown macules) on one side of the midline and sexual precocity in females. Multiple bones are involved, and the cardiac output may be elevated, as in patients with Paget's disease of bone.

Pregnancy

The effects of pregnancy on the normal circulation and the relationship between pregnancy and cardiovascular disease are discussed in detail in Chapter 53. Here it should be pointed out that in pregnancy cardiac output rises slowly to a peak averaging 40 per cent above control and is accompanied by an increase in blood volume and a reduction in systemic vascular resistance. The elevation of cardiac output is related only in part to the augmented total metabolism characteristic of pregnancy, because the output reaches a peak between the twentieth and twenty-fourth weeks of gestation, yet the combined oxygen needs of mother and fetus continue to climb to reach a peak at term; hormonal effects appear to be responsible in part. This physiological increase in cardiac output does not lead to congestive failure, except when the pregnancy is superimposed on underlying cardiac disease or is added to another major cardiovascular burden.

Hyperkinetic Heart Syndrome

Gorlin and coworkers described a group of patients with increased cardiac output of no discernible cause; cardiac indices averaged 6.4 liters/min/sq meter, with slightly elevated systolic and pulse pressures, normal mean arterial pressure, and low systemic vascular resistance.[90,91] Most were young men with a hyperkinetic precordium, often with third and fourth heart sounds, systolic ejection clicks, midsystolic murmurs along the left sternal border, electrocardiograms suggestive of left ventricular hypertrophy, and radiological evidence of plethoric lung fields. The high value for oxygen consumption (177 ml/min/sq meter) in Gorlin's early report suggested that anxiety contributed to the elevated cardiac output. Indeed, it had been pointed out earlier by Hickam et al. that anxiety can lead to significant increases in oxygen consumption and cardiac output.[92] However, it is now clear that in some patients with this syndrome cardiac output is elevated even after sedation and in the presence of normal oxygen consumption (Fig. 24–5).

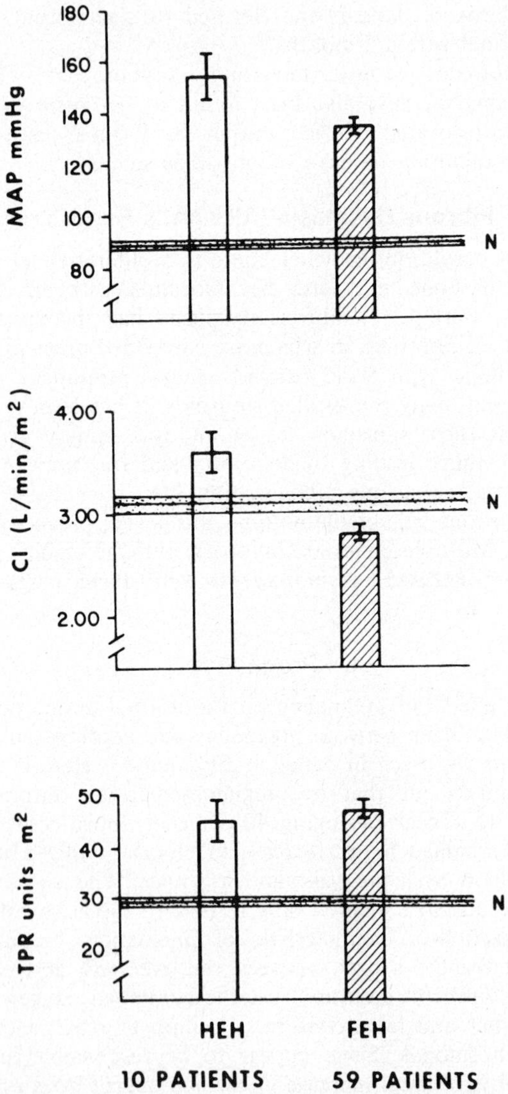

FIGURE 24–5 Hemodynamic characteristics of hyperkinetic essential hypertension. Both mean arterial pressure (MAP) and cardiac index (CI) were significantly higher in the 10 hypertensive patients with hyperkinetic circulation than in the 59 patients with fixed essential hypertension. HEH and FEH = hyperkinetic and fixed essential hypertension, respectively; N = normal values for laboratory; TPR = total peripheral resistance. Bars indicate standard error. (From Ibrahim, M. M., et al.: Hyperkinetic heart in severe hypertension: A separate clinical hemodynamic entity. Am. J. Cardiol. *35*:667, 1975.)

TABLE 24–2 IDIOPATHIC HYPERKINETIC HEART SYNDROME: PRESENTING MANIFESTATIONS

Clinical Findings
Young males
Generally asymptomatic
Systolic cardiac murmurs
Overactivity of heart and pulses
Labile hypertension in 50% of patients
LVH by ECG in most patients
Hemodynamic Findings
Increased cardiac index
Decreased A – V O_2 difference
Normal O_2 consumption
Normal heart rate
Increased LV ejection rate
Increased pulse pressure
Decreased SVR

LVH = left ventricular hypertrophy; SVR = systemic vascular resistance. (Modified from Gillum, R. F., Teichholz, L. E., Herman, M. V., et al.: The idiopathic hyperkinetic heart syndrome: Clinical course and long-term prognosis. Am. Heart J. *102*:728, 1981.)

These patients generally receive medical attention because of palpitations, tachycardia, cardiac awareness, atypical chest pain, an unconvincing history of fatigue, dyspnea, or tachypnea. Various diagnoses have been attached to these patients, including neurasthenia, anxiety neurosis, Da Costa syndrome, effort syndrome, and soldier's heart.[93] A similar condition has been described by Frohlich and coworkers as "hyperdynamic beta-adrenergic circulatory state," since treatment with propranolol resulted in improvement.[94]

The elevated systolic arterial pressure and cardiac output and lowered systemic vascular resistance characteristic of this condition are restored to normal by beta-adrenergic blockade. Therapy with a beta-adrenergic blocking agent has been effective in some patients; indeed, cardiac output has been maintained at normal levels for 2 years with doses of 80 to 160 mg/day and promptly returned to the previously elevated levels when the drug was discontinued (Fig. 24–6 and Table 24–2).[95]

There has been some speculation that the hyperkinetic heart syndrome is related to hypertrophic obstructive cardiomyopathy, in that a hyperkinetic precordium, systolic murmur, and elevated cardiac output are present in both conditions (Chap. 41). However, the resemblance between these two conditions is superficial, and no definitive link between them has been proved. Although it has been proposed that hypertrophic obstructive cardiomyopathy may be a complication of the hyperkinetic syndrome, the authors have not encountered any patient in whom this transition occurred, nor has it been satisfactorily documented by others.

Recently, two studies have been reported describing the long-term follow-up of patients who had been diagnosed as having the hyperkinetic heart syndrome.[96,97] In one study,[96] 14 patients were observed for 5 years. Half the group received propranolol, and the remaining 7 patients received placebo. There was symptomatic improvement in the treated group, and symptoms recurred when propranolol was stopped. However, neither propranolol-treated nor placebo-treated patients developed echocardiographic evidence of left ventricular hypertrophy. In the second study,[97] 19 patients initially diagnosed as having hyperkinetic heart syndrome were followed for periods of 11 to 25 years. One

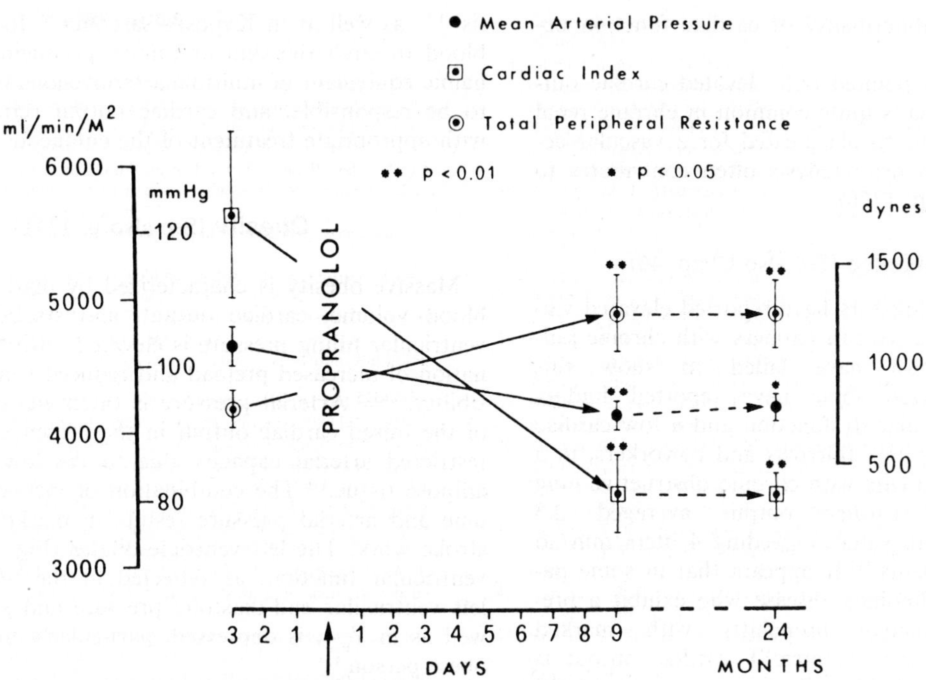

FIGURE 24–6 Average changes in mean arterial pressure, cardiac index, and total peripheral resistance induced by short-term (9 days) and long-term (24 months) treatment with propranolol in hyperkinetic patients. Statistical comparison is made between values in the control and in the treated state. (From Guazzi, M., et al.: Long-term treatment of the hyperkinetic heart syndrome with propranolol. Am. J. Med. Sci. *270*:465, 1975.)

patient died of complicating severe mitral stenosis. Of the remaining patients, in general, the initial physical findings had disappeared or decreased. Two patients developed sustained hypertension. It was concluded that the long-term prognosis of the condition is excellent, and beta blockade was recommended only for those with significant symptoms or hypertension.

An abnormally elevated cardiac output at rest may be responsible for the elevation of arterial pressure in some patients with essential hypertension (Chap. 26). Although this is generally associated with early or labile hypertension,[98] an elevated cardiac output has been observed in some patients with fixed, severe hypertension as well.[99] Presumably, the augmented sympathetic drive to the heart and vascular bed is responsible for both elevated cardiac output and elevated vascular resistance in this subset of patients.

Hepatic Disease

Increased cardiac output has been reported to occur in patients with cirrhosis of the liver,[100–103] and it has been speculated that it may represent the effect of arteriovenous shunting (e.g., vascular spiders) within the liver and other organs. Microarteriovenous fistulas in the lung are usually responsible for arterial hypoxemia and the shunting in the lung[101,102,104–106]; less commonly, collateral vessels between the portal and pulmonary veins are responsible for the right-to-left shunting and cyanosis. In some cases pulmonary arteriovenous shunting may result in 10 to 20 per cent of mixed venous blood traversing the lungs without gas exchange.[101]

Hepatocellular failure, regardless of etiology, increases the cardiac output and induces systemic vasodilatation. The increase in cardiac output may be striking, with elevations of two to four times the normal value at rest.[100] In patients with acute hepatitis the hyperkinetic state reverses when the hepatitis subsides. The mechanism responsible for the widespread arteriolar dilatation and the resulting hyperkinetic state is not clear. Hypoxemia can contribute to the high cardiac output, as in patients with severe anemia, but does not appear to be a sufficient explanation. Diminished deactivation of vasodilator substances and estrogens may be important.

Renal Disease (See also Chap. 52)

Cardiac output has been reported to increase in some[107–109] but not all[110] patients with acute glomerulonephritis. In a report of six patients with acute glomerulonephritis,[107] cardiac output was increased to an average of 5.4 liters/min/sq meter. Oxygen consumption also increased, as did mean arterial and pulmonary wedge pressures, whereas systemic vascular resistance was normal and the arterial–mixed venous oxygen difference was reduced. Since the patients were in the oliguric stage of their disease, it appears that the combination of hypervolemia, resulting from abnormal salt and water retention, and the increased metabolic rate (high oxygen consumption) was responsible for the high–cardiac output state.

The *pulmonary edema* that occurs in some patients with acute nephritis is not usually a reflection of left ventricular failure, but rather it may be a consequence of the hypervolemia. In addition, left ventricular work may be strikingly elevated as a consequence of the augmentation of cardiac output and arterial pressure; this is associated with an elevation of left ventricular end-diastolic pressure as the ventricle moves to the steep portion of its diastolic pressure-volume curve (Chap. 14). This condition has been termed the *congested state* by Eichna to contrast it with heart fail-

68. Akbarian, M., Yankopoulos, N. A., and Abelmann, W. H.: Hemodynamic studies in beriberi heart disease. Am. J. Med. *41*:197, 1966.
69. Akram, H., Maslowski, A. H., Smith, B. L., and Nichols, M. G.: The haemodynamic, histopathological and hormonal features of alcoholic beriberi. Q. J. Med. *50*:359, 1981.
70. Carson, P.: Alcoholic cardiac beriberi. Br. Med. J. *284*:1817, 1982.
71. Editorial: Cardiovascular beriberi. Lancet *1*:1287, 1982.
72. Akbarian, M., and Dreyfus, P. M.: Blood trans-ketolase activity in beriberi heart disease. J.A.M.A. *20*:77, 1968.
73. Baker, H., and Frank, O.: Clinical Vitaminology: Methods and Interpretation. New York, Wiley Interscience, 1968.
74. Baker, H., quoted in Sauberlich, H. E.: Biochemical alterations in thiamine deficiency—their interpretation. Am. J. Clin. Nutr. *20*:543, 1967.
75. Brin, M.: Erythrocyte transketolase in early thiamine deficiency. Ann. N.Y. Acad. Sci. *98*:528, 1962.
76. Brin, M.: The use of the erythrocyte in the functional evaluation of vitamin adequacy. *In* Bishop, L., and Surgenor, D. M. (eds.): The Red Blood Cell. New York, Academic Press, 1964, p. 45.
77. Jeffrey, F. E., and Abelmann, W. H.: Recovery of proved Shoshin beriberi. Am. J. Med. *50*:123, 1971.
78. Whittemore, R., and Caddell, J. L.: Metabolic and nutritional diseases. *In* Moss, A. J., et al. (eds.): Heart Disease in Infants, Children and Adolescents. 2nd ed. Baltimore, Williams and Wilkins Co., 1977, pp. 590 and 591.
78a. Yui, Y., Fujiwara, H., Mitsui, H., et al.: Furosemide-induced thiamine deficiency. Jpn. Circ. J. *42*:744, 1978.
79. Edholm, O. G., and Howarth, S.: Studies on the peripheral circulation in osteitis deformans. Clin. Sci. *12*:277, 1953.
80. Heistad, D. D., Abboud, F. M., Schmid, P. G., Mark, A. L., and Wilson, W. R.: Regulation of blood flow in Paget's disease of the bone. J. Clin. Invest. *55*:69, 1975.
81. DeDeuxchaisnes, C. N., and Krane, S. M.: Paget's disease of bone: Clinical and metabolic observations. Medicine (Balt.) *43*:233, 1964.
82. Woodhouse, N. J. Y., Crosbie, W. A., and Mohamedally, S. M.: Cardiac output in Paget's disease: Response to long-term salmon calcitonin therapy. Br. Med. J. *4*:686, 1975.
83. Rhodes, B. A., Gregson, N. D., and Hamilton, C. R., Jr.: Absence of anatomic arteriovenous shunts in Paget's disease of bone. N. Engl. J. Med. *287*:686, 1972.
84. Crosbie, W. A., Mohamedally, S. M., and Woodhouse, N. J. Y.: Effect of salmon calcitonin on cardiac output, oxygen transport, and bone turnover in patients with Paget's disease. Clin. Sci. Molec. Med. *48*:537, 1975.
85. Henley, J. W., Croxson, R. S., and Ibbertson, H. K.: The cardiovascular system in Paget's disease of bone—the response to therapy with calcitonin and diphosphonate. N. Z. Med. J. *84*(Abstr.):161, August, 1976.
86. Howarth, S.: Cardiac output in osteitis deformans. Clin. Sci. *12*:271, 1953.
87. Rutishauser, E., Veyrat, R., and Rouiller, C.: La vascularization de l'os pagétique, étude anatomo-pathologique. Presse Méd. *62*:654, 1954.
88. Lequime, J., and Denolin, H.: Circulatory dynamics in osteitis deformans. Circulation *12*:215, 1955.
89. McIntosh, H. D., Miller, D. E., Gleason, W. L., and Goldner, J. L.: The circulatory dynamics of polyostotic fibrous dysplasia. Am. J. Med. *32*:393, 1962.
90. Gorlin, R., Brachfeld, N., Turner, J. O., Messer, J. V., and Salazar, E.: The idiopathic high cardiac output state. J. Clin. Invest. *38*:2144, 1959.
91. Gorlin, R.: The hyperkinetic heart syndrome. J.A.M.A. *182*:823, 1962.
92. Hickam, J. B., Cargill, W. H., and Golden, A.: Cardiovascular reactions to emotional stimuli. Effect on cardiac output, arteriovenous oxygen difference, arterial pressure, and peripheral resistance. J. Clin. Invest. *27*:290, 1947.
93. Editorial: The hyperkinetic heart. Lancet *2*:967, 1982.
94. Frohlich, E. D., Tarazi, R. C., and Dustan, H. P.: Hyperdynamic beta adrenergic circulatory state: Increased beta receptor responsiveness. Arch. Intern. Med. *123*:1, 1969.
95. Guazzi, M., Polese, A., Magrini, F., Fiorentini, C., and Olivari, M. T.: Long-term treatment of the hyperkinetic heart syndrome with propranolol. Am. J. Med. Sci. *270*:465, 1975.
96. Fiorentini, C., Olivarai, M. T., Moruzzi, P., and Guazzi, M. D.: Long-term follow-up of the primary hypertrophic heart. Am. J. Med. *71*:221, 1981.
97. Gillum, R. F., Teicholz, L. E., Herman, M. V., and Gorlin, R.: The idiopathic hyperkinetic heart syndrome: Clinical course and long-term prognosis. Am. Heart J. *102*:728, 1981.
98. Julius, S., and Esler, M.: Autonomic nervous cardiovascular regulation in borderline hypertension. Am. J. Cardiol. *36*:685, 1975.
99. Ibrahim, M. M., Tarazi, R. C., Dustan, H. P., Bravo, E. L., and Gifford, R. W.: Hyperkinetic heart in severe hypertension: A separate clinical hemodynamic entity. Am. J. Cardiol. *35*:667, 1975.
100. Kowalski, J. J., and Abelmann, W. H.: The cardiac output at rest in Laennec's cirrhosis. J. Clin. Invest. *32*:1025, 1953.
101. Wechsler, R. L., Myers, J. D., Dekker, A., Carey, L., and Stilley, J. W.: Cardiovascular effects of severe liver disease. Am. J. Dig. Dis. *21*:114, 1976.
102. Wolfe, J. D., Tashkin, D. P., Holly, F. E., Brachman, M. B., and Genovesi, M. G.: Hypoxemia of cirrhosis. Am. J. Med. *63*:746, 1977.
103. Murray, J. F., Dawson, A. M., and Sherlock, S.: Circulatory changes in chronic liver disease. Am. J. Med. *24*:358, 1958.
104. Karlish, A. J., Marshall, R., Reid, L., and Sherlock, S.: Cyanosis with cirrhosis: A case with pulmonary arteriovenous shunting. Thorax *22*:555, 1967.
105. Hales, M.: Multiple small arteriovenous fistulae of the lungs. Am. J. Pathol. *32*:927, 1956.
106. Berthelot, P., Walker, M. B., Sherlock, S., and Reid, L.: Arterial changes in the lungs in cirrhosis of the liver: Lung spider nevi. N. Engl. J. Med. *274*:291, 1966.
107. Binak, K., Sirmaci, N., Ucak, D., and Harmanci, N.: Circulatory changes in acute glomerulonephritis at rest and during exercise. Br. Heart J. *37*:833, 1975.
108. McCrary, W. W.: The heart in glomerulonephritis. Pediatrics *69*:1176, 1966.
109. DeFanzio, V., Christensen, R. C., Regan, T. J., Baer, L. M., Morita, Y., and Hellems, H. K.: Circulatory changes in acute glomerulonephritis. Circulation *20*:190, 1959.
110. Eichna, L. W., Farber, S. T., Berger, A. R., Rader, B., Smith, W. W., and Albert, R. E.: Non-cardiac circulatory congestion simulating congestive heart failure. Trans. Assoc. Am. Phys. *67*:72, 1954.
111. Eichna, L. W.: Circulatory congestion and heart failure. Circulation *22*:864, 1960.
112. Harvey, R. M., Ferrer, M. I., Richards, D. W., and Cournand, A.: Influence of chronic pulmonary disease on the heart and circulation. Am. J. Med. *10*:719, 1951.
113. Burrows, B., Kettel, L. J., Niden, A. H., Rabinowitz, M., and Diener, C. F.: Patterns of cardiovascular dysfunction in chronic obstructive lung disease. N. Engl. J. Med. *286*:912, 1972.
114. Fowler, N. O., Westcott, R. N., Scott, R. C., and Hess, E.: The cardiac output in chronic cor pulmonale. Circulation *6*:888, 1952.
115. Williams, J. F., Childress, R. H., Boyd, D. L., Higgs, L. M., and Behnke, R. H.: Left ventricular function in patients with chronic obstructive pulmonary disease. J. Clin. Invest. *47*:1143, 1968.
116. Baum, G. L., Schwartz, A., Llamas, R. M., and Castillo, C.: Left ventricular function in chronic obstructive lung disease. N. Engl. J. Med. *285*:361, 1971.
117. Frank, M. J., Weisse, A. B., Moschos, C. B., and Levinson, G. E.: Left ventricular function, metabolism, and blood flow in chronic cor pulmonale. Circulation *47*:798, 1973.
118. Cobb, L. A., Kramer, R. J., and Finch, C. A.: Circulatory effects of chronic hypervolemia in polycythemia vera. J. Clin. Invest. *39*:1722, 1960.
119. Grahame-Smith, D. G.: The carcinoid syndrome. *In* Bondy, P. K., and Rosenberg, L. E. (eds.): Metabolic Control and Disease. 8th ed. Philadelphia, W. B. Saunders Co., 1980, p. 1703.
120. Schwaber, J. R., and Lukas, D. S.: Hyperkinemia and cardiac failure in the carcinoid syndrome. Am. J. Med. *32*:846, 1962.
121. Voight, G. C., Kronthal, H. L., and Crounse, R. G.: Cardiac output in erythroderma skin disease. Am. Heart J. *72*:615, 1966.
122. Shuster, S.: High output cardiac failure from skin disease. Lancet *1*:1338, 1963.
123. Hecht, H. H., Candiolo, B. M., Malkinson, F. D., Nair, K. G., and Saqueton, A. C.: On cardio-cutaneous syndromes. Trans. Assoc. Am. Phys. *80*:91, 1967.
124. DeVitiis, O., Fazio, S., Petito, M., Maddalena, G., Contaldo, F., and Mancini, M.: Obesity and cardiac function. Circulation *64*:477, 1981.
125. Masserli, F. H., Ventura, H. O., Reisin, E., Dreslinski, G. R., Dunn, F. G., MacPhee, A. A., and Frohlich, E. D.: Borderline hypertension and obesity: Two prehypertensive states with elevated cardiac output. Circulation *66*:55, 1982.
126. Masserli, F. H.: Cardiovascular effects of obesity and hypertension. Lancet *1*:1165, 1982.
127. Backman, L., Freyschuss, U., Hallberg, D., and Melcher, A.: Reversibility of cardiovascular changes in extreme obesity. Acta Med. Scand. *205*:367, 1979.

25 PULMONARY HYPERTENSION

by William Grossman, M.D., Joseph S. Alpert, M.D., and Eugene Braunwald, M.D.

NORMAL PULMONARY CIRCULATION

During the passage of blood through the lungs, hemoglobin molecules are normally oxygenated to nearly their full capacity and the blood is cleansed of much particulate matter and bacteria. The lung, in addition to functioning as a blood oxygenator and filter, plays a dominant role in achieving acid-base balance by excreting carbon dioxide, thereby helping to maintain an optimum blood pH.[1] Normally, the pulmonary vascular bed offers remarkably little resistance to flow. Pulmonary hypertension results when reductions in the caliber of the pulmonary vessels or increases in pulmonary blood flow occur.

PULMONARY BLOOD FLOW, PRESSURE, AND RESISTANCE

NORMAL ADULT CIRCULATION. *Pulmonary blood flow* refers to the volume of blood per unit of time that passes from the pulmonary artery through the alveolar capillaries and into the pulmonary veins. However, it must be remembered that the lungs have a dual circulation and receive both systemic venous blood (the "pulmonary blood flow") through the pulmonary artery and arterial blood through the bronchial circulation. The bronchial arteries ramify normally into a capillary network drained by bronchial veins, some of which empty into the pulmonary veins, whereas the remainder empty into the systemic venous bed. Therefore the bronchial circulation constitutes a physiological "right-to-left" shunt. The function of the bronchial circulation is to provide nutrition to the airways. Normally blood flow through this system is quite low, amounting to approximately 1 per cent of cardiac output[2]: the resulting desaturation of left atrial blood is usually trivial. However, in some forms of pulmonary disease, e.g., advanced bronchiectasis or cystic fibrosis, and in the presence of congenital cardiovascular malformations that cause cyanosis, the blood flow through the bronchial circulation can increase significantly and account for nearly 30 per cent of the cardiac output.[3] In pulmonary disease, significant right-to-left shunting through the bronchial circulation may result in arterial desaturation. In cyanotic congenital heart disease, bronchial blood flow may participate in gas exchange and improve systemic oxygenation.

The normal pulmonary artery pressure in an individual living at sea level has a peak systolic value of 18 to 25 mm Hg, an end-diastolic value of 6 to 10 mm Hg, and a mean value ranging from 12 to 16 mm Hg (Chap. 9).* Definite pulmonary hypertension is present when pulmonary artery systolic and mean pressures exceed 30 and 20 mm Hg, respectively. Mean pulmonary venous pressure is usually 6 to 10 mm Hg; therefore, the normal arteriovenous pressure

*All pressures discussed here are in reference to atmospheric pressure at the level of the heart. True transmural pressures are more physiologically meaningful, especially when pulmonary parenchymal disease is present, but these are rarely measured.

pulmonary artery pressure rose substantially after 3 days of hypoxia and had doubled by day 14. These hemodynamic changes were associated with (1) abnormal extension of muscle into peripheral arteries where it is not normally present, (2) increased wall thickness of the muscular arteries, and (3) reduction in the number of arteries expressed as an increase in the ratio of alveoli to arteries. In a follow-up study,[22] it was found that these hypoxia-induced chronic vascular changes were more extensive in infants than in adult rats. Furthermore, after recovery under normoxic conditions for 3 months, residual vascular changes were present in all animals studied, but again were more severe in the younger rats.

Changes in alveolar oxygenation directly affect the oxygenation of blood in small pulmonary arteries and arterioles by direct gaseous diffusion from the alveoli, respiratory bronchioles, and alveolar ducts in the pulmonary arterioles,[23–25] even though the latter are "upstream" in relation to the alveoli. This fact, taken together with evidence for a reduction in pulmonary arterial blood volume during hypoxia,[26] supports the view that the small pulmonary arteries and arterioles are the main sites of vasoconstriction and increased resistance during hypoxia.[26,27] While alveolar oxygen tension is a major physiological determinant of pulmonary arteriolar tone, a reduction in the oxygen tension in the mixed venous blood flowing through the small pulmonary arteries and arterioles may also lead to pulmonary arterial vasoconstriction.[15,28]

Acidemia appears to potentiate the effects of hypoxemia (Fig. 46–6, p. 1577), whereas alkalosis may be protective.[29–31] Thus, two potent stimuli for vasodilatation in the systemic arteriolar bed cause vasoconstriction of pulmonary arteries and arterioles. Although *hypercapnia* can be shown to increase pulmonary vascular resistance in some experimental preparations, the effects are variable and probably not important in humans.[15]

With regard to *neural regulation* of pulmonary vascular resistance, it should be pointed out that morphological studies have demonstrated that the media and adventitia of the large elastic pulmonary arteries and of the large pulmonary veins are supplied by nerve fibers that may influence the distensibility of these capacitance vessels.[2,13] Although neural regulation of pulmonary vascular resistance can be demonstrated[32] and may be particularly important in fetal life, its importance in the normal human adult is uncertain.

Chemical and hormonal regulation of pulmonary vascular resistance is a complex and as yet incompletely understood subject, with roles having been reported for catecholamines, acetylcholine, prostaglandins, histamine, bradykinin, serotonin, and angiotensin.[2,13,23,33–60] The exact site of action of these agents within the pulmonary vascular tree (i.e., arterioles, venules, capillaries, and so on) is uncertain at present.

There is controversy concerning the effects of *alpha-adrenergic agonists* on the pulmonary vascular bed. Several studies have shown that norepinephrine causes increases in pulmonary arterial and wedge pressures with no change in pulmonary blood flow or pulmonary vascular resistance.[48–51] Systemic arterial pressure increases markedly, and this presumably accounts for the increase in pulmonary venous pressure. In one study an increase in pulmonary vascular resistance with norepinephrine was reported,[52] and there is experimental evidence for alpha-adrenergic–mediated constriction of small pulmonary arteries and veins induced by either the injection of norepinephrine or the stimulation of sympathetic nerves.[53]

The alpha blocker phentolamine has been shown to lower pulmonary vascular resistance.[54] In addition, tolazoline (Priscoline), which also exhibits alpha-adrenergic blocking action, may exert a strong pulmonary vasodilating effect in some patients. Tolazoline was first reported in the pharmacological literature as a vasodepressor agent having effects comparable to those of histamine. Subsequently, it was shown to antagonize the actions of alpha-adrenergic agonists. Like phentolamine, it is an imidazoline compound, and both these agents have vasodepressor effects independent of their alpha-adrenergic antagonistic properties. In fact, there is some evidence that the pulmonary vasodilator effect of tolazoline is mediated through histamine-2 receptors.[55] Tolazoline has been reported to produce a transient fall in pulmonary vascular resistance in patients with pulmonary hypertension having a major reversible component.[56] Dresdale et al. described a patient with primary pulmonary hypertension in whom mean pulmonary arterial pressure fell from 70 to 31 mm Hg after administration of tolazoline.[57] The wedge pressure was not measured, but cardiac output rose. When 1 mg/kg of tolazoline is injected into the pulmonary artery of patients with pulmonary hypertension, a reduction of pulmonary resistance identifies a vasoconstrictive component of the elevated pulmonary artery pressure.[58]

Beta-adrenergic stimulation with isoproterenol has been shown repeatedly to cause pulmonary *vasodilatation*.[6] In contrast, beta-adrenergic blockade does not produce any change in pulmonary vascular resistance, suggesting that there is no tonic activation of beta receptors for maintenance of the normal low pulmonary vascular resistance. *Acetylcholine* is also a potent relaxant of pulmonary arteries and arterioles[33–35] and transiently lowers pulmonary vascular resistance in patients with elevated pulmonary vascular resistance with a major reversible component.

Lung tissue is particularly active in the synthesis, metabolism, and release of a number of the *prostaglandins*, some of which may play a role in the regulation of pulmonary vascular resistance. Prostaglandins I_2 and E are active pulmonary vasodilators, whereas $F_{2\alpha}$ and A_2 are pulmonary vasoconstrictors.[36] The role of these prostaglandins and their precursors in the regulation of pulmonary vascular tone in humans is uncertain at present. However, the prostaglandin synthesis inhibitor (indomethacin) produced a substantial increase in pulmonary vascular resistance and a decline in cardiac output.[37] If inhibition of prostaglandin synthesis leads to an *increase* in pulmonary vascular resistance, it might be expected that specific prostaglandin in fusion might have a vasodilatory effect on the pulmonary vasculature. This was examined in two studies of patients with pulmonary hypertension (primary in nine cases and secondary to thromboembolism and obstructive airway disease in the other two cases) who received an intravenous infusion of PGI_2 (prostacyclin).[38,39] Pulmonary arterial pressure and pulmonary vascular resistance fell toward normal; however, systemic vascular resistance decreased as well (with resultant systemic hypotension in three of the four cases), and the ratio of pulmonary to systemic vascular resistance remained unchanged or increased in all cases. This suggests that PGI_2 acted as a general vasodilator, without selective pulmonary vascular action.

Histamine, a vasodilator in the systemic circulation, is primarily a vasoconstrictor in the pulmonary vascular bed. Since large doses of chlorpheniramine and other antihistamines or histamine depletors attenuate the hypoxia-induced pulmonary vasoconstrictor response, it has been suggested that histamine may actually be the chemical mediator of hypoxia-induced vasoconstriction in animals.[40–44] This suggestion is supported by the observation that the periarterial mast cells in the rat and guinea pig lung lose their granules and apparently release histamine during hypoxia.[27] However, other experimental findings are contradictory,[13] and as a consequence, the role of histamine in the regulation of the pulmonary circulation in man remains unclear. Perhaps this confusion can be resolved by the recent finding that histamine may have both pulmonary vasoconstrictor (H_1-receptor) and vasodilator (H_2-receptor) actions.[59–61] In at least one study, histamine acted as a pulmonary vasoconstrictor in the presence of normal oxygenation and as a vasodilator under hypoxic conditions.[59] As mentioned above, tolazoline may act through stimulation of the H_2-receptors.[55]

Serotonin is a potent pulmonary vasoconstrictor in experimental animals[46] but apparently has little or no effect in humans.[47] In this regard, it should be noted that in patients with hepatic metastases of malignant carcinoid of the bowel, large quantities of serotonin are produced and changes in the endocardium and valves of the right side of the heart may occur (p. 1430), but these patients do not exhibit pulmonary hypertension. *Angiotensin II*, generated in the lung by means of enzymatic conversion of angiotensin I, is thought to be a potent pulmonary vasoconstrictor.[27] However, its role in the normal regulation of pulmonary vascular resistance in humans is unknown.

RESPONSE TO ENVIRONMENTAL FACTORS

Life at *high altitude* is associated with pulmonary hypertension of variable severity, reflecting the range of reactivities of different persons to the pulmonary vasoconstrictive effect of hypoxia.[15,62–64] As discussed earlier, pulmonary arterial pressure normally declines rapidly following birth at sea level. However, the fall in pulmonary artery pressure of infants born at high altitude may be slower in onset and of lesser magnitude.[65] Mean pulmonary arterial pressure in normal adults living 10,000 feet above sea level is approximately 25 mm Hg[66] and increases to over 50 mm Hg with exercise. The relationship between *cigarette smoking* and chronic obstructive lung diseases is clear.[67–69] Since many patients with chronic obstructive lung diseases exhibit pulmonary hypertension (Chap. 46),[70,71] cigarette smoking may be considered an indirect stimulus to the development of pulmonary hypertension.

SECONDARY PULMONARY HYPERTENSION

A classification of conditions associated with pulmonary hypertension is given in Table 25–1. As can be seen, pulmonary hypertension results when there is increased resistance to blood flow at any of a number of sites within the circulation, the pulmonary vascular bed itself representing only one of these potential sites. In addition to increased resistance to blood flow (Table 25–1, I–III), markedly increased flow alone may cause pulmonary hypertension, even when resistance to flow is normal at every point in the circulation. Hypoventilation and its various causes (Table 25–1, IV) have been listed as a separate category of conditions associated with pulmonary hypertension, although this is somewhat arbitrary, and it might well be argued that these conditions all produce pulmonary hypertension by hypoxic pulmonary vasoconstriction and thus represent a subcategory of increased resistance to flow through the pulmonary vascular bed (Table 25–1, II).

Increased Resistance to Pulmonary Venous Drainage

PATHOPHYSIOLOGY. Increased resistance to pulmonary venous drainage is a mechanism common to several conditions of diverse etiology in which pulmonary arterial hypertension occurs. Altered resistance to pulmonary venous drainage may be the result of diseases affecting the left ventricle or pericardium, mitral or aortic valvular disease, or rare entities such as cor triatriatum, left atrial myxoma, or pulmonary veno-occlusive disease (see below).

The magnitude of pulmonary hypertension depends, in part, on the performance of the right ventricle. In response to an acute stress, such as pulmonary embolism, the normal right ventricle of an adult living at sea level can tolerate systolic pulmonary pressures of 45 to 50 mm Hg, above which right ventricular failure supervenes. Systolic pressures of 80 to 100 mm Hg can be generated only by a hypertrophied right ventricle that undergoes normal perfusion. If right ventricular infarction or ischemia has occurred,[72–74] or if the right and left ventricles are both affected by a myopathic process, right ventricular failure will occur at lower levels of pulmonary vascular pressures, and significant pulmonary hypertension may not develop despite an increase in pulmonary vascular resistance.

In the presence of a healthy, nonischemic right ventricle, an increase in left atrial pressure from subnormal levels up to 7 mm Hg results in a fall in both pulmonary vascular resistance and the pressure gradient across the lungs.[5] These reductions may reflect distention of a population of compliant small vessels or recruitment of additional vascular channels or both. With further increases in left atrial pressure, pulmonary arterial pressure rises pari passu with pulmonary venous pressure, i.e., at a constant pulmonary blood flow, the pressure gradient between the pulmonary artery and veins and the pulmonary vascular resistance remains constant.[5] Finally, when pulmonary venous pressure ally develops following surgical correction of *tetralogy of Fallot* is unclear. In the patient with tetralogy of Fallot, pulmonary vascular thrombotic lesions are common and, if extensive, may predispose to pulmonary hypertension when operation—either complete correction or creation of a left-to-right shunt—causes a sudden increase in pulmonary blood flow.[2,182]

Sickle cell anemia may be complicated by in situ pulmonary thrombosis and infarction, although, as discussed in Chapter 49, this does not usually lead to pulmonary hypertension. There are two case reports of cor pulmonale associated with hemoglobin SC disease,[184,185] but the prevalence of pulmonary hypertension in individuals with this condition is unknown.

Intravenous drug abuse may lead to diffuse pulmonary vascular occlusion and pulmonary hypertension, as in the case of a 25-year-old man who injected himself with crushed, dissolved pentazocine intravenously has been reported.[186] After 1 month he developed chest pain, shortness of breath, and fatigue and was found to have a pulmonary artery pressure of 72/30 mm Hg (mean 46 mm Hg) with a right atrial pressure of 14 mm Hg. Analysis of lung biopsy material implicated embolization of the cellulose filter material in the tablet with subsequent severe tissue reaction and granuloma formation. Prednisone therapy led to improvement in the clinical state and gradual lowering of the pulmonary artery pressure.

A patient in whom moderately severe pulmonary hypertension developed in association with *alveolar proteinosis* has been reported.[187] Hypoxemia seemed to be the mediating factor, and the patient showed substantial reduction in pulmonary artery pressure (60/25 mm Hg to 32/14 mm Hg) in response to oxygen inhalation. Pulmonary arterial involvement with pulmonary hypertension has been reported to occur in approximately 25 per cent of patients with *Takayasu's disease.*[188,189] The pulmonary pressure elevations are usually only moderate, but striking abnormalities may be present on lung scan or pulmonary angiogram (Fig. 25–8).

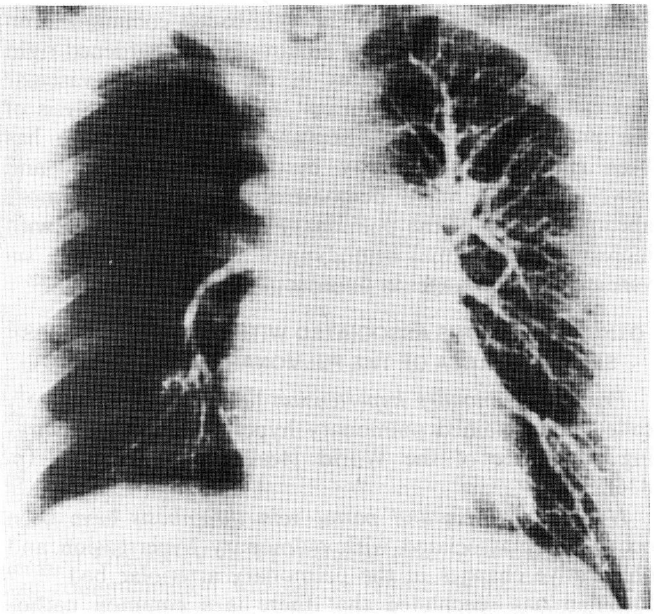

FIGURE 25–8 Pulmonary angiogram from a 27-year-old Japanese woman with Takayasu's disease and pulmonary hypertension. There is marked narrowing of the right pulmonary artery and no appearance of its branches. (Reprinted with permission from Kawai, C.: Pulmonary pulseless disease: Pulmonary involvement in so-called Takayasu's disease. Chest *73*:651, 1978.)

PRIMARY (UNEXPLAINED) PULMONARY HYPERTENSION

In some patients with pulmonary hypertension, no cause is discernible, in which case the pulmonary hypertension is termed idiopathic, essential, unexplained,[157] or, most frequently, *primary.* In contrast to systemic hypertension, in which the etiology is primary (essential) in a large percentage of patients (Chap. 26), primary hypertension in the pulmonary circuit is uncommon. Primary pulmonary hypertension (PPH) is often readily suspected on clinical examination, but the diagnosis should be made only after detailed examination of the heart and lungs, i.e., ordinarily after cardiac catheterization and pulmonary angiography have revealed no specific cause for the pulmonary hypertension.

ETIOLOGY

Although a number of theories have been advanced to explain the origin of PPH, none has as yet gained clear ascendancy. Indeed, were the etiology of the pulmonary hypertension clear, the designation "primary" would not be appropriate.

Recurrent occult venous thrombosis with pulmonary embolism may be extremely difficult to exclude as the cause of pulmonary hypertension. A number of patients with chronic, recurrent thromboembolic disease develop pulmonary hypertension and cor pulmonale slowly, with no overt clinical manifestation of pulmonary embolism (p. 1597). Early in the course such patients may exhibit pulmonary angiographic findings characteristic of emboli, but late in the course such findings may be absent. Therefore, it has been argued that PPH may result from recurrent episodes of asymptomatic pulmonary embolism.[190] In support of this theory is the common autopsy finding of clinically unrecognized organizing or recanalizing pulmonary emboli in patients considered during life to have had PPH.[190–192] Moreover, one can produce experimental pulmonary arterial lesions in animals resembling those seen in patients with PPH by intravenous injection of autologous thrombi or other material (e.g., plant spores or polystyrene beads).[193–197] The fact that PPH occasionally develops or worsens post partum also supports a thromboembolic or an amniotic fluid embolic etiology.[192,193]

An alternative explanation relates the development of PPH to *thrombosis* in situ in small pulmonary arteries, with resultant widespread pulmonary vascular obstruction. In support of this theory, various defects in coagulation, including abnormal platelet function and defective fibrinolysis, have been demonstrated in patients with

PPH.[191,193,198–203] A relationship between microangiopathic hemolytic anemia, thrombocytopenia, and PPH has also been suggested.[201] The development of PPH in young women taking contraceptive pills has been thought to be related to the hypercoagulable state that these agents induce.

On the other hand, numerous pathological studies have demonstrated clear-cut morphological differences in the pulmonary vascular bed of patients with thromboembolic or thrombotic pulmonary hypertension, compared with changes noted in patients with PPH. These findings argue *against* recurrent pulmonary thromboembolism or in situ thrombosis as the etiology of PPH.[191–193,199,200] In patients with thromboembolic or thrombotic pulmonary hypertension, thrombi of varying sizes and in various stages of organization can generally be demonstrated in pulmonary arteries and arterioles. By contrast, in patients with PPH, pulmonary arterioles exhibit intimal fibrosis of the onion-skin type, medial hypertrophy, fibrinoid necrosis and arteritis, dilatation, and plexiform lesions (Figs. 25–9 and 25–10); thrombi in pulmonary arteries and arterioles, when present, are small and of recent origin. It seems, therefore, that despite their similar clinical and hemodynamic features, PPH and recurrent silent venous thromboembolism can be distinguished pathologically. Although it is possible that a fraction of patients considered on clinical grounds to be suffering from PPH may be found at autopsy to have had chronic thromboembolism, this does not provide a clue to the etiology of PPH; instead, it suggests that PPH may occasionally be falsely diagnosed during life. Obviously, it is of great clinical importance to differentiate these two conditions, since effective treatment for chronic pulmonary thromboembolism is available.

Several *congenital defects* have been proposed as causes of PPH. A deficiency in the media of the pulmonary arterial bed resulting in intimal thickening and proliferation with consequent obstruction of small pulmonary vessels has been suggested as the underlying defect.[204] Persistence of the fetal pulmonary arterial architecture,[205] increased systemic-pulmonary arterial collaterals,[206–208] and a generalized degenerative pulmonary arteriopathy[209] have also been proposed, although the latter two lesions are felt to be secondary to the pulmonary hypertension itself,[192,199,200] and none has been found in the systemic arteries of patients with PPH.

The occurrence of an arteritis and of fibrinoid necrosis in the walls of the smaller pulmonary arteries, and the frequent presence of Raynaud's phenomenon in patients with PPH, has led some authorities to suggest that PPH may be a form of *collagen-vascular or autoimmune disease.*[210,211] Since Raynaud's phenomenon is an expression of vasospasm in digital arteries, its presence in 10 to 30 per cent of patients with PPH suggests that vasospasm in pulmonary arteries may be present as well. Interestingly, in families of patients with PPH, other members not affected by the disease may exhibit Raynaud's phenomenon. Pulmonary hypertension occurs frequently in patients with the so-called CREST syndrome, a variant of scleroderma (calcinosis, Raynaud's phenomenon, esophageal dysfunction, sclerodactyly, and telangiectasia). The histological changes in the pulmonary vessels in patients with this syndrome resemble those seen in patients with PPH and are similar to those seen in the pulmonary vessels of about 10 per cent of patients with the more usual forms of scleroderma.[133]

Takayasu's arteritis (giant cell) frequently involves the pulmonary vessels (Fig. 25–8), but the pathological changes resemble those seen in systemic arteries (p. 1558). In the vast majority of these patients, the aorta and major arch vessels are involved as well. This condition can also be distinguished from PPH by virtue of the fact that the occlusive changes occur in the large and intermediate vessels rather than in the more distal vessels characteristic of PPH.[189]

A number of cases of PPH coexisting with postnecrotic *hepatic cirrhosis* have been reported, suggesting that a vasculitis might be responsible for the pulmonary hypertension.[212–216] *Polyarteritis nodosa* and *hypersensitivity to a variety of drugs,* including penicillin, chloramphenicol, and the sulfonamides, have also been suggested as etiologies for PPH,[200,217] although allergic vasculitis is unlikely to affect only the pulmonary vasculature.[192] Occasionally a patient with PPH has been erroneously diagnosed as suffering from polyarteritis nodosa limited to the lungs.[192,218]

Pulmonary hypertension has developed in a number of individuals who had ingested the anorexigenic drug *aminorex fumarate.*[219–221] The clinical course of these patients was similar to that of patients with PPH, although in some instances regression of pulmonary hypertension upon withdrawal of the drug was reported.[222] Although causation has not been demonstrated definitively, the circumstantial evidence in favor of this relationship is impressive.[193] Since only 0.2 per cent of individuals ingesting the drug develop pulmonary hypertension, some other factor such as a genetic predisposition or an idiosyncratic reaction must be involved.

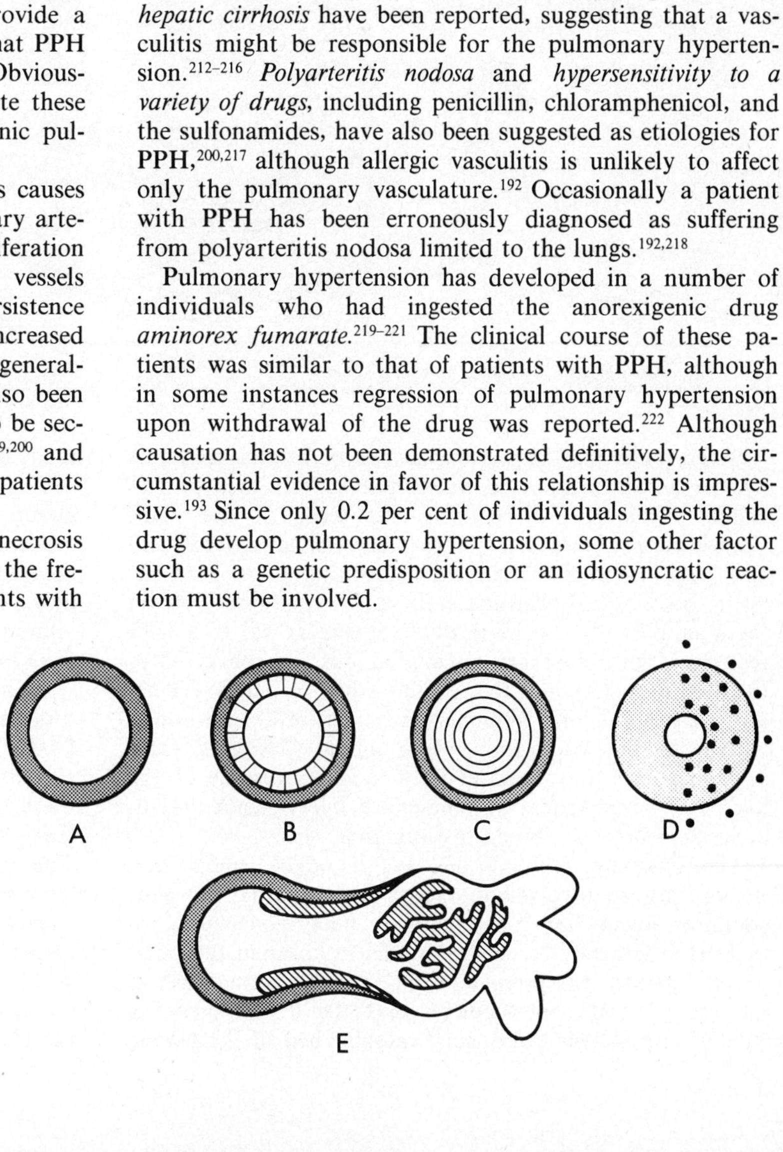

FIGURE 25–9 Plexogenic pulmonary arteriopathy. Arteries with (*A*) medial hypertrophy, (*B*) cellular intimal proliferation, (*C*) concentric-laminar intimal fibrosis, (*D*) fibrinoid necrosis with or without arteritis, and (*E*) plexiform lesions. (From Wagenvoort, C. A., and Wagenvoort, N.: Pathology of Pulmonary Hypertension. New York, copyright 1977, reprinted by permission of John Wiley and Sons, Inc.)

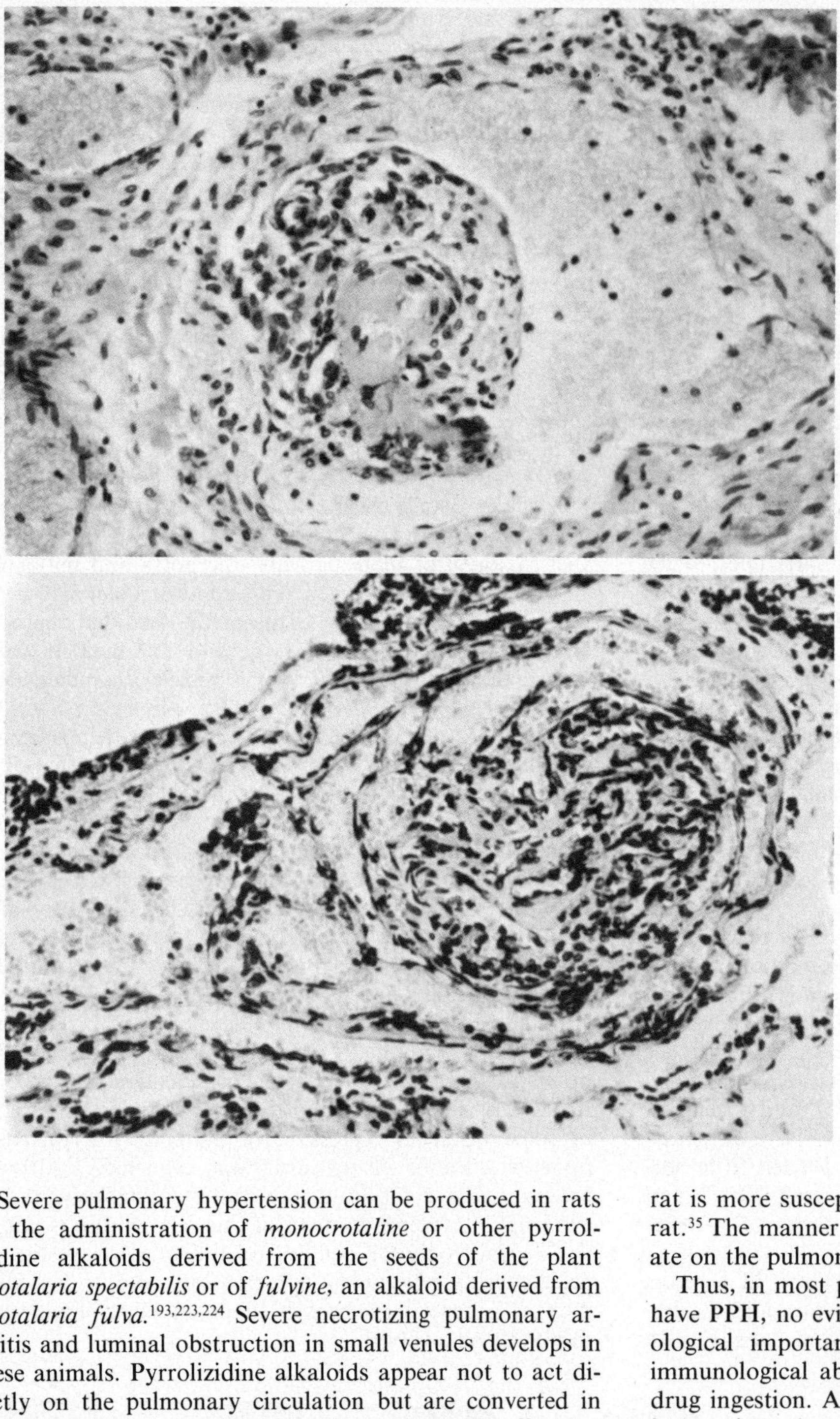
A
B

FIGURE 25–10 *A*, Early plexiform lesion of muscular pulmonary artery in a 13-year-old girl with unexplained plexogenic pulmonary arteriopathy. There is active proliferation of cells in a fibrin clot (hematoxylin and eosin, ×225). *B*, Full-grown plexiform lesion in muscular pulmonary artery in a 28-year-old woman with unexplained plexogenic pulmonary arteriopathy (hematoxylin and eosin, ×225). (From Wagenvoort, C. A., and Wagenvoort, N.: Pathology of Pulmonary Hypertension. New York, copyright 1977, reprinted by permission of John Wiley and Sons, Inc.)

Severe pulmonary hypertension can be produced in rats by the administration of *monocrotaline* or other pyrrolizidine alkaloids derived from the seeds of the plant *Crotalaria spectabilis* or of *fulvine*, an alkaloid derived from *Crotalaria fulva*.[193,223,224] Severe necrotizing pulmonary arteritis and luminal obstruction in small venules develops in these animals. Pyrrolizidine alkaloids appear not to act directly on the pulmonary circulation but are converted in the liver to metabolites that exhibit a hepatotoxic effect before they affect the pulmonary vascular bed.[225] Although natives of the West Indies who ingest *Crotalaria fulva* in "bush tea" may develop veno-occlusive disease of the liver,[193,226] no instances of pulmonary hypertension in humans have been attributed to *Crotalaria.*

The following observations suggest that *female hormones* may be involved in the genesis of PPH: (1) This condition occurs most frequently in pubertal females, (2) there is a tendency for exacerbations to occur in the postpartum period, (3) there may be an association between the use of oral contraceptives and the development of PPH,[227] and (4) the pulmonary vascular bed of the female rat is more susceptible to hypoxia than is that of the male rat.[35] The manner in which this endocrine effect may operate on the pulmonary vascular bed is obscure.

Thus, in most patients considered on clinical grounds to have PPH, no evidence can be adduced to support the etiological importance of thromboembolism, congenital or immunological abnormalities, collagen-vascular disease, or drug ingestion. Although pulmonary hypertension can truly be said to be primary in such patients, a number of factors have been identified that may shed some light on the mechanisms underlying the development of pulmonary hypertension, even in these patients. It is well known that there is considerable interindividual variation in the reactivity of the pulmonary vascular bed. Vasoconstrictive stimuli, such as hypoxia or acidosis, can produce marked pulmonary hypertension in one person and be essentially without effect in another. The pulmonary arterial pressor response to hypoxia is particularly great in individuals with blood group A.[35] This variability in the responsivity of the pulmonary vascular bed undoubtedly accounts for the fact that only a minority of individuals develop pulmonary edema on exposure to high altitude (p. 568). In addition, the severity of pulmonary hypertension and the level of pulmonary vascular resistance vary considerably among individuals with congenital heart disease and comparably sized ventricular septal defects. Presumably, there is a *genetic basis for these differences in pulmonary vascular reactivity,* just as there appears to be a genetic basis for the increased reactivity of the systemic vascular bed in essential systemic hypertension (pp. 863 and 1636).

The finding of increased pulmonary vascular reactivity and pulmonary vasoconstriction in patients with PPH, suggests that a marked *vasospastic or constrictive tendency* underlies the development of PPH in predisposed individuals.[192,193,228,229] The autonomic nervous system has been considered a factor in the development of PPH through stimulation of the pulmonary vascular bed by either neuronally released or circulating catecholamines. In some patients with PPH, the response to pulmonary vasodilators such as tolazoline, acetylcholine, or isoproterenol is a reduction in both pulmonary artery pressure and pulmonary vascular resistance,[228–236] supporting the notion of the importance of the autonomic nervous system in maintaining an elevated level of pulmonary vascular resistance. Other patients, however, are unresponsive to pulmonary vasodilating agents.[56,237] Samet and Bernstein reported an interesting case of a patient with PPH who, when examined initially, exhibited marked pulmonary vasodilatation in response to an infusion of acetylcholine.[238] Three years later, on repeat catheterization, the pulmonary hypertension was more severe, and the patient did not respond to acetylcholine infusion. This observation suggests that patients with PPH initially may have increased pulmonary vasomotor tone. As the disease progresses, functional changes give way to fixed, anatomical lesions unaffected by pharmacological intervention.

Familial cases of PPH have been reported with autosomal dominant inheritance;[203,235,239–241] other than from a positive family history, there is no way to distinguish these patients from those with the sporadic form of the disease. They may represent instances of the genetic transmission of extreme pulmonary vascular reactivity. The interplay between certain environmental factors such as hypoxia and a genetic predisposition for pulmonary vascular reactivity may also underlie the development of PPH. The reactivity of the pulmonary vascular bed of cattle to hypoxia has been shown clearly to be genetically determined.[18] In addition, it has been reported that the incidence of PPH increases at high altitude and that children with this condition improve when they move to lower altitudes;[192] conversely, patients with PPH may deteriorate if they ascend to higher altitudes.[3]

PATHOLOGICAL FINDINGS

Several pathological findings are common to almost all patients with PPH: (1) intimal thickening of the smaller pulmonary arteries and arterioles with fibrosis, producing a characteristic "onionskin" configuration (Fig. 25–11); (2) increased thickness of the media of muscular pulmonary arteries and muscularization of arterioles; (3) necrotizing arteritis in the walls of muscular pulmonary arteries with fibrinoid necrosis of the media of such vessels[191–194, 242]; and (4) *plexiform lesions,* i.e., dilated, thin-walled side branches of muscular pulmonary arteries probably resulting from endothelial proliferation (Figs. 25–9 and 25–10). These lesions are responsible for the term *plexogenic pulmonary arteriopathy,* which was accepted by a working party of the World Health Organization[193] and which is now frequently used to characterize the pathological changes in this condition. Although characteristic of PPH, these anatomical changes are not pathognomonic of the disease and are also found in patients with pulmonary hypertension secondary to cardiac shunts (p. 833).

The pathological diagnosis of PPH can be made when the above-mentioned features, particularly the plexiform lesions, occur in the absence of congenital cardiac shunts and when there is no evidence of old or fresh pulmonary emboli, such as eccentric intimal proliferation, recanalizing channels, and intraluminal fibrous webs. The pattern of elastic tissue of the pulmonary trunk is of the adult variety in PPH, consistent with the belief that the pulmonary hypertension was acquired during adult life.[243] A number of pathological findings are *secondary* to the pulmonary hypertension itself, i.e., in situ thromboses in small pulmonary arteries, atherosclerosis of the major pulmonary arterial trunks, and marked right ventricular hypertrophy.

Recently, Reid and coworkers examined the lungs of a number of patients with PPH using quantitative pathological techniques and electron microscopy.[199,244] These investigators noted thickening of the basement membranes and of the endothelial cells of small (< 40 μm), nonmuscular pulmonary arterioles. The endothelial cells also contained increased numbers of organelles and pinocytotic vesicles, suggesting heightened metabolic activity; indeed, in some

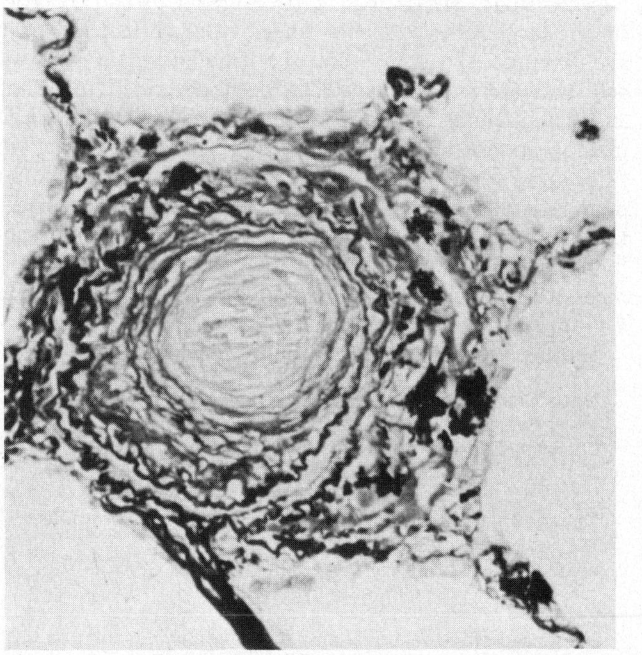

FIGURE 25–11 Transverse section of muscular pulmonary artery from a case of primary pulmonary hypertension in a man 50 years of age. There is intimal fibroelastosis of the "onionskin" type, with atrophy and disruption of the underlying media (elastic/van Gieson, ×375.) (From Harris, P., and Heath, D.: The Human Pulmonary Circulation. 2nd ed. New York, Churchill Livingstone, 1977.)

nonmuscular pulmonary arterioles, proliferation of endothelial cells obliterated the vascular lumen.[244] Quantitative analysis of the vessel population in patients with PPH demonstrated a distinct reduction in the number of small, nonmuscular pulmonary arterioles. Residual, nonfunctioning "ghost vessels" seemed to remain in place of these small arterioles. At more proximal levels of the pulmonary vascular bed, there was considerable hypertrophy of smooth muscle of the media of small muscular pulmonary arteries.[199]

A *tentative* pathophysiological scheme for PPH consistent with the observed findings, but not yet firmly established, is presented in Figure 25–12. In an individual who is susceptible—whether on a genetic or an acquired basis—stimuli for pulmonary vasoconstriction result in excessive responses and transient pulmonary hypertension. Frequent episodes of pulmonary vasoconstriction and the resultant pulmonary hypertension eventually cause hypertrophy of the smooth muscle in the media of these vessels and perhaps thickening and proliferation of the endothelial cells in the nonmuscular vessels. Ultimately, the vessels are reduced in number, and the residua of these destroyed vessels can be seen histologically as "ghost vessels." Destruction of large numbers of pulmonary arterioles reduces the cross-sectional area of the pulmonary vascular bed, thus producing a permanent increase in pulmonary vascular resistance and fixed pulmonary hypertension. The latter, in turn, damages other blood vessels and initiates a vicious cycle, with progressively rising pulmonary arterial pressure.

CLINICAL FEATURES

NATURAL HISTORY AND SYMPTOMATOLOGY. In one large series, patients ranged from 16 to 69 years of age (average 33 years),[192] and the female-to-male ratio was 4:1. However, cases have also been described in infants and young children, and in these younger individuals, a female preponderance is not evident. Most patients with PPH come to medical attention relatively late in the course of the disease, after symptoms have developed and after a latent, asymptomatic phase with progressive pulmonary hypertension has passed. Since there is currently no convenient way to identify such individuals, the duration of this asymptomatic phase is unknown.

Some patients with PPH, followed by means of serial catheterization over a number of years, exhibit some hemodynamic improvement if they are given pulmonary vasodilating agents when they are first seen.[228,229] During later stages of the disease, however, such drugs have no effect on the pulmonary vascular bed.[229,238] Late in the course of the disease, patients develop right ventricular failure, and exertional syncope may occur, presumably because of a low fixed cardiac output and hypoxemia. PPH is a fatal disease in almost all instances; the duration of symptoms varies, but on the average death occurs approximately 3 years after the onset of symptoms. The course may be more precipitous in some patients, particularly in children, whereas a few patients have lived for as long as 30 years after the onset of symptoms.[2,245] In one reported case, PPH appeared to regress.[246]

Patients with PPH commonly complain of exertional dyspnea, syncope, precordial chest pain, weakness, and, later, dyspnea at rest.[191,233,242,247] These symptoms probably all result from low cardiac output or hypoxemia or both. Precordial chest pain may also be secondary to ischemia of the right ventricular subendocardium or distention of the pulmonary artery or both.[248–250] The pain may radiate to the neck but not characteristically to the arms. Palpitations are also common and may be caused by ventricular tachyarrhythmias, which occur not infrequently in the late stages of PPH. Occasionally, cough and hemoptysis occur. These latter symptoms may be due to rupture of dilated plexiform lesions, to in situ pulmonary arterial thromboses, or to episodes of pulmonary embolism occurring late in the course of the disease. Pulmonary embolism occurs frequently as a *result* of severe right ventricular failure, and it may intensify the pulmonary hypertension. However, as has already been pointed out, the clinical distinction between these two pathogenetic sequences—(1) PPH → right ventricular failure → pulmonary thrombotic and/or embolic disease → further pulmonary hypertension → more severe right ventricular failure as opposed to (2) pulmonary thrombotic and/or embolic disease → secondary pulmonary hypertension → right ventricular failure—may be difficult to make.

PHYSICAL EXAMINATION. Examination of patients with PPH discloses findings consistent with pulmonary hypertension and right ventricular pressure overload: a large *a* wave in the jugular venous pulse; a low-volume, carotid arterial pulse with a normal upstroke; a left parasternal (right ventricular) heave; a systolic pulsation produced by a dilated, tense pulmonary artery in the second left interspace; an ejection click and flow murmur in the same area; a closely split second heart sound with a prominent pulmonic component; a fourth heart sound of right ventricular origin; and, late in the course, signs of right ventricular failure (hepatomegaly, peripheral edema, and ascites) may be present. Patients with severe pulmonary hypertension may also have prominent *v* waves in the jugular venous pulse, owing to tricuspid regurgitation; a third heart sound of right ventricular origin; a high-pitched early diastolic murmur of pulmonic regurgitation; and a holosystolic murmur of tricuspid regurgitation.[191,242,247] Cyanosis is a late finding in PPH and may be due to a patent foramen ovale with a right-to-left shunt occurring secondary to elevation of right atrial pressure. Other causes for cyanosis include a markedly reduced cardiac output with systemic

Vasoconstriction or vasospasm in susceptible individuals
↓
Decreased flow in small pulmonary arterioles and reactive pulmonary hypertension
↓
Damage to and eventual loss of small pulmonary arterioles (replaced by ghost vessels)
↓ ↑
Pulmonary hypertension
↓
Decreased cross-sectional area in pulmonary vascular bed at level of small pulmonary arterioles
↑
Development of plexiform lesions with further reduction of vascular cross-sectional area

FIGURE 25–12 Possible pathogenesis of primary pulmonary hypertension.

vasoconstriction, intrapulmonary right-to-left shunting via vascular anastomoses, and ventilation-perfusion mismatches in the lung itself.[247] Rarely, the left laryngeal nerve becomes paralyzed as a consequence of compression by a dilated pulmonary artery.[232]

LABORATORY FINDINGS

Hematological and Chemical Studies. Results of these studies are usually normal in patients with PPH. If there is arterial oxygen desaturation, polycythemia may be present. A number of investigators have reported hypercoagulable states, abnormal platelet function, defects in fibrinolysis, and other abnormalities of coagulation in patients with PPH.[191,193,198,200] Abnormal liver function tests can indicate right ventricular failure with resultant systemic venous hypertension.

Electrocardiography. The electrocardiogram in PPH will exhibit right atrial and right ventricular enlargement, and a direct correlation between the magnitude of the QRS-T angle and the level of pulmonary arterial pressure has been reported.[191]

Roentgenography. X-ray examination of the chest in patients with PPH shows enlargement of the main pulmonary artery and its major branches, with marked tapering of peripheral arteries.[251] The right ventricle and atrium may also be enlarged. Fluoroscopic examination may disclose exaggerated pulsations of secondary pulmonary arterial branches, reflecting an elevation in pulmonary arterial pulse pressure. However, in contrast to the plethoric peripheral lung fields in patients with left-to-right shunts, oligemia is noted in these lung regions in patients with PPH (Fig. 25–13). It has been suggested that survival in PPH correlates inversely with the size of the main pulmonary artery[252]—a reasonable suggestion, since the latter correlates with the height of the pulmonary arterial pressure.

Pulmonary Function Tests. Pulmonary function tests are usually normal; rarely, a defect in diffusion capacity is present and may be the result of increased capillary-to-alveolar distance secondary to hypertrophy of vascular endothelial cells.[244] Some patients have increased residual volumes and reduced maximum voluntary ventilation.[191,232,232a] Arterial blood gas analysis usually reveals evidence of hyperventilation with low pCO_2 and elevated pH, whereas arterial pO_2 is normal or slightly reduced.

Echocardiography. This technique demonstrates enlarged right ventricular dimensions, small or normal left ventricular dimensions, and a thickened interventricular septum; the septal/posterior left ventricular wall ratio may be abnormally increased, as in hypertrophic obstructive cardiomyopathy (Chap. 5), but the other echocardiographic signs characteristic of that condition are not present. The E-F slope of the anterior mitral valve leaflet is reduced, presumably because of the diminished flow rate across the mitral valve, whereas the diastolic motion of the posterior mitral leaflet is normal. Systolic prolapse of the mitral valve is frequently present, as is abnormal septal motion of the ventricular septum, presumably due to right ventricular dilatation or tricuspid and pulmonic regurgitation or both.[253]

Lung Scan. Perfusion lung scans in patients with PPH are usually either normal or demonstrate small, nonspecific, subsegmental defects. Lung scanning may be hazardous late in the course of the disease because the macroaggregated albumin particles employed in scanning may significantly reduce the already critically narrowed cross-sectional area of the pulmonary vascular bed.[254]

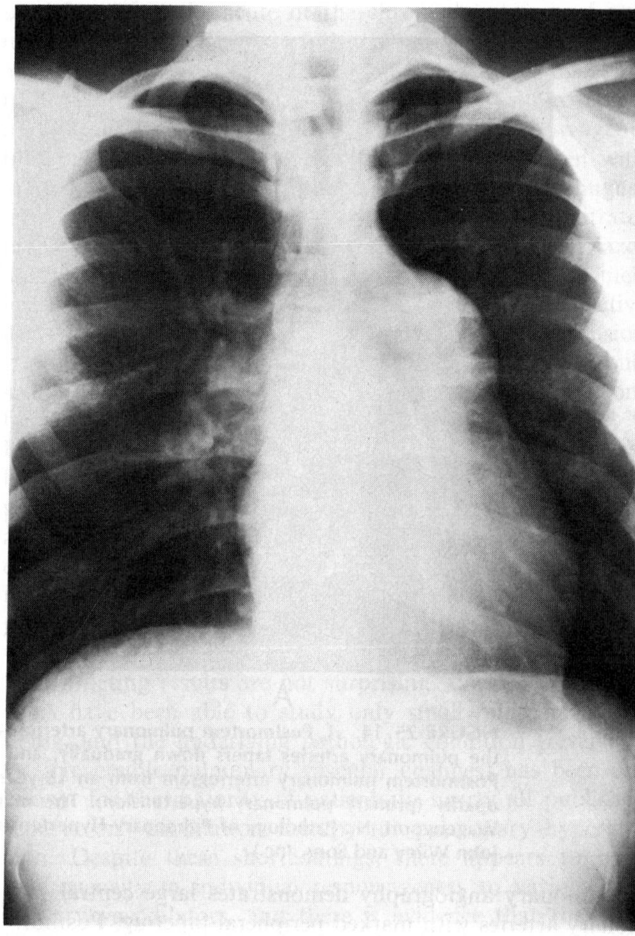

FIGURE 25–13 Frontal chest roentgenogram of a 15-year-old boy with PPH. Note the enlarged main pulmonary artery and the radiolucent lung fields. (Courtesy of Dr. Lloyd E. Hawes.)

Catheterization and Angiography. The diagnosis of PPH cannot be confirmed without performing catheterization and pulmonary angiography. Some patients may be too ill for one or both of these procedures (see below), and in such individuals, the diagnosis must remain tentative and be based primarily on exclusion, following clinical evaluation and noninvasive tests. Right-heart catheterization reveals elevated pulmonary arterial and right-ventricular systolic pressures that may approach, equal, or sometimes even exceed systemic arterial levels; right atrial pressure may also be increased. The calculated pulmonary vascular resistance is extremely high, approaching or sometimes even exceeding systemic vascular resistance. When tricuspid regurgitation is absent, the *a* wave in the right atrial pressure tracing is predominant; when it is present, the height of the *v* wave may equal or exceed that of the *a* wave. Left ventricular, left atrial, and pulmonary capillary wedge pressures are low or normal, but it is often difficult to record the pulmonary capillary wedge pressure. A patent foramen ovale with a small right-to-left shunt is frequently present.

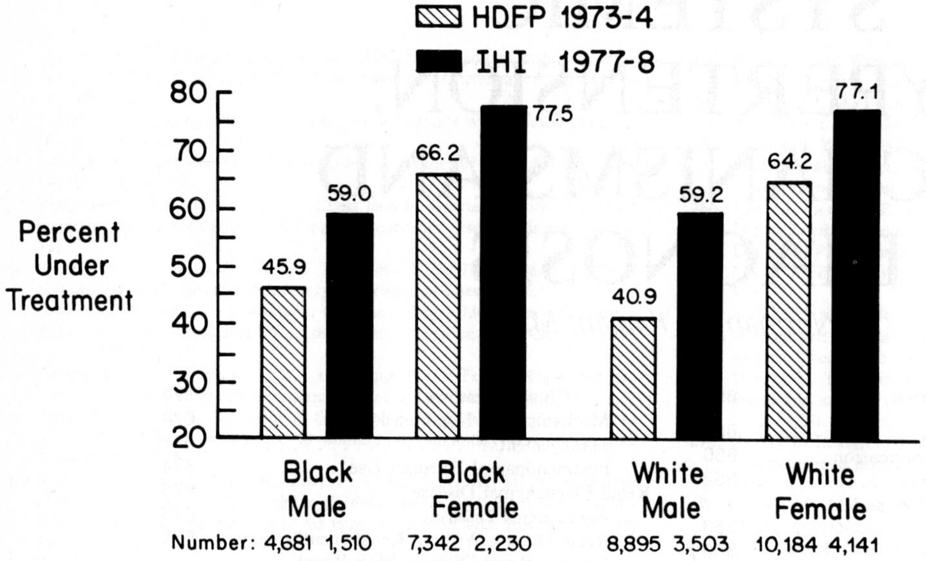

FIGURE 26–1 · Percentage of hypertensives in three U.S. communities whose blood pressure was under treatment in 1973–74 (HDFP) and in 1977–78 (IHI). (From Apostolides, A. Y., et al.: Impact of hypertension information on high blood pressure control between 1973 and 1978. Hypertension *2*:708, 1980, by permission of the American Heart Association, Inc.)

have reduced the overall cardiovascular risk status of the American population, including declines in smoking, in consumption of saturated fats, and in physical inactivity.[3] In addition, a significant part of this reduction likely reflects improvements in the management of millions of patients with hypertension[4] (Fig. 26–1).

As impressive as these improvements are, major problems persist: (1) many hypertensive individuals are at risk because their disease remains undiagnosed and untreated; (2) most hypertension remains idiopathic, primary, or "essential," and without knowledge of causes, prevention of the disease is not possible; (3) in most cases, it is difficult for patients to comply with antihypertensive therapy indefinitely. This and the succeeding chapter attempt to provide guidance for the clinician in handling these problems of management. In this chapter, the mechanisms most likely responsible for primary and secondary hypertension are presented so that diagnostic evaluation can be more sharply focused. In Chapter 27, therapy will be systematically presented, with emphasis on nonpharmacological approaches as well as the rational use of drugs, with the goal of improving patient compliance with lifelong management.

GENERAL CONSIDERATIONS

To provide the background for the physician to deal efficiently and effectively with hypertensive patients, the following general questions will be examined initially:

- At what level is blood pressure considered to be abnormally high?
- How common is hypertension?
- What are the frequencies of various hypertensive diseases?
- What are the risks of uncontrolled hypertension?

Thereafter, the pathophysiology of the primary as well as the major forms of secondary hypertensive diseases will be discussed. Although Chapter 27 deals exclusively with therapy, the coverage of secondary diseases in this chapter will be accompanied by brief descriptions of their specific therapies.

Definition of Hypertension

More and more people are having their blood pressure taken. As more asymptomatic people are being found to have elevated blood pressure, the need to identify those with sufficiently elevated levels to justify therapy has become an increasing problem in clinical practice. The problem largely revolves around the wide variation in blood pressure throughout the day and night, both in persons whose levels remain normal and in those with high levels[5] (Fig. 26–2). In some cases, this variation accompanies physical activity and emotional stress, but in others it is without obvious cause. In a few patients, markedly high readings clearly indicate serious disease requiring immediate treatment. But in most, initial readings are not so high as to indicate immediate danger, and the diagnosis should be substantiated by repeated readings. The reason for such care is obvious: the diagnosis of hypertension imposes heavy psychological and socioeconomic burdens and implies a commitment to lifelong therapy.

DOCUMENTATION OF HYPERTENSION

In deciding what is normal or abnormal for an individual, these guidelines should be followed:

1. Multiple readings should be taken using appropriate techniques (Table 26–1). These guidelines complement the recommendations made in 1980 by an American Heart Association expert committee.[6]

2. Although the logical approach is to average the multiple readings in deciding whether hypertension is or is not present, even a single high reading should not be disre-

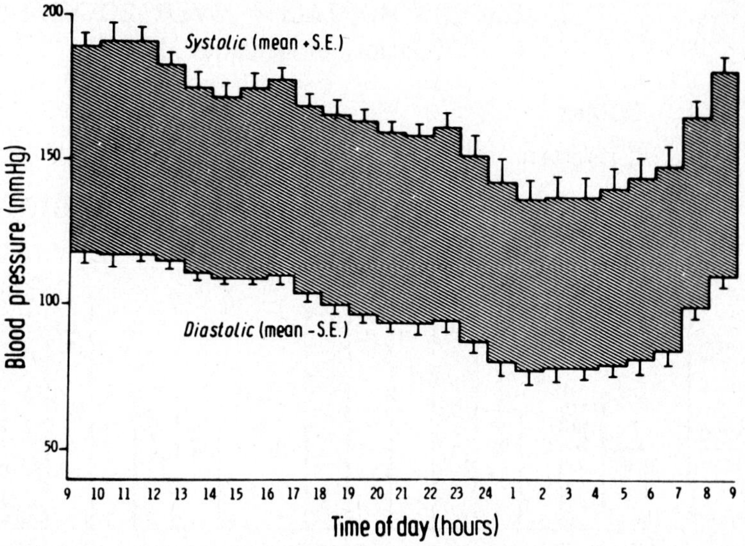

FIGURE 26–2 The hourly mean systolic and diastolic blood pressures of 20 previously untreated ambulant hypertensive subjects recorded continuously by means of intraarterial cannulation. (From Millar-Craig, M. W., et al.: Circadian variation of blood pressure. Lancet *1*:795, 1978.)

garded. Single, casual readings have been found to relate closely to the subsequent development of cardiovascular disease, both in the Framingham Study[7] and by actuarial analysis.[8]

3. Relatively small elevations, if left untreated, are associated with significant morbidity and mortality. The data shown in Figure 26–3 from life insurance actuarial experience were based on one set of readings obtained under rather uncontrolled conditions, but they are supported by the more careful observations from Framingham, showing increases in cardiovascular morbidity and mortality with each increment in blood pressure.[7]

4. As clearly shown by the Framingham data, systolic elevations pose a risk equal to or greater than diastolic elevations.[7] Even isolated systolic hypertension is a risk, particularly for stroke[9] (Table 26–2), but we remain uncertain about both the value of and the techniques for its treatment. The need for greater certainty with regard to the management of such patients is obvious, since as many as one-third of people over 65 have isolated systolic hypertension.[10]

A particular problem may cause falsely high readings in the elderly. Markedly sclerotic vessels may not be occluded until very high pressures are exerted by sphygmoma-

TABLE 26–1 GUIDELINES IN MEASURING BLOOD PRESSURE

I. Conditions for the patient
  A. Posture
    1. For initial reading, patient should be supine for 5 minutes; take blood pressure in both arms and, in patients below age 20, one leg. Thereafter take readings immediately and 2 minutes after the patient stands.
    2. For routine follow-up, patient should sit quietly for 5 minutes and the arm should be supported at the level of the heart.
    3. For patients receiving therapy, occasionally check for postural changes.
  B. Circumstances
    1. No caffeine for preceding hour.
    2. No smoking for preceding 15 minutes.
    3. No exogenous adrenergic stimulants, e.g., phenylephrine in nasal decongestants or eye drops for pupillary dilation.
    4. A quiet, warm setting.
    5. Home readings under varying circumstances, may be preferable and more accurate in predicting subsequent cardiovascular morbidity.*
II. Equipment
  A. Cuff size: preferably the bladder should encircle and cover two thirds of the length of the arm; if not, place the bladder over the brachial artery; if bladder is too small, spuriously high readings may result.†
  B. Manometer: anaeroid gauges should be calibrated every 6 months against a mercury manometer.
  C. For infants, use equipment employing ultrasound, e.g., the Doppler method.
III. Technique
  A. Number of readings
    1. Initially, take three readings, separated by as much time as is practical, on three different days.
    2. Thereafter, or with higher initial readings, take at least two readings.
    3. Anticipate considerable variability; readings must vary by at least 10 mm Hg to be significantly different; if variation exceeds 10 mm Hg, take additional readings.
  B. Performance
    1. Inflate the bladder quickly to a pressure of 20 mm Hg above the systolic, as recognized by disappearance of the radial pulse.
    2. Deflate the bladder 3 mm Hg every second.
    3. Record the Korotkoff phase V (disappearance) except in children, in whom use of phase IV (muffling) is advocated
    4. If Korotkoff sounds are weak, have the patient raise the arm and open and close the hand 5 to 10 times, after which the bladder should be inflated quickly.

*Ibrahim, M. M., et al.: Electrocardiogram in evaluation of resistance of antihypertensive therapy. Arch. Intern. Med. *137*:1125, 1977. Copyright 1977, American Medical Association.

†Nielsen, P. E., and Janniche, H.: The accuracy of auscultatory measurement of arm blood pressure in very obese subjects. Acta Med. Scand. *195*:403, 1974.

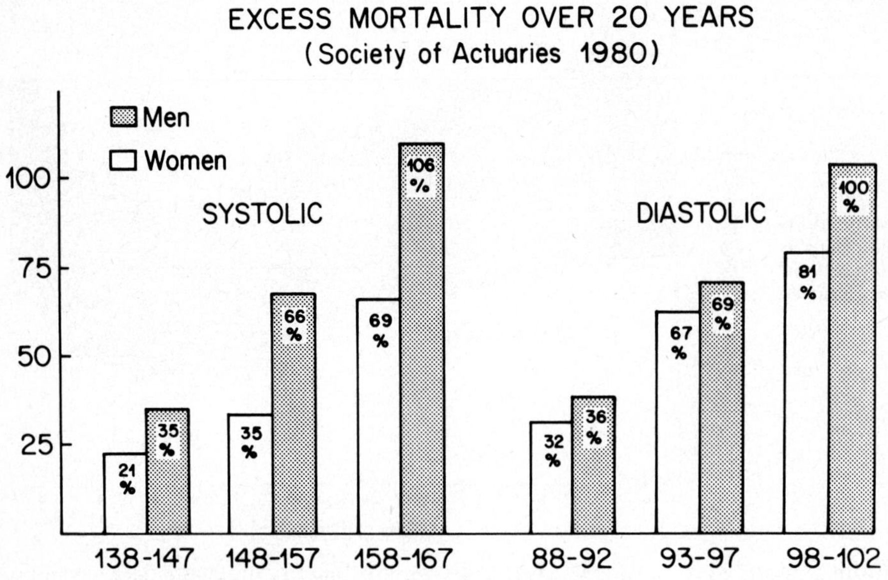

FIGURE 26–3 Excess mortality observed over 20 years by initial systolic and diastolic blood pressures among 4.5 million men and women who obtained life insurance. (From Society of Actuaries: Blood Pressure Study, 1979. Recording and Statistical Corp., 1980.)

nometry, so that indirect readings may be considerably higher than those found on direct intraarterial measurement.[11] In patients with high readings but no hypertensive retinopathy, cardiac hypertrophy, or other evidence of longstanding hypertension, "pseudohypertension" should be suspected before treatment is begun.

5. If the pressures taken repeatedly are coming down, home recordings may be particularly useful to document the course of changes in blood pressure. Home readings will likely be 5 to 10 mm Hg lower than those taken in the office and often show a progressive fall with time.[12]

6. For the individual patient, the diagnosis of definite hypertension should be made when most readings are at a level known to be associated with a significantly higher cardiovascular risk without treatment. Life insurance actuarial data indicate that mortality is increased significantly when blood pressure levels are above the following:

Men below age 45	140/90 mm Hg
Men above age 45	140/95 mm Hg
Women at any age	150/95 mm Hg

Although these limits are below the "official" level designated by the World Health Organization, i.e., 160/95, they may, in fact, be too high: in Framingham, persons with casual blood pressure measurements between 140/90 and 160/95 had a doubled risk of cardiovascular disease over the subsequent 18 years.[7]

Even lower levels may, in the future, be used to define hypertension. When the risk for major coronary events by the level of diastolic blood pressure was determined for over 7000 white American men ages 40 to 59, a 52 per cent increase in relative risk was noted for those in the middle quintile, whose diastolic pressures were between 80 and 87, compared to patients with diastolic pressures below 80 mm Hg[13] (Table 26–3). These men had no clinical evidence of heart disease at entry and were followed for 8.6 years. On the basis of these findings, those with diastolic pressures above 85 mm Hg should be advised that they may be at increased risk and counseled to follow better health habits, hopefully to lessen the progression toward definite hypertension.

BORDERLINE HYPERTENSION

In view of the usual changeability of the blood pressure, the term "labile" is inappropriate for describing diastolic pressures that exceed 90 mm Hg only occasionally. Instead, the term "borderline" should be used. In many patients, initial diastolic readings are above 90 mm Hg but subsequent readings, taken soon after, will be well below this value. In the Hypertension Detection and Follow-up Program, 29 per cent of blacks and 39 per cent of whites displayed this pattern.[14] In a screening program, 52 per cent of the adults whose initial readings were over 90 mm Hg had subsequent readings below this value, with such lability most prevalent in young white men.[15] Even a larger number of children with initially high readings will be nor-

TABLE 26–2 RISK OF STROKE OVER 24 YEARS OF FOLLOW-UP IN FRAMINGHAM (MEN AND WOMEN, AGES 50 TO 79, WITH DIASTOLIC BLOOD PRESSURE BELOW 95 MM HG)

	Men		Women	
Systolic BP	*Population at Risk (Person-Years)*	*Age Adjusted Rate/1000 in 2 Years*	*Population at Risk (Person-Years)*	*Age Adjusted Rate/1000 in 2 Years*
140	6,735	5.3	7,827	3.8
140 to 159	1,816	7.4	2,894	6.6
160	544	21.0	1,295	9.6

Data from Kannel, W. B., et al.: Systolic blood pressure, arterial rigidity and risk of stroke. J.A.M.A. *245*:1225, 1981.

TABLE 26–3 THE 8.6-YEAR RISK FOR MAJOR CORONARY EVENTS IN 7054 WHITE MEN BY DIASTOLIC BLOOD PRESSURE AT ENTRY

DIASTOLIC BP AT ENTRY*	ADJUSTED RATE OF MAJOR CORONARY EVENTS PER 1000	RELATIVE RISK	ABSOLUTE EXCESS RISK PER 1000
Below 80 (Quintiles 1 and 2)	66.0	1.0	—
80 to 87 (Quintile 3)	100.6	1.52	34.6
88 to 95 (Quintile 4)	109.4	1.66	43.4
Above 95 (Quintile 5)	143.3	2.17	77.3

*The blood pressure ranges varied slightly for various 5-year age groups: 40 to 44, 45 to 49, and so on.

Data from The Pooling Project Research Group. J. Chron. Dis. *31*:201, 1978.

mal on repeat examinations. One large survey found fewer than 1 per cent with persistent elevations, although 13 per cent had high readings initially.[16]

It is probably best to advise such patients that their blood pressure level is "borderline" and should be checked annually while they follow general hygienic measures. Long-time tracking of patients with such transient hypertension has not been sufficient to provide firm data regarding the likelihood that persistent hypertension will develop. The available evidence suggests that this likelihood is greater, but long-term followup studies have shown that persistently elevated blood pressure develops in only about 20 per cent of such cases.[17]

HYPERTENSION IN CHILDREN AND ADOLESCENTS
(See also pp. 891 and 1055)

The caution advised in handling adults with transient or borderline hypertension is even more necessary in dealing with children. Now that the blood pressure of large numbers of normal children have been measured and the data have been made available,[18] those with single readings above the 95th percentile might be considered abnormal. However, the Task Force on Blood Pressure Control in Children has wisely warned against premature labeling of such children as hypertensive, since long-time tracking of those with such levels is only now being carried out.[19] Those with levels above the 95th percentile on at least three separate occasions are considered to have "sustained elevated blood pressure," whereas those with only one such reading are said to have "high normal blood pressure."[18] Appropriate management for asymptomatic children with sustained elevated blood pressure has not been settled. Although most maintain similarly high readings over three- to four-year periods, many become normotensive.[20] Such patients should be carefully followed, with particular emphasis placed on weight reduction in the hope of preventing progression of the disease.

Frequency of Hypertension

As we have come to recognize the usual—and often considerable—variability of blood pressure, we also recognize the wisdom of the late Sir George Pickering, who repeatedly warned against artificially classifying patients as "normotensive" or "hypertensive" on the basis of a single reading.[21] Obviously, the level chosen to divide the population greatly affects the number of people considered hypertensive. In a large screening program of a representative population, the percentage of hypertensive individuals was 18 per cent using 160/95 mm Hg as the dividing line but rose to 38 per cent if the level 140/90 was used.[22]

Most surveys have assigned 160/95 mm Hg as the minimum blood pressure level denoting hypertension for adults. The levels used to define hypertension in the previous section are lower, but this diagnosis should be based on multiple readings taken under more controlled circumstances. Even using the higher number, which is likely to underestimate the number of younger people at risk, hypertension is common, and its frequency increases with the age of the population (Fig. 26–4). The incidence of hypertension among blacks is greater at every age beyond adolescence and a given level of hypertension tends to induce more vascular damage in blacks than in whites, even though systemic hemodynamics are similar in the two races.[23]

Among the large number of people with hypertension, it is helpful to know whether some secondary process, hopefully curable by operation or more easily controlled by a specific drug, is likely to be present. In this way, the clinician can determine whether more definitive diagnostic testing is in order (Table 26–4). In many of the secondary forms, the hypertension is often obviously related to the underlying disease and therefore of little diagnostic or therapeutic concern. Our attention will be directed toward those forms that more often enter into the differential diagnosis of hypertension because of their frequency or their lack of readily apparent distinguishing features.

Most surveys to determine the relative proportion of various secondary diseases are biased by the prior selection process, with only the increasingly suspect population "funneled" to an investigator interested in that disease. By this means, estimates as high as 20 per cent for certain secondary forms of hypertension have been published, but these should not be applied to the population at large.

Two surveys highlight the problem: Among 236 patients referred to a medical center for an extensive evaluation to detect secondary diseases, 16 per cent were found to have renovascular hypertension and 12 per cent primary aldosteronism.[24] On the other hand, markedly lower figures were obtained when an estimate was made of the total number of hypertensive patients seen at the Mayo Clinic and related to the number of surgical procedures performed over a three-year period.[25] Only 0.18 per cent underwent surgery for renovascular hypertension, and 0.01 per cent for primary aldosteronism. Although these figures are too low, since not all patients were adequately tested and not all those identified underwent surgery, they may be closer

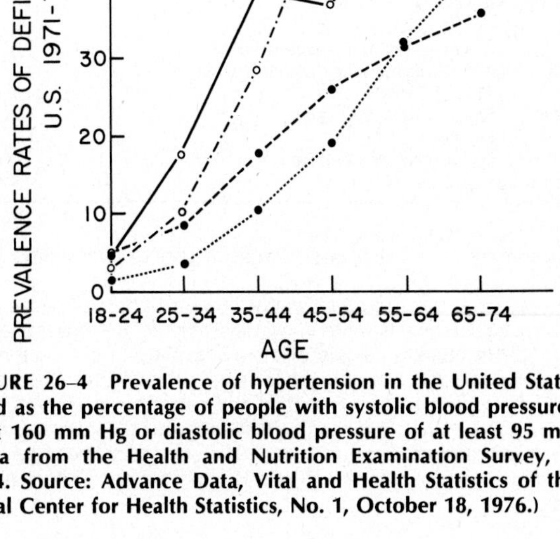

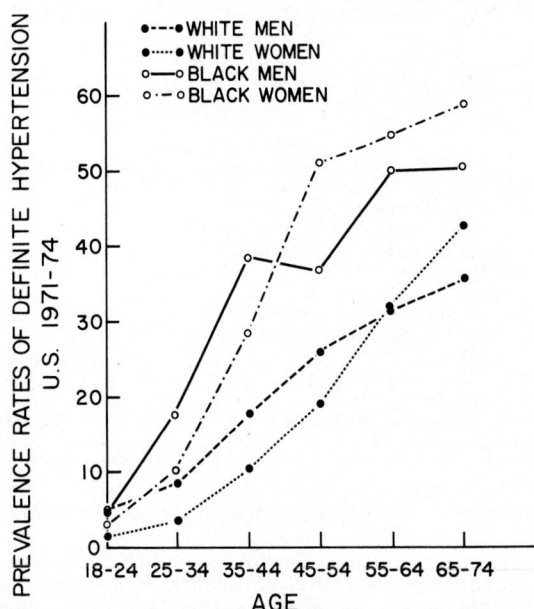

FIGURE 26–4 Prevalence of hypertension in the United States defined as the percentage of people with systolic blood pressure of at least 160 mm Hg or diastolic blood pressure of at least 95 mm Hg. (Data from the Health and Nutrition Examination Survey, 1971–1974. Source: Advance Data, Vital and Health Statistics of the National Center for Health Statistics, No. 1, October 18, 1976.)

TABLE 26–4 TYPES OF HYPERTENSION

I. Systolic and diastolic hypertension
- A. Primary, essential, or idiopathic
- B. Secondary
  1. Renal
     - a. Renal parenchymal disease
       - (1) Acute glomerulonephritis
       - (2) Chronic nephritis
       - (3) Polycystic disease
       - (4) Connective tissue diseases
       - (5) Diabetic nephropathy
       - (6) Hydronephrosis
     - b. Renovascular
     - c. Renin-producing tumors
     - d. Renoprival
     - e. Primary sodium retention (Liddle's syndrome, Gordon's syndrome)
  2. Endocrine
     - a. Acromegaly
     - b. Hypothyroidism
     - c. Hypercalcemia
     - d. Hyperthyroidism
     - e. Adrenal
       - (1) Cortical
         - (a) Cushing's syndrome
         - (b) Primary aldosteronism
         - (c) Congenital adrenal hyperplasia
       - (2) Medullary: pheochromocytoma
     - f. Extraadrenal chromaffin tumors
     - g. Carcinoid
     - h. Exogenous hormones
       - (1) Estrogen
       - (2) Glucocorticoids
       - (3) Mineralocorticoids: licorice, carbenexolone
       - (4) Sympathomimetics
       - (5) Tyramine-containing foods and MAO inhibitors
  3. Coarctation of the aorta
  4. Pregnancy-induced hypertension
  5. Neurological disorders
     - a. Increased intracranial pressure
       - (1) Brain tumor
       - (2) Encephalitis
       - (3) Respiratory acidosis: lung or CNS disease
     - b. Quadriplegia
     - c. Acute porphyria
     - d. Familial dysautonomia
     - e. Lead poisoning
     - f. Guillain-Barré syndrome
  6. Acute stress, including surgery
     - a. Psychogenic hyperventilation
     - b. Hypoglycemia
     - c. Burns
     - d. Pancreatitis
     - e. Alcohol withdrawal
     - f. Sickle cell crisis
     - g. Postresuscitation
     - h. Postoperative
  7. Increased intravascular volume
  8. Drugs and other substances

II. Systolic hypertension
- A. Increased cardiac output
  1. Aortic valvular regurgitation
  2. AV fistula, patent ductus
  3. Thyrotoxicosis
  4. Paget's disease of bone
  5. Beriberi
  6. Hyperkinetic circulation
- B. Rigidity of aorta

to what primary care practitioners might expect to find among their patients.

Estimates more likely to be indicative of the numbers of cases usually seen in clinical practice are shown in Table 26–5.[26-28] Berglund et al.[26] surveyed a random sample of the 47- to 54-year-old men in Göteborg, Sweden, who were found to have a blood pressure above 175/115 mm Hg, so that both women and milder hypertensives were excluded. Even though secondary forms are more common among those with more severe hypertension, 94 per cent of these patients with diastolic readings above 115 mm Hg had primary (essential) hypertension.

TABLE 26–5 FREQUENCY OF VARIOUS DIAGNOSES IN HYPERTENSIVE SUBJECTS

Diagnosis	Berglund	Rudnick	Danielson
Essential hypertension	94%	94%	95.3%
Chronic renal disease	4%	5%	2.4%
Renovascular disease	1%	0.2%	1.0%
Coarctation	0.1%	0.2%	
Primary aldosteronism	0.1%		0.1%
Cushing's syndrome		0.2%	0.1%
Pheochromocytoma			0.2%
Oral contraceptive–induced	(Men only)	0.2%	0.8%
Number of patients	689	665	1000

From Berglund, G., et al.: Br. Med. J. *2*:554, 1976; Rudnick, K. V., et al.: Can. Med. Assoc. J. *117*:492, 1977; Danielson, M., and Dammström, B.: Acta Med. Scand. *209*:451, 1981.

A closer approximation of usual medical practice is the survey by Rudnick et al.[27] in which the patients were middle-class whites seen in a family practice in Hamilton, Canada, from 1965 to 1974. As in all three of these surveys, many of the patients underwent intravenous pyelography in addition to a history, physical examination, and routine urine and blood tests. Although a few with secondary diseases may have been missed in each of these surveys, the closeness of these data strongly support the view that in 95 per cent of all hypertensives there will be no recognizable cause.

The Changing Nature of Childhood Hypertension. Even among children, secondary hypertension is less common than indicated by previous surveys of hospital-based populations. As more apparently normal children are being screened and more are found to be hypertensive, the clinical presentation of childhood hypertension is changing from that of a rare and serious disease, usually related to renal damage, to a fairly common and usually asymptomatic process, in most cases without recognizable cause.[19] Many prepubertal hypertensive children do not have underlying secondary diseases, whereas most recognized after puberty have idiopathic hypertension.

The Need for Selectivity in Screening Tests. Because of the relatively low frequency of these various secondary diseases, selectivity in performing the various screening and diagnostic tests is warranted. The presence of features "inappropriate" for hypertension (Table 26–6) indicates the need for additional tests. However, for 9 of the 10 hypertensive patients in whom these features are absent, a hematocrit, urine analysis, automated blood biochemical profile (including plasma glucose, potassium, creatinine, and cholesterol), and an electrocardiogram are all that is required.

Although some would include other tests, the greater the number of screening tests done for relatively rare diseases, the more likely a false-positive result will arise. Based on Bayes' theorem (p. 273), which relates the predictive value of tests to their sensitivity and specificity of detection and the prevalence of the disease, and using a prevalence rate of 2 per cent for renovascular hypertension, an intravenous pyelogram (IVP) suggestive of renal hypertension has only a 10 per cent predictive value for that diagnosis.[29]

The practitioner is well-advised to limit the application of the IVP and other screening tests to those relatively few patients with suspicious features on initial history, physical examination, and laboratory testing, so that the predictive value of a positive test will justify its

TABLE 26–6 FEATURES OF "INAPPROPRIATE" HYPERTENSION

1. Onset before age 20 or after age 50 years
2. Level of blood pressure > 180/110 mm Hg
3. Organ damage
   - a. Funduscopic findings of Grade 2 or higher
   - b. Serum creatinine > 1.5 mg/100 ml
   - c. Cardiomegaly (on x-ray or echocardiogram) or left ventricular hypertrophy (on electrocardiogram)
4. Features indicative of secondary causes
   - a. Unprovoked hypokalemia
   - b. Abdominal bruit
   - c. Variable pressures with tachycardia, sweating, tremor
   - d. Family history of renal disease
5. Poor response to therapy that is usually effective

use. Thus, among children, in whom renal hypertension is much more prevalent, addition of the IVP to "routine" testing enabled recognition of all those cases due to secondary causes.[30] However, in adults without features suggestive of renovascular hypertension (i.e., young age, severe hypertension, abdominal bruit), an abnormal IVP is more likely to be a false-positive result rather than a true-positive, indicative of a specific diagnosis.[4]

Natural History of Untreated Hypertension

Knowledge about the natural history of the disease must be gleaned from what has already been reported. Since the efficacy of antihypertensive therapy has been proved, simply observing large numbers of hypertensives for prolonged periods without instituting suitable therapy is no longer ethical. However, useful information about the shorter-term effects of untreated hypertension (3 to 5 years) has been obtained from the placebo-treated controls in recently completed trials of therapy for mild hypertension.

SYMPTOMS AND SIGNS

Because uncomplicated hypertension is almost always asymptomatic, people may be unaware for as long as 10 to 20 years that their elevated blood pressure is causing progressive cardiovascular damage. Only if blood pressure measurements are made frequently and people are made aware that, even if they are asymptomatic, hypertension is harmful will the remaining 50 per cent of Americans with hypertension that is unrecognized or inadequately treated be managed effectively.

Symptoms often attributed to hypertension, i.e., headache, nosebleed, tinnitus, dizziness, and fainting, may be seen just as commonly among normotensive people.[31] Headache is usually considered the most frequent and bothersome symptom. Some believe it to be related to the disease,[32] while others believe that it is largely nonspecific, often psychogenic, and more likely to be identified among hypertensive patients because they are more likely to be asked about the symptom. In a survey among people still unaware that they had hypertension, 16 per cent had headaches; among patients aware of their hypertension, receiving no therapy, and otherwise similar to those who were unaware, 74 per cent had headaches, mostly attributable to anxiety.[33] After reviewing the literature and his own experience in Australia, Bauer concludes that "headache appears to be a signal of a sociopsychological disorder rather than a truly hypertensive symptom. It is often precipitated or aggravated by the recognition of hypertension. . . . Symptomatic relief does not relate to blood pressure lowering, but to reassurance, suggestion, and cessation of analgesic abuse."[34]

Nocturia and postural unsteadiness were the only other symptoms more commonly noted among untreated hypertensives in the British series.[32]

COURSE OF THE DISEASE WITHOUT TREATMENT

As noted in Table 26–3, the presence of even minimal hypertension is accompanied by significant increases in coronary disease and mortality. Careful observations of the Framingham cohort clearly portray the increased risks for various types of cardiovascular diseases over many years among those with hypertension (Fig. 26–5).

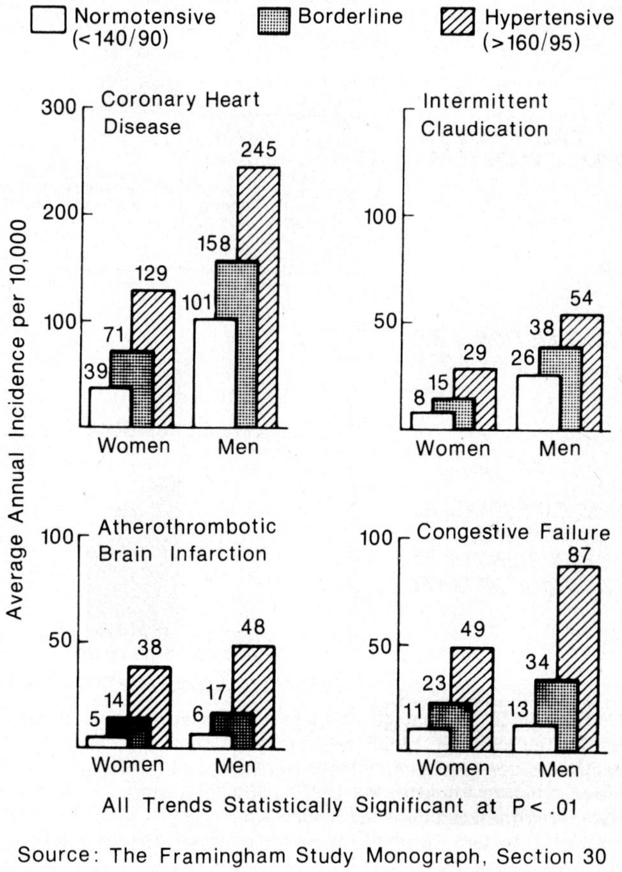

FIGURE 26–5 Risks of coronary heart disease, intermittent claudication, atherothrombotic brain infarction, and congestive failure for women and men ages 45 to 74 in the Framingham cohort, based upon the blood pressure status at each biennial exam over an 18-year follow-up (From Kannel, W. B., and Sorlie, P.: Hypertension in Framingham. *In* Paul, O. (ed.): Epidemiology and Control of Hypertension. Miami, Symposia Specialists, 1975, p. 558.)

But these figures may be misleading, since they seem to imply that most hypertensives, including those with minimally elevated pressures, will get into trouble, and rather quickly. Remember that the actuarial data shown in Figure 26–3 are percentages of *excess* mortality, relative to the experiences of the entire insured population. The fact that men whose initial diastolic pressure was in the range of 88 to 92 mm Hg had a 36 per cent increased mortality does not mean that 36 per cent of these men died, from hypertension or any other cause. Similarly, the data shown in Table 26–3, which includes part of the Framingham cohort, indicate that those white men with diastolic pressures of 80 to 87 mm Hg had a 52 per cent greater relative risk of having a major coronary event over an 8.6-year period but not that 52 per cent did, in fact, have such an event. A large majority of hypertensives portrayed in both sets of data did not die or suffer a coronary event.

Nonetheless, because there are so many people with hypertension, the fact that even a minority of them will suffer a premature cardiovascular catastrophe in the course of their disease makes hypertension a major societal problem. In fact, when the death rates for various levels of diastolic blood pressure are multiplied by the proportion of people in the population who have these various levels, the majority of excess deaths attributable to hypertension are clearly

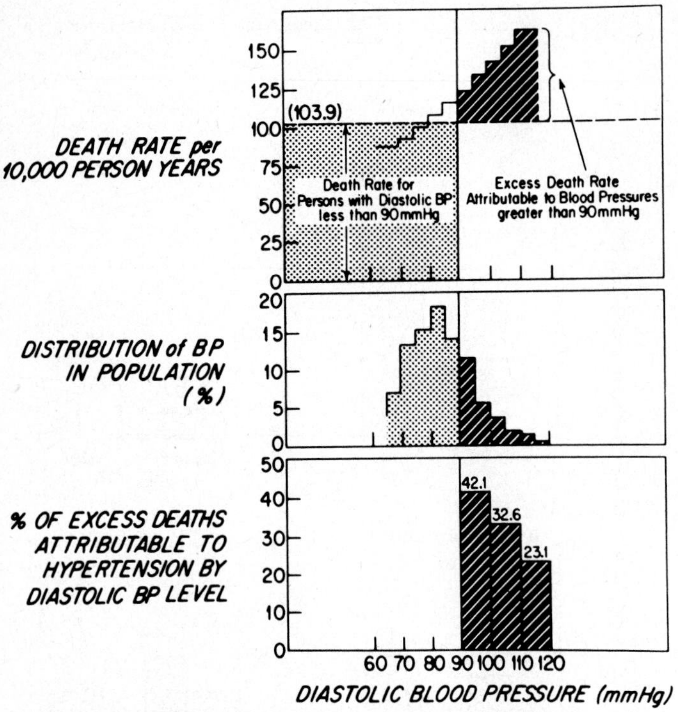

FIGURE 26–6 **Percentage of excess deaths attributable to hypertension by diastolic blood pressure level (*bottom*), based on the death rate observed in Framingham (*top*) and the distribution of the blood pressure found in the HDFP population (*middle*). (From The Hypertension Detection and Follow-up Program. Circ. Res. *40*:I–106, 1977, by permission of the American Heart Association, Inc.)**

shown to occur among those with the minimally elevated pressures[35] (Fig. 26–6).

As the public and the medical profession have become aware of the overall societal consequences of even "mild" hypertension, enthusiasm for its early recognition and aggressive treatment has been generated. This enthusiasm for therapy was apparent even before definitive evidence was available that treatment would relieve some of these risks. In 1978, prior to publication of the results of any large-scale trials of therapy for mild hypertension, 92 per cent of physicians surveyed in New York indicated that they prescribed antihypertensive drugs for asymptomatic patients with a diastolic pressure of 90 to 104 mm Hg.[36]

A closer look at the issue of deciding upon the need for therapy will be provided in the next chapter. However, further consideration of the natural course of hypertension—as it applies to the individual patient—is needed in order to answer a basic question: Is the blood pressure high enough to justify medical intervention? Unless the risk is high enough to mandate some form of intervention there seems no need to identify and label the person as hypertensive, since psychological and socioeconomic burdens accompany this label; unless risks clearly outweigh these burdens, caution is obviously advised. A cogent view of this issue has been offered by Geoffrey Rose[37]:

> As doctors we are trained to feel responsible for patients—that is, to care for the sick; and from that position accepting responsibility for those with major risk factors is not too difficult a transition. They are almost patients. A general practitioner, say, makes a routine measurement of a man's blood pressure and finds it raised. Thereafter both the man and the doctor will say that he 'suffers' from high blood pressure. He walked in a healthy man but he walks out a patient, and his newfound status is confirmed by the giving and receiving of tablets. An inappropriate label has been accepted because both public and professional feel that if the man were not a patient the doctor would have no business treating him. In reality the care of the symptomless hypertensive person is preventive medicine, not therapeutics.

Rose would certainly not deny the benefits of preventive medicine but he goes on to emphasize the need for great caution in applying preventive measures to large groups of people:

> If a preventive measure exposes many people to a small risk, the harm it does may readily—as in the case of clofibrate—outweigh the benefits, since these are received by relatively few. . . . We may thus be unable to identify that small level of harm to individuals from long-term intervention that would be sufficient to make that line of prevention unprofitable or even harmful. Consequently we cannot accept long-term mass preventive medication.[37]

We are thus left with a dilemma: for the mass of hypertensives, even those with the least elevated pressures, there is an increased risk; for the individual hypertensive, the risk may not justify the labeling or treatment of the condition.

ASSESSMENT OF INDIVIDUAL RISK

Guidelines to help the practitioner resolve this dilemma in dealing with the individual patient are available, based upon the overall assessment of cardiovascular risk and the biological aggressiveness of the hypertension. These guidelines are intended to apply only to those with "mild" hypertension, as defined in the HDFP as diastolic pressure between 90 and 104 mm Hg; those with diastolic levels persistently above 105 mm Hg have been shown to be at high enough risk from the hypertension per se to justify immediate intervention.[38]

Overall Cardiovascular Risk. The Framingham study and other epidemiological surveys have clearly defined certain risk factors for premature cardiovascular disease beyond hypertension (see Chap. 35). For varying levels of blood pressure, the Framingham data show the increasing likelihood of a vascular event over the next eight years for both men and women at various ages as more and more risk factors are added (Fig. 26–7). Notice that a 40-year-old man with a systolic blood pressure of 195 mm Hg who is otherwise at low risk would have a 4.6 per cent chance of developing a vascular event in the next eight years. A man of the same age with the same pressure but with all the additional risk factors has a 70.8 per cent chance. Obviously the higher the overall risk, the more intensive the interventions should be.

Target Organ Damage. The biological aggressiveness of a given level of hypertension varies between individuals. This inherent propensity to induce vascular damage can be ascertained best by examination of the eyes, heart, and kidney.

Funduscopic Examination. As described by Keith, Wagener, and Barker in 1939, vascular changes in the fundus reflect both hypertensive neuroretinopathy and arteriosclerotic retinopathy.[39] The two processes first induce narrowing of the arteriolar lumen (Grade 1) and then sclerosis of the adventitia and/or thickening of the arteriolar

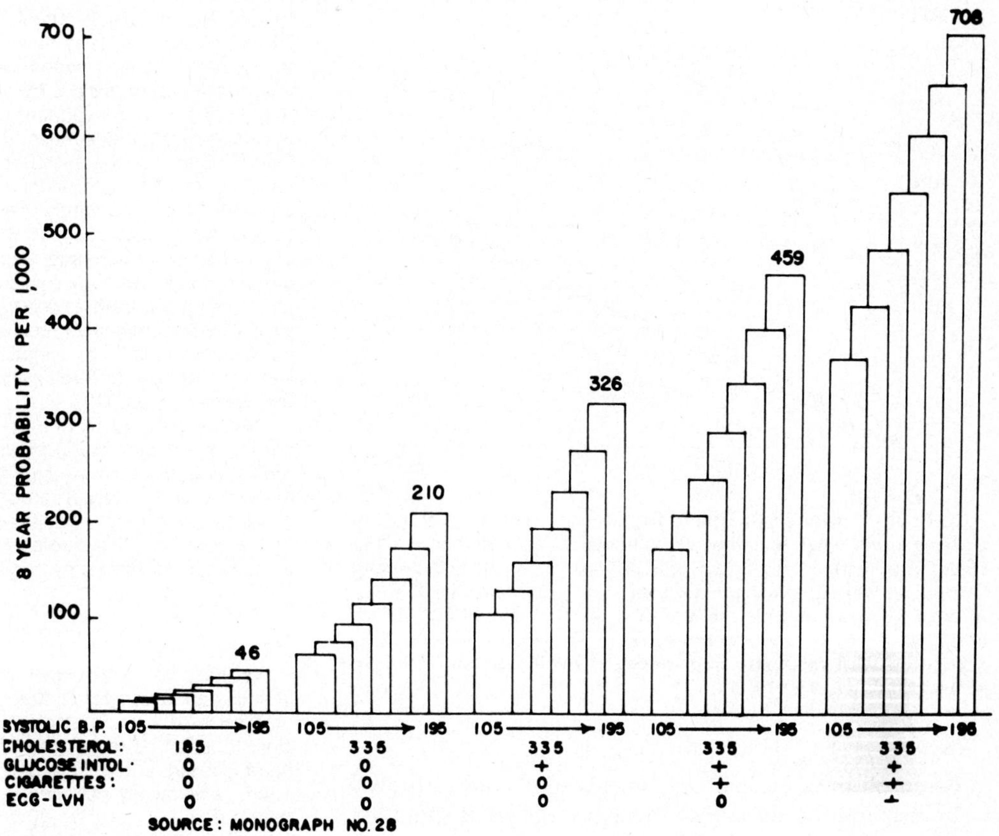

FIGURE 26–7 The 8-year risk of cardiovascular disease for 40-year-old men in Framingham according to progressively higher systolic blood pressure at specified levels of other risk factors. (From Kannel, W. B.: *In* Genest, J., et al. (eds.): Hypertension: Physiopathology and Treatment. Copyright © 1977 McGraw-Hill Book Company. Used with the permission of McGraw-Hill Book Company.)

wall, visible as arteriovenous nicking (Grade 2). With progressive arteriosclerosis, the vein becomes invisible below the arteriole and then completely obstructed. Progressive hypertension induces rupture of small vessels, seen as hemorrhages and exudates (Grade 3) and eventually papilledema (Grade 4) (see Fig. 2–2, p. 18).

Among 855 50-year old men followed for 12.5 years, attenuated arterioles and focal narrowing were found to be closely related to the presence of hypertension and subsequent mortality from strokes, whereas crossing defects were more predictive of mortality from arteriosclerotic diseases.[40]

Cardiac Involvement. Evidence of cardiac involvement includes the following:

1. Left ventricular hypertrophy on electrocardiography, based on increased voltage of QRS complexes, intrinsicoid deflection over V_5 or V_6 greater than 0.06 sec, and ST-segment depression greater than 0.5 mm (Chap. 7).

2. Left ventricular enlargement on x-ray (Chap. 6) or echocardiography (Chap. 5). Echocardiograms are more sensitive in recognizing early cardiac involvement; in 234 patients with mild to moderate hypertension (mean BP = 150/95 mm Hg), 61 per cent had an echocardiographic abnormality.[41]

3. Changes indicative of coronary artery disease.

4. Manifestations of left ventricular failure.

In Framingham, electrocardiographic evidence of left ventricular hypertrophy was a serious prognostic sign: 32 per cent of men with this finding succumbed to a cardiovascular catastrophe within five years, and congestive failure occurred 10 times more commonly.[7]

Renal Function. Renal dysfunction, too subtle to be recognized, is likely responsible for the development of most hypertension. As will be discussed, increased renal retention of salt and water may be a mechanism initiating idiopathic hypertension, but the increase is so small that it escapes detection. With detailed study, including arteriography[42] and biopsy,[43] both structural damage and functional derangement can be found in almost all hypertensive individuals, even in those with apparently early, mild disease. In patients with longstanding hypertension, creatinine clearance may be decreased, albumin may be found in the urine, and a loss of concentrating ability may be manifested by nocturia. As hypertension-induced nephrosclerosis proceeds, the plasma creatinine level begins to rise, and eventually renal insufficiency with uremia develops in 10 to 20 per cent of patients. Prognosis can be closely related to the degree of renal damage[44] (Fig. 26–8).

Renin as a Prognostic Guide. In 1972, data were published showing that a group of hypertensives with low levels of plasma renin activity (PRA) had a more benign course, with no heart attacks or strokes uncovered on retrospective analysis.[45] Subsequently, many investigators have examined the relationship between renin levels and cardiovascular complications, and with very few exceptions, patients with low PRA have been found to have no more benign a course than do those with normal PRA.[46] Indeed, in a five-year prospective study, patients with initially low renin levels suffered as many heart attacks and strokes as those with normal levels, but when a cardiovascular complication appeared, initially low renin levels tended to rise.[47] This sequence may provide a rational explanation for the finding in the retrospective study of Brunner et al.,[45] since patients whose initially low renin levels rose after a complication would not have been recognized retrospectively.

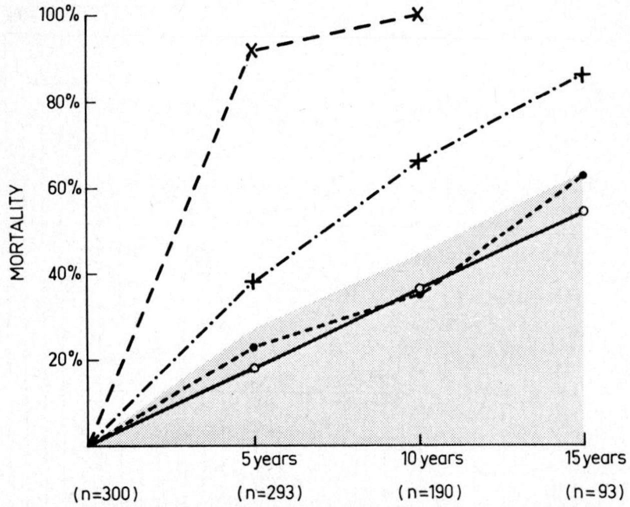

FIGURE 26–8 Mortality graph of hypertensive patients with normal and impaired renal function, all followed and treated in a single clinic. The shaded area is the mortality curve for all 300 patients. ○—○ = Normal renal function; ●- - -● = proteinuria; X·---X = BUN of 21 to 44 mg/100 ml; X- - -X = BUN above 45 mg/100 ml. (From Bauer, G. E., and Humphrey, T. J.: The natural history of hypertension with moderate impairment of renal function. Clin. Sci. Molec. Med. *45*:191s, 1973.)

Based on these various assessments of overall cardiovascular risk and the severity of the hypertension, it should be possible to determine the approximate status and prognosis for individual patients.

The Short-Term Course of Low-Risk Hypertension. The data on the four-year experiences of over 1600 "low-risk" hypertensives who served as the controls in the Australian Therapeutic Trial document the validity of this assessment.[48] For patients to enter this placebo-versus-drug trial—the largest yet reported—the second set of diastolic pressures had to be between 95 and 109 mm Hg and they had to be free of all identifiable cardiovascular disease. They can therefore be considered "low-risk" hypertensives.

Over the next four years, in the majority of these patients, who were given placebo tablets but neither nondrug nor drug therapy, blood pressures dropped progressively, from an average of 157/102 to 144/91 mm Hg. The diastolic pressure was below 95 mm Hg in 47.5 per cent at the end of the trial. The fall in blood pressure was not related to any recognizable change in the patient's status. Similar decreases occurred in those whose weight went up or down or stayed the same.[49] It is of great interest that no excess morbidity or mortality occurred among those whose diastolic pressures stayed below 100 mm Hg.

These results strongly support the view that certain patients can be characterized as being at relatively low risk and can therefore safely do without drug therapy long enough to allow one to observe the course of their blood pressure and, if indicated, the effectiveness of nondrug therapies. The large number of patients whose pressures fell and the large average degree of fall may seem surprising, but unlike most other trials, none of these patients started with any identifiable cardiovascular disease or complications of their hypertension. Moreover, placebo may be more effective than no therapy. Similar results were observed in a smaller trial of male patients free of target organ damage who had diastolic pressures below 110 mm Hg and were followed for three years and given no placebo pills.[50] About half the nontreated group exhibited a fall in diastolic pressure, and relatively little trouble developed in those with pressures initially below 100 mm Hg.

The Potential for Progression. As comforting as these data are about the short-term benignity of "low-risk" hypertension, it should be noted that the diastolic blood pressure rose above 110 mm Hg in 12.2 per cent of the nondrug-treated patients in the Australian trial[48] and in 17.2 per cent of those in the Oslo trial.[50] Levels above 110 mm Hg demand immediate attention, so that continual monitoring of the blood pressure levels is obviously needed for all patients with even the mildest "low-risk" hypertension.

A Synthesis of Risk. Taken altogether, the data indicate that the degree of risk from hypertension can be categorized with reasonable accuracy, taking into account the level of the blood pressure, the biological nature of the hypertension as assessed from target organ function, and the coexistence of other risks. Although there is increased risk for the hypertensive population as a whole, most of the trouble will develop in those with higher levels of pressure, considerable target organ damage, and other risk factors. For them, immediate and "aggressive" reduction of pressure seems indicated. But for the majority, who are at relatively low risk, the more reasonable approach is to continue to monitor the blood pressure while encouraging healthy habits, i.e., weight control, moderate sodium restriction, isotonic exercise, and relaxation, in hopes of slowing progression of the disease (Chap. 27).

This approach justifies the screening and identification of all persons with elevated blood pressure. Since there is no certain way to predict the course of the blood pressure, all hypertensives should be followed and the recognition of their hypertension used as motivation to follow good health habits. In this way, no harm should be done and a potentially considerable benefit gained, if progression of the disease can be slowed by nondrug therapies.

COMPLICATIONS OF HYPERTENSION

For those with "high-risk" hypertension, premature development of various cardiovascular diseases is engendered by the acceleration of atherosclerosis, the pathological hallmark of uncontrolled hypertension. If untreated, about half of hypertensive patients die of coronary heart disease, a third of stroke, and 10 to 15 per cent of renal failure. Those with rapidly accelerating hypertension die more frequently of renal failure.[4]

It is easy to underestimate the role of hypertension in producing the underlying vascular damage that leads to these cardiovascular catastrophes. Hypertension as a cause of death is recorded on fewer than 20 per cent of death certificates even though the physician is aware of its presence.[51] Death is attributed to stroke or myocardial infarction instead of to the hypertension that was largely responsible. Moreover, hypertension may not persist after a myocardial infarction or stroke.

In general, the vascular complications of hypertension can be considered to be either "hypertensive" or "atherosclerotic" (Table 26–7). Those listed as "hypertensive" are more directly caused by the increased level of the blood pressure per se and can be prevented by lowering this level. Those listed as "atherosclerotic" have more multiple causations (Chap. 35), and although hypertension may represent quantitatively the most significant of the known risk factors, lowering the blood pressure may not, by itself, prevent progression of the atherosclerotic process. As shown in Figure 26–9, the translation of elevated pressure into vascular damage may proceed by numerous pathways, some well defined (shown as solid lines) and others still uncertain (shown as dotted lines).[52]

The path from hypertension to vascular disease likely involves two interrelated processes: pulsatile flow and smooth muscle cell replication. Applying the physical principles of stress, O'Rourke[53] concludes that "one would expect that pulse pressure and maximal dP/dt would be more important in causing arterial degeneration and damage than mean arterial pressure. . . . Structural damage to the aortic media can be attributed to increases in mean pressure, pulse pressure and

TABLE 26–7 VASCULAR COMPLICATIONS OF HYPERTENSION

HYPERTENSIVE	ATHEROSCLEROTIC
Malignant phase	Coronary heart disease
Hemorrhagic stroke	Sudden death
Congestive heart failure	Other arrhythmias
Nephrosclerosis	Atherothrombotic stroke
Aortic dissection	Peripheral vascular disease

From Smith, W. M.: Treatment of mild hypertension. Results of a ten-year intervention trial. Circ. Res. *25*(Suppl. I):98, 1977, by permission of the American Heart Association, Inc.

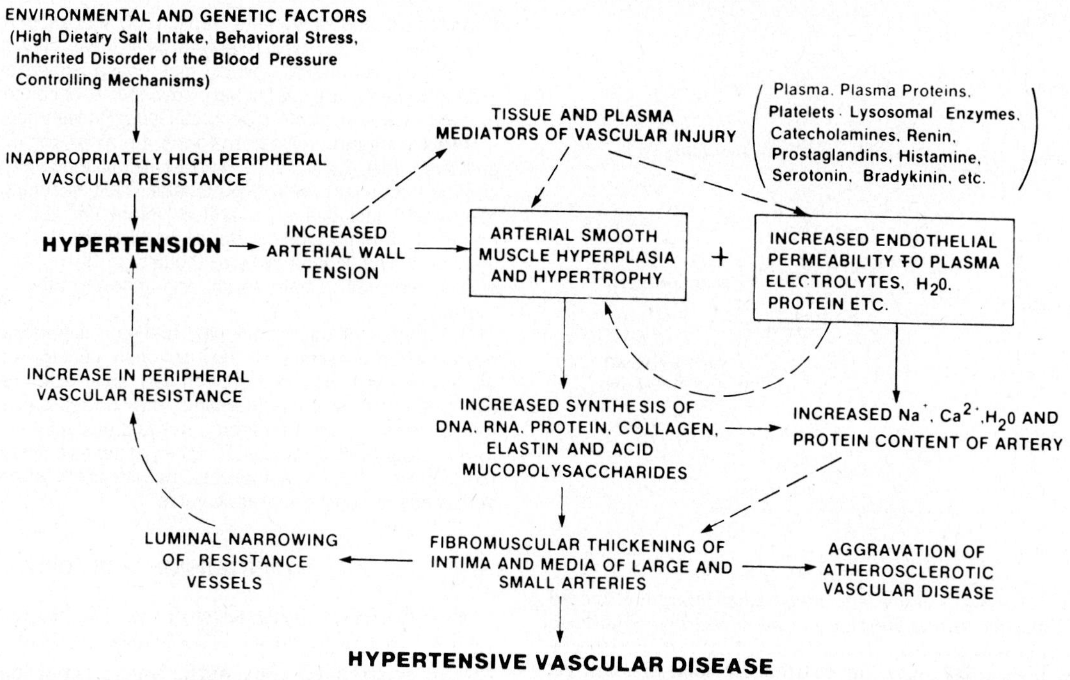

FIGURE 26–9 A unified concept of the causes and results of hypertensive vascular disease. (From Hollander, W.: Role of hypertension in atherosclerosis and cardiovascular disease. Am. J. Cardiol. *38*:786, 1976.)

dP/dt. These changes can be held responsible for medionecrosis, aneurysm formation, and for the later complications of aortic dissection and cerebral hemorrhage. Pulsatile stresses on the aortic wall are also responsible for the early intimal and subintimal changes of atheroma so that the same factors operating in hypertension can explain the increased incidence of atheroma in hypertension."

The critical importance of pulsatile flow in causing damage to vessel walls has been shown by Palmer in studies of hypertensive turkeys susceptible to aortic dissection.[54] A specific connection between these mechanical forces and the reaction by the arterial wall, which may lead to the development of atheroma, has been demonstrated in tissue taken from patients with coarctation of the aorta: arterial smooth muscle cells previously exposed to high pressure in vivo have a shorter in vitro life span, suggesting that they have already undergone an increased number of replications in response to the high pressure.[55]

Regardless of how the damage occurs, hypertension is a major factor in cardiovascular disease, as is most clearly shown in the data from Framingham (Fig. 26–5). Let us examine more closely these various cardiovascular diseases, the incidence of which is so clearly increased by hypertension.

Ischemic Heart Disease (See also p. 1216). Hypertension increases left ventricular wall tension, leading to structural, biochemical, and physiological changes in the myocardium (Fig. 26–10). These, in concert with accelerated atherosclerosis in coronary vessels, lead to ischemic heart disease manifested as angina, myocardial infarction, and sudden death. Left atrial and ventricular enlargement and dysfunction are recognized in most patients with uncomplicated hypertension, particularly by means of echocardiography.[41,56] When such overt abnormalities appear, risk of a coronary event sharply increases, as is clearly shown by the Framingham study.[7] In the 26-year Manitoba study, a rise in the level of systolic blood pressure was even more strongly associated with the incidence of ischemic heart disease than was an initially high level.[57] Moreover, survival after infarction was related to the preexisting level of the blood pressure[58] (Fig. 26–11). The improved prognosis offered by beta-adrenergic blocking drugs after myocardial infarction[59] may in part reflect their antihypertensive effects.

After myocardial infarction, hypertension may recede and never return to its previous level. In 58 hypertensive patients, blood pressure returned to normal in 37 after infarction and remained normal for up to eight weeks.[60] On the other hand, if hypertension persists, it poses a major risk of death.[61]

Congestive Heart Failure. The relationships between hypertension and congestive heart failure were clearly demonstrated in the Framingham study[62]: Hypertension was present in 75 per cent of all patients with congestive heart failure; the incidence of failure increased in both men and women at all ages as systolic or diastolic pressure increased; despite treatment, 50 per cent of those who developed congestive heart failure died within five years.

The bases for these relationships are shown in Figure 26–10. Heart

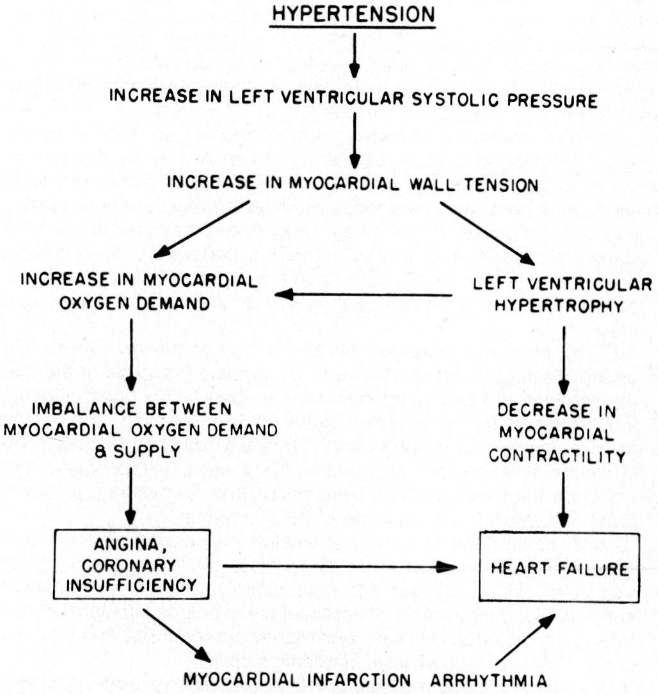

FIGURE 26–10 Adverse effects of hypertension on myocardial function. (From Hollander, W.: Role of hypertension in atherosclerosis and cardiovascular disease. Am. J. Cardiol. *38*:786, 1976.)

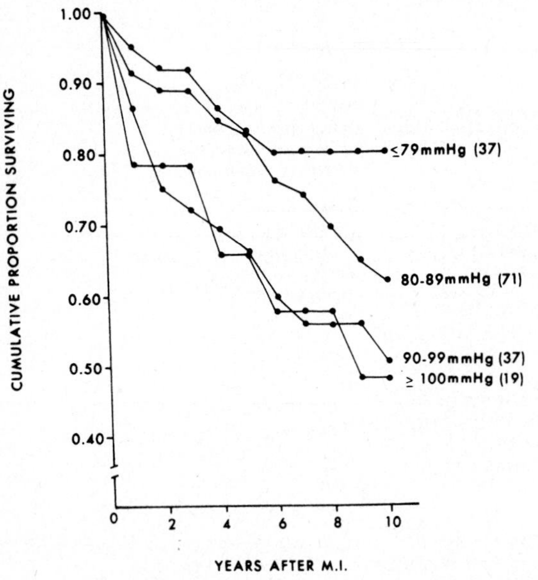

FIGURE 26–11 Survival curves after myocardial infarction according to the last diastolic blood pressure before infarction. (Number of patients shown in parentheses.) (From Rabkin, S. W., et al.: Prognosis after acute myocardial infarction: Relation to blood pressure values before infarction in a prospective cardiovascular study. Am. J. Cardiol. *40*:604, 1977.)

failure is preceded by left ventricular hypertrophy and functional impairment, with a decreased ejection rate and a prolonged tension-time index.[63] After heart failure occurs, aggressive reduction of blood pressure may be lifesaving[64]; however, the presence of hypertension in severe heart failure may be masked by the fall in blood pressure that accompanies a markedly reduced cardiac output. This sequence may be mistaken for idiopathic congestive cardiomyopathy, usually with concentric hypertrophy.[65]

Large-Vessel Disease. Occlusive vascular disease of both proximal and peripheral arteries is increased in patients with hypertension (Fig. 26–5). Presumably by accentuating atherosclerosis and medial necrosis, hypertension is also a predisposing factor in aneurysm and dissection of the aorta.[66] If the pressure is high with aortic dissection, therapy should include rapid lowering of systolic blood pressure to 100 to 120 mm Hg with a parenteral antihypertensive agent (Chap. 44).

Cerebral Vascular Disease. Hypertension is an even more potent risk factor for cerebrovascular accidents than for coronary or renal vascular disease. In Framingham, brain infarcts occurred 5 to 30 times more commonly in hypertensive than in normotensive subjects[67] (Fig. 26–5). Systolic pressures are even more predictive than are diastolic pressures,[68] and isolated systolic hypertension, so commonly seen in the elderly, is associated with a two to four times greater incidence of strokes compared with normotensive people of the same age.[9]

In hypertensive patients, strokes most commonly arise from atherothrombotic infarcts of smaller penetrating branches of the middle cerebral and basilar arteries. Intracerebral hemorrhage, although less common, is more lethal. Subarachnoid bleeding also occurs more commonly in hypertensives. Transient ischemic attacks (TIA), temporary episodes of focal cerebral dysfunction, develop more commonly on the background of hypertension and, in concert with carotid bruits, are indicative of an increased risk of stroke.[69]

More subtle defects in cerebral function may accompany hypertension. When 20 men with newly discovered, untreated diastolic blood pressures above 105 mm Hg were compared to 20 normotensive subjects matched for age, educational level, and occupational status, those with hypertension were significantly slower in reaction time and in performance of other tests of attention span.[70]

Lowering the blood pressure prevents initial and recurrent strokes.[71] Unless the pressure is very high and causing immediate damage, a gradual reduction of longstanding hypertension is wise, allowing cerebral autoregulation to maintain normal perfusion. As shown by Strandgaard and coworkers, rapid reduction of chronically elevated pressures to levels well tolerated by normal individuals may invoke cerebral hypoperfusion,[72] which may cause ischemic brain damage.[73] Elderly patients are particularly susceptible because the mechanism of cerebral autoregulation becomes sluggish with age.[74]

Renal Damage. Hypertension is the most common cause of progressive renal insufficiency, and some evidence of renal damage is common in patients with hypertension. This evidence, reflecting nephrosclerosis, includes an elevated serum uric acid level, present in one-third of untreated hypertensives.[75] Levels of a lysosomal enzyme, N-acetyl-β-D-glucosaminidase, thought to be of renal origin, are frequently elevated in both serum and urine of patients with mild hypertension.[76]

The course of the relationship between hypertension and the kidneys is often uncertain: as they progress, primary renal diseases, frequently cause hypertension. As we shall see, renal dysfunction, although clinically not bothersome, may be the basic defect of primary hypertension, and the degree of renal dysfunction is closely related to the prognosis[44] (Fig. 26–8). Antihypertensive treatment will protect the kidneys, allowing some patients with even far-advanced renal insufficiency to survive for many years.[77]

HYPERTENSION IN BLACKS

Blacks have hypertension more frequently than do whites, and they suffer more morbidity and mortality from it.[78] In particular, they suffer more renal damage, leading to a significantly greater prevalence of end-stage renal disease requiring chronic dialysis.[79]

Hypertension seen in blacks has been characterized as having a relatively greater component of fluid volume excess, including a higher prevalence of low levels of plasma renin activity[80] and their greater responsiveness to diuretic therapy.[81] These and other features suggestive of volume excess may reflect larger degrees of one or more of the abnormalities in sodium transport across cell membranes that will be described in the next section, Mechanisms of Primary Hypertension. Black hypertensives have been found to have greater suppression of ouabain-insensitive Na-K pump activity than white hypertensives[82]—a defect which, if generalized, would result in higher intracellular sodium concentrations.

Perhaps blacks, who originally lived in hot, arid climates in which avid sodium conservation was necessary for survival, have evolved the physiological machinery that offers protection in their original habitat, in which the diet was relatively low in sodium, but that makes them susceptible to "sodium overload" when they migrate to areas where sodium intake is excessive. This view is supported by the experience of the Xhosa people in Southern Africa: when they migrated to urban areas, their blood pressures began to rise in association with their increased dietary intake of sodium.[83]

A complete annotated bibliography through late 1981 relative to hypertension among blacks has recently been published.[84]

HYPERTENSION IN WOMEN

Unlike blacks, women in general suffer less cardiovascular morbidity and mortality than men for any degree of hypertension (Fig. 26–5). Moreover, hypertension is less common in women than in men before the age of menopause (Fig. 26–4). Perhaps the lower frequency and severity of hypertension reflect the lower blood volume and viscosity afforded women by their monthly menses.

HYPERTENSION IN THE ELDERLY

We have previously noted the high frequency and risks of systolic hypertension among the elderly. As more people live longer, more predominantly systolic and combined systolic and diastolic hypertension will be seen among people over age 65. These individuals may have certain special needs:

— To a large extent, the progressive rise in systolic pressure reflects a loss of compliance within the major arteries due to permanent sclerosis; therapy may be either ineffectual, since vasodilation may not be possible, or poorly tolerated, since a shrinkage of fluid volume or decrease in cardiac output may diminish blood flow to the brain.

— Baroreceptor sensitivity often decreases with age, so that the buffering provided by this reflex with changes in posture and the like may be lost; old people may experience a greater rise in blood pressure upon standing[85] as well as the propensity for postural hypotension.[74]

— More elderly patients with significant hypertension of recent onset will have chronic renal disease or atherosclerotic renovascular disease as a cause of their hypertension.[86]

Now that we have reviewed the background of hypertension, let us examine what is known about the causes of the form of this condition responsible for 95 per cent of all cases, idiopathic or primary hypertension, in which the cause is unknown. At least some new clues have come to light.

MECHANISMS OF PRIMARY (ESSENTIAL) HYPERTENSION

Without knowledge of the specific cause, we can begin by considering those factors known to affect the blood pressure (Fig. 26–12). Although other forces may be involved, *cardiac output* and *peripheral resistance* are the primary determinants. The interplay of various derangements in factors affecting cardiac output and peripheral resistance may precipitate the disease; these may differ in both type and degree in different patients. Looking for a single defect in all patients with essential hypertension may be a mistake. Note the sage advice presented in an editorial in *Lancet*:

> Blood pressure is a measurable end-product of an exceedingly complex series of factors including those which control blood-vessel caliber and responsiveness, those which control fluid volume within and outside the vascular bed, and those which control cardiac output. None of these factors is independent; they interact with each other and respond to changes in blood pressure. It is not easy, therefore, to dissect out cause and effect. Few factors which play a role in cardiovascular control are completely normal in hypertension: indeed, normality would require explanation since it would suggest a lack of responsiveness to increased pressure.[87]

The search for such defects to unravel the pathogenesis of essential hypertension may be misguided for another reason—it may not be a distinct disease caused by specific abnormalities. George Pickering was the most persistent and eloquent advocate of the concept that essential hypertension was only a quantitative deviation from the norm, so that people were rather arbitrarily called "hypertensive" if they were on the higher portion of a unimodal distribution curve, rather than being a separate portion of a biomodal curve.[21] The distribution of large populations is unimodal (Fig. 26–6), but such curves do not exclude the possiblity that those who become hypertensive are, in fact, qualitatively different.

Before presenting a specific hypothesis that includes such qualitative differences, let us examine the hemodynamic patterns of cardiac output and peripheral resistance that have been measured in patients with hypertension. One caution is needed: the pathogenesis of the disease is likely a slow and gradual process. By the time the blood pressure is high, the initiating faults may no longer be apparent, since they may have been "normalized" by the compensatory interactions alluded to in the *Lancet* editorial.

Nonetheless, when a group of untreated, young hypertensive patients was initially studied, cardiac output was normal or slightly increased and peripheral resistance was normal[88] (Fig. 26–13). Over the next 10 years, cardiac output fell and peripheral resistance rose. A similar conversion from initially high cardiac output to increased peripheral resistance has been found by others.[89]

Although this "traditional" pattern is found in some patients, it may not be usual or obligatory. On the one hand, in a few patients a high-output state may be present even

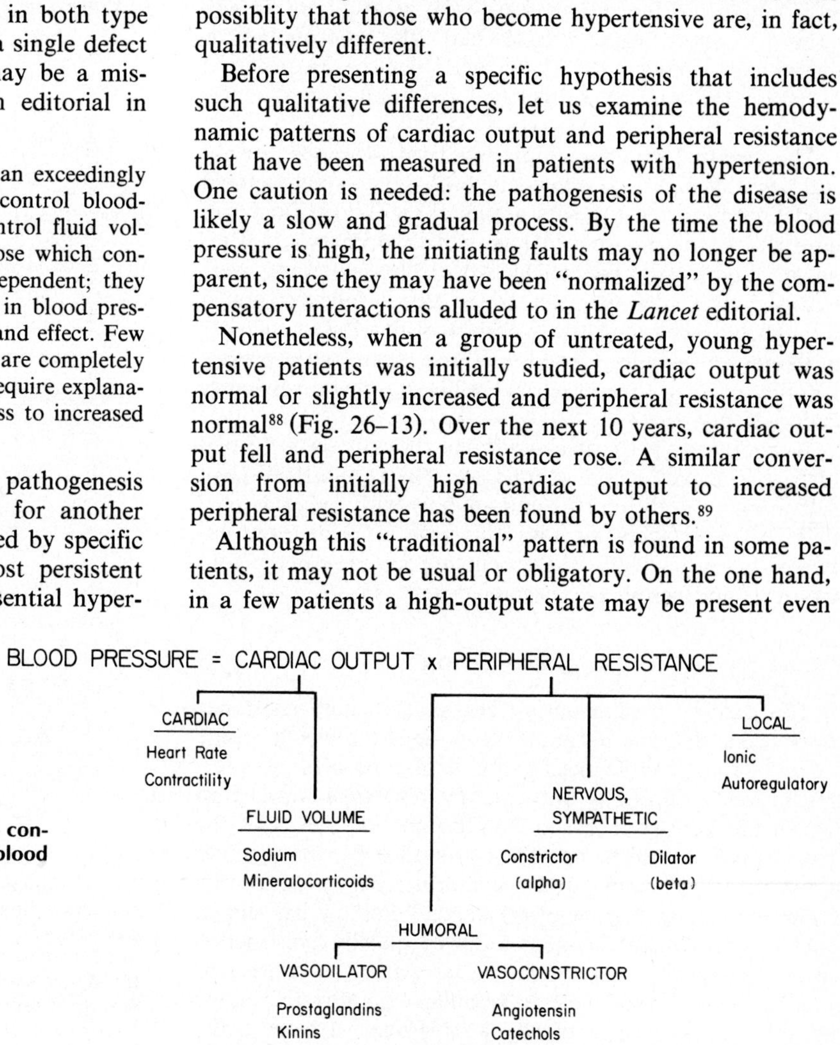

FIGURE 26–12 Some of the factors involved in the control of blood pressure that affect the basic equation: blood pressure = cardiac output × peripheral resistance.

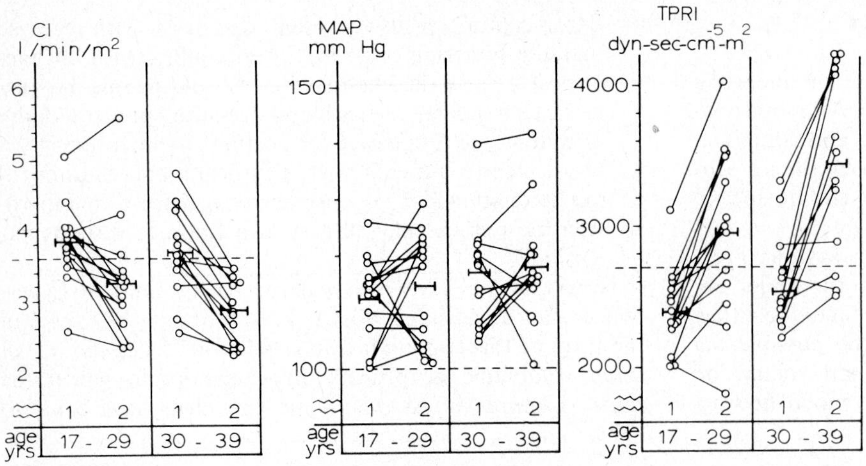

FIGURE 26–13 A 10-year follow-up study of the hemodynamics at rest in 28 untreated patients with essential hypertension. Cardiac index (CI), mean arterial pressure (MAP), and total peripheral resistance index (TPRI) at first (1) and second (2) study. Values between brackets (I__I) are mean values. The broken horizontal lines represent the upper limits of normal. (From Lund-Johansen, P.: Hemodynamic alterations in hypertension—spontaneous changes and effects of drug therapy. Acta Med. Scand. Suppl. *603*:1, 1977.)

after 20 years[90]; on the other, peripheral resistance is often abnormally high, even in those patients with initially high outputs. The expected response to increased cardiac output is vasodilation with a fall in peripheral resistance. Thus, "normal" resistance in the presence of a high cardiac output is actually abnormally elevated, constituting the primary mechanism of the hypertension.[91] Those patients with persistently expanded blood volume who would be expected to have relatively low peripheral resistance have an even higher resistance than those with greatly reduced volumes.[92] In short, Tarazi advises that "the spectrum of hemodynamic changes associated with volume disturbances in hypertension is too wide to be forced under one hypothesis alone."[92]

The eventual primacy of the factor of increased peripheral resistance can be shown in both human and animal models of hypertension with an initial increase in fluid volume and cardiac output. Patients with primary aldosteronism, completely controlled with spironolactone, were followed after administration of the aldosterone antagonist was discontinued, and the syndrome was allowed to recur in its natural manner.[93] The initial overexpansion of plasma volume returned toward normal while peripheral resistance progressively rose.

In another hypertensive syndrome thought to be related mainly to excess blood volume, i.e., the administration of salt loads to both humans and animals with reduced renal mass, there is again an initial increase in cardiac output, but within a few weeks the output returns to near the control level and peripheral resistance rises[94] (Fig. 26–14).

AUTOREGULATION

The pattern of high output changing to high resistance does occur in some instances. How does the change come about? One possible mechanism is the process of autoregulation, a property intrinsic to resistance vessels, in which an increase in blood flow beyond the needs of the tissue leads to vasoconstriction. As this decreases blood flow and brings supply and demand into balance, it results in an increase in peripheral resistance.[94] Folkow has shown that this functional change is followed quickly by structural alterations that thicken the vessel walls.[95] In concert or independently, an increase in vascular reactivity to pressor stimuli may also be involved. In experimental models, the increased sensitivity of vascular smooth muscle to pressor stimuli appears before the blood pressure rises and may thus be a primary mechanism for increased peripheral resistance.[96]

To summarize the observational data, cardiac output and fluid volume may be elevated initially, but the hypertension is maintained by an increased peripheral resistance that may reflect, first, functional tightening and, then, structural thickening of vessel walls.

Before looking for specific causes for this hemodynamic

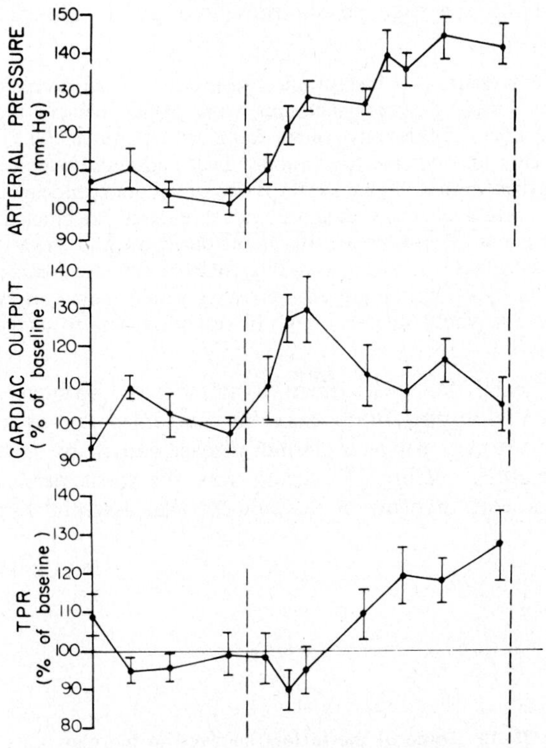

FIGURE 26–14 Arterial pressure, cardiac output, and total peripheral resistance in six partially nephrectomized dogs infused with 0.9 per cent saline. After an 8-day control period, partial nephrectomy was performed, indicated by the broken vertical line. Saline was infused continuously for the next 13 days. (From Coleman, T. G., et al.: Whole-body circulatory autoregulation and hypertension. Circ. Res. *29*(Suppl. II):76, 1971, by permission of the American Heart Association, Inc.)

pattern, the genetic predisposition for hypertension should be recognized.

GENETIC PREDISPOSITION (See also p. 1636)

Familial correlations relative to blood pressure levels have been found in infants as young as 6 months of age, supporting a genetic mechanism.[97] In studies of twins and family members in which the degree of familial aggregation of the blood pressure is compared to the closeness of genetic sharing, the genetic contribution has been estimated to be as low as 30 per cent to as high as 60 per cent.[98] The blood pressure of parents was much more closely related to that of their natural children than to that of their adopted children.[99] Since both the natural and the adopted children shared the same environment, these data support a predominant role for heredity in the familial resemblance regarding blood pressure.

The debate concerning the roles of heredity and environment may be largely academic, but it could have important practical implications. First, the children and siblings of hypertensives should be more carefully screened. Second, they should be vigorously advised to avoid environmental factors known to aggravate hypertension and increase cardiovascular risks, i.e., obesity, smoking, inactivity, and sodium.

The Inherited Defect. If heredity does indeed play a role, what is inherited? Children of hypertensive parents have shown a greater blood pressure response to psychological stress, which was further accentuated after they ingested 10 additional grams of sodium chloride for two weeks.[100] Although exposure to high levels of stress may induce hypertension regardless of the genetic substrate, it is obvious that not all who are exposed to stress develop hypertension. A genetically determined heightened response to stress and sodium would be in keeping with the findings of Falkner et al.[100]

Enhancement of stress-mediated rises in blood pressure by extra dietary sodium noted in these studies is in keeping with the accentuation of pressor responsiveness to exogenous norepinephrine[101] and angiotensin[102] after increased sodium intake. The enhanced pressor sensitivity to these hormones may reflect an increase in their vascular receptors induced by high sodium intake.[103]

The evidence for a role of excessive dietary sodium intake in the pathogenesis of hypertension is summarized in Table 26–8. We are all consuming more sodium than we need and likely a great deal more than our ancestors consumed up until fairly recent times. The increase in sodium probably occurred when food sources began to be harvested, stored, and processed instead of grown or caught and eaten fresh.[104]

TABLE 26–8 EVIDENCE FOR A ROLE OF SODIUM IN PRIMARY (ESSENTIAL) HYPERTENSION

1. In large populations, the prevalence of hypertension tends to increase with increasing levels of sodium intake.
2. Multiple, scattered groups who consume little sodium (less than 50 mmol/day) have little or no hypertension. When they consume more sodium, hypertension appears.
3. Animals given sodium loads, if genetically predisposed, develop hypertension.
4. Some people, when given large sodium loads over short periods, develop an increase in vascular resistance and blood pressure.
5. An increased concentration of sodium is present in the vascular tissue and blood cells of most hypertensives.
6. Sodium restriction, to a level of 60 to 90 mmol per day, will lower blood pressure in most people. The antihypertensive action of diuretics requires an initial natriuresis.

TABLE 26–9 ABNORMAL ERYTHROCYTE Na^+/K^+ FLUX TEST IN NORMOTENSIVE CHILDREN OF NORMOTENSIVE OR HYPERTENSIVE PARENTS

	Parents' Blood Pressure		
	Both Normotensive	*One Hypertensive*	*Both Hypertensive*
Number of children	86	97	19
Number with + test	3	52	14
Per cent + test	3.5%	53.6%	73.6%
Per cent expected with autosomal dominant gene	0	50.0%	75.0%

Data from Meyer, P., et al.: Inheritance of abnormal erythrocyte cation transport in essential hypertension. Br. Med. J. *282*:1114, 1981.

Before proceeding with this hypothesis, note should be taken of perhaps the most provocative and far-reaching evidence of a genetic defect that may interact directly with excess dietary sodium intake. This comes from studies on the movement (or flux) of sodium and potassium across red blood cell membranes.[105] These studies have shown an abnormal Na-K flux in half the normotensive children with one parent hypertensive and in three-fourths of the children with both parents hypertensive (Table 26–9), closely fitting an autosomal dominant mode of inheritance. As we shall see, such a defect in sodium transport could lead directly to hypertension.

But the primary hypothesis to be developed here involves additional steps. The hypothesis proposes that a genetic abnormality exposes some of the population to the pro-hypertensive effects of one or more environmental factors. The person predisposed by an inherited defect might not develop hypertension if the environmental factor were avoided. Both the genetic defect and the environmental factor are needed. Similarly, the degree of hypertension that develops could reflect varying degrees of exposure to the environmental factor(s). Homozygotes might also develop more hypertension than heterozygotes, or there may be more than one genetic defect, so that the end result could vary markedly with the interplay of multiple genetic and environmental factors.

As complicated as the eventual situation may be, the hypothesis to be developed will propose only one of two possible genetic defects involving sodium transport and two major environmental factors. The genetic defects involve the renal excretion of sodium and the transport of sodium across cell membranes; the environmental factors are excess dietary sodium intake and stress. This hypothesis, based on evidence still incomplete, may turn out to be wrong or incomplete, but at this time it seems both logical and parsimonious.

Let us go back, then, to the idea that the effects of stress plus excess dietary sodium are responsible for activation of the sympathetic nervous system in people somehow genetically predisposed to develop hypertension. Evidence for an increased degree of sympathetic nervous activation in hypertensives is summarized in Table 26–10.

TABLE 26–10 EVIDENCE FOR SYMPATHETIC NERVOUS ACTIVATION IN PRIMARY (ESSENTIAL) HYPERTENSION

1. In animals, acute hypertension can be induced by the release of catecholamines in response to discrete brain lesions.
2. In rats bred to become hypertensive spontaneously, alerting stimuli invoke greater discharges from central autonomic centers.
3. Some hypertensive people have high plasma catecholamine levels that correlate with the blood pressure.
4. Hypertensives with high plasma catechols (and high plasma renin levels) display greater suppressed hostility on psychometric testing.
5. Some hypertensives overrespond to stress; and people exposed to high levels of psychogenic stress develop more hypertension.
6. Drugs that inhibit adrenergic nervous activity lower the blood pressure.

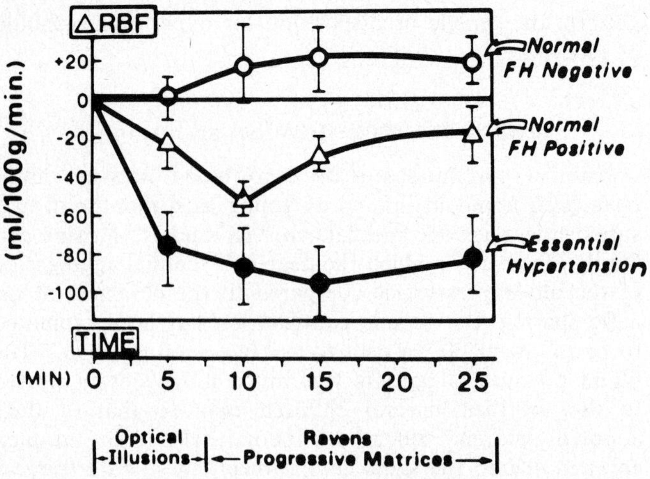

FIGURE 26–16 The response of renal blood flow (RBF) to the mild emotional stress provoked by performing a nonverbal IQ test, Ravens Progressive Matrices, in normotensives with either a negative or a positive family history and in patients with essential hypertension. (From Hollenberg, N. K., et al.: Essential hypertension: Abnormal renal vascular and endocrine responses to a mild psychological stimulus. Hypertension *3*:11, 1981, by permission of the American Heart Association, Inc.)

SYMPATHETIC NERVOUS ACTIVATION

Increased sympathetic nervous activity could raise blood pressure in a number of ways—alone or in concert with catecholamine stimulation of renin release—by causing arteriolar and venous constriction, by increasing cardiac output or by altering the normal renal pressure-volume relationship.[106] Renin release is directly stimulated by sympathetic discharge. Although plasma renin activity is usually normal in patients early in the course of hypertension, such "normal" levels may be inappropriately high, since both the higher level of blood pressure and the relatively overfilled vascular bed should serve to shut off the release of renin. The combination of high catecholamines and renin-angiotensin levels may then result in a disturbed pressure-natriuresis.

PRESSURE-NATRIURESIS

When the normal kidney is exposed to higher arterial pressure, it quickly excretes extra sodium and water, the process of pressure-natriuresis. Guyton and coworkers have long argued that this process must be defective in a hypertensive, because if it were normal, whatever caused the pressure to rise would be countered by enhanced natriuresis, which would shrink fluid volume and restore normal pressure.[107] This resetting of the pressure-natriuresis curve has been explained by increased resistance within the renal efferent arterioles[108] (Fig. 26–15), which could arise from exposure to increased amounts of or increased sensitivity to angiotensin II or catecholamines.[109] The greater degree of efferent arteriolar constriction would increase the fraction of blood filtered (filtration fraction), increasing the peritubular oncotic pressure and thereby exerting a greater force for reabsorption of tubular sodium.

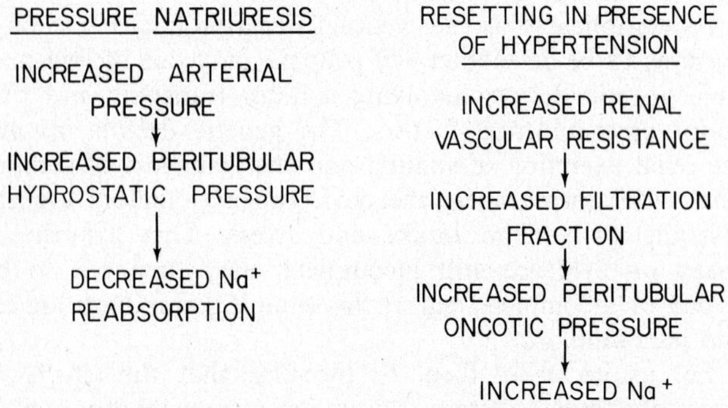

FIGURE 26–15 Origin of pressure natriuresis (*left*) and its resetting in the presence of essential hypertension (*right*). (From Brown, J. J., et al.: Renal abnormality of essential hypertension. Lancet *2*:320, 1974.)

Both human[110] and animal[111] data have shown increased renal efferent arteriolar constriction early in the course of hypertension. Studies in humans by Hollenberg et al.,[110] using radioxenon to measure renal blood flow, have shown excessive sympathetically mediated, reversible intrarenal vasoconstriction in early hypertension and, to a lesser degree, in normotensives with a positive family history for hypertension (Fig. 26–16). In animal studies by Click et al.,[111] direct visualization of renal tissue in hypertensive hamsters demonstrated a greater degree of constriction of efferent than of afferent arterioles upon exposure to either norepinephrine or angiotensin.

Plasma Volume. The reset pressure-natriuresis curve would eventuate in a relatively greater volume within the circulation for the level of blood pressure. A relatively expanded plasma volume has been measured in at least 80 per cent of hypertensive patients compared with the expected and observed progressive decrease in volume with increasing blood pressure among normotensive subjects[112] (Fig. 26–17).

This relatively increased plasma volume, inappropriately high for the level of blood pressure, would overfill the vascular bed. Although there may be an absolute increase in plasma or extracellular fluid volume, the vascular bed is also likely to be somewhat smaller in response to the vasoconstrictive action of the increased levels of cathecholamines and angiotensin.

Natriuretic Hormone. When plasma volume is expanded, renal excretion of sodium is increased, in part by the action of a circulating natriuretic hormone, which has still not been identified as to structure but is widely recognized as to function.[113] Natriuretic substances have been shown to be present in the blood and urine of both normal subjects and hypertensives whose blood volume is

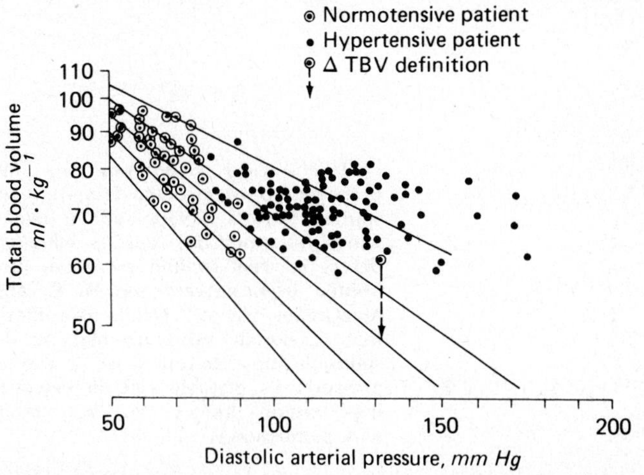

FIGURE 26–17 The relation between diastolic blood pressure and total blood volume (TBV) in 48 normotensive (open circles) and 106 hypertensive (solid circles) subjects. Only 20 per cent of the hypertensive patients fell within the 95 per cent confidence limits of the normal curve. The ΔTBV represents the degree of the pressure-volume disturbance. (Reprinted from London, G. M., et al.: Volume-dependent parameters in essential hypertension. Kidney Int. *11*:204, 1977, with permission.)

expanded.[114,115] In animals, the hormone appears to come from the hypothalamus.[116] Increased circulating levels of an endogenous inhibitor of NaK-ATPase, which shares immunological determinants with the cardiac glycoside digoxin and which has been called "endoxin," have been measured in both volume-expanded dogs[117] and hypertensive monkeys.[118] This may well be the putative natriuretic hormone. Another natriuretic factor has been extracted from cardiac atrial tissue.[118a]

The hormone increases natriuresis by inhibiting NaK-ATPase activity in the kidney, thereby reducing active sodium reabsorption. Plasma levels of an inhibitor of renal NaK-ATPase were 25 times higher when normal subjects were on a high-sodium diet (when increased amounts of a natriuretic hormone are expected) than when they were on a low-sodium diet.[119] In the plasma of patients with essential hypertension the concentration of an inhibitor of renal NaK-ATPase activity is raised.[120] The natriuresis provoked by the inhibition of renal NaK-ATPase would counter the forces that initially increased renal sodium reabsorption at the onset of the process, which eventually leads to hypertension, so that the tendency toward continually expanding fluid volume would be thwarted. Such an enhanced natriuresis has long been recognized to accompany human hypertension.[4]

Beyond its renal site of action, there is mounting evidence that natriuretic hormone acts upon NaK-ATPase activity elsewhere, such as in leukocytes[121] and, most importantly, vascular smooth muscle.[122] This inhibition of extrarenal NaK-ATPase would diminish the active extrusion of sodium from cells by the Na-K pump mechanism. Evidence for reduced NaK-ATPase activity includes the following four observations: (1) Hypertensives have been found to have a reduced rate constant for active sodium efflux from white blood cells (WBCs), a process that is ouabain-sensitive and therefore considered to reflect NaK-ATPase activity.[121] (2) The active sodium efflux rate was reduced most in those with the lowest plasma renin levels, who might be expected to have the greatest effective expansion of vascular volume (and the highest levels of natriuretic hormone).[123] (3) After therapy with diuretics, which should shrink vascular volume and diminish the stimulus for natriuretic hormone, the abnormality in active sodium efflux from hypertensives' WBCs was corrected.[124] (4) Moreover, a decrease in sodium efflux rate was induced in the WBCs of normotensives by incubation of their cells in the serum from hypertensives.[125]

Until now, these observations in human hypertensive subjects in support of an extrarenal site of impaired sodium efflux by natriuretic hormone–induced inhibition of NaK-ATPase activity have been limited to WBCs, since it has not been possible to examine vascular tissue. In dogs and rats with nongenetic volume-expanded hypertension, suppression of Na-K pump activity has been measured in the blood vessels and heart,[126] and the suppression appears to arise from a circulating, heat-stable, ouabain-like agent evoked from the brain by volume expansion[127]—all characteristics that fit what is known about natriuretic hormone.

On the other hand, Overbeck and associates, using ouabain-sensitive rubidium uptake as a measure of Na-K pump activity have repeatedly found *increased* Na-K pump activity in the arterial tissue of rats with various forms of hypertension, including both nongenetic and genetic volume-expanded models.[128] These investigators conclude that the increased pump activity may reflect a compensatory increase in the number of active sarcolemmal pumps, perhaps in response to increased passive permeability of vascular smooth muscle to sodium, which develops in various experimental models.[129] This sequence has been shown to occur in rat aortic smooth muscle cells in culture after exposure to angiotensin II: sodium uptake increased about threefold, and presumably as a consequence of the increased intracellular sodium, Na-K pump activity almost doubled.[130] Thus, whenever intracellular sodium concentration is increased, Na-K pump activity may be stimulated in a compensatory manner, thereby obscuring the effect of a pump inhibitor such as natriuretic hormone, which previously blocked sodium efflux and was responsible for the initial rise in intracellular sodium.

Effects on Blood Pressure. Despite this possible sidetrack, the mounting evidence for the presence of a natriuretic hormone that inhibits NaK-ATPase in volume-expansion forms of hypertension fulfills the prediction made in 1969 by Dahl and coworkers, based upon their studies on parabiotic rats.[131] A logical connection between the suppression of NaK-ATPase and the development of hypertension involves an increase in intracellular sodium, an increase previously recognized in the arteries[132] and red[133] and white[121] blood cells of hypertensive patients.

INTRACELLULAR SODIUM AND CALCIUM

The next step in this sequence was provided by Blaustein[134] when he showed that an increase in intracellular sodium enhances a sodium-calcium exchange mechanism and thereby increases intracellular calcium. Blaustein calculated that a rise of 0.5 mmol/liter in intracellular sodium could give rise to an increase in intracellular calcium of 4 to 40 μmol/liter—enough to increase the resting tone of vascular smooth muscle by 50 per cent.

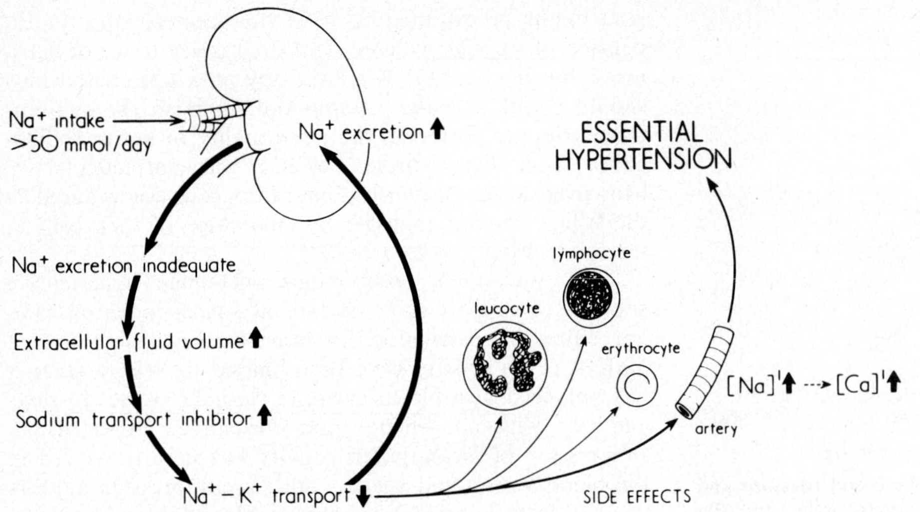

FIGURE 26–18 Hypothesis for the pathogenesis of essential hypertension, starting with a dietary sodium intake above 50 mmol/day and an inherited defect in renal sodium excretion. (Reprinted from deWardener, H. E., and MacGregor, G. A.: Dahl's hypothesis that a saluretic substance may be responsible for a sustained rise in arterial pressure: Its possible role in essential hypertension. Kidney Int. *18*:1, 1980, with permission.)

The increase in intracellular calcium is translated into an increase in vascular resistance by its binding to a myofilament regulatory protein and stimulation of myosin phosphorylation.[135] Indirect support for such calcium-mediated vasoconstriction in primary hypertensives comes from the lowering of their blood pressure, but not that of normotensives, by calcium entry–blocking drugs.[136] In the same study, the blood pressure of both normotensives and hypertensives was lowered by nitroprusside, which is thought not to inhibit calcium entry.

THE COMPLETE HYPOTHESIS

The complete hypothesis incorporates a great deal of what is known about experimental and clinical primary hypertension. The major portion of this hypothesis was formulated by deWardener and MacGregor (Fig. 26–18). They proposed that the increased fluid volume that stimulates natriuretic hormone was induced by an inherited defect in sodium excretion, acting in concert with excessive dietary sodium intake. The basis for their proposal for an inherited decrease in renal sodium excretion was the experimental evidence from kidney transplantation involving both the Dahl[137] and the Milan[138] hypertensive rats, which showed that the blood pressure "follows the kidney": When a kidney is taken from a hypertensive donor rat and transplanted into a normotensive host rat, the blood pressure of the host rises. The reverse also occurs, i.e., a kidney implanted from a normotensive rat lowers the blood pressure of a hypertensive host.

This proposal, however, skips the rather convincing evidence of a resetting of the pressure-natriuresis curve and does not require the mediation of stress-induced activation of the sympathetic nervous system. Therefore, although it is less parsimonious, the scheme portrayed in Figure 26–19 is presented as a more complete representation of the currently available clinical and experimental evidence for the pathogenesis of essential hypertension.

Additional Sodium Transport Defects. Most of this hypothesis (and deWardener's as well) can be bypassed by the direct insertion in the scheme of a defect in membrane permeability to sodium, as shown in the bottom right corner of Figure 26–19. Such a defect was proposed by Losse et al. in 1960,[133] but the current enthusiasm for its role

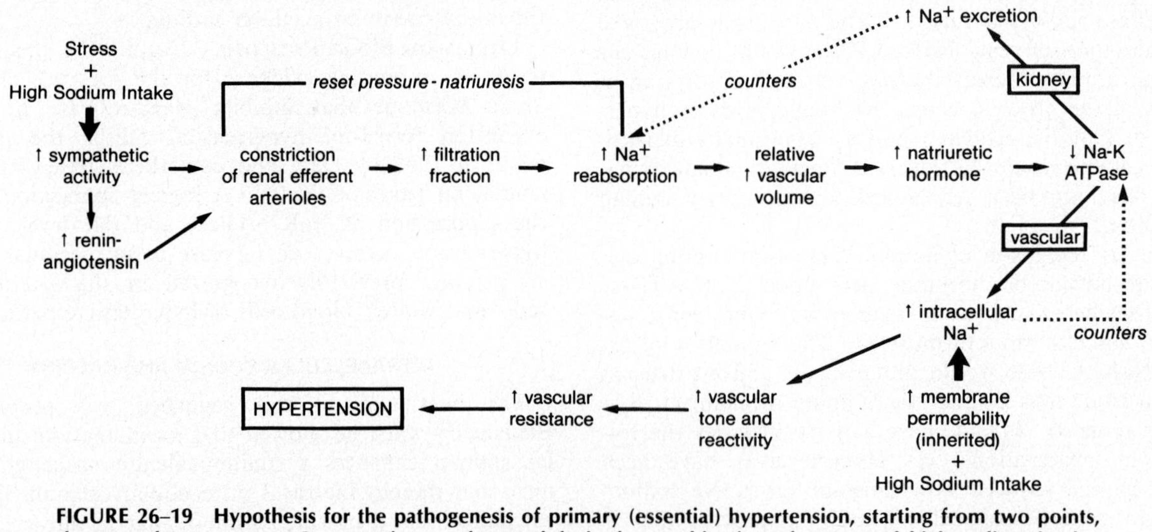

FIGURE 26–19 Hypothesis for the pathogenesis of primary (essential) hypertension, starting from two points, shown as heavy arrows. One, starting on the top left, is the combination of stress and high sodium intake, which induces an increase in natriuretic hormone and thereby inhibits sodium transport. The other, starting at the bottom right, invokes an inherited defect in sodium transport plus a high sodium intake to induce an increase in intracellular sodium.

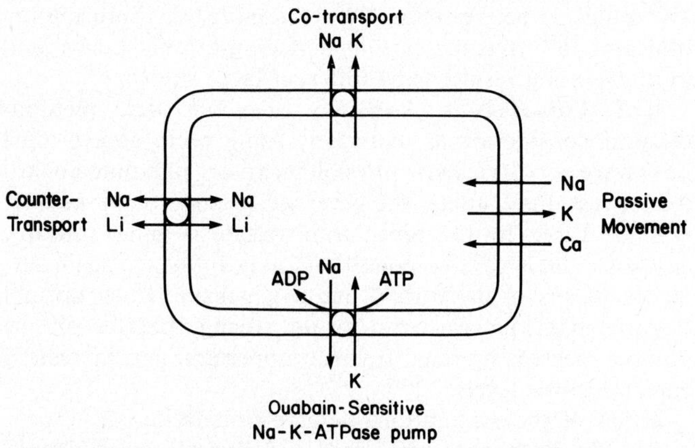

FIGURE 26–20 Schematic representation of four sodium transport mechanisms that have been demonstrated in red blood cells.

arose from the demonstration of alterations in transport mechanisms other than the active, ouabain-sensitive NaK-ATPase pump that is suppressed by natriuretic hormone. The four transport systems shown in Figure 26–20 are only some of those which may be involved in maintaining the marked concentration gradient of sodium between extracellular fluid (with 140 mmol/liter of sodium) and intracellular fluid (with 7 to 10 mmol/liter).[139] The NaK-ATPase pump is likely the primary physiological regulator, whereas the others may operate mainly in the presence of a sodium load.[140] Defects in the other three transport mechanisms in red blood cells shown in Figure 26–20 have been found in the majority of hypertensives tested: passive movement was shown to be increased by Wessels in 1967,[141] the Na-K cotransport mechanism was first found to be suppressed by Garay and Meyer in 1979,[142] and the Na-Li countertransport system was first reported to be increased by Canessa et al. in 1980.[143] About three-fourths of patients have been reported to have either reduced Na-K cotransport or increased Na-Li countertransport[144]; however, the two are often not found together,[145] and they are thought to reflect two different transport proteins.[146]

The decreased Na-K cotransport could result in an increased intracellular sodium concentration and thereby lead into the remainder of the scheme shown at the bottom of Figure 26–19. Moreover, a preliminary report has indicated that a similar cotransport mechanism exists in vascular smooth muscle cells.[147]

These defects may be specifically responsible for the pathogenesis of hypertension or may simply be in vitro markers for another process. Of considerable interest is the evidence that they are inherited, being present in about half the normotensive children of hypertensive parents[148] (Table 26–9). Support for a genetic connection comes from the finding of similar reductions in sodium efflux (i.e., the cotransport mechanism) in the red blood cells of three types of genetically hypertensive rats.[149] Moreover, a higher proportion of black Africans than white Frenchmen have the defect, in keeping with the different frequency of hypertension in the two populations.[150]

Problems with the Sodium Transport Concept. Although the preceding evidence for an inherited defect that could so easily interact with dietary sodium intake to induce hypertension is attractive, discrepancies have already begun to appear. Thus, although countertransport was increased in the red blood cells of hypertensives in both Paris and Boston, the cotransport was reduced in the Parisians but increased in the Bostonians.[146] Other investigators have been unable to find alterations in cotransport in the red cells of patients with essential hypertension compared to normotensives.[151,152] The considerable overlap in cotransport noted by some has brought the use of the test as a genetic marker into question.[153] Moreover, an increased passive influx of Na^+ into ouabain-treated red cells was found in 19 of 21 American white hypertensives but no such defect was found in the cells of 32 American black hypertensives.[153a]

Some of these discrepancies may be methodological in origin as well as reflections of variability in drug intake, plasma potassium levels and one or more of a host of factors, such as obesity, that may alter red cell sodium transport.[154] Moreover, the human may be similar to the rat[149] in having multiple genetically determined defects in sodium transport.

Beyond these discrepancies, the applicability of what goes on in the non-nucleated red cell under the highly artificial conditions of the assays used to measure cotransport to what is happening in human vascular tissue obviously remains to be proved, and it will take years to show that the defect serves as a genetic marker by foretelling the appearance of hypertension among normotensives with the defect. But as techniques to measure sodium transport become simpler, we may find one or another that will provide, at the least, a readily available marker of an individual's predisposition to hypertension and, hopefully, an insight into what causes this condition.

Other Hypotheses

At present, the "sodium transport" hypothesis is the most attractive unifying hypothesis for the pathogenesis of hypertension. As shown in Figure 26–19, it encompasses most of the other hypotheses given currency in the recent past—autoregulation, renal pressure-natriuresis, sympathetic-stress, and renin-angiotensin. But before leaving the mechanisms of primary hypertension, let us look at other possible mechanisms and associations with other conditions. In view of the probable role of the renin-angiotensin system both in primary and in some cases of secondary hypertension, further discussion of this system is in order.

THE RENIN-ANGIOTENSIN-ALDOSTERONE SYSTEM

The proteolytic enzyme renin cleaves a substrate protein in plasma to liberate the decapeptide angiotensin I. This inactive prohormone is in turn converted into the potent octapeptide hormone angiotensin II by a converting enzyme. Angiotensin II performs two major related roles: one involves control of blood pressure by constricting arterial vessels, the other control of body fluid volume by increasing renal retention of salt and water (Fig. 26–21). The two effects are the result of multiple actions. In addition, recall the evidence for a direct connection between angiotensin and the previously described sodium transport hypothesis shown in cultured rat aortic smooth muscle cells.[130] When angiotensin II was added to these cells, their perme-

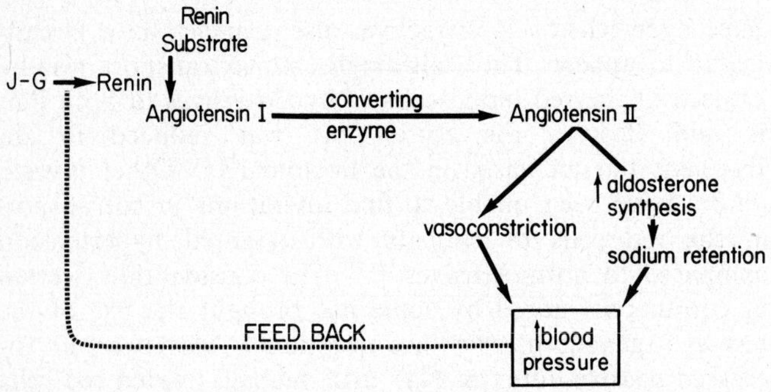

FIGURE 26–21 Overall scheme of the renin-angiotensin mechanism.

ability to sodium was increased threefold and intracellular sodium concentration rose proportionally. Angiotensin may thereby short-circuit part of the scheme shown in Figure 26–19 and induce hypertension by a direct effect on sodium transport.

Increases in renin-angiotensin are directly responsible for renovascular hypertension and are associated with a variety of other hypertensive diseases to be considered subsequently. As noted earlier, inappropriately high levels of angiotensin may be one of the switches that turns on the pathogenetic mechanism. Measuring plasma renin activity (PRA) may also provide a marker for different elements of the hypertensive spectrum.

THE NATURE OF RENIN. Although recognized in 1898, the various forms of renin remain poorly characterized:

1. The human kidney contains at least two forms of renin, most with a molecular weight (MW) of 40,000 but some with a higher MW, around 55,000.[155] Some renal renin is inactive and is biochemically similar to the inactive renin in plasma.[156]

2. In plasma, there appear to be at least three forms of renin: normal, active (MW $\simeq$ 40,000); big, active (MW $\simeq$ 54,000); and big, inactive (MW $\simeq$ 54,000). The third, inactive form can be activated in vitro by acidification or exposure to cold or proteolytic enzymes such as kallikrein.[157,158] The active component is measured by assays using a pH of 5.5 to 7.4, whereas both active and inactive forms are measured by assays using a pH below 4.0. The latter are preferably called assays of plasma renin concentration or total renin activity.

3. Tissue isorenins have also been described, particularly in the brain,[159] where all the components of the system have been identified.[160] A protein having the molecular weight of renin and that is immunologically cross-reactive with renal renin has been said to be synthesized by arterial smooth muscle cells in culture.[161]

4. Another protease enzyme, tonin, purified from rat submaxillary glands, cleaves angiotensin II directly from renin substrate.[162]

Why bother with all these forms of renin, particularly since some are found only after extreme and unphysiological manipulations? Although they may be largely laboratory curiosities, certain hints as to their possible clinical importance have surfaced, suggesting that big or inactive forms of renin may be physiologically potent as precursors of normal or active renin.[163] Furthermore, this information indicates the need for care in performing renin assays and in interpreting results from different laboratories.[164]

USE OF RENIN ASSAYS. Beyond these methodological considerations, clinicians using renin assays must be aware that various physiological or pharmacological maneuvers may affect the level of plasma renin activity (PRA) (Table 26–11). Since renin release is under multiple controls, these various conditions may influence renin levels by means of more than one mechanism. Thus, upright posture may increase renin by decreasing effective plasma volume, decreasing renal perfusion pressure, and increasing catecholamine levels.

A few of these conditions deserve elucidation:

Age. In both normotensive[165] and hypertensive[80] people, renin levels progressively decline with advancing age, an important factor in the choice of normal controls for comparison with hypertensive patients.

Race. Blacks, both normotensive and hypertensive, have lower renin levels than whites.[80] Values obtained from nor-

TABLE 26–11 CLINICAL CONDITIONS AFFECTING RENIN LEVELS

DECREASED PRA	INCREASED PRA
Expanded fluid volume	***Shrunken fluid volume***
Salt loads, oral or IV	Salt deprivation
Primary salt retention (Liddle's syndrome, Gordon's syndrome)	Fluid losses
Mineralocorticoid excess	Diuretic-induced
Primary aldosteronism	GI losses
Congenital adrenal hyperplasia	Hemorrhage
Cushing's syndrome	Salt-wasting renal disease
Licorice excess	Decreased effective plasma volume
Deoxycorticosterone (DOC), 18-hydroxy-DOC excess	Upright posture
	Adrenal insufficiency
	Cirrhosis with ascites
	Nephrotic syndrome
Catecholamine deficiency	***Decreased renal perfusion pressure***
Autonomic dysfunction	Therapy with peripheral vasodilators
Therapy with adrenergic neuronal blockers	Renovascular hypertension
Therapy with beta-adrenergic blockers	Accelerated-malignant hypertension
Hyperkalemia	Chronic renal disease (renin-dependent)
Decreased renin substrate (?)	Juxtaglomerular hyperplasia (Bartter's syndrome)
Androgen therapy	
Decrease of renal tissue	***Catecholamine excess***
Hyporeninemic hypoaldosteronism	Pheochromocytoma
Chronic renal disease (volume-dependent)	Stress: hypoglycemia, trauma
Anephric state	Exercise
Increasing age	Hyperthyroidism
	Caffeine
Unknown	***Hypokalemia***
Low-renin essential hypertension	
	Increased renin substrate
	Pregnancy
	Estrogen therapy
	Autonomous renin hypersecretion
	Renin-secreting tumors
	Acute damage to juxtaglomerular cells
	Acute renal failure
	Acute glomerulonephritis
	Unknown
	High-renin essential hypertension

From Kaplan, N. M.: Clinical Hypertension. 3rd ed. Baltimore, Williams and Wilkins Co., 1982, p. 220.

mal blacks should probably be used when defining the renin status of hypertensive blacks.

Posture. A few minutes of standing will markedly elevate renin levels.[166] Posture can conveniently be used as a stimulus for renin testing and must be taken into account in clinical use of the procedure. If "basal" levels are being examined, patients should be supine for at least an hour.

Dietary sodium intake. Renin levels will increase in patients ingesting less that 75 mEq of sodium per day.

Natural variation. Without any obvious cause, renin secretion varies from minute to minute and displays a diurnal rhythm.[167]

Exogenous factors. Some drugs affect renin levels by means of obvious effects on the blood pressure and body fluid volume. Estrogens routinely increase PRA by their activation of the hepatic synthesis of renin substrate, so that more angiotensin is generated for any given level of renin. Inhibitors of prostaglandin synthesis (e.g., aspirin and indomethacin) will blunt the renin response to diuretic stimulation.[168] The amount of caffeine in two or three cups of coffee will increase PRA, presumably by activation of catecholamine release.[169]

The patient's *sex* and the *level of the blood pressure* may also affect renin responsiveness; women and patients with higher diastolic levels responded less well to diuretics and upright posture.[170]

The lesson to be learned from all this is that renin secretion and PRA levels can be altered by a multitude of factors, some easily recognized and avoided and others still not identified. Even when the same assay procedure and testing conditions are used in the same patients without any recognizable changes in their conditions, renin status may change. Twenty-two of 85 patients initially found to have a low renin level in response to a low-salt diet plus upright posture had a normal renin level when retested.[171] Differences in renin status appear when different stimuli are used. When nine different stimuli were used in the same 47 hypertensive patients, only 28 per cent had consistently normal levels, and none of the testing procedures provided maximal detection of both low- and high-renin states.[172] The prudent clinician will take as many of the known variables into account as possible and recognize the vagaries of PRA, taking care neither to ascribe more certainty to a given level than is justified nor to make important diagnostic, prognostic, or therapeutic decisions based upon small differences.

RENIN LEVELS IN ESSENTIAL HYPERTENSION. Many studies have reaffirmed Helmer's original findings[173] that among patients with uncomplicated essential hypertension, about 30 per cent have low values, 60 per cent normal, and 10 per cent high.

The percentage of cases of low-renin hypertension progressively increases as the age of the population increases. Although this may represent a different underlying hypertensive process, more likely it simply reflects a progressive decline in functioning juxtaglomerular cells or in their responsiveness, a process that occurs in normal subjects as well but is accentuated in hypertensive individuals, in whom nephrosclerosis is usually more advanced.[174]

The separation of patients into low, normal, and high categories is in large part artifactual. The dividing line between low and normal is arbitrary and depends upon the type of analysis applied to the data. Renin levels in essential hypertension follow a continuous distribution curve, with a predominance of lower values because of the larger proportion of blacks and older people in the hypertensive population[175] (Fig. 26–22). As shown in this schematic view, PRA measurements can be useful for recognizing certain hypertensive syndromes with distinctly low or high levels. For the majority of patients with essential hypertension, little is to be gained from a determination of their renin status.

The concept that renin profiling could identify the relative contributions of vasoconstriction and volume to the underlying hypertensive process has been proposed.[176] According to this bipolar vasoconstriction-volume analysis of hypertension, arteriolar vasoconstriction by angiotensin II is predominantly responsible for the hypertension in patients with "high renin," and volume expansion is predominantly responsible in those with "low renin." When renin levels and the relative proportions of volume and vasoconstriction have actually been measured, no such relation has been found.[92,177] In fact, as renin levels increased, peripheral resistance progressively decreased—the reverse effect of that predicted by this proposal.[177]

THE ROLE OF RENIN IN ESSENTIAL HYPERTENSION. Foregoing the confusion as to the actual significance of renin levels, let us reexamine the question whether or not the renin-angiotensin-aldosterone mechanism plays a role in the pathogenesis of essential hypertension. The available evidence suggests a limited role at most. As an example, renin levels were *lower* in a group of "pre-hypertensive" young adults with sustained higher levels of blood pressure.[178] However, some argue that the role for renin is much greater.[176]

As we have seen, most patients with essential hypertension have normal levels of PRA. Since high pressure in the renal afferent arterioles should suppress the release of re-

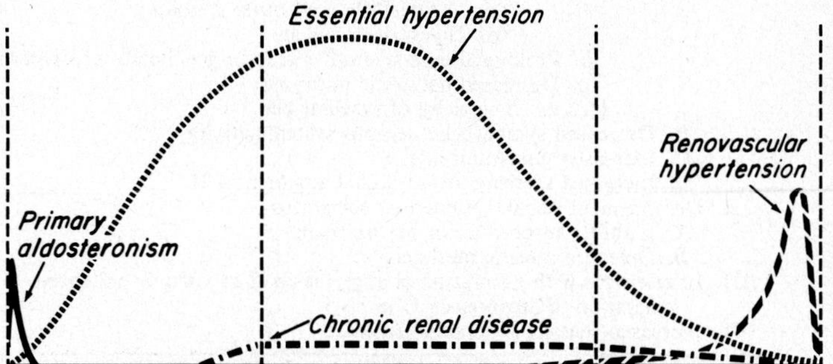

FIGURE 26–22 Schematic representation of plasma renin activity in various hypertensive diseases. The expected number of patients with each type of hypertension is indicated along with their proportion of low, normal, or high renin levels. (From Kaplan, N. M.: Renin profiles: The unfulfilled promises. J.A.M.A. *238*:611, 1977. Copyright 1977, American Medical Association.)

nin from the juxtaglomerular cells through the baroreceptor mechanism, the presence of normal renin levels may be considered inappropriate. Thus, the normal negative feedback between blood pressure and renin release may be imperfect in hypertension, resulting in inappropriately high renin levels, which may contribute to the hypertension. Support for a possible role of renin in such patients comes from the fall in their blood pressure when they are given an inhibitor of the enzyme that converts the inactive angiotensin I to the active angiotensin II.[179] This same enzyme is also responsible for the inactivation of the vasodepressor bradykinin, so the fall in blood pressure could reflect bradykinin accumulation and not necessarily indicate a role for renin.

A number of possible explanations for these "inappropriately" normal renin levels have been provided:

1. Renin release cannot be normally turned off: When exogenous angiotensin II was infused into normal-renin and high-renin hypertensives, their plasma renin levels were not suppressed normally.[180]

2. Renin release is being driven by heightened adrenergic stimulation: Esler et al.[181] found increased neural stimulation of renin release in patients with high-renin hypertension, as reflected in higher basal levels of plasma norepinephrine, greater responsiveness of PRA to the adrenergically mediated stimulus of upright posture, and a greater degree of suppression by beta-adrenergic blockade.

3. Renin release is abnormally sensitive to adrenergic stimulation: Morganti et al.[182] found that patients with high renin levels had normal plasma levels of norepinephrine and similar rises after the head-up tilt test. They conclude, therefore, that the degree of neural stimulation is not different but rather that the sensitivity of renin responsiveness is increased.

4. The adrenal aldosterone response to angiotensin II is decreased: Some patients with either normal or high renin levels show a subnormal rise in plasma aldosterone in response to endogenous and exogenous angiotensin II.[183] If aldosterone and the body fluid volume that it regulates are poorly responsive to angiotensin, it would require higher levels to "close the volume-renin-aldosterone feedback loop, potentially resulting in greater vasoconstrictor activity."[184]

On the other hand, those with low renin levels, which seem more appropriate to primary hypertension, may owe their low levels to increased sensitivity of adrenal receptors to angiotensin, so that less renin-angiotensin would be needed to maintain fluid volume; when given exogenous angiotensin, low-renin patients show a supernormal rise in plasma aldosterone.[185]

We are left with no clear definition of the role of renin-angiotensin in essential hypertension. In patients with natural or induced high renin levels, renin-angiotensin probably has a considerable influence. In the majority of hypertensive patients, with normal or low renin levels, the effect of renin-angiotensin on hypertension is probably only minimal.

LOW-RENIN ESSENTIAL HYPERTENSION. The presence of low or suppressed renin levels in 30 per cent of the hypertensive population, as previously argued, most likely represents a Gaussian distribution curve that is shifted toward the low side by the larger proportion of blacks and older people and not indicative of a peculiar form of hypertension. Nonetheless, the known presence of low renin levels in other hypertensive diseases associated with mineralocorticoid excess or volume expansion (Table 26–12) has prompted an extensive search for such a mechanism in low-renin essential hypertension. In addition, some believe that patients with low renin levels may have a better prognosis and special therapeutic needs.

Diagnosis. The possible mechanisms for low-renin hypertension go beyond volume expansion with or without mineralocorticoid excess (Table 26–12), although an expanded body fluid volume is a logical explanation for

TABLE 26–12 LOW-RENIN HYPERTENSION

Possible Mechanisms	Clinical Expression
I. "Physiologic" inhibition of renin release	
A. Increased pressure at the juxtaglomerular apparatus and/or increased sodium at macula densa	
1. Elevated perfusion pressure	Primary hypertension
2. Expanded effective plasma volume	
a. Renal sodium retention	
(1) Primary	Liddle's syndrome
(2) Secondary to increased mineralocorticoid activity	
(a) Aldosterone	Primary aldosteronism
(b) Deoxycorticosterone (DOC)	Congenital adrenal hyperplasia, adrenal tumors
(c) 18-OH-DOC and other steroids	
(d) Glycyrrhizinic acid	Licorice, carbenoxolone toxicity
b. Prolonged excessive salt intake in genetically predisposed	
c. Decreased natiuretic hormone	
3. Decreased capacity of vascular bed	
B. Decreased sympathetic nervous system activity	Diabetes mellitus, adrenergic blocking drugs
C. Increased potassium intake	
D. Increased systemic or intrarenal angiotensin II	
II. Derangement of juxtaglomerular apparatus	
A. Inability to produce or release renin	Chronic renal disease, (?) primary hypertension
B. Defect in sensing mechanism	(?) Primary hypertension
III. Interference with generation of angiotensin II in vitro or enhanced generation of angiotensin II in vivo	
IV. Increased sensitivity to angiotensin II	(?) Primary hypertension

From Kaplan, N. K.: Clinical Hypertension. 3rd ed. Baltimore, Williams and Wilkins Co., 1982.

low-renin hypertension. Even though such expansion has been reported, the majority of careful analyses have failed to indicate any abnormality. In one of the better studies, total exchangeable sodium was shown to be the same in low-renin hypertensives as in normal-renin hypertensives and normotensive controls, whereas it was appropriately expanded in untreated primary aldosteronism.[186]

If volume expansion were responsible for low-renin hypertension, a logical mechanism would be an excess in mineralocorticoid hormone. Despite initial claims that an excess of one or another mineralocorticoid is present, subsequent study has failed to document either the excess or the mineralocorticoid potency of the putative hormone.[187] Perhaps most meaningful is the observation that the plasma in low-renin hypertension, unlike that of patients with known mineralocorticoid excess, displays no excessive competition for binding to mineralocorticoid receptors,[188] suggesting that the search for such a hormone may prove to be futile.

Prognosis. As noted earlier in this chapter, one retrospective study showed that patients with low-renin hypertension had no myocardial infarcts or strokes over a 7-year interval, whereas 11 per cent of normal-renin and 14 per cent of high-renin patients had experienced one of these cardiovascular complications.[45] A number of subsequent studies have failed to document an improved prognosis in low-renin hypertension.[46] The only prospective study has found equal numbers of myocardial infarcts and strokes among those with initially low renin levels as among those with initially normal levels.[47] A rise in renin levels was noted after a vascular complication, providing a plausible explanation for those few retrospective studies which have reported a lower incidence of complications in low-renin hypertensives.

Therapy. In keeping with their presumed volume excess, patients with low-renin essential hypertension have been found to have a greater fall in blood pressure when given diuretics than do normal-renin patients.[189] However, others report no difference between the response to diuretics in the two groups.[190]

If low-renin hypertensive patients do respond better to diuretics, the response does not necessarily indicate a greater volume load. By definition, patients with low renin are less responsive to stimuli that increase renin levels, including diuretics, so that they experience a lower rise in PRA with diuretic therapy. Less renin and angiotensin could result in less compensatory vasoconstriction and aldosterone secretion, so that volume depletion would proceed and the blood pressure would fall further in low-renin hypertensive patients given a diuretic.

In the aggregate, the evidence that patients with low renin are unique in the spectrum of essential hypertension seems slim. For now, the prudent clinician should assume that the determination of renin status has little to offer in deciding on the management of patients with essential hypertension.

VASOPRESSIN

High endogenous levels of this hormone have been incriminated in certain experimental models of hypertension, but measurements in humans do not substantiate a relation between even very high plasma levels and hypertension.[191]

VASODEPRESSOR DEFICIENCY

In addition to an excess of the various pressor hormones, a deficiency of one or more vasodepressor hormones may be involved in experimental and clinical hypertension.

Bradykinin. This nonapeptide is cleaved from a protein substrate, kininogen, by the action of the enzyme kallikrein. It is difficult to measure bradykinin levels, and its role remains undefined. Decreased urinary excretion of kallikrein was found in some patients with essential hypertension.[192] However, subsequent study has found no evidence of systemic deficiency of kallikrein or bradykinin in patients with essential hypertension.[193]

Prostaglandins. These ubiquitous fatty-acid derivatives have profound pharmacological effects, but their involvement in human disease remains unproved. Recently, prostaglandins that act at their site of synthesis have been shown to produce physiologically important effects, so that the search for circulating prostaglandins may be futile. Prostacyclin, synthesized within the vessel wall, is vasodilatory; thromboxane A, released from platelets, is vasoconstrictive.[194]

The major site of prostaglandin action relative to hypertension may be in the kidney. PGE_2 is synthesized mainly in the renal medulla by medullary interstitial cells. When PGE_2 or the precursor, arachidonic acid, is infused into the renal artery, renal vasodilation, increased renal blood flow, and natriuresis follow. Thus, PGE_2 may protect against ischemia. When renal blood flow is compromised, both renin and prostaglandins are released. By this mechanism the kidney can raise systemic blood pressure via renin-angiotensin without diminishing renal blood flow, since intrarenal prostaglandins would counteract the effects of intrarenal angiotensin.[195] A deficiency of PGE_2 might then lead to hypertension by impairing renal function and permitting fluid retention as well as by accentuating the ill effects of renin-angiotensin. Decreased levels of urinary PGE_2 have been measured in hypertensive patients and have been related to decreased renal blood flow and urinary sodium excretion.[196]

Renomedullary Lipids. In addition to the acidic prostaglandins, two lipids from renomedullary interstitial cells have been identified which exert definite antihypertensive effects in animals.[196a] One is neutral, the other highly polar. The polar vasodepressor substance appears to be an alkyl ether analog of phosphatidylcholine. The role of these renomedullary lipids in human pathophysiology is not yet known.

OTHER POSSIBLE MECHANISMS

The preceding does not exhaust the list of suggested mechanisms for essential hypertension. Excesses or deficiencies of various minerals and changing ratios among dietary sodium, calcium, and potassium have also been postulated. Of these various claims, the evidence for a lower dietary calcium intake among hypertensives is most impressive.[197] Yet the blood pressure has been found to correlate directly with both serum and urinary levels of calcium.[198] Hypertensives may have a renal leak of calcium, compensated for by increased secretion of parathyroid hormone. A possible role of endogenous opioid peptides in the regulation of blood pressure has been noted in animals,[199] but there are no data pertaining to humans. Support for these and other postulated mechanisms is meager, and the overall scheme shown in Figure 26–19 seems more than adequate to explain the pathogenesis of essential hypertension. However, a number of associations between essential hypertension and other conditions have been noted and may offer additional insights into the potential causes and possible prevention of the disease.

Associations With Other Conditions

OBESITY. Despite the possible overestimation of blood pressure levels in the obese because of the use of small sphygmomanometer cuffs, true hypertension is more common among these individuals and adds to their risk of developing ischemic heart disease.[200] The association of excessive weight gain with the development of hypertension has been particularly obvious in children and young adults.[19] It is hoped that the prevention of obesity will reduce the incidence of hypertension.

The manner in which obesity causes hypertension likely involves the mass of fat per se.[201] In terms of hemodynamics, overweight hypertensives may have an inappropriately increased cardiac output and a relatively restricted arterial capacity.[202] It is of interest that the red cells of a group of obese *normotensive* Pima Indians showed reduced NaK-ATPase activity[203] in a manner analogous to that shown in Figure 26–19 to be possibly involved in the pathogenesis of hypertension.

Weight reduction as a means of treating established hypertension is discussed in Chapter 27.

ALCOHOL INTAKE. In the Framingham cohort, the prevalence of hypertension in those who drank more than an average of two ounces of ethanol or three mixed drinks a day was higher than in those who drank less[204] (Fig. 26–23). In other studies, a linear correlation between alcohol consumption and blood pressure has been observed, which is independent of age, adiposity, and smoking.[205] Despite their increased propensity for developing hypertension, those who drink one or two ounces of alcohol a day have less coronary heart disease than either teetotalers or heavier drinkers.[206]

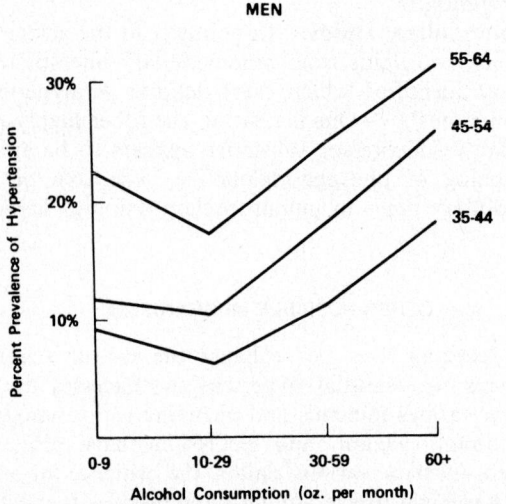

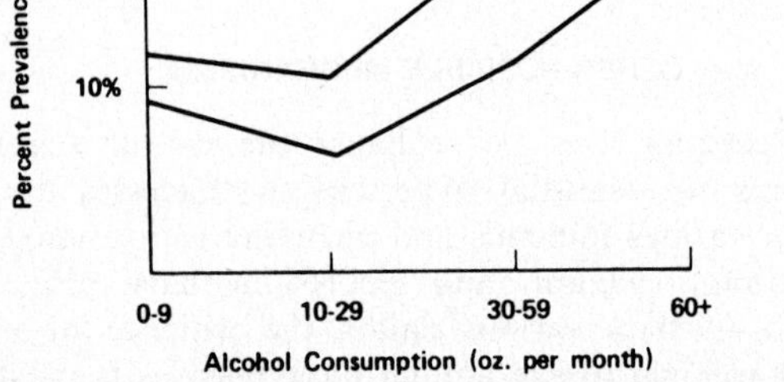

FIGURE 26–23 Prevalence of hypertension in various age groups in Framingham study plotted against their average alcohol consumption. (From Kannel, W. B., and Sorlie, P.: Hypertension in Framingham. *In* Paul, O. (ed.): Epidemiology and Control of Hypertension. Miami, Symposia Specialists, 1975.)

SMOKING. Cigarette smoking raises the blood pressure, probably through the nicotine-induced release of norepinephrine from adrenergic nerves.[207] Yet when smokers quit, a trivial rise in blood pressure may occur, probably reflecting a gain in weight.[208]

DIABETES MELLITUS (See also p. 1738). Hypertension is present in about two-thirds of longstanding diabetics with the intercapillary glomerulosclerosis described by Kimmelstiel and Wilson, and the prevalence of essential hypertension in the overall diabetic population is somewhat increased.[209] This may be related to an exaggerated pressor responsiveness to norepinephrine observed in a group of diabetics without renal insufficiency.[210]

When hypertensive, diabetics may confront some interesting problems. With progressive renal insufficiency and autonomic neuropathy, they may have few functioning juxtaglomerular cells and a reduced ability to stimulate the release of renin. As a result, very low renin levels are frequently observed, with a tendency toward the syndrome of hyporeninemic hypoaldosteronism. If hypoglycemia develops because of too much insulin or other drugs, severe hypertension may occur as a result of stimulated sympathetic nervous activity.

When treated for hypertension, diabetics are also susceptible to some special problems. Diuretics may exacerbate their carbohydrate intolerance, probably by inducing potassium deficiency. Those who are brittle and prone to hypoglycemia may have problems if they are given beta blockers, since their protective catecholamine response would be blunted, and severe hypoglycemia might develop without warning.

POLYCYTHEMIA (See also p. 1684). Polycythemia vera is frequently associated with hypertension. More common is a "pseudo" or "stress" polycythemia with a high hematocrit and increased blood viscosity but contracted plasma volume as well as normal red cell mass and serum erythropoietin levels.[211] Such patients may also have elevated plasma fibrinogen levels.[212] Cerebral blood flow was reduced in patients with hematocrits between 47 and 58 per cent and rose significantly after venesection.[213] Reduction of the blood pressure may normalize the hematocrit and blood viscosity.[211]

GOUT. Hyperuricemia is present in 25 to 50 per cent of individuals with untreated essential hypertension—about five times the frequency among normotensive persons.[214] In 71 male hypertensives, asymptomatic hyperuricemia was associated with decreased renal blood flow, presumably a reflection of nephrosclerosis.[75] When diuretics are used, the uric acid level rises further; however, even after prolonged exposure, patients with diuretic-induced hyperuricemia do not seem to develop urate deposition, so that treatment for the elevated uric acid level is usually unnecessary.[215] Nonetheless, gout may be precipitated in those who are genetically susceptible.

OTHER DISEASES. Cancer mortality has been found to be increased among hypertensives without relation to therapy or other known risk factors.[216] On the other hand, a lower death rate from cancer among hypertensives was reported from England.[217]

Other diseases and conditions have been found more commonly in patients with essential hypertension, including uterine fibromyoma, color blindness, and increased intraocular pressure.[4] In addition, a number of diseases themselves induce hypertension, and these will now be discussed.

SECONDARY FORMS OF HYPERTENSION

These will be considered in the approximate order of their frequency based on the data shown in Table 26–5: oral contraceptive use, renal parenchymal disease, renovascular hypertension (and renin-secreting tumors), adrenal causes of hypertension (primary aldosteronism, Cushing's syndrome, pheochromocytoma, and congenital adrenal hyperplasia), and a miscellaneous group. Of the less common forms listed in Table 26–4, only those recently elucidated will be discussed.

Oral Contraceptive Use

The use of estrogen-containing oral contraceptive pills may be the most common cause of secondary hypertension. Most women who take them experience a slight rise in blood pressure, and about 5 per cent will develop hypertension (i.e., a blood pressure above 140/90 mm Hg) within five years of pill use—more than twice the incidence seen among women of the same age who do not use the pill.[218] Although the hypertension is usually mild, it may persist after the pill is discontinued, may be severe, and is almost certainly a factor in the increased cardiovascular mortality seen in young women who take oral contraceptives. Despite these facts, the pill has provided effective and safe birth control for millions of women and the need for oral contraceptives remains.[219]

The dangers of the pill need to be put into proper perspective. While it is true that use of the pill is associated with increased morbidity and mortality, overall mortality from cardiovascular diseases has been progressively declining among women in the United States, at a rate equal to that noted among American men. Although the relative rates of coronary and cerebral vascular diseases are increased three- to seven fold among users of the pill—and much of this effect persists even after the pill is stopped—the absolute number of women affected is small, particularly among those below age 35 who do not smoke.[220] The excess annual death rate attributable to pill use for women under 35 who do not smoke is one per 77,000, whereas for women 35 to 44 who smoke the excess is one per 2,000. Thus, for most, the pill—particularly the currently used low-estrogen and progestogen forms—seems safe for the purposes of temporary birth control.

Hypertension is likely one of the major contributors to the cardiovascular complications from the pill, in concert with an increased tendency for the blood to clot, changes in lipid and carbohydrate metabolism, an increase in coronary artery smooth muscle tone, and proliferation of fibroblasts and smooth muscle cells in vessel walls.[221] The propensity toward a rise in blood pressure is accentuated by heavy alcohol intake: among women taking the pill, consumption of more than 10 ounces of ethanol a week was associated with a systolic blood pressure 8 mm Hg higher than that among those drinking 0.1 to 1.1 ounces a week.[222]

INCIDENCE. The best data on the incidence of pill-induced hypertension have come from a large, ongoing study by the Royal College of General Practitioners. They found a 2.6 times greater incidence of hypertension among 23,000 pill-users compared to 23,000 nonusers, resulting in a 5 per cent incidence over five years of pill use.[218] The incidence of hypertension increased with long duration of pill use, being only slightly higher than that among the controls during the first year but rising to almost three times higher by the fifth year.

Similar data have come from a survey of 13,358 American women, with new cases of hypertension occurring over a three-year period at a rate of 6.8 per 1,000 among pill-users compared to 1.2 per 1,000 among nonusers.[223] In a much smaller but more carefully performed prospective study of 186 Scottish women, during the first two years of pill use the systolic pressure rose in 164 (by more than 25 mm Hg in 8) and the diastolic pressure rose in 150 (by more than 20 mm Hg in two).[224] After three years, the mean rise in 83 of these women was 9.2 mm Hg (Fig. 26–24). Use of smaller amounts of estrogen than the 50 μg taken by most of these women may induce less hypertension: In six women whose blood pressure returned to normal when they were not on oral contraceptives, mean blood pressure was considerably higher (172/112) with the 50-μg estrogen pill than the level of 155/95 recorded with a 30-μg estrogen pill.[225] Obviously more data are needed to document the possibility that lower-dose pills are safer.

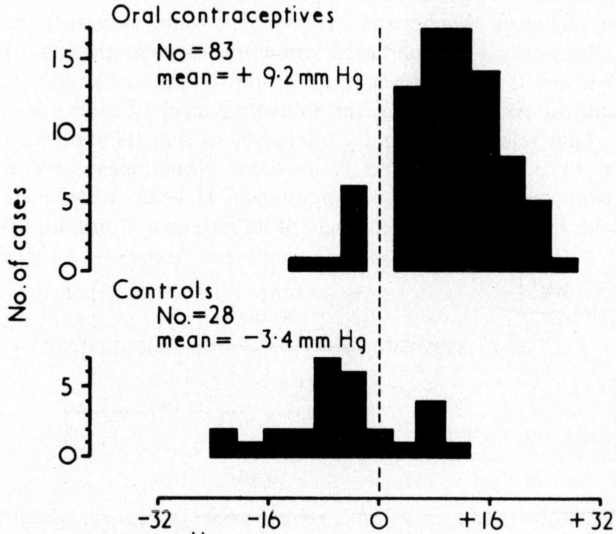

FIGURE 26–24 Changes in systolic blood pressure after three years in 83 women taking oral contraceptives and in 28 controls using mechanical methods of contraception. (Weir, J. R., et al.: Blood pressure in women taking oral contraceptives. Br. Med. J. *1*:533, 1974.)

CLINICAL FEATURES

Predisposing Factors. Any woman taking estrogens may develop hypertension, but the likelihood is much greater among those over age 35 and in those who are obese. A positive family history of hypertension is present in about half. The presence of hypertension during a prior pregnancy increases the likelihood but not enough to preclude pill use in such women who require contraception. One in 20 women with prior pregnancy-induced hypertension became hypertensive while on the pill over a three-year period—twice the rate among nulliparous women taking the same contraceptive.[226] Interestingly, women with sustained hypertension did not experience a further rise in blood pressure during a one-year period of pill use.[227]

Course of the Hypertension. In most women, the hypertension is mild, but in some it may accelerate rapidly and cause severe renal damage. When the pill is discontinued, blood pressure falls to normal within three to six months in about one-half of cases. Whether the pill caused permanent hypertension in the other half or just uncovered essential hypertension at an earlier time remains unknown. Among 14 women whose hypertension receded when the pill was discontinued, seven developed spontaneous hypertension during the subsequent six years.[228] In a few patients, the hypertension rapidly accelerates and causes extensive renal damage, very rarely a full-blown hemolytic uremic syndrome.[229] Even when the hypertension recedes after the pill is stopped, considerable renal damage may persist.[230]

MECHANISMS OF HYPERTENSION. The pill likely causes hypertension by renin-aldosterone–mediated volume expansion. Increases in body weight, plasma volume, and cardiac output were measured in 30 women given an oral contraceptive for two to three months, even though their blood pressure rose very little over this short interval.[231]

Estrogens and the synthetic progestogens used in oral contraceptive pills both cause sodium retention. This likely results from the following sequence (Fig. 26–25). (1) Estrogen increases the hepatic synthesis of renin substrate. (2) In the presence of increased substrate, more angiotensin is generated from whatever level of renin is present in the circulation. As a result of the increased level of angiotensin II, renin release is partially inhibited, so that its concentration in peripheral blood is lowered. Nonetheless, overall plasma renin activity and angiotensin II levels remain elevated. (3) The increased levels of angiotensin stimulate adrenal synthesis of aldosterone. (4) Aldosterone causes sodium retention. At the same time, systemic and renal vasoconstriction is induced by the angiotensin, and renal blood flow is shifted downward.[232] Significant elevations of blood pressure may occur only in those with the greatest degree of vascular sensitivity to the increased levels of angiotensin.

When women with pill-induced hypertension are given the angiotensin antagonist saralasin, blood pressure falls in those whose blood pressure subsequently becomes normal when the pill is stopped.[233] Thus, the overall evidence strongly supports a renin-angiotensin-aldosterone mechanism in pill-induced hypertension, with a greater sensitivity to this mechanism in the 5 per cent of women who develop overt hypertension.

The amount of progestogen may also influence the development of vascular disease: In the original Royal College data, more hypertension was seen with higher doses of progestogen.[218] Subsequently, more vascular disease has been noted with the use of 250 μg of levonorgestrel than with 150 μg of this progestogen.[234]

MANAGEMENT. The use of estrogen-containing oral contraceptives should be restricted in women over age 35, particularly if they are already hypertensive, smoke, have hypercholesterolemia, and are obese. Women given the pill should be properly monitored as follows: (1) the supply should be limited initially to three months and thereafter to six months; (2) the patient should be required to return for a blood pressure check before an additional supply is provided; and (3) if blood pressure has risen, an alternative contraceptive should be offered.[235]

If the pill remains the only acceptable contraceptive, the elevated blood pressure can be reduced with appropriate therapy. In view of the probable role of aldosterone, use of a diuretic-spironolactone combination seems appropriate. In those who stop taking the pill, evaluation for secondary hypertensive diseases should be postponed for at least three months to allow the renin-aldosterone changes to remit. If the hypertension does not recede, additional workup and therapy may be needed.

POSTMENOPAUSAL ESTROGEN USE. Millions of women use estrogen for its potential benefits after menopause. These "replacement" doses do not induce hypertension as often as in those who use estrogen for contraception,[236] even though they do induce the various changes in the renin-aldosterone mechanism seen with the pill.[237] In fact, lower blood pressures have been reported

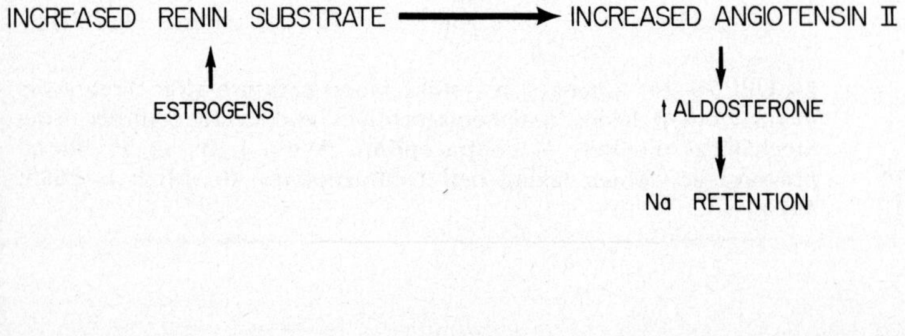

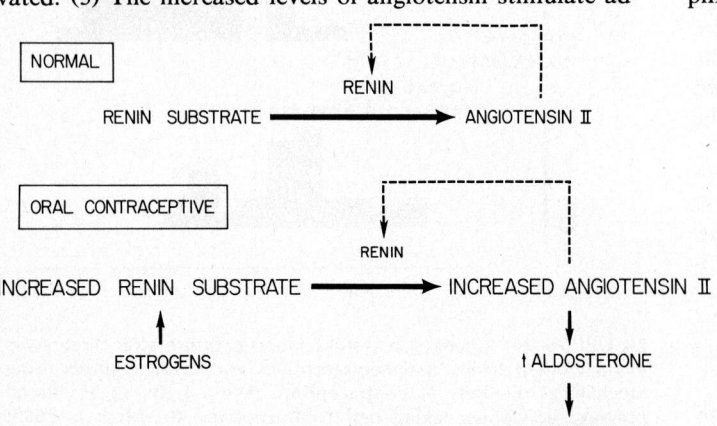

FIGURE 26–25 Schematic representation of the changes in the renin-angiotensin system induced by oral contraceptives containing estrogen. The dotted lines show the feedback inhibition of renin release by angiotensin II.

among postmenopausal estrogen users.[238] Moreover, two case-control studies have shown a significantly *lower* mortality rate from coronary heart disease among postmenopausal estrogen users than nonusers.[239,240]

Renal Parenchymal Disease

(See also Chapter 52)

Beyond the oral contraceptive pill, renal parenchymal disease, mainly chronic glomerulonephritis, is the most common form of secondary hypertension, responsible for 2 to 4 per cent of cases of hypertension seen in unselected adult populations (Table 26–5). As chronic renal disease worsens, hypertension usually appears and contributes further to the deterioration of renal function. In addition, primary hypertension is a common *cause* of progressive renal damage. In the United States, it is responsible for at least one of every six patients with end-stage renal disease (ESRD) entering chronic dialysis or renal transplantation programs.[79] Their higher prevalence of hypertension is likely responsible for the significantly higher rate of ESRD among American blacks; with hypertension as the underlying cause in one-third to one-half of these cases.

Not only does hypertension cause renal failure and renal failure cause hypertension, but more subtle renal dysfunction may be involved in the 95 per cent of patients with primary (essential) hypertension. As discussed earlier (pp. 864 to 867), the kidneys may initiate the hemodynamic cascade that eventuates in primary hypertension. As that disease progresses, some renal dysfunction is demonstrable in most patients, and progressive renal damage is the end result and the cause of death in at least 10 per cent of hypertensives. As we have already seen, and shall document further in Chapter 27, early therapy will protect against nephrosclerosis, so that there is hope that the control of hypertension will slow the progression and reduce the frequency of end-stage renal disease.

In considering hypertension with renal parenchymal disease, we shall follow a sequence of progressively worsening renal damage:

1. Acute renal diseases that are often reversible.
2. Unilateral and bilateral diseases without renal insufficiency.
3. Chronic renal disease with renal insufficiency.
4. Hypertension in the anephric state and after renal transplantation.

ACUTE RENAL DISEASES

Hypertension may appear with any sudden, severe insult to the kidneys that markedly impairs either the excretion of salt and water, leading to volume expansion, or the reduction of renal blood flow, setting off the renin-angiotensin mechanism. Bilateral ureteral obstruction is an example of the former; sudden bilateral renal artery occlusion, as by emboli, is an example of the latter. Relief of either may dramatically reverse severe hypertension. Some of the collagen diseases may also produce rapidly progressive renal damage. The more common acute processes are glomerulonephritis and oliguric renal failure.

Acute Glomerulonephritis. The classic syndrome of type-specific poststreptococcal nephritis appearing after pharyngitis has become much less common, but acute glomerulonephritis is involved in a variety of diseases of diverse causes and courses. Moreover, although the epidemic poststreptococcal disease is still usually self-limited,[241] recent reports have documented a progressive smoldering course in some patients that may lead to renal insufficiency.[242] Patients with sporadic disease may have underlying, previously unrecognized chronic renal disease, and they frequently have progressive renal disease with hypertension.[243] Typically, hypertension accompanies the oliguria and fluid retention of the acute injury. Renal damage is usually obvious based on urinary findings, but these may be minimal, and hypertension of a severe nature may be the overriding feature. Although the hypertension probably reflects fluid expansion, peripheral resistance has been found to be increased.[244] Absolute renin levels are usually not very high but may be inappropriately elevated in the presence of overexpansion of fluid volume and hypertension.[245]

Regardless of the mechanism, the hypertension is best relieved by fluid and sodium restriction and by appropriate doses of potent diuretics such as furosemide. Dialysis and parenteral antihypertensive drugs may be needed if encephalopathy supervenes. In milder cases, the hypertension recedes as the edema is relieved. However, some patients have a rapidly progressive course, often with prolonged anuria.

Acute Oliguric Renal Failure. More commonly, acute renal failure appears after shock develops in patients in whom renin levels are already high, such as cirrhotics with ascites or at the end of pregnancy. The release of even more renin by decreased blood pressure and effective circulating blood volume may flood the renal vasculature and cause such intense renal vasoconstriction that renal function shuts down.[246] A hemolytic-uremic syndrome may accompany the acute renal failure.[247]

Hypertension in this setting is usually not an important problem and can be controlled by preventing volume overload. High doses of furosemide may be helpful, but dialysis is often needed. Although this may allow recovery even after prolonged oliguria, up to 50 per cent of patients with acute renal failure die, usually from complications of the underlying disease responsible for the renal failure.[248]

Vasculitis. Rapidly progressive renal deterioration with severe hypertension occurs not infrequently in the course of scleroderma and other forms of vasculitis (see Chap. 47). Therapy with antihypertensives, particularly angiotensin-converting enzyme inhibitors, may reverse the process.[249]

RENAL DISEASE WITHOUT RENAL INSUFFICIENCY

Although an entire kidney may be removed without obvious effect and no rise in blood pressure, hypertension may be associated with unilateral and bilateral renal parenchymal diseases in the absence of significant renal insufficiency. Such hypertension may reflect other unrecognized processes, but most likely it is caused by activation of the renin-angiotensin mechanism. However, in some patients whose hypertension has been relieved by correction of a renal defect, the levels of renin have not been found to be high.

Unilateral Renal Parenchymal Disease. Congenital hypoplasia and acquired infections may affect only one kidney, causing a reduction in size and function. Most of these small kidneys do not cause hypertension, and when they are indiscriminately removed, hypertension is relieved in only about 25 per cent of patients.[250] Of that 25 per cent, most have arterial occlusive disease, either as the primary cause of the renal atrophy or secondary to irregular scarring of the parenchyma.[251] In many of these cases, high levels of renin can be found in the venous blood from the shrunken kidney,[252] while in some, renal vein renin tests have been falsely negative.[253]

Renal tumors, including rare juxtaglomerular cell tumors, Wilms' tumors, and hypernephromas, may be accompanied by renin-induced hypertension.[254]

Hydronephrosis. Either unilateral or bilateral ureteral obstruction may cause hypertension, and relief of the obstruction may also relieve the hypertension. In most patients with curable hypertension from hydronephrosis, renin levels are increased.[255]

Polycystic Kidney Disease. Although patients with adult polycystic kidney disease usually progress to renal insufficiency, some retain reasonably normal glomerular filtration rates (GFR) and display no azotemia during their course. Hypertension, although more common in those with renal failure, is present in perhaps half of those with a normal GFR and likely reflects variable degrees of both renin excess and fluid retention.[256]

Chronic Pyelonephritis. The relationship between pyelonephritis and hypertension is multifaceted: pyelonephritis, either unilateral or bilateral, may cause hypertension[257]; hypertensive individuals may be more susceptible to renal infection.[258] In patients with hypertension but fairly normal renal function, renin levels are usually high,[259] probably from interstitial scarring with obstruction of intrarenal vessels.

CHRONIC RENAL DISEASES WITH RENAL INSUFFICIENCY

As dialysis and transplantation prolong the lives of more patients with renal insufficiency, their hypertension must be dealt with over much longer periods. Hypertension in most patients with renal insufficiency is predominantly caused by volume overload. With proper attention to salt and water intake and adequate dialysis, control of the blood pressure is usually not particularly difficult. Unfortunately, some patients are much more fragile, alternating between low and high pressures, and some are much more resistant, presumably because of a greater contribution of high renin levels to their hypertension. With judicious use of available therapy, hypertension should not be a major problem for most patients with renal insufficiency. However, in concert with various mechanisms for vascular damage,[260] hypertension remains a major risk factor for the increasing prevalence of cardiovascular disease in these patients.

Mechanisms for Hypertension. Volume excess is the predominant mechanism for hypertension, and this may involve increases in pressor sensitivity to sodium,[261] redistribution of more fluid into the intravascular space,[261] and inhibition of sodium transport via NaK-ATPase pumps.[262] Some degree of renin-mediated vasoconstriction is probably involved in many and may be unmasked by therapy with angiotensin-converting enzyme inhibitors.[263] In addition, adrenergic hyperactivity may contribute, although this too may be apparent only after therapy.[264]

This admixture of mechanisms for the clinical syndrome has also been observed in experimental studies of renal hypertension. However, confusion has arisen largely because models appropriate for renovascular hypertension have been used inappropriately to study the "renoprival" hypertension of chronic renal disease. When appropriate models are used, *volume* is the predominant mechanism for the hypertension of renal insufficiency and *renin* the predominant mechanism for renovascular hypertension. In Figure 26–26, the effects of removing sodium and water and their reinfusion are shown in four groups of rats, including a normal group and a group without kidneys.[265] The anephric animals are exquisitely sensitive to volume changes. In the next group, animals with one kidney removed and the artery to the other partially clamped (the one kidney–one clip Goldblatt model), the pressure is also responsive to volume, but it remains above normal even after excess volume is removed, presumably reflecting the persistence of excess renin. This is a model for *renovascular hypertension plus renal insufficiency.* In the fourth group, one renal artery is clamped and the other kidney is intact (two kidney–one clip Goldblatt model). This is the model for *renovascular hypertension* most frequently seen in humans. When volume is initially reduced, blood pressure rises even further, probably because even more renin is secreted. After volume is restored, the blood pressure changes little.

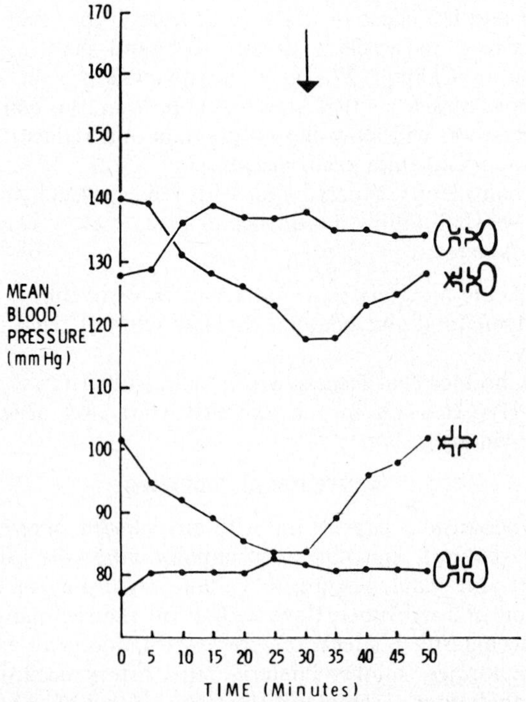

FIGURE 26–26 Effects on blood pressure in four different groups of rats by removal of sodium by peritoneal dialysis at time zero and the reinfusion of an equal amount of saline at the time indicated by the arrow. The symbols at the right (from the top) define the groups of animals studied as follows: one renal artery clipped and the other left untouched; one renal artery clipped and the other kidney removed; both kidneys removed; sham bilateral nephrectomy. (From Swales, J. D., et al.: Dual mechanism for experimental hypertension. Lancet *2*:1181, 1971.)

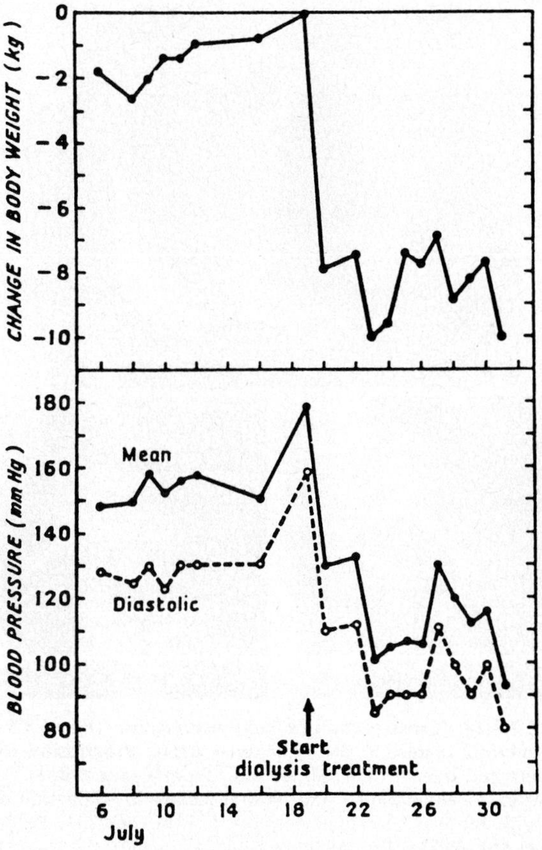

FIGURE 26–27 Effect of decrease in body fluid volume because of dialysis upon the blood pressure of a patient with chronic renal disease. (From Blumberg, A., et al.: Extracellular volume in patients with chronic renal disease treated for hypertension by sodium restriction. Lancet *2*:69, 1967.)

In the typical patient with chronic renal failure, as in the one kidney–one clip Goldblatt model, the decreased functioning renal mass is unable to handle the usual sodium and water intake, so that intravascular volume progressively expands and raises the blood pressure. When the excess volume is removed by dialysis, blood pressure falls promptly and impressively[266] (Fig. 26–27).

In a few—perhaps 10 per cent of the total group of hypertensives with chronic renal failure—hypersecretion of renin is the predominant mechanism[267]; while most of these patients may respond to treatment with antihypertensive agents, a few require nephrectomy.[268] The predominant role of excess renin may be identified by the blood pressure reduction with the angiotensin antagonist saralasin or the converting enzyme inhibitor captopril.[263] Even in those individuals with mainly volume-dependent or controllable hypertension, renin almost certainly plays some role. Their renin levels, although not inordinately high, cannot be suppressed by volume expansion to the low levels observed in normal controls.[269]

SPECIAL CIRCUMSTANCES. A few special circumstances relating to hypertension in chronic renal disease will now be considered. Use of antihypertensive therapy for patients with renal disease is covered in Chapters 27 and 51.

Diabetic Nephropathy. Hypertension often accompanies the syndrome of diabetic nephropathy caused by intercapillary glomerulosclerosis. The hypertension may reflect both advancing renal insufficiency with the inability to handle volume loads and extensive structural narrowing of the peripheral vasculature—the hallmark of long-standing diabetes. Moreover, intrarenal hypertension may accelerate the progress of the glomerulosclerosis.[270] As common as it is, hypertension may not be as severe or as likely to progress to an accelerated-malignant phase in diabetics with nephropathy for two reasons: first, these patients often have a diminished intravascular volume due to the hypoalbuminemia of the nephrotic syndrome; second, they have low renin levels, presumably due to hyalinization of juxtaglomerular cells.[271]

Hyporeninemic Hypoaldosteronism. Renin levels may become so low that the syndrome of hyporeninemic hypoaldosteronism develops. Although this pattern may accompany other forms of chronic renal disease, it is found most commonly among diabetics, since they are unable to mobilize either the aldosterone or the insulin needed to transfer potassium from the blood to the tissues and are thus particularly vulnerable to hyperkalemia.[272]

Whether diabetic or not, patients with this syndrome are usually recognized by a degree of hyperkalemia out of proportion to the degree of renal damage. The low renin levels are inadequate to stimulate aldosterone, and renal potassium excretion falls. Renin suppression in these patients may also reflect the expansion of fluid volume so common in advanced renal disease. Caution is obviously needed in treating such patients with either supplemental potassium or potassium-sparing diuretics.

Hypercalcemia. Whenever blood calcium is above normal, blood pressure usually rises; however, patients with chronic renal disease are particularly vulnerable to this condition. Marked hypertensive reactions have occurred when these patients are inappropriately given "therapeutic" calcium loads to offset the low plasma levels commonly seen in renal insufficiency or as a test for hyperparathyroidism.[273]

Analgesic Nephropathy. Permanent renal damage may supervene after prolonged exposure to analgesics, particularly phenacetin. In some countries, notably Australia, this is a common form of chronic renal disease.[274] Until late in their course, these patients have a greater propensity for salt-wasting and therefore may have less severe hypertension. However, in Australians, severe hypertension has been noted in 50 to 86 per cent of patients with analgesic nephropathy. Among those with malignant hypertension, a higher prevalence of renal artery stenosis and, at times, of active sloughing of renal papillae was observed.[274] Although aspirin alone seems to cause renal dysfunction rarely, it may reversibly depress glomerular filtration if given to patients with underlying renal disease or during sodium restriction, presumably because of the increased dependency of renal perfusion upon renal prostaglandins under these circumstances.[275]

HYPERTENSION IN THE ABSENCE OF RENAL TISSUE. In the absence of functioning renal tissue, blood pressure is mainly dependent upon body fluid volume. Without either the vasoconstrictor effects of renal renin or the vasodepressor actions of various renal hormones, blood pressure may be particularly labile and sensitive to changes in adrenergic activity. When the kidneys are removed for control of severe hypertension, blood pressure becomes normal, but hypertension may return with excess fluid loads or, as described below, after renal transplantation. The sympathetic nerves may be important in controlling the blood pressure; high levels of catecholamines may be responsible for hypertension in patients without renal tissue, and autonomic insufficiency may be a cause for dialysis-related hypotension.[276]

HYPERTENSION AFTER RENAL TRANSPLANTATION. A variety of problems may give rise to hypertension after renal transplantation, including stenosis of the renal artery at the site of anastomosis, rejection reactions, high doses of adrenal steroids, and excess renin derived from the retained diseased kidneys. Even when these causes were excluded, hypertension was found in 20 per cent of patients one year after transplantation.[277] Higher blood pressures correlated with older age, heavier body weight, and higher serum creatinine levels. Less hypertension was found in those receiving higher doses of prednisone, suggesting that glucocorticoids play a minimal role in posttransplant hypertension but not excluding their role in individual patients. More hypertension was observed when the kidney came from a cadaver than from a living related donor.

Unfortunately, renin measurements in these patients may not always reflect the ischemia, probably because volume expansion is also present and tends to suppress renin release. The response to the angiotensin antagonist saralasin may be a better indicator of the role of the renin-angiotensin system.[278] Whatever the mechanism, the hypertension that occurs in both chronic dialysis and renal transplant patients adds to their considerable susceptibility to accelerated cardiovascular disease, so that the elevated blood pressure in these patients should be treated intensively.

Renovascular Hypertension

(See also Chapter 52)

PREVALENCE. Fewer than 2 per cent of adults with hypertension have renovascular hypertension, the prevalence in different series varying from less than 1 to as high as 20 per cent, depending on the extent of patient selection.[4] Higher prevalence figures sometimes reflect the inclusion of patients with renovascular disease in whom the hypertension is not caused by renal ischemia. As people grow older, atherosclerotic disease of the renal arteries becomes increasingly common, in both normotensive and hypertensive patients.[279] Obviously, the diagnosis must be based upon evidence that the renovascular lesion is the cause of the hypertension.

Renovascular hypertension is seen in children, usually as a result of congenital dysplasia of the renal arteries. Infants have been found to develop the syndrome from thrombosis of the renal artery following catheterization of the umbilical artery.[280] In adults, the two major types of renovascular disease tend to appear at different times in different sexes. Atherosclerotic disease (Fig. 26–28) affecting mainly the proximal third of the main renal artery is seen mostly in men ages 40 to 70. Fibroplastic disease (Fig. 26–29) involving mainly the distal two-thirds and branches of the renal arteries appears most commonly in women ages 20 to 50. Overall, about two-thirds of cases

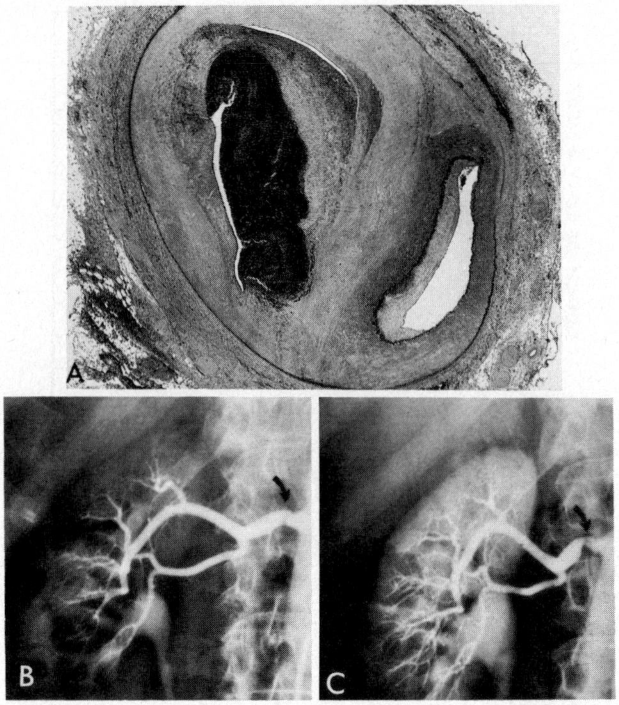

FIGURE 26–28 Cross section (*A*) and arteriograms (*B* and *C*) of an atherosclerotic plaque in the right renal artery. Progression from *B* to *C* occurred over a one-year period. (From Stewart, B. H., et al.: Correlation of angiography and natural history in evaluation of patients with renovascular hypertension. J. Urol. *104*:231, Baltimore, Williams and Wilkins Co., 1970.)

are caused by atherosclerotic disease and one-third by fibroplastic disease. The nonatherosclerotic stenoses involve all layers of the renal artery, but the most common is medial fibroplasia.[281] In addition, there are a number of other intrinsic and extrinsic causes of renovascular hypertension.[4] An interesting association between increased mobility of the right kidney and fibroplastic involvement of the right renal artery has been noted.[282] With repeated stretching of the renal artery, structural changes might be produced, leading to renal artery stenosis sufficient to cause renovascular hypertension.

Among blacks, less atherosclerosis develops in the main renal arteries and the incidence of renovascular hypertension is lower.[283] Among diabetic hypertensive individuals, despite their greater propensity for vascular disease, the incidence of atherosclerotic renal artery stenosis is not increased.[284] The sudden onset or worsening of hypertension among elderly patients may represent renovascular hypertension.

MECHANISMS

Since Goldblatt, in searching for the mechanism underlying essential hypertension, produced renovascular hypertension in the dog in 1934, the pathophysiology of this disease has been studied extensively. Confusion was introduced by the use of one-kidney models, which, as previously noted (p. 876), are more appropriate to the study of renoprival hypertension. Although some controversy remains, the sequence of changes in the two-kidney (one-clip) model and in patients with renovascular hypertension almost certainly starts with the release of increased amounts of renin when enough ischemia is induced to di-

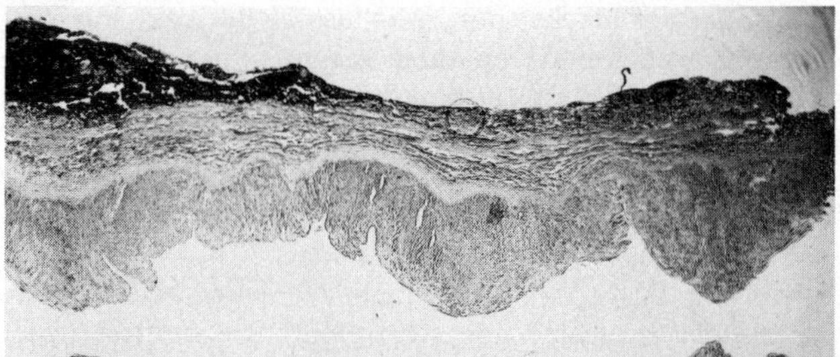

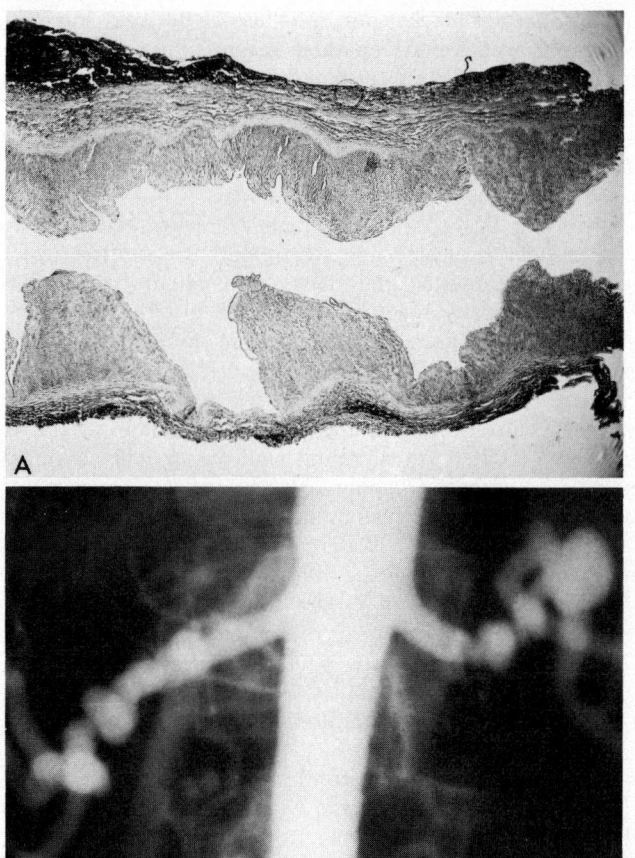

FIGURE 26–29 Fibromuscular dysplasia with medial fibroplasia. *A*, Longitudinal section of the vessel with multiple stenoses and mural aneurysms. *B*, The arteriogram shows bilateral multifocal stenoses with mural aneurysms. (From Harrison, E. G., and McCormack, L. J.: Pathologic classification of renal arterial disease in renovascular hypertension. Mayo Clin. Proc. *46*:161, 1971.)

minish pulse pressure in the renal afferent arterioles (Fig. 26–30). In people, as in animals, reduction of renal perfusion pressure by 50 per cent leads to an immediate and persistent increase in renin secretion from the ischemic kidney with suppression of secretion from the contralateral one.[285] Not only are renin levels markedly elevated but blockade of angiotensin activity with the antagonist saralasin or the converting enzyme inhibitor will correct the hypertension.[286] With time, renin levels fall, blood pressure fails to respond to short infusions of angiotensin antagonists, and the hemodynamic pattern changes to include an expanded volume and increased cardiac output.

The sequence shown in Figure 26–30 is most likely responsible: the increased angiotensin stimulates aldosterone, causing volume expansion, and partially inhibits renin release. Despite the changed pattern, renin is almost certainly still responsible, although its chronic effects may involve more of its secondary stimulation of aldosterone and, thereby, volume expansion. In addition, angiotensin acts centrally to increase thirst and exert pressor actions. Lesions in the third ventricle of rats blocked the induction of renovascular hypertension.[287]

In patients with proved renovascular hypertension of many years' duration, excess renin secretion persists,[288] so that the experimental data are confirmed clinically. However, more than simply renin excess and its consequences may be involved: experimentally, the sympathetic nervous system is activated,[289] although catecholamine levels are not measurably higher in patients with unilateral renal hypertension.[290] When hypertension in rats is reversed by removal of the renal artery clip, the blood pressure drops further than if the ischemic kidney is removed, suggesting that vasodepressors may be involved.[291] In dogs, inhibition of prostaglandin synthesis does not alter the development of renovascular hypertension,[292] but renal prostaglandins may be responsible for the increase in sodium and water excretion that follows the initial volume retention.

In both animals and man, when renovascular hypertension induces extensive nephrosclerosis in the contralateral kidney, a different picture may evolve. Relief of the stenosis may not relieve the hypertension; rather, the contralateral kidney becomes the culprit, with the stenotic kidney's vessels having been protected from the high pressure. With removal of the contralateral kidney, the hypertension may recede.[293]

Variants. Most renovascular hypertension appears as partial obstruction of one main renal artery. However, only a branch need be involved, and segmental disease was found in 11 per cent of cases in one series.[294] On the other hand, apparent complete occlusion of the renal artery, if slow in developing, will allow development of enough col-

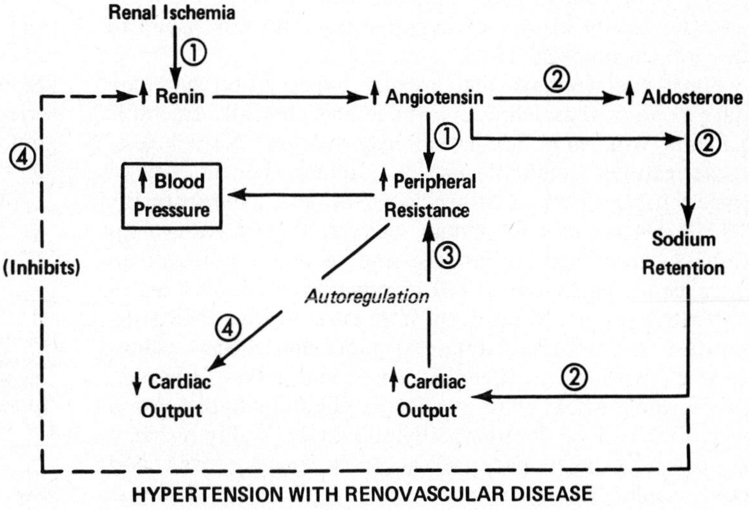

FIGURE 26–30 Stepwise hemodynamic changes in development of renovascular hypertension. The circled numbers represent the likely sequence of hemodynamic and hormonal changes in each phase of the disease: 1 = the immediate consequences of renal ischemia, 2 = changes that occur in a few days, and 3 and 4 = changes that eventually develop as the disease becomes chronic.

lateral flow to preserve the viability of the kidney. Thereby, the seemingly nonfunctioning kidney may be responsible for continued renin secretion and hypertension. If recognized, such totally occluded vessels can sometimes be repaired, with return of renal function and relief of hypertension.[295]

The process is often bilateral, although usually one side is clearly predominant. In the Cooperative Study, 25 per cent of the subjects had bilateral atherosclerotic or fibroplastic disease.[296] The possibility should be suspected, particularly if rapidly progressive oliguric renal failure develops without evidence of obstructive uropathy.

DIAGNOSIS

The presence of certain clinical features indicates the need for a screening test for renovascular hypertension in perhaps 10 per cent of all hypertensives. A positive screening test—or very strong clinical features—calls for more definitive confirmatory tests.

Clinical Features. Renovascular hypertension may be suspected on the following clinical grounds:

— The presence of an abdominal bruit, particularly if a diastolic component is present and if the bruit is heard lateral to the midline. Bruits confined to systole and heard mostly in older patients and that are loudest in the epigastrium and in the middle usually reflect atherosclerosis in the abdominal aorta.
— Onset of hypertension before age 30, particularly in white women who are slender.
— Sudden onset of hypertension after age 50, particularly in white men.
— Onset of hypertension after renal trauma.
— Severe, rapidly accelerating hypertension that is difficult to control.
— Evidence of rapidly deteriorating renal function.

The clinical picture of the two major forms of renovascular disease differ, as confirmed by the Cooperative Study on Renovascular Hypertension[297]: "Patients with atherosclerotic lesions were older, had a higher systolic blood pressure and more frequent arterial disease in areas outside of the kidney, and were more likely to develop target-organ damage than patients with essential hypertension. By contrast, patients with fibromuscular hyperplasia were young, predominantly female, more likely to have no family history of hypertension, and less prone to develop cardiomegaly."

Some patients have renovascular hypertension but may have none of these clinical features and clinically resemble patients with mild idiopathic hypertension. Nonetheless, these features should be used to exclude the majority of hypertensives from additional work-up and to identify the 10 per cent or so who should undergo a complete evaluation. As described earlier, the routine performance of an intravenous pyelogram (IVP) or other screening test on all hypertensives would result in more false-positive than true-positive results,[29] mandating even more unnecessary examinations, with their attendant costs and risks. However, those who present with rapidly accelerating hypertension with Grade 3 or 4 retinopathy should be highly suspect; among 123 such patients, at least 23 per cent had renovascular hypertension.[298] Once again, this was less common among blacks, but in at least 4 per cent this curable cause was found for their severe hypertension. The high frequency of renovascular hypertension in this series may reflect a greater propensity for the development of hypertensive encephalopathy on the background of renovascular hypertension than with other forms of hypertension in patients, as has been noted in animals.[299]

Screening Tests. No additional work-up need be done if the patient is clearly not a candidate for surgical treatment or transluminal angioplasty. This should be decided before, not after, subjecting the patient to either screening or confirmatory tests for renovascular hypertension. The diagnosis need not be made if therapy will be medical, since the same treatment protocol will be followed whether the hypertension is idiopathic or renovascular in origin. It may turn out that transluminal angioplasty will be an alternative to surgery for poor-risk patients, so that more of the latter will deserve evaluation.

Patients who are *less* likely candidates for surgical treatment include those with the following features:

— Hypertension of over 2 years' duration.
— Age over 55.
— Coexisting diseases (particularly atherosclerosis) that increase operative mortality.
— Relatively mild hypertension that is easily manageable with drugs.
— Inconclusive diagnostic studies.

On the other hand, patients with many of these features who are unwilling or unable to follow medical therapy, whose blood pressure level does not respond to adequate therapy, or who have marked stenosis of a renal artery or rapidly advancing renal damage may be considered for surgery and should be subjected to further study.

For screening among populations with an expected prevalence of perhaps 5 per cent (taking only those with clinical features suggestive of renovascular hypertension), an easy and safe procedure that results in very few false-negatives is needed. A certain number of false-positive results must be expected; considering that about 20 per cent of all adults will have primary (essential) hypertension, at least 20 per cent of patients with renovascular hypertension would be expected to have positive screening tests but would not be cured through repair of the stenosis, and these are therefore classified as "false-positives."

The four procedures commonly used as screening tests for renovascular hypertension were compared in a large population of hypertensives, 64 of whom turned out to have surgically reversible renovascular hypertension[300] (Table 26–13). Based upon this and numerous other published series, including the Cooperative Study, the following guidelines seem appropriate.

TABLE 26–13 SCREENING TESTS FOR RENAL VASCULAR HYPERTENSION

	Essential Hypertension	Renovascular Hypertension
Number of patients	199	64
Systolic/diastolic bruit	1%	39%
Abnormal IVP	2%	76%
Upright PRA > 30 ng/ml/3 hr	5%	27%
Depressor response to saralasin	2 of 13	12 of 23

From Grim, C. E., et al.: Sensitivity and specificity of screening tests for renal vascular hypertension. Ann. Intern. Med. *91*:617, 1979.

Bruit. Almost half of patients with renovascular hypertension have a systolic and diastolic bruit. If one is heard, additional evaluation is indicated; if one is not heard, the diagnosis is certainly not excluded.

Intravenous Pyelography. Rapid-sequence IVP should be performed when clinical features suggest renovascular hypertension. Based on the three major criteria for features suggestive of renal ischemia (Table 26–14), results were false-positive in 11.4 per cent of 771 patients with essential hypertension and false-negative in 17 of 138 patients with proved renovascular hypertension.[301]

If the rates of sensitivity and specificity of the IVP from the Cooperative Study on Renovascular Hypertension are used and a prevalence of renovascular hypertension of 2 per cent in the general population is assumed (i.e., 10 per cent of all hypertensives), an abnormal IVP would be only 10 per cent predictive of the diagnosis, according to Bayes' theorem[29] (p. 273). However, if prior screening had increased the prevalence of the disease in the population tested to 10 per cent, a positive IVP would now be 40 per cent predictive. A negative IVP offers greater than 99 per cent assurance that renovascular hypertension is not present.

The IVP is readily available and provides additional information concerning renal parenchymal disease. As digital subtraction angiography becomes more readily available (p. 191), it will be possible to view the renal arteries and the IVP simultaneously, so there may be better reason to do the procedure in more patients.[302] The IVP is usually safe; 1.7 per cent of 33,000 patients had an adverse reaction, of which only 5 per cent were severe and there was one death.[303] However, the elderly who have severe hypertension, renal insufficiency, or diabetes are at much greater risk of incurring acute renal failure.[304]

Renography and Split-Function Studies. Isotopic renography can be substituted for the IVP, although it is somewhat less accurate. If the expensive equipment and skilled personnel are available, the renogram provides data concerning renal blood flow quickly and with less discomfort and risk to the patient but with less discrimination between vascular and parenchymal disease than is obtained with the IVP.

Split-function tests have been virtually abandoned, since the other procedures provide equally satisfactory evidence of the functional significance of renovascular disease with much less inconvenience and discomfort to the patient.

Peripheral Blood Renin Assays. By themselves, peripheral blood PRA levels are of only limited value in screening for renovascular hypertension. Most hypertensives with high PRA do not have renovascular hypertension (Table 26–15), and at least one-third of patients with proved renovascular hypertension have normal peripheral blood PRA.[252] Better discrimination may be provided by obtaining the blood after the patient has been upright for one or more hours and by relating the PRA level to the 24-hour urine sodium determination. Thirteen of 14 patients with high PRA detected by this technique were cured by operation; of 10 with normal PRA, five failed to respond to corrective surgery.[305] If the peripheral blood PRA is elevated, when obtained under appropriate conditions, additional work-up for renovascular hypertension is indicated. However, if the criterion for abnormality is set high enough to exclude most false-positives, as in the series of Grim et al. (Table 26–13), many false-negatives will be noted and the procedure becomes a poor screening test.

TABLE 26–14 FEATURES OF IVP SUGGESTIVE OF RENOVASCULAR HYPERTENSION

1. Disparity in renal size > 1.5 cm
2. Delayed appearance time of contrast medium of one or more minutes
3. Late hyperconcentration of contrast medium
4. Suggestive but less specific features:
   a. Ureteral and pelvic notching
   b. Decreased volume of the collecting system
   c. Parenchymal atrophy
   d. Nonfunctioning kidney, with normal retrograde pyelogram
   e. Defect in renal silhouette suggestive of segmental infarction
   f. Renal ptosis > 7.5 cm

TABLE 26–15 HIGH-RENIN HYPERTENSION

I. Increased renin substrate
   A. Estrogen intake, pregnancy-induced
   B. Cortisol excess
II. Increased renal renin secretion
   A. Renal artery stenosis
   B. Renin-secreting tumors
   C. Intrarenal ischemia
      1. Accelerated-malignant hypertension
      2. Renal parenchymal disease
III. Unknown—Essential hypertension (10 per cent)

Blood Pressure Response to Saralasin. Renin-mediated hypertension may be easier to identify by observing the blood pressure response to infusion of the angiotensin antagonist saralasin. In a series of 1036 hypertensive patients, Streeten and Anderson found false-positive responses in about 5 per cent and false-negative responses in about 12 per cent.[306] Note, however, the much lower discrimination achieved in the study by Grim et al. (Table 26–13).

The procedure must be done carefully. In order to accentuate the differences between patients with high and normal renin, a mild state of volume contraction is required. This can be achieved with 40 mg of intravenous furosemide followed by 2 hours of upright posture. The same volume contraction minimizes the pressor response seen if saralasin is given to patients with low renin levels, since this antagonist also has agonist effects. To prevent both marked pressor responses in those with low renin and marked depressor responses in those with high renin, the infusion of saralasin should begin with a low dose, 0.05 to 0.10 $\mu g/kg/min$, and gradually be increased until a response occurs, to a maximum of 10 $\mu g/kg/min$.

The other available blocker of angiotensin activity, the converting-enzyme inhibitor captopril, lacks the discriminatory power of saralasin as a testing agent, since it lowers the blood pressure of most hypertensives with normal as well as high renin levels.[179]

Confirmatory Tests. If renovascular hypertension is suspected, from either an abnormal screening test or a strongly suggestive clinical setting, the diagnosis must be established and the nature of the disease defined before operation, regardless of the outcome of screening tests. Some perform renal arteriography first, others determine the renal vein renin ratio. If the degree of clinical suspicion is high, both tests may be performed at the same time; however, patients should not receive renin-suppressing antihypertensive drugs, including all adrenergic blocking agents, for at least a few days before the renal vein catheter study, whereas these drugs may be needed to lower blood pressure enough to minimize the risks of arteriography. Therefore, if the patient is on effective therapy, arteriography may be done first. If results are negative, renal vein renin levels need not be determined. On the other hand, arteriography is a more dangerous procedure and may not be needed if the renin ratio is normal. These guidelines are further beclouded by the increasing recognition that some patients without lateralizing renin ratios may be cured by surgery (see later).

As digital subtraction angiography becomes more readily available and accurate, it may be possible to visualize the renal arteries (and obtain an IVP) with much less morbidity. However, at the present time, it is not possible to exclude or completely define renovascular disease—particularly branch lesions—by using this procedure. Renal arteriography still has a place. One could argue that in patients for whom definitive examination of the renal arterial architecture is needed, a transfemoral arteriogram remains the procedure of choice.

Renal Vein Renin Ratio. This procedure has been used widely since Helmer and Judson showed in 1960 that functionally significant renovascular disease could be recognized by the finding of high levels of renin activity in blood obtained by percutaneous catheterization of the renal veins[307] (Fig. 26–31). According to a survey of published data, 93 per cent of patients with a lateralizing ratio—i.e., greater than 1.5 to 2.0 between the abnormal and contralateral sides—were cured or improved by operation[308] (Table 26–16). However, when patients who had other features suggestive of renovascular hypertension but who did not have a lateralizing ratio greater than 2.0 were subjected to operation, 57 per cent were also cured or improved. Use of a ratio of 1.5 would decrease the number of false-negatives but would increase the number of false-positive tests. When patients with essential hypertension were tested, 19 per cent had a renal vein renin ratio of 1.5 or higher.[309] Although this may reflect asymmetrical nephrosclerosis, it probably results from the common practice of using a single catheter and sequentially sampling the renal veins. Renin secretion is episodic, and by the time the catheter is switched, significantly more or less renin may be coming from one renal vein than from the other.

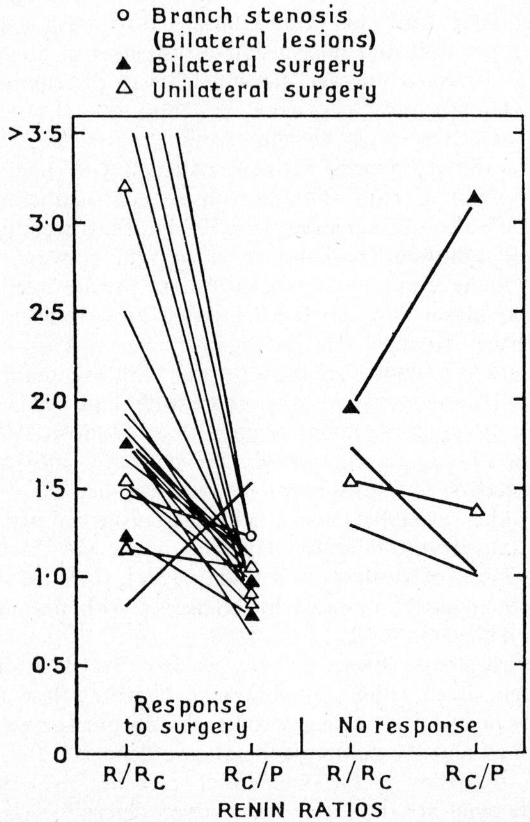

FIGURE 26–31 Relation between renal vein renin ratio (R/R_c) and R_c/P in 25 patients with renovascular hypertension, classified according to response to surgery. R_c = nonstenotic or less involved renal vein; P = peripheral blood PRA. (From Stockigt, J. R., et al.: Renal-vein renin in various forms of renal hypertension. Lancet *1*: 1194, 1972.)

TABLE 26–16 OPERATIVE RESULTS IN HYPERTENSIVE PATIENTS WITH UNILATERAL STENOSIS OF A MAIN RENAL ARTERY WITH RESPECT TO RENAL VEIN RENIN RATIOS

		Patients with Lateralizing Renal Vein Renin Ratios		Patients without Lateralizing Renal Vein Renin Ratios	
	Number of Patients	*Cured or Improved*	*Failed*	*Cured or Improved*	*Failed*
Summary of literature review	412	267	19	64	62
Present data	56	24	3	24	5
Totals	468	291 (93%)	22 (7%)	88 (57%)	67 (43%)

Data from Marks, L. S., et al.: Renovascular hypertension: Does the renal vein renin ratio predict operative results? J. Urol. *115*:365, 1976. Copyright 1976, The Williams and Wilkins Co., Baltimore.

To enhance the reliability of the procedure and accentuate the difference between the two sides, renin secretion should be stimulated by prior volume contraction using a low-salt diet and diuretics or converting enzyme inhibitor.[310] To insure further that surgical cure is probable, renin secretion from the contralateral kidney should be completely suppressed, as shown by a renin level identical to that in the inferior caval blood (Fig. 26–31).

Renovascular disease is bilateral in 25 per cent of patients, but usually one side is more involved, and an abnormal renin ratio is usually found.[311] Care should be taken to obtain blood draining any area in which segmental or branch arterial disease may be present.

Renal Arteriography. Ultimately the renal vasculature must be visualized to prove the diagnosis and to decide upon the feasibility and type of operation. The transfemoral approach is preferred, allowing selective visualization of each artery and its branches. Films can be taken with the patient upright to unravel vessels involved with medial fibroplasia that are often long and curled. Care must also be taken not to miss atherosclerotic lesions in the renal artery where it originates from the aorta. Sometimes arterial spasm from irritation by the catheter may give the false appearance of a lesion.

Although the arteriogram is needed to diagnose renovascular disease, it provides little help in deciding upon surgical curability. In the Cooperative Study, neither the degree of stenosis, the presence of poststenotic dilatation, nor the presence of collateral circulation was of much value in predicting the success of operation for individual patients.[296] Patients with stenosis of greater than 90 per cent may require operation to prevent complete occlusion.

THERAPY

Unfortunately, little is known about the natural history of untreated renovascular disease so it is difficult to assess the results of therapy. No properly controlled study comparing medical versus surgical treatment is available, although one is in progress at Vanderbilt Medical School.[312] Advances in medical therapy have made it easier to control the hypertension and the availability of transluminal angioplasty offers another "curative" approach, but current evidence supports surgical repair as being more likely to provide relief of hypertension and preserve renal function. Among 41 patients randomly allocated to medical therapy in the ongoing Vanderbilt trial, 17 showed deterioration of renal function or loss of renal size, despite acceptable blood pressure control in 15 of the 17.[312]

Operation should be considered in patients with proved, functionally significant renovascular disease if their general status and life expectancy are reasonably good. Better results follow repair of fibroplastic disease, in part because these patients tend to be younger and healthier. In various series, about 5 per cent of patients die during or after surgery; about 90 per cent of those with fibroplastic disease are cured or improved after one year, and about 70 per cent of those with atherosclerotic disease are similarly helped.[313,314] Vascular repair should always be attempted. Although initial results with nephrectomy may be as good, the other renal artery is obviously susceptible to the same process.[315]

The response to surgery may be predicted based on the response to the angiotensin-converting enzyme inhibitor captopril, which also provides effective medical therapy for those unable to undergo an operation.[316]

More and more patients may be subjected to transluminal angioplasty as cumulative experience seems to document its safety and effectiveness.[317] In patients with marked renal insufficiency from stenosis of a solitary kidney or bilateral disease, vessels have been successfully dilated.[318] On the other hand, most patients above 60 years of age who are subjected to surgical treatment improve,[319] so this remains the preferable approach for most patients.

We have, then, easier ways to recognize renovascular disease and more effective ways to relieve renovascular hypertension. As our sights are focused on the 5 to 10 per cent of patients likely to have this condition, we should be able to diagnose and treat many of them, with the expectation of relieving a considerable burden of severe hypertension.

Renin-Secreting Tumors

Made up of juxtaglomerular cells or hemangiopericytomas, these tumors have been found mostly in young patients with severe hypertension, very high renin levels both in peripheral blood and in the kidney harboring the tumor, and secondary aldosteronism manifested by hypokalemia.[320] The tumor can usually be recognized by selective renal angiography, usually done because of the suspicion of renovascular hypertension. More commonly, children with Wilms' tumors may have hypertension and high renin levels that revert to normal after nephrectomy.[321]

Adrenal Causes of Hypertension

(See also Chapter 51)

Three adrenal causes of hypertension will now be considered—primary excesses of aldosterone, cortisol, and catecholamines—which together constitute less than 1 per cent of all hypertensive diseases. In addition, congenital adrenal hyperplasia will be discussed. Each can usually be recognized with relative ease, and patients suspected of having these disorders can be screened by means of readily available tests. However, specific identification of the particular adrenal disease responsible for each type of hormonal excess, which is necessary before decisions concerning therapy can be made, can be difficult.

PRIMARY ALDOSTERONISM (See also p. 1733)

First recognized almost 30 years ago, this disease is relatively rare (Table 26–5), although it may be found fairly often in selected populations.[24,322,323]

Pathophysiology. Primary aldosterone excess usually arises from solitary benign adenomas. As diagnostic tests improve and become more readily available, larger numbers of patients with minimal features are recognized and found to have bilateral adrenal hyperplasia, the number varying from one-fifth[323] to more than half[322] of the cases of aldosteronism. The validity of defining the condition in these patients with bilateral hyperplasia as "idiopathic hyperaldosteronism" has been strongly denied by investigators from the MRC Blood Pressure Unit.[324,325] Their argument is persuasive, and I agree with their conclusion that "idiopathic hyperaldosteronism is at the upper end of a wider-than-normal distribution of aldosterone in essential hypertension, from which it has been separated wrongly."[325] Nonetheless, there is evidence that such patients may be responding to an unknown stimulus to aldosterone secretion, including suppression of their high aldosterone levels by the serotonin antagonist cyproheptadine.[326]

Some other variants are seen: a few patients have familial glucocorticoid-suppressible hyperaldosteronism[327]; a few extraadrenal tumors may hypersecrete aldosterone[328]; exogenous mineralocorticoids may cause "pseudoaldosteronism," including the glycyrrhizinic acid in licorice from candy[329] or chewing tobacco[330] and nasal sprays mistakenly containing mineralocorticoid instead of glucocorticoid.[331]

Whatever the source, excess aldosterone causes hypertension and hypokalemia, here defined as a plasma potassium level below 3.2 mEq/liter (Fig. 26–32). Very rarely, the syndrome has been recognized in normotensive individuals.[332] Not so rarely, hypokalemia may be absent or only intermittent, but in most patients with adenomas, persistent hypokalemia is almost invariable.[328]

The hypertension begins as a volume overload but soon converts, as do apparently all forms of hypertension, to increased peripheral resistance.[93] The degree of hypertension can be significant, with a mean pressure in one group of 136 patients of 205/123 mm Hg.[328] Malignant hypertension may supervene,[333] and in the large series from Scotland, four of the 136 patients had histological evidence of malignant hypertension on renal biopsy.[328] Furthermore, 23 per cent of their patients had a serious vascular complication

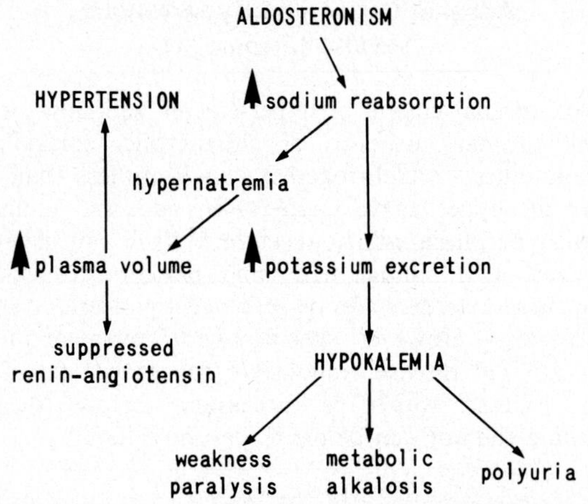

FIGURE 26–32 Pathophysiology of primary aldosteronism. (From Kaplan, N. M.: Primary aldosteronism. *In* Astwood, E. B., and Cassidy, C. E. (eds.): Clinical Endocrinology. Vol. II. New York, 1968, p. 468, by permission of Grune and Stratton.)

such as stroke or myocardial infarction. Thus, the hypertension can be serious.

In association with the increased pressure and expanded volume, renin secretion is suppressed. This finding has been almost invariable with the syndrome, but the overwhelming majority of hypertensive patients with suppressed renin do not have primary aldosteronism (Table 26–12).

Hypokalemia results from the aldosterone-mediated increase in renal potassium wastage. Although hypokalemia may not be recognized until diuretics or salt loads are ingested, the effects may be striking, with muscular weakness, polyuria, metabolic alkalosis, impaired carbohydrate tolerance, and blunting of circulatory reflexes.

Diagnosis. No serious consideration need be given the diagnosis of primary aldosteronism unless hypertension and hypokalemia coexist. If the rare normokalemic patient with the disease is thereby missed, little will be lost as long as the patient is protected by appropriate treatment for the hypertension. Since this will likely include a diuretic, significant hypokalemia will soon become manifest, making the diagnosis obvious.

Potassium-Wasting. The first step in evaluating the hypokalemic hypertensive should be the determination of potassium excretion in a 24-hour urine sample collected while the patient is hypokalemic, receiving no supplemental potassium or diuretic, and ingesting a normal sodium intake (i.e., urinary sodium excretion is above 100 mEq/day) (Fig. 26–33). If urinary potassium under these circumstances is less than 30 mEq/day, mineralocorticoid excess is highly unlikely, and the work-up can be aborted; if the value is above 30, further evaluation is warranted.

In most hypertensive patients hypokalemia is caused by the prior use of diuretics. Losses may be large and may require prolonged potassium supplementation. On the other hand, severe hypokalemia appearing soon after the initiation of diuretic therapy may presage primary aldosteronism.

Renin Suppression. If urinary potassium-wasting has been documented, the patient should receive potassium supplementation for a period of 3 to 6 weeks to bring the plasma potassium level within the normal range and maintain it, so that subsequent studies will be unaffected by hypokalemia. One or another mild stimulus to renin secretion should be applied to demonstrate suppression. By whatever technique, renin levels are almost invariably and significantly suppressed in patients with primary aldosteronism.

Aldosterone Excess. Increased levels of aldosterone can be found in urine or blood. When urine is used, the

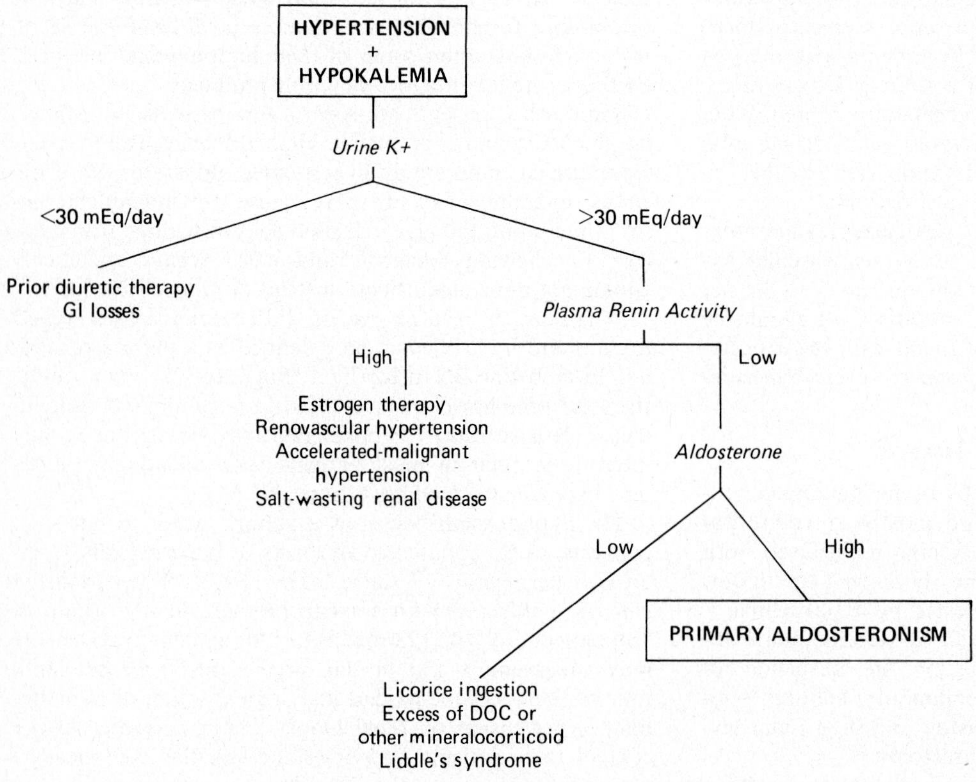

FIGURE 26–33 Flow diagram for the differential diagnosis of hypertension with hypokalemia. (From Kaplan, N. M.: Clinical Hypertension. 3rd ed. Baltimore, Williams and Wilkins Co., 1982, p. 306.)

24-hour collection should contain over 100 mEq of sodium to insure that high aldosterone levels are not simply secondary to sodium restriction. Various techniques to suppress endogenous aldosterone secretion have been used to insure further that the aldosterone excess is primary. These include infusions of saline, injections of DOCA, and oral administration of fludrocortisone (Florinef).

One of the easiest and most reliable procedures is the saline suppression test of plasma aldosterone[334] in which 2 liters of normal saline are infused over a four-hour interval. The plasma aldosterone level remains high in those with primary aldosteronism but is suppressed to below 6 ng/100 ml in patients with essential hypertension or secondary aldosteronism.

Once the diagnosis is established, a less direct approach may be used to document the diagnosis and to prepare the patient for surgery, i.e., the response to high doses of the aldosterone antagonist spironolactone.[335] It may also be useful in predicting the response to operation; in one study the decrease in blood pressure with spironolactone was closely correlated to the subsequent response to operation in 44 patients tested.[336]

Bilateral Adrenal Hyperplasia. Various maneuvers are available to differentiate patients with apparent aldosterone excess due to bilateral adrenal hyperplasia from those with an adrenal adenoma.[4] The differential diagnosis should be made, and only those patients with a tumor should be subjected to operation, since it may not be possible to determine the type of pathologic condition at operation without removing both adrenal glands.

Now that computerized axial tomography (CAT) is capable of identifying adrenal lesions as small as 1.0 cm, this procedure has become the best initial test to identify the type of adrenal disease.[337] If it fails to define an adrenal adenoma when the clinical situation is strongly suggestive, bilateral adrenal vein catheterization with venography and analysis of venous steroid levels should be attempted.[323] Rather than false-negative tests, there will likely be more problems with false-positive CAT scans, i.e., finding nonfunctioning adrenal tumors, which are present in a considerable number of normotensive and hypertensive people.[338]

Therapy. Once the diagnosis of primary aldosteronism is made and the type of adrenal disorder has been established, the choice of therapy is fairly easy: patients with a solitary adenoma require resection of the tumor; those with bilateral hyperplasia should be treated with spironolactone and a thiazide diuretic.[336] Fortunately, the doses of spironolactone required for chronic therapy are usually low enough to avoid bothersome side effects. Triamterene[339] and amiloride[340] (p. 533) will also control the disease if spironolactone is poorly tolerated. When an adenoma is resected, about 75 per cent of patients will become normotensive, while the other 25 per cent remain hypertensive, either from preexisting essential hypertension or from renal damage due to prolonged secondary hypertension.[341]

CUSHING'S SYNDROME (See also p. 1732)

Hypertension occurs in about 80 per cent of patients with Cushing's syndrome. If left untreated, it can cause congestive heart failure and death.[342] As with hypertension of other endocrine causes, the longer hypertension is present, the less likely it will be to disappear when the disease is cured.[341]

Mechanism of Hypertension. Blood pressure may increase for a number of reasons:

1. The secretion of a mineralocorticoid, DOC or aldosterone, may also be increased along with cortisol.
2. The excess cortisol exerts a sufficient intrinsic salt-retaining effect to expand volume and lead to hypertension.
3. Cortisol stimulates the synthesis of renin substrate, which in turn causes more angiotensin to be generated. The angiotensin antagonist saralasin lowered the blood pressure of seven of nine patients with Cushing's syndrome.[343]
4. Vascular reactivity to pressor substances, including norepinephrine, increases.

Diagnosis. The syndrome should be suspected in patients with central obesity, thin skin, muscle weakness, and osteoporosis. If clinical features are suggestive, the diagnosis can be either ruled out or virtually assured by the simple, overnight *dexamethasone suppression test.*[344] In normal subjects, the level of plasma cortisol in a sample drawn at 8 A.M. after a bedtime dose of 1 mg of dexamethasone should be below 7 μg/100 ml. If the level is higher, additional workup is in order to establish both the diagnosis of cortisol excess and the pathological type. Patients who are under stress or depressed may fail to show suppression. Measurement of urine free cortisol levels is almost as good a screening test: most patients who do not have Cushing's syndrome excrete less than 100 μg/24 hours.

The next procedure should be a longer dexamethasone suppression test, using 0.5 mg every 6 hours and then 2.0 mg every 6 hours, each for 2 days. Urinary 17-hydroxycorticoid (17-HOCS) or free cortisol excretion should be measured on the second day of each dose. Patients with Cushing's syndrome will fail to suppress urinary 17-HOCS to below 2.5 mg/day on the 0.5-mg dose; if Cushing's syndrome is caused by an excess pituitary ACTH drive with bilateral adrenal hyperplasia, urinary 17-HOCS will be suppressed to below 50 per cent of the control value on the 2.0 mg dose.[344] As plasma ACTH assays become more reliable, they provide additional differentiation between pituitary and ectopic ACTH excess on the one hand and adrenal tumors with ACTH suppression on the other.

If hormonal excess is documented, the source of the adrenal disease should be documented further by CAT scans of the pituitary, chest, and abdomen.[345]

Therapy. In about two-thirds of patients with Cushing's syndrome, the process begins with overproduction of ACTH by the pituitary, which leads to bilateral adrenal hyperplasia. Although pituitary hyperfunction may reflect a hypothalamic disorder, the majority of patients have discrete pituitary adenomas that can usually be resected by selective transsphenoidal microsurgery.[346] In children with fairly mild disease, conventional high-voltage pituitary irradiation is often curative.[347] High-energy proton-beam irradiation has also been used. Only rarely is bilateral adrenalectomy necessary. Medical therapy is almost never curative.

If an adrenal tumor is present, it should be surgically removed. With earlier diagnosis and more selective surgical therapy, it is hoped that more patients with Cushing's syndrome will be cured without the need for lifelong glucocorticoid replacement therapy and with permanent relief of their hypertension.

Pheochromocytoma (See also p. 1734)

The wild fluctuations in blood pressure and dramatic symptoms of pheochromocytoma usually alert both the patient and the physician to the possibility of this diagnosis. However, the fluctuations may be missed or, as occurs in half the patients, the hypertension may be persistent. The symptoms may be ascribed to psychoneurosis by practitioners desensitized to "spells," which usually represent menopausal hot flushes or anxiety-induced hyperventilation. Unfortunately, if the diagnosis is missed, severe complications may arise from very high blood pressure and damage to the heart by catecholamines. Stroke and hypertensive crises with encephalopathy and retinal hemorrhages occur most commonly, probably because extremely high levels of pressure develop suddenly in vessels unprepared by chronic hypertension. Fortunatey, a simple and inexpensive test will detect the disease with virtual certainty, so that diagnostic indecision may be minimized.

PATHOPHYSIOLOGY. Pheochromocytomas may arise wherever the sympathogonia from the primitive neural crest come to lie. These cells differentiate into ganglion cells, neuroblasts, and chromaffin cells. Tumors develop from each of these cell types; ganglioneuromas and neuroblastomas usually occur in children and are recognized by the excretion of large amounts of homovanillic acid (HVA), which is a metabolite of dopamine, the immediate precursor of norepinephrine. Paragangliomas may arise in chemoreceptor tissue, where they are called chemodectomas; along the sympathetic chain, including the organ of Zuckerkandl; and in the urinary bladder. A pheochromocytoma was found in 10 of 18 patients with neurofibromatosis and hypertension.[347a]

The majority of pheochromocytomas, about 90 per cent, arise in the adrenal medulla; 10 per cent of these are bilateral and another 10 per cent are malignant. Multiple adrenal tumors are particularly common in patients with simple familial pheochromocytoma and multiple endocrine adenomatosis, Type II, in association with medullary carcinoma of the thyroid (Sipple's syndrome); or with mucosal ganglioneuromas in addition (Type IIB or III). Diffuse medullary hyperplasia may precede the development of tumors, and the tumors may, in fact, reflect extreme degrees of nodular hyperplasia.[348]

Secretion from nonfamilial pheochromocytomas varies considerably, with small tumors tending to secrete larger proportions of active catecholamines. If the predominant secretion is epinephrine, which is formed only in the adrenal medulla, the symptoms reflect its effects—mainly systolic hypertension due to increased cardiac output, tachycardia, sweating, flushing, and apprehension. If norepinephrine is predominantly secreted, as from some of the adrenal tumors and from almost all the extraadrenal tumors, the symptoms include both systolic and diastolic hypertension from peripheral vasoconstriction but less tachycardia, palpitations, and anxiety.

DIAGNOSIS. Many more hypertensive patients have variable blood pressures and "spells" than the 0.2 per cent or so who harbor a pheochromocytoma. A number of stresses and some rather rare diseases may involve transient catecholamine release (Table 26–17). Other causes of recurrent spells of paroxysmal hypertension may not be related to increased sympathetic nervous activity.

TABLE 26–17 DIFFERENTIAL DIAGNOSIS OF PHEOCHROMOCYTOMA

Recurrent spells
Anxiety with hyperventilation
Menopause
Hypoglycemia*
Angina
Paroxysmal tachycardia
Lead poisoning
Migraine and cluster headaches
Diencephalic seizures
Familial dysautonomia
Acrodynia*
Porphyria*
Carcinoid*
Paroxysmal hypertension
Acute pulmonary edema
Acute myocardial infarction
Stroke
Brain tumor*
Rebound after abrupt cessation of clonidine and other antihypertensives*
Hypertensive crises associated with MAO inhibitors*
Intake of sympathomimetic drugs*
Autonomic dysreflexia (quadriplegia)*
Hypertension and hypermetabolism
Thyrotoxicosis
Diabetes mellitus
Eclampsia

*Reported to cause increased levels of catecholamines.

TABLE 26–18 CONDITIONS IN WHICH PATIENTS SHOULD BE SCREENED FOR PHEOCHROMOCYTOMA

Paroxysmal hypertension
OR
Persistent hypertension, if accompanied by
Headache
Sweating
Palpitations
Nervousness
Weight loss
Hypermetabolism
Orthostatic hypotension
Severe pressor response in association with
Induction of anesthesia
Pregnancy or delivery
Surgery
Histamine for gastric analysis
Intake of phenothiazines, tricyclic antidepressants, or adrenal glucocorticoids
Saralasin testing for angiotensin-mediated hypertension
Family history of pheochromocytoma, medullary carcinoma of the thyroid, or hyperparathyroidism
Neurocutaneous lesions

A pheochromocytoma should be suspected in patients with hypertension that is either paroxysmal or persistent and accompanied by certain symptoms and signs, as listed in Table 26–18. In addition, children and patients with rapidly accelerating hypertension should be screened. Those whose tumors secrete predominantly epinephrine are prone to postural hypotension from a contracted blood volume and blunted sympathetic reflex tone. Suspicion should be heightened if activities such as bending over, exercise, or palpation of the abdomen cause repetitive spells that begin abruptly, advance rapidly, and subside within minutes.

High levels of catecholamines may induce acute myocarditis, which may progress to cardiomyopathy and left ventricular failure.[349] In the patient described by Baker et al., the decreased cardiac output that resulted from myocardial damage kept the blood pressure normal.[349] Acute myocardial infarction also occurs with increased frequency.[350] Opiates given to such patients may raise the pressure through release of catecholamines.[351]

LABORATORY CONFIRMATION

Screening. The easiest and best procedure is either a 24-hour or spot urine assay for total metanephrines.[352] This catecholamine metabolite is least affected by various interfering substances including antihypertensive drugs. Among 50 patients seen at the Mayo Clinic, the metanephrine test gave the lowest number of false-negatives (4 per cent) when compared with vanillylmandelic acid (VMA) assays (29 per cent), urinary catecholamines (21 per cent), or basal plasma catecholamines (47 per cent).[353] The ranges for these three urinary tests are shown in Table 26–19.

Urinary metanephrine excretion will be increased if patients are taking sympathomimetic drugs or MAO inhibitors and will be decreased for the next few days after use of x-ray contrast media containing methylglucamine (e.g., Renografin, Hypaque). Therefore, the urine should be collected before an IVP or other such procedure is done.

Plasma catecholamine assays are now becoming available and may provide a way to confirm the diagnosis but will not serve as a screening test, since they result in too

TABLE 26–19 URINARY TESTS FOR PHEOCHROMOCYTOMA

COMPOUND	URINARY EXCRETION (MG/DAY OR μG/MG CREATININE)	
	Normal Adults	*Pheochromocytoma*
Free catecholamines	<0.1	0.1 to 10.0
Metanephrine + normetanephrine	<1.2	1.0 to 100.0
Vanillylmandelic acid	<6.5	5 to 600

many false-positive values.[345] If plasma levels are equivocal, measurement of a plasma norepinephrine level 3 hours after a single 0.3-mg oral dose of the adrenergic inhibitor clonidine has been shown to separate the nonpheochromocytoma patients, whose levels are suppressed, from those with the disease, who do experience suppression.[355]

Localization of the Tumor. Once the diagnosis has been made, medical therapy should be given and the tumor localized, if possible, by CAT scan, which usually demonstrates the typically large tumors with ease. It is hoped that radioisotopes that localize in chromaffin tissue will become available to be of additional help in those few patients in whom localization is not possible by current techniques.[348]

THERAPY. Once diagnosed and localized, pheochromocytomas should be resected. Great care should be taken in preparing patients for operation and managing them through the procedure.[356] The most important part of their preoperative management is adequate adrenergic blockade over enough time to overcome vasoconstriction and allow the reduced blood volume to reexpand. If the tumor is unresectable, chronic medical therapy with the alpha blocker phenoxybenzamine (Dibenzyline) or the inhibitor of catechol synthesis α-methyl-tyrosine (Demser) can be used.

Congenital Adrenal Hyperplasia

Two distinct enzymatic defects may induce hypertension: (1) 11-hydroxylase deficiency, which leads to virilization (from excessive androgens) and hypertension with hypokalemia (from excessive DOC), which may not become manifest until adult life[357]; and (2) 17-hydroxylase deficiency, which causes similar hypertension from excess DOC but also failure of secondary sexual development because sex hormones are also deficient.[358] Affected children are hypertensive, but the defect in sex hormone synthesis may not become obvious until after puberty. Thereafter, affected males display ambiguity of sexual development and females fail to mature or menstruate.

Miscellaneous Causes of Hypertension

A host of other causes of hypertension are known (see Table 26–4). One that is likely becoming more common is ingestion of various drugs[359]—prescribed (e.g., Danazol[360]), over-the-counter (e.g., phenylpropanolamine[361]), and illicit (e.g., cocaine).

Coarctation of the Aorta

(See also Chapters 29 and 30)

Congenital narrowing of the aorta may occur at any level of the thoracic or abdominal aorta. It is usually found just beyond the origin of the left subclavian artery or distal to the insertion of the ligamentum arteriosum. The coarctation may be localized or more diffuse. Other cardiac anomalies usually accompany the latter, and over half of those afflicted die during the first year of life, although operative treatment of both the coarctation and associated anomalies may reduce this mortality rate.[362] With less severe postductal lesions, damage is more insidious, and symptoms may not appear until the teens or later. To diminish the development of congestive failure, endocarditis, and stroke, the obstruction should be recognized and corrected before the age of 5 years.[363] The pathogenesis of the hypertension may be more complicated than simple mechanical obstruction: the renin-angiotensin levels may be inappropriately high-normal[364] and the sympathetic nervous system may be activated.[365] Hypertension in the arms and weak or absent femoral pulses are the classic features of coarctation. The lesion may be detected by cross-sectional echocardiography[366] (p. 975). Aortography proves the diagnosis. Immediately after surgical repair, the blood pressure may transiently rise even further, and mesenteric arteritis may develop. These changes may reflect very high levels of renin-angiotensin[367] and catecholamines.[368] The latter may persist for up to six months after operation.

HYPERPARATHYROIDISM

Hypertension occurs in one-fourth to one-half of patients with hyperparathyroidism and is found commonly in patients with other hypercalcemic states.[369] As more and more patients are found to be hypertensive and undergo routine testing of serum calcium, asymptomatic hypercalcemia associated with hyperparathyroidism is not infrequently recognized. Moreover, thiazide diuretics—the most frequently used drugs in the treatment of hypertension—may accentuate previously borderline hypercalcemia. Hypercalcemia was found in 1.9 per cent of patients receiving thiazides compared to 0.6 per cent in the remainder in a community screening program.[370] Of 15 persistently hypercalcemic hypertensive individuals, 14 turned out to have hyperparathyroidism.

The mechanism by which hypercalcemia elevates the blood pressure is unknown. Calcium directly increases the contractility of vascular smooth muscle and may activate the sympathetic nervous system.[369] Interestingly, parathyroid function may be enhanced in essential hypertension, as a homeostatic response to a urinary calcium leak.[371]

HYPERTENSION AFTER CARDIAC SURGERY

Transient hypertension may develop postoperatively for various reasons: pain, physical and emotional excitement, hypoxia, hypercapnia, and excessive volume loads[372] (Table 26–20). More severe hypertension has been noted following various cardiovascular surgical procedures:

— *Coronary bypass surgery.* The incidence, exceeding 33 per cent, is far higher than after other major cardiac or noncardiac surgery. The problem appears more commonly on the background of

TABLE 26–20 HYPERTENSION ASSOCIATED WITH CARDIAC SURGERY

Preoperative
- Anxiety, angina, and the like
- Discontinuation of antihypertensive therapy
- "Rebound" from discontinuing beta-blocking agents in patients with coronary artery disease

Intraoperative
- Induction of anesthesia
  - Specific drugs
  - Hypertension due to tracheal intubation and nasopharyngeal, urethral, or rectal manipulation
- Precardiopulmonary bypass (during sternotomy and chest retraction)
- Cardiopulmonary bypass
- Postcardiopulmonary bypass (during surgery)

Postoperative
- Early—within 2 hours
  - Obvious cause: Hypoxia, hypercarbia, ventilatory difficulties, hypothermia, shivering, arousal from anesthesia
  - No obvious cause: After myocardial revascularization; less frequently after valve replacement; early (Sealy type I) hypertension after resection of aortic coarctation
- Intermediate—12 to 36 hours after surgery: Sealy type II after repair of aortic coarctation
- Late—weeks to months: After aortic valve replacement by homografts

From Estafanous, F. G., and Tarazi, R. C.: Systemic arterial hypertension associated with cardiac surgery. Am. J. Cardiol. *46*:685, 1980.

preexisting hypertension, greater than 50 per cent obstruction of the left main coronary artery, or the preoperative use of beta blockers.[373] The hemodynamic pattern of increased peripheral resistance could be explained by the markedly high plasma catecholamine and renin activity measured in such patients. Since many of these patients will have been receiving beta-blocker therapy that has been discontinued, the postoperative hypertension may to some extent reflect a rebound phenomenon. Therapy is often required, and intravenous nitroprusside and stellate ganglion or thoracic epidural block are effective.[372]

— *Aortic valve replacement.* Transient hypertension may give way to more permanent hypertension. In one series, 53 per cent of 116 patients were hypertensive five years after surgery, and hypertension was a major determinant of late failure of the homograft valve.[374]

— *Closure of an atrial septal defect.*[375]

PREGNANCY-INDUCED HYPERTENSION

(See also Chapter 53)

A small percentage of women enter pregnancy with hypertension. A larger number develop hypertension during pregnancy. With a diastolic blood pressure exceeding 84 mm Hg at any time during gestation, fetal mortality increases, even more so if accompanied by proteinuria[376] (Fig. 26–34). About 10,000 fetal deaths in the United States every year are attributable to hypertension.[377] Although the cause of pregnancy-induced hypertension is unknown, it can be recognized early and managed with relative ease, to the advantage of both mother and baby.

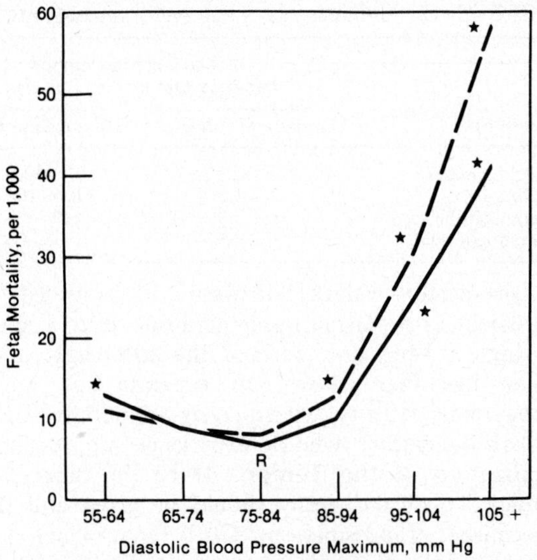

FIGURE 26–34 Fetal mortality in relation to the maximal diastolic blood pressure recorded during 38,636 pregnancies by the Collaborative Perinatal Project. The solid line represents the total series; the broken line represents the patients with concomitant proteinuria of any degree. Asterisks designate mortality significantly higher than in patients with normal maximal diastolic values (R). (From Friedman, E. A., and Neff, R. K.: Hypertension–hypotension in pregnancy. Correlation with fetal outcome. J.A.M.A. *239*:2249, 1978.)

DEFINITIONS

Blood pressure falls during the course of normal pregnancy to levels lower than those found in nonpregnant women[378] (Fig. 26–35), so that different criteria are needed for the diagnosis of hypertension. In most cases, these involve a rise in blood pressure of 30/15 mm Hg or more, or an absolute level greater than 140/90 on two or more occasions taken at least 6 hours apart. As with other forms of hypertension, the blood pressure may vary by 20 to 40 mm Hg within short intervals for no apparent reason.[379]

The types of hypertension seen include the following:

1. *Preeclampsia*: Hypertension with proteinuria and/or edema developing after the 20th week of gestation.

2. *Eclampsia*: The above, plus convulsions not caused by coincidental neurological disease.

3. *Chronic hypertension of whatever cause*: Most of these patients turn out to have essential hypertension that may not have been recognized prior to pregnancy and that is often masked by the usual fall in blood pressure during the midtrimester. Women with pressures above 110/75 at weeks 17 to 20 have a greater chance of developing pregnancy-induced hypertension.[380]

4. *Preeclampsia superimposed on chronic hypertension.*

MECHANISMS

The hemodynamic changes of normal pregnancy are described in Chapter 53. When preeclampsia begins, peripheral resistance rises, vascular reactivity to pressor agents

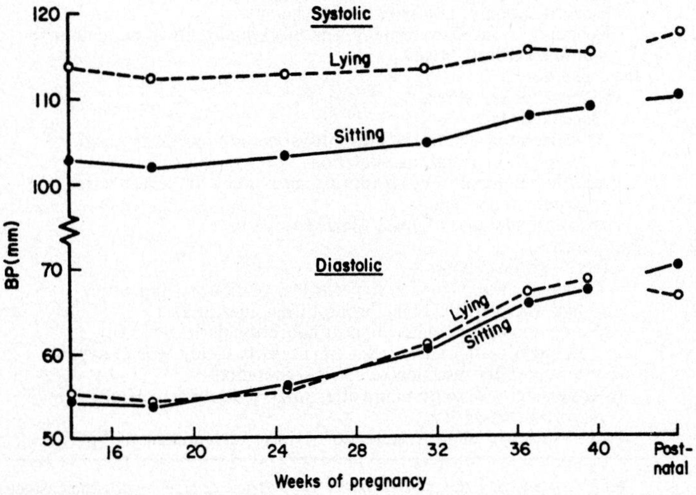

FIGURE 26–35 Mean blood pressures of 226 primigravidas seen at St. Mary's Hospital, London. Included are all the patients seen at or before 20 weeks of pregnancy over an 18-month interval. (From MacGillivray, I., et al.: Blood pressure survey in pregnancy. Clin. Sci. *37*:395, 1969.)

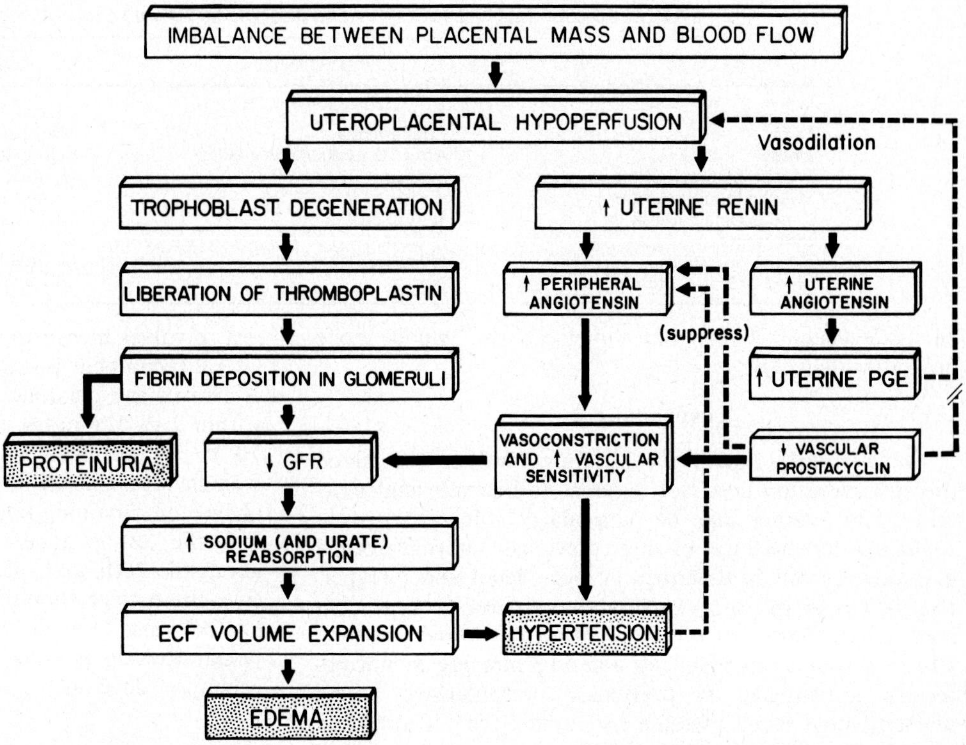

FIGURE 26–36 A unified working hypothesis for the pathophysiology of pregnancy-induced hypertension. The solid lines lead to the three primary manifestations: proteinuria, edema, and hypertension. The dotted lines indicate attempts to counteract the underlying defect of uteroplacental hypoperfusion. (From Kaplan, N. M.: Clinical Hypertension. 3rd ed. Baltimore, Williams and Wilkins Co., 1982, p. 367).

increases, plasma volume falls, and renal function diminishes.[381] Although the hypoperfused uterus may produce more renin, the levels of renin, angiotensin, and aldosterone in the maternal circulation all fall when the syndrome is full-blown. A unified working hypothesis has been constructed to explain these changes (Fig. 26–36); although parts of this scheme remain unproved, it serves as a useful model. The basic problem seems to be an imbalance between placental mass and blood flow.[382] In some women predisposed to preeclampsia, placental blood flow is impaired, as in those with diabetes or preexisting chronic hypertension. In others, placental mass is increased, as in those with multiple births and hydatidiform moles. In those with the greatest predisposition, young primigravidas, both a relatively greater placental mass and an inadequately developed blood supply may be involved.[383]

Whatever the basic reason, when the uteroplacental structure is hypoperfused, the cascade of events shown in Figure 26–36 is set into motion. Events shown on the left are well documented; those on the right are less so, but they have received support from recent investigations.

When the uterus is hypoperfused, it secretes more renin, which generates more angiotensin within the placental circulation. In response to moderately increased levels of angiotensin, uteroplacental blood flow increases,[384] possibly as a result of the action of angiotensin to liberate increased amounts of vasodilatory prostaglandins,[385] in particular prostacyclin.[386] The vasodilation provides an appropriate compensatory response to hypoperfusion, but this compensation may be inadequate in the preeclamptic patient: prostacyclin levels in amniotic fluid,[387] urine,[388] and fetal and maternal blood vessels[389] are lower in those with preeclampsia than in normal pregnancy. If an inability to synthesize prostaglandins is involved, it may also explain another aspect of developing preeclampsia—increased pressor sensitivity to exogenous angiotensin.[390]

Normal pregnant women are relatively resistant to the pressor effects of angiotensin. High levels of prostaglandins could explain this resistance in normal pregnancy.[391] Decreased prostaglandin (PG) levels, as would be expected after administration of the inhibitor of PG synthesis indomethacin, caused normal pregnant women to become much more sensitive to angiotensin.[390] Women who develop preeclampsia show increased pressor sensitivity to angiotensin well before their blood pressure rises.[390] Thus, uteroplacental prostaglandins, including prostacyclin, which enters the systemic circulation,[392] may mediate the vasodilated, low-pressure state of normal pregnancy and a decrease in these vasodepressor hormones may be involved in the pathogenesis of preeclampsia. Prostaglandins may be involved in another manner: plasma levels of free-radical oxidation products generated during prostaglandin biosynthesis are increased in preeclampsia; these free radicals may induce tissue injury.[393]

OTHER THEORIES

As attractive as this scheme appears, other theories are favored by some, including (1) a primary alteration in platelet function leading to slow intravascular coagulation with fibrin deposition[394]; and (2) an immunological basis, which could explain the increased incidence of preeclampsia in first pregnancies, its familial tendency, and its association with an enlarged placenta.[395] The familial tendency is compatible with a single recessive gene.[396]

Clinical Features

The distinction between preeclampsia and chronic hypertension should be made, since the former is a self-limited disease that is a threat only to the first pregnancy and should be treated more conservatively, with less pharmacological intervention. In most patients, the distinction can

TABLE 26–21 DIFFERENCES BETWEEN PREECLAMPSIA AND CHRONIC HYPERTENSION

	Preeclampsia	Chronic Hypertension
Age	Young (<20)	Older (>30)
Parity	Primigravida	Multipara
Onset	After 20 weeks of pregnancy	Before 20 weeks of pregnancy
Weight gain and edema	Sudden	Gradual
Systolic blood pressure	<160	>160
Funduscopic findings	Spasm, edema	Arteriovenous nicking, exudates
Proteinuria	Present	Absent
Plasma uric acid	Increased	Normal
Blood pressure after delivery	Normal	Elevated

be made (Table 26–21), but sometimes this can be done only after delivery.

HYPERTENSION

As previously noted, the absolute level of the blood pressure elevation need not be great to increase fetal mortality. The mother may be particularly vulnerable to encephalopathy because of her previously normal blood pressure. As will be described in more detail under Hypertensive Crises (p. 892), cerebral blood flow is kept constant over a fairly narrow range of mean arterial pressure, which is roughly between 60 and 110 mm Hg in normotensive individuals. A previously normotensive young woman whose blood pressure rises acutely to 150/100 may exceed the upper limit of autoregulation, resulting in a breakthrough of cerebral blood flow that leads to cerebral edema, convulsions, and all the clinical manifestations of eclampsia.

OTHER FEATURES

Proteinuria and Renal Damage. Even traces of proteinuria add significantly to the seriousness of the clinical situation (Fig. 26–34). Renal damage may be reflected in a falling creatinine clearance rate and a rising plasma uric acid concentration.

Edema. Some pedal edema is seen in over half of normal pregnant women, but a sudden weight gain of more than 2 pounds in one week and the subsequent appearance of more generalized edema commonly forewarns of preeclampsia.

Additional Features. On funduscopic examination, sequential constriction of the retinal arterioles is seen first, followed by retinal edema causing a retinal sheen. The presence of arteriovenous nicking and exudates suggests a chronic hypertensive process. If any of the following clinical features is present and does not improve, delivery within 24 hours should be considered: diastolic blood pressure above 110 mm Hg, headaches, visual scotomas, proteinuria 2+ or greater, or epigastric pain.

Management

PREVENTION. The only sure preventative against the syndrome of pregnancy-induced hypertension is prevention of pregnancy among teenagers. Once pregnant, primigravidas should be watched carefully, particularly if they are young or diabetic or have a family history of preeclampsia.

A simple test to predict subsequent preeclampsia has been described[397] and has been found to have fair specificity and sensitivity.[398] The supine pressor test, or "roll-over" test, involves measuring the blood pressure first in the left lateral recumbent position and then in the supine position. A rise in the diastolic pressure of 20 mm Hg or greater within 2 to 5 minutes is considered positive and predicts a 70 to 90 per cent chance of subsequent preeclampsia; women with a negative test have a greater than 90 per cent chance of remaining normotensive.

If the test is done on a normotensive primigravida at about the 28th week of pregnancy and if the result is positive, the patient should be instructed to restrict her activity, be seen frequently, and be warned that immediate hospitalization may be necessary if early features of preeclampsia develop.

TREATMENT

Once the blood pressure rises, the patient's physical activity should be restricted, preferably through admission to a high-risk pregnancy unit where she can be carefully observed. Remarkable results have been achieved in such a low-cost hospital setting.[399] Most women became normotensive without medication and safely carried their fetus to maturity. As a result, perinatal mortality fell to 9 per 1000—lower than that noted among infants born to women without preeclampsia on the general obstetric ward at the same hospital.[399]

ANTIHYPERTENSIVE THERAPY. Only if the diastolic pressure does not fall below 110 mm Hg on modified bedrest is antihypertensive drug therapy used. Diuretics and salt restriction are avoided, particularly since there is increasing evidence that preeclampsia is associated with a shrunken plasma volume.[381] Methyldopa (Aldomet) or hydralazine (Apresoline) has been usually chosen, the former for more chronic oral use and the latter for more acute parenteral use. In a randomly controlled trial, half of a group of hypertensive women, most with chronic, preexisting hypertension, received methyldopa, while the other half were left untreated. Their children were closely followed for 7½ years and the following differences were noted: the treated sons were lighter and shorter; sons whose mothers were started on methyldopa between 16 and 20 weeks' gestation had smaller heads but no difference in intelligence quotients.[400] Thus, there may be some developmental problems, particularly if methyldopa is started during the midtrimester. Since methyldopa acts centrally to influence the metabolism of the neurotransmitter dopamine, the safety of other drugs has been investigated.

Beta blockers initially received a bad press, with scattered reports of fetal hypoglycemia, bradycardia, and respiratory depression.[401] However, a properly controlled comparison showed that therapy with oxprenolol was equally effective as methyldopa and was associated with fewer fetal difficulties.[402] Another, less well controlled study of metoprolol had similar results.[403]

If the patient enters pregnancy while receiving antihypertensive drugs, including diuretics, the medications are usually continued, based on the idea that the mother should be protected and that the fetus will not suffer from any sudden hemodynamic shifts such as occur when therapy is first begun. Among women with chronic hypertension but who were not undergoing treatment, therapy with either hydralazine or methyldopa significantly reduced the incidence of preeclampsia compared to the course among a placebo-treated group.[404] Thus, those with chronic hypertension should probably be started on therapy early in their pregnancy.

MANAGEMENT OF ECLAMPSIA. With appropriate care of preeclampsia, eclampsia hardly ever supervenes; when it does, however, maternal mortality may reach 14 per cent and fetal mortality 27 per cent.[405] Among those women who die, contraction band necrosis of the myocardium, indicative of coronary artery spasm, is frequently noted and may be a contributing factor.[406]

Susceptible patients are given magnesium sulfate ($MgSO_4$) prophylactically, and blood pressure is brought under control with antihypertensive agents. Diazoxide, although favored by some, will cause labor to cease, since it relaxes uterine muscles. If convulsions have already occurred, they can be halted with $MgSO_4$, and delivery should be delayed until the blood pressure is controlled and fluid and electrolyte balance is achieved. With this approach, there have been no maternal deaths and fetal survival has been excellent in 154 consecutive cases.[399]

CONSEQUENCES. The long-term prognosis of women with pregnancy-induced hypertension is excellent. When some 200 women who had had eclampsia were followed for up to 44 years, the distribution of blood pressures was identical to that in the general population.[396] Chesley concludes that "eclampsia neither is a sign of latent essential hypertension nor causes hypertension."

POSTPARTUM HYPERTENSION

After delivery, women may develop transient or persistent hypertension. In many, early essential hypertension may have been masked by the hemodynamic changes of pregnancy. However, some women develop postpartum heart failure that may be related to hypertension or may be a primary cardiomyopathy[407] (see Chapter 52). A small number of others develop rapidly progressive acute oliguric renal failure associated with severe hypertension.[408]

HYPERTENSION IN CHILDREN AND ADOLESCENTS

(See also Chapter 31)

The linkage between hypertension in children and adolescents and that in adults is being strengthened, but long-term tracking studies are not available to document the natural history of the process. As an example, taken from the description of abnormal sodium transport in the pathogenesis of primary hypertension earlier in this chapter, half of the normotensive children of hypertensive parents have the abnormality but it will take another 20 or more years to determine whether the abnormality presages the development of hypertension. Regardless, a great deal of work is being done to define the frequency, mechanisms, natural history, and treatment of hypertension in childhood. Many of these aspects are covered in Chapter 31, and only a few will be highlighted here.

BLOOD PRESSURE MEASUREMENTS

The grids shown on page 1057, published in 1977 by a task force of the NHLBI, have been widely accepted as the "official" new standards for the distribution of blood pressure levels in normal male and female children, ages 2 to 17 years. However, other surveys have found the normal levels to be lower by an average of 5 to 10 mm Hg and few children to be definitely hypertensive.[409] The most obvious reason for these lower levels is the use of more than one blood pressure measurement in most of these studies.

The need to take more than one reading was shown as follows: in the Muscatine survey, 13 per cent of the 6,622 schoolchildren had elevated blood pressure on the first examination but less than 1 per cent had persistent elevations[410]; in Dallas, 8.9 per cent of 10,641 eighth-graders had levels at or above the 95th percentile on the first screening but only 1.2 per cent had hypertension on reexamination.[411]

In a number of studies, repeated measurements are being taken to assess the tracking of blood pressure levels. Correlations as high as 0.7 are noted over one year. Although lesser degrees of correlation are noted over long periods of time, the tracking of both systolic and diastolic pressures does persist for up to eight years.[412] Thus, the long-term course of blood pressure can be predicted with increasing confidence during early childhood. The need for repeated blood pressure measurements for all children is now established, with particular emphasis on families with hypertension, premature deaths, or other risk factors for cardiovascular disease.

ESSENTIAL OR PRIMARY HYPERTENSION

The studies by Zinner et al., in addition to providing long-term tracking data, reconfirm their previous findings of familial aggregation of both blood pressure and the excretion of kallikrein in the urine.[412] Low levels of this vasodilator could represent a causal mechanism for primary (essential) hypertension.

As noted before, about half the normotensive children of hypertensive parents have a rate of Na^+/K^+ flux within the range seen in patients with established, primary hypertension.[105] Whether those children will develop hypertension remains to be seen. If so, a new tool of great value in unraveling the mechanisms of hypertension may be available.

In the meantime, the levels of blood pressure in children have been shown to be related to various factors (Table 26–22). Perhaps the most important, beyond prior levels of blood pressure, is body weight, shown in various studies to be more closely related than age. In hopes of preventing subsequent hypertension, prevention of childhood obesity is being increasingly advocated, along with a reduction in the high levels of sodium intake. Of interest, the blood pressures of healthy black children are not higher—and may be lower—than those seen in white children.[413,414] Thus, the reasons for the much greater incidence of hypertension in black adults must be sought among factors

TABLE 26–22 EPIDEMIOLOGICAL FACTORS RELATED TO BLOOD PRESSURE LEVELS IN CHILDREN AND ADOLESCENTS

Genetic
Parental and sibling blood pressure levels
Erythrocyte sodium flux
Urinary kallikrein level
Environmental
Socioeconomic status
Rural vs. urban residence
Migration from developing to developed area
Pulse rate
Mixed genetic and environmental
Body mass and muscular development
Salt
Stress

From Lieberman, E.: *In* Kaplan, N. M. (ed.): Clinical Hypertension. 3rd ed. Baltimore, Williams and Wilkins Co., 1982, p. 420.

with long "incubation" or which are active mainly beyond adolescence. When asymptomatic children with persistently elevated pressures are studied, most turn out to have no recognizable secondary cause. In Muscatine, 23 of the 41 with high pressures were obese; of the 18 lean subjects, 13 had essential hypertension.[410]

The hemodynamic profile in children with primary hypertension is complex and variable. In a study of the cardiac output, fluid volumes, and intraarterial blood pressure in 42 young hypertensives (ages 15 to 25), there was no clear relation of the blood pressure to either cardiac output or blood volume.[415] Thus, hypertension in children does not usually fit a "hyperdynamic" pattern with high cardiac output and fast pulse rates.

The role of the sympathetic nervous and angiotensin mechanisms in blood pressure elevation among children remains unknown. Plasma renin and aldosterone levels tend to be *low* in those with the higher levels of blood pressure,[416] particularly among blacks.[417] Plasma catecholamine levels are usually normal,[416] but they may show a greater cardiovascular response to mental and other types of stress.[418]

The potential harm of even relatively small elevations in blood pressure may be found in careful studies of heart size and function. In 114 hypertensive high school students, heart size and contractile functions as determined by echocardiography were significantly increased in comparison to findings in normotensives of the same age.[419]

SECONDARY HYPERTENSION

As more experience is gained, the need for extensive laboratory work-up for the majority of postpubertal children with relatively mild hypertension continues to be deemphasized.[19] Only those with fairly severe hypertension or an abnormality on initial screening laboratory studies need to undergo additional testing, including an IVP. As shown years ago by Londe and coworkers,[419] most hypertension in children has no apparent cause but, when the diastolic is above 120 mm Hg, perhaps 95 per cent will have secondary hypertension. Thus, it may be appropriate to investigate more thoroughly only those with abnormalities on the physical examination or on urine analysis and those with a blood pressure that is 10 mm Hg or more above the 95th percentile.

THERAPY

The proper therapy for children with hypertension remains uncertain. In general, the guidelines for adult hypertension provided in Chapter 27 seem appropriate for the young, although a longer trial of weight reduction and sodium restriction seems indicated before drug treatment is begun. The long-term effects of various antihypertensive agents need to be more carefully assessed.

HYPERTENSIVE CRISES

Having considered the various forms of hypertension—both idiopathic and secondary—in children and adults, we will now turn to the life-threatening complication of all hypertensive diseases, hypertensive crisis.

Definitions

A number of clinical circumstances may require rapid reduction of the blood pressure (Table 26–23).

Hypertensive crisis: The presence of a blood pressure level so high that immediate vascular necrosis threatens. A mean arterial pressure above 150 mm Hg is enough to produce vascular damage within hours in experimental animals.[420] In humans, a diastolic pressure above 140 mm Hg is usually associated with acute vascular damage, although some may suffer seriously from lower levels and others manage to withstand even higher levels without apparent harm. As we shall see, the rapidity of the rise may be more important than the degree in producing acute vascular damage.

TABLE 26–23 CIRCUMSTANCES REQUIRING RAPID REDUCTION OF BLOOD PRESSURE

1. Hypertensive encephalopathy from any cause
   a. Essential hypertension
   b. Renal parenchymal diseases: acute and chronic glomerulonephritis
   c. Renal vascular disease
   d. Toxemia of pregnancy
2. Uncontrolled hypertension
   a. Malignant hypertension
   b. Pheochromocytoma
   c. Intake of catecholamine precursors in patients taking MAO inhibitors
   d. Head injuries
   e. Severe burns
   f. Rebound hypertension after cessation of antihypertensive drugs
3. Severe to moderate hypertension accompanying
   a. Acute left ventricular failure
   b. Intracranial hemorrhage
   c. Dissecting aneurysm of the aorta
   d. Postoperative bleeding at vascular suture lines
   e. Severe epistaxis

From Kaplan, N. M.: Clinical Hypertension. 3rd ed. Baltimore, Williams and Wilkins Co., 1982, p. 194.

Hypertensive encephalopathy: The association of headache, irritability, alterations in consciousness, and other manifestations of central nervous dysfunction with sudden and marked elevations in blood pressure. Symptoms can be reversed by a reduction in the pressure.

Accelerated hypertension: Retinal hemorrhages and exudates, usually with diastolic pressures above 140 mm Hg. This usually represents a sudden increase in chronically elevated blood pressure.

Malignant hypertension: Papilledema and diastolic pressures usually above 140 mm Hg. Accelerated hypertension usually precedes malignant hypertension. Without reduction of the pressure, death rapidly ensues, usually because of destruction of the kidneys.

Incidence

In about 1 per cent of patients with essential hypertension, the disease progresses to an accelerated or malignant phase. Presumably, if left untreated, many more patients would follow this pattern, since the incidence had been higher before effective therapies became available,[421] and it seems to be decreasing steadily. Ten per cent of patients with diastolic pressure below 115 mm Hg experienced a rise in pressure to above 125 when given placebos over a 5-year period[38]; if therapy had not been started, some would likely have progressed to malignant hypertension.

Any hypertensive disease can initiate malignant hypertension. Some, including pheochromocytoma and renovascular hypertension, do so at a higher rate than does essential hypertension. However, since hypertension is idiopathic in over 90 per cent of all patients, the largest number of hypertensive crises appear when there is preexisting essential hypertension.

Pathophysiology

Two distinct but usually concurrent processes are involved. One is functional, i.e., the dilatation of cerebral arterioles, allowing excessive cerebral blood flow that leads to hypertensive encephalopathy. The other is structural, i.e., acute damage to the arteriolar wall, resulting in fibri-

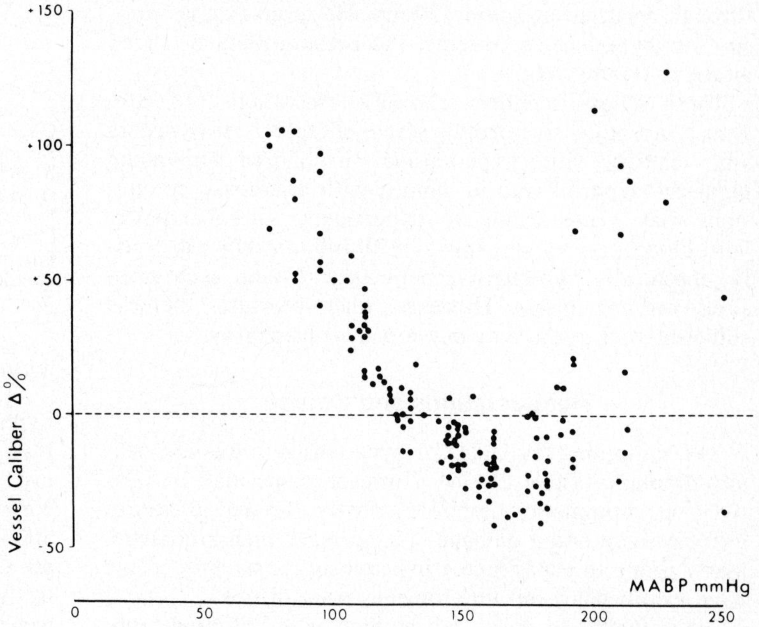

FIGURE 26–37 Change observed in the caliber of pial arterioles with a caliber less than 50 μ in 8 cats when blood pressure was raised by intravenous infusion of angiotensin II. Calculation is based on the percentage of change from the caliber at a mean arterial blood pressure (MABP) of 135 mm Hg. (From MacKenzie, E. T., et al.: Effects of acutely induced hypertension in cats on pial arteriolar caliber, local cerebral blood flow, and the blood-brain barrier. Circ. Res. *39*:33, 1976, by permission of the American Heart Association, Inc.)

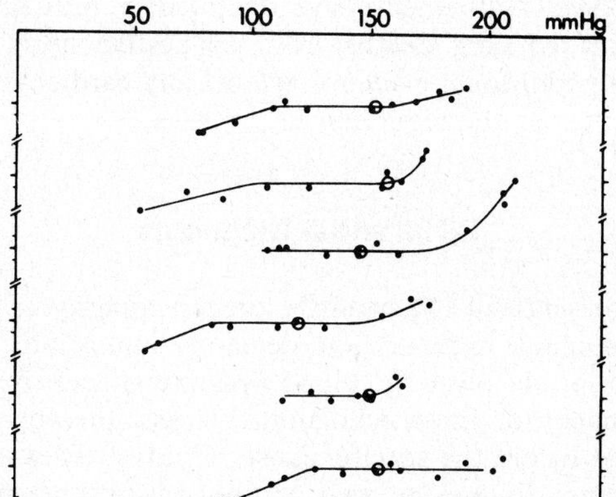

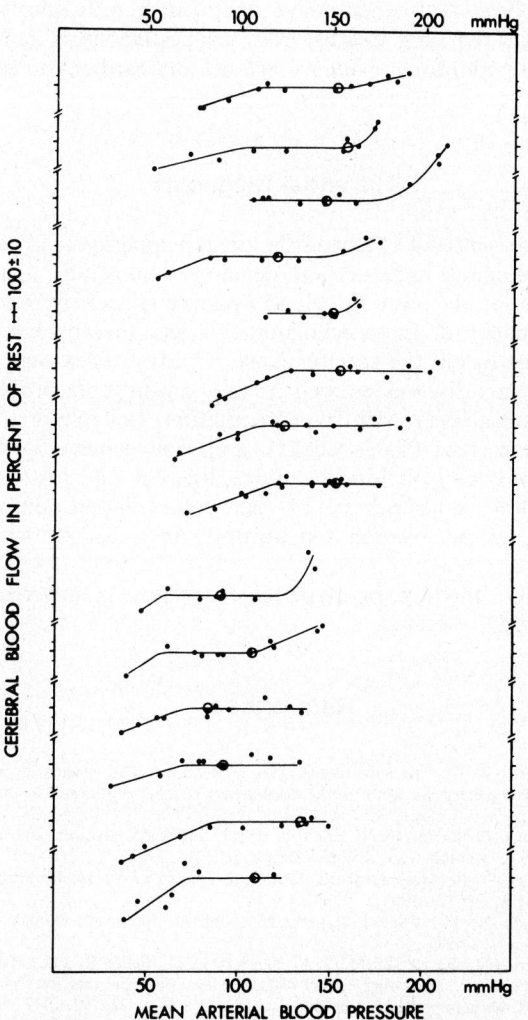

FIGURE 26–38 Curves of cerebral blood flow with varying levels of blood pressure in 14 patients: 8 hypertensive (*top*) and 6 normotensive (*bottom*). Each patient's habitual pressure is indicated by the open circle. The curves reflect autoregulation, with a shift upward or to the right in the hypertensives. Both lower and upper limits of autoregulation are shown. Note the breakthrough of CBF when the upper limit is exceeded. (From Johansson, B., et al.: On the pathogenesis of hypertensive encephalopathy. Circ. Res. *35*(Suppl.):I–167, 1974, by permission of the American Heart Association, Inc.)

noid necrosis. Both processes are most likely the consequences of very high blood pressure and may develop without apparent involvement of the renin-angiotensin or other hormonal mechanisms.[420]

Studies done in animals and man by Strandgaard and associates have elucidated the mechanism of encephalopathy. First, they directly measured the caliber of pial arterioles over the cerebral cortex in cats whose blood pressures were varied over a wide range by infusion of vasodilators or angiotensin II[422] (Fig. 26–37). As the pressure fell, the arterioles became dilated; as the pressure rose, the arterioles became constricted. Thus a constant cerebral blood flow was maintained by means of autoregulation. However, when mean arterial pressure rose above 180 mm Hg, the tightly constricted vessels could no longer withstand the pressure and suddenly became dilated. This began in an irregular manner, first in areas with less muscular tone and then diffusely, producing generalized vasodilatation. This breakthrough of cerebral blood flow hyperperfuses the brain under high pressure, causing leakage of fluid into the perivascular tissue, and resulting in cerebral edema and the syndrome of hypertensive encephalopathy.

In human subjects, they repetitively measured cerebral blood flow by an isotopic technique while lowering or raising the blood pressure with vasodilators or vasoconstrictors in a manner similar to that in the animal studies.[423] Curves depicting cerebral blood flow demonstrate autoregulation with a constancy of flow over mean pressures in normotensive persons from about 60 to 120 mm Hg and in hypertensive patients from about 110 to 180 mm Hg (Fig. 26–38). This shift to the right in the hypertensive patients is the result of structural thickening of the arterioles as an adaptation to the chronically elevated pressures.[424]

When pressures were raised beyond the upper limit of autoregulation, the same "breakthrough" with hyperperfusion occurred as was seen in the animal studies (Fig. 26–38). In previously normotensive people, whose vessels have not been altered by prior exposure to high pressure, breakthrough occurred at about 120 mm Hg mean arterial pressure; in hypertensive patients, the breakthrough occurred at about 180 mm Hg.

These studies confirm clinical observations. In previously normotensive people, severe encephalopathy occurs with relatively little hypertension. In children with acute glomerulonephritis and in women with eclampsia, convulsions may occur owing to hypertensive encephalopathy with blood pressures as low as 150/100 mm Hg. Obviously, chronically hypertensive patients withstand such pressures without duress. However, when pressures increase sufficiently, they too may develop encephalopathy.

Manifestations and Course

The symptoms and signs of hypertensive crises are usually dramatic (Table 26–24). However, some may be relatively asymptomatic, despite markedly elevated pressures and extensive organ damage. Young black men are particularly prone to experience a hypertensive crisis with severe renal insufficiency but little obvious prior distress.

When the blood pressure is so high as to induce encephalopathy or accelerated-malignant hypertension, the following clinical features are frequently seen:

1. Renal insufficiency with protein and red cells in the urine and azotemia. Acute oliguric renal failure may develop.
2. Elevated levels of plasma renin activity from the diffuse intrarenal ischemia, resulting in secondary aldosteronism, often manifested by hypokalemia. Although not causal, the secondarily elevated renin and aldosterone levels most likely exacerbate the hypertensive process, so that a vicious cycle is established: severe hypertension → intrarenal vascular damage → increased renin secretion → increased hypertension by the vasoconstrictor action of angiotensin II and by its stimulation of aldosterone, causing additional volume overload.
3. Microangiopathic hemolytic anemia with red cell fragmentation and intravascular coagulation.

If left untreated, patients die quickly from brain damage or more gradually from renal damage. Before effective therapy was available, fewer than 25 per cent of patients with malignant hypertension were alive after one year and only 1 per cent after five years.[425] With therapy, over 70 per cent survive for one year and about 50 per cent for five years.[426] Death in patients with severe hypertension is usually from stroke or renal failure if it occurs in the first few years after onset.[426] If therapy keeps patients alive for longer than five years, death will likely be caused by coronary disease. Although this could reflect some ill effect of antihypertensive therapy on the coronary vessels, it is likely that high pressure per se plays an important role in causing strokes and renal damage and a lesser role in causing coronary artery disease in which the primary mechanism is atherosclerosis and in which other important risk factors are involved. Antihypertensive treatment is particularly effective in reducing deaths from congestive heart failure, providing additional evidence against any cardiotoxic effect of the drugs or the reduction in pressure.

TABLE 26–24 CLINICAL CHARACTERISTICS OF HYPERTENSIVE CRISIS

Blood pressure: Usually > 140 mm Hg diastolic
Funduscopic findings: Hemorrhages, exudates, papilledema
Neurological status: Headache, confusion, somnolence, stupor, visual loss, focal deficits, seizures, coma
Cardiac findings: Prominent apical impulse, cardiac enlargement, congestive failure
Renal: Oliguria, azotemia
Gastrointestinal: Nausea, vomiting

From Kaplan, N. M.: Clinical Hypertension. 3rd ed. Baltimore, Williams and Wilkins Co., 1982.

TABLE 26–25 DISEASES TO BE DIFFERENTIATED FROM A HYPERTENSIVE CRISIS

Acute left ventricular failure
Uremia from any cause, particularly with volume overload
Cerebral vascular accident
Subarachnoid hemorrhage
Brain tumor
Head injury
Epilepsy (postictal)
Collagen diseases, particularly lupus, with cerebral vasculitis
Encephalitis
Overdose and withdrawal from narcotics, amphetamines, and so on
Acute anxiety with hyperventilation syndrome

From Kaplan, N. M.: Clinical Hypertension. 3rd ed. Baltimore, Williams and Wilkins Co., 1982, p. 200.

Differential Diagnosis

The presence of hypertensive encephalopathy or accelerated-malignant hypertension demands immediate, aggressive therapy to lower the blood pressure effectively. Except in pregnancy or in catecholamine excess, therapy may be instituted before the specific cause is known. However, certain serious diseases as well as one psychogenic problem, i.e., acute anxiety with hyperventilation, can mimic a hypertensive crisis (Table 26–25), and management of these conditions may obviously require different diagnostic and therapeutic approaches. In particular, blood pressure should not be lowered too abruptly in a patient with a stroke.

Specific therapy of hypertensive crises is covered in Chapter 27.

References

1. Roberts, W. C.: The hypertensive diseases. Evidence that systemic hypertension is a greater risk factor to the development of other cardiovascular diseases than previously suspected. Am. J. Med. *59*:523, 1975.
2. National Center for Health Statistics: Births, marriages, divorces, and deaths for 1981. Monthly Vital Statistics Report *30* (12):1, 1982.
3. Kannel, W. B.: Meaning of the downward trend in cardiovascular mortality. J.A.M.A. *247*:877, 1982.
4. Kaplan, N. M.: Clinical Hypertension. 3rd ed. Baltimore, Williams and Wilkins Co., 1982.
5. Pickering, T. G., Harshfield, G. A., Kleinert, H. D., Blank, S., and Laragh, J. H.: Blood pressure during normal daily activities, sleep and exercise. Comparison of values in normal hypertensive subjects. J.A.M.A. *247*:992, 1982.
6. Kirkendall, W. M., Feinleib, M., Freis, E. D., and Mark, A. L.: Recommendations for human blood pressure determination by sphygmomanometers. Hypertension *3*:510A, 1981.
7. Dawber, T. R.: The Framingham Study. The Epidemiology of Atherosclerotic Disease. Cambridge, Massachusetts, Harvard University Press, 1980.
8. Society of Actuaries and Association of Life Insurance Medical Directors of America: Blood Pressure Study, 1979. Recording and Statistical Corp., 1980.
9. Kannel, W. B., Wolf, P. A., McGee, D. L., Dawber, T. R., McNamara, P., and Castelli, W. P.: Systolic blood pressure, arterial rigidity and risk of stroke. The Framingham study. J.A.M.A. *245*:1225, 1981.
10. Gifford, R. W., Jr.: Isolated systolic hypertension in the elderly. J.A.M.A. *247*:781, 1982.

11. Spence, J. D., Sibbald, W. J., and Cape, R. D.: Pseudohypertension in the elderly. Clin. Sci. Molec. Med. *55*:399s, 1978.
12. Laughlin, K. D., Fisher, L., and Sherrard, D. J.: Blood pressure reductions during self-recording of home blood pressure. Am. Heart J. *298*:629, 1979.
13. The Pooling Project Research Group: Relationship of blood pressure, serum cholesterol, smoking habit, relative weight and ECG abnormalities to incidence of major coronary events: Final report of the pooling project. J. Chron. Dis. *31*:201, 1978.
14. Hypertension Detection and Follow-up Program Cooperative Group: Blood pressure studies in 14 communities. A two-stage screen for hypertension. J.A.M.A. *237*:2385, 1977.
15. Carey, R. M., Reid, R. A., Ayers, C. R., Lynch, S. S., McLain, W. L., III, and Vaughan, E. D., Jr.: The Charlottesville blood-pressure survey. Value of repeated blood-pressure measurements. J.A.M.A. *236*:847, 1976.
16. Rames, L. K., Clarke, W. R., Connor, W. E., Reiter, M. A., and Lauer, R.M.: Normal blood pressures and the evaluation of sustained blood pressure elevation in childhood. The Muscatine (Iowa) study. Pediatrics *61*:245, 1978.
17. Julius, S., Hansson, L., Andren, L, Gudbrandsson, T., Sivertsson, R., and Svensson, A.: Borderline hypertension. Acta Med. Scand. *208*:481, 1980.
18. National Heart, Lung, and Blood Institute: Report of the Task Force on Blood Pressure Control in Children. Pediatrics *59* (Suppl.):797, 1977.
19. Lieberman E.: Hypertension in childhood and adolescence. *In* Kaplan, N. M. (ed.): Clinical Hypertension. 3rd ed. Baltimore, Williams and Wilkins Co., 1982, p. 411.
20. Voors, A. W., Webber, L. S., and Berenson G. S.: Time course study of blood pressure in children over a three-year period. Bogalusa heart study. Hypertension *2* (Suppl. I):I–202, 1980.
21. Pickering, G.: Hypertension: Definitions, natural histories and consequences. Am. J. Med. *52*:570, 1972.
22. Itskovitz, H. S., Kochar, M. S., Anderson, A. J., and Rim, A. A.: Patterns of blood pressure in Milwaukee. J.A.M.A. *238*:864, 1977.
23. Messerli, F. H., DeCarvalho, J. G. R., Christie, B., and Frohlich, E. D.: Essential hypertension in black and white subjects. Am. J. Med. *67*:27, 1979.
24. Grim, C. E., Weinberger, M. H., Higgins, J. T., and Kramer, N. J.: Diagnosis of secondary forms of hypertension. A comprehensive protocol. J.A.M.A. *237*:1331, 1977.
25. Tucker, R. M., and Labarthe, D. R.: Frequency of surgical treatment for hypertension in adults at the Mayo Clinic from 1973 through 1975. Mayo Clin. Proc. *52*:549, 1977.
26. Berglund, G., Andersson, O., and Wilhelmsen, L.: Prevalence of primary and secondary hypertension: Studies in a random population sample. Br. Med. J. *2*:554, 1976.
27. Rudnick, K. V., Sackett, D. L., Hirst, S., and Holmes, C.: Hypertension in family practice. Canad. Med. Assoc. J. *3*:492, 1977.
28. Danielson, M., and Dammström, B.: The prevalence of secondary and curable hypertension. Acta Med. Scand. *209*:451, 1981.
29. Fagan, T. J.: Nomogram for Bayes theorem. N. Engl. J. Med. *293*:257, 1975.
30. Aschinberg, L. C., Zeis, P. M., Miller, R. A., John, E. G., and Chan, L. L.: Essential hypertension in childhood. J.A.M.A. *238*:322, 1977.
31. Weiss, N. S.: Relation of high blood pressure to headache, epistaxis, and selected other symptoms. N. Engl. J. Med. *287*:631, 1972.
32. Bulpitt, C. J., Dollery, C. T., and Carne, S.: Change in symptoms of hypertensive patients after referral to hospital clinic. Br. Heart J. *38*:121, 1976.
33. Stewart, I. McD. G., and Lond, M. D.: Headache and hypertension. Lancet *1*:1261, 1953.
34. Bauer, G. E.: Hypertension and headache. Aust. N.Z.J. Med. *6*:492, 1976.
35. Hypertension Detection and Follow-Up Program Cooperative Group: The Hypertension Detection and Follow-Up Program. A progress report. Circ. Res. *40*:I–106, 1977.
36. Thompson, G. E., Alderman, M. H., Wassertheil-Smoller, S., Rafter, J. G., and Samet, R.: High blood pressure diagnosis and treatment: Consensus recommendations vs. actual practice. Am. J. Public Health *71*:413, 1981.
37. Rose, G.: Strategy of prevention: Lessons from cardiovascular disease. Br. Med. J. *282*:1847, 1981.
38. Veterans Administration Cooperative Study Group on Antihypertensive Agents: Effects of treatment on morbidity in hypertension. II. Results in patients with diastolic blood pressure averaging 90 through 114 mm Hg. J.A.M.A. *213*:1143, 1970.
39. Keith, N. M., Wagener, H. P., and Barker, N. W.: Some different types of essential hypertension: Their course and prognosis. Am. J. Med. Sci. *268*:336, 1974.
40. Svardsudd, K., Wedel, H., Aurell, E., and Tibblin, G.: Hypertensive eye ground changes. Acta Med. Scand. *204*:159, 1978.
41. Savage, D. D., Drayer, J. I. M., Henry, W. L., Mathews, E. C., Ware, J. H., Gardin, J. M., Cohen, E. R., Epstein, S. E., and Laragh, J. H.: Echocardiographic assessment of cardiac anatomy and function in hypertensive subjects. Circulation *59*:623, 1979.
42. Hollenberg, N. K., and Adams, D. F.: The renal circulation in hypertensive disease. Am. J. Med. *60*:773, 1976.
43. Wollam, G. L., and Gifford, R. W., Jr.: The kidney as a target organ in hypertension. Geriatrics *31*:71, 1976.
44. Bauer, G. E., and Humphrey, T. J.: The natural history of hypertension with moderate impairment of renal function. Clin. Sci. Molec. Med. *45*:191s, 1973.
45. Brunner, H. R., Laragh, J. H., Baer, L., Newton, M. A., Goodwin, F. T., Krakoff, L. R., Bard, R. H., and Buhler, F. R.: Essential hypertension: Renin and aldosterone, heart attack and stroke. N. Engl. J. Med. *286*:441, 1972.
46. Kaplan, N. M.: The prognostic implications of plasma renin in essential hypertension. J.A.M.A. *231*:167, 1975.
47. Birkenhager, W. H., Kho, T. L., Schalekamp, M.A.D.H., Kolsters, G., Wester, A., and De Leeuw, P. W.: Renin levels and cardiovascular morbidity in essential hypertension. A prospective study. Acta Clin. Belg. *32*:168, 1977.
48. Management Committee: The Australian therapeutic trial in mild hypertension. Lancet *1*:1261, 1980.
49. Management Committee: Untreated mild hypertension. Lancet *1*:185, 1982.
50. Helgeland, A.: Treatment of mild hypertension: A five year controlled drug trial. The Oslo Study. Am. J. Med. *69*:725, 1980.
51. Schweitzer, M. D., Gearing, F. R., and Perera, G. A.: The epidemiology of primary hypertension. J. Chron. Dis. *18*:847, 1965.
52. Hollander, W.: Role of hypertension in atherosclerosis and cardiovascular disease. Am. J. Cardiol. *38*:786, 1976.
53. O'Rourke, M. D.: Pulsatile arterial hemodynamics in hypertension. Aust. N.Z.J. Med. *6*:40, 1976.
54. Palmer, R. F.: Vascular compliance and pulsatile flow as determinants of vascular injury. *In* Laragh, J. H., Buhler, F. R., and Seldin, D. W. (eds.): Frontiers in Hypertension. New York, Springer-Verlag, 1981.
55. Bierman, E. L., Brewer, C., and Baum, D.: Hypertension decreases replication potential of arterial smooth muscle cells: Aortic coarctation in humans as model. Proc. Soc. Exp. Biol. Med. *166*:335, 1981.
56. Dunn, F. G., Chandraratna, P., DeCarvalho, J. G. R., Basta, L. L., and Frohlich, E. D.: Pathophysiologic assessment of hypertensive heart disease with echocardiography. Am. J. Cardiol. *39*:789, 1977.
57. Rabkin, S. W., Mathewson, F. A. L., and Tate, R. B.: Longitudinal blood pressure measurements during a 26-year observation period and the risk of ischemic heart disease. Am. J. Epidemiol. *109*650, 1979.
58. Rabkin, S. W., Mathewson, F. A. L., and Tate, R. B.: Prognosis after acute myocardial infarction: Relation to blood pressure values before infarction in a prospective cardiovascular study. Am. J. Cardiol. *40*:604, 1977.
59. Beta-Blocker Heart Attack Trial Research Group: A randomized trial of propranolol in patients with acute myocardial infarction. I. Mortality results. J.A.M.A. *247*:1707, 1982.
60. Astrup, J., Bisgaard-Frantzen, H. O., Nielsen, S. L., and Rossing, N.: Blood pressure–lowering effect of acute myocardial infarction. Lancet *2*:903, 1976.
61. Kannel, W. B., Sorlie, P. Castelli, W. P., and McGee, D.: Blood pressure and survival after myocardial infarction: The Framingham study. Am. J. Cardiol. *45*:326, 1980.
62. McKee, P. A., Castelli, W. P., McNamara, P. M., and Kannel, W. B.: The natural history of congestive heart failure: The Framingham study. N. Engl. J. Med. *285*:1441, 1971.
63. Tarazi, R. C., and Levy, M. N.: Cardiac responses to increased afterload. Hypertension *4* (Suppl. II):II-8, 1982.
64. Breckinridge, A.: Vasodilators in heart failure. Br. Med. J. *284*:765, 1982.
65. Goodwin, J. D.: Congestive and hypertrophic cardiomyopathies. A decade of study. Lancet *1*:731, 1970.
66. Roberts, W. C.: Aortic dissection: Anatomy, consequences, and causes. Am. Heart J. *101*:195, 1981.
67. Kannel, W. B., Dawber, T. R., Sorlie, P., and Wolf, P. A.: Components of blood pressure and risk of atherothrombotic brain infarction: The Framingham study. Stroke *7*:327, 1976.
68. Rabkin, S. W., Mathewson, F. A. L., and Tate, R. B.: Predicting risk of ischemic heart disease and cerebrovascular disease from systolic and diastolic blood pressures. Ann. Intern. Med. *88*:342, 1978.
69. Wolf, P. A., Kannel, W. B., Sorlie, P., and McNamara, P.: Asymptomatic carotid bruit and risk of stroke. The Framingham study. J.A.M.A. *245*:1442, 1981.
70. Boller, F., Vrtunski, P. B., Mack, J. L., and Kin, Y.: Neuropsychological correlates of hypertension. Arch. Neurol. *34*:701, 1977.
71. Whisnant, J. P., Cartlidge, N. E. F., and Elveback, L. R.: Carotid and vertebral-basilar transient ischemic attacks: Effect of anticoagulants, hypertension, and cardiac disorders on survival and stroke occurrence—A population study. Ann. Neurol. *3*:107, 1978.
72. Strandgaard, S.: Autoregulation of cerebral blood flow in hypertensive patients. The modifying influence of prolonged antihypertensive treatment on the tolerance to acute, drug-induced hypotension. Circulation *53*:720, 1976.
73. Ledingham, J. G. G., and Rajagopalan, B.: Cerebral complications in the treatment of accelerated hypertension. Quart. J. Med. *48*:25, 1979.
74. Wollner, L., McCarthy, S. T., Soper, N. D. W., and Macy, D. J.: Failure of cerebral autoregulation as a cause of brain dysfunction in the elderly. Br. Med. J. *1*:1117, 1979.
75. Messerli, F. H., Frohlich, E. D., Dreslinski, G. R., Suarez, D. H., and Aristimuno, G. G.: Serum uric acid in essential hypertension: An indicator of renal vascular involvement. Ann. Intern. Med. *93*:817, 1980.
76. Simon, G., and Altman, S.: Increased serum *N*-acetyl-*β*-*D*-glucosaminidase activity in human hypertension. Clin. Exp. Hyper. Theory Practice *A4* (3):355, 1982.
77. Woods, J. W., Blythe, W. B., and Huffines, W. D.: Management of malignant hypertension complicated by renal insufficiency. N. Engl. J. Med. *241*:10, 1974.
78. Cruickshank, J. D., and Beevers, D. G.: Epidemiology of hypertension: Blood pressure in blacks and whites. Clin. Sci. *62*:1, 1982.
79. Rostand, S. G., Kirk, K. A., Rutsky, E. A., and Pate, B. A.: Racial differences in the incidence of treatment for end-stage renal disease. N. Engl. J. Med. *306*:1276, 1982.

80. Kaplan, N. M., Kem, D. C., Holland, O. B., Kramer, N. J., Higgins, J., and Gomez-Sanchez, C. E. The intravenous furosemide test: A simple way to evaluate renin responsiveness. Ann. Intern. Med. *84*:639, 1976.
81. Holland, O. B., and Fairchild, C.: Renin classification for diuretic and beta-blocker treatment of black hypertensive patients. J. Chron. Dis. *35*:179, 1982.
82. Woods, K. O., Beevers, D. G., and West, M.: Familial abnormality of erythrocyte cation transport in essential hypertension. Br. Med. J. *282*:1186, 1981.
83. Sever, P. S., Peart, W. S., Gordon, D., and Beighton, P.: Blood-pressure and its correlates in urban and tribal Africa. Lancet *2*:60, 1980.
84. Gibson, G. S., and Gibbons, A.: Hypertension among blacks. An annotated bibliography. Hypertension *4* (1):I-1, 1982.
85. Berkman, M., Magnier, J. P., Tran, M. D., and Thillaud, P.: Orthostatic increase in blood pressure in the elderly. Am. Heart J. *97*:131, 1979.
86. Maxwell, M. H., Bleifer, K. H., Franklin, S. S., and Varady, P. D.: Cooperative study of renovascular hypertension: Demographic analysis of the study. J.A.M.A. *220*:1195–1204, 1972.

MECHANISMS OF PRIMARY HYPERTENSION

87. Editorial: Catecholamines in essential hypertension. Lancet *1*:1088, 1977.
88. Lund-Johansen, P.: Hemodynamic alterations in hypertension—spontaneous changes and effects of drug therapy. Acta Med. Scand. Suppl. *603*:1, 1977.
89. Weiss, Y. A., Safar, M. E., London, G. M., Simon, A. C., Levenson, J. A., and Milliez, P. M.: Repeat hemodynamic determinations in borderline hypertension. Am. J. Med. *64*:382, 1978.
90. Ibrahim, M. M., Tarazi, R. C., Dustan, H. P., Bravo, E. L., and Gifford, R. W., Jr.: Hyperkinetic heart in severe hypertension: A separate clinical hemodynamic entity. Am. J. Cardiol. *35*:667, 1975.
91. Korner, P. H.: Circulatory regulation in hypertension. Br. J. Clin. Pharmacol. *13*:95–105, 1982.
92. Tarazi, R. C.: Hemodynamic role of extracellular fluid in hypertension. Circ. Res. *38* (Suppl. II):73, 1976.
93. Wenting, G. J., Man In'T Veld, A. J., and Schalekamp, M. A. D. H.: Time-course of vascular resistance changes in mineralocorticoid hypertension of man. Clin. Sci. *61*:97, 1981.
94. Coleman, T. J., Samar, R. E., and Murphy, W. R.: Autoregulation versus other vasoconstrictors in hypertension. Hypertension *1*:324, 1979.
95. Folkow, B.: Physiological aspects of primary hypertension. Physiol. Rev. *62*: 347–504, 1982.
96. Hermsmeyer, K., Abel, P. W., and Trapani, A. J.: Norepinephrine sensitivity and membrane potentials of caudal arterial muscle in DOCA-salt, Dahl, and SHR hypertension in the rat. Hypertension *4* (Suppl. II):II-49–II-51,1982.
97. Levine, R. S., Hennekens, C. H., Duncan, R. C., Robertson, E. G., Gourley, J., Cassady, J. C., and Gelband, H.: Blood pressure in infant twins: Birth to 6 months of age. Hypertension *2* (Suppl. I):I-29, 1980.
98. Havlik, R. J., and Feinleib, M.: Epidemiology and genetics of hypertension. Hypertension *4* (Supp. III):III-121–III-127, 1982.
99. Biron, P., Mongeau, J. G., and Bertrand, D.: Familial aggregation of blood pressure in 558 adopted children. Canad. Med. Assoc. J. *115*:773, 1976.
100. Falkner, B., Onesti, G., and Hayes, P.: The role of sodium in essential hypertension in genetically hypertensive adolescents. *In* Onesti, G., and Kim, K. E., (eds.): Hypertension in the Young and the Old. New York, Grune and Stratton, 1981, p. 29.
101. Johansson, B.: Vascular smooth muscle reactivity. Ann. Rev. Physiol. *43*:359, 1981.
102. Kaplan, N. M., and Silah, J. G.: Effect of angiotensin II on blood pressure in humans with hypertensive disease. J. Clin. Invest. *43*:659, 1964.
103. Wright, G. B., Alexander, R. W., Ekstein, L. S., and Gimbrone, M. A., Jr.: Sodium, divalent cations, and guanine nucleotides regulate the affinity of the rat mesenteric artery angiotensin II receptor. Circ. Res. *50*:462, 1982.
104. Blackburn, H., and Prineas, R.: Diet and hypertension: Anthropology, epidemiology and public health implications. *In* Paoletti, R., and Gotto, A. (eds.): Advances in Cardiovascular Diseases (*in press*).
105. Meyer, P., Garay, R. P., Nazaret, C., Dagher, G., Bellet, Z. M., Broyer, M., and Feingold, J.: Inheritance of abnormal erythrocyte cation transport in essential hypertension. Br. Med. J. *282*:1114, 1981.
106. Abboud, F. M.: The sympathetic system in hypertension. Hypertension *4* (Suppl. II):II-208, 1982.
107. Guyton, A. C., Coleman, T. G., Cowley, A. W., Jr., Scheel, K. W., Manning, R. D., Jr., and Norman, R. A., Jr.: Arterial pressure regulation. Overriding dominance of the kidneys in long-term regulation and in hypertension. Am. J. Med. *52*:584, 1972.
108. Brown, J. J., Lever, A. F., Robertson, J. I. S., and Schalekamp, M. A. D. H.: Renal abnormality of essential hypertension. Lancet *2*:320, 1974.
109. Kaplan, N. M.: The Goldblatt Memorial Lecture. Part II: The role of the kidney in hypertension. Hypertension *1*:456, 1979.
110. Hollenberg, N. K., Williams, G. H., and Adams, D. F.: Essential hypertension: Abnormal renal vascular and endocrine responses to a mild psychological stimulus. Hypertension *3*:11, 1981.
111. Click, R. L., Joyner, W. L., and Gilmore, J. P.: Reactivity of glomerular afferent and efferent arterioles in renal hypertension. Kidney Int. *15*:109, 1979.
112. London, G. M., Safer, M. E., Weiss, Y. A., Corvol, P. L., Lehner, J. P., Menard, J. M., Simon, A. C., and Milliez, P. L.: Volume-dependent parameters in essential hypertension. Kidney Int. *11*:204, 1977.
113. de Wardener, H. E., and MacGregor, G. A.: The natriuretic hormone and essential hypertension. Lancet *1*:1450–1454, 1982.
114. Sealey, J. E., Kirshma, D., and Laragh, J. H.: Natriuretic activity in plasma and urine of salt-loaded man and sheep. J. Clin. Invest. *48*:2210, 1969.
115. Licht, A., Stein, S., McGregor, C. W., Bourgoignie, J. J., and Bricker, N. S.: Progress in isolation and purification of an inhibitor of sodium transport obtained from dog urine. Kidney Int. *21*:339, 1982.
116. Clarkson, E. M., Koutsaimanis, K. G., Davidman, M., Du Bois, M., Penn, W. P., and deWardener, H. E.: The effect of brain extracts on urinary sodium excretion of the rat and the intracellular sodium concentration of renal tubule fragments. Clin. Sci. Molec. Med. *47*:201, 1974.
117. Plunket, W. C., Hutchins, P. M., Gruber, K. A., and Buckalew, V. M.: Evidence for a vascular sensitizing factor in plasma of saline-loaded dogs. Hypertension *4*:581–589, 1982.
118. Gruber, K. A., Rudel, L. L., and Bullock, B. C.: Increased circulating levels of an endogenous digoxin-like factor in hypertensive monkeys. Hypertension *4*:348, 1982.
118a. Keeler, R.: Atrial natriuretic factor has a direct, prostaglandin-independent action on kidneys. Can. J. Physiol. Pharmacol. *60*:1078–1082, 1982.
119. deWardener, H. E., Clarkson, E. M., Bitensky, L., MacGregor, G. A., Alaghband-Zadeh, J., and Chayen, J.: Effect of sodium intake on ability of human plasma to inhibit renal Na^+-K^+ adenosine triphosphatase in vitro. Lancet *1*:411, 1981.
120. Hamlyn, J. M., Ringel, R., Schaeffer, J., Levinson, P. D., Hamilton, B. P., Kowarski, A. A., and Blaustein, M. P.: A circulating inhibitor of (Na^+K)-ATPase associated with essential hypertension. Nature (in press) 1983.
121. Edmondson, R. P. S., Thomas, R. D., Hilton, P. J., Patrick, J., and Jones, N. F.: Abnormal leucocyte composition and sodium transport in essential hypertension. Lancet *2*:1003, 1975.
122. Haddy, F. J., Pamnani, M., Clough, D., and Huot, S.: Role of a humoral sodium-potassium pump inhibitor in experimental low renin hypertension. Life Sci. *30*:571, 1982.
123. Edmondson, R. P. S., and MacGregor, G. A.: Leucocyte cation transport in essential hypertension: Its relation to the renin-angiotensin system. Br. Med. J. *282*:1267, 1981.
124. Poston, L., Jones, R. B., Richardson, P. J., and Hilton, P. J.: The effect of antihypertensive therapy on abnormal leucocyte sodium transport in essential hypertension. Clin. Exp. Hypertension *3*:693, 1981.
125. Poston, L., Sewell, R. B., Wilkinson, S. P., Richardson, P. J., Williams, R., Clarkson, E. M., MacGregor, G. A., and de Wardener, H. E.: Evidence for a circulating sodium transport inhibitor in essential hypertension. Br. Med. J. *282*:847, 1981.
126. Pamnani, M. B., Clough, D. L., Huot, S. J., and Haddy, F. J.: Sodium-potassium pump activity in experimental hypertension. In Vanhoutte, P. M., and Leusen, I. (eds.) Vasodilation. New York, Raven Press, 1981.
127. Songu-Mize, E., Bealer, S. T., and Caldwell, R. W.: Effect of AV3V lesions on development of DOCA-salt hypertension and vascular Na^+-pump activity. Hypertension *4*:575–580, 1982.
128. Brock, T. A., Smith, J. F., and Overbeck, H. W.: Relationship of vascular sodium-potassium pump activity to intracellular sodium in hypertensive rats. Hypertension *4* (Suppl. II):II-43, 1982.
129. Friedman, S. M.: Evidence for an enhanced transmembrane sodium (Na^+) gradient induced by aldosterone in the incubated rat tail artery. Hypertension *4*:230, 1982.
130. Brock, T. A., Lewis, L. J., and Smith, J. B.: Angiotensin increases Na^+ entry and Na^+/K^+ pump activity in cultures of smooth muscle from rat aorta. Proc. Natl. Acad. Sci. USA *79*:1438, 1982.
131. Dahl, L. K., Knudsen, K. D., and Iwai, J.: Humoral transmission of hypertension: Evidence from parabiosis. Circ. Res. *25*:I-21, 1969.
132. Tobian, L., Jr., and Binton, J. T.: Tissue cations and water in arterial hypertension. Circulation *5*:754, 1952.
133. Losse, H., Wermeyer, H., and Wessels, F.: The water and electrolyte content of erythrocytes in arterial hypertension. Klin. Wschr. *38*:393, 1960.
134. Blaustein, M. P.: Sodium ions, calcium ions, blood pressure regulation, and hypertension: A reassessment and a hypothesis. Am. J. Physiol. *232*:C165–C173, 1977.
135. Murphy, R. A.: Myosin phosphorylation and crossbridge regulation in arterial muscle. Hypertension *4* (Suppl. II):II-3, 1982.
136. Hulthen, U. L., Bolli, P., Amann, F. W., Kiowski, W., and Bühler, F. R.: Enhanced vasodilation in essential hypertension by calcium channel blockade with verapamil. Hypertension *4* (Suppl. II):II-31, 1982.
137. Dahl, L. K., and Heine, M.: Primary role of renal homografts in setting chronic blood pressure levels in rats. Circ. Res. *36*:692, 1975.
138. Bianchi, G., Baer, P. G., Fox, U., and Guidi, E.: The role of the kidney in the rat with genetic hypertension. Postgrad. Med. J. *53*(Suppl. 2):123, 1977.
139. Tosteson, D. C.: Cation countertransport and cotransport in human red cells. Fed. Proc. *40*:1429, 1981.
140. Meyer, P., and Garay, R. P.: Hypertension as a membrane disease. Eur. J. Clin. Invest. *11*:337, 1981.
141. Wessels, F., Junge-Hulsing, G., and Losse, H.: Untersuchungen zur Natriumpermeabilität der Erythrozyten bei Hypertonikern mit familiärer Hochdruckbelastung. Z. Kreislaufforsch. *56*:374, 1967.
142. Garay, R. P., and Meyer, P.: A new test showing abnormal net $Na^+$and K^+ fluxes in erythrocytes of essential hypertensive patients. Lancet *1*:349, 1979.
143. Canessa, M., Adragna, N., Solomon, H. S., Connolly, T. M., and Tosteson, D.

C.: Increased sodium-lithium countertransport in red cells of patients with essential hypertension. N. Engl. J. Med. *302*:772, 1980.
144. Garay, R. P.: Cation transport in essential hypertension. Lancet *1*:501, 1982.
145. Cusi, D., Barlassina, C., Ferrandi, M., Lupi, P., Ferrari, P., and Bianchi, G.: Familial aggregation of cation transport abnormalities and essential hypertension. Clin. Exp. Hypertens. *3*:871, 1981.
146. Canessa, M., Bize, I., Solomon, H., Adragna, N., Tosteson, D. C., Dagher, G., Garay, R. P., and Meyer, P.: Na countertransport and cotransport in human red cells: Function, dysfunction, and genes in essential hypertension. Clin. Exp. Hypertens. *3*:783, 1981.
147. Tuck, M. L., Garay, R. P., and Meyer, P.: Identification of the Na^+, K^+ cotransport system in vascular smooth muscle cells: Effects of catecholamines on cation transport. Clin. Res. *30*:340A, 1982 (abstr).
148. Woods, J. W., Falk, R. J., Pittman, A. W., Klemmer, P. J., Watson, B. S., and Namboodiri, K.: Increased red-cell sodium-lithium countertransport in normotensive sons of hypertensive parents. N. Engl. J. Med. *306*:592, 1982.
149. De Mendonca, M., Knorr, A., Grichois, M., Ben-Ishay, D., Garay, R. P., and Meyer, P.: Erythrocytic sodium ion transport systems in primary and secondary hypertension of the rat. Kidney Int. *21*:11(S-69), 1982.
150. Garay, R. P., Nazaret, C., Dagher, G., Bertrand, E., and Meyer, P.: A genetic approach to the geography of hypertension: Examination of Na^+-K^+ cotransport in Ivory Coast Africans. Clin. Exp. Hypertens. *3*:861, 1981.
151. Swarts, H. G. P., Bonting, S. L., de Pont, J. J. H. H. M., Stekhoven, F. M. A. H. S., Thien, T. A., and Van't Laar, A.: Cation fluxes and Na^+-K^+–activated ATPase activity in erythrocytes of patients with essential hypertension. Hypertension *3*:641, 1981.
152. Walter, U., and Distler, A.: Abnormal sodium efflux in erythrocytes of patients with essential hypertension. Hypertension *4*:205, 1982.
153. Davidson, J. S., Opie, L. H., and Keding, B.: Sodium-potassium cotransport activity as genetic marker in essential hypertension. Br. Med. J. *284*:539, 1982.
153a. Etkin, N. L., Mahoney, J. R., Forsthoefel, M. W., Gillum, R. F., and Eaton, J. W.: Racial differences in hypertension-associated red cell sodium permeability. Nature *297*:588, 1982.
154. Cumberbatch, M., and Morgan, D. B.: Relations between sodium transport and sodium concentration in human erythrocytes in health and disease. Clin. Sci. *60*:555, 1981.
155. Inagami, T.: Renin. *In* Soffer, R. L. (ed.): Biochemical Regulation of Blood Pressure. New York, John Wiley & Sons, 1981.
156. Atlas, S. A., Sealey, J. E., Hesson, T. E., Kaplan, A. P., Menard, J., Corvol, P., and Laragh, J. H.: Biochemical similarity of partially purified inactive renins from human plasma and kidney. Hypertension *4* (Suppl. II):II–86, 1982.
157. Sealey, J. E., Atlas, S. A., and Laragh, J. H.: Prorenin and other large molecular weight forms of renin. Endocr. Rev. *4*:365, 1980.
158. Hsueh, W. A.: Inactive renin in human plasma. Is it prorenin? Mineral Electrolyte Metab. *7*:169, 1982.
159. Ganten, D., and Speck, G.: The brain renin-angiotensin system: A model for the synthesis of peptides in the brain. Biochem. Pharmacol. *27*:2379, 1978.
160. Fishman, M. C., Zimmerman, E. A., and Slater, E. E.: Renin and angiotensin: The complete system within the neuroblastoma X glioma cell. Science *214*:921, 1981.
161. Re, R., Fallon, J. T., Dzau, V., Quay, S., and Haber, E.: Renin synthesis by canine aortic smooth muscle cells in culture. Life Sciences *30*:99, 1982.
162. Ikeda, M., Gutkowska, J., Thibault, G., Boucher, R., and Genest, J.: Purification of tonin by affinity chromatography. Hypertension *3*:81, 1981.
163. Day, R. P., Luetscher, J. A., and Zager, P. G.: Big renin: Identification, chemical properties and clinical implications. Am. J. Cardiol. *37*:667, 1976.
164. Preibisz, J. J., Sealey, J. E., Aceto, R. M., and Laragh, J. H.: Plasma renin activity measurements: An update. Cardiovasc. Rev. Rep. *3*:787, 1982.
165. Crane, M. G., and Harris, J. J.: Effect of aging on renin activity and aldosterone excretion. J. Lab. Clin. Med. *87*:947, 1976.
166. Sassard, J., Vincent, M., Annat, G., and Bizollon, C. A.: A kinetic study of plasma renin and aldosterone during changes of posture in man. J. Clin. Endocrinol. Metab. *42*:20, 1976.
167. Katz, F. H., Romfh, P., and Smith, J. A.: Episodic secretion of aldosterone in supine man: Relationship to cortisol. J. Clin. Endocrinol. Metab. *35*:178, 1972.
168. Rumpf, K. W., Frenzel, S., Lowitz, H. D., and Scheler, F.: The effect of indomethacin on plasma renin activity in man under normal conditions and after stimulation of the renin-angiotensin system. Prostaglandins *10*:611, 1975.
169. Robertson, D., Frolich, J. C., Carr, R. K., Watson, J. T., Hollifield, J. W., Shand, D. G., and Oates, J. A.: Effects of caffeine on plasma renin activity, catecholamines and blood pressure. N. Engl. J. Med. *298*:181, 1978.
170. McDonald, R. H., Jr., Corder, C. N., Vagnucci, A. H., and Shuman, J.: The multiple factors affecting plasma renin activity in essential hypertension. Arch. Intern. Med. *138*:557, 1978.
171. Crane, M. G., Harris, J. J., and Johns, V. J., Jr.: Hyporeninemic hypertension. Am. J. Med. *52*:457, 1972.
172. Holle, R., Levy, S. B., and Stone, R. A.: A composite analysis of renin classification methods. Arch. Intern. Med. *138*:1514, 1978.
173. Helmer, O. M.: Renin activity in blood from patients with hypertension. Canad. Med. Assoc. J. *90*:221, 1964.
174. Swales, J. D.: Low-renin hypertension: Nephrosclerosis? Lancet *1*:75, 1975.
175. Kaplan, N. M.: Renin profiles: The unfulfilled promises. J.A.M.A. *238*:611, 1977.
176. Laragh, J. H., Letcher, R. L., and Pickering, T. G.: Renin profiling for diagnosis and treatment of hypertension. J.A.M.A. *241*:151, 1979.
177. Fagard, R., Amery, A., Reybrouck, T., Lijnen, P., Billiet, L., and Joossens, J. V.: Plasma renin levels and systemic hemodynamics in essential hypertension. Clin. Sci. Molec. Med. *52*:591, 1977.
178. Kotchen, T. A., Guthrie, G. P., Jr., Cottrill, C. M., McKean, H. E., and Kotchen, J. M.: Low renin-aldosterone in "prehypertensive" young adults. J. Clin. Endocrinol. Metab. *54*:808, 1982.
179. Case, D. B., Wallace, J. M., Keim, H. J., Weber, M. A., Sealey, J. E., and Laragh, J. H.: Possible role of renin in hypertension as suggested by renin-sodium profiling and inhibition of converting enzyme. N. Engl. J. Med. *296*:641, 1977.
180. Williams, G. H., Hollenberg, N. M., Moore, T. J., Dluhy, R. G., Bavli, S. Z., Solomon, H. S., and Mersey, J. H.: Failure of renin suppression by angiotensin II in hypertension. Circ. Res. *42*:46, 1978.
181. Esler, M., Zweifler, A., Randall, O., Julius, S., and DeQuattro, V.: The determinants of plasma-renin activity in essential hypertension. Ann. Intern. Med. *88*:746, 1978.
182. Morganti, A., Pickering, T. G., Lopez-Ovejero, J. A., and Laragh, J. H.: High and low renin subgroups in essential hypertension: Differences and similarities in their renin and sympathetic responses to neural and nonneural stimuli. Am. J. Cardiol. *46*:306, 1980.
183. Dluhy, R. G., Bavli, S. Z., Leung, F. K., Solomon, H. S., Moore, T. J., Hollenberg, N. K., and Williams, G. H.: Abnormal adrenal responsiveness and angiotensin II dependence in high renin essential hypertension. J. Clin. Invest. *64*:1270, 1979.
184. Williams, G. H., Hollenberg, N. K., Moore, T. J., Swartz, S. L., and Dluhy, R. G.: The adrenal receptor for angiotensin II is altered in essential hypertension. J. Clin. Invest. *63*:419, 1979.
185. Wisgerhof, M., and Brown, R. D.: Increased adrenal sensitivity to angiotensin II in low-renin essential hypertension. J. Clin. Invest. *61*:1456, 1978.
186. Lebel, M., Brown, J. J., Kremer, D., Robertson, J. I. S., Schalekamp, M., Davies, D. L., Lever, A. F., Tree, M., Beevers, D. G., Frazier, R., Morton, J. J., and Wilson, A.: Sodium and the renin-angiotensin system in essential hypertension and mineralocorticoid excess. Lancet *2*:308, 1974.
187. Gomez-Sanchez, C. E.: The role of steroids in human essential hypertension. Biochem. Pharmacol. *31*:893, 1982.
188. Baxter, J. D., Schambelan, M., Matulich, D. T., Spindler, B. J., Taylor, A. A., and Bartter, F. C.: Aldosterone receptors and the evaluation of plasma mineralocorticoid activity in normal and hypertensive states. J. Clin. Invest. *58*:579, 1976.
189. Vaughan, E. D., Jr., Laragh, J. H., Gavras, I., Buhler, F. E., Gavras, H., Brunner, H. R., and Baer, L.: Volume factor in low and normal renin essential hypertension. Am. J. Cardiol. *32*:523, 1973.
190. Holland, O. B., Gomez-Sanchez, C., Fairchild, C., and Kaplan, N. M.: Role of renin classification for diuretic treatment of black hypertensive patients. Arch. Intern. Med. *139*:1365, 1979.
191. Padfield, P. L., Brown, J. J., Lever, A. F., Morton, J. J., and Robertson, J. I. S.: Blood pressure in acute and chronic vasopressin excess. N. Engl. J. Med. *304*:1067, 1981.
192. Margolius, H. S., Horwitz, D., Pisano, J. J., and Keiser, H. R.: Relationships among urinary kallikrein, mineralocorticoids and human hypertensive disease. Fed. Proc. *35*:203, 1976.
193. Holland, O. B., Chud, J. M., and Braunstein, H.: Urinary kallikrein excretion in essential and mineralocorticoid hypertension. J. Clin. Invest. *65*:347, 1980.
194. Moncada, S., and Vane, J. R.: Arachidonic acid metabolites and the interactions between platelets and blood vessel walls. N. Engl. J. Med. *300*:1142, 1979.
195. Romero, J. C., and Strong, C. G.: The effect of indomethacin blockade of prostaglandin synthesis on blood pressure of normal rabbits and rabbits with renovascular hypertension. Circ. Res. *40*:35, 1977.
196. Weber, P. C., Siess, W., Sherer, B., Held, E., Witzgall, H., and Lorenz, R.: Arachidonic acid metabolites, hypertension and arteriosclerosis. Klin. Wochenschr. *60*:479–488, 1982.
196a. Muirhead, E. E., Byers, L. W., Desiderio, D. M., Brooks, B., and Brosius, W. M.: Antihypertensive lipids from the kidney: Alkyl ether analogs of phosphatidylcholine. Fed. Proc. *40*:2285–2290, 1981.
197. McGarron, D. A., Morris, C. D., and Cole, C.: Dietary calcium in human hypertension. Science *217*:267–269, 1982.
198. Kesteloot, H., and Geboers, J.: Calcium and blood pressure. Lancet *1*:813, 1982.
199. Lang, R. E., Bruckner, U. B., Kempf, B., Rascher, W., Sturm, V., Unger, T., Speck, G., and Ganten, D.: Opioid peptides and blood pressure regulation. Clin. Exper. Hyper. Theory and Practice *A4*:249–269, 1982.
200. Rabkin, S. W., Mathewson, F. A. L., and Hsu, P. H.: Relation of body weight to development of ischemic heart disease in a cohort of young North American men after a 26 year observation period: The Manitoba study. Am. J. Cardiol. *39*:452, 1977.
201. Siervogel, R. M., Roche, A. F., Chumlea, W. C., Morris, J. G., Webb, P., and Knittle, J. L.: Blood pressure, body composition, and fat tissue cellularity in adults. Hypertension *4*:382, 1982.
202. Messerli, F. H.: Cardiovascular effects of obesity and hypertension. Lancet *1*:1165, 1982.
203. Klimes, I., Nagulesparan, M., Unger, R. H., Aronoff, S. L., and Mott, D. M.: Reduced Na^+,K^+ -ATPase activity in intact red cells and isolated membranes from obese man. J. Clin. Endocrinol. Metab. *54*:721, 1982.
204. Kannel, W. B., and Sorlie, P.: Hypertension in Framingham. *In* Paul, O. (ed.):

Epidemiology and Control of Hypertension. Miami, Symposia Specialists, 1975, p. 553.
205. Cooke, K. M., Frost, G. W., Thornell, I. R., and Stokes, G. S.: Alcohol consumption and blood pressure. Med. J. Aust. *1*:65, 1982.
206. Klatsky, A. L., Friedman, G. D., and Siegelaub, A. B.: Alcohol and mortality. Ann. Intern. Med. *95*:139, 1981.
207. Cryer, P. E., Haymond, M. W., Santiago, J. V., and Shah, S. D.: Norepinephrine and epinephrine release and adrenergic mediation of smoking-associated hemodynamic and metabolic events. N. Engl. J. Med. *295*:573, 1976.
208. Gordon, T., Kannel, W. B., Dawber, T. R., and McGee, D.: Changes associated with quitting cigarette smoking: The Framingham study. Am. Heart J. *90*:322, 1975.
209. Christlieb, A. R., Warram, J. H., Krolewski, A. S., Busick, E. J., Ganda, O. M. P., Asmal, A. C., Soeldner, J. S., and Bradley, R. F.: Hypertension: The major risk factor in juvenile-onset insulin-dependent diabetics. Diabetes *30* (Suppl. 2):90, 1981.
210. Beretta-Piccoli, C., and Weidmann, P.: Exaggerated pressor responsiveness to norepinephrine in nonazotemic diabetes mellitus. Am. J. Med. *71*:829, 1981.
211. Chrysant, S. G., Frohlich, E. D., Adamopoulos, P. N., Stein, P. D., Whitcomb, W. H., Allen, E. W., and Neller, G.: Pathophysiologic significance of "stress" or relative polycythemia in essential hypertension. Am. J. Cardiol. *37*:1069, 1976.
212. Letcher, R. L., Chien, S., Pickering, T. G., Sealey, J. E., and Laragh, J. H.: Direct relationship between blood pressure and blood viscosity in normal and hypertensive subjects. Role of fibrinogen and concentration. Am. J. Med. *70*:1195, 1981.
213. Humphrey, P. R. D., Marshall, J., Russell, R. W. R., Wetherley-Mein, G., DuBoulay, G. H., Pearson, T. C., Symon, L., and Zilkha, E.: Cerebral bloodflow and viscosity in relative polycythaemia. Lancet *2*:873, 1979.
214. Breckenridge, A.: Hypertension and hyperuricaemia. Lancet *1*:15, 1966.
215. Editorial: Hypertension and uric acid. Lancet *1*:365, 1981.
216. Raynor, W. J., Jr., Shekelle, R. B., Rossof, A. H., Maliza, C., and Paul, O.: High blood pressure and 17-year cancer mortality in the Western Electric Health Study. Am. J. Epidemiol. *113*:371, 1981.
217. Gillis, G. R., Hole, D., MacLean, D. S., Hawthorne, V. M., Watt, H. D., and Watkinson, G.: High blood-pressure and cancer? Lancet *2*:612, 1975.

SECONDARY FORMS OF HYPERTENSION

218. Oral Contraceptive Study of the Royal College of General Practitioners: Hypertension. *In* Oral Contraceptives and Health. New York, Pitman Publishing Corp., 1974, p. 37.
219. Zelnik, M., Kim, Y. J., and Kantner, J. F.: Probabilities of intercourse and conception among U.S. teenage women, 1971 and 1976. Fam. Plan. Perspect. *11*:177, 1979.
220. Royal College of General Practitioners Oral Contraception Study: Further analyses of mortality in oral contraceptive users. Lancet *1*:541, 1981.
221. Stadel, B. V.: Oral contraceptives and cardiovascular disease. N. Engl. J. Med. *305*:672, 1981.
222. Wallace, R. B., Barrett-Connor, E., Criqui, M., Wahl, P., Hoover, J., Hunninghake, D., and Heiss, G.: Alteration in blood pressures associated with combined alcohol and oral contraceptive use—the Lipid Research Clinics Prevalance Study. J. Chron. Dis. *35*:251, 1982.
223. Fisch, I. R., and Frank, J.: Oral contraceptives and blood pressure. J.A.M.A. *237*:2499, 1977.
224. Weir, R. J.: When the pill causes a rise in blood pressure. Drugs *16*:522, 1978.
225. Weir, R. J.: Effect on blood pressure of changing from high to low dose steroid preparation in women with oral contraceptive induced hypertension. Scott. Med. J. *27*:212–215, 1982.
226. Pritchard, J. A., and Pritchard, S. A.: Blood pressure response to estrogen-progestin oral contraceptive after pregnancy-induced hypertension. Am. J. Obstet. Gynecol. *129*:733, 1977.
227. Spellacy, W. N., and Birk, S. A.: The effects of mechanical and steroid contraceptive methods on blood pressure in hypertensive women. Fertil. Steril. *25*:467, 1974.
228. Woods, J. W.: Oral contraceptives and hypertension. Lancet *2*:653, 1967.
229. Hauglustaine, B., VanDamme, B., Vanrenterghem, Y., and Michielsen, P.: Recurrent hemolytic uremic syndrome during oral contraception. Clin. Nephrol. *15*:148, 1981.
230. Boyd, W. N., Burden, R. P., and Aber, G. M.: Intrarenal vascular changes in patients receiving oestrogen-containing compounds—A clinical, histological, and angiographic study. Quart. J. Med. (n.s.) *44*:415, 1975.
231. Walters, W. A. W., and Lim, Y. L.: Haemodynamic changes in women taking oral contraceptives. J. Obstet. Gynecol. Brit. Commonw. *77*:1007, 1970.
232. Hollenberg, N. K., Williams, G. H., Burger, B., Chenitz, W., Hooshmand, I., and Adams, D. F.: Renal blood flow and its response to angiotensin II. Circ. Res. *38*:35, 1976.
233. Streeten, D. H. P., Anderson, G. H., Jr., and Dalakos, T. G.: Angiotensin blockade: Its clinical significance. Am. J. Med. *60*:817, 1976.
234. Kay, C. R.: Progestogens and arterial disease—Evidence from the Royal College of General Practitioners' study. Am. J. Obstet. Gynecol. *142*:762, 1982.
235. Kaplan, N. M.: Complications of the birth control pill. *In* Isselbacher, K. J., Adams, R. D., Braunwald, E., Martin, J. P., Petersdorf, R. G., and Wilson, J. D. (eds.): Update I. Harrison's Principles of Internal Medicine. New York, McGraw-Hill Book Co., 1981, p. 57.
236. Pfeffer, R. I., Kurosaki, T. T., and Charlton, S. K.: Estrogen use and blood pressure in later life. Am. J. Epidemiol. *110*:469, 1979.
237. Pallas, K. G., Holzwarth, G. J., Stern, M. P., and Lucas, C. P.: The effect of conjugated estrogens on the renin-angiotensin system. J. Clin. Endocrinol. Metab. *44*:1061, 1977.
238. Barrett-Connor, E., Brown, W. V., Turner, J., Austin, M., and Criqui, M. H.: Heart disease risk factors and hormone use in postmenopausal women. J.A.M.A. *241*:2167, 1979.
239. Bain, C., Willett, W., Hennekens, C. H., Rosner, B., Belanger, C., and Speizer, F. E.: Use of postmenopausal hormones and risk of myocardial infarction. Circulation *64*:42, 1981.
240. Ross, R. K., Mack, T. M., Henderson, B. E., Paganini-Hill, A., and Arthur, M.: Menopausal oestrogen therapy and protection from death from ischaemic heart disease. Lancet *1*:858, 1981.
241. Kurtzman, N. A.: Does acute poststreptococcal glomerulonephritis lead to chronic renal disease? N. Engl. J. Med. *298*:795, 1978.
242. Garcia, R., Rubio, L., and Rodriguez-Iturbe, B.: Long-term prognosis of epidemic poststreptococcal glomerulonephritis in Maracaibo: Follow-up studies 11 to 12 years after the acute episode. Clin. Nephrol. *15*:291, 1981.
243. Schact, R. G., Gallo, G. R., Gluck, M. C., Iqbal, M. S., and Baldwin, D. S.: Irreversible disease following acute poststreptococcal glomerulonephritis in children. J. Chron. Dis. *32*:515, 1979.
244. Birkenhager, W. H., Schalekamp, M. A. B. H., Schalekamp-Kuyken, M., Kolsters, P. A., Kolsters, G., and Krauss, X. H.: Interrelations between arterial pressure, fluid-volume, and plasma-renin concentration in the course of acute glomerulonephritis. Lancet *1*:1086, 1970.
245. Rodriguez-Iturbe, B., Baggio, B., Colina-Chourio, J. J., Favaro, S., Garcia, R., Sussana, F., Castillo, L., and Borsatti, A.: Studies on the renin-aldosterone system in the acute nephritic syndrome. Kidney Int. *19*:445, 1981.
246. Levinsky, N. G.: Pathophysiology of acute renal failure. N. Engl. J. Med. *296*:1453, 1977.
247. Ponticelli, C., Rivolta, E., Imbasciati, E., Rossi, E., and Mannucci, P. M.: Hemolytic uremic syndrome in adults. Arch. Intern. Med. *140*:353, 1980.
248. Harrington, J. T., and Cohen, J. J.: Current concepts. Acute oliguria. N. Engl. J. Med. *292*:89, 1975.
249. Traub, Y. M., Shapiro, A. P., Osial, T. A., Jr., Rodnan, G. P., Medsger, T. A., Leb, D. E., and Christy, W. C.: Response of patients with renal involvement by progressive systemic sclerosis to antihypertensive therapy. Clin. Sci. *61*:395a, 1981.
250. Smith, H. W.: Unilateral nephrectomy in hypertensive disease. J. Urol. *76*:685, 1956.
251. Gifford, R. W., Jr., McCormack, L. J., and Poutasse, E. F.: The atrophic kidney: Its role in hypertension. Mayo Clin. Proc. *40*:834, 1965.
252. Stockigt, J. R., Noakes, C. A., Collins, R. D., Schambelan, M., and Biglieri, E. G.: Renal-vein renin in various forms of renal hypertension. Lancet *1*:1194, 1972.
253. Lamberton, R. P., Noth, R. H., and Glickman, M.: Frequent falsely negative renal vein renin tests in unilateral renal parenchymal disease. J. Urol. *125*:477, 1981.
254. Dahl, T., Eide, I., and Fryjordet, A.: Hypernephroma and hypertension. Acta Med. Scand. *209*:121, 1981.
255. Weidmann, P., Beretta-Piccoli, C., Hirsch, D., Reubi, F. C., and Massry, S. G.: Curable hypertension with unilateral hydronephrosis. Studies on the role of circulating renin. Ann. Intern. Med. *87*:437, 1977.
256. Nash, D. A., Jr.: Hypertension in polycystic kidney disease without renal failure. Arch. Intern. Med. *137*:1571, 1977.
257. Meyer, P., Luscher, T., Rufener, J., Pouliadis, G., Vetter, H., Greminger, P., Siengenthaler, W., and Vetter, W.: Prävalenz der Hypertonie bei Röntgenologischen Zeichen der Pyelonephritis im intravenosen Pyelogramm. Schweiz. Med. Wschr. *111*:482, 1981.
258. Shapiro, A. P., Sapira, J. D., and Scheib, E. T.: Development of bacteriuria in hypertensive population. A 7-year follow-up study. Ann. Intern. Med. *74*:861, 1971.
259. Holland, N. H., Kotchen, T., and Bhathena, D.: Hypertension in children with chronic pyelonephritis. Kidney Int. *8*:S-43, 1975.
260. Ayus, J. C., Frommer, J. P., and Young, J. B.: Cardiac and circulatory abnormalities in chronic renal failure. Semin. Nephrol. *1*:112, 1981.
261. Koomans, H. A., Roos, J. C., Boer, P., Geyskes, G. G., and Mees, E. J. D.: Salt sensitivity of blood pressure in chronic renal failure. Evidence for renal control of body fluid distribution in man. Hypertension *4*:190, 1982.
262. Swaminathan, R., Glegg, G., Cumberbatch, M., Zareian, Z., and McKenna, F.: Erythrocyte sodium transport in chronic renal failure. Clin. Sci. *62*:489, 1982.
263. Brunner, H. R., Wauters, J., McKinstry, D., Waeber, B., Turini, G., and Gavras, H.: Inappropriate renin secretion unmasked by captopril (SQ 14 225) in hypertension of chronic renal failure. Lancet *2*:704, 1978.
264. Henrich, W. L., Mitchell, H., Anderson, S., Cronin, R., and Pettinger, W. A.: Effect of antihypertensive therapy on plasma catecholamines in renal failure patients. Clin. Nephrol. *16*:131, 1981.
265. Swales, J. D., Queiroz, F. P., Thurston, H., Medina, A., and Holland, J.: Dual mechanism for experimental hypertension. Lancet *2*:1181, 1971.
266. Blumberg, A., Hegstrom, R. M., Nelp, W. B., and Scribner, B. H.: Extracellular volume in patients with chronic renal disease treated for hypertension by sodium restriction. Lancet *2*:69, 1967.
267. Weidmann, P., and Maxwell, M. H.: The renin-angiotensin-aldosterone system in terminal renal failure. Kidney Int. *8*:S-219, 1975.

268. Lee, C., Neff, M. S., Slifkin, R. F., and Leiter, E.: Bilateral nephrectomy for hypertension in patients with chronic renal failure on a dialysis program. J. Urol. *119*:20, 1978.
269. Warren, D. J., and Ferris, T. F.: Renin secretion in renal hypertension. Lancet *1*:159, 1970.
270. Hostetter, T. H., Rennke, H. G., and Brenner, B. M.: The case for intrarenal hypertension in the initiation and progression of diabetic and other glomerulopathies. Am. J. Med. *72*:375, 1982.
271. Christlieb, A. R.: Nephropathy, the renin system, and hypertensive vascular disease in diabetes mellitus. Cardiovasc. Med. *3*:417, 1978.
272. Perez, G. O., Lespier, L., Knowles, R., Oster, J. R., and Vaamonde, C. A.: Potassium homeostasis in chronic diabetes mellitus. Arch. Intern. Med. *137*:1018, 1977.
273. Weidmann, P., Massry, S. G., Coburn, J. W., Maxwell, M. H., Atleson, J., and Kleeman, C. R.: Blood pressure effects of acute hypercalcemia. Studies in patients with chronic renal failure. Ann. Intern. Med. *76*:741, 1972.
274. Kincaid-Smith, P.: Analgesic abuse and the kidney. Kidney Int. *17*:250, 1980.
275. Muther, R. S., Potter, D. M., and Bennett, W. M.: Aspirin-induced depression of glomerular filtration rate in normal humans: Role of sodium balance. Ann. Intern. Med. *94*:317, 1981.
276. Textor, S. C., Gavras, H., Tifft, C. P., Bernard, D. B., Idelson, B., and Brunner, H.: Norepinephrine and renin activity in chronic renal failure. Evidence for interacting roles in hemodialysis hypertension. Hypertension *3*:294, 1981.
277. Jacquot, C., Idatte, J. M., Bedrossian, J., Weiss, Y., Safar, M., and Bariety, J.: Long-term blood pressure changes in renal homotransplantation. Arch. Intern. Med. *138*:233, 1978.
278. Zawada, E. T., Maxwell, M. H., Marks, L. S., Lee, D. B. N., and Kaufman, J. J.: The diagnostic and therapeutic uses of saralasin in renal transplant hypertension. J. Urol. *123*:148, 1980.
279. Eyler, W. R., Clark, M. D., Garman, J. E., Rian, R. L., and Meininger, D.: Angiography of the renal areas including a comparative study of renal arterial stenoses in patients with and without hypertension. Radiology *78*:879, 1962.
280. Plumer, L. B., Kaplan, G. W., and Mendoza, S. A.: Hypertension in infants—a complication of umbilical arterial catheterization. J. Pediat. *89*:802, 1976.
281. Harrison, E. G., Jr., and McCormack, L. J.: Pathologic classification of renal arterial disease in renovascular hypertension. Mayo Clin. Proc. *46*:161, 1971.
282. de Zeeuw, D., Burema, J., Donker, A. J. M., van der Hem, G. K., and Mandema, E.: Nephroptosis and hypertension. Lancet *1*:213, 1977.
283. Keith, T. A., III: Renovascular hypertension in black patients. Hypertension *4*:438, 1982.
284. Munichoodappa, C., D'Elia, J. A., Libertino, J. A., Gleason, R. E., and Christlieb, A. R.: Renal artery stenosis in hypertensive diabetics. J. Urol. *121*:555, 1979.
285. Fiorentini, C., Guazzi, M. D., Olivari, M. T., Bartorelli, A., Necchi, G., and Magrini, F.: Selective reduction in renal perfusion pressure and blood flow in man: Humoral and hemodynamic effects. Circulation *63*:973, 1981.
286. Barger, A. C.: The Goldblatt Memorial Lecture. Part I: Experimental renovascular hypertension. Hypertension *1*:447, 1979.
287. Buggy, J., Fink, G. D., Johnson, A. K., and Brody, M. J.: Prevention of the development of renal hypertension by anteroventral third ventricular tissue lesions. Circ. Res. *40* (Suppl. I):110, 1977.
288. Winer, B. M., Lubbe, W. F., Simon, M., and Williams, J. A.: Renin in the diagnosis of renovascular hypertension. J.A.M.A. *202*:139, 1967.
289. Katholi, R. W., Whitlow, P. L., Winternitz, S. R., and Oparil, S.: Importance of the renal nerves in established two-kidney, one clip Goldblatt hypertension. Hypertension *4* (Suppl. II):II–166, 1982.
290. Weidmann, P., Schiffl, H., Ziegler, W. H., Glück, Z., Meier, A., and Keusch, G.: Catecholamines, sodium and renin in unilateral renal hypertension in man. Mineral Electrolyte Metab. *7*:97, 1982.
291. Russell, G. I., Bing, R. F., Thurston, H., and Swales, J. D.: Surgical reversal of two-kidney one-clip hypertension during inhibition of the renin-angiotensin system. Hypertension *4*:69, 1982.
292. Dietz, J. R., Davis, J. O., DeForrest, J. M., Freeman, R. H., Echtenkamp, S. F., and Seymour, A. A.: Effects of indomethacin in dogs with acute and chronic renovascular hypertension. Am. J. Physiol. *240*:H533, 1981.
293. Thal, A. P., Grage, T. B., and Vernier, R. L.: Function of the contralateral kidney in renal hypertension due to renal artery stenosis. Circulation *27*:36, 1963.
294. Bookstein, J. J.: Segmental renal artery stenosis in renovascular hypertension. Radiology *90*:1073, 1968.
295. Zinman, L., and Libertino, J. A.: Revascularization of the chronic totally occluded renal artery with restoration of renal function. J. Urol. *118*:517, 1977.
296. Bookstein, J. J., Abrams, H. L., Buenger, R. E., Reiss, M. D., Lecky, J. W., Franklin, S. S., Bleifer, K. W., Varady, P. D., and Maxwell, M. H.: Radiologic aspects of renovascular hypertension. Part 3. Appraisal of arteriography. J.A.M.A. *21*:368, 1972.
297. Simon, N., Franklin, S. S., Bleifer, K. W., and Maxwell, M. H.: Clinical characteristics of renovascular hypertension. J.A.M.A. *220*:1209, 1972.
298. Davis, B. A., Crook, M. E., Vestal, R. E., and Oates, J. A.: Prevalence of renovascular hypertension in patients with grade III or IV hypertensive retinopathy. N. Engl. J. Med. *301*:1273, 1979.
299. Mueller, S. M., and Luft, F. C.: The blood-brain barrier in renovascular hypertension. Stroke *13*:229, 1982.
300. Grim, C. E., Luft, F. C., Weinberger, M. H., and Grim, C. M.: Sensitivity and specificity of screening tests for renal vascular hypertension. Ann. Intern. Med. *91*:617, 1979.
301. Bookstein, J. J., Abrams, H. L., Buenger, R. E., Lecky, J., Franklin, S. S., Reiss, M. D., Bleifer, K. H., Klatte, E. C., Varady, P. D., and Maxwell, M. H.: Radiologic aspects of renovascular hypertension. Part 2. The role of urography in unilateral renovascular disease. J.A.M.A. *220*:1225, 1972.
302. Hillman, B. J., Ovitt, T. W., Capp, M. P., Prosnitz, E. H., Osborne, R. W., Goldstone, J., Zukoski, C. F., and Malone, J. M.: The potential impact of digital video substraction angiography on screening for renovascular hypertension. Radiology *142*:577, 1982.
303. Witten, S. M.: Reactions to urographic contrast media. J.A.M.A. *231*:974, 1975.
304. Teruel, J. L., Marcen, R., Onaindia, J. M., Serrano, A., Quereda, C., and Ortuno, J.: Renal function impairment caused by intravenous urography. A prospective study. Arch. Intern. Med. *141*:1271, 1981.
305. Vaughan, E. D., Jr., Buhler, F. R., Laragh, J. H., Sealey, J. E., Baer, L., and Bard, R. H.: Renovascular hypertension: Renin measurements to indicate hypersecretion and contralateral suppression, estimate renal plasma flow, and score for surgical curability. Am. J. Med. *55*:402, 1973.
306. Streeten, D. H. P., and Anderson, G. H., Jr.: Outpatient experience with saralasin. Kidney Int. *15*:S–44, 1979.
307. Helmer, O. M., and Judson, W. E.: The presence of vasoconstrictor and vasopressor activity in renal vein plasma of patients with arterial hypertension. *In* Skelton, F. R. (ed.): Hypertension: Proceedings of the Council for High Blood Pressure Research, Vol. 8. New York, American Heart Association, 1960, p. 38.
308. Marks, L. S., Maxwell, M. H., Varady, P. D., Lupu, A. N., and Kauffman, J. J.: Renovascular hypertension: Does the renal vein renin ratio predict operative results? J. Urol. *115*:365, 1976.
309. Maxwell, M. H., Marks, L. S., Varady, P. D., Lupu, A. N., and Kauffman, J. J.: Renal vein renin in essential hypertension. J. Lab. Clin. Med. *86*:901, 1975.
310. Re, R., Novelline, R., Escourrou, M. T., Athanasoulis, C., Burton, J., and Haber, E.: Inhibition of angiotensin-converting enzyme for diagnosis of renal-artery stenosis. N. Engl. J. Med. *298*:582, 1978.
311. Foster, J. H., Dean, R. H., Pinkerton, J. A., and Rhamy, R. K.: Ten years' experience with the surgical management of renovascular hypertension. Ann. Surg. *177*:755, 1973.
312. Dean, R. H., Kieffer, R. W., Smith, B. M., Oates, J. A., Nadeau, J. H. J., Hollifield, J. W., and DuPont, W. D.: Renovascular hypertension. Arch. Surg. *116*:1408, 1981.
313. Kaufman, J. J.: Renovascular hypertension: The UCLA experience. J. Urol. *121*:139, 1979.
314. Novick, A. C., Straffon, R. A., Stewart, B. H., Gifford, R. W., and Vidt, D.: Diminished operative morbidity and mortality in renal revascularization. J.A.M.A. *246*:749, 1981.
315. Jones, E. O. P., Wilkinson, R., and Taylor, R. M. R.: Contralateral renal artery fibromuscular dysplasia after nephrectomy for renal artery stenosis. Br. Med. J. *1*:825, 1978.
316. Atkinson, A. B., Brown, J. J., Cumming, A. M. M., Fraser, R., Lever, A. F., Leckie, B. J., Morton, J. J., and Robertson, J. I. S.: Captopril in renovascular hypertension: Long-term use in predicting surgical outcome. Br. Med. J. *284*:689, 1982.
317. Mahler, F., Probst, P., Haertel, M., Weidmann, P., and Krneta, A.: Lasting improvement of renovascular hypertension by transluminal dilatation of atherosclerotic and nonatherosclerotic renal artery stenoses. Circulation *65*:611, 1982.
318. Madias, N. E., Kwon, Q. J., and Millan, V. G.: Percutaneous transluminal renal angioplasty. A potentially effective treatment for preservation of renal function. Arch. Intern. Med. *142*:693, 1982.
319. Delin, K., Aurell, M., Granerus, G., Holm, J., and Schersten, T.: Surgical treatment of renovascular hypertension in the elderly patient. Acta Med. Scand. *211*:169, 1982.
320. Conn, J. W., Cohen, E. L., Lucas, C. P., McDonald, W. J., Mayor, G. H., Blough, W. M., Jr., Eveland, W. C., Bookstein, J. J., and Lapides, J.: Primary reninism. Hypertension, hyperreninemia, and secondary aldosteronism due to renin-producing juxtaglomerular cell tumors. Arch. Intern. Med. *130*:682, 1972.
321. Sheth, K. J., Tang, T. T., Blaedel, M. E., and Good, T. A.: Polydipsia, polyuria, and hypertension associated with renin-secreting Wilms' tumor. J. Pediat. *92*:921, 1978.
322. Streeten, D. H. P., Tomycz, N., and Anderson, G. H., Jr.: Reliability of screening methods for the diagnosis of primary aldosteronism. Am J. Med. *67*:403, 1979.
323. Weinberger, M. H., Grim, C. E., Hollified, J. W., Kem, D. C., Ganguly, A., Kramer, N. J., Yune, H. Y., Wellman, H., and Donohue, J. P.: Primary aldosteronism. Ann. Intern. Med. *90*:386, 1979.
324. Davies, D. L., Beevers, D. G., Brown, J. J., Cumming, A. M. M., Fraser, R., Lever, A. F., Mason, P. A., Morton, J. J., Robertson, J. I. S., Titterington, M., and Tree, M.: Aldosterone and its stimuli in normal and hypertensive man: Are essential hypertension and primary hyperaldosteronism without tumour the same condition? J. Endocrinol. *81*:12, 1979.
325. Padfield, P. L., Davies, D., Lever, A. F., Robertson, J. I. S., Brown, J. J., Fraser, R., and Morton, J. J.: The myth of idiopathic hyperaldosteronism. Lancet *2*:83, 1981.
326. Gross, M. D., Grekin, R. J., Gniadek, T. C., and Villareal, J. Z.: Suppression of aldosterone by cyproheptadine in idiopathic aldosteronism. N. Engl. J. Med. *305*:181, 1981.
327. Ganguly, A., Grim, C. E., Bergstein, J., Brown, R. D., and Weinberger, M.

H.: Genetic and pathophysiologic studies of a new kindred with glucocorticoid-suppressible hyperaldosteronism manifest in three generations. J. Clin. Endocrinol. Metab. *53*:1040, 1981.
328. Ferriss, J. B., Beevers, D. G., Brown, J. J., Davies, D. L., Fraser, R., Lever, A. F., Mason, P., Neville, A. M., and Robertson, J. I. S.: Clinical, biochemical and pathological features of low renin ("primary") hyperaldosteronism. Am. Heart J. *95*:375, 1978.
329. Ibsen, K. K.: Liquorice consumption and its influence on blood pressure in Danish school-children. Dan. Med. Bull. *28*:124, 1981.
330. Blachley, J. D., and Knochel, J. P.: Tobacco chewer's hypokalemia: Licorice revisited. N. Engl. J. Med. *302*:784, 1980.
331. Mantero, F., Armanini, D., Opocher, G., Fallo, F., Sampieri, L., Cuspidi, B., Ambrosi, C., and Faglia, G.: Mineralocorticoid hypertension due to a nasal spray containing 9α-fluoroprednisolone. Am. J. Med. *71*:352, 1981.
332. Kono, T., Ikeda, F., Oseko, F., Imura, H., and Tanimura, H.: Normotensive primary aldosteronism: Report of a case. J. Clin. Endocrinol. Metab. *52*:1009, 1981.
333. Kaplan, N. M.: Primary aldosteronism with malignant hypertension. N. Engl. J. Med. *269*:1282, 1963.
334. Kem, D. C., Weinberger, M. H., Mayes, D. M., and Nugent, C. A.: Saline suppression of plasma aldosterone in hypertension. Arch. Intern. Med. *128*:380, 1971.
335. Spark, R. F., and Melby, J. C.: Aldosteronism in hypertension. The spironolactone response test. Ann. Intern. Med. *69*:685, 1968.
336. Ferriss, J. B., Beevers, D. G., Brody, K., Brown, J. J., Davies, D. L., Fraser, R., Kremer, D., Lever, A. F., and Robertson, J. I. S.: The treatment of low-renin ("primary") hyperaldosteronism. Am. Heart J. *96*:97, 1978.
337. Abrams, H. L., Siegelman, S. S., Adams, D. F., Sanders, R., Feinberg, H. J., Hessel, S. J., and McNeil, B. J.: Computed tomography versus ultrasound of the adrenal gland: A prospective study. Radiology *143*:121, 1982.
338. Kaplan, N. M.: The steroid content of adrenal adenomas and measurements of aldosterone production in patients with essential hypertension and primary aldosteronism. J. Clin. Invest. *46*:728, 1967.
339. Ganguly, A., and Weinberger, M. H.: Triamterene-thiazide combination: Alternative therapy for primary aldosteronism. Clin. Pharmacol. Ther. *30*:246, 1981.
340. Griffing, G. T., Cole, A. G., Aurecchia, S. A., Sindler, B. A., Komanicky, P., and Melby, J. C.: Amiloride in primary hyperaldosteronism. Clin. Pharmacol. Ther. *31*:56, 1982.
341. O'Neal, L. W., Kissane, J. M., and Hartroft, P. M.: The kidney in endocrine hypertension. Arch. Surg. *100*:498, 1970.
342. Ross, E. J., and Linch, D. C.: Cushing's syndrome—killing disease: Discriminatory value of signs and symptoms aiding early diagnosis. Lancet *2*:646–649, 1982.
343. Dalakos, T. G., Elias, A. N., Anderson, G. H., Jr., Streeten, D. H. P., and Schroeder, E. T.: Evidence for an angiotensinogenic mechanism of the hypertension of Cushing's syndrome. J. Clin. Endocrinol. Metab. *46*:114, 1978.
344. Crapo, L.: Cushing's syndrome: A review of diagnostic tests. Metabolism *28*:955, 1979.
345. White, F. E., White, M. C., Drury, P. L., Fry, I. K., and Besser, G. M.: Value of computed tomography of the abdomen and chest in investigation of Cushing's syndrome. *284*:771, 1982.
346. Bigos, S. T., Somma, M., Rasio, E., Eastman, R. C., Lanthier, A., Johnston, H. H., and Hardy, J.: Cushing's disease: Management by transsphenoidal pituitary microsurgery. J. Clin. Endocrinol. Metab. *50*:348, 1980.
347. Jennings, A. S., Liddle, G. W., and Orth, D. N.: Results of treating childhood Cushing's disease with pituitary irradiation. N. Engl. J. Med. *297*:957, 1977.
347a. Kalff, V., Shapiro, B., Lloyd, R., Sisson, J. C., Holland, K., Nakajo, M., and Beierwaltes, W. H.: The spectrum of pheochromocytoma in hypertensive patients with neurofibromatosis. Arch. Intern. Med. *142*:2092–2098, 1982.
348. Valk, T. W., Frager, M. S., Gross, M. D., Sisson, J. C., Wieland, D. M., Swanson, D. P., Mangner, T. J., and Beierwaltes, W. H.: Spectrum of pheochromocytoma in multiple endocrine neoplasia. A scintigraphic portrayal using ^{131}I-metaiodobenzylguanidine. Ann. Intern. Med. *94*:762, 1981.
349. Baker, G., Zeller, N. H., Weitzner, S., and Leach, J. K.: Pheochromocytoma without hypertension presenting as cardiomyopathy. Am. Heart J. *83*:688, 1972.
350. Gupta, K. K.: Phaeochromocytoma and myocardial infarction. Lancet *1*:281, 1975.
351. Chaturvedi, N. C., Walsh, M. J., Boyle, D. M., and Barber, J. M.: Diamorphine-induced attack of paroxysmal hypertension in phaeochromocytoma. Br. Med. J. *2*:538, 1974.
352. Kaplan, N. M., Kramer, N. J., Holland, O. G., Sheps, S. G., and Gomez-Sanchez, C.: Single-voided urine metanephrine assays in screening for pheochromocytoma. Arch. Intern. Med. *137*:190, 1977.
353. Remine, W. H., Chong, G. C., Van Heerden, J. A., Sheps, S. G., and Harrison, E. G., Jr.: Current management of pheochromocytoma. Ann. Surg. *179*:740, 1974.
354. Bravo, E. L., Tarazi, R. C., Gifford, R. W., Jr. and Stewart, B. H.: Circulating and urinary catecholamines in pheochromocytoma. N. Engl. J. Med. *301*:682, 1979.
355. Bravo, E. L., Tarazi, R. C., Fouad, F. M., Vidt, D. G., and Gifford, R. W., Jr.: Clonidine-suppression test. A useful aid in the diagnosis of pheochromocytoma. N. Engl. J. Med. *305*:623, 1981.
356. Manger, W. M., and Gifford, R. W., Jr.: Hypertension secondary to pheochromocytoma. Bull. N.Y. Acad. Med. *58*:139, 1982.
357. Cathelineau, G., Brerault, J., Fiet, J., Julien, R., Dreux, C., and Canivet, J.: Adrenocortical 11β-hydroxylation defect in adult women with postmenarchial onset of symptoms. J. Clin. Endocrinol. Metab. *51*:287, 1980.
358. Biglieri, E. G., Herron, M. A., and Brust, N.: 17-Hydroxylation deficiency in man. J. Clin. Invest. *45*:1946, 1966.
359. Messerli, F. H., and Frohlich, E. D.: High blood pressure. A side effect of drugs, poisons, and food. Arch. Intern. Med. *139*:682, 1979.
360. Bretza, J. A., Novey, H. S., Vaziri, N. D., and Warner, A. S.: Hypertension. A complication of danazol therapy. Arch. Intern. Med. *140*:1379, 1980.
361. Horowitz, J. D., Howes, L. G., Christophidis, N., Louis, W. J., Lang, W. J., Fennessy, M. R., and Rand, M. J.: Hypertensive responses induced by phenylpropanolamine in anorectic and decongestant preparations. Lancet *1*:60, 1980.
362. Shinebourne, E. A., Tam, A. S. Y., Elsee, A. M., Paneth, M., Lennox, S. C., Cleland, W. P., Lincoln, C., Joseph, M. C., and Anderson, R. H.: Coarctation of the aorta in infancy and childhood. Br. Heart J. *38*:375, 1976.
363. Liberthson, R. R., Pennington, D. G., Jacobs, M. L., and Daggett, W. M.: Coarctation of the aorta: Review of 234 patients and clarification of management problems. Am. J. Cardiol. *43*:835, 1979.
364. Alpert, B. S., Bain, H. H., Balfe, J. W., Kidd, B. S. L., and Olley, P. M.: Role of the renin-angiotensin-aldosterone system in hypertensive children with coarctation of the aorta. Am. J. Cardiol. *43*:828, 1979.
365. Warren, D. J., and Smith, R. S.: Inappropriate renin secretion and abnormal cardiovascular reflexes in coarctation of the aorta. Br. Heart J. *45*:733, 1981.
366. Weyman, A. E., Caldwell, R. L., Hurwitz, R. A., Girod, D. A., Dillon, J. C., Feigenbaum, H., and Green, D.: Cross-sectional echocardiographic detection of aortic obstruction. Part 2. Coarctation of the aorta. Circulation *57*:498, 1978.
367. Rocchini, A. P., Rosenthal, A., Barger, A. C., Castaneda, A. R., and Nadas, A. S.: Pathogenesis of paradoxical hypertension after coarctation resection. Circulation *54*:382, 1976.
368. Benedict, C. R., Grahame-Smith, D. G., and Fisher, A.: Changes in plasma catecholamines and dopamine beta-hydroxylase after corrective surgery for coarctation of the aorta. Circulation *57*:598, 1978.
369. Vlachakis, N. D., Frederics, R., Velasquez, M., Alexander, N., Singer, F., and Maronde, R. F.: Sympathetic system function and vascular reactivity in hypercalcemic patients. Hypertension *4*:452, 1982.
370. Christensson, T., Hellstrom, K., and Wengle, B.: Hypercalcemia and primary hyperparathyroidism. Arch. Intern. Med. *137*:1138, 1977.
371. McCarron, D. A., Pingree, P. A., Rubin, R. J., Gaucher, S. M., Molitch, M., and Krutzik, S.: Enhanced parathyroid function in essential hypertension: A homeostatic response to a urinary calcium leak. Hypertension *2*:162, 1980.
372. Estafanous, F. G., and Tarazi, R. C.: Systemic arterial hypertension associated with cardiac surgery. Am. J. Cardiol. *46*:685, 1980.
373. Whelton, P. K., Flaherty, J. T., MacAllister, N. P., Watkins, L., Potter, A., Johnson, D., Russel, R. P., and Walker, W. G.: Hypertension following coronary artery bypass surgery. Role of preoperative propranolol therapy. Hypertension *2*:291, 1981.
374. Layton, C., Brigden, W., McDonald, L., Monro, J., McDonald, A., and Weaver, J.: Systemic hypertension after homograft aortic valvar replacement. A cause of late homograft failure. Lancet *2*:1343, 1973.
375. Cockburn, J. S., Benjamin, I. S., Thompson, R. M., and Bain, W. H.: Early systemic hypertension after surgical closure of atrial septal defect. J. Thorac. Cardiovasc. Surg. *16*:1, 1975.
376. Friedman, E. A., and Neff, R. K.: Hypertension-hypotension in pregnancy. Correlation with fetal outcome. J.A.M.A. *239*:2249, 1978.
377. Chesley, L. C.: Hypertensive Disorders in Pregnancy. New York, Appleton-Century-Crofts, 1978.
378. MacGillivray, I., Rose, G. A., and Rowe, B.: Blood pressure survey in pregnancy. Clin. Sci. *37*:395, 1969.
379. Sawyer, M. M., Lipshitz, J., Anderson, G. D., Dilts, P. V., and Halperin, L.: Diurnal and short-term variation of blood pressure: Comparison of pre-eclamptic, chronic, hypertensive, and normotensive patients. Obstet. Gynecol. *58*:291, 1981.
380. Gallery, E. D. M., Hunyor, S. N., Ross, M., and Gyory, A. Z.: Predicting the development of pregnancy-associated hypertension: The place of standard blood-pressure measurement. Lancet *1*:1273, 1977.
381. Gallery, E. D. M.: Pregnancy-associated hypertension: Interrelationships of volume and blood pressure changes. Clin. Exper. Hyper.—Hyper. in Pregnancy *B1*:39, 1982.
382. Lunnell, N. O., Nylund, L. E., Lewander, L. E., and Sarby, B.: Uteroplacental blood flow in pre-eclampsia measurements with indium-113m and a computer-linked gamma camera. Clin. Exper. Hyper.—Hyper. in Pregnancy *B1*:105, 1982.
383. Gant, N. F., Madden, J. D., Chand, S., Worley, R. J., Strong, J. D., and MacDonald, P. C.: Metabolic clearance rate of dehydroisandrosterone sulfate. V. Studies of essential hypertension complicating pregnancy. Obstet. Gynecol. *47*:319, 1976.
384. Ferris, T. F., Stein, J. H., and Kauffman, J.: Uterine blood flow and uterine renin secretion. J. Clin. Invest. *51*:2827, 1972.
385. Terrango, N. A., Terrango, D.A., Pacholczyk, D., and McGiff, J. C.: Prostaglandins and the regulation of uterine blood flow in pregnancy. Nature *249*:57, 1974.
386. Downing, I., Shepherd, G. L., and Lewis, P. J.: Kinetics of prostacyclin synthetase in umbilical artery microsomes from normal and pre-eclamptic pregnancies. Br. J. Clin. Pharmac. *13*:195, 1982.
387. Bodzenta, A., Thompson, J. M., Poller, L., Burslem, R. W., and Wilcox, F. L.:

Prostacyclin-like and kallikrein activity of amniotic fluid in pre-eclampsia. Br. J. Obstet. Gynecol. *88*:1217, 1981.
388. Goodman, R. P., Killam, A. P., Brash, A. R., and Branch, R. A.: Prostacyclin production during pregnancy: Comparison of production during normal pregnancy and pregnancy complicated by hypertension. Am. J. Obstet. Gynecol. *142*:817, 1982.
389. Remuzzi, G., Marchesi, D., Zoja, C., Muratore, D., Mecca, G., Misiani, R., Rossi, E., Barbato, M., Capetta, P., Donati, M. B., and de Gaetano, G. Reduced umbilical and placental vascular prostacyclin in severe pre-eclampsia. Prostaglandins *20*:105, 1980.
390. Gant, N. F., Worley, R. J., Everett, R. B., and MacDonald, P. C.: Control of vascular responsiveness during human pregnancy. Kidney Int. *18*:253, 1980.
391. Pipkin, F. B., Hunter, J. C., Turner, S. R., and O'Brien, P. M. S.: Prostaglandin E_2 attenuates the pressor response to angiotensin II in pregnant subjects but not in nonpregnant subjects. Am. J. Obstet. Gynecol. *142*:168, 1982.
392. Gerber, J. G., Payne, N. A., Murphy, R. C., and Nies, A. S.: Prostacyclin produced by the pregnant uterus in the dog may act as a circulating vasodepressor substance. J. Clin. Invest. *67*:632, 1981.
393. Wickens, D., Wilkins, M. H., Lunec, J., Ball, G., and Dormandy, L. T.: Free-radical oxidation (peroxidation) products in plasma in normal and abnormal pregnancy. Ann. Clin. Biochem. *18*:158, 1981.
394. Whigham, K. A. E., Howie, P. W., Drummond, A. H., and Prentice, C. R. M.: Abnormal platelet function in pre-eclampsia. Br. J. Obstet. Gynecol. *85*:28, 1978.
395. Scott, J. S., Jenkins, D. M., and Need, J. A.: Immunology of pre-eclampsia. Lancet *1*:704, 1978.
396. Chesley, L. C.: Hypertension in pregnancy: Definitions, familial factor, and remote prognosis. Kidney Int. *18*:234, 1980.
397. Gant, N. D., Chand, S., Worley, R. J., Whalley, P. J., Crosby, U. D., and MacDonald, P. C.: A clinical test useful for predicting the development of acute hypertension in pregnancy. Am. J. Obstet. Gynecol. *120*:1, 1974.
398. Kuntz, W. D.: Supine pressor (roll-over) test: An evaluation. Am. J. Obstet. Gynecol. *137*:764, 1980.
399. Pritchard, J. A.: Management of preeclampsia and eclampsia. Kidney Int. *18*:259, 1980.
400. Cockburn, J., Ounsted, M., Moar, V. A., and Redman, C. W. G.: Final report of study on hypertension during pregnancy: The effects of specific treatment on the growth and development of the children. Lancet *1*:647, 1982.
401. Habib, A., and McCarthy, J. S.: Effects on the neonate of propranolol administered during pregnancy. J. Pediatr. *91*:808, 1977.
402. Gallery, E. D. M., Saunders, D. M., Hunyor, S. N., and Gyory, A. Z.: Randomized comparison of methyldopa and oxprenolol for treatment of hypertension in pregnancy. Br. Med. J. *1*:1591, 1979.
403. Sandstrom, B.: Adrenergic beta-receptor blockers in hypertension of pregnancy. Clin. Exper. Hyper.—Hyper. in Pregnancy. *B1*:127, 1982.
404. Welt, S. I., Dorminy, J. H., Jelovsek, F. R., Crenshaw, M. C., and Gall, M. D.: The effect of prophylactic management and therapeutics on hypertensive disease in pregnancy: Preliminary studies. Obstet. Gynecol. *57*:557, 1981.
405. Lopez-Llera, M.: Complicated eclampsia. Fifteen years' experience in a referral medical center. Am. J. Obstet. Gynecol. *142*:28, 1982.
406. Bauer, T. W., Moore, G. W., and Hutchins, G. M.: Morphologic evidence for coronary artery spasm in eclampsia. Circulation *65*:255, 1982.
407. Brockington, I. F.: Postpartum hypertensive heart failure. Am. J. Cardiol. *27*:650, 1971.
408. Strauss, R. G., and Alexander, R. W.: Postpartum hemolytic uremic syndrome. Obstet. Gynecol. *47*:169, 1976.
409. Fixler, D. E., Kautz, J. A., and Dana, K.: Systolic blood pressure differences among pediatric epidemiological studies. Hypertension *2* (Suppl. I):I–3, 1980.
410. Rames, L. K., Clarke, W. R., Connor, W. E., Reiter, M. A., and Lauer, T. M.: Normal blood pressures and the evaluation of sustained blood pressure elevation in childhood: the Muscatine study. Pediatrics *61*:245, 1978.
411. Fixler, D. E., Laird, W. P., Fitzgerald, V., Stead, S., and Adams, R.: Hypertension screening in schools: Results of the Dallas study. Pediatrics *63*:32, 1979.
412. Zinner, S. H., Margolius, H. S., Rosner, B., and Kass, E. H.: Stability of blood pressure rank and urinary kallikrein concentration in childhood: An eight year follow-up. Circulation *58*:908, 1978.
413. Harlan, W. R., Coroni-Huntley, J., and Leaverton, P. E.: Blood pressure in childhood. The National Health Examination Survey. Hypertension *1*:559, 1979.
414. Reed, W. L.: Racial differences in blood pressure levels of adolescents. Am. J. Public Health *71*:1165, 1981.
415. Fouad, F. M., Tarazi, R. C., Dustan, H. P., and Bravo, E. L.: Hemodynamics of essential hypertension in young subjects. Am. Heart J. *96*:646, 1978.
416. Sinaiko, A. R., Gillum, R. F., Jacobs, D. R., Sopko, G., and Prineas, R. J.: Renin-angiotensin and sympathetic nervous system activity in grade school children. Hypertension *4*:299, 1982.
417. Voors, A. W., Webber, L. S., and Berenson, G. S.: Racial contrasts in cardiovascular response tests for children from a total community. Hypertension *2*:686, 1980.
418. Falkner, B., Kushner, H., Onesti, G., and Angelakos, E. T.: Cardiovascular characteristics in adolescents who develop essential hypertension. Hypertension *3*:521, 1981.
419. Goldring, D., Hernandez, A., Choi, S., Lee, J. Y., Londe, S., Lindgren, F. T., and Burton, R. M.: Blood pressure in a high school population. II. Clinical profile of the juvenile hypertensive. J. Pediatr. *95*:298, 1979.
420. Beilin, L. J., and Goldby, F. S.: High arterial pressure versus humoral factors in the pathogenesis of the vascular lesions of malignant hypertension. Clin. Sci. Molec. Med. *52*:111, 1977.
421. Lee, T. H., and Alderman, M. H.: Malignant hypertension: Declining mortality rate in New York City, 1958 to 1974. N.Y. State J. Med. *78*:1389, 1978.
422. MacKenzie, E. T., Strandgaard, S., Graham, D. I., Jones, J. V., Harper, A. M., and Farrar, J. K.: Effects of acutely induced hypertension in cats on pial arteriolar caliber, local cerebral blood flow, and the blood-brain barrier. Circ. Res. *39*:33, 1976.
423. Strandgaard, S., Olesen, J., Skinhoj, E., and Lassen, N. A.: Autoregulation of brain circulation in severe arterial hypertension. Br. Med. J. *1*:507, 1973.
424. Jones, J. V., Fitch, W., Mackenzie, E. T., Strandgaard, S., and Harper, A. M.: Lower limit of cerebral blood flow autoregulation in experimental renovascular hypertension in the baboon. Circ. Res. *39*:555, 1976.
425. Hodge, J. V., McQueen, E. C., and Smirk, F. H.: Results of hypotensive therapy in arterial hypertension. Br. Med. J. *1*:1, 1961.
426. Barnett, A. J., and Silberberg, F. G.: Long-term results of treatment of severe hypertension. Med. J. Aust. *2*:960, 1973.

27 SYSTEMIC HYPERTENSION: THERAPY

by Norman M. Kaplan, M.D.

INTRODUCTION

In the United States, the general attitude toward the therapy of hypertension has rapidly swung, like a pendulum, from overly conservative to one that is likely too liberal. Occurring over the past 10 years, this dramatic change has come about through the confluence of a number of factors, including (1) increasing awareness in the medical community and among the public of the dangers of untreated hypertension—the "silent killer;" (2) the availability of effective, safe, and easily tolerated medications; and (3) the documentation of protection against cardiovascular damage through reduction of blood pressure with drug therapy. Protection by therapy was shown first for malignant hypertension in the late 1950s,[1] then, in 1967, for diastolic levels between 115 and 129 mm Hg,[2] for diastolic levels between 104 and 115 in 1970,[3] and, most recently, for levels above 90[4] or 95.[5] As noted in Chapter 26 (see Fig. 26–6, p. 856), the proportion of the hypertensive population brought under the therapeutic umbrella has increased markedly as the criterion for the acceptable lower limit for treatment has been reduced: over 70 per cent of the total hypertensive population is in the "mild" category, with diastolic blood pressure between 90 and 104 mm Hg, and this group comprises about 30 million Americans.

The high degree of risk associated with diastolic pressures above 105 and the marked protection against that risk afforded by antihypertensive drug therapy demonstrated in the Veterans Administration Cooperative Study[3] strongly support the validity of active pharmacotherapy for persons with pressures at that level—assuming that such pressures have been shown to persist after the initial observation. Recall the tendency for many such high readings to fall upon repeat measurements.[6] Although only diastolic levels are being referred to, an even closer relation to eventual risk has been shown for systolic levels in the Framingham study.[7] Specific coverage of therapy for predominantly systolic hypertension is provided later in this chapter. For now, the focus is on the majority of patients, i.e., those with diastolic pressures between 90 and 104 mm Hg.

CURRENT ENTHUSIASM TOWARD THERAPY

As we shall see, the evidence that drug therapy is needed to protect an individual against mild hypertension is neither as conclusive nor as encompassing as many have assumed.[8] Even so, the medical community has been more than willing to accept the evidence in support of treatment for a larger proportion of the hypertensive population: In a survey of physicians in New York carried out in 1978, *before* publication of the results of any large-scale trials showing that treatment was of value in mild hypertension, 92 per cent indicated that they would treat patients whose diastolic pressure was 90 to 104 mm Hg.[9]

Two reasons have been given to explain this enthusiastic acceptance of the need for active drug therapy in mild hypertension, even in advance of proof of its efficacy.[10] First is the belief that such an approach would be *preventive*, based on the demonstrated benefits of therapy for more severe hypertension. The second is a *sociological* premise, based on two widely held attitudes: (1) "technological optimism—the disposition to employ technologies in the belief that the benefits that flow from them will outweigh whatever unforeseen and undesirable effects ensue, and that these effects will themselves be manageable by existing or potential technological means"; and (2) "therapeutic activism—physicians prefer to take the risk of treating when intervention may not be called for to the potential error of not treating when treatment is needed."[10]

This enthusiasm to treat may involve almost 60 million Americans, if all those with diastolic pressures above 90 mm Hg are included.[11] Over 27 million new prescriptions for antihypertensive drugs were

TABLE 27–1 GUIDE TO THERAPY
WHEN DIASTOLIC BLOOD PRESSURE IS 90 TO 104 mm Hg*

Under 45 years of age	1	Target organ damage	2
Black	1	Parent with major cardiovascular event	1
Male	1		
All diastolic pressures > 95	1	Hypercholesterolemia	1
Systolic pressures > 165	1	Smoker	1

Drug therapy if diastolic blood pressure is:
100 to 104 with 2 points or more
95 to 99 with 3 points or more
90 to 94 with 4 points or more

*Recommended by Dr. Edward Freis.

written in 1981; with regard to sales in the United States, seven of the top 20 drugs were antihypertensive agents. It should be noted that this enthusiasm—referred to as "early and aggressive treatment" in widely seen advertisements—is not shared by physicians elsewhere; in England, most physicians withhold therapy until diastolic pressures exceed 100 mm Hg.[12]

A MORE MODERATE VIEW

Based upon a careful analysis of evidence available as of late 1982, a more moderate position than that currently taken by most American physicians would seem to be warranted. Results of another large therapeutic trial now being conducted in England[13] may provide more evidence in favor of earlier and more aggressive therapy, but the results of the Hypertension Detection and Follow-up Program (HDFP)[4] and of the Australian trial[5] do not prove the need for routine drug therapy for all those with mild hypertension. Let us examine the evidence in support of a more moderate position: "that such therapy should be provided selectively, quickly to those at high risk, but only after a period of observation plus non-drug therapy for the majority. Hopefully, such selectivity in using drug therapy will protect those in immediate need while at the same time postponing or perhaps removing the need for such therapy in many more patients."[14]

THE DEGREE OF RISK

The overall increase in long-term cardiovascular risk from even a mild degree of hypertension has been amply documented (see Fig. 26–3, p. 852). But, as noted in the preceding chapter, the majority of patients with mild hypertension do not suffer apparent harm over a few years. Recall the experience of the 1600 patients who served as controls in the Australian trial[5]: the majority of those patients who entered the trial with diastolic pressures between 95 and 109 mm Hg experienced a lowering of blood pressures over the next four years, and those whose pressures stayed below 100 mm Hg had no excess morbidity or mortality (Fig. 27–1). On the other hand, remember that in 12.2 per cent of this placebo-treated group, blood pressures progressed to 110 mm Hg or higher, indicating the *need for continued surveillance* of all patients identified as hypertensive. These Australian patients were free of identifiable cardiovascular damage at the time of entry into the trial. Therefore, their relatively benign short-term experience should not be extrapolated to those patients with more biologically aggressive disease, evidenced by target organ damage.

The need to consider factors other than blood pressure that contribute to cardiovascular risk has been cogently demonstrated by Alderman and Madhavan.[15] Using the risk factors found in the Framingham study to be major predictors of the development of cardiovascular disease, they calculated the likelihood of such complications appearing over a 15-year interval in men and women aged 35 who had similar blood pressure levels but were at varying degrees of overall risk (Fig. 27–2). Note that a "high-risk" man with a systolic blood pressure of 195 has an 86 per cent likelihood of developing cardiovascular disease, whereas a "low-risk" man of the same age and with the same blood pressure has a 15 per cent chance and a similar "low-risk" woman only a 6 per cent chance.

The Framingham data can be used to calculate the probable risk for adults with any combination of factors, to provide some objective evidence for each individual as to the urgency of the need for active intervention. Some years ago, Dr. Edward Freis formulated a simple guide to drug therapy for patients with diastolic pressures of 90 to 104, assigning points to many of the known factors associated with increased risk and choosing therapy based on total score (Table 27–1). The purpose of these assessments is to limit the immediate use of drug therapy to that part of the population with mild hypertension who are most in need, i.e., taking more precise aim rather than scatter-shooting at many to protect a few.

This rationale is based on two more assumptions: (1) drug therapy may not be needed for many whose blood pressure responds to time and nondrug therapies and (2) drug therapy may invoke its own inherent risks. Following this line of reasoning, we will next examine the evidence that drug therapy offers protection to such patients.

PROTECTION BY THERAPY

The drug-treated half of the Australian patients had 30 per cent less morbidity and mortality than did the placebo-treated half over the three years of the trial, associated with an average 6 mm Hg lower diastolic blood pressure (88 versus 94).[5]

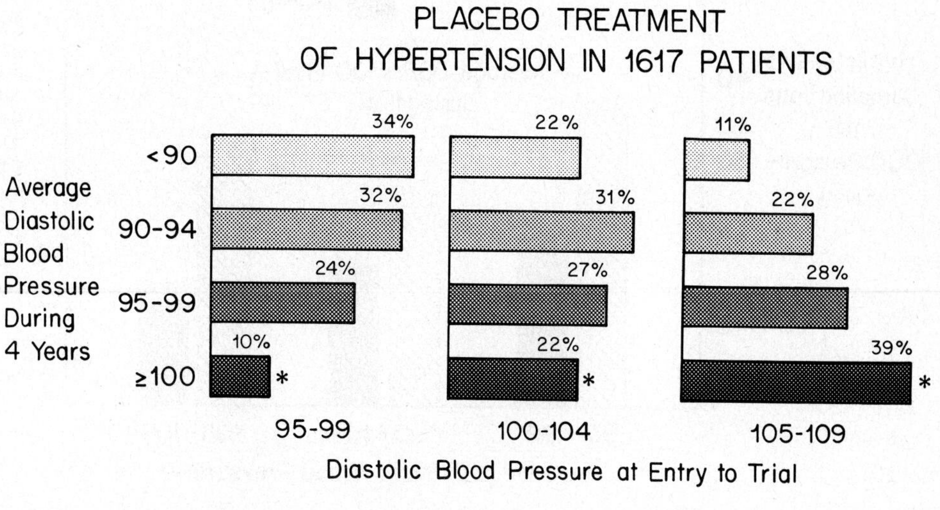

FIGURE 27-1 Average diastolic blood pressure levels during the four years of the Australian therapeutic trial of the 1617 patients randomly assigned to placebo therapy. Patients were divided into three groups based on their initial diastolic blood pressure upon entry into the trial. The excess morbidity and mortality observed in the placebo group occurred in those whose diastolic BP averaged 100 mm Hg or higher (noted by asterisks). (Drawn from Report of the Management Committee. Lancet *1*:1261, 1980.)

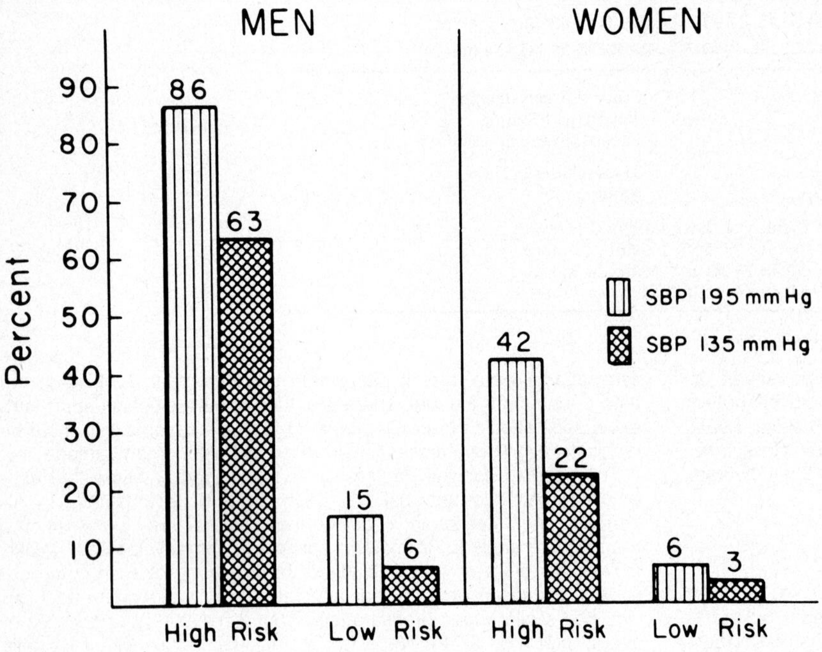

FIGURE 27–2 Risk of developing cardiovascular disease in 15 years for 35-year-old men and women, according to systolic blood pressure (SBP) level and risk status in the Framingham cohort. High risk = Left ventricular hypertrophy (LVH) by ECG, cigarette smoker, blood cholesterol level of 310 mg/100 ml, and glucose intolerance. Low risk = No LVH by ECG, nonsmoker, blood cholesterol of 235 mg/100 ml, and no glucose intolerance. (From Alderman, M.H., and Madhaven, S.: Management of the hypertensive patient: A continuing dilemma. Hypertension *3*:192, 1981, by permission of the American Heart Association, Inc.)

In the HDFP, the 11,000 patients whose initial pressures were between 90 and 104 were all offered therapy, but half were more intensively treated (the Stepped-Care group) than the other half (the Referred-Care group). At the end of the five-year study, the Stepped-Care group had a 20 per cent lower overall mortality rate than did the Referred-Care group, associated with a 5 mm Hg lower average diastolic blood pressure (83 versus 88 mm Hg).[4] These results, along with similar data from a smaller study done in Oslo,[16] have been considered definitive proof of the value of "early and aggressive" therapy of all patients with mild hypertension. However, closer examination of these results suggests that they should not be applied to the universe of mild hypertensives.

The HDFP Data. As for the HDFP data, the 20 per cent reduction in overall and cardiovascular mortality was accompanied by a 13 per cent reduction in mortality from noncardiovascular diseases. This decrease likely reflects the more intensive overall medical care provided the Stepped-Care group and suggests that the program was "as much a trial of medical care as of antihypertensive drugs."[17] Some may assume that the 20 per cent difference in mortality rates means that 20 per cent of the less actively treated group died and could have been protected by further reduction in their blood pressure. In fact, the 20 per cent reduction in mortality represents an actual difference in survival of less than 1.5 per cent between the two groups, with 94 per cent of the Stepped-Care and 92.5 per cent of the Referred-Care alive at the end of the five years. The 1.5 per cent difference is a 20 per cent relative difference in the rates for the two groups, but the smaller number is a more accurate representation of the actual number of people who would benefit from therapy.

The Australian Trial. In the Australian trial, the development of cardiovascular disease, referred to as trial end points, was continually monitored, and when a statistically significant difference of 30 per cent was noted, the trial was stopped, providing strong evidence for the value of drug therapy. When the data are closely scrutinized, two additional conclusions can be reached. First, as noted earlier, the overall 30 per cent excess in morbidity occurred only among the placebo-treated patients whose diastolic blood pressure averaged above

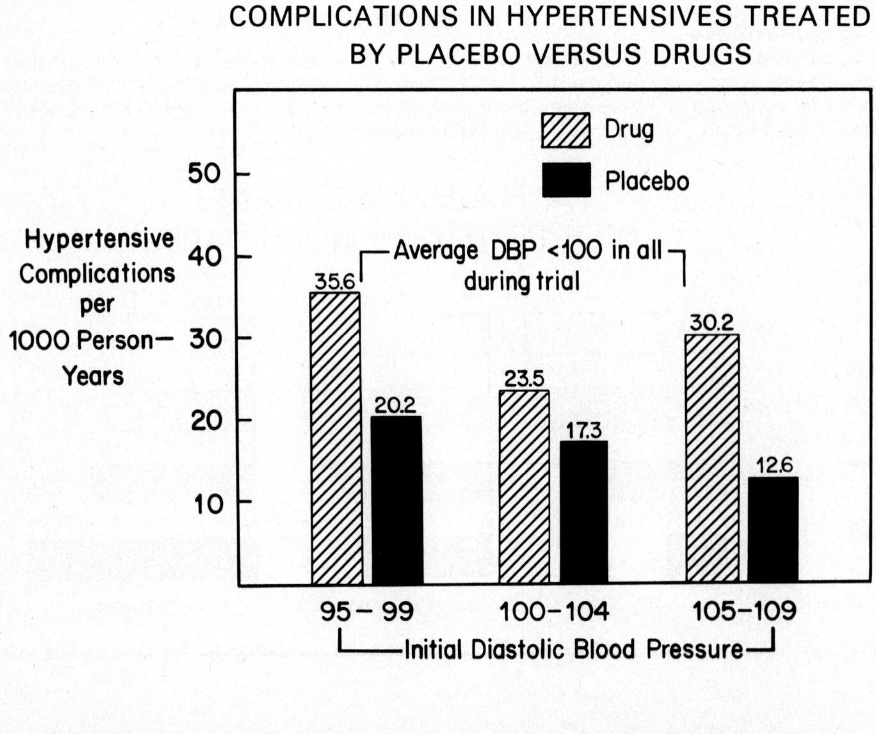

FIGURE 27-3 Cardiovascular complications per 1000 person-years among those receiving drugs and those receiving placebo during the Australian therapeutic trial. Note that for those whose average diastolic blood pressure (DBP) was below 100, regardless of the initial DBP range, complication rates were lower in those not on drugs. More of those from each initial DBP group who were on drugs achieved an end DBP below 100. (Drawn from Report of the Management Committee. Lancet *1*:1261, 1980.)

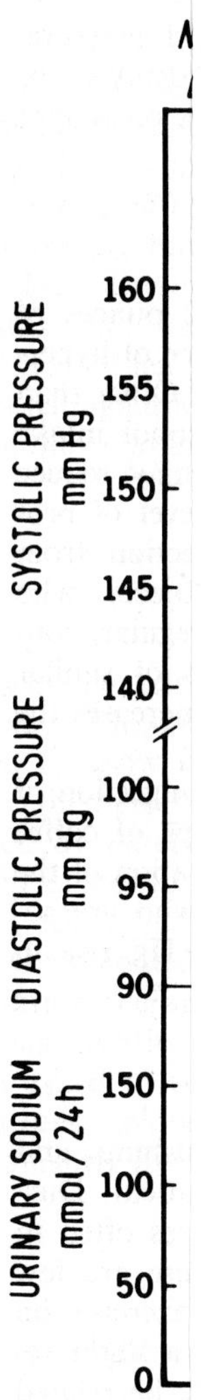

100 mm Hg. When the average diastolic pressures of the entire placebo-treated population throughout the trial is portrayed (Fig. 27–1), the majority (78 per cent) are shown to be below 100 mm Hg, even among those who started with pressure readings between 105 and 109 mm Hg. Thus the excess complications occurred in the 22 per cent of the placebo-treated group whose average diastolic pressure was above 100 mm Hg throughout the four years of the study.

Second, for those whose DBP was below 100 mm Hg, there were *fewer* complications among those on placebo than among those on drug therapy. As shown in Figure 27–3, the patients are again divided into three groups based on their initial level of diastolic pressure and only those whose average pressure was below 100 during the four years of the trial are portrayed. Since more of the drug-treated patients in each subdivision had an average diastolic pressure below 100 during the trial, there are more of them in each set. Since the numbers of patients and their duration of exposure to risk differ between the two groups, the obvious interpretation may be misleading, but it is hard to deny that interpretation: those given drugs had *more* cardiovascular complications than those with comparable blood pressures who were not receiving antihypertensive drugs. This interpretation, in turn, can be explained in various ways: (1) More of the drug-treated patients who averaged the same diastolic blood pressure during the trial as the placebo-treated group started with higher pressures; even though all patients were free of identifiable cardiovascular disease at the start of the trial, those with higher initial pressures might have been more likely to experience clinical complications despite the lowering of their pressure. (2) Although drugs are effective in protecting against complications, they are not able to remove the excess risk entirely. (3) Drugs are inherently toxic and patients with uncomplicated hypertension whose diastolic pressure stays below 100 are better off not receiving drug therapy.

The third interpretation may not be valid, but it cannot be dismissed. As we shall see, every group of antihypertensive drugs may adversely affect one or more cardiovascular risk factors, thereby diminishing, if not ablating, the potential benefits of the reductions of blood pressure. For example, diuretics tend to raise plasma cholesterol levels by 15 mg/dl—an effect recognized only after they had been used in the treatment of millions of hypertensives for almost 20 years.[18] Recall the warning by Geoffrey Rose, quoted in Chapter 26, (p. 856) that "if a preventive measure exposes many people to a small risk, the harm it does may readily . . . outweigh the benefits since those are received by relatively few."[19]

Overall Guidelines for the Use of Drug Therapy

The preceding discussion has attempted to establish three premises: (1) the relative risk for cardiovascular disease is based upon more than just the blood pressure, and by using simple clinical tools, it is possible to establish each individual's relative risk status; (2) for most mild hypertensives, the short-term risk is minimal, and the use of nondrug therapies (plus the spontaneous fall in pressure observed in some) may be adequate to relieve even that small degree of risk; and (3) drug therapy may pose inherent long-term risks along with the bother of more obvious and immediate side effects.

Based upon these premises, the author believes that the following guidelines are appropriate for deciding upon the institution of therapy, once the presence of hypertension has been confirmed by multiple blood pressure readings:

1. Patients with diastolic blood pressure above 100 mm Hg, particularly if it is accompanied by target organ damage or other major cardiovascular risks, should begin drug therapy immediately.

2. Patients with diastolic levels below 100 mm Hg who are otherwise at low risk should be encouraged to lose weight if obese, reduce sodium intake, exercise regularly, relax, and drink alcohol only in moderation. (More specific details about these nondrug therapies are provided later in this chapter.)

3. Patients whose diastolic pressure remains below 100 mm Hg should not be given drugs and should be observed at least every six months. If the diastolic pressure rises to and remains above 100, the patient should be treated with appropriate drugs.

4. When drug therapy is given, the diastolic blood pressure should be reduced to the low 80s, if that goal can be reached without bothersome side effects.

OTHER VIEWPOINTS

This more cautious approach is similar to that espoused by many outside the United States. A committee representing the World Health Organization and the International Society of Hypertension, after analyzing the published data from trials of the treatment of mild hypertension, offered this conclusion in early 1982: "The first line of treatment for people with mild hypertension should be observation, perhaps combined with general health measures such as weight reduction and restriction of salt intake."[13]

Although this viewpoint may reflect the consensus of most experts outside the U.S., many in the U.S. would argue for more widespread and earlier use of drug therapy.[20] Their arguments include the following: the assessment of relative risk is by no means certain, and most patients fall into an intermediate risk group; various nondrug therapies have not been shown to be either practical or effective for large groups of patients over prolonged periods; drug therapy will lower blood pressure, and providing it to most patients will avoid errors based on incorrect assessments of risk and will satisfy the widespread assumption that if their problem is not serious enough to be treated with medication, it is not serious enough to mandate changes in longstanding habits of life style. Furthermore, the HDFP found that patients with mild hypertension and no evidence of target organ damage achieved significant protection from stroke morbidity and mortality,[21] supporting the view that the overall benefit of more intensive drug therapy outweighs the potential hazards.

THE QUESTION OF PROTECTION FROM CORONARY DISEASE

Amid these arguments, an additional factor has given some authorities pause in advocating drug therapy for mild hypertension; i.e., an apparent lack of protection from the major cardiovascular risk, coronary artery disease. In the earlier trials, including those by the VA[2,3] and USPHS,[22] the reduction in the incidence of coronary disease offered by therapy was not statistically significant. In the Australian trial, fewer cases of fatal coronary artery disease occurred in the drug-treated group than in those treated with placebo (2 versus 8), but the difference in nonfatal coronary events (70 versus 88) was, once again, not statistically significant. In the HDFP, deaths from myocardial infarction were reduced by 46 per cent but deaths from "ischemic heart disease" were 9 per cent higher in the more actively treated Stepped-Care group.

The difficulty in showing protection from coronary artery disease likely reflects several factors: the advanced age of the study populations and the early age of onset of coronary atherosclerosis, the relatively short duration of the studies, and the multiple etiologies of coronary artery disease. Hypertension probably plays a less direct role in causing coronary artery disease than in causing heart failure, stroke, and renal damage. Coronary atherosclerosis is accentuated by high blood lipid levels, smoking, stress, and a sedentary life style.

Nonetheless, a noncontrolled study involving men with more severe hypertension, i.e., diastolic pressures above 115 mm Hg, did show a significant decrease in nonfatal and fatal coronary artery disease among 635 treated patients compared to 391 untreated ones.[23] Moreover, preliminary data from the HDFP report a "substantial" decrease in four indices of coronary artery disease among the Stepped-Care group compared to the less intensively treated Referred-Care group.[24] These include a lower incidence of angina by history and of myocardial infarction by history, Rose Questionnaire, and electrocardiography.

Further evidence comes from a study of left ventricular hypertro-

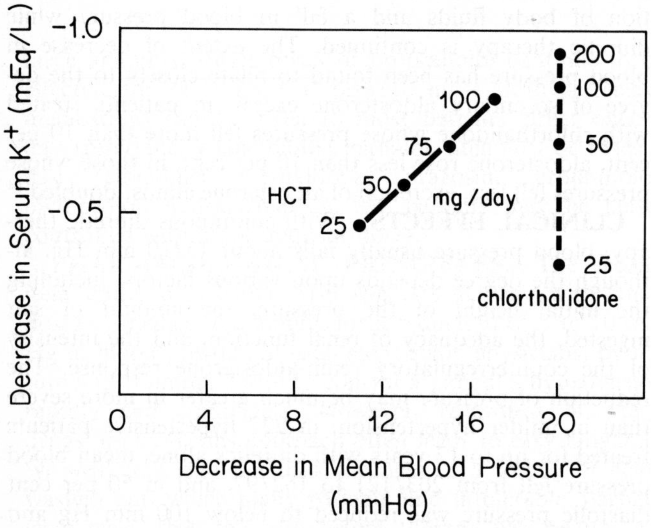

FIGURE 27-7 Effects of varying doses of hydrochlorothiazide (HCT) and chlorthalidone on the blood pressure and serum potassium in two groups of hypertensives. The different doses of chlorthalidone and HCT were given for 6- to 8-week periods in random order. (Data on HCT from Degnbol, B., et al.: The effect of different diuretics on elevated blood pressure and serum potassium. Acta Med. Scand. *193*:407, 1973; data on chlorthalidone from Tweeddale, M. G., et al.: Antihypertensive and biochemical effects of chlorthalidone. Clin. Pharmacol. Ther. *22*:519, 1977.)

respond to the lower doses of the various diuretics listed in Table 27-4, an amount equivalent to 25 mg of hydrochlorothiazide. Larger doses will have some additional antihypertensive effect but at the price of additional potassium wastage[66] (Fig. 27-7). With chlorthalidone, maximal antihypertensive effectiveness is achieved with 25 mg a day.[67] For uncomplicated hypertension, a moderately long-acting thiazide is a logical choice and a single morning dose of hydrochlorothiazide will provide a 24-hour antihypertensive effect.[68] When a short-acting drug (furosemide, 40 mg given twice daily) was compared to a longer acting drug (hydrochlorothiazide, 50 mg given twice daily), blood pressure was lowered significantly only with the longer acting drug.[69]

With renal insufficiency, manifested by a serum creatinine level above 2.5 mg/100 ml or creatinine clearance below 25 ml/min, thiazides are usually not effective, and multiple doses of furosemide or a single dose of metolazone will be needed.[70]

SIDE EFFECTS (Fig. 27-8). A number of biochemical changes often accompany successful diuresis, including a decrease in plasma potassium and increases in uric acid and cholesterol.

Hypokalemia. Serum potassium falls an average of 0.6 mmol/liter after institution of continuous, daily diuretic therapy for hypertension.[71] Among 158 hypertensives given diuretics for two years, plasma potassium levels fell to between 3.0 and 3.3 mmol/liter in 29 per cent and to between 2.6 and 2.9 mmol/liter in 7 per cent.[72] Although this fall in serum concentration may not reflect a significant decrease in total body potassium,[73] it may precipitate potentially hazardous ventricular ectopic activity, even in patients not known to be susceptible because of concomitant digitalis therapy or myocardial irritability.[74] The arrhythmogenic effect of diuretic-induced hypokalemia may become manifest only at times of stress, when catecholamines may lower the plasma potassium level another 0.5 to 1.0 mMol/liter.[74a] Acute myocardial infarction is one such stress wherein a high frequency of ventricular arrhythmias has been noted in patients with diuretic-induced hypokalemia.[74b] The degree of diuretic-induced hypokalemia may diminish with time despite continued therapy.[75] This may reflect a decrease in the secretion of potassium after the higher initial rate of tubular fluid flow down the nephron, which sweeps more potassium into the urine.[76]

Most patients are unaware of mild diuretic-induced hypokalemia, although it may contribute to leg cramps, polyuria, and muscle weakness. But subtle interference with antihypertension therapy may accompany even mild hypokalemia; volume retention and a rise in plasma angiotensin are seen experimentally.[77] In addition to increasing the propensity to ventricular ectopic activity, hypokalemia may precipitate serious arrhythmias in patients receiving digitalis (see Chap. 16). The occasional loss of carbohydrate tolerance and the frequent rise in plasma lipids seen with diuretic use may reflect a suppression of insulin secretion by hypokalemia.

Prevention of hypokalemia is preferable to correction of

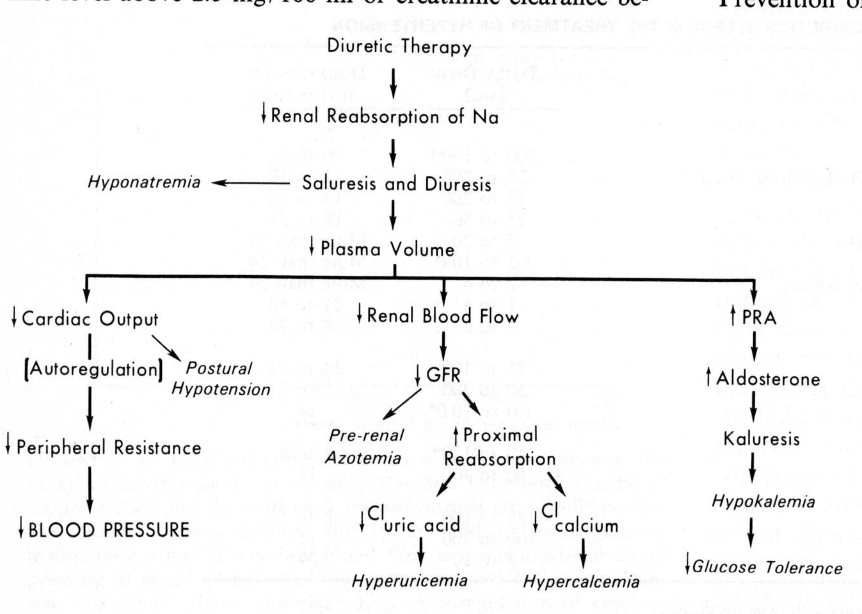

FIGURE 27-8 Desired antihypertensive action and various side effects of diuretics are shown to arise from the changes induced by a reduction in plasma volume.

potassium deficiency. The following maneuvers should help prevent diuretic-induced hypokalemia.

- Use the smallest amount of diuretic needed (Fig. 27–7).
- Use a moderately long-acting (12- to 18-hour) diuretic, since longer acting drugs (e.g., chlorthalidone) may increase potassium loss.[27]
- Restrict sodium intake to 60 to 100 mEq a day (i.e., 2 sodium).
- Increase dietary potassium intake.
- Restrict concomitant use of laxatives.
- Use a combination of a thiazide with a potassium-sparing agent. If the latter is prescribed, avoid supplemental potassium, since dangerous hyperkalemia may supervene if these drugs are given together.
- The concomitant use of a beta blocker may diminish potassium loss, presumably by blunting the diuretic-induced rise in renin-aldosterone, but hypokalemia may still occur with the combination.[78]

If hypokalemia is to be treated, the above maneuvers should be instituted along with some form of supplemental potassium. Potassium chloride is preferred for correction of the associated alkalosis. Despite the occasional appearance of mucosal lesions by gastroscopy after very large doses,[78a] a resin-matrix, slow-release tablet of KCl is both safe and effective, and most patients prefer it to liquid preparations. If tolerated, KCl can be given as a salt substitute; thereby, extra potassium will be provided at little expense while sodium intake is reduced.[79] Caution is necessary when supplemental KCl is given to older patients with borderline renal function in whom hyperkalemia may be induced.

In some patients, concomitant diuretic-induced magnesium deficiency will prevent the restoration of intracellular deficits of potassium[80] so that hypomagnesemia should be corrected.

Hyperuricemia. The serum uric acid level is elevated in as many as one-third of untreated hypertensive patients, particularly in those who are obese.[81] With chronic diuretic therapy, hyperuricemia appears in another third of patients, probably as a consequence of increased proximal tubular reabsorption accompanying volume contraction.[82] Even more marked hyperuricemia may develop when an adrenergic blocking drug is added to the diuretic.[81]

Diuretic-induced hyperuricemia only rarely precipitates acute gout or chronic nephropathy, but, based on observation of patients with idiopathic hyperuricemia, the potential for such complications remains. Assuming that urate excretion is diminished, patients with serum uric acid levels persistently above 10 mg/dl should probably be treated with a uricosuric drug such as probenecid. Although allopurinol is often used, it is more likely to cause side effects and seems a less rational choice, since the problem is a failure to excrete uric acid and not its overproduction.

Hyperlipidemia. Serum triglyceride and, to a lesser degree, serum cholesterol levels often rise after diuretic therapy.[18,83] Fortunately, the rise in lipids can be prevented by a "prudent" low-saturated fat diet.[84]

Hypercalcemia. A slight rise in serum calcium, less than 0.5 mg/dl, is frequently seen with effective diuretic therapy, at least in part because increased calcium reabsorption accompanies the increased sodium reabsorption in the proximal tubule induced by contraction of extracellular fluid volume. The rise is of little clinical importance except in patients with previously unrecognized hyperparathyroidism, who may experience a much more marked rise.

Hyperglycemia. Diuretics may impair glucose tolerance[85] and rarely may precipitate diabetes, perhaps by direct suppression of insulin secretion from the diuretic-induced hypokalemia.

Other Problems. A surprisingly high rate of impotence (22.6 per cent) was found among men taking 10 mg a day of bendrofluazide, compared to a rate of 10.1 per cent among those on placebo and 13.2 per cent among those on propranolol in the large Medical Research Council (MRC) trial.[86] This high rate may reflect the rather large dose of diuretic, perhaps through hypokalemia. Although inhibitors of prostaglandin synthesis (e.g., indomethacin) will blunt the diuretic effect of loop diuretics, no such interference occurs with thiazides.[87]

OTHER DIURETICS

Loop Diuretics. As described in Chapter 26, loop diuretics are usually needed in the treatment of hypertensive patients with renal insufficiency, defined as a serum creatinine above 2.5 mg/dl. Furosemide has been most widely used, although metolazone may work as well and requires only a single daily dose.[70] Many use furosemide in the management of uncomplicated hypertension, but, as noted earlier, this drug seems to provide less antihypertensive effect when given once or twice a day than do longer acting diuretics.

Potassium-Sparing Agents. These drugs are not diuretics but are usually employed in combination with a diuretic. Of the three currently available, one (spironolactone) is an aldosterone antagonist, while the other two (dyrenium and amiloride) are direct inhibitors of potassium secretion. In combination with a thiazide diuretic, they will diminish the amount of potassium wasting; although they are more expensive than thiazides alone, they may decrease the total cost of therapy by reducing the need to monitor and treat potassium depletion.

Diuretics Under Investigation. Of a number of diuretics currently under investigation, most are similar to agents now available. Indapamide may also inhibit calcium entry.[88]

AN OVERVIEW OF DIURETICS IN HYPERTENSION

Diuretics have been effective for the treatment of millions of hypertensive patients during the past 25 years. They will reduce diastolic pressure and maintain it below 90 mm Hg in about half of all hypertensive patients, providing the same degree of effectiveness as beta blockers and most other antihypertensive drugs.[89] In two groups that constitute a rather large portion of the hypertensive population, the elderly[90] and blacks,[91] diuretics alone are more effective than beta blockers. One diuretic tablet per day is usually all that is needed, minimizing cost and maximizing adherence to therapy.

The side effects of diuretic therapy are usually benign and, except for the potential hazards of hypokalemia, are of little clinical significance. Patients tolerate them better than[92] or as well as[86] the other drugs: in the large MRC trial in which patients were randomly given either a diuretic or a beta blocker, the percentage of patients who withdrew from therapy because of side effects during the first two years was almost identical for the two drugs.[86]

Some investigators view the hemodynamic changes induced by diuretic therapy as hazards.[57] However, objective evidence does not support the potential vasculotoxic effects of diuretic-induced increases in plasma renin activity.[93] Unless the patient undergoes excessive diuresis and is dehydrated, the hemodynamic changes incurred with chronic diuretic therapy are exactly what is needed, i.e., little, if any, fall in cardiac output and a reduction in peripheral and renal vascular resistance.[60] Thus the recommendation that a diuretic be the first drug in the therapy of virtually all hypertensive patients seemed logical.[56] However, the disquieting evidence that diuretics may be associated with additional risks for coronary disease[59a] has led to the idea that adrenergic blocking drugs be considered as initial therapy.[59b] If an adrenergic blocking drug is chosen for initial therapy, a tendency for volume retention should be recognized and moderate sodium restriction strongly encouraged. If fluid retention occurs or the blood pressure is inadequately controlled, the addition or substitution of a diuretic should be considered.

ADRENERGIC BLOCKING DRUGS

A number of adrenergic blocking drugs are available including some that act centrally upon vasomotor center activity, peripherally upon neuronal catecholamine discharge, or by blocking alpha and/or beta receptors (Table 27–5); some act at multiple sites. Figure 27–9, a schematic view of the ending of an adrenergic nerve and the effector cell with its receptors, depicts how some of these drugs act. When the nerve is stimulated, norepinephrine, which is synthesized and stored in granules, is released into the synaptic cleft. It binds to postsynaptic alpha and beta receptors and thereby initiates various intracellular processes. In the vascular smooth muscle, alpha stimulation causes constriction and beta stimulation causes relaxation. In the central vasomotor centers, sympathetic outflow is inhibited by alpha stimulation; the effect of beta stimulation is unknown.

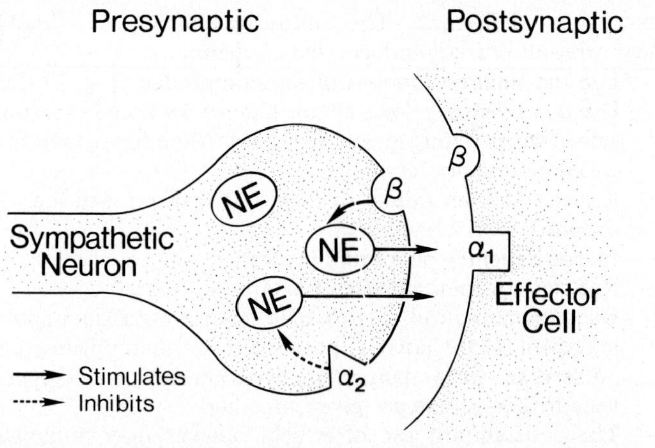

FIGURE 27-9 Simplified schematic view of the adrenergic nerve ending showing that norepinephrine (NE) is released from its storage granules when the nerve is stimulated and enters the synaptic cleft to bind to alpha$_1$ and beta receptors on the effector cell (postsynaptic). In addition, a short feedback loop exists, in which NE binds to alpha$_2$ and beta receptors on the neuron (presynaptic), either to inhibit or to stimulate further release.

An important aspect of sympathetic activity involves the feedback of norepinephrine to alpha and beta receptors located on the neuronal surface, i.e., presynaptic receptor.[94] Presynaptic alpha-receptor activation inhibits further norepinephrine release, whereas presynaptic beta-receptor activation stimulates further norepinephrine release. These presynaptic receptors probably play a role in the action of some of the drugs to be discussed.

Elucidation and quantitation of the various actions of these drugs remain incomplete. The listing in Table 27–5 is based upon the predominant site of action according to currently available data. The beta-adrenergic receptor blockers almost certainly act upon central vasomotor mechanisms, but most of their effect probably depends on peripheral actions.

TABLE 27–5 ADRENERGIC BLOCKERS

Drugs that Act Within the Neuron
Reserpine
Guanethidine (Ismelin)
Bethanidine (Tenathan)
Debrisoquine
Drugs that Act Upon Receptors
Predominantly Central Agonists
Methyldopa (Aldomet)
Clonidine (Catapres)
Guanabenz (Wytensin)
Lofexidine
Predominantly Peripheral Antagonists
Alpha
Pre- and postsynaptic:
Phenoxybenzamine (Dibenzyline)
Phentolamine (Regitine)
Postsynaptic: Prazosin (Minipress)
Beta
Atenolol (Tenormin)
Metoprolol (Lopressor)
Nadolol (Corgard)
Pindolol (Visken)
Propranolol (Inderal)
Timolol (Blocadren)
Acebutolol, sotalol, etc.
Alpha and Beta: Labetolol

Drugs That Act Within the Neuron

Reserpine, guanethidine, and related compounds act to inhibit the release of norepinephrine from peripheral adrenergic neurons, each in a different manner, totally unlike the feedback suppression of norepinephrine release that may be involved in the effects of the alpha-agonists methyldopa, clonidine, and guanabenz.

RESERPINE. Reserpine, the most active and widely used of the derivatives of the rauwolfia alkaloids, depletes the postganglionic adrenergic neurons of norepinephrine by inhibiting its uptake into storage vesicles, exposing it to degradation by cytoplasmic monoamine oxidase. The peripheral effect is predominant, although the drug enters the brain and depletes central catecholamine stores as well. This probably accounts for the sedation and depression seen with reserpine use.

The drug has certain advantages; only one dose a day is needed; in combination with a diuretic, the antihypertensive effect is significant, with a mean decrease in diastolic pressure of 16.7 mm Hg noted in one study[95] and an effect equal to or greater than that noted with methyldopa or propranolol in another;[96] little postural hypotension is noted; and many patients experience no side effects. The drug has a flat dose-response curve, so that a dose of only 0.05 mg a day will give almost as much antihypertensive effect as 0.125 or 0.25 mg a day but fewer side effects.[97]

The psychological depression that occurs in perhaps 2 per cent of patients may be severe but difficult to recognize and treat. The specter of breast cancer associated with reserpine raised in 1974 has not been substantiated.[98] Although it remains popular in some places, the use of reserpine has declined progressively.

GUANETHIDINE. Guanethidine and a series of related guanidine compounds, including bethanidine and debrisoquine, act by inhibiting the release of norepinephrine from the adrenergic neurons, perhaps by a local anesthetic-like effect on the neuronal membrane. In order to act, the drug must be actively transported into the nerve through an amine pump. Various drugs, in particular tricyclic antidepressants, amphetamines, and ephedrine, will competitively block the uptake of guanethidine into the nerves and thereby antagonize its effects.

Its low lipid solubility prevents guanethidine from entering the brain, so that sedation, depression, and other side effects on the central nervous system are not seen. Initially, the predominant hemodynamic effect is to decrease cardiac output; after continued use, peripheral resistance declines. Blood pressure is reduced further when the patient is upright, owing to gravitational pooling of blood in the legs, since compensatory sympathetic nervous system–mediated vasoconstriction is blocked. This results in the most common side effect, postural hypotension. Patients should be advised to arise slowly, sleep with the head of the bed elevated, and wear elastic hose to minimize this potential problem.

Unlike reserpine, guanethidine has a steep dose-response curve, so that it can be successfully used in treating hypertension of any degree in daily doses of 10 to 300 mg. Like reserpine, it has a long biological half-life and may be given once daily. As other drugs have become available, guanethidine has been relegated mainly to the treatment of severe hypertension. Now that the combination of beta blockers and vasodilator drugs has become the most widely prescribed treatment for severe hypertension, the use of guanethidine will probably decline further.

Bethanidine and debrisoquine are similar to guanethidine but have a shorter duration of action and, perhaps, fewer side effects.[99]

Drugs That Act Upon Receptors

PREDOMINANTLY CENTRAL AGONISTS

METHYLDOPA (ALDOMET). Since the late 1960's, methyldopa had been the most widely used of the adrenergic blockers, but its use has fallen off as beta blockers have become more popular. At first it was thought that methyldopa entered the catecholamine biosynthetic pathway by inhibiting dopa-decarboxylase. Later it was believed to act by inducing the synthesis of alpha-methylnorepinephrine in peripheral sympathetic nerves, which would serve as a weak or false neurotransmitter. Finally, the primary site of action has been found to be within the central nervous system, where alpha-methylnorepinephrine is released from adrenergic neurons and stimulates central alpha receptors, reducing the sympathetic outflow from the central nervous system.[100]

The blood pressure falls mainly from a decrease in peripheral resistance with little effect upon cardiac output. However, as is true with all adrenergic blockers, patients with borderline cardiac function may be thrown into congestive failure by removal of adrenergic support. On the other hand, when 10 hypertensives were treated with methyldopa, the degree of left ventricular hypertrophy as seen by echocardiography was reduced in four patients within 12 weeks, although blood pressure was not significantly altered.[101] Renal blood flow is well maintained, and significant postural hypotension is unusual. Therefore, the drug has been widely used in hypertensive patients with renal insufficiency or cerebral vascular disease; smaller doses are needed in the presence of renal insufficiency. Renin levels usually decrease, but the reduction in blood pressure is dependent neither upon initially high plasma renin activity nor upon a subsequent fall in this level.

On the basis of pharmacokinetic data, the drug has been prescribed in three or four doses a day. However, it need be given no more than twice daily.[50] The dosage range is from 250 to 3000 mg a day, with most patients responding to 750 to 1500 mg. As in the case of the other adrenergic blockers and peripheral vasodilators, methyldopa is best used in combination with a diuretic.

Side effects include some that are common to centrally acting drugs that reduce sympathetic outflow: sedation, dry mouth, orthostatic hypotension, impotence, and galactorrhea. However, methyldopa causes some unique side effects that are probably of an autoimmune nature, since a positive antinuclear antibody test is seen in about 10 per cent of patients who take the drug, a positive Coombs' test in about 25 per cent, and abnormal liver function tests in about 8 per cent. Less commonly, these laboratory abnormalities presage serious trouble: myocarditis;[102] hemolytic anemia in about 0.2 per cent; and acute hepatitis or chronic hepatic injury,[103] which may be related to the binding of a reactive metabolite with liver cell macromolecules.[104]

CLONIDINE (CATAPRES). Although they differ in structure, clonidine shares many features with methyldopa: it most likely acts in the same central sites, has similar antihypertensive efficacy, and causes many of the same bothersome but less serious side effects (e.g., sedation, dry mouth) but does not induce the autoimmune side effects.

This imidazoline derivative acts as an alpha-adrenergic receptor agonist and lowers blood pressure by stimulating the postsynaptic alpha receptors in the vasomotor centers of the brain.[100] Sympathetic outflow from the brain is thereby reduced, resulting in a decrease in basal heart rate and cardiac output and a fall in peripheral resistance. Since the baroreceptor reflex is left intact, blood pressure responds appropriately to upright posture and exercise, so that hypotension is rarely a problem. Renal blood flow is well maintained, and renin secretion is reduced. The decrease in renin is not necessary for the decrease in blood pressure but may be responsible for an immediate effect in patients with high renin levels.[105]

As an alpha-receptor agonist, the drug also acts upon presynaptic alpha receptors and inhibits norepinephrine release (Fig. 27–9), and plasma catecholamine levels fall.[106] The drug has a fairly short biological half-life, so that when it is discontinued, the inhibition of norepinephrine release disappears within about 12 to 18 hours, and plasma catecholamine levels rise. This is probably responsible for a rapid rebound of the blood pressure to pretreatment levels and the occasional appearance of withdrawal symptoms, including tachycardia, restlessness, and sweating. Rarely, the blood pressure increases beyond the pretreatment level. Similar overshoots have been reported after the discontinuation of a variety of other antihypertensives,[107] including methyldopa, but since that drug has a longer biological half-life, the blood pressure does not usually rise until about 48 hours later and then more gradually. If the rebound requires treatment, clonidine may be reintroduced or alpha-receptor antagonists may be given.

By itself, clonidine will often induce fluid retention, so that it should generally be used with a diuretic and be given in two doses a day. After control has been achieved with two daily doses of clonidine and a diuretic, it may be maintained with a single bedtime dose.

GUANABENZ. This drug differs in structure but shares many characteristics with both methyldopa and clonidine, acting primarily as a central alpha-agonist. However, it may differ in *not* causing reactive fluid retention,[108] so that it may turn out to be effective without the need for a concomitant diuretic.

LOFEXIDINE AND GUANFACINE. These drugs, similar to clonidine, are under clinical investigation.[109,109a]

Predominantly Peripheral Antagonists

ALPHA-RECEPTOR ANTAGONISTS. Prior to 1977, the only alpha blockers used to treat hypertension were *phenoxybenzamine* (Dibenzyline) and *phentolamine* (Regitine). These drugs are effective in acutely lowering blood pressure, but their effects are offset by an accompanying increase in cardiac output, and side effects are frequent and bothersome. Their limited effect may reflect their blockade of presynaptic alpha receptors, which interferes with the feedback inhibition of norepinephrine release (Fig. 27–9). Increased catecholamine release would then blunt the action on postsynaptic alpha receptors. Their use has largely been limited to the treatment of patients with pheochromocytoma.

Prazosin (Minipress) is a selective antagonist of the postsynaptic alpha receptors. Although this drug was introduced as a peripheral vasodilator, subsequent study has clearly shown its primary effect to be that of a postsynaptic alpha blocker.[110] By blocking alpha-mediated vasoconstriction, prazosin induces a fall in peripheral resistance. Since the presynaptic alpha receptor is left unblocked, the feedback loop for the inhibition of norepinephrine release is intact, an action which is almost certainly responsible for the greater antihypertensive effect of the drug and the absence of concomitant tachycardia, tolerance, and renin release. The inhibition of norepinephrine release may also account for the propensity toward postural hypotension. However, this is noted mainly with the first dose, and a greater initial effect on receptors in the veins, leading to an abrupt loss of sympathetic venous tone with venous pooling, has been invoked to explain this first-dose hypotension.[111] This problem can be mitigated by limiting the first dose to 0.5 mg to 1.0 mg.

Prazosin is about as effective as methyldopa and is similarly aided by concomitant use of a diuretic. It can be safely and effectively used in patients with renal insufficiency. The addition of small doses of prazosin has been found to be particularly effective in the management of severe hypertension refractory to other medications.[112] The ability of the drug to dilate the venous capacitance bed and reduce preload while also lowering systemic resistance has prompted its successful use in the treatment of severe congestive heart failure[113] (see Chap. 16).

Side effects, beyond first-dose hypotension, include persistent postural hypotension, dizziness, weakness, fatigue, and headaches. However, most patients find the drug easy to take, with little (if any) sedation, dry mouth, or impotence.

BETA-RECEPTOR ANTAGONISTS (see also pp. 1349–1350). In the past few years, beta blockers have been used increasingly, becoming the most popular form of antihypertensive therapy, after diuretics. Their popularity reflects their relative effectiveness and freedom from bothersome side effects. However, they are no more effective in lowering blood pressure than are other adrenergic blocking agents such as reserpine,[95] and side effects occur in up to 25 per cent of hypertensive patients who take them.[14] Some of these side effects, including bradycardia, bronchospasm, and peripheral vasospasm, may be quite bothersome. However, for the majority of patients who do not develop such side effects, beta blockers are usually easier to take than are other adrenergic blocking drugs, since somnolence, dry mouth, and impotence are rarely encountered. Moreover, more cardioselective beta blockers are now available, and their use will reduce, although not eliminate, some of the serious side effects.[114]

Beta blockers may have an important advantage over other antihypertensives, i.e., protection from coronary disease and the risk of angina, myocardial infarction, and sudden death. Such protection has been shown in patients, both hypertensive and normotensive, after an initial myocardial infarction with a variety of beta blockers (see Chap. 38). However, no data are available regarding the prevention of initial episodes of coronary disease, except for the results of the HDFP and Australian trials described earlier in this chapter, which involved a variety of antihypertensive drugs. Beta blockers may provide protection beyond their antihypertensive effects: their antianginal and antiarrhythmic actions are well documented, and they inhibit both the aggregation of platelets and their synthesis of the vasoconstrictor thromboxane.[115] Whether or not beta blockers provide clinically important primary cardioprotection, they can be used for their known antihypertensive effects, with the possibility of protection from coronary events viewed as a bonus—greatly desired but not yet proved.

The Variety of Beta Blockers. The beta blockers now being used in the United States are listed in Table 39–5 (p. 1350). Among the first to be widely used was practolol, which has since been withdrawn because it resulted in an oculomucocutaneous syndrome that caused blindness and peritoneal fibrosis. This reaction appears to be a hypersensitivity response[116] and may be unique to practolol, the only beta blocker to possess an acetanilid side chain. Similar reactions to the other beta blockers have been extremely unusual.

Propranolol was first used in the treatment of hypertension in 1964, and as many as 15 beta blockers are now available in some European countries. Pharmacologically, these beta blockers differ considerably with respect to degree of absorption, protein binding, and bioavailability. But the three most important differences affecting their clinical use are cardioselectivity, intrinsic sympathomimetic activity, and lipid solubility. Despite all these differences, they all seem to be effective antihypertensives, and about equally so.[117]

Cardioselectivity. As seen in Table 39–5 (p. 1350), atenolol and metoprolol are relatively cardioselective, having a greater blocking effect on the $beta_1$-receptors in the heart than on the $beta_2$-receptors in the bronchi, peripheral blood vessels, and elsewhere. Such cardioselectivity can be easily shown using small doses in acute studies; with the rather high doses used to treat hypertension, part of this effect is lost. Nonetheless, atenolol and metoprolol cause less clinically bothersome $beta_2$-mediated side effects.[114] Two randomized crossover trials demonstrate the advantages: the rise in plasma triglyceride and fall in HDL-cholesterol levels were less with atenolol and metoprolol than with propranolol[118]; metoprolol did not impair glucose metabolism in noninsulin-dependent diabetes but propranolol did.[119]

Intrinsic Sympathomimetic Activity (ISA). Pindolol has the greatest ISA, interacting with beta receptors to cause a measurable agonist response, but at the same time, blocking the greater agonist effects of endogenous catecholamines. As a result, while in usual doses pindolol lowers the blood pressure to about the same degree as other beta blockers, it causes a smaller decline in heart rate, cardiac output, and renin levels.[120] However, with higher doses, less antihypertensive effect and even a paradoxical rise in blood pressure may be noted, presumably because of the considerable agonist effect. Although the clinical relevance of this difference remains to be proved, a drug with high ISA may prove useful when a beta blocker is needed for patients in whom bradycardia or peripheral vascular disease is a problem.

Lipid Solubility. Atenolol and nadolol are the least lipid-soluble of the beta blockers listed in Table 39–5 (p. 1350). This translates into some clinically important advantages: (1) because they are not taken up and metabolized in the liver, they reach and maintain stable plasma concentrations quickly, requiring fewer dose titrations; (2) since they escape hepatic inactivation, they remain as active drugs in the plasma much longer, allowing once-a-day dosage; and (3) because they do not enter the brain as readily, they may cause fewer central nervous system (CNS) side effects. When 33 patients who experienced such side effects (depression, insomnia, nightmares) while on propranolol were switched to atenolol, the symptoms were relieved in 24.[121] On the other hand, since these drugs are removed mainly through renal excretion, high blood levels may accumulate in patients with renal insufficiency.

Mode of Action. Despite these and other differences, the various beta blockers now available seem about equipotent as antihypertensive agents.[117] How they lower the blood pressure remains uncertain, although a number of possible mechanisms are likely to be involved (Fig. 27–10). Cardiac output falls 15 to 20 per cent, renin release is reduced about 60 per cent, and central nervous beta-adrenergic blockade may reduce sympathetic discharge. Recall, too, that blockade of presynaptic beta receptors should inhibit catechol release (Fig. 27–9). Although propranolol decreases plasma clearance of norepinephrine and thereby raises plasma norepinephrine levels,[122] no obvious inhibition of sympathetic nervous function has been demonstrable.[123] On the other hand, in rats, propranolol antagonizes the enhancement of sympathetic nerve transmission by angiotensin II, apparently through the release of prostaglandins.[124] Other CNS effects may also be involved; again in rats, brain serotonergic activity was reduced after treatment with metoprolol.[125]

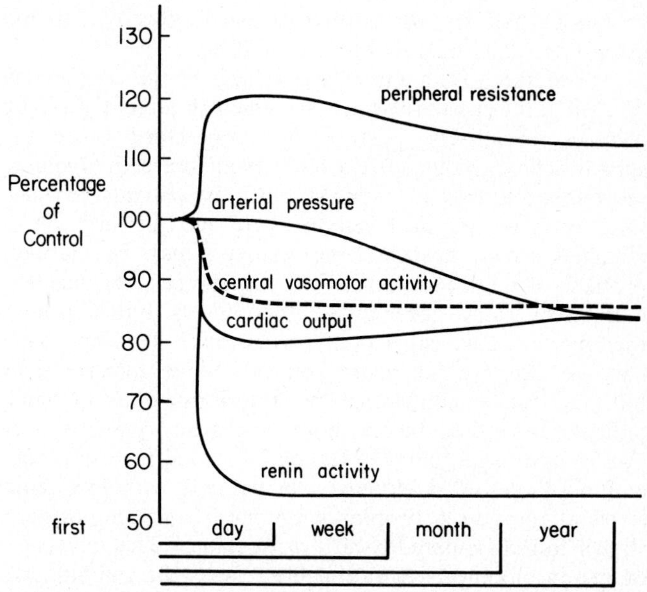

FIGURE 27-10 Schematic representation of the multiple actions of beta-blocker therapy over variable periods of time. The solid lines have been measured; the dotted line of central vasomotor activity has not. (Adapted from Birkenhager, W. H., et al.: Therapeutic effects of β-adrenoceptor blocking agents in hypertension. *In* Frick, P., et al.: Advances in Internal Medicine and Pediatrics. No. 39. Berlin, Springer-Verlag, 1977, pp. 117–134.)

At the same time that beta blockers are lowering blood pressure through various means, their blockade of peripheral beta receptors inhibits vasodilation, leaving alpha receptors open to catechol-mediated vasoconstriction. As a result, peripheral resistance rises and stays up.[126] Although evidence for a parallel decrease in alpha-mediated vasoconstriction has been found,[127] a decrease in peripheral blood flow is a common problem with beta-blocker therapy in cold climates.

Clinical Effects. Even in small doses, beta blockers begin to lower the blood pressure within a few hours, although their maximal effect may not be noted for some weeks.[128] Even though progressively higher doses have usually been given, careful study has shown a near-maximal effect from smaller doses: in a double-blind crossover study involving 24 patients, 40 mg of propranolol twice a day provided the same antihypertensive effects as 80, 160, or 240 mg twice a day.[129] The degree of blood pressure reduction is at least comparable to that noted with other antihypertensive drugs. By itself, a beta blocker will lower the diastolic blood pressure to below 90 mm Hg in about half the patients with mild to moderate hypertension; when combined with a diuretic, the percentage rises to about 80 per cent.[95] Duration of action is well beyond the drug's plasma half-life. With propranolol, which has a 3-

to 6-hour half-life, the antihypertensive effect of 240 mg given once daily persisted for up to 28 hours.[54]

One of the attractions of these drugs is the consistency of their antihypertensive action, which is altered little by changes in activity, posture, or temperature. Since the sympathetic nervous system is blocked, the hemodynamic responses to stress are reduced, but most patients can perform ordinary physical activities without difficulty. With maximal stress, however, the response may be blunted, probably enough to interfere with athletic performance.[130]

Beta blockers have been proposed as initial monotherapy for most cases of hypertension.[131] This approach may be effective for many younger, white hypertensives but may not be suitable for the majority of older or black patients. As noted before, both blacks and patients over age 50 have been found to respond less well to beta-blocker monotherapy.[90,91] Moreover, in patients with low renin levels at the outset, propranolol alone has sometimes been shown to induce paradoxical *hypertension.*[132] This unexpected rise in blood pressure probably reflects the combination of fluid retention and alpha-adrenergic–mediated peripheral and renal vasoconstriction that occurs in the face of blockade of $beta_2$-receptors in the vascular bed. In patients with normal or high renin, the inhibition of renin by propranolol probably counteracts both these antagonistic actions. If beta-blocker therapy is given with a diuretic, the potential problems of fluid retention and paradoxical hypertension will be avoided without the need to determine a patient's renin status.

Special Uses for Beta Blockers

Coexisting Coronary Disease. Even without proof that beta blockers protect patients from initial coronary events, the antiarrhythmic and antianginal effects of the drug make them especially valuable in hypertensive patients with coexisting coronary disease.

Patients Needing Antihypertensive Vasodilator Therapy. If a diuretic and an adrenergic blocker are inadequate to control blood pressure, the addition of a vasodilator is a logical third step. When used alone, vasodilators induce reflex sympathetic stimulation of the heart. The simultaneous use of beta blockers prevents this undesirable increase in cardiac output, which not only bothers the patient but also dampens the antihypertensive effect of the vasodilator.

Patients With Hyperkinetic Hypertension. Some hypertensive patients have increased cardiac output that may persist for many years. Beta blockers should be particularly effective in such patients, but a reduction in exercise capacity may restrict their use in young athletes.[130]

Patients With Marked Anxiety. The somatic manifestations of anxiety—tremor, sweating, and tachycardia—can be helped. In one controlled study, the performance of 24 musicians was found to improve when they took 40 mg of oxprenolol before the concert.[133] The undesirable effects of methods commonly used to control anxiety, i.e., alcohol and tranquilizers, were not observed.

Patients Taking Tricyclic Antidepressants and Antipsychotic Agents. The effects of guanethidine, clonidine, and other adrenergic neuronal blocking drugs may be blunted by these agents; beta blockers should not be affected. Moreover, they may counteract the tachycardia and arrhythmias sometimes seen with the tricyclics (see Chap. 56). Sedation and depression rarely develop as side effects of beta blockers and other central nervous system problems are rare except with very high doses.

Patients in Whom Diuretics are Contraindicated. Diuretics can exacerbate diabetes and gout. Although these problems can be managed, use of a beta blocker without a diuretic is rational and will likely be effective. As previously described, fluid retention and a subsequent loss of antihypertensive efficacy less commonly follow beta-blocker therapy than they do therapy with other nondiuretic antihypertensive drugs.

Side Effects. Most of the side effects of beta blockers relate to their major pharmacological action, the blockade of beta receptors. Those which are less cardioselective are likely to cause more of the $beta_2$-mediated side effects. The experience of a group of English clinicians in treating a large number of hypertensives with either a nonselective drug (propranolol) or a more selective one (atenolol) documents this difference[114] (Table 27–6). With propranolol, 9.7 per cent of patients had to discontinue the drug, whereas with atenolol, only 2.2 per cent had to discontinue its use.

If patients with preexisting bronchospasm are excluded, the most common problem is peripheral vasospasm. Fatigue likely reflects the decrease in cerebral blood flow that may accompany successful lowering of the blood pressure by any drug[55] (see Figure 27–6). More direct effects on the central nervous system—depression, insomnia, bad dreams, and hallucinations—occur in some patients. Of all the side effects, these are most dose-dependent. The remainder are likely to develop, if at all, with small doses and do not tend to increase in frequency with higher doses, presumably because smaller doses provide as much beta blockade as will occur in most tissues. The more frequent side effects of other adrenergic blocking drugs—sedation, depression, dry mouth, impotence, and postural hypotension—are very rare. Thus, if patients escape the rather serious side effects, they are likely to tolerate the drugs well, and most prefer these to all others.[128]

The reduction in cardiac output, one of the pharmacological effects of beta blockers, might be expected to induce *congestive heart failure* rather frequently. However, with the reduction in arterial pressure the demands upon

TABLE 27–6 ADVERSE EFFECTS WITH PROPRANOLOL (390 PATIENTS, 10 YEARS) AND ATENOLOL (543 PATIENTS, 4 YEARS)

	Percentage of Patients	
	Propranolol	*Atenolol*
Heart failure	0.8	0.4
Peripheral vascular disturbances:		
Cold extremities	2.5	2.8
Worsening claudication	2.8	1.3
Bronchospasm	5.1	3.3
Central nervous system disturbances:		
Vivid dreams, hallucinations	2.5	0.9
Dizziness, ataxia	0.4	1.1
Depression	0.8	0.7
Fatigue	3.9	3.9
Impotence	0.2	0.2
Total adverse effects	24.1	16.9

From Zacharias et al.: Atenolol in hypertension: A study of long-term therapy. Postgrad. Med. J. *53* (Suppl. 3):102, 1977.

the heart are lowered even more, so that failure was noted in only 0.8 per cent of Zacharias' patients during their 10 years on propranolol (Table 27–6), a number below that expected in patients with hypertension for this length of time.

Diabetics may have additional problems with nonselective beta blockers such as propranolol. The responses to hypoglycemia, both the symptoms and the counterregulatory hormonal changes that raise blood sugar levels, are partially dependent upon sympathetic nervous activity. Diabetics susceptible to hypoglycemia may have more serious reactions when taking propranolol. However, the majority of more stable diabetics can take the drug without difficulty, while the more cardioselective beta blockers, such as metoprolol, are preferable for diabetics with more brittle disease.[119]

When propranolol is discontinued suddenly, *angina pectoris* may appear for the first time or, if present previously, may be intensified (p. 1350).[134] Patients with hypertension are more susceptible to coronary disease, so they should be weaned gradually. Blood pressure may also rebound to high levels.[107] These effects may reflect a state of supersensitivity or an increase in the number of beta receptors induced during the prior beta blockade, leading to augmented responsiveness to normal levels of endogenous catecholamines. The withdrawal syndrome can be prevented by use of a small dose (30 mg a day) for 2 weeks before complete withdrawal.[135] If patients require immediate cessation of oral therapy, they can be protected by continuous propranolol infusion.[136]

Patients with *renal insufficiency* may take beta blockers without additional hazard, although a 20 per cent fall in renal blood flow and glomerular filtration rate has been measured with noncardioselective beta blockers, presumably from $beta_2$-mediated renal vasoconstriction.[137] Dosage of the lipid-insoluble atenolol and nadolol should be reduced in patients with renal insufficiency.

Caution is advised in patients suspected of having *pheochromocytoma,* since unopposed alpha-adrenergic action may precipitate a serious hypertensive crisis if this disease is present. The use of beta blockers during *pregnancy* has been beclouded by scattered case reports of various fetal problems. However, two prospective studies found that the use of beta blockers to treat hypertension during pregnancy did not lead to an increase in fetal morbidity.[138,139]

Perturbations of *lipoprotein metabolism* may accompany the use of beta blockers. After 8 weeks of propranolol therapy, serum HDL-cholesterol was reduced by 13 per cent and total triglycerides increased by 24 per cent.[140] Less marked changes were noted with the cardioselective agents atenolol and metoprolol than with propranolol.[118]

Impotence has been reported only rarely. In the large MRC trial, the frequency of impotence, as determined by questionnaire, was 10.1 per cent among those on placebo and 13.2 per cent among those on propranolol.[86]

The metabolism and bioavailability of beta blockers—particularly the lipid-soluble ones, such as propranolol, which are metabolized in the liver—may be affected by various factors that alter liver blood flow and enzymatic activity. As examples, decreases in hepatic extraction and/or metabolism, leading to higher blood levels of propranolol, have been reported with concomitant cimetidine therapy[141] ; increases in liver metabolism, leading to lower blood levels of active drug, have been found after consumption of alcohol.[142] Moreover, some people (about 10 per cent of those tested in England) have a genetically determined deficiency in drug oxidation, which leads to unusually high concentrations of lipid-soluble beta blockers and may be responsible for a greater propensity to develop side effects when usual doses are given.[143]

An Overview of Beta Blockers in Hypertension. Beta blockers will likely continue to be the most popular of the adrenergic inhibitors in the treatment of hypertension. They may be particularly effective in those with high-renin states, such as renovascular hypertension. In some with ordinary hypertension, they may be effective when used alone. If a beta blocker is chosen, a more cardioselective, lipid-insoluble one (see Table 39–5, p. 1350) offers the likelihood of greater patient adherence to therapy, since only one dose a day will be needed and side effects will likely be minimized.

ALPHA- AND BETA-RECEPTOR ANTAGONISTS. The combination of an alpha and a beta blocker may often prove to be effective for patients resistant to one drug alone. There are promising reports of a drug, labetolol, which combines both alpha- and beta-blocking actions, in a ratio of approximately 1:3. The fall in pressure results mainly from a decrease in peripheral resistance, with little or no fall in cardiac output.[144] Side effects have been minimal, although 9 of 47 patients developed a positive antinuclear factor. Intravenous labetolol has been used successfully to treat hypertensive emergencies, particularly those resulting from catecholamine excess.[145]

VASODILATORS

If a diuretic and adrenergic blocker do not control the blood pressure, a peripheral vasodilator is an appropriate third drug. Hydralazine (Apresoline) is the only agent of this type now available for routine use. Minoxidil is even more potent but is usually reserved for patients with severe, refractory hypertension associated with renal insufficiency. Diazoxide and nitroprusside are given intravenously for hypertensive crises and will be discussed at the end of this chapter.

HYDRALAZINE. First introduced in 1953, hydralazine has regained popularity since it was recognized that beta blockers could be used to prevent its side effects and enhance its efficacy[59] (Fig. 27–11). Since the early 1970's, hydralazine in combination with a diuretic and a beta blocker has been used increasingly to treat more severe hypertension. The drug acts directly to relax the smooth muscle in precapillary resistance vessels with little or no effect on postcapillary venous capacitance vessels. As a result, blood pressure falls but, in doing so, a number of reactive processes are activated that blunt the decrease in pressure and cause side effects. However, when a diuretic is used to overcome the tendency for fluid retention and a beta blocker is used to prevent the reflex increase in sympathetic activity and rise in renin, the vasodilator is more effective and causes few, if any, side effects (Fig. 27–12).

The drug need be given only twice a day,[53] and its daily dosage should be kept below 400 mg to prevent the lupus-like syndrome that appears in 10 to 20 per cent of patients who receive more. This reaction, although uncomfortable to the patient, is completely reversible and does not cause

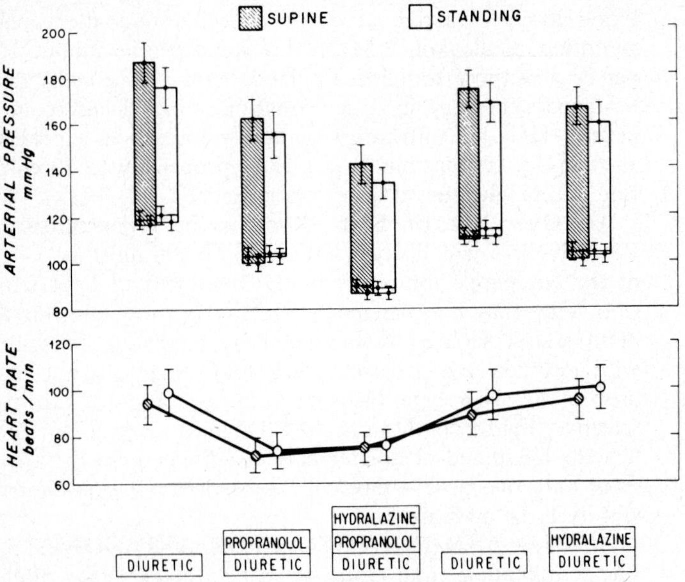

FIGURE 27-11 Arterial pressures and heart rates of 23 hypertensive patients treated with four drug regimens. The combination of hydralazine and propranolol provided the greatest effect on blood pressure without a rise in heart rate. (From Zacest, R., et al.: Treatment of essential hypertension with combined vasodilatation and beta-adrenergic blockade. N. Engl. J. Med. *286*:617, 1972, by permission of the New England Journal of Medicine.)

permanent injury. In fact, *lower* subsequent blood pressure and improved survival has been noted among 42 patients with this toxic reaction when compared to matched-patients given hydralazine but who did not experience the reaction.[146] The reaction is very rare with daily doses of 200 mg or less and is more common in slow acetylators of the drug.

Without the protection conferred by concomitant use of an adrenergic blocker, numerous other side effects—tachycardia, flushing, headache, and precipitation of angina—are seen; with the combination, most patients experience few or no side effects.

MINOXIDIL. This drug, unrelated to other vasodilators, acts in a manner similar to hydralazine but is even more effective. It has been found to be particularly useful in managing patients with severe hypertension and renal insufficiency.[147] Even more than with hydralazine, diuretics and adrenergic blockers must be used with minoxidil to prevent the reflex increase in cardiac output and fluid retention. Unfortunately, the drug also causes hair to grow profusely, and the facial hirsutism discourages some women from taking the drug. Previous concerns that the drug leads to pulmonary hypertension and causes right atrial lesions, as it does in dogs, have been shown to be unfounded.[147] However, pericardial effusions have appeared in about 3 per cent of those given minoxidil and are likely related to the renal insufficiency that is usually present but are sometimes seen in patients without renal or cardiac failure.[148]

CALCIUM-ENTRY BLOCKERS

(See also p. 1350–1353)

One or more of these agents will probably be approved for use in the treatment of hypertension. Of those currently available for treatment of coronary disease, nifedipine has the most attractive hemodynamic profile: it has the greatest peripheral vasodilatory action with little effect on cardiac conduction. Initial trials have shown nifedipine to be effective, both by sublingual and by oral routes.[149,149a,149b] Verapamil is also effective,[150] and both agents tend to reduce blood pressure significantly only in those patients with hypertension.[151]

The antihypertensive effect of these agents may be so fast and so marked as to precipitate coronary ischemic

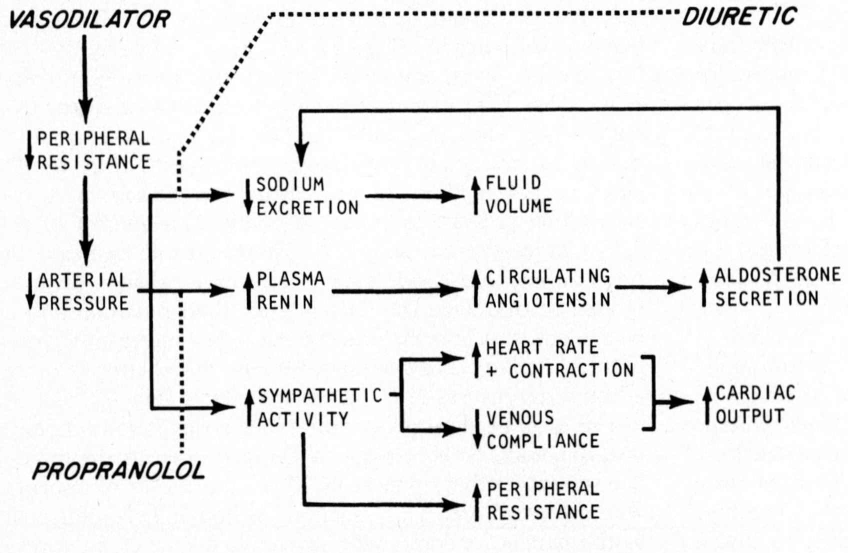

FIGURE 27-12 The primary and secondary effects of vasodilator therapy in essential hypertension and the manner by which diuretic and beta-adrenergic blocker therapy can overcome the undesirable secondary effects. (Adapted from Koch-Weser, J.: Vasodilator drugs in the treatment of hypertension. Arch. Intern. Med. *133*:1017, 1974. Copyright 1974, American Medical Association.)

changes on ECG.[152] But of potentially greater concern are the possible diffuse effects of these agents on various secretory processes that involve calcium entry.[153] Verapamil has been found to dampen the release of gonadotropin and thyrotropin from the pituitary,[154] but the clinical significance of these hormonal changes remains uncertain.

As the basic mechanisms of action of various antihypertensive agents are being unraveled, inhibition of calcium entry may turn out to be common to many: both beta-[155] and alpha-adrenergic[156] blocking drugs may work in this manner, as may direct-acting vasodilators.[157]

RENIN-ANGIOTENSIN BLOCKERS

Activity of the renin-angiotensin system may now be inhibited in four ways (Fig. 27–13), three of which can be applied clinically. The first, use of adrenergic blockers to inhibit the release of renin, was discussed earlier in this chapter. The second, direct inhibition of renin activity by antirenin antibodies, is not now clinically feasible. The fourth, blockade of angiotensin's actions by a competitive blocker, is used, in the form of saralasin, as a diagnostic test for renovascular hypertension and was described on page 881. The third, inhibition of the enzyme that converts the inactive decapeptide angiotensin I to the active octapeptide angiotensin II, is now feasible with the use of the orally effective converting enzyme inhibitor (CEI) *captopril* (Capoten).[158] Captopril is likely the first of a family of CEI's, the second of which (MK-421) is already being investigated.[159] Introduced for use only in patients resistant or intolerant to other medications, captopril has now been found to be both effective in and well tolerated by patients with mild hypertension.[160] In these patients, as in those with more severe hypertension, a diuretic is usually needed to achieve an adequate response.

MODE OF ACTION. Captopril was synthesized as a specific inhibitor of the converting enzyme that breaks the peptidyldipeptide bond in angiotensin I. It binds to three sites on the converting enzyme, thereby preventing the enzyme from attaching to and splitting the angiotensin I structure. Since angiotensin II cannot be formed and angiotensin I is inactive, the CEI paralyzes the workings of the renin-angiotensin system, thereby removing the effects of endogenous angiotensin II as both a vasoconstrictor and a stimulant to aldosterone synthesis. In about 70 per cent of hypertensives, the blood pressure falls and, in almost all, the levels of aldosterone are reduced.[161]

The same enzyme which converts angiotensin I to angiotensin II is also responsible for inactivation of the vasodepressor hormone bradykinin. By inhibiting the breakdown of bradykinin, CEI may increase the concentration of a vasodepressor hormone while it decreases the concentration of a vasoconstrictor hormone.[162] At the same time, levels of vasodilatory prostaglandins may also be increased. However it works, captopril lowers blood pressure mainly by reducing peripheral resistance, with little if any effect upon heart rate, cardiac output, or body fluid volumes.

CLINICAL USE. The antihypertensive response to captopril is greatest in those patients whose hypertension is being generated by high levels of angiotensin II, such as those with renovascular hypertension or scleroderma. Similarly, the response in those with lesser contributions by angiotensin II will be enhanced by concomitant use of a diuretic, which will raise endogenous angiotensin II levels.

In multiple clinical trials, the mean decrease in blood pressure was 11 per cent in those who started with low renin, 14 per cent in those with normal renin, and 19 per cent in those with high renin.[163] Among 40 patients with an average initial blood pressure of 174/110 mm Hg, captopril alone lowered the blood pressure by 23/14 mm Hg; captopril plus hydrochlorothiazide lowered it by 51/20 mm Hg.[164]

The initial dose of captopril may precipitate a rather dramatic but transient fall in blood pressure, but the full effect may not be seen for 7 to 10 days.[161] The initial dosage is usually 25 mg three times a day, which is then gradually increased to a maximum of 150 mg three times a day. Since much of the drug is excreted by the kidneys, smaller doses are usually adequate in patients with renal insufficiency. The response to captopril is usually well maintained, perhaps because its marked suppression of aldosterone mitigates the tendency toward volume expansion that often antagonizes the effects of other hypertensives. However, half the patients in one series[165] required larger doses or more diuretic to maintain long-term control.

Captopril has been found to be effective in reducing afterload in the treatment of severe congestive heart failure (see p. 539).

SIDE EFFECTS. Among 81 patients, captopril caused

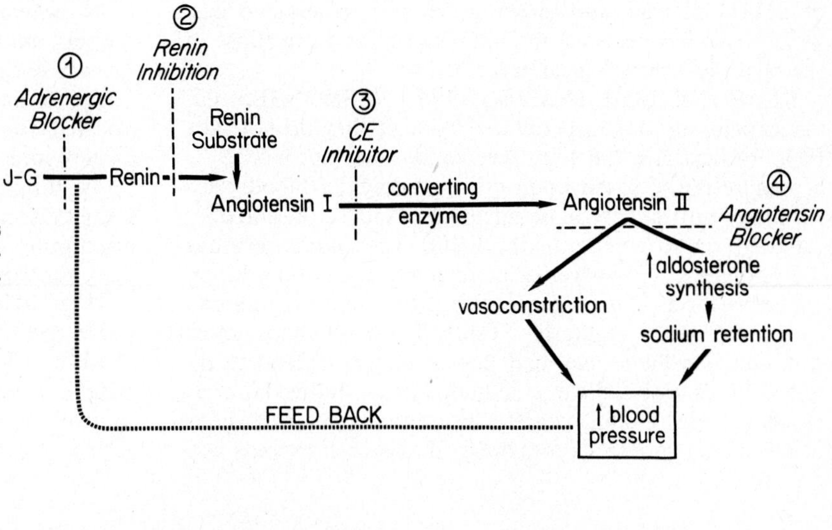

FIGURE 27-13 The four sites of action of inhibitors of the renin-angiotensin system. (J-G = juxtaglomerular apparatus.) (From Kaplan, N. M.: Clinical Hypertension, 3rd ed. Baltimore, Williams and Wilkins Co., 1982, p. 223.)

side effects in 47 per cent, necessitating withdrawal in 23 per cent.[166] About 20 per cent develop a skin rash or some disturbance in taste. Fortunately, two more serious complications are much less common: membranous glomerulopathy (in about 1 per cent) and bone marrow suppression with leukopenia (in perhaps 0.3 per cent). Changes in renal biopsy specimens similar to those found after captopril have been observed in hypertensives who have never taken the drug,[167] but a cause-and-effect relationship with overt renal damage has been clearly demonstrated.[168] Leukopenia has occurred within three months of the onset of therapy but has been slowly progressive and is reversible if recognized and the drug discontinued.[169]

SPECIAL CONSIDERATIONS IN THERAPY

CHOICE OF DRUGS. The stepped-care approach has used a diuretic first, an adrenergic blocker second, and a vasodilator third. As previously discussed, an adrenergic blocker may be as effective as and safer than a diuretic for initial therapy. Whether used as first or second drug, effectiveness differs little among the adrenergic blockers: along with a diuretic, all these agents will lower blood pressure to below 90 mm Hg in about 80 per cent of hypertensive patients. The choice is then logically made based on ease of administration and freedom from side effects. Certain trade-offs may be required: reserpine and guanethidine may be given in only one dose per day, but the side effects may be intolerable; methyldopa, despite its efficacy, may cause some unique and serious problems; if poor patient compliance is anticipated, clonidine should be avoided; prazosin may provide more "physiological" control of the blood pressure but may cause bothersome postural hypotension; beta blockers are probably most convenient for most patients but may cause serious side effects even after careful exclusion of patients known to be susceptible. Although the evidence for protection from coronary events afforded by beta blockers is not yet conclusive, the possibility of this advantage, added to the relative freedom from bothersome side effects, makes a beta blocker—preferably one that is cardioselective—the usual choice for the second drug. Patients who cannot take a beta blocker can be given clonidine or prazosin.

If a third drug is needed, hydralazine will usually be added, although prazosin or clonidine may also be effective if a beta blocker is the second drug. The combination of a beta blocker and either of these adrenergic drugs, which have mechanisms of action that differ from those of the beta blocker, is logical and effective.

REASONS FOR INADEQUATE RESPONSE. Often patients do not respond well because they do not take their medications. On the other hand, what appears to be a poor response based upon office readings of blood pressure may turn out to be an adequate response (as corroborated by improvements in the ECG) when home readings are evaluated.[170] However, a number of factors may be responsible for a poor response even if the appropriate medication is taken regularly (Table 27–7). Perhaps most common is volume overload due to either inadequate diuretic or excessive dietary sodium intake. If the latter is suspected, the sodium content in an overnight or 24-hour urine sample should be measured. If this level exceeds 100 mEq/day, some restriction of dietary salt should be prescribed. Larger doses or more potent diuretics may bring resistant hypertension under control.[171] However, there are a few patients whose blood pressure is resistant to therapy because of overly vigorous diuresis, which contracts vascular volume and activates both renin and catecholamines.[172] This is most likely to occur in patients with obligatory salt-wasting due to interstitial renal disease.

TABLE 27–7 CAUSES OF POOR RESPONSE TO ANTIHYPERTENSIVE DRUGS

1. Inadequate drugs (? poor adherence)
   a. Doses too low
   b. Inappropriate combinations
   c. Rapid inactivation (hydralazine, propranolol)
   d. Antagonism from other drugs
      (1) Sympathomimetics
      (2) Antidepressants
      (3) Adrenal steroids
      (4) Estrogens
2. Associated diseases
   a. Renal insufficiency
   b. Renovascular hypertension
   c. Pheochromocytoma
3. Volume overload
   a. Inadequate diuretic
   b. Excessive sodium intake
   c. Fluid retention from reduction of blood pressure
   d. Progressive renal damage
4. Volume depletion → increased renin → vasoconstriction
   a. Renal salt-wasting
   b. Overly aggressive diuretic therapy

ANESTHESIA IN HYPERTENSIVE PATIENTS. Most anesthesiologists suggest that hypertensive patients be well controlled by means of medications prior to anesthesia and surgery. On the basis of careful hemodynamic measurements in patients receiving various antihypertensive medications, Prys-Roberts et al. found "no evidence that any antihypertensive drugs other than reserpine in any way predisposed to adverse circulatory changes, either in the patient's response to anesthesia or during recovery."[173] Patients receiving beta blockers may have slightly higher blood pressures during anesthesia but fewer problems with tachycardia, increases in pressure during intubation, or electrocardiographic evidence of myocardial ischemia.[174]

TREATMENT OF CHILDREN. Almost nothing is known about the effects of various antihypertensive medications given to children over long periods of time. Since most of the adrenergic blockers act upon the central nervous system, their effects upon growth hormone, gonadotropins, and other hormones involved in maturation and growth should be ascertained. However, in the absence of adequate data, a stepped-care approach similar to that advocated for adults is advised.[175] The doses of drugs are largely interpolated from those used in adults on a mg/kg basis. Emphasis has been placed upon the need for weight reduction in hypertensive children who are obese, thereby attempting to control hypertension without the need for drug therapy.

HYPERTENSION DURING PREGNANCY. (See pages 888 to 891.)

THE ELDERLY WITH SYSTOLIC HYPERTENSION. Here again, almost no data are available as to the indications for therapy and the appropriate choice of drugs. If both systolic and diastolic pressures are elevated, elderly patients should be handled in a manner similar to that for younger persons; they seem to respond as well and have no more problems with medications.[176] In view of the reduced effectiveness of the baroreceptor reflex and the failure of cerebral autoregulation that may occur in the elderly,[177] drugs with a propensity to cause postural hypotension should be avoided, and all drugs should be given in slowly increasing doses to prevent excessive lowering of the pressure.

Isolated systolic hypertension presents a risk, particularly of strokes.[178] It is likely that judicious lowering of the pressure will protect against and not precipitate cardiovascular catastrophes. Admittedly, most systolic pressure elevations are due to structural hardening of the arterial walls, and the vessels may not be able to dilate as well as the constricted, more compliant vessels of young people. The goal of therapy should be relaxed; a systolic pressure of 160 mm Hg seems reasonable for people over 60 years of age. It is hoped that data on the effectiveness of therapy for isolated systolic hypertension will be forthcoming.

Some elderly people may have very high blood pressure as measured by the sphygmomanometer but may have less or no hypertension when direct intraarterial readings are made.[179] Presumably the pseudohypertension is related to the failure of the sphygmomanometer cuff to collapse the rigid artery beneath the cuff. For those patients with vessels that feel rigid and who have few retinal or cardiac findings of hypertension, as would be expected with high sphygmomanometer readings, direct intraarterial measurements should be made before therapy is begun.

Prescription of a thiazide diuretic plus moderate sodium restriction seems the logical first step. As a second step, small doses of methyldopa or clonidine seem preferable to beta blockers, which appear to be less effective in the elderly, or prazosin, which may cause postural hypotension. Hydralazine may be tolerated as a second step, presumably because of reduced baroreceptor reflex sensitivity to vasodilation.

HYPERTENSION WITH RENAL INSUFFICIENCY. In the presence of renal insufficiency, hypertension is usually predominantly caused by volume excess, and most patients can be successfully treated with salt restriction and diuretics.[180] When serum creatinine exceeds 2.5 mg/dl, thiazides are usually relatively ineffective, and either metolazone or high doses of furosemide are required.[70] A few patients with chronic renal disease have a more resistant form of hypertension, usually associated with—and perhaps caused by—high levels of plasma renin activity. Although a few of these patients will require bilateral nephrectomy to control their hypertension, medical therapy with beta blockers, minoxidil,[147] or captopril[158] has been increasingly effective, not only in controlling the hypertension but in halting the deterioration of renal function.[181] With appropriate therapy, hypertension can be controlled in most patients, and even in some patients with far-advanced renal insufficiency, long-term therapy can halt the deterioration.

HYPERTENSION WITH CONGESTIVE HEART FAILURE. Cardiac output may fall so markedly in hypertensive patients who are in heart failure that their blood pressure is reduced, obscuring the degree of hypertension; often, however, the diastolic pressure is raised by intense vasoconstriction while the systolic pressure falls as a result of the reduced stroke volume. Lowering the blood pressure may, by itself, relieve the heart failure, but often diuretics and digitalis are needed. Antihypertensive drugs that primarily decrease cardiac output, particularly beta blockers, which remove the heart's needed sympathetic support, may be dangerous in the presence of heart failure. Prazosin has been found to be particularly effective,[113] presumably because it dilates veins and reduces preload as well.

HYPERTENSION WITH ISCHEMIC HEART DISEASE. The coexistence of coronary artery disease makes antihypertensive therapy even more essential, since relief of the hypertension may ameliorate the coronary disease. Beta blockers are particularly useful if angina or arrhythmias are present, and calcium-entry blockers will probably also find a major use in such patients.

HYPERTENSION WITH DIABETES MELLITUS. Diuretics may worsen diabetic control, probably because they induce potassium depletion.[71] Brittle diabetics on insulin should not be given nonselective beta blockers, since these drugs may prevent the outpouring of catecholamines that counteracts a precipitous fall in blood sugar levels, thereby preventing the recognition of impending hypoglycemia and delaying the rebound rise in the blood sugar.

HYPERTENSION WITH PSYCHIATRIC ILLNESS. Patients who are anxious and emotionally labile may benefit from the calming effects of beta blockers upon the somatic manifestations of anxiety.[133] However, caution is advised in using high doses of beta blockers, which may induce nightmares and hallucinations. If antidepressant or antipsychotic medications are needed, they will not blunt the effects of beta blockers as they may those of guanethidine, methyldopa, or clonidine.

THERAPY FOR HYPERTENSIVE CRISES

When diastolic blood pressure exceeds 140 mm Hg, rapidly progressive damage to the arterial vasculature is demonstrable experimentally, and a surge of cerebral blood flow may rapidly lead to encephalopathy[55] (see Fig. 27–6). Since previously normotensive patients may develop encephalopathy at much lower levels of blood pressure, such an elevated pressure must be quickly lowered.

A number of drugs for this purpose are now available (Table 27–8), and others, such as labetolol[145] are under investigation. If diastolic pressure exceeds 140 mm Hg, and the patient has any complications such as a stroke or congestive failure, a constant infusion of nitroprusside is most effective and will almost always lower the pressure to the desired level. Constant monitoring, preferably with an intraarterial line, is mandatory; a slightly excessive dose may abruptly lower the pressure to levels that will induce shock. The potency and rapidity of action of nitroprusside make it the treatment of choice for life-threatening hypertension. Cyanide toxicity from prolonged therapy can be prevented by intravenous hydroxycobalamin.[182] Occasionally, as in therapy for aortic dissection, beta-adrenergic blockade with propranolol may enhance the efficacy and safety of nitroprusside.[183]

With less serious hypertension, intravenous diazoxide is effective and usually safe. The use of 300-mg doses given by rapid bolus injection may lower the pressure too much

TABLE 27–8 DRUGS FOR TREATMENT OF HYPERTENSIVE CRISIS (IN ORDER OF RAPIDITY OF ONSET OF ACTION)

	Adult Dosage	Time Course of Action: Onset	Maximum	Duration	Advantages	Disadvantages	Side Effects
Nitroprusside (Nipride)	50 mg/500 ml 5% glucose in water IV	< 1 min	1 to 2 min	2 to 5 min	Effective instantly, continuously, and consistently	Requires constant monitoring of BP and dose	Nausea
Diazoxide (Hyperstat)	150 to 300 mg by rapid IV injection	1 min	2 to 4 min	4 to 12 hr	Effective rapidly and consistently	Fixed dosage; occasional hypotension	Tachycardia, nausea, flushing
Hydralazine (Apresoline)	10 to 50 mg IM	10 to 20 min	20 to 40 min	3 to 6 hr	Ease of administration; maintains renal blood flow	Increases cardiac output	Tachycardia, nausea, headache
Reserpine (Serpasil)	0.5 to 5.0 mg IM	1½ to 3 hr	3 to 4 hr	6 to 24 hr	Gradual and prolonged effect	Delayed onset of action; sedative; cumulative effect may cause hypotension	Sedation, nasal congestion
Methyldopa (Aldomet)	250 to 1000 mg IV	2 to 3 hr	3 to 5 hr	6 to 12 hr	Gradual and prolonged effect	Not always effective; delayed onset of action	Sedation, lack of effect

and cause cerebral or myocardial ischemia. Such excessive hypotension can be avoided by either repeated injections of 150 mg each or slow infusions, with little delay in reducing the pressure to safe levels.[184]

The other drugs listed in Table 27–8 are less satisfactory for rapid reduction of very high blood pressure. However, in less emergent situations oral therapy may be adequate.[185] Intramuscular hydralazine is widely used to treat preeclampsia. With any of these agents, intravenous furosemide is often needed to lower the blood pressure further and prevent retention of salt and water.

Once the patient is out of immediate danger, oral therapy, usually consisting of a combination of diuretic, beta blocker, and hydralazine, should be initiated. Under these circumstances, the gradual, gentle approach toward lowering the pressure, advocated earlier in this chapter for most hypertensive patients, seems inappropriate. Fortunately, fewer patients in a hypertensive crisis are being seen, presumably because more hypertensive patients are being recognized and treated before the disease enters this malignant course. It is hoped that the continued successful treatment of many more hypertensives will lead to similar increases in prevention of the other, more subtle, but more frequent, long-range sequelae of hypertension.

References

1. Dustan, H. P., Schneckloth, R. E., Corcoran, A. C., and Page, I. H.: The effectiveness of long-term treatment of malignant hypertension. Circulation *18*: 644, 1958.
2. Veterans Administration Cooperative Study Group on Antihypertensive Agents: Effects of treatment on morbidity in hypertension. Results in patients with diastolic blood pressures averaging 115 through 129 mm Hg. J.A.M.A. *202*:116, 1967.
3. Veterans Administration Cooperative Study Group on Antihypertensive Agents: Effects of treatment on morbidity in hypertension. II. Results in patients with diastolic blood pressure averaging 90 through 114 mm Hg. J.A.M.A. *213*:1143, 1970.
4. Hypertension Detection and Follow-up Program Cooperative Group: Five-year findings of the Hypertension Detection and Follow-up Program. I. Reduction in mortality of persons with high blood pressure, including mild hypertension. J.A.M.A. *242*:2562, 1979.
5. Report of the Management Committee: The Australian therapeutic trial in mild hypertension. Lancet *1*:1261, 1980.
6. Laughlin, K. D., Fisher, L., and Sherrard, D. J.: Blood pressure reductions during self-recording of home blood pressure. Am. Heart J. *98*:629, 1979.
7. Kannel, W. B., Dawber, T. R., and McGee, D. L.: Perspectives on systolic hypertension. Circulation *61*:1179, 1980.
8. Kaplan, N. M.: Whom to treat: The dilemma of mild hypertension. Am. Heart J. *101*:867, 1981.
9. Thomson, G. E., Alderman, M. H., Wassertheil-Smoller, S., Rafter, J. G., and Samet, R.: High blood pressure diagnosis and treatment: Consensus recommendations vs actual practice. Am. J. Public Health *71*:413, 1981.
10. Guttmacher, S., Teitelman, M., Chapin, G., Garbowski, G., and Schnall, P.: Ethics and preventive medicine: The case of borderline hypertension. Hastings Center Reports *11*:12, 1981.
11. Frohlich, E. D.: Continued gains in hypertension. Am. J. Cardiol. *47*:375, 1981.
12. Taylor, L., Foster, M. C., and Beevers, D. G.: Divergent views of hospital staff on detecting and managing hypertension. Br. Med. J. *1*:715, 1979.
13. W.H.O./I.S.H. Mild Hypertension Liaison Committee. Trials of the treatment of mild hypertension. Lancet *1*:149, 1982.
14. Kaplan, N. M.: The therapy of hypertension. *In* Clinical Hypertension. 3rd ed. Baltimore, Williams and Wilkins Co., 1982, p. 108.
15. Alderman, M. H., and Madhavan, S.: Management of the hypertensive patient: A continuing dilemma. Hypertension *3*:192, 1981.
16. Helgeland, A.: Treatment of mild hypertension: A five year controlled drug trial. Am. J. Med. *69*:725, 1980.
17. Peart, W. S., and Miall, W. E.: M.R.C. mild hypertension trial. Lancet *1*:104, 1980.
18. Ames, R. P., and Hill, P.: Increases in serum-lipids during treatment of hypertension with chlorthalidone. Lancet *1*:721, 1976.
19. Rose, G.: Strategy of prevention: Lessons from cardiovascular disease. Br. Med. J. *282*:1847, 1981.
20. Moser, M.: On the management of "mild hypertension." Arch. Intern. Med. *141*:1587, 1981.
21. Hypertension and Follow-up Program Cooperative Group: Five-year findings of the hypertension detection and follow-up program. III. Reduction in stroke incidence among persons with high blood pressure. J.A.M.A. *247*:633, 1982.
22. Smith, W. M.: Treatment of mild hypertension. Results of a ten-year intervention trial. Circ. Res. *40* (Suppl. I):I-98, 1977.
23. Wilhelmsen, L., Berglund, G., Sannerstedt, R., Hansson, L., Andersson, O., Sievertsson, R., and Wikstrand, J.: Effect of treatment of hypertension in the primary preventive trial, Göteborg, Sweden. J. Clin. Pharmacol. *7* (Suppl. 2):261, 1979.
24. Hypertension Detection and Follow-up Program Cooperative Group: Beneficial effect of the hypertension detection and follow-up program stepped care regime on indices of coronary artery and myocardial disease. Am. J. Cardiol. *49*:912, 1982 (abstract).
25. Rowlands, D. B., Glover, D. R., Ireland, M. A., McLeay, R. A. B., Stallard, T. J., Watson, R. D. S., and Littler, W. A.: Assessment of left-ventricular mass and its response to antihypertensive treatment. Lancet *1*:467, 1982.

NONDRUG THERAPY

26. MacGregor, G. A., Markandu, N. D., Best, F. E., Elder, D. M., Cam, J. M., Sagnella, G. A., and Squires, M.: Double-blind randomised crossover trial of moderate sodium restriction in essential hypertension. Lancet *1*:351, 1982.
27. Ram, C. V. S., Garrett, B. N., and Kaplan, N. M.: Moderate sodium restriction and various diuretics in the treatment of hypertension. Arch. Intern. Med. *141*:1015, 1981.
28. Landmann-Suter, R., and Struyvenberg, A.: Initial potassium loss and hypokalemia during chlorthalidone administration in patients with essential hyperten-

sion: The influence of dietary sodium restriction. Eur. J. Clin. Invest. *8*:155, 1978.
29. Warren, S. E., Vieweg, W. V. R., and O'Connor, D. T.: Sympathetic nervous system activity during sodium restriction in essential hypertension. Clin. Cardiol. *3*:348, 1980.
30. Kaplan, N. M., Simmons, M., McPhee, C., Carnegie, A., Stefanu, C., and Cade, S.: Two techniques to improve adherence to dietary sodium restriction in the treatment of hypertension. Arch. Intern. Med. *42*:1638, 1982.
31. Linas, S. L.: Mechanism of hyperreninemia in the potassium-depleted rat. J. Clin. Invest. *68*:347, 1981.
32. Knochel, J. P.: Neuromuscular manifestations of electrolyte disorders. Am. J. Med. *72*:521, 1982.
33. MacGregor, G. A., Smith, S. J., Markandu, N. D., Banks, R. A., and Sagnella, G. A.: Moderate potassium supplementation in essential hypertension. Lancet *2*:567–570, 1982.
34. Iimura, O., Kijima, T., Kikuchi, K., Miyama, A., Ando, T., Nakao, T., and Takigami, Y.: Studies on the hypotensive effect of high potassium intake in patients with essential hypertension. Clin. Sci. *61*:77s, 1981.
35. Hovell, M. F.: The experimental evidence for weight-loss treatment of essential hypertension: A critical review. Am. J. Public Health *72*:359, 1982.
36. Reisin, E., Abel, R., Modan, M., Silverberg, D. S., Eliahou, H. E., and Modan, B.: Effect of weight loss without salt restriction on the reduction of blood pressure in overweight hypertensive patients. N. Engl. J. Med. *298*:1, 1978.
37. Cooke, K. M., Frost, G. W., Thornell, I. R., and Stokes, G. S.: Alcohol consumption and blood pressure. Med. J. Aust. *1*:65, 1982.
38. Klatsky, A. L., Friedman, G. D., and Siegelaub, A. B.: Alcohol and mortality. Ann. Intern. Med. *95*:139, 1981.
39. Castelli, W. P., Gordon, T., Hjortland, M. C., Kagan, A., Doyle, J. T., Hames, C. G., Hulley, S. B., and Jukel, W. J.: Alcohol and blood lipids. Lancet *2*:153, 1977.
40. Gruchow, H. W., Hoffmann, R. G., Anderson, A. J., and Barboriak, J. J.: Effects of drinking patterns on the relationship between alcohol and coronary occlusion. Atherosclerosis *43*:393, 1982.
41. Robertson, D., Frölich, J. C., Carr, R. K., Watson, J. T., Hollifield, J. W., Shand, D. G., and Oates, J. A.: Effects of caffeine on plasma renin activity, catecholamines and blood pressure. N. Engl. J. Med. *298*:181, 1978.
41a. Freestone, S., and Ramsay, L. E.: Effect of coffee and cigarette smoking on the blood pressure of untreated and diuretic-treated hypertensive patients. Am. J. Med. *73*:348–353, 1982.
42. Hoel, B. L., Lorensten, E., and Lund-Larsen, P. G.: Hemodynamic responses to sustained hand-grip in patients with hypertension. Acta Med. Scand. *188*: 491, 1970.
43. Black, H. R.: Nonpharmacologic therapy for hypertension. Am. J. Med. *66*: 837, 1979.
44. Roman, O., Camuzzi, A. L., Villalon, E., and Klenner, C.: Physical training program in arterial hypertension. Cardiology *67*:230, 1981.
45. Jacobson, E.: Variation of blood pressure with skeletal muscle tension and relaxation. Ann. Intern. Med. *12*:1194, 1939.
46. Patel, C., Marmot, M. G., and Terry, D. J.: Controlled trial of biofeedback-aided behavioural methods in reducing mild hypertension. Br. Med. J. *282*: 2005, 1981.
47. Stamler, J., Farinaro, E., Mojonnier, L. M., Hall, Y., Moss, D., and Stamler, R.: Prevention and control of hypertension by nutritional-hygienic means. J.A.M.A. *243*:1819, 1980.

ANTIHYPERTENSIVE DRUG THERAPY

48. Haynes, R. B., Mattson, M. E., Chobanian, A. V., Dunbar, J. M., Engebretson, T. O., Jr., Garrity, T. F., Leventhal, H., Levine, R. J., and Levy, R. L.: Management of patient compliance in the treatment of hypertension. Hypertension *4*:415, 1982.
49. Haynes, R. B., Sackett, D. L., Taylor, D. W., Roberts, R. S., and Johnson, A. L.: Manipulation of the therapeutic regimen to improve compliance: Conceptions and misconceptions. Clin. Pharmacol. Ther. *22*:125, 1977.
50. Wright, J. M., Orozco-Gonzalez, M., Polak, G., and Dollery C. T.: Duration of effect of single daily dose methyldopa therapy. Br. J. Clin. Pharmacol. *13*: 847–854, 1982.
51. Jain, A. K., Ryan, J. R., Vargas, R., and McMahon, F. G.: Efficacy and acceptability of different dosage schedules of clonidine. Clin. Pharmacol. Ther. *21*:382, 1977.
52. Wilkinson, P. R., Dixon, N., and Hunter, K. R.: Twice-daily propranolol treatment for hypertension. J. Intern. Med. Res. *2*:220, 1974.
53. Silas, J. H., Ramsay, L. E., and Freestone, S.: Hydralazine once daily in hypertension. Br. Med. J. *284*:1602, 1982.
54. Watson, R. D. S., Stallard, T. J., and Littler, W. A.: Influence of once-daily administration of β-adrenoceptor antagonists on arterial pressure and its variability. Lancet *1*:1210, 1979.
55. Strandgaard, S.: Autoregulation of cerebral blood flow in hypertensive patients. Circulation *53*:720, 1976.
56. The Joint National Committee on Detection, Evaluation, and Treatment of High Blood Pressure: The 1980 report of the Joint National Committee on detection, evaluation, and treatment of high blood pressure. Arch. Intern. Med. *140*:1280, 1980.
57. Laragh, J. H.: Vasoconstriction-volume analysis for understanding and treating hypertension: The use of renin and aldosterone profiles. Am. J. Med. *55*:261, 1973.
58. Dustan, H. P., Tarazi, R. C., and Bravo, E. L.: Dependence of arterial pressure on intravascular volume in treated hypertensive patients. N. Engl. J. Med. *286*:861, 1972.
59. Zacest, R., Gilmore, E., and Koch-Weser, J.: Treatment of essential hypertension with combined vasodilation and beta-adrenergic blockade. N. Engl. J. Med. *286*:617, 1972.
59a. Multiple Risk Factor Intervention Trial Research Group: Multiple risk factor intervention trial. Risk factor changes and mortality results. J.A.M.A. *248*: 1465–1477, 1982.
59b. Kaplan, N. M.: Mild hypertension: When and how to treat. Arch. Intern. Med. 1983 (in press).
60. Freis, E. D.: Salt in hypertension and the effects of diuretics. Ann. Rev. Pharmacol. Toxicol. *19*:13, 1979.
61. Lake, C. R., Ziegler, M. G., Coleman, M. D., and Kopin, I. J.: Hydrochlorothiazide-induced sympathetic hyperactivity in hypertensive patients. Clin. Pharmacol. Ther. *26*:428, 1979.
62. Webster, J., Dollery, C. T., Hensby, C. N., and Friedman, L. A.: Antihypertensive action of bendroflumethiazide: Increased prostacyclin production? Clin. Pharmacol. Ther. *28*:751, 1980.
63. Bennett, W. M., McDonald, W. J., Kuehnel, E., Hartnett, M. N., and Porter, G. A.: Do diuretics have antihypertensive properties independent of natriuresis? Clin. Pharmacol. Ther. *22*:499, 1977.
64. Weber, M. A., Drayer, J. I. M., Rev, A., and Laragh, J. H.: Disparate patterns of aldosterone response during diuretic treatment of hypertension. Ann. Intern. Med. *87*:558, 1977.
65. Beevers, D. G., Hamilton, M., and Harpur, J. E.: The long-term treatment of hypertension with thiazide diuretics. Postgrad. Med. J. *47*:639, 1971.
66. Degnbol, B., Dorph, S., and Marner, T.: The effect of different diuretics on elevated blood pressure and serum potassium. Acta Med. Scand. *192*:407, 1973.
67. Tweeddale, M. G., Ogilvie, R. L., and Ruedy, J.: Antihypertensive and biochemical effects of chlorthalidone. Clin. Pharmacol. Ther. *22* (Part 1):519, 1977.
68. Lutterodt, A., Nattel, S., and McLeod, P. J.: Duration of antihypertensive effect of a single daily dose of hydrochlorothiazide. Clin. Pharmacol. Ther. *27*:324, 1980.
69. Anderson, J., Godfrey, B. E., Hill, D. M., Munro-Faure, A. D., and Sheldon, J.: A comparison of the effects of hydrochlorothiazide and of furosemide in the treatment of hypertensive patients. Quart. J. Med. *40*:541, 1971.
70. Dargie, H. J., Allison, M. E. M., Kennedy, A. C., and Gray, M. J. B.: High dosage metolazone in chronic renal failure. Br. Med. J. *4*:196, 1972.
71. Morgan, D. B., and Davidson, C.: Hypokalaemia and diuretics: An analysis of publications. Br. Med. J. *280*:905, 1980.
72. Sandor, F. F., Pickens, P. T., and Crallan, J.: Variations of plasma potassium concentrations during long-term treatment of hypertension with diuretics without potassium supplements. Br. Med. J. *284*:711, 1982.
73. Kassirer, J. P., and Harrington, J. T.: Diuretics and potassium metabolism: A reassessment of the need, effectiveness and safety of potassium therapy. Kidney Int. *11*:505, 1977.
74. Holland, O. B., Nixon, J. V., and Kuhnert, L.: Diuretic-induced ventricular ectopic activity. Am. J. Med. *70*:762, 1981.
74a. Struthers, A. D., Reid, J. L., Lawrie, C. B., and Rodger, J. C.: β-adrenoceptor–linked Na/K ATPase. Drugs, 1983 (in press).
74b. Nordrehaug, J. E.: Malignant arrhythmias in relation to serum potassium values in patients with an acute myocardial infarction. Acta Med. Scand. (Suppl.) *647*:101–107, 1981.
75. Lemieux, G., Beauchemin, M., Vinay, P., and Gougoux, A.: Hypokalemia during the treatment of arterial hypertension with diuretics. Can. Med. Assoc. J. *122*:905, 1980.
76. Good, D. W., and Wright, F. S.: Luminal influences on potassium secretion: Sodium concentration and fluid low rate. Am. J. Physiol. *236*:F192, 1979.
77. Hollenberg, N. K., Williams, G., Burger, B., and Hooshmand, I.: The influence of potassium on the renal vasculature and the adrenal gland, and their responsiveness to angiotensin II in normal man. Clin. Sci. Molec. Med. *49*:527, 1975.
78. Skehan, J. D., Barnes, J. N., Drew, P. J., and Wright, P.: Hypokalaemia induced by a combination of a beta-blocker and a thiazide. Br. Med. J. *284*:83, 1982.
78a. McMahon, F. G., Ryan, J. R., Akdamar, F., and Ertan, A.: Upper gastrointestinal lesions after potassium chloride supplements: A controlled clinical trial. Lancet *2*:1059–1061, 1982.
79. Sopko, J. A., and Freeman, R. M.: Salt substitutes as a source of potassium. J.A.M.A. *238*:608, 1977.
80. Sheehan, J., and White, A.: Diuretic-associated hypomagnesaemia. Br. Med. J. *285*:1157–1159, 1982.
81. Helgeland, A., Hjermann, I., Holme, I., and Leren, P.: Serum triglycerides and serum uric acid in untreated and thiazide-treated patients with mild hypertension. Am. J. Med. *64*:34, 1978.
82. Weinman, E. J., Eknoyan, G., and Suki, W. N.: The influence of the extracellular fluid volume on the tubular reabsorption of uric acid. J. Clin. Invest. *55*:283, 1975.
83. Goldman, A. I., Steele, B. W., Schnaper, H. W., Fitz, A. E., Frolich, E. D., and Perry, H. M., Jr.: Serum lipoprotein levels during chlorthalidone therapy. J.A.M.A. *244*:1691, 1980.

84. Grimm, R. H., Leon, A. S., Hunninghake, D. B., Lenz, K., Hannan, P., and Blackburn, H.: Effects of thiazide diuretics on plasma lipids and lipoproteins in mildly hypertensive patients. Ann. Intern. Med. *94*:7, 1981.
85. Amery, A., Berthaux, P., Bulpitt, C., Deruyttere, M., de Schaepdryver, A., Dollery, C., Fagard, R., Forette, F., Hellermans, J., Lund-Johansen, P., Mutsers, A., and Tuomilehto, J.: Glucose intolerance during diuretic therapy. Lancet *1*:681, 1978.
86. Medical Research Council Working Party on Mild to Moderate Hypertension: Adverse reactions to bendrofluazide and propranolol for the treatment of mild hypertension. Lancet *2*:539, 1981.
87. Williams, R. L., Davies, R. O., Berman, R. S., Holmes, G. I., Huber, P., Gee, W. L., Lin, E. T., and Benet, L. Z.: Hydrochlorothiazide pharmacokinetics and pharmacologic effect: The influence of indomethacin. J. Clin. Pharmacol. *22*:32, 1982.
88. Guidi, G., Guintoli, F., Saba, G., Diamanti, G., Checchi, M., Gabbani, S. A., Birindelli, A., and Saba, P.: Clinical investigation on efficacy of indapamide as an antihypertensive agent. Curr. Ther. Res. *31*:601, 1982.
89. Berglund, G., and Andersson, O.: Beta-blockers or diuretics in hypertension? A six year follow-up on blood pressure and metabolic side effects. Lancet *1*: 744, 1981.
90. Buhler, F. R., Burkart, F., Lutold, B. E., Kung, M., Marbet, G., and Pfisterer, M.: Antihypertensive beta blocking action as related to renin and age: A pharmacologic tool to identify pathogenetic mechanisms in essential hypertension. Am. J. Cardiol. *36*:653, 1975.
91. Veterans Administration Cooperative Study Group on Antihypertensive Agents: Comparison of propranolol and hydrochlorothiazide for the initial treatment of hypertension. I. Results of short-term titration with emphasis on racial differences in response. J.A.M.A. *248*:1996–2003, 1982.
92. Beilin, L. J., Bulpitt, C. J., Coles, E. C., Dollery, C. T., Gear, J. S. S., Harper, G., Johnson, B. F., Munro-Faure, A. D., and Turner, S. C.: Long-term antihypertensive drug treatment and blood pressure control in three hospital hypertension clinics. Br. Heart J. *43*:74, 1980.
93. Kaplan, N. M.: The prognostic implications of plasma renin in essential hypertension. J.A.M.A. *231*:167, 1975.
94. Langer, S. Z., and Shepperson, N. B.: Prejunctional modulation of noradrenaline release by α_2-adrenoceptors: Physiological and pharmacological implications in the cardiovascular system. J. Cardiovasc. Pharmacol. *4* (Suppl. 1):S35, 1982.
95. Veterans Administration Cooperative Study Group on Antihypertensive Agents. Propranolol in the treatment of essential hypertension. J.A.M.A. *237*: 2303, 1977.
96. Finnerty, F. A., Gyftopoulos, A., Berry, C., and McKenney, A.: Step 2 regimens in hypertension. J.A.M.A. *241*:579, 1979.
97. Participating Veterans Administration Medical Centers: Low dose *v* standard dose of reserpine. J.A.M.A. *248*:2471–2477, 1982.
98. Curb, J. D., Hardy, R. J., Labarthe, D. R., Borhani, N. O., and Taylor, J. O.: Reserpine and breast cancer in the hypertension detection and follow-up program. Hypertension *4*:307, 1982.
99. Corder, C. N.: Bethanidine dose, plasma levels, and antihypertensive effects. J. Clin. Pharmacol. *18*:249, 1978.
100. Häusler, G.: Central α-adrenoceptors involved in cardiovascular regulation. J. Cardiovasc. Pharmacol. *4*:S72, 1982.
101. Fouad, F. M., Nakashima, Y., Tarazi, R. C., and Salcedo, E. E.: Reversal of left ventricular hypertrophy in hypertensive patients treated with methyldopa. Am. J. Cardiol. *49*:795, 1982.
102. Seeverens, H., deBruin, C. D., and Jordans, J. G. M.: Myocarditis and methyldopa. Acta Med. Scand. *211*:233, 1982.
103. Rodman, J. A., Deutsch, D. J., and Gutman, S. I.: Methyldopa hepatitis. Am. J. Med. *60*:941, 1976.
104. Dybing, E., Nelson, S. D., Mitchell, J. R., Sasame, H. A., and Gillette, J. R.: Oxidation of α-methyldopa and other catechols by cytochrome P-450–generated superoxide anion: Possible mechanisms of methyldopa hepatitis. Molec. Pharmacol. *12*:911, 1976.
105. Weber, M. A., Case, D. B., Baer, L., Sealey, J. E., Drayer, J. I. M., Lopez-Ovejero, J. A., and Laragh, J. H.: Renin and aldosterone suppression in the antihypertensive action of clonidine. Am. J. Cardiol. *38*:825, 1976.
106. Metz, S. A., Halter, J. B., Porte, D., Jr., and Robertson, R. P.: Suppression of plasma catecholamines and flushing by clonidine in man. J. Clin. Endocrinol. Metab. *46*:83, 1978.
107. Houston, M. C.: Abrupt cessation of treatment in hypertension: Consideration of clinical features, mechanisms, prevention and management of the discontinuation syndrome. Am. Heart J. *102*:415, 1981.
108. Bosanac, P., Dubb, J., Walker, B., Goldberg, M., and Agus, Z. S.: Renal effects of guanabenz: A new antihypertensive. J. Clin. Pharmacol. *16*:631, 1976.
109. Fagan, T. C., Bloomfield, S. S., Cowart, T. D., Corns-Hurwitz, R. H., Lipicky, R. J., Conradi, E. C., Hsu, C., Grossman, W. J., Harmon, G. E., Degenhart, W. J., Sinkfield, A. W., and Gafney, T.: Antihypertensive effects of lofexidine in patients with essential hypertension. Br. J. Clin. Pharmacol. *13*:405, 1982.
109a. Safar, M. E., Loria, Y., Weiss, Y. A., and Boutier, J. R.: Antihypertensive effects and plasma levels of guanfacine in man. J. Clin. Pharmacol. *22*:385–390, 1982.
110. Davey, M. J.: The pharmacology of prazosin, an alpha 1-adrenoceptor antagonist and the basis for its use in the treatment of essential hypertension. Clin. Exper. Hyper. *A4*:47, 1982.
111. Jauernig, R. A., Moulds, R. F. W., and Shaw, J.: The action of prazosin in human vascular preparation. Arch. Intern. Pharmacodyn. *231*:81, 1978.
112. Heagerty, A. M., Russell, G. I., Bing, R. F., Thurston, H., and Swales, J. D.: The addition of prazosin to standard triple therapy in the treatment of severe hypertension. Br. J. Clin. Pharmacol. *13*:539, 1982.
113. Miller, R. R., Awan, N. A., Maxwell, K. S., and Mason, D. T.: Sustained reduction of cardiac impedance and preload in congestive heart failure with the antihypertensive vasodilator prazosin. N. Engl. J. Med. *297*:303, 1977.
114. Zacharias, F. J., Cuthbertson, P. J. R., Prestt, J., Cowen, K. J., Johnson, T. B. W., Thompson, J., Vickers, J., Simpson, W. T., and Tuson, R.: Atenolol in hypertension: A study of long-term therapy. Postgrad. Med. J. *53*(Suppl. 3):102, 1977.
115. Campbell, W. B., Johnson, A. R., Callahan, K. S., and Graham, R. M.: Antiplatelet activity of beta-adrenergic antagonists: Inhibition of thromboxane synthesis and platelet aggregation in patients receiving long-term propranolol treatment. Lancet *2*:1382, 1981.
116. Amos, H. E., Lake, B. G., and Artis, J.: Possible role of antibody specific for a practolol metabolite in the pathogenesis of oculomucocutaneous syndrome. Br. Med. J. *1*:402, 1978.
117. Wilcox, R. G.: Randomised study of six beta-blockers and a thiazide diuretic in essential hypertension. Br. Med. J. *2*:383, 1978.
118. Day, J. L., Metcalfe, J., and Simpson, C. N.: Adrenergic mechanisms in control of plasma lipid concentrations. Br. Med. J. *284*:1145, 1982.
119. Groop, L., Tötterman, K. J., Harno, K., and Gordin, A.: Influence of beta-blocking drugs on glucose metabolism in patients with non-insulin dependent diabetes mellitus. Acta Med. Scand. *211*:7, 1982.
120. Fitzgerald, J. D.: The effect of different classes of beta-antagonists on clinical and experimental hypertension. Clin. Exper. Hyper. *A4*:101, 1982.
121. Henningsen, N. C., and Mattiasson, I.: Long-term clinical experience with atenolol—a new selective β-1-blocker with few side-effects from the central nervous system. Acta Med. Scand. *205*:61, 1979.
122. Esler, M., Jackman, G., Leonard, P., Skews, H., Bobik, A., and Jennings, G.: Effects of propranolol on noradrenaline kinetics in patients with essential hypertension. Br. J. Clin. Pharmacol. *12*:375, 1981.
123. O'Connor, D. T., and Preston, R. A.: Propranolol effects on autonomic function in hypertensive men. Clin. Cardiol. *5*:340, 1982.
124. Jackson, E. K., and Campbell, W. B.: A possible antihypertensive mechanism of propranolol: Antagonism of angiotensin II enhancement of sympathetic nerve transmission through prostaglandins. Hypertension *3*:23, 1981.
125. Hallberg, H., Almgren, O. L., and Svensson, T. H.: Reduced brain serotonergic activity after repeated treatment with β-adrenoceptor antagonists. Psychopharmacology *76*:114, 1982.
126. Lund-Johansen, P.: Hemodynamic consequences of long-term beta-blocker therapy: A 5-year follow-up study of atenolol. J. Cardiovasc. Pharmacol. *1*: 487, 1979.
127. Bolli, P., Amann, F. W., Burkart, F., and Bühler, F. R.: Role of α-adrenoceptor–mediated vasoconstriction for antihypertensive β-blockade. J. Cardiovasc. Pharmacol *4*:S162, 1982.
128. Kristensen, B. O., Brons, M., Christensen, C. K., Geday, E., Jacobsen, F. K., Jensen, S. N., and Linde, N. C.: Antihypertensive effect of atenolol (100 mg once a day) and methyldopa (250 mg thrice a day). Acta Med. Scand. *209*: 267, 1981.
129. Serlin, M. M., Orme, M. L'E., Baber, N. A., Sibeon, R. G., Laws, E., and Breckenridge, A.: Propranolol in the control of blood pressure: A dose-response study. Clin. Pharmacol. Ther. *27*:586, 1980.
130. Lundborg, P., Aström, H., Bengtsson, C., Fellenius, E., Von Schenck, H., Svensson, L., and Smith, U.: Effect of β-adrenoceptor blockade on exercise performance and metabolism. Clin. Sci. *61*:299, 1981.
131. Laragh, J. H.: Modern system for treating high blood pressure based on renin profiling and vasoconstriction-volume analysis: A primary role for beta blocking drugs such as propranolol. Am. J. Med. *61*:797, 1976.
132. Drayer, J. I. M., Keim, H. J., Weber, M. A. A., Case, D. B., and Laragh, J. H.: Unexpected pressor responses to propranolol in essential hypertension. Am. J. Med. *60*:897, 1976.
133. James, I. M., Griffith, D. N. W., Pearson, R. M., and Newbury, P.: Effect of oxprenolol on stage-fright in musicians. Lancet *2*:952, 1977.
134. Frishman, W. H., Christodoulou, J., Weksler, B., Smithen, C., Killip, T., and Scheidt, S.: Abrupt propranolol withdrawal in angina pectoris: Effects on platelet aggregation and exercise tolerance. Am. Heart J. *95*:169, 1978.
135. Rangno, R. E., Nattel, S., and Lutterodt, A.: Prevention of propranolol withdrawal mechanism by prolonged small dose propranolol schedule. Am. J. Cardiol. *49*:828, 1982.
136. Smulyan, H., Weinberg, S. E., and Howanitz, P. J.: Continuous propranolol infusion following abdominal surgery. J.A.M.A. *247*:2539, 1982.
137. Wilkinson, R.: β-blockers and renal function. Drugs *23*:195, 1982.
138. Gallery, E. D. M., Saunders, S. M., Hunyor, S. N., and Györy, A. Z.: Randomised comparison of methyldopa and oxprenolol for treatment of hypertension in pregnancy. Br. Med. J. *1*:1591, 1979.
139. Sandstrom, B.: Adrenergic beta-receptor blockers in hypertension of pregnancy. Clin. Exper. Hyper. *B1*:127, 1982.
140. Leren, P., Foss, P. O., Helgeland, A., Hjermann, I., Holme, I., and Lund-Larsen, P. G.: Effect of propranolol and prazosin on blood lipids. Lancet *2*:4, 1980.
141. Feely, J., Wilkinson, G. R., and Wood, A. J. J.: Reduction of liver blood flow and propranolol metabolism by cimetidine. N. Engl. J. Med. *304*:692, 1981.
142. Sotaniemi, E. A., Anttila, M., Rautio, A., Stengard, J., Saukko, P., and Järvensivu, P.: Propranolol and sotalol metabolism after a drinking party. Clin. Pharmacol. Ther. *29*:705, 1981.

143. Alvan, G., vonBahr, C., Seideman, P., Sjöqvist, F.: High plasma concentration of β-receptor blocking drugs and deficient debrisoquine hydroxylation. Lancet *1*:333, 1982.
144. Lund-Johansen, P., and Bakke, O. M.: Haemodynamic effects and plasma concentrations of labetolol during long-term treatment of essential hypertension. Br. J. Clin. Pharmacol. *7*:169, 1979.
145. Cumming, A. M. M., Brown, J. J., Lever, A. F., and Robertson, J. I. S.: Intravenous labetalol in the treatment of severe hypertension. Br. J. Clin. Pharmacol. *13*(Suppl. 1):93s–96s, 1982.
146. Perry, H. M., Jr., Camel, G. H., Carmody, S. E., Ahmed, K. A., and Perry, E. F.: Survival in hydralazine-treated hypertensive patients with and without late toxicity. J. Chron. Dis. *30*:519, 1977.
147. Hagstam, K., Lundgren, R., Wieslander, J.: Clinical experience of long-term treatment with minoxidil in severe arterial hypertension. Scand. J. Urol. Nephrol. *16*:57, 1982.
148. Houston, M. C., McChesney, J. A., and Chatterjee, K.: Pericardial effusion associated with minoxidil therapy. Arch. Intern. Med. *141*:69, 1981.
149. Husted, S. E., Nielsen, H. K., Christensen, C. K., and Pedersen, O. L.: Long-term therapy of arterial hypertension with nifedipine given alone or in combination with a beta-adrenoceptor blocking agent. Eur. J. Clin. Pharmacol. *22*:101, 1982.
149a. Bonaduce, D., Ferrara, N. Petretta, M., Romano, E., Postiglione, M., Rengo, F., and Condorelli, M.: Hemodynamic study of nifedipine administration in hypertensive patients. Am. Heart J. *105*:865, 1983.
149b. Hornung, R. S., Gould, B. A., Jones, R. I., Sonecha, T. N., and Raftery, E. B.: Nifedipine tablets for systemic hypertension: A study using continuous ambulatory intraarterial recording. Am. J. Cardiol. *51*:1323, 1983.
150. Anavekar, S. N., Christophidis, N., Louis, W. J., and Doyle, A. E.: Verapamil in the treatment of hypertension. J. Cardiovasc. Pharmacol. *2*:287, 1981.
151. Krebs, R., Graefe, K.-H., and Ziegler, R.: Effects of calcium-entry antagonists in hypertension. Clin. Exper. Hyper. *A4*:271, 1982.
152. Yagil, Y., Kobrin, I., Leibel, B., and Ben-Ishay, D.: Ischemic ECG changes with initial nifedipine therapy of severe hypertension. Am. Heart J. *103*:310, 1982.
153. Rubin, R. P.: Actions of calcium antagonists on secretory cells. *In* Weiss, G. B. (ed.): New Perspectives on Calcium Antagonists. Bethesda, American Physiological Society, 1981, p. 147.
154. Barbarino, A., and De Marinis, L.: Calcium antagonists and hormone release. II. Effects of verapamil on basal, gonadotropin-releasing hormone– and thyrotropin–releasing hormone–induced pituitary hormone release in normal subjects. J. Clin. Endocrinol. Metab. *51*:749, 1980.
155. Lindemann, J. P., Bailey, J. C., and Watanabe, A. M.: Potential biochemical mechanisms for regulation of the slow inward current: Theoretical basis for drug action. Am. Heart J. *103*:746, 1982.
156. Atlas, D., and Adler, M.: α-Adrenergic antagonists as possible calcium channel inhibitors. Proc. Natl. Acad. Sci. *78*:1237, 1981.
157. Weiss, G. B.: Sites of action of calcium antagonists in vascular smooth muscle. *In* Weiss, G. B. (ed.): New Perspectives on Calcium Antagonists. Bethesda, American Physiological Society, 1981, p. 83.
158. Vidt, D. G., Bravo, E. L., and Fouad, F. M.: Captopril. N. Engl. J. Med. *306*: 214, 1982.
159. Gavras, H., Biollaz, J., Waeber, B., Brunner, H. R., Gavras, I., and Davies, R. O.: Effects of the new oral angiotensin converting enzyme inhibitor MK-421 in human hypertension. Clin. Exper. Hyper. *A4*:303, 1982.
160. Vlasses, P. H., Rotmensch, H. H., Swanson, B. N., Mojaverian, P., and Ferguson, R. K.: Low-dose captopril. Its use in mild to moderate hypertension unresponsive to diuretic treatment. Arch. Intern. Med. *142*:1098, 1982.
161. Atlas, S. A., Case, D. B., Sealey, J. E., Laragh, J. H., and McKinstry, D. N.: Interruption of the renin-angiotensin system in hypertensive patients by captopril induces sustained reduction in aldosterone secretion, potassium retention and natriuresis. Hypertension *1*:274, 1979.
162. Swartz, S. L., Williams, G. H., Hollenberg, N. K., Moore, T. J., and Dluhy, R. G.: Converting enzyme inhibition in essential hypertension: The hypotensive response does not reflect only reduced angiotensin II formation. Hypertension *1*:106, 1979,
163. Jenkins, A. C., and McKinstry, D. N.: Review of clinical studies of hypertensive patients treated with captopril. Med. J. Aust. (Suppl.)*2*:32, 1979.
164. Karlberg, B. E., Asplund, J., Nilsson, O. R., Wettre, S., and Öhman, P. K.: Captopril, an orally active converting enzyme inhibitor, in the treatment of primary hypertension. Acta Med. Scand. *209*:245, 1981.
165. Tarazi, R. C., Bravo, E. L., and Fouad, F. M.: Late resistance to captopril. *In* Laragh, J. H., Buhler, F. R., and Seldin, D. W. (eds.): Frontiers in Hypertension Research. New York, Springer-Verlag, 1981.
166. Waeber, B., Gavras, I., Brunner, H. R., and Gavras, H.: Safety and efficacy of chronic therapy with captopril in hypertensive patients: An update. J. Clin. Pharmacol. *21*:508, 1981.
167. Captopril Collaborative Study Group: Does captopril cause renal damage in hypertensive patients? Lancet *1*:988, 1982.
168. Case, D. B., Atlas, S. A., Mouradian, J. A., Fishman, R. A., Sherman, R. L., and Laragh, J. H.: Proteinuria during long-term captopril therapy. J.A.M.A. *244*:346, 1980.
169. Erslev, A. J., Alexander, J. C., Caro, J., and Boyd, R. L.: Hematologic side effects of captopril and associated risk factors. Cardiovasc. Rev. Rep. *3*:660, 1982.
170. Ibrahim, M. M., Tarazi, R. C., Dustan, H. P., and Gifford, R. W., Jr.: Electrocardiogram in evaluation of resistance to antihypertensive therapy. Arch. Intern. Med. *137*:1125, 1977.
171. Gavras, H., Waeber, B., Kershaw, G. R., Liang, C., Textor, S. C., Brunner, H. R., Tifft, C. P., and Gavras, I.: Role of reactive hyperreninemia in blood pressure changes induced by sodium depletion in patients with refractory hypertension. Hypertension *3*:441, 1981.
172. Cohn, J. N.: Paroxysmal hypertension and hypovolemia. N. Engl. J. Med. *275*:643, 1966.
173. Prys-Roberts, C., Meloche, R., and Föex, P.: Studies of anaesthesia in relation to hypertension. I. Cardiovascular responses of treated and untreated patients. Br. J. Anaesth. *43*:122, 1971.
174. Prys-Roberts, C., Föex, P., Biro, G. P., and Roberts, J. G.: Studies of anaesthesia in relation to hypertension. V. Andrenergic beta-receptor blockade. Br. J. Anaesth. *45*:671, 1973.
175. Lieberman, E.: Hypertension in childhood and adolescence. *In* Kaplan, N. M. (ed.): Clinical Hypertension. 3rd ed. Baltimore, Williams and Wilkins Co., 1982, pp. 411–435.
176. Management Committee: Treatment of mild hypertension in the elderly. Med. J. Aust. *2*:398, 1981.
177. Wollner, L., McCarthy, S. T., Soper, N. D. W., and Macy, D. J.: Failure of cerebral autoregulation as a cause of brain dysfunction in the elderly. Br. Med. J. *1*:1117, 1979.
178. Gifford, R. W., Jr.: Isolated systolic hypertension in the elderly. J.A.M.A. *247*:781, 1982.
179. Spence, J. D., Sibbald, W. J., and Cape, R. D.: Pseudohypertension in the elderly. Clin. Sci. Molec. Med. *55*:399s, 1978.
180. Bank, N., Lief, P. D., and Piczon, O.: Use of diuretics in treatment of hypertension secondary to renal disease. Arch. Intern. Med. *138*:1524, 1978.
181. Friedlaender, M. M., Rubinger, D., and Popovtzer, M. M.: Improved renal function in patients with primary renal disease after control of severe hypertension. Am. J. Nephrol. *2*:12, 1982.
182. Cottrell, J. E., Casthely, P., Brodie, J. D., Patel, K., Klein, A., and Turndorf, H.: Prevention of nitroprusside-induced cyanide toxicity with hydroxycobalamin. N. Engl. J. Med. *298*:809, 1978.
183. Niarchos, A. P., and Kritikou, P. E.: Cardiovascular effects of sodium nitroprusside in hypertensive patients before and during acute beta-adrenergic blockade. J. Clin. Pharmacol. *19*:31, 1979.
184. Garrett, B. N., and Kaplan, N. M.: Efficacy of slow infusion of diazoxide in the treatment of severe hypertension without organ hypoperfusion. Am. Heart J. *103*:390, 1982.
185. Alpert, M. A., and Bauer, J. H.: Rapid control of severe hypertension with minosidil. Arch. Intern. Med. *142*:2099–2104, 1982.

28 HYPOTENSION AND SYNCOPE

by Burton E. Sobel, M.D., and Robert Roberts, M.D.

The *sudden* development of hypotension, particularly when it occurs in a recumbent patient, is usually associated with impaired systemic perfusion and may be an important feature of shock, as discussed in detail in Chapter 18. In contrast, *chronic hypotension*, with systolic pressure in the range of 85 to 110 mm Hg is not pathological and may actually be associated with a longer life expectancy than a "normal" arterial pressure. This chapter deals with a variety of syndromes responsible for *episodic hypotension* and its cardinal clinical manifestation, syncope.

REGULATION OF ARTERIAL PRESSURE

Systemic arterial pressure is closely related to the product of cardiac output and systemic vascular resistance. *Cardiac output* is the product of heart rate and stroke volume, the latter being determined by interactions between preload, afterload, and contractility, as described in Chapter 14. Thus, the cardiac causes of sudden hypotension relate to abrupt reductions in ventricular rate, as occurs with atrioventricular block, or in stroke volume, as may occur in hypovolemia (reduced preload); to critical aortic stenosis (augmented afterload); or to massive myocardial infarction (impaired ventricular function). *Vascular resistance* varies inversely with the fourth power of the radius of the resistance vessels, the arterioles, and therefore is determined by the intrinsic physical characteristics of these vessels, i.e., the ratio of lumen to wall thickness; the degree of extravascular support and compression; and the extent of contraction of the smooth muscle in the vascular wall. The last-named is in turn influenced by (1) metabolic and mechanical autoregulatory mechanisms that act to maintain *nearly* constant perfusion of each vascular bed—there is substantial evidence that adenosine is a principal metabolic mediator of vascular resistance (p. 1244); (2) neurogenic vasoconstrictor influences, operating through the action of adrenergic neurotransmitter norepinephrine on alpha-adrenergic receptors in vascular smooth muscle; (3) neurogenic vasodilator influences, operating through the action of acetylcholine on muscarinic receptors, or norepinephrine on $beta_2$ receptors, and perhaps of histamine, serotonin, and other transmitters; and (4) circulating and locally released vasoactive substances, including catecholamines, angiotensin II, bradykinin, and prostaglandins. The vascular causes of hypotension may involve any of these four mechanisms (Table 28–1).

The autonomic nervous system plays a major role in the maintenance of arterial pressure because it influences both cardiac output and the degree of constriction of the vessels of resistance (arterioles) and capacitance (venules and veins). The afferent limbs of the autonomic reflex arcs that acutely regulate arterial pressure arise in stretch receptors in the aortic arch, the carotid sinuses, ventricles, and atria. Impulses are transmitted along afferent fibers in the glossopharyngeal and vagus nerves to extensive central connections in the medulla. Synapses connect not only the sympathetic and parasympathetic nuclei and efferent arcs but also the cerebral cortex and hypothalamic nuclei, which control hormonal secretion via the pituitary gland (Fig. 28–1).

A sudden reduction of arterial and intraventricular pressure diminishes the stimulation of pressoreceptors, which in turn reflexly activates sympathetic outflow and inhibits parasympathetic activity. As a result, vascular smooth muscle in arterioles and veins constricts, whereas heart rate and myocardial contractility are augmented. In addition, as arterial pressure falls, adrenal medullary secretion increases, along with the output of antidiuretic hormone (ADH), adrenocorticotropic hormone (ACTH), renin, and aldosterone; all these effects restore the arterial pressure toward control levels. Opposite changes occur if arterial pressure rises suddenly. Thus, the operation of these baro-

TABLE 28–1 IMPORTANT CAUSES OF PROLONGED OR INTERMITTENT HYPOTENSION

1. Cardiac dysfunction
   a. Disturbances of rate and rhythm
      (1) Conduction abnormalities
      (2) Diverse dysrhythmias, including severe bradycardia and paroxysmal tachycardias
   b. Obstruction to flow
      (1) Aortic or pulmonary valvular stenosis
      (2) Hypertrophic obstructive cardiomyopathy
      (3) Atrial myxoma
      (4) Primary pulmonary hypertension
      (5) Pulmonary peripheral branch stenosis
      (6) Pulmonary emboli
      (7) Cardiac tamponade
      (8) Mitral or tricuspid stenosis
      (9) Cor triatriatum
      (10) Tetralogy of Fallot
      (11) Eisenmenger's syndrome
   c. Impaired ventricular function
      (1) Myocardial infarction
      (2) Cardiomyopathy

2. Vascular or neurological dysfunction
   a. Vasovagal
   b. Postural hypotension
      (1) Idiopathic
      (2) Acquired
      (3) Familial
   c. Hyperventilation
   d. Carotid sinus hypersensitivity
   e. Glossopharyngeal neuralgia, micturition, deglutition, or post-tussive syncope

3. Metabolic and endocrine disturbances
   a. Pheochromocytoma
   b. Serotonin-secreting tumors
   c. Hyperbradykininemia

4. Drug toxicity
   a. Vasodilators
   b. Adrenergic antagonists
   c. Diuretics
   d. Phenothiazines
   e. Barbiturates and other CNS depressants
   f. Vincristine and other neuropathic drugs
   g. Quinidine and other drugs with negative chronotropic effects
   h. Digitalis

receptors and a number of hormonal systems normally serve to buffer the body from a variety of influences that would otherwise produce marked alterations in arterial pressure.

In a resting supine adult, the level of sympathetic discharge to the vasculature is low.[1] Assumption of the upright posture is accompanied by venous pooling of approximately 700 ml of blood in the legs.[1,2] Systemic arterial pressure is maintained by venous and arterial constriction mediated by sympathetic stimulation. Even modest reflex changes of this type markedly facilitate maintenance of venous return and stroke volume.[1] The initial gravitational effects associated with upright posture are compensated not only by reflex arteriolar and venous constriction but also by acceleration of heart rate and by mechanical factors that limit venous pooling in the lower extremities, including venous valves, "milking" of veins in the lower extremities by contractions of the leg musculature (Fig. 28–2), and reduced intrathoracic pressure that facilitates venous return. The increased sympathetic activity is reflected in a rise in concentration of plasma catecholamines.[3] As a consequence of these compensatory mechanisms, when a normal person assumes the upright posture, there is only a transient decline in systolic arterial blood pressure, generally of 5 to 15 mm Hg. Diastolic pressure tends to rise, and mean arterial pressure remains essentially unchanged; cardiac output and stroke volume decline; and there is reflex tachycardia and vasoconstriction, the latter reflected in a rise in systemic vascular resistance. In patients with orthostatic hypotension, by definition the decline in arterial pressure with assumption of the upright posture is more profound and persistent. Depending on the severity and duration of the hypotension, it may be accompanied by symptoms of impaired cerebral perfusion such as dizziness, presyncope, or syncope.

Hypotension may be a manifestation of impairment of any element in (1) the afferent limb, including the carotid, aortic, ventricular, and atrial baroreceptors; (2) the central

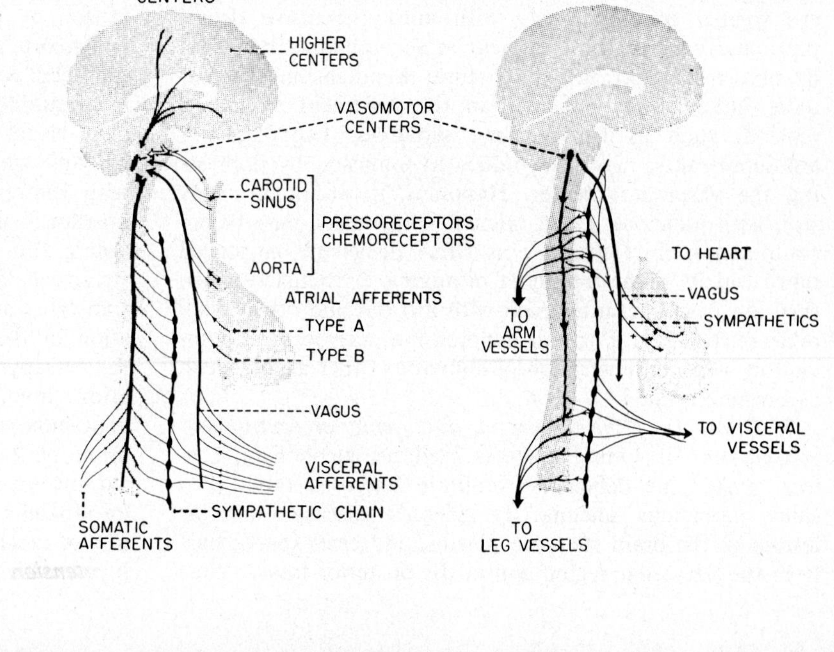

FIGURE 28–1 The vasomotor centers in the medulla receive afferent impulses from many different areas of the body, including the higher centers of the nervous system, heart, blood vessels, viscera, and somatic pain receptors. Efferent impulses descend via the spinal cord in the intermediolateral column and initiate sympathetic impulses to the blood vessels throughout the organism. (From Rushmer, R. F.: Cardiovascular Dynamics. Philadelphia, W. B. Saunders Co., 1961, p. 153.)

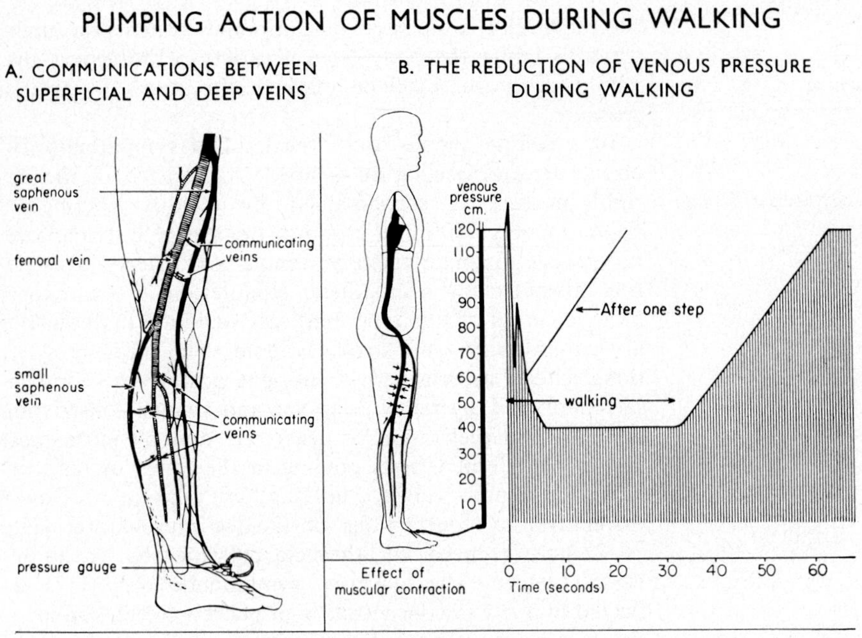

FIGURE 28–2 The venous blood from the leg may return to the heart via superficial or deep channels. Even a single step is associated with a marked reduction in venous pressure that is maintained with walking. With resumption of standing, pressure returns only gradually to control values. (From Rushmer, R. F.: Cardiovascular Dynamics, Philadelphia, W. B. Saunders Co., 1961, p. 176.)

vasomotor centers; (3) the cortical or spinal outflow efferent tracts; (4) the peripheral sympathetic or parasympathetic nerves; (5) mechanical factors that normally limit pooling in the peripheral veins; (6) intravascular blood volume; and (7) the heart's ability to maintain cardiac output.

CAUSES OF ORTHOSTATIC HYPOTENSION

Clinically, the causes of orthostatic hypotension may be classified as follows:[4]

1. *Chronic idiopathic hypotension,* a primary degenerative disorder impairing the function of the autonomic nervous system (discussed below).
2. *Vasoactive drugs,* including essentially all antihypertensive but particularly ganglionic blocking agents; depletors of catecholamines such as reserpine; and drugs that block the neuronal release of catecholamines, such as guanethidine (Chap. 27). In patients with hypertension who are treated too vigorously with antihypertensive drugs, particularly when the treatment is accompanied by dehydration and hypovolemia, postural hypotension is common. Other drugs not used in the treatment of hypertension, such as tranquilizers, sedatives, hypnotics, or antidepressants, may also induce hypotension by depressing the vasomotor center. Hypotension, although rarely seen with judicious use of calcium antagonists, may be encountered more frequently as these drugs are employed more widely in the treatment of angina, particularly when they are used in combination with nitrates and other vasodilators (p. 1351). Postural hypotension may occur in association with administration of numerous other agents, such as bromocriptine.[5]
3. *Disorders of the peripheral, autonomic, or central nervous system,* including diabetes mellitus, alcoholism, uremia, pyridoxine deficiency, multiple sclerosis, tabes dorsalis, pernicious anemia, Parkinson's disease, vascular lesions in the brain stem, neoplasms, and cysts (particularly in the parasellar region and in the posterior fossa), Wernicke's encephalopathy, syringomyelia, and a number of demyelinating disorders.
4. *Cardiovascular deconditioning* after any prolonged illness with prolonged recumbency, especially in elderly patients.
5. *Diseased or varicose veins* causing pooling of blood in the lower extremities.
6. *The supine hypotensive syndrome of pregnancy* (p. 1764), resulting from obstruction of the inferior vena cava with reduction in venous return and decline in cardiac output.
7. *Infiltration of vessel walls,* which may preclude a physiological response to sympathetic stimulation, e.g., amyloidosis.
8. *Surgically induced sympathectomy* with abolition of vasopressor reflex responses.

CHRONIC IDIOPATHIC ORTHOSTATIC HYPOTENSION. This syndrome, the *Bradbury-Eggleston syndrome,* which most often occurs in older men, has also been termed *primary autonomic insufficiency* and is characterized by postural hypotension without a compensatory tachycardia, hypohidrosis, impotence, and disturbed sphincter control.[6] Hypertension in the supine position and postprandial hypotension are relatively common. Dizziness, visual disturbances, presyncope, and syncope accompanying standing or walking are typical signs and occur with distressing regularity, especially when the upright posture is assumed suddenly and during the early morning hours; the course is usually progressive. The *Shy-Drager syndrome* (also known as multiple system atrophy) is a somewhat similar disorder but exhibits prominent degeneration of the central nervous system, with involvement of the extrapyramidal tracts and basal ganglia.[7,8] The degeneration involves the dorsal nucleus of the vagus and pigmented brain stem nuclei, intermediate and lateral columns of the spinal cord, and sympathetic ganglia;[9,10] in a variant form the pathological findings resemble those of Parkinson's disease, with dementia, extrapyramidal signs, loss of facial expressions, and tremor. *Secondary orthostatic hypotension* occurs in a number of neurological disorders that involve the autonomic nervous system, including alcoholic and diabetic neuropathy, subacute combined sclerosis, spinal cord transection, syringomyelia, and tabes dorsalis.

The postural hypotension in chronic idiopathic orthostatic hypotension and in many of the forms of secondary orthostatic hypotension[11] is due primarily to impairment of peripheral vasoconstriction, acceleration of heart rate, and maintenance of cardiac output in response to the assumption of the upright posture.[3,12–14] There is a greater than normal decline in arterial pressure during the Valsalva maneuver, with a reduced or absent arterial pressure overshoot following release, as well as a paradoxical decline in arterial pressure during exercise.

Kontos et al. found that patients with idiopathic orthostatic hypotension do not exhibit vasoconstriction in the forearm and hands in response to intraarterial administration of tyramine, whereas the vasoconstrictor responses to intraarterial administration of norepinephrine are augmented. These findings strongly suggest that sympathetic nerve endings are depleted of and unable to take up norepinephine. Depletion of norepinephrine from sympathetic nerve endings was confirmed by histochemical demonstration of the absence of catecholamine-specific fluorescence in sympathetic vasomotor nerves.[15,16]

Excretion of norepinephrine and its synthesis from precursors are reduced in this condition.[17–20] Plasma renin release and aldosterone secretion in response to assumption of the erect posture or to salt restriction are also blunted,[15,17–19] possibly contributing to the difficulty in augmenting plasma volume to compensate adequately for the impaired reflex control of vasomotor tone. Thus, blood volume in patients with these disorders is normal or only slightly increased.

While recumbent, patients with idiopathic orthostatic hypotension and multiple central nervous system defects have *normal* plasma levels of norepinephrine that fail to increase normally after standing or exertion. In contrast, patients with peripheral autonomic insufficiency *without* signs of central nervous system defects have *low* levels of plasma norepinephrine while recumbent that also fail to increase normally after standing or exercise. Both groups have low levels of plasma dopamine beta-hydroxylase. These findings are consistent with other pathological and pharmacological observations, suggesting that patients with idiopathic orthostatic hypotension and central nervous system disease are unable to activate appropriately an otherwise intact sympathetic nervous system, whereas in patients without signs of central nervous system disease, the defect affects peripheral sympathetic nerves.[10]

Since the fundamental disorder is not amenable to therapy, the *treatment* of patients with chronic idiopathic hypotension and the Shy-Drager syndrome must be symptomatic.[20a] This involves (1) a high-salt diet and judicious and monitored administration of mineralocorticoids such as fludrocortisone to expand plasma volume; (2) hydroxyamphetamine, dihydroergotamine,[21,21a] L-dopa,[8] or other directly or indirectly acting sympathomimetic agents; combined with (3) a monoamine oxidase inhibitor, such as tranylcypromine, to augment norepinephrine concentration at nerve endings;[18,22–24] (4) propranolol, a nonselective beta blocker that may prevent adrenergically mediated vasodilation and result in unopposed vasoconstriction;[8,25] (5) indomethacin, which acts presumably by inhibiting synthesis of vasodilatory prostaglandins;[8] and (6) mechanical support by elastic stockings or, in severe cases, an antigravity suit (Fig. 28–3). The *prognosis* for survival is approximately 10 years following the development of symptoms in patients without other evident neurological disease, but it is only about 5 years in patients with associated abnormalities of the central nervous system.

Familial Dysautonomia. Familial dysautonomia (Riley-Day syndrome) is a progressive disorder inherited in a pattern consistent with an autosomal recessive trait limited primarily to Ashkenazi Jews.[26] It is characterized by the appearance at or soon after birth of autonomic instability with both postural hypotension and hypertensive episodes due to defective reflex control of vascular tone. Other features include fever; impaired perception of pain, temperature, and taste; lack of fungiform papillae on the tongue; impaired lacrimation; diminished or absent deep tendon reflexes; ataxia; loss of the histamine-flare response; feeding difficulties; and susceptibility to viral pneumonia in infancy.[26,27]

Tissue norepinephrine stores are normal or elevated;[28] the concentrations of plasma catecholamines are normal in patients who are recumbent and at rest but fail to increase normally with exercise or assumption of the upright posture. Plasma dopamine beta-hydroxylase activity and the excretion of vanillylmandelic acid (VMA) are often reduced, consistent with impaired release of catecholamines from sympathetic nerve endings.[28] The cardiovascular response to infused

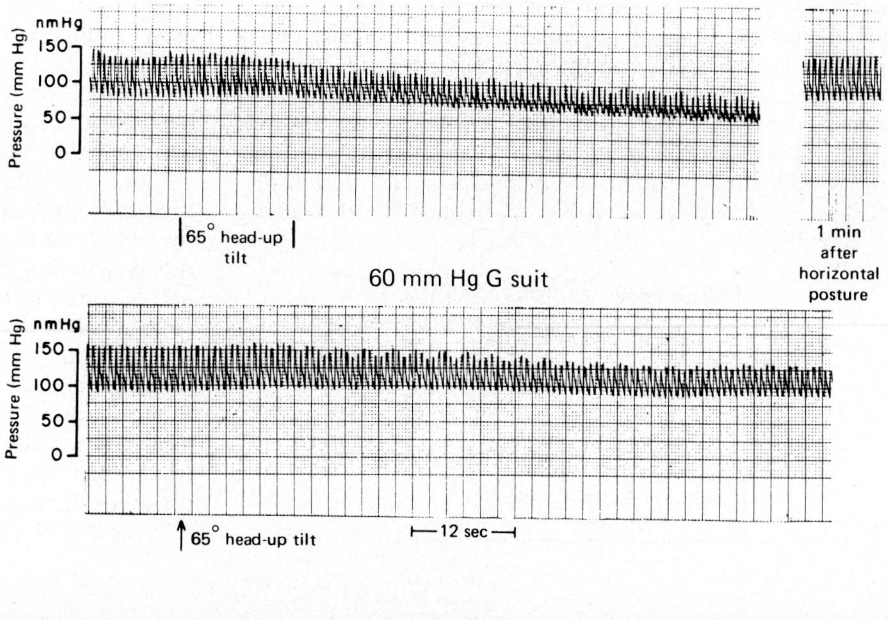

FIGURE 28–3 Direct recording of intraarterial blood pressure in a patient with orthostatic hypotension. *Top panel,* Drop in blood pressure accompanying a change from horizontal to head-up tilt position (140/85 to 85/65 mm Hg), with recovery accompanying return to the horizontal position. *Bottom panel,* Minimal change in blood pressure (155/90 to 125/90 mm Hg) with the same postural changes but with the patient wearing an antigravity suit. (From Fowler, N. O.: Cardiac Diagnosis and Treatment. 3rd ed. Hagerstown, Md., Harper and Row, 1980, p. 1210.)

norepinephrine is exaggerated, suggesting receptor hypersensitivity or reduced uptake of the neurotransmitter by nerve endings or both.

Patients with familial dysautonomia synthesize and store norepinephrine in sympathetic nerve endings and release catecholamines from the adrenal medulla in response to stress induced by hypoglycemia.[29] Thus, the hypertensive episodes that frequently accompany even mild anxiety and are associated with increases in plasma norepinephrine may, like the response to infused catecholamines, reflect increased reactivity of vascular receptors to released adrenal catecholamines.

Although the specific abnormality responsible for familial dysautonomia remains unidentified,[26,27] defective release of norepinephrine from the nerve endings is a prominent pathophysiological component. Although it may reflect abnormalities in the afferent or efferent sympathetic system, demonstrable degeneration in the reticular formation of the brain stem suggests a primary abnormality in the central nervous system. However, in some patients the defect may be confined to the peripheral autonomic nervous system. In these patients at rest and in the recumbent position, circulating concentrations of catecholamines are low and do not rise in response to stress.[10]

Unfortunately, no specific treatment is available, and the disease progresses to death in early adult life. Symptomatic treatment involves the general measures described previously for management of postural hypotension as well as the administration of parasympathomimetic agents, such as bethanechol chloride (Urecholine), to facilitate lacrimation, reduce gastric distention and vomiting, improve esophageal motility, and improve bladder control.

Metabolic Abnormalities. Metabolic or endocrine disturbances leading to reduction of plasma volume, altered adrenergic function, or vasodilatation may underlie persistent or episodic hypotension. These include diabetes mellitus, primary systemic amyloidosis, and acute porphyria. The hypovolemia seen with adrenocortical insufficiency, hypoaldosteronism, and salt-wasting nephritis is the primary cause of hypotension in these conditions, although altered vascular responses to catecholamines may contribute in Addison's disease, and diminished levels of angiotensin may play a role in conditions in which plasma renin activity is low.[30]

Depletion of plasma volume is characteristically associated with pheochromocytoma and is a primary cause of postural hypotension in this disorder (p. 1734). However, epinephrine-induced vasodilatation contributes in some patients with epinephrine-secreting tumors. Rarely, circulatory instability results from high concentrations of circulating bradykinins. Hyperbradykininemia, a disorder that is sometimes familial, is characterized by severe tachycardia and a narrowed pulse pressure. The cause is an enzyme deficiency resulting in impaired destruction of the circulating peptides.[31] Kinins may also play a role in the hypotension and syncope sometimes seen with the carcinoid syndrome.

SYNCOPE

Syncope refers to loss of consciousness due to the impairment (usually temporary) of cerebral perfusion.[32] The metabolism of the brain, in contrast to that of many other organs, is exquisitely dependent on perfusion. In contrast to skeletal muscle, for example, storage of high-energy phosphate in the brain is limited, and energy supply depends largely on the oxidation of glucose extracted from the blood. Consequently, cessation of cerebral flow leads to loss of consciousness within approximately 10 seconds (Table 28–2).[33]

TABLE 28–2 FACTORS POTENTIALLY AFFECTING CEREBRAL PERFUSION SELECTIVELY

1. Metabolic causes
Hypercapnia
Hypotension
2. Decreased effective perfusion pressure
Cerebral vascular disease (usually atherosclerotic)
Arterial spasm
Increased intracranial pressure
Cerebral venospasm

A typical syncopal episode is characterized by hypotension, pallor, diaphoresis, and loss of consciousness in a motionless patient with depressed, shallow respirations and intact sphincter tone. If postural hypotension is the cause, cerebral blood flow is usually restored promptly, and consciousness is regained when the patient falls or is placed in a horizontal position. Although syncope is most often associated with the upright posture because it is frequently a manifestation of postural hypotension, it may result from conduction disturbances or other arrhythmias causing profound, sudden reductions in cardiac output in which case postural associations may be lacking.

Faintness or presyncope, a less severe but etiologically similar phenomenon, is characterized by sudden weakness, the inability to stand, visual difficulty, and the sensation of impending loss of consciousness. At this stage, frank loss of consciousness can often be averted if cerebral perfusion is restored, as by the assumption of the supine posture.

REFLEX-MEDIATED VASOMOTOR INSTABILITY. Inappropriate or excessive activation of vasomotor reflexes may initiate syncope in syndromes such as *carotid sinus hypersensitivity*. Pressure on the carotid artery was observed to slow the heart by Czermak in 1866, a reflex phenomenon shown by Hering to be initiated by pressure on the carotid sinus rather than on the vagus nerve. Under physiological conditions, afferent impulses from the carotid sinuses are transmitted via the glossopharyngeal nerve to vasomotor and cardioinhibitory centers in the medulla. The efferent limb of the carotid sinus reflex comprises vagal and cervical sympathetic fibers (Fig. 28–4).[34,35] Afferent impulses from the carotid sinus impinge on the medulla with a frequency dependent on the pressure and rate of change of pressure in the walls of the vessel. Increased pressure leads to an increased frequency of afferent stimulation of the central vasomotor (pressor) center. Consequently, parasympathetic outflow increases, sympathetic outflow is reduced, and systemic vasodilatation and bradycardia ensue.

A clinical syndrome, the hypersensitive carotid sinus syndrome, has been recognized as a cause of hypotension, bradycardia, dizziness, presyncope, and syncope.[35,35a] Two major forms of hypersensitive carotid sinus syndromes have been well delineated.[36] The most common, the *vagal* or *cardioinhibitory* type, occurring in approximately 70 per cent of patients with this syndrome, is manifested by sinus bradycardia, sinus arrest, atrioventricular block, a combination of these disturbances, or even asystole (Fig. 28–5). The second, or *vasodepressor type*, is manifested by marked hypotension without significant bradycardia or atrioventricular (AV) block. Many patients exhibit a combination of both the cardioinhibitory and the vasodepressor syndromes.[37] Carotid sinus hypersensitivity usually occurs in the elderly and is more frequent in men than in women. Arteriosclerosis, hypertension, diabetes mellitus, and local pathological changes such as scars, lymph nodes, and tumors involving the carotid body[36] predispose to a hyperactive carotid sinus. Episodes are often precipitated by turning the head or pressure on the carotid sinus area, such as during shaving. Attacks can be initiated and the diagnosis thereby confirmed by manual pressure on the carotid sinus. Occasionally, cervical lymphadenopathy, scar tissue, or a carotid body tumor may be responsible.[36] Usually, however, the underlying increased sensitivity of the

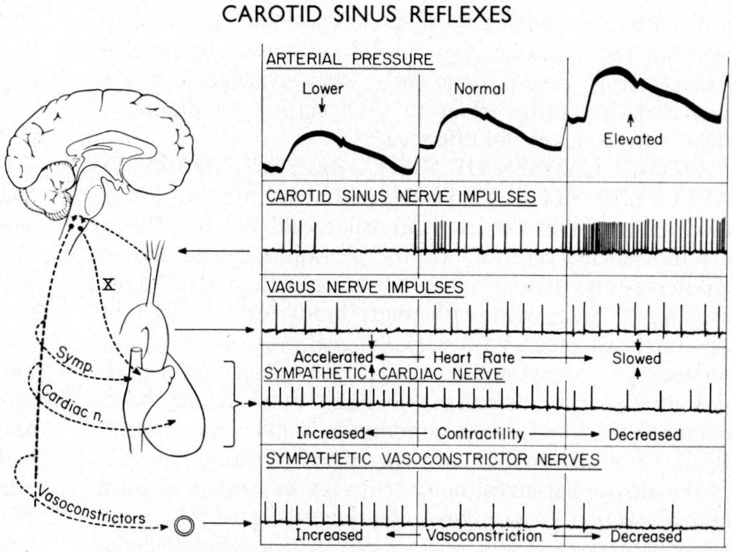

FIGURE 28–4 Relationship between carotid sinus discharge and arterial blood pressure. With a drop in blood pressure (first panel), the frequency of baroreceptor impulses decreases, afferent vagal impulses decrease, and efferent sympathetic nerve impulses increase. The sympathetic vasoconstrictor fiber impulse traffic is active, and an increase in peripheral resistance occurs, resulting in a rise in blood pressure. With an increase in blood pressure, the opposite occurs, resulting in vasodilatation and a drop in blood pressure. (From Rushmer, R. F.: Cardiovascular Dynamics. Philadelphia, W. B. Saunders Co., 1961, p. 150.)

carotid sinus to pressure accompanying specific movements of the neck or a tight collar is not associated with an overt anatomic lesion. Electrophysiological study usually reveals normal intrinsic function of the sinoatrial node and atrioventricular conduction system.[38]

Diagnosis is confirmed by applying manual pressure to the carotid artery in the region of the carotid sinus with the patient supine and the head in a neutral position.[39] Pressure should be applied only lightly at first on only one side and for a maximum of 20 seconds at a time while the electrocardiogram and blood pressure are monitored. Normal subjects exhibit mild sinus bradycardia, sometimes with first-degree atrioventricular block. Ventricular asystole with a duration of 3 seconds or more or a decrease in systolic arterial blood pressure exceeding 50 mm Hg is a definitively abnormal response. Complications of carotid sinus stimulation are rare but potentially catastrophic and include cardiac standstill and hemiplegia.[40] The risk is greatest in elderly, hypertensive patients with cerebral or extracranial vascular occlusive disease. Emergency treatment with closed chest cardiac compression, intravenous atropine, epinephrine, and norepinephrine is indicated.

Other coexisting causes of syncope or episodes mimicking syncope must be excluded, since documentation of a hypersensitive carotid sinus does not prove that it is responsible for the syncopal episode in an individual case.[40] Impaired cerebral perfusion due to cerebral vascular disease may also be responsible for syncope associated with extrinsic pressure on the vessels of the neck,[37] and this condition must be differentiated from the hypersensitive carotid sinus syndrome.

If the syndrome is caused by an anatomically identifiable lesion, such as a carotid sinus tumor, excision is required. In the usual case in which no anatomical cause is recognizable and when symptoms are infrequent, reassurance, precautions to avoid rapid movements, and avoidance of tight collars usually constitute effective therapy.[37] Frequent symptoms should be evaluated by ambulatory electrocardiographic monitoring. If associated with severe bradycardia, they may be prevented by ventricular[37] or

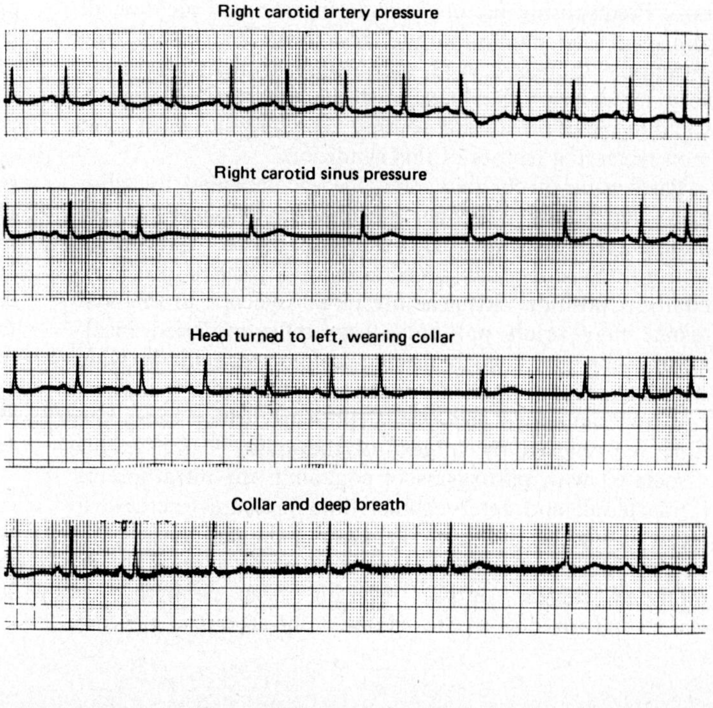

FIGURE 28–5 Electrocardiographic tracings obtained from a patient with the hypersensitive carotid sinus syndrome who presented with attacks of dizziness associated with wearing a tight collar (cardioinhibitory type). Right carotid pressure or sudden turning of the head while wearing a tight collar produced suppression of the sinoatrial node with a junctional escape rhythm. (From Fowler, N. O.: Cardiac Diagnosis and Treatment. 3rd ed. Hagerstown, Md., Harper and Row, 1980, p. 1208.)

atrioventricular pacing.[37a] Surgical resection[37] or denervation[41] of the hypersensitive carotid sinus may be required for refractory cases, particularly when syncope is due to vasodilatation rather than to bradycardia. Irradiation of the carotid sinus is not effective.[36]

OTHER CAUSES OF SYNCOPE SECONDARY TO AFFERENT STIMULATION. Afferent impulses associated with pain in the ear, soft palate, larynx, or pharynx are transmitted centrally via the glossopharyngeal and vagal nerves and may also give rise to reflex hypotension and syncope[42,43] associated with sinus bradycardia,[43] sinus arrest, or heart block.[44] *Glossopharyngeal neuralgia* is characterized by paroxysmal pain usually localized to the posterior pharynx or external auditory canal. It may be accompanied by syncope, secondary to bradycardia and systemic vasodilatation. It may be caused by tumor invasion of the glossopharyngeal nerve and may be treated by intracranial section of the glossopharyngeal nerve.[45] Syncope, often with associated severe vertigo, which follows pleural or peritoneal taps and prostatic massage, may be responsible for similar cardiovascular changes.

Syncope[46–49] or occasionally severe bradycardia without syncope[48] may be provoked by swallowing, usually in association with esophageal tumor,[46] diverticulum,[47] or spasm,[48] but sometimes occurs in patients without overt esophageal disease (*deglutition syncope*).[49] Attacks can be reproduced by inflation of a balloon at the level of an esophageal diverticulum in some patients and in others can be prevented by administration of atropine or by local anesthesia of the vagus nerve in the neck with procaine.[50,51] In some cases afferent impulses may be transmitted via the glossopharyngeal nerve, which also supplies the posterior pharynx and a portion of the esophagus. Treatment requires correction of overt esophageal disease. Palliation and reduction of recurrent syncope may be achieved with the use of an artificial pacemaker in selected patients.

Another reflex-mediated syndrome, *postmicturition syncope*, occurs typically in healthy young to middle-aged men, usually when the patient arises from bed to void. Syncope occurs during or immediately after micturition, and recovery is rapid and complete. Recurrent episodes are rare. Predisposing factors include ingestion of alcohol, diminished food intake, fatigue, and upper respiratory tract infection.[52] Increased vagal stimulation at night, vagal sensory input from the bladder during micturition and the standing position during voiding represent the most common triggering factors of this syndrome.[53]

Paroxysms of coughing may be accompanied by giddiness, vertigo, or syncope, particularly in short, stocky, middle-aged men with chronic lung disease (*post-tussive syncope*). Syncope may occur even with patients in the recumbent position. Sequelae are rare.[54] Syncope in this syndrome may result not only from reflex-mediated mechanisms but also from hydraulic factors, particularly when it follows a paroxysm of coughs, in which case it may result from increased intracranial pressure, which can sometimes be relieved by surgery of the spine.[54,55] In syncope associated with paroxysms of coughing, the intrathoracic, intraarterial, and cerebrospinal fluid pressures increase to levels as high as 300 mm Hg. During the paroxysm, pressure within the cerebral vessels declines because of the diminished cardiac output resulting from inhibition of venous return due to the elevated intrathoracic pressure and secondary to the increased intracranial pressure reflecting the rise in cerebrospinal fluid pressure. Accordingly, cerebral perfusion declines precipitously (Table 28–2).

VASOVAGAL HYPOTENSION AND SYNCOPE (VASODEPRESSOR SYNCOPE, THE COMMON FAINT). This type of syncope is the most frequently encountered form, accounting for more than 55 per cent of cases in some series.[56] It is often precipitated by the sight of blood; the sudden loss of blood, such as that occurring with phlebotomy; a sudden stressful or painful experience, such as arterial puncture or venipuncture; surgical manipulation; or severe trauma. Vasodepressor syncope is most likely to occur in association with hunger, fatigue, or crowding, particularly in a hot room. Premonitory signs and symptoms are common, including pallor, yawning, sighing, hyperventilation, epigastric discomfort, nausea, diaphoresis, blurred vision, impaired hearing, a vague feeling of unawareness, mydriasis, and sometimes a rapid heart rate. It generally occurs with the patient in an upright position, and if the patient sits or lies down promptly, frank syncope may be aborted.[56a]

Pathophysiology. Despite intensive study of the phenomenon, its etiology has not been elucidated definitively.[57–60] Early in the process, peripheral vasodilatation appears to predominate. Blood pressure declines modestly while blood flow to the limbs, cardiac output, and heart rate remain essentially constant.[58–60] Later, resistance in the skeletal muscular beds is reduced, and skeletal blood flow rises markedly while flow through other vascular beds such as the cutaneous, mesenteric, renal, and cerebral declines as arterial pressure falls rapidly. Although cardiac output does not usually decline markedly in vasodepressor syncope, the pathophysiological mechanism must involve more than arteriolar dilation (or failure of normal arteriolar constriction in the upright position), since in normal individuals the fall in peripheral vascular resistance induced by vasodilatation would be compensated for by a compensatory increase in heart rate and cardiac output, which would limit the reduction of arterial pressure. In patients with vasodepressor syncope, however, cardiac output and heart rate fail to rise, presumably owing to some impairment of venous return, perhaps because of venous dilatation or failure of normal venous constriction. In addition, there appears to be a diminished rise in plasma renin, and presumably this reduces angiotensin-mediated vasoconstriction.

The marked vasodilatation in skeletal muscle beds may be mediated, in part, by reflexes triggered by stimulation of intracardiac receptors[61,62] in a cycle that may involve hypotension due to peripheral vasodilatation, reflex-increased sympathetic stimulation of the heart, increased intramyocardial wall tension and stimulation of intracardiac receptors, and reflex-potentiated vasodilatation.[63] The vasodilatation may also be exacerbated by efferent cholinergic sympathetic stimulation of the arterioles in skeletal muscle.[59] With syncope the electroencephalogram shows slow wave activity of large amplitude.

The hyperventilation that generally precedes and accompanies vasodepressor syncope results in a decline in arterial pCO_2, which in turn produces cerebral vasoconstriction, thereby further impairing cerebral perfusion. Later, heart rate, arterial pressure, central venous pressure, and cardiac output decline precipitously.

During the recovery period, oliguria is common, mediated by increased secretion of antidiuretic hormone (ADH).[64] This finding suggests that some of the other clinical features of the syndrome, including pallor and nausea, may be mediated in part by posterior pituitary hormones.[65]

Management. Vasovagal syncope appearing for the first time demands a thorough diagnostic evaluation, since the syncope may be caused by conditions such as valvular or subvalvular aortic stenosis, hypertrophic obstructive cardiomyopathy, carotid sinus hypersensitivity, or another unrecognized cardiac or neurological abnormality. Therapy consists of placing the patient in the recumbent position with the lower extremities elevated (reverse Trendelenburg). Removal of the offending stimuli, inhalation of spirits of ammonia, and stimulation of the face with cold water usually suffice in treatment of the acute episode. Treatment with vasopressors is not usually required. Consciousness is usually regained rapidly, with a somewhat slower regression of bradycardia. Rarely, if recovery is delayed, atropine may be helpful.

CARDIAC CAUSES OF SYNCOPE. The common denominator in syncope of cardiac cause is a transient, marked diminution of cardiac output due to an arrhythmia or reduced stroke volume.[66,67] The association of syncope and bradycardia, first described by Gerbezius in 1719 and later by Morgagni in 1769[68] and by Adams in 1827,[69] was clarified by Stokes in 1846, who recognized the etiological connections between a change in heart rate and cerebral manifestations.[70] The mechanism underlying syncope even among patients with complete heart block is often a superimposed arrhythmia (such as transient asystole or ventricular fibrillation)[71] at the time of loss of consciousness[71] rather than the heart block per se. Thus, the generic term "arrhythmia-induced syncope" may be more useful.[72]

More than 50,000 new cases of complete heart block occur annually in the United States,[72] and approximately 50 per cent of patients with acquired, complete heart block experience syncope. The causes of complete heart block are listed in Table 28–3 and discussed in detail in Chapter 22.

Arrhythmias Causing Syncope (see also Chapter 22). Arrhythmia-induced syncope may result from asystole, severe bradycardia, or tachyarrhythmia and generally conforms to one of the following categories:

TABLE 28–3 CAUSES OF COMPLETE HEART BLOCK

1. Structural abnormalities of the conduction system
   a. Congenital heart block
   b. Infectious diseases such as diphtheria, syphilis, toxoplasmosis, mumps, rheumatic fever
   c. Collagen diseases
   d. Valvular heart disease
   e. Degenerative disease (Lev's disease, Lenegre's disease, Friedreich's ataxia, progressive muscular dystrophy, myotonic dystrophy, Duchenne's dystrophy)
   f. Coronary artery disease with or without infarction
   g. Tumors
   h. Endocrine and metabolic disorders (gout with urate deposition in the conduction system, hypo- and hyperthyroidism, hemochromatosis, Addison's disease)
   i. Trauma
   j. Diseases of unknown etiology (Reiter's syndrome, sarcoidosis, amyloidosis, Paget's disease)
2. Electrolyte disturbances such as hyperkalemia, acidosis, hypomagnesemia
3. Drug toxicity: Examples include digitalis, quinidine, lidocaine, aprindine, phenytoin (Dilantin), and amitriptyline (Elavil)

1. Transitory, complete interruption of atrioventricular conduction with asystole during the "preautomatic pause" or "pacemaker warm-up" interval.

2. Asystole developing in the presence of persistent complete heart block, owing to failure of the intra- or infranodal pacemaker, accompanied by a preautomatic pause in other potential pacemakers.

3. Paroxysmal ventricular tachycardia or fibrillation precipitated by ischemia due to the slow heart rate in patients with complete heart block.

4. Paroxysmal ventricular tachycardia or fibrillation in patients with normal atrioventricular conduction, recognized increasingly more often with the use of ambulatory electrocardiographic monitoring.

5. Supraventricular tachy- or bradyarrhythmias leading to decreased cardiac output secondary to the rate itself or to the deleterious effects of the arrhythmia on myocardial perfusion already compromised by coronary artery disease.

6. Asystole due to atrial standstill with failure of automaticity in subsidiary pacemakers, commonly seen in patients with the sick sinus syndrome.[73]

7. Combinations of conduction disturbances and supraventricular arrhythmia, commonly associated with the sick sinus syndrome (p. 693).

Hemodynamic Abnormalities Predisposing to Syncope. Systemic vascular resistance ordinarily declines as a consequence of arteriolar dilatation secondary to the accumulation of vasodilator metabolites during exercise. Normally, this vasodilatation is more than compensated for by the augmentation of cardiac output and arterial pressure during heavy exertion (Chap. 8). However, in those severe forms of heart disease in which cardiac output rises proportionately less than vascular resistance falls, arterial pressure declines, sometimes to hazardous levels. Thus, exertional hypotension and syncope are characteristic features of virtually all forms of heart disease in which cardiac output is relatively fixed and fails to rise normally or even declines during exertion. It is most characteristic of severe valvular aortic stenosis and other forms of obstruction to left ventricular outflow and of coronary artery disease in which global ischemia occurs during exertion.

The mechanism responsible for exertional hypotension and syncope in patients with lesions producing right or left outflow tract obstruction probably involves peripheral vasodilatation as well as decreased cardiac output, the former reflexes resulting from high intraventricular pressure acting on ventricular baroreceptors with blunting of the compensatory carotid and aortic baroreceptor-mediated reflexes.[74,75] Patients with aortic valvular stenosis have been shown to exhibit an excessive reduction of forearm vascular resistance with exertion, with a return of the physiological vasoconstrictor response after correction of the aortic valve lesion.[74] In patients in whom syncope can be ascribed to obstruction to left ventricular outflow, surgical intervention is ordinarily necessary (p. 1103). Syncope in patients with prosthetic cardiac valves is an ominous phenomenon, often indicative of the need for urgent reoperation to relieve a mechanical obstruction caused by serious dysfunction of the prosthetic valve or formation of a thrombus.

When left ventricular outflow tract obstruction is dynamic, as in hypertrophic obstructive cardiomyopathy (Chap. 41), it is exacerbated by increased contractility, decreased chamber dimensions, or decreased afterload and distending pressure. Thus, drugs with positive inotropic effects such as digitalis or arterial or venous vasodilators such as nitroglycerin may precipitate hypotension.[76]

Sustained hypotension associated with ischemic heart disease is usually due to severely impaired ventricular function, but episodic hypotension or syncope often results from conduction disturbances or arrhythmia. Sometimes, marked hypotension accompanies angina pectoris or acute myocardial infarction, owing to increased parasympathetic activity, particularly with ischemia of the inferior wall (Chap. 37). Afferent reflexes from atrial and ventricular myocardium or from the coronary vessels themselves elicit increased parasympathetic outflow, bradycardia, and hypotension, which, coupled with the decreased contractility resulting from ischemia, may precipitate syncope.[13,77,78]

Pedunculated left atrial myxoma (p. 1459) or a large thrombus may obstruct the left ventricular inflow tract and suddenly reduce cardiac output. An important clinical clue to the diagnosis is the association of syncope with specific postures (such as sitting or leaning forward) because of movement of a pedunculated or migratory tumor or clot into the left ventricular inflow tract.

Systemic hypotension may be a critical complication in patients with *congenital heart disease* characterized by right-to-left shunting (Chaps. 29 and 30). When pulmonary blood flow is reduced with right-to-left shunting through an intracardiac communication associated with obstruction to right ventricular outflow or severe pulmonary hypertension, marked arterial hypoxemia occurs; this serves as a potent vasodilatory stimulus.

Hypotension may also result from obstruction to outflow due to lesions *extrinsic* to the heart, such as massive pulmonary embolus (Chap. 46), Takayasu's disease (Chap. 45), and supravalvular aortic stenosis (Chaps. 29 and 30), all of which interfere with ventricular emptying. Syncope is a manifestation of primary pulmonary hypertension (Chap. 25) and rarely of pulmonary valvular stenosis (Chaps. 29 and 30); it may accompany cardiac tamponade (Chap. 43).

DIFFERENTIAL DIAGNOSIS OF SYNCOPE. Syncope and presyncope must be differentiated from a variety of other acute episodes. It is critical, for example, to distinguish syncopal episodes from epileptic seizures, particularly the akinetic type. In general, syncope due to vasomotor failure or impaired cardiac output occurs when the patient is in the upright position, although syncopal episodes secondary to cardiac arrhythmia may occur in any position. Syncope occurs most commonly in young women or elderly males and, in contrast to epilepsy, in most instances (1) is of gradual onset *without* aura; (2) is *not* associated with injury from falling; (3) is *not* associated with convulsive movements, biting of the lips, or urinary incontinence; (4) is *brief*, with a rapid return to consciousness; and (5) is *not* followed by a state of confusion.

Epileptic seizures, in contrast, can occur with the patient in any position and are sudden in onset; the warning aura, if it occurs at all, lasts only a few seconds. Injury from falling is frequent, as are convulsive movements with the eyes upturned. The period of unconsciousness usually lasts for minutes, and there is often urinary incontinence, biting of the lips, and a prolonged postictal state of mental confusion and drowsiness.

Attacks of *cerebral ischemia* due to cerebral arteriosclerosis may produce transient ischemic attacks characterized by neurological deficits that tend to resemble each other from attack to attack. These are often visual disturbances, hemiparesis, hemianesthesia, slurred speech, and impaired consciousness.

Anxiety attacks may produce dizziness but not frank syncope. They are usually characterized by, and can be reproduced by, hyperventilation, which results in reduction of cerebral blood flow; are not accompanied by cardiac arrhythmia; and are not relieved by recumbency. *Hysterical fainting* occurs most frequently in persons with hysterical personalities and is not accompanied by any changes in blood pressure, heart rate, or skin color. *Hypoglycemia* is manifested by confusion, sinus tachycardia, jitteriness, and other symptoms of sympathetic stimulation, ultimately leading to loss of consciousness. Loss of consciousness with this entity proceeds gradually but is often prolonged, constituting frank coma. When caused by a tumor of the islets of Langerhans, it occurs with and can be reproduced by prolonged fasting, but when hypoglycemia is reactive, it tends to occur 3 to 5 hours after meals. The diagnosis is confirmed by the finding of reduced blood glucose.

APPROACH TO DIAGNOSIS OF POSTURAL HYPOTENSION AND SYNCOPE

The cause of postural hypotension or syncope is often obvious, after a thorough history and physical examination and laboratory tests selected on the basis of positive findings have been done. In taking the patient's history, the examiner must determine the onset, frequency, and duration of premonitory symptoms; circumstances surrounding the attacks (such as relationship to meals, alcohol ingestion, cough, micturition, defecation, or movements of the head and neck); associated symptoms such as nausea, vomiting, chest pain, or dyspnea; medications utilized; the presence of potentially predisposing disorders such as diabetes mellitus, chronic illness with weight loss, prolonged bed rest, blood loss, or plasma volume depletion. Exclusion of the simple faint is important, since this condition usually requires no treatment and only minor investigation.

Physical examination should focus on the following:

1. Evaluation of blood pressure with the patient recumbent and standing after the patient has been recumbent for at least 3 minutes;
2. Evaluation of blood pressure in both arms and legs;
3. Recognition of bruits in the carotid, subclavian, supraorbital, and temporal vessels;
4. Detection of cyanosis, clubbing, and other signs of congenital heart disease; and
5. Assessment of the heart rate and blood pressure response to carotid sinus pressure and simulated movements precipitating syncope.

Accurate measure of blood pressure with the patient recumbent and sitting is all that is required to detect postural hypotension. The patient should be recumbent for at least 3 minutes before assuming an upright posture. If acceleration of heart rate accompanies postural hypotension, the syncope is more likely to be drug-induced, secondary to prolonged deconditioning, or due to old age rather than

TABLE 28–4 EVALUATION OF AUTONOMIC FUNCTION

Procedure	Mechanism and Normal Pathway Tested	Normal Response	Usual Clinical Implications of Abnormal Response
Standing (sometimes simulated in the laboratory with the use of a tilt table)	Systemic venous pooling of blood leads to a reduction of cardiac output, decreased baroreceptor discharge, and consequent vasomotor center stimulation in the central nervous system, sympathetic discharge, and end-organ response and vasoconstriction	≤ 20 mm Hg decrease of systolic arterial blood pressure associated with modest tachycardia and an increase of ≥ 140 pg/ml of plasma norepinephrine	Exaggerated hypotension suggests the presence of a lesion affecting the afferent, central, or efferent adrenal system or end-organ unresponsiveness
Deep breathing	Afferent, central, and efferent vagal system	≥ 10 beat/min variation in heart rate or R-R interval measured electrocardiographically	Impaired vagal function due to afferent, central, or efferent component lesions or end-organ unresponsiveness
Valsalva maneuver	Increased intrathoracic pressure diminishes systemic venous return to the heart after transitory augmentation of pulmonary venous return. Cardiac output declines, eliciting systemic hypotension, decreased baroreceptor discharge, and afferent, central, and efferent sympathoadrenal discharge with tachycardia. Sustained sympathoadrenal discharge results in a post-Valsalva overshoot of blood pressure and consequent modest bradycardia	A 4-phase response, including transitory initial blood pressure elevation, ≥ 50% decrease of systemic arterial blood pressure with tachycardia during the maneuver, and a blood pressure overshoot with modest tachycardia after release of Valsalva	Sympathetic lesion (afferent, central, efferent) or end-organ unresponsiveness
Hyperventilation	Vasomotor center responsivity and efferent sympathoadrenal system	A decrease of arterial pressure of 10 to 20 mm Hg	A central lesion
Cold pressor test (immersion of an extremity in ice water for 1 to 3 minutes)	Centrally mediated sympathoadrenal discharge as well as afferent pain fiber stimulation, spinal cord reflex arcs, efferent sympathetic discharge, and end-organ response	≥ 15 mm Hg increase in both systolic and diastolic blood pressure	A central or efferent sympathetic lesion
Inhalation of amyl nitrite	Systemic arterial vasodilatation leads to reduction of systemic arterial blood pressure, decreased baroreceptor discharge, afferent and central nervous system stimulation, and efferent sympathetic discharge	Tachycardia in response to systemic arterial hypotension	Central or efferent sympathetic lesion
Induction of hyperthermia	Augmentation of core temperature by 1°C leads to centrally mediated sympathetic stimulation involving cholinergic postganglionic neurons	Sweating	Central or efferent sympathetic lesions. End-organ unresponsiveness can be excluded with a direct sweat test with 5 to 15 mg of pilocarpine HCl or electrical stimulation
Administration of atropine (0.02 mg/kg)	Efferent parasympathetic fibers, including vagal fibers	An increase of heart rate by ≥ 20% or resting rate	Central or efferent parasympathetic impairment
Administration of tyramine (200 to 6000 μg doses incrementally)	Release of catecholamine stores from adrenergic nerves	Increased systemic blood pressure by ≤ 20 mm Hg/1000 μg bolus	Postganglionic sympathetic lesion
Norepinephine bitartrate (0.05 to 0.07 μg/kg/min)	End-organ response (peripheral vasculature)	An increase of systolic and diastolic blood pressures of approximately 20 mm Hg	Exaggerated hypertension implies the presence of a postganglionic sympathetic lesion or denervation hypersensitivity
Responses of the pupil to conjunctival sac instillations of 1 to 2 drops of epinephrine HCl (1:1000) or 4% phenylephrine or indirect-acting agents such as hydroxamphetamine (1%) or cocaine (4%)	End-organ response	No effect with dilute solutions of direct-acting agents; mydriasis with indirect-acting agents	Exaggerated response to epinephrine implies the presence of a postganglionic sympathetic lesion (denervation hypersensitivity). Absence of mydriasis to indirect-acting agents but not to cocaine implies a preganglionic or central lesion. A sympathetic lesion can be confirmed by absence of mydriasis induced by homatropine (5%), a cholinergic antagonist

Modified from Henrich, W. L.: Autonomic insufficiency. Arch. Intern. Med. *142*:339, 1982.

because of degenerative or familial orthostatic hypotension. Detection of bruits in the vessels of the neck may suggest vascular obstruction. Since hypotensive episodes due to congenital heart disease in adults are usually caused by intracardiac shunts, cyanosis and clubbing may be important clues. Carotid hypersensitivity is established by maneuvers that reproduce the patient's symptoms and by simulation of movements potentially precipitating syncope in a given case, such as turning movements of the head. Assessment of the blood pressure in both arms and legs is particularly helpful in detecting differences due to obstructive vascular disease such as Takayasu's disease.

Test of autonomic function may be particularly helpful (Table 28–4). In addition, assessment of the following may be useful:

1. Twenty-four–hour (ambulatory) electrocardiographic recordings (p. 632): Many patients with underlying cardiac causes of syncope have normal electrocardiograms between attacks, although some exhibit abnormalities such as premature ventricular contractions, atrial arrhythmias, or minor conduction defects. These abnormalities in themselves do not confirm the cause of syncope. Often it is necessary to monitor the patient for 24 hours, preferably during his or her usual activities. Short runs of ventricular tachycardia, transient complete heart block, or asystole may be demonstrable. If the patient develops syncope or presyncope during the recording, and the electrocardiogram reveals an arrhythmia that can account for the symptoms, appropriate treatment is instituted; this usually consists of drugs for tachyarrhythmias and permanent pacing for bradyarrythmias. If, on the other hand, the recording is normal even though the patient concurrently develops syncope, arrhythmias can be excluded as a cause of symptoms. If the patient remains asymptomatic during a recording that shows arrhythmias, it may be desirable to repeat the 24-hour electrocardiogram, commence a trial of antiarrhythmic therapy, or carry out the electrophysiological studies described below. The last-named, in any case, are indicated when patients are asymptomatic during the recording, when the recording is normal or nearly so, and when no other medical or neurological cause of syncope or presyncope is evident.

2. Electrophysiological evaluation with programmed atrial and ventricular stimulation: This technique may be very helpful in establishing the diagnosis and selecting treatment for tachy- and bradyarrhythmias and intermittent conduction disturbances leading to syncope[79–81] (p. 634). Induction of the responsible arrhythmia by programmed ventricular stimulation and suppression of inducibility by specific pharmacological agents provide an objective means of selecting appropriate therapy. When the cause of syncope is obscure, inducibility of recurrent atrial or ventricular tachycardia accompanied by syncope or presyncope strongly suggests that the arrhythmia occurs spontaneously and is responsible for the syncope.[79,80] The presence of uni- or bifascicular block with stress-induced complete heart block by atrial pacing, a prolonged His-ventricular (HV) interval on His bundle recordings, or the demonstration of prolonged sinoatrial node recovery in patients with symptoms of hypotension or syncope may implicate conduction system disease, requiring a permanent artificial pacemaker.[82]

3. Determination of levels of plasma electrolytes, catecholamines (with the patient supine and upright), dopamine beta-hydroxylase, and urinary vanillylmandelic acid (VMA): Under physiological conditions, plasma catecholamine concentrations increase several-fold with assumption of the upright position. In contrast, among patients with idiopathic orthostatic hypotension or diabetic neuropathy, the response is markedly blunted or absent. In these patients, basal plasma dopamine beta-hydroxylase levels are low, and values do not increase with assumption of an upright posture. Urinary VMA and plasma catecholamines are elevated markedly in patients with pheochromocytoma; rarely, the tumor may secrete predominantly epinephrine, eliciting paradoxical hypotension.

4. Determination of plasma aldosterone and mineralocorticoids: Among patients with primary or secondary adrenal cortical insufficiency or hypoaldosteronism, concentrations of plasma and urinary mineralocorticoids are low.

5. Glucose tolerance test: A normal glucose tolerance test with normal plasma insulin responses will exclude functional hypoglycemia or an insulin-secreting tumor.

6. Electroencephalography: This test frequently detects abnormalities in patients with epilepsy, even when these studies are performed between attacks.

7. Ophthalmotonometry and cerebral angiography: These tests are sometimes necessary to identify a cerebral or extracranial vascular lesion.

8. Physiological stress tests, such as carotid sinus stimulation and tilt-table tests, with evaluation of the plasma catecholamine response: In patients with orthostatic hypotension or recurring vasovagal fainting episodes without obvious cause, it may be necessary to assess the hemodynamic and catecholamine responses to tilting, since hypotension without a physiological compensatory elaboration of catecholamines is common in this entity.

A combined approach that employs meticulous acquisition of historical data, thorough physical examination, and judicious utilization of selected laboratory procedures will generally delineate even the most obscure causes of recurrent hypotension and syncope.

References

1. Folkow, B.: Nervous control of the blood vessels. Physiol. Rev. *35*:629, 1955.
2. Hickam, J. B., and Pryor, W. W.: Cardiac output in postural hypotension. J. Clin. Invest. *30*:410, 1951.
3. Cryer, P. E., and Weiss, S.: Reduced plasma norepinephrine response to standing in autonomic dysfunction. Arch. Neurol. *33*:275, 1976.
4. Hines, S., and Houston, M.: The clinical spectrum of autonomic dysfunction. Am. J. Med. *70*:1091, 1981.
5. Linch, D. C., Shaw, K. M., Mohleman, M. F., and Ross, E. J.: Bromocriptine induced postural hypotension in acromegaly. Lancet *2*:320, 1978.
6. Bradbury, S., and Eggleston, C.: Postural hypotension: A report of three cases. Am. Heart J. *1*:73, 1925.
7. Shy, G. M., and Drager, G. A.: A neurological syndrome associated with orthostatic hypotension. A clinical pathological study. Arch. Neurol. *2*:511, 1960.
8. Cohen, J. I. (ed.): Postural hypotension. Johns Hopkins Med. J. *148*:127, 1981.
9. Bannister, R.: Degeneration of the autonomic nervous system. Lancet *2*:175, 1971.
10. Ziegler, M. G., Lake, C. R., and Kopin, I. J.: The sympathetic nervous system defect in primary orthostatic hypotension. N. Engl. J. Med. *296*:293, 1977.
11. Hilsted, J., Parving, H.-H., Christensen, N. J., Benn, J., and Galbo, H.: Hemodynamics in diabetic orthostatic hypotension. J. Clin. Invest. *68*:1427, 1981.
12. Bannister, R., Ardill, L., and Fentem, P.: Defective autonomic control of blood vessels in idiopathic orthostatic hypotension. Brain *90*:725, 1967.
13. Abboud, F. M., Heistad, D. D., Mark, A. L., and Schmid, P. G.: Reflex control of the peripheral circulation. Prog. Cardiovasc. Dis. *18*:371, 1976.

14. Bannister, R.: Chronic autonomic failure with postural hypotension. Lancet. *2*: 404, 1979.
15. Kontos, H. A., Richardson, D. W., and Norvell, J. E.: Norepinephrine depletion in idiopathic orthostatic hypotension. Ann. Intern. Med. *82*:336, 1975.
16. Bannister, R., Crowe, R., Eames, R., and Brunstock, G.: Adrenergic innervation in autonomic failure. Neurology *31*:1501, 1981.
17. Luft, R., and von Euler, U. S.: Two cases of postural hypotension showing a deficiency in release of norepinephrine and epinephrine. J. Clin. Invest. *32*: 1065, 1953.
18. Hickler, R. B., Thompson, G. R., Fox, L. M., et al.: Successful treatment of orthostatic hypotension with 9-alpha-fluorohydrocortisone. N. Engl. J. Med. *261*:788, 1959.
19. Goodall, M., Harlan, W. R., Jr., and Alton, H.: Noradrenaline release and metabolism in orthostatic (postural) hypotension. Circulation *36*:489, 1967.
20. Goodall, M. C. C., Harlan, W. R., Jr., and Alton, H.: Decreased noradrenaline (norepinephrine) synthesis in neurogenic orthostatic hypotension. Circulation *38*:592, 1968.
20a. Wilcox, C. S.: Current therapy for orthostatic hypotension. J. Cardiovasc. Med. *8*:292, 1983.
21. Fouad, F. M., Tarazi, R. C., and Bravo, E. L.: Dihydroergotamine in idiopathic orthostatic hypotension: Short-term intramuscular and long-term oral therapy. Clin. Pharmacol. Ther. *30*:782, 1981.
21a. Chobanian, A. V., Tifft, C. P., Faxon, D. P., Creager, M. A., and Sackel, H.: Treatment of chronic orthostatic hypotension with ergotamine. Circulation *67*: 602, 1983.
22. Diamond, M. A., Murray, R. H., and Schmid, P. G.: Idiopathic postural hypotension: Physiological observations and report of a new mode of therapy. J. Clin. Invest. *49*:1341, 1970.
23. Lubke, K. O.: A controlled study with Dihydergot on patients with orthostatic dysregulation. Cardiology *61*(Suppl. 1):333, 1976.
24. Nanda, R. N., Johnson, R. H., and Keogh, H. J.: Treatment of neurogenic orthostatic hypotension with a monoamine oxidase inhibitor and tyramine. Lancet *2*:1164, 1976.
25. Brevetti, G., Chiariello, M., Giudice, P., De Michele, G., Mansi, D., and Campanella, G.: Effective treatment of orthostatic hypotension by propranolol in the Shy-Drager syndrome. Am. Heart J. *102*:938, 1981.
26. Riley, C. M., Day, R. L., Greeley, D. M., and Langford, W. E.: Central autonomic dysfunction with defective lacrimation. I. Report of 5 cases. Pediatrics *3*: 468, 1949.
27. Dancis, J., and Smith, A. A.: Familial dysautonomia. N. Engl. J. Med. *274*: 207, 1966.
28. Ziegler, M. G., Lake, C. R., and Kopin, I. J.: Deficient sympathetic nervous response in familial dysautonomia. N. Engl. J. Med. *294*:630, 1976.
29. Smith, A. A., and Dancis, J.: Catecholamine release in familial dysautonomia. N. Engl. J. Med. *277*:61, 1967.
30. Williams, G. H., Cain, J. P., Dluhy, R. G., and Underwood, R. H.: Studies of the control of plasma aldosterone concentration in normal man. I. Response to posture, acute and chronic volume depletion, and sodium loading. J. Clin. Invest. *51*:1731, 1972.
31. Streeten, D. H. P., Kerr, L. P., Prior, J. C., Kerr, C., and Dalakos, T. G.: Hyperbradykininism: A new orthostatic syndrome. Lancet *2*:1048, 1972.
32. McHenry, L. C., Jr., Fazekas, J. F., and Sullivan, J. F.: Cerebral hemodynamics of syncope. Am. J. Med. Sci. *241*:173, 1961.
33. Rossen, R., Kabat, H., and Anderson, J. P.: Acute arrest of cerebral circulation in man. A.M.A. Arch. Neurol. Psychiatry *50*:510, 1943.
34. Hering, H. E.: Die Sinus Reflexe vom Sinus Caroticus werden durch einen Nerven (Sinusvert) vermittelt, der ein Ast des Nervus glossopharyngeus ist. Munch. Med. Wschr. *71*:1265, 1924.
35. Weiss, S., and Baker, J. P.: The carotid sinus reflex in health and disease: Its role in the causation of fainting and convulsions. Medicine *12*:297, 1933.
35a. Leatham, A.: Carotid sinus syncope. Br. Heart J. *47*:409, 1982.
36. Gardner, R. S., Magovern, G. J., Park, S. B., Cushing, W. J., Liebler, G. A., and Hughes, R.: Carotid sinus syndrome: New surgical considerations. Vasc. Surg. *9*:204, 1975.
37. Peretz, D. I., Gerein, A. N., and Miyahishima, R. T.: Permanent demand pacing for hypersensitive carotid sinus syndrome. Can. Med. Assoc. J. *108*:1131, 1973.
37a. Morley, C. A., Perrins, E. J., Grant, P., Chan, S. L., McBrien, D. J., and Sutton, R.: Carotid sinus syncope treated by pacing. Analysis of persistent symptoms and role of atrioventricular sequential pacing. Br. Heart J. *47*:411, 1982.
38. Walter, P. F., Crawley, I. S., and Dorney, E. R.: Carotid sinus hypersensitivity and syncope. Am. J. Cardiol. *42*:396, 1978.
39. Lown, B., and Levine, S. A.: The carotid sinus: Clinical value of its stimulation. Circulation *23*:766, 1961.
40. Lesser, L. M., and Wenger, N. K.: Carotid sinus syncope. Heart Lung *5*:453, 1976.
41. Trout, H. H., III, Brown, L. I., and Thompson, J. E.: Carotid sinus syndrome: Treatment by carotid sinus denervation. Ann. Surg. *189*:575, 1979.
42. Lee, Y. T., Lee, T. K., and Tsai, H. C.: Glossopharyngeal neuralgia as the cause of cardiac syncope: A case report with a review of literature. J. Formosan Med. Assoc. *4*:103, 1975.
43. Khero, B. A., and Millins, C. B.: Cardiac syncope due to glossopharyngeal neuralgia. Arch. Intern. Med. *128*:806, 1971.
44. Kong, Y., Heyman, A., Entman, M. L., and McIntosh, H. D.: Glossopharyngeal neuralgia associated with bradycardia, syncope, and seizures. Circulation *30*:109, 1964.
45. Dykman, T. R., Montgomery, E. B., Gerstenberger, P. D., Zeiger, H. E., Clutter, W. E., and Cryer, P. E.: Glossopharyngeal neuralgia with syncope secondary to tumor: Treatment and pathophysiology. Am. J. Med. *71*:165, 1981.
46. Waddington, J. K. B., Matthews, H. R., Evans, C. C., and Ward, D. W.: Carcinoma of the esophagus with swallow syncope. Br. Med. J. *3*:232, 1975.
47. Wik, B., and Hillestead, L.: Deglutition syncope. Br. Med. J. *3*:747, 1975.
48. Tolman, K. G., and Ashworth, W.: Syncope induced by dysphagia correction by esophageal dilatation. Am. J. Dig. Dis. *16*:1026, 1971.
49. Levin, B., and Posner, J. B.: Swallow syncope. Neurology *22*:1086, 1972.
50. Weiss, S., and Ferris, E. B.: Adams-Stokes syndrome with transient complete heart block of vasovagal reflex origin. Arch. Intern. Med. *54*:931, 1934.
51. James, A. H.: Cardiac syncope after swallowing. Lancet *1*:771, 1958.
52. Haldane, J. H.: Micturition syncope. Can. Med. Assoc. J. *101*:712, 1969.
53. Godec, C. J., and Cass, A. S.: Micturition syncope. J. Urol. *126*:551, 1981.
54. Larson, S. J., Sances, A., Baker, J. B., and Reigel, D.: Herniated cerebellar tonsils and cough syncope. J. Neurosurg. *40*:524, 1974.
55. Corbett, J. J., Butler, A. B., and Kaufman, B.: Sneeze syncope, basilar invagination and Arnold-Chiari type I malformation. J. Neurol. Neurosurg. Psychiatry *39*:381, 1976.
56. Wayne, H. H.: Syncope, physiological considerations and an analysis of the clinical characteristics in 510 patients. Am. J. Med. *30*:418, 1961.
56a. Day, S. C., Cook, F., Funkenstein,, H., and Goldman, L.: Evaluation and outcome of emergency room patients with transient loss of consciousness. Am. J. Med. *73*:15, 1983.
57. Barcroft, H., Edholm, O. G., McMichael, J., and Sharpey-Schafer, E. P.: Posthemorrhagic fainting: Study by cardiac output and forearm flow. Lancet *1*:489, 1944.
58. Weissler, A. M., Warren, J. V., Estes, E. H., Jr., McIntosh, H. D., and Leonard, J. J.: Vasodepressor syncope: Factors influencing cardiac output. Circulation *15*:875, 1957.
59. Glick, G., and Yu, P. N.: Hemodynamic changes during spontaneous vasovagal reactions. Am. J. Med. *34*:42, 1963.
60. Epstein, S. E., Stampfer, M., and Beiser, G. D.: Role of the capacitance and resistance vessels in vasovagal syncope. Circulation *37*:524, 1968.
61. Aviado, D. M., Jr., and Schmidt, C. F.: Cardiovascular and respiratory reflexes from the left side of the heart. Am. J. Physiol. *196*:726, 1959.
62. Friedberg, C. K.: Syncope: Pathological physiology: Differential diagnosis and treatment (II). Mod. Concepts Cardiovasc. Dis. *40*:61, 1971.
63. Martin, A. K., Hackel, D. B., and Sieber, H. O.: Intraventricular pressure changes in dogs during hemorrhagic shock. Fed. Proc. *22*:252, 1963.
64. Brun, C., Knudsen, E. O. E., and Raaschou, F.: Kidney function and circulatory collapse, postsyncopal oliguria. J. Clin. Invest. *25*:568, 1946.
65. Stead, E. A., Jr., Kunkel, P., and Weiss, S.: Effect of pitressin in circulatory collapse induced by sodium nitrate. J. Clin. Invest. *18*:673, 1939.
66. Wright, K. E., Jr., and McIntosh, H. D.: Syncope: A review of pathophysiological mechanisms. Progr. Cardiovasc. Dis. *13*:580, 1971.
67. MacMurray, F. G.: Stokes-Adams disease: A historical review. N. Engl. J. Med. *256*:643, 1957.
68. Morgagni, J. B.: The seats and causes of disease. *In* Major, H. H. (ed.): Classic Descriptions of Disease. Oxford, Blackwell Scientific Publications, 1948, p. 346.
69. Adams, R.: Cases of diseases of the heart, accompanied with pathological observations. Dublin Hosp. Rep. *4*:353, 1827.
70. Stokes, W.: Observations on some cases of permanently slow pulse. Dublin Q. J. Med. Sci. *2*:73, 1846.
71. Parkinson, J., Papp, C., and Evans, W.: The electrocardiogram of the Stokes-Adams attack. Br. Heart J. *3*:171, 1941.
72. Pomerantz, B., and O'Rourke, R. A.: The Stokes-Adams syndrome. Am. J. Med. *46*:941, 1969.
73. Moss, A. J., and Davis, R. J.: Brady-tachy syndrome. Prog. Cardiovasc. Dis. *16*:439, 1974.
74. Mark, A. L., Kioschos, J. M., Abboud, F. M., Heistadt, D., and Schmid, P. G.: Abnormal vascular responses to exercise in patients with aortic stenosis. J. Clin. Invest. *52*:1138, 1973.
75. Flamm, M. D., Braniff, B. A., Kimball, R., and Hancock, E. W.: Mechanism of effort syncope in aortic stenosis. Circulation *35*:II–109, 1967.
76. Braunwald, E., Brockenbrough, E. D., and Frye, R. L.: Studies on digitalis. V. Comparison of the effects of ouabain on left ventricular dynamics in valvular aortic stenosis and hypertrophic subaortic stenosis. Circulation *26*:166, 1962.
77. Jarisch, A., and Zotterman, Y.: Depressor reflexes from the heart. Acta Physiol. Scand. *16*:31, 1948.
78. Eckberg, D. L., Drabinsky, M., and Braunwald, E.: Defective cardiac parasympathetic control in patients with heart disease. N. Engl. J. Med. *285*:877, 1971.
79. DiMarco, J. P., Garan, H., Harthorne, W., and Ruskin, J. N.: Intracardiac electrophysiologic techniques in recurrent syncope of unknown cause. Ann. Intern. Med. *95*:542, 1981.
80. Josephson, M. D., and Seides, S. F.: Clinical Cardiac Electrophysiology: Techniques and Interpretations. Philadelphia, Lea and Febiger, 1979, p. 44.
81. Kapoor, W. N., Karpf, M., Maher, Y., Miller, R. A., and Levey, G. S.: Syncope of unknown origin: The need for a more cost-effective approach to its diagnostic evaluation. J.A.M.A. *247*:2687, 1982.
82. Hauer, R. N. W., Lie, K. I., Liem, K. L., and Durrer, D.: Long term prognosis in patients with bundle branch block complicating acute anteroseptal infarction. Am. J. Cardiol. *49*:1581, 1982.

PART III

DISEASES OF THE HEART, PERICARDIUM, AORTA, AND PULMONARY VASCULAR BED

29 CONGENITAL HEART DISEASE IN INFANCY AND CHILDHOOD

by William F. Friedman, M.D.

INTRODUCTION

DEFINITION. Congenital cardiovascular disease is defined as an abnormality at birth in cardiocirculatory structure or function.

Congenital cardiovascular malformations result generally from altered embryonic development of a normal structure or failure of such a structure to progress beyond an early stage of embryonic or fetal development. The aberrant patterns of flow created by an anatomical defect may, in turn, significantly influence the structural and functional development of the rest of the circulation. For instance, the presence in utero of mitral atresia may not permit normal development of the left ventricle, aortic valve, and ascending aorta. Similarly, speculation exists that constriction of the fetal ductus arteriosus may result directly in right ventricular dilatation and tricuspid regurgitation in the fetus and newborn, contribute importantly to the development of pulmonary arterial aneurysms in the presence of ventricular septal defect and absent pulmonic valve, or, further, result in an alteration in the number and caliber of fetal and newborn pulmonary vascular resistance vessels. In this same regard, postnatal events may markedly influence the clinical presentation of a specific "isolated" malformation. The infant with Ebstein's malformation of the tricuspid valve may improve dramatically as the magnitude of tricuspid regurgitation diminishes with normal fall in pulmonary vascular resistance after birth; the infant with hypoplastic left heart syndrome or interrupted aortic arch may not exhibit circulatory collapse, and the baby with pulmonic atresia or severe stenosis may not become cyanotic until normal spontaneous closure occurs of a patent ductus arteriosus. Ductal constriction many days after birth may also be a central factor in some infants in the development of coarctation of the aorta. Still later in life the patient with a ventricular septal defect may experience spontaneous closure of the abnormal communication, or develop right ventricular outflow tract obstruction and/or aortic regurgitation, or pulmonary vascular obstructive disease. These selected examples serve to emphasize that anatomical and physiological changes in the heart and circulation may continue indefinitely from prenatal life in association with any specific congenital cardiocirculatory lesion.

It should be recognized further that certain congenital defects are not apparent on gross inspection of the heart or circulation. Examples include the electrophysiological pathways for ventricular preexcitation or interruptions in the cardiac conduction system giving rise to paroxysmal supraventricular tachycardia or congenital complete heart block, respectively. Similarly, abnormalities in the development of myocardial autonomic innervation or in the ultrastructure of myocardial cells may ultimately prove to contribute to asymmetrical septal hypertrophy and left ventricular outflow tract obstruction. These examples make clear that occasional difficulties arise in distinguishing between congenital anomalies that are readily apparent at or shortly after birth and lesions that may have as their basis a subtle or undetectable abnormality that is present at birth.

INCIDENCE. The true incidence of congenital cardiovascular malformations is difficult to determine accurately, partly because of the difficulties in definition discussed above. It has been estimated that approximately 0.8 per cent of live births are complicated by a cardiovascular malformation.[1] This figure does not take into account what may be the two most common cardiac anomalies: the congenital, nonstenotic bicuspid aortic valve[2] and the leaflet abnormality associated with mitral valve prolapse.[3] Moreover, the widely quoted 0.8 per cent incidence figure fails to include small preterm infants, almost all of whom have persistent patent ductus arteriosus, or the prevalence of cardiovascular abnormalities in stillborn infants. Thus, it is clear that past statistical analyses have seriously underestimated the incidence of congenital heart disease.

Precise data concerning frequency of individual congenital lesions are also lacking, and the results of many analyses differ, depending upon the source (living or dead) and the selection of the study population.[4] Table 29–1 is a compilation from both clinical and pathological studies that approximates the frequency of occurrence of specific cardiovascular malformations.[5,6]

Taken in toto, children with congenital heart disease are predominantly male. Moreover, specific defects may show a definite sex preponderance; patent ductus arteriosus and atrial septal defect are more common in females, whereas valvular aortic stenosis, coarctation of the aorta, tetralogy of Fallot, and transposition of the great arteries are more common in males.

TABLE 29–1 FREQUENCY OF OCCURRENCE OF CARDIAC MALFORMATIONS AT BIRTH

Disease	Percentage
Ventricular septal defect	30.5
Atrial septal defect	9.8
Patent ductus arteriosus	9.7
Pulmonic stenosis	6.9
Coarctation of the aorta	6.8
Aortic stenosis	6.1
Tetralogy of Fallot	5.8
Complete transposition of the great arteries	4.2
Persistent truncus arteriosus	2.2
Tricuspid atresia	1.3
All others	16.5

Data based on 2310 cases.

Extracardiac anomalies occur in approximately 25 per cent of infants with significant cardiac disease,[7] and their presence may significantly increase mortality. Often the extracardiac anomalies are multiple, in part involving the musculoskeletal system; one third of infants with both cardiac and extracardiac anomalies have some established syndrome.

ETIOLOGY. Malformations appear to result from an interaction between multifactorial genetic and environmental systems too complex to allow a single specification of etiology.[8] In most instances, a causal factor cannot be identified. Maternal rubella, ingestion of thalidomide early during gestation, and chronic maternal alcohol abuse are environmental insults known to interfere with normal cardiogenesis in man.[9–12] *Rubella syndrome* consists of cataracts, deafness, microcephaly, and, either singly or in combination, patent ductus arteriosus, pulmonic valvular and/or arterial stenosis, and atrial septal defect. *Thalidomide* is associated with major limb deformities and occasionally with cardiac malformations without predilection for a specific lesion. The *fetal alcohol syndrome* consists of microcephaly, micrognathia, microphthalmia, prenatal growth retardation, developmental delay, and cardiac defects. The latter—often defects of the ventricular septum—occur in approximately 45 per cent of affected infants. *Maternal lupus erythematosus* during pregnancy has recently been linked to congenital complete heart block (p. 1014). Animal experiments have incriminated hypoxia, deficiency or excess of several vitamins, intake of several categories of drugs, and ionizing irradiation as teratogens capable of causing cardiac malformations.[10] The precise relationship of these animal teratogens to human malformations is not clear.

The genetic aspects of congenital heart disease are discussed extensively in Chapter 47. A single gene mutation may be causative in the familial forms of atrial septal defect with prolonged AV conduction, mitral valve prolapse, ventricular septal defect, congenital heart block, situs inversus, pulmonary hypertension, the combination of supravalvular aortic stenosis and peripheral pulmonary arterial stenosis, and the syndromes of Noonan, LEOPARD, Holt-Oram, Ellis–van Creveld, and Kartagener. Table 29–

TABLE 29–2 SYNDROMES WITH ASSOCIATED CARDIOVASCULAR INVOLVEMENT

Syndrome	Major Cardiovascular Manifestations	Major Noncardiac Abnormalities
Heritable and Possibly Heritable		
Ellis–van Creveld	Single atrium or atrial septal defect	Chondrodystrophic dwarfism, nail dysplasia, polydactyly
TAR (thrombocytopenia-absent radius)	Atrial septal defect, tetralogy of Fallot	Radial aplasia or hypoplasia, thrombocytopenia
Holt-Oram	Atrial septal defect (other defects common)	Skeletal upper limb defect, hypoplasia of clavicles
Kartagener	Dextrocardia	Situs inversus, sinusitis, bronchiectasis
Laurence-Moon-Biedl-Bardet	Variable defects	Retinal pigmentation, obesity, polydactyly
Noonan	Pulmonic valve dysplasia	Webbed neck, pectus excavatum, cryptorchidism
Tuberous sclerosis	Rhabdomyoma, cardiomyopathy	Phakomatosis, bone lesions, hamartomatous skin lesions
Multiple lentigenes (LEOPARD)	Pulmonic stenosis	Basal cell nevi, broad facies, rib anomalies
Rubinstein-Taybi	Patent ductus arteriosus (others)	Broad thumbs and toes, hypoplastic maxilla, slanted palpebral fissures
Familial deafness	Arrhythmias, sudden death	Sensorineural deafness
Friedreich's ataxia	Cardiomyopathy and conduction defects	Ataxia, speech defect, degeneration of spinal cord dorsal columns
Muscular dystrophy	Cardiomyopathy	Pseudohypertrophy of calf muscles, weakness of trunk and proximal limb muscles
Weber-Osler-Rendu	Arteriovenous fistulas (lung, liver, mucous membranes)	Multiple telangiectasias
Cystic fibrosis	Cor pulmonale	Pancreatic insufficiency, malabsorption, chronic lung disease
Sickle cell anemia	Cardiomyopathy, mitral regurgitation	Hemoglobin SS
Conradi-Hünermann	Ventricular septal defect, patent ductus arteriosus	Asymmetrical limb shortness, early punctate mineralization, large skin pores
Cockayne	Accelerated atherosclerosis	Cachectic dwarfism, retinal pigment abnormalities, photosensitivity dermatitis
Progeria	Accelerated atherosclerosis	Premature aging, alopecia, atrophy of subcutaneous fat, skeletal hypoplasia
Apert	Ventricular septal defect	Craniosynostosis, midfacial hypoplasia, syndactyly
Incontinentia pigmenti	Patent ductus arteriosus	Irregular pigmented skin lesions, patchy alopecia, hypodontia
Connective Tissue Disorders		
Cutis laxa	Peripheral pulmonic stenosis	Generalized disruption of elastic fibers, diminished skin resilience, hernias
Ehlers-Danlos	Arterial dilatation and rupture, mitral regurgitation	Hyperextensible joints, hyperelastic and friable skin
Marfan	Aortic dilatation, aortic and mitral incompetence	Gracile habitus, arachnodactyly with hyperextensibility, lens subluxation
Osteogenesis imperfecta	Aortic incompetence	Fragile bones, blue sclerae
Pseudoxanthoma elasticum	Peripheral and coronary arterial disease	Degeneration of elastic fibers in skin, retinal angioid streaks
Inborn Errors of Metabolism		
Pompe's disease	Glycogen storage disease of heart	Acid maltase deficiency, muscular weakness
Homocystinuria	Aortic and pulmonary artery dilatation, intravascular thrombosis	Cystathionine synthetase deficiency, lens subluxation, osteoporosis
Mucopolysaccharidoses:		
Hurler; Hunter	Multivalvular and coronary and great artery disease, cardiomyopathy	Hurler: Deficiency of α-L-iduronidase, corneal clouding, coarse features, growth and mental retardation Hunter: Deficiency of L-idurano-sulfate sulfatase, coarse facies, clear cornea, growth and mental retardation
Morquio; Scheie; Maroteaux-Lamy	Aortic incompetence	Morquio: Deficiency of N-acetylhexosamine sulfate sulfatase, cloudy cornea, normal intelligence, severe bone changes involving vertebrae and epiphyses Scheie: Deficiency of α-L-iduronidase, cloudy cornea, normal intelligence, peculiar facies Maroteaux-Lamy: Deficiency of arylsulfatase B, cloudy cornea, osseous changes, normal intelligence
Chromosomal Abnormalities		
Trisomy 21 (Down's syndrome)	Endocardial cushion defect, atrial or ventricular septal defect, tetralogy of Fallot	Hypotonia, hyperextensible joints, mongoloid facies, mental retardation
Trisomy 13 (D)	Ventricular septal defect, double-outlet right ventricle	Single midline intracerebral ventricle with midfacial defects, polydactyly, nail changes, mental retardation
Trisomy 18 (E)	Ventricular septal defect, patent ductus arteriosus, pulmonic stenosis	Clenched hand, short sternum, low arch dermal ridge pattern on fingertips, mental retardation
Cri du chat (short-arm deletion-5)	Ventricular septal defect	Cat cry, microcephaly, antimongoloid slant of palpebral fissures, mental retardation
XO (Turner)	Coarctation of aorta	Short female, broad chest, lymphedema, webbed neck
XXXY and XXXXX	Patent ductus arteriosus	XXXY: Hypogenitalism, mental retardation, radial-ulnar synostosis XXXXX: Small hands, incurving of fifth fingers, mental retardation

Modified from Friedman, W. F.: Congenital heart disease. *In* Isselbacher, K. J., Adams, R. D., Braunwald, E., Petersdorf, R. G., and Wilson, J. D. (eds.): Harrison's Principles of Internal Medicine. 10th ed. New York, McGraw-Hill Book Co., 1983, p. 1383.

TABLE 29–3 RECURRENCE RISK IN SIBLINGS OF PROBANDS WITH CONGENITAL HEART LESIONS

Defect	Affected Siblings (%)
Ventricular septal defect	4.4
Patent ductus arteriosus	3.4
Tetralogy of Fallot	2.7
Atrial septal defect	3.2
Pulmonic stenosis	2.9
Aortic stenosis	2.2
Atrioventricular canal	2.6
Transposition of great arteries	1.9
Coarctation of aorta	1.8

Modified from Nora, J. J., et al.: Etiologic aspects of cardiovascular disease and pre-disposition detectable in the infant and child. *In* Friedman, W. F., et al. (eds.): Neonatal Heart Disease. New York, Grune and Stratton, 1973, p. 279.

2 provides a partial list of syndromes in which cardiovascular anomalies may be manifestations of the pleiotropic effects of single genes or examples of gross chromosomal defects. Less than 5 to 10 per cent of all cardiac malformations can be accounted for by chromosomal aberrations or genetic mutations or transmission.

The finding that, with some exceptions, only one of a pair of monozygotic twins is affected by congenital heart disease indicates that the vast majority of cardiovascular malformations are not inherited in a simple manner.[13] Family studies indicate a two- to five-fold increase in the incidence of congenital heart disease in siblings of affected patients or in the offspring of an affected parent. Malformations are often concordant or partially concordant within families.[13a] Table 29–3 provides the recurrence risks observed in 3400 siblings of probands with various congenital heart lesions. Because the incidence of congenital heart disease in the offspring or siblings of an index patient is only 2 to 5 per cent, it is rarely wise to discourage the parents of one affected child from having additional children if either parent is free of a cardiovascular anomaly.[14] Moreover, the low recurrence rate and the increasing possibilities for effective treatment for nearly all cardiac lesions usually justify a positive approach to family counseling. When two or more members of the family are affected, the recurrence risk may be quite high, and a pedigree should be obtained before further counseling. If a dominant or recessive mendelian pattern is established, the mendelian laws apply, and the risk of recurrence in each pregnancy is equal.

Prevention. The feasibility of preventive programs will depend upon what is learned in the future about the cause of the 90 per cent or more of cardiovascular anomalies for which no cause is currently known. Strict testing in animals of new drugs that may be teratogenic when taken during pregnancy may be expected to reduce the chances of another thalidomide tragedy. In this regard, the dictum cannot be emphasized too strongly that no medication should be taken during pregnancy without prior consultation with a physician. Physicians dealing with pregnant women should be aware of known teratogens as well as of drugs that may have a functional rather than a structural damaging influence on the fetal and newborn heart and circulation and should recognize that drugs abound for which there is inadequate information concerning their teratogenic potential. Similarly, appropriate use of radiological equipment and techniques for reducing gonadal and fetal radiation exposure should always be employed to reduce the potential hazards of this likely cause of birth defects.

Detection of abnormal chromosomes in fetal cells obtained from amniotic fluid (Chap. 47) may occasionally predict cardiac malformation as one component of the multiple system involvement that may exist in Down's, Turner's, or trisomy 13–15 (D1) and 16–18 (E) syndrome. Similarly, identification in such cells of the enzyme disorders observed in the mucopolysaccharidoses, homocystinuria, or type II glycogen storage disease may allow one to predict the ultimate presence of cardiac disease. Lastly, immunization of children with rubella vaccine may be anticipated to minimize the effects of maternal rubella and its cardiac consequences.

Embryology

Correlation of anatomical features of malformed hearts and embryonic cardiac morphology allows a developmental analysis of various anomalies. Detailed accounts of the normal development of the cardiovascular system are provided elsewhere.[15–17] In brief, during the first month of gestation the primitive, straight cardiac tube is formed, comprising the sinuatrium, the primitive ventricle, the bulbus cordis, and the truncus arteriosus in series (Fig. 29–1). In the second month of gestation this tube doubles over on itself to form two parallel pumping systems, each with two chambers and a great artery. The two atria develop from the sinuatrium; the atrioventricular canal is divided by the endocardial cushions into tricuspid and mitral orifices; and the right and left ventricles develop from the primitive ventricle and bulbus cordis. Differential growth of myocardial cells causes the straight cardiac tube to bear to the right, and the bulboventricular portion of the tube doubles over on itself, bringing the ventricles side by side (Fig. 29–2). Migration of the atrioventricular canal to the right and of the ventricular septum of the left serves to align each ventricle with its appropriate atrioventricular valve. At the distal end of the cardiac tube the bulbus cordis divides into a subaortic muscular conus and a subpulmonic muscular conus; the subpulmonic conus elongates, and the subaortic conus reabsorbs, allowing the aorta to move posteriorly and connect with the left ventricle.

A host of anomalies may result from defects in this basic developmental pattern. Thus, double-inlet left ventricle (p. 1012) is observed

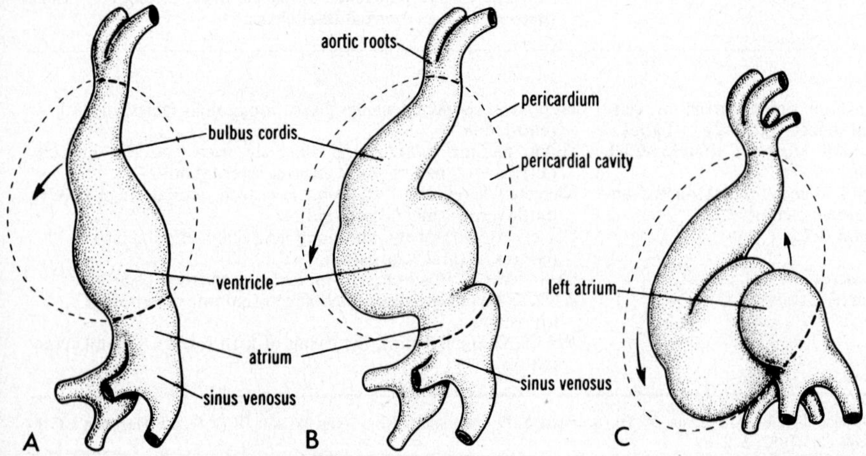

FIGURE 29–1 Formation of the cardiac loop as seen from the left side at 32 days *(A)*, 34 days *(B)*, and 38 days *(C)*. Dashed line indicates parietal pericardium. The atrium gradually assumes an intrapericardial position. (From Langman, J., and van Mierop, L. H. S.: Development of the cardiovascular system. *In* Moss, A. J., and Adams, F. H. (eds.): Heart Disease in Infants, Children and Adolescents. Baltimore, Williams and Wilkins, 1968.)

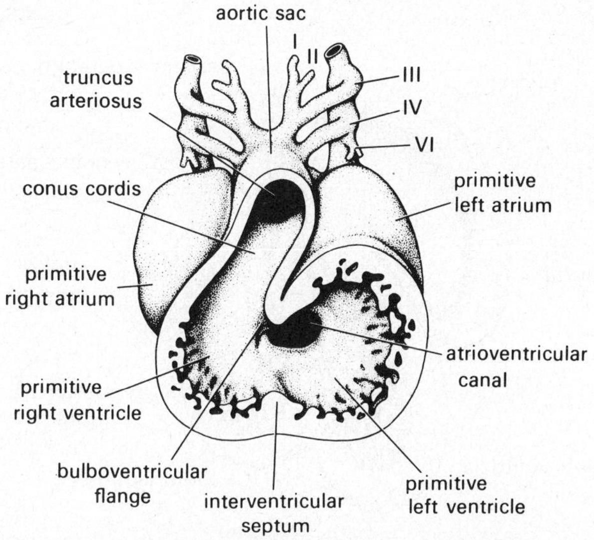

FIGURE 29–2 Frontal section through the heart of 5-mm embryo showing the side-by-side primitive ventricles and the single opening of the atrium into the ventricles. (From Langman, J., and van Mierop, L. H. S.: Development of the cardiovascular system. *In* Moss, A. J., and Adams, F. H. (eds.): Heart Disease in Infants, Children and Adolescents. Baltimore, Williams and Wilkins, 1968.)

if the tricuspid orifice does not align over the right ventricle. The various types of persistent truncus arteriosus (p. 969) result from failure of the truncus to divide into main pulmonary artery and aorta. Double-outlet anomalies of the right ventricle (p. 1005) are produced by failure of either the subpulmonic or subaortic conus to resorb, whereas resorption of the subpulmonic instead of the subaortic conus may be central to transposition of the great arteries (p. 997).

The primitive sinuatrium is separated into right and left atria by the downgrowth from its roof of the septum primum toward the atrioventricular canal, thereby creating an inferior intraatrial ostium primum opening (Fig. 29–3). Multiple perforations form in the anterosuperior portion of the septum primum as the septum secundum begins to develop to the right of the former. The coalescence of these perforations forms the ostium secundum. The septum secundum completely separates the atrial chambers except for a central opening—the fossa ovalis—which is covered by tissue of the septum primum forming the valve of the foramen ovale. Fusion of the endocardial cushions anteriorly and posteriorly divides the atrioventricular canal into tricuspid and mitral inlets (Fig. 29–4). The inferior portion of the atrial septum, the superior portion of the ventricular septum, and portions of the septal leaflets of both the tricuspid and mitral valves are formed from the endocardial cushions. The integrity of the atrial septum depends on growth of the septum primum and septum secundum and proper fusion of the endocardial cushions. Atrial septal defects (p. 958) and varying degrees of endocardial cushion defect (p. 961) are the result of developmental deficiencies of this process.

Partitioning of the ventricles occurs as cephalad growth of the main ventricular septum results in its fusion with the endocardial cushions and the infundibular or conus septum. Defects in the ventricular septum may occur owing to a deficiency of septal substance; malalignment of septal components in different planes, preventing their fusion; or an overly long conus, keeping the septal components apart. Isolated defects (p. 963) probably result from the former mechanism, while the latter two appear to generate the ventricular defects seen in tetralogy of Fallot (p. 990) and transposition complexes (p. 967).

The lungs arise from the primitive foregut and are drained early in embryogenesis by channels from the splanchnic plexus to the cardinal and umbilicovitelline veins. An outpouching from the posterior left atrium forms the common pulmonary vein, which communicates with the splanchnic plexus, establishing pulmonary venous drainage to the left atrium. The umbilicovitelline and anterior cardinal vein communications atrophy as the common pulmonary vein is incorporated into the left atrium. Anomalous pulmonary venous connections (p. 1008) to the umbilicovitelline (portal) venous system or to the cardinal system (superior vena cava) result from failure of the common pulmonary vein to develop or establish communications to the splanchnic plexus. Cor triatriatum (p. 984) results from a narrowing of the common pulmonary vein–left atrial junction.

The truncus arteriosus is connected to the dorsal aorta in the embryo by six pairs of aortic arches. Partition of the truncus arteriosus into two great arteries is a result of the fusion of tissue arising from the back wall of the vessel and the truncus septum. Rotation of the truncus coils the aorticopulmonary septum and creates the normal spiral relationship between aorta and pulmonary artery. Semilunar valves and their related sinuses are created by absorption and hollowing out of tissue at the distal side of the truncus ridges. Aorticopulmonary septal defect (p. 969) and persistent truncus arteriosus (p. 969) represent varying degrees of partitioning failure.

Although the six aortic arches appear sequentially, portions of the arch system and dorsal aorta disappear at different times during embryogenesis (Fig. 29–5). The first, second, and fifth sets of paired arches regress completely. The proximal portions of the sixth arches become the right and left pulmonary arteries and the distal left sixth arch becomes the ductus arteriosus. The third aortic arch forms the connection between internal and external carotid arteries, while the left fourth arch becomes the arterial segment between left carotid and subclavian arteries; the proximal portion of the right subclavian

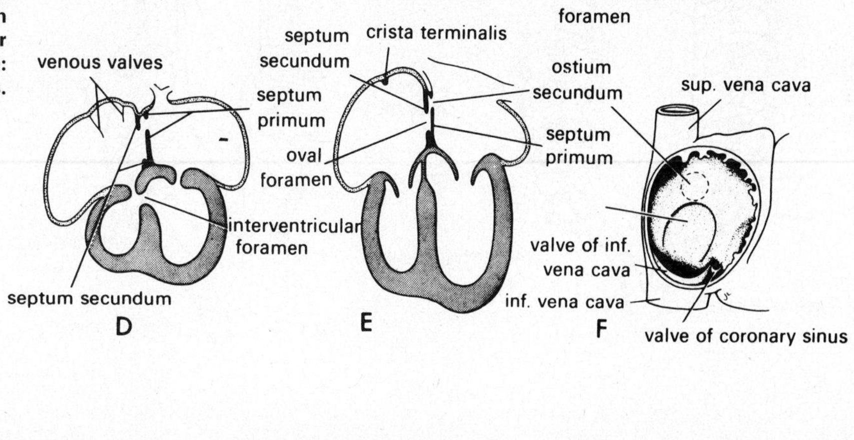

FIGURE 29–3 Diagrammatic representation of the atrial septa at 30 days *(A)*, at 33 days *(B)*, at 33 days (seen from the right side) *(C)*, at 37 days *(D)*, and in the newborn *(E)*; the newborn atrial septum viewed from the right *(F)*. (From Langman, J., and van Mierop, L. H. S.: Development of the cardiovascular system. *In* Moss, A. J., and Adams, F. H. (eds.): Heart Disease in Infants, Children and Adolescents. Baltimore, Williams and Wilkins, 1968.)

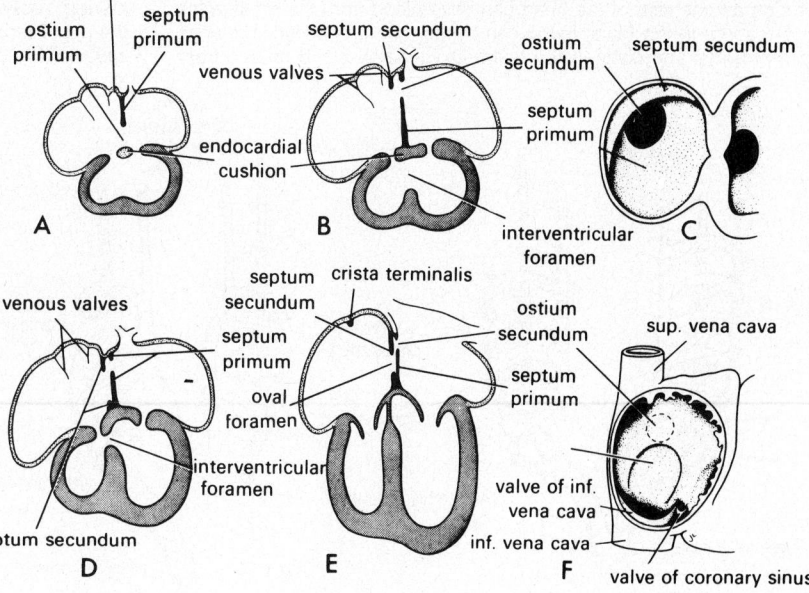

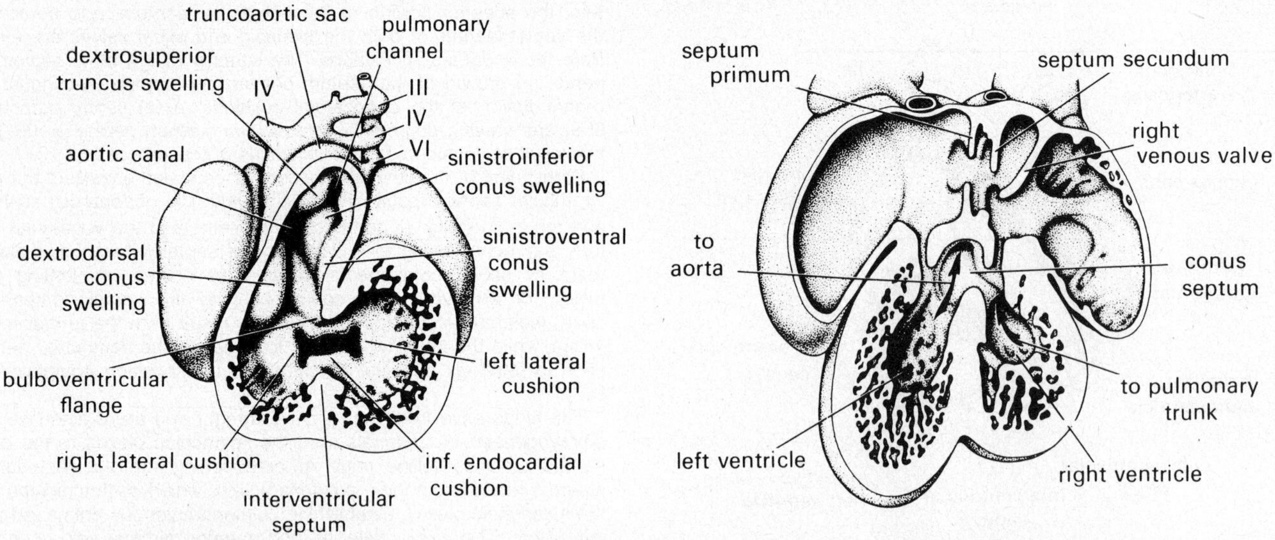

FIGURE 29–4 **Frontal section through the heart of a 9-mm embryo (*left panel*) and 15-mm embryo (*right panel*). At 9 mm, development is noted of the cushions in the atrioventricular canal, and the truncus and conus swellings are visible. At 15 mm, the conus septum is completed; note the septation in the atrial region. (From Langman, J., and Van Mierop, L. H. S.: Development of the cardiovascular system. *In* Moss, A. J., and Adams, F. H. (eds.): Heart Disease in Infants, Children and Adolescents. Baltimore, Williams and Wilkins, 1968.)**

artery forms from the right fourth arch. An abnormality in regression of the arch system in a number of sites can produce a wide variety of arch anomalies, whereas a failure of regression results generally in a double aortic arch malformation (p. 1013).

Fetal and Transitional Circulations

Although the illness created by the presence of a cardiac malformation is almost always recognized only after an affected baby is born, important effects on the circulation have existed from early in pregnancy until the time of delivery.[18] Thus, knowledge of the changes in cardiocirculatory structure, function, and metabolism that accompany development is central to a systematic comprehension of congenital heart disease.

Dynamic alterations occur in the circulation during the transition from fetal to neonatal life when the lungs, rather than the placenta, take over the function of gas exchange.[19] The single fetal circulation consists of parallel pulmonary and systemic pathways (Fig. 29–6) in contrast to the two-circuit system in the newborn and adult in whom the pulmonary vasculature exists in series with the systemic circulation. Prenatal survival is not endangered by major cardiac anomalies as long as one side of the heart can drive blood from the great veins to the aorta; in the fetus, blood can bypass the nonfunctioning lungs both proximal and distal to the heart. Oxygenated blood returns from the placenta through the umbilical vein and enters the portal venous system. A variable amount of this stream bypasses the hepatic microcirculation and enters the inferior vena cava via the ductus venosus. Inferior vena caval blood is composed of flow from the ductus venosus, hepatic vein, and lower body venous drainage, which is summarily deflected to a significant extent across the foramen ovale into the left atrium. Almost all superior vena caval blood passes directly through the tricuspid valve entering the right ventricle. Most of the blood that reaches the right ventricle bypasses the high-resistance, unexpanded lungs and passes through the ductus arteriosus into the descending aorta. The output of the right and left ventricles contributes to the total fetal cardiac output in an approximate ratio of 2/3 to 1/3. The major portion of blood ejected from the left ventricle supplies the brain and upper body, with lesser flow to the coronary arteries; the balance passes across the aortic isthmus to the descending aorta where it joins with the large stream from the ductus arteriosus before flowing to the lower body and placenta.

In fetal life pulmonary arteries and arterioles are surrounded by a fluid medium, have relatively thick walls and small lumina, and resemble comparable arteries in the systemic circulation. The low pulmonary blood flow in the fetus (7 to 10 per cent of the total cardiac output) is the result of high pulmonary vascular resistance. Fetal pulmonary vessels are highly reactive to changes in oxygen tension or in the pH of blood perfusing them as well as to a number of other physiological and pharmacological influences.

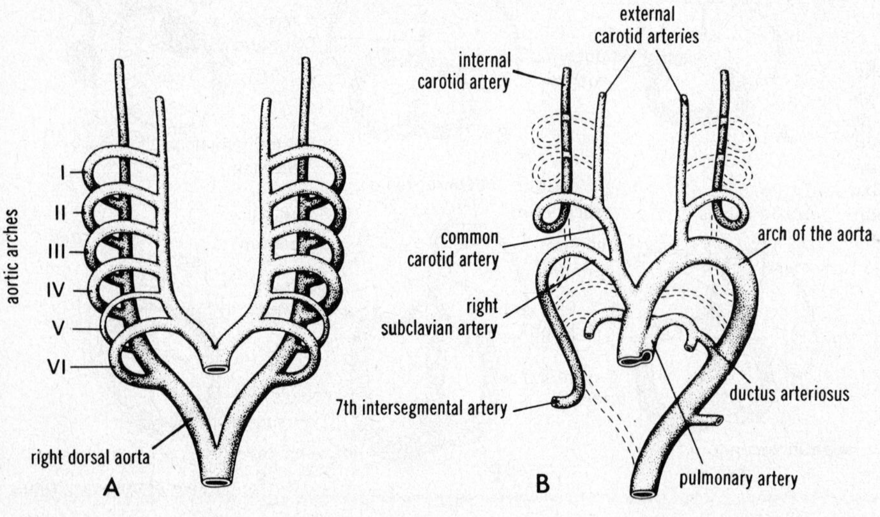

FIGURE 29–5 ***A,*** **Aortic arches and dorsal aortas before transformation into the definitive vascular pattern. *B,* Aortic arches and dorsal aortas after transformation. The obliterated components are indicated by broken lines. (From Langman, J., and van Mierop, L. H. S.: Development of the cardiovascular system. *In* Moss, A. J., and Adams, F. H. (eds.): Heart Disease in Infants, Children and Adolescents. Baltimore, Williams and Wilkins, 1968.)**

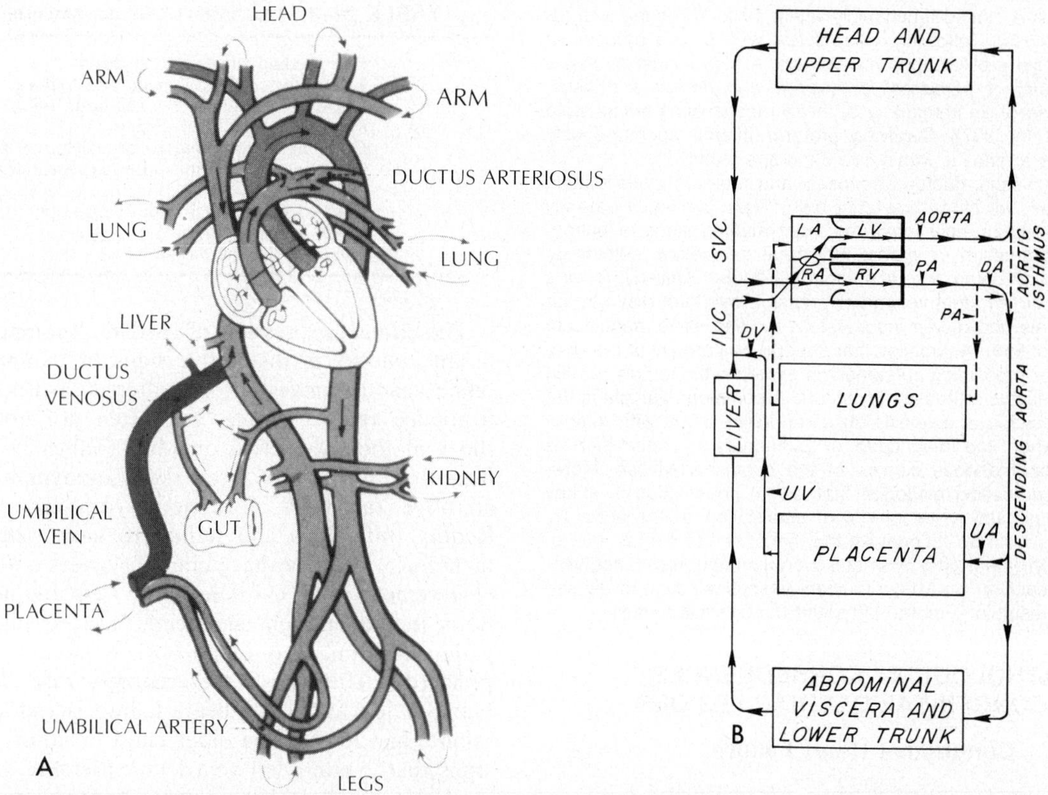

FIGURE 29–6 *A*, The fetal circulation. Shading shows the relative oxygenation of the blood, and arrows indicate its direction of flow. *B*, Prenatally, a fraction of umbilical venous (UV) blood enters the ductus venosus (DV) and bypasses the liver. This relatively well-oxygenated blood flows across the foramen ovale to the left heart, preferentially perfusing the coronary arteries, head, and upper trunk. Superior vena caval (SVC) blood is ejected by the right heart into the pulmonary artery (PA) and ductus arteriosus (DA). This stream circulates to the placenta as well as to the abdominal viscera and lower trunk. Dashed lines indicate diminished blood flow to and from the lungs and across the aortic isthmus. IVC = inferior vena cava, RA = right atrium, LA = left atrium, RV = right ventricle, LV = left ventricle, PA = pulmonary artery. (From Kaplan, S.: Congenital heart disease. *In* Vaughan, V. C., and McKay, R. J. (eds.): Nelson Textbook of Pediatrics. 10th ed. Philadelphia, W. B. Saunders Co., 1975.)

Although fetal somatic growth may be unimpaired, the hemodynamic effects in utero of many cardiac malformations may alter the development and structure of the fetal heart and circulation.[18] Thus, total anomalous pulmonary venous connection in utero may result in underdevelopment of the left atrium and left ventricle (p. 983), and premature closure of the foramen ovale may result in hypoplasia of the left ventricle (p. 983). Moreover, postnatally the caliber of the aortic isthmus may be reduced (p. 973) in the presence of lesions in utero that create left ventricular hypertrophy and impede filling because of reduced compliance of that chamber or that interfere with left ventricular filling directly (e.g., mitral stenosis) or indirectly by diverting a proportion of left ventricular output away from the ascending aorta while increasing right ventricular output and ductus arteriosus flow (e.g., endocardial cushion defect with left ventricular–right atrial shunt or aortic or subaortic stenosis with ventricular septal defect). Similarly, obstruction in utero to right ventricular outflow is associated with an increase in proximal aortic flow and diameter and almost never with aortic coarctation (p. 973). In these and other examples it is important to recognize that malformations compatible with fetal survival may nonetheless result in abnormal development of the circulation in utero and also affect circulatory adjustments after birth.

Compared to the adult heart, the fetal and newborn heart is unique with respect to its ultrastructural appearance,[20] its mechanical and biochemical properties,[21–23] and its autonomic innervation.[22–25] During late fetal and early neonatal development there is maturation of the biochemical composition of the heart's energy-utilizing myofibrillar proteins and of ATP and creatine phosphate energy-producing proteins.[23] Moreover, fetal and neonatal myocardial cells are small in diameter and reduced in density, so that the young heart contains relatively more noncontractile mass (primarily mitochondria, nuclei, and surface membranes) than later in postnatal life. As a result, force generation and the extent and velocity of shortening are decreased, and stiffness and water content of ventricular myocardium are increased in the fetal and early newborn periods. The diminished function of the young heart is reflected in its limited ability to increase cardiac output in the presence of either a volume load or a lesion that increases resistance to emptying.[26] Although functional integrity exists of efferent and afferent cardiac autonomic pathways early in life, fetal and newborn myocardium lacks the complete development of sympathetic but not cholinergic innervation. Thus, adaptation to cardiocirculatory stress in fetal or early newborn life may be less effective than in the adult.

Normally, the fundamental change that occurs at birth is a division of the single parallel fetal circulation into separate, independent circulations. Inflation of the lungs at the first inspiration produces a marked reduction in pulmonary vascular resistance owing partly to the sudden suspension in air of fetal pulmonary vessels previously supported by fluid media. The reduced extravascular pressure assists new vessels to open and already patent vessels to enlarge. The rapid decrease in pulmonary vascular resistance is related more importantly to vasodilatation due to the increase in oxygen tension to which pulmonary vessels are exposed than to physical expansion of alveoli with gas. Pulmonary arterial pressure falls, and pulmonary blood flow increases greatly. Systemic vascular resistance rises when clamping of the umbilical cord removes the low-resistance placental circulation. Increased pulmonary blood flow increases the return of blood to the left atrium and raises left atrial pressure, which in turn closes the foramen ovale. The shift in oxygen dependence from the placenta to the lungs produces a sudden increase in arterial blood oxygen tension, which, in concert with alterations in the local prostaglandin milieu, initiates constriction of the ductus arteriosus.[27] Pulmonary pressure falls further as the ductus constricts. In mature infants the ductus arteriosus is closed functionally within 10 to 15 hours, with total anatomical closure following within a few weeks by a process of thrombosis, intimal proliferation, and fibrosis. A high incidence exists in preterm infants of persistent patency of the ductus arteriosus, probably because of an immaturity of those mechanisms responsible for constriction (p. 967). Surviving preterm infants spontaneously close the ductus arteriosus within 4 to 6 months of birth.

The ductus venosus, ductus arteriosus, and foramen ovale remain potential channels for blood flow after birth, Thus, persistent patency of the ductus venosus may mask the most marked signs of pulmonary venous obstruction in infants with total anomalous pulmonary venous connection below the diaphragm (p. 1008). Similarly, lesions producing right or left atrial volume or pressure overload may stretch the foramen ovale and render incompetent the flap valve mechanism for its closure (p. 958). Anomalies that depend on patency of the ductus arteriosus for preserving pulmonary or systemic blood flow remain latent until the ductus arteriosus constricts. A common example is the sudden intensification of cyanosis observed in the infant with tetralogy of Fallot when the magnitude of pulmonary hypoperfusion is unmasked by spontaneous closure of the ductus arteriosus. Moreover, there is increasing evidence that ductal constriction is a key factor in the postnatal development of coarctation of the aorta (p. 973). Lastly, it should be recognized that because the ductus arteriosus is potentially patent after birth and the pulmonary resistance vessels are hyperreactive, hypoxic pulmonary vasoconstriction of diverse etiologies may result in a right-to-left shunt through the ductus.

PATHOLOGICAL CONSEQUENCES OF CONGENITAL CARDIAC LESIONS

Congestive Heart Failure

Although the basic mechanisms of cardiac failure, as outlined in Chapter 13, are the same for all ages, the pediatric cardiologist should recognize clearly that the common causes, time of onset, and often the approach to treatment vary with age.[28–30,30a] Infants under one year of age with cardiac malformations account for 80 to 90 per cent of pediatric patients who develop congestive failure. Moreover, cardiac decompensation in the infant is a medical emergency necessitating immediate treatment if the patient is to be saved.

In the preterm infant, especially under 1500 grams birthweight, persistent patency of the ductus arteriosus is the most common cause of cardiac decompensation, and other forms of structural heart disease are rare. In the fullterm newborn the earliest important causes of heart failure are the hypoplastic left heart and coarctation of the aorta syndromes, paroxysmal atrial tachycardia, cerebral or hepatic arteriovenous fistula, and myocarditis. Among the lesions commonly producing heart failure beyond age 1 to 2 weeks, when diminished pulmonary vascular resistance allows substantial left-to-right shunting, are ventricular septal and endocardial cushion defects, transposition of the great arteries, truncus arteriosus, and total anomalous pulmonary venous connection, often with pulmonary venous obstruction. Although heart failure is most usually the result of a structural defect or of myocardial disease, it should be recognized that the newborn myocardium may be depressed severely by such abnormalities as hypoxemia and acidemia, anemia, septicemia, marked hypoglycemia, hypocalcemia, and polycythemia. In the older child, heart failure is often due to acquired disease (Chap. 31) or is a complication of open-heart surgical procedures. In the acquired category are rheumatic and endomyocardial diseases, infective endocarditis, hematological and nutritional disorders, and severe cardiac arrhythmias.

TABLE 29–4 FEATURES OF HEART FAILURE IN INFANTS

Poor feeding and failure to thrive
Respiratory distress—mainly tachypnea
Rapid heart rate (160 to 180 beats/min)
Pulmonary rales or wheezing
Cardiomegaly and pulmonary edema on x-ray
Hepatomegaly (peripheral edema unusual)
Gallop sounds
Color—ashen pale or faintly cyanotic
Excessive perspiration
Diminished urine output

The clinical expression of cardiac decompensation in the infant consists of distinctive signs of pulmonary and systemic venous congestion and altered cardiocirculatory performance that resemble, but often are not identical to, those of the older child or adult (Table 29–4).[31] These reflect the interplay between the hemodynamic burden and adaptive responses. Common symptoms and signs are feeding difficulties and failure to gain weight and grow, tachypnea, tachycardia, pulmonary rales and rhonchi, liver enlargement, and cardiomegaly. Less frequent manifestations include peripheral edema, ascites, pulsus alternans, gallop rhythm, and inappropriate sweating. Pleural and pericardial effusions are exceedingly rare. The distinction between left and right heart failure is less obvious in the infant than it is in the older child or adult, since most lesions that create a left ventricular pressure or volume overload also result in left-to-right shunting of blood through the foramen ovale and/or patent ductus arteriosus as well as pulmonary hypertension due to elevated pulmonary venous pressures. Conversely, augmented filling or elevated pressure of the right ventricle in the infant reduces left ventricular compliance disproportionately when compared to the older child or adult and gives rise to signs of both systemic and pulmonary venous congestion.[22]

Fatigue and dyspnea on exertion express themselves as a feeding problem in the infant. Characteristically, the respiratory rate in heart failure is rapid (50 to 100 breaths/min). In the presence of left ventricular failure, interstitial pulmonary edema reduces pulmonary compliance and results in tachypnea and retractions. Excessive pulmonary blood flow via significant left-to-right shunts may further decrease lung compliance. Moreover, upper airway obstruction may be produced by selective enlargement of cardiovascular structures. In patients with large left-to-right shunts and left atrial and main pulmonary artery enlargement, the left main stem bronchus may be compressed, resulting in emphysematous expansion of the left upper or lower lobe or left lower lobe collapse.[32] Respiratory distress with grunting, flaring of the alae nasi, and intercostal retractions is observed when failure is severe and especially when pulmonary infection precipitates cardiac decompensation, which is often the case. Under these circumstances pulmonary rales may be due to the infection or failure or both. A resting heart rate with little variability is characteristic of heart failure. Hepatomegaly is seen regularly in infants in failure, although liver tenderness is uncommon. Cardiomegaly may be assessed roentgenographically, but it must be recognized that in the normal newborn infant the cardiac diameter may be as much as 60 per cent of the thoracic diameter, and the large thymus gland in infants interferes occasionally with evaluation of heart size.

Echocardiography provides a good estimate of cardiac chamber dimensions, and values may be compared to data derived from normal infants.[33–36]

Cardiac decompensation may progress with extreme rapidity in the first hours and days of life, producing a clinical picture of advanced cardiogenic shock and a profoundly obtunded infant. The presence of marked hepatomegaly and gross cardiomegaly usually allows distinction from noncardiac causes of diminished systemic perfusion.

Cyanosis

(See also page 7)

Cyanosis is produced by an increased amount of reduced hemoglobin in cutaneous vessels in excess of 3 gm/dl. Peripheral cyanosis usually reflects an abnormally great extraction of oxygen from normally saturated arterial blood, commonly the result of peripheral cutaneous vasoconstriction. Central cyanosis is a result of arterial blood oxygen unsaturation, most often in patients with congenital heart disease caused by shunting of systemic venous blood into the arterial circuit. Infants especially may appear cyanotic when in heart failure because of both peripheral and central factors; the latter may include severe impairment of pulmonary function that commonly exists with alveolar hypoventilation, ventilation-perfusion inequality, or impaired oxygen diffusion. In patients with central cyanosis due to arterial oxygen unsaturation, the degree of cutaneous discoloration depends upon the absolute amount of reduced hemoglobin, the magnitude of the right-to-left shunt relative to systemic flow, and the oxyhemoglobin saturation of venous blood. The last of these depends in turn upon the tissue extraction of oxygen. Commonly, cyanosis appears or intensifies with physical activity or exercise as the saturation of systemic venous blood declines concurrent with an increase in right-to-left shunting across a defect as peripheral vascular resistance decreases. Oxygen transfer to the tissues is affected by shifts in the oxygen-hemoglobin dissociation relationship, which may be altered by blood pH and levels of red blood cell 2,3 diphosphoglycerate concentration.[37]

CLUBBING AND POLYCYTHEMIA. Prominent accompaniments of arterial hypoxemia are polycythemia and clubbing of the digits. The latter is associated with an increased number of capillaries with increased blood flow through extensive arteriovenous aneurysms and an increase of connective tissue in the terminal phalanges of the fingers and toes. Polycythemia is a physiological response to chronic hypoxemia that stimulates erythrocytosis. The extremely high hematocrits observed in patients with arterial oxygen unsaturation cause a progressive increase in blood viscosity, especially beyond packed red blood cell volumes of 60 per cent. Both the hematocrit and the circulating whole blood volume are increased in polycythemia accompanying cyanotic congenital heart disease; the hypervolemia is the result of an increase in red cell volume. The augmented red blood cell volume provoked by hypoxemia provides an increased oxygen-carrying capacity and enhanced oxygen supply to the tissues. The compensatory polycythemia is often of such severity that it becomes a liability and produces adverse physiological effects such as thrombotic lesions in diverse organs and a hemorrhagic diathesis.[38] In this regard, oral steroid contraceptives are contraindicated in the adolescent cyanotic female because of the enhanced risk of cerebral thrombosis. Red cell volume reduction and replacement with plasma or albumin (erythrophoresis) lowers blood viscosity and increases systemic blood flow and systemic oxygen transport and thus may be helpful in the management of patients with severe hypoxic polycythemia (hematocrit $\geq$ 65 per cent). A final hematocrit of 55 to 63 per cent should be achieved; the higher level is necessary in patients with low initial oxygen saturation in order to avoid a severe reduction in arterial oxygen content. Acute phlebotomy without fluid replacement is contraindicated.

CEREBRAL AND PULMONARY COMPLICATIONS. Cerebral vascular accidents and brain abscesses occur particularly in cyanotic patients with substantial arterial desaturation.[39–41] *Cerebral thrombosis* is most common under age 2 years in severely cyanotic children, even in the presence of relatively low hematocrits, and occurs especially in a clinical setting in which oxygen requirements are raised by fever or, if blood viscosity is increased, by dehydration.

Brain abscesses are an important complication of cyanotic heart disease.[40,41] They are rare under 18 months of age and commonly are of insidious onset marked by headache, low-grade fever, vomiting, and a change in personality. Seizures or paralysis less frequently heralds the onset of a brain abscess. Abscess must be suspected in any cyanotic child with focal neurological signs. Morbidity and mortality are related inversely to oxygen saturation levels. Brain abscess is thought to occur in approximately 2 per cent of the population with cyanotic congenital heart disease; a mortality rate of 30 to 40 per cent is often related to delay in diagnosis and treatment.

Paradoxical embolus is a rare complication of cyanotic heart disease, usually observed only at necropsy.[42] Emboli arising in systemic veins may pass directly to the systemic circulation, since right-to-left intracardiac shunts allow venous blood to bypass the normal filtering action of the lungs.

Retinopathy consisting of dilated tortuous vessels progressing to papilledema and retinal edema is occasionally observed in cyanotic patients and appears to be related to decreased arterial oxygen saturation and/or to erythrocytosis but not to hypercapnea.

Hemoptysis is an uncommon but major complication in cyanotic patients with congenital heart disease and occurs most often in the presence of pulmonary vascular obstructive disease or in patients with an extensive bronchial collateral circulation or pulmonary venous congestion.[43] Massive hemoptysis almost always represents rupture of a dilated bronchial artery.

SQUATTING. After exertion, patients with cyanotic heart disease, especially tetralogy of Fallot, typically assume a squatting posture in order to obtain relief from breathlessness.[44] Squatting appears to improve arterial oxygen saturation by increasing systemic vascular resistance, thereby diminishing the right-to-left shunt, and also by the pooling of markedly desaturated blood in the lower extremities. In addition, systemic venous return and therefore pulmonary blood flow may increase.

HYPOXIC SPELLS. Hypercyanotic or hypoxemic

spells commonly complicate the clinical course in younger children with certain types of cyanotic heart disease, especially tetralogy of Fallot (p. 990).[44,45] The spells are characterized by anxiety, hyperpnea, and a sudden marked increase in cyanosis; they are the result of an abrupt reduction in pulmonary blood flow. Unless terminated, the hypercyanotic episodes may lead to convulsions and may even be fatal. The sudden reduction in pulmonary blood flow may be precipitated by fluctuations in arterial pCO_2 and pH, a sudden fall in systemic or increase in pulmonary vascular resistance, or an acute increase in the severity of right ventricular outflow tract obstruction either by augmented contraction of the hypertrophied muscle in the right ventricular outflow tract or by a decrease in right ventricular cavity volume due to tachycardia. *Treatment* consists of oxygen administration, placing the child in the knee-chest position, and administration of morphine sulfate. Additional medications that may prove of value include the intravenous administration of sodium bicarbonate to correct the accompanying acidemia, alpha-adrenergic receptor stimulants such as neosynephrine or methoxamine to raise peripheral resistance and diminish right-to-left shunting, and beta-adrenergic blocking agents that reduce cardiac sympathetic tone and depress cardiac contractility directly and that increase ventricular volume by reducing heart rate.

Acid-base Imbalance

Disturbances in blood gas and acid-base equilibrium are noted particularly in infants with either congestive heart failure or cyanosis.[46] Large-volume left-to-right shunts, especially with pulmonary edema, may be associated with moderate respiratory acidemia and a lowering of arterial oxygen tensions, reflecting an increase in the alveolar-arterial oxygen tension gradient and ventilation-perfusion imbalance. Interference with carbon dioxide transport implies moderate to severe failure in these infants. Lesions associated with a reduced systemic cardiac output, such as severe coarctation of the aorta or critical aortic stenosis in infancy, present often with cardiac failure complicated by a severe metabolic acidemia and relatively high values of arterial oxygen tension. The latter finding, even in the presence of right-to-left shunting across a patent ductus arteriosus, is a result of diminished systemic perfusion and an elevated pulmonary-to-systemic blood flow ratio. Respiratory acidemia and depressed levels of oxygen tension are observed in infants with obstruction to pulmonary venous return and right-to-left atrial shunting. Infants with severe hypoxemia due to lesions such as transposition of the great arteries or pulmonic atresia often show metabolic acidemia and marked reductions in carbon dioxide tension secondary to hyperventilation resulting from hypoxic stimulation of peripheral chemoreceptors.

Impaired Growth

Impaired growth and physical development and delayed onset of adolescence are common features of many cyanotic and, to a lesser extent, acyanotic forms of congenital heart disease.[47] Mental development is rarely affected. In general, the severity of growth disturbance depends upon the anatomical lesion and its functional effect. Most children with mild defects grow normally. Weight gain is commonly slower than linear growth in acyanotic patients with large left-to-right shunts, whereas in cyanotic congenital heart disease height and weight usually parallel each other. Boys appear to be more retarded in growth than girls, especially in the second decade. Skeletal maturity (i.e., bone age) is delayed in cyanotic children in relation to the severity of hypoxemia. In some children, prenatal factors such as intrauterine infection and chromosomal or other hereditary and nonhereditary syndromes are responsible for growth retardation. In other patients, extracardiac malformations may contribute to poor weight gain and linear growth. Additional explanations for the mechanisms of growth interference have implicated malnutrition as a result of anorexia and inadequate nutrients and caloric intake, hypermetabolic state, acidemia and cation imbalance, tissue hypoxemia, diminished peripheral blood flow, chronic cardiac decompensation, malabsorption or protein loss, recurrent respiratory infections, and endocrine or genetic factors. In some instances, the underdevelopment is influenced little by operative correction of the underlying cardiac anomaly. Among factors that may be responsible for persistent growth retardation postoperatively are age at operation, hemodynamically significant residual lesions, and sequelae or complications of operation. As a general rule, it is unwise preoperatively to guarantee to the parents of a child with heart disease that surgery will result in accelerated growth and development.

Pulmonary Hypertension

(See also Chapter 25)

Pulmonary hypertension is a common accompaniment of many congenital cardiac lesions, and the status of the pulmonary vascular bed is often the principal determinant of the clinical manifestations, course, and whether surgical treatment is feasible.[48] Increases in pulmonary arterial pressure result from elevations of pulmonary blood flow and/or resistance, the latter due sometimes to an increase in vascular tone, but usually the result of obstructive, obliterative structural changes within the pulmonary vascular bed.[49]

Normally, pulmonary vascular resistance falls rapidly immediately after birth owing to onset of ventilation and subsequent release of hypoxic pulmonary vasoconstriction. Subsequently the medial smooth muscle of pulmonary arterial resistance vessels thins gradually.[50] This latter process is delayed often by several months in infants with large aorticopulmonary or ventricular communications, at which time levels of pulmonary vascular resistance are still somewhat elevated. In patients with high pulmonary arterial pressure from birth, failure of normal growth of the pulmonary circulation may occur, and anatomical changes in the pulmonary vessels in the form of proliferation of intimal cells and intimal and medial thickening often progress, so that in the older child or adult vascular resistance may ultimately become fixed by obliterative changes in the pulmonary vascular bed. The causes of pulmonary vascular obstructive disease remain unknown, although increased pulmonary blood flow, increased pulmonary arterial blood pressure, elevated pulmonary venous pressure, polycythemia, systemic hypoxia, acidemia, and the nature of the bronchial circulation have all been implicated. There are many patients with pulmonary vascular obstruction whose cardiac anomaly places them at particular risk quite early in life, precluding survival to adulthood. Patients at particularly high risk for the development of significant pulmonary vascular obstruction are those with certain forms of cyanotic congenital heart disease, such as complete transposition of the great arteries with or without ventricular septal defect or patent ductus arteriosus, single ventricle without pulmonary stenosis, double outlet right ventricle, and truncus arteriosus. Other conditions in which pulmonary vascular obstruction appears to progress rapidly include large ventricular septal defect, as well as the less common conditions of unilateral pulmonary artery absence, congenital left-to-right shunts in an environment of high altitude or in association with the Down's syndrome of trisomy 21, and complete atrioventricular canal defects, even unassociated with a chromosomal anomaly.

Intimal damage appears to be related to shear stresses, since endothelial cell damage occurs at high-flow shear rates. A reduction in pulmonary arteriolar lumen size due to either thickened medial muscle or vasoconstriction increases the velocity of flow. Shear stress also increases as blood viscosity rises; therefore, infants with hypoxemia and high hematocrits as well as increased pulmonary blood flow are at increased risk of developing pulmonary vascular disease. In patients with left-to-right shunts, pulmonary arterial hypertension, if not present in infancy or childhood, may never occur or may not develop until the third or fourth decade or later. Once developed, intimal proliferative changes with hyalinization and fibrosis are not reversible by repair of the underlying cardiac defect. In severe pulmonary vascular obstructive disease, arteriovenous malformations may develop and predispose to massive hemoptysis.

Most vexing is the variability among patients with the same or similar cardiac lesions in both the time of appearance and rate of progression of their pulmonary vascular obstructive process. While genetic influences may be operative (an example is the apparent acceleration of pulmonary vascular disease in patients with congenital heart disease and trisomy 21), evidence is now accumulating for important pre- and postnatal modifiers of the pulmonary vascular bed that appear, at least in part, to be lesion-dependent. Thus, a quantitative variability exists in the pulmonary vascular bed related to the *number,* not just the size and wall structure, of arterial vessels within the pulmonary circulation.[51] Modeling of the blood vessels occurs proximal to and within terminal bronchioles (pre- and intra-acinar vessels, respectively) continuously from before birth. The intra-acinar vessels, in particular, increase in size and number from late fetal life throughout childhood with minimal muscularization of their walls. The ensuing increase in the cross-sectional area of the pulmonary arterial circulation allows the cardiac output to rise substantially without an increase in pulmonary arterial pressure. If, however, the presence of a cardiac lesion interferes with the normal growth and multiplication of these most peripheral arteries, the resulting elevation of pulmonary vascular resistance may first be related to failure of the intra-acinar pulmonary circulation to develop fully, and then secondarily to the morphological changes of obliterative vascular disease—medial thickening, intimal proliferation, hyalinization and fibrosis, and angiomatoid and plexiform lesions, and, ultimately, arterial necrosis.[49]

Since pulmonary vascular obstructive disease may be the factor limiting a decision concerning the advisability of operation, it is important to quantify and compare pulmonary-to-systemic flow and resistance in patients with severe pulmonary hypertension. Moreover, the reactivity of the pulmonary vascular bed should be evaluated. A marked reduction in pulmonary vascular resistance with infusion of tolazoline or the inhalation of oxygen suggests that the resistance is not fixed and may fall after successful operation. Some defects between the left and right sides of the heart should be closed in order to eliminate a sizable left-to-right shunt, which may in turn result in a significant drop in pulmonary arterial pressure. Conversely, little or no benefit and high mortality rates may be expected from closure of defects associated with bidirectional or predominantly right-to-left shunts in patients with high resistance and obstructive pulmonary hypertension.

The clinical manifestations of pulmonary hypertension associated with a large left-to-right shunt reflect the specific malformation responsible. When pulmonary vascular resistance is elevated and a significant right-to-left shunt exists, the patient is cyanotic, and polycythemia and clubbing are noted. A dominant *a* wave in the jugular venous pulse may be seen reflecting vigorous right atrial contraction due to diminished compliance of the right ventricle. In some instances there are large systolic *c-v* waves, which suggest tricuspid regurgitation. A prominent right ventricular parasternal lift and palpable systolic expansion of the pulmonary artery are present. A soft pulmonary systolic ejection murmur preceded by an ejection sound and followed by a markedly accentuated pulmonic component of the second heart sound are often audible on auscultation; an early diastolic decrescendo blowing murmur of pulmonary regurgitation may be heard. If right ventricular failure and dilatation supervene, the systolic murmur of tricuspid regurgitation may be audible at the lower left sternal border. Right ventricular enlargement may be evident on the chest roentgenogram and electrocardiogram. The former examination also reveals a conspicuously enlarged pulmonary artery, prominent hilar pulmonary vascular markings, and attenuated peripheral vessels. The site of the underlying defect may be localized by means of cardiac catheterization and angiocardiography. Pressures in the right side of the heart are essentially identical to systemic pressures in cyanotic patients if the shunt is at the ventricular or aorticopulmonary levels, but they are usually lower than systemic pressures in patients with an intra-atrial shunt. No specific treatment has proved beneficial for obstructive pulmonary vascular disease.

Infective Endocarditis

(See also Chapter 33)

Infective endocarditis is uncommon under age 2 years and thereafter most often affects children with tetralogy of Fallot (especially after systemic-pulmonary anastomosis), ventricular septal defect, aortic stenosis, and patent ductus arteriosus. Postsurgical patients with prosthetic heterograft or homograft valves or conduits are at particular risk. A causative organism can be isolated in approximately 90 per cent of children, usually either alpha-streptococci (usually

Strep. viridans) or *Staphylococcus aureus.*[52] Fungal endocarditis is quite rare in the pediatric age group. Mortality appears to be highest when coagulase-positive staphylococcus is the offending organism and when the endocarditis involves the left, rather than the right, side of the heart. Most recent data suggest 75 to 80 per cent overall survival.[52,53] Factors predisposing to endocarditis may be identified in approximately one third of cases; these include cardiovascular surgery with infection during the perioperative period; respiratory tract infections; and ear, nose, throat, and dental procedures. Less often, contamination during a surgical procedure or cardiac catheterization or an infection involving the skin, genitourinary tract, or other organ system has been the cause.

Although routine antimicrobial prophylaxis is recommended for all children with congenital heart disease and for the majority of patients after operative repair of the lesion, it should be recognized that many different microbes are responsible for the disease and that an effective preventive approach may center ultimately on active immunization rather than antibiotics. Currently, antibiotic prophylaxis is recommended for all dental procedures except minor readjustments of braces, oral trauma, and other procedures such as tonsillectomy, gastrointestinal surgery, and genitourinary surgery, or diagnostic procedures such as proctosigmoidoscopy and cystoscopy (Table 29–5).[54] The risk of endocarditis is undoubtedly related both to the magnitude of bacteremia and to the type of underlying heart disease. Since infection on a prosthetic heart valve or conduit may be devastating, combinations of antibiotics given parenterally are advisable in these patients.

Chest Pain

(See also pages 5 and 1335)

Angina pectoris is an uncommon symptom of cardiac disease in infants and children, occurring in association with anomalous pulmonary origin of a coronary artery or occasionally in association with severe aortic stenosis, pulmonic stenosis, or pulmonary hypertension due to pulmonary vascular obstruction. Cardiac pain in the infant with anomalous coronary artery (p. 971) most usually takes the

TABLE 29–5 PROPHYLACTIC ANTIBIOTICS FOR PROTECTION FROM BACTERIAL ENDOCARDITIS

For Dental Procedures and also for Tonsillectomy, Adenoidectomy, and Bronchoscopy

I. For most patients: **PENICILLIN**	**a) Intramuscular** plus **Oral** **Adults**: 600,000 units or procaine penicillin G mixed with 1,000,000 units or aqueous crystalline penicillin G intramuscularly 30–60 minutes prior to procedure, followed by 500 mg penicillin V orally every 6 hours for 8 doses. **Children**: 30,000 units aqueous penicillin G/kg mixed with 600,000 units of procaine penicillin intramuscularly (not to exceed adult dose). For children less than 60 lbs the dose of penicillin V is 250 mg every 6 hours for 8 doses. **b) Oral only** **Adults**: 2.0 gm of penicillin V 30–60 minutes prior to procedure and then 500 mg every 6 hours for 8 doses. **Children less than 60 lbs**: 1.0 gm of penicillin V orally 30 minutes to one hour prior to procedure and then 250 mg orally every 6 hours for 8 doses.
II. For those allergic to penicillin (may also be selected for those receiving oral penicillin as continuous rheumatic fever prophylaxis): **ERYTHROMYCIN**	**Adults**: 1.0 gm orally one and one-half to two hours prior to procedure and then 500 mg every 6 hours for 8 doses (or Regimen IV). **Children**: 20 mg/kg orally one and one-half to two hours prior to procedure and then 10 mg/kg (not to exceed adult dosage) every 6 hours for 8 doses (or Regimen IV).
III. For those patients at higher risk of infective endocarditis (especially those with prosthetic heart valves) who are not allergic to penicillin: **PENICILLIN** plus **STREPTOMYCIN**	**Adults**: IM penicillin as outlined above in I.a, **plus** streptomycin 1.0 gm IM, both given 30–60 minutes before procedure; then penicillin V 500 mg orally every 6 hours for 8 doses. **Children**: Timing of doses is same as for adults. Aqueous penicillin dose is 30,000 units/kg mixed with 600,000 units procaine penicillin. Streptomycin dose is 20 mg/kg (not to exceed adult dosage). For children less than 60 lbs, the dose of penicillin V is 250 mg every 6 hours for 8 doses.
IV. For higher risk patients (especially those with prosthetic heart valves) who are allergic to penicillin: **VANCOMYCIN** intravenously and **ERYTHROMYCIN** orally	**Adults**: Vancomycin 1 gm IV over 30–60 minutes, begun 30–60 minutes before procedure; then erythromycin 500 mg orally every 6 hours for 8 doses. **Children**: Timing of doses is same as for adults. Dose of vancomycin is 20 mg/kg. Dose of erythromycin is 10 mg/kg every 6 hours for 8 doses (not to exceed adult dose).

For Gastrointestinal and Genitourinary Tract Surgery and Instrumentation and also for Any Surgery of Infected Tissues

I. For most patients: **PENICILLIN** or **AMPICILLIN** plus **STREPTOMYCIN** or **GENTAMICIN**	**Adults**: 2 million units of aqueous penicillin G IM or IV **or** 1.0 gm ampicillin IM or IV **plus** gentamicin 1.5 mg/kg (not to exceed 80 mg) IM or IV **or** streptomycin 1.0 gm IM. This should be given 30–60 minutes before procedure. Repeat every 8 hours for 2 additional doses if gentamicin is used, or every 12 hours for 2 additional doses if streptomycin is used. **Children**: Same timing of medications as adult schedule. Dosages are aqueous penicillin G 30,000 units/kg **or** ampicillin 50 mg/kg; gentamicin 2.0 mg/kg (not to exceed adult dosage).
II. For patients allergic to penicillin: **VANCOMYCIN** plus **STREPTOMYCIN**	**Adults**: 1.0 gm vancomycin IV given over 30–60 minutes **plus** 1.0 gm streptomycin IM, each given 30–60 minutes before procedure. Doses may be repeated in 12 hours. **Children**: Timing as above. Doses are vancomycin 20 mg/kg and streptomycin 20 mg/kg (not to exceed adult dosage).

NOTE: In patients with significantly compromised renal function, antibiotic dosages may need to be modified. Intramuscular injections may be contraindicated in patients receiving anticoagulants.

Adapted from The Report of the Committee on Rheumatic Fever and Bacterial Endocarditis, American Heart Association, 1977.[54]

form of irritability and crying during feeding or straining at bowel movement. In children with severe left or right ventricular outflow tract obstruction chest pain commonly follows effort and is identical to angina observed in adults. Cardiac pain associated with *pulmonary vascular obstruction* may be anginal in nature but often is evanescent and pleuritic in type. Atypical forms of chest pain associated with the syndrome of *mitral valve prolapse* are much less usual in children than adults. A sensation of chest discomfort or cardiac awareness is frequently interpreted as pain by the parents of children with cardiac arrhythmias. Careful questioning serves to identify palpitations rather than pain as the symptom and often elicits an additional history of anxiety, pallor, and sweating. Pain due to *pericarditis* is commonly of acute onset, is associated with fever, and can be identified by specific physical, roentgenographic, and echocardiographic findings.

Most commonly, chest pain in children is *musculoskeletal* in origin and may be reproduced upon upper extremity movement or by palpation; often, chest wall pain is the result of *costochondritis*. Lastly, children, like adults, may suffer chest pain of nonspecific pattern owing to *anxiety* in the presence or absence of hyperventilation; often a history is elicited of a family member or friend who had died recently or suffered myocardial infarction.

Syncope
(See also Chapter 28)

Syncope is an unusual feature of heart disease in children; its presence suggests specific diagnoses, the most common being an arrhythmia. The symptom is observed in children with complete atrioventricular block that is less often of congenital origin than a sequela of cardiac operation. Syncope due to abrupt episodes of either bradycardia or tachycardia occurs in association with the sick sinus syndrome. The latter is most commonly produced in children after surgical procedures involving the region of the sinoatrial node, e.g., atrial septal defect closure or Mustard's procedure for transposition of the great arteries (p. 1001). Syncope is an occasional but ominous symptom if associated with severe aortic stenosis, pulmonary vascular obstruction, or a left atrial myxoma that transiently occludes left ventricular inflow.

Sudden Death
(See also Chapter 23)

In contrast to adults, children seldom die suddenly and unexpectedly from cardiovascular disease. Arrhythmias, hypoxemia, and coronary insufficiency secondary to left ventricular outflow tract obstruction are the most frequent causes of death.[55] Sudden death is most often reported in patients with aortic stenosis or hypertrophic obstructive cardiomyopathy, the Eisenmenger syndrome of pulmonary vascular obstruction, myocarditis, congenital complete heart block, primary endocardial fibroelastosis, anomalies of the coronary arteries, and cyanotic congenital heart disease with pulmonic stenosis or atresia. A relationship exists between strenuous exercise and sudden demise in patients with aortic stenosis or obstructive cardiomyopathy, thus providing justification for restricting patients with these lesions from gymnastic activities and strenuous competitive sports.

APPROACH TO THE HIGH-RISK INFANT

Approximately one-third of all infants born with congenital heart disease will die in the first months of life without prompt recognition, accurate diagnosis, or treatment of their life-threatening anomaly. Heart failure and cyanosis are the two cardinal signs of the high-risk infant with heart disease, and this section will provide an approach for the management of each.

Heart Failure
(See also Chapter 16)

Care of the infant with heart failure must include careful consideration of the underlying structural or functional disturbance. The general aims of treatment are to achieve an increase in cardiac performance, augment peripheral perfusion, and decrease pulmonary and systemic venous congestion. It must be emphasized, however, that under many conditions medical management cannot control the effects of the abnormal loads imposed by a host of congenital cardiac lesions. Under these circumstances cardiac catheterization and operative intervention may be urgently required.[56] Thus, initial therapy is aimed at stabilizing the infant for diagnostic hemodynamic and angiocardiographic study as soon as possible. In almost all situations the decision to intervene surgically or to continue medical management requires a definitive anatomical diagnosis.

Table 29–6 lists supportive and pharmacological measures in the treatment of the newborn with heart failure. Digitalis glycosides and certain diuretic agents provide the most important elements of medical therapy, but it is important to recognize that the dosage regimen of drugs administered to young patients must be adjusted to take into account the age and size of the patient and the maturity-dependent pharmacological properties of cardioactive drugs.[57,58] Since this is especially true in early infancy, Table 29–7 provides the dosages of digoxin and diuretics commonly employed. Digoxin is the glycoside used exclusively to treat pediatric patients in most cardiac centers, since it is readily absorbed, is available in convenient dosage form, and is excreted rapidly from the body. Premature infants are more sensitive to digitalis than are full-term newborns who, in turn, are more sensitive than older infants. Infants absorb and excrete digoxin as well as adults

TABLE 29–6 TREATMENT OF CONGESTIVE HEART FAILURE

I. Rest (occasional sedation)
   - Semi-Fowler position
   - Temperature and humidity control
   - Oxygen

II. Diet—Decrease NaCl load, recognize danger of aspiration

III. Medications
   - Correct hypoglycemia, anemia, or acidemia, if present
   - Treat infection, if contributing factor
   - Diuretics
   - Digitalis
   - Occasional need for catecholamine infusion, mechanical ventilation, peritoneal dialysis, afterload reduction, prostaglandin infusion or blocker

IV. Surgery

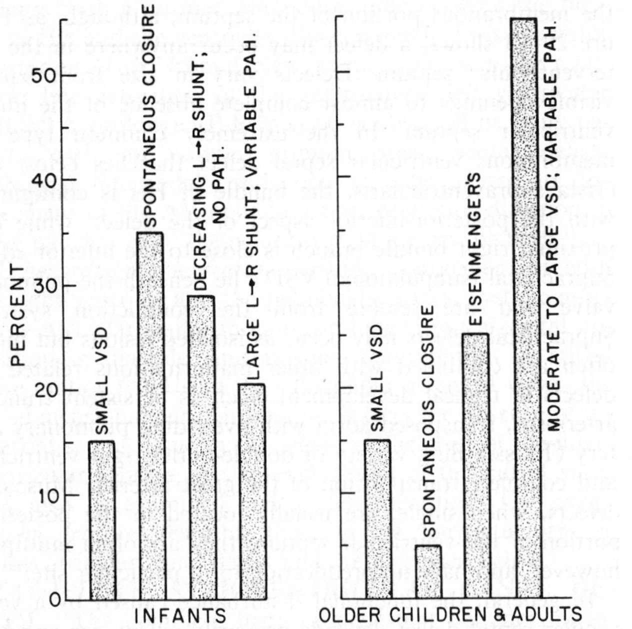

FIGURE 29–14 Natural history of ventricular septal defect. Approximate percentages are depicted for the various events that may occur in infants *(left)* and older children and adults *(right)* with VSD. PAH = pulmonary arterial hypertension, L-R = left to right. (From Friedman, W. F., and Pitlick, P. T.: Ventricular septal defect in infancy—University of California, San Diego (Specialty Conference). West. J. Med. *120*:295, 1974.)

the systemic and pulmonary circulations. In such patients the magnitude of the left-to-right shunt varies inversely with pulmonary vascular resistance.

A wide spectrum exists in the natural history of VSD, ranging from spontaneous closure to congestive cardiac failure and death in early infancy (Fig. 29–14). Within this spectrum are possible development of pulmonary vascular obstruction, right ventricular outflow tract obstruction, aortic regurgitation, and infective endocarditis.[98–107]

INFANCY. It is unusual for a VSD to cause difficulties in the immediate postnatal period, although congestive heart failure during the first 6 months of life is a frequent occurrence. Early diagnosis is helpful in order to ensure more careful observation of the affected infant.[107] The examining physician usually suspects the diagnosis because of a harsh systolic murmur at the lower left sternal border. The electrocardiogram and chest roentgenogram are within normal limits in the immediate neonatal period because appreciable left-to-right shunting occurs only after the pulmonary vascular resistance decreases as the pulmonary vessels lose their fetal characteristics. It is desirable to follow these infants continually. A VSD that either decreases in size or closes completely during the first year of life presents no problems to the practicing physician. Spontaneous closure occurs by age 3 years in approximately 40 per cent of patients born with VSD; occasional patients, however, do not experience spontaneous closure until age 8 to 10 years.[103] Closure is more common in patients born with a small VSD; nonetheless, approximately 7 per cent of infants with a large defect and congestive heart failure early in life may also experience spontaneous closure. Partial rather than complete closure is common in patients with both large and small VSD's.[98] Anatomically, reduction of the VSD is often based on adherence of the tricuspid valve to the VSD, hypertrophy of septal muscle, or ingrowth of fibrous tissue; rarely, VSD closure is the result of prolapse of an aortic cusp[108] or infective endocarditis.[109] Some defects close when an aneurysm forms in the ventricular septum. On auscultation a click may be heard in early systole as the aneurysm tenses toward the right; the septal aneurysm may be detected by echocardiography as an anterior systolic bulge in the right ventricular outflow tract. A persistent minute VSD is not life-threatening unless bacterial endocarditis develops. With proper precautions the incidence of this complication is less than 1 per cent.

If a moderate or large defect maintains its size after birth, the net left-to-right shunt increases during the first month of life as pulmonary vascular resistance falls. *Physical examination* during this time usually reveals a thrill along the lower left sternal border, and the holosystolic murmur of flow across the interventricular defect is accompanied by a low-pitched diastolic rumble at the apex, reflecting increased flow across the mitral valve. *Chest roentgenograms* reveal increased pulmonary vascular markings; evidence of left or biventricular hypertrophy may be observed on the electrocardiogram. Infants with a large left-to-right shunt tend to do poorly, with recurrent upper and lower respiratory tract infections, failure to gain weight, and congestive heart failure. Congestive heart failure may be severe and intractable despite intensive medical management.[105,106] For these infants we currently recommend primary intracardiac repair of the VSD rather than surgical banding of the pulmonary artery[107,110] in order to reduce pulmonary blood flow and alleviate heart failure. Primary VSD closure may be performed in infancy employing cardiopulmonary bypass, profound hypothermia and cardiocirculatory arrest, or a combination of the two techniques. Mortality is less than 10 per cent if the defect is single but approaches 25 per cent if multiple defects are present.[111–114]

Fortunately, medical treatment often is successful in controlling congestive heart failure. Nevertheless, these infants should be referred for cardiac catheterization to evaluate pulmonary vascular resistance and to detect associated defects that may require operation, such as patent ductus arteriosus and coarctation of the aorta.

It is of utmost importance to identify patients who may develop irreversible pulmonary vascular obstructive disease (the Eisenmenger reaction).[115–117] Retrospective analyses of children who develop this complication indicate that infants with systemic or near systemic pressures in the pulmonary artery at the time of initial hemodynamic study are most at risk. Recatheterization before age 18 months and a second determination of pulmonary vascular resistance should be performed in these patients in order to decide whether surgical intervention is necessary to prevent development of fixed obliterative changes in the pulmonary vessels. It is likely that multiple factors are involved in the development of pulmonary vascular disease (p. 832 and 950). The anatomically large VSD allows some or all of the systemic pressure to be transmitted to the pulmonary arteries, thereby retarding regression of their muscular media. Medial hypertrophy in the first months of life is responsible for higher pulmonary vascular resistance than would be anticipated for the amount of pulmonary blood flow. The shearing forces created by the high velocity of flow through narrowed pulmonary arterioles cause endothelial damage that is progressive. While an evalation in left atrial pressure may contribute to the rise in pulmonary vascular resistance, it is not an essential factor, since pulmonary venous pressures can be low in patients who later develop pulmonary vascular disease. Nonetheless, pulmonary venous hypertension may also contribute to pulmonary arterial vasoconstriction and thus to increased shear forces. In this same regard, pulmonary vasoconstriction enhancing the risk of pulmonary vascular obstruction may also be caused by hypoxia due to either high altitude or lung disease. At high altitude, large VSD's have higher pulmonary vascular resistances and smaller shunts than at low altitude.

CHILDHOOD. Beyond the first year of life a variable clinical picture emerges in children with VSD.[98-107] If a small defect is present, the child is usually asymptomatic, the electrocardiogram is generally normal, and the chest roentgenogram shows normal or only a mild increase in pulmonary vascular markings. Effort intolerance and fatigue are associated with moderate left-to-right shunts. These children exhibit cardiomegaly with a forceful left ventricular impulse and a prominent systolic thrill along the lower left sternal border. The second heart sound is normally split, with moderate accentuation of the pulmonic component; a third heart sound and rumbling diastolic murmur that reflects increased flow across the mitral valve are audible at the cardiac apex. The characteristic murmur resulting from flow across the defect is harsh and holosystolic, is best heard along the third and fourth interspaces to the left of the sternum, and is widely transmitted over the precordium. A basal midsystolic ejection murmur due to increased flow across the pulmonic valve may also be heard. The electrocardiogram reveals left or combined ventricular hypertrophy, and the chest roentgenogram shows cardiomegaly, left atrial enlargement, and vascular engorgement.

RIGHT VENTRICULAR OUTFLOW TRACT OBSTRUCTION. With time, the clinical picture changes in 8 to 15 per cent of patients with VSD and a moderate to large left-to-right shunt early in life. It begins to resemble more closely the tetralogy of Fallot (p. 990), i.e., subvalvular right ventricular outflow tract obstruction due to progressive hypertrophy of the crista supraventricularis develops. Depending on the severity of the latter process, it may result ultimately in reduced blood flow and a right-to-left shunt across the VSD. As right ventricular outflow tract obstruction develops, the holosystolic VSD murmur is replaced by the crescendo-decrescendo ejection systolic murmur of pulmonic stenosis, and the pulmonary closure sound becomes softer. Right ventricular hypertrophy is evident on the electrocardiogram, while the chest x-ray shows a reduction in pulmonary vascular markings and a smaller heart size with a right ventricular configuration. Infundibular hypertrophy may progress quite rapidly within the first year of life, but the typical evolution to a clinical picture of cyanotic tetralogy of Fallot often takes 1 to 4 years. In those infants who develop right ventricular outflow obstruction the incidence of spontaneous closure or reduction in size of a ventricular septal defect is low.

AORTIC REGURGITATION (AR). This is a well-described complication of VSD that occurs in approximately 5 per cent of patients.[118-123] It is usually noted after age 5 years when a physician detects the early diastolic blowing murmur and wide pulse pressure of aortic regurgitation while following a patient with a VSD. In such patients, AR may become the predominant hemodynamic abnormality. It is of interest that VSD with AR is rare in Europe and America, with an incidence of approximately 4 per cent of all cases of isolated VSD, whereas in Japan the incidence is substantially higher (approximately 10 per cent). In the Japanese, in particular, AR is the result of herniation of an aortic leaflet (usually the right coronary) through a subpulmonic supracristal VSD. In these patients, closure of the VSD may be all that is required to relieve aortic regurgitation. In many patients, however, especially in the western world, the VSD is below the crista supraventricularis. While aortic leaflet herniation, especially of the right or noncoronary cusp, may occur in some of these patients, quite often AR results from a primary abnormality of the valve, usually one defective commissure. In the latter situation, plication of the elongated leaflet may lessen, but not abolish, the aortic regurgitation; in some patients prosthetic aortic valve replacement may be necessary to provide hemodynamic relief. In most patients with VSD and AR, the VSD is small to moderate in size, and mild right ventricular outflow tract obstruction exists. The latter is caused either by subpulmonic infundibular stenosis or projection of the herniated aortic cusp into the right ventricular outflow tract. The distinction between types of VSD with AR can usually be made by selective left ventricular angiocardiography to define the site of the interventricular communication in combination with retrograde aortography to assess the anatomy and competence of the aortic valve (Fig. 29–15).

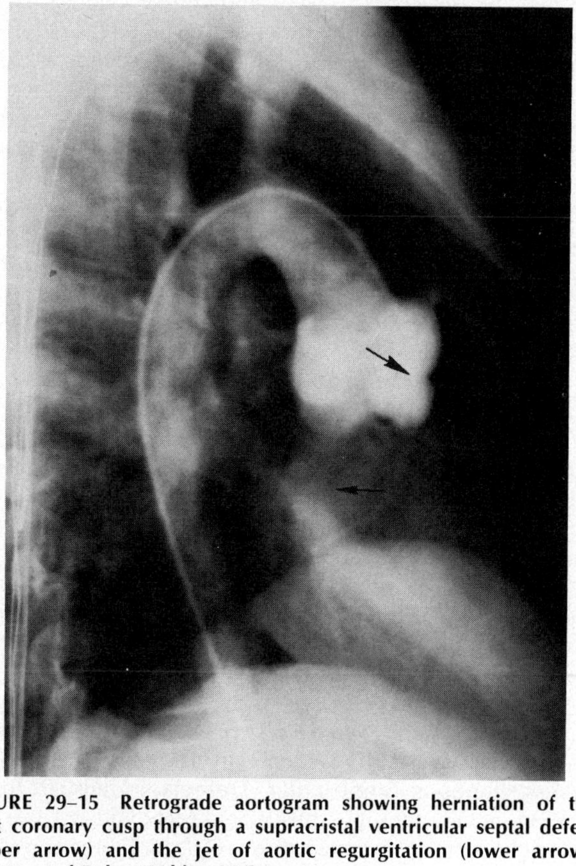

FIGURE 29–15 Retrograde aortogram showing herniation of the right coronary cusp through a supracristal ventricular septal defect (upper arrow) and the jet of aortic regurgitation (lower arrow). (Courtesy of Robert White, M.D.)

Currently, optimal management of the patient with VSD and AR is controversial. In patients with a large, hemodynamically significant left-to-right shunt, repair of the VSD is indicated, but AR is repaired only if at least moderate aortic regurgitation exists. If a supracristal VSD without AR is identified at cardiac catheterization in early childhood, a sensible argument for prophylactic closure of the VSD can be put forth to prevent the potential complication of aortic valve incompetence. In the presence of moderate or severe AR, valvuloplasty is preferred to valve replacement, in recognition of the fact that the severity of aortic regurgitation may increase in subsequent years and that reoperation with valve replacement may be necessary. Operation should probably be deferred in asymptomatic patients with a subcristal VSD and an insignificant left-to-right shunt in whom AR is not severe. If the defect is supracristal in the same clinical setting, its closure may not alleviate the mild degree of aortic incompetence but may retard its progression.

It is rarely necessary to restrict the activities of a child with an isolated VSD in any way. Subacute bacterial endocarditis is always a threat, and antibiotic prophylaxis for dental procedures and minor surgery is indicated.[124] Respiratory infections require prompt evaluation and treatment. These children should be seen at least once or twice yearly to detect changes in the clinical picture that suggest the development of pulmonary vascular obliterative changes.

PULMONARY VASCULAR OBSTRUCTION. If a child who previously had a loud murmur and thrill associated with poor growth suddenly has a growth spurt, fewer respiratory infections, and a diminution of the intensity of the cardiac murmur and disappearance of the thrill, he or she may be developing severe obliterative changes in the pulmonary vascular bed. An increase in intensity of the pulmonic component of the second heart sound, a reduction in heart size on chest roentgenograms, and more pronounced right ventricular hypertrophy on the electrocardiogram are also noted. These changes occur because the increased pulmonary vascular resistance causes a decrease in the left-to-right shunt. If these changes are suspected, cardiac catheterization should be repeated; if they are confirmed, prompt surgical repair is indicated before an inoperable predominant right-to-left shunt ensues. If operation is performed under age 2 years, pulmonary vascular resistance may be expected to fall to normal levels.[117] In older patients the degree to which pulmonary vascular resistance is elevated before operation is a critical factor determining prognosis. If the pulmonary vascular resistance is one third or less of the systemic value, progressive pulmonary vascular disease after operation is unusual. However, if a moderate-to-severe increase in pulmonary vascular resistance exists preoperatively, either no change or progression of pulmonary vascular disease is common postoperatively. Moreover, the presence of increased pulmonary vascular resistance results in a higher immediate postoperative mortality rate for closure of VSD. These observations make it clear that a large VSD should be approached surgically very early in life when pulmonary vascular disease is still reversible or has not yet developed.

Miscellaneous Ventricular Defects. Unusual forms of VSD include multiple muscular defects and left ventricular–right atrial communications. Defects in the muscular ventricular septum frequently are multiple small fenestrations that produce a large net left-to-right shunt.[98] Their recognition is a necessary preliminary to successful operation, since incomplete repair may result in post-operative cardiac failure and death. A shunt from the left ventricle to right atrium may occur with a VSD in the most superior portion of the ventricular septum, since the tricuspid valve is lower than the mitral valve. The clinical, electrocardiographic, and radiological findings in these patients do not differ appreciably from those of a simple VSD, although right atrial enlargement may provide a clue to correct diagnosis of left ventricular–right atrial communication. The pathophysiology of single or common ventricle (p. 1012) resembles that of a large VSD, although these defects are dissimilar embryologically. The single chamber frequently is the morphological left ventricle; transposition of the great arteries is quite common. There may be no detectable cyanosis if selective streaming and increased pulmonary blood flow rather than complete mixing occurs. Pulmonary hypertension invariably is present unless pulmonic stenosis exists. It is imperative to differentiate a single ventricle from a large VSD by echocardiography[125] and angiography[126] because corrective operation of the former malformation has had only limited success.

MANAGEMENT. Whenever clinical findings suggest a moderate shunt but no pulmonary hypertension, elective hemodynamic evaluation should be advised between ages 3 and 6 years. Of prime importance in the hemodynamic evaluation is a determination of pressure and blood flow in the pulmonary artery.[107,127] We do not recommend surgical treatment for children who have normal pulmonary arterial pressures with small shunts (pulmonary-systemic flow ratios of less than 1.5 to 2.0:1). In such patients the remaining risk of infective endocarditis[124] does not exceed the risk of operation. Moreover, although the inherent risk of operation is small, the possibility of postoperative heart block, infection, or other complications of operation and cardiopulmonary bypass dictates a conservative approach when the cardiac defect may be well tolerated for life.

With larger shunts, elective operation may be advised before the child enters school, thus minimizing any subsequent distinction of these patients from their normal classmates.[127a] A total assessment of the psychosocial dynamics of the family and child is obviously helpful in determining the proper age for elective operation in each patient.

Complete heart block is the most significant surgically induced conduction system abnormality, occurring immediately following surgery in less than 1 per cent of patients. Late-onset complete heart block is occasionally a problem, especially in the 10 to 25 per cent of patients whose postoperative electrocardiographic findings show complete right bundle branch block with left anterior hemiblock.[128] When the latter electrocardiographic pattern is observed in patients with transient complete heart block in the early postoperative period, electrophysiological studies should be conducted at postoperative cardiac catheterization. It would appear that patients presenting postoperatively with right bundle branch block and left anterior hemiblock fall into two different populations, defined by either peripheral damage to the conduction system or damage to the bundle of His or its proximal branches.[129] The former has not been associated with transient postoperative complete heart block, and these patients have been found to have a generally benign course. Trifascicular damage may be demonstrated in the latter population by a prolonged H-V interval, which implies a higher risk of complete heart block later in life. Although the prophylactic use of permanent pacemakers in asymptomatic patients with evidence of trifascicular damage is not currently recommended, this group certainly requires careful follow-up and continued study.

Intense treadmill exercise studies in patients who preoperatively had normal or only moderately elevated pulmonary vascular resistance and essentially normal postoperative cardiac catheterization data may uncover late abnormalities in circulatory function.[130] Despite normal cardiac output at rest, an impaired cardiac output response to exercise is noted in some. Moreover, despite a normal pulmonary arterial pressure at rest, markedly abnormal increases in pulmonary arterial pressure may be noted during exercise. These findings may be related to abnormal left ventricular function after closure of the VSD and/or to persistent pathological changes in the pulmonary arterioles or to abnormal pulmonary vascular reactivity.[131,132] A direct relation exists between age at operation and the magnitude of the pulmonary arterial pressure response to intense exercise, suggesting that early operation may prevent permanent impairment of the functional capacity of the myocardium and pulmonary vascular bed.

Occasionally a child may come to medical attention who has already developed pulmonary vascular obstruction and a net right-to-left shunt across the VSD. Symptoms may consist of exertional dyspnea, chest pain, syncope, and hemoptysis; the right-to-left shunt leads to cyanosis, clubbing, and polycythemia. At present there is little to offer this group of patients other than continuing support to the patient and family.

Patent Ductus Arteriosus

The ductus arteriosus exists normally in the fetus as a widely patent vessel connecting the pulmonary trunk and the descending aorta just distal to the left subclavian artery (Fig. 29–5). In the fetus most of the output of the right ventricle bypasses the unexpanded lungs via the ductus arteriosus and enters the descending aorta where it travels to the placenta, the fetal organ of oxygenation. Until recently it was assumed that during fetal life the ductus arteriosus was a passively open channel that constricted postnatally by means of undefined molecular mechanisms in response to the abrupt rise in arterial pO_2 accompanying the first breath of life.[133] Evidence now exists that even in utero the size of the ductus arteriosus lumen may be influenced by vasoactive substances, particularly prostaglandins.[61,134,135] Thus, inhibition of prostaglandin synthesis causes profound constriction of the ductus arteriosus in the mammalian fetus that may be reversed by administration of vasodilatory E-type prostaglandins. Initial contraction and functional closure of the ductus arteriosus immediately after birth may be related to both the sudden increase in arterial oxygen saturation that accompanies ventilation and the synthesis, release, or inhibition of vasoactive substances. Intimal proliferation and fibrosis proceed more gradually, so that anatomical closure may take as long as several weeks for completion.

The ductus arteriosus is a unique structure after birth, since its patency may, on the one hand, result in cardiac decompensation but may, on the other hand, provide the only life-sustaining conduit to preserve systemic or pulmonary arterial blood flow in the presence of certain cardiac malformations.[59] Appreciable left-to-right shunting across the patent ductus arteriosus frequently complicates the clinical course of infants born prematurely.[27,136] The ductal shunt has been implicated specifically in the deterioration of pulmonary function in infants with the respiratory distress syndrome in whom severe congestive heart failure is often unresponsive to digitalis and diuretics.

A distinction should be made between patency of the ductus arteriosus in the *preterm* infant, who lacks the normal mechanisms for postnatal ductal closure because of immaturity, and the full-term newborn, in whom patency of the ductus is a true congenital malformation, related most likely to a primary anatomical defect of the elastic tissue within the wall of the ductus.[137] In the former circumstance, delayed spontaneous closure of the ductus may be anticipated if the infant does not succumb to the cardiopulmonary difficulties caused by the ductus itself or to some lethal complication of prematurity, such as hyaline membrane disease, intraventricular hemorrhage, or necrotizing enterocolitis. In similar fashion, some full-term newborns have persistent patency of the ductus arteriosus for weeks or months because their relative hypoxemia contributes to vasodilatation of the channel. In the latter category are infants born at high altitude; those born with congenital malformations causing hypoxemia, such as pulmonic atresia with and without ventricular septal defect; or malformations in which ductal flow supplies the systemic circulation, such as hypoplastic left heart syndrome, interruption of the aortic arch, or some examples of coarctation of the aorta syndrome. In the clinical settings in which the ductus preserves pulmonary blood flow, the essentially inevitable spontaneous closure of the vessel is associated with profound clinical deterioration. The latter may be reversed medically by infusion of vasodilatory prostaglandins intravenously or via an aortic catheter at the level of the ductus. By dilating the constricted ductus arteriosus, this results in a temporary increase in arterial blood oxygen tension and oxygen saturation and correction of acidemia.[59,138] These infants can then undergo operation, usually a systemic-pulmonary anastomosis, under more optimal circumstances. Pharmacological dilation of the ductus arteriosus may also be effective in the preoperative restoration of systemic blood flow and the alleviation of heart failure, especially in infants with aortic coarctation, and in infants with complete transposition of the great arteries in whom intercirculatory mixing is augmented.[59]

PREMATURE INFANTS. In most, if not all, preterm infants under 1500 grams birthweight, persistence of a patent ductus arteriosus is prolonged, and in approximately one third of these infants a large aorticopulmonary shunt is responsible for significant cardiopulmonary deterioration.[139–143] Radiographic and echocardiographic signs of significant left-to-right shunting usually precede the appearance of physical findings suggesting ductal patency.[144] A significant increase in the cardiothoracic ratio is seen on sequential radiographs as well as increased pulmonary arterial markings progressing to perihilar and generalized

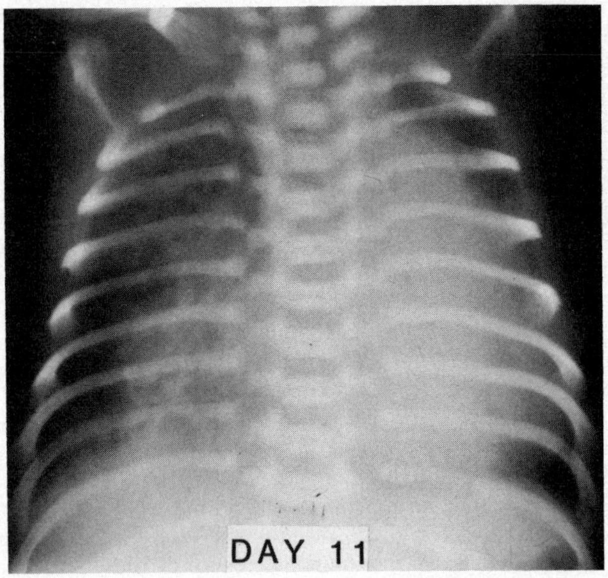

FIGURE 29–16 Chest roentgenogram in 11-day preterm infant with a large patent ductus arteriosus revealing cardiomegaly, pulmonary hypervascularity, and pulmonary edema. (From Higgins, C. B., et al.: Patent ductus arteriosus in preterm infants with idiopathic respiratory distress syndrome. Radiographic and echocardiographic evaluation. Radiology *124*:189, 1977.)

pulmonary edema (Fig. 29–16). Serial echocardiographic evaluations that demonstrate increases in left ventricular end-diastolic and left atrial dimensions, especially when correlated with the aforementioned radiographic signs, are highly accurate in detecting a large shunt (Fig. 29–17).[145,146] The clinical findings include bounding peripheral pulses, an infraclavicular and interscapular systolic murmur (occasionally a continuous murmur), precordial hyperactivity, hepatomegaly, and either multiple episodes of apnea and bradycardia or respirator dependency.

Management of the preterm infant with a patent ductus arteriosus varies, depending upon the magnitude of shunting and the severity of hyaline membrane disease, since the ductus may contribute importantly to mortality in the respiratory distress syndrome. Intervention in an asymptomatic infant with a small left-to-right shunt is unnecessary, since the patent ductus arteriosus will almost invariably undergo spontaneous closure and will not require late surgical ligation and division. Those infants who demonstrate unmistakable signs of a large ductal left-to-right shunt during the course of the respiratory distress syndrome are often unresponsive to medical measures to control congestive heart failure and require closure of the patent ductus arteriosus in order to survive. These infants are best managed within the first 2 to 7 days of life either by pharmacological inhibition of prostaglandin synthesis to constrict and close the ductus[136,139–143,147] or by surgical ligation.[27,148] Early intervention is advised in order to reduce the likelihood of bronchopulmonary dysplasia related to prolonged respirator and oxygen dependency. Less often, indications for pharmacological or surgical closure of the ductus consist of life-threatening episodes of apnea and bradycardia or a prolonged failure to gain weight and grow.

FULL-TERM INFANTS AND CHILDREN. In full-term newborns and older infants and children, patency of the ductus arteriosus occurs particularly in females and in the offspring of pregnancies complicated by first-trimester rubella. Although most frequent in isolated form, the anomaly may coexist with other malformations, particularly coarctation of the aorta, ventricular septal defect, pulmonic stenosis, and aortic stenosis. Flow across the ductus is determined by the pressure relationship between the aorta and the pulmonary artery and by the cross-sectional area and length of the ductus itself.[149] Most commonly, pulmonary pressures are normal, and a persistent gradient and shunt from aorta to pulmonary artery exist throughout the cardiac cycle. Physical examination reveals a char-

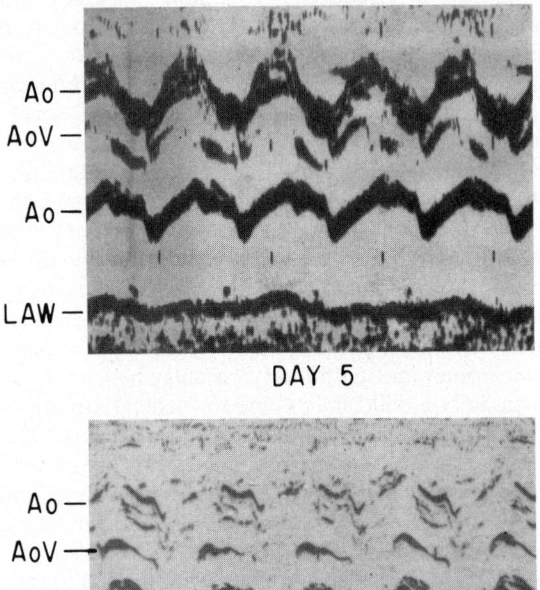

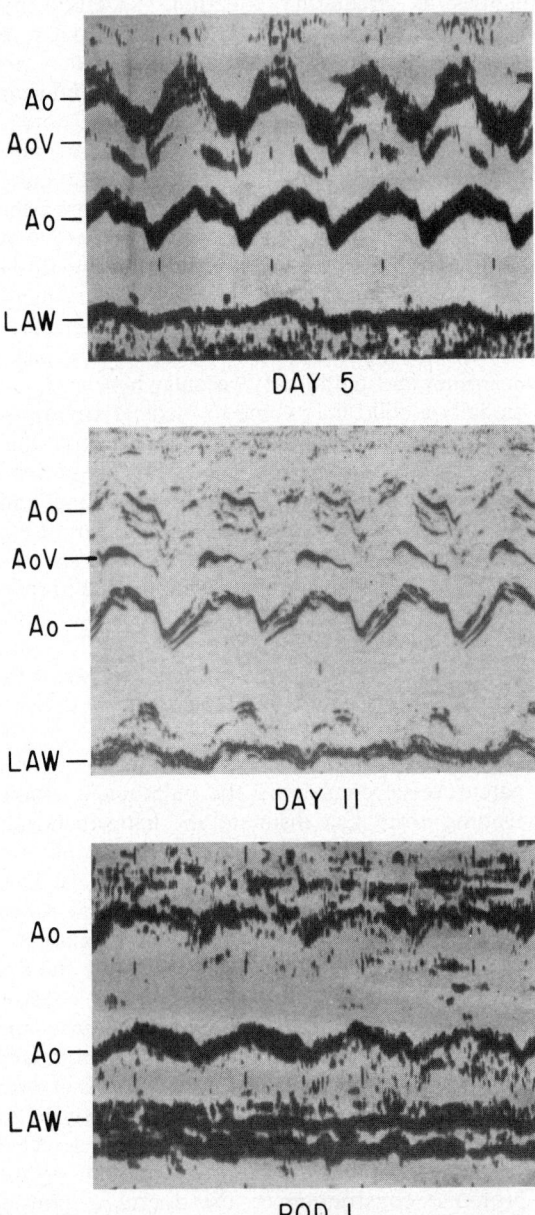

FIGURE 29–17 Serial echocardiograms in a preterm infant. On day 5, left atrial dimensions are normal but are increased on day 11, indicating the presence of a large left-to-right shunt across the ductus arteriosus. One day after ductus ligation (POD 1) left atrial dimensions have returned to normal. Ao = aorta, AoV = aortic valve, LAW = left atrial wall. (From Higgins, C. B., et al.: Patent ductus arteriosus in preterm infants with idiopathic respiratory distress syndrome. Radiographic and echocardiographic evaluation. Radiology *124*:189, 1977.)

acteristic thrill and a continuous "machinery" murmur with a late systolic accentuation at the upper left sternal border. The left atrium and left ventricle enlarge to accommodate the increased pulmonary venous return, and flow murmurs across the mitral and aortic valves may be detected. With significant left-to-right shunting, the runoff of blood through the ductus causes a widened systemic pulse pressure and bounding peripheral pulses. The hemodynamic abnormality is reflected electrocardiographically by left ventricular and occasionally left atrial hypertrophy, and radiologically by left atrial hypertrophy, and radiologically by left atrial and ventricular enlargement, and prominent ascending aorta and pulmonary artery, and pulmonary vascular engorgement. The clinical diagnosis may be difficult when the findings do not conform to the classic presentation.[150,151] As mentioned above, disappearance of the diastolic component of the murmur is common in premature infants because higher pulmonary arterial diastolic pressures exist at that age. In older patients both heart failure and pulmonary hypertension are associated with a reduction in the pressure gradient across the ductus arteriosus and result in atypical systolic murmurs. When severe pulmonary vascular obstructive disease results in reversal of flow through the ductus and preferential shunting of unoxygenated blood to the descending aorta, the toes, rather than the fingers, may show cyanosis and clubbing.

The full-term infant with patent ductus arteriosus may survive for a number of years, although occasionally a large defect results in heart failure and pulmonary edema early in life. The leading causes of death in older children are bacterial endocarditis and heart failure. Beyond the third decade severe pulmonary vascular obstruction has been known to cause aneurysmal dilatation, calcification, and rupture of the ductus.[150]

Cardiac catheterization is indicated when additional lesions or pulmonary hypertension is suspected, except in the preterm infant, in whom the risk of cardiac catheterization is high and the syndrome created by ductal patency can be recognized easily by noninvasive studies.[144,151] In the absence of severe pulmonary vascular disease with predominant left-to-right shunting the anatomical presence of a patent ductus is generally considered sufficient indication for operation.[150a] Ligation or division of the ductus carries a low risk, whether performed electively in the asymptomatic child or at any age if symptoms are present. The operative risk is reduced if heart failure can be compensated by medical measures before surgery. Operation should be deferred for several months in patients treated successfully for bacterial endarteritis because the ductus may remain somewhat edematous and friable. Rarely, when the infection will not subside with intensive antibiotic treatment, surgical ligation may be necessary to eradicate the infection.

Aorticopulmonary Septal Defect

Aorticopulmonary window or fenestration, partial truncus arteriosus, and aortic septal defect are other designations applied to this relatively uncommon anomaly. Septation of the aortopulmonary trunk occurs by fusion of the conotruncal ridges (see Fig. 29–4). The right and left sixth aortic arches, destined to become the pulmonary arteries, join the pulmonary artery to complete great artery development (see Fig. 29–5). Congenital defects between the ascending aorta and the pulmonary artery result from faulty development of this area during embryonic life. The typical aortopulmonary septal defect results because of incomplete fusion of the distal aortal-pulmonary septum.[152] Malalignment of the conotruncal ridges results in unequal partitioning of the aortopulmonary trunk, which may result in partial or complete fusion of the right pulmonary artery to the aorta. The usual defect consists of a communication between the aorta and pulmonary artery just above the semilunar valves. Persistent patency of the ductus arteriosus is an associated lesion in 10 to 15 per cent of cases. Less common accompanying cardiovascular lesions include ventricular septal defect, coarctation of the aorta, and right aortic arch. Aorticopulmonary septal defects are usually large and are accompanied by severe pulmonary arterial hypertension.

On *physical examination* the pulses are typically bounding, like those of a large patent ductus arteriosus. However, the murmur is rarely continuous, and a basal systolic murmur is most common.[153] Cardiomegaly is present, and pulmonary hypertension is reflected in a loud and palpable sound of pulmonary valve closure. Aorticopulmonary septal defect should be suspected whenever a large shunt into the pulmonary artery is demonstrated at catheterization.[153,154] Distinction from patent ductus and persistent truncus arteriosus is facilitated by selective angiocardiography with the injection of contrast material into the left ventricle and/or the root of the aorta (Fig. 29–18).[155] Although occasional patients may survive to adulthood with uncorrected aorticopulmonary septal defect, most will die during childhood unless surgical treatment is undertaken. Operative correction is indicated in children with large left-to-right shunts; total cardiopulmonary bypass is required, and the defect is closed usually via a transaortic approach with a prosthetic patch.[154–156,156a]

Persistent Truncus Arteriosus

Persistent truncus arteriosus is a rare but serious anomaly in which a single vessel forms the outlet of both ventri-

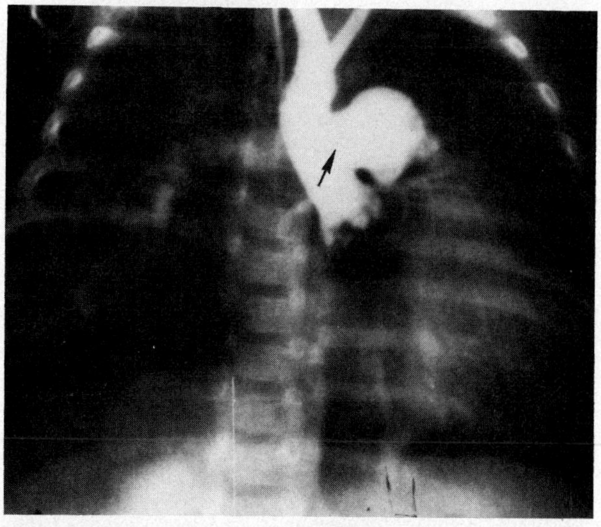

FIGURE 29–18 Aortic root injection of contrast material in the frontal view produces simultaneous opacification of aorta and pulmonary artery through a large aorticopulmonary septal defect (arrow). (Courtesy of Robert White, M.D.)

cles and gives rise to the systemic, pulmonary, and coronary arteries.[157,158] The defect results from failure of septation of the embryonic truncus by the infundibular truncal ridges (see Fig. 29–4). It is always accompanied by a ventricular septal defect and frequently by a right-sided aortic arch. The ventricular septal defect is due to the absence or underdevelopment of the distal portion of the pulmonary infundibulum. The truncal valve is usually tricuspid but is quadricuspid in approximately one third of patients and, rarely, bicuspid. Truncal valve regurgitation and truncal valve stenosis are each seen in 10 to 15 per cent of patients. There may be a single coronary artery, displacement of the coronary ostia (usually the left ostium posteriorly), or a single posterior descending coronary artery arising from the right coronary or, less often, from the left circumflex artery, especially in patients with a single coronary artery.[159]

Truncus malformations may be classified either anatomically according to the mode of origin of pulmonary vessels from the common trunk or from a functional point of view, based on the magnitude of blood flow to the lungs.[160] In the common type (type I) of truncus arteriosus malformation a partially separate pulmonary trunk of varying length exists because of the presence of an incompletely formed aorticopulmonary septum (Fig. 29–19). The pulmonary trunk is usually very short and gives rise to left and right pulmonary arteries. When the aorticopulmonary septum is absent, there is no discrete main pulmonary artery component, and both pulmonary artery branches arise directly from the truncus. In type II, each pulmonary artery arises separately but close to the other from the posterior aspect of the truncus. In type III, each pulmonary artery arises from the lateral aspect of the truncus. Less commonly, one pulmonary artery branch may be absent, with collateral arteries supplying the lung that does not receive a pulmonary artery branch from the truncus. Truncus arteriosus malformation should not be confused with "pseudotruncus arteriosus," which is the severe form of tetralogy of Fallot with pulmonary atresia in which the single aorta arises from the heart accompanied by a remnant of atretic pulmonary artery.

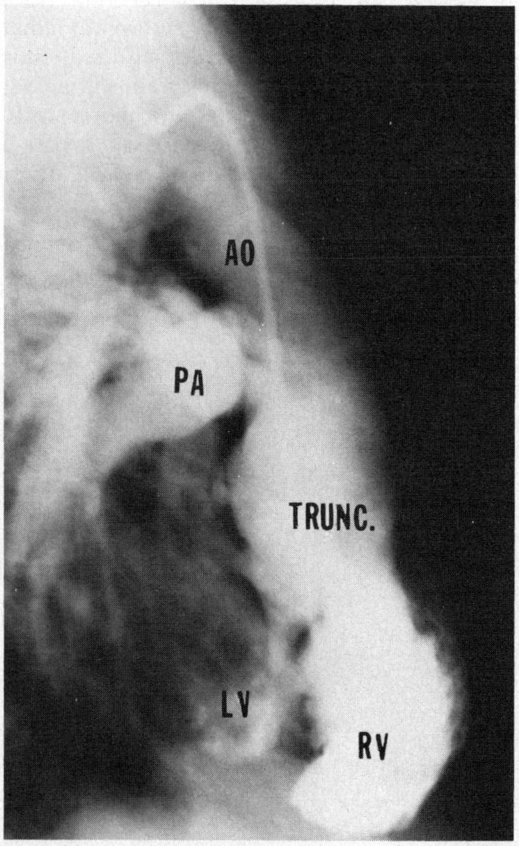

FIGURE 29–19 Right ventriculogram in the lateral view in a patient with type I truncus arteriosus. The contrast agent enters the left ventricle (LV) across a ventricular septal defect. The pulmonary artery (PA) arises directly from the persistent truncus arteriosus (TRUNC). AO = aorta; RV = right ventricle. (Courtesy of Robert White, M.D.)

Pulmonary blood flow is governed by the size of the pulmonary arteries and the pulmonary vascular resistance. In infancy, pulmonary blood flow is usually excessive, since pulmonary vascular resistance is not greatly increased. Thus, despite an obligatory admixture of systemic and pulmonary venous blood in the common trunk, only minimal cyanosis is present. Rarely, pulmonary blood flow is restricted by hypoplastic or stenotic pulmonary arteries arising from the truncus. Pulmonary vascular obstruction does not appear to restrict pulmonary blood flow before 1 to 2 years of age.[161] Hence, the infant with truncus arteriosus usually presents with mild cyanosis coexisting with the cardiac findings of a large left-to-right shunt. Symptoms of heart failure and poor physical development usually appear in the first weeks or months of life. The most frequent physical findings include cardiomegaly, a systolic ejection sound accompanied by a thrill, a loud single second heart sound, a harsh systolic murmur, and a low-pitched mid-diastolic rumbling murmur and bounding pulses.

Truncal valve incompetence is suggested by the presence of a diastolic decrescendo murmur at the base of the heart.[162] The physical findings are quite different if pulmonary blood flow is restricted by either high pulmonary vascular resistance or pulmonary arterial stenosis: cyanosis is prominent, congestive failure is rare, and only a short systolic ejection may be audible accompanied occasionally by continuous murmurs posteriorly of bronchial collateral flow. Left ventricular hypertrophy alone or in combination with right ventricular hypertrophy is present electrocardiographically when a prominent left-to-right shunt exists; right ventricular hypertrophy is observed in patients with restricted pulmonary blood flow. The radiographic findings depend upon the hemodynamic circumstances. Gross cardiomegaly with left or combined ventricular enlargement, left atrial enlargement, and a small or absent main pulmonary artery segment with pulmonary vascular engorgement are the usual radiographic features. A right aortic arch is common (25 to 30 per cent of patients). When pulmonary blood flow is reduced, both heart size and pulmonary vascular markings are less prominent.

The *echocardiographic* features of truncus arteriosus include the detection of a large truncal root overriding the ventricular septum, an increase in the right ventricular dimension, and mitral valve–truncal root continuity.[163] The dimension of the left atrium determined echocardiographically provides a good index of pulmonary flow. Differentiation between truncus arteriosus and tetralogy of Fallot by ultrasound may be difficult unless pulmonic valve echoes are observed in the latter anomaly.[67] Diagnosis should be suspected at cardiac catheterization if the catheter fails to enter the central pulmonary arteries from the right ventricle. Selective angiocardiography and retrograde aortography are necessary to establish a precise diagnosis and to reveal the common trunk arising from the heart and the origin of the pulmonary arteries from the truncus.

The early fatal course as well as early development of pulmonary vascular obstructive disease in patients surviving infancy is responsible for the poor prognosis associated with truncus arteriosus. In infants and young children with large left-to-right shunts, surgical banding of one or both pulmonary arteries has been employed to reduce pulmonary flow.[164] Corrective operation is preferred before age 1 to 2 years if the patient is free of severe pulmonary vascular obstructive disease.[165–167,167a]

Operation consists of closure of the ventricular septal defect, leaving the aorta arising from the left ventricle; the pulmonary arteries are excised from their truncus origin and a valve-containing prosthetic conduit is used to establish continuity between the right ventricle and the pulmonary arteries. Truncal valve regurgitation significantly enhances the risk of corrective surgery, since valve replacement is associated with significantly increased surgical mortality. Patients with only one pulmonary artery are especially prone to early development of severe pulmonary vascular disease but otherwise are not at increased risk from surgery. With truncus arteriosus defects, the possible inequalities of pressure and flow between the two pulmonary arteries often make precise calculation of pulmonary resistance difficult.[161] Corrective operation may be performed in patients with at least one adequate pulmonary artery having low distal pressure or arteriolar resistance. Conversely, significant systemic arterial desaturation in a patient with two pulmonary arteries and with neither pulmonary artery stenosis nor a previous pulmonary artery band signifies that high pulmonary vascular resistance exists and that the condition is probably inoperable. It is not yet clear how often and at what age the conduit between the right ventricle and pulmonary artery must be replaced with a larger prosthesis either because of growth of the patient and/or obstruction caused by the new outflow tract.

CORONARY ARTERIOVENOUS FISTULA

Coronary arteriovenous fistula is an unusual anomaly that consists of a communication between one of the coronary arteries (rarely both) and an intracardiac chamber.[168] Connections between the coronary system and a cardiac chamber appear to represent persistence of embryonic intertrabecular spaces and sinusoids. The majority of these fistulas drain into the right ventricle, right atrium, or coronary sinus; fistulous communication to the pulmonary artery, left atrium, or left ventricle is much less frequent.[169] Most often the shunt through the fistula is of small magnitude, and myocardial blood flow is not compromised.[170] Potential complications include pulmonary hypertension and congestive heart failure if a large left-to-right shunt exists, bacterial endocarditis, rupture or thrombosis of the fistula or an associated arterial aneurysm, and myocardial ischemia distal to the fistula due to decreased coronary blood flow.

The majority of patients are asymptomatic and are referred because of a cardiac murmur that is loud, superficial, and continuous at the lower or midsternal border. The site of maximal intensity of the murmur is related to the site of drainage and is usually different from the second left intercostal space—the classic site of the continuous murmur of persistent ductus arteriosus—except when the fistula drains into the pulmonary artery or right ventricle. In the latter situation the murmur is louder in diastole than in systole because of compression of the fistula by contracting myocardium. The electrocardiogram and chest x-ray are quite often normal and rarely show selective chamber enlargement or myocardial ischemia.

Retrograde thoracic aortography or coronary arteriography can be employed to identify the size and anatomical features of the fistulous tract (Fig. 29–20), which may be closed by suture obliteration in most cases.[171] Indications for operation are not precise. In the presence of a large left-to-right shunt and symptoms of heart failure, the decision to operate is clearly justified. Most often the fistula is closed in asymptomatic patients in order to prevent future symptoms or complications. The risk of death or substantial morbidity following closure of a coronary artery–cardiac chamber fistula is quite low.

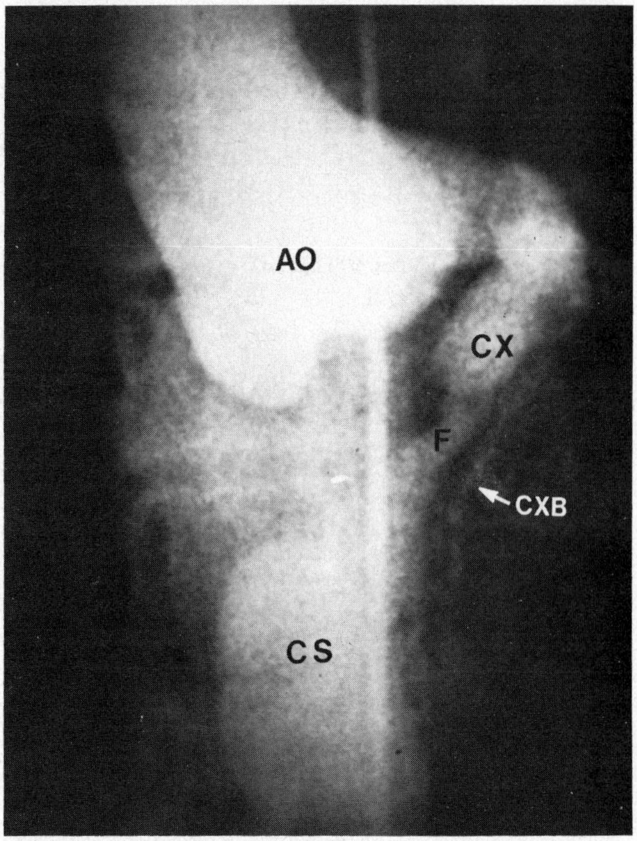

FIGURE 29–20 Coronary arteriovenous fistula draining into the coronary sinus in the frontal projection. AO = aorta, CX = circumflex coronary artery, CXB = circumflex coronary artery branch, F = fistula, CS = coronary sinus.

ANOMALOUS PULMONARY ORIGIN OF THE CORONARY ARTERY

This rare malformation occurs in approximately 0.4 per cent of patients with congenital cardiac anomalies. In almost all patients the left coronary artery originates from the posterior sinus of the pulmonary artery.[172–174]

Unusual cases have been reported in which the right coronary artery, or the entire coronary artery system, originates from the main pulmonary trunk.[172] Embryologically the distal coronary artery system is formed by 9 weeks from solid angioblastic buds that extend throughout the epicardium to form the major coronary artery branches. Proximally the coronary network forms a ring around the truncus arteriosus, joining with coronary buds from the primitive aortic sinuses as the truncus partitions to form the great arteries. The varieties of anomalous pulmonary origin of the coronary artery are the result of displacement in this proximal process.

During fetal life pulmonary artery pressure is slightly greater than aortic pressure, and perfusion of the left coronary artery is antegrade. After birth, when pulmonary artery pressure falls below aortic pressure, perfusion of the left coronary artery from the pulmonary artery ceases, and the direction of flow in the anomalous vessel reverses. Blood flows from the aorta to the right coronary artery, then through collateral channels to the left coronary artery, and finally to the pulmonary artery. In effect, the left coronary artery behaves as a fistulous communication between the aorta and pulmonary artery. If

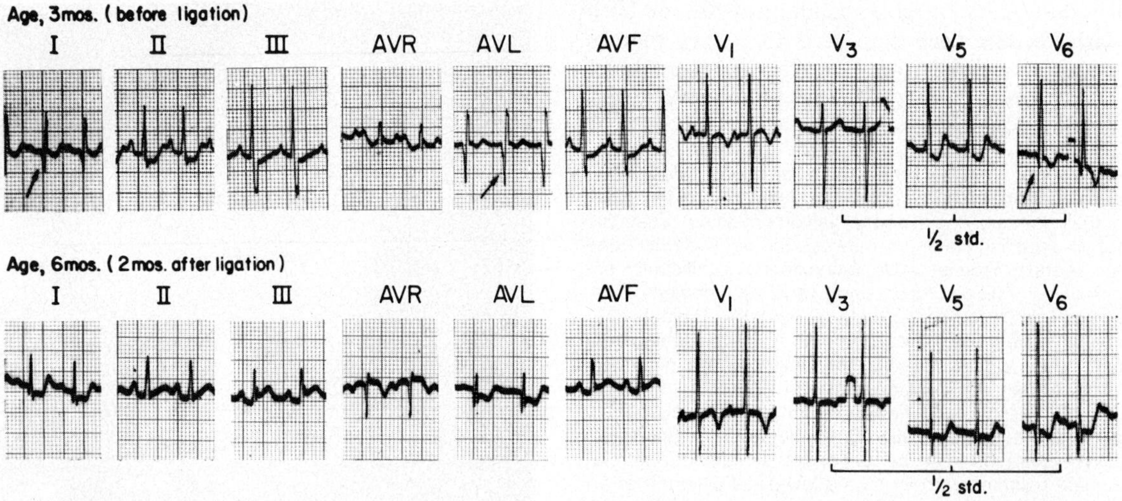

FIGURE 29–21 Typical electrocardiogram of an infant with anomalous left coronary artery before *(above)* and after *(below)* ligation of the anomalous left coronary artery. Arrows point to the abnormal Q waves. (Courtesy of Delores A. Danilowicz, M.D.)

adequate collateral channels exist or develop between the two coronary artery circulations, total myocardial perfusion through the right coronary artery increases. In 10 to 15 per cent of patients myocardial ischemia never develops because extensive intercoronary collaterals allow survival to adolescence or adulthood. In fact, if collateral blood flow is considerable, the patient may develop the clinical manifestations of a large arteriovenous shunt and a continuous or diastolic murmur. Older children or adults usually present with a continuous murmur or with mitral regurgitation resulting from dysfunction of ischemic or infarcted papillary muscles. In some instances the coronary anomaly is unsuspected until a previously well adolescent or adult experiences angina, heart failure, or sudden death.

By far the most common clinical presentation are those infants who suffer a myocardial infarction and develop congestive heart failure. The infant syndrome usually becomes manifest at age 2 to 4 months with angina-like symptoms that may occasionally be misinterpreted as colic. Feeding and defecation are often accompanied by dyspnea, irritability and crying, pallor, diaphoresis, and occasional loss of consciousness. The diagnosis of anomalous origin of the coronary artery is supported by the electrocardiographic demonstration of deep Q waves in association with ST-segment alterations and T-wave inversions in leads I, aV_1, V_5, and V_6 (Fig. 29–21). Chest roentgenograms show moderate to severe enlargement of the left atrium and ventricle. Aortography or coronary angiography is the definitive diagnostic procedure and demonstrates the retrograde drainage of the coronary vessel into the pulmonary artery (Fig. 29–22). It should be recognized that ventricular arrhythmias may complicate the course of hemodynamic study. Management of these infants depends, in part, upon the magnitude of shunting into the pulmonary artery, which may be determined by oximetry, indicator dilution curves, or angiography.

Medical treatment is indicated in all infants with myocardial infarction for congestive heart failure, arrhythmias, and cardiogenic shock. In patients with a small left-to-right shunt or no shunt at all, the prognosis is exceedingly poor with conservative management, justifying an attempt to reestablish a two coronary artery system. The operations that have been employed include reimplanting the left coronary artery into the aortic root, or anastomosis of the left coronary artery with the subclavian artery or with the aorta via a graft.[175,176] If clinical deterioration occurs in infants in whom a sizable left-to-right shunt exists into the pulmonary artery, simple ligation of the left coronary artery at its origin prevents retrograde flow and allows perfusion of the left ventricle with blood supplied through anastomoses with the right coronary artery. If medical management stabilizes the infant with significant intercoronary collaterals, operation should be postponed to allow the patient to grow, since increased size of the vessels

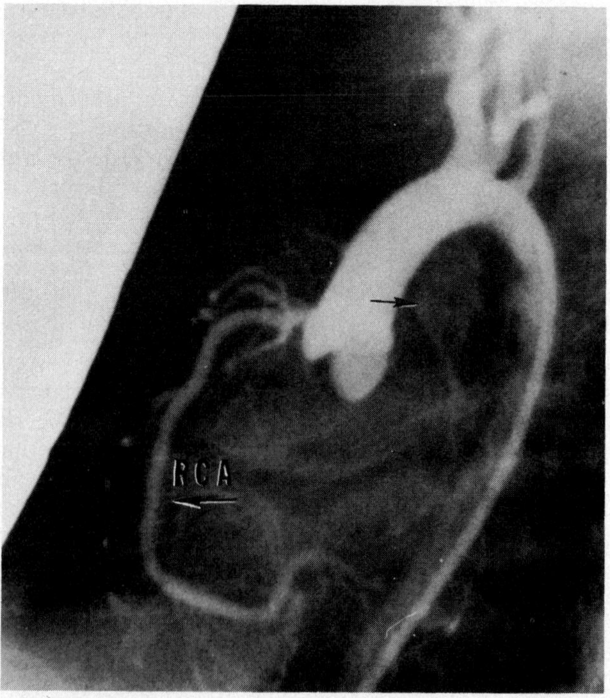

FIGURE 29–22 Lateral view of anomalous left coronary artery. Retrograde aortogram fills the right (RCA) and then the left coronary artery through collateral channels. The left coronary artery enters the main pulmonary artery (upper arrow). (Courtesy of Robert Freedom, M.D.)

enhances the likelihood of successful coronary arterial bypass surgery. The outcome of surgery and ultimate prognosis are influenced significantly by the degree of myocardial damage suffered preoperatively. In rare patients it is necessary to consider aneurysmectomy or mitral valve replacement.

AORTIC SINUS ANEURYSM AND FISTULA

Congenital aneurysm of an aortic sinus of Valsalva, particularly the right coronary sinus, is an uncommon anomaly occurring more often in males. The malformation consists of a separation, or lack of fusion, between the media of the aorta and the annulus fibrosis of the aortic valve.[177] The receiving chamber of the aorticocardiac fistula usually is the right ventricle, but occasionally, when the noncoronary cusp is involved, the fistula drains into the right atrium.

Five to 15 per cent of aneurysms originate in the posterior or noncoronary sinus; rarely is the left aortic sinus involved. Associated anomalies are common and include bicuspid aortic valve, ventricular septal defect, and coarctation of the aorta.

It is not clear whether the aneurysm itself is present at birth, although the deficiency in the aortic media would appear to be congenital. Reports in children are infrequent, since progressive aneurysmal dilatation of the weakened area develops but may not be recognized until the third or fourth decade of life when rupture into a cardiac chamber occurs.

The *unruptured aneurysm* generally does not produce a hemodynamic abnormality, although pressure on the intracardiac conduction system by an unruptured aneurysm may be a rare cause of complete atrioventricular block; myocardial ischemia may rarely be caused by coronary arterial compression.[177] Rupture often is of abrupt onset, causes chest pain, and creates continuous arteriovenous shunting and volume loading of both right and left heart chambers, which results in heart failure.[178-180] An additional complication is bacterial endocarditis, which may originate either on the edges of the aneurysm or on those areas in the right side of the heart that are traumatized by the jetlike stream of blood flowing through the fistula.

The presence of this anomaly should be suspected in a patient with a history of chest pain of recent onset, symptoms of diminished cardiac reserve, bounding pulses, and a loud superficial continuous murmur accentuated in diastole when the fistula opens into the right ventricle as well as a thrill along the right or left lower parasternal border. The *physical findings* may occasionally be difficult to distinguish from those produced by a coronary arteriovenous fistula. *Electrocardiography* shows biventricular hypertrophy, and chest roentgenography demonstrates generalized cardiomegaly. Two dimensional and pulsed Doppler *echocardiographic* studies may detect the wall of the aneurysms and disturbed flow within the aneurysm, respectively.[181,182] *Cardiac catheterization* reveals a left-to-right shunt at the ventricular or, less commonly, the atrial level; the diagnosis may be established definitively by retrograde thoracic aortography (Fig. 29–23). Preoperative medical management consists of measures to relieve cardiac failure and to treat coexistent arrhythmias or endocarditis, if present. At operation the aneurysm is closed and amputated, and the aortic wall is reunited with the heart, either by direct suture or with a prosthesis.[179,179a] Every effort should be made to preserve the aortic valve in children, since patch closure of the defect combined with prosthetic valve replacement greatly enhances the risk of operation in small patients.

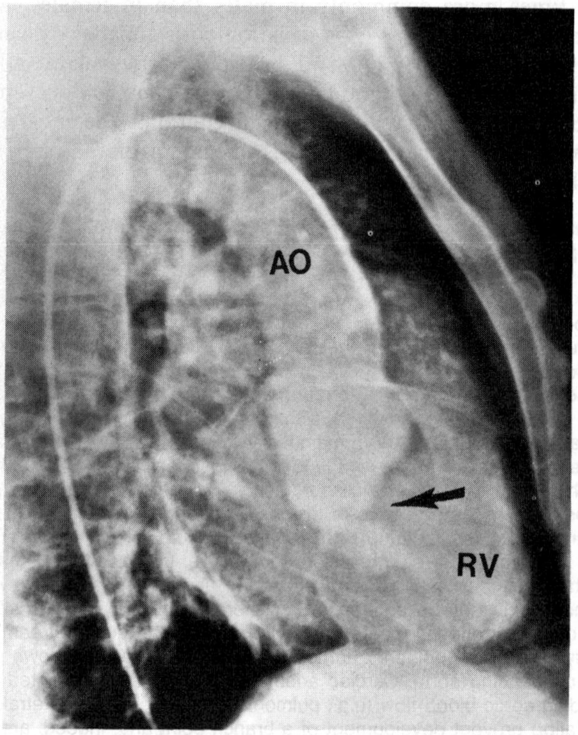

FIGURE 29–23 A retrograde aortogram shows the fistulous connection between the noncoronary sinus of Valsalva and the right ventricle (RV) (arrow). AO = aorta. (Courtesy of Robert White, M.D.)

VALVULAR AND VASCULAR LESIONS WITH OR WITHOUT RIGHT-TO-LEFT SHUNT

Aortic Arch Obstruction

The conventional anatomical and clinical division into pre- and postductal coarctation or infantile and adult types, respectively, is misleading, since the anatomical localization is inaccurate and the age-dependency of clinical presentation does not hold true (i.e., the adult type is seen often in the first weeks of life). A spectrum of anatomical lesions exists, causing obstruction of the aortic arch or proximal portion of the descending aorta. These range from a localized coarctation or constriction of the lumen, most commonly located just distal to the origin of the left subclavian artery and related closely to the attachment of the ductus arteriosus with the aorta, to diffuse narrowing or interruption of a portion of the aortic arch. In this chapter, aortic arch obstruction is divided into three types: (1) localized juxtaductal coarctation, (2) hypoplasia of the aortic isthmus, and (3) aortic arch interruption. *Pseudocoarctation* is a term used synonymously with "kinking," or "buckling," of the aorta, which is a subclinical form of localized juxtaductal coarctation of the aorta.[183]

Localized Juxtaductal Coarctation

MORPHOLOGY. This lesion consists of a localized shelflike thickening and infolding of the posterolateral aortic wall opposite the ductus arteriosus; the wall of the aorta into which the ductus or ligamentum arteriosum inserts is not involved.[184] Juxtaductal coarctation occurs two to

Experimental hypervitaminosis D produced in the pregnant rabbit has caused craniofacial abnormalities and malformations resembling those of supravalvular aortic stenosis in the offspring.[254-256] In humans, with one exception, chromosome studies have consistently revealed normal karyotypes. Most often supravalvular aortic stenosis is a feature of the distinctive syndrome described above. However, peripheral pulmonary artery stenosis and the aortic anomaly are also seen in familial and sporadic forms unassociated with the other features of the syndrome.[259] Genetic studies suggest that the familial anomaly is transmitted as an autosomal dominant with variable expression. Some family members may have supravalvular pulmonic stenosis either as an isolated lesion or in combination with the supravalvular aortic anomaly. Unlike the other forms of aortic stenosis, there appears to be no sex predilection.

Three anatomical types of supravalvular aortic stenosis are recognized, although some patients may have findings of more than one type. Most common is the hourglass type, in which marked thickening and disorganization of the aortic media produce a constricting annular ridge at the superior margin of the sinuses of Valsalva. The membranous type is the result of fibrous or fibromuscular semicircular diaphragm with a small central opening stretched across the lumen of the aorta. Uniform hypoplasia of the ascending aorta characterizes the hypoplastic type.

Because the coronary arteries arise proximal to the site of outflow obstruction in supravalvular aortic stenosis, they are subjected to the elevated pressure that exists within the left ventricle. These vessels are often dilated and tortuous, and premature coronary arteriosclerosis has been observed. Moreover, if the free edges of some or all of the aortic cusps adhere to the site of supravalvular stenosis, coronary artery inflow may be reduced. The formation of thoracic aortic aneurysms has been described in several patients.

Most often, patients with supravalvular aortic stenosis syndrome are mentally retarded and resemble one another in their facial features. The typical appearance is similar to the "elfin" facies observed in the severe form of idiopathic infantile hypercalcemia and is characterized by a high prominent forehead, epicanthal folds, underdeveloped bridge of the nose and mandible, overhanging upper lip, strabismus, and anomalies of dentition (Fig. 29–31). Recognition of this distinctive appearance, even in infancy, should alert the physician to the possibility of underlying multiple system disease. In addition, a positive family history in a patient with a normal appearance and clinical signs suggesting left ventricular outflow obstruction should lead to the suspicion of either supravalvular aortic stenosis or hypertrophic obstructive cardiomyopathy. Patients with supravalvular aortic obstruction appear to be subject to the same risks of unexpected sudden death and infective endocarditis as those with valvular aortic stenosis.

With few exceptions, the major *physical findings* resemble those observed in patients with valvular aortic stenosis. Among these exceptions are accentuation of aortic valve closure due to elevated pressure in the aorta proximal to the stenosis, an infrequent systolic ejection sound, and the especially prominent transmission of a thrill and murmur into the jugular notch and along the carotid vessels. Uncommonly, there is an early diastolic, decrescendo, blowing murmur of aortic regurgitation due to the fusion of one or more cusps to the area of stenosis. The narrowing of the peripheral pulmonary arteries that often coexists in these patients frequently produces a late systolic or continuous murmur that may help distinguish this anomaly from valvular aortic stenosis. This differentiation is reinforced by the frequent finding of a significant disparity between the arterial pressures in the upper extremities in supravalvular aortic stenosis; the systolic pressure in the right arm tends to be the higher of the two and occasionally exceeds that in the femoral arteries. The disparity in pulses may relate to the tendency of a jet stream to adhere to a vessel wall (Coanda effect) and selective streaming of blood into the innominate artery.[260,261]

Electrocardiography generally reveals left ventricular hypertrophy when obstruction is severe. However, biventricular, or even right ventricular, hypertrophy may be found if significant narrowing of peripheral pulmonary arteries coexists. In a number of patients without significant right-sided lesions the vectorcardiogram has shown displacement of the maximum transverse QRS loop rightward and posteriorly and a tendency for initial forces to be directed leftward, perhaps reflecting posterobasal left ventricular hypertrophy or a manifestation of left posterior hemiblock.[262] Radiographically, in contrast to valvular and discrete subvalvular aortic stenosis, poststenotic dilation of the ascending aorta is rarely seen. Usually the sinuses of Valsalva are dilated and ascending aorta and the aortic arch are of normal size or appear small. Retrograde aortic catheterization is the most valuable technique for localizing the site of obstruction to the supravalvular area and determining the degree of hemodynamic abnormality (Fig. 29–32).

The supravalvular aortic lumen may be widened by the insertion of an oval- or diamond-shaped fabric patch in those patients with a normal ascending aorta. If the aorta is hypoplastic, this operation merely displaces the pressure gradient distally without abolishing the obstruction. Under these circumstances, repair may require replacement or widening of the entire hypoplastic aorta with an appropriate prosthesis. Operation may be recommended when relatively little hypoplasia of the ascending aorta and arch

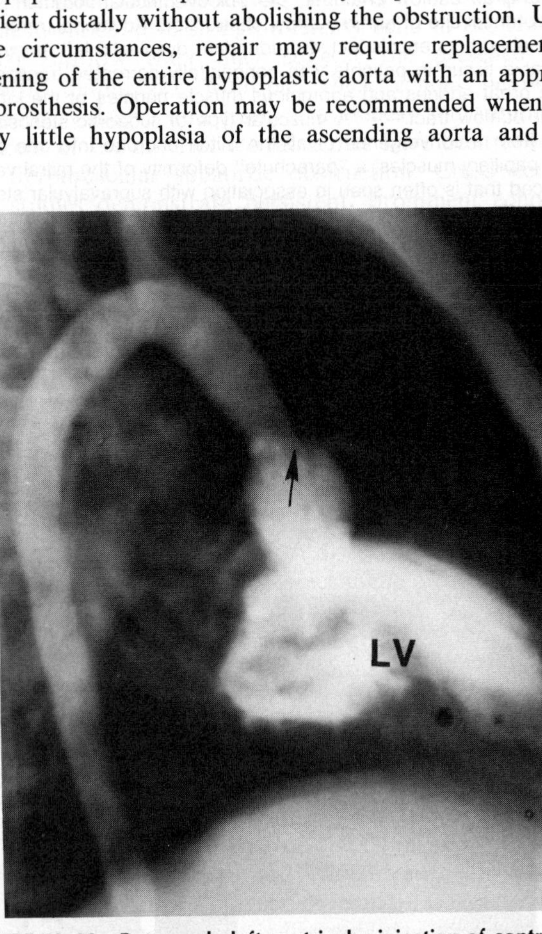

FIGURE 29–32 Retrograde left ventricular injection of contrast material in a patient with supravalvular aortic stenosis showing dilated sinuses of Valsalva and an aortic constriction just above the sinuses (arrow). LV = left ventricle.

exists and when the obstruction is discrete and severe, i.e., with a systolic gradient exceeding 75 mm Hg.

Hypoplastic Left Heart Syndrome

This designation is used to describe a group of closely related cardiac anomalies characterized by underdevelopment of the left cardiac chambers, atresia or stenosis of the aortic and/or the mitral orifices, and hypoplasia of the aorta.[263,264] These anomalies are an especially common cause of heart failure in the first week of life. The left atrium and ventricle often exhibit *endocardial fibroelastosis.* Pulmonary venous blood traverses a patent foramen ovale and a dilated and hypertrophied right ventricle acts as the systemic, as well as the pulmonary, ventricle; the systemic circulation receives blood via a patent ductus arteriosus (Fig. 29–33). The diagnosis should be considered in infants, particularly males, with the sudden onset of heart failure, systemic hypoperfusion, and nonspecific murmur. Electrocardiography frequently reveals right axis deviation, right atrial and ventricular enlargement, and ST and T-wave abnormalities in the left precordial leads. Chest roentgenography may show only slight enlargement shortly after birth, but with clinical deterioration there is marked cardiomegaly and increased pulmonary venous and arterial vascular markings.

The echocardiographic findings may be diagnostic and include a diminutive aortic root and left ventricular cavity and absence or poor visualization of aortic and mitral valve echoes, which, when seen, are of diminished amplitude and mobility.[265,266]

Medical therapy directed at cardiac decompensation,

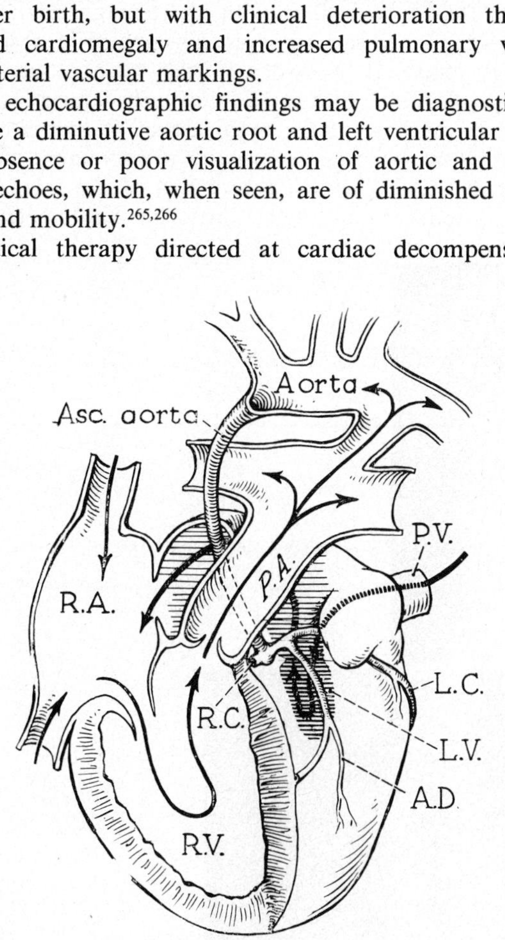

FIGURE 29–33 Hypoplastic left heart with aortic hypoplasia, aortic valve atresia, and a hypoplastic mitral valve and left ventricle. R.A. = right atrium; R.V. = right ventricle; R.C. = right coronary; P.A. = pulmonary artery; P.V. = pulmonary vein; L.C. = left coronary artery; L.V. = left ventricle; A.D. = anterior descending coronary artery. (From Neufeld, H. N., et al.: Diagnosis of aortic atresia by retrograde aortography. Circulation *25*:278, 1962, by permission of the American Heart Association, Inc.)

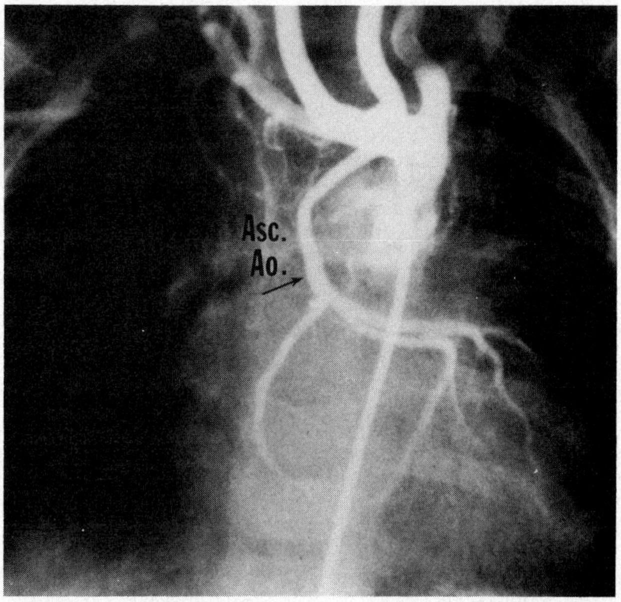

FIGURE 29–34 Retrograde aortogram showing marked hypoplasia of the ascending aorta (Asc. Ao.) (arrow) in an infant with hypoplastic left heart syndrome. (From Freedom, R. M., et al.: Aortic atresia with normal left ventricle: Distinctive angiocardiographic findings. Cath. Cardiovasc. Diag. *3*:283, 1977.)

hypoxemia, and metabolic acidemia rarely allows survival beyond the first days of life. Constriction of the patent ductus arteriosus and limited flow through a restrictive patent foramen ovale are the principal factors responsible for early death.[263,267] At present the anatomical lesions are not correctable (Fig. 29–34). Some centers are attempting staged surgical management in an effort to provide long-term palliation.[268,269] The first stage consists of creating an unobstructed communication between the right ventricle and aorta, usually with a prosthetic conduit connecting the pulmonary artery to the aorta; pulmonary blood flow and pressure are limited by a controlled opening in the conduit to the distal pulmonary artery. A large interatrial communication must also be assured in stage I. In stage II, an interatrial baffle is created to provide continuity between left atrium and tricuspid valve; the pulmonary arterial circulation is provided by anastomosis of the right atrium to the pulmonary arteries.

AORTIC REGURGITATION

Congenital aortic valve regurgitation is an extremely rare isolated congenital cardiac lesion.[270] Most often aortic regurgitation occurs in association with congenital valvular aortic stenosis in which the valve commissures are fused inhibiting cusp mobility, subvalvular aortic stenosis in which the aortic ring is dilated and the valve cusps are deformed, coarctation of the aorta when the aortic ring is dilated and the aortic valve is bicuspid, ventricular septal defect (see p. 965), and endocardial fibroelastosis.[271] Aortic valve regurgitation may also accompany aortic sinus aneurysm or be secondary to dilatation of the ascending aorta in patients with Marfan syndrome, cystic medial necrosis, or osteogenesis imperfecta in which the aortic lesions are manifestations of the underlying connective tissue disorder (Chap. 48).

Severe aortic regurgitation may also occur through channels other than the aortic valve.[272] Thus, aortico–left ventricular tunnel is a rare anomaly that must be distinguished from congenital aortic valve regurgitation, since the approach to management of the former does not usually include consideration for prosthetic valve replacement.

The aortico–left ventricular tunnel is an abnormal channel beginning in the ascending aorta above the right coronary orifice and ending in the left ventricle below the right aortic cusp. The channel usually passes behind the right ventricular infundibulum and through the ventricular septum.

Aortography is necessary to establish a precise diagnosis. In infants and children with congenital aortic valve insufficiency the severity of regurgitation increases with time, and valve replacement, rather than plication, is almost always necessary to correct the lesion. Operation should be deferred until symptoms and signs dictate its necessity.[273] Conversely, closure of an aortico–left ventricular communication is advisable before progressive dilation of the aortic annulus creates secondary changes in the aortic valve itself which may necessitate aortic valve replacement.

PULMONARY VEIN ATRESIA AND STENOSIS

Pulmonary vein atresia is a quite rare anomaly in which the pulmonary veins do not connect with the heart or with a major systemic vein.[274] The lesion is incompatible with life, but infants may survive for days, probably because communications exist between the pulmonary veins and the bronchial or esophageal veins that allow limited egress for pulmonary venous blood. Pulmonary vein stenosis may occur as a focal stenosis at the atrial junction or generalized hypoplasia of one or more pulmonary veins. There is an extremely high incidence of associated cardiac malformations, including atrial septal defect, tetralogy of Fallot, tricuspid and mitral atresia, and endocardial cushion defect. The severe pulmonary vein obstruction imposed by pulmonary vein abnormalities causes severe cyanosis, congestive cardiac failure, and early death. Focal stenosis of one or more pulmonary veins at the atrial junction, recognized on angiography, may be relieved surgically.

COR TRIATRIATUM

In this malformation failure of resorption of the common pulmonary vein results in a left atrium divided by an abnormal fibromuscular diaphragm into a posterosuperior chamber receiving the pulmonary veins and an anteroinferior chamber giving rise to the left atrial appendage and leading to the mitral orifice.[274,275] The communication between the divided atrial chambers may be large, small, or absent depending on the size of the opening(s) in the subdividing diaphragm, which determines the degree of obstruction to pulmonary venous return.[276] Elevations of both pulmonary venous pressure and pulmonary vascular resistance result in severe pulmonary artery hypertension. The diagnosis should be suspected at cardiac catheterization if the pulmonary arterial wedge pressure is higher than a simultaneous left atrial pressure. The diagnosis is established by visualizing the obstructing lesion angiographically (Fig. 29–35). Although rare, it is important to recognize the malformation because it may be easily correctable at operation.[276,277]

MITRAL STENOSIS

Anatomical types of mitral stenosis include the parachute deformity of the valve, in which shortened chordae tendineae converge and insert into a single large papillary muscle; thickened leaflets with shortening and fusion of the chordae tendineae; an anomalous arcade of obstructing papillary muscles; accessory mitral valve tissue; and a supravalvular circumferential ridge of connective tissue arising at the base of the atrial aspect of the mitral leaflets.[278,279] Associated cardiac defects are common, including endocardial fibroelastosis, coarctation of the aorta, patent ductus arteriosus, and left ventricular outflow tract ob-

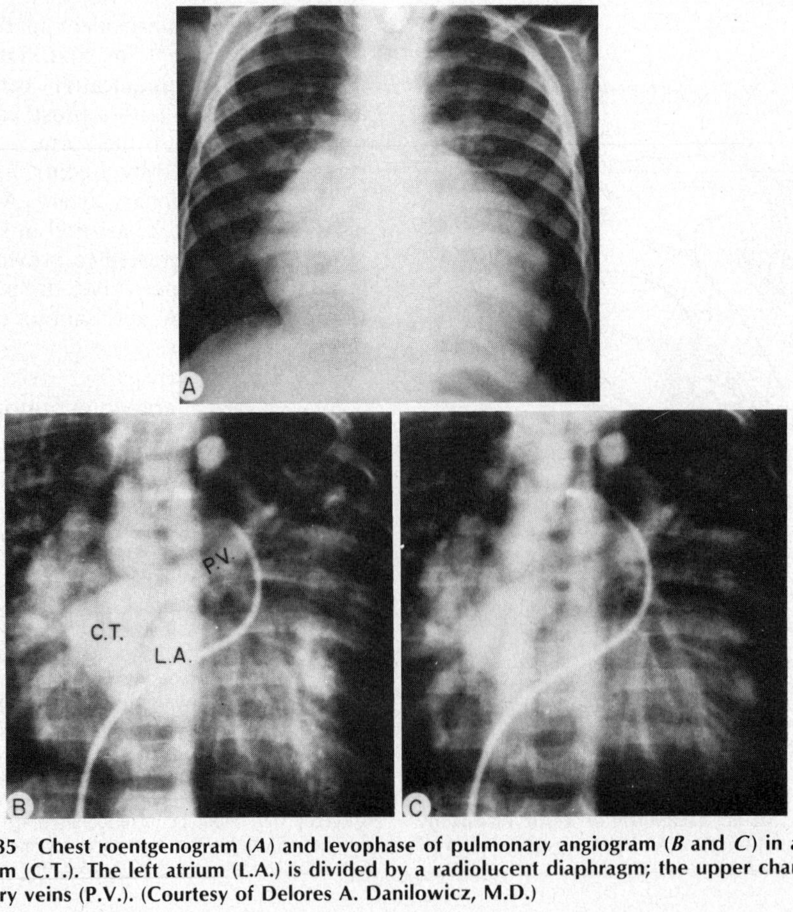

FIGURE 29–35 Chest roentgenogram (*A*) and levophase of pulmonary angiogram (*B* and *C*) in an infant with cor triatriatum (C.T.). The left atrium (L.A.) is divided by a radiolucent diaphragm; the upper chamber receives the pulmonary veins (P.V.). (Courtesy of Delores A. Danilowicz, M.D.)

struction. The clinical and hemodynamic consequences of isolated congenital mitral stenosis are similar to those of acquired mitral obstruction with modifications imposed by coexisting anomalies.[278,280,281] The prognosis is poor; symptoms attributable to pulmonary vein obstruction begin usually in infancy and the majority of patients expire before age one year.

MITRAL REGURGITATION

The syndrome of *mitral valve prolapse* is discussed on pages 1089 to 1094. This condition is generally quite benign in children. However, occasional difficulties exist with infective endocarditis, arrhythmias, atypical chest pain, and sudden death.

Isolated congenital mitral regurgitation of hemodynamic significance is an unusual lesion in infants and children. Most often, congenital malformations of the mitral valve producing insufficiency are encountered in association with endocardial cushion defect, congenitally corrected transposition of the great arteries, endocardial fibroelastosis, anomalous pulmonary origin of the coronary artery, congenital subaortic stenosis, hypertrophic obstructive cardiomyopathy, and coarctation of the aorta. Mitral valve dysfunction is also seen commonly in a variety of metabolic disorders (e.g., the mucopolysaccharidoses), primary and secondary cardiomyopathies, connective tissue disease (e.g., rheumatoid arthritis, Marfan syndrome, Ehlers-Danlos syndrome, pseudoxanthoma elasticum), and rheumatic and nonrheumatic inflammatory diseases of the myocardium[281] (see Chap. 48).

The various anatomical lesions that result in isolated congenital mitral regurgitation include prolapse of one or both mitral leaflets, cleft or perforated mitral leaflet, inadequate leaflet tissue, double orifice of the mitral valve, anomalous insertion of chordae tendineae (anomalous mitral arcade), redundant leaflet tissue, displacement inferiorly of the ring of the inferior leaflet into the left ventricle, and abnormal length of chordae tendineae.[282-288] The clinical and hemodynamic findings in patients with isolated congenital mitral incompetence resemble those observed in acquired mitral regurgitation. Mitral annuloplasty (which is preferred) or prosthetic valve replacement are procedures reserved for infants or children who are at least moderately symptomatic despite comprehensive medical management, often with repeated episodes of pulmonary infection, or cardiac failure with anorexia and retarded growth and development.[287,287a] Operative candidates are shown at hemodynamic and angiographic study to have pulmonary hypertension, a regurgitant fraction in excess of 50 per cent, and a marked increase in left ventricular end-diastolic volume.

PULMONARY ARTERIOVENOUS FISTULA

Abnormal development of the pulmonary arteries and veins in a common vascular complex is responsible for this rare congenital anomaly. A variable number of pulmonary arteries communicate directly with branches of the pulmonary veins; in some cases the fistula receives systemic arterial branches.[289] The majority of patients have an associated Weber-Osler-Rendu syndrome; additional associated problems include bronchiectasis and other malformations of the bronchial tree, and absence of the right lower lobe. Venoarterial shunting depends upon the extent of the fistulous communications and may result in cyanosis and secondary polycythemia. Patients with hereditary hemorrhagic telangiectasis are often anemic owing to repeated blood loss and may have less obvious cyanosis. Systolic and continuous murmurs are audible over areas of the fistula(s). Rounded opacities of variable size in one or both lungs on chest roentgenogram may suggest the presence of the lesion. Pulmonary angiography reveals the site and extent of the abnormal communication. Unless the lesions are widespread throughout both lungs, surgical treatment aimed at removing the lesions with preservation of healthy lung tissue is indicated to avoid the complications of massive hemorrhage, bacterial endocarditis, and rupture of arteriovenous aneurysms.

PERIPHERAL PULMONARY ARTERY STENOSIS

Stenosis of the pulmonary artery may be single or multiple and occur anywhere from the main pulmonary trunk to the smaller peripheral arterial branches. Associated defects are observed in the majority of patients and include pulmonic valvular stenosis, ventricular septal defect, tetralogy of Fallot, and supravalvular aortic stenosis.

The most important cause of significant pulmonary artery stenoses producing symptoms in the newborn is intrauterine rubella infection.[290] Diagnosis is facilitated in these infants by finding elevations of the IgM fraction and rubella antibody titer. Other cardiovascular malformations seen commonly in association with congenital rubella include patent ductus arteriosus, pulmonic valve stenosis, and atrial septal defect. Generalized systemic arterial stenotic lesions may also be a feature of the rubella embryopathy, often involving large and medium-sized vessels such as the aorta and coronary, cerebral, mesenteric, and renal arteries. Cardiovascular lesions are but one manifestation of intrauterine rubella infection, since cataracts, microphthalmia, deafness, thrombocytopenia, hepatitis, and blood dyscrasias are also common. Thus, the clinical picture in infants with rubella syndrome depends upon the severity of the cardiovascular lesions and the associated abnormalities of other organs and systems.

Obstruction within the pulmonary arterial tree may be classified into four types: (1) stenosis of the main pulmonary trunk or the main left or right branch; (2) narrowing at the bifurcation of the pulmonary artery, extending into both right and left branches; (3) multiple sites of peripheral branch stenosis; and (4) a combination of main and peripheral stenosis. Pulmonary artery obstruction may be produced by localized narrowing, diffuse constrictions, or rarely, by a membrane or diaphragm. Post-stenotic dilatation is usual when the stenosis is localized, but may be absent or minimal with elongated constriction. It should be recognized that a physiological branch pulmonary artery stenosis is often present in the normal newborn in whom both right and left main pulmonary arteries are small and arise almost perpendicular from a large main pulmonary artery.[291] The branch vessels increase in size with growth and become less angulated in their take-off from the main pulmonary artery.

The degree of obstruction is the principal determinant of clinical severity; the type of obstruction determines the feasibility of direct surgical relief. The clinical features vary; most infants and children are asymptomatic.[292,293] An ejection systolic murmur at the upper left sternal border that is well transmitted to the axillae and back is most common. The presence of an ejection sound suggests that pulmonic valve stenosis coexists. The pulmonic component of the second heart sound may be slightly accentuated, but occasionally is extremely loud if multiple peripheral stenoses exist. A continuous murmur is audible, expecially in patients with main or branch stenosis, and particularly if an associated cardiovascular anomaly produces increased pulmonary blood flow. Electrocardiography shows right ventricular hypertrophy when obstruction is severe; left axis deviation with counterclockwise orientation of the frontal QRS vector is common in the rubella syndrome and when the lesion coexists with supravalvular

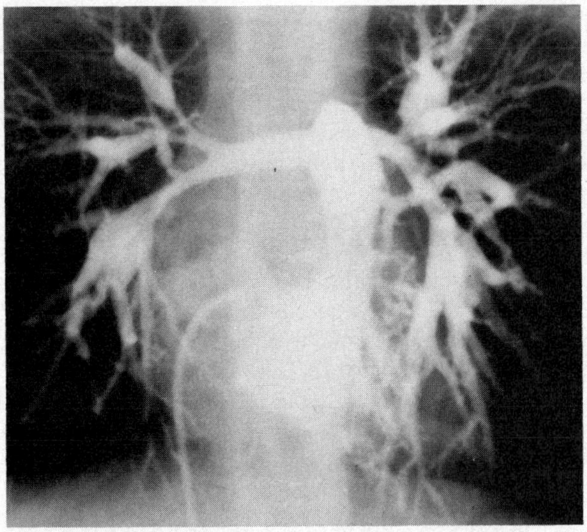

FIGURE 29–36 Right ventricular angiocardiogram showing multiple sites of peripheral pulmonic stenosis and post-stenotic dilatation of the peripheral pulmonic arteries.

aortic stenosis. Mild or moderate stenosis usually produces a normal chest roentgenogram; detectable differences in vascularity between regions of the lungs or dilated pulmonary artery segments are uncommon. When obstruction is bilateral and severe, right atrial and ventricular enlargement may be observed.

Diagnosis is confirmed by observing pressure gradients within the pulmonary arterial system at cardiac catheterization; selective pulmonary angiography defines the exact location, extent, and distribution of the lesion (Fig. 29–36). Mild to moderate unilateral or bilateral stenosis does not require surgical relief; numerous stenotic areas are not amenable to correction. Well-localized obstruction of severe degree in the main pulmonary artery or its major branches may be alleviated with a patch graft or bypassed with a tubular conduit. The natural history of peripheral pulmonary stenosis is not clear.[292] Obstruction may increase by discrepant growth between a stenotic area and normal portions of the pulmonary artery tree, or as a result of an increase in cardiac output, especially during adolescence. Rarely, hypertrophy is progressive of right ventricular infundibular muscle and results in hypercyanotic spells.

Pulmonic Stenosis with Intact Ventricular Septum

Valvular pulmonic stenosis, resulting from fusion of the valve cusps during mid to late intrauterine development, is the most common form of isolated right ventricular obstruction and occurs in approximately 7 per cent of patients with congenital heart disease. Hypertrophy of the septal and parietal bands narrowing the right ventricular infundibulum often accompanies the pulmonic valve lesion, especially if it is severe. Fused cusps of varying thickness and rigidity form a fibrous dome in the most severe forms. Pulmonic valve dysplasia, especially common in patients with Noonan's syndrome (p. 1614), produces obstruction in the absence of adherent leaflets because leaflets are thickened, rigid, and myxomatous and are limited in their lateral movement because of the presence of tissue pads within the pulmonic valve sinuses.[294,295]

INFANCY. The clinical presentation and course of circulation in the newborn with pulmonic stenosis depends on the severity of obstruction and the degree of development of the right ventricle and its outflow tract, the tricuspid valve, and the pulmonary arterial tree.[296–298] The greater the degree of pulmonic valve stenosis, the more closely the manifestations resemble those observed with pulmonary atresia and intact ventricular septum (see p. 988). Severe pulmonic stenosis is characterized by cyanosis due to right-to-left shunting through the foramen ovale, cardiomegaly, and diminished pulmonary blood flow in the absence of persistent patency of the ductus arteriosus. Hypoxemia and metabolic acidemia, rather than right ventricular failure, are the main clinical disturbances in the symptomatic infant. Distinction of these babies from those with tetralogy of Fallot or tricuspid or pulmonary atresia is usually possible, since infants with tetralogy generally do not have roentgenographic evidence of cardiomegaly; infants with tricuspid and pulmonary atresia show a preponderance of left ventricular forces by electrocardiography in contrast to the right ventricular hypertrophy observed usually with critical pulmonic stenosis in the absence of right ventricular hypoplasia. Cardiac catheterization and angiographic studies establish a precise diagnosis (Fig. 29–37). Pulmonary valvotomy is the operative procedure of choice, but a systemic-to-pulmonary arterial shunt may also be necessary in infants with underdevelopment of the right ventricular cavity.[296]

CHILDHOOD. The clinical profile of patients with valvular pulmonic stenosis beyond infancy is generally distinctive.[299] The severity of obstruction is the most important determinant of the clinical course. In the presence of a normal cardiac output a peak systolic transvalvular pressure gradient between 50 and 80 mm Hg or a peak systolic right ventricular pressure between 75 and 100 mm Hg is considered to be moderate stenosis; levels below and above that range are classified as mild and severe, respectively. Patients with mild pulmonic stenosis are generally asymptomatic and are discovered during routine examination. In patients with more significant obstruction the severity of stenosis may increase with time. Progression may be relative and reflect disproportionate physical growth of the patient, infundibular narrowing due to progressive hypertrophy of the right ventricular outflow tract, or fibrosis of the valve cusps. Symptoms, when present, vary from mild exertional dyspnea and mild cyanosis to signs and symptoms of heart failure depending upon the degree of obstruction and the level of myocardial compensation. Exertional fatigue, syncope, and chest pain are related to an inability to augment pulmonary blood flow during exercise in some patients with moderate or severe obstruction.

The severity of obstruction is often suggested by the physical findings. Right ventricular hypertrophy reduces compliance of that chamber and a forceful right atrial contraction is necessary to augment right ventricular filling. Prominent *a*-waves in the jugular venous pulse, a fourth heart sound, and occasionally, presystolic pulsations of the liver reflect a vigorous atrial contraction and suggest the presence of severe stenosis. Cardiomegaly and a right ventricular parasternal lift accompany moderate or severe obstruction. A systolic thrill is palpable along the upper left sternal border in all but the mildest forms of stenosis. The

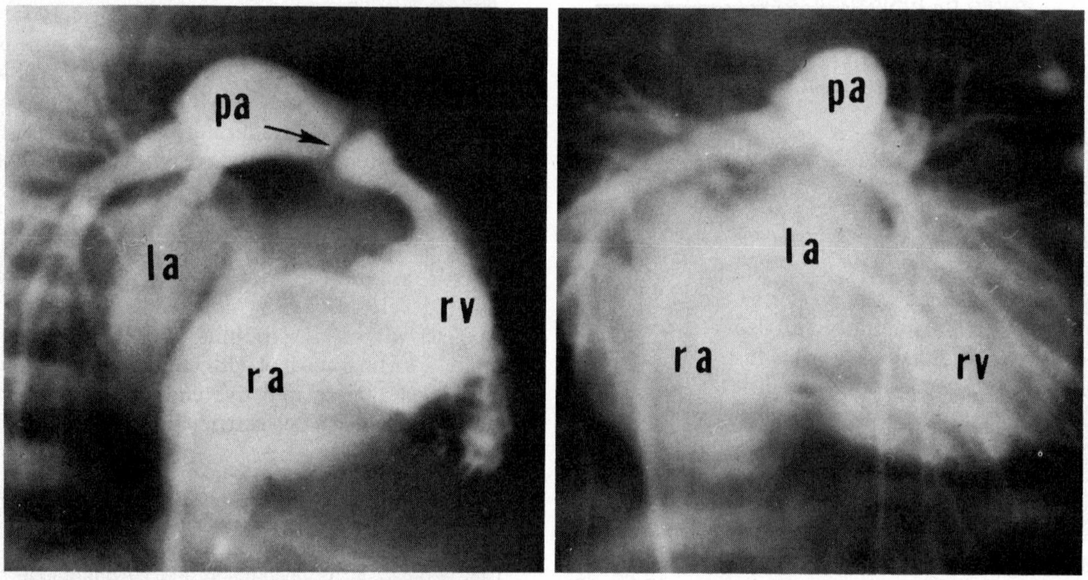

FIGURE 29–37 Right ventriculogram in an infant with critical pulmonic stenosis shows the thickened, nonmobile pulmonic valve (arrow) in the lateral projection (*left*). Both the lateral and frontal (*right*) projections show regurgitation of contrast material across the tricuspid valve into the right atrium (ra), with subsequent shunting across the foramen ovale to the left atrium (la). rv = right ventricle; pa = pulmonary artery. (Courtesy of Norman Talner, M.D.)

first heart sound is normal and is followed by a systolic ejection sound at the upper left sternal edge produced by sudden opening of the stenotic valve; an ejection sound is not heard in patients with pulmonic valve dysplasia. The ejection sound typically is louder during expiration; when it is inaudible or occurs less than 0.08 second from the onset of the Q wave on electrocardiogram, severe obstruction is suggested. Right ventricular ejection is prolonged in patients with moderate or severe stenosis and the sound of pulmonic valve closure is delayed and soft. The characteristic feature of valvular pulmonic stenosis on auscultation is a harsh, diamond-shaped systolic ejection murmur heard best at the upper left sternal border. The systolic murmur becomes louder and its crescendo occurs later in systole, obscuring the aortic component of the second sound with more severe degrees of valvular obstruction, since these patients have a greater prolongation of right ventricular systole. The holosystolic decrescendo murmur of tricuspid regurgitation may accompany severe pulmonic stenosis, especially in the presence of congestive heart failure. Cyanosis, reflecting venoarterial shunting through a patent foramen ovale, is absent with mild stenosis and infrequent with moderate obstruction. However, cyanosis may not be apparent in patients with severe obstruction if the atrial septum is intact.

Electro- and *vectorcardiography* may be helpful in assessing the degree of obstruction to right ventricular output.[300] In mild cases the electrocardiogram is often normal, whereas moderate and severe stenoses are associated with right axis deviation and right ventricular hypertrophy. A tall QR wave in the right precordial leads with T-wave inversion and ST-segment suppression (right ventricular "strain") reflects severe stenosis. When an rSR′ pattern is observed in lead V_1 (20 per cent of patients) generally lower right ventricular pressures are found than in patients with a pure R wave of equal amplitude. High amplitude P waves in leads II and V_1 indicating right atrial enlargement are associated with severe stenosis. The vectorcardiogram shows clockwise rotation of the QRS loop in the horizontal plane with a leftward anterior direction of initial forces, followed by a broad limb directed to the right anteriorly. Chest roentgenography in patients with mild or moderate pulmonic stenosis often shows a heart of normal size and normal pulmonary vascularity. Poststenotic dilatation of the main and left pulmonary arteries is often evident. Right atrial and right ventricular enlargement are observed in patients with severe obstruction and resultant right ventricular failure. The pulmonary vascularity may be reduced in patients with severe stenosis, right ventricular failure, and/or a venoarterial shunt at the atrial level. Echocardiography may be of limited value because of technical difficulties in imaging the pulmonic valve.[301] Complete opening of the pulmonic valve with atrial systole ("*a*" wave of a pulmonic valve echogram) may be seen with severe stenosis. Moreover, prolongation beyond 480 msec of the interval between the onset of the QRS complex of the electrocardiogram and the point of pulmonic valve cusp closure reflects the prolonged right ventricular ejection time associated with severe obstruction.

Cardiac catheterization and *angiocardiography* with right ventricular injection localizes the site of obstruction, evaluates its severity, and documents the coexistence of additional cardiac malformations (Fig. 29–38). The resting cardiac output is usually normal, even in cases of severe stenosis, and most children show the ability to increase cardiac output with exercise.[302,303] Right ventricular dysfunction occurs especially when venoarterial shunting is significant and produces systemic arterial desaturation.[304,305] In patients with critical stenosis, care must be taken during hemodynamic study that the cardiac catheter does not dangerously occlude the stenotic valve opening. The angiographic appearance of a typical valvular pulmonic stenosis differs from that of a dysplastic valve. The former is thickened and domes during systole, returning to a normal con-

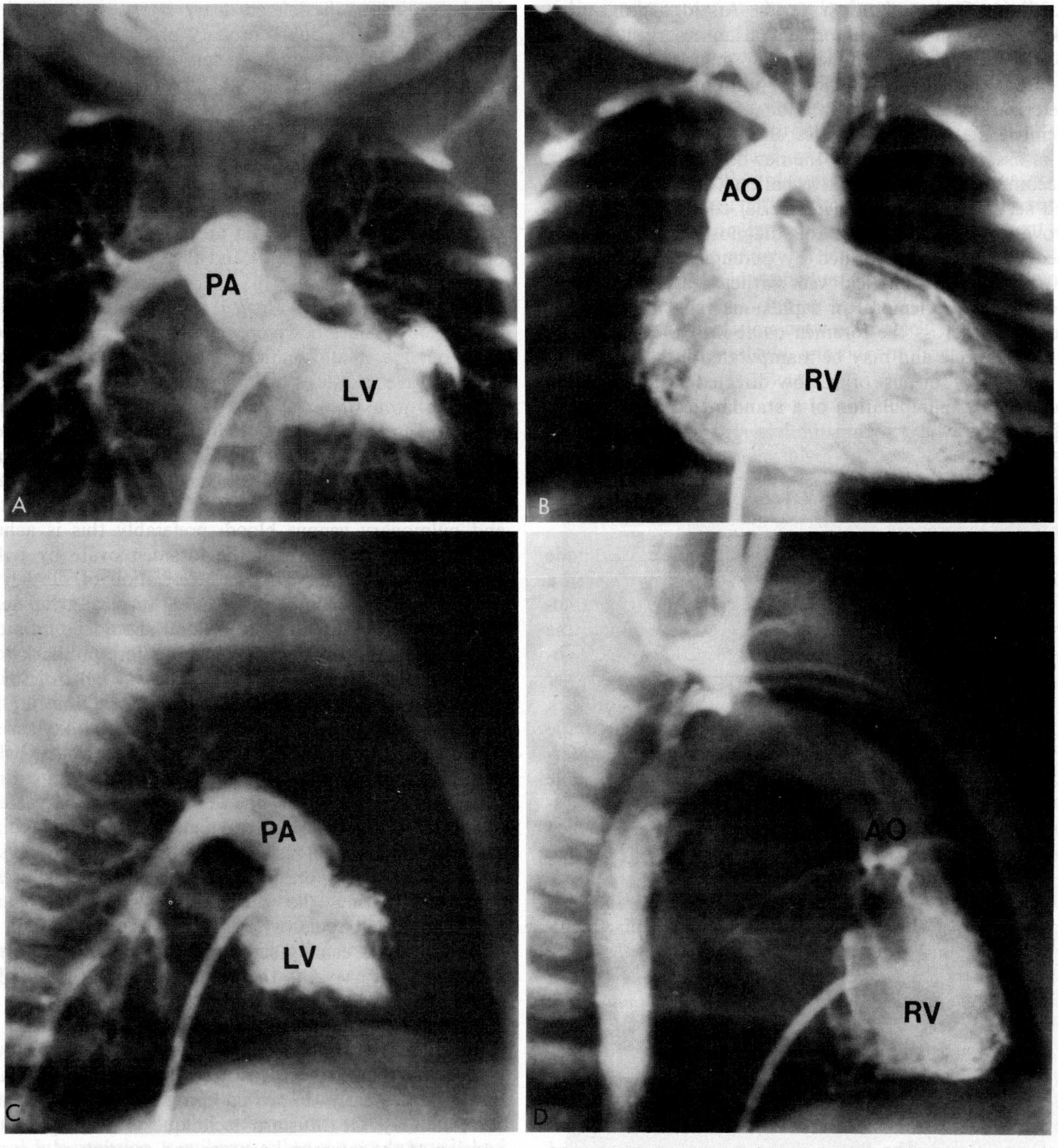

FIGURE 29–59 Frontal (*A* and *B*) and lateral (*C* and *D*) views of selective left (*A* and *C*) and right (*B* and *D*) ventricular angiograms in a patient with complete transposition of the great arteries and an intact ventricular septum. LV = left ventricle; PA = pulmonary artery; RV = right ventricle; AO = aorta. (Courtesy of Robert White, M.D.)

mortality less than 5 per cent. Clinical improvement is usually quite dramatic. In some patients postoperative complications are observed that are directly related to the intraatrial repair (shunts across the intraatrial patch and obstruction to either systemic or pulmonary venous return or both.[413,414] There is a high incidence of early and late postoperative dysrhythmias that are more likely to have their basis in injury to the sinoatrial node and/or its arterial supply than in disruption of internodal tracts or damage to the atrioventricular node.[415,416] Tricuspid regurgitation is a less common complication of operation and may be related in some patients to a preexisting abnormality of the tricuspid valve,[417] whereas in most it is related to right ventricular dysfunction. Although the assessment of right ventricular contractility is difficult, it has been suggested that the right ventricular pump function is impaired prior to Mustard operation and does not return to normal following successful surgery.[418,419] It is not yet clear whether the right ventricle can perform as a systemic pumping chamber for the duration of a normal life span.[420]

In the unusual infant with an intact ventricular septum and a significant patent ductus arteriosus, an early intra-

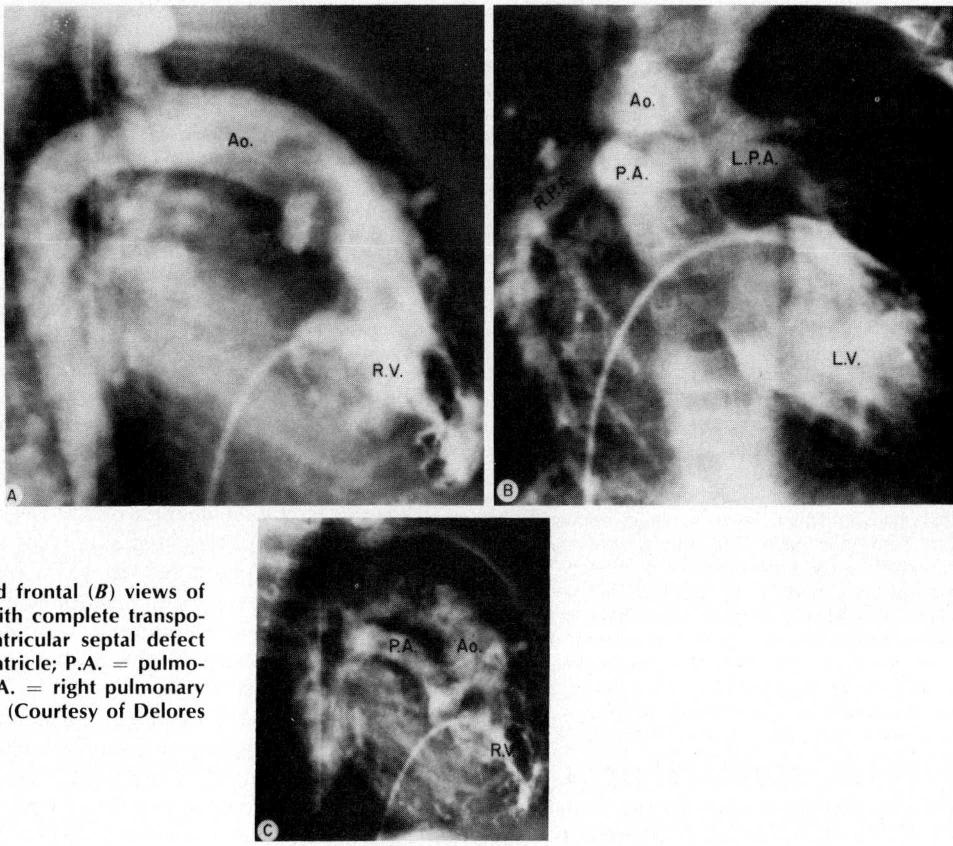

FIGURE 29–60 Lateral (*A* and *C*) and frontal (*B*) views of selective ventriculograms in a child with complete transposition of the great arteries and a ventricular septal defect (V.S.D.). Ao. = aorta; R.V. = right ventricle; P.A. = pulmonary artery; L.V. = left ventricle; R.P.A. = right pulmonary artery; L.P.A. = left pulmonary artery. (Courtesy of Delores A. Danilowicz, M.D.)

atrial corrective operation with closure of the ductus is indicated at 4 to 6 months of age to prevent the likely progression of pulmonary vascular disease.[404] Debate exists concerning the optimal management of patients with a large ventricular septal defect. In some centers pulmonary artery banding is advocated early in life, followed by definitive intracardiac repair at 1 to 2 years of age. Others favor a one-stage intraatrial repair with patch closure of the ventricular septal defect prior to age 6 months. Experience is accumulating with a one-stage operation designed to close the ventricular septal defect; transpose both coronary arteries to the posterior artery; and transsect, contrapose, and anastomose the aorta and pulmonary arteries (Jatene operation).[421,422] The arterial switch anatomical correction may be complicated by coronary ostial stenosis, acquired supravalvular aortic and/or pulmonary stenosis, and aortic incompetence. Infants with transposition of the great arteries plus a ventricular septal defect and left ventricular outflow tract obstruction may require a systemic–pulmonary artery anastomosis when a pronounced diminution in pulmonary blood flow exists. A later corrective procedure for these patients bypasses the left ventricular outflow obstruction and employs an intracardiac ventricular baffle connecting the left ventricle to the aorta and an extracardiac prosthetic conduit between the right ventricle and the distal end of a divided pulmonary artery (Rastelli procedure).[423] In patients with significant pulmonary vascular obstructive disease the risk of definitive repair (intraatrial baffle and closure of the ventricular septal defect) is great. In this group of patients a "palliative" Mustard procedure leaving the ventricular septal defect open often provides good, short-term, symptomatic improvement by increasing arterial oxygen tension and reducing the stimulus to progressive polycythemia.[424]

Congenitally Corrected Transposition of the Great Arteries

This term is applied to two distinctly different anomalies, anatomically corrected transposition or malposition of the great arteries and physiologically corrected, levo- or L-transposition of the great arteries.

Morphology. Anatomically corrected malposition of the great arteries is a rare form of congenital heart disease in which the great arteries are abnormally related to each other and to the ventricles but arise, nonetheless, above the anatomically correct ventricles.[425,426] Because of this, the term *malposition*, rather than *transposition*, is preferable. The anomaly results from either leftward looping of the ventricular segment of the embryonic heart tube in the situs solitus heart, or rightward looping in the situs inversus heart. In this unusual malformation the aorta is to the left (levo- or L-malposition) and the pulmonary artery is to the right. When no other defect exists, the circulation proceeds normally. When an associated lesion prompts cardiac catheterization, diagnosis of the abnormal relationships between the great arteries may be made by biplane angiocardiography. Anomalies commonly associated with anatomically corrected malposition of the great arteries include ventricular septal defect, left juxtaposition of the atrial appendages, tricuspid atresia or stenosis, and valvular and subvalvular pulmonic stenosis.

Invariably, the term *congenitally corrected transposition* is applied to the patient in whom a functional correction of the circulation exists by virtue of the relationships between the ventricles and great arteries.[427,428] Corrected or L-transposition occurs when the primitive cardiac tube loops to the left, instead of to the right, during embryogenesis.[429] The anatomical right ventricle comes to lie on the left and receives oxygenated blood from the left atrium; this blood is ejected into an anteriorly placed, left-sided aorta. The anatomical left ventricle lies to the right and connects the right atrium to a posteriorly placed pulmonary artery. This arrangement of the great arteries and ventricles (in contrast to the uncorrected, complete, or D-transposition) permits functional correction, so that systemic venous blood passes into the pulmonary trunk while arterialized pulmonary venous blood flows into the aorta. In the heart with congenitally corrected transposition, the venae cavae and coronary sinus drain into a right atrium that is normal in position and structure. Venous blood flows from the right atrium, designated as the "venous atrium," across an atrioventricular valve that has the structure of a normal mitral valve and into the right-sided "venous ventricle." The venous ventricle, however, has the morphological characteristics of a normal left ventricle, i.e., its interior lining is trabeculated, it has no crista supraventricularis, and the atrioventricular valve is in continuity with the posteriorly placed semilunar valve. It ejects blood into the pulmonary trunk, which arises posterior to the ascending aorta. Oxygenated blood returns from the lungs to the left atrium, which is normal in position and structure; from here it flows into the left-sided "arterial ventricle" across an atrioventricular valve that has the structure of a normal tricuspid valve. The interior lining of the arterial ventricle has the morphological characteristics of a normal right ventricle (i.e., it has course trabeculations and a crista supraventricularis), and the tricuspid atrioventricular valve is not in continuity with the anteriorly placed semilunar valve. The arterial ventricle ejects blood into the aorta, which arises anterior to the pulmonary trunk. In addition to inversion of the cardiac ventricles, there is inversion of the conduction system and coronary arteries. Commonly associated anatomical lesions include atrial and/or ventricular septal defects; single ventricle with an outlet chamber with or without pulmonic stenosis; left atrioventricular valve regurgitation, usually because of an Ebstein's malformation of the left-sided tricuspid valve; ventricular septal defect and pulmonic stenosis; and dextrocardia.[430]

CLINICAL MANIFESTATIONS. The clinical presentation, course, and prognosis of patients with congenital functionally corrected transposition vary, depending on the nature and severity of the complicating intracardiac anomalies. Patients in whom corrected transposition exists as an isolated anomaly present no functional alterations and have no symptoms.

The physical findings in congenitally corrected transposition are those of the associated lesions with two exceptions: (1) a single accentuated second heart sound is usually present in the second left intercostal space, representing closure of the aortic valve lying lateral and anterior to the pulmonic valve; and (2) there is a high incidence of cardiac dysrhythmias. Because of the inversion of the heart's conduction system the electrocardiogram may provide important clues in the diagnosis. An abnormal direction of initial (septal) depolarization from right to left causes leftward, anterior, and superior orientation of the initial QRS forces and reversal of the precordial Q-wave pattern (Q waves are present in the right precordial leads and absent in the left [Fig. 29–61]).

LABORATORY EXAMINATION. In addition to inversion of the conduction system, the His bundle is elongated because of the greater distance between the atrioventricular node and the base of the ventricular septum.[432] The His bundle is located beneath the pulmonic valve in the position of mitral pulmonary continuity; thus, it is subject to significant excursions during mitral valve closure. This arrangement may be a causal factor in the arrhythmias and atrioventricular conduction disturbances commonly observed in these patients. First-degree atrioventricular (AV) block occurs in about 50 per cent, and complete AV block occurs in 10 to 15 per cent of patients. Other degrees of AV dissociation may be observed as well as paroxysmal supraventricular tachycardia and ventricular extrasystoles. In some patients, Kent bundle connections provide the anatomical substrate for preexcitation.[433] Roentgenographic examination characteristically reveals absence of the normal pulmonary artery segment and a smooth convexity of the left supracardiac border produced by the displaced ascending aorta (Fig. 29–62). The latter may be visualized by radionuclide scintillation scans of the central circulation.[434] The main pulmonary trunk is medially displaced and absent from the cardiac silhouette; the right pulmonary hilus is often prominent and elevated compared to the left, producing a right-sided "waterfall" appearance.

Real-time *cross-sectional echocardiography* may suggest the diagnosis of corrected transposition.[34,406] By tracing the great arteries back to their ventricles of origin in the short-axis plane, one would find that the anterior leftward great artery (the aorta) arises from the left-sided ventricle and is not in continuity with the left-sided atrioventricular valve. Because the ventricular septum lies in the anteroposterior plane parallel to the echo beam, it may not be visualized. In apical-basal, four-chamber echo views, the right and left ventricular morphology and the inverted atrioventricular valves may be ascertained correctly. The latter views may

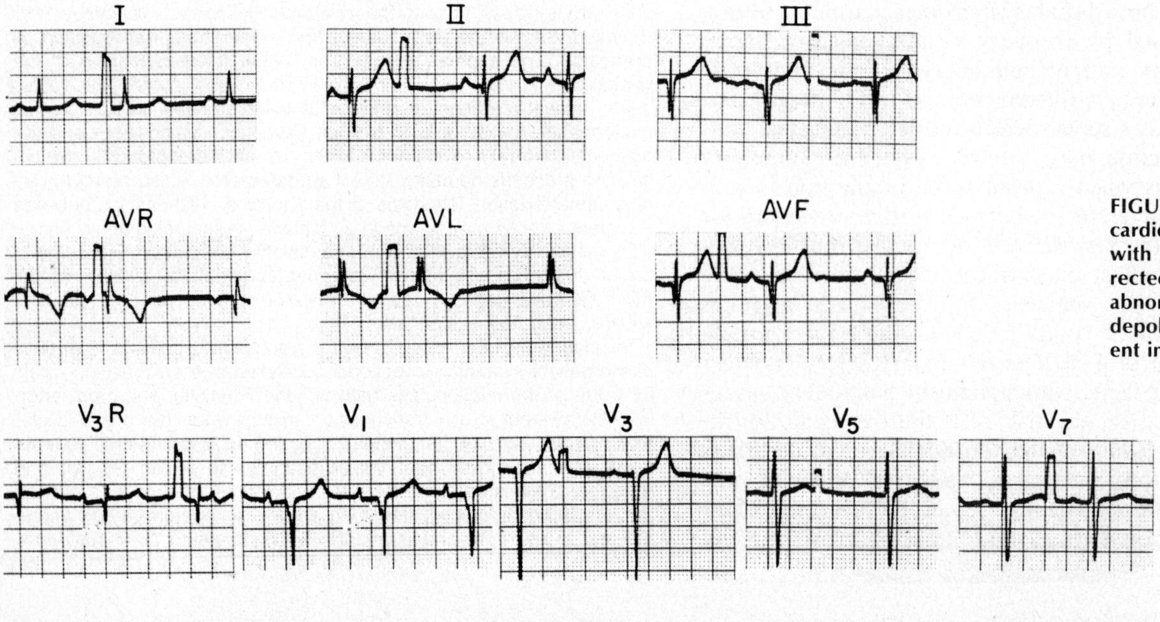

FIGURE 29–61 Electrocardiogram in a patient with congenitally corrected transposition. The abnormality of initial depolarization is apparent in V_3R and V_1.

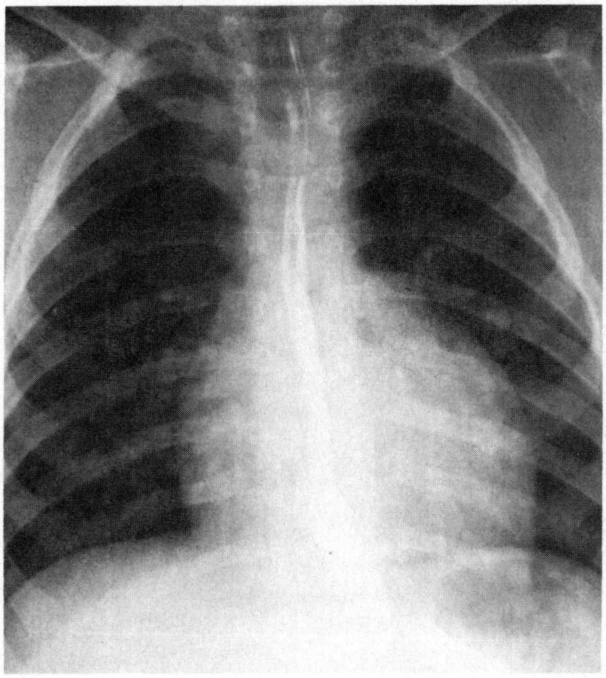

FIGURE 29–62 Chest roentgenogram in a child with congenitally corrected transposition of the great arteries. The smooth convexity of the left superior cardiac border is formed by the displaced ascending aorta. The main pulmonary artery is medially displaced and absent from the cardiac silhouette.

also allow detection of inferior displacement of the left-sided tricuspid valve when Ebstein's anomaly coexists.[34]

At *cardiac catheterization* the diagnosis should be suspected when the venous catheter enters a posterior and midline main pulmonary trunk. Retrograde arterial catheter passage establishes the typical position of the ascending aorta at the upper left cardiac border. Hemodynamic abnormalities depend upon the lesions associated with corrected transposition. Selective *angiocardiography* allows visualization of the transposed great arteries and morphological differentiation of the two ventricles (Fig. 29–63).[435] The ventricles tend to lie side by side, with the ventricular septum oriented in an anteroposterior direction. Selective aortography demonstrates the inverted coronary arterial pattern that is invariably present in corrected transposition. The competence of the left atrioventricular valve may be determined by injection of contrast material into the arterial ventricle.[436] When a left-sided Ebstein's malformation exists, the leaflets are displaced distal to the true valve annulus. The level of the annulus may be determined by visualization of the circumflex branch of the left coronary artery, which courses posteriorly in the AV groove.

Specific problems have attended operative repair of the lesions associated with congenitally corrected transposition, owing primarily to the course of the AV conduction system and the coronary arterial pattern.[437,438] Intraoperative electrophysiological mapping of the course of the conduction system has reduced, but not abolished, the risk of surgically induced heartblock. The AV bundle is located anteriorly and in relation to the anterolateral quadrant of the pulmonary outflow tract. Thus, when a ventricular septal defect is present, the bundle is usually related to the anterior and superior margins of the defect and lies beneath the pulmonic valve. In corrected transposition, the coronary arteries have a course appropriate to their ventricles, i.e., the anterior descending and circumflex arteries supply the morphological left ventricle, and the right coronary artery supplies the morphological right ventricle. However, because the great arteries are transposed, the noncoronary sinus is the anterior sinus of the aortic valve. Occasionally, the inversion of the coronary arterial system may limit and preclude an incision into the venous ventricle, thereby interfering with exposure of intracardiac defects in the usual manner. The disadvantage in approaching intracardiac anomalies using an incision in the morphological right ventricle is that this is the systemic ventricle. Surgical risks are especially high in patients in whom significant regurgitation exists from the arterial ventricle to the arterial atrium.

Double-Outlet Right Ventricle

Other designations applied to this lesion include origin of both great arteries from the right ventricle, partial transposition, complete transposition of the aorta and levo-position of the pulmonary artery, complete dextroposition of the aorta, and the Taussig-Bing complex. An abnormal relationship exists in this malformation between the aorta and the pulmonary trunk, which both arise from the right ventricle.[439,440] The only outlet from the left ventricle is a ventricular septal defect. The anatomical classification of the various types of double-outlet right ventricle takes into account the location of the ventricular septal defect, the presence or absence of pulmonic stenosis, and whether or not dextro- or levo-malposition of the great arteries is present.[441] An increased incidence of the anomaly occurs in infants with the trisomy 18 syndrome. The most common associated anomalies are pulmonic stenosis, coarctation of the aorta, and patent ductus arteriosus. Less often associated are anomalous pulmonary venous connection, endocardial cushion defect, and atrial septal defect. The most common extracardiac malformations are asplenia and visceral heterotaxy.

The pathological features in most patients include side-by-side pulmonic and aortic valves and discontinuity between the mitral and aortic valves.[442] The latter exists because muscular infundibulum is usual beneath both semilunar valves. The ventricular septal defect may be remote from or related closely to one or both semilunar valves (Fig. 29–64).[443] When the interventricular defect is subpulmonic, with or without a straddling pulmonary trunk, the complex is designated "Taussig-Bing." In most patients the interventricular septal defect is below the crista supraventricularis and is subaortic in location. Least often the defect is either remote from both semilunar valves ("uncommitted") or underlies both ("doubly committed").

The *clinical and physiological picture* is determined by the size and location of the ventricular septal defect and the presence or absence of pulmonic stenosis. In the Taussig-Bing form of double-outlet right ventricle, the malformation resembles physiologically and clinically complete transposition with ventricular septal defect and pulmonary hypertension. When the ventricular septal defect is subaortic, the stream of blood from the left ventricle is directed preferentially to the aorta. Thus, there may be little or no detectable cyanosis, and these patients usually clinically resemble those with an isolated, large ventricular septal defect and pulmonary hypertension. The most important determinant of the natural history in both these types of double-outlet right ventricle is the progression of pulmonary vascular obstruction. In contrast, when there is pulmonary outflow tract obstruction, which is often severe and found commonly in those patients in whom the ventricular septal defect is subaortic, clinical findings are similar to those of cyanotic tetralogy of Fallot. In some patients, especially without pulmonic stenosis, the electrocardiogram shows a superiorly oriented counterclockwise frontal plane QRS loop in addition to right ventricular hypertrophy.[444] The pattern appears to result from relative hypoplasia of the anterosuperior left bundle and preferential activation of the posteroinferior left ventricular wall. Recent reports suggest that the presence of the latter electrocardiographic pattern in patients with double-outlet right ventricle should raise the possibility of a coexistent

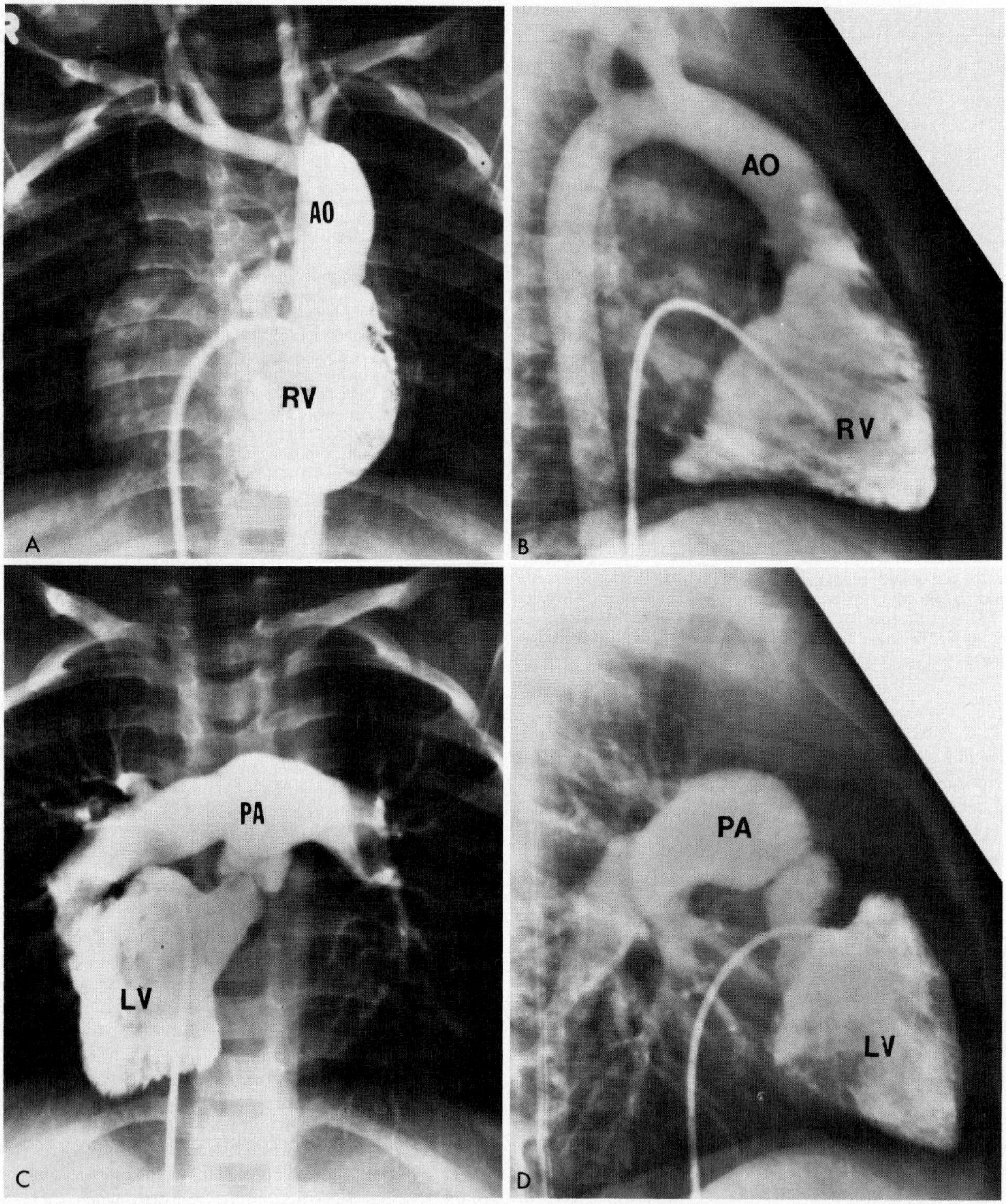

FIGURE 29–63 Congenitally corrected (levo-)transposition of the great arteries in a 4-year-old boy. *A*, Anteroposterior ventriculogram in left-sided ventricle with mesocardia. The morphological right ventricle (RV) is left-sided, indicating an L-ventricular loop (inverted ventricles in situs solitus). The aorta (AO) originates above the morphological right ventricle and is thus transposed and in the classic levo-transposition position. *B*, Lateral ventriculogram in left-sided ventricle (same frame as *A*). The aorta originates anteriorly above the morphological right ventricle (RV). *C*, Anteroposterior ventriculogram in right-sided morphological left ventricle (LV). The transposed pulmonary artery (PA) arises from this ventricle, and the ventricular septum appears intact. Pulmonic valve thickening is also evident. The aorta (*A*) is to the left of the pulmonary artery. Note that the ventricular septum in the L-ventricular loop is visualized best in the anteroposterior views. *D*, Lateral ventriculogram in right-sided ventricle (same frame as *C*). The pulmonary artery is posterior to the aorta, and supravalvular pulmonic narrowing is seen. (From Freedom, R. M., et al.: The differential diagnosis of levo-transposed or malposed aorta. An angiocardiographic study. Circulation *50*:1040, 1974, by permission of the American Heart Association, Inc.)

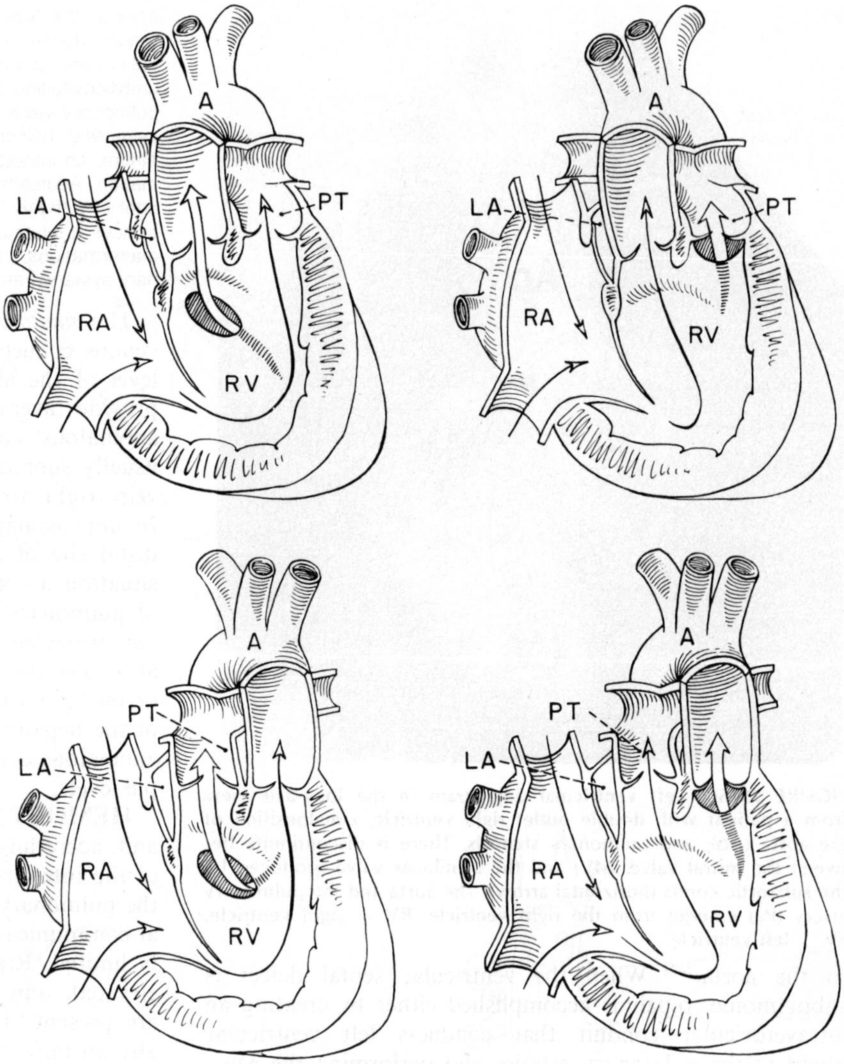

FIGURE 29–64 Double-outlet right ventricle (RV) with side-by-side relation of great arteries is illustrated in the top two panels. A subaortic ventricular septal defect (VSD) below the crista supraventricularis (*top left*) favors delivery of left ventricular blood to the aorta (A). Location of the VSD above the crista (*top right*) favors streaming to the pulmonary trunk (PT). When the great arteries are malposed (*bottom two panels*), streaming continues to depend on the relationship between a particular great artery and the VSD. The subcristal VSD (*bottom left*) favors delivery of left ventricular blood to the pulmonary trunk. The supracristal VSD depicted at the bottom right lies below the malpositioned aorta, which receives most of the left ventricular output. LA = left atrium; RA = right atrium; PT = pulmonary trunk. (From Sridaromont, S., et al.: Double outlet right ventricle: Hemodynamic and anatomic correlations. Am. J. Cardiol. *38*:85, 1976.)

endocardial cushion defect or abnormality of the mitral valve.[442] Two-dimensional *echocardiography* may reliably distinguish double-outlet right ventricle from other lesions causing cyanosis, such as tetralogy of Fallot and transposition of the great arteries. In the short-axis view, imaging is simultaneous with both great arteries in an anterior location; the ventricular septum is identified posteriorly. Atrioventricular valve–semilunar valve discontinuity and great artery relations are then defined by a variety of axial ultrasonic imaging views.[331,331a]

In each of the different types of double-outlet right ventricle, precise delineation of the malformation depends on careful angiocardiographic analysis. The diagnosis can be established with confidence when the angiographic findings include simultaneous opacification of both great vessels from the right ventricle, aortic and pulmonic valves at the same transverse level, and separation of the aortic valve from the aortic leaflet of the mitral valve by the crista supraventricularis (Fig. 29–65).[445] The position of the ventricular septal defect and the relationships between the great arteries must be defined in order to plan surgical procedures appropriately (Fig. 29–66).[446,447]

In double-outlet right ventricle with subaortic ventricular septal defect, repair is accomplished by creating an intraventicular baffle that conducts left ventricular blood

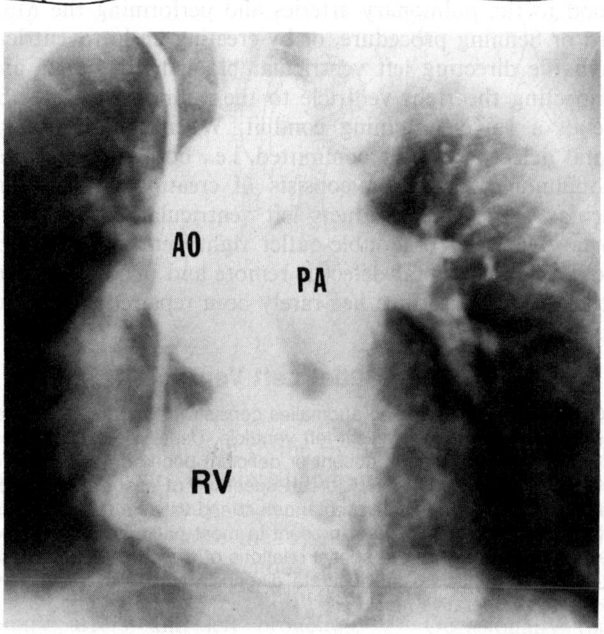

FIGURE 29–65 Simultaneous opacification of both great arteries from a right ventricular injection of contrast material in a patient with double-outlet right ventricle (RV). The aortic and pulmonic valves are at the same transverse level. AO = aorta; PA = pulmonary artery. (Courtesy of Robert White, M.D.)

echocardiography. *In* Clinical and Pathological Correlations in Adolescent and Adult Heart Disease. Boston, Little, Brown and Co., 1983.
35. Mercier, J. C., DiSessa, T. G., Jarmakani, J., and Friedman, W. F.: Two dimensional echocardiographic assessment of left ventricular volumes and ejection fraction. Circulation *65*:962, 1982.
36. Williams, R. G., and Tucker, C. R.: Echocardiographic Diagnosis of Congenital Heart Disease. Boston, Little, Brown and Co., 1977.
37. Lister, G., and Talner, N. S.: Oxygen transport in congenital heart disease. *In* Engle, M. A. (ed.): Pediatric Cardiovascular Disease. Philadelphia, F. A. Davis, 1981, p. 129.
38. Rosenthal, A., Nathan, D. G., Marty, A. T., Button, L. N., Miettinen, O. S., and Nadas, A. S.: Acute hemodynamic effects of red cell volume reduction, polycythemia of cyanotic congenital heart disease. Circulation *42*:297, 1970.
39. Voigt, G. C., and Wright, J. R.: Cyanotic congenital heart disease and sudden death. Am. Heart J. *87*:773, 1974.
40. Fischbein, C. A., Rosenthal, A., Fischer, E. G., Nadas, A. S., and Welch, K.: Risk factors for brain abscess in patients with congenital heart disease. Am. J. Cardiol. *34*:97, 1974.
41. Shaher, R. M., and Deuchard, D. C.: Hematogenous brain abscess in cyanotic congenital heart disease. Am. J. Med. *52*:349, 1972.
42. Corrin, C.: Paradoxical embolism. Br. Heart J. *26*:549, 1964.
43. Haroutunian, L. M., and Neill, C. A.: Pulmonary complications of congenital heart disease: Hemoptysis. Am. Heart J. *84*:540, 1972.
44. Guntheroth, W. G., Morgan, B. C., and Mullens, G. L.: Physiologic studies of paroxysmal hyperpnea in cyanotic congenital heart disease. Circulation *31*: 1965.
45. Bonchek, L. I., Starr, A., Sunderland, C. O., and Menashe, V. D.: Natural history of tetralogy of Fallot in infancy. Circulation *48*:392, 1973.
46. Talmer, N. S.: Congestive heart failure in the infant. Pediatr. Clin. North Am. *18*:1011, 1971.
47. Rosenthal, A., and Castaneda, A. R.: Growth and development after cardiovascular surgery in infants and children. *In* Rosenthal, A., Sonnenblick, E. H., and Lesch, M. (eds.): Postoperative Congenital Heart Disease. New York, Grune and Stratton, 1975, p. 119.
48. Vogel, J. H. K.: Pulmonary hypertension. *In* Moss, A. J., Adams, F. H., and Emmanouilides, G. C. (eds.): Heart Disease in Infants, Children and Adolescents. 2nd ed. Baltimore, Williams and Wilkins, 1977, p. 629.
49. Heath, D., and Edwards, J. E.: The pathology of hypertensive pulmonary vascular disease. Circulation *18*:533, 1958.
50. Levin, D. L., Rudolph, A. M., Heymann, M. A., and Phibbs, R. H.: Morphological development of the pulmonary vascular bed in the fetal lamb. Circulation *53*:144, 1976.
51. Rabinovitch, M., and Reid, L. M.: Quantitative structural analysis of the pulmonary vascular bed in congenital heart defects. *In* Engle, M. A. (ed.): Pediatric Cardiovascular Disease. Philadelphia, F. A. Davis, 1981, p. 149.
52. Kaplan, E. L., and Taranta, A. V.: Infective Endocarditis. An American Heart Association Symposium. Dallas, The American Heart Association, Inc., 1977.
53. Durack, D. T.: Current practice in prevention of bacterial endocarditis. Br. Heart J. *37*:478, 1975.
54. Kaplan, E. J.: Prevention of bacterial endocarditis. Circulation *56*:139A, 1977.
55. Lambert, E. C., Menon, V. A., Wagner, H. R., and Vlad, P.: Sudden unexpected death from cardiovascular disease in children. Am. J. Cardiol. *34*:89, 1974.
56. Nadas, A. S., Fyler, D. C., and Castaneda, A. R.: The critically ill infant with congenital heart disease. Mod. Conc. Cardiovasc. Dis. *42*:53, 1973.
57. Rutkowski, M. M., Cohen, S. N., and Doyle, E. F.: Drug therapy of heart disease in pediatric patients. II. The treatment of congestive heart failure in infants and children with digitalis preparation. Am. Heart J. *86*:270, 1973.
58. Cohen, S. N., Doyle, E. F., and Rutkowski, M. M.: Drug therapy of heart disease in pediatric patients. I. Congestive heart failure in infancy and concepts of developmental pharmacology. Am. Heart J. *86*:133, 1973.
59. Freed, M. D., Hegmann, M. A., Lewis, A. B., Roehl, S. L., and Kensey, R. C.: Prostaglandin E_1 in infants with ductus arteriosus dependent congenital heart disease. Circulation *64*:899, 1981.
60. Lewis, A. B., Freed, M. D., Hegmann, M. A., Roehl, S. L., and Kensey, R. C.: Side effects of therapy with prostaglandin E_1 in infants with critical congenital heart disease. Circulation *64*:893, 1981.
61. Friedman, W. F., Kurlinski, J., Jacob, J., DiSessa, T. G., Gluck, L., Merritt, T. A., and Feldman, B. H.: Inhibition of prostaglandin and prostacyclin synthesis in clinical management of PDA. Semin. Perinatol. *4*:125, 1980.
62. Benson, L. N., Bohn, D., Edwards, J. F., Fortune, R. L., Price, S. A., Williams, W. G., and Rowe, R. D.: Nitroglycerin therapy in children with low cardiac index after heart surgery. Cardiovasc. Med. *4*:2, 1979.
63. Dillon, T. R., Janos, G. G., Meyer, R. A., Benzing, G., III, and Kaplan, S.: Vasodilator therapy for congestive heart failure. J. Pediatr. *96*:623, 1980.
64. Kirkpatrick, S. E., Corrin, A., Higgins, C. B., and Nyhan, W. F.: Differential diagnosis of congenital heart disease in the newborn. West. J. Med. *128*:127, 1978.
65. Friedman, W. F., Sahn, D. J., and Hirschklau, M. J.: A review: Newer, noninvasive cardiac diagnostic methods. Pediatr. Res. *11*:190, 1977.
66. Kleinman, C. S., Donnerstein, R. L., Talner, N. S., and Hobbins, J. C.: Fetal echocardiography for evaluation of in utero congestive heart failure. N. Engl. J. Med. *306*:568, 1982.
67. DiSessa, T. G., and Friedman, W. F.: Echocardiography in congenital heart disease. Cardiol. Clin. North Am. (*in press*)
68. Stanger, P., Heymann, M. A., Tarnoff, H., Hoffman, J. I. E., and Rudolph, A. M.: Complications of cardiac catheterization of neonates, infants and children. Circulation *50*:595, 1974.
69. Hoffman, J. I. E., Rudolph, A. M., and Danilowicz, D.: Left to right atrial shunts in infants. Am. J. Cardiol. *38*:68, 1972.
70. Hunt, C. E., and Lucas, R. V., Jr.: Symptomatic atrial septal defect in infancy. Circulation *42*:1042, 1973.
71. Craig, R. J., and Seltzer, A.: Natural history and prognosis of atrial septal defect. Circulation *37*:805, 1968.
72. Davea, J. E., Cheitlin, M. D., and Bedynek, J. L.: Sinus venosus atrial septal defect. Am. Heart J. *85*:177, 1973.
73. Tanden, R., and Edwards, J. E.: Atrial septal defect in infancy. Common association with other anomalies. Circulation *49*:1005, 1974.
74. Leachman, R. D., Cokkinos, D. V., and Cooley, D. A.: Association of ostium secundum atrial septal defects with mitral valve prolapse. Am. J. Cardiol. *38*: 167, 1976.
75. Levin, A. R., Spach, M. S., Boineau, J. P., Canent, R. V., Jr., Capp, M. P., and Jewett, P. H.: Atrial pressure flow dynamics and atrial septal defects (secundum type). Circulation *37*:476, 1968.
76. O'Toole, J. D., Reddy, I., Curtiss, E. I., and Shaver, J. A.: The mechanism of splitting of the second heart sound in atrial septal defect. Circulation *41*:1047, 1977.
77. Clark, E. B., and Kugler, J. D.: Preoperative secundum atrial septal defect with coexisting sinus node and atrioventricular node dysfunction. Circulation *65*:976, 1982.
78. Taketa, R. M., Sahn, D. J., Simon, A. L., Pappelbaum, S. J., and Friedman, W. F.: Catheter positions in congenital cardiac malformations. Circulation *51*: 749, 1975.
79. Cohn, L. H., Morrow, A. G., and Braunwald, E.: Operative treatment of atrial septal defect: Clinical and hemodynamic assessments in 175 patients. Br. Heart J. *29*:725, 1967.
80. Levin, A. R., Liebson, P. R., Ehlers, K. H., and Daimant, B.: Assessment of left ventricular function in atrial septal defect. Pediatr. Res. *9*:894, 1975.
81. Ebstein, S. E., Beiser, G. D., Goldstein, R. E., Rosing, D. R., Redwood, D. R., and Morrow, A. G.: Hemodynamic abnormalities in response to mild and intense upright exercise following operative correction of an atrial septal defect or tetralogy of Fallot. Circulation *42*:1065, 1973.
82. Ugarte, M., Enriques de Salamanca, F., and Quero, M.: Endocardial cushion defects and anatomical study of 54 specimens. Br. Heart J. *38*:674, 1976.
83. Bharati, S., and Lev, M.: The spectrum of common atrioventricular orifice. Am. Heart J. *86*:553, 1973.
84. Borkon, A. M., Pieroni, D. R., Varghese, P. J., Ho, C. S., and Rowe, R. D.: The superior QRS axis in ostium primum ASD. Am. Heart J. *92*:15, 1975.
85. Goodman, D. J., Harrison, D. C., and Cannom, D. S.: Atrioventricular conduction in patients with incomplete endocardial cushion defect. Circulation *49*: 630, 1974.
86. Jacobsen, J. R., Gillette, P. C., Corbett, B. N., Rabinovitch, M., and McNamara, D. G.: Intracardiac electrography in endocardial cushion defects. Circulation *54*:599, 1976.
87. Waldo, A. L., Kaiser, G. A., Bowman, F. O., Jr., and Malm, J. R.: Etiology of prolongation of the PR interval in patients with an endocardial cushion defect. Circulation *43*:19, 1973.
88. Bierman, F. Z., and Williams, R. G.: Subxyphoid two-dimensional imaging of the interatrial septum in infants and neonates with congenital heart disease. Circulation *60*:80, 1979.
89. Lange, L. W., Sahn, D. J., Allen, H. D., and Goldberg, S. J.: Subxyphoid cross-sectional echocardiography in infants and children with congenital heart disease. Circulation *59*:513, 1979.
90. Baron, M. G.: Abnormalities of the mitral valve and endocardial cushion defect. Circulation *45*:672, 1972.
91. Rastelli, G. C., Ongley, P. A., Kirklin, J. W., and McGoon, D. C.: Surgical repair of the complete former persistent common atrioventricular canal. J. Thorac. Cardiovasc. Surg. *55*:299, 1968.
92. Elliott, L. P., Bargeron, L. M., Bream, P. R., Soto, B., and Curry, G. C.: Axial cineangiography in congenital heart disease. Circulation *46*:1084, 1977.
93. Newfeld, E. A., Sher, M., Paul, M. H., and Nikaido, H.: Pulmonary vascular disease and complete atrioventricular canal defect. Am. J. Cardiol. *39*:721, 1977.
94. Mair, D. D., and McGoon, D. C.: Surgical correction of atrioventricular canal during the first year of life. Am. J. Cardiol. *40*:66, 1977.
95. Carpentier, A.: Surgical anatomy and management of the mitral component of atrioventricular canal defects. *In* Anderson, R. H., and Shinebourne, E. A. (eds.): Paediatric Cardiology. London, Churchill-Livingstone, 1978, p. 477.
96. Ebert, P. A., and Gordon, D. A.: Complete atrioventricular canal malformation: Further classification of the anatomy of the common leaflet and its relationship to the VSD in surgical correction. Ann. Thorac. Surg. *25*:134, 1978.
97. McCabe, J. C., Engle, M. A., Gay, W. A., Jr., and Ebert, P. A.: Surgical treatment of endocardial cushion defect. Am. J. Cardiol. *39*:72, 1977.
97a. Kawaguchi, A., Broda, J., Gingel, R., Roland, J-M., Pieroni, D., and Subramanian, S.: Surgical repair of complete atrioventricular canal. A new concept. J. Am. Coll. Cardiol. *1*:651, 1983.
98. Friedman, W. F., Mehrizi, A., and Pusch, A. L.: Multiple muscular ventricular septal defects. Circulation *32*:35, 1964.
99. Bloomfield, D. K.: Natural history of ventricular septal defect in patients surviving infancy. Circulation *29*:914, 1964.

100. Keith, J. D., Rose, V., Collins, G., and Kidd, V. S. L.: Ventricular septal defect. Incidence, morbidity and mortality in various age groups. Br. Heart J. *33*: 81, 1971.
101. Dickinson, D. F., Arnold, R., and Wilkinson, J. L.: Ventricular septal defects in children born in Liverpool. Evaluation of natural course and surgical implications in an unselected population. Br. Heart J. *46*:47, 1981.
102. Collins, G., Calder, L., Rose, V., Kidd, L., and Keith, J. D.: Ventricular septal defect: Clinical and hemodynamic changes in the first five years of life. Am. Heart J. *84*:695, 1972.
103. Hoffman, J. I. E.: Natural history of congenital heart disease. Circulation *37*: 97, 1968.
104. Weidman, W. H., Blount, S. G., Jr., DuShane, J. W., Gersony, W. M., Hayes, C. J., and Nadas, A. S.: Clinical course in ventricular septal defect. Natural history study. Circulation *56* (Suppl.):I-56, 1977.
105. Lister, G., Hellenbrand, W. E., Kleinman, C. S., and Talner, N. S.: Physiologic effects of increasing hemoglobin concentration in left to right shunting in infants with ventricular septal defects. N. Engl. J. Med. *306*:502, 1982.
106. Beekman, R. H., Rocchini, A. P., and Rosenthal, A.: Hemodynamic effects of hydralazine in infants with a large ventricular septal defect. Circulation *65*:523, 1982.
107. Friedman, W. F., and Pitlick, P. T.: Ventricular septal defect in infancy—University of California, San Diego (Specialty Conference). West. J. Med. *120*:295, 1974.
108. Alpert, B. S., Cook, D. H., Varghese, P. J., and Rowe, R. D.: Spontaneous closure of small ventricular septal defects: A ten-year follow-up. Pediatrics *63*: 204, 1979.
109. Blumenthal, S., Griffiths, S. P., and Morgan, B. C.: Bacterial endocarditis in children with heart disease. (A review based on the literature and experience with 58 cases.) Pediatrics *26*:993, 1960.
110. Kirklin, J. W.: Pulmonary artery banding in babies with large ventricular septal defect. Circulation *43*:321, 1971.
111. Sigmann, J. M., Perry, B. L., Behrendt, M., Stern, A. M., Kirsh, M. M., and Sloan, H. E.: Ventricular septal defect: Results after repair in infancy. Am. J. Cardiol. *39*:66, 1977.
112. Agosti, J., and Subramanian, S.: Corrective treatment of isolated ventricular septal defect in infancy. J. Pediatr. Surg. *10*:785, 1975.
113. Dooley, K. J., Paresi-Buckley, L., Fyler, D. C., and Nadas, A. S.: Results of pulmonary arterial banding in infancy. Am. J. Cardiol. *36*:484, 1975.
114. Sade, R. M., Williams, R. G., and Castaneda, A. R.: Corrective surgery for congenital cardiovascular defects in early infancy. Am. Heart J. *90*:656, 1975.
115. Friedli, B., Kidd, B. S. L., Mustard, W. T., and Keith, J. D.: Ventricular septal defect with increased pulmonary vascular resistance. Am. J. Cardiol. *22*: 403, 1974.
116. Hislop, A., Haworth, S. G., Shinebourne, E. A., and Reid, L.: Quantitative structural analysis of pulmonary vessels in isolated ventricular septal defect in infancy. Br. Heart J. *37*:1014, 1975.
117. DuShane, J. W., and Kirklin, J. W.: Late results of the repair of ventricular septal defect on pulmonary vascular disease. *In* Kirklin, J. W. (ed.): Advances in Cardiovascular Surgery. New York, Grune and Stratton, 1973, p. 9.
118. Plauth, W. H., Braunwald, E., Rockhoff, S. D., Mason, D. T., and Morrow, A. G.: Ventricular septal defect and aortic regurgitation. Am. J. Med. *39*:552, 1965.
119. Van Praagh, R., and McNamara, J. J.: Anatomic types of ventricular septal defect with aortic insufficiency: Diagnostic and surgical considerations. Am. Heart J. *75*:604, 1968.
120. Sanfelippo, P. M., DuShane, J. W., McGoon, D. C., and Danielson, G. K.: Ventricular septal defects and aortic insufficiency: Surgical considerations and results of operation. Ann. Thorac. Surg. *17*:213, 1974.
121. Trusler, G. A., Moes, C. A. F., and Kidd, B. S. L.: Repair of ventricular septal defect with aortic insufficiency. J. Thorac. Cardiovasc. Surg. *66*:394, 1973.
122. Kawashima, Y., Danno, M., Shimizu, Y., Matsuda, H., Miyamoto, T., Fugita, T., Kozuka, T., and Manabe, H.: Ventricular septal defects associated with aortic insufficiency. Anatomic classification and method of operation. Circulation *47*:1057, 1973.
123. Keane, J. F., Plauth, W. H., Jr., and Nadas, A. S.: Ventricular septal defect with aortic regurgitation. Natural history study. Circulation *56* (Suppl.):I-72, 1977.
124. Gersony, W. M., and Hayes, C. J.: Bacterial endocarditis in patients with pulmonary stenosis, aortic stenosis, or ventricular septal defect. Natural history study. Circulation *56* (Suppl.):I-84, 1977.
125. Sutherland, G. R., Godman, M. J., Smallhorn, J. F., Guiterras, P., Anderson, R. H., and Hunter, S.: Ventricular septal defect. Two-dimensional echocardiographic and morphological correlations. Br. Heart J. *47*:316, 1982.
126. Elliott, L. P., Bargeron, L. M., Jr., Soto, B., and Bream, P. R.: Axial cineangiography in congenital heart disease. Radiol. Clin. North Am. *18*:515, 1980.
127. Levin, A. E., Spach, M. S., Canent, R. V., Jr., Boano, J. P., Capp, M. P., Jain, V., and Barr, R. C.: Ventricular pressure flow dynamics in ventricular septal defect. Circulation *35*:430, 1967.
127a. deLeval, M.: Ventricular septal defects. *In* Stark, J., and deLeval, M. (eds.): Surgery for Congenital Heart Defects, New York, Grune and Stratton, Inc., 1983, p. 271.
128. Godman, M. J., Roberts, N. K., and Izukawa, T.: Late postoperative conduction disturbances after repair of ventricular septal defect in tetralogy of Fallot. Circulation *49*:214, 1974.
129. Okarama, E. O., Guller, B., Molony, J. D., and Weidman, W. H.: Etiology of right bundle-branch block pattern after surgical closure of ventricular-septal defects. Am. Heart J. *90*:14, 1975.
130. Maron, B. J., Redwood, D. R., Hirschfield, J. W., Jr., Goldstein, R. E., Morrow, A. G., and Ebstein, S. E.: Postoperative assessment of patients with ventricular septal defect and pulmonary hypertension. Response to intense upright exercise. Circulation *48*:864, 1973.
131. Jarmakani, A. M., Graham, T. P., Jr., and Canent, R. V.: Left ventricular contractile state of children with successfully corrected ventricular septal defect. Circulation (Suppl.) *46*:102, 1972.
132. Graham, T. P., Jr., Atwood, G. F., Boucek, R. J., Jr., Cordell, D., and Boerth, R. C.: Right ventricular volume characteristics in ventricular septal defect. Circulation *54*:800, 1976.
133. Heymann, M. A., and Rudolph, A. M.: Control of the ductus arteriosus. Physiol. Rev. *55*:62, 1975.
134. Friedman, W. F., and Molony, D.: Prostaglandins and the perinatal period. Adv. Pediatr. *25*:151, 1978.
135. Friedman, W. F., Printz, M. P., Skidgel, R. A., Benson, L. N., and Zednikova, M.: Prostaglandins and the ductus arteriosus. *In* Oates, J. A. (ed.): Prostaglandins and the Cardiovascular System, vol. 10: Samuelsson, B., and Paoletti, R. (eds.). Advances in Prostaglandin, Thromboxane and Leukotriene Research. New York, Raven Press, 1982, p. 277.
136. Mahony, L., Carnero, V., Brett, C., Heymann, M. A., and Clyman, R. I.: Prophylactic indomethacin therapy for patent ductus arteriosus in very low birth weight infants. N. Engl. J. Med. *306*:506, 1982.
137. Gittenberger-DeGroot , A. C.: Persistent ductus arteriosus: Most probably a primary congenital malformation. Br. Heart J. *39*:610, 1977.
138. Lange, P., Freed, M. D., Rosenthal, A., Castaneda, A. R., and Nadas, A. S.: The use of prostaglandin E in an infant with interruption of the aortic arch. J. Pediatr. *91*:805, 1977.
139. Jones, R. W. A., and Pickering, D.: Persistent ductus arteriosus complicating the respiratory distress syndrome. Arch. Dis. Child. *52*:274, 1977.
140. Friedman, W. F., Hirschklau, M. J., Printz, M. P., Pitlick, P. T., and Kirkpatrick, S. E.: Pharmacologic closure of patent ductus arteriosus in the premature infant. N. Engl. J. Med. *295*:526, 1976.
141. Merritt, T. A., Gluck, L., Higgins, C., Friedman, W. F., and Nyhan, W. L.: Management of the premature infant with patent ductus arteriosus. West. J. Med. *128*:212, 1978.
142. Jacob, J., Gluck, L., DiSessa, T. G., Kulovich, M., Kurlinski, J., Merritt, T., and Friedman, W. F.: The contribution of PDA in the neonate with severe RDS. J. Pediatr. *96*:79–87, 1980.
143. Merritt, T. A., Harris, J. P., and Roghmann, K.: Early closure of the patent ductus arteriosus in very low birth weight infants: A controlled trial. J. Pediatr. *99*:281, 1981.
144. Higgins, C. B., Rausch, J., Friedman, W. F., Hirschklau, M. J., Kirkpatrick, S. E., Goergen, T., and Reinke, R. T.: Patent ductus arteriosus in preterm infants with idiopathic respiratory distress syndrome. Radiographic and echocardiographic evaluation. Radiology *124*:189, 1977.
145. Sahn, D. J., Vaucher, Y., Williams, D. E., Allen, H. D., Goldberg, S. E., and Friedman, W. F.: Echocardiographic detection of large left to right shunts and cardiomyopathies in infants and children. Am. J. Cardiol. *38*:73, 1976.
146. Hirschklau, M. J., DiSessa, T. G., Higgins, C. B., and Friedman, W. F.: Echocardiographic pitfalls in the premature infant with large patent ductus arteriosus. J. Pediatr. *92*:474, 1978.
147. Friedman, W. F., Heymann, M. A., and Rudolph, A. M.: Commentary: New thoughts on an old problem—patent ductus arteriosus in the premature infant. J. Pediatr. *90*:338, 1977.
148. Eggert, L. D., Jung, A. J., McGough, E. C., and Ruttenberg, H. D.: Surgical treatment of patent ductus arteriosus in pre-term infants. Pediatr. Cardiol. *2*: 15, 1982.
149. Jarmakani, M. M., Graham, T. P., Jr., Canent, R. V., Jr., Spach, M. S., and Capp, M. P.: Effect of site of shunt on left heart volume characteristics in children with ventricular septal defect and patent ductus arteriosus. Circulation *40*: 411, 1969.
150. Berlind, S., Bojs, G., Korsgran, M., and Varnaukas, E.: Severe pulmonary hypertension accomapnying patent ductus arteriosus. Am. Heart J. *73*:460, 1967.
151. Bessenger, F. B., Jr., Blieden, L. C., and Edwards, J. E.: Hypertensive pulmonary vascular disease associated with patent ductus arteriosus. Circulation *52*: 157, 1975.
152. Neufeld, H. N., Lesser, R. G., Adams, P., Jr., Anderson, R. C., Lillehiei, C. W., and Edwards, J. E.: Aorticopulmonary septal defect. Am. J. Cardiol. *9*:12, 1962.
153. Parker, B. M., Burford, T. H., Carlsson, E. C., and Buchner, E. F.: The diagnosis of aortico-pulmonary septal defect. Am. Heart J. *65*:534, 1963.
154. Richardson, J. V., Doty, D. B., and Rossi, N. P.: The spectrum of anomalies of aorto-pulmonary septation. J. Thorac. Cardiovasc. Surg. *78*:21, 1979.
155. Blieden, L. C., and Moller, J. H.: Aorticopulmonary septal defect. An experience in 17 patients. Br. Heart J. *36*:630, 1974.
156. Doty, D. B., Richardson, J. V., Falkovsky, G. E., Gordanova, M. I., and Burakovsky, V. I.: Aorto-pulmonary septal defect: Hemodynamics, angiography and operation. Ann. Thorac. Surg. *32*:244, 1981.
156a. Stark, J.: Aorto-pulmonary window. *In* Stark, J., and deLeval, M. (eds.): Surgery for Congenital Heart Defects, New York, Grune and Stratton, Inc., 1983, p. 483.
157. Van Praagh, R.: Classification of truncus arteriosus communis. Am. Heart J. *92*: 129, 1976.

158. Crupi, G., Macartney, F. J., and Anderson, R. H.: Persistent truncus arteriosus: A study of 66 autopsy cases with special reference to definition and morphogenesis. Am. J. Cardiol. *40*:569, 1977.
159. Shrivastava, F., and Edwards, J. E.: Coronary arterial origin and persistent truncus arteriosus. Circulation *55*:551, 1977.
160. Calder, L., Van Praagh, R., Sears, W. P., Corwin, R., Levy, A., Keith, J. D., and Paul, M. H.: Truncus arteriosus communis. Am. Heart J. *92*:23, 1976.
161. Marceletti, C., McGoon, D. C., and Mair, D. D.: The natural history of truncus arteriosus. Circulation *54*:108, 1976.
162. Gelband, H., Van Meter, S., and Gersony, W. M.: Truncal valve abnormalities in infants with persistent truncus arteriosus. Circulation *45*:397, 1972.
163. Chung, K. J., Alexson, C. G., Manning, J. A., and Gramiak, R.: Echocardiography in truncus arteriosus. Circulation *48*:281, 1973.
164. McFall, R. C., Mair, D. D., Feldt, R. H., Ritter, D. G., and McGoon, D. C.: Truncus arteriosus and previous pulmonary arterial banding: Clinical and hemodynamic assessment. Am. J. Cardiol. *38*:626, 1976.
165. Turley, K. A., Tucker, W. Y., and Ebert, P. A.: The changing role of palliative procedures in the treatment of infants with congenital heart disease. J. Thorac. Cardiovasc. Surg. *79*:194, 1980.
166. Peetz, D., Spicer, R. L., Crowley, D. C., Sloan, H., and Behrendt, D. M.: Correction of truncus arteriosus in the neonate using a non-valved conduit. J. Thorac. Cardiovasc. Surg. *83*:743, 1982.
167. Wallace, R. B., Rastelli, G. C., Ongley, P. A., Titus, J. L., and McGoon, D. C.: Complete repair of truncus arteriosus defect. J. Thorac. Cardiovasc. Surg. *57*:95, 1969.
167a. deLeval, M.: Persistent truncus arteriosus. *In* Stark, J., and deLeval, M. (eds.): Surgery for Congenital Heart Defects, New York, Grune and Stratton, Inc., 1983, p. 417.
168. Morgan, J. R., Forker, A. D., O'Sullivan, M. J., and Fosburg, R. G.: Coronary arterial fistulas. Am. J. Cardiol. *34*:32, 1972.
169. Baim, D. S., Klein, H., and Silverman, J. F.: Bilateral coronary artery–pulmonary artery fistulas. Circulation *65*:810, 1982.
170. Liberthson, R. R., Sagar, K., Berkoben, J. P., Weintraub, R. M., and Levine, F. H.: Congenital coronary arteriovenous fistula. Circulation *59*:849, 1979.
171. Ruttenhouse, E. A., Doty, D. B., and Ehrenhaft, J. L.: Congenital coronary artery–cardiac chamber fistula. Review of operative management. Ann. Thorac. Surg. *20*:468, 1975.
172. Wesselhoeft, H., Fawcett, J. S., and Johnson, A. L.: Anomalous origin of the left coronary artery from the pulmonary trunk: Its clinical spectrum, pathology, and pathophysiology based on a review of 140 cases with 7 further cases. Circulation *38*:403, 1968.
173. Kimbris, D., Iskandrian, A. S., Segal, E. L., and Bemis, C. E.: Anomalous aortic origin of coronary arteries. Circulation *58*:606, 1978.
174. Askenazij, J., and Nadas, A. S.: Anomalous left coronary artery originating from the pulmonary artery. Circulation *51*:976, 1975.
175. Arciniegas, E., Farooki, Z. Q., Hakimi, M., and Green, E. W.: Management of anomalous left coronary artery from the pulmonary artery. Circulation *62* (Suppl. 1):180, 1980.
176. Stephenson, L. W., Edmunds, L. H., Jr., Friedman, S., Meijboon, E., Gewitz, M., and Weinberg, P.: Subclavian–left coronary artery anastomosis for anomalous origin of the left coronary artery from the pulmonary artery. Circulation *64* (Suppl. 2):130, 1981.
177. Fishbein, M. C., Obma, R., and Roberts, W. C.: Unruptured sinus of Valsalva aneurysm. Am. J. Cardiol. *35*:918, 1975.
178. Boutefeu, J. M., Morat, P. R., Hahn, C., and Hauf, E.: Aneurysms of the sinus of Valsalva. Report of seven cases in review of the literature. Am. J. Med. *65*:18, 1978.
179. Myer, J., Wukasch, D. C., Holman, G. L., and Cooley, D. A.: Aneurysm and fistula of the sinus of Valsalva. Clinical considerations and surgical treatment of 45 patients. Ann. Thorac. Surg. *19*:170, 1975.
179a. deLeval, M.: Congenital anomalies of sinuses of Valsalva and coronary arteries. *In* Stark, J., and deLeval, M. (eds.): Surgery for Congenital Heart Defects. New York, Grune and Stratton, Inc., 1983, p. 487.
180. Kakos, G. S., Kilman, J. W., Williams, T. E., and Hosier, D. M.: Diagnosis and management of sinus of Valsalva aneurysm in children. Ann. Thorac. Surg. *17*:474, 1974.
181. Engle, P. J., Held, J. S., Bel-Kahn, J. V. D., and Spitz, H.: Echocardiographic diagnosis of congenital sinus of Valsalva aneurysm. Circulation *63*:705, 1981.
182. Yokoi, K., Kambe, T., and Nishimura, K.: Ruptured aneurysm of the right sinus of Valsalva: Two post-Doppler echocardiographic studies. J. Clin. Ultrasound *9*:505, 1981.
183. Smyth, P. T., and Edwards, J. E.: Pseudocoarctation, kinking or buckling of the aorta. Circulation *46*:1027, 1972.
184. Hutchins, G. M.: Coarctation of the aorta explained as a branch point of the ductus arteriosus. Am. J. Pathol. *63*:203, 1971.
185. Rudolph, A. M., Heymann, M. A., and Spitznas, U.: Hemodynamic considerations of the development of narrowing of the aorta. Am. J. Cardiol. *30*:514, 1972.
186. Talner, N. S., and Berman, M. A.: Postnatal development of obstruction in coarctation of the aorta: Role of the ductus arteriosus. Pediatrics *56*:562, 1975.
187. Bruins, C.: Competition between aortic isthmus and ductus arteriosus; reciprocal influence of structure and flow. Eur. J. Cardiol. *8*:87, 1978.
188. Heymann, M. A., Berman, W., Jr., Rudolph, A. M., and Whitman, V.: Dilatation of the ductus arteriosus by prostaglandin E_1 in aortic arch abnormalities. Circulation *59*:169, 1979.
189. Connors, J. P., Hartmann, A. F., Jr., and Weldon, C. S.: Consideration in the surgical management of infantile coarctation of the aorta. Am. J. Cardiol. *36*: 489, 1975.
190. Fishman, N. H., Bronstein, N. H., Berman, W., Jr., Roe, B. B., Edmunds, L. H., Jr., Robinson, S. J., and Rudolph, A. M.: Surgical management of severe aortic coarctation/interrupted aortic arch in neonates. J. Thorac. Cardiovasc. Surg. *71*:35, 1976.
191. Rocchini, A. P., Rosenthal, A., Barger, A. C., Castaneda, A. R., and Nadas, A. S.: Pathogenesis of paradoxical hypertension after coarctation resection. Circulation *54*:382, 1976.
192. Godwin, G. D., Herfkens, R. J., Brundage, D. H., and Lipton, N. J.: Evaluation of coarctation of the aorta by computed tomography. J. Comput. Assist. Tomogr. *5*:153, 1981.
192a. Steele, P. M., Fuster, V., Weidman, W. H., Feldt, R., and McGoon, D. C.: Isolated coarctation of the aorta: Long-term operative results. J. Am. Coll. Cardiol. *1*:651, 1983.
192b. Hammon, J. W., Jr., Graham, T. P., Jr., Boucek, R. J., Jr., Parrish, M. D., and Bender, H. W.: Repair of coarctation of the aorta in infancy: Improved results with prostaglandin E_1 infusion and subclavian flap angioplasty. J. Am. Coll. Cardiol. *1*:663, 1983.
193. Beekman, R. H., Rocchini, A. P., Behrendt, D. M., and Rosenthal, A.: Re-operation for coarctation of the aorta. Am. J. Cardiol. *48*:1108, 1981.
194. Alpert, B. S., Bain, H. H., Balfe, J. W., Kidd, B. S. L., and Olley, P. M.: Role of the renin-angiotensin-aldosterone system in hypertensive children with coractation of the aorta. Am. J. Cardiol. *43*:828, 1979.
195. Igler, F. O., Boerboom, L. E., Werner, P. H., Donegan, J. H., and Kampine, J. P.: Coarctation of the aorta and narrow receptor resetting. Circulation Res. *48*:365, 1981.
196. Nanton, M. A., and Olley, P. M.: Residual hypertension after coarctectomy in children. Am. J. Cardiol. *37*:769, 1976.
197. Maron, B. J., Humphries, J., Rowe, R. D., and Mellits, E. D.: Prognosis of surgically corrected coarctation of the aorta. Circulation *47*:119, 1973.
198. Freed, M. D., Rocchini, A., Rosenthal, A., Nadas, A. S., and Castaneda, A. R.: Exercise-induced hypertension after surgical repair of coarctation of the aorta. Am. J. Cardiol. *43*:253, 1979.
199. Van Woezik, E. V. M., Kline, H. W., and Krediet, P.: Normal internal calibers of ostia, great arteries and aortic isthmus in children. Br. Heart J. *39*:860, 1977.
200. Graham, T. P., Jr., Atwood, G. F., Boerth, R. C., Boucek, R. J., Jr., and Smith, C. W.: Right and left heart size and function in infants with symptomatic coarctation. Circulation *56*:641, 1977.
201. Trusler, G. A., and Freedom, R. M.: Surgical approach to the management of interruption of the aorta. *In* Godman, M. J., and Marquis, R. M. (eds.): Paediatric Cardiology, vol. 2. Edinburgh, Churchill-Livingstone, 1979, p. 268.
202. Dekker, A. O., Gittenberger-de-Groot, A. C., and Roozendaal, H.: The ductus arteriosus and associated cardiac anomalies in interruption of the aortic arch. Pediatr. Cardiol. *2*:185, 1982.
203. Jaffee, R. B.: Complete interruption of the aortic arch. II. Characteristic angiographic features with emphasis on collateral circulation to the descending aorta. Circulation *53*:161, 1976.
204. Moulton, A. L., and Bowman, F. O., Jr.: Primary definitive repair of type-B interrupted aortic arch, ventricular septal defect and patent ductus arteriosus. J. Thorac. Cardiovasc. Surg. *82*:501, 1981.
205. Sturm, J. T., van Heeckeren, P., and Borkart, G.: Surgical treatment of interrupted aortic arch in infancy with expanded polytetrafluoroethylene grafts. J. Thorac. Cardiovasc. Surg. *81*:245, 1981.
206. Friedman, W. F., and Benson, L. B.: Congenital aortic stenosis. *In* Adams, F. H., and Emmanouilides, G. C. (eds.): Moss' Heart Disease in Infants, Children and Adolescents. 3rd ed. Baltimore, Williams and Wilkins, 1983.
206a. Donner, R., Carabello, B. A., Black, I., and Spann, J. F.: Left ventricular wall stress in compensated aortic stenosis in children. Am. J. Cardiol. *51*:946, 1983.
207. Friedman, W. F., and Pappelbaum, S. J.: Indications for hemodynamic evaluation and surgery in congenital aortic stenosis. Pediatr. Clin. North Am. *18*: 1207, 1971.
208. Friedman, W. F.: Congenital aortic valve disease: Natural history, indications and results of surgery. *In* Morse, D., and Goldberg, H. (eds.): Important Topics in Congenital, Valvular, and Coronary Artery Disease. Mt. Kisco, N.Y., Futura Publishing Co., 1975, p. 43.
209. Cueto, L., and Moller, J. H.: Hemodynamics of exercise in children with isolated aortic valvular disease. Br. Heart J. *35*:93, 1973.
210. Buckberg, G., Eber, L., Herman, N., and Gorlin, R.: Ischemia in aortic stenosis: Hemodynamic prediction. Am. J. Cardiol. *35*:778, 1975.
211. Lewis, A. L., Heymann, M. A., Stanger, P., Hoffman, J. I. E., and Rudolph, A. M.: Evaluation of subendocardial ischemia in valvar aortic stenosis in children. Circulation *49*:978, 1974.
212. Lakier, J. B., Lewis, A. B., Heymann, M. A., Stanger, P., Hoffman, J. I. E., and Rudolph, A. M.: Isolated aortic stenosis of the neonate: Natural history and hemodynamic considerations. Circulation *50*:801, 1974.
213. Broderick, T. W., Higgins, C. B., and Friedman, W. F.: Critical aortic stenosis in neonates. Radiology *129*:393, 1978.
214. Keane, J. F., Bernhard, W. F., and Nadas, A. S.: Aortic stenosis surgery in infancy. Circulation *52*:1138, 1975.
215. Edmunds, L. H., Jr., Wagner, H. R., and Heymann, M. A.: Aortic valvulotomy in neonates. Circulation *61*:421, 1980.
216. Braunwald, E., Goldblatt, A., Aygen, M. M., Rockoff, S. D., and Morrow, A. G.: Congenital aortic stenosis. I. Clinical and hemodynamic findings in 100 patients. Circulation *27*:426, 1963.

217. Johnson, A. M.: Aortic stenosis, sudden death, and the left ventricular baroreceptors, Br. Heart J. *33*:1, 1971.
218. Wagner, H. R., Weidman, W. H., Ellison, R. C., and Miettinen, O. S.: Indirect assessment of severity in aortic stenosis. Natural history study. Circulation *56* (Suppl.):I-20, 1977.
219. Halloran, K. H.: A telemetered exercise electrocardiogram in congenital aortic stenosis. Pediatrics *47*:31, 1971.
220. Chandramouli, B., Ehruka, D. A., And Lauer, R. M.: Exercise-induced electrocardiographic changes in children with congenital aortic stenosis. J. Pediatr. *87*:725, 1975.
221. Gamboa, R., Hugenholtz, P. G., and Nadas, A. S.: Comparison of electrocardiograms in congenital arotic stenosis. Br. Heart J. *27*:344, 1965.
222. Reeve, R., Kawamata, K., and Selzer, A.: Reliability of vectorcardiography in assessing the severity of congenital aortic stensos. Circulation *34*:92, 1966.
223. Nanda, N. C., Gramiak, R., Shah, P. M. Steward, S., and DeWeese, J. A.: Echocardiography in the diagnosis of idiopathic hypertrophic subaortic stenosis coexisting with aortic valve disease. Circulation *50*:752, 1974.
224. Williams, D. E., Sahn, D. J., and Friedman, W. F.: Cross-sectional echocardiographic localization of the sites of left ventricular outlfow tract obstruction. Am. J. Cardiol. *37*:250, 1976.
225. Hagan, A. D., DiSessa, T. G., and Friedman, W. F.: Reliability of echocardiography in diagnosing and quantitating valvular aortic stenosis. J. Cardiovasc. Med. *5*:391, 1980.
226. Aziz, K. U., van Grondelle, A., Paul, M. H., and Muster, A. J.: Echocardiographic assessment of the relation between left ventricular wall and cavity dimensions and peak systolic pressure in children with aortic stenosis. Am. J. Cardiol. *40*:775, 1977.
227. Young, J. B., Quinones, M. A., Waggoner, A. D., and Miller, R. R.: Diagnosis and quantification of aortic stenosis with pulsed Doppler echocardiography. Am. J. Cardiol. *45*:987, 1980.
228. Hohn, A. R., Van Praagh, S., Moore, A. A. D., Vlad, P., and Lambert, E. C.: Aortic stenosis. Circulation *31* (Suppl. III):4, 1965.
229. Bentivoglio, L. G., Sagarminaga, J., and Uricchio, J.: Congenital bicuspid aortic valve: A clinical and hemodynamic study. Br. Heart J. *22*:321, 1960.
230. El-Said, G., Gallioto, F. J., Mullens, C. E., and McNamara, D. G.: Natural hemodynamic history of congenital aortic stenosis in childhood. Am. J. Cardiol. *30*:6, 1972.
231. Hurwitz, R. A.: Aortic valve stenosis in childhood: Clinical and hemodynamic history. J. Pediatr. *82*:228, 1973.
232. Friedman, W. F., Modlinger, J., and Morgan, J.: Serial hemodynamic observations in asymptomatic children with valvar aortic stenosis. Circulation *43*:91, 1971.
233. Cohen, L. S., Friedman, W. F., and Braunwald, E.: Natural history of mild congenital aortic stenosis elucidated by serial hemodynamic studies. Am. J. Cardiol. *30*:1, 1972.
234. Bandy, G. E., and Vogel, J. H. K.: Progressive congenital valvular aortic stenosis. Chest *60*:189, 1971.
235. Friedman, W. F., Novak, V., and Johnson, A. D.: Congenital aortic stenosis in adults. *In* Roberts, W. C. (ed.): Congenital Heart Disease in Adults. Philadelphia, F. A. Davis, 1979, p. 235.
236. Wagner, H. R., Ellison, R. C., Keane, J. F., Humphries, J. O., and Nadas, A. S.: Clinical course in aortic stenosis. Natural history study. Circulation *56* (Suppl.):I-47, 1977.
237. Fisher, R. D., Mason, D. T., and Morrow, A. G.: Results of operative treatment in congenital aortic stenosis. J. Thorac. Cardiovasc. Surg. *59*:218, 1970.
238. Sandor, E. G. S., Olley, P. M., Trusler, G. A., Williams, W. G., Rowe, R. D., and Morch, J. E.: Long-term follow-up with patients after valvotomy for congenital valvular aortic stenosis in children. J. Thorac. Cardiovasc. Surg. *80*:171, 1980.
239. Conkle, D. M., Jones, M., and Morrow, A. G.: Treatment of congenital aortic stenosis: An evaluation of the late results of the aortic valvotomy. Arch. Surg. *107*:649, 1973.
240. Presbitero, P., Sommerville, J., Chion, R. R., and Ross, D.: Open aortic valvotomy for congenital aortic stenosis. Last results. Br. Heart J. *47*:26, 1982.
241. DiSessa, T. G., Hagan, A. D., Isabel-Jones, J. B., and Friedman, W. F.: Two-dimensional echocardiographic evaluation of discrete subaortic stenosis from the apical long axis view. Am. Heart J. *101*:774, 1981.
242. Williams, D. E., Sahn, D. J., and Friedman, W. F.: Cross-sectional echocardiographic localization of the sites of left ventricular outflow tract obstruction. Am. J. Cardiol. *37*:250, 1976.
243. Bloom, K. R., Meyer, R. A., Bove, K. E., and Kaplan, S.: The association of fixed and dynamic left ventricular outflow obstruction. Am. Heart J. *89*:586, 1975.
244. Freedom, R. M., Dische, M. R., and Rowe, R. D.: Pathologic anatomy of subaortic stenosis and atresia in the first year of life. Am. J. Cardiol. *39*:1035, 1977.
245. Newfeld, E. A., Muster, A. J., Paul, M. H., Idriss, F. S., and Riker, W. L.: Discrete subvalvular aortic stenosis in childhood. Am. J. Cardiol. *38*:53, 1976.
246. Reis, R. L., Peterson, L. M., Mason, D. T., Simon, A. L., and Morrow, A. G.: Congenital fixed subvalvular aortic stenosis. An anatomical classification and correlations with operative results. Circulation *43*(Suppl. I):I-11, 1971.
247. Champsaur, G., Trusler, G. A., and Mustard, W. T.: Congenital discrete subvalvar aortic stenosis. Surgical experience and long-term followup in 20 pediatric patients. Br. Heart J. *35*:443, 1973.
248. Somerville, J., Stone, S., and Roth, D.: Fate of patients with fixed subaortic stenosis after surgical removal. Br. Heart J. *43*:629, 1980.
249. Maron, B. J., Redwood, D. R., Roberts, W. C., Henry, W. L., Morrow, A. G., and Epstein, S. E.: Tunnel subaortic stenosis. Circulation *54*:404, 1976.
250. Ergin, M. A., Cooper, R., LaCourte, M., Golinko, R., and Griepp, R. B.: Experience with left ventricular apicoaortic conduits for complicated left ventricular outflow obstruction in children and young adults. Ann. Thorac. Surg. *32*:369, 1981.
251. Edwards, J. E.: Pathology of left ventricular outflow tract obstruction. Circulation *31*:586, 1965.
252. Ferencz, C.: Atrioventricular defect of membranous septum: Left ventricular–right atrial communication of the malformed mitral valve simulating aortic stenosis. Bull. Johns Hopkins Hosp. *100*:209, 1957.
253. Schon, J. D., Sellers, R. D., and Anderson, R. C.: The developmental complex of parachute mitral valve, supravalvular ring of left atrium, subaortic stenosis, and coarctation of aorta. Am. J. Cardiol. *11*:714, 1963.
254. Friedman, W. F., and Roberts, W. C.: Vitamin D and the supravalvar aortic stenosis syndrome: The transplacental effects of vitamin D on the aorta of the rabbit. Circulation *34*:77, 1966.
255. Friedman, W. F.: Vitamin D embryopathy. Adv. Teratol. *3*:85, 1968.
256. Friedman, W. F., and Mills, L. F.: The relationship between vitamin D and the craniofacial and dental anomalies of the supravalvular aortic stenosis syndrome. Pediatrics *43*:12, 1969.
257. Garcia, R. E., Friedman, W. F., Kaback, M. M., and Rowe, R. D.: Idiopathic hypercalcemia and supravalvular aortic stenosis: Documentation of a new syndrome. N. Engl. J. Med. *271*:117, 1964.
258. Taylor, A. B., Stern, P. H., and Bell, N. H.: Abnormal regulation of circulating 25-hydroxy vitamin D in the William's syndrome. N. Engl. J. Med. *306*:972, 1982.
259. Kahler, R. L., Braunwald, E., Plauth, W. H., Jr., and Morrow, A. G.: Familial congenital heart disease. Am. J. Med. *40*:384, 1966.
260. French, J. W., and Guntheroth, W. G.: An explanation of asymmetric upper extremity blood pressure in supravalvular aortic stenosis: The Coanda effect. Circulation *42*:31, 1970.
261. Goldstein, R. E., and Epstein, S. E.: Mechanism of elevated innominate artery pressures in supravalvular aortic stenosis. Circulation *42*:23, 1970.
262. Gaum, W. E., Chou, T. C., and Kaplan, S.: The vectorcardiogram and electrocardiogram in supravalvular aortic stenosis and coarctation of the aorta. Am. Heart J. *84*:620, 1972.
263. Noonan, J. A.: Hypoplastic left ventricle. *In* Moss, A. J., Adams, F. H., and Emmanouilides, G. C. (eds.): Heart Disease in Infants, Children and Adolescents. 2nd ed. Baltimore, Williams and Wilkins, 1977, p. 430.
264. Moodie, E. S., Gallen, W. J., and Friedberg, D. Z.: Congenital aortic atresia. Report of long survival and some speculations about surgical approaches. J. Thorac. Cardiovasc. Surg. *63*:726, 1972.
265. Meyer, R. A., and Kaplan, S.: Echocardiography in the diagnosis of hypoplasia of the left to right ventricles in the neonate. Circulation *41*:55, 1972.
266. Bass, J. L., Ben-Shaghar, G., and Edwards, J. E.: Comparison of M mode echocardiography and pathologic findings in the hypoplastic left heart syndrome. Am. J. Cardiol. *45*:79, 1980.
267. Miller, G. A. H.: Aortic atresia: Diagnostic catheterization in the first week of life. Br. Heart J. *33*:367, 1971.
268. Norwood, W. I., Lang, P., Castaneda, A. R., and Campbell, D. M.: Experience with operations for hypoplastic left heart syndrome. J. Thorac. Cardiovasc. Surg. *82*:511, 1981.
269. Behrendt, D. M., and Rocchini, A.: An operation for hypoplastic left heart syndrome: Preliminary report. Ann. Thorac. Surg. *32*:284, 1981.
270. Frahm, C. J., Braunwald, E., and Morrow, A. G.: Congenital aortic regurgitation. Am. J. Med. *31*:63, 1961.
271. Carter, J. B., Sethi, S., Lee, G. B., and Edwards, J. E.: Prolapse of semilunar cusps as causes of aortic insufficiency. Circulation *43*:922, 1971.
272. Somerville, J., English, T., and Ross, D. N.: Aortico-left ventricular tunnel. Clinical features and surgical management. Br. Heart J. *36*:321, 1974.
273. Turley, K., Silverman, N. H., Teitel, D., Mavroudis, C., Snider, R., and Rudolph, A.: Repair of aortico–left ventricular tunnel in the neonate: Surgical, anatomic, and echocardiographic considerations. Circulation *65*:1015, 1982.
274. Lucas, R. V., Jr., and Schmidt, R. E.: Anomalous venous connection, pulmonary and systemic. *In* Moss, A. J., Adams, F. H., and Emmanouilides, G. C., (eds.): Heart Disease in Infants, Children and Adolescents. 2nd ed. Baltimore, Williams and Wilkins, 1977, p. 437.
275. Marin-Garcia, J., Tandon, R., Lucas, R. V., Jr., and Edwards, J. E.: Cor triatriatum: Study of 20 cases. Am. J. Cardiol. *35*:59, 1975.
276. Richardson, J. V., Doty, D. B., Siewers, R. D., and Zuberbuhler, J. R.: Cor triatriatum. J. Thorac. Cardiovasc. Surg. *81*:232, 1981.
277. Jacobstein, M. D., and Hirschfeld, S. S.: Concealed left atrial membrane: Pitfalls in the diagnosis of cor triatriatum and supravalve mitral stenosing ring. Am. J. Cardiol. *49*:780, 1982.
278. Macartney, F. J., Bain, H. H., Ionescu, M. I., Deverall, P. B., and Scott, O.: Angiocardiographic/pathologic correlations in congenital mitral valve anomalies. Eur. J. Cardiol. *4*:191, 1976.
279. Ruckman, R. N., and Van Praagh, R.: Anatomic types of congenital mitral stenosis: Report of 49 autopsy cases with consideration of diagnosis and surgical implications. Am. J. Cardiol. *42*:592, 1978.
280. Smallhorn, J., Tommasini, G., Deanfield, J., Douglas, J., and Macartney, F.: Congenital mitral stenosis. Anatomical and functional assessment by echocardiography. Br. Heart J. *45*:527, 1981.
281. Perloff, J. K.: Evolving concepts of mitral valve prolapse. N. Engl. J. Med. *307*:369, 1982.

282. Carney, E. K., Braunwald, E., Roberts, W. C., Aygen, M., and Morrow, A. G.: Congenital mitral regurgitation. Am. J. Med. *33*:223, 1962.
283. Vlad, P.: Mitral valve anomalies in children. Circulation *33*:465, 1971.
284. Ruschhaupt, D. G., Bharati, S., and Lev, M.: Mitral valve malformation of Ebstein type in absence of corrected transposition. Am. J. Cardiol. *38*:109, 1976.
285. Sahn, D. J., Allen, H. D., Goldberg, S. J., and Friedman, W. F.: Mitral valve prolapse in children. Circulation *53*:651, 1976.
286. Macartney, F. J., Bain, H. H., Ionescu, M. I., Deverall, P. B., and Scott, O.: Angiocardiographic/pathologic correlations in congenital mitral valve anomalies. Eur. J. Cardiol. *4*:191, 1976.
287. Galioto, F. M., Jr., Midgley, F. M., Shapiro, S. R., Perry, L. W., and Scott, L. T.: Mitral valve replacement in infants and children. Pediatrics *67*:230, 1981.
287a. Carpentier, A.: Congenital malformations of the mitral valve. *In* Stark, J., and deLeval, M. (eds.): Surgery for Congenital Heart Defects. New York, Grune and Stratton, Inc., 1983, p. 467.
288. Carpentier, A., Branchini, B., Cour, J. C., Asfaou, E., Villani, M., Deloche, A., Relland, J., D'Allaines, C., Blondeau, P., Piwnica, A., Parenzan, L., and Brom, G.: Congenital malformations of the mitral valve in children: Pathology and surgical treatment. J. Thorac. Cardiovasc. Surg. *72*:854, 1976.
289. Dines, D. E., Arms, R. A., Bernatz, P. D., and Gomes, M. R.: Pulmonary arteriovenous fistulas. Mayo Clin. Proc. *49*:460, 1974.
290. Venables, A. W.: The syndrome of pulmonary stenosis complicating maternal rubella. Br. Heart J. *27*:49, 1965.
291. Danilowicz, D. A., Rudolph, A. M., Hoffman, J. I. E., and Heymann, M. A.: Physiologic pressure differences between main and branch pulmonary arteries in infants. Circulation *45*:410, 1972.
292. Eldredge, W. J., Tingelstad, J. B., Robertson, L. W., Mauck, H. P., and McCue, C. M.: Observations on the natural history of pulmonary artery coarctation. Circulation *45*:404, 1972.
293. Barrillon, A., Havy, G., Scebat, L., Baragan, J., and Gerbaux, A.: Congenital pressure gradients between main pulmonary artery and the primary branches. Br. Heart J. *36*:669, 1974.
294. Koretzky, E., Moller, J. H., Korns, M. E., Schwartz, C. J., and Edwards, J. E.: Congenital pulmonary stenosis resulting from dysplasia of valve. Circulation *40*:43, 1969.
295. Collins, E., and Turner, G.: The Noonan's syndrome—a review of the clinical and genetic features of 27 cases. J. Pediatr. *83*:941, 1973.
296. Srinivasan, V., Konyer, A., Broda, J. J., and Subramanian, S.: Critical pulmonary stenosis in infants less than three months of age: A reappraisal of closed transventricular pulmonary valvotomy. Ann. Thorac. Surg. *34*:46, 1982.
297. Danilowicz, D., Hoffman, J. I. E., and Rudolph, A. M.: Serial studies of pulmonary stenosis in infancy and childhood. Br. Heart J. *37*:808, 1975.
298. Gersony, W. M., Bernhard, W. F., Nadas, A. S., and Gross, R. E.: Diagnosis and surgical treatment of infants with critical pulmonary outflow obstruction. Circulation *35*:765, 1967.
299. Mody, M. R.: The natural history of uncomplicated valvular pulmonary stenosis. Am. Heart J. *90*:317, 1975.
300. Ellison, R. C., and Miettinen, O. S.: Interpretation of rSR' in pulmonic stenosis. Am. Heart J. *88*:7, 1974.
301. LeBlanc, M. H., and Paquet, M.: Echocardiographic assessment of valvular pulmonary stenosis in children. Br. Heart J. *46*:363, 1981.
302. Stone, F. M., Betthinger, F. B., Jr., Lucas, R. V., Jr., and Moller, J. H.: Pre- and postoperative rest and exercise hemodynamics in children with pulmonary stenosis. Circulation *49*:1102, 1974.
303. Moller, J. H., Rao, S., and Lucas, R. V., Jr.: Exercise hemodynamics of pulmonary valvular stenosis: Study of 64 children. Circulation *46*:1018, 1972.
304. Nazawa, M., Marks, R. A., Isabel-Jones, J., and Jarmakani, J. M.: Right and left ventricular volume characteristics in children with pulmonary stenosis and intact ventricular septum. Circulation *53*:884, 1976.
305. Graham, T. P., Jr., Bender, H. W., Atwood, G. F., Page, D. L., and Fell, C. G. R.: Increase in right ventricular volume following valvulotomy for pulmonary atresia or stenosis with intact ventricular septum. Circulation *49* (Suppl.):II-69, 1974.
306. Neugent, E. W., Freedom, R. M., Nora, J. J., Ellison, R.C., Rowe, R. D., and Nadas, R. S.: Clinical course in pulmonary stenosis. Circulation *56* (Suppl.):I-38, 1977.
307. Wennevold, A., and Jacobsen, J. R.: Natural history of valvular pulmonary stenosis in children below the age of two years: Long-term follow-up with serial heart catheterizations. Eur. J. Cardiol. *8*:371, 1978.
308. Finnigan, P., Ihenacho, H. N. C., Singh, S. O., and Abrams, L. D.: Hemo-dynamic studies at rest and during exercise in pulmonary stenosis after surgery. Br. Heart J. *36*:913, 1974.
309. Trusler, G. A., Freedom, R. N., Patel, R., and Williams, W. G.: The surgical management of pulmonary atresia with intact ventricular septum. *In* Godman, M. J. and Marquis, R. N. (eds.): Paediatric Cardiology, vol. 2. Edinburgh, Churchill-Livingstone, 1979, p. 305.
310. Ellis, K., Casarella, W. J., Hayes, C. J., Gersony, W. M., Bowman, F. O., Jr., and Malm, J. R.: Pulmonary atresia with intact ventricular septum: New developments in diagnosis and treatment. Am. J. Roentgenol. *116*:501, 1972.
311. Patel, R. G., Freedom, R. M., Moes, C. A. F., Bloom, K. R., Olley, P. M., Williams, W. B., Trusler, G. A., and Rowe, R. D.: Right ventricular volume determinations in 18 patients with pulmonary atresia and intact ventricular septum. Analysis of factors influencing right ventricular growth. Circulation *61*: 428, 1980.
312. Zuberbuhler, J. R., and Anderson, R. H.: Morphological variations in pulmonary artresia with intact ventricular septum. Br. Heart J. *41*:281, 1979.
313. Bharati, S., McAllister, H. A., Jr., Chiemmongkoltip, P., and Lev, M.: Congenital pulmonary atresia with tricuspid insufficiency: Morphologic study. Am. J. Cardiol. *40*:70, 1977.
314. Rudolph, A. M., Heymann, M. A., Fischman, N., and Lakier, J. B.: Formalin infiltration of the ductus arteriosus. N. Engl. J. Med. *299*:1263, 1975.
315. Forster, J. W., and Humphreys, J. O.: Right ventricular anomalous muscle bundle: Clinical and laboratory presentation and natural history. Circulation *43*:115, 1971.
316. Danilowicz, D., and Ishmael, R.: Anomalous right ventricular muscle bundle: Clinical pitfalls and extracardiac anomalies. Clin. Cardiol. *4*:146, 1981.
317. Rowland, T. W., Rosenthal, A., and Castaneda, A. R.: Double chamber right ventricle: Experience in 17 cases. Am. Heart J. *89*:455, 1975.
318. Engle, M. A.: Cyanotic congenital heart disease. Am. J. Cardiol. *37*:283, 1976.
319. Kirklin, J. W., and Karp, R. B.: The tetralogy of Fallot: From a surgical view-point. Philadelphia, W. B. Saunders Co., 1970.
320. Rayo, B. N., Anderson, R. C., and Edwards, J. E.: Anatomic variations in tetralogy of Fallot. Am. Heart J. *81*:361, 1971.
321. Faller, K., Haworth, S. G., Taylor, J. F. N., and Macartney, F. J.: Duplicate sources of pulmonary blood supply and pulmonary atresia with ventricular septal defect. Br. Heart J. *46*:263, 1981.
322. Rabinovitch, M., DeLeon, V. H., Castaneda, A. R., and Reid, L.: Growth and development of the pulmonary vascular bed in patients with tetralogy of Fallot with or without pulmonary atresia. Circulation *64*:1234, 1981.
323. Nihill, M. R., Mullins, C. E., and MacNamara, D. G.: Visualization of the pulmonary arteries in pseudo-truncus by pulmonary vein wedge angiography. Circulation *58*:140, 1978.
324. Sondheimer, H. M., Oliphant, M., Schneider, B., Kavey, R. E. W., Blackman, M. S., and Parker, F. B.: Computerized axial tomography of the chest for visualization of absent pulmonary arteries. Circulation *65*:1020, 1982.
325. Chesler, E., Matisonn, R., and Beck, W.: The assessment of the arterial supply to the lungs in pseudotruncus arteriosus and truncus arteriosus type IV in relation to surgical repair. Am. Heart J. *88*:542, 1974.
326. McGoon, M. D., Fulton, R. E., Davis, G. D., Ritter, D. G., Neill, C. A., and White, R. I., Jr.: Systemic collateral and pulmonary artery stenosis in patients with congenital pulmonary valve atresia and ventricular septal defect. Circulation *56*:474, 1977.
327. Fellows, K. E., Freed, M. D., Keane, J. F., Van Praagh, R., Bernard, W. R., and Castaneda, A. C.: Results of routine preoperative coronary angiography and tetralogy of Fallot. Circulation *51*:561, 1977.
328. Morgan, B. C., Guntheroth, W. G., Blume, R. S., and Fyler, D. C.: A clinical profile of paroxysmal hyperpnea in cyanotic congenital heart disease. Circulation *31*:66, 1965.
329. Morris, D. C., Felner, J. M., Schlant, R. C., and French, R. H.: Echocardiographic diagnosis of tetralogy of Fallot. Am. J. Cardiol. *36*:908, 1975.
330. Seward, J. B., Tajik, A. J., Hagler, D. J., and Ritter, D. G.: Peripheral venous contrast echocardiography. Am. J. Cardiol. *39*:202, 1977.
331. DiSessa, T. G., Hagan, A. D., Pope, C., and Friedman, W. F.: Two-dimensional echocardiographic characteristics of double outlet right ventricle. Am. J. Cardiol. *44*:1146, 1979.
331a. Matina, D., van Doesburg, N. H., Fouron, J-C., Guerin, R., and Davignon, A.: Subxiphoid two-dimensional echocardiographic diagnosis of double-chamber right ventricle. Circulation *67*:885, 1983.
332. Fellows, K. E., Smith, J., and Keane, J. S.: Preoperative angiocardiography in infants with tetrad of Fallot. Am. J. Cardiol. *47*:1279, 1981.
333. Kirklin, J. W., Blackstone, E. H., Pacifico, A. D., Brown, R. N., and Bargeron, L. M.: Routine primary repair versus two stage repair of tetralogy of Fallot. Circulation *60*:373, 1979.
334. Castaneda, A. R., Freed, M. D., Williams, R. G., and Norwood, W. I.: Repair of tetralogy of Fallot in infancy: Early and late results. J. Thorac. Cardiovasc. Surg. *74*:372, 1977.
335. Sunderland, C. O., Matarazzo, R. G., Lees, M. H., Menashe, V. D., Bonchek, L. I., Rosenberg, J. A., and Starr, A.: Total correction of tetralogy of Fallot in infancy: Postoperative hemodynamic evaluation. Circulation *48*:398, 1973.
336. Tucker, W. Y., Turley, K., Ullyot, D. J., and Ebert, P. A.: Management of symptomatic tetralogy of Fallot in the first year of life. J. Thorac. Cardiovasc. Surg. *78*:490, 1979.
337. Garson, A., Jr., Gorry, G. A., McNamara, D. G., and Cooley, D. A.: The surgical decision in tetralogy of Fallot: Weighing risks and benefits with decision analysis. Am. J. Cardiol. *45*:108, 1980.
338. Cole, R. B., Muster, A. J., Fixler, D. E., and Paul, M. H.: Long-term results of aortopulmonary anastomosis for tetralogy of Fallot. Circulation *43*:263,1971.
339. Roberts, W. C., Freisinger, G. C., Cohen, L. S., Mason, D. T., and Ross, R. S.: Acquired pulmonic atresia: Total obstruction to right ventricular outflow after systemic to pulmonary arterial anastomoses for cyanotic congenital cardiac disease. Am. J. Cardiol. *24*:335, 1969.
340. Marbarger, J. P., Sandza, J. G., Hartmann, A. F., and Weldon, C. S.: Blalock-Taussig anastomosis: The preferred shunts in infants and newborns. Circulation *58*(Suppl. 1):73, 1978.
340a. deLeval, M.: Systemic pulmonary and cavopulmonary shunts. *In* Stark, J., and deLeval, M. (eds.): Surgery for Congenital Heart Defects. New York, Grune and Stratton, Inc., 1983, p. 175.
341. Grinnell, V. S., Mehringer, C. M., Stanley, P., and Lurie, P. R.: Transaortic occlusion of collateral arteries to the lung by detachable valved balloons in the patient with tetralogy of Fallot. Circulation *65*:1276, 1982.
342. Piehler, J. M., Danielson, G. K., McGoon, D. C., Wallace, R. V., and Mair, D. D.: Management of pulmonary atresia with ventricular septal defect and hypoplastic pulmonary arteries by right ventricular outflow construction. J. Thorac. Cardiovasc. Surg. *80*:552, 1980.

343. Rocchini, A., Rosenthal, A., Keane, J. F., Castaneda, A. R., and Nadas, A. S.: Hemodynamics after surgical repair of right ventricle to pulmonary artery conduit. Circulation *54*:951, 1976.
344. Richardson, J. P., and Clarke, C. P.: Tetralogy of Fallot. Risk factors associated with complete repair. Br. Heart J. *38*:926, 1976.
345. Jarmakani, J. M., Nakazawa, M., Isabel-Jones, J., and Marx, R. A.: Right ventricular function in children with tetralogy of Fallot before and after aortic to pulmonary shunt. Circulation *53*:556, 1976.
346. Graham, T. P., Jr., Cordell, D., Atwood, J. F., Bouseck, R. J., Jr., Boerth, R. C., Bender, H. W., Nelson, J. H., and Vaughn, W. K.: Right ventricular volume characteristics before and after palliative and reparative operations in tetralogy of Fallot. Circulation *54*:417, 1976.
347. Borow, K. M., Green, L. H., Castaneda, A. R., and Keane, J. F.: Left ventricular function after repair of tetralogy of Fallot and its relationship to age at surgery. Circulation *61*:1150, 1980.
348. Kavey, R. E. W., Blackman, M. S., and Sondheimer, H. M.: Incidence and severity of chronic ventricular dysrhythmias after repair of tetralogy of Fallot. Am. Heart J. *103*:342, 1982.
349. Quattelbaum, P. G., Varghese, P. J., Neill, C. A., and Donahoo, J. S.: Sudden death among postoperative patients with tetralogy of Fallot. Circulation *54*:289, 1976.
350. Pacifico, A. D., Kirklin, J. W., and Blackstone, E. H.: Surgical management of pulmonary stenosis in tetralogy of Fallot. J. Thorac. Cardiovasc. Surg. *74*:382, 1977.
351. Garson, A., Jr., and McNamara, D. G.: Post-operative tetralogy of Fallot. *In* Engle, M. A. (ed.): Pediatric Cardiovascular Disease. Philadelphia, F. A. Davis, 1981, p. 407.
352. James, F. W., Kaplan, S., Schwartz, D. C., Chou, T. C., Sandker, M. J., and Naylor, V.: Response to exercise in patients after total correction of tetralogy of Fallot. Circulation *54*:671, 1976.
353. Wessel, H. U., Cunningham, W. J., Paul, M. H., Muster, A. J., and Idriss, F. S.: Exercise performance in tetralogy of Fallot after intracardiac repair. J. Thorac. Cardiovasc. Surg. *80*:582, 1980.
354. Yabek, S. M., Jarmakani, J. M., and Roberts, N.: Postoperative trifascicular block complicating tetralogy of Fallot repair. Pediatrics *58*:236, 1976.
355. Niederhauser, H., Simonin, P., and Friedli, B.: Sinus node function and conduction system after complete repair of tetralogy of Fallot. Circulation *52*:214, 1975.
356. Katz, N. M., Blackstone, E. H., Kirklin, J. W., Pacifico, A. D., and Bargeron, L. M.: Late survival and symptoms after repair of tetralogy of Fallot. Circulation *65*:403, 1982.
357. Rocchini, A. P.: Hemodynamic abnormalities and response to supine exercise in patients after operative correction of tetrad of Fallot after early childhood. Am. J. Cardiol. *48*:325, 1981.
357a. Tamer, D., Wolff, G. S., Ferrer, P., Pickoff, A. S., Casta, A., Mehta, A. V., Garcia, O., and Gelband, H.: Hemodynamics and intracardiac conduction after operative repair of tetralogy of Fallot. Am. J. Cardiol. *51*:552, 1983.
358. Nasrallah, A., Williams, R. L., and Nouri, S.: Absent pulmonary valve and tetralogy of Fallot: Clinical and angiographic considerations with review of the literature. Cardiovasc. Dis. Bull. Texas Heart Inst. *1*:392, 1974.
359. Lakier, J. B., Stanger, P., Heymann, M. A., Hoffman, J. I. E., and Rudolph, A. M.: Tetralogy of Fallot with absent pulmonary valve: Natural history and hemodynamic considerations. Circulation *50*:167, 1974.
360. Emmanouilides, G. C., Thanopoulos, B., Siassi, B., and Fishbein, M.: Agenesis of ductus arteriosus associated with the syndrome of tetralogy of Fallot and absent pulmonary valve. Am. J. Cardiol. *37*:403, 1976.
361. Stafford, E. G., Mair, D. D., McGoon, D. C., and Danielson, G. K.: Tetralogy of Fallot with absent pulmonary valve. Surgical considerations and results. Circulation *47*(Suppl.):III-24, 1973.
362. Litwin, S. B., Rosenthal, A., and Fellows, K.: Surgical management of young infants with tetralogy of Fallot, absence of the pulmonary valve, and respiratory distress. J. Thorac. Cardiovasc. Surg. *65*:552, 1973.
363. Byrne, J. P., Hawkins, J. A., Battiste, C. E., and Khoury, G. H.: Palliative procedures in tetralogy of Fallot in absent pulmonary valve: A new approach. Ann. Thorac. Surg. *33*:499, 1982.
364. Dunnigan, A., Oldham, H. N., and Benson, D. W.: Absent pulmonary valve syndrome in infancy: Surgery reconsidered. Am. J. Cardiol. *48*:117, 1981.
365. Anderson, R. H., Wilkerson, J. L., Gerlis, L. M., Smyth, A., and Becker, A. E.: Atresia of the right atrioventricular orifice. Br. Heart J. *39*:414, 1977.
365a. Rao, P. S. (ed.): Tricuspid Atresia. Mt. Kisco, N.Y. Futura Publishing Co., Inc. 1982.
366. Dick, M., Fyler, D. C., and Nadas, A. S.: Tricuspid atresia, clinical course in 101 patients. Am. J. Cardiol. *36*:327, 1975.
367. Sauer, U., and Hall, D.: Spontaneous closure or critical decrease in size of the ventricular septal in tricuspid atresia: Surgical implications. Herz. *5*:369, 1980.
368. Bharati, S., and Lev, M.: Conduction system in tricuspid atresia with and without regular D-transposition. Circulation *56*:423, 1977.
369. Koiwaya, Y., Watanabe, K., and Hirata, T.: Contrast two-dimensional echocardiography in diagnosis of tricuspid atresia. Am. Heart J. *101*:507, 1981.
370. Williams, W. G., Rubis, L., Fowler, R. S., Rao, M., Trusler, G. A., and Mustard, W. T.: Tricuspid atresia: Results of treatment in 160 children. Am. J. Cardiol. *38*:235, 1976.
371. Kyger, E. R., Reul, G. J., Jr., Sandiford, F. M., Wukash, E. C., Holman, G. L., and Cooley, D. A.: Surgical palliation of tricuspid atresia. Circulation *52*:685, 1975.
372. Tatooles, C. J., Ardekani, R., Miller, R. A., and Serratto, M.: Operative repair of tricuspid atresia. Thorac. Surg. *6*:499, 1976.
372a. Peterson, R. J., Franch, R. H., Fajman, W. A., and Jones, R. H.: Noninvasive determination of exercise cardiac function following the Fontan operation. J. Am. Coll. Cardiol. *1*:663, 1983.
373. Bjork, V. O., Olin, C. L., Bjarke, B. B., and Thoren, C. A.: Right atrial–right ventricular anastomosis for correction of tricuspid atresia. J. Thorac. Cardiovasc. Surg. *77*:452, 1979.
374. Doty, B. D., Marvin, W. J., and Lauer, R. M.: Modified Fontan procedure. J. Thorac. Cardiovasc. Surg. *81*:470, 1981.
375. LaCorte, M. A., Dick, M., Scheer, G., LaFarge, C. G., and Fyler, D. C.: Left ventricular function in tricuspid atresia. Circulation *52*:996, 1975.
376. Shachar, G. B., Fuhrman, B. P., Wang, Y., Lucas, R. V., and Lock, J.: Rest and exercise hemodynamics after the Fontan procedure. Circulation *65*:1043, 1982.
377. William, D. B., Kiernan, P. D., Schaff, H. V., and Danielson, G. K.: The hemodynamic response to dopamine and nitroprusside following right atrium–pulmonary artery bypass (Fontan procedure). Ann. Thorac. Surg. *34*:51, 1982.
378. Ehren, B. L., Mills, M., and Lower, R. R.: Congenital tricuspid insufficiency: Definition and review. Chest *69*:637, 1976.
379. Watson, H.: Natural history of Ebstein's anomaly of tricuspid valve in childhood and adolescence: An international cooperative study of 505 cases. Br. Heart J. *36*:417, 1974.
380. Guiliani, E. R., Fuster, V., Brandenberg, R. O., and Mair, D. D.: Ebstein's anomaly: The clinical features and natural history of Ebstein's anomaly of the tricuspid valve. Mayo Clin. Proc. *54*:163, 1979.
381. Bucciarelli, R. L., Nelson, R. M., Egan, E. A., Eitzman, D. Z., and Gessner, I. H.: Transient tricuspid insufficiency in the newborn: A form of myocardial dysfunction in stressed newborns. Pediatrics *59*:330, 1977.
382. Boucek, R. J., Jr., Graham, T. P., Jr., Morgan, J. P., Atwood, G. F., and Boerth, R. C.: Spontaneous resolution of massive congenital tricuspid insufficiency. Circulation *54*:795, 1976.
383. Freedom, R. M., Culham, J. A. G., Olley, P. M., Moes, C. A. F., and Rowe, R. D.: The differentiation of functional from organic pulmonary atresia: The role of aortography. Am. J. Cardiol. *41*:914, 1978.
384. Kastor, J. A., Goldreier, B. N., Josephson, M. E., Perloff, J. K., Scharf, D. L., Manchester, J. H., Shelbourne, J. C., and Hirshfield, J. W., Jr.: Electrophysiologic characteristics of Ebstein's anomaly of the tricuspid valve. Circulation *52*:987, 1975.
385. Lowe, K. G., Smith, D. E., Robertson, P. G. C., and Watson, H.: Scalar vector and intracardiac electrocardiograms in Ebstein's anomaly. Br. Heart J. *30*:617, 1968.
386. Marcus, F. I., Fontaine, G. H., Frank, R., and Grosgogedt, Y.: Right ventricular dysplasia: A report of 24 adult cases. Circulation *65*:384, 1982.
387. Gussenhoven, W. J., Spitaels, S.E.C., Bom, N., and Becker, A. E.: Echocardiographic criteria for Ebstein's anomaly of tricuspid valve. Br. Heart J. *43*:31, 1980.
388. Farooki, Z. Q., Henry, G. J., and Green, E. W.: Echocardiographic spectrum of Ebstein's anomaly of tricuspid valve. Circulation *53*:63, 1976.
389. Milner, S., Myer, R. A., Venables, A. W., Korfhagen, J., and Kaplan, S.: Mitral and tricuspid valve closure in congenital heart disease. Circulation *53*:513, 1976.
390. Hirschklau, M. J., Sahn, D. J., Hagan, A. D., Williams, D. E., and Friedman, W. F.: Cross-sectional echocardiographic features of Ebstein's anomaly of the tricuspid valve. Am. J. Cardiol. *40*:400, 1977.
391. Kerber, R. E., Markus, M. L., and Wolffson, P. M.: Demonstration of Ebstein's anomaly by simultaneous catheter tip localization of tricuspid valve and right coronary artery visualization: A new method. Chest *68*:99, 1975.
392. Marcial-Barbero, M., Verginelli, G., Awad, M., Ferriera, S., Ebaid, M., and Zerbini, E. J.: Surgical treatment of Ebstein's anomaly. J. Thorac. Cardiovasc. Surg. *78*:416, 1979.
393. Danielson, G. K., Maloney, J. D., and Devloo, R. A. E.: Surgical repair of Ebstein's anomaly. Mayo Clin. Proc. *54*:185, 1979.
394. Paul, M. H.: D-Transposition of the great arteries. *In* Moss, A. J., Adams, F. H., and Emmanouilides, G. C. (eds.): Heart Disease in Infants, Children and Adolescents. 2nd ed. Baltimore, Williams and Wilkins, 1977, p. 301.
395. Thiene, G., Razzolini, R., and Dalla-Volta, S.: Aorto-pulmonary relationship, arterio-ventricular alignment, and ventricular septal defects in complete transposition of the great arteries. Eur. J. Cardiol. *4*:13, 1976.
396. Mair, D. D., and Ritter, D. G.: Factors influencing systemic arterial oxygen saturation in complete transposition of the great arteries. Am. J. Cardiol. *31*:742. 1973.
397. Lakier, J. B., Stanger, P., Heymann, M. A., Hoffman, J. I. E., and Rudolph, A. M.: Early onset of pulmonary vascular obstruction in patients with aortopulmonary transposition and intact ventricular septum. Circulation *51*:875,1975.
398. Clarkson, P. M., Neutze, J. M., Wardill, J. C., and Barratt-Boyes, B. G.: The pulmonary vascular bed in patients with complete transposition of the great arteries. Circulation *53*:539, 1976.
399. Newfeld, E. A., Paul, M. H., Muster, A. J., and Idriss, F. S.: Pulmonary vascular disease in complete transposition of the great arteries: A study of 200 patients. Am. J. Cardiol. *34*:75, 1974.
400. Aziz, K. U., Paul, M. H., and Rowe, R. D.: Bronchopulmonary circulation in D-transposition of the great arteries: Possible role and genesis of accelerated pulmonary vascular disease. Am. J. Cardiol. *39*:432, 1977.
401. Muster, A. J., Paul, M. H., Van Grondell, E. A., and Conway, J. J.: Asymmetric distribution of the pulmonary blood flow between the right and left lungs in D-transposition of the great arteries. Am. J. Cardiol. *38*:352, 1976.
402. Dick, M., Heidelberger, K., Crowley, D., Rosenthal, A., and Hees, P.: Quantitative morphimetric analysis of the pulmonary arteries in two patients with D-transposition of the great arteries and persistence of the fetal circulation. Pediatr. Res. *15*:1397, 1981.

403. Sansa, M., Tonkin, I. L., Bargeron, L. M., and Elliott, L. P.: Left ventricular outflow tract obstruction in transposition of the great arteries. Am. J. Cardiol. *44*:88, 1979.
404. Waldman, J. D., Paul, M. H., Newfeld, E. A., Muster, A. J., and Idriss, F. S.: Transposition of the great arteries with intact ventricular septum and patent ductus arteriosus. Am. J. Cardiol. *39*:232, 1977.
405. Tonkin, I. L., Kelley, M. J., Bream, P. R., and Elliott, L. P.: The frontal chest film as a method of suspecting transposition complexes. Circulation *53*:1016, 1976.
406. Thompson, K., and Serwer, G. A.: Echocardiographic features of patients with and without residual defects after Mustard's procedure for transposition of the great vessels. Circulation *64*:1032, 1981.
407. Hirschfeld, S., Meyer, R., Schwartz, D. C., Korthagen, J., and Kaplan, S.: Measurement of right and left ventricular systolic time intervals by echocardiography. Circulation *51*:304, 1975.
408. Gutgesell, H. P.: Echocardiographic estimation of pulmonary artery pressure in transposition of the great arteries. Circulation *57*:1151, 1978.
409. DiSessa, T. G., Childs, W., Ti, C. C., and Friedman, W. F.: Systolic anterior motion of the mitral valve in a one day old infant with transposition of the great vessels. J. Clin. Ultrasound *6*:186, 1978.
410. Mahony, L., Turley, K., Ebert, P., and Heymann, M. A.: Long-term results after atrial repair of transposition of the great arteries in early infancy. Circulation *66*:253, 1982.
411. Parenzan, L., Locatelli, C. T., Alfieri, O., and Giorgio, I.: The Senning operation for transposition of the great arteries. J. Thorac. Cardiovasc. Surg. *76*:305, 1978.
412. Stark, J.: Surgical treatment of patients with transposition of the great arteries. Bull. Johns Hopkins Med. J. *140*:181, 1977.
412a. Stark, J.: Concordant transpoition—Mustard operation. *In* Stark, J., and deLeval, M. (eds.): Surgery for Congenital Heart Defects. New York, Grune and Stratton, Inc., 1983, p. 331.
413. Gutgesell, H. P., Garson, A., and McNamara, D. G.: Prognosis for the newborn with transposition of the great arteries. Am. J. Cardiol. *44*:96, 1979.
414. Graham, T. P., Jr.: Hemodynamic residua and sequelae following intra-atrial repair of transposition of the great arteries: A review. Pediatr. Cardiol. *2*:203, 1982.
415. Arciniegas, E., Farooki, Z. Q., Hakimi, M., Perry, B. L., and Green, E. W.: Results of the Mustard operation for dextro-transposition of the great arteries. J. Thorac. Cardiovasc. Surg. *81*:580, 1981.
416. Gillette, P. C., Kuglar, J. D., Garson, A., Jr., Gutgesell, H. P., Duff, D. F., and McNamara, D. G.: Mechanisms of cardiac arrhythmias after the Mustard operation for transposition of the great arteries. Am. J. Cardiol. *45*:1225, 1980.
417. Huhta, J. C., Edwards, W. D., Danielson, G. K., and Feldt, R. H.: Abnormalities of the tricuspid valve in complete transposition of the great arteries with ventricular septal defect. J. Thorac. Cardiovasc. Surg. *83*:569, 1982.
418. Borow, K. M., Keane, J. F., Castaneda, A. R., and Fried, M. D.: Systemic ventricular function in patients with tetralogy of Fallot, ventricular septal defect and transposition of the great arteries repaired during infancy. Circulation *64*:878, 1981.
419. Graham, T. P., Jr., Atwood, G. F., Boucek, R. J., Jr., Boerth, R. C., and Bender, H. W., Jr.: Abnormalities of right ventricular function following Mustard operation for transposition of the great arteries. Circulation *52*:678, 1975.
420. Benson, L. N., Bonet, J., Olley, P. M., Trusler, G., Rowe, R. D., and Morch, J.: Assessment of right ventricular function during supine bicycle exercise after Mustard's operation. Circulation *65*:1052, 1982.
421. Freedom, R. M., Culham, J. A. G., Olley, P. M., Rowe, R. D., Williams, W. G., and Trusler, G. A.: Anatomic correction of transposition of the great arteries: Pre- and post-operative cardiac catheterization with angiocardiography in five patients. Circulation *63*:905, 1981.
422. Yacoub, M. H., Berhard, A., Radley-Smith, R., Lange, P., Sievers, H., and Heintzen, P.: Supravalvular pulmonary stenosis after anatomic correction of transposition of the great arteries: Causes and prevention. Circulation *66* (Suppl. 1):193, 1982.
423. Moulton, A. L., deLeval, M. R., Macartney, F. J., Taylor, J. F. N., and Stark, J.: Rastelli procedure for transposition of the great arteries, ventricular septal defect, and left ventricular outflow tract obstruction. Early and late results in 41 patients. Br. Heart J. *45*:20, 1981.
424. Mair, D. D., Ritter, D. G., Danielson, G. K., Wallace, R. B., and McGoon, D. C.: The palliative Mustard operation; rationale and results. Am. J. Cardiol. *37*:762, 1976.
425. Van Praagh, R., Durnin, R. E., Jockin, H., Wagner, H. R., Korns, M., Garabedian, H., Endo, M., and Calder, A. L.: Anatomically corrected malposition of the great arteries. Circulation *51*:20, 1975.
426. Kirklin, J. W., Pacifico, A. D., Bargeron, L. M., Jr., and Soto, B.: Cardiac repair and anatomically corrected malposition of the great arteries. Circulation *48*:153, 1973.
427. Berry, W. B., Roberts, W. C., Morrow, A. G., and Braunwald, E.: Corrected transposition of the aorta and pulmonary trunk: Clinical, hemodynamic, and pathologic findings. Am. J. Med. *36*:35, 1964.
428. Freedberg, D. Z., and Nadas, A. S.: Clinical profile of patients with congenital corrected transposition of the great arteries. N. Engl. J. Med. *282*:1053, 1970.
429. Allwork, S. P., Bentall, H. H., Becker, A. E., Cameron, H., Gerlis, L. M., Wilkinson, J. L., and Anderson, R. H.: Congenitally corrected transposition of the great arteries. Morphologic study of 32 cases. Am. J. Cardiol. *38*:910, 1976.
430. Bjarke, B. B., and Kidd, B. S. L.: Congenitally corrected transposition of the great arteries: A clinical study of 101 cases. Acta Paediatr. Scand. *65*:153, 1976.
431. Victorika, B. E., Miller, B. L., and Gessner, H.: Electrocardiogram and vectorcardiogram and ventricular inversion (corrected transposition). Am. Heart J. *86*:734, 1973.
432. Waldo, A. L., Pacifico, A. D., Bargeron, L. M., Jr., James, T. N., and Kirklin, J. W.: Electrophysiological delineation of specialized AV conduction system in patients with corrected transposition of the great vessels and ventricular septal defect. Circulation *52*:435, 1975.
433. Bharati, B., Rosen, K., Steinfield, L., Miller, R. A., and Lev, M.: The anatomic substrate for pre-excitation in corrected transposition. Circulation *62*:831, 1980.
434. Hagan, A. D., Friedman, W. F., Ashburn, W. L., and Alazraki, N.: Further applications of scintillation scanning techniques to the diagnosis and management of infants and children with congenital heart disease. Circulation *45*:858, 1972.
435. Freedom, R. M., Harrington, D. P., and White, R. I., Jr.: The differential diagnosis of levotransposed or malposed aorta: An angiocardiographic study. Circulation *50*:1040, 1974.
436. Henry, J. G., Gordon, S., and Timmis, G. C.: Corrected transposition of great vessels in Ebstein's anomaly of tricuspid valve. Br. Heart J. *41*:249, 1979.
437. Marcelletti, C., Maloney, J. D., Ritter, D. G., Danielson, G. K., McGoon, D. C., and Wallace, R. B.: Corrected transposition in ventricular septal defect: Surgical experience. Ann. Surg. *191*:751, 1980.
438. deLeval, M. R., Bastos, P., Stark, J., Taylor, J. F. N., Macartney, F. J., and Anderson, R. H.: Surgical technique to reduce the risk of heart block following closure of ventricular septal defect in atrioventricular discordance. J. Thorac. Cardiovase. Surg. *78*:515, 1979.
439. Cameron, A. H., Acerete, F., Quero, M., and Castro, M. C.: Double outlet right ventricle. Study of 27 cases. Br. Heart J. *38*:1124, 1976.
440. Sridaromont, S., Feldt, R. H., Ritter, D. G., Davis, G. D., and Edwards, J. E.: Double outlet right ventricle: Hemodynamic and anatomic correlations. Am. J. Cardiol. *38*:85, 1976.
441. Van Praagh, R., Perez-Trevino, C., Reynolds, J. L., Moes, C. A. F., Keith, J. D., Roy, D. L., Belcort, C., Weinberg, P. M., and Parisi, L. F.: Double outlet right ventricle with subaortic ventricular septal defect and pulmonary stenosis. Am. J. Cardiol. *35*:42, 1975.
442. Sondheimer, H. M., Freedom, R. M., and Olley, P. M.: Double outlet right ventricle: Clinical spectrum and prognosis. Am. J. Cardiol. *39* :709, 1977.
443. Goor, A. A., and Edwards, J. E.: The spectrum of transposition of the great arteries with special reference to developmental anatomy of the conus. Circulation *48*:406, 1973.
444. Goitein, K. J., Neches, W. H., Park, S. C., Matthews, R. A., Lennox, C. C., and Zuberbuhler, J. R.: Electrocardiogram in double chamber right ventricle. Am. J. Cardiol. *45*:604, 1980.
445. Sridaromont, S., Ritter, D. G., Feldt, R. H., Davis, G. D., and Edwards, J. E.: Double outlet right ventricle: Anatomic and angiocardiographic correlations. Mayo Clin. Proc. *53*:555, 1978.
446. Pitlick, P., French, J., Guthaner, D., Shumway, N., and Baum, D.: Results of intraventricular baffle procedure for ventricular septal defect in double outlet right ventricle or D-transposition of the great arteries. Am. J. Cardiol. *47*:307, 1981.
447. Stewart, S.: Double outlet right ventricle. A collective review with a surgical viewpoint. J. Thorac. Cardiovasc. Surg. *71*:355, 1976.
447a. Stark, J.: Double-outlet ventricles. *In* Stark, J., and deLeval, M. (eds.): Surgery for Congenital Heart Defects. New York, Grune and Stratton, 1983, p. 397.
448. Kirklin, J. K., and Castaneda, A. R.: Surgical correction of double-outlet right ventricle with non-committed ventricular septal defect. J. Thorac. Cardiovasc. Surg. *73*:399, 1977.
449. Brandt, P. W. T., Calder, A. L., Barratt-Boyes, B. G., and Neutze, J. M.: Double outlet left ventricle: Morphology, cineangiographic diagnosis, and surgical treatment. Am. J. Cardiol. *38*:897, 1976.
450. Van Praagh, R., and Weinberg, P. M.: Double outlet left ventricle. *In* Moss, A. J., Adams, F. H., and Emmanouilides, G. C. (eds.): Heart Disease in Infants, Children and Adolescents. 2nd ed. Baltimore, Williams and Wilkins, 1977, p. 367.
451. Murphy, E. A., Gillis, D. A., and Sridhara, K. S.: Intraventricular repair of double outlet left ventricle. Ann. Thor. Surg. *31*:364, 1981.
452. Clarke, D. R., Stark, J., De Leval, M., Pincott, J. R., and Taylor, J. S. N.: Total anomalous pulmonary venous drainage in infancy. Br. Heart J. *39*:436, 1977.
453. Gathman, G. E., and Nadas, A. S.: Total anomalous pulmonary venous connection: Clinical and physiologic observations in 75 pediatric patients. Circulation *42*:143, 1970.
454. Gersony, W. M., Bowman, F. O., Jr., Steeg, C. N., Hayes, C. J., Jesse, M. J., and Malm, J. R.: Management of total anomalous pulmonary venous drainage in early infancy. Circulation *43*(Suppl.):I-19, 1971.
455. Turley, K., Tucker, W. Y., Ullyot, D. J., and Ebert, P. A.: Total anomalous pulmonary venous connection in infancy. Influence of age and type of lesion. Am. J. Cardiol. *45*:92, 1980.
456. Duff, D. N., Nyhill, M. R., and McNamara, D. G.: Infradiaphragmatic total anomalous pulmonary venous return. Review of clinical and pathological findings and results of operation in 28 cases. Br. Heart J. *39*:619, 1977.
457. Jensen, J. B., and Blount, S. G., Jr.: Total anomalous pulmonary venous return: A review and report of the older surviving patient. Am. Heart J. *82*:387, 1971.

458. Delisle, G., Endo, M., Calder, A. L., Zuberbuhler, J. R., Rochenmacher, S., Alday, L. E., Mangini, O., Van Praagh, S., and Van Praagh, R.: Total anomalous pulmonary venous connection: Report of 93 autopsy cases with emphasis on diagnostic and surgical considerations. Am. Heart J. *91*:99, 1976.
459. Elliott, L. P., and Edwards, J. E.: The problem of pulmonary venous obstruction in total anomalous pulmonary venous connection to the left innominate vein. Circulation *25*:913, 1962.
460. Byrun, C. J., Dick, M., Behrendt, D. M., and Rosenthal, A.: Repair of total anomalous pulmonary venous connection in patients younger than six months old: Late post-operative hemodynamic and electrophysiologic status. Circulation *66* (Suppl. 1):208, 1982.
461. Newfeld, E. A., Wilson, A., Paul, M. H., and Reisch, J. S.: Pulmonary vascular disease in total anomalous pulmonary venous drainage. Circulation *61*:103, 1980.
462. Snider, A. R., Roge, C. L., Schiller, N. B., and Silverman, N.: Congenital left ventricular inflow obstruction evaluated by two-dimensional echocardiography. Circulation *61*:848, 1980.
463. Haworth, S. G., Reid, L., and Simon, G.: Radiological features of the heart and lungs in total anomalous pulmonary venous return in early infancy. Clin. Radiol. *28*:561, 1977.
464. Smallhorn, J. F., Sutherland, G. R., Tommasini, G., Hunter, S., Anderson, R. H., and Macartney, F. J.: Assessment of total anomalous pulmonary venous connection by two-dimensional echocardiography. Br. Heart J. *46*:613, 1981.
464a. Stark, J.: Anomalies of the pulmonary venous return. *In* Stark, J., and deLeval, M. (eds.): Surgery for Congenital Heart Defects. 1983, Grune and Stratton, Inc., p. 235.
465. Matthew, R., Thilenius, O. G., Replogle, R. L., and Arcilla, R. A.: Cardiac function in total anomalous pulmonary venous return before and after surgery. Circulation *55*:361, 1977.
466. Nakazawa, M., Jarmakani, J. M., Gyepes, M. T., Prochazka, J. V., Yabek, S. M., and Marks, R. A.: Pre- and postoperative ventricular function in infants and children with right ventricular volume overload. Circulation *55*:479, 1977.
467. Healey, J. E.: An anatomic survey of anomalous pulmonary veins: Their clinical significance. J. Thorac. Cardiovasc. Surg. *23*:433, 1952.
468. Kuiper-Oosterwal, C. H., and Moulaert, A.: The scimitar syndrome in infancy and childhood. Eur. J. Cardiol. *1*:55, 1973.
469. Van Praagh, R.: Terminology of congenital heart disease: Glossary and commentary. Circulation *56*:139, 1977.
470. Stanger, P., Rudolph, A. M., and Edwards, J. E.: Cardiac malpositions: An overview based on a study of 65 necropsy specimens. Circulation *56*:159, 1977.
471. Van Praagh, R., Weinberg, P. M., and Van Praagh, S.: Malposition of the heart. *In* Moss, A. J., Adams, F. H., and Emmanouilides, G. (eds): Heart Disease in Infants, Children and Adolescents. 2nd ed. Baltimore, Williams and Wilkins, 1977, p. 394.
472. Shinebourne, E. A., Macartney, F. J., and Anderson, R. H.: Sequential chamber localization—Logical approach to diagnosis in congenital heart disease. Br. Heart J. *38*:327, 1976.
473. de la Cruz, M. V., Berrazueta, J. R., Arteaga, M., Atti, E. F., and Soni, J.: Rules for diagnosis of arterioventricular discordance and spatial identification of ventricles. Crossed great arteries and transposition of the great arteries. Br. Heart J. *38*:341, 1976.
474. Nasser, W. K.: Congenital absence of the left pericardium. Am. J. Cardiol. *26*: 466, 1970.
475. Morgan, J. R., Rogers, A. K., and Forker, A. D.: Congenital absence of the left pericardium: Clinical findings. Ann. Intern. Med. *74*:370, 1971.
476. Pernot, C., Hoeffel, J. C., and Henry, M.: Radiologic patterns of congenital malformation of the pericardium. Radiol. Clin. (Basel) *44*:505, 1975.
477. Payvandi, M. N., and Kerber, R. E.: Echocardiography in congenital and acquired absence of the pericardium. Circulation *53*:86, 1976.
478. Rastelli G., Kirklin, J. W., and Titus, J. L.: Anatomic observations on complete form of persistent common atrioventricular canal with special reference to atrioventricular valves. Mayo Clin. Proc. *41*:296, 1966.
479. Soto, B., Pacifico, A. D., and DiSciascio, G.: Univentricular heart: An angiographic study. Am. J. Cardiol. *49*:787, 1982
480. Shimazaki, Y., Kawashima, Y., Mori, T., Matsuda, H., Kitamura, S., and Yokota, K.: Ventricular function of single ventricle after ventricular septation. Circulation *61*:653, 1980.
481. Van Praagh, R., and Van Praagh, S.: What is a ventricle? The single ventricle trap. Pediatr. Cardiol. *2*:79, 1982.
482. Ritter, D. G., Seward, J. B., Moodie, D., and Danielson, G. K.: Univentricular heart (common ventricle): Pre-operative diagnosis. Herz *4*:198, 1979.
483. Marin-Garcia, J., Tandon, R., Moller, J. H., and Edwards, J. E.: Common (single) ventricle with normally related great arteries, with great vessels. Circulation *39*:565, 1974.
484. Tandon, R., Becker, A. E., Moller, J. H., and Edwards, J. E.: Double inlet left ventricle. Straddling tricuspid valve. Br. Heart J. *36*:747, 1974.
485. Macartney, F. J., Partridge, J. B., Scott, O., and Deverall, P. B.: Common or single ventricle: angiographic and hemodynamic study of 42 patients. Circulation *53*:543, 1976.
486. Rigby, M. L., Anderson, R. H., Gibson, D., Jones, O. D. H., Joseph, M. C., and Shinebourne, E. A.: Two-dimensional echocardiographic categorization of the univentricular heart. Ventricular morphology, type, and mode of atrioventricular connection. Br. Heart J. *46*:603, 1981.
487. Ritter, D. G.: Echocardiograms in common (single) ventricle: Angiographic, anatomic correlation. Am. J. Cardiol. *39*:217, 1977.
488. Seward, J. B., Tajik, A. J., Haggler, D. J., and Ritter, D. G.: Contrast echocardiography in single or common ventricle. Circulation *55*:513, 1977.
489. Danielson, G. K., McGoon, D. C., Maloney, J. D., and Ritter, G. D.: Surgical septation of univentricular heart with outlet chamber. Herz *4*:262, 1979.
490. Krongrad, E., and Malm, J. R.: Intra-operative mapping in patients with univentricular heart. Herz *4*:232, 1979.
491. Danielson, G. K., Giuliani, E. R., and Ritter, D. G.: Successful repair of common ventricles associated with complete atrioventricular canal. J. Thorac. Cardiovasc. Surg. *67*:152, 1974.
492. Cabral, R. J. M., Miller, D. C., Oyer, P. E., Stinson, E., Reitz, E. A., and Shumway, N. E.: A surgical approach for single ventricle incorporating total right atrium–pulmonary artery diversion. J. Thorac. Cardiovasc. Surg. *79*:202, 1980.
493. Eklof, O., Elstrom, G., Ericksson, B. O., Michaelsson, M., Stevenson, O., Soderlund, S., Thoren, C., and Wallgren, G.: Arterial anomalies causing compression of the trachea and/or the esophagus. Acta Paediatr. Scand. *60*:81, 1971.
494. Shuford, W. H., Sybers, R. G., and Weens, H. S.: The angiographic features of double aortic arch. Am. J. Roentgenol. *116*:126, 1972.
495. Park, C. D., Waldhausen, J. A., Friedman, S., Aberdeen, I., and Jamson, J.: Tracheal compression by the great arteries in the mediastinum: Report of 39 cases. Arch. Surg. *103*:626, 1971.
496. Koopot, R., Nikaido, H., and Idriss, F. S.: Surgical management of anomalous left pulmonary artery causing tracheo-bronchial obstruction: Pulmonary artery sling. J. Thorac. Cardiovasc. Surg. *69*:239, 1975.
496a. deLeval, M.: Vascular rings. Stark, J., and deLeval, M. (eds.): Surgery for Congenital Heart Defects, New York, Grune and Stratton, Inc., 1983, p. 227.
497. Said, R. M., Rosenthal, A., Fellows, K., and Castaneda, A. R.: Pulmonary artery sling. J. Thorac. Cardiovasc. Surg. *69*:333, 1975.
498. Anderson, R. H., Wenick, A. C. G., Losekoot, T. G., and Becker, A. E.: Congenitally complete heart block. Circulation *56*:90, 1977.
499. Chemeides, L., Truex, R. C., Vetter, V., Rashkind, W. J., Gallioto, F. M., and Noonan, J.: Association of maternal systemic lupus erythematosus with congenital complete heart block. N. Engl. J. Med. *297*:1204, 1977.
500. McCue, C. M., Mantakas, M. E., Tingelstad, J. B., and Ruddy, S.: Congenital heart block in newborns of mothers with connective tissue disease. Circulation *56*:82, 1977.
501. Michaelsson, M., and Engle, M. A.: Congenital complete heart block: An international study of the natural history. Cardiovasc. Clin. *4*:85, 1972.
502. Scarpelli, E. M., and Rudolph, A. M.: The hemodynamics of congenital heart block. Progr. Cardiovasc. Dis. *6*:327, 1964.
503. Thilenius, O. G., Chiemmongkoltip, P., Cassels, D. E., and Arcilla, R. A.: Hemodynamic studies in children with congenital atrioventricular block. Am. J. Cardiol. *30*:13, 1972.
504. Benrey, J., Gillette, P. C., Nasraloah, A. T., and Hallman, G. L.: Permanent pacemaker implantation in infants, children, and adolescents. Circulation *53*: 245, 1976.
505. Kleinman, C. S., Donnerstein, R. L., DeVore, G. R., Jaffee, C. C., Lynch, D. C., Berkowitz, R. L., Talner, N. S., and Hobbins, J. C.: Fetal echocardiography for evaluation of in utero congestive heart failure. N. Engl. J. Med. *306*:568, 1982.
506. Harrigan, J. T., Kangos, J. J., and Sikka, A.: Successful treatment of fetal congestive heart failure secondary to tachycardia. N. Engl. J. Med. *304*:1527, 1981.
507. Radford, D. J., Izukawa, T., and Rowe, R. D.: Congenital paroxysmal atrial tachycardia. Arch. Dis. Child. *51*:613, 1976.
508. Gillette, P. C.: The mechanisms of supraventricular tachycardia in children. Circulation *54*:133, 1976.
509. Whitman, V., Friedman, Z., Berman, W., Jr., and Maisels, M. J.: Supraventricular tachycardia in newborn infants: An approach to therapy. J. Pediatr. *91*:304, 1977.
510. Brechenmacher, C., Coumel, P., and James, T. N.: Intractable tachycardia in infancy. Circulation *53*:377, 1976.
511. Porter, C. J., Gillette, P. C., Garson, A., Hesslein, P. S., Carpawich, P. P., and McNamara, D. G.: Effects of verapamil on supraventricular tachycardia. Am. J. Cardiol. *48*:487, 1981.

30 CONGENITAL HEART DISEASE IN THE ADULT

by Kenneth M. Borow, M.D., Joseph S. Alpert, M.D., and Eugene Braunwald, M.D.

GENERAL PRINCIPLES

During the past 25 years our ability to diagnose and treat congenital heart disease has advanced rapidly. Until recently, the only patients to survive to adulthood were those with simple, uncomplicated defects. This is no longer the case. Palliative or corrective surgical procedures have been developed for almost all congenital cardiac anomalies, leading to an increase in the population of adult cardiac patients. As the effects of coronary atherosclerosis and systemic hypertension are superimposed upon cardiac malformations that have undergone varying degrees of surgical correction, the pathophysiology of congenital heart disease in the adult may become even more complicated. It is therefore of increasing importance that clinicians understand the anatomy, diagnostic approaches, and natural history of those congenital cardiac defects found most frequently in the adult population.

RELATIVE INCIDENCE IN ADULTS AND CHILDREN. The relative incidence of the various congenital heart lesions in adults differs from that in children. Complex congenital lesions are considerably more common in children than in adults. Ventricular septal defect is the most common cardiovascular malformation diagnosed in children, while stenosis of a congenital bicuspid aortic valve and atrial septal defect are the lesions most frequently found in adults. In infants the most common cardiac lesion producing cyanosis is transposition of the great arteries, while in the adult population it is tetralogy of Fallot.

Occasionally, congenital heart disease remains undetected until the patient reaches adulthood. Two factors contribute to this delay in diagnosis: First, in children, a cardiovascular malformation may go unrecognized or may be mistaken for a functional murmur because of the subtle manner in which it expresses itself, the classic example being the small or moderate-sized isolated atrial septal defect. Second, medical attention may be inadequate, particularly for individuals who grow up in medically underserved areas, and as a consequence, cardiovascular anomalies of even moderate severity may go undetected.

GENETICS AND CONGENITAL HEART DISEASE (see also pages 942 and 1613). As an increasing number of individuals with congenital heart disease reach childbearing age, the need for detailed information regarding the etiology of such diseases becomes more apparent. Nora and Nora reported that the cause of congenital heart disease is predominantly genetic in 8 per cent of cases and predominantly environmental in 2 per cent. In the remaining 90 per cent, a complex interaction between genetic and environmental factors is thought to exist.[1] Not surprisingly, the greater the number of affected first-degree relatives with congenital heart disease within the family, the greater the risk of recurrence.[1–3] The recurrence risk is somewhat higher if the affected first-degree relative is a parent rather than a sibling. When two first-degree relatives are affected, the recurrence risk for the next child becomes two to three times as great compared to the case when only one first-degree relative is affected.[1–3] If one parent has a congenital cardiac defect, the chance of his offspring having the same lesion is approximately 2 to 4 per cent (Table 30–1). Surgical repair of a woman's congenital heart defect does not affect her risk of having affected children.[4]

TABLE 30–1 AFFECTED OFFSPRING, GIVEN ONE PARENT WITH A CONGENITAL HEART DEFECT

ANOMALY	AFFECTED OFFSPRING Number	%
Ventricular septal defect	7/174	4.0
Persistent ductus arteriosus	6/139	4.3
Atrial septal defect	5/199	2.5
Tetralogy of Fallot	6/141	4.2
Pulmonic stenosis	4/111	3.6
Coarctation of the aorta	7/253	2.7
Aortic stenosis	4/103	3.9

Adapted from Nora, J. J., and Nora, A. H.: The evolution of specific genetic and environmental counseling in congenital heart disease. Circulation *57*:205, 1978. By permission of the American Heart Association, Inc.

Surgically Corrected Congenital Heart Defects

The adult with a surgically corrected congenital heart defect is now emerging as a new type of patient in cardiology practice.[5–7] Three categories of such patients exist: (1) asymptomatic individuals who have undergone complete repair of their defects, (2) asymptomatic or symptomatic patients with residual defects or complications despite surgical correction, and (3) symptomatic patients who had previously undergone palliative procedures.

The clinical course of asymptomatic patients in whom congenital cardiac malformations are totally corrected early in life appears to be a relatively stable one.[5] Many of these individuals are independent, socially well-adjusted, and free of anxiety concerning their cardiac condition. Patients who undergo correction of their defect in childhood are significantly less anxious in this regard than are those whose lesion is corrected during adult life.

Patients with residual defects or complications following repair may be asymptomatic or symptomatic.[5,8] Conditions frequently associated with altered hemodynamics postoperatively include: (1) ostium secundum atrial septal defect that has been closed, with residual mitral regurgitation due to associated mitral valve prolapse (p. 1089); (2) ventricular septal defect or tetralogy of Fallot with residual left-to-right shunt from a leak in the patch closing the septal defect; (3) congenital aortic stenosis with inadequate relief of the obstruction, restenosis of the valve, or significant aortic regurgitation; (4) persistent or recurrent systemic hypertension after coarctectomy; and (5) severe pulmonic regurgitation or residual right ventricular outflow tract obstruction after repair of pulmonic stenosis or tetralogy of Fallot. Such patients may remain asymptomatic or minimally symptomatic for many years. The ultimate effect of the residual cardiac abnormality depends on the specific lesion as well as its severity. Patients with residual cardiac abnormalities are, in general, less well adjusted socially and emotionally than are individuals without residual cardiac problems. Many of these patients have considerable difficulty obtaining life and health insurance policies and even employment.[9]

A modest number of patients who have undergone palliative procedures such as Blalock-Taussig, Potts, or Waterston systemic-to-pulmonary artery anastomoses survive to reach adult life.[10] The cardiac reserve of these patients is usually limited, often severely. Physically, such individuals may be underdeveloped, with chest deformities such as pectus carinatum. Although these patients generally adapt to their condition, marked limitations in lifestyle are common. In some of these patients, complete correction is feasible during adult life, albeit at a higher risk than in childhood or adolescence; in others, the presence of irreversible changes in the pulmonary vascular bed or the complex nature of the malformation prohibits complete correction.

Taussig and associates have reviewed the long-term consequences of the Blalock-Taussig operation.[10] Their findings might be considered representative of those resulting from palliative procedures in patients with complex anomalies. One hundred and sixty-nine patients, mostly children, diagnosed clinically as having tetralogy of Fallot underwent a subclavian–pulmonary artery anastomosis only. At least 119 of these patients (70 per cent) were still alive and 62 (35 per cent) were not seriously disabled 20 to 28 years after their operation. Examination of the entire cohort of 685 patients originally treated with a Blalock-Taussig anastomosis for tetralogy of Fallot, including those without additional operation and those with subsequent palliative and corrective operative procedures, has revealed a vast improvement in their quality of life. Over 50 per cent of them have married and two-thirds of them have had children. Thirty-five per cent of the patients graduated from college and almost 70 per cent are earning substantial incomes. Approximately 70 per cent of these patients have repaid in taxes the cost to society of their medical treatment and rehabilitation.[10] However, a number of serious complications have also occurred. Infective endocarditis, most commonly due to streptococcus and staphylococcus, occurred 80 times in 71 of the patients. Sixteen (23 per cent) of these 71 affected patients died.

Over the past 25 years, more than 500,000 patients with functionally significant congenital cardiac malformations have attained adulthood.[9] The magnitude of this success is due primarily to the medical and surgical advances since the early 1960s.

ENDOCARDITIS PROPHYLAXIS (see also pages 951 and 1175). Surgical treatment may increase, decrease, or leave unchanged an individual's risk of endocarditis.[11,12] The incidence of postoperative endocarditis is so low in patients in whom a persistent ductus arteriosus or atrial septal defect has been closed that prophylaxis can be omitted. The risk of endocarditis after operation in persons with completely repaired ventricular septal defects and tetralogy of Fallot is also markedly reduced. On the other hand, patients with residual, hemodynamically insignificant left-to-right shunts following repair of a ventricular septal defect may be at even higher risk of endocarditis than they were preoperatively, despite the satisfactory physiological result. The risk of endocarditis also increases in patients who undergo prosthetic replacement of any valve or in whom a prosthetic conduit is inserted,[13] whereas the risk remains unchanged following aortic valvulotomy for congenital aortic stenosis or repair of coarctation of the aorta. Pulmonic stenosis carries a low risk of endocarditis both before and after valvulotomy. Because patients frequently feel so well after corrective and occasionally after palliative operations, it may be difficult to convince them of the importance of prophylactic antibiotics.

Pregnancy in Patients with Congenital Heart Disease (See also page 1769)

Most congenital cardiac malformations do not interfere with the *initiation* of pregnancy.[4,14–18] However, some of these parturients abort or give birth to premature, nonviable infants.[4] In a few cardiovascular malformations, pregnancy presents a definite danger to the mother. Among patients with severe pulmonary hypertension or marginally compensated cardiac failure, mortality is high during pregnancy. In women with small or moderate-sized left-to-right shunts (i.e., pulmonary-to-systemic flow ratios less than 2:1) and only modest pulmonary hypertension (i.e., pulmonary artery systolic pressure less than 50 mm Hg), pregnancy is generally well tolerated. In patients with larger left-to-right shunts, left ventricular failure may occur, while in those with more severe pulmonary hypertension, further elevation of pulmonary arterial pressure may occur during pregnancy.

In a review of the obstetrical experience of 28 women with unrepaired *coarctation of the aorta,* there was no maternal mortality and the spontaneous abortion rate was 25 per cent.[14] Most of the remaining pregnancies were uncomplicated, and the infants were normal. Because of the increased cardiac output associated with the second and third trimesters of pregnancy, parturients with unrepaired coarctation of the aorta may experience a significant increase in systolic arterial pressure, and antihypertensive therapy may be of some benefit. Nitroprusside infusion is often useful in treating acute elevations in blood pressure during delivery and the immediate postpartum period. In a small fraction of patients with coarctation of the aorta, aortic dissection or rupture occurs during pregnancy, but it is likely that in these cases intrinsic disease of the ascending aorta with cystic necrosis was present prior to pregnancy. Fortunately, this complication is so rare in women with unrepaired coarctation of the aorta followed in modern obstetrical practice that there seems to be little rationale for elective coarctectomy during pregnancy.[4,14] Rarely, the bacteremia that accompanies labor results in endocarditis or endarteritis in patients with coarctation.

Maternal and fetal mortality rates are high among patients with uncorrected *tetralogy of Fallot.* As is the case with other forms of cyanotic congenital heart disease, the infants tend to be small for their gestational age. Palliative surgical procedures carried out prior to pregnancy in these patients may decrease maternal and infant risk. Pregnancy after successful total correction of tetralogy of Fallot seems to pose little threat to either mother or child.[16] Patients with *congenital heart block* tolerate pregnancy without difficulty, although Stokes-Adams attacks have been reported to commence shortly after delivery.[17] Insertion of a temporary transvenous pacemaker may be helpful for maintaining stable hemodynamics at the time of delivery in women with marked bradycardia due to congenital heart block. In patients with permanent pacemakers inserted for either congenital or acquired complete heart block, improved hemodynamics may be achieved if the pacing rate is increased immediately prior to labor and delivery.

Pregnancy is contraindicated in women with severe *pulmonary vascular disease.*[18] If early termination of the pregnancy is not possible, close fetal and maternal monitoring as well as judicious medical care is required throughout the prenatal period. Maternal and fetal risk become maximal during labor and delivery. Uterine contractions, especially when associated with the application of forceps, may have an adverse effect on pulmonary and systemic hemodynamics.[19] Management of these patients should include inhalation of high concentrations of oxygen and epidural anesthesia. Serial arterial blood gas determinations may be useful in detecting changes in shunt flow associated with an acute increase in pulmonary vascular resistance or a sudden fall in systemic vascular resistance. Increased maternal risk extends at least several days into the immediate postpartum period.

SPECIFIC MALFORMATIONS

Valvular Aortic Stenosis
(See also pages 976 and 1095)

Congenital abnormalities of the aortic valve occur in 1 to 2 per cent of the general adult population. The most common cause of congenital valvular aortic stenosis is the bicuspid valve with peripheral fusion of the leaflets and diminished effective orifice size. A valve that is functionally normal early in life may become thickened, fibrotic, calcified, and stenotic during adulthood. Valvular aortic stenosis may be associated with coarctation of the aorta and, less frequently, ventricular septal defect or isolated pulmonic stenosis.[20]

In the young or middle-aged adult, isolated valvular aortic stenosis is usually congenital rather than rheumatic in origin.[21,22] By age 45, approximately 50 per cent of all bicuspid valves show some degree of stenosis.[20,23] The frequency and severity of valvular narrowing increase with age, in part reflecting progressive calcium deposition within the leaflets.[24] In many patients, the congenitally bicuspid aortic valve becomes regurgitant as well as stenotic. The noninfected congenitally bicuspid aortic valve is also an important cause of pure aortic regurgitation severe enough to require valve replacement.[25] All patients with congenital abnormalities of the aortic valve require antibiotic prophylaxis against infective endocarditis.

Pathophysiology. Left ventricular systolic hypertension acts as a stimulus for concentric hypertrophy (p. 1097). Left ventricular compliance is frequently decreased, resulting in elevations of left ventricular end-diastolic and left atrial mean pressures and symptoms of pulmonary congestion. Because of increased left ventricular muscle mass and high intracavity systolic pressure, left ventricular ischemia may occur even in the absence of significant coronary artery disease. In some patients with severe stenosis, cardiac output may not increase appropriately during exercise, reflecting severe mechanical obstruction at the valvular level and/or intrinsic abnormalities of the left ventricular contractile state. This can result in exercise-induced syncope or presyncope.

Symptoms. The major symptoms of congenital valvular aortic stenosis in the adult include angina pectoris, syncope, and congestive heart failure.[26] Sudden death during exercise can occur in patients with severe disease but is rarely the presenting event in a previously undiagnosed or asymptomatic adult.[27] Hemodynamic and clinical compensation are usual until middle age. However, from the time of onset of symptoms, the average survival in patients with unrepaired severe valvular aortic stenosis is less than five years.[26]

Physical Examination. The predominant physical finding in adults with congenital valvular aortic stenosis is a harsh systolic ejection murmur, loudest along the right upper sternal edge and radiating along the carotid arteries. In mild to moderate valvular aortic stenosis, an ejection click caused by abrupt cessation of movement of the thickened, doming leaflets is frequently present. In contrast to the click found in pulmonic stenosis, it does not vary in intensity with respiration. As the severity of the valvular aortic stenosis increases, the murmur becomes longer and louder and peaks later in systole. Examination of the carotid pulse demonstrates the characteristic findings of a delayed upstroke, low anacrotic shoulder, systolic shudder, and prolonged ejection time (see Figure 3–22, p. 56). The apical precordial impulse is often heaving and sustained, with a palpable atrial presystolic tap.

Noninvasive Studies. The *ECG* shows a variable degree of left ventricular hypertrophy. Approximately 75 per cent of adult patients with severe valvular aortic stenosis (left ventriculo-aortic pressure gradient greater than 75 mm Hg) exhibit left ventricular hypertrophy with strain. This finding is less common in patients with mild to moderate obstruction.

On *chest x-ray,* poststenotic dilatation of the ascending aorta (see Figure 6–52, p. 185) is common, but this finding does not correlate well with the severity of the obstruction. Calcification of the aortic valve becomes evident more frequently after the third decade of life. Overall heart size is usually normal until left ventricular failure occurs, although the left ventricle may be prominent in patients with only moderate obstruction (gradient of approximately 50 mm Hg) even without failure.

On *M-mode echocardiography,* the bicuspid aortic valve is often thickened, with an eccentric closure line reflecting the asymmetry of the valve leaflets (see Figure 5–48, p. 115). Rather than opening fully with ventricular systole, the leaflets frequently show a doming pattern. When this occurs, leaflet excursion seen on an M-mode study may not accurately reflect the severity of the stenosis. This problem can be solved in part by the use of two-dimensional echocardiography to demonstrate leaflet doming on the long-axis parasternal view and the presence of only two leaflets on the short-axis parasternal view[28] (Fig. 30–1). Pulsed Doppler echocardiography (p. 94) can also be useful in quantifying the severity of aortic stenosis and associated regurgitation.[29,30]

Surgical Treatment. The decision to operate for congenital valvular aortic stenosis in adults depends on multiple factors, including the magnitude and type of symptoms, the calculated aortic valve area at cardiac catheterization, and the state of left ventricular function.[27,31,31a] Our general criteria are a peak systolic ejection gradient exceeding 75 mm Hg in association with a normal forward cardiac output and an aortic valve area less than approximately 0.7 cm^2 (0.4 cm^2/m^2 body surface area). In patients with reduced forward cardiac output, the peak systolic ejection gradient may be low, reflecting underlying myocardial dysfunction or afterload mismatch. In such patients, calculation of the aortic valve area is vital for determining the hemodynamic significance of the left ventricular outflow tract obstruction. The young adult with severe valvular aortic stenosis but without calcification of the valve may be a candidate for aortic valvulotomy. However, residual or recurrent stenosis as well as valvular incompetence is a frequent complication of this procedure.[27,32,33] In the older patient, aortic valve replacement is often necessary owing to leaflet fibrosis and calcification.

Atrial Septal Defect (See also page 958)

This malformation frequently permits survival into middle age and beyond.[34,35] The diagnosis of atrial septal defect (ASD) may be difficult because the associated physical

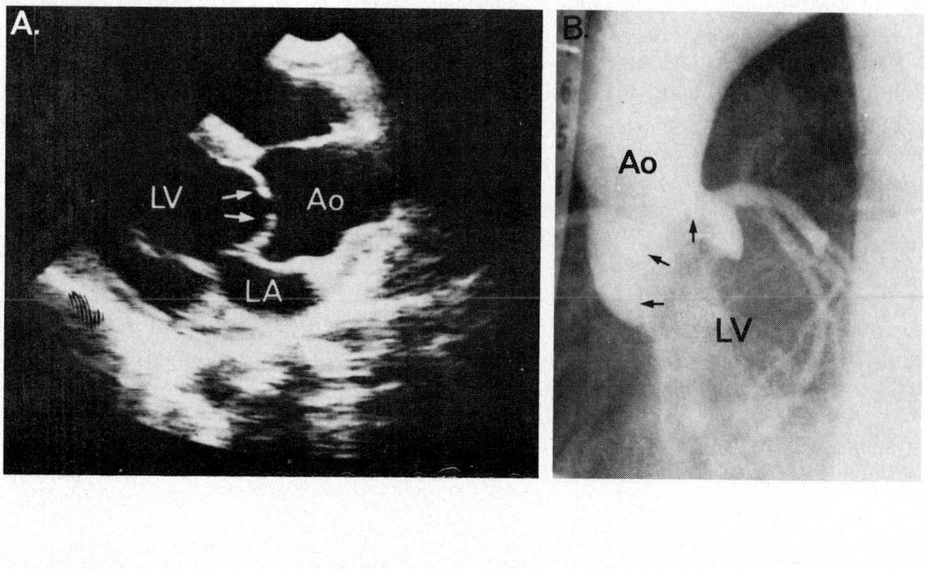

FIGURE 30–1 Echocardiographic and angiographic findings in a young adult with valvular aortic stenosis. *A,* Two-dimensional echocardiographic study with the transducer in the long-axis parasternal position demonstrating leaflet doming and thickening (arrows). *B,* Aortogram from the same patient showing doming of the aortic valve leaflets. The negative shadow in the proximal aortic root (Ao) is caused by a jet of nonopacified blood from the left ventricle (LV) as it exits through the stenotic aortic valve. LA = left atrium.

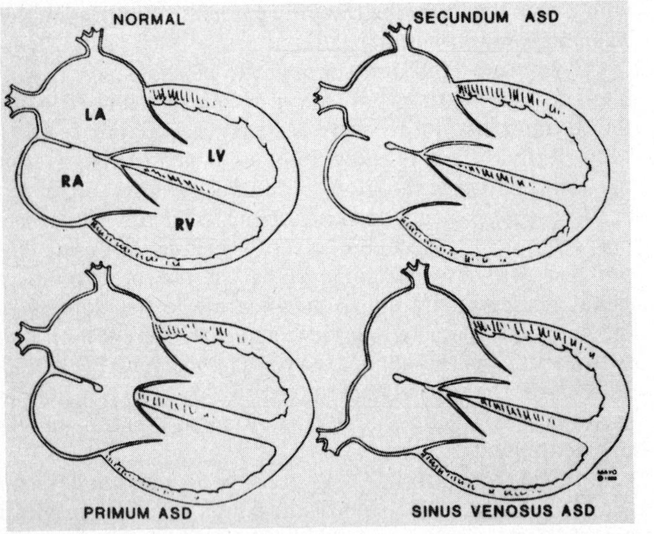

FIGURE 30–2 Normal atrial septum and anatomical sites of the three types of atrial septal defects (ASD) as visualized by the two-dimensional echocardiographic technique utilizing a subcostal position. (From Nasser, F. N., et al.: Diagnosis of sinus venosus atrial septal defect by two-dimensional echocardiography. Mayo Clin. Proc. *56*:571, 1981.)

findings may be subtle and the patient asymptomatic. Moreover, ASD may not be recognized in adults because of the presence of associated conditions, such as coronary artery disease or chronic obstructive pulmonary disease. One characteristic of ASD that sets it apart from many other significant congenital heart lesions is the prolonged period during which the patient remains asymptomatic or almost so. Serious limitation of exercise capacity may develop secondary to progressive pulmonary vascular disease, but this usually does not occur until the fourth or fifth decade of life.[34,34a] Three types of ASD are seen in adults: ostium secundum, ostium primum, and sinus venosus (Fig. 30–2). Ostium secundum ASD is by far the most common type.

PATHOPHYSIOLOGY. Blood flow through the ASD occurs primarily during late ventricular systole, early diastole, and atrial systole. The magnitude of the left-to-right shunt depends on the size of the defect, on the relationship between the compliance of the two ventricles, and indirectly on the relationship between pulmonary and systemic vascular resistance. The net effect in a patient with an uncomplicated ASD is volume overload of the right atrium and right ventricle with consequent enlargement of these chambers without dilatation of the left cardiac chambers. Some patients with ASD will have mild to modest elevations of pulmonary artery pressure on the basis of a high transpulmonary blood flow rather than elevated pulmonary vascular resistance.

The mechanism of heart failure in patients with ASD was first studied in 1956 by Dexter,[36] who noted that all four cardiac chambers are in communication during diastole. Ordinarily, a left-to-right shunt occurs at that time because the right ventricle offers less resistance to inflowing blood than does the left ventricle, despite equality of pressures in all four chambers. The right ventricle is more compliant than the left, so that when both atria and ventricles are in communication, blood follows the path of least resistance, i.e., into the more compliant right ventricle. According to this concept, when a patient with ASD develops right ventricular hypertrophy as a consequence of a superimposed pressure overload from pulmonary hypertension, resistance to right ventricular filling is increased and the left-to-right shunt declines. As these processes continue, the right ventricle may become less compliant than the left, with resultant right-to-left shunting and the development of cyanosis.

Left ventricular failure in adults with ASD is usually the result of one or a combination of associated conditions that affect the left ventricle, such as ischemic heart disease, systemic hypertension, aortic valvular disease, or mitral regurgitation.[35–39] Left ventricular failure reduces chamber compliance, thus increasing the magnitude of the left-to-right shunt. If the right ventricle cannot accept an increase in the quantity of blood shunted from left to right, the diastolic pressures in all four cardiac chambers increase. As a consequence of the defect in the atrial septum, this increase in diastolic pressure produces systemic venous congestion. For these reasons, left ventricular failure in patients with ASD can elevate systemic venous pressure and result in the clinical signs usually associated with right heart failure.

The issue of whether left ventricular dysfunction occurs frequently in patients with uncomplicated ASD remains controversial. Older studies suggested that intrinsic abnormalities of left ventricular function do exist in some patients,[41] but these findings have been questioned.[38,40–42] Bonow et al. demonstrated that left ventricular ejection fraction at rest measured by radionuclide angiography was usually normal in adults with ASD without evidence of hemodynamically severe right or left ventricular failure. However, an abnormal response of the ejection fraction to exercise was common. Impairment of the left ventricular response to exercise resolved after operative closure of the defect. This study suggests that left ventricular dysfunction in patients with ASD may result from reversible mechanical factors related to right ventricular volume overload with abnormal displacement of the ventricular septum and perhaps compromise of left ventricular preload rather than to intrinsic, irreversible impairment of left ventricular contractility.

CLINICAL FINDINGS

Symptoms. Most patients over age 40 are symptomatic.[38,39] Dyspnea on exertion, fatigue, and symptoms secondary to supraventricular tachyarrhythmias are the most frequent complaints. Life expectancy is shortened in ASD, although many patients reach advanced years.[43,44] Even young adults who develop pulmonary hypertension usually survive beyond the age of 40 years. When patients succumb to ASD, the cause of death is usually right heart failure.[45] Other fatal complications include pulmonary embolism, in situ pulmonary thrombosis, bronchopulmonary infection, paradoxical embolism, brain abscess, and rupture of the pulmonary artery.

Pulmonary hypertension rarely occurs before age 20 in patients who reside at sea level; however, those who live at high altitudes may develop this complication earlier.[34] Patients with pulmonary hypertension usually complain of dyspnea and fatigue, effort cyanosis, and/or hemoptysis. Chest pain resembling angina may also occur.

TABLE 30–2 ELECTROCARDIOGRAPHIC PATTERNS ASSOCIATED WITH CONGENITAL HEART DISEASE

CARDIAC DEFECT	ELECTROCARDIOGRAPHIC PATTERN: Atrial Flutter/Fibrillation	Supraventricular Tachycardia	Ventricular Arrhythmia	Atrioventricular Block	Preexcitation Syndrome	Abnormal P-wave Orientation	Right Atrial Overload	Left Atrial Overload	Left Axis Deviation	Left Bundle Branch Block	Right Bundle Branch Block	Right Ventricular Volume Overload	Right Ventricular Pressure Overload	Left Ventricular Volume Overload	Left Ventricular Pressure Overload	Biventricular Overload	Abnormal Q Waves or Myocardial Infarction Pattern
Atrial septal defect (secundum)	++	+	0	+	0	+	++	+	0	0	+	+++	+	0	0	0	0
Prolapsed mitral valve syndrome	+	+	+	0	+	0	0	+	0	0	0	0	0	+	0	0	0
Aortic stenosis	0	0	+	+	0	0	0	+	+	+	0	0	0	0	+++	0	0
Idiopathic hypertrophic subaortic stenosis	+	0	++	0	+	0	0	++	++	++	0	0	0	0	+++	0	++
Pulmonary stenosis	0	0	0	0	0	0	++	0	0	0	+	+	+++	0	0	0	0
Ventricular septal defect	+	0	0	0	0	0	0	+	+	0	0	0	0	+++	0	+	0
Patent ductus arteriosus	+	0	0	0	0	0	0	++	+	+	0	0	0	+++	0	+	0
Tetralogy of Fallot	0	0	+	0	0	0	++	0	+	0	+	0	+++	0	0	+	0
Coarctation of aorta	+	0	0	0	0	0	0	+	+	0	0	0	0	0	++	0	0
Eisenmenger's syndrome	+	0	+	0	0	0	++	0	0	0	+	0	+++	0	0	+	0
Atrial septal defect (primum)	++	+	0	++	0	0	+	+	+++	0	+	+++	+	+	0	+	0
Corrected transposition*	+	+	0	+++	+	0	+	+	+	0	0	0	0	+	+	+	+++
Ebstein's anomaly	++	+++	0	+	++	0	+++	0	+	0	+++	+	0	0	0	0	0
Tricuspid atresia	+	+	+	0	0	0	+++	+	+++	+	0	0	0	+	+	0	+
Congenital anomalies of coronary arteries	+	0	++	0	0	0	0	++	++	+	0	0	0	+	+	0	+++
Transposition of great arteries (postop)	+	++	0	+	0	0	+	0	0	0	0	0	+++	0	0	0	0

+++ = Almost always seen (characteristic of defect).
++ = Commonly seen with defect.
+ = Sometimes seen with defect (especially with associated defects or advancing age).
0 = Rarely seen with defect.

*The precordial QRS progression in corrected transposition may mimic left ventricular hypertrophy, usually with ST-segment abnormalities. True hypertrophy of the left-sided ventricle can occur in corrected transposition from associated left atrioventricular valvular regurgitation, ventricular septal defect, and so on.

From Ellison, R. C., and Sloss, L. J.: Electrocardiographic features of congenital heart disease in the adult. *In* Roberts, W. C. (ed.): Congenital Heart Disease in Adults. Philadelphia, F. A. Davis Co., 1979, p. 267.

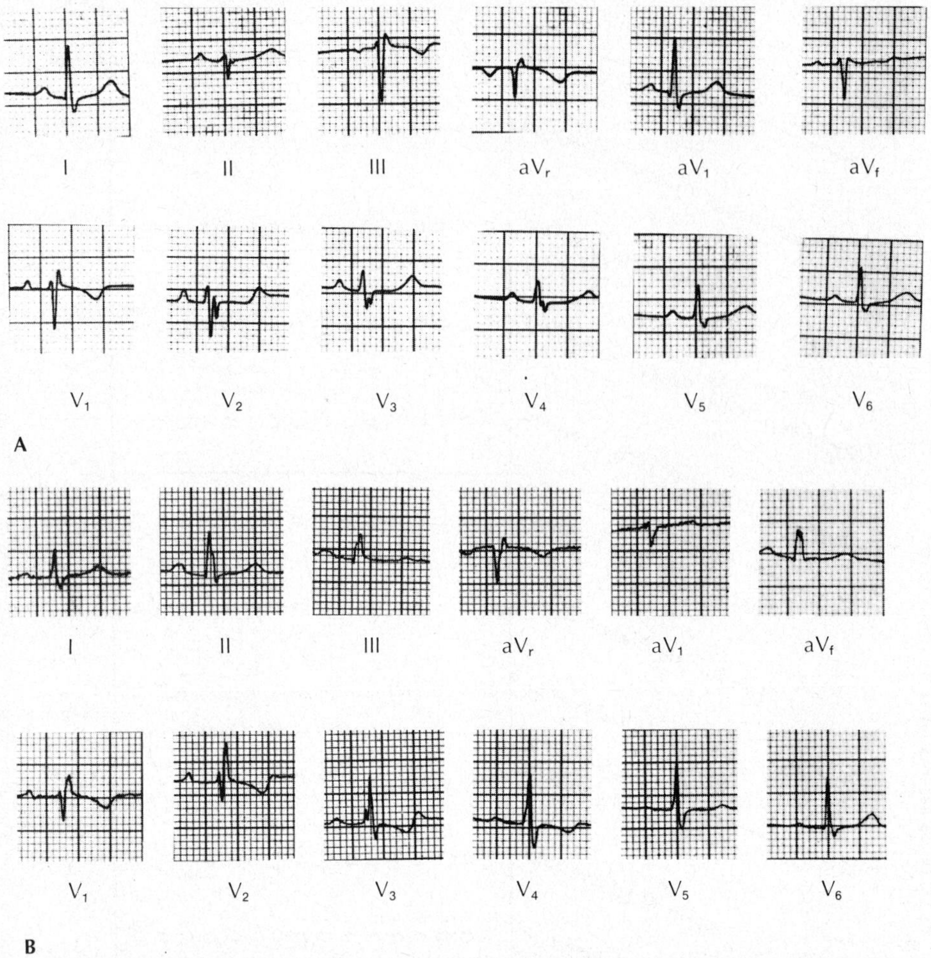

FIGURE 30–3 Representative 12-lead electrocardiograms (ECG) in adults with congenital heart disease. *A*, ECG of a 36-year-old woman with an ostium primum atrial septal defect, a large atrial left-to-right shunt with normal pulmonary pressures, and trivial mitral valve dysfunction. The P-R interval is upper normal. The P waves show evidence of mild right atrial overload in the precordial leads. There is a superior QRS axis and rather subtle evidence of volume-overload right ventricular hypertrophy ("incomplete right bundle branch block" pattern). *B*, ECG of a 52-year-old woman with a large left-to-right shunt via an ostium secundum atrial septal defect; pulmonary pressures are normal. The tracing shows borderline first-degree atrioventricular block and findings typical of volume-overload right ventricular hypertrophy. The P wave shows slight evidence of right atrial overload in the precordial leads, and the QRS axis is normal. *C*, ECG of a 21-year-old man with severe valvular pulmonic stenosis. Right ventricular peak systolic pressure is considerably higher than systemic levels. The P wave reflects right atrial overload, and the P-R interval is at the upper limit of normal. There is marked right-axis deviation and right ventricular hypertrophy with "strain." Left ventricular forces are not apparent. *D*, ECG of a 45-year-old man who presented with cyanosis and congestive heart failure of recent onset. Catheterization revealed a large persistent ductus arteriosus, pulmonary hypertension, and a bidirectional shunt. The tracing shows predominant right atrial and lesser left atrial overload. There is prolongation of the QRS complex with left anterior fascicular block and biventricular hypertrophy. (From Ellison, R. C., and Sloss, L. J.: Electrocardiographic features of congenital heart disease in the adult. *In* Roberts, W. C. (ed.): Congenital Heart Disease in Adults. Philadelphia, F. A. Davis Co., 1979, p. 119.)

Illustration continues on opposite page.

Physical Examination. Adults with ASD are usually normal in appearance, although a gracile habitus is relatively common. Occasionally the left precordium is prominent or even bulging. Cyanosis and digital clubbing may be seen in individuals with pulmonary hypertension and right-to-left shunts. Skeletal malformations characteristic of the autosomal dominant Holt-Oram syndrome may be present and consist of the inability to appose the thumb (which may have an accessory phalanx or be rudimentary) and a variety of other osseous changes involving the upper extremities (p. 1616).[46] The major differences in the cardiac examination between children and adults with ASD are that in the adult there is usually more marked widening of the two components of the second heart sound and the mid-diastolic rumble due to increased flow across the tricuspid valve is less common.

Patients with severe pulmonary hypertension often have fourth heart sounds originating from the right ventricle and may also demonstrate murmurs of pulmonic and/or tricuspid regurgitation, a pulmonic ejection sound, and an accentuated pulmonic component of the second heart sound.[46a] There is an association between ostium secundum ASD and mitral valve prolapse,[39,47–49] and findings typical of both conditions are often found on physical examination. A murmur of clinically significant mitral regurgitation may be present in older patients with mitral valve abnormalities.

Electrocardiographic Findings (Table 30–2). Atrial

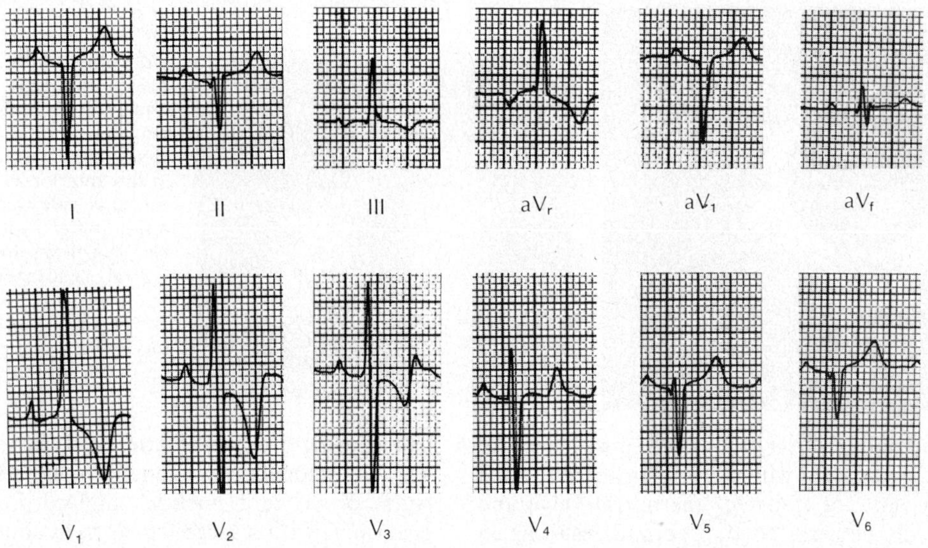

C

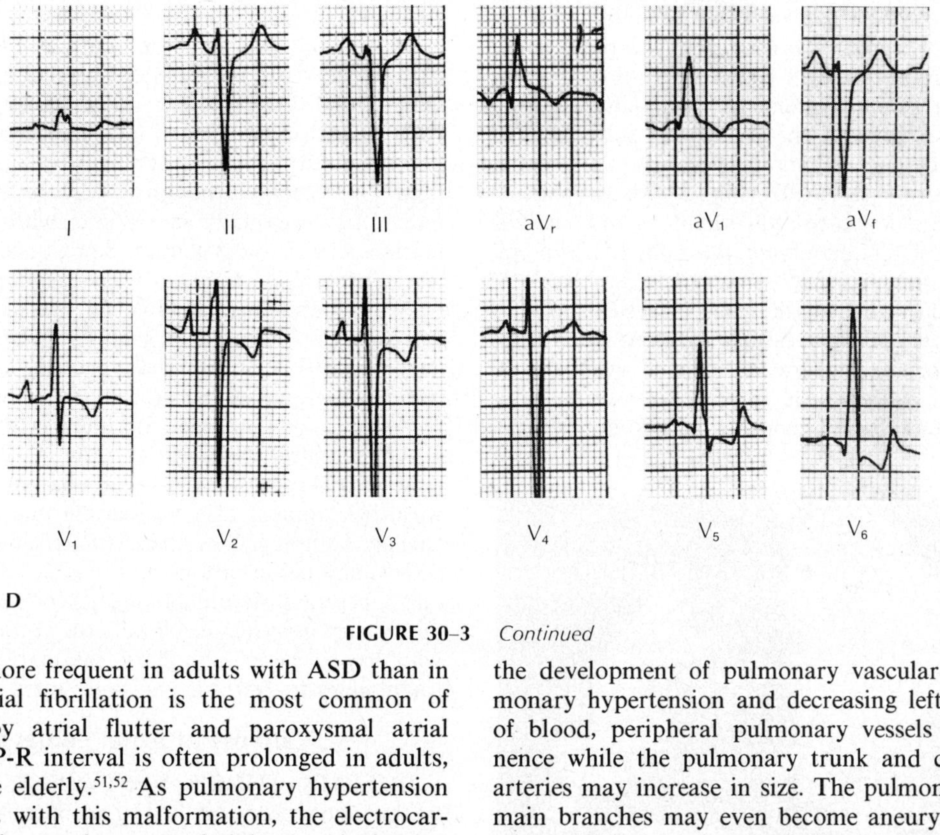

D

FIGURE 30–3 *Continued*

arrhythmias are more frequent in adults with ASD than in children.[43,44,50] Atrial fibrillation is the most common of these, followed by atrial flutter and paroxysmal atrial tachycardia. The P-R interval is often prolonged in adults, particularly in the elderly.[51,52] As pulmonary hypertension develops in adults with this malformation, the electrocardiogram reflects the development of right ventricular hypertrophy. Coexisting conditions, such as ischemic or hypertensive heart disease, which are common in adults, produce distinctive alterations that are superimposed on those already present on the ECG recording. Patients with ostium primum and secundum defects can frequently be distinguished electrocardiographically: The latter usually have a normal QRS axis, while the former usually manifest left-axis deviation (Fig. 30–3*A* and *B*).[52,53] Patients with sinus venosus atrial septal defects frequently have an ectopic atrial rhythm.

Roentgenographic Findings. The peripheral pulmonary vascular bed may be plethoric in adults with ASD and large left-to-right shunt (see Fig. 6–28, p. 166). With the development of pulmonary vascular obstruction, pulmonary hypertension and decreasing left-to-right shunting of blood, peripheral pulmonary vessels lose their prominence while the pulmonary trunk and central pulmonary arteries may increase in size. The pulmonary artery and its main branches may even become aneurysmal, with calcification of the vessel wall similar to that of the aortic wall in patients with systemic hypertension.

Echocardiographic Findings (see also page 120). The M-mode echocardiogram usually shows right ventricular dilatation, often associated with paradoxical or flattened movement of the ventricular septum. In the absence of mitral regurgitation, the left ventricle frequently appears decreased in size. This may reflect diminished left ventricular preload as well as an alteration in left ventricular geometry due to right ventricular dilatation.[41,54] Mitral valve prolapse may be present. Two-dimensional echocardiography can be useful in determining which anatomical type of ASD is present.[55,56] Visualization of the interatrial septum from the subcostal transducer position is particularly helpful for

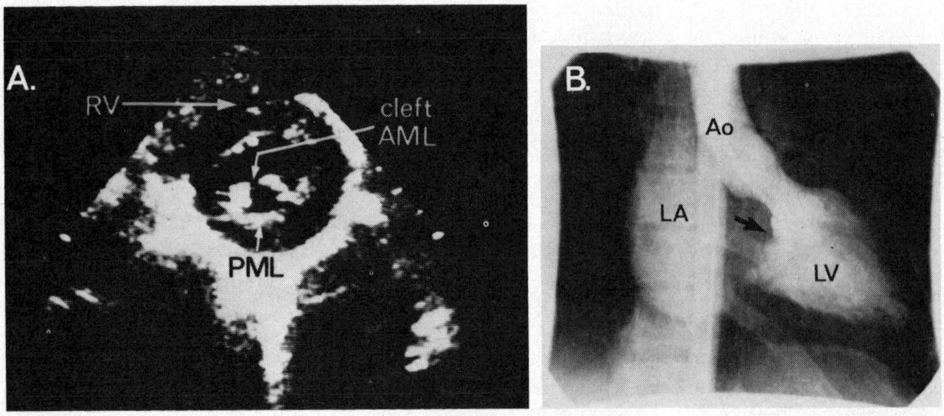

FIGURE 30–4 Studies from a 27-year-old patient with a primum atrial septal defect and cleft mitral valve. *A*, Two-dimensional echocardiographic study performed with the transducer in the short-axis parasternal position. The cleft in the anterior leaflet of the mitral valve (AML) is indicated (arrow). PML = posterior mitral leaflet; RV = right ventricle. *B*, Left ventriculogram showing the typical "gooseneck deformity" of the left ventricular (LV) outflow tract. The mitral valve cleft is indicated (arrow). Moderate mitral regurgitation is present. LA = left atrium; Ao = aorta.

distinguishing a secundum from a sinus venosus type of defect (Fig. 30–2). Patients with a primum ASD often have a cleft in the anterior leaflet of the mitral valve and abnormal chordal attachments to the septum, resulting in a characteristic two-dimensional echo pattern (Fig. 30–4).

Contrast injections of either indocyanine dye or saline into a peripheral arm vein can enhance the ability to diagnose an ASD.[57–60] In patients with a left-to-right shunt across the interatrial septum, a contrast-free area may be noted in the right atrium because of blood shunted from the left atrium washing out the "contrast" substance. In patients with right-to-left shunts, it is possible to visualize contrast echoes across the ASD (Fig. 30–5). In patients suspected of having a left-to-right shunt, a radionuclide scan can be helpful in quantifying the pulmonary-to-systemic blood flow ratio (p. 359).[61] It is not unreasonable to send a young adult patient with typical physical findings of an ASD to surgery without cardiac catheterization if (1) there is evidence of right ventricular volume overload, (2) the anterior leaflet of the mitral valve appears normal, (3) right-to-left shunting is not evident on two-dimensional echocardiographic evaluation, (4) there is no electrocardiographic evidence of pulmonary hypertension, and (5) results of a radionuclide angiocardiographic study are consistent with a large left-to-right shunt.[62]

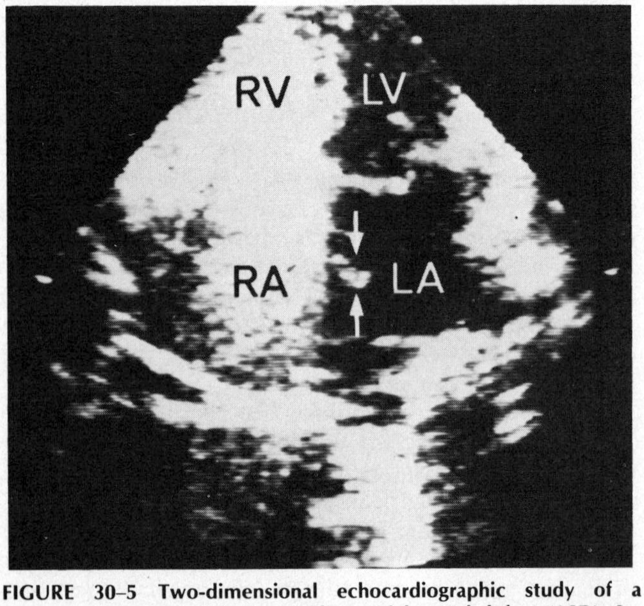

FIGURE 30–5 Two-dimensional echocardiographic study of a 53-year-old patient with a secundum atrial septal defect (ASD). Saline was injected into a peripheral arm vein, resulting in contrast echoes in the right atrium (RA) and right ventricle (RV). In addition, contrast echoes are seen crossing the ASD (arrows) into the left atrium (LA), confirming the presence of a right-to-left shunt at the atrial level. LV = left ventricle.

Surgical Treatment. Since it is impossible to predict whether pulmonary hypertension will develop in a patient with ASD, we recommend closure of defects (even in asymptomatic patients) for adults under 45 years of age with left-to-right shunts that result in a pulmonary-to-systemic blood flow ratio exceeding 1.5:1.0.[35,63,63a] Even elderly patients with large shunts have been shown to benefit from operation.[43,44,64] The risk of this procedure is very low (less than 1 per cent), although it is somewhat higher in older individuals, especially in patients with pulmonary hypertension and/or heart failure. Some residual right ventricular dysfunction frequently persists postoperatively in patients operated upon after the age of 40 years. Surgical correction is indicated in such patients as long as pulmonary blood flow substantially exceeds systemic blood flow (ratio $>2:1$), unless severe left ventricular dysfunction is responsible for the shunt. In adults with ASD and moderate pulmonary hypertension, the net left-to-right shunt may be quite small; however, it may increase considerably with development of a myocardial infarction and left ventricular failure. Under these circumstances, closure of the defect may be hazardous and may lead to pulmonary edema. Operation should not be performed in patients with pulmonary-to-systemic blood flow ratios less than 1.5:1.0 who have severe pulmonary vascular obstructive disease (pulmonary-to-systemic resistance ratio $\geq 0.7:1.0$).

Variants of Atrial Septal Defect

LUTEMBACHER'S SYNDROME. This term refers to the combination of ASD and mitral stenosis.[65] The latter is almost invariably rheumatic in origin. Lutembacher's syndrome is more common in adults than in children; only rarely does congenital mitral stenosis coexist with ASD.[65] Patients with this syndrome are invariably symptomatic, complaining of exertional dyspnea, fatigue, and palpitations. Orthopnea and paroxysmal nocturnal dyspnea are rare, and hemoptysis does not appear to occur. The ASD exerts a protective effect on the mitral stenosis by decompressing the left atrium and the pulmonary venous system, resulting in a large left-to-right shunt. Severe pulmonary congestion or edema does not occur in these patients unless the ASD is repaired without relief of the mitral stenosis.

The findings on *physical examination* suggest both lesions, i.e., a parasternal right ventricular heave and widely split second heart sound are uniformly present and a loud first heart sound and opening snap are also frequently heard. The *electrocardiogram* usually reveals right ventricular hypertrophy, while the chest roentgenogram shows pulmonary plethora and right atrial and ventricular enlargement. Elevated right atrial pressure with prominent *v* waves is a constant finding in patients with Lutembacher's syndrome.[65] The systemic flow index is usually low, while pulmonary blood flow is markedly elevated; thus, the pulmonary-to-systemic blood flow ratio is quite high.

PATENT FORAMEN OVALE. Patency of the foramen ovale is common,[66] with "pencil patent" foramina (0.6 to 1.0 cm in diameter) occurring in 6 per cent and "probe patent" foramina (0.2 to 0.5 cm in diameter) occurring in 29 to 35 per cent of adults at autopsy.[67] Patency of the foramen ovale produces no abnormality on physical examination, electrocardiogram, or chest roentgenogram.[66] Its presence may be deduced by means of a dilution curve obtained from injecting indicator dye into a systemic vein or the inferior vena cava and sampling from a systemic artery (p. 290) during a Valsalva maneuver; early appearance of the indicator dye is diagnostic of a right-to-left shunt. Contrast echocardiography can be used in a similar manner. This defect is significant only in that it is a potential route for paradoxical embolism.[66] Left-to-right shunts do not usually occur.

ANOMALOUS PULMONARY VENOUS DRAINAGE (see also page 1011). Partial anomalous pulmonary venous drainage occurs when one or more (but not all) of the pulmonary veins drain into the right atrium or systemic venous circulation rather than into the left atrium.[68-70] This malformation is often associated with an ASD of the sinus venosus type. When partial anomalous venous return is associated with ASD, the natural history, physical examination, electrocardiogram, and chest roentgenogram are usually indistinguishable from those for patients with isolated ASD. Patients with partial anomalous venous drainage and an *intact* atrial septum usually show respirophasic variation of the second heart sound and can thereby be distinguished from patients with associated ASD. Systolic flow murmurs across the pulmonary outflow tract and diastolic murmurs across the tricuspid orifice are common in patients with anomalous pulmonary venous return and an intact atrial septum. Electrocardiographic and roentgenographic findings are identical to those in patients with ASD. When the entire right lung drains into the inferior vena cava (the "scimitar syndrome"), the anomalous vein can sometimes be identified on the plain chest roentgenogram.

Identification of this anomaly may be difficult. Techniques that have been successful in establishing this diagnosis at the time of catheterization include differential indicator-dye dilution curves from the right and left main pulmonary arteries, careful probing of the atrial septum with a catheter, and pulmonary angiography and selective injection of contrast media into an anomalous pulmonary vein that has been entered by a catheter during cardiac catheterization.[68] Right heart pressures are usually normal. In most patients with anomalous pulmonary venous return and an intact atrial septum, the left-to-right shunt is usually modest in size (i.e., pulmonary-to-systemic blood flow ratio less than 2:1). Pulmonary hypertension rarely develops in these patients. Surgical correction consists of incorporating the site of drainage of the anomalous vein into the left atrium and closing the ASD, if it is present. Operation is usually indicated when the pulmonary-to-systemic blood flow ratio exceeds 1.5:1.0.[69]

Total anomalous pulmonary venous return (p. 1008) is rarely seen in adults.

Ventricular Septal Defect (See also page 963)

Ventricular septal defect (VSD) is the most common congenital malformation reported in infants and children. However, in adults, VSD is surpassed in frequency by ASD, a change that can be related to three factors: First—and most importantly—a significant number of VSD (even those with large left-to-right shunts) close spontaneously during infancy or childhood; occasionally, spontaneous closure occurs during adulthood.[71] Second, patients with VSD may die of heart failure early in life. Finally, many patients with VSD now undergo surgical closure of the defect during childhood.

Patients with moderate or large VSD without pulmonary vascular obstructive disease experience significant left-to-right shunting with volume overload of the left atrium and ventricle. Left ventricular hypertrophy is noted early in life. Although symptoms of left ventricular failure may develop in infants with VSD, left heart failure is generally *not* part of the natural history of this congenital defect in patients over 2 years of age unless aortic regurgitation or infective endocarditis supervene (see below).[71] Maron and coworkers,[72] and Lueker et al.[73] used exercise testing to evaluate postoperative cardiovascular function in adult patients with surgically closed VSD. In several patients they found normal hemodynamic measurements at rest but abnormal values with vigorous exercise, and they concluded that postoperative left ventricular function may be abnormal in patients who undergo closure of a large VSD at an older age. However, both studies assessed left ventricular function in patients whose defects were repaired during the 1960s when the myocardial preservation techniques used were inferior to those currently available. How much effect intraoperative myocardial ischemia had on postoperative left ventricular performance in these patients is unknown.

Recently, rest and exercise ventricular performance were compared using equilibrium gated radionuclide angiography in 34 patients (mean age 27 years) with hemodynamically documented VSD.[73a] The response of left ventricular ejection fraction to dynamic exercise was abnormal in patients who previously underwent surgical closure of VSD as well as in patients with residual defects. This again raises the issue of whether lifelong left ventricular volume overload may be detrimental to myocardial function.

Complications that accompany VSD in adult life include aortic regurgitation, infective endocarditis, pulmonary hypertension, infundibular pulmonic stenosis, and heart failure.[74]

Aortic regurgitation was noted in 5.5 per cent of all patients with a VSD followed in the Natural History Study of Congenital Heart Disease.[75] In most cases the VSD was either infracristal (membranous) or subpulmonic. No patient under 2 years of age had this combination of lesions, supporting the impression that the aortic regurgitation is an acquired problem. Of the 34 patients over 11 years of

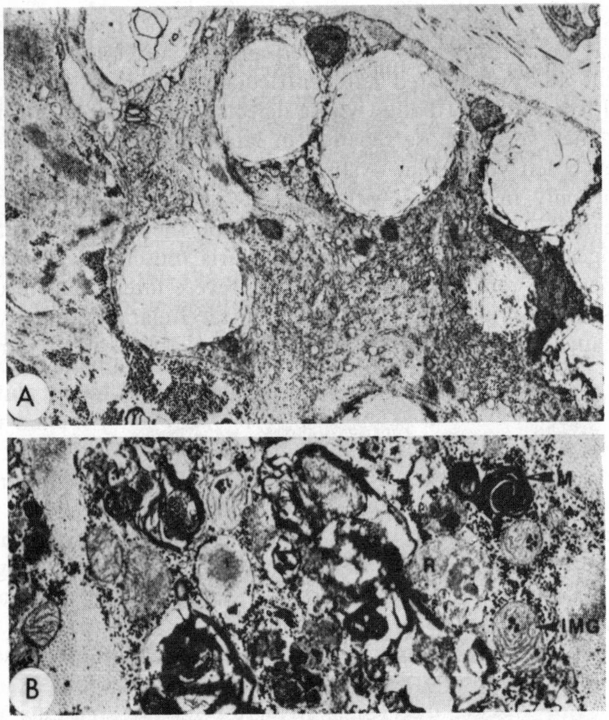

FIGURE 30–8 *A,* Electron micrograph of degenerated cardiac muscle cells from a 33-year-old man with tetralogy of Fallot. Normal myofibrillar structure has been completely lost, and the cells contain large lipid droplets, vesicles of sarcoplasmic reticulum, masses of Z-band material, glycogen particles, and actin filaments. Electron-dense lamellae are present at the periphery of the lipid droplets. (×16,000, reduced by 18 per cent.) *B,* Portion of a muscle cell from a 36-year-old man with valvular and infundibular pulmonic stenosis and an atrial septal defect. The cell contains numerous myelin figures (M), residual bodies (R) of lysosomal origin, and deposits of intramitochondrial glycogen (IMG). Extramitochondrial glycogen and myofibrils are normal. (×27,000 reduced by 18 per cent.) (From Jones, M., and Ferrans, V. J.: Myocardial degeneration in congenital heart disease. Am. J. Cardiol. *39*:1051, 1977.)

ples obtained from children with tetralogy of Fallot (Figs. 30–7 and 30–8).[87] It is possible that such degenerative changes in the myocardium affect cardiac function adversely and are, in part, the cause of heart failure and arrhythmias in older patients with tetralogy of Fallot.

Adults with tetralogy complain frequently of severe headaches, dizziness, and episodes of exertional chest pain that resemble angina pectoris in character.[86] Their chronic hypoxemia stimulates release of increased amounts of erythropoietin, resulting in polycythemia. A hematocrit exceeding 65 per cent is associated with marked increases in blood viscosity and resistance to blood flow and substantially increases the possibility of intravascular thrombosis, thrombotic strokes, and paradoxical emboli. These patients are also at risk for brain abscesses and attacks of acute gouty arthritis, the latter resulting from a high turnover of erythrocyte nucleic acid and subsequent hyperuricemia. Women with unrepaired tetralogy of Fallot tolerate pregnancy poorly, and there is an increased incidence of fetal demise as well as of small-for-gestational-age babies.[89]

Laboratory Findings. The *electrocardiogram* is characterized by right-axis deviation, right ventricular hypertrophy, and, in older patients, a right ventricular conduction abnormality. By middle age, the patient with uncorrected tetralogy may develop atrial fibrillation or flutter.

The *roentgenographic* appearance of tetralogy of Fallot (Fig. 29–43, p. 991), which is classic for infants and children (i.e., a small, boot-shaped heart and pulmonary hypovascularity), is less typical in adults, who often have less distinctive cardiac silhouettes and normal-sized hearts on the posteroanterior chest roentgenogram; right ventricular enlargement is frequently but not invariably noted on the lateral view. Pulmonary vascularity is normal or even increased in almost half the adult patients, particularly those who are acyanotic.[86] Adults with tetralogy of Fallot usually have well-developed systemic-to-pulmonary collateral vessels that can be visualized during angiography and that may account for the long survival of some adults who do not undergo palliative or corrective surgical procedures for this defect.[86,90]

M-mode echocardiography (Fig. 24–44, p. 991) can be used to document the abnormal relationship between the aortic annulus and the interventricular septum. The VSD can occasionally be visualized as dropout of septal echoes. A *two-dimensional echocardiographic* examination gives information regarding the presence and degree of aortic overriding, the extent and location of the infundibular obstruction, the size of the pulmonic valve and main pulmonary artery, and the degree of right ventricular hypertrophy.

The major information to be obtained at *cardiac catheterization and angiography* includes the size of the pulmonary annulus and pulmonary arteries and the severity of right ventricular outflow tract obstruction. In patients with prior surgical systemic–to–pulmonary artery shunts, kinking of the pulmonary artery may have occurred at the anastomotic site, resulting in peripheral pulmonic stenosis. Angiography is also useful in locating collateral vessels, defining the coronary artery anatomy, and determining the significance of associated or acquired anomalies.

Surgical Treatment. Potential risks of palliative shunts include continued right-to-left shunting at the ventricular level with paradoxical emboli, endocarditis, and the development of pulmonary vascular obstructive disease. As a general rule, the adult patient with tetralogy of Fallot and a palliative shunt should undergo total operative repair. Total repair of tetralogy of Fallot can be undertaken in adults with a mortality rate comparable to that reported for children.[91,92,92a] Surgery usually consists of right infundibulectomy, pulmonary valvulotomy, patch closure of the ventricular septal defect with direction of the left ventricular outflow tract into the aorta, and a right ventricular outflow tract patch. Postoperative bleeding from extensive collateral vessels and impaired postoperative cardiac function may pose special problems in adults. Residual obstruction to right ventricular outflow and/or pulmonary regurgitation as well as VSD are the most common anatomical problems after repair.[91–94] Electrophysiological abnormalities include right bundle branch block; left anterior hemiblock; prolonged intra-atrial, AV nodal, and His-Purkinje conduction times; and complete heart block.[95–97] Several studies have shown a correlation between resting or exercise-induced ventricular arrhythmias, abnormal hemodynamics, and sudden death.[95–98] Ventricular ectopic activity may be a late developing phenomenon and may increase in severity with longer postoperative intervals.[98] Postoperative patients with tetralogy of Fallot who have ventricular arrhythmias should be treated aggressively with antiarrhythmic drugs.[96,98,98a]

Pulmonic Stenosis (See also page 986)

Pulmonic stenosis is among the more common congenital cardiac malformations in adults.[99] Prior to the development of surgical treatment, survival to age 50 and beyond was uncommon. However, even some infants with severe pulmonic stenosis have been known to survive into adult life without surgical correction. This undoubtedly reflects the tendency for the stenotic pulmonic valve orifice to enlarge somewhat as body size increases. On the other hand, a congenitally deformed pulmonic valve may become more fibrotic, thickened, and calcified in later adult life, thus reducing valve mobility and effective valve area. Also, the development of subvalvular muscular hypertrophy (i.e., infundibular stenosis), may occur and contributes further to the obstruction to right ventricular outflow. This occurs most often in older children and adults with valvular stenosis and can pose major difficulties in the early postoperative period unless resection of the infundibulum is carried out along with pulmonic valvulotomy.

Clinical Findings. Most adult patients with mild (right ventricular systolic pressure less than 75 mm Hg) to moderate (pressure between 75 and 100 mm Hg) pulmonic stenosis are asymptomatic. In adults with severe stenosis, dyspnea and fatigue secondary to an inadequate response of cardiac output to exercise are the most common symptoms.[100,101] Orthopnea does not occur in these patients, since their pulmonary venous pressure is normal; a small right-to-left shunt through a patent foramen ovale is common. Eventually, patients with more severe grades of pulmonic stenosis develop tricuspid regurgitation and frank right ventricular failure, which may ultimately become intractable and lead to death. Exertional syncope or lightheadedness occasionally occurs in patients with severe pulmonic stenosis, but sudden death is extremely rare.[100]

Chest pain resembling angina pectoris occasionally develops in children but is observed most frequently in adults with severe pulmonic stenosis in whom right ventricular oxygen requirements are greatly increased.[100,101] Patchy fibrosis of the hypertrophied right ventricle is a common finding in such patients at postmortem examination.

The physical findings, electrocardiogram (Fig. 30–3*C*), echocardiogram, and roentgenogram in adults are similar to those in children (p. 987). Calcification of the pulmonic valve, when present on roentgenography, is a sign of longstanding obstruction and is therefore usually seen only in adults.[101] With valvular calcification, the pulmonic ejection sound—an important auscultatory feature of mild or moderate pulmonic stenosis—disappears. It has been suggested that lung size, airway dimensions and conductance, and pulmonary diffusing capacity are reduced in adults with severe pulmonic stenosis.[102]

Treatment. It is generally agreed that symptomatic adults with pulmonic stenosis should undergo pulmonic valvulotomy.[4] Moreover, there is a consensus that when right ventricular systolic pressure at rest is less than 75 mm Hg, pulmonic stenosis is well tolerated, and such asymptomatic patients rarely if ever require surgical treatment.[100] More controversial is the question of whether asymptomatic adults with moderate or severe pulmonic stenosis (i.e., right ventricular systolic pressures exceeding 77 mm Hg) should undergo pulmonic valvulotomy. Johnson et al. reported two patients with severe pulmonic stenosis who were in their fifties.[100] These authors advised that surgical therapy be reserved for adults with symptomatic pulmonic stenosis. In general, since operative treatment by a skilled surgical team entails little risk, patients with right ventricular systolic pressures exceeding 75 mm Hg in the basal state should probably undergo surgery, regardless of symptoms.[103] Exercise capacity generally improves in symptomatic patients after successful surgery. When valvulotomy is performed, postoperative pulmonic regurgitation is common. Older patients, who seldom tolerate moderate or severe pulmonic regurgitation, may require pulmonic valve replacement.

PULMONARY ARTERY STENOSIS (see also page 985). **Stenosis of the pulmonary artery (the main vessel or a branch, single or multiple)** is commonly associated with other congenital malformations, including ASD and VSD, supravalvular aortic stenosis, persistent ductus arteriosus, tetralogy of Fallot, and the congenital rubella syndrome. Occasionally, the malformation occurs in an isolated form. Since pulmonary arterial stenosis is usually not lethal, an increasing number of patients with peripheral pulmonary artery stenosis are being recognized in adult life. The principal complication is right ventricular pressure overload. Poststenotic dilatation of peripheral pulmonary arterial branches occasionally leads to the formation of thin-walled aneurysms that can rupture and produce significant hemoptysis.[104,105] If the pulmonic valve is normal in these patients, pulmonic ejection sounds are absent, and splitting of the second heart sound is usually normal. The systolic murmurs are typically crescendo-decrescendo and are widely distributed over the thorax. Occasionally, stenosis in a pulmonary arterial branch gives rise to a continuous murmur. This occurs most frequently when moderate to severe pulmonary artery hypertension is present proximal to the area of narrowing and reflects the existence of a pressure gradient across the stenotic site throughout the cardiac cycle.

If stenosis of the pulmonary arterial branch is sufficiently close to the main pulmonary artery, and if there are no further peripheral branch stenoses, a graft can be constructed to bypass the obstruction from the main pulmonary artery to the branch distal to the stenosis. Alternatively, patch grafts may be placed to enlarge the lumen at sites of obstruction. If the area of peripheral pulmonary artery stenosis extends into the lung parenchyma, effective surgical repair may not be possible.[106]

Idiopathic Dilatation of the Pulmonary Artery

This malformation is characterized by congenital dilatation of the main pulmonary artery and its branches in the absence of any apparent anatomical or physiological cause. It may be the result of a defect in the normal development of the pulmonary arterial elastic tissue. Patients with this disorder are asymptomatic. *Physical examination* may reveal a palpable pulmonary arterial impulse in the second left intercostal space, a pulmonic ejection sound, and a midsystolic murmur heard best in the second left intercosystolic pressure may occur, followed on the second or third day by a rise in diastolic pressure.[124] This hypertension that occurs within 24 hours of repair is associated with evidence of hyperactivity of the sympathetic nervous system, such as a decreased response to cold pressor stimuli[124] and markedly elevated plasma norepinephrine levels.[125] The paradoxical hypertension that occurs two to three days postoperatively is associated with a marked transient rise in plasma renin activity and is probably best treated with converting enzyme inhibitors or angiotensin II blocking agents.[124,126,127] Development of chronic persistent postoperative hypertension appears to be a function of age at the time of repair.

Optimal timing for surgery is one to five years of age. Even with early "correction," development of valvular stenosis or regurgitation secondary to a bicuspid aortic valve, residual stenosis at the coarctation site, or persistent hypertension at rest and particularly during exercise, despite apparently successful coarctectomy, may increase late mortality.[128]

OTHER FORMS OF CYANOTIC CONGENITAL HEART DISEASE

Cyanotic adults with congenital heart disease fall into two categories. The first includes patients with obligatory right-to-left shunts in whom cyanosis generally commences in infancy and often progresses (Table 30–3). Common examples are patients with tetralogy of Fallot or Ebstein's anomaly of the tricuspid valve. The number of patients with congenital tricuspid atresia (p. 994) who survive to adulthood is increasing due to successful palliative surgery

TABLE 30–3 CYANOTIC CONGENITAL HEART DISEASE IN ADULTS

I. Lesions Relatively Frequently Encountered
A. Reduced pulmonary blood flow
1. Tetralogy of Fallot (pulmonic stenosis with ventricular septal defect)
2. Pulmonic atresia with ventricular septal defect
3. Pulmonic stenosis with atrial right-to-left shunt
B. Increased pulmonary vascular resistance
1. Ventricular septal defect with Eisenmenger reaction
2. Patent ductus arteriosus with Eisenmenger reaction
3. Atrial septal defect with Eisenmenger reaction
II. Lesions Less Frequently Encountered
A. Reduced pulmonary blood flow
1. Single ventricle with pulmonic stenosis or atresia
2. Tricuspid atresia with pulmonic stenosis or atresia or small ventricular septal defect
3. Transposition with pulmonic stenosis or atresia
B. Increased pulmonary vascular resistance
1. Single ventricle with Eisenmenger reaction
2. Transposition with Eisenmenger reaction
3. Truncus arteriosus
C. Ebstein's anomaly with atrial right-to-left shunt
III. Lesions Rarely Encountered
A. Double-outlet right ventricle with or without pulmonic stenosis
B. Congenital pulmonary arteriovenous fistula
C. Congenital vena caval to left atrial communication
D. Mitral atresia
E. Double-outlet left ventricle
F. Asplenia or polysplenia syndromes
G. Total anomalous pulmonary venous return

From Graham, T. P., Jr., and Friesinger, G. C.: Complex cyanotic congenital heart disease in adults. *In* Roberts, W. C. (ed.): Congenital Heart Disease in Adults. Philadelphia, F. A. Davis Co., 1979, p. 383.

TABLE 30–4 CONGENITAL CARDIAC LESIONS THAT CAN BE COMPLICATED BY THE EISENMENGER REACTION

Aortic Shunts
Patent ductus arteriosus
Aorticopulmonary septal defect
Truncus arteriosus
Pulmonic atresia, ventricular septal defect, and large "bronchial" collateral vessels
Ventricular Shunts
Ventricular septal defect
Single ventricle
Transposition of the great arteries with ventricular septal defect
Double-outlet right ventricle
Tricuspid atresia and ventricular septal defect without pulmonic stenosis
Mitral atresia and ventricular septal defect or single ventricle
Atrioventricular canal
Atrial Shunts
Atrial septal defect: secundum, primum, sinus venosus
Common atrium
Total anomalous pulmonary venous return
Partial anomalous pulmonary venous return
Transposition with atrial septal defect

From Graham, T. P., Jr.: The Eisenmenger reaction and its management. *In* Roberts, W. C. (ed.): Congenital Heart Disease in Adults. Philadelphia, F. A. Davis Co., 1979, p. 531.

during childhood and the development of a physiological repair using the Fontan procedure.[129–132] Rarely, patients with anomalies such as transposition of the great arteries, pulmonary atresia, truncus arteriosus, and single ventricle survive to adult life (Table 30–3).[133,134] In a few instances, surgical correction of these lesions during adult life has been successful.[135]

The second category includes patients in whom the right-to-left shunt occurs as a consequence of pulmonary vascular disease. While the term *Eisenmenger's complex* refers to VSD, pulmonary vascular disease, and right-to-left shunting of blood,[135,136] the term *Eisenmenger's syndrome* is used to describe any communication between the systemic and pulmonary circulation that produces pulmonary vascular disease of such severity that right-to-left shunting occurs (Table 30–4). Most of these patients become cyanotic in adolescence or early adult life; the cyanosis and disability are generally progressive. Significant clubbing and polycythemia are usually present in adults with Eisenmenger's syndrome.

Surgical intervention is generally contraindicated in patients with Eisenmenger's syndrome because elevated pulmonary vascular resistance persists or worsens after surgical closure of the defect[136,137]; frequently the result is severe right ventricular failure. Although the long-term outlook for patients with Eisenmenger's syndrome who are not operated upon is guarded because survival beyond the age of 50 years is unusual, it is often true that these patients may lead reasonably active and productive lives through early adulthood.

Death often occurs suddenly in these patients, although symptomatic arrhythmias do not usually pose a problem. Heart failure is a common complication of adults with Eisenmenger's syndrome, but it can usually be controlled by medical therapy and is not severely disabling. Although chest pain, syncopal attacks, and hemoptysis have been traditionally considered to be ominous prognostic signs, more recent studies have questioned this observation.

However, pregnancy is often life-threatening in patients with Eisenmenger's syndrome.[138]

EBSTEIN'S ANOMALY OF THE TRICUSPID VALVE

(See also page 996)

The principal abnormality of Ebstein's anomaly is downward displacement of a malformed tricuspid valve into an underdeveloped right ventricle with reduced pumping capacity.[139,140] The presence of a portion of the right ventricle between the atrioventricular groove and the downward displaced origin of the septal and posterior leaflets of the tricuspid valve results in a direct communication between the right atrium and the "atrialized" right ventricle. The degree of hemodynamic compromise to right ventricular function depends on the amount of right ventricular tissue above the tricuspid valve as well as the extent of adherence of the valve tissue to the right ventricular wall. The atrialized portion of the right ventricle is usually hypokinetic, contributing little to the ventricle's forward stroke volume. Tricuspid regurgitation, a problem frequently associated with Ebstein's anomaly, further compromises effective right ventricular output.[141] Many patients with Ebstein's anomaly have a concomitant interatrial communication (an atrial septal defect or patent foramen ovale) that allows right-to-left shunting of blood.

Cyanosis occurs in about three fourths of adult patients with this malformation and may appear or become worse with exercise, fatigue, or exposure to cold. In the other one fourth, right ventricular pumping capacity is almost normal. The severity of the anatomical abnormalities associated with Ebstein's anomaly is variable, with a considerable proportion of these patients surviving into adult life.[141,142] Patients with milder forms of Ebstein's anomaly may even have a normal life expectancy.[143]

Many patients remain asymptomatic until the third or fourth decade. Right ventricular failure, characterized by dyspnea, fatigue, weakness, and peripheral edema, usually marks the beginning of a downhill course for patients with Ebstein's anomaly; heart failure is the most common cause of death.[141,142] Syncope secondary to atrial and ventricular arrhythmias and precordial discomfort are also ominous signs. Palpitations are common, since patients with Ebstein's anomaly are prone to atrial and ventricular arrhythmias. Wolff-Parkinson-White syndrome (type B) occurs in 10 to 25 per cent of patients with this malformation.[141,144,145] Sudden death, presumably secondary to arrhythmias, occurs in as many as 20 per cent of adults with Ebstein's anomaly.[144] Paradoxical embolism and brain abscess are other common complications.

Two-dimensional echocardiography is useful in confirming the diagnosis of Ebstein's anomaly of the tricuspid valve as well as in assessing the significance of associated lesions (Fig. 30–11). Pulsed Doppler echocardiography is helpful in detecting tricuspid valvular regurgitation.[146]

Surgical treatment of Ebstein's anomaly has met with variable success. Operative approaches have included annuloplasty or replacement of the tricuspid valve, plication of the free wall of the atrialized portion of the right ventricle, right atrial reduction, and closure of the ASD.[147–150] If the right ventricle has sufficient capacity to accept the entire cardiac output, operative results may be salutary. If the right ventricle is diminutive and has a low compliance and pumping capacity, replacement of the tricuspid valve and closure of the interatrial communication result in severe, low-output right ventricular failure. Because of the rapid clinical deterioration that usually commences after the onset of right ventricular failure, surgical intervention should be considered for patients with this complication.

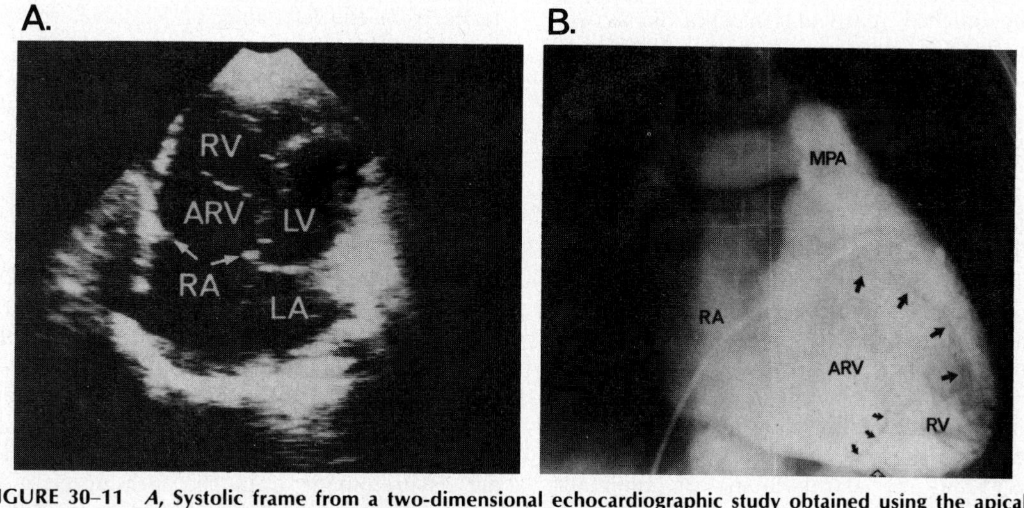

FIGURE 30–11 *A*, Systolic frame from a two-dimensional echocardiographic study obtained using the apical transducer position in a mildly cyanotic 25-year-old woman with a holosystolic murmur and multiple systolic clicks. Portions of the tricuspid valve are displaced downward into the right ventricle (RV). The arrows delineate the level of the atrioventricular (AV) groove. The portion of the RV between the AV groove and the downward displaced origin of the tricuspid valve leaflets is termed the "atrialized right ventricle" (ARV), an area that is hemodynamically right atrium (RA) but electrophysiologically RV. The true RA is enlarged. Both the left atrium (LA) and the left ventricle (LV) are decreased in size. Mitral valve prolapse is present. In other panels, right-to-left bowing of the interatrial septum was present, suggesting that the atrial septal defect was relatively small. Pulsed Doppler echocardiographic study confirmed the presence of tricuspid regurgitation. *B*, Right ventriculogram from the same patient demonstrating downward displacement of the large, sail-like anterior (straight solid arrows) and smaller posterior (curved solid arrows) leaflets of the tricuspid valve. A notch (open arrow) is apparent at the site of the anomalous insertion of the tricuspid valve. The RV is moderately hypoplastic. Pulmonic stenosis is not present. MPA = main pulmonary artery.

RIGHT VENTRICULAR DYSPLASIA

Right ventricular dysplasia is characterized by partial or total replacement of a portion of right ventricular musculature with fatty and fibrous tissue.[151–154] In its extreme, called *Uhl's anomaly,* there is apposition of endocardial and epicardial layers of the affected area.[155,156] Right ventricular dysplasia is more common in males and may be associated with mitral valve prolapse.[151] Adults with this lesion present frequently with palpitations or syncope. Ventricular tachycardia, usually with a left bundle branch block configuration, may be the predominant dysrhythmia. In a report of 24 patients with this condition, mean age at the time of hospitalization was 39 years.[151]

The cardiac examination in adults is often normal except for the right-sided fourth heart sound. Chest roentgenogram shows normal pulmonary blood flow with, at most, mild cardiomegaly. Two-dimensional echocardiography, which demonstrates right ventricular enlargement with normal left ventricular chamber size, can be helpful in distinguishing right ventricular dysplasia from other lesions such as Ebstein's anomaly of the tricuspid valve, atrial septal defect, anomalous pulmonary venous drainage, or congenital absence of the left pericardium.[151] At cardiac catheterization, angiography shows increased right ventricular size. In some cases, segmental motion abnormalities with systolic expansion of the infundibular area may be present.[151]

The pathogenesis and natural history of right ventricular dysplasia are unknown. Symptoms usually depend on the rate of the patient's tachyarrhythmia. Many patients with ventricular tachycardia respond to antiarrhythmic drug treatment; some require surgery, consisting of one or more ventricular incisions. The location of these incisions is based on the results of ventricular epicardial mapping performed during induced ventricular tachycardia as well as during either sinus or atrial paced rhythm.[151,152] Death resulting from ventricular fibrillation is infrequent.

CORONARY ARTERY ANOMALIES AND CORONARY ARTERIOVENOUS FISTULA

(See also page 971)

Four anomalies involving the coronary circulation are of particular significance in adults: (1) origin of one coronary artery from the pulmonary artery; (2) origin of both coronary arteries from the right sinus of Valsalva; (3) origin of both coronary arteries from the left sinus of Valsalva; and (4) coronary arteriovenous fistula.

When *both coronary arteries originate from the pulmonary artery,* death usually occurs soon after birth.[157] Patients with origin of the right coronary artery from the pulmonary artery may be asymptomatic or minimally symptomatic as long as right ventricular oxygen demands remain normal. However, as might be anticipated, pulmonary hypertension of any etiology is tolerated poorly in such individuals. This anomaly has been noted as an incidental autopsy finding in patients dying of other causes.

Approximately 15 per cent of patients with anomalous origin of the left coronary artery from the pulmonary are able to reach adulthood largely because of effective intercoronary collaterals that reduce the hazards of myocardial ischemia.[157–161] These individuals may have a history of transient exertional chest pain and left ventricular failure. Other adults with this malformation complain of angina and left ventricular failure; they may present with mitral regurgitation or sudden death.[162,163] Adults may exhibit continuous or diastolic murmurs along either sternal border or at the base of the heart; these arise as a consequence of flow through the collaterals and through reversal of flow in the anomalous coronary artery. In addition, these patients frequently have murmurs of mitral regurgitation because of ischemic injury to papillary muscles. Surgical treatment consists of placement of a saphenous vein graft connecting the left coronary artery to the aorta and ligation of the pulmonary arterial ostium of the left coronary artery.[163–165] Alternatively, the anomalous left coronary artery may be reimplanted into the aorta[166] or the left subclavian artery may be anastomosed to the anomalous left coronary artery.[167]

Origin of both coronary arteries from the right or left sinus of Valsalva has been recognized with increasing frequency since the widespread employment of coronary arteriography.[168] This anomaly has been noted in a little over 1 per cent of a large number of patients who underwent coronary arteriography. Patients with origin of both coronary arteries from the right sinus of Valsalva are prone to sudden death.[169] Cheitlin et al. noted 9 unexplained sudden deaths among 33 patients (27 per cent) in whom both coronary arteries arose from the right sinus of Valsalva, and they suggested that the mechanism of death was acute myocardial ischemia.[169] The latter was considered to develop when increased cardiac output resulted in dilatation of the aorta and pulmonary artery, thereby stretching and narrowing the left coronary artery, the proximal portion of which was already narrowed because of the acute angle the vessel had to make in its leftward passage behind the pulmonary artery.

In patients with anomalous origin of both coronary arteries from the left sinus of Valsalva, the proximal right coronary artery may be compromised by a mechanism similar to that described for the left coronary artery when it arises from the right sinus of Valsalva. Chest pain, presumably angina pectoris, and one example of a subendocardial myocardial infarction have been noted in patients with this malformation.[169–172]

Congenital coronary arteriovenous fistulas occur between either the right or the left coronary artery and the right atrium, coronary sinus, or right ventricle. The right coronary artery is involved more frequently than the left, but both can be affected.[173] Hemodynamic disturbances consist of a left-to-right shunt of variable magnitude and myocardial ischemia. Most patients with this anomaly who are not operated upon survive to adulthood, although their life expectancy is usually reduced.[173] The majority of patients are asymptomatic until the fifth or sixth decade, when signs and symptoms of left ventricular failure occur secondary to the left-to-right shunt.[173,174] The development of heart failure is related to the magnitude and duration of the left-to-right shunt, which may increase as the fistula increases in size over a period of time. The continuous murmur characteristic of this anomaly may change to a systolic murmur in those adults who develop congestive heart failure with elevated right heart pressures. Adults with this malformation may demonstrate ischemic ST-segment changes in the precordial leads. Surgical closure of the fistula is indicated in patients with moderately large left-to-right shunts (pulmonary-to-systemic blood flow ratios exceeding 1.5:1.0); this procedure generally relieves manifestations of diminished cardiac reserve.[175]

CONGENITAL PULMONARY ARTERIOVENOUS FISTULAS
(See also page 985)

Pulmonary arteriovenous fistulas arise through abnormal development of pulmonary arteries and veins from a common vascular complex.[176] These fistulas usually involve the lower lobes or the right middle lobe; they can be solitary or multiple and of varying size.[177] The fistula replaces the normal capillary bed and usually consists of a tangle of tortuous vessels or several large and, on occasion, aneurysmal vascular trunks.[176] Pulmonary arteriovenous fistulas may coexist with systemic telangiectasias as part of the "Osler-Weber-Rendu" disease,[176] in which there are multiple small telangiectasias in the skin, oral and nasal mucosa, gastrointestinal tract, liver, central nervous system, and kidneys. The physiological consequences of pulmonary arteriovenous fistulas depend principally on the quantity of venous blood that is shunted into the systemic circulation; if this amount is sufficiently large, cyanosis can result. Usually only a modest increase in cardiac output occurs in contrast to the marked increase that may occur with a systemic arteriovenous fistula.[176,177]

Complications include rupture of the fistulous vessels, with resultant hemoptysis or hemothorax, paradoxical embolism, cerebral abscess, and infectious endarteritis.[176] Cardiac failure rarely if ever occurs in adults with this malformation. Pulmonary arteriovenous fistulas are usually discovered during routine chest roentgenography in asymptomatic individuals. A solitary fistula or multiple fistulas confined to one lobe can be treated by means of lobectomy; patients with fistulas in multiple lobes are usually not considered to be surgical candidates. Catheter embolization by mechanical occluding devices can also be employed in selected cases to obliterate a pulmonary arteriovenous fistula.[178]

Isolated varicose dilatation of one or more of the pulmonary veins without an arteriovenous communication is a rare malformation.[179] Hemoptysis is the principal complication.

CONGENITAL ANEURYSMS OF THE SINUS OF VALSALVA
(See also page 973)

Congenital absence of the media in the aortic wall behind a sinus of Valsalva may result in aneurysmal dilatation of the sinus,[180] which may enlarge over a period of years. Nonruptured aneurysms usually cause no cardiac dysfunction and are noted as incidental findings at autopsy,[181] but they may occasionally cause heart block as a result of compression of the atrioventricular conduction system. Rupture of an aneurysm of the sinus Valsalva occurs more commonly in males than in females.[182] This complication develops in adult life, generally between the ages of 18 and 30 years. When the fistula to a cardiac chamber produced by rupture of the aneurysm causes a large left-to-right shunt, patients often report the sudden onset of chest pain of epigastric discomfort and dyspnea. These symptoms may persist or may gradually resolve, even without specific therapy. A loud, continuous murmur accompanied by a thrill along the lower sternum is commonly found. The diagnosis is aided by both M-mode and two-dimensional echocardiography[183,184] and is established by aortography. Successful surgical obliteration of a ruptured aneurysm of the sinus of Valsalva results in dramatic relief of symptoms.[185]

CONGENITAL HEART BLOCK (See also page 1014)

Congenital heart block may be caused by a variety of lesions affecting the atrioventricular node or bundle of His.[186] Adults with congenital heart block without associated malformations may be asymptomatic for many years because of the presence of a stable accelerated junctional pacemaker under autonomic control, which allows for some increase in heart rate during exercise. This permits a reasonably normal hemodynamic response to exercise and other stresses.[187]

Hereditary congenital heart block, inherited as an autosomal dominant trait, has been noted in some families.[188] It is of considerable interest that mothers with systemic lupus erythematosus and other connective tissue diseases give birth to children with a surprisingly high incidence of congenital heart block. This observation suggests that environmental as well as genetic factors may be important in the etiology of this arrhythmia.[189,190] In general, patients with familial congenital heart block with wide QRS complexes and/or associated cardiac malformations have a poorer prognosis than do patients without these features. A number of serious complications have been noted in adults with congenital heart block, including malignant ventricular tachyarrhythmias (both with exercise testing and on Holter monitoring), Stokes-Adams attacks, and decreasing cardiac output.[17,191] Exercise stress testing and Holter monitoring should be carried out in these patients, since they may disclose an indication for antiarrhythmic therapy and/or permanent pacing, e.g., tachyarrhythmias, prolonged asystole, or marked ventricular slowing. Exercise intolerance secondary to bradycardia is also an indication for permanent pacing.

References

1. Nora, J. J., and Nora, A. H.: The evolution of specific genetic and environmental counseling in congenital heart disease. Circulation *57*:205, 1978.
2. Smith, C.: Recurrence risks for multifactorial inheritance. Am. J. Hum. Genet. *23*:578, 1971.
3. Czeizel, A., Pornoi, A., Peterffy, E., and Tarcal, E.: Study of children of parents operated on for congenital cardiovascular malformations. Br. Heart J. *47*:290, 1982.
4. Whittemore, R., Hobbins, J. C., and Engle, M. A.: Pregnancy and its outcome in women with and without surgical treatment of congenital heart disease. Am. J. Cardiol. *50*:641, 1982.
5. McNamara, D. G., and Latson, L. A.: Long-term followup of patients with malformations for which definitive surgical repair has been available for 25 years or more. Am. J. Cardiol. *50*:560, 1982.
6. Graham, T. P.: Assessing the results of surgery for congenital heart disease—A continuing process. Circulation *65*:1049, 1982.
7. Rashkind, W. J.: Historical aspects of surgery for congenital heart disease. J. Thorac. Cardiovasc. Surg. *84*:619, 1982.
8. Graham, T. P.: Ventricular performance in adults after operation for congenital heart disease. Am. J. Cardiol. *50*:612, 1982.
9. Manning, J. A.: Insurability and employability of young cardiac patients. *In* Engle, M. A.: Pediatric Cardiovascular Disease. Philadelphia, F. A. Davis, 1981, p. 117.
10. Taussig, H. B., Kallman, C. H., Nagel, D., Baumgardner, R., Momberger, N., and Kirk, H.: Long-time observations on the Blalock-Taussig operation. VIII. Twenty to 28-year followup on patients with a tetralogy of Fallot. Johns Hopkins Med. J. *137*:13, 1975.
11. Johnson, D. H., Rosenthal, A., and Nadas, A. S.: A 40-year review of bacterial endocarditis in infancy and childhood. Circulation *41*:581, 1975.
12. Johnson, C. M., and Rhodes, K. H.: Pediatric endocarditis. Mayo Clin. Proc. *57*:86, 1982.

13. McGoon, D. C.: Long-term effects of prosthetic materials. Am. J. Cardiol. *50*: 621, 1982.
14. Deal, K., and Wooley, C. F.: Coarctation of the aorta and pregnancy. Ann. Intern. Med. *78*:706, 1973.
15. Blake, S., O'Neill, H., and MacDonald, D.: Haemodynamic effects of pregnancy in patients with heart failure. Br. Heart J. *47*:495, 1982.
16. Ralstin, J. H., and Dunn, M.: Pregnancies after surgical correction of tetralogy of Fallot. J.A.M.A. *235*:2627, 1976.
17. Reid, J. M., Coleman, E. N., and Doig, W.: Complete congenital heart block —Report of 35 cases. Br. Heart J. *48*:236, 1982.
18. Pirlo, A., and Herren, A. L.: Eisenmenger's syndrome and pregnancy. A case report and review of the literature. Anesth. Rev. *6*:9, 1979.
19. Midwall, J., Jaffin, H., Herman, M. V., and Kupersmith, J.: Shunt flow and pulmonary hemodynamics during labor and delivery in the Eisenmenger's syndrome. Am. J. Cardiol. *42*:299, 1978.
20. Roberts, W. C.: The congenitally bicuspid aortic valve. A study of 85 autopsy patients. Am. J. Cardiol. *26*:72, 1970.
21. Roberts, W. C.: The structure of the aortic valve in clinically isolated aortic stenosis—An autopsy study of 162 patients over 15 years of age. Circulation *42*:91, 1970.
22. Borow, K. M.: Congenital aortic stenosis in the adult. J. Cardiovasc. Med. (in press).
23. Fenoglio, J. J., McAllister, H. A., DeCastro, C. M., Davia, J. E., and Cheitlin, M. D.: Congenital bicuspid aortic valve after age 20. Am. J. Cardiol. *39*:164,1977.
24. Wagner, S., and Selzer, A.: Patterns of progression of aortic stenosis—A longitudinal hemodynamic study. Circulation *65*:709, 1982.
25. Roberts, W. C., Morrow, A. G., McIntosh, C. L., Jones, M., and Epstein, S. E.: Congenitally bicuspid aortic valve causing severe, pure aortic regurgitation without superimposed infective endocarditis. Am. J. Cardiol. *47*:206, 1980.
26. Rappaport, E.: Natural history of aortic and mitral valve disease. Am. J. Cardiol. *35*:221, 1975.
27. Hossack, K. F., Heutze, J. M., Iowe, J. B., and Barratt-Boyes, B. G.: Congenital valvar aortic stenosis—Natural history and assessment of operation. Br. Heart J. *43*:561, 1980.
28. DeMaria, A. N., Bommer, W., Joye, J., Lee, G., Bouteller, J., and Mason, D. T.: Value and limitation of cross-sectional echocardiography of the aortic valve in the diagnosis and quantification of valvar aortic stenosis. Circulation *62*: 304, 1980.
29. Young, J. B., Quinones, M. A., Waggoner, A. D., and Miller, R. R.: Diagnosis and quantification of aortic stenosis with pulsed Doppler echocardiography. Am. J. Cardiol. *45*:987, 1980.
30. Ciobanu, M., Abbasi, A. S., Allen, M., Herman, A., and Spellberg, R.: Pulsed Doppler echocardiography in the diagnosis and estimation of severity of aortic insufficiency. Am. J. Cardiol. *49*:339, 1982.
31. Friedman, W. F.: Indications for and results of surgery in congenital aortic stenosis. Adv. Cardiol. *17*:2, 1976.
31a. Stark, J., and deLeval, M. (eds.): Surgery for Congenital Heart Defects. New York, Grune and Stratton, Inc., 1983, p. 71–94.
32. Jones, M., Barnhart, G. R., and Morrow, A. G.: Late results after operation for left ventricular outflow tract obstruction. Am. J. Cardiol. *50*:569, 1982.
33. Prebiterc, P., Somerville, J., Revel-Chion, R., and Ross, D.: Open aortic valvotomy for congenital aortic stenosis—Late results. Br. Heart J. *47*:26, 1982.
34. Hamilton, W. T., Haffajee, C. I., Dalen, J. E., Dexter, L., and Nadas, A. S.: Atrial septal defect secundum: Clinical profile with physiologic correlates in children and adults. *In* Roberts, W. C. (ed.): Congenital Heart Disease in Adults. Philadelphia, F. A. Davis Co., 1979, p. 267.
34a. Konstam, M. A., Idoine, J., Wynne, J., Grossman, W., Cohn, L., Beck, J. R., Kozlowski, J., and Holman, B. L.: Right ventricular function in adults with pulmonary hypertension with and without atrial septal defect. Am. J. Cardiol. *51*:1144, 1983.
35. Breyer, R. H., Monson, D. O., Ruggie, N. T., Weinberg, M., and Najafi, H.: Atrial septal defect—Repair in patients over 35 years of age. J. Cardiovasc. Surg. *20*:583, 1979.
36. Dexter, L.: Atrial septal defect. Br. Heart J. *18*:209, 1956.
37. Popio, K. A., Gorlin, R., Teichholz, L. E., Cohn, P. F., Bechtel, D., and Herman, M. V.: Abnormalities of left ventricular function and geometry in adults with an atrial septal defect: Ventriculographic, hemodynamic and echocardiographic studies. Am. J. Cardiol. *36*:302, 1975.
38. Carabello, B. A., Gash, A., Mayers, D., and Spann, J. F.: Normal left ventricular systolic function in adults with atrial septal defect and left heart failure. Am. J. Cardiol. *49*:1868, 1982.
39. Liberthson, R. R., Boucher, C. A., Fallon, J. T., and Buckley, M. J.: Severe mitral regurgitation—A common occurrence in the aging patient with secundum atrial septal defect. Clin. Cardiol. *4*:229, 1981.
40. Bonow, R. O., Borer, J. S., Rosing, D. R., Bacharach, S. L., Green, M. V., and Kent, K. M.: Left ventricular functional reserve in adult patients with atrial septal defect: Pre- and postoperative studies. Circulation *63*:1315, 1981.
41. Hung, J., Uren, R. F., Richmond, D. R., and Kelly, D. T.: The mechanism of abnormal septal motion in atrial septal defect: Pre- and postoperative study of radionuclide ventriculography in adults. Circulation *63*:142, 1981.
42. Wanderman, K. L., Ovsyshcher, I., and Gueron, M.: Left ventricular performance in patients with atrial septal defect: Evaluation with noninvasive methods. Am. J. Cardiol. *41*:487, 1978.
43. Nasrallah, A. T., Hall, R. J., Garcia, E., Lechman, R. D., and Cooley, D. A.: Surgical repair of atrial septal defect in patients over 60 years of age: Long-term results. Circulation *53*:329, 1976.
44. St. John Sutton, M. G., Tajik, A. J., and McGoon, D. C.: Atrial septal defect in patients ages 60 years or older: Operative results and long-term postoperative followup. Circulation *64*:402, 1981.
45. Liberthson, R. R., Boucher, C. A., Strauss, H. W., Dinsmore, R. E., McKusick, K. A., and Pohost, G. M.: Right ventricular function in adult atrial septal defect—Preoperative and postoperative assessment and clinical implications. Am. J. Cardiol. *47*:56, 1981.
46. Moguilevsky, H. C., O'Reilly, M. V., Dizadji, H., and Shaffer, A. B.: Atrial septal defect associated with skeletal anomalies (Holt-Oram syndrome). Chest *57*:230, 1970.
46a. Fisher, J., Platia, E. V., Weiss, J. L., and Brinker, J. A.: Atrial septal defect in the adult: Clinical findings before and after surgery. Cardiovasc. Rev. Rep. *4*:396, 1983.
47. Pocock, W. A., and Barlow, J. B.: An association between the billowing posterior mitral leaflet syndrome and congenital heart disease, particularly atrial septal defect. Am. Heart J. *81*:720, 1971.
48. Nagata, S., Nimura, Y., Sakakibara, H., Beppu, S., Yung-Dae, P., Kawazoe, K., and Fujita, T.: Mitral valve lesion associated with secundum atrial septal defect—analysis by real time two dimensional echocardiography. Br. Heart J. *49*:51, 1983.
49. Schreiber, T. L., Feigenbaum, H., and Weyman, A. E.: Effect of atrial septal defect repair on left ventricular geometry and degree of mitral valve prolapse. Circulation *61*:888, 1980.
50. Kuzman, W. J., and Yuskis, A. S.: Atrial septal defects in the older patient simulating acquired valvular heart disease. Am. J. Cardiol. *15*:303, 1976.
51. Anderson, P. A. W., Rogers, M. C., Canent, R. V., Jr., and Spach, M. S.: Atrioventricular conduction in secundum atrial septal defects. Circulation *48*: 27, 1973.
52. Ellison, R. C., and Sloss, L. J.: Electrocardiographic features of congenital heart disease in the adult. *In* Roberts, W. C. (ed.): Congenital Heart Disease in Adults. Philadelphia, F. A. Davis Co., 1979, p. 267.
53. Hynes, J. K., Tajik, A. J., Seward, J. B., Fuster, V., Ritter, D. G., Brandenburg, R. O., Puga, F. J., Danielson, G. K., and McGoon, D. C.: Partial atrioventricular canal defect in adults. Circulation *66*:284, 1982.
54. Weyman, A. E., Wann, S., Feigenbaum, H., and Dillon, J. C.: Mechanisms of abnormal septal motion in patients with right ventricular volume overload. Circulation *54*:179, 1976.
55. Nasser, F. N., Tajik, A. J., Seward, J. B., and Hagler, D. J.: Diagnosis of sinus venosus atrial septal defect by two-dimensional echocardiography. Mayo Clin. Proc. *56*:568, 1981.
56. Beppu, S., Nimura, Y., and Sakakibara, H.: Mitral cleft in ostium primum atrial septal defect assessed by cross-sectional echocardiography. Circulation *62*:1099, 1980.
57. Fraker, T. D., Harris, P. J., Behar, V. S., and Kisslo, J. A.: Detection and exclusion of interatrial shunts by two dimensional echocardiography and peripheral venous injection. Circulation *59*:379, 1979.
58. Bourdillon, P. D. V., Foale, R. A., and Rickards, A. F.: Identification of atrial septal defects by cross-sectional contrast echocardiography. Br. Heart J. *44*: 401, 1980.
59. Gullace, G., Savoia, M. T., Ravizza, P., Knuppel, M., and Ranzi, C.: Detection of atrial septal defect with left-to-right shunt by inferior vena cava contrast echocardiography. Br. Heart J. *47*:445, 1982.
60. Valdes-Cruz, L. M., Pieroni, D. R., Jones, M., Roland, J. A., Shematek, J. P., Allen, H. D., Goldberg, S. J., and Sahn, D. J.: Residual shunting in the early postoperative period after closure of atrial septal defect. J. Thorac. Cardiovasc. Surg. *84*:73, 1982.
61. Botvinick, E. H., and Schiller, N.: The complementary role of M-mode echocardiography and scintigraphy in the evaluation of adults with suspected left-to-right shunts. Circulation *62*:1070, 1980.
62. Borow, K. M.: Under what circumstances can cardiac surgery be undertaken without catheterization? J. Cardiovasc. Med. *8*:84, 1983.
63. Anderson, M., Lyngborg, K., Moller I., and Wennwold, A.: The natural history of small atrial septal defects: Long-term followup with serial heart catheterizations. Am. Heart J. *92*:302, 1976.
63a. Steele, P. M., Fuster, V., Ritter, D. G., and McGoon, D. W.: Secundum atrial septal defect with pulmonary vascular obstructive disease: Long-term followup and prediction of outcome after surgical correction. J. Am. Coll. Cardiol. *1*:663, 1983.
64. Forfang, K., Simonsen S., Anderson, A., and Efskind, L.: Atrial septal defect of secundum type in the middle-aged. Am. Heart J. *94*:44, 1977.
65. Steinbrunn, W., Cohn, D. E., and Selzer, A.: Atrial septal defect associated with mitral stenosis: The Lutembacher syndrome revisited. Am. J. Med. *48*: 295, 1970.
66. Meister, S. B., Grossman, W., Dexter, L., and Dalen, J. E.: Paradoxical embolism: Diagnosis during life. Am. J. Med. *53*:292, 1972.
67. Thompson, T., and Evans, W.: Paradoxical embolism. Quart. J. Med. *23*:135, 1930.
68. Alpert, J. S., Dexter, L., Vieweg, W. V. R., Haynes, F. W., and Dalen, J. E.: Anomalous pulmonary venous return with intact atrial septum: Diagnosis and pathophysiology. Circulation *56*:870, 1977.
69. Kalke, B. R., Carlson, R. G., Ferlic, R. M., Sellers, R. D., and Lillehei, C. W.: Partial anomalous pulmonary venous connection. Am. J. Cardiol. *20*:91, 1967.
70. Bauer, A., Korfer, R., and Bircks, W.: Left-to-right shunt of atrial level due to anomalous venous connection of the left lung. J. Thorac. Cardiovasc. Surg. *84*: 626, 1982.

71. Weidman, W. H., DuShane, J. W., and Ellison, R. C.: Clinical course in adults with ventricular septal defect. Circulation *56*:178, 1977.
72. Maron, B. J., Redwood, D. R., Hirshfeld, J. W., Jr., Goldstein, R. E., Morrow, A. G., and Epstein, S. E.: Postoperative assessment of patients with ventricular septal defect and pulmonary hypertension. Response to intense upright exercise. Circulation *48*:864, 1973.
73. Lueker, R. D., Vogel, J. H. K., and Blount, S. G.: Cardiovascular abnormalities following surgery for left-to-right shunts. Circulation *40*:785, 1969.
73a. Jablonsky, G., Hilton, J. D., Liu, P. P., March, J. E., Druck, M. N., Bar-Shlomo, B., and McLaughlin, P. R.: Rest and exercise ventricular function in adults with congenital ventricular septal defects. Am. J. Cardiol. *51*:293, 1983.
74. Corone, P., Doyon, F., Gaudeau, S., Guerin, F., Vernant, P., Ducam, H., Rumeau-Rouquette, C., and Gaudeau, P.: Natural history of ventricular septal defect: A study involving 790 cases. Circulation *55*:908, 1977.
75. Keane, J. F., Plauth, W. H., and Nadas, A. S.: Ventricular septal defect with aortic regurgitation. Circulation *56*:172, 1977.
76. Friedman, W. F., and Heiferman, M. F.: Clinical problems of postoperative pulmonary vascular disease. Am. J. Cardiol. *50*:631, 1982.
77. Rabinovitch, M., Castaneda, A. R., and Reid, L.: Lung biopsy with frozen section as a diagnostic and in patients with congenital heart defects. Am. J. Cardiol. *47*:77, 1981.
78. Allan, H. D., Anderson, R. C., Noren, G. R., and Moller, J. H.: Postoperative followup of patients with ventricular septal defect. Circulation *50*:465, 1974.
79. Sutherland, G. R., Godman, M. J., Smallhorn, J. F., Gutierras, P., Anderson, R. H., and Hunter, S.: Ventricular septal defects—Two-dimensional echocardiographic and morphological correlations. Br. Heart J. *47*:316, 1982.
80. Stevenson, J. G., Kawabori, I., Dooley, T., and Guntheroth, W. G.: Diagnosis of ventricular septal defect by pulsed Doppler echocardiography. Circulation *58*:322, 1978.
81. Blake, R. S., Chung, E. E., Wesley, H., and Hallidie-Smith, K. A.: Conduction defects, ventricular arrhythmias and late death after surgical closure of ventricular septal defect. Br. Heart J. *47*:305, 1982.
82. Vetter, V. L., and Horowitz, L. N.: Electrophysiologic residua and sequelae of surgery for congenital heart defects. Am. J. Cardiol. *50*:588, 1982.
83. Anderson, R. H., Allwork, S. P., Ho, S. Y., Lenox, C. C., and Zuberbuhler, J. R.: Surgical anatomy of tetralogy of Fallot. J. Thorac. Cardiovasc. Surg. *81*:887, 1981.
84. Danilowicz, D., and Ishmael, R.: Anomalous right ventricular muscle bundle—Clinical pitfalls and extracardiac anomalies. Clin. Cardiol. *4*:146, 1981.
84a. Matina, D., van Doesburg, N. H., Fouron, J., Guerin, R., and Davignon, A.: Subxiphoid two-dimensional echocardiographic diagnosis of double-chambered right ventricle. Circulation *67*:885, 1983.
85. Goitein, K. J., Neches, W. H., Park, S. C., Mathews, R. A., Lenox, C. C., and Zuberbuhler, J. R.: Electrocardiogram in double chamber right ventricle. Am. J. Cardiol. *45*:604, 1980.
86. Higgins, C. B., and Mulder, D. G.: Tetralogy of Fallot in the adult. Am. J. Med. *29*:837, 1972.
87. Jones, M., and Ferrans, V. J.: Myocardial degeneration in congenital heart disease: Comparison of morphologic findings in young and old patients with congenital heart disease associated with muscular obstruction to right ventricular outflow. Am. J. Cardiol. *39*:1051, 1977.
88. Borow, K. M., Green, L. H., Castaneda, A. R., and Keane, J. F.: Left ventricular function after repair of tetralogy of Fallot and its relationship to age at surgery. Circulation *61*:1150, 1980.
89. Bertranou, E. G., Blackstone, E. H., Hazelrig, J. B., Turner, M. E., and Kirklin, J. W.: Life expectancy without surgery in tetralogy of Fallot. Am. J. Cardiol. *43*:458, 1978.
90. Abraham, K. A., Cherian, G., Rao, V. D., Sukumar, I. P., Krishnaswami, S., and John, S.: Tetralogy of Fallot in adults: A report of 147 patients. Am. J. Med. *66*:811, 1979.
91. Fuster, V., McGoon, D. C., Kennedy, M. A., Ritter, D. G., and Kirklin, J. W.: Long-term evaluation (12 to 22 years) of open heart surgery for tetralogy of Fallot. Am. J. Cardiol. *46*:635, 1980.
92. Katz, N. M., Blackstone, E. H., Kirklin, J. W., Pacifico, A. D., and Bargeron, L. M.: Late survival and symptoms after repair of tetralogy of Fallot. Circulation *65*:403, 1982.
92a. Hu, D. C., Seward, J. B., Puga, F. J., Fuster, V., and Tajik, A. J.: Total correction of tetralogy of Fallot at age 40 and older: Long-term followup. J. Am. Coll. Cardiol. *1*:651, 1983.
93. Uretzky, G., Puga, F. J., Danielson, G. K., Hagler, D. J., and McGoon, D. C.: Reoperation after correction of tetralogy of Fallot. Circulation *66*:I-202, 1982.
94. Ebert, P. A.: Second operation for pulmonary stenosis or insufficiency after repair of tetralogy of Fallot. Am. J. Cardiol. *50*:637, 1982.
95. Deanfield, J. E., McKenna, W. J., Hallidie-Smith, K. A.: Detection of late arrhythmia and conduction disturbance after correction of tetralogy of Fallot. Br. Heart J. *44*:248, 1980.
95a. Tamer, D., Wolff, G. S., Ferrer, P., Pickoff, A. S., Casta, A., Mehta, A. V., Garcia, O., and Gelband, H.: Hemodynamics and intracardiac conduction after operative repair of tetralogy of Fallot, Am. J. Cardiol. *51*:552, 1983.
96. Gillette, P. C., Yeoman, M. A., Mullins, C. E., and McNamara, D. G.: Sudden death after repair of tetralogy of Fallot. Circulation *56*:566, 1977.
97. Wessel, H. U., Bostanier, C. K., Paul, M. H., Berry, T. E., Cole, R. B., and Muster, A. J.: Prognostic significance of arrhythmia in tetralogy of Fallot after intracardiac repair. Am. J. Cardiol. *46*:843, 1980.
98. Garson, A., Gillette, P. C., Gutgesell, H. P., and McNamara, D. G.: Stress-induced ventricular arrhythmia after repair of tetralogy of Fallot. Am. J. Cardiol. *46*:1006, 1980.
98a. Deanfield, J. E., Ho, S., Anderson, R. H., McKenna, W. J., Allwork, S. P., and Hallidie-Smith, K. A.: Late sudden death after repair of tetralogy of Fallot—a clinicopathologic study. Circulation *67*:626, 1983.
99. Hoffman, J. E., and Christianson, R.: Congenital heart disease in a cohort of 19,502 births with long-term followup. Am. J. Cardiol. *42*:641, 1978.
100. Johnson, L. W., Grossman, W., Dalen, J. E., and Dexter, L.: Pulmonic stenosis in the adult: Long-term followup results. N. Engl. J. Med. *287*:1159, 1972.
101. Covarrubias, E. A., Sheikh, M. U., Isner, J. M., Gomes, M., Hufnagel, C. A., and Roberts, W. C.: Calcific pulmonic stenosis in adulthood. Chest *75*:399, 1979.
102. DeTroyer, A., Yernault, J. C., and Englert, M.: Lung hypoplasia in congenital pulmonary valve stenosis. Circulation *56*:647, 1977.
103. Møller, I., Wennevold, A., and Lyngborg, K. E.: The natural history of pulmonary stenosis. Long-term followup with serial heart catheterizations. Cardiology *58*:193, 1973.
104. Delaney, T. B., and Nadas, A. S.: Peripheral pulmonic stenosis. Am. J. Cardiol. *13*:451, 1964.
105. Roberts, N., and Moes, C. A. F.: Supravalvular pulmonic stenosis. J. Pediart. *82*:838, 1973.
106. Cohn, L. H., Sanders, J. H., Jr., and Collins, J. J., Jr.: Surgical treatment of congenital unilateral pulmonary arterial stenosis with contralateral pulmonary hypertension. Am. J. Cardiol. *38*:257, 1976.
107. John, S., Muralidharan, S., Mani, G. K., Krishnaswami, S., and Sukumar, I. P.: The adult ductus. J. Thorac. Cardiovasc. Surg. *82*:314, 1981.
108. Campbell, M.: Natural history of patent ductus arteriosus. Br. Heart J. *30*:4, 1968.
109. Dexter, L.: Pulmonary vascular disease in acquired and congenital heart disease. Arch. Intern. Med. *139*:922, 1979.
110. Borow, K. M., Hessel, S. J., and Sloss, L. J.: Fistulous aneurysm of ductus arteriosus. Br. Heart J. *45*:467, 1981.
111. Stevenson, J. G., Kawabori, I., and Guntheroth, W. G.: Noninvasive detection of pulmonary hypertension in patent ductus arteriosus by pulsed Doppler echocardiography. Circulation *60*:355, 1979.
112. Porstmann, W., Hieronymi, K., Wierny, L., and Warnke, H.: Nonsurgical closure of oversized patent ductus arteriosus with pulmonary hypertension: Report of a case. Circulation *50*:376, 1974.
113. Sato, K., Fujino, M., Kozuka, T., Naito, Y., Kitamura, S., Nakano, S., Ohyama, C., and Kawashima, Y.: Transfemoral plug closure of patent ductus arteriosus. Experiences in 61 cases treated without thoracotomy. Circulation *51*:337, 1975.
114. Serfas, D., and Borow, K. M.: Coarctation of the aorta. J. Cardiovasc. Med. (in press).
115. Rosenquist, G. C.: Congenital mitral valve disease associated with coarctation of the aorta. A spectrum that includes parachute deformity of the mitral valve. Circulation *49*:985, 1974.
116. Rippe, J. M., Sloss, L. J., Angoff, G., and Alpert, J. S.: Mitral valve prolapse in adults with congenital heart disease. Am. Heart J. *97*:561, 1979.
117. Liberthson, R. R., Pennington, D. G., Jacobs, M. L., and Dagget, W. M.: Coarctation of the aorta—Review of 234 patients and clarification of management problems. Am. J. Cardiol. *43*:835, 1979.
118. Campbell, M.: Natural history of coarctation of the aorta. Circulation *41*:1067, 1970.
119. Alpert, B. S., Bain, H. H., Balfe, J. W., Kidd, B. S. L., and Olley, P. M.: Role of the renin-angiotensin-aldosterone system in hypertensive children with coarctation of the aorta. Am. J. Cardiol. *43*:828, 1979.
120. Samanek, M., Goetzova, J., Fiserova, J., and Skovranek, J.: Differences in muscle blood flow in upper and lower extremities of patients after correction of the aorta. Circulation *54*:377, 1976.
121. Simon, A. B., and Zloto, A. E.: Coarctation of the aorta. Longitudinal assessment of operated patients. Circulation *50*:456, 1974.
122. Shested, J., Baandrup, U., and Mikkelsen, E.: Different reactivity and structure of the prestenotic and poststenotic aorta in human coarctation—Implications for baroreceptor function. Circulation *65*:1060, 1982.
123. Weyman, A. E., Caldwell, R. L., Hurwitz, R. A., Girod, D. A., Dillon, J. C., Feigenbaum, H., and Green, D.: Cross-sectional echocardiographic detection of aortic obstruction: Coarctation of the aorta. Circulation *57*:498, 1978.
123a. Glancy, D. L., Morrow, A. G., Simon, A. L., and Roberts, W. C.: Juxtaductal aortic coarctation—analysis of 84 patients studied hemodynamically, angiographically, and morphologically after age 1 year. Am. J. Cardiol. *51*:537, 1983.
124. Rocchini, A. P., Rosenthal, A., and Barger, C. A.: Pathogenesis of paradoxical hypertension after coarctation resection. Circulation *54*:382, 1976.
125. Benedict, C. R., Grahame-Smith, D. G., and Fisher, A.: Changes in plasma catecholamine and dopamine beta-hydroxylase after corrective surgery for coarctation of the aorta. Circulation *57*:598,1978.
126. Farrell, B. G., Parker, F. B., Poirier, R. A., Anderson, G., Streeter, D. H. P., and Blackman, M.: Angiotensin blockade in postoperative paradoxical hypertension of coarctation of the aorta. Surg. Forum *30*:189, 1979.
127. Casta, A., Conti, V. R., Talabi, A., and Brouhard, B. H.: Effective use of captopril in postoperative paradoxical hypertension of coarctation of the aorta. Clin. Cardiol. *5*:551, 1982.
128. Freed, M. D., Rocchini, A., and Rosenthal, A.: Exercise-induced hypertension after surgical repair of coarctation of the aorta. Am. J. Cardiol. *43*:253, 1979.
129. Laks, H., Williams, H. G., Hellenbrand, W. E., Freedom, R. M., Talner, N. S., Rowe, R. D., and Trusler, G. A.: Results of right atrial to right ventricular

and right atrial to pulmonary artery conduits for complex congenital heart disease. Ann. Surg. *192*:382, 1980.
130. Patterson, W., Baxley, W. A., Karp, R. B., Soto, B., and Bargeron, L. L.: Tricuspid atresia in adults. Am. J. Cardiol. *49*:142, 1982.
131. Shackar, G. B., Fuhrnan, B. P., Wang, Y., Lucas, R. V., and Lock, J. E.: Rest and exercise hemodynamics after the Fontan procedure. Circulation *65*:1043, 1982.
132. Neveux, J. Y., Dreyfus, G., Leca, F., Marchand, M., and Bex, J. P.: Modified technique for correction of tricuspid atresia. J. Thorac. Cardiovasc. Surg. *82*: 457, 1981.
133. Graham, T. P., Jr., and Friesinger, G. C.: Complex cyanotic congenital heart disease in adults. *In* Roberts, W. C. (ed.): Congenital Heart Disease in Adults. Philadelphia, F. A. Davis Co., 1979, p. 383.
134. Benson, L. N., Bonet, J., McLaughlin, P., Olley, P. M., Feiglin, D., Druck, M., Truoler, G., Rowe, R. D., and March, J.: Assessment of right ventricular function during supine bicycle exercise after Mustard's operation. Circulation *65*:1052, 1982.
135. Prusty, S., and Ross, D. N.: Adult cyanotic congenital heart disease. Thorax *30*:650, 1975.
136. Graham, T. P., Jr.: The Eisenmenger reaction and its management. *In* Roberts, W. C. (ed.): Congenital Heart Disease in Adults. Philadelphia, F. A. Davis Co., 1979, p. 531.
137. Brammell, H. L., Vogel, J. H. K., Pryor, R., and Blount, S. G., Jr.: The Eisenmenger syndrome: A clinical and physiologic reappraisal. Am. J. Cardiol. *28* :679, 1971.
138. Arias, F.: Maternal death in a patient with Eisenmenger's syndrome. Obstet. Gynecol. *50*:765, 1977.
139. Anderson, K. R., Zuberbuhler, J. R., Anderson, R. H., Becker, A. E., and Lie, J. T.: Morphologic spectrum of Ebstein's anomaly of the heart. Mayo Clin. Proc. *54*:174, 1979.
140. Anderson, K. R., and Lie, J. T.: Pathologic anatomy of Ebstein's anomaly of the heart revisited. Am. J. Cardiol. *41*:739, 1978.
141. Giuliani, E. R., Fuster, V., Brandenburg, R. O., and Mair, D. D.: Ebstein's anomaly: The clinical features and natural history of Ebstein's anomaly of the tricuspid valve. Mayo Clin. Proc. *54*:163, 1979.
142. Seward, J. B., Tajik, A. J., Feist, D. J., and Smith, H. C.: Ebstein's anomaly in an 85-year-old man. Mayo Clin. Proc. *54*:193, 1979.
143. Cabin, H. S., Wood, T. P., Smith, J. D., and Roberts, W. C.: Ebstein's anomaly in the elderly. Chest *80*:212, 1981.
144. Hansen, J. F., Leth, A., Dorph, S., and Wennevold, A.: The prognosis in Ebstein's disease of the heart — Long-term followup of 22 patients. Acta Med. Scand. *201*:331, 1977.
145. Watson, H.: Natural history of Ebstein's anomaly of tricuspid valve in childhood and adolescence. An international cooperative study of 505 cases. Br. Heart J. *36*:417, 1974.
146. Waggoner, A. D., Quinones, M. A., Young, J. B., Brandon, T. A., Shah, A. A., Verani, M. S., and Miller, R. R.: Pulsed Doppler echocardiographic detection of right-sided valve regurgitation. Am. J. Cardiol. *47*:279, 1981.
147. Bove, E. L., and Kirsh, M. M.: Valve replacement for Ebstein's anomaly of the tricuspid valve. J. Thorac. Cardiovasc. Surg. *78*:229, 1979.
148. Danielson, G. K., Maloney, J. D., and Devloo, R. A.: Surgical repair of Ebstein's anomaly. Mayo Clin. Proc. *54*:185, 1979.
149. Caralps, J. M., Aris, A., Bonnin, J. O., Solanes, H., and Torner, M.: Ebstein's anomaly: Surgical treatment with tricuspid valve replacement without right ventricular plication. Ann. Thorac. Surg. *31*:277, 1981.
150. Danielson, G. K., and Fuster, V.: Surgical repair of Ebstein's anomaly. Ann. Surg. *196*:499, 1982.
151. Marcus, F. I., Fontaine, G. H., Guiraudon, G., Frank, R., Laurenceau, J. L., Malergue, C., and Grosgogeat, Y.: Right ventricular dysplasia — A report of 24 adult cases. Circulation *65*:384, 1982.
152. Olsson, S. B., Edvardsson, N., Emanuelsson, H., and Enestrom, S.: A case of arrhythmogenic right ventricular dysplasia with ventricular fibrillation. Clin. Cardiol. *5*:591, 1982.
153. Frank, R., Fontaine, G., Vedel, J., Miolet, G., Sol, C., Guiraudon, G., Grosgogeat, Y. H.: Electrocardiologie de genetic case de dysplasie ventriculaire droite arythmogene. Arch. Mal Coeur *71*:963, 1978.
154. Vedel, J., Frank, R., Fontaine, G., Dobrinski, G., Guiraudon, G., Brocheriou C., and Grosgogeat, Y.: Tachycardies ventriculaires recidivantes et ventricule droit papyrace de l'adulte (à propos de deux observations anatomo-cliniques). Arch. Mal Coeur *71*:973, 1978.
155. Uhl, H. S.: A previously undescribed congenital malformation of the heart — Almost total absence of the myocardium of the right ventricle. Bull. Johns Hopkins Hosp. *91*:197, 1952.
156. Vecht, R. J., Carmichael, J. S., Gopal, R., and Phillip, G.: Uhl's anomaly. Br. Heart J. *41*:676, 1979.
157. Blake, H. A., Manion, W. C., Mattingly, T. W., and Baroldi, G.: Coronary artery anomalies. Circulation *30*:927, 1964.
158. Chaitman, B. R., Lesperance, J., Sahiel, J., and Bourassa, M. G.: Clinical, angiographic and hemodynamic findings in patients with anomalous origin of coronary arteries. Circulation *53*:122, 1976.
159. Wright, N. L., Baue, A. E., Baum, S., Blakemore, W. S., and Zinsser, H. F.: Coronary artery steal due to an anomalous left coronary artery origin from the pulmonary artery. J. Thorac. Cardiovasc. Surg. *54*:461, 1970.
160. Askenazi, J., and Nadas, A. S.: Anomalous left coronary artery originating from the pulmonary artery. Report on 15 cases. Circulation *51*:976, 1975.
161. Moodie, D. S., Cook, S. A., Gill, C. C., and Napoli, C. A.: Thallium-201 myocardial imaging in young adults with anomalous left coronary artery arising from the pulmonary artery. J. Nucl. Med. *21*:1076, 1980.
162. Harthorne, J. W., Scannell, J. A., and Dinsmore, R. E.: Anomalous origin of the left coronary artery: Remediable cause of sudden death in adults. N. Engl. J. Med. *275*:660, 1966.
163. Arciniegas, E., Farooki, Z. Q., Hakimi, M., and Green, E. W.: Management of anomalous left coronary artery from the pulmonary artery. Circulation *62* (Suppl.):I-180, 1980.
164. Stephenson, L. W., Edmunds, L. H., Freedman, S., Meyboom, E., Geurtz, M., and Weinberg, P.: Subclavian–left coronary artery anastomosis (Meyer operation) for anomalous origin of the left coronary artery from the pulmonary artery. Circulation *64*(Suppl.):II-130, 1981.
165. Wilson, C. L., Dlabal, P. W., and McGuire, S. A.: Surgical treatment of anomalous left coronary artery from pulmonary artery — Followup in teenagers and adults. Am. Heart J. *98*:440, 1979.
166. Grace, R. R., Angelini, P., and Cooley, D. A.: Aortic implantation of anomalous left coronary artery arising from pulmonary artery. Am. J. Cardiol. *39*:608, 1977.
167. Monro, J. L., Sharratt, G. P., and Conway, N.: Correction of anomalous origin of left coronary artery using left subclavian artery. Br. Heart J. *40*:79, 1978.
168. Kimbiris, D., Iskandrian, A. S., Segal, B. L., and Bemis, C. E.: Anomalous aortic origin of the coronary arteries. Circulation *58*:606, 1978.
169. Cheitlin, M. D., DeCastro, C. M., McAllister, H. A.: Sudden death as a complication of anomalous left coronary origin from the anterior sinus of Valsalva. A not-so-minor congenital anomaly. Circulation *50*:780, 1974.
170. Liberthson, R. R., Dinsmore, R. E., and Fallon, J. T.: Aberrant coronary artery origin from the aorta. Circulation *59*:748, 1979.
171. Liberthson, R. R., Zaman, L., Weyman, A., Kiger, R., Dinsmore, R. E., Leinbach, R. C., Strauss, H. W., and Buckley, M. J.: Aberrant origin of the left coronary artery from proximal right coronary artery. Diagnostic features and pre- and postoperative course. Clin. Cardiol. *5*:377, 1982.
172. Sharbaugh, A. H., and White, R. S.: Single coronary artery: Analysis of the anatomic variation, clinical importance and report of five cases. J.A.M.A. *230*: 243, 1974.
173. Liberthson, R. R., Sagar, K., Berkoben, J. P., Weintraub, R. M., and Levine, F. H.: Congenital coronary arteriovenous fistula: Report of 13 patients, reviews of the literature and delineation of management. Circulation *59*:849, 1979.
174. Barnes, R. J., Cheung, A. C. S., and Wu, R. W. Y.: Coronary artery fistula. Br. Heart J. *31*:299, 1969.
175. Jaffe, R. B., Glancy, L., Epstein, S. E., Brown, B. G., and Morrow, A. G.: Coronary arterial–right heart fistulae: Long-term observations in seven patients. Circulation *47*:133, 1973.
176. Moyer, J. H., Glantz, G., and Brest, A. N.: Pulmonary arteriovenous fistulas. Am. J. Med. *32*:417, 1962.
177. Sahn, S. H., Bluth, I., and Schub, H.: Pulmonary arteriovenous fistula. Dis. Chest *44*:542, 1963.
178. Taylor, R. B., Cockerill, E. M., Manfredi, F., and Klatte, E. C.: Therapeutic embolization of the pulmonary artery in pulmonary arteriovenous fistula. Am. J. Med. *64*:360, 1978.
179. Nelson, W. P., Hall, R. J., and Garcia, E.: Varicosities of the pulmonary veins simulating arteriovenous fistulas. J.A.M.A. *195*:13, 1966.
180. Edwards, J. E., and Burchell, H. B.: Specimen exhibiting the essential lesion in aneurysm of the aortic sinus. Proc. Staff Meet. Mayo Clin. *31*:407, 1956.
181. Fishbein, M. C., Obma, R., and Roberts, W. C.: Unruptured sinus of Valsalva aneurysm. Am. J. Cardiol. *35*:918, 1975.
182. Kwittken, J., Christopoulos, P., Dua, N. K., and Bruno, M. S.: Congenital and acquired aortic sinus aneurysm. Arch. Intern. Med. *115*:684, 1965.
183. Matsumoto, M., Matsuo, H., Beppu, S., Yoshioka, Y., Kawashima, Y., Nimura, Y., and Abe, H.: Echocardiographic diagnosis of ruptured aneurysms of sinus of Valsalva: Report of two cases. Circulation *53*:382, 1976.
184. Engel, P. J., Held, J. S., Vander Bel Kahn, J., and Spitz, H.: Echocardiographic diagnosis of congenital sinus of Valsalva aneurysm with dissection of the interventricular septum. Circulation *63*:75, 1981.
185. Tanabe, T., Yokota, A., and Sugie, S.: Surgical treatment of aneurysms of the sinus of Valsalva. Ann. Thorac. Surg. *27*:133, 1979.
186. Ohkawa, S., Sugiura, M., Itoh, Y., Kitano, K., Hiraoka, K., Veda, K., and Murakami, M.: Electrophysiologic and histologic correlations in chronic complete atrioventricular block. Circulation *64*:215, 1981.
187. Corne, R. A., and Mathewson, F. A. L.: Congenital complete atrioventricular heart block: A 25-year followup study. Am. J. Cardiol. *29*:412, 1972.
188. Lynch, H. T., Mohiuddin, S., Moran, J., Kaplan, A., Sketch, M., Zencka, A., and Runco, V.: Hereditary progressive atrioventricular conduction defect. Am. J. Cardiol. *36*:297, 1975.
189. McCue, C. M., Mantakas, M. E., Tingelstad, J. B., and Ruddy, S.: Congenital heart block in newborns of mothers with connective tissue disease. Circulation *56*:82, 1977.
190. Chameides, L., Truex, R. C., Vetter, V., Rashkind, W. J., Galioto, F. M., Jr., and Noonan, J. A.: Association of maternal systemic lupus erythematosus with congenital complete heart block. N. Engl. J. Med. *297*:1204, 1977.
191. Winkler, R. B., Freed, M. D., and Nadas, A. S.: Exercise-induced ventricular ectopy in children and young adults with complete heart block. Am. Heart J. *99*:87, 1980.

31 ACQUIRED HEART DISEASE IN INFANCY AND CHILDHOOD

by William F. Friedman, M.D.

Since most of the topics discussed in this chapter are given more substantial coverage elsewhere in this text, the emphasis herein will be placed on features of acquired heart disease that are relatively unique to infancy and childhood, although the disease processes per se may not recognize age-related boundaries. Acute rheumatic fever and rheumatic heart disease have been excluded from this chapter, since these conditions are discussed extensively in Chapter 48. The hyperlipidemias are discussed in Chapters 35 and 47.

NONRHEUMATIC INFLAMMATORY DISEASE

Infective Myocarditis
(See also Chapter 41)

Infectious processes causing inflammatory disease of the heart may occur at any age, even during fetal life. Etiological agents include bacteria, viruses, fungi, protozoa, helminths, rickettsia, and spirochetes. As a general rule, very few of the generalized illnesses caused by these agents feature significant involvement of the heart. Myocardial involvement may be demonstrated histologically, but in most cases little or no expression of cardiac inflammation will be detected clinically. Important exceptions are infections due to certain viruses, diphtheria, and trypanosomes; these are discussed individually below.

Viral Myocarditis. Coxsackie B and rubella viruses are the most common causative agents in infective myocarditis of the newborn. The rubella embryopathy and its associated cardiovascular malformations are discussed on page 942. Active *rubella myocarditis* occurs in utero and may cause varying degrees of myocardial damage.[1] Invariably, however, other cardiovascular manifestations of the rubella syndrome dominate the clinical picture.

Coxsackie B typically causes outbreaks of epidemic myocarditis but may occur in the isolated infant in the newborn nursery, commonly with a fatal outcome.[2,3] The illness is of sudden onset and is characterized by fever, tachycardia, signs of systemic hypoperfusion, cyanosis, and occasionally cardiac failure. In some infants signs and symptoms of encephalomyelitis and hepatitis predominate. The diagnosis is suggested by electrocardiographic findings of atrial and/or ventricular arrhythmias, generalized ST-segment and T-wave changes, and low-voltage QRS complexes, accompanied by the appearance of marked generalized cardiomegaly and pulmonary vascular congestion on the chest roentgenogram. Echocardiography reveals dilatation of both ventricles and depressed indices of cardiac performance. Echocardiography is especially helpful in excluding congenital structural anomalies. The diagnosis is strongly suggested or confirmed when virus can be isolated from pericardial fluid, pharyngeal secretions, or feces, and elevations occur in type-specific–neutralizing, hemagglutination-inhibiting, or complement-fixing antibody.[4] Digitalis, diuretics, and general supportive measures are of limited benefit. Although increased sensitivity to the toxic effects of the glycosides is common, digitalis should be administered cautiously and continued until heart size is normal, since cardiac failure may recur when the drug is discontinued.

Numerous viral agents have been identified as a cause of myocarditis in childhood beyond infancy.[5–7] The most common are Coxsackie A and B (Fig. 31–1), influenza, adenovirus, and ECHO virus. Moreover, myocarditis, usually of mild degree, may be associated with the common viral infectious diseases of childhood, including mumps, measles, infectious mononucleosis, varicella, and variola. Although the diagnosis is generally one of exclusion, it may be

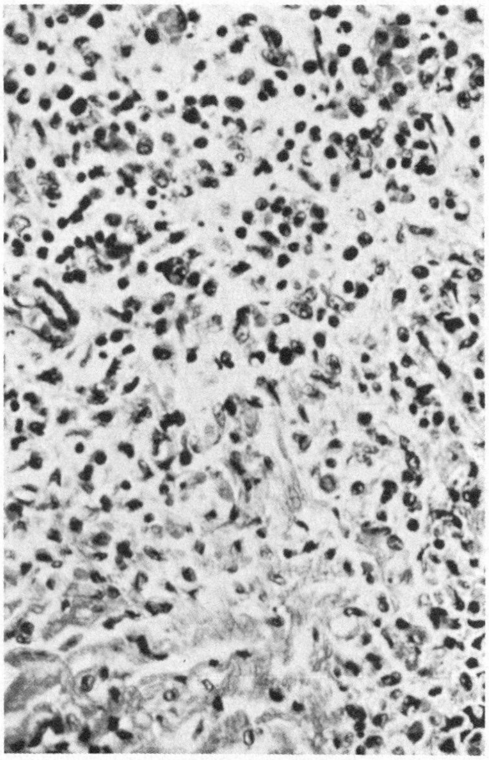

FIGURE 31–1 Photomicrograph of Coxsackie B_2 viral myocarditis. The major features are myocardial necrosis, edema, and heavy infiltrate of lymphocytes and large mononuclear cells. (× 400.) (From Gore, I., and Kline, I. K.: Pericarditis and myocarditis. *In* Gould, S. E. (ed.): Pathology of the Heart and Blood Vessels. 3rd ed. Springfield, Ill., Charles C Thomas, 1968, p. 740.)

suggested by the presence of cardiomegaly without significant murmurs, poor quality heart sounds, a gallop rhythm, an unexplained arrhythmia, and the electrocardiographic findings mentioned above. Important differential diagnostic possibilities include endocardial fibroelastosis, glycogen storage disease with cardiac involvement, anomalous pulmonary origin of a coronary artery, critical aortic stenosis in infancy, and coarctation of the aorta or hypoplastic left heart syndromes.

The vast majority of these children recover from the acute episode of myocarditis with little or no sequelae. On occasion patients may retain a permanent conduction defect or mild cardiac enlargement as a result of the acute illness. Rarely a child may progress from the acute episode to a chronic cardiomyopathy, characterized by signs of left ventricular dysfunction and mitral valve insufficiency. Unfortunately, there are no predictive criteria to identify the latter situation.[8]

Diphtheritic Myocarditis. Diphtheria usually occurs in unimmunized children, especially in the western United States. Myocarditis results from the effect of the endotoxin on the heart rather than from cardiac invasion by the bacillus[9] (Fig. 31–2). Cardiac involvement occurs in approximately 10 per cent of affected patients and is the most common cause of death in this disease. Myocarditis is most reliably indicated by electrocardiographic changes, which range from ST-segment and T-wave changes to arrhythmias and conduction disturbances, including complete heart block.[10] Occasionally, the electrocardiographic pattern of myocardial infarction may emerge. The electrocardiogram is a fair indicator of the extent of myocardial involvement and of prognosis. The latter is generally favorable if only ST-segment and T-wave changes are observed in the absence of conduction system disturbances. Right or left bundle branch block and complete atrioventricular block are associated with mortality rates of 50 to 80 per cent. The electrocardiographic findings may be accompanied by evidence of myocardial dysfunction and ventricular chamber dilatation on cardiac ultrasound.

Treatment for diphtheritic myocarditis is generally unsatisfactory. All patients should receive diphtheria antitoxin and intravenous penicillin after appropriate skin testing. Although corticosteroids have been used in the treatment of the myocardial problem, their value is debatable. Digitalis, diuretics, and antiarrhythmic medications are usually indicated. If the child recovers from the acute episode of diphtheritic myocarditis, the prognosis is quite good.

Myocarditis Due to Trypanosomal Infection. Chagas' disease (p. 1438) is a chronic parasitosis caused by *Trypanosoma cruzi*, transmitted to humans by the bite of insects in the reduviid family. In the United States the disease is seen mostly in the southern states; endemic infection occurs in Latin America. Its most important clinical manifestation is a late-developing, chronic myocarditis and, much less frequently, an early acute myocarditis that is fatal in up to 10 per cent of cases.[11] In patients surviving the acute

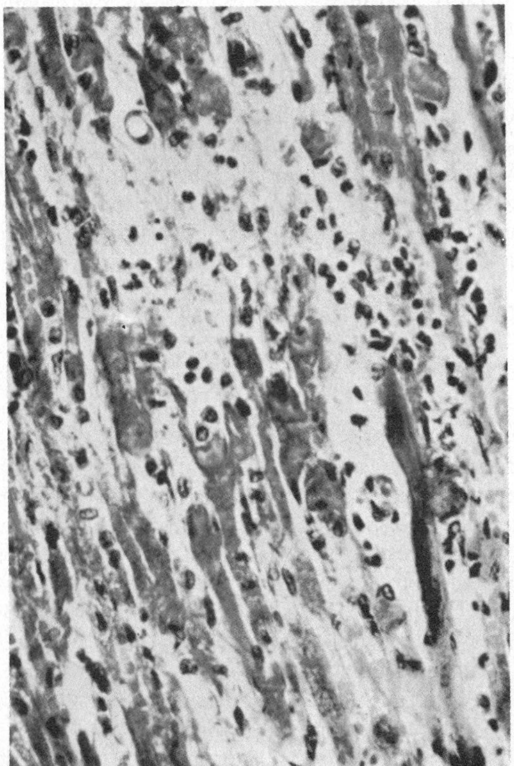

FIGURE 31–2 Photomicrograph of diphtheritic myocarditis. Prominent features are interstitial edema, hyaline degeneration of myocardial fibers, and cellular infiltrate consisting of lymphocytes, plasma cells, and histiocytes. (× 400.) (From Gore, I., and Kline, I. K.: Pericarditis and myocarditis. *In* Gould, S. E. (ed.): Pathology of the Heart and Blood Vessels. 3rd ed. Springfield, Ill., Charles C Thomas, 1968, p. 743.)

stage, cardiomyopathy may occur after an interval of 10 to 30 years.[12] Diagnosis of the acute illness is supported by findings of edema and adenitis in the region of the insect bite, associated with low-grade intermittent fever, sweating, muscular pain, and at times, diarrhea and vomiting; weeks or months later, cardiomegaly, gallop rhythm, and conduction disturbances may be noted. Xenodiagnosis (examination of the excreta of laboratory-bred insects fed on the patient) or complement-fixation tests provide confirmation.

Trypanosoma rhodesiense, which causes African sleeping sickness, may also produce myocardial hemorrhage, interstitial edema, mononuclear infiltration, and myocardial degeneration.[13] Cardiac involvement is usually relatively mild, and the clinical picture is dominated by evidence of encephalitis.

Infective Pericarditis

Numerous infectious agents may be responsible for infective pericarditis. Viral and tuberculous inflammatory pericardial disease is discussed in detail in Chapter 43. Of special concern in infancy and childhood is disease due to pyogenic bacteria.[14–16] Purulent pericarditis occurs most often in the first two decades of life and is especially common in children under 6 years of age. Acute bacterial pericarditis is usually fatal if misdiagnosed or improperly treated. The most common pathogens are *Staphylococcus aureus, Streptococcus pneumoniae, Hemophilus influenzae,* and *Neisseria meningitides.* Unusual organisms causing purulent pericarditis include *Escherichia coli, Pseudomonas, Salmonella, Klebsiella, Proteus,* and *Bacteroides. Hemophilus influenzae,* in particular, affects infants and young children, usually in association either with upper respiratory infection and croup or with lower respiratory pneumonia or bronchitis.

Presenting clinical signs and symptoms vary depending on the age of the patient, the responsible organism, and the site(s) of associated infection. The latter two require identification if therapy is to be effective. Fever, tachycardia, dyspnea, and chest pain are invariably present. Pericardial exudate resulting from the acute suppurative process commonly produces signs of life-threatening cardiac tamponade. Physical findings suggestive of purulent pericarditis include neck vein distention and hepatomegaly, pulsus paradoxicus, and/or systemic hypotension with a narrow pulse pressure, muffled and distant heart sounds, marked cardiomegaly, and a point of maximal cardiac impulse well within the area of percussed dullness. Although the presence of a pericardial friction rub points clearly to pericardial involvement, this sign occurs infrequently.

An enlarged, globular cardiac configuration on chest x-ray and electrocardiographic findings of diminished QRS amplitude and abnormalities of the ST segment (usually elevated) and T waves (often inverted) usually focus attention on the pericardium. Echocardiographic evaluation (p. 130) is superior to scintillation scanning in diagnostic reliability for establishing the diagnosis of pericardial effusion. Culture and examination of pericardial fluid obtained by pericardiocentesis are essential for diagnosis and treatment. Unless effective surgical drainage is combined with antibiotic treatment the mortality rate is high. Operation should consist of creation of a subxiphoid pericardial window with placement of a drainage tube, or anterior pericardiectomy with tube drainage.[17] Early aggressive diagnosis and treatment reduce the risk of death substantially (10 to 20 per cent). Pericardial constriction is uncommon, but all patients should be followed carefully for this complication.

Postpericardiotomy Syndrome

(See also p. 1514)

In the first year after cardiac operation in which the pericardium is opened, and rarely in the second or third postoperative year, a febrile illness may occur, consisting of a pericardial and pleural inflammatory reaction with effusion and often with pulmonary parenchymal involvement. The illness occurs in approximately 25 per cent of children undergoing pericardiotomy and is usually self-limiting; infants undergoing open-heart surgery are affected rarely. It is characterized by fever; chest, neck, or shoulder pain that becomes worse with inspiration; anorexia; and laboratory findings of leukocytosis and an elevated erythrocyte sedimentation rate.[18] Recurrences are uncommon and usually mild. Physical, electrocardiographic, roentgenographic, and echocardiographic signs of pericardial involvement vary with the magnitude of the effusion. Cardiac tamponade, while not usual, occurs with sufficient frequency to warrant careful observation of the patient.

Viral infection and an autoimmume reaction have been implicated in the pathogenesis.[19] Serum antibodies and a rise in titer are found frequently against adenovirus, Coxsackie virus, and cytomegalovirus. Elevations in levels of heat-reactive antibody are common.

The syndrome must be distinguished from infective endocarditis and the postperfusion syndrome of atypical lymphocytosis and hepatomegaly, which occurs approximately 3 to 6 weeks after extracorporeal circulation and is caused by cytomegalovirus infection.[20]

Treatment of the postpericardiotomy syndrome depends upon the degree of patient discomfort and the magnitude of pericardial and/or pleural effusion. In some patients signs of cardiac tamponade will require pericardiocentesis.[21] Bed rest and salicylates or indomethacin lessen patient discomfort and diminish the production of pleural or pericardial fluid. Corticosteroids are indicated for severe illness and promptly relieve fever and symptoms. Antibiotics are not useful in treatment. Prolonged therapy is rarely necessary because of the self-limited nature of this postoperative complication.

PRIMARY CARDIOMYOPATHIES

Obstructive cardiomyopathies are discussed in Chapter 41. The important nonobstructive disorders in this category, of special concern in infants and children, are the familial and nonfamilial forms of endocardial fibroelastosis.[22–26]

ENDOCARDIAL FIBROELASTOSIS. Various designations have been applied to this condition, including endocardial sclerosis, fetal endocarditis, fetal endomyocardial fibrosis, and elastic tissue hyperplasia.[22] In recent years familial cases have been encountered more commonly than has the isolated form. The data provided by family studies fit neither an autosomal recessive nor a multifactorial mode of inheritance. Although the reasons are obscure, a marked reduction has been observed in the past decade of isolated, nonfamilial, endocardial fibroelastosis. No definite cause for this condition has been established, although a host of theories have been proposed; inadequate subendocardial blood flow and/or pre- or postnatal inflammation or infection are currently considered the most likely pathogenetic pathways.[8,24,25]

Pathologically, both primary and secondary forms of endocardial fibroelastosis (EFE) have been recognized.[26] In the *secondary* variety, focal areas of opaque fibroelastotic thickening of the mural endocardium or cardiac valves are observed in association with other types of cardiac malformations. Underlying cardiovascular anomalies are almost always obstructive lesions, particularly of the left side of the heart, and these create cardiac hypertrophy and an imbalance in the myocardial oxygen supply-demand relationship. Thus, secondary EFE occurs quite commonly in aortic stenosis, coarctation of the aorta, and hypoplastic left heart syndrome.

This discussion focuses on the *primary* form of EFE, which invariably involves the left ventricle and mitral and aortic valves without significant associated cardiac defects. Primary EFE commonly produces a marked dilatation of the left ventricle; rarely, a "contracted" type of primary EFE is observed, in which the left ventricle is relatively hypoplastic or normal in size. In the latter situation the right and left atrium and the right ventricle are markedly enlarged and hypertrophied, with minimal or no endocardial sclerosis. In the common, dilated type of primary EFE, microthrombi may be found adherent to the endocardium. The diffuse endocardial hyperplasia may be several millimeters thick (Fig. 31–3). The aortic and mitral valve leaflets are thickened and distorted; mitral regurgitation is especially common. The papillary muscles and chordae tendineae are involved in the fibroelastic process and are shortened and distorted.

Primary EFE is a disease of infancy; symptoms develop usually between 4 and 10 months of age, although rarely they may be present shortly after birth. Clinical features reflect left ventricular dysfunction and congestive heart failure.[27,28] Noted initially are fatigue and breathlessness during feeding, failure to thrive, irritability, pallor, increased sweating, peripheral cyanosis, cough, wheezing, or grunting. Symptoms are usually rapidly progressive. Examination of the infant reveals tachycardia, cardiomegaly, a gallop rhythm, and hepatosplenomegaly. Cardiac murmurs may be absent; approximately 40 per cent of infants have the characteristic apical systolic murmur of mitral regurgitation.

Chest roentgenography reveals marked, generalized cardiomegaly with normal or congested pulmonary vascular markings. A typical electrocardiographic finding is left ventricular hypertrophy with inverted T waves in the left precordial leads; less usual are tracings suggestive of myocardial infarction, varying degrees of atrioventricular block, or arrhythmias. Echocardiographic features include an increase in left atrial and left ventricular dimensions, reduced left ventricular septal and posterior wall motion, reduced ejection fraction, and abnormal mitral valve motion. The diagnosis of primary EFE is usually made easily by the characteristic clinical findings but is, nonetheless, one of exclusion. Differential diagnosis includes anomalous pulmonary origin of the left coronary artery, myocarditis, hypertrophic obstructive cardiomyopathy, anomalies causing left ventricular outflow tract obstruction, and glycogen storage disease of the heart. In general, the first four of these entities differ appreciably from fibroelastosis in their electrocardiographic or echocardiographic features; the skeletal muscle biopsy in glycogen storage disease is diagnostic.

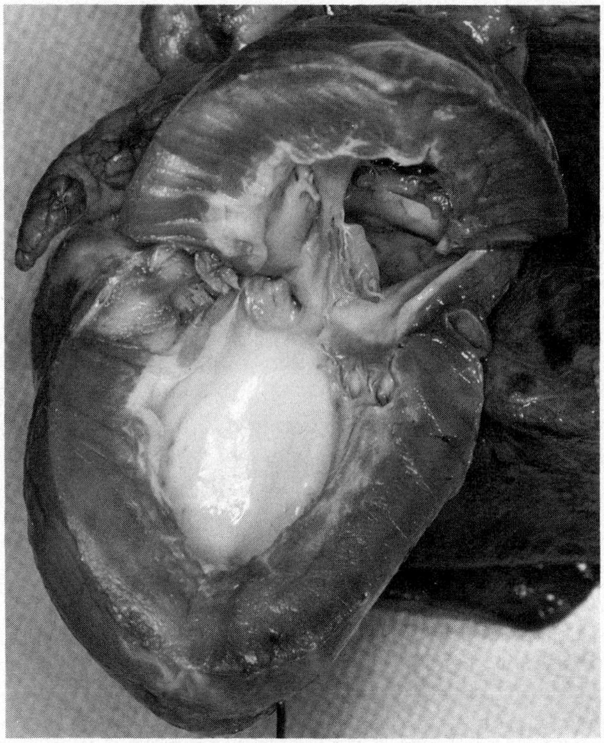

FIGURE 31–3 Diffuse left ventricular endocardial fibroelastosis. There is myocardial hypertrophy and obliteration of the papillary muscles as well as encroachment of the sclerotic subendocardial process onto the base of the aortic cusps. (From Tingelstaad, J. B., et al.: The electrocardiogram in the contracted type of primary endocardial fibroelastosis. Am. J. Cardiol. *27*:304, 1971.)

Hemodynamic studies reveal evidence of left ventricular dysfunction.[29] This includes elevations in left ventricular end-diastolic and left atrial pressures, moderate pulmonary hypertension, widened arteriovenous oxygen differences, and reduced left ventricular stroke volume and cardiac output. Angiography usually demonstrates a markedly dilated left ventricle, a reduced ejection fraction, and varying degrees of mitral regurgitation. The configuration of the left ventricular chamber is usually globular or spherical; dyskinetic or akinetic patterns of contraction are uncommon. Endomyocardial catheter biopsy techniques (p. 297) are difficult to use in infants but, when employed, will show a diagnostic invasion of the endocardium and subendocardium by fibroelastic tissue.[30] The *contracted form* of primary EFE produces a clinical picture of left-sided obstructive disease, particularly if the mitral valve is small. Left atrial pressure is elevated, with pulmonary artery pressures at or near systemic arterial levels.

The optimal management of patients with primary EFE consists of early and prolonged treatment with digitalis. Glycoside therapy should be continued for many years after the disappearance of symptoms, since cessation of the drug may result in acute cardiac failure, even when the heart size has returned to normal. The results of pericardial poudrage and mitral valve replacement in seriously afflicted infants have been disappointing, and operative procedures are not recommended.

SECONDARY CARDIOMYOPATHIES

The designation "secondary" cardiomyopathy refers to intrinsic myocardial disease that is secondary to or associated with systemic disease or diseases of other organs or in other systems. Myocardial disease coexisting with collagen vascular disorders (Chap. 48), neuromuscular disorders (Chap. 50), neoplasms (Chap. 49), acute glomerulonephritis (Chap. 52), and thalassemia (Chap. 49) is discussed elsewhere in this text. Additional secondary cardiomyopathies of special interest to those caring for infants and children are those associated with glycogen storage disease, neonatal thyrotoxicosis, infantile beriberi, protein-calorie malnutrition, tropical endomyocardial fibrosis, and the mucocutaneous lymph node syndrome. Attention in this chapter will be directed to each of these latter disorders.

Glycogen Storage Disease and Infants of Diabetic Mothers

Glycogen storage disease is the result of a deficiency of one or more of the enzymes involved in the biosynthesis and degradation of glycogen.[31] The heart is involved in three of the eight types of glycogen storage disease—types II, III, and IV. Type III (Forbes' or Cori's disease) is a result of deficiency in the debranching enzyme amylo-1,6-glucosidase; type IV (Andersen's disease) is caused by a deficiency in the branching enzyme alpha-1,4 glucan-6 glucosyltransferase. Most cases of glycogen storage causing cardiomegaly occur in type II (Pompe's disease), which results from a deficiency of alpha-1,4-glucosidase (acid maltase), a lysosomal enzyme that hydrolyzes glycogen into glucose. This disease is a hereditary error of metabolism transmitted through a single recessive autosomal gene. Generalized glycogenosis takes place but occurs especially in heart, skeletal muscle, and liver. The glycogen within cardiac muscle cells is biochemically normal but is present in excessive amounts, both within lysosomes and free in the cytoplasm.[32] As a result, the heart enlarges, often to a marked degree, and congestive heart failure supervenes. Usually glycogen deposition within the myocardium is uniform, although occasionally the interventricular septum is especially involved, producing subpulmonic obstruction or a constellation of features indistinguishable from hypertrophic obstructive cardiomyopathy. Selective angiography has revealed a distinctive trabeculation of the left ventricle in some infants.[33]

Clinical signs of type II glycogen storage disease usually become prominent in the early neonatal period.[34] Characteristic symptoms include failure to thrive, progressive hypotonia, lethargy, and a weak cry. Prominent early features include nonspecific cardiac murmurs, cardiomegaly, signs of congestive heart failure, macroglossia, poor skeletal muscle tone, and weakness. The electrocardiogram shows extremely tall, broad QRS complexes with a short P-R interval (commonly less than 0.09 sec) (Fig. 31–4). The short P-R interval may be the result of facilitated atrioventricular conduction due to myocardial glycogen deposition. Less often, deep Q waves are observed over the mid or left precordium as well as T-wave inversion and ST-segment elevation. Chest roentgenograms show an enlarged globular heart associated with pulmonary vascular congestion (Fig. 31–5). In rare patients with cardiac glycogenosis the cardiac murmur suggests left ventricular outflow tract obstruction and/or mitral regurgitation; the echocardiographic, hemodynamic, and angiographic features in this subgroup are indistinguishable from those in infants with hypertrophic obstructive cardiomyopathy. Diagnosis is confirmed by demonstrating the enzymatic deficiency in lymphocytes, skeletal muscle, or liver. Skeletal muscle biopsy reveals histological and histochemical evidence of glycogen deposition.

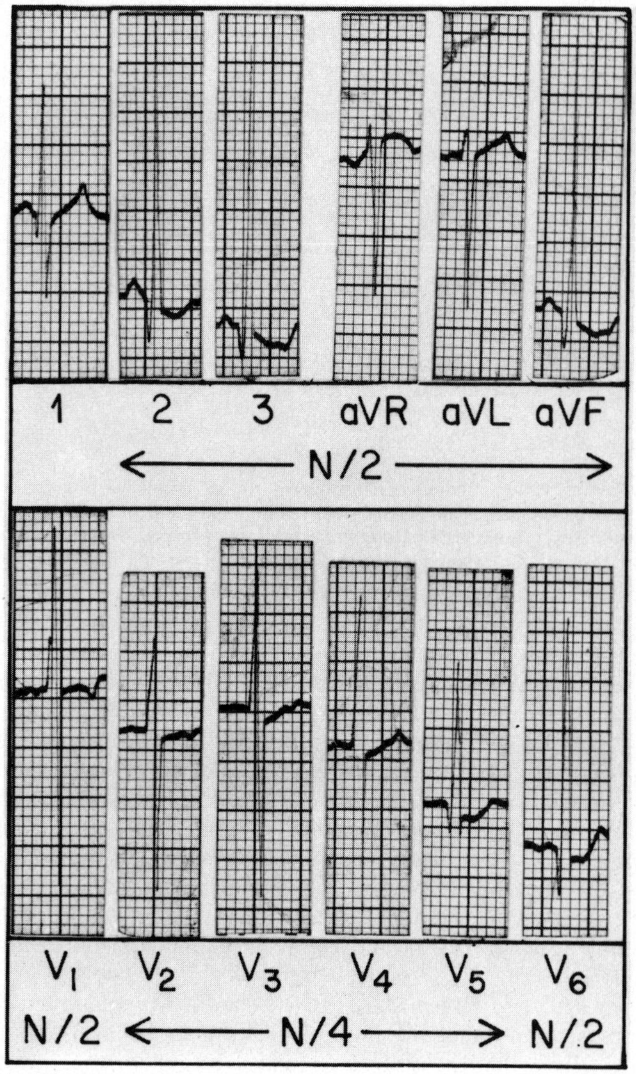

FIGURE 31–4 Electrocardiogram in an infant with glycogen storage disease showing a short PR interval and left ventricular hypertrophy.

Cardiac glycogenosis may be confused with other entities that cause cardiac failure in the early months of life, including endocardial fibroelastosis, anomalous pulmonary origin of the left coronary artery, fixed and dynamic forms of left ventricular outflow tract obstruction, coarctation of the aorta, and myocarditis. The short P-R interval and the skeletal muscle hypotonia in glycogen storage disease help distinguish this disorder from *endocardial fibroelastosis.* Infants with an *aberrant left coronary artery* usually have a

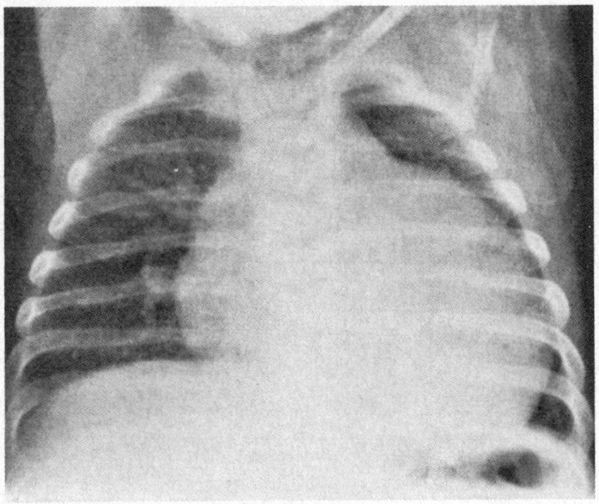

FIGURE 31–5 Chest roentgenogram of an infant with glycogen storage disease showing massive cardiomegaly and pulmonary edema. (From Taussig, H.: Congenital Malformations of the Heart. Vol. 2. 2nd ed. Commonwealth Fund, Harvard University, Boston, 1960, p. 901.)

distinctive electrocardiographic pattern of anterolateral myocardial infarction. In infants with *coarctation of the aorta* the pulse and blood pressure discrepancies between the upper and lower extremities point to the proper diagnosis (p. 975). *Myocarditis* is usually of abrupt onset in a previously healthy child and is not associated with marked hypotonia; the generally low-voltage electrocardiogram does not show the short P-R interval. Occasionally the skeletal muscle hypotonia and the macroglossia in infants with glycogen storage disease raise the possibilities of amyotonia congenita and cretinism or mongolism, respectively.

Cardiac glycogenosis leads to progressive impairment of myocardial function; Pompe's disease is uniformly fatal usually within the first year of life. Death is quite often the result of either cardiac failure or complications of respiratory management such as pneumonia or aspiration.

Infants born of diabetic mothers who are not afflicted with the enzyme disorder of glycogen storage disease occasionally display two basic forms of cardiomyopathy, both of which are usually transient.[34,35] It has been suggested that suboptimal metabolic control of maternal diabetes during pregnancy increases the incidence of these abnormalities.[36,37] In some of these infants, hypertrophy and hyperplasia of myocardial cells constitute a diffuse process, producing reversible signs and symptoms that resemble those of congestive cardiomyopathy. In other infants, the clinical findings are indistinguishable from hypertrophic obstructive cardiomyopathy. The natural history in this latter group has, in general, been one of gradual spontaneous regression of obstructive murmurs, cardiomegaly, and electrocardiographic and echocardiographic abnormalities typical of hypertrophic obstructive cardiomyopathy.

Neonatal Thyrotoxicosis

Long-acting thyroid-stimulating hormone, a 7S $gamma_2$ globulin, traverses the placental barrier and stimulates the fetal thyroid gland when maternal hyperthyroidism exists.[38] Infants are often born prematurely or are small for gestational age. Jitteriness and irritability are noted early. Cardiac findings include tachycardia, bounding pulses, systolic hypertension, and a precordial systolic murmur.[38–40] Frequently, congestive heart failure is present, and occasionally, the presenting finding is an episode of paroxysmal atrial tachycardia. A neonatal goiter may be observed, especially if the mother received iodine therapy during pregnancy.

Diagnosis should be anticipated whenever a history of hyperthyroidism exists in the mother. Neonatal thyrotoxicosis occurs in the offspring of about 1 to 2 per cent of these women. A maternal level of long-acting thyroid-stimulating hormone should be obtained before delivery in anticipation of the problem arising in the newborn infant, since high levels are often observed in both mother and offspring. A maternal level in excess of 300 per cent implies neonatal thyrotoxicosis, but a low value does not ensure that the newborn will not be affected. Thyroxine levels are increased in the newborn.

The infant who presents with heart failure may be treated with digitalis and propylthiouracil or carbamizole. However, the latter two drugs will not be completely effective for many weeks. Propranolol is usually the drug of choice. Supportive measures such as sedation and minimal manipulation may be helpful. Exchange transfusion or corticosteroid treatment is of no proven benefit.

Infants usually improve between the second and third months of life, although lack of attention to the problem or inadequate therapy may result in a fatal outcome.

Infantile Beriberi

(See also page 814)

Thiamine (vitamin B_1) deficiency occurs mainly in regions of southeast Asia, India, Brazil, and Africa, in which the dietary staple is polished rice or cassava. Thiamine functions as a coenzyme in decarboxylation of alpha-keto acids and in the utilization of pentose in the hexose monophosphate shunt. A reduction in myocardial energy production causes symptoms in the infant, usually between one and four months of age, who is breastfed by a thiamine-deficient mother.[41] Such infants are usually edematous, irritable, pale, and anorectic. Hoarseness or aphonia is common, owing to involvement of the recurrent laryngeal nerve; blepharoptosis occurs in one third of infants. Typically, cardiac involvement manifests as dilatation of the right ventricle and prominent signs of systemic venous congestion. Electrocardiographic findings are nonspecific, and radiological findings consist principally of right ventricular dilatation. Infantile beriberi may be rapidly fatal but responds quickly and well to administration of thiamine (25 to 50 mg intravenously initially, with reduction of the dose to 10 mg/day for several days, and then orally for several weeks). Dramatic amelioration occurs within a few days of the cardiac findings. Cure is complete with no known sequelae.

Protein-Calorie Malnutrition

(See also page 1742)

This is a major public health problem in underdeveloped areas of the tropics.[42,43] In infants, inadequate diet results in a state of emaciation termed "marasmus;" "kwashiorkor" is a designation applied to this syndrome in children beyond one year of age. The disease results from a deficiency of protein relative to calories, although the latter and other essential nutrients are often lacking as well. General muscle wasting, loss of subcutaneous fat, and atrophy of most organs, including the heart, are typical in marasmic infants. In both marasmus and kwashiorkor, thinning and atrophy of cardiac muscle fibers and interstitial edema or vacuolization of the myocardial fibers are noted.[44] As the condition progresses, listlessness becomes prominent. Cardiovascular collapse is precipitated easily in these infants by the stress of infection.

In both infancy and childhood the principal physical findings reflect systemic hypoperfusion and consist principally of hypothermia, hypotension, tachycardia, and low-amplitude peripheral pulsations. Peripheral edema is prominent, as are wasting of the skeletal musculature, exfoliative dermatitis, and gray or reddish discoloration of the hair. Changes seen on electrocardiogram and on radiographic examination are nonspecific.

Treatment should be directed at correcting fluid and electrolyte imbalance, eradication of infection, and management of such associated problems as anemia and parasitic infestation.[45] Care is required in the correction of dehydration or severe anemia, since volume overload of the heart is easily produced. Supplements of potassium and magnesium are often required, and because of deficiencies in these elements, digitalis should probably be avoided or used with extreme caution. If the infant or child survives the initial phase, a well-balanced diet will effect an impressive recovery over several months' duration.

Tropical Endomyocardial Fibrosis

Endomyocardial fibrosis is a rare, acquired, progressive disease, usually involving children and young adults from Africa, Southeast Asia, and South America. This cardiomyopathy of unknown etiology is characterized by focal, endocardial fibrosis of one or rarely both ventricles.[46] Conjecture exists as to whether or not tropical endomyocardial fibrosis, which is not associated with eosinophilia, and Löffler's endocarditis with eosinophilia (Chap. 41) are the same disorders described from tropical and temperate climates, respectively.[47] Endocardial fibrosis is located almost exclusively in the inflow tracts of the ventricles and commonly involves one or the other atrioventricular valve. Partial obliteration of either cardiac chamber results in reduced ventricular compliance with impairment of filling. The fibrotic process often involves the chordae tendineae, resulting in mitral and/or tricuspid regurgitation. Plaques of heaped-up fibrous tissue without elastic fibers are especially common within the left ventricle. Endomyocardial fibrosis involving the right ventricle may have to be differentiated from Ebstein's anomaly of the tricuspid valve (p. 996), and endomyocardial fibrosis involving the left ventricle may have to be differentiated from rheumatic mitral regurgitation.

When left ventricular disease predominates, the clinical findings often resemble those of mitral stenosis or regurgitation. When endocardial involvement of the right ventricle is more severe than that of the left ventricle, the patient usually presents with findings of markedly elevated systemic venous pressure and tricuspid regurgitation.

Treatment is supportive, and survival usually depends on the extent of endocardial and valvular involvement and is better when right ventricular disease predominates. Mean survival after the onset of symptoms is approximately 24 months. Specific treatment does not exist, and corticosteroid therapy has not proved efficacious. Surgical excision (decortication) of affected tissue, with prosthetic valve replacement has been associated with clinical improvement.[48,49] However, children most severely affected by this disease reside in regions of the tropics and subtropics where cardiac surgery is not readily available.

Mucocutaneous Lymph Node Syndrome

The mucocutaneous lymph node syndrome in infancy (Kawasaki's disease) has been accepted as a new syndrome by most Japanese pediatricians.[50] The clinical and pathological findings are strikingly similar to those of polyarteritis nodosa of infancy, and important questions and controversy exist about whether the two disorders are one and the same.[51,52] In excess of 18,000 cases have been reported and the disorder is being recognized with increasing frequency in North America and Europe.[53]

The syndrome is a febrile illness of children that occurs before the age of 10 and usually before the age of 2 years. Patients commonly present with fever and ocular and oral manifestations followed in 5 days by a rash and indurative edema of the hands and feet, with palmar and plantar erythema. Finally, after about 2 weeks, cutaneous desquamation occurs. Diagnostic criteria include (1) a fever lasting five days or more that is unresponsive to antibiotics; (2) bilateral congestion of the ocular conjunctiva; (3) peripheral limb changes that include an indurative peripheral edema and erythema of the palms and feet, followed later in the course of the illness by a membranous desquamation of the fingertips; (4) changes in the lips and mouth, including dry, erythematous, and fissured lips, injected oropharyngeal mucosa, and a strawberry tongue; and (5) a polymorphous exanthema of the trunk without crusts or vesicles. Diagnosis is accepted when the first criterion and at least three of the remainder are present.

In addition to the mucous membrane and cutaneous effects, multiple organ system involvement has been noted. Noncardiovascular complications of the illness include arthritis, cerebrospinal fluid pleocytosis, pulmonary infiltrates, and hydrops of the gallbladder. The illness is often accompanied by cervical adenopathy, diarrhea, leukocytosis with a predominance of neutrophils, thrombocytosis, sterile pyuria and proteinuria, elevated liver transaminases, an elevation in the erythrocyte sedimentation rate and alpha-2-globulin, and a positive C-reactive protein.

Based on pathologic data, progression of the disease may be divided into four stages.[54] In stage I, lasting 1 to 9 days, acute perivasculitis of the small arteries is evident and involves the vasa vasorum of the major coronary arteries. Pericarditis, interstitial myocarditis, and endocardial inflammation are also seen; these changes consist chiefly of neutrophilic, eosinophilic, and lymphocytic infiltrations. In stage II, of 12 to 25 days' duration, panvasculitis involves the major coronary arteries. It affects the intima, media, and adventitia and results in aneurysm and thrombus formation. In stage III, of 28 to 31 days' duration, granulating thrombi and marked intimal thickening cause partial

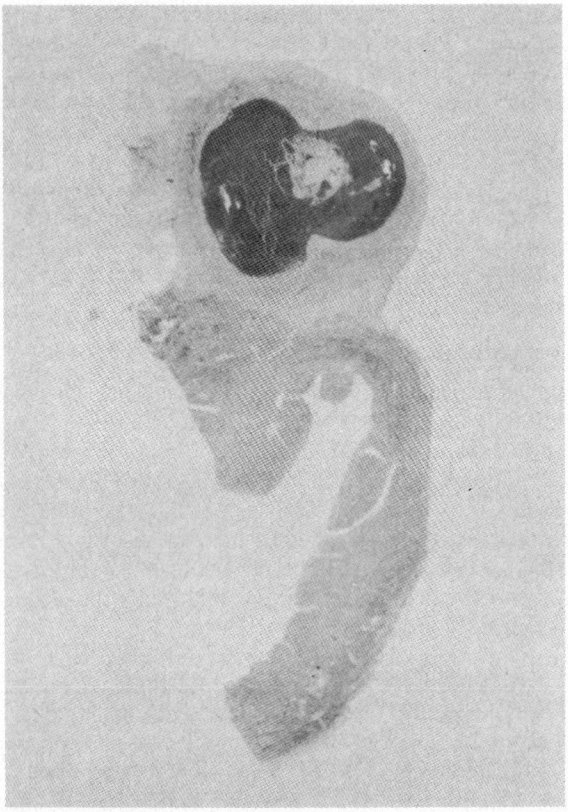

FIGURE 31–6 Low-power photomicrograph of a coronary artery aneurysm with recent occlusive thrombosis in a patient with mucocutaneous lymph node syndrome. (From Landing, B. H., and Larson, E. J.: Are infantile periarteritis nodosa with coronary artery involvement and fatal mucocutaneous lymph node syndrome the same? Comparison of 20 patients from North America with patients from Hawaii and Japan. Pediatrics *59*:651, 1977. Copyright American Academy of Pediatrics, 1977.)

or total occlusion of the major coronary arteries. Stage IV follows and may be of many years' duration, in which healing occurs, consisting of myocardial scarring, calcification, and recanalization of occluded arteries.

The syndrome has an associated mortality of 1 to 2 per cent, secondary to complications from coronary artery involvement, with a majority of deaths occurring in the third or fourth week of the illness.[55] Autopsy examination has almost uniformly demonstrated coronary arterial aneurysms, with occlusion due to thromboendarteritis (Fig. 31–6). Occasional findings include rupture of coronary arterial aneurysms, myocardial infarction, diffuse endocardial sclerosis, and aneurysms of peripheral arteries.

It appears that the disease has often been misdiagnosed in the United States as scarlet fever, Stevens-Johnson syndrome, Rocky Mountain spotted fever, rheumatoid arthritis, scleroderma, or lupus erythematosus.

Infants and children with this syndrome should be watched closely for signs of cardiac involvement. A significant number of patients show evidence of myocarditis or pericarditis, or both, in the early phases of the disease.[56,57] Electrocardiographic evidence of myocarditis with low voltage and nonspecific ST-T wave changes, are seen in 45 per cent of patients, echocardiographic evidence of poor left ventricular function in 25 per cent, pericardial effusion in 9 per cent, cardiomegaly on chest radiographs in 25 per cent, and a gallop rhythm in 12 percent. Aneurysms of the coronary arteries with narrowing, tortuosity, and obstruction are almost invariably present on aortography and coronary angiography[58,59] (Fig. 31–7). Excellent success has been achieved in visualizing these lesions with two-dimensional cross-sectional echocardiography (Fig. 31–8).[59,59a] Although the incidence of residual cardiac abnormalities following recovery from the acute illness phase is not known, estimates from 25 to 60 per cent have been

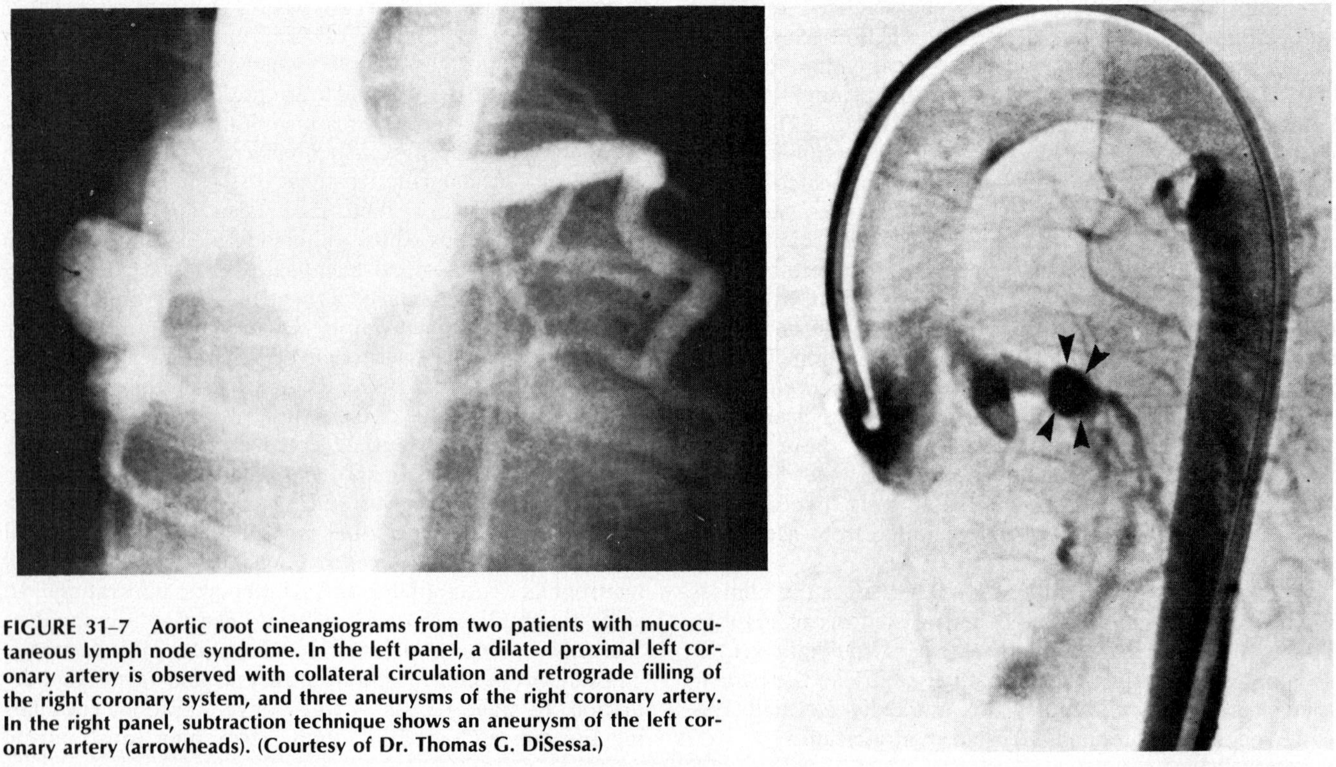

FIGURE 31–7 Aortic root cineangiograms from two patients with mucocutaneous lymph node syndrome. In the left panel, a dilated proximal left coronary artery is observed with collateral circulation and retrograde filling of the right coronary system, and three aneurysms of the right coronary artery. In the right panel, subtraction technique shows an aneurysm of the left coronary artery (arrowheads). (Courtesy of Dr. Thomas G. DiSessa.)

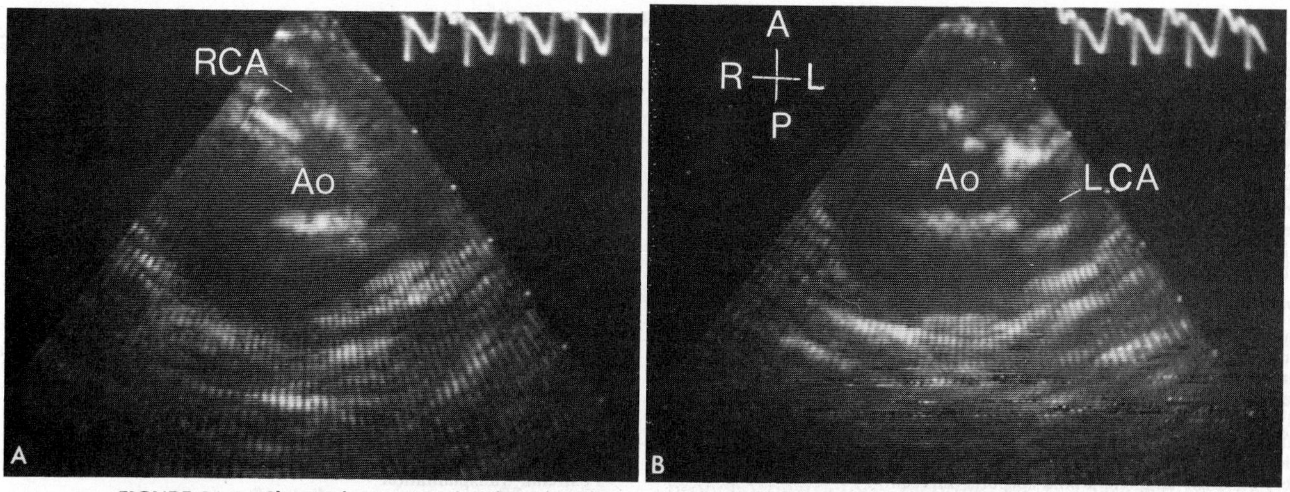

FIGURE 31–8 Short-axis cross-sectional echocardiographic views of aneurysms of the proximal right coronary artery (RCA) (*A*) and proximal left coronary artery (LCA) (*B*) in a 3-year-old boy with mucocutaneous lymph node syndrome. The right ventricular outflow tract is anterior (A) to the aorta (Ao) and the left atrium is posterior (P). R = right; L = left.

suggested.[60,61,61a] Associated findings may include compromise of left ventricular function secondary to the coronary arterial involvement and papillary muscle dysfunction with mital regurgitation. It has been suggested that corticosteroid therapy is detrimental during the acute illness. Salicylate treatment (30 mg/kg/day) is advisable for all patients in the acute phases of the illness. In patients who develop coronary arterial involvement, aspirin therapy is maintained indefinitely (5 to 10 mg/kg/day). In as many as 50 per cent of patients followed serially by means of coronary arteriography, it has been noted that the arterial aneurysms tend to regress.[61] Most children survive the acute phase of the illness, although the state of the coronary arteries in these survivors is usually not known. Two-dimensional echocardiography is indicated in all children with evidence of significant cardiac involvement; coronary angiography is suggested in those with proven coronary arterial aneurysm(s) or obstruction. The prognosis for these children should be guarded, and some may be candidates for coronary arterial bypass surgery.[61b,61c]

SYSTEMIC HYPERTENSION

(See also page 891)

Unfortunately, physicians usually consider hypertension a disease of adults and not of children. Thus, all too frequently, blood pressure is not recorded during the pediatric physical examination. It should be emphasized that elevations in systemic blood pressure may occur in as much as 2 per cent of the pediatric population, and that undetected or untreated hypertension may lead to unfortunate consequences.[62–64] Three points in particular require recognition:

1. Causes of hypertension in infants and children differ markedly from those in adults. Most children have secondary rather than essential forms of hypertension (Table 31–1), so that a premium should be placed on finding a remedial cause.

2. Offspring of hypertensive parents are known to have an increased susceptibility to blood pressure elevation (Chap. 47).

3. Children with elevated blood pressure require the same surveillance and treatment as do adults.

Accurate blood pressure measurements require cuffs of different sizes because of the variation in arm size from infancy through adolescence.[65] To measure blood pressure correctly, the inner rubber bag should be wide enough to cover two thirds of the length and three fourths of the circumference of the upper arm or thigh while leaving the antecubital or popliteal fossa free. A cuff that is too small is apt to produce spuriously high readings. In infants under age 2 years the flush technique may be used, although a Doppler instrument is preferred. Since disappearance of the Korotkoff sound may cause underestimation of the diastolic pressure, both muffling (the fourth Korotkoff sound) and the disappearance of the sound (the fifth Korotkoff sound) should be recorded. The fourth Korotkoff sound is the more accurate measure of diastolic pressure in most prepubertal children; beyond adolescence the fifth sound more closely reflects diastolic pressure.[67,68]

The normal ranges of blood pressure relative to age are illustrated in Figures 31–9 to 31–11 and serve as a guide in judging unsafe levels. Since considerable variation exists in most children's pressures, it should be recognized that a single blood pressure recording at, or higher than, the 90th percentile at a single point in time may not be an abnormal finding. In an apparently healthy child measurements should be repeated serially; further investigation is warranted if the blood pressure persists at or above the 95th percentile. In contrast, definite or severe hypertension, i.e., pressures well beyond the broad limits of normal, require prompt investigation and treatment.[69] Particularly urgent attention must be paid to those children whose systolic and diastolic pressures are remarkably high, i.e., equal to or greater than 180 and 110 mm Hg, respectively. Other findings identifying the patient at risk include localized neurological signs and/or local or generalized seizures; blurred vision or such eye ground changes as retinal hemorrhage, exudate, papilledema, or retinal arterial constriction; renal or abdominal pain; evidence of left ventricular hypertrophy or cardiac decompensation; renal dysfunction; palpation of an abdominal mass

TABLE 31–2 DRUGS COMMONLY USED IN PEDIATRIC CARDIOLOGY

Drug	Route of Administration	Dosage
Acetaminophen (Tylenol)	PO or PR	< 1 year 60 mg (q4h) 1 to 3 years 120 mg (q4h) > 3 years 120 to 240 mg (q4h)
Acetylsalicylic acid (Aspirin)	PO or PR	30 to 100 mg/kg/day (q4h)
ε-Aminocaproic acid (Amicar)	IV	Total 100 mg/kg; ¼ total dose (q1h)
Aminophylline	PO, PR, or IV	12 mg/kg/day (q6h)
Ammonium chloride	PO	75 mg/kg/day (q6h)
Atropine	IV, SC, or PO	0.01 to 0.03 mg/kg (q4–6h)
Bicarbonate sodium	IV	1 to 2 mEq/kg/5 min
Bishydroxycoumarin (Dicumarol)	PO	Loading dose: 50 to 100 mg Maintenance dose: 10 to 50 mg/day (Regulate according to prothrombin times)
Bretylium	IV	5 mg/kg/dose over 10 minutes, then 50 to 100 μg/kg/min
Calcium chloride	IV	1 to 4 ml of 10% solution; for cardiac arrest, 10 mg/kg/dose
Calcium gluconate	IV PO	2 to 6 ml of 10% solution; for cardiac arrest, 10 mg/kg/dose 500 mg/kg/day (q6h)
Chlorothiazide (Diuril)	PO	20 to 40 mg/kg/day (q12h)
Chlorthalidone	PO	1 to 2 mg/kg/day (q12h)
Cholestyramine (Questran)	PO	250 to 1500 mg/kg/day (q6–12h)
Clofibrate (Atromid S)	PO	0.5 to 1.5 mg/day in divided doses
Clonidine (Catapres)	PO	0.002 to 0.008 mg/kg/day in divided doses
Codeine	PO	0.5 to 1.5 mg/kg/dose (q3h)
Dexamethasone (Decadron)	IV	0.2 to 0.4 mg/kg/dose (q6h) for cerebral edema
Diazoxide	IV	3 to 5 mg/kg/dose over 30 sec (q2–6h) (careful of severe hypotension)
Digitalis (Digoxin)		Loading dose: Premature infants 0.030 mg/kg IV or IM Term infants Oral: Up to 2 wk: 0.03 mg/kg 2 wk to 6 mo: 0.06 mg/kg 6 mo to 2 yr: 0.045 mg/kg Beyond 2 yr: 0.03 mg/kg Parenteral: 75% of oral dose Maintenance dose: 1/3 to 1/4 of loading dose, given in two divided doses/24 hr
Dobutamine	IV	2 to 10 μg/kg/min
Dopamine	IV	1 gm in 250 ml D_5W; 2 to 20 μg/kg/min
Edrophonium chloride (Tensilon)	IV	0.05 to 0.2 mg/kg/dose
Ephedrine sulfate	IM or PO	0.8 to 1.6 mg/kg/day (q6h)
Epinephrine (Adrenalin)	IV	For cardiac arrest: single dose: 0.1 to 1.0 ml of 1:1000; 0.1 to 1.0 μg/min infusion
Ethacrynic acid (Edecrin)	IV	1.0 mg/kg/day
Ethylenediaminetetraacetic acid (EDTA) disodium salt	IV	20 mg/ml: 10 to 50 mg/kg (q12h)
Furosemide (Lasix)	IV or IM PO	1 to 2 mg/kg/dose 1 to 4 mg/kg/day

TABLE 31–2 DRUGS COMMONLY USED IN PEDIATRIC CARDIOLOGY (*Continued*)

Drug	Route of Administration	Dosage
Glucagon	IV	0.05 to 0.10 mg/kg/hr
Glucose 50%	IV	1 mg/kg/dose
Glucose 50% + Insulin	IV	1 gm glucose/kg (50% solution) with insulin, 1 unit/3 gm glucose
Guanethidine sulfate (Ismelin)	PO	0.2 to 1.0 mg/kg/day (q6h)
Heparin	IV	100 units/kg (q4h)
Hydralazine hydrochloride (Apresoline)	IV PO	0.8 to 3.0 mg/kg/day (q4–6h) 0.75 to 7.5 mg/kg/day (q6–8h)
Hydrochlorothiazide	PO	1 to 3 mg/kg/day (q12h)
Hydrocortisone sodium succinate (Solu-Cortef)	IV	For shock: 50 to 75 mg/kg (q6h)
Indomethacin	IV	0.2 mg/kg/dose
Innovar (Fentanyl citrate & Droperidol)	IV	0.01 to 0.02 ml/kg
Isoproterenol hydrochloride (Isuprel hydrochloride)	IV	0.05 to 0.25 μg/kg/min
Lidocaine (Xylocaine hydrochloride)	IV	Single dose: 1 mg/kg; 20 to 50 μg/kg/min infusion
Magnesium sulfate, 3%	IV	For neonatal seizure: single dose: 2 to 6 ml
Mannitol	IV	For cerebral edema: 1 to 2 gm/kg Repeated doses: 250 mg/kg (q4h) For hemoglobinuria: single dose: 0.5 gm/kg; 5% solution infusion if necessary
Meperidine hydrochloride (Demerol)	IM or IV	1 mg/kg/dose (q3h)
Meralluride (Mercuhydrin)	IM	< 1 yr: single dose: 0.1 to 0.3 ml 1 to 5 yr: single dose: 0.3 to 0.7 ml > 5 yr: single dose: 1 ml
Mercaptomerin sodium (Thiomerin sodium)	IM	Same as Meralluride
Metaraminol (Aramine metaraminol bitartrate)	IV	Single dose: 0.1 mg/kg or 50 mg/500 ml; titrate to effect infusion
Methyldopa (Aldomet)	PO or IV	10 to 40 mg/kg/day (q6–8h)
Methylprednisolone (Solu-Medrol)	IV	For shock: 30 mg/kg/dose For cerebral edema: 4 to 5 mg/kg/dose
Minoxidil	PO	0.05 to 2.0 mg/kg/day
Morphine sulfate	SC	0.1 to 0.2 mg/kg/dose (q3h)
Naloxone hydrochloride (Narcan)	IM or IV	0.01 mg/kg/dose
Nitroprusside, sodium	IV	0.5 to 8.0 μg/kg/min initial rate; titrate to effect
Norepinephrine (Levophed bitartrate)	IV	0.1 to 1.0 μg/kg/min
Pentobarbital (Nembutal)	PO or IM	2 to 3 mg/kg/dose
Phenobarbital	PO or IM	3 to 5 mg/kg/day (q8h)
Phenoxybenzamine	IV	0.5 to 1.0 mg/kg
Phentolamine	IV	0.05 to 0.10 mg/kg

Table continues on following page

TABLE 31–2 DRUGS COMMONLY USED IN PEDIATRIC CARDIOLOGY (*Continued*)

Drug	Route of Administration	Dosage
Phenylephrine (Neo-Synephrine hydrochloride)	IV	10 mg/100 ml D_5W; 1 to 10 μg/kg/min, titrate to effect
Phenytoin (Dilantin)	PO or IV	For seizures: 5 to 10 mg/kg/day (q8h) For arrhythmias: 1 to 5 mg/kg/5 min
Potassium chloride	PO IV	1 to 2 mEq/kg/day 0.5 mEq/kg/hr not to exceed 2 mEq/kg, as 40 to 80 mEq/l solution
Potassium gluconate (Kaon) and Potassium triplex	PO	1 to 2 mEq/kg/day
Procainamide hydrochloride (Pronestyl)	PO IM IV	40 to 60 mg/kg/day (q4–6h) 5 to 8 mg/kg (q6h) 1 mg/kg/dose over 5 min
Propranolol hydrochloride (Inderal)	PO IV IM	1.0 to 6.0 mg/kg/day (divide q6h) 0.01 to 0.15 mg/kg (q6–8h) 0.5 to 1.0 mg/kg (q4–6h)
Promethazine	PO	1 to 2 mg/kg/day (q6–8h)
Prostaglandin E_1	IV	0.1 μg/kg/min, reduce to 0.01 μg/kg/min to maintain effect
Protamine sulfate	IV	3 mg for every 200 units of heparin
Quinidine gluconate	PO IM or IV	10 to 30 mg/kg/day (q4–8h) 2 to 10 mg/kg/dose (q3–6h)
Quinidine sulfate	PO	3 to 12 mg/kg/dose (q3h)
Reserpine (Serpasil)	PO IM	0.01 to 0.02 mg/kg/day (q12h) 0.07 mg/kg (q12h)
Sodium polystyrene sulfonate (Kayexalate)	PR	1 gm/kg mixed with 70% sorbitol
Spironolactone	PO	1 to 3 mg/kg/day (q6–12h)
Succinylcholine chloride (Anectine chloride)	IM IV	2 mg/kg/dose 1 mg/kg/dose
Tolazoline (Prixoline)	IV	1 mg/kg/dose, then 1 to 3 mg/kg/hr
Triamterene	PO	2–4 mg/kg/day
Trimethaphan camsylate (Arfonad)	IV	50 mg in 100 ml D_5W, titrate to effect
Tris (Hydroxymethyl) aminomethane (THAM)	IV	(0.3M) weight (kg) × base deficit = dose in ml
Tubocurarine chloride (curare)	IM or IV	Initial dose: 0.3 to 0.5 mg/kg Subsequent dose: 0.1 mg/kg
Verapamil	IV	0.1 to 0.2 mg/kg/dose over 2 min
Vitamin K (Aquamephyton)	IM or IV	Single dose (neonate): 1 mg
Warfarin sodium crystalline (Coumadin)	PO or IM	Initial dose: 0.5 mg/kg Maintenance dose: 1 to 5 mg/day (Regulate according to prothrombin times)

TABLE 31–3 FASTING LIPID LEVELS IN SCHOOL CHILDREN

A. Cholesterol

	Males				Females			
Age	*5%*	*50%*	*95%*	*N*	*5%*	*50%*	*95%*	*N*
5	109	150	189	60	120	155	200	58
6	121	154	200	193	119	154	198	197
7	122	154	199	194	125	159	202	164
8	125	159	194	188	117	161	203	165
9	125	158	213	165	122	161	206	202
10	129	163	206	187	125	159	205	197
11	122	159	202	198	126	161	204	194
12	119	159	213	221	116	158	210	222
13	116	153	205	184	125	158	200	181
14	117	150	187	168	120	157	203	182
15	113	148	190	146	121	157	203	188
16	118	148	192	108	121	151	200	134
17	108	145	189	91	118	164	209	110

B. Triglyceride

	Males				Females			
Age	*5%*	*50%*	*95%*	*N*	*5%*	*50%*	*95%*	*N*
5	23	46	99	60	26	48	92	58
6	26	47	95	193	27	47	94	197
7	27	43	102	194	26	50	106	164
8	24	43	91	188	26	50	97	165
9	25	49	92	165	29	52	110	202
10	23	46	108	187	30	51	110	197
11	24	48	103	198	29	61	140	194
12	28	53	119	221	33	61	123	222
13	26	52	113	184	34	61	127	181
14	30	50	106	168	33	56	123	182
15	26	52	111	146	33	58	111	188
16	31	63	108	108	34	59	112	134
17	31	58	132	91	34	65	140	110

N = Number of children studied.
From Carter, G. A., et al.: Coronary heart disease risk factors: Identification and management. *In* Shen, J. T. (ed.): Clinical Practice of Adolescent Medicine. New York, Appleton-Century-Crofts, 1979.

be treated. Guidelines for abnormal levels in the first two decades of life are provided in Table 31–3.

Hyperlipidemia is defined as an increase in the plasma concentration of cholesterol or triglycerides, or both, above these normal values, but it should be recognized that the latter may be changed as a result of future studies. Diagnosis should be reserved for those children with elevated cholesterol or triglyceride levels on two or more separate determinations from venous blood samples after a 12-hour fast; the laboratory in which the tests are performed must be unquestionably accurate and reliable.

In the absence of mass screening programs or incorporation of this test as part of routine pediatric practice, serum lipid levels should be analyzed in all children from families with hyperlipidemia or with histories that include hypertension, myocardial infarction stroke, or peripheral vascular disease among parents or grandparents before age 50 years.[72,74,75] Differentiation is necessary between acquired hyperlipidemia and one of the familial, and presumably genetic, hyperlipidemias.

Homozygous familial hypercholesterolemia causes severe atherosclerosis of the coronary arteries and myocardial infarction in childhood; rarely it causes atherosclerosis of the aortic valve, leading to critical aortic stenosis that requires surgical treatment.[76]

References

1. Ainger, L. E., Lawyer, N. G., and Fitch, C. W.: Neonatal rubella myocarditis. Br. Heart J. *28*:691, 1966.
2. Ayuthya, T. S. N., Jayavasu, J., and Pongpanich, B.: Coxsackie group B virus in primary myocardial disease in infants and children. Am. Heart J. *88*:311, 1974.
3. Suckling, P. V., and Vogelpoel, L.: Coxsackie myocarditis of the newborn. Lancet *2*:421, 1970.
4. Lerner, A. M., and Wilson, F. M.: Virus myocardiopathy. Progr. Med. Virol. *15*:63, 1973.
5. Oda, T., Hamamoto, K. and Morinaga, H.: Clinical aspects of non-rheumatic myocarditis in children. Jap. Circ. J. *43*:443, 1979.
6. Wink, K., and Schmitz, H.: Cytomegalovirus myocarditis. Am. Heart J. *100*: 667, 1980.
7. Arita, M., Ueno, Y., and Masuyama, Y.: Complete heart block in mumps myocarditis. Br. Heart J. *46*:342, 1981.
8. Noren, G. R., Kaplan, E. L., and Staley, N. A.: Non-rheumatic inflammatory cardiovascular disease. *In* Moss, A. J., Adams, F. H., and Emmanouilides, G. C. (eds.): Heart Disease in Infants, Children and Adolescents. Baltimore, Williams and Wilkins Co., 1977, p.p. 559–576.
9. Morgan, B. C.: Cardiac complications of diphtheria. Pediatrics *32*:549, 1963.
10. Srivastava, S. C., Puri, D. S., and Lumba, S. T.: An electrocardiographic study of myocarditis and diphtheria. J. Assoc. Phys. India *14*:365, 1966.
11. Prata, A.: Chagas' heart disease. Cardiologia *52*:79, 1968.
12. Rosenbaum, M. B.: Chagasic myocardiopathy. Progr. Cardiovasc. Dis. *7*:199, 1964.
13. Koten, J. W., and DeRaadt, P.: Myocarditis and *Trypanosoma rhodesiense* infections. Trans. R. Soc. Trop. Med. Hyg. *63*:485, 1969.
14. Gersony, W. M., and McCracken, G. H., Purulent pericarditis in infancy. Pediatrics *42*:24, 1967.
15. Okoroma, E. O., Terry, L. W., and Scott, L. T.: Acute bacterial pericarditis in children: Report of 25 cases. Am. Heart J. *90*:709, 1975.

16. VanReken, D., Strauss, A., Hernandez, A., and Feigin, R. D.: Infectious pericarditis in children. J. Pediatr. *85*:165, 1974.
17. Lajos, T. Z., Black, H. E., Cooper, R. G., and Wanka, J.: Pericardial decompression. Ann. Thorac. Surg. *19*:47, 1975.
18. Livelli, F. B., Johnson, R. A., McEnany, M. T., Block, P. C., and DeSanctis, R. W.: Unexplained in-hospital fever following cardiac surgery: Natural history, relationship to post-pericardiotomy syndrome, and a prospective study of therapy. N. Engl. J. Med. *57*:968, 1978.
19. Engle, M. A., Ehlers, K. H., O'Laughlin, J. E., Linday, L. A., and Fried, R.: The post-pericardiotomy syndrome: Iatrogenic illness with immunologic and virologic components. *In* Engle, M. A. (ed.): Pediatric Cardiovascular Disease. Philadelphia, F. A. Davis, 1981, p. 381.
20. Paloheimo, J. A., Van Essen, R., Klemola, E., Kaarinen, L., and Siltanen, P.: Sub-clinical cytomegalovirus infections and cytomegalovirus mononucleosis after open heart surgery. Am. J. Cardiol. *22*:624, 1968.
21. Shabetai, R.: Diagnosis and treatment of pericardial effusion. J. Cardiovasc. Med. *6*:2, 1981.
22. Greenwood, R. D., Nadas, A. S., and Fyler, D. C.: The clinical course of primary myocardial disease in infants and children. Am. Heart J. *92*:549, 1976.
23. Goodwin, J. F.: The frontiers of cardiomyopathy. Br. Heart J. *48*:1, 1982.
24. Schryer, M. J. P., and Karnauchow, P. N.: Endocardial fibroelastosis: Etiologic and pathogenic considerations in children. Am. Heart J. *88*:557, 1974.
25. Factor, S. M.: Endocardial fibroelastosis: Myocardial and vascular alterations associated with viral-like nuclear particles. Am. Heart J. *96*:791, 1978.
26. Moller, J. N., Lucas, R. V., Adams, P., Anderson, R. C., Jorgens, J., and Edwards, J. R.: Endocardial fibroelastosis. A clinical and anatomic study of 47 patients with emphasis on its relationship to mitral insufficiency. Circulation *30*:759, 1964.
27. Lambert, E. C., and Vlad, P.: Primary endomyocardial disease. Pediatr. Clin. North Am. *5*:1057, 1958.
28. Sellers, F. J., Keith, J. D., and Manning, J. A.: The diagnosis of primary endocardial fibroelastosis. Circulation *29*:49, 1964.
29. McLaughlin, T. G., Schiebler, G. L., and Krovetz, L. J.: Hemodynamic findings in children with endocardial fibroelastosis. Am. Heart J. *75*:162, 1968.
30. Neustein, H. B., Lurie, P. R., and Fugita, M.: Endocardial fibroelastosis found on transvascular endomyocardial biopsy in children. Arch. Pathol. Lab. Med. *103*:214, 1979.
31. Howell, R. R.: Glycogen storage diseases. *In* Stanbury, J. B., Wyngaarden, J. B., and Frederickson, D. S. (eds.): The Metabolic Basis of Inherited Disease, 3rd ed. New York, McGraw-Hill Book Co., 1972, pp. 149–173.
32. Bordiuk, J. N., Logato, M. J., Lovelace, R. E., and Blumenthal, S.: Pompe's disease: Electron myographic, electron microscopic and cardiovascular aspects. Arch. Neurol. (Chicago) *23*:113, 1970.
33. Dickenson, E. F., Houlsby, W. T., and Wilkinson, J. L.: Unusual angiographic appearance of the left ventricle in two cases of Pompe's disease (glycogenosis type 2). Br. Heart J. *41*:238, 1979.
34. Wolfe, R. R., and Way, G. L.: Cardiomyopathies in infants of diabetic mothers. Johns Hopkins Med. J. *140*:177, 1977.
35. Gutgesell, H. P., Speer, M. E., and Rosenberg, H. S.: Characterization of the cardiomyopathy in infants with diabetic mothers. Circulation *51*:441, 1980.
36. Miller, E., Hare, J. W., Cloherty, J. P., Dunn, P. J., Gleason, R. E., and Kitzmiller, J. L.: Elevated maternal hemoglobin A_{1C} in early pregnancy and major congenital anomalies in infants of diabetic mothers. N. Engl. J. Med. *304*:1331, 1981.
37. Eriksson, U., Dahlstrom, E., Larsson, K. S., and Wellerstrom, C.: Increased incidence of congenital malformations in the offspring of diabetic rats and their prevention by maternal insulin therapy. Diabetics *31*:1, 1982.
38. Whittemore, R., and Caddell, J. L.: Metabolic and nutritional diseases. *In* Moss, A. J., Adams, F. H., and Emmanouilides, G. C. (eds.): Heart Disease in Infants, Children and Adolescents. 2nd ed. Baltimore, Williams and Wilkins Co., 1977, pp. 579–602.
39. Sunshine, P., Kusumoto, H., and Kriss, J. P.: Survival time in circulating long-acting thyroid stimulator in neonatal thyrotoxicosis. Pediatrics *36*:869, 1965.
40. Eason, E., Costom, B. and Papageorgiou, A. N.: Hypertension in neonatal thyrotoxicosis. J. Pediatr. *100*:766, 1982.
41. Sanstead, H. H.: Clinical manifestations of certain vitamin deficiencies. *In* Goodhart, M. S., and Shils, M. E. (eds.): Modern Nutrition in Health and Disease. 5th ed. Philadelphia, Lea and Febiger, 1973, p. 593.
42. Sanstead, H. H.: Mineral metabolism and protein malnutrition. *In* Olson, R. E. (ed.): Protein Calorie Malnutrition. New York, Academic Press, 1975, p. 213.
43. Cadell, J. L.: Diseases of the cardiovascular system. *In* Jelliffe, B. B. (ed.): Diseases of Children in the Subtropics and Tropics. London, Edward Arnold, Ltd., 1970, p. 398.
44. Nutter, D. O., Murray, T. G., Heymsfield, S. B., and Fuller, E. O.: The effect of chronic protein-calorie undernutrition in the rat on myocardial function and cardiac function. Circulation Res. *45*:144, 1979.
45. Waterlow, J. C., and Alleyne, G. A. O.: Protein malnutrition in children: Advances in the last ten years. Adv. Protein Chem. *25*:117, 1971.
46. Roberts, W. C., and Ferrans, V. J.: Pathological aspects of certain cardiomyopathies. Circ. Res. *34* (Suppl. II):II–128, 1974.
47. Roberts, W. C., Buja, L. M., and Ferrans, V. J.: Löffler's fibroplastic parietal endocarditis, eosinophilic leukemia, and Davies' endomyocardial fibrosis: The same disease at different stages? Pathol. Microbiol. (Basel) *35*:90, 1970.
48. Lepley, D., Jr., Aris, A., Korns, M. E., Walker, J. A., and D'Cunha, R. M.: Endomyocardial fibrosis: A surgical approach. Ann. Thorac. Surg. *18*:626, 1974.
49. Metras, D., Coulibaly, A. O., Schauvet, J., Ekra, A., Bertrand, E., and Castaneda, A. R.: Endomyocardial fibrosis. J. Thorac. Cardiovasc. Surg. *83*:52, 1982.
50. Kawasaki, T., Kosaki, S., and Okawa, S.: A new infantile, acute febrile mucocutaneous lymph node syndrome prevailing in Japan. Pediatrics *54*:71, 1974.
51. Tanaka, N., Sekimoto, K., and Naoe, S.: Kawasaki disease: Relationship with infantile periarteritis nodosa. Arch. Pathol. Lab. Med. *100*:81, 1976.
52. Landing, B. H., and Larson, E. J.: Are infantile periarteritis nodosa with coronary artery involvement and fatal mucocutaneous lymph node syndrome the same? Comparison of 20 patients from North America with patients from Hawaii and Japan. Pediatrics *59*:651, 1977.
53. DiSessa, T. G., Klitzner, T., Hiraishi, S., Welsh, M., and Kangarloo, H.: Cardiovascular effects of Kawasaki's disease. J. Cardiovasc. Med. *6*:1159, 1981.
54. Hiraishi, S., Yashiro, K., Oguchi, K., and Nakazawa, K.: Clinical course of cardiovascular involvement in the mucocutaneous lymph node syndrome. Am. J. Cardiol. *47*:323, 1981.
55. Kegel, S. M., Dorsey, T. J., Rowen, M., and Taylor, W. F.: Cardiac death in mucocutaneous lymph node syndrome. Am. J. Cardiol. *40*:282, 1977.
56. Meade, R. H., and Brandt, L.: Manifestation of Kawasaki disease in New England outbreak of 1980. J. Pediatr. *100*:558, 1982.
57. Onouchi, Z., Shimazu, S., Takamatsu, T., and Hamaoka, K.: Aneurysms of the coronary arteries in Kawasaki disease: An angiographic study of 30 cases. Circulation *66*:6, 1982.
58. Chung, K., Brandt, L., Fulton, D. R., and Kreidberg, M. B.: Cardiac and coronary arterial involvement in infants and children with mucocutaneous lymph node syndrome. Am. J. Cardiol. *50*:136, 1982.
59. Yoshida, H., Maeda, T., and Taniguchi, N.: Subcostal two-dimensional echocardiographic imaging of peripheral right coronary artery in Kawasaki disease. Circulation *65*:956, 1982.
59a. Grenadier, E., Allen, H. D., Goldberg, S. J., Valdes-Cruz, L. M., Sahn, D. J., Lima, C. O., and Barron, J. V.: Left ventricular wall motion abnormalities in Kawasaki's disease. J. Am. Coll. Cardiol. *1*:714, 1983.
60. Glanz, S., Bittner, S. J., Berman, M. A., Dolan, T. F., Jr., and Talner, N. S.: Regression of coronary artery aneurysms in infantile polyarteritis nodosa. N. Engl. J. Med. *294*:939, 1976.
61. Kato, H., Ichinose, E., Matsunaga, S., Suzuki, K., and Rikatake, N.: Fate of coronary aneurysms in Kawasaki disease: Serial coronary angiography and long-term follow-up study. Am. J. Cardiol. *49*:1758, 1982.
61a. Anderson, T., Meyer, R. A., and Kaplan, S.: Long term evaluation of cardiac size and function in patients with Kawasaki disease. J. Am. Coll. Cardiol. *1*: 714, 1983.
61b. Suma, K., Takeuchi, Y., Shiroma, K., Tsuji, T., Inoue, K., Yoshikawa, T., Koyama, Y., Narumi, J., Asai, T., and Kusakawa, S.: Early and late postoperative studies in coronary arterial lesions resulting from Kawasaki's disease in children. J. Thorac. Cardiovasc. Surg. *84*:224, 1982.
61c. Kitamura, S., Kawachi, K., Harima, R., Sakakibara, T., Hirose, H., and Kawashima, Y.: Surgery for coronary heart disease due to mucocutaneous lymph node syndrome (Kawasaki disease). Am. J. Cardiol. *51*:444, 1983.
62. New, M. I., and Levine, L. S.: Hypertension in childhood and adolescence. Cardiovasc. Rev. *3*:115, 1982.
63. Lieberman, E.: Diagnostic evaluation of hypertensive children. Pediatr. Ann. *6*: 390, 1977.
64. McCrory, W. W.: What should blood pressure be in children? Pediatrics *70*: 143, 1982.
65. Levine, R. S., Hennekens, C. H., Klein, B., Gourley, J., Briese, F. W., Hokanson, J., Gelband, H., and Jesse, M. J.: Tracking correlations of blood pressure levels in infancy. Pediatrics *61*:1, 1978.
66. Luciani, J.-C., Baldet, P., Dumas, R., and Jean R.: Etude du systeme rénine-angiotensine dans deux cas de tumeur de Wilms avec hypertension artérielle sévère. Arch. Franç. Pédiatr. *36*:230, 1979.
67. Berenson, G. S., Webber, L. S., and Voors, A. W.: Diagnosing hypertension in children. J. Cardiovasc. Med., *6*:273, 1982.
68. Blumenthal, S., Epps, R. P., Heavenrich, R., Lauer, R. M., Lieberman, E., Mirkin, B., Mitchell, S. C., Naito, V. B., O'Hare, D., Smith, W. McF., Tarazi, R. C., and Upson, D.: Report of the task force on blood pressure control in children. Pediatrics *59* (Suppl.):797, 1977.
69. McLean, L. G.: Therapy of acute severe hypertension in children. J. A. M. A. *239*:755, 1978.
70. Fleischmann, L. E.: Management of hypertensive crises in children. Pediatr. Ann. *6*:410, 1977.
71. Lee, J., Lauer, R. M., and Clarke, W. R.: Coronary risk factors in children. *In* Engle, M. A., (ed.): Pediatric Cardiovascular Disease. Philadelphia, F. A. Davis, 1981, p. 1.
72. Schrott, H. G., Clark, W. R., Abrahams, P., Wiebe, D. A., and Lauer, R. M.: Coronary artery disease mortality in relatives of hypertriglyceridemic school children: The Muscatine study. Circulation *65*:300, 1982.
73. Berwick, D. M., Cretin, S., and Keeler, E.: Cholesterol, children, and heart disease: An analysis of alternatives. Pediatrics *68*:721, 1981.
74. Levy, R. I., and Rifkind, B. M.: Diagnosis and management of hyperlipoproteinemia in infants and children. Am. J. Cardiol. *31*:547, 1973.
75. Neill, C. A., Ose, L., and Kwiterovich, P. O., Jr.: Hyperlipidemia: Clinical clues in the first two decades of life. Johns Hopkins Med. J. *140*:171, 1977.
76. Forman, M. B., Kinsley, R. M., DuPlessis, J. P ., Dansky, R., Milner, S., and Levin, S. E.: Surgical correction of combined supravalvular and valvular aortic stenosis in homozygous familial hypercholesterolemia. SA Med. J. *1*:579, 1982.

32 VALVULAR HEART DISEASE

by Eugene Braunwald, M.D.

MITRAL STENOSIS

ETIOLOGY AND PATHOLOGY

The predominant cause of mitral stenosis is rheumatic fever[1] (p. 1647). Far less frequently, it is congenital, and this form is observed almost exclusively in infants and young children (p. 984). Rarely, mitral stenosis is a complication of malignant carcinoid (p. 1430), systemic lupus erythematosus,[1a] rheumatoid arthritis,[2] and the mucopolysaccharidoses of the Hunter-Hurley phenotype.[3] It has been suggested, though without proof, that many viruses, especially Coxsackie virus, may be responsible for chronic valvular heart disease.[4] Mitral stenosis, generally on a rheumatic basis, may be associated with atrial septal defect in Lutembacher's syndrome (p. 1032). Left atrial tumor, particularly myxoma (p. 1460); ball valve thrombus in the left atrium; and a congenital membrane in the left atrium, i.e., cor triatriatum (p. 984), may also obstruct left atrial outflow and therefore may simulate mitral stenosis. Although calcification of the mitral annulus usually causes mitral regurgitation (p. 1074), when subvalvular or intravalvular extension is extensive, mitral stenosis may result.[5]

Approximately 25 per cent of all patients with rheumatic heart disease have pure mitral stenosis, and an additional 40 per cent have combined mitral stenosis and regurgitation.[6] Two-thirds of all patients with rheumatic mitral stenosis are female.

Rheumatic fever results in four forms of fusion of the mitral valve apparatus leading to stenosis: (1) commissural, (2) cuspal, (3) chordal, and (4) combined.[3] Thickening of the commissures alone occurs in 30 per cent, of the cusps alone in 15 per cent, and of the chordae alone in 10 per cent; in the remainder, thickening of more than one of these structures is involved. Characteristically, mitral valve cusps fuse at their edges, and fusion of the chordae results in thickening and shortening of these structures. The stenotic mitral valve is typically funnel-shaped, and the orifice is frequently shaped like a "fish mouth" or buttonhole, with calcium deposits in the valve leaflets sometimes extending to involve the valve ring, which may become quite thick[7] (Figs. 32–1 and 48–5, p. 1647). The thickened leaflets may be so adherent and rigid that they cannot open or shut, reducing or rarely even abolishing the first heart sound (S_1) and leading to combined mitral stenosis and regurgitation.[8,9] There is a correlation between the severity of calcification and the transvalvular gradient.[10] When rheumatic fever results exclusively or predominantly in contraction and fusion of the chordae tendineae, dominant mitral regurgitation results.

It probably takes a minimum of two years after the onset of acute rheumatic fever for severe mitral stenosis to develop, and most patients in temperate climates remain asymptomatic for at least a decade more.[11] Symptoms commence most commonly in the third or fourth decade, although mild mitral stenosis in the aged is becoming a more frequent finding. In the tropics, particularly in underdeveloped areas, the disease advances more rapidly, and severe mitral stenosis may be present in early adolescence.[12] The debate continues about whether the anatomical changes result from a smoldering rheumatic process or whether once the valve has been deformed by the initial episode, the constant trauma produced by the turbulent blood flow leads to progressive fibrosis, thickening, and calcification of the valve apparatus.[13]

Enlargement of the left atrium and resultant elevation of the left main stem bronchus, calcification of the left atrial wall, the development of mural thrombi, and obliterative changes in the pulmonary vascular bed (p. 830) may all result from chronic mitral stenosis.

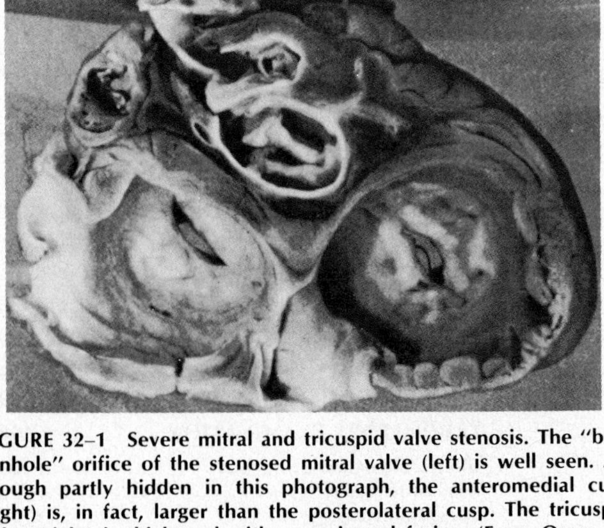

FIGURE 32–1 Severe mitral and tricuspid valve stenosis. The "buttonhole" orifice of the stenosed mitral valve (left) is well seen. Although partly hidden in this photograph, the anteromedial cusp (right) is, in fact, larger than the posterolateral cusp. The tricuspid valve (right) is thickened with commissural fusion. (From Oram, S.: Clinical Heart Disease. London, William Heinemann Medical Books, Ltd., 1971, p. 323.)

PATHOPHYSIOLOGY

In normal adults the mitral valve orifice is 4 to 6 cm^2. When the orifice is reduced to approximately 2 cm^2, which is considered mild mitral stenosis, blood can flow from the left atrium to the left ventricle only if propelled by an abnormal pressure gradient. When the mitral valve opening is reduced to 1 cm^2, which is considered critical mitral stenosis, a left atrioventricular pressure gradient of approximately 20 mm Hg (and therefore, in the presence of a normal left ventricular diastolic pressure, a mean left atrial pressure of approximately 25 mm Hg) is required to maintain normal cardiac output at rest (Figs. 32–2 and 32–3). The elevated left atrial pressure in turn raises pulmonary venous and capillary pressures, resulting in exertional dyspnea (p. 493). The first bouts of dyspnea in patients with mitral stenosis are usually precipitated by exercise, emotional stress, infection, or atrial fibrillation, all of which increase the rate of blood flow across the mitral orifice and result in further elevation of the left atrial pressure.[14,15]

In order to assess the severity of obstruction of the mitral valve (and, for that matter, of any valve), it is essential to measure both the transvalvular pressure gradient (Fig. 32–2) and the flow rate (Figure 9–8, p. 288). The latter depends not only on cardiac output but on heart rate as well. An increase in heart rate shortens diastole proportionately more than systole and diminishes the time available for flow across the mitral valve. Therefore, at any given level of cardiac output, tachycardia augments the transmitral valvular pressure gradient and elevates left atrial pressures further.[16] This explains the sudden development of dyspnea and pulmonary edema in previously asymptomatic patients who experience atrial fibrillation with a rapid ventricular rate[17,18] and the equally rapid improvement in these patients when the ventricular rate is slowed by means of cardiac glycosides and/or beta-adrenergic blocking agents, even when the cardiac output per minute remains constant. Hydraulic considerations dictate that at any given orifice size the transvalvular gradient is a function of the square of the transvalvular flow rate (p. 293 and Fig. 32–3).[19,20] Thus, a doubling of flow rate will quadruple the pressure gradient, so that a stress such as exercise in patients with moderate or severe stenosis will cause marked elevation of left atrial pressure.[21]

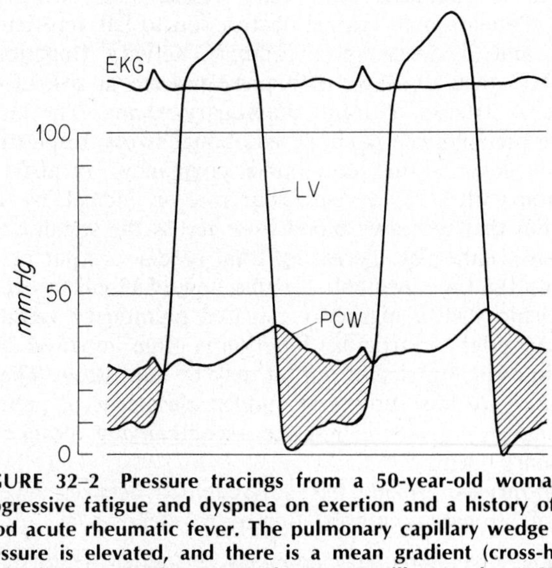

FIGURE 32–2 **Pressure tracings from a 50-year-old woman with progressive fatigue and dyspnea on exertion and a history of childhood acute rheumatic fever. The pulmonary capillary wedge (PCW) pressure is elevated, and there is a mean gradient (cross-hatched area) of 22 mm Hg between pulmonary capillary wedge (PCW) and left ventricular (LV) pressures throughout diastole. The calculated mitral valve area was reduced to 0.8 cm^2.**

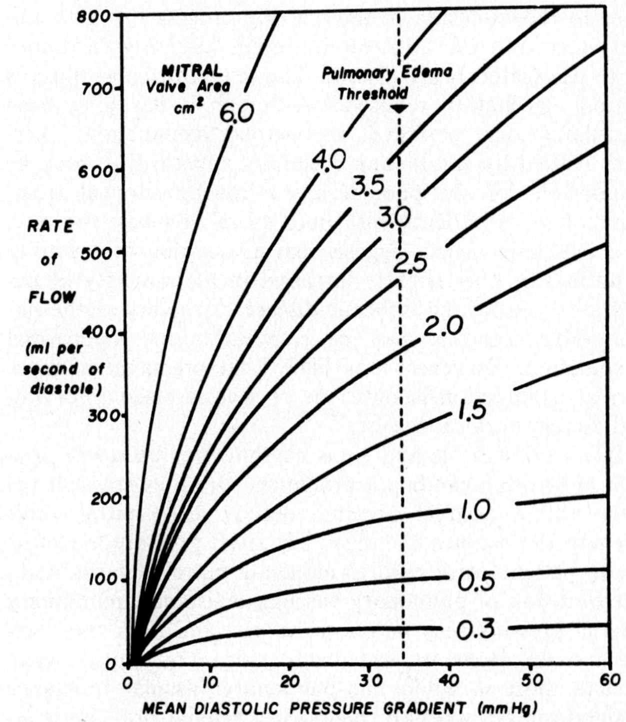

FIGURE 32–3 **Chart illustrating the relation between mean diastolic gradient across the mitral valve and rate of flow across the mitral valve per second of diastole, as predicted by the Gorlin formula. Note that when the mitral valve area is 1.0 cm^2 or less, very little additional flow can be achieved by an increased pressure gradient. (Reproduced with permission from Wallace, A. G.: Pathophysiology of cardiovascular disease. *In* Smith, L. H., Jr., and Thier, S. O. [eds.]: Pathophysiology: The Biological Principles of Disease. The International Textbook of Medicine. Vol. 1. Philadelphia, W. B. Saunders Co., 1981, p. 1192.)**

Atrial contraction augments the presystolic transmitral valvular gradient by approximately 30 per cent in patients with mitral stenosis. Withdrawal of atrial transport when atrial fibrillation develops decreases cardiac output by about 20 per cent. At any level of cardiac output, effective atrial contraction maintains lower levels of mean left atrial pressure than would be present in atrial fibrillation.[22] In addition, the more rapid ventricular rate that is common in atrial fibrillation raises the transvalvular pressure gradient. Thus, hemodynamic considerations indicate the desirability of maintaining sinus rhythm in patients with mitral stenosis.[17,23]

INTRACARDIAC AND INTRAVASCULAR PRESSURES

Left ventricular diastolic pressure is normal in patients with pure mitral stenosis; coexisting mitral regurgitation, aortic valve lesions, systemic hypertension, ischemic heart disease, or cardiomyopathy may all be responsible for elevations of left ventricular diastolic pressure. In approximately 85 per cent of patients with pure mitral stenosis, the end-diastolic volume is within the normal range, whereas it is reduced in the remainder.[24] In approximately one-third of patients the ejection fraction is below normal, most likely owing to chronic reduction in preload and perhaps to the extension of the scarring process from the mitral valve into the adjacent posterior basal myocardium[25] or to associated heart disease. The left ventricular mass is normal or slightly reduced.[26] Although it has long been postulated that persistent myocardial dysfunction,[27] perhaps caused by smoldering rheumatic myocarditis, may be responsible for the poor results following surgical treatment of some patients with pure mitral stenosis, the bulk of available evidence suggests that myocardial contractility is normal or only slightly impaired in the majority of patients.[28,29] Associated ischemic disease or rigidity of the mitral valve complex may be responsible for myocardial dysfunction. However, it is likely that preoperative myocardial dysfunction is only one of several reasons for unsatisfactory surgical results.[30]

In mitral stenosis and sinus rhythm, the *left atrial pressure pulse* often exhibits a prominent atrial contraction (*a*) wave and a gradual pressure decline after mitral valve opening (*y* descent); the mean left atrial pressure is elevated. In patients with mild to moderate mitral stenosis without elevation of pulmonary vascular resistance, pulmonary arterial pressure may be normal at rest and rises only during exercise. However, in patients with severe mitral stenosis and those in whom the pulmonary vascular resistance is significantly increased, pulmonary arterial pressure is elevated when the patient is at rest, and in cases of extreme elevation of the pulmonary vascular resistance it may exceed the systemic arterial pressure (Chap. 25). Further elevations of left atrial and pulmonary vascular pressures occur during exercise or tachycardia or both. With moderate elevation of pulmonary artery pressure, right ventricular performance is maintained.[31] An elevation of pulmonary arterial systolic pressure exceeding 70 mm Hg represents a serious impedance to emptying of the right ventricle, and when this level is exceeded in patients with rheumatic heart disease, right ventricular end-diastolic and right atrial pressures often rise.

The *clinical and hemodynamic features* of mitral stenosis of any given severity are dictated largely by the levels of cardiac output and pulmonary vascular resistance.[32] The response to a given degree of mitral obstruction may be characterized on one end of the hemodynamic spectrum by a normal cardiac output and a high left atrioventricular pressure gradient or, at the opposite end of the spectrum, by a markedly reduced cardiac output and low transvalvular pressure gradient. In some patients with moderately severe stenosis (mitral valve area = 1.0 to 1.5 cm^2) cardiac output may be normal, not only at rest but during exertion as well. In these patients, marked elevation of left atrial and pulmonary capillary pressures leads to symptoms of severe pulmonary congestion. However, in the majority of patients with severe mitral stenosis, cardiac output is subnormal at rest and rises subnormally during exertion, thus reducing the pulmonary venous pressure and the severity of symptoms of pulmonary congestion more than would be the case if the output rose normally. In patients with severe stenosis (mitral valve area < 1.0 cm^2), particularly when pulmonary vascular resistance is elevated, cardiac output is usually depressed at rest and fails to rise during exertion. These patients frequently have prominent symptoms secondary to a low cardiac output (p. 495).

Pulmonary hypertension in patients with mitral stenosis results from (1) passive backward transmission of the elevated left atrial pressure; (2) arteriolar constriction, which presumably is triggered by left atrial and pulmonary venous hypertension (reactive pulmonary hypertension); and (3) organic obliterative changes in the pulmonary vascular bed, which may be considered to be a complication of longstanding and severe mitral stenosis (Chap. 25). In time, severe pulmonary hypertension results in right-sided failure and tricuspid and sometimes pulmonic regurgitation. However, it has been suggested that these changes in the pulmonary vascular bed may also be considered to exert a protective effect; the elevated precapillary resistance makes the development of symptoms of pulmonary congestion less likely by tending to prevent blood from surging into the pulmonary capillary bed and damming up behind the stenotic mitral valve, although this protection occurs at the expense of a decreased cardiac output.[33] Patients with severe mitral stenosis manifest a marked reduction in lung compliance, an increase in the work of breathing, and a redistribution of pulmonary blood flow from the bases to the apices (p. 1785).

The combination of mitral valve disease and atrial inflammation secondary to rheumatic carditis causes left atrial dilatation, fibrosis of the atrial wall, and disorganization of the atrial muscle bundles. The last leads to disparate conduction velocities and inhomogeneous refractory periods. Premature atrial activation due either to an automatic focus or to reentry may stimulate the left atrium during the vulnerable period and may thus precipitate a bout of atrial fibrillation. Chronic atrial fibrillation results in turn in diffuse atrophy of the muscle, which causes further inhomogeneity of refractoriness and conduction and leads to irreversible atrial fibrillation.[34]

CLINICAL MANIFESTATIONS

(Table 32–1)

History

The principal symptom of mitral stenosis is dyspnea, largely the result of reduced compliance of the lungs (p. 1785). Vital capacity is reduced, presumably owing to the presence of engorged pulmonary vessels and interstitial edema. Patients with critical obstruction to left ventricular inflow and dyspnea upon ordinary activity (functional Class III) generally have orthopnea and are at risk of experiencing attacks of frank pulmonary edema. The latter may be precipitated by effort, emotional stress, respiratory infection, fever, sexual intercourse, pregnancy,[35] or atrial fibrillation with a rapid ventricular rate or, indeed, by any condition that increases blood flow across the stenotic mitral valve, either by increasing total cardiac output or by reducing the time available for this flow of blood to occur. In patients with a markedly elevated pulmonary vascular resistance, right ventricular function is often impaired, and a rise in right ventricular output may be impossible. Therefore, they are less subject to sudden elevations of pulmonary capillary pressure and the accompanying attacks of pulmonary edema.[15,36]

Hemoptysis. Wood has differentiated between several kinds of *hemoptysis* complicating mitral stenosis.[15]

1. So-called pulmonary apoplexy, a sudden hemorrhage which, while often profuse, is rarely life-threatening.[37,38] This results from the rupture of thin-walled, dilated bronchial veins as a consequence of a sudden rise in left atrial

TABLE 32–1 DIAGNOSIS OF MITRAL VALVE DISEASE

	Mitral Stenosis	Mitral Regurgitation
Sex	Women > Men	Men > Women
Severity of rheumatic fever	Less severe	Often fulminating
Presystolic murmur	Present	Absent
First sound	Loud unless calcification	*Never loud*
Apical systolic murmur	Usually absent	Pansystolic or late
Mid-diastolic murmur	Long, not necessarily loud	*If present, short*
Opening snap of mitral valve	Present unless heavy calcification, pulmonary hypertension, or aortic regurgitation	Rarely present
Third sound	*Never present*	Commonly present and loud
Cardiac impulse	Tapping ("closing snap"); right ventricular type if pulmonary vascular resistance raised	Left ventricular type; right ventricular type if pulmonary vascular resistance raised
Radial pulse	Small volume	Small volume but collapsing
Systemic emboli	Common	Less common
Left atrial size	Enlarged but rarely aneurysmal	May be aneurysmal; systolic
Left ventricle	*Normal or poor filling,* aorta hypoplastic	*Enlarged, rapidly filling,* and hyperdynamic
Electrocardiogram	RVH if pulmonary vascular resistance raised	LVH; RVH if pulmonary vascular resistance raised
Hemodynamic data	a. LAP may be greatly raised b. Gradient across valve in diastole c. PVR may be severely raised	a. Less severely raised as a rule b. No gradient usually c. PVR not commonly greatly raised

RVH = right ventricular hypertrophy; LVH = left ventricular hypertrophy; LAP = left atrial pressure; PVR = pulmonary vascular resistance.
Modified from Oram, S.: Clinical Heart Disease. London, William Heinemann Medical Books, 1981, p. 335.

pressure. After several years of pulmonary venous hypertension, the walls of these veins thicken appreciably, and this form of hemoptysis tends to disappear.

2. Blood-stained sputum associated with attacks of nocturnal dyspnea.

3. Pink, frothy sputum characteristic of acute pulmonary edema due to rupture of alveolar capillaries.

4. Pulmonary infarction, a late complication of mitral stenosis associated with heart failure.

5. Blood-stained sputum complicating chronic bronchitis; the edematous bronchial mucosa in patients with chronic mitral stenosis increases the likelihood of chronic bronchitis, a common complication of mitral stenosis, particularly in Great Britain.

Chest Pain. A small fraction, perhaps 15 per cent, of patients with mitral stenosis experience chest discomfort that is indistinguishable from angina pectoris.[14,15] This symptom may be caused by right ventricular hypertension[39] or by coincidental coronary atherosclerosis, or it may be secondary to coronary obstruction caused by coronary embolization.[40] In many such patients, however, a satisfactory explanation cannot be uncovered even after complete hemodynamic and angiographic studies.

Thromboembolism. This is an important complication of mitral stenosis.[41,42] Prior to the development of surgical treatment, systemic embolism developed in at least 20 per cent of patients at some time during the course of their disease, and in the past as many as 10 to 15 per cent of this group died as a consequence. Before the era of anticoagulant therapy and surgical treatment, approximately one-fourth of all fatalities in patients with mitral valve disease were secondary to embolism. The tendency for embolization correlates inversely with cardiac output and directly with age and the size of the left atrial appendage; 80 per cent of patients in whom systemic emboli develop are in atrial fibrillation. When embolization occurs in patients in sinus rhythm, the possibility of underlying infective endocarditis should be considered. There is no simple correlation between the incidence of embolism on one hand and the size of the mitral orifice or the level of pulmonary vascular resistance on the other. Indeed, embolism may be the first symptom of mitral stenosis and may occur in patients with mild mitral stenosis even prior to the development of dyspnea. Patients older than age 35 years and having atrial fibrillation, especially with a low cardiac output and dilation of the left atrial appendage, are at the highest risk from emboli and therefore should be considered for prophylactic anticoagulant treatment.

Since thrombi are found in the left atrium in only a minority of patients with a history of recent embolism at operation, it is likely that only fresh clots are discharged from the atria into the systemic circulation. Approximately half of all clinically apparent emboli are found in the cerebral vessels. Coronary embolism may lead to myocardial infarction or angina pectoris or both, and renal emboli may be responsible for the development of systemic hypertension. Emboli are recurrent and multiple in approximately 25 per cent of patients subject to this complication. Rarely, massive thrombosis develops in the left atrium, resulting in a pedunculated ball-valve thrombus, which may aggravate obstruction to left atrial outflow when a specific body position is assumed, or it may cause sudden death.[43]

Infective Endocarditis. This complication tends to occur less frequently on a rigid, thickened, calcified valve and is therefore more common in patients with mild than with severe mitral stenosis.

Other Symptoms. Compression of the left recurrent laryngeal nerve by a greatly dilated left atrium, enlarged tracheobronchial lymph nodes, and dilated pulmonary artery causes hoarseness (Ortner's syndrome).[44] A history of repeated hemoptysis is common in patients with pulmonary hemosiderosis, and longstanding elevation of pulmonary venous pressure is present in patients with pulmonary ossification. Systemic venous hypertension, hepatomegaly, edema, ascites, and hydrothorax are all signs of severe mitral stenosis with elevated pulmonary vascular resistance and right heart failure.

Physical Examination

Patients with severe mitral stenosis, a low cardiac output, and systemic vasoconstriction often exhibit the so-called mitral facies, characterized by pinkish-purple patches on the cheeks.[15] The *arterial pulse* is usually normal, but in patients in whom the stroke volume is reduced, the pulse may be small in volume. The *jugular venous pulse* usually exhibits a prominent *a* wave in patients with sinus rhythm and elevated pulmonary vascular resistance (Fig. 3–35, p. 63). In atrial fibrillation, the *x* descent of the jugular pulse disappears, and there is only one crest, a prominent *v* or *c-v* wave, per cardiac cycle and a slow *y* descent. *Palpation* of the cardiac apex usually reveals an inconspicuous left ventricle;[45] the presence of either a palpable presystolic expansion wave or an early diastolic rapid filling wave *excludes* significant mitral stenosis. The presence of a readily palpable, tapping first heart sound (S_1) suggests that the anterior mitral valve leaflet is pliable. When the patient is in the left lateral recumbent position, the low-pitched diastolic rumbling murmur of mitral stenosis is often palpable as a thrill at the apex. Often a right ventricular lift is palpable in the left parasternal region in patients with pulmonary hypertension. A markedly enlarged right ventricle may displace the left ventricle posteriorly and produce a prominent apex beat that can be confused with a left ventricular lift. A pulmonic closure sound (P_2) may be palpable in the second left intercostal space in patients with mitral stenosis and pulmonary hypertension.

AUSCULTATION. The auscultatory (and phonocardiographic) features of mitral stenosis (some of which are illustrated in Figures 3–14, p. 50, and Figures 32–4 and 32–5) include an accentuated S_1 with prolongation of the Q-S_1 interval (p. 43), correlating with the level of the left atrial pressure.[8] Accentuation of S_1 occurs when the mitral valve is flexible[46] and is due in part to the rapidity with which left ventricular pressure rises at the time of mitral valve closure as well as to the wide closing excursion of the valve leaflets. Marked calcification or thickening of the mitral valve leaflets or both reduce the amplitude of S_1, probably because of diminished movement of the leaflets. As pulmonary artery pressure rises, P_2 at first becomes accentuated and widely transmitted and can often be readily heard and recorded at both the mitral and the aortic areas. With further elevation of pulmonary artery pressure, splitting of S_2 narrows because of reduced compliance of the pulmonary vascular bed, which shortens the "hang-out interval" (p. 47). Finally, S_2 becomes single and accentuated. Other signs of pulmonary hypertension include a nonvalvular pulmonic ejection sound (See Figure 3–13, p. 49) that diminishes during inspiration, owing to dilatation of the pulmonary artery; the systolic murmur of tricuspid

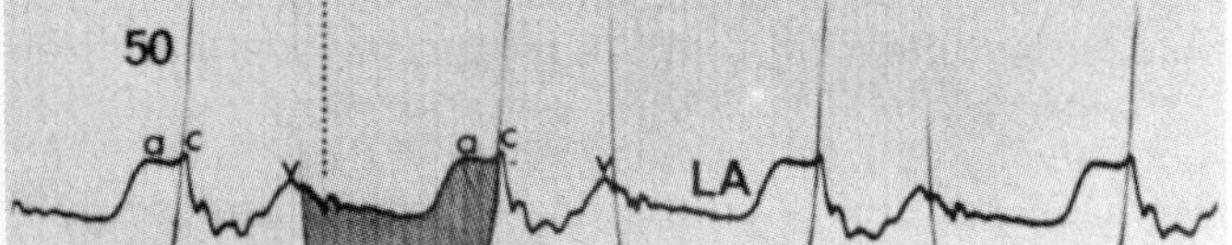

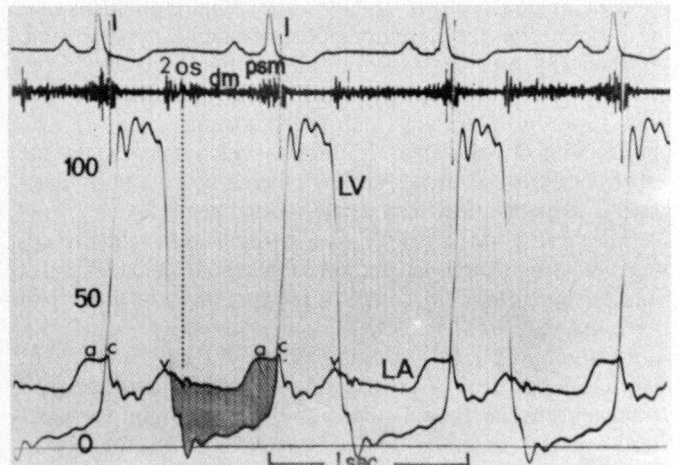

FIGURE 32–4 The auscultatory complex of mitral stenosis. An apical phonocardiogram demonstrates the accentuated first sound (1), opening snap (os), rumbling diastolic murmur (dm), and crescendo presystolic murmur (psm) in relation to simultaneous left ventricular (LV) and left atrial (LA) pressures. The first sound is coincident with the left atrial *c* wave, and the opening snap coincides with a notch (dotted line) on the downslope (*y* descent) of the left atrial *v* wave. The presystolic murmur exhibits a crescendo after the *a* wave peak, during a decline in the atrioventricular pressure gradient (shaded area). (Time lines = 0.04 sec.) (From Criley, J. M., et al.: Departures from the expected auscultatory events in mitral stenosis. *In* Likoff, W. [ed.]: Cardiovascular Clinics. Vol. 5, No. 2, Valvular Heart Disease. Philadelphia, F. A. Davis, 1973, p. 192.)

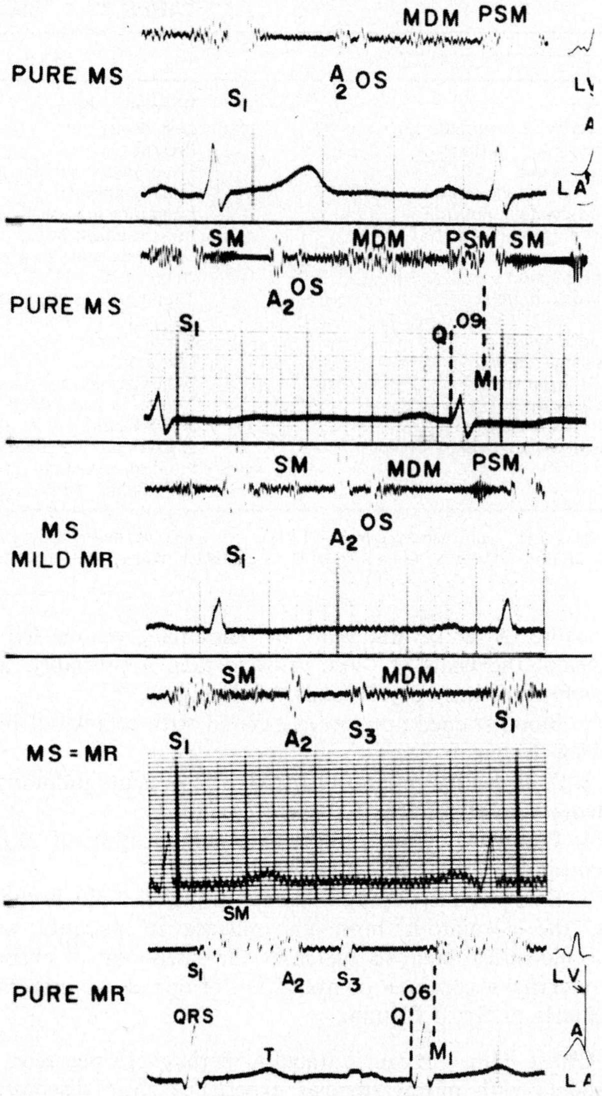

FIGURE 32–5 Representative phonocardiograms at the cardiac apex ranging from pure mitral stenosis (MS) to pure mitral regurgitation (MR), with illustrative left ventricular (LV) and left atrial (LA) pressure pulses at the two extremes. The first sound (S_1) gets progressively softer, the holosystolic murmur (SM) of mitral regurgitation becomes more prominent, the opening snap (OS) is replaced by a third heart sound (S_3), and the presystolic murmur (PSM) softens and vanishes, whereas the mid-diastolic murmur (MDM) shortens and finally disappears. (From Reichek, N., et al.: Clinical aspects of rheumatic valvular disease. *In* Sonnenblick, E. S., and Lesch, M. [eds.]: Valvular Heart Disease. New York, Grune and Stratton, 1974, p. 143, by permission of Grune and Stratton, Inc.)

regurgitation; a Graham Steell murmur of pulmonic regurgitation; and an S_4 originating from the right ventricle.[47] An S_3 originating from the left ventricle is absent, unless significant mitral or aortic regurgitation coexists.

The *opening snap* (OS) of the mitral valve appears to be due to a sudden tensing of the valve leaflets by the chordae tendineae after the valve cusps have completed their opening excursion[48] and is best heard at the apex and with the diaphragm of the stethoscope.[49–52] It can usually be differentiated from P_2, since the OS occurs later, unless right bundle branch block is present. The mitral valve cannot be totally rigid if it produces an OS, which is usually accompanied by an accentuated S_1. Calcification confined to the top of the mitral valve does not preclude an OS, although calcification of the body and tip does.[53] In patients with combined mitral stenosis and regurgitation, the OS may be followed by an S_3. The mitral OS follows A_2 by 0.04 to 0.12 sec, and the A_2-OS interval varies inversely with left atrial pressure[51,52] (p. 49). Although a short A_2-OS interval is a reliable indicator of severe stenosis, the converse is not necessarily the case, since the time interval between the actual opening of the mitral valve and the OS can be prolonged in the presence of valvular calcification and tight stenosis.[48] The (Q-S_1)–(A_2-OS) correlates better with the height of the left atrial pressure than does either measurement alone.[49]

The diastolic murmur of mitral stenosis is a low-pitched, rumbling murmur, best heard at the apex and with the bell of the stethoscope. When this murmur is soft, it is limited to the apex, but when louder, it may radiate to the axilla or the lower left sternal area. Although the intensity of the diastolic murmur is not closely related to the severity of stenosis, the *duration* of the murmur is a guide to the severity of mitral narrowing, and in patients with combined mitral stenosis and regurgitation, a long diastolic murmur always signifies the presence of significant stenosis and, in general, persists for as long as the gradient across the mitral valve exceeds approximately 3 mm Hg. The murmur usually commences immediately after the mitral OS. In mild mitral stenosis, the murmur is brief but commences again in presystole. In severe stenosis, the murmur is holodiastolic, with presystolic accentuation.

Although a *presystolic murmur* is usually present in patients with sinus rhythm in whom transvalvular blood flow is accelerated by atrial contraction, such a murmur may also occur in patients with atrial fibrillation, in whom it results from the increased velocity of blood flow across a mitral valve orifice that begins to narrow after the onset of left ventricular contraction[54–56] (see Figure 4–18, p. 80). Since, in patients with atrial fibrillation, this murmur results from motion of the mitral valve leaflets, a flexible mitral valve is required for its generation; its absence in a patient with moderate or severe obstruction suggests either a rigid calcified valve or a markedly reduced cardiac output.

The *diastolic rumbling murmur* of mitral stenosis may be masked by the presence of obesity, pulmonary emphysema, and a low cardiac output with a low flow rate across the mitral valve. The rumble may be sharply localized and thus missed unless one uses palpation to detect the apex of the left ventricle and to pinpoint the area at which auscultation should be carried out. In so-called "silent" mitral stenosis, there is usually marked right ventricular enlargement, so that the right ventricle occupies the cardiac apex, and cardiac output is reduced, so that the murmur either is not audible at all or can be heard only in the mid- or posterior axillary line.[57] Auscultation of the murmur is facilitated by use of the bell of the stethoscope, placing the patient in the left lateral position and auscultating during expiration after a few sit-ups or other maneuvers described below.

Dynamic Auscultation. The diastolic murmur and OS of mitral stenosis are often reduced during inspiration and augmented during expiration[58]—the opposite of what occurs when these findings are secondary to tricuspid stenosis. During inspiration the A_2-OS interval widens, and three sequential sounds (A_2, P_2, and OS) are frequently audible. Sudden standing and the resultant reduction of venous return lower left atrial pressure and widen the A_2-OS interval[59]; this maneuver is useful in distinguishing an A_2-OS combination from a split S_2, which narrows. In contrast, A_2-OS is significantly narrowed during exercise.[60] The diastolic rumbling murmur of mitral stenosis is reduced during the strain of a Valsalva maneuver, and there is a delayed return to prestrain levels during the overshoot, six to eight beats after release. Amyl nitrite, coughing, isometric or isotonic exercise, and sudden squatting are all useful in accentuating a faint or equivocal murmur of mitral stenosis. Progressive narrowing of A_2-OS on serial examinations suggests an increase in the severity of stenosis, whereas widening of A_2-OS after mitral commissurotomy indicates that the severity of stenosis has been reduced significantly.

DIFFERENTIAL DIAGNOSIS. It is important to recognize that a variety of conditions other than mitral stenosis may exhibit auscultatory findings that can be confused with mitral stenosis, and these are summarized in Table 32–2. In addition to the findings listed in the table, the *Carey-Coombs* murmur of acute rheumatic fever (p. 1649) is a sign of active mitral valvulitis and can be confused with the murmur of mitral stenosis. It is a soft, early diastolic murmur, usually varies from day to day, and is higher pitched than the diastolic rumbling murmur of established mitral stenosis. In pure, severe *mitral regurgitation*—indeed, in any condition in which there is increased flow across a nonstenotic mitral valve—there may also be a loud, short, diastolic murmur following an S_3. *Left atrial myxoma* may produce auscultatory findings similar to those in rheumatic mitral valvular stenosis (p. 1460).

A *pansystolic murmur of tricuspid regurgitation* and an S_3 originating from the right ventricle may be audible in the fourth intercostal space in the left parasternal region in patients with severe mitral stenosis. These signs, secondary to pulmonary hypertension, may be confused with the findings of mitral regurgitation.[61] However, the inspiratory augmentation of the murmur and of the S_3 and the prominent *v* wave in the jugular venous pulse aid in establishing that the murmur originates from the tricuspid valve. A decrescendo diastolic murmur along the left sternal border in patients with mitral stenosis and pulmonary hypertension is usually due to aortic regurgitation and rarely represents a Graham Steell murmur of pulmonary regurgitation[62] (p. 1122); the latter, when present, characteristically increases during inspiration.

TABLE 32–2 CONDITIONS OTHER THAN MITRAL STENOSIS THAT MAY SIMULATE AUSCULTATORY FINDINGS IN MITRAL STENOSIS

Auscultatory Event	Condition Other Than Mitral Stenosis	Explanation of Event
Loud and snapping first sound	Hyperkinetic states	High left ventricular dP/dt at time of mitral closure
Early diastolic opening snap	Myxoma of left atrium	Tumor movement into ventricle Abrupt checking of tumor (tumor plop)
	Constrictive pericarditis	Checking of ventricular filling by pericardium
	Tricuspid stenosis	Stenotic valve
Diastolic rumbling murmur	Aortic regurgitation (Austin Flint murmur)	Preclosure of mitral valve (?) Regurgitant stream (?) Fluttering of mitral valve
	Dilated ventricle Myocarditis Cardiomyopathy	Preclosure of mitral valve (?) Centrifugal displacement of papillary muscles
	Hypertrophic, restrictive ventricle Hypertrophic obstructive cardiomyopathy Aortic valve disease	Impaired filling of left ventricle (?) Impaired opening of mitral valve
	Tricuspid stenosis	Narrow orifice
	Myxoma of left atrium	Narrow orifice
	Augmented atrioventricular flow Mitral regurgitation Left-to-right shunts	Preclosure of valve (?) Centrifugal displacement of papillary muscles
Crescendo presystolic murmur	Aortic regurgitation (Austin Flint murmur)	Preclosure of mitral valve opposing atrial systole
	Hypertrophic, restrictive ventricle	Summation of S_4 and S_1 may simulate presystolic murmur
	Tricuspid stenosis	Narrow orifice
	Myxoma of left atrium	Narrow orifice

Modified from Criley, J. M., et al.: Departures from the expected auscultatory events in mitral stenosis. *In* Likoff, W. (ed.): Cardiovascular Clinics. Vol. 5, No. 2, Valvular Heart Disease. Philadelphia, F. A. Davis, 1973, p. 213.

LABORATORY EXAMINATION

ELECTROCARDIOGRAM. The electrocardiogram and vectorcardiogram are relatively insensitive techniques for the detection of mild mitral stenosis, but they do show characteristic changes in patients with moderate or severe obstruction. Left atrial enlargement (P-wave duration in lead II >0.12 sec, terminal negative P force in lead V_1 > .003 mv/sec, P-wave axis between +45 and −30 degrees) is a principal electrocardiographic feature of mitral stenosis (Fig. 7–11*A*, p. 208) and is found in 90 per cent of patients with significant mitral stenosis and sinus rhythm.[63,64] The electrocardiographic signs of left atrial enlargement correlate more closely with left atrial volume than with left atrial pressure[65] and often regress following successful valvulotomy.[15] When atrial fibrillation is present, the fibrillatory waves are coarse, i.e., greater than 0.1 mv in amplitude in V_1, also suggesting the presence of atrial enlargement.[66] The development of atrial fibrillation correlates with the preexistent electrocardiographic diagnosis of left atrial enlargement and is related to the size and the extent of fibrosis of the left atrial myocardium,[67] the duration of atriomegaly, and the age of the patient.[68]

Electrocardiographic evidence of right ventricular hypertrophy depends on the level of right ventricular systolic pressure; this finding is infrequent in patients with right ventricular systolic pressures less than 70 mm Hg.[63] However, approximately half of all patients with right ventricular systolic pressures between 70 and 100 mm Hg manifest the electrocardiographic criteria for right ventricular hypertrophy, including both a mean QRS axis that is greater than 80 degrees in the frontal plane and an R:S ratio greater than 1.0 in V_1.[69] In other patients with this degree of pulmonary hypertension, there is no frank evidence of right ventricular hypertrophy, but the R:S ratio fails to increase from right to midprecordial leads. When right ventricular systolic pressures exceed 100 mm Hg, electrocardiographic evidence of right ventricular hypertrophy is found quite consistently. The mean QRS axis averages +150 degrees, and there is a Q-R morphology in the right precordial leads, accompanied by inverted or biphasic T waves.[70]

The *QRS axis in the frontal plane* often correlates with the severity of valve obstruction and with the level of pulmonary vascular resistance in pure mitral stenosis; thus, a mean frontal axis between 0 and +60 degrees suggests that the mitral valve area exceeds 1.3 cm^2, whereas an axis greater than 60 degrees generally indicates that the valve area is less than 1.3 cm^2. In patients in whom pulmonary vascular resistance is greater than 650 dynes-sec-cm^{-5}, the mean axis usually exceeds +110 degrees.[69]

VECTORCARDIOGRAM. The characteristic *vectorcardiographic finding* in mitral stenosis is right ventricular hypertrophy Type C (Figure 7–17, p. 213) characterized by counterclockwise rotation in the horizontal plane and a terminal deflection directed to the right, posteriorly, and superiorly.[63,69–72] In other patients with mitral stenosis without frank right ventricular hypertrophy, QRS loops with posterior and rightward terminal appendages are evident without conduction delays.[63,69] There is vectorcardiographic evidence of right ventricular hypertrophy Type A (Figure 7–17, p. 213) in only 10 per cent of patients with mitral stenosis, but when present it indicates that both the hypertrophy and the stenosis are severe. Vectorcardiograms showing right ventricular hypertrophy Type B (Figure 7–17), are infrequent in mitral stenosis.

Rotation of the P loop in the frontal plane, with superior orientation of the terminal P forces and a wide angle between the initial and terminal P vectors, occurs in about one-fourth of patients with pure mitral stenosis and may be the only evidence of left atrial enlargement.[73] The terminal portion of the P loop is usually directed posteriorly and inferiorly, and the T loop is often directed leftward and posterosuperiorly and is discordant with respect to the QRS loop, resulting in a diphasic T wave with initial negativity and terminal positivity in lead V_1.[64]

RADIOLOGICAL FINDINGS (see also p. 163). Although the cardiac silhouette may be normal in the frontal projection, with the exception of an enlarged atrial appendage (Fig. 6–3*A*, p. 149), in patients with hemodynamically significant mitral stenosis, left atrial enlargement is almost invariably evident on the lateral and left anterior oblique views.[74,75] The size of the left atrium does *not* correlate with the severity of obstruction. However, extreme left atrial enlargement rarely occurs in pure mitral stenosis; when it is present, mitral regurgitation is usually severe. Enlargement of the pulmonary artery, right ventricle, and right atrium (as well as the left atrium) is commonly seen in severe mitral stenosis (Figure 6–2, p. 148, and Figure 6–13, p. 156). Occasionally, calcification of the mitral valve is evident on the chest roentgenogram (see Figure 6–9, p. 154), but, more commonly, fluoroscopy is required to detect valvular calcification.

Radiological changes in the lung fields (see Figure 6–26, p. 165) are useful in assessing the height of pulmonary venous pressure and thereby the severity of mitral stenosis. Interstitial edema, an indication of severe obstruction, is manifest as Kerley B lines (dense, short, horizontal lines most commonly seen in the costophrenic angles).[76] This finding is present in 30 per cent of patients with resting pulmonary artery wedge pressures below 20 mm Hg and in 70 per cent of patients with pressures exceeding 20 mm Hg. Severe, longstanding mitral obstruction often results in Kerley A lines (straight, dense lines up to 4 cm in length and running toward the hilum) as well as the findings of pulmonary hemosiderosis[77] and rarely of parenchymal ossification.

Angiograms exposed in the right and left anterior oblique projections afford the best views of the mitral valve.[78] Although, ideally, contrast medium should be injected into the left atrium, it is often possible to achieve good visualization of the left side of the heart by injecting a large volume of contrast medium into the main pulmonary artery. Such left atrial or pulmonary angiograms provide an assessment of left atrial size, may demonstrate thickening and reduced motion of the valve leaflets (Figure 6–54, p. 187), and may outline large intraluminal thrombi.[79] In most catheterization laboratories today, left cine ventriculography is the primary (and often the sole) angiographic procedure for assessment of mitral valve motion. Although this technique allows visualization of only the ventricular aspect of the leaflet in patients with pure mitral stenosis, it makes possible simultaneous assessment of left ventricular contractile function and of the subvalvular mitral apparatus.[80]

ECHOCARDIOGRAPHY (see also p. 109). Mitral stenosis can ordinarily be readily diagnosed by M-mode echocardiography (Figure 3–14, p. 50, and Figure 5–38, p. 110), but this technique does not allow a precise determination of its severity. Echoes of a thickened, calcified stenotic rheumatic valve demonstrate increased acoustic impedance and fusion of the mitral valve leaflets and poor leaflet separation in diastole.[81,82] Normally, the posterior leaflet of the mitral valve moves posteriorly during early diastole, but in more than 90 per cent of patients with mitral stenosis, both leaflets move anteriorly at this time (Fig. 32–6). The E–F slope is reduced,[81–86] but this finding is not pathognomonic of mitral stenosis, since it may occur in other conditions in which left ventricular compliance and the velocity of left ventricular filling are reduced,[86] or in which there is substantial right ventricular pressure overload.[87] However, in these other conditions the posterior leaflet of the mitral valve moves normally, emphasizing the importance of recording the motion of this structure in order to establish the diagnosis of mitral stenosis by echocardiography.[81] Reduction of the E–F slope does not correlate with the severity of obstruction. However, the maximal diastolic separation of the anterior and posterior leaflets,[85] their rate of diastolic apposition,[82,86] and the slope of motion of the left ventricular posterior wall during diastole[87] appear to correlate more closely with the mitral valve area. The ratio $Q-C/A_2-E$ (where C and E represent mitral valve closure and opening, respectively, Q is the onset of the QRS complex, and A_2 the closure of the aortic valve) correlates well with the left atrial pressure.[88] Cross-

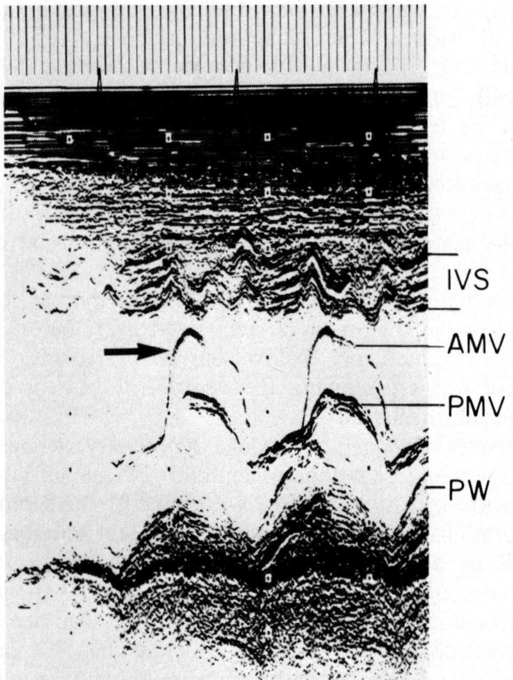

FIGURE 32–6 Mitral valve echogram in a patient with rheumatic mitral stenosis demonstrating limitation and concordance of motion of anterior (AMV) and posterior (PMV) leaflets, with thickening of the posterior leaflet typical of fibrosclerotic rheumatic mitral stenosis. Note that the PMV moves anteriorly (upward) during diastole. Also, there is a diminished E–F slope and slurring of the rapid and slow filling phases of mitral valve motion. The posterior wall (PW) of the left ventricle exhibits a continuous upward motion during diastole (i.e., diastolic filling), suggesting at least moderately severe mitral stenosis. In addition, high-frequency diastolic vibrations of the anterior leaflet (arrow) are noted, indicative of concomitant aortic regurgitation. (IVS = interventricular septum.)

sectional[81,84,89,90] echocardiography is more accurate than M-mode echocardiography in determining mitral orifice size (Figure 5–39, p. 110).

Other important echocardiographic findings in patients with pulmonary hypertension and mitral stenosis include a small or absent *a* wave in the pulmonic valve echogram (Figure 5–37, p. 109). The left atrium is usually enlarged, and the left ventricular cavity is normal or reduced in size. M-mode echocardiography is also useful in detecting mitral annular calcification, which may accompany mitral stenosis and in which a band of dense echoes is present in the region of the mitral annulus, in contrast to the thin and delicate echoes recorded from the normal mitral annulus. Two-dimensional echocardiography may be helpful in the preoperative recognition of left atrial thrombus,[91] although the demonstration of a thrombus by the finding of neovascularity on coronary arteriography is probably a more accurate technique.[92]

MANAGEMENT

Medical Treatment

Patients with rheumatic heart disease should receive penicillin prophylaxis for beta-hemolytic streptococcal infections, as outlined on p. 1655, and prophylaxis for bacterial endocarditis, as summarized on p. 1175. Adolescents and young adults should be advised to avoid physically strenuous occupations. Anemia and infections should be treated promptly and aggressively in patients with valvular heart disease.

In symptomatic patients with mitral valve disease, considerable improvement can be expected with oral diuretics and the restriction of sodium intake. Digitalis glycosides do not alter the hemodynamics and usually do not benefit patients with mitral stenosis and sinus rhythm[93] but are helpful in the treatment of right-sided heart failure. However, as pointed out below, cardiac glycosides are of greatest value in slowing the ventricular rate in patients with atrial fibrillation.

Measures designed to reduce pulmonary venous pressure, including sedation, assumption of the upright posture, and aggressive diuresis, are used to treat hemoptysis. If operation is not to be carried out, oral anticoagulants should be administered to patients with mitral stenosis who have suffered systemic emboli, as well as patients who are at high risk of embolization, i.e., those who are in atrial fibrillation, especially if they are older than 40 years and have a greatly enlarged left atrium.

Treatment of Arrhythmias. Frequent premature atrial contractions often presage atrial fibrillation, and the administration of antiarrhythmic drugs, as outlined on p. 700, may be effective in preventing this complication. However, once atrial fibrillation has developed, these agents may be ineffective in restoring sinus rhythm or even in maintaining sinus rhythm following electrical cardioversion, because of pathological changes that occur in the atrium secondary to the arrhythmia itself.[34] After electrical cardioversion, sinus rhythm can often be maintained with antiarrhythmic drugs in young patients with mild mitral stenosis without marked left atrial enlargement who have been in atrial fibrillation less than 6 months and who have been treated with adequate doses of quinidine. In any event, if elective cardioversion (pharmacological or electrical) is to be attempted in the patient with mitral stenosis and atrial fibrillation, a preparatory 3- to 4-week course of anticoagulation should be given to minimize the risk of systemic embolism when sinus rhythm has resumed. Immediate treatment of atrial fibrillation should be directed toward reducing the ventricular rate by means of digitalis and, if possible, toward reestablishing sinus rhythm by a combination of pharmacological treatment and cardioversion (p. 700). However, it must be appreciated that in 1 to 2 per cent of patients with mitral stenosis, systemic embolism develops following electrical or pharmacological cardioversion. Paroxysmal atrial fibrillation and repeated conversions, spontaneous or induced, carry the risk of embolization.[94] Following reversion to sinus rhythm, administration of quinidine or a similar antiarrhythmic agent should be continued indefinitely in order to diminish the likelihood of recurrent fibrillation. In patients who cannot be converted or maintained in sinus rhythm, the ventricular rate at rest should be maintained at approximately 60 to 65 beats/min with digitalis. If this is not possible, small doses of a beta blocker, such as propranolol (10 to 20 mg four times a day), may be added. Repeat cardioversion is not indicated if the patient has not sustained sinus rhythm while on adequate doses of quinidine.

In patients with rheumatic heart disease and heart failure and/or atrial fibrillation, anticoagulant therapy is helpful in preventing venous thrombosis and pulmonary embolism, in reducing the frequency of systemic embolism in patients who have experienced one or more previous embolic episodes, and in reducing the frequency of thromboembolism in patients with prosthetic heart valves. However, there is no firm evidence that anticoagulant therapy reduces the incidence of pulmonary or systemic embolism in patients in sinus rhythm in whom embolic episodes have not previously occurred and who are not in heart failure.

Natural History

The development of effective surgical treatment has obscured our understanding of the natural history of mitral stenosis and, for that matter, of all valvular lesions.[95] Although few meaningful data are available, it appears that after a latent period of 10 to 20 years following an attack of rheumatic fever during which the patient is asymptomatic, it takes approximately 5 to 10 years for most patients to progress from mild disability (i.e., early Class II) to total disability (i.e., Class IV). In the presurgical era, Olesen found 62 per cent 5-year and 38 per cent 10-year survival among patients in New York Heart Association functional Class III but only a 15 per cent 5-year survival rate in patients in Class IV.[96] Among asymptomatic medically treated patients (Class I) with mitral stenosis followed medically, 40 per cent had deteriorated or died within 10 years. Among mildly symptomatic patients (Class II), the comparable number was 80 per cent.[97] In medically treated patients with mitral stenosis or with combined mitral stenosis and regurgitation, Munoz et al. found a 45 per cent 5-year survival rate.[36] In a comparable group of patients subjected to mitral commissurotomy, the 5-year survival rate was substantially better. In an unselected mix of patients with mitral stenosis of varying severity, 80 per cent of the patients were alive after 5 years and 60 per cent after 10 years of medical treatment.[98]

Surgical Treatment

INDICATIONS FOR OPERATION. Patients with mitral stenosis who are asymptomatic or minimally symptomatic frequently remain so for years. However, once symptoms become more severe, the disease progresses relatively rapidly to death, and operation should therefore be carried out in patients with severe mitral stenosis (i.e., a mitral valve orifice size < 1.0 cm^2/m^2 body surface area [BSA]).

There has been considerable debate concerning the need for routine cardiac catheterization in determining whether operation is indicated.[99–101] Although a careful clinical evaluation and noninvasive assessment, particularly using two-dimensional echocardiography, can provide sufficient information to permit an informed decision in the majority of patients, the consequences of valvular surgery, particularly valve replacement, are so profound that I recommend routine preoperative catheterization and angiography in the majority of patients with mitral stenosis who are potential surgical candidates. These studies are particularly helpful in patients (1) with heart murmurs and other findings suggesting the presence of valve lesions in addition to mitral stenosis, (2) with associated chronic obstructive pulmonary disease, (3) in whom left atrial myxoma must be excluded, and (4) who are more than 45 years old and/or who have angina-like chest pain and in whom associated coronary artery disease must be excluded. Critical narrowing of one or more coronary vessels occurs in approximately one-fourth of all patients with severe mitral stenosis; it is more common in men over the age of 45 years who have angina and who have risk factors for coronary artery disease.[102,103] I believe that preoperative catheterization can usually be omitted in the young (< 35 years) patient without angina who has typical symptoms and classic findings of pure mitral stenosis on physical examination and by noninvasive tests, including two-dimensional echocardiography.

Care of mildly symptomatic patients (Class II) must be individualized. If there are no obvious contraindications to operation, left- and right-heart catheterization should be performed to determine the size of the valve orifice. In general, surgery can be deferred in patients with mild stenosis (i.e., mitral valve orifice size > 1.0 cm^2/m^2 BSA), whereas it should be recommended for those with moderate or severe stenosis (i.e., mitral valve orifice size < 1.0 cm^2/m^2 BSA). However, this plan is subject to qualification. For instance, operation might well be deferred in a retired woman in her seventies with modest needs for elevated cardiac output and a mitral valve orifice of 0.8 cm^2/m^2 BSA, whereas a 25-year-old laborer whose family's economic well-being depends on his continued physical exertion might be an excellent candidate for operation, though the mitral valve orifice size is 1.2 cm^2/m^2 BSA.

Because of the high rate of recurrence, operation is also indicated in patients with mitral stenosis in whom systemic embolism has previously occurred, even if they are otherwise asymptomatic and even though there is no definitive evidence that the incidence of recurrent emboli will be significantly reduced. In these cases, anticoagulants should be administered up to the time of operation. Although the risk of operation is higher in patients with advanced disease characterized by severe pulmonary hypertension and right-sided heart failure, surviving patients nearly always show striking clinical and hemodynamic improvement, with a marked reduction in pulmonary vascular pressures. In the pregnant patient with mitral stenosis, operative treatment should be carried out only if serious pulmonary congestion occurs despite intensive medical treatment (p. 1777).

There is no evidence that surgical treatment improves the prognosis of patients with no or only slight functional impairment. Therefore, valvulotomy is *not* indicated in patients who are entirely asymptomatic, except in unusual circumstances. For example, I recently saw a 33-year-old woman with moderately severe mitral stenosis who had hemoptysis and pulmonary edema during the second trimester of a pregnancy at age 31. She then became asymptomatic but wishes to have another child. Hemodynamic study showed a pulmonary wedge pressure of 17 mm Hg and a mitral orifice area of 1.7 cm^2/m^2 BSA. Prophylactic mitral commissurotomy was undertaken in this patient, since it was virtually certain that another pregnancy would result in serious heart failure.

SURGICAL TECHNIQUES. Three basically different operative approaches are available for the treatment of rheumatic mitral stenosis:[104–112] (1) closed mitral commissurotomy; (2) open commissurotomy, i.e., commissurotomy carried out under direct vision with the aid of cardiopulmonary bypass; and (3) mitral valve replacement. *Closed mitral commissurotomy,* performed with the aid of a transventricular dilator, is generally preferred to simple transatrial finger fracture.[109,112] It is an effective operation, provided that mitral regurgitation, atrial thrombosis, or valvular calcification is not serious and that chordal fusion and shortening are not severe. Unfortunately, few patients satisfy all these criteria, and they are difficult to identify preoperatively. Therefore, if this procedure is carried out at all, it is with "pump standby"; if the surgeon is unable to achieve a satisfactory result, the patient is placed on cardiopulmonary bypass, and the commissurotomy is carried out under direct vision. This procedure is rarely used in the United States today, but is more popular in developing nations, where the expense of open-heart surgery is an important factor and where patients with mitral valve disease are younger.[113] In any event, echocardiography is useful in selecting suitable candidates without valvular calcification or dense fibrosis.[90,114]

Most surgeons prefer to carry out *direct-vision* or *open commissurotomy.*[115,116] Cardiopulmonary bypass is established, and in order to obtain a dry, quiet heart, body temperature is usually lowered, the heart is arrested, and the aorta is occluded intermittently (Chap. 55). Thrombi are removed from the atrium and its appendage, and the latter is often amputated in order to remove a potential source of postoperative emboli. The commissures are incised, and, when necessary, fused chordae are separated, the underlying papillary muscle is split, and the valves are debrided of calcium; mild or even moderate mitral regurgitation may be corrected with suture plication or annuloplasty. Left atrial and ventricular pressures are measured after bypass has been discontinued to confirm that the commissurotomy has, in fact, been effective.[107] In patients with atrial fibrillation, conversion to sinus rhythm is carried out at the completion of the operation.

The mortality rate after mitral commissurotomy, whether open or closed, ranges from 1 to 3 per cent, depending on the condition of the patient and the skill of the surgical team.[115] In general, open commissurotomy provides better hemodynamic relief of mitral valve obstruction than does the closed procedure,[117] and the risk of dislodging thrombi from the atrium or calcium from the mitral valve is also less.[115,116] However, it must be recognized that mitral commissurotomy, whether open or closed, is a palliative rather than a curative operation, and even when successful, it merely "turns the clock back." Thus, it does not result in a normal mitral valve but in one resembling the valve as it existed perhaps a decade earlier. Since the valve is not normal postoperatively, turbulent flow may persist in the paravalvular region, and this may well play a role in restenosis. These changes are analogous to the development of obstruction in a congenitally bicuspid aortic valve and are not usually the result of recurrent rheumatic fever.

Mitral Re-stenosis. This condition can be diagnosed with certainty only on the basis of three satisfactory hemodynamic investigations: a preoperative study; a second study following a satisfactory operation in which an increase in the size of the valvular orifice can be demonstrated; and a third one after the reappearance of symptoms, when a reduction in size relative to the earlier postoperative study is noted. Based on clinical grounds alone, the incidence of "re-stenosis" has been estimated to range widely, from 2 to 60 per cent;[118] approximately 10 per cent of patients who have undergone mitral commissurotomy require reoperation within 5 years, but that fraction increases to 60 per cent by 10 years.[119] However, the need for reoperation does not necessarily imply re-stenosis. More often, recurrent symptoms are due to an inadequate first operation, with residual stenosis; the presence or development of mitral regurgitation, either at operation or as a consequence of infective endocarditis; the progression of aortic valve disease; or the development of ischemic heart disease. In a study in which the size of the mitral valve orifice was estimated using cross-sectional echocardiography in 18 patients who had undergone successful mitral commissurotomy, no change in the mitral valve area occurred over a 10- to 14-year period in 13 patients, whereas in 5 (28 per cent) true re-stenosis developed.[119] Approximately 10 per cent of patients returning to the hospital with persistent or recurrent symptoms 6 years after operation have true re-stenosis.[120]

Thus, in properly selected patients, mitral commissurotomy results in a significant increase in the size of the mitral orifice and, at a low risk, favorably alters the clinical course of an otherwise progressive disease. Pulmonary artery pressure falls promptly and decisively when mitral obstruction is effectively relieved.[121–124] Some patients maintain clinical improvement for many (10 to 15) years of follow-up; indeed, fully one-fourth of the patients in functional Class III preoperatively maintain their improvement for 15 years.[33] When a second operation is required because of symptometic deterioration, the valve is often calcified and more seriously deformed than at the time of the first operation, and adequate reconstruction may not be possible. Accordingly, mitral valve replacement is then usually necessary. Also, in patients with combined mitral stenosis and regurgitation, and in those with extensive calcification involving the commissures of the valve, mitral replacement rather than commissurotomy is often required. The operative mortality following mitral valve replacement ranges from 5 to 8 per cent in most hospitals, and as described below (p. 1088), the long-term fate of the prosthetic valves is not yet clear; also, the hazards of lifelong anticoagulant treatment in patients with mechanical prostheses cannot be neglected. Therefore, in patients in whom preoperative evaluation suggests that valve replacement may be required, the threshold for operation should be higher than in patients believed to require commissurotomy alone.

MITRAL REGURGITATION

ETIOLOGY AND PATHOLOGY

The mitral valve apparatus involves the mitral annulus, the mitral leaflets per se, the chordae tendineae, and the papillary muscles. Abnormalities of any of these structures may cause mitral regurgitation (Table 32–3).[1,125–127] The mitral valve prolapse syndrome, an important cause of mitral regurgitation, is discussed in a separate section (p. 1089).

ABNORMALITIES OF VALVE LEAFLETS. Mitral regurgitation due to involvement of the valve leaflets occurs most commonly in chronic rheumatic heart disease and is more frequent in men than in women. It is a consequence of shortening, rigidity, deformity, and retraction of one or both cusps of the mitral valve as well as shortening and fusion of the chordae tendineae and papillary muscles.[128] Destruction of the mitral valve leaflets can also be a consequence of penetrating and nonpenetrating trauma (p. 1535) and of infective endocarditis (Chap. 33). Retraction of the mitral valve cusps during the healing phase of endocarditis can also cause mitral regurgitation.

ABNORMALITIES OF THE MITRAL ANNULUS

Dilatation. In a normal adult the mitral annulus measures approximately 10 cm in circumference. During systole, contraction of the surrounding left ventricular muscle causes the annulus to constrict, and this constriction contributes importantly to valve closure. Mitral regurgitation secondary to dilatation of the mitral annulus (Fig. 32–7) can occur in any form of heart disease characterized by severe dilatation of the left ventricle. It is often difficult to differentiate this secondary from the primary forms of mitral regurgitation (Table 32–4), but it is notable that regurgitation secondary to dilatation of the annulus is usually less severe than primary valvular regurgitation.

Calcification. Idiopathic calcification of the mitral annulus is one of the most common cardiac abnormalities

TABLE 32–3 CAUSES OF MITRAL REGURGITATION

I. Disorders of the Mitral Valve Leaflets
- A. Loss of contracture of valvular tissue
  - Rheumatic fever
  - Infection—bacterial, viral, fungal
  - External and direct trauma
  - Spontaneous rupture
  - Systemic lupus erythematosus
  - Methysergide-induced
- B. Incomplete or abnormal valvular development
  - Anterior leaflet clefts with AV cushion defect
  - Isolated clefts or perforations
  - Absence of leaflets
  - Redundancy of leaflets
  - Congenital fusion of commissures
  - Anomalous leaflet attachment
  - Ebstein's malformation with corrected transposition of the great arteries
- C. Defects of the connective tissue
  - Ehlers-Danlos syndrome
  - Hurler's syndrome
  - Marfan's syndrome
  - Pseudoxanthoma elasticum
  - Osteogenesis imperfecta

II. Disorders of the Mitral Annulus
- A. Calcification
  - Degenerative
  - Associated with coronary atherosclerosis, hypertension, and rheumatic heart disease
  - Marfan's syndrome
- B. Destruction of the annulus fibrosus
  - Bacterial valve ring abscesses
  - Rheumatic fever
  - Rheumatoid arthritis
- C. Dilatation of the annulus fibrosus
  - Connective tissue disorder
  - Left ventricular dilatation
- D. Disruption of ring of prosthetic valve

III. Disorders of the Chordae Tendineae
- A. Rupture of chordae tendineae
  - Idiopathic
  - Bacterial endocarditis
  - Trauma
  - Marfan's syndrome
  - Ehlers-Danlos syndrome
  - Rheumatic fever
  - Myocardial infarction
  - Hypertrophic obstructive cardiomyopathy
- B. Thickened or poorly defined chordae tendineae in association with
  - Congenital mitral stenosis
  - Congenital mitral regurgitation
  - AV cushion defect
  - Hypoplastic left heart syndrome
  - Parachute mitral valve complex
  - Supravalvular ring of left atrium
  - Carcinoid syndrome
  - Hurler's syndrome
- C. Elongated chordae tendineae
  - Marfan's syndrome
  - Ehlers-Danlos syndrome
  - Idiopathic
- D. Arising from an unusual location in association with AV cushion defect
  - Corrected transposition of great vessels
  - Congenital mitral regurgitation

IV. Disorders of the Papillary Muscles
- A. Dysfunction or rupture of papillary muscle
  - Myocardial infarction—ischemia, fibrosis, rupture
  - Bacterial abscess
  - Trauma
  - Anomalous coronary artery
  - Polyarteritis
  - Aortic stenosis
  - Syphilis
  - Sarcoidosis
  - Amyloidosis
  - Mucocutaneous lymph node syndrome
  - Myocardial disease
  - Myocarditis
  - Temporal disturbance of activation and contraction
- B. Malalignment
  - Endocardial fibroelastosis
  - Idiopathic hypereosinophilic syndrome
  - Dilatation of the left ventricle
  - Hypertrophic obstructive cardiomyopathy
  - Massive left atrial enlargement
  - Ventricular aneurysm
- C. Congenital abnormality in development
  - Absent papillary muscle
  - Congenital mitral stenosis
  - Anomalous mitral arcade

Modified from Silverman, M. E., and Hurst, J. W.: The mitral complex: Clues to its afflictions. *In* Likoff, W. (ed.): Cardiovascular Clinics. Vol. 5, No. 2, Valvular Heart Disease. Philadelphia, F. A. Davis, 1973, pp. 37, 40, 45, and 48.

found at autopsy; in most hearts this degenerative change is of little functional consequence.[128,129] However, when severe it may be an important cause of mitral regurgitation in the elderly, and in contrast to rheumatic fever, this cause is more common in women than in men.[130] In addition to the idiopathic form, degenerative calcification of the mitral annulus is accelerated by systemic hypertension, aortic stenosis, and diabetes, as well as by an intrinsic defect in the fibrous skeleton of the heart, such as occurs in the Marfan and Hurler syndromes. In these two conditions, the mitral annulus not only is calcified but also is dilated, further contributing to mitral regurgitation. The incidence of mitral annular calcification is also increased in patients with hypertrophic obstructive cardiomyopathy[131] and in patients with chronic renal failure with secondary hyperparathyroidism.[132]

When annular calcification is severe, a rigid, curved bar or ring of calcium encircles the mitral orifice, and calcific spurs may project into the adjacent left ventricular myocardium;[133-136] the bulk of the calcium is located in the subvalvular region. The calcification may immobilize the

TABLE 32–4 PRIMARY AND SECONDARY FORMS OF CHRONIC MITRAL REGURGITATION

Anatomic or Hemodynamic Feature	Primary	Secondary
Mitral valve	Mitral valve apparatus abnormal anatomically and functionally	Normal structural anatomy
Left ventricle	Enlarged	Markedly enlarged
Left atrium	Markedly enlarged	Enlarged
Pulmonary venous redistribution and pulmonary edema	Late in the course	Early
Left ventricular end-diastolic volume	Increased	Markedly increased
Left ventricular end-diastolic pressure	Normal until late in the course	Elevated early
Cardiac output	Normal, with decreases late in the course	Reduced early
Ejection fraction	Increased or normal (> 0.5)	Depressed (< 0.4)

Modified from Haffajee, C. I.: Chronic mitral regurgitation. *In* Dalen, J. E., and Alpert, J. S. (eds.): Valvular Heart Disease. Boston, Little, Brown, and Co., 1981, p. 97.

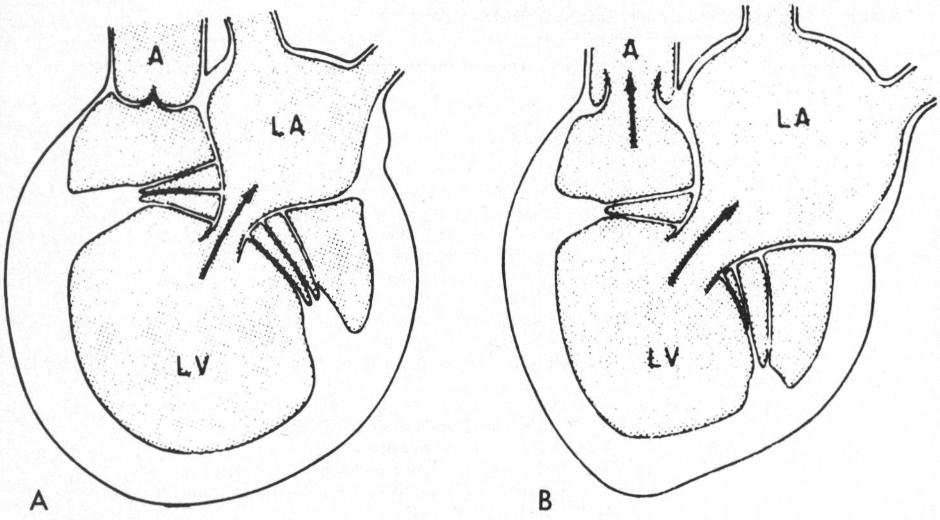

FIGURE 32–7 Proposed mechanism of regurgitation in left ventricular dilatation. The papillary muscles are displaced laterally and perhaps downward from the ring, permitting leaflet separation and regurgitation during early systole (*A*) and during ejection (*B*). (From Kremkau, E. L., et al.: Acquired, nonrheumatic mitral regurgitation: Clinical management with emphasis on evaluation of myocardial performance. Prog. Cardiovasc. Dis. *15*:414, 1973, by permission of Grune and Stratton, Inc.)

basal portion of the mitral leaflets, preventing their normal excursion in diastole and coaptation in systole and aggravating the mitral regurgitation that results from loss of the normal sphincteric action of the mitral ring. Rarely, when severe calcification encroaches on or protrudes into the mitral orifice, obstruction to left ventricular filling may occur. Calcification of the aortic valve cusps is an associated finding in approximately 50 per cent of patients with severe annular calcification, but this rarely causes aortic stenosis. In patients with severe regurgitation, calcium may invade the conduction system, leading to atrioventricular and/or intraventricular conduction defects.[126] Occasionally, calcific deposits extend into the coronary arteries. The annulus may also become thick and rigid as a consequence of rheumatic involvement, and when this process is severe, it also can interfere with valve closure.

ABNORMALITIES OF THE CHORDAE TENDINEAE. These are important causes of mitral regurgitation (Table 32–3).[137–139] The chordae may be congenitally abnormal, or they may rupture as a consequence of infective endocarditis, trauma, rheumatic fever, or myxomatous proliferation;[140] in most cases no cause for chordal rupture is apparent, other than increased mechanical strain.[141] Patients with idiopathic rupture of mitral chordae tendineae frequently exhibit pathological fibrosis of the papillary muscles, and it is possible that the dysfunction of the papillary muscles may have caused stretching and ultimately rupture of the chordae.[142] Chordal rupture may also result from acute left ventricular dilatation, regardless of etiology. Depending on the number and rate of chordal rupture, the resultant mitral regurgitation may be mild, moderate, or severe on the one hand or acute, subacute, or chronic on the other.

INVOLVEMENT OF THE PAPILLARY MUSCLES. Diseases of the left ventricular papillary muscles frequently cause mitral regurgitation (Table 32–3).[143] Since these muscles are perfused by the terminal portion of the coronary vascular bed,[144] they are particularly vulnerable to ischemia, and any disturbance in coronary perfusion may result in papillary muscle dysfunction (Fig. 32–8). When ischemia is transient, it results in temporary papillary muscle dysfunction and may cause transient episodes of mitral regurgitation during attacks of angina pectoris (p. 1339). When ischemia is severe and persistent, as in acute myocardial infarction, it produces papillary muscle necrosis and permanent mitral regurgitation (Fig. 32–9). The posterior papillary muscle, which is supplied by the posterior descending branch of the right coronary artery, becomes

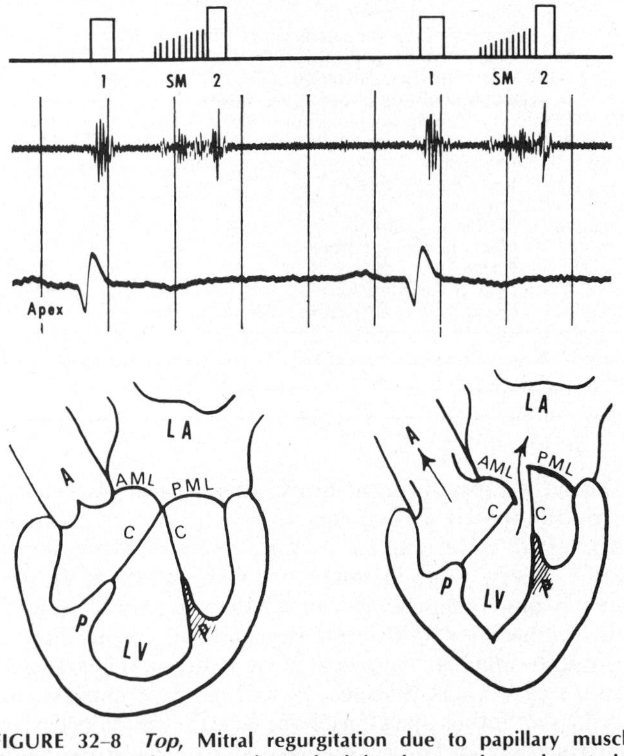

FIGURE 32–8 *Top,* Mitral regurgitation due to papillary muscle dysfunction. At the onset of systole (left), the anterior and posterior mitral valve leaflets (AML and PML) approximate. Later in systole (right), the anterior papillary muscle (P, nonhatched) contracts while the posterior papillary muscle (P, hatched) fails to contract because of ischemia or infarction. Part of the posterior leaflet is allowed to prolapse into the left atrium (LA) during systole, producing regurgitation. This process may involve either papillary muscle. C = chordae tendineae; LV = left ventricle; A = aorta.

Bottom, Late systolic murmur (SM) that developed in a patient following an inferior myocardial infarction and is probably due to weakening of the posterior papillary muscle with prolapse of the mitral leaflet into the atrium during late systole. (From Ravin, A., et al.: Auscultation of the Heart. 3rd ed. Chicago, Year Book Medical Publishers, 1977, p. 99.)

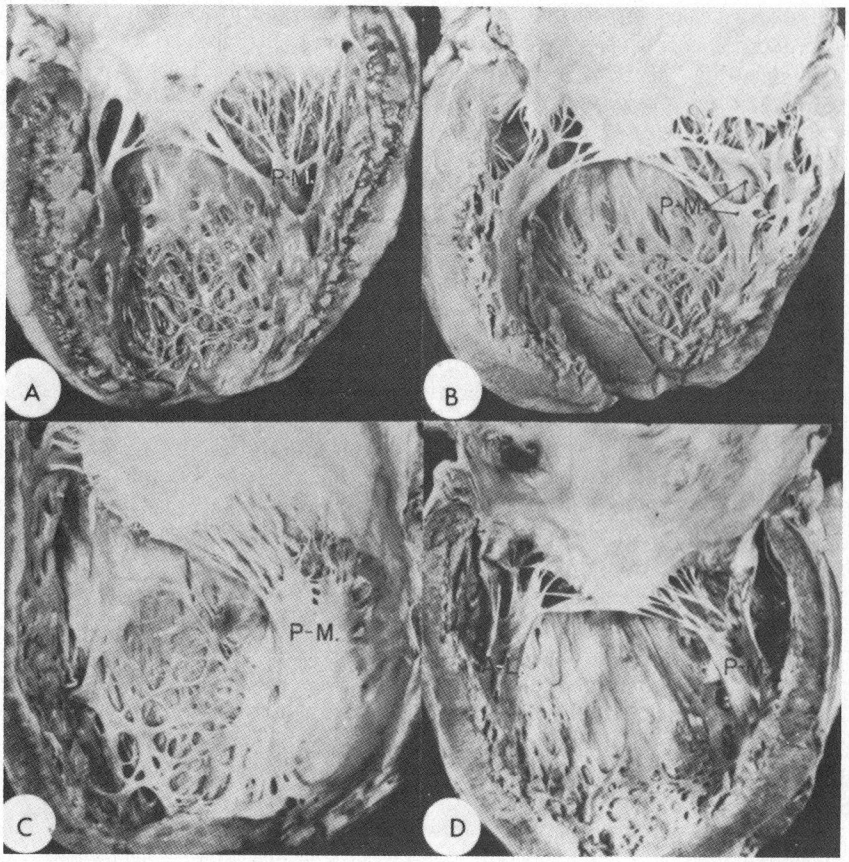

FIGURE 32–9 Myocardial infarction involving the papillary muscles. *A*, Light discoloration of the left ventricular wall in relation to the posteromedial (P-M) papillary muscle represents extensive acute myocardial infarction; the muscle was also infarcted but intact. *B*, Healed myocardial infarction of the distribution shown in *A*. In addition to thinning and scarring of the free wall of the left ventricle, atrophy of the posteromedial papillary muscle has resulted from healing of the infarction. *C*, Infarction of the inferior wall of the left ventricle with aneurysm formation. The endocardium over the infarct site is thickened. The related posteromedial papillary muscle is also involved in the process of infarction. *D*, Healed myocardial infarction of extensive nature in which both anterolateral (A-L) and posteromedial (P-M) papillary muscles are atrophic as the result of infarction and secondary scarring. (From Vlodaver, Z., and Edwards, J. E.: Mitral insufficiency in subjects 50 years of age or older. *In* Edwards, J. E. [ed.]: Clinical-Pathologic Correlations #2, Philadelphia, F. A. Davis, 1973, p. 158.)

ischemic and infarcted more frequently than does the anterolateral papillary muscle, which is supplied by diagonal branches of the left anterior descending coronary artery and often by marginal branches from the left circumflex artery as well. Ischemia of the papillary muscle is caused most commonly by coronary artery disease, but it may also occur in severe anemia, shock, coronary arteritis of any etiology, and anomalous left coronary artery. In pa-

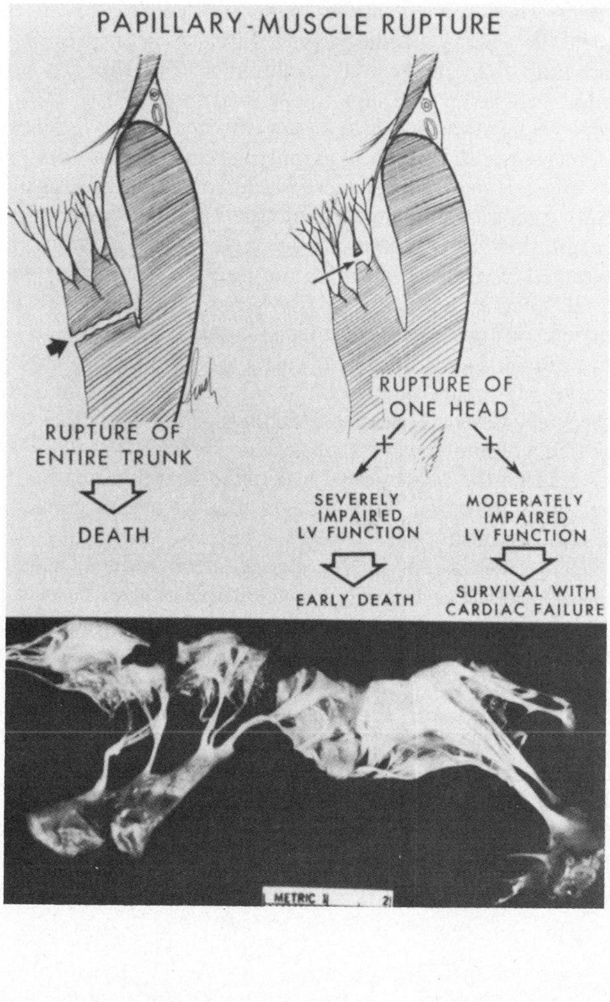

FIGURE 32–10 *Top*, Diagrammatic representation of the types of, and possible consequences of, papillary muscle rupture during acute myocardial infarction. It is likely that rupture of the entire trunk (*left*) is incompatible with survival in any patient, since a major portion of the support to both valve leaflets is destroyed. With rupture of an apical head (*right*), survival would appear to depend on the extent to which left ventricular function has been impaired by the infarct. With severe impairment, the additional burden of even modest mitral regurgitation may be intolerable, and death will ensue. If the left ventricle is less severely compromised, survival is possible for weeks or months, but congestive heart failure will invariably develop.

Bottom, Rupture of a portion of one papillary muscle during acute myocardial infarction in a 51-year-old man who underwent mitral valve replacement 3 months after the onset of infarction. Preoperatively, pulmonary arterial pressure was 60/28 mm Hg (mean = 40); pulmonary arterial wedge pressure, mean = 28, v = 42; left ventricular pressure = 74/17 mm Hg; and cardiac index = 1.7 liters/min/sq meter. The excised mitral valve shows the ventricular aspects of the leaflets. The leaflets are normal, but the posteromedial papillary muscle is necrotic and fibrotic, and a portion of it is entwined in chordae tendineae at the margin of the anterior mitral leaflet. (From Roberts, W. C., et al.: Nonrheumatic valvular cardiac disease. A clinicopathologic survey of 27 different conditions causing valvular dysfunction. *In* Likoff, W. [ed.]: Cardiovascular Clinics. Vol. 5, No. 2, Valvular Heart Disease. Philadelphia, F. A. Davis, 1973, p. 395.)

tients with healed myocardial infarcts, mitral regurgitation is frequent and is caused by dyskinesis of the left ventricular myocardium at the base of a papillary muscle.[145]

Left ventricular dilatation of any cause, including ischemia, can alter the spatial relationships between the papillary muscles and the chordae tendineae and thereby result in mitral regurgitation (Fig. 32–7). Although *necrosis of a papillary muscle* is a frequent complication of myocardial infarction,[146] frank rupture of a papillary muscle is far less common. Total rupture of a papillary muscle is usually fatal because of extremely severe regurgitation, whereas rupture of one or two of the apical heads of a muscle, which results in a lesser degree of mitral regurgitation, makes survival possible, depending on the functional capacity of the left ventricle (Fig. 32–10).

Some degree of mitral regurgitation is found in approximately 30 per cent of those patients with coronary artery disease who are being considered for coronary bypass surgery[145] and is secondary to ischemic damage of the papillary muscles or dilatation of the mitral valve ring or both.[148,149] The incidence and severity of regurgitation vary inversely with the left ventricular ejection fraction and directly with the left ventricular end-diastolic pressure.

A variety of other disorders of papillary muscles may also be responsible for the development of mitral regurgitation (Table 32–3). These include congenital malposition; absence of one papillary muscle, resulting in the so-called parachute mitral valve syndrome (p. 1089); and involvement or infiltration of papillary muscles by a variety of processes, including abscesses, granulomas, neoplasms, amyloidosis and sarcoidosis.[126]

Other causes of mitral regurgitation, discussed in greater detail elsewhere, include a variety of congenital anomalies (p. 985), obstructive cardiomyopathy (p. 1409), prolapse of the mitral valve (p. 1089), trauma (p. 1535), and left atrial myxoma (p. 1466).

PATHOPHYSIOLOGY

Since the regurgitant mitral orifice is in parallel with the aortic valve, the resistance to ventricular emptying (left ventricular afterload) is reduced in mitral regurgitation. Consequently, as the left ventricle decompresses into the left atrium—both during isometric contraction and early during ejection—the left ventricular volume declines. Indeed, Eckberg et al. found that in patients with mitral regurgitation almost one-half the regurgitant volume is ejected into the left atrium before the aortic valve opens.[150]

The volume of mitral regurgitant flow depends on the size of the regurgitant orifice as well as on the pressure gradient between the left ventricle and left atrium;[151–153] both of these factors—orifice size and pressure gradient—are labile. Left ventricular systolic pressure and therefore the left ventricular–left atrial gradient are dependent on systemic vascular resistance and forward stroke volume,[151] and in patients in whom the mitral annulus is not calcific or rigid, the cross-sectional area of the mitral annulus may be altered by many interventions.[154] Thus, increases of both preload[155] and afterload and depressions of contractility increase left ventricular size and enlarge the mitral regurgitant orifice. In mitral regurgitation caused by conditions in which the mitral valve apparatus is not rigid, such as ventricular dilatation due to ischemic heart disease, hypertensive heart disease or cardiomyopathy, dysfunction of papillary muscles, and rupture of chordae tendineae, the volume of regurgitant flow is influenced significantly by left ventricular dimensions, which in turn affect the regurgitant orifice. When ventricular size is reduced by treatment with cardiac glycosides, diuretics and particularly vasodilators, the volume of regurgitant flow may become diminished, as reflected in the height of the *v* wave in the left atrial pressure pulse (Figure 16–19, p. 540) and in the intensity and duration of the systolic murmur. Conversely, left ventricular dilatation may increase mitral regurgitation.

In experiments in which the acute effects of equally severe mitral and aortic regurgitation on the left ventricle were compared, left ventricular end-diastolic pressure, volume, and radius rose with both lesions, but far less so with mitral regurgitation.[156,157] Peak left ventricular wall tension rose markedly when aortic regurgitation was induced but either did not change greatly or actually declined with mitral regurgitation. According to Laplace's law (p. 431), myocardial wall tension is related to the product of intraventricular pressure and ventricular radius. Since mitral regurgitation reduces both late systolic ventricular pressure and radius, left ventricular wall tension declines markedly (and proportionately to a greater extent than left ventricular pressure), permitting the velocity of myocardial fiber shortening to increase.

At any given left ventricular end-diastolic and aortic systolic pressures, mitral regurgitation reduces the tension developed by the left ventricular myocardium. The reduced load on the ventricle allows a greater proportion of the contractile energy of the myocardium to be expended in shortening than in tension development and explains how the left ventricle can adapt to the load imposed by chronic mitral regurgitation. Thus, it appears to be the reduction in left ventricular tension in mitral regurgitation that allows the left ventricle to increase its total output and ultimately accounts for the finding that patients with mitral regurgitation can sustain large regurgitant volumes for prolonged periods while maintaining forward cardiac output at normal levels for many years. Although the left ventricle initially compensates for the development of acute mitral regurgitation, in part by emptying more completely,[151] as regurgitation persists or increases, the function of the left ventricle deteriorates, and left ventricular end-diastolic volume increases progressively (Fig. 32–11). This may enlarge the regurgitant orifice and thereby create a vicious cycle in which "mitral regurgitation begets more mitral regurgitation."

A large volume of mitral regurgitation induced experimentally produces increased myocardial oxygen consumption only slightly,[158] because myocardial fiber shortening, which is elevated in mitral regurgitation, is not as important a determinant of myocardial oxygen consumption[159] (p. 1238) as are the three major factors.[159] One of these, tension, may be reduced, whereas the other two, contractility and heart rate, are little affected in this condition. In addition, the duration of left ventricular systolic tension is reduced in mitral regurgitation. These experimental observations correlate with the low incidence of clinical manifestations of myocardial ischemia in patients with severe

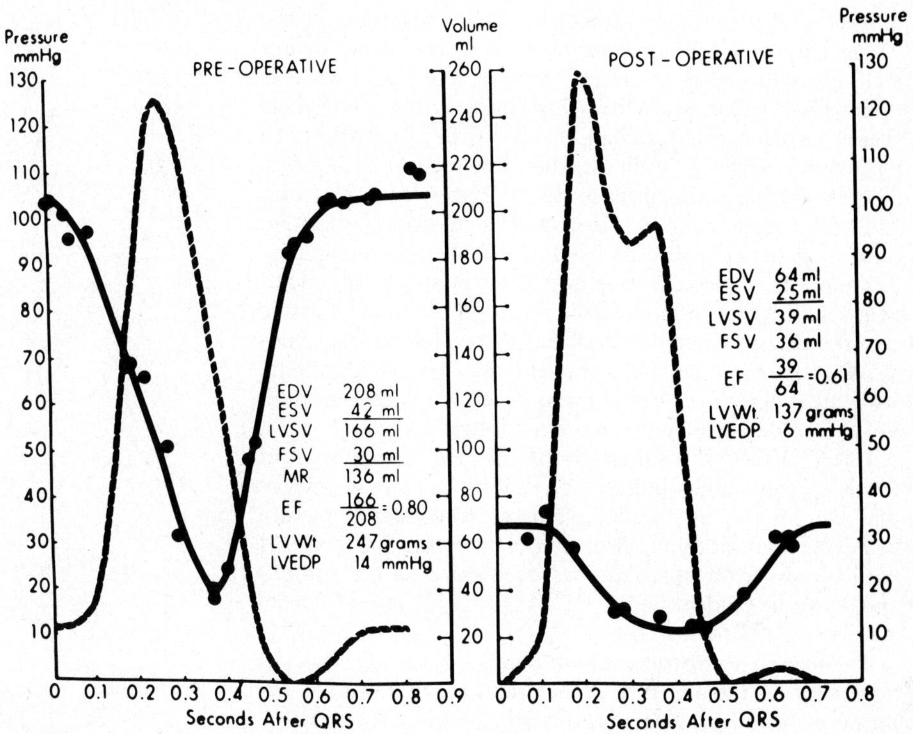

FIGURE 32–11 Preoperative and postoperative (after 1 year) quantitative volume measurements in a patient with severe mitral regurgitation. Postoperative study documented the absence of regurgitation, marked reduction in end-diastolic volume, and regression of hypertrophy. (From Rackley, C. E., and Hood, W. P., Jr.: Quantitative angiography evaluation and pathophysiologic mechanisms in valvular heart disease. *In* Sonnenblick, E. S., and Lesch, M. [eds.]: Valvular Heart Disease. New York, Grune and Stratton, 1974, p. 124, by permission of Grune and Stratton, Inc.)

mitral regurgitation, compared with that occurring in patients with aortic stenosis or regurgitation or both, in which myocardial oxygen demands are augmented.

In patients with chronic regurgitation, both left ventricular end-diastolic volume and mass are increased, with the degree of hypertrophy appropriate to the left ventricular dilatation, so that the ratio of left ventricular mass to end-diastolic volume is normal (Figure 13–7, p. 452).[26] In acute mitral regurgitation, on the other hand, the left ventricle dilates rapidly; and before the myocardium becomes hypertrophied, the ratio of left ventricular mass to end-diastolic volume is reduced, i.e., the left ventricle is thin-walled (Table 14–1, p. 474).

Patients with severe mitral regurgitation may actually exhibit small elevations in ejection phase indices of myocardial contractility (p. 480), such as ejection fraction, extent, and velocity of circumferential fiber shortening (VCF) when they are in the compensated state as a consequence of reduced afterload.[160,161] However, by the time patients become symptomatic,[162] peak and mean VCF have usually declined to normal levels. As mitral regurgitation persists, the tendency for a low impedance leak, which tends to increase myocardial shortening, is counteracted by the impairment of myocardial function characteristic of chronic overload. However, even in patients with overt heart failure secondary to valvular regurgitation, the ejection fraction and fractional fiber shortening may be only slightly reduced.[161,163] Therefore, *normal* values for the ejection phase indices of myocardial performance in patients with severe mitral regurgitation may actually reflect impaired myocardial function, whereas a moderately reduced value (e.g., an ejection fraction of 40 to 50 per cent) generally signifies severe, not moderate, impairment of contractility. An ejection fraction under 40 per cent in patients with marked mitral regurgitation represents advanced myocardial dysfunction; such patients are high operative risks and may not experience marked improvement following mitral valve replacement, perhaps because of the increase in left ventricular afterload that occurs with abolition of the regurgitant leak.[164] In patients with chronic mitral regurgitation, there is often an increase in left ventricular compliance, so that ventricular end-diastolic volume may be increased with little or no elevation of end-diastolic pressure.[165]

End-systolic Volume. Preoperative myocardial contractility is an important determinant of the risk of cardiac failure in the perioperative period and of the level of left ventricular function postoperatively. Therefore, it is not surprising that end-systolic volume has emerged as a useful index for evaluating left ventricular function in patients with valvular regurgitation (p. 475). Indeed, this value was found to be more useful as a predictor of outcome than the ejection fraction, end-diastolic volume, or end-diastolic pressure.[166,167,167a] Patients with severe mitral regurgitation with a normal preoperative end-systolic volume (< 30 ml/m^2) retained normal left ventricular function postoperatively, whereas marked enlargement of the end-systolic volume (> 90 ml/m^2) signified a high perioperative mortality and residual left ventricular dysfunction. Patients with mitral regurgitation and modest enlargement of end-systolic volume (between 30 and 90 ml/m^2) usually tolerate operation satisfactorily but may have reduced left ventricular function postoperatively. For any level of end-systolic volume, patients with mitral regurgitation have more severe left ventricular dysfunction than do patients with aortic regurgitation. This finding reflects the lower afterload in mitral regurgitation and correlates with the clinical observation that patients with mitral regurgitation have a less favorable response to surgical intervention than do those with aortic regurgitation.[168,169]

Effective (forward) *cardiac out ut* is usually depressed in seriously symptomatic patients, whereas total left ventricular output (the sum of forward and regurgitant flow, which can be measured by radionuclide ventriculography)[170] is usually elevated. The atrial contraction (*a*) wave in the left atrial pressure pulse is usually not as prominent in mitral regurgitation as in mitral stenosis, but the *v* wave is often much taller, since it is inscribed during ventricular systole, when the left atrium is filled with blood from the pulmonary veins as well as from the left ventricle (Fig. 32–12). During early diastole, as the distended left atrium suddenly empties, the *y* descent is particularly rapid. However, in patients with combined mitral stenosis and regurgitation, the *y* descent is gradual. Although a left atrioventricular pressure gradient persisting throughout diastole signifies the presence of significant associated mitral stenosis, a brief, early diastolic gradient may occur in patients with pure, severe regurgitation as a result of the torrential flow of blood across a normal-sized mitral orifice.

LEFT ATRIAL COMPLIANCE. The compliance of the left atrium (and pulmonary venous bed) is an important determinant of the hemodynamic and clinical picture in mitral regurgitation. Three major subgroups of patients with severe mitral regurgitation based on left atrial compliance have been identified[157,171,172] (Fig. 32–13) and are characterized as follows:

1. Normal or Reduced Compliance. There is little enlargement of the left atrium but marked elevation of the mean left atrial pressure, particularly of the *v* wave,[26,173,174] and pulmonary congestion is a prominent symptom. In most cases, severe mitral regurgitation has developed suddenly, as occurs with rupture of chordae tendineae, infarction of one of the heads of a papillary muscle, or perforation of a mitral leaflet as a consequence of trauma or endocarditis. Sinus rhythm is usually present; the left atrial wall frequently exhibits striking hypertrophy, is capable of contracting vigorously, and facilitates left ventricular filling. Thickening of the walls of the pulmonary veins and proliferative changes in the pulmonary arteries as well as marked elevation of pulmonary vascular resistance usually develop over the course of 6 to 12 months.

2. Markedly Increased Compliance. At the opposite end of the spectrum from patients in the first group are those with severe, longstanding mitral regurgitation with massive enlargement of the left atrium and normal or only slightly elevated left atrial pressure. The atrial wall contains only a small remnant of muscle surrounded by a great deal of fibrous tissue. Longstanding mitral regurgitation in these patients has altered the physical properties of the left atrial wall and thereby displaced the atrial pressure-volume curve, allowing a normal or almost normal pressure to exist in a greatly enlarged left atrium. Pulmonary artery pressure and pulmonary vascular resistance are normal or only slightly elevated at rest. Atrial fibrillation and a low cardiac output are almost invariably present.[171]

3. Moderately Increased Compliance. This, the most common subgroup, consists of patients between the ends of the spectrum represented by groups 1 and 2; these patients have severe chronic regurgitation and exhibit variable degrees of enlargement of the left atrium, associated with significant elevation of the left atrial pressure.

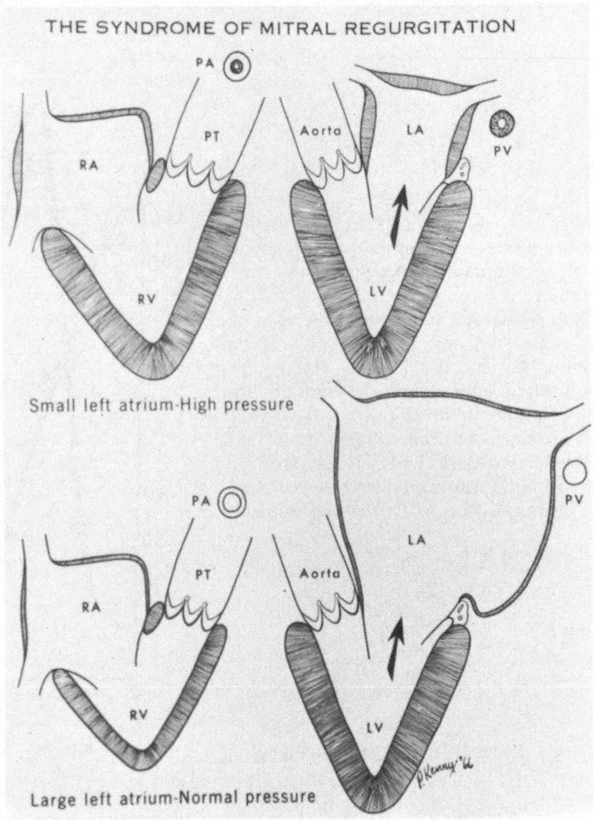

FIGURE 32–13 Diagram depicting the two extremes of the spectrum in pure mitral regurgitation. When severe mitral regurgitation appears suddenly in individuals with previously normal or near-normal hearts, the left atrium (LA) is relatively small and the high pressure within it is reflected back into the pulmonary vessels and right ventricle (RV). The anatomical indicator of this latter physiological event is severe hypertrophy of the left atrial and right ventricular walls and marked intimal proliferation and medial hypertrophy of the pulmonary arteries (PA), arterioles, and veins (PV). At the other extreme, the left atrial cavity is of giant size and its wall is thin. It is thus able to "absorb" the left ventricular (LV) pressure without reflecting it back into the pulmonary vessels or right ventricle. As a consequence, pulmonary vessels remain normal, and the right ventricular wall does not thicken. PT = pulmonary trunk; RA = right atrium. (From Roberts, W. C., et al.: Nonrheumatic valvular cardiac disease. A clinicopathologic survey of 27 different conditions causing valvular dysfunction. *In* Likoff, W. [ed.]: Cardiovascular Clinics. Vol. 5, No. 2, Valvular Heart Disease. Philadelphia, F. A. Davis, 1973, p. 403.)

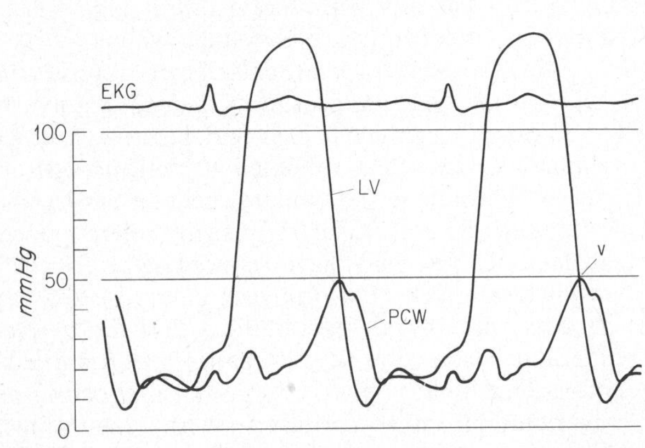

FIGURE 32–12 Pressure tracings from a 59-year-old man with shortness of breath on exertion, a loud systolic murmur, and evidence of ruptured chordae tendineae on echocardiogram. The pulmonary capillary wedge (PCW) pressure is elevated (mean = 25 mm Hg), with a markedly increased regurgitant (*v*) wave peaking at 50 mm Hg. In addition, left ventricular end-diastolic pressure is elevated to 27 mm Hg. These findings are consistent with severe mitral regurgitation.

CLINICAL MANIFESTATIONS

(See Table 32–1, p. 1067)

History

The symptoms of patients with chronic mitral regurgitation are a function of the severity of regurgitation, its rate of progression, the level of pulmonary artery pressure, and the presence of associated valvular or coronary artery disease in patients with chronic rheumatic mitral regurgitation.[175] Since symptoms do not develop until the left ventricle fails, the time interval between the initial attack of rheumatic fever (when one has occurred) and the development of symptoms tends to be longer than in mitral stenosis and often exceeds two decades. The incidence of acute pulmonary edema is lower in chronic mitral regurgitation than in mitral stenosis, presumably because sudden surges in left atrial pressure are less frequent.[14] Similarly, although hemoptysis and systemic embolization do occur in mitral regurgitation, they are less common than in mitral stenosis. On the other hand, chronic weakness and fatigue secondary to a low cardiac output are more prominent.

Patients with mild mitral regurgitation may remain asymptomatic for their entire lives, and the majority of patients with mitral regurgitation of rheumatic origin have only mild disability, unless regurgitation progresses as a result of chronic rheumatic activity, infective endocarditis, or rupture of chordae tendineae.[176] The development of atrial fibrillation affects the course adversely but not as dramatically as it does in mitral stenosis, since rapid ventricular rate often caused by this arrhythmia does *not* elevate left atrial pressure as markedly in mitral regurgitation.

In patients with severe chronic mitral regurgitation with a greatly enlarged left atrium and with relatively mild left atrial hypertension (group 2 with increased left atrial compliance, described above), pulmonary vascular resistance does not usually rise. Instead, the major symptoms, i.e., fatigue and exhaustion, are related to a low cardiac output. In contrast, in patients with acute mitral regurgitation with a normal-sized left atrium (group 1 with normal or reduced left atrial compliance, described above), the left atrial pressure rises abruptly, possibly leading to pulmonary edema, marked elevation of pulmonary vascular resistance, and right-sided heart failure. The last, characterized by congestive hepatomegaly, ankle edema, and ascites, however, is also observed, both in patients with longstanding severe mitral regurgitation and in patients with acute regurgitation and elevated pulmonary vascular resistance. Angina pectoris is rare unless coronary artery disease coexists.

Natural History. This is variable and depends on a combination of the volume of regurgitation, the state of the myocardium, and the etiology of the underlying disorder. Asymptomatic patients with mild mitral regurgitation usually remain stable for many years;[177] severe regurgitation develops in only a small percentage of these, in some cases because of intervening infective endocarditis[176] or rupture of chordae tendineae. Regurgitation tends to progress more rapidly in patients with connective tissue diseases, such as Marfan's syndrome, than in those with chronic regurgitation on a rheumatic basis. In an unselected group of patients with mitral regurgitation who were treated medically, approximately 80 per cent survived 5 years after the diagnosis had been established and almost 60 per cent survived 10 years;[98] patients with combined mitral stenosis and regurgitation had a poorer prognosis, with only 67 per cent surviving 5 years and 30 per cent surviving 10 years after the diagnosis. Munoz et al., in studying a group of patients with greater disability, found that medically treated patients with severe mitral regurgitation had a 5-year survival rate of only 45 per cent.[36] Among medically treated patients with mitral regurgitation, the arteriovenous oxygen difference and ventricular end-diastolic volume were significant (inverse) predictors of survival.[178]

Physical Examination

Palpation of the arterial pulse is helpful in differentiating aortic stenosis from mitral regurgitation, both of which may produce a prominent systolic murmur at the base of the heart; the carotid arterial upstroke is sharp in mitral regurgitation[179] and delayed in aortic stenosis; the volume of the pulse may be normal in both conditions or reduced in the presence of heart failure.

The cardiac impulse is brisk, hyperdynamic, and displaced to the left[14] (Fig. 3–28, p. 59), and a prominent left ventricular filling wave is frequently palpable in early diastole. A presystolic apical impulse is rarely palpable, except in patients with acute regurgitation. Systolic expansion of the enlarged left atrium may result in a late systolic thrust in the parasternal region, which may be confused with right ventricular enlargement (p. 30).[180] Rarely, a greatly enlarged left atrium may be palpable in the third left intercostal space during systole.[14]

AUSCULTATION. With severe, chronic mitral regurgitation due to defective valve cusps, S_1, produced by valve closure, is usually diminished. Wide splitting of S_2 is common and results from the shortening of left ventricular ejection and an earlier A_2 as a consequence of reduced resistance to left ventricular outflow. When pulmonary hypertension is present, P_2 is louder than A_2. The abnormal increase in the flow rate across the mitral orifice during the rapid filling phase is usually associated with an S_3, the auscultatory counterpart of a palpable rapid filling wave (Fig. 3–1, p. 41). A left ventricular S_3, i.e., one that is not augmented by inspiration, excludes predominant mitral stenosis (unless aortic regurgitation, ischemic heart disease, or another cause of an S_3 is present).

The *systolic murmur* is the most prominent physical finding in mitral regurgitation; it must be differentiated from the systolic murmur heard in aortic stenosis, tricuspid regurgitation, and ventricular septal defect (Table 32–5). In most cases of severe mitral regurgitation, the *systolic murmur* commences immediately after the soft S_1 (Fig. 32–5) and continues beyond and may obscure A_2 because of the persistence of the pressure difference between the left ventricle and left atrium (Fig. 4–2, p. 69). The holosystolic murmur of chronic mitral regurgitation is usually constant in intensity, blowing, high-pitched, and loudest at the apex (Fig. 4–11, p. 74) with radiation to the axilla and left infrascapular area; however, radiation toward the sternum or the aortic area may occur with abnormalities of the posterior leaflet. The murmur shows little change even in the presence of large beat-to-beat variations of left ventricular stroke volume, as occur in atrial fibrillation,[181] in contrast

TABLE 32–5 HELPFUL POINTS IN DIFFERENTIAL DIAGNOSIS OF MITRAL REGURGITATION, VENTRICULAR SEPTAL DEFECT, TRICUSPID REGURGITATION, AND AORTIC STENOSIS

Physical, Roentgenographic, or Electrocardiographic Feature	Mitral Regurgitation	Ventricular Septal Defect	Tricuspid Regurgitation	Aortic Stenosis
Systolic murmur	Harsh and pansystolic	Harsh and pansystolic	Pansystolic	Ejection, crescendo-decrescendo
Primary location of murmur	Apex	Left sternal border	Left sternal border	Base of heart; occasionally apical
Radiation of murmur	Axilla; occasionally base and neck	Left precordium	Little	Carotids
Thrill	Occasionally present at apex	Usually present at left sternal border	Rare	Occasionally present at base
Murmur with inspiration	No change	No change	Increases	No change
Valsalva maneuver	May increase	Increases or no change	No change	Decreases
Venous pressure	Often normal	Slightly elevated with prominent *a* and *v* waves	Elevated, with very prominent *v* waves	Usually normal
Pulsatile liver	No	No	Yes	No
Pulmonary component of S_2	Normal; occasionally increased	Normal or loud; usually delayed	Usually increased	Normal
Apical impulse	Hyperkinetic; occasional heaving	Hyperkinetic	Weak or normal	Forceful and sustained
ECG	Left ventricular hypertrophy; left atrial hypertrophy	Biventricular hypertrophy	Right ventricular hypertrophy, occasional right atrial hypertrophy	Left ventricular hypertrophy with associated ST-T changes
Chest roentgenogram	Moderately enlarged heart, marked left atrial enlargement	Enlarged left and right ventricles	Enlarged right ventricle	Normal heart size or left ventricular hypertrophy

Reproduced with permission from Haffajee, C. I.: Chronic mitral regurgitation. *In* Dalen, J. E., and Alpert, J. S. (eds.): Valvular Heart Disease. Boston, Little, Brown and Co., 1981, p. 97.

to most midsystolic (ejection) murmurs, such as in aortic stenosis, which vary greatly in intensity with stroke volume and therefore with the duration of diastole.[182] There is little correlation between the intensity of the systolic murmur and the severity of mitral regurgitation. Indeed, in patients with severe mitral regurgitation due to left ventricular dilatation or paraprosthetic valvular regurgitation or in those who have marked emphysema, obesity, or chest deformity, the systolic murmur may be soft or even absent.[183]

Pansystolic and late systolic murmurs are both characteristic of mitral regurgitation. When the murmur is confined to late systole, the regurgitation is usually mild and may be secondary to prolapse of the mitral valve or papillary muscle dysfunction, conditions that cause late systolic regurgitation. These causes of mitral regurgitation are frequently associated with a normal S_1 because initial closure of the mitral valve cusps may be unimpaired. The systolic murmur is usually of no more than Grade 3/6 intensity, is a mid to late diamond-shaped murmur (Fig. 32–8), or exhibits late systolic accentuation and radiates more frequently to the lower left sternal border than to the axilla.[143] The murmur of papillary muscle dysfunction is particularly variable; it may become accentuated or holosystolic during acute myocardial ischemia and often disappears when ischemia is relieved.[184] The response of a mid- to late-systolic murmur to a number of maneuvers, as described on page 1091, helps to establish the diagnosis of prolapse of the mitral valve.

DYNAMIC AUSCULTATION. The holosystolic murmur of rheumatic mitral regurgitation shows little variation during respiration. However, sudden standing and amyl nitrite inhalation usually diminish the murmur (Table 32–6), whereas squatting and methoxamine or phenylephrine augment it. The murmur is reduced during the strain of the Valsalva maneuver and shows a left-sided response, i.e., a transient overshoot, six to eight beats following release. The murmur is usually intensified by isometric exercise, differentiating it from the systolic murmurs of valvular aortic stenosis and hypertrophic obstructive car-

TABLE 32–6 EFFECT OF VARIOUS INTERVENTIONS ON SYSTOLIC MURMURS

Intervention	Hypertrophic Obstructive Cardiomyopathy	Aortic Stenosis	Mitral Regurgitation	Mitral Prolapse
Valsalva	↑	↓	↓	↑ or ↓
Standing	↑	↑ or unchanged	↓	↑
Handgrip or squatting	↓	↓ or unchanged	↑	↓
Supine position with legs elevated	↓	↑ or unchanged	Unchanged	↓
Exercise	↑	↑ or unchanged	↓	↑
Amyl nitrite	↑ ↑	↑	↓	↑
Isoproterenol	↑ ↑	↑	↓	↑

↑ ↑ = Markedly increased.

Modified from Paraskos, J. A.: Combined valvular disease. *In* Dalen, J. E., and Alpert, J. S. (eds.): Valvular Heart Disease. Boston, Little, Brown and Co., 1981, p. 365.

diomyopathy, both of which are reduced by this intervention. The murmur of mitral regurgitation due to left ventricular dilatation decreases in intensity and duration with effective therapy with cardiac glycosides, diuretics, rest, and particularly vasodilators.

The holosystolic murmur of mitral regurgitation resembles that produced by a ventricular septal defect. However, the latter is usually loudest at the left sternal border rather than the apex and is often accompanied by a parasternal thrill. The murmur of mitral regurgitation may also be confused with that of tricuspid regurgitation, which is usually heard best along the left sternal border, is augmented during inspiration, and is accompanied by a prominent *v* wave and *y* descent in the jugular venous pulse.

When the chordae tendineae to the posterior leaflet of the mitral valve rupture, the regurgitant jet is often directed anteriorly, so that it impinges on the atrial septum adjacent to the aortic root and causes a systolic murmur most prominent at the base of the heart, which can be confused with that of aortic stenosis. The acoustic energy derived from the mitral regurgitant jet may be transmitted to the aorta by the impact of the jet on the portion of the left atrial wall adjacent to the aortic root.[185] On the other hand, when the chordae to the anterior leaflet rupture, the jet is usually directed to the posterior wall of the left atrium, and the murmur may be transmitted to the spine or even to the top of the head.[186] Because the *v* wave is markedly elevated in acute mitral regurgitation, the pressure gradient between the left ventricle and atrium declines at the end of systole, and the murmur may not be holosystolic but decrescendo, ending well before A_2 (Figure 4–16, p. 77). It is usually lower pitched and softer than the murmur of chronic mitral regurgitation. Pulmonary hypertension, common in acute mitral regurgitation, may increase the intensity of P_2 and the murmurs of pulmonary and tricuspid regurgitation, and right-sided S_4 may develop.

Patients with rheumatic disease of the mitral valve exhibit a spectrum of abnormalities, ranging from pure stenosis to pure regurgitation[187] (Fig. 32–5). The presence of an S_3, a rapid left ventricular filling wave and left ventricular impulse on palpation, and a soft S_1 all favor predominant regurgitation, whereas an accentuated S_1, a prominent OS with a short A_2-OS interval, and a soft short systolic murmur all point to predominant stenosis. Elucidation of the predominant valvular lesion may be complicated by the presence of a holosystolic murmur of tricuspid regurgitation in patients with pure mitral stenosis and pulmonary hypertension; this murmur, as has already been noted, may sometimes be heard at the apex when the right ventricle is greatly enlarged and may therefore be mistaken for the murmur of mitral regurgitation. Many patients with severe tricuspid regurgitation have a low cardiac output and an inaudible or barely audible diastolic murmur of mitral stenosis, further complicating the clinical diagnosis. An S_3 originating from the right ventricle in patients with mitral stenosis and pulmonary hypertension may falsely suggest the presence of mitral regurgitation. On the other hand, systolic expansion of the left atrium, as occurs in severe mitral regurgitation, often produces a late systolic parasternal expansion that may be confused with right ventricular hypertrophy and falsely attributed to mitral stenosis.

Laboratory Examination

ELECTROCARDIOGRAM AND VECTORCARDIOGRAM. The principal *electrocardiographic* findings in patients with mitral regurgitation are left atrial enlargement and atrial fibrillation.[62,188,189] Electrocardiographic evidence of left ventricular enlargement occurs in about half the patients with severe mitral regurgitation. Approximately 15 per cent exhibit electrocardiographic evidence of right ventricular hypertrophy, a change which reflects the presence of pulmonary hypertension of sufficient severity to counterbalance not only the normally larger but actually hypertrophied left ventricle. The *vectorcardiogram* often shows left ventricular hypertrophy, with initial forces directed to the right and anteriorly, whereas the maximal QRS vector is directed to the left, posteriorly, and inferiorly, with an increased magnitude usually exceeding 2.0 mv; the T loop is usually discordant with respect to the QRS.[69–71] Vectorcardiographic evidence of combined right and left ventricular hypertrophy or right ventricular hypertrophy Type C, Figure 7–17, p. 213) is less common[63,190] and, as is the case for the electrocardiogram, reflects severe pulmonary hypertension.

RADIOLOGICAL FINDINGS (See also p. 163) Cardiomegaly with left ventricular, and particularly with left atrial, enlargement is a common finding in patients with chronic severe mitral regurgitation.[78,191] However, there is little correlation between left atrial size and pressure. Acute valvular regurgitation, even if severe, often does not increase overall cardiac size and may produce only mild left atrial enlargement despite marked elevation of left atrial pressure, as already noted. Changes in the lung fields are less prominent in mitral regurgitation than in mitral stenosis, but interstitial edema with Kerley B lines is frequently seen with acute regurgitation or with progressive left ventricular failure.

In patients with combined stenosis and regurgitation, overall cardiac enlargement and particularly left atrial dilatation are prominent findings. However, it is usually difficult to determine which lesion is predominant from the plain chest roentgenogram, since it may be difficult to distinguish between right and left ventricular enlargement. Predominant mitral stenosis is suggested by relatively mild cardiomegaly with significant changes in the lung fields, whereas predominant regurgitation is more likely when the heart is greatly enlarged and the changes in the lungs are relatively slight. When the left atrium is aneurysmally dilated, regurgitation is almost always the dominant lesion. Calcification of the mitral valve occurs in patients with stenosis, regurgitation, or mixed lesions.

Calcification of the mitral annulus, an important cause of mitral regurgitation in the elderly, is most prominent in the posterior third of the cardiac silhouette[78] and is best visualized on films exposed in the lateral or right anterior oblique projection, in which it appears as a dense, coarse, C-shaped opacity (Figure 6–24, p. 163).

The diagnosis of mitral regurgitation can be established by means of left *ventricular angiocardiography,*[192] the prompt appearance of contrast material in the left atrium following its injection into the left ventricle indicating the presence of mitral regurgitation. The injection should be rapid enough to permit left ventricular opacification but slow enough to avoid the development of premature ventricular contractions, which can induce spurious regurgitation.

The regurgitant volume can be determined from the difference between the total left ventricular stroke volume, estimated angiocardiographically, and the simultaneous measurement of the effective forward stroke volume by Fick's method. The results of such studies suggest that in patients with severe regurgitation, the regurgitant volume is of the same magnitude as, or may even exceed, the effective forward stroke volume.

Qualitative, but clinically useful estimates of the severity of regurgitation may be made by (cine)angiographic observation of the degree of opacification of the left atrium and pulmonary veins following the injection of contrast material into the left ventricle. Mitral regurgitation secondary to rheumatic heart disease is characterized angiographically by a central regurgitant jet and by thickened leaflets that exhibit reduced motion, whereas in regurgitation due to other causes, particularly dilatation of the mitral annulus or ruptured chordae and papillary muscles, the systolic jet may be eccentric, and the valves consist of thin filaments

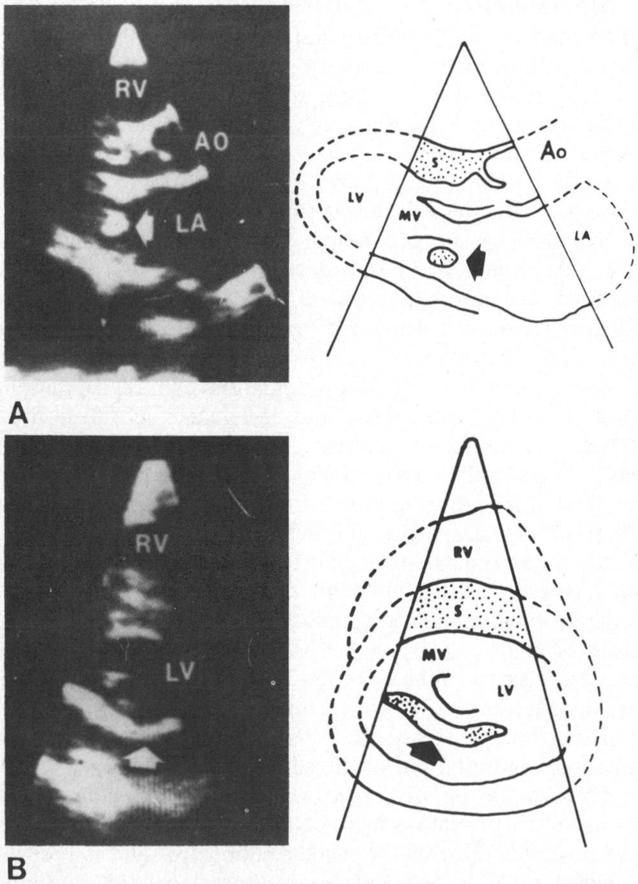

FIGURE 32–14 Long-axis (*A*) and short-axis (*B*) sector scans from a patient with mitral annular calcification (arrows). Atrioventricular junction in *A* was identified by the differing wall motion of the left atrium and the left ventricle, as seen on real-time recording and by location of the mitral valve. The extent of calcification can be appreciated only on the short-axis view. Ao = aorta; LA = left atrium; RV = right ventricle; LV = left ventricle; MV = mitral valve; S = interventricular septum. (Reproduced with permission from Kronzon, I., Mitchell, J., Shapiro, J., et al.: Two-dimensional echocardiography in mitral annulus calcification. Am. J. Radiol. *134*: 355, 1980.)

that display excessive motion.[170] The etiology of the regurgitation, e.g., prolapse of the mitral valve, and a flail leaflet are often distinguishable angiographically (Figure 32–8, p. 1094).

ECHOCARDIOGRAPHY (see also p. 111). M-mode and two-dimensional echocardiography are more useful in determining the etiology than in estimating the severity of mitral regurgitation.[193,194] Severe mitral regurgitation results in enlargement of the left atrium and left ventricle,[195] with increased motion of both of these chambers. With acute mitral regurgitation, there may be little increase in the internal diameter of either of these chambers, but increased systolic motion is particularly prominent. The underlying cause of the regurgitation—e.g., rupture of chordae tendineae,[196] mitral valve prolapse (Figs. 5–41 to 5–43, p. 112; Fig. 32–14), flail leaflets (Figure 5–44, p. 113), and vegetations, Figure 5–45, p. 113)—can sometimes be determined, and the echocardiogram may also show calcification of the mitral annulus as a band of dense echoes between the mitral apparatus and the posterior wall of the heart (Fig. 32–14).[134,196a]

Two-dimensional echocardiography may be useful in the detection of significant mitral regurgitation by demonstrating failure of the leaflets to close,[197] and flail leaflets[198] and valvular prolapse may also be identified by this technique[199] (Figs. 5–42 and 5–43, p. 112). Pulsed Doppler echocardiography (Figure 5–12, p. 95) can reveal mitral regurgitant flow and may be useful in assessing its severity.[200,201,201a]

RADIOISOTOPE ANGIOGRAPHY. Gated pool imaging or first-pass angiography may reveal an increased end-diastolic volume; the regurgitant fraction can be estimated from the ratio of left ventricular to right ventricular stroke volume;[167,202] in patients with mitral regurgitation and impaired left ventricular function, ejection fraction fails to rise normally during exercise.[203] Radionuclide angiograms are useful for interval follow-up of patients. Progressive increases in ventricular end-diastolic or end-systolic volumes often suggest that surgical treatment is necessary (see below).

MANAGEMENT

MEDICAL TREATMENT

This includes all the measures used in the treatment of heart failure, as outlined in Chapter 16. Digitalis glycosides clearly play a more important role in the management of mitral regurgitation than of mitral stenosis. Afterload reduction is also of conspicuous benefit in the management of mitral regurgitation—both the acute and the chronic forms.[204] By reducing the impedance to ejection into the aorta, the volume of blood regurgitating into the left atrium is reduced, causing left atrial pressure and, in particular, the elevated *v* wave, to decline (Figure 16–19, p. 540). In addition, decreasing left ventricular volume reduces the size of the mitral annulus and thereby the regurgitant orifice.[205] Afterload reduction with intravenous nitroprusside may be life-saving in acute mitral regurgitation due to rupture of the head of a papillary muscle occurring in the course of an acute myocardial infarction. It may permit stabilization of the patient's condition and thereby allow operation to be carried out with the patient in an optimal condition. When surgical treatment is contraindicated, chronic afterload reduction with oral hydralazine or prazosin may improve the clinical state for months or even years in patients with severe mitral regurgitation.

Antiarrhythmic therapy with quinidine or procainamide may be helpful in suppressing frequent atrial or ventricular premature contractions as well as in maintaining sinus rhythm following electrical or pharmacological conversion from atrial fibrillation. Appropriate prophylaxis to prevent infective endocarditis (p. 1175) is indicated.

Left-heart catheterization, selective left ventricular angiocardiography, and coronary arteriography are indicated in patients with significant functional disability despite optimal medical management. The objectives of these studies are to (1) confirm the presence of regurgitation and estimate its severity; (2) aid in the identification of patients with primary myocardial disease and relatively mild, functional mitral regurgitation secondary to ventricular dilatation who are not likely to benefit greatly from operation and in whom the operative risk is relatively high; (3) detect and assess the severity of any associated valve lesions; and (4) determine the presence and assess the extent of coronary artery disease.

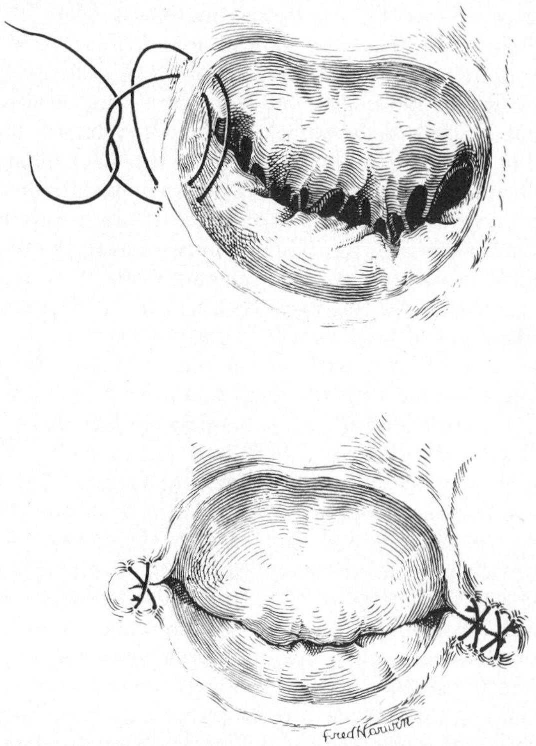

FIGURE 32–15 Commissural plication of the regurgitant mitral valve annulus. (From Starr, A., and Macmanus, Q.: Acquired valvular heart disease. *In* Efflet, D. B. [ed.]: Blades' Surgical Diseases of the Chest. 4th ed. St. Louis, The C. V. Mosby Co., 1978, p. 513.)

SURGICAL TREATMENT

When operative treatment is under consideration, the chronic, often slowly progressive nature of the disease must be weighed against the immediate risks and long-term uncertainties attendant upon surgery. Surgical mortality depends on the patient's hemodynamic and clinical state, particularly the function of the left ventricle, the presence of associated conditions such as renal, hepatic, or pulmonary disease, as well as on the experience of the surgical team. It does not appear to depend significantly on which of the currently widely used tissue or mechanical valve prostheses is employed.

In selected patients with pure or predominant mitral regurgitation—i.e., patients who have severe noncalcific mitral regurgitation, a dilated mitral annulus, absence of severe subvalvular chordal thickening, and no major loss of leaflet substance—an annuloplasty, often using a rigid or semirigid prosthetic ring (i.e., a Carpentier ring),[206] direct suture repair of the valve (Fig. 32–15), or replacement of torn chordae tendineae has been successful. A relatively small number of surgeons, particularly in Europe, have reported a relatively low operative mortality rate, in the range of 5 per cent, with long-term clinical improvement in the majority of survivors.[207] The results of these "plastic" operations have, in general, been more favorable in children and adolescents with pliable valves and in patients with severe coronary artery disease and mitral regurgitation secondary to annular dilatation, papillary muscle dysfunction or rupture, or chordal rupture than in adults with primary valvular deformity and thickening.[208,209,209a] Most surgeons, however, particularly in the United States, have found that regurgitant valves are not amenable to direct repair in the majority of cases. Instead, mitral valve replacement has emerged as the principal surgical approach to pure mitral regurgitation or combined mitral stenosis and regurgitation.

Results. Mortality rates of 1 to 4 per cent in patients with predominant mitral stenosis and of 2 to 7 per cent in patients with pure or predominant regurgitation who undergo isolated mitral valve replacement operated upon electively in functional Class II or III are now common in many centers.[210–213] Age per se is no barrier to successful surgery; mitral valve replacement can be carried out in patients more than 70 years of age with the same or only slightly higher risk as in younger patients,[214] if their general health status is adequate. Surgical treatment substantially improves survival in patients with symptomatic mitral regurgitation. Factors such as an age of less than 60 years, a preoperative New York Heart Association functional Class of II, a cardiac index exceeding 2.0 liters/min/m^2, a left ventricular end-diastolic pressure less than 12 mm Hg, and a normal ejection fraction all correlate with improved immediate as well as long-term survival. Patients with moderate impairment of the ejection fraction (30 to 50 per cent), in particular, exhibit improved survival following surgical compared with medical treatment.[178] In other series, only age and preoperative ejection fraction predicted long-term survival following mitral valve replacement.[213]

Emergency surgical treatment of acute left ventricular failure caused by acute mitral regurgitation due to myocardial infarction and rupture of the head of a papillary muscle, by trauma to the mitral valve, or by endocarditis is associated with a much higher mortality rate than is the elective surgical treatment of chronic mitral regurgitation. However, unless such patients with acute, severe endocarditis and heart failure are treated aggressively, a fatal outcome is almost certain. If, on the other hand, the condition of patients with mitral regurgitation secondary to acute infarction can be stabilized by medical treatment, it is preferable to defer operation until 4 to 6 weeks after infarction. Vasodilator treatment may be useful during this period. However, medical management should not be prolonged if multisystem (renal or pulmonary or both) failure occurs. Surgical mortality is also higher in patients with refractory heart failure (functional Class IV), in those in whom a previously implanted prosthetic valve must be replaced because of thromboembolism or valve dysfunction,[215] and in those with active infective endocarditis (of a natural or prosthetic valve). Despite the higher surgical risks, the efficacy of early operation has been established in patients with infective endocarditis complicated by medically uncontrollable congestive heart failure, recurrent emboli, or both[216,217] (p. 1171). Since fungal endocarditis responds poorly to medical management, it is now the practice to recommend valve replacement in these cases *before* the onset of heart failure or embolization.

In most patients with mitral regurgitation, the symptomatic state and thus the quality of life improve following valve replacement. Severe pulmonary hypertension is relieved almost uniformly,[121–124] and left ventricular end-diastolic volume and mass are reduced (Fig. 32–11). However, in contrast to patients with aortic or mitral stenosis, whose cardiac function and cardiac symptoms generally improve following operation, patients with mitral regurgitation who had marked left ventricular dysfunction preoperatively sometimes remain symptomatic following a technically satisfactory operation. Furthermore, long-term survival in patients with predominant mitral regurgitation who undergo mitral valve replacement may be poorer than in those with pure stenosis or mixed stenotic and regurgitant lesions, presumably because left ventricular dysfunction may be quite advanced and largely irreversible by the time patients with pure regurgitation become seriously symptomatic.[212,218] Since, as indicated earlier (p. 1084), mitral regurgitation reduces ventricular afterload, abolition of regurgitation raises afterload and thereby may interfere with left ventricular emptying, causing a reduction of the ejection fraction[165,213] and an increase of end-systolic volume; these hemodynamic changes may be particularly troublesome during the early postoperative period, when vasodilator treatment may be effective. However, even though it is clearly desirable to operate upon patients with mitral regurgitation before they develop marked left ventricular dysfunction, and despite these limitations of the results of surgical treatment in patients with severe left ventricular failure, operation is still indicated in the majority of these patients, since conservative therapy has little to offer.

The etiology of the mitral regurgitation also plays an important role in the outcome following surgical treatment. In patients in whom mitral dysfunction is secondary to ischemic heart disease, the 5-year survival rate is about 30 per cent, whereas in rheumatic mitral regurgitation it is much better, approximately 70 per cent. Furthermore, occlusive coronary artery disease coexisting with, but not the primary cause of mitral dysfunction is associated with decreased perioperative and long-term postoperative survival as well.[212] However, some improvement from mitral valve replacement can be expected even in patients with mitral regurgitation secondary to ischemic heart disease who are medically unresponsive and in congestive heart failure, as long as the cardiac index and ejection fraction exceed 1.5 liters/min/m^2 and 35 per cent, respectively. When left ventricular dysfunction is more severe, however, the risk of operative mortality becomes prohibitive.[219]

INDICATIONS FOR OPERATION. In view of the advances in surgical techniques, the reduction in operative mortality, the continuous improvement of artificial valves as well as the poor long-term results in many patients whose mitral regurgitation is corrected after a long history of heart failure, a more aggressive stance concerning the desirability of operation is in order. Only a few years ago many cardiologists, including the author, recommended operation for patients with chronic severe mitral regurgitation only if they were in functional Class III or IV,[220] i.e., with symptoms at rest or on ordinary activity despite intensive medical treatment; however, it is now my policy to recommend operation also for patients with severe mitral regurgitation who are in Class II, i.e., who become distinctly symptomatic only on heavy exertion, particularly if cardiomegaly and an elevated left ventricular end-systolic volume (> 30 ml/m^2 BSA) persist despite aggressive medical therapy. However, patients with mitral regurgitation who are asymptomatic or only mildly symptomatic are not considered to be candidates for surgical treatment at this time, since they may live for many years with little deterioration in their condition.

ARTIFICIAL CARDIAC VALVES

(see Table 32–7)

MECHANICAL PROSTHESES (Fig. 32–16). Two major types of artificial valves are currently available in models designed for both the atrioventricular (mitral and tricuspid) and the aortic positions—mechanical prostheses and tissue valves. The first series of successful replacements of the mitral and aortic valves was accomplished by Harken et al.[221] and Starr in 1960,[222] and at the present time, the *Starr-Edwards caged-ball valve,* in which the sewing ring and struts are cloth-covered to reduce the incidence of thromboembolism, is still widely used.[223,224] An alternative, the *Smeloff-Cutter valve,* has a double-cage design that is somewhat superior hydrodynamically, since the diameter of the valve orifice is equal to or slightly larger than the ball diameter, which is not the case for the Starr-Edwards valve.

Two types of tilting-disk valves are widely employed. The *Björk-Shiley valve* consists of a low-profile stellite valve housing covered with a Teflon fabric sewing ring. Its design allows an excellent ratio between the diameter of the valve orifice and tissue annulus. It contains a suspended tilting disk occluder made of pyrolytic carbon (Pyrolyte), which opens to an angle of 60 degrees, providing central laminar flow.[212,225] The *Lillehei-Kaster pivoting disk valve* consists of a titanium valve housing with a Teflon fabric sewing ring in which a pyrolite disk is suspended. In the open position, this disk swings to an angle of 80 degrees, providing a large central flow orifice.[226] A recently developed valve, the *St. Jude valve,* is made of pyrolytic carbon; two semicircular disks pivot between open and closed positions without the need for supporting struts. Although experience with this valve in patients dates back only to 1977, it appears to possess favorable flow characteristics and causes a lower transvalvular gradient at any outer diameter and cardiac output.[227]

All of these prosthetic valves have an excellent record of durability—up to 20 years in the case of the caged-ball valves. However, problems with thromboembolism persist despite the fact that the cloth covering of the sewing ring

TABLE 32–7 ADVANTAGES AND DISADVANTAGES OF COMMONLY USED PROSTHESES

Type	Name-Model	Advantages	Disadvantages
Caged ball (non–cloth-covered)	Starr-Edwards 1260, 6120 Smeloff-Cutter	1. Predictable performance 2. Abundant long-term experience 3. Inaudible	1. Thromboembolism 2. Anticoagulation 3. Bulky cage design
Caged ball (Cloth-covered)	Starr-Edwards 2400, 6400	1. Very low incidence of thromboembolism	1. Anticoagulation 2. Bulky cage design 3. Noise 4. Hemolysis 5. Poor hemodynamics in small sizes
Tilting disk	Björk-Shiley Lillehei-Kaster	1. Excellent hemodynamics 2. Very low profile 3. Durability	1. Anticoagulation 2. Thromboembolism 3. Noise
	St. Jude	1. Outstanding hemodynamics 2. Very low profile	1. Anticoagulation 2. Uncertainty about durability and actual incidence of thromboembolism
Porcine xenograft	Hancock Carpentier-Edwards	1. Very low incidence of thromboembolism 2. Central flow 3. No hemolysis 4. Inaudible 5. Anticoagulants usually unnecessary	1. Uncertain durability 2. Poor hemodynamic performance in small sizes (standard models)
Bovine pericardium	Ionescu-Shiley	1. Very low incidence of thromboembolism 2. Central flow 3. No hemolysis 4. Inaudible 5. Anticoagulants usually unnecessary 6. Excellent hemodynamics in aortic position	1. Uncertain durability 2. Gradients in mitral position

Reproduced with permission from Bonchek, L. E.: The basis for selecting a valve prosthesis. *In* McGoon, D. C. (ed.): Cardiovascular Clinics. Cardiac Surgery. Philadelphia, F. A. Davis Co., 1982, p. 103.

and struts has reduced the incidence of this complication considerably. Although the St. Jude valve results in a relatively low incidence of nonfatal emboli—possibly lower than that of the caged-ball valves[212,227]—the Björk-Shiley valve has been associated with massive thrombosis, despite anticoagulation; this uncommon, though potentially catastrophic, complication may be related to the limited excursion of the disk that results when a large valve is inserted into a relatively small ventricle.[228]

All prosthetic valves, regardless of design or placement (mitral, tricuspid, or aortic), require long-term anticoagulation because of the hazard of thromboembolism. Without anticoagulation the incidence of thromboembolism increases three- to sixfold;[229] the risk of thromboembolism is greatest in the first postoperative year. Anticoagulation with sodium warfarin should begin about 2 days after operation in order to achieve a prothrombin time in the range of 20 to 25 seconds (about twice the control value). This relatively conservative approach reduces the risk of anticoagulant hemorrhage, yet does not appear to be associated with a greater frequency of thromboembolism than a prothrombin time of 30 to 35 seconds. It must be recognized that the administration of warfarin carries its own morbidity and mortality, estimated at 0.2 and 2.2 per 100 patient-years, respectively,[229] and despite treatment with

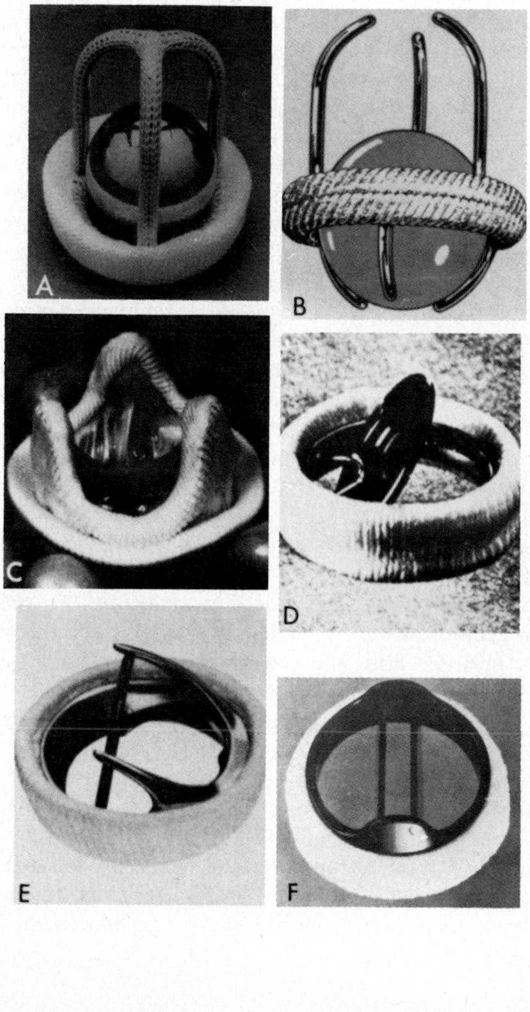

FIGURE 32–16 *A*, Model 2400 Starr-Edwards aortic prosthesis. The valve is totally cloth-covered, except for a thin track on the inside of the struts. *B*, Smeloff-Cutter. *C*, Hancock porcine bioprosthesis. *D*, Björk-Shiley. *E*, Lillehei-Kaster. *F*, St. Jude prosthesis with two semicircular tilting leaflets. (*A* and *F* reproduced with permission from Bonchek, L. I.: Current status of cardiac valve replacement: Selection of a prosthesis and indications for operation. Am. Heart J. *101*: 96, 1981.)

anticoagulants, the incidence of thromboembolic complications is still about 0.2 (fatal) and 1 to 2 (nonfatal) per 100 patient-years.

Although their value has not been definitively established, in some centers acetylsalicylic acid, 0.6 gm twice daily, or dipyridamole, 25 to 50 mg three times daily,[229,229a] is also given to inhibit platelet aggregation.

TISSUE VALVES. Largely to overcome the complication of thromboembolism that is inherent in all prosthetic valves, considerable effort has been devoted to the development of nonthrombogenic tissue valves.[230] The first of these to be widely used were chemically sterilized homografts. Unfortunately, these exhibited a high incidence of breakdown within 3 years.[231] Fresh antibiotic-treated or frozen-irradiated homografts were then developed; these were somewhat more durable but also proved to have a significant late failure rate due to collagen dissolution of the valve cusp,[232] possibly representing a subtle form of rejection. The use of homograft valves has been restricted by continuing uncertainty about their durability, and difficulty of inserting unmounted grafts into the aortic position, and the problems inherent in their procurement.

To overcome these difficulties, *porcine heterografts* were developed and used clinically beginning in 1965. At first, these valves were sterilized with formalin, which dissolved the collagen cross linkages in the valve cusps and resulted in a high failure rate.[233] Carpentier et al. then developed the process of fixation and sterilization of porcine heterografts using a dilute solution of glutaraldehyde, which appears to promote the stability of the collagen cross linkages, so that after their exposure to this agent the valves become essentially inert collagen shells with little, if any, antigenicity.[234] The valves were then mounted on a semiflexible stent made of a stellite ring and flexible struts of polypropylene.[235] This form of the Hancock porcine bioprosthetic cardiac valve (Fig. 32–16) was the first quality-controlled, mass-produced tissue valve and has been widely used in the mitral, tricuspid, and aortic positions. The Carpentier-Edwards porcine valve is mounted on a stent made of Elgiloy—an alloy of spring steel. Heterologous (bovine) glutaraldehyde-fixed pericardium[236–238] has also been utilized for fabrication of cardiac valves mounted on a titanium frame. They have been employed successfully for more than 5 years with a record of durability, incidence of thromboembolism, and hemodynamic performance comparable to that of the porcine valves, although at this time the total experience with the latter is far greater than with all the other tissue valves combined. Homologous dura mater[239] has been used successfully in a similar manner, but there is little experience with this valve in the United States.

Tissue valves have succeeded in reducing the risk of thromboembolism.[211,229,240–243] The majority of the thromboembolic episodes with the xenograft in the mitral position occur in the first 6 to 12 postoperative weeks, and therefore it appears desirable to treat these patients with anticoagulants for this period of time.[243] Treatment is then gradually discontinued over a 2- to 10-week period[244] unless thrombogenic factors not related to the prosthesis persist, such as chronic atrial fibrillation,[244a] the finding of a clot in the atrium at operation, a markedly dilated left atrium, a calcified left atrial wall, or a postoperative thromboembolic event; with any of the aforementioned conditions, anticoagulation is continued permanently. With this approach, the incidence of thromboembolic complications is extremely low, approximately 2 per 100 patient-years, comparable to that of anticoagulant-treated patients receiving the Björk-Shiley prostheses in the mitral position[243] over a 2-year follow-up period. The incidence of postoperative emboli following implantation of a porcine bioprosthesis into the mitral position is three times as high in patients with atrial fibrillation (despite anticoagulation) as in patients in sinus rhythm. It is unlikely that *any* replacement of the mitral valve can be associated with a thromboembolism rate much below 0.5 per cent per year, since some of the emboli in patients with longstanding mitral valve disease are derived from the left atrium rather than from the valve itself.[245] The incidence of embolization in patients who have experienced repeated emboli from a prosthetic mitral valve may be reduced by replacement with a tissue valve.

HEMODYNAMICS OF VALVE REPLACEMENTS. It must be recognized that all valve replacements—mechanical prostheses as well as tissue valves—have an effective in vitro orifice size that is smaller than a normal human valve.[246] After insertion, tissue ingrowth and endothelialization reduce the in vivo effective orifice size further,[247] and therefore most valve devices currently available must be considered to be at least mildly stenotic.[248] However, postoperative hemodynamic measurements of the rigid prostheses show reasonably good function, with effective valve orifice averaging 1.7 to 2.0 cm^2 and mitral valvular gradients of 4 to 8 mm Hg at rest. Although definitive comparisons have not been carried out, the cloth-covered Starr-Edwards valve appears to be intrinsically slightly more stenotic than the tilting-disk (Björk-Shiley or Lillehei-Kaster) valves; the St. Jude valve, in turn, may be slightly superior to the latter.[227] In hemodynamic studies, the recently modified porcine and the Ionescu bovine pericardial mitral valves behave in a fashion similar to that of an artificial prosthetic valve of the same diameter,[249,250] although subtle, late hemodynamic deterioration with the porcine bioprosthesis has been reported.[243] Serious hemodynamic obstruction of an artificial valve in the mitral position is quite uncommon, unless the valve is placed in a small left ventricular cavity or a small mitral annulus or unless the prosthesis chosen is too large.

SELECTION OF AN ARTIFICIAL VALVE. The characteristics of both tissue and prosthetic valves are almost evenly matched, and the choice between the two is difficult. It is important that the relative advantages and disadvantages of the various valves be explained to the patient, who should be a participant in the final decision. As indicated, there appear to be no significant differences insofar as hemodynamics are concerned, except that in patients with an unusually small left ventricular cavity or mitral annulus, the low-profile (tilting-disk) prosthetic, St. Jude, or tissue valve may be superior to the more bulky, caged-ball valve.[251] The hazard of thromboembolism, albeit lower than a decade ago, is still considerably higher with prosthetic than with tissue valves. Therefore, a tissue valve is preferred over a prosthesis in patients in whom anticoagulation is difficult to control or is especially hazardous—for example, in vigorous young adults whose vocations or avocations place them at particular risk for bleeding. Because of the uncertainties surrounding their long-term durability,[252,252a] I believe that a mechanical prosthetic valve is still the most desirable in patients under the age of 65 years without contraindications to anticoagulants. Patients with coexisting disease who are prone to hemorrhage or who are unwilling, unreliable, or unlikely to take anticoagulants on a regular basis or patients over the age of 65 years in whom the question of durability is less important and who are at a greater risk of hemorrhage while taking anticoagulants should receive a bioprosthesis. The high incidence of bioprosthetic valve failure in children and adolescents[253,254] and in patients on chronic hemodialysis[211] prohibits their use in these patients. In young adults (> 20 and < 35 years), the failure of bioprosthetic valves is somewhat higher than it is in older adults; this serves as a relative, not an absolute, contraindication in this age group.

Female patients with artificial mitral valves can tolerate the hemodynamic load of pregnancy well, but there is an increased risk of thromboembolism in such patients with prosthetic valves when anticoagulation is interrupted and an increased risk of fatal fetal hemorrhage in those in whom it is continued.[255] There may also be a risk of fetal malformation caused by the possible teratogenic effect of warfarin.[256] These problems represent powerful arguments for the use of tissue valves in all women of childbearing age.[257] In the case of a pregnant woman in whom a prosthetic valve is already in place, the risk to the fetus if the mother receives oral anticoagulants appears to be lower than is the risk to the mother if anticoagulants are discontinued.[258] It is therefore advisable in a pregnant patient with a prosthetic valve to use heparin during the first trimester and again after week 37 of gestation. Oral anticoagulants may be used in the interim period, provided that prothrombin times are monitored frequently. Anticoagulation with heparin should be discontinued with the onset of labor and then reinstituted 24 hours after uncomplicated delivery and continued until the desired effects of oral anticoagulation can be achieved.[256]

When noncardiac surgery is required in patients with prosthetic mitral valves who are receiving anticoagulants, the risk is minimal when the drug regimen is stopped 1 to 3 days preoperatively and for a similar period postoperatively. It may be desirable, however, to protect the patient with low molecular weight dextran during the perioperative period.

A distinct advantage of the rigid prostheses is their predictable performance and durability; some have now been in place and functioning successfully since 1961.[222] Although, with the exception of children and patients on chronic hemodialysis, the mechanical performance of the porcine xenograft preserved by glutaraldehyde has been excellent in the majority of patients for periods of up to 12 years[242,243] (at the time of this writing), there have been an increasing number of reports of valve breakdown after 5 years. Pathological changes in these valves include degeneration, deposition of fibrin on the inflow and outflow surfaces, inflammatory cell infiltrates, focal disruption of the fibrocollagenous structure, and ultimately calcification.[259-262] Although the fraction of all implanted valves that have failed to date has been very small (less than 1 per cent), these pathological observations indicate that the porcine bioprosthesis may not be totally inert in the human circulation, suggesting that replacement of the valve might ultimately become necessary in a significant, although as yet unknown, number of patients. The incidence of infection appears to be approximately equal with all available mechanical and tissue valves. Hemolysis is now rarely a serious problem, but when it does occur it is most conspicuous with the cloth-covered Starr-Edwards valve.

Artificial valves have characteristic auscultatory and phonocardiographic characteristics[263] (Figure 3–19, p. 52). Echocardiography, phonocardiography, and cineradiography[264] are extremely useful in the identification of artificial valve dysfunction.[265-267] Two-dimensional echocardiography is particularly promising in the follow-up of patients who demonstrate clinical deterioration in the postoperative period following porcine heterograft implantation. This technique may prove capable of distinguishing between failure of the bioprosthesis (abnormal structure or valve motion) and left ventricular dysfunction.[268,269]

THE MITRAL VALVE PROLAPSE SYNDROME

ETIOLOGY AND PATHOLOGY

The mitral valve prolapse (MVP) syndrome—which has been given many names, including the systolic click–murmur syndrome, Barlow's syndrome, billowing mitral valve syndrome, ballooning mitral cusp syndrome, floppy valve syndrome, and redundant cusp syndrome,[270-274]—is a common but variable clinical syndrome resulting from diverse pathogenic mechanisms of the mitral valve apparatus. The MVP syndrome has become recognized as one of the most prevalent cardiac valvular abnormalities, affecting as much as 5 to 10 per cent of the population.[275-277] It had been thought for many years that midsystolic clicks and late systolic murmurs, the auscultatory hallmarks of this syndrome, were of extracardiac origin. However, in 1961 it was postulated,[278] and 2 years later Barlow and associates demonstrated that these auscultatory findings are frequently associated with prolapse of the mitral valve, often with regurgitation.[279] Strong support for this formulation came from cineangiography and intracardiac phonocardiography and echocardiography.[274]

The many causes of or conditions associated with prolapse of mitral valves into the left atrium during ventricular systole are shown in Table 32–8. Prominent among these is myxomatous proliferation of the mitral valve, in which the spongiosa component of the valve, i.e., the middle layer of the leaflet composed of loose, myxomatous material, is unusually prominent[280,280a] and the quantity of acid mucopolysaccharide is increased secondary to a fundamental but as yet undefined abnormality of collagen metabolism.[281] The concordance between inadequate production of type III collagen with echocardiographic findings of MVP in patients with type IV Ehlers-Danlos syndrome suggests that this abnormality of collagen is responsible.[282] Mucopolysaccharide infiltration and fragmentation of valvular collagen are common findings.[283] A reduction of type III and AB collagen has also been found in a patient with MVP without the Ehlers-Danlos syndrome.[284]

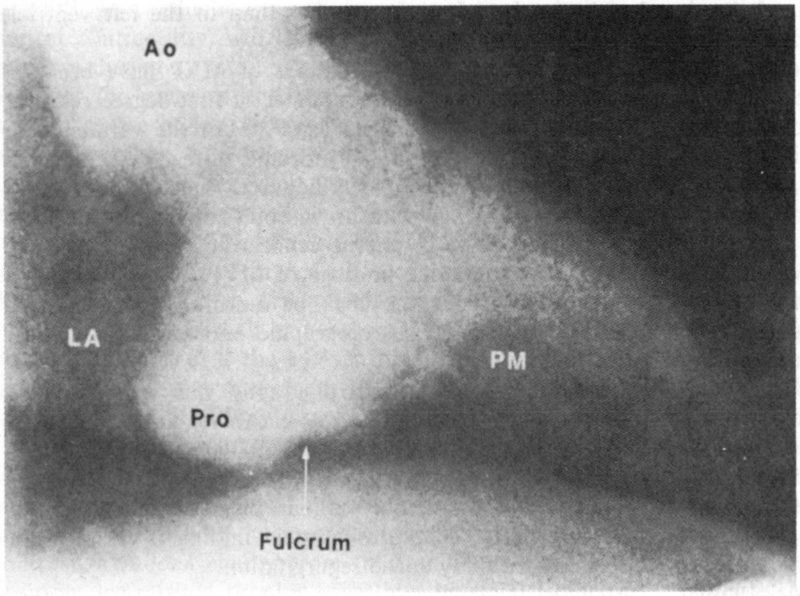

FIGURE 32–18 Systolic frame of left ventricular angiogram demonstrating prolapse (Pro) of the mitral valve. The posteromedial commissural scallop of the posterior mitral leaflet extends posteriorly and inferiorly to the fulcrum. PM = papillary muscle. (From Cohen, M. V., et al.: Angiographic-echocardiographic correlation in mitral valve prolapse. Am. Heart J. *97*:46, 1979.)

and little or no mitral regurgitation have normal left ventricular hemodynamics. An increased rate of circumferential fiber shortening may be observed in the presence of significant mitral regurgitation, as in patients with regurgitation of other etiologies.[357] Ejection fraction at rest determined by radionuclide angiography is normal in patients having MVP without associated mitral regurgitation. However, a subgroup of these patients do not exhibit a normal increase in ejection fraction during exercise, suggesting that a cardiomyopathic process may be responsible for the reduced cardiac reserve.[358]

Natural History

The outlook for MVP in children is excellent, a large majority remaining asymptomatic for many years without any change in clinical or laboratory manifestations.[359,360]

Progressive mitral regurgitation occurs in about 15 per cent of patients over a 10- to 15-year period; the incidence of this complication is significantly greater in patients with both murmurs and clicks than in those with an isolated click.[360] In many patients, rupture of chordae tendineae or infective endocarditis is responsible for the intensification of the mitral regurgitation.[273] When mitral regurgitation is severe, valve replacement may be required; indeed MVP is an important cause of pure mitral regurgitation in patients requiring mitral valve replacement.[313] Patients with the MVP syndrome are also at risk of developing infective endocarditis,[273,361,362] although the incidence appears to be extremely low in patients with only a midsystolic click. When encountered in the elderly, MVP is often a cause of heart failure.[363]

Acute hemiplegia, transient ischemic attacks, cerebellar infarcts, amaurosis fugax, and retinal arteriolar occlusions all appear to occur more frequently in patients with the MVP syndrome, suggesting that cerebral emboli are unusually common in this condition.[364–368] These neurological complications are often associated with shortened platelet survival[367] and platelet coagulant hyperactivity.[365] Loss of endothelial continuity and tearing of the endocardium overlying the myxomatous valve may initiate platelet aggregation and the formation of mural platelet-fibrin complexes.[368a] The paroxysmal arrhythmias that occur in the MVP syndrome may contribute to the likelihood of embolization. Indeed, it is possible that cerebral embolization secondary to MVP may be a significant cause for unexplained strokes and other cerebral and retinal complications in young people with undetected cerebrovascular disease.[364,365] Similarly, myocardial infarction in patients with MVP and normal coronary arteries may be secondary to embolization.[368b]

Treatment

Asymptomatic patients (or those whose principal complaint is anxiety) with no arrhythmias evident on a routine extended electrocardiographic tracing and on prolonged auscultation, with normal ST segments and without evidence of serious mitral regurgitation should be reassured about the favorable prognosis but should have follow-up examinations every 2 or 3 years. Patients with a long systolic murmur may show progression of mitral regurgitation and should be examined more frequently, at intervals of approximately 12 months. Since infective endocarditis is a well-recognized complication of MVP,[273] *endocarditis prophylaxis* is advisable in patients with a typical systolic murmur and characteristic echocardiographic features. Although opinions on this point are not unanimous, prophylaxis is probably also advisable in patients with a midsystolic click without a systolic murmur, since bacterial endocarditis has been reported in such patients and it is well established that the systolic murmur may be intermittent or provoked.[273]

Patients with a history of palpitations, lightheadedness, dizziness, or syncope or those who have arrhythmias on clinical examination or on a routine electrocardiogram should undergo ambulatory (24-hour) electrocardiographic monitoring or treadmill exercise testing or both. Propranolol is the drug of choice for many ventricular arrhythmias, and either propranolol or phenytoin is useful in patients with prolongation of the Q-T interval. Aprindine (a drug not yet released for general use in the United States at this time) has resulted in a striking reduction in the number of premature ventricular extrasystoles and in the frequency and duration of ventricular tachycardia in patients with the MVP syndrome[369] and may be considered in patients who do not respond to other antiarrhythmic drugs. Stellate ganglion blockade followed by thoracic sympathectomy and even mitral valve replacement have been proposed for the treatment of refractory ventricular tachycardia; however, the results are insufficient to evaluate the effectiveness of these modes of therapy.

Beta-adrenergic blockade may be useful in the treatment of chest discomfort, both in patients with associated coronary artery disease and in those with normal coronary vessels in whom the symptoms may be due to regional ischemia secondary to MVP.[370] Nitrates should be used with caution, since the reduction of cardiac size induced by these drugs may intensify the prolapse and the resultant ischemia of the base of the papillary muscles.

Patients with symptoms of reduced functional cardiac reserve should be treated like other patients with severe mitral regurgitation (p. 1084), and those with severe regurgitation who are not responsive to medical management may require mitral valve replacement.[313] In patients with angina on effort and/or ischemic electrocardiographic changes and abnormalities on a thallium perfusion scan during exercise, coronary arteriography should be performed, and treatment should take into account the responsiveness of symptoms to medical management and the coronary anatomy, as outlined in Chapter 39. In patients with MVP who have had any of the aforementioned cerebral events and in whom no other etiology is apparent, anticoagulant therapy and/or drugs that interfere with platelet function, such as aspirin and dipyridamole, should be given.

Although this discussion has focused attention on complications of the MVP syndrome, it should not be forgotten that, on the whole, this is a benign condition and that the vast majority of patients with this syndrome remain asymptomatic for their entire lives and require, at most, observation every few years and reassurance.

AORTIC STENOSIS

ETIOLOGY AND PATHOLOGY

Obstruction to left ventricular outflow is localized most commonly at the aortic valve, discussed in this section. However, obstruction may also occur above the valve (supravalvular stenosis [p. 981]) or below the valve (discrete subvalvular aortic stenosis [p. 980]) or may be caused by hypertrophic obstructive cardiomyopathy (p. 1409). In an analysis of the hearts of 543 patients with valvular disease, Roberts found isolated aortic stenosis to be the most common lesion.[371] Valvular aortic stenosis without accompanying mitral valve disease is more common in men and very rarely occurs on a rheumatic basis but instead is usually either congenital or degenerative in origin[371–374] (Figs. 32–19 and 32–20).

CONGENITAL AORTIC STENOSIS (See also p.1026). Congenital malformations of the aortic valve may be unicuspid, bicuspid, or tricuspid or may be a dome-shaped diaphragm (Fig. 32–20).[128] *Unicuspid valves* produce severe obstruction in infancy[375] and are the most frequent malformations found in fatal valvular aortic stenosis in children under the age of 1 year.[376] Congenitally *bicuspid valves* may be stenotic with commissural fusion at birth, but more commonly they are not responsible for serious narrowing of the aortic orifice during childhood;[377–379] their abnormal architecture induces turbulent flow, which traumatizes the leaflets and ultimately leads to fibrosis, increased rigidity, and calcification of the leaflets and narrowing of the aortic orifice[380] (Fig. 32–21). Infective endocarditis may develop on a congenitally bicuspid valve, which then becomes regurgitant. Rarely, a congenitally bicuspid valve is purely regurgitant in the absence of antecedent infection. It should be emphasized that in a majority of cases, a bicuspid valve is not stenotic at birth and that the changes causing stenosis resemble those occurring in senile, degenerative calcific stenosis of a tricuspid aortic valve except that in the congenitally bicuspid valve these changes occur several decades earlier.

A third form of a congenitally malformed valve is *tricuspid*, with the cusps of unequal size and some commissural fusion. Although many of these valves retain normal func-

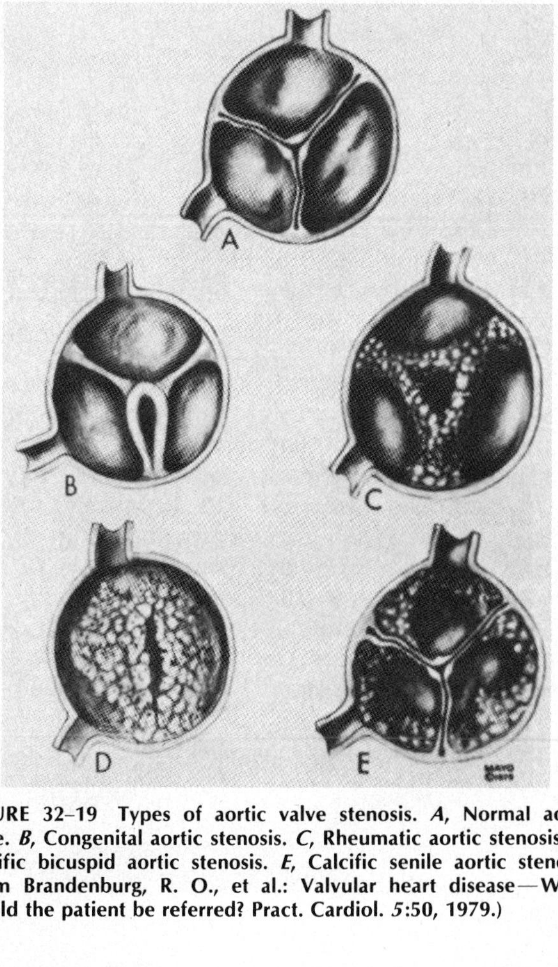

FIGURE 32–19 Types of aortic valve stenosis. *A*, Normal aortic valve. *B*, Congenital aortic stenosis. *C*, Rheumatic aortic stenosis. *D*, Calcific bicuspid aortic stenosis. *E*, Calcific senile aortic stenosis. (From Brandenburg, R. O., et al.: Valvular heart disease—When should the patient be referred? Pract. Cardiol. *5*:50, 1979.)

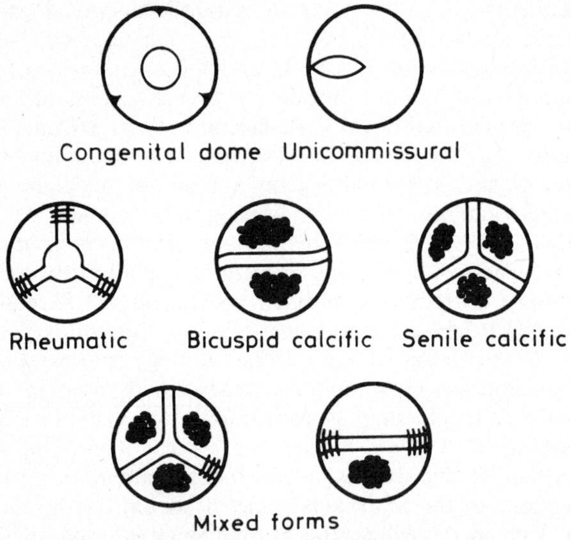

FIGURE 32–20 Schematic representation of the types of aortic valve stenosis, viewed from above. (Reproduced with permission from Davies, M. J.: Pathology of Cardiac Valves. London, Butterworths, 1980.)

tion throughout life, it has been postulated that the turbulent flow produced by the mild congenital architectural abnormality may lead to fibrosis and ultimately to calcification and stenosis.[371] Tricuspid stenotic aortic valves in adults may be congenital, rheumatic, or degenerative in origin.

ACQUIRED AORTIC STENOSIS. *Rheumatic aortic stenosis* results from adhesions and fusion of the commissures and cusps and vascularization of the leaflets and the valve ring, leading to retraction and stiffening of the free borders of the cusps, with calcific nodules present on both surfaces and an orifice that is reduced to a small round or triangular opening. As a consequence, the rheumatic valve is often regurgitant as well as stenotic (Figs. 32–20, 32–21, and 32–22 and 48–5, p. 1647). The heart frequently exhibits other stigmata of rheumatic heart disease, especially mitral valve involvement. In *degenerative (senile) calcific aortic stenosis,* the cusps are immobilized by a deposit of calcium along their flexion lines at their bases. This common cause of aortic stenosis in adults appears to result from years of normal mechanical stress on the valve. Although degenerative calcification may extend in the direc-

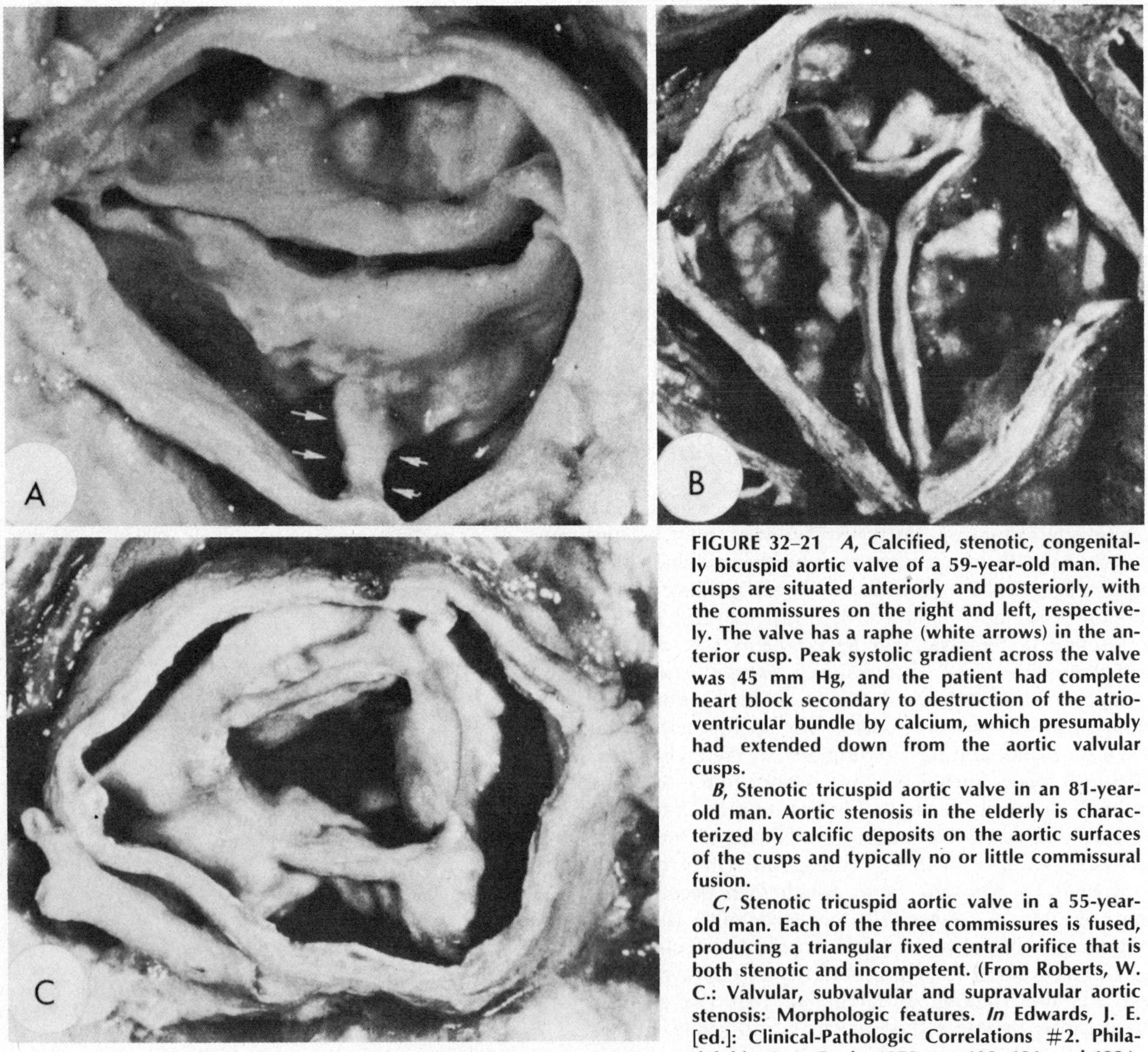

FIGURE 32–21 *A,* Calcified, stenotic, congenitally bicuspid aortic valve of a 59-year-old man. The cusps are situated anteriorly and posteriorly, with the commissures on the right and left, respectively. The valve has a raphe (white arrows) in the anterior cusp. Peak systolic gradient across the valve was 45 mm Hg, and the patient had complete heart block secondary to destruction of the atrioventricular bundle by calcium, which presumably had extended down from the aortic valvular cusps.

B, Stenotic tricuspid aortic valve in an 81-year-old man. Aortic stenosis in the elderly is characterized by calcific deposits on the aortic surfaces of the cusps and typically no or little commissural fusion.

C, Stenotic tricuspid aortic valve in a 55-year-old man. Each of the three commissures is fused, producing a triangular fixed central orifice that is both stenotic and incompetent. (From Roberts, W. C.: Valvular, subvalvular and supravalvular aortic stenosis: Morphologic features. *In* Edwards, J. E. [ed.]: Clinical-Pathologic Correlations #2. Philadelphia, F. A. Davis, 1973, pp. 100, 106, and 108.)

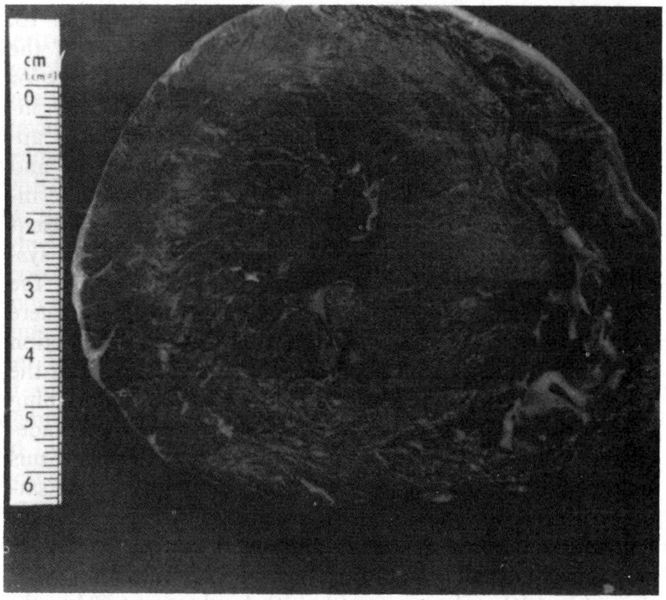

FIGURE 32–22 Heart from a man aged 62 years, who died suddenly with aortic valve stenosis (bicuspid calcific). The total heart weight was 610 gm. The left ventricular cavity is small, and the wall thickness is 3 cm. (Reproduced with permission from Davies, M. J.: Pathology of Cardiac Valves. London, Butterworths, 1980.)

tion of the cusps, no commissural fusion is present.[128] Degenerative "wear and tear" appears to be the most likely cause of this form of aortic stenosis, which is commonly accompanied by calcifications of the mitral annulus and coronary arteries but rarely by aortic regurgitation. The stenosis is produced by the calcific deposits that prevent the cusps from opening normally during systole (Fig. 32–21). In *atherosclerotic aortic valvular stenosis*, severe atherosclerosis involves the aorta and other major arteries; this form of aortic stenosis occurs most frequently in patients with severe hypercholesterolemia[381] and is observed in children with homozygous Type II hyperlipoproteinemia (p. 1630). *Rheumatoid involvement* of the valve is a rare cause of aortic stenosis and results in nodular thickening of the valve leaflets and involvement of the proximal part of the aorta (p. 1658). *Ochronosis* is another rare cause of aortic stenosis.[382]

Roberts studied hearts with aortic stenosis in patients between 15 and 65 years of age and found that almost 40 per cent were tricuspid. Since there was thickening of the mitral valve and a history of acute rheumatic fever in half of these cases, it is likely that the aortic stenosis was rheumatic in etiology; in the remainder it was either congenital or degenerative in origin. In 90 per cent of hearts examined at autopsy in patients with aortic stenosis who were older than 65 years, the valves were tricuspid, with nodular calcific deposits on the aortic aspects of the cusps, but without commissural fusion.[371]

Hemodynamically significant aortic stenosis leads to severe concentric left ventricular hypertrophy,[383] with heart weights as great as 1000 gm (Fig. 32–22). The interventricular septum often bulges into and encroaches on the right ventricular cavity. When left ventricular failure supervenes, the left ventricle dilates,[383] the left atrium enlarges, and changes secondary to backward failure occur in the pulmonary vascular bed, right side of the heart, and systemic venous bed.

Pathophysiology

The left ventricle responds to the sudden production of severe obstruction to outflow by dilatation and reduction of stroke volume. However, in adults with aortic stenosis, the obstruction usually develops and increases gradually over a prolonged period. In infants and children with congenital aortic stenosis, the valve orifice shows little change as the child grows, thereby intensifying obstruction quite gradually. Left ventricular function can be well maintained in experimentally produced, chronic, gradually developing subcoronary aortic stenosis.[384] Left ventricular output is maintained by the presence of left ventricular hypertrophy, which may sustain a large pressure gradient across the aortic valve for many years without a reduction in cardiac output, left ventricular dilatation, or the development of symptoms (Figs. 32–23 and 9–7, p. 288). A peak systolic pressure gradient exceeding 50 mm Hg in the presence of a normal cardiac output or an effective aortic orifice less than about 0.4 cm^2/m^2 of body surface area, i.e., less than approximately one-fourth of the normal orifice, is generally considered to represent critical obstruction to left ventricular outflow (Fig. 32–24).[385]

As contraction of the left ventricle becomes progressively more isometric, the left ventricular pressure pulse exhibits a rounded, rather than flattened, summit. The elevated left ventricular end-diastolic pressure, which is characteristic of severe aortic stenosis, does not necessarily signify the presence of left ventricular dilatation or failure but often reflects diminished compliance of the hypertrophied left ventricular wall; usually it results from both processes.

In patients with severe aortic stenosis, large *a* waves usually appear in the left atrial pressure pulse because of the combination of enhanced contraction of a hypertrophied left atrium and diminished left ventricular compliance. Atrial contraction plays a particularly important role in filling of the left ventricle in aortic stenosis.[23] It raises left ventricular end-diastolic pressure without producing a concomitant elevation of mean left atrial pressure.[386] This "booster pump" function of the left atrium prevents the pulmonary venous and capillary pressures from rising to levels that would produce pulmonary congestion, while at the same time maintaining left ventricular end-diastolic pressure at the elevated level necessary for effective left

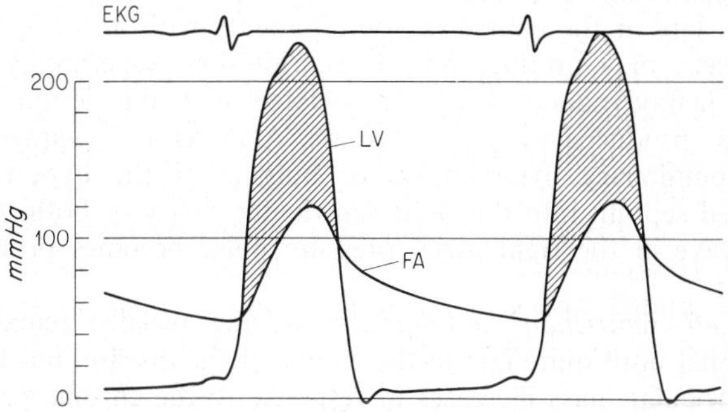

FIGURE 32–23 Pressure tracings from a 77-year-old man with a history of recent syncopal attacks. A mean pressure gradient of 90 mm Hg (cross-hatched area) between left ventricular (LV) pressure and arterial pressure measured at the right femoral artery (FA) is demonstrated. In addition, the arterial pressure curve has a markedly delayed upstroke with a reduced rate of rise. The calculated aortic valve area was narrowed to 0.5 cm^2.

TABLE 32–9 CONDITIONS FREQUENTLY CONFUSED WITH AORTIC STENOSIS

CONDITION	DISTINGUISHING FEATURES
Dilated aorta (hypertension, syphilis) with systolic murmur in second right intercostal space	No single or paradoxical S_2; A_2 normal or loud; murmur often short
Bruit arising in carotid or subclavian arteries (benign supraclavicular bruit, arterial occlusive disease)	Bruit louder in neck or supraclavicular fossae and may be obliterated by subclavian artery compression; bruit may be shorter; normal S_2
Pulmonic valvular stenosis	Murmur reaches A_2; more frequent systolic ejection click; P_2 faint and delayed; A_2 normal; right ventricular enlargement; occasional large jugular *a* wave
Severe aortic regurgitation	Widened pulse pressure; visible carotid pulse; A_2 may be normal
Minimal valvulitis or calcification	Normal A_2; normal respiratory motion of S_2; no left ventricular enlargement
Mitral regurgitation	Pansystolic or ejection murmur; normal respiratory variation of S_2; normal A_2; S_1 may be faint; S_3 gallop common if severe; aortic stenosis murmur often of grunting quality at cardiac apex; murmur usually well heard in left axilla, decreased by amyl nitrite inhalation (which increases murmur of aortic stenosis) and increased by administration of phenylephrine; no aortic valve calcification on fluoroscopy

From Fowler, N. O.: Aortic stenosis: Left ventricular outflow tract obstruction. *In* Fowler, N. O. (ed.): Cardiac Diagnosis and Treatment. 3rd ed. Hagerstown, Md., Harper and Row, 1980, p. 550.

either side of the sternum or in the suprasternal notch and is frequently transmitted along the carotid arteries.

Rarely, evidence of right ventricular failure with systemic venous congestion, hepatomegaly, and edema precedes left ventricular failure, probably owing to the so-called Bernheim effect, which results from the hypertrophied ventricular septum bulging into and encroaching on the right ventricular cavity and leads to impairment of right ventricular filling. In such cases, the jugular venous pressure is elevated and the *a* wave is prominent.

AUSCULTATION (Table 32–5). S_1 is normal or soft and S_4 is prominent, presumably because atrial contraction is vigorous and the mitral valve is partially closed during presystole.[414,415] S_2 may be single because calcification and immobility of the aortic valve make A_2 inaudible, because P_2 is buried in the prolonged aortic ejection murmur, or because prolongation of left ventricular systole makes A_2 coincide with P_2. Paradoxical splitting of S_2, which suggests associated left ventricular dysfunction, may also occur. With left ventricular failure and secondary pulmonary hypertension, P_2 may become accentuated. When the valve is rigid, A_2 may be inaudible, but when the valve is flexible, A_2 may be snapping and accentuated (Figure 3–22, p. 56).

An *aortic ejection sound* occurs simultaneously with the halting upward movement of the aortic valve. It is dependent on mobility of the valve cusps[416] and disappears when they become severely calcified. Thus, it is common in children with congenital aortic stenosis but rare in elderly adults with acquired calcific aortic stenosis and rigid valves. This sound occurs approximately 0.06 sec after the onset of S_1, has a frequency similar to S_1, and is heard most readily with the diaphragm of the stethoscope along the left sternal border, although it is often well transmitted to the apex, where it may be confused with S_1 (and the S_1 may be mistaken for an S_4). In contrast to a pulmonic ejection sound, aortic ejection sounds usually do not vary with respiration and usually occur later.

TABLE 32–10 COMPARISONS OF VALVULAR AORTIC STENOSIS, HYPERTROPHIC OBSTRUCTIVE CARDIOMYOPATHY, AND DISCRETE (CONGENITAL) SUBAORTIC STENOSIS

FEATURES	HYPERTROPHIC OBSTRUCTIVE CARDIOMYOPATHY	VALVULAR AORTIC STENOSIS	DISCRETE SUBAORTIC STENOSIS
Family history	Or familial	Extremely uncommon	Extremely uncommon
Symptoms	Dyspnea, angina, syncope	Dyspnea, angina, syncope	Dyspnea, angina, syncope
Arterial pulse	Quick upstroke, jerky; prominent tidal wave	Anacrotic	Normal or anacrotic
Cardiac impulse	Double thrust	Left ventricular	Left ventricular
Systolic ejection murmur	Maximal internal to apex beat; late onset	Maximal at aortic area (or apex)	Maximal at aortic area and apex; early onset
Reversed split of second heart sound	Rare	Common	Occasional
Systolic click	Occasional	Frequent unless calcified	Rare
Aortic valve closure	Audible	Audible unless heavily calcified	Inaudible
Aortic diastolic murmur	Rare	Not uncommon	Frequent
Mitral systolic murmur	Very common	Occasional	Common
Mitral diastolic murmur	Not uncommon	Not uncommon	Rare
Prominent *a* wave in jugular venous pulse	May be striking	Unimpressive unless pulmonary hypertension	Unimpressive
Atrial sound	Very common	Common	Common
Aortic valve calcification	Never seen	Very common after age 40	Absent
Left heart catheterization	Gradient across left ventricular outflow tract may be extremely variable or absent	Gradient constant across aortic valve	Subvalvular gradient
Dilatation of ascending aorta	Absent	Common	Common

From Cleland, W., et al.: Medical and Surgical Cardiology. Oxford, Blackwell Scientific Publications, 1969, p. 967.

The *midsystolic murmur* of aortic stenosis is heard best at the base of the heart but is often well transmitted along the carotid vessels and to the apex. Cessation of the murmur before A_2 is usually helpful in differentiating it from a pansystolic mitral murmur, but it may be falsely considered to be a pansystolic murmur because it may end with S_2, which represents pulmonic valve closure, A_2 being soft or even inaudible (Figures 3–22, p. 56, 4–1, p. 69, and 4–7, p. 72). In patients with calcified aortic valves, the murmur is harsh and rasping at the base, but high-frequency components selectively radiate to the apex (the so-called Gallavardin phenomenon), where it may actually be more prominent and where it may be mistaken for the murmur of mitral regurgitation. Frequently, there is a "quiet area" between the base and apex where the murmur is diminished in intensity, supporting the erroneous impression that the apical and basal murmurs have different origins. In general, the more severe the stenosis, the longer the duration of the murmur and the later in systole its peak intensity.[417]

In patients with degenerative or atherosclerotic aortic stenosis, there may be heavy valvular calcification, but obstruction may not be severe because the commissural fusion characteristic of congenital and rheumatic aortic stenosis is absent. The nonfused calcified cusps vibrate freely, resulting in a softer, more musical murmur, more prominent at the apex than the murmur of congenital or rheumatic aortic stenosis.[417] High-pitched decrescendo diastolic murmurs secondary to aortic regurgitation are common in many patients with dominant aortic stenosis.

Dynamic Auscultation (Table 32–6). The murmur of valvular aortic stenosis is augmented by the inhalation of amyl nitrite or with squatting or lying flat and is reduced in intensity during the Valsalva strain (which increases the murmur of hypertrophic obstructive cardiomyopathy or with vasopressors, moderate isometric exercise, or standing.[418] It varies in intensity from beat to beat when the duration of diastolic filling varies, as in atrial fibrillation or following a premature contraction, and this characteristic is helpful in differentiating aortic stenosis from mitral regurgitation, in which the murmur is usually unaffected (Figure 4–8, p. 70). An aortic diastolic murmur is frequently present in patients with valvular aortic stenosis. In hypertrophic obstructive cardiomyopathy, the murmur is delayed in onset and may continue up to A_2; the carotid artery characteristically rises sharply (Table 32–9) and is bisferiens. Palpation of the carotid pulse is also extremely helpful in differentiating between valvular aortic stenosis, on the one hand, and hypertrophic obstructive cardiomyopathy and mitral regurgitation, on the other, since the arterial pulse generally rises slowly in aortic stenosis but sharply in the other two conditions. However, confusion can arise in the young patient with congenital aortic stenosis, in whom sudden upward displacement ("doming") of the pliant aortic leaflet or leaflets with ventricular systole may result in a brisk initial upstroke in the carotid pulse, coincident with the systolic ejection click.

When the left ventricle fails in aortic stenosis and the cardiac output falls, the murmur becomes softer or disappears altogether, and the slowly rising pulse is more difficult to appreciate. Stated simply, the clinical picture changes to that of severe left ventricular failure with a low cardiac output and pulmonary edema. Thus, occult aortic stenosis may be a cause of intractable heart failure, and critical aortic stenosis should be actively sought in patients with severe heart failure of unknown cause, since operative treatment may be life-saving and may result in substantial clinical improvement.[419]

LABORATORY EXAMINATION

ELECTROCARDIOGRAM. The principal electrocardiographic change is left ventricular hypertrophy, which is found in approximately 85 per cent of patients with severe aortic stenosis[70] (Figure 7–14*A*, p. 210). The absence of left ventricular hypertrophy does not exclude the presence of critical aortic stenosis, and the relationship between the absolute voltages in precordial leads and the severity of obstruction, which is quite good in children with congenital aortic stenosis, is not as good in adults. T-wave inversion and ST-segment depressions in leads having upright QRS complexes are common. ST-segment depressions greater than 0.3 mv in patients with aortic stenosis suggest that severe ventricular hypertrophy is present. The progressive development of ST-segment and T-wave abnormalities suggests that hypertrophy has progressed. Occasionally, a "pseudoinfarction" pattern is present, characterized by a loss of r waves in the right precordial leads and an early vector directed posteriorly in the horizontal plane of the vectorcardiogram, simulating anteroseptal infarction.[420] A good correlation has been reported between the sum of the QRS amplitude in 12 leads and the height of the left ventricular systolic pressure.[421] There is evidence of left atrial enlargement in more than 80 per cent of patients with severe isolated aortic stenosis;[422] the principal manifestation is prominent late negativity of the P wave in V_1 rather than an increased duration in lead II, suggesting that hypertrophy rather than dilatation is present. Atrial fibrillation is an uncommon and late sign of pure aortic stenosis[423] and, when present in a patient who is not greatly disabled, should suggest the possibility of mitral valvular disease or ischemic heart disease.

The extension of calcific infiltrates from the aortic valve into the conduction system may cause various forms and degrees of atrioventricular and intraventricular block in 5 per cent of patients with calcific aortic stenosis;[424,425] almost 10 per cent of all instances of left anterior hemiblock are secondary to aortic valvular disease.[426]

Vectorcardiogram. In patients with severe aortic stenosis, the vectorcardiogram usually shows an increase in the maximal spatial voltage and counterclockwise inscription of the loop in the transverse plane, with the major forces in the left posterior quadrant. In the left sagittal plane, the QRS loop is usually directed posteriorly and superiorly.[427]

Graphic Recordings. The indirect carotid, jugular, and apical pulse tracings, systolic time intervals, and phonocardiographic findings in aortic stenosis are discussed in Chapters 3 and 4.

RADIOLOGICAL FINDINGS. Routine radiological examination may be entirely normal despite the presence of critical aortic stenosis. The heart is usually of normal size or slightly enlarged, with a rounding of the left ventricular border and apex (Figure 6–27, p. 165), unless regurgitation or left ventricular failure is present and causes substantial cardiomegaly.[428] Poststenotic dilatation of the ascending aorta is a common finding. Calcification of the aortic valve is found in almost all adults with hemodynamically significant aortic stenosis;[428a] it may have to be sought on fluoroscopy (or the echocardiogram) rather than on the roentgenogram. This is an important finding; indeed, the *absence* of calcium in the region of the aortic valve on careful fluoroscopic examination in a patient older than 35 years essentially rules out severe aortic stenosis. The converse is not true, however, and in patients over the age of 60 years, severe calcification of the aortic valve may occur with only mild obstruction. The left atrium may be slightly enlarged, and there may be radiological signs of pulmonary venous hypertension. However, when left atrial enlargement is marked, particularly if the atrial appendage is prominent, the presence of associated mitral valvular disease should be suspected.

Angiographic studies of the aortic valve are best performed by injecting contrast medium into the left ventricle and filming in the 30-degree right anterior oblique and 60-degree left anterior oblique projections. These examinations often make it possible to ascertain the number of cusps of the stenotic valve and to demonstrate doming of a thickened valve and a systolic jet. However, it must be appreciated that there is some hazard of the rapid injection of a large volume of contrast material into a high-pressure left ventricle.

ECHOCARDIOGRAPHY (see also p. 114). The normal range of opening of the aortic valve is 1.6 to 2.6 cm, and normally the aortic valve leaflets are barely visible in systole. In patients with severe aortic stenosis, thickened leaflets and a barely discernible aortic orifice in systole can often be recognized on the M-mode echocardiogram (Figure 5–47, p. 114). However, a reduced aortic valve opening may also be seen in other conditions, such as heart failure, in which there is decreased blood flow across the aortic valve. In patients with a bicuspid aortic valve, the valve cusps are asymmetrical, resulting in their eccentric position within the aortic root.[429] Dense, multiple echoes within the aortic root in the area of the aortic leaflets suggest valvular calcification and support the diagnosis of aortic stenosis. Systolic vibrations of the interventricular septum are common in congenital aortic stenosis.[430] Although M-mode echocardiography can be used to diagnose calcific aortic stenosis, detect marked elevations in left ventricular end-diastolic pressure by prolongation of the A-C interval (Figure 5–35, p. 107), detect dilatation of the aorta, and estimate the severity of left ventricular hypertrophy as well as assess left ventricular function,[431] it cannot establish the severity of obstruction directly; the ratio of left ventricular wall thickness to chamber radius at end diastole, however, correlates well with left ventricular systolic pressure.[432] Two-dimensional echocardiography may also be helpful in determining the severity of the stenosis, although the accuracy of this technique is limited in patients with an intermediate degree of obstruction (Figure 5–48, p. 115).[433–435]

MANAGEMENT

Medical Treatment

Patients with aortic stenosis should be apprised of the hazards of endocarditis, and the necessity for endocarditis prophylaxis should be explained (p. 1175). Patients who are asymptomatic should be advised to report the development of any symptoms to their physician. Those with known or suspected critical obstruction should be cautioned to avoid vigorous athletic and physical activity. However, such restrictions do not apply to patients with mild obstruction. It is important to recognize that with the passage of time there is a tendency for the obstruction to become progressively more severe in patients with aortic stenosis.[436] Thus, in children and young adults, mild aortic stenosis often progresses to severe obstruction in adulthood, and in adults, moderate stenosis may progress to severe obstruction in later life. Therefore, asymptomatic patients with aortic stenosis should be followed carefully; in doing so, it is essential to look for signs of possible progression.[437] Repeated clinical examinations and electrocardiographic and echocardiographic studies at intervals of 6 to 12 months are indicated in asymptomatic patients with significant aortic stenosis.

There is no need to use digitalis glycosides unless there is evidence of an increase in ventricular volume or a reduced ejection fraction on angiographic, echocardiographic, or radionuclide examination. Although diuretics are beneficial when there is abnormal accumulation of fluid, they must be used with caution, since hypovolemia may reduce the elevated left ventricular end-diastolic pressure, lower cardiac output, and produce orthostatic hypotension. Beta-adrenergic blockers can depress myocardial function and induce left ventricular failure and should be used only with great caution, if at all, in patients with aortic stenosis.

Atrial arrhythmias occur in less than 10 per cent of patients with severe aortic stenosis, perhaps because of the late occurrence of left atrial enlargement in this condition. When such an arrhythmia is observed in a patient with aortic stenosis, the possibility of associated mitral valve disease should be considered. In light of the adverse hemodynamic effects of loss of atrial booster pump function with atrial fibrillation in patients with aortic stenosis,[386] an effort should be made to prevent the development of this arrhythmia by means of pharmacological prophylaxis when premature atrial contractions are frequent. When atrial fibrillation does occur, the rapid ventricular rate may cause angina or electrocardiographic evidence of myocardial ischemia or both; in some cases, loss of the atrial "kick" and a sudden fall in cardiac output may cause serious hypotension. Therefore, this arrhythmia should be treated promptly (p. 700), and a search for previously unrecognized mitral valve disease should be undertaken.

Cardiac catheterization should be carried out in children in whom clinical examination and noninvasive tests suggest critical obstruction, regardless of whether or not symptoms are present. Adults considered to have severe aortic stenosis should have catheterization if any symptoms develop. The purpose of catheterization in patients with aortic stenosis is to localize the site and document the severity of the obstruction, to determine the state of left ventricular function, to ascertain the presence or absence of associated valvular disease, and, in patients with angina pectoris, to determine the status of the coronary circulation.[393]

Natural History

In contrast to mitral stenosis, which leads to symptoms almost immediately after its development, patients with severe aortic stenosis may be asymptomatic for many years despite the presence of severe obstruction. The systolic pressure gradient can exceed 150 mm Hg, and the peak left ventricular systolic pressure can reach approximately 300 mm Hg with relatively little increase in overall heart size on radiographic examination, with normal left ventricular end-diastolic and end-systolic volumes. Patients with severe chronic aortic stenosis tend to be free of cardiovascular symptoms until relatively late in the course of the disease. In Rapaport's series, 40 per cent of patients treated medically survived for 5 years and 20 per cent for 10 years after diagnosis.[98] In another series of patients with hemodynamically significant valvular aortic stenosis treated medically, the 5-year survival rate was 64 per cent. However, once patients with aortic stenosis become symptomatic with angina or syncope, the average survival is 2 to 3 years, whereas with congestive heart failure it is 1½ years[401] (Fig. 32–25). Sudden death, like syncope, in patients with severe aortic stenosis may be due to cerebral hypoperfusion followed by arrhythmia.[438,439] Among symptomatic patients with moderate or severe aortic stenosis not subjected to operation, mortality rates from onset of symptoms was approximately 25 per cent at 1 year and 50 per cent at 2 years; more than half of the deaths were sudden. Asymptomatic patients have an excellent prognosis without mortality.[440] The obstruction tends to progress more rapidly in patients with degenerative calcific disease than in those with congenital or rheumatic disease.[441]

Surgical Treatment

INDICATIONS FOR OPERATION. The most critical decision in the management of patients with aortic stenosis—indeed, of all patients with valvular heart disease—concerns the advisability and timing of surgical treatment. The indications for as well as the techniques and results of operation depend on the patient's age and the nature of the valvular deformity. In children and adolescents with noncalcific congenital aortic stenosis, who most commonly have bicuspid aortic valves, simple commissural incision under direct vision usually leads to substantial hemodynamic improvement at a low risk, i.e., a mortality rate of less than 2 per cent (p. 980).[442] Therefore, this procedure is indicated not only in symptomatic patients but also in asymptomatic children and adolescents with critical aortic stenosis, i.e., a calculated effective orifice less than 0.4 cm^2/m^2 BSA. Despite the salutary hemodynamic results following this procedure, the valve is not rendered entirely normal anatomically, and the turbulent flow around it may lead to further deformation, calcification, the development of regurgitation, and re-stenosis after 10 to 20 years, probably requiring reoperation and valve replacement at some later date.

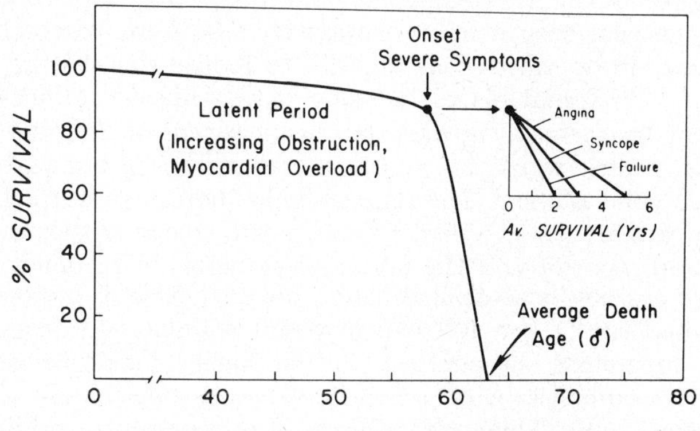

FIGURE 32–25 Natural history of aortic stenosis without operative treatment. (From Ross, J., Jr., and Braunwald, E.: Aortic stenosis. Circulation *38*(Suppl. 5):61, 1968, by permission of the American Heart Association, Inc.)

In most adults with calcific aortic stenosis, satisfactory valvular function *cannot* be restored, even by deliberate sculpturing procedures carried out under direct vision, and valve replacement will ultimately be necessary.[443] Replacement of the aortic valve should be carried out in patients with hemodynamic evidence of severe obstruction (aortic valve orifice < 0.75 cm^2 or < 0.4 cm^2/m^2 BSA) and symptoms believed to result from aortic stenosis as well as in asymptomatic patients with serious left ventricular dysfunction and progressive cardiomegaly. Although a prospective randomized controlled study has not been carried out, the long-term mortality in patients undergoing operation in the latter group appears to be lower than that in medically treated patients without operation.[444] As artificial valves and surgical skills continue to improve, it is likely that patients with severe aortic stenosis will become candidates for operation at earlier stages in the natural history of their disease. At the present time, the author does not recommend prophylactic replacement of a critically narrowed aortic valve in asymptomatic patients without evidence of progressive left ventricular dysfunction.

RESULTS. Successful replacement of the aortic valve has resulted in substantial clinical and hemodynamic improvement in patients with aortic stenosis, aortic regurgitation, or combined lesions.[445–453] In patients without frank left ventricular failure, the operative risk ranges from 5 to 10 per cent in most centers. Symptoms secondary to elevations of left atrial pressure and myocardial ischemia are relieved in virtually all patients. Hemodynamic results are equally impressive; elevated end-diastolic and end-systolic volumes show significant reductions. Ventricular performance returns to normal[454] more frequently in patients with aortic stenosis than in those with aortic regurgitation.[455] The increased left ventricular mass is reduced toward (but not quite to) normal within 18 months following aortic valve replacement in patients with aortic stenosis, regurgitation, or mixed lesions.[395,456]

When operation is carried out in patients with frank left ventricular failure or a depressed ejection fraction, the operative risk is higher, and the mortality ranges from 10 to 25 per cent, depending on the skill of the surgical team and the severity of depression of left ventricular function.[457] A depressed relation between ejection fraction and wall stress is a poor prognostic index (Figure 13–9, p. 453), as is a depressed level of dP/dt max at any given left ventricular end-diastolic pressure.[447] Furthermore, a number of factors are now recognized to exert an adverse effect on *long-term* survival; these include a history of acute myocardial infarction, heart failure, advanced functional disability, radiographic evidence of cardiac enlargement, elevations of left atrial and pulmonary artery pressures, and a depressed cardiac output,[444] as well as age and the presence of ventricular arrhythmias.[433] Obviously, it is desirable to perform surgery before these events occur, but even in the most desperate situations, such as cardiac arrest or pulmonary edema from aortic stenosis, emergency operation may be life-saving.[458] Certainly, in view of the extremely poor prognosis of such patients when they are treated medically, there is usually little choice but to advise immediate surgical treatment.[459] Many symptomatic patients with calcific aortic stenosis are elderly, and particular attention must be directed to the adequacy of their hepatic, renal, and pulmonary function. However, the results of aortic valve replacement are satisfactory in patients more than 70 years of age, and if the patient's general condition permits, age, per se, should not be considered a contraindication to operation.[460] In patients with aortic stenosis and obstructive coronary artery disease, aortic valve replacement and myocardial revascularization should be performed together.[461,462] Although the risk of aortic valve surgery is increased by the association of coronary artery disease, the operative mortality in patients undergoing the combined procedure is not necessarily higher than that of isolated aortic valve replacement in this group.[463] The ability to avoid serious myocardial ischemia in the perioperative period is a major factor that has served to reduce operative mortality. After the patient has been placed on cardiopulmonary bypass, the heart is protected by means of hypothermic cardiac arrest alone or combined with cardioplegia. The calcified valve must be removed with great care to avoid embolization of calcified fragments into the systemic circulation.

Characteristics of Artificial Valves

(Fig. 32–16)

The general issues surrounding replacement of the aortic valve are similar to those already discussed in relation to mitral valve replacement (p. 1086), with a number of qualifications: (1) thromboembolic complications are less common following replacement of the aortic than of the mitral valve, which may be related, in part, to the fact that after operation, patients with aortic valvular disease are rarely left with enlarged, fibrillating atria, where clots readily form; (2) the aortic annulus is smaller than the mitral annulus, increasing the likelihood of stenosis of the artificial valve; and (3) the hydraulic stress placed on the aortic valve is greater than that placed on the mitral valve, which *may* lead to a somewhat higher risk of valve dysfunction.

MECHANICAL PROSTHESES. As is the case for prosthetic mitral valves, the Starr-Edwards caged-ball valve is the "benchmark" in aortic valve replacement. Model No. 1260 now has a record of durability extending back to 1965;[464] the addition of a cloth covering has decreased the incidence of thromboembolism[465] but has increased the likelihood of valve dysfunction. Tilting-disk valves (Björk-Shiley and Lillehei-Kaster) in the aortic valve position have resulted in a low incidence of thromboembolism, but just as in the mitral valve position, total thrombosis of these valves has been reported in a few instances.[210,214,466] The overall embolic rate for prosthetic aortic valve replacement in patients treated with anticoagulants ranges from 1 to 5 per 100 patient-years, with fatal emboli occurring in approximately 0.2 per 100 patient-years.[229]

Since the Starr-Edwards caged-ball valve intrudes on the diameter of the ascending aorta, obstruction may be produced not only by the orifice of the prosthetic valve itself but also by encroachment of the valve on the lumen of the aortic annulus. To avoid this obstruction, patching with a prosthetic gusset may be required. The Smeloff-Cutter double-caged valve[467] provides a slightly more effective orifice-to-diameter ratio than that provided by the Starr-Edwards prosthesis. The Björk-Shiley, Lillehei-Kaster, and St. Jude disk valves employ semicentral or central flow rather than the circumferential flow of the ball valves, improve the effective orifice area, and do not obstruct the aorta above the annulus. These valves therefore result in larger effective orifice areas, at any annulus diameter, than do the caged-ball valves. They are preferable to the Starr-Edwards and Smeloff-Cutter valves in patients with unusually small aortic annuli. All these valves, including the Magovern-Cromie sutureless caged-ball valve,[468] have excellent records of durability. Experience with the St. Jude valve suggests that it has a larger effective orifice for any size of aortic orifice, and it may therefore prove to be the prosthetic valve of choice in patients with a small aortic root.[227,451]

TISSUE VALVES. As is the case when they are placed in the mitral position (p. 1088), homografts that are sterilized by a variety of techniques and used to replace the aortic valve initially had a relatively high incidence of breakdown, but this problem has been largely corrected; procurement and preparation still present problems, and with some exceptions[446] their use has been largely abandoned. The glutaraldehyde-treated porcine heterograft has a good record of durability.[211–213,469] However, this valve is slightly stenotic, because of a residual bar of right ventricular muscle on the inferior aspect of the right coronary cusp, which becomes increasingly obstructive as the diameter of the valve is reduced. Indeed, significant transvalvular gradients have been documented in the 21 and 23 mm sizes of the conventional Hancock porcine aortic valve.[470] The heterograft has been modified by replacing the muscular cusp with a nonmuscular cusp from a second porcine aortic valve. This appears to reduce the obstruction[212,449,450,471] and places the ratio of the effective orifice-to-annulus diameter in the same range as that of the prosthetic valves, which are most favorable from a hemodynamic point of view. The Ionescu-Shiley bovine pericardial bioprosthesis has excellent hemodynamic characteristics in the aortic position.[238] The porcine heterograft in the aortic valve position is associated with a low incidence of thromboembolism (1 per 100 patient-years) without anticoagulant treatment, in contrast to the higher incidence of thromboembolism with prosthetic valves despite the use of anticoagulants. Thus, the incidence of thromboembolism in patients not treated with anticoagulants is comparable to the incidence of complications due simply to anticoagulant therapy.

SELECTION OF AN ARTIFICIAL VALVE. In choosing a replacement for the aortic valve, one must relate the patient's specific anatomical factors, age, and clinical features to the durability, thromboembolic potential, and hemodynamic properties of the replacement valve. If durability is the principal concern, as in a relatively young (< 45 years) patient, the Starr-Edwards and Smeloff-Cutter valves have the best records of performance. However, the Björk-Shiley and Lillehei-Kaster valves also appear to be extremely promising in this regard, since they have been in use for 13 years. There is least experience with the St. Jude valve (6 years at this writing) but it, too, looks promising. The porcine heterografts also have a good durability record (more than 11 years at the time of this writing), but as already discussed (p. 1089), reports of valve deterioration are beginning to appear, and there is some concern about their long-term durability, particularly in children and young adults.

Thromboembolic complications are markedly reduced with all tissue valves, and the need for long-term anticoagulation, which presents its own risks, is thereby obviated. Therefore, in patients for whom long-term anticoagulation is contraindicated or difficult or in whom the threat of bleeding is unusually high, a tissue valve is indicated. Since the question of their durability has not been answered, but since anticoagulants present a greater hazard in the elderly, tissue valves may be most appropriate in patients over the age of 65 years. In patients with small aortic annuli, the caged-ball valves are inappropriate. The small-diameter, tilting-disk, and the St. Jude valves result in less obstruction, although the modified Hancock porcine heterograft and the Ionescu-bovine pericardial heterograft may prove to be as effective hemodynamically.

As has already been pointed out (p. 1086), all valve replacements, when functioning in vivo, must be considered to be intrinsically stenotic. This problem may be most serious in patients with aortic stenosis, in whom the annulus into which the prosthesis is inserted is usually smaller than in patients with regurgitation, and the surgeon may be forced to select an artificial valve of relatively small size. As a consequence, aortic valve replacement may not abolish obstruction but merely convert severe to mild or moderate obstruction. When the smaller models of the porcine xenograft or mechanical prosthesis are placed into the aortic position, effective orifice areas of about 1.0 to 1.3 cm^2 are common. In such patients, peak transvalvular gradients as high as 40 mm Hg during exercise have been recorded,[470] and it is possible that the poor late results observed in a minority of patients may be the delayed effects of moderate stenosis of the prosthesis. In patients who do not exhibit clinical improvement postoperatively, it is important to evaluate both prosthetic and left ventricular function. This can be accomplished by means of right- and eft-heart catheterization, left ventricular angiocardiography, and cross-sectional echocardiography. Rarely, reoperation to correct a malfunctioning artificial valve is necessary.

AORTIC REGURGITATION

ETIOLOGY AND PATHOLOGY

Aortic regurgitation may be caused by primary disease of either the aortic valve leaflets or the wall of the aortic root or both (Table 32–11).

VALVULAR DISEASE. *Rheumatic fever* is a common cause of primary disease of the valve leading to regurgitation.[3,472] The cusps become infiltrated with fibrous tissues and retract, a process that prevents cusp apposition during diastole and that usually leads to regurgitation into the left ventricle through a defect in the center of the valve. Often the associated fusion of the commissures may also restrict the opening of the valve, resulting in combined aortic stenosis and regurgitation (Fig. 32–26*B*); some mitral valve involvement is common. Other primary valvular causes of aortic regurgitation include *infective endocarditis* (Chap. 33), in which the infection may destroy the valve or cause a perforation of a leaflet, or the vegetations may interfere with proper coaptation of the cusps. *Trauma* (p. 1564) resulting in a tear of the ascending aorta and loss of commissural support can cause prolapse of an aortic cusp. Although the most common complication of a *bicuspid valve* is stenosis in adult life, the larger of the two cusps of a congenitally *bicuspid valve* may prolapse[473] and cause regurgitation in childhood; more commonly, progressive regurgitation of a congenitally bicuspid valve develops in the third and fourth decades[474,475] (as may the aortic cusps in patients with Marfan's syndrome, Ehlers-Danlos syndrome, cystic medionecrosis of the aorta, myxomatous proliferation of the aortic valve, and related diseases of connective tissue). Less common causes of aortic regurgitation include rupture of a congenitally fenes-

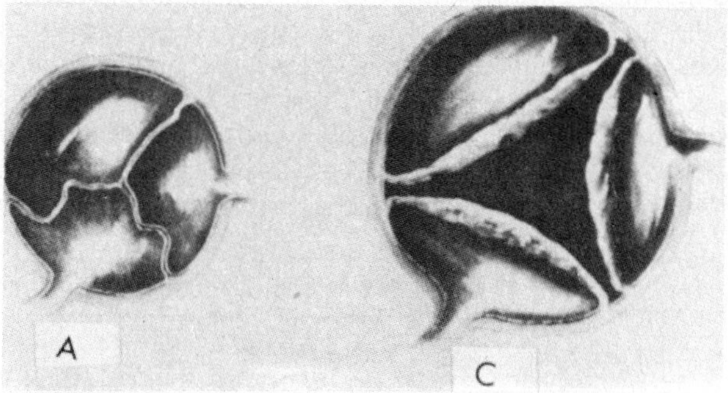

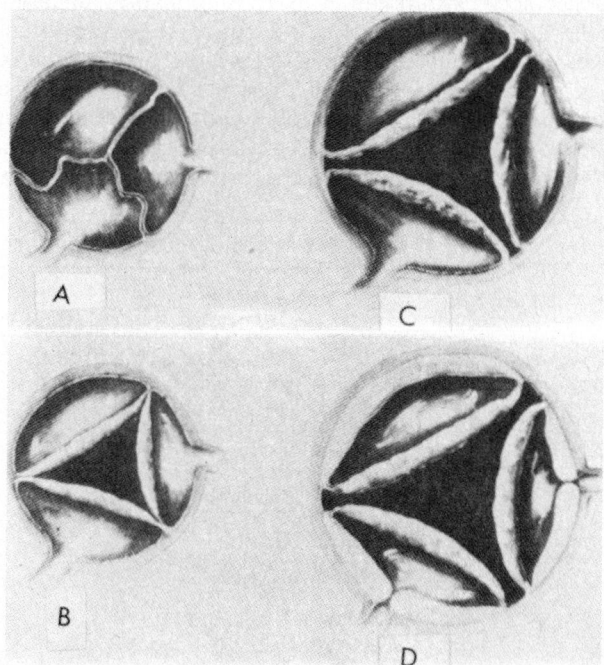

FIGURE 32–26 Variations in the aortic valve. *A*, The normal valve. *B*, Shortening of the cusps characteristic of rheumatic aortic regurgitation. The caliber of the aorta is normal. *C*, Dilatation of the aorta, as occurs in syphilitic aortitis and other conditions in which dilatation is responsible for aortic regurgitation. The main feature results from bowing of the leaflets. Commissural separation is illustrated and may also be present. *D*, In addition to the features shown in *C*, there is atherosclerosis of the aorta, as occurs in syphilitic aortitis, with consequent coronary ostial narrowing. (From Roberts, W. C.: Valvular, subvalvular and supravalvular aortic stenosis: Morphologic features. In Edwards, J. E. [ed.]: Clinical-Pathologic Correlations #2. Philadelphia, F. A. Davis, 1973, p. 133.)

TABLE 32–11 MECHANISMS OF AORTIC REGURGITATION

1. Cusp abnormality	Perforation	Bacterial endocarditis
	Reduction in area	Rheumatic disease Rheumatoid disease Ankylosing spondylitis
2. Aortic root distortion (aortitis)		Ankylosing spondylitis Nonspecific urethritis Nonspecific aortitis Rheumatoid disease Syphilis
3. Loss of commissural support		Fallot-type VSD Dissection tears of aorta
4. Aortic root dilatation	Aortitis (inflammatory)	Syphilis All other aortitis
	"Aortopathy" (non-inflammatory)	Marfan Familial Idiopathic Ehlers-Danlos Pseudoxanthoma elasticum

Reproduced with permission from Davies, M. J.: Pathology of Cardiac Valves. London, Butterworths, 1980.

trated valve[476] in the presence of hypertension,[477] systemic lupus erythematosus,[477,478] rheumatoid arthritis,[479] ankylosing spondylitis,[480] and Whipple's disease.[480a] Isolated congenital aortic regurgitation is an uncommon lesion on necropsy studies, but when present, it is usually associated with a bicuspid valve.[481]

AORTIC ROOT DISEASE. A variety of diseases produce aortic regurgitation by causing marked dilatation of the ascending aorta (Fig. 32–26*C*). These conditions, discussed in detail in Chapter 45, include annuloaortic ectasia, cystic medionecrosis of the aorta (either isolated or associated with classic Marfan's syndrome), osteogenesis imperfecta, syphilitic aortitis, ankylosing spondylitis, Behçet's disease,[481a] psoriatic arthritis, arthritis associated with ulcerative colitis, relapsing polychondritis, Reiter's syndrome, giant cell arteritis, and systemic hypertension.[482–490]

Table 32–12 presents a comparison of the findings in four important conditions in which dilation of the aorta causes aortic regurgitation. In each of these, the aortic annulus may become greatly dilated, the aortic leaflets separate, and aortic regurgitation may ensue. Dissection of the diseased aortic wall may occur and may aggravate the aortic regurgitation. Dilatation of the aortic root may also have secondary effects on the aortic valve, since it results in tension and bowing of the individual cusps, which may thicken, retract, and become too short to close the aortic orifice. This leads to intensification of the aortic regurgita-

Table 32–12 CARDIOVASCULAR MANIFESTATIONS OF CONDITIONS CAUSING AORTIC REGURGITATION

	Syphilis	Ankylosing Spondylitis	Rheumatoid Arthritis	Marfan's Syndrome
Average age	50	45	70	30
Predominant sex	Men	Men	Women	Men
Aortic regurgitation	++++	++++	+	++++
Mitral regurgitation	0	++	+	+++
Conduction disturbances	+	++++	++	+
Serology (STS)	+	0	0	0
Morphology of aorta				
Thickened adventitia	++++	++++	+	+
Degenerated media	+++	+++	0	++++
Intimal proliferation	+++	+++	0	+
Vasa vasorum abnormal	++++	++++	0	0
Calcium	++	+	0	0
Aneurysms	+++	0	0	+++
Rupture	+	0	0	+
Dissection	0	0	0	+
Limited to sinuses	0	+	0	0
Morphology of aortic valve				
Cusp thickening				
Diffuse	0	+	0	0
Focal	+	0	+	+
Cusp calcification	0	0	0	0
Shortening	0	+	0	0
Commissural abnormality	+	+	0	0

From Roberts, W. C., et al.: Nonrheumatic valvular cardiac disease: A clinicopathologic survey of 27 different conditions causing valvular dysfunction. *In* Likoff, W. (ed.): Cardiovascular Clinics. Vol. 5, No. 2, Valvular Heart Disease. Philadelphia, F. A. Davis, 1973, p. 424.

tion, which increases left ventricular stroke volume, further dilating the ascending aorta and thus leading to a vicious cycle.

Aortic regurgitation, regardless of its etiology, produces dilatation and hypertrophy of the left ventricle, dilatation of the mitral valve ring, and sometimes hypertrophy and dilatation of the left atrium. Endocardial pockets frequently develop in the left ventricular cavity at sites of impact of the regurgitant jet.

PATHOPHYSIOLOGY

In contrast to mitral regurgitation, in which a fraction of the left ventricular stroke volume is delivered into the low-pressure left atrium, in aortic regurgitation the entire left ventricular stroke volume is ejected into a high-pressure chamber, i.e., the aorta (although the low aortic diastolic pressure does facilitate ventricular emptying during early systole). Whereas in mitral regurgitation the reduction of wall tension (i.e., reduced afterload) allows more complete systolic emptying (p. 1078), in aortic regurgitation the increase in left ventricular end-diastolic volume provides major hemodynamic compensation.[383,489,491,491a,491b,491c]

Severe aortic regurgitation may occur with a normal effective forward stroke volume and a normal ejection fraction (total [forward plus regurgitant] stroke volume/end-diastolic volume), together with an elevated left ventricular end-diastolic pressure and volume (Figs. 32–27 and 32–28). In accord with Laplace's law (p. 431), left ventricular dilatation increases the left ventricular systolic tension required to develop any level of systolic pressure. The increased wall stress leads to replication of sarcomeres in series, elongation of fibers, and sufficient wall thickening to maintain systolic wall stress at normal levels; the ratio of ventricular wall thickness to cavity radius remains normal.[492] This contrasts with the events in aortic stenosis, i.e., replication of sarcomeres in parallel (p. 452) and an increased ratio of wall thickness to cavity radius (p. 454).

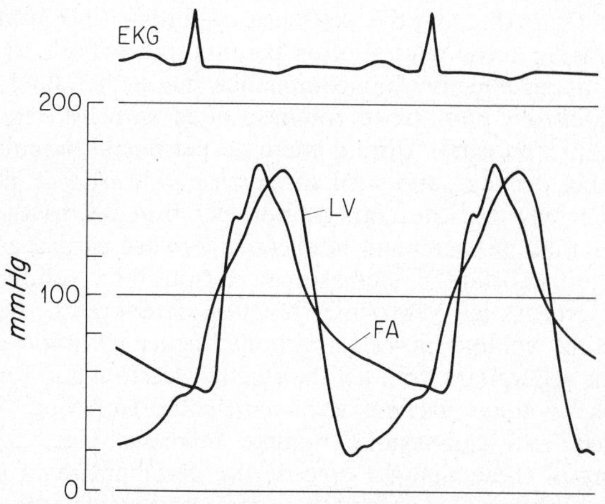

FIGURE 32–27 Pressure curves obtained from a 63-year-old man with symptoms of left ventricular failure and a loud decrescendo diastolic murmur. The femoral arterial (FA) pressure tracing demonstrates a widened pulse pressure of 115 mm Hg and equalization with left ventricular (LV) pressure late in diastole. The LV pressure curve exhibits a steady pressure increase throughout diastole, culminating in a markedly elevated end-diastolic pressure of 45 mm Hg. These findings are indicative of severe aortic regurgitation.

In aortic regurgitation, left ventricular mass is usually greatly elevated (Fig. 32–28), often to levels even higher than in isolated aortic stenosis[383] and sometimes exceeding 1000 gm.

Patients with severe chronic aortic regurgitation have the largest end-diastolic volumes of any form of heart disease[26] (Fig. 32–28) (resulting in the so-called *cor bovinum*), but end-diastolic pressure is not uniformly elevated (i.e., left ventricular compliance often becomes increased), and there is a wide scatter in the relationship between end-diastolic volume and end-diastolic pressure.[383] In the more severe cases of aortic regurgitation, the regurgitant flow may exceed 20 liters/min, so that the total left ventricular output approaches 30 liters/min,[26] a level that can be achieved only by a trained endurance runner during maximal exer-

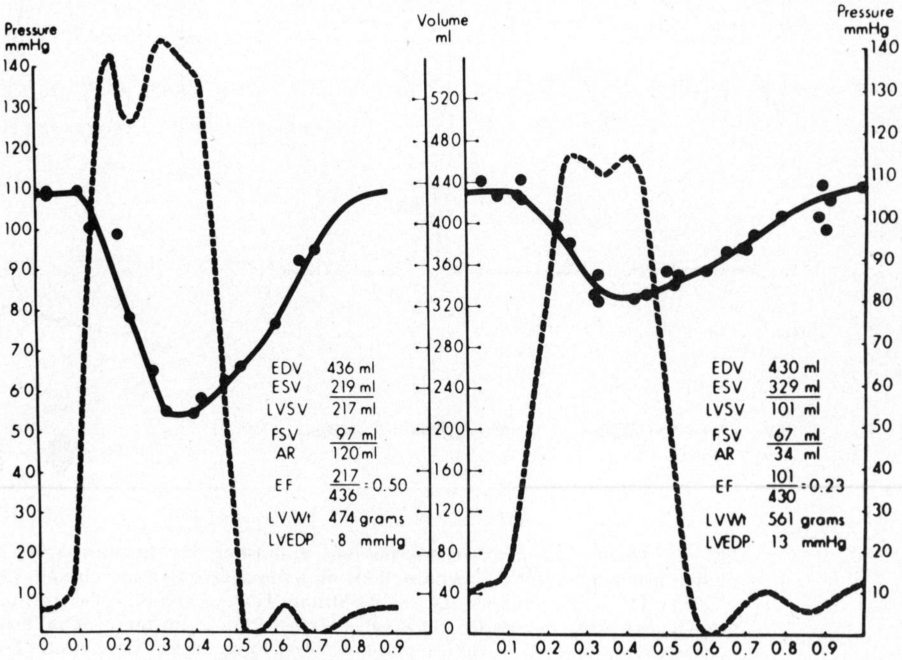

FIGURE 32–28 Left ventricular pressure and volume curves in two patients with volume overload due to aortic regurgitation. On the left graph, left ventricular stroke volume (LVSV) is 217 ml, regurgitant volume (AR) is 120 ml, and ejection fraction (EF) is 0.50. On the right graph, left ventricular stroke volume is 101 ml, regurgitant volume is 34 ml, and ejection fraction is 0.23. The patient on the left was clinically asymptomatic, whereas the patient on the right experienced severe clinical heart failure. (From Rackley, C. E., and Hood, W. P., Jr.: Quantitative angiography evaluation and pathophysiologic mechanisms in valvular heart disease. *In* Sonnenblick, E. S., and Lesch, M. [eds.]: Valvular Heart Disease. New York, Grune and Stratton, 1974, p. 122, by permission of Grune and Stratton, Inc.)

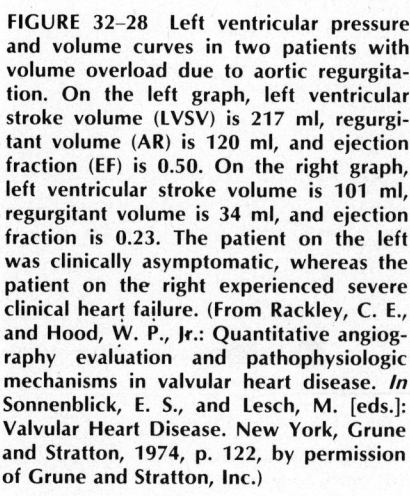

cise. Thus, the adaptive response to chronic and gradually increasing aortic regurgitation permits the ventricle to function as an effective low-compliance pump, handling large end-diastolic and stroke volumes, often with little increase in filling pressure. During exercise, peripheral vascular resistance declines, and with an increase in heart rate, diastole shortens and the regurgitation per beat decreases,[493,494] facilitating an increment in effective forward cardiac output without substantial increases in end-diastolic volume and pressure. As left ventricular function deteriorates, the end-diastolic volume increases without further elevation of the aortic regurgitant volume; the ejection fraction and forward stroke volume decline, and ventricular emptying is impaired, i.e., end-systolic volume increases (Fig. 32–28). Many of these changes precede the development of symptoms. In advanced stages there may be considerable elevation of the left atrial, pulmonary artery wedge, pulmonary arterial, right ventricular, and right atrial pressures and lowering of the effective cardiac output, even at rest.

As is the case for mitral regurgitation (p. 1079), the end-systolic volume is a sensitive index of myocardial function in patients with aortic regurgitation and correlates with operative mortality and postoperative left ventricular dysfunction.[166] Both the immediate and the long-term results are excellent in patients with normal left ventricular end-systolic volumes (< 30 ml/m²), poor in patients in whom this index is elevated (> 90 ml/m²), and variable in patients with intermediate values. In general, however, for any given preoperative level of impairment of left ventricular function, the outlook for left ventricular function in the postoperative period is better in patients with aortic than with mitral regurgitation.

When *acute* aortic regurgitation is induced experimentally, preload, wall tension, and myocardial oxygen consumption all rise substantially,[158,491] a situation contrasting with that produced by acutely induced mitral regurgitation (p. 1078). In patients with chronic severe aortic regurgitation, myocardial oxygen requirements are also augmented by the increase in left ventricular mass. Since the major portion of coronary blood flow occurs during diastole, when arterial pressure is lower than normal, coronary perfusion pressure is reduced.[495] The result—a combination of increased oxygen demand and reduced supply—sets the stage for the development of myocardial ischemia, especially during exercise.[496] The heightened activity of the adrenergic nervous system as a compensatory mechanism in patients with chronic aortic regurgitation is reflected in an abnormal increase in plasma catecholamine content during exercise, accompanied by a reduction in cardiac norepinephrine stores.[497] Symptomatic patients with severe chronic aortic regurgitation generally exhibit a depression of the relations between end-systolic pressure and stress and end-systolic volume. This depression of myocardial function, combined with the increased demands placed on the left ventricle, augments left ventricular end-diastolic volume and ultimately pressure, causing symptoms of pulmonary congestion.[498] Symptomatic patients with aortic regurgitation demonstrate a failure of the normal decline in end-systolic volume or rise in ejection fraction during exercise, as determined by radionuclide angiography.[499] However,

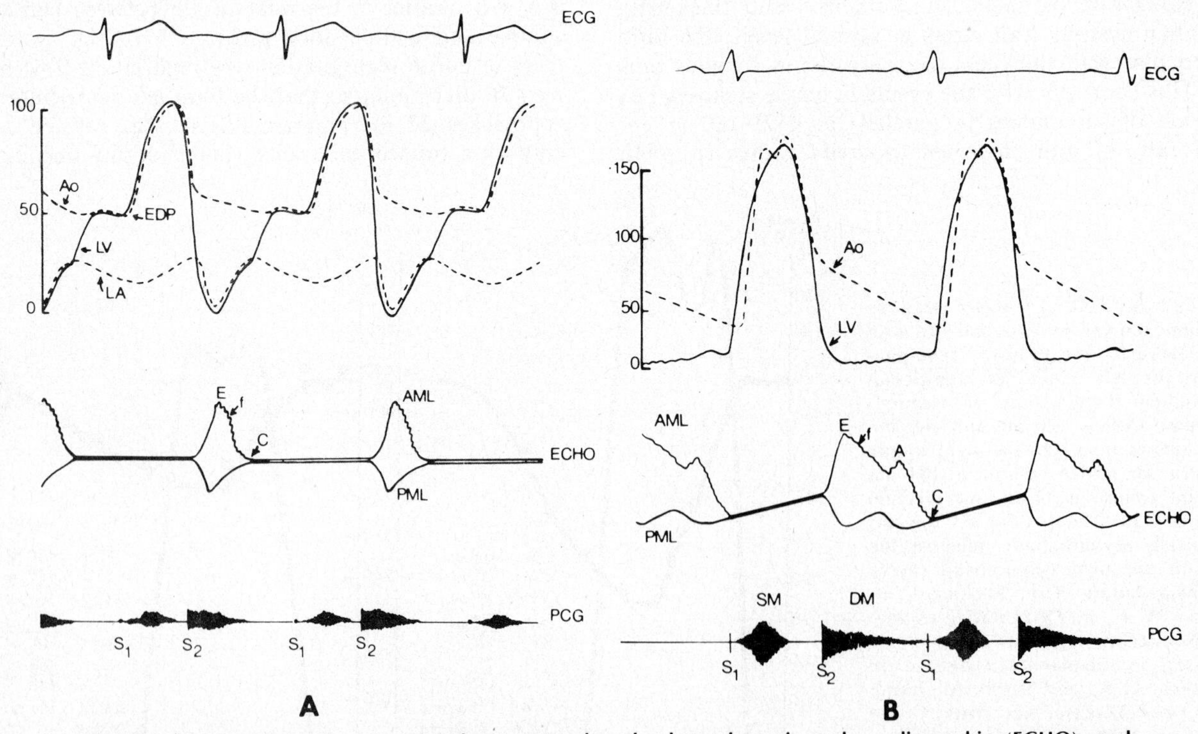

FIGURE 32–29 Schematic representations contrasting the hemodynamic, echocardiographic (ECHO), and phonocardiographic (PCG) manifestations of acute severe (*A*) and chronic severe (*B*) aortic regurgitation. Ao = aorta; LV = left ventricle; LA = left atrium; EDP = end-diastolic pressure; f = flutter of anterior mitral valve leaflet; AML = anterior mitral valve leaflet; PML = posterior mitral leaflet; SM = systolic murmur; DM = diastolic murmur; C = closure point of mitral valve. (From Morganroth, J. et al.: Acute severe aortic regurgitation. Ann. Intern. Med. *87*:225, 1977.)

Table 32–13 DIFFERENCES BETWEEN ACUTE AND CHRONIC SEVERE AORTIC REGURGITATION

CLINICAL FEATURES	*Acute*	*Chronic*
Congestive heart failure	Early and sudden	Late and insidious
Arterial pulse		
Rate per minute	Increased	Normal
Rate of rise	Normal	Increased
Systolic pressure	Normal to decreased	Increased
Diastolic pressure	Normal to decreased	Decreased
Pulse pressure	Near normal	Increased
Contour of peak	Single	Bisferiens
Pulsus alternans	Common	Uncommon
Left ventricular (LV) impulse	Nearly normal to moderately displaced, not hyperdynamic	Displaced hyperdynamic
Auscultation		
S_1	Soft to absent	Normal
Aortic component of S_2	Soft	Normal or decreased
Pulmonic component of S_2	Normal or increased	Normal
S_3	Common	Uncommon
S_4	Consistently absent	Usually absent
Aortic systolic murmur	Grade 3 or less	Grade 3 or more
Aortic regurgitant murmur	Short, medium-pitched	Long, high-pitched
Austin Flint	Mid-diastolic	Presystolic, mid-diastolic, or both
Peripheral arterial auscultatory signs	Absent	Present
Electrocardiogram	Normal LV voltage with minor repolarization abnormalities	Increased LV voltage with major repolarization abnormalities
Chest roentgenogram		
Left ventricle	Normal to moderately increased	Markedly increased
Aortic root and arch	Usually normal	Prominent
Pulmonary venous vascularity	Increased	Normal

HEMODYNAMIC FEATURES	*Acute*	*Chronic (Without Left Ventricular Failure)*
Left ventricular (LV) compliance	Normal	Normal or increased
Regurgitant volume	Increased	Increased
LV end-diastolic pressure	Markedly increased	Normal or increased
LV ejection velocity	Not significantly increased	Markedly increased
Aortic systolic pressure	Not increased	Increased
Aortic diastolic pressure	Normal to decreased	Markedly decreased
Systemic arterial pulse pressure	Slightly to moderately increased	Markedly increased
Ejection fraction	Normal or decreased	Normal
Effective stroke volume	Decreased	Normal
Effective cardiac output	Decreased	Usually normal
Heart rate	Increased	Normal
Peripheral vascular resistance	Usually increased	Normal

ECHOCARDIOGRAPHIC FEATURES	*Acute*	*Chronic*
Mitral valve		
Closure point	Premature	Normal
Opening point	Delayed	Normal
E–F slope	Decreased	Normal
Fluttering	Usually present	Usually present
Left ventricle		
Internal dimension (end diastole)	Normal	Increased
Septal and free wall thickness	Normal	Normal
Septal and free wall motion	Normal	Increased
Left ventricular mass	Normal	Increased

From Morganroth, J., et al.: Acute severe aortic regurgitation. Ann. Intern. Med. *87*:224, 228, and 230, 1977.

abnormal left ventricular function can be discerned even in subgroups of asymptomatic patients with normal ejection fractions; this dysfunction is reflected in failure of the normal increase in ejection fraction during exercise[500,501] or a depressed end-systolic pressure-volume relation.[501] These techniques are likely to prove of great value in the identification of those patients with severe chronic aortic regurgitation, who, although asymptomatic or almost so, are at greater risk of developing left ventricular failure and therefore are candidates for consideration of surgical treatment.

ACUTE AORTIC REGURGITATION (Table 32–13). In contrast to the pathophysiological events in chronic aortic regurgitation described above, in which the left ventricle has had the opportunity to adapt to the increased load, in *acute* regurgitation (caused most commonly by infective endocarditis, aortic dissection, and trauma) the regurgitant blood fills a ventricle of normal size that cannot accommodate the combined large regurgitant volume and inflow from the left atrium. Since total stroke volume cannot rise markedly, forward stroke volume declines, left ventricular diastolic pressure rises rapidly to high levels,[489] and the left ventricle operates on a less compliant (steep) portion of its pressure-volume curve (Figure 12–12, p. 428).[491]

The hemodynamic findings in acute aortic regurgitation contrast with those in chronic aortic regurgitation.[502] For a similarly severe degree of aortic regurgitation, the patient with acute regurgitation has a much smaller aortic pulse pressure and effective forward cardiac output, a smaller left ventricular chamber size, and a higher heart rate than the patient with chronic aortic regurgitation. In addition, as left ventricular pressure rises rapidly above left atrial pressure during early diastole, the mitral valve closes prematurely in diastole (Fig. 32–29).[488,502,503] This protects the pulmonary venous bed from backward transmission of the greatly elevated end-diastolic pressure. Premature closure of the mitral valve, together with the tachycardia that shortens diastole, reduces the time interval during which the mitral valve is open.[503] Left ventricular and aortic systolic pressures exhibit little change. Since aortic diastolic pressure cannot decline below the elevated left ventricular end-diastolic pressure, the systemic arterial pulse pressure widens relatively little.

CLINICAL MANIFESTATIONS

History

In patients with *chronic,* severe aortic regurgitation, there is a long period during which the left ventricle gradually undergoes enlargement while the patient remains asymptomatic or almost so.[504–506] Symptoms of reduced cardiac reserve or myocardial ischemia develop, most often in the fourth or fifth decades and usually only after considerable cardiomegaly and myocardial dysfunction have occurred. When symptoms do develop, exertional dyspnea, orthopnea, and paroxysmal nocturnal dyspnea are the principal complaints. Syncope is rare, and although angina pectoris is less frequent than in patients with aortic stenosis, nocturnal angina, often accompanied by diaphoresis, which occurs when the heart rate slows and arterial diastolic pressure falls to extremely low levels, may be particularly troublesome; these episodes may be accompanied by abdominal discomfort, presumably caused by splanchnic ischemia. Patients with severe aortic regurgitation often complain of an uncomfortable awareness of the heart beat, especially on lying down, and disagreeable thoracic pain due to pounding of the heart against the chest wall. Tachycardia, occurring with emotional stress or exertion, may produce palpitations and head pounding; premature ventricular contractions are particularly distressing because of the great heave of the volume-loaded left ventricle during the postpremature beat. These complaints may be present for many years before symptoms of left ventricular dysfunction develop.

In light of the limited ability of the left ventricle to tolerate *acute* regurgitation, patients with this valvular lesion often develop sudden clinical manifestations of cardiovascular collapse, with weakness, severe dyspnea, and hypotension; angina is uncommon (Table 32–12).[502,502a]

Physical Examination

In patients with chronic severe aortic regurgitation, the head frequently bobs with each heartbeat (*de Musset's sign*),[507] and the pulses are of the waterhammer or collapsing type with abrupt distention and quick collapse (*Corrigan's pulse*). This pulse is readily visible in the carotid arteries and can be best appreciated by palpation of the radial artery with the patient's arm elevated. A bisferiens pulse may be present (Figure 3–24, p. 57) and is more readily recognized in the brachial and femoral than in the carotid arteries. A variety of auscultatory findings provide confirmation of a wide pulse pressure. *Traube's sign* refers to booming systolic and diastolic sounds heard over the femoral artery, *Müller's sign* consists of systolic pulsations of the uvula, and *Duroziez's sign* consists of a systolic murmur heard over the femoral artery when it is compressed proximally and a diastolic murmur when it is compressed distally. Capillary pulsations, i.e., *Quincke's sign,* can be detected by pressing a glass slide on the patient's lip or by transmitting a light through the patient's fingertips.

Systolic arterial pressure is elevated, and diastolic pressure is abnormally low. *Hill's sign* refers to popliteal cuff systolic pressure exceeding brachial cuff pressure by more than 60 mm Hg. Korotkoff sounds often persist to zero even though intraarterial pressure rarely falls below 30 mm Hg. The point of change in intensity of the Korotkoff sounds, i.e., the muffling of these sounds in phase IV, correlates with the diastolic pressure. As heart failure supervenes, peripheral vasoconstriction may occur and arterial diastolic pressure may rise. However, this finding should not be interpreted as a reduction in the severity of the aortic regurgitation.

The apical impulse is diffuse and hyperdynamic and is displaced laterally and inferiorly; there may be systolic retraction over the parasternal region (see Figure 2–6, p. 27). A rapid ventricular filling wave is often palpable at the apex, as is a systolic thrill at the base of the heart or suprasternal notch and over the carotid arteries, resulting from the augmented stroke volume. In many patients, a carotid shudder is palpable or may be recorded.[508]

AUSCULTATION. In *chronic* severe aortic regurgitation, a soft S_1 and prolongation of the P-R interval are frequently present. A_2 is soft or absent, and P_2 may be obscured by the early diastolic murmur.[509] Thus, S_2 is variable; it may be absent or single or exhibit narrow or paradoxical splitting. A systolic ejection sound, presumably related to abrupt distention of the aorta by the augmented stroke volume, is frequently audible. An S_3 gallop correlates with an increased left ventricular end-systolic volume and has been suggested as a sign useful in considering patients with severe regurgitation for surgical treatment (Fig. 32–30).[510]

The aortic regurgitant murmur is one of high frequency that begins immediately after A_2 (see Figures 3–24, p. 57, and 4–22 and 4–23, p. 82). It may be distinguished from the murmur of pulmonic regurgitation (p. 1122) by its earlier onset, i.e., immediately after A_2 rather than after P_2, and often by the presence of a widened pulse pressure. The murmur is heard best through the diaphragm of the stethoscope while the patient is sitting up and leaning forward, with the breath held in deep expiration. In severe aortic regurgitation, the murmur reaches an early peak and then has a dominant decrescendo pattern throughout diastole.

The severity of the regurgitation correlates better with the *duration* than with the *intensity* of the murmur. In mild aortic regurgitation, the murmur may be limited to

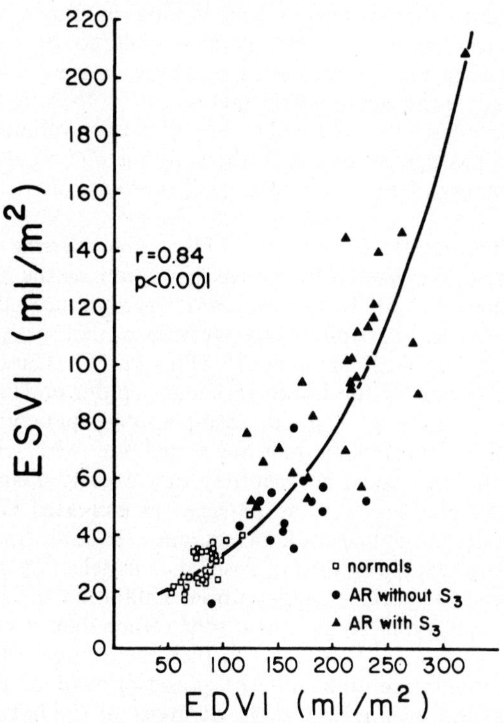

FIGURE 32–30 Exponential curvilinear relationship between the end-diastolic and end-systolic volume index (EDVI and ESVI, respectively) in 31 normal subjects and 42 patients with aortic regurgitation (AR). The latter group consists of 28 patients with and 14 without an S_3 gallop. Note higher values for EDVI and ESVI in patients with than without an S_3. (From Abdulla, A. M., Frank, M. J., Erdin, R. A., Jr., and Canedo, M. I.: Circulation *64*:464, 1981, by permission of the American Heart Association, Inc.)

the early phase of diastole and is typically high-pitched; in moderately severe and severe regurgitation, the murmur is holodiastolic and may have a rough quality. When the murmur is musical ("cooing dove" murmur), it usually signifies eversion or perforation of an aortic cusp. In severe aortic regurgitation and left ventricular decompensation, equilibration of aortic and left ventricular diastolic pressures in late diastole abolish this component of the regurgitant murmur. The murmur is best heard along the left sternal border in the third and fourth intercostal spaces when regurgitation is due to primary valvular disease, but it is often more readily audible along the right sternal border when it is due mainly to dilatation of the ascending aorta.[511] Murmurs in the latter position may be overlooked if auscultation along the right sternal border is not carried out routinely.

A mid- and late-diastolic apical rumble, the *Austin Flint murmur*, is common in severe aortic regurgitation and may occur in the presence of a normal mitral valve (Figures 4–22, p. 82, and 32–31). This murmur appears to be created by rapid antegrade flow across a mitral orifice[494] that may be being narrowed by the rapidly rising left ventricular diastolic pressure caused by severe aortic reflux.[512,513] The Austin Flint murmur may be difficult to differentiate from that due to mitral stenosis, but the presence of an opening snap and a loud S_1 in mitral stenosis and the absence of these findings in aortic regurgitation are helpful clues. As the left ventricular end-diastolic pressure rises, the Austin Flint murmur commences and terminates earlier, and in acute aortic regurgitation with premature diastolic closure of the mitral valve, the presystolic portion of the Austin Flint murmur is eliminated. A short, midsystolic murmur, grades 1 to 4/6, related to the increased ejection rate and stroke volume, may be audible at the base of the heart and transmitted to the carotid vessels. It may be higher pitched and less rasping than the murmur of aortic stenosis but is often accompanied by a thrill.

Dynamic Auscultation. The diastolic murmur of aortic regurgitation may be accentuated when the patient sits up and leans forward or by any intervention that raises the arterial pressure, such as infusion of a vasopressor drug, squatting, or isometric exercise; it is reduced by interventions that lower the systolic pressure, such as amyl nitrite inhalation and the strain of the Valsalva maneuver.[514] The Austin Flint murmur, like the murmur of aortic regurgitation, is augmented by isometric exercise and vasopressors and is reduced by amyl nitrite inhalation (Fig. 32–31).[514]

ACUTE AORTIC REGURGITATION. These patients often appear gravely ill, with tachycardia, severe peripheral vasoconstriction and cyanosis, and sometimes pulmonary congestion and edema (Table 32–13).[502,502a] The peripheral signs of aortic regurgitation are often not impressive and certainly not as dramatic as in patients with chronic aortic regurgitation.[503] Duroziez's murmur, pistol shot sounds over the peripheral arteries, and bisferiens pulses are absent. The arterial pulse may exhibit pulsus alternans. The normal pulse pressure may lead to serious underestimation of the severity of the valvular lesion. The left

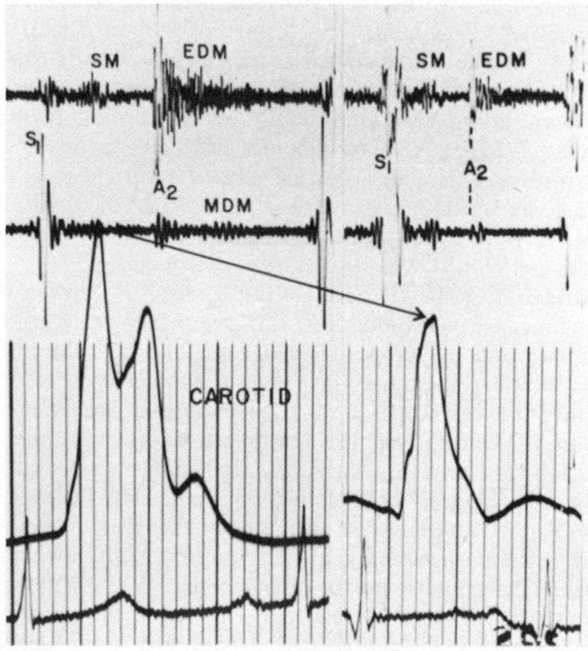

FIGURE 32–31 Response of the Austin Flint mid-diastolic murmur (MDM) to inhalation of amyl nitrite. *A*, Control tracing showing the midsystolic murmur (SM) of rapid flow, the early diastolic murmur (EDM) of aortic regurgitation, and the mid-diastolic murmur (MDM) of Austin Flint. Note the bisferiens carotid pulse. *B*, Test tracing showing loss of the bisferiens pulse as aortic regurgitation diminishes, together with a decrease in intensity of the early diastolic murmur and disappearance of the mid-diastolic Austin Flint murmur. (From Reichek, N., et al.: Clinical aspects of rheumatic valvular disease. Prog. Cardiovasc. Dis. *15*:521, 1973, by permission of Grune and Stratton.)

ventricular impulse is normal or nearly so, and the rocking motion of the chest characteristic of chronic aortic regurgitation is not apparent. S_1 may be soft or absent because of premature closure of the mitral valve.[515] Instead, the sound of mitral valve closure is heard occasionally in mid diastole. However, closure of the mitral valve may be incomplete, and diastolic mitral regurgitation may occur.[516] Evidence of pulmonary hypertension, with an accentuated P_2 and an S_3 and S_4, is frequently present. The early diastolic murmur of acute aortic regurgitation is lower pitched and shorter than that of chronic aortic regurgitation, since as left ventricular end-diastolic pressure rises, the pressure gradient between the aorta and the left ventricle is rapidly reduced. The Austin Flint murmur, if present, is brief and ceases when left ventricular pressure exceeds left atrial pressure in diastole.

LABORATORY EXAMINATION

ELECTROCARDIOGRAM. *Chronic* aortic regurgitation results in left axis deviation and a pattern of left ventricular diastolic volume overload, characterized by an increase in initial forces (prominent Q waves in leads I, aV_1, and V_3 to V_6) and a relatively small r wave in V_1. With the passage of time, these initial forces diminish, but the total QRS amplitude increases. The T waves may be tall and upright in left precordial leads early in the course, but more commonly they are inverted, with ST-segment depressions.[517,518] Left intraventricular conduction defects occur late in the course. When aortic regurgitation is caused by an inflammatory process, P-R prolongation may result. In *acute* aortic regurgitation, the electrocardiogram may (Figure 7–14*B*, p. 210) or may not show left ventricular hypertrophy, despite the presence of left ventricular failure, depending upon the severity and duration of the regurgitation. However, nonspecific ST-segment and T-wave changes are common.

RADIOLOGICAL FINDINGS (p. 164). Cardiac size is a function of the duration and severity of regurgitation and the state of left ventricular function. In *acute* aortic regurgitation, there may be little cardiac enlargement, but marked enlargement is a common finding in *chronic* regurgitation. Typically, the left ventricle enlarges in an inferior and leftward direction, causing a significant increase in the long axis (Figure 6–4*A*, p. 150) but sometimes little or no increase in the transverse diameter of the heart. Calcification of the aortic valve is uncommon in patients with pure aortic regurgitation but is often present in patients with combined stenosis and regurgitation. As is the case with aortic stenosis, the presence of distinct left atrial enlargement in the absence of heart failure should suggest the possibility of mitral valve disease. Dilatation of the ascending aorta is more marked than in aortic stenosis and may involve the entire aortic arch, including the aortic knob. Severe, aneurysmal dilatation of the aorta should suggest that aortic root disease (e.g., Marfan's syndrome, cystic medionecrosis, or annuloaortic ectasia) is responsible for the aortic regurgitation.

For angiographic assessment of aortic regurgitation, contrast material should be injected rapidly (i.e., 25 to 35 ml/sec) into the aortic root, and filming should be carried out in the right and left anterior oblique projections. Opacification may be improved by filming during a Valsalva maneuver. In acute aortic regurgitation, there is only a slight increase in ventricular end-diastolic volume, but with the passage of time both the end-diastolic volume and the thickness of the ventricular wall increase, often in parallel.

ECHOCARDIOGRAM (p. 114). The severity of regurgitation is reflected in increased motion of the septum and posterior wall. In *chronic aortic regurgitation,* the left ventricular end-diastolic diameter and extent of systolic shortening are both augmented[519] (Fig. 32–32). There is increased motion of the interventricular septum and posterior left ventricular wall in compensated patients, but shortening is normal or reduced in patients with left ventricular failure. Serial studies may detect early changes in left ventricular function, as reflected in increased end-diastolic and end-systolic diameters and reduced fractional shortening, which may be of assistance in selecting the optimal time for surgical intervention. Dilatation of the aortic root may point to an aortic root rather than a valvular origin of the reflux (Fig. 32–33). Increased thickness of the interventricular septum and the posterior wall of the left ventricle and an increase in the diameter of the left atrium may be detected.[520]

In *acute aortic regurgitation* (Table 32–13 and Fig. 32–29), the echocardiogram reveals a reduction in amplitude of the opening movement of the mitral valve, premature closure (see Figure 5–34, p. 106) and delayed opening of the mitral valve,[521] and a reduction in the E–F slope, indicating that the left ventricle is operating on the steep portion of its pressure-volume curve. Left ventricular end-

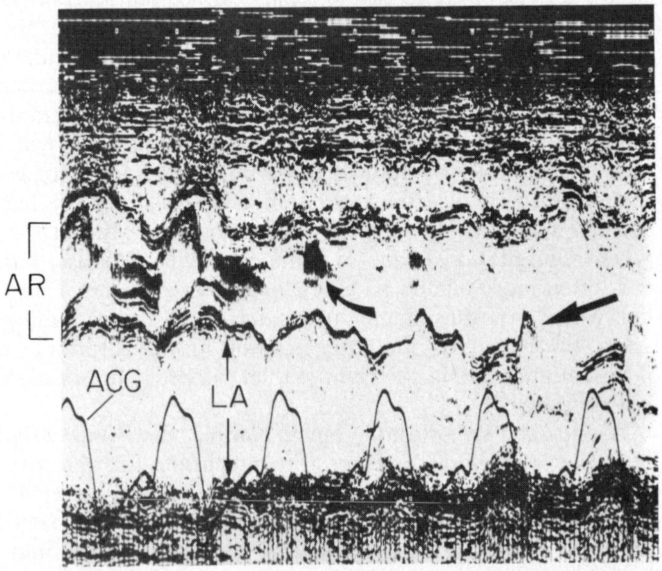

FIGURE 32–32 Echocardiogram in severe aortic regurgitation. A markedly dilated aortic root (AR) is apparent on the left, appearing anterior to a slightly enlarged left atrium (LA). The left ventricle (at the right of the tracing) is dilated and demonstrates vigorous symmetrical contractile motion of the posterior wall and interventricular septum. Projecting anterior to the mitral valve is an abnormal diastolic echo (curved arrow) suggestive of a partially disrupted aortic valve cusp prolapsing into the left ventricular outflow tract. ACG = apexcardiogram.

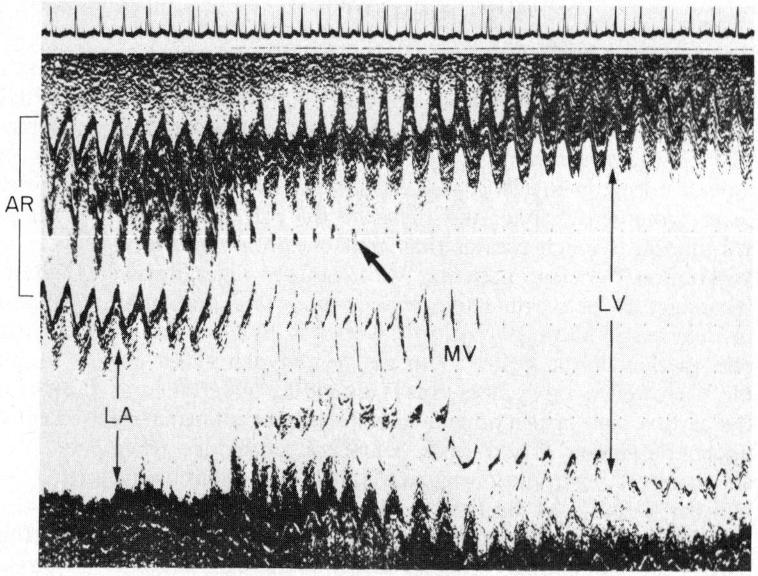

FIGURE 32–33 An echocardiographic sweep from the aortic root (AR) across the left ventricular (LV) outflow tract to the mitral valve (MV) in this patient with vegetative infective endocarditis demonstrates high-frequency diastolic vibrations in the region of the aortic cusps. In addition, a regurgitant aortic jet has caused the anterior mitral leaflet to vibrate with a similar frequency in diastole (arrow).

diastolic dimensions are not markedly increased, and fractional shortening is normal. This contrasts with the findings in chronic aortic regurgitation, in which end-diastolic dimensions and wall motion are increased. Occasionally, with equilibration of aortic and left ventricular pressures in diastole, premature opening of the aortic valve may be detected.[522] Sometimes the echocardiogram may identify the cause of acute regurgitation by revealing echoes due to a partially disrupted aortic valve cusp (Fig. 32–32), vegetations of infective endocarditis (Fig. 32–33), or aneurysmal dilatation of the aortic root. Rarely, in patients with regurgitation due to a flail aortic valve leaflet, its fluttering may be recognized.

High-frequency, diastolic fluttering of the anterior leaflet of the mitral valve during diastole (Figs. 32–34 and 5–34, p. 106) is an important echocardiographic finding in both acute and chronic aortic regurgitation;[523] it does not occur, however, when the mitral valve is rigid. This sensitive sign, which, unlike the Austin Flint rumble, occurs even in mild aortic regurgitation, results from the movement imparted to the anterior leaflet of the mitral valve by the jet of blood regurgitating from the aorta.

Two-dimensional echocardiography is extremely useful in determining the etiology of aortic regurgitation[524] (Fig. 32–35). In patients with severe reflux, short-axis views characteristically display an abnormal indentation of the mitral valve in early diastole caused by the regurgitant jet.[525]

Echocardiography has also proved useful in assessing left ventricular function in order to allow appropriate selection of patients for operation (see below).

RADIONUCLIDE TECHNIQUES. Radionuclide angiography, by allowing determination of the regurgitant fraction and of the left ventricular/right ventricular stroke volume ratio, provides an accurate noninvasive quantitation of aortic regurgitation.[526,526a] As indicated above, these techniques are of value in the assessment of left ventricular function in patients with aortic regurgitation.[499–501]

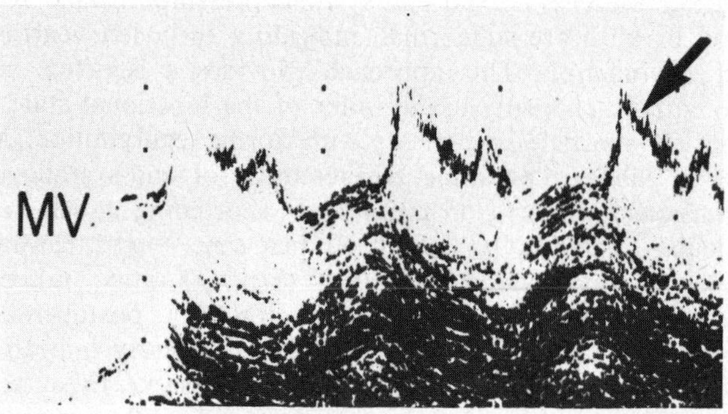

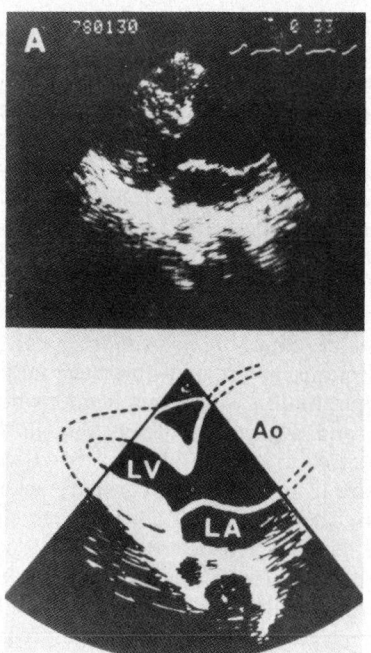

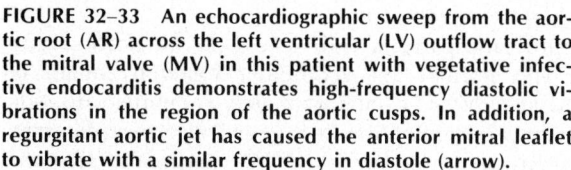

FIGURE 32–34 Echocardiogram in aortic regurgitation. High-frequency diastolic vibrations (arrow) of the anterior mitral valve leaflet (MV) are typical of aortic regurgitation.

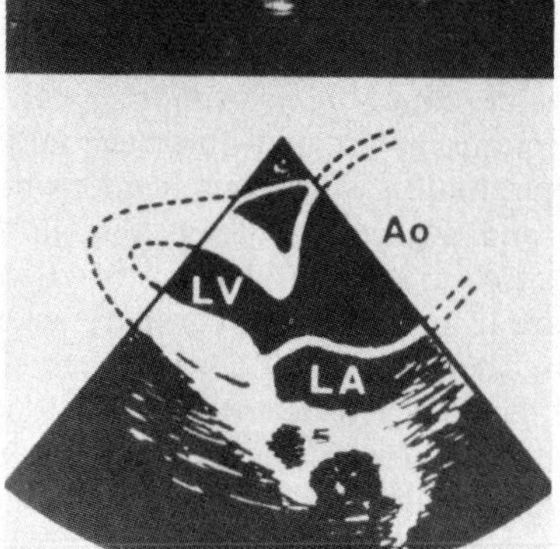

FIGURE 32–35 Panel *A*, Long-axis view of the aortic root (Ao) in end systole by two-dimensional echocardiography. The unusually dilated aortic root is visualized. (Reproduced with permission from Imaizumi, T., Orita, Y., Koiwaya, Y., et al.: Utility of two-dimensional echocardiography in the differential diagnosis of the etiology of aortic regurgitation. Am. Heart J. *103*:887, 1982.)

MANAGEMENT

ACUTE AORTIC REGURGITATION. Since early death due to left ventricular failure is frequent in patients with severe *acute aortic regurgitation* despite intensive medical management, prompt surgical intervention is indicated. Even a normal ventricle cannot sustain the burden of acute severe volume overload, and therefore the risk of *acute* regurgitation is much greater than that of chronic aortic regurgitation.[502,503] In patients with severe regurgitation secondary to active infective endocarditis, operation may be deferred to allow 10 days to 2 weeks of intensive antibiotic therapy if the patient remains hemodynamically stable.[527] However, valve replacement should be undertaken at the earliest sign of hemodynamic instability or immediately upon completion of a 2-week course of antibiotics when acute, severe regurgitation has developed. The cautious use of vasodilators may be helpful in stabilizing the patient's condition but is no substitute for prompt surgery in the patient with pulmonary edema, severe pulmonary congestion, and/or an obvious low forward cardiac output state.

NATURAL HISTORY. Management of patients with *chronic aortic regurgitation* must take into account the natural history of the lesion.[528] Severe or moderately severe chronic aortic regurgitation is associated with a generally favorable prognosis for many years. Approximately 75 per cent of patients survive for 5 years and 50 per cent for 10 years after diagnosis.[98] However, as is the case for aortic stenosis, once the patient becomes symptomatic, the condition often deteriorates rapidly. Without surgical treatment, death usually occurs within 4 years after the development of angina and within 2 years after the onset of heart failure.[529,530]

Medical Treatment

Although there is no unanimity of opinion on this subject, the author believes that cardiac glycosides should be employed in patients with severe aortic regurgitation and left ventricular dilatation even in the absence of symptoms. If present, systemic arterial diastolic hypertension should be treated, since it increases the regurgitant flow; however, drugs that impair left ventricular function, such as propranolol, should be avoided. Atrial fibrillation and bradyarrhythmias are poorly tolerated and should be prevented if possible. Since these and other cardiac arrhythmias and infections are poorly tolerated in patients with free aortic regurgitation, such complications must be treated promptly and vigorously. Even though nitroglycerin and other nitrates are not as helpful in relieving anginal pain as they are in patients with coronary artery disease or aortic stenosis, they are worth a trial when this symptom occurs. Patients with aortic regurgitation secondary to syphilitic aortitis (p. 1562) should receive a full course of penicillin therapy. Although patients with left ventricular failure secondary to aortic regurgitation require surgical treatment, they also respond, at least temporarily, to treatment with digitalis glycosides, salt restriction, and diuretics. The response to vasodilator therapy is often impressive (see Figure 16–20, p. 541). Hemodynamic studies have shown beneficial effects of intravenous hydralazine,[531,532] sublingual nifedipine,[533] and oral prazosin.[533b] This form of therapy may be particularly helpful in stabilizing patients with acute lesions or those with decompensated chronic regurgitation who are awaiting operation. Preliminary observations on the long-term effects of therapy suggest that the initial hemodynamic improvement may be maintained in some patients.[531] If the severity of aortic regurgitation can be reduced on a long-term basis, then it is possible that regression of left ventricular changes and alteration of the natural history might occur.

Asymptomatic patients with severe *chronic* aortic regurgitation and normal left ventricular function should be examined at intervals of approximately 6 months. In addition to clinical examination, x-ray, and electrocardiogram, serial noninvasive assessments of left ventricular size and performance should be carried out using echocardiography or radionuclide angiography or both.

Surgical Treatment

INDICATIONS FOR OPERATION. There is general agreement that operative correction is indicated in patients with severe *chronic* aortic regurgitation who have become symptomatic. Irreversible changes in left ventricular function are present in a subset of such patients; even after successful surgical correction of aortic regurgitation, this subset of patients may develop congestive heart failure or have persistent cardiomegaly as well as depressed left ventricular function.[533–540] Postoperative left ventricular function is usually excellent in patients who are asymptomatic and have normal systolic function preoperatively.[538] Therefore, in order to minimize the risk of postoperative dysfunction, every effort should be made to operate on the patient before serious left ventricular dysfunction occurs.[535–540] Although quantitative biplane ventriculography is the most precise method for assessing left ventricular performance, it cannot be readily employed in serial fashion. Instead, serial echocardiograms, or radionuclide ventriculograms or both should be obtained to detect changes in left ventricular size and function. These examinations can provide valuable information concerning progressive deterioration in left ventricular function at rest. Radionuclide angiography, in particular (p. 362), is a safe, simple, and noninvasive method that allows repeated evaluation of ejection fraction and end-systolic volume at rest and during exercise.[499–501]

In some asymptomatic patients with chronic severe aortic regurgitation in whom both left ventricular end-diastolic pressure and ejection fraction are normal at rest, the ejection fraction measured by radionuclide angiography during exercise or the end-systolic pressure–volume relation or both are subnormal, indicating early left ventricular dysfunction. This approach provides a sensitive and potentially clinically useful index of the functional state of the left ventricle in patients with aortic regurgitation. M-mode echocardiographic measurement of end-systolic dimensions exceeding 55 mm,[536,538,539] shortening of left ventricular diameter less than 30 per cent,[535] and elevated levels of end-diastolic radius/wall thickness ratios and end-systolic stress[533,533a] all correlate with poor postoperative left ventricular function. By providing an early indication of diminished left ventricular functional reserve, these techniques help to identify patients who, while still asymptomatic, require surgical intervention.

OPERATIVE PROCEDURES. The surgical treatment of aortic regurgitation and of combined aortic stenosis and regurgitation is valve replacement. Since the aortic annulus in patients with severe aortic regurgitation is usually not as narrow as it is in patients with aortic stenosis, a larger artificial valve can be inserted, and postoperative obstruction to left ventricular outflow is not a problem, as it may be in some patients with stenosis. Occasionally, when a leaflet has been torn from its attachments to the aortic annulus by trauma, surgical repair may be possible. In patients in whom aortic regurgitation is due to aneurysmal dilatation of the annulus and the ascending aorta, regurgitation may occasionally be reduced or eliminated by narrowing the annulus or by excising a portion of the aorta. More often, effective treatment in these patients requires replacement of the aortic valve and excision of the aneurysmal portion of the aorta and its replacement with a graft, sometimes with reimplantation of the coronary arteries. This more extensive procedure is associated with a higher operative risk than is aortic valve replacement alone.

Aortic valve replacement is discussed on page 1103. In general, results in patients with aortic regurgitation are similar to those in patients with aortic stenosis, with a large fraction of patients exhibiting striking clinical improvement. Reductions in heart size and in left ventricular diastolic volume and mass occur in the majority of patients.[541,541a,541b] However, as already indicated, the extent of improvement in left ventricular function may not be as salutary as in patients with aortic stenosis,[534–540] perhaps reflecting the fact that ventricular dysfunction is more advanced in patients with aortic regurgitation by the time they become symptomatic and are referred for surgical treatment.[541c,541d] As is the case for aortic stenosis, the operative risk of aortic valve replacement in patients with aortic regurgitation depends on the general condition of the patient, the state of left ventricular function,[541,542] and the skill of the surgical team; the mortality rate ranges from 5 to 10 per cent in most medical centers. A late mortality of approximately 5 per cent per year is observed in survivors in whom cardiac enlargement was marked and left ventricular dysfunction was prolonged preoperatively. By extending the indications for operation to symptomatic patients with normal left ventricular function as well as to asymptomatic patients with early left ventricular dysfunction, it is likely that both early and late results will improve. It is likely that with the continued improvement of surgical techniques and results, it will become possible to extend the recommendation for operative treatment to asymptomatic patients with severe regurgitation and normal or nearly normal cardiac function. However, the risk of operation and the uncertainties of function of artificial valves suggests that the time for such a policy has not yet arrived.[543]

DISEASES OF THE TRICUSPID AND PULMONIC VALVES

TRICUSPID STENOSIS

Etiology and Pathology

Tricuspid stenosis is almost always rheumatic in origin. Other causes of obstruction to right atrial emptying are unusual and include tricuspid atresia (p. 994), right atrial tumors (which may produce a clinical picture suggesting rapidly progressive tricuspid stenosis [p. 1459]), and the carcinoid syndrome (which usually produces tricuspid regurgitation [p. 1430] but which may occasionally produce stenosis). Rarely, obstruction to right ventricular inflow can be due to pericardial constriction, extracardiac tumors, and vegetations.

Rheumatic tricuspid stenosis almost never occurs as an isolated lesion but generally accompanies mitral valve disease;[544–547] in many patients the aortic valve is also involved. Tricuspid stenosis is present at autopsy in 14 per cent of patients with rheumatic heart disease but is of clinical significance in only about 5 per cent.[548]

Organic tricuspid valve disease is more common in India than in North America or Western Europe and has been reported to occur in the hearts of more than one-third of patients with rheumatic heart disease studied at autopsy in that country.[549] The anatomical changes of rheumatic tricuspid stenosis resemble those of mitral stenosis (Fig. 32–1), with fusion and shortening of the chordae tendineae and fusion of the leaflets at their edges producing a diaphragm with a fixed central aperture.[128] As is the case for mitral stenosis, tricuspid stenosis is more common in women and, in the United States, is seen most commonly in persons between the ages of 20 and 60 years. Again, as in mitral valve disease, stenosis, regurgitation, or some combination of the two may exist.

The right atrium is often greatly dilated, and its walls are thickened. There may be evidence of severe passive congestion, with enlargement of the liver and spleen.

Pathophysiology

A diastolic pressure gradient between the right atrium and ventricle—the hemodynamic expression of tricuspid stenosis—is augmented when the transvalvular blood flow increases during exercise or inspiration and is reduced when flow declines during expiration. A mean diastolic pressure gradient exceeding 5 mm Hg is usually sufficient to elevate mean right atrial pressure to levels that result in systemic venous congestion and, unless sodium intake has been restricted or diuretics have been given, is associated with jugular venous distention, ascites, and edema.

In patients with sinus rhythm, the right atrial *a* wave may be extremely tall (Fig. 32–36) and may even approach the level of the right ventricular systolic pressure. Resting cardiac output is usually markedly reduced and fails to rise during exercise, accounting for the normal or only slightly elevated left atrial, pulmonary arterial, and right ventricular systolic pressures, despite the presence of accompanying mitral valve disease.

A small mean diastolic pressure gradient across the tricuspid valve as low as 2 mm Hg is sufficient to establish the diagnosis of tricuspid stenosis. Therefore, whenever this diagnosis is suspected, right atrial and ventricular

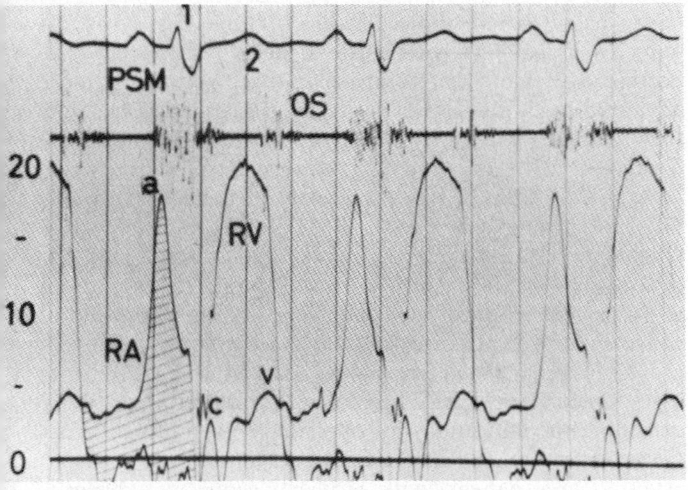

FIGURE 32–36 Phonocardiogram and right heart pressures in a patient with tricuspid stenosis. The giant right atrial *a* wave (a) nearly equals right ventricular (RV) systolic pressure and produces a large diastolic gradient (shaded area). A presystolic murmur (PSM), loud first heart sound (1), and early diastolic opening snap (OS) simulate the findings in mitral stenosis. (Time lines = 0.2 sec.) (From Criley, J. M., et al.: Departures from the expected auscultatory events in mitral stenosis. *In* Likoff, W. [ed.]: Valvular Heart Disease. Philadelphia, F. A. Davis, 1973, p. 214.)

pressures should be recorded simultaneously, using two catheters or a single catheter with a double lumen, with one lumen opening on either side of the tricuspid valve. The effects of respiration on any pressure difference should be examined.

Clinical Manifestations

HISTORY. The low cardiac output characteristic of tricuspid stenosis causes fatigue, and patients often complain of discomfort due to hepatomegaly, swelling of the abdomen, and anasarca. These symptoms, which are secondary to an elevated systemic venous pressure, are out of proportion to the degree of dyspnea.[546] Some patients complain of a fluttering discomfort in the neck, caused by giant *a* waves in the jugular venous pulse. Despite the coexistence of mitral stenosis, the symptoms characteristic of this valve lesion, i.e., hemoptysis, paroxysmal nocturnal dyspnea, and acute pulmonary edema, are usually absent. Indeed, the absence of the symptoms of pulmonary congestion in a patient with obvious mitral stenosis should suggest the possibility of tricuspid stenosis.

PHYSICAL EXAMINATION. Because of the high frequency with which mitral stenosis occurs in patients with tricuspid stenosis, the diagnosis of tricuspid stenosis is commonly overlooked, since the physical findings are attributed to mitral stenosis, and therefore a high index of suspicion is required to detect the tricuspid valve lesion. In the presence of sinus rhythm (which is surprisingly common), the *a* wave in the jugular venous pulse is tall, sharp, and flicking and on first impression may be confused with an arterial pulsation; a presystolic hepatic pulsation is often palpable. The *y* descent is slow and barely appreciable, indicating the absence of normal rapid, early right ventricular filling. The lung fields are clear, and despite engorgement of the neck veins and the presence of ascites and anasarca, the patient is normally comfortable while lying flat. A parasternal (right ventricular) lift is inconspicuous, and pulmonic valve closure is not palpable, but occasionally the pulsations of a greatly enlarged right atrium may be felt to the right of the sternum. Thus, on inspection and palpation the combination of a prominent *a* wave in the jugular venous pulse in a patient with mitral stenosis without the clinical signs of pulmonary hypertension or right ventricular enlargement should suggest the diagnosis of tricuspid stenosis. This suspicion is strengthened when a diastolic thrill of tricuspid stenosis is felt at the lower left sternal edge, particularly during inspiration.[14]

The auscultatory findings of mitral stenosis are usually prominent and often overshadow the more subtle signs of tricuspid stenosis. A tricuspid valvular opening snap (OS) may be audible but is often difficult to distinguish from a mitral OS. However, the tricuspid OS usually follows the mitral OS, and is localized to the lower left sternal border, whereas the mitral OS is usually most prominent at the apex and is more widely distributed. The diastolic murmur of tricuspid stenosis is commonly heard best along the lower left parasternal border in the fourth intercostal space and is usually softer, higher pitched, and shorter in duration than the murmur of mitral stenosis. The presystolic component has a scratchy quality, commences earlier (0.06 sec after the P wave in tricuspid stenosis compared with 0.12 in mitral stenosis), and has a crescendo-decrescendo configuration, diminishing before S_1. The diastolic murmur and OS of tricuspid stenosis are both augmented by inspiration, the Mueller maneuver, assumption of the right lateral decubitus position, leg-raising, inhalation of amyl nitrite, prompt squatting, and both isotonic and isometric exercise. They are reduced during expiration or the strain of the Valsalva maneuver and return to control levels immediately (i.e., within two to three beats) after Valsalva release.

Laboratory Examination

ELECTROCARDIOGRAM. In the absence of atrial fibrillation, tricuspid stenosis is suggested by the presence of electrocardiographic evidence of right atrial enlargement disproportionate to the degree of right ventricular hypertrophy. The P-wave amplitude in leads II and V_1 exceeds 0.25 mv (p. 207), and there may be depression of the P-R segment resulting from increased magnitude of the atrial T wave. Since most patients with tricuspid stenosis have mitral valve disease, the electrocardiographic signs of biatrial enlargement (p. 208) with abnormally tall, broad P waves in leads II, III, and aV_f and prominent positive and negative deflections in V_1 are commonly found. Right atrial dilatation may rotate the ventricular septum and affect QRS morphology in a manner so that the large volume of the right atrium between the exploring electrode and the ventricles reduces the amplitude of the QRS complex in lead V_1 (which often has a Q wave), whereas the QRS complex is much taller in V_2.[64]

RADIOLOGICAL FINDINGS. The key radiological findings in tricuspid stenosis are marked cardiomegaly, with conspicuous enlargement of the right atrium (i.e., prominence of the right heart border), which extends into a dilated superior vena cava and azygos vein, but without dilatation of the pulmonary artery. The vascular changes

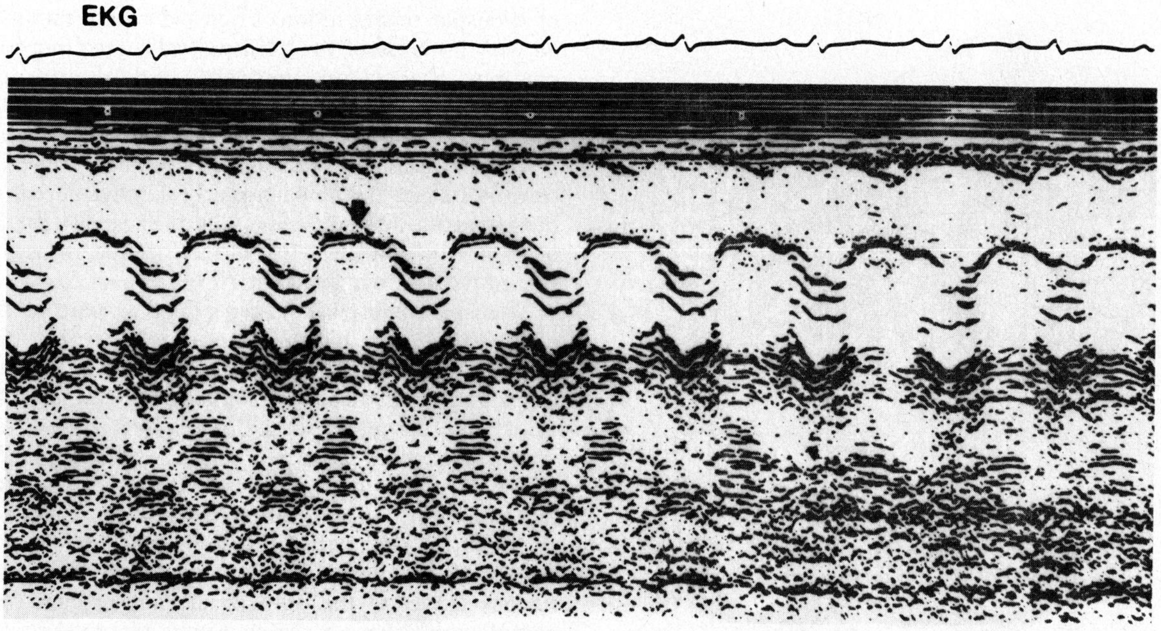

FIGURE 32–37 M-mode echocardiogram of a patient with carcinoid involvement of the tricuspid valve. The flat E–F slope (arrow) is consistent with tricuspid stenosis. (Reproduced with permission from Strickman, N. E., et al.: Carcinoid heart disease: A clinicial, pathologic and therapeutic update. *In* Harvey, W. P., et al. (eds.): Current Problems in Cardiology. Copyright © 1982 by Year Book Medical Publishers, Inc., Chicago.)

in the lungs characteristic of mitral valve disease may be masked, with little or no interstitial edema or vascular redistribution.

Angiography carried out following injection of contrast material into the right atrium and filming in the 30-degree right anterior oblique projection is useful for evaluating the appearance of the tricuspid valve. Thickening and decreased mobility of the leaflets, a jet through the constricted orifice, and thickening of the right atrial wall are characteristic findings.

ECHOCARDIOGRAM (see also p. 115). Although the motion of the normal tricuspid valve is similar to that of the normal mitral valve, it is more difficult to image. The changes in the echocardiogram in tricuspid stenosis resemble those observed in mitral stenosis. Thus, there is a reduction in the E–F slope of the anterior leaflet and usually paradoxical motion of the septal leaflet in diastole (Fig. 32–37).[550,550a] Calcification and thickening of the tricuspid valve often results in multiple and disorganized echoes. In the presence of elevated right ventricular end-diastolic pressure, there is prolongation of the A-C interval, and the time difference between the electrocardiographic P-R interval and the echocardiographic A-C interval is abbreviated. Two-dimensional echocardiography is useful in estimating the size of the tricuspid orifice.[551,552]

Management

Although the fundamental approach to the management of severe tricuspid stenosis is surgical treatment, intensive sodium restriction and diuretic therapy may diminish the symptoms secondary to the accumulation of excess salt and water. A prolonged preparatory period of diuresis may diminish hepatic congestion and thereby improve hepatic function sufficiently to diminish the risks of subsequent operation.

Surgical treatment of tricuspid stenosis should be carried out at the time of mitral commissurotomy or valve replacement in patients with tricuspid stenosis in whom mean diastolic pressure gradients exceed 5 mm Hg and tricuspid orifices are less than approximately 2.0 cm^2. Since tricuspid stenosis is almost always accompanied by significant tricuspid regurgitation, simple finger fracture valvulotomy often does not result in significant hemodynamic improvement but may merely substitute severe regurgitation for stenosis. However, open commissurotomy in which the stenotic tricuspid valve is converted into a functionally bicuspid one may result in substantial improvement. The commissures between the anterior and septal leaflets and between the posterior and septal leaflets are opened; it is not advisable to open the commissure between the anterior and posterior leaflets for fear of producing severe regurgitation.[208] If open commissurotomy does not restore reasonably normal valve function, the tricuspid valve may have to be replaced.[553,553a] A tissue valve such as a porcine heterograft (p. 1087) is generally preferred to a mechanical prosthesis in the tricuspid valve position.

TRICUSPID REGURGITATION

Etiology and Pathology

The most common cause of tricuspid regurgitation is not intrinsic involvement of the valve itself but *dilatation of the right ventricle* and of the tricuspid annulus, which may be complications of right ventricular failure of any cause (Fig. 32–38). Functional tricuspid regurgitation is observed in patients with right ventricular hypertension secondary to any form of cardiac and pulmonary vascular disease, most commonly mitral valve disease, right ventricular infarction,[554,555] congenital heart disease (e.g., pulmonic stenosis and pulmonary hypertension secondary to Eisenmenger's syndrome), primary pulmonary hypertension, and

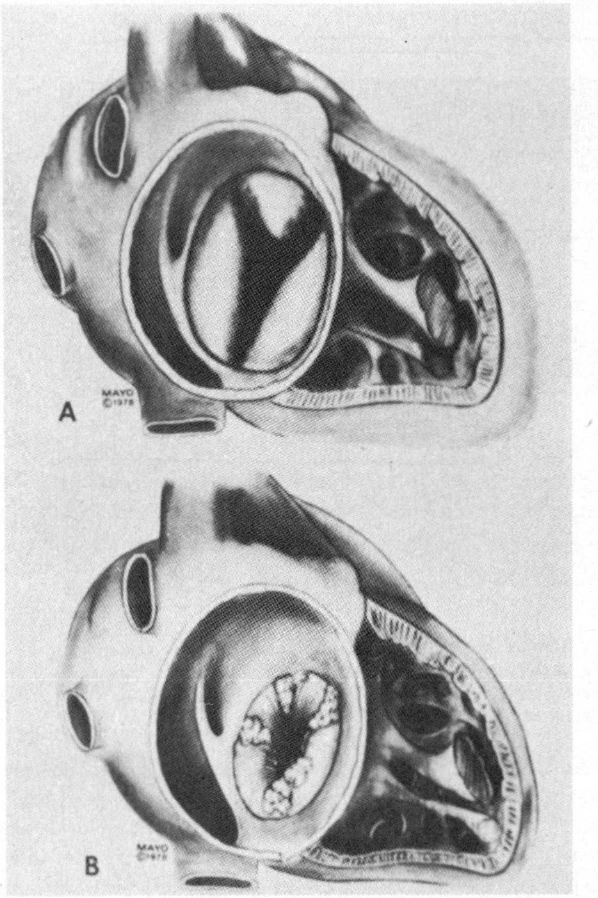

FIGURE 32–38 Types of tricuspid incompetence. *A*, Functional tricuspid incompetence secondary to dilatation of the right ventricle. *B*, Organic rheumatic tricuspid incompetence. (From Brandenburg, R. O., et al.: Valvular heart disease—When should the patient be referred? Pract. Cardiol. *5*:50, 1979.)

cor pulmonale. Severe tricuspid regurgitation has been reported to be the presenting manifestation in thyrotoxicosis.[556] In infants, tricuspid regurgitation may complicate right ventricular failure secondary to neonatal pulmonary diseases and pulmonary hypertension with persistence of the fetal pulmonary circulation.[557] In all these cases, tricuspid regurgitation reflects the presence of, and in turn aggravates, severe right ventricular failure. All of these forms of functional regurgitation may diminish or disappear as the right ventricle decreases in size. Tricuspid regurgitation can also occur as a consequence of dilatation of the annulus in Marfan's syndrome, in which it is not associated with right ventricular dilatation secondary to pulmonary hypertension.

A variety of disease processes can affect the tricuspid valve apparatus *directly* and lead to regurgitation. Thus, organic tricuspid regurgitation may occur on a congenital basis, as a part of Ebstein's anomaly (p. 996), common atrioventricular canal, when the tricuspid valve is involved in the formation of an aneurysm of the ventricular septum,[558] or as an isolated congenital lesion.[438] Rheumatic fever may attack the tricuspid valve directly, and when it does so, it usually leads to both regurgitation and stenosis (Fig. 32–38*B*). Infarction, rupture, or ischemia of the papillary muscles of the right ventricle in coronary artery disease[554,555] and in perinatal asphyxia[555] is an important cause of tricuspid regurgitation. Tricuspid regurgitation associated with prolapse of the tricuspid valve resulting from myxomatous changes in the valve and chordae tendineae usually, but not always, accompanies prolapse of the mitral valve[559] and may be associated with atrial septal defect.[560] Other causes include trauma[561] (p. 1535), infective endocarditis (Chap. 33),[562] particularly staphylococcal endocarditis in drug addicts, and surgical excision that has been necessary in patients with infective endocarditis unresponsive to medical management.[563,564]

Tricuspid regurgitation can occur as part of the *carcinoid syndrome* (p. 1430), which leads to focal or diffuse deposits of fibrous tissue on the endocardium of the valvular cusps and cardiac chambers and on the intima of the great veins and coronary sinus. The white, fibrous carcinoid plaques are most extensive on the right side of the heart, where they are usually deposited on the ventricular surfaces of the tricuspid valve and cause the cusps to adhere to the underlying right ventricular wall, thereby producing tricuspid regurgitation.[565–568] In addition, deposition of the fibrous tissue on the right atrial endocardium reduces its compliance.[569] Less common causes of tricuspid regurgitation include cardiac tumors, particularly right atrial myxoma (p. 1459); endomyocardial fibrosis (p. 1428); and, rarely, constrictive pericarditis. Tricuspid regurgitation may also occur rarely as an isolated congenital lesion.[570]

Clinical Manifestations

HISTORY. In the absence of pulmonary hypertension, tricuspid regurgitation is generally well tolerated. However, when pulmonary hypertension and tricuspid regurgitation coexist, cardiac output declines, and the manifestations of right-sided heart failure, become intensified. Thus, the symptoms of tricuspid regurgitation result from a reduced cardiac output and from ascites, painful congestive hepatomegaly, and massive edema. Occasionally, patients complain of throbbing pulsations in the neck due to jugular venous distention, which intensify on effort.[14] In the many patients with tricuspid regurgitation who have mitral valve disease, the symptoms of the latter predominate. Symptoms of pulmonary congestion may abate as tricuspid regurgitation develops, but they are replaced by weakness, fatigue, and other manifestations of a depressed cardiac output.

PHYSICAL EXAMINATION (Figures 3–32, p. 62, 3–37, p. 64, and 4–13, p. 75). Evidence of weight loss, cachexia, cyanosis, and jaundice is often present on inspection. Atrial fibrillation is common. There is jugular venous distention, the normal x and x^1 descents disappear, and a prominent systolic ("s") wave, i.e., a *c-v* wave, is apparent. The descent of this wave, the y descent, is sharp and becomes the most prominent event in the venous pulse, unless there is coexisting tricuspid stenosis. The right ventricular impulse is hyperdynamic and thrusting in quality. Occasionally, a right atrial systolic impulse may be observed or palpated along the right lower sternal edge.[14] In patients with combined mitral valve disease and tricuspid regurgitation, a relatively quiet zone may be present between the apex and the left sternal edge. Systolic pulsations of an enlarged tender liver are commonly present initially (see Figure 15–5, p. 497), but in chronic tricuspid regurgitation with congestive cirrhosis, the liver may be firm and nontender. Ascites and edema are frequent.

Auscultation (Table 32–5). This usually reveals an S_3 originating from the right ventricle, i.e., one which is accentuated by inspiration; when tricuspid regurgitation is associated with pulmonary hypertension, P_2 is accentuated as well. The pansystolic murmur of tricuspid regurgitation is high-pitched and loudest in the fourth intercostal space in the parasternal region but occasionally in the subxiphoid area. When tricuspid regurgitation is mild, the murmur may be short. With acute tricuspid regurgitation, due to infective endocarditis or trauma, the murmur is usually of low intensity and limited to the first half of systole. When the right ventricle is greatly dilated and occupies the anterior surface of the heart, the murmur may be most prominent at the apex and difficult to distinguish from that produced by mitral regurgitation; this may also occur in tricuspid regurgitation secondary to Ebstein's malformation.

The response of the murmur to respiration and other maneuvers is of considerable aid in establishing the diagnosis of tricuspid regurgitation. It is usually augmented during inspiration.[14,571,572] (Rivero-Carvello's sign), but when the failing ventricle can no longer increase its stroke volume, the inspiratory augmentation is lost. Under these circumstances, respiratory variation may be elicited by standing and thereby reducing venous return. The murmur also increases during inspiration, the Mueller maneuver (forced inspiration against a closed glottis), exercise, leg-raising, and amyl nitrite inhalation as well as after a prolonged diastole, and it demonstrates an immediate overshoot after release of the Valsalva strain. It is reduced in intensity and duration in the standing position and during the strain of the Valsalva maneuver. Rarely, tricuspid regurgitation is silent except for the selective appearance of a soft systolic murmur during inspiration.[573]

Increased atrioventricular flow may cause a short early diastolic flow rumble in the left parasternal region following S_3 (see Figure 3–37, p. 64).

Laboratory Examination

Radiological Findings. Marked cardiomegaly secondary to the condition responsible for the dilatation of the right ventricle is usually evident. The right atrium is prominent (Figures 6–2, p. 148). Evidence of elevated right atrial pressure may include distention of the azygos vein and the presence of pleural effusion. Ascites with upward displacement of the diaphragm may be present. Rarely, with prolonged elevation of right ventricular pressure, the tricuspid ring may calcify. The findings of pulmonary arterial and venous hypertension are common. Fluoroscopy may reveal systolic pulsation of the right atrium.

Electrocardiogram. This is usually nonspecific and characteristic of the lesion causing tricuspid regurgitation. Incomplete right bundle-branch block, Q waves in lead V_1 (Figure 7–12, p. 209), and atrial fibrillation are commonly found.

Echocardiogram (see also p. 116). The right ventricle is usually dilated, and there is evidence of right ventricular diastolic overload, with paradoxical motion of the ventricular septum similar to that in atrial septal defect.[574] Exaggerated motion and delayed closure of the tricuspid valve are evident in patients with Ebstein's anomaly. In patients with tricuspid regurgitation secondary to right ventricular dilatation and pulmonary hypertension, the pulmonic valve echogram shows a diminished or absent *a* deflection (Figure 5–37, p. 109). *Prolapse of the tricuspid valve* may be evident on M-mode echocardiography,[575] and simultaneous echocardiographic studies of the tricuspid valve and phonocardiography may reveal a nonejection systolic click that occurs at the onset of prolapse, originating from the right side of the heart, since it is delayed during inspiration. Two-dimensional echocardiography is particularly useful in the diagnosis of tricuspid prolapse; it reveals the leaflet or leaflets lying above the tricuspid valve ring, i.e., in the right atrium, in systole.[559,576] Cross-sectional echocardiography also allows measurement of right atrial size (which is always increased in the presence of moderate or severe tricuspid regurgitation) as well as detection of paradoxical motion of the ventricular septum.[444]

Contrast echocardiography involving rapid injection of saline or indocyanine green dye into an antecubital vein during two-dimensional echocardiography (p. 95) is both sensitive and specific for tricuspid regurgitation.[577] The injection produces microcavities that are readily visible on echocardiography and normally travel as a bolus through the circulation. In tricuspid regurgitation, these microcavities can be seen to travel back and forth across the tricuspid orifice and to pass into the inferior vena cava and hepatic veins during systole (Fig. 32–39).[578] Tricuspid regurgitation secondary to carcinoid heart disease shows thickened, retracted valve leaflets,[567,568] whereas that due to endocarditis may reveal vegetations on the valve.[562]

HEMODYNAMIC AND ANGIOGRAPHIC FINDINGS. The right atrial and right ventricular end-diastolic pressures are characteristically elevated in tricuspid regurgitation, whether the condition is due to organic disease of the tricuspid valve or is secondary to right ventricular systolic overload (e.g., pulmonary hypertension and pulmonic stenosis). The right atrial pressure tracing reveals absence of the *x* descent, a prominent *v* or *c-v* wave ("ventricularization" of the atrial pressure); thus the right atrial pressure pulse increasingly resembles the right ventricular pressure pulse as the severity of tricuspid regurgitation increases (Fig. 32–40).[579,580] A rise or no change in right atrial pressure on deep inspiration, rather than the usual fall, is characteristic of tricuspid regurgitation.[571] Pulmonary artery (or right ventricular) systolic pressure may offer a rough guide as to whether the tricuspid regurgitation is primary (disease of the valve or its supporting structures) or secondary. Pulmonary artery or right ventricular systolic pressure less than 40 mm Hg favors a primary etiology, whereas when the systolic pressure is greater than 60 mm Hg, the tricuspid regurgitation could be primary or secondary to right ventricular dilatation and failure. In some cases of tricuspid regurgitation, abnormalities in the right atrial pressure contour may be mild or absent. A more sensitive and precise tool for assessing tricuspid regurgitation is the indicator dilution technique.[581] Injection of indicator substance (e.g., indocyanine green) into the right ventricle with sampling in both the right atrium and a peripheral artery allows detection of the "early appearance" of indicator in the right atrium as well as quantitation of the relative magnitudes of forward versus regurgitant flows (Fig. 32–41).

of the pulmonic valve ring, retraction and fusion of the valve cusps, and obstruction to right ventricular outflow.[566] Obstruction in the region of the pulmonic valve may be extrinsic to the valve apparatus and may be produced by cardiac tumors or aneurysm of the sinus of Valsalva.[592]

By far the most common cause of *pulmonic regurgitation* is dilatation of the valve ring secondary to pulmonary hypertension (of any etiology) or to dilatation of the pulmonary artery, either idiopathic[593,594] or consequent to a connective tissue disorder such as Marfan's syndrome.[595] Less frequently it results from a variety of lesions directly affecting the pulmonic valve. These include congenital malformations, such as absent, malformed, fenestrated, or supernumerary leaflets.[126] These anomalies may occur as isolated lesions but more often are associated with other congenital anomalies, particularly tetralogy of Fallot, ventricular septal defect, and pulmonic valvular stenosis.[596–603] Pulmonic regurgitation may occur as a consequence of infective endocarditis[604] or following surgical correction of valvular or subvalvular stenosis or surgical removal of the valve for treatment of endocarditis; less common causes include carcinoid syndrome, rheumatic involvement,[591] injury produced by a pulmonary artery flow-directed catheter,[605] and syphilis.[593]

Clinical Manifestations

Like tricuspid regurgitation, isolated pulmonic regurgitation may be tolerated for many years without difficulty unless it complicates or is complicated by pulmonary hypertension, in which case it is usually accompanied by and aggravates right ventricular failure. In most patients the clinical manifestations of the primary disease are severe and usually overshadow the pulmonic regurgitation, which often results only in incidental auscultatory findings. *Physical examination* reveals a hyperdynamic right ventricle, producing palpable systolic pulsations in the left parasternal area and an enlarged pulmonary artery that often results in palpable systolic pulsations in the second left intercostal space; sometimes systolic and diastolic thrills are felt in the same area. A tap reflecting pulmonic valve closure is usually easily palpable in the second left intercostal space in patients with pulmonary hypertension and secondary pulmonic regurgitation.

AUSCULTATION. In patients with congenital absence of the pulmonic valve, P_2 is not audible, but this sound is accentuated in patients with pulmonic regurgitation secondary to pulmonary hypertension, particularly when the dilated pulmonary artery is near the chest wall. There may be wide splitting of S_2 due to prolongation of right ventricular ejection accompanying the augmented stroke volume.[606] A nonvalvular systolic ejection click due to the sudden expansion of the pulmonary artery by the augmented right ventricular stroke volume frequently initiates a midsystolic ejection murmur, most prominent in the second left intercostal space. An S_3 and S_4 originating from the right ventricle are often audible, most readily in the fourth intercostal space at the left parasternal area, and are augmented by inspiration.

In the absence of pulmonary hypertension, the diastolic murmur of pulmonic regurgitation is low-pitched and is usually heard best at the third and fourth left intercostal spaces adjacent to the sternum (Figure 4–24, p. 83). The murmur commences when the pulmonary artery and right ventricular pressures diverge, approximately 0.04 sec after P_2. It is diamond-shaped in configuration and brief, reaching a peak intensity when the gradient between these pressures is maximal and ending with equilibration of the pressures.[607] The murmur becomes louder during inspiration and following inhalation of amyl nitrite.

When pulmonary artery systolic pressure exceeds approximately 70 mm Hg, dilatation of the pulmonic annulus results in a regurgitant jet of high velocity that is responsible for the so-called Graham Steell murmur of pulmonic regurgitation. This murmur is a high-pitched, blowing decrescendo murmur beginning immediately after P_2 and is most prominent in the left parasternal region in the second to fourth intercostal spaces (see Figure 4–24, p. 83). Thus, although it resembles the murmur of aortic regurgitation, it is usually accompanied by the findings of severe pulmonary hypertension, i.e., an accentuated P_2 or fused S_2, an ejection sound, and a systolic murmur of tricuspid regurgitation. Sometimes a low-frequency presystolic murmur is present, i.e., a right-sided Austin Flint murmur originating from the tricuspid valve that is analogous to the more common left-sided Austin Flint murmur originating from the mitral valve[608] (p. 1111).

The Graham Steell murmur of pulmonic regurgitation secondary to pulmonary hypertension usually increases in intensity with inspiration, exhibits little change after amyl nitrite inhalation or vasopressors, is diminished during the Valsalva strain, and returns to baseline intensity almost immediately after release of the Valsalva strain. This murmur resembles and may be confused with the diastolic blowing murmur of aortic regurgitation. However, indicator dilution studies[609] and retrograde thoracic aortography[610] have established that a diastolic blowing murmur along the left sternal border in patients with rheumatic heart disease and pulmonary hypertension—even in the absence of peripheral signs of aortic regurgitation—is usually due to aortic and not pulmonic regurgitation.

Laboratory Examination

ELECTROCARDIOGRAM. In the absence of pulmonary hypertension, pulmonic regurgitation often results in an electrocardiogram that reflects right ventricular diastolic overload, i.e., an rSr' (or rsR') configuration in the right precordial leads. Pulmonic regurgitation secondary to pulmonary hypertension is usually associated with electrocardiographic evidence of right ventricular hypertrophy.

RADIOLOGICAL FINDINGS. Both the pulmonary artery and the right ventricle are usually enlarged,[611] but these signs are nonspecific. Fluoroscopy may demonstrate pronounced pulsation of the main pulmonary artery. Pulmonic regurgitation can be diagnosed by observing opacification of the right ventricle following injection of contrast material into the main pulmonary artery (Figure 32–43). The diagnosis is supported by noting superimposition of the pulmonary artery and right ventricular pressure curves during mid and late diastole. Indicator dilution techniques

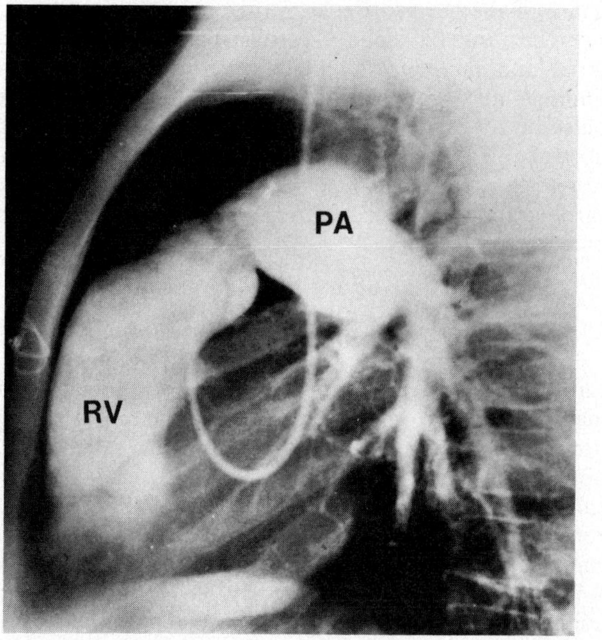

FIGURE 32–43 Pulmonic valvular regurgitation. Contrast medium has been injected into the main pulmonary artery (PA) and regurgitates back into an enlarged right ventricle (RV). (From Carlsson, E., et al.: The radiological diagnosis of cardiac valvar insufficiencies. Circulation *55*:921, 1977, by permission of the American Heart Association, Inc.)

with injections into the pulmonary artery and sampling from the right ventricle,[612] as well as intracardiac phonocardiography,[593,613] can also be helpful in establishing the diagnosis in mild cases.

ECHOCARDIOGRAM. This shows right ventricular dilatation and, in patients with pulmonary hypertension, right ventricular hypertrophy as well. Diastolic fluttering of the tricuspid valve leaflets, similar to that of the mitral valve leaflets in aortic regurgitation, is often noted. Abnormal motion of the septum characteristic of volume overload of the right ventricle in diastole may be evident. The motion of the pulmonic valve may point to the etiology of the pulmonic regurgitation.[614] Absence of *a* waves and systolic notching of the posterior leaflet suggest pulmonary hypertension; large *a* waves indicate pulmonic stenosis. The pulsed Doppler technique is extremely accurate in detecting pulmonary regurgitation. Abnormal Doppler signals in the right ventricular outflow tract whose velocity is sustained throughout diastole are observed in patients in whom dilatation of the valve ring (functional regurgitation) is the cause. When the velocity falls during diastole, the pulmonary artery pressure is normal, and the regurgitation is caused by an abnormality of the valve itself.[614]

Management

Pulmonic regurgitation *per se* is seldom severe enough to require specific treatment. Cardiac glycosides are useful in the management of right ventricular dilatation or failure. Treatment of the primary condition responsible for the pulmonary hypertension, such as surgical treatment of mitral valvular disease, often ameliorates the pulmonic regurgitation. Surgical treatment of primary pulmonic regurgitation directed specifically at the pulmonic valve is required only occasionally because of intractable right heart failure, and in this case valve replacement may be carried out.[601]

MULTIVALVULAR DISEASE

Multivalvular involvement is common, particularly in patients with rheumatic heart disease, and a variety of clinical and hemodynamic syndromes can be produced by different combinations of valvular abnormalities. Development of pulmonic and tricuspid regurgitation secondary to dilatation of the pulmonic valve ring and tricuspid annulus, respectively, and as a consequence of disease involving the mitral or aortic valve or both, has already been discussed (pp. 1117 and 1121), as has the combination of *organic* tricuspid and mitral valvular disease (p. 1117). As a general rule, clinical manifestations produced by the more proximal (upstream) of two valvular lesions, i.e., the mitral valve in patients with combined mitral and aortic valvular disease and the tricuspid valve in patients with combined tricuspid and mitral valvular disease, are more prominent than those produced by the distal lesion.

It is important to recognize multivalvular involvement preoperatively, since failure to correct all significant valvular disease at the time of operation increases mortality considerably. In patients with multivalvular disease, the relative severity of each lesion may be difficult to estimate by clinical examination and noninvasive techniques, because one lesion may mask the manifestations of the other. For this reason, patients suspected of multivalvular involvement and in whom surgical treatment is under consideration should undergo (in addition to careful clinical examination and noninvasive work-up, with emphasis on two-dimensional echocardiography), right- and left-heart catheterization and angiography. If there is any question concerning the presence of significant aortic stenosis in patients undergoing an operation on the mitral valve, the aortic valve should be inspected, since overlooking this condition can lead to a high perioperative mortality. Similarly, it is useful to palpate the tricuspid valve at the time of operation on the mitral valve.

Mitral Stenosis and Aortic Regurgitation

Approximately two-thirds of patients with severe mitral stenosis have an early blowing diastolic murmur along the left sternal border with a normal pulse pressure; in 90 per cent of these patients the murmur is due to aortic regurgitation and is usually of little clinical importance. However, approximately 10 per cent of patients with mitral stenosis have severe rheumatic aortic regurgitation,[505] which can usually be recognized by the peripheral signs of a widened pulse pressure, left ventricular dilatation and increased wall motion on echocardiography, and signs of left ventricular enlargement on radiological and electrocardiographic examinations.

On clinical examination of patients with obvious aortic regurgitation, errors may be made in that mitral stenosis may be missed or, conversely, may be falsely diagnosed. An accentuated S_1 and an opening snap in a patient with aortic regurgitation should suggest the possibility of mitral valvular disease. On the other hand, an Austin Flint murmur may be considered to be a mitral diastolic rumbling murmur of mitral stenosis. These two murmurs may be distinguished at the bedside by means of amyl nitrite inhalation, which diminishes the Austin Flint murmur (Fig. 32–31, p. 1111) but augments the murmur of mitral stenosis (p. 1069); isometric handgrip and squatting augment the diastolic murmur of aortic regurgitation and the Austin Flint murmur. Echocardiography is of decisive value in the detection of both lesions.

Mitral Stenosis and Aortic Stenosis

When mitral and aortic stenosis coexist, the mitral obstruction masks many of the clinical manifestations of aortic stenosis. The cardiac output tends to be reduced further than in patients with isolated aortic stenosis, and the atrial booster pump mechanism, so important in filling the ventricle in aortic stenosis (p. 1097), has little impact when mitral stenosis is present. The reduction in cardiac output lowers both the transaortic valvular pressure gradient and the left ventricular systolic pressure, diminishes the incidence of angina, and retards the development of aortic calcification and left ventricular hypertrophy.[615,616] On the other hand, clinical manifestations associated with mitral stenosis, such as pulmonary congestion and hemoptysis, atrial fibrillation, and systemic embolization, occur more frequently than in patients with isolated aortic stenosis. On physical examination, presystolic distention of the left ventricle and an S_4, common in pure aortic stenosis, are usually not present. The midsystolic murmur may be reduced in intensity and duration because of the reduced stroke volume. The *electrocardiogram* may fail to demonstrate left ventricular hypertrophy, but left atrial enlargement is common in patients in sinus rhythm. The *chest roentgenogram* is usually typical of mitral stenosis except for calcium in the region of the aortic valve. The two-dimensional *echocardiogram* is of the greatest value because stenosis of both valves may be evident. The indirect *carotid pulse* tracing reveals a delayed upstroke.

It is vital to recognize the presence of hemodynamically significant aortic valvular disease (stenosis and/or regurgitation) preoperatively in patients who are to undergo surgical correction of mitral stenosis, since isolated mitral valvulotomy may be hazardous in such patients; this operation can impose a sudden hemodynamic load on the left ventricle that may lead to acute pulmonary edema.

Aortic Stenosis and Mitral Regurgitation

The combination of severe aortic stenosis and mitral regurgitation is hazardous but fortunately relatively uncommon. Obstruction to left ventricular outflow, on the one hand, augments the volume of mitral regurgitant flow,[151] whereas the presence of mitral regurgitation, on the other, diminishes the ventricular preload necessary for maintenance of the left ventricular stroke volume in aortic stenosis. The result is reduced cardiac output and marked left atrial and pulmonary venous hypertension. The physical findings may be confusing because the delayed arterial pulse of aortic stenosis may be counteracted by the sharp upstroke of mitral regurgitation, and it may be difficult to recognize two distinct systolic murmurs. On echocardiography the left ventricle is usually larger than in pure aortic stenosis.

Aortic Regurgitation and Mitral Regurgitation

In this relatively frequent combination[617] the clinical features of aortic regurgitation usually predominate, and it may be difficult to determine whether the mitral regurgitation is due to organic involvement of this valve or dilatation of the mitral valve ring secondary to left ventricular enlargement. This combination of lesions also occurs as a consequence of dilatation of the mitral and aortic annuli in connective tissue diseases such as Marfan's syndrome. When both valvular leaks are severe, this combination of lesions is poorly tolerated. The normal mitral valve ordinarily serves as a "backup" to the aortic valve, and premature (diastolic) closure of the mitral valve limits the volume of reflux that occurs in patients with acute aortic regurgitation.[489] With combined regurgitant lesions, regardless of the etiology of the mitral lesion, blood may reflux from the aorta through both chambers of the left heart into the pulmonary veins. Physical and laboratory examination will usually show evidence of both lesions.

When mitral regurgitation occurs in patients with aortic valvular disease (stenosis and/or regurgitation) secondary to left ventricular dilatation, it often regresses following aortic valve replacement. If severe, it may be corrected by annuloplasty at the time of aortic valve replacement; replacement of an intrinsically normal mitral valve with regurgitation due to a dilated annulus is neither necessary nor advisable.

Surgical Treatment of Multivalvular Disease

DOUBLE VALVE REPLACEMENT. Combined aortic and mitral valve replacement is usually associated with a higher risk and poorer survival than is replacement of one of these two valves.[618,619] Thus, in one representative series, operative mortality was 10.8 per cent for mitral valve replacement, 9.0 per cent for aortic valve replacement, and 18.6 per cent for combined mitral and aortic valve replacement; the 5-year survival was 71 per cent for mitral valve replacement, 70 per cent for aortic valve replacement, and 47 per cent for combined mitral and aortic valve replacement.[620] Some surgeons, however, have reported no increased mortality or lower survival in patients undergoing double compared with single valve replacement.[621]

TRIPLE VALVE REPLACEMENT. Hemodynamically significant disease involving the mitral, aortic, and tricuspid valves is uncommon. Patients with these lesions often present in advanced heart failure with marked cardiomegaly, and surgical correction of all three valvular lesions is imperative. Attempts to shorten the duration of operation by leaving one severely impaired valve in place after a double valve replacement are usually unsatisfactory.[208] However, triple valve replacement is a long and complex operation that has been reported to be associated with a mortality rate of 18 per cent in patients in functional Class III and 40 per cent in Class IV.[622] However, even this high risk must often be accepted because of the otherwise dismal prognosis in these patients.

Patients who survive triple valve replacement usually show substantial clinical improvement in the early postoperative period,[623,624] and postoperative catheterization studies show marked reductions in pulmonary arterial and capillary pressures.[625] However, some patients succumb to arrhythmias[624a] or congestive heart failure in the late postoperative period despite normally functioning prostheses. The cause of cardiac failure in this situation is not known, but it has been speculated that it may be related to intraoperative myocardial ischemia, microemboli from the multiple prostheses, or continued subclinical episodes of rheumatic myocarditis.[621]

References

MITRAL STENOSIS

1. Roberts, W. C.: Morphologic features of the normal and abnormal mitral valve. Am. J. Cardiol. *51*:1005, 1983.

1a. Evans, D. T. P., and Sloman, J. G.: Mitral stenosis and mitral incompetence due to Libman-Sacks endocarditis and mitral valve replacement. Aust. N.Z. J. Med. *11*:526, 1981.

2. Roberts, W. C., Kehoe, J. A., Carpenter, D. F., and Golden, A.: Cardiac valvular lesions in rheumatoid arthritis. Arch. Intern. Med. *122*:121, 1968.

3. Johnson, G. L., Vine, D. L., Cottrill, C. M., and Noonan, J. A.: Echocardiographic mitral valve deformity in the mucopolysaccharidoses. Pediatrics *67*:401, 1981.

4. Chandy, K. G., John, T. J., and Cherian, G.: Coxsackieviruses and chronic valvular heart disease. Am. Heart J. *100*:578, 1980.

5. Osterberger, L. E., Goldstein, S., Khaja, F., and Lakier, J. B.: Functional mitral stenosis in patients with massive annular calcification. Circulation *64*: 472, 1981.

6. Kumar, A., Sinha, M., and Sinha, D. N. P.: Chronic rheumatic heart diseases in Rancho. Angiology *33*:141, 1982.

7. Rusted, I. E., Schiefly, C. H., and Eduardo, J. E.: Studies of the mitral valve. II. Certain anatomic features of the mitral valve and associated structures in mitral stenosis. Circulation *14*:398, 1956.

8. Wells, B.: The assessment of mitral stenosis by phonocardiography. Br. Heart J. *16*:261, 1954.

9. Craige, E.: Phonocardiographic studies in mitral stenosis. N. Engl. J. Med. *257*: 650, 1957.

10. Lachman, A. S., and Roberts, W. C.: Calcific deposits in stenotic mitral valves. Circulation *57*:808, 1978.

11. Bowe, J. C., Bland, F., Sprague, H. B., and White, P. D.: Course of mitral stenosis without surgery: ten and twenty year perspectives. Ann. Intern. Med. *52* :741, 1960.

12. Tendon, R., Potti, S., Mathur, V. S., and Ray, S. B.: Critical mitral stenosis in children. Indian Pediatr. *9*:171, 1972.

13. Selzer, A., and Cohn, K. E.: Natural history of mitral stenosis: A review. Circulation *45*:878, 1972.

14. Reichek, N., Shelburne, J. C., and Perloff, J. R.: Clinical aspects of rheumatic valvular disease. Prog. Cardiovasc. Dis. *15*:491, 1973.

15. Wood, P.: An appreciation of mitral stenosis. Br. Med. J. *1*:1051 and 1113, 1954.

16. Arandi, D. T., and Carleton, R. A.: The deleterious role of tachycardia in mitral stenosis. Circulation *36*:511, 1967.

17. Mitchell, J. H., and Shapiro, W.: Atrial function and the hemodynamic consequences of atrial fibrillation in man. Am. J. Cardiol. *23*:556, 1969.

18. Selzer, A.: Effects of atrial fibrillation upon the circulation in patients with mitral stenosis. Am. Heart J. *59*:518, 1960.

19. Gorlin, R., and Gorlin, S. G.: Hydraulic formula for calculation of the area of stenotic mitral valve, other cardiac valves and central circulatory shunts. Am. Heart J. *41*:1, 1951.

20. Cohen, M. V., and Gorlin, R.: Modified orifice equation for the calculation of mitral valve area. Am. Heart J. *84*:839, 1972.

21. Nakhjavan, F. K., Katz, M. R., Maranhao, V., and Goldberg, H.: Analysis of influence of catecholamine and tachycardia during supine exercise in patients with mitral stenosis and sinus rhythm. Br. Heart J. *31*:753, 1969.

22. Thompson, M. E., Shaver, J. A., and Leon, D. T.: Effect of tachycardia on atrial transport in mitral stenosis. Am. Heart J. *94*:297, 1977.

23. Stott, D. K., Marpole, D. G. F., Bristow, J. D., Kloster, F. E., and Griswold, H. E.: The role of left atrial transport in aortic and mitral stenosis. Circulation *41*:1031, 1970.

24. Kennedy, J. W., Yarnall, S. R., Murray, J. A., et al.: Quantitative angiocardiography. IV. Relationships of left atrial and ventricular pressure and volume in mitral valve disease. Circulation *41*:817, 1970.

25. Heller, S. J., and Carleton, R. A.: Abnormal left ventricular contraction in patients with mitral stenosis. Circulation *42*:1099, 1970.

26. Dodge, H. T., Kennedy, J. W., and Petersen, J. L.: Quantitative angiographic methods in the evaluation of valvular heart disease. Prog. Cardiovasc. Dis. *16*: 1, 1973.

27. Harvey, R. M., Ferrer, M. I., Samet, P., Bader, R. A., Bader, M. E., Cournand, A., and Richards, D. W.: Mechanical and myocardial factors in rheumatic heart disease in mitral stenosis. Circulation *11*:531, 1955.

28. Bolen, J. L., Lopes, M. G., Harrison, D. C., and Alderman, E. L.: Analysis of left ventricular function in response to afterload changes in patients with mitral stenosis. Circulation *52*:894, 1975.

29. Ahmed, S. S., Regan, T. J., Fiore, J. J., and Levinson, G. E.: The state of the left ventricular myocardium in mitral stenosis. Am. Heart J. *94*:28, 1977.

30. Selzer, A., and Cohn, K. E.: The "myocardial factor" in valvular heart disease. *In* Likoff, W. (ed.): Cardiovascular Clinics. Vol. 5, No. 2, Valvular Heart Disease. Philadelphia, F. A. Davis, 1973, p. 171.

31. Wroblewski, E., Spann, J. F., and Bove, A. A.: Right ventricular performance in mitral stenosis. Am. J. Cardiol. *47*:51, 1981.

32. Hugenholtz, P. G., Ryan, T. J., Stein, S. W., and Abelmann, W. H.: The spectrum of pure mitral stenosis. Hemodynamic studies in relation to clinical disability. Am. J. Cardiol. *10*:773, 1962.

33. Dalen, J. E., and Alpert, J. S.: Valvular Heart Disease. Boston, Little, Brown and Co., 1981, 473 pp.

34. Noble, R. J., and Fisch, C.: Factors in the genesis of atrial fibrillation in rheumatic valvular disease. *In* Likoff, W. (ed.): Cardiovascular Clinics. Vol. 5, No. 2, Valvular Heart Disease. Philadelphia, F. A. Davis, 1973, p. 97.

35. Ueland, K.: Rheumatic heart disease and pregnancy. *In* Elkayam, U., and Gleicher, N. (eds.): Cardiac Problems in Pregnancy. New York, Alan R. Liss, 1982, p. 80.

36. Munoz, S., Gallardo, J., Diaz-Gorrin, J. R., and Medina, O.: Influence of surgery on the natural history of rheumatic mitral and aortic valve disease. Am. J. Cardiol. *35*:234, 1975.

37. Diamond, M. A., and Genovese, P. D.: Life-threatening hemoptysis in mitral stenosis: Emergency mitral valve replacement resulting in rapid sustained cessation of pulmonary bleeding. J.A.M.A. *215*:441, 1971.

38. Schwartz, R., Meyerson, R. M., Lawrence, L. T., and Nichols, H. T.: Mitral stenosis, massive pulmonary hemorrhage and emergency valve replacement. N. Engl. J. Med. *275*:755, 1966.

39. Ross, R. S.: Right ventricular hypertension as a cause of precordial pain. Am. Heart J. *61*:134, 1961.

40. Baxter, R. H., Reid, J. M., McGuiness, J. B., and Stevenson, J. G.: Relation of angina to coronary artery disease in mitral and aortic valve disease. Br. Heart J. *40*:918, 1978.

41. Nielson, G. H., Galea, E. G., and Hossack, K. F.: Thromboembolic complications of mitral valve disease. Aust. N. Z. J. Med. *8*:372, 1978.

42. Daley, R., Mattingly, T. W., Holt, C. L., Bland, E. F., and White, P. D.: Systemic arterial embolism in rheumatic heart disease. Am. Heart J. *42*:566, 1951.

43. Lie, J. T., and Entman, M. L.: "Hole-in-one" sudden death: Mitral stenosis and left atrial thrombus. Am. Heart J. *91*:798, 1976.

44. Sharma, N. G. K., Kapoor, C. P., Mahambre, L., and Borkar, M. P.: Ortner's syndrome. J. Indian Med. Assoc. *60*:427, 1973.

45. Mounsey, P.: Inspection and palpation of the cardiac impulse. Prog. Cardiovasc. Dis. *10*:187, 1967.

46. McCall, B. W., and Price, J. L.: Movement of mitral valve cusps in relation to first heart sound and opening snap in patients with mitral stenosis. Br. Heart J. *29*:417, 1967.

47. Perloff, J. K.: Auscultatory and phonocardiographic manifestations of pulmonary hypertension. Prog. Cardiovasc. Dis. *9*:303, 1967.

48. Kalmanson, D., Veyrat, C., Bernier, A., Witchitz, S., and Chiche, P.: Opening snap and isovolumic relaxation period in relation to mitral valve flow in patients with mitral stenosis: Significance of the A_2-OS interval. Br. Heart J. *38*: 135, 1976.

49. Craige, E.: Phonocardiographic studies in mitral stenosis. N. Engl. J. Med. *257*: 650, 1957.

50. Mounsey, P.: The opening snap of mitral stenosis. Br. Heart J. *15*:135, 1953.

51. Yigitbasi, O., Nalbantgil, I., Birand, A., and Terek, A.: O-I/II A-OS formula for predicting left atrial pressure in mitral stenosis. Br. Heart J. *32*:547, 1970.

52. Ebringer, R., Pitt, A., and Anderson, S. T.: Haemodynamic factors influencing opening snap interval in mitral stenosis. Br. Heart J. *32*:350, 1970.

53. Chandraratna, P. A. N., Aronow, W. S., and Lurie, M.: Cross-sectional echocardiographic observations on the mechanism of preservation of the opening snap in calcific mitral stenosis. Chest *78*:822, 1980.

54. Criley, J. M., Chambers, R. D., Blaufuss, A. H., and Friedman, N. J.: Mitral stenosis: Mechanico-acoustical events. *In* Leon, D. F., and Shaver, J. A. (eds.): Physiological Principles of Heart Sounds and Murmurs. New York, American Heart Association Monograph No. 46, 1975, pp. 149–159.

55. Toutouzas, P., Koidakis, A., Velimezis, A., and Avgoustakis, D.: Mechanisms of diastolic rumble and presystolic murmur in mitral stenosis. Br. Heart J. *36*: 1096, 1974.

56. Tavel, M. E., and Bonner, A. J., Jr.: Presystolic murmur in atrial fibrillation: Fact or fiction? Circulation *54*:167, 1976.

57. Harvey, W. P.: Silent valvular heart disease. *In* Likoff, W. (ed.): Cardio-

vascular Clinics. Vol. 5, No. 2, Valvular Heart Disease. Philadelphia, F. A. Davis, 1973, p. 77.

58. Delman, A. J., and Stein, E.: Rheumatic mitral stenosis. *In* Dynamic Cardiac Auscultation and Phonocardiography. Philadelphia, W. B. Saunders Co., 1979, p. 849.
59. Surawicz, B.: Effect of respiration and upright position on the interval between the two components of the second heart sound and that between the second sound and mitral opening snap. Circulation *16*:422, 1957.
60. Delman, A. J., Gordon, G. M., Stein, E., and Escher, D. J. W.: The second sound–mitral opening snap (A2-OS) interval during exercise in the evaluation of mitral stenosis. Circulation *33*:399, 1966.
61. Aravanis, C., and Michaelides, G.: Tricuspid insufficiency masquerading as mitral insufficiency in patients with severe mitral stenosis. Am. J. Cardiol. *20*: 417, 1967.
62. McArthur, J. D., Sukumar, I. P., Munis, S. C., Krishnaswami, S., and Cherian, G.: Reassessment of Graham Steell murmur using platinum electrode technique. Br. Heart J. *36*:1023, 1974.
63. Cooksey, J. D., Dunn, M., and Massie, E.: Clinical Vectorcardiography and Electrocardiography. 2nd ed. Chicago, Year Book Medical Publishers, 1977, p. 272.
64. Rios, J. C., and Goo, W.: Electrocardiographic correlates of rheumatic valvular disease. *In* Likoff, W. (ed.): Cardiovascular Clinics, Vol. 5, No. 2, Valvular Heart Disease. Philadelphia, F. A. Davis, 1973, p. 248.
65. Kasser, I., and Kennedy, J. W.: The relationship of increased left atrial volume and pressure to abnormal P waves on the electrocardiogram. Circulation *39*: 339, 1969.
66. Mounsey, P.: The atrial electrocardiogram as a guide to prognosis after mitral valvulotomy. Br. Heart J. *21*:617, 1961.
67. Bailey, G. W., Braniff, B. A., Hancock, E. W., and Cohn, K. E.: Relationship of left atrial pathology to atrial fibrillation in mitral valvular disease. Ann. Intern. Med. *69*:13, 1968.
68. Probst, P., Goldschlager, N., and Selzer, A.: Left atrial size and atrial fibrillation in mitral stenosis: Factors influencing their relationship. Circulation *48* :1282, 1973.
69. Cueto, J., Toshima, J., Armyo, G., Tuna, N., and Lillehei, C. W.: Vectorcardiographic studies in acquired valvular disease with reference to the diagnosis of right ventricular hypertrophy. Circulation *33*:588, 1967.
70. Taymor, R. C., Hoffman, I., and Henry, E.: The Frank vectorcardiogram in mitral stenosis. Circulation *30*:865, 1964.
71. Walston, A., Harley, A., and Pipberger, H. V.: Computer analysis of the orthogonal electrocardiogram and vectorcardiogram in mitral stenosis. Circulation *50*:472, 1974.
72. Donoso, E., Jick, S., Braunwald, E., Lamelas, M., and Grishman, A.: The spatial vectorcardiogram in mitral valve disease. Am. Heart J. *53*:760, 1957.
73. Gooch, A. S., Calatayud, J. B., Gorman, P. A., Saunders, J. L., and Caceres, C. A.: Leftward shift of the terminal P forces in the ECG associated with left atrial enlargement. Am. Heart J. *71*:727, 1966.
74. Chen, J. T. T., Behar, V. S., Morris, J. J., Jr., McIntosh, H. D., and Lester, R. G.: Correlation of roentgen findings with hemodynamic data in pure mitral stenosis. Am. J. Roentgenol. Radium Ther. Nucl. Med. *102*:280, 1968.
75. Amplatz, K.: The roentgenographic diagnosis of mitral and aortic valvular disease. Am. Heart J. *64*:556, 1962.
76. Melhem, R. E., Dunbar, J. D., and Booth, R. W.: "B" lines of Kerley and left atrial size in mitral valve disease: Their correlation with mean left atrial pressure as measured by left atrial puncture. Radiology *76*:65, 1961.
77. Fleischner, F. G., and Reiner, L.: Linear x-ray shadows in acquired pulmonary hemosiderosis and congestion. N. Engl. J. Med. *250*:900, 1954.
78. Van Houten, F. X., Adams, D. F., and Abrams, H. C.: Radiology of valvular heart disease. *In* Sonnenblick, E. H., and Lesch, M. (eds.): Valvular Heart Disease. New York, Grune and Stratton, 1974, p. 1.
79. Parker, B. M., Friedenberg, M. J., Templeton, A. W., and Burford, T. H.: Preoperative angiocardiographic diagnosis of left atrial thrombi in mitral stenosis. N. Engl. J. Med. *273*:136, 1965.
80. Akius, C. W., Kirklin, J. K., Block, P. C., Buckley, M. J., and Austen, W. G.: Preoperative evaluation of subvalvular fibrosis in mitral stenosis. A predictive factor in conservative vs. replacement surgical therapy. Circulation *60*(Suppl. I):71–76, 1978.
81. Parisi, A. F., and Tow, D. C.: Noninvasive Approaches to Cardiovascular Diagnosis. New York, Appleton-Century-Crofts, 1979, p. 113.
82. Thuillez, C., Theroux, P., Bourassa, M., Blanchard, M., Peronneau, P., Guermonprez, J.-L., Diebold, B., and Waters, D. D.: Pulsed Doppler echocardiographic study of mitral stenosis. Circulation *61*:381, 1980.
83. Henry, W. L., and Kastl, D. G.: Echocardiographic evaluation of patients with mitral stenosis. Am. J. Med. *62*:813, 1977.
84. Wann, L. S., Weyman, A. E., Feigenbaum, H., Dillon, J. C., Johnston, K. W., and Eggleton, R. C.: Determination of mitral valve area by cross-sectional echocardiography. Ann. Intern. Med. *88*:337, 1978.
85. Fisher, M. L., Parisi, A. F., Plotnick, G. D., DeFelice, C. E., Carliner, N. H., and Fortuin, N. J.: Assessment of severity of mitral stenosis by echocardiographic leaflet separation. Arch. Intern. Med. *139*:402, 1979.
86. Shiu, M. F., Crowther, A., Jenkins, B. S., and Webb-Peploe, M. M.: Echocardiographic and exercise evaluation of results of mitral valvotomy operations. Br. Heart J. *41*:139, 1979.
87. Wise, J. R., Jr.: Echocardiographic evaluation of mitral stenosis using diastolic posterior left ventricular wall motion. Circulation *61*:1037, 1980.
88. Palomo, A. R., Quinones, M. A., Waggoner, A. D., Kumpuris, A. G., and Miller, R. R.: Echo-phonocardiographic determination of left atrial and left ventricular filling pressures with and without mitral stenosis. Circulation *61*: 1043, 1980.
89. Motro, M., Schneeweiss, A., Lehrer, E., Rath, S., and Neufeld, H. N.: Correlation between cardiac catheterization and echocardiography in assessing the severity of mitral stenosis. Int. J. Cardiol. *1*:25, 1981.
90. Naito, M., Morganroth, J., Mardelli, T. J., Chen, C. C., and Dreifus, L. S.: Rheumatic mitralstenosis: Cross-sectional echocardiographic analysis. Am. Heart J. *100*:34, 1980.
91. Schweizer, P., Bardos, P., Erbel, R., Meyer, J., Merx, W., Messmer, B. J., and Effert, S.: Detection of left atrial thrombi by echocardiography. Br. Heart J. *45*: 148, 1981.
92. Colman, T., de Ubago, J. L. M., and Figueroa, A.: Coronary arteriography and atrial thrombosis in mitral valve disease. Am. J. Cardiol. *47*:973, 1981.
93. Beiser, G. D., Epstein, S. E., Stampfer, M., Robinson, B., and Braunwald, E.: Studies on digitalis. XVIII. Effects of ouabain on the hemodynamic response to exercise in patients with mitral stenosis in normal sinus rhythm. N. Engl. J. Med. *278*:131, 1968.
94. Levine, H. J.: Which atrial fibrillation patients should be on chronic anticoagulation? J. Cardiovasc. Med. *6*:483, 1981.
95. Kloster, F. E., and Morris, C. D.: Natural history of valvular heart disease. Circulation *65*:1283, 1982.
96. Olesen, K. H.: The natural history of 271 patients with mitral stenosis under medical treatment. Br. Heart J. *24*:349, 1962.
97. Rowe, J. C., Bland, E. F., Sprague, H. B., and White, P. D.: The course of mitral stenosis whout surgery: Ten- and twenty-year perspectives. Ann. Intern. Med. *52*:741, 1960.
98. Rapaport, E.: Natural history of aortic and mitral valve disease. Am. J. Cardiol. *35*:221, 1975.
99. Sutton, M. J. St.J., Oldershaw, P., Sacchetti, R., Paneth, M., Lennox, S. C., Gibson, R. V., and Gibson, D. G.: Valve replacement without preoperative cardiac catheterization. N. Engl. J. Med. *305*:1233, 1981.
100. Brandenburg, R. O.: No more routine catheterization for valvular heart disease? N. Engl. J. Med. *305*:1277, 1981.
101. O'Rourke, R. A.: Preoperative cardiac catheterization. Its need in most patients with valvular heart disease. J.A.M.A. *248*:745, 1982.
102. Chun, P. K. C., Gertz, E., Davia, J. E., and Cheitlin, M. D.: Coronary atherosclerosis in mitral stenosis. Chest *81*:36, 1982.
103. Ramsdale, D. R., Faragher, E. B., Bennett, D. H., Bray, C. L., Ward, C., and Beton, D. C.: Preoperative prediction of significant coronary artery disease in patients with valvular heart disease. Br. Med. J. *284*:223, 1982.
104. Cohn, L. H., and Collins, J. J., Jr.: Surgical treatment of mitral stenosis. A medical milestone. N. Engl. J. Med. *289*:1035, 1973.
105. Gobel, F. L., Andrew, D. J., Witherspoon, J. M., Lillehei, R. C., Castaneda, A., and Wang, Y.: The hemodynamic results of instrumental and digital valvotomy in patients with mitral stenosis. Circulation *39*:317, 1969.
106. Appelbaum, A., Kouchoukos, N. T., Blackstone, E. H., and Kirklin, J. W.: Early risks of open heart surgery for mitral valve disease. Am. J. Cardiol. *37*: 201, 1976.
107. Mullin, E. M., Jr., Glancy, D. L., Higgs, L. M., Epstein, S. E., and Morrow, A. G.: Current results of operation for mitral stenosis: Clinical and hemodynamic assessments in 124 consecutive patients treated by closed commissurotomy, open commissurotomy or valve replacement. Circulation *46*: 298, 1972.
108. Ellis, L. B., Harken, D. E., and Black, H.: A clinical study of 1,000 consecutive cases of mitral stenosis two to nine years after mitral valvuloplasty. Circulation *19*:803, 1959.
109. Logan, A., and Turner, R.: Surgical treatment of mitral stenosis with particular reference to the transventricular approach with a mechanical dilator. Lancet *2*:874, 1959.
110. Cohn, P. F.: Mitral valve surgery. Circulation *63*:965, 1981.
111. Bryant, L. R., and Trinkle, J. K.: Mitral valvotomy in the valve replacement era. Ann. Surg. *173*:1024, 1971.
112. Olinger, G. N., Rios, F. W., and Maloney, J. F., Jr.: Closed valvulotomy for calcific mitral stenosis. J. Thorac. Cardiovasc. Surg. *62*:357, 1971.
113. Commerford, P. J., Hastie, T., and Beck, W.: Closed mitral valvotomy: Actuarial analysis of results in 654 patients over 12 years and analysis of preoperative predictors of long-term survival. Ann. Thorac. Surg. *33*:473, 1982.
114. Dernevik, L., Brorsson, L., Wallentin, I., and William-Olsson, G.: Improved results of closed commissurotomy for mitral stenosis using ultrasonocardiography as selection ground. Acta Med. Scand. *210*:283, 1981.
115. Gross, R. I., Cunningham, J. N., Jr., Snively, S. L., Catinella, F. P., Nathan, I. M., Adams, P. X., and Spencer, F. C.: Long-term results of open radical mitral commissurotomy: Ten year followup study of 202 patients. Am. J. Cardiol. *47*:821, 1981.
116. Smith, W. M., Neutze, J. M., Barratt-Boyes, B. G., and Lowe, J. B.: Open mitral valvotomy. Effect of preoperative factors on result. J. Thorac. Cardiovasc. Surg. *82*:738, 1981.
117. Aryanpur, I., Shakibi, J., Yazdanyar, A., Mehranpur, M., Paydar, M., Azar, H., Motlagh, F. A., Tarbiat, S., and Siassi, B.: Closed versus open mitral commissurotomy in children with rheumatic mitral stenosis. J. Thorac. Cardiovasc. Surg. *76*:223, 1978.
118. Aora, R., Khalilullah, M., Gupta, M. P., and Padmavati, S.: Mitral restenosis. Incidence and epidemiology. Indian Heart J. *30*:265, 1978.
119. Heger, J. J., Wann, L. S., Weyman, A. E., Dillon, J. C., and Feigenbaum, H.:

Long-term changes in mitral valve area after successful mitral commissurotomy. Circulation *59*:443, 1979.
120. Higgs, L. M., Glancy, D. L., O'Brien, K. P., Epstein, S. E., and Morrow, A. G.: Mitral restenosis: An uncommon cause of recurrent symptoms following mitral commissurotomy. Am. J. Cardiol. *26*:34, 1970.
121. Ward, C., and Hancock, B. W.: Extreme pulmonary hypertension caused by mitral valve disease. Natural history and results of surgery. Br. Heart J. *37*:74, 1975.
122. Braunwald, E., Braunwald, N. S., Ross, J., Jr., and Morrow, A. G.: Effects of mitral valve replacement on the pulmonary vascular dynamics of patients with pulmonary hypertension. N. Engl. J. Med. *273*:509, 1965.
123. Dalen, J. E., Matloff, J. M., Evans, G. L., Hoppin, F. G., Jr., Bhardwaj, P., Harken, D. E., and Dexter, L.: Early reduction of pulmonary vascular resistance after mitral valve replacement. N. Engl. J. Med. *277*:387, 1967.
124. Zener, J. C., Hancock, E. W., Shumway, N. E., and Harrison, D. C.: Regression of extreme pulmonary hypertension after mitral valve surgery. Am. J. Cardiol. *30*:820, 1972.

MITRAL REGURGITATION

125. Silverman, M. E., and Hurst, J. W.: The mitral complex: Clues to its afflictions. *In* Likoff, W. (ed.): Cardiovascular Clinics. Vol. 5, No. 2, Valvular Heart Disease. Philadelphia, F. A. Davis, 1973, p. 36.
126. Roberts, W. C., Dangel, J. C., and Bulkley, B. H.: Nonrheumatic valvular cardiac disease: A clinicopathologic survey of 27 different conditions causing valvular dysfunction. *In* Likoff, W. (ed.): Cardiovascular Clinics. Vol. 5, No. 2, Valvular Heart Disease. Philadelphia, F. A. Davis, 1973, p. 334.
127. Perloff, J. D., and Roberts, W. C.: The mitral apparatus. Functional anatomy of mitral regurgitation. Circulation *46*:227, 1972.
128. Davies, M. J.: Pathology of Cardiac Valves. London, Butterworths, 1980.
129. Bloor, C. M.: Valvular heart disease in the elderly. J. Am. Geriatr. Soc. *30*:466, 1982.
130. Korn, D., DeSanctis, R. W., and Sell, S.: Massive calcification of the mitral annulus. N. Engl. J. Med. *267*:900, 1962.
131. Wanderman, K. L., and Margulis, G.: Coexistence of hypertrophic obstructive cardiomyopathy and mitral annular calcification: Proposed etiologic relationship. Isr. J. Med. Sci. *15*:422, 1979.
132. DePace, N. L., Rohrer, A. H., Kotler, M. N., Brezin, J. H., and Parry, W. R.: Rapidly progressive, massive mitral annular calcification. Occurrence in a patient with chronic renal failure. Arch. Intern. Med. *141*:166, 1981.
133. Papa, L. A., Raniolo, J., and Schiff, S.: Mitral anular calcification: Clinical and echocardiographic findings. J.A.O.A. *81*:471, 1982.
134. Zanolla, L., Marino, P., Nicolosi, G. L., Peranzoni, P. F., and Poppi, A.: Two-dimensional echocardiographic evaluation of mitral valve calcification. Sensitivity and specificity. Chest *82*:154, 1982.
135. Mellino, M., Salcedo, E. E., Lever, H. M., Vasudevan, G., and Kramer, J. R.: Echographic-quantified severity of mitral anulus calcification: Prognostic correlation to related hemodynamic, valvular, rhythm, and conduction abnormalities. Am. Heart J. *103*:222, 1982.
136. Kronzon, I., Mitchell, J., Shapiro, J., Winer, H. E., and Newman, P.: Two-dimensional echocardiography in mitral annulus calcification. Am. J. Roentgenog. *134*:355, 1980.
137. Scott-Jupp, W., Barnett, N. L., Gallagher, P. J., Monro, J. L., and Ross, J. K.: Ultrastructural changes in spontaneous rupture of mitral chordae tendineae. J. Pathol. *133*:185, 1981.
138. Selzer, A., Kelly, J. J., Jr., Vannitamby, M., Walker, P., Gerbode, F., and Kerth, W. J.: The syndrome of mitral insufficiency due to isolated rupture of the chordae tendineae. Am. J. Med. *43*:822, 1967.
139. Luther, R. R., and Meyers, S. N.: Acute mitral insufficiency secondary to ruptured chordae tendineae. Arch. Intern. Med. *134*:568, 1974.
140. Caulfield, J. B., Page, D. L., Kastor, J. A., and Sanders, C. A.: Dissolution of connective tissue in ruptured chordae tendineae. Circulation *40*:57, 1969.
141. Godley, R. W., Wann, L. S., Rogers, E. W., Feigenbaum, H., and Weyman, A. E.: Incomplete mitral leaflet closure in patients with papillary muscle dysfunction. Circulation *63*:565, 1981.
142. Gallagher, P. J., Caves, P. K., and Stinson, E. B.: Pathological changes in spontaneous rupture of chordae tendineae. Ann. Cir. Gynaecol. *66*:135, 1977.
143. Burch, G. E., DePasquale, N. P., and Phillips, J. H.: The syndrome of papillary muscle dysfunction. Am. Heart J. *75*:399, 1968.
144. Estes, E. H., Jr., Dalton, F. M., Entman, M. L., et al.: The anatomy and blood supply of the papillary muscle of the left ventricle. Am. Heart J. *71*:356, 1966.
145. Gahl, K., Sutton, R., Pearson, M., Caspari, P., Lairet, A., and McDonald, L.: Mitral regurgitation in coronary heart disease. Br. Heart J. *39*:13, 1977.
146. Becker, A. E., and Anderson, R. H.: Mitral insufficiency complicating acute myocardial infarction. Eur. J. Cardiol. *2*:351, 1975.
147. Morrow, A. G., Cohen, L. S., Roberts, W. C., Braunwald, N. S., and Braunwald, E.: Severe mitral regurgitation following acute myocardial infarction and ruptured papillary muscle. Hemodynamic findings and results of operative treatment in four patients. Circulation *37*(Suppl. II):124, 1968.
148. Bulkley, B. H., and Roberts, W. C.: Dilatation of the mitral annulus. Am. J. Med. *59*:457, 1975.
149. Balu, V., Hershowitz, S., Masud, A. R. Z., Bhayana, J. N., and Dean, D. C.: Mitral regurgitation in coronary artery disease. Chest *81*:550, 1982.
150. Eckberg, D. L., Gault, J. H., Bouchard, R. L., Karliner, J. S., and Ross, J., Jr.: Mechanics of left ventricular contraction in chronic severe mitral regurgitation. Circulation *47*:1252, 1973.
151. Braunwald, E., Welch, G. H., Jr., and Sarnoff, S. J.: Hemodynamic effects of quantitatively varied experimental mitral regurgitation. Circ. Res. *5*:539, 1957.
152. Selzer, A., and Katayama, F.: Mitral regurgitation: Clinical patterns, pathophysiology and natural history. Medicine (Baltimore) *51*:337, 1972.
153. Pierpont, G. L., and Talley, R. C.: Pathophysiology of valvar heart disease. Arch. Intern. Med. *142*:998, 1982.
154. Yellin, E. L., Yoran, C., Sonnenblick, E. H., Gabbay, S., and Frater, R. W. M.: Dynamic changes in the canine mitral regurgitant orifice area during ventricular ejection. Circ. Res. *45*:677, 1979.
155. Yoran, C., Yellin, E. L., Becker, R. M., Gabbay, S., Frater, R. W. M., and Sonnenblick, E. H.: Dynamic aspects of acute mitral regurgitation: Effects of ventricular volume, pressure and contractility on the effective regurgitant orifice area. Circulation *60*:170, 1979.
156. Urschel, C. W., Covell, J. W., Sonnenblick, E. H., Ross, J., Jr., and Braunwald, E.: Myocardial mechanics in aortic and mitral valvular regurgitation: The concept of instantaneous impedance as a determinant of the performance of the intact heart. J. Clin. Invest. *47*:867, 1968.
157. Braunwald, E.: Mitral regurgitation: Physiological, clinical and surgical considerations. N. Engl. J. Med. *281*:425, 1969.
158. Urschel, C. W., Covell, J. W., Graham, T. P., Clancy, R. L., Ross, J., Jr., Sonnenblick, E. H., and Braunwald, E.: Effects of acute valvular regurgitation on the oxygen consumption of the canine heart. Circ. Res. *23*:33, 1968.
159. Braunwald, E.: Control of myocardial oxygen consumption: Physiologic and clinical considerations. Am. J. Cardiol. *27*:416, 1971.
160. Sasayama, S., Takahashi, M., Osakada, G., Hirose, K., Hamashima, H., Nishimura, E., and Kawai, C.: Dynamic geometry of the left atrium and left ventricle in acute mitral regurgitation. Circulation *60*:177, 1979.
161. Ross, J., Jr.: Left ventricular function and the timing of surgical treatment in valvular heart disease. Ann. Intern. Med. *94*:498, 1981.
162. Ronan, J. A., Jr., Steelman, R. B., DeLeon, A. C., Jr., Waters, T. J., Perloff, J. K., and Harvey, W. P.: The clinical diagnosis of acute severe mitral insufficiency. Am. J. Cardiol. *27*:284, 1971.
163. Vokonas, P. S., Gorlin, R., Cohn, P. F., Herman, M. V., and Sonnenblick, E. H.: Dynamic geometry of the left ventricle in mitral regurgitation. Circulation *48*:786, 1973.
164. Osbakken, M. D., Bove, A. A., and Spann, J. F.: Left ventricular regional wall motion and velocity of shortening in chronic mitral and aortic regurgitation. Am. J. Cardiol. *47*:1055, 1981.
165. Wong, C. Y. H., and Spotnitz, H. M.: Systolic and diastolic properties of the human left ventricle during valve replacement for chronic mitral regurgitation. Am. J. Cardiol. *47*:40, 1981.
166. Borow, K., Green, L. H., Mann, T., Sloss, L. J., Braunwald, E., Collins, J. J., Cohn, L., and Grossman, W.: End-systolic volume as a predictor of postoperative left ventricular performance in volume overload from valvular regurgitation. Am. J. Med. *68*:655, 1980.
167. Boucher, C. A., Bingham, J. B., Osbakken, M. D., Okada, R. D., Strauss, W. H., Block, P. C., Levine, F. H., Phillips, H. R., and Pohost, G. M.: Early changes in left ventricular size and function after correction of left ventricular volume overload. Am. J. Cardiol. *47*:991, 1981.
167a. Zile, M. R., Gaasch, W. H., Carroll, J. D., and Levine, H. J.: Chronic mitral regurgitation: Predictive value of preoperative echocardiographic indices of LV function and wall stress. J. Am. Coll. Cardiol. *1*:625, 1983 (Abstr.).
168. Peterson, C. R., Herr, R., Crisera, R. V., Starr, A., Bristow, D., and Griswold, H. E.: The failure of hemodynamic improvement after valve replacement surgery. Ann. Intern. Med. *66*:1, 1967.
169. Barnhorst, D. A., Oxman, H. A., Connolly, D. C., Pluth, J. R., Danielson, G. K., Wallace, R. B., and McGoon, D. C.: Long-term followup of isolated replacement of the aortic or mitral valve with the Starr-Edwards prosthesis. Am. J. Cardiol. *35*:228, 1975.
170. Konstam, M. A., Wynne, J., Holman, B. L., Brown, E. J., Neil, J. M., and Kozlowski, J.: Use of equilibrium (gated) radionuclide ventriculography to quantitate left ventricular output in patients with and without left-sided valvular regurgitation. Circulation *64*:578, 1981.
171. Braunwald, E., and Awe, W. C.: The syndrome of severe mitral regurgitation with normal left atrial pressure. Circulation *27*:29, 1963.
172. Roberts, W. C., Braunwald, E., and Morrow, A. G.: Acute severe mitral regurgitation secondary to ruptured chordae tendineae. Clinical, hemodynamic and pathologic considerations. Circulation *33*:58, 1966.
173. Cohen, L. S., Mason, D. T., and Braunwald, E.: Significance of an atrial gallop sound in mitral regurgitation: A clue to the diagnosis of ruptured chordae tendineae. Circulation *35*:112, 1966.
174. Kennedy, J. W., Baxley, W., and Dodge, H. T.: Hemodynamics of acute ruptured chordae tendineae. Circulation *34*:142, 1966.
175. Fowler, N. O.: Cardiac Diagnosis and Treatment. Hagerstown, Md., Harper and Row, 1980, pp. 541–660.
176. Allen, H., Harris, A., and Leatham, A.: Significance and prognosis of an isolated late systolic murmur. Br. Heart J. *36*:525, 1974.
177. Leatham, A., and Brigden, W.: Mild mitral regurgitation and the mitral prolapse fiasco. Am. Heart J. *99*:659, 1980.
178. Hammermeister, K. E., Fisher, L., Kennedy, J. W., Samuels, S., and Dodge, H. T.: Prediction of late survival in patients with mitral valve disease from clinical, hemodynamic, and quantitative angiographic variables. Circulation *57*:341, 1978.

179. Elkins, R. C., Morrow, A. G., Vasko, J. S., and Braunwald, E.: The effects of mitral regurgitation on the pattern of instantaneous aortic blood flow. Clinical and experimental observations. Circulation *36*:45, 1967.
180. Basta, L. L., Wolfson, P., Eckberg, D. L., and Abboud, F. M.: The value of left parasternal impulse recordings in the assessment of mitral regurgitation. Circulation *48*:1055, 1973.
181. Perloff, J. K., and Harvey, W. P.: Auscultatory and phonocardiographic manifestations of pure mitral regurgitation. Prog. Cardiovasc. Dis. *5*:172, 1962.
182. Karliner, J. S., O'Rourke, R. A., Kearney, D. J., and Shabetai, R.: Haemodynamic explanation of why the murmur of mitral regurgitation is independent of cycle length. Br. Heart J. *35*:397, 1973.
183. Aravanis, C.: Silent mitral insufficiency. Am. Heart J. *70*:620, 1965.
184. Dusall, J. C., Pryor, R., and Blount, S. G.: Systolic murmur following myocardial infarction. Am. Heart J. *87*:577, 1974.
185. Antman, E. M., Angoff, G. H., and Sloss, J. J.: Demonstration of the mechanism by which mitral regurgitation mimics aortic stenosis. Am. J. Cardiol. *42*:1044, 1978.
186. Merendino, K. A., and Hessel, E. A.: The murmur on top of the head in acquired mitral insufficiency. J.A.M.A. *199*:392, 1967.
187. Perloff, J. K.: Combined mitral stenosis and regurgitation: An auscultatory evaluation of their relative significance. *In* Segal, B., and Likoff, W. S. (eds.): The Theory and Practice of Auscultation. Philadelphia, F. A. Davis, 1964, p. 448.
188. Bentoviglio, L. G., Uricchio, J. F., Waldow, A., Likoff, W., and Goldberg, H.: An electrocardiographic analysis of mitral regurgitation. Circulation *18*:572, 1956.
189. Morris, J. J., Estes, E. H., Whalen, R. E., Thompson, H. K., and McIntosh, H. D.: P wave analysis in valvular heart disease. Circulation *29*:242, 1964.
190. Hamer, J.: The vectorcardiogram in mitral valve disease. Br. Heart J. *32*:149, 1970.
191. Priest, E. A., Finlayson, J. K., and Short, D. S.: The x-ray manifestations in the heart and lungs of mitral regurgitation. Prog. Cardiovasc. Dis. *5*:219, 1962.
192. Wexler, L., Silverman, J. F., DeBusk, R. F., and Harrison, D. C.: Angiographic features of rheumatic and nonrheumatic mitral regurgitation. Circulation *44*: 1080, 1971.
193. Mourant, A. J., Weaver, J., and Johnston, K.: Echocardiographic findings in rheumatic mitral valve disease with chordal rupture. J. Clin. Ultrasound *10*:79, 1982.
194. Kotler, M. N., Mintz, G. S., Parry, W. R., and Segal, B. L.: M-mode and two-dimensional echocardiography in mitral and aortic regurgitation: Pre- and postoperative evaluation of volume overload of the left ventricle. Am. J. Cardiol. *46*:1144, 1980.
195. Burgess, J., Clark, R., and Kamigaki, M.: Echocardiographic findings in different types of mitral regurgitation. Circulation *48*:97, 1973.
196. Sweatman, T., Selzer, A., Kamageki, M., and Cohn, K.: Echocardiographic diagnosis of mitral regurgitation due to ruptured chordae tendineae. Circulation *46*:580, 1972.
196a. Nair, C. K., Aronow, W. S., Sketch, M. H., Mohiuddin, S. M., Pagano, T., Esterbrooks, D. J., and Hee, T. T.: Clinicial and echocardiographic characteristics of patients with mitral annular clacification. Am. J. Cardiol. *51*:992, 1983.
197. Wann, L. S., Feigenbaum, H., Weyman, A. E., and Dillon, J. C.: Cross-sectional echocardiographic detection of rheumatic mitral regurgitation. Am. J. Cardiol. *41*:1258, 1978.
198. Child, J. S., Skorton, D. J., Taylor, R. D., Krivokapich, J., Abbasi, A. S., Wong, M., and Shah, P. D.: M-mode and cross-sectional echocardiographic features of flail posterior mitral leaflets. Am. J. Cardiol. *44*:1383, 1979.
199. Mintz, G. S., Kotler, M. N., Segal, B. L., and Parry, W. R.: Two-dimensional echocardiographic recognition of ruptured chordae tendineae. Circulation *57*: 244, 1978.
200. Abbasi, A. S., Allen, M. W., DeCristofaro, D., and Ungar, I.: Detection and estimation of the degree of mitral regurgitation by range-gated pulsed Doppler echocardiography. Circulation *61*:143, 1980.
201. Pearlman, A. S.: Assessing valvular regurgitation by pulsed Doppler echocardiography. J. Cardiovasc. Med. *6*:251, 1981.
201a. Patel, A. K., Rowe, G. G., Thomsen, J. H., Dhanani, S. P., Kosolcharoen, P. and Lyle, L.E.W.: Detection and estimation of rheumatic mitral regurgitation in the presence of mitral stenosis by pulsed Doppler echocardiography. Am. J. Cardiol. *51*:986, 1983.
202. Thompson, R., Ross, I., and Elmes, R.: Quantification of valvular regurgitation by cardiac gated pool imaging. Br. Heart J. *46*:629, 1981.
203. Boucher, C. A., Okada, R. D., and Pohost, G. M.: Current status of radionuclide imaging in valvular heart disease. Am. J. Cardiol. *46*:1153, 1980.
204. Greenberg, B. H., Massie, B. M., Brundage, B. H., Botvinick, E. H., Parmley, W. W., and Chatterjee, K.: Beneficial effects of hydralazine in severe mitral regurgitation. Circulation *58*:273, 1978.
205. Yoran, C., Yellin, E. L., Becker, R. M., Gabbay, S., Frater, R. W. M., and Sonnenblick, E. H.: Mechanism of reduction of mitral regurgitation with vasodilator therapy. Am. J. Cardiol. *43*:773, 1979.
206. Chopra, P. S., Rowe, G. G., Young, W. P., Loring, L. L., Hamann, R. C., and Kahn, D. R.: Carpentier ring annuloplasty in severe noncalcific mitral insufficiency. Arch. Surg. *112*:1469, 1977.
207. Kay, J. H., Zubiate, P., Mendez, M. A., Vanstrom, N., and Yokoyama, T.: Mitral valve repair for significant mitral insufficiency. Am. Heart J. *96*:253, 1978.
208. Spencer, F. C.: Acquired heart disease. *In* Schwartz, S. I., Shires, G. T., Spencer, F. C., and Storer, E. H. (eds.): Principles of Surgery. 2nd ed. New York, McGraw-Hill Book Co., 1979, p. 813.
209. Kay, J. H., Zubiate, P., Mendez, M. A., Vanstrom, N., Yokoyama, T., and Gharavi, M. A.: Surgical treatment of mitral insufficiency secondary to coronary artery disease. J. Thorac. Cardiovasc. Surg. *79*:12, 1980.
209a. Radley-Smith, R., and Yacoub, M. H.: Evaluation of long term results of valve conserving operations for severe mitral regurgitation in children. J. Am. Coll. Cardio. *1*:587, 1983 (Abstr.).
210. Dalby, A. J., Firth, B. G., and Forman, R.: Preoperative factors affecting the outcome of isolated mitral valve replacement: A 10 year review. Am. J. Cardiol. *47*:826, 1981.
211. Cohn, L. H., Mudge, G. H., Pratter, F., and Collins, J. J., Jr.: Five- to eight-year followup of patients undergoing porcine heart-valve replacement. N. Engl. J. Med. *304*:258, 1981.
212. Bonchek, L. I.: Current status of cardiac valve replacement: Selection of a prosthesis and indications for operation. Am. Heart J. *101*:96, 1981.
213. Phillips, H. R., Levine, F. H., Carter, J. E., Boucher, C. A., Osbakken, M. D., Okada, R. D., Akins, C. W., Daggett, W. M., Buckley, M. J., and Pohost, G. M.: Mitral valve replacement for isolated mitral regurgitation: Analysis of clinical course and late postoperative left ventricular ejection fraction. Am. J. Cardiol. *48*:647, 1981.
214. Jamieson, W. R. E., Thompson, D. M., and Munro, A. I.: Cardiac valve replacement in elderly patients. Can. Med. Assoc. J. *123*:628, 1980.
215. Cohn, L. H., Koster, J. K., VandeVanter, S., and Collins, J. J.: The in-hospital risk of rereplacement of dysfunctional mitral and aortic valves. Circulation *66* (Suppl. I):I–153, 1982.
216. Levitsky, S., Mammana, R. B., Silverman, N. A., Weber, F., Hiro, S., and Wright, R. N.: Acute endocarditis in drug addicts: Surgical treatment for gram-negative sepsis. Circulation *66*(Suppl. I):I–135, 1982.
217. Dinubile, M. J.: Surgery in active endocarditis. Ann. Intern. Med. *96*:650, 1982.
218. Schuler, G., Peterson, K. L., Johnson, A., Francis, G., Dennish, G., Utley, J. R., Dailey, P. O., Ashburn, W., and Ross, J., Jr.: Temporal response of left ventricular performance to mitral valve surgery. Circulation *59*:1218, 1979.
219. Gann, D., Colin, C., Hildner, F. J., Samet, P., Yahr, W. Z., Byrd, C., and Greenberg, J. J.: Mitral valve replacement in medically unresponsive congestive heart failure due to papillary muscle dysfunction. Circulation *56*(Suppl. II):101, 1977.
220. Fowler, N. O., and VanDerBel-Kahn, J. M.: Indications for surgical replacement of the mitral valve. With particular reference to common and uncommon causes of mitral regurgitation. Am. J. Cardiol. *44*:148, 1979.
221. Harken, D. E., Soroff, M. S., and Taylor, M. C.: Partial and complete prostheses in aortic insufficiency. J. Thorac. Cardiovasc. Surg. *40*:744, 1960.
222. Starr, A., and Edwards, M. L.: Mitral replacement: Clinical experience with a ball-valve prosthesis. Ann. Surg. *154*:726, 1961.
223. Teply, J. F., Grunkemeier, G. L., Sutherland, H. D'A., Lambert, L. E., Johnson, V. A., and Starr, A.: The ultimate prognosis after valve replacement: An assessment at twenty years. Ann. Thorac. Surg. *32*:111, 1981.
224. Fuster, V., Pumphrey, C. W., McGoon, M. D., Chesebro, J. H., Pluth, J. R., and McGoon, D. C.: Systemic thromboembolism in mitral and aortic Starr-Edwards prostheses: A 10- to 19-year followup. Circulation *66*(Suppl. I):I–157, 1982.
225. Björk, V. O.: A new tilting disc valve prosthesis. Scand. J. Thorac. Cardiovasc. Surg. *3*:1, 1969.
226. Zwart, H. H. J., Hicks, G., Schuster, B., Nathan, M., Tabrah, F., Wenzke, F., Ahmed, T., and DeWall, R. A.: Clinical experience with the Lillehei-Kaster valve prosthesis. Ann. Thorac. Surg. *28*:158, 1979.
227. Nicoloff, D. M., Emery, R. W., Arom, K. V., Northrup, W. F., Jorgensen, C. R., Wang, Y., and Lindsay, W. G.: Clinical and hemodynamic results with the St. Jude medical cardiac valve prosthesis. A three-year experience. J. Thorac. Cardiovasc. Surg. *82*:674, 1981.
228. Copans, H., Lakier, J. B., Kinsley, R. H., Colsen, P. R., Fritz, V. U., and Barlow, J. B.: Thrombosed Björk-Shiley mitral prostheses. Circulation *61*:169, 1980.
229. Edmunds, L. H., Jr.: Thromboembolic complications of current cardiac valvular prostheses. Ann. Thorac. Surg. *34*:96, 1981.
229a. Shattel, L.F.B.: The prevention of prosthetic valve thromboembolism. Uses and limitations of anti-platelet drugs. Int. J. Cardiol. *3*:87, 1983.
230. Ionescu, M. I.: Tissue Heart Valves. London, Butterworths, 1979.
231. Ross, D. N.: Homograft replacement of the aortic valve. Lancet *2*:487, 1962.
232. Barrett-Boyes, B. G., Roche, A. H. G., and Whitlock, R. M. L.: Six-year review of results of freehand aortic valve replacement using an antibiotic sterilized homograft valve. Circulation *55*:353, 1977.
233. Buch, S., Kosek, J. C., and Angell, W. W.: Deterioration of formalin-treated aortic heterografts. J. Thorac. Cardiovasc. Surg. *69*:673, 1970.
234. Carpentier, A., Lemaigre, G., and Robert, L.: Biological factors affecting long-term results of valvular heterografts. J. Thorac. Cardiovasc. Surg. *58*:467, 1969.
235. Reis, R. L., Hancock, W. D., Yarbrough, J. W., et al.: The flexible stent: A new concept in the fabrication of tissue heart valve prostheses. J. Thorac. Cardiovasc. Surg. *62*:683, 1971.
236. Ionescu, M. I., Tandon, A. P., Mary, D. A. S., et al.: Heart valve replacement with the Ionescu-Shiley pericardial xenograft. J. Thorac. Cardiovasc. Surg. *73*: 31, 1977.
237. Becker, R. M., Sandor, L., Tindel, M., and Frater, R. W. M.: Medium-term followup of the Ionescu-Shiley heterograft valve. Ann. Thorac. Surg. *32*:120, 1981.

238. Silverton, N. P., Tandon, A. P., and Ionescu, M. I.: Mitral valve replacement without long term anticoagulation using the Ionescu-Shiley pericardial xenograft. J. Am. Coll. Cardiol. *1*:700, 1983.
239. Puig, L. B., Verginelli, G., Iryia, K., et al.: Homologous dura mater cardiac valves. J. Thorac Cardiovasc. Surg. *69*:722, 1975.
240. Reitz, B. A., Stinson, E. B., Griepp, R. B., and Shumway, N. E.: Tissue valve replacement of prosthetic heart valves with thromboembolism. Am. J. Cardiol. *41*:512, 1978.
241. Cevese, P. G., Gallucci, V., Morea, M., Volta, S. D., Fasoli, G., and Casarotto, D.: Heart valve replacement with the Hancock Bioprosthesis. Analysis of long-term results. Circulation *56*(Suppl. II):111, 1976.
242. Oyer, P. E., Stinson, E. B., Reitz, B. A., Miller, D. C., Rossiter, S. J., and Shumway, N. E.: Long-term evaluation of the porcine xenograft bioprosthesis. J. Thorac. Cardiovasc. Surg. *78*:343, 1979.
243. DiSesa, V. J., Collins, J. J., Jr., and Cohn, L. H.: Mitral valve replacement with the porcine bioprosthesis. *In* Ionescu, M. I., and Cohn, L. H. (eds.): The Mitral Valve. London, Butterworths, 1983 (in press).
244. Angell, W. W., Angell, J. D., Sywak, A., and Kosek, J. C.: The tissue valve as a superior cardiac valve replacement. Surgery *82*:875, 1977.
244a. Janusz, M. T., Jamieson, W. R. E., Burr, L. H., Miyagishima, R. T., and Tyers, F. O.: Thromboembolic risks and role of anticoagulants in patients in chronic atrial fibrillation following mitral valve replacement with porcine bioprostheses. J. Am. Coll. Cardiol. *1*:587, 1983.
245. Hetzer, R., Hill, J. D., Kerth, W. J., Ansbro, J., Adappa, M. G., Rodvien, R., Kamm, B., and Gerbode, F.: Thromboembolic complications after mitral valve replacement with Hancock xenograft. J. Thorac. Cardiovasc. Surg. *75*:651, 1978.
246. Ubago, J. L., Figueroa, A., Colman, T., Ochoteco, A., and Duran, C. G.: Hemodynamic factors that affect calculated orifice areas in the mitral Hancock xenograft valve. Circulation *61*:388, 1980.
247. Rahimtoola, S.: The problem of valve prosthesis—patient mismatch. Circulation *58*:20, 1978.
248. Holen, J., H ie, J., and Semb, B.: Obstructive characteristics of Björk-Shiley, Hancock, and Lillehei-Kaster prosthetic mitral valves in the immediate postoperative period. Acta Med. Scand. *204*:5, 1978.
249. Hannah, H., and Reis, R. L.: Current status of porcine heterograft prostheses. Circulation *54*(Suppl. III):27, 1976.
250. Luri, A. J., Miller, R. R., Maxwell, K. S., Grehl, T. M., Vismara, L. A., Hurley, E. J., and Mason, D. T.: Hemodynamic assessment of the glutaraldehyde-preserved porcine heterograft in the aortic and mitral positions. Circulation *56* (Suppl. II):104, 1977.
251. Roberts, W. C.: Complications of cardiac valve replacement: Characteristic abnormalities of prostheses pertaining to any specific site. Am. Heart J. *103*: 113, 1982.
252. Kirklin, J. W.: The replacement of cardiac valves. N. Engl. J. Med. *304*:291, 1981.
252a. Schoen, F. J., Collins, J. J., Jr., and Cohn, L. W.: Long-term failure rate and morphologic correlations in porcine bioprosthetic heart valves. Am. J. Cardiol. *51*:957, 1983.
253. Miller, D. C., Stinson, E. B., Oyer, P. E., Billingham, M. E., Pitlick, P. T., Reitz, B. A., Jamieson, S. W., Baumgartner, W. A., and Shumway, N. E.: The durability of porcine xenograft valves and conduits in children. Circulation *66* (Suppl. I): I–172, 1982.
254. Attie, F., Kuri, J., Zanoniani, C., Renteria, V., Buendia, A., Ovseyevitz, J., Lopez-Soriano, F., Garcia-Cornejo, M., and Martinez-Rios, M. A.: Mitral valve replacement in children with rheumatic heart disease. Circulation *64*:812, 1981.
255. Taguchi, K.: Pregnancy in patients with a prosthetic heart valve. Surg. Gynecol. Obstet. *145*:206, 1977. Managing pregnant patients with a heart valve prosthesis. Contemp. Ob. Gyn. *11*:82, 1978.
256. Harrison, E. C., Roschke, J., Ferenczi, G., and Mitani, G. H.: Managing Pregnant Patients with a heart valve prosthesis. Contemp. Obstet. Gynecol. *11*:82, 1978.
257. Oakley, C., and Doherty, P.: Pregnancy in patients after valve replacement. Br. Heart J. *38*:1140, 1976.
258. Limet, R., and Grondin, C. M.: Cardiac valve prostheses, anticoagulation and pregnancy. Ann. Thorac. Surg. *23*:337, 1977.
259. Spray, T. L., and Roberts, W. C.: Structural changes in porcine xenografts used as substitute cardiac valves. Gross and histologic observations in 51 glutaraldehyde-preserved Hancock valves in 41 patients. Am. J. Cardiol. *40*:319, 1977.
260. Fishbein, M. C., Gissen, S. A., Collins, J. J., Jr., Barsamian, E. M., and Cohn, L. H.: Pathologic findings after cardiac valve replacement with glutaraldehyde-fixed porcine valves. Am. J. Cardiol. *40*:331, 1977.
261. Rose, A. G., Forman, R., and Bowen, R. M.: Calcification of glutaraldehyde-fixed porcine xenograft. Thorax *33*:111, 1978.
262. Thandroyen et al.: Severe calcification of glutaraldehyde preserved porcine xenografts. Am. J. Cardiol. *45*:1980.
263. Smith, N. D., Raizada, V., and Abrams, J.: Auscultation of the normally functioning prosthetic valve. Ann. Intern. Med. *95*:594, 1981.
264. Cunha, C. L. P., Giuliani, E. R., Callahan, J. A., and Pluth, J. R.: Echophonocardiographic findings in patients with prosthetic heart valve malfunction. Mayo Clin. Proc. *55*:231, 1980.
265. Stein, P. D., Sabbah, H. N., Lakier, J. B., Magilligan, D. J., Jr., and Goldstein, S.: Frequency of the first heart sound in the assessment of stiffening of mitral bioprosthetic valves. Circulation *63*:200, 1981.
266. Morris, D. C.: Management of patients with prosthetic heart valves. Curr. Probl. Cardiol. *7*: Aug., 1982.
267. Griffiths, B. E., Charles, R., and Coulshed, N.: Echophonocardiography in diagnosis of mitral paravalvular regurgitation with Bjork-Shiley prosthetic valve. Br. Heart J. *43*:325, 1980.
268. Schapira, J. N., Martin, R. P., Fowles, R. E., Rakowski, H., Stinson, E. B., French, J. W., Shumway, N. E., and Popp, R. O.: Two-dimensional echocardiographic assessment of patients with bioprosthetic valves. Am. J. Cardiol. *43*:510, 1979.
269. Alam, M., Madrazo, A. C., Magilligan, D. J., and Goldstein, S.: M-mode and two dimensional echocardiographic features of porcine valve dysfunction. Am. J. Cardiol. *43*:502, 1979.

MITRAL VALVE PROLAPSE

270. Cheitlin, M. D.: Mitral valve prolapse. Circulation *59*:610, 1979.
271. Abrams, J.: Mitral valve prolapse: A plea for unanimity. Am. Heart J. *92*:413, 1976.
272. Barlow, J. B., and Pocock, W. A.: Mitral valve prolapse, the specific billowing mitral leaflet syndrome, or an insignificant non-ejection systolic click. Am. Heart J. *97*:277, 1979.
273. Lucas, R. V., and Edwards, J. E.: The floppy mitral valve. Curr. Probl. Cardiol. *7*: July, 1982.
274. Jeresaty, R. M.: Mitral Valve Prolapse. New York, Raven Press, 1979, 251 pp.
274a. Chesler, E., King, R. A., and Edwards, J. E.: The myxomatous mitral valve and sudden death. Circulation *67*:632, 1983.
275. Devereaux, R. B., Perloff, J. K., Reichek, N., and Josephson, M. D.: Mitral valve prolapse. Circulation *54*:3, 1976.
276. Procacci, P. M., Savran, S. V., Schreiter, S. L., and Bryson, A. L.: Prevalence of clinical mitral valve prolapse in 1,169 young women. N. Engl. J. Med. *294*: 1086, 1976.
277. Markiewicz, W., Stoner, J., London, E., Hunt, S. A., and Popp, R. L.: Mitral valve prolapse in one hundred presumably healthy young females. Circulation *53*:464, 1976.
278. Reid, J. V.: Mid-systolic clicks. S. Afr. Med. J. *35*:353, 1961.
279. Barlow, J. B., Pocock, W. A., Marchand, P., and Denny, M.: The significance of the late systolic murmurs. Am. Heart J. *66*:443, 1963.
280. Olsen, E. G. J., and Al-Rufaie, H. K.: The floppy mitral valve. Study on pathogenesis. Br. Heart J. *44*:674, 1980.
280a. Pyeritz, R. E., and Wappel, M. A.: Mitral valve dysfunction in the Marfan syndrome. Am. J. Med. *74*:797, 1983.
281. Davies, M. J., Moore, B. P., and Braimbridge, M. V.: The floppy mitral valve. Study of incidence, pathology and complications in surgical, necropsy and forensic material. Br. Heart J. *40*:368, 1978.
282. Jaffe, A. S., Geltman, E. M., Rodey, G. E., and Uitto, J.: Mitral valve prolapse: A consistent manifestation of Type IV Ehlers-Danlos syndrome. The pathogenetic role of the abnormal production of Type III collagen. Circulation *64*:121, 1981.
283. King, B. D., Clark, M. A., Baba, N., Kilman, J. W., and Wooley, C. F.: "Myxomatous" mitral valves: Collagen dissolution as the primary defect. Circulation *66*:288, 1982.
284. Hammer, D., Leier, C. V., Baba, N., Vasko, J. S., Wooley, C. F., and Pinnell, S. R.: Altered collagen composition in a prolapsing mitral valve with ruptured chordae tendineae. Am. J. Med. *67*:863, 1979.
285. Gravanis, M. B., and Campbell, W. G., Jr.: The syndrome of prolapse of the mitral valve. Arch. Pathol. Lab. Med. *106*:369, 1982.
286. Child, J. S., Cabeen, W. R., Jr., and Roberts, N. K.: Mitral valve prolapse complicated by ruptured chordae tendineae. West. J. Med. *129*:160, 1978.
287. Malcolm, A. D., Chayen, J., Cankovic-Darracott, S., Jenkins, B. S., and Webb-Peploe, M. M.: Biopsy evidence of left ventricular myocardial abnormality in patients with mitral leaflet prolapse and chest pain. Lancet *1*:1052, 1979.
288. Malcolm, A. D.: Myocardial mysteries surrounding mitral leaflet prolapse. Am. Heart J. *100*:265, 1980.
289. Rizzon, P., Biasco, G., Brindicei, G., and Mauro, F.: Familial syndrome of midsystolic click and late systolic murmur. Br. Heart J. *35*:245, 1973.
290. O'Rourke, R. A., and Crawford, M. H.: The systolic click-murmur syndrome: Clinical recognition and management. Curr. Probl. Cardiol. *1*:1–60, 1976.
291. Cabeen, W. R., Jr., Reza, M. J., Kovick, R. B., and Stern, M. S.: Mitral valve prolapse and conduction defects in Ehlers-Danlos syndrome. Arch. Intern. Med. *137*:1227, 1977.
292. Lebwohl, M. G., Distefano, D., Prioleau, P. G., Uram, M., Yannuzzi, L. A., and Fleischmajer, R.: Pseudoxanthoma elasticum and mitral valve prolapse. N. Engl. J. Med. *307*:228, 1982.
293. Strasberg, B., Kanakis, C., Dhingra, R. C., and Rosen, K. M.: Myotonia dystrophica and mitral valve prolapse. Chest *78*:845, 1980.
294. Sanyal, S. K., Johnson, W. W., Dische, M. R., Pitner, S. E., and Beard, C.: Dystrophic degeneration of papillary muscle and ventricular myocardium. A basic for mitral valve prolapse in Duchenne's muscular dystrophy. Circulation *62*:430, 1980.
295. Mason, J. W., Koch, F. H., Billingham, M. E., and Winkle, R. A.: Cardiac biopsy evidence for a cardiomyopathy associated with symptomatic mitral valve prolapse. Am. J. Cardiol. *42*:557, 1978.
296. Pickering, N. J., Brody, J. I., and Barrett, M. J.: Von Willebrand syndrome and mitral valve prolapse. Linked mesenchymal dysplasias. N. Engl. J. Med. *305*:131, 1981.

297. Beardsley, T. L., and Foulks, G. N.: An association of keratoconus and mitral valve prolapse. Ophthalmology *89*:35, 1982.
298. Channick, B. J., Adlin, E. V., Marks, A. D., et al.: Hyperthyroidism and mitral valve prolapse. N. Engl. J. Med. *305*:497, 1981.
299. Jeresaty, R. M.: Mitral valve prolapse–click syndrome in atrial septal defect. Chest *67*:132, 1975.
300. Somerville, J., Kaku, S., and Saravalli, O.: Prolapsed mitral cusps in atrial septal defect. An erroneous radiological interpretation. Br. Heart J. *40*:58, 1978.
301. Rippe, J. M., Sloss, J. J., Angoff, G., and Alpert, J. S.: Mitral valve prolapse in adults with congenital heart disease. Am. Heart J. *97*:561, 1979.
302. Zema, M. J., Chiaramida, S., DeFilipp, G. J., Goldman, M. A., and Pizzarello, R. A.: Somatotype and idiopathic mitral valve prolapse. Cathet. Cardiovasc. Diagn. *8*:105, 1982.
303. Udoshi, M. B., Shah, A., Fisher, V. J., and Dolgin, M.: Incidence of mitral valve prolapse in subjects with thoracic skeletal abnormalities—A prospective study. Am. Heart J. *97*:303, 1979.
304. Bon Tempo, C. P., Ronan, J. A., Jr., de Leon, A. C., Jr., and Twigg, H. L.: Radiographic appearance of the thorax in systolic click-late systolic murmur syndrome. Am. J. Cardiol. *36*:27, 1975.
305. Weinrauch, L. A., McDonald, D. G., DeSilva, R. A., Hawkins, E. T., Leland, O. S., and Shubrooks, S. J., Jr.,: Mitral valve prolapse in rheumatic mitral stenosis. Chest *72*:752, 1977.
306. Gottdiener, J. S., Sherber, H. S., and Harvey, W. P.: Mid-systolic click and mitral valve prolapse following mitral commissurotomy. Am. J. Med. *64*:295, 1978.
307. Barlow, J. B., Pocock, W. A., and Obel, I. W. P.: Mitral valve prolapse: Primary, secondary, both or neither? Am. Heart J. *102*:140, 1981.
308. Crawford, M. H.: Mitral valve prolapse due to coronary artery disease. Am. J. Med. *62*:447, 1977.
309. Chesler, E., Matisonn, R. E., Lakier, J. B., Pocock, W. A., Obel, I. W. P., and Barlow, J. B.: Acute myocardial infarction with normal coronary arteries. A possible manifestation of the billowing mitral leaflet syndrome. Circulation *54*: 203, 1976.
310. Imaizumi, T., Chandraratna, P. A. N., Whayne, T. F., Jr., Schechter, E., and Bhatia, S. K.: Transmural myocardial infarction. With the prolapsing mitral-leaflet syndrome and normal coronary arteries. Arch. Intern. Med. *138*:1354, 1978.
311. Tutassaura, H., Gerein, A. N., and Miyagishima, R. T.: Mucoid degeneration of the mitral valve. Clinical review, surgical management and results. Am. J. Surg. *132*:276, 1976.
312. Brown, O. R., DeMots, H., Kloster, F. E., Roberts, A., Menashe, V. D., and Beals, R. K.: Aortic root dilatation and mitral valve prolapse in Marfan's syndrome. Circulation *52*:651, 1975.
313. Guy, F. C., MacDonald, R. P. R., Fraser, D. B., and Smith, E. R.: Mitral valve prolapse as a cause of hemodynamically important mitral regurgitation. Can. J. Surg. *23*:166, 1980.
314. Goghlan, H. C., Phares, P., Cowley, M., Copley, D., and James, T. N.: Dysautonomia in mitral valve prolapse. Am. J. Med. *67*:236, 1979.
315. Gaffney, F. A., Karlsson, E. S., Campbell, W., Schutte, J. E., Nixon, J. V., Willerson, J. T., and Blomqvist, C. G.: Autonomic dysfunction in women with mitral valve prolapse syndrome. Circulation *59*:894, 1979.
316. Boudoulas, H., Reynolds, J. C., Mazzaferri, E., and Wooley, C. F.: Metabolic studies in mitral valve prolapse syndrome. A neuroendocrine-cardiovascular process. Circulation *61*:1200, 1980.
316a. Puddu, P. E., Pasternac, A., Tubau, J. F., Krol, R., Farley, L., and de Champlain, J.: QT Interval prolongation and increased plasma catecholamine levels in patients with mitral valve prolapse. Am. Heart J. *105*:422, 1983.
317. Leor, R., and Markiewicz, W.: Neurocirculatory asthenia and mitral valve prolapse—Two unrelated entities? Isr. J. Med. Sci. *17*:1137, 1981.
318. Tei, C., Shah, P. M., Cherian, G., Wong, M., and Ormiston, J. A.: The correlates of an abnormal first heart sound in mitral valve prolapse syndromes. N. Engl. J. Med. *307*:334, 1982.
319. Alexander, M. D., Bloom, K. R., Hart, P., D'Silva, F., and Murgo, J. P.: Atrial septal aneurysm: A cause of midsystolic click. Report of a case and review of the literature. Circulation *63*:1186, 1981.
320. Wei, J. Y., and Fortuin, N. J.: Diastolic sounds and murmurs associated with mitral valve prolapse. Circulation *63*:559, 1981.
321. Delman, A. J., and Stein, E.: Mitral valve prolapse. *In* Dynamic Cardiac Auscultation and Phonocardiography. Philadelphia, W. B. Saunders Co., 1979, p. 888.
322. Liedtke, A. J., Gault, J. H., Leaman, D. M., and Blumenthal, M. S.: Geometry of left ventricular contraction in the systolic click syndrome. Circulation *47*:27, 1973.
323. Towne, W. D., Patel, R., Cruz, J., Kramer, N., and Chawla, K. K.: Effects of gravitational stresses on mitral valve prolapse. I. Changes in auscultatory findings produced by progressive passive head-up tilt. Br. Heart J. *40*:482, 1978.
324. Winkle, R. A., Goodman, D. J., and Popp, R. L.: Simultaneous echocardiographic-phonocardiographic recordings at rest and during amyl nitrite administration in patients with mitral valve prolapse. Circulation *51*: 522, 1975.
325. Combs, R. L., Shah, P. M., Klorman, R. S., and Klorman, R.: Effects of induced psychological stress on click and rhythm in mitral valve prolapse. Am. Heart J. *99*:714, 1980.
326. Braunwald, E., Oldham, H. N., Jr., Ross, J., Jr., Linhart, J. W., Mason, D. T., and Fort, L., III: The circulatory response of patients with idiopathic hypertrophic subaortic stenosis to nitroglycerin and to the Valsalva maneuver. Circulation *29*:422, 1964.
327. Swartz, M. H., Teichholz, L. E., and Donoso, E.: Mitral valve prolapse. A review of associated arrhythmias. Am. J. Med. *62*:377, 1977.
328. Josephson, M. E., Horowitz, L. N., and Kastor, J. A.: Proximal supraventricular tachycardia in patients with mitral valve prolapse. Circulation *57*: 111, 1978.
329. Wei, J. Y., Bulkley, B. H., Schaeffer, A. H., Greene, H. L., and Reid, P. R.: Mitral valve prolapse syndrome and recurrent ventricular tachyarrhythmias. Ann. Intern. Med. *89*:6, 1978.
330. Bharati, S., Granston, A. S., Liebson, P. R., Loeb, H. S., Rosen, K. M., and Lev, M.: The conduction system in mitral valve prolapse syndrome with sudden death. Am. Heart J. *101*:667, 1981.
331. Ritchie, J. L., Hammermeister, K. E., and Kennedy, J. W.: Refractory ventricular tachycardia and fibrillation in a patient with prolapsing mitral leaflet syndrome: Successful control with overdrive pacing. Am. J. Cardiol. *37*: 314, 1976.
332. Winkle, R. A., Lopes, M. G., Popp, R. L., and Hancock, E. W.: Life-threatening arrhythmias with mitral valve prolapse syndrome. Am. J. Med. *60*: 961, 1976.
332a. Hochreiter, C., Kramer, H. M., Kligfield, P., Kramer-Fox, R., Devereaux, R. B., and Borer, J. S.: Arrhythmias in mitral valve prolapse. Effect of additional mitral regurgitation. J. Am. Coll. Cardiol. *1*:607, 1983 (Abstr.).
333. Gelfand, M. L., and Kloth, H.: Bradyarrhythmia in mitral valve prolapse treated with a pacemaker. Bull. N. Y. Acad. Med. *54*:889, 1978.
334. Wit, A. L., Fenoglio, J. J., Wagner, B. M., and Bassett, A. L.: Electrophysiological properties of cardiac muscle in the anterior mitral valve leaflet and the adjacent atrium in the dog. Possible implications for the genesis of atrial dysrhythmias. Circ. Res. *32*:731, 1973.
335. Perloff, J. K.: Evolving concepts of mitral valve prolapse. N. Engl. J. Med. *307*:369, 1982.
336. Wit, A. L., Fenoglio, J. J., Hordof, A. J., and Reemtsma, K.: Ultrastructure and transmembrane potentials of cardiac muscle in the human anterior mitral valve leaflet. Circulation *59*:1283, 1979.
337. Campbell, R. W. F., Godman, M. G., Fiddler, G. I., Marquis, R., and Julian, D. G.: Ventricular arrhythmias in syndrome of balloon deformity of mitral valve. Definition of possible high risk group. Br. Heart J. *38*:1053, 1976.
338. Gallagher, J. J., Gilbert, M., and Svenson, R. H.: Wolff-Parkinson-White syndrome. The problem, evaluation and surgical correction. Circulation *57*: 767, 1975.
339. Bekheit, S. G., Ali, A. A., Deglin, S. M., and Jain, A. C.: Analysis of QT interval in patients with idiopathic mitral valve prolapse. Chest *81*:620, 1982.
340. Jeresaty, R. M.: Sudden death in the mitral valve prolapse–click syndrome. Am. J. Cardiol. *37*:317, 1976.
341. Woodley, D., Chambers, W., Starke, H., Dzindzio, B., and Forker, A. D.: Intermittent complete atrioventricular block masquerading as epilepsy in the mitral valve prolapse syndrome. Chest *72*:369, 1977.
342. Leichtman, D., Nelson, R., Gobel, F. L., Alexander, C. S., and Cohn, J. N.: Bradycardia with mitral valve prolapse. A potential mechanism of sudden death. Ann. Intern. Med. *85*:453, 1976.
343. Popp, R. L., Brown, O. R., Silverman, J. F., and Harrison, D. C.: Echocardiographic abnormalities in the mitral valve prolapse syndrome. Circulation *49*:428, 1974.
344. Weiss, A. N., Mimbs, J. W., Ludbrook, P. A., and Sobel, B. E.: Echocardiographic detection of mitral valve prolapse. Circulation *52*:1091, 1975.
345. Morganroth, J., Jones, R. H., Chen, C. C., and Naito, M.: Two-dimensional echocardiography in mitral, aortic and tricuspid valve prolapse. The clinical problem, cardiac nuclear imaging considerations and a proposed standard for diagnosis. Am. J. Cardiol. *46*:1164, 1980.
346. Morganroth, J., Mardelli, T. J., Naito, M., and Chen, C. C.: Apical cross-sectional echocardiography. Standard for the diagnosis of idiopathic mitral valve prolapse syndrome. Chest *79*:23, 1981.
347. Sahn, D. J., Wood, J., Allen, H. D., Peoples, W., and Goldberg, S. J.: Echocardiographic spectrum of mitral valve motion in children with and without mitral valve prolapse: The nature of false positive diagnosis. Am. J. Cardiol. *39*:422, 1977.
348. DeMaria, A. N., Neumann, A., Lee, G., and Mason, D. T.: Echocardiographic identification of the mitral valve prolapse syndrome. Am. J. Med. *62*:819,1977.
349. Ogawa, S., Hayashi, J., Sasaki, H., Tani, M., Akaishi, M., Mitamura, H., Sano, M., Hoshino, T., Handa, S., and Nakamura, Y.: Evaluation of combined valvular prolapse syndrome of two-dimensional echocardiography. Circulation *65*:174, 1982.
350. Gooch, A. S., Maranhao, V., Scampardonis, G., Cha, S. D., and Yang, S. S.: Prolapse of both mitral and tricuspid leaflets in systolic murmur–click syndrome. N. Engl. J. Med. *287*:1218, 1972.
351. Rodger, J. C., and Morley, P.: Abnormal aortic valve echoes in mitral prolapse. Echocardiographic features of floppy aortic valve. Br. Heart. J. *47*: 337, 1982.
352. Klein, G. J., Kostuk, W. J., Boughner, D. R., and Chamberlain, M. J.: Stress myocardial imaging in mitral leaflet prolapse syndrome. Am. J. Cardiol. *42*: 746, 1978.
353. Butman, S., Chandraratna, P. A. N., Milne, N., Olson, H., Lyons, K., and Aronow, W. S.: Stress myocardial imaging in patients with mitral valve prolapse: Evidence of a perfusion abnormality. Cathet. Cardiovasc. Diagn. *8*: 243, 1982.

354. Scampardonis, G., Yang, S. S., Maranhao, V., Goldberg, H., and Booch, A. S.: Left ventricular abnormalities in prolapsed mitral leaflet syndrome. Review of eighty-seven cases. Circulation *48*:287, 1973.
355. Ranganathan, N., Silver, M. D., Robinson, T. I., and Wilson, J. K.: Idiopathic prolapse mitral leaflet syndrome. Angiographic-clinical correlations. Circulation *54*:707, 1976.
356. Cohen, M. V., Shah, P. K., and Spindola-Franco, H.: Angiographic-echocardiographic correlation of mitral valve prolapse. Am. Heart J. *97*:43, 1979.
357. Cipriano, P. R., Kline, S. A., and Baltaxe, H. A.: An angiographic assessment of left ventricular function in isolated mitral valvular prolapse. Invest. Radiol. *15*:293, 1980.
358. Gottdiener, J. S., Borer, J. S., Bacharach, S. L., Green, M. V., and Epstein, S. E.: Left ventricular function in mitral valve prolapse: Assessment with radionuclide cineangiography. Am. J. Cardiol. *47*:7, 1981.
359. Bisset, G. S., III, Schwartz, D. C., Meyer, R. A., James, F. W., and Kaplan, S.: Clinical spectrum and long-term followup of isolated mitral valve prolapse in 119 children. Circulation *62*:423, 1980.
360. Bisset, G. S., III: Mitral valve prolapse in children. Primary Cardiol. *8*:71, 1982.
361. Mills, P., Rose, J., Hollingsworth, J., Amara, I., and Craige, E.: Long-term prognosis of mitral valve prolapse. N. Engl. J. Med. *297*:13, 1977.
362. Corrigall, D., and Popp, R.: Mitral valve prolapse and infective endocarditis. Am. J. Med. *63*:215, 1977.
363. Tresch, D. D., Siegel, R., Keelan, M. H., Jr., Gross, C. M., and Brooks, H. L.: Mitral valve prolapse in the elderly. J. Am. Geriatr. Soc. *27*:421, 1979.
364. Barnett, H. J. M., Boughner, D. R., Taylor, D. W., Cooper, P. E., Kostuk, W. J., and Nichol, P. M.: Further evidence relating mitral-valve prolapse to cerebral ischemic events. N. Engl. J. Med. *302*:139, 1980.
365. Caltrider, N. D., Irvine, A. R., Kline, H. J., and Rosenblatt, A.: Retinal emboli in patients with mitral valve prolapse. Am. J. Ophthalmol. *90*:534, 1980.
366. Walsh, P. N., Kansu, T. A., Corbett, J. J., Savino, P. J., Goldburgh, W. P., and Schatz, N. J.: Platelets, thromboembolism and mitral valve prolapse. Circulation *63*:552, 1981.
367. Hanson, M. R., Conomy, J. P., and Hodgman, J. R.: Brain events associated with mitral valve prolapse. Stroke *11*:499, 1980.
368. Cheitlin, M. D.: Thromboembolic studies in the patient with the prolapsed mitral valve. Has Salome dropped another veil? Circulation *60*:46, 1979.
368a. Schnee, M. A., and Bucal, A. A.: Fatal embolism in mitral valve prolapse. Chest *83*:285, 1983.
368b. Makino, H., and Al-Sadir, J.: Myocardial infarction in patients with mitral valve prolapse and normal coronary arteries. J. Am. Coll. Cardiol. *1*:661, 1983.
369. Troup, P. J., and Zipes, D. P.: Aprindine treatment of recurrent ventricular tachycardia in patients with mitral valve prolapse. Am. Heart J. *97*:322, 1979.
370. Winkle, R. A., and Harrison, D.: Propranolol for patients with mitral valve prolapse. Am. Heart J. *93*:422, 1977.

AORTIC STENOSIS

371. Roberts, W. C.: Valvular, subvalvular and supravalvular aortic stenosis. Morphologic features. Cardiovasc. Clin. *5*:97, 1973.
372. Roberts, W. C.: Anatomically isolated aortic valvular disease. The case against its being of rheumatic origin. Am. J. Med. *49*:151, 1970.
373. Roberts, W. C.: The congenitally bicuspid aortic valve. A study of 85 autopsy cases. Am. J. Cardiol. *26*:72, 1970.
374. Roberts, W. C., Perloff, J. K., and Constantino, T.: Severe valvular aortic stenosis in patients over 65 years of age. A clinicopathologic study. Am. J. Cardiol. *27*:497, 1971.
375. Roberts, W. C., and Morrow, A. G.: Congenital aortic stenosis produced by a unicommissural valve. Br. Heart J. *27*:505, 1965.
376. Moller, J. H., Nakib, A., Elliott, R. S., and Edwards, J. E.: Symptomatic congenital aortic stenosis in the first year of life. J. Pediatr. *67*:728, 1966.
377. Fenoglio, J. J., Jr., McAllister, H. A., Jr., DeCastro, C. M., Davis, J. E., and Cheitlin, M. D.: Congenital bicuspid aortic valve after age 20. Am. J. Cardiol. *29*:164, 1977.
378. Mills, P., Leech, G., Davies, M., and Leatham, A.: The natural history of a non-stenotic bicuspid aortic valve. Br. Heart J. *40*:951, 1978.
379. Emanuel, R., Withers, R., O'Brien, K., Ross, P., and Feizi, O.: Congenitally bicuspid aortic valves. Clinicogenetic study of 41 families. Br. Heart J. *40*:1402, 1978.
380. Braunwald, E., Goldblatt, A., Aygen, M. M., Rockoff, S. D., and Morrow, A. G.: Congenital aortic stenosis: Clinical and hemodynamic findings in 100 patients. Circulation *27*:426, 1963.
381. Narang, N. K., Andrew, A. M. R., Chaudhury, H. R., and Gaba, B. S.: Aortic stenosis due to familial hypercholesterolemic xanthomatosis. A case report with brief review of literature. Indian Heart J. *30*:189, 1978.
382. Gould, L., Reddy, C. V. R., DePalma, D., DeMartino, A., and Kalish, P. E.: Cardiac manifestations of ochronosis. J. Thorac. Cardiovasc. Surg. *72*:788, 1976.
383. Kennedy, J. W., Twiss, R. D., Blackmon, J. R., et al.: Quantitative angiocardiography. III. Relationships of left ventricular pressure volume and mass in aortic valve disease. Circulation *38*:838, 1968.
384. Carabello, B. A., Mee, R., Collins, J. J., Jr., Kloner, R. A., Levin, D., and Grossman, W.: Contractile function in chronic gradually developing subcoronary aortic stenosis. Am. J. Physiol. *240*:H80, 1981.
385. Morrow, A. G., Roberts, W. C., Ross, J., Jr., Fisher, D. R., Behrendt, D. M., Mason, D. T., and Braunwald, E.: Clinical staff conference. Obstruction to left ventricular outflow. Current concepts of management and operative treatment. Ann. Intern. Med. *69*:1255, 1968.
386. Braunwald, E., and Frahm, C. J.: Studies on Starling's law of the heart. IV. Observations on the hemodynamic functions of the left atrium in man. Circulation *24*:633, 1961.
387. Sasayama, S., Ross, J., Jr., Franklin, D., Bloor, C. M., Bishop, S., and Dilley, R. B.: Adaptations of the left ventricle to chronic pressure overload. Circ. Res. *38*:172, 1976.
388. Gunther, S., and Grossman, W.: Determinants of ventricular function in pressure overload hypertrophy in man. Circulation *59*:679, 1979.
389. Ross, J., Jr.: Afterload mismatch and preload reserve: A conceptual framework for the analysis of ventricular function. Prog. Cardiovasc. Dis. *18*:255, 1976.
389a. Donner, R., Carabello, B. A., Black, I., and Spann, J. F.: Left ventricular wall stress in compensated aortic stenosis in children. Am. J. Cardiol. *51*:946, 1983.
389b. DePace, N. L., Ren, J-F., Iskandrian, A. S., Kotler, M. N., Hakki, A-H., and Segal, B. L.: Correlation of echocardiographic wall stress and left ventricular pressure and function in aortic stenosis. Circulation *67*:854, 1983.
390. Fifer, M. A., Gunther, S., Grossman, W., Mirsky, I., Carabello, B., and Barry, W. H.: Myocardial contractile function in aortic stenosis as determined from the rate of stress development during isovolumic systole. Am. J. Cardiol. *44*: 1318, 1979.
391. Carabello, B. A., Green, L. H., Grossman, W., Cohn, L. H., Koster, J. K., and Collins, J. J., Jr.: Hemodynamic determinants of prognosis of aortic valve replacement in critical aortic stenosis and advanced congestive heart failure. Circulation *62*:42, 1980.
392. Huber, D., Grimm, J., Koch, R., and Krayenbuehl, H. P.: Determinants of ejection performance in aortic stenosis. Circulation *64*:126, 1981.
393. Johnson, A. D., Engler, R. L., LeWinter, M., Karliner, J., Peterson, K., Tauji, I. J., and Daily, P. O.: The medical and surgical management of patients with aortic valve disease. A Symposium. West. J. Med. *126*:460, 1977.
394. Peterson, K. J., Tsuji, J., Johnson, A., DiDonna, J., and LeWinter, M.: Diastolic left ventricular pressure-volume and stress-strain relations in patients with valvular aortic stenosis and left ventricular hypertrophy. Circulation *58*: 77, 1978.
395. Schwarz, F., Flameng, W., Schaper, J., Langebartels, F., Sesto, M., Hehrlein, F., and Schlepper, M.: Myocardial structure and function in patients with aortic valve disease and their relation to postoperative results. Am. J. Cardiol. *41*: 661, 1978.
396. Bertrand, M. E., LaBlanche, J. M., Tilmant, P. Y., Thieuleux, F. P., Delforge, M. R., and Carre, A. G.: Coronary sinus blood flow at rest and during isometric exercise in patients with aortic valve disease. Mechanism of angina pectoris in presence of normal coronary arteries. Am. J. Cardiol. *47*:199, 1981.
397. Vinten-Johansen, J., and Weiss, H. R.: Oxygen consumption in subepicardial and subendocardial regions of the canine left ventricle—The effect of experimental acute valvular aortic stenosis. Circ. Res. *46*:139, 1980.
398. Hakki, A.-H., Kimbiris, D., Iskandrian, A. S., Segal, B. L., Mintz, G. S., and Bemis, C. E.: Angina pectoris and coronary artery disease in patients with severe aortic valvular disease. Am. Heart J. *100*:441, 1980.
399. Contratto, A. W., and Levine, S. A.: Aortic stenosis with special reference to angina pectoris and syncope. Ann. Intern. Med. *10*:1636, 1936.
400. Ross, J., Jr., and Braunwald, E.: The influence of corrective operations on the natural history of aortic stenosis. Circulation *37*(Suppl. V):61, 1968.
401. Frank, S., Johnson, A., and Ross, J., Jr.,: Natural history of valvular aortic stenosis. Br. Heart J. *35*:41, 1973.
402. Fallen, E. L., Elliott, W. C., and Gorlin, R.: Mechanisms of angina in aortic stenosis. Circulation *36*:480, 1967.
403. Storstein, O., and Enge, I.: Angina pectoris in aortic valvular disease and its relation to coronary pathology. Acta Med. Scand. *205*:275, 1979.
404. Holley, K. E., Bahn, R. C., McGoon, D. C., and Mankin, H. T.: Spontaneous calcific embolization associated with calcific aortic stenosis. Circulation *27*:197, 1963.
405. Flamm, M. D., Braiff, B. A., Kimball, R., and Hancock, E. W.: Mechanism of effort syncope in aortic stenosis. Circulation *36*(Suppl. II):109, 1967.
406. Schwartz, L. S., Goldfischer, J., Sprague, G. J., and Schwartz, S. P.: Syncope and sudden death in aortic stenosis. Am. J. Cardiol. *23*:647, 1969.
407. Shoenfeld, Y., Eldar, M., Bedazovsky, B., Levy, M. J., and Pinkhas, J.: Aortic stenosis associated with gastrointestinal bleeding. A survey of 612 patients. Am. Heart J. *100*:179, 1980.
408. Love, J. W.: The syndrome of calcific aortic stenosis and gastrointestinal bleeding: Resolution following aortic valve replacement. J. Thorac. Cardiovasc. Surg. *83*:779, 1982.
409. Pleet, A. B., Massey, E. W., and Vengrow, M. E.: TIA, stroke, and the bicuspid aortic valve. Neurology *31*:1540, 1981.
410. Brockmeier, L. B., Adolph, R. J., Gustin, B. W., Holmes, J. C., and Sacks, J. G.: Calcium emboli to the retinal artery in calcific aortic stenosis. Am. Heart J. *101*:32, 1981.
411. Wood, P.: Aortic stenosis. Am. J. Cardiol. *1*:553, 1958.
412. Cooper, T., Braunwald, E., and Morrow, A. G.: Pulsus alternans in aortic stenosis: Hemodynamic observations in 50 patients studied by left heart catheterization. Circulation *18*:64, 1958.
413. Perloff, J. K.: Clinical recognition of aortic stenosis. The physical signs and

differential diagnosis of the various forms of obstruction to left ventricular outflow. Prog. Cardiovasc. Dis. *10*:323, 1968.
414. Goldblatt, A., Aygen, M. M., and Braunwald, E.: Hemodynamic-phonocardiographic correlations of the fourth heart sound in aortic stenosis. Circulation *26*: 92, 1962.
415. Caulfield, W. H., deLeon, A. C., Perloff, J. K., and Steelman, R. B.: The clinical significance of the fourth heart sound in aortic stenosis. Am. J. Cardiol. *28*:179, 1971.
416. Hancock, E. W.: The ejection sound in aortic stenosis. Am. J. Med. *40*:569, 1966.
417. Morton, B. C.: Natural history and management of chronic aortic valve disease. Can. Med. Assoc. J. *126*:477, 1982.
418. Delman, A. J., and Stein, E.: Valvular aortic stenosis. *In* Dynamic Cardiac Auscultation and Phonocardiography. Philadelphia, W. B. Saunders Co., 1979, p. 795.
419. Morgan, D. J. R., and Hall, R. J. C.: Occult aortic stenosis as cause of intractable heart failure. Br. Med. J. *1*:784, 1979.
420. Kini, P. M., Eddelman, E. E., and Pipberger, H. V.: Electrocardiographic differentiation between left ventricular hypertrophy and anterior myocardial infarction. Circulation *42*:875, 1970.
421. Siegel, R. J., and Roberts, W. C.: Electrocardiographic observations in severe aortic valve stenosis: Correlative necropsy study to clinical, hemodynamic, and ECG variables demonstrating relation of 12-lead QRS amplitude to peak systolic transaortic pressure gradient. Am. Heart J. *103*:210, 1982.
422. Gooch, A. S., Calatayud, J. B., Rogers, P. A., and Garman, P. A.: Analysis of the P wave in severe aortic stenosis. Dis. Chest *49*:459, 1966.
423. Myler, R. K., and Sanders, C. A.: Aortic valve disease and atrial fibrillation: Report of 122 patients with electrocardiographic, radiographic and hemodynamic observations. Arch. Intern. Med. *121*:530, 1968.
424. Thompsom, R., Mitchell, A., Ahmed, M., Towers, M., and Yacoub, M.: Conduction defects in aortic valve disease. Am. Heart J. *98*:3, 1979.
425. Dhingra, R. C., Amat-y-Leon, F., Pietras, R. J., Wyndham, C., Deedwania, P. C., Wu, D., Denes, P., and Rosen, K. M.: Sites of conduction disease in aortic stenosis. Significance of valve gradient and calcification. Ann. Intern. Med. *87*: 275, 1977.
426. Rosenbaum, M., Elizari, M., and Lazari, J.: Los Hemibloques. Buenos Aires, Paidos, 1968, p. 363.
427. Bell, H., Pugh, D., and Dunn, M.: Vectorcardiographic evolution of left ventricular hypertrophy. Br. Heart J. *30*:70, 1968.
428. Klatte, E. C., Tampas, J. P., Campbell, J. A., and Lurie, P. R.: The roentgenographic manifestations of aortic stenosis and aortic valvular insufficiency. Am. J. Roentgenol. Radium Ther. Nucl. Med. *88*:57, 1962.
428a. Siegel, R. J., Maurer, G., Nivatpumin, T., and Shah, P. K.: Accurate non-invasive assessment of critical aortic valve stenosis in the elderly. J. Am. Coll. Cardiol. *1*:639, 1983.
429. Nanda, N. C., Gramiak, R., Manning, J., Mahoney, E. B., Lipchik, E. O., and DeWeese, J. A.: Echocardiographic recognition of the congenital bicuspid aortic valve. Circulation *49*:870, 1974.
430. Vukas, M., Wallentin, I., and Hjalmarson, A.: Analysis of systolic vibrations of interventricular septum in patients with aortic valvular stenosis. Acta Med. Scand. *210*:397, 1981.
431. McDonald, I. G.: Echocardiographic assessment of left ventricular function in aortic valve disease. Circulation *53*:860, 1976.
432. Reichek, N., and Devereaux, R. B.: Reliable estimation of peak left ventricular systolic pressure by M-mode echographic–determined end-diastolic relative wall thickness: Identification of severe valvular aortic stenosis in adult patients. Am. Heart J. *103*:202, 1982.
433. DeMaria, A. N., Bommer, W., Joye, J., Lee, G., Bouteller, J., and Mason, D. T.: Value and limitations of cross-sectional echocardiography of the aortic valve in the diagnosis and quantification of valvular aortic stenosis. Circulation *62*:304, 1980.
434. Godley, R. W., Green, D., Dillon, J. C., Rogers, E. W., Feigenbaum, H., and Weyman, A. E.: Reliability of two-dimensional echocardiography in assessing the severity of valvular aortic stenosis. Chest *79*:657, 1981.
435. Weyman, A. E.: Cross-sectional echocardiographic assessment of aortic obstruction. Acta Med. Scand. (Suppl. 627):120, 1979.
436. Cohen, L. S., Friedman, W. F., and Braunwald, E.: Natural history of mild congenital aortic stenosis elucidated by serial hemodynamic studies. Am. J. Cardiol. *30*:1, 1972.
437. Cheitlin, M. D., Gertz, E. W., Brundage, B. H., Carlson, C. J., Quash, J. A., and Bode, R. S., Jr.: Rate of progression of severity of valvular aortic stenosis in the adult. Am. Heart J. *98*:689, 1979.
438. Hammarsten, J. F.: Syncope in aortic stenosis. Arch. Intern. Med. *87*:274, 1951.
439. Morrow, A. G., Goldblatt, A., and Braunwald, E.: Congenital aortic stenosis. II. Surgical treatment and the results of operation. Circulation *27*:450, 1963.
440. Chizner, M. A., Pearle, D. L., and deLeon, A. C., Jr.: The natural history of aortic stenosis in adults. Am. Heart J. *99*:419, 1980.
441. Wagner, S., and Selzer, A.: Patterns of progression of aortic stenosis: A longitudinal hemodynamic study. Circulation *65*:709, 1982.
442. Spencer, F. C.: Congenital heart disease. *In* Schwartz, S. I., Shires, G. T., Spencer, F. C., and Storer, E. H. (eds.): Principles of Surgery. 2nd ed. New York, McGraw-Hill Book Co., 1979, p. 755.
443. Henry, W. L., Bonow, R. O., Borer, J. S., Kent, K. M., Ware, J. H., Redwood, D. R., Itscoitz, S. B., McIntosh, C. L., Morrow, A. G., and Epstein, S. E.: Evaluation of aortic valve replacement in patients with valvular aortic stenosis. Circulation *61*:814, 1980.
444. Copeland, J. G., Griepp, R. B., Stinson, E. B., and Shumway, N. E.: Long-term followup after isolated aortic valve replacement. J. Thorac. Cardiovasc. Surg. *74*:875, 1977.
445. Krayenbuehl, H. P., Turina, M., Hess, O. M., Rothlin, M., and Senning, A.: Pre- and postoperative left ventricular contractile function in patients with aortic valve disease. Br. Heart J. *41*:204, 1979.
446. Rahimtoola, S. H.: Outcome of aortic valve surgery. Circulation *60*:1191, 1979.
447. Mirsky, I., Henschke, C., Hess, O. M., and Krayenbuehl, H. P.: Prediction of postoperative performance in aortic valve disease. Am. J. Cardiol. *48*:295, 1981.
448. Khanna, S. K., Ross, J. K., and Monro, J. L.: Homograft aortic valve replacement: Seven years' experience with antibiotic-treated valves. Thorax *36*: 330, 1981.
449. Rossiter, S. J., Miller, D. C., Stinson, E. B., Oyer, P. E., Reitz, B. A., Moreno-Cabral, R. J., Mace, J. G., Robert, E. W., Tsagaris, T. J., Sutton, R. B., Alderman, E. L., and Shumway, N. E.: Hemodynamic and clinical comparison of the Hancock modified orifice and standard orifice bioprostheses in the aortic position. J. Thorac. Cardiovasc. Surg. *80*:54, 1980.
450. DiSesa, V. J., Collins, J. J., Jr., and Cohn, L. H.: Valve replacement in the small annulus aorta: Performance of the Hancock modified-orifice bioprosthesis. *In* Cohn, L. H., and Gallucci, V.: Cardiac Bioprostheses. New York, Yorke Medical Books, 1982, p. 552.
451. Gill, C. C., King, H. C., Lytle, B. W., Cosgrove, D. M., Golding, L. A. R., and Loop, F. D.: Early clinical evaluation of aortic valve replacement with the St. Jude medical valve in patients with a small aortic root. Circulation *66* (Suppl. I):I–147, 1982.
452. Cheung, D., Flemma, R. J., Mullen, D. C., Lepley, D., Jr., Anderson, A. J., and Weirauch, E.: Ten-year followup in aortic valve replacement using the Björk-Shiley prosthesis. Ann. Thorac. Surg. *32*:138, 1981.
453. Acar, J., Ducimetiere, P., Cadilhac, M., Jallut, H., and Vahanian, A.: Prognosis of surgically treated chronic aortic valve disease. Predictive indicators of early postoperative risk and long-term survival, based on 439 cases. J. Thorac. Cardiovasc. Surg. *82*:114, 1981.
454. Croke, R. P., Pifarre, R., Sullivan, H., Gunnar, R., and Loeb, H.: Reversal of advanced left ventricular dysfunction following aortic valve replacement for aortic stenosis. Ann. Thorac. Surg. *24*:38, 1977.
455. Pantely, G., Morton, M., and Rahimtoola, S. H.: Effects of successful, uncomplicated valve replacement on ventricular hypertrophy, volume and performance in aortic stenosis and in aortic incompetence. J. Thorac. Cardiovasc. Surg. *75*:383, 1978.
456. Kennedy, J. W., Doces, J., and Stewart, D. K.: Left ventricular function before and following aortic valve replacement. Circulation *56*:944, 1977.
457. O'Tolle, J. D., Geiser, E. A., Reddy, S., Curtiss, E. I., and Landfair, R. M.: Effect of preoperative ejection fraction on survival and hemodynamic improvement following aortic valve replacement. Circulation *58*:1175, 1978.
458. Sanders, J. H., Jr., Cohn, L. H., Dalen, J. E., and Collins, J. J., Jr.: Emergency aortic valve replacement. Am. J. Surg. *135*:495, 1976.
459. Smith, N., McAnulty, J. H., and Rahimtoola, S. H.: Severe aortic stenosis with impaired left ventricular function and clinical heart failure: Results of valve replacement. Circulation *58*:255, 1978.
460. Kay, P. H., and Paneth, M.: Aortic valve replacement in the over seventy age group. J. Cardiovasc. Surg. *22*:312, 1981.
461. Richardson, J. V., Kouchoukos, N. T., Wright, J. O., and Karp, R. B.: Combined aortic valve replacement and myocardial revascularization: Results in 220 patients. Circulation *59*:75, 1979.
462. Kirklin, J. W., and Kouchoukos, N. T.: Aortic valve replacement without myocardial revascularization. Circulation *63*:252, 1981.
463. MacManus, Q., Grunkemeier, G., Lambert, L., Dietl, C., and Starr, A.: Aortic valve replacement and aorto-coronary bypass surgery. Results with perfusion of proximal and distal coronary arteries. J. Thorac. Cardiovasc. Surg. *75*:865, 1978.
464. Starr, A., Pierie, U. R., Raible, D. A., et al.: Cardiac valve replacement. Experience with the durability of silicone rubber. Circulation *34*(Suppl. I):1, 1966.
465. Bonchek, L. I., and Starr, A.: Ball valve prostheses: Current appraisal of late results. Am. J. Cardiol. *35*:843, 1975.
466. Yoganathan, A. P., Corcoran, W. H., Harrison, E. C., and Carl, J. R.: The Björk-Shiley aortic prosthesis: Flow characteristics, thrombus formation and tissue overgrowth. Circulation *58*:70, 1978.
467. Sarma, R., Roschke, E. J., Harrison, E. C., Edmiston, W. A., and Lau, F. Y. K.: Clinical experience with the Smeloff-Cutter aortic valve prosthesis: An 8-year followup study. Am. J. Cardiol. *40*:338, 1977.
468. Magovern, G. J., Liebler, G. A., Cushing, W. J., Park, S. G., and Burkholder, J. A.: A thirteen-year review of the Magovern-Cromie aortic valve. J. Thorac. Cardiovasc. Surg. *73*:64, 1977.
469. Stinson, E. B., Griepp, R. B., Oyer, P. E., and Shumway, N. E.: Long-term experience with porcine aortic valve xenografts. J. Thorac. Cardiovasc. Surg. *73*:54, 1977.
470. Morris, D. C., King, S. B., III, Douglas, J. S., Jr., Wickliffe, C. W., and Jones, E. L.: Hemodynamic results of aortic valvular replacement with the porcine xenograft valve. Circulation *56*:841, 1977.
471. Wright, J. T. M.: A pulsatile flow study comparing the Hancock porcine xenograft aortic valve prostheses models 242 and 250. Med. Instrum. *11*:114, 1977.

AORTIC REGURGITATION

472. Stapleton, J. F., and Harvey, W. P.: A clinical analysis of aortic incompetence. Postgrad. Med. *46*:156, 1969.
473. Carter, J. B., Sethi, S., Lee, G. B., and Edward, J. E.: Prolapse of semilunar cusps as causes of aortic insufficiency. Circulation *43*:922, 1971.
474. Frahm, C. J., Braunwald, E., and Morrow, A. G.: Congenital aortic regurgitation. Clinical and hemodynamic findings in four patients. Am. J. Med. *31*:63, 1961.
475. Roberts, W. C., Morrow, A. G., McIntosh, C. L., Jones, M., and Epstein, S. E.: Congenitally bicuspid aortic valve causing severe, pure aortic regurgitation without superimposed infective endocarditis. Am. J. Cardiol. *47*:206, 1981.
476. Morain, S. V., Casanegra, P., Maturana, G., and Dubernet, J.: Spontaneous rupture of a fenestrated aortic valve. Surgical treatment. J. Thorac. Cardiovasc. Surg. *73*:716, 1977.
477. Puchner, T. C., Huston, J. H., and Hellmuth, G. A.: Aortic valve insufficiency in arterial hypertension. Am. J. Cardiol. *5*:758, 1960.
478. Thandroyen, F. T., Matisonn, R. E., and Weir, E. K.: Severe aortic incompetence caused by systemic lupus erythematosus. S.A. Med. J. *54*:166, 1978.
479. Devlin, A. B., Goldstraw, P., and Caves, P. K.: Aortic valve replacement in rheumatoid aortic incompetence. Thorax *33*:612, 1978.
480. Schilder, D. P., Harvey, W. P., and Hufnagel, C. A.: Rheumatoid spondylitis and aortic insufficiency. N. Engl. J. Med. *255*:11, 1956.
480a. Bostwick, D. G., Bensch, K. G., Burke, J. S., Billingham, M. E., Miller, D. C., Smith, J. C., and Keren, D. F.: Whipple's disease presenting as aortic insufficiency. N. Engl. J. Med. *305*:995, 1981.
481. Darvill, F. R., Jr.: Aortic insufficiency of unusual etiology. J.A.M.A. *184*:753, 1963.
481a. Rae, S. A., Vandenburg, M., and Scholtz, C. L.: Aortic regurgitation and false aneurysm formation in Behçet's disease. Postgrad. Med. J. *56*:438, 1980.
482. Emanuel, R., Ng, R. A. L., Marcomichelakis, J., Moores, E. C., Jefferson, K. E., Macfaul, P. A., and Withers, R.: Formes frustes of Marfan's syndrome presenting with severe aortic regurgitation. Clinicogenetic study of 18 families. Br. Heart J. *39*:190, 1977.
483. Roberts, W. C., Hollingsworth, J. F., Bulkley, B. H., Jaffe, R. B., Epstein, S. E., and Stinson, E. B.: Combined mitral and aortic regurgitation in ankylosing spondylitis: Angiographic and anatomic features. Am. J. Med. *56*:237, 1974.
484. Reid, G. D., Patterson, M. W. H., Patterson, A. C., and Cooperberg, P. L.: Aortic insufficiency in association with juvenile ankylosing spondylitis. J. Pediatr. *95*:78, 1979.
485. Paulus, H. E., Pearson, C. M., and Pitts, W., Jr.: Aortic insufficiency in five patients with Reiter's syndrome: A detailed clinical and pathologic study. Am. J. Med. *53*:464, 1972.
486. Hollingworth, P., Hall, P. J., Knight, S. C., and Newman, R.: Lone aortic regurgitation, sacroiliitis, and HLA B27: Case history and frequency of association. Br. Heart J. *42*:229, 1979.
487. Heppner, R. L., Babitt, H. I., Bianchine, J. W., and Warbasse, J. R.: Aortic regurgitation and aneurysm of sinus of Valsalva associated with osteogenesis imperfecta. Am. J. Cardiol. *31*:654, 1973.
488. Waller, B. F., Zoltick, J. M., Rosen, J. H., Katz, N. M., Gomes, M. N., Fletcher, R. D., Wallace, R. B., and Roberts, W. C.: Severe aortic regurgitation from systemic hypertension (without aortic dissection) requiring aortic valve replacement. Analysis of four patients. Am. J. Cardiol. *49*:473, 1982.
489. Welch, G. H., Jr., Braunwald, E., and Sarnoff, S. J.: Hemodynamic effects of quantitatively varied experimental aortic regurgitation. Circ. Res. 5:546, 1957.
490. Soorae, A. S., McKeown, F., and Cleland, J.: Aortic valve replacement for severe aortic regurgitation caused by idiopathic giant cell aortitis. Thorax *35*: 60, 1980.
491. Belenkie, I., and Rademaker, A.: Acute and chronic changes after aortic valve damage in the intact dog. Am. J. Physiol. *241*:H95, 1981.
491a. Iskandrian, A. S., Hakki, A-H., Manno, B., Amenta, A., and Kane, S. A.: Left ventricular function in chronic aortic regurgitation. J. Am. Coll. Cardiol. *1*:1374, 1983.
491b. Boucher, C. A., Wilson, R. A., Kanarek, D. J., Hutter, A. M., Jr., Okada, R. D., Liberthson, R. R., Strauss, H. W., and Pohost, G. M.: Exercise testing in asymptomatic or minimally symptomatic aortic regurgitation: Relationship of left ventricular ejection fraction to left ventricular filling pressure during exercise. Circulation *67*:1091, 1983.
491c. Johnson, L. L., Powers, E. R., Tzall, W. R., Feder, J., Sciacca, R. R., and Cannon, P. J.: Left ventricular volume and ejection fraction response to exercise in aortic regurgitation. Am. J. Cardiol. *51*:1379, 1983.
492. Grossman, W., Jones, D., and McLaurin, L. P.: Wall stress and patterns of hypertrophy in the human left ventricle. J. Clin. Invest. *56*:56, 1975.
493. Judge, T. P., Kennedy, J. W., Bennett, L. J., Willis, R. E., Murray, J. A., and Blackman, J. R.: Quantitative hemodynamic effects of heart rate on aortic regurgitation. Circulation *44*:355, 1971.
494. Laniado, S., Yellin, E. L., Yoran, C., Strom, J., Hori, M., Gabbay, S., Terdiman, R., and Frater, R. W. M.: Physiologic mechanism in aortic insufficiency. I. The effect of changing heart rate on flow dynamics. II. Determinants of Austin Flint murmur. Circulation *66*:226, 1982.
495. Falsetti, H. L., Carroll, R. J., and Cramer, J. A.: Total and regional myocardial blood flow in aortic regurgitation. Am. Heart J. *97*:485, 1979.
496. Uhl, G. S., Boucher, C. A., Oliveros, R. A., and Murgo, J. P.: Exercise-induced myocardial oxygen supply-demand imbalance in asymptomatic or mildly symptomatic aortic regurgitation. Chest *80*:686, 1981.
497. Maurer, W., Ablasser, A., Tschada, R., Hausen, M., Saggau, W., and Kubler, W.: Myocardial catecholamine metabolism in patients with chronic aortic regurgitation. Circulation *66*(Suppl. I):I–139, 1982.
498. Osbakken, M., Bove, A. A., and Spann, J. F.: Left ventricular function in chronic aortic regurgitation with reference to end-systolic pressure, volume and stress relations. Am. J. Cardiol. *47*:193, 1981.
499. Dehmer, G. J., Firth, E. G., Hillis, L. D., Corbett, J. R., Lewis, S. E., Parkey, R. W., and Willerson, J. T.: Alterations in left ventricular volumes and ejection fraction at rest and during exercise in patients with aortic regurgitation. Am. J. Cardiol. *48*:17, 1981.
500. Lewis, S. M., Riba, A. L., Berger, H. J., Davies, R. A., Wackers, F. J. T., Alexander, J., Sands, M. J., Cohen, L. S., and Zaret, B. L.: Radionuclide angiographic exercise left ventricular performance in chronic aortic regurgitation: Relationship to resting echographic ventricular dimensions and systolic wall stress index. Am. Heart J. *103*:498, 1982.
501. Schuler, G., Olshausen, K. V., Schwarz, F., Mehmel, H., Hofmann, M., Hermann, H.-J., Lange, D., and Kubler, W.: Noninvasive assessment of myocardial contractility in asymptomatic patients with severe aortic regurgitation and normal left ventricular ejection fraction at rest. Am. J. Cardiol. *50*:45, 1982.
502. Morganroth, J., Perloff, J. K., Zeldis, S. M., and Dunkman, W. B.: Acute severe aortic regurgitation. Pathophysiology, clinical recognition and management. Ann. Intern. Med. *82*:223, 1977.
502a. Perlofff, J. K.: Acute severe aortic regurgitation: Recognition and management. J. Cardiovasc. Med. *8*:209, 1983.
503. Mann, T., McLaurin, L. P., Grossman, W., and Craige, E.: Assessing the hemodynamic severity of acute aortic regurgitation due to infective endocarditis. N. Engl. J. Med. *293*:108, 1975.
504. Spagnuolo, M., Kloth, H., Taranta, A., Doyle, E., and Pasternack, B.: Natural history of rheumatic aortic regurgitation: Criteria predictive of death, congestive heart failure and angina in young patients. Circulation *44*:368, 1971.
505. Segal, J., Harvey, W. P., and Hufnagel, C. A.: Clinical study of one hundred cases of severe aortic insufficiency. Am. J. Med. *21*:200, 1956.
506. Bland, E. F., and Wheeler, E. O.: Severe aortic regurgitation in young people. A long-term perspective with reference to prognosis. N. Engl. J. Med. *256*: 667, 1957.
507. Sapira, J. D.: Quincke, deMusset, Duroziez and Hill: Some aortic regurgitations. South. Med. J. *74*:459, 1981.
508. Alpert, J. S., Vieweg, W. V. R., and Hagan, A. D.: Incidence and morphology of carotid shudders in aortic valve disease. Am. Heart J. *92*:435, 1976.
509. Sabbah, H. N., Khaja, F., Anbe, D. T., and Stein, P. D.: The aortic closure sound in pure aortic insufficiency. Circulation *56*:859, 1977.
510. Abdulla, A. M., Frank, M. J., Erdin, R. A., Jr., and Canedo, M. I.: Clinical significance and hemodynamic correlates of the third heart sound gallop in aortic regurgitation. A guide to optimal timing of cardiac catheterization. Circulation *64*:464, 1981.
511. Harvey, W., Corrado, M. A., and Perloff, J. K.: "Right-sided" murmurs of aortic insufficiency. Am. J. Med. Sci. *245*:53, 1963.
512. Fortuin, N. J., and Craige, E.: On the mechanism of the Austin Flint murmur. Circulation *45*:558, 1972.
513. O'Brien, K. P., and Cohen, L. S.: Hemodynamic and phonocardiographic correlates of the Austin Flint murmur. Am. Heart J. *77*:603, 1969.
514. Delman, A. J., and Stein, E.: Aortic regurgitation. *In* Dynamic Cardiac Auscultation and Phonocardiography. Philadelphia, W. B. Saunders Co. 1979, pp. 811–824.
515. Spring, D. A., Folts, J. D., Young, W. P., and Rowe, G. G.: Premature closure of the mitral and tricuspid valves. Circulation *45*:663, 1972.
516. Wong, M.: Diastolic mitral regurgitation. Hemodynamic and angiographic correlation. Br. Heart J. *31*:468, 1969.
517. Perloff, J. K., and Singer, D.: Electrocardiogram of free aortic insufficiency. Circulation *26*:786, 1962.
518. Estes, E. H.: Left ventricular hypertrophy in acquired heart disease: A comparison of the vectorcardiogram in aortic stenosis and aortic insufficiency. *In* Hoffman, I. (ed.): Vectorcardiography. Amsterdam, North Holland Publishing Co., 1976.
519. Paoloni, H. J., Wilcken, D. E. L., and Dadd, M. J.: The role of echocardiography in the assessment of chronic aortic regurgitation. Aust. N.Z.J. Med. *7* :491, 1977.
520. Abdulla, A. M., Frank, M. J., Canedo, M. I., and Stefadouros, M. A.: Limitations of echocardiography in the assessment of left ventricular size and function in aortic regurgitation. Circulation *61*:148, 1980.
521. Pridie, R. B., Benham, R., and Oakley, C. M.: Echocardiography of the mitral valve in aortic valve disease. Br. Heart J. *33*:296, 1971.
522. Weaver, W. F., Wilson, C. S., Rourke, T., and Caudill, C. C.: Mid-diastolic aortic valve opening in severe acute aortic regurgitation. Circulation *55*:112, 1977.
523. Winsberg, F., Gabor, G. E., Hernberg, J. G., et al.: Fluttering of the mitral valve in aortic insufficiency. Circulation *41*:225, 1970.
524. Imaizumi, T., Orita, Y., Koiwaya, Y., Hirata, T., and Nakamura, M.: Utility of two-dimensional echocardiography in the differential diagnosis of the etiology of aortic regurgitation. Am. Heart J. *103*:887, 1982.
525. Rowe, D. W., Pechacek, L. W., DeCastro, C. M., Garcia, E., and Hall, R. J.: Initial diastolic indentation of the mitral valve in aortic insufficiency. J. Clin. Ultrasound *10*:53, 1982.
526. Manyari, D. E., Nolewajka, A. J., and Kostuk, W. J.: Quantitative assessment

of aortic valvular insufficiency by radionuclide angiography. Chest *81*:170, 1982.

526a. Steingart, R. M., Yee, C., Weinstein, L., and Scheuer, J.: Radio-nuclide ventriculographic study of adaptations to exercise in aortic regurgitation. Am. J. Cardiol. *51*:483, 1983.

527. Utley, J. R., Mills, J., and Roe, B. B.: The role of valve replacement in the treatment of fungal endocarditis. J. Thorac. Cardiovasc. Surg. *69*:255, 1975.

528. Goldschlager, N., Pfeifer, J., Cohn, K., Pepper, R., and Selzer, A.: The natural history of aortic regurgitation. A clinical and hemodynamic study. Am. J. Med. *54*:577, 1973.

529. Dexter, L.: Evaluation of the results of cardiac surgery. *In* Jones, A. M. (ed.): Modern Trends in Cardiology. Vol. 2. New York, Appleton-Century-Crofts, 1969, p. 311.

530. Massell, B. F., Ameccua, F. J., and Czohiczer, G.: Prognosis of patients with pure or predominant aortic regurgitation in the absence of surgery. Circulation *34*(Suppl. II):164, 1966.

531. Greenberg, B. H.: Aortic insufficiency: Vasodilator therapy. Primary Cardiol. *8*: 35, 1982.

532. Greenberg, B. H., DeMots, H., Murphy, E., and Rahimtoola, S. H.: Mechanism for improved cardiac performance with arteriolar dilators in aortic insufficiency. Circulation *63*:263, 1981.

533. Fioretti, P., Benussi, B., Scardi, S., Klugmann, S., Brower, R. W., and Camerini, F.: Afterload reduction with nifedipine in aortic insufficiency. Am. J. Cardiol. *49*:1728, 1982.

533a. Gaasch, W. H., Carroll, J. D., Levine, H. J., and Criscitiello, M. G.: Chronic aortic regurgitation: Prognostic value of left ventricular end-systolic dimensions and end-diastolic radius/thickness ratio. J. Am. Coll. Cardiol. *3*:775, 1983.

533b. Jebavy, P., Koudelkova, E., and Henzlova, M.: Unloading effects of prazosin in patients with chronic aortic regurgitation. Am. Heart J. *105*:567, 1983.

534. Kumpuris, A. G., Quinones, M. A., Waggoner, A. D., Kanon, D. J., Nelson, J. G., and Miller, R. R.: Importance of preoperative hypertrophy, wall stress and end-systolic dimension as echocardiographic predictors of normalization of left ventricular dilatation after valve replacement in chronic aortic insufficiency. Am. J. Cardiol. *49*:1091, 1982.

535. Cunha, C. L. P., Giuliani, E. R., Fuster, V. Seward, J. B., Brandenburg, R. O., and McGoon, D. C.: Preoperative M-mode echocardiography as a predictor of surgical results in chronic aortic insufficiency. J. Thorac. Cardiovasc. Surg. *79*: 256, 1980.

536. Henry, W. L., Bonow, R. O., Rosing, D. R., and Epstein, S. E.: Observations on the optimum time for operative intervention for aortic regurgitation. II. Serial echocardiographic evaluation of asymptomatic patients. Circulation *61*: 484, 1980.

537. Toussaint, C., Cribier, A., Cazor, J. L., Soyer, R., and Letac, B.: Hemodynamic and angiographic evaluation of aortic regurgitation 8 and 27 months after aortic valve replacement. Circulation *64*:456, 1981.

538. Bonow, R. O., Rosing, D. R., Kent K. M., and Epstein, S. E.: Timing of operation for chronic aortic regurgitation. Am. J. Cardiol. *50*:325, 1982.

539. Henry, W. L., Bonow, R. O., Borer, J. S., Ware, J. H., Kent, K. M., Redwood, D. R., McIntosh, C. L., Morrow, A. G., and Epstein, S. E.: Observations on the optimum time for operative intervention for aortic regurgitation. I. Evaluation of the results of aortic valve replacement in symptomatic patients. Circulation *61*:471, 1980.

540. O'Rourke, R. A., and Crawford, M. H.: Timing of valve replacement in patients with chronic aortic regurgitation (Editorial). Circulation *61*:493, 1980.

541. Gaasch, W. H., Andrias, C. W., and Levine, H. J.: Chronic aortic regurgitation. The effect of aortic valve replacement on left ventricular volume, mass and function. Circulation *58*:825, 1978.

541a. Carroll, J. D., Gaasch, W. H., Naimi, S., and Levine, H. J.: Regression of myocardial hypertrophy: Electrocardiographic-echocardiographic correlations after aortic valve replacement in patients with chronic aortic regurgitation. Circulation *65*:980, 1982.

541b. Bonow, R. O., Rosing, D. R., Maron, B. J., Jones, M., McIntosh, C. L., and Epstein, S. E.: Reversal of left ventricular dysfunction after valve replacement in patients with aortic regurgitation. Influence of duration of preoperative left ventricular dysfunction. J. Am. Coll. Cardiol. *1*:639, 1983 (Abstr.).

541c. Pomar, J. L., Garcia-Dorado, D., Almazan, A., Betriu, A., Chaitman, B. R., and Pelletier, C.: Determinants of clinical status following valve replacement for pure aortic regurgitation. J. Am. Coll. Cardiol. *1*:586, 1983 (Abstr.).

541d. Carroll, J. D., Gaasch, W. H., Zile, M. R., and Levine, H. J.: Serial changes in left ventricular function after correction of chronic aortic regurgitation. Dependence on early changes in preload and subsequent regression of hypertrophy. Am. J. Cardiol. *51*:476, 1983.

542. Thompson, R., Ahmed, M., Seabra-Gomes, R., Ilsley, C., Rickards, A., Towers, M., and Yacoub, M.: Influence of preoperative left ventricular function on results of homograft replacement of the aortic valve for aortic regurgitation. J. Thorac. Cardiovasc. Surg. *77*:411, 1979.

543. Rahimtoola, S. H.: Valve replacement should *not* be performed in all asymptomatic patients with severe aortic incompetence. J. Thorac. Cardiovasc. Surg. *79*:163, 1980.

TRICUSPID AND PULMONIC VALVE DISEASE

544. Smith, J. A., and Levine, S. A.: Clinical features of tricuspid stenosis. Am. Heart. J. *23*:739, 1942.

545. Morgan, J. R., Forker, A. D., Coates, J. R., and Myers, W. S.: Isolated tricuspid stenosis. Circulation *44*:729, 1971.

546. Perloff, J. K., and Harvey, W. P.: The clinical recognition of tricuspid stenosis. Circulation *22*:346, 1960.

547. Killip, T., III, and Lukas, D. S.: Tricuspid stenosis. Clinical features in twelve cases. Am. J. Med. *24*:836, 1958.

548. Kitchin, A., and Turner, R.: Diagnosis and treatment of tricuspid stenosis. Br. Heart J. *26*:354, 1964.

549. Mahapatra, R. K., Agarwal, J. B., and Wasir, H. S.: Rheumatic tricuspid stenosis. Indian Heart J. *30*:138, 1978.

550. Joyner, C. R., Hey, B. E., Jr., Johnson, J., and Reid, J. M.: Reflected ultrasound in the diagnosis of tricuspid stenosis. Am. J. Cardiol. *19*:66, 1967.

550a. Daniels, S. J., Mintz, G. S., and Kotler, M. N.: Rheumatic tricuspid valve disease. Two-dimensional echocardiographic, hemodynamic, and angiographic correlations. Am. J. Cardio. *51*:492, 1983.

551. Mardelli, T. J., Morganroth, J., Chen, C. C., Naito, M., and Vergel, J.: Tricuspid valve prolapse diagnosed by cross-sectional echocardiography. Chest *79*: 201, 1981.

552. Veyrat, C., Kalmanson, D., Farjon, M., Manin, J. P., and Abitbol, G.: Noninvasive diagnosis and assessment of tricuspid regurgitation and stenosis using one and two dimensional echo-pulsed Doppler. Br. Heart J. *47*:596, 1982.

553. Péterffy, A., Jonassoh, R., and Henze, A.: Haemdynamic changes after tricuspid valve surgery. Scand J. Thorac. Cardiovasc. Surg. *15*:161, 1981.

553a. Throburn, C. W., Morgan, J. J., Shanahan, M. X., and Chang, V. P.: Long-term results of tricuspid valve replacement and the problem of prosthetic valve thrombosis. Am. J. Cardiol. *51*:1128, 1983.

554. Zone, D. D., and Botti, R. E.: Right ventricular infarction with tricuspid insufficiency and chronic right heart failure. Am. J. Cardiol. *37*:445, 1976.

555. McAllister, R. G., Jr., Friesinger, G. C., and Sinclair-Smith, B. C.: Tricuspid regurgitation following inferior myocardial infarction. Arch. Intern. Med. *136*: 95, 1976.

556. Dougherty, M. J., and Craige, E.: Apathetic hyperthyroidism presenting as tricuspid regurgitation. Chest *63*:767, 1973.

557. Nelson, R. M., Bucciarelli, R. L., Eitzman, D. V., Egan, E. A., II, and Gessner, I. H.: Serum creatine phosphokinase MB fraction in newborns with transient tricuspid insufficiency. N. Engl. J. Med. *298*:146, 1978.

558. Esaghpour, E., Kawai, N., and Linhart, J. W.: Tricuspid insufficiency associated with aneurysm of the ventricular septum. Pediatrics *61*:586, 1978.

559. Chen, C. C., Morganroth, J., Mardelli, J. T., and Naito, M.: Tricuspid regurgitation in tricuspid valve prolapse demonstrated with contrast cross-sectional echocardiography. Am. J. Cardiol. *46*:983, 1980.

560. Chandraratna, P. A. N., Littman, B. B., and Wilson, D.: The association between atrial septal defect and prolapse of the tricuspid valve. An echocardiographic study. Chest *73*:839, 1978.

561. Bardy, G. H., Talano, J. V., Meyers, S., and Lesch, M.: Acquired cyanotic heart disease secondary to traumatic tricuspid regurgitation. Am. J. Cardiol. *44*:1401, 1979.

562. Ginzton, L. E., Siegel, R. J., and Criley, J. M.: Natural history of tricuspid valve endocarditis: A two-dimensional echocardiographic study. Am. J. Cardiol. *49*:1853, 1982.

563. Arbulu, A., and Asfaw, I.: Tricuspid valvulectomy without prosthetic replacement. Ten years of clinical experience. J. Thorac. Cardiovasc. Surg. *82*: 684, 1981.

564. Sethia, B., and Williams, B. T.: Tricuspid valve excision without replacement in a case of endocarditis secondary to drug abuse. Br. Heart J. *40*:579, 1978.

565. Gutierrez, F. R., McKnight, R. C., Jaffe, A. S., Ludbrook, P. A., Biello, D., and Weldon, C. S.: Double porcine valve replacement in carcinoid heart disease. Chest *81*:101, 1982.

566. Lie, J. T.: Carcinoid tumors, carcinoid syndrome, and carcinoid heart disease. Primary Cardiol. *8*:163, 1982.

567. Come, P. C., Come, S. E., Hawley, C. R., Gwon, N., and Riley, M. F.: Echocardiographic manifestations of carcinoid heart disease. J. Clin. Ultrasound *10*:233, 1982.

568. Baker, B. J., McNee, V. D., Scovil, J. A., Bass, K. M., Watson, J. W., and Bissett, J. K.: Tricuspid insufficiency in carcinoid heart disease: An echocardiographic description. Am. Heart J. *101*:107, 1981.

569. Roberts, W. C., and Sjoerdsma, A.: The cardiac disease associated with the carcinoid syndrome (carcinoid heart disease). Am. J. Med. *36*:5, 1964.

570. Pernot, C., Hoeffel, J. C., Henry, M., and Piwurca, A.: Case report of congenital tricuspid insufficiency. Cathet. Cardiovasc. Diagn. *4*:71, 1978.

571. Lingamneni, R., Cha, S. D., Maranhao, V., Booch, A. S., and Goldberg, H.: Tricuspid regurgitation: Clinical and angiographic assessment. Cathet. Cardiovasc. Diagn. *5*:7, 1979.

572. Cha, S. D., Gooch, A. S., and Maranhao, V.: Intracardiac phonocardiography in tricuspid regurgitation: Relation to clinical and angiographic findings. Am. J. Cardiol. *48*:578, 1981.

573. Sepulveda, G., and Lukas, D. S.: The diagnosis of tricuspid insufficiency: Clinical features in 60 cases with associated mitral valve disease. Circulation *11*: 552, 1955.

574. Seides, S. F., DeJoseph, R. L., Brown, A. E., and Damato, A. N.: Echocardiographic findings in isolated, surgically created tricuspid insufficiency. Am. J. Cardiol. *35*:679, 1975.

575. Chandraratna, P. A., Lopez, J. M., Fernandez, J. J., and Cohen, L. S.: Echocardiographic detection of tricuspid valve prolapse. Circulation *51*:823, 1975.

576. Lieppe, W., Behar, V. S., Scallion, R., and Kisslo, J. A.: Detection of tricuspid regurgitation with two-dimensional echocardiography and peripheral vein injections. Circulation *57*:128, 1978.
577. Meltzer, R. S., van Hoogenhuyze, D., Serruys, P. W., Haalebos, M. M. P., Hugenholtz, P. G., and Roelandt, J.: Diagnosis of tricuspid regurgitation by contrast echocardiography. Circulation *63*:1093, 1981.
578. Tei, C., Shah, P. M., and Ormiston, J. A.: Assessment of tricuspid regurgitation by directional analysis of right atrial systolic linear reflux echoes with contrast M-mode echocardiography. Am. Heart J. *103*:1025, 1982.
579. McCord, M. C., and Blount, S. G., Jr.: The hemodynamic pattern in tricuspid valve disease. Am. Heart J. *44*:671, 1952.
580. Rubeiz, G. A., Nassar, M. E., and Dagher, I. K.: Study of the right atrial pressure pulse in functional tricuspid regurgitation and normal sinus rhythm. Circulation *30*:190, 1964.
581. Hansing, C. E., and Rowe, G. G.: Tricuspid insufficiency. A study of hemodynamics and pathogenesis. Circulation *45*:793, 1972.
582. Pepino, C. J., Nichols, W. W., and Selby, J. H.: Diagnostic tests for tricuspid insufficiency: How good? Cathet. Cardiovasc. Diagn. *5*:1, 1979.
583. Lingameni, R., Cha, S. D., Maranhao, V., Gooch, A. S. and Goldberg, H.: Tricuspid regurgitation: Clinical and angiographic assessment. Cathet. Cardiovasc. Diagn. *5*:7, 1979.
584. Ubago, J. L., Figueroa, A., Colman, T., Ochoteco, A., Rodriguez, M., and Duran, C. M. G.: Right ventriculography as a valid method for the diagnosis of tricuspid insufficiency. Cathet. Cardiovasc. Diagn. *7*:433, 1981.
585. Carpentier, A., Deloche, A., and Dauptain, J.: A new reconstructive operation for correction of mitral and tricuspid insufficiency. J. Thorac. Cardiovasc. Surg. *61*:1, 1971.
586. Peterffy, A., Jonasson, R., Szamosi, A., and Henze, A.: Comparison of Kay's and DeVega's annuloplasty in surgical treatment of tricuspid incompetence. Clinical and haemodynamic results in 62 patients. Scand. J. Thorac. Cardiovasc. Surg. *14*:249, 1980.
587. Duran, C. M. G., Pomar, J. L., Colman, T., Figueroa, A., Revuelta, J. M., and Ubago, J. L.: Is tricuspid valve repair necessary? J. Thorac. Cardiovasc. Surg. *80*:849, 1980.
588. Carpentier, A., Deloche, A., Hanania, G., Furman, J., Sellier, P., Piwnica, A., and Dubost, C.: Surgical management of acquired tricuspid valve disease. J. Thorac. Cardiovasc. Surg. *67*:53, 1974.
589. Breyer, R. H., McClenathan, J. H., Michaelis, L. L., McIntosh, C. L., and Morrow, A. G.: Tricuspid regurgitation. A comparison of nonoperative management, tricuspid annuloplasty, and tricuspid valve replacement. J. Thorac. Cardiovasc. Surg. *72*:867, 1976.
590. Korr, K. S., Levinson, H., Bough, E. W., Gheorghiade, M., Stone, J., McEnany, M. T., and Shulman, R. S.: Tricuspid valve replacement for cardiogenic shock after acute right ventricular infarction. J.A.M.A. *244*:1958, 1980.
591. Vela, J. E., Conteras, R., and Sosa, F. R.: Rheumatic pulmonary valve disease. Am. J. Cardiol. *23*:12, 1969.
592. Seymour, J., Emaneul, R., and Patterson, N.: Acquired pulmonary stenosis. Br. Heart J. *30*:776, 1968.
593. Runco, V., and Levin, H. S.: The spectrum of pulmonic regurgitation. *In* Physiologic Principles of Heart Sounds and Murmurs. American Heart Association Monograph No. 46, 1975, p. 175.
594. Brayshaw, J. R., and Perloff, J. K.: Congenital pulmonary insufficiency complicating idiopathic dilatation of the pulmonary artery. Am. J. Cardiol. *10*: 282, 1962.
595. Childers, R. W., and McCrea, P. C.: Absence of the pulmonary valve. A case occurring in the Marfan's syndrome. Circulation *29*:598, 1964.
596. Hamby, R. I., and Gulotta, S. J.: Pulmonic valvular insufficiency: Etiology, recognition and management. Am. Heart J. *74*:110, 1967.
597. Harris, B. C., Shaver, J. A., Kroetz, F. W., and Leonard, J. J.: Congenital pulmonary valvular insufficiency complicating tetralogy of Fallot. Intracardiac sound and pressure correlates. Am. J. Cardiol. *23*:864, 1969.
598. Holmes, J. C., Fowler, N. O., and Kaplan, S.: Pulmonary valvular insufficiency. Am. J. Med. *44*:851, 1968.
599. Osman, M. Z., Meng, C. C. L., and Girdany, B. R.: Congenital absence of the pulmonary valve: Report of eight cases with review of the literature. Am. J. Roentgenol. *106*:58, 1969.
600. Layton, C. A., McDonald, A., McDonald, L., Towers, M., Weaver, J., and Yacoub, M.: The syndrome of absent pulmonary valve. Total correction with aortic valvular homografts. J. Thorac. Cardiovasc. Surg. *63*:800, 1972.
601. Emery, R. W., Landes, R. G., Moller, J. H., and Nicoloff, D. M.: Pulmonary valve replacement with a porcine aortic heterograft. Ann. Thorac. Surg. *27*: 148, 1979.
602. Hurwitz, L. E., and Roberts, W. C.: Quadricuspid semilunar valve. Am. J. Cardiol. *31*:623, 1973.
603. Collins, N. P., Braunwald, E., and Morrow, A. G.: Isolated congenital pulmonic valvular regurgitation. Am. J. Med. *28*:159, 1960.
604. Levin, H. S., Runca, V., Wooley, C. F., and Ryan, J. M.: Pulmonic regurgitation following staphylococcal endocarditis. An intracardiac phonocardiographic study. Circulation *30*:411, 1964.
605. O'Toole, J. D., Wurtzbacher, J. J., Wearner, N. E., and Jain, A. C.: Pulmonary valve injury and insufficiency during pulmonary-artery catheterization. N. Engl. J. Med. *301*:1167, 1979.
606. Jacoby, W. J., Tucker, D. H., and Sumner, R. G.: The second heart sound in congenital pulmonary valvular insufficiency. Am. Heart J. *69*:603, 1965.
607. Bousvaros, G. A., and Deuchar, D. C.: The murmur of pulmonary regurgitation which is not associated with pulmonary hypertension. Lancet *2*: 962, 1961.
608. Green, E. W., Agruss, N. S., and Adolph, R. J.: Right-sided Austin Flint murmur. Documentation by intracardiac phonocardiography, echocardiography and postmortem findings. Am. J. Cardiol. *32*:370, 1973.
609. Braunwald, E., and Morrow, A. G.: A method for detection and estimation of aortic regurgitant flow in man. Circulation *17*:505, 1958.
610. Runco, V., Molnar, W., Meckstroth, C. V., and Ryan, J. M.: The Graham Steell murmur versus aortic regurgitation in rheumatic heart disease. Results of aortic valvulography. Am. J. Med. *31*:71, 1961.
611. Pernot, C., Hoeffel, J. C., Henry, M., Worms, A. M., Stehlin, H., and Louis, J. P.: Radiological patterns of congenital absence of the pulmonary valve in infants. Radiology *102*:619, 1972.
612. Collins, N. P., Braunwald, E., and Morrow, A. G.: Detection of pulmonic and tricuspid valvular regurgitation by means of indicator solutions. Circulation *20*: 561, 1959.
613. Levin, H. S., Runco, V., Wooley, C. F., and Ryan, J. M.: Intracardiac phonocardiography in organic pulmonic insufficiency. Circulation *24*:980, 1961.
614. Miyatake, K., Okamoto, M., Kinoshita, N., Matsuhisa, M., Nagata, S., Beppu, S., Park, Y.-D., Sakakibara, H., and Nimura, Y.: Pulmonary regurgitation studied with the ultrasonic pulsed Doppler technique. Circulation *65*:969, 1982.

MULTIVALVULAR DISEASE

615. Honey, M.: Clinical and hemodynamic observations on combined mitral and aortic stenosis. Br. Heart J. *23*:545, 1961.
616. Schattenberg, T. T., Titus, J. L., and Parkin, T. W.: Clinical findings in acquired aortic valve stenosis. Effect of disease of other valves. Am. Heart J. *73*: 322, 1967.
617. Melvin, D. B., Tecklenberg, P. L., Hollingsworth, J. F., Levine, F. H., Glancy, D. L., Epstein, S. E., and Morrow, A. G.: Computer-based analysis of preoperative and postoperative prognostic factors in 100 patients with combined aortic and mitral valve replacement. Circulation *48*(Suppl. III):58, 1973.
618. Nitter-Hauge, S., Frøysaker, T., Enge, I., and Rostad, H.: Clinical and haemodynamic observations after combined aortic and mitral valve replacement with the Björk-Shiley tilting disc valve prosthesis: Early and late results in 25 patients. Scand. J. Thorac. Cardiovasc. Surg. *13*:25, 1979.
619. Baxley, W. A., and Soto, B.: Hemodynamic evaluation of patients with combined mitral and aortic prostheses. Am. J. Cardiol. *45*:42, 1980.
620. Isom, O. W., Spencer, F. C., Glassman, E., Teiko, P., Boyd, A. D., Cunningham, J. N., and Reed, G. E.: Long-term results in 1375 patients undergoing valve replacement with the Starr-Edwards cloth-covered steel ball prosthesis. Ann. Surg. *186*:310,1977.
621. Cohn, L. H., Koster, J. K., Mee, R. B. B., and Collins, J. J., Jr.: Long-term followup of the Hancock bioprosthetic heart valve. A 6-year review. Circulation *60*(Suppl. II):93, 1979.
622. Stephenson, L. W., Kouchoukos, N. T., and Kirlin, J. W.: Triple valve replacement: An analysis of eight years' experience. Ann. Thorac. Surg. *23*:327, 1977.
623. MacManus, Q., Grunkemeier, G., and Starr, A.: Late results of triple valve replacement: A 14-year review. Ann. Thorac. Surg. *25*:402, 1978.
624. Péterffy, A., Jonasson, R., and Björk, V. O.: Ten years' experience of surgical management of triple valve disease. Early and late results in thirty-four consecutive cases. Scand. J. Thorac. Cardiovasc. Surg. *13*:191, 1979.
624a. Vatterott, P. J., Gersh, B. J., Fuster, V., Schaff, H. V., Danielson, G. K., Pluth, J. R., and McGoon, D. C.: Long-term followup (2–20 years) of patients with triple valve replacement. J. Am. Coll. Cardiol. *1*:586, 1983 (Abstr.).
625. Rhodes, G. R., McIntosh, C. L., Redwood, D. R., Itscoitz, S. B., and Epstein, S. E.: Clinical and hemodynamic results following triple valve replacement: Mechanical vs. procine xenograft prostheses. Circulation *56*(Suppl. II):122, 1977.

33 INFECTIVE ENDOCARDITIS

by Louis Weinstein, M.D., Ph.D.

HISTORY

Probably the first description of endocarditis was recorded by Lazare Riviere in 1646.[1] His patient sought his attention because of "palpitation of the heart." Riviere "found the pulse, small, irregular, with every variety of irregularity." The patient developed severe dyspnea and edema of the legs, gradually became more ill, produced bloody sputum, and died. The following findings were noted at autopsy: "In the left ventricle of the heart, round carunculae were found like the substance of the lungs, the larger of which resembled a cluster of hazel nuts and filled up the opening of the aorta."

In 1883, Eichorst published the first clinical classification of the different forms of endocarditis.[1] He defined the different presentations of the disease as *acute* (septic), *subacute* (endocarditis verrucosa), and *chronic* (endocarditis retrahens). With the possible exception of the last, this classification remains standard. In his Gulstonian lectures in 1885,[2] Osler pointed out that about 75 per cent of patients who developed bacterial endocarditis had underlying damage to the cardiac valves. He described the clinical and pathological features of the disease in detail and commented that "micrococci are constant elements in the vegetations." Interest in subacute bacterial endocarditis among physicians in the United States was stimulated by the publication of the classic paper of Libman and Celler in 1910.[3] They reported their observations in 43 cases of the disease and presented detailed descriptions of the causative organisms.

No effective means of treatment were available, however. Sulfonamides were used to treat bacterial endocarditis after their introduction in 1937, but results were poor; only 4 to 6 per cent of patients were said to have been cured.[4,5] These drugs probably played a much more important role in reducing the risk of valvular infections by controlling extracardiac disease produced by the pneumococcus, *Streptococcus pyogenes*, gonococcus, and bacteremia caused by sensitive organisms.

A new era in the natural history of infective endocarditis began in 1943 and 1944 with the reports by Florey and Florey[6] and Loewe et al.[7] of the successful cure of the subacute form of the disease with penicillin. As more and more antimicrobial agents have become available over the ensuing years, it has become possible to treat a broader variety of etiologically different types of infective endocarditis effectively. In more recent years a number of other features—microbiological, immunological, and therapeutic—have altered the course and management of this disease. Among these are the increasingly frequent involvement of unusual organisms, the increase in infections of the right side of the heart (related primarily to the wide use of intravenously administered illicit drugs such as heroin), the longer life spans of patients, a striking change in the types of cardiac disease on which valvular infection is superimposed, and a striking increase in and knowledge of the immunological phenomena that contribute to complications of infective endocarditis. An important new aspect of this disease has been the development of and increasing experience with cardiac surgery, which may be responsible for valvular infections (prosthesis) or be the critical maneuver in the cure of the infection (both natural and prosthetic valves) or which may be responsible for the management of potential complications such as intractable congestive failure or intracardiac complications such as abscesses, aneurysms, and the like.

The incidence of infective endocarditis in the United States in 1936 was reported by Hedley to have been 4000 to 5000 cases, or 4.2 per 100,000 of the population.[8] Approximately 70 per cent of all cases were of the subacute variety. These data in the preantibiotic era are comparable to the experience in Great Britain, where an annual average of 964 cases of bacterial endocarditis was reported in the years 1924 to 1944.[9]

Kaye and his colleagues noted a marked decrease in the incidence of infective endocarditis.[10] They suggested that the factors responsible for this were (a) widespread use of antibiotics in all types of infections, (b) chemoprophylaxis for patients with rheumatic or congenital heart disease, and (c) the tendency to refer patients with valvular infections to "referral" teaching hospitals. A fall in the number of cases admitted to large municipal hospitals has been reported by Finland[11] and Afremow.[12] However, Cherubin and Neu noted no change in the incidence of the disease over a period of 30 years (1938 to 1967).[13] In contrast, Lerner and Weinstein suggested that there has been a definite *increase* in the frequency of this disease over the past 25 years.[14] When the increase in the number of factors proven to predispose to the development of infective endocarditis is considered, it seems likely to this author that the incidence of the disease has increased and continues to do so. Thus, although there is still some controversy concerning the present incidence of infective endocarditis, there is general agreement that there has been a change in its distributions at various levels.

Though involving primarily young adults in the preantibiotic era, the disease now affects chiefly older individuals, as emphasized by analysis of data obtained from study at necropsy. Thus, the mean age of patients with subacute bacterial endocarditis has increased from 32 years of age in the 1930's and 1940's [16] to 40 to 42 years in the 1950's[17,18] and to 50 to 54 years in the 1960's.[15-20] Endocarditis remains an uncommon disease in the first decade of life but is becoming increasingly common in the 60- to 80-year age group.[14] Endocarditis affecting infants under the age of two years is usually of the acute variety and attacks normal valves, with a predilection for the tricuspid valve. There is a striking difference in the sex distribution of infective endocarditis. A male-female ratio of 2 to 1 was noted by Lerner and Weinstein.[14] However, in patients 51 to 60 years of age, this ratio increased to 9:1.

The etiological agents responsible for all types of bacterial endocarditis have changed since the advent of penicillin therapy. The number of acute cases due to pneumococcus, gonococcus, meningococcus, and group A hemolytic streptococci decreased strikingly in the first decade of antibiotic therapy; there was a relative, but not absolute, increase in nonhemolytic streptococcal cases. In the second decade of the antibiotic era, an increase in cases due to *Staphylococcus aureus* became apparent.[14a]

MICROBIOLOGY OF ENDOCARDITIS

Infective endocarditis has usually been classified primarily as acute or subacute according to the nature of the responsible organism. Thus, when *Staphylococcus aureus, Streptococcus pneumoniae, Neisseria meningitidis, Neisseria gonorrhoeae, Strep. pyogenes,* and *Hemophilus influenzae* are the causative agents, the endocarditis is considered acute. In contrast, when viridans streptococcus or *Staph. epidermidis* is recovered from the blood, the infection is called subacute. This clinical differentiation remains important because the presenting manifestations, the duration of the course, the nature of the complications, and the final outcome differ greatly, even when appropriate antimicrobial therapy and other therapeutic modalities are applied. It has become clear, however, that there is an appreciable number of instances in which no relation to the invading organism exists. For this reason, Lerner and Weinstein suggested that the designations *acute* and *subacute* be abolished, because disease that is originally acute may be converted to subacute status by appropriate therapy, while subacute disease may suddenly become life-threatening when serious complications develop.[14] In addition, they and others[21-23] have studied patients with valvular infections caused by *Staph. aureus* with a consistently subacute course as well as other patients infected with *Streptococcus viridans* in whom clinical behavior was entirely acute; this has been true especially in some instances of enterococcal disease.

The microbiology of infective endocarditis is summarized in Table 33–1.

MICROBIOLOGY OF INFECTIONS OF PROSTHETIC VALVES

Infections of prosthetic valves have involved a large number of microbes, some of which have been associated only with this kind of disease. The bulk of microorganisms responsible for invasion of cardiac prostheses is, however, the same as those that cause infection of natural valves. For example, *Staph. aureus, Staph. epidermidis,* various streptococci, *Hemophilus, Brucella,* and *Candida* are known to invade prosthetic as well as natural valves. Among those that have been involved primarily in infection of valvular prostheses are gram-negative bacteria such as *Serratia, Acinetobacter calcoaceticus, Pseudomonas cepacia, Ps. aeruginosa, Ps. multophilia, Flavobacterium, Bacteroides, Edwardsiella tarda,* and *Eikenella corrodens.* Gram-positive organisms that invade prosthetic rather than natural valves include groups B, D, and K streptococci. *Staph. epidermidis* affects patients with prostheses more often than it does those who have not had valves replaced, and it is the most frequent cause of disease early after operation. When prosthetic infection occurs late, both staphylococci and streptococci are commonly involved; however, *Staph. epidermidis* is much more common than *Staph. aureus* in necropsied cases. Most instances of endocarditis due to *Propionibacterium acnes, Bacteroides,* and *Eikenella corrodens* have occurred in individuals with cardiac prostheses.

Valvular disease caused by the atypical mycobacteria *Mycobacterium chelonei* and *M. gordonae* has been observed only when cardiac bioprostheses (porcine valves [Table 33–1]) have been present.

The recent striking increase in the incidence of endocarditis caused by yeasts and fungi is attributable almost entirely to the presence of valvular prostheses, to the increased number of patients addicted to drugs administered intravenously, and to long-term antimicrobial therapy. The organisms most commonly involved are *Candida, Aspergillus,* and *Histoplasma.* Among the species of *Candida* recovered from infected prostheses have been *albicans, parapsilosis, tropicalis, stellatoidea,* and *krusei* (Table 33–1).

An appreciable number of infections involving prosthetic valves—especially those caused by unusual bacteria, yeasts, and fungi—are probably superinfections induced by antimicrobial chemoprophylaxis or therapy. Organisms may also be introduced into the bloodstream during intravenous injection of drugs in addicted persons.

Cumulative experience indicates that aortic valve prostheses are more frequently infected than prostheses replacing other valves. One study of prosthetic endocarditis demonstrated infection in 3 per cent of patients in whom the aortic valve was replaced versus 1 per cent of those with mitral valve prostheses.[111] Infection of combined mitral and aortic valve prostheses is not uncommon. Complications of infected prostheses include ruptured mycotic aneurysms, ruptured aorta, ruptured aneurysm of the sinus of Valsalva, perivalvular abscess, myocardial abscess, pericardio-mediastinal fistula, abscess of the atrioventricular ring, and thrombosis of the prosthesis.

TABLE 33–1 MICROBIOLOGY OF ENDOCARDITIS

	GRAM-POSITIVE COCCI
Streptococcus viridans	Responsible for 50% of all cases of endocarditis, 70% of subacute disease. Three instances of progressive, invasive disease.[24] Predisposing factors: trauma; dental manipulations (extractions, flossing, gingivectomy, periapical abscess, Water-Pik). May produce disease in edentulous patients.[25] Usually produces subacute disease, rarely acute.
Enterococcus	Member of group D streptococci. May produce α, β, or γ hemolysis. Species: *Strep. liquefaciens, Strep. zymogenes, Strep. faecalis, Strep. faecium, Strep. durans.* Source of organisms: GU and GI tracts and oral cavity. Causes 3–17% of cases of endocarditis. Course of the disease acute or subacute.
Streptococcus bovis	Member of group D, but not an enterococcus. Responsible for about 50% of cases caused by group D streptococci.[26] Fails to grow in medium containing 6.5% saline. Sensitive to penicillin G. Survival rate higher than with enterococcus. High degree of association of endocarditis with cancer of the colon, Crohn's disease, ulcerative colitis.[27-30]
Peptostreptococcus	Anaerobe—causes 3–8.5% of cases.[17] Requires culture under anaerobic conditions (thioglycollate broth). Produces mostly subacute disease, occasionally acute.
Streptococcus pyogenes (group A, "beta-hemolytic")	Currently an uncommon cause of endocarditis, probably because of high rate of successful treatment of pharyngitis, cellulitis, and other extracardiac foci of infection. Although organism usually produces "beta-hemolysis," some strains may be alpha-hemolytic on surface of blood agar. Clinical course of valvular infection is acute. May produce intracardiac complications, e.g., rupture of valve leaflets.
Streptococcus pneumoniae	Frequency of endocarditis decreasing because of highly successful therapy of pneumonia and other extracardiac infections caused by this organism. Current incidence about 5 to 6%.[31] Disease is usually acute. High frequency of destructive intracardiac complications. Increased risk of valvular infection in patients with multilobar pulmonary involvement and bacteremia.
Other Species of Streptococci	*Strep. mutans.*[32] *Group G.*[33] *Group C*—uncommon, acute disease, with destruction of valves.[34] Organism may be "tolerant" to penicillin G.[35] *Strep. constellatus*—only one case reported.[36] *Group B*[37]—involves mitral valve most commonly; next is aortic valve. *Groups D, G,* and *K.*[38] Group L.[39]
Nutritionally-Deficient Streptococci ("satelliting" streptococci)	Uncommon. Require pyridoxine for growth. Thioglycollate broth plus pyridoxine is good medium. Colonies group around colonies of *Staph. aureus* (satelliting). Grow in ordinary broth, but cannot be subcultured from these or agar.[40]
Staphylococcus aureus	Commonest organism producing acute endocarditis. Predisposing factors: cardiac surgery, intravenous abuse of drugs, infections of the skin, osteomyelitis, peripheral sepsis, rheumatic carditis (rare). No underlying cardiac disease in 50 to 60% of cases. No murmurs in presence of endocarditis in about 1/3 of patients. High frequency of intracardiac complications: rupture of valvular leaflets, septal abscesses, aneurysm of sinus of Valsalva, myocardial abscesses. Disseminated extracardiac infections common. Proved staphylococcal bacteremia in absence of evidence of endocarditis is associated with risk of valvular infection in 30 to 65% of cases.[41] Most strains are resistant to penicillin G. Treatment with a penicillinase-resistant penicillin or an active cephalosporin is required. Some strains are "methicillin-resistant" ("tolerant") and fail to be killed by penicillins and cephalosporins. Replacement of infected valve with a prosthesis is often required. Average fatality rate about 50%.
Staphylococcus epidermidis ("*albus*")	Incidence has increased over the past 25 years. Occasionally involves normal valves; most patients have underlying valvular disease. Common in "main-line" drug addicts. Thought to be commonest organism infecting prosthetic valves. Produces subacute and chronic endocarditis. High incidence of recurrence after "appropriate" antimicrobial therapy. May require replacement of involved valve. Organism variably sensitive to antibiotics. Fatality rate high.[42]
	GRAM-POSITIVE BACILLI
Erysipelothrix insidiosa	Acquired from fish, birds, cats. May involve normal heart. Disease is acute. Fatality rate 50%.[43]
Lactobacillus	Dental procedures predisposing factor. May be no underlying cardiac disease.[44,45]
Listeria monocytogenes	Rare. Involves natural and prosthetic valves. High incidence of systemic embolization.[46]
Corynebacteria	Aerobic diphtheroids and anaerobic *Propionibacterium acnes.* Uncommon cause of endocarditis.[47,48]
Corynebacterium diphtheriae	Rare cause of endocarditis. Only 8 cases (1944–1980). Not all strains produce toxin. Increased susceptibility with congenital heart disease.[49,50]
Bacillus cereus	Only two reported cases. Has involved only prosthetic valves.[51]
Bacillus subtilis	Only one reported case. Drug addict—right heart involved.[52]
Rothia dentocariosa	Only two reported cases of endocarditis. Produces subacute disease.[53,54]
	GRAM-NEGATIVE COCCI
Neisseria gonorrhoeae	Caused 10 to 14% of cases in preantibiotic era[55]; now uncommon. Not always related to genital infection. Aortic and mitral valves involved most often. High incidence of infection of right heart. Arthritis in 50% of cases. No underlying heart disease in most patients. One patient with prolapsed mitral valve described.[56] Frequent intra- and extracardiac complications requiring surgery. Recent increase in number of penicillin-resistant strains.
Neisseria meningitidis	Rare. Always secondary to bacteremia, with or without meningitis. Acute endocarditis.
Other Gram-negative Cocci	*N. flava, N. catarrhalis, N. pharyngis, N. mucosa,*[14] *Megasphaera elsdenii* (anaerobe).[57]
	GRAM-NEGATIVE BACILLI
Escherichia coli	Responsible for about 3 to 10% of endocarditis. For a recent detailed review, see Ref. 58. Murmur not always present. Mitral valve most often involved.[59]
Enterobacter	Uncommon. Manipulation of genitourinary tract predisposing factor is 50% of cases.[60]
Klebsiella pneumoniae	Very rare. Preceding infection of urinary tract.[61]
Proteus	Rare. Both indole-positive and indole-negative strains involved. Infection of urinary tract predisposing factor.[62]
Pseudomonas aeruginosa	Most common in drug addicts. In nonaddicted, occurs most often during therapy of another infection (superinfection). Emboli produce necrosis of walls of blood vessels. Tricuspid valve commonly involved. Infection of more than one valve not rare.[63,64]
Other Species of *Pseudomonas*	*Ps. multophilia,*[65] *Ps. cepacia.*[66]
Salmonella	Uncommon cause of endocarditis. Most patients over 50 years old. Underlying cardiac disease in most instances. Course often acute. GI tract source of organism in $<50\%$ of patients. Fatality rate high, even when treated.[67]
Hemophilus	Responsible for about 0.5% of cases of endocarditis. Three species involved: *H. influenzae,*[68] *H. parainfluenzae,*[69] and *H. aphrophilus.*[70] High frequency of embolization with *H. parainfluenzae.*

TABLE 33–1 MICROBIOLOGY OF ENDOCARDITIS *(Continued)*

Brucella	Rare. Species involved: *Br. abortus, Br. suis, Br. melitensis.* Underlying heart disease in most cases. Mitral valve most often involved. Occasionally acute. Bulky vegetations.[71]
Pasteurella	Rare. Usual source is animal bite or scratch. Cats and dogs carry organism. Three species: *P. multocida* (commonest),[72] *P. pneumotropica, P. hemolytica.*
Acinetobacter	May involve normal heart. Acute or subacute disease. Cardiac failure and embolization in > 50% of cases. Fatality rate 50–75%.[73]
Serratia	75% of cases in drug addicts. Infection of prosthetic valves common. Subacute course commonest. Large emboli in most instances. Fatality rate about 70%.[74]
Campylobacter (Vibrio)	One species, *fetus.* May involve normal heart. Dental manipulation a predisposing factor. Aortic valve usually affected.[75]
Streptobacillus moniliformis	Rare. Endocarditis occurs during course of rat bite fever.[76]
Cardiobacterium hominis	Uncommon. Organism present in pharynx of 70% of normal people. Usually involves abnormal valves. Course subacute. Emboli in 50% of cases.[77]
Actinobacillus actinomycetemcomitans	Most common in middle-aged and older men. Normal valves involved in 2/3 of cases. Course subacute. Organism grows slowly.[78]
Flavobacterium	Only one case reported. Ulceration of aortic valve.[79]
Edwardsiella tarda	Single case report.[80]
Citrobacter diversus	Single case.[81]
	YEASTS AND FUNGI
Yeasts	Species of *Candida* involved: *C. albicans, C. parapsilosis, C. guilliermondii, C. krusei, C. stellatoidea, C. tropicalis* (commonest cause in drug addicts). One third of cases follow cardiac surgery. 20% related to superinfection. Course subacute. Emboli in 50% of patients—occlude large arteries. Blood cultures negative in 75% of cases.[82–84] *Torulopsis glabrata.*[85]
Histoplasma capsulatum	Uncommon. Most cases in eastern U.S., Ohio, and Mississippi Valley. Involves natural and prosthetic valves. Embolus to large artery may be first sign. Cultures of blood usually negative.[86]
Aspergillus	Various species involved. All cases in debilitated or immunocompromised patients or those treated with antibiotics. Prosthetic valves most commonly involved. Infection or mural endocardium common. Blood cultures rarely positive.[87]
Other Yeasts and Fungi	*Penicillium, Phialophora, Hormodendrum, Paecilomyces, Curvilacea, Saccharomyces, Mucor, Torulopsis glabrata, Trichosporon cutaneum, Cryptococcus, Rhodotorula.*[88–90]
	OTHER ORGANISMS
Mycobacterium chelonei	Porcine bioprostheses involved. Organisms cultured from the valves prior to insertion.[91]
Mycobacterium gordonae	An atypical mycobacterium—one instance of infection of a prosthetic valve.[92]
Mycobacterium tuberculosis	Usually involves only natural valves as a complication of disseminated tuberculosis.[93] Infection of homograft valves reported.[94]
Coxiella burnetii (Q fever)	All cases of endocarditis have occurred in the course of Q fever. Very few reported from the United States; all others in Australia and New Zealand. Duration of Q fever before development of endocarditis—1 to 20 years. Diagnosis made by detection of rising titer of phase-1 complement-fixing antibody.[95]
Actinomyces israelii (bovis)	Infection by this organism very rare.[96] Both natural and prosthetic valves involved.
Nocardia israelii	Very rare.[97] Both natural and prosthetic valves involved.
Bacteroides	Several species involved. Only 11 reported cases. Usually subacute but may be acute. Infects both prosthetic and natural valves.[98,99]
Fusobacterium	Only 10 reported cases. May be fulminant.[98]
Chlamydia psittaci	Infection not proved by isolation of the organism. Contact with birds important. Diagnosis made by staining endocardial biopsies with fluorescein-labeled specific antibody.[100]
Chlamydia trachomatis	Infection or aortic valve in one case; complicated by pericarditis.[101]
Cell Wall–Deficient Organisms	Possible but not proved cause of endocarditis. Thought to be responsible for fever persisting despite appropriate therapy. Commonest in drug addicts and in patients undergoing cardiac surgery.[102,103]
Polymicrobial Infection	Incidence from 1 in 250 to 1 in 10.[104,105] More than 2 organisms in some cases.[14] Mostly mixtures of gram-positive cocci, or these with gram-negative rods or yeast.
Virus	Indirect evidence. One case of serologically proved coxsackievirus B endocarditis.[106]
	ENDOCARDITIS ASSOCIATED WITH DRUG ADDICTION
Staph. aureus	Incidence higher than in nonaddicted patients. Right side of heart involved more often. Commonest organism.[107]
Streptococci	*Strep. viridans, Strep. faecalis,* enterococcus.[108]
Other Bacteria	Various species of *Pseudomonas,* aerobic and anaerobic diphtheroids. *Staph. epidermidis, Hemophilus, Strep. pneumoniae,* anaerobes and gram-negative organisms.[109,110]
Yeasts and Fungi	*Histoplasma, Saccharomyces, Paecilomyces, Mucor, Cryptococcus, Candida, Aspergillus.* 5% of patients.[105]
Polymicrobial Infection	Reported to range from 1 case in 250 up to as high as 5%. Mixtures of different streptococci, other gram-positive cocci with gram-negative rods, gram-negative bacilli, and/or yeasts and fungi.[104,105]

PATHOLOGY OF ENDOCARDITIS

Vegetations are common to all types of infective endocarditis and are situated most frequently on the valvular leaflets and less often on the endocardium of the ventricles or of the left atrium (McCallum's patch of rheumatic carditis) and on pulmonary or other arteries. When fresh, the vegetations are pink, red, yellow, or green but change to gray as they heal. These lesions are usually larger and much more friable than those of rheumatic fever; small particles are easily broken off and become disseminated in the blood stream as emboli. The largest vegetations develop in the course of fungal infections of the valves; emboli that arise from these are large enough to occlude large arteries, a distinguishing characteristic of this type of endocarditis (Fig. 33–1). Occasionally, the vegetations formed during infection by *Staph. aureus* are larger than those associated with alpha-streptococci. In some instances of infection of prosthetic valves and, less often, when staphylococci or some gram-negative organisms are involved, valvular lesions may be of such a size that they obstruct the valve orifice, sharply reduce cardiac output, and lead to congestive heart failure.

Infective endocarditis involves the left side of the heart much more frequently than the right, affecting the mitral, aortic, or both valves, in that order.[112] Disease of the pul-

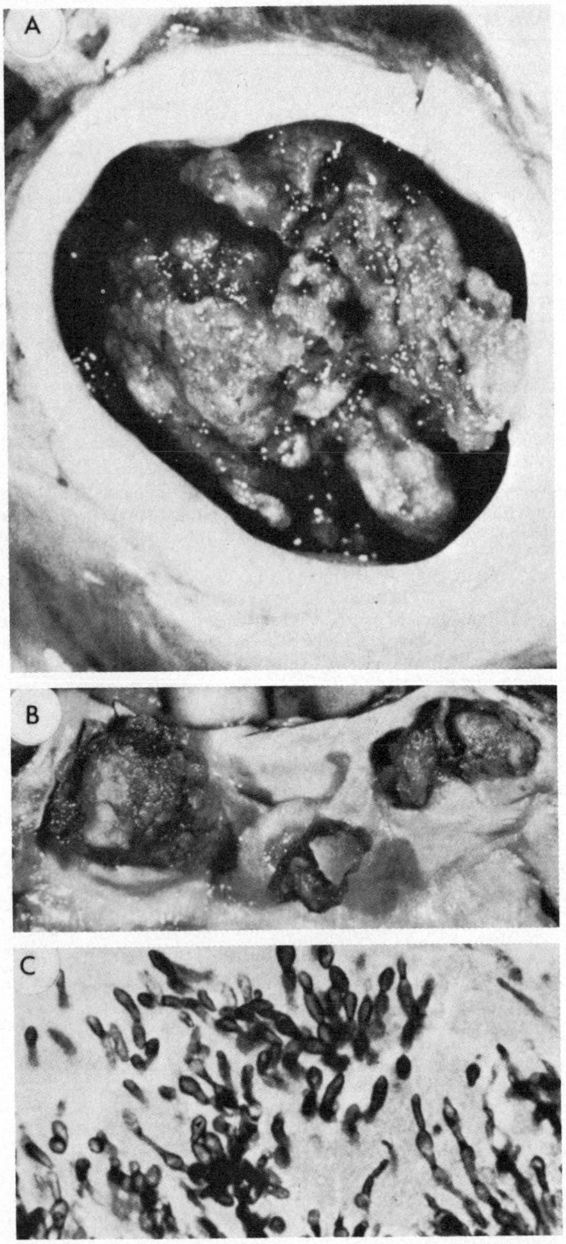

FIGURE 33–1 *Candida parapsilosis* **endocarditis involving the aortic valve led to an embolus to the left anterior descending coronary artery with a large transmural acute myocardial infarct two months before death.** ***A,*** **Aortic valve viewed from above. The large vegetations appear to obstruct the valve orifice.** ***B,*** **Opened valve showing vegetations on each cusp.** ***C,*** **Photomicrograph of vegetation showing pseudomycelia of** ***C. parapsilosis.*** **(Methenamine silver stain.) (From Roberts, W. C., and Buchbinder, N. A.: Healed left-sided infective endocarditis. A clinicopathological study of 59 patients. Am. J. Cardiol.** ***40*****:876, 1976.)**

monic and tricuspid valves is relatively uncommon; however, the latter has increased over the past 15 years with the rise in drug addiction. Although much more common in acute than in subacute valvular infections, vegetations on the mitral valve may extend along the chordae tendineae to the apex of the papillary muscles. This may lead to rupture of these structures, especially in acute infections. Rupture is rare in subacute endocarditis unless the infection has remained untreated for a prolonged period. This is also the case when aortic valvular vegetations spread by contiguity along the ventricular endocardium or when ulcerated lesions appear on the ventricular surface of the anterior mitral cusp.

Necrosis of the affected valve may lead to aneurysms and/or perforation of the cusps. This occurs most often in acute infective endocarditis, especially that caused by *Staph. aureus,* but only rarely in subacute valvular infections. In addition to aneurysms of the sinus of Valsalva, these lesions, when present at the base of the aorta, may extend into the pericardial space between the aorta and pulmonary artery and produce a hemorrhagic, pyogenic, or fibrinous pericarditis (Fig. 33–2). The infectious process may invade the interventricular septum. Septal perforation may follow when endocarditis is acute.

Arnett and Roberts have described both the gross and histological abnormalities in the active and healed stages of various types of infective endocarditis.[113] In a study of 45 cases of *active left-sided endocarditis,* as well as a review of autopsy reports, Buchbinder and Roberts[114] noted that myocardial lesions were present in 88 to 100 per cent of cases. Evidence of bacterial endocarditis involving previously normal valves was found in as many as 42 per cent of patients. Heart failure due to valvular dysfunction occurred in 59 to 74 per cent of patients studied at autopsy. Papillary muscle necrosis that did not lead to mitral regurgitation was present in 58 per cent. Pericarditis produced by direct extension of inflammation into the pericardium was noted in 8 per cent of patients. Of 31 individuals with infection of the aortic valve, 12 had ring abscesses, an indication of severe destruction of valvular cusps.

Studies of the gross pathology of *healed left-sided endocarditis* revealed that half had anatomical lesions readily attributable to healed infective endocarditis.[115] Unequivocal residua of valvular infection were more common in purely incompetent than in stenotic or mixed valvular disease. Half of the patients had either cuspal perforation, probably secondary to ring abscesses, ruptured chordae tendineae, or aneurysms. The most common organism was alpha-streptococcus. The mitral or aortic valve, or both, were either stenotic or purely incompetent. Patients with valvular perforations and ruptured chordae tendineae usually had pure regurgitation. Three individuals with ring abscesses

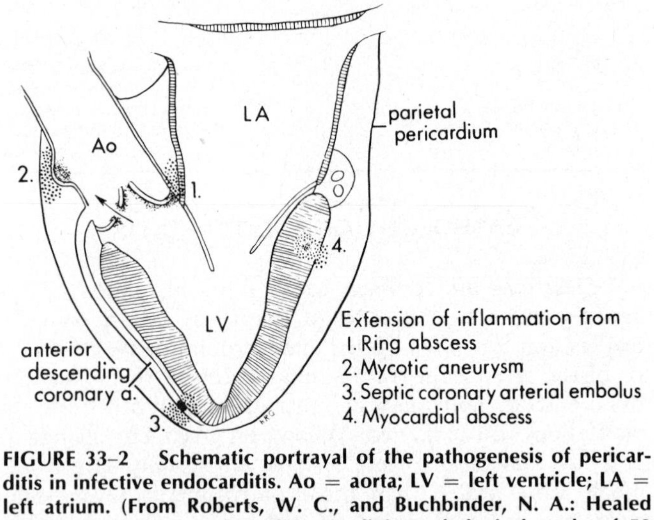

FIGURE 33–2 Schematic portrayal of the pathogenesis of pericarditis in infective endocarditis. Ao = aorta; LV = left ventricle; LA = left atrium. (From Roberts, W. C., and Buchbinder, N. A.: Healed left-sided infective endocarditis. A clinicopathological study of 59 patients. Am. J. Cardiol. ***40*****:876, 1976.)**

had competent valves. All of the stenotic valves were diffusely fibrotic; most contained calcific deposits. Diffuse or focal fibrosis was present in incompetent valves. Autopsy findings suggested that the left-sided valves had been anatomically normal in 15 per cent of patients prior to the development of endocarditis. Forty-one per cent of patients had underlying rheumatic heart disease and 29 per cent had a congenital cardiac lesion.

The pathoanatomy of right-sided bacterial endocarditis in 12 patients was reported by Roberts and Buchbinder.[116] Bacteria were present on the tricuspid or pulmonary valve in 7 cases. Among the lesions observed were ruptured chordae tendineae, necrosis of the papillary muscles, and suppurative or nonsuppurative myocarditis. In 9 of 12 patients the vegetations in the right side of the heart did not extend to involve the basal attachments of the leaflets to the annuli. Mural lesions were observed in 3 cases; in 2, they were present on the right ventricular endocardium.

Pathology of Prosthetic Valve Endocarditis. Excellent studies of the gross pathology of endocarditis involving *prosthetic valves* have been recorded by Arnett and Roberts[117] and Anderson et al.[118] The former studied 22 necropsied patients with infections of rigid-frame valvular prostheses replacing aortic valves in 15 and mitral valves in 7 cases (Fig. 33–3). Endocarditis developed within two months after operation in 8, and 2 months or longer postoperatively in 14 patients. The organism recovered most often was located behind the site of attachment of the prosthesis to the valve ring. It spread to adjacent structures in 13 patients, 11 of whom had aortic prostheses. In most cases, the prosthetic valve was detached. Conduction defects, including left bundle branch or complete block, were present in 7 individuals. These were observed most often when aortic prostheses were present, suggesting that conduction abnormalities were related to the presence of abscess or necrosis in the upper area of the interventricular septum.

Among 22 patients with endocarditis involving valvular prostheses studied by Anderson et al. at autopsy, 95 per cent had cardiac hypertrophy and 73 per cent had dilated left ventricles.[118] Dysfunction of the prosthesis was present in 17 per cent and was due to ulceration of a cusp, paravalvular leak, entrapment of the poppet by a thrombus, perforation of a ring abscess into the right ventricle, or mitral stenosis (most common). Fifty-seven per cent of patients experienced infection of the aortic annulus, while involvement of the mitral annulus was observed in 43 per cent. Fibrinous or purulent pericarditis, aortic stenosis due to exuberant vegetations, and embolic myocarditis (abscess and focal necrosis) were also noted. In no instance did infection of a prosthesis spread to the other valves. In two persons with first-degree block, the atrioventricular node was extensively involved by the inflammatory process that had extended from an abscess of the aortic ring; the bundle of His was intact. Among the extracardiac findings were peripheral (85 per cent), splenic (59 per cent), renal (50 per cent), and cerebral (45 per cent) emboli.

The pathological features of infected *Hancock porcine bioprostheses* have been described by Bartolloti et al.[119] (Fig. 33–4). The vegetations were friable, small to massive, and present on the inflow surface of the valve. Infected cusps were torn, frayed, or perforated. Ring abscess or valvular calcification was uncommon. Among the histological findings were deposition of fibrin on the inflow surface of the valve and breakdown of collagen. Moderate to marked subendothelial inflammation was present in some instances. Macrophages, neutrophils, and clusters of bacteria within the tissue of the cusps were noted in all cases. Granulomas were present when fungi were involved. The following features that distinguish endocarditis involving porcine valves from that of infection of rigid-frame prostheses have been pointed out by Ferrans et al.[120]: (a) infection can involve the porcine valve itself as well as fibrin, organized thrombi, and fibrous tissue of the patient, and

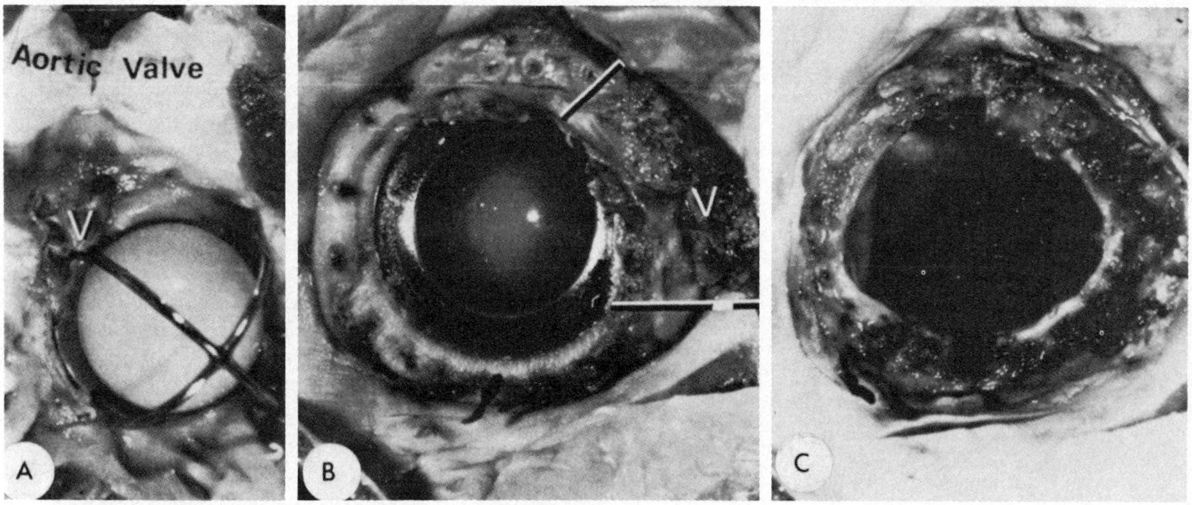

FIGURE 33–3 Prosthetic mitral valve endocarditis caused by *Staphylococcus epidermidis.* The infection appeared 10 years after replacement of both mitral and tricuspid valves. At necropsy, only the mitral prosthesis was infected. *A,* Infected mitral valve prosthesis viewed from the left ventricle. Vegetative material (V) is present on the prosthetic annulus just below the aortic valve. *B,* Prosthesis as viewed from the left atrium showing vegetations (V) at the junction of the prosthetic and natural valve annuli. *C,* Same view after removal of the prosthesis, showing even greater extension of the infection at the site of attachment of the prosthesis. (From Arnett, E. N., and Roberts, W. C.: Prosthetic valve endocarditis. Clinicopathological analysis of 22 necropsy patients with comparison of observations in 74 necropsy patients with active infective endocarditis involving natural left-sided cardiac valves. Am. J. Cardiol. *38*:281, 1976.)

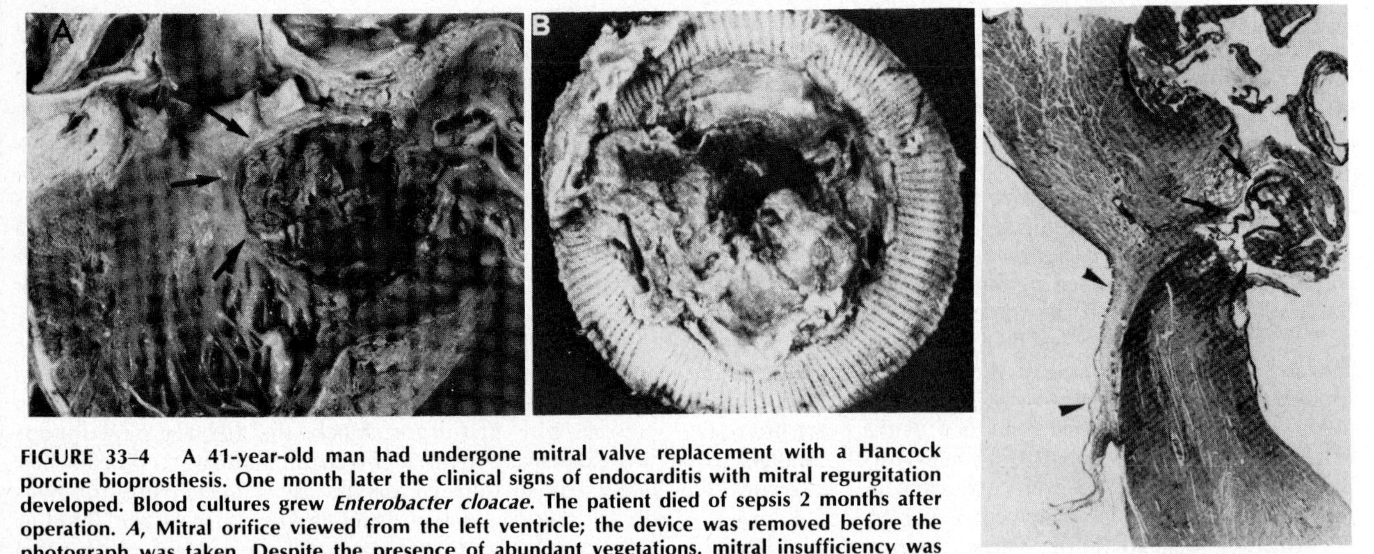

FIGURE 33–4 A 41-year-old man had undergone mitral valve replacement with a Hancock porcine bioprosthesis. One month later the clinical signs of endocarditis with mitral regurgitation developed. Blood cultures grew *Enterobacter cloacae*. The patient died of sepsis 2 months after operation. *A*, Mitral orifice viewed from the left ventricle; the device was removed before the photograph was taken. Despite the presence of abundant vegetations, mitral insufficiency was found. This dysfunction was caused by prosthetic detachment owing to a ring abscess (arrows). *B*, Atrial view of the explanted heterograft with moderate thrombotic vegetations. *C*, Histological examination of the conducting tissue revealed a spared atrioventricular node (arrowheads) and bundle and an extensive ring abscess (arrows) on the left side of the central fibrous body. (Elastic van Gieson stain, orig. mag. × 3.) (From Bortolotti, U., et al.: Pathological study of infective endocarditis on Hancock porcine bioprostheses. J. Thorac. Cardiovasc. Surg. *81*:934, 1981. Reproduced with permission.)

destroy the valve; (b) ring abscesses are uncommon; (c) perforation of cusps does not occur; (d) valvular stenosis is common; and (e) paravalvular leaks are uncommon.

Histological Changes. Histological abnormalities of subacute infective endocarditis were described by Libman and Friedberg. They noted that the vegetations consisted essentially of platelet-fibrin thrombi containing colonies of bacteria on and below the surface and suggested that the

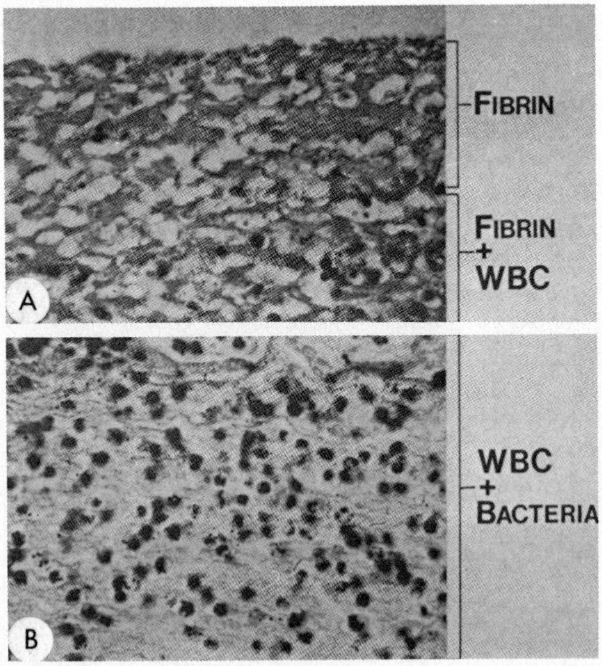

FIGURE 33–5 Infective vegetation. Photomicrographs of an infective vegetation. *A*, Note fibrin and a few leukocytes near the surface. *B*, Deeper, toward the base in the vegetation, are numerous leukocytes and stainable bacteria. Note the lack of vascular channels. (From Applefeld, M. M., and Woodward, T. E.: Infective endocarditis: A clinical overview. *In* Harvey, W. P., et al. (eds.): Current Problems in Cardiology. Vol. 2, No. 5. Copyright © 1977 by Year Book Medical Publishers, Inc., Chicago. Reproduced with permission of the publishers and courtesy of Dr. William C. Roberts.)

thrombus was derived from the inflamed valve that had undergone destructive change (Fig. 33–5). The inflammatory reaction consisted chiefly of mononuclear cells, lymphocytes, and histiocytes; very few polymorphonuclear cells were present. Not uncommonly, giant cells containing phagocytized bacteria were present. The cusp underlying the vegetation was the site of a destructive process that was either localized or extended to both surfaces. Healing was an early and prominent feature. At this stage, most of the bacteria had disappeared. In addition to inflammatory cells, the cusp contained numerous capillaries and fibroblasts. When healing was prolonged, the vegetations became calcified.

The myocardium may show a variety of lesions. These are usually diffuse or localized collections of lymphocytes and mononuclear cells and are the so-called Bracht-Wachter lesions that replace the muscle itself. Diffuse or localized collections of polymorphonuclear cells, with or without myocardial necrosis or miliary abscesses, are observed occasionally. Gross suppuration is absent. Muscle fibers may show degenerative changes, often with small scars in various stages of healing. The small coronary branches show swelling and proliferation of the endothelial cells of capillaries and arterioles, arteriolitis, or necrosis of the media or adventitia; perivascular cellular infiltrates and scars may be present. A large branch of a coronary artery may contain an embolus or reveal a mycotic aneurysm.

Among the lesions noted in cases of right-sided endocarditis have been myocardial abscesses containing colonies of bacteria, septic emboli (extramural or intramural) in one or more coronary arteries, foci of necrosis in the ventricular wall or papillary muscles, calcification of individual myocardial fibers, and acute pneumonia with pulmonary infarcts or abscesses.[116] The histopathological findings observed during necropsy of patients with left-sided infective endocarditis were foci of myocardial fibrosis in the ventricular papillary muscles, ventricular free wall, or both.[115] In about 20 per cent of cases, there was greater than 75 per cent cross-sectional narrowing of coronary arterial lumina.

The microanatomy of acute bacterial endocarditis is entirely different from that of the subacute form of the disease. In the former, the histological picture is of a rapidly progressive destructive lesion, with no features that indicate any attempt at healing, such as the presence of fibroblasts or organization. In untreated cases, the fibrin-platelet thrombus contains only polymorphonuclear leukocytes and large numbers of bacteria. The affected underlying valve is the site of necrosis. These features satisfy the criteria for the term *ulcerative endocarditis* that has been applied to this type of disease and explain the predisposition to tearing of the valvular leaflets, rupture of papillary muscles and chordae tendineae, the formation of aneurysms, and the frequency of intracardiac spread of infection—common complications of this type of disease.

Portals of Entry and Predisposing Factors

The most important factor predisposing to infection of cardiac valves is invasion of the bloodstream by any of the organisms suspected to be involved in this disease. The bacteremias or fungemias that initiate infective endocarditis may be persistent or transient, may arise in the course of a variety of manipulations in patients without a predisposing infected site, or may be a consequence of spread into the circulation from an area of established infection.

Transient Bacteremias. It is remarkable that transient bacteremias occur following various types of manipulation of areas in which organisms are normally present, such as the mouth, upper airway, skin, external genital tract, and intestine. An excellent review of transient bacteremia has been published recently by Everett and Hirschman,[121] a summary of which is presented here:

The reported incidence of transient bacteremia associated with extraction of teeth has varied from 18 to 85 per cent. The organisms are most commonly streptococci, usually of the alpha type, but occasionally enterococci. They are rarely present in the blood for longer than 15 to 20 minutes, but this may be prolonged when multiple teeth are removed; the number of bacteria in the blood is small and ranges from as few as 5 to as many as 50 to 60 per ml. In addition to streptococci, "diphtheroids," *Staph. epidermidis*, and anaerobic members of the normal oral microflora have also been recovered. Peterson and Peacock noted transient bacteremia in 35 per cent of 101 youngsters who had nondiseased primary teeth removed, in 53 per cent of those in whom diseased primary and permanent teeth were extracted, and in 61 per cent undergoing removal of healthy permanent teeth.[122] Among dental procedures other than extraction associated with transient bacteremia are rocking of teeth, chewing of paraffin or hard candy, scaling of gums, brushing of teeth, periodontal operations, dental prophylaxis, use of unwaxed dental floss, and employment of oral irrigation devices (Water-Pik). It must be emphasized that infective endocarditis may occur in edentulous individuals.[123]

Tonsilloadenoidectomy is the procedure involving the airway most commonly associated with bacteremia; from 28 to 38 per cent of patients subjected to this operation experience transient bacterial invasion of the bloodstream. Other manipulations in this area that may lead to bacteremia are bronchoscopy (the rigid but not the fiberoptic instrument), orotracheal intubation, and nasal operations. Among the organisms present in the circulation have been *Staph. aureus*, streptococci, *Hemophilus* species, *Strep. pneumoniae*, and *Staph. epidermidis*. A recent study of nasotracheal suctioning by LeFrock et al. demonstrated bacteremia lasting up to 15 minutes[124] in 17.6 per cent of 68 patients who underwent this procedure.

Barium enema may be accompanied by transient bacteremia. LeFrock and his associates reported that in 11.4 per cent of patients who underwent this study, bacteria appeared transiently in the blood.[125] In another study LeFrock and his colleagues noted that 10 per cent of patients who underwent sigmoidoscopy had transient bacteremia; viridans streptococci were present in 90 per cent of these.[126] Shull et al. carried out fiberoptic gastroscopy in 50 patients; after the procedure, 4 exhibited bacteremia that lasted from 5 to 30 minutes.[127] This incidence is lower than that following sigmoidoscopy, presumably because of the diameter and greater flexibility of the fiberoptic colonoscope.[128] Transient bacteremia also occurs with percutaneous biopsy of the liver.[129]

A large variety of urological procedures have resulted in transient bacterial invasion of the blood[130] with incidence as follows: internal urethrotomy, 75 per cent; urethral dilatation of external urethrotomy, 85.9 per cent; transurethral prostatectomy, 12.3 per cent in general, but 10.8 per cent when urine was sterile and 57.5 per cent when organisms were present in the urine; removal of indwelling catheter from patients with infected urine, 26.3 per cent; retropubic prostatectomy, 7.4 to 12.8 per cent when urine has been sterile and 82.4 per cent when bacteriuria has been a problem; cystoscopy, 0 to 17 per cent; urethral catheterization, 8 per cent. Gram-negative bacilli are the commonest transient intruders.

Most studies of transient bacteremia from various gynecological procedures have produced negative results. Invasion of the bloodstream does not occur during parturition. However, a recent study has indicated that about 85 per cent of patients who underwent a suction abortion experienced transient bacteremia; the bacteria were present only intermittently in some; in others, the bacteremia persisted for as long as one hour after the abortion was completed. In a few instances, organisms were recovered from the blood following only bimanual pelvic examination.[131]

Cirrhosis. Snyder et al. reported that infective endocarditis[132] among patients admitted to the hospital was 3.4 times more frequent when cirrhosis was present than when it was absent.

Drug Addiction and Surgery. Addiction to the intravenous use of drugs has become an increasingly important factor predisposing to the development of infective endocarditis. This is also true of cardiac surgery, especially the insertion of prosthetic valves; the appearance of a paravalvular leak, probably because it produces hemodynamic abnormalities, favors the deposition of platelet-fibrin thrombi on which organisms may be implanted. Prolonged use of polyethylene catheters or any type of "long line" is associated with an increased risk of endocarditis related to either colonization of the tip of the catheter or entry of organisms at the site where the tube enters the skin.

Burns. Burned patients appear to be more susceptible to infective endocarditis. In the study by Baskin et al., the infection involved the right side of the heart in 18 patients, the left in 9, and both sides in 8.[133] The disease was acute in 22 and subacute in 13. Murmurs were detectable in only two instances. The commonest organism present on the valves was *Staph. aureus* (77 per cent).

Pacemakers. An uncommon source of infection of the heart is the transvenous cardiac pacemaker.[134] Sustained staphylococcal bacteremia (at least 12 hours) may develop 2 weeks to 10 months after insertion of the apparatus. About 5 to 6 per cent of cases of endocarditis have been associated with infection in the subcutaneous pocket into which the pacemaker is inserted. Of seven cases reported up to 1975, the tricuspid valve was infected in four, the mitral endocardium of the left atrium in two, and the right ventricle in one. Myocardial abscess resulting from contamination of the wire is even less common.

Other Predisposing Factors. A number of other infectious and noninfectious predisposing factors have been reported by Garvey and Neu.[135] Among these are neoplastic disease, nonmalignant hematological disorders, "collagen-vascular" disease, diabetes mellitus, chronic active viral hepatitis, preexisting renal failure, treatment with corticosteroids (50 per cent of patients), antitumor chemotherapy and radiation (20 per cent of cases), perinephric abscess, obstruction of the common bile duct, perforation of the bowel (*Clostridium perfringens* endocarditis), and infections of sternal wounds produced in the course of cardiac surgery.

Hyperalimentation is also associated with an increased risk of fungal endocarditis.

Extracardiac Foci of Infection. Foci of infection *outside* the heart may serve as sources of bacteremia that lead to the development of endocarditis. Among such lesions are mild to severe infections of the skin ("pimple," boils), especially if they are mishandled by squeezing or inappropriate surgical incision. The organism most often responsible for disease in this situation is *Staph. aureus.* Pneumonia, particularly that caused by *Strep. pneumoniae*, was a relatively common predisposing factor in the preantibiotic era. Disease of the lung caused by *Strep. pyogenes* and other highly invasive organisms such as *H. influenzae* may also serve as a source of bacteremia and subsequent infective endocarditis.

Among other extracardiac lesions are acute hematogenous osteomyelitis, acute pyelonephritis, meningococcemia with or without meningitis, brucellosis, Q fever, rat-bite fever, and a variety of immunosuppressive disorders including the vasculitides when they are complicated by bacteremia, and superinfection by bacteria or fungi induced by therapy with antibiotics. Garvey and Neu[135] and Rosen and Armstrong [136] have noted that a significant number of the patients with infections of normal valves were immunosuppressed because of major underlying disease or treatment with corticosteroids or radiation. These individuals were older, and involvement of the right side of the heart was more likely than in those who were immunologically competent. They were also more susceptible to invasion of the valves by gram-negative bacilli and fungi. In about one-third of cases, the presence of infective endocarditis was not suspected during life. The fatality rate was 57 per cent in this group and only 28 per cent in patients who were without immunological abnormalities.

Infective endocarditis is a subtle and often lethal complication of *hemodialysis.*[137] The source of the organisms has been infection or manipulation of access sites and dental procedures, most commonly involving *Staph. aureus.* The incidence of infection is lower in patients with arteriovenous fistulas than in those with arteriovenous cannulas. Although *Pseudomonas aeruginosa* is a frequent cause of infection of access sites, it produces endocarditis uncommonly. Cure of the cardiac infection requires, in addition to antimicrobial therapy, removal of the shunt.

A rare predisposing factor in the pathogenesis of infective endocarditis is penetration of the heart by a foreign body.[138] Cardiac catheterization may rarely be associated with a transient bacteremia that leads to the development of infective endocarditis.

UNDERLYING HEART DISEASE

RHEUMATIC HEART DISEASE. Although chronic rheumatic heart disease was the underlying lesion in from 80 to 90 per cent of cases of subacute bacterial endocarditis for many years,[18] this has not been so since antimicrobial agents have become available. This may be related to the decreased incidence of acute rheumatic fever and to the highly successful prevention of recurrences of the disease. At present, only about 40 to 60 per cent of instances of infective endocarditis are superimposed on preexisting rheumatic heart disease.[14] The long-held concept that patients with pure mitral stenosis, atrial fibrillation, and congestive heart failure were at extremely low risk of developing endocarditis does not appear to be as important as it was in the past.

Uncommonly, both acute or subacute bacterial endocarditis and acute rheumatic carditis may be present simultaneously. The differential diagnosis of acute rheumatic fever and infective endocarditis may, in some instances, be difficult because (1) blood cultures may occasionally be positive in the former and negative in the latter, (2) both conditions feature fever and leukocytosis, and (3) petechiae may be present in both. Blood cultures should be obtained in patients in whom fever persists despite treatment with adequate doses of salicylate. If four or more cultures yield an organism, the possibility of superimposed infective endocarditis must be seriously considered and appropriate antimicrobial therapy instituted.

CONGENITAL HEART DISEASE. Although probably more frequently the basis for endocarditis in children, congenital heart disease is also important in adults. Gelfman and Levine[139] reported in 1942 that endocarditis occurred in about 6.5 per cent of 453 youngsters over the age of 2 years with congenital heart disease studied at necropsy; the incidence has been recorded to be as high as 16 per cent.[140,141] In patients younger than 2 years, valvular infection is less commonly superimposed on anatomical defects of the heart. In the first weeks or months of life, this disease is usually a complication of an episode of overwhelming sepsis; murmurs are usually absent, diagnosis is difficult, and the fatality rate is inordinately high.

Patent ductus arteriosus, ventricular septal defect, and tetralogy of Fallot are the congenital lesions most commonly associated with infective endocarditis[142]; aortic or pulmonic stenosis is less frequent. The frequency of infection in patients with ventricular septal defect (Fig. 33–6) has been estimated to be 1 in 470 patient years, or 2.1 per 100 cases in 10 years.[143] When ventricular septal defect and aortic regurgitation coexist, the incidence of endocarditis increases to about 24 per cent. In patients with the tetralo-

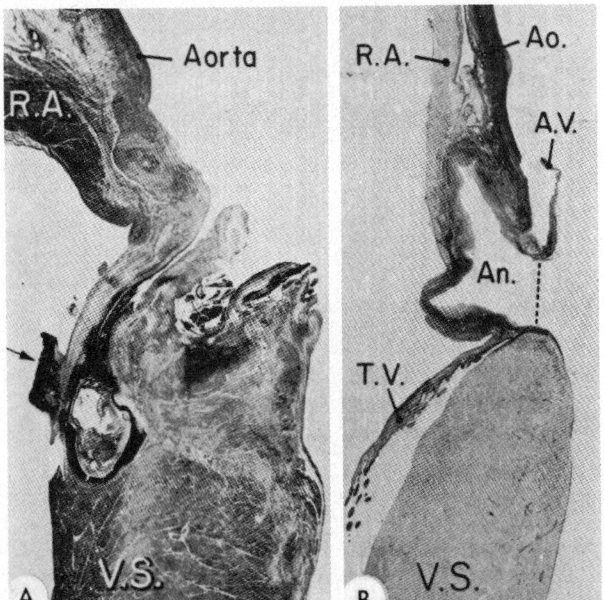

FIGURE 33–6 Photomicrographs of longitudinal sections of ventricular septum (V.S.) at two levels. *A*, Section showing extension of the infective process through the entire thickness of the muscular V.S. A small vegetation (arrow) is apparent on the endocardium of the right side of the heart. R.A. = right atrium. *B*, Section includes aneurysm (An.) of membranous portion of V.S. The dashed line represents the normal site of the ventricular septum. T.V. = tricuspid valve leaflet; A.V. = aortic valve cusp; Ao. = aorta. (From Roberts, W. C., and Buchbinder, N. A.: Healed left-sided infective endocarditis. A clinicopathological study of 59 patients. Am. J. Cardiol. *40*: 876, 1976.)

gy of Fallot in whom an anastomosis has been created between the systemic and pulmonary circulations, infective endocarditis occurs more frequently than in any other form of congenital heart disease. The aortic valve may, at times, become infected in patients with the tetralogy of Fallot or pulmonary atresia. The aortic root and descending aorta are larger than normal, and the aortic abnormalities induce turbulence of blood flow in the aortic root, which may produce sufficient trauma to the normal endocardium to cause deposition of a platelet-fibrin thrombus, the focus for bacterial invasion,[144] and aortic regurgitation may ensue.

Atrial septal defects are rarely infected, probably because of the absence of large interatrial pressure gradients.[143] However, endocarditis involving the mitral valve has occurred in patients with ostium primum defects. Two other congenital cardiac lesions that predispose to the development of valvular infection are bicuspid aortic valves and coarctation of the aorta. Endocarditis tends to develop most frequently in congenital lesions that produce significant pressure gradients.[145] In cases of coarctation of the aorta the infectious process is usually situated on the poststenotic side and on an accompanying bicuspid aortic valve.[146] The pulmonic valve is most often involved when the tetralogy of Fallot is present.[144] The left pulmonary artery in the area of the ductal orifice is the site most often infected in patients with patent ductus arteriosus.

ATHEROSCLEROSIS AND CALCIFICATION. Kerr suggested that, as the population aged, atherosclerotic heart disease would probably become a significant lesion predisposing to the development of infective endocarditis.[19] It has since become clear that certain factors associated with aging play an important role in the pathogenesis of this infection and account for the increase in the incidence of bacterial disease of the heart in the older age group. Atheromatous deposits on the aortic valve have been noted at autopsy in 25 per cent of patients over 40 years of age who have succumbed to endocarditis. The incidence of valvular atheromas, excrescences, and nodules increases progressively with age; these lesions are most prominent in areas where the change in pressure and turbulence of flow are greatest, such as the left side of the heart, in general, and the aortic valve, in particular.[147] Watanakunakorn has described five older patients with calcification of the mitral valve annulus (p. 1074) who developed endocarditis.[148] The organisms involved were gram-negative cocci and *Staph. aureus.* He pointed out that (a) murmurs may not be present, (b) significant narrowing of the mitral orifice was absent, and (c) vegetations were most commonly present on the *posterior* leaflet of the mitral valve. An analysis of the frequency of calcification of the valves in a population without endocarditis showed that about 5 per cent of uninfected persons between 50 and 70 years of age have calcified mitral valves. In those older than 90 years, the incidence of calcification of the valves is about 60 per cent.

HYPERTROPHIC OBSTRUCTIVE CARDIOMYOPATHY. The incidence of infective endocarditis in patients with this condition is usually considered to be in the range of 5 to 10 per cent, but in one recent report was as high as 50 per cent.[149] Wang and his associates have reported that the aortic valve is infected most often, followed by the mitral valve alone or both valves simultaneously.[150] They suggested that the infectious process originates on the ventricular aspect of the anterior portion of the anterior mitral leaflet. This area is frequently thickened and becomes susceptible to bacterial invasion as a result of the trauma produced by the abutting action of the anterior mitral leaflet against the thickened septum (p. 1411). Infection may then extend to the chordae tendineae and produce tears. In 10 patients with discrete membranous subaortic stenosis and endocarditis, the infection was noted to involve the aortic valve in all, the aorta above the aortic valve in 6, the mitral valve in 4, and the membranous ridge in 3. The high incidence of endocarditis of the aortic valve and wall in this condition compared to valvular infection in hypertrophic cardiomyopathy suggested that there is a more prominent jet stream in discrete membranous stenosis than in hypertrophic cardiomyopathy, and that this causes more damage to the aortic leaflets and wall. Aortic regurgitation is also a more common complication of endocarditis in the discrete, membranous form than in hypertrophic obstructive cardiomyopathy. Infection of the aortic wall has not been reported with hypertrophic obstructive cardiomyopathy but is common in the membranous type of disease and may be complicated by mycotic aneurysms, which may rupture.

MARFAN SYNDROME AND MITRAL VALVE PROLAPSE. Up until 1974, 21 cases of infective endocarditis occurring in patients with the *Marfan syndrome* (p. 1665) had been reported.[151] The mitral valve is infected most often. Although the aortic valve is commonly abnormal in this disease, it is rarely the site of infection. The *mitral valve prolapse syndrome* (p. 1089) has been identified as a predisposing condition in the development of infective endocarditis.[152,152a] *Staph. aureus* is commonly involved; in some instances, alpha-streptococci and enterococci have been recovered from the blood.[153]

CARDIAC SURGERY. Cardiac surgery represents an iatrogenic type of underlying heart disease that predisposes to the development of infective endocarditis. Before 1957, about 1 per cent of patients subjected to operations on the heart developed infection. During the next 10 years, the incidence of this complication rose considerably, especially in cases in which valvular prostheses were implanted. The incidence of endocarditis complicating placement of Starr-Edwards valves has been recorded to be as high as 10 per cent.[154,155] However, as experience with cardiac surgery has increased, the frequency of infection has fallen to 3 to 3.5 per cent with valve replacement and to about 1 per cent with other types of operation on the heart. Stein et al. pointed out that the type of surgical procedure played a role in determining the incidence of endocarditis.[156] They noted infection in only 0.6 per cent of patients undergoing closed-heart operations, in 0.9 per cent of those undergoing open cardiac procedures, and in 3.3 per cent of those in whom prosthetic valves were placed. Infected suture material appears to be an important contributing factor. Decrease in the effectiveness of removal of organisms from the bloodstream by phagocytosis, which has been shown to be impaired by use of cardiopulmonary bypass, may also play an important role in increasing susceptibility to valvular infection.

Several studies have indicated that *infection of prosthetic valves* may occur at various times after operation.[157] Most reports divide the cases into early or late. "Early" has been defined as within one to three weeks and "late" as longer than one, two, or three months. It has been suggested that evidence of infection in the first one or two weeks postoperatively usually indicates extracardiac infection, and that the later fever develops, the more likely prosthetic valvular endocarditis is present.[158] Although this is true in many instances, there are a number of cases in which fever developing in the first few days after operation has been found to be the first manifestation of infection of the prosthesis.[159] In sharp contrast are the occasional cases in which endocarditis does not appear until five or more years after the device has been implanted (Fig. 33–3). A study by Wilson et al. indicated that, in a group of 45 patients, infection of the prosthesis became apparent within two months in 36 per cent, while in the remaining 64 per cent, the disease did not become manifest until more than two months after operation.[157] In early cases, the commonest organisms were *Staph. aureus* (44 per cent) and gram-negative bacilli (38 per cent); in late cases, *Strep. viridans* and gram-negative bacilli were commonest. In a similar study of 38 patients by Dismukes et al., 50 per cent of patients developed infection in less than 60 days (early) and the other 50 per cent after 60 days (late).[38] Again, *Staph. aureus* was most frequently involved in the early and streptococci in the late episodes. A study of 122 cases of postcardiotomy endocarditis by Starkebaum et al. indicated that the disease appeared within two weeks in 27 per cent[160]; 70 per cent occurred with 2 months. "The findings were consistent with the hypothesis that the incubation period of postcardiotomy endocarditis is short."

Certain types of cardiac surgery impose a higher risk of infective endocarditis than does the implantation of a prosthesis. Kaplan et al. have reported that 8 per cent of patients with tetralogy of Fallot developed endocarditis following the Pott's procedure (i.e., aortopulmonary shunt). Intracardiac infection also appears to be increased in patients operated on for tricuspid atresia.[161] The highest risk of infective endocarditis is associated with operative procedures on patients with transposition of the great arteries. Valvular infections have not been a notable complication in coronary bypass operations.

Among the conditions predisposing to invasion of prosthetic valves by organisms in the *early* postoperative period are infected surgical wounds in the chest and urinary catheters. Sources of infection include contamination of blood by the oxygenator and of the blood used to prime the pump; the connecting tubes on the large venous and arterial cannulas; direct contamination by hands, instruments, or room air; reactivation of latent infection in patients with episodes of endocarditis prior to placement of the prosthetic valve; and contamination of the prosthesis. Predisposing conditions in the convalescent period include bacteremia from sites of infection in the chest wound or at the cannulation site, infected pleural fluid, postoperative pneumonia, tracheostomy, contaminated indwelling catheters, and superinfections related to prophylaxis or therapy with antimicrobial agents. Other conditions predisposing to *late* endocarditis are infections of the urinary tract, dental procedures, disease of the upper airway, ingrown toenails, use of the nasal cautery and pilonidal cyst. The primary factor involved in both early and late convalescence is bacteremia resulting from dental, dermatological, gastrointestinal, and genitourinary procedures or minor surgical operations. In addition to these, Dismukes et al. reported that cystoscopy, excision of a carbuncle, uterine dilatation and curettage, paravalvular leaks that developed immediately postoperatively, and preexisting endocarditis (same organism) predisposed to infection of the prosthetic valves.[38]

There is an increasing number of instances of infective endocarditis involving otherwise *normal valves,* particularly in cases of the acute disease. For example, 40 to 60 per cent of patients with infections caused by *Staph. aureus* have previously normal cardiac valves. This is also true in an appreciable number of instances in which *Strep. pyogenes, Strep. pneumoniae, N. meningitidis,* and *N. gonorrhoeae* are involved. In recent years, endocarditis affecting normal valves has occurred more frequently because of the increase in the number of individuals using intravenous illicit drugs.

Seven cases of bacterial endocarditis following penetration of the heart by *foreign bodies* have been recorded.[138]

MYOCARDIAL INFARCTION. Infective endocarditis may occur as a complication of myocardial infarction.[162] The location of the infection is determined by the site of necrosis of the muscle, and the predisposing factor is the development of a platelet-fibrin clot over the infarcted area. The infection may be situated on the left side of the septum in cases of anteroseptal infarction or on the endocardium over the site of damage in the left ventricle. In addition, development of an *aneurysm* in which a clot forms provides a potential area of invasion for organisms.

NONVALVULAR INFECTIVE ENDOCARDITIS. Nonvalvular infective endocarditis may occur in *ventricular septal defect* (Fig. 33–6). Although the tricuspid valve may be infected occasionally, three other sites are involved more commonly. One is the point of impact of the jet stream on the right ventricular endocardium; the resulting injury leads to the formation of a small platelet-fibrin thrombus on which bacteria may be implanted. Infection may also develop on the right side of the septal opening; the Venturi effect created by the flow of blood from an area of high (left ventricle) to one of lower pressure (right ventricle) leads to the deposition of a clot around the opening on the right side of the septum. Much less common is infection of the left ventricular side of the defect. The risk of infection is reduced when the septal opening is large, because this does not produce an interventricular pressure gradient.

A rare form of nonvalvular infection of the heart is infected *atrial myxoma.* A patient described by Graham et al. is one of four similar cases, three of which had *Staph. aureus* infections.[163] Embolization to the central nervous system occurred in every instance. Infection of an atrial myxoma by *Histoplasma capsulatum* has been described.[164]

Single or multiple *myocardial abscesses* may develop in the course of bacteremias unrelated to valvular infection. *Staph. aureus* and *N. meningitidis* are among the organisms involved. Several instances of subacute bacterial endocarditis in patients with *rheumatic valvular disease* in which the infection did not involve any of the affected valves have been noted. In these cases, the infectious process was superimposed on McCallum's patch, an area of endocardial injury in the left atrium induced by the acute rheumatic process.

TABLE 33–2 LOCI OF LESIONS IN ENDOCARDITIS

CONDITION	HIGH-PRSSURE SOURCE	ORIFICE	LOW-PRESSURE SINK	LOCATION OF LESIONS	SATELLITE LESIONS
Coarctation of aorta	Central aorta	Coarctation	Distal aorta	Downstream wall	Lateral wall of aorta peripheral to stenotic lesion
Patent ductus arteriosus	Aorta	Ductus	Pulmonary artery	Pulmonary artery	Pulmonic valve
Arteriovenous fistula	Artery	Fistula	Vein	Fistula and vein	
Ventricular septal defect	Left ventricle	Defect	Right ventricle	Right ventricular surface defect	Pulmonary artery
Aortic regurgitation	Aorta	Closed aortic valves	Left ventricle	Ventricular surface aortic valve	Mitral chordae
Mitral regurgitation	Left ventricle	Closed mitral valves	Left atrium	Atrial surface mitral valve	Atrium
Pulmonic regurgitation	Pulmonary artery	Closed pulmonic valves	Right ventricle	Ventricular surface pulmonic valve	
Tricuspid regurgitation	Right ventricle	Closed tricuspid valves	Right atrium	Atrial surface tricuspid valve	

Adapted from Rodbard, S.: Blood velocity and endocarditis. Circulation *27*:18, 1963, by permission of the American Heart Association, Inc.

PATHOGENESIS

Subacute Endocarditis

Since Osler's[2] classic description of endocarditis, many investigators have tried to explain the fact that infected endocardial vegetations consistently occur in the same location. Four mechanisms are responsible for the initiation and localization of the *subacute* infection: (1) a previously damaged cardiac valve or a hemodynamic situation in which damage results from a jet effect, produced by blood flowing from a zone of high to one of relatively low pressure, as in mitral regurgitation or ventricular septal defect (Table 33–2); (2) a sterile platelet-fibrin thrombus; (3) bacteremia, often transient; and (4) a high titer of agglutinating antibody against the infecting organism.

THE JET AND VENTURI EFFECTS. Of 1024 patients with infective endocarditis studied by Lepeschkin at autopsy, mitral valves were involved in 86 per cent, aortic valves in 55 per cent, tricuspid valves in 19.6 per cent, and pulmonic valves in 1.1 per cent.[165] By correlating the impact of pressure on these valves with the frequency of involvement of the corresponding valves, Lepeschkin presented a strong argument for *mechanical stress* as a critical factor in the evolution of endocarditis. By injecting a bacterial aerosol into the air stream passing through an agar Venturi tube, Rodbard elegantly demonstrated how high pressure drives an infected fluid into a low-pressure sink to establish a characteristic pattern of colony distribution; a collar of maximal deposition consistently appeared in the low-pressure sink immediately beyond the orifice (Fig. 33–7).[145] This model helps to explain the distribution of lesions often complicating various cardiac valvular and septal defects (Table 33–2). The early observation that in infective endocarditis the atrial side of the valve and adjacent segment of atrium are characteristically involved in patients with mitral regurgitation is also explained; a Venturi effect is produced when blood is driven from a high-pressure source (the left ventricle) through an orifice (the nearly closed but regurgitant mitral valve) into a low-pressure sink (the atrium). A jet effect on the atrial wall establishes the other site of potential involvement, McCallum's patch (Fig. 33–8).

The sites of aortic valvular infection are established in a similar way. Some degree of aortic regurgitation is crucial. The high-pressure source is the aorta, and the low-pressure sink is the left ventricle. Vegetations are typically found on the ventricular surface of the aortic leaflets. Satellite lesions, which may be found on the chordae tendineae, are the result of a high-velocity regurgitant stream from an incompetent aortic valve—a situation analogous to the jet effect in mitral regurgitation. In a ventricular septal defect with a small orifice and left-to-right shunt, a Venturi effect often leads to the development of lesions around the orifice on the right ventricular side of the opening. Secondary lesions may be present on the right ventricular wall opposite the defect, the site of impact of the jet. Similar hemodynamic relations in tricuspid regurgitation, arteriovenous fistula, coarctation of the aorta, and patent ductus arteriosus can be used, in each instance, to predict the location of the endothelial lesions. Table 33–2 presents the distribution of endocardial infections in common cardiovascular disorders.

Attenuation of the jet and Venturi effects is seen in congestive heart failure and atrial fibrillation and helps to ex-

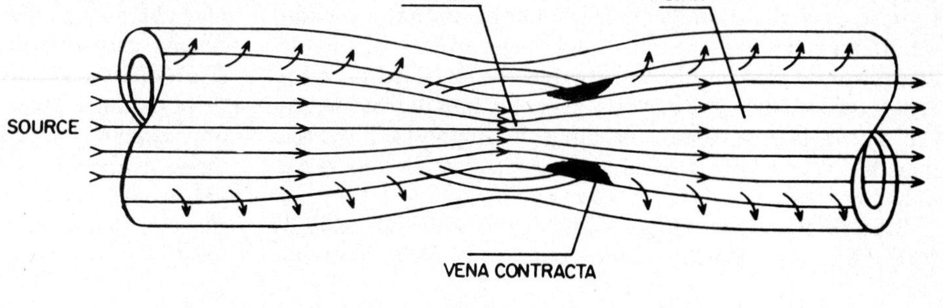

FIGURE 33–7 Venturi model of high-pressure source driving a bacterial aerosol into a low-pressure sink. Characteristic distribution of bacterial colonies is shown at the vena contracta. (From Rodbard, S.: Blood velocity in endocarditis. Circulation *27*:18, 1963, by permission of the American Heart Association, Inc.)

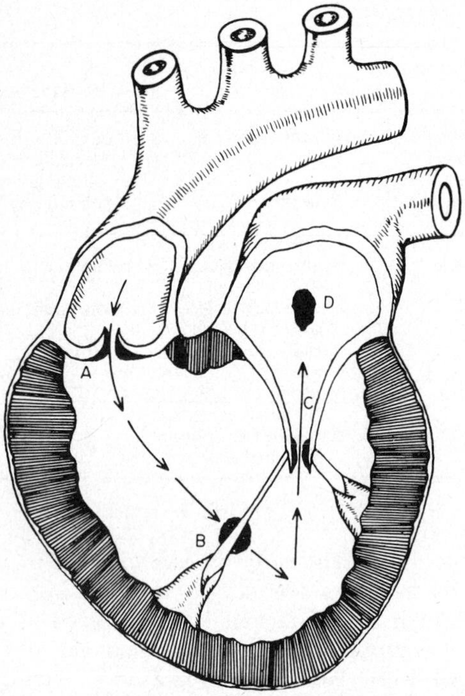

FIGURE 33–8 High-velocity streams in mitral and aortic regurgitation and sites of endocarditis lesions. Arrow at left indicates a high arterial pressure that generates regurgitant flow from aorta to ventricle. The vena contracta and endocarditic lesions appear at the ventricular surface of the aortic valve (A). The stream through the incompetent aortic valve may produce lesions on the chordae tendineae of the aortic leaf of the mitral valve (B). If the mitral valves cannot seat properly during ventricular systole, the regurgitant stream (arrow at right) will pass to the sink of the left atrium, and the endocarditic lesion will tend to become engrafted on the atrial surface of the mitral valve (C). The atrial endocardium in line with the regurgitant stream may produce a fibrous area, MacCallum's patch (D), which may become another site of endocarditic lesions. (Adapted from Rodbard, S.: Blood velocity in endocarditis. Circulation *27*:18, 1963, by permission of the American Heart Association, Inc.)

plain the long recognized infrequency of infective endocarditis in these settings.[166] Likewise, defects with surface areas large enough to abolish a gradient and those in which smaller volumes minimize the gradient are not associated with endocarditis. These findings probably explain the rarity of endocarditis in isolated atrial septal defects and the greater threat of infection in small than in large ventricular septal defects. The lesion responsible for the initiation of endocarditis is occasionally too small to produce enough turbulence to create an audible murmur.

THE PLATELET-FIBRIN THROMBUS. Turbulence and the jet effect traumatize the endothelial surface and initiate a series of events that may lead to the establishment of an infected focus. Collagen is exposed, and platelet deposition occurs in a manner analogous to the formation of the primary platelet plug of normal hemostasis after vascular injury. Central to these events is the role of the sterile platelet-fibrin thrombus, or so-called nonbacterial thrombotic endocarditis. The nonspecific nature of the sterile platelet-fibrin thrombus is emphasized by the fact that it can be produced as a result of numerous types of stress or injury.

BACTEREMIA AND AGGLUTINATING ANTIBODIES. As already pointed out (p. 1143), transient bacteremias occur frequently in normal persons. They are usually without clinical importance, even when sterile platelet-fibrin thrombi are situated on the cardiac valves. In most cases, the failure of implantation of organisms on such sites is related to the small number and low invasive capability of circulating organisms. A major factor, probably involved in initiating subacute valvular infection because it permits large numbers of bacteria to adhere to the sterile platelet-fibrin thrombus, is *circulating antibody*, especially agglutinins. By clumping the organisms, the antibody produces an inoculum large enough to induce bacterial multiplication and infection—a phenomenon much more important in the pathogenesis of subacute than of acute endocarditis.

Evidence of the importance of antibody may be found in studies of the development of endocarditis in horses[167] undergoing immunization with pneumococci. Infected vegetations appeared late in the course of immunization, coincidentally with the highest titers of antibody. The exact mechanism by which pathogens ultimately adhere to the platelet-fibrin thrombus is unknown. One possibility is that the platelet-covered lesion somehow provides a favorable surface.

Acute Endocarditis

The pathoanatomical mechanisms involved in the development of acute bacterial endocarditis are quite different from those in the subacute form. In 50 to 60 per cent of acute cases, previously *normal* valves are the sites of infection. It appears, therefore, that the presence of a sterile platelet-fibrin thrombus is unnecessary in the pathogenesis of this form of the valvulitis. Because the organisms responsible for the acute infection (*Staph. aureus, Strep. pneumoniae, N. meningitidis* or *gonorrhoeae, Strep. pyogenes,* and *H. influenzae*) are highly invasive, only small numbers are required to establish infection. Thus, the critical requirement in the pathogenesis of acute endocarditis is bacteremia caused by an invasive organism. It should be pointed out, however, that acute infective endocarditis may also occur in patients with underlying acquired or congenital valvular damage and that, in these patients, sterile platelet-fibrin thrombi may develop and facilitate infection just as is the case in subacute endocarditis.

The exact mechanism by which pathogenic bacteria invade normal valve leaflets has now been determined. Recent studies have indicated that specific properties of various bacteria determine their ability to adhere to the surface of cardiac valves. Gould et al.[168] and Holmes and Ramirez[169] examined the capacity of a number of organisms to adhere to canine and human valvular leaflets in vitro. The degree of adherence was found to vary with the type of organism studied, being highest with enterococci and *Staph. aureus,* followed by viridans streptococci, *Staph. epidermidis,* and *P. aeruginosa* and lowest with *Escherichia coli* and *Klebsiella pneumoniae.* These data are of potentially great clinical importance because they probably explain the relative frequency with which certain bacteria, especially *Staph. aureus,* invade previously normal valves. Of equal clinical interest is the demonstration of the poor adherence of *E. coli* and *K. pneumoniae,* which may very well account for the low incidence of endocarditis caused by these organisms, despite the well-known high frequency with which they produce bacteremia.

In subacute bacterial endocarditis, the inducing bacteremia frequently originates not from an infectious process but from trauma to areas where the causative organisms normally reside as components of the indigenous flora, such as the teeth, urogenital tract, or intestine. In acute endocarditis, the inducing bacteremia originates in an active infection, usually at a site remote from the heart, such as the skin, lungs, or genitourinary tract. In an appreciable number of instances, however, there is no demonstrable portal of entry of the organisms into the bloodstream; this may be the case when *Staph. aureus* is the causative agent.

CLINICAL MANIFESTATIONS

Four mechanisms may be involved in the clinical manifestations of infective endocarditis: (1) the infectious process on the involved valve, (2) embolization, (3) metastatic infection, and (4) deposition of abnormal globulins and circulating immune complexes at various sites remote from the heart. All these are not present in every patient, and there are also striking qualitative and quantitative differences in their roles in the acute and subacute forms of the disease.[170]

Modes of Onset

SUBACUTE ENDOCARDITIS

Incubation Period. The exact "incubation period" of subacute infective endocarditis is very difficult to define. However, an extensive review of the literature by Starkebaum et al.,[160] based on a study of the time elapsing between exposure to a situation that might induce transient bacteremia and the development of the first manifestations of valvular infection, suggested that the median "incubation period" is about one week. Symptoms appeared within two weeks in about 84 per cent of the patients. Thus, the "incubation period" of subacute bacterial endocarditis is often shorter than realized. Procedures carried out more than two weeks before onset of symptoms are not likely to be causally related.

Manifestations of Infection. In many instances, the onset of subacute infective endocarditis is characterized by the *general manifestations of infection* without any signs or symptoms suggesting disease of the heart or any other organ. Common complaints include persistent low-grade fever, lassitude, anorexia, fatigue, loss of weight, sleepiness, and a grippe-like syndrome. Libman and Friedberg pointed out that this infection may simulate a number of disorders that suggest involvement of extracardiac sites, as follows: (a) headache, generalized pain, malaise, and respiratory symptoms resembling influenza; (b) fever, cough, loss of weight, weakness, pain in the chest, and even hemoptysis, suggesting the possibility of tuberculosis; (c) elevated temperature and arthralgia or arthritis suggestive of acute rheumatic fever; (d) diarrhea, fever, headache, and drowsiness, symptoms similar to those of typhoid fever; (e) intermittent chills and fever, resembling malaria (common in persons who are treated with salicylates intermittently to control fever and who experience rigor as the temperature begins to rise); (f) dyspnea, precordial discomfort, palpitation, and, at times, peripheral edema (frequently in patients in whom valvular infection has been present for weeks or months and in whom congestive heart failure finally develops); (g) fever and pain in the right upper abdomen consistent with hepatic or subdiaphragmatic infection; (h) fever, abdominal pain, and urinary symptoms with or without hematuria; (i) a clinical picture suggesting carcinoma of the stomach, characterized by vomiting, postprandial distress, and anorexia, or a syndrome suggestive of appendicitis.[171]

Development of Complications. Other modes of onset of subacute infective endocarditis are related to the development of complications of the disease that often appear before therapy is initiated, especially when the infection has not been treated for weeks or months. Some of these are embolic, some are due to progressive involvement of the valve, while others result from the development and activity of immunological disorders.[172]

Embolic Complications. Manifestations of this type of onset include (a) *sudden occlusion of the middle cerebral artery* leading to hemiplegia; (b) a clinical picture of *acute meningitis*, in which the spinal fluid is sterile but contains an increased number of cells, concentration of protein and a normal sugar content; (c) manifestations consistent with diffuse encephalitis; (d) sudden development of pain in either the right of left upper abdominal quadrant due to gross infarction of either the kidney or the spleen; (e) hematuria without pain, caused by small, multiple infarcts of the kidney, interstitial nephritis, or diffuse proliferative glomerulonephritis; (f) unilateral blindness of acute onset caused by embolic occlusion of the retinal artery; and (g) myocardial infarction caused by embolic occlusion of one of the coronary arteries. The first manifestation of endocarditis involving the right side of the heart, particularly the tricuspid valve, may be the development of "pneumonia" which is actually an embolic pulmonary infarct. The appearance of multiple areas of infiltration in the lungs in a patient with fever and a murmur should alert the physician immediately to the possibility of infection of the right side of the heart.

Progressive Involvement of the Valves. The modes of onset related to continued activity of the infectious process on the affected valve in untreated persons are a change in the character of a murmur and the development of progressive cardiac failure due to valvular dysfunction induced by slow destruction and fibrosis of the involved valve.

Immunological Disorders. An increasing number of patients with infective endocarditis in whom the diagnosis is delayed for weeks or months may have, as the first manifestation suggesting the possibility of subacute disease, findings related to the development of immunological phenomena. Some individuals may first come to medical attention because of the weakness, anorexia, and anemia associated with renal failure due to interstitial nephritis or proliferative glomerulonephritis resulting from the deposition of immune complexes in the kidney. Others may complain of arthralgias or arthritis probably related to the presence of the same type of complexes in the synovia. An occasional patient may complain of increasing difficulty with "palpitations." This may be immunological in origin, as suggested by the presence of Bracht-Wächter bodies in the myocardium, or may be the result of spread of infection from the valve to the conducting system in the interventricular septum. That the initial presentation of subacute endocarditis may be related to the development of immunological reactions is supported by the observation that the Osler node and probably the Roth spot may be, in part, due to vasculitis (see below).

Lumbar Pain. Persistent pain in the lumbar area has become an increasingly common early complaint of patients with subacute endocarditis. This is not due to vertebral osteomyelitis, as evidenced by failure to demonstrate any changes in the vertebral bodies over months of radiographic examination, and by the rapid disappearance of the pain after effective antimicrobial therapy is initiated.

Prosthetic Valvular Infections. The onset of infection involving prosthetic valves is often difficult to recognize because there may be no signs or symptoms, with the exception of fever, that clearly indicate the presence of this disease.

Drug Users. The mode of onset of infective endocarditis in persons who use illicit drugs intravenously is not sufficiently suggestive to permit a diagnosis; however, two features may indicate the presence of valvular infection in these patients. In those in whom the tricuspid valve is involved, the appearance of repeated episodes of pulmonary infarction is suggestive of the diagnosis. In persons with fungal infection of the mitral or aortic valves, the first manifestation may be embolic occlusion of a major artery, most often in one of the legs, because of the large size of the vegetations characteristic of this type of disease. In these cases, diagnosis is often established by embolectomy and isolation of the organism from the clot.

ACUTE ENDOCARDITIS

The mode of onset of acute infective endocarditis is distinctly different from that of the subacute form. Patients are usually previously well and become ill rapidly, with manifestations of severe infection. There are usually no signs indicating the presence of valvular disease in the early stage. Unlike subacute endocarditis, complications related directly to the rapidly advancing destructive process occur commonly within a week or less after infection and are often reflected by the rapid development of heart failure, especially when the aortic valve is involved. Because the thrombi on the affected valve are moderately large and soft, embolization is often the first manifestation of the disease, and patients may first be seen by a physician because of multiple petechiae or purpuric lesions of the skin, acute onset of neurological signs, or, if the infection involves the right side of the heart, "pneumonia" or single or multiple abscesses of the lung.

Signs and Symptoms

Elevation of the temperature is by far the most common sign of infective endocarditis; it has been reported in 100 per cent of cases by some investigators. However, the type and course of the fever are variable; normal or subnormal temperatures may be present in from 3 to 15 per cent of cases.[173] Absence of fever is not uncommon in elderly individuals with the subacute form of infection. This may be so because, with increasing age, basal (96.7°F or 36°C) and maximal (98.6°F or 37°C) daily temperatures tend to become lower than in young individuals. It is probably for this reason that older patients with subacute infective endocarditis have "normal" temperatures. The writer has seen a number of cases of this disease in patients in their 70's who have been thought to be free of fever. However, when the course of the daily temperatures is charted over a period, variations ranging from 96.8°F (36°C) in the early morning to 98.6°F (37°C) in the late afternoon are noted, representing fever in such individuals. Absence of an elevated temperature should not preclude obtaining blood cultures when other signs and symptoms suggest endocarditis.

Other conditions in which fever may be absent in the face of subacute endocarditis are massive intracerebral or subarachnoid hemorrhage, cardiac failure, uremia, and administration of antimicrobial drugs in doses sufficient to decrease elevated temperatures but inadequate to eradicate the valvular infection. Repeated short courses of antimicrobial therapy, interspersed with periods during which treatment is withheld in patients with undiagnosed endocarditis, produce a characteristic pattern of repetitive episodes of remission and relapse of fever; this course should alert physicians to the possibility of the disease in any patient in whom a murmur is audible. With few exceptions, the maximal daily temperature of patients with acute infective endocarditis is higher (102 to 104°F or 39 to 40°C) than when the disease is subacute. Shaking chills are strikingly infrequent in the subacute infection unless salicylates are administered at inappropriate intervals; rigor will usually appear as the antipyretic activity disappears and the temperature begins to increase. In sharp contrast, patients with the acute form of infective endocarditis frequently experience high-grade fever in the range of 102 to 104°F (39 to 40°C) or higher early in the disease; shaking chills are common even when salicylates are not given.

Cardiac Murmurs

It was accepted dogma for many years that absence of a murmur ruled out the possibility of infective endocarditis, especially the subacute form of the disease. However, it is now apparent that up to 10 per cent of patients with subacute bacterial endocarditis do not have a detectable murmur when they first come to medical attention. In most instances, a murmur appears at some time during the period of treatment; less frequently, a murmur may not be detected until two to three months after therapy has been discontinued; in a rare patient, a murmur may never appear, even many years after cure of the infection.

Murmurs are not present in about one-third of patients with acute valvular infections involving the left side of the heart.[172,174] One of 167 patients with subacute and 7 of 54 patients with acute endocarditis were reported by Pankey to be free of murmurs.[175] He noted that changes in the character of the murmur occurred in 16.7 per cent of the subacute cases. This has not been the experience of this writer, who, in studies of more than 900 patients with subacute valvular infections, has found changing murmurs to be very uncommon. A change in a murmur occurs much more frequently in patients with acute valvular infections. One-third of cases of endocarditis of the right side of the heart, especially the tricuspid valve, and all with infection of the mural endocardium are free of murmurs. Basal systolic murmurs, caused either by the flow of blood from the left ventricle into a widened tortuous aorta or by atherosclerotic changes in the aortic valve, often pose a problem in the diagnosis of infective endocarditis, especially the subacute form, since the physician detects no change in the character of the murmur, the presence of which he may have been aware of for a long time. It must be stressed that, in older patients with unexplained fever who are known to have had a murmur for many years, the possibility of subtle bacterial endocarditis must always be entertained, even in the occasional instance in which blood cultures are negative. With respect to infective endocarditis, *no murmur can be considered "innocent."* Personal experience has taught that the discovery of a so-called "flow" or systolic "ejection" murmur that remains unchanged over long periods of observation has resulted in failure to consider the possibility of valvular infection.

Anemia is a universal feature of both acute and subacute infective endocarditis; *pallor* of the skin and mucous membranes is common. Libman and Friedberg called attention to rare patients who exhibited erythema of the nose and surrounding skin, especially the cheeks, bearing a slight resemblance to the facial lesion in systemic lupus erythematosus.[21]

Characteristic Diagnostic Lesions ("Peripheral Stigmata")

Five lesions involving the skin and its appendages and the eye have, for many years, been considered the classic peripheral manifestations of subacute bacterial endocarditis: *petechiae, subungual hemorrhages, Osler nodes, Janeway lesions,* and *Roth spots.* Because of the long course of the active disease in the pre-antibiotic era, these peripheral lesions were much more common than now, when effective antibiotic therapy usually rapidly brings the disease under control.[173] There has been a decrease in the incidence of *petechiae,* especially in the subacute form of the disease, from about 85 per cent before antimicrobial agents were available to 19 to 40 per cent at present.[14,17,19,172,174] Libman and Friedberg pointed out that petechiae with pale centers are of greater diagnostic importance than those with yellow centers.[171] These lesions are often present in the conjunctivae and are detectable, in some cases, only when the upper eyelids are everted. They also tend to occur most prominently on the skin on the dorsa of the hands and feet but are also commonly seen on the anterior chest and abdominal wall, oral and pharyngeal mucosa, and soft palate. Purpuric lesions develop occasionally and are rarely associated with thrombocytopenia. The presence of petechiae is not always diagnostic of infective endocarditis, since these lesions develop in patients with various types of hematological disorders (especially when the number of circulating platelets is markedly reduced), systemic lupus erythematosus, scurvy, renal insufficiency, bacteremia without endocarditis (staphylococcal, streptococcal, meningococcal, and gonococcal), atrial myxoma, and verrucous endocardiosis ("marantic endocarditis"). Over 50 per cent of patients who undergo cardiopulmonary bypass develop conjunctival petechiae in the immediate postoperative period, in the absence of infection, presumably owing to fat microemboli.[176] Because these persons are especially susceptible to valvular infection, physicians must be aware of this "false-positive" sign.

Subungual ("splinter") hemorrhages are uncommon in patients with bacterial endocarditis. At present they are observed more frequently in general hospital populations than in individuals with valvular infections[177] and are often related to advanced age and trauma. The characteristic features of a splinter hemorrhage are its linear form and the fact that its distal end does not reach the anterior edge of the nail bed; the latter distinguishes this lesion from a true splinter. The number of fingers involved is variable and ranges from a single nail bed with only one hemorrhage to several fingers, each of which contains several "splinters." In some cases, the toes may be involved, either alone or together with the fingers. In trichinosis, subungual hemorrhages are very common, and each nail bed contains numerous lesions.

Osler nodes are small, raised, nodular, red to purple, painful, tender lesions that are present most often in the pulp spaces of the terminal phalanges of the fingers. They may also be present on the back of the toes, soles of the feet, and the thenar and hypothenar eminences. They are less common on the sides of the fingers, the forearms, and the ears and rarely occur on the trunk. The most characteristic feature of these lesions is their tenderness. At times, patients can anticipate the development of Osler nodes because of an antecedent peculiar, local "sensation" or pain at a site in which the lesion later appears. They may be fleeting in some cases and disappear within a few hours after they have developed; however, they usually persist for four to five days but remain tender for only two to three days and rarely become necrotic. Although almost completely restricted to the subacute type of endocarditis, Osler nodes are present rarely in the acute form of valvular infection. There has been a striking decrease in the incidence of Osler nodes over the past 30 years.

Janeway lesions are small (1 to 4 mm in diameter), irregular, flat, erythematous, nontender, painless macules present most often on the thenar and hypothenar eminences of the hands and the soles of the feet of patients with subacute infective endocarditis. They appear less often on the tips of the fingers and plantar surfaces of the toes; rarely, they take the form of a diffuse macular erythematous rash over the extremities and trunk. The lesions on the hands and feet blanch with pressure and with elevation of the extremities. When present in cases of acute valvular infection, the lesions tend to be purple in color and hemorrhagic.

Clubbing of fingers and/or toes was present in virtually all patients with subacute bacterial endocarditis 25 to 30 years ago but is now quite uncommon.

Ocular signs are occasionally present in patients with infective endocarditis, especially the subacute type. In addition to the conjunctival petechiae, these lesions may also appear in the sclera and in the retina, where they are circular or flame-shaped. The *Roth spot,* as first described, is located in the retina and has the appearance of a "cotton-wool" exudate; it consists of aggregations of cytoid bodies.[178] Histological study of these lesions has shown them to be composed of perivascular collections of lymphocytes in the nerve layer of the retina that may or may not be surrounded by edema and hemorrhage. Because the association of these lesions with infective endocarditis was first recognized by Litten,[179] they are referred to as "Litten's sign" in the French literature. The boat-shaped hemorrhage in the retina, erroneously called a Roth spot, was first described by Doherty and Trubek, who attributed it to recurrent crops of petechiae.[180] They noted that these lesions often appeared over a period of only a few hours. Both the cytoid bodies and hemorrhagic spots have decreased in incidence over the years and are now present in less than 5 per cent of cases. Round white spots are occasionally present in the retina; they are noted more often in the acute than in the subacute form of the disease. Optic neuritis occurs occasionally.

Splenomegaly is still a relatively frequent sign in patients with endocarditis but is not as common as in the preantibiotic era, when it occurred in 80 to 90 per cent of cases. The spleen may be only slightly enlarged and barely palpable; in the acute form of the disease it may be large, soft, painful, and tender.

A number of other signs and symptoms, some of which are uncommon or rare, may be present in infective endocarditis. Among these are pericardial friction rub, manifestations of congestive heart failure, cardiac arrhythmias of various types, hematuria (in the absence of renal infarction), cough that may occur early and be very distressing, hoarseness, arthritis, and pain and tenderness of the long bones and of the sternum (especially when anemia is severe).

BACTERIA-FREE STAGE

The "bacteria-free stage" of endocarditis, first described by Libman in 1913,[181] is now very rare as a result of early diagnosis and treatment of the disease. However, this syndrome is still seen, albeit uncommonly, in patients in whom the disease remains unsuspected and untreated for months. The outstanding features of this form of valvular infection include congestive heart failure, diaphoresis, pain in the joints, swelling of the legs, and severe pain in the thighs. Fever is absent in most cases but develops when embolism occurs. Organisms are usually not present in the embolus. Although all patients have lesions of the mitral or aortic valves, new murmurs do not develop; in fact, they may disappear. The kidney is usually involved; macroscopic hematuria is common, even in the absence of infarction. Renal insufficiency is frequent and is the cause of death in about one third of cases. Anemia is universal. The white blood count is usually low, and granulocytopenia may develop. The spleen is enlarged to such an extent that it dominates the clinical picture. Petechiae are much less common than in the active stage of the disease, but purpuric lesions are more frequent. Osler nodes are uncommon. Two of the most frequent signs of the bacteria-free stage of endocarditis are marked tenderness of the sternum and a striking brown pigmentation of the face and back of the hands.

The criteria for the diagnosis of this syndrome are absence of manifestations indicating active valvular infection, during which bacteremia may have been present; negative blood cultures but organisms still present in the vegetations; renal insufficiency; severe progressive anemia; embolic phenomena; striking splenomegaly; brown pigmentation of the face; and absence of fever. Patients with this syndrome have survived for as long as three years and usually die from renal insufficiency or congestive heart failure.

COMPLICATIONS

Cardiac Complications

HEART FAILURE. Congestive heart failure resulting from acute aortic regurgitation is currently the leading cause of death from infective endocarditis. This may occur over a varying period of time in untreated cases of the subacute form of the disease. In sharp contrast, cardiac failure may appear with startling rapidity in acute endocarditis when the aortic valve is infected and may become so severe within a week after the onset of infection that replacement of the valve becomes an emergency procedure. In a review of 144 cases of infective endocarditis, Mills et al. noted congestive failure in 55 per cent.[182] Eighty per cent of those with failure had regurgitant aortic valves and/or enterococcal infection. Cardiac decompensation occurred in about 50 per cent of patients with mitral valve regurgitation and in less than 20 per cent of those with congenital heart disease or infection of the tricuspid valve. Nearly 95 per cent of patients who experienced cardiac failure within six months after the onset of endocarditis had premonitory manifestations within one month after infection. Heart failure seldom developed de novo after six months. The organisms involved were (in order of frequency) enterococcus, *Strep. pneumoniae, Staph. aureus,* and *Strep. viridans.* Review of collected studies of congestive heart failure complicating infective endocarditis indicates an incidence ranging from 15 to 65 per cent. Aortic or mitral valve regurgitation may develop as early as one month after infection and nearly always within six months; in some instances, it may not occur until as long as one year after the appearance of endocarditis. Although it had been suggested that myocarditis is the basis of cardiac failure, it now seems clear that the primary cause is valvular destruction.

Another complication responsible for heart failure, said to be common in patients with severe aortic regurgitation, is the impact of the jet stream created by the regurgitant aortic valve on the mitral valve, leading to the development of a secondary lesion that varies in character from erosion to perforation of a cusp; the regurgitant stream may occasionally cause rupture of the chordae tendineae.[183] Severe involvement of the mitral valve accentuates the left ventricular overload imposed by the aortic regurgitation and markedly exaggerates the heart failure.

Hemodynamically important valvular stenosis may result from infective endocarditis when the vegetations are unusually large, as in fungal infection, and obstruct the flow of blood to and from the left ventricle.[184,185] One of the reasons for the development of congestive heart failure in patients with the Starr-Edwards prosthesis is progressive obstruction of the valvular outlet during the course of infection; this is most common when the invading organism is *Candida* or *Aspergillus,* because of the characteristically large vegetations. The hemodynamic changes in aortic regurgitation produced by infective endocarditis have been evaluated by Mann and his colleagues.[186] They noted that the mean pulse pressure, left ventricular end-diastolic volume, and stroke volume were significantly smaller in patients who developed aortic regurgitation acutely than in those with the chronic condition (p. 1111).

OTHER CARDIAC COMPLICATIONS. A number of intracardiac complications related directly to the valvular involvement may develop in the course of infective endocarditis and are much more common in the acute than in the subacute form of the disease.[170,172] Some, but not all, are associated with rapid or progressive congestive heart failure, a change in the character of an existing murmur, or the appearance of a murmur not previously detected. Some of the complications result from disruption of the valves and their supporting structures (Fig. 33–9). Among these are fenestration or tears of a leaflet, detachment of one or more areas of a valve from its annulus, and rupture of the chordae tendineae or papillary muscles. Another group of intracardiac complications includes the formation of fistulas, aneurysms (particularly of the sinus of Valsalva) that often involve the fibrous atrioventricular body, perforation of valve cusps, septal and other abscesses, and acute pericarditis with cardiac tamponade. In studies correlating anatomical and electrocardiographic abnormalities in 24 patients with aortic valve endocarditis, Roberts and Somerville found prolonged P-R intervals unrelated to digitalis therapy in 18 and atrioventricular dissociation in 4.[187] In 4 of 6 with prolonged P-R intervals and in 3 of 4 with normal conduction and left bundle branch block, aneurysms had invaded the interventricular septum; 4 out of 6 patients with prolonged conduction died suddenly.

Abscesses. One of the most serious intracardiac complications of bacterial endocarditis is the development of abscesses (Fig. 33–10) that are thought to be present in about 20 per cent of patients who succumb to valvular infections.[188,189] Abscesses tend to occur most often when *Staph. aureus* and enterococci are involved and are rare when infection is caused by *Strep. viridans.* Multiple myocardial abscesses may be present, especially when coagulase-positive staphylococci cause the disease and when antimicrobial therapy is not instituted until relatively late in the course of infection. A single large abscess may be present and rupture into the pericardial sac, causing rapid death from the resulting pyohemopericardium (Fig. 33–2). Septal abscesses are not uncommon in patients with acute staphylococcal endocarditis. In some instances, these completely destroy the involved area and produce a left-to-right shunt.

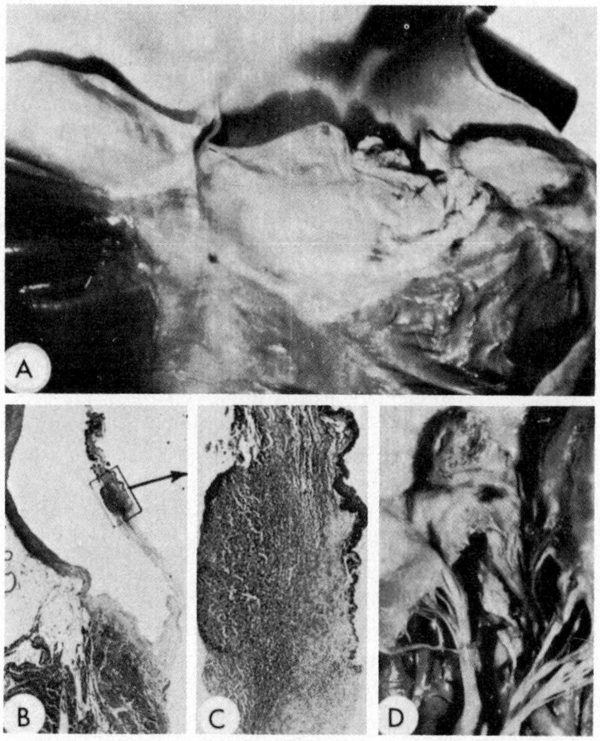

FIGURE 33–9 *Staphylococcus aureus* endocarditis involving pulmonic (*A, B,* and *C*) and mitral (*D*) valves. The vegetation on the pulmonic valve caused tearing of one leaflet. *B,* Histological section through portion of pulmonic valve cusp. *C,* Higher power view of a portion of the infected cusp shown in *B.* (From Roberts, W. C., and Buchbinder, N. A.: Right-sided valvular infective endocarditis. Am. J. Med. *53*:7, 1972.)

Abscesses of the interventricular septum secondary to in-

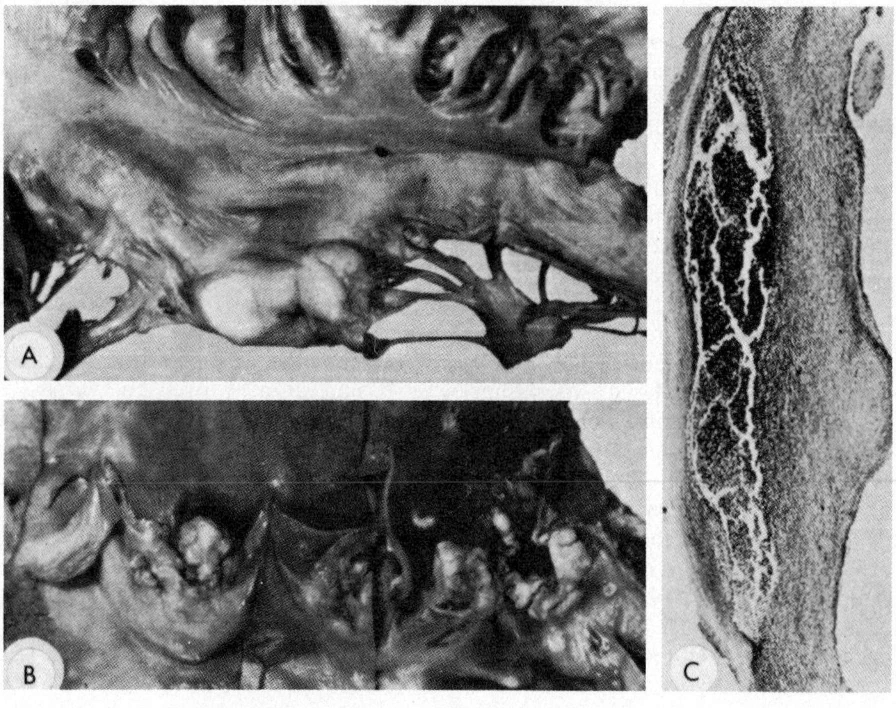

FIGURE 33–10 Pneumococcal endocarditis involving tricuspid (*A*) and aortic (*B*) valves. The vegetation on the tricuspid valve is small, whereas the vegetations on the aortic valve are large and cause extensive destruction of the cusps. *C,* Histological section of a portion of the tricuspid leaflet showing abscess formation. (From Roberts, W. C., and Buchbinder, N. A.: Right-sided valvular infective endocarditis. Am. J. Med. *53*:7, 1972.)

fection of the mitral valve are usually located in the lower part of the septum. The presence of this complication may be suspected on the basis of serial changes in the electrocardiogram, consisting of a gradual increase in atrioventricular conduction time and eventually left bundle branch block; the right bundle is much less frequently involved. Recognition of this entity during life is of great importance because surgical removal of the abscess and its replacement by a patch may be life-saving. A much more serious threat, because it is less often manageable surgically and is usually not suspected clinically, is an abscess involving the upper end of the septum that develops as a result of contiguous spread from an acutely infected aortic valve. In these cases, the electrocardiographic changes are not as characteristic as in the lower septal lesions; the diagnosis is usually overlooked. However, the appearance of various types of arrhythmias, including varying degrees of heart block, especially complete block, should alert the physician to the possibility of this type of abscess. Surgical removal is required for cure.

A specific type of *intracardiac abscess* involving the valvular ring has been described by Arnett and Roberts in 27 patients who succumbed to infective endocarditis.[190] The aortic annulus was involved most often, and abscess of the atrioventricular ring was observed in a few instances. This complication was not related to the age or sex of the patients, the status of the valves prior to the development of endocarditis, the nature of the infecting organism, or treatment with antimicrobial agents. The following criteria were found to be of value in the diagnosis of abscesses of valvular rings: (a) infection of the aortic valve, (b) recent appearance of regurgitation, (c) the presence of pericarditis, (d) a high degree of atrioventricular block (complete in five cases and Mobitz type II in one case), and (e) short duration of symptoms followed by the rapid development of severe disability and death.

Pericarditis. This is a rare complication of the subacute type of infective endocarditis and is not the result of bacterial invasion of the pericardial space in the vast majority of cases. It probably represents an immunological reaction, possibly deposition of immune complexes, in most instances. In contrast, the pericarditis that occasionally complicates the acute type of valvular infection is often purulent and results from hematogenous deposition of organisms in the pericardial space or from rupture of a myocardial abscess into the sac (Fig. 33–2). Other causes of pericarditis in patients with infective endocarditis include erosion of a mycotic aneurysm of the sinus of Valsalva, extension of infection from the aortic valve into the pericardial wedge between the root of the aorta and the pulmonary artery, uremia, and reactivation of rheumatic fever during the course of endocarditis.

Myocarditis. Although its pathogenesis is unclear at the moment, many observers consider myocarditis one of the important complications of infective endocarditis.[191,192] Whether it is the result of ischemic damage secondary to occlusion of the coronary arteries by emboli, damage produced by bacterial toxins, myocardial invasion by organisms, or the activity of immune complexes, or whether it may have a variety of causes, is as yet undetermined. The typical lesions associated with the myocarditis are the so-called Bracht-Wächter bodies (see earlier). Diffuse collections of lymphocytes or localized of diffuse aggregations of polymorphonuclear leukocytes, with or without myocardial necrosis or miliary abscesses, are occasionally present. The myocardium may show areas of degeneration. Proliferation of the cells of capillaries and arterioles, arteriolitis or necrosis of the media or adventitia, and perivascular cellular infiltrations are detectable in some cases.

EMBOLIZATION. Next to complications involving the heart itself, arterial embolization is the most common potentially serious complication of infective endocarditis; its incidence has decreased over the past 30 years. Emboli were clinically detected in 70 to 97 per cent of patients in the preantibiotic era but are now found in only 15 to 35 per cent.[9,14,17,19,193] The most common sites are the spleen, kidneys, coronary vessels, and brain, although almost every tissue and organ may be involved. Splenic emboli have been discovered at autopsy in 44 per cent of cases but are suspected only rarely during life. Renal infarcts have been detected in as many as 56 per cent of patients studied at necropsy but are recognized clinically less often.[15] Bell has reported embolic glomerular lesions in the kidneys of 52 per cent of patients with subacute and in 7 per cent with acute bacterial endocarditis.[194] Myocardial infarction, often undetected by electrocardiography, has been found in 40 to 60 per cent of autopsied patients with valvular infections and is due to embolization of the coronary arterial bed. When the aortic valve is infected, infarction of the myocardium often leads to the development of congestive heart failure.[9,195–197] Major cerebral emboli have been observed in almost one third of patients with endocarditis at autopsy.[170]

The middle cerebral artery and its branches are most frequently involved, and hemiplegia is the most frequent consequence.[170,198] Jochman's dictum, "In hemiplegia in young adults or children always think of subacute bacterial endocarditis," is as applicable today as when it was first stated in 1914.[199] Three per cent of all emboli to the brain arise from infections of the cardiac valves.[200] Embolic occlusion of cerebral vessels may be the presenting sign of endocarditis. The clinical manifestations resulting from this are discussed below. Embolization of the vascular supply of the spinal cord is rare; it usually produces girdle pain and paraplegia.[201] Weakness, peripheral neuropathy, nerve tenderness, sensory disturbances, and localized pain may develop when emboli invade supplying peripheral nerves.[202–204]

Unilateral blindness due to embolization of the retinal artery, infarction of the retina with formation of a hole, and mononeuropathy may complicate valvular infections.[205]

It is important to emphasize that embolic occlusion of large arteries (e.g., the femoral) is rare when bacteria cause endocarditis; the most likely cause is fungal valvular disease or atrial myxoma. Large vegetations may also be present in an occasional case caused by *Staph. aureus.* It is well known that embolic phenomena may occur weeks to months after the infectious process on the valve has been eradicated. Most likely this is related to the fact that as long as six months may be required before the vegetations on the affected valve become completely covered by endothelium.

Metastatic Infections

In the acute infection, especially that due to *Staph. aureus,* an abscess develops at every site at which an embolus is deposited. In most patients who succumb to staphylococcal endocarditis, abscesses are present in almost every organ and tissue. If such lesions are not present at other sites, they are practically always detected in the kidneys and myocardium; the abscesses are usually small. The clinical course of staphylococcal endocarditis complicated by multiple diffuse abscesses may often be sufficiently characteristic to be diagnostic. The distinguishing features are (a) defervescence early during antimicrobial therapy; (b) return of fever either during treatment or after it has been discontinued; (c) failure to respond to the drug given initially or to the administration of another "effective" agent; and (d) negative blood cultures. If organisms are recovered from the blood, they are frequently still sensitive to the drug employed at the beginning of treatment.

In sharp contrast to this, metastatic infection following deposition of emboli in the course of subacute endocarditis, particularly that caused by *Strep. viridans*, is distinctly rare, probably because the number of organisms in the embolus is small, the bacteria have a low invasive capability, and most patients with this type of infection have high titers of specific bactericidal antibody that, in the presence of normal serum levels of complement, rapidly kills the few streptococci that are deposited. Thus, although infarction of the myocardium, brain, kidneys, and spleen develop in patients with subacute endocarditis, abscesses in these organs—suppurative myocarditis, pyogenic meningitis, splenic abscess, or pyelonephritis—are very rare. However, a sterile meningitis, with the biochemical and cellular characteristics of so-called aseptic meningitis, or a syndrome consistent with diffuse encephalitis with an abnormal or normal cerebrospinal fluid may occur in the subacute type of valvular infection and provide the first clue to the diagnosis, especially in cases in which an audible murmur is not present.

MYCOTIC ANEURYSMS. Mycotic aneurysms are a major complication of infective endocarditis. Although they have probably not decreased in incidence over the years, as indicated by the results of studies of autopsied cases, they are now detected clinically less often and are not as frequently fatal as they were in the past. They have been reported to occur in about 2.5 per cent of patients with valvular infections[206] and constitute 2.5 to 6.2 per cent of *all* aneurysms involving the brain. These lesions usually develop during the active phase of the infectious process but may not become manifest for months to years after it has been eradicated. They are most common when relatively noninvasive organisms such as *Strep. viridans* are involved and are less frequent when *Staph. aureus* is the causative agent. Several mechanisms may be involved in their pathogenesis. Among these are injury produced by deposition of immune complexes in the arterial wall, embolic occlusion of the vasa vasorum and sterile infarction of a blood vessel (usually in subacute endocarditis), and direct invasion by organisms or deposition of bacteria-laden emboli followed by infarction and the formation of an abscess in the vascular wall (common in acute infections). When mycotic aneurysms develop in the course of endocarditis due to *Staph. aureus*, there is a high incidence of rupture at the area of involvement of the blood vessel. Although any artery may be the site of an aneurysm, the vessels most often involved are those in the brain; the sinuses of Valsalva; ligated ductus arteriosus; the abdominal aorta and its branches; and the coronary and pulmonary arteries.[15,207] The development of aneurysms is usually silent; clinical manifestations appear usually after the lesions have started to leak slowly or rupture and produce gross hemorrhages. When present in the brain, their pressure effects may produce headache or cranial nerve palsies. Areas in which mycotic aneurysms pose the greatest threat to life are the brain, abdominal aorta, the superior mesenteric, splenic, and coronary arteries, and ligated ductus arteriosus.

Neurological Complications

Neurological complications are some of the most life-threatening complications of infective endocarditis in both treated and untreated patients. The reported incidence of these phenomena has ranged from 9 to 80 per cent, with an average of about 15 to 30 per cent. They have been classified into three groups: (1) vascular phenomena due to embolization, (2) rupture of mycotic aneurysms, and (3) acute meningitis or meningocerebritis. Ziment[208] grouped the neurological manifestations of endocarditis on the basis of their etiology as follows:

Toxic—headache, impaired concentration, drowsiness, insomnia, vertigo, and irritability.

Psychiatric—neurosis, psychosis, confusion, disorientation, emotional instability, delirium, auditory and visual disturbances, apathy, and altered personality.

Cerebrovascular—hemi-, di-, para-, or quadriplegia, sensory and motor aphasia, aphonia, stupor, and coma.

Meningoencephalitis—acute brain syndrome.

Cranial nerves—visual disturbances, palsies of various cranial nerves, pseudobulbar palsy, and sensory impairment.

Dyskinesia—tremor, ataxia, parkinsonism, seizures, chorea, hemifacial dyskinesia, hiccupping, and myoclonus.

Spinal cord or peripheral nerves—girdle pain, weakness, paraplegia, paresis, sensory disturbances, myalgia, and peripheral neuropathy.

The brain may be the site of embolic abscesses in about 1 per cent of cases of subacute and in about 25 per cent of patients with acute infective endocarditis. Subdural empyema has also occurred. Ziment noted that encephalomalacia and endarteritis due to vasculitis of the cerebral arteries may be present. Petechiae and purpuric lesions may develop in the brain; they appear mostly in the white matter adjacent to the lateral ventricles but also in the gray matter along the aqueduct and in the corpus callosum. Meningeal or cerebral edema is present in some cases but usually produces no signs or symptoms. In addition to embolic retinal arterial occlusion, multiple retinal and conjunctival hemorrhages may develop. Other ocular complications of infective endocarditis are papilledema, iridocyclitis, panophthalmitis (usually in acute endocarditis), nystagmus, conjugate deviation of the eyes, and paresis of the third cranial nerves.

A study of the neurological complications observed in 281 cases of infective endocarditis admitted to the Massachusetts General Hospital has been reported by Pruitt et al.[209] Eighty-four patients (39 per cent) experienced neurological dysfunction during the course of the disease. The sex distribution of the cases was even; ages ranged from 3 months to 89 years, with most patients older than 50 years. The fatality rate was 58 per cent in those with manifestations of nervous system disorders, but only 20 per cent in persons with no neurological abnormalities. It was noted that neurological complications were most common with valvular infections caused by *Staph. aureus*, followed by streptococci, *Strep. pneumoniae*, and *Enterobacter*. Disturbances in function of the nervous system were noted in 79 of 84 patients with underlying cardiac valvular disease but in none with nonvalvular congenital heart disease.

Embolic cerebral infarction is the commonest neurological complication of infective endocarditis. It occurs in 6 to 31 per cent of patients with this disease and is associated more often with infection of the mitral than of the aortic valve. The infarctions are both macroscopic and microscopic. Emboli are present in other organs simultaneously with those in the brain in about half of cases. Cerebral infarction tends to occur within 2 weeks after the onset of valvular infection when highly invasive organisms such as *Staph. aureus*, enterococci, and *E. coli* are involved; staphylococci are responsible for about 70 per cent of these. When other bacteria, principally streptococci, produce the disease, cerebral infarctions develop in a biphasic manner and occur either 2 to 4 weeks or 1 to 3 months after the onset of the endocarditis. The fatality rate of cerebral infarction complicating infective endocarditis ranges from 17 to 81 per cent in patients who experience embolic strokes; approximately three fourths die within one year after onset of their valvular infection.[209]

Mycotic aneurysms of cerebral arteries are present in 2 to 10 per cent of patients with infective endocarditis and account for 2.5 to 6.2 per cent of all intracranial aneurysms.[209] A study of 85 cases of endocarditis in which the presence of cerebral mycotic aneurysms was demonstrated by angiography, indicated a fatality rate of 80 per cent in cases in which the lesions ruptured, and 30 per cent in those in which it remained intact; the overall death rate was 46 per cent.[210] Multiple aneurysms were present in 15 patients (17.6 per cent); in three, the second aneurysm did not appear until after treatment of the first. Angiographic examination showed that single aneurysms tended to be peripheral to the first bifurcation of a major intracranial artery; 20 of the lesions were at or proximal to that point. Sixty-five per cent of the aneurysms ruptured spontaneously; they disappeared in 10 cases.

Cerebral abscesses were noted at necropsy in 9 of the 218 patients (4.1 per cent); these lesions were not detected during life. In 8 cases, the abscesses were microscopic (< 1 cm^3). In 6 cases, multiple microabscesses in the brain were associated with similar lesions in other organs.

Neurological dysfunction of various types has been noted to be the presenting manifestation in a large number of cases of infective endocarditis.[209] Evidence of a major cerebral embolic episode involving mainly the middle cerebral arteries was the commonest problem that brought individuals to medical attention. Other manifestations included focal and/or generalized seizures (11 per cent), signs of cerebral embolus and hemorrhage, personality change, weakness of the lower extremities, subdural hemorrhage, and cortical blindness and obtundation without a focal defect. Among the disturbances of the nervous system developing after admission to the hospital were those listed above as well as multiple cerebral microemboli, microscopic brain abscesses, visual disturbances, cranial or peripheral neuropathy, mycotic aneurysms, cerebral infarcts in the "watershed areas" due to hypotension, and psychiatric disturbances.

Cerebrospinal fluid has been normal in 28 per cent of the patients with neurological manifestations.[209] Polymorphonuclear leukocytes were predominant in cases caused by *Staph. aureus*, gram-negative bacilli, and *Strep. pneumoniae*. In the other instances, the meningitis was considered aseptic; these were associated, in most instances, with valvular disease produced by relatively avirulent bacteria such as *Strep. viridans*. Thirteen per cent of the patients had hemorrhagic cerebrospinal fluid.

MUSCULOSKELETAL SYSTEM. Churchill, Geraci, and Hunder noted involvement of the musculoskeletal system in 44 per cent of patients with infective endocarditis.[211] In 27 per cent, symptoms and signs of dysfunction of the muscles or joints were the first or among the first complaints. The commonest manifestation was arthralgia. The shoulder joint was most commonly involved, followed, in descending order of frequency, by the knees, hips, wrists, ankles, and metatarsophalangeal and metacarpophalangeal joints. Multiple joints were affected in some cases. Objective evidence of arthritis was present in about one third of the cases. The ankle was most often involved, followed by the knees, wrists, sternoclavicular joints, elbows, metatarsophalangeal and metacarpophalangeal joints, and shoulder, hip, and acromioclavicular joints. Migrating polyarthritis was present in some instances. Pain in the lumbar area of the back, diffuse myalgias, and synovitis were also noted. Acute arthritis or arthralgia is present in 33 per cent of cases of gonococcal and 50 per cent of meningococcal endocarditis.

Renal Involvement

Involvement of the kidney is relatively common in patients with either acute or subacute infective endocarditis. Five types of renal lesions may develop.[212,213] Two are caused by embolization. While large bland infarcts of the kidney, associated with gross hematuria, were quite common 25 to 30 years ago, they now occur only infrequently.[174] However, multiple small infarcts are a relatively frequent finding at autopsy. One or more large abscesses or, more often, multiple microabscesses are commonly present in the kidneys of patients who die from acute valvular infections caused by *Staph. aureus*. The other lesions are all the result of immunological reactions and include interstitial nephritis and either acute or chronic proliferative glomerulonephritis. The acute form of the latter has been reported by Bell in 64 per cent of patients with subacute and 28 per cent of those with acute infective endocarditis.[194]

Immunological Phenomena

Immunoglobulins. Specific agglutinating, complement-fixing, and bactericidal antibodies and cryoglobulins are present in the serum of patients with infective endocarditis, especially the subacute form. *Hypergammaglobulinemia* has been demonstrated by Cordeiro et al.,[214] who noted an early increase in 19S and 7S globulins followed by a rise in $alpha_2$ globulin. Immunoglobulins with specific affinities for the renal glomerular basement membrane, vascular walls, and myocardium of normal individuals were present. In patients with subacute endocarditis, gamma globulin was fixed in the sarcolemma and myofibrils of the myocardium; in the walls of blood vessels, especially in the intima and subintima; and in the basal layer of the glomeruli of the kidney.

The first report of the presence of *rheumatoid factor* in the blood of patients with subacute infective endocarditis was that of Williams and Kunkel.[215] They demonstrated positive latex fixation reactions in about 50 per cent of cases of the subacute type of endocardial infection, with high titers in most instances. The reactive factor was 19S globulin. With successful treatment, titers of circulating rheumatoid factor fell rapidly; even when very high, they reached zero within about 2 months after therapy was initiated. The latex fixation test is positive in about 50 per cent of patients with valvular infections present for 6 or more weeks. In addition to the duration of disease, the degree of elevation of serum levels of gamma G immunoglobulin is an important factor in determining positivity of this test. Other immunological abnormalities detected in some patients with infective endocarditis are antinuclear antibody and depression of total hemolytic complement as well as both C_3 and C_4.[216]

Sheagren et al. have reported that elevated titers of rheumatoid factor may also develop in patients with acute infective endocarditis.[217] They noted that 13 (24 per cent) of 55 parenteral drug users with valvular infections caused by *Staph. aureus* had circulating antibody of this type at some point in the course of their disease.

The presence of *circulating immune complexes* has been demonstrated by Bayer and his colleagues in 97 per cent of patients with infective endocarditis.[218] Blood levels of the complexes were greater than 12 μg/ml in all instances and were significantly higher than in patients with sepsis without endocarditis. Circulating immune complexes were correlated with long duration of valvular infection, extravascular manifestations of the disease, and hypocomplementemia. In general, the complexes disappeared from the circulation within 6 weeks following successful antimicrobial or surgical treatment; this was concurrent with the resolution of extravascular signs, eradication of the bacteria from the bloodstream, and an increase in serum concentration of complement. In some patients, the concentration of the complexes in the blood did not fall until the infected valve was removed surgically.

Two studies have defined the type of endocardial disease associated with circulating immune complexes (IC). McKenzie and his colleagues[219] detected IC in 75 per cent of patients with valvular infections. This correlated with a subacute course and associated cutaneous vasculitis, glomerulonephritis, involvement of joints, and tissue deposits of immunoglobulins and complement. There was no correlation of IC with acute endocarditis, major embolic phenomena, Osler's nodes, Janeway lesions, or clinical evidence of renal disease. Serial determinations of IC were found to be important in monitoring the activity of the disease in patients whose blood cultures were negative, and in those with continued extravalvular manifestations of activity of the disease. Assessment of IC was of value in evaluating the need for replacement of valves. Kauffman et al.[220] studied four types of cases: endocarditis, septicemia without endocardial disease, endocardial lesions with nonseptic fever, and uncomplicated preexisting endocardial defects. IC was positive in 63 per cent of patients with endocarditis on admission. It occurred in 7 to 12 per cent of the others. The incidence of positive IC was higher when preexisting endocardial lesions were present, when endocarditis was caused by nonvirulent organisms, and when valvular infection had been present for more than 4 weeks. No differences were detected between left- and right-sided endocarditis. The levels of IC were higher when renal involvement was present. Higher mean peak levels were not detected when petechiae, subungual hemorrhages, Osler's nodes, Janeway lesions, or embolization developed.

Immunological phenomena play a critical role throughout the course of subacute infective endocarditis. A prime factor involved in the pathogenesis of this syndrome is the gradual development of *specific agglutinating antibody* as a result of repeated episodes of transient bacteremia over a period of years. It is believed that this finally stimulates development of a sufficient level of agglutinin to cause conglutination of the small number of organisms present in a transient bacteremia and leads to deposition of a bacterial inoculum of sufficient size to initiate infection in the sterile platelet-fibrin clot. Until a high concentration of this antibody develops in the circulation over a period of years, usually as a result of multiple intrusions of organisms (most often *Strep. viridans*) infection does not occur, because the bacteria are few in number, have low invasive capability, remain in the bloodstream for a short time (usually no more than 5 to 10 minutes), and are rapidly eliminated by effective humoral and cellular clearing mechanisms. In the absence of technical problems (discussed below), blood cultures are negative in patients with valvular infection as a result of another immunological factor—specific bactericidal antibody.

Clinical Manifestations of Immunological Origin. Several of the manifestations present during the early stage of subacute bacterial endocarditis are probably immunological in origin. *Roth spots* resemble the cytoid bodies that may appear in systemic lupus erythematosus and other vasculitides. *Janeway lesions* may represent an immunological reaction.[216] It has also been postulated that the pathology of *Osler nodes* is strongly suggestive of an Arthus reaction. Howard has demonstrated a perivasculitis in many tiny vessels in the malpighian layers, without evidence of emboli or bacteria in these lesions.[221] Alpert et al.[222] have isolated *Staph. aureus* and *Candida* from these lesions and have suggested, as did Kerr,[15,19] that Osler nodes "are in all probability caused by minute emboli." The arthralgias of infective endocarditis are now also thought to be caused by deposition of immune complexes in the synovia; however, this has not been proved.

Among other clinical manifestations of infective endocarditis that may be related to disposition of immune complexes are sterile pericarditis, dermal vasculitis, deposition of immunoglobulin in blood vessels of normal skin, and leukocytoclastic angiitis of skin (purpuric lesions).[223,224] The best proved example of the operation of immunological reactions in the pathogenesis of complications of both acute and subacute valvular infection is acute, subacute, and chronic proliferative glomerulonephritis. These have been demonstrated in endocarditis caused by viridans streptococci as well as *Staph. aureus*.[225,226] Gutman and his associates noted discrete deposits of fibrin containing IgG and complement in the basement membrane and/or in the mesangial region of the glomeruli. Antibody eluted from the kidney of a patient with subacute endocarditis who died of renal failure was shown by Levy and Hong to combine specifically with the bacteria cultured from the blood.[227] The elute also contained antiglomerular antibody and activated complement in the destroyed basement membrane. Lumpy-bumpy glomerular fluorescence, when stained for IgG and β_1C, has been demonstrated in patients with subacute endocarditis.[228]

ENDOCARDITIS INVOLVING THE RIGHT SIDE OF THE HEART

Infective endocarditis involving the right side of the heart occurs in about 5 per cent of cases[229,230] (Figs. 33–9 and 33–10), but there has been a sharp increase in this type of cardiac disease in recent years. This is, for the most part, due to infection of the tricuspid valve in users of illicit drugs. Many of these infections are caused by *Staph. aureus, Pseudomonas,* yeasts, and fungi.

Two thirds of the cases of right-sided endocarditis studied at the Mayo Clinic were acute, with prominent pulmonary manifestations; murmurs, splenomegaly, or multiple cutaneous and renal abscesses were present in about one third of cases.[229] Blood cultures were usually positive. *Staph. aureus* was isolated in half the cases; *Strep. pneumoniae, N. gonorrhoeae,* streptococci *(viridans, faecalis, and pyogenes),* and gram-negative bacilli have also been recovered. Hearts with congenital malformations or normal ones are most often involved. Infections of skin wounds, respiratory tract *(Strep. pneumoniae),* and urethra; prostatic massage; dental sepsis; normal parturition; septic abortion; and narcotic addiction are among the reported pathogenetic factors.[229,230] In 80 per cent of the cases with tricuspid valve involvement a murmur was not heard, and the diagnosis was not suspected during life.[229] Renal involvement, most commonly abscesses or diffuse pyelonephritis, was detected in 65 per cent of patients. Glomerular and tubular hemorrhage and focal embolic glomerulonephritis have also been noted. In congenital lesions with exclusive or predominant left-to-right shunts, defects of the interventricular septum, or patent ductus arteriosus complicated by endocarditis, emboli are deposited almost exclusively in the lungs early in the course of the disease and may produce hemoptysis, pleurisy, or pneumonia;[231] peripheral embolization may occur later.

Myocarditis is one of the complications of endocarditis involving the right side of the heart. Histologically, this consists of small foci of perivascular collections of polymorphonuclear leukocytes or diffuse infiltrates with the same type of cell or miliary abscesses. The lungs are the primary site for the deposition of emboli, resulting in the development of single or multiple *pulmonary infarcts.* If the infecting organisms are relatively avirulent (e.g., *Strep. viridans*), the infarcted areas will only rarely be infected. In contrast, when a highly invasive bacterium such as *Staph. aureus* is the causative agent, the infarcts are almost always infected and are rapidly converted to abscesses. Other pulmonary complications include pneumonia, thrombosis, and septic arteritis of the branches of the pulmonary artery. Among the *renal complications* of endocarditis involving the right side of the heart are suppurative nephritis, focal or diffuse proliferative glomerular nephritis, or tubular hemorrhages.

The sequential appearance of repeated episodes of "pneumonia" (infarcts of the lung) followed by hepatomegaly, often associated with a mild degree of jaundice, and finally the development of progressive renal failure in patients with persistent fever, should raise the possibility of infection of the right heart, even in the absence of a murmur. Blood cultures are frequently negative when relatively noninvasive organisms are involved. However, when infectious process is caused by *Staph. aureus,* blood culture is often positive *after* the development of infected pulmonary infarcts, which become the source of bacteria entering the systemic circulation. Causes of death in untreated persons with involvement of the right heart, and even in some who receive appropriate therapy, are multiple pulmonary infarcts and abscesses, cardiac failure, and post-operative hemorrhages in patients subjected to surgery for patent ductus arteriosus.

INFECTIVE ENDOCARDITIS IN CHILDREN

(See also p. 951)

Kerr noted that only about 2 to 3 per cent of cases of infective endocarditis occur during the first decade of life.[15] Only 5 cases in over 400 instances of valvular infection were noted by Cates and Christie.[9] The subacute form of the disease has been identified in babies as young as 8 and 10 months of age,[15] and mycotic endocarditis has been observed in a 7-week-old premature infant. Although bacterial endocarditis is exceedingly uncommon in neonates, a recent report[141] has described three babies (one aged 7 weeks and two only 7 hours old) who died of infective endocarditis. The diagnosis was made only at autopsy. The tricuspid valve was involved in two and the mitral valve in one of the neonates. The responsible bacteria were *Staph. epidermidis* in one, *E. coli* in another; no organisms were recovered from the third baby. All the infants had had catheters inserted into the umbilical or other veins.

An analysis by Zakrzewski and Keith of 50 cases of infective endocarditis in children has indicated that underlying rheumatic heart disease is a very uncommon predisposing factor[232]; the commonest one appears to be the tetralogy of Fallot, followed in order of frequency by aortic stenosis, patent ductus arteriosus, and pulmonic stenosis. There is a striking difference in the factors that predispose to valvular infection in children and adults. In children, these include severe burns, osteomyelitis, asthma, bronchitis, infection of the urinary tract, otitis media, thrombophlebitis, pneumonia, pansinusitis, diarrhea, dermatitis, circumcision, and acute rheumatic fever.

A difference in the frequency of specific organisms responsible for endocarditis in children was noted by Zakrzewski and Keith in a comparison of cases studied from 1952 to 1961 and those observed between 1958 and 1962.[232] *Staph. aureus* was responsible for 37 per cent and *Strep. viridans* for 32 per cent in the first period; in the latter one, *Staph. aureus* and *epidermidis* caused 72 per cent, while *Strep. viridans* was involved in about 20 per cent; the marked increase in staphylococcal valvular disease is undoubtedly related to the greater frequency of cardiac surgery.

Infective endocarditis in infants less than 2 years of age, most of whom were only a few weeks or months old, was characterized by a number of features that distinguish it from that involving older children[143]; all cases were of the acute type and involved more than one valve. Congenital heart disease was present in only 8 per cent. About 60 per cent had infection of the mitral valve; the tricuspid valve was affected in 32 per cent, the aortic valve in 17 per cent, and the pulmonic valve in 6.5 per cent. Embolic phenomena were present in only 18 per cent. In every instance, there was evidence of disease at extracardiac sites. Among these were infections of the skin, enteritis, empyema, osteomyelitis, and tuberculosis. Diagnosis of endocarditis in these infants was usually made post mortem. Valvular infections in older children were caused most commonly by *Staph. aureus*; next most frequent were *Strep. viridans* and *Staph. epidermidis*; together, these three organisms were responsible for 80 per cent of the cases. Other bacteria involved included *Pseudomonas, E. coli, H. influenzae,* and *K. pneumoniae*; enterococci rarely caused the disease. Although before 1958 rheumatic heart disease was the underlying lesion in 50 per cent of the older children, in the following years this disorder was rarely a predisposing factor. Osler nodes were not observed in any of these children.

An extensive review of 149 instances of bacterial endocarditis in 141 children studied at the Children's Hospital Medical Center in Boston during the period 1933 to 1972 has been presented by Johnson, Rosenthal, and Nadas.[233] Six of the patients had two and one had three episodes of the disease. Predisposing factors, in order of frequency, included infected extracardiac foci (urinary tract infection, meningitis, and osteomyelitis), dental manipulation, cardiac surgery, catheterization, and orthopedic and otolaryngological surgical procedures. The commonest underlying types of heart disease were congenital (118 cases) and rheumatic (14 cases). There were no significant disorders of the heart in 17 patients. The most frequent underlying lesion was the tetralogy of Fallot; the others, in order of incidence, were ventricular septal defects, aortic stenosis, rheumatic heart disease, patent ductus arteriosus, and transposition of the great arteries. Blood cultures were sterile in 19 children. Presenting clinical manifestations consisted of fever (87 per cent), splenomegaly (65 per cent), petechiae (42 per cent), and heart failure (34 per cent). In 21 per cent, heart murmurs were present and underwent changes during the course of the disease. The most frequent complication was congestive heart failure; others included central nervous system disorders, pulmonary emboli, and aortic regurgitation.

A study of 33 autopsies of patients who had endocarditis during the first decade of life disclosed that rheumatic rather than congenital heart disease was the commonest underlying cardiac lesion. The left side of the heart was involved more often than the right; peripheral septic foci and pneumonia were the most frequent sources of infection.[234]

Fifty children (aged 6 months to 16 years) with endocarditis were studied at the Mayo Clinic over a 30-year period.[140] Thirty-seven had congenital heart disease, 4 had a history of rheumatic carditis, 17 had undergone cardiac surgery, 8 had had some type of instrumentation or noncardiac surgical procedure within 2 weeks before developing valvular infection, and 11 had an obvious extracardiac bacterial infection. A cardiac murmur was present in all but one. Microscopic hematuria, neurologic deficits, or other embolic phenomena and abnormal funduscopic findings were present in some patients. *Staph. aureus* was the most common infecting organism. Viridans streptococci were next most common. The rest were produced by other gram-positive organisms or gram-negative bacilli. The fatality rate was significantly higher in younger children. Older ones had a better outcome, as did those (any age) with viridans streptococcal infection. The results of this study indicated that pediatric endocarditis occurs primarily in children with congenital heart disease. The mortality is high, despite antibiotic therapy. The findings of persistent unexplained fever and bacteremia in a child with congenital heart disease should suggest the presence of endocarditis.

PROSTHETIC VALVE ENDOCARDITIS

The clinical features of infection of prosthetic valves are, for the most part, the same as those that characterize endocarditis involving natural valves. Infection of the surgical wound in the sternum, or sternal osteomyelitis, is a common predisposing factor. Variations in the period of time elapsing between operation and the onset of prosthetic infection were discussed earlier (p. 1146). The development of fever associated with or following detection of a new murmur suggestive of a paravalvular leak suggests the presence of endocarditis.

Several complications are peculiar to prosthetic valvular endocarditis. One is associated primarily with the presence of a ball-type prosthesis, especially the Starr-Edwards valve (Fig. 33–3), and consists of the gradual development of congestive heart failure due to progressive obstruction of the outlet of the valve by growth of bacteria or, more commonly, yeasts or fungi. Another complication of endocarditis of prosthetic valves, shared by patients addicted to intravenously administered drugs, is an increased incidence of embolization of large arteries due to the greater frequency of fungal colonization and infection. Persistent elevation of temperature in patients with valvular prostheses, in the absence of either a change in an existing murmur or the development of a new one, together with sterile cultures of blood, is highly suggestive of an abscess in the annulus, frequently at the site of one or more of the sutures anchoring the prosthesis. Rarely, diffuse invasion of the annulus may lead to almost complete tearing away of the prosthesis. Synthetic materials used to close septal defects may also become infected. The clinical features of endocarditis associated with this last condition are not specific, and the complications that develop do not specifically suggest infection of the synthetic materials.

ENDOCARDITIS DURING PREGNANCY AND THE PUERPERIUM

Libman and Friedberg pointed out that bacterial endocarditis may occur during pregnancy or shortly after childbirth.[171] They suggested that, in the presence of pelvic inflammatory disease, a transient bacteremia occurring during labor and delivery might be followed by subacute endocarditis in women with underlying cardiac disease. If the uterus becomes infected during the puerperium (puerperal sepsis), especially when the infection is exogenous in origin, the endocarditis may be of the acute type, because of the high frequency with which *Strep. pyogenes* is the responsible organism. When endocarditis develops as a complication of endogenous puerperal sepsis, it is likely to be subacute and caused by relatively noninvasive organisms such as *Strep. viridans.* Although there is currently no evidence that the fetus is infected during the course of endocarditis occurring during pregnancy, it is entirely possible that this may occur if the infective organism is highly pathogenic. When the disease is caused by *Staph. aureus, Strep. pyogenes, Strep. pneumoniae, N. gonorrhoeae,* or *H. influenzae,* especially if bacteremia is present, fetal infection may develop and lead to the death of the baby or spontaneous abortion.

RELAPSE AND RECURRENCE OF INFECTIVE ENDOCARDITIS

Early or intercurrent relapses are defined as the development of manifestations of infection together with positive blood cultures that appear during or shortly after (<3 months) completion of treatment with antimicrobial agents. Among the factors responsible are (a) superinfection (by an organism different from the one initially present) often associated with the use of "broad-spectrum" antibiotics; (b) spread, via the circulation, of a drug-resistant bacterium or fungus from an extracardiac site such as a colonized intravenous catheter, suppurative thrombophlebitis, or infection of the urinary tract; (c) the development of resistance of the organism initially responsible for the disease; and (d) the appearance of "cell wall–deficient" organisms ("persisters"), especially when drugs that inhibit the synthesis of the bacterial cell wall (penicillins, cephalosporins) are administered. This last factor has been suggested, but its importance in intercurrent relapses remains to be proved.

A syndrome that appears to be an early relapse but is actually due to an intra- or extracardiac complication occurs occasionally in patients with endocarditis caused by *Staph. aureus.* As pointed out above (p. 1155), the development of abscesses in one or more other organs is usually accompanied by a return of fever and bacteremia after a period of what appears to be a satisfactory therapeutic response; however, this is not due to relapse of infection in the affected valve.

Late relapse is defined as return of all the features of active endocarditis three to six months after antimicrobial treatment has led to apparent "cure" of the infection. The causative agent of the relapse may be different from the one initially responsible for the valvular disease. In some instances, however, it is identical to the one originally recovered from the blood. Late relapse is relatively common in patients with endocarditis caused by yeasts or fungi. The reasons for this are (a) relative insensitivity of the organism to the drug used for treatment, (b) failure of the antifungal agent to penetrate the valvular lesion to a depth great enough to eradicate all the organisms, and (c) spread of the infection to sites in the heart contiguous to the affected valve. Late relapses are also quite common when endocarditis involves prosthetic valves, and the causative agent is often the one initially involved. However, in some instances, the initial bacterial infection may be followed, either during treatment or within six months by invasion of the prosthesis by a fungus or yeast, especially when combined "broad-spectrum" antimicrobial therapy is given.

Recurrent Endocarditis. This is defined as the reappearance of all the cardinal manifestations of infective endocarditis and positive blood cultures later than six months after cure of the initial episode. It may be caused by the same organism that produced the first episode but is often due to a different bacterium or fungus. A mechanism that may be responsible for recurrent endocarditis has been suggested by Cordeiro and Pimental.[235] They noted that bacteria frequently persist in healed valvular lesions for longer than 10 months after a clinical "cure" had been accomplished by means of appropriate chemotherapy and compared this situation with "inactive" tuberculosis. The incidence of recurrent endocarditis has been reported to range from 2 to 4 per cent;[19] however, higher frequencies have been recorded when the period of follow-up study has been long. Morgan and Bland noted second episodes in 8.5 per cent of their patients.[20] Patients with prosthetic valves may experience recurrent infections over a period of months or years. This writer has studied one patient who experienced a mixture of five relapses and recurrences. The first involved a natural valve; the others were infections of various types of valvular prostheses, each of which was removed. A different organism was responsible for each of the episodes.

Recurrent endocarditis was noted by Welton and his associates in 18 of 58 patients (31 per cent). In addition to drug abuse, prior heart disease and periodontitis were each related to recurrence. Patients with two or more of these three risk factors were more likely to have a recurrence than those with only one risk factor, and the fatality rate was higher with recurrences than with initial episodes of endocarditis.[235]

LABORATORY FINDINGS

Elevation of erythrocyte sedimentation rate is the most common and almost universal abnormal laboratory finding in infective endocarditis.[14] *Anemia* is present in from 50 to 80 per cent of patients with this disease when they first come to medical attention. In those with subacute infection, the loss of hemoglobin is gradual and may reach strikingly low levels when the process is prolonged. In the acute form, the anemia may progress with striking rapidity and become pronounced within one to two weeks after onset. In both instances, the characteristics of the anemia are those observed in all types of infection. In rare instances, an acute hemolytic process may develop in both acute and subacute endocarditis.

In subacute infective endocarditis the *white blood count,* in most instances, does not exceed 7,000 to 8,000/mm^3. However, in almost all cases, there is a shift to the left, and a varying percentage of immature forms is the rule. In contrast, leukocytosis, with white blood counts ranging from 15,000 to 20,000/mm^3 or higher, is usual when the acute disease is present; there is usually a shift to the left. It must be stressed, however, that a normal white blood count and even leukopenia may be present in the acute infection.

Hyperstimulation of the reticuloendothelial system, as evidenced by an *increase in the number of plasma cells in the bone marrow,* is common in subacute endocarditis. In rare cases, the number of these cells in the marrow is so great that a diagnosis of multiple myeloma or disseminated tuberculosis is suspected. Large lymphocytic cells—histiocytes—are detectable in the capillary blood in 15 to 25 per cent of the subacute cases. These are usually not present in the peripheral blood but are demonstrable in blood obtained from the tip of a finger or the lobe of the ear.

Although *thrombocytopenia* due to disseminated intravascular coagulation occurs as a rare complication of acute bacterial endocarditis, this may appear as an infrequent, isolated finding in both the subacute and acute types of valvular infection. The presence of some types of immunological abnormalities in both acute and subacute endocarditis is an important finding that may be helpful in diagnosis (p. 1149).

The *urine* is normal in uncomplicated cases of infective endocarditis. In some instances, *proteinuria* may be the only abnormality and is often related to the presence of fever. Red blood cells in the urine usually indicate renal infarction. *Hematuria, red blood cell casts,* and *proteinuria* suggest acute proliferative glomerulonephritis.

Unless patients have problems with water loss through sweating or vomiting or develop glomerulonephritis, renal infarcts, or interstitial nephritis, BUN, creatinine, and serum electrolyte levels are normal. In the early stages of bacteremia and endocarditis due to gram-negative organisms, alkalosis may develop; this appears to be due to hyperventilation induced, in an unknown manner, by stimulation of the respiratory center and loss of CO_2.

DIAGNOSIS

CLINICAL FEATURES. The characteristic features, especially of the subacute form of infective endocarditis, have undergone such remarkable changes over the past 30 years that if present-day physicians relied on the clinical diagnostic criteria established in the years preceding 1950, the disease would not be suspected in 90 per cent or more of the cases.[14,22,82,174] Thus, as already pointed out, Osler nodes, Janeway lesions, and Roth spots have become quite uncommon. Even subungual hemorrhages and petechiae are seen only occasionally.

The most striking feature of "modern" infective endocarditis is the increasing frequency with which *cardiac murmurs are absent* in both acute and subacute forms of the disease. Fifty years ago, the absence of a murmur was considered to rule out subacute endocarditis. It has now become apparent that an increasing number of patients with this type of infection have no detectable murmur when first seen; the diagnosis is usually suspected on the basis of multiple positive blood cultures, in the absence of any other source of infection and, quite often, the development of an embolic complication. In most of these individuals, a murmur develops during the course of treatment; in a few, it does not become detectable until two to three months after cure is accomplished and is not related to recurrence of the infection; in a rare instance, a murmur may never develop. The increased number of patients who do not have murmurs when they first come to medical attention is due, in part, to the higher frequency of acute endocarditis involving the left side of the heart and acute or subacute infection of the tricuspid valve. These forms of endocarditis are characterized by absence of a murmur in about one third of cases early in the course of the disease. In most, a murmur usually appears at some time during or after treatment.

Most physicians are still under the impression that a change in the character of the murmur is common in infective endocarditis and that this is a diagnostic feature of the disease. This is rarely the case in subacute valvular infection. It is, however, fairly common in patients in whom the process is acute, especially when it is caused by *Staph. aureus.* The cause of the change is practically always destruction of the valve and its supporting structures. Very common in patients with staphylococcal endocarditis involving the aortic valve is the sudden appearance of a loud diastolic blowing murmur related to the development of aortic regurgitation. Less common, but also responsible for a change in murmur in the acute disease, is rupture of the chordae tendineae or papillary muscles or separation of a leaflet of the valve from the annulus. In patients with prosthetic valves, the appearance of a murmur or a change in one already present is often associated with a paravalvular leak that may or may not be induced by infection.

One of the most difficult diagnostic problems is presented by the older patient known to have had a grade 2 or 3 basal systolic murmur for years, who develops fever, whose blood culture may or may not be positive, and who presents with none of the peripheral manifestations of infective endocarditis. This type of murmur is usually caused by calcific, degenerative changes in the aortic valve or may be due only to the widening and tortuosity of the aorta associated with aging. Often the diagnosis of valvular infection is not considered seriously in such individuals, especially when blood cultures are negative. A similar problem is encountered with younger patients in whom a grade 2 "ejection" or "flow" murmur is considered "innocent," whereas, in fact, it represents a valvular abnormality on which either acute or subacute infection may become superimposed.

The availability of effective antimicrobial agents has resulted in an important diagnostic problem, which, if not appreciated, may lead to potentially life-threatening complications of subacute infective endocarditis. Typically, the patient seeks medical attention because of fever. Despite detection of a murmur, blood cultures are not carried out, but oral therapy with an antibiotic is initiated. In the individual with valvular infection caused by an organism susceptible to the drug administered, defervescence often occurs within 4 to 5 days. However, when the fever is a manifestation of endocarditis, it usually returns in about 7 to 10 days after treatment has been discontinued. This usually leads to another visit to the physician, who often makes a diagnosis of "viral infection" and reinstitutes treatment with the antibiotic that had previously reduced the elevated temperature. Such short periods of exposure to one or more antimicrobial agents may be repeated several times before it becomes apparent that the patient is becoming increasingly ill, or until an embolic episode, heart failure, or some other complication develops, when the patient is finally hospitalized, blood samples are cultured, and the diagnosis is established. It must be emphasized that each recurrence of fever, because it represents the recrudescence of the valvular infection, adds to the valvular damage. This course of events in a patient with fever and cardiac murmur is so highly suggestive of infective endocarditis that a full course of antimicrobial therapy with bactericidal agents should be instituted even when multiple blood cultures prove to be sterile.

BLOOD CULTURES. The sine qua non for the diagnosis of infective endocarditis is recovery of the causative organism from the blood.

Whether or not bacteria or other infectious agents are grown depends on a number of factors, some of which are technical and some of which involve specific clinical and immunological phenomena.[236] It is now clear that the bacteremia of endocarditis is qualitatively continuous but quantitatively discontinous, i.e., organisms are probably always present but their numbers vary considerably. This is illustrated by the study of Beeson et al.,[239] who showed that only about 3 per cent of blood cultures of patients with subacute valvular infections contained more than 100 organisms/ml. Only 2 of 19 blood cultures were found to be positive by Mallen et al.[238] The incidence of positive blood cultures, as recorded by various observers, has varied considerably. Werner and his colleagues obtained positive cultures in 95 per cent of 789 cultures in 206 patients.[239] The first culture of the blood of individuals with streptococcal endocarditis was positive in 95 per cent of the cases; one of the first two cultures yielded the causative agent in 98 per cent. When infection was caused by organisms other than streptococcus, positive cultures were obtained in only 82 per cent. The bacteremia was commonly of "low magnitude"; only 17 per cent of the blood samples contained more than 100 organisms/ml. Others have reported an incidence of positive blood cultures ranging from 53 to 74 per cent.[240,241] Belli and Waisbren noted that the organism responsible for the valvular infection could be isolated from one of the three initial blood cultures in only 82 per cent of their patients.[241] Differences in the colony counts in blood collected from different arterial and venous sites were noted by Beeson and his coworkers.[237] In general, mixed venous blood entering the heart contained about 35 per cent fewer colonies than did arterial blood. Despite this, a number of other observers have noted no advantage in culture of arterial over venous blood in establishing the presence of clinically significant bacteremia in cases of infective endocarditis.

A unique approach in determining the site of infection in patients with valvular infection caused by *Pseudomonas* has been recorded by Pazan and his colleagues,[242] who catheterized the left brachial artery, right atrium, right pulmonary artery, right ventricle, superior vena caval–right atrial junction, pulmonary artery, and ascending aorta; blood obtained from each of these sites was cultured quantitatively. The largest number of organisms was recovered during "pull-back" from the pulmonary artery. There was no consistent "step-up" over the mitral valve. There was a "step-up" in the number of bacteria between the superior and inferior vena cava and the right atrium. This suggested infection and regurgitation of the tricuspid valve, which was confirmed by dye dilution curves, phonocardiography, and angiography.

In a rare instance, culture of bone marrow may identify the organism responsible for endocarditis when the blood is sterile. It must be emphasized, however, that a single positive culture is not diagnostic; instead, a minimum of three, all of which yield the same agent, is required before a causal relation between the recovered bacterium and the disease can be considered suggestive. This is also true for positive cultures of the urine in the absence of bacteremia; in the uncommon case in which this occurs, there are usually no sedimentary abnormalities indicating infection of the urinary tract.

In patients with fungal endocarditis, especially when the causative agent is *Aspergillus* blood cultures are frequently negative. However, the fungus responsible for the valvular infection may often be recovered from an embolus that lodges in a large artery—a relatively frequent occurrence in this type of disease.

Cultures of the blood of patients with infective endocarditis have been reported to be sterile in from 2.5 to 65 per cent.[243] A number of factors are responsible for this. Some are technical in nature, while others involve the type of disease, the kind of patient affected, the characteristics of the organism responsible for the infection, and the use of antimicrobial agents.

Renal insufficiency has been common in persons with negative cultures of blood. These cases are identical to the "bacteria-free stage" of the disease described by Libman in which organisms, although absent from the blood, are still present on the infected valves.[21] Lerner and Weinstein confirmed the relation between renal failure and negative blood cultures.[14] However, later studies have indicated that the important factor involved in the sterility of the blood is the duration of untreated disease and that specific bactericidal antibody is responsible for the absence of organisms. Although bacteria are still present in the vegetations, they are rapidly eradicated by this antibody when they enter the circulation.

An analysis of 1500 cases of infective endocarditis by Cannady and Sandford showed that cultures of the blood were sterile in from 2.5 to 31 per cent.[243] They pointed out that among the factors involved in this were mural endocarditis, bacteria with special growth requirements, and nonbacterial organisms such as *Coxiella burnetii* and *Chlamydia*.

Negative Cultures. One of the increasingly important reasons for the greater frequency of negative blood cultures in patients with infective endocarditis is treatment with one or more antimicrobial agents before the diagnosis is established.[244–246] As short a period of exposure to an antibiotic as two days may make it impossible to retrieve organisms from the blood, despite the fact that they are still present on the vegetations. It is difficult to indicate how long a period is required after therapy has been discontinued before blood cultures will again become positive. This does not depend entirely on the time required for the antimicrobial agent to be excreted for three reasons: (1) animal studies in which fibrin clots were used as models of the basic lesion of endocarditis—the sterile platelet-fibrin thrombus—have shown that all antimicrobial agents persist in a mass of fibrin for as long as 12 or more hours after they are no longer detectable in the blood[247,248]; (2) some antibiotics persist in the circulation for fairly long periods; and (3) exposure to an antibacterial drug may completely eradicate the organisms lying on the surface of the platelet-fibrin thrombus but may fail to kill all those buried in the fibrin mass, which, when therapy is discontinued, require a varying time to resume multiplication until they reach the surface of the lesion, from which they are shed into the bloodstream. The longer the exposure to drug, the greater the time required for this to occur.

It is impossible to state categorically, in any patient, how long it would take for blood rendered sterile by an antimicrobial agent to yield organisms after cessation of treatment. In some instances, especially when the period of treatment has been only two to three days, cultures may become positive 48 hours after the drug has been withdrawn. In contrast, when an antiinfective compound has been administered for longer periods, cultures may not become positive until a week or more after its use has been discontinued. Because of this, patients who are suspected on clinical grounds of having infective endocarditis and who have been treated must no longer receive the drug. Culturing of the blood should be initiated 24 to 48 hours after therapy has been withdrawn. If results are negative, cultures should be repeated until 7 to 10 days have elapsed. If the blood is still sterile at that time, a factor other than the antimicrobial therapy, the presence of an unusual organism, or a diagnosis other than infective endocarditis should be considered. When subacute bacterial endocarditis is present, there is no real danger in delaying therapy for as long as a week, since (1) if, as in the bulk of instances, fever is absent, the patient has already been partially treated, and (2) early death is not related to the infectious process but rather to a potentially lethal embolic episode—an unpredictable event that is not prevented by the most effective antimicrobial therapy. This is not true in most cases of acute endocarditis, in which a delay of 24 to 48 hours in initiating treatment may be seriously life-threatening.

In a number of cases, technical factors, including the use of inadequate quantities of blood or medium, improper timing of the culture, too small a number of specimens, and inappropriate incubation, are responsible for failure to recover the causative agent from patients with infective endocarditis. Because the number of organisms in the blood is small and variable, the optimal quantity drawn should be no less than 10 ml, in order to furnish an inoculum adequate to initiate bacterial growth. Many patients, especially those who have had the subacute form of the disease, have low to moderate concentrations of antibody or have received treatment with minimal doses of an orally administered antibiotic; therefore, the quantity of medium into which a single specimen of blood is innoculated should be 100 ml. The optimal ratio of blood to medium is about 1:10. This may dilute the quantity of circulating antibody or antibiotic sufficiently to inhibit antibacterial activity. Clearly the quantity of blood drawn cannot always be 10 ml, particularly since several cultures are required to establish the diagnosis; this presents the greatest problem in young children. In this case, the ratio of blood to medium should still be at least 1:10. It must be stressed, however, that the quantity of blood obtained should be maximum for a given clinical situation.

Techniques. There has been considerable discussion concerning the optimal time for drawing blood and the number of cultures required to establish the presence of endocarditis. A single positive culture is of no diagnostic value because, regardless of the nature of the organism recovered, it may represent contamination. The minimal number of cultures of the blood required to establish the presence of infective endocarditis has been reported by Belli and Waisbren to be five.[241] Probably the best time for obtaining a blood culture is two hours before the temperature begins to rise. This is based on the well-established observation that this is the period required for bacterial endotoxin to stimulate the production of endogenous pyrogen by neutrophilic leukocytes and macrophages. However, this is not always practical. The writer uses the following approach to timing and number of blood cultures: Temperature is monitored, from a normal level, every hour until about 1°F of fever is present. At this point, a specimen of blood is drawn every 5 to 10 minutes until six samples have been obtained. In most instances, three or more of these will be positive; a similar approach the following day usually yields the same results. If the first six cultures are all negative, all succeeding sets of the same number are usually also sterile.

All blood obtained must be cultured aerobically and anaerobically. Because about 10 per cent of cases of infective endocarditis are caused by microaerophilic streptococci and a small number are caused by strict anaerobes such as *Peptostreptococcus, Peptococcus*, or *Bacteroides*, it is imperative that the blood be incubated anaerobically. Some organisms, e.g., *N. gonorrhoeae, N. meningitidis*, and *Brucella abortus*, grow best in an atmosphere of 5 to 10 per cent CO_2. The presence of *H. influenzae* in the blood will be overlooked unless Levinthal liquid medium or chocolate agar is used for culture. If cell wall–deficient organisms are suspected, culture of the blood in an osmotically stable medium is required; on repeated subculture, these bacteria may revert to the parent cell wall–containing form. A series of negative blood cultures in patients with a clinical picture highly suggestive of infective endocarditis should suggest the possibility that nutritionally variant strains of streptococci may be involved. These organisms grow in the initial culture of blood in liquid media. Although their presence in the broth can be demonstrated on Gram stain, they fail to multiply when subcultured on solid media, unless this is supplemented with thiol compounds (cysteine or thioglycollate broth). These are also known as "satelliting" streptococci because, if a streak of *Staph. aureus* is placed on the agar, the organisms grow in close proximity to the area in which the staphylococcus grows. Another type of streptococcus responsible for an occasional instance of subacute valvular infection requires pyridoxine for growth. The optimal solution to the problem of negative blood cultures in cases in which nutritionally fastidious and all other streptococci as well as most of the other bacteria may be involved is the use of a medium containing cysteine and pyridoxine. It should be emphasized that *Pseudomonas* will not grow in unvented bottles. Special media or tissue cultures are required to identify *Coxiella burnetii* and *Chlamydia*, rare causes of endocarditis. The use of a medium containing broth and soft agar (Castaneda principle) increases the yield of fungi.

Inappropriate periods of incubation may be responsible for "negative" blood cultures when some organisms are involved. Although most bacteria grow in cultures of blood within a few days to a week, some require a considerably longer period. Cultures for *Brucella* may not become positive until after four to six weeks of incubation. Growth of many common organisms may be delayed for a week or longer in cases in which antibiotics have been administered. Most of the fungi involved in endocarditis grow slowly and may multiply more rapidly when incubated at room temperature than at 37°C. *Aspergillus* frequently cannot be recovered from cultures until they have been incubated for as long as 20 days. In most cases, these organisms cannot be recovered from the blood, no matter how long the period of incubation.

Serological Tests. A positive serological test may be of value in establishing the diagnosis of infective endocarditis. Examples of this are *Coxiella burnetii, Chlamydia, Brucella, Cryptococcus*, and *Candida*.

The importance of serological tests for teichoic acid in establishing the diagnosis of valvular infection caused by *Staph. aureus* has been demonstrated.[249]

Concomitant elevation of IgG and IgM antibody levels has been demonstrated by Wheat et al.[250] in 50 per cent of patients with endocarditis or complicated bacteremia. These antibodies were detected in only about 5 per cent of cases of other types of staphylococcal infections, and in about 3 per cent of normal persons. Studies of antibody to bacterial peptidoglycan in the serum of patients with endocarditis or bacteremia due to *Staph. aureus* have been carried out by Zeiger et al.[251] Patients treated with beta-lactam antibiotics had higher antigen-binding levels than healthy individuals or those receiving exclusively vancomycin. Serological studies in patients with candidal endocarditis have indicated that persisting or rising levels of precipitating or agglutinating antibodies, or both, whether or not associated with candidemia, signal invasion of prosthetic valves by the organism.[252] Although humoral antibodies to *Candida* increase after operations on the heart in some patients, even in the absence of clinical evidence of endocarditis, serial immunological studies are of value in patients with clinical manifestations of valvular infection by *Candida*, especially in patients whose blood cultures fail to grow the yeast.[253] Scheld et al.,[254] using an experimental model of candidal endocarditis in rabbits, found the enzyme-linked immunoabsorbent assay (ELISA) was much more sensitive than culturing of blood or determination of fever. This assay is more highly specific and more sensitive than the currently available techniques for demonstrating antibodies for *Candida*.

SCINTILLATION SCANNING. Scanning of the heart with gallium-67 appears to be of diagnostic value in some instances of bacterial endocarditis. Scintillation scanning of the precordial region 2 to 7 days after the intravenous administration of 3 mc of the radionuclide has been reported to yield positive results in seven individuals, three of which were confirmed by postmortem imaging at autopsy.[255] The scans were negative at 48 hours and positive from 3 to 8 days following injection. Fifteen patients without endocarditis, who served as controls, showed no uptake of the isotope in the region of the myocardium 48 hours or more after it was injected. A ventricular abscess in a patient was first suspected on the basis of a positive gallium-67 scan[256]; the disadvantages of this approach to the diagnosis of infective endocarditis are an insufficient degree of resolution to indicate the site of infection, the length of time (48 hours) required for localization of the radionuclide, and a 40 per cent incidence of false-negative results.[257]

ELECTROCARDIOGRAPHY. Changes in the electrocardiogram are not diagnostic in uncomplicated infective endocarditis. However, as pointed out earlier (p. 1153), this approach is helpful in that incomplete or complete heart block, bundle branch block, and premature ventricular contractions are associated with septal abscesses or myocarditis. The anatomical relation of the noncoronary cusp of the aortic valve and the mitral annulus to the conduction apparatus has been considered responsible for the development of abnormalities of conduction and is of some value in localizing the site of the lesion. Miller and Casey have expressed the importance of obtaining serial electrocardiograms in patients with the diagnosis of infective endocarditis: "Electrocardiographic evidence of an infarction or heart block is associated with a poor prognosis. New conduction defects indicate abscess or aneurysm formation and may suggest the need for surgical intervention."[257]

RADIOGRAPHY. Radiological findings in patients with endocarditis involving the left side of the heart are usually not impressive until destruction of the affected valve is so far advanced that congestive failure develops.[258] There are no diagnostic radiographic abnormalities in cases in which the right side of the heart is involved until pulmonary infarction, with or without infection, develops.

Echocardiography (See also page 116)

Echocardiography provides another approach to the diagnosis of infective endocarditis and some of its intracardiac complications. An increasing number of studies have pointed out the limits of this diagnostic technique, as well as the features that permit recognition of the specific valve involved and the characteristics of specific complications.[259]

The value of echocardiography in staphylococcal infection of the aortic valve has been reported by Fox and his colleagues.[260] "Shaggy" echoes were recorded from the aortic leaflets in diastole as well as irregular diastolic densities in the left ventricular outflow tract, suggesting that the infection caused flailing of the aortic leaflets. Echocardiographic detection of flail aortic leaflets and premature closure of the mitral valve indicated the need for immediate replacement of the aortic valve.

Of 14 patients with endocarditis involving the aortic valve studied by Berger et al.,[261] 12 had vegetations demonstrated by two-dimensional echocardiography; in the others, the presence of the disease was identified anatomically. This technique was found to be superior to the M-mode in determining the size, shape, and movement of the vegetations. The echocardiographic (two-dimensional) characteristics of aortic valvular endocarditis were noted to include (a) globular, polypoid masses, (b) elongated lesions with chaotic movement, and (c) a cord-like structure. Serial echocardiography carried out after completion of antimicrobial therapy in seven patients disclosed no change in the vegetations in five and complete disappearance in two. The authors made the following important statement: "In those patients with negative two-dimensional echocardiograms, the vegetations were 3 mm in diameter or less at surgery or autopsy. Vegetations that were visualized on two-dimensional echocardiography were found to be at least 5 mm in diameter at the time of operation." Two echocardiographic features characteristic of aortic valvular endocarditis are (a) thick, uneven cusp echoes that may be present only in systole or diastole or, less commonly, in both, and (b) normal systolic excursion of all cusps, regardless of their involvement in the disease.

Echocardiography has also been found to be of value in identification of abscesses of various valvular ring abscesses. Using both M-mode and two-dimensional techniques in a patient with a suspected mitral ring abscess, Nakamura et al.[262] observed a round, dense, echo mass between the posterior mitral leaflet and the posterior wall of the left ventricle. The diagnosis was confirmed at surgery. They pointed out that the two-dimensional procedure was superior to the M-mode. The diagnosis of an aortic root abscess, the presence of which was not suspected clinically, was established only by two-dimensional echocardiography by Wong and his colleagues.[263] They noted an abscess cavity and a vegetation posterior and lateral to the root that deformed the left atrial cavity. The lesion was confirmed by cardiac catheterization and at surgery.

Scanlan et al.[264] expressed the same opinion and emphasized that wide-angle two-dimensional echocardiography was the only noninvasive technique of value in direct visualization of ring abscesses complicating infection of the aortic valve. The presence of the abscesses was identified by the demonstration of an echo-free cavity in the tissues around the valve. The lesions extended into the perivalvular space, the left ventricular myocardium, and the myocardium or contiguous fibrous structures.

An extensive study by Andy and his colleagues of the efficacy of echocardiography in the detection of infective endocarditis and its complications, especially in relation to involvement of specific valves, indicated that vegetations on the tricuspid valve, as visualized by echocardiography, were always larger than those on the mitral valve.[265] No patients with tricuspid regurgitation demonstrated torn cusps. Wide-angle two-dimensional echocardiograms were found by Berger and his colleagues[266] to be superior to the M-mode technique in identifying endocarditis involving the tricuspid and pulmonic valves. The use of multiple transducer positions led to better visualization of the valves. Studies carried out after the completion of antimicrobial therapy in seven patients showed that the vegetations were unchanged in three, decreased in mass in the same number, and had disappeared in one.

Two-dimensional echocardiography has also been noted to be useful in establishing the diagnosis of isolated pulmonic valve endocarditis[267] and in demonstrating infection in cases of intraventricular septal defect.

Since size is critical to detection of the valvular vegetations in patients with infective endocarditis, echocardiography might be expected to give positive results more often when infections are caused by fungi because of the characteristically large valvular lesions. The features of aortic valvular disease caused by *Candida parapsilosis* have been described by Gomes and his associates[268] and include clusters of abnormal echoes visible intermittently in the aortic root; thickening of the valve leaflets, with abnormal "shaggy" echoes in both systole and diastole; and normal excursion of the leaflets except when damage is extensive.

Eighty-seven patients with clinical evidence of infective endocarditis studied by Stewart et al.[269] were divided into two groups on the basis of positive and negative echocardiography (M-mode and two-dimensional). The individuals in whom one or more vegetations were demonstrated by the noninvasive technique were found to be at a higher risk of developing complications (emboli, congestive cardiac failure, and need for surgery) than those in whom echocardiography demonstrated no vegetations. The authors stressed the important point that "although the detection of vegetations by echocardiography in patients with clinical syndrome of endocarditis clearly identifies a subgroup at risk of complications, decisions regarding clinical management made solely on the basis of the presence or absence of vegetative lesions are hazardous. Management of such patients must continue to be based on the clinical integration of multiple factors."

The effectiveness of M-mode and two-dimensional echocardiography in detecting masses in patients suspected, on clinical grounds, of having endocarditis was studied by Martin et al.[270] No individual without evidence of valvular infection had any echocardiographic abnormalities. Of 36 confirmed cases of endocarditis studied by the M-mode technique, 5 (14 per cent) had a demonstrable mass; in 12 there was a nonspecific abnormality, and in 19 no mass was detected. When two-dimensional echocardiography was used, the frequency with which a mass was found increased to 81 per cent; this technique was found to be more useful in cases in which a mass was present on a prosthetic mitral or aortic valve.

Hickey and his colleagues[271] have reported that "M-mode echocardiography can reliably detect vegetations in patients with bacterial endocarditis even in the presence of pre-existing valvular lesions, and may permit the identification of a subset of high risk patients who may need early surgery." Those in whom vegetations were not detected echocardiographically appeared to be less likely to develop serious complications than those in whom valvular deposits were demonstrable. In contrast, Markiewicz et al.[272] suggested that caution must be exercised in the interpretation of findings of "vegetations" by echocardiography in cases in which preexisting valvular disease is present.

An interesting study of the value of echocardiography in the diagnosis of endocarditis in 11 patients with negative blood cultures in whom the presence of the disease was established during cardiac surgery was carried out by Rubenson et al.[273] Both natural (5 cases) and prosthetic valves (6 cases) were involved. Valvular masses were identified by echocardiography in 8 cases. The other three had prosthetic aortic valves that showed the diastolic mitral valve vibration characteristic of aortic regurgitation. In 3 instances, the illness was poorly defined clinically. The authors emphasize the point that, in these individuals, echocardiography was a prime factor in identifying the presence of endocarditis.

Dillon et al.[274] have suggested that initial and serial echocardiographic studies carried out over the course of treatment not only play an important role in diagnosis but are also of value in evaluation of the size of vegetations and the state of valvular function while antimicrobial therapy is being administered. Strom et al.[275] have reported the results of an interesting study of the correlation between the findings demonstrated by echocardiography and those identified at the time of cardiac surgery. Only 84 per cent of 32 valves thought to be involved when examined echocardiographically before operation were found to carry vegetations at the time of surgery. The presence of a myocardial abscess, suspected in five patients on the basis of the findings present during the noninvasive studies, was proved in only one during cardiac surgery.

As discussed above, one of the important points to remember about the use of echocardiography in the diagnosis of infective endocarditis is related to the size of the vegetations on the affected valve. Clearly the larger the lesions, the more likely their presence is to be detected by echocardiography. Thus, this technique produces positive results in fungal valvular infections most often because, as a rule, the vegetations are large. The technique is of less value, but still useful, in acute endocarditis caused by *Staph. aureus*, in which endocardial lesions are often of moderate size. The primary difficulty of echocardiographic diagnosis arises in patients with the subacute form of the disease, because of the very small size of the vegetations associated with infection by viridans streptococci and other relatively avirulent organisms.

In addition to the demonstration of vegetative lesions, echocardiography is of great value in determining hemodynamic abnormalities related to the complications associated with valvular infections (Chap. 5).

MANAGEMENT OF INFECTIVE ENDOCARDITIS

Prior to the antibiotic era, attempts to treat infective endocarditis were relatively unsuccessful. For the most part, physicians were limited to observation and study of the "natural history" of this almost invariably fatal disease. The development of highly potent antimicrobial agents followed by refinements of and advances in the techniques of cardiac surgery have so altered this heretofore "hopeless" situation that today young physicians are often perplexed when defervescence fails to occur within 24 to 48 hours after initiation of treatment, and older physicians are upset by a fatal outcome when, not long ago, they were amazed if their patients recovered.

Antimicrobial Therapy

Although penicillin—the first antibiotic effective in the management of infective endocarditis—still remains the agent of choice in the majority of cases, the increasing involvement of uncommon bacterial species and fungi in the pathogenesis of the disease has posed difficult and, at times, insurmountable therapeutic problems and underscores the need for careful application of sensitive microbiological techniques not only to isolate all organisms involved but also to identify them and evaluate their susceptibility to a wide range of antimicrobial agents.

Selection of Drugs. The choice of specific antimicrobial therapy for infective endocarditis depends strictly on the nature of the organism recovered from the blood and its susceptibility to various drugs. Usually treatment need not be immediate in the subacute form of infection, since most of these patients have been ill for several weeks to as long as 3 or more months before the diagnosis is established. Therefore, a delay in instituting treatment of two or three days until definitive microbiological data become available is of little or no prognostic importance. If death occurs before therapy is begun in such cases, it is most often due, not to the infectious process, but rather to one of its sequelae, such as rupture of a mycotic aneurysm or embolic occlusion of a coronary artery—complications not prevented by chemotherapy.

In sharp contrast to this, it is imperative that there be no delay in treatment in acute bacterial endocarditis, especially when it involves a highly destructive organism such as *Staph. aureus*, because of the rapidity with which valve leaflets, papillary muscles, or chordae tendineae may rupture or myocardial and/or septal abscesses may develop. In the absence of bacteriological evidence, the etiology of acute endocarditis may, at times, be suspected on the basis of the circumstances in which it developed. For example, a staphylococcal skin infection in a patient with endocarditis should implicate this organism as the cause of the valvular infection. Examination of stained smears of petechial lesions or of the "buffy coat" of the peripheral blood may reveal the causative organism one or two days before results of blood cultures are available. Despite the urgent need for treatment in these cases, administration of antimicrobial agents should be withheld until sufficient blood cultures have been obtained, a procedure that usually involves a delay of no more than one hour. If the clinical features of the disease are mild, if the duration of manifestations has been short, or if there is no demonstrable primary extracardiac focus of infection, it may be safe to wait 24 hours, the time usually required to recover the causative organism. However, chemotherapy must be started before the results of sensitivity tests become available; if these tests indicate that a drug other than the one being given is preferable, the appropriate agent should be substituted.

Antibacterial Effectiveness. It is very important that, in addition to its antimicrobial activity, the agent selected pose minimal risk of untoward effects, be administered by a route acceptable to the patient, and present no problems with respect to the physiological, biochemical, and anatomical characteristics of the host.[276] In general, bactericidal drugs appear to be more effective than bacteriostatic ones not only in eradicating the valvular infection but also in reducing the risk of relapse after therapy has been completed.

To determine the effectiveness of chemotherapy, it is often helpful to measure the antibacterial activity of the patient's serum against the organism recovered from the blood. This is readily accomplished by adding a standard inoculum from an overnight culture of the organism to serial, twofold dilutions of serum obtained at various intervals after administration of a dose of antibiotics.[277] Inhibition of bacterial growth, both bacteriostatic and bactericidal, by dilutions of 1:8, 1:16, or higher usually indicates a potentially favorable therapeutic response.[278] Although this is standard practice in the treatment of infective endocarditis, its importance in evaluating the response to treatment has been questioned on the basis of experiments demonstrating that the quantity of antibiotic penetrating a fibrin clot and the duration of antibacterial activity depend on only two factors: the peak serum concentration and the degree of protein-binding of the drug.[243,248] Thus, it is clear that antibacterial effects usually persist at the site of infection for many hours after they are no longer demonstrable in the blood. In addition, it has been reported that in some instances, there may be no correlation between serum antibacterial activity and therapeutic outcome.[279]

Dosage Considerations. Despite the fact that antimicrobial agents have been used for more than 30 years in the treatment of infective endocarditis, no firm data are available concerning the proper daily dose of any of these drugs. Regimens vary greatly and depend on the experience of the physician. Thus, doses of penicillin ranging from as low as 4 to 6 million units to as high as 20 to 30 million units per day have been administered to patients with subacute disease when the responsible agent has been a highly susceptible strain of alpha-streptococcus or other organism. Unfortunately there is no proof that either of these extremes of dosage is necessary or ideal. For this reason, the doses of antibiotics recommended below for the management of valvular infections are necessarily based on published experiences and are perforce empirical.

In terms of generating the highest levels and longest duration of antimicrobial activity, Barza et al. have shown that the bolus injection of an antibiotic is more effective than is a constant intravenous infusion.[280] Although the question of what constitutes an optimal interval between doses in the management of infective endocarditis still remains unsettled, experimental data obtained from studies of the penetration and persistence of antimicrobial activity in fibrin, combined with 35 years of experience treating both acute and subacute infective endocarditis, have convinced this author that an interval of 6 hours between doses of a parenterally administered drug is effective in most adults; it is possible that this might be extended in older individuals, because of decreased renal tubular secretory function; however, in children, a shorter interval (3 to 4 hours) between doses may be required to maintain effective concentrations of drug in the infected platelet-fibrin thrombus, because of the high level of tubular secretory function that leads to rapid urinary excretion of penicillins and cephalosporins.

Duration of Therapy. The duration of therapy required to cure infective endocarditis is, for the most part, empirical and therefore often controversial. Although many physicians continue treatment for only 4 weeks, there is an increasing tendency to extend this to 6 weeks despite the lack of statistically significant evidence that this leads to a higher percentage of cures or reduces the incidence of relapse in most cases, especially when the organisms are highly susceptible to the antibiotic used. It remains to be proved whether 6 weeks of exposure to an antibiotic is required when the infection is caused by uncommon bacterial species, by strains less sensitive to antimicrobial agents, or by fungi. The observation that the risk of superinfection is directly related to the length of time over which an antibiotic is administered, especially when the drug used has a "broad spectrum" of activity,[281] suggests that there may actually be some danger in prolonging therapy beyond 4 weeks. Attempts have also been made to limit the duration of treatment to 2 weeks in patients with subacute bacterial endocarditis caused by such noninvasive organisms as *Strep. viridans*.[282] Although cure has been reported in some instances, this approach can not yet be recommended until considerably more data regarding rate of cure and risk of relapse become available.

Routes of Administration. Most physicians experienced in the treatment of subacute infective endocarditis recommend parenteral administration of antibiotics, usually by the intravenous route. However, in a number of cases, successful treatment of this disease with oral penicillin has been reported. The stimulus for this approach has been the desire to avoid the pain of intramuscular or intravenous injection and to eliminate such complications as thrombophlebitis and sterile or infected abscesses in muscle. Antimicrobial agents that have been administered orally include buffered penicillin G and phenoxymethylpenicillin (penicillin V).[282–285] In many instances, oral treatment with one of the penicillins has been combined with the intramuscular injection of streptomycin. Therapy with this regimen has also been continued for only 2 weeks in a number of cases.[282] While high rates of cure have been reported by several investigators,[282–285] relapses have occurred in a relatively small number of cases. This type of therapy must be restricted to patients with *subacute* bacterial endocarditis caused by organisms that are highly susceptible to the antibiotic used; it has no place and is extremely dangerous in treatment of the acute type of valvular infections. Although Burman et al.[286] have recently reported a cure of refractory staphylococcal endocarditis with rifampin and erythromycin, it must be pointed out that this approach is potentially dangerous and should not be used except in the most unusual circumstances.

A recent review by Phillips and Watson of oral therapy for infective endocarditis points out that "despite much discussion, no final conclusion has been reached about the optimum duration of oral treatment."[287] Short courses (2 weeks) have been reported to be effective, while some investigators have recommended therapy for as long as 6 or more weeks. Despite the reports of success with oral antibiotics, many physicians prefer to treat this disease parenterally. The following objections to oral administration have been raised.[288]

1. Large groups of patients treated with parenteral antibiotics have experienced no relapses, an important consideration, since each recrudescence of valvular infection not only adds an increment of permanent damage to an already functionally poor valve but also presents a risk of death.
2. Orally administered antibiotics may be irregularly absorbed, especially in patients who are quite ill; this necessitates constant monitoring of blood levels of the antibiotic, a technique not available in most "routine" diagnostic microbiological laboratories.
3. Patients may fail to take each dose of drug unless under the continuous watchful eye of the physician or nurse.
4. Gastrointestinal irritation leading to nausea, vomiting, and diarrhea is associated with the oral use of antibiotics in some persons.
5. The risk of superinfections, even rapidly fatal ones, is not eliminated when antibiotics are taken orally.

Although 4 weeks of intravenous or intramuscular injection of an antimicrobial agent causes discomfort in most individuals, vast clinical experience has indicated that, with proper attention and encouragement from the physician, almost all patients accept this form of treatment with minimal complaint.

Problems of Therapy. A fairly common therapeutic problem arises when the clinical picture is highly suggestive of subacute bacterial endocarditis but the blood cultures are repeatedly sterile. Because of the high fatality rate when the disease is not treated, therapy is usually based on experience and clinical judgment. Initially therapy should be directed at possible enterococcal infection, as discussed below (p.1169). Cannady and Sandford[243] have made the following suggestions regarding therapy of patients with suspected endocarditis when blood cultures have failed to yield an organism: If there is no satisfactory response after 2 weeks of empirical treatment, administration should be continued for an additional 14 days, during which cultures and serological tests may indicate the presence of infection caused by fungi, *Chlamydia, Rickettsia,* or *Brucella.* If all these studies are negative, treatment should be discontinued and the patient reevaluated. These investigators also point out that the most difficult problem involves the compromised host who has received many antibiotic regimens or the patient with a prosthetic heart valve. The latter may have fungal endocarditis and may well be a candidate for empirical therapy with amphotericin B, but surgical removal of the infected valve may be necessary to cure the disease.

It must be emphasized that these suggestions apply only to individuals with the *subacute* form of valvular infection. There is no place for delay in the management of the acute disease, which progresses rapidly and leads to potentially lethal intra- and extracardiac complications. Negative cultures of the blood are rarely, if ever, a problem in acute infections involving the left side of the heart. In endocarditis involving the right side of the heart, organisms may not be recovered from the peripheral circulation until pulmonary infarction and infection occur, after which cultures of the blood become positive. However, if embolization to the lungs does not occur and the blood remains sterile, therapy must be undertaken as soon as possible and should be directed against organisms known to be most often responsible for this kind of disease, especially coagulase-positive staphylococcus. When the enterococcus may be the causative agent, the use of a penicillinase-resistant penicillin plus an aminoglycoside is recommended; an optimal choice is nafcillin or oxacillin (12 gm/day, in divided doses) plus gentamicin or tobramycin (80 mg every 8 hours).

ANTICOAGULANTS

The use of anticoagulants in patients with infective endocarditis has been and remains controversial.[289] It is clear that anticoagulants are of no benefit in the management of valvular infections because these drugs do not prevent separation of small fragments from the valvular thrombus and the vegetations do not increase in size if antimicrobial therapy is effective. Anticoagulation may cause bleeding at the site of deposition of an embolus. It is this author's view that when a condition such as phlebothrombosis of the extremities or pelvis results in pulmonary embolism, with or without infarction, and requires anticoagulation with heparin or coumadin, the presence of infective endocarditis does not absolutely contraindicate the use of these drugs. When embolization from the infected valve occurs, the situation must be reevaluated relative to the risks of hemorrhage at the sites where emboli have been deposited and of a fatal pulmonary infarct; anticoagulation is very likely to be of no value in this situation. When the phlebothrombosis involves the extremities or pelvis, the issue can be resolved by surgical occlusion of the vena cava. That anticoagulation was of no danger in patients with subacute endocarditis was suggested by Loewe et al., who treated all their patients with heparin and penicillin.[7]

TREATMENT OF ENDOCARDITIS CAUSED BY SPECIFIC ORGANISMS (Table 33–3)

Gram-Positive Cocci

STREPTOCOCCI. Of the organisms responsible for subacute infective endocarditis, *Streptococcus viridans* is the commonest. Although the majority of these bacteria are highly sensitive to penicillin G, it must be emphasized that all strains in this group do not constitute a single species, and all are not susceptible to this antibiotic. Among these are enterococci as well as vitamin B_6 (pyridoxal hydrochloride)–dependent streptococci.

Treatment of streptococcal (viridans) endocarditis with a combination of penicillin and streptomycin or gentamicin has been recommended on the basis of in vitro synergy of the drugs.[290] However, this author's experience with over 900 cases given penicillin alone does not support this recommendation; all the patients survived, and none relapsed over the six months following discontinuation of treatment. Two recent reports have confirmed this experience.[291,292]

For patients sensitized to penicillin, several approaches are available: one involves desensitization to this drug—a

TABLE 33–3 CHEMOTHERAPY OF INFECTIVE ENDOCARDITIS

Symbols:

AMB = Amphotericin B
AMK = Amikacin
AMP = Ampicillin
CARB = Carbenicillin
CFM = Cefamandole
CFX = Cefoxitin
CL = Clindamycin
CM = Chloramphenicol
CP = Cephalothin
CY = Cycloserine
EM = Erythromycin
ETH = Ethambutol
FC = 5-Fluorocytosine
GM = Gentamicin
INH = Isoniazid
KN = Kanamycin
MNZ = Metronidazole
NF = Nafcillin
OX = Oxacillin
PCN = Penicillin G
RF = Rifampin
RST = Results of Sensivity Tests
SM = Streptomycin
SN/TMP = Sulfamethoxazole plus trimethoprim
TBM = Tobramycin
TC = Tetracycline
TIC = Ticarcillin
VC = Vancomycin
Third Generation Cephalosporins = They may eventually prove valuable in the therapy of infective endocarditis, but current experience with them is too limited to evaluate them effectively.

	Drug		
Organism	*1st Choice*	*2nd Choice*	*3rd Choice*
Alpha-streptococcus	PCN	CP	AMP
Strep. bovis	PCN	CP	AMP
Pyridoxine-dependent streptococci	PCN + GM or TBM	PCN + SM	—
Enterococcus	PCN + GM, TBM, or SM	AMP	VC
Other streptococci	RST	—	—
Strep. pneumoniae	PCN[1]	CP	EM
Peptostreptococcus	PCN[2]	RST	RST
Staph. aureus	PCN,[2,3] CP, OX	NF	EM
Methicillin-resistant *Staph. aureus*	VC	RST	—
Staph. epidermidis	RST	—	—
Micrococcus	RST	—	—
Aerobic diphtheroids	PCN[3]	PCN + GM	EM
Listeria monocytogenes	PCN	EM	CP
Lactobacillus acidophilus	PCN + SM	RST	—
Lactobacillus plantarum	PCN	CP	RST
Bacillus subtilis	RST	—	—
Bacillus cereus	EM	GM, TBM	TC, CL, or CM
Nocardia israelii	SM + SN/TMP	AMP + SN/TMP	TC + CY or SN/TMP
Escherichia coli	CP	AMP	GM or TBM
Klebsiella pneumoniae	CP	GM, TBM	CM + SM
Enterobacter species	RST	—	—
Proteus mirabilis	AMP	CP	PCN
Pseudomonas aeruginosa	TMB + CARB or TIC	GM + CARB or TIC	AMK
Pseudomonas cepacia	SN/TMP + KN	RST	—
Serratia marcescens	AMK	SN/TMP	RST
Vibrio fetus	CM	EM	RST
Hemophilus influenzae	AMP[3,4]	CFM	CM
Hemophilus parainfluenzae	AMP	CM	GM, CP, or CARB
Hemophilus aphrophilus	CM	GM	PCN, CP, or RF
Cardiobacterium hominis	PCN	RST	—
Brucella—all types	TC + SM	CM + SM	RF
Salmonella—all species	RST[5]	—	—
Pasteurella multicoda	PCN	TC	—
Acinetobacter	SN/TMP	KN or TBM	GM
Actinobacillus actinomycetemcomitans	AMP + GM	AMP + SM	RST
Flavobacterium	RF	CL	SN/TMP or VC
Streptobacillus moniliformis	PCN	EM	CP
Neisseria meningitidis	PCN	EM	CM
Neisseria gonorrhoeae	PCN[6]	CFX sh,14,15 EM	
Nonpathogenic *Neisseria*	RST	—	—
Bacteroides fragilis	CL + CARB or TIC	CARB or TIC	MNZ
Bacteroides melaninogenicus	PCN	CARB	RST
Propionibacterium acnes	EM	PCN[7]	RST
Mycobacterium tuberculosis	INH + ETH + SM[8]	ETH + RF + SM[8]	RST
Mycobacterium chelonei	INH + ETH + RF[9]	RST	—
Yeasts and Fungi	AMB + FC[10]	—	—
Chlamydia trachomatis or *psittaci*	TC	CM	—
Coxiella burnetii (Q fever)	TC	CM	—

[1] Rare strains of the pneumococcus are resistant to penicillin.
[2] May require as much as 40 to 80 million units of penicillin G per day.
[3] Only if organism is sensitive to penicillin.
[4] Increasing number of strains are resistant to ampicillin.
[5] Ampicillin and chloramphenicol are the most effective agents; some strains are resistant to one or both of these agents. Infection caused by *Salmonella typhi* has been shown to respond favorably to large doses of sulfamethoxazole/trimethoprim in some cases.
[6] Some strains are totally resistant to penicillin G.
[7] Many strains are resistant to penicillin G.
[8] One gm of streptomycin daily for one month followed by 1 gm every Monday and Thursday for two months, and then discontinued.
[9] The combination of isoniazid plus rifampin produces hepatoxicity more often then does either drug alone.
[10] Before 5-fluorocytosine is given, organism must be examined for sensivity to the drug.

simple and minimally dangerous procedure that is often not necessary because of the availability of other effective antimicrobial agents. An adequate substitute for penicillin G in these cases is intravenous cephalothin, 2 gm every 4 hours. (The risk of cross-reactivity between these agents has been less than 1 per cent in the experience of this author.) Another cephalosporin, cefazolin, has been reported by Quinn et al. to be effective in the treatment of staphylococcal endocarditis.[293] However, relapses have been noted when this antibiotic has been used.[294] Vancomycin (2 gm/day) has been reported to be effective in some instances of this type of endocarditis.[295] Most strains of *Strep. viridans* susceptible to penicillin are sensitive to erythromycin, 1 gm given intravenously every 6 hours. In endocarditis caused by alpha-streptococci, clindamycin is thought to be a "third-line" drug for use in patients who have previously had a serious reaction to both penicillins and cephalosporins,[296] because relapse has occurred after therapy was discontinued.

Since the first report that treatment of enterococcal endocarditis with penicillin plus streptomycin was more effective than the use of either agent alone,[297] a considerable body of information has accumulated concerning the mechanism by which these antibiotics act synergistically. Moellering and his colleagues have demonstrated that drugs that inhibit the synthesis of bacterial cell walls (penicillins, cephalosporins, vancomycin, cycloserine, bacitracin) allow entry of aminoglycosides (streptomycin, gentamicin, tobramycin, amikacin) into the cell, resulting in death of the organisms.[298,299] Failure to achieve synergism against the enterococcus can be correlated with resistance to the aminoglycoside being used[299]; and a therapeutic effect can be produced by substitution of another aminoglycoside.[300] Thus, if the organism is resistant to 2000 μg/ml of streptomycin, the addition of this compound will not, in most instances, yield synergistic activity. It must be emphasized that, although usually synergistic in vitro, the combination of cephalothin plus streptomycin or gentamicin is therapeutically ineffective.

A number or regimens have been found to be of value in the management of endocarditis caused by enterococci. Among these are penicillin G (20 million units intravenously every 6 hours) plus streptomycin (0.5 gm intramuscularly every 12 hours) or gentamicin or tobramycin (3 to 5 mg/kg in three equally divided doses at 8-hour intervals). A combination that has proved to be more effective than penicillin plus an aminoglycoside in vitro is nafcillin plus gentamicin or tobramycin; the intravenous dose of nafcillin is 1 gm every 3 hours or 2 gm every 4 hours. Some strains of enterococci are quite sensitive to ampicillin; the dose of this drug for subacute endocarditis is 8 to 12 gm/day, in three or four equally divided and spaced intravenous injections, together with gentamicin or tobramycin. In patients sensitized to penicillins, the administration of 4 gm/day of erythromycin (1 gm intravenously every 6 hours) has proved to be highly effective when the organism is sensitive to this dosage. Vancomycin (0.5 gm every 6 hours) has been reported to be effective in the management of this type of disease.[295] Rather than resort to the use of other antibiotics, some have preferred to desensitize penicillin-sensitive individuals and then administer this agent together with an aminoglycoside or vancomycin. Optimal therapy of infections caused by vitamin B_6–dependent streptococci has been found to be a combination of penicillin G and streptomycin.[301] Doses should be in the same range as those used for the therapy of disease caused by the enterococcus.

Strep. bovis is highly sensitive to penicillin G.[302] Therapy for endocarditis caused by this organism is the same as that for disease caused by alpha-streptococci sensitive to this antibiotic. Valvular infection produced by *Peptostreptococcus* (anaerobic streptococcus) responds well to the administration of penicillin G. However, these organisms are generally relatively insensitive to this drug, and disease caused by them requires the use of "massive" doses of the order of 15 to 20 million units every 6 hours intravenously. Because this quantity may produce seizures and cardiac arrhythmia with death, the following precautions must be taken: The dose must be reduced in the presence of any degree of renal insufficiency, because this is associated with decreased excretion of the drug and accumulation in the brain to levels that may be epileptogenic. In addition, because the commercially available penicillin is the potassium salt (1 million units of penicillin contains about 1.5 mEq/liter of K^+), potentially lethal hyperkalemia may develop. Patients with either localized or generalized disease of the brain may develop jacksonian epilepsy or generalized convulsions. The plasma level of sodium must be kept within normal limits, since hyponatremia increases the susceptibility to convulsions.[303,304]

STAPHYLOCOCCI. Despite the use of antimicrobial agents effective against *Staph. aureus* in vitro, the clinical results of therapy of endocarditis caused by this organism are relatively poor, when compared to subacute disease produced by alpha-streptococci. In patients not sensitized to penicillins, this group of agents is first choice. However, because about 15 per cent of infections caused by *Staph. aureus* that occur outside hospitals and over 90 per cent that develop during hospitalization are caused by penicillin-resistant strains, initial therapy must consist of a penicillinase-resistant drug such as nafcillin, oxacillin, or cephalothin. The minimal dose of these agents should be 12 gm/day (2 gm every 4 hours intravenously). If in vitro studies indicate that the organism isolated from the blood is susceptible to penicillin G, therapy with this agent may be substituted. The dose of this drug is empirical; this author recommends 20 to 30 million units given intravenously in four equally divided and spaced doses per day. Failure to respond raises the question of a methicillin-resistant" or tolerant" strain (p. 1171). Some of these organisms are tolerant" not only to the penicillins but also to the cephalosporins. Vancomycin is useful in many of these cases.

The fatality rate from staphylococcal endocarditis in 25 patients treated with a single antibiotic (penicillin G, methicillin, nafcillin, cephalothin, or vancomycin) was noted to be 40 per cent. It was identical in 15 individuals who received combined therapy (nafcillin plus gentamicin, penicillin plus gentamicin, or methicillin plus gentamicin).[305] A recent prospective study has indicated that treatment with a single effective antibiotic (a penicillinase-resistant penicillin or a cephalosporin) is curative, and that the addition of an aminoglycoside does not increase the rate of cure.[306]

A number of other approaches to the management of

valvular infections caused by *Staph. aureus* have been employed, especially in patients sensitized to the penicillins. Despite some variability in results,[307] vancomycin (0.5 gm every 6 hours intravenously) should be considered a potentially effective alternative in patients with staphylococcal endocarditis sensitized to penicillins and cephalosporins. This drug is clearly the agent of choice for infection by strains of *Staph. aureus*, which are resistant to practically all the antimicrobial compounds currently available, and for patients highly sensitized to the penicillins and cephalosporins. Clindamycin has been found to be ineffective in the therapy of staphylococcal endocarditis in patients sensitized to penicillin,[296] and the results with cefazolin are equivocal.[293,296]

The results of the therapy of endocarditis caused by coagulase-positive staphylococci are not as good as those reported in cases of the disease produced by streptococci, regardless of the antibiotic employed. A varying fatality rate, in excess of that of alpha-streptococcal infection, has characterized the treatment of staphylococcal infection. This is largely related to the intracardiac complications described earlier (p. 1153).

In the author's experience, even large doses of the most active antimicrobial drugs fail to cure the infection in patients in whom a large number of abscesses develop either before or after therapy has been initiated. An important determinant of the eventual outcome of this disease is failure to institute treatment early in the course of the disease; a delay of as little as 4 to 5 days may increase the risk of a fatal outcome.

Despite the low invasive capacity of *Staph. epidermidis*, the prognosis for recovery from endocarditis produced by this organism is generally poor, even when patients are treated with an antibiotic that is considered to be sensitive to it on the basis of in vitro study. A common course of events in this type of valvular infection is relapse after discontinuation of treatment. This may occur several times, in spite of repeated administration of an effective drug, and may finally lead to congestive failure. At this point, replacement of the affected valve with a prosthesis is indicated.

Yeasts and Fungi

Over a decade of use has demonstrated the effectiveness of amphotericin B in the management of infections caused by a large variety of yeasts and fungi. Therapy with this agent has been beneficial in histoplasmosis, cryptococcosis, and candidiasis. However, experience indicates that the treatment of fungal infections of the heart presents a number of problems that are unique to this organ, and are quite different from those encountered when this kind of disease involves other organs. Although sporadic reports have suggested that candidal endocarditis has been eradicated by administration of amphotericin B alone, the diagnosis in these cases has been based largely on the demonstration of candidemia, a finding not always diagnostic of cardiac or systemic disease.[308,309]

The relatively poor results of chemotherapy of fungal infections of cardiac valves has prompted consideration of adjunct therapy, i.e., surgical removal of the infected site. In 1961, Kaye and his colleagues reported an instance of candidal endocarditis resistant to amphotericin B that was ultimately cured by débridement of an infected tricuspid valve.[310] Experience since then has emphasized the intolerably high frequency of primary drug failure and underscores the need for surgical intervention in infections not only of natural valves but especially of prosthetic valves.[311] It must be pointed out, however, that not even this combined therapeutic approach results in an acceptable rate of cure. When the diagnosis of fungal endocarditis is established, treatment with amphotericin B must be initiated promptly. After about a week of administration of the antibiotic, it is best to remove the infected valve, replace it with a prosthesis, and continue chemotherapy for at least 6 to 8 weeks. When this fails, it has been the practice in some instances to replace the prosthetic valve with a new one. However, even this has failed to eradicate the disease in many cases.

Another approach to this problem has been suggested recently. In individuals in whom endocarditis is limited to the tricuspid valve, total valvulectomy without prosthetic replacement has been carried out.[312] Patients apparently get along fairly well following operation. Administration of amphotericin B was continued for a number of weeks until there was a clinical impression of eradication of the infectious process. A prosthesis was then inserted, and treatment continued. It must be emphasized that, of all types of endocarditis, the prognosis for recovery is poorest in those due to yeasts and fungi.

Several regimens have been recommended for intravenous therapy with amphotericin B.[313,314] One involves administration of 0.25 mg/kg the first day, followed by an increase of 0.25 mg/kg each day until a dose of 1 mg/kg/day is reached. This is continued until the completion of therapy. In severe infections, such as is the case in fungal endocarditis, the daily dose may be increased to 1.5 mg/kg/day. Another approach involves the administration of 1 mg the first day and 5 mg the second day, followed by daily increases of 5 to 10 mg until 1 mg/kg/day is being administered. The sclerosing activity of the drug and the immediate unpleasant side effects associated with its administration have prompted the use of a regimen designed to minimize the frequency and possibly the intensity of these reactions. This involves the intravenous infusion of 1.5 mg/kg every other day[313]; the individual daily dose must not exceed 90 mg. This procedure appears to be pharmacologically sound. Peak serum levels are usually higher with treatment on alternate days.

Because of lack of precise information, choice of the period over which amphotericin is given is empirical but is commonly 6 to 8 weeks. In some instances, this has been extended. It may be necessary to administer a second or even third course of the antibiotic, if relapse follows discontinuation of therapy.

A compound of potential value in the management of fungal diseases is 5-fluorocytosine, a drug that can be administered orally. In most instances, this agent is being used, together with amphotericin B, for the treatment of fungal endocarditis when the responsible organism is susceptible to both drugs. This combination is of no value if the organism is resistant to 5-fluorocytosine. In some instances in which the organism is susceptible, the latter has been given alone for varying periods of time, often many months, after "cure" has been accomplished by combined therapy.

When given orally, 5-fluorocytosine is well absorbed from the gastrointestinal tract and reaches clinically effective concentrations.[315-317] Blood levels may be 'cidal for some strains of *Candida* but only 'static for others.[317] The dose of the drug is 50 to 150 mg/kg given at 6-hour intervals; this must be reduced in the presence of renal insufficiency. The most frequent side effects are hepatotoxicity and depression of the bone marrow, which are usually reversible when the drug is discontinued. Nausea and vomiting are fairly common.

Assessment of cure of fungal endocarditis should be made with caution because symptoms of the disease may remain suppressed for long periods.[318] A more accurate view of this situation is that it is "stabilized." Patients should be followed from the time chemotherapy is discontinued, because relapse may occur as long as 2 years after completing treatment. Blood cultures are usually negative. Antibodies to *Candida* may be absent in the presence of infection, and their detection does not identify an active infectious process, because precipitins to *Candida* are present in 40 per cent of individuals who undergo cardiac surgery and are not infected, as well as in those in whom there has been an apparent cure.[253]

Surgical Therapy

Despite the emphasis on the medical management of infective endocarditis over the past 40 years, it must be pointed out that the first spontaneous cure of an infection of the cardiovascular system was accomplished by Touroff and Vessell in 1940 when they ligated an infected patent ductus arteriosus.[319] After a hiatus of many years, during which the prognosis of endocarditis changed from almost complete hopelessness to a high expectancy of recovery as more and more highly effective antimicrobial agents became available, surgical approaches have again become the ultimate therapeutic modality in patients in whom all other forms of treatment have been unsuccessful. However, as is often the case with progress in medicine, the development of new methods of management, while solving one set of problems, has frequently created new ones that are often more difficult to solve than the ones they replace. This is unquestionably the case in the surgical treatment of infective endocarditis. On the one hand, successful surgical manipulation of the uninfected heart has been responsible for an appreciable increment in the incidence of cardiovascular infections (p. 1141). On the other hand, while it is often the final successful approach to the eradication of valvular infections, surgical intervention raises difficult questions in relation not only to its advisability and indications but also, once such a course has been accepted as necessary, to the time when it should be undertaken.[319a]

One of the most critical and unquestioned indications for surgical intervention in cases of infective endocarditis is the development of intractable cardiac failure due to disruption of valve leaflets or their supporting structures. It must be pointed out, however, that the mere appearance of even severe decompensation of the heart does not always necessitate surgical therapy. In some instances this condition may be well controlled by medical management alone. However, when all conventional measures have failed, or decompensation progresses despite intensive treatment of heart failure, surgical repair should be undertaken without delay; temporizing may lead to failure, even when the surgical manipulation itself has been entirely successful. The role of intractable congestive failure in death from infective endocarditis is emphasized by the fact that this is the most common cause of fatality in this disease. Involvement of the aortic valve is most often the cause of this problem,[320-322] but severe mitral regurgitation, although less common, has also required replacement of the damaged valve with a prosthesis.[323,324] It has become increasingly clear that the *presence of active infection is not a contraindication to cardiac surgery* in patients whose valves and their supporting structures have been severely injured or destroyed by infection.[325,326]

A study of ten patients with acute aortic valve regurgitation requiring urgent valvular replacement led Wise and his colleagues to distinguish two syndromes—acute and chronic.[327] In their opinion, only the acute form required immediate surgical intervention. The clinical features that indicated the presence of this syndrome (p. 1111) were (a) diastole of shorter duration than systole, (b) low cardiac output, (c) soft murmurs, (d) lack of appreciable enlargement of the left ventricle on radiographic or electrocardiographic study, and (e) diminished intensity of the first heart sound secondary to high left ventricular diastolic pressure. Although an important degree of aortic regurgitation can usually be detected on physical examination, determination of the significance of mitral valve incompetence in the course of infective endocarditis may require cardiac catheterization.

The fatality rate in emergency aortic valve replacement has been reported to be about 33 per cent but it is probably declining[320-322]; it is far less when it is carried out electively.[320] The necessity of surgical intervention in patients with perforation of the aortic valve leading to regurgitation during the course of endocarditis is emphasized by a report of eight patients in whom operation was not carried out and all of whom died; of seven individuals with the same lesion who underwent repair of the perforation or replacement of the valve, only three succumbed.[328] Griffin et al. have stressed the need for immediate insertion of a prosthesis when severe cardiac failure complicates valvular infections.[329] They also suggested that this procedure be performed early in patients with mild decompensation of the heart because of a significant risk of sudden death from embolic myocardial infarction or the development of potentially lethal arrhythmias.

INDICATIONS. The following are the important indications for cardiac surgery in patients with infective endocarditis: (1) *Congestive failure* that does not respond to intensive medical management. Active infection is not a contraindication. (2) *No response of the infectious process* on the involved valve despite appropriate, intensive antimicrobial therapy for about one week. An additional benefit in this situation is removal of the bulk of the bacterial load. (3) *Repeated embolic occlusions,* especially when vital areas such as brain, eyes, coronary arteries, and kidneys are involved. In this situation, the problem that arises involves a decision as to when surgery should be performed. Should this be after the first, second, third, or more embolic episode? There are no data that indicate the answer to this question. (4) *Presence of a septal abscess.* (5) *Relapse of infection* (3 months or less after "cure"). It is this writer's practice to treat the first relapse over the same length carditis, they have also been observed occasionally in patients with the subacute type of disease.[14]

Cardiac decompensation increases the incidence of failure of antimicrobial therapy and of early and late death. Lerner and Weinstein reported that 6 months after completion of treatment, the survival rate was four times greater in patients with normal than in those with abnormal cardiac function.[14] This has also been observed by others.[345,349] That this problem has become more prominent since the advent of effective chemotherapy is substantiated by experiences at the Philadelphia General Hospital between 1933 and 1938 and 1950 and 1960.[350] Uncontrolled infection was responsible for 64 per cent and heart failure for 6 per cent of the deaths in the preantibiotic era; cardiac decompensation occurred in 61 per cent of the fatal cases—a tenfold increase—in the later period.

Several observers have noted that *myocarditis* is common and is probably an important factor in determining the prognosis of endocarditis.[192,351,352] The presence of myocardial abscesses involving either the septum or walls of the ventricles increases the risk of death. However, if these are recognized early and are removed surgically, the prognosis improves.

Although the presence of *myocardial infarction* is seldom detected during life, it is a relatively common autopsy finding.[9,353-355] Coronary occlusions, even those of minor degree, but especially when multiple, threaten the prognosis not only because they are, in themselves, potentially lethal but also because they may provoke cardiac decompensation.[9] Jackson and Allison have presented strong evidence in support of the role of myocardial infarction in the congestive heart failure that occurs in infective endocarditis; they found the incidence of embolic coronary lesions to be much higher than that of dynamic aortic regurgitation (with or without perforation or rupture of a valve) in persons dying of heart failure.[356]

The development of *renal dysfunction* during or after recovery from infective endocarditis is an ominous prognostic sign, especially if heart failure is also present. It has been suggested that "severe renal damage, particularly proliferative glomerulonephritis, may prove fatal, in spite of penicillin therapy."[9] About 5 to 10 per cent of the deaths in treated endocarditis are associated with renal failure.[9,20] Many observers have documented the finding that even severe uremia may be reversed by intensive antimicrobial therapy.

When *embolic phenomena* supervene, the prognosis for survival depends greatly on the site at which the emboli are deposited, the time in the course of the disease when they develop, and whether or not they produce suppuration.[20,172] Thus, embolization of the coronary arteries or vital areas of the brain and lung (if cardiac failure is present) is a considerably greater threat to survival than involvement of other organs. Systemic emboli have been found in 60 and 45 per cent, respectively, of fatal cases of acute and subacute endocarditis studied at the Massachusetts General Hospital.[20] Cerebral vessels were involved in over 60 per cent. Embolization may occur longer than 6 months after successful treatment of the cardiac infection but is rarely fatal at that time.[345,352,357,358]

Mycotic aneurysms often begin to develop in the early stages of infective endocarditis but may not rupture until many weeks or months after apparent recovery.[9,19] The degree of danger with which they are associated depends on their location; tears do not mean inevitable death. Pearce and Guze noted that, when cerebral emboli and mycotic aneurysms are not immediately fatal, the prognosis for recovery is good.[346] Of 20 patients with mycotic aneurysms studied by Cates and Christie, 17 died; the cerebral vessels were involved in all but one of the fatal cases.[9] Aneurysms of the sinus of Valsalva are said to occur in 10 to 15 per cent.[20,175] In addition to the cerebral arteries, which are the commonest and most dangerous sites, aneurysms have been found in the abdominal aorta, superior mesenteric artery, sinus of Valsalva, mitral valve, splenic artery, ligated ductus arteriosus, and coronary arteries.[146,359-362] Karchmer[363] has pointed out that improvement in the prognosis of infective endocarditis rests on "anticipating complications, recognizing them as they occur, and referring patients promptly to a major medical center when an operation is essential."

PROSTHETIC VALVULAR INFECTIONS. The prognosis in infection of prosthetic valves is determined, in general, by the same factors that influence the outcome in patients with endocarditis involving natural valves. In addition, it is also dependent on whether complications develop, such as obstruction of the valvular outlet (Starr-Edwards valve), paravalvular leaks, or separation of the prosthesis to a degree that causes congestive heart failure or severe bleeding as a result of improper control with anticoagulants. The fatality rate in infections that developed when a previously infected natural valve was replaced with a prosthesis was found to be 28 per cent by Boyd et al.[364] and was 90 per cent in patients treated for 4 to 6 weeks without control of the infection or surgical intervention. In those with uncontrolled disease who were operated upon within 10 days, the survival rate was 83 per cent. A review of the literature indicated that the average fatality rate in individuals with infected intracardiac prostheses was about 70 per cent.[365] It is clear from these and other recorded experiences that early recognition of infection of prosthetic valves and prompt medical and surgical treatment greatly improve the possibility of survival.[366]

Young and his co-workers studied 163 episodes of infective endocarditis in which 32 cardiac operations were performed during the active stage of the disease.[367] Cardiac failure was the primary reason for surgical intervention in 88 per cent. *Staphylococcus* and enterococcus were the organisms most often involved. Postoperative complications were rare. There were no instances of continued infection, prosthetic dehiscence, or advanced heart block; one patient developed a paravalvular leak and another a systemic embolus. Eleven individuals were moribund prior to surgery. The authors emphasized that there is a "high medical and surgical mortality in patients with IE and that delayed operative intervention may be a major causative factor resulting in a high surgical mortality." They also pointed out that these experiences "justify an aggressive surgical approach in patients with valve dysfunction and heart failure." Kaplan[368] studied 63 patients who had been subjected to cardiac surgery before developing infective endocarditis. Fifty-five per cent had had a prosthetic valve inserted; most of these had underlying rheumatic heart disease. Most of the patients studied had congenital heart disease with systemic artery-to-pulmonary artery shunts. In this group, the highest risk of developing endocardial infection was in those who were cyanotic and had palliative pulmonary artery-to-systemic artery shunts. In discussing the prognosis of infective endocarditis, Scalia et al.[369] stressed the point that early surgical intervention affects favorably the prognosis, especially in cases of isolated aortic valve involvement." In a study of the prognosis of endocarditis involving prosthetic valves in 48 patients studied between 1962 and 1978, Masur and Johnson[370] indentified a fatality rate of 69 per cent, with 20 per cent of the deaths associated with embolization to the central nervous system. A fatal outcome that exceeded 75 per cent was noted when the aortic valve was involved, when a nonstreptococcal organism was the causative agent, when new or increased regurgitant murmurs developed, and when significant congestive failure supervened. The fatality rate was lowest when the prosthesis was invaded by streptococci (29 per cent) and when a mitral valve had been replaced (47 per cent). Cohn and his colleagues have reported that, of 128 patients who underwent porcine heart-valve replacement (aortic 47, mitral 62, combined mitral-aortic 19), only 5 (4 per cent) developed infective endocarditis over the following 5 to 8 years.[371]

PREVENTION

Although there are still no statistically valid data to establish the effectiveness of chemoprophylaxis in infective endocarditis, anecdotal experiences are sufficient to support it. In general, all individuals known to have disease of the heart, particularly that involving the valves, should be considered candidates for prophylaxis. This includes patients with congenital heart disease (excluding uncomplicated secundum atrial septal defect and ligated and divided patent ductus arteriosus), acquired lesions (rheumatic, atherosclerotic, calcific), prolapsing mitral valve with regurgitation ("click murmur"), hypertrophic obstructive cardiomyopathy, calcified mitral annulus, and an intracardiac prosthesis or "patch," or those who, after a previous episode of valvular infection, are subjected to dental manipulations (extraction, deep scaling, and gingivectomy) or surgery involving the respiratory, gastrointestinal, urinary, or genital tracts.

The value of prophylaxis is uncertain in procedures that may be associated with a transient bacteremia associated with an indwelling vascular catheter, transvenous pacemakers, arteriovenous shunts, ventriculoatrial shunts, barium enema, sigmoidoscopy, colonoscopy, and biopsy of the liver. Available evidence does not prove its necessity in these situations. Nevertheless, some physicians recommend chemoprophylaxis, despite the probably very small risk of the development of endocarditis. Kaye[372] has made the comment that optimal antimicrobial prophylaxis administered to patients undergoing various procedures known to be associated with transient bacteremia could be expected to prevent only a few cases of endocarditis.

Selection of appropriate prophylactic antibiotics requires knowledge both of the organisms most likely to invade the blood during procedures producing transient bacteremia and of those most often responsible for infection of cardiac valves. For example, the bacteria present in the blood after dental manipulation or operations on the upper respiratory tract are, for the most part, *Strep. viridans*; however, enterococci or staphylococci may also invade the circulation. Transient bacteremia associated with procedures involving the urinary, gastrointestinal, and genital tracts are usually characterized by the presence of various species of streptococci, gram-negative bacteria, and occasionally *Bacteroides. Staph. aureus* is a common culprit in cardiac surgery involving extracorporeal circulation. When incision and drainage of an abscess or débridement of contaminated tissue is carried out, the choice of the prophylactic agent is based on the type of organism recovered from the infected site.

Prophylaxis

A variety of approaches to prophylaxis have been recommended for patients undergoing dental manipulation or operations on the upper respiratory tract. One involves the administration of 250 mg of phenoxymethyl penicillin (penicillin V) orally three or four times a day for 2 days before, the day of, and for 2 days after surgery. In addition, a dose of 600,000 or 1.2 million units of procaine penicillin G is given intramuscularly on the day of operation. An alternate program recommends the intramuscular injection of 1 million units of penicillin G one hour before and one hour after surgical manipulation. It has been suggested by some that patients receive a daily injection of the same dose of antibiotic for 2 days after operation. This author prefers to use erythromycin because, in his experience, this drug is active against most strains of *Strep. viridans*, enterococcus, and penicillin-sensitive or penicillin-resistant *Staph. aureus*. This program involves the administration of 1 gm of erythromycin orally one hour before the procedure and 0.5 gm one hour after the surgery, followed by 0.5 gm every 6 hours for a total of four doses. Another regimen employed by others, especially for patients sensitized to penicillin, involves the administration of 0.5 gm of erythromycin every 6 hours for 2 days before, on the day of, and for 2 days after dental surgery. In the author's opinion, this program is excessive prophylaxis for a transient bacteremia that persists, as a rule, no longer than 20 minutes.

AMERICAN HEART ASSOCIATION GUIDELINES. A committee of the American Heart Association has made a number of recommendations for chemoprophylaxis in patients with underlying cardiac disease (Table 29–5, p. 952).[373] They have pointed out that "since there have been no controlled clinical trials, adequate data for comparing various methods for prevention of endocarditis in man are not available." Its recommendations are as follows: For all dental procedures associated with bleeding or surgery or instrumentation of the upper respiratory tract, two regimens are suggested. The first involves the intramuscular injection of 1 million units of penicillin G mixed with 600,000 units of procaine penicillin G 30 to 60 minutes prior to the procedure. This is followed by 500 mg of phenoxymethyl penicillin (penicillin V) orally every 6 hours for 8 doses. The regimen for children is the same, but the dose of penicillin is reduced to 30,000 units/kg and that of procaine penicillin is unchanged; the oral dose of penicillin V is reduced to 250 mg every 6 hours for eight doses. The second involves only oral administration of antibiotics. Adults are given 2 gm of penicillin V orally 30 to 60 minutes before the procedure and 500 mg of the same drug every 6 hours for eight doses postoperatively. The same regimen is used for children over 60 pounds in weight; for those under 60 pounds, the preoperative dose of penicillin V is 1 gm and the postoperative dose is 250 mg at the same interval and number of doses as for adults. A third recommended regimen includes the same doses of the various penicillins, as described above for parenteral prophylaxis, with the addition of 1 gm of streptomycin (20 mg/kg for children) postoperatively. The following programs are recommended for patients allergic to penicillin: Adults, 1 gm of vancomycin intravenously 30 to 60 minutes preoperatively followed by 500 mg of erythromycin orally every 6 hours for eight doses. The doses of vancomycin and erythromycin for children are reduced to 20 mg/kg and 10 mg/kg, respectively.

The American Heart Association's recommendations for

prophylaxis for surgery or instrumentation of the genitourinary and gastrointestinal tracts are as follows: Adults are given 2 million units of penicillin G or 1 gm of ampicillin plus gentamicin (1.5 mg/kg but no more than 80 mg) intramuscularly or intravenously *or* 1 gm of streptomycin 30 to 60 minutes prior to the procedure. When gentamicin is used, a similar dose of this drug plus penicillin or ampicillin is given every 8 hours for two doses. When streptomycin has been given prior to the procedure, a similar dose is given together with penicillin every 12 hours for two doses. The program for children is similar, but the doses of penicillin G, ampicillin, gentamicin, and streptomycin are reduced to 30,000 units/kg, 50 mg/kg, 2 mg/kg, and 20 mg/kg, respectively. Adults sensitive to penicillin are given 1 gm of vancomycin intramuscularly preoperatively. Although this may not be necessary, a second course of these drugs may be given 12 hours after operation. The dose of both vancomycin and streptomycin for children sensitized to penicillin is 20 mg/kg.

Dismukes[374] has reported the results of a review of published data indicating the level of risk of transient bacteremia associated with procedures involving the airway, gastrointestinal tract, and urologic manipulation. On the basis of the frequency and four types of organisms recovered from the blood stream, he recommended specific antimicrobial prophylaxis for procedures involving various organ systems. The data in the paper differ, in some respects, from those presented by the American Heart Association,[373] which, as both he and others have pointed out, are based on the results of animal studies.

Keys[375] has suggested chemoprophylactic procedures that represent a modification of those recommended by the American Heart Association,[373] which he says are "inconvenient, painful and expensive" and "may not be enforced in actual practice." He also emphasizes the point with which this author (L.W.) (with the exception of the word "secure") fully agrees, that "although experimental studies in animals have provided a secure foundation for our concepts of antimicrobial prophylaxis, carefully conducted clinical trials of various programs are urgently needed." In commenting about chemoprophylaxis in patients susceptible to the risk of transient bacteremia in the course of dental manipulation, Oakley and Somerville[376] made the statement that "it is a sobering thought that a rise in the standard of oral hygiene in this country would probably help more than any other measure to reduce the incidence of streptococcal infective endocarditis. If we can accomplish this and prophylaxis, too, then endocarditis should become a rare disease."

Despite specific recommendations for antimicrobial prophylaxis in patients with underlying heart disease subjected to procedures associated with transient bacteremia, the problem remains unsolved because of a lack of acceptable data to support it. The present state of the art has best been defined by Schadelin[377] in the following statement: "Prophylactic antibiotic coverage of all interventions with a high risk of bacteremia is accepted practice in patients with valvular heart disease. A true cost-benefit ratio, however, has not been possible to demonstrate due to the low risk involved in these procedures and, therefore, the current recommendations rely on experimental work with animals. Full application of these findings in patients is difficult and even so incapable of preventing the majority of cases of infective endocarditis."

Prophylaxis for Surgery. The effectiveness of the chemoprophylaxis for "open-heart" surgery has been studied by a number of investigators. One report has indicated no difference in the incidence of infection when penicillin G, methicillin, or a placebo was administered.[378] A similar observation has been made in patients given penicillin G plus streptomycin, oxacillin, or a placebo prophylactically.[379] A study comparing methicillin and cephalothin demonstrated that none of 492 persons receiving the cephalosporin but 11 of 129 given methicillin developed endocarditis.[380] Other investigations comparing cephalothin with cloxacillin and gentamicin given before, during, and after operation have failed to show any significant reduction in the risk of prosthetic infection.[379] A recent prospective double-blind study involving 200 patients in whom prosthetic valves were implanted and who were given cephalothin for 2 or 6 days produced no convincing evidence that the longer period of prophylaxis had an advantage over the shorter one.[380]

Infective endocarditis that develops early in the postoperative period is often caused by *Staph. aureus* or *Staph. epidermidis.* Organisms less frequently responsible are streptococci, gram-negative bacteria, and fungi. Because there is no chemoprophylactic program that will protect against invasion by all organisms, prudence suggests that it be directed primarily against the staphylococcus. For this reason, the antibiotics used most frequently have been oxacillin, nafcillin, or cephalothin, the latter protecting against invasion not only by staphylococci but also by common gram-negative bacilli such as *E. coli, Proteus mirabilis*, and *K. pneumoniae.* An acceptable regimen for these antibiotics is 2 gm intravenously 2 hours before operation, 1 gm intraoperatively, and 1 gm every 4 hours for no more than 2 to 3 days in order to minimize the risk of superinfection. The author prefers cephalothin because of its activity against most staphylococci and streptococci as well as against the common gram-negative bacteria. Vancomycin, 1 gm intravenously 2 hours before surgery followed by the same dose every 12 hours for 2 days, may be used in persons sensitized to the penicillins or cephalosporins.

A prophylactic program for patients with underlying cardiac disease who undergo surgical or other manipulation of the genitourinary or gastrointestinal tract must include drugs that inhibit multiplication of many gram-positive and gram-negative bacteria. The program recommended by the American Heart Association, although not supported by data, proving its efficacy, may be used.[373] This involves administration of 1 gm of ampicillin plus 1.5 mg/kg of gentamicin intramuscularly or intravenously 30 to 60 minutes prior to the procedure. The same doses of the antibiotics are repeated 8 and 16 hours after operation.

All individuals with cardiac diseases known to predispose to endocarditis who have active extracardiac infections and who must undergo some type of surgical procedure should be treated before an operation is performed. The drugs selected are those to which the causative organism is sensitive, and conventional therapeutic doses should be administered. It may be necessary only to bring the infectious process under control when there is an urgent need for surgery; whenever possible, however, it is probably best to eradicate the infection completely before the surgical procedure is undertaken.

It must be emphasized that the chemoprophylactic programs currently used to prevent recurrences of rheumatic fever may not eliminate the risk of the development of infective endocarditis. For this reason, all patients on such programs who are subjected to manipulations of the oral cavity or upper respiratory, urinary, or gastrointestinal tracts must receive additional prophylaxis, as described above.

References

1. Major, R. H.: Notes on the history of endocarditis. Bull. Hist. Med. *17*:351, 1945.
2. Osler, W.: Malignant endocarditis. Gulstonian Lectures. Lancet *1*:459, 1885.
3. Libman, E., and Celler, H. L.: The etiology of subacute infective endocarditis. Am. J. Med. Sci. *140*:516, 1910.
4. Lichtman, S. S.: Treatment of subacute bacterial endocarditis: Current results. Ann. Intern. Med. *19*:787, 1943.
5. Kelson, S. R.: Observations on the treatment of subacute bacterial (streptococcal) endocarditis since 1939. Ann. Intern. Med. *22*:75, 1945.
6. Florey, M. E., and Florey, H. W.: General and local administration of penicillin. Lancet *1*:387, 1943.
7. Loewe, L., Rosenblatt, P., Greene, H. J., and Russel, M.: Combined penicillin and heparin therapy of subacute bacterial endocarditis. J.A.M.A. *124*:144, 1944.
8. Hedley, O. F.: Rheumatic heart disease in Philadelphia hospitals. III. Fatal rheumatic heart disease and subacute bacterial endocarditis. Pub. Health Rep. *55*:1707, 1940.

9. Cates, J. E., and Christie, R. V.: Subacute bacterial endocarditis. A review of 442 patients treated in 14 centres appointed by the Penicillin Trials Committee of the Medical Research Council. Q. J. Med. *20*:93, 1951.
10. Kaye, D., McCormack, R. C., and Hook, E. W.: Bacterial endocarditis: Changing pattern since introduction of penicillin therapy. Antimicrob. Agents Chemother. *3*:37, 1961.
11. Finland, M., and Barnes, M. W.: Changing etiology of bacterial endocarditis in the antibacterial era: Experiences at Boston City Hospital 1933–1965. Ann. Intern. Med. *72*:341, 1970.
12. Afremow, M. L.: Review of 202 cases of bacterial endocarditis. III. Med. J. *107*:67, 1955.
13. Cherubin, C. E., and Neu, H. C.: Infective endocarditis at the Presbyterian Hospital in New York City from 1938–1967. Am. J. Med. *51*:83, 1971.
14. Lerner, P. I., and Weinstein, L.: Infective endocarditis in the antibiotic era. N. Engl. J. Med. *274*:199, 259, 323, 387, 1966.
14a. Brandenburg, R. O., Guiliani, E. R., Wilson, W. R., and Geraci, J. E.: Infective endocarditis –A 25-year overview of diagnosis and therapy. J. Am. Coll. Cardiol. *1*:280, 1983.
15. Kerr, A., Jr.: Bacterial endocarditis—revisited. Mod. Con. Cardiovasc. Dis. *33*:831, 1964.
16. Hamburger, M.: Acute and subacute bacterial endocarditis. Arch. Intern. Med. *112*:1, 1963.
17. Wedgwood, J.: Early diagnosis of subacute bacterial endocarditis. Lancet *2*:1058, 1955.
18. Kelson, S. R., and White, P. D.: Notes on 250 cases of subacute bacterial (streptococcal) endocarditis studied and treated between 1927 and 1939. Ann. Intern. Med. *22*:40, 1940.
19. Kerr, A., Jr.: Subacute bacterial endocarditis. *In* Pullen, R. L. (ed.): Springfield, Ill., Charles C Thomas, 1955. (No. 274, Am. Lecture Series, Monograph of Bannerstone Division of Am. Lectures in Internal Medicine.)
20. Morgan, W. L., and Bland, E. F.: Bacterial endocarditis in antibiotic era. Circulation *19*:753, 1959.

MICROBIOLOGY AND PATHOLOGY

21. Libman, E., and Friedberg, C. K.: Subacute Bacterial Endocarditis. New York, Oxford University Press, 1941.
22. Uwaydah, M. M., and Weinberg, A. N.: Bacterial endocarditis—a changing pattern. N. Engl. J. Med. *273*:1231, 1965.
23. Kaye, D., McCormack, R. C., and Hook, E. W.: Bacterial endocarditis: The changing patterns since introduction of penicillin therapy. *In* Antimicrobial Agents and Chemotherapy. American Society of Microbiology. Washington, D.C., 1961, pp. 37–46.
24. Hosea S. H.: Virulent *Streptococcus viridans* bacterial endocarditis. Am. Heart J., *101*:174, 1981.
25. Cameron, I. W.: Subacute bacterial endocarditis in an edentulous patient: A case report. Br. Dent. J. *130*:404, 1971.
26. Moellering, R. C., Jr., Watson, B. K., and Kunz, L. J.: Endocarditis due to group D streptococci. Comparison of disease caused by *Streptococcus bovis* with that produced by enterococci. Am. J. Med. *57*:239, 1974.
27. Keusch, G. T.: Opportunistic infections in colon carcinoma. Am. J. Clin. Nutr. *27*:1481, 1974.
28. Klein, R. S., Recco, R. A., Catalano, M. T., Edberg, S. C., Casey, J. I., and Steigbigel, N. H.: Association of *Streptococcus bovis* with carcinoma of the colon. N. Engl. J. Med. *297*:800, 1977.
29. Rose, D. F., Richman, H., and Localio, S. A.: Bacterial endocarditis associated with colorectal carcinoma. Ann. Surg. *179*:190, 1974.
30. Reid, T. M. S.: Group D streptococcal endocarditis. Scott. Med. J. *22*:13,1977.
31. Wilson, L. M.: Etiology of bacterial endocarditis: Before and since introduction of antibiotics. Ann. Intern. Med. *58*:946, 1963.
32. Harder, E. J., Wilkowske, C. J., Washington, J. A., III, and Geraci, J. E.: *Streptococcus mutans* endocarditis. Ann. Intern. Med. *80*:364, 1974.
33. Bouza, E., Meyer, R. A., and Busch, D. F.: Group G streptococcal endocarditis. Am. J. Clin. Pathol. *70*:108, 1978.
34. Davies, M. K., Ireland, M. A., and Clarke, D. B.: Infective endocarditis from group C streptococci causing stenosis of both the aortic and mitral valves. Thorax *36*:69–71, 1981.
35. Portnoy, D., Wink, I., Richards, G. K., and Blanc, M. Z.: Bacterial endocarditis due to a penicillin-tolerant group C streptococcus. CMA J. *122*:69–75, 1980.
36. Levin, R. M., Pulliam, L., Mondry, C., Levy, D., Hadley, W. K., and Grossman, M.: Penicillin-resistant *Streptococcus constellatus* as a cause of endocarditis. Am. J. Dis. Child. *136*:42–45, 1982.
37. Eickoff, T. C., Klein, J. O., Daly, A. K., Ingall, D., and Finland, M.: Neonatal sepsis and other infections due to group B beta-hemolytic streptococci. N. Engl. J. Med. *271*:1221, 1974.
38. Dismukes, W. E., Karchmer, A. W., Buckley, M. J., Austen, W. G., and Swartz, M. N.: Prosthetic valve endocarditis. Circulation *48*:365, 1973.
39. Bevanger, L., and Stamnes, T. I.: Group L streptococci as the cause of bacteraemia and endocarditis. Acta Pathol. Microbiol. Scand. *87*:301–302, 1979.
40. Roberts, K. B., and Sidlak, M. J.: Satellite streptococci: A major cause of "negative" blood cultures in bacterial endocarditis? J.A.M.A. *241*:2293, 1979.
41. Wilson, R., and Hamburger, M.: Fifteen years' experience with staphylococcus septicemia in large city hospital: Analysis of fifty-five cases in Cincinnati General Hospital 1940–1954. Am. J. Med. *22*:437, 1957.
42. Keys, T. F., and Hewitt, W. L.: Endocarditis due to micrococci and *Staphylococcus epidermidis*. Arch. Intern. Med. *132*:216, 1973.
43. Simberkoff, M. S., and Rahal, J. J., Jr.: Acute and subacute endocarditis due to *Erysipelothrix rhusiopathiae*. Am. J. Med. Sci. *266*:53, 1978.
44. Axelrod, J., Keusch, G. T., Bottone, E., Cohen, S. M., and Hirschman, S. Z.: Endocarditis caused by *Lactobacillus plantarum*. Ann. Intern. Med. *78*:33, 1973.
45. Dupont, B., and Lapreste, C. L.: Maladie d'Osler à lactobacille. Nouv. Presse Med. *6*:3627, 1977.
46. Bayer, A. S., Chow, A. N., and Guze, L. B.: *Listeria monocytogenes* endocarditis: Report of a case and review of the literature. Am. J. Med. Sci. *273*:319, 1977.
47. Kaplan, K., and Weinstein, L.: Diphtheroid infections in man. Ann. Intern. Med. *70*:919, 1969.
48. Murray, B. E., Karchmer, A. W., and Moellering, R. C., Jr.: Diphtheroid prosthetic valve endocarditis. A study of clinical features and infecting organisms. Am. J. Med. *69*:838–848, 1980.
49. Gaurd, R. W.: Non-toxigenic *Corynebacterium diphtheriae* causing subacute bacterial endocarditis. Pathology *11*:533, 1979.
50. Love, J. W., Medina, D., Anderson, S., and Braniff, B.: Infective endocarditis due to *Corynebacterium diphtheriae*: Report of a case and review of the literature. Johns Hopkins Med. J. *148*:41, 1981.
51. Block, C. S., Levy, M. L., and Fritz, V. U.: *Bacillus cereus* endocarditis. A case report. S. Afr. Med. J. *53*:556, 1978.
52. Reller, L. B.: Endocarditis caused by *Bacillus subtilis*. Am. J. Clin. Pathol. *60*:714, 1973.
53. Schafer, F. J., Wing, E. J., and Norden, C. W.: Infectious endocarditis caused by *Rothia dentocariosa*. Ann. Intern. Med. *91*:747, 1979.
54. Pape, J., Singer, C., Kiehn, T. E., Lee, B. J., and Armstrong, D.: Infective endocarditis caused by *Rothia dentocariosa*. Ann. Intern. Med. *91*:746, 1979.
55. Thayer, W. S.: Bacterial or infective endocarditis. Edinburgh Med. J. *38*:237–265, 207–334, 1931.
56. Sugar, A. M., Utsinger, P. D., and Santoro, J.: Gonococcal endocarditis in a patient with mitral valve prolapse. Study of host immunology and organism characteristics. Am. J. Med. Sci. *283*:165–168, 1982.
57. Brancaccio, M., and Legendre, G. G.: *Megasphaera elsdenii* endocarditis. J. Clin. Microbiol. *10*:72–74, 1979.
58. Cohen, P. S., Maguire, J. H., and Weinstein, L.: Infective endocarditis caused by gram-negative bacteria: A review of the literature, 1945–1977. Prog. Cardiovasc. Dis. *22*:205–242, 1980.
59. Hansing, C. E., Allen, V. D., and Cherry, J. D.: *Escherichia coli* endocarditis: A review of the literature and a case study. Arch. Intern. Med. *120*:472–477, 1967.
60. Carruthers, M. M.: Endocarditis due to enteric bacilli other than *Salmonellae*: Case reports and literature review. Am. J. Med. Sci. *273*:203, 1977.
61. Satterwhite, T. K., McGee, Z. A., Schaffner, W., et al.: Infection of an avulsed papillary muscle tip stimulating bacterial endocarditis. Am. Heart J. *86*:107–111, 1973.
62. Rosen, P., and Armstrong, D.: Infective endocarditis in patients treated for malignant neoplastic disease (a postmortem study). Am. J. Clin. Pathol. *59*:241–250, 1978.
63. Carruthers, M. M., and Kanokvechayant, R.: *Pseudomonas aeruginosa* endocarditis: Report of a case, with review of the literature. Am. J. Med. *55*:811, 1973.
64. Reyes, M. P., Palutke, W. A., Wylin, R. F., Lerner, A. M., Arbulu, A. M., Pursel, S. E., and Schatz, I. J.: *Pseudomonas* endocarditis in the Detroit Medical Center, 1969–1973. Medicine *52*:173, 1973.
65. Yu, V. L., Rumans, L. W., Wing, E. J., et al.: *Pseudomonas maltophilia* causing heroin-associated infective endocarditis. Arch. Intern. Med. *138*:1667–1671, 1978.
66. Noriega, E. R., Rubinstein, E., Simberkoff, M. S., et al.: Subacute and acute endocarditis due to *Pseudomonas cepacia* in heroin addicts. Am. J. Med. *59*:29–36, 1975.
67. Rubin, R. H., and Weinstein, L.: Salmonenosis. Microbiologic Pathologic and Clinical Features. New York, Stratton Intercontinental Medical Book Corporation, 1977.
68. Emmerson, A. M., Perinpanayagam, R. M., and Barnado, D. E.: *Haemophilus* endocarditis. Postgrad. Med. J. *57*:117–119, 1981.
69. Jemsek, J. G., Greenberg, S. B., Gentry, L. O., Welton, D. E., and Mattox, K. L.: *Haemophilus parainfluenzae* endocarditis: Two cases and review of the literature in the past decade. Am. J. Med. *66*:51, 1979.
70. Root, T. E., Silva, E. A., Edwards, L. D., and Topp, J. H.: *Hemophilus aphrophilus* endocarditis with a probable dental focus of infection. Chest *80*:109, 1981.
71. Golden, B., Layman, T. E., Koontz, F. P., et al.: *Brucella suis* endocarditis. S. Med. J. *63*:392–395, 1970.
72. Lehmann, V., Knutsen, S. B., Ragnhildstveit, E., et al.: Endocarditis caused by *Pasteurella multocida*. Scand. J. Infect. Dis. *9*:247–248, 1977.
73. Block, P. C., Desanctis, R. W., Weinberg, A. W., et al.: Prosthetic valve endocarditis. J. Thorac. Cardiovasc. Surg. *60*:541–548, 1970.
74. Mills, J., and Drew, D.: *Serratia marcescens* endocarditis. A regional illness associated with intravenous drug use. Ann. Intern. Med. *84*:29, 1976.
75. Schmidt, U., Chmel, H., Kaminski, Z., and Sen, P.: The clinical spectrum of *Campylobacter fetus* infections: Report of five cases and review of the literature. Q. J. Med. *49*:431, 1980.
76. McCormack, R. C., Kaye, D., and Hook, E. W.: Endocarditis due to *Strepto-*

bacillus moniliformis. A report of two cases and review of the literature. J. Am. Med. Assoc. *200*:183, 1967.
77. Weiner, M., and Werthamer, S.: *Cardiobacterium hominis* endocarditis — Characterization of the unusual organisms and review of the literature. Am. J. Clin. Pathol. *63*:131, 1975.
78. Geraci, J. E., Wilson, W. R., and Washington, J. A., III: Infective endocarditis caused by *Actinobacillus actinomycetemcomitans.* Mayo Clin. Proc. *55*:415, 1980.
79. Schiff, J., Suter, L. S., Gourley, R. D., et al.: *Flavobacterium* infection as a cause of bacterial endocarditis: Report of a case, bacteriological studies and review of the literature. Ann. Intern. Med. *55*:499, 1961.
80. LeFrock, L. J., Klainer, A. S., and Zuckerman, K.: *Edwardsiella tarda* bacteremia. S. Med. J. *69*:188, 1976.
81. McCullough, D., Menzies, R., and Corhere, B. M.: Endocarditis due to *Citrobacter diversus* developing resistance to cephalothin. N. Z. Med. J. *85*:182, 1977.
82. Walsh et al.: Fungal infections of the heart: Analysis of 51 autopsied patients. Am. J. Cardiol. *45*:357, 1980.
83. Parker, J. C.: The potentially lethal problem of cardiac candidosis. Am. J. Clin. Pathol. *73*:356, 1980.
84. Brandstetter, R. D., and Brause, B. D.: *Candida parapsilosis* endocarditis. Recovery of the causative organism from an addict's own syringe. J.A.M.A. *243*:1073, 1980.
85. Hollway, H. D., Keipper, V., and Kaiser, A. B.: *Torulopsis glabrata* endocarditis. J.A.M.A. *140*:2088, 1980.
86. Hartley, R. A., Remsberg, J. R. S., and Sinaly, N. P.: *Histoplasma* endocarditis: Case report and review of the literature. Arch. Intern. Med. *119*: 527, 1967.
87. Baret, R. J., Prince, A. S., and Neu, H. C.: *Aspergillus* endocarditis in children: Case report and review of the literature. Pediatrics *68*:73, 1981.
88. Gaynes, R. P., Gardner, P., and Causey, W.: Prosthetic valve endocarditis caused by *Histoplasma capsulatum.* Arch. Intern. Med. *141*:1533, 1981.
89. Del Rossi, A. J., Morse, D., Spagna, P. M., and Lemole, G. M.: Succesful management of *Penicillium* endocarditis. J. Thorac. Cardiovasc. Surg. *80*:945, 1980.
90. Arnold, A. G., Gribbin, B., DeLeval, M., Macartney, F., and Slack, M.: *Trichosporon capitatum* causing recurrent fungal endocarditis Thorax *36*:478, 1981.
91. Tyras, D. H., Kaiser, G. C., Barnes, H. B., Laskowski, L. F., and Marr, J. J.: Atypical mycobacteria and the xenograft valve. J. Thorac. Cardiovasc. Surg. *75*:331, 1978.
92. Lohr, D. C., Goeken, J. A., Doty, D. B., and Donta, S.: *Mycobacterium gordonae* infection of a prosthetic valve. J.A.M.A. *239*:1528, 1978.
93. Baker, R. D.: Endocardial tuberculosis. Arch. Pathol. *19*:621, 1935.
94. Anyanwu, C. H., Nassau, E., and Yacoub, M.: Miliary tuberculosis following homograft valve replacement. Thorax *31*:101, 1976.
95. Tobin, M. J., Cahill, N., Geарty, G., Maurer, B., Blake, S., Daly, K., and Hone, R.: Q fever endocarditis. Am. J. Med. *72*:396, 1982.
96. Waters, E. W., Romansky, M. J., Johnson, A. C., and Conway, S. J.: *Actinomyces bovis* endocarditis: An uncommon and complex problem. *In* Sylvester, J. C. (ed.): Antimicrobial Agents and Chemotherapy — 1962. Proceedings of the Second Interscience Conference on Antimicrobial Agents and Chemotherapy. American Society of Microbiology, 1963, p. 517.
97. Vlachakis, N. D., Gazes, P. C., and Hairston, P.: Nocardial endocarditis following mitral valve replacement. Chest *63*:276, 1975.
98. Nastro, I. J., and Finegold, S. M.: Endocarditis due to anaerobic gram-negative bacilli. Am. J. Med. *54*:482, 1973.
99. Fredericka, D. N.: Endocarditis and brain abscess due to *Bacteroides oralis.* J. Infect. Dis. *145*:918, 1982.
100. Jones, R. B., Priest, J. B., and Kuo, C. C.: Subacute chlamydial endocarditis. J.A.M.A. *247*:655, 1982.
101. Van der Bel-Kahn, J. M., Watanakunakorn, C., Menefee, N. G., Long, H. D., and Dicter, R.: *Chlamydia trachomatis* endocarditis. Am. Heart J. *95*:627, 1978.
102. Mattman, L. H., and Mattman, P. E.: L-forms of *Streptococcus fecalis* in septicemia. Arch. Intern. Med. *115*:315, 1965.
103. Piepkorn, M. W., and Reichenbach, D. D.: Infective endocarditis associated with cell wall–deficient bacteria. Electron microscopic findings in four cases. Hum. Pathol. 9:163, 1978.
104. Dale, A. J., and Geraci, J. E.: Mixed cardiac valvular infections: Report of case and review of literature. Proc. Staff Meet. Mayo Clin. *36*:288, 1965.
105. Saravolatz, L. D., Burch, K. H., Quinn, E. L., et al.: Polymicrobial infective endocarditis. Am. Heart J. *95*:163, 1978.
106. Bharucha, P. E., and Nair, K. G.: Coxsackie B_1 endocarditis. Clin. Pediatr. *14*:188, 1975.
107. Sklaver, A. R., Hoffman, T. A., and Greenman, R. I.: Staphylococcal endocarditis in addicts. South. Med. J. *71*:638, 1978.
108. Reiner, N. E., Gopalakrishna, K. V., and Lerner, P. I.: Enterococcal endocarditis in heroin addicts. J.A.M.A. *235*:1861, 1976.
109. Dreyer, N. P., and Fields, B. N.: Heroin-associated infective endocarditis. Ann. Intern. Med. *78*:699, 1973.
110. Rosenblatt, J. E., Dahlgran, J. G., Fishback, R. S., and Talky, F. P.: Gram-negative bacterial endocarditis in narcotic addicts. Calif. Med. *118*:1, 1973.
111. Bailey, I. K., and Richards, J. G.: Infective endocarditis in a Sydney teaching hospital — 1962–1971. Aust. N. Z. Med. *5*:413, 1975.
112. Pankey, G. A.: The prevention and treatment of bacterial endocarditis. Am. Heart J. *98*:102, 1979.
113. Arnett, E. N., and Roberts, W. C.: Acute infective endocarditis: A clinicopathologic analysis of 137 necropsy patients. Curr. Probl. Cardiol. *1*:3, 1976.
114. Buchbinder, N. A., and Roberts, W. C.: Left-sided valvular active endocarditis. Am. J. Med. *53*:20, 1972.
115. Roberts, W. C., and Buchbinder, N. A.: Healed left-sided infective endocarditis. A clinicopathological study of 59 patients. Am. J. Cardiol. *40*:876, 1976.
116. Roberts, W. C., and Buchbinder, N. A.: Right-sided valvular infective endocarditis. Am. J. Med. *53*:7, 1972.
117. Arnett, E. N., and Roberts, W. C.: Prosthetic valve endocarditis. Clinicopathological analysis of 22 necropsy patients with comparison of observations in 74 necropsy patients with active infective endocarditis involving natural left-sided cardiac valves. Am. J. Cardiol. *38*:281, 1976.
118. Anderson, D. J., Buckley, B. H., and Hutchins, G. M.: A clinicopathologic study of prosthetic valve endocarditis in 22 patients: Morphologic basis for diagnosis and therapy. Am. Heart J. *94*:325, 1977.
119. Bortolotti, U., Thiene, G., Milano, A., Panizzon, G., Valente, M., and Gallucci, V.: Pathological study of infective endocarditis on Hancock porcine bioprostheses. J. Thorac. Cardiovasc. Surg. *81*:934–942, 1981.
120. Ferrans, V. J., Boyce, S. W., Billingham, M. E., Spray, T. L., and Roberts, W. C.: Infection of glutaraldehyde-preserved porcine valve heterografts. Am. J. Cardiol. *43*:1123–1135, 1979.
121. Everett, E. D., and Hirschman, J. V.: Transient bacteremia and endocarditis: A review. Medicine *56*:61, 1977.
122. Peterson, L. J., and Peacock, R.: The incidence of bacteremia in pediatric patients following tooth extraction. Circulation *53*:676, 1976.
123. Goodman, J. S., Kolhouse, J. F., and Koenig, M. G.: Recurrent endocarditis due to *Streptococcus viridans* in an edentulous" man. South. Med. J. *66*:352, 1973.
124. LeFrock, J. L., Klainer, A. S., Wu, W. H., and Turndorf, H.: Transient bacteremia associated with nasotracheal suctioning. J.A.M.A. *236*:1610, 1977.
125. LeFrock, J. L., Ellis, C. A., Klainer, A., and Weinstein, L.: Transient bacteremia associated with barium enema. Arch. Intern. Med. *135*:835, 1975.
126. LeFrock, J. L., Ellis, C. A., Turchik, J. B., and Weinstein, L.: Transient bacteremia associated with sigmoidoscopy. N. Engl. J. Med. *289*:469, 1973.
127. Shull, H. J., Green, B. M., Allen, S. R., Dunn, G. D., and Schenker, S.: Bacteremia with upper gastrointestinal endoscopy. Ann. Intern. Med. *83*:212, 1975.
128. Rafoth, A. J., Sorenson, R. M., and Bond, J. H.: Bacteremia following colonoscopy. Gastrointest. Endosc. *22*:32, 1975.
129. LeFrock, J. L., Ellis, C. A., Turchik, J. B., Zawacki, J. K., and Weinstein, L.: Transient bacteremia associated with percutaneous liver biopsy. J. Inf. Dis. *131* (Suppl.):104, 1975.
130. Sullivan, N. M., Sutter, V. L., Mims, M. M., Marsh, V. H., and Finegold, S. M.: Clinical aspects of bacteremia after manipulation of the genitourinary tract. J. Inf. Dis. *127*:49, 1973.
131. Ritvo, R., Monroe, P., and Andriole, V. T.: Transient bacteremia due to suction abortion. Implications for SBE prophylaxis. Yale J. Biol. Med. *50*:471, 1977.
132. Snyder, N., Atterbury, C. E., Correia, J. P., and Conn, H. F.: Increased concurrence of cirrhosis and bacterial endocarditis. Gastroenterology *73*:1107, 1977.
133. Baskin, T. W., Rosenthal, A., and Pruitt, B. A., Jr.: Acute bacterial endocarditis: A silent source of sepsis in the burn patient. Ann. Surg. *184*:618, 1976.
134. Lemire, G. G., Morin, J. E., and Dobell, A. R. C.: Pacemaker infections: A 12-year review. Can. J. Surg. *18*:181–184, 1975.
135. Garvey, G. J., and Neu, H. C.: Infective endocarditis — an envolving disease. A review of endocarditis at the Columbia-Presbyterian Medical Center, 1968–1973. Medicine *57*:105, 1978.
136. Rosen, P., and Armstrong, D.: Infective endocarditis in patients treated for malignant neoplastic disease. Am. J. Clin. Pathol. *60*:241, 1973.
137. Cross, A. S., and Steigbigel, R. T.: Infective endocarditis and access site infections in patients on hemodialysis. Medicine *55*:453, 1976.
138. Markowitz, S. M., Szentpetery, S., Lower, R. R., and Duma, R. J.: Endocarditis due to accidental penetrating foreign bodies. Am. J. Med. *60*:571, 1976.

UNDERLYING HEART DISEASE AND PATHOGENESIS

139. Gelfman, R., and Levine, S. A.: The incidence of acute and subacute bacterial endocarditis in congenital heart disease. Am. J. Med. Sci. *204*:324, 1942.
140. Johnson, C. M., and Rhodes, H. K.: Pediatric endocarditis. Mayo Clin. Proc. *57*:86–94, 1982.
141. McGuinness, G. A., Schieken, R. M., and Maguire, G. F.: Endocarditis in the newborn. Am. J. Dis. Child. *134*:577–580, 1980.
142. Shah, P., Singh, W. S. A., Rose, V., and Keith, J. D.: Incidence of bacterial endocarditis in ventricular septal defects. Circulation *34*:127, 1966.
143. Hallidie-Smith, K. A., Olsen, E. G. J., Oakley, C. M., Goodwin, J. F., and Cleland, W. P.: Ventricular septal defect and aortic regurgitation. Thorax *24*:257, 1969.
144. Blumenthal, S., Griffiths, S. P., and Morgan, B. C.: Bacterial endocarditis in children with heart disease. Pediatrics *26*:933, 1960.
145. Rodbard, S.: Blood velocity and endocarditis. Circulation *27*:18, 1963.
146. Glenn, F., Stewart, H. J., Engle, M. A., Lukas, D. S., Artusio, J., Steinberg, I. S., and Holswade, G. R.: Coarctation of aorta complicated by bacterial endocarditis and an aneurysm of the sinus of Valsalva. Circulation *17*:432, 1958.

147. Korn, D., DeSanctis, R. W., and Sell, S.: Massive calcification of the mitral annulus: a clinicopathologic study of fourteen cases. N. Engl. J. Med. *267*:900, 1962.
148. Watanakunakorn, C.: *Staphylococcus aureus* endocarditis on the calcified mitral annulus fibrosus. Am. J. Med. Sci. *266*:219, 1973.
149. Chagnac, A., Rudniki, C., and Loebel, H.: Infectious endocarditis in idiopathic hypertrophic subaortic stenosis. Report of three cases and review of the literature. Chest *81*:346–349, 1982.
150. Wang, K., Gobel, F. L., and Gleason, D. F.: Bacterial endocarditis in idiopathic hypertrophic subacute stenosis. Am. Heart J. *89*:359, 1975.
151. Soman, V. R., Breton, G., Hershkowitz, M., and Mark, H.: Bacterial endocarditis of mitral valve in Marfan's syndrome. Br. Heart J. *36*:1247, 1974.
152. Lachman, A. S., Branwell-Jones, D. M., Lakier, J. B., Pocock, W. A., and Barlow, J. B.: Infective endocarditis in the billowing mitral leaflet syndrome. Br. Heart J. *37*:326, 1975.
152a. Clemens, J. E., Horowitz, R. I., Jaff ee, C. C., Feinstein, A. R., and Stanton, B. F.: A controlled evaluation of the risk of bacterial endocarditis in persons with mitral valve prolapse. N. Engl. J. Med. *307*:776, 1982.
153. Nolan, C. M., Kane, J. J., and Grunow, W. A.: Infective endocarditis and mitral prolapse. A comparison with other types of endocarditis. Arch. Intern. Med. *141*:447–450, 1981.
154. Amoury, R. A., Bowman, F. O., Jr., and Malm, J. R.: Endocarditis associated with intracardiac prostheses. J. Thorac. Cardiovasc. Surg. *51*:36, 1966.
155. Yeh, T. J., Anabtani, I. N., Cornett, V. E., White, A., Stern, W. H., and Ellison, R. G.: Bacterial endocarditis following open-heart surgery. Ann. Thorac. Surg. *3*:29, 1967.
156. Stein, P. D., Harken, D. E., and Dexter, L.: The nature and prevention of prosthetic valve endocarditis. Am. Heart J. *71*:393, 1966.
157. Wilson, W. R., Jaumun, P. M., Danielson, G. K., Giuliani, E. R., Washington, J. A., III, and Geraci, J. E.: Prosthetic valve endocarditis. Ann. Intern. Med. *82*:751, 1975.
158. Sande, M. A., Johnson, W. D., Jr., Hook, E. W., and Kaye, D.: Sustained bacteremia in patients with prosthetic valves. N. Engl. J. Med. *286*:1067, 1972.
159. Weinstein, L.: Infected prosthetic valves: A diagnostic and therepeutic dilemma. N. Engl. J. Med. *286*:1108, 1972.
160. Starkebaum, M., Durack, D., and Beeson, P.: The "incubation period" of subacute bacterial endocarditis. Yale J. Biol. Med. *50*:49–58, 1977.
161. Kaplan, E., Helmsworth, J. A., Ahearn, E. N., Benzing, G., III, Daoud, G., and Schwartz, D. C.: Results of palliative procedures for tetralogy of Fallot in infants and young children. Ann. Thorac. Surg. *5*:489, 1968.
162. Persuad, V.: Two unusual cases of mural endocarditis with a review of the literature. Am. J. Clin. Pathol. *53*:832, 1970.
163. Graham, H. V., von Hartitzch, B., and Medina, J. R.: Infected atrial myxoma. Am. J. Cardiol. *38*:658, 1976.
164. Rogers, E. W., Weyman, A. E., Nobel, R. J., and Burns, S. C.: Left atrial myxoma infected with *Histoplasma capsulatum*. Am. J. Med. *64*:683, 1978.
165. Lepeschkin, E.: On the relation between the site of valvular involvement in endocarditis and the blood pressure resting on the valve. Am. J. Med. Sci. *224*:318, 1952.
166. Allen, A. C.: Mechanism of localization of vegetations of bacterial endocarditis. Arch. Pathol. *27*:399, 1939.
167. Wadsworth, A. B.: A study of the endocardial lesions developing during pneumococcus infection in horses. J. Med. Res. *34*:279, 1919.
168. Gould, K., Ramirez-Ronda, C. H., Holmes, R. K., and Sanford, J. P.: Adherence of bacteria to heart valves *in vitro*. J. Clin. Invest. *56*:1364, 1975.
169. Holmes, R. K., and Ramirez-Ronda, C. H.: Adherence of bacteria to the endothelium of heart valves. Infective Endocarditis, an American Heart Association Monograph. No. 52, 1977, pp. 12–13.

CLINICAL MANIFESTATIONS

170. Weinstein, L., and Schlesinger, J. J.: Pathoanatomic, pathophysiologic and clinical correlations in endocarditis. N. Engl. J. Med. *291*:832, 1122, 1974.
171. Libman, E., and Friedberg, C. K.: Subacute Bacterial Endocarditis. 2nd ed. New York, Oxford University Press, 1948.
172. Weinstein, L., and Rubin, R. H.: Infective endocarditis—1973. Progr. Cardiovasc. Dis. *16*:239, 1973.
173. Weinstein, L.: Infective endocarditis: Past, present and future. J. R. Coll. Phys. Lond. *6*:161, 1972.
174. Weinstein, L.: Modern infective endocarditis. J.A.M.A. *233*:260, 1975.
175. Pankey, G. A.: Acute bacterial endocarditis at University of Minnesota Hospitals, 1939–1959. Am. Heart J. *64*:583, 1962.
176. Willerson, J. T., Moellering, R. C., Jr., Buckley, M. J., and Austen, W. G.: Conjunctival petechiae after open-heart surgery. N. Engl. J. Med. *284*:539, 1971.
177. Kilpatrick, Z. M., Greenberg, P. A., and Sanford, J. P.: Splinter hemorrhages —their clinical significance. Arch. Intern. Med. *115*:730, 1965.
178. Roth, M.: Ueber Netzhautaffectionen bei Wundfiebern. Dtsch. Z. Chir. *1*:471, 1872.
179. Litten, M.: Ueber akute maligne Endocarditis und die dabei vorkommender Retinalveränderungen. Charit. Ann. *3*:137, 1878.
180. Doherty, W. B., and Trubek, M.: Significant hemorrhagic retinal lesions in bacterial endocarditis (Roth's spots). J.A.M.A. *97*:308, 1931.
181. Libman, E.: The clinical features of cases of subacute bacterial endocarditis that have spontaneously become bacteria-free. Am. J. Med. Sci. *146*:625, 1913.
182. Mills, J., Utley, J., and Abbott, J.: Heart failure in infective endocarditis: Predisposing factors, course and treatment. Chest *66*:151, 1974.
183. Gonzalez-Lavin, L., Lise, M., and Ross, D.: The importance of the "jet lesion" in bacterial endocarditis involving the left heart: Surgical considerations. J. Thorac. Cardiovasc. Surg. *59*:185, 1970.
184. Roberts, W. C., Ewy, G. A., Glancy, D. L., and Marcus, F. I.: Valvular stenosis produced by active infective endocarditis. Circulation *36*:449, 1967.
185. Sacks, P. V., Lakier, J. B., and Barlow, J. B.: Severe aortic stenosis produced by bacterial endocarditis. Br. Med. J. *3*:97, 1969.
186. Mann, T., McLaurin, L., Grossman, W., and Graige, E. E.: Assessing the hemodynamic severity of acute regurgitation due to infective endocarditis. N. Engl. J. Med. *293*:108, 1975.
187. Roberts, N. K., and Somerville, J.: Pathological significance of electrocardiographic changes in aortic valve endocarditis. Br. Heart J. *31*:395, 1969.
188. Gopalakrishna, K. V., Kwan, K., and Shah, A.: Metastatic myocardial abscess due to group F streptococci. Am. J. Med. Sci. *274*:329, 1977.
189. Kim, H-S., Weilbacher, D. G., Lie, J. T., and Titus, J. L.: Myocardial abscesses. Am. J. Clin. Pathol. *70*:18, 1978.
190. Arnett, E. N., and Roberts, W. C.: Valve ring abscess in active infective endocarditis. Frequency, location and clues to clinical diagnosis from the study of 95 necropsy patients. Circulation *54*:140, 1976.
191. Perry, E. L., Fleming, R. G., and Edwards, J. E.: Myocardial lesions in subacute bacterial endocarditis. Ann. Intern. Med. *36*:126, 1952.
192. Blankenhorn, M. A., and Gall, E. A.: Myocarditis and myocardiosis: Clinicopathologic appraisal. Circulation *13*:217, 1956.
193. Vogler, W. R., and Dorney, E. R.: Bacterial endocarditis in congenital heart disease. Am. Heart J. *64*:198, 1962.
194. Bell, E. T.: Glomerular lesions associated with endocarditis. Am. J. Pathol. *8*:639, 1932.
195. Pfeifer, J. F., Lipton, M. J., Oury, J. H., Angell, W. W., and Hulgren, H. N.: Acute coronary embolism complicating bacterial endocarditis: Operative treatment. Am. J. Cardiol. *37*:920, 1976.
196. Menzies, C. J. G.: Coronary embolism with infarction in bacterial endocarditis. Br. Heart J. *23*:464, 1961.
197. Brunson, J. G.: Coronary embolism in bacterial endocarditis. Am. J. Pathol. *29*:689, 1953.
198. Horder, T. J.: Infective endocarditis: With an analysis of 150 cases and with special reference to the chronic form of the disease. Q. J. Med. *2*:289, 1909.
199. Jochman, G.: Lehrbuch der Infektionskrankheiten für Ärtze und Studierende. Berlin, Julius Springer, 1914, pp. 144–148.
200. McDevitt, E.: Treatment of cerebral embolism. Mod. Treat. *2*:52, 1965.
201. Harrington, A. W.: Embolism of the spinal cord. Glasgow Med. J. *103*:28, 1925.
202. Harrison, M. J. G., and Hampton, J. R.: Neurological presentation of bacterial endocarditis. Br. Med. J. *2*:148, 1967.
203. Kernohan, J. W., Woltman, H. W., and Barnes, A. R.: Involvement of the nervous system associated with endocarditis: Neuropsychiatric and neuropathological observations in forty-two cases of fatal outcome. Arch. Neurol. Psych. *42*:789, 1939.
204. Jones, H. R., Jr., and Siekert, R. G.: Embolic mononeuropathy and bacterial endocarditis. Arch. Neurol. *19*:535, 1968.
205. Schocket, S., and Braver, D.: Cilioretinal artery occlusion in a patient with suspected bacterial endocarditis. South. Med. J. *63*:1, 1970.
206. Roach, M. R., and Drake, C. G.: Ruptured cerebral aneurysms caused by microorganisms. N. Engl. J. Med. *273*:240, 1963.
207. Kauffman, S. L., Lynfield, J., and Hennigar, G. R.: Mycotic aneurysms of the intrapulmonary arteries. Circulation *35*:90, 1967.
208. Ziment, I.: Nervous system complications in bacterial endocarditis. Am. J. Med. *47*:593, 1969.
209. Pruitt, A. A., Rubin, R. H., Karchmer, A. W., and Duncan, G. W.: Neurologic complications of bacterial endocarditis. Medicine *57*:329, 1978.
210. Bohmfalk, G. L., Story, J. L., Wissinger, J. P., and Brown, W. E.: Bacterial intracranial aneurysm. J. Neurosurg. *48*:369, 1978.
211. Churchill, M. A., Geraci, J. E., and Hunder, G. G.: Musculoskeletal manifestations of bacterial endocarditis. Ann. Intern. Med. *87*:754, 1977.
212. Baehr, G.: Renal complications of endocarditis. Trans. Assoc. Am. Phys. *46*:87, 1931.
213. Villarreal, H., and Sokoloff, L.: The occurrence of renal insufficiency in subacute bacterial endocarditis. Am. J. Med. Sci. *220*:655, 1950.
214. Cordeiro, A., Costa, H., and Lagenha, F.: Editorial. Immunologic phase of subacute bacterial endocarditis. A new concept and general considerations. Am. J. Cardiol. *16*:477, 1965.
215. Williams, R. C., and Kunkel, H. G.: Rheumatoid factor, complement and conglutinin aberrations in patients with subacute bacterial endocarditis, J. Clin. Invest. *41*:666, 1962.
216. Williams, R. C.: Bacterial endocarditis—an analysis of immunopathology of infective endocarditis. An American Heart Association Symposium (No. 52) 1977, pp. 20–23.
217. Sheagren, J. N., Tuazon, C., Griffin, C., and Padmore, N.: Rheumatoid factor in acute bacterial endocarditis. Arthritis Rheum. *19*:887, 1976.
218. Bayer, A. S., Theofilopoulos, A. N., Eisenberg, R., Dixon, F. J., and Guze, J. B.: Circulating immune complexes in infective endocarditis. N. Engl. J. Med. *295*:1500, 1976.
219. McKenzie, P. E., Hawke, D., Woodroffe, A. J., Thompson, A. J., Seymour, A. E., and Clarkson, A. R.: Serum and tissue immune complexes in infective endocarditis. J. Clin. Lab. Immunol., *4*:125–132, 1980.

220. Kauffman, R. H., Thompson, J., Valentijn, R. M., et al.: The clinical implications and the pathogenetic significance of circulating immune complexes in infective endocarditis. Am. J. Med. *71*:17–25, 1981.
221. Howard, E. J.: Osler's nodes. Am. Heart J. *59*:633, 1960.
222. Alpert, J. S., Krous, H. F., Dalen, J. E., O'Rourke, R. A., and Bloor, C. M.: Pathogenesis of Osler's nodes. Ann. Intern. Med. *85*:471, 1976.
223. Davis, J. A., Weisman, M. H., and Dail, D. H.: Vascular disease in infective endocarditis: Report of immune-mediated events in skin and brain. Arch. Intern. Med. *138*:480, 1978.
224. Rubenfeld, S., and Kyung-Whan, M.: Leucocytoclastic angiitis in subacute bacterial endocarditis. Arch. Dermatol. *113*:1073, 1977.
225. Tu, W. H., Shearn, M. A., and Lee, J. C.: Acute diffuse glomerulonephritis in acute staphylococcal endocarditis. Ann. Intern. Med. *71*:335, 1969.
226. Gutman, R. A., Striker, G. E., Gilliland, B. C., and Cutler, R. E.: The immune complex glomerulonephritis of bacterial endocarditis. Medicine *51*:1, 1972.
227. Levy, R. L., and Hong, R.: The immune nature of subacute bacterial endocarditis (SBE) nephritis. Am. J. Med. *64*:645, 1973.
228. Keslin, M. H., Messner, R. P., and Williams, R. C., Jr.: Glomerulonephritis with subacute bacterial endocarditis. Arch. Intern. Med. *132*:578, 1973.
229. Bain, R. C., Edwards, J. E., Scheiffey, C. H., and Geraci, J. E.: Right-sided bacterial endocarditis and endarteritis: Clinical and pathologic study. Am. J. Med. *24*:98, 1958.
230. Bashour, F. A., and Winchell, C. P.: Right-sided bacterial endocarditis. Am. J. Med. Sci. *240*:411, 1960.
231. Altschule, M. D.: Subacute bacterial endocarditis of the right heart. Med. Sci. *15*:50, 1964.
232. Zakrzewski, T., and Keith, J.: Bacterial endocarditis in infants and children. J. Pediatr. *67*:1179, 1965.
233. Johnson, D H., Rosenthal, A., and Nadas, A. S.: A forty-year review of bacterial endocarditis in infancy and childhood. Circulation *51*:581, 1975.
234. Mendelsohn, G., and Hutchins, G. M.: Infective endocarditis during the first decade of life. Am. J. Dis. Child. *133*:619, 1979.
235. Welton, D. E., Young, J. B., Gentry, W. O., Raizner, A. E., Alexander, J. K., Chahine, R. A., and Miller, R. R.: Recurrent infective endocarditis. Am. J. Med. *66*:932, 1979.
236. Pankey, G. A.: The prevention and treatment of bacterial endocarditis. Am. Heart J. *98*:102, 1979.
237. Beeson, P. B., Brannon, E. S., and Warren, J. V.: Observations on the sites of removal of bacteria from the blood in patients with bacterial endocarditis. J. Exp. Med. *81*:9, 1945.
238. Mallen, M. S., Hube, E. L., and Brenes, M.: Comparative study of blood cultures made from artery, vein and bone marrow in patients with subacute bacterial endocarditis. Am. Heart J. *33*:692, 1947.
239. Werner, A. S., Cobbs, C. G., Kaye, D., and Hook, E. W.: Studies on the bacteremia of bacterial endocarditis. J.A.M.A. *202*:127, 1967.
240. Kelson, S. E., and White, P. D.: Notes on 250 cases of subacute bacterial (streptococcal) endocarditis studied and treated between 1927 and 1929. Ann. Intern. Med. *22*:40, 1945.
241. Belli, J., and Waisbren, B. A.: The number of blood cultures necessary to diagnose most cases of bacterial endocarditis. Am. J. Med. Sci. *232*:284, 1956.
242. Pazan, G. J., Person, K. L., Guff, F. W., Shaver, J. A., and Ho, M.: Determination of site of infection in endocarditis. Ann. Intern. Med. *82*:746, 1975.
243. Cannady, P. B., Jr., and Sandford, J. P.: Negative blood cultures in infective endocarditis: A review. South. Med. J. *69*:1420, 1976.
244. Pesanti, E. L., and Smith, I. M.: Infective endocarditis with negative blood cultures. An analysis of 52 cases. Am. J. Med. *66*:43, 1979.
245. Pazin, G. J., Saul, S., and Thompson, M. E.: Blood culture positivity. Suppression by outpatient antibiotic therapy in patients with bacterial endocarditis. Arch. Intern. Med. *142*:263, 1982.
246. Van Scoy, R. E.: Culture-negative endocarditis. Mayo Clin. Proc. *57*:149, 1982.
247. Weinstein, L., Daikos, G., and Perrin, T. S.: Studies on the relationship of tissue fluid and blood levels of penicillin. J. Lab. Clin. Med. *38*:715, 1951.
248. Barza, M., Samuelson, T., and Weinstein, L.: Penetration of antibiotics into fabrin loci *in vivo*: II. Comparison of nine antibiotics: Effect of dose and degree of protein binding. J. Inf. Dis. *129*:66, 1974.
249. Nagel, J. G., Tuazon, C. U., Cardella, T. A., and Sheagren, J. N.: Teichoic acid serologic diagnosis of staphylococcal endocarditis. Use of gel diffusion and counterimmunoelectrophoretic methods. Ann. Intern. Med. *82*:13, 1975.
250. Wheat, L. J., Kohler, R. B., Tabarah, Z. A., and White, A.: IgM antibody response to staphylococeal infection. J. Infect. Dis. *144*:307, 1981.
251. Zeiger, A. R., Tuazon, C. U., and Sheagren, J. N.: Antibody levels to bacterial peptidoglycan in human sera during the time course of endocarditis and bacteremic infections caused by *Staphylococcus aureus*. Infect. Immun. *33* (Suppl.):795, 1981.
252. Seelig, M. S., Speth, C. P., Kozinn, P. J., Taschdjian, C. L., Toni, E. F., and Goldberg, P.: Patterns of *Candida* endocarditis following cardiac surgery: Importance of early diagnosis and therapy (an analysis of 91 cases). Progr. Cardiovasc. Dis. *17*:125, 1974.
253. Parsons, E. R., and Nassau, E.: *Candida* serolo gy in open-heart surgery. J. Med. Microbiol. *7*:415, 1974.
254. Scheld, W. M., Brown, R. S., Jr., Harding, S. A., and Sande, M. A.: Detection of circulating antigen in experimental *Candida albicans* endocarditis by an enzyme-linked immunoabsorbent assay. J. Clin. Microbiol. *12*:679, 1980.
255. Wiseman, J., Rouleau, J., Rigo, P., Strauss, H. W., and Pitt, B.: Gallium-67 myocardial imaging for the detection of bacterial endocarditis. Radiology, *120*:135, 1976.
256. Spies, S. M., Myers, S. M., Barresi, V., Grais, I. M., and DeBoer, A.: A case of myocardial abscess evaluated by radionuclide techniques: A case report. J. Nucl. Med. *18*:1089, 1977.
257. Miller, M. H., and Casey, J. I.: Infective endocarditis: New diagnostic techniques. Am. Heart J. *96*:123, 1978.
258. Ellis, K., Jaffe, C., Malm, J. R., and Bowman, F. O., Jr.: Infective endocarditis: Roentgenographic considerations. Radiol. Clin. North Am. *11*:415, 1973.
259. Stewart, J. A., Silimperi, D., Harris, P., Wise, N. K., Fraker, T. D., Jr., and Kisslo, J. A.: Echocardiographic documentation of vegetative lesions in infective endocarditis: Clinical implications. Circulation *61*:374, 1980.
260. Fox, S., Kotler, M. N., Segal, B. L., and Parry, W.: Echocardiographic diagnosis of acute aortic valve endocarditis. Arch. Intern. Med. *137*:85, 1977.
261. Berger, M., Gallerstein, P. E., Benhuri, P., Balla, R., and Goldberg, E.: Evaluation of aortic valve endocarditis by two-dimensional echocardiography. Chest *80*:61, 1981.
262. Nakamura, K., Suzuki, S., Satomi, G., Hayashi, H., and Hirosawa, K.: Detection of mitral ring abscess by two-dimensional echocardiography. Circulation *65*:816, 1982.
263. Wong, A. M., Oldershaw, P., and Gibson, D. G.: Echocardiographic demonstration of aortic root abscess after infective endocarditis. Br. Heart J. *46*:584, 1981.
264. Scanlan, J. G., Seward, J. B., and Tajik, A. J.: Valve ring abscess in infective endocarditis: Visualization with wide-angle two-dimensional echocardiography. Am. J. Cardiol. *49*:1794, 1982.
265. Andy, J. J., Sheikh, M. U., Nayab, A., Barores, B. O., Fox, L. M., Curry, C. L., and Roberts, W. C.: Echocardiographic observations in opiate addicts with infective endocarditis. Am. J. Cardiol. *40*:17, 1977.
266. Berger, M., Delfin, L. A., Helveh, M., and Goldberg, E.: Two-dimensional echocardiographic findings in right-sided infective endocarditis. Circulation *61*:855, 1980.
267. Dander, B., Richetti, B., and Poppi, B.: Echocardiographic diagnosis of isolated pulmonary valve endocarditis. Br. Heart J. *47*:298, 1982.
268. Gomes, J. A., Calderon, J., Lajam, F., Sakurai, H., Friedman, H. S., and Tatz, J. S.: Echocardiographic detection of fungal vegetations in *Candida parapsilosis* endocarditis. Am. J. Med. *61*:273, 1976.
269. Stewart, J. A., Silimperi, D., Harris, P., Wise, N. K., Fraker, T. D., and Kisslo, J. A.: Echocardiographic documentation of vegetative lesions in infective endocarditis: Clinical implications. Circulation *61*:374, 1980.
270. Martin, R. P., Meltzer, R. S., Louria, B., Stinson, B., Stinson, E. B., Makowski, H., and Popp, R. L.: Clinical utility of two-dimensional echocardiography in infective endocarditis. Am. J. Cardiol. *46*:379, 1980.
271. Hickey, A. J., Wolfers, J., and Wilcken, D. E. L.: Reliability and clinical relevance of detection of vegetations by echocardiography in bacterial endocarditis. Br. Heart J. *46*:624, 1981.
272. Markiewicz, W., Peled, B., Alroy, G., Pollack, S., Brook, G., Rapoport, J., and Kerner, H.: Echocardiography in infective endocarditis. Lack of specificity in patients with valvular pathology. Eur. J. Cardiol. *10*:247, 1979.
273. Rubenson, D. A., Tucker, C. R., Stinson, E. B., London, E. J., Oyer, P., Moreno-Cabral, R., and Popp, R. L.: The use of echocardiography in diagnosing culture-negative endocarditis. Circulation *64*:641, 1981.
274. Dillon, T., Meyer, R. A., Korfhagen, J. C., Kaplan, S., and Chung, K. J.: Management of infective endocarditis using endocardiography. J. Pediatr. *96*:552, 1980.
275. Strom, J., Becker, R., Davis, R., Matsomoto, M., Frishman, W., Sonnenblick, E. H., and Frater, R. W. M.: Echocardiographic and surgical correlations in bacterial endocarditis. Circulation *62*:164, 1980.

MANAGEMENT

276. Weinstein, L., and Dalton, A. C.: Host determinants of response to antimicrobial agents. N. Engl. J. Med. *279*:467, 524, 580, 1968.
277. Schlichter, J. G., MacLean, H., and Milzer, A.: Effective penicillin therapy in subacute bacterial endocarditis and other chronic infections. Am. J. Med. Sci. *217*:600, 1949.
278. Hall, B., and Dowling, H. F.: Negative blood cultures in bacterial endocarditis: A decade's experience. Med. Clin. North Am. *50*:159, 1966.
279. Cooper, R., and Mills, J.: Serratia endocarditis. A follow-up report. Arch. Intern. Med. *140*:199, 1980.
280. Barza, M., Brusch, J., Bergeron, M. G., and Weinstein, L.: Penetration of antibiotics into fibrin loci *in vivo*. III. Intermittent versus continuous infusion and effect of probenecid. J. Inf. Dis. *129*:73, 1974.
281. Weinstein, L., Goldfield, M., and Chang, T-W.: Infections occurring during chemotherapy: A study of their frequency, type and predisposing factors. N. Engl. J. Med. *251*:247, 1954.
282. Tan, J. S., Kaplan, S., Terhune, C. A., Jr., and Hamburger, M.: Successful two-week treatment schedule for penicillin-susceptible *Streptococcus viridans* endocarditis. Lancet *2*:1340, 1971.
283. Walker, W. F., and Hamburger, M.: Penicillin-sensitive streptococcal endocarditis. Arch. Intern. Med. *100*:359, 1957.
284. Goodman, S., Berry, R. H., Benjamin, J. E., Schiro, H. S., and Hamburger, M.: Subacute bacterial endocarditis treated with oral penicillin. Arch. Intern. Med. *104*:625, 1959.

285. Hamburger, M., Kaplan, S., and Walker, W. F.: Subacute bacterial endocarditis caused by penicillin-sensitive streptococci. J.A.M.A. *175*:554, 1961.
286. Burman, N. D., Joffe, H. S., and Watson, C.: Oral antibiotic cure of staphylococcal endocarditis. Postgrad. Med. J. *49*:920, 1973.
287. Phillips, B., and Watson, G. H.: Oral treatment of subacute bacterial endocarditis in children. Arch. Dis. Child. *52*:235, 1977.
288. Weinstein, L., and Schlesinger, J.: Treatment of infective endocarditis—1973. Progr. Cardiovasc. Dis. *6*:275, 1973.
289. Kanis, J. A.: The use of anticoagulants in bacterial endocarditis. Postgrad. Med. J. *50*:312, 1974.
290. Wolfe, J. C., and Johnson, W. D.: Penicillin-sensitive streptococcal endocarditis. *In vitro* and clinical observations on penicillin-streptomycin therapy. Ann. Intern. Med. *81*:178, 1974.
291. Karchmer, A. W., Moellering, R. C., Jr., Maki, D. G., and Swartz, M. N.: Single-antibiotic therapy for streptococcal endocarditis. J.A.M.A. *241*:1801, 1979.
292. Malacoff, R. F., Frank, E., and Andriole, V. T.: Streptococcal endocarditis (nonenterococcal, non-group A). J.A.M.A. *241*:1807, 1979.
293. Quinn, E. L., Pohlod, D., Madhaven, T., Burch, K., Fisher, E., and Cox, F.: Clinical experience with cefazolin and other cephalosporins in bacterial endocarditis. J. Inf. Dis. *128* (Suppl.):S386, 1973.
294. Bryant, R. E., and Alford, R. H.: Unsuccessful treatment of staphylococcal endocarditis with cefazolin. J.A.M.A. *237*:569, 1977.
295. Geraci, J. E., and Wilson, W. R.: Vancomycin therapy for infective endocarditis. Rev. Infect. Dis. *3*:S250, 1981.
296. Hinthom, D. R., Baker, L. H., Romig, D. A., Voth, D. W., and Liu, C.: Endocarditis treated with clindamycin: Relapse and liver dysfunction. South. Med. J. *70*:823, 1977.
297. Hunter, T. H.: Use of streptomycin in the treatment of bacterial endocarditis. Am. J. Med. *2*:436, 1974.
298. Moellering, R. C., Jr., and Weinberg, A. N.: Studies on antibiotic synergism against enterococci. J. Clin. Invest. *50*:2580, 1971.
299. Standiford, H. D., de Maine, J. B., and Kirby, W. M. M.: Antibiotic synergism of enterococci. Arch. Intern. Med. *126*:255, 1970.
300. Moellering, R. C., Jr., Wennersten, C., and Weinberg, A. N.: Synergy of penicillin and gentamicin against enterococci. J. Infect. Dis. *124* (Suppl.):207, 1971.
301. Carey, R. A., Brause, B. D., and Roberts, R. B.: Antimicrobial therapy of vitamin B_6-dependent streptococcal endocarditis. Arch. Intern. Med. *87*:150, 1977.
302. Thornsberry, C., Baker, C. N., and Facklain, R. R.: Antibiotic susceptibility of *Streptococcus bovis* and other group D causing endocarditis. Antimicrob. Agents Chemother. *5*:228, 1974.
303. Weinstein, L., Lerner, P. I., and Chew, W. H.: Clinical and bacteriologic studies of the effect of massive doses of penicillin G on infections caused by gram-negative bacilli. N. Engl. J. Med. *271*:525, 1964.
304. Smith, H., Lerner, P. I., and Weinstein, L.: Neurotoxicity and "massive" intravenous therapy with penicillin. Arch. Intern. Med. *120*:47, 1967.
305. Watanakunakorn, C., and Baird, I. M.: Prognostic factors in *Staphylococcus aureus* endocarditis and results of therapy with penicillin and gentamicin. Am. J. Med. Sci. *273*:133, 1977.
306. Abrams, B., Sklaver, A., Hoffman, T., and Greenman, R.: Single or combination therapy of staphylococcal endocarditis in intravenous drug abusers. Ann. Intern. Med. *90*:789, 1979.
307. Gopal, V., Bisno, A. L., and Silverblatt, F. J.: Failure of vancomycin treatment in *Staphylococcus aureus* endocarditis. J.A.M.A. *236*:1604, 1976.
308. Menda, K. B., and Gorbach, S. L.: Favorable experience with bacterial endocarditis in heroin addicts. Ann. Intern. Med. *78*:25, 1973.
309. Mayrer, A. R., Brown, A., Weintraub, R. A., Ragni, M., and Postic, B.: Successful medical therapy for endocarditis due to *Candida parapsilosis.* Chest *73*:546, 1978.
310. Kay, J. H., Bernstein, S., Feinstein, D., and Biddle, M.: Surgical cure of *Candida albicans* endocarditis with open heart surgery. N. Engl. J. Med. *264*:907, 1961.
311. Kay, J. H., Bernstein, S., Tsuji, H. K., Redington, J. V., Milgram, M., and Brem, T.: Surgical treatment of *Candida* endocarditis. J.A.M.A. *203*:621, 1968.
312. Arbulu, A., Thomas, N. W., and Wilson, R. F.: Valvulectomy without prosthetic replacement. A life-saving operation for tricuspid *Pseudomonas* endocarditis. J. Thorac. Cardiovasc. Surg. *64*:103, 1972.
313. Bindschadler, D. D., and Bennett, J. E.: A pharmacologic guide to the clinical use of amphotericin B. J. Inf. Dis. *120*:427, 1969.
314. Drutz, D. J., Spickard, A., Rogers, D. E., and Koenig, M. G.: Treatment of disseminated mycotic infections: A new approach to amphotericin B therapy. Am. J. Med. *45*:405, 1968.
315. Fass, R. J., and Perkins, R. L.: 5-Fluorocytosine in the treatment of cryptococcal and *Candida* mycoses. Ann. Intern. Med. *74*:535, 1971.
316. Vandevelde, A. G., Mauceri, A. A., and Johnson, J. E., III: 5-Fluorocytosine in the treatment of mycotic infections. Ann. Intern. Med. *77*:43, 1972.
317. Record, C. O., Skinner, J. M., Sleight, P., and Speller, D. C. E.: *Candida* endocarditis treated with 5-fluorocytosine. Br. Med. J. *1*:262, 1971.
318. Galgiani, J. N., and Stevens, D. A.: Fungal endocarditis: Need for guidelines in evaluating therapy. J. Thorac. Cardiovasc. Surg. *73*:293, 1977.
319. Touroff, A. S. W., and Vessell, H.: Subacute *Streptococcus viridans* endarteritis complicating patent ductus arteriosus. J.A.M.A. *115*:1270, 1940.
319a. Croft, C.H., Woodward, W., Elliott, A., Commerford, P. J., Barnard, C. N., and Beck, W.: Analysis of surgical versus medical therapy in active complicated native valve infective endocarditis Am. J. Cardiol. *51*:1650, 1983.
320. Hancock, E. W., Shumway, N. E., and Remington, J. S.: Valve replacement in active bacterial endocarditis. J. Infect. Dis. *123*:106, 1971.
321. Kaiser, G. C., Williams, V. L., Thurmann, M., and Hanlon, C. R.: Valve replacement in cases of aortic insufficiency due to active endocarditis. J. Thorac. Cardiovasc. Surg. *54*:491, 1967.
322. Wise, J. R., Jr., Cleland, W. P., Halldie-Smith, K. A., Bentall, H. H., Goodwin, J. F., and Oakley, C. M.: Urgent aortic-valve replacement for acute aortic regurgitation due to infective endocarditis. Lancet *2*:115, 1971.
323. Robicsek, F., Payne, R. B., Daugherty, H. K., and Sanger, P. W.: Bacterial endocarditis of the mitral valve treated by excision and replacement. Ann. Surg. *166*:854, 1967.
324. Khonsari, S., Bahabozurgui, S., Cook, W. A., and Frater, R. W. M.: Urgent open-heart surgery for endocarditis of mitral valve. N.Y. State J. Med. *71*:2650, 1971.
325. Jung, J. Y., Saab, S. B., and Almond, C. H.: The case for early surgical treatment of left-sided primary infective endocarditis. A collective review. J. Thorac. Cardiovasc. Surg. *70*:509, 1975.
326. Stinson, E. B., Griepp, R. B., Vosti, K., Copeland, J. G., and Shumway, N. E.: Operation treatment of active endocarditis. J. Thorac. Cardiovasc. Surg. *71*:659, 1976.
327. Wise, J. R., Jr., Cleland, W. P., Haldie-Smith, K. A., et al.: Urgent aortic-valve replacement for acute regurgitation due to infective endocarditis. Lancet *2*:115, 1971.
328. Fowler, N. O., Hamgurger, M. H., and Bove, K. E.: Aortic valve perforation. Am. J. Med. *42*:539, 1967.
329. Griffin, F. M., Jr., Jones, G., and Cobbs, C. G.: Aortic insufficiency in bacterial endocarditis. Ann. Intern. Med. *76*:23, 1972.
330. Robinson, M. J., Greenberg, J. J., Korn, M., and Rywlin, A. M.: Infective endocarditis at autopsy: 1965–1969. Am. J. Med. *52*:492, 1972.
331. Walker, S. R., Shumway, N. E., and Merigan, T. C.: Man agement of infected cardiac valve prostheses. J.A.M.A. *208*:531, 1969.
332. Watanakunakorn, C., and Hamburger, M.: *Staphylococcus epidermidis* endocarditis complicating a Starr-Edwards prosthesis: A therapeutic dilemma. Arch. Intern. Med. *126*:1014, 1970.
333. Okies, J. E., Viroslav, J., and Williams, T. W., Jr.: Endocarditis after cardiac valve replacement. Chest *59*:198, 1971.
334. Block, P. C., DeSanctis, R. W., Weinberg, A. N., and Austen, W. G.: Prosthetic valve endocarditis. J. Thorac. Cardiovasc. Surg. *60*:540, 1970.
335. Dorney, E. R., and King, S. R.: Bacterial endocarditis following prosthetic valve surgery: Early and late occurrence. Circulation *41* (Suppl. 3):150, 1970.
336. Wilson, W. R., Danielson, G. K., Givliani, E. R., Washington, J. A., III, Jaumin, P. M., and Geraci, J. E.: Valve replacement in patients with active infective endocarditis. Circulation *58*:585, 1978.
337. Richardson, J. V., Karp, R. B., Kirklin, J. W., and Dismukes, W. E.: Treatment of infective endocarditis: A 10-year comparative analysis. Circulation *58*: 589, 1978.
338. Rapaport, E.: Editorial. The changing role of surgery in the management of infective endocarditis. Circulation *58*:598, 1978.
339. Simberkoff, M. S., Isom, W., Smithivast, T., Noriega, E. R., and Rahal, J. J., Jr.: Two-stage tricuspid valve replacement for mixed bacterial endocarditis. Arch. Intern. Med. *133*:212, 1974.
340. Robin, E., Thoms, N. W., Arbulu, A., Ganguly, S. N., and Magnisalis, K.: Hemodynamic consequences of total removal of the tricuspid valve without prosthetic replacement. Am. J. Cardiol. *35*:481, 1975.
341. Sethia, B., and Williams, B. T.: Tricuspid valve excision without replacement in a case of endocarditis secondary to drug abuse. Br. Heart J. *40*:579, 1978.
342. Arbulu, A., and Asfaw, I.: Tricuspid valvulectomy with prosthetic replacement. J. Thorac. Cardiovasc. Surg. *82*:684, 1981.
343. Bogart, D. B., Hodges, G. R., Lewis, H. D., Jr., and Fixley, M. S.: Prosthetic valve endocarditis: Reviewing the problem. Postgrad. Med. *62*:119, 1977.

PROGNOSIS

344. Wallach, J. B., Glass, M., Lakash, L., and Angrist, A. A.: Bacterial endocarditis in aged. Ann. Intern. Med. *42*:1206, 1955.
345. Bunn, P., and Lunn, J.: Late follow up of 64 patients with subacute bacterial endocarditis treated with penicillin. Am. J. Med. Sci. *243*:549, 1962.
346. Pearce, M. L., and Guze, L. B.: Some factors affecting prognosis in bacterial endocarditis, Ann. Intern. Med. *55*:270, 1961.
347. Cummings, V., Furman, S., Dunset, M., and Rubin, I. L.: Subacute bacterial endocarditis in older age group. J.A.M.A. *172*:137, 1960.
348. McNeill, K. M., Strong, J. E., Jr., and Lockwood, W. R.: Bacterial endocarditis: An analysis of factors affecting long-term survival. Am. Heart J. *95*:448, 1978.
349. Wedgwood, J.: Prognosis in subacute bacterial endocarditis. Lancet *2*:922, 1957.
350. Robinson, M. J., and Ruedy, J.: Sequelae of bacterial endocarditis. Am. J. Med. *32*:922, 1962.
351. Guze, L. B., and Pearce, M. L.: Hospital-acquired bacterial endocarditis. Arch. Intern. Med. *112*:56, 1963.
352. Zeman, F. D.: Subacute bacterial endocarditis in aged. Am. Heart J. *29*:661, 1945.
353. Menzies, C. J.: Coronary embolism with infarction in bacterial endocarditis. Br. Heart J. *23*:464, 1961.

354. Marietta, J. S.: Acute bacterial endocarditis and coronary embolism. Texas State J. Med. *56*:426, 1960.
355. Brunson, J. G.: Coronary embolism in bacterial endocarditis. Am. J. Pathol. *29*:689, 1953.
356. Jackson, J. F., and Allison, F., Jr.: Bacterial endocarditis. South. Med. J. *54*:1331, 1961.
357. Priest, W. S., and Smith, J. M.: Effect of healed subacute bacterial endocarditis on cardiac dynamics. Arch. Intern. Med. *95*:646, 1955.
358. Mendelson, C. E., Cahue, A., Katz, L. N., and Brams, W. A.: Long-term outlook for healed subacute bacterial endocarditis. J.A.M.A. *160*:437, 1956.
359. Hoffman, F. G., and Robinson, J. J.: Aneurysm of mitral valve associated with bacterial endocarditis. Am. Heart J. *63*:826, 1962.
360. Blum, L.: Development of current concept of mycotic aneurysm. N.Y. State J. Med. *64*:1317, 1964.
361. Poblacion, D., McKenty, J., and Campbell, M.: Mycotic aneurysm of the superior mesenteric artery complicating subacute bacterial endocarditis: Successful resection. Canad. Med. Assoc. J. *90*:744, 1964.
362. Case Records of the Massachusetts General Hospital (Case 43371). N. Engl. J. Med. *257*:515, 1957.
363. Karchmer, A. W.: Active infective endocarditis: When to operate. J. Cardiovasc. Med. *6*:1015, 1981.
364. Boyd, A. A., Spencer, F. C., Isom, O. W., Cunningham, J. N., Reed, G. E., Acinapura, A. J., and Tice, D. A.: Infective endocarditis: An analysis of 54 surgically treated patients. J. Thorac. Cardiovasc. Surg. *73*:23, 1977.
365. Sandza, J. G., Clark, R. E., Ferguson, T. B., Connors, J. P., and Weldon, C. S.: Replacement of prosthetic heart valves. J. Thorac. Cardiovasc. Surg. *74*:864, 1977.
366. Utley, J. R., Mills, J., and Roe, B. B.: The role of valve replacement in the treatment of fungal endocarditis. J. Thorac. Surg. *69*:255, 1975.
367. Young, J. B., Welton, D. E., Raizner, A. E., et al.: Surgery in infective endocarditis. Circulation *60* (Suppl. I):177, 1979.
368. Kaplan, E. L., Rich, H., Gersony, W., and Manning, J.: A collaborative study of infective endocarditis in the 1970's. Emphasis on infections in patients who have undergone cardiovascular surgery. Circulation *59*:327, 1979.
369. Scalia, D., Bortolotti, U., Milano, A., Stritoni, P., Panizzon, G., Valfre, C., Mazzucco, A., and Gallucci, V.: Surgical treatment of infectious endocarditis in the active phase. Experience in 40 cases. G. Ital. Cardiol. *11*:643, 1981.
370. Masur, H., and Johnson, W. D., Jr.: Prosthetic valve endocarditis. J. Thorac. Cardiovasc. Surg. *80*:31, 1980.
371. Cohn, L. H., Mudge, G. H., Pratter, F., and Collins, J. J., Jr.: Five to eight-year follow-up of patients undergoing porcine heart-valve replacement. N. Engl. J. Med. *304*:258, 1981.
372. Kaye, D. (ed.): Prophylaxis of Endocarditis. Baltimore, University Park Press, 1976, p. 245.
373. Kaplan, E. L., Anthony, B. F., Bisno, A., Durack, D., Houser, H., Millard, H. D., Sanford, J., Shulman, S. T., Stillerman, M., Taranta, A., and Wenger, N.: Prevention of bacterial endocarditis. Circulation *56*:139A, 1977.
374. Dismukes, W. E.: Who needs endocarditis prophylaxis? J. Cardiovasc Med. *6*: 347, 1981.
375. Keys, T. F.: Antimicrobial prophylaxis for patients with congenital or valvular heart disease. Mayo Clin. Proc., *57*:171, 1982.
376. Oakley, C., and Somerville, W.: Prevention of infective endocarditis. Br. Heart J. *45*:233, 1981.
377. Schadelin, J.: Praktische probleme der endokarditis prophylaxe. Schweiz. Med. Wochenschr. *111*:646, 1981.
378. Fekety, F. R., Cluff, L. E., Sabiston, D. C., Seidl, L. F., Smith, J. W., and Thoburn, R.: A study of antibiotic prophylaxis in cardiac surgery, J. Thorac. Cardiovasc. Surg. *57*:757, 1969.
379. Goodman, J. S., Schaffner, W., Collins, H. A., Battersky, E. J., and Koenig, M. G.: Infection after cardiovascular surgery. Clinical study including examination of antimicrobial prophylaxis. N. Engl. J. Med. *278*:117, 1968.
380. Myerowitz, P. D., Caswell, K., Lindsay, W. G., and Demetre, M. N.: Antibiotic prophylaxis for open heart surgery. J. Thorac. Cardiovasc. Surg. *73*:625, 1977.
381. Hill, D. G., and Yates, A. K.: Prophylactic antibiotics in open heart surgery, N.Z. Med. J. *81*:414, 1975.
382. Goldman, D. A., Hopkins, C. C., Karchmer, A. W., Abel, R. M., McEnany, M. T., Akins, C., Buckley, M. J., and Moellering, R. C., Jr.: Cephalothin prophylaxis in cardiac valve surgery. J. Thorac. Cardiovasc. Surg. *73*:470, 1977.

34 PRINCIPLES OF THE PATHOGENESIS OF ATHEROSCLEROSIS

by Robert W. Wissler, Ph.D., M.D.

The purpose of this chapter is to provide an understanding of the pathological processes that lead to progressive atherosclerotic plaques in the coronary arteries. In addition, it is hoped that it will furnish information of value in the clinician's attempts to prevent the development of clinically important plaques, retard their progression, and perhaps make possible their regression. It also presents some of the increasing evidence indicating that plaque formation is not only a largely preventable pathological process but also a substantially reversible one. The process has been found to be multifaceted in its origins as well as in its anatomical, biochemical, and pathophysiological manifestations.[1,2] An attempt will also be made to elucidate the relationship between coronary atherosclerotic plaques and the development of ischemic heart disease, including classic acute myocardial infarction, sudden death (usually as a result of acute-onset ventricular fibrillation), and chronic angina pectoris.

Atherosclerosis is a special type of thickening and hardening of the medium-sized and large arteries that accounts for a large proportion of heart attacks and cases of ischemic heart disease.[3] It also accounts for many strokes (those due to cerebral ischemia and infarction), numerous instances of peripheral vascular disease, and most aneurysms of the lower abdominal aorta, which can rupture and cause sudden fatal hemorrhage.

A geographically unevenly distributed pathological condition, atherosclerosis manifests itself as a progressive process, resulting in clinical disease in groups making up only about one-fourth of the world's total population. It is largely limited to the more industrialized countries, especially in the temperate zones of North America, Europe, and the Soviet Union. It is rare to find a high rate of heart attacks due to atherosclerosis in Asia (including China, Japan, India, and most of Southeast Asia), much of the Near East, Africa, or South and Central America. Many epidemiological and geographical pathological studies spanning the last half century have linked the remarkable contrast in clinical heart attack rate and mortality to the level of serum cholesterol in these populations and, in turn, to life styles, in particular, dietary habits.[4–6] Additional risk factors considered in these and many other studies include the incidence of hypertension, cigarette smoking, and diabetes as well as the effects of factors generally beyond control, such as sex, age, hemodynamic forces, and genetic mechanisms. Hardness of water consumed, a sedentary life style, and emotional stress have also been surveyed repeatedly and offer interesting correlations which may help us understand the factors influencing the response of the arterial wall to injury.[7] In Chapter 35 the environmental "risk factors" for the development of atherosclerosis are considered in detail, and in Chapter 47 the genetic aspects of lipoprotein metabolism as they pertain to atherosclerosis are explained.

In this chapter, the major emphasis is on the arterial wall. Its pathophysiological response to the many alterations in constituents, both cellular and fluid, will be considered. Salient aspects of the dynamics of blood flow which appear to be important in the initiation, progression, and regression of the advanced atherosclerotic plaque, particularly in coronary arteries, will be presented.

In arteries of all sizes, the transected wall shows three major microscopic layers: the intima, the media, and the adventitia.[8]

INTIMA. The major constituents of the normally thin intima are endothelium, basement membrane, an occasional smooth muscle myointimal cell, a few collagen and/or elastic fibers, and an infrequent blood-derived mononuclear cell.[9] In arteries where it is prominent, the intimal elastic membrane or lamina (IEM or IEL) defines the limit of the intima. The multilayered cushion of myointimal cells formed in arteries at all ages in many species, including human, may be a pathological finding.[10] It is not clear whether these cushions predispose toward or protect against atherosclerosis.[11] It is likely that hemodynamic stimulation can lead to fibrous lesions (diffuse intimal thickening) and hence to atheromatous lesions when the blood lipids are elevated.[12]

The arterial endothelium probably both admits and discharges macromolecules of the size of low-density lipoproteins (LDL) (p. 1211).[13] Their concentration in the lymph from the arterial wall has been found to be about one-tenth that in the bloodstream.[14,15] Although most plasma proteins can enter the artery in this concentration,[16] lipoproteins and fibrinogen are particularly likely to accumulate in the intima.[17]

"Large pore" transendothelial vesicle chains allow entrance into the arterial wall.[13,18] Additional quantitative study is needed to determine the effect on this transverse channel of dilatation of arteries or increased tension on arterial wall.[19] Other risk factors may also be important in altering endothelial permeability.[1,20]

Another factor suspected of being involved in controlling endothelial permeability is the glycocalyx—the thin, fuzzy layer of complex carbohydrate on the luminal side of the endothelial cell that localizes ruthenium red dye or lectins, such as concanavalin-A. This layer is remarkably thin in those areas of the artery prone to the development of atherosclerotic plaques and at sites where plaques develop in some experimental animals.[21,22]

MEDIA. The media of the mammalian artery—both the large elastic artery, such as the aorta, or the medium-sized muscular artery, such as the coronary artery—is formed by multiple layers of smooth muscle cells (SMC), usually two cells wide, separated by a prominent elastic membrane.[9] Each of these recurring structures, which contain an elastic membrane in the center and a SMC on each side, is called a "lamellar unit." In a given species, the number of these units in each artery appears to be highly predictable relative to the size of the animal and many other factors.[1,23,24] The apparent interstitial "space" between the cells and the regularly recurring elastic membranes contain variable quantities of collagen, elastin, and glycosaminoglycans.

At present, both circumstantial evidence and careful in vitro studies of the arterial SMC indicate that it can synthesize collagen, elastin, and glycosaminoglycans.[25–29] These multiple cell products, which appear prominent when the SMC reacts to certain pathological stimuli, led us a number of years ago to dub it the "malfunctional medial mesenchymal cell." At that time we suggested that it should be considered the most prominent and important cell in the process of atherogenesis (Fig. 34–1).[25] No new evidence has come to light to revise this assumption, but it must be borne in mind that the blood-derived monocyte (or macrophage) is probably present, at least in small numbers, in most atheromatous lesions. These cells, as well as platelets, can exert a strong influence on the atherosclerotic process during various stages of development and regression of the plaque.[2,30–32]

Significant new observations about the functional anatomy of the artery are being reported with increasing frequency.[33] It now appears likely that relationships between cells, collagen, and elastin in the media are orderly and beautifully designed, permitting the strength and relative inflexibility of collagen to interact in the best possible way with elastin.[34] This yields a highly functional vessel that can adapt to varying demands and pathophysiological conditions.[24,33] The SMC probably acts as the major monitor of this adaptability, since it can vary its synthesis of the various fiber proteins and matrix carbohydrates in response to different physical and chemical stimuli.

ADVENTITIA. The adventitia of the artery is important to arterial function. Its mainly collagenous structure provides the major mechanical support when the media is badly weakened owing to advanced atherosclerosis. It is also important because it provides the media of larger arteries with much of its nutrition by means of the vasa vasorum, as well as with lymphatic drainage and innervation of the arteries. The predominant cell of the adventitia is the fibroblast.

Penetrating branches of the vasa vasorum, terminating at about the twenty-ninth lamellar unit of the media, are consistently found in large arteries of large mammals and humans.[23,24] This finding may help to explain the more severe atherosclerosis usually observed in the abdominal aor-

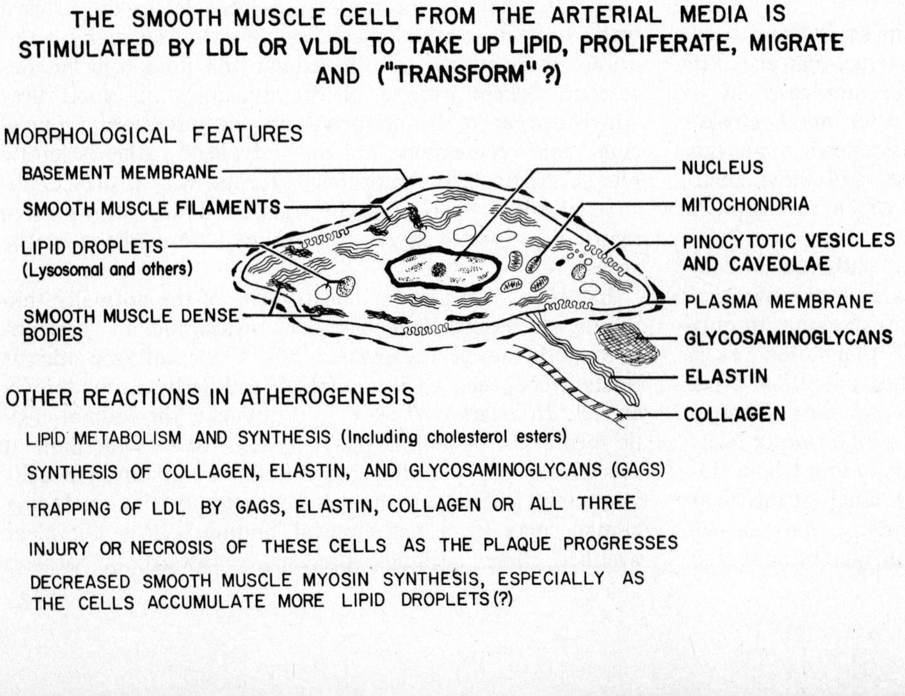

FIGURE 34–1 The major morphological features of the "multifunctional medial mesenchymal cell," the principal cell type involved in atherogenesis, along with a listing of some of its functions that are particularly important in atherosclerosis. (Modified from Wissler, R. W., et al.: Abnormalities of the arterial wall and its metabolism in atherogenesis. Prog. Cardiovasc. Dis. *18*:5, 1976, by permission of Grune and Stratton.)

ta of *Homo sapiens.* Wolinsky and Glagov have suggested that the absence of penetrating vasa vasorum in the human abdominal aorta and the unusual physical stresses to which this part of the artery is exposed may make it particularly vulnerable to atherogenesis.

MAJOR FEATURES OF ATHEROSCLEROTIC LESIONS

Human atherosclerosis produces its effects largely in the medium-sized muscular arteries (such as the coronary, carotid, basilar, and vertebral). It also affects arteries supplying the lower extremities and the larger arteries (such as the aorta and iliac). It should not be confused with many of the minor intimal and medial forms of *arterio*sclerosis, which rarely produce clinical effects, or with the clinically important forms of sclerosis of small arteries (arteriolosclerosis) that often appear in hypertension and diabetes (Fig. 34–2).

The feature that sets *athero*sclerosis apart from other forms of arteriosclerosis is the lipid, which in the advanced plaque is often represented by a central necrotic core that is rich in cholesterol esters and is often accompanied by visible cholesterol crystals. This part of the lesion, which on gross examination is usually soft and grumous, is responsible for the name of the disease process, derived from the Greek stem "athera," meaning gruel or porridge.

LOCALIZATION. The distribution of atherosclerotic plaques in the arterial tree of human subjects follows certain patterns (Fig. 34–3). In general, the abdominal aorta, for reasons just discussed, is much more extensively involved than is the thoracic aorta, and aortic lesions tend to be much more prominent near ostia of major branches.[24] Renal arteries are usually spared from stenosing plaques, except at their ostia;[35] coronary arteries show the most intense atherosclerotic involvement within the first 6 cm.[36] The severity of involvement of the coronary artery is, on the average, less than that of the abdominal aorta in most age groups and is somewhat more severe and extensive than that of the adjacent thoracic aorta, from which these arteries are derived—a phenomenon that may be related to the peculiarities of blood flow in the coronary artery.[37] Other interesting aspects of plaque distribution are beyond

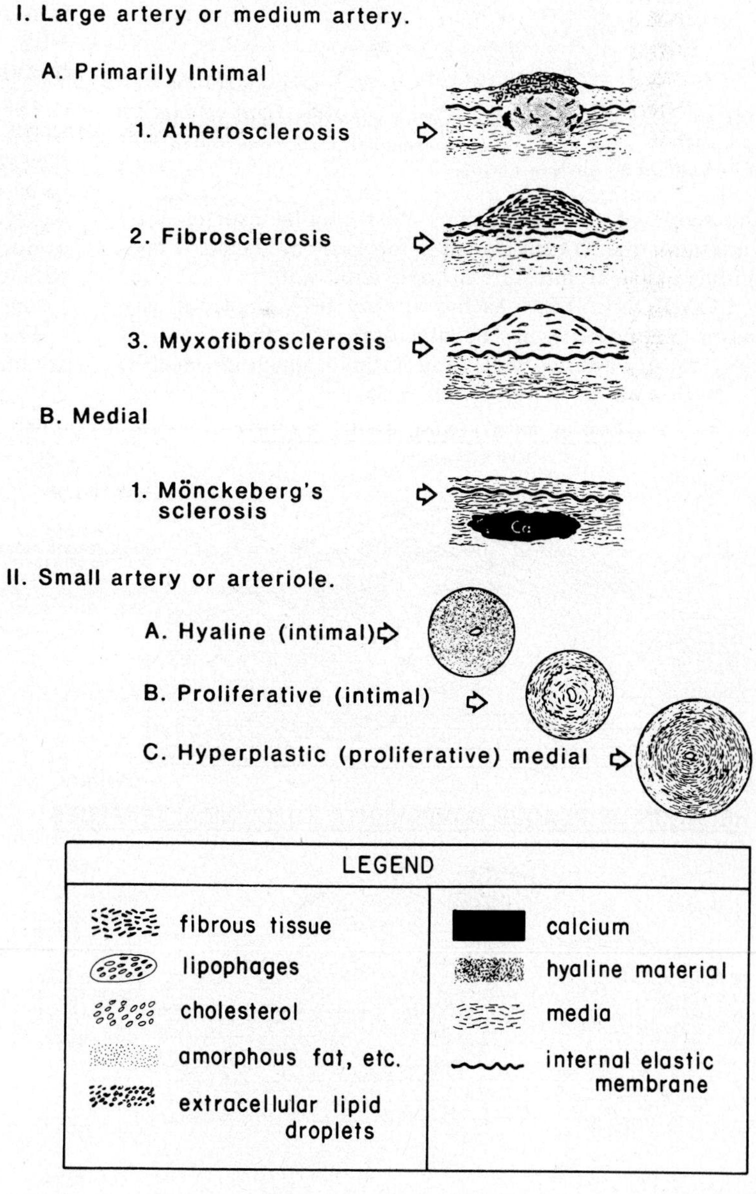

FIGURE 34–2 A classification of arteriosclerosis represented diagrammatically to contrast the features of atherosclerosis with other commonly observed forms of arteriosclerosis. *Fibrosclerosis* is used to describe the commonly observed benign collagen-rich intimal thickenings that show little or no lipid or necrosis. *Myxofibrosclerosis* is a term we have used to describe lipid-poor lesions that are rich in glycosaminoglycans. They are frequently observed in large arteries of patients with diabetes and in arteries distal to a point of severe stenosis or mechanical occlusion.

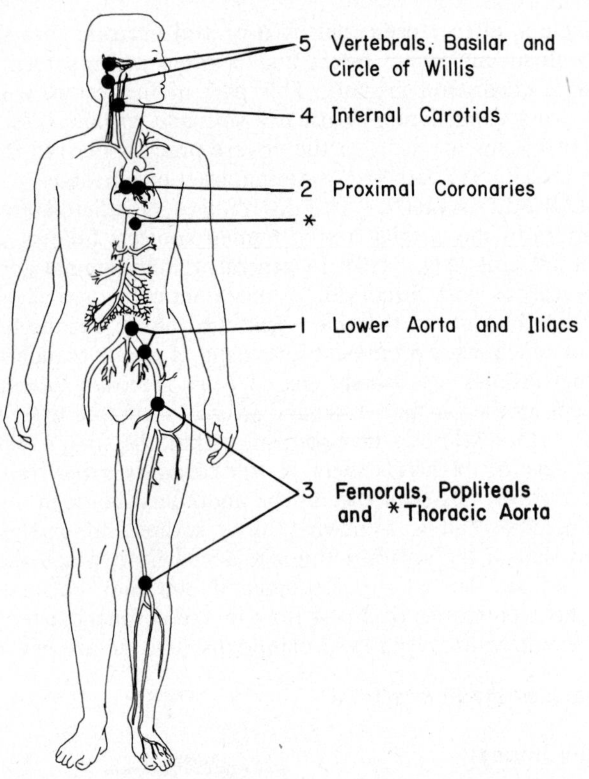

FIGURE 34–3 Sites of predilection for clinically significant atherosclerosis, in usual rank order. Substantial exceptions can occur, often without an obvious reason.

the scope of this discussion; most can be explained by variations due to hemodynamic forces or by localized conditions of the architecture of the arterial wall.[24]

COMPONENTS. As has already been suggested, the major components of the atherosclerotic plaque are its cells, mostly arterial SMC, and its lipid, much of which is extracellular (Fig. 34–4*A*). The relative proportions of these two major components, along with the fibrous proteins and complex carbohydrate products of the SMC, vary greatly from plaque to plaque. These proportions also vary during the sequence of development or regression of a given plaque. Unfortunately, however, at our present stage of technology, it is virtually impossible to quantitate these major components in the human plaque at any specific time, short of surgical removal or examination at autopsy.

CLINICAL EFFECTS. The clinical effects of advanced plaques of most medium-sized arteries, which include the main coronary vessels, are due to either their space-occupying characteristics, which lead to stenosis, or their thrombogenic qualities, which often appear related to fracture or rupture of the fibrous cap and the resulting ulceration of the plaque surface (Fig. 34–4*B*). This frequently results in an obstructing thrombus, which in a major coronary artery can—and often does—form over a well-developed atheromatous plaque and lead to acute sudden coronary occlusion and myocardial infarction.

It has recently been proposed that the eccentric, largely intimal, advanced atheromatous plaque found in most muscular arteries may have quite different functional effects relative to stenosis, thrombosis, spasm, and susceptibility to regression than do the rather rare concentric, transmural plaques which are sometimes observed.[38,39]

The major clinical effects of plaques in the aorta (and sometimes in the iliac arteries) are usually not the result of their space-occupying features. They are much more likely to be caused by thinning of the media beneath the plaques, weakening of the wall, aneurysm formation and rupture, or formation of a mural thrombus over ulcerated areas, with embolization to more distal radicles of the arterial system.

The composition and clinical consequences of the plaque are not necessarily functions of how long it has been in the

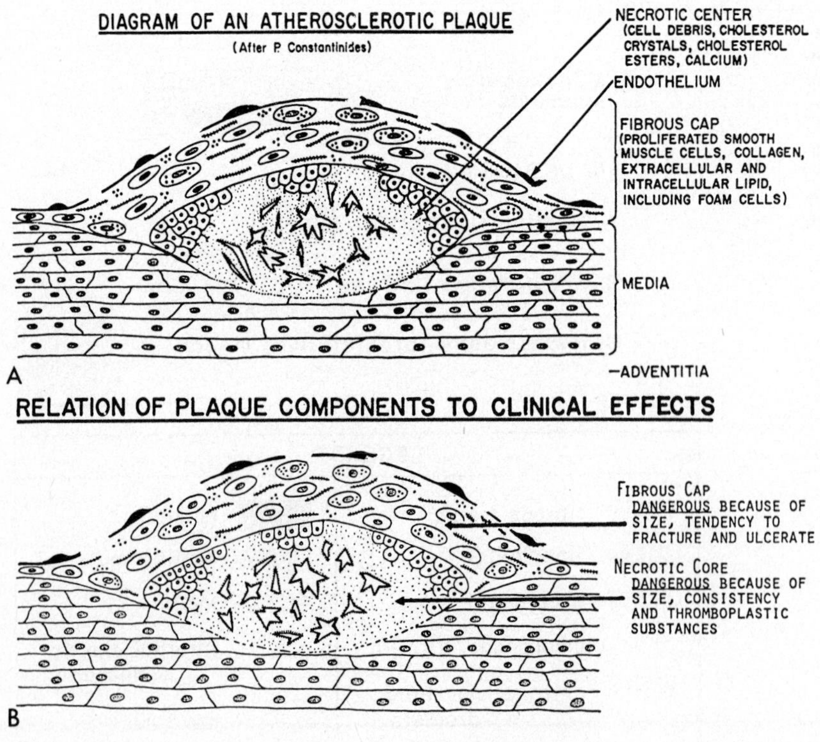

FIGURE 34–4 *A*, Major components of the advanced (clinically important) atherosclerotic plaque. *B*, Characteristics of the advanced plaque that account for its clinical effects in medium-sized (muscular) arteries. (Modified from Wissler, R. W., and Vesselinovitch, D.: Animal models of regression. *In* Schettler, G., et al. (eds.): Atherosclerosis IV. Berlin, Springer-Verlag, 1977, p. 377.)

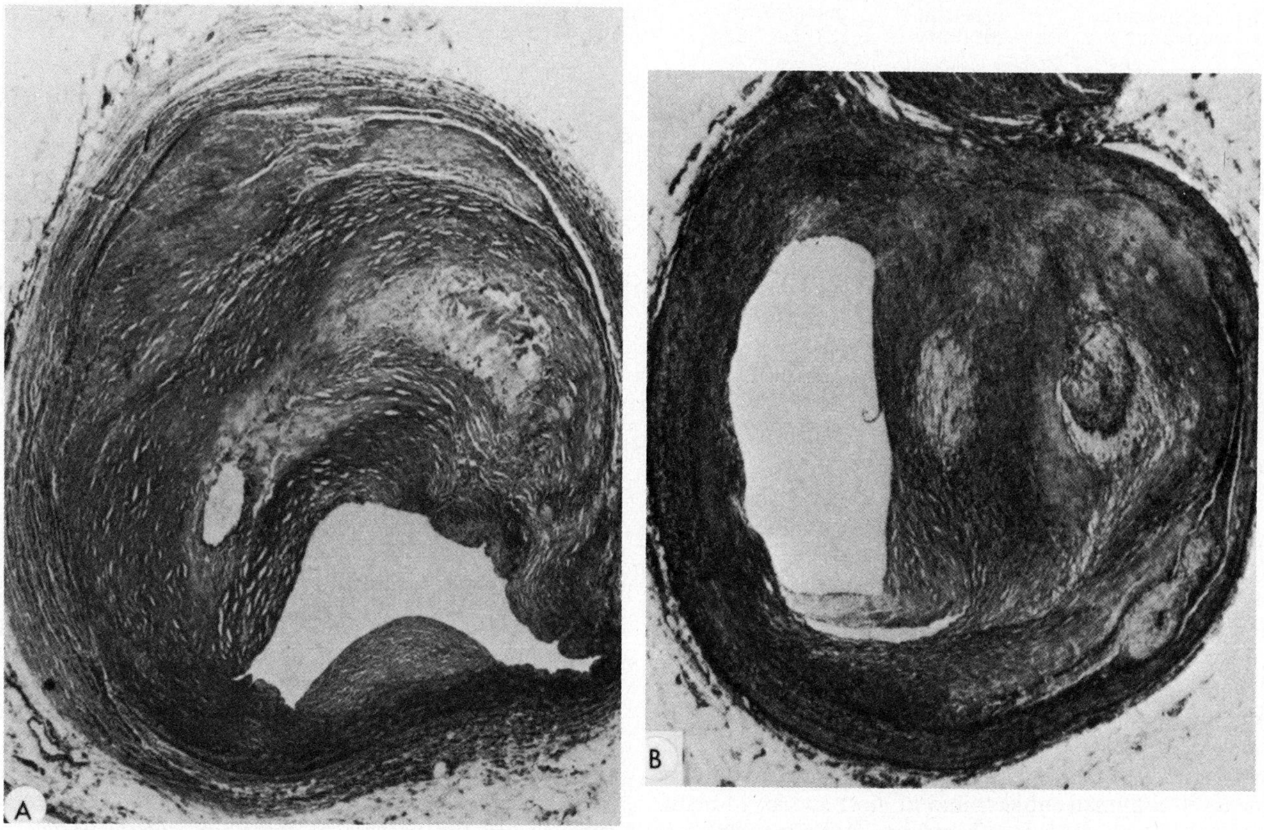

FIGURE 34–5 *A*, An advanced plaque in the coronary artery of a 29-year-old woman with heterozygous familial hypercholesterolemia (Type II disease) who died with ischemic heart disease. *B*, Plaque in severe coronary artery atherosclerosis in 71-year-old man who died suddenly of left ventricular free-wall rupture. Note the resemblance in principal components (necrotic core and fibrous cap) to the severe atherosclerosis in *A*. (From Roberts, W. C.: The coronary arteries in coronary heart disease: Morphologic observations. Pathobiol. Annu. *5*:249, 1975.)

process of formation. In fact, the few well-illustrated reports of plaques in relatively young individuals who are victims of fatal heart attacks and who have displayed severe, genetically controlled elevations in LDL levels show the same lesion components in about the same proportions as those plaques which usually occur in older individuals (Fig. 34–5).[40,41]

THEORIES OF PATHOGENESIS

Historically, pathologists who have studied the mechanisms by which the atherosclerotic plaque develops have approached the problem from two points of view. One of these, often believed to have been proposed by Virchow, holds that a principal factor in the progression of the plaque is the increased passage and accumulation of plasma constituents from the arterial lumen into the arterial intima, i.e., a type of low-grade inflammatory edema (insudation). The second, often associated with Rokitansky, specifies that small mural thrombi on areas of arterial intimal injury (hemodynamic and otherwise) occur early in atherogenesis (encrustation) and that the organization of these thrombi by SMC as well as their gradual growth plays a definitive role in the progression of the plaque.

The two concepts described differ principally in that the latter, the encrustation formulation, attributes much more weight to the environmental factors which cause arterial endothelial injury and trigger thrombus formation of the type frequently seen in arteries, i.e., thrombi of the "white" (platelet, fibrin, and leukocyte) variety. These encrusted white thrombi are thought by some to form much of the space-occupying substance of the developing plaque. According to this hypothesis, the lipid in the plaque is a more or less passive and secondary product of the spongelike action of the thrombus and the breakdown of platelets and leukocytes.

The insudation theory, on the other hand, more easily accommodates the role of elevated levels of serum lipoproteins in carrying cholesterol into the artery wall. It has gradually become the predominant theory within the scientific community, especially in the United States.

In general, all theories of pathogenesis of atherosclerosis support the notion that plaque development begins rather early in life, with the process then continuing over a period of many years (Fig. 34–6).[42] There are indications of periods of quiescence and even regression interspersed with periods of progression, until the disease reaches a point at which it becomes clinically important.[43]

Insudation and Encrustation

ROLE OF SERUM CHOLESTEROL. The emergence of the insudation theory is the result of two major developments: one positive and one negative. The positive one is the accumulation of consistent evidence indicating that a sustained elevation in the level of serum cholesterol

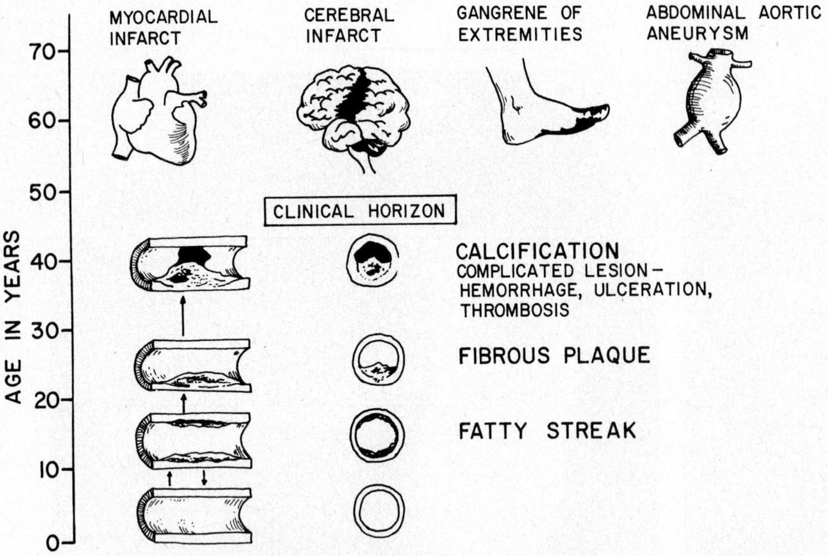

FIGURE 34–6 The natural history of atherosclerosis. Plaques usually develop slowly and insidiously over many years, and they generally progress from a fatty streak to a fibrous plaque and then to a complicated plaque that is likely to lead to clinical effects. Not shown is the concept that this pathological process can probably be accelerated by arterial endothelial injury. In addition, the degree of elevation of either blood pressure or levels of serum cholesterol may help to determine the severity of endothelial injury. (Modified from McGill, H. C., Jr., et al.: Natural history of human atherosclerotic lesions. *In* Sandler, M., and Bourne, G. H. (eds.): Atherosclerosis and Its Origin. New York, Academic Press, 1963, p. 42.)

leads to classic progressive atherosclerotic lesions. This elevation may be endogenously induced as a result of genetic factors or of metabolic disease such as "lipoid" nephrosis and hypothyroidism, or it may be exogenously produced by the long-term effects of a high-fat, high-cholesterol diet. However, the inverse of this relationship appears to be equally true, i.e., if the serum cholesterol is maintained at a low level in human subjects and in most species of mammals, then atherosclerosis is a rare development. The evidence supporting these relationships comes from many types of studies: epidemiological, geographical, and pathological (autopsy) studies of the natural history of the plaque. In fact, no population has been identified in which progressive atherosclerosis develops if the serum cholesterol level is low. These relationships are also supported by clinicopathological studies, experimental animal studies and, more recently, investigations in cell biology and molecular pathology.[1,2,44] These results, in general, reinforce each other and provide strong evidence that the significant class of substances accumulating in the arterial intima in excessive amounts during insudation comprises cholesterol-rich lipoproteins. If these macromolecules are derived from serum having an elevated cholesterol content, the influx tends to support the eventual development of a progressive, and ultimately an advanced, atherosclerotic plaque of the type that leads to clinical manifestations, including ischemic heart disease.[1]

ENDOTHELIAL DAMAGE AND PLATELET ADHESION. Pathologists who have studied the natural history of human atherosclerosis generally support the concept of organization of thrombi over advanced plaques as a mechanism of plaque growth. On the other hand, they have failed to find evidence of sufficient encrustation to support organization of arterial mural thrombi as a major pathogenetic mechanism for early atherogenesis.[36] This negative reaction to the classic encrustation theory is supported by the recent experimental evidence that clearly shows that even extensive endothelial damage to normal arteries following balloon catheterization or other intima-destroying experimental manipulations does not support the development of a progressive mural thrombus and does not lead to a typical atheromatous plaque.[45,46] As will be considered later, platelets do accumulate along with some fibrin and leukocytes, and some SMC proliferation does occur under these conditions. However, unless sustained hypercholesterolemia is present, these proliferative lesions tend to regress and heal, and the arterial intima is restored nearly to normal (Fig. 34–7).[2,47]

Much more work needs to be done, but in general it now appears likely that these two previously divergent theories are in the process of combining into a unified concept for the pathogenesis of atherosclerosis, which proposes that the insudation of hyperlipidemic serum, with its cholesterol-rich low-density lipoprotein fractions, is an

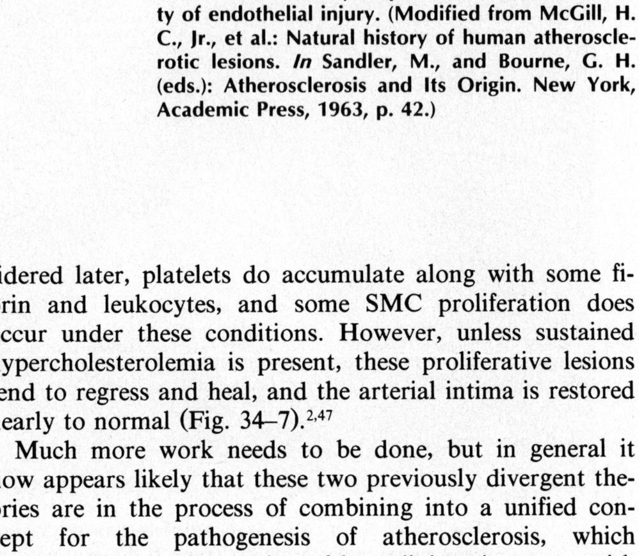

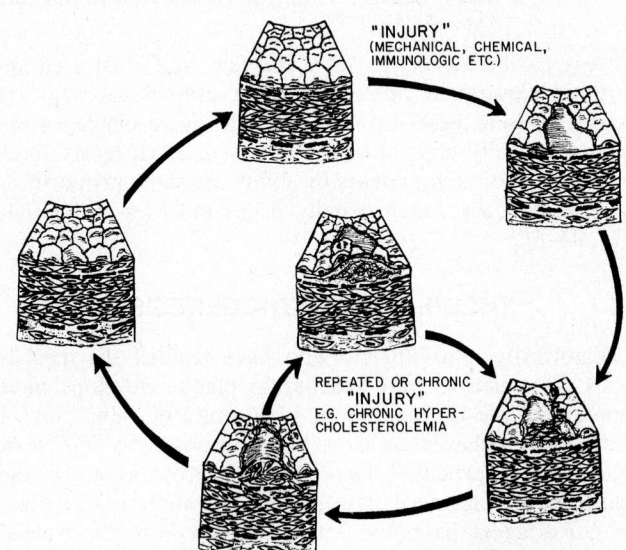

FIGURE 34–7 Endothelial injury acts as a triggering mechanism to promote the sticking and spreading of platelets. This in turn releases the "platelet factor" that stimulates migration of arterial smooth muscle cells from the arterial media and proliferation of these cells in the intima and media. The process is represented as being almost completely reversible when only one episode of endothelial damage occurs; it is progressive when repeated or continuous endothelial injury occurs, as is likely with elevation of serum low-density lipoprotein or other chronic endothelial injuries. (Slightly modified from Ross, R., and Glomset, J. A.: The pathogenesis of atherosclerosis. N. Engl. J. Med. *295*:420, 1976, reprinted by permission of the New England Journal of Medicine.)

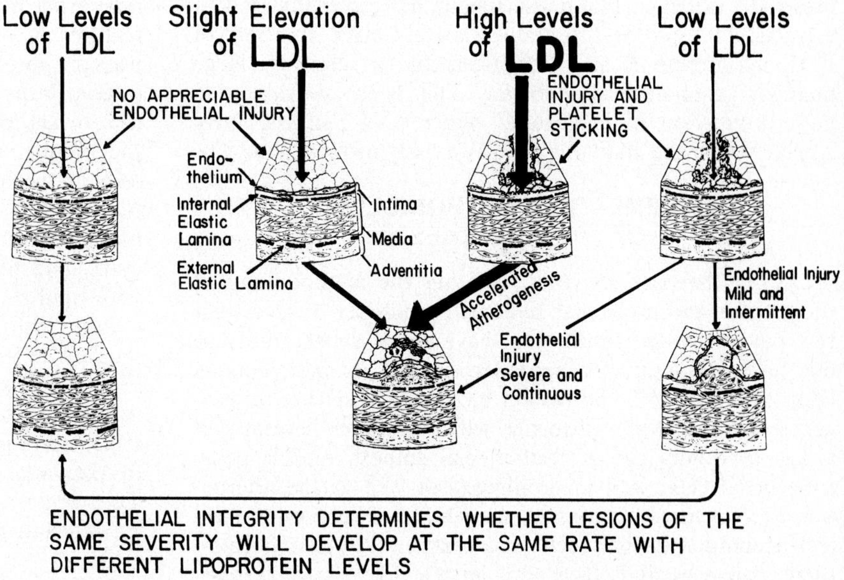

FIGURE 34–8 Several of the pathways of interaction between elevated levels of low-density lipoprotein and arterial endothelial injury to produce a progressive atherosclerotic plaque. Although in extreme instances of continuous and severe endothelial damage, progressive plaque formation can occur even when the low-density lipoprotein levels are low (*extreme right*), this does not negate the protective effect of low levels of low-density lipoproteins if the endothelium is not being damaged severely (*extreme left*) or is damaged slightly and not very often. (Modified from Ross, R., and Glomset, J. A.: The pathogenesis of atherosclerosis. N. Engl. J. Med. *295*:420, 1976, reprinted by permission of the New England Journal of Medicine.)

important element in atherogenesis and, under most conditions, is the *predominant* factor in determining whether or not progressive plaques develop. It also suggests that endothelial injury often plays a major part in accelerating atherogenesis because it results in encrustation of platelets and monocytes, which in turn expose the intimal and medial arterial SMC to the peptides that stimulate cell proliferation (liberated by these cell fragments and cells). This element of endothelial dysfunction may also help determine where plaques develop most frequently and prominently. It helps to explain the occasional exceptional or paradoxical case in which severe, clinically important atherosclerotic plaques develop in young people who do not seem to have sufficiently elevated lipoproteins or other risk factors commonly recognized, such as cigarette smoking or untreated hypertension (Fig. 34–8).

Another reason for including *arterial endothelial damage and platelet sticking* in theories of atherogenesis is the increasing evidence that hypercholesterolemia itself leads to increased endothelial permeability and endothelial damage, thus creating a "vicious cycle" that can sustain and augment endothelial injury from some other cause and lead to progressive plaque formation.[48–51] Furthermore, it now appears that one mechanism by which cigarette smoking and hypertension act as risk factors at the cellular level is by means of the endothelial dysfunction they produce.[52–55]

The Initial Lesion

One of the current problems in explaining the morphogenesis of the atherosclerotic process is the emerging doubt whether or not the classic grossly evident "fatty streak" is the precursor lesion in the histogenetic sequence of atherosclerosis. There has long been some controversy about this slightly raised, poorly defined yellow streak in which most of the lipid can be seen on microscopic examination to be within cells of the intima and inner media. First, it is commonly seen in infants and young children in virtually all the populations of the world, whether or not progressive atherosclerosis develops in that population. To some extent, this is true in many other species of mammals also—even though few of them are likely to develop progressive atherosclerosis unless other measures are taken. Furthermore, Mitchell and Schwartz have presented evidence from autopsies indicating that the locations of aortic fatty streaks in young individuals did not coincide with those of the progressive and advanced plaques in the aortas of older persons.[56] More recently, Smith et al. and others, as a result of extensive biochemical and immunochemical studies, have also questioned the role of the fatty streak, as usually defined and described, in the process of atherogenesis.[16,57–61]

It is evident that this problem needs further study. A preliminary study of young Americans who succumbed to sudden accidental death has recently been extended. It has been shown that "fatty streaks" include a variety of lesions that differ considerably in their staining characteristics.[62] Even though all are yellow, poorly demarcated, and only slightly raised in the formalin-fixed state, some contain most of the stainable lipid within the cytoplasm of the myointimal cells, whereas in others most of the lipid is in extracellular pools; in many, it occurs in both locations. Many reveal stainable lipid in and around the in situ medial cells of the inner media, and occasionally the positive staining of fat with oil red O is limited to the more or less intact internal elastic lamella. Of particular interest in this study has been the finding that most of the stainable lipid is extracellular and that few foam cells are seen in these aortic fatty streaks from accidental death victims in the 15 to 35 age group studied.[63]

More definitive postmortem studies are planned to ascertain whether any of these or other variable features of fatty streaks can be correlated with known major risk factors. Assessment of risk factors can be obtained from retrospective investigation of the history of accidental sudden death victims in their late teens, twenties, or early thirties when much of the evidence indicates that rapid progression of atherosclerosis in the human aorta is most likely to occur.

Smith and coworkers have suggested that the lesions most likely to progress are those identified as "gelatinous," owing to their appearance in unfixed specimens. They have presented evidence that these lesions are especially rich in extracellular lipid and contain relatively large amounts of LDL apoprotein B and fibrinogen and a relatively large quantity of cholesterol linoleate. This is in contrast to a high proportion of cholesterol oleate in the classic fatty streak, where the stainable lipid is mostly intracellular.[59,60]

THE EMERGING PATHOBIOLOGY OF ATHEROGENESIS

During the past 25 years, utilizing the methodology of the cellular and molecular biologist, a number of investigators have provided results that have added substantially to our understanding of atherosclerosis and its pathogenesis (Fig. 34–9).[1,2,30,64,65] The results have indicated that atherogenesis is a complex disorder which involves several cell types, especially the arterial medial smooth muscle cells, endothelial cells, and macrophages, as well as the interaction of two major processes, namely, lipid (cholesterol ester) accumulation and cell proliferation. Without both of these processes, it is clear that progressive atherosclerosis of clinical significance will not develop. Many of these seminal discoveries during this period of rapid progress have come from studies of human plaques at various stages of development through the use of transmission electron microscopy and chemical (biochemical and physicochemical) and histochemical, as well as immunohistochemical, approaches.

THE INTERACTION OF ARTERIAL CELLS AND LIPOPROTEINS

Beginning in the early 1960's, a number of ultrastructural studies revealed that the predominant cells in the human atherosclerotic plaque are modified medial SMC's, the features of which are diagrammed in Figure 34–1.[25,66–69] It was proposed that these cells accumulated as a result of migration and proliferation from the inner media. Classic fibroblasts, believed previously to be the dominant cells of the plaque, were not generally identified, although some cells of the human lesion were admittedly difficult to identify. A few had ultrastructural features associated with blood-derived leukocytes, including lymphocytes, granulocytes, and monocytes; many of the last-named were filled with lipid droplets. From the outset there was some doubt —and still is—about whether most of the lipid-filled "foam" cells, which generally make up a small proportion of the cells of the human plaque, are derived from blood monocytes or whether they are mostly modified SMC's which have lost some of their mature features as a reaction to the large quantities of lipid which they had imbibed. This important question needs further study using improved and more definitive cell markers for these types of cells.

These ultrastructural studies of the human plaque have indeed been embellished by a few immunohistochemical studies which utilized fluorescein or horseradish peroxidase–labeled antibody to smooth muscle myosin to indicate that most plaque cells resemble arterial medial SMC's immunohistochemically.[64,70,71] The Campbells from Melbourne have made very good use of both ultrastructural studies and immunohistochemistry as well as in vitro approaches to establish the concept of phenotypic modulation.[72–75] Their astute observations have helped to illuminate some of the structural and functional changes from normal medial cells displayed by plaque SMC.

The other key advance of the 1960's which has helped

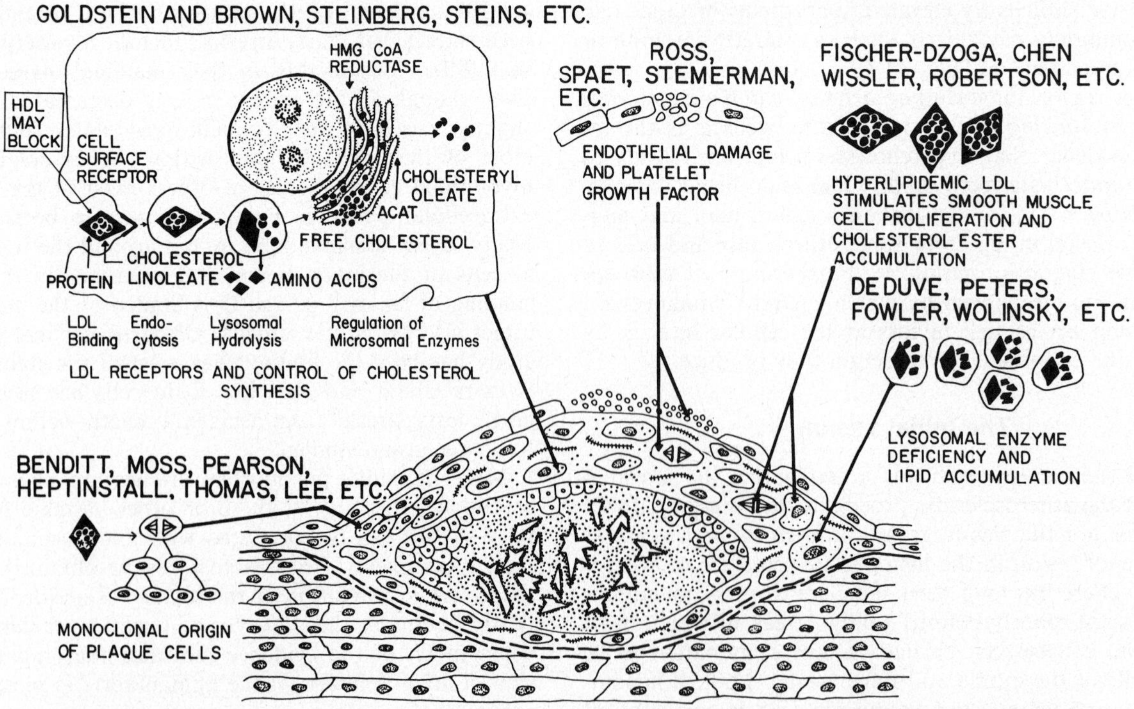

FIGURE 34–9 Some of the major recent developments in understanding a few of the cellular pathobiological reactions that appear to be important in the pathogenesis (and regression) of the atherosclerotic plaque. (Modified from Wissler, R. W.: Coronary atherosclerosis and ischemic heart disease. *In* Zülch, K. J., et al. (eds.): Brain and Heart Infarct. Berlin, Springer-Verlag, 1977, p. 206.)

TABLE 34–1 NEW RELATIONSHIPS OF LIPOPROTEIN FRACTIONS TO ATHEROGENESIS

Current Lipoprotein Designations	Predominant Apo Protein (s)	Functions and Presumed Functions in Atherogenesis
Chylomicrons	Apo B 240 Apo E	May furnish cholesterol and triglycerides for atherogenesis at the arterial cell surface due to action of lipoprotein lipase (LPL) (Zilversmit) and via other remnants (Mahley, Getz)
VLDL	Apo B 335, Apo E Apo C-1 to C-III	Very little evidence of atherogenic effect except via LPL activity
Broad-beta VLDL	Apo B 240 Apo E	Highly atherogenic remnant particles derived from chylomicrons in subjects (especially dogs) fed a high-cholesterol, high-fat ration (Mahley)
H-LDL*† LDL I†	Apo B 335	Perhaps the most consistently atherogenic fraction in human species (FH) and lipogenic and mitogenic in other primates (Fless, Scanu, Fischer-Dzoga); when altered by endothelial cells or by malondialdehyde, it is avidly taken up by macrophages in vitro (Scanu, Rudel)
LDL II†		May support build up of cholesterol in arterial SMC
LDL III†	Apo B 335	Little direct evidence of atherogenicity with the exception of mitogenic effect of particle after neuraminidase treatment (Fless, Scanu, et al.)
LDL IV†		Probably identical with LPa; epidemiological evidence supports atherogenicity
HDL_C	Apo E	Probably especially important in cholesterol excretion
HDL_1	Apo A-I Apo A-II	High-affinity receptors for hepatic apo E may help in cholesterol excretion
HDL_2	Apo E Apo A-I Apo A-II Apo C	Serum level correlated with protection against atherosclerosis in numerous species, including humans Precursor to HDL_1
HDL_3	Apo A-I Apo A-II Apo C	Precursor to HDL_2, but the level is not predictive

*LDL from hyperlipidemic serum (enlarged cholesterol-rich particle).
†LDL fractions as designated by Fless and Scanu.

to foster the modern era of atherosclerosis research was the demonstration by numerous methods that most of the cholesterol and cholesterol esters in human plaques at various stages of development was probably derived from low-density lipoprotein (LDL) or very low-density lipoprotein (VLDL) that gained entrance to the intima and the inner media from the bloodstream (Fig. 34–9).[76–81] As modern work on the pathogenesis of atherosclerosis has progressed, it has become increasingly evident that in addition to LDL from hyperlipidemic serum, several other lipoprotein fractions may be important in depositing cholesterol and cholesterol esters in the artery. Those receiving most attention are listed in Table 34–1. It has now become clear that the LDL particles are not a homogeneous family and that the large, cholesterol-rich LDL from hyperlipidemic serum (H-LDL) may have a number of important features which distinguish it from LDL derived from subjects with normal basal levels of LDL.[82,83] Furthermore, recent work by Fless and Scanu using rhesus monkeys has yielded important new evidence of heterogeneity of LDL. They have utilized single-spin, gradient-density centrifugation to produce LDL I, II, III, and IV, each of which appears to have distinctive qualities.[84–86] Some of those fractions most relevant to atherogenesis will be discussed later.

As the interactions between various cells and lipoproteins are studied further, it has become evident that LDL which is altered in the test tube or by platelet[87] or endothelial cell[88] action also has distinguishing features which decrease its avidity for apo B receptors on the smooth muscle cells and increase its binding and internalization for macrophages.[31,89] Furthermore, as more is understood about the artery wall lipases, a new concept has been developed by Zilversmit[90] which relates VLDL and chylomicron metabolism to atherogenesis. It has also become clear from the work of Mahley and coworkers that broad β-VLDL resulting from hyperresponses to an atherogenic ration may have a definitive role in promoting progressive atherogenesis in certain species, such as the dog.[91]

All of these new discoveries and new concepts must be evaluated in relation to the established body of evidence indicating that in the human atheromatous lesion the major apoprotein of LDL (apo B) can regularly be identified by immunohistochemical means, both intracellularly and extracellularly. Furthermore, apo B appears to be the only apoprotein which increases as the plaque develops in size and severity from the early, nonelevated lesion, in which lipid stained with oil red O is barely discernible, to the most advanced lesions with large, necrotic, lipid-rich cores surrounded by "foam" cells and overlaid by a thick, fibrous cap (see Fig. 34–4*A*).[76–81]

ROLE OF PLATELETS AND ENDOTHELIAL DAMAGE

During the 1970's, another aspect of the pathogenesis of atherosclerosis began to receive attention. Using "balloon catheter" injury as an experimental method to produce denudation of the arterial intima and modern pathobiological methods to study cells, Ross and coworkers discovered that sticking of platelets to the damaged arterial intimal surfaces and disintegration of platelets were important contributors to the development of arterial SMC proliferation.[74-76] These studies followed the work of Mustard and coworkers, who pioneered the elucidation of the platelet-endothelial phenomena that occur on the arterial intimal surface, where atherosclerosis is likely to develop.[92] They, along with others, have in more recent studies demonstrated that some of the risk factors for atherogenesis lead to an increased tendency for platelets to agglutinate and to be consumed rapidly.[93-100]

Ross recognized that platelets liberate a potent peptide (or peptides) that promotes proliferation of arterial SMC's in vitro.[2,32,47,101] This observation was combined with important in vivo studies which demonstrated that factors which inhibit platelet sticking, spreading, and disintegration over areas of damaged arterial endothelium also inhibit SMC proliferation in these areas. These studies led Ross, Harker, and Glomset to utilize nonhuman primate experimental models and to coordinate these findings with observations in human subjects with metabolic disorders, especially homocystinemia, and with their in vitro study of the proliferative response of arterial SMC in tissue culture.[2,32,47,101-104] These investigators have proposed that the proliferative response of the SMC's in atherosclerotic plaques that develop over injured arterial intima is mainly due to the "platelet factor," which appears to be liberated from adherent and disintegrating platelets (Fig. 34–7). This work by the Seattle group has been reviewed in light of other observations that support the importance of endothelial injury in some cases of human atherosclerosis and in some types of experimental plaque formation.[2,32]

Recent advances in the understanding of the platelet-derived growth factor have included the purification of this active peptide[105-107] and the demonstration that it supports SMC migration as well as proliferation,[108] that it interacts with mesenchymal cells to increase pinocytosis,[109] and that it binds specifically with a receptor on the surface of cells it stimulates.[110,111]

One of the paradoxes about endothelial injury and atherogenesis which is the subject of intensive investigation is the observation first reported by Minick, Stemerman, and Insull.[112] They found that the most severe rabbit atherogenesis did not occur in the balloon catheter–denuded areas which were carpeted by platelets, but rather in the areas where endothelial cells had recently grown over the denuded areas. Further study has indicated that, in part at least, this increased atherogenesis in the reendothelialized areas may be correlated with the increased binding of lipoprotein lipid by proteoglycans associated with this newly covered area,[113] and that these areas are prone to increased cholesterol synthesis and decreased hydrolysis.[114]

The recognition that arterial endothelial damage is important in some cases of atherogenesis has additional implications which support the role of LDL in atherogenesis. One of the weaknesses of the so-called "lipid theory" of the pathogenesis of atherosclerosis has been the occasional exceptional case, in which advanced atherosclerosis with clinical effects occurs at an early age and in the absence of major risk factors (hypercholesterolemia, hypertension, and cigarette smoking). It now appears that a number of these exceptional or paradoxical cases may fall into a specific category, represented diagrammatically in the right-hand portion of Figure 34–8. If accelerated and advanced plaque formation can occur even when LDL (cholesterol) levels are low, while arterial endothelial injury is *severe* and *sustained* or *repeated frequently*, this would offer a rational explanation for a number of clinical reports and recent experimental results.[115-119] Recognition of the importance of arterial endothelial injury in the absence of hypercholesterolemia, cigarette smoking, and hypertension should encourage the search for better clinical tests to help the practicing physician detect and correct endothelial injury as a major risk factor when it is a predominant part of atherogenesis or when it is an important adjunct of hypercholesterolemia (Table 34–2).[120] Thus far, platelet survival time seems to be the best available laboratory test for measuring severe endothelial damage.[102] Unfortunately, this is a rather cumbersome invasive procedure that requires the removal of blood, separation of the patient's own

TABLE 34–2 FACTORS WHICH HAVE BEEN SHOWN TO INJURE ARTERIAL ENDOTHELIUM AND TO PRODUCE INCREASED PERMEABILITY TO MACROMOLECULES, INCLUDING LIPOPROTEINS

Substance or Physical Condition	Mechanism Involved	Clinical Condition
Hemodynamic forces; tension, stretching, shearing, eddy currents	Separation or damage to endothelial cells, increased permeability, platelet sticking, stimulation of smooth muscle cell proliferation	Hypertension
Angiotensin II	"Trap-door" effect	Hypertension
Carbon monoxide or decreased O_2 saturation	Destruction of endothelial cells	Cigarette smoking
Catecholamines (epinephrine, norepinephrine, serotonin, bradykinin)	Hypercontraction, swelling and loss of endothelial cells, platelet agglutination	Stress, cigarette smoking
Metabolic products	Endothelial cell damage	Homocystinemia, uremia, and so on
Endotoxins and other similar bacterial products	Endothelial cell destruction, platelet sticking	Acute bacterial infections
Ag-Ab complexes, immunological defects	Platelet agglutination	Serum sickness, transplant rejection, immune complex diseases, lupus erythematosus
Virus diseases	Endothelial cell infection and necrosis	Viremias
Mechanical trauma to endothelium	Platelet sticking, increased local permeability	Catheter injury
Hyperlipidemia with increase in circulating lipoproteins (cholesterol, triglycerides, phospholipids) and free fatty acids	Platelet agglutination in areas of usually hemodynamic damage, over "fatty streaks"	Chronic nutritional imbalance (high-fat and high-cholesterol diets), familial hypercholesterolemia, diabetes, nephrosis, hypothyroidism

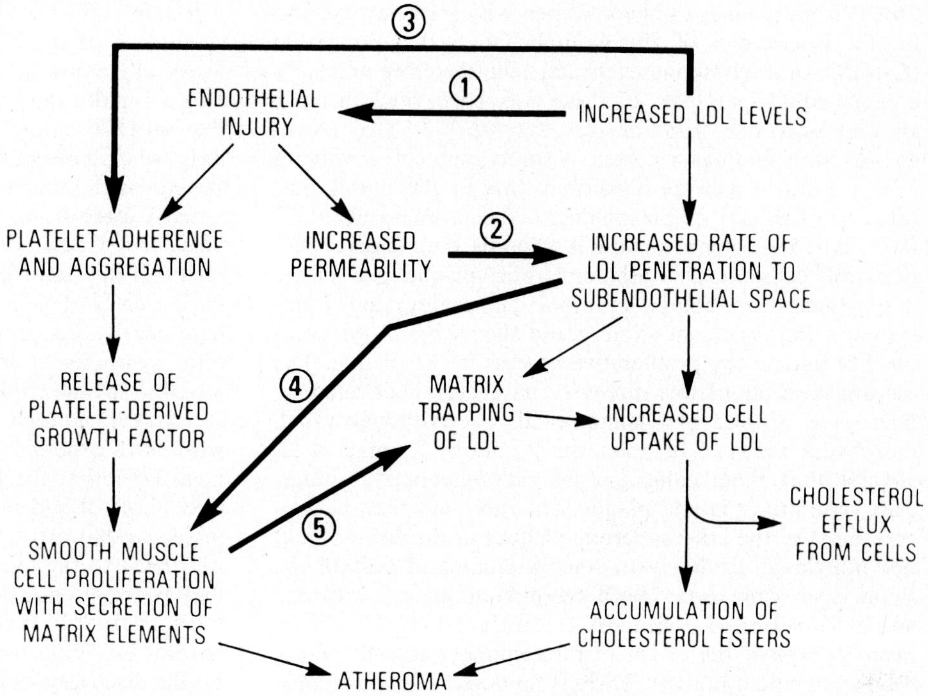

FIGURE 34–10 This diagram indicates the probable interactions between the two major pathogenetic mechanisms proposed for atherogenesis. The steps involved according to the endothelial injury formulation are on the left, and those for the lipid-cholesterol formulation are on the right. The interactions are numbered as follows: (1) LDL in high concentrations induces endothelial injury; (2) endothelial injury increases influx of LDL; (3) hyperlipoproteinemia stimulates platelet aggregation; (4) high LDL levels stimulate proliferation of arterial SMC which are in the stationary phase; and (5) SMC-produced extracellular matrix binds and traps LDL molecules, which in turn may permit increased cellular uptake of LDL. (From Steinberg, D.: Metabolism of lipoproteins at the cellular level in relation to atherogenesis. *In* Miller, N. E., and Lewis, B. (eds.): Lipoproteins, Atherosclerosis and Coronary Heart Disease. Amsterdam, Elsevier, 1981, p. 31.)

platelets, and labeling of these platelets with an appropriate radioactive isotope. A simpler but reliable noninvasive procedure, such as radioimmunoassay for circulating platelet factor 4, may ultimately be useful to detect widespread endothelial damage and platelet sticking in the absence of other risk factors.[121]

As the concepts of lipoprotein insudation and arterial endothelial injury advance and become more clearly understood, it becomes increasingly evident that we are dealing with strongly interacting pathogenetic mechanisms. These interactions have been recently summarized in a highly useful diagrammatic form by Steinberg.[122] He has indicated (Fig. 34–10) the ways in which elevated levels of LDL (or β-VLDL) and the various forms of endothelial injury may interact to support the progression of the atherosclerotic plaque. In the last analysis, it now seems likely that both of these pathological processes may be active in plaque formation.

ROLE OF MACROPHAGES

Another area of study which has had a recent upsurge, relative to the pathobiology and pathogenesis of atherosclerosis, is the evaluation of the role of the macrophages in the developing atherosclerotic lesion. This is not a new area of interest, since the proposal of a special function for the blood-derived macrophage in certain well-defined experimental atheromatous lesions has existed for many years.[123] Because of the evidence which, in general, indicates that the fibroblast and the arterial SMC have, under most circumstances, limited capacities for lipid accumulation, there has been a general trend to search for a "scavenger cell" of another type which could correspond to the appearance of the limited number of foam cells in most human atherosclerotic lesions.

The macrophage fulfills this role, since it has a very large capacity to take up and store altered low-density[89] or diet-induced β-VLDL lipoproteins.[31] Furthermore, it has been demonstrated that LDL can be altered in several ways to a suitable form to be inbibed by macrophages which might be active during atherogenesis. These include malondialdehyde alterations of LDL by platelets,[87] conversion of LDL to a special form by endothelial cells,[88] and the formation of quantities of β-VLDL by cholesterol and fat feeding.[91] The macrophage and its functions are complex, and at the present time, although no one doubts its role as a scavenger, it is difficult to be certain whether its scavenger function is more likely to inhibit lesion progression by removing lipid as well as furnishing collagenases and elastases, or whether it is a major force in producing more lipid accumulation and SMC proliferation by depositing altered LDL lipid (by means of foam cell death) and secreting a growth factor or factors which stimulate arterial SMC proliferation. Unfortunately, none of these functions has been well documented in human atherosclerotic lesions.

IN VITRO STUDIES

Recently, some of the most promising and most exciting developments in the investigation of the pathogenesis of atherosclerosis have come from the use of in vitro as well as microdissection methods to study the pathobiology of cells of the arterial wall.[1,64,120,124] A variety of methods have been utilized in these studies, ranging from the biochemical and cell kinetic investigations of small fragments of arterial media or atherosclerotic plaques derived from humans or animals, to the study and growth of cells from explants of arterial media or subcultures of these outgrowths, to the study of dispersed cells or homogenates from small, carefully selected, microdissected samples of human or animal lesions.

Each of these approaches has yielded valuable new insights into the atherosclerotic process, but none is more surprising or innovative than the reports of Benditt and coworkers. These investigators found that many foci of

SMC's from plaques of black women who are heterozygotic for the isoenzymes of glucose-6-phosphate dehydrogenase (G-6-PD) and whose mesenchymal cells therefore normally contain equal quantities of these two isoenzymes, usually showed only one form of this enzyme.[125–128] This corresponds with findings reported in similar subjects involving benign tumors such as fibroleiomyoma in the uterus and other neoplasms.[129–131] This finding of isoenzymatically similar cells is interesting because it suggests that these collections of cells in the atherosclerotic plaque are either monoclonal or monotypic in origin. The analogy to neoplasia raises important questions about the nature of the stimuli that initiate the proliferative process in the plaque. The essential aspects of this discovery have been confirmed by Pearson et al. and by Thomas et al.[132–135] Although much more work needs to be done, the studies by Thomas et al. suggest that these collections of isoenzymatically similar cells arise rather late in plaque formation and that, in general, most of the atherosclerotic plaques in the aorta of any one individual are likely to contain clumps of cells of the same isoenzymic type. Both these findings, if confirmed and extended, tend to support a "natural selection" mechanism to explain the origin of these monotypic cells rather than a somatic mutation. There is no doubt that this painstaking effort and the rationale behind it have stimulated further research into the fundamental nature of the processes controlling cell proliferation in the atherosclerotic plaque.

Other significant recent findings have come from the investigations by Goldstein and Brown at the University of Texas, using in vitro techniques.[31,89,91,136–138] These scientists have discovered the defective control mechanisms in the mesenchymal cells of patients suffering from familial hypercholesterolemia. They have established the importance of receptors to apo B on the surfaces of peripheral cells as well as their role in regulating cholesteryl ingress into the cell and the rates at which cholesterol ester is hydrolyzed and free cholesterol is esterified. This fascinating series of studies and the genetic principles involved are reviewed in Chapter 47.

Mahley et al. have extended this approach to the study of the enhanced avidity of arginine-rich apoproteins (Apo E) for receptors on mesenchymal and some parenchymal cells.[139] This too, appears to be only an initial step in discovering the pathobiology of plaque formation using in vitro methods, since clearly it is necessary to extend these studies to include the quantitative variations that occur in the more or less normal mesenchymal cells of most individuals who acquire this disease process. Furthermore, much is still to be learned about the alternate routes by which cholesterol gains entrance to the cytoplasm of arterial SMC when apolipoprotein receptors are absent. The Mahley group, combined with Goldstein, Brown, and others,[138] has gone far to clarify the genetic aspects of familial dysbetalipoproteinemia (i.e., type 3 hyperlipoproteinemia). Mahley and his colleagues have provided a clear-cut view of the comparative pathology of atherogenesis in a number of species. Specifically, they have documented the importance of β-VLDL in atherogenesis and demonstrated that SMC really can develop into foam cells in the dog.[139] The mechanisms of egress—short of cell death—of excess cholesterol and cholesteryl ester from the cells of the atherosclerotic lesion are an almost untouched area of research.

ROLE OF HIGH-DENSITY LIPOPROTEIN. The interaction of the high-density lipoprotein (HDL) fraction (especially some of its components) with arterial SMC's is also a rapidly developing field of investigation. It appears that rat HDL apo C-III (or human HDL apo A-I), particularly when present with certain phospholipids, facilitates the egress of substantial quantities of cholesterol and cholesterol ester from the cytoplasm of cultured lipid-laden SMC's.[140–143] Scanu, Byrne, and Milhovilovic have recently reviewed this complex area.[144] Innerarity, Pitas, and Mahley have clearly demonstrated a modulating effect of canine high-density lipoproteins rich in apo E on the cholesteryl ester synthesis in macrophages usually stimulated by β-VLDL.[145] These studies of cultured cells are supported by a substantial amount of epidemiological work and some work with experimental animals.[146–149] They have led to the hypothesis that the HDL fraction, which is relatively poor in cholesterol and rich in phospholipid, acts as a protective molecule that can transport cholesterol from peripheral tissues back to the liver, where, if conditions are favorable, it may be excreted rather than re-utilized in the production of more LDL.[150,151] Knowledge of HDL contribution to cholesterol excretion has been substantially increased recently by the discovery of the hepatic apo E receptor and its relationship to apo B, E hepatic receptor.[152]

One of the most interesting new aspects of research to confirm the protective effect of a relatively high level of HDL in the circulation is the positive correlation between regular physical exercise, such as that recommended to strengthen the cardiorespiratory system, and the favorable ratio between HDL and LDL that seems to accompany this type of activity.[153–155] This phenomenon has now been demonstrated clearly in nonhuman primates.[156] So far, the reasons for this correlation at the cellular or basic biochemical level are not clear, but this appears to be a rich field for further study and may ultimately provide a more compelling justification for regular, vigorous exercise to prevent atherogenesis.

We have already described the work of Ross and colleagues relative to the emerging pathobiology of arterial SMC proliferation in vitro as part of their study of the role of endothelial injury and "platelet factor" in the development of the atherosclerotic plaque.[101–104] Ross' observations[2,32] play a prominent role in a number of studies yielding new findings about endogenous factors in the mammal that may exert important influences on the proliferation of mesenchymal cells in health and disease.[157] Knowledge in this fast-changing field will be substantially advanced when the mechanism of action and the interrelationships of these potent stimulators of cell proliferation are better defined.

EFFECT OF LDL ON SMOOTH MUSCLE CELLS. Apparently quite separate from the platelet, macrophage, and endothelial cell factors and equally incompletely understood is the SMC proliferation–stimulating effect of LDL obtained from hyperlipidemic rhesus monkey or rabbit serum, first reported from our laboratory in 1968.[158] This effect is apparently due to a narrow fraction of LDL, not present in normal serum (H-LDL) and over a wide range is not dose dependent on LDL cholesterol concentration.[159–161] It apparently is also not related to the type of food fat fed, even though the latter may affect plaque cell proliferation in vivo.[162]

This growth-stimulating effect of LDL from hyperlipidemic monkey serum is distinct from and additive to the effects of the platelet factor.[163,164] Chen et al. have also demonstrated similar effects using LDL from hyperlipidemic rabbit serum and subcultures from rabbit aortic medial cells.[165,166] Robertson has reported that subcultures of human arterial SMC exposed to LDL from hyperlipidemic human serum are stimulated to increased mitotic activity and increased incorporation of ^{3}H thymidine.[167,168] Serum and LDL from homozygous type II patients have been tested on stationary outgrowths from aortic media explants of rhesus monkeys.

Myasnikov et al., in the Soviet Union, demonstrated as early as 1966 the cell growth–stimulating effect of hyperlipidemic serum from patients with atherosclerosis.[169] This followed their earlier demonstration of similar effects with rabbit hyperlipidemic serum and aortic cells.[170]

Estradiol and HDL from normal serum block the mitosis-stimulating effect of LDL from hyperlipidemic serum.[171,172] This general effect of LDL from hyperlipidemic serum on arterial SMC proliferation has recently been clarified somewhat by the work of Fless and Scanu.[85,86] They have found that it is possible to identify and isolate fractions of rhesus monkey LDL, which they have designated LDL I, II, III, and IV. LDL I, usually present in rather small amounts in normal monkey serum, will stimulate quiescent arterial SMC to proliferate. It is similar to, but probably not identical with, the predominant LDL fraction (H-LDL), which is elevated in hyperlipidemic rhesus monkey serum. LDL II, III, and IV have no such cell proliferation stimulatory effect in their native form, but LDL III from normal monkey serum becomes active when it is suitably treated with sialidase from *Clostridium perfringens.* These recently reported results make it possible to study the entire question of the mechanism of stimulation of arterial SMC proliferation by LDL from hyperlipidemic serum under carefully controlled conditions.

Stimulatory effects of serum from diabetic animals and humans, first demonstrated by Ledet,[173–178] and from untreated hypertensive animals, reported by Fischer-Dzoga and Pick and others,[179–184] are other possible mechanisms by which risk factors increase arterial SMC proliferation. These observed effects do not seem to be related to proliferation stimulated by insulin or glucose content of the serum. Further work is indicated to determine whether these serum factors are major contributors to the hyperplasia of arterial smooth muscle cells.

Some effects of various types of lipoproteins on the lipid and cholesterol metabolism of subcultures of arterial smooth muscle cells have been described in detail in Chapter 47. Studies by Chen et al., by Bates and Wissler, and more recently by St. Clair et al.[185–191] indicate that the LDL from hyperlipidemic serum is able to promote accumulation of cholesteryl esters in arterial smooth muscle cells. This may be due to qualitative differences between LDL from hyperlipidemic serum and normolipidemic serum, to an HDL/LDL imbalance, or to some other mechanism. This phenomenon supports the importance of elevated LDL levels in atherogenesis.

In vitro studies using cultured endothelial cells and other modern cell biological studies promise to yield important data.[192–195] They have been used to investigate antihemophilic and von Willebrand factors and to develop knowledge about the metabolism of endothelium as it relates to atherosclerosis.[13,195–200] Since synthesis and deposition of extracellular products of the arterial SMC, such as collagen, elastin, and glycosaminoglycans, may be influenced by the same factors as are atherosclerotic plaques, further study is needed.[25,27–29]

Factors that allow egress of lipid from these cells are also important in determining the extent of necrosis and ulceration. The elegant in vitro systems now available will continue to be applied to further investigation of the mechanisms of lipid accumulation, cell proliferation, cell necrosis, synthesis of fiber proteins, and lipid egress, all of which are important in atherosclerosis research.

EXPERIMENTAL MODELS OF ATHEROSCLEROSIS

The inaccessibility of tissues and the gradual development of the disease process over decades in humans, as well as the difficulties of conducting controlled studies of large groups of free-living people, make reliable animal models of atherosclerosis relevant and especially valuable. Experimental counterparts of the human disease process are becoming much more highly developed, and their similarities to, as well as their differences from, the lesions in people are becoming better documented. Animal models are thus making a growing contribution to an understanding of the pathogenesis or the regression of atheromatous lesions.[123,201–205]

Although all of the commonly used animal models have contributed valuable information, some are much more useful for the study of advanced disease.[201] The swine and the macaque monkey models appear to provide a much closer approximation to the clinically demonstrable disease process than do some of the older models. Although the dog has generally been reported to be relatively resistant to diet-induced disease, it has been possible to produce advanced disease and to study successfully the regression of canine lesions subsequent to induction of severe hypercholesterolemia by means of an atherogenic ration and thyroid suppression.[206,207] Recently, the dog has proved to be valuable in the study of atherogenicity of hydrogenated coconut oil.[208,209] Using either of these means of induction, Mahley et al. have demonstrated that the development of significant atherosclerosis in the dog correlates well with hypercholesterolemias which have unusually high levels of cholesterol-rich and apo B–rich lipoproteins with a density of 1.006 gm/ml or below (so called broad-beta or beta-rich VLDL).[210]

Studies of the Monkey

The rhesus monkey (*Macaca mulatta*) has been the most frequently utilized species of the nonhuman primate models, since it has virtually no spontaneous atheromatous disease but develops progressive atherosclerosis with "clinical" complications soon after being fed a mixed and well-balanced commercial monkey ration supplemented with saturated fat and cholesterol (Fig. 34–11).[30,202,204,211–219]

Ingestion of Coconut Oil. In pioneering studies, Taylor et al. showed that rhesus monkeys developed lesions which were essentially similar to human plaques in distribution and in plaque components.[11,220–226] Unlike in nonprimate models, there appeared to be little small artery involvement, little loading of the reticuloendothelial system (RES), and relatively little monocyte-derived foam cell lesion component. Subsequently, studies in this laboratory showed that substitution in the ration of coconut oil for part of the butterfat augmented the process.[64,123,211,227]

In studies with the cebus monkey, we have observed that coconut oil is more effective than butterfat in inducing an elevation of serum LDL levels. The atherosclerotic lesions produced by it seem to exhibit more cell proliferation, a larger necrotic center, and more evidence of irritation or low-grade inflammation of the artery wall, based on mononuclear cell infiltrates in the adventitia.[211,228] Since coconut oil is increasingly used often as a "hidden" ingredient labeled only as "vegetable fat," the special atherogenicity of this food fat is a cause for concern.[208–211,229]

TABLE 34–3 PROBABLE MECHANISMS OF ACTION OF RISK FACTORS AT THE CELLULAR LEVEL

Hypercholesterolemia (Whether due to high-cholesterol-calorie-saturated fat *diet** or metabolically induced,* including inherited types	Increased levels of circulating low-density lipoproteins (LDL) damage endothelium and carry cholesterol into artery wall, especially if high-density lipoprotein (HDL) levels are low; lipid (cholesterol) is "trapped," accumulates in smooth muscle cells, or is bound to their extracellular products; leads to cell proliferation and/or necrosis, increased collagen formation, and so on
Hypertension	Increased endothelial permeability to LDL *due to* 1. Increased artery wall tension 2. "Trap-door effect" of and endothelial damage from angiotensin 3. Platelet sticking (norepinephrine-induced?) with release of vasoactive amines 4. Especially bad when added to hypercholesterolemia 5. Serum "factor" stimulates arterial smooth muscle cell (SMC) proliferation
Cigarette smoking	*Damage to cells of artery wall due* to 1. Circulating CO 2. Platelet agglutination (norepinephrine-induced?) 3. ↑lipid mobilization (norepinephrine-induced?), leading to hyperlipemia and increased lipid in artery wall
Diabetes	CHO-induced hyperlipemia (VLDL) along with an increase of glycosaminoglycans in the intima that binds lipoproteins; factors in the serum of diabetics that are not related to lipoproteins, insulin, or sugar stimulate arterial smooth muscle cell (SMC) proliferation
Sedentary living and obesity	Appear to increase the tendency toward elevated serum LDL with relatively low serum levels of HDL, increased incidence of diabetes and hypertension, poor cardiac reserve, and increased work for the heart

*May also stimulate platelet sticking and clotting tendency so that superimposed thrombosis is more likely to occur.

bran along with its naturally occurring gums and fibers.[295] We must also be alert to the existence of unrecognized risk factors that may produce chronic and substantial damage to the arterial endothelium.

The current spectrum of promising interventions in the process of atherosclerosis is presented in Figure 34–13. The natural history of the development of lesions during an individual's lifetime offers an opportunity at almost all ages for prevention or treatment. The major problem for the general public, for public health professional personnel and officers, and for the practicing physician is still the early detection of risk factors before the catastrophic and life-threatening effects of severe atherosclerosis ensue.

Here, too, the advancement of knowledge is swift and promising. For many years, the absence of coronary thrombi in most people who died suddenly with advanced coronary atherosclerosis presented a dilemma.[296–298] Now it appears that there are actually two or more pathogenic mechanisms in acute heart attacks, although, in almost all cases, both should be regarded as results of severe coronary atherosclerosis.[299–301] One is the classic development of *thrombosis of the coronary artery and transmural myocardial infarction,* which usually does not lead to sudden death and which benefits from prompt medical attention and hospitalization. In this instance, attempts are made to limit the size of the infarct, and modern coronary care is provided.[302]

The second is the *sudden onset of ventricular fibrillation* at home, at work, or in the community as a result of electrical instability of cardiac rhythm triggered by mechanisms that are not always clear (Chap. 23). These victims will die suddenly unless promptly rescued by individuals trained in cardiopulmonary resuscitation (CPR). This must be followed by prompt attention from trained emergency medical care teams equipped with modern defibrillation and life-support devices and medication. We now know that many of these victims are not likely to develop electrocardiographic or enzymatic evidence of myocardial infarction if resuscitation and defibrillation are successful.[303] However, this type of heart attack tends to recur, and

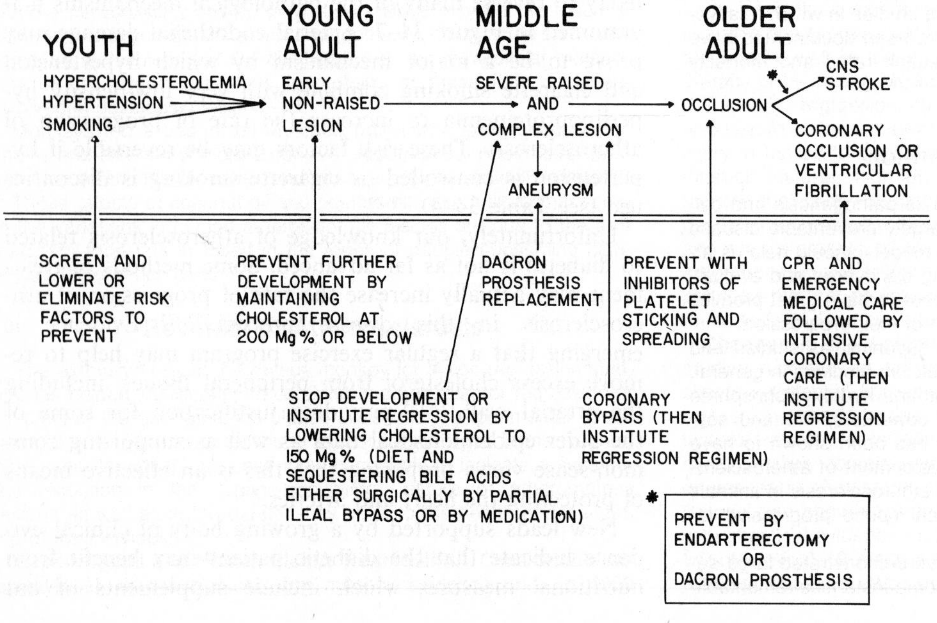

FIGURE 34–13 A spectrum of the available methods of intervention in human atherosclerosis, beginning early in life with an emphasis on prevention and later employing measures designed to retard or reverse the development of progressive plaques. As clinical effects of lesions develop, therapy should be designed to prolong life and facilitate regression of the plaques. (Modified from Wissler, R. W., and Vesselinovitch, D.: Regression of atherosclerosis in experimental animals and man. Verh. Dtsch. Ges. Inn. Med. (Munich) *81*:857, 1975.)

these patients should be considered to be prone to the serious effects of atherosclerosis. They not only should be protected from subsequent episodes of ventricular fibrillation by means of the most reliable and effective medications available but also should undergo therapy to slow the progress of the lesion, which, it is hoped, will in some instances result in regression of the underlying disease.

Chronic angina is another clinical effect of atherosclerosis that does not always seem to fit into the commonly accepted concept of risk factors leading to lipid-filled plaques, which, in turn, lead to coronary thrombosis and finally myocardial infarction. For one thing, females show a propensity for angina, and, in addition, these patients appear to have a lower rate of myocardial infarction than would be expected in individuals with severe atherosclerosis without angina.[304] Are the coronary atherosclerotic lesions different in these patients with chronically recurring angina than in those who develop acute myocardial infarction? Is there greater involvement of the small artery? Does this type of heart disease have a different set of risk factors that are more endogenously determined, such as coronary arterial spasm? Recent observations point to the role of spasm near areas of especially severe coronary atherosclerosis possibly triggered by products released by adherent platelets in these highly damaged and diseased areas.[305–307] The spasms demonstrated angiographically in these studies have correlated well with the onset of symptoms of angina.

In general, it appears that the atherosclerosis in patients with angina is qualitatively similar to that in other patients but may be more diffuse in distribution and more fibrous in character. Also, the small coronary radicles are not involved in most patients. We have not learned to identify other risk factors for the syndrome, if indeed, any exist. We therefore have much to learn about this manifestation of atherosclerosis.

Patients who have had a myocardial infarction or who have undergone coronary bypass surgery, endarterectomy, or balloon arterioplasty must have skillful and diligent medical management with emphasis on removing all recognizable risk factors. The areas of severe disease, the junctions with grafts, and the areas of arterial manipulation are particularly vulnerable to progression of the atherosclerotic process. In those especially vulnerable patients who already have evidence of advanced atherosclerosis, it is important that every effort be made to retard or to produce regression of the atherogenic process.

Acknowledgments

The author is grateful to Gertrud Friedman, Gwen Matthews, and Denise Wooten for their diligent and skillful work in helping to prepare this revision. He also wishes to acknowledge the help of Mr. Gordon Bowie in preparing much of the accompanying illustrative material. Many colleagues and coworkers have also helped greatly in the studies in this laboratory which have sustained our interest in the pathogenesis of atherosclerosis and have helped us to contribute in a modest way to the concepts of pathogenesis and regression herein described. Special recognition is extended to Draga Vesselinovitch, Sandra Bates, Jayme Borensztajn, Robert Chen, Katti Fischer-Dzoga, Robin Fraser, Godfrey Getz, Seymour Glagov, Masako Mitsumata, Ruth Pick, Leon Resnekov, Arthur Rubenstein, Angelo Scanu, Thomas Schaffner, Yoji Yoshida, and Christopher Zarins, as well as to our technical and scientific associates, Manuela Bekermeier, Blanche Berger, Tim Bridenstine, Gabrielle Chassagne, Laurence Frazier, Laura Harris, Randolph Hughes, and Rose Jones.

The studies in this laboratory referred to and summarized in this chapter were supported in part by funds from U.S. Public Health Service grants HL 15062, HL 17648, HL 12308, and HL 6894 as well as the Cardiovascular Research Foundation of The University of Chicago.

References

1. Wissler, R. W., Vesselinovitch, D., and Getz, G. J.: Abnormalities of the arterial wall and its metabolism in atherogenesis. Prog. Cardiovasc. Dis. *18*: 341, 1976.
2. Ross, R., and Glomset, J. A.: The pathogenesis of atherosclerosis. N. Engl. J. Med. *295*:369, 420, 1976.
3. Arteriosclerosis, 1981. Report of the Working Group on Arteriosclerosis of the National Heart, Lung and Blood Institute. Vol. 1, DHHS–NIH Publication No. 81–2034, Washington, 1981.
4. Stamler, J.: Diet-related risk factors for human atherosclerosis: Hyperlipidemia, hypertension, hyperglycemia—Current status. *In* Sirtori, C., Ricci, G., and Gorini, G. (eds.): Diet and Atherosclerosis. (Adv. Exp. Med. Biol., Vol. 60.) New York, Plenum Press, 1975, p. 125.
5. Keys, A.: Coronary heart disease—The global picture. Atherosclerosis *22*:149, 1975.
6. Intersociety Commission for Heart Disease Resources Report: Primary prevention of the atherosclerotic diseases. Circulation *62*:A–55, 1970.
7. Kuller, L. H.: Epidemiology of cardiovascular diseases: Current perspectives Am. J. Epidemiol. *104*:425, 1976.
8. Meyer, W. W., Walsh, S. Z., and Lind, J.: Functional morphology of arteries during fetal and post-natal development. *In* Schwartz, C. J., Werthessen, N. T., and Wolf, S. (eds.): Structure and Function of the Circulation. Vol. I. New York, Plenum Press, 1980, p. 95.
9. Hess, R., and Staubli, W.: Ultrastructure of vascular changes. *In* Schettler, F. G., and Boyd, G. S. (eds.): Atherosclerosis: Pathology, Physiology, Aetiology, Diagnosis and Clinical Management. Amsterdam, Elsevier Publishing Co., 1969, p. 49.
10. McGill, H. C.: The lesion. *In* Schettler, G., and Weizel, A. (eds.): Atherosclerosis III. Berlin, Springer-Verlag, 1974, p. 27.
11. Taylor, C. B., Trueheart, R. E., and Cox, G. E.: Atherosclerosis in rhesus monkeys. III. The role of increased thickness of arterial walls in atherogenesis. Arch. Pathol. *76*:14, 1963.
12. Zarins, C. K., Bomberger, R. A., and Glagov, S.: Local effects of stenoses: Increased flow velocity inhibits atherogenesis. Circulation *64*:II–221, 1981.
13. Gimbrone, M. A., Jr.: Vascular endothelium and atherosclerosis. *In* Moore, S. (ed.): Vascular Injury and Atherosclerosis. New York, Marcel Dekker, 1981, p. 25.
14. Reichl, D., Simons, L. A., Myant, N. B., Pflug, J. J., and Mills, G. L.: The lipids and lipoproteins of human peripheral lymph with observations on the transport of cholesterol from plasma and tissues into lymph. Clin. Sci. Mol. Med. *45*:313, 1973.
15. Scott, P. J., and Hurley, P. J.: The distribution of radio-iodinated serum albumin and low density lipoprotein in tissues and the arterial wall. Atherosclerosis *11*:77, 1970.
16. Smith, E. B., and Slater, R. W.: Relationship between low density lipoprotein in aortic intima and serum lipid levels. Lancet *1*:463, 1972.
17. Day, C. E., and Levy, R. S.: Control of the precipitation reaction between low density lipoproteins and polyions. Artery *1*:150, 1975.
18. Stein, O., Stein, Y., and Eisenberg, S.: Radioautographic study of the transport of ^{125}I-labeled serum lipoproteins in rat aorta. Z. Zellforsch Mikrosk. Anta. *138*:223, 1973.
19. Esterly, J., and Glagov, S.: Altered permeability of the renal artery of the hypertensive rat: An electron microscopic study. Am. J. Pathol. *43*:619, 1963.
20. Wissler, R. W.: Progression and regression of atherosclerotic lesions. *In* Chandler, A. B., Eurenius, K., McMillan, G. C., Nelson, C. B., Schwartz, C. J., and Wessler, S. (eds.): The Thrombotic Process in Atherogenesis. New York, Plenum Press, 1978, p. 77.
21. Gerrity, R., Richardson, M., Somer, J. B., Bell, F. P., and Schwartz, C. J.: Endothelial cell morphology in areas of in vivo Evans Blue uptake in the aorta of young pigs. Am. J. Pathol. *89*:313, 1977.
22. Weber, G., Fabbrini, P., and Resi, L.: On the presence of a concanavallin-A reactive coat over the endothelial aortic surface and its modifications during early experimental cholesterol atherogenesis in rabbits. Virchows Arch. Abt. A. Path. Anat. *259*:299, 1973.
23. Wolinsky, H., and Glagov, S.: Comparison of abdominal and thoracic aortic medial structure in mammals. Deviation of man from the usual pattern. Circ. Res. *25*:677, 1969.
24. Glagov, S.: Hemodynamic risk factors: Mechanical stress, mural architecture, medial nutrition and the vulnerability of arteries to atherosclerosis. *In* Wissler, R. W., and Geer, J. C. (eds.): The Pathogenesis of Atherosclerosis. Baltimore, The Williams and Wilkins Co., 1972, p. 164.
25. Wissler, R. W.: The arterial medial cell, smooth muscle or multifunctional mesenchyme? J. Atheros. Res. *8*:201, 1968.
26. Fischer-Dzoga, K., Jones, R. M., Vesselinovitch, D., and Wissler, R. W.: Ultrastructural and immunohistochemical studies of primary cultures of aortic medial cells. Exp. Mol. Pathol. *18*:162, 1973.

27. Ross, R., and Klebanoff, S. J.: The smooth muscle cell. I. In vivo synthesis of connective tissue proteins. J. Cell Biol. *50*:159, 1971.
28. Ross, R.: The smooth muscle cell. II. Growth of smooth muscle in culture and formation of elastic fibers. J. Cell Biol. *50*:172, 1971.
29. Wight, T. N., and Ross, R.: Proteoglycans in primate arteries. II. Synthesis and secretion of glycosaminoglycans by arterial smooth muscle cells in culture. J. Cell Biol. *67*:675, 1975.
30. Wissler, R. W.: Atherosclerosis: Its pathogenesis in perspective. *In* Homberger, F. (ed.): Comparative Pathology of the Heart. (Advances in Cardiology, Vol. 13.) Basel, Karger, 1974, p.10.
31. Goldstein, J. L., Ho, Y. K., Brown, M. S., Innerarity, T. L., and Mahley, R. W.: Cholesteryl ester accumulation in macrophages resulting from receptor-mediated uptake and degradation of hypercholesterolemic canine β-very low density lipoproteins. J. Biol. Chem. *255*:1839, 1980.
32. Ross, R.: Atherosclerosis: A problem of the biology of arterial wall cells and their interactions with blood components. Arteriosclerosis *1*:293, 1981.
33. Clark, J. M., and Glagov, S.: Structural integration of the arterial wall. I. Relationships and attachments of medial smooth muscle cells in normally distended and hyperdistended aortas. Lab. Invest. *40*:587, 1979.
34. Glagov, S.: Relation of structure to function in arterial walls. Artery *5*:295, 1979.
35. Glagov, S., and Ozoa, A.: Significance of the relatively low incidence of atherosclerosis in the pulmonary, renal and mesenteric arteries. Ann. N.Y. Acad. Sci. *149*:940, 1968.
36. Strong, J. P., Eggen, D. A., and Oalmann, M. C.: The natural history, geographic pathology, and epidemiology of atherosclerosis. *In* Wissler, R. W., and Geer, J. C. (eds.): The Pathogenesis of Atherosclerosis. Baltimore, The Williams and Wilkins Co., 1972, p. 20.
37. Glagov, S., Rowley, D. A., Cramer, D. B., and Page, R. G.: Heart rate during 24 hours of usual activity for 100 normal men. J. Appl. Physiol. *29*:799, 1970.
38. Wissler, R. W., and Vesselinovitch, D.: Atherosclerosis—Relationship to coronary blood flow. Sixth Triennial Australian National Heart Foundation Conference on Physiology and Pathology of Coronary Heart Disease, Canberra, Australia, February 1982. Am. J. Cardiol. (in press).
39. Wissler, R. W., and Vesselinovitch, D.: New concepts of factors involved in the natural history and regression of atherosclerosis. First World Vascular Day and 7th International Symposium of the International Society for Angiography and Angiology, Berlin, West Germany. Periodica Angiologica, 1982.
40. Roberts, W. C.: The status of the coronary arteries in fatal ischemic heart disease. Cardiovasc. Clin. *7*:1, 1975.
41. Roberts, W. C.: The coronary arteries in coronary heart disease: Morphologic observations. Pathobiol. Ann. *5*:249, 1975.
42. McGill, H. C., Jr., Geer, J. C., and Strong, J. P.: Natural history of human atherosclerotic lesions. *In* Sandler, M., and Bourne, G. H. (eds.): Atherosclerosis and its origin. New York, Academic Press, 1963, p. 42.
43. Constantinides, P.: Experimental Atherosclerosis. Amsterdam, Elsevier Publishing Co., 1965.
44. Brown, M. S., Kovanen, P. T., and Goldstein, J. L.: Regulation of plasma cholesterol by lipoprotein receptors. Science *212*:628, 1981.
45. Stemerman, M. B., and Ross, R.: Experimental atherosclerosis I. Fibrous plaque formation in primates, an electron microscopic study. J. Exp. Med. *136*: 769, 1972.
46. Bjorkerud, S., and Bondjers, G.: Repair responses and tissue lipid after experimental injury to the artery. Ann. N.Y. Acad. Sci. *275*:180, 1976.
47. Ross, R.: Atherosclerosis and the arterial smooth muscle cell. Science *180*: 1332, 1973.
48. Getz, G. S., Wissler, R. W., Hughes, R. H., Graber, C., and Tantraj, S.: Metabolism of lipids in the atherosclerotic rhesus monkey aorta. Proc. Inst. Med. Chicago *27*:106, 1968.
49. Adams, C. M., Morgan, R. S., and Bayliss, O. B.: The differential entry of ^{123}I-albumin into mildly and severely atheromatous rabbit aortas. Atherosclerosis *11*:119, 1970.
50. Ross, R., and Harker, L.: Hyperlipidemia and atherosclerosis. Science *193*:1094, 1976.
51. Stemerman, M. B.: Effects of moderate hypercholesterolemia on rabbit endothelium. Arteriosclerosis *1*:25, 1981.
52. Wanstrup, J., Kjeldsen, K., and Astrup, P.: Acceleration of spontaneous intimal-subintimal changes in rabbit aorta by prolonged moderate carbon monoxide exposure. Acta Pathol. Microbiol. Scand. *75*:353, 1969.
53. Kjeldsen, K., Astrup, P., and Wanstrup, J.: Ultrastructural intimal changes in the rabbit aorta after a moderate carbon monoxide exposure. Atherosclerosis *16*:67, 1972.
54. Robertson, A. L., Jr., and Khairallah, P. A.: Arterial endothelial permeability and vascular disease: The "trap-door" effect. Exp. Mol. Pathol. *18*:241, 1973.
55. Schwartz, S. M.: Assessment of angiotensin endothelial injury by incident light microscopy. Fed. Proc. *35*:208, 1976.
56. Mitchell, J. R. A., and Schwartz, C. J.: Arterial Disease. Oxford, Blackwell Scientific Publishers, 1965.
57. Smith, E. B., Slater, R. S., and Chu, P. K.: The lipids in raised fatty and fibrous lesions in human aorta. A comparison of changes at different stages of development. J. Atheros. Res. *8*:399, 1968.
58. Smith, E. B., Slater, R. S., and Crothers, D. C.: Quantitative interrelationships between plasma constituents and normal and atherosclerotic human intimal tissue. *In* Schettler, G., and Weizel, A. (eds.): Atherosclerosis III. Berlin, Springer-Verlag, 1974, p. 96.
59. Smith, E. B., and Slater, R. S.: Lipids and low density lipoproteins in intima in relation to its morphological characteristics. *In* Atherogenesis: Initiating Factors (Ciba Found. Symp. No. 12). Amsterdam, Elsevier Publishing Co., 1973, p. 39.
60. Smith, E. B.: Molecular interactions in human atherosclerotic plaques. Am. J. Pathol. *86*:665, 1977.
61. Panganamala, R. V., Geer, J. C., Sharma, H. A., and Cornwell, D. G.: The gross and histologic appearance and the lipid composition of normal intima and lesions from human coronary arteries and aorta. Atherosclerosis *20*:93, 1974.
62. Wissler, R. W., McAllister, H. A., Jr., and Vesselinovitch, D.: A histopathological study of the fatty streak in aortas and coronary arteries of young American military personnel. Am. J. Pathol. *78*:64a, 1975.
63. Yang, C., Schaffner, T., and Wissler, R. W.: Enzyme histochemical and histopathological features of human atherosclerotic plaques in young Americans. Unpublished observations.
64. Wissler, R. W.: Development of the atherosclerotic plaque. *In* Braunwald, E. (ed.): The Myocardium: Failure and Infarction. New York, HP Publishing Co., 1974, p. 155.
65. Getz, G. S., Vesselinovitch, D., and Wissler, R. W.: A dynamic pathology of atherosclerosis. Am. J. Med. *46*:657, 1969.
66. Haust, M. D., More, R. H., and Movat, H. Z.: The role of the smooth muscle cell in the fibrogenesis of atherosclerosis. Am. J. Pathol. *37*:377, 1960.
67. Geer, J. C., McGill, H. C., Jr., and Strong, J. P.: Fine structure of human atherosclerotic lesions. Am. J. Pathol. *38*:263, 1961.
68. McGill, H. C., and Geer, J. C.: The human lesion, fine structure. *In* Jones, R. J. (ed.): Evolution of the Atherosclerotic Plaque. Chicago, University of Chicago Press, 1963, p. 65.
69. Geer, J. C., and Haust, M. D.: Smooth Muscle Cells in Atherosclerosis. (Monographs on Atherosclerosis, Vol. 2.) Basel, Karger, 1972.
70. Knieriem, H. J., Kao, V. C., and Wissler, R. W.: Actinomyosin and myosin and the deposition of lipids and serum lipoproteins. Arch. Pathol. *84*:118, 1967.
71. Becker, C. G., and Murphy, G. E.: Demonstration of contractile protein in endothelium and cells of the heart valves, endocardium, intima, arteriosclerotic plaques, and Aschoff bodies of rheumatic heart disease. Am. J. Pathol. *55*:1, 1969.
72. Chamley, J. H., Groschel-Stewart, U., Campbell, R. G., and Burnstock, G.: Distinction between smooth muscle, fibroblasts and endothelial cells in culture by the use of fluoresceinated antibodies against smooth muscle actin. Cell Tissue Res. *177*:445, 1977.
73. Campbell, G. R., Uehara, Y., Mark, G., and Burnstock, G.: Fine structure of smooth muscle cells grown in tissue culture. J. Cell Biol. *49*:21, 1971.
74. Chamley-Campbell, J., Campbell, G. R., and Ross, R.: The smooth muscle cell in culture. Physiol. Rev. *59*:1, 1979.
75. Campbell, G. R., Chamley-Campbell, J. H., and Burnstock, G.: Differentiation and phenotypic modulation of arterial smooth muscle cells. *In* Schwartz, C. J., Werthessen, N. T., and Wolf, S. (eds.): Structure and Function of the Circulation. (Vol. III) New York, Plenum Press, 1981, p. 357.
76. Hanig, M., Shainoff, J. R., and Lowry, A. D.: Flotational lipoproteins extracted from human atherosclerotic aortas. Science *124*:176, 1956.
77. Gero, S., Gergely, J., Jakab, L., Szekely, J., and Virac, S.: Comparative immunoelectrophoretic studies on homogenates of aorta, pulmonary arteries and inferior vena cava of atherosclerotic individuals. J. Atheros. Res. *1*:88, 1961.
78. Tracy, R. E., Merchant, E. B., and Kao, V.: On the antigenic identity of human serum beta and alpha-w lipoproteins and their identification in aortic intima. Circ. Res. *9*:472, 1961.
79. Watts, H. F.: Role of lipoproteins in the formation of atherosclerotic lesions. *In* Jones, R. J. (ed.): Evolution of the Atherosclerotic Plaque. Chicago, University of Chicago Press, 1963, p. 117.
80. Kao, V. C. Y., and Wissler, R. W.: A study of the immunohistochemical localization of serum lipoproteins and other plasma proteins in human atherosclerotic lesions. Exp. Mol. Pathol. *4*:465, 1965.
81. Hollander, W., Kramsch, D. M., and Inuoue, G.: The metabolism of cholesterol, lipoproteins and acid mucopolysaccharides in normal and atherosclerotic vessels. *In* Miras, C. H., Howard, A. N., and Paoletti, R. (eds.): Progress in Biochemical Pharmacology. (Vol. 4.) Basel, Karger, 1968, p. 270.
82. Fless, G., Wissler, R. W., and Scanu, A. M.: Study of abnormal plasma low density lipoprotein in rhesus monkeys with diet-induced hyperlipidemia. Biochemistry *15*:5799, 1976.
83. Rudel, L. L., Pitts, L. L., II, and Nelson, C. A.: Characterization of plasma low density lipoproteins of nonhuman primates fed dietary cholesterol. J. Lip. Res. *18*:211, 1977.
84. Fless, G., and Scanu, A. M.: Isolation and characterization of the three major low density lipoproteins from normolipidemic rhesus monkeys (*Macaca mulatta*). J. Biol. Chem. *254*:8653, 1979.
85. Fless, G. M., Kirchhausen, T., Fischer-Dzoga, K., Wissler, R. W., and Scanu, A. M.: Relationship between the properties of apo B containing low-density lipoproteins (LDL) of normolipidemic rhesus monkey and their mitogenic action on arterial smooth muscle cells grown in vitro. *In* Gotto, A. M., Jr., Smith, L. C., and Allen, B. (eds.): Proceedings of the 5th International Symposium on Atherosclerosis. New York, Springer Verlag, 1980, p. 607.
86. Fless, G. M., Kirchhausen, T., Fischer-Dzoga, K., Wissler, R. W., and Scanu, A. M.: Serum low density lipoproteins with mitogenic effect on cultured aortic smooth muscle cells. Atherosclerosis *41*:171, 1982.
87. Fogelman, A. M., Shechter, I., Seager, J., Hokom, M., Child, J. S., and Edwards, P. A.: Malondialdehyde alterations of low density lipoprotein leads to

cholesteryl ester accumulation in human monocyte-macrophages. Proc. Natl. Acad. Sci. USA *77*:2214, 1980.
88. Henriksen, T., Mahoney, E. M., and Steinberg, D.: Enhanced macrophage degradation of low density lipoprotein previously incubated with cultured endothelial cells: Recognition by receptors for acetylated low density lipoproteins. Proc. Natl. Acad. Sci. USA *78*:6499, 1981.
89. Goldstein, J. L., Ho, Y. K., Basu, S. K., and Brown, M. S.: A binding site on macrophages that mediates the uptake and degradation of acetylated low-density lipoprotein producing massive cholesterol deposition. Proc. Natl. Acad. Sci. *76*:333, 1979.
90. Zilversmit, D. B.: Atherogenesis: A postprandial phenomenon. Circulation *60*: 473, 1979.
91. Mahley, R. W., Innerarity, T. L., Brown, M. S., Ho, Y. K., and Goldstein, J. L.: Cholesteryl ester synthesis in macrophages: Stimulation by β-very low density lipoproteins from cholesterol-fed animals of several species. J. Lipid Res. *21*:970, 1980.
92. Mustard, J. F., Packham, M. A., and Kinlough-Rathbone, R. L.: Platelets, atherosclerosis and clinical complications. *In* Moore, S. (ed.): Vascular Injury and Atherosclerosis. New York, Marcel Dekker, 1981, p. 79.
93. Mustard, J. F.: Increased activity of the clotting mechanism during alimentary lipemia: Its significance with regard to thrombosis and atherosclerosis. Can. Med. Assoc. J. *77*:308, 1957.
94. Murphy, E. A., and Mustard, J. F.: Coagulation tests and platelet economy in atherosclerotic and control subjects. Circulation *25*:114, 1962.
95. Farbiszewski, R., and Worowski, K.: Enhancement of platelet aggregation and adhesiveness by beta lipoprotein. J. Atheros. Res. *8*:988, 1968.
96. Carvalho, A. C. A., Colman, R. W., and Lees, R. S.: Platelet function in hyperlipoproteinemia. N. Engl. J. Med. *290*:434, 1974.
97. Nordøy, A., and Rødset, J. M.: Platelet function and platelet phospholipids in patients with hyperlipoproteinemia. Acta Med. Scand. *189*:385, 1971.
98. Sullivan, J. M., Heinle, R. A., and Gorlin, R.: Studies of platelet adhesiveness, glucose tolerance and serum lipoprotein patterns in patients with coronary artery disease. Am. J. Med. Sci. *264*:475, 1972.
99. Nordøy, A., and Rødset, J. M.: The influence of dietary fats on platelets in man. Acta Med. Scand. *190*:27, 1971.
100. Mustard, J. F., and Murphy, E. A.: Effect of smoking on blood coagulation and platelet survival in man. Br. Med. J. *1*:846, 1963.
101. Ross, R., Glomset, J., Kariya, B., and Harker, L.: A platelet-dependent serum factor that stimulates the proliferation of arterial smooth muscle cells in vitro. Proc. Natl. Acad. Sci. USA *71*:1207, 1974.
102. Harker, L. A., Slichter, S. J., Scott, C. R., and Ross, R.: Homocystinemia: Vascular injury and arterial thrombosis. N. Engl. J. Med. *291*:537, 1974.
103. Harker, L. A., Ross, R., Schlicter, S. J., and Scott, C. R.: Homocystine-induced arteriosclerosis. The role of endothelial cell injury and platelet response in its genesis. J. Clin. Invest. *58*:731, 1976.
104. Harker, L. A., Ross, R., and Glomset, J.: Role of the platelet in atherogenesis. Ann. N.Y. Acad. Sci. *275*:321, 1976.
105. Antoniades, H. N., Scher, C. D., and Stiles, C. D.: Purification of human platelet-derived growth factor. Proc. Natl. Acad. Sci. *76*:1809, 1979.
106. Heldin, C. H., Westermark, B., and Wasteson, A.: Platelet derived growth factor. Isolation by a large scale procedure and analysis by subunit composition. Biochem J. *193*:907, 1981.
107. Raines, E. W., and Ross, R.: Platelet-derived growth factor. I. High yield purification and evidence for multiple forms. J. Biol. Chem. *257*:5154, 1982.
108. Grotendorst, G. R., Seppa, H., Kleinman, H. K., and Martin, G. R.: Attachment of smooth muscle cells to collagen and their migration toward platelet-derived growth factor. Proc. Natl. Acad. Sci. *78*:3669, 1981.
109. Davies, P. F., and Ross, R.: Mediation of pinocytosis in cultured arterial smooth muscle and endothelial cells by platelet-derived growth factor. J. Cell Biol. *79*:663, 1978.
110. Bowen-Pope, D. F., and Russell, R.: Platelet-derived growth factor. II. Specific binding to cultured cells. J. Biol. Chem. *257*:5161, 1982.
111. Glenn, K., Bowen-Pope, D. F., and Ross, R.: Platelet-derived growth factor. III. Identification of a platelet-derived growth factor receptor by affinity labeling. J. Biol. Chem. *257*:5172, 1982.
112. Minick, C. R., Stemerman, M. B., and Insull, W., Jr.: Role of endothelium and hypercholesterolemia in intimal thickening and lipid accumulation. Am. J. Pathol. *95*:131, 1979.
113. Falcone, D. J., Hajjar, D. P., and Minick, C. R.: Enhancement of cholesterol and cholesteryl ester accumulation in re-endothelialized aorta. Am. J. Pathol. *99*:81, 1980.
114. Hajjar, D. P., Falcone, D. J., Fowler, S., and Minick, C.: Endothelium modifies the altered metabolism of the injured aortic wall. Am. J. Pathol. *102*:28, 1981.
115. Jensen, G., and Sigurd, B.: Systemic lupus erythematosus and acute myocardial infarction. Chest *64*:653, 1973.
116. Tsakraklides, V. G., Glieden, L. C., and Edwards, J. E.: Coronary atherosclerosis and myocardial infarction associated with systemic lupus erythematosus. Am. Heart J. *87*:637, 1974.
117. Bulkley, B. H., and Roberts, W. C.: The heart in systemic lupus erythematosus and the changes induced in it by corticosteroid therapy. Am. J. Med. *58*:243, 1975.
118. More, S.: Thromboatherosclerosis in normolipemic rabbits: A result of continued endothelial damage. Lab. Invest. *29*:478, 1973.
119. Friedman, R. J., Moore, S., and Singal, D. P.: Repeated endothelial injury and induction of atherosclerosis in normolipemic rabbits by human serum. Lab. Invest. *32*:404, 1975.
120. Wissler, R. W.: Coronary atherosclerosis and ischemic heart disease. *In* Zülch, K. J., Kaufman, W., Hossmann, K. A., and Hossman, V. (eds.): Brain and Heart Infarct. Berlin, Springer-Verlag. 1977, p. 206.
121. Kaplan, K. L., and Owen, J.: Plasma levels of beta-thromboglobulin and platelet factor 4 as indices of platelet activation in vivo. Blood *57*:199, 1981.
122. Steinberg, D.: Metabolism of lipoproteins at the cellular level in relation to atherogenesis. *In* Miller, N. E., and Lewis, B. (eds.): Lipoproteins, Atherosclerosis and Coronary Heart Disease. Amsterdam, Elsevier Publishing Co., 1981, p. 31.
123. Wissler, R. W., and Vesselinovitch, D.: Experimental models of human atherosclerosis. Ann. N.Y. Acad. Sci. *149*:907, 1968.
124. Wissler, R. W.: The emerging cellular pathobiology of atherosclerosis. Artery *5*: 409, 1979.
125. Benditt, E. P., and Benditt, J. M.: Evidence for a monoclonal origin of human atherosclerotic plaques. Proc. Nat. Acad. Sci. USA *70*:1753, 1973.
126. Benditt, E. P.: Implications of the monoclonal character of human atherosclerotic plaques. Am. J. Pathol. *86*:693, 1977.
127. Benditt, E. P.: The origin of atherosclerosis. Sci. Am. *236*:74, 1977.
128. Benditt, E. P., and Gown, A. M.: Atheroma: The artery wall and the environment. Int. Rev. Exp. Pathol. *21*:56, 1980.
129. Lindner, D., and Gartler, S. M.: Glucose-6-phosphate dehydrogenase mosaicism: Utilization as a cell marker in the study of leiomyomas. Science *150*:67, 1965.
130. Fialkow, P. J.: Use of genetic markers to study cellular origin and development of tumors in human females. Adv. Cancer Res. *15*:191, 1972.
131. Fialkow, P. J.: The origin and development of human tumors studied with cell markers. N. Engl. J. Med. *291*:26, 1974.
132. Pearson, T. A., Wang, A., and Solex, K.: Clonal characteristics of fibrous plaques and fatty streaks from human aortas. Am. J. Pathol. *81*:379, 1975.
133. Pearson, T. A., Kramer, E. D., Solez, K., and Heptinstall, R. H.: The human atherosclerotic plaque. Am. J. Pathol. *86*:657, 1977.
134. Thomas, W. A., Janakidevi, K., Florentin, R. A., and Reiner, J. M.: The reversibility of the human atherosclerotic plaque. *In* Hauss, W. H., Wissler, R. W., and Lehmann, R. (eds.): International Symposium: State of Prevention and Therapy in Human Arteriosclerosis and in Animal Models. Opladen. Westdeutscher Verlag. Vol. *63*:1978, p. 73.
135. Thomas, W. A., Reiner, J. M., Florentin, R. A., Janakidevi, K., and Lee, K. J.: Arterial smooth muscle cells in atherogenesis: Births, deaths and clonal phenomena. *In* Schettler, G., Goto, G., Hata, Y., and Klose, G. (eds.): Atherosclerosis IV. Berlin, Springer-Verlag, 1977, p. 16.
136. Goldstein, J. L., and Brown, M. S.: The low density lipoprotein pathway and its relation to atherosclerosis, Ann. Rev. Biochem. *46*:897, 1977.
137. Goldstein, J. L., and Brown, M. S.: Familial hypercholesterolemia—Pathogenesis of receptor disease. Johns Hopkins Med. J. *143*:8, 1978.
138. Schneider, W. T., Kovanen, P. T., Brown, M. S., Goldstein, J. L., Utermann, G., Weber, W., Havel, R. J., Kotite, L., Kane, J., Innerarity, T. L., and Mahley, R. W.: Familial dysbetalipoproteinemia. Abnormal binding of mutant apoprotein E to low density lipoprotein receptors of human fibroblasts and membranes from liver and adrenal of rats, rabbits, and cows. J. Clin. Invest. *68*:1075, 1981.
139. Mahley, R. W.: Atherogenic hyperlipoproteinemia. The cellular and molecular biology of plasma lipoproteins altered by dietary fat and cholesterol. Med. Clin. North Am. *66*:375, 1982.
140. Jackson, R. L., Stein, O., Gotto, A. N., and Stein, Y.: A comparative study on the removal of cellular lipids from Landschütz ascites cells by human plasma apolipoproteins. J. Biol. Chem. *250*:7204, 1975.
141. Stein, Y., Glange, M. C., Fainaru, M., and Stein, O.: The removal of cholesterol from aortic smooth muscle cells in culture and Landschütz ascites cells by fractions of human high-density lipoproteins. Biochim. Biophys. Acta *380*:106, 1975.
142. Stein, O., Vanderhoek, J., and Stein, Y.: Cholesterol content and sterol synthesis in human skin fibroblasts and rat aortic smooth muscle cells exposed to lipoprotein-depleted serum and high density apolipoprotein/phospholipid mixtures. Biochim. Biophys. Acta *431*:347, 1976.
143. Stein, Y., and Stein, O.: Interaction between serum lipoproteins and cellular components of the arterial wall. *In* Scanu, A. M., Wissler, R. W., and Getz, G. S. (eds.): The Biochemistry of Atherosclerosis. New York, Marcel Dekker, 1979, p. 313.
144. Scanu, A. M., Byrne, R. E., and Mihovilovic, M.: Functional roles of plasma high density lipoproteins. CRC Crit. Rev. Biochem. *13*:109, 1982.
145. Innerarity, T. L., Pitas, R. E., and Mahley, R. W.: Modulating effects of canine high density lipoproteins on cholesteryl ester synthesis induced by β-very low density lipoproteins in macrophages. Arteriosclerosis *2*:114, 1982.
146. Miller, G. J., and Miller, N. E.: Plasma-high-density-lipoprotein concentration and development of ischaemic heart disease. Lancet *1*:16, 1975.
147. Castelli, W. P., Doyle, J. T., Gordon, T., Hames, C., Hulley, S. B., Kagan, A., McGee, D., Vicic, W. J., and Zukel, W. J.: HDL cholesterol levels (HDLC) in coronary heart disease (CHD)—Cooperative lipoprotein phenotyping study. Circulation *52*(Suppl. II):97, 1975.
148. Miller, N. W., Weinstein, D. B., and Steinberg, D.: Uptake and degradation of high density lipoprotein—Comparison of fibroblasts from normal subjects and from homozygous familial hypercholesterolemic subjects. J. Lipid Res. *19*:644, 1978.
149. Hayes, K. C., Hojnacki, J. L., and Nicolosi, R. J.: High density lipoproteins in nonhuman primates. *In* Day, C. E., and Levy, R. S. (eds.): High Density Lipoproteins. New York, Plenum Press, 1981.

150. Carew, T. E., Koschinsky, T., Hayes, S. B., and Steinberg, D.: A mechanism by which high density lipoproteins may slow the atherogenic process. Lancet *1*: 1315, 1976.
151. Miller, N. W., Nestel, P. J., and Clifton-Bligh, P.: Relationships between plasma lipoprotein cholesterol concentrations and the pool size and metabolism of cholesterol in man. Atherosclerosis *23*:535, 1976.
152. Mahley, R. W., Hui, D. Y., Innerarity, T. L., and Weisgraber, K. H.: Two independent lipoprotein receptors on hepatic membranes of the dog, swine, and man: The apo-B, E and apo-E receptors. J. Clin. Invest. *68*:1197, 1981.
153. Krauss, R. M., Lindgren, F. T., Wood, P. D., Haskell, W. L., Albers, J. J., and Cheung, M. C.: Differential increases in plasma high density lipoprotein subfractions and apolipoproteins (APO-LP) in runners. Circulation *56*(Suppl. III):100, 1977.
154. Wood, P. D., Haskell, W. L., Klein, H., Lewis, S., Stern, M. P., and Farquhar, J. W.: The distribution of plasma lipoproteins in middle-aged male runners. Metabolism *25*:1249, 1976.
155. Erkelens, D. W., Albers, J. J., Hazzard, W. R., Frederick, R. C., and Bierman, E. L.: Moderate exercise increases high density lipoprotein cholesterol in myocardial infarction survivors. Clin. Res. *26*:158a, 1978.
156. Kramsch, D., Aspen, A. J., Abramowitz B. M., Kreimendahl, T., and Hood, W. B., Jr.: Reduction of coronary atherosclerosis by moderate conditioning exercise in monkeys on an atherogenic diet. N. Engl. J. Med. *305*:1485, 1981.
157. Wissler, R. W., Fischer-Dzoga, K., Bates, S. R., and Chen, R. M.: Arterial smooth muscle cells in tissue culture. *In* Schwartz, C. J., Werthessen, N. T., and Wolf, S. (eds.): Structure and Function of the Circulation, (Vol. III.) New York, Plenum Press, 1981, p. 427.
158. Kao, V. C. Y., Wissler, R. W., and Dzoga, K.: The influence of hyperlipemic serum on the growth of medial smooth muscle cells on Rhesus monkey aorta in vitro. Circulation *38*(Suppl. VI):12, 1968.
159. Fischer-Dzoga, K., Wissler, R. W., and Scanu, A. M.: The lipoproteins and arterial smooth muscle cells: cellular proliferation and morphology. *In* Manning, G. W., and Haust, M. D. (eds.): Atherosclerosis: Metabolic, Morphologic and Clinical Aspects (Advances in Experimental Medicine and Biology Vol. 82). New York, Plenum Press, 1977, p. 915.
160. Fischer-Dzoga, K., Chen, R., and Wissler, R. W.: Effects of serum lipoproteins on the morphology, growth and metabolism of arterial smooth muscle cells. *In* Wagner, W. D., and Clarkson, T. B. (eds.): Arterial Mesenchyme and Arteriosclerosis. New York, Plenum Press, 1974, p. 299.
161. Fischer-Dzoga, K., and Wissler, R. W.: Stimulation of proliferation in stationary primary cultures of monkey aortic smooth muscle cell. II. Effect of varying concentrations of hyperlipemic serum and low density lipoproteins of varying dietary fat origins. Atherosclerosis *24*:515, 1976.
162. Fischer-Dzoga, K., Fraser, R., and Wissler, R. W.: Stimulation of proliferation in stationary primary cultures of monkey and rabbit aortic smooth muscle cells. I. Effects of lipoprotein fractions of hyperlipemic serum and lymph. Exp. Mol. Pathol. *24*:346, 1976.
163. Fischer-Dzoga, K., and Wissler, R. W.: Response of arterial smooth muscle cells to hyperlipemia. *In* Schettler, G., Goto, Y., Hata, Y., and Klose, G. (eds.): Atherosclerosis IV. Berlin, Springer-Verlag, 1977, p. 624.
164. Fischer-Dzoga, K., Kuo, Y.-F., and Wissler, R. W.: The proliferative effect of platelets and hyperlipidemic serum on stationary primary cultures. Atherosclerosis *47*:35, 1983.
165. Chen, R. M., Getz, G. S., Fischer-Dzoga, K., and Wissler, R. W.: The role of hyperlipidemic serum on the proliferation and necrosis of aortic medial cells in vitro. Exp. Mol. Pathol. *26*:359, 1977.
166. Chen, R. M., Fischer-Dzoga, K., and Wissler, R. W.: Influence of lysosomal enzyme stability in hyperlipemic serum-induced metabolic changes of monkey aortic medial cells. *In* Schettler, G., Goto, Y., Hata, Y., and Klose, G. (eds.): Atherosclerosis IV. Berlin, Springer-Verlag, 1977, p. 649.
167. Robertson, A. L., Jr.: The artery and process of arteriosclerosis. Pathogenesis. *In* Wolf, S., (ed.): Advances in Experimental Medicine and Biology. Vol. 16A. New York, Plenum Press, 1971, p. 229.
168. Robertson, A. L.: Functional characterization of arterial cells involved in spontaneous atheroma. *In* Schettler, G., and Weizel, A. (eds.): Atherosclerosis III. Berlin, Springer-Verlag, 1974, p. 175.
169. Myasnikov, A. L., Block, Y. E., and Pavlov, V. M.: Influence of lipemic serums of patients with atherosclerosis on tissue cultures of adult human aortas. J. Atheros. Res. *6*:224, 1966.
170. Myasnikov, A. L., and Block, Y. E.: Influence of some factors in lipoidosis and cell proliferation in aorta tissue cultures of adult rabbits. J. Atheros. Res. *5*:33, 1965.
171. Fischer-Dzoga, K., Vesselinovitch, D., and Wissler, R. W.: The effect of estrogen on the rabbit aortic medial tissue culture cells. Am. J. Pathol. *74*:52a, 1974.
172. Yoshida, Y., Fischer-Dzoga, K., and Wissler, R. W.: Effects of normolipemic HDL on proliferation of monkey aortic smooth muscle cells induced by hyperlipemic LDL. Circulation *56*(Suppl. III):100, 1977.
173. Ledet, T., Fischer-Dzoga, K., and Wissler, R. W.: Diabetic macroangiopathy: in vitro study of the proliferation of the aortic smooth muscle cells. Am. J. Pathol. *74*:50a, 1974.
174. Ledet, T., Fischer-Dzoga, K., and Wissler, R. W.: Growth of rabbit aortic smooth muscle cells cultured in media containing diabetic and hyperlipemic serum. Diabetes *25*:207, 1976.
175. Ledet, T.: Diabetic cardiomyopathy: Quantitative histological studies of the heart from young juvenile diabetics. Acta Pathol. Microbiol. Scand. (Sect. A) *84*:421, 1976.
176. Ledet, T.: Growth hormone stimulating the growth of arterial medial cells in vitro: absence of effect of insulin. Diabetes *25*:1011, 1976.
177. Ledet, T.: Growth of rabbit aortic smooth muscle cells in serum from patients with juvenile diabetes. Acta Pathol. Microbiol. Scand. (Sect. A) *84*:508, 1976.
178. Ledet, T.: Growth hormone antiserum suppresses the growth effect of diabetic serum. Studies of rabbit aortic medial cell cultures. Diabetes *26*:798, 1977.
179. Fischer-Dzoga, K., Pick, R., and Kuo, Y.: In vitro response of aortic smooth muscle cells to serum of hypertensive monkeys. Circulation *56*(Suppl. III):100, 1977.
180. Belfiore, F., Napoli, E., Lo Vecchio, L., and Rabuazzo, A. M.: Serum acid phosphatase activity in diabetes mellitus. Am. J. Med. Sci. *266*:139, 1973.
181. Wolinsky, H., Goldfischer, S., Schiller, B., and Kasak, L. E.: Lysosomes in aortic smooth muscle cells: effects of hypertension. Am. J. Pathol. *73*:727, 1973.
182. Wolinsky, H., Goldfischer, S., Schiller, B., and Kasak, L. E.: Modification of the effects of hypertension on lysosomes and connective tissue in the rat aorta. Circ. Res. *34*:233, 1974.
183. Wolinsky, H., Goldfischer, S., Daly, M. M., Kasak, L. E., and Coltoff-Schiller, B.: Arterial lysosomes and connective tissue in primate atherosclerosis and hypertension. Circ. Res. *36*:553, 1975.
184. Fushimi, H., and Tarui, S.: Beta-glycosidases and diabetic microangiopathy. I. Decreases of beta-glycosidase activities in diabetic rat kidney. J. Biochem. *79*: 265, 1976.
185. Chen, R.: Effects of Hyperlipemic Rabbit Serum and its Lipoproteins on Proliferation and Lipid Metabolism of Rabbit Aortic Medial Cells In Vitro. Doctoral Thesis, The University of Chicago, 1973.
186. Chen, R. M., and Fischer-Dzoga, K.: Effect of hyperlipemic serum lipoproteins on the lipid accumulation and cholesterol flux of rabbit aortic medial cells. Atherosclerosis *28*:339, 1977.
187. Chen, R. M., Getz, G. S., Fischer-Dzoga, K., and Wissler, R. W.: Effect of hyperlipemic serum and its lipoproteins on the lipid metabolism of rabbit aortic medial cells in vitro. Unpublished observation.
188. Chen, R. M., and Yang, F. P.: Effect of Metformin on the metabolism of rabbit aortic cells in vitro. Fed. Proc. *37*:934, 1978.
189. Bates, S. R.: Effect of hyperlipemic serum on cholesterol accumulation in monkey aortic medial cells. Fed. Proc. *35*:208, 1976.
190. Bates, S. R., and Wissler, R. W.: Effect of hyperlipemic serum on cholesterol accumulation in monkey aortic medial cells. Biochim. Biophys. Acta *450*:78, 1976.
191 St. Clair, R. W., Smith, B. P., and Wood, L. L.: Stimulation of cholesterol esterification in rhesus monkey arterial smooth muscle cells. Circ. Res. *40*:166, 1977.
192. Jaffe, E. A., Nachman, R. L., Becker, C. G., and Minick, C. R.: Culture of human endothelial cells derived from umbilical veins. Identification by morphological and immunological criteria. J. Clin. Invest. *52*:2745, 1973.
193. Thorgeirsson, G., and Robertson, A. L., Jr.: The vascular endothelium—Pathobiologic significance. Am. J. Pathol. *93*:803, 1978.
194. Schwartz, S. M., Gajdusek, C., and Owens, G. K.: Vessel wall growth control. *In* Nossel, H., and Vogel, H. J. (eds.): Pathobiology of the Endothelial Cell. New York, Academic Press, 1982, p. 63.
195. Gimbrone, M. A., Jr.: Culture of vascular endothelium. Progr. Hemost. Thromb. *3*:1, 1976.
196. Jaffe, E. A., Hoyer, L. W.,and Nachman, R. L.: Synthesis of antihemophilic factor antigen by cultured human endothelial cells. J. Clin. Invest. *52*:2757, 1973.
197. Jaffe, E. A., Hoyer, L. W., and Nachman, R. L.: Synthesis of von Willebrand factor by cultured human endothelial cells. Proc. Nat. Acad. Sci. USA *71*: 1906, 1974.
198. Jagannathan, S. N., Connor, W. E., and Lewis, L. J.: Cholesterol metabolism in human endothelial cells in culture. *In* Manning, G. W., and Haust, M. D. (eds.): Atherosclerosis: Metabolic, Morphologic and Clinical Aspects. New York, Plenum Press, 1977, p. 244.
199. Booyse, F. M., Quarfoot, A. J., Bell, S., Fass, D. N., Lewis, J. C., Mann, K. G., and Bowie, E. J. W.: Cultured aortic endothelial cells from pigs with von Willebrand disease: in vitro model for studying the molecular defect(s) of the disease. Proc. Nat. Acad. Sci. USA *74*:5702, 1977.
200. Gimbrone, M. A., Jr., and Alexander, R. W.: Prostaglandin production by vascular endothelial and smooth muscle cells in cutlure. *In* Silver, M. J., et al. (eds.): Prostaglandins in Hematology. New York, Spectrum, 1977, p. 121.
201. Wissler, R. W., and Vesselinovitch, D.: Differences between human and animal atherosclerosis. *In* Schettler, G., and Weizel, A. (eds.): Atherosclerosis III. Berlin, Springer-Verlag, 1974, p. 319.
202. Wissler, R. W., and Vesselinovitch, D.: Atherosclerosis in nonhuman primates. *In* Brandley, C. A., Corneliu, C. E., and Simpson, C. F. (eds.): Advances in Veterinary Science and Comparative Medicine. Vol. 21. (Cardiovascular Pathophysiology). New York, Academic Press, 1977, p. 351.
203. Wissler, R. W., and Vesselinovitch, D.: Animal models of regression. *In* Schettler, G., Goto, Y., Hata, Y., and Klose, G. (eds.): Atherosclerosis IV. Berlin, Springer-Verlag, 1977, p. 377.
204. Strong, J. P.: Atherosclerosis in Primates. (Prim. Med. Vol. 9.) Basel, Karger, 1976.
205. Gresham, G. A.: Primate Atherosclerosis. (Monogr. Atheros. Vol. 7.) Basel, Karger, 1976.
206. Bevans, M., Davidson, J. D., and Kendall, F. F.: Regression of lesions in canine arteriosclerosis. Arch. Pathol. *51*:288, 1951.
207. Mahley, R. W., Innerarity, T. L., Weisgraber, K. H., and Fry, D. L.: Canine

hyperlipoproteinemia and atherosclerosis. Accumulation of lipid by aortic medial cells in vivo and in vitro. Am. J. Pathol. *87*:205, 1977.
208. Lazzarini-Robertson, A., Butkus, A., Ehrhart, L. A., and Lewis, L. A.: Experimental arteriosclerosis in dogs. Evaluation of anatomopathological findings. Atherosclerosis *15*:307, 1972.
209. McCullagh, K. G., and Ehrhart, L. A.: Increased arterial collagen synthesis in experimental canine atherosclerosis. Atherosclerosis *19*:13, 1974.
210. Mahley, R. W., Weisgraber, K. H., and Innerarity, T.: Canine lipoproteins and atherosclerosis. II. Characterization of the plasma lipoproteins associated with atherogenic and nonatherogenic hyperlipidemia. Circ. Res. *35*:722, 1974.
211. Wissler, R. W.: Recent progress in studies of experimental primate atherosclerosis. *In* Miras, C. J., Howard, A. N., and Paoletti, R. (eds.): Progress in Biochemical Pharmacology. Vol. 4. Basel, Karger, 1968, p. 378.
212. Scott, R. F., Morrison, E. S., Jarmolych, J., Nam, S. C., Kroms, M., and Coulston, F.: Experimental atherosclerosis in rhesus monkeys. I. Gross and light microscopy features and lipid values in serum and aorta. Exp. Mol. Pathol. *7*:11, 1967.
213. Scott, R. F., Jones, R., Daoud, A. S., Zumbo, O., Coulston, F., and Thomas, W. A.: Experimental atherosclerosis in rhesus monkeys. II. Cellular elements of proliferative lesions and possible role of cytoplasmic degeneration in pathogenesis as studied by electron microscopy. Exp. Mol. Pathol. *7*:34, 1967.
214. Armstrong, M. L., Connor, W. E., and Warner, E. D.: Tissue cholesterol concentration in the hypercholesterolemic rhesus monkey. Arch. Pathol. *87*:81, 1969.
215. Tucker, C. F., Catsulis, C., Strong, J. P., and Eggen, D. A.: Regression of early cholesterol-induced aortic lesions in rhesus monkeys. Am. J. Pathol. *65*: 493, 1972.
216. Armstrong, M. L., and Warner, E. D.: Morphology and distribution of diet-induced atherosclerosis in rhesus monkeys. Arch. Pathol. *92*:295, 1971.
217. Manning, P. J., Clarkson, T. B., and Lofland, H. B.: Cholesterol absorption, turnover, and excretion rates in hypercholesterolemic rhesus monkeys. Exp. Mol. Pathol. *14*:75, 1971.
218. Manning, P. J., and Clarkson, T. B.: Development, distributions and lipid content of diet-induced atherosclerotic lesions of rhesus monkeys. Exp. Mol. Pathol. *17*:38, 1972.
219. Eggen, D. A.: Cholesterol metabolism in rhesus monkey, squirrel monkey and baboon. J. Lipid Res. *15*:139, 1974.
220. Taylor, C. B., Cox, G. E., Counts, M., and Yogi, N.: Fatal myocardial infarction in the rhesus monkey with diet-induced hypercholesterolemia. Am. J. Pathol. *35*:674, 1959.
221. Taylor, C. B., Cox, G. E., Manalo-Estrella, P., Southworth, J., Patton, D. E., and Cathcart, C.: Atherosclerosis in rhesus monkeys. II. Arterial lesions associated with hypercholesteremia induced by dietary fat and cholesterol. Arch. Pathol. *74*:16, 1962.
222. Taylor, C. B., Trueheart, R. E., and Cox, G. E.: Atherosclerosis in rhesus monkeys. III. The role of increased thickness of arterial walls in atherogenesis. Arch. Pathol. *76*:14, 1963.
223. Cox, G. E., Trueheart, R. W., Kaplan, J., and Taylor, C. B.: Atherosclerosis in rhesus monkeys. IV. Repair of arterial injury—an important secondary atherogenic factor. Arch. Pathol. *76*:166, 1963.
224. Taylor, C. B., Manalo-Estrella, P., and Cox, G. E.: Atherosclerosis in rhesus monkeys. V. Marked diet-induced hypercholesteremia with xanthomatosis and severe atherosclerosis. Arch. Pathol. *76*:239, 1963.
225. Taylor, C. B., Patton, D. E., and Cox, G. E.: Atherosclerosis in rhesus monkeys. VI. Fatal myocardial infarction in a monkey fed fat and cholesterol. Arch. Pathol. *76*:404, 1963.
226. Taylor, C. B.: Experimentally induced arteriosclerosis in nonhuman primates . *In* Roberts, J. C., Jr., and Straus, R. (eds.): Comparative Atherosclerosis. New York, Harper and Row, 1965, p. 215.
227. Vesselinovitch, D., Wissler, R. W., Schaffner, T. J., and Borensztajn, J.: The effects of various diets on atherogenesis in rhesus monkeys. Atherosclerosis *35*: 189, 1980.
228. Wissler, R. W., Frazier, L. W., Hughes, R. H., and Rasmussen, R. A.: Atherogenesis in the cebus monkey. I. A comparison of three food fats under controlled dietary conditions. Arch. Pathol. *74*:312, 1962.
229. Malmros, H., and Sternby, N. H.: Induction of atherosclerosis in dogs by a thiouracil-free semi-synthetic diet containing cholesterol and hydrogenated coconut oil. *In* Miras, C. J., Howard, A. N., and Paoletti, R. (eds.): Progress in Biochemical Pharmacology. Vol. 4. Basel, Karger, 1968, p. 482.
230. Vesselinovitch, D., Getz, G. J., Hughes, R. H., and Wissler, R. W.: Atherosclerosis in the rhesus monkey fed three food fats. Atherosclerosis *20*: 303, 1974.
231. Gresham, G. A., and Howard, A. N.: The independent production of atherosclerosis and thrombosis in the rat. Br. J. Exp. Pathol. *41*:395, 1960.
232. Imai, H., Lee, K. T., Pastori, S., Panlillo, E., Florentin, R., and Thomas, W. A.: Atherosclerosis in rabbits. Architectural and subcellular alterations of smooth muscle cells of aortas in response to hyperlipemia. Exp. Mol. Pathol. *5*:273, 1966.
233. Florentin, R. A., and Nam, S. C.: Dietary-induced atherosclerosis in miniature swine. Exp. Mol. Pathol. *8*:263, 1968.
234. Kritchevsky, D., Tepper, S. A., Vesselinovitch, D., and Wissler, R. W.: Cholesterol vehicle in experimental atherosclerosis. Part 11. Peanut oil. Atherosclerosis *14*:53, 1971.
235. Kritchevsky, D., Tepper, S. A., Vesselinovitch, D., and Wissler, R. W.: Cholesterol vehicle in experimental atherosclerosis. Part 13. Randomized peanut oil. Atherosclerosis *17*:225, 1973.
236. Kritchevsky, D., Muher, J. J., Marai, L., and Kuskis, A.: Aglycerol structure of peanut oils of different atherogenic potential. Lipids *12*:775, 1977.
237. Kritchevsky, D., Tepper, S. A., Kim, H. K., Story, J. A., Vesselinovitch, D., and Wissler, R. W.: Experimental atherosclerosis in rabbits fed cholesterol-free diets. 5. Comparison of peanut, corn, butter and coconut oils. Exp. Mol. Pathol. *24*:375, 1976.
238. Kritchevsky, D., Tepper, S. A., Scott, D. A., Klurfeld, D. M., Vesselinovitch, D., and Wissler, R. W.: Cholesterol vehicle in experimental atherosclerosis. 18. Comparison of North American, African and South American Peanut Oils. Atherosclerosis *38*:291, 1981.
239. Jones, R. M., Hughes, R., Vesselinovitch, D., and Wissler, R. W.: Ultrastructural changes in the aortas of rhesus monkeys fed large quantities of food fats for short periods. Fed. Proc. *31*:273, 1972.
240. Stary, H. C.: Cell proliferation and ultrastructural changes in regressing atherosclerotic lesions after reduction of serum cholesterol. *In* Schettler, G., and Weizel, A. (eds.): Atherosclerosis III. Berlin, Springer-Verlag, 1974, p. 187.
241. Strong, J. P.: Reversibility of fatty streaks in rhesus monkey. Primates Med. *9*: 300, 1976.
242. Armstrong, M. L., Warner, F. D., and Connor, W. E.: Regression of coronary atheromatosis in rhesus monkeys. Circ. Res. *27*:59, 1970.
243. Vesselinovitch, D., Wissler, R. W., Hughes, R., and Borensztajn, J.: Reversal of advanced atheroscleroris in rhesus monkeys. I. Light microscopic studies. Atherosclerosis *23*:155, 1976.
244. Bond, M. G., Bullock, B. C., Clarkson, T. B., and Lehner, N. D.: The effect of plasma cholesterol concentrations on "regression" of primate atherosclerosis. Am. J. Pathol. *82*:69a, 1976.
245. Armstrong, M. L.: Regression of atherosclerosis. *In* Paoletti, R., and Gotto, A. M., Jr. (eds.): Atherosclerosis Reviews. Vol. 1. New York, Raven Press, 1976, p. 137.
246. Katz, L. N., Stamler, J., and Pick, R.: Nutrition and Atherosclerosis. Philadelphia. Lea and Febiger, 1958.
247. Wissler, R. W., and Vesselinovitch, D.: Studies of regression of advanced atherosclerosis in experimental animals and man. *In* Atherogenesis (Proceedings of the 1st International Symposium). Ann. N.Y. Acad. Sci. *275*: 363, 1976.
248. Vartiainen, T., and Kanerva, K.: Arteriosclerosis and wartime. Ann. Med. Intern. Fenn. *36*:748, 1947.
249. Wilens, S. L.: The resorption of arterial atheromatous deposits in wasting disease. Am. J. Pathol. *23*:793, 1947.
250. Vesselinovitch, D., and Wissler, R. W.: Comparison of primates and rabbits as animal models in experimental atherosclerosis. *In* Manning, G. W., and Haust, M. D. (eds.): Atherosclerosis: Metabolic, Morphologic and Clinical Aspects. (Advances in Experimental Medicine and Biology, Vol. 82.) New York, Plenum Press, 1977, p. 614.
251. Fritz, K. E., Augustyn, J. M., Jarmolych, J., Daoud, A. S., and Lee, K. T.: Regression of advanced atherosclerosis of swine (Chemical studies). Arch. Pathol. Lab. Med. *100*:380, 1976.
252. Armstrong, M. L., and Megan, M. B.: Lipid depletion in atheromatous coronary arteries in rhesus monkeys after regression diets. Circ. Res. *30*:675, 1972.
253. Wartman, A., Lampe, T. L., McCann, D. S., and Boyle, A. J.: Plaque reversal with MgEDTA in experimental atherosclerosis: Elastin and collagen metabolism. J. Atheros. Res. *7*:331, 1967.
254. Kjeldsen, K., Astrup, P., and Wanstrup, J.: Reversal of rabbit atheromatosis by hyperoxia. J. Atheros. Res. *10*:173, 1969.
255. Vesselinovitch, D., Wissler, R. W., Fischer-Dzoga, K., Hughes, R., and DuBien, L.: Regression of atherosclerosis in rabbits. I. Treatment with low fat diet, hyperoxia and hypolipidemic agents. Atherosclerosis *19*:259, 1974.
256. Daoud, A. S., Jarmolych, J., Augustyn, J. M., Fritz, K. E., Singh, J. K., and Lee, K. T.: Regression of advanced atherosclerosis in swine. Arch. Pathol. Lab. Med. *100*:372, 1976.
257. Vesselinovitch, D., Wissler, R. W., and Schaffner, T.: Quantitation of lesions during progression and regression of atherosclerosis in rhesus monkeys. *In* Naito, H. (ed.): Nutrition and Heart Disease. New York, S.P. Medical and Scientific Books, 1982, p. 121.
258. Vesselinovitch, D., and Wissler, R. W.: Correlation of types of induced lesions with regression of coronary atherosclerosis in two species of macaques. *In* Noseda, G., Fragiacomo, C., Fumagalli, R., and Paoletti, R. (eds.): Lipoproteins and Coronary Atherosclerosis. Amsterdam, Elsevier Publishing Co., 1982, p. 401.
259. Armstrong, M. L., and Megan, M. B.: Arterial fibrous proteins in cynomolgus monkeys after atherogenic and regression diets. Circ. Res. *36*:256, 1975.
260. Armstrong, M. L.: Connective tissue in regression. *In* Paoletti, R., and Gotto, A. M. (eds.): Atherosclerosis Reviews. Vol. 3. New York, Raven Press, 1978 p. 147.
261. Armstrong, M. L.: Connective tissue changes in regression. *In* Schettler, G., Goto, Y., Hata, Y., and Klose, G. (eds.): Atherosclerosis IV. Berlin, Springer-Verlag, 1977, p. 405.
262. Weber, G., Fabbrini, P., Resi, L., Jones, R., Vesselinovitch, D., and Wissler, R. W.: Regression of arteriosclerotic lesions in rhesus monkey aortas after regression diet: Scanning and transmission electron microscope observations of the endothelium. Atherosclerosis *26*:535, 1977.
263. Wissler, R. W., and Vesselinovitch, D.: The combined effects of cholestyramine and probucol on regression of atherosclerosis in rhesus monkey aortas. J. Appl. Pathol., July, 1983.
264. Wissler, R. W.: Current status of regression studies. *In* Paoletti, R., and

Gotto, A. M. (eds.): Atherosclerosis Reviews. Vol. 3. New York, Raven Press, 1978, p. 213.
265. Borensztajn, J., Foreman, K., Wissler, R. W., von Zutphen, H., Vesselinovitch, D., and Hughes, R.: Egress of aortic cholesterol and cholesterol ester during regression of atherosclerosis in rhesus monkeys. Circulation *52*(Suppl. II):269, 1975.
266. Slater, H. R., Packard, C. J., Bicker, S., and Shepherd, J.: Effects of cholestyramine on receptor-mediated plasma clearance and tissue uptake of human low density lipoproteins in the rabbit. J. Biol. Chem. *255*:10210, 1980.
267. Zelis, R., Mason, D. T., Braunwald, E., and Levy, R. I.: Effects of hyperlipoproteinemias and their treatment on the peripheral circulation. J. Clin. Invest. *49*:1007, 1970.
268. Buchwald, H. L., Moore, R. B., and Varco, R. L.: Surgical treatment of hyperlipidemia. III. Clinical status of the partial ileal bypass operation. Circulation *49*(Suppl. I):22, 1974.
269. Baltaxe, H. A., Amplatz, K., Varco, R. L., and Buchwald, H.: Coronary arteriography in hypercholesterolemic patients. Am. J. Roentgenol. Radium Ther. Nucl. Med. *105*:784, 1969.
270. Knight, L., Scheibel, R., Amplatz, K., Varco, R. L., and Buchwald, H.: Radiographic appraisal of the Minnesota partial ileal bypass study. Surg. Forum *23*:141, 1972.
271. Blankenhorn, D. H., Brooks, S., II., Selzer, R. H., Crawford, D. W., and Chin, H. P.: Assessment of atherosclerosis from angiographic images. Proc. Soc. Exp. Biol. Med. *145*:1298, 1974.
272. Crawford, D. W., Beckenbach, E. S., Blankenhorn, D. H., Selzer, R. H., and Brooks, S. H.: Grading of coronary atherosclerosis: Comparison of a modified IAP visual grading method and a new quantitative angiographic technique. Atherosclerosis *19*:231, 1974.
273. Blankenhorn, D. H.: Studies of regression/progression of atherosclerosis in man. *In* Manning, G. W., and Haust, M. D. (eds.): Atherosclerosis: Metabolic, Morphologic and Clinical Aspects. (Advances in Experimental Medicine and Biology, Vol. 82.) New York, Plenum Press, 1977, p. 453.
274. Buchwald, H., Moore, R. B., and Varco, R. L.: The partial ileal bypass operation in treatment of hyperlipemias. *In* Kritchevsky, D., Paoletti, R., and Holmes, W. (eds.): Lipids, Lipoproteins and Drugs. (Advances in Experimental Medicine and Biology, Vol 63.) New York, Plenum Press, 1975, p. 221.
275. Barndt, R., Jr., Blankenhorn, D. H., Crawford, D. W., and Brooks, S. H.: Regression and progression of early femoral atherosclerosis in treated hyperlipoproteinemic patients. Ann. Intern. Med. *86*:139, 1977.
276. Malinow, M. R.: Regression of atherosclerosis in humans: Fact or myth? Circulation *64*:1, 1981.
277. Blankenhorn, D. H.: Discussion, Chapter 23. *In* Bond, W. G., and Insull, W., Jr. (eds.): Clinical Diagnosis of atherosclerosis. Quantitative Methods of Evaluation. Mock, M. B.: Review of clinical studies on the quantification and progression of atherosclerosis. New York, Springer-Verlag, 1983.
278. Dorr, A. E., Gundersen, K. Schneider, J. C., Spencer, T. W., and Martin, W. B.: Colestipol hydrochloride in hypercholesterolemic patients: effect on serum cholesterol and mortality. J. Chron. Dis. *31*:5, 1978.
279. Turpeinen, D.: Effect of cholesterol-lowering diet on mortality from coronary heart disease and other causes. Circulation *59*:1, 1979.
280. Malinow, M. R., McLaughlin, P., Naito, H. K., Lewis, L. A., and McNulty, W. P.: Effect of alfalfa meal on shrinkage (regression) of atherosclerotic plaques during cholesterol feeding in monkeys. Atherosclerosis *30*:27, 1978.
281. Malinow, M. R., McLaughlin, P., Papworth, L., Stafford, C., Kohler, G. O., Livingston, A. L., and Cheeke, P. R.: Effect of alfalfa saponins on intestinal cholesterol absorption in rats. Am. J. Clin. Nutr. *30*:2061, 1977.
282. Kramsch, D. M., Chan, C. T., Aspen, A. J., and Wells, H.: Prevention and therapy of induced atherosclerosis in rabbits and monkeys by anticalcemic drugs regardless of serum cholesterol levels. *In* Hauss, W. H., Wissler, R. W., and Lehmann, R. (eds.): International Symposium: State of Prevention and Therapy in Human Arteriosclerosis and in Animal Models. Opladen, Westdeutscher Verlag, Vol. 63, 1978, p. 153.
283. Kramsch, D. M., Aspen, A. J., and Apstein, C. S.: Suppression of experimental atherosclerosis by the Ca^{++}-antagonist lanthanum. J. Clin. Invest. *65*:967, 1980.
284. Kim, D. N., Lee, K. T., Reiner, J. M., and Thomas, W. A.: Effect of a soy protein product on serum and tissue cholesterol concentrations in swine fed high-fat, high-cholesterol diets. Exp. Mol. Pathol. *29*:385, 1978.
285. Hamilton, R. M. G., and Carroll, K. K.: Plasma cholesterol levels in rabbits fed low fat, low cholesterol diets. Effects of dietary proteins, carbohydrates and fiber from different sources. Atherosclerosis *24*:47, 1976.
286. Harris, W. S., Connor, W. E., and McMurry, M. P.: The comparative reductions of the plasma lipids and lipoproteins by dietary polyunsaturated fats: Salmon oil versus vegetable oil. Metabolism *32*:179, 1983.
287. Harris, W. S., and Connor, W. E.: The effects of salmon oil upon plasma lipids, lipoproteins, and triglyceride clearance. Trans. Assoc. Am. Physicians *43*:148, 1980.
288. Goodnight, S. J., Jr., Harris, W. S., Connor, W. E., and Illingworth, D. R.: Polyunsaturated fatty acids, hyperlipidemia, and thrombosis. Arteriosclerosis *2*: 87, 1982.
289. Veterans Administration Cooperative Study Group on Antihypertensive Agents: Effects of treatment on morbidity in hypertension. J.A.M.A. *213*: 1143, 1970.
290. Hypertension Detection and Follow-up Program Cooperative Group. Five-year findings of the Hypertension Detection and Follow-up Program. I. Reduction in mortality of persons with high blood pressure, including mild hypertension. J.A.M.A. *242*:2562, 1979.
291. Rogot, E.: Smoking and mortality among U.S. veterans. J. Chron. Dis. *27*:189, 1974.
292. The University Group Diabetes Program: A study of the effects of hypoglycemic agents on vascular complications in patients with adult-onset diabetes. I. Design, method and baseline results. Diabetes *19*(Suppl. II):747, 1970.
293. Stamler, J.: Atherosclerotic coronary heart disease. *In* Sussman, K. E., and Metz, R. J. S. (eds.): Diabetes Mellitus. 4th ed. New York, American Diabetes Association, 1975, p. 229.
294. Morris, J. N., Heady, J. A., Raffle, P. A. B., Roberts, C. G., and Parks, J. W.: Coronary heart disease and physical activity of work. Lancet *2*:1054, 1111, 1953.
295. Kirby, R. W., Anderson, J. W., Sieling, B., Rees, E. D., Chen, W. L., Miller, R. W., and Kay, R. M.: Oat-bran intake selectively lowers serum low-density lipoprotein cholesterol concentrations of hypercholesterolemic men. Am. J. Clin. Nutr. *34*:824, 1981.
296. Spain, D. M., Bradess, V. A., Matero, A., and Taiter, R.: Sudden death due to coronary atherosclerotic heart disease. J.A.M.A. *207*:1347, 1969.
297. Friedman, M., Manwaring, J. H., Rosenman, R. H., Donlon, G., Ortega, P., and Grube, S. M.: Instantaneous and sudden deaths. Clinical and pathological differentiation in coronary artery disease. J.A.M.A. *225*:1319, 1973.
298. Miller, R. D., Burchell, H. B., and Edwards, J. E.: Myocardial infarction with and without coronary occlusion. Arch. Intern. Med. *88*:597, 1951.
299. Schwartz, C. J., and Gerrity, R. G.: The anatomic pathology of sudden unexpected cardiac death. Circulation *52*(Suppl. III):78, 1975.
300. Wissler, R. W.: Current concepts of coronary thrombosis as related to atherosclerosis in myocardial infarction. *In* Manning, G. W., and Haust, M. D. (eds.): Atherosclerosis: Metabolic, Morphologic and Clinical Aspects. (Advances in Experimental Medicine and Biology, Vol. 82.) New York, Plenum Press, 1977, p. 86.
301. Buja, L. M., Hillis, L. D., Petty, C. S., and Willerson, J. T.: The role of coronary arterial spasm in ischemic heart disease. Arch. Pathol. Lab Med. *105*: 221, 1981.
302. Chandler, A. B., Chapman, I., Erhardt, L. R., Roberts, W. C., Schwartz, C. J., Sinapius, D., Spain, D. M., Sherry, S., Ness, P. M., and Simon, T. L.: Coronary thrombosis in myocardial infarction. Report of a workshop on the role of coronary thrombosis in the pathogenesis of acute myocardial infarction. Am. J. Cardiol. *34*:823, 1974.
303. Baum, R. S., Alvarez, H., III, and Cobb, L. A.: Survival after resuscitation from out-of-hospital ventricular fibrillation. Circulation *50*:1231, 1974.
304. Gorlin, R.: Coronary Artery Disease. Philadelphia, W. B. Saunders Co., 1976.
305. Maseri, A., L'Abbate, A., Baroldi, G., Chierchia, S., Marzilli, M., Ballestra, A. M., Severi, S., Parodi, O., Biagini, A., Distante, A., and Pesola, A.: Coronary vasospasm as a possible cause of myocardial infarction. A conclusion derived from the study of "preinfarction" angina. N. Engl. J. Med. *299*:1271, 1978.
306. Maseri, A., Severi, S., De Nes, M., L'Abbate, A., Chierchia, S., Marzilli, M., Ballestra, A. M., Parodi, O., Biagini, A., and Distante, A.: "Variant" angina: One aspect of a continuous spectrum of vasospastic myocardial ischemia. Pathogenetic mechanisms, estimated incidence and clinical and coronary arteriographic findings in 138 patients. Am. J. Cardiol. *42*:1019, 1978.
307. Kligfield, P.: New concepts in ischemic heart disease: The role of coronary artery spasm. New York, Science and Medicine Publishing Co., 1979.

35 RISK FACTORS FOR CORONARY ARTERY DISEASE AND THEIR MANAGEMENT

by Robert I. Levy, M.D., and Manning Feinleib, M.D., Dr. P.H.

During the past half century, epidemiologists and vital statisticians have observed wide variations in the rate of occurrence of coronary artery disease (CAD) in regard to time, place, and person. CAD and its major clinical manifestation, myocardial infarction, was a medical rarity prior to the First World War.[1] This was due in part to the fact that myocardial infarction was only first described in 1912. During the 1920's and 1930's, it was recognized with increasing frequency as being a common problem among white men in urban areas of North America and Europe, particularly among the more affluent. By 1940, CAD was the leading cause of death in the United States and several other countries, and its frequency continued to increase through the 1950's.

In the late 1940's and early 1950's, several studies of free-living populations were begun to discern the factors associated with the occurrence of CAD and how the disease evolves and terminates in a total population. Clinical impressions were soon confirmed—CAD did not occur randomly in the population. Its rate of occurrence varied greatly according to such demographical factors as age, race, and sex. Personal attributes detectable by simple medical examination—high serum cholesterol, high blood pressure, hyperglycemia, and obesity—were found to increase the frequency of the disease. Personal habits which the patient could easily recognize himself—cigarette smoking, lack of exercise, and nutritional habits—were also investigated. More recently, some specific environmental hazards—carbon disulfide and oral contraceptives—have been associated with increased occurrence of CAD. Underlying these factors, familial and genetic effects are believed to play an inceptive role, in concert with their complex interrelationships with social and psychological factors.

EPIDEMIOLOGICAL STUDIES

Epidemiologists have used a variety of strategies to study the precursors of CAD, but two have been paramount: (1) comparison of CAD rates and associated characteristics of large population groups, such as differences between countries, racial groups, religious groups, or occupations; and (2) studies of characteristics of individuals and the relation of the development of CAD in these individuals to these characteristics. The first strategy is usually based on disease rates derived from vital statistics on mortality and from relatively crude data on group characteristics, e.g., diet. Data on vital statistics are prone to many uncertainties: varying fashions in the certification of causes of death; lack of standardization of evidence to be used in establishing diagnoses; and incompleteness of reporting. Yet these data, being based on large numbers, can document major differences in the death rates from CAD in different populations. More detailed clinical and autopsy studies have generally confirmed the major trends established by data on vital statistics.[2,3] Certain trends in vital statistics can be accounted for by deliberate changes in the manner of classifying data on death certificates, such as the major change introduced with the eighth revision of the International Classification of Diseases in the manner of coding hypertension.[4] This resulted in an apparent sharp rise in the death rates from CAD (or Ischemic Heart Disease, as it is officially designated in the ICD) from 1967 to 1968 and a compensating sharp decline in deaths attributed to hypertension.

The limitations of data on the relevant characteristics of populations are also legion, and only gross estimates of incidence can be obtained for such important factors as diet, cigarette smoking, or quality of medical care. Furthermore, large populations differ from one another in multiple unmeasurable characteristics that may play important roles in determining the overall rates of occurrence of CAD. Thus, comparisons between populations must be considered circumspectly; they may, however, suggest important clues for further research, corroborate broad hypotheses, or be useful for didactic purposes.

As observations and hypotheses regarding the occurrence and etiology of CAD accumulated during the 1920's and 1930's, the need to use a more organized and better controlled approach to studying its precursors and natural history became evident. Long-term prospective, population-based studies of individuals were considered the optimal strategy to acquire the necessary data. It was recognized that representative samples of several thousand persons would be needed; that these people would have to be examined while they were ostensibly healthy (i.e., before clinically overt CAD had become manifest); that carefully standardized examination procedures, questionnaires, and laboratory methods were required; and that diligent and careful surveillance of the entire group must be maintained for many years. With this general approach, numerous epidemiological studies involving tens of thousands of people have been undertaken in a variety of populations during the last three decades.

The Framingham Heart Study is perhaps the best known of these,[5] but major contributions have been made by many others, including those in the National Cooperative Pooling Project,[6,7] the Tecumseh Study,[8] the Western Collaborative Group Study,[9] the Seven Countries Study,[10] the Evans County Study,[11] the Puerto Rico Study,[12] the Ni-Hon-San Study of Japanese Men,[13] the Göteborg Study,[14] and the Paris Study.[15]

These prospective epidemiological studies started out by examining several thousand men who were free from clinical evidence of heart disease. (The Framingham, Tecumseh, and Evans County studies are among the few that studied women.) Each study attempted to include representative samples of populations defined by location or occupation. Considering the difficulties of such undertakings, all achieved satisfactorily high rates of cooperation. Each participant was examined for a variety of characteristics, including weight, blood pressure, blood composition, smoking habits, and electrocardiographical evidence of CAD. In some studies, many other variables were investigated, such as diet, exercise, behavioral characteristics, and social factors. Each study then followed the participants for several years, using repeated examinations and other surveillance procedures to document all deaths and all new cardiovascular disease developing in the cohorts.

Despite the large size and careful design of these studies, they cannot be considered to be formal scientific experiments. The variation in baseline characteristics occurred naturally, without any manipulation by the investigators, and was beyond their control and ken. There was no element of randomization in determining who had a high level and who had a low level of a particular trait. At best, these were "natural experiments" rather than controlled experiments. Because the factors, largely unknown, that may have led to the particular distribution of characteristics in the subjects might also be related to the occurrence of disease through other independent pathways, clear-cut causal relationships cannot be established by such studies.

Well-designed scientific experiments of causal hypotheses generally require, at the minimum, manipulation of the level of the causal factor (exposure) and random allocation of exposure to the participants in the study. This type of design is the one employed currently in the various prophylactic trials and intervention studies conducted by the National Heart, Lung, and Blood Institute to test various components of the "risk factor hypothesis." The hypothesis, therefore, must be considered to be resting on naturally occurring associations between traits and disease states, rather than being the outcome of controlled experimentation. Thus, we prefer to speak of the various traits studied in these epidemiological studies as "risk factors" or "predictors of disease," rather than as causes or etiological factors in the disease process. Although this may appear academic and overly cautious in view of the volume of evidence that has accumulated for some risk factors, it will serve to remind us that firm experimental confirmation is not yet available.

DEMOGRAPHICAL VARIATIONS IN FREQUENCY OF CAD

The frequency of occurrence of CAD and its mortality are known to vary according to the characteristics of person, place, and time. Comparison of mortality data based on age and sex for different places and over several decades provides insight into the evolution of CAD as the major health problem of most developed countries during the last 50 years.

In describing the demographical features of the occurrence of CAD, it would be desirable to have data for mortality (deaths from CAD) as well as morbidity (nonfatal CAD events). However, when dealing with national populations, only mortality data derived from routine death certificates are usually available. Morbidity data must be derived from special surveys (such as the Household Interview Survey), examinations (such as the Health and Nutrition Examination Survey), or searches of records (such as the Hospital Discharge Survey).[16-18]

When comparing mortality data for different subgroups of a population, one may first consider the absolute number of deaths from a specified cause occurring during a stated time period. Since the number of deaths obviously depends on the size of the population, its age structure, and other characteristics of the group, however, vital statisticians use various calculated rates to take these factors into account. The crude death rate for a specified cause is the absolute number of deaths from the specified cause during a year, divided by the size of the population at midyear. Thus, during 1979, there were a total of 551,365 deaths attributed to CAD in the United States. The estimated midyear population was 224,567,000, yielding a crude mortality rate for CAD of 245.5 per 100,000.[19] One may calculate mortality rates for specific subgroups of the population if one knows the numerator (the number of deaths in the specific subgroup from the cause of interest) and the denominator (the size of the specific subgroup). Thus, Table 35–1 shows the age-, sex-, and race-specific mortality rates from CAD in the U.S. from 1950 to 1977.

Occasionally, it may be necessary to compare mortality rates for populations of diverse age and sex distributions, e.g., in comparing the trends in the mortality rates of different countries or in one country at different points in time. To do this, vital statisticians commonly employ adjusted mortality rates or standardized ones. These are weighted averages of the age- and sex-specific mortality rates, using a standard, albeit arbitrary, set of weightings. Most commonly, a specified historical distribution of population is used as the standard weight, e.g., the 1940 distribution of population in the U.S. These standardized rates are also shown in Table 35–1.

Age. The mortality of CAD shows a striking relationship to age in each sex and race group. Although quite rare in younger white women, the disease is aready a ma-

TABLE 35–1 ISCHEMIC HEART DISEASE DEATH RATES PER 100,000 POPULATION IN THE UNITED STATES

	White							
	Men				*Women*			
Age Group	1950*	1960*	1968†	1977†	1950*	1960*	1968†	1977†
35–44	77.5	86.0	87.6	59.8	13.2	12.7	16.3	11.1
45–54	323.1	352.5	350.0	266.9	66.6	61.9	72.8	56.5
55–64	812.9	901.3	945.2	715.1	267.5	277.6	283.7	216.9
65–74	1608.2	1909.2	2119.3	1642.8	838.9	916.3	998.3	704.8
Age-adjusted	259.5	305.3	336.5	264.7	120.6	137.8	160.8	119.0
	Nonwhite							
	Men				*Women*			
Age Group	1950*	1960*	1968†	1977†	1950*	1960*	1968†	1977†
35–44	74.3	87.8	134.9	91.3	48.1	46.7	68.6	36.6
45–54	254.2	297.0	419.4	315.9	165.7	168.0	222.9	144.7
55–64	554.1	723.7	998.1	786.3	366.7	482.3	623.6	423.0
65–74	943.1	1340.2	1920.2	1435.5	656.8	807.0	1362.1	945.8
Age-adjusted	164.0	219.5	316.9	245.3	112.6	145.8	213.2	152.3

*7th Revision ICD Code 420.
†8th Revision ICD Code 410–413.
Crude comparability ratio $\frac{8th}{7th}$ = 1.1457.

jor cause of death for men aged 35 to 44 years. The mortality of CAD rapidly increases, so that by age 55 to 64, 35 per cent of all deaths among men are due to this single cause.

Sex. As shown in Table 35–1, the male mortality rates from CAD are much higher than those for females, for both whites and nonwhites. The ratios of the mortality rates of men to those of women are much higher for whites than nonwhites, however, and in both groups are higher at the younger ages than at older ages. Thus, among whites, in 1979, the male mortality rate from CAD was 5.2 times greater than in females at ages 35 to 44 and was 2.4 times as great at ages 65 to 74, whereas among nonwhites the respective ratios were 2.8 and 1.6. As an approximation, the female rates lag behind the male rates by about 10 years among whites and by about 7 years among nonwhites.

Race. The differences in the mortality of CAD between whites and nonwhites have not been wholly consistent during the last 30 years. Nonwhite men tended to have lower rates than white men prior to 1968, but since then they have had higher rates up to the age of 65. Nonwhite women have tended to have higher rates than white women throughout this period.

Among specific ethnic groups in the United States, Japanese men in Hawaii and California and men in Puerto Rico have been found to have about half the amount of CAD as Caucasians.[20]

Geography. Mortality rates from CAD vary both between different countries and within countries. Figure 35–1 shows the mortality rates in the United States. Marked regional differences can be noted. High mortality rates occur in those states along the southeastern Atlantic Coast and in the industrialized states of the Midwest and Northeast. The lowest rates are found in the Great Plains and mountain states. These rather clear regional differences have not been adequately explained, although some relationships have been found with ecological factors. Climatic variables have also been implicated to some degree: Extremes of temperature and snowfall have been related to increased mortality rates.[21] Altitude, either directly or via other factors, may play a role; areas at highest altitudes tend to have lower rates of CAD.[22]

A positive association has been reported between the *hardness of drinking water* and local mortality rates from heart disease in the U.S., Great Britain, and Canada, but inconsistent relationships have been found with the content of trace elements in the water.[23–25] One constituent of water in particular that has been studied extensively is artificial fluoride. In a study of all U.S. cities with more than 25,000 people between 1945 and 1969, no association was found between the introduction of artificial fluoride to the water supply and changes in mortality of heart disease.[26]

International differences in mortality of CAD are also striking (Table 35–2). It should be noted, however, that reliable data are lacking for most of the countries of Asia, Africa, and Latin America. It is believed that CAD is uncommon in most nonindustrialized countries, so that it is safe to assume, on the basis of the data available, that there is at least a 10-fold variation in the international rates of death from CAD. As with the regional differences within the United States, these international differences have not been satisfactorily explained. Comparative autopsy studies and standardized investigations in different countries show that these differences are not simply artifacts of varying practices in death certification.[2,3,10,26] It might be speculated that these differences can be accounted for by genetic factors. Thus, one is struck by the finding that after Finland, the next seven countries with highest mortality from CAD are the major English-speaking countries of the world. However, studies of migrants and of people of similar ethnic backgrounds in different countries point to *environmental* factors as being of major importance.[13,27,28] Furthermore, there have been marked changes in mortality rates from CAD over time that cannot be explained by sudden changes in the genetic structure of the populations.[29,30,31]

The mortality from CAD in Japan and the experience of the Japanese in different areas of the world provide interesting material for speculation about the possible roles of

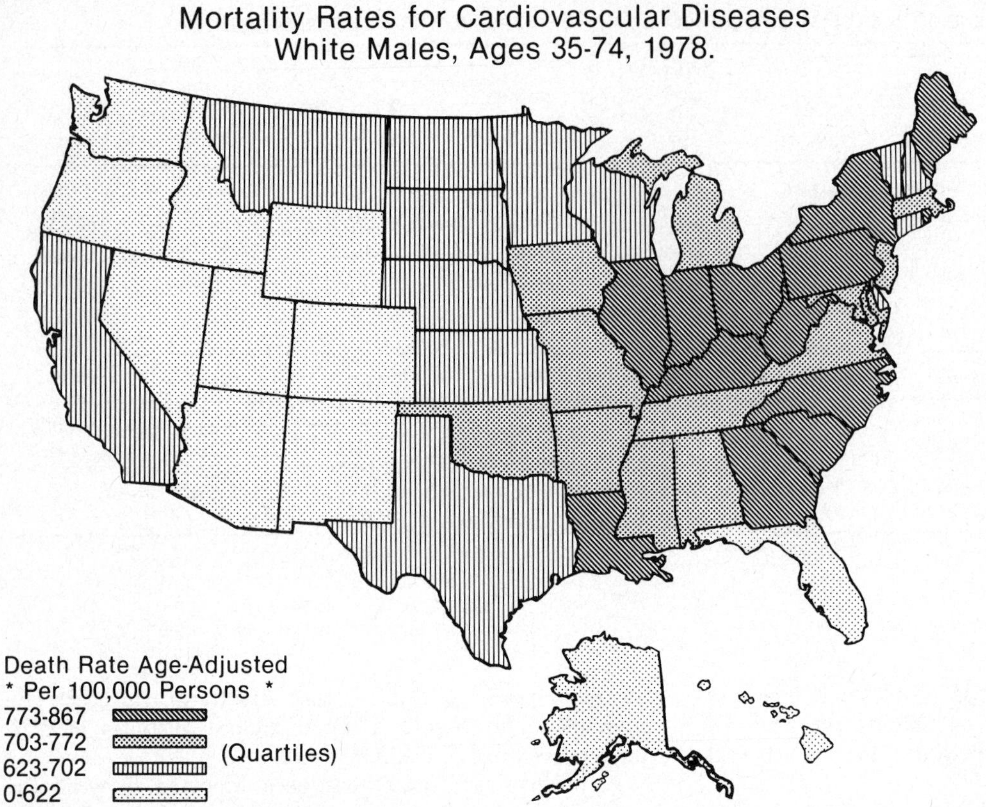

FIGURE 35–1 Mortality rates for cardiovascular diseases, white males, ages 35 to 74, 1978.

genetics and environment. The low CAD rates in Japan, even after some allowance for differences in death certification, indicate that industrialization need not be automatically associated with high rates of heart disease. However, Japanese in Hawaii and California have almost twice the rate of CAD as do Japanese in Japan, but still only about half the CAD rate of U.S. Caucasians. Thus, the experience of Japanese in the United States indicates that although environmental factors may play a major role, they cannot account for all the differences between certain groups.[13,20,32]

Time Trends. Table 35–1 also shows that mortality rates from CAD have varied over time. After a general increase in mortality rates for all age-sex-race groups in the U.S. through the 1950's, there was a leveling off of the rates for most subgroups through the 1960's. Since 1968, however, there has been a steady and dramatic decline in the death rate for each subgroup. The U.S. adjusted mor-

TABLE 35–2 DEATH RATES FOR CORONARY HEART DISEASE AND ALL CAUSES IN 1977 FOR SELECTED COUNTRIES: MEN, AGES 55 TO 64*

	Coronary Heart Disease		All Causes	
Country	*1977*	*Per cent Change 1969–1977*	*1977*	*Per cent Change 1969–1977*
Finland	996.9**	−3.8	2398.6**	−12.3
Northern Ireland	925.0	+11.4	2199.1	−0.1
Scotland	899.8	−0.3	2265.1	−8.5
Australia	730.9	−20.2	1815.6	−15.1
New Zealand	766.6†	−10.0	1887.2†	−6.4
U.S.A. (White)	715.1	−22.2	1848.9	−16.1
England and Wales	710.8	+0.3	1877.4	−13.2
Canada	697.0**	−5.6	1834.4**	−1.5
Israel	513.0	−24.5	1518.5	−8.5
Norway	570.5	−9.1	1466.3	−9.7
Denmark	578.2	+7.0	1613.6	−3.2
Sweden	563.6	+15.8	1411.8	−1.9
Netherlands	519.8	+2.4	1584.9	−7.9
German Federal Republic	462.5	−0.4	1806.6	−17.0
Hungary	477.3††	+11.4	2125.0††	+8.1
Austria	442.8	+0.3	1857.5	−15.5
Italy	326.6††	+6.1	1804.4††	−7.6
Switzerland	321.1	+5.9	1460.0	−15.9
Japan	94.8	−22.4	1284.8	−25.6

*Per 100,000 population.
**Rates for 1975.
†Rates for 1976.
†† Rates for 1974.

tality rate from CAD has fallen 26.5 per cent from 1968 to 1978 (Fig. 35–2). In most other countries, CAD rates are continuing to increase or are showing considerably smaller declines. The reasons for the decline in the U.S. are still speculative, but there is some evidence that much of it can be associated with changes in habits and life styles that may decrease the average person's risk for CAD.[30–36]

ATHEROSCLEROTIC RISK FACTORS

In order to uncover individual characteristics that are related to the occurrence of CAD, it is necessary to turn from studies of vital statistics to studies of individual people. Epidemiological studies of free-living populations followed for many years have identified specific characteristics of people and some personal habits that are strongly related to the chance of developing CAD. These bodily characteristics and personal habits have been called "risk factors" for CAD.

An example of the relationship between risk factors and the chance of developing disease is given in Figure 35–3. This figure is based on data from the Framingham Heart Study, but its main features have been confirmed in virtually all the studies cited previously.[37–40] Figure 35–3 shows the probability of developing CAD in 8 years according to sex and age. For each sex, three risk categories are shown, as defined by four characteristics of the individual: systolic blood pressure, serum cholesterol level, cigarette smoking, and evidence of glucose intolerance. The wide differences in the chances of developing CAD among these risk categories is a measure of our ability to identify, while they are still healthy, those men and women who are most prone to develop clinical disease.

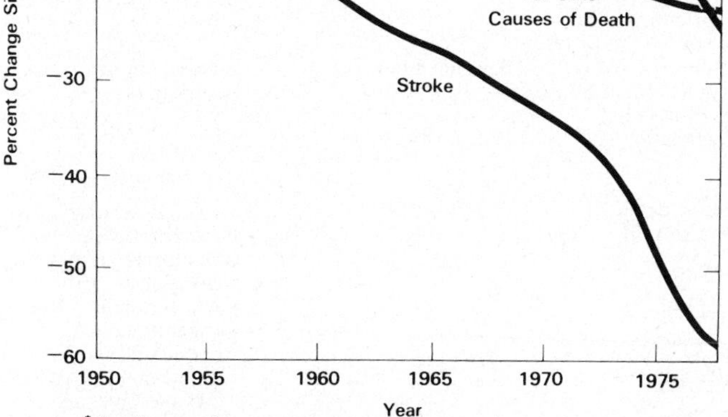

FIGURE 35–2 Per cent change in death rates since 1950 for CAD, stroke, and all other causes, ages 35 to 74, United States, 1950 to 1978. (From Levy, R. I.: Declining mortality in coronary heart disease. Arteriosclerosis 1:312, 1981.)

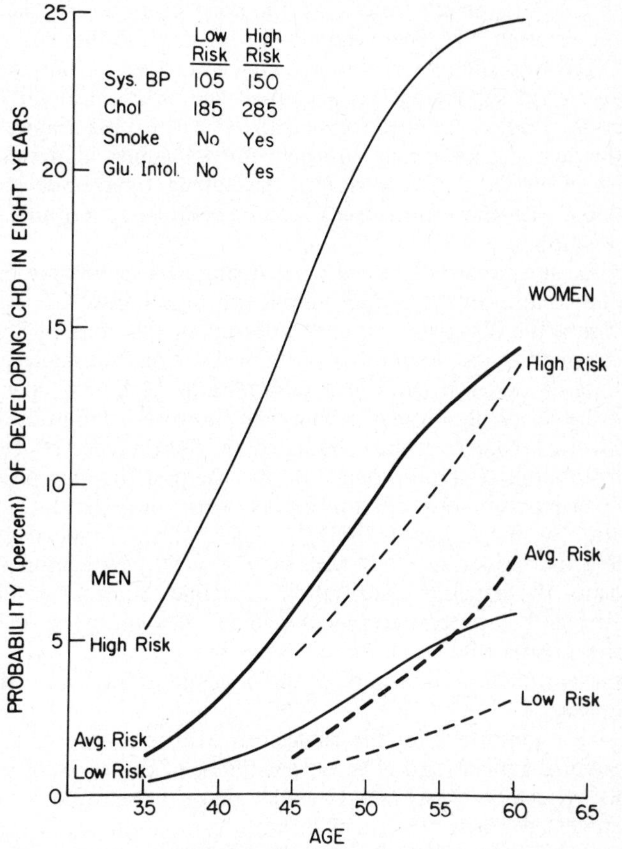

FIGURE 35–3 Probability of developing CAD in eight years according to age, sex, and risk category (The Framingham Heart Study).

Figure 35–3 shows the combined effects of all four risk factors for CAD, determined by using a multivariate logistic regression model (discussed later). Similar analyses have been done for each factor separately. These show that each of the four risk factors indicated makes a separate and significant contribution to the risk of developing CAD. Following is a brief discussion of each of the major risk factors taken individually and then a consideration of their cumulative effects.

Blood Lipids (See also p. 1628)

Among the numerous recognized risk factors for the development of atherosclerosis, one of the best documented is the association between blood lipids and CAD.[6] The evidence of the association between serum cholesterol level and CAD is extensive and unequivocal.[41–44] It is derived from a variety of sources, including (1) production of atherosclerotic lesions in animals by use of hypercholesterolemia-inducing diets; (2) the nature and dynamics of the human atherosclerotic plaque (see Chapter 34); (3) the occurrence of hyperlipidemia in groups of subjects with clinically manifested atherosclerotic disease; (4) the study of genetic hyperlipidemias associated with premature CAD; and (5) epidemiological studies of populations with differing serum cholesterol levels. Although triglyceride levels have been associated with CAD in several cross-sectional studies, prospective studies remain inconclusive in their indictment of serum triglycerides as a coronary risk factor.[45–47] In sharp contrast, evidence from several prospective studies clearly establishes that in an otherwise healthy population, the risk

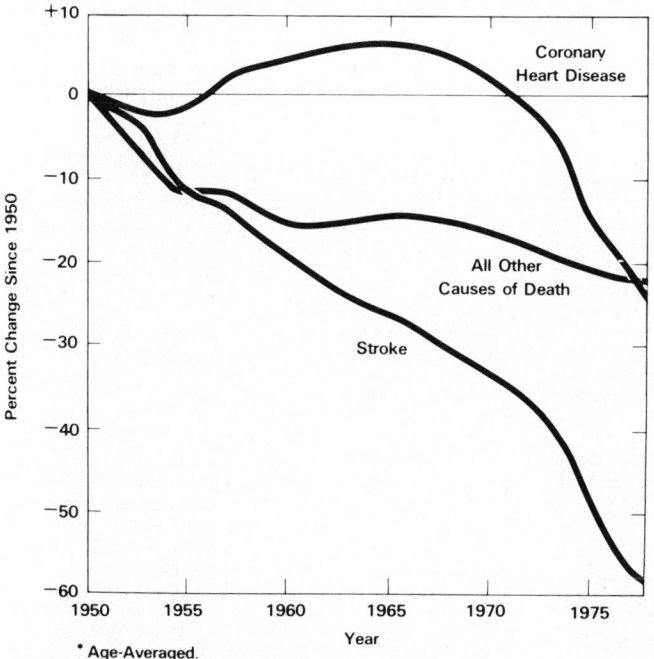

of CAD is directly related to the concentration of plasma cholesterol.[10,48,49] The accuracy of predicting the risk of CAD according to cholesterol concentrations is, however, greater in the young (younger than age 65) than in the elderly. One of the most important results of these studies is the demonstration that subjects with the highest cholesterol levels are at a greater risk of developing CAD, but even those with the lowest levels are not completely immune to the disease.[50]

As indicated later in this discussion, it has become evident that even more information can be obtained by measuring the plasma cholesterol in terms of the units of lipid transport—the lipoproteins—than by simply calculating total cholesterol. Until long-term data in relation to specific levels of lipoprotein accumulate, however, definition of cardiovascular risk must be based on the evidence relating to total cholesterol obtained during the past three decades.

The continuous relationship between cholesterol levels and the incidence of CAD is of the utmost importance. When considering CAD risk, there is little justification for using the gaussian distribution to define "normal" levels. It must be appreciated that the higher the cholesterol level, the greater the need for concern; but no single level of plasma cholesterol separates those at risk from those who are not.

It is important for the clinician to realize that for differential diagnosis and effective treatment of disorders of lipid transport associated with marked elevations of cholesterol or triglycerides, or both, systems currently exist that use arbitrary limits (usually the 90th or 95th percentile) of cholesterol, low-density lipoprotein, and triglycerides. A clear distinction should exist between these arbitrary limits used to define "types" of hyperlipoproteinemia and the concept of cholesterol as a risk factor.

TRANSLATING HYPERCHOLESTEROLEMIA INTO HYPERLIPOPROTEINEMIA. The major plasma lipids, including cholesterol and triglyceride, do not circulate freely in solution in the blood but rather are transported in the form of lipoprotein complexes (Table 35–3).[51] The major lipoprotein families—chylomicrons, very low-density lipoproteins (VLDL), low-density lipoproteins (LDL), and high-density lipoproteins (HDL)—are usually conveniently classified in terms of physicochemical properties such as density or electrophoretic mobility.[52] Sufficient elevation in the concentration of any of the lipoprotein families can result in hypercholesterolemia. Similarly, hypertriglyceridemia can result from increased concentrations of chylomicrons, VLDL, or IDL (intermediate-density lipoproteins) alone or in various combinations.

Plasma concentrations of LDL correlate closely with plasma concentrations of cholesterol, as would be expected, since 60 to 75 per cent of the total plasma cholesterol is normally transported in this lipoprotein. They thus have more or less the same predictive capability.

HDL, which normally accounts for 20 to 25 per cent of the total plasma cholesterol, is also a potent risk factor for CAD. Whereas LDL cholesterol is directly related to risk, however, HDL shows an indirect relationship. In spite of numerous studies in the past that demonstrated this inverse relationship between HDL and atherosclerosis, HDL is only now becoming part of a standard coronary risk profile. Gordon et al. have shown that in both men and women older than the age of 50 years, HDL cholesterol has the strongest relationship to CAD.[53] They suggest that HDL should be integrated into the risk profile for CAD, together with LDL and VLDL, and that this inclusion would greatly improve our ability to predict CAD.

THE LIPOPROTEINS

Chylomicrons. Chylomicrons are composed primarily of triglycerides and originate from exogenous dietary fat in the intestine. Seventy to 100 gm of dietary fat are trans-

TABLE 35–3 BIOCHEMICAL AND CLINICAL FEATURES OF LIPOPROTEINS

Family	Origin	Function	Catabolism	Plasma Appearance	Clinical Features of Elevated Level
Chylomicrons	Intestine, from dietary fat	Transport of dietary fat	Lipoprotein lipase at tissue sites; chylomicron remnant cleared by liver	Creamy supernate; clear infranate	Eruptive xanthoma; lipemia retinalis; organomegaly; pancreatitis
VLDL	Liver and small bowel, from carbohydrates, free fatty acids, medium-chain triglycerides	Transport of endogenus trigylcerides	Complex; probably requires lipoprotein lipase for degradation	Turbid serum	Glucose intolerance; hyperuricemia
IDL	VLDL	Unknown	Unclear; degradation to LDL	Turbid serum	Glucose intolerance; hyperuricemia; premature atherosclerosis; tuboeruptive, tendinous, and palmar planar xanthoma
LDL	VLDL; IDL (? alternative source)	Unknown	Primary site and removal unclear	Clear	Premature atherosclerosis; corneal arcus; tendinous and tuberous xanthoma; xanthelasma
HDL	? Intestine ? Liver	? Facilitates cholesterol ester and triglyceride metabolism	? Liver	Clear	No associated abnormality

ported from the intestine to sites of utilization and storage each day. Chylomicrons are usually absent in plasma after 12 to 14 hours of fasting. Their presence in fasting plasma should always be considered abnormal. When present, these large particles produce turbidity and, upon standing in a cold test tube 24 to 40 hours, will rise as a creamy layer to the top of the tube. When chylomicronemia is present, the cholesterol/triglyceride ratio in the plasma can be as high as 1:20. Even marked chylomicronemia has not been associated with premature CAD.

Very Low-Density Lipoproteins (VLDL). VLDL are composed primarily of triglyceride, derived endogenously from the liver and small intestine. The cholesterol/triglyceride ratio in this class of lipoproteins is normally about 1:5. Between 15 and 25 gm of VLDL glyceride are released into the bloodstream daily. Diets high in carbohydrate will invariably increase triglyceride levels, at least transiently. Other factors that contribute to the lability of VLDL triglyceride levels include changes in weight, alcohol intake, stress, and exercise.

Although sustained elevation of VLDL has sometimes been associated with premature atherosclerosis, epidemiological evidence of the relationship of plasma triglycerides to CAD is less clear.[47,54–59] One of the difficulties is in distinguishing an elevated level of triglycerides as a separate risk factor from the hypertension, obesity, and glucose intolerance that often accompany it.

Intermediate-Density Lipoproteins (IDL). Intermediate-density lipoproteins are essentially a transitional form in the catabolism of VLDL to LDL. Their average cholesterol content is 30 per cent, and the triglyceride content is 40 per cent. There is evidence that IDL may be identical in form to the abnormal lipoprotein that characterizes Type III hyperlipoproteinemia, but further confirmation of this is needed. In Type III hyperlipoproteinemia, excess levels of IDL-like particles are associated with premature coronary and peripheral vessel disease.[59]

Low-Density Lipoproteins (LDL). It is now known that LDL are the product of the intravascular metabolism of the glyceride-rich lipoprotein, VLDL.[60,61] One of the major functions of VLDL is to transport glyceride through the plasma. It is then catabolized rapidly to an intermediate form (IDL) and ultimately to LDL. Thus, subjects with increased LDL in the plasma are accumulating the remnants of the metabolism of VLDL. The increase may be due either to overproduction of VLDL (which is uncommon) or to a defective clearance of LDL.

LDL as a molecule is approximately 50 per cent cholesterol by weight. Thus, a patient with an elevated level of LDL will usually have an increased level of cholesterol. The other lipoproteins—chylomicrons, VLDL, and HDL—also contain cholesterol, but in lesser amounts than LDL. The major reason for measuring LDL is that this lipoprotein has been most directly associated with CAD.[54,63] In a population with "normal" levels of LDL, a comparison of levels below 119 mg/dl with levels above 150 mg/dl (equivalent to a plasma cholesterol level of approximately 230 mg/dl) reveals a clear difference in the rates of cardiovascular events.[64] Subjects with high levels of LDL more often have CAD, measured as either overt heart attacks or other events, such as angina. Thus, even in a normal population, the higher levels of LDL carry a greater risk of vascular disease.

High-density Lipoproteins (HDL). Exciting recent findings have focused attention on the high-density lipoproteins. The role of HDL in lipid transport is unclear. It may serve to remove cholesterol from tissues or, alternatively, to accept it during VLDL metabolism in vivo. Unlike the atherogenic LDL, HDL has been *inversely* associated with CAD risk.[65–67] Moreover, the negative correlation between HDL cholesterol and CAD is independent of other risk factors.[53,64,67] Earlier reports that healthy men have higher levels of HDL than men with CAD were largely ignored, inexplicably, until a 1975 review of the evidence thrust HDL into the forefront of lipoprotein research.[65] Mounting epidemiological findings support the tempting hypothesis that increased concentrations of HDL may be a protective factor in the development of vascular disease. The cause and effect of the inverse relationship between HDL and CAD remains unclear, however. Levels of HDL have been correlated positively with exercise and moderate ingestion of alcohol and inversely related to obesity, smoking, poor control of diabetes, and the use of progestin-containing contraceptives.[68,69] The results of a recent study show that the prevalence of CAD at HDL levels of 30 mg/dl was *double* that at 60 mg/dl.[66] Mean values of HDL cholesterol were lower in subjects with CAD. *These findings provide a cogent reason to determine whether elevated cholesterol levels are due to increases in LDL or HDL.* Familial excesses of HDL or deficiencies of LDL have been associated with decreased risk of CAD.[70]

DISTRIBUTION OF PLASMA LIPIDS AND LIPOPROTEINS. The variability in plasma lipids and lipoproteins precludes the establishment of universally acceptable limits. What may be considered normal for one population group may not necessarily be applicable to another. Even within a country, these "normal" limits may vary from one region to another and are markedly age- and sex-dependent.

The relative contribution of genetic and environmental factors to the distribution curve for concentration of cholesterol cannot be assessed with certainty in any population. However, studies of families and twins have shown that genetic components (including polygenic effects as well as the mutant allele responsible for familial hypercholesterolemia) may account for as much as 40 per cent of the total variability. On the other hand, environmental factors, although not clearly understood, also markedly influence the variability in the distribution of concentrations of cholesterol between populations. For example, immigrants who come to the U.S. from countries where the mean level of cholesterol is low usually acquire the high levels characteristic of North America. Nutritional factors have important effects upon the metabolism of lipids and probably play a dominant role in the pathogenesis of the mild hypercholesterolemia so commonly found in Western populations.

The Lipid Research Clinics (LRC) Program recently completed a series of surveys that have yielded data of interest to both epidemiologists and clinicians. These surveys were conducted to determine the prevalence of hyperlipidemias and the distribution of various levels of lipids and lipoproteins in 11 North American populations.[71,72] The resulting data are of particular interest because of the size and diversity of the populations studied: Triglyceride and cholesterol levels were determined for more than 70,000 in-

TABLE 35–4 TOTAL PLASMA CHOLESTEROL (mg/dl) IN 11 FREE-LIVING NORTH AMERICAN WHITE POPULATIONS*

	Males (n = 3580)			Females (n = 3413)		
		Percentiles			Percentiles	
Age	*Mean* ± *SEM*	*10th*	*90th*	*Mean* ± *SEM*	*10th*	*90th*
5–9	155.3 ± 1.8	131	183	164.0 ± 1.8	135	189
10–14	160.9 ± 1.5	132	191	160.1 ± 1.5	131	191
15–19	153.1 ± 1.4	123	183	159.5 ± 1.6	126	198
20–24	162.2 ± 2.5	126	197	170.3 ± 2.5	132	220
25–29	178.7 ± 2.1	137	223	179.5 ± 1.7	142	217
30–34	193.1 ± 1.8	152	237	179.2 ± 1.7	141	215
35–39	200.6 ± 1.9	157	248	189.6 ± 2.1	149	233
40–44	205.2 ± 1.9	161	251	197.5 ± 1.9	156	241
45–49	213.4 ± 1.9	171	258	206.2 ± 2.0	162	256
50–54	213.2 ± 1.9	168	263	217.3 ± 2.4	171	267
55–59	215.0 ± 2.2	172	260	228.7 ± 2.4	182	278
60–64	216.6 ± 3.3	170	262	232.2 ± 3.7	186	282
65–69	221.0 ± 3.8	174	275	234.1 ± 4.0	179	282
70+	210.3 ± 3.4	160	253	224.5 ± 2.8	181	268

*From Lipid Research Clinics Population Studies Data Book. Vol. 1. The Prevalence Study. Washington, D.C., U.S. Department of Health and Human Services, Public Health Service. NIH Publ. No. 80-1527, 1980.

TABLE 35–5 PLASMA TRIGLYCERIDES (mg/dl) IN 11 FREE-LIVING NORTH AMERICAN WHITE POPULATIONS*

	Males (n = 3580)			Females (n = 3413)		
		Percentiles			Percentiles	
Age	*Mean* ± *SEM*	*10th*	*90th*	*Mean* ± *SEM*	*10th*	*90th*
5–9	51.9 ± 1.7	34	70	63.8 ± 2.5	37	103
10–14	63.4 ± 1.6	37	94	72.0 ± 1.7	44	104
15–19	78.2 ± 2.4	43	125	72.8 ± 1.9	40	112
20–24	89.3 ± 3.7	50	146	87.3 ± 2.9	42	135
25–29	104.2 ± 4.2	51	171	87.4 ± 2.8	45	137
30–34	122.1 ± 3.7	57	214	86.0 ± 2.8	45	140
35–39	140.8 ± 5.5	58	250	98.3 ± 3.2	47	170
40–44	152.4 ± 6.9	69	252	98.1 ± 2.6	51	161
45–49	143.4 ± 5.9	65	218	112.5 ± 3.4	55	180
50–54	153.4 ± 5.5	75	244	116.0 ± 3.4	58	190
55–59	134.3 ± 4.2	70	210	133.1 ± 4.8	65	229
60–64	130.6 ± 8.7	65	193	132.1 ± 9.1	66	210
65–69	138.6 ± 11.1	61	227	136.5 ± 6.8	64	221
70+	132.8 ± 7.2	71	202	128.3 ± 6.5	68	189

*From Lipid Research Clinics Population Studies Data Book. Vol. 1. The Prevalence Study. Washington, D.C., U.S. Department of Health and Human Services, Public Health Service. NIH Publ. No. 80-1527, 1980.

TABLE 35–6 PLASMA LDL CHOLESTEROL (mg/dl) IN 11 FREE-LIVING NORTH AMERICAN WHITE POPULATIONS*

	Males (n = 3540)			Females (n = 3413)		
		Percentiles			Percentiles	
Age	*Mean* ± *SEM*	*10th*	*90th*	*Mean* ± *SEM*	*10th*	*90th*
5–9	92.5 ± 1.8	69	117	100.4 ± 2.1	73	125
10–14	96.8 ± 1.4	73	123	97.4 ± 1.3	73	126
15–19	94.4 ± 1.3	68	123	95.7 ± 1.5	66	129
20–24	103.3 ± 2.4	73	138	103.7 ± 2.2	65	141
25–29	116.7 ± 1.9	75	157	110.2 ± 1.6	75	148
30–34	126.4 ± 1.6	88	166	111.3 ± 1.5	77	146
35–39	133.2 ± 1.7	92	176	119.7 ± 2.0	81	161
40–44	135.6 ± 1.6	98	173	125.1 ± 1.8	84	165
45–49	143.7 ± 1.8	106	185	129.4 ± 1.9	89	173
50–54	142.3 ± 1.7	102	185	138.1 ± 2.3	94	186
55–59	145.8 ± 2.1	103	191	146.1 ± 2.4	97	199
60–64	146.3 ± 3.1	106	188	152.0 ± 3.6	105	191
65–69	150.4 ± 3.5	104	199	153.8 ± 4.1	99	205
70+	142.9 ± 2.9	100	182	148.6 ± 2.7	108	189

*From Lipid Research Clinics Population Studies Data Book. Vol. 1. The Prevalence Study. Washington, D.C., U.S. Department of Health and Human Services, Public Health Service. NIH Publ. No. 80-1527, 1980.

dividuals, and lipoprotein determinations were done for approximately 25 per cent of that group. Although the populations studied were not necessarily statistically representative of the entire North American population, they were well-defined, diverse target groups that (1) spanned a range of ethnic, geographical, socioeconomic, occupational, and age groups; and (2) were studied according to highly standardized procedures. Tables 35–4 to 35–7 give the means and selected percentiles of the distributions of plasma lipids and lipoproteins determined in the LRC Study.[73]

THE EVALUATION OF HYPERLIPOPROTEINEMIA

The lack of specificity of hypercholesterolemia and hypertriglyceridemia makes their translation into hyperlipoproteinemia useful for both differential diagnosis and treatment. Five patterns (types) of hyperlipoproteinemia have been described (Table 35–8).[51,54,74] Each is a "shorthand" or jargon term that describes which lipoproteins are increased in the plasma. Since all the lipoprotein families have a relatively fixed composition, and since two of them refract light and produce turbidity, defining hyperlipoproteinemia usually only requires a look at the standing plasma (after storage overnight at 4°C) and an accurate and precise measurement of cholesterol and triglyceride levels (see Table 35–3). Hyperchylomicronemia can be differentiated from increased VLDL (both of which produce hypertriglyceridemia) by noting the appearance of the plasma. A creamy layer over a clear infranatant is generally diagnostic of Type I. In cases of hyperbetalipoproteinemia (Type IIA), the cholesterol level is elevated, and the plasma is clear. Turbid plasma may be observed in Types IIB, III, IV, and V. There may be a separate creamy layer of chylomicrons in Types III and V.

Sometimes, additional procedures such as ultracentrifugation or the determination of concentrations of HDL (or both) may be necessary to establish the type of lipoprotein. Electrophoresis is not usually necessary for the translation of hyperlipidemia into hyperlipoproteinemia. Frequently, the type of lipoprotein can be related to the patient's history and the clinical features of the disease.

TABLE 35–7 PLASMA HDL CHOLESTEROL (mg/dl) IN 11 FREE-LIVING NORTH AMERICAN WHITE POPULATIONS*

	Males (n = 3573)			Females (n = 3407)		
		Percentiles			Percentiles	
Age	*Mean* ± *SEM*	*10th*	*90th*	*Mean* ± *SEM*	*10th*	*90th*
5–9	55.8 ± 1.0	43	70	53.2 ± 1.0	38	67
10–14	54.9 ± 0.7	40	71	52.2 ± 0.7	40	64
15–19	46.1 ± 0.6	34	59	52.3 ± 0.7	38	68
20–24	45.4 ± 1.0	32	57	53.3 ± 1.0	37	72
25–29	44.7 ± 0.7	32	58	56.0 ± 0.8	39	74
30–34	45.5 ± 0.6	32	59	56.0 ± 0.7	40	73
35–39	43.5 ± 0.6	31	58	55.0 ± 0.8	38	75
40–44	44.2 ± 0.6	31	60	57.8 ± 0.9	39	79
45–49	45.5 ± 0.6	33	60	59.4 ± 1.0	41	82
50–54	44.1 ± 0.6	31	58	62.0 ± 1.0	41	84
55–59	47.6 ± 0.9	31	54	62.2 ± 1.1	41	85
60–64	51.5 ± 1.3	34	69	63.8 ± 1.4	44	87
65–69	51.1 ± 1.5	33	74	63.3 ± 1.8	38	85
70+	50.5 ± 1.7	33	70	60.7 ± 1.4	38	82

*From Lipid Research Clinics Population Studies Data Book. Vol. 1. The Prevalence Study. Washington, D.C., U.S. Department of Health and Human Services, Public Health Service. NIH Publ. No. 80-1527, 1980.

TABLE 35–8 TYPES OF HYPERLIPOPROTEINEMIA

	Features	Secondary Causes
Type I	Increased chylomicrons	Insulinopenic diabetes mellitus Dysglobulinemia Lupus erythematosus
Type IIA	Increased LDL	Nephrotic syndrome Hypothyroidism
Type IIB	Increased LDL and VLDL	Obstructive liver disease Porphyria Multiple myeloma
Type III	Increased IDL	Hypothyroidism Dysgammaglobulinemia
Type IV	Increased VLDL	Diabetes mellitus Nephrotic syndrome Pregnancy Hormone use Glycogen storage disease Alcoholism Gaucher disease Niemann-Pick disease
Type V	Increased chylomicrons and VLDL	Insulinopenic diabetes mellitus Nephrotic syndrome Alcoholism Myeloma Idiopathic hypercalcemia

Simple quantitative techniques can determine whether an elevated cholesterol level is due to an increased amount of LDL or to other lipoproteins. In the absence of chylomicrons, only three forms of lipoproteins are present in the plasma—VLDL, LDL, and HDL. Since VLDL is the primary triglyceride-carrying form in the fasting patient, one can approximate its concentration by dividing the amount of plasma triglyceride by 5 (based on the triglyceride/cholesterol ratio of VLDL).[75] HDL cholesterol can be measured directly with a very simple precipitation technique.[76] LDL may be calculated by using a formula based on cholesterol (C) and triglyceride (TG) values:

$$C - LDL = \text{total } C - [TG/5 + (C - HDL)].$$

A few facts must be remembered for measurement of lipid or lipoprotein levels to be most useful:

1. Reliable measurements of plasma lipids are not routinely obtained in many laboratories. Results from laboratories that employ convenience techniques, or even multiphasic automated procedures, are often imprecise and inaccurate. Many large automated laboratories are employing techniques that yield values 10 to 40 per cent higher than those obtained with the standard Abel-Kendall procedure for determining cholesterol. The particular method being used must be known, and allowance must be made for any systematic difference in accuracy that occurs in comparison with the standard procedure.

2. The concentrations of lipids and lipoproteins increase with age. A value for cholesterol that is acceptable in a person 40 to 50 years old might be alarmingly high in a 10-year-old child. Hyperlipoproteinemia of one type or another is usually somewhat arbitrarily defined in terms of the level of a lipid or lipoprotein. The diagnosis of Type II or hyperbetalipoproteinemia, for example, requires the finding of an age-adjusted level of LDL cholesterol that is greater than the 95th percentile. Hyperprebetalipoproteinemia (Type IV) requires a value for plasma triglyceride that is greater than the 95th percentile as well as the absence of chylomicrons. It must be appreciated, however, that the presence of a level of LDL cholesterol or triglyceride lower than the cut-off points used to define hyperlipoproteinemia does not indicate absence of risk. As already noted, a continuous relationship has been shown between the level of plasma (and LDL) cholesterol and the risk of occurrence of atherosclerotic events.

3. Chylomicrons normally appear in the blood 2 to 10 hours after a meal; thus, a fasting specimen (12 to 16 hours after eating) is necessary to exclude this potentially confounding influence.

4. Concentrations of lipoproteins are under dynamic metabolic control and are easily affected by diet, illness, drugs, and weight gain and loss. The level of lipoproteins in the blood changes dramatically immediately after a myocardial infarction, and these fluctuations continue about 6 weeks. The levels of plasma cholesterol and LDL may fall as much as 60 per cent in the first few days.

5. Samples should be obtained from patients in a steady state who are on a regular diet. If the results are abnormal, at least two confirmatory samples should be obtained before therapy is recommended.

6. To conclude a diagnostic work-up of hyperlipoproteinemia, possible secondary causes must be ruled out (Fig. 35–4).[51,54] Dietary excess may be a causal factor. Consumption of large quantities of eggs, butter, milk, cheese, and organ meat will increase levels of LDL. Other factors that can raise levels of lipid include hypothyroidism, nephrotic syndrome, multiple myeloma, porphyria, liver disease, and alcoholism. If these disorders are ruled out, and primary hyperlipoproteinemia is diagnosed, family screening should be performed to uncover possible genetic transmission as well as to detect others at risk for CAD.

TYPING HYPERLIPOPROTEINEMIA

As already noted, equal degrees of hypercholesterolemia and hypertriglyceridemia may result from elevation of the levels of different lipoproteins. By identifying the specific lipoprotein that is abnormal, one can assume a more rational approach to diagnosis and management. There are two equally important questions to be considered: "How much cholesterol or triglyceride is present in the plasma," and "How are these lipids distributed in the lipoproteins?"

Studies of the lipoprotein apoproteins, i.e., the protein moieties to which the lipids are bound, have helped clarify the role of lipoproteins in the transport of lipids. Quantification of the apolipoproteins is rapidly becoming a practical immunochemical technique which promises to facilitate the diagnosis of hyperlipoproteinemia and, potentially, the assessment of the risk of developing CAD.[77]

In 1967, a system for classification of the hyperlipoproteinemias was introduced. It was adopted by the WHO in 1971, with minor modifications. Two main shortcomings were soon detected in the everyday use of this system: (1) Its value in genetic analysis is limited; and (2) elaborate techniques and equipment, not readily available in every clinical laboratory, are required to define some types specifically and to distinguish between types. Nevertheless, judicious application of this typing system in the classification of patients with clearly elevated levels of plasma lipids can greatly clarify diagnosis and rationalize the therapeutic approach.

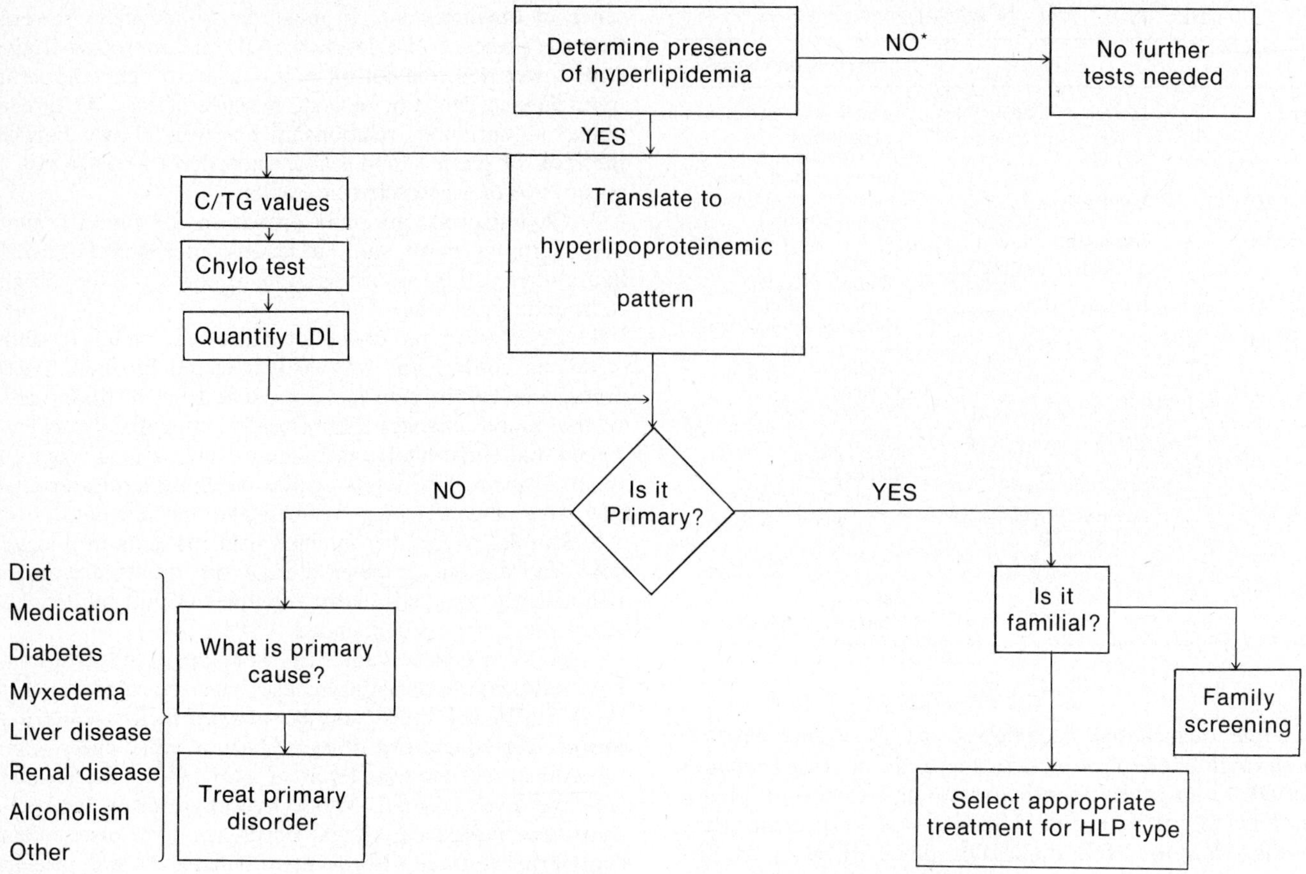

FIGURE 35–4 Schema used in diagnosis of hyperlipoproteinemia.

It should be realized that the "types" of hyperlipoproteinemia are not disease entities but are, instead, groups of disorders that affect similarly the concentrations of plasma lipids and lipoproteins and result in similar patterns of lipoproteins (see Table 35–8). Therefore, classifying a patient as being one of the hyperlipoproteinemic types is not making a clinical diagnosis per se, but rather it is defining a lipoprotein pattern that may result from different underlying disorders.

A clear distinction must be made between *primary* and *secondary* hyperlipoproteinemia in the patient who has elevated levels of plasma lipids and lipoproteins, since this distinction has important therapeutic and prognostic consequences. Treatment of secondary hyperlipoproteinemias is usually aimed at the underlying cause, and the abnormal pattern of lipoproteins resolves when the basic disorder is corrected. The prognosis for the patient with secondary hyperlipoproteinemia clearly depends on the prognosis associated with the basic disease.

Table 35–8 details some of the major causes of secondary hyperlipoproteinemias and delineates the association between the hyperlipoproteinemic patterns and these disorders. Observation of heterogeneity within the primary disorders portends a new classification system based on the specific underlying biochemical defects.

Type I.[78] Familial Type I hyperlipoproteinemia is transmitted as a recessive trait and is characterized by excess levels of chylomicrons in fasting plasma (measured 14 hours or more following a meal).[78] The excess of chylomicrons observed in Type I can also be secondary to insulinopenic diabetes, dysglobulinemia, or lupus erythematosus. The pattern results from the body's inability to clear exogenous triglyceride from the plasma. Patients with Type I have a deficient amount of the enzyme lipoprotein lipase, which originates in the adipose cell and muscle and is involved in the catabolism of circulating triglycerides. An identical clinical syndrome has been described in a family lacking apolipoprotein CII, the apoprotein catalyst involved in the intravascular hydrolysis of triglyceride by lipoprotein lipase.[79,80]

Primary Type I hyperlipoproteinemia often occurs in childhood with recurrent bouts of abdominal pain. Other clinical features include pancreatitis, eruptive xanthomas, hepatosplenomegaly, and lipemia retinalis. Despite a marked increase in the level of triglyceride and, sometimes, cholesterol, this pattern has *not* been associated with an increased risk of developing vascular disease.

Type II.[78] Type II (hyperbetalipoproteinemia) is characterized by elevated levels of LDL, either alone (Type IIA) or associated with increased VLDL (Type IIB).[78] The level of cholesterol generally ranges from 300 to 600 mg/dl. In its most common primary form, the disorder is diagnosable at birth. (Levels of LDL are elevated.) Primary Type II is often familial and is inherited most commonly as an autosomal dominant trait, so that there is a 50 per cent chance that each sibling and child of a victim will be affected. Since Type II is associated with a high risk of developing premature vascular disease, sampling of all first-degree relatives of patients found to have primary hyperbetalipoproteinemia is always indicated.[63] Hypercholesterolemia may also be secondary to dietary excess, obstructive liver disease, hypothyroidism, nephrosis, porphyria, myxedema, or multiple myeloma. Clinical features of familial Type II (familial hypercholesterolemia) sometimes include tendon xanthomas at the elbows, extensor surfaces of the hands, and the Achilles tendons; premature corneal arcus (arcus in a Caucasian younger than age 55); and xanthelasma. Tuberous xanthomas may also occur, but these are less frequent. They may develop in late adolescence or adulthood in patients with heterozygous forms of the disease. In a study of more than 1000 relatives of 116 kindred affected with primary Type II, the probability of developing fatal or nonfatal CAD by age 40 in heterozygous Type II men was 16 per cent; by age 60, the risk rose to 56 per cent (Fig. 35–5).[63] In women, the risk lagged by more than a decade but was found to increase with age. In the more severe homozygous case, xanthomas can be observed at birth or in early childhood, accompanied by pronounced elevation of LDL. CAD develops early and progresses rapidly, and patients rarely survive to adulthood.

Accumulating evidence suggests that primary hyperbetalipoproteinemia is heterogeneous and represents a multiplicity of disorders. In addition to familial hypercholesterolemia (just described), there is also familial combined hyperlipoproteinemia, in which parents and siblings may have increased levels of LDL accompanied by excesses of other lipoprotein fractions (p. 1634).

In recent years, the basic defect in familial hypercholesterolemia has been partially elucidated. Brown and Goldstein have shown that fibroblasts and lymphocytes from patients with familial hypercholesterolemia have a defective receptor-mediated uptake of LDL (p. 1629).[81] Homozygous patients are divided into three major groups, according to the type of defect in function of the receptors: (1) those with receptor-negative cells unable to bind LDL with high affinity; (2) those with receptor-defective cells that bind LDL with a strength of only about 10 per cent of normal; and (3) those with a defect in internalization (i.e., LDL is bound normally to cells but is not internalized into them). The homozygous state is characterized by a lack of functional receptors for LDL. In heterozygous patients with familial hypercholesterolemia, the values for degradation of LDL are about halfway between those of normal persons and homozygous patients with familial hypercholesterolemia. It should be noted, however, that no routine receptor assay for clinical laboratory use is yet available.

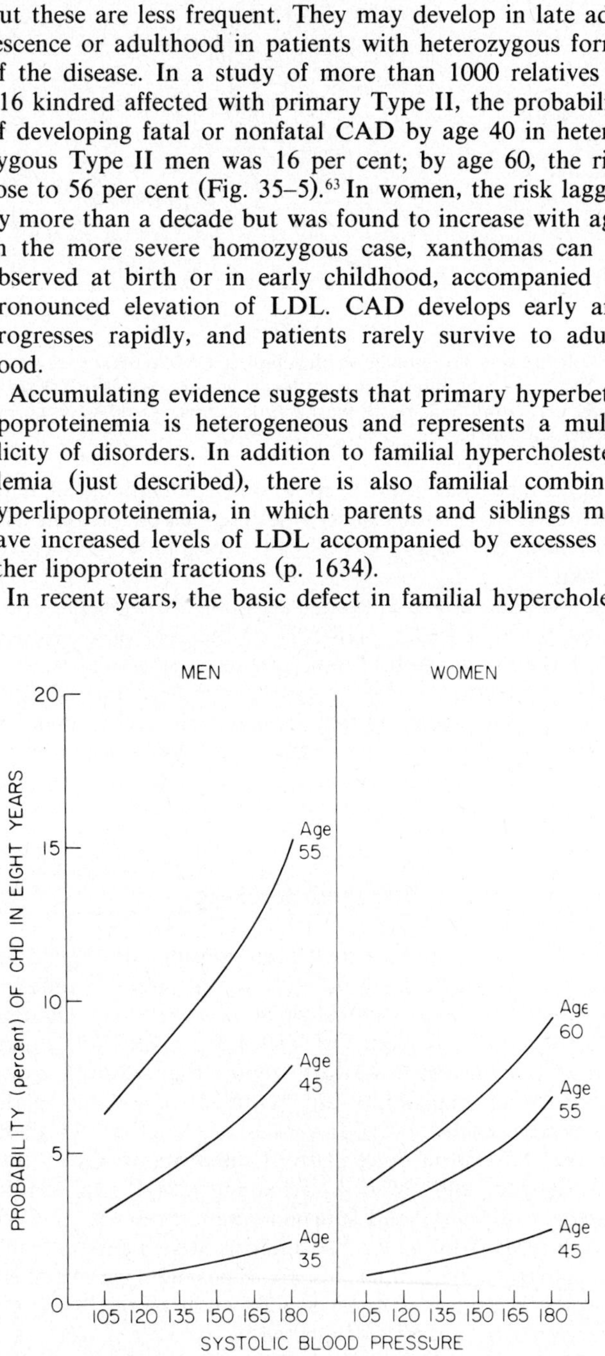

FIGURE 35–5 Cumulative probability by decade of developing fatal or nonfatal CAD. (From Stone, N. J., et al.: Coronary artery disease in 116 kindred with familial Type II hyperlipoproteinemia. Circulation *49*:482, 1974, by permission of the American Heart Association, Inc.)

Type III.[78] Like Type II, Type III is associated with an increased risk of developing premature vascular disease.[78] Patients with this disorder manifest, at a relatively young age, an increased incidence of intermittent claudication, angina pectoris, myocardial infarction, or other evidence of atherosclerosis.[54]

Type III is an uncommon disorder characterized by an increased concentration of IDL. This lipoprotein, not seen in normal fasting plasma, has flotation properties that overlap with VLDL but, on paper electrophoresis, migrates as a broad band with beta mobility. Neither of these diagnostic criteria, however, has proved specific enough when used alone for diagnosis without first ascertaining the associated clinical findings. A chemical method of diagnosis based on a detailed description of the clinical and biochemical features of Type III has been proposed.[82,83] More recently, a diagnostic assay for apolipoprotein E (one of the seven known lipoprotein apoproteins) has also been proposed, but its usefulness remains to be demonstrated.[84,85]

Clinically, primary Type III can be recognized by the discovery of unusual orange-yellow deposits in the palmar creases. Tuboeruptive xanthomas are also common. Peripheral vascular disease is as prevalent as CAD, but in men it is much more common and occurs earlier than in women.[83] Type III patients are exquisitely sensitive to caloric balance, dietary carbohydrate, estrogens, and clofibrate. Primary Type III is a fascinating disorder of lipid transport that responds readily to therapy.

Type IV.[78] The distinguishing abnormality in lipoproteins in Type IV is an increased accumulation of VLDL, always accompanied by hypertriglyceridemia. The level of cholesterol is generally normal.[78] The pattern is a very common one, but diagnosis of the familial form or forms is complicated because of the influence that diet, stress, intake of alcohol, environmental factors, and fluctuations in body weight have on levels of triglycerides.

Type IV is often associated with glucose intolerance. Obesity and hyperuricemia are often present, and eruptive xanthomas occasionally occur in patients with severely increased levels of VLDL. Familial Type IV usually does not manifest itself until adulthood and is frequently secondary to other disorders, particularly diabetes mellitus. It is also found frequently in women between the ages of 20 and 50 years who are using oral contraceptives.[86]

Although primary Type IV has been observed in a high proportion of young subjects with CAD, this has been counterbalanced by the greater prevalence of Type IV among clinically "normal" adults as well.[47,57,87,88] A further difficulty in clarifying the association between Type IV and CAD is separating the risk resulting from excess VLDL from the often concomitant risk factors of obesity, glucose intolerance, and elevated blood pressure.

Type V.[78] Type V is a mixed pattern of chylomicronemia and increased levels of VLDL.[78] Levels of triglyceride in the plasma are grossly elevated, ranging from 1000 to 6000 mg. The clinical features of the disorder are the same as in Type I, except that they do not manifest themselves until adulthood. The glucose intolerance and hyperuricemia associated with Type IV are common in Type V and are more acute. Excess intake of alcohol can also aggravate the disorder. Type V is a relatively uncommon pattern and may be secondary to insulinopenic diabetes mellitus, nephrosis, myeloma, or alcoholism.

A descriptive analysis of a population of primary Type V subjects confirmed the distinctiveness of this lipoprotein abnormality.[89] A high incidence of hyperuricemia, diabetes, pancreatitis, and xanthomatosis was found among the 32 propositi studied, but less striking excesses were found among affected relatives: Evaluation of the 32 families failed to provide any evidence of excessive CAD.

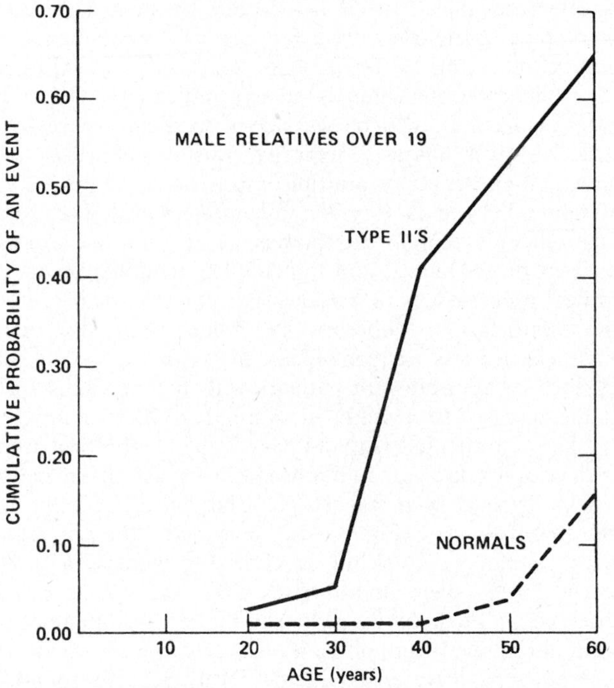

FIGURE 35–6 Probability of developing CAD within 8 years according to systolic blood pressure levels in persons with cholesterol levels measuring 235 mg/dl who are nonsmokers and have normal glucose tolerance.

Blood Pressure

(See also Chap. 26)

Elevated blood pressure, either systolic or diastolic, is predictive of an increased risk of developing CAD.[90] Both systolic and diastolic blood pressure have a continuous, unimodal distribution in the population when measured under usual office conditions. Although there is some skewing of the distribution toward high values, there is no evidence of bimodality. Thus, although the level of blood pressure appears to have a major genetic determination,[91,92] it occurs as a continuously distributed trait with no clear cut-off points to differentiate qualitatively distinct entities. Furthermore, the curve of the risk of morbidity and mortality from CAD, as well as the risk of other atherosclerotic diseases, shows a smooth, direct relationship to the levels of blood pressure over the entire range of values. As with the concentration of plasma cholesterol, there is no cut-off point at which risk suddenly changes from low to high values.

Blood pressure is often subject to marked changes, not only over the years but also within the span of a few minutes. Posture, exercise, emotional stress, ambient temperature, and a variety of other factors affect blood pressure. A major contribution of the prospective epidemiological studies was the confirmation that casual measurements of blood pressures, obtained under usual office conditions, were potent predictors of the risk of developing CAD.[90] The gradient of risk as it relates to blood pressure is illustrated in Figure 35–6. As an individual predictor, blood pressure has been found to be more reliable than the level of cholesterol or cigarette smoking. Although blood pressure normally tends to rise with age, elevated blood pressure is still a risk factor in the elderly. The common notion that elderly people tolerate hypertension better than younger ones has little basis in the epidemiological data. Furthermore, the relationship between blood pressure and the risk of developing CAD is as strong in women as it is in men.[90]

In several studies, systolic blood pressure has been found to be a better predictor of the risk of developing CAD than is diastolic blood pressure. Since the two are highly correlated in the general population, their relative merits as risk predictors may be academic. Yet it would be imprudent to dismiss isolated systolic hypertension as being a normal concomitant of aging, unrelated to the risk of developing CAD.

Tobacco Smoking

Tobacco smoking has long been considered a health hazard that is particularly harmful to the lungs. Numerous investigations have demonstrated, however, that cigarette smoking is also a major risk factor for myocardial infarction and death due to CAD.[93–98] More than 12 million person-years of experience are represented by the major prospective epidemiological studies of the effects of smoking that have been done in the United States, Great Britain, Canada, and Sweden. Total mortality, total cardiovascular mortality, and mortality and incidence of CAD were increased by about 1.6 times in male cigarette smokers compared with nonsmokers. Pipe and cigar smokers, however, were found to have only slight increases in total cardiovascular deaths and morbidity.[93]

Most prospective studies with sufficient data tend to show that the risk of developing CAD is directly related to the number of cigarettes smoked per day (Table 35–9). Furthermore, and of major importance for the prevention

TABLE 35–9 RELATIVE RISK OF CAD AND CIGARETTE SMOKING IN MEN

	Number of Cigarettes Smoked Per Day			
	None	*< 20*	*20*	*> 20*
Framingham Heart Study[5]				
Ages 45–54	1.00	1.29	1.67	2.15
55–64	1.00	1.15	1.32	1.51
65–74	1.00	1.12	1.24	1.39
Western Collaborative Group Study[9]				
Ages 39–49	1.00	1.29	1.56	1.95
50–59	1.00	1.33	1.77	2.35

of CAD, those who discontinue smoking assume a lesser risk than those who continue to smoke.[99,100] For CAD, as opposed to lung cancer and emphysema, the excess risk in ex-smokers seems to decline within a year or two of discontinuation of the habit but tends to remain slightly greater than the risk assumed by nonsmokers.[43,101] Discontinuation of the smoking habit may be followed by a slight increase in weight and uric acid levels but has no discernible effect on other CAD risk factors.[102] Although the ex-smokers in these epidemiological studies are a self-selected group, the improvement in their mortality rates is not due to differences in baseline risk factors from those in persons who continue to smoke.[103] Switching to filter cigarettes does not seem to offer any protection against the subsequent risk of CAD.[104] Unfortunately, the few randomized trials on smoking intervention that have been reported to date have not been consistent. Some failed to show any marked improvement in CAD rates among the smokers who have stopped, whereas the Multiple Risk Factor Intervention Trial showed that high-risk men who discontinue this habit had a marked reduction in mortality.[105,106,106a]

A few other questions have arisen about the consistency of the data relating cigarette smoking to the development of CAD. There is some indication from the Framingham Study that the harmful effects of cigarettes may diminish as one gets older (see Table 35–9).[100,101] However, other studies, such as the Western Collaborative Group Study, show no decrease in the effect of smoking with age.[107]

The relationship of cigarette smoking to development of CAD among women is somewhat more complex. In relation to myocardial infarction, women show about the same gradient of risk correlated with the amount of smoking as do men.[108,109] Because of the smaller number of cases available for study, however, these gradients do not usually achieve the high level of statistical significance that they do for men. The effects in women are further obscured by the inconsistent relationship found between cigarette smoking and the occurrence of angina pectoris.[101,107,110,111] Since the most frequent manifestation of CAD in women is angina, the total rates of occurrence of CAD in women fail to show a relationship to cigarette smoking.[108]

Nevertheless, the overwhelming evidence supports a strong and definite relationship between cigarette smoking and CAD. A variety of mechanisms have been suggested for the adverse effects of cigarette smoking on the heart and blood vessels. The results of each of the hypothesized mechanisms could also be reversed upon discontinuation of the smoking habit. Among these mechanisms is the effect of nicotine and carbon monoxide upon the heart, the coronary arteries, and the blood. Specific changes include increased myocardial demand for oxygen, induced by nicotine; interference with oxygen supply by carboxyhemoglobin; increased adhesiveness of platelets; and lowering of the threshold for ventricular fibrillation. Cigarette smoking has also been found to be associated with decreased levels of HDL cholesterol, compared with those in nonsmokers and ex-smokers.[68,112]

Abnormal Glucose Tolerance

Clinically overt diabetes mellitus has long been recognized as a precursor of vascular disease, and this association has been confirmed in prospective epidemiological studies.[113–118] These studies have also shown that hyperglycemia and glucose intolerance, as measured from levels of blood sugar obtained 1 hour after administration of a standardized oral glucose load, or even as indicated by high casually measured levels of blood sugar, are associated with increased risk of developing CAD.[116–118] Men with glucose intolerance have about a 50 per cent greater chance of developing CAD than men with no evidence of glucose intolerance, whereas in women the risk is more than doubled—virtually eliminating the differential in rates of CAD between men and women.[59,108] Although early-onset diabetes appears to be primarily involved in mortality from renal disease, adult-onset diabetes is associated with death from CAD.[119] In adults, both insulin-dependent and non–insulin-dependent diabetics appear to be at increased risk for development of CAD.[116,118,120]

In the Coronary Drug Project, in which the effects of several lipid-lowering agents on mortality and coronary conditions in men who had previously suffered a myocardial infarction were studied, the prognostic importance of the level of plasma glucose was examined.[121] It was found that a high fasting level of glucose is a significant predictor of subsequent risk of myocardial infarction even after adjustment for many other risk factors and concomitant variables is made.

The mechanism associating hyperglycemia and increased risk of CAD is obscure, although several aspects have been investigated.[113] Hyperlipidemia, particularly hypertriglyceridemia, is often linked with diabetes.[122] Both hyperlipidemia and hyperglycemia tend to be associated with obesity and thereby indirectly with hypertension. A variety of interrelationships between glucose intolerance and levels of insulin have been observed, which may suggest several mechanisms related to the initiation or promotion of atherosclerosis. They involve the real or potential effects of insulin or glucose or both on the synthesis and/or catabolism of cellular and extracellular elements in the arterial wall. Still other associations have been noted between hyperglycemia and the increased adhesiveness of platelets and other abnormalities of coagulation. Thus, several complex mechanisms may be involved, separately or in concert.

The relationship between the methods for control of hyperglycemia and the risk of developing CAD is exceedingly confused and controversial at the present time. The University Group Diabetes Program has investigated the effects of several oral hypoglycemic agents and of two regimens of insulin usage on the vascular complications in patients with adult-onset diabetes.[123,124] When compared with the placebo group, no significant benefits were found for any of the treatment modalities. There has been considerable controversy over these results, but it would appear that no current regimen used to control hyperglycemia has an appreciable effect on the atherosclerotic complications of diabetes.[113,125]

Other Risk Factors

GOUT. Gouty arthritis has been associated with a doubling of the risk of developing CAD.[126] There also appears to be a moderate association between CAD and level of uric acid in the absence of clinical gout.[127] However, elevated levels of uric acid tend also to be associated with higher levels of blood pressure, elevated levels of serum cholesterol and triglyceride, and obesity.[128] These may reflect interrelated metabolic processes.

MENOPAUSE AND ORAL CONTRACEPTIVES. The marked difference in risk between women and men has already been noted. Undoubtedly, part of this difference can be attributed to hormonal factors, but the relationship of the risk of developing CAD to specific hormones has not yet been established. Among women, however, both the menopause and the use of oral contraceptive agents appear to be related to an increased risk of developing CAD. Women in their 40's and 50's who have undergone menopause have been found to have three times the incidence of CAD as do women of these ages who are still menstruating.[129] Although menopause is associated with changes in other risk factors as well, these do not account entirely for the increased risk of developing CAD.

The use of oral contraceptive drugs has recently been suspected of having a marked influence on the occurrence of CAD in premenopausal women.[130–133] The risk of myocardial infarction in young women using oral contraceptives who already have associated adverse risk factors, particularly hypertension and diabetes, is greatly enhanced. In some studies, women who smoked cigarettes and who also used oral contraceptives were at extremely high risk, pointing to a strong interaction between the effects of both these hazards.[134] Oral contraceptives also tend to produce an increase in blood pressure (p. 873) and an alteration of serum levels of lipoproteins[135] as well as disturbances in clotting and enhancement of thromboembolic changes. Oral contraceptives containing high doses of progestin tend to lower levels of HDL cholesterol, whereas those containing high doses of estrogen tend to raise levels of HDL.[69]

The effect of estrogens on the risk of developing CAD is a somewhat controversial issue. In postmenopausal women, exogenous estrogens had no discernible effect on the risk of developing CAD in most studies[136–138] but did lower risk in some.[139] Stilbestrol used in men for the treatment of prostatic cancer, conjugated equine estrogens given to men in the Coronary Drug Project to lower levels of serum cholesterol, and noncontraceptive estrogens used by young women, however, all tended to *increase* the risk of developing CAD.[140–143]

VASECTOMY. Recent experimental work in two species of monkeys found that arteries of vasectomized animals developed more severe atherosclerotic plaques than did the vessels of control animals.[144] This effect seemed to be independent of plasma lipid levels, and it was postulated that the mechanism responsible involved endothelial damage from circulatory antibodies to sperm antigens. Studies of vasectomized men, however, have failed to show any increased risk of CAD in these men compared with nonvasectomized men matched for a variety of risk factors.[145,145a] Neither is there any consistent evidence at present for a significant excess of sex hormone concentrations in men with CAD.[146]

OBESITY. Although obesity has long been known to predispose to CAD,[147] its *independent effect* has been questioned,[148,149] since several studies have shown that the relationship of CAD to obesity is virtually entirely accounted for by the relationship of obesity to other risk factors.[59,150] However, when populations are followed for many years, obesity has been found to be a risk factor for CAD independent of its association with other risk factors.[151,151a]

There has been little agreement regarding how to define or measure obesity in epidemiological studies.[149] Measurement of body fat requires elaborate techniques (e.g., total body immersion to estimate body density) and is not adaptable to population studies.[152] Measurement of the thickness of the subcutaneous fat at several body sites has been recommended but has not been employed uniformly. Thus, measurements of overweight rather than of obesity or fatness have generally been employed. Whatever criterion for overweight is used, it tends to confound weight due to muscular development (e.g., as found in football players) with that due to fat accumulation. Two general criteria of overweight have been used: (1) relative weight, as determined by distribution of weight according to height, such as the Metropolitan Life Insurance Company standards or the Framingham Relative Weight based on median weight for each inch of height[153]; and (2) indices derived from the mathematical relationship between height and weight.[154] Of the latter, the body mass index (weight divided by the square of height) has been found to be most useful as a measure of relative obesity.

Overweight has been found in many studies to be highly associated with hypertension, glucose intolerance, and adverse lipid profiles.[56] Furthermore, in both metabolic ward and epidemiological studies, a direct cause-and-effect relationship has been found between change in weight and an alteration of these risk factors.[68,155,156] Therefore, it should not be surprising that when obesity is considered in combination with these traits as a predictor of the incidence of CAD, its effects as an independent contributor are overshadowed by the possibly more direct influence of the other risk factors,[59,150] and its independent contribution to CAD risk requires many years of follow-up to detect.[151] Nevertheless, although the association between obesity and the risk of developing CAD may operate through the effects of obesity on other characteristics, the role of obesity as a risk variable should not be denigrated. Furthermore, recent studies have found that obesity may indeed be an independent contributor in populations with low levels of other risk factors, e.g., Japanese men in Hawaii, and in younger individuals.[157,158]

PHYSICAL ACTIVITY. The evidence of a beneficial effect of physical activity on the development of CAD is gradually accumulating, although controversial aspects still exist.[159–167,167a] Despite the problems inherent in self-selection of physically active jobs and leisure activities, documentation of quantitative levels of physical activity, and adjustment for variations of other risk factors, the bulk of evidence supports the hypothesis that regular physical exercise may have a protective effect on developing CAD. However, there is little agreement regarding whether moderate amounts of exercise will suffice (threshold model) or whether more strenuous and prolonged exercise is needed to obtain any benefit. There is also no agreement about whether exercise improves myocardial function and coronary circulation directly or whether its protective effect acts through the alteration of other risk factors.[168–171]

TYPE OF PERSONALITY BEHAVIOR (See also p. 1826). In the late 1950's, Friedman and Rosenman put forward the concept of a behavior pattern which they called Type A and which they believed was related to the occurrence of CAD.[9,172] In the past 20 years, many investigators have confirmed in varying degrees the existence of a "coronary-prone behavior pattern."[173–175] Rosenman has described the Type A behavior pattern as follows.[176]

> We conceive of the Type A behavior pattern as being a particular action-emotion complex that is possessed and exhibited by an individual who is engaged in a relatively chronic and excessive struggle to obtain an unlimited number of things from the environment in the shortest period of time and/or against the opposing efforts of other persons or things in the same environment. This chronic struggle might consist of attempts to achieve or to do more and more in less and less time or other conflicts with one or more persons. Since the Type A subject rarely despairs of losing the chronic struggle, such individuals sharply differ from those with fear or anxiety or other simple neurotic states. Type A's exhibit enhanced personality traits of aggressiveness, ambitiousness and competitiveness. They are often preoccupied with deadlines and are work-oriented. In this interplay, Type A's exhibit chronic impatience and usually a strong sense of time urgency. The converse Type B individual is mainly free of such enhanced personality traits and generally feels no pressing conflict with either time or other persons and is therefore free of any habitual sense of time urgency.
>
> The 20th century environment that is associated with the CHD incidence has generally encouraged Type A behavior because it appears to offer special rewards to those who can perform rapidly and aggressively. Moreover, with increasing urbanization and technological progress as well as increasing population density, our civilization presents unique new challenges never experienced by earlier and less time-conscious generations. Type A behavior does not stem solely from individual personality but emerges when certain challenges or conditions of the milieu arise to elicit this complex of responses in susceptible individuals.[176]

The Western Collaborative Group Study, after 8.5 years of follow-up of 3154 men who had been characterized as having the Type A pattern of behavior, found that Type A men had twice the risk of developing CAD as did Type B men.[9] Similar risks have recently been found for Type A women.[174,177] Personality type appears to act independently of such risk factors as high blood pressure, smoking, and high cholesterol levels.[178] The severity of atherosclerotic involvement of coronary vessels observed angiographically is positively associated with Type A behavior.[178]

Other Psychological and Social Risk Factors. Jenkins has presented comprehensive reviews of the evidence supporting psychological and social risk factors for coronary disease.[180] For some factors, the evidence is highly suggestive, whereas for others the evidence is weak or inconsistent. Sociological indices such as socioeconomic status, occupation, religious affiliation, education, and marital status have been widely studied, but conflicting results have been obtained. Social mobility and incongruity of status (defined as the simultaneous possession of the identifying markings of different social classes) have been suspected to be related to the incidence of CAD. Recent studies, however, have tended to add to the confusion rather than to clarify matters. It would seem that these sociological concepts are more complex than they first appeared, at least with respect to their association with CAD.

A family of symptoms and behavior referred to as "anxiety" and "neuroticism" is, according to a variety of studies, related to CAD.[180] Studies comparing patients having CAD with patients suffering from other diseases failed to discriminate whether the anxiety preceded the CAD or resulted from it. Yet many of these studies, and the few with prospective data, tend to show that anxiety, depression, irritability, and sleeplessness—which may reflect "emotional drain"—are related to CAD.

Problems, dissatisfaction, and stress associated with life changes have been difficult to study. The available evidence is not consistent, although some of the reported relationships are provocative. For example, social support systems seem to protect the individual from the health hazards associated with stressful life situations, a fact that gives hope of developing more effective coping behavior for dealing with life's stresses.[32] The possible adverse effects of retirement and stressful job situations upon risk of CAD have recently been highlighted.[181,182] Much more research is needed in this area.

FAMILY HISTORY. Familial and genetic factors may play an important role in the determination of some major risk factors—in particular, hypertension, glucose intolerance, and levels of lipoprotein.[183] It is also clear that some risk factors have their onset in childhood.[184] It appears that there may be a familial or genetic predisposition toward CAD per se that is independent of the other known risk factors.[185,185a]

DIETARY CHOLESTEROL AND SATURATED FAT. Striking correlations have been found between average intake of fat and average levels of serum cholesterol in epidemiological studies comparing Western and non-Western populations. In the Seven Countries Study, the relationship of diet to the level of serum cholesterol was studied in men between the ages of 40 and 59.[10,186] A direct correlation was found between the intake of saturated fat, on the one hand, and the incidence of CAD and hypercholesterolemia, on the other. The populations of Greece and Yugoslavia derive an average of 30 per cent of total calories from fat, compared with 40 per cent in the American diet. These differences in fat intake were interpreted as being major factors in the three- to fivefold difference between these countries in the incidence of CAD. Another study that reported direct correlations between intake of fat and levels of serum cholesterol compared Japanese men living in Japan with those in Hawaii and California.[187] The mean percentage of calories derived from fat ranged from 15 per cent in Japan to 36.7 per cent in California. Serum cholesterol levels were lowest in Japan (180 mg/dl), higher in Hawaii (218 mg/dl), and highest in California (225 mg/dl). Data from studies of Seventh-Day Adventists show that those adhering to a vegetarian diet have one-third the mortality rate from CAD of nonvegetarians, but whether or not this difference is mediated through differences in serum lipid levels is not yet clear.[188]

It is interesting that a clear correlation is lacking when individuals *within* populations are studied. In Framingham, no correlation was found between individual diets, levels of serum cholesterol measured concomitantly, and subsequent risk of developing CAD.[189] An analysis of the association between daily dietary intake and levels of serum lipids in the Tecumseh population did not exclude the existence of a relationship between dietary cholesterol and the amount of serum cholesterol, although obesity was found to be more highly correlated with lipid levels than were specific dietary factors.[190] In contrast, the 20-year follow-up report of the Western Electric Study has revealed highly correlated results between diet score (intake of dietary cholesterol, saturated fat, and polyunsaturated fatty acids) and serum cholesterol levels, and between change in diet score and change in serum cholesterol levels and has demonstrated a positive prospective association between mean baseline diet score and 19-year risk of death from CAD.[191] Forthcoming data from the Lipid Research Clinics (LRC) prevalence studies should clarify further the association between individual dietary habits and levels of plasma cholesterol. A preliminary report from the LRC program indicates a significant fall (5 to 10 per cent) in the level of cholesterol in the U.S. population in the last decade.[192] This finding is consistent with U.S. Department of Agriculture reports of declining consumption of butter and other animal fats and oils and the increased use of vegetable oils.

The evidence from other types of studies is also illuminating. Numerous metabolic ward investigations involving controlled dietary manipulation show a strong and direct correlation between dietary and serum lipids. Mean levels of serum cholesterol responded predictably to the intake of saturated and polyunsaturated fat and dietary cholesterol.[193–195] Innumerable animal studies performed over the past 60 years provide further evidence that cholesterol-feeding diets raise levels of serum cholesterol, leading to atherosclerosis. The disease will regress following termination of the diet, however.[196]

Concentrations of LDL are directly related to the ingestion of dietary saturated fats and cholesterol, whereas polyunsaturated fats have been shown to depress levels of LDL.

Carbohydrate Consumption. A change in the American diet consisting of the consumption of large amounts of sucrose and glucose and smaller amounts of fiber and more purified foods has been incriminated as a causal factor in the development of CAD, hyperlipidemia, obesity, and diabetes mellitus. The evidence from a number of sources suggests an association but does not yet prove causality.

The average per capita consumption of sugar in the U.S. is 50 kg per year. Epidemiological correlations suggest that this factor may be involved in the mortality rates for CAD, but there is no conclusive proof, and opinions are divided.[197] Evidence from animal studies does not suggest a correlation between the consumption of dietary sucrose or carbohydrates and the development of atherosclerosis.

Studies involving feeding of carbohydrates generally show that a short-term increase in the consumption of dietary carbohydrates provokes a marked rise in the level of plasma triglycerides.[198,199] This induction of hypertriglyceridemia has been shown to be transitory, however; in general, its effects on serum lipids are confusing, owing in part to inadequate experimental designs.

Moreover, there are divergent views regarding which type of carbohydrate is the most hypertriglyceridemic. Studies also show that most population groups with a low incidence of CAD derive 65 to 85 per cent of their total energy from whole grain and potatoes. Current studies of the effects of fiber on the metabolism of lipids show clear indications of changes in the absorption of carbohydrate and lipid.[200,201] At the present time, the evidence is far from conclusive, and further work is needed to separate fact from hypothesis.

Salt Intake. (See also Chap. 26) Studies have shown that diets high in sodium can produce hypertension in genetically predisposed animals. The role of sodium in the etiology of hypertension in humans, however, has not been established. Some epidemiological studies have suggested a strong association between sodium and the prevalence of hypertension, but other factors such as intake of potassium, body weight, and physical activity complicate the assessment of this association.[202,203]

In the treatment of hypertension, restriction of sodium is beneficial for some patients, but a recent study has shown that weight reduction may be more important.[204] Although it is unknown whether or not limiting the intake of salt will prevent hypertension, it would be prudent to recommend restraint in the consumption of sodium. Specifically, this would include avoiding overly salted prepared foods, refraining from adding salt to cooked foods, reducing the amount of sodium added to baby foods, and cooking with small amounts of salt.

Alcohol Consumption. The evidence relating daily consumption of alcohol to the development of CAD is conflicting. A number of recent studies report negative associations and suggest a possible preventive result from moderate daily intake of alcohol.[205–209] Other investigators have found either a positive association or no apparent overall association.[210–212]

The effect of the consumption of alcohol on lipid transport is well known, but the emphasis of earlier studies was principally on its effect on triglycerides. The Cooperative Lipoprotein Phenotyping Study and the LRC Prevalence Study have reported significant positive associations between alcohol intake and HDL cholesterol levels.[213,214] Alcohol intake has also been reported to be positively associated with blood pressure.[207,209]

Coffee Ingestion. Although large doses of caffeine have been associated with distinct cardiovascular changes (tachycardia, arrhythmias, and extrasystoles), there is no definitive proof that the ingestion of coffee increases the risk of cardiovascular disease. Evidence from both case control and prospective studies is conflicting.[215–217] Although the data on caffeine as an independent risk factor for CAD are mixed, they do suggest that coffee plays a role in association with other existing factors, such as hypertension.

Trace Metals. Ecologic studies comparing different regions or communities have demonstrated an inverse relationship between the hardness of drinking water and local cardiovascular mortality rates.[23,218] ("The harder the water, the softer the arteries.") Hardness of water is not a specific chemical element but is a complex characteristic measured by titration with a chelating agent. Efforts to identify specific chemical components that are related to mortality from CAD have produced conflicting results. Protective effects have been attributed to magnesium, chromium, selenium, and zinc, whereas harmful effects have been suspected for cadmium, manganese, and lead. At the present time, it cannot be recommended that the hardness or trace metal content of drinking water be altered in an effort to decrease the incidence of CAD.

Miscellaneous Risk Factors. A variety of other factors have been suspected as being related to the occurrence of CAD, and some have received corroboration from one or two studies. Vital capacity was found to have an inverse relation to CAD in the Framingham Study.[108] Blood groups have been investigated in several populations.[219,220] There have been some consistent findings that Type O individuals are at lesser risk than those with Type A blood. Although coagulation factors play a role in the formation of thrombi and in the atherosclerotic process, there is scant evidence linking clotting abnormalities to the risk of developing CAD, other than the previously mentioned association between CAD and contraceptive pills.[221] It has been speculated that increased blood viscosity may play a role in the development of thrombotic processes and may exacerbate the potential for development of ischemia.[222] This might explain the associations reported between elevated hematocrit and risk of CAD.[223] Increased severity of atherosclerosis in patients with nephrotic syndrome or in those undergoing long-term dialysis has not been consistently found.[224–227]

The role of immunological factors is obscure. There has been some discussion that autoimmune thyroiditis may be a risk factor.[228] On the other hand, patients with rheumatoid arthritis tend to have a lower incidence of CAD, which has been attributed by some to aspirin therapy and its inhibition of the aggregation of platelets.[229] Another uncommon but apparently strong risk factor is post–radiation treatment for mediastinal tumors.[230] Another factor about which there is some speculation is ear-lobe creases.[231]

Environmental Factors. Evidence regarding the impact of environmental factors on cardiovascular disease is inconclusive.[232] Water softness, trace metals, carbon monoxide, noise exposure, and physical and psychosocial stress have been associated with cardiovascular effects, but the available data are inadequate and inconsistent.

Only in the case of two industrial chemicals, carbon disulfide and aliphatic nitrates, has the association been established. Studies of the effects of cold snaps and snowstorms on the incidence of ischemic heart disease have failed to show any association in relation to either age or preexisting heart disease.[233,234] In most studies of external environmental effects, it has proved difficult to separate these risk factors from other concomitant conditions that vary from place to place.

Undoubtedly, other risk factors exist. Several studies comparing the incidence of heart disease in different groups have shown that the currently known risk factors cannot explain all the differences that have been found. For example, the male-female differences are not accounted for. Differences between Japanese and Puerto Rican men compared with Caucasian men cannot be attributed to variations in smoking, blood pressure, or levels of cholesterol.[20] Thus, the search for additional risk factors or for new relationships among existing ones must continue.

Multivariate Risk Functions For CAD

The preceding discussion clearly indicates that many attributes of individuals are related to their risk of developing CAD. It has also been stated that most risk factors make independent contributions to the prediction of the risk; i.e., they supply additional information beyond that provided by a knowledge of the other risk factors possessed by the individual. In order to describe the cumulative effect of numerous factors acting simultaneously and in order to assess the relative contribution of each factor, statisticians have explored several multivariate methods of describing these relationships. An initial approach was to divide each risk factor into two or three levels (e.g., hypertensive-normotensive) and to subclassify the study population into several subgroups on the basis of the combined levels of three or four risk factors. Although this method is feasible when only a few risk factors are involved—and is a desirable method for studying specific interactions—it is readily apparent that as the number of subgroups increases geometrically, the number of observations in any one subgroup can become quite small.

Other approaches included discriminant function analysis and multiple regression techniques. A linear multiple regression function for predicting the risk of disease (P = probability of developing disease in a stated period of time) from a knowledge of the levels of several risk factors ($X_1, X_2, \ldots, X_k$) takes the following form:

$$P = \beta_0 + \beta_1 X_1 + \beta_2 X_2 + \ldots + \beta_k X_k$$

where the betas are appropriate coefficients to be estimated from the data set. This states that risk is a weighted sum of the values of the individual risk factors. Two deficiencies of this model soon became apparent. (1) For some individuals, the estimated value of P could be negative, and for others it could be greater than 1. (Since P is an estimate of probability, it should always lie between 0 and 1.) (2) A linear relationship did not adequately describe the curvilinear relationship that existed for some of the risk factors.

An improved model was developed in which the logarithm of the odds of developing disease (log $P/1 - P$) was used as the dependent variable. This has been called the "multiple logistical model." An example is given in Figure 35–2, with six curves defined by sex and three specified levels (designated high, low, and average) for each of four risk factors. The six curves then allow for the independent effect of variation in age. The curvilinear estimates of risk are apparent, and these must lie between 0 and 1.

Another explicit numerical example of the multivariate approach to risk is given in Table 35–10. This shows the probability of developing CAD in 8 years for both 45-year-old men and 65-year-old men according to five other risk factors: systolic blood pressure, total serum cholesterol, cigarette smoking, evidence of glucose intolerance, and electrocardiographic evidence of left ventricular hypertrophy. Similar tables for men of other ages and for women have also been published.[37,235] Approximate estimates for these groups can be obtained from Table 35–10 by interpolating between the ages shown, or, for women, by using estimates for men 10 years younger. These tables emphasize that the risk of developing CAD is a continuous graded function of the level of the risk factors of blood pressure and cholesterol. This probably also applies to the other risk factors, but we do not have appropriate scales or sufficient data for glucose intolerance and left ventricular hypertrophy (on the electrocardiogram). These gradients of risk hold for other populations, although the absolute levels may differ.[38–40] This latter point suggests that other risk factors which are not included in the tables also contribute to the likelihood of developing disease. One factor that has recently been introduced into the quantitative risk model is the Type A pattern of behavior.[9] One would increase the probabilities shown in Table 35–10 by 20 per cent for a Type A individual and decrease them by 20 per cent for a Type B person.

Two other observations should be made about the use of these tables. Although these estimates have been confirmed in studies of other groups, new functions will have to be estimated as new or additional risk factors are introduced to allow for a possible overlap of effects or for interactions. Thus, for example, use of data on levels of specific lipoproteins may modify or even eliminate the importance of total cholesterol in the risk function.[66] In addition, data on certain risk factors in the model produce similar information. For example, knowledge of diastolic blood pressure does not enhance the ability of a model to predict the occurrence of disease if systolic blood pressure is already contained in the equation. Likewise, indices of obesity do not seem to make any significant contribution to the model, presumably because the effects of obesity operate through its associations with the other included risk factors.

Thus, the multivariate risk function is a useful concept for quantifying the combined effect of a group of interrelated risk factors. It emphasizes that risk must be assessed as a multifactorial phenomenon with a continuous gradient of response. With currently available data, it is possible to identify, for each age group, the 10 per cent at greatest risk (among whom a quarter to a third of all new cases of CAD will occur). This provides relatively powerful predictive ability for use in screening programs and for advising individual patients.

MANAGEMENT OF RISK FACTORS

Having identified the patient who is at relatively high risk of developing CAD because of the presence of adverse risk factors, the physician must consider possible approaches to the management of these risk factors. There is no doubt that many can be changed, but the question of whether modification of these risk factors will reduce the

TABLE 35–10 PROBABILITY OF DEVELOPING CORONARY ARTERY DISEASE IN 8 YEARS*

45-YEAR-OLD MAN†

LVH—ECG Negative

		Does Not Smoke Cigarettes							*Smokes Cigarettes*					
	CHOL	*SBP 105*	*120*	*135*	*150*	*165*	*180*	CHOL	*SBP 105*	*120*	*135*	*150*	*165*	*180*
Glucose intolerance absent	185	20	24	29	35	42	51	185	32	39	46	56	67	81
	210	25	30	36	44	53	64	210	40	48	58	69	83	99
	235	31	38	45	55	66	79	235	50	60	72	86	103	122
	260	39	47	56	68	81	97	260	62	74	89	106	126	149
	285	48	58	70	84	100	119	285	76	92	109	130	153	181
	310	60	72	87	104	123	146	310	94	113	134	158	186	217
	CHOL	*SBP 105*	*120*	*135*	*150*	*165*	*180*	CHOL	*SBP 105*	*120*	*135*	*150*	*165*	*180*
Glucose intolerance present	185	25	30	36	44	53	64	185	40	48	58	69	83	99
	210	31	38	45	55	66	79	210	50	60	72	86	102	122
	235	39	47	56	68	81	97	235	62	74	89	106	126	149
	260	48	58	70	84	100	119	260	76	91	109	130	153	181
	285	60	72	87	103	123	146	285	94	112	134	158	186	217
	310	75	89	107	127	150	177	310	116	138	163	191	223	259

LVH—ECG Positive

		Does Not Smoke Cigarettes							*Smokes Cigarettes*					
	CHOL	*SBP 105*	*120*	*135*	*150*	*165*	*180*	CHOL	*SBP 105*	*120*	*135*	*150*	*165*	*180*
Glucose intolerance absent	185	41	50	60	72	86	102	185	65	78	93	111	132	157
	210	51	62	74	89	106	126	210	81	96	115	136	161	189
	235	64	76	91	109	130	153	235	100	118	141	166	195	227
	260	79	94	112	134	158	186	260	122	145	171	200	234	270
	285	97	116	138	163	191	223	285	149	176	206	240	277	318
	310	120	142	167	196	229	266	310	181	212	246	284	326	370
	CHOL	*SBP 105*	*120*	*135*	*150*	*165*	*180*	CHOL	*SBP 105*	*120*	*135*	*150*	*165*	*180*
Glucose intolerance present	185	51	62	74	88	105	126	185	81	96	115	136	161	189
	210	64	76	91	109	129	153	210	99	118	140	166	195	227
	235	79	94	112	133	158	186	235	122	145	171	200	233	270
	260	97	116	137	162	191	223	260	149	176	206	240	277	318
	285	119	142	167	196	229	265	285	181	211	246	284	325	370
	310	146	172	202	235	272	313	310	217	252	291	333	378	425

*Sixteen-year follow-up of the Framingham Study. Probability is shown in thousandths.

†Men aged 45 years have an average systolic blood pressure of 131 mm Hg and an average serum cholesterol of 235 mg/dl. Sixty-seven per cent smoke cigarettes, 1.3 per cent have definite LVH according to electrocardiographic findings, and 3.8 per cent have glucose intolerance. At these average values, the probability of developing coronary heart disease in 8 years is 60/1000.

Table continues on opposite page.

incidence of CAD is still under a great deal of scientific investigation. The evidence is strongest that curtailment of cigarette smoking is associated with a fairly rapid decline in the incidence of heart attacks, to levels approaching those associated with people who have never smoked.[83,95–106] There is fairly strong evidence that effective treatment of moderate and high degrees of hypertension will result in lower mortality, particularly from strokes and congestive heart failure. Recently, the efficacy of treating even mild hypertension has been demonstrated, suggesting benefit for both cerebrovascular disease and CAD.[236,237] There is still less certitude about the effects of modifying adverse levels of cholesterol, and this, too, is under intense study.[106,238] The management strategies recommended in the next section are based on recent assessments by several panels of experts of the available evidence and of current theories on the pathogenesis of atherosclerosis. As the results of the ongoing studies of interventions accumulate, more specific strategies may be developed.

In the management of the high-risk patient, the active participation of the patient and his family may be even more important than the role of the physician. It is well recognized that changing established life styles is difficult, but new techniques have appeared to guide the physician in helping the patient to help himself.[239] The physician should not hesitate to call on trained professionals and paraprofessionals who are knowledgeable about the techniques of behavior modification used for health maintenance. This may be particularly important in the management of obesity and the cigarette habit, as described further on.

Adverse risk factors may be managed with respect to the natural history of the disease process. Three phases may be defined: (1) efforts to prevent the occurrence of adverse risk factors; (2) management of established adverse risk factors before the occurrence of clinically manifest CAD; and (3) management of risk factors after CAD develops. Phase 1, the primary prevention of adverse risk factors, generally must start early in life, preferably in childhood, if it is to be effective in preventing or delaying the atherosclerotic process. Phase 3 is usually referred to as secondary prevention of subsequent coronary events. In secondary prevention the patient has already developed CAD, and the risk factors just described play a smaller role in determining the patient's progress than they do before the occurrence of manifest disease. In the Coronary Drug Project, an analysis of the factors influencing prognosis after recovery from myocardial infarction indicates that the major determinants of long-term survival are the state of the myocardium and its functional ability.[240] The traditional risk factors, particularly the level of serum cholesterol, did demonstrate some predictive ability in this

TABLE 35–10 PROBABILITY OF DEVELOPING CORONARY ARTERY DISEASE IN 8 YEARS* Continued

65-Year-old Man**														
	Does Not Smoke Cigarettes							*Smokes Cigarettes*						
	LVH—ECG Negative													
	CHOL	*SBP 105*	*120*	*135*	*150*	*165*	*180*	CHOL	*SBP 105*	*120*	*135*	*150*	*165*	*180*
Glucose intolerance absent	185	67	80	96	115	136	151	185	105	124	147	174	204	237
	210	69	83	99	118	140	165	210	107	128	151	178	209	243
	235	71	85	102	121	143	169	235	111	131	155	183	214	249
	260	73	88	104	124	147	174	260	114	135	159	187	219	254
	285	75	90	107	128	151	178	285	117	139	164	192	224	260
	310	77	93	110	131	155	183	310	120	142	168	197	230	266
	CHOL	*SBP 105*	*120*	*135*	*150*	*165*	*180*	CHOL	*SBP 105*	*120*	*135*	*150*	*165*	*180*
Glucose intolerance present	185	83	99	118	140	165	194	185	128	152	179	209	243	281
	210	85	102	121	144	169	199	210	132	156	183	214	249	287
	235	88	105	125	148	174	204	235	135	160	188	220	255	294
	260	90	108	128	151	178	209	260	139	164	193	225	261	300
	285	93	111	131	155	183	214	285	143	168	197	230	267	307
	310	95	114	135	160	188	219	310	146	173	202	236	273	314
	LVH—ECG Positive													
	CHOL	*SBP 105*	*120*	*135*	*150*	*165*	*180*	CHOL	*SBP 105*	*120*	*135*	*150*	*165*	*180*
Glucose intolerance absent	185	132	156	184	215	250	288	185	198	231	268	308	351	397
	210	136	160	188	220	256	295	210	203	237	274	314	358	404
	235	139	164	193	226	262	301	235	208	242	280	321	365	412
	260	143	169	198	231	268	308	260	213	248	286	328	373	419
	285	147	173	203	237	274	314	285	219	254	293	335	380	427
	310	151	178	208	242	280	321	310	224	260	299	342	387	435
	CHOL	*SBP 105*	*120*	*135*	*150*	*165*	*180*	CHOL	*SBP 105*	*120*	*135*	*150*	*165*	*180*
Glucose intolerance present	185	161	189	221	256	295	337	185	237	274	315	359	405	453
	210	165	193	226	262	302	344	210	243	281	322	366	412	461
	235	169	198	231	268	308	351	235	248	287	329	373	420	468
	260	173	203	237	274	315	359	260	254	293	335	380	428	476
	285	178	208	243	280	322	366	285	260	300	342	388	435	484
	310	183	214	248	287	328	373	310	266	306	349	395	443	491

**Men aged 65 years have an average systolic blood pressure of 143 mm Hg and an average serum cholesterol of 236 mg/dl. Forty-five per cent smoke cigarettes, 7.9 per cent have definite LVH according to electrocardiographic findings, and 9.6 per cent have glucose intolerance. At these average values, the probability of developing coronary heart disease in 8 years is 145/1000.

From Gordon, T., Sorlie, P., and Kannel, W. B.: Coronary heart disease, atherothrombotic brain infarction, intermittent claudication—a multivariate analysis of some factors related to their incidence: Framingham Study, 16-year followup. *In* Kannel, W. B., and Gordon, T. (eds.): The Framingham Study. An Epidemiological Investigation of Cardiovascular Disease. Section 27, 1971.

group of approximately 2800 post–myocardial infarction patients, but their relatively minor role indicates that it is unlikely that much benefit from intervention aimed at traditional risk factors will be demonstrated in patients with preexisting myocardial damage. In these patients, the extent of damage to the heart will be the most decisive factor affecting prognosis.

It matters little whether we refer to Phase 2 as primary prevention of clinical disease, as most do, or as secondary prevention of the effects of established risk factors, as others prefer. From either point of view, it is clear that intervention aimed at adverse risk factors would appear to have the most beneficial effect if done before the occurrence of CAD. Again, however, the ability of modification of risk factors to arrest or reverse the atherosclerotic process and thereby decrease the morbidity in high-risk patients has not been fully established. In fact, the recently completed Multiple Risk Factor Intervention Trial, involving 12,866 high-risk men aged 35 to 57 years, failed to demonstrate a mortality benefit over a 6-year period from a special intervention program consisting of stepped-care treatment for hypertension, counseling for cigarette smoking, and dietary advice for lowering blood cholesterol levels.[106a] It is uncertain whether this is because risk factor intervention does not affect coronary heart disease mortality or more likely because the current secular trends in coronary heart disease mortality and risk factor changes in the control group or an unfavorable response in a subgroup with hypertension and an abnormal electrocardiogram at baseline prevented demonstration of a positive response.

Evidence for the Reversibility of the Atherosclerotic Process

(See also p. 1196)

The notion that atherosclerosis is a reversible process that might be affected by a reduced intake of dietary fat was first suggested in the 1920's. Obtaining experimental proof of this hypothesis has been problematic, however. Most direct evidence for the regression of atherosclerosis comes from animal studies that cannot be duplicated in humans, but that do offer encouraging results for further investigation.[241]

In a study by Armstrong et al. of four groups of nonhuman primates, one group was maintained on a low-cholesterol chow, whereas the three other groups were fed a high-cholesterol, high-fat human chow.[242] One of the three high-fat diet groups was sacrificed after 12 months, and extensive coronary arteriosclerosis was found in these monkeys (measured by amounts of luminal narrowing, internal thickening, and lipid in the vessels). The other two high-fat groups were changed to (1) a low-fat, low-cholesterol chow, and (2) a diet high in unsaturated fat and low in cholesterol. When both groups were sacrificed 1 year later, not only had the progression of the vascular disease been arrested, but actual evidence of regression throughout the coronary system was found as well.

Other animal studies have focused on the fate of the arterial connective tissue in regression.[243,244] The change in the protein content of plaques is less well established at present.

The evidence of the reversibility of the atherosclerotic process in humans is more ambiguous, owing in part to the difficulties in *collecting* this type of evidence. Perhaps the main problem is determining the extent and degree of atherosclerosis in living humans. If one relies on secondary prevention trials of lipid lowering, it is necessary for asymptomatic arteriosclerosis first to become symptomatic —a process that may take many years. As the data from the Coronary Drug Project show, an enormous number of subjects must sustain a sufficient number of coronary events before the efficacy of the lowering of cholesterol can be assessed meaningfully. Primary prevention data are still limited, although the results of current studies such as the Lipid Research Clinics' Coronary Primary Prevention Trial should prove enlightening.

For the data on regression in humans that *are* available at present, there are often problems of interpretation.[245-247] Thus, in the case of Starzl's patient with homozygous Type II hyperlipoproteinemia who received a portacaval shunt, regression of atherosclerotic lesions was found to have accompanied the reduction of plasma cholesterol, but the patient died suddenly from advanced myocardial disease.

Two caveats must be remembered in attempting to relate the evidence from animal studies to that from studies of humans. First, the human atherosclerotic lesion develops differently from the experimentally induced atherosclerosis in animals. Consequently, the finding of regression in animals cannot be generalized in toto to humans. Second, atherosclerosis in humans may be due to a multiplicity of causes and not just to hypercholesterolemia, as is the experimental atherosclerosis induced in animals. Future studies will need to focus on the interaction of other cardiovascular risk factors in the reversal of the atherosclerotic process.

Intervention in Childhood

From the previous discussion, it should be apparent that the most effective measures for the management of adverse risk factors will be aimed at the prevention of their occurrence. This will probably require one to start early in childhood to establish good health habits and a life style that avoids adverse risk factors. Although there is much to be learned about the onset of high blood pressure and elevated levels of cholesterol in youth, there are certain risk factors that might be avoided at an early age. It is usually easier to establish good habits early than to change them later. Intervention for obesity, lack of exercise, and cigarette smoking can begin in childhood. Proper nutrition in childhood without the intake of excess calories, engaging in vigorous but nonviolent sports, and prevention of cigarette smoking are likely to decrease greatly the rates of coronary artery disease in adulthood.

More active management may be considered for some children. Thus, children in families with a strong history of premature CAD or with markedly adverse risk factors may be considered for fuller evaluation and periodic follow-up. In the absence of any direct evidence for the efficacy of intervention aimed at risk factors during childhood, the individual physician must exercise careful judgment in recommending long-term therapy that may possibly have side effects or may produce undue anxiety.

General Nutritional Guidelines

A few prudent nutritional guidelines should now become evident. Each is founded on good nutritional practices that promise to help develop and maintain health and promote optimal nutrition. As detailed later in this chapter, some of these guidelines become *rules* when dealing with subjects obviously at risk, i.e., with hyperlipoproteinemia, hypertension, diabetes, or obesity, or a combination of these factors.

1. Avoidance of weight gain and overt obesity is a lifelong task that requires cognizance of the fact that caloric intake does count and that caloric balance must be individualized to meet demands for energy. Maintenance of ideal weight should be the starting point of any prudent diet.
2. In the United States today, our diet is characterized by the ingestion of 40 to 45 per cent of calories as fat, much of it saturated and of animal origin, containing 400 to 700 mg of cholesterol per day. Moderate reduction of the amount of fat, especially of saturated fat, coupled with a prudent decrease in intake of cholesterol, can lower the average American's blood level of cholesterol (and LDL) by 5 to 15 per cent. These reductions can usually be achieved simply by avoiding or limiting the intake of foods high in saturated fat and cholesterol and by replacing them, when necessary, with complex carbohydrates and polyunsaturated vegetable fats and oils.

Intake of cholesterol may be curbed by avoiding excessive consumption of foods rich in cholesterol, e.g., liver and other organ meats, shrimp (limit to once or twice monthly), and egg yolks (limit to 3 per week).

Intake of saturated fat may be controlled by decreasing the amount of animal fat, e.g., butter, whole milk, cheese, heavily marbled (usually more expensive grade) meats, cold cuts and sausage, vegetable fats so hydrogenated that they become as saturated as animal fats, and most "nondairy" products (such as nondairy sour cream containing highly saturated coconut oil).

Polyunsaturated fats may be substituted for saturated fats at the table and in most recipes. These sources provide the vegetable oils: corn, cottonseed, soybean, safflower, sunflower, and walnut. The liquids on the grocery shelf labeled "vegetable oil" are usually soybean oil or a mixture of soybean and cottonseed oil. It is important to note that the commercial use of vegetable oil often involves coconut oil, especially in nondairy and bakery items such as frostings and crackers. Advising the patient to read nutritional labels on food products prior to purchase is important.

Although it has not yet been proved in humans that reduction of the intake of cholesterol will reduce cardiovascular risk, there is little likelihood that such dietary changes will do harm. Such measures will indeed lower the level of plasma cholesterol. In fact, over the past 10 years, a 4 to 8 per cent average fall in blood levels of cholesterol in Americans of all ages is temporarily associated with a decrease in fat, especially saturated fat and cholesterol, in the diet.[33,62,248,249]

More specific nutritional guidelines have been released by the Senate Select Committee on Nutrition.[250] How rigidly these should be followed must depend for the moment on each individual physician's index of suspicion and certitude in regard to the relationship of diet to cardiovascular disease. These guidelines include a decrease in the intake of fat to less than 30 per cent of calories (and only 10 per cent of the fat should be saturated), reduction to ideal body weight, reduction of intake of salt (and avoidance of salt-rich foods such as processed items, soups, and cheeses), reduction of consumption of cholesterol to less than 300 mg/day, and an increase in the intake of dietary carbohydrates (not refined) to 50 to 60 per cent of calories.

Management of Hyperlipoproteinemia

Hyperlipoproteinemia can be effectively controlled with dietary manipulation and a variety of powerful hypolipidemic drugs. The first objective of treatment is to lower elevated levels of lipoproteins to or as near the normal range as possible.[251,252,252a] Treatment of hyperlipoproteinemia is based on the selection of diet or drug therapy, or both, aimed at either decreasing production or increasing removal of the lipoprotein fractions that are elevated.

DIET THERAPY. A dietary prescription for hyperlipoproteinemia must be formulated on an individual basis and is partly dependent on the clinical situation. In America today, mild to moderate hypercholesterolemia (increased levels of LDL) is frequently related to dietary habits (ingestion of excess amounts of cholesterol and saturated fats). Excessive consumption of any food with an associated weight gain may lead to hypertriglyceridemia through an increase in the level of VLDL; this is particularly true in individuals with already elevated levels of triglycerides. Even moderate weight reduction in hypertriglyceridemic overweight patients usually leads to lower levels of VLDL. Common sense dictates that the first step in the evaluation and management of hyperlipoproteinemia is a careful dietary history and detailed dietary instruction, ideally provided by a dietitian. In many patients with primary hyperlipoproteinemia, the levels of plasma lipids will return to normal if a dietary regimen is followed. The recommended dietary guidelines for the treatment of hyperlipoproteinemia are outlined in Table 35–11.[253]

Increased Number of Chylomicrons. Since chylomicrons are derived from dietary fat, their plasma concentration can be lowered effectively by decreasing the intake of fat from the usual 70 to 120 gm per day to 25 gm per day, supplemented by medium-chain triglycerides. Both saturated and unsaturated long-chain fatty acids must be restricted in the diet. Such treatment results within days in clearing of the lipemia, with associated correction of the hyperlipidemia, cessation of the abdominal attacks, and regression of eruptive xanthomas and hepatosplenomegaly. Maintenance of sufficiently low levels of triglyceride will prevent recurrence of abdominal pain. There is no effective drug for the treatment of Type I.

Correction of the combined chylomicronemia and increase in VLDL found in Type V is often achieved by reduction to ideal weight, followed by a maintenance

TABLE 35–11 DIETS FOR TYPES I–V HYPERLIPOPROTEINEMIA

	Type I	Type IIA	Type IIB and Type III	Type IV	Type V
Diet Prescription	Low fat, 25–35 gm	Low cholesterol, polyunsaturated fat increased	Low cholesterol Approximately: 20% cal Protein 40% cal Fat 40% cal CHO	Controlled CHO (approximately 45% of calories) Moderately restricted cholesterol	Restricted fat, 30% of calories Controlled CHO, 50% of calories Moderately restricted cholesterol
Calories	Not restricted	Not restricted	Achieve and maintain "ideal" weight, i.e., reduction diet if necessary	Achieve and maintain ideal" weight, i.e., reduction diet if necessary	Achieve and maintain ideal" weight, i.e. reduction diet if necessary
Protein	Total protein intake is not limited	Total protein intake is not limited	High protein	Not limited other than control of patient's weight	High protein
Fat	Restricted to 25–35 gm Kind of fat not important	Saturated fat intake limited Polyunsaturated fat intake increased	Controlled to 40% calories (polyunsaturated fats recommended in preference to saturated fats)	Not limited other than control of patient's weight (polyunsaturated fats recommended in preference to saturated fats)	Restricted to 30% of calories (polyunsaturated fats recommended in preference to saturated fats)
Cholesterol	Not restricted	As low as possible; the only source of cholesterol is the meat in the diet	Less than 300 mg—the only source of cholesterol is the meat in the diet	Moderately restricted to 300–500 mg	Moderately restricted to 300–500 mg
Carbohydrate	Not limited	Not limited	Controlled—concentrated sweets are restricted	Controlled—concentrated sweets are restricted	Controlled—concentrated sweets are restricted
Alcohol	Not recommended	May be used with discretion	Limited to 2 servings (substituted for carbohydrate)	Limited to 2 servings (substituted for carbohydrate)	Not recommended

regimen in which intake of both fat and carbohydrate is restricted. Alcohol is strictly forbidden, for it can grossly exacerbate the hypertriglyceridemia seen in Type V.

Increased Levels of VLDL. Increased levels of VLDL are associated with factors such as obesity, stress, glucose intolerance, and hyperinsulinemia. In the majority of patients, weight reduction and achievement of ideal weight will be sufficient to control excess VLDL. Further decreases may be attained by reducing the intake of the precursors of VLDL triglyceride, namely, carbohydrates and alcohol. Cholesterol is moderately restricted (300 to 500 mg per day), and polyunsaturated fats are preferred.

Increased Levels of IDL. As with increased levels of VLDL, weight reduction is the most important step in controlling excess IDL. Maintenance of ideal weight through a balanced diet containing protein, fat, and carbohydrates in the proportions of 20:40:40 is recommended. Cholesterol is restricted to less than 300 mg per day, and the P/S ratio* is raised to 2:1.

Increased Levels of LDL. An effective means of lowering the high level of LDL in Type II patients is a low-cholesterol (< 300 mg per day), high P/S (2:1) diet. Strict adherence, as in metabolic wards, usually reduces total levels of plasma cholesterol and LDL by 15 to 25 per cent. In the free-living population, reductions of 10 to 20 per cent are often observed. The dietary changes enhance the rate of clearance of LDL from the bloodstream. No direct relationship exists between changes in body weight and LDL.

Multiple Increases in Lipoproteins. When more than one lipoprotein is increased, the above recommendations for the treatment of elevations of individual lipoproteins are additive. For example, in patients with increased levels of VLDL and LDL (Type IIB), the former may be controlled with caloric restriction, and the latter with a diet low in cholesterol and high in polyunsaturated fats.

DRUG THERAPY. A number of potent hypolipidemic drugs are available for the treatment of hyperlipoproteinemia.[254–257,257a] Because of the heterogeneity of the disorders, no one drug is effective in controlling all lipoprotein increases. All have side effects, and patients should be carefully monitored for potential drug toxicity.[258]

The currently available drugs can control hyperlipoproteinemia by one of two mechanisms: (1) decreasing production of lipoproteins or (2) increasing clearance of lipoproteins. Clofibrate and nicotinic acid belong to the former category, whereas cholestyramine, colestipol, dextrothyroxine, and possibly probucol are in the latter group (Table 35–12).

Nicotinic Acid. Nicotinic acid is primarily indicated in states characterized by increased levels of VLDL. It is also useful in decreasing IDL and LDL, and increasing levels of HDL. The initial dose is 100 mg orally three times a day, with increases of 300 mg/day every 4 to 7 days until the maintenance dose of 3 to 9 gm per day is reached.

Side effects include cutaneous flushing and pruritus in the vast majority of patients. These effects usually decrease rapidly after the first few days of administration of the medication, even when dosage is greatly increased. Other transient effects include nausea, vomiting, and diarrhea. More serious side effects are abnormal liver function tests, abnormal glucose tolerance, and hyperuricemia. Nicotinic acid should therefore be used with extreme caution, if at all, in patients with liver disease, diabetes mellitus, or gout.

Clofibrate. Clofibrate has been especially useful in states characterized by increased levels of VLDL and IDL. It has limited value in controlling increases in LDL and sometimes, in fact, increases levels of LDL. It is prepared

*Polyunsaturated/saturated ratio.

TABLE 35–12 APPROVED HYPOLIPIDEMIC AGENTS

	To Decrease Lipoprotein Synthesis	Enhanced Intravascular Lipoprotein Catabolism		To Increase Lipoprotein Catabolism		
	Nicotinic Acid	*Clofibrate*	*Gemfibrozil*	*Colestipol Cholestyramine*	*D-Thyroxine*	*Probucol*
Primary indication	↑ VLDL; ↑ IDL (Types III, IV, and V)	↑ IDL (Type III)	↑ VLDL (Types IV and V)	↑ LDL (Type II)	↑ LDL (Type II)	↑ LDL (Type II)
Other indications	↑ LDL (Type II)	↑ VLDL (Types IV and V)	? ↑ IDL (Type III)		↑ IDL (Type III)	
Initial dose	100 mg t.i.d.	1 gm b.i.d.		8 gm b.i.d.	2 mg q.i.d.	250 mg b.i.d.
Maintenance dose	1–3 gm t.i.d.	1 gm b.i.d.	600 mg b.i.d.	8–16 gm b.i.d.	4–8 mg q.d.	500 mg b.i.d.
Major side effects	Flushing Pruritus Nausea Diarrhea	Nausea Diarrhea	Nausea GI discomfort	Constipation Nausea	Mild hypermetabolism ↑ Angina and cardiac irritability in patients with heart disease	Diarrhea Nausea
Other side effects	Glucose intolerance Hyperuricemia Hepatotoxicity	Myositis Ventricular ectopy Abnormal liver function tests Cholelithiasis	? ↑ Glucose intolerance ? Cholelithiasis	Hyperchloremic acidosis Biliary tract calcification Steatorrhea	Glucose intolerance Neutropenia	?
Drug interactions	↑ Vasodilatation by ganglioplegic antihypertensive agents	↑ Hypoprothrombinemic effect of warfarin sodium	Potentiates effect of anticoagulants	↓ Absorption of phenylbutazone, thiazides, tetracycline, phenobarbital, thyroid, digitalis, and warfarin sodium	↑ Hypoprothrombinemic effect of warfarin	?

in 500-mg capsules and is administered orally in a total dose of 1.5 to 2 gm per day, in two divided doses.

The drug has not usually produced serious side effects. However, in the Coronary Drug Project, the drug was associated with a twofold increase in cholelithiasis and a significant increase in arrhythmias, new angina, thromboembolism, and intermittent claudication in patients who had had a myocardial infarction.[258] In a recently completed primary prevention trial, treatment with clofibrate was associated with an increase in overall mortality, although a significant decline in suspected and proven myocardial infarction was noted.[259]

Cholestyramine. Cholestyramine is a highly effective bile acid sequestrant that is indicated for the treatment of states characterized by excess LDL. It may actually increase levels of VLDL and IDL in subjects with excesses of these lipoproteins. It is manufactured as a powder and is taken orally mixed with a liquid such as fruit juice or lemonade. The initial dose is 16 gm per day, given in two to four divided doses at meals. This may be raised by 4 to 8 gm every 2 to 3 weeks until a maximum dose of 32 gm per day is reached.

The most frequent side effects involve the gastrointestinal system, but these usually respond to a reduction in dosage.

Colestipol. Colestipol is a bile acid sequestrant whose effect on plasma cholesterol is similar to that of cholestyramine. It is indicated for treatment of the same states as cholestyramine.[261]

Colestipol is available in water-insoluble beads. The usual dose is 4 to 5 gm three times per day, although doses up to 10 gm three times per day have been used.

D-Thyroxine. D-Thyroxine is indicated for controlling increased levels of LDL. However, because it has been associated with serious potential cardiotoxic effects in patients with CAD, its role as a primary hypolipidemic agent must be considered limited. The initial dose is 2 mg per day orally, increased by 1 to 2 mg per month to a maintenance dose of 4 to 8 mg per day.

The drug was withdrawn from the Coronary Drug Project because of excess morbidity and mortality in patients with symptoms or signs of CAD who were in the D-thyroxine treatment group.[260]

Probucol and Gemfibrozil. Probucol has only recently been approved by the Food and Drug Administration for use in patients with hyperlipidemia.[262–264] Its mechanism of action is unclear. Experience with the drug is limited, so that its potential usefulness and side effects are not well defined. Serious side effects have thus far been few. In a dosage of 500 mg b.i.d., the drug appears to be most effective in subjects with mild to moderate elevations of LDL. The potential value of probucol in the prevention or control of CAD is limited by its consistent reduction of HDL levels greater or equal to its reduction of LDL concentrations.[264] In this regard, *gemfibrozil,* the most recently approved lipid-lowering drug, apparently increases levels of HDL while lowering concentrations of VLDL and LDL.[265] As with probucol, experience with this new drug is limited, and its mechanisms of action and potential usefulness are still unclear.

Combination Chemotherapy. The combination of hypolipidemic agents that act by alternate mechanisms has proved highly effective in some cases. For example, cholestyramine and nicotinic acid can function synergistically to reduce extremely high levels of LDL in Type II homozygotes and in some heterozygotes. Other combinations of drugs are still being investigated. Since all hypolipidemic agents have side effects, and the efficacy of their use in the control of cardiovascular disease is still uncertain, combination hypolipidemic therapy should usually be instituted with caution.[266]

OTHER THERAPY. *Partial ileal bypass* can significantly lower levels of LDL.[267] As with the bile acid sequestrants, levels of VLDL and IDL either are unaffected or may increase. The use of the bypass procedure for Type II subjects with or greatly at risk for CAD has been recommended by some. At present, the authors recommend it only for high-risk subjects with the heterozygous form of primary Type II who are unable to follow other therapies of their own accord (e.g., drug therapy). In the Type II homozygote, ileal bypass has not proved effective.[268]

Portacaval shunt dramatically lowered levels of LDL in one subject with homozygous Type II hyperlipoproteinemia, with an associated disappearance of angina and coronary atherosclerosis. Its use in other homozygous Type II subjects has been much less dramatic, however, usually lowering levels of LDL by only 10 to 20 per cent.[269]

Recently, *plasma exchange* on a monthly basis has been used with some effectiveness in controlling the levels of LDL and decreasing xanthomatosis and possibly coronary artery disease in homozygous Type II individuals.[270]

When to Treat

Dietary advice aimed at normalizing body weight and reducing levels of plasma lipids should be offered to any individual with a total plasma cholesterol greater than 240 mg per 100 ml. All patients with strong family histories (CAD, stroke, or arteriosclerotic peripheral vascular disease) should receive dietary advice, even though their levels of plasma lipids may be only moderately elevated. Therapeutic goals should be a level of cholesterol less than 220 mg per 100 ml and a value for triglycerides below 250 mg per 100 ml.

Since all the currently available lipid-lowering drugs have unproven efficacy but proven side effects, the use of drugs should usually be considered only after at least 6 months of unrelenting effort by the physician and dietitian has failed to achieve therapeutic goals. Even then, it should be considered only for the following groups: (1) patients with clinically manifest CAD; (2) patients with strong family histories of CAD, hyperlipidemia, or both; and (3) patients with one or more of the other established risk factors besides the hyperlipidemia, e.g., hypertension, diabetes, or cigarette smoking.

Management of Hypertension

(See also Chap. 27)

The logistic risk model described previously indicates that the risk of developing CAD is related to blood pressure in a continuous graded manner. As shown in Figure 35–6, the higher the blood pressure, the greater the risk. There is no discrete level of blood pressure that marks a discontinuous transition from low risk to high risk. Furthermore, levels of blood pressure are distributed in a smooth, continuous, unimodal curve in the general population.[271] Despite these observations, it has become rather firmly entrenched in medical thinking that there are operational cut-off points that can define an optimal strategy for managing elevated blood pressure. The strategy described here is that recommended by the National Committee on Detection, Evaluation, and Treatment of High Blood Pressure.[272]

As stated previously, approximately 40 per cent of the adult population in the United States meets the usual criterion for having hypertension, i.e., mean blood pressure on two occasions of greater than 140/90 mm Hg. Although the level of blood pressure has been found to be associated with a number of personal characteristics (family history, obesity, renal disease, sex, and race), there is little that our present state of knowledge can contribute to the primary prevention of hypertension per se. If we therefore concede that hypertension represents a disease state already in process, we must rely on secondary prevention to abort its progression and prevent its sequelae. The key modalities of secondary prevention in this case are early detection and effective treatment.

Every adult should have his blood pressure measured at least annually by a competent and properly trained observer. The Joint National Committee recommends that all adults (age 18 and older) with diastolic pressures 95 mm Hg or greater on initial measurement should be remeasured within 3 months. A diagnosis of hypertension is confirmed when this average of multiple measurements on at least two subsequent visits is 90 mm Hg or greater. The efficacy of a systematic antihypertensive treatment program in reducing mortality of persons with high blood pressure has been clearly demonstrated by the Hypertension Detection and Follow-up Program.[236] In this community-based, randomized clinical trial involving 10,940 persons with high blood pressure, 5-year mortality from all causes was 17 per cent lower for the group receiving a systematic stepped-care program than for the group referred to usual community medical therapy. Even among those with diastolic blood pressure between 90 to 104 mm Hg at entry into the study, mortality was 20 per cent lower among those receiving the stepped-care regimen. It therefore seems likely that systematic management of "mild" hypertension, as outlined in Chapter 27, has great potential for reducing overall mortality. Details of the stepped-care approach are given in Chapter 27.

Changing Cigarette Smoking Habits

Cigarette smoking has definitely been implicated as a major contributor to cardiovascular mortality and morbidity.[95,96,273] Cigarette smokers have a risk that is 60 per cent or more higher than that of nonsmokers in respect to total mortality, cardiovascular mortality, and coronary artery disease mortality and incidence.[93,95–97] There is also massive evidence that in ex-smokers and cigarette smokers who switch to cigars or pipes, risk is lowered to about the level of those who never smoked.[93,99,100]

Two limitations of the evidence, however, must be conceded. In persons older than the age of 65, cigarette smoking has not shown up as a major risk factor for coronary artery disease, although it is still a major contributor to morbidity from lung cancer and chronic bronchitis and emphysema.[95,96] The second anomaly is the lack of a consistent relationship between cigarette smoking and angina pectoris.[101,107,110,111] This issue has been used to obscure the definite and consistent relationship between cigarette smoking and other forms of atherosclerotic disease and mortality.

Since the appearance of the Surgeon General's report in 1964, there have been marked changes in the cigarette smoking habits of Americans. By 1975, the proportion of men smoking cigarettes had declined by 25 per cent, from 53 per cent in 1964 to 39 per cent in 1975.[274] The number of pounds of cigarette tobacco consumed per capita had declined by 19 per cent, although the number of cigarettes sold per capita remained essentially constant. This is true because of the increased use of filter-tip cigarettes, which contain less tobacco than regular cigarettes.

Despite the widespread warning that cigarette smoking is a health hazard, and despite the vigorous public health campaigns to educate the general population about the harmful effects of smoking, many people continue to smoke. Teenaged boys continue to assume the habit as frequently now as they did in 1964, whereas teenaged girls and younger women smoked considerably more in the 1970's than their peers did in the 1960's. Many public health activists are urging legislative measures to curb cigarette smoking, including prohibition of smoking in many public areas and segregation of smokers from nonsmokers in planes and restaurants. Indeed, such rulings are already in effect in many areas.

As a group, physicians have shown a much greater decline in cigarette smoking than has the general population.[275] Thus, many physicians are able to serve as appropriate role models for patients who wish to discontinue smoking. However, simply informing patients of the ill effects of smoking and advising them to quit will not influence many who have been enjoying the habit for years. The physician who shows genuine concern about and understanding of his patient's smoking problem, who spends time with the patient to explain that cessation of smoking will have beneficial effects, and who offers helpful, practical advice and reinforcement may achieve considerable success.[273,276]

The American Heart Association Ad Hoc Committee on Cigarette Smoking and Cardiovascular Diseases has made some practical recommendations for actively encouraging the elimination of cigarette smoking.[273] The Committee advises the following:

1. Do not allow patients or nurses in physicians' offices to smoke.
2. Always raise the question of smoking in connection with the finding of vascular or pulmonary disease and in general health examinations.
3. Locate and refer patients to smoking cessation clinics when necessary.
4. Obtain help from the family in the endeavors to cease smoking.
5. Check on compliance with advice periodically.

Management of Obesity

Although obesity has not been established firmly as an independent risk factor for CAD (p. 1218), it has long been associated with the development of vascular disease. As such, it represents a major health problem for 30 to 50 per cent of the adult population of the United States.[277] The management of obesity poses a formidable challenge, however, and studies have shown that although obesity is preventable, it is almost incurable. Regardless of the weight-reducing method used, most people will fail to lose weight or to maintain weight loss for any length of time. The rates of recidivism are high, with most obese patients regaining the weight they lost within 1 to 6 years.

The procedures for the management of obesity that are most widely accepted by the medical community include: (1) diet, (2) exercise, (3) behavior modification, (4) surgical intervention, (5) pharmacological intervention, and (6) psychotherapy. Of these, behavior modification appears to hold the most promise because it deals directly with the cause of obesity, namely, eating behavior, and focuses on changing eating habits permanently so that weight loss may be maintained on a long-term basis.[278]

One of the difficulties in weight reduction lies in the creation of a negative caloric balance, that is, expending more energy than is being ingested. The vast majority of sources agree that the creation of a negative energy balance is the only reliable way to lose weight.[279,280] This can be achieved through reduction of caloric intake or increasing the caloric expenditure, or a combination of both. The results of numerous studies evaluating the effects of diet combined with exercise versus diet alone show that significantly more weight is lost by the group following both restricted caloric intake and regular exercise.[281,282] However, without concomitant behavioral changes, the attrition rate in clinical treatment programs is discouragingly high, as are the chances of recidivism.

The difficulties in weight reduction have helped popularize a number of recent diets based on the premise that weight can be lost by changing the composition of the diet without reducing the quantity of food consumed. Diets such as the high protein, high-fat, or low-carbohydrate plans are some of the most popular, but the evidence shows that these diets may have serious side effects and can be dangerous. Moreover, weight is frequently regained rapidly once the diet is terminated. Medical authorities agree that a good reducing diet should do the following:

1. Provide for adequate basic nutrition.
2. Create the desired degree of negative caloric balance.
3. Adapt as closely as possible to the tastes of the individual dieter.
4. Be palatable, socially acceptable, easy to obtain, and inexpensive.
5. Protect the dieter from hunger, satisfy his need for food, and result in a minimum of fatigue.
6. Help create new eating habits that can contribute to the maintenance of a lower body weight, once it is achieved.

None of the existing methods for treatment of obesity assures success, partly because treatment programs often fail to reinforce new eating habits and neglect the long-term maintenance of weight. Thus, alterations in diet and exercise should be viewed within the context of overall behavioral modification.

Exercise

There is a growing enthusiasm in Americans for various forms of leisure-time physical activity. The direct evidence for a protective effect of physical activity in regard to development of CAD is still rather weak. Judging from the recent public enthusiasm for jogging, cycling, tennis, and similar activities, however, many people believe that this is a pleasant way to achieve better health and improve the "quality of life."

Most individuals with sedentary occupations will probably benefit from a regular program of moderate exercise. Paul Dudley White was a vocal advocate of regular exercise in the form of bicycle riding and walking. Modern enthusiasts have urged more vigorous pursuits such as jogging and running. It is not possible at the current state of knowledge to formulate with any scientific basis an exercise program that will be optimal for most people.[163]

The physician should be prepared to urge all who wish to embark on exercise programs to do so, but only after observing a few obvious precautions. It has been recommended that anyone older than the age of 35 who has not engaged in regular exercise for a number of years should undergo a medical examination before starting an exercise program. The examination would include evaluation of the heart and lungs, a resting electrocardiogram, and assessment of the coronary risk factors. Many also advocate a treadmill exercise test. Those with evidence of possible CAD should be encouraged to engage in a carefully graded exercise program, but they should be warned not to increase their activity too rapidly.

A gradual increase in the level of physical activity over a period of weeks or even months is probably desirable for all who have previously been sedentary. The use of proper equipment for the chosen activity will help to prevent muscle, bone, and joint problems. Patients should be advised to consult a reliable book concerning appropriate equipment, warm-up exercises, and training methods. In general, the patient can avoid many of the acute aches and pains that often afflict the novice sports enthusiast by not overdoing it too early.

Psychosocial Tension

The recognition that psychosocial factors may play a role in the induction of CAD has only recently begun to receive support from epidemiological studies. Most clinicians have probably had occasion to warn a patient to "take it easy or you'll have a heart attack." This is usually accompanied by advice to relax more, slow down a little, take a vacation, or develop a new hobby. Such advice is clearly intended to help the anxious, overworked, harried patient to change a life style that the physician believes to be associated with an increased risk of developing acute CAD. Since psychosocial tension may arise from a wide variety of stressful interactions and can be handled differently by different individuals, it is impossible to give specific advice for its management.

A few patterns have been sufficiently well defined, however, and evidence of their association with CAD has begun to appear, so that some help may be offered the high-risk patient. It should be borne in mind that no studies have yet been done that demonstrate that modification of these patterns will reduce the risk of heart disease.

Epidemiological studies have shown that the Type A behavior is a predictor of increased risk of developing CAD.[173] It is this type of behavior that generates the admonition to "take it easy." Friedman and Rosenman have provided some guidelines that may be useful for some patients.[172] These include techniques for providing positive reinforcement of non-Type A behavior and suggestions for avoiding situations that elicit Type A behavior. In one prospective study on a group of postinfarction patients, it was shown that advice and counseling designed to diminish the intensity of Type A behavior reduced the rate of reinfarction.[283]

More general indices of psychosocial tension that have been related to incidence of CAD, such as status incongruity, lack of peer support systems, and geographical and cultural mobility, have not yet yielded clues for effective intervention strategies. To the extent that these situations are accompanied by depression, anxiety, or other psychological manifestations, the sympathetic physician should provide appropriate counseling.

Acknowledgment

The authors wish to acknowledge with gratitude Ms. Irene Kuraeff for her diligent and skillful work in helping to prepare this chapter.

References

1. White, P. D.: Perspectives. Prog. Cardiovasc. Dis. *14*:250–255, 1971.
2. McGill, H. D., Jr. (ed.): Geographic Pathology of Atherosclerosis. Baltimore, The Williams and Wilkins Co., 1968.
3. Puffer, R. R., and Griffith, G. W.: Patterns of urban mortality. Report of the Inter-American Investigation of Mortality. Pan American Health Organization Scientific Publ. No. 151, 1967.
4. Klebba, A. J., and Dolman, A. B.: Comparability of mortality statistics for the seventh and eighth revision of the International Classification of Diseases. United States. Vital and Health Statistics: Series 2, No. 66. Washington, D. C., DHEW Publ. No. (HRA) 76-1340, 1976.
5. Kannel, W. B., McGee, D., and Gordon, T.: A general cardiovascular risk profile: The Framingham Study. Am. J. Cardiol. *38*:46, 1976.
6. Inter-society Commission for Heart Disease Resources: Primary prevention of the atherosclerotic diseases. Circulation *42*:A55, 1970.
7. Stamler, J., and Epstein, F. H.: Coronary heart disease: Risk factors as guides to preventive action, Prev. Med. *1*:27, 1972.
8. Epstein, F. H., Napier, J. A., Block, W. D., Hayner, N. S., Higgins, M. P., Johnson, B. C., Keller, J. B., Mitzner, H. L., Montoye, H. J., Ostrander, L. D., and Ullman, B. M.: The Tecumseh Study. Design, progress and prospectives. Arch. Environ. Health *21*:402, 1970.
9. Rosenman, R. H., Brand, R. J., Sholtz, R. I., and Friedman, M.: Multivariate prediction of coronary heart disease during 8.5 year follow-up in the Western Collaborative Group Study. Am. J. Cardiol. *37*:903, 1976.
10. Keys, A.: Coronary heart disease in seven countries. Circulation *41*(Suppl. 1):I-1–I-211, 1970.
11. Hames, C. J.: Evans County cardiovascular and cerebrovascular epidemiologic study—Introduction. Arch. Intern. Med. *128*:833, 1971.
12. Garcia-Palmieri, M. R., Costas, R., Jr., Cruz-Vidal, M., Cortes-Alicea, M., Colon, A. A., Feliberti, M., Ayala, A. M., Patterne, D., Subrino, R., Torres, R., and Nazario, E.: Risk factors and prevalence of coronary heart disease in Puerto Rico. Circulation *42*:541, 1970.
13. Marmot, M. G., Syme, S. L., Kagan, A., Kato, H., Cohen, J. B., and Belsky, J.: Epidemiologic studies of coronary heart disease and stroke in Japanese men living in Japan, Hawaii and California: Prevalence of coronary and hypertensive heart disease and associated risk factors. Am. J. Epidemiol. *102*:514, 1975.
14. Tibblin, G., Wilhelmsen, L., and Werko, L.: Risk factors for myocardial infarction and death due to ischemic heart disease and other causes. Am. J. Cardiol. *35*:514, 1975.
15. Ducimetiere, P., Richard, J. L., Cambien, F., Rakotovao, R., and Claude, J. R.: Coronary heart disease in middle-aged Frenchmen. Comparisons between Paris Prospectives Study, Seven Countries Study, and Pooling Project. Lancet *1*:1346, 1980.
16. Health Interview Survey Procedure. Vital and Health Statistics. Series 1, No. 11. Washington, D. C., DHEW Publ. No. (HSM) 73-1311, 1957–1974.
17. Plan and Operation of the Health and Nutrition Examination Survey (United States). Vital and Health Statistics: Series 1, No. 10. Washington, D. C., DHEW Publ. No. (HSM) 73-1310, 1971–1973.
18. Uniform Hospital Abstract: Minimum basic data set. A report of the United States National Committee on Vital and Health Statistics. Vital and Health Statistics: Series 4, No. 14, Washington, D.C., DHEW Publ. No. (HSM) 73-1451, 1973.
19. Monthly Vital Statistics Report. National Center for Health Statistics, Washington, D. C., Vol. 31, No. 6, September 30, 1982.
20. Gordon, T., Garcia-Palmieri, M. R., Kagan, A., Kannel, W. B., and Schiffman, J.: Differences in coronary heart disease in Framingham, Honolulu and Puerto Rico. J. Chronic Dis. *27*:329, 1974.
21. Rogot, E., and Padgett, S. J.: Associations of coronary and stroke mortality with temperature and snowfall in selected areas of the United States, 1962–1966. Am. J. Epidemiol. *103*:565, 1976.
22. Fabsitz, R., and Feinleib, M.: Geographic patterns in county mortality rates from cardiovascular diseases. Am. J. Epidemiol. *111*:325, 1980.
23. Comstock, G. W.: Water hardness and cardiovascular diseases. Am. J. Epidermiol. *110*:375, 1979.
24. Sharrett, A. R.: Water hardness and cardiovascular disease. Circulation *63*:247A, 1980.
25. Masisoni, R., Pisa, Z., and Clayton, D.: Myocardial infarction and water hardness in the WHO myocardial infarction registry network. Bull. WHO *57*:291, 1979.
26. Rogot, E., Sharrett, A. R., Feinleib, M., and Fabsitz, R. R.: Trends in urban mortality in relation to fluoridation status. Am. J. Epidemiol. *106*:104, 1978.
27. Reid, D. D., Cornfield, J., Markush, R. E., Seigal, D., Pederson, E., and Haenzel, W.: Studies of disease among migrants and native populations in Great Britain, Norway and the United States. III. Prevalence of cardio-respiratory symptoms among migrants and native born in the United States. Nat. Cancer Inst. Monogr. *19*:321, 1966.
28. Medalie, J. H., Kahn, H. A., Neufeld, H. N., Riss, E., Goldbourt, U., Perlstein, T., and Oron, D.: Myocardial infarction over a five-year period. I. Prevalence, incidence and mortality experience. J. Chronic Dis. *24*:63, 1973.
29. Anderson, T. W.: Mortality from ischemic heart disease. Changes in middle-aged men since 1900. J.A.M.A. *224*:336, 1973.
30. Levy, R. I.: Declining mortality in coronary heart disease. Arteriosclerosis *1*:312, 1981.
31. Patrick, C. H., Palesch, Y. Y., Feinleib, M., and Brody, J. A.: Sex differences in declining cohort death rates from heart disease. Am. J. Public Health *72*:161, 1982.
32. Marmot, M. G., and Syme, S. L.: Acculturation and coronary heart disease in Japanese-Americans. Am. J. Epidemiol. *104*:225, 1976.
33. Havlik, R. J., and Feinleib, M.: Proceedings of the Conference on the Decline in Coronary Heart Disease Mortality. U.S. Department of Health, Education, and Welfare, NIH Publ. No. 79-1610, 1979, p. 399.
34. Feinleib, M., Havlik, R. J., and Thom, T. J.: The changing pattern of ischemic heart disease. J. Cardiovasc. Med. *7*:139, 1982.
35. Strong, J. P., and Guzman, M. A.: Decrease in coronary atherosclerosis in New Orleans. Lab. Invest. *43*:297, 1980.
36. Dwyer, T., and Netzel, B. S.: A comparison of trends of coronary heart disease mortality in Australia, U.S.A. and England and Wales with reference to three major risk factors—hypertension, cigarette smoking and diet. Int. J. Epidemiol. *9*:65, 1980.
37. Gordon, T., Sorlie, P., and Kannel, W. B.: The Framingham Study. An Epidemiological Investigation of Cardiovascular Disease. Section 27. Coronary Heart Disease, Antherothrombotic Brain Infarction, Intermittent Claudication—A Multivariate Analysis of Some Factors Related to their Incidence: Framingham Study, 16-Year Follow-up. Washington, D.C., U.S. Government Printing Office, 1971.
38. McGee, and Gordon, T.: The results of the Framingham Study applied to four other U.S.-based epidemiologic studies of cardiovascular disease. The Framingham Study—Section 31. Washington, D.C., DHEW Publication No. (NIH) 76-1083, 1976.
39. Brand, R. J., Rosenman, R. H., Sholtz, R. I., and Friedman, M.: Multivariate prediction of coronary heart disease in the Western Collaborative Group Study compared to the findings of the Framingham Study. Circulation *53*:348, 1976.
40. Keys, A., Aravanis, C., Blackburn, H., Buchem, F. S. P., Buzina, R., Djordjevic, B. S., Fidanza, F., Karvonen, M. J., Menotti, A., Puddu, V., and Taylor, H. L.: Probability of middle-aged men developing coronary heart disease in 5 years. Circulation *45*:815, 1972.
41. Arteriosclerosis 1981. Report of the Working Group on Arteriosclerosis of the National Heart, Lung, and Blood Institute. Vols. 1 and 2. Washington, D.C., U.S. Department of Health and Human Services, Public Health Service, NIH Publ. No. 81–2034 and 82–2035, 1981 and 1982.
42. Dawber, T. R., Kannel, W. B., Revotskie, N., and Kagan, A.: The epidemiology of coronary heart disease. The Framingham enquiry. Proc. Roy. Soc. Med. *551*:265, 1962.
43. Stamler, J.: Diet, serum lipids, and coronary heart disease: The epidemiologic evidence. *In* Levy, R. I., Rifkind, B. M., Dennis, B. H., and Ernst. N. (eds.):

Nutrition, Lipids, and Coronary Heart Disease—A Global View. New York, Raven Press, 1979.
44. Kannel, W. B., Castelli, W. P., and Gordon, T.: Cholesterol in the prediction of atherosclerotic disease. New perspectives based on the Framingham Study. Ann. Intern. Med. *90*:85, 1979.
45. Albrink, M. M., Meigs, J. W., and Man, E. B.: Serum lipids, hypertension and coronary artery disease. Am. J. Med. *31*:4, 1961.
46. Carlson, L. A.: Serum lipids in men with myocardial infarction. Acta Med. Scand. *167*:399, 1960.
47. Hulley, S. B., Rosenman, R. H., Bawol, R. D., and Brand, R. J.: Epidemiology as a guide to clinical decisions. N. Engl. J. Med. *307*:1383, 1980.
48. Kannel, W. B., Castelli, W. P., Gordon, T., and McNamara, P.: Serum cholesterol, lipoproteins and the risk of coronary heart disease. The Framingham Study. Ann. Intern. Med. *74*:1, 1971.
49. Kinch, S. H., Doyle, J. T., and Hilleboe, H. E.: Risk factors in ischaemic heart disease. Am. J. Public Health *53*:438, 1963.
50. Stamler, J.: Lifestyles, major risk factors, proof and public policy. Circulation *58*:3, 1978.
51. Fredrickson, D. S., Levy, R. I., and Lees, R. S.: Fat transport in lipoproteins—an integrated approach to mechanisms and disorders. N. Engl. J. Med. *276*:32, 1967.
52. Hatch, F. T., and Lees, R. S.: Practical methods for plasma lipoprotein analysis. Adv. Lipid Res. *6*:1, 1968.
53. Gordon, T., Castelli, W. P., Hjortland, M., Kannel, W. B., and Dawber, T.: High density lipoprotein as a protective factor against coronary artery disease: The Framington Study. Am. J. Med. *62*:707, 1977.
54. Fredrickson, D. S., and Levy, R. I.: Familial hyperlipoproteinemia. *In* Stanbury, J. B., Wyngaarden, J. B., and Fredrickson, D. S. (eds.): The Metabolic Basis of Inherited Disease. 3rd ed. New York, McGraw-Hill Book Co., 1972.
55. Brown, D. F., Kinch, S. H., and Doyle, J. T.: Serum triglycerides in health and in ischemic heart disease. N. Engl. J. Med. *273*:947, 1965.
56. Levy, R. I., and Glueck, C. J.: Hypertriglyceridemia, diabetes mellitus and coronary vessel disease. Arch. Intern. Med. *123*:220, 1969.
57. Heinle, R. A., Levy, R. I., Fredrickson, D. S., and Gorlin, R.: Lipid and carbohydrate abnormalities in patients with angiographically documented coronary artery disease. Am. J. Cardiol. *24*:178, 1969.
58. Carlson, L. A., and Bottiger, L. D.: Ischemic heart disease in relation to fasting values of plasma triglycerides and cholesterol. Lancet *1*:865, 1972.
59. Tatami, R., Mabuchi, H., Veda, K., Veda, R., Haba, T., Kametani, T., Ito, S., Koizumi, J. U., Ohta, M., Miyamoto, S., Nakayama, A., Kanaya, H., Oiwake, H., Genda, A., and Takeda, R.: Intermediate-density lipoprotein and cholesterol-rich very low density lipoprotein in angiographically determined coronary artery disease. Circulation *64*:1174, 1981.
60. Levy, R. I., Bilheimer, D. W., and Eisenberg, S.: The structure and metabolism of chylomicrons and very low density lipoproteins (VLDL). *In* Smellie, R. M. S. (ed.): Plasma Lipoproteins. New York, Academic Press, 1971.
61. Havel, R. J.: Mechanisms of hyperlipoproteinemia. Adv. Exp. Med. Biol. *26*:57, 1972.
62. Levy, R. I.: Cholesterol, lipoproteins, apoproteins, and heart disease: Present status and future prospects. Clin. Chem. *27*:653, 1981.
63. Stone, N. J., Levy, R. I., Fredrickson, D. S., and Verter, J.: Coronary artery disease in 116 kindred with familial type II hyperlipoproteinemia. Circulation *49*:476, 1974.
64. Rhoads, G. C., Gulbrandsen, C. L., and Kagan, A.: Serum lipoproteins and coronary heart disease in a population of Hawaii Japanese men. N. Engl. J. Med. *294*:293, 1976.
65. Miller, G. J., and Miller, N. E.: Plasma high density lipoprotein concentration and development of ischemic heart disease. Lancet *1*:16, 1975.
66. Castelli, W. P., Doyle, J. T., Gordon, T., Haines, C. G., Hjortland, M., Hulley, S. B., Kagan, A., and Zukel, W. J.: HDL cholesterol and other lipids in coronary heart disease. The Cooperative Lipoprotein Phenotyping Study. Circulation *55*:767, 1977.
67. Miller, N. E., Thelle, D. S., Forde, O. H., and Mjos, O. D.: The Tromso Heart-Study. High density lipoprotein and coronary heart disease: A prospective case-control study. Lancet *1*:965, 1977.
68. Tyroler, H. A. (ed.): Epidemiology of plasma high-density lipoprotein cholesterol levels. The Lipid Research Clinics Program Prevalence Study. Circulation *62*(Suppl.):4, 1980, 1.
69. Bradley, D. D., Wingred, J., Petitti, D. B., Krauss, R. M., and Ramcharan, S.: Serum high-density-lipoprotein cholesterol in women using oral contraceptives, estrogens and progestins. N. Engl. J. Med. *299*:17–20, 1978.
70. Glueck, C. J., Gartside, P., Fallat, R. W., Sielski, J., and Steiner, P. M.: Longevity syndromes: Familial hypobeta and familial hyperalpha lipoproteinemia. J. Lab. Clin. Med. *88*:941, 1976.
71. Lipid Research Clinics (LRC) Program Epidemiology Committee: Plasma lipid distributions in 11 North American populations: The Lipid Research Clinics Program Prevalence Study. Circulation *60*:427, 1979.
72. Rifkind, B. M., Tamir, I., Heiss, G., Wallace, R. B., and Tyroler, H. A.: Distribution of high-density and other lipoproteins in selected Lipid Research Clinics Prevalence Study populations: A brief survey. Lipids *14*:105, 1979.
73. Lipid Research Clinics Population Studies Data Book. Vol. 1. The Prevalence Study. Washington, D.C., U.S. Department of Health and Human Services, Public Health Service. NIH Publ. No. 80-1527, 1980.
74. WHO Bulletin. Classification of hyperlipidemias and hyperlipoproteinemias. Circulation *45*:501, 1972.
75. Friedewald, W. T., Levy, R. I., and Fredrickson, D. S.: Estimation of the concentration of low-density lipoprotein cholesterol in plasma, without use of the preparative ultracentrifuge. Clin. Chem. *18*:499, 1972.
76. Lipid Research Clinics Program. Manual of Laboratory Operations, Vol. 1, Washington, D.C., DHEW Publ. No. (NIH) 75-628, 1974.
77. Schaefer, E. J., Eisenberg, S., and Levy, R. I.: Lipoprotein apoprotein metabolism. J. Lipid Res. *19*:667, 1978.
78. Rifkind, B. M., and Levy, R. I. (eds.): Hyperlipidemia: Diagnosis and Therapy. New York, Grune and Stratton, 1977.
79. Breckenridge, W. C., Little, J. A., Steiner, G., Chow, A., and Poapst, M.: Hypertriglyceridemia associated with deficiency of apolipoprotein C-II. N. Engl. J. Med. *298*:1265, 1978.
80. Cox, D. W., Breckenridge, W. C., and Little, J. A.: Inheritance of apolipoprotein C-II deficiency with hypertriglyceridemia and pancreatitis. N. Engl. J. Med. *299*:1421, 1978.
81. Brown, M. S., and Goldstein, J. L.: Familial hypercholesterolemia: A genetic defect in the low-density lipoprotein receptor. N. Engl. J. Med. *294*(25):1386, 1976.
82. Fredrickson, D. S., Morganroth, J., and Levy, R. I.: Type III hyperlipoproteinemia: An analysis of two contemporary definitions. Ann. Intern. Med. *82*:150, 1975.
83. Morganroth, J., Levy, R. I., and Fredrickson, D. S.: The biochemical, clinical and genetic features of Type III hyperlipoproteinemia. Ann. Intern. Med. *82*:158, 1975.
84. Kushwaha, R. S., Hazzard, W. R., Wahl, P. W., and Hoover, J. J.: Type III hyperlipoproteinemia: Diagnosis in whole plasma by apolipoprotein-E immunoassay. Ann. Intern. Med. *86*:509, 1977.
85. Ghiselli, G., Gascon, P., and Brewer, H. B., Jr.: Type III hyperlipoproteinemia associated with apolipoprotein E deficiency (letter). Science *214*:1239, 1980.
86. Wallace, R. B., Hoover, J., Sandler, D., and Rifkind, B. M.: Altered plasma-lipids associated with oral contraceptive or estrogen consumption. Lancet *2*:11, 1977.
87. Goldstein, J. L., Hazzard, W. R., Schrott, H. G., Bierman, E. L., and Motulsky, A. G.: Hyperlipidemia in coronary heart disease. I. Lipid levels in 500 survivors of myocardial infarction. J. Clin. Invest. *52*:1533, 1973.
88. Wood, P. D., Stern, M. P., Silvers, A., Reaven, G. M., and Von der Groeben, J.: Prevalence of plasma lipoprotein abnormalities in a free-living population of the Central Valley, California. Circulation *45*:114, 1972.
89. Greenberg, B. H., Blackwelder, W. C., and Levy, R. I.: Primary Type V hyperlipoproteinemia. A descriptive study of 32 families. Ann. Intern. Med. *87*:526, 1977.
90. Kannel, W. B.: Role of blood pressure in cardiovascular disease: The Framingham Study. Angiology *26*:1, 1975.
91. Feinleib, M., Garrison, R., Borhani, N., Rosenman, R., and Christian, J.: Studies of hypertension in twins. *In* Paul, O. (ed.): Epidemiology and Control of Hypertension. Miami, Symposia Specialists, 1975, pp. 3–20.
92. Feinleib, M.: Genetics and familial aggregation of blood pressure. *In* Onesti, G., and Klimt, C. (eds.): Hypertension Determinants. Complications and Intervention. The Fifth Hahnemann International Symposium on Hypertension. New York, Grune and Stratton, 1979, pp. 35–48.
93. Feinleib, M., and Williams, R. R.: Relative risks of myocardial infarction, cardiovascular disease and peripheral vascular disease by type of smoking. Proc. Third World Conf. Smoking and Health *1*:243, 1976.
94. Aronow, W. S.: Effect of cigarette smoking and of carbon monoxide on coronary heart disease. Chest *70*:514, 1976.
95. The Health Consequences of Smoking. Washington, D.C., U.S. Public Health Service, 1973.
96. The Health Consequences of Smoking. Washington, D.C., U.S. Public Health Service, 1971.
97. Wilhelmsson, C., Vedin, J. A., Elmfeldt, D., Tibblin, G., and Wilhelmsen, L.: Smoking and myocardial infarction. Lancet *1*:415, 1975.
98. Report of the Surgeon General: Smoking and Health. U.S. Department of Health, Education and Welfare, Public Health Service Publ. No. 79-50066, 1979.
99. Rogot, E.: Smoking and general mortality among U.S. veterans, 1954–1969. Washington, D.C., DHEW Publ. No. (NIH) 74-544, 1974.
100. Gordon, T., Kannel, W. B., McGee, D., and Dawber, T. R.: Death and coronary attacks in men after giving up cigarette smoking. A report from the Framingham study. Lancet *2*:1345, 1974.
101. Doyle, J. T., Dawber, T. R., Kannel, W. B., Kinch, S. H., and Kahn, H. A.: The relationship of cigarette smoking to coronary heart disease. The second report of the combined experience of the Albany, N.Y., and Framingham, Mass. studies. J.A.M.A. *190*:886, 1964.
102. Friedman, G. D., and Siegelaub, A. B.: Changes after quitting cigarette smoking. Circulation *61*:716, 1980.
103. Friedman, G. D., Petitti, D. B., Bawol, R. D., and Siegelaub, A. B.: Mortality in cigarette smokers and quitters. Effect of base-line differences. N. Engl. J. Med. *304*:1407, 1981.
104. Castelli, W. P., Garrison, R. J., Dawber, T. R., McNamara, P. M., Feinleib, M., and Kannel, W. B.: The filter cigarette and coronary heart disease: The Framingham Study. Lancet *2*:109, 1981.
105. Rose, G., and Hamilton, P. J. S.: A randomised controlled trial of the effect on middle-aged men of advice to stop smoking. J. Epidemiol. Community Health *32*:275, 1978.
106. Hjermann, I., Velve-Byre, K., Holme, I., and Leren, P.: Effect of diet and

smoking intervention on the incidence of coronary heart disease. Report from the Oslo Study Group of a randomised trial in healthy men. Lancet *2*:1303, 1981.

106a. Multiple Risk Factor Intervention Trial Research Group: Multiple Risk Factor Intervention Trial. Risk factor changes and mortality results. J.A.M.A. *248*: 1465, 1982.

107. Jenkins, C. D., Rosenman, R. H., and Zyzanski, S. J.: Cigarette smoking: Its relationship to coronary heart disease and related risk factors in the Western Collaborative Group Study. Circulation *38*:1140, 1968.

108. Shurtleff, D.: Some characteristics related to the incidence of cardiovascular disease and death: The Framingham Study, 18-year follow-up. Washington, D.C., DHEW Publ. No. (NIH) 74-599, Section No. 30, 1974.

109. Slone, D., Shapiro, S., Rosenberg, L., Kaufman, D. W., Hartz, S. C., Rossi, A. C., Stolley, P. D., and Miettinen, O. S.: Relation of cigarette smoking to myocardial infarction in young women. N. Engl. J. Med. *298*:1273–1276, 1978.

110. Shapiro, S., Weinblatt, E., Frank, C. W., and Sager, S. V.: Incidence of coronary heart disease in a population insured for medical care (HIP): Myocardial infarction, angina pectoris, and possible myocardial infarction. Am. J. Public Health *59*(Suppl.):1, 1969.

111. Mulcahy, R., and Hickey, N.: Cigarette smoking habits of patients with coronary heart disease. Br. Heart J. *28*:404, 1966.

112. Garrison, R. J., Kannel, W. B., Feinleib, M., Castelli, W. P., McNamara, P. M., and Padgett, S. J.: Cigarette Smoking and HDL cholesterol. The Framingham Offspring Study. Atherosclerosis *30*:17, 1978.

113. Ostrander, L. D., and Epstein, F. H.: Diabetes, hyperglycemia and atherosclerosis: New research directions. *In* Fajans, S. (ed.): Diabetes Mellitus. Washington, D.C., DHEW Publ. No. (NIH) 76-854, 1976.

114. Sharkey, T. P.: Diabetes mellitus—present problems and new research. The heart and vascular disease. J. Am. Diet. Assoc. *58*:336, 1971.

115. Report of the National Commission on Diabetes. Washington, D.C., DHEW Publ. No. (NIH) 76-1022, 1975.

116. Garcia, M. J., McNamara, P. M., Gordon, T., and Kannel, W. B.: Morbidity and mortality of diabetes in the Framingham population. Sixteen year follow-up study. Diabetes *23*:105, 1976.

117. Ostrander, L. D., Jr., Block, W. D., Lamphiear, D. E., and Epstein, F. H.: Altered carbohydrate and lipid metabolism and coronary heart disease among men in Tecumseh, Michigan. *In* Camerini-Davalos, R. A., and Cole, H. S. (eds.): Vascular and Neurological Changes in Early Diabetes. New York, Academic Press, 1973, p. 73.

118. Fuller, J. N., Shipley, M. J., Rose, G., Jarrett, R. J., and Keen, N.: Coronary heart disease risk and impaired glucose tolerance. The Whitehall Study. Lancet *1*:1373, 1980.

119. Knowles, H. C., Jr.: Magnitude of the renal failure problem in diabetic patients. Kidney International, Vol. 6, No. 4, Suppl. 1. New York, Springer-Verlag, 1974.

120. Vigorita, V. J., Moore, G. W., and Hutchins, G. N.: Absence of correlation between coronary arterial atherosclerosis and severity or duration of diabetes mellitus of adult onset. Am. J. Cardiol. *46*:535, 1980.

121. Coronary Drug Project Research Group, Baltimore: The prognostic importance of plasma glucose levels and the use of oral hypoglycemic drugs after myocardial infarction in men. Diabetes *26*:453, 1977.

122. Sosenko, J. N., Breslow, J. L., Niettinen, O. S., and Gabbay, K. N.: Hyperglycemia and plasma lipid levels. A prospective study of young insulin-dependent diabetic patients. N. Engl. J. Med. *302*:650, 1980.

123. University Group Diabetes Program: A study of the effects of hypoglycemic agents on vascular complications in patients with adult-onset diabetes. II. Mortality results. Diabetes *19*(Suppl. 2):785, 1970.

124. Knatterud, G. L., Klimt, C. R., Levin, M. E., Jacobson, M. E., and Goldner, M. G.: Effects of hypoglycemic agents in vascular complications in patients with adult-onset diabetes. VII. Mortality and selected nonfatal events with insulin treatment. J.A.M.A. *240*:37, 1978.

125. Carlstrom, S.: Treatment with sulphonylurea drugs and cardiovascular disease. Proc. Ninth Congr. Int. Diabetes Federation. Amsterdam, Excerpta Medica, 1977, pp. 426–433.

126. Hall, A. P.: Correlations among hyperuricemia, hypercholesterolemia, coronary disease and hypertension. Arthritis Rheum. *8*:846, 1965.

127. Fessel, W. J.: High uric acid as an indicator of cardiovascular disease: Independence from obesity. Am. J. Med. *68*:401, 1980.

128. Persky, V. W., Dyer, A. R., Idris-Soven, E., Stamler, J., Shekelle, K. B., Schoenberger, J. A., Berkson, D. M., and Lindberg, H. A.: Uric acid: a risk factor for coronary heart disease? Circulation *59*:969, 1979.

129. Kannel, W. B., Hjortland, M. C., McNamara, P. M., and Gordon, T.: Menopause and risk of cardiovascular disease: The Framingham Study. Ann. Intern. Med. *85*:447, 1976.

130. Mann, J. I., and Inman, W. H. W.: Oral contraceptives and death from myocardial infarction. Br. Med. J. *2*:245, 1975.

131. Jick, H., Dinan, B., and Rothman, K. J.: Oral contraceptives and nonfatal myocardial infarction. J.A.M.A. *239*:1403, 1978.

132. Layde, P. M., Beral, V., and Kay, C. R.: Further analysis of mortality in oral contraceptive users. Royal College of General Practitioners' Oral Contraception Study. Lancet *1*:549, 1981.

133. Slone, D., Shapiro, S., Kaufman, D. W., Rosenberg, L., Niettinen, O. S., and Stolley, P. D.: Risk of myocardial infarction in relation to current and discontinued use of oral contraceptives. N. Engl. J. Med. *305*:420, 1981.

134. Vessey, M. P., McPherson, K., and Yeates, D.: Mortality in oral contraceptive users. Lancet *1*:549, 1981.

135. Wallace, R. B., Hoover, J., Barrett-Conner, E., Rifkind, B. M., Hunninghake, D. B., Mackenthun, A., and Heiss, G.: Altered plasma lipid and lipoprotein levels associated with oral contraceptive and estrogen use. Lancet *2*:111, 1979.

136. Rosenberg, L., Armstrong, B., and Jick, H.: Myocardial infarction and estrogen therapy in post-menopausal women. N. Engl. J. Med. *294*:1256, 1976.

137. Pfeffer, R. I., Whipple, G. H., Kurosaki, T. T., and Chapman, J. M.: Coronary risk and estrogen use in post-menopausal women. Am. J. Epidemiol. *107*:479, 1978.

138. Barrett-Conner, E., Brown, W. V., Turner, J., Austin, M., and Criqui, M.: Heart disease risk factors and hormone use in postmenopausal women. J.A.M.A. *241*:2167, 1979.

139. Ross, R. K., Paganini-Hill, A., Mack, T. M., Arthur, N., and Henderson, B. E.: Menopausal oestrogen therapy and protection from death from ischaemic heart disease. Lancet *1*:858, 1981.

140. Byar, D. P.: The Veterans Administration Cooperative Urological Research Group's studies on cancer of the prostate. Cancer *32*:1126, 1973.

141. The Coronary Drug Project Research Group: The Coronary Drug Project. Initial findings leading to modification of its research protocol. J.A.M.A. *226*:652, 1973.

142. The Coronary Drug Project Research Group: The Coronary Drug Project. Findings leading to discontinuation of the 2.5 mg/day estrogen group. J.A.M.A. *226*:652, 1973.

143. Jick, H., Dinan, B., and Rothman, K. J.: Noncontraceptive estrogens and nonfatal myocardial infarction. J.A.M.A. *239*:1407, 1978.

144. Clarkson, T. B., and Alexander, N. J.: Does vasectomy increase the risk of atherosclerosis? J. Cardiovasc. Med. *5*:999, 1980.

145. Walker, A. M., Jick, H., Hunter, J. R., Danford, A., Watkins, R. N., Alhadeff, L., and Rothman, K. J.: Vasectomy and non-fatal myocardial infarction. Lancet *1*:13, 1981.

145a. Goldacre, M. J., Holford, T. R., and Vessey, M. P.: Cardiovascular disease and vasectomy. Findings from two epidemiologic studies. N. Engl. J. Med. *308*: 805, 1983.

146. Heller, R. F., Jacobs, H. S., Vermeulen, A., and Deslypere, J. P.: Androgens, oestrogens, and coronary heart disease. Br. Med. J. *282*:438, 1981.

147. Lew, E. A., and Garfinkel, L.: Variations in mortality by weight among 750,000 men and women. J. Chronic Dis. *32*:563, 1979.

148. Keys, A.: Coronary heart disease—the global picture. Atherosclerosis *22*:149, 1975.

149. Keys, A.: Overweight and the risk of heart attack and sudden death. *In* Bray, G. A. (ed.): Obesity in Perspective. Vol. 2, Part 2. Washington, D. C., DHEW Publ. No. (NIH) 75-708, 1976, p. 215.

150. Gordon, T., and Kannel, W. B.: Obesity and cardiovascular disease: The Framingham Study. Clin. Endocrinol. Metab. *5*:367, 1976.

151. Hubert, N., Feinleib, M., McNamara, P. M., and Castelli, W. P.: Obesity as an independent risk factor for cardiovascular disease in Framingham. Presented at the Twenty-Second Annual Cardiovascular Epidemiology Meeting, March 1982, San Antonio, Texas.

151a. Hubert, H. B., Feinleib, M., McNamara, P. M., and Castelli, W. P.: Obesity as an independent risk factor for cardiovascular disease. A 26-year follow-up of participants in the Framingham Heart Study. Circulation *67*:968, 1983.

152. Grande, F.: Assessment of body fat in man. *In* Bray, G. A. (ed.): Obesity in Perspective. Vol. 2, Part 2. Washington, D.C., DHEW Publ. No. (NIH) 76-852, 1976, pp. 189–203.

153. Bray, G. A.: Standard for definitions of overweight and obesity. *In* Bray, G. A. (ed.): Obesity in Perspective. Vol. 1, Part 1, Chap. 2. Washington, D.C., DHEW Publ. No. (NIH) 75-708, 1976, p. 7.

154. Keys, A., Fidanza, F., Karvonen, M. J., Kimura, N., and Taylor, H. L.: Indices of relative weight and obesity. J. Chronic Dis. *25*:322, 1972.

155. Ashley, F. W., and Kannel, W. B.: Relation of weight change to changes in atherogenic traits: The Framingham Study. J. Chronic Dis. *27*:103, 1974.

156. Streja, D. A., Boyko, E., and Rabkin, S. W.: Changes in plasma high-density lipoprotein cholesterol concentration after weight reduction in grossly obese subjects. Br. Med. J. *281*:770, 1980.

157. Kagan, A., Gordon, T., Rhoads, G. G., and Schiffman, J. C.: Some factors related to coronary heart disease incidence in Honolulu Japanese men: The Honolulu Heart Study. Int. J. Epidemiol. *4*:271, 1975.

158. Rabkin, S. W., Mathewson, F. A. L., and Hsu, P.: Relation of body weight to development of ischemic heart disease in a cohort of young North American men after a 26 year observation period: The Manitoba Study. Am. J. Cardiol. *39*:452, 1977.

159. Paffenbarger, R. S., and Hale, W. E.: Work activity and coronary heart mortality. N. Engl. J. Med. *292*:545, 1975.

160. Paffenbarger, R. S., Hale, W. E., Brand, R. J., and Hyde, R. T.: Work-energy level, personal characteristics and fatal heart attack: A birth cohort effect. Am. J. Epidemiol. *105*:200, 1977.

161. Cooper, K. H., Pollock, M. L., Martin, R. P., White, S. R., Linnerud, A. L., and Jackson, A.: Physical fitness levels vs. selected coronary risk factors. A cross-sectional study. J.A.M.A. *236*:166, 1976.

162. Hickey, N., Mulcahy, R., Bourke, G. J., Graham, J., and Wilson-Davis, K.: Study of coronary risk factors related to physical activity in 15,171 men. Br. Med. J. *3*:507, 1975.

163. Fox, S. M., and Naughton, J. P.: Physical activity and the prevention of coronary heart disease. Prev. Med. *1*:92, 1972.

164. Wyndham, C. H.: The role of physical activity in the prevention of ischemic heart disease. S. Afr. Med. J. *36*:7, 1979.

165. Siegel, A. J., Hennekens, C. H., Rosner, B., and Karlson, L. K.: Paternal his-

tory of coronary-heart disease reported by marathon runners. N. Engl. J. Med. *301*:90, 1979.
166. Noakes, T. D., Opie, C. H., Rose, A. G., and Kleynhans, P. H. T.: Autopsy-proved coronary atherosclerosis in marathon runners. N. Engl. J. Med. *301*:86, 1979.
167. Morris, J. N., Everitt, M. G., Pollard, R., Chave, S. P. W., and Semmence, A. M.: Vigorous exercise in leisure-time: Protection against coronary heart disease. Lancet *2*:1207, 1980.
167a. Gibbons, L. W., Blair, S. N., Cooper, K. H., and Smith, M: Association between coronary heart disease risk factors and physical fitness in healthy adult women. Circulation *67*:977, 1983.
168. Wood, P. D., and Haskell, W. L.: The effect of exercise on plasma high density lipoproteins. Lipids *14*:417, 1979.
169. Hartung, G. H., Foreyt, J. P., Mitchell, R. E., Vlasek, I., and Gotto, A. M., Jr.: Relation of diet to high-density-lipoprotein cholesterol in middle-aged marathon runners, joggers, and inactive men. N. Engl. J. Med. *302*:357, 1980.
170. Soman, V. R., Koivisto, V. A., Deibert, D., Felig, P., and DeFronzo, R. A.: Increased insulin sensitivity and insulin binding to monocytes after physical training. N. Engl. J. Med. *301*:1200, 1979.
171. Williams, R. S., Logue, E. E., Lewis, J. L., Barton, T., Stead, N. W., Wallace, A. G., and Pizzo, S. V.: Physical conditioning augments the fibrinolytic response to venous occlusion in healthy adults. N. Engl. J. Med. *302*:987, 1980.
172. Friedman, H., and Rosenman, R. H.: Type A Behavior and Your Heart. New York, Alfred A. Knopf, 1974.
173. Dembroski, T. M., Feinlieb, M., Haynes, S. G., Shields, J. L., and Weiss, S. M. (eds.): Proceedings of the forum on coronary-prone behavior. Washington, D. C., DHEW Publ. No. (NIH) 78-1451, 1978.
174. Haynes, S. G., Feinleib, M., and Kannel, W. B.: The relationship of psychosocial factors to coronary heart disease in the Framingham Study. III. Eight-year incidence of coronary heart disease. Am. J. Epidemiol. *111*:37, 1980.
175. Review Panel on Coronary-Prone Behavior and Coronary Heart Disease. Coronary-prone behavior and coronary heart disease: A critical review. Circulation *63*:1199, 1981.
176. Rosenman, R. H.: History and definition of the Type A coronary-prone behavior pattern. *In* Dembroski, T. M., Feinleib, M., Haynes, S. G., Shields, J. L., and Weiss, S. M. (eds.): Proceedings of the forum on coronary-prone behavior. Washington, D.C., DHEW Publ. No. (NIH) 78-1451, 1978, p. 13.
177. Haynes, S. G., Feinleib, M., Levine, S., Scotch, N., and Kannel, W. B.: The relationship of psychosocial factors to coronary heart disease in the Framingham Study. II. Prevalence of coronary heart disease. Am. J. Epidemiol. *107*:384, 1978.
178. Haynes, S. G., and Feinleib, M.: Type A behavior and the incidence of coronary heart disease in the Framingham Heart Study. Adv. Cardiol. *29*:85, 1982.
179. Frank, K. A., Heller, S. S., Kornfeld, D. S., Sporn, A. A., and Weiss, M. B.: Type A behavior pattern and coronary angiographic findings. J.A.M.A. *240*:761, 1978.
180. Jenkins, C. D.: Recent evidence supporting psychologic and social risk factors for coronary disease. N. Engl. J. Med. *294*:987, 1976.
181. Casscells, W., Hennekens, C. H., Evans, D., Rosener, B., DeSilva, R. A., Lown, B., Davies, J. E., and Jesse, M. J.: Retirement and coronary mortality. Lancet *1*:1288, 1980.
182. Haynes, S. G., and Feinleib, M.: Women, work and coronary heart disease: Prospective findings from the Framingham Heart Study. Am. J. Public Health *70*:133, 1980.
183. Report from the National Heart and Lung Institute Task Force on Genetic Factors in Atherosclerotic Disease. Washington, D.C., DHEW Publ. No. (NIH) 76-922, 1976.
184. Lee, J., Lauer, R. M., and Clarke, W. R.: Coronary risk factors in children. *In* Engle, M. E. (ed.): Pediatric Cardiovascular Disease, Philadelphia, F.A. Davis, 1981.
185. Snowden, D. B., McNamara, P. M., Garrison, R. J., Feinleib, M., Kannel, W. B., and Epstein, F. H.: Predicting coronary heart disease in siblings—a multivariate assessment: The Framingham Heart Study. Am. J. Epidemiol. *115*:217, 1982.
185a. Neufeld, H. N., and Goldbourt, U.: Coronary heart disease: Genetic aspects. Circulation *67*:943, 1983.
186. The diet and all-cause death rate in the Seven Countries Study. Lancet *2*:58, 1981.
187. Kato, H., Tillotson, J., Nichaman, M., Rhoads, G., and Hamilton, H.: Epidemiologic studies of coronary heart disease and stroke in Japanese men living in Japan, Hawaii, and California: Serum lipids and diet. Am. J. Epidemiol. *97*:372, 1973.
188. Phillips, R. L., Lemon, F. R., Beeson, L., and Kuzman, J. W.: Coronary heart disease mortality among Seventh-Day Adventists with differing dietary habits: A preliminary report. Am. J. Clin. Nutr. *31*:S191, 1978.
189. The Framingham Study. An Epidemiological Investigation of Cardiovascular Disease. Section 23. The Framingham Diet Study: Diet and the regulation of serum cholesterol. Washington, D.C., U.S. Government Printing Office, 1970.
190. Nichols, A. B., Ravenscroft, C., Lamphiear, D. E., and Ostrander, L. D., Jr.: Daily nutritional intake and serum lipid levels. The Tecumseh Study. Am. J. Clin. Nutr. *29*:1384, 1976.
191. Shekelle, R. B., Shryock, A. M., Paul, O., Lepper, M., Stamler, J., Liu, S., and Raynor, W. J.: Diet, serum cholesterol, and death from coronary heart disease. The Western Electric Study. N. Engl. J. Med. *304*:65, 1981.
192. NIH release first data from Lipid Research Clinic Program. J. Am. Oil Chemists' Soc. *54*:717A, 1977.
193. Ahrens, E. H., Jr., Insull, W., Blomstrand, R., Hirsch, J., Tsaltas, T. T., and Peterson, M. L.: The influence of dietary fats on serum-lipid levels in man. Lancet *1*:943, 1957.
194. Keys, A., Anderson, J. T., and Grande, F.: Serum cholesterol response to changes in the diet. Metabolism *4*:747, 1965.
195. Mattson, F. H., Erickson, B. A., and Kligman, A. M.: Effect of dietary cholesterol on serum cholesterol in man. Am. J. Clin. Nutr. *25*:589, 1972.
196. Kuller, L. H.: Epidemiology of cardiovascular disease: Current perspectives. Am. J. Epidemiol. *104*:425, 1976.
197. Connor, W. E., and Connor, S. E.: Sucrose and carbohydrate. *In* Present Knowledge in Nutrition. 4th ed. New York, Nutrition Foundation, Inc., 1976, p. 33.
198. Bierman, E. L., and Porte, D., Jr.: Carbohydrate intolerance and lipidemia. Ann. Intern. Med. *68*:926, 1968.
199. Glueck, C. J., Levy, R. I., and Fredrickson, D. S.: Immunoreactive insulin, glucose tolerance and carbohydrate inducibility in types II, III, and IV hyperlipoproteinemia. Diabetes *18*:739, 1969.
200. Jenkins, D. J. A., Leeds, A. R., Gassull, M. A., Cochet, B., and Alberti, K. G.: Decrease in postprandial insulin and glucose concentrations by guar and pectin. Ann. Intern. Med. *86*:20, 1977.
201. Kritchevsky, D.: Dietary fiber and other dietary factors in hypercholesterolemia. Am. J. Clin. Nutr. *30*:979, 1977.
202. Report of the Hypertension Task Force. Vol. 8. Current Research and Recommendations from the Task Force Subgroups on (1) Renin-Angiotensin-Aldosterone; (2) Salt and Water. U.S. DHEW, Public Health Service, NIH Publ. No. 79-1630, 1979.
203. Page, L. B.: Epidemiologic evidence on etiology of human hypertension and its possible prevention. Am. Heart J. *91*:527, 1976.
204. Reisin, E., Abel, R., Modan, M., Silverberg, D. S., Eliahou, H. E., and Modan, B.: Effect of weight loss without salt restriction and the reduction of blood pressure in overweight hypertensive patients. N. Engl. J. Med. *298*:1, 1978.
205. Shurtleff, D.: Some characteristics related to the incidence of cardiovascular disease and death: Framingham Study, 16-year follow-up. *In* Kannel, W. B., and Gordon, T. (eds.): The Framingham Study, Section 26, Washington, D.C., U.S. Government Printing Office, 1970.
206. Yano, K., Rhoads, G. G., and Kagan, A.: Coffee, alcohol and risk of coronary heart disease among Japanese men living in Hawaii. N. Engl. J. Med. *297*:405, 1977.
207. Hennekens, C. H., Willett, W., Rosner, B., Cole, D. S., and Mayrent, S. L.: Effects of beer, wine, and liquor in coronary deaths. J.A.M.A. *242*:1973, 1979.
208. Marmot, M. G., Rose, G., Shipley, M. J., and Thomas, B. J.: Alcohol and mortality: A U-shaped curve. Lancet *1*:580, 1981.
209. Kozarevic, D., McGee, D., Vojrodic, N., Racic, Z., Dawber, T. R., Gordon, T., and Zukel, W.: Frequency of alcohol consumption and morbidity and mortality: The Yugoslavia Cardiovascular Disease Study. Lancet *1*:613, 1980.
210. Wilhelmsen, L., Wedel, H., and Tibblin, G.: Multivariate analysis of risk factors for coronary heart disease. Circulation *48*:950, 1973.
211. Stason, W. B., Neff, R. K., Miettinen, O. S., and Jick, H.: Alcohol consumption and nonfatal myocardial infarction. Am. J. Epidemiol. *104*:603, 1976.
212. Dyer, A. R., Stamler, J., Paul, O., Berkson, D. M., Lepper, M. N., McKean, H., Shekelle, R. B., Lindburg, H. A., and Garside, D.: Alcohol consumption, cardiovascular risk factors and mortality in two Chicago epidemiologic studies. Circulation *56*:1067, 1977.
213. Castelli, W. P., Gordon, T., Hjortland, M. C., Kagan, A., Doyle, J. T., Hames, C. G., Hulley, S. B., and Zukel, W. B.: Alcohol and blood lipids. The Cooperative Lipoprotein Phenotyping Study. Lancet *2*:154, 1977.
214. Gordon, T., Ernst, N., Fisher, M., and Rifkind, B. M.: Alcohol and high-density lipoprotein cholesterol. Circulation *64*(Suppl III):III–63, 1981.
215. Dawber, T. R., Kannel, W. B., and Gordon, T.: Coffee and cardiovascular disease: Observations from the Framingham Study. N. Engl. J. Med. *291*:871, 1974.
216. Boston Collaborative Drug Surveillance Program: Coffee drinking and acute myocardial infarction. Lancet *2*:1278, 1972.
217. Jick, H., Miettinen, O. S., Neff, R. K., Shapiro, S., Heinonen, O. P., and Slone, D.: Coffee and myocardial infarction. N. Engl. J. Med. *289*:63, 1973.
218. Crawford, M. D., Clayton, D. G., Stanley, F., and Shaper, A. G.: An epidemiological study of sudden death in hard and soft water areas. J. Chronic Dis. *30*:69, 1977.
219. Medalie, J. H., Levene, C., Papier, L., Goldbourt, U., Dreyfuss, F., Oron, D., Neufeld, H., and Riss, E.: Blood groups, myocardial infarction, and angina pectoris among 10,000 adult males. N. Engl. J. Med. *285*:1348, 1971.
220. Garrison, R. J., Havlik, R. J., Harris, R. B., Feinleib, M., Kannel, W. B., and Padgett, S. J.: ABO blood group and cardiovascular disease. The Framingham Study. Atherosclerosis *25*:311, 1976.
221. Meade, T. W., North, W. R. S., Chakrabarti, R., Stirling, Y., Haines, A. P., Thompson, S. G., and Brozovic, M.: Haemostatic function and cardiovascular death: Early results of a prospective study. Lancet *1*:1050, 1980.
222. Dintenfass, L.: Viscosity factors in hypertensive and cardiovascular disease. Cardiovasc. Med. *2*:337, 1977.
223. Sorlie, P. D., Garcia-Palmieri, M. R., Costas, R., Jr., and Havlik, R. J.: Hematocrit and risk of coronary heart disease: The Puerto Rico Heart Health Program. Am. Heart J. *101*:456, 1981.
224. Curry, R. C., Jr., and Roberts, W. C.: Status of the coronary arteries in the nephrotic syndrome. Analysis of 20 necropsy patients aged 15 to 35 years

to determine if coronary atherosclerosis is accelerated. Am. J. Med. *63*:183, 1977.
225. Wass, V. J., Jarrett, R. J., Chilvers, C., and Cameron, J. S.: Does the nephrotic syndrome increase the risk of cardiovascular disease? Lancet *2*:664, 1979.
226. Lundsgaard-Hansen, P.: Intensive plasmapheresis as a risk factor for arteriosclerotic cardiovascular disease? Vox Sang. *33*:1, 1977.
227. Nicholls, A. J., Gatto, G. R. D., Edward, N., Engeset, J., and Macleod, M.: Accelerated atherosclerosis in long-term dialysis and renal-transplant patients: Fact or fiction? Lancet *1*:276, 1980.
228. Editorial: Thyroiditis, autoimmunity, and coronary risk factors. Lancet *2*:173, 1977.
229. Davis, R. F., and Engleman, E. G.: Incidence of myocardial infarction in patients with rheumatoid arthritis. Arthritis Rheum. *17*:527, 1974.
230. Rodgers, D. L.: Precocious myocardial infarction after radiation treatment for Hodgkin's disease. Chest *70*:675, 1976.
231. Doering, C., Ruhsenberger, C., and Phillips, D. S.: Ear-lobe creases and heart disease. J. Am. Geriatr. Soc. *25*:183, 1977.
232. Report of the American Heart Association Task Force on Environment and the Cardiovascular System (W. R. Harlan, Chairman). Impact of the Environment on Cardiovascular Disease. Circulation *63*:244A, 1981.
233. Anderson, T. W., and Rochard, C.: Cold snaps, snowfall and sudden death from ischemic heart disease. Can. Med. Assoc. J. *121*:1580, 1979.
234. Glass, R. I., Wiesenthal, A. M., Zack, M. M., and Preston, M.: Risk factors for myocardial infarction associated with the Chicago snowstorm of January 13–15, 1979. J.A.M.A. *245*:164, 1981.
235. Coronary Risk Handbook. Estimating risk of coronary heart disease in daily practice. New York, American Heart Association, 1973.
236. Five-year findings of the Hypertension Detection and Follow-up Program: I. Reduction in mortality of persons with high blood pressure, including mild hypertension. J.A.M.A. *242*:2562, 1979.
237. Report of the Management Committee. The Australian therapeutic trial in mild hypertension. Lancet *1*:1261, 1980.
238. Lipid Research Clinics Program: The Coronary Primary Prevention Trial: Design and implementation. J. Chronic Dis. *32*:609, 1979.
239. Pomerleau, O., Bass, F., and Crown, V.: Role of behavior modification in preventive medicine. N. Engl. J. Med. *292*:1277, 1975.
240. The Coronary Drug Project Research Group: The Coronary Drug Project: Factors influencing long-term prognosis after recovery from myocardial infarction. Three-year findings of the Coronary Drug Project. J. Chronic Dis. *27*:267, 1974.
241. Clarkson, T. B., Lehner, D. M., Wagner, W. D., St. Clair, R. W., Bond, M. G., and Bullock, B. C.: A study of atherosclerosis regression in *Macaca mulatta*. I. Design of experiment and lesion induction. Exp. Mol. Pathol. *30*:360, 1979.
242. Armstrong, M. L., Warner, E. D., and Connor, W. E.: Regression of coronary atheromatosis in rhesus monkeys. Circ. Res. *25*:59, 1970.
243. Armstrong, M. L., and Megan, M. B.: Arterial fibrous proteins in cynomolgus monkeys after atherogenic and regression diets. Circ. Res. *36*:256, 1975.
244. Vesselinovitch, D., Wissler, R. W., Hughes, R., and Borensztajn, J.: Reversal of advanced atherosclerosis in rhesus monkeys. Atherosclerosis *23*:155, 1976.
245. Starzl, T. E., Chase, H. P., Putnam, C. W., and Nora, J. J.: Follow-up of patient with portacaval shunt for the treatment of hyperlipidaemia. Lancet *2*:714, 1974.
246. Starzl, T. E., Chase, H. P., Putnam, C. W., Nora, J. J., Fennell, R. H., Jr., and Porter, K. A.: Portacaval shunt in hyperlipidaemia. Lancet *2*:1263, 1974.
247. Barndt, R., Jr., Blankenhorn, D. H., Crawford, D. W., and Brooks, S. H.: Regression and progression of early femoral atherosclerosis in treated hyperlipoproteinemic patients. Ann. Intern. Med. *86*:139, 1977.
248. Glueck, C. J., Mattson, F., and Bierman, E. L.: Sounding boards: Diet and coronary heart disease: Another view. N. Engl. J. Med. *298*:1471, 1978.
249. Status Report: Current Findings of the Lipid Research Clinics Program. Press conference given at NIH, Bethesda, Maryland, July 13, 1977. (Also cited in Clinical Trends in Cardiology, Vol. 7, No. 1, p. 1, 1977.)
250. Select Committee on Nutrition and Human Needs, United States Senate: Dietary Goals for the United States. 2nd ed. Washington, D.C., U.S. Government Printing Office, 1977.
251. Levy, R. I., and Rifkind, B. M.: Lipid-lowering drugs and hyperlipidemia. Drugs *6*:12, 1973.
252. Levy, R. I., Fredrickson, D. S., Shulman, R., Bilheimer, D. W., Breslow, J. L., Stone, N. J., Lux, S. E., Sloan, H. R., Krauss, R. M., and Herbert, P. N.: Dietary and drug treatment of primary hyperlipoproteinemia. Ann. Intern. Med. *77*:267, 1972.
252a. Heath, G. W., Ehasni, A. A., Hagberg, J. M., Hinderliter, J. M., and Goldberg, A. P.: Exercise training improves lipoprotein lipid profiles in patients with coronary artery disease. Am. Heart J. *105*:889, 1983.
253. Fredrickson, D. S., Levy, R. I., Bonnell, M., and Ernst, N.: Dietary Management of Hyperlipoproteinemia. Washington, D.C., DHEW Publ. No. (NIH) 75-110, 1974.
254. Gotto, A. M., Jr.: Drug treatment of hyperlipidemia. Mod. Med. February 15, 1978, p. 92.
255. Levy, R. I.: Drugs used in the treatment of hyperlipoproteinemia. *In* Goodman, A. G. (ed.): Goodman and Gilman's The Pharmacological Basis of Therapeutics. 6th ed. New York, Macmillan, 1980, pp. 834–847.
256. Levy, R. I.: Hyperlipoproteinemia and its management. J. Cardiovasc. Med. *5*:435, 1980.
257. Kane, J. P., Malloy, M. J., Tun, P., Phillips, N. R., Freedman, D. D., Williams, M. L., Rowe, J. S., and Havel, R. J.: Normalization of low-density-lipoprotein levels in heterozygous familial hypercholesterolemia with a combined drug regimen. N. Engl. J. Med. *304*:251, 1981.
257a. Mabuchi, H., Sakai, T., Sakai, Y., Yoshimura, A., Watanabe, A., Wakasugi, T., Koizumi, J., and Takeda, R.: Reduction of serum cholesterol in heterozygous patients and familial hypercholesterolemia. Additive effects of compactin and cholestyramine. N. Engl. J. Med. *308*:609, 1983.
258. The Coronary Drug Project: Clofibrate and niacin in coronary heart disease. J.A.M.A. *213*:360, 1975.
259. Report from the Committee of Principal Investigators: A cooperative trial in the primary prevention of ischaemic heart disease using clofibrate. Br. Heart J. *40*:1069, 1978.
260. Kuo, P. T., Hayase, K., Kostis, J. B., and Moreyra, A. E.: Use of combined diet and colestipol in long-term (7–7½ years) treatment of patients with type II hyperlipoproteinemia. Circulation *59*:199, 1979.
261. The Coronary Drug Project: Findings leading to further modifications of its protocol with respect to dextrothyroxine. J.A.M.A. *220*:996, 1972.
262. The Medical Letter on Drugs and Therapeutics: Probucol for hypercholesterolemia. Vol. 19, No. 10, May 20, 1977.
263. Heel, R. C., Brogden, R. N., Speight, T. M., and Avery, G. S.: Probucol: A review of its pharmacological properties and therapeutic use in patients with hypercholesterolemia. Drugs *15*:409, 1978.
264. Simons, L. A., Balasubramanian, S., and Beins, D. M.: Metabolic studies with probucol in hypercholesterolaemia. Atherosclerosis *40*:299, 1981.
265. Royal Society of Medicine: Gemfibrozil: A new lipid-lowering agent. Proc. R. Soc. Med. *69*(Suppl. *2*):1, 1976.
266. Levy, R. I., and Rifkind, B. M.: Lipid lowering drugs and hyperlipidaemia. *In* Avery, G. S. (ed.): Cardiovascular Drugs, Vol. 1: Antiarrhythmic, Antihypertensive and Lipid Lowering Drugs. Sydney, Australia, ADIS Press Australasia Pty., Ltd., 1977, p. 1.
267. Buchwald, H., Moore, R. B., and Varco, R. L.: Surgical treatment of hyperlipidemia. Circulation *49*(v29 Suppl. 1):1, 1974.
268. Thompson, G. R., and Gotto, A. M.: Ileal bypass in the treatment of hyperlipoproteinemia. Lancet *2*:35, 1973.
269. Starzl, T. E., Putnam, C. W., and Koep, L. J.: Portacaval shunt and hyperlipidemia. Arch. Surg. *113*:71, 1978.
270. Thompson, G. R., Myant, N. B., Kilpatrick, D., Oakley, C. M., Raphael, M. J., and Steiner, R. E.: Assessment of long-term plasma exchange for familial hypercholesterolaemia. Br. Heart J. *43*:680, 1980.
271. Pickering, G.: High Blood Pressure. New York, Grune and Stratton, 1968.
272. Hypertension Detection and Follow-up Program Cooperative Group: Five-year findings of the Hypertension Detection and Follow-up Program. J.A.M.A. *242*: 2562, 1979.
273. Kannel, W. B., Doyle, J. T., Fredrickson, D. T., and Harlan, W. R.: Report of the Ad Hoc Committee on Cigarette Smoking and Cardiovascular Diseases for Health Professionals. Circulation *57*:406A, 1978.
274. Adult use of tobacco — 1975. Atlanta, Georgia. Center for Disease Control, Bureau of Health Education, June, 1976.
275. Statistical Abstract of the United States, 1975, p. 751.
276. Hymowitz, N.: The practicing physician and smoking cessation. J. Med. Soc. N.J. *74*:139, 1977.
277. Bray, G. A. (ed.): Obesity in America. Washington, D.C., DHEW Publ. No. (NIH) 79-359, 1979.
278. Stuart, R. B.: Behavioral control of overeating: A status report. *In* Bray, G. (ed.): Obesity in Perspective. Washington, D.C., DHEW Publ. No. 75-708, 1973.
279. Young, C. M.: Dietary treatment of obesity. *In* Bray, G. (ed.): Obesity in Perspective. Washington, D.C., DHEW Publ. No. 75-708, 1973.
280. Hashim, S. A., and Porikos, K.: Food intake behavior in man: Implications for treatment of obesity. Clin. Endocrinol. Metab. *5*:503, 1976.
281. Hursch, L. M.: Exercise in weight reduction. Nebr. Med. J. *61*:158, 1976.
282. Bjorntorp, P.: Exercise in the treatment of obesity. Clin. Endocrinol. Metab. *5*:431, 1976.
283. Friedman, M., Thorensen, G. B., Gill, J. J., et al.: Recurrent Coronary Prevention Project Study: Methods, baseline results and preliminary findings. Circulation *66*:83, 1982.

36 CORONARY BLOOD FLOW AND MYOCARDIAL ISCHEMIA

by Eugene Braunwald, M.D., and Burton E. Sobel, M.D.

Hypoxia, or *hypoxemia,* is a state of reduced oxygen supply to tissue despite adequate perfusion; *anoxia* is the absence of oxygen supply despite adequate perfusion; *ischemia* is the condition of oxygen deprivation accompanied by inadequate removal of metabolites consequent to reduced perfusion. Although clinical manifestations of coronary insufficiency generally reflect the effects of ischemia, under selected experimental and clinical conditions, deprivation of oxygen can be separated from reduced washout of metabolites. For example, in isolated hearts perfused at high flow rates with media equilibrated with a gas mixture poor in oxygen, anoxia without ischemia results, since washout of metabolites is not hindered. An analogous situation is seen in patients with cyanotic congenital heart disease, as well as in those with cor pulmonale and marked hypoxemia but with a normal coronary circulation. In contrast, the reduction of regional myocardial perfusion in the presence of hyperbaric oxygen may produce localized ischemia with limitation of the removal of metabolites, without concomitant impairment of oxygen delivery to cuffs of cells surrounding myocardial capillaries.

Neither ischemia nor hypoxia can be defined in absolute terms, since the blood flow and quantity of oxygen required to support myocardium under one set of conditions will not necessarily pertain under another. In man, blood flow of 60 to 90 ml/min per 100 gm of myocardium is generally required under basal physiological conditions. On the other hand, when the mechanical activity of the heart and its metabolic requirements are markedly reduced, myocardial viability may be maintained by perfusion at much lower rates, approximately 10 to 20 ml/min per 100 gm, or even with complete interruption of perfusion for periods of up to 100 minutes. Examples of conditions that reduce oxygen needs include ventricular fibrillation, asystole, cardiopulmonary bypass, and hypothermia with or without cardiopulmonary bypass. Another example of lowered cardiac oxygen needs occurs following the administration of nitroglycerin and other nitrates, which reduce the preload and afterload, and of beta-adrenergic blockers, which lower heart rate and contractility. This reduction of oxygen needs is perhaps the *principal* mechanism by which these agents relieve anginal pain (p. 1349).

The importance of defining ischemia in *relative* rather than absolute terms is underscored by the use of a variety of stress tests to detect or assess the severity of coronary artery disease. Whether the endpoint is angina, deviation of the ST-segment on the electrocardiogram (Chap. 8), relative diminution of accumulation of ^{201}Tl in myocardial "perfusion images," regional wall motion disorders or diminution of ejection fraction detectable with gated blood pool images (Chap. 11), the underlying principle is the same. Induction of stress by exercise, atrial pacing, hand grip, or any other means leads to a transitory disparity in the balance between oxygen supply and demand. Although this balance may be adequate under conditions of rest, the disparity becomes manifest when stress is imposed.

CONTROL OF MYOCARDIAL OXYGEN CONSUMPTION

The heart is an aerobic organ; that is, it relies almost exclusively on the oxidation of substrates for the generation of energy, and it can develop only a small oxygen debt.

Therefore, in a steady state, determination of the heart's $\dot{V}O_2$ provides an accurate measure of its total metabolism.

It has been known for many years that the total metabolism of the arrested, quiescent heart is only a small fraction of that of the working organ. The $\dot{V}O_2$ of the beating canine heart ranges from 8 to 15 ml/min per 100 gm, while the $\dot{V}O_2$ of the noncontracting heart is approximately 1.5 ml/min per 100 gm.[1,2] This quantity of oxygen is required for those physiological metabolic processes not directly associated with contraction. Increases in the frequency of depolarization in the noncontracting heart are accompanied by only very small increases of $M\dot{V}O_2$. Indeed, the quantity of oxygen required for electrical activation of the heart is approximately only 0.5 per cent of the total oxygen consumed by the normal working heart; thus, the oxygen cost of electrical depolarization is trivial in relation to the cost of contractile activity.[3]

In 1915 Evans and Matsuoka concluded from studies on the Starling heart-lung preparation that "there is a relation between the tension set up on contraction and the metabolism of the contractile tissue."[4] Subsequently, experimental techniques for regulating the external performance of the heart improved enormously. In 1955, in a systematic investigation of the relative effects of aortic pressure, stroke volume, and heart rate on $M\dot{V}O_2$, it became apparent that it is not possible to estimate the energy needs of the myocardium simply from the external work produced by the heart when work is calculated in the classic manner as the product of developed pressure and stroke volume. As a corollary, it was shown that myocardial efficiency, i.e., the ratio of the work performed to the oxygen consumed, varies widely depending on the hemodynamic conditions.[5,6] These investigations suggested that the tension-time index, i.e., the area under the left ventricular pressure curve, is an important determinant of the $M\dot{V}O_2$ (Fig. 36–1). Subsequently, it was emphasized that the tension in the wall of the

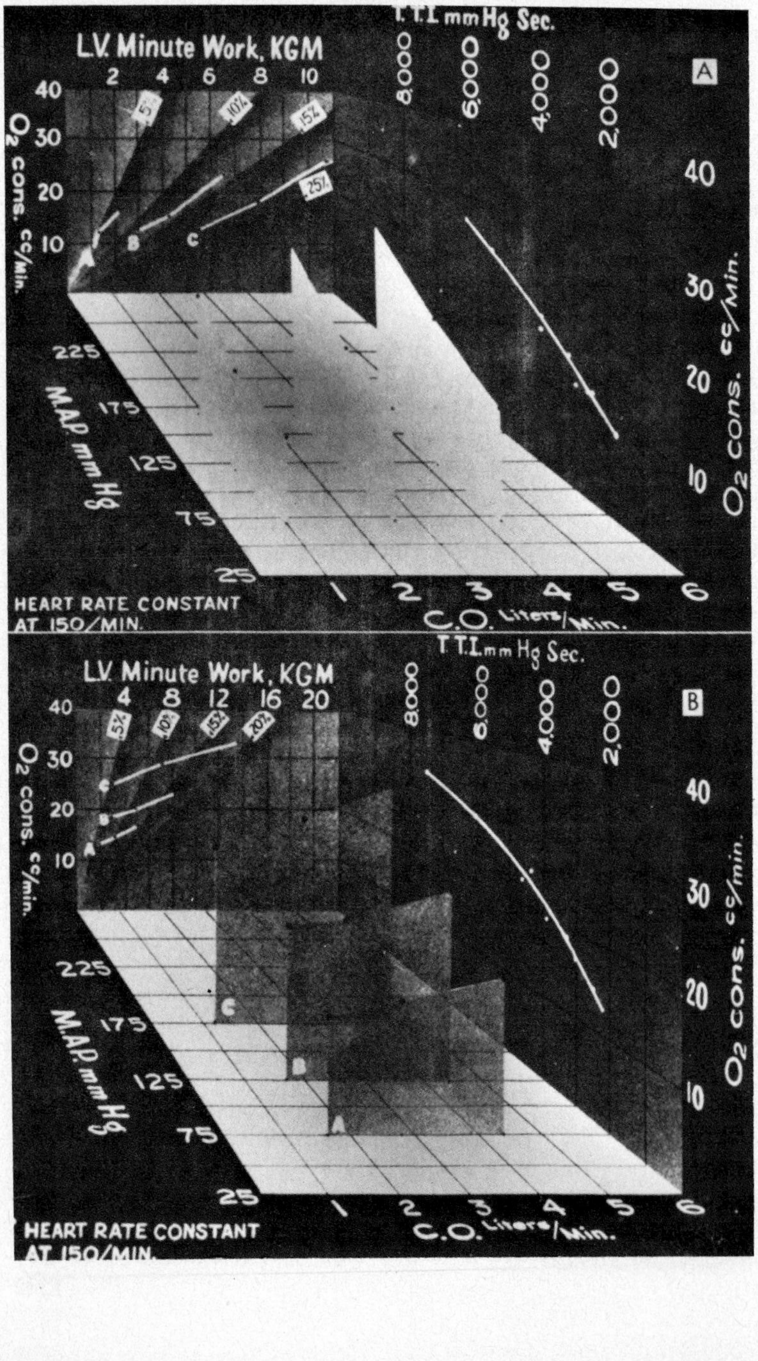

FIGURE 36–1 Summary of the interrelationships between various hemodynamic variables and myocardial oxygen consumption. In both top and bottom panels, the *base grids* show the experimental conditions, cardiac output (C.O.), and aortic pressure (M.A.P.) at which each determination of oxygen consumption was made. The height above the base grid of each experimental point represents its oxygen consumption. The *rear grids* show the plot of left ventricular minute work against myocardial oxygen consumption. The shaded lines on the rear grid labeled with percentage figures are isoefficiency lines. The *right grids* show the relation between the tension-time index (T.T.I.) in mm Hg-sec and myocardial oxygen consumption.

A, Three pressure runs at low, medium, and high levels of cardiac output. Note the negligible change in external efficiency as aortic pressure is increased within any given run. *B*, Three flow runs at low, medium, and high mean levels of aortic pressure. Note the increase in external efficiency within the course of any given flow run. (From Sarnoff, S. J., Braunwald, E., Welch, G. H., Jr., Case, R. B., Stainsby, W. N., and Macruz, R.: Hemodynamic determinants of oxygen consumption of the heart with special reference to the tension-time index. Am. J. Physiol. *192*:148, 1958.)

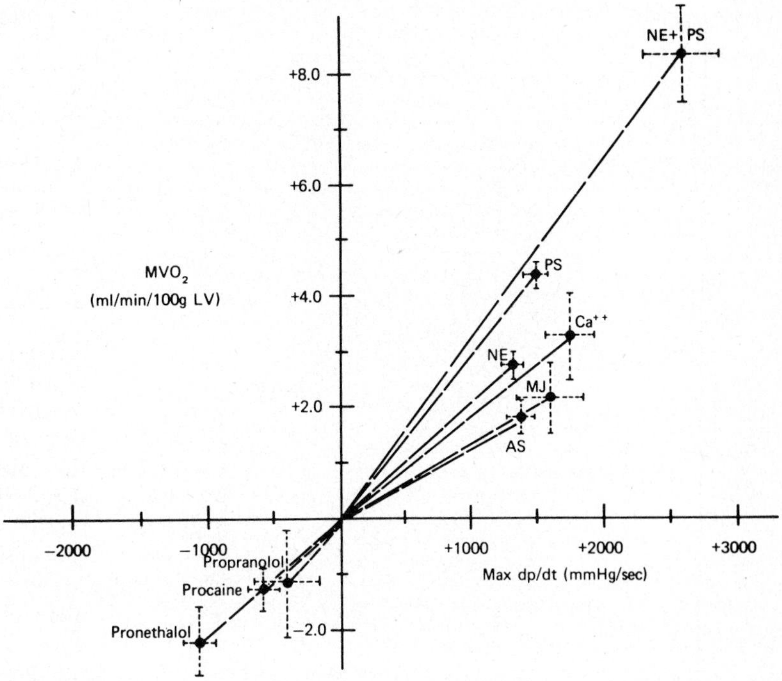

FIGURE 36–2 Relation between changes in maximal intraventricular dP/dt and myocardial oxygen consumption ($M\dot{V}O_2$). Each point represents the average of a series of experiments ± SE. AS = acetylstrophanthidin; MJ = noncatecholamine nonglycoside positive inotropic agent; Ca^{++} = calcium; NE = norepinephrine; PS = paired electrical stimulation. (From Braunwald, E.: Control of myocardial oxygen consumption: Physiologic and clinical considerations. Am. J. Cardiol. *27*:416, 1971.)

ventricle is a direct function of the radius and the intraventricular pressure and is inversely related to ventricular wall thickness. Also, tension in the myocardial wall is a more definitive determinant of myocardial energy utilization than is developed pressure.[7] Later studies demonstrated that velocity of myocardial contraction—a reflection of the heart's contractile state—is an additional, important determinant of $M\dot{V}O_2$ (Fig. 36–2).[8]

Recent reexamination of the determinants of $M\dot{V}O_2$ has emphasized that it correlates closely with the left ventricular systolic pressure-volume area, which consists of the sum of the area within the systolic pressure-volume loop, i.e., the external mechanical work, and the end-systolic elastic potential energy in the ventricular wall.[9,10] Rooke and Feigl have provided impressive evidence that $M\dot{V}O_2$ is also influenced by stroke volume (and therefore stroke work), although less so than by pressure development.[2] They have also provided an experimental basis for the use of the systolic pressure-rate product (plus an estimate of the oxygen consumption of the noncontracting heart) as a clinically useful index of $M\dot{V}O_2$. These observations are consistent with Fenn's classic observations on skeletal muscle which showed that the energy release (a variable related to $\dot{V}O_2$) is proportional to the sum of tension development and external work of the muscle.[11,12] Thus, both skeletal muscle and myocardium have the capacity to adjust their energy costs to external conditions imposed *after* stimulation.

EFFECT OF INOTROPIC AGENTS. The effect on $M\dot{V}O_2$ of positive inotropic stimuli, such as cardiac glycosides or catecholamines, is the end result of their influence on two major determinants of $M\dot{V}O_2$ which change in opposite directions: tension, which declines as a consequence of a reduction in heart size, and myocardial contractility, which is augmented. In the failing, dilated ventricle, the increased contractility reduces the left ventricular end-diastolic pressure and volume. On the basis of the Laplace relation (p. 431), this reduction in ventricular volume leads to a decline in intramyocardial tension, which tends to reduce $M\dot{V}O_2$. However, the decrease in $M\dot{V}O_2$ that might be expected to result from falling tension in the ventricular wall is offset by the increase in contractility, which tends to augment $M\dot{V}O_2$. The net result of these opposing effects is to produce no change, a small increase, or a small decrease in $M\dot{V}O_2$. Thus, the change in $M\dot{V}O_2$ that follows a stimulation of contractility depends on the extent to which intramyocardial tension is reduced in relation to the extent to which the contractile state is augmented.[13] In the absence of heart failure, drugs that stimulate myocardial contractility elevate $\dot{V}O_2$, since heart size and, therefore, wall tension are not reduced and do not offset the effect on metabolism of the stimulation of contractility.

The conclusion that myocardial contractility is an important determinant of $M\dot{V}O_2$ is supported by observations on the effects of reducing contractility. Thus, in animal experiments reductions in contractility and in the velocity of contraction produced by cardiac depressant drugs, including propranolol, and procainamide, were shown to reduce $M\dot{V}O_2$ when wall tension was held constant, or almost so.[14]

The results of experiments in which the relative effects on $M\dot{V}O_2$ of changes in tension development and in myocardial contractility were assessed in the same heart are summarized in Figure 36–3.[15] The three diagonal parallel lines are $M\dot{V}O_2$ isopleths, showing the levels of tension and V_{max} associated with 20, 40, and 60 μ liters/beat per 100 gm, respectively. The reciprocal relation between tension and velocity is evident. A given level of $M\dot{V}O_2$ can be achieved with a relatively high level of V_{max} and low peak developed tension, or a low level of V_{max} and a relatively high level of tension. The broken lines near the center of the figure illustrate the increases in peak developed tension and V_{max} required to increase $M\dot{V}O_2$ by 50 per cent. Such an increase could be achieved either by increasing V_{max} at a constant developed tension, as shown by the vertical arrow, or by increasing peak developed tension at a constant V_{max}, as shown by the horizontal arrow. From these stud-

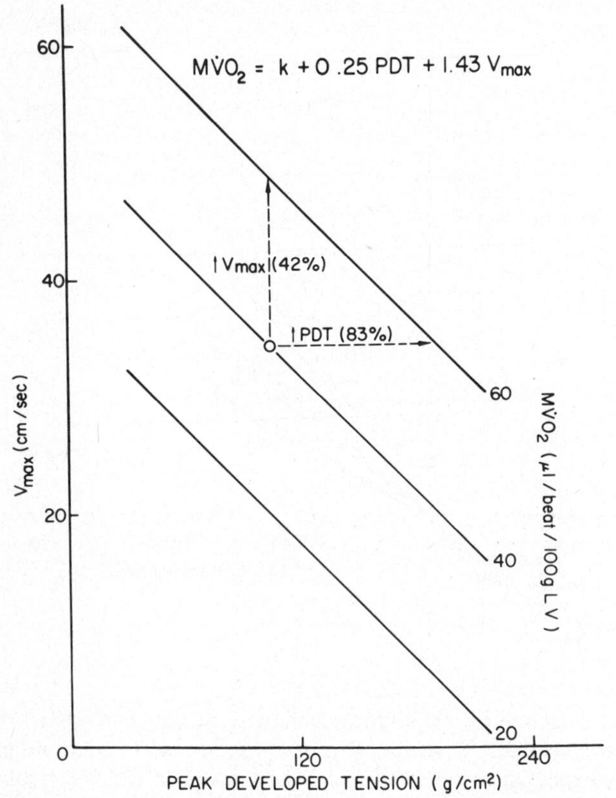

FIGURE 36–3 $M\dot{V}O_2$ isopleths as a function of V_{max} and peak developed tension (PDT). Isopleths were calculated from the equation at the top of the figure, which was derived by multiple regression analysis of a series of experiments in dogs. Broken lines indicate the effect on $M\dot{V}O_2$ of hypothetical increases in PDT at a constant V_{max} (horizontal lines) and in V_{max} at a constant PDT (vertical line). (From Graham, T. P., Jr., Covell, J. W., Sonnenblick, E. H., Ross, J., Jr., and Braunwald, E.: Control of myocardial oxygen consumption: Relative influence of contractile state and tension development. J. Clin. Invest. *47*:375, 1968.)

ies it was concluded that the quantitative effects on $M\dot{V}O_2$ of changes in contractility and tension development are both substantial and of the same order of magnitude.

It is important to emphasize that in these experiments heart rate was purposely held constant, since heart rate itself is an important determinant of $M\dot{V}O_2$. An augmentation of rate elevates the level of $M\dot{V}O_2$ per minute by increasing the frequency of tension development per unit of time, as well as by increasing contractility.[5,16]

TABLE 36–1 DETERMINANTS OF MYOCARDIAL OXYGEN CONSUMPTION

1. Tension development
2. Contractile state
3. Heart rate
4. Shortening against a load (Fenn effect)
5. Maintenance of cell viability in basal state
6. Depolarization
7. Activation
8. Maintenance of active state
9. Direct metabolic effect of catecholamines
10. Fatty acid uptake

Although the exact costs of maintenance of the active state of the myocardium have not yet been clearly defined, they are likely to be relatively low. In studies on isolated papillary muscles, $\dot{V}O_2$ was found to be a function of the tension that is developed and the velocity of shortening of the unloaded muscle. Shortening against a load requires oxygen above and beyond that required for the development of tension. Almost the entire increase in $M\dot{V}O_2$ produced by the administration of catecholamines results from the increased contractile activity produced, rather than from a direct stimulating effect of the catecholamines on myocardial metabolism. Severe valvular regurgitation does not increase myocardial consumption significantly when myocardial tension is held constant because of the low oxygen cost of the additional muscle shortening associated with valvular regurgitation[5,17] (Table 36–1). $M\dot{V}O_2$ is influenced also by the substrate utilized. Specifically, it varies directly with the fraction of energy derived from the metabolism of fatty acids, which in turn varies directly with the arterial concentration of fatty acids and inversely with that of glucose and insulin.[18]

REGULATION OF CORONARY BLOOD FLOW (Fig. 36–4)

ANATOMICAL FACTORS. Coronary blood flow is influenced by anatomical, hydraulic, mechanical, and metabolic factors.[6,19,20,20a] During diastole, when the aortic valve is closed, aortic diastolic pressure is transmitted without impediment through the dilated sinuses of Valsal-

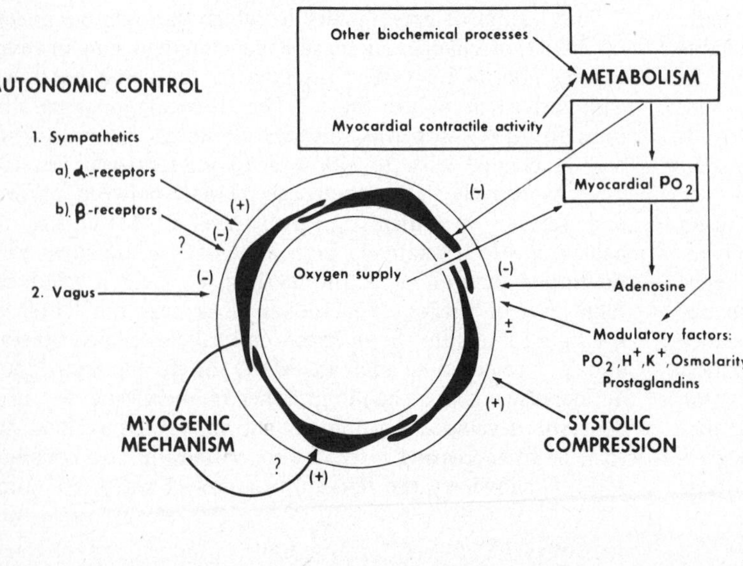

FIGURE 36–4 Schematic representation of principal factors influencing coronary blood flow. (+) = factors that reduce arteriolar lumen by compression or by contraction of vascular smooth muscle (ring of four overlapping cells). (−) = factors that relax vascular smooth muscle. Force exerted by blood pressure to stretch the vessel is not shown. Note that metabolic factors can act either via adenosine or other metabolites or by some direct effect on the vessel wall. (From Berne, R. M., and Rubio, R.: Coronary circulation. *In* Berne, R. M., Sperelakis, N., and Geiger, S. R. (eds.): Handbook of Physiology. Section 2, The Cardiovascular System. Bethesda, Md., American Physiological Society, 1979, p. 897.)

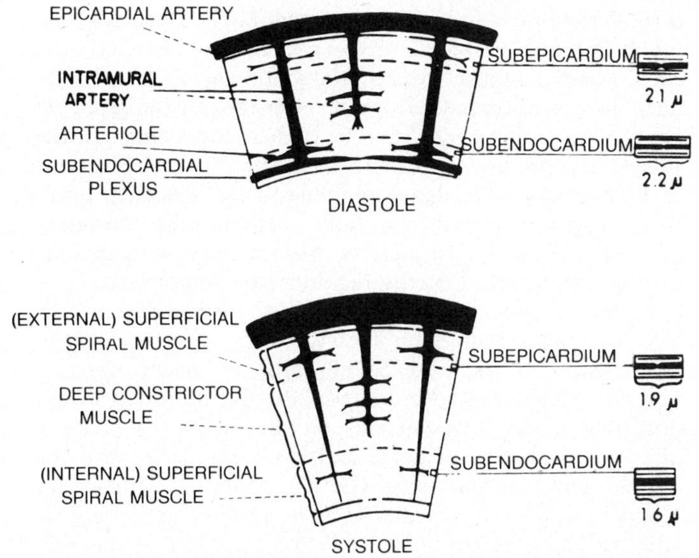

FIGURE 36–5 Cross-section of the left ventricular wall in systole and diastole. Factors involved in the susceptibility of the subendocardium to the development of ischemia include the greater dependence of this region on diastolic perfusion and the greater degree of shortening, and therefore of energy expenditure, of this region during systole. (From Bell, J. R., and Fox, A. C.: Pathogenesis of subendocardial ischemia. Am. J. Med. Sci. *268*:2, 1974.)

va to the ostia themselves. The sinuses then act as miniature reservoirs, facilitating maintenance of relatively uniform coronary inflow through diastole.[21] Both the left and right coronary arteries course across the epicardial surface of the heart. Major vessels and their branches give rise to smaller penetrating vessels approximately at right angles (Fig. 36–5).[22] The dense capillary network of about 4000 capillaries/sq mm cross-section of the heart[23] is not uniformly patent, since precapillary sphincters appear to serve a regulatory function,[24] depending on the flow needs of the myocardium.

Anastomotic connections without an intervening capillary bed exist between portions of the same coronary artery and between different coronary arteries. The distribution and extent of these collateral vessels differ markedly between species, as well as among different individuals of the same species. In canine hearts, an extensive epicardial network of collateral vessels is common, but epicardial collateral vessels are not prominent in porcine hearts. In human hearts, the distribution and extent of collateral vessels are quite variable.[25] Under physiological conditions, such vessels are generally less than 40 μ in diameter and appear to have little or no functional role. However, when myocardial perfusion is compromised by obstructions affecting major vessels, these collateral vessels enlarge over several weeks and blood flow through them increases.[26–28] Under these conditions, perfusion via collaterals may equal or exceed perfusion via the obstructed vessel.

The functional significance of collateral vessels varies widely.[29] At best, collaterals may maintain the viability of myocardium in the presence of total occlusion. However, myocardial perfusion through collaterals cannot increase sufficiently to meet the augmented requirements of the myocardium during the stress of exercise. Therefore, when cardiac muscle is supplied entirely or largely by collateral vessels, it often becomes ischemic if its oxygen demands increase above basal levels.

PERFUSION PRESSURE. As in any vascular bed, blood flow in the coronary bed depends on the driving pressure and the resistance offered by this bed. However, the coronary circulation differs from other circulations in that the resistance offered by the bed is influenced considerably by phasic systolic extravascular compression of the myocardium. The effective driving or perfusion pressure is the pressure gradient between the coronary arteries and the coronary sinus. However, effective perfusion pressure is not constant throughout the cardiac cycle. When the aortic valve is open and ejected blood flows rapidly past the coronary ostia, perfusion pressure is reduced slightly below aortic pressure because of the Venturi effect. In addition, phasic changes in right atrial pressure occurring during the cardiac cycle modify the effective perfusion pressure gradient, albeit only slightly, except in the presence of a tall *v* wave, as in tricuspid regurgitation.

FACTORS EXTRINSIC TO THE VASCULAR BED. Coronary vascular resistance is influenced both by factors *extrinsic* to the bed, particularly compressive forces within the myocardium (intramyocardial pressure acting on the intramyocardial vessels), and by metabolic, neural, and humoral factors *intrinsic* to the bed causing changes in the cross-sectional area of coronary resistance vessels. Intramyocardial pressure is determined primarily by the ventricular pressure throughout the cardiac cycle.[30–32] Because ventricular pressure is so much higher in systole than it is in diastole, myocardial compressive forces acting on intramyocardial vessels are much greater during this phase of the cardiac cycle. Accordingly, a large proportion of coronary blood flow to the left ventricle occurs during diastole. Since an increase in heart rate diminishes the total amount of diastolic time per minute (and increases myocardial oxygen demands), tachycardia may compromise coronary perfusion. This "throttling" effect of systole on myocardial perfusion[19] is particularly important when systolic intraventricular pressure is elevated but coronary perfusion pressure is not, as in the case of obstruction to left ventricular outflow by valvular or subvalvular aortic stenosis, or in severe aortic regurgitation.

The dramatic impact of left ventricular compression on coronary blood flow can be demonstrated experimentally with a beating heart perfused at constant pressure and ventricular asystole induced transiently by vagal stimulation. During asystole, coronary blood flow suddenly increases by approximately 50 per cent because of relief of the compressive effect.[20] Since compressive forces exerted by the right ventricle are ordinarily far less than those of the left ventricle, perfusion of the right ventricle is not interrupted during systole (Fig. 36–6).

The systolic compressive effect just discussed is much greater in subendocardial compared with subepicardial zones of the heart.[31] Under physiological conditions, marked transitory disparities exist between endocardial and epicardial wall stresses and, correspondingly, between endocardial and epicardial flow throughout the cardiac cycle. Nevertheless, under physiological conditions, the ratio of endo- to epicardial flow averaged throughout the cardiac cycle is approximately 1:1 as a consequence of preferential dilatation of the subendocardial vessels.[32,33] Inter-

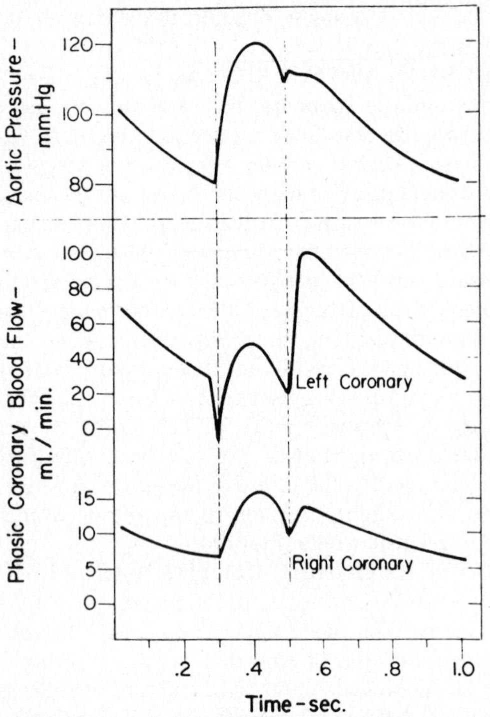

FIGURE 36–6 Phasic right and left coronary artery blood flow in relation to aortic blood pressure. (From Berne, R. M., and Levy, M. D.: Cardiovascular Physiology, 2nd ed. St. Louis, The C. V. Mosby Co., 1972.)

ventions that reduce the perfusion pressure gradient during diastole (as occurs with coronary obstruction, elevation of ventricular diastolic pressure, and tachycardia) lower the ratio of subendocardial to subepicardial flow and may cause the subendocardium to become ischemic.

The combination of a greater wall stress, and hence greater resistance to flow, and higher metabolic demands results in lower coronary vascular tone in the subendocardium than in the subepicardium. As a consequence, the reserve for vasodilatation is also less in the subendocardium than in the subepicardium, and as perfusion is reduced the deeper layers of myocardium become ischemic before the more superficial ones. This phenomenon is manifested by reduced intracellular oxygen tension and contractility and increased production of lactate initially in the inner layers of the ventricular wall.[31,34,35]

The susceptibility of the subendocardium to ischemia by the combination of limited reserve for vasodilation, extrinsic compression from the higher wall stress to which it is subjected,[36] and the resultant high metabolic demands accounts for ST segment depression on the electrocardiogram characteristically associated with transient episodes of angina pectoris (Fig. 7–29, p. 222). Injury currents from the subendocardium, resulting in ST segment depression, accompany the maldistribution of transmural flow and metabolic impairment of subendocardial tissue under these circumstances, even though net transmural flow may remain near normal.[37] These considerations provide the basis for the recognition of myocardial ischemia by ST-segment depression during exercise stress testing (Chap. 8). When perfusion is limited, the adaptive changes of the subendocardial zone include its greater potential for glycolytic metabolism[38] due to higher glycolytic enzyme activity and, consequently, higher lactate production rates[39] when coronary flow is restricted. However, even though the glycogen content of subendocardium is higher than that of the subepicardium under aerobic conditions,[40] concentrations of high-energy phosphate compounds are generally lower than those in the mid- and subepicardium when coronary flow is restricted,[41] because of the inability of anaerobic metabolism to fulfill energy requirements completely.

Hoffman, Buckberg, Griggs, and their collaborators have developed indices for the evaluation of subendocardial ischemia in the absence of coronary artery obstruction.[35,42–44] They reasoned that the driving force for subendocardial blood flow depends on the integrated pressure difference between the aorta and left ventricle, termed the *diastole pressure–time index* (DPTI), while the demand for blood flow, i.e., myocardial O_2 consumption, is closely related to the area beneath the systolic portion of the ventricular pressure curve, i.e., the *systolic pressure–time index* (SPTI). The ratio DPTI/SPTI has been used as an index of the relation between subendocardial oxygen supply and demand. This ratio can be reduced by (1) opening an arteriovenous fistula or patent ductus arteriosus or inducing aortic regurgitation to diminish aortic diastolic pressure; (2) increasing preload or afterload, causing left ventricular dysfunction, or reducing left ventricular compliance; these maneuvers all raise left ventricular diastolic pressure; and (3) inducing tachycardia to shorten diastole.[45,46] These investigators found that with reduction of the DPTI/SPTI below a critical value of approximately 0.7, the endocardial/epicardial blood flow ratio also decreased.

These observations can explain a number of clinical findings, such as the development of angina and the electrocardiographic and biochemical evidence of ischemia caused by tachycardia in patients with aortic stenosis. Indeed, myocardial lactate production has been observed to occur during beta-adrenergic receptor stimulation with isoproterenol in patients with aortic stenosis,[47] when left ventricular systolic pressure, contractility, heart rate, and, therefore, myocardial oxygen demand rise. When adrenergic stimulation was carried out in dogs with experimentally produced aortic stenosis, the myocardial lactate concentration and the lactate-pyruvate ratio rose while the reduction of ATP stores was more prominent in the inner than the outer half of the ventricle,[35] again indicating that the subendocardium is more vulnerable to ischemia and therefore becomes dependent on anaerobic metabolism more readily than does the subepicardium.

In experimentally produced aortic regurgitation, diastolic coronary blood flow falls but systolic flow rises, so the total coronary flow does not change;[48] however, with severe reductions in aortic diastolic pressure the subendocardial region exhibits biochemical evidence of anaerobic metabolism. Although metabolically stimulated coronary dilatation in the subendocardial region can maintain blood flow despite considerable reduction in aortic diastolic pressure, this compensation is often incomplete with very severe aortic regurgitation. As the DPTI/SPTI declines, the subendocardial lactate-pyruvate ratio rises, providing evidence of anaerobic metabolism by the myocardium. These experiments are clinically relevant when it is considered that angina pectoris occurs in more than one third of patients with severe aortic regurgitation in the absence of coronary artery disease[49] (p. 1110). Other conditions in which subendocardial ischemia occurs include marked systemic hypotension, regardless of etiology (Chap. 18), and pulmonary embolism; in these conditions the ischemia results from a combination of lowered coronary perfusion pressure, tachycardia, and increased subendocardial tension secondary to sympathetic stimulation of myocardial contractility.

In the presence of coronary obstruction the *effective* pressure perfusing the subendocardial region is reduced to the gradient between the diastolic coronary pressure *distal* to the obstruction and the left ventricular end-diastolic pressure; the DPTI no longer reflects the driving force for subendocardial blood flow. Since maldistribution of transmural blood flow compromises the subendocardial tissue, antianginal drugs may be effective if they improve the ratio of subendocardial to subepicardial flow even if they do not augment net transmural perfusion.[31] Analysis of the washout of ^{86}Rb and fractional uptake of radioactive labeled microspheres has shown that both nitroglycerin and propranolol redistribute blood flow to the subendocardium.[50,51] Whether or not this phenomenon reflects the direct effects of the drugs on the coronary vascular bed or, as is more likely, the reduction of extravascular compressive forces induced by a lowering of ventricular diastolic pressure resulting from a reduction of preload (nitroglycerin) or a reduction of ischemia consequent to diminishing myocardial oxygen needs (propranolol), the net result is a decline in extrinsic resistance with an augmentation of subendocardial perfusion.

INTRINSIC FACTORS. Coronary resistance is influenced markedly by changes in the tone of the vascular bed, changes that are mediated by neural, metabolic, pharmacological, and myogenic factors.[52]

The coronary arteries are richly innervated by sympathetic and parasympathetic nerves.[20] Both alpha- and beta-2 receptor activity has been demonstrated in the coronary vascular bed of the intact unanesthetized dog.[53,54] Intravenous administration of norepinephrine induces a brief fall, followed by a sustained rise, in coronary vascular resistance, accompanied by a decline in coronary sinus pO_2 (Fig. 36–7).[55] The early vasodilatation can be eliminated by beta-adrenergic blockade and presumably results from the augmented myocardial oxygen needs consequent to stimulation of myocardial beta receptors; the later increase in coronary vascular resistance can be prevented by alpha-adrenergic receptor blockade and presumably results from stimulation of alpha receptors in the coronary vascular bed.

Baroreceptor activity affects coronary vascular resistance reflexly. In the dog with sectioned vagal nerves, occlusion of the carotid arteries to produce baroreceptor hypotension induces an increase in heart rate and blood pressure, accompanied by a reduction in coronary vascular resistance.[56] When the reflex tachycardia and myocardial contractility (which would be expected to increase $M\dot{V}O_2$ and lower coronary vascular resistance) are blocked with propranolol, an increase in coronary vascular resistance is observed,

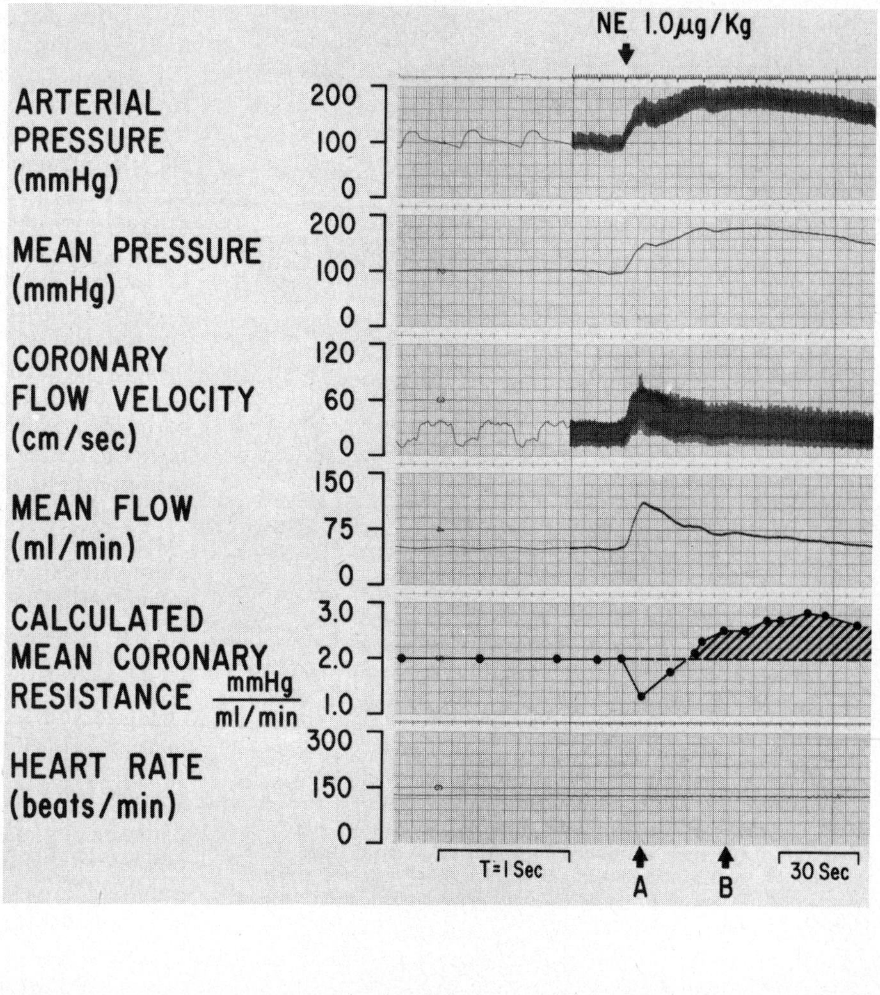

FIGURE 36–7 Effects of intravenously administered norepinephrine (NE) in the intact unanesthetized dog with heart rate held constant. Coronary vascular resistance fell initially (A) and then showed a sustained increase (B). (From Vatner, S. F., Higgins, C. B., and Braunwald, E.: Effects of norepinephrine on coronary circulation and left ventricular dynamics in the conscious dog. Circ. Res. *34*: 812, 1974, by permission of the American Heart Association, Inc.)

which can be prevented by cardiac sympathectomy. It may be concluded that with intact sympathetic nerves and beta receptors, the coronary dilatation consequent to carotid occlusion is due to heightened cardiac metabolic activity induced reflexly by baroreceptor hypotension. When this augmentation of myocardial beta-receptor–mediated activity is prevented with beta blockade, reflex coronary *vasoconstriction* secondary to carotid hypotension is unmasked.[57] Stimulation of the distal ends of the vagi produces coronary vasodilatation,[57,58] an effect that is mediated by the release of acetylcholine from vagal nerve endings and that can be blocked by atropine.[20]

There is also evidence for *tonic* coronary constriction mediated by the sympathetic nerves.[59] Acute surgical denervation of the heart produces a fall in coronary vascular resistance with a decrease in arteriovenous oxygen extraction.[60] Coronary vascular resistance in patients as well as in dogs[61] with innervated hearts declines by almost 25 per cent in response to alpha-adrenergic blockade, suggesting that basal coronary constrictor tone mediated by alpha receptors was released. However, resistance does not diminish when patients with cardiac transplants receive alpha-adrenergic blockade, suggesting that cardiac denervation had previously released the coronary constrictor tone. In the unanesthetized dog, stimulation of the carotid sinus nerves results in a substantial reduction in coronary vascular resistance (Fig. 36–8),[59] an effect which can be prevented by alpha-receptor blockade, suggesting that sympathetic coronary constrictor tone is present in the resting conscious dog and that coronary vasodilatation attendant upon electrical stimulation of the carotid sinus nerves results from a reduction in this resting vasoconstrictor tone. Coronary vasodilatation resulting from stimulation of the carotid sinus nerves occurs also during exercise, suggesting that alpha-receptor–mediated constrictor tone persists in the coronary vascular bed during exercise, despite the coexisting metabolic vasodilatation. This conclusion is supported by studies using alpha-adrenergic blocking drugs which have shown that the increase in coronary blood flow and oxygen delivery to the myocardium during normal exercise is limited by alpha-adrenergic vasoconstriction.[62,63]

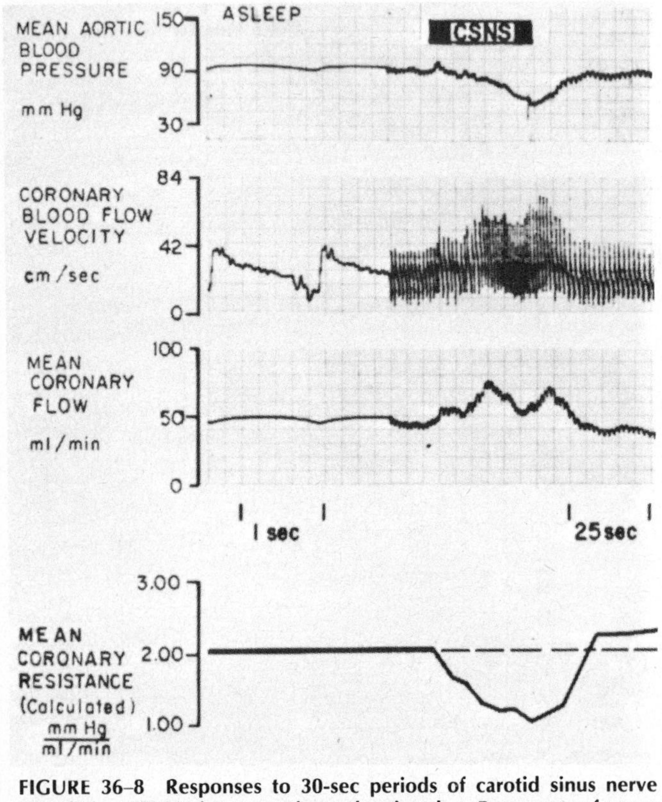

FIGURE 36–8 Responses to 30-sec periods of carotid sinus nerve stimulation (CSNS) in a conscious, sleeping dog. Responses of mean arterial pressure, phasic and mean coronary blood flow, and calculated mean coronary resistance are shown. (From Vatner, S. F., Franklin, D., and Braunwald, E.: Effects of anesthesia and sleep on circulatory response to carotid sinus nerve stimulation. Am J. Physiol. *220*:1249, 1971.)

Efferent neural influences on the coronary vascular bed may also be activated reflexly by cardiopulmonary parasympathetic receptors. Stimulation of parasympathetic receptors leads to reflex systemic and coronary vasodilatation.[64] Chemoreceptor activation can also cause coronary dilatation, a reflex that is mediated by the vagi and can be abolished by atropine.[20] Intracoronary injection of veratrum alkaloids, as well as other metabolically active substances, induces reflex bradycardia and hypotension (the Bezold-Jarisch reflex),[65,66] the afferent limb of which involves the vagus nerves. The effects of efferent vagus nerve activity causing *coronary* vasodilatation[67] have been documented, indicating that the Bezold-Jarisch reflex involves coronary efferent as well as afferent parasympathetic components.[64]

Coronary beta-adrenergic receptors are similar to those in other vessels and conform to the beta-2 category.[68] Administration of a beta-1 agonist stimulates myocardial contractility and heart rate, with the enhanced production of metabolites eliciting coronary vasodilatation. Administration of propranolol, on the other hand, might be expected to reduce coronary blood flow and elevate coronary vascular resistance by two separate mechanisms: (1) blocking the effect of beta-1 receptors and thereby reducing $M\dot{V}O_2$ and the metabolic vasodilatation consequent thereto; and (2) blocking coronary vasodilator influences mediated by activation of beta-2 receptors. However, despite these theoretical considerations and the demonstration of the activity of beta-adrenergic agonists and antagonists in vitro,[69] under physiological conditions direct effects of beta-adrenergic antagonists on the coronary vascular bed are not prominent.

AUTOREGULATION. When sudden alterations in coronary perfusion pressure are imposed on an experimental preparation in which myocardial oxygen demands are held constant, the abrupt changes in coronary blood flow are only transitory, with flow promptly returning toward the previous steady-state level.[70] This phenomenon, termed autoregulation (Fig. 36–9), tends to maintain regional coronary perfusion within a relatively narrow range, regardless of transitory changes in perfusion pressure. Demonstration of autoregulation in intact animals is difficult because modification of coronary perfusion pressure also changes both $M\dot{V}O_2$ and extrinsic compression of the coronary vessels. However, under experimental conditions in which perfusion pressure is altered but ventricular pressure, cardiac contractility, and heart rate—the principal determinants of $M\dot{V}O_2$—are maintained constant, autoregulation is clearly evident. Several mechanisms have been implicated, including myogenic and metabolic factors as well as tissue pressure.[19,20]

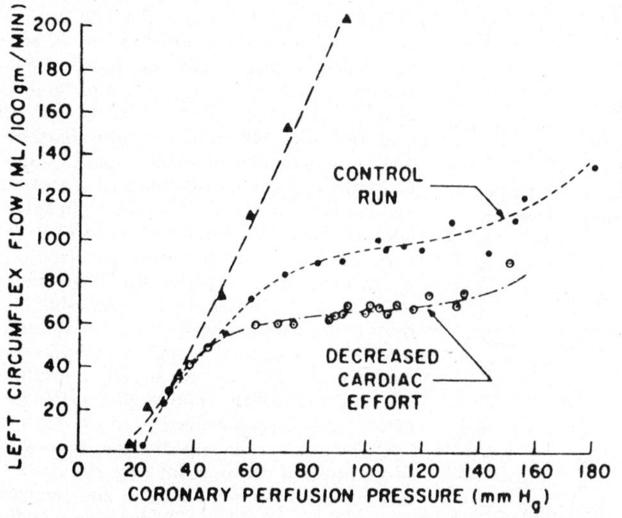

FIGURE 36–9 Relation between left circumflex coronary flow and coronary perfusion pressure. Coronary perfusion pressure has been altered independently of aortic pressure, which is maintained essentially constant. Triangles represent the immediate change in flow with various sudden increases in perfusion pressure from a pressure of 40 mm Hg. Closed circles along the middle curve represent the readjusted steady-state flow levels over a range of perfusion pressures after autoregulation has occurred. Note the relative independence of flow from coronary perfusion pressure between approximately 70 and 130 mm Hg. When cardiac effort was reduced by lowering aortic pressure (open circles), the steady-state level of left circumflex flow was also reduced but again remained relatively independent of coronary perfusion pressure over a broad range of perfusion pressure changes. (From Mosher, P., et al.: Control of coronary blood flow by an autoregulatory mechanism. Circ. Res. *14*:250, 1964, by permission of the American Heart Association, Inc.)

Myogenic Factors. Stretch of vascular smooth muscle resulting from an increase in perfusion pressure stimulates the muscle to contract.[70a] The consequent augmentation of resistance tends to return blood flow toward normal despite the higher perfusion pressure. Although the myogenic mechanism, sometimes called the Bayliss effect, appears to be a general characteristic of vascular smooth muscle,[71] its role in the regulation of coronary blood flow is probably a modest one.[20]

Metabolic Factors. It is likely that changes in regional myocardial metabolism are important determinants of autoregulation (and therefore coronary blood flow). Several mediators have been implicated, including oxygen, carbon dioxide, and vasodilator metabolites, such as adenosine, that accumulate in hypoperfused regions of myocardium. For example, a reduction in coronary arterial perfusion pressure, causing an immediate decrease in flow, might be expected to cause an increased myocardial oxygen extraction and a reduction in myocardial oxygen tension; the resultant hypoxia then causes coronary vasodilatation,[72,73] presumably because oxygen acts on vascular smooth muscle directly, possibly by altering the electrochemical potential of the muscle cells. Direct vasodilating effects of diminished oxygen tension have been demonstrated in the coronary, femoral, and other vessels.[74–76] Molecular oxygen diffusing across the walls of the vessels appears to be a primary determinant of constrictor tone of precapillary sphincters under physiological conditions.[77,78] Thus, diminution of oxygen tension increases the number of capillaries perfused within a predefined region of myocardium, presumably by relaxation of these sphincters.[79] In this manner coronary blood flow would be expected to remain constant despite a reduction of perfusion pressure. Transitory augmentation of the concentration of potassium in extracellular fluid, an early consequence of myocardial ischemia, may also modify the transmembrane potential of vascular smooth muscle cells and result in vasodilatation.

Degradation of adenine nucleotides under conditions in which ATP utilization exceeds the capacity of myocardial cells to resynthesize high-energy phosphate compounds (a process dependent on oxidative phosphorylation in mitochondria) results in the efflux of purine bases that cannot be reutilized readily by the heart. Accordingly, adenosine and its metabolites, inosine and hypoxanthine, appear in interstitial fluid and in the coronary sinus venous effluent. *Adenosine* is a powerful vasodilator[80,81] that is considered to be an important, perhaps *the critical, mediator* linking metabolically induced vasodilatation to diminish coronary perfusion (Fig. 36–10). Concentrations of adenosine in the venous effluent are much lower than those in interstitial fluid, in part because capillary endothelium rapidly converts adenosine to inosine and hypoxanthine.[82] However, when the enzyme responsible for this conversion, adenosine deaminase, is inhibited by administration of 8-azaguanine, prominent increases occur in the concentration of adenosine in the effluent.[75] If, at a constant level of myocardial metabolism, adenosine were being released at a constant rate, an elevation of coronary perfusion pressure and the resultant increase in coronary blood flow would augment the washout of adenosine, reduce its concentration, and thus increase coronary vascular resistance. Such a mechanism could provide a feedback to account for pressure-independent autoregulation of coronary blood flow and could also explain the close correlation between the metabolic activity of the heart and the level of coronary blood flow.[83] It is also possible that adenosine interacts with hypoxia in causing coronary relaxation.[84]

It appears that adenosine acts on the surface of vascular smooth muscle cells, presumably at a receptor site on the cell membrane; presumably adenosine blocks entry of Ca^{++} into these cells and thereby causes vasodilatation.[20] In addition to its potent vasodilating action, adenosine exerts a generally depressant activity on cardiac automaticity and atrioventricular conduction and attenuates the effects of adrenergic influences on myocardial contractility.[85]

Despite its importance, adenosine is almost certainly not the only metabolic factor involved. Prostaglandins, kinins,[86] potassium, and a number of metabolites alter coronary vascular resistance profoundly and may play a role in mediating vasodilatation in response to hypoxia. The infusion of at least two prostaglandins synthesized in the heart (PGI_2 and PGE_2) can cause coronary vasodilatation,[87] and the inhibition of prostaglandin synthesis with indomethacin causes an increase in coronary vascular resistance in humans.[88]

When coronary perfusion pressure falls to below 60 to 70 mm Hg, the coronary vessels become maximally dilated and flow becomes pressure-dependent[19]; i.e., coronary autoregulation is lost (Fig. 36–9). This observation explains the importance of maintaining coronary perfusion pressure in patients with acute myocardial infarction (Chap. 38). In patients with cardiogenic shock, the reduc-

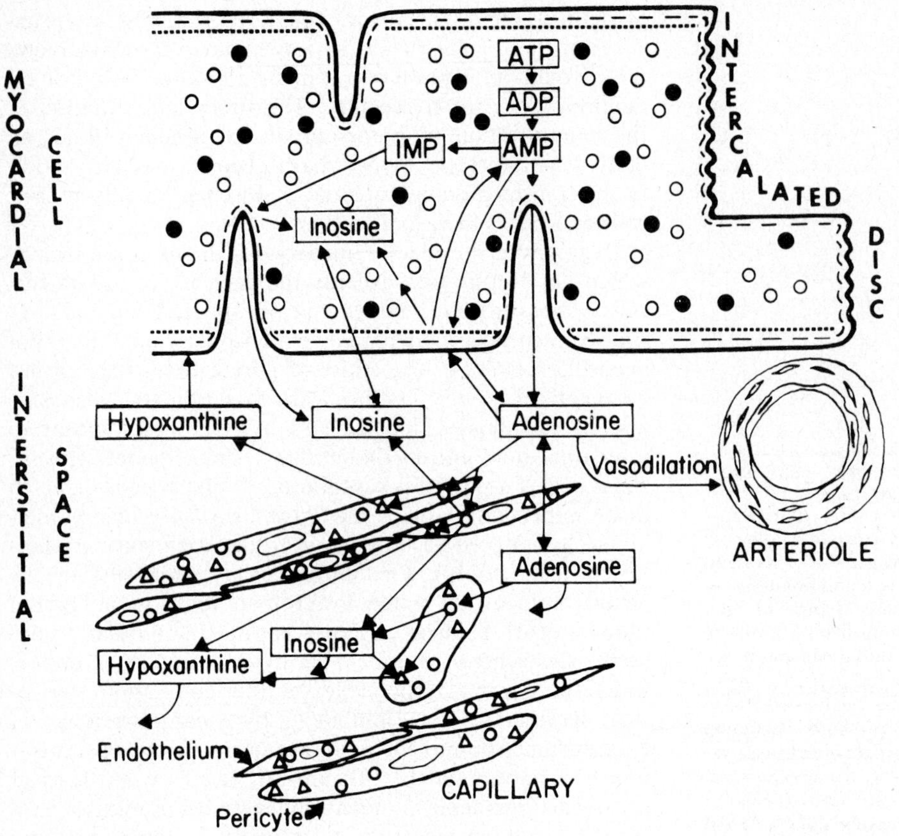

FIGURE 36–10 Schematic drawing depicting a myocardial cell, interstitial space, an arteriole, and a capillary with the localization of enzymes involved in the formation and fate of adenosine. Adenosine formed by 5′-nucleotidase from AMP (which in turn arises from ATP) can enter the interstitial space. There it can induce arteriolar dilation and reenter the myocardial cell, where it is either phosphorylated to AMP by adenosine kinase or deaminated to inosine by adenosine deaminase, or it can enter the capillaries and leave the tissue. A large fraction of adenosine that crosses the capillary wall is deaminated to inosine, which in turn is split to hypoxanthine and ribose-1-PO_4 by nucleoside phosphorylase located in the endothelial cells, pericytes, and erythrocytes. Most of the adenosine is taken up by the myocardial cells, and that escaping into the circulation is largely in the form of inosine and hypoxanthine. Since adenylic acid deaminase (which deaminates AMP to IMP) is in low concentration in heart muscle, the major degradative pathway from AMP is via dephosphorylation to adenosine.

○ = Adenosine deaminase; ● = adenylic acid deaminase; △ = nucleoside phosphorylase; (---) = 5′-nucleotidase; (·····) = adenosine kinase. (From Berne, R. M., and Rubio, R.: Coronary circulation. *In* Berne, R. M., Sperelakis, N., and Geiger, S. R. (eds.): Handbook of Physiology, Section 2. The Cardiovascular System, Bethesda, Md., American Physiological Society, 1979, p. 924.)

tion of perfusion pressure below this level lowers coronary blood flow even through nonobstructed vessels and may reduce collateral blood flow to the peri-infarction zone, thereby enlarging the infarct.[89]

As noted, with organic occlusive lesions or spasm in major coronary arteries the effective myocardial perfusion pressure is the low pressure existing *distal* to the obstruction, and autoregulation in the distal bed may be compromised because it is already maximally dilated in the basal state. As a consequence, perfusion of this distal bed becomes dependent entirely on perfusion pressure. Under these circumstances, augmentation of cardiac oxygen requirements *without* an increase in perfusion pressure results in or intensifies ischemia. Since blood flow to regions supplied by normal vessels can be increased (because regional vasodilatation in these regions is possible), while blood flow to the compromised zone cannot (because it is already maximally dilated), disparities in regional perfusion can become intensified. In addition, vasodilatation in the normal zones may reduce perfusion pressure to the ischemic zones and deprive them further of blood flow, a phenomenon sometimes termed "coronary steal."

PHARMACOLOGICAL AGENTS. Alpha-adrenergic agonists can cause constriction of both coronary conduction vessels, i.e., the large epicardial arteries, as well as coronary resistance vessels, i.e., the small intramural arteries and arterioles[90] (Fig. 36–5). This effect tends to be minimized by the passive distention of the vessels consequent to an elevation of intravascular pressure as well as by the metabolically induced coronary vasodilatation consequent to an imbalance between oxygen supply and demand resulting from the coronary constriction and from any increase in $M\dot{V}O_2$ accompanying the arterial hypertension induced by these drugs. Directly acting coronary vasodilators, such as nitroglycerin and isosorbide dinitrate,[27,28] augment perfusion of ischemic zones, as reflected by increased clearance of ^{133}Xe in patients with coronary artery disease[90]; these drugs have been shown to dilate coronary conductance vessels, coronary collaterals, and even atherosclerotic stenoses,[91–93] as well as to reduce the ventricular diastolic tension which tends to limit flow to the subendocardium; they have a lesser effect on resistance vessels.[92] The effects of calcium antagonists, such as verapamil or nifedipine, on coronary perfusion appear to reflect primarily direct action on the large epicardial conductance vessels as well as on the resistance vessels.[93] These agents increase blood flow to normal as well as ischemic myocardium.[94] Dipyridamole dilates the distal (resistance) vessels; since these are also acted upon by the endogenous vasodilator (adenosine), this agent is of little if any value in the treatment of myocardial ischemia. Prostaglandin I_2, which inhibits platelet aggregation, also decreases coronary vascular resistance,[87] whereas thromboxane A_2, which aggregates platelets, is also a potent coronary vasoconstrictor.

Factors Limiting Coronary Perfusion

The normal coronary vascular bed has the capacity to reduce its resistance to approximately 25 per cent of basal levels during the stress of maximal exercise; i.e., a four- to fivefold increase in coronary blood flow can occur during maximal exercise, which is generally accompanied by an increase in arterial pressure and a marked tachycardia. It is then not surprising that, in the basal state, the cross-sectional area of a proximal coronary artery can be reduced by up to approximately 80 per cent of normal, and vasodilatation of the coronary resistance vessels distal to the obstruction can maintain blood flow without the development of ischemia at rest (p. 261). However, since coronary blood flow cannot rise with this degree of obstruction in the proximal coronary bed, any stimulus that increases $M\dot{V}O_2$, such as exercise- or pacing-induced tachycardia, will elicit ischemia. With lesser degrees of obstruction, the distal bed is not maximally dilated in the basal state and, although the capacity for further dilatation exists, this capacity is subnormal and ischemia may develop, depending on the extent to which myocardial oxygen demands are augmented. When obstruction of a proximal coronary artery reduces the lumen to less than approximately 20 per cent of normal, ischemia will be present even in the basal state, despite maximal dilatation of the resistance vessels (unless the myocardium distal to the obstructed vessel is perfused by collateral vessels). Transient severe obstruction, as may occur in coronary spasm, will result in brief periods of ischemia, chest pain, electrocardiographic changes, and myocardial dysfunction. When it persists, myocardial necrosis ensues.

Basic considerations of fluid mechanics indicate that the pressure drop across a stenosis varies directly with the length of the stenosis and inversely with the fourth power of the radius (Bernoulli's theorem). Stenosis resistance changes relatively little with mild degrees of vascular narrowing but rises progressively and precipitously with severe obstruction; indeed, resistance almost triples as stenosis severity increases from 80 to 90 per cent.[95] As a consequence, with even a slight change in the severity of stenosis—as might occur when the resistance of the distal bed and therefore the pressure distending the narrowed coronary artery declines, as during exercise or following dipyridamole—the perfusion pressure distal to the obstruction may become reduced and subendocardial perfusion impaired.[96]

Myocardial ischemia and its consequences may occur as a result of fixed, atherosclerotic lesions or may be secondary to transitory reduction of myocardial blood flow caused by coronary spasm or platelet aggregates.[97] The clinical sequelae of myocardial ischemia, whether produced by an increase in $M\dot{V}O_2$ in the face of fixed obstruction or by a reduction in myocardial oxygen supply resulting from coronary spasm or transient aggregation of platelets, may be manifest clinically as angina pectoris, electrical instability, characteristic electrocardiographic changes, and depression of myocardial function.

EFFECTS OF ISCHEMIA ON MYOCARDIAL CONTRACTILITY

EFFECTS ON VENTRICULAR CONTRACTION. In 1935 Tennant and Wiggers demonstrated that after ligation of a coronary artery the contraction of cardiac muscle supplied by this vessel ceases, and the affected area appears cyanotic, dilated, and bulging.[98] More recent studies by Vatner have shown that in the basal state there is no reserve in blood flow; any given reduction in flow, even one as small as 10 to 20 per cent, results in an approximately similar per cent reduction of myocardial segment shortening. A reduction of blood flow of 80 per cent results in akinesis, while a 95 per cent reduction causes systolic bulging (dyskinesis).[99] Patients with coronary artery disease and a previous myocardial infarction exhibit impaired left ventricular function; in the presence of angina, transient episodes of myocardial ischemia cause left ventricular systolic and diastolic dysfunction.[100] The duration of impaired function may be quite prolonged, and postischemic depression ("stunning") of the myocardium, with impaired mechanical performance, high-energy phosphate stores, and abnormal ultrastructure may persist for a week or longer following a brief—15-minute—period of coronary occlusion, which is not enough to cause myocardial necrosis.[101] Myocardial ischemia may be associated with elimination of the normal contractile performance in a *localized area* of myocardium, resulting in an asynergic contraction.[102] Figure 36–11 shows the immediate regional myocardial functional responses to an acute coronary occlusion: paradoxical motion in the central ischemic zone, reduced contraction in the adjacent area, and compensatory hyperfunction of the uninvolved normal myocardium, the latter mediated in part by its dilation and the operation of the Frank-Starling mechanism.

Regional loss of myocardial contractile activity, whether sustained or transient, if sufficiently widespread, may depress overall left ventricular function, producing reductions of stroke volume, stroke work, cardiac output, and ejection fraction and elevation of end-diastolic volume and pressure.[103] Clinical evidence of heart failure occurs when regional asynergy is so severe and extensive that the uninvolved myocardium cannot sustain the excess load it must sustain. Hemodynamic evidence of left ventricular failure develops when contraction ceases in 20 to 25 per cent of the left ventricle; with loss of 40 per cent or more of left ventricular myocardium, severe pump failure ensues and, if this loss is acute, fatal or near-fatal cardiogenic shock usually develops (p. 591).

Since the heart has virtually no stores of oxygen, its high rate of energy expenditure results in a sudden, striking decline of myocardial oxygen tension within seconds of coronary occlusion, coincident with the loss of contractility. The marginal zone contracts weakly, whereas the nonischemic myocardium exhibits a compensatory increase in its force of contraction. The rapid decline in contractility induced by ischemia cannot be attributed to alterations in excitability.[104] Although ischemia does not produce major changes in the amplitude and upstroke velocity of the action potential, the duration of the plateau phase of the action potential is shortened, which may signify a reduction in the slow inward current, carried largely by calcium.

It is possible that the concentrations of high-energy phosphate compounds in critical locations—such as the sarcoplasmic reticulum, a locus of calcium binding and release, or the sarcolemma, where ion fluxes and cell volume may be affected—are reduced by ischemia, even when the overall intracellular concentration of these compounds is still normal or near normal.

A final possibility is that ischemia reduces the release of Ca^{++} from the sarcolemma, the sarcoplasmic reticulum, or both, and thereby interferes with the interaction of Ca^{++} with the contractile proteins.[105,106] As outlined in Chapter 13, contraction is normally initiated by the rapid release of

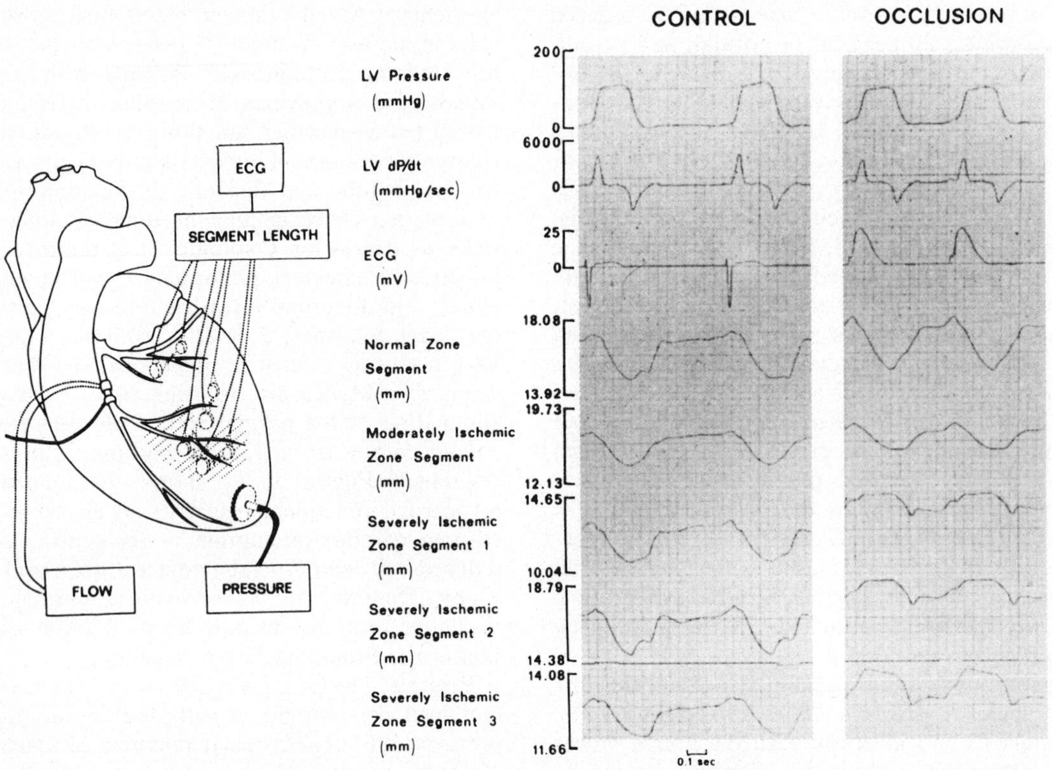

FIGURE 36–11 Effects of coronary occlusion on left ventricular (LV) pressure, LV dP/dt, and the epicardial electrogram in the severely ischemic zone, and on left ventricular dimensions in a normal segment of myocardium, a moderately ischemic segment (at the border between the normal and severely ischemic segment), and in three severely ischemic segments. The experimental preparation is illustrated on the left; an occluding cuff and flow meter are placed around the left anterior descending coronary artery, and crystals for ultrasonographic measurement of cardiac dimensions are sewn into the left ventricle. With coronary occlusion, only a slight decline in left ventricular systolic pressure and a slight elevation in left ventricular end-diastolic pressure occur, but there is a marked rise in the ST segment in the ischemic zone. The normal zone exhibits increased excursion per cardiac cycle with an increase in end-diastolic dimensions. Shortening of the segmental length per contraction decreases in the moderately ischemic zone. There is frank paradoxical pulsation in all three severely ischemic zones. (From Vatner, S. F., and Baig, H.: The effects of inotropic stimulation on ischemic myocardium in conscious dogs. Trans. Assoc. Am. Phys. *91*:283, 1978.)

Ca^{++} from the sarcoplasmic reticulum,[107] and this release is triggered by a rise in the local concentration of Ca^{++} in the vicinity of the sarcoplasmic reticulum. According to this concept, when the Ca^{++} concentration in the cytoplasm reaches a critical level, a massive release of Ca^{++} from the sarcoplasmic reticulum occurs, leading to muscle contraction.[108] Changes in intracellular pH may influence this Ca^{++} trigger mechanism—i.e., a fall in intracellular pH, as occurs in ischemia, may reduce the sensitivity of the sarcoplasmic reticulum to the local concentrations of Ca^{++}.

As discussed on p. 413, once Ca^{++} is released from the sarcoplasmic reticulum, it combines with specific receptor sites on the regulator protein, troponin, which ultimately leads to muscle tension and shortening. The high intracellular $[H^+]$ induced by ischemia may compete with Ca^{++} for the receptors on the troponin molecules. Thus, the actin-myosin interaction is impaired and it has been postulated that as a result of these two processes, i.e., reduction of the sensitivity of the sarcoplasmic reticulum to any given concentration of Ca^{++} and competition between H^+ and Ca^{++} for the troponin receptor sites, contractility is reduced.[105,109,110]

This concept of the critical importance of intracellular $[H^+]$ is supported by the observations that the functional changes induced by primary acidosis in the face of adequate myocardial oxygenation are similar to those produced by ischemia.[111] Furthermore, the reversal of acidosis by the administration of alkali improves contractile performance.[112] In addition to the role played by intracellular $[H^+]$, minor reductions of ATP may be important. Even a small reduction of intracellular ATP to levels that are still well above those required for the contractile process can be responsible for the changes in ion transport, which ultimately lead to a reduction in the delivery of Ca^{++} to the contractile sites.

In summary, it is likely that the abnormalities of contraction caused by ischemia result from the reduced release of Ca^{++} by the sarcoplasmic reticulum, ultimately making less Ca^{++} available to the contractile sites, as well as from the accumulation of intracellular H^+ and its interference with the interaction of Ca^{++} and the contractile proteins. Further exploration is needed of the roles of reduced transsarcolemmal passage of Ca^{++} during the plateau of the action potential and of lowered intracellular oxygen tension on stores of high-energy phosphate compounds in critical locations within the myocardial cell.

EFFECTS ON VENTRICULAR RELAXATION. Myocardial ischemia and infarction alter not only the contractile properties of the heart but also the diastolic pressure-volume relations of the left ventricle.[113] Myocardial ischemia impairs ventricular relaxation, as evidenced by a decreased peak negative maximal rate of pressure decline (negative dP/dt) and ventricular wall thinning and prolongs the isovolumetric relaxation period.[113-118] In turn, this impairment in ventricular relaxation increases the resistance to ventricular filling.[119,120] The combination of increased diastolic stiffness, decreased rate of wall thinning, and slow active pressure decay all contribute to the upward shift of the ventricular pressure-volume relationship observed during pacing-induced angina.[116] The mechanism responsible for the ischemia-induced impairment of myocardial relaxation has not been fully elucidated, but it has been proposed that reductions of myocardial high-energy stores impair the rate of uptake of Ca^{++} from the neighborhood of the myofilaments into the sarcoplasmic reticulum, thus prolonging contraction. Ca^{++} channel blockade will antagonize this process and by diminishing Ca^{++} influx into the cell will lower cytosolic $[Ca^{++}]$, restoring rapid relaxation. On the other hand, caffeine, an agent known to prolong Ca^{++} availability, potentiates the ischemia-induced impairment of ventricular relaxation.[121]

Ischemia thus causes impairment of cardiac contraction and incomplete ventricular emptying (systolic failure) and an elevation of ventricular end-diastolic volume. In addition, it impairs ventricular relaxation and shifts the diastolic pressure-volume curve upward (diastolic failure). The combination of systolic and diastolic failure, leads to elevated ventricular filling pressures,[115,122] ultimately causing symptoms of pulmonary congestion.

RECOGNITION OF MYOCARDIAL ISCHEMIA

ELECTROCARDIOGRAPHIC TECHNIQUES. It has been known for more than a half century that ST-segment elevation is an electrocardiographic sign of coronary artery occlusion.[123] Within 30 to 60 seconds after occlusion in dogs with open chests, epicardial leads from within the area of cyanosis show ST-segment elevation, reaching a maximum 5 to 7 minutes after occlusion. ST-segment elevation in the central area of cyanosis is usually more marked than at the periphery.[124,125] With the use of small intracavitary electrodes, simultaneous ST-segment elevation is noted on the endocardial surface, although it is less marked than that recorded on the epicardium.[124]

The electrophysiological basis of ST-segment changes in myocardial ischemia is discussed on page 223; an altered ion transport across the myocardial cell membrane apparently is the underlying cause. In the nonischemic myocardium, cell volume is regulated within narrow limits by a "sodium pump" located on the plasma membrane.[126] This active, metabolically dependent pump maintains a high extracellular $[Na^+]$ as well as high intracellular $[K^+]$ and colloids, thus stabilizing cell volume.[127] It has been postulated that with ischemia, the availability of energy necessary for this pumping is reduced. According to this concept, Na^+, accompanied by Cl^- and H_2O, accumulates intracellularly and K^+ begins to leak into the extracellular space.[128] The cells eventually lose all control of volume and have an electrolyte distribution similar to that of the extracellular fluid.[126] The reduction in intracellular $[K^+]$ or the accumulation of extracellular K^+ or both are critical in the generation of the elevated ST segment,[129] since small changes in the ratio of intracellular to extracellular $[K^+]$ have a marked effect on the polarity of cellular membranes.[130]

The magnitude of epicardial ST-segment elevation correlates, in general, with the decrease in blood flow, lactate accumulation, and depletion of high-energy phosphate compounds in the underlying myocardium.[131] In addition, ST-segment elevation is associated with a reduction in oxygen tension in the affected tissue below 65 per cent of control,[132] and the magnitude of the elevation correlates well with intramyocardial oxygen tension.[133] Measurements with a mass spectrometer have shown that intramyocardial ST-segment elevations correspond to changes in myocardial gas tensions.[134] Also, epicardial ST-segment elevations shortly after coronary artery occlusion correlate closely with subsequent depletion of myocardial creatine phosphokinase (CPK) activity and with histological evidence of necrosis in the subjacent myocardium.[135-137] It is now clear that the distribution of epicardial ST-segment elevation provides a reasonable index of the extent of myocardial ischemia and that the intramyocardial ST segment is a more sensitive index than the epicardial. However, it must be appreciated that ST-segment elevation is not specific for myocardial ischemia, since the ST segment is also affected by changes in temperature, by drugs (including the digitalis glycosides and quinidine), by sympathetic stimulation of the heart,[138] by epicardial injury due to pericarditis, and by localized intraventricular conduction defects.[139]

ALTERATIONS IN CELLULAR ELECTROPHYSIOLOGY INDUCED BY ISCHEMIA. Ischemia-induced ventricular tachyarrhythmias can be caused by increased automaticity (p. 622), triggered activity (p. 620), and reentry (p. 629). However, knowledge of the effects of acute ischemia on the electrophysiology of the human heart is limited. Although studies in animal models provide major insights, these models may differ from the clinical condition in several aspects, including the nature of the occlusive coronary artery lesion, the presence of multiple lesions, and differences in collateral blood flow. After acute coronary artery ligation *in the dog*, ventricular arrhythmias occur in three phases[140,141]:

1. An early phase begins almost immediately after coronary ligation, frequently culminates in ventricular fibrillation within 3 to 6 minutes, and usually lasts less than 30 minutes. Within minutes after coronary occlusion, marked alterations occur in the electrophysiological properties of ventricular myocardial cells, with shortening of action potential duration and decreased amplitude, upstroke velocity, and resting potential.[142] Extracellular recordings from the epicardial surface of the ischemic zone show marked loss of amplitude and delay and fractionation of recorded electrograms, suggesting that activation in myocardium is irregular and that the effects of ischemia are not uniform.[143] Available evidence suggests that reentry is responsible for ventricular tachycardia and ventricular fibrillation early during ischemia, while the cause of ventricular premature beats is less clear but may be related to the triggering of automatic activity by the current of injury.[144] This early arrhythmic phase observed in experimental animals could be related to the "prehospital" phase of arrhythmias observed in patients, which is also marked by a high incidence of ventricular fibrillation and sudden death. The arrhythmias

of the early phase are intimately rate-related.[140,143,145] Thus, vagally induced cardiac slowing can avert or abort ectopic ventricular rhythms.[143,145] Conversely, ectopic ventricular rhythm can be induced by cardiac pacing.[140]

There is evidence that regional myocardial sympathetic stimulation contributes to the early malignant phase of ventricular arrhythmia after the onset of ischemia. Sympathectomy and beta-adrenergic blockade mitigate both the regional augmentation of cyclic AMP and the frequency and severity of the early phase of ventricular arrhythmias.[146,147] On the other hand, the effectiveness of antiarrhythmic drugs such as quinidine, lidocaine, or aprindine during the early phase is controversial.[148–150]

2. After a period of quiescence, a delayed arrhythmic phase begins at about 6 to 9 hours following coronary occlusion in the dog and lasts for 24 to 72 hours. During this period spontaneous polymorphic ventricular rhythms occur, but ventricular fibrillation is uncommon. Multiple electrophysiological mechanisms are probably involved in the delayed arrhythmic phase, particularly abnormal automaticity of subendocardial Purkinje fibers.[151,152] This phase may partly correspond to ventricular tachycardia and "accelerated idioventricular rhythms" (p. 1286) commonly seen on the second and third days following infarction in humans. Antiarrhythmic drugs such as quinidine, procainamide, lidocaine, and disopyramide suppress these arrhythmias by reducing automaticity.

3. By 72 hours after coronary ligation in the dog, the spontaneous polymorphic ventricular rhythms have nearly subsided, but the heart is still prone to ventricular tachyarrhythmias and, occasionally, ventricular fibrillation. These arrhythmias may be easily induced by rapid cardiac pacing or programmed premature stimulation[153] and are the result of reentrant circuits in the subepicardial layer of the infarction, including the boundary zone between the infarction and surrounding viable myocardium. This late phase of ventricular vulnerability may correspond to the "post-coronary care unit" ventricular arrhythmias and late in-hospital ventricular fibrillation. Antiarrhythmic drugs, such as lidocaine or procainamide, seem to abolish these late reentrant arrhythmias by further depression or block of the already slowed conduction in the reentrant circuit.[154,155]

Mechanics of Arrhythmias. There has been considerable interest in the mechanism of ventricular arrhythmias that occur with release of coronary occlusion and reperfusion,[156] as opposed to occlusion arrhythmias. Ventricular fibrillation is likely to occur abruptly without warning following reperfusion, whereas it is often heralded by ventricular ectopic beats with increasing frequency following occlusion. The most likely explanation for reperfusion arrhythmias is that chemical and electrical gradients caused by washout of metabolites and electrolytes that have accumulated in the ischemic zone are responsible for the electrophysiological derangement.[157,158] Reperfusion is accompanied by changes in regional concentrations of K^+, Ca^{++}, H^+, catecholamines, and lysophosphoglycerides; the last are derived from degradation of membrane phospholipids in cells undergoing infarction.[159] There may be some relevance of reperfusion arrhythmias in experimental animals to such clinical syndromes as the abrupt onset of ventricular fibrillation in patients who are undergoing surgical, thrombolytic, or spontaneous reperfusion after thrombotic coronary occlusion, and the malignant arrhythmias that can accompany Prinzmetal's angina; the release of coronary spasm may be a common cause of reperfusion and its attendant arrhythmias.

The biochemical correlates of ischemia-induced electrophysiological changes are not clearly identified. Ischemia depresses the energy-dependent membrane sodium-potassium pumping system, which leads to a gain in intracellular sodium and loss of intracellular potassium with consequent elevation of extracellular potassium concentration in the vicinity of the sarcolemma.[160,161] As a result of anaerobic metabolism, intracellular pH declines. Ischemia also results in release of norepinephrine from adrenergic nerve endings and an increase of tissue levels of cyclic AMP.[162] It has been postulated that in the ischemic zone, high concentrations of extracellular K^+ may depolarize the cells to the extent that the rapid Na^+ channel is inactivated, and high concentrations of catecholamines may stimulate the slow current carried principally by Ca^{++}, resulting in slow response action potentials. The latter could explain the slowed conduction and reentrant ventricular arrhythmias associated with ischemia. However, it must be acknowledged that while this hypothesis is attractive, its validity has not been established, and indeed has been questioned.[150,157,163]

The concept that slow response action potentials are responsible for ischemia-induced electrophysiological disturbances loses much of its plausibility in the later stage of myocardial infarction. The extracellular K^+ concentration is probably not as high as in the early stage of ischemia. Besides, total catecholamines in the ischemic region decline to a very low level on the day after coronary occlusion.[164] However, ischemic myocardium still shows markedly depressed action potentials, slow conduction, and a high propensity for reentrant rhythms.[165] In the later stage of ischemia, ischemic myocardial cells have been found to be exquisitely sensitive to the depressant effect of tetrodotoxin, a specific blocker of the fast Na^+ channel, and not to verapamil and D600, which are blockers of the slow Ca^{++} channel.[165] These observations suggest that poor membrane responses of ischemic myocardial cells are related to depression of the fast Na^+ channel. The clinical relevance of studies of ischemia-induced ionic conductance changes relates to the choice of ideal antiarrhythmic therapy following ischemia. Thus, the antiarrhythmic effect of lidocaine on ischemia-induced reentrant ventricular arrhythmias is due to selective depression of ischemic myocardial cells forming part of the reentrant pathway.[154,155] The finding that the effect of lidocaine on depressed ischemic cells is similar to that of tetrodotoxin suggests that lidocaine acts by further depressing the tenuous Na^+ channel in ischemic cells.[154,155]

EFFECTS OF ISCHEMIA ON MYOCARDIAL METABOLISM

HIGH-ENERGY PHOSPHATE METABOLISM. During the first minutes of severe ischemia, the production of high-energy phosphates (the sum of ATP and creatine phosphate (CP)) declines and is greatly exceeded by the utilization; hence tissue stores decline progressively, with CP stores falling more rapidly than ATP stores. CP is depleted by transferring its high-energy phosphate to ADP in an attempt to maintain ATP stores. In the presence of normal aerobic mitochondrial function, ADP is converted to ATP (through the myokinase reaction), but in the absence of normal oxidative phosphorylation it is converted to AMP (Fig. 36–12), which in turn is broken down to adenosine and ultimately to inosine, hypoxanthine, and xanthine (Fig. 36–10).[166] Reimer and Jennings have shown that when ATP was reduced below 20 per cent of control values the ability to regenerate high-energy phosphate, preserve cell volume, and maintain ionic regulation were lost. When ATP fell below 10 per cent of control, damage to the sarcolemma occurred.[167] When tissue is *reversibly* injured by ischemia (i.e., its viability can be maintained by reperfusion), ATP stores are usually greater than 60 per cent of control and electronmicroscopy may reveal only glycogen loss, nuclear chromatin clumping, intermyofibrillar edema, and mitochondrial swelling but no sarcolemma damage or amorphous dense bodies in the mitochondria. Reduction of ATP below 30 per cent is usually associated with visible sarcolemmal damage and irreversible injury (i.e., the tissue is not viable despite reperfusion).[168,169]

The technique of phosphorus-31 nuclear magnetic resonance spectroscopy (^{31}PNMR) (Chap. 11B) is providing important new information concerning high-energy phosphate stores and intracellular pH in ischemic myocardium. Multiple sequential measurements can be made on the same tissue and correlated with mechanical activity.[169] This technique has demonstrated that the magnitude of intracellular acidosis and associated increase in inorganic phosphate correlate inversely with postischemic structure and recovery of function. ATP but not CP content correlates with return of contractile function after reperfusion.[170]

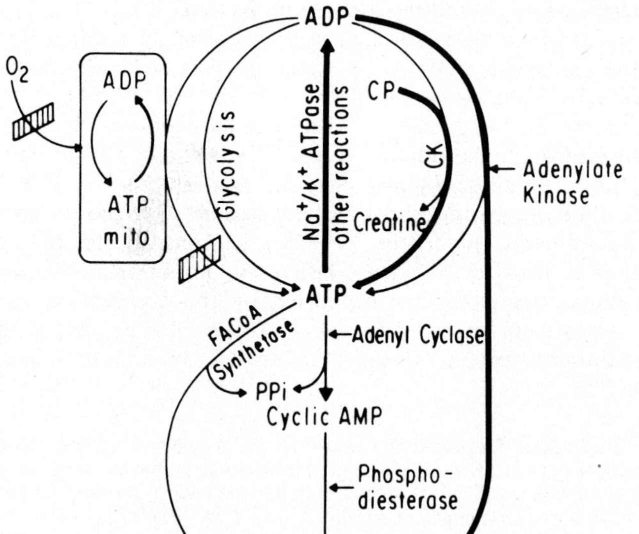

FIGURE 36–12 The major metabolic pathways of adenine nucleotide degradation during myocardial ischemia are illustrated. The quantitatively most important pathways are indicated by the solid arrows. (Reproduced with permission from Jennings, R. B., Reimer, K. A., Hill, M. L., and Mayer, S. E.: Total ischemia in dog hearts, in vitro. 1. Comparison of high energy phosphate production, utilization, and depletion, and of adenine nucleotide catabolism in total ischemia in vitro vs. severe ischemia in vivo. Circ. Res. *49*:892, 1981, by permission of the American Heart Association, Inc.)

Carbohydrate metabolism. Under normal aerobic conditions, myocardium derives its energy primarily from oxidative phosphorylation, a process localized to the mitochondria. Although many types of substrate can be utilized, oxidation of fatty acids predominates. Oxidative phosphorylation is regulated to a large extent by the phosphate potential: (ATP)/(ADP) $\times$ (P_i). When oxygen availability is limited, the rate of ATP synthesis declines and high-energy phosphate stores decline. Depletion of purine nucleotide pools is prompt. It persists for hours to days after even brief intervals of ischemia, in part because of the limited capacity of myocardium for de novo purine synthesis. The reduction in the phosphate potential and the prevailing concentrations of intermediates such as glucose-6-phosphate alter the activity of enzymes involved in intermediary metabolism. During hypoxia, glycolytic flux increases because of enhanced uptake of glucose and also phosphorylation, reflecting (1) decline of glucose-6-phosphate and release of inhibition of hexokinase; (2) release of inhibition of phosphofructokinase (PFK) by citrate and ATP; and (3) activation of PFK by inorganic phosphate. Glycogenolysis accelerates because of transformation of phosphorylase b, an inactive form of the enzyme under physiological conditions, to the active, phosphorylated form, phosphorylase a. Later, glycogenolysis is potentiated by activation of phosphorylase b itself, by accumulating metabolites such as adenosine monophosphate, and by release of inhibition by glucose-6-phosphate (Fig. 36–13).

The augmentation of glycolytic flux so characteristic of hypoxia and of the initial response to ischemia may contribute to maintenance of viability of the heart by providing ATP. The importance of glycolysis in the generation of energy is reflected in the observation that inhibition of glycolysis with iodoacetate results in cessation of beating of the anoxic heart even though the agent does not influence the apparent function of the well-oxygenated heart. Augmentation of glycolytic flux by provision of glucose or prior augmentation of glycogen stores confers some resistance to the deterioration of function induced by anoxia or ischemia. Nevertheless, even with insulin present in the perfusion medium, anaerobic metabolism can supply less than half the energy requirement for maintenance of viability of the nonworking, isolated, perfused, anoxic heart. Thus, anaerobic metabolism alone cannot maintain myocardial ATP stores indefinitely in the nonworking heart, let alone in myocardium with markedly greater energy requirements associated with contractile function.

Under aerobic conditions, carbohydrate metabolism proceeds via oxidation through the Krebs (tricarboxylic acid) cycle. However, when anoxia supervenes, the lack of oxygen inhibits Krebs cycle activity and the metabolism of glucose can proceed only via anaerobic glycolysis. When the cause of anoxia is ischemia, lactate accumulates, since oxidation of pyruvate is precluded by the inhibition of the Krebs cycle, and washout of metabolites is reduced because of the limited perfusion. The initial burst of glycolytic activity accompanying hypoxia with or without ischemia appears to depend on allosteric effects of adenine nucleotides and other regulators of enzymes such as phosphorylase b, hexokinase, and phosphofructokinase.[173] However, under conditions of limited perfusion sufficient to induce hypoxia, the rapidly increasing concentration of lactic acid within the cell, the decline of pH, and the accumulation of other metabolites inhibit glycolytic flux at the phosphofructokinase and glyceraldehyde-3-phosphate dehydrogenase[172,173] steps, among others (Fig. 36–11).

In isolated perfused hearts, lactate exerts a deleterious effect on glycolytic flux independent of pH[174] by inhibiting the glyceraldehyde-phosphate dehydrogenase reaction, which is responsible for conversion of glyceraldehyde-3-phosphate to 1,3-diphosphoglyceric acid. On the other hand, acidosis itself inhibits glycolytic flux,[174,175] left ventricular performance, and the malate-aspartate cycle.[174–176] This and other similar cycles provide a shuttle via intermediates to which the mitochondrial membranes are permeable, permitting transport of reducing equivalents formed in the cytosol across the mitochondrial membranes and thereby allowing their oxidation by the respiratory chain. Persistent or prolonged ischemia results in inhibition of the shuttle reactions because of accumulation of reducing equivalents in the mitochondria (due to the lack of oxygen as a terminal electron and hydrogen receptor), with consequent accumulation of reducing equivalents and hydrogen ions in the cytosol as well.

The acidosis and accumulation of metabolites contribute directly to inhibition of glycolytic flux.[177] Thus, because glycolytic flux in ischemic tissue becomes limited relatively soon after the initial burst of activity, it is capable of meeting only a significantly smaller proportion of energy requirements than in anoxic tissue. The decline of high-energy phosphate stores is therefore faster, perhaps contributing to the more

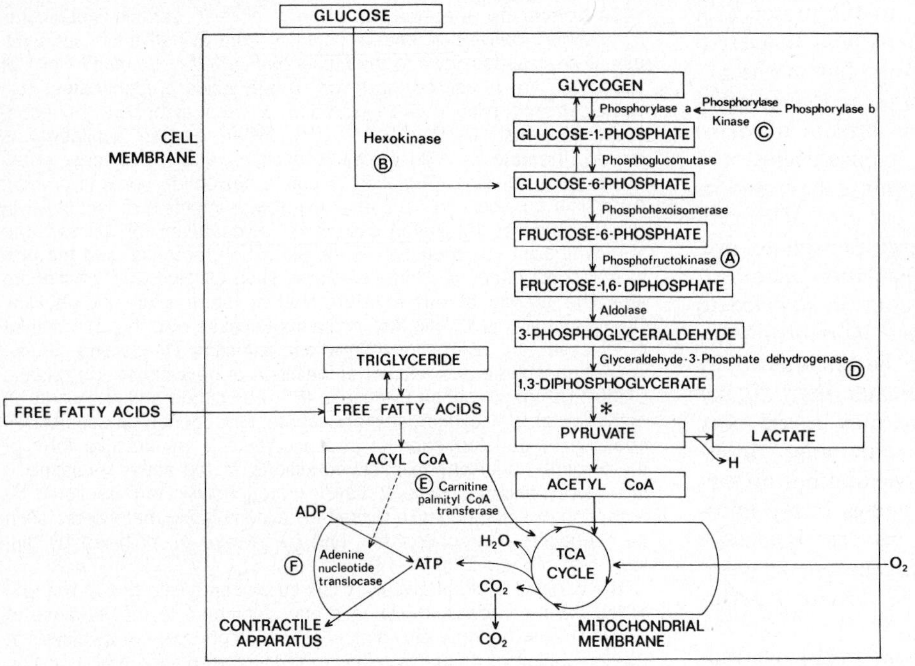

FIGURE 36–13 Effects of ischemia on glycolysis and free fatty acid metabolism. Ischemia increases intracellular lactate concentration; this accumulation inhibits several enzymes in the glycolytic pathway: Phosphofructokinase (A); hexokinase (B); and phosphorylase kinase (C), which prevents activation of phosphorylase b to phosphorylase a and therefore suppresses conversion of glycogen to glucose-1-phosphate. Glyceraldehyde-3-phosphate dehydrogenase (D) is suppressed by an elevation of intracellular lactate. (* denotes that the glycolytic pathway has been condensed at this point.) Ischemia increases the intracellular concentration of acyl CoA esters, in part because the intracellular accumulation of lactate inhibits carnitine palmityl coenzyme A transferase (E), the enzyme that catalyzes the transfer of acyl CoA from the cell cytoplasm to the mitochondria. Acyl CoA esters inhibit the effective exchange of ADP and ATP between the cytoplasm of the cell and the mitochondria by suppressing the activity of adenine nucleotide translocase (F). The antilipolytic agents are effective because they prevent a build-up of acyl CoA esters within the cytoplasm, and 1-carnitine exerts a salutary effect on ischemic myocardium by reversing the inhibition of adenine nucleotide translocase, thus allowing continued movement of ADP and ATP between the cell cytoplasm and the mitochondria. (TCA = tricarboxylic acid.) (Reproduced with permission from Hillis, L. D., and Braunwald, E.: Myocardial ischemia. N. Engl. J. Med. *296*:971, 1034, and 1093; 1977.)

rapid development of irreversible injury in ischemic compared with anoxic myocardium.

The above-described changes in carbohydrate metabolism induced by myocardial ischemia account for the relationship between lactate production and the severity of impaired perfusion; this relationship may be exploited diagnostically. Under normal aerobic conditions, myocardium extracts lactate from the arterial blood with extraction fractions in the range of 20 per cent. Extraction persists despite acceleration of ventricular rate by pacing.[178] However, when myocardial ischemia is present at rest or develops in response to stress induced by pacing or other physiological stimuli, lactate extraction declines or is replaced by net lactate production[179] (p. 1344). In general, both decreased lactate extraction and an increase in lactate production are accompanied by an increase in coronary venous lactate/pyruvate ratios, compared with values in arterial blood. Unfortunately, relationships between the concentrations of lactate in coronary sinus blood and in extracellular fluid, cytosol, and mitochondrial compartments are complex and are influenced by nonspecific factors such as acid-base balance, adrenergic stimulation of the heart, substrate availability, permeability of cell membranes to lactate and pyruvate, concomitant disorders such as diabetes mellitus, and prevailing levels of plasma free fatty acids. Furthermore, net lactate extraction is a relatively insensitive index of changes occurring in localized regions of the heart. Accordingly, the diagnostic sensitivity and specificity of altered lactate extraction for the detection or assessment of severity of ischemia are somewhat limited.

Differences Between Ischemia and Anoxia. Although differences between anoxia and ischemia have been alluded to above, it is useful to summarize them at this point. Not only is oxidative metabolism reduced during ischemia, as it is in anoxia, but the anaerobic production of ATP also proceeds at less than maximal capacity. In the ischemic working heart the concentration of lactic acid rises and the intracellular pH falls rapidly as the acid products of glycolysis accumulate. In contrast, in the anoxic heart perfusion results in the washout of the acid products of glycolysis, thereby retarding the rate of development of intracellular acidosis. The increased lactate production is not sustained by the ischemic heart, which has a glycolytic rate about one fourth that of the anoxic heart in a steady state. This is unrelated to a reduction of substrate availability, because the addition of insulin and glucose to the perfusion medium fails to stimulate glycolysis to the extent observed in anoxia or under normal aerobic conditions. While insulin and elevated glucose in the perfusate are able to increase glucose transport and augment the intracellular glucose concentration, they do not prevent ischemia from inhibiting glucose utilization.

The lower glycolytic flux in the ischemic as compared to the anoxic heart probably results in part from the inhibition by intracellular acidosis of PFK (Fig. 36–11), a key enzyme in the glycolytic chain. The reduction of glycolytic flux through the inhibition of PFK results in the accumulation of glucose-6-phosphate, and this inhibits hexokinase, further decreasing the phosphorylation of glucose. As a consequence, glycolysis provides less energy to the ischemic than to the anoxic heart. The importance of intracellular pH is further supported by the observation that pretreatment of rat myocardium to an alkaline pH of 7.9 maintains tension during a subsequent period of hypoxia.[180]

Fatty Acid Metabolism. Under normal aerobic conditions, 60 to 90 per cent of myocardial energy requirements is met by oxidation of free fatty acids (FFA),[181] which are trapped in cells in the form of fatty (acyl) esters containing coenzyme A (acyl-CoA). The preferential utilization of FFA by myocardium appears to depend on the high activity of several enzyme systems, including the acyl-CoA–carnitine transferase systems that facilitate continuing transport of acyl-CoA from the cytosol to the mitochondria in a series of steps in which acyl-CoA and acyl-carnitine are interconverted.

After fatty acids are taken up by myocardial cells and undergo esterfication with CoA, the acyl-CoA intermediates generally remain trapped in the cell. Acyl-CoA may be incorporated into triglycerides in the cytosol or oxidized after transport through the mitochondrial membrane. Under aerobic conditions, oxidation predominates since the products formed (two carbon moieties called acetyl groups) are readily incorporated as intermediates into the citric acid cycle and oxidized to CO_2 and water. Oxidation of fatty acids inhibits glucose uptake, glycolytic flux, and glycogenolysis. The increased production of acetyl-CoA accompanying fatty acid oxidation inhibits pyruvate dehydrogenase,[182] thereby limiting the flow of carbohydrate metabolism through the citric acid cycle. Accumulation of glucose-6-phosphate inhibits hexokinase, decreasing phosphorylation of glucose. The decreased phosphorylation, coupled with direct inhibition of membrane transport of glucose mediated by fatty acids, contributes to the overall reduction of carbohydrate metabolism when fatty acid availability is high and oxygenation adequate.[183]

Striking changes in fatty acid metabolism result from myocardial ischemia. The limited supply of oxygen inhibits beta-oxidation—as does the increased ratio of NADH/NAD and the reduced concentration of flavoproteins.[173] With more prolonged ischemia, oxidation of fatty acids is inhibited by another mechanism: inhibition or loss of long-chain acyl-carnitine transferase enzyme activity, necessary for transport of cytosolic acyl-CoA to the mitchondria prior to oxidation.[184] Accordingly, intracellular concentrations of acyl-CoA increase and acetyl-CoA content declines.[185,186] The increased acyl-CoA accompanied by increased production of glycerol, a byproduct of the enhanced glycolytic flux induced by ischemia, leads to increased synthesis of triglycerides,[187] which accumulate in the ischemic myocardium.

Accumulation of acyl-CoA may be deleterious because it inhibits further formation of CoA esters of fatty acids. Thus, fatty acids entering the cell cannot be esterified and trapped and are therefore prone to egress promptly. Furthermore, oxidation of fatty acids entering the cell cannot proceed without initial esterification with CoA. Accordingly, accumulation of fatty acid labeled with carbon-11, which can be monitored externally in vivo by positron tomography, is diminished in ischemic or hypoxic zones.[188,189] Restored metabolism accompanying reperfusion implemented promptly enough to maintain cell viability is reflected by a return of myocardial accumulation of fatty acid toward normal[190,191] (Fig. 36–14).

Accumulation of acyl-CoA esters also inhibits activity of an enzyme in the inner mitochondrial membrane, adenine nucleotide translocase—important in myocardial energy metabolism[192] and required for transport of ATP synthesized in the mitochrondria to the cytosol. Although definitive information is not yet available, inhibition of the translocase and consequent failure of repletion of cytosolic ATP may be one factor accounting for the prompt decline of creatine phosphate in ischemic myocardium. Creatine kinase facilitates phosphorylation of ADP to form ATP, with concomitant conversion of creatine phosphate to creatine when cytosolic ATP concentrations decline. Thus, cytosolic creatine phosphate content declines as the cell compensates for diminished transport of ATP from mitochrondria to cytosol. Accordingly, the effects of limited oxygen availability in ischemic myocardium on fatty acid metabolism may result in impaired energy production not only by direct limitation of oxidation of fatty acids, but also because of deleterious effects of the accumulating acyl-CoA intermediates on cellular function.

Detection of altered fatty acid metabolism is the basis for recognition of ischemic myocardium in experimental animals and patients after intravenous administration of cyclotron-produced, positron-emitting, ^{11}C-labeled fatty acids. In isolated perfused hearts, transitory diminution of perfusion leads to a reversible reduction of ^{11}C-palmitate accumulation, reflecting decreased uptake and oxidation of fatty acids in the perfusate.[193,194,194a,194b,194c] The uptake of tracer is independent of flow per se, as long as metabolic activity of the myocardium remains constant. In dogs subjected to coronary occlusion, diminished accumulation of ^{11}C-palmitate is evident in computer-reconstructed images obtained by positron-emission, transaxial tomography. Because this technique permits quantitative delineation of the distribution of the tracer in a cross-section of the heart after intravenous administration, the diminution of ^{11}C-palmitate uptake detectable tomographically corresponds quantitatively to biochemical and morphometric criteria of infarction.[195] Reduced flow alone does not diminish uptake of a substrate if intermediary metabolism is not altered, since the extraction fraction increases. Thus, transitory ischemia without reduction of either myocardial oxygen consumption or fatty acid utilization would not be manifested tomographically by decreased ^{11}C-palmitate uptake.[196] However, prolonged ischemia, with impairment of oxidative metabolism but without necrosis, would give rise to a zone

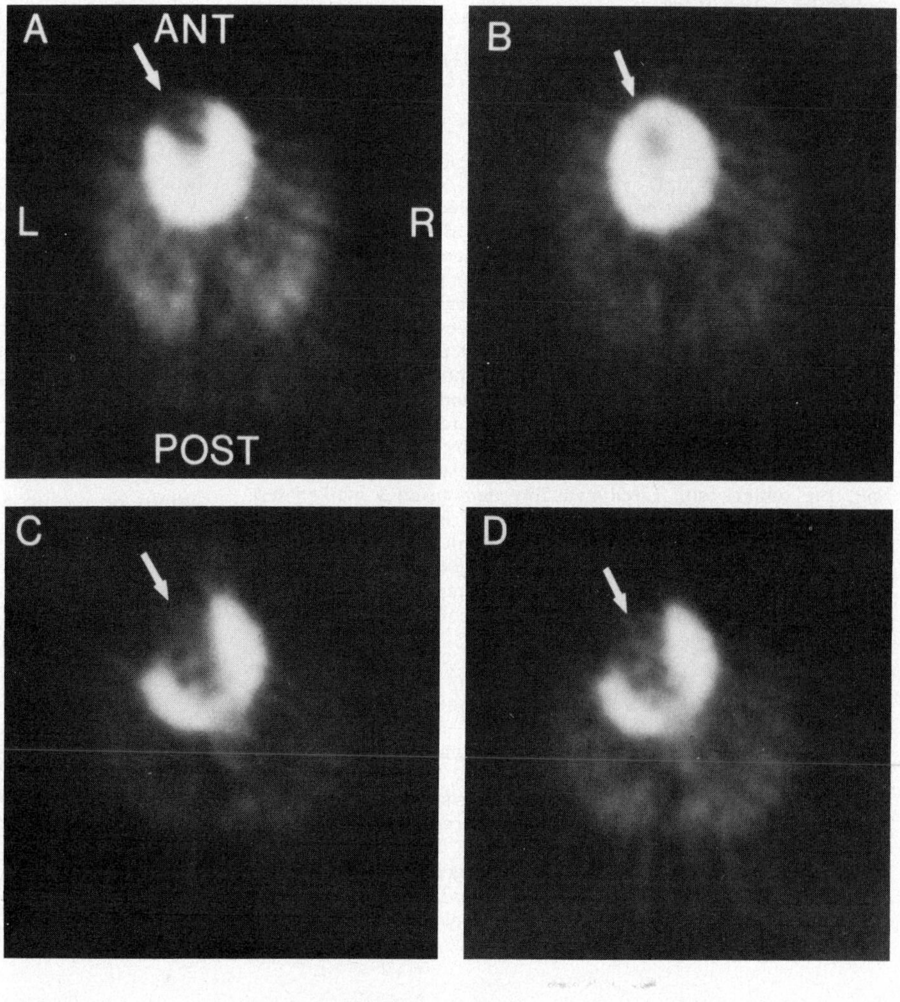

FIGURE 36–14 Transverse cardiac positron emission tomographic reconstructions obtained after intravenous administration of ^{11}C-palmitate in dogs. Reconstructions depicted are those obtained one hour after experimentally induced left anterior descending coronary artery thrombosis (*A*) and again after thrombolysis in the same dog (*B*). Normal myocardium extracts palmitate uniformly, whereas the ischemic zone exhibits diminished accumulation of tracer (arrow). The tomogram in panel *B* demonstrates substantial restoration of metabolism in the previously compromised anterior myocardium. In the lower panel, a tomogram six hours after onset of thrombosis and prior to the administration of streptokinase is shown (*C*) with a repeat tomogram (*D*) from the same dog one hour after intracoronary thrombolysis with streptokinase (confirmed angiographically). In contrast to the restoration of metabolism observed in dogs in which reperfusion was induced early after thrombosis, animals subjected to thrombolysis later than six hours after occlusion exhibited no significant restoration of metabolism despite angiographically documented lysis of coronary thrombi. (From Sobel, B. E., and Bergmann, S. R.: Coronary thrombolysis: Some unresolved issues. Am. J. Med. *72*:1, 1982. Reprinted with permission of Yorke Publishing Corporation.)

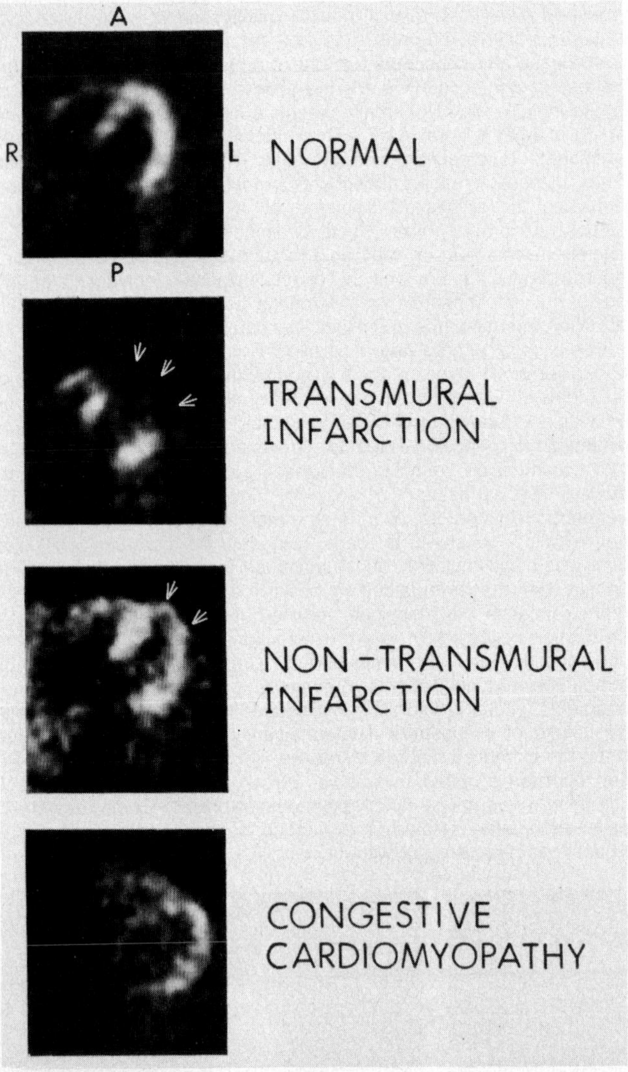

FIGURE 36–15 Cardiac positron emission tomographic reconstructions obtained at the midventricular level after the intravenous injection of ^{11}C-palmitate, in a normal subject, patients with transmural and nontransmural infarction, and a patient with congestive cardiomyopathy. The horseshoe-shaped region depicts a 1.5 cm thick cross-section of the left ventricular myocardium. Accumulation of palmitate is homogeneous throughout each cross-section in the left ventricle in the normal subject. A homogeneous, intense depression of the accumulation of palmitate indicated by the arrow is found in the subject with anterior transmural infarction. The region of nontransmural infarction indicated by the arrow involves only a portion of the thickness of the anterolateral left ventricular wall. The subject with cardiomyopathy demonstrates marked left ventricular enlargement with marked spatial heterogeneity of the accumulation of palmitate within the left ventricular myocardium. A = anterior, P = posterior, L = left, R = right. (From Geltman, E. M., and Sobel, B. E.: Cardiac positron tomography. Chest, in press. Reprinted with permission of the American College of Chest Physicians.)

of decreased accumulation of the tracer evident by tomography. The two conditions (prolonged ischemia without necrosis and infarction per se) can be readily differentiated with the use of serial studies. Prolonged and persistent diminution of oxidative metabolism and hence persistently impaired regional uptake of ^{11}C-palmitate detectable tomographically are tantamount to necrosis in view of the well-established irreversibility of injury sustained by myocardium rendered ischemic for 2 hours or more[197] (Fig. 36–15).

Protein Metabolism. Characteristic changes in synthesis and degradation of myocardial proteins accompany ischemia. Synthesis decreases because of inhibition of peptide chain initiation and elongation.[198] Efflux of alanine reflects not only its diminished utilization in protein synthesis but also augmented synthesis by transamination of pyruvate, a precursor accumulating because of impaired carbohydrate exudation.[199] Thus, alanine release from the ischemic heart is analogous to lactate production.

Release of another amino acid, phenylalanine, has been employed in experimental preparations in which reincorporation into protein is prevented by pretreatment with cycloheximide (an inhibitor of protein synthesis) to provide an index of protein degradation under a variety of conditions, including normal oxygenation, anoxia, and simulated ischemia. The process of protein degradation requires energy derived from oxidative metabolism under physiological conditions based on observations with such preparations, since the rate of protein degradation declines by as much as 80 per cent in isolated hearts subjected to severe ischemia.[200] Although proteolysis mediated by lysosomal hydrolases has been implicated as a factor leading to irreversible injury in myocardium undergoing ischemic injury, increases in free and total lysosomal hydrolase activity do not occur until several hours after the onset of ischemia.[201] Accordingly, it appears likely that the early loss of functional sarcolemmal integrity accompanied by electrophysiological manifestations, subsequent impairment of cell volume regulation, and leakage of cytoplasmic constituents reflects primary damage to the cell membrane itself. Only later during the evolution of ischemic injury, when tissue pH is markedly diminished and reparative processes have already begun, do activation and liberation of lysosomal enzymes appear to be prominent. These and related observations suggest that the irreversible nature of injury sustained by ischemic myocardium is not due to proteolysis or activation of lysosomal enzymes, even though activation of these enzymes may account for the release of relatively late markers of cell death and result in protein degradation late in the evolution of necrosis.

Under physiological conditions, the myocardium extracts glutamic acid from arterial blood and produces ammonia and glutamine which appear in the coronary venous effluent. When ischemia supervenes, ammonia derived from amino acids that cannot be incorporated into protein under these conditions is incorporated into alanine and glutamine with a consequent increase in their concentrations in the coronary sinus effluent. The increased production of alanine has been viewed as analogous to the increased production of lactate. Both are markers of ischemia. In the case of alanine, transamination of pyruvate serves as a sink for ammonia that would otherwise accumulate. In the case of lactate, the pyruvate serves as a sink for hydrogen ions.

OXIDATIVE PHOSPHORYLATION. The importance of oxidative phosphorylation, i.e., the coupling of ATP synthesis to aerobic respiration, for the metabolic integrity of myocardium is underscored by some simple quantitative considerations. Complete oxidation of one mole of glucose gives rise to the net production of 36 moles of ATP. In contrast, only 2 moles of ATP are produced from complete anaerobic metabolism of 1 mole of glucose. Thus, even if the profound derangements in intermediary metabolism associated with increased production of reducing equivalents accompanying anaerobic glycolysis could be corrected, an 18-fold increase in glycolytic flux would be required for myocardium to synthesize comparable quantities of ATP via anaerobic compared to aerobic metabolism. The failure of energy production to keep pace with demand in ischemic cells is manifest by a prompt decline in the concentration of creatine phosphate, a major constituent of myocardial high-energy phosphate stores.[202]

The dependence of myocardial viability on the availability of oxygen has stimulated careful assessment of the gradients of oxygen present within ischemic zones of the heart, based on analysis of the oxidation-reduction state of specific components of the electron transport chain and different spectra reflecting changes in the oxygenation of myoglobin.[203] Results obtained with optical techniques applied to the infarcted heart in vitro suggest that individual cells, and possibly individual mitochondria, are either fully aerobic or fully anaerobic in regions of myocardium subjected to ischemia. Thus, at any given instant, borders between anoxic and oxygenated tissue are very sharp. This phenomenon is in part a reflection of the very high affinity of mitochondria for oxygen. In response to ischemia, the mitochondria remain oxidized, despite very low levels of tissue oxygen tension, and become reduced only when virtually the last remaining oxygen has been utilized within a region. However, it should be recognized that the sharp, anatomically definable, border zones detectable at a given instant with these optical techniques do not imply the absence of a time-dependent, potentially large mass of jeopardized but not yet irreversibly injured ischemic myocardium, susceptible to favorable influence by selected interventions. In fact, as ischemia persists, the locations of the discrete borders shift, judging from morphological observations in canine hearts subjected to coronary occlusion.

The percentage of transmural necrosis ultimately developing within a zone of myocardium rendered ischemic by coronary occlusion maintained for 40 minutes, 3 hours, 6 hours, and 24 hours, followed by reperfusion for 2 to 4 days, varies from 38 to 85 per cent with a "wavefront" of necrosis progressing from subendocardial to epicardial tissue.[204] Obviously, a cell may be able to tolerate severe ischemia for a brief interval although it will become necrotic after a prolonged insult. A cell with similar energy requirements will be able to tolerate a milder degree of ischemia for a longer period before becoming necrotic.[205] The extent to which ischemic myocardium may be protected by metabolic, pharmacological, or physiological interventions designed to improve the balance between myocardial oxygen supply and demand (Chap. 38) cannot be inferred from the sharpness of the border of oxygenation at a specific instant during the evolution of injury. In fact, the location of the transmural wavefront of irreversible injury is a function of the duration as well as the severity of limitation of oxygen supply and of the rate of accumulation of noxious metabolites in specific regions.

ACTIVATION OF LYSOSOMAL ENZYMES. Most tissues contain latent lysosomal hydrolases capable of mediating proteolysis under certain conditions. Lysosomal hydrolases are activated by an acid pH, although mammalian cells contain neutral proteases as well. Relatively late reparative processes in myocardium undergoing infarction are accompanied by consistent increases in lysosomal hydrolase activity in tissue extracts as well as in the circulation, suggesting that activation of proteases with dissolution of cellular debris is a component of the response to irreversible injury. However, the extent to which activation of lysosomal hydrolases contributes to early manifestations of ischemia or irreversibility remains controversial. What is clear is that much of the lysosomal activity in the heart undergoing infarction comes from cells participating in the response to inflammation, such as polymorphonuclear leukocytes rather than myocardial cells per se.

Calcium Metabolism in Ischemia

Myocardial injury induced by ischemia is associated with complexes of calcium in the tissue detectable by electron microscopy.[205–207] The interaction between myocardial ischemia and myoplasmic [Ca^{++}] is complex, as illustrated in Figure 36–16. Ischemia, however produced, is characterized by a reduction of myocardial ATP stores, which interferes with the transsarcolemmal Na^+-K^+ exchange, which in turn elevates intracellular [Na^+], raising intracellular [Ca^{++}] through an enhanced Na^+-Ca^{++} exchange. Lowered ATP stores also reduce Ca^{++} uptake by the sarcoplasmic reticulum and reduce extrusion of Ca^{++} from cells. The resultant augmented intracellular [Ca^{++}] causes mitochondrial Ca^{++} overload, which depresses ATP production further. Activation of intracellular Ca^{++} ATPases augments ATP usage and activates sarcolemmal phospholipases, which release membrane phospholipid degradation products whose detergent properties impair the integrity of the cell membrane.[208,209] Calcium-channel blockers interfere with Ca^{++} influx through voltage-dependent channels.

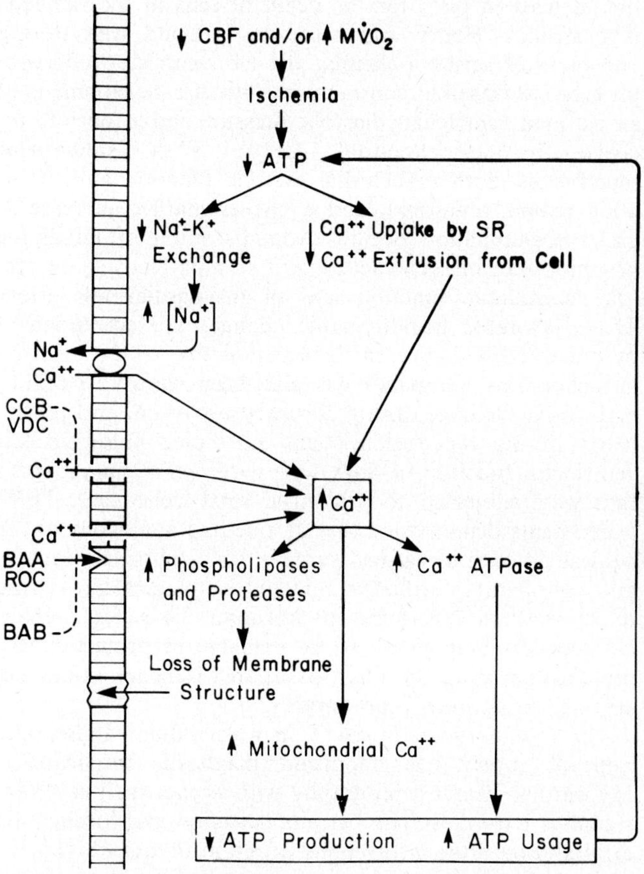

FIGURE 36–16 Interactions between myocardial ischemia and [Ca^{++}]. A reduction of coronary blood flow (CBF), sometimes accompanied by an increase in myocardial oxygen requirements ($M\dot{V}O_2$), causes myocardial ischemia, which in turn reduces cellular ATP stores. This reduction interferes with the transsarcolemmal Na^+-K^+ exchange, which elevates intracellular [NA^+], raising intracellular [Ca^{++}] through an enhanced Na^+-Ca^{++} exchange. Lowered ATP stores also reduce Ca^{++} uptake by the sarcoplasmic reticulum (SR) and reduce extrusion of Ca^{++} from cells. The resultant augmented intracellular [Ca^{++}] causes mitochondrial Ca^{++} overload, which depresses ATP production further; activation of intracellular Ca^{++} ATPases, which augment ATP usage; and activation of sarcolemmal phospholipases and proteases, which impair the integrity of the cell membrane. Calcium-channel blockers (CCB) interfere with Ca^{++} influx through voltage-dependent channels (VDA). Beta-adrenergic agonists (BAA) recruit additional receptor-operated channels (ROC). Beta-adrenergic blockers (BAB) reduce Ca^{++} influx by interfering with the recruitment of ROC. (Reproduced with permission from Braunwald, E.: Mechanism of action of calcium channel blocking agents. N. Engl. J. Med. *307*:1618, 1982.)

Beta-adrenergic agonists recruit additional receptor-operated channels, and beta-adrenergic blockers reduce Ca^{++} influx by interfering with the recruitment of receptor-operated channels. Thus, one would expect beta blockers and Ca^{++}-channel blockers to have similar effects in the treatment of ischemia. Indeed, both groups of compounds delay ischemia-induced necrosis and, particularly when combined with reperfusion, reduce the extent of myocardial necrosis.[210,211]

The hypothesis that the entry of Ca^{++} into ischemic cells may be harmful is based on the observation that after a period of myocardial ischemia and subsequent reperfusion the accumulation of excess Ca^{++} in the mitochondria may interfere with their capacity to generate ATP. The destructive chain of metabolic events provoked by increased intracellular [Ca^{++}] appears to be responsible, at least in part, for the death of cells in the ischemic myocardium. Henry and associates[212] found that during one hour of severe ischemia, the left ventricle undergoes progressive ischemic contracture, with the development of an elevated ventricular diastolic pressure and a fourfold increase in mitochondrial Ca^{++}. With subsequent reperfusion, both myocardial systolic function and relaxation remain abnormal, and a further marked increase in Ca^{++} accumulation occurs. Administration of nifedipine prevents ischemic contracture and permits recovery of systolic contractile function and of myocardial relaxation. These favorable hemodynamic changes are accompanied by a marked reduction in the accumulation of Ca^{++} in the mitochondria. Verapamil has also been shown to reduce myocardial damage during coronary occlusion, and particularly during reperfusion,[213] and nifedipine preserved left ventricular function in dogs with cardiopulmonary bypass that were subjected to prolonged total ischemia.[214] These experiments demonstrate that in a setting analogous to the clinical practice of cardiac surgery, Ca^{++}-channel blockers give considerable hemodynamic and histological protection to the ischemic-reperfused myocardium. Thus, Ca^{++}-channel blockers may prove to be valuable in protecting the myocardium from the Ca^{++}-associated ischemic injury occurring during open heart surgery.

The accumulation of Ca^{++} in myocardium undergoing ischemic injury has important diagnostic implications. Myocardial infarct scintigraphy with agents such as ^{99m}Tc-stannous pyrophosphate permits detection and localization of infarction after intravenous injection of tracer. The tissue's avidity for the tracer appears to depend on the accumulation of Ca^{++} (p. 380).

RELEASE OF ENZYMES IN DETECTION OF ACUTE MYOCARDIAL INFARCTION

Acute myocardial infarction is detected on the basis of clinical, electrocardiographic, biochemical, and radiographic phenomena, considered in detail in Chapter 37. Since biochemical markers of ischemic injury have become important clinical tools, some considerations required for their proper interpretation merit particular attention. Loss of functional integrity of the sarcolemma is a primary common denominator underlying liberation of cytoplasmic constituents into the circulation, such as transaminase (SGOT, AST), lactic dehydrogenase (LDH), and creatine kinase (CK).[215,216] Species of lower molecular weight, such as myoglobin, are liberated, but elevated concentrations persist in the circulation only briefly because of rapid renal clearance. Furthermore, myoglobin released from hypoperfused skeletal muscle may cloud interpretation of elevated values in plasma.[217]

Accurate assessment of myocardial infarction based on analysis of plasma enzyme time-activity curves has been facilitated by the demonstration that one isoenzyme of creatine kinase, MB CK, is localized virtually exclusively in myocardium as opposed to other tissues in humans.[216-218] Under carefully defined conditions in experimental animals, depletion of myocardial CK activity correlates with infarct size estimated independently by morphometric techniques or with the use of radioactively labeled microspheres.[219] The corollary of these observations, namely, that increases in plasma enzyme activity reflect infarct size, has been recognized for many years.[220]

Based on review of many clinical studies[221] and observations in conscious experimental animals,[222] it has become clear that release of myocardial cytosolic enzymes into the circulation is tantamount to cell death when the cause of enzyme release is myocardial ischemia. Accordingly, infarct size has been estimated from analysis of plasma enzyme CK time-activity curves,[223-225] and recently from curves obtained by quantitative assay of plasma samples for MB CK activity.[226] Despite obvious imperfections, enzymatic estimates of infarct size have correlated with biochemical and morphological analyses of infarction in hearts of experimental animals, morbidity and mortality in patients, histochemical assessment of necrosis among patients who succumb to acute myocardial infarction,[227] early and late ventricular arrhythmia, and impairment of ventricular function.[228-230] Time-activity curves are influenced by regional myocardial perfusion, local degradation of enzyme in the heart, the ratio of enzyme released compared to that destroyed,[231] inactivation of enzyme in lymph,[232] exchange of enzyme between vascular and extravascular compartments,[224] and potential variation in the rate of inactivation and removal of enzyme once it has reached the circulation.[232] Thus, the pattern of enzyme release and its overall magnitude may be influenced by interventions resulting in early reperfusion and accelerated washout. Nevertheless, analysis of plasma time-activity curves of MB CK and other biochemical markers of ischemic injury has proved useful in quantitative assessment of the progress and extent of myocardial infarction in the clinical setting and should prove useful in dating the onset of effective reperfusion.[225]

MODIFICATION OF ISCHEMIC INJURY

A variety of interventions have been shown in animal experiments to modify the severity of ischemic injury, and in some instances parallel changes in infarct size have been observed. The theoretical basis for these interventions and the experimental results are discussed below. The clinical application of these observations is discussed on p. 1318.

The potency of any intervention designed to limit infarct size is inversely related to the interval between the onset of the ischemic stimulus and the time the intervention is applied.[234] In the normothermic working dog heart no intervention can be expected to exert a significant beneficial effect if it is begun more than six hours after the onset of severe ischemia, because by this time all tissue in the distribution of the occluded vessel has become irreversibly injured.

INTERVENTIONS THAT INCREASE MYOCARDIAL INJURY AFTER CORONARY ARTERY OCCLUSION (TABLE 36–2)

The extent and severity of myocardial ischemic injury, and ultimately of myocardial infarction after coronary occlusion, depend on the balance between oxygen supply and demand in the jeopardized myocardium. Certain interventions known to increase myocardial oxygen consumption also increase the severity and extent of myocardial injury in the presence of residual coronary blood flow. In the dog without heart failure, isoproterenol, digitalis (in the absence of heart failure), and amrinone[235,236] have a deleterious effect on ischemic myocardium. Also, pacing-induced tachycardia increases ischemic damage,[236,237] and a similar observation in patients has been reported.[238] Hypoxemia,[239] anemia,[240] and hypotension, regardless of how produced,[241] increase myocardial ischemic injury after coronary occlusion, since in all of these conditions the delivery of oxygen to the ischemic tissue is reduced; similarly, hypoglycemia augments ischemic injury.[242] Hyperthermia impairs mechanical performance of the ischemic myocardium;[243] through its direct stimulation of myocardial oxygen consumption and heart rate, it exerts an adverse effect on myocardial oxygen balance.

The positive inotropic and chronotropic effects of isoproterenol improve the function of normal myocardium and elevate $M\dot{V}O_2$. When isoproterenol is administered in the presence of global myocardial ischemia, however, myocardial function deteriorates rapidly.[244–246] The effects of isoproterenol on myocardial function in the presence of regional ischemia, a situation in which the myocardium is perfused heterogeneously, are more complex. In the conscious dog with regional myocardial ischemia, isoproterenol elicits a spectrum of reactions in areas with different degrees of ischemia.[247] Specifically, myocardial function deteriorates in severely ischemic zones but improves in normal and moderately ischemic zones. These changes in myocardial function in response to isoproterenol correlate with changes in myocardial blood flow; severely ischemic sites exhibit no increase in blood flow and a deterioration of function occurs during infusion of isoproterenol, as a result of an increase in $M\dot{V}O_2$, whereas normal or moderately ischemic areas show an improvement of both myocardial function and regional blood flow. The positive chronotropic and inotropic actions of isoproterenol cause an increase in infarct size in anesthetized dogs with open chests,[219] and myocardial lactate production increases when isoproterenol is given to patients with acute myocardial infarction.[248]

An increase in the concentration of circulating fatty acids also aggravates ischemia following coronary occlusion[249]; the augmentation of myocardial oxygen requirements[250] in the presence of limited oxygen supply, intensifies ischemia, depresses myocardial contractility, and, in all likelihood, precipitates arrhythmias.[251]

TABLE 36–2 SOME INTERVENTIONS THAT INCREASE MYOCARDIAL INJURY AFTER CORONARY ARTERY OCCLUSION

Increase Myocardial Oxygen Requirements
- Isoproterenol
- Digitalis and amrinone (in the absence of heart failure)
- Tachycardia
- Hyperthermia

Decrease Myocardial Oxygen Supply
- Directly
  - Hypoxemia
  - Anemia
- Through collateral vessels, reducing coronary perfusion pressure
  - Hemorrhage
  - Sodium nitroprusside
  - Minoxidil
  - Other vasodilators (including isoproterenol)
  - Coronary vasoconstriction (indomethacin)

Decrease substrate availability
- Hypoglycemia

INTERVENTIONS THAT REDUCE MYOCARDIAL INJURY AFTER CORONARY ARTERY OCCLUSION (TABLE 36–3)

The balance between myocardial oxygen supply and demand in the ischemic myocardium can be improved by augmenting oxygen supply and/or reducing demand. Several studies in animals have shown that early reperfusion results in smaller infarction than if the occlusion is sustained. As might be expected, the extent of salvage depends on the duration of occlusion.[204,252,253] Reperfusion after less than 15 to 20 minutes of coronary occlusion salvages essentially all of the ischemic tissue. With longer periods of ischemia, a wavefront of necrosis beginning in the subendocardium and moving progressively outward, i.e., to the epicardium and laterally, occurs. When reperfusion is carried out after six hours of coronary occlusion, most of the jeopardized myocardium becomes necrotic and no tissue is salvaged. In some experiments histological evidence of hemorrhagic necrosis has been noted with coronary artery reperfusion.[254,255] This does not appear to be associated with extension of infarction but rather with acceleration of necrosis of tissue that had already been irreversibly injured. The inhalation of an *oxy-*

TABLE 36–3 SOME INTERVENTIONS THAT REDUCE EXPERIMENTAL MYOCARDIAL INJURY FOLLOWING CORONARY OCCLUSION

Increasing myocardial oxygen supply
- Directly
  - Coronary artery reperfusion (surgery, thrombolysis)
  - Elevating arterial pO_2
  - Fluorocarbons
- Through collateral vessels
  - Elevation of coronary perfusion pressure by methoxamine, neosynephrine, or norepinephrine
  - Intra-aortic balloon counterpulsation
- Coronary vasodilatation (calcium blockers, nitroglycerin, prostacyclin)

Decreasing myocardial oxygen demand
- Beta-adrenergic blockers
- Cardiac glycoside in the failing heart
- Intra-aortic balloon counterpulsation
- Decreasing afterload in hypertensive individuals
- Inhibiting calcium influx
- Hypothermia

Increasing plasma osmolality
- Mannitol
- Hypertonic glucose

Augmenting anaerobic metabolism (presumed)
- Glucose-insulin-potassium
- Hypertonic glucose

Enhancing transport to the ischemic zone of substrate utilized in energy production (presumed)

Protecting against autolytic and heterolytic processes (presumed)
- Glucocorticoids
- Cobra venom factor
- Aprotinin
- Nonsteroidal anti-inflammatory agents—ibuprofen

gen-rich gas mixture exerts a slight beneficial effect on the ischemic myocardium, also presumably by enhancing delivery of O_2 to ischemic tissue through collaterals.[256] This may be greatly enhanced by combining inhalation of 100 per cent oxygen with fluorocarbon mixtures, i.e., so-called artificial blood, which greatly augments O_2 delivery.[257]

Intra-aortic balloon counterpulsation (p. 593) reduces the severity of ischemic injury, presumably by reducing $M\dot{V}O_2$, as a consequence of lowering systolic wall tension, while simultaneously augmenting oxygen delivery by increasing aortic diastolic (coronary perfusion) pressure. In experimental animals, *beta-adrenergic blockers* appear to prolong the survival of severely ischemic tissue, judging from changes in ST segments, QRS complexes, myocardial creatine kinase activity, and electronmicroscopic, histochemical, and histological criteria.[258] In addition, it appears to improve the ratio of subendocardial to subepicardial blood flow in both ischemic and normal areas of myocardium in dogs with coronary occlusion, despite failing to alter net transmural blood flow to ischemic zones. Beta blockade appears to be more useful in delaying than preventing cell death and is especially effective in limiting infarct size in animals subjected to coronary occlusion and reperfusion.[259,260] As discussed above (p. 1253), an influx of Ca^{++} into the myocardial cell is associated with and may play a role in cell necrosis. It has been observed that the Ca^{++} channel blockers verapamil,[207,210,213] nifedipine,[261] and diltiazem[261a] reduce the severity of ischemic injury as well as infarct size.

A number of *metabolic interventions* may also improve the energy balance of ischemic myocardium. As fatty acid oxidation is impaired by ischemia, glucose becomes the principal source of energy.[262] In the ischemic dog heart, oxidative phosphorylation and cardiac function are enhanced by the infusion of glucose-insulin-potassium (GIK),[263] whereas, in the anoxic, isolated heart, both electrical and mechanical function improve and recovery occurs more rapidly when glucose is added to the perfusate.[169,264] Other beneficial effects that have been attributed either to glucose alone or to glucose-insulin-potassium include an increase in contractility due to the hyperosmolar action of glucose,[265] a reduction in the concentration and myocardial uptake of circulating free fatty acids (which reduces $M\dot{V}O_2$, p. 1250), a restoration of the intracellular potassium concentration, thus stabilizing the membrane potential[266,267] and reducing the frequency of serious ventricular dysrhythmias. In the open-chest dog, administration of GIK begun 30 minutes after coronary occlusion and maintained for 24 hours reduces the extent of myocardial necrosis that eventually develops.[268] Hypertonic glucose without insulin and potassium also reduces myocardial necrosis, but its salutary effect is not as great as that of GIK. In the baboon, GIK infusion after acute coronary occlusion preserves myocardial energy stores, with greater amounts of ATP, creatine phosphate, and glycogen in the ischemic zones of treated than in those of untreated animals.[269]

In the dog with experimentally produced coronary occlusion, myocardial ischemic injury is reduced by other agents that inhibit myocardial extraction of free fatty acids (i.e., antilipolytic agents, such as beta-pyridyl carbinol, and lipid-free albumin infusion), thus indirectly favoring glucose metabolism.[270] Injury is also reduced by sodium dichloroacetate,[271] which enhances the utilization of glucose relative to that of free fatty acids and by L-carnitine, which, by reversing the inhibition of adenine nucleotide translocase in vitro, prevents the depletion of cytoplasmic high-energy phosphate stores (Fig. 36–11).[272]

A number of agents that limit the inflammatory or immune response reduce myocardial ischemic injury in the laboratory animal, and some have been used in limited numbers of patients (Chap. 38). The activation of the complement system via its alternate pathway, a shift that characterizes ischemic tissue, releases leukotactic factors and increases capillary permeability, leading to interstitial edema. As a result, the microvasculature is compressed, further diminishing blood flow to the ischemic area.[273] *Cobra venom factor,* a protein that enzymatically cleaves C3 and prevents the effects of the complement system, reduces myocardial injury.[274] Similarly, the kallikrein system enhances leukotactic activity, capillary permeability, interstitial edema, and proteolytic activity, and *aprotinin,* an inhibitor of this system, diminishes ischemic injury.[275] A single large dose of a *glucocorticosteroid* also reduces myocardial infarct size in the dog with coronary occlusion.[276–278] These compounds limit myocardial necrosis, presumably by stabilizing lysosomal and other cellular membranes,[279] but they may also increase blood flow to the ischemic myocardium. Regardless of the effect of corticosteroids on the extent of myocardial ischemic injury, there is also evidence that when multiple doses are employed they may inhibit healing of the infarct, increasing the risk of ventricular rupture or aneurysm formation.[278–282] *Ibuprofen,* a nonsteroidal anti-inflammatory compound, has also been shown to reduce infarct size in experimental animals,[283] but, like corticosteroids, interferes with infarct healing and scar formation.[284]

Mannitol reduces the extent of ischemic injury and improves the function of the ischemic myocardium. This hyperosmotic agent reduces cell swelling and also presumably improves collateral blood flow to the ischemic myocardium.[285]

Hyaluronidase also reduces myocardial necrosis[286] in the dog and rabbit.[287] The depolymerization of mucopolysaccharides caused by hyaluronidase may increase the supply of nutrients to the myocardium or increase the washout of damaging metabolites.[288] This agent decreases ST-segment elevations in dogs with coronary occlusion and decreases the ultimate extent of damage, estimated electrocardiographically, biochemically, and morphologically.

For decades *nitroglycerin* was avoided in patients with acute myocardial infarction because nitroglycerin-induced reductions in systemic arterial pressure and concomitant reflex increases in heart rate were believed to intensify ischemic injury.[289] However, use of this drug has recently been reassessed, and it has been shown in the dog that intravenous nitroglycerin, administered at a rate sufficient to cause a mild diminution in systemic arterial pressure, reduces the magnitude and extent of ischemic injury,[290,291] and that this injury can be further lessened if the blood pressure decrease and reflex tachycardia induced by nitroglycerin are abolished by the simultaneous infusion of methoxamine and phenylephrine. In addition, the administration of nitroglycerin shortly after coronary artery occlusion partially reverses the ventricular fibrillation threshold, whereas nitroglycerin and phenylephrine in combination restore this threshold to normal.[292,293] Nitroglycerin is presumed to act by augmenting perfusion of the border of the ischemic zone[293] by dilating collaterals and by reducing myocardial oxygen demands by lowering preload and afterload.

References

1. McKeever, W. P., Gregg, D. E., and Canney, P. C.: Oxygen uptake of the nonworking left ventricle. Circ. Res. *6*:612, 1958.
2. Rooke, G. A., and Feigl, E. O.: Work as a correlate of canine left ventricular oxygen consumption, and the problem of catecholamine oxygen wasting. Circ. Res. *50*:273, 1982.
3. Klocke, F. J., Braunwald, E., and Ross, J., Jr.: Oxygen cost of electrical activation of the heart. Circ. Res. *18*:357, 1966.
4. Evans, C. L., and Matsuoka, Y.: The effect of various mechanical conditions on the gaseous metabolism and efficiency of the mammalian heart. J. Physiol. *49*:378, 1915.
5. Sarnoff, S. J., Braunwald, E., Welch, G. H., Jr., Case, R. B., Stainsby, W. N., and Macruz, R.: Hemodynamic determinants of oxygen consumption of the heart with special reference to the tension-time index. Am. J. Physiol. *192*:148, 1958.
6. Braunwald, E., Sarnoff, S. J., Case, R. B., Stainsby, W. N., and Welch, G. H., Jr.: Hemodynamic determinants of coronary flow: Effect of changes in aortic pressure and cardiac output on the relationship between myocardial oxygen consumption and coronary flow. Am. J. Physiol. *192*:157, 1958.
7. Rodbard, S., Williams, C. B., and Rodbard, D.: Myocardial tension and oxygen uptake. Circ. Res. *14*:139, 1964.
8. Sonnenblick, E. H., Ross, J., Jr., Covell, J. W., and Braunwald, E.: Velocity of contraction as a determinant of myocardial oxygen consumption. Am. J. Physiol. *209*:919, 1965.
9. Suga, H., Hayashi, T., Suehiro, S., Hisano, R., Shirahata, M., and Ninomiya, I.: Equal oxygen consumption rates of isovolumic and ejecting contractions with equal systolic pressure-volume areas in canine left ventricle. Circ. Res. *49*:1082, 1981.
10. Suga, H., Hisano, R., Hirata, S., Hayashi, T., and Ninomiya, I.: Mechanism of higher oxygen consumption rate: Pressure-loaded vs. volume-loaded heart. Am. J. Physiol. *242*(Heart Circ. Physiol. 11):H942, 1982.
11. Fenn, W. O.: A quantitative comparison between the energy liberated and the work performed by the isolated sartorius muscle of the frog. J. Physiol. (Lond.) *58*:175, 1923.
12. Rall, J. A.: Sense and nonsense about the Fenn effect. Am. J. Physiol. *242* (Heart Circ. Physiol. 11):H1, 1982.
13. Covell, J. W., Braunwald, E., Ross, J., Jr., and Sonnenblick, E. H.: Studies on digitalis. XVI. Effects on myocardial oxygen consumption. J. Clin. Invest. *45*:1535, 1966.
14. Graham, T. P., Jr., Ross, J., Jr., Covell, J. W., Sonnenblick, E. H., and Clancy, R. L.: Myocardial oxygen consumption in acute experimental cardiac depression. Circ. Res. *21*:123, 1967.
15. Graham, T. P., Jr., Covell, J. W., Sonnenblick, E. H., Ross, J., Jr., and Braunwald, E.: Control of myocardial oxygen consumption: Relative influence of contractile state and tension development. J. Clin. Invest. *47*:375, 1968.
16. Boerth, R. C., Covell, J. W., Pool, P. E., and Ross, J., Jr.: Increased myocardial oxygen consumption and contractile state associated with increased heart rate in dogs. Circ. Res. *24*:725, 1969.
17. Urschel, C. W., Covell, J. W., Graham, T. P., Clancy, R. L., Ross, J., Jr., Sonnenblick, E. H., and Braunwald, E.: Effects of acute valvular regurgitation on the oxygen consumption of the canine heart. Circ. Res. *23*:33, 1968.
18. Vik-Mo, H., and Mjos, O. E.: Influence of free fatty acids on myocardial oxygen consumption and ischemic injury. Am. J. Cardiol. *48*:361, 1981.
19. Braunwald, E., Ross, J., Jr., and Sonnenblick, E. H.: Regulation of coronary blood flow. *In* Mechanisms of Contraction of the Normal and Failing Heart, 2nd Ed. Boston, Little, Brown, 1976, p. 200.
20. Berne, R. M., and Rubio, R.: Coronary circulation. *In* Berne, R. M., Sperelakis, N., and Geiger, S. R. (eds.): Handbook of Physiology; Section 2, The Cardiovascular System. Bethesda, American Physiological Society, 1979, p. 897.
20a. Feigl, E. O.: Coronary physiology. Physiol. Rev. *63*:1, 1983.
21. Gorlin, R.: Coronary anatomy. *In* Coronary Artery Disease. Philadelphia, W. B. Saunders Co., 1976, p. 40.
22. Bell, J. R., and Fox, A. C.: Pathogenesis of subendocardial ischemia. Am. J. Med. Sci. *268*:2, 1974.
23. Wearn, J. T.: Morphological and functional alterations of the coronary circulation. Harvey Lect. *35*:243, 1940.
24. Provenza, D. V., and Scherlis, S.: Coronary circulation in dog's heart: Demonstration of muscle sphincters in capillaries. Circ. Res. *7*:318, 1959.
25. Fulton, W. F. M.: The Coronary Arteries. Springfield, Ill., Charles C Thomas, 1965.
26. Schaper, W.: The physiology of the collateral circulation in the normal and hypoxic myocardium. Rev. Physiol. Biochem. Pharmacol. *63*:102, 1971.
27. Fam, W. M., and McGregor, M.: Effect of coronary vasodilator drugs on retrograde flow in areas of chronic myocardial ischemia. Circ. Res. *15*:355, 1964.
28. Cohen, M. V., Downey, J. M., Sonnenblick, E. H., and Kirk, E. S.: The effects of nitroglycerin on coronary collaterals and myocardial contractility. J. Clin. Invest. *52*:2836, 1973.
29. Kolibash, A. J., Bush, C. A., Wepsic, R. A., Schroeder, D. P., Tetalman, M. R., and Lewis, R. P.: Coronary collateral vessels: Spectrum of physiologic capabilities with respect to providing rest and stress myocardial perfusion, maintenance of left ventricular function and protection against infarction. Am. J. Cardiol. *50*:230, 1982.
30. Downey, J. M., and Kirk, E. S.: Inhibition of coronary blood flow by a vascular waterfall mechanism. Circ. Res. *36*:753, 1975.
31. Moir, T. W.: Subendocardial distribution of coronary blood flow and the effect of antianginal drugs. Circ. Res. *30*:621, 1972.
32. Gregg, D. E., Khouri, E. M., and Rayford, C. R.: Systemic and coronary energetics in the resting unanesthetized dog. Circ. Res. *16*:102, 1965.
33. Klocke, F. J.: Coronary blood flow in man. Prog. Cardiovasc. Dis. *19*:117, 1976.
34. Sonnenblick, E. H., and Kirk, E. S.: Effects of hypoxia and ischemia on myocardial contraction: Alterations in the time course of force and ischemia-dependent inhomogeneity of contractility. Cardiology *56*:302, 1971/72.
35. Griggs, D. M., Jr., Chen, C. C., and Tchokoev, V. V.: Subendocardial metabolism in experimental aortic stenosis. Am. J. Physiol. *224*:607, 1973.
36. Sabbah, H. N., and Stein, P. D.: Effect of acute regional ischemia on pressure in the subepicardium and subendocardium. Am. J. Physiol. *242*(Heart Circ. Physiol. 11):H240, 1982.
37. Brazier, J., Cooper, N., and Buckberg, G.: The adequacy of subendocardial oxygen delivery: The interaction of determinants of flow, arterial oxygen content and myocardial oxygen need. Circulation *49*:968, 1974.
38. Lundsgaard-Hansen, P., Meyer, C., and Riedwyl, H.: Transmural gradients of glycolytic enzyme activities in left ventricular myocardium. I. The normal state. Pfluegers Arch. *297*:89, 1967.
39. Rovetto, M. J., Whitmer, J. T., and Neely, J. R.: Comparison of the effects of anoxia and whole heart ischemia on carbohydrate utilization in isolated working rat hearts. Circ. Res. *32*:699, 1973.
40. Jedeikin, L. A.: Regional distribution of glycogen and phosphorylase in the ventricles of the heart. Circ. Res. *14*:202, 1964.
41. Allison, T. B., Ramey, C. A., and Holsinger, J. W., Jr.: Transmural gradients of left ventricular tissue metabolites after circumflex artery ligation in dogs. J. Mol. Cell. Cardiol. *9*:837, 1977.
42. Buckberg, G. D., Fixler, D. E., Archie, J. P., and Hoffman, J. I. E.: Experimental subendocardial ischemia in dogs with normal coronary arteries. Circ. Res. *30*:67, 1972.
43. Hoffman, J. I. E.: Determinants and prediction of transmural myocardial perfusion. Circulation *58*:381, 1978.
44. Oliveros, R. A., Boucher, C. A., Haycraft, G. L., and Beckmann, C. H.: Myocardial oxygen supply-demand ratio. A validation of peripherally vs. centrally determined values. Chest *75*:693, 1979.
45. Becker, L. C.: Effect of tachycardia on regional left ventricular blood flow after coronary artery occlusion. Am. J. Cardiol. *35*:122, 1975.
46. Neill, W. A., Oxendine, J., Phelps, N., and Anderson, R. P.: Subendocardial ischemia provoked by tachycardia in conscious dogs with coronary stenosis. Am. J. Cardiol. *35*:30, 1975.
47. Fallen, E. L., Elliott, W. C., and Gorlin, R.: Mechanisms of angina in aortic stenosis. Circulation *36*:480, 1967.
48. Griggs, D. M., Jr., and Chen, C. C.: Coronary hemodynamics and regional myocardial metabolism in experimental aortic insufficiency. J. Clin. Invest. *53*:1599, 1974.
49. Segal, J., Harvey, W. P., and Hufnagel, C.: A clinical study of one hundred cases of severe aortic insufficiency. Am. J. Med. *21*:200, 1956.
50. Becker, L. C., Fortuin, N. J., and Pitt, B.: Effect of ischemia and antianginal drugs on the distribution of radioactive microspheres in the canine left ventricle. Circ. Res. *28*:263, 1971.
51. Mathes, P., and Rival, J.: Effect of nitroglycerin on total and regional coronary blood flow in the normal and ischaemic canine myocardium. Cardiovasc. Res. *5*:54, 1971.
52. Belloni, F. L.: The local control of coronary blood flow. Cardiovasc. Res. *13*:63, 1979.
53. Pitt, B., Elliot, E. C., and Gregg, D. E.: Adrenergic receptor activity in the coronary arteries of the unanesthetized dog. Circ. Res. *21*:75, 1967.
54. Vatner, S. F., Hintze, T. H., and Macho, P.: Regulation of large coronary arteries by beta-adrenergic mechanisms in the conscious dog. Circ. Res. *51*:56, 1982.
55. Vatner, S. F., Higgins, C. B., and Braunwald, E.: Effects of norepinephrine on coronary circulation and left ventricular dynamics in the conscious dog. Circ. Res. *34*:812, 1974.
56. Szentivanyi, M., and Juhasz-Nagy, N.: Physiological role of the coronary constrictor fibers. Q. J. Exp. Physiol. *48*:93, 1963.
57. Hackett, J. G., Abboud, F. M., Mark, A. L., Schmid, P. G., and Heistad, D. D.: Coronary vascular responses to stimulation of chemoreceptors and baroreceptors. Circ. Res. *21*:8, 1972.
58. Higgins, C. B., Vatner, S. F., and Braunwald, E.: Parasympathetic control of the heart. Pharmacol. Rev. *25*:119, 1973.
59. Vatner, S. F., Franklin, D., VanCitters, R. L., and Braunwald, E.: Effects of carotid sinus nerve stimulation on the coronary circulation of the conscious dog. Circ. Res. *27*:11, 1970.
60. Brachfeld, N., Monroe, R. G., and Gorlin, R.: Effects of pericoronary denervation on coronary hemodynamics. Am. J. Physiol. *199*:174, 1960.
61. Macho, P., and Vatner, S. F.: Effects of prazosin on coronary and left ventricular dynamics in conscious dogs. Circulation *65*:1186, 1982.
62. Heyndrickx, G. R., Muylaert, P., and Pannier, J. L.: Alpha-adrenergic control of oxygen delivery to myocardium during exercise in conscious dogs. Am. J. Physiol. *242*(Heart Circ. Physiol. 11):H805, 1982.
63. Murray, P. A., and Vatner, S. F.: Alpha adrenoceptor attenuation of the coro-

nary vascular response to severe exercise in the conscious dog. Circ. Res. *45*: 654, 1979.
64. Feigl, E. O.: Reflex parasympathetic coronary vasodilation elicited from cardiac receptors in the dog. Circ. Res. *37*:175, 1975.
65. Bezold, A., and Hirt, L.: Über die physiologischen Wirkungen des essigsauren Veratrins. Unters. Physiol. Lab. Würzburg *1*:75, 1867.
66. Jarisch, A., and Zotterman, Y.: Depressor reflexes from the heart. Acta Physiol. Scand. *16*:31, 1948.
67. Feigl, E. O.: Parasympathetic control of coronary blood flow in dogs. Circ. Res. *25*:509, 1969.
68. Hamilton, F. N., and Feigl, E. O.: Coronary vascular sympathetic beta-receptor innervation. Am. J. Physiol. *230*:1569, 1976.
69. Ross, G.: Adrenergic responses of the coronary vessels. Circ. Res. *39*:461, 1976.
70. Driscol, T. E., Moir, T. W., and Eckstein, R. W.: Vascular effects of changes in perfusion pressure in the nonischemic and ischemic heart. Circ. Res. *15* (Suppl. I):I-94, 1964.
70a. Øien, A. H., and Aukland, K.: A mathematical analysis of the myogenic hypothesis with special reference to autoregulation of renal blood flow. Circ. Res. *52*:241, 1983.
71. Bayliss, W. M.: On the local reaction of the arterial wall to changes in arterial pressure. J. Physiol. (Lond.) *28*:220, 1902.
72. Coffman, J. D., and Gregg, D. E.: Oxygen metabolism and oxygen debt repayment after myocardial ischemia. Am. J. Physiol. *201*:881, 1961.
73. Berne, R. M., Blackmon, J. R., and Gardner, T. H.: Hypoxemia and coronary flow. J. Clin. Invest. *36*:1101, 1957.
74. Weglicki, W. B., Rubenstein, C. J., Entman, M. L., Thompson, H. K., Jr., and McIntosh, H. D.: Effects of hyperbaric oxygenation on myocardial blood flow and myocardial metabolism in the dog. Am. J. Physiol. *216*:1219, 1969.
75. Rubio, R., Berne, R. M., and Katori, M.: Release of adenosine in reactive hyperemia of the dog heart. Am. J. Physiol. *216*:56, 1969.
76. Detar, R., and Bohr, D. F.: Oxygen and vascular smooth muscle contraction. Am. J. Physiol. *214*:241, 1968.
77. Duling, B. R.: Microvascular responses to alterations in oxygen tension. Circ. Res. *31*:481, 1972.
78. Duling, B. R.: Changes in microvascular diameter and oxygen tension induced by carbon dioxide. Circ. Res. *32*:370, 1973.
79. Martini, J., and Honig, C. R.: Direct measurement of intercapillary distance in beating rat heart in situ under various conditions of O_2 supply. Microvasc. Res. *1*:244, 1969.
80. Rubio, R., and Berne, R. M.: Release of adenosine by the normal myocardium and its relationship to the regulation of coronary resistance. Circ. Res. *25*:407, 1969.
81. Bardenheuer, H., and Schrader, J.: Relationship between myocardial oxygen consumption, coronary flow and adenosine release in an improved isolated working heart preparation of guinea pigs. Circ. Res. *52*:263, 1983.
82. Rubio, R., Berne, R. M., and Dobson, J. G., Jr.: Sites of adenosine production in cardiac and skeletal muscle. Am. J. Physiol. *225*:938, 1973.
83. McKenzie, J. E., Steffen, R. P., and Haddy, F. J.: Relations between adenosine and coronary resistance in conscious exercising dogs. Am. J. Physiol. *242*:H24, 1982.
84. Gellai, M., Norton, J. M., and Detar, R.: Evidence for direct control of coronary vascular tone by oxygen. Circ. Res. *32*:279, 1973.
85. Belardinelli, L., Vogel, S., Linden, J., and Berne, R. M.: Anti-adrenergic action of adenosine on ventricular myocardium in embryonic chick hearts. J. Molec. Cell. Cardiol. *14*:291, 1982.
86. Needleman, P., Marshall, G. R., and Sobel, B. E.: Hormone interactions in the isolated rabbit heart: Synthesis and coronary vasomotor effects of prostaglandins, angiotensin, and bradykinin. Circ. Res. *37*:802, 1975.
87. Bergman, G., Atkinson, L., Richardson, P. J., Daly, K., Rothman, M., Jackson, G., and Jewitt, D. E.: Prostacyclin: Haemodynamic and metabolic effects in patients with coronary artery disease. Lancet *1*:569, 1981.
88. Friedman, P. L., Brugada, P., Kuck, K. H., Bar, F. W. H. M., and Wellens, H. J. J.: Coronary vasoconstrictor effect of indomethacin in patients with coronary artery disease. N. Engl. J. Med. *305*:1171, 1981.
89. DeBoer, L. W. V., Rude, R. E., Davis, R. F., Maroko, P. R., and Braunwald, E.: Extension of myocardial necrosis into normal epicardium following hypotension during experimental coronary occlusion. Cardiovasc. Res. *16*:423, 1982.
90. Vatner, S. F., Pagani, M., Manders, T., and Pasipoularides, A. D.: Alpha adrenergic vasoconstriction and nitroglycerin vasodilation of large coronary arteries in the conscious dog. J. Clin. Invest. *65*:5, 1980.
91. Feldman, R. L., Marx, J. D., Pepine, C. J., and Conti, C. R.: Analysis of coronary responses to various doses of intracoronary nitroglycerin. Circulation *66*:321, 1982.
92. Macho, P., and Vatner, S. F.: Effects of nitroglycerin and nitroprusside on large and small coronary vessels in conscious dogs. Circulation *64*:1101, 1981.
93. Hintz, T. H., and Vatner, S. F.: Comparison of effects of nifedipine and nitroglycerin on large and small coronary arteries and cardiac function in conscious dogs. Circulation Res. *52*:I-139, 1983.
94. Engle, H.-J., and Lichten, P. R.: Beneficial enhancement of coronary blood flow by nifedipine: Comparison with nitroglycerin and beta blocking agents. Am. J. Med. *71*:658, 1981.
95. Klocke, F. J.: Measurements of coronary blood flow and degree of stenosis: Current clinical implications and continuing uncertainties. J. Am. Coll. Cardiol. *1*:31, 1983.
96. Gould, K. L.: Dynamic coronary stenosis. Am. J. Cardiol. *45*:286, 1980.
97. Hillis, L. D., and Braunwald, E.: Coronary artery spasm. N. Engl. J. Med. *299*: 695, 1978.
98. Tennant, R., and Wiggers, C. J.: The effect of coronary occlusion on myocardial contractions. Am. J. Physiol. *112*:351, 1935.
99. Vatner, S. F.: Correlation between acute reductions in myocardial blood flow and function in conscious dogs. Circ. Res. *47*:201, 1980.
100. Herman, M. V., Heinle, R. A., Klein, M. D., and Gorlin, R.: Localized disorders in myocardial contraction: Asynergy and its role in congestive heart failure. N. Engl. J. Med. *277*:222, 1967.
101. Braunwald, E., and Kloner, R. A.: The stunned myocardium: Prolonged, postischemic ventricular dysfunction. Circulation *66*:1146, 1982.
102. Osakada, G., Hess, O. M., Gallather, K. P., Kemper, W. S., and Ross, J., Jr.: End-systolic dimension-wall thickness relations during myocardial ischemia in conscious dogs. Am. J. Cardiol. *51*:1750, 1983.
103. Parker, J. O., Ledwich, J. R., West, R. O., and Case, R. B.: Reversible cardiac failure during angina pectoris: Hemodynamic effects of atrial pacing in coronary artery disease. Circulation *39*:745, 1969.
104. Kardesch, M., Hogancamp, C. E., and Bing, R. J.: The effect of complete ischemia on the intracellular electrical activity of the whole mammalian heart. Circ. Res. *6*:715, 1958.
105. Katz, A. M.: Effects of ischemia on the contractile processes of heart muscle. Am. J. Cardiol. *32*:456, 1973.
106. Chesnais, J. M., Coraboeuf, E., Sauviat, M. P., and Vassas, J. M.: Sensitivity to H, Li and Mg ions of the slow inward sodium current in frog atrial fibres. J. Mol. Cell. Cardiol. *7*:627, 1975.
107. Sandow, A.: Excitation-contraction coupling in skeletal muscle. Pharmacol. Rev. *17*:265, 1965.
108. Fabiato, A., and Fabiato, F.: Contractions induced by a calcium-triggered release of calcium from the sarcoplasmic reticulum of single skinned cardiac cells. J. Physiol. *249*:469, 1975.
109. Katz, A. M., and Hecht, H. H.: The early "pump" failure of the ischemic heart. Am. J. Med. *47*:497, 1969.
110. Braunwald, E., Ross, J., Jr., and Sonnenblick, E. H.: Mechanisms of Contractions in the Normal and Failing Heart, 2nd Ed. Boston, Little, Brown, 1976, p. 357.
111. Williamson, J. R., Schaffer, S. W., Ford, C., and Safer, B.: Contribution of tissue acidosis to ischemic injury in the perfused rat heart. Circulation *53*(Suppl. 1):3, 1976.
112. Regan, T. J., Effros, R. M., Haider, B., Oldewurtel, H. A., Ettinger, P. O., and Ahmed, S. S.: Myocardial ischemia and cell acidosis: Modification by alkali and the effects on ventricular function and cation composition. Am. J. Cardiol. *37*:501, 1976.
113. Barry, W. H., Brooker, J. Z., Alderman, E. L., and Harrison, D. C.: Changes in diastolic stiffness and tone of the left ventricle during angina pectoris. Circulation *49*:255, 1974.
114. Hess, O. M., Osakada, G., Lavelle, J. F., Gallagher, K. P., Kemper, W. S., and Ross, J., Jr.: Diastolic myocardial wall stiffness and ventricular relaxation during partial and complete coronary occlusions in the conscious dog. Circulation Res. *52*:387, 1983.
115. Grossman, W., and McLaurin, L. P.: Diastolic properties of the left ventricle. Ann. Intern. Med. *84*:316, 1976.
116. Bourdillon, P. D., Lorell, B. H., Mirsky, I., Paulus, W. J., Wynne, J., and Grossman, W.: Increased regional myocardial stiffness of the left ventricle during pacing-induced angina in man. Circulation *67*:316, 1983.
117. Carroll, J. D., Hess, O. M., Hirzel, H. O., and Krayenbuehl, H. P.: Exercise-induced ischemia: The influence of altered relaxation on early diastolic pressures. Circulation *67*:521, 1983.
118. Kay, H. R., Levine, F. H., Grotte, G. J., Rosenthal, S., Austen, W. G., and Buckley, M. J.: Isovolumic relaxation as a critical determinant of postischemic ventricular function. J. Surg. Res. *26*:659, 1979.
119. McLaurin, L. P., Rolett, E. L., and Grossman, W.: Impaired left ventricular relaxation during pacing-induced ischemia. Am. J. Cardiol. *32*:751, 1973.
120. Linhart, J. W., Hildner, F. J., Barold, S. S., Lister, J. W., and Samet, P.: Left heart hemodynamics during angina pectoris induced by atrial pacing. Circulation *40*:483, 1969.
121. Paulus, W. J., Serizawa, T., and Grossman, W.: Altered left ventricular diastolic properties during pacing-induced ischemia in dogs with coronary stenoses. Potentiation by caffeine. Circ. Res. *50*:218, 1982.
122. McCans, J. L., and Parker, J. O.: Left ventricular pressure-volume relationships during myocardial ischemia in man. Circulation *48*:775, 1973.
123. Pardee, H. E. B.: An electrocardiographic sign of coronary artery obstruction. Arch. Intern. Med. *26*:244, 1920.
124. Rakita, L., Borduas, J. L., Rothman, S., and Prinzmetal, M.: Studies on the mechanism of ventricular activity. XII. Early changes in the RS-T segment and QRS complex following acute coronary artery occlusion: Experimental study and clinical applications. Am. Heart J. *48*:351, 1954.
125. Ekmekci, A., Toyoshima, H., Dowczynski, J. K., Nagaya, T., and Prinzmetal, M.: Angina pectoris. IV. Clinical and experimental difference between ischemia with S-T elevation and ischemia with S-T depression. Am. J. Cardiol. *7*:412, 1961.
126. Leaf, A.: Cell swelling: A factor in ischemic tissue injury. Circulation *48*:455, 1973.
127. Flores, J., DiBona, D. R., Beck, C. H., and Leaf, A.: The role of cell swelling in ischemic renal damage and the protective effect of hypertonic solute. J. Clin. Invest. *51*:118, 1972.
128. Opie, L. H., Owen, P., Thomas, M., and Samson, R.: Coronary sinus lactate measurements in assessment of myocardial ischemia: Comparison with changes in lactate/pyruvate and beta-hydroxybutyrate/acetoacetate ratios and with release of hydrogen, phosphate and potassium ions from the heart. Am. J. Cardiol. *32*:295, 1973.

129. Johnson, E. A.: First electrocardiographic sign of myocardial ischemia: An electrophysiological conjecture. Circulation *53*(Suppl. I):82, 1976.
130. Holland, R. P., and Brooks, H.: The QRS complex during myocardial ischemia: An experimental analysis in the porcine heart. J. Clin. Invest. *57*: 541, 1976.
131. Karlsson, J., Templeton, G. H., and Willerson, J. T.: Relationship between epicardial S-T segment changes and myocardial metabolism during acute coronary insufficiency. Circ. Res. *32*:725, 1973.
132. Sayen, J. J., Peirce, G., Katcher, A. H., and Sheldon, W. F.: Correlation of intramyocardial electrocardiograms with polarographic oxygen and contractility in the nonischemic and regionally ischemic left ventricle. Circ. Res. *9*:1268, 1961.
133. Angell, C. S., Lakatta, E. G., Weisfeldt, M. L., and Shock, N. W.: Relationship of intramyocardial oxygen tension and epicardial ST segment changes following acute coronary artery ligation: Effects of coronary perfusion pressure. Cardiovasc. Res. *9*:12, 1975.
134. Khuri, S. F., Flaherty, J. T., O'Riordan, J. B., Pitt, B., Brawley, R. K., Donahoo, J. S., and Gott, V. L.: Changes in intramyocardial ST segment voltage and gas tensions with regional myocardial ischemia in the dog. Circ. Res. *37*:455, 1975.
135. Braunwald, E., and Maroko, P. R.: ST-segment mapping: Realistic and unrealistic expectations. Circulation *54*:529, 1976.
136. Maroko, P. R., Kjekshus, J. K., Sobel, B. E., Covell, J. W., Ross, J., Jr., and Braunwald, E.: Factors influencing infarct size following experimental coronary artery occlusions. Circulation *43*:67, 1971.
137. Hillis, L. D., Askenazi, J., Braunwald, E., Radvany, P., Muller, J. E., Fishbein, M. C., and Maroko, P. R.: Use of changes in epicardial QRS complex to assess interventions which modify the extent of myocardial necrosis following coronary artery occlusion. Circulation *54*:591, 1976.
138. Kralios, F. A., Martin, L., Burgess, M. J., and Millar, K.: Local ventricular repolarization changes due to sympathetic nerve-branch stimulation. Am. J. Physiol. *228*:1621, 1975.
139. Muller, J. E., Maroko, P. R., and Braunwald, E.: Evaluation of precordial electrocardiographic mapping as a means of assessing changes in myocardial ischemic injury. Circulation *52*:16, 1975.
140. Elharrar, V., and Zipes, D. P.: Cardiac electrophysiological alterations during myocardial ischemia. *In* Levy, M. N., and Vassalle, M. (Eds.): Excitation and Neural Control of the Heart. Baltimore, Williams and Wilkins, 1982, pp. 149–180.
141. Mehra, R., Zeiler, R. H., Gough, W. B., and El-Sherif, N.: Reentrant ventricular arrhythmias in the late myocardial infarction period. 9. Electrophysiologic-anatomic correlation of reentrant circuits. Circulation *67*:11, 1983.
142. Downar, E., Janse, M. J., and Durrer, D.: The effect of acute coronary artery occlusion on subepicardial transmembrane potentials in the intact porcine heart. Circulation *56*:217, 1977.
143. El-Sherif, N., Scherlag, B. J., and Lazzara, R.: Electrode catheter recording during malignant ventricular arrhythmias following experimental acute myocardial ischemia. Evidence for reentry, due to conduction delay and block in ischemic myocardium. Circulation *51*:1003, 1975.
144. Janse, M. J., and Kleber, A. G.: Electrophysiological changes and ventricular arrhythmias in the early phase of regional myocardial ischemia. Circ. Res. *49*: 1069, 1981.
145. Kent, F. K., Smith, E. R., Redwood, D. R., and Epstein, S. E.: Electrical stability of acutely ischemic myocardium. Influence of heart rate and vagal stimulation. Circulation *47*:291, 1973.
146. Schaal, S. F., Wallace, A. G., and Sealy, W. C.: Protective influence of cardiac denervation against arrhythmias of myocardial infarction. Cardiovasc. Res. *3*: 241, 1969.
147. Corr, P. B., Witkowski, F. X., and Sobel, B. E.: Mechanisms contributing to malignant dysrhythmias induced by ischemia in the cat. J. Clin. Invest. *61*: 109, 1978.
148. Hope, R. R., Williams, D. O., El-Sherif, N., Lazzara, R., and Scherlag, B. J.: The efficacy of antiarrhythmic agents during acute myocardial ischemia and the role of heart rate. Circulation *50*:507, 1974.
149. Kupersmith, J., Ontman, E. M., and Hoffman, B. F.: In vivo electrophysiological effects of lidocaine in canine acute myocardial infarction. Circ. Res. *36*:84, 1975.
150. Elharrar, J., Gaum, W. E., and Zipes, D. P.: Effect of drugs on conduction delay and incidence of ventricular arrhythmias induced by acute coronary occlusion in dogs. Am. J. Cardiol. *39*:544, 1977.
151. Friedman, P. L., Stewart, J. R., and Wit, A. L.: Spontaneous and induced cardiac arrhythmias in subendocardial Purkinje fibers after extensive myocardial infarction in dogs. Circ. Res. *33*:612, 1973.
152. Horowitz, L. N., Spear, J. F., and Moore, E. N.: Subendocardial origin of ventricular arrhythmias in 24-hour-old experimental myocardial infarction. Circulation *53*:56, 1976.
153. El-Sherif, N., Hope, R. R., Scherlag, B. J., and Lazzara, R.: Re-entrant ventricular arrhythmias in the late myocardial infarction period. 2. Patterns of initiation and termination of reentry. Circulation *55*:702, 1977.
154. El-Sherif, N., Scherlag, B. J., Lazzara, R., and Hope, R. R.: Reentrant ventricular arrhythmias in the late myocardial infarction period. 4. Mechanism of action of lidocaine. Circulation *56*:395, 1977.
155. Lazzara, R., Hope, R. R., El-Sherif, N., and Scherlag, B. J.: Effects of lidocaine on hypoxic and ischemic cardiac cells. Am. J. Cardiol. *41*:872, 1978.
156. Murdock, D. K., Loeb, J. M., Euler, D. E., and Randall, W. C.: Electrophysiology of coronary reperfusion. A mechanism for reperfusion arrhythmias. Circulation *61*:175, 1980.
157. Downar, E., Janse, M. S., and Durrer, D.: The effect of "ischemic" blood on transmembrane potentials of normal porcine ventricular myocardium. Circulation *55*:455, 1977.
158. Sobel, B. E., Corr, P. B., Robinson, A. K., Goldstein, R. A., Witkowski, F. X., and Klein, M. S.: Accumulation of lysophosphoglycerides with arrhythmogenic properties in ischemic myocardium. J. Clin. Invest. *61*:109, 1978.
159. Corr, P. B., Cain, M. E., Witkowski, F. X., Price, D. A., and Sobel, B. E.: Potential arrhythmogenic electrophysiological derangements in canine Purkinje fibers induced by lysophosphoglycerides. Circ. Res. *44*:822, 1979.
160. Schwartz, A., Wood, J. M., Allen, J. C., Barret, E., Entman, M. L., Goldstein, M. A., Sordahl, L. Z., Suzuki, M., and Lewis, R. M.: Biochemical and morphologic correlates of cardiac ischemia. 1. Membrane systems. Am. J. Cardiol. *32*:46, 1973.
161. Cherry, G., and Myers, M. B.: The relationship to ventricular fibrillation of early tissue sodium and potassium shifts and coronary vein potassium levels in experimental myocardial infarction. J. Thorac. Cardiovasc. Surg. *61*:587, 1971.
162. Podzuweit, T., Dalby, A. J., Cherry, G. W., and Opie, L. H.: Tissue levels of cyclic AMP in ischemic and non-ischemic myocardium following coronary artery ligation. J. Mol. Cell. Cardiol. *10*:81, 1978.
163. Kuppersmith, J., Shaing, H., Litwak, R. S., and Harman, M. V.: Electrophysiologic effects of verapamil in canine myocardial ischemia. Am. J. Cardiol. *37*:149, 1976.
164. Griffith, J., and Leung, F.: The sequential estimation of plasma catecholamines and whole blood histamine in myocardial infarction. Am. Heart J. *82*:171, 1971.
165. El-Sherif, N., and Lazzara, K.: Reentrant ventricular arrhythmias in the late myocardial infarction period. 7. Effect of verapamil and D-600 and role of the "slow channel." Circulation *60*:3, 1979.
166. Jennings, R. B., Reimer, K. A., Hill, M. L., and Mayer, S. E.: Total ischemia in dog hearts in vitro. I. Comparison of high energy phosphate production, utilization and depletion, and of adenine nucleotide catabolism in total ischemia in vitro vs. severe ischemia in vivo. Circ. Res. *49*:892, 1981.
167. Reimer, K. A., Jennings, R. B., and Hill, M. L.: Total ischemia in dog hearts, in vitro. 2. High energy phosphate depletion and associated defects in energy metabolism, cell volume regulation, and sarcolemmal integrity. Circ. Res. *49*: 901, 1981.
168. Rude, R. E., DeBoer, L. W. V., Ingwall, J. S., Kloner, R. A., Hale, S. L., Davis, M., Maroko, P. R., and Braunwald, E.: Prediction of biochemical derangement in ischemic myocardium following experimental coronary artery occlusion. Am. J. Cardiol. *45*:415, 1980.
169. Ingwall, J. S.: Phosphorus nuclear magnetic resonance spectroscopy of cardiac and skeletal muscles. Am. J. Physiol. *242* (Heart Circ. Physiol. 11):H729, 1982.
170. Flaherty, J. T., Weisfeldt, M. L., Bulkley, B. H., Gardner, T. J., Gott, V. L., and Jacobus, W. E.: Mechanisms of ischemic myocardial cell damage assessed by phosphorus-31 nuclear magnetic resonance. Circulation *65*:561, 1982.
171. Pernot, A-C., Ingwall, J. S., Menasche, P., Grousset, C., Bercot, M., Pinwnica, A., and Fossel, E. T.: Evaluation of high-energy phosphate metabolism during cardioplegic arrest and reperfusion: A phosphorus-31 nuclear magnetic resonance study. Circulation *67*:1296, 1983.
172. Sobel, B. E., and Mayer, S. E.: Cyclic adenosine monophosphate and cardiac contractility. Circ. Res. *32*:407, 1973.
173. Rovetto, M. J., Lamberton, W. F., and Neely, J. R.: Mechanisms of glycolytic inhibition in ischemic rat hearts. Circ. Res. *37*:742, 1975.
174. Williamson, J. R., Schaffer, S. W., Ford, C., and Safer, B.: Contribution of tissue acidosis to ischemic injury in the perfused rat heart. Circulation *53*(Suppl. I):I–3, 1976.
175. Ng, M. L., Levy, M. N., and Zieske, H. A.: Effects of changes of pH and of carbon dioxide tension on left ventricular performance. Am. J. Physiol. *213*: 115, 1967.
176. Williamson, J. R., Safer, B., LaNoue, K. F., Smith, C. M., and Walajtys, E.: Mitochondrial-cytosolic interactions in cardiac tissue: Role of the malate aspartate cycle in the removal of glycolytic NADH from the cytosol. Symp. Soc. Exp. Biol. *27*:241, 1973.
177. LaNoue, K. F., and Williamson, J. R.: Interrelationships between malate-aspartate shuttle and critic acid cycle in rat heart mitochondria. Metabolism *20*: 119, 1971.
178. Most, A. S., Gorlin, R., and Soeldner, J. S.: Glucose extraction by the human myocardium during pacing stress. Circulation *45*:92, 1972.
179. Opie, L. H., Owen, P., Thomas, M., and Samson, R.: Coronary sinus lactate measurements in assessment of myocardial ischemia: Comparison with changes in lactate/pyruvate and beta-hydroxybutyrate/acetoacetate ratios and with release of hydrogen, phosphate and potassium ions from the heart. Am. J. Cardiol. *32*:295, 1973.
180. Regan, T. J., Effros, R. M., Haider, R., Oldewurtel, H. A., Ettinger, P. O., and Ahmed, S. S.: Myocardial ischemia and cell acidosis: Modification by alkali and the effects on ventricular function and cation composition. Am. J. Cardiol. *27*:501, 1976.
181. Neely, J. R., and Morgan, H. E.: Relationship between carbohydrate and lipid metabolism and the energy balance of heart muscle. Annu. Rev. Physiol. *36*: 413, 1974.
182. Crass, M. F., III, McCaskill, E. S., and Shipp, J. C.: Glucose-free fatty acid interactions in the working heart. J. Appl. Physiol. *29*:87, 1970.
183. Neely, J. R., Bowman, R. H., and Morgan, H. E.: Effects of ventricular pressure development and palmitate on glucose transport. Am. J. Physiol. *216*: 804, 1969.
184. Wood, J. M., Sordahl, L. A., Lewis, R. M., and Schwartz, A.: Effect of chronic myocardial ischemia on the activity of carnitine palmityl-coenzyme A transferase of isolate canine heart mitochondria. Circ. Res. *32*:340, 1973.

185. Bremer, J., and Wojtczak, A. B.: Factors controlling the rate of fatty acid β-oxidation in rat liver mitochondria. Biochim. Biophys. Acta *280*:515, 1972.
186. Neely, J. R., Rovetto, M. J., Whitmer, J. T., and Morgan, H. E.: Effects of ischemia on ventricular function and metabolism in the isolated working rat heart. Am. J. Physiol. *225*:651, 1973.
187. Brachfeld, N., Ohtaka, Y., Klein, I., and Kawade, M.: Substrate preference and metabolic activity of the aerobic and the hypoxic turtle heart. Circ. Res. *31*:453, 1972.
188. Lerch, R. A., Bergmann, S. R., Ambos, H. D., Welch, M. J., Ter-Pogossian, M. M., and Sobel, B. E.: Effect of flow-independent reduction of metabolism on regional myocardial clearance of ^{11}C-palmitate. Circulation *65*:731, 1982.
189. Sobel, B. E.: The diagnostic promise of positron tomography. Am. Heart J. *103*:673, 1982.
190. Bergmann, S. R., Lerch, R. A., Fox, K. A. A., Ludbrook, P. A., Welch, M. J., Ter-Pogossian, M. M., and Sobel, B. E.: Temporal dependence of beneficial effects of coronary thrombolysis characterized by positron tomography. Am. J. Med. *73*:573, 1982.
191. Sobel, B. E., and Bergmann, S. R.: Coronary thrombolysis: Some unresolved issues. Am. J. Med. *72*:1, 1982.
192. Shrago, E., Shug, A., and Elson, C.: Regulation of cell metabolism by mitochondrial transport systems. *In* Hanson, R. W., and Mehlman, M. A. (eds.): Gluconeogenesis: Its Regulation in Mammalian Species. New York, John Wiley & Sons, 1976, p. 221.
193. Weiss, E. S., Hoffman, E. J., Phelps, M. E., Welch, M. J., Henry, P. D., Ter-Pogossian, M. M., and Sobel, B. E.: External detection and visualization of myocardial ischemia with ^{11}C-substrates in vitro and in vivo. Circ. Res. *39*:24, 1976.
194. Ter-Pogossian, M. M., Klein, M. S., Markham, J., Roberts, R., and Sobel, B. E.: Regional assessment of myocardial metabolic integrity in vivo by positron-emission tomography with ^{11}C-labeled palmitate. Circulation *61*:242, 1980.
194a. Geltman, E. M., and Sobel, B. E.: Cardiac positron tomography. Chest *83*: 553, 1983.
194b. Schelbert, H. R., Phelps, M. E., and Shine, K. I.: Imaging metabolism and biochemistry—a new look at the heart. Am. Heart J. *105*:522, 1983.
194c. Schelbert, H. R., Henze, E., Schon, H. R., Keen, R., Hansen, H., Selin, C., Huang, S-C., Barrio, J. R., and Phelps, M. E.: C-11 palmitate for the noninvasive evaluation of regional myocardial fatty acid metabolism with positron computed tomography. III. In vivo demonstration of the effects of substrate availability on myocardial metabolism. Am. Heart J. *105*:492, 1983.
195. Weiss, E. S., Ahmed, S. A., Welch, M. J., Williamson, J. R., Ter-Pogossian, M. M., and Sobel, B. E.: Quantification of infarction in cross sections of canine myocardium in vivo with positron emission transaxial tomography and ^{11}C-palmitate. Circulation *55*:66, 1977.
196. Fox, K. A. A., Nomura, H., Sobel, B. E., and Bergmann, S. R.: Consistent substrate utilization despite reduced flow in hearts with maintained work. Am. J. Physiol. (in press).
197. Rude, R. E., Kloner, R. A., DeBoer, L. W. V., Hale, S. L., Davis, M. A., Maroko, P. R., and Braunwald, E.: A predictive index of subendocardial ischemic damage following coronary artery occlusion. Circulation *60*(Suppl. 2):96, 1979.
198. Kao, R., Rannels, E., and Morgan, H. E.: Effects of anoxia and ischemia on protein synthesis in perfused rat hearts. Circ. Res. *38*(Suppl. I):I–124, 1976.
199. Taegtmeyer, H., Peterson, M. B., Ragavan, V. V., Ferguson, A. G., and Lesch, M.: De novo alanine synthesis in isolated oxygen-deprived rabbit myocardium. J. Biol. Chem. *252*:5010, 1977.
200. Rannels, D. E., McKee, E. E., and Morgan, H. E.: Regulation of protein synthesis and degradation in heart and skeletal muscle. *In* Litwack, G. (ed.): Biochemical Actions of Hormones. New York, Academic Press, 1976.
201. Weissman, G., Hoffstein, S., Gennaro, D., and Fox, A. C.: Lysosomes in ischemic myocardium, with observations on the effects of methyl-prednisolone. *In* Lefer, A. M., Kelliher, G. J., and Rovetto, M. J. (eds.): Pathophysiology and Therapeutics of Myocardial Ischemia. New York, Spectrum Publications, Inc., 1977, p. 367.
202. Williamson, J. R., Steenbergern, C., Rich, T., Deleeuw, G., Barlow, C., and Chance, B.: The nature of ischemic injury in cardiac tissue. *In* Lefer, A. M., Kelliher, G. J., and Rovetto, M. J. (eds.): Pathophysiology and Therapeutics of Myocardial Ischemia. New York, Spectrum Publications, Inc., 1977, p. 193.
203. Chance, B.: Discussion. Circ. Res. *38*(Suppl. I):I–69, 1976.
204. Reimer, K. A., Lowe, J. E., Rasmussen, M. M., and Jennings, R. B.: The wavefront phenomenon of ischemic cell death. I. Myocardial infarct size vs duration of coronary occlusion in dogs. Circulation *56*:786, 1977.
205. Fleckenstein, A.: Calcium Antagonism in Heart and Smooth Muscle. New York, John Wiley and Sons, 1983.
206. Shen, A. C., and Jennings, R. B.: Kinetics of calcium accumulation in acute myocardial ischemic injury. Am. J. Pathol. *67*:441, 1972.
207. Braunwald, E.: Mechanism of action of calcium channel blocking agents. N. Engl. J. Med. *307*:1618, 1982.
208. Corr, P. B., Gross, R. W., and Sobel, B. E.: Arrhythmogenic amphiphilic lipids and the myocardial cell membrane. J. Molec. Cell. Cardiol. *14*:619, 1982.
209. Sedlis, S. P., Corr, P. B., Sobel, B. E., and Ahumada, G. G.: Lysophosphatidyl choline potentiates Ca^{++} accumulation in rat cardiac myocytes. Am. J. Physiol. *13*:H32, 1983.
210. Kloner, R. A., DeBoer, L. W. V., Carlson, N., and Braunwald, E.: The effect of verapamil on myocardial ultrastructure during and following release of coronary artery occlusion. Exp. Molec. Pathol. *36*:277, 1982.
211. Braunwald, E., Muller, J. E., Kloner, R. A., and Maroko, P. R.: Role of beta-adrenergic blockade in the therapy of patients with myocardial infarction. Am. J. Med. *784*:113, 1983.
212. Henry, P. D., Shuchleib, R., Davis, J., Weiss, E. S., and Sobel, B. E.: Myocardial contracture and accumulation of mitochondrial calcium in ischemic rabbit heart. Am. J. Physiol. (Heart Circ. Physiol.) *2*:H677, 1977.
213. DeBoer, L. W. V., Strauss, H. W., Kloner, R. A., Rude, R. E., David, R. F., Maroko, P. R., and Braunwald, E.: Autoradiographic method for measuring the ischemic myocardium at risk: Effects of verapamil on infarct size after experimental coronary artery occlusion. Proc. Natl. Acad. Sci. *77*:6119, 1980.
214. Clark, R. E., Christlieb, I. Y., and Ferguson, T. B.: Laboratory and initial clinical studies of nifedipine, a calcium antagonist for improved myocardial preservation. Ann. Surg. *193*:719, 1981.
215. Sobel, B. E., Roberts, R., and Larson, K. B.: Considerations in the use of biochemical markers of ischemic injury. Circ. Res. *38*(Suppl. I):I–99, 1976.
216. Ahumada, G., Roberts, R., and Sobel, B. E.: Evaluation of myocardial infarction with enzymatic indices. Prog. Cardiovasc. Dis. *18*:405, 1976.
217. Stone, M. J., Willerson, J. T., Gomez-Sanchez, C. E., and Waterman, M. R.: Radioimmunoassay of myoglobin in human serum: Results in patients with acute myocardial infarction. J. Clin. Invest. *56*:1334, 1975.
218. Wagner, G. S., Roe, C. R., Limbird, L. E., Rosati, R. A., and Wallace, A. G.: The importance of identification of the myocardial specific isoenzyme of creatine phosphokinase (MB form) in the diagnosis of acute myocardial infarction. Circulation *47*:263, 1973.
219. Braunwald, E., and Maroko, P. R.: Limitation of infarct size. Curr. Probl. Cardiol. *3*:51, 1978.
220. Nachlas, M. M., Friedman, M. M., and Cohen, S. P.: A method for the quantitation of myocardial infarcts and the relation of serum enzyme levels to infarct size. Surgery *55*:700, 1964.
221. Sobel, B. E., and Shell, W. E.: Diagnostic and prognostic value of serum enzyme changes in patients with acute myocardial infarction. *In* Yu, P. N., and Goodwin, J. F. (eds.): Progress in Cardiology 4. Philadelphia, Lea and Febiger, 1975, p. 165.
222. Ahmed, S. A., Williamson, J. R., Roberts, R., Clark, R. E., and Sobel, B. E.: The association of increased plasma MB CPK activity and irreversible ischemic myocardial injury in the dog. Circulation *54*:187, 1976.
223. Shell, W. E., Kjekshus, J. K., and Sobel, B. E.: Quantitative assessment of the extent of myocardial infarction in the conscious dog by means of analysis of serial changes in serum creatine phosphokinase activity. J. Clin. Invest. *50*: 2614, 1971.
224. Sobel, B. E., Markam, J., Karlsberg, R. P., and Roberts, R.: The nature of disappearance of creatine kinase from the circulation and its influence on enzymatic estimation of infarct size. Circ. Res. *41*:836, 1977.
225. Geltman, E. M., Ehsani, A. A., Campbell, M. K., Schechtman, K., Roberts, R., and Sobel, B. E.: The influence of location and extent of myocardial infarction on long-term ventricular dysrhythmia and mortality. Circulation *60*: 805, 1979.
226. Roberts, R., Gowda, K. S., Ludbrook, P. A., and Sobel, B. E.: Specificity of elevated serum MB creatine phosphokinase activity in the diagnosis of acute myocardial infarction. Am. J. Cardiol. *36*:433, 1975.
227. Bleifeld, W., Mathey, D., Hanrath, P., Buss, H., and Effert, S.: Infarct size estimated from serial serum creatine phosphokinase in relation to left ventricular hemodynamics. Circulation *55*:303, 1977.
228. Mathey, D., Bleifeld, W., Hanrath, P., and Effert, S.: Attempt to quantitate relation between cardiac function and infarct size in acute myocardial infarction. Br. Heart J. *36*:271, 1974.
229. Norris, R. M., Whitlock, R. M. L., Barratt-Boyes, C., and Small, C. W.: Clinical measurement of myocardial infarct size. Modification of a method for the estimation of total creatine phosphokinase release after myocardial infarction. Circulation *51*:614, 1975.
230. Yasmineh, W. G., Pyle, R. B., Cohn, J. N., Nicoloff, D. M., Hanson, N. Q., and Steele, B. W.: Serial serum creatine phosphokinase MB isoenzyme activity after myocardial infarction. Studies in the baboon and man. Circulation *55*: 733, 1977.
231. Vatner, S. F., Baig, H., Manders, W. T., and Maroko, P. R.: Effects of coronary artery reperfusion on myocardial infarct size calculated from creatine kinase. J. Clin. Invest. *61*:1048, 1978.
232. Clark, G. L., Robison, A. K., Gnepp, D. R., Roberts, R., and Sobel, B. E.: Effects of lymphatic transport of enzyme on plasma CK time-activity curves after myocardial infarction. Circ. Res. *43*:162, 1978.
233. Sobel, B. E., Markam, J., and Roberts, R.: Factors influencing enzymatic estimates of infarct size. Am. J. Cardiol. *39*:130, 1977.
234. Rude, R. E., Muller, J. E., and Braunwald, E.: Efforts to limit the size of myocardial infarcts. Ann. Intern. Med. *95*:736, 1981.
235. Maroko, P. R., Kjekshus, J. K., Sobel, B. E., Watanabe, T., Covell, J. W., Ross, J., Jr., and Braunwald, E.: Factors influencing infarct size following experimental coronary artery occlusion. Circulation *43*:67, 1971.
236. Kloner, R. A., and Braunwald, E.: Review—Observations on experimental myocardial ischemia. Cardiovasc. Res. *14*:371, 1980.
237. Shell, W. E., and Sobel, B. E.: Deleterious effects of increased heart rate on infarct size in the conscious dog. Am. J. Cardiol. *31*:474, 1973.
238. Richman, S.: Adverse effect of atropine during myocardial infarction: Enhancement of ischemia following intravenously administered atropine. J.A.M.A. *228*:1414, 1974.
239. Radvany, P., Maroko, P. R., and Braunwald, E.: Effect of hypoxemia on the extent of myocardial necrosis after experimental coronary occlusion. Am. J. Cardiol. *35*:795, 1975.

240. Yoshikawa, H., Powell, W. J., Jr., Bland, J. H. L., and Lowenstein, E.: Effect of acute anemia on experimental myocardial ischemia. Am. J. Cardiol. *32*:670, 1973.
241. DeBoer, L. W. V., Rude, R. E., Davis, R. F., Maroko, P. R., and Braunwald, E.: Extension of myocardial necrosis into normal epicardium following hypotension during experimental coronary occlusion. Cardiovasc. Res. *16*:423, 1982.
242. Libby, P., Maroko, P. R., and Braunwald, E.: The effect of hypoglycemia on myocardial ischemic injury during acute experimental coronary artery occlusion. Circulation *51*:621, 1975.
243. Liedtke, A. J., and Hughes, H. C.: Hyperthermic insult to ischemic myocardium: Implications of fever as an energy draining process in myocardial infarct. Clin. Res. *24*:227A, 1976.
244. Vatner, S. F., McRitchie, R. J., Maroko, P. R., Patrick, T. A., and Braunwald, E.: Effects of catecholamines, exercise, and nitroglycerin on the normal and ischemic myocardium in conscious dogs. J. Clin. Invest. *54*:563, 1974.
245. Maroko, P. R., Libby, P., and Braunwald, E.: Effect of pharmacologic agents on the function of the ischemic heart. Am. J. Cardiol. *32*:930, 1973.
246. Davidson, S., Maroko, P. R., and Braunwald, E.: Effects of isoproterenol on contractile function of the ischemic and anoxic heart. Am. J. Physiol. *227*:439, 1974.
247. Vatner, S. F., Millard, R. W., Patrick, T. A., and Heyndrickx, G. R.: Effects of isoproterenol on regional myocardial function, electrogram, and blood flow in conscious dogs with myocardial ischemia. J. Clin. Invest. *57*:1261, 1976.
248. Mueller, H., Ayres, S. M., Gregory, J. J., Giannelli, S., Jr., and Grace, W. J.: Hemodynamics, coronary blood flow, and myocardial metabolism in coronary shock: Response to 1-norepinephrine and isoproterenol. J. Clin. Invest. *49*: 1885, 1970.
249. Shug, A., and Shrago, E.: A proposed mechanism for fatty acid effects on energy metabolism of the heart. J. Lab. Clin. Med. *81*:214, 1973.
250. Mjøs, O. D., Kjekshus, J. K., and Lekven, J.: Importance of free fatty acids as a determinant of myocardial oxygen consumption and myocardial ischemic injury during norepinephrine infusion in dogs. J. Clin. Invest. *53*:1290, 1974.
251. Kjekshus, J. K., and Mjøs, O. D.: Effect of free fatty acids on myocardial function and metabolism in the ischemic dog heart. J. Clin. Invest. *51*:1767, 1972.
252. Schaper, J., and Schaper, W.: Reperfusion of ischemic myocardium: Ultrastructural and histochemical aspects. J. Am. Coll. Cardiol. *1*:1037, 1983.
253. Ellis, S. G., Henschke, C. I., Sandor, T., Wynne, J., Braunwald, E., and Kloner, R. A.: Time course of functional and biochemical recovery of myocardium salvaged by reperfusion. J. Am. Coll. Cardiol. *1*:1047, 1983.
254. Higginson, L. A. J., Beanlands, D. S., Nair, R. C., Temple, V., and Sheldrick, K.: The time course and characterization of myocardial hemorrhage after coronary reperfusion in the anesthetized dog. Circulation *67*:1024, 1983.
255. Lang, T. W., Corday, E., Gold, H., Meerbaum, S., Rubins, S., Constantini, C., Hirose, S., Osher, J., and Rosen, V.: Consequences of reperfusion after coronary occlusion: Effects on hemodynamic and regional myocardial metabolic function. Am. J. Cardiol. *33*:69, 1974.
256. Maroko, P. R., Radvany, P., Braunwald, E., and Hale, S. L.: Reduction of infarct size by oxygen inhalation following acute coronary occlusion. Circulation *52*:360, 1975.
257. Glogar, D. H., Kloner, R. A., Muller, J., DeBoer, L. W. V., and Braunwald, E.: Fluorocarbons reduce myocardial ischemic damage after coronary occlusion. Science *211*:1439, 1981.
258. Braunwald, E., Muller, J. E., Kloner, R. A., and Maroko, P. R.: Role of beta-adrenergic blockade in the therapy of patients with myocardial infarction. Am. J. Med. *74*:113, 1983.
259. Lange, R., Kloner, R. A., and Braunwald, E.: First ultra-short-acting-beta-adrenergic blocking agent: Its effect on size and segmental wall dynamics of reperfused myocardial infarcts in dogs. Am. J. Cardiol. *51*:1759, 1983.
260. Hammerman, H., Kloner, R. A., Briggs, L. L., and Braunwald, E.: Combination therapy for early treatment of myocardial infarction: Beta blockade plus reperfusion. Clin. Res. *31*:524a, 1983.
261. Henry, P. R., Shuchleib, R., Borda, L. J., Roberts, R., Williamson, J. R., and Sobel, B. E.: Effects of nifedipine on myocardial perfusion and ischemic injury in dogs. Circ. Res. *43*:372, 1978.
261a. Drury, J. K., Haendchen, R. V., Meerbaum, S., Fishbein, M. C., Y-Rit, J., and Corday, E.: Diltiazem improves function and reduces infarct size after acute coronary occlusion. J. Am. Coll. Cardiol. *1*:692, 1983.
262. Opie, L. H.: Metabolism of free fatty acids, glucose and catecholamines in acute myocardial infarction: Relation to myocardial ischemia and infarct size. Am. J. Cardiol. *36*:938, 1975.
263. Calva, E., Mujica, A., Bisteni, A., and Sodi-Pallares, D.: Oxidative phosphorylation in cardiac infarct: Effect of glucose-KCl-insulin solution. Am. J. Physiol. *209*:371, 1965.
264. Henry, P. D., Sobel, B. E., and Braunwald, E.: Protection of hypoxic guinea pig hearts with glucose and insulin. Am. J. Physiol. *226*:390, 1974.
265. Wildenthal, K., Mierzwiak, D. S., and Mitchell, J. H.: Acute effects of increased serum osmolality on left ventricular performance. Am. J. Physiol. *216*: 898, 1969.
266. Regan, T. J., Harman, M. A., Lehan, P. H., Burke, W. M., and Oldewurtel, H. A.: Ventricular arrhythmias and K^+ transfer during myocardial ischemia and intervention with procaine amide, insulin, or glucose solution. J. Clin. Invest. *46*:1657, 1967.
267. Sodi-Pallares, D., Bisteni, A., Medrano, G. A., Testelli, M. R., and DeMicheli, A.: The polarizing treatment of acute myocardial infarction: Possibility of its use in other cardiovascular conditions. Dis. Chest. *43*:424, 1963.
268. Maroko, P. R., Libby, P., Sobel, B. E., Bloor, C. M., Sybers, H. D., Shell, W. E., Covell, J. W., and Braunwald, E.: Effect of glucose-insulin-potassium infusion on myocardial infarction following experimental coronary artery occlusion. Circulation *45*:1160, 1972.
269. Opie, L. H., Bruyneel, K., and Owen, P.: Effects of glucose, insulin, and potassium infusion on tissue metabolic changes within the first hour of myocardial infarction in the baboon. Circulation *52*:49, 1975.
270. Kjekshus, J. K.: Effect of lipolytic and inotropic stimulation on myocardial ischemic injury. *In* Hjalmarson, A., and Werko, L. (eds.): Experimental and Clinical Aspects on Preservation of the Ischemic Myocardium. Sweden, Molndal, 1976, p. 35.
271. Mjøs, O. D.: Effect of reduction of myocardial free fatty acid metabolism relative to that of glucose on the ischemic injury during experimental coronary artery occlusion in dogs. *In* Hjalmarson, A., and Werko, L. (eds.): Experimental and Clinical Aspects on Preservation of the Ischemic Myocardium. Sweden, Molndal, 1976, p. 29.
272. Folts, J. D., Shug, A. S., Koke, J. R., and Bittar, N.: Protection of the ischemic dog myocardium with L-carnitine. Clin. Res. *24*:217A, 1976.
273. Flores, J., DiBona, D. R., Beck, C. H., and Leaf, A.: The role of cell swelling in ischemic renal damage and the protective effect of hypertonic solute. J. Clin. Invest. *51*:118, 1972.
274. Maroko, P. R., Carpenter, C. B., Chiariello, M., Fishbein, M. C., Radvany, P., Knostman, J. B., and Hale, S. L.: Reduction by cobra venom factor of myocardial necrosis following coronary artery occlusion. J. Clin. Invest. *61*: 661, 1978.
275. Diaz, P. E., Fishbein, M. C., Davis, M. A., Askenazi, J., and Maroko, P. R.: Effect of kallikrein inhibitor aprotinin on myocardial ischemic injury following coronary artery occlusion in the dog. Am. J. Cardiol. *40*:541, 1977.
276. Libby, P., Maroko, P. R., Bloor, C. M., Sobel, B. E., and Braunwald, E.: Reduction of experimental myocardial infarct size by corticosteroid administration. J. Clin. Invest. *52*:599, 1973.
277. Masters, T. N., Harbold, N. B., Jr., Hall, D. G., Jackson, R. D., Mullen, D. C., Daugherty, H. K., and Robicsek, F.: Beneficial metabolic effects of methylprednisolone sodium succinate in acute myocardial ischemia. Am. J. Cardiol. *37*:557, 1976.
278. Hammerman, H., Kloner, R. A., Hale, S. L., Schoen, F. J., and Braunwald, E.: Is scar thinning and LV topographic alterations induced by antiinflammatory agent of functional significance? Clin. Res. (abst.), in press.
279. Weissman, G.: Corticosteroids and membrane stabilization. Circulation *53* (Suppl. 1):171, 1976.
280. Kloner, R. A., Fishbein, M. C., Lew, H., Maroko, P. R., and Braunwald, E.: Mummification of the infarcted myocardium by high dose corticosteroids. Circulation *57*:56, 1978.
281. Roberts, R. deMello, V., and Sobel, B. E.: Deleterious effects of methylprednisolone in patients with myocardial infarction. Circulation *53*(Suppl. 1):1, 1976.
282. Maclean, D., Maroko, P. R., Fishbein, M. C., and Braunwald, E.: Effects of corticosteroids on myocardial infarct size and healing following experimental coronary occlusion. Am. J. Cardiol. *39*:280, 1977.
283. Jugdutt, B. I., Hutchins, G. M., Bulkley, B. H., and Becker, L. C.: Salvage of ischemic myocardium by ibuprofen during infarction in the conscious dog. Am. J. Cardiol. *46*:74, 1980.
284. Brown, E. J., Kloner, R. A., Schoen, F. J., Hammerman, H., Hale, S., and Braunwald, E.: Scar thinning due to ibuprofen administration following experimental myocardial infarction. Am. J. Cardiol. *51*:877, 1983.
285. Willerson, J. T., Watson, J. T., and Platt, M. R.: Effect of hypertonic mannitol and intraaortic counterpulsation on regional myocardial blood flow and ventricular performance in dogs during myocardial ischemia. Am. J. Cardiol. *37*: 514, 1976.
286. Maroko, P. R., Libby, P., Bloor, C. M., Sobel, B. E., and Braunwald, E.: Reduction by hyaluronidase of myocardial necrosis following coronary artery occlusion. Circulation *46*:430, 1972.
287. Wetstein, L., Simson, M. B., Haselgrove, J., Barlow, C. H., and Harken, A. H.: Mechanism of action of hyaluronidase in decreasing myocardial ischemia post coronary occlusion in the isolated perfused rabbit heart. Am. Heart J. *104*: 529, 1982.
288. Askenazi, J., Hillis, L. D., Diaz, P. E., Davis, M. A., Braunwald, E., and Maroko, P. R.: The effects of hyaluronidase on coronary blood flow following coronary artery occlusion in the dog. Cir. Res. *40*:566, 1977.
289. Epstein, S. E., Borer, J. S., Kent, K. M., Redwood, D. R., Goldstein, R. E., and Levitt, B.: Protection of ischemic myocardium by nitroglycerin: Experimental and clinical results. Circulation *53*(Suppl. 1): 191, 1976.
290. Smith, E. R., Redwood, D. R., McCarron, W. E., and Epstein, S. E.: Coronary artery occlusion in the conscious dog: Effects of alterations in arterial pressure produced by nitroglycerin, hemorrhage, and alpha-adrenergic agonists on the degree of myocardial ischemia. Circulation *47*:51, 1973.
291. Myers, R. W., Scherer, J. L., Goldstein, R. A., Goldstein, R. E., Kent, K. M., and Epstein, S. E.: Effects of nitroglycerin and nitroglycerin-methoxamine during acute myocardial ischemia in dogs with preexisting multivessel coronary occlusive disease. Circulation *51*:632, 1975.
292. Kent, K. M., Smith, E. R., Redwood, D. R., and Epstein, S. E.: Beneficial electrophysiologic effects of nitroglycerin during acute myocardial infarction. Am. J. Cardiol. *33*:513, 1974.
293. Forman, R., Eng, C., and Kirk, E. S.: Comparative effect of verapamil and nitroglycerin on collateral blood flow. Circulation *67*:1200, 1983.

37 ACUTE MYOCARDIAL INFARCTION: PATHOLOGICAL, PATHOPHYSIOLOGICAL, AND CLINICAL MANIFESTATIONS

by Joseph S. Alpert, M.D., and Eugene Braunwald, M.D.

Approximately one-third of all deaths in the United States are due to ischemic heart disease, and, of these, one-half are attributable to acute myocardial infarction (AMI). Approximately one-half of patients with AMI die suddenly, i.e., within 1 hour of onset (Chap. 23). Most of the remainder, annually approximately one-half million patients, are admitted to hospitals with AMI.[1] The mortality rates during hospitalization and during the year following infarction are approximately 15 and 10 per cent, respectively, with at least half of the post-hospitalization deaths occurring suddenly before the victim can be returned to the hospital. In addition to this high probability of death within the first year after myocardial infarction (MI), excessive mortality risk continues for a prolonged period. Indeed, a three- to fourfold excess in the risk of death persists even 10 years after infarction.[2] Recently, a modest though significant reduction in the death rate from coronary artery disease has been noted (p. 1208).[3] The cause of this decreased mortality is unknown, but it may be the result, in part, of a decreased incidence of AMI, improved treatment, or both.

PATHOLOGY OF MYOCARDIAL INFARCTION

Almost all myocardial infarctions result from atherosclerosis of the coronary arteries. The genesis of the coronary atherosclerotic lesion is a complex and controversial issue (see Chap. 34), and a number of risk factors have been associated with the development of atherosclerosis (see Chap. 35). However, regardless of the etiology and pathogenesis of the atherosclerotic process, the end result is plaques that cause luminal narrowing of the coronary arterial tree and thus reduce the blood supply to the myocardium. Below a certain critical level of blood flow, myocardial cells develop ischemic injury, a process described in detail in Chapter 36. When severe ischemia is prolonged, irreversible damage, i.e., myocardial infarction, occurs.

Since the coronary luminal narrowing affects the major coronary arteries and their various branches to a different extent, MI usually occurs focally in specific regions of the heart. The location and size of a particular infarction depend on a number of different factors: (1) the location and severity of the atherosclerotic narrowings in the coronary arterial tree; (2) the presence, site, and severity of coronary arterial spasm; (3) the size of the vascular bed perfused by the narrowed vessels; (4) the extent of development of collateral blood vessels; and (5) the oxygen needs of the poorly perfused myocardium.

GROSS PATHOLOGICAL CHANGES OF MYOCARDIAL INFARCTION

Myocardial infarction may be divided into two major types: *transmural infarcts*, in which myocardial necrosis involves the full thickness of the ventricular wall, and *subendocardial (nontransmural) infarcts*, in which the necrosis involves the subendocardium, the intramural myocardium, or both without extending all the way through the ventricular wall to the epicardium.

Gross changes do not appear in the myocardium until 6 hours after the onset of myocardial infarction.[4] Initially, the myocardium in the affected region appears pale, bluish, and slightly swollen. Eighteen to 36 hours after the onset of the infarct, the myocardium appears tan or reddish-purple, with a serofibrinous exudate evident on the epicardium in transmural infarcts. These changes persist for approximately 48 hours; the infarct then turns gray, and fine yellow lines, secondary to neutrophilic infiltration, appear at its periphery. This zone gradually widens and during the next few days extends throughout the infarct.

Eight to 10 days following infarction, the thickness of the cardiac wall in the area of the infarct is reduced as necrotic muscle is removed by mononuclear cells. The cut surface of an infarct of this age is yellow, surrounded by a reddish-purple band of granulation tissue (Fig. 37–1) that extends through the necrotic tissue by 3 to 4 weeks. Commencing at this time and extending over the next 2 to 3 months, the infarcted area gradually acquires a gelatinous, ground-glass, gray appearance, eventually converting into a shrunken, thin, firm scar, which whitens and firms progressively with time;[5–7] this process begins at the periphery of the infarct and gradually moves centrally. The endocardium below the infarct increases in thickness and becomes gray and opaque.

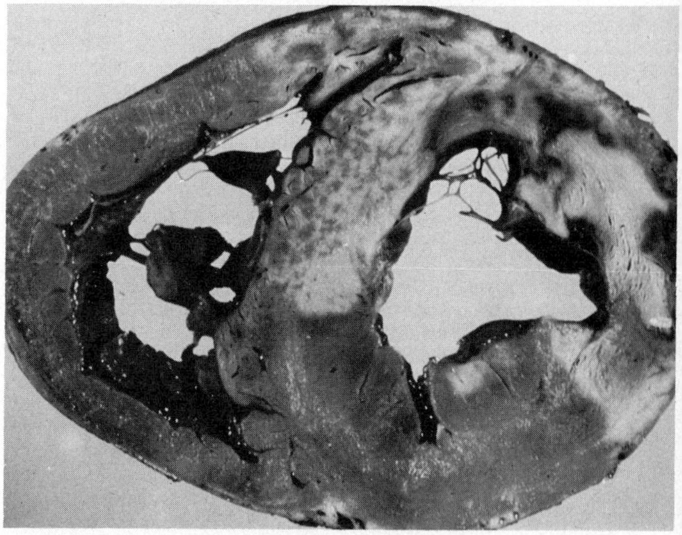

FIGURE 37–1 Acute myocardial infarct. Cross section of the heart shows myocardial infarct about 1 week old, involving the posterior half of the interventricular septum and the posterior lateral left ventricular walls. This infarct is secondary to occlusion of the left circumflex coronary artery. The myocardium has a mottled appearance, and the margins of the infarct are well demarcated. In the central portion of the infarct involving the posterior papillary muscle, there is evidence of hemorrhage. (From Bloor, C. M.: Cardiac Pathology. Philadelphia, J. B. Lippincott Co., 1978.)

HISTOLOGICAL AND ULTRASTRUCTURAL CHANGES

On light microscopy, severe ischemia, which is potentially reversible, causes cloudy swelling, as well as hydropic, vascular, and fatty degeneration.[8] For many years it was believed that no light microscopic changes could be seen in infarcted myocardium until 8 hours

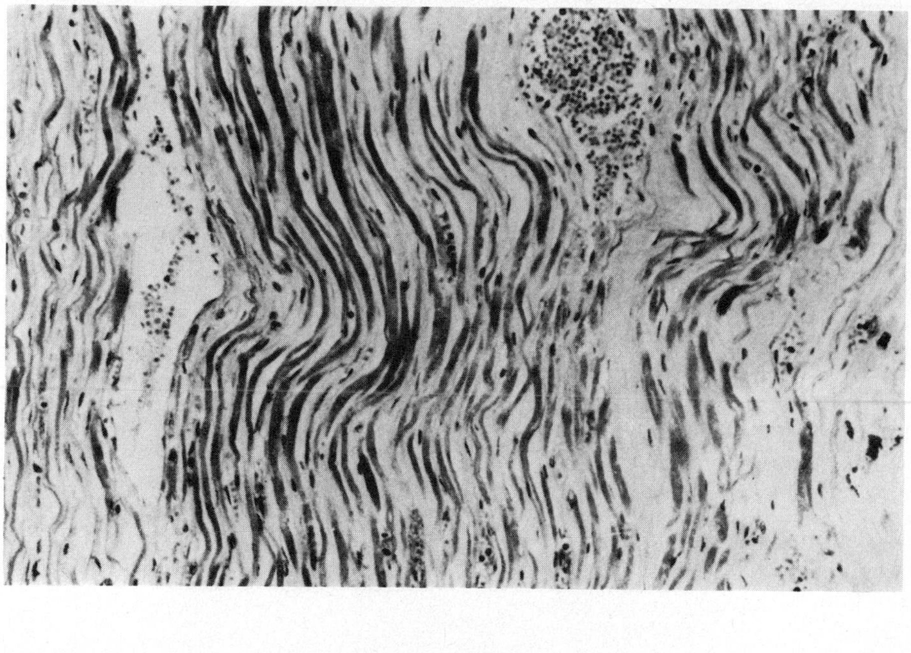

FIGURE 37–2 Wavy and stretched appearance of necrotic muscle cells in an acute myocardial infarct. The wavy myocardial fibers have pyknotic nuclei and hypereosinophilic cytoplasm. (Hematoxylin and eosin, × 128). (Reproduced with permission from Willerson, J. T., Hillis, L. D., and Buja, L. M. [eds.]: Pathogenesis and pathology of ischemic heart disease. *In* Ischemic Heart Disease. Clinical and Pathophysiological Aspects. New York, Raven Press, 1982, p. 46.)

after interruption of blood flow. Bouchardy and Majno, however, have called attention to a wavy pattern of myocardial cells that occurs shortly after the onset of infarction (Fig. 37–2), a pattern that is probably the result of agonal contraction of myocardial cells.[9,10] With careful light microscopy, contraction bands and small spaces between myocardial cells are also revealed.[11] After 8 hours, edema of the interstitium becomes evident, as do increased fatty deposits in the muscle fibers, along with infiltration of neutrophilic polymorphonuclear leukocytes and red blood cells. Muscle cell nuclei become pyknotic and then undergo karyolysis, and small blood vessels undergo necrosis.

By 24 hours there is clumping of the cytoplasm and loss of cross striations, with appearance of focal hyalinization and irregular cross bands in the involved myocardial fibers. The nuclei become pyknotic and sometimes even disappear. The myocardial capillaries in the involved region dilate, and polymorphonuclear leukocytes accumulate, first at the periphery and then in the center of the infarct. During the first 3 days, the interstitial tissue becomes edematous and red blood cells may extravasate. Generally, on about the fourth day after infarction, removal of necrotic fibers begins, again commencing at the periphery. Later, lymphocytes, macrophages, and fibroblasts infiltrate between myocytes, which become fragmented. At 8 days the necrotic muscle fibers have become dissolved; by about 10 days the number of polymorphonuclear leukocytes is reduced, and granulation tissue first appears at the periphery. Ingrowth of blood vessels and fibroblasts continues, along with removal of necrotic muscle cells, until the fourth to sixth week following infarction, by which time much of the necrotic myocardium has been removed. This process continues along with increasing collagenization of the infarcted area. By the sixth week, the infarcted area has usually been converted into a firm connective tissue scar with interspersed intact muscle fibers.[6]

A variety of *histochemical* approaches have been used to detect myocardial changes compatible with infarction before routine microscopic changes become evident at 6 hours. These include estimation of glycogen, using a periodic acid–Schiff stain (PAS) and succinic dehydrogenase activity. Glycogen stores may become depleted within 3 to 4 hours after the onset of severe myocardial ischemia. However, the reliability of these procedures diminishes with lengthening of the interval between death and the examination of the myocardium.[4]

One of the most useful histochemical methods is the nitro-blue tetrazolium staining technique; the heart is sliced transversely into several sections. These sections are washed and incubated in buffered tetrazolium solution, which is reduced to a dark blue compound, formazan, in viable zones of myocardium. Reduction of tetrazolium is accomplished by endogenous substrates, coenzymes, and dehydrogenases; these are absent or deficient in necrotic areas of myocardium, which therefore remain uncolored and hence identifiable. This reaction can distinguish infarcted myocardium 6 to 8 hours after the start of infarction.[11]

Although the *alterations in cardiac ultrastructure* to be described are based on animal experiments and are not directly applicable to clinical diagnosis, they provide important information concerning the process of myocardial infarction. The earliest ultrastructural changes in cardiac muscle following ligation of a coronary artery, noted within 20 minutes, consist of reduction in the size and number of glycogen granules, development of intracellular edema, and swelling and distortion of the transverse tubular system, the sarcoplasmic reticulum, and the mitochondria (Fig. 37–3).[12–17] When these changes are relatively mild, they are compatible with reversible ischemic injury. Changes after 60 minutes of occlusion include myocardial cell swelling, mitochondrial abnormalities such as swelling and internal disruption, aggregation and margination of nuclear chromatin, and relaxation of myofibrils.[11] After 20 minutes to 2 hours of ischemia, changes in some cells become irreversible, and there is progression of these alterations; additional changes include indistinct, tight junctions at the intercalated disks, swollen sacs of the sarcoplasmic reticulum at the level of the A band, greatly enlarged mitochondria with few cristae, thinning and fractionation of myofilaments, disappearance of the heterochromatin, rarefaction of the euchromatin and peripheral aggregation of chromatin in the nucleus, disorientation of myofibrils, and clumping of mitochondria. Cells irreversibly damaged by ischemia are usually swollen, with an enlarged sarcoplasmic space; the sarcolemma may peel off the cells, defects in the plasma membrane may appear, and the mitochondria are fragmented.

The swollen mitochondria obtained from ischemic myocardium contain deposits of calcium phosphate and amorphous matrix densities;[18] many of these changes become more intense when blood flow is restored.[14,19] However, it appears unlikely that the structural and functional deterioration of mitochondria—the hallmark of ischemic injury—is the primary mediator of myocardial cell death. In experimental infarction, reflow into an area rendered ischemic for 40 to 60 minutes results in violent cell swelling with vacuolization of myocardial cell cytoplasm and marked swelling of mitochondria. Cell membranes are lifted off the myofibrils, and subsarcolemmal blebs appear. The speed with which these morphological changes occur during early postischemic reflow suggests that ischemia produces a defect of volume regulation in myocardial cells.

Three patterns of myocardial necrosis are recognized. *Coagulation necrosis*[20] results from severe, persistent ischemia and is usually present in the central region of infarcts, which results in the arrest of muscle cells in the relaxed state and the passive stretching of ischemic muscle cells. On light microscopy the myofibrils are stretched, many with unclear pyknosis, with vascular congestion and healing by phagocytosis of necrotic muscle cells. There is evidence of mitochondrial damage with prominent amorphous (flocculent) densities but no calcification.

Coagulative myocytolysis[9,21,22] (also termed contraction band necrosis)[23] results primarily from severe ischemia followed by reflow.[12] It is

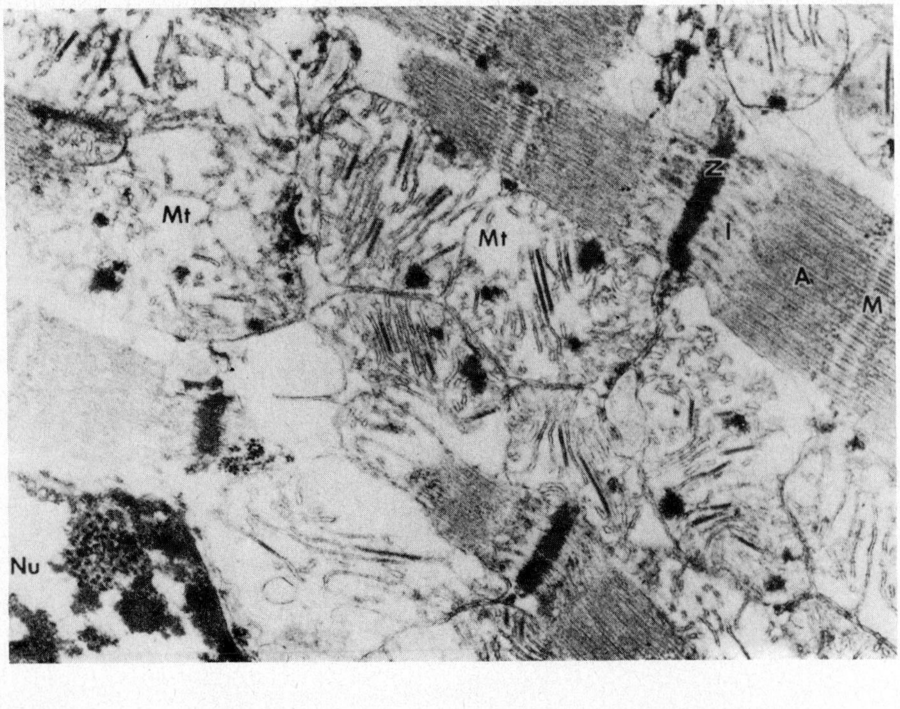

FIGURE 37–3 Electron micrograph of a muscle cell from the center of an infarct produced by permanent coronary occlusion in the dog. The myofibrils are fixed in a relaxed state and exhibit I, A, M, and Z bands. There is slight edema and no glycogen. (The clusters of granules resembling glycogen probably are ribosomes.) The mitochondria (Mt) are swollen and have linear densities and amorphous matrix (flocculent) densities. The nucleus (Nu) has clumped chromatin along the nuclear membrane and large lucent areas. (Tissue fixed with glutaraldehyde and osmium. Epoxy section stained with uranyl acetate and lead citrate, × 19,500). (Reproduced with permission from Willerson, J. T., Hillis, L. D., and Buja, L. M. [eds.]: Pathogenesis and pathology of ischemic heart disease. *In* Ischemic Heart Disease. Clinical and Pathophysiological Aspects. New York, Raven Press, 1982, p. 47.)

caused by increased Ca^{++} influx into dying cells, resulting in the arrest of cells in the contracted state. It is seen in the periphery of large infarcts or constitutes the entire infarct in patients subjected to iatrogenic reperfusion (by surgery or thrombolysis). Its presence in a large segment of some infarcts suggests that reperfusion through spontaneous thrombolysis or the release of spasm or both have occurred. It is characterized by hypercontracted myofibrils with contraction bands and mitochondrial damage, frequently with calcification, marked vascular congestion, and healing by lysis of muscle cells.

Myocytolysis results from prolonged moderate ischemia and, like coagulative myocytolysis, is also frequently seen at the borders of an infarct as well as in patchy areas of infarction in patients with chronic ischemic heart disease. It is characterized by edema and cell swelling, early lysis of myofibrils, late lysis of nuclei, no neutrophilic response, and healing by lysis and phagocytosis of necrotic myocytes.[7,21]

Relation of Myocardial Infarction to Coronary Arterial Obstruction

Myocardial infarction usually occurs in hearts with more than one severely narrowed coronary artery.[24,25] One-third to two-thirds of patients with AMI have critical obstruction (less than 25 per cent of luminal area), whereas the remainder is equally divided between patients having one-vessel disease and those having two-vessel disease.[26,27] Most transmural infarcts occur distal to a totally occluded coronary artery. However, the converse is not the case, in that total occlusion of a coronary artery is not always associated with myocardial infarction. Collateral blood flow and other factors—such as the level of myocardial metabolism, the presence and location of stenoses in other coronary arteries, the rate of development of the obstruction, and the quantity of myocardium supplied by the obstructed vessel—all influence the viability of myocardial cells distal to the occlusion. In many series of patients studied at necropsy or by coronary arteriography, a small number (< 5 per cent) of patients with MI are found to have normal coronary vessels. In these patients, an embolus that has lysed or a prolonged episode of severe coronary spasm may have been responsible for the reduction in coronary flow.

Obstruction of the left anterior descending coronary artery usually causes infarction or threatens the viability of the anterior and apical regions of the left ventricle; portions of the septum, anterolateral wall, papillary muscles, and inferoapical wall of the left ventricle may also be involved. Obstruction of the left circumflex artery can cause infarction of the lateral or inferoposterior wall of the left ventricle, whereas occlusion of the right coronary artery usually results in infarction of the inferoposterior wall of the left ventricle, the inferior portions of the septum, and the posteromedial papillary muscle. The size of the infarction and its location depend on the distribution of the obstructed coronary vessels. Thus, with occlusion of a dominant right coronary artery, which supplies the posterior descending artery and posterior left ventricular wall, the inferoposterior wall of the left ventricle becomes infarcted, whereas the same region of the myocardium becomes involved with occlusion of the left circumflex coronary artery in the presence of a dominant left coronary artery. Rather frequently, when an area of the ventricle is perfused by collateral vessels, an infarct occurs at a distance from a coronary occlusion. For example, following the gradual obliteration of the lumen of the right coronary artery, the inferior wall of the left ventricle may be maintained viable by collateral vessels arising from the left anterior descending coronary artery. In this circumstance, an occlusion of the left anterior descending artery may cause an infarct of the diaphragmatic wall.

Transmural infarctions are found at postmortem examination to be associated with fresh or organizing thrombosis of the coronary artery supplying the infarcted region in slightly more than half of the cases;[27] as discussed below, a much larger percentage of these patients are thought to have thrombi at the onset of infarct. Transmural infarcts are more frequently localized to the zone of distribution of a single coronary artery. Nontransmural infarctions (either subendocardial or multifocal), however, frequently occur in the setting of severely narrowed but still patent coronary arteries, often in patients with pulmonary embolism, hypertension, hypotension, anemia, aortic stenosis, operative procedures, or cerebrovascular accidents.[28,29] In the presence of severe atherosclerotic narrowing of the coronary arteries, these and other conditions associated with increased myocardial metabolic demands or decreased myocardial oxygen delivery or both are capable of producing patchy, nontransmural myocardial necrosis.

CORONARY ARTERIAL THROMBI. Coronary arterial thrombi, which are approximately 1 cm in length in most cases,[25] adhere to the luminal surface of an artery and are composed of platelets, fibrin, erythrocytes, and leukocytes. The composition of the thrombus may vary at different levels: A white thrombus is composed of platelets, fibrin, or both distally, and a red thrombus is composed of erythrocytes, fibrin, platelets, and leukocytes proximally. Early thrombi are usually small and nonocclusive and are composed almost exclusively of platelets.

In patients with MI, coronary thrombi are usually superimposed on or adjacent to atherosclerotic plaques; the mechanism by which thrombosis occurs in these stenotic areas remains controversial. It has been suggested that degenerative changes in the atherosclerotic intima damage supportive perivascular tissue with resultant rupture of a plaque, sometimes accompanied by intramural hemorrhage.[12,30,31] This process may enlarge the volume of the plaque so that it occludes the arterial lumen without the occurrence of thrombosis, or the hemorrhage may disrupt the intima covering the plaque, thereby exposing collagen to flowing blood, a strong stimulus for thrombus formation.[25] Another possible mechanism for coronary thrombosis is ulceration or erosion of an atherosclerotic plaque with resultant exposure of collagen and other thrombogenic materials to the bloodstream.[26] Coronary spasm in the vicinity of an atherosclerotic plaque may be responsible for the development of a platelet fibrin thrombus.[31a] Platelet aggregates, in turn, may release thromboxane A_2, a potent vasoconstrictor, which may be responsible for the development or enhancement of coronary spasm.

THE CORONARY ARTERIAL BED IN MYOCARDIAL INFARCTION. Roberts has pointed out that (1) in patients with *fatal* ischemic heart disease, the lumina of at least two of the three major coronary arteries are usually narrowed by more than 75 per cent by atherosclerotic plaques; (2) the atherosclerotic process is limited to the epicardial arteries and spares the intramural vessels; and (3) the degree of luminal narrowing by atherosclerotic plaques is similar irrespective of the type of fatal coronary event.[32,33] There has been little dispute about these points. On the other hand, there has been some controversy about the relationship between coronary occlusion and myocardial infarction. In the three decades following Herrick's description of the condition,[34] the clinical manifestations of myocardial infarction were felt to stem from sudden coronary arterial occlusion, usually due to thrombosis; hence the terms *coronary thrombosis* and *acute myocardial infarction* became almost synonymous. One weakness of this concept was shown by Blumgart, Schlesinger, and their colleagues, who demonstrated that *coronary occlusion could occur in the absence of infarction,* when the collateral circulation was adequate to maintain myocardial nutrition.[24,35] Equally important, Friedberg and Horn observed that *infarction could occur in the absence of coronary occlusion.*[28] The patients whom they described had severe coronary arterial narrowing, and the areas of patchy, subendocardial infarction which occurred were felt to have developed secondary to relative insufficiency of coronary blood flow. Miller, Burchell, and Edwards then expanded on these observations, demonstrating that predominantly subendocardial infarcts were rarely associated with coronary occlusion, whereas transmural infarctions were frequently so.[36]

In order to define the precise relationship between coronary thrombosis and MI, it is important to know the time course of thrombus formation in relation to the onset of infarction. Unfortunately, estimates of the age of coronary thrombi and myocardial infarction by histological criteria may be quite imprecise.[32,37,38] Recent studies in which coronary arteriography was performed on patients within the first few hours after the onset of myocardial infarction have demonstrated that the coronary artery supplying the area of evolving infarction is totally occluded in the majority of these individuals.[39–44] If fibrinolytic agents are infused into the occluded artery, patency is achieved in a high percentage of cases. Angiography performed after fibrinolytic therapy usually demonstrates residual high-grade stenotic lesions at the site where coronary arterial occlusion had existed. Fresh thrombi have been recovered from the majority of patients with acute myocardial infarction undergoing emergency coronary bypass surgery.[43]

It is now clear that a transmural MI is usually (in more than 90 per cent of cases) caused by coronary thrombosis, as postulated by early investigators.[34] It is still not clear whether and how often coronary spasm plays an important role in the pathophysiological sequence leading from coronary atherosclerosis to MI.[31a] Less frequently, perhaps in one-third to one-half of cases, coronary thrombosis is responsible for regional subendocardial infarction, i.e., in the distribution of a single coronary artery. Rarely, coronary thrombosis causes multifocal or circumferential infarction. The converse, however, is not often the case. It is well established that coronary thrombosis or acute coronary occlusion of any cause may not be associated with MI. The extent of coronary collaterals will determine whether acute coronary occlusion causes a transmural infarct (sparse collaterals), a subendocardial infarct (moderate collaterals), or no infarct (extensive collaterals).[12] However, coronary thrombosis is one—perhaps the most important, but not the only—cause of acute coronary occlusion; other causes include coronary spasm, as well as rupture of, or hemorrhage into, an atherosclerotic plaque. Alterations in platelet function and an imbalance of the thromboxane A_2—prostacyclin system can play a role both in the development of coronary thrombosis and in coronary vasospasm.[12,26,45]

Nonatherosclerotic Causes of Acute Myocardial Infarction

Numerous pathological processes other than atherosclerosis can, on occasion, involve the coronary arteries and result in myocardial infarction (Table 37–1).[46] For example, coronary arterial occlusions can be the result of embolization of a coronary artery. Emboli most frequently lodge in the distribution of the left anterior descending coronary artery, commonly in the distal epicardial and intramural branches.[25] The causes of coronary embolism are numerous: infective and marantic endocarditis (Chap. 33), mural thrombi, prosthetic valves, and calcium deposits from manipulation of calcified valves at operation. In situ thrombosis of coronary arteries can occur secondary to chest-wall trauma (Chap. 44). Syphilitic aortitis may produce marked narrowing or occlusion of one or both coronary ostia,[47] whereas Takayasu's arteritis may result in obstruction of the coronary arteries (Chap. 48).[48] Necrotizing arteritis, polyarteritis nodosa, mucocutaneous lymph node syndrome (Kawasaki's disease) (p. 1053),[49,50] systemic lupus erythematosus,[51] and syphilis can cause coronary artery obstruction. Therapeutic levels of mediastinal radiation can cause thickening and hyalinization of the walls of coronary arteries, with subsequent infarction (p. 1690).[52] MI may also be the result of coronary arterial involvement in amyloidosis (Fig. 41–19, p. 1424), Hurler syndrome, pseudoxanthoma elasticum, and homocystinuria (Chap. 48).[53–55]

Involvement of the small coronary arteries (0.1 to 1.0 mm in diameter) by a number of disease processes may produce intimal and medial hyperplasia, necrosis, dissection, and thrombosis,[56] resulting in occlusions that produce *focal* areas of infarction and ultimately of fibrosis. Depending on the location and extent of the fibrotic reaction, arrhythmias, conduction defects, heart block, and heart failure can occur.

Myocardial Infarction with Angiographically Normal Coronary Vessels

Approximately 4 per cent of all patients with AMI and perhaps four times that percentage of patients with this diagnosis under the age of 35 years do not have coronary atherosclerosis demonstrated by coronary arteriography or at autopsy. Perhaps half the patients of this group, in turn, have a variety of other lesions involving the coronary vessels or myocardium (Table 37–1), whereas the others have no detectable coronary obstructive lesions.[57–60] Patients with AMI and normal coronary arteries tend to be young and to have relatively few coronary risk factors; usually they have no history of angina pectoris prior to the infarction.[58] The infarction in these patients is usually not preceded by any prodrome, but the clinical, laboratory, and electrocardiographic features of AMI are otherwise indistinguishable from those present in the overwhelming majority of patients with AMI who have classic obstructive atherosclerotic coronary artery disease.[61] In patients without coronary obstruction, the prognosis for survival of the

TABLE 37–1 SOME CAUSES OF MYOCARDIAL INFARCTION WITHOUT CORONARY ATHEROSCLEROSIS

Coronary Artery Disease Other Than Atherosclerosis

- Arteritis
  - Luetic
  - Granulomatous (Takayasu's disease)
  - Polyarteritis nodosa
  - Mucocutaneous lymph node (Kawasaki's) syndrome
  - Disseminated lupus erythematosus
  - Rheumatoid arthritis
  - Ankylosing spondylitis
- Trauma to coronary arteries
  - Laceration
  - Thrombosis
  - Iatrogenic
- Coronary mural thickening with metabolic diseases or intimal proliferative disease
  - Mucopolysaccharidoses (Hurler's disease)
  - Homocystinuria
  - Fabry's disease
  - Amyloidosis
  - Juvenile intimal sclerosis (idiopathic arterial calcification of infancy)
  - Intimal hyperplasia associated with contraceptive steroids or with the postpartum period
  - Pseudoxanthoma elasticum
  - Coronary fibrosis caused by radiation therapy
- Luminal narrowing by other mechanisms
  - Spasm of coronary arteries (Prinzmetal's angina with normal coronary arteries)
  - Spasm after nitroglycerin withdrawal
  - Dissection of the aorta
  - Dissection of the coronary artery

Emboli to Coronary Arteries

- Infective endocarditis
- Prolapse of mitral valve
- Mural thrombus from left atrium, left ventricle
- Prosthetic valve emboli
- Cardiac myxoma
- Associated with cardiopulmonary bypass surgery and coronary arteriography
  - Paradoxical emboli
  - Papillary fibroelastoma of the aortic valve ("fixed embolus")

Congenital Coronary Artery Anomalies

- Anomalous origin of left coronary from pulmonary artery
- Left coronary artery from anterior sinus of Valsalva
- Coronary arteriovenous and arteriocameral fistulae
- Coronary artery aneurysms

Myocardial Oxygen Demand-Supply Disproportion

- Aortic stenosis, all forms
- Incomplete differentiation of the aortic valve
- Aortic insufficiency
- Carbon monoxide poisoning
- Thyrotoxicosis
- Prolonged hypotension

Hematological (in situ Thrombosis)

- Polycythemia vera
- Thrombocytosis
- Disseminated intravascular coagulation
- Hypercoagulability
- Hypercoagulability, thrombosis, thrombocytopenic purpura

Miscellaneous

- Myocardial contusion
- Myocardial infarction with normal coronary arteries

Modified from Cheitlin, M., et al.: Myocardial infarction without atherosclerosis. J.A.M.A. *231*:951, 1975. Copyright 1975, American Medical Association.

acute event is usually excellent, but a few fatalities have occurred, and it has therefore been possible to document the presence of this syndrome at autopsy.[60,62] In 10 such patients, infarcts ranged from 5 to 33 per cent (mean of 18 per cent) of the left ventricle.[62] In patients who recover, areas of localized dyskinesis and hypokinesis can often be demonstrated by left ventricular angiography.

The long-term prognosis for patients who have survived an AMI with normal coronary vessels on arteriography appears to be substantially better than for patients with MI and obstructive coronary artery disease.[57–63] Following recovery from the initial infarct, recurrent infarction, heart failure, and death are unusual in patients with normal coronary arteries. Indeed, most of these individuals have normal exercise electrocardiograms,[64] and only a minority develop angina pectoris.

Numerous theories have been proposed to explain the occurrence of AMI in patients with normal coronary arteriograms. Suggested causes include coronary emboli, perhaps from a small mural thrombus, a prolapsed mitral valve[64a] (p. 1091), or a myxoma; coronary artery spasm;[65] coronary artery disease in vessels too small to be visualized by coronary arteriography or coronary arterial thrombosis with subsequent recanalization (Table 37–1); a variety of hematological disorders causing in situ thrombosis in the presence of normal coronary arteries,[60] such as polycythemia vera, sickle cell anemia, disseminated intravascular coagulation, thrombocytosis, and thrombotic thrombocytopenic purpura; augmented oxygen needs; hypotension secondary to sepsis, blood loss, or pharmacological agents; and anatomical changes, such as anomalous origin of a coronary artery and coronary arteriovenous fistula.[46,58,64–70] Eliot and coworkers examined the hearts of 10 patients who had died of a recent MI and in whom minimal or no coronary disease was present.[62] No thromboembolic material was seen in the coronary arterial tree despite the fact that the infarcts were only 2 days old in five patients and 3 or 4 days old in three others.

Collateral Circulation

Normal hearts contain an extensive network of interarterial anastomotic blood vessels, greater than 60 μm in diameter, involving epicardial, intramyocardial, and subendocardial connections. This collateral circulation exists at birth and apparently grows in size along with the rest of the coronary circulation but is beyond the limit of resolution of coronary arteriographic techniques and is not seen in living subjects without disease. In patients with coronary artery disease, these preexisting channels progressively enlarge, presumably as a consequence of the release of local vasodilators; flow through the collaterals will occur when pressure differences exist across these channels.[35,71–73] The coronary collateral circulation is particularly well developed in patients with (1) coronary occlusive disease, especially when it is severe, with the reduction of the luminal cross-sectional area by more than 75 per cent in one or more major vessels; (2) chronic hypoxia, as occurs in severe anemia, chronic obstructive pulmonary disease, and cyanotic congenital heart disease; and (3) left ventricular hypertrophy, which intensifies coronary collaterals.

There is considerable variability in the development of collateral channels that exists among patients with comparable degrees of coronary artery disease. Although the increases in the collateral circulation in patients with ischemic heart disease are due primarily to enlargement of already existing anastomoses, the possibility exists that new anastomotic channels are formed during the reparative phase following AMI. In animals, collateral development occurs rapidly after experimental coronary artery obstruction; Blumgart et al. noted maximum increases in collateral circulation in pigs 12 to 21 days after the production of severe coronary arterial stenoses,[73] whereas Gregg observed that a spontaneous and progressive increase in collateral blood flow was present 12 hours after coronary occlusion in dogs.[74] Eckstein noted marked increases in collateral circulation in dogs rendered anemic for 4 weeks.[72] The time course for development of collateral vessels in humans is not known. However, in an interesting case report of a 14-year-old boy who had suffered a traumatic right coronary arteriovenous fistula, collateral vessels were visible on a coronary angiogram 9 days later. Two weeks after repair of the fistula, angiographic evidence of collateral vessels was no longer evident.[75]

Collateral blood vessels are frequently noted on coronary arteriograms of patients with severe obstructive coronary vascular disease (p. 332). However, considerable debate has centered on the issue of whether collateral vessels are truly functional.[76] A number of angiographic studies have attempted to examine the functional state of these collateral vessels by quantifying left ventricular function in patients with and without evidence of collateral circulation. In several investigations, no differences in overall left ventricular performance were noted in patients with obstructive coronary artery disease, regardless of whether or not collateral vessels were present.[71,77,78] On the other hand, significantly better left ventricular function has been noted in regions of the left ventricle in the distribution of obstructed coronary vessels, supplied by collateral vessels, than in regions without collateral vessels,[79] and congestive heart failure and cardiomegaly have been reported to occur with greater frequency in patients with coronary artery disease who lack collateral vessels than in those patients who have them.[80] Also supporting the argument in favor of a functional role for coronary collateral vessels is the finding that in patients with coronary occlusion the area of myocardial necrosis is frequently smaller than the area supplied by the occluded coronary artery when collaterals are present. Indeed, it is rather common for patients with abundant collaterals to have totally occluded coronary arteries without evidence of infarction in the distribution of that coronary vessel; thus, the survival of the myocardium distal to such occlusions must be dependent on collateral blood flow.

Of interest also are reports on patients who suffered traumatic lacerations of the heart requiring ligation of the left anterior descending coronary artery but who did not develop clinical or, in one instance, postmortem evidence of myocardial necrosis.[81] Again, collateral circulation must have supplied sufficient blood flow to the myocardium distal to the ligation to have prevented MI. In addition, among patients with total coronary occlusion and AMI, the response of precordial ST-segment elevation to beta-adrenergic blockade is distinctly superior when collaterals enter the myocardium perfused by the occluded vessel.[82]

In conclusion, collateral coronary vessels, present from birth, frequently enlarge and may become functional in the presence of severe myocardial hypoxia or ischemia and following acute coronary occlusion and MI. Although blood flow through collaterals may be capable of contributing importantly to the maintenance of the resting energy requirements of the heart, and although the collaterals may limit infarct size in the face of total coronary occlusion and thereby contribute to patient survival, blood flow through collaterals is not sufficient to meet the needs of the myocardium when the latter are augmented by stress or to prevent myocardial necrosis in the majority of instances.[71]

Right Ventricular and Atrial Infarction

MI most commonly involves the left ventricle and interventricular septum; however, approximately one-third of patients with inferior infarction have some involvement of the right ventricle.[83–85,85a] Among these patients, right ventricular infarction occurs exclusively in those with transmural infarction of the inferoposterior wall and the posterior portion of the septum. The incidence of clinically significant right ventricular infarction is considerably lower than the incidence rate found at autopsy. Although right ventricular infarction almost invariably develops in association with infarction of the adjacent septum and left ventricular myocardium, *isolated* infarction of the right ventricle occurs in 3 to 5 per cent of autopsy-proved cases of myocardial infarction.

Right ventricular infarction, regardless of whether or not it is combined with involvement of the left ventricle, is generally associated with obstructive lesions of the right coronary artery. However, right ventricular infarction occurs less commonly than would be anticipated from the frequency of atherosclerotic lesions involving the right coronary artery.[86] This discrepancy can probably be explained by the lower oxygen demands of the right ventricle, since right ventricular infarcts occur more commonly in conditions associated with increased right ventricular oxygen needs.[87] Moreover, the intercoronary collateral system of the right ventricle is richer than that of the left, and the thinness of the right ventricular wall allows the chamber to derive some nutrition from blood within the right ventricular cavity. Rarely, a mural thrombus overlying a right ventricular infarct produces pulmonary embolism. Abnormal right ventricular wall motion, cavity dilatation, tricuspid regurgitation,[88] and cardiogenic shock with normal left but elevated right ventricular filling pressures have been documented in patients with infarction of the right ventricle.[83,84,86,89,89a]

Atrial infarction occurs in 7 to 17 per cent of autopsy-proved cases of myocardial infarction,[49,87,90–92] is often seen in conjunction with left ventricular infarction, can result in rupture of the atrial wall, and is more common on the right than the left side.[92] Infarcts occur more frequently in the atrial appendages than in the lateral or posterior walls of the atria. These differences in incidence might be explained by the considerably higher oxygen content of left atrial blood, which may nourish the thin atrial wall despite obstructive disease involving the coronary arterial system perfusing it. Since right atrial infarction is usually associated with obstructive disease of the sinus node artery, it is frequently accompanied by atrial arrhythmias.

Myocardial Rupture

RUPTURE OF THE FREE WALL (Table 37–2). Rupture of the free wall of the infarcted ventricle occurs in

TABLE 37–2 CLINICAL FEATURES OF CARDIAC RUPTURE

Factors Indicating Increased Risk of Cardiac Rupture

1. Recurrent chest pain without electrocardiographic changes suggestive of another infarct or extension
2. Sustained hypertension after myocardial infarction
3. First myocardial infarction; no or only recent history of angina
4. Less than 5 days since myocardial infarction
5. Patient 80 years or older

Signs and Symptoms Suggesting Cardiac Rupture

Terminal Signs

1. Pericardial blood and tamponade
2. Electromechanical dissociation
3. Failure of closed chest resuscitation to produce peripheral pulses

Preterminal Signs and Symptoms

1. Pericardial blood
2. Recurrent severe chest pain without evidence of new infarct
3. M-complex in electrocardiogram
4. Pericardial fluid on echocardiography

From Bates, R. J., et al.: Cardiac rupture—Challenge in diagnosis and management. Am. J. Cardiol. *40*:429, 1977.

up to 10 per cent of patients dying in the hospital of AMI. Thinness of the apical wall, marked intensity of necrosis at the terminal end of the blood supply, poor collateral flow, the shearing effect of muscular contraction against an inert and stiffened necrotic area, and aging of the myocardium with laceration in the myocardial microstructure have all been proposed as the local factors that lead to rupture.[93–95]

This serious complication of AMI

1. Occurs more frequently in women than in men with infarction and more frequently in the elderly;

2. Is more common in hypertensive than normotensive patients;[96]

3. Occurs approximately seven times more frequently in the left than the right ventricle and seldom occurs in the atria;

4. Usually involves the anterior or lateral walls of the ventricle in the area of the terminal distribution of the left anterior descending coronary artery;

5. Is usually associated with transmural infarction involving at least 20 per cent of the left ventricle;

6. Occurs between 1 day and 3 weeks, but most commonly 3 to 5 days, following the infarct;

7. Is usually preceded by infarct expansion, i.e., thinning and a disproportionate dilatation within the softened necrotic zone;[97]

8. Most commonly results from a distinct tear in the myocardial wall or a dissecting hematoma that perforates a necrotic area of myocardium (Fig. 37–4);

9. Usually occurs near the junction of the infarct and the normal muscle;

10. Occurs less frequently in the center of the infarct, but when rupture occurs here, it is usually during the second rather than the first week following the infarct;

11. Rarely occurs in a hypertrophied ventricle or in an area of excellent collateral vessels.[93]

Rupture of the free wall of the left ventricle usually leads to hemopericardium and immediate death from cardiac tamponade. Occasionally, rupture of the free wall of the ventricle occurs as the first clinical manifestation in patients with undetected or silent myocardial infarction, and then it may be considered a form of "sudden cardiac death" (Chap. 23).

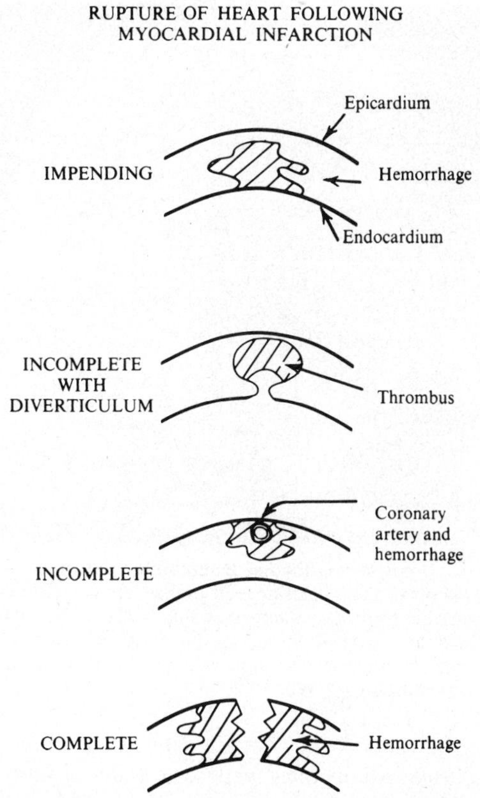

FIGURE 37–4 Range of complications that may follow an intramural hemorrhage in a patient with myocardial infarction. (From Datta, B. N., et al.: Incomplete rupture of the heart with diverticulum formation. Pathology *7*:179, 1975.)

Incomplete rupture of the heart may occur when organizing thrombus and hematoma, together with pericardium, seal a rupture of the left ventricle and thus prevent the development of hemopericardium (Figs. 37–5 and 37–6). With time, this area of organized thrombus and pericardium can become a small, left ventricular diverticulum or a large, false (pseudo) aneurysm which maintains communication with the cavity of the left ventricle.[98] In con-

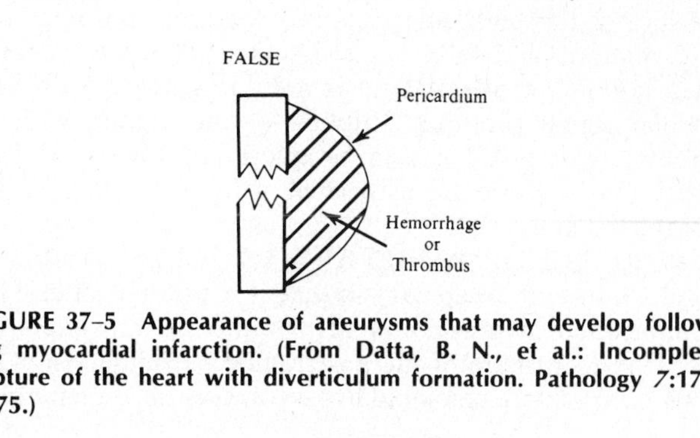

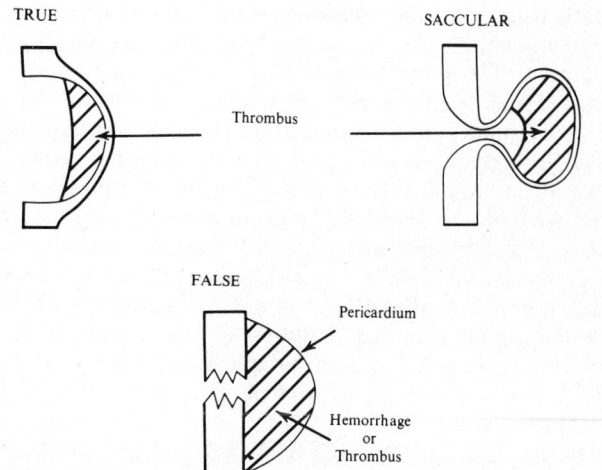

FIGURE 37–5 Appearance of aneurysms that may develop following myocardial infarction. (From Datta, B. N., et al.: Incomplete rupture of the heart with diverticulum formation. Pathology *7*:179, 1975.)

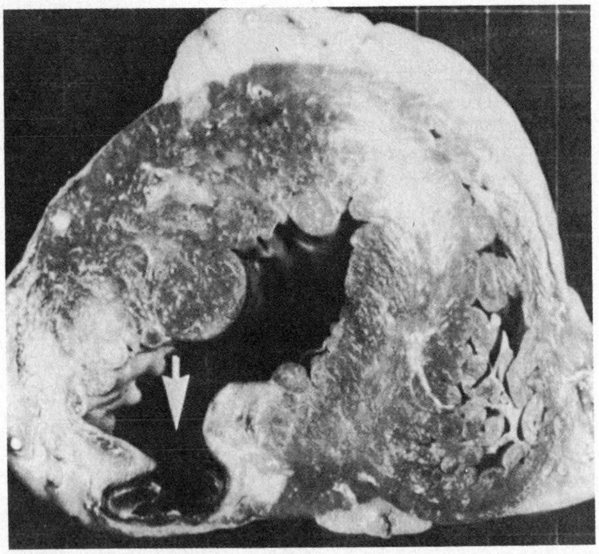

FIGURE 37-6 Heart slice showing incomplete rupture with diverticulum formation in the posterior wall of the left ventricle (arrow). Its lumen contains thrombus. Note scarring of the walls of the left ventricle. Coronary arteries have barium in their lumens. (From Datta, B. N., et al.: Incomplete rupture of the heart with diverticulum formation. Pathology 7:179, 1975.)

trast to true aneurysms, which always contain some myocardial elements in their walls, the walls of false aneurysms are composed of pericardium and organized hematoma and lack any elements of the original myocardial wall. False aneurysms can become quite large, even equaling the true ventricular cavity in size, and they communicate with the left ventricular cavity through a narrow neck. Frequently, false aneurysms contain significant amounts of old and recent thrombus, superficial portions of which can result in arterial emboli. False aneurysms can drain off a portion of each ventricular stroke volume just like true aneurysms. However, in contrast to true aneurysms, false aneurysms do have a tendency to rupture, even in late stages.[98]

RUPTURE OF THE INTERVENTRICULAR SEPTUM. Although rupture of the interventricular septum is said to be less common than rupture of the free wall,[93,96,99–101] our experience has been otherwise, perhaps because death usually is not immediate, and patients can reach a referral center where treatment of this complication is common. The perforation is usually single and ranges in length from one to several centimeters. The size of the defect determines the magnitude of the left-to-right shunt and the extent of hemodynamic deterioration, which in turn affects the likelihood of survival. As in rupture of the free wall of the ventricle, transmural infarction underlies rupture of the ventricular septum. Anterior and anterolateral myocardial infarctions are somewhat more common than inferior or inferolateral infarcts in patients with ventricular septal rupture.[99] Rupture of the septum with an anterior infarction tends to be apical in location, whereas inferior infarctions are associated with perforation of the basal septum.

RUPTURE OF PAPILLARY MUSCLES. Partial or total rupture of a papillary muscle is a rare but often fatal complication of transmural MI.[101a] Inferior wall infarction can lead to rupture of the posteromedial papillary muscle. This occurs more commonly than rupture of the anterolateral muscle, a consequence of anterolateral MI; rupture of a right ventricular papillary muscle is rare but can cause massive tricuspid regurgitation and right ventricular failure. Complete transection of a left ventricular papillary muscle is incompatible with life because the sudden massive mitral regurgitation which develops cannot be tolerated.[102–104] Rupture of a portion of a papillary muscle which results in severe, though not necessarily overwhelming, mitral regurgitation is much more frequent (Fig. 32–9 and 32–10, p. 1077).

In a small number of patients, rupture of more than one cardiac structure is noted at postmortem examination; all possible combinations of rupture of the free left ventricular wall, the interventricular septum, and a papillary muscle have been described.[99]

ANEURYSM. A ventricular aneurysm, which is a circumscribed, noncontractile outpouching of the left ventricle, develops in 12 to 15 per cent of patients who survive a myocardial infarction.[105] The wall of the aneurysm is thin in comparison with the rest of the left ventricle (Fig. 37–5), and it is usually composed of fibrous tissue as well as necrotic muscle, occasionally mixed with viable myocardium.[106] Aneurysm formation presumably occurs when intraventricular tension stretches the noncontracting infarcted heart muscle, thus producing infarct expansion,[97,107] a relatively weak, thin layer of necrotic muscle, and fibrous tissue that bulges with each systole. With the passage of time, the wall of the aneurysm becomes more densely fibrotic, but it continues to bulge with systole, thus "stealing" some of the left ventricular stroke volume during each systole.[108]

Aneurysms range from 1 to 8 cm in diameter and usually involve the left ventricle.[105] They occur approximately four times more often at the apex and in the anterior wall than in the inferoposterior wall.[105] The overlying pericardium is usually densely adherent to the wall of the aneurysm, which may even become partially calcified after several years. Rarely, a true left ventricular aneurysm ruptures soon after its development. Late rupture, when the aneurysm has become stabilized by the formation of dense fibrous tissue in its wall, almost never occurs.[98,105]

Mural thrombosis is found at autopsy or operation in 15 to 77 per cent of left ventricular aneurysms. Approximately half the patients with mural thrombi at autopsy also have evidence of systemic emboli.[105,109,110]

CARDIOGENIC SHOCK (p. 591). This is the most severe and most commonly fatal complication of AMI. Page et al., who studied 20 such patients at autopsy, found that all exhibited necrosis of at least 40 per cent of the left ventricle. In contrast, 35 per cent or less of the left ventricle had been destroyed in all but 1 of 14 patients who succumbed without having been in cardiogenic shock.[111] Similar findings were reported by Alonso et al.: Patients with cardiogenic shock had lost an average of 51 per cent of the left ventricular myocardium (range: 35 to 68 per cent), whereas in a group of infarcted patients who died suddenly from arrhythmias and who had never been in cardiogenic shock, necrosis averaged 23 per cent (range: 14 to 31 per cent) of the left ventricle.[86] Patients with rupture of the ventricular septum or of a papillary muscle can also present with cardiogenic shock. These patients often have smaller infarcts than do those with cardiogenic shock sec-

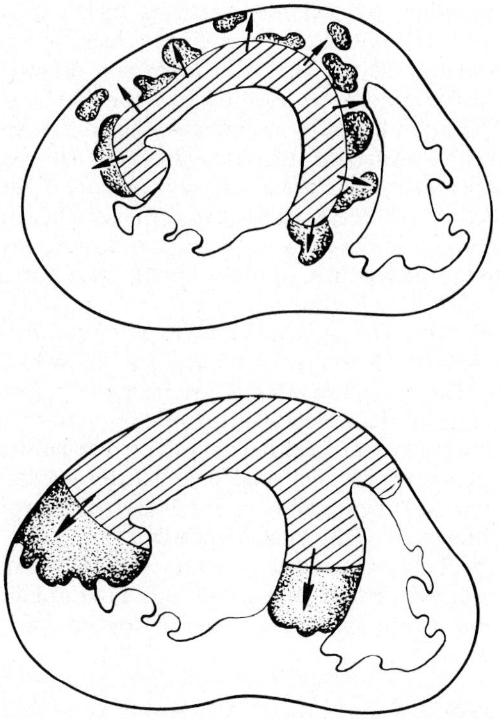

FIGURE 37–7 Two types of extension of myocardial infarction. Type A (top) was observed at the edges of an infarct, usually subepicardially. Type B (bottom) occurred at the lateral margins. (From Alonso, D. R., et al.: Pathophysiology of cardiogenic shock: Quantification of myocardial necrosis, clinical, pathologic and electrocardiographic correlation. Circulation *48*:588, 1973, by permission of the American Heart Association, Inc.)

ondary to ventricular failure without a mechanical lesion. The prognosis is better in such patients, since the smaller infarct allows their left ventricle to support the circulation once the mechanical defect has been corrected surgically.

At autopsy, patients with cardiogenic shock consistently demonstrate marginal extension of recent areas of infarction (Fig. 37–7).[111–114] Moreover, focal areas of necrosis are also frequently found in regions of the left and right ventricles that are not adjacent to the major area of recent infarction.[111] Such extensions and focal lesions are probably the result of the shock state itself, since they can also be found in the hearts of patients dying of noncardiogenic shock.

The shock state in patients with AMI would therefore appear to be the result of a vicious cycle, demonstrated in Figure 37–8. According to this formulation, coronary obstruction leads to myocardial ischemia which impairs myocardial contractility and ventricular performance; this, in turn, reduces arterial pressure and therefore coronary perfusion pressure, leading to further ischemia and extension of necrosis until the left ventricle has insufficient contracting myocardium to sustain life. Stasis in the smaller arteries and arterioles distal to a major proximal occlusion may result in secondary microvascular obstruction, further impairing myocardial perfusion. The progressive nature of the myocardial insult in this syndrome is reflected in the stuttering and progressive evolution of elevations in the plasma enzyme–time activity curves of markers specific for myocardial injury.[114]

At autopsy, more than two-thirds of patients with cardiogenic shock demonstrate stenosis of 75 per cent or more of the luminal diameter of all three major coronary vessels, usually including the left anterior descending coronary artery.[115] Almost all patients with cardiogenic shock are found to have thrombosis of the artery supplying the major region of recent infarction.[111,112]

LEFT VENTRICULAR THROMBUS AND ARTERIAL EMBOLISM. Mural thrombi are common in patients succumbing to AMI.[115a] In one report, 44 per cent of 924 patients dying of AMI were found to have mural thrombi attached to the endocardium overlying the infarct;[116] thrombi are more common in patients with large than small infarcts and therefore are probably more frequently found in nonsurvivors than in survivors. They are almost universally located in the left ventricle, particularly at its apex; with extensive transmural infarction of the septum, however, mural thrombi may overlie infarcted myocardium in both ventricles. As noted earlier, mural thrombus in a ventricular aneurysm or pseudoaneurysm is rather common. Mural thrombi can be recognized pre mortem by two-dimensional echocardiography in approximately one-third of all patients with acute transmural anterior or apical infarctions (Figure 5–68, p. 127); they are extremely rare in patients with inferior-posterior infarcts.[110]

Although a mural thrombus adheres to the endocardium overlying the infarcted myocardium, superficial portions of it can become detached and produce systemic arterial emboli. In one study, systemic emboli were noted at autopsy in 10 per cent of 500 patients who died of acute myocardial infarction; half of the emboli were cerebral.[117] The other half usually lodged in the kidney or spleen or at the bifurcation of the aorta or iliac or femoral arteries; rarely, intestinal infarction results from embolization of the superior mesenteric artery. Occasionally, embolism from a mural

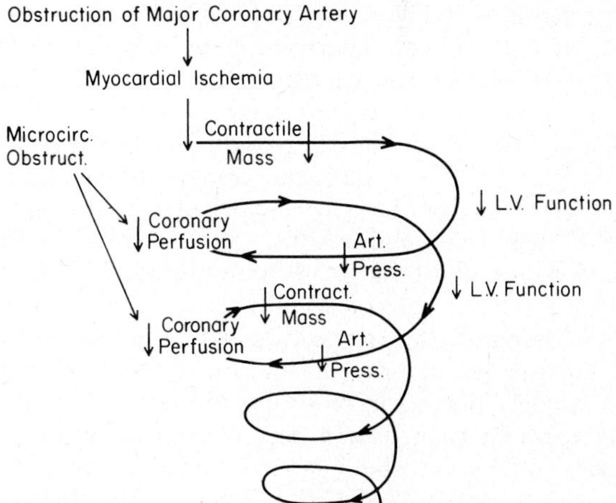

FIGURE 37–8 The sequence of events in the vicious cycle in which coronary artery obstruction leads to cardiogenic shock and progressive circulatory deterioration. (Reproduced with permission from Braunwald, E., and Alpert, J. S. *In* Petersdorf, R., et al. [eds.]: Harrison's Principles of Internal Medicine, New York, McGraw-Hill Book Co., 1983.)

thrombus is the presenting symptom, with the underlying myocardial infarction either silent or overlooked.

VENOUS THROMBOSIS AND EMBOLISM. Almost all pulmonary emboli originate from thrombi in the veins of the lower extremities (Chap. 46); much less commonly, they originate from mural thrombi overlying an area of infarction in the right atrium or ventricle. Bed rest and heart failure predispose to venous thrombosis and subsequent pulmonary embolism, and both of these factors occur commonly in patients with AMI, particularly those with large infarctions. In one autopsy study, major pulmonary emboli were present (though not always responsible for a fatal outcome) in 11 per cent of patients dying of AMI.[11]

Several decades ago, at a time when patients with AMI were subjected to prolonged periods of bed rest, significant pulmonary embolism was found in more than 20 per cent of patients with autopsy-proved myocardial infarction,[118] and massive pulmonary embolism accounted for 10 per cent of deaths from MI.[116] In recent years, with early mobilization and the widespread use of low-dose anticoagulant prophylaxis (Chap. 38), pulmonary embolism has become a rare cause of death in this condition.

PERICARDITIS (see also p. 1503). Transmural myocardial infarction, by definition, extends to the epicardial surface and is responsible for producing a local pericarditis in approximately 50 per cent of patients and diffuse, fibrinous, or serofibrinous pericarditis in about 15 per cent. This complication generally occurs between the second and fourth days following the infarction. In some patients with diffuse pericarditis, pericardial effusion may be large, but tamponade is rare. Occasionally, hemorrhagic effusion with cardiac tamponade develops in patients with post–myocardial infarction pericarditis who are treated with anticoagulants.[119]

Dressler's syndrome (p. 1513), or the *post–myocardial infarction syndrome*,[120,121] usually occurs 2 to 10 weeks after infarction. The incidence of this syndrome is difficult to define because it often blends imperceptibly with the more common early post–myocardial infarction pericarditis. At autopsy, patients with this syndrome usually demonstrate localized fibrinous pericarditis[122] containing polymorphonuclear leukocytes.[123] The post–myocardial infarction syndrome is probably the result of an autoimmune antibody response against certain pericardial and myocardial antigens exposed to the immune system at the time of infarction.[124]

PATHOPHYSIOLOGY OF ACUTE MYOCARDIAL INFARCTION

SYSTOLIC VENTRICULAR FUNCTION. The fundamental pathological alteration underlying left ventricular dysfunction in AMI is loss of functioning segments of myocardium.[124a] Depression of cardiac function in myocardial infarction is directly related to the extent of left ventricular damage.[125,125a] Cessation of blood flow to a region of myocardium produces four sequential abnormal contraction patterns[126] (Figure 10–48, p. 339): (1) *dyssynchrony,* dissociation in the time course of contraction of adjacent segments of myocardial segments; (2) *hypokinesis,* reduction in the extent of shortening; (3) *akinesis,* cessation of shortening; and (4) *dyskinesis,* paradoxical expansion, systolic bulging.[108,127] If a sufficient amount of myocardium undergoes ischemic injury, left ventricular pump function becomes depressed, and cardiac output, stroke volume, blood pressure, and peak dp/dt are reduced.[125,127] The paradoxical systolic expansion of an area of ventricular myocardium decreases the stroke output of the left ventricle. With the passage of time, edema and cellular infiltration and ultimately fibrosis increase the stiffness of the infarcted myocardium back to and beyond control values.[128] Increasing stiffness in the infarcted zone of myocardium improves left ventricular function, since it prevents systolic paradoxical wall motion.

Areas with reduced and absent wall motion are universally seen in patients with transmural AMI. Rackley and collaborators have demonstrated a linear relationship between specific parameters of left ventricular function and clinical symptoms.[129] The earliest abnormality is a reduction in diastolic distensibility, which can be observed with infarcts that involve only 8 per cent of the total left ventricle on angiographic examination. When the abnormally contracting segment exceeds 10 per cent, the ejection fraction is reduced; with 15 per cent involvement, elevations of left ventricular end-diastolic pressure and volume occur. Clinical heart failure accompanies areas of abnormal contraction exceeding 25 per cent, and cardiogenic shock, often fatal, accompanies loss of more than 40 per cent of the left ventricular myocardium.[129]

Unless extension of the infarct occurs, some improvement in abnormal wall motion takes place during the healing phase, as recovery of function occurs in initially reversibly injured myocardium. Regardless of the age of the infarct, patients who continue to demonstrate abnormal wall motion of 20 to 25 per cent of the left ventricle manifest hemodynamic signs of left ventricular failure.[130] Physical signs and symptoms of left ventricular failure also increase proportional to increasing areas of abnormal left ventricular wall motion.[127] These findings are of interest in view of the experimental work of Pfeffer et al., who produced infarcts of varying sizes and studied their left ventricular performance 3 weeks later.[125] Rats with relatively small infarcts (< 30 per cent of the left ventricle) had no detectable impairment of function; those with moderate-sized infarcts (31 to 46 per cent) exhibited normal baseline measurements but inadequate responses to hemodynamic stresses; rats with large infarcts (> 46 per cent) uniformly exhibited left ventricular failure. Patients with AMI often also show reduced myocardial contractile function in noninfarcted zones of myocardium.[131] This may result from obstruction of the coronary artery supplying this region of the ventricle, which is perfused by collaterals from the vessel that becomes occluded, a condition that has been termed *ischemia at a distance.*[132]

DIASTOLIC VENTRICULAR FUNCTION. As pointed out on page 1246, myocardial ischemia alters not only the systolic performance but also the diastolic characteristics of the left ventricle, ultimately raising its diastolic pressure at any given volume.[128,133–135] As outlined on page 1247, left ventricular diastolic properties are altered in infarcted and ischemic myocardium, leading initially to an increase but later to a reduction in left ventricular compliance. Patients who have recovered from an AMI frequently continue to manifest decreased left ventricular compliance secondary to the fibrous scar that remains in the left ventricle.

Pathophysiology of Left Ventricular Failure

In patients with AMI, heart failure is characterized by left ventricular diastolic and therefore pulmonary venous hypertension, leading to pulmonary congestion. The two mechanisms responsible for the pulmonary venous hypertension are (1) reduced ventricular diastolic compliance with resultant augmented resistance to left ventricular filling; and (2) reduced ventricular systolic function with resultant increases in end-diastolic volume and pressure. Both of these mechanisms are responsible for elevation of the left ventricular diastolic pressure, which is often associated with a depression of cardiac output. Clinical manifestations of both expressions of left ventricular failure become more common as the extent of the injury to the left ventricle increases.[129]

Cardiogenic Shock. The severest clinical expression of left ventricular failure, cardiogenic shock, is associated with extensive damage to the left ventricular myocardium.[111,112,112a] Patients who die as a consequence of cardiogenic shock often develop this complication of MI while in the hospital. These individuals often have a stepwise increase or progression of myocardial necrosis from marginal extension of their infarct in an ischemic zone bordering on the infarction.[136] Deterioration in left ventricular function secondary to apparent extension of infarction may, in some cases, result from *expansion* of the necrotic zone of myocardium without actual extension of the necrotic process.[137] Shearing forces that develop during ventricular systole can disrupt necrotic myocardial muscle bundles, with resultant expansion and thinning of the akinetic zone of myocardium, which in turn results in deterioration of overall left ventricular function.[138]

Alonso et al. described pathological evidence of marginal extensions of infarction in 18 of 22 patients dying of cardiogenic shock (Fig. 37–7).[112] Infarction of this ischemic periinfarction zone can be precipitated by a number of factors that adversely affect the supply of oxygen or the metabolic demand in the zone of myocardium, including a reduction of coronary perfusion pressure and an augmentation of myocardial oxygen demand resulting from the local release of catecholamines from ischemic adrenergic nerve endings in the heart as well as from circulating endogenous or infused catecholamines. Much recent work focuses on the development of strategies for limiting infarct size and prevention of infarct extension, thereby preventing the vicious downward spiral into irreversible cardiogenic shock (Fig. 37–8).[139] The experimental basis for these efforts is described on page 1255, and their clinical application is discussed on page 1318.

Swan, Forrester, and their associates have examined the cardiac output and wedge pressure together and have identified four major subsets of patients with AMI (Table 37–3): patients with normal perfusion and without pulmonary congestion (normal cardiac output and normal wedge pressure), patients with normal perfusion and pulmonary congestion (normal cardiac output and elevated wedge pressure), patients with decreased perfusion but without pulmonary congestion (reduced cardiac output and normal wedge pressure), and patients with decreased perfusion and pulmonary congestion (reduced cardiac output and elevated wedge pressure).[140] Although this classification is useful, it must be appreciated that patients frequently pass from one category to another with therapy and, sometimes, even apparently spontaneously.

The hemodynamic subsets of AMI usually reflect the clinical status of the patients.[141] Hypoperfusion usually becomes evident clinically when the cardiac index falls below approximately 2.2 liters/min/sq meter, whereas pulmonary congestion is noted when the wedge pressure exceeds approximately 20 mm Hg. However, approximately 25 per cent of patients with cardiac indices less than 2.2 liter/min/sq meter and 15 per cent of patients with elevated pulmonary capillary wedge pressures are not recognized clinically. Discrepancies in hemodynamic and clinical classification of patients with AMI arise for a variety of reasons. Patients may exhibit "phase lags" as clinical pulmonary congestion develops or resolves, symptoms secondary to chronic obstructive pulmonary disease may be confused with those resulting from pulmonary congestion, or longstanding left ventricular dysfunction may mask signs of hypoperfusion secondary to compensatory vasoconstriction.[140]

If the cardiac index is plotted as a function of the pulmonary capillary wedge pressure (a modified Starling relationship) in patients with AMI, a wide range of left ventricular performances is apparent (Fig. 37–9). It is clear from this figure that mortality in AMI increases in association with the severity of the hemodynamic deficit. In addition, one-third of patients with AMI have normal resting left ventricular hemodynamics.[140]

Certain patients present a hemodynamic pattern that is

TABLE 37–3 HEMODYNAMIC SUBSETS IN ACUTE MYOCARDIAL INFARCTION

Clinical Subset	Cardiac Index *(liter/min/sq meter)*	Pulmonary Capillary Wedge Pressure *(mm Hg)*	Mortality *(%)*
I. No pulmonary congestion or peripheral hypoperfusion	2.7 ± 0.5	12 ± 7	2.2
II. Isolated pulmonary congestion	2.3 ± 0.4	23 ± 5	10.1
III. Isolated peripheral hypoperfusion	1.9 ± 0.4	12 ± 5	22.4
IV. Both pulmonary congestion and hypoperfusion	1.6 ± 0.6	27 ± 8	55.5

From Forrester, J. S., et al.: Medical therapy of acute myocardial infarction by application of hemodynamic subsets. N. Engl. J. Med. *295*:1404, 1976. Reprinted by permission.

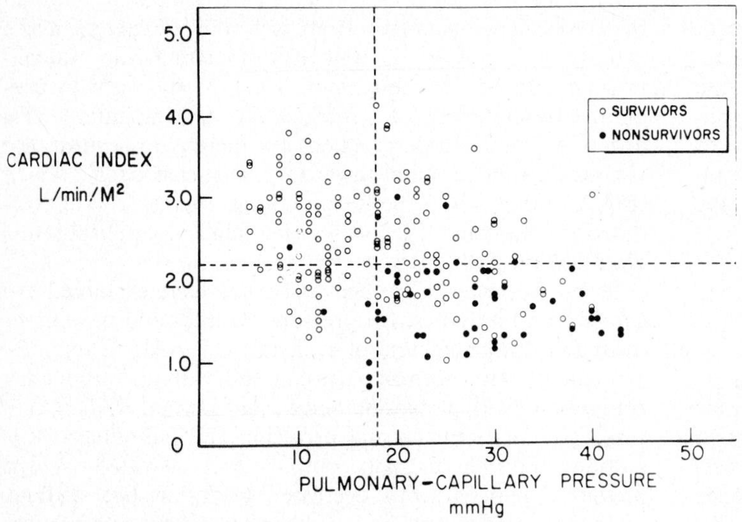

FIGURE 37–9 Relation between pulmonary-capillary pressure and cardiac index in 200 patients with acute myocardial infarction. The dotted lines are placed at the levels of 18 mm Hg for pulmonary-capillary pressure and 2.1 liters per minute per square meter for cardiac index. There is a wide degree of variability in left ventricular performance in patients with acute myocardial infarction, and mortality rate increases as cardiac performance deteriorates. (Reproduced with permission from Forrester, J. S., et al.: Medical therapy of acute myocardial infarction by application of hemodynamic subsets. N. Engl. J. Med. *295*:1356, 1976.)

a variant of group 1 (normal or nearly normal pulmonary artery occlusive pressure and cardiac output).[141a] These patients exhibit a hyperkinetic state characterized by sinus tachycardia and hypertension in addition to normal wedge pressure and cardiac output. Presumably, the increased heart rate and blood pressure are the result of inappropriate activation of the sympathetic nervous system, possibly secondary to augmented release of catecholamines or anxiety or both. It is important to recognize this variant of group 1, since such individuals may benefit from therapy with beta-adrenergic blocking agents (p. 1321).

Physiological assessment of left ventricular function refines the information obtained by clinical means.[141] Among patients with AMI who are clinically uncomplicated (Killip Class I, p. 1280), approximately 50 per cent have a reduced cardiac output and 75 per cent have an elevated ventricular filling pressure. Patients with one or both of these hemodynamic abnormalities have a worse prognosis than those without any hemodynamic disturbance, even though they may be clinically uncomplicated.[141] Similarly, the prognosis of patients in Killip Class IV (cardiogenic shock) is a function of the hemodynamic status. Rackley et al. reported that in such patients a filling pressure greater than 29 mm Hg was associated with a mortality of 100 per cent; a filling pressure greater than 15 mm Hg and a cardiac index less than 2.0 liter/min/sq meter with a mortality of 93 per cent; and a filling pressure less than 15 mm Hg and a cardiac index less than 2.0 liters/min/sq meter with a mortality of 63 per cent.[141] Thus, it is clear that hemodynamics vary widely among patients with AMI having similar clinical presentations, and for this reason measurement of pertinent hemodynamic variables may be of great value in patients with complications.[142]

Classifications of patients with AMI by hemodynamic subsets has therapeutic relevance, as discussed in Chapter 38. For example, patients with normal wedge pressures and hypoperfusion often benefit from infusion of fluids, since the peak value of stroke volume is usually not attained until left ventricular filling pressure reaches 20 to 24 mm Hg.[141] However, a low level of left ventricular filling pressure does not imply that left ventricular damage is necessarily slight. Such patients may be relatively hypovolemic and/or may have suffered a right ventricular infarct with or without severe left ventricular damage.[143]

The relation between ventricular filling pressure and cardiac index with an increase in preload produced by an infusion of saline or dextran can provide valuable hemodynamic information, in addition to that obtained from baseline measurements. For example, the ventricular function curve rises steeply (marked increase in cardiac index, small increase in filling pressure) in patients with normal left ventricular function and hypovolemia, whereas the curve rises gradually or remains flat in those patients with a combination of hypovolemia and depressed cardiac function. The slope of the ventricular function curve, obtained 2 or 3 days following the infarction, correlates well with the ejection fraction determined 4 to 6 weeks later.[141]

HEMODYNAMIC FINDINGS IN RIGHT VENTRICULAR INFARCTION (Table 37–4). A characteristic hemodynamic pattern has been observed in patients

TABLE 37–4 FEATURES OF RIGHT VENTRICULAR INFARCTION

1. Inferior-posterior myocardial infarction
2. Clinical findings may include:
   A. Normal or depressed right ventricular function
   B. Shock
   C. Tricuspid regurgitation
   D. Ruptured ventricular septum
3. Hemodynamic measurements
   A. Abnormally elevated right atrial pressure
   B. Normal right ventricular and pulmonary artery systolic pressures
   C. Increased ratio of right ventricular to left ventricular filling pressure
   D. Depressed right ventricular function curve
4. Scintigraphy
   A. Uptake in right ventricular free wall
   B. Increased right ventricular dimensions and decreased wall motion
5. Echocardiography
   A. Increased right ventricular dimension
   B. Absence of pericardial effusion
6. Cardiac enzymes
   A. Increased magnitude of enzyme values to left ventricular dysfunction
7. Cardiac catheterization
   A. Involvement of right or left circumflex coronary arteries
   B. Right ventricular akinesis
8. Differential diagnosis
   A. Hypotension with acute myocardial infarction
   B. Pericardial tamponade
   C. Constrictive pericarditis
   D. Pulmonary embolus

Reproduced with permission from Rackley, C. E., Russell, R. O., Jr., Mantle, J. A., Rogers, W. J., Papapietro, S. E., and Schwartz, K. M.: Right ventricular infarction and function. Am. Heart J. *101*:215, 1981.

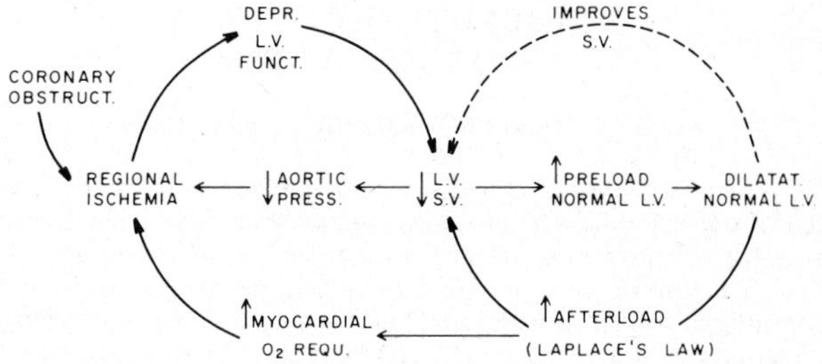

FIGURE 37–10 Changes in circulatory regulation in ischemic heart disease. DEPR. L.V. FUNCT., depressed left ventricular function; S.V., stroke volume; DILATAT., dilatation; O_2 REQU., oxygen requirements. Solid lines indicate that the effect is produced or intensified; broken lines indicate that it is diminished. (Reproduced with permission from Braunwald, E.: Regulation of the circulation. N. Engl. J. Med. *290*:1420, 1974.)

with right ventricular infarction[141b,141c] (which, as stated above, frequently accompanies inferior left ventricular infarction or less commonly occurs in isolated form): elevated right-heart filling pressures (central venous, right atrial, and right ventricular end-diastolic pressures) with normal or modestly elevated left ventricular filling pressures.[143] Right ventricular systolic and pulse pressures are decreased, and cardiac output is depressed. Many patients with the combination of normal left ventricular filling pressure and depressed cardiac index in fact have right ventricular infarcts (with accompanying inferior left ventricular infarcts). The hemodynamic picture may superficially resemble that seen in patients with pericardial disease (Chap. 42):[143] i.e., elevated right ventricular filling pressure; well-preserved, steep, right atrial *y* descent; and an early diastolic dip and plateau (square root sign) in the right ventricular pressure tracing. Moreover, Kussmaul's sign (inspiratory rise in mean right atrial pressure) and pulsus paradoxus (inspiratory fall > 10 mm Hg in systolic arterial blood pressure) may be present in patients with right ventricular infarction (Chap. 42). Echocardiography is helpful in the differential diagnosis,[89a] since in right ventricular infarction, in contrast to pericardial tamponade, no significant amounts of pericardial fluid are seen. Loss of atrial transport in patients with right ventricular infarction can result in marked decreases in stroke volume and arterial blood pressure.[144] The hemodynamic importance of right ventricular infarction in patients with inferior infarction is reflected in the observations of Marmor et al., who noted that although infarct size (reflected in CK release curves) was similar in patients with anterior and inferior infarcts, the former had more severe depression of the left ventricular ejection fraction and the latter had more severe depression of the right ventricular ejection fraction.[145]

CIRCULATORY REGULATION IN MYOCARDIAL INFARCTION

The abnormality in circulatory regulation that is present in AMI is diagrammed in Figure 37–10.[146] The process begins with an anatomical or functional obstruction in the coronary vascular bed, which results in regional myocardial ischemia and, if the ischemia persists, in infarction. If the infarct is of sufficient size, it depresses overall left ventricular function so that left ventricular stroke volume falls and filling pressures rise. The hemodynamic deterioration is more severe if an atrioventricular conduction disturbance develops or if mitral regurgitation or ventricular septal rupture occurs. A marked depression of left ventricular stroke volume ultimately lowers aortic pressure and reduces coronary perfusion pressure; this condition may intensify myocardial ischemia and thereby initiate the aforementioned vicious cycle (see Fig. 37–9). The inability of the left ventricle to empty also leads to an increased preload—that is, it dilates the well-perfused, normally functioning portion of the left ventricle. This compensatory mechanism tends to restore stroke volume to normal levels. However, the dilatation of the left ventricle also elevates ventricular afterload, because Laplace's law dictates that at any given arterial pressure the dilated ventricle must develop a higher wall tension (p. 431). The increased afterload not only depresses left ventricular stroke volume but also elevates myocardial oxygen consumption, which in turn intensifies regional myocardial ischemia. When regional myocardial dysfunction is limited and the function of the remainder of the left ventricle is normal, compensatory mechanisms will sustain overall left ventricular function. If a large portion of the left ventricle becomes necrotic, pump failure occurs, i.e., overall left ventricular function becomes so depressed that the circulation cannot be sustained despite the dilatation of the remaining viable portion of the ventricle.

Some of the consequences of treating pump failure, discussed in Chapter 38, should be considered. The favorable effect of raising a depressed arterial pressure results from the increased coronary perfusion pressure and the subsequent augmented blood flow across the stenotic areas and through the collateral vessels. This improvement of coronary blood flow may limit the size of the infarction by improving oxygen delivery to the periinfarction zone. In this manner, myocardial fiber shortening may be augmented, thereby increasing stroke volume and cardiac output and elevating arterial pressure.

However, there are also some unfavorable effects of increasing arterial pressure because this intervention usually necessitates an elevation of left ventricular intracavitary pressure (unless it is achieved by a circulatory assist device, such as an intraaortic balloon). The increased afterload causes cardiac dilatation; intramyocardial tension rises, not only because of the higher intraventricular pressure but also because of the cardiac dilatation (p. 431). The increased wall tension augments myocardial oxygen needs and reduces myocardial fiber shortening (p. 1237). These changes can cause further ischemia of the marginally viable myocardium adjacent to that supplied exclusively by the occluded vessel. Thus, cardiac function may deteriorate further.

It is obvious that the circulation is delicately balanced in patients with AMI. Unless the loss of viable myocardium is so extensive that it precludes survival, or is so small that the patient's survival is not threatened, the outcome may well depend on the physician's appreciation of the interaction of the many factors that influence circulatory performance and their judicious manipulation.

PATHOPHYSIOLOGY OF OTHER ORGAN SYSTEMS

ALTERATIONS IN PULMONARY FUNCTION

Significant changes in the pulmonary function and arterial blood gases of patients with AMI are described in Chapter 54. Hypoxemia is a frequent consequence, with its severity, in general, proportional to that of left ventricular failure. Thus, there is an inverse relation between arterial oxygen tension and pulmonary artery diastolic pressure in patients with AMI (Figs. 37–11 and 54–7, p. 1788), suggesting that increased pulmonary capillary hydrostatic pressure leads to interstitial edema, which results in arteriolar and bronchiolar compression that ultimately causes perfusion of poorly ventilated alveoli with resultant hypoxemia.[147,148] In addition to hypoxemia, hyperventilation often occurs in patients with AMI and may cause hypocapnia and respiratory alkalosis, particularly in restless, anxious patients with pain. Intrapulmonary shunting of blood has been noted in patients in whom left ventricular failure complicates AMI. With improvement in heart failure, hypoxemia and intrapulmonary shunting diminish.

In patients with MI, particularly when complicated by left ventricular failure or cardiogenic shock, the affinity of hemoglobin for oxygen is reduced, i.e., the P_{50} is increased.[149,150] The increase in P_{50} results from increased levels of erythrocyte 2,3-diphosphoglycerate (2,3-DPG), is maximal after 24 hours, and constitutes an important compensatory mechanism, responsible for an estimated 18 per cent increase in oxygen release from oxyhemoglobin in patients with cardiogenic shock.[149]

With a double radioisotope indicator dilution technique, a positive correlation has been demonstrated between pulmonary extravascular (interstitial) water content, left ventricular filling pressure, and the clinical signs and symptoms of left ventricular failure.[147] Over a period of 2 to 4 days following AMI, both the pulmonary extravascular water content and the wedge pressure decline. Presumably the increased pulmonary extravascular water represents a transudate secondary to increased pulmonary capillary pressure.

The increase in pulmonary extravascular water may also be responsible for the alterations in pulmonary mechanics observed in patients with AMI, i.e., reductions of airway conductance, pulmonary compliance, forced expiratory volume and midexpiratory flow rate, and an increase in closing volume—the last presumably related to the widespread closure of small, dependent airways during the first 3 days following AMI.[151] Recovery of left ventricular function or diuresis reduces abnormally elevated values for closing volumes to normal. Presumably, competition for space between arteries and small airways in the bronchovascular sheath accounts for some of the elevation in airway resistance, particularly at left atrial pressures under 15 mm Hg. Higher left atrial pressures produce increases in airway resistance secondary to interstitial, alveolar, and peribronchial edema.

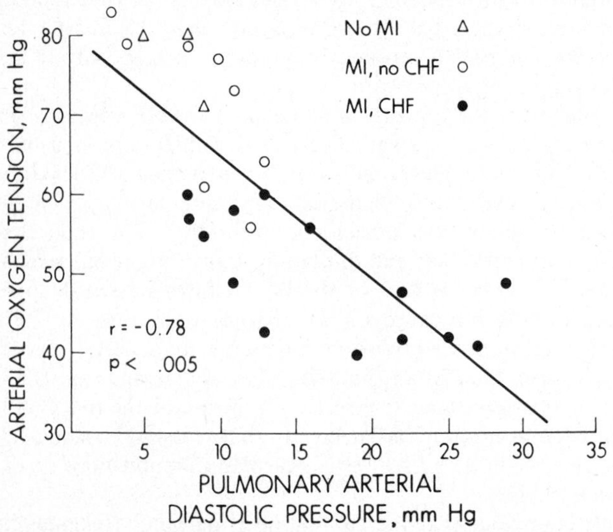

FIGURE 37–11 Arterial oxygen tension during the breathing of air, plotted in relation to pulmonary arterial diastolic pressure in patients with and without myocardial infarction (MI) and congestive heart failure (CHF). (From Fillmore, S. J., et al.: Blood-gas changes and pulmonary hemodynamics following acute myocardial infarction. Circulation *45*:583, 1972, by permission of the American Heart Association, Inc.)

Increased pulmonary venous pressure also results in redistribution of pulmonary blood flow from the bases to the apices of the lung in patients with AMI,[152] altering the relationship between ventilation and perfusion (p. 1786). However, at follow-up examination 3 to 25 weeks after MI, the ventilation/perfusion relationship has usually returned to normal or almost so.

ALTERATIONS IN ENDOCRINE FUNCTION (Fig. 37–12)

Pancreas. Hyperglycemia and impaired glucose tolerance are common in patients with AMI. Although the absolute levels of blood insulin are often in the normal range in patients with uncomplicated AMI, they are usually inappropriately low for the level of blood sugar elevation, and there may be relative insulin resistance as well.[153] Patients with cardiogenic shock often demonstrate marked hyperglycemia and depressed levels of circulating insulin, often with complete suppression of insulin secretion in response to tolbutamide.[154] These abnormalities in insulin secretion and the resultant impaired glucose tolerance appear to be secondary to a reduction in pancreatic blood flow as a consequence of splanchnic vasoconstriction, which accompanies severe left ventricular failure. In addition, increased activity of the sympathetic nervous system with augmented circulating catecholamines[155] inhibits insulin secretion[156,157] and augments glycogenolysis, also contributing to the elevation of blood sugar.[158]

Since hypoxic heart muscle derives a considerable portion of its energy from the metabolism of glucose (Chap. 36), and since insulin is essential for the uptake of glucose by the myocardium as well as for myocardial protein synthesis and inhibition of lysosomal activity, the deleterious effects of insulin deficiency are clear.[159]

Adrenal Gland. Excessive secretion of catecholamines produces many of the characteristic signs and symptoms of AMI. The plasma and urinary catecholamine levels are highest during the first 24 hours after the onset of chest pain,[158] with the greatest rise in plasma catecholamine secretion occurring during the first hour after the onset of MI,[160] when it may be in the range observed in racing car drivers immediately upon completion of a race.[161] These high levels of circulating catecholamines in patients with AMI correlate with the occurrence of serious arrhythmias[157,162-164] and result in the stimulation of myocardial oxygen consumption, both directly and indirectly, as a consequence of catecholamine-induced elevation of circulating free fatty acids.[160] As might be anticipated, the concentration of circulating catecholamines correlates with both the incidence of cardiogenic shock and the mortality rate.[157] Circulating catecholamines enhance platelet aggregation; when this occurs in the coronary microcirculation, the release of the potent vasoconstrictor thromboxane A_2 may further impair cardiac perfusion.[158]

Plasma and urinary 17-hydroxycorticosteroids and ketosteroids, as well as aldosterone, are also markedly elevated in patients with AMI.[158,165,166] Their concentrations correlate directly with the peak level of serum glutamic oxaloacetic transaminase, implying that the stress imposed by larger infarcts is associated with greater secretion of adrenal steroids. Glucocorticosteroids also contribute to the impairment of glucose tolerance; although it has been suggested that the secretion of glucocorticoids is increased, it is inadequate to meet the demands for the stress imposed by a massive AMI, particularly if it is accompanied by cardiogenic shock.[158]

Hematological Function (see also p. 1699). AMI generally occurs in the presence of extensive coronary and systemic atherosclerotic plaques, which may serve as the site for the formation of platelet aggregates, a sequence which has been suggested as the initial step in the process of coronary thrombosis, coronary occlusion, and subsequent MI. Approximately one-third of patients with AMI demonstrate shortened platelet survival times.[167] Types III and IV hyperlipoproteinemia, frequently present in patients with AMI, can also be responsible for shortening platelet survival. Findings suggestive of a hypercoagulable state as a risk factor for AMI are discussed on page 1695.

Elevated levels of serum fibrinogen degradation products, an end product of thrombosis[168]—as well as release of distinctive proteins when platelets are activated, i.e., platelet factor 4[169]—have been reported in some patients with AMI. The interpretation of the coagulation tests in patients with AMI may be complicated by elevated blood levels of catecholamines, concomitant shock, and/or pulmonary em-

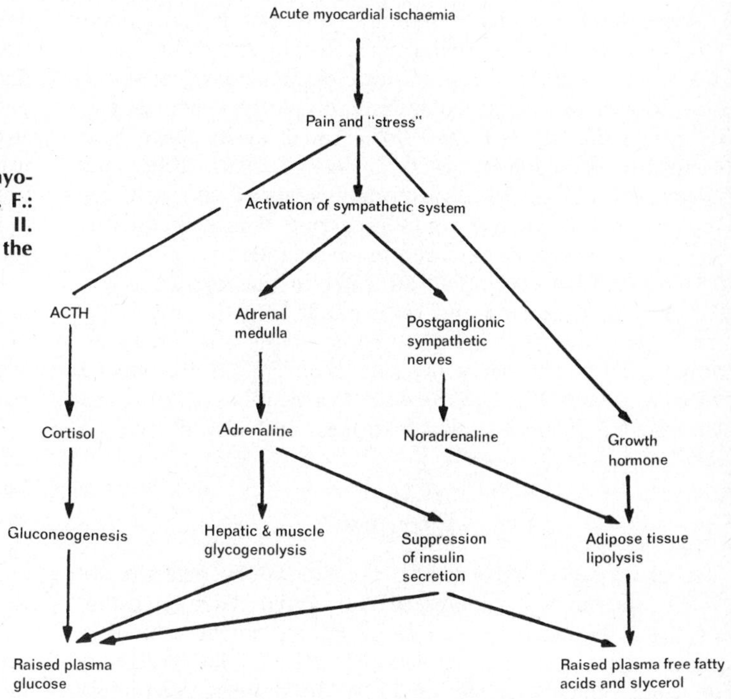

FIGURE 37–12 Principal hormonal and metabolic effects of myocardial infarction. (Reproduced with permission from Oliver, M. F.: Metabolic response during impending myocardial infarction. II. Clinical implications. Circulation *45*:491, 1972 by permission of the American Heart Association, Inc.)

bolism, conditions which are all capable of altering various tests of platelet and coagulation function.[170] Thus, it is not yet clear whether the above-mentioned changes are the causes or consequences of AMI.

An elevation of *blood viscosity* also occurs in patients with AMI.[171] During the first few days after infarction, this is mainly attributable to hemoconcentration, but later the increases in plasma viscosity and red cell aggregation correlate with elevated serum concentrations of $alpha_2$ globulin and fibrinogen, which are nonspecific reactions to tissue necrosis and which are also responsible for the elevated sedimentation rate characteristic of AMI.[172] The high values of blood viscosity are observed most frequently in patients with complications, such as left ventricular failure, cardiogenic shock, and thromboembolism.

Alterations in Renal Function. Both prerenal azotemia and acute renal failure can complicate the marked reduction of cardiac output that occurs in cardiogenic shock. These conditions are discussed on pages 587 and 1752.

CLINICAL FEATURES OF ACUTE MYOCARDIAL INFARCTION

PRECIPITATING FACTORS

In most patients with AMI, no precipitating factor can be identified. An early study noted the following patient activities at the onset of AMI: heavy physical exertion, 13 per cent; modest or usual exertion, 18 per cent; surgical procedure, 6 per cent; rest, 51 per cent; and sleep, 8 per cent.[173] Another study showed similar results except that only 2 per cent of patients experienced MI during heavy physical exertion.[174] Others, however, have reported that a significant number of AMI's occur within a few hours of severe physical exertion.[175,176] It has been pointed out that the *severe exertion* which preceded an infarction was often performed at times when the patient was unduly fatigued or emotionally stressed.[177] Thus, although adequate control studies have not been carried out, there is suggestive evidence that heavy exercise may play a precipitating role in some patients. Such infarctions are presumably the result of marked increases in myocardial oxygen consumption in the presence of severe coronary arterial narrowing. Supporting this hypothesis is the finding that fatal MI occurring during heavy exertion is often associated with severe coronary arterial narrowing but no occlusion.[176]

Surgical procedures associated with acute blood loss have also been noted as frequent precursors of MI (p. 1818). Reduced myocardial perfusion secondary to hypotension and increased myocardial oxygen demands secondary to fever, tachycardia, and agitation are presumably responsible for the myocardial necrosis. Other factors reported as predisposing to MI include respiratory infections, hypoxemia of any cause, pulmonary embolism, hypoglycemia, administration of ergot preparations, serum sickness, allergy, and wasp stings.[178–181] In patients with Prinzmetal's angina (p. 1360), MI may develop in the territory of the coronary artery, which repeatedly undergoes spasm. Rarely, munition workers exposed to high concentrations of nitroglycerin may develop myocardial infarction when they are withdrawn from this exposure, suggesting that it is caused by vasospasm.[182] Unstable angina (accelerating angina) and rest angina (p. 1355) may culminate as infarction of the myocardium, again in the distribution of the affected vessel.[183]

Considerable evidence has accumulated that *emotional stresses* may be a precipitating factor in the initiation of AMI.[184] A number of reports have documented that upsetting life events occur commonly in patients who subsequently suffer an MI (p. 1827).[185] Such events have been quantified and scored as *Life Change Units.* Rahe and coworkers noted, on retrospective analysis, a significant buildup in Life Change Units in patients who subsequently suffered myocardial infarction or died suddenly.

Trauma may precipitate an AMI in one of two ways. Myocardial contusion and hemorrhage into the myocardium may actually cause cell necrosis, or the injury may involve a coronary artery, causing occlusion of that vessel with resultant MI (Chap. 44). *Neurological disturbances* (transient ischemic attacks or strokes) may also precipitate AMI.[186]

HISTORY

Despite recent advances in the laboratory detection of AMI, the history remains of substantial value in establishing a diagnosis. A *prodromal history* can be elicited in 20 to 60 per cent of patients with AMI.[186,187] The prodrome is usually characterized by chest discomfort, resembling classic angina pectoris (described on pp. 5 and 1355), but it occurs at rest or with less activity than usual and can therefore be classified as unstable angina (p. 1355). However, the latter is often not disturbing enough to induce the patient to seek medical attention, and if he does, he is not usually hospitalized. Among patients who are hospitalized for unstable angina, fewer than 15 per cent develop AMI (p. 1359).

The pain of AMI is variable in intensity; in most patients it is severe and, in some instances, intolerable. The pain is prolonged, usually lasting for more than 30 minutes and frequently for a number of hours. The discomfort is described as constricting, crushing, oppressing, or compressing; often the patient complains of something sitting on or squeezing the chest. Although usually described as a squeezing, choking, viselike, or heavy pain, it may also be characterized as a stabbing, knifelike, boring, or burning discomfort. The pain is usually retrosternal in location, spreading frequently to both sides of the anterior chest, with predilection for the left side. Often the pain radiates down the ulnar aspect of the left arm, producing a tingling sensation in the left wrist, hand, and even fingers. Some patients note only a dull ache or numbness of the wrists in association with severe substernal or precordial discomfort. In some instances, the pain of AMI may begin in the epigastrium and simulate a variety of abdominal disorders, a fact which often causes MI to be misdiagnosed as "indigestion." In other patients the discomfort of AMI radiates to the shoulders, upper extremities, neck, jaw, and interscapular region, again usually favoring the left side. In patients with preexisting angina pectoris, the pain of infarction usually resembles that of angina with respect to quality and location. However, it is generally much more severe, lasts longer, and is not relieved by rest and nitroglycerin.

In some patients, particularly the elderly, AMI is manifest clinically not by chest pain but rather by symptoms of acute left ventricular failure and chest tightness or by overwhelming weakness, accompanied by diaphoresis, nausea, vomiting, and diarrhea.[186] The pain of AMI may have disappeared by the time the physician first encounters the patient (or the patient reaches the hospital), or it may persist for many hours. Opiates—in particular, morphine—usually relieve the pain, although a persistent soreness, pressure, or dull ache may remain for several hours or more despite intensive treatment with analgesics. Both angina pectoris and the pain of AMI are thought to arise from nerve endings in ischemic or injured, but not necrotic, myocardium.[188] Thus, in MI, stimulation of nerve fibers in an ischemic zone of myocardium surrounding the necrotic central area of infarction probably gives rise to the pain.

The pain of AMI may simulate the pain of *acute pericarditis,* which is usually associated with some pleuritic features, i.e., it is aggravated by respiratory movements and coughing and often involves the shoulder, ridge of the trapezius, and neck. *Pleural pain* is usually sharp, knifelike, and aggravated by each breath, which distinguishes it from the deep, dull, steady pain of AMI. *Pulmonary embolism* (Chap. 46) generally produces pain laterally in the chest, is often pleuritic in nature, and may be associated with hemoptysis. The pain due to *acute dissection of the aorta* (Chap. 45) is usually localized in the center of the chest, is extremely severe, persists for many hours, and often radiates to the lower back and sometimes into the legs. Often one or more major arterial pulses are absent. Pain arising from the *costochondral and chondrosternal articulations* may be associated with localized swelling and redness; it is usually sharp and "darting" and is characterized by marked localized tenderness.

Nausea and vomiting occur frequently in patients with AMI and severe chest pain, presumably owing to activation of a vagal reflex. These occur more commonly in patients with inferior MI than in those with anterior MI. Occasionally a patient complains of diarrhea or a violent urge to evacuate the bowels during the acute phase of MI. Moreover, nausea and vomiting are common side effects of opiates. When the pain of AMI is epigastric in location and is associated with nausea and vomiting, the clinical picture may easily be confused with that of acute cholecystitis, gastritis, or peptic ulcer. Other symptoms include feelings of profound weakness, dizziness, palpitations, cold perspiration, and a sense of impending doom. On occasion, symptoms arising from an episode of cerebral embolism or other systemic arterial embolism are the first signs of an AMI. Rarely, patients with inferior infarction report intractable hiccupping, a finding which has been attributed to diaphragmatic irritation by the infarct.[189] The aforementioned symptoms may or may not be accompanied by chest pain.[190]

Approximately one-quarter of nonfatal MI are unrecognized by the patient and are discovered only on subsequent routine electrocardiographic[191,192] or postmortem examinations. Of these unrecognized infarctions, approximately half are truly silent, with the patients unable to recall any symptoms whatsoever referable to the infarction. The other half of patients with so-called silent infarction can recall an event characterized by symptoms compatible with acute infarction when leading questions are posed after the abnormal electrocardiogram is discovered. Unrecognized or silent infarction rarely occurs in patients with antecedent angina pectoris, and it is more common in patients with diabetes and hypertension.

In an analysis of atypical presentations of AMI, Bean[193] lists the following: (1) congestive heart failure—beginning de novo or worsening of established failure; (2) classic angina pectoris without a particularly severe or prolonged attack; (3) atypical location of the pain; (4) central nervous system manifestations, resembling those of stroke, secondary to a sharp reduction in cardiac output in a patient with cerebral arteriosclerosis; (5) apprehension and nervousness; (6) sudden mania or psychosis; (7) syncope; (8) overwhelming weakness; (9) acute indigestion; and (10) peripheral embolism.

Pericarditis secondary to transmural AMI (p. 1503) may produce pain as early as the first day and as late as 6 weeks after MI and may be confused with pain resulting from persistent ischemia or extension of the infarct or both. Although transitory pericardial friction rubs are very common among patients with transmural infarction within the first 48 hours, the pain or electrocardiographic changes occur much less often. The discomfort of pericarditis usually becomes worse during a deep inspiration, but it may be somewhat relieved when the patient sits up and leans forward (Chap. 43).

Angina developing within the first 10 days following AMI is disconcerting to patients and physicians alike. In most patients, it responds to rest, nitroglycerin, beta-adrenergic blockade, and calcium channel antagonists,[194] just as does classic angina. In a minority of patients, postinfarction angina may be refractory to treatment and is provoked by minimal activity, meals, or emotional upset. When accompanied by ST-T–wave changes in the same area where Q waves have appeared, it is probably due to coronary spasm.[195,196]

It is frequently difficult to distinguish postinfarction angina from infarct extension. The latter is usually associated with more severe and prolonged discomfort, *persistent* electrocardiographic changes (ST-T changes or QRS changes or both), and reelevation of serum enzymes.

PHYSICAL EXAMINATION

GENERAL APPEARANCE. Patients suffering an AMI usually appear anxious and in considerable distress. An anguished facial expression is common, and—in contrast to patients with angina pectoris, who often lie, sit, or stand quite still, realizing that all forms of activity increase the discomfort—patients suffering an AMI are often restless and move about in an effort to find a comfortable position. They may massage or clutch their chests and frequently describe their pain with a clenched fist held against the sternum (a sign of ischemic pain popularized by Dr. Samuel A. Levine). In patients with left ventricular failure and sympathetic stimulation, cold perspiration and skin pallor may be evident; they usually sit or are propped up in bed, gasping for breath. Between breaths, they may complain of chest discomfort or a feeling of suffocation. Cough productive of frothy, pink, or blood-streaked sputum is common.

Patients in cardiogenic shock often lie listlessly, making few, if any, spontaneous movements. The skin is cool and clammy, with a bluish or mottled color over the extremities, and there is marked facial pallor with severe cyanosis of the lips and nailbeds. Depending on the degree of cerebral perfusion, the patient in shock may converse normally or may evidence confusion and disorientation.

VITAL SIGNS. The heart rate may vary from a marked bradycardia to rapid regular or irregular tachycardia, depending on the underlying rhythm and the degree of left ventricular failure. Most commonly, the pulse is rapid and regular initially (sinus tachycardia at 100 to 110 beats/min), slowing as the patient's pain and anxiety are relieved; premature ventricular beats are common, occurring in more than 95 per cent of patients evaluated early after the onset of symptoms.

The majority of patients with uncomplicated AMI are normotensive, although the reduced stroke volume accompanying the tachycardia may cause a small decline in systolic pressure and an elevation of diastolic pressure. In a minority of previously normotensive patients, a hypertensive response occurs, with the arterial pressure exceeding 160/90 mm Hg, presumably as a consequence of adrenergic discharge secondary to pain and agitation. The arterial pressure rarely exceeds 200/110 mm Hg. It is rather common for previously hypertensive patients to become normotensive without treatment following AMI, although approximately two-thirds of these previously hypertensive patients eventually regain their elevated levels of blood pressure, generally 3 to 6 months after infarction. In patients with massive infarcts, arterial pressure falls acutely, owing to left ventricular dysfunction and venous pooling secondary to administration of morphine or nitrates or both; as recovery occurs, the arterial pressure tends to return to preinfarction levels. Patients in cardiogenic shock (p. 591), by definition, have systolic pressures below 90 mm Hg. However, hypotension does not necessarily signify cardiogenic shock, since some patients with inferior infarction, in whom the Bezold-Jarisch reflex is activated, may also have systolic blood pressure below 90 mm Hg.[197,198] These patients do not demonstrate peripheral manifestations of hypoperfusion; their prognosis is generally good and their hypotension eventually resolves spontaneously, although this resolution can be accelerated by atropine and assumption of the Trendelenburg position. Other patients who are initially only slightly hypotensive may demonstrate gradually falling blood pressures with progressive reduction in cardiac output over several days as they gradually develop cardiogenic shock as a consequence of increasing ischemia and extension of infarction (Fig. 37–8).

Most patients with AMI develop *fever,* a nonspecific response to tissue necrosis, within 24 to 48 hours of the onset of infarction. Body temperature often begins to rise within 4 to 8 hours after the onset of infarction, and rectal temperature often reaches 101 to 102° F. Fever usually resolves by the seventh or eighth day following infarction.

The *respiratory rate* may be slightly elevated soon after the development of an AMI; in patients without heart failure, it results from anxiety and pain, since it returns to normal with treatment of physical and psychological discomfort. In patients with left ventricular failure, the respiratory rate correlates with the severity of failure; patients with pulmonary edema may have respiratory rates exceeding 40 per minute. However, the respiratory rate is not necessarily elevated in patients with cardiogenic shock.

Cheyne-Stokes (periodic) respiration (p. 449) may occur in elderly individuals with cardiogenic shock and heart failure, particularly after opiate therapy and in the presence of cerebrovascular disease.

THE FUNDI. Hypertension, diabetes, and generalized atherosclerosis commonly accompany AMI, and since these conditions may produce characteristic changes in the fundus, a careful funduscopic examination may provide information concerning the underlying vascular status; this is particularly useful in patients unable to provide a detailed history.

JUGULAR VENOUS PULSE. The height and contour of the jugular venous pulse reflect right atrial and right ventricular diastolic pressures (p. 20). Since these pressures are usually normal or only slightly elevated in patients with AMI (even in the presence of mild to moderate left ventricular failure), it is not surprising that the jugular venous pulse does not appear to be abnormal. The *a* wave may be prominent in patients with pulmonary hypertension secondary to left ventricular failure or reduced compliance.[199] In contrast, right ventricular infarction (whether or not it accompanies left ventricular infarction) often results in marked jugular venous distention and, when it is complicated by necrosis of right ventricular papillary muscles, tall *v* waves of tricuspid regurgitation are evident. In patients with AMI and cardiogenic shock, the jugular venous pressure is usually elevated. In patients with AMI, hypotension, and hypoperfusion, who may specifically resemble those with cardiogenic shock but who have flat neck veins, it is likely that the depression of left ventricular performance may be related, at least in part, to hypovolemia, but the differentiation can be made only by assessing left ventricular performance.

CAROTID PULSE. Palpation of the carotid arterial pulse provides a clue to the left ventricular stroke volume; a small pulse suggests a reduced stroke volume, whereas a sharp, brief upstroke is often observed in patients with mitral regurgitation or ruptured ventricular septum with a left-to-right shunt. Pulsus alternans reflects severe left ventricular dysfunction.

THE CHEST. Moist rales are audible in patients who develop left ventricular failure and/or a reduction of left ventricular compliance after AMI. As noted, the prognosis is related to the fraction of the lung field over which rales are heard (Table 37–5). Diffuse wheezing may be present in patients with severe left ventricular failure. Cough with hemoptysis, suggesting pulmonary embolism with infarction, may also occur.

THE HEART. Despite severe symptoms and extensive myocardial damage, the findings on examination of the heart may be surprisingly unremarkable in patients with AMI. Palpation of the precordium may yield normal findings but more commonly reveals a presystolic pulsation, synchronous with an audible fourth heart sound, reflecting a vigorous left atrial contraction filling a ventricle with reduced compliance. In the presence of left ventricular systolic dysfunction, an outward movement of the left ventricle may be palpated in early diastole, coincident with a third heart sound. When the anterior or lateral portion of the ventricle is dyskinetic, an abnormal systolic pulsation is present in the third, fourth, or fifth interspaces to the left of the sternum. In some patients, this abnormal paradoxical precordial impulse is clearly separable from the point of maximal impulse, which is more lateral and to the left. In other patients, the abnormal impulse is a diffuse, rippling, precordial movement, approximately 5 to 10 cm in diameter, not clearly separable from the point of maximal impulse. Patients with longstanding hypertension or previous infarction with left ventricular hypertrophy often demonstrate a laterally displaced, sustained point of maximum impulse.

Auscultation. The heart sounds, particularly the first sound, are frequently muffled[200] and occasionally inaudible immediately after the infarct, and their intensity increases as healing occurs.[201] A soft first sound may also reflect prolongation of the P-R interval. Patients with marked ventricular dysfunction or left bundle branch block may have paradoxical splitting of the second heart sound (p. 47). Individuals with postinfarction angina also may develop transient, paradoxically split second heart sounds during anginal episodes because of prolongation of the left ventricular preejection period.

A *fourth heart sound* is almost universally present in patients with AMI and is usually best heard between the left sternal border and the apex. This sound reflects a reduction in left ventricular compliance (p. 51) and is associated with an elevation of left ventricular end-diastolic pressure, even in the absence of left ventricular systolic dysfunction. It is of little diagnostic value, since it is commonly audible in most patients with chronic ischemic heart disease as well as in many normal subjects older than 45 years.

A *third heart sound* reflects extensive left ventricular

TABLE 37–5 KILLIP CLASSIFICATION OF PATIENTS WITH ACUTE MYOCARDIAL INFARCTION

	Definition	Patients with Acute Myocardial Infarction Admitted to CCU in This Category (%)	Approximate Mortality (%)
Class I	Absence of rales over the lung fields and absence of S3	30–40	8
Class II	Rales over 50 per cent or less of the lung fields or the presence of an S3	30–50	30
Class III	Rales over more than 50 per cent of the lung fields (frequently pulmonary edema)	5–10	44
Class IV	Shock	10	80–100

Adapted from Killip, T., and Kimball, J. T.: Treatment of myocardial infarction in a coronary care unit. A two year experience with 250 patients. Am. J. Cardiol. *20*:457, 1967.

dysfunction. It is usually heard in patients with large infarctions. This sound is heard best at the apex, with the patient in the left lateral recumbent position, and is more common in patients with transmural anterior infarctions than in those with inferior or nontransmural infarctions[202]; patients with a third heart sound often have elevated left ventricular filling pressure. The mortality of patients who manifest a third heart sound during the acute phase of MI is 40 per cent, contrasted with 15 per cent for patients without such a sound.[202] A third sound may be caused not only by left ventricular failure but also by increased inflow into the left ventricle, as occurs in mitral regurgitation or ventricular septal defect. Third and fourth heart sounds emanating from the left ventricle are heard best at the apex; in patients with right ventricular infarcts that originate from this chamber, these sounds may be heard along the left sternal border and are intensified by inspiration.

Systolic murmurs, transient or persistent, are commonly audible in patients with AMI and generally result from mitral regurgitation secondary to papillary muscle dysfunction. A new, prominent holosystolic murmur at the apex, accompanied by a thrill, may represent rupture of a head of a papillary muscle (p. 1076); the findings in rupture of the interventricular septum are similar, although the murmur and thrill are usually most prominent along the left sternal border. The systolic murmur of tricuspid regurgitation (caused by right ventricular failure due to pulmonary hypertension or right ventricular infarction or by infarction of a right ventricular papillary muscle) is also heard along the left sternal border but is characteristically intensified by inspiration and is accompanied by a prominent *v* wave in the jugular venous pulse. In evaluating systolic murmurs in patients with chest pain, it is important to note that aortic stenosis is a common cause of ischemic pain (p. 1099) and that, like coronary artery disease, it occurs most commonly in middle-aged and elderly men. Therefore, the diagnosis of aortic stenosis should be considered in patients suspected of having suffered an MI who have a systolic murmur at the base of the heart. Rarely, *diastolic murmurs* are produced by blood flowing through a severe coronary arterial stenosis.

Pericardial friction rubs are audible in up to 20 per cent of patients with AMI and in a high percentage of patients with transmural infarcts.[203] Rubs are notorious for their evanescence and, hence, are probably even more common than reported; frequent auscultation in patients with transmural infarction often results in the discovery of a rub which might otherwise have gone unnoticed. Although friction rubs may be heard by 24 hours or as late as 2 weeks after the onset of infarction, most commonly they are noted on the second or third day. Occasionally, in patients with extensive infarction, a loud rub may be heard for many days. Delayed onset of the rub and the associated discomfort of pericarditis (as late as three months postinfarction) are characteristic of the postmyocardial infarction syndrome (p. 1514).[120-124]

Pericardial rubs are most readily audible along the left sternal border or just inside the point of maximal impulse and occur after either anterior or inferoposterior transmural infarction. Loud rubs may be audible over the entire precordium and even over the back. Occasionally, only the systolic portion of a rub is heard; it may be confused with a systolic murmur, and the diagnosis of rupture of the ventricular septum or mitral regurgitation may be considered. The presence of a pericardial friction rub does not exclude the presence of a significant pericardial effusion.

THE ABDOMEN. As noted above, in patients with AMI (particularly inferior infarcts) with diaphragmatic irritation, the pain may localize in the epigastrium or the right upper quadrant. Pain in the abdomen associated with nausea, vomiting, restlessness, and even abdominal distention is often interpreted by patients as a sign of "indigestion,"[193] resulting in self-medication with antacids, and it may suggest an acute abdominal process to the physician. A normal abdominal examination aids in ruling this out and in pointing to the correct diagnosis. Right heart failure, characterized by hepatomegaly and a positive abdominojugular reflux, is unusual in patients with acute left ventricular infarction but does occur in patients with severe and usually prolonged left ventricular failure or right ventricular infarction.

THE EXTREMITIES. Coronary atherosclerosis is often associated with systemic atherosclerosis, and it is therefore common for patients with AMI to have a history of intermittent claudication and to demonstrate physical findings of peripheral vascular disease. Thus, diminished peripheral arterial pulses, loss of hair, and atrophic skin in the lower extremities are frequently noted in patients with coronary artery disease. Peripheral edema is a manifestation of right ventricular failure and, like congestive hepatomegaly, is unusual in patients with acute left ventricular infarction. Cyanosis of the nailbeds is common in patients with severe left ventricular failure and is particularly striking in patients with cardiogenic shock.

NEUROPSYCHIATRIC EXAMINATION. Except for the altered mental status which occurs in patients with AMI who have a markedly reduced cardiac output and cerebral hypoperfusion, the neurological examination is normal unless the patient has suffered cerebral embolism secondary to a mural thrombus. Indeed, an underlying MI is common in patients with cerebral embolic stroke. There is an increased coincidence of cerebrovascular accidents and AMI. In a prospective study of patients with cerebrovascular accidents admitted to the hospital within 72 hours of the onset, 12.7 per cent has an associated AMI; in contrast, in a series of patients with AMI, only 1.7 per cent suffered a stroke. The coincidence was confined to patients with large myocardial infarcts as reflected in markedly elevated serum creatine kinase concentrations.[204] The coincidence between these two conditions may be explained by systemic hypotension due to MI precipitating a cerebral infarction and the converse, as well as by mural emboli from the heart causing cerebral emboli.

As discussed in Chapter 57, patients with AMI often exhibit alterations of the emotional state, including intense anxiety, denial, and depression.

LABORATORY EXAMINATIONS

ENZYMES. Irreversibly injured myocardial cells release a number of enzymes into the circulation, where they can be measured by specific chemical reactions (p. 1254).[205] Increased activities of many enzymes have been found in

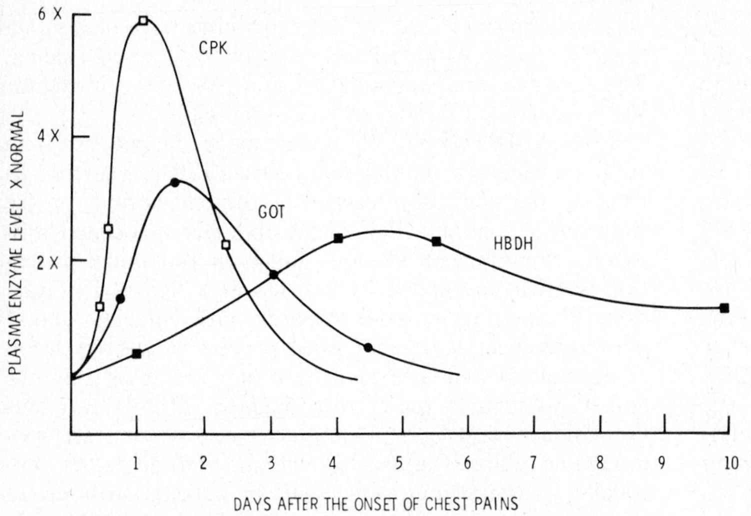

FIGURE 37–13 Typical plasma profiles for creatine kinase (CPK), glutamate oxalocetate transaminase (GOT), and hydroxybutyrate dehydrogenase (HBDH, LDH) activities following the onset of acute myocardial infarction. (From Hearse, D. J.: Myocardial enzyme leakage. J. Mol. Med. *2*: 185, 1977.)

the serum or plasma of patients with AMI.[206] Following experimental MI, a small, but significant, myocardial venoarterial difference of enzyme activity can be measured,[207] and elevated plasma levels of enzymes correlate with corresponding depletion of these same enzymes from infarcted tissue.[208] Determinations of serum activity of creatine kinase (CK), glutamic oxaloacetic transferase (GOT), and lactic dehydrogenase (LDH) have become standard in the laboratory diagnosis of AMI. Although only one of these enzymes need be elevated to establish the diagnosis of AMI, most hospitals continue to measure all three because of the different time patterns of release.

Serum glutamic oxaloacetic transferase (SGOT) activity usually exceeds the normal range within 8 to 12 hours following the onset of chest pain; peak SGOT levels occur 18 to 36 hours after infarction and fall to normal within 3 to 4 days (Fig. 37–13). Elevated SGOT activity has been found in 97 per cent of 119 autopsy-proved cases of myocardial infarction.[209] False-positive elevations of this enzyme occur in patients with primary liver disease, hepatic congestion, and skeletal muscle disease and following intramuscular injections, pulmonary embolism, and various forms of shock.[205] Elevated levels of SGOT have also been noted in patients with pericarditis and epicardial involvement.

LDH activity rises and falls more slowly than SGOT and exceeds the normal range by 24 to 48 hours after the onset of AMI, reaches a peak 3 to 6 days after the onset of pain, and returns to normal levels 8 to 14 days after the infarction. In one study, elevations in serum LDH activity occurred in 86 per cent of 282 patients with the clinical diagnosis of AMI and in all 39 patients with autopsy-proved infarction.[209] Like SGOT, the total LDH, while sensitive, is not specific; false-positive elevations occur in patients with hemolysis, megaloblastic anemia, leukemia, liver disease, hepatic congestion, renal disease, a variety of neoplasms, pulmonary embolism, myocarditis, skeletal muscle disease, and shock.[205]

LDH has five isoenzymes, which are numbered in the order of the rapidity of their migration toward the anode of an electrophoretic field. LDH_1 moves most rapidly, whereas LDH_5 is the slowest. Fractionation of serum LDH into its five isoenzymes increases diagnostic accuracy, since the heart contains principally LDH_1, whereas liver and skeletal muscle contain primarily LDH_4 and LDH_5. Thus, LDH_5 is commonly elevated in patients with congestive hepatomegaly. Most conditions causing elevated serum total LDH activity, such as liver or skeletal muscle disease or injury, are readily distinguished from AMI by analysis of LDH isoenzymes. Increased serum LDH_1 activity precedes elevation of serum total LDH and usually occurs within 8 to 24 hours after infarction.[210] Elevations of LDH and in the ratio of LDH_1 to total LDH occur in more than 95 per cent of patients with AMI.[205,211] Since hemolysis also raises serum LDH_1 activity, particular care must be taken in the withdrawal and handling of the blood specimens. LDH_1 reduces alpha-ketobutyric acid more readily than the more slowly moving isoenzymes of LDH; therefore, this property of the enzyme is termed hydroxybutyric dehydrogenase (HBD) activity,[205] and serum activity of alpha-HDB is often measured in patients with AMI. However, HBD should not be called a specific enzyme because its measurement actually reflects LDH_1 activity.

Serum CK activity exceeds the normal range within 6 to 8 hours following the onset of AMI, peaks at about 24 hours, and declines to normal within 3 to 4 days after the onset of chest pain (Fig. 37–13).[205] CK values in women are normally about two-thirds of those in men. Although elevation of the serum CK is the most sensitive enzymatic detector of AMI that can be used routinely,[205,210–213] 15 per cent false-positive results will occur in patients with muscle disease, alcohol intoxication, diabetes mellitus, skeletal muscle trauma, vigorous exercise, convulsions, intramuscular injections, and pulmonary embolism.[205] However, serum CK activity is normal in patients with heart failure and hepatic disease.

Three isoenzymes of CK (MM, BB, and MB) have been identified by electrophoresis. Extracts of brain and kidney contain predominantly the BB isoenzyme, skeletal muscle contains principally MM, and both MM and MB isoenzymes are present in cardiac muscle. The MB isoenzymes of CK may also be present in minor quantities in the small intestine, tongue, diaphragm, uterus, and prostate.[213,214] Despite these small amounts of CK-MB isoenzyme in tissues other than heart, elevated serum activity of CK-MB may be considered for practical purposes to be the result of AMI (except in the case of trauma or surgery on the above-mentioned organs, which contain small quantities of the enzyme). Thus, measurement of serum CK-MB isoenzyme appears to be a most useful test for myocardial necrosis.[214-216] The development of radioimmunoassay for the measurement of serum CK-MB has been helpful in increasing the accuracy, sensitivity, and specificity of this test.[217] In addition to AMI secondary to coronary obstruction, other forms of injury to cardiac muscle—such as those resulting from myocarditis, trauma, cardiac catheterization, and cardiac surgery—may also produce elevated serum CK-MB activity.[218-220] These latter causes of elevations of serum CK-MB values can usually be readily distinguished from AMI by the clinical setting. In approximately 15 per cent of patients with AMI, the CK-MB may be elevated despite a normal total CK.[221,221a] Therefore, total CK is not a sensitive adequate screening test. Serial measurement of CK-MB and application of the methods devised by Sobel and Shell (p. 1254)[205,208] allow prediction of infarct size determined at necropsy;[222] infarct size estimated by this method varies inversely with ejection fraction[223] and with survival[224] (Fig. 38–8, p. 1319).

Other Chemical Measurements. Numerous nonspecific manifestations may be recognized in patients with AMI. Although they are not generally employed in establishing the diagnosis, awareness of their coexistence with infarction is important in order to avoid misinterpretation or erroneous diagnosis of other disorders.

Hyperglycemia occurs frequently following AMI, not only in diabetic patients, in whom ketoacidosis may be precipitated, but also (with a lower frequency) in nondiabetics, in whom several weeks may elapse before carbohydrate tolerance returns to normal.[225] The plasma urea and creatinine concentrations are normal, except in patients with severe left ventricular failure, in whom reduced renal perfusion and glomerular filtration may result in azotemia (p. 1750). Hypokalemic alkalosis may be present in patients who develop an AMI while receiving thiazide or loop diuretics for antecedent hypertension or heart failure.

Serum lipids are often determined shortly after admission in patients with AMI. However, the results may be misleading, since numerous factors that can alter the values are operating at the time of the patient's admission to the hospital; for example, stress increases serum cholesterol, whereas recumbency decreases it.[226,227] Serum triglycerides are affected by caloric intake, intravenous glucose, and recumbency.[227] Therefore, it is best to defer determinations of serum lipid levels until 4 to 8 weeks after the infarction has occurred.

Release of *myoglobin* into the circulation from injured myocardial cells can be demonstrated within a few hours after the onset of infarction, and myoglobinemia is common in patients with AMI. Peak levels of serum myoglobin are reached considerably earlier (3 to 20 hours, mean = 11.4 hours after onset of infarction) than peak values of serum CK.[228] However, the time of earlier appearance of myoglobin in the serum, its peak level, and the duration of detectable myoglobin release do *not* correlate well with these same parameters for serum CK and with clinical estimates of the severity of infarction. Myoglobin appears in the serum in multiple short bursts which last for only an hour or two; in contrast to CK, myoglobin (which has a molecular weight of only 17,000) is readily excreted into the urine. This pattern of myoglobin release suggests that MI may be occurring in a series of short bursts rather than as a single episode.[228] The clinical value of serial determinations of myoglobin in AMI is limited because of the brief duration of its elevation and the lack of specificity resulting from the fact that myoglobin is a constituent of skeletal muscle and is readily detected in the serum following damage to skeletal muscle.

Alterations in serum concentrations of various *trace metals* have been noted during AMI. Elevations in serum concentration of copper and nickel have been observed which seem to parallel elevations in the sedimentation rate.[229,230] Significant decreases in serum zinc,[231] iron,[232] and magnesium[233] concentration occur within a day after infarction. The significance of alterations in serum concentrations of trace metals after infarction is currently unknown.

Hematological Manifestations. An increase in the *white blood count* occurs frequently following AMI; it may be a response to tissue necrosis or increased secretion of adrenal glucocorticoids or both. The elevation of the white count usually develops within 2 hours after the onset of chest pain, reaches a peak 2 to 4 days following infarction, and returns to normal in 1 week; the peak white blood cell count usually ranges between 12 and 15 $\times$ 10^3 per cubic millimeter but occasionally rises to as high as 20 $\times$ 10^3 per cubic millimeter. Often there is an increase in the percentage of polymorphonuclear leukocytes and a shift of the differential count to band forms. The *erythrocyte sedimentation rate* (ESR) is usually normal during the first day or two after infarction, even though fever and leukocytosis may be present. It then rises to a peak on the fourth or fifth day and may remain elevated for several weeks. The increase in the ESR is secondary to elevated plasma alpha$_2$ globulin and fibrinogen,[234] but the peak does not correlate well with the size of the infarction or with the prognosis. The *hematocrit* often increases during the first few days following infarction as a consequence of hemoconcentration.[171]

ELECTROCARDIOGRAPHIC FINDINGS

(See also p. 222)

In the majority of patients with AMI, some change can be documented when serial electrocardiographic tracings are compared. However, many factors limit the ability of the electrocardiogram to diagnose and localize myocardial infarcts: the extent of myocardial injury, the age of the infarct, its location, the presence of conduction defects, the presence of previous infarcts or acute pericarditis, changes in electrolyte concentrations, and the administration of cardioactive drugs. Nonetheless, the standard 12-lead electrocardiogram remains a clinically useful method for the detection and localization of transmural infarction.[235]

Although there is general agreement on electrocardiographic and vectorcardiographic criteria for the recognition of infarction of the anterior and inferior myocardial walls (Table 7–5, p. 230), there is less agreement on criteria for lateral and posterior infarcts.[236] Although most patients continue to demonstrate the electrocardiographic changes from an infarction for the rest of their lives, in a substantial minority the typical changes disappear and the electrocardiogram returns to normal after a number of months or, more commonly, years.[237]

The electrocardiographic diagnosis of subendocardial (nontransmural) MI is often difficult and is usually characterized by persistent ST-segment depression or T-wave inversion or both. However, ST-segment and T-wave changes are quite nonspecific and may occur in a variety of conditions, including stable and unstable angina pectoris, ventricular hypertrophy, acute and chronic pericarditis, myocarditis, early repolarization, electrolyte imbalance, shock, metabolic disorders, and following the administration of digitalis (Chap. 7).[236] Serial electrocardiograms may be of considerable aid in differentiating these conditions from subendocardial infarction: Transient changes favor angina or electrolyte disturbances, whereas persistent changes argue for infarction if other causes such as shock, administration of a glycoside, and metabolic disorders can be eliminated. In the final analysis, the diagnosis of subendocardial infarction rests more on the combination of clinical findings and the elevation of serum enzymes than on the electrocardiogram.

Right ventricular infarction is difficult to diagnose by the electrocardiogram, presumably because the right ventricular myocardial mass is small in comparison with the left.

However, ST-segment elevation in right precordial leads (V_1, V_{4R}) has been noted to be a relatively sensitive and specific sign of right ventricular infarction.[238,239] The presence of *atrial infarction* can occasionally be suspected from the electrocardiogram;[240,241] the most common electrocardiographic patterns are depression or elevation of the PQ segment, alterations in the contour of the P wave and abnormal atrial rhythms, including atrial flutter, atrial fibrillation, wandering atrial pacemaker, and AV nodal rhythm.[236]

The relative values of vectorcardiography and conventional scalar electrocardiography in the recognition of MI continue to be debated.[242-244] Table 7–5 (p. 230) lists a number of currently accepted vectorcardiographic criteria for the diagnosis and localization of MI.

ARRHYTHMIAS IN ACUTE MYOCARDIAL INFARCTION

The genesis and diagnosis of arrhythmias are presented in Chapters 19 and 21 and their treatment in Chapters 20 and 38. Discussed in this section is the role of arrhythmias in complicating the course of patients with AMI.

Some abnormality of cardiac rhythm has been noted in 72 to 96 per cent of patients with acute myocardial infarction treated in coronary care units (Table 37–6).[186,245,246] Moreover, many arrhythmias occur prior to hospitalization, before the patient is monitored.[247,247a] Thus, the overall incidence of rhythm disturbance in AMI may actually be as high as 100 per cent. However, these data are difficult to interpret, since ambulatory electrocardiographic monitoring has also disclosed arrhythmias in a high percentage of asymptomatic, middle-aged, actively employed men.[248]

Sinus Bradycardia (also see p. 690). Sinus bradycardia is the most common arrhythmia occurring during the early phases of AMI, and it is particularly frequent in patients with inferior infarction.[247-251] Observations in mobile coronary care units indicate that 40 per cent of patients with AMI have electrocardiographic evidence of sinus bradycardia within the first hour after the onset of symptoms; however, 4 hours after infarction commences, the incidence of sinus bradycardia has declined to 20 per cent. This arrhythmia occurs more frequently in patients with infarcts involving the inferior and posterior walls than in those with infarcts affecting the anterior and lateral walls. It is a manifestation of the Bezold-Jarisch reflex,[251a] is mediated by the vagi, and occurs during thrombolytic reperfusion, particularly of the right coronary artery.[252]

The clinical significance of this arrhythmia is under debate. There is evidence, on the one hand, that sinus bradycardia is an important risk factor during the very early phase of AMI and predisposes the patient to the development of repetitive ventricular arrhythmias and hypotension.[251] On the other hand, it has been suggested on the basis of data obtained in experimental infarction and from some clinical observations that the increased vagal tone that produces sinus bradycardia during the early phase of AMI may actually be protective, perhaps because it reduces myocardial oxygen demands.[250] Thus the acute mortality rate appears to be lower in patients with sinus bradycardia than in patients without this arrhythmia (Table 37–5).

Sinus Tachycardia (p. 689). Almost one-third of patients with an AMI will develop sinus tachycardia at some time during the first few days after the infarction.[246,253] The most common causes of sinus tachycardia are anxiety, persistent pain, and left ventricular failure. Other causes include fever, pericarditis, hypovolemia, atrial infarction, pulmonary embolism, and the administration of cardioaccelerator drugs such as atropine, epinephrine, or isoproterenol. Sinus tachycardia is particularly common in patients with anterior infarction. It is an undesirable rhythm in patients with AMI, since it results in an augmentation of myocardial oxygen consumption, as well as a reduction in the time available for coronary perfusion. Persistent sinus tachycardia may signify persistent heart failure and under these circumstances is a poor prognostic sign associated with an excess mortality.

Atrial Premature Contractions (p. 694). Atrial premature contractions are relatively common after MI, occurring in up to half of all patients.[246,253,254] Atrial premature contractions, and the atrial tachyarrhythmias (paroxysmal supraventricular tachycardia, atrial flutter, and atrial fibrillation) which they often herald, may be caused

TABLE 37–6 ARRHYTHMIAS DETECTED BY ECG MONITORING IN A CORONARY CARE UNIT IN 1000 CONSECUTIVE PATIENTS WITH INFARCTION 1967–71

Arrhythmia	Incidence (%)	Mortality (%)	Association with Ventricular Fibrillation (%)
All ventricular ectopics	57	19	14
i. Salvos (runs)	17	35	26
ii. Bigemini	7	36	22
iii. R on T	6	41	40
iv. VPBs not i, ii or iii	36	15	8
Ventricular tachycardia	10	55	52
Ventricular fibrillation	8	61	
Accelerated idioventricular rhythm	9	19	12
Atrial fibrillation	11	28	
Atrial flutter	3	24	
Paroxysmal supraventricular tachycardia	3	37	
Sinus tachycardia	41	26	11
Sinus bradycardia	25	9	8
All cases		18	8

Reproduced with permission from Norris, R. M., and Singh, B. N.: Arrhythmias in acute myocardial infarction. *In* Norris, R. M. (ed.): Myocardial Infarction. Its Presentation, Pathogenesis and Treatment. Edinburgh, Churchill Livingstone, 1982, p. 55.

by atrial distention secondary to increases in left ventricular diastolic pressure, by pericarditis with its associated atrial epicarditis, or, less commonly, by ischemic injury to the atria and sinus node. Atrial premature beats per se are not associated with an increase in mortality, and cardiac output is unaffected.[255] The importance of atrial premature beats is that they often reflect an elevation of atrial (usually left atrial) pressure and that they may presage sustained supraventricular tachyarrhythmias which may impair cardiac performance. However, occasionally an atrial premature beat may initiate ventricular tachycardia[256] or even ventricular fibrillation[257] in the presence of AMI.

Paroxysmal Supraventricular Tachycardia (also see p. 702). This arrhythmia occurs in 2 to 5 per cent of patients with AMI.[258] Its deleterious effects result from the elevation of myocardial oxygen consumption and the impairment of ventricular performance consequent to the rapid ventricular rate; it is associated with an increase in mortality.

Atrial Flutter (also see p. 697). Atrial flutter is the least common atrial arrhythmia associated with AMI, occurring in only 1 to 3 per cent of all patients.[246,247,253,255] As in patients who develop this arrhythmia in the absence of infarction, atrial flutter is usually associated with 2:1 atrioventricular block. Since the atrial rate ranges from 250 to 350 beats/min, the ventricular rate is usually 125 to 175 beats/min. Atrial flutter is usually transient and is a consequence of augmented sympathetic stimulation of the atria, often occurring in patients with left ventricular failure[246] or pulmonary emboli. Atrial flutter often intensifies hemodynamic deterioration.

Atrial Fibrillation. Atrial fibrillation is far more common than flutter, occurring in 10 to 15 per cent of patients with AMI.[247,253-255,258] As with atrial premature contractions and atrial flutter, fibrillation is usually transient and tends to occur in patients with left ventricular failure but is also observed in patients with pericarditis and ischemic injury to the atria; it occurs more frequently following anterior than inferior infarction. The increased ventricular rate and the loss of the atrial contribution to left ventricular filling—i.e., the atrial kick—result in a significant reduction in cardiac output. As might be anticipated, both atrial fibrillation and flutter are associated with an increased mortality.

Junctional Rhythms (also see p. 702). Sustained junctional rhythms fall into three categories:

1. *AV junctional rhythm* at a rate of 35 to 60 beats/min in which the AV junctional tissue simply assumes the role of the dominant pacemaker when the sinus node is depressed.

2. *Accelerated junctional rhythm* in which increased rhythmicity of the junctional tissue usurps the role of pacemaker, usually at a rate of 70 to 130 beats/min.

These two arrhythmias usually develop and terminate gradually and are characterized by QRS complexes which resemble those of normally conducted beats. Retrograde P waves may be evident, or atrioventricular dissociation may occur, with the junctional rate slightly in excess of the underlying sinus rate. Disagreement exists concerning the prognostic implications of these arrhythmias; some observers attach a poor prognosis to these arrhythmias, whereas others feel that they are benign.[246,254,259] However, in patients with relatively slow junctional rhythm, the process is generally a benign protective escape rhythm and is commonly seen among patients with a slow sinus rate in the presence of inferior myocardial infarction.

3. *Paroxysmal junctional tachycardia* usually manifests rates between 160 and 220 beats/min.[246,254] This arrhythmia is uncommon in AMI, occurring in only 1 to 2 per cent of patients. In contrast to accelerated junctional rhythms, episodes of paroxysmal junctional tachycardia commence and terminate abruptly, thereby resembling other forms of paroxysmal supraventricular tachycardia, and they often occur in the presence of left ventricular failure, ischemia of the conduction system, or digitalis excess.[254] When intraventricular conduction defects are present, it may be difficult to distinguish paroxysmal atrial or junctional tachycardia from ventricular tachycardia. The hemodynamic and prognostic significance of paroxysmal junctional tachycardia is similar to that for paroxysmal atrial tachycardia except that the atrial kick is lost with the junctional rhythm.

Ventricular Premature Beats (VPB's) (see also p. 719). Although VPB's are very frequent, indeed, almost universal[260,261] in the presence of AMI, the value of the so-called warning arrhythmias in the prediction of ventricular fibrillation is not clear. It was believed that warning arrhythmias—defined as frequent VPB's (more than five per minute), VPB's with multiform configuration, early coupling (the "R-on-T" phenomenon), and repetitive patterns in the form of couplets or salvos—presage ventricular fibrillation. However, it is now clear that they are present in as many patients who develop fibrillation as who do not.[186] Several reports have shown that primary ventricular fibrillation (see below) occurs without antecedent warning arrhythmias in 40 to 83 per cent of cases.[262-265] On the other hand, frequent and complex VPB's are commonly observed in patients with AMI who never develop ventricular fibrillation.[262,263]

The prognostic significance of early coupling ("R-on-T" phenomenon) has been reassessed in several experimental[265,266] and clinical[263] studies which have shown that ventricular tachyarrhythmias in patients with AMI are often initiated by a VPB that does *not* fall on an antecedent T wave. As a matter of fact, a majority of ventricular tachycardias in patients with AMI appear to be initiated by a *late*-coupled VPB.[267,268] In two clinical reports on electrocardiographic antecedents of primary ventricular fibrillation, 45 per cent[262] and 41 per cent[263] of episodes of ventricular fibrillation, respectively, were initiated by a late-coupled VPB. However, in one study[269] frequent VPB's showing the R-on-T phenomenon did appear to herald the development of ventricular fibrillation but not of ventricular tachycardia. Thus, the prognostic value, if any, of various forms of VPB's in AMI still requires clarification.

In the post–myocardial infarction period, the prognostic significance of VPB's, particularly frequent ones, appears to be less controversial. Although there is little correlation between ventricular arrhythmias occurring in the early hours or days of AMI and those observed in the late postinfarction period,[270,271] frequent VPB's or ventricular tachycardia *following* hospital discharge do appear to be associated with increased risk of sudden death (p. 783).[272,273]

Ventricular Tachycardia (also see p. 721). Ventricular

tachycardia is generally defined as three or more consecutive ventricular ectopic beats occurring at a frequency exceeding 120 beats/min. The reported incidence of ventricular tachycardia in AMI is in the range of 10 to 40 per cent.[186,246] When this arrhythmia occurs within the first 24 hours, it is usually precipitated by a late VPB and is transient and benign. Ventricular tachycardia occurring late in the course of AMI is more common in patients with transmural infarction and left ventricular dysfunction, is sustained, usually induces marked hemodynamic deterioration, and is associated with a relatively high hospital mortality rate—40 to 50 per cent[246] (Table 37–6). However, the relative contribution to the high mortality rate of this arrhythmia per se, compared with that of the underlying impairment of left ventricular performance due to large infarction, is not clear.[274] In addition, the long-term mortality in patients who exhibit ventricular tachycardia in the late hospital phase of AMI is greatly increased.[275]

Accelerated Idioventricular Rhythm (Fig. 21–37, p. 725). Commonly defined as a ventricular rhythm with a rate of 60 to 110 (or 125) beats/min,[276,277] this arrhythmia is seen in 8 to 20 per cent of patients with AMI, usually in the first 2 days, and seems to be equally common in anterior and inferior infarctions. About half of all episodes of accelerated idioventricular rhythm manifest as an escape rhythm occurring during slowing of the sinus rhythm or gradual speeding of the ventricular pacemaker; the other half of accelerated idioventricular rhythms is initiated by a premature beat.[278] Most episodes are of short duration, and the arrhythmia may terminate abruptly, slow gradually before termination, or be overdriven by acceleration of the basic cardiac rhythm. Variation of the rate is common and may take the form of gradual acceleration, gradual slowing, or a grossly irregular rate. In a few instances, the rate may suddenly double, resulting in rapid ventricular tachycardia and suggesting the presence of a fast ectopic focus with exit block.[278] Accelerated idioventricular rhythms in patients with AMI probably results from enhanced automaticity of Purkinje fibers. In contrast to rapid ventricular tachycardia, accelerated idioventricular rhythms are thought not to affect prognosis.[186,277,278] However, accelerated idioventricular rhythms are frequently associated with episodes of rapid ventricular tachycardia, and in many patients increased automaticity is manifest at times as accelerated idioventricular rhythms and at other times as ventricular tachycardia.

Ventricular Fibrillation (also see p. 728). Ventricular fibrillation occurs in 4 to 18 per cent of patients with AMI treated in coronary care units.[262–264] It occurs with equal incidence in patients with anterior and with inferior transmural infarctions[253] and is rare in patients with nontransmural infarction. This arrhythmia may occur in three settings in hospitalized patients with AMI. Its occurrence as a mechanism of sudden death is discussed in Chapter 23. *Primary* ventricular fibrillation, responsible for more than 80 per cent of all instances of this arrhythmia,[264] occurs suddenly and unexpectedly in patients with no or few signs or symptoms of left ventricular failure. Approximately 60 per cent of episodes occur within 4 hours and 80 per cent within 12 hours of the onset of symptoms.[264] *Secondary* ventricular fibrillation, on the other hand, is the final phase of a progressive downhill course with left ventricular failure and cardiogenic shock.[253] So-called *late* ventricular fibrillation usually occurs 1 to 6 weeks following AMI. Coronary care unit survivors with anteroseptal infarction complicated by right or left bundle branch block are particularly vulnerable to this complication.[279] The prognosis, both immediate and late, is best in the primary form, worst in the secondary form, and intermediate in the late ventricular fibrillation group.

Asystole. This arrhythmia has been reported to occur in 1 to 14 per cent of patients with AMI admitted to coronary care units.[246,253] This wide variation in incidence reflects differences in the definition of this event. The lower incidence rates include only patients who develop asystole either as a primary event or following abnormalities of atrioventricular or intraventricular conduction, whereas the higher rates include patients who develop asystole as a terminal complication. In either event, the mortality is very high, ranging upward from 90 per cent.[246]

HEMODYNAMIC CONSEQUENCES OF CARDIAC ARRHYTHMIAS. Patients with significant left ventricular dysfunction have a relatively fixed stroke volume and depend on changes in heart rate to alter cardiac output. However, there is a narrow range over which the cardiac output is maximal, with significant reductions occurring at faster and lower rates.[280] Thus, all forms of bradycardia and tachycardia may depress the cardiac output in patients with AMI. Although the optimal rate insofar as cardiac output is concerned may exceed 100 per minute, it is important to consider that heart rate is one of the major determinants of myocardial oxygen consumption (p. 1238) and that at more rapid heart rates myocardial energy needs can be elevated to levels that adversely affect ischemic myocardium. Therefore, in patients with AMI, the optimal rate is usually somewhat lower, in the range of 80 to 90 beats/min.

A second factor to consider in assessing the hemodynamic consequences of a particular arrhythmia is the loss

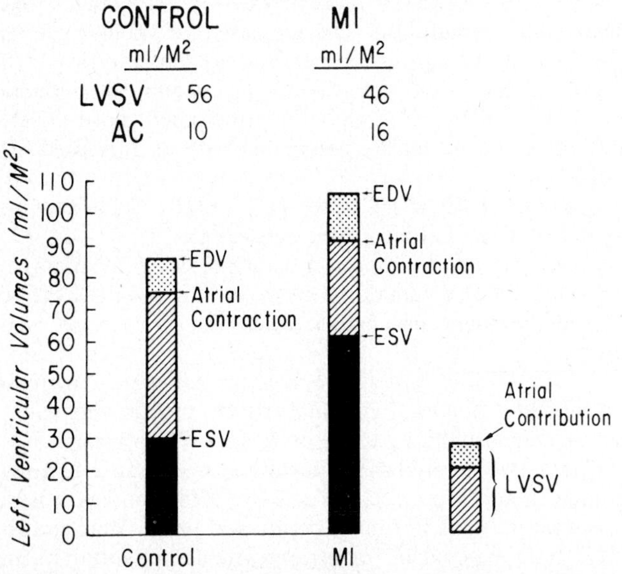

FIGURE 37–14 Average end-diastolic volumes (EDV), end-systolic volumes (ESV), left ventricular stroke volumes (LVSV), and atrial contribution (AC) in a control group of patients and in patients after myocardial infarction (MI). (From Rahimtoola, S. H., et al.: Left atrial transport function in myocardial infarction. Am. J. Med. *59*:686, 1975.)

of atrial transport function, i.e., the atrial "kick."[281] Studies in patients without AMI have demonstrated that loss of atrial transport decreases left ventricular output by 15 to 20 per cent.[282] However, in patients with reduced diastolic left ventricular compliance of any etiology (including AMI), atrial systole is of greater importance for left ventricular filling. In patients with AMI, atrial systole boosts end-diastolic volume by 15 per cent, end-diastolic pressure by 29 per cent, and stroke volume by 35 per cent (Fig. 37–14).[283]

Conduction Disturbances

Ischemic injury can produce blocks at any level of the atrioventricular or intraventricular conduction system. Such blocks may occur in the atrioventricular node, producing various grades of AV block; in either main bundle branch, producing right or left bundle branch block; and in the anterior and posterior divisions of the left bundle, producing left anterior or left posterior (fascicular) divisional blocks (Table 37–7). Disturbances of conduction can, of course, occur in various combinations. The mechanisms and recognition of intraventricular conduction disturbances are discussed in Chapter 7 and of atrioventricular conduction disturbances in Chapter 21.

First-degree AV Block (Fig. 21–42, p. 730). First-degree AV block occurs in 4 to 14 per cent of patients with AMI admitted to coronary care units. His bundle electrocardiographic studies have shown that almost all patients with first-degree AV block have disturbances in conduction *above* the bundle of His, i.e., intranodal. The localization of the site of block is of considerable importance, since the development of complete heart block and ventricular asystole is restricted almost exclusively to those patients with first-degree block in whom the conduction disturbance is *below* the bundle of His,[284] and this occurs more commonly in patients with anterior infarction and in those with associated bifascicular block.[285,286]

Second-degree AV Block

Mobitz Type I, or Wenckebach (Fig. 21–43, p. 731). Mobitz type I block occurs in 4 to 10 per cent of patients with AMI admitted to coronary care units[246,285] and accounts for about 90 per cent of all patients with second-degree AV block. This type of block (1) generally occurs within the AV node; (2) is usually associated with narrow QRS complexes; (3) is presumably secondary to ischemic injury; (4) commonly occurs in patients with inferior myocardial infarction; (5) is usually transient and does not persist for more than 72 hours after infarction; (6) may be intermittent; and (7) rarely progresses to complete AV block. First-degree and type I second-degree AV block do not appear to affect survival, are most commonly associated with inferior wall infarction, and are caused by ischemia of the AV node.

Mobitz Type II (Fig. 21–44, p. 732). This is a rare conduction defect following AMI, occurring in only 10 per cent of all cases of second-degree block;[246] thus, the overall incidence of Mobitz type II block after infarction is less than 1 per cent. In contrast to Mobitz type I block, type II second-degree block (1) usually originates from a lesion in the conduction system below the bundle of His;[285] (2) is associated with a wide QRS complex; (3) often, but not invariably, reflects trifascicular block with impaired conduction distal to the bundle of His; (4) often progresses suddenly to complete atrioventricular block; and (5) is almost always associated with anterior rather than inferior infarction.

Complete (Third-degree) AV Block. The atrioventricular conduction system has a dual blood supply, the AV branch of the right coronary artery and the septal perforating branch from the left anterior descending coronary artery. Therefore, complete AV block can occur in patients with either anterior or inferior infarction. Complete AV block develops in 5 to 8 per cent of patients with AMI. As with other forms of AV block, the prognosis depends on the anatomical location of the block in the conduction system and the size of the infarction.

In general, complete heart block in patients with inferior infarction results from an intranodal lesion and develops gradually, often progressing from first-degree and type I second-degree block. The escape rhythm is often junctional with a narrow QRS complex in 60 per cent of cases and a wide QRS in the remaining 40 per cent. This form of complete AV block is usually transient and resolves in 1 week. The mortality is approximately 20 to 25 per cent.[286,287]

In patients with anterior infarction, third-degree AV block often occurs with dramatic suddenness, 12 to 24 hours after the onset of the infarct. It is usually preceded by intraventricular block, not lower degrees of AV block. Such patients have escape rhythms with wide QRS complexes and rates less than 40 beats/min; ventricular asystole may occur quite suddenly in these patients. The mortality in this group of patients is extremely high, approximately 70 to 80 per cent.[288–291]

The prognosis for patients with AV block complicating AMI depends on the extent and secondarily on the anatomical site of the myocardial injury. Thus, patients with inferior infarction often have concomitant ischemia or infarction of the AV node secondary to hypoperfusion of the AV nodal artery. However, the His-Purkinje system usually escapes injury in such individuals. As noted above, junctional escape rhythms with narrow QRS complexes occur commonly in this setting. Hemodynamic derangements are often mild in these patients, and mortality is only slightly increased.[292] In patients with anterior infarction, AV block usually develops as a result of extensive

TABLE 37–7 INCIDENCE AND PROGNOSES OF CONDUCTION BLOCKS IN ACUTE MYOCARDIAL INFARCTION

Type of Conduction Block	Incidence of Conduction Block (%)	Patients with Conduction Block Who Develop Complete AV Block (%)	Mortality (%)
None		6	15
LAH	5	3	27
LPH	1	0	42
RBBB + LAH	5	46	45
RBBB + LPH	1	43	57
RBBB	2	43	46
LBBB	5	20	44

Adapted from Mullins, C. B., and Atkins, J. M.: Prognoses and management of ventricular conduction blocks in acute myocardial infarction. Mod. Concepts Cardiovasc. Dis. *45*:129, 1976, by permission of the American Heart Association, Inc.

septal necrosis that involves the bundle branches; the high mortality in this group of patients with slow idioventricular rhythms and wide QRS complexes is the consequence of extensive myocardial necrosis resulting in severe left ventricular failure and often shock.[292]

Intraventricular Block (Table 37–7). Intraventricular conduction disturbances, i.e., block within one or more of the three subdivisions (fascicles) of the His-Purkinje system (the anterior and posterior divisions of the left bundle and the right bundle, p. 217) occur in 10 to 20 per cent of patients with AMI. The right bundle branch and the left posterior division have a dual blood supply from the left anterior descending and right coronary artery, whereas the left anterior division is supplied by septal perforators originating from the left anterior descending coronary artery. Not all conduction blocks observed in patients with AMI can be considered to be complications of infarcts, since almost half are already present at the time the first electrocardiogram is recorded, and they may represent antecedent disease of the conduction system.

Preexisting bundle branch block or divisional block is less often associated with the development of complete heart block in patients with AMI than are newly acquired conduction defects. First-degree AV block adds to the risk of intraventricular conduction defects progressing to complete AV block.[293,294]

Left anterior divisional block (Fig. 7–24, p. 218) occurs in 3 to 5 per cent of patients with AMI,[295,296] and, as noted in Table 37–7, mortality is increased in these patients, though not as much as in patients with other forms of conduction block. Since left anterior divisional block may be difficult to diagnose in the presence of inferior wall infarction, it may be helpful to employ the vectorcardiogram to establish this diagnosis.

Left posterior divisional block occurs in only 1 per cent of patients with AMI admitted to coronary care units. The posterior fascicle is larger than the anterior fascicle, and, in general, a larger infarct is required to block it. As a consequence, mortality is markedly increased (Table 37–7).[295] Complete AV block is not a frequent complication of *either* form of isolated divisional block.

Right bundle branch block occurs in approximately 2 per cent of patients with AMI and frequently leads to AV block because it is often a new lesion, associated with anteroseptal infarction. The mortality is high even if complete AV block does not occur (Table 37–7).[246,293,295–297]

Bidivisional (Bifascicular) Block. The combination of right bundle branch block with either left anterior or posterior divisional block or the combination of left anterior and posterior divisional blocks (i.e., left bundle branch block) is known as bidivisional block (p. 219). If new block occurs in two of the three divisions of the conduction system, the risk of developing complete AV block is quite high.[246,295] Mortality is also high because of the occurrence of severe pump failure secondary to the extensive myocardial necrosis required to produce such an extensive intraventricular block.[298] Left bundle branch block occurs in approximately 5 per cent of patients with AMI (Table 37–7). Although the latter defect progresses to complete AV block only half as frequently as does right bundle branch block, it is associated with as high a mortality as right bundle branch block and the other two forms of bifascicular block,[246,293,295] and with a high late mortality.[186] Patients with intraventricular conduction defects, particularly right bundle branch block, account for the majority of patients who develop ventricular fibrillation late in their hospital stay. However, the high mortality in these patients occurs even in the absence of AV block and appears to be related to cardiac failure and massive infarction rather than to the conduction disturbance.

Roentgenographic and Radionuclide Studies

Roentgenography (see also p. 160). The initial chest roentgenogram in patients with AMI is almost invariably a film portably obtained in the emergency room or the coronary care unit. Two findings are common: signs of left ventricular failure and cardiomegaly. Although the pulmonary vascular markings on the roentgenogram generally reflect the left ventricular end-diastolic pressure, significant discrepancies may occur because of what have been termed *diagnostic lags* and *post-therapeutic phase lags.* In the former, patients may have elevated left ventricular filling pressures and normal chest roentgenograms, and, because of the time required for pulmonary edema to accumulate after left ventricular filling pressure has become elevated, 12 hours may elapse before the radiographic findings reflect the hemodynamic status. The post-therapeutic phase lag represents the longer time interval, generally 1 or 2 days, required for pulmonary edema to resorb and the radiographic signs of pulmonary congestion to clear after left ventricular filling pressure has returned toward normal.[299–301]

Cardiomegaly in a patient with AMI usually signifies prior infarction or another form of antecedent heart disease with subsequent left ventricular dilatation, and it is usually associated with significantly impaired left ventricular function.[302] The converse is not true, however, in that patients may have increased end-diastolic volumes and still demonstrate a normal-sized heart on roentgenographic examination. The degree of congestion and the size of the left side of the heart on the initial chest film are highly useful independent predictors for defining groups of patients with AMI who are at increased risk of dying within the first year after the acute event.[303]

Radioisotopic Studies. All major forms of cardiac imaging—radionuclide angiography, perfusion scintigraphy, infarct avid scintigraphy, and positive emission tomography—are useful in detecting AMI, in assessing infarct size, in determining the effects of the infarct on ventricular function, and in establishing prognosis. The application of these techniques is discussed in Chapter 11A.[304–306]

Echocardiography (See also p. 127)

Although *M-mode echocardiography* is a sensitive technique for examining regional left ventricular wall motion,[306a] it is limited to the imaging of small segments of the interventricular septum and posterior left ventricular wall; rarely, small segments of the anterior wall can be imaged as well. Therefore, abnormalities of regional wall motion and even left ventricular aneurysms, particularly those involving the anterior wall, may be missed completely.[307] Despite this obvious shortcoming, some useful information

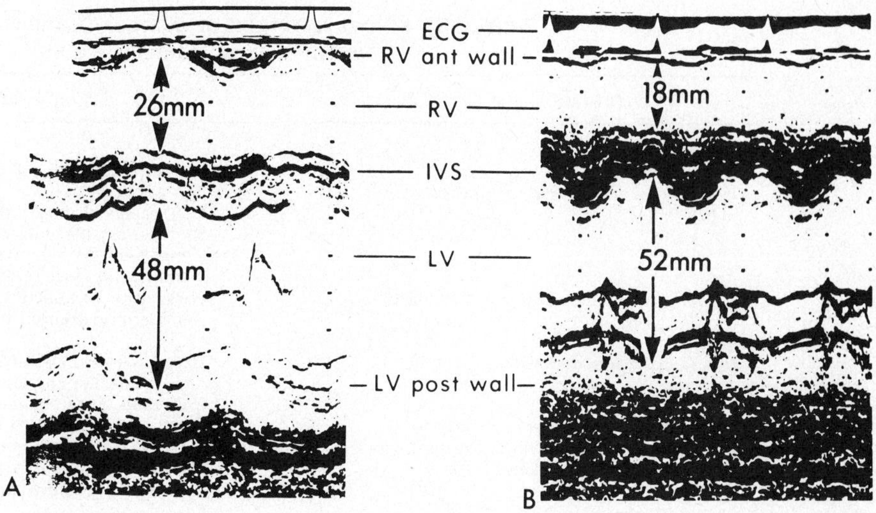

FIGURE 37–15 Echocardiograms. *A,* Patient with RV infarction and dilatation. *B,* Patient with LV inferior infarction and normal RV dimensions. (From Sharpe, D. N., et al.: The noninvasive diagnosis of right ventricular infarction. Circulation *57*:483, 1978, by permission of the American Heart Association, Inc.)

can be obtained from patients with acute or old MI, particularly in the diagnosis of complications of MI (Table 37–8). Abnormalities of left ventricular wall motion, usually corresponding to the electrocardiographic site of infarction, may be recognized in the majority of patients with transmural infarction, and exaggerated normal motion can be found in noninfarcted areas in approximately one-third of patients.[308] An increased internal diameter of the left ventricle, determined by echocardiography, correlates closely with clinical, hemodynamic, and angiographic signs of heart failure.[309] The echocardiographic distance between the E-point of the anterior mitral valve and the septum has been shown to correlate well with the global left ventricular ejection fraction in patients with AMI.[310]

M-mode echocardiography is also useful in detecting small pericardial effusions in patients with postinfarction pericarditis.[311] A number of changes—including increased amplitude of upper septal wall motion; dilatation of the right ventricle; and abnormal mitral valve motion in diastole, suggesting increased mitral valve flow—have been noted in the echocardiograms of patients with rupture of the ventricular septum after MI. Although not specific, this combination of echocardiographic findings provides a useful clue to the diagnosis of septal rupture.[312,313] M-mode echocardiography can also be employed in the noninvasive diagnosis of right ventricular infarction. Findings include an increased right ventricular end-diastolic diameter and an increased ratio of right ventricular to left ventricular end-diastolic diameter (Fig. 37–15).[314]

Two-dimensional echocardiography can provide both longitudinal and transverse views of the left ventricle, and a much larger fraction of the ventricular wall—including significant portions of the left ventricular apical, anterior, septal, inferior, and posterior walls—can be imaged[315] by this method than by the M-mode technique. Areas of abnormal regional wall motion are observed almost universally in patients with AMI (Fig. 37–16).[316,317] Left ventricular function, estimated from two-dimensional echocardiograms, correlates well and sometimes predicts the clinical course. The detection of wall-motion disorders outside the infarct zone predicts the development of heart failure or cardiogenic shock. In many patients, regional abnormalities of left ventricular wall motion detected during AMI improve during the recovery phase. In addition, in patients with AMI who develop a loud systolic murmur, two-dimensional echocardiography can detect and localize a ventricular septal defect, as well as detect mitral regurgitation and elucidate its cause.[318–321]

Systolic Time Intervals and Apexcardiograms

(See also Chap. 4)

Systolic time intervals (preejection period [PEP] and left ventricular ejection time [LVET]) have been employed to

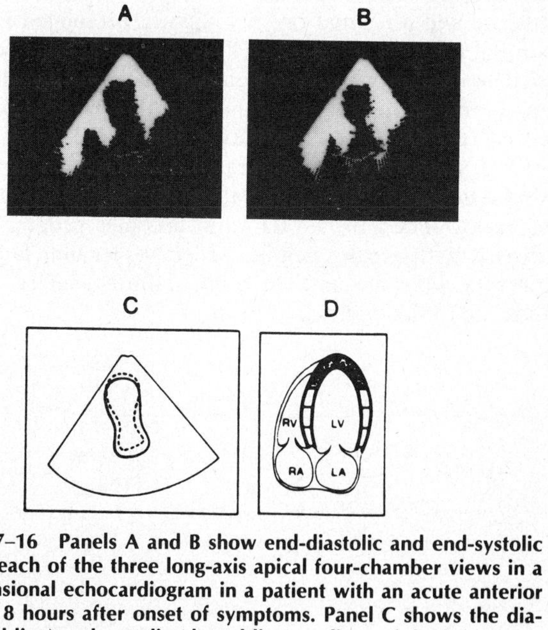

FIGURE 37–16 Panels A and B show end-diastolic and end-systolic frames of each of the three long-axis apical four-chamber views in a two-dimensional echocardiogram in a patient with an acute anterior infarction, 8 hours after onset of symptoms. Panel C shows the diastolic (solid line) and systolic (dotted line) outlines of the left ventricle. There is extensive asynergy. In Panel D the dotted segments represent the visually estimated asynergic area of the left ventricular wall, calculated at 37 per cent. Ao = aorta; LA = left atrium; LV = left ventricle; RV = right ventricle; RA = right atrium. (Reproduced with permission from Visser, C. A., Kan, G., Lie, K. I., Becker, A. E., and Durrer, D.: Apex two dimensional echocardiography. Alternative approach to quantification of acute myocardial infarction. Br. Heart J. *47*:461, 1982.)

TABLE 37–8 COMPLICATIONS OF ACUTE MYOCARDIAL INFARCTION DETECTED BY ECHOCARDIOGRAPHY

Complication	Echocardiographic Manifestations
Early	
Arrhythmias	Not applicable
Heart block and/or marked bradycardia	Not applicable
Shock	Large areas of noncontractile LV myocardium Right ventricular infarction: impaired RV wall motion; increased RV size with or without abnormal septal motion; absence of pericardial fluid
Pulmonary edema (congestive heart failure)	Large areas of noncontractile LV myocardium and/or anatomical complications (e.g., ventricular septal defect)
Subacute	
Infarct extension/expansion	Expansion demonstrated by disproportionate transmural diastolic thinning and associated regional ventricular dilation on two-dimensional echocardiography (2DE)
Severe mitral regurgitation secondary to papillary muscle dysfunction or rupture	Rupture demonstrated by visualization of untethered mitral valve leaflet on 2DE
Acute ventricular septal defect	2DE visualization of septal rent; negative contrast effect after IV fluid injection
Subacute to late	
Ventricular aneurysm	Localized interruption in the diastolic configuration of LV wall; orifice to aneurysm is wide
Ventricular pseudoaneurysm	Demonstration of narrow neck leading into the false aneurysm cavity
Thromboembolism	Visualization of LV thrombus

Reproduced with permission from Strauss, W. E., and Parisi, A. F.: Echocardiography. *In* Morganroth, J., Parisi, A., and Pohost, G. M. (eds.): Noninvasive Cardiac Imaging. Copyright © 1983 by Year Book Medical Publishers, Inc., Chicago.

estimate the state of left ventricular function in patients with AMI, but considerable disagreement exists concerning the value of these measurements in this condition.[322–325] Because of the adrenergic hyperactivity commonly present in patients with AMI, comparison of systolic time intervals in patients with AMI with those obtained from patients with chronic, stable, left ventricular dysfunction is not valid. In general, patients with AMI demonstrate an abnormally short LVET, reflecting a reduction of stroke volume and a normal or only slightly prolonged PEP. The normal or nearly normal PEP should, in reality, be considered to be abnormally prolonged, since a markedly shortened PEP is normally obtained in the presence of excess adrenergic activity. Patients with AMI and normal PEP/LVET ratios demonstrate fewer clinical signs of left ventricular failure than do patients with abnormally elevated ratios. The PEP/LVET ratio becomes progressively increased with greater degrees of left ventricular failure, and patients who succumb to pump failure usually have the most abnormally elevated ratios.

Serial measurements of systolic time intervals usually reflect the changes in left ventricular function that frequently occur during the course of an acute myocardial infarction. Thus, the PEP/LVET ratio rises in patients with infarct extension.

Apexcardiography can be employed to gain information about left ventricular systolic and diastolic function (p. 58). Abnormalities of the *a* wave and systolic wave of the apexcardiogram correlate with measurements of left ventricular function obtained at the time of cardiac catheterization (Fig. 37–17).[326] Moreover, paradoxical motion of the left ventricle secondary to an aneurysm can be identified by apexcardiography. Thus, Khan and Haywood recorded serial apexcardiograms in 40 patients with AMI and in 21 patients with angiographically proved left ventricular aneurysms. Increased amplitude of the *a* wave and an abnormal morphology of the systolic wave (presence of an abnormally shaped systolic wave or a secondary systolic bulge) of the apexcardiogram correlated well with akinesia or dyskinesia or both identified angiographically.[326]

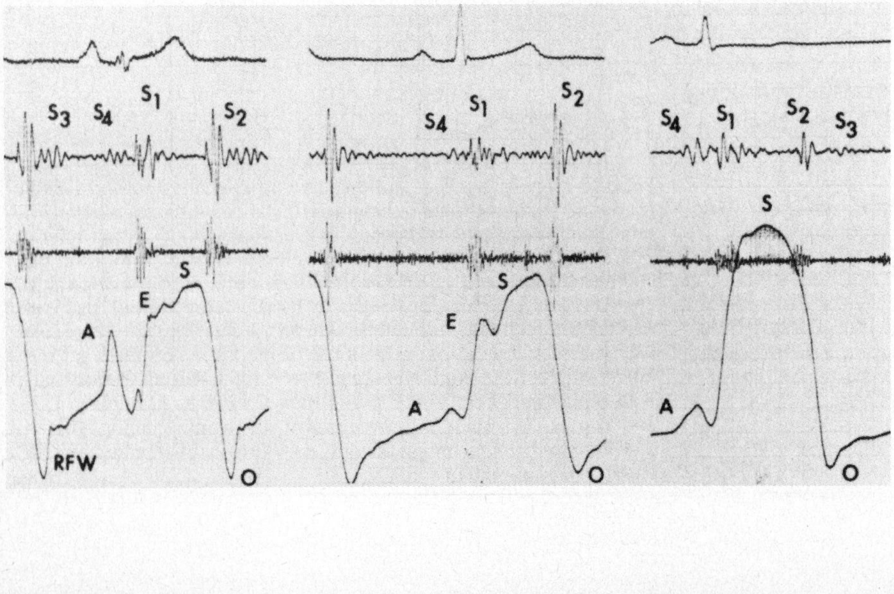

FIGURE 37–17 Examples of abnormal apexcardiograms frequently seen in acute myocardial infarction. Note tall *a* wave and prominent secondary systolic wave (S) (systolic bulge) in left panel, normal *a* wave and bifid systolic wave corresponding to E point and secondary systolic wave in middle panel, and *a* wave normal in height and monophasic secondary systolic wave in panel on right. S_2, second heart sound; and RFW, rapid filling wave. (From Khan, A. H., et al.: Value of serial apex cardiograms during and after myocardial infarction. Chest *70*:367, 1976.)

Hemodynamics and Angiography

Hemodynamic monitoring in the coronary care unit has become widespread in recent years.[140,141,327–330] A balloon-tipped catheter is advanced, usually with fluoroscopic guidance, from a peripheral vein through the right heart and into the pulmonary artery (Chap. 9). Judicious positioning of the catheter allows recording of the pulmonary arterial pressure when the balloon is deflated and of the pulmonary capillary wedge pressure when the balloon is inflated.[327] Blood may be sampled from the tip of the catheter in the pulmonary artery and, in certain models, from a second lumen opening into the right atrium. In addition, some models of pulmonary artery balloon catheters have a thermistor near the tip for recording thermodilution cardiac output.[331] Thus, a single catheter in the right heart can yield the following information: saturation of blood in the pulmonary artery and right atrium, pressures in the pulmonary artery, pulmonary wedge position, and right atrium and cardiac output. A good correlation has been found between pulmonary artery occlusive pressure (which is equal to pulmonary capillary pressure) and left ventricular diastolic pressure in patients with AMI.[332]

Pulmonary arterial systolic pressure is distinctly elevated in patients with AMI and in individuals with chronic obstructive pulmonary disease or pulmonary embolism. Patients with significant mitral regurgitation complicating MI may demonstrate tall *v* waves in the pulmonary capillary wedge positions (p. 1080) (Fig. 37–18). Patients with rupture of the interventricular septum have increased right ventricular and pulmonary arterial blood oxygen saturation, as well as wide pulmonary arterial pulse pressures.[140] These patients may also demonstrate tall *v* waves in the pulmonary wedge pressure tracing.[333]

In the past, central venous or right atrial pressure was used to gauge the degree of left ventricular failure in patients with MI. This estimate is fraught with error, since central venous pressure actually reflects *right* rather than left ventricular function (Figure 38–3, p. 1312). Right ventricular function, and therefore systemic venous pressure, may be normal or nearly so in patients with significant left ventricular failure.[140] Conversely, patients with right ventricular failure due to right ventricular infarction or pulmonary embolism may exhibit elevated right atrial and central venous pressures despite normal left ventricular function.[334] Low values for right atrial and central venous pressures imply hypovolemia, whereas elevated right atrial pressures usually result from right ventricular failure secondary to left ventricular failure, pulmonary hypertension, or right ventricular infarction, or, less commonly, from tricuspid regurgitation or pericardial tamponade.

Both the prognosis and the clinical status are related to the cardiac output. Patients with normal cardiac output after MI have an expected mortality as low as 1 per cent;[141] prognosis worsens as cardiac output declines. Patients with cardiac indices in the range of 2.7 to 4.3 liters/min/sq meter usually have no clinical signs of impaired perfusion, whereas patients with cardiac indices ranging from 1.8 to 2.2 liters/min/sq meter demonstrate early signs of hypoperfusion (cool skin and decreasing urine output and mental acuity). Patients whose cardiac index is less than 1.8 liters/min/sq meter are usually in shock. The pulmonary artery occlusive pressure reflects the state of left ventricular filling, its compliance, and its ability to empty. As pulmonary pressure rises, progressive increases in pulmonary congestion occur. Increasing degrees of pulmonary congestion can also be monitored through changes in the physical examination (development of tachypnea, rales, wheezing, or pleural effusion) or on the chest roentgenogram.

Patients with intraventricular conduction defects or heart block or both after anterior infarction have lower cardiac indices and higher pulmonary capillary wedge pressures than do patients without these conduction disturbances. On the other hand, patients with these conduction defects and inferior myocardial infarction usually do not demonstrate such hemodynamic abnormalities. The difference in hemodynamic measurements between these two groups is the result of the more extensive myocardial necrosis in patients with anterior infarction.[292]

HEMODYNAMIC FINDINGS IN VENTRICULAR SEPTAL RUPTURE AND MITRAL REGURGITATION. It may be difficult, on clinical grounds, to distinguish between acute mitral regurgitation and rupture of the ventricular septum in patients with AMI who suddenly

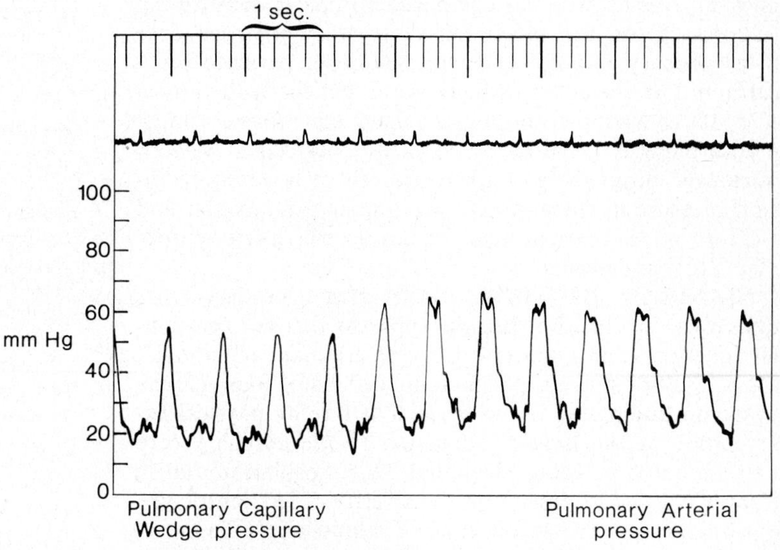

FIGURE 37–18 Acute mitral regurgitation secondary to ruptured chord from infarcted papillary muscle in a 45-year-old man. Tracing shows mitral regurgitation, tall *v* waves in pulmonary capillary wedge and pulmonary artery tracings. (Courtesy of Ira S. Ockene, M.D.)

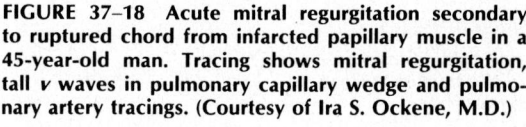

develop a loud systolic murmur.[335] One approach to the differentiation is first-pass radionuclide ventriculography (p. 356). In addition, a right-heart catheterization with a balloon-tipped catheter can readily distinguish between these two complications. Patients with ventricular septal rupture demonstrate a "step-up" in oxygen saturation in blood samples from the right ventricle and pulmonary artery compared with those from the right atrium; patients with acute mitral regurgitation lack this step-up; they may demonstrate tall *v* waves in both the pulmonary capillary and the pulmonary arterial pressure tracings (Fig. 37–18). Cardiac output is usually significantly decreased in both conditions.

Left Ventricular Function after Myocardial Infarction. As noted, angiographic or echocardiographic evidence of abnormal regional left ventricular wall motion is very commonly present after AMI;[336] some improvement in function occurs during uncomplicated convalescence, whereas extension (or possibly expansion) of the infarction increases the segment of the left ventricle that is hypokinetic or akinetic.[337] Patients who have suffered a transmural MI often demonstrate increased left ventricular end-diastolic volume and pressure and reduced ejection fraction, velocity of circumferential fiber shortening, and cardiac index.[338,339] Some degree of mitral regurgitation is present in almost half of all patients following transmural infarction. Discrete aneurysmal bulges are seen on the left ventriculogram in about one-fifth of such patients.[336,340] Patients in cardiogenic shock invariably demonstrate markedly abnormal hemodynamics, with elevated pulmonary capillary wedge pressure (> 15 mm Hg), reduced cardiac index (< 2.3 liters/min/sq meter), and severely reduced ejection fractions.[341]

PROGNOSIS (Table 37–9)

Both short-term and long-term survival following an AMI depends on a number of factors;[341a,341b,341c] the most important are the state of left ventricular function and the severity of the obstructive lesions in the coronary vascular bed perfusing residual viable myocardium. At one extreme, the prognosis is best for the patient with normal intrinsic coronary vessels who has completed an infarct constituting less than 5 per cent of the left ventricle as a consequence of a coronary embolus and who has no jeopardized myocardium. At the other extreme is the patient with a massive infarct who is in cardiogenic shock and whose residual myocardium is perfused by markedly obstructed vessels; obviously, progression of atherosclerosis or lowering perfusion pressure in these vessels will impair the function and viability of the residual myocardium on which left ventricular function depends.

CLINICAL FACTORS. Soon after coronary care units were instituted, it became apparent that left ventricular function is an important early determinant of survival. Thus, Killip studied patients divided into four groups based on findings of left ventricular failure by physical examination at the time of admission to the coronary care unit; as noted in Tables 37–3 and 37–5, hospital mortality from MI depends directly on the severity of left ventricular dysfunction present at the time of admission.[342] Similarly, Peel[343] and Norris[344] and their collaborators developed prognostic indices for patients with AMI. Although they used historical, electrocardiographic, and radiological data to predict hospital mortality, evidence of left ventricular failure heavily weights these indices in the direction of poor prognosis.

Certain demographic and historical factors are associated with a poor prognosis after infarction, including male sex, age greater than 60 years and a history of diabetes mellitus, hypertension, prior angina pectoris, and previous myocardial infarction. The last factor may contribute to a poor prognosis, since it indicates loss of viable myocardium preceding the reference infarct.

INFARCT EXTENSION. Extension occurs in 10 to 30 per cent of patients with AMI during the first 10 days.[344a] It is generally defined as reelevation or reappearance of CK-MB in the serum after the initial peak. Neither chest pain nor the electrocardiogram provides accurate markers for recognizing infarct extension. The majority of patients with cardiogenic shock have developed infarct extension.[112] In the prospective study of patients, it was found that mortality in those experiencing extension is more than double that noted in patients in whom extension did not occur.[345–348] Marmor reported that infarct extension occurred most frequently in obese females and was most common in patients with nontransmural infarction.[348] Presumably, the higher mortality associated with infarct extension is related to the larger mass of myocardium whose function becomes compromised.

HEMODYNAMICS. Physiological evidence of compromised left ventricular function also correlates with hospital mortality in AMI,[349] as already discussed (Table 37–

TABLE 37–9 FACTORS ASSOCIATED WITH POOR PROGNOSIS AFTER MYOCARDIAL INFARCTION

Left Ventricular Function
- Clinical evidence of heart failure
- Hemodynamic evidence of heart failure
- Invasive and/or noninvasive demonstration of poor left ventricular systolic function

Electrocardiogram
- Persistent, repetitive, ventricular ectopic activity
- Atrioventricular and intraventricular conduction defects
- Persistent ST-segment depression or elevation (the latter without pericarditis)
- Persistent T-wave inversions
- Abnormal Q waves in multiple leads
- Atrial fibrillation
- Left ventricular hypertrophy

Chest Roentgenogram
- Cardiomegaly

Age > 60 Years
Male Sex
Presence of Additional Diseases
- Previous myocardial infarction or angina
- Post–myocardial infarction angina
- Diabetes mellitus
- Hypertension

Laboratory Data
- Markedly elevated cardiac enzymes (e.g., GOT > 250 Karmen units; CK > 2000 IU)
- Elevated blood urea nitrogen
- Absence of collateral blood vessels to region of reduced perfusion by angiography

Psychological Aspects
- Psychosis

3). Thus, patients with hemodynamic (elevated pulmonary capillary wedge pressure or depressed cardiac index or both) or ventriculographic (depressed ejection fraction and elevated end-systolic volume by radionuclide angiography) evidence of left ventricular failure have a worse prognosis than patients without these findings.[350,351,351a] The *chest roentgenogram* is also prognostic, since patients with cardiomegaly or increased heart volume after infarction do not fare as well as individuals without these features.[303] Since impaired ventricular function is generally a manifestation of the cumulative extent of myocardial damage sustained, one important determinant of prognosis is, therefore, *infarct size.* Thus, patients with markedly elevated plasma enzyme levels (CK > 2000 IU) often manifest left ventricular failure with concomitant poor prognosis. Furthermore, prognosis for as long as 4 years after an initial infarction is related to infarct size estimated from plasma CK time-activity curves at the time of the acute episode (Figure 38–8, p. 1319).[224] A large defect or multiple defects on a thallium-201 perfusion scintigram, obtained very early in the course of AMI, also presumably related to infarct size, is associated with a high incidence of mortality or subsequent cardiac events.[351,351a] Similarly, patients with largest infarcts on technetium-99m scintigrams have the poorest prognosis.[305,352]

ELECTROCARDIOGRAM. Patients whose electrocardiogram demonstrates persistent advanced (e.g., Mobitz type II, second-degree, or third-degree atrioventricular block) or new intraventricular conduction abnormalities (bifascicular or trifascicular) in the course of an AMI have a worse prognosis than do patients without these abnormalities (Table 37–7). Other electrocardiographic findings that augur poorly for the postinfarction patient are repetitive ventricular ectopic activity (Table 37–6) (couplets, runs), persistent horizontal or downsloping ST-segment depression and Q waves in multiple leads, atrial arrhythmias (especially atrial fibrillation), and voltage criteria for left ventricular hypertrophy.

ST-segment depressions in leads other than those with acute Q waves are also a poor prognostic sign; for example, patients with acute inferior wall infarcts who demonstrate ST-segment depressions in precordial leads have a worse prognosis than do patients without this finding. There is controversy concerning whether these ST-segment depressions reflect reciprocal electrical changes, associated disease of the left anterior descending coronary artery, or, most likely, a larger inferior infarct.[353–355,355a] Similarly, patients who develop angina during the first 10 days following infarction, with new electrocardiographic changes distant from the acute infarct, i.e., angina "at a distance," have a distinctly worse prognosis than do patients having postinfarct angina with ischemia in the infarct zone.[356]

TRANSMURAL VERSUS SUBENDOCARDIAL INFARCTION. Patients with myocardial infarction are usually classified into two groups on the basis of electrocardiographic criteria: *transmural and subendocardial (nontransmural) infarction.* Transmural infarctions demonstrate definite Q waves, loss of R-wave voltage, or both, whereas subendocardial infarctions are characterized by only ST- or T-wave changes on their electrocardiograms. Of course, subendocardial and even transmural infarction can occur in the absence of electrocardiographic changes.

Earlier workers noted a more favorable clinical course in patients with nontransmural infarctions compared with individuals having transmural infarcts,[357–359] and it is agreed that the acute mortality in patients with subendocardial infarcts is approximately half that in patients with transmural infarcts.[347,360] However, it is now clear that nontransmural infarctions are not benign conditions.[361–363] Thus, 60 per cent of patients with subendocardial infarction have critical obstruction in two or three of the major coronary arteries, and approximately 20 per cent go on to develop an acute transmural infarction within 3 months of the subendocardial infarct.[361] In one series almost half of the patients with subendocardial infarction developed unstable angina during a follow-up period averaging 11 months.[364] In another, the incidence of infarct extension or early recurrent infarction was high.[361] Hutter et al. have reported high early and late reinfarction rates in patients with subendocardial infarctions and comparable late mortalities in patients with subendocardial and transmural infarctions.[360]

The correlation between the electrocardiographic findings of transmural and subendocardial myocardial infarction and their pathological counterparts is not good.[361a] Indeed, many patients with pathological transmural infarctions have no Q waves or have loss of R waves on the electrocardiogram and vice versa. Consequently, it has been suggested that the electrocardiographic terms transmural and subendocardial be changed to "Q-wave" and "non–Q-wave infarctions."

Notwithstanding the terminology, non–Q-wave infarctions (whether they represent subendocardial infarcts or not) may be considered relatively unstable conditions associated with a low initial mortality rate, a high risk of later infarction, and a high late mortality rate. The recognition in differences between the natural histories of these two forms of infarction suggests a more aggressive diagnostic approach, perhaps followed by early surgical treatment in suitable patients who have sustained an acute non–Q-wave infarction.

LATE POSTINFARCT ASSESSMENT. Following recovery from AMI—i.e., by 2 to 4 weeks after the event —long-term prognosis can be evaluated by ambulatory electrocardiographic monitoring and exercise testing.[364a] The development of ST-segment abnormalities, typical angina or exercise limitation by dyspnea at low levels of exercise (heart rate < 120 beats/min or exercise duration < 6 minutes on the Bruce protocol [p. 266]), and a major (> 2 mm) ST-segment depression and a stress-induced fall in blood pressure at any level of exercise signify a poor prognosis (p. 274 and 1389).[351,365,365a,365b,366] Radionuclide angiography,[366a] as well as coronary arteriography and left ventriculography, can provide additional important prognostic information, but the invasive tests are ordinarily carried out only if the patient is symptomatic or if the noninvasive tests suggest a poor prognosis and if the results of these examinations would alter the management (p. 1327) (Chap. 39).[361,368] Recent evidence indicates that electrical instability, as reflected in frequent, multiple, or complex ventricular extrasystoles, and left ventricular dysfunction, as reflected in a depressed left ventricular ejection fraction (< 40 per cent) 10 days after the occurrence of an AMI, are independent risk factors; the presence of both risk factors was associated with an increased 15-month mortality.[369,370]

References

1. May, G. S., Furberg, C. D., Eberlein, K. A., and Gerard, B. J.: Secondary prevention after myocardial infarction: a review of short term acute phase trials. Prog. Cardiovasc. Dis. *25*:335, 1983.
2. Blackburn, H.: Progress in the epidemiology and prevention of coronary heart disease. *In* Yu, P. N., and Goodwin, J. F. (eds.): Progress in Cardiology. Philadelphia, Lea and Febiger, 1974, p. 1.
3. Feinleib, M., Havlik, R. J., and Thom, T. J.: The changing pattern of ischemic heart disease. J. Cardiovasc. Med. *7*:139, 1982.

PATHOLOGY

4. Bloor, C. M.: Cardiac Pathology. Philadelphia, J. B. Lippincott Co., 1978, p. 176.
5. Mallory, G. K., White, P. D., and Salcedo-Salger, J.: The speed of healing of myocardial infarction: A study of the pathological anatomy in seventy-two cases. Am. Heart J. *18*:647, 1939.
6. Fishbein, M. C., Maclean, D., and Maroko, P. R.: The histopathological evolution of myocardial infarction. Chest *73*:843, 1978.
7. Buja, L. M., and Willerson, J. T.: Clinicopathologic correlates of acute ischemic heart disease syndromes. Am. J. Cardiol. *47*:343, 1981.
8. Schlesinger, M. J., and Reiner, L.: Focal myocytolysis of the heart. Am. J. Pathol. *31*:443, 1955.
9. Bouchardy, B., and Majno, G.: Histopathology of early myocardial infarcts. Am. J. Pathol. *74*:301, 1974.
10. Derias, N. W., and Adams, C. W. M.: The non-specific nature of the myocardial wave fiber. Histopathology *3*:241, 1979.
11. Kloner, R. A., Ganote, C. E., Whalen, D. A., Jr., and Jennings, R. B.: Effect of a transient period of ischemia on myocardial cells: Fine structure during the first few minutes of reflow. Am. J. Pathol. *74*:399, 1974.
12. Willerson, J. T., Hillis, L. D., and Buja, L. M.: Ischemic Heart Disease. New York, Raven Press, 1982, 374 pp.
13. Sybers, H. D., Maroko, P. R., Ashraf, M., Libby, P., and Braunwald, E.: The effect of glucose-insulin-potassium on cardiac ultrastructure following acute experimental coronary occlusion. Am. J. Pathol. *70*:401, 1973.
14. Jennings, R. B., and Ganote, C. E.: Structural change in myocardium during acute ischemia. Circ. Res. *35*(Suppl. 3):156, 1974.
15. Kloner, R. A., Rude, R. E., Carlson, N., Maroko, P. R., Karaffa, S., DeBoer, L. W. V., and Braunwald, E.: Ultrastructural evidence of microvascular damage and myocardial cell injury after coronary artery occlusion: Which comes first? Circulation *62*:945, 1980.
16. Kloner, R. A., and Braunwald, E.: Review—Observations on experimental myocardial ischemia. Cardiovasc. Res. *14*:371, 1980.
17. Kloner, R. A., DeBoer, L. W. V., Carlson, N., and Braunwald, E.: The effect of verapamil on myocardial ultrastructure during and following release of coronary artery occlusion. Exp. Mol. Pathol. *36*:277, 1982.
18. Caulfield, J., and Klionsky, B.: Myocardial ischemia and early infarction: An electron microscopic study. Am. J. Pathol. *35*:489, 1959.
19. Shen, A. C., and Jennings, R. B.: Kinetics of calcium accumulation in acute myocardial ischemic injury. Am. J. Pathol. *67*:441, 1972.
20. Kloner, R. A., Fishbein, M. C., Hare, C. M., and Maroko, P. R.: Early ischemic ultrastructural and histochemical alterations in the myocardium of the rat following coronary artery occlusion. Exp. Mol. Pathol. *30*:129, 1979.
21. Baroldi, G.: Different types of myocardial necrosis in coronary heart disease: A pathophysiologic review of their functional significance. Am. Heart J. *89*: 742, 1975.
22. Hagler, H. K., Sherwin, L., and Buja, L. M.: Effect of different methods of tissue preparation on mitochondrial inclusions of ischemic and infarcted canine myocardium: Transmission and analytical electron microscopic study. Lab. Invest. *40*:529, 1979.
23. Hutchins, G. M., and Bulkley, B. H.: Correlation of myocardial contraction band necrosis and vascular patency: A study of coronary artery bypass graft anastomoses at branch points. Lab Invest. *36*:642, 1977.
24. Blumgart, H. L., Schlesinger, M. J., and Davis, D.: Studies on the relation of the clinical manifestations of angina pectoris, coronary thrombosis, and myocardial infarction to the pathologic findings with particular reference to the significance of the collateral circulation. Am. Heart J. *19*:1, 1940.
25. Roberts, W. C.: Coronary arteries in fatal acute myocardial infarction. Circulation *45*:215, 1972.
26. Betriu, A., Castaner, A., Sanz, G. A., Pare, J. C., Roig, E., Coll, S., Magrina, J., and Navarro-Lopez, F.: Angiographic findings 1 month after myocardial infarction: A prospective study of 259 survivors. Circulation *65*:1099, 1982.
27. Silver, M. D., Baroldi, G., and Mariani, F.: The relationship between acute occlusive coronary thrombi and myocardial infarction studied in 100 consecutive patients. Circulation *61*:219, 1980.
28. Friedberg, C. K., and Horn, H.: Acute myocardial infarction not due to coronary artery occlusion. J.A.M.A. *112*:1675, 1939.
29. Allison, R. B., Rodriguez, F. L., Higgins, E. A., Jr., Leddy, J. P., Abelmann, W. H., Ellis, L. B., and Robbins, S. L.: Clinicopathologic correlations in coronary atherosclerosis. Four hundred thirty patients studied with post-mortem coronary angiography. Circulation *27*:170, 1963.
30. Paterson, J. C.: Capillary rupture with intimal hemorrhage as a causative factor in coronary thrombosis. Arch. Pathol. *25*:474, 1938.
31. Paterson, J. C.: Relation of physical exertion and emotion to precipitation of coronary thrombi. J.A.M.A. *112*:895, 1939.

31a. Dalen, J. E., Ockene, I. S., and Alpert, J. S.: Coronary spasm, coronary thrombosis and myocardial infarction. Am. Heart J. *104*:1119, 1982.

32. Roberts, W. C.: The coronary arteries in fatal coronary events. *In* Chung, E. K. (ed.): Controversies in Cardiology. New York, Springer-Verlag, 1976, p. 1.
33. Chandler, A. B., Chapman, I., Erhardt, L. R., Roberts, W. C., Schwartz, C. J., Sinapius, D., Spain, D. M., Sherry, S., Ness, P. M., and Simon, T. L.: Coronary thrombosis in myocardial infarction. Report of a workshop on the role of coronary thrombosis in the pathogenesis of acute myocardial infarction. Am. J. Cardiol. *34*:823, 1974.
34. Herrick, J. B.: Clinical features of sudden obstruction of the coronary arteries. J.A.M.A. *59*:2015, 1912.
35. Blumgart, H. L., Schlesinger, M. J., and Zoll, P. M.: Angina pectoris, coronary failure, and acute myocardial infarction; Role of coronary occlusions and collateral circulation. J.A.M.A. *116*:91, 1941.
36. Miller, R. D., Burchell, H. B., and Edwards, J. E.: Myocardial infarction with and without acute coronary occlusion; A pathologic study. Arch. Intern. Med. *88*:597, 1951.
37. Chandler, A. B.: Relationship of coronary thrombosis to myocardial infarction. Mod. Concepts Cardiovasc. Dis. *44*:1, 1975.
38. Barold, G.: Pathological anatomy of myocardial infarction. *In* Wilhelmsen, L., and Hjalmarson, A. (eds.): Acute and Long-Term Medical Management of Myocardial Ischemia. Sweden, Mölndal, 1978, p. 41.
39. Ganz, W., Buchbinder, N., Marcus, H., Mondkar, A., Maddahi, J., Charuzi, Y., O'Connor, L., Shell, W., Fishbein, M. C., Kass, R., Miyamoto, A., and Swan, H. J. C.: Intracoronary thrombolysis in evolving myocardial infarction. Am. Heart J. *101*:4, 1981.
40. Mathey, D. G., Kuck, K. H., Tilsner, V., Krebber, H. J., and Bleifeld, W.: Nonsurgical coronary artery recanalization in acute myocardial infarction. Circulation *63*:489, 1981.
41. Rentrop, P., Blanke, H., Karsch, K. R., Kaiser, H., Kostering, H., and Leitz, K.: Selective intracoronary thrombolysis in acute myocardial infarction and unstable angina pectoris. Circulation *63*:307, 1981.
42. Markis, J. E., Malagold, M., Parker, J. A., Silverman, K. J., Barry, W. H., Als, A. V., Paulin, S., Grossman, W., and Braunwald, E.: Myocardial salvage after intracoronary thrombolysis with streptokinase in acute myocardial infarction. N. Engl. J. Med. *305*:777, 1981.
43. DeWood, M. A., Spores, J., and Notske, R.: Prevalence of total coronary occlusion during the early hours of transmural myocardial infarction. N. Engl. J. Med. *303*:897, 1980.
44. Gagnon, R. M., Morissette, M., Bensimon, H., Beaudet, R., Poirier, N., Noel, C., Presant, S., and Lemire, J.: The role of coronary thrombosis in myocardial infarction: Further evidence shown by intracoronary thrombolysis with streptokinase. Cathet. Cardiovasc. Diagn. *8*:393, 1982.
45. Oliva, P. B.: Pathophysiology of acute myocardial infarction, 1981. Ann. Intern. Med. *94*:236, 1981.
46. Cheitlin, M. D., McAllister, H. A., and deCastro, C. M.: Myocardial infarction without atherosclerosis. J.A.M.A. *231*:951, 1975.
47. Connolley, J. E., Eldridge, F. L., Calvin, J. W., and Stemmer, E. A.: Proximal coronary artery obstruction. N. Eng. J. Med. *271*:213, 1964.
48. Roberts, W. C., MacGregor, R. R., DeBlanc, H. J., Beiser, G. D., and Wolff, S. M.: The prepulseless phase of pulseless disease, or pulseless disease with pulses. Am. J. Med. *46*:313, 1969.
49. Laurie, W., and Woods, J. D.: Infarction (ischemic fibrosis) in the right ventricle of the heart. Acta Cardiol. *18*:399, 1963.
50. Kegel, S. M., Dorsey, T. J., Rowen, M., and Taylor, W. F.: Cardiac death in mucocutaneous lymph node syndrome. Am. J. Cardiol. *40*:282, 1977.
51. Liberthson, R. R., Homcy, C., Fallon, J. T., Gross, S., Leppo, J., and Miller, L.: Systemic lupus erythematosis and heart disease. Primary Cardiol. *9*:77, 1983.
52. Cohn, K. E., Stewart, J. R., Fajardo, L. F., and Hancock, E. W.: Heart disease following radiation. Medicine *46*:281, 1967.
53. Perloff, J. K.: Coronary artery disease—Antidote to a stereotype. Am. J. Cardiol. *30*:437, 1972.
54. Bonfiglio, T. A., Botti, R. E., and Hagstrom, J. W. C.: Coronary arteritis, occlusion, and myocardial infarction due to lupus erythematosus. Am. Heart J. *83*:153, 1972.
55. Huang, S., Kumar, G., Steele, H. D., and Parker, J. O.: Cardiac involvement in pseudoxanthoma elasticum. Am. Heart J. *74*:680, 1967.
56. James, T. N.: Small arteries of the heart. Circulation *56*:2, 1977.
57. Thompson, S. I., Vieweg, W. V. R., Alpert, J. S., and Hagan, A. D.: Incidence and age distribution of patients with myocardial infarction and normal coronary arteriograms. Cathet. Cardiovasc. Diagn. *3*:1, 1977.
58. Rosenblatt, A., and Selzer, A.: The nature and clinical features of myocardial infarction with normal coronary arteriograms. Circulation *55*:578, 1977.
59. Glover, M. V., Kuber, M. T., Warren, S. E., and Vieweg, W. V. R.: Myocardial infarction before age 36: Risk factor and arteriographic analysis. Am. J. Cardiol. *49*:1600, 1982.

59a. Ciraulo, D. A., Bresnahan, G. F., Frankel, P. S., Isely, P. E., Zimmerman, W. R., and Chesne, R. B.: Transmural myocardial infarction with normal coronary angiograms and with single vessel coronary obstruction. Clinical-angiographic features and five-year follow-up. Chest *83*:196, 1983.

60. Achuff, S. C., Bell, W. R., and Bulkley, B. H.: Thromboses in previously normal coronary arteries. Primary Cardiol. *8*:137, 1982.
61. Khan, A. H., and Haywood, L. J.: Myocardial infarction in nine patients with radiologically patent coronary arteries. N. Engl. J. Med. *291*:428, 1974.

62. Eliot, R. S., Baroldi, G., and Leone, A.: Necropsy studies in myocardial infarction with minimal or no coronary luminal reduction due to atherosclerosis. Circulation *49*:1127, 1974.
63. Eslami, B., Russell, R. O., Jr., Bailey, M. T., Oberman, A., Tieszen, R. L., and Rackley, C. E.: Acute myocardial infarction in the absence of coronary arterial insufficiency. Ala. J. Med. Sci. *12*:322, 1975.
64. Arnett, E. N., and Roberts, W. C.: Acute myocardial infarction and angiographically normal coronary arteries: An unproven combination. Circulation *53*:395, 1976.
64a. Makino, H., and Al-Sadir, J.: Myocardial infarction in patients with mitral valve prolapse and normal coronary arteries. J. Am. Coll. Cardiol. *1*:661, 1983.
65. Braunwald, E.: Editorial. Coronary spasm and acute myocardial infarction—New possibility for treatment and prevention. N. Engl. J. Med. *299*:1301, 1978.
66. Sasse, L., Wagner, R., and Murray, F. E.: Transmural myocardial infarction during pregnancy. Am. J. Cardiol. *35*:448, 1975.
67. Chesler, E., Matisonn, R. E., Lakier, J. B., Pocock, W. A., Obel, I. W. P., and Barlow, J. B.: Acute myocardial infarction with normal coronary arteries. A possible manifestation of the billowing mitral leaflet syndrome. Circulation *54*: 203, 1976.
68. Regan, T. J., Wu, C. F., Weisse, A. B., Moschos, C. B., Ahmed, S. S., and Lyons, M. D.: Acute myocardial infarction in toxic cardiomyopathy without coronary obstruction. Circulation *51*:453, 1975.
69. Hallman, G. L., Cooley, D. A., and Singer, D. B.: Congenital anomalies of the coronary arteries. Surgery *59*:133, 1966.
70. James, T. N.: Angina without coronary disease. Circulation *42*:189, 1970.
71. Gorlin, R.: Coronary collaterals. *In* Coronary Artery Disease. Philadelphia, W. B. Saunders Co., 1976, p. 59.
72. Eckstein, R. W.: Development of interarterial coronary anastomoses by chronic anemia: Disappearance following correction of anemia. Circ. Res. *3*:306, 1955.
73. Blumgart, H. L., Zoll, P. M., Paul, M. H., and Norman, L. R.: The effect of experimental acute coronary occlusion on stimulation of intercoronary collateral anastomoses. Trans. Assoc. Am. Phys. *68*:155, 1955.
74. Gregg, D. E.: Coronary Circulation in Health and Disease. Philadelphia, Lea and Febiger, 1950.
75. Siepser, S. L., Kaltman, A. J., Mills, N., Pughkem, T., and Fox, A. C.: Coronary collateral flow after traumatic fistula between right coronary artery and right atrium. N. Engl. J. Med. *287*:754, 1972.
76. Wiggers, C. J.: The functional importance of coronary collaterals. Circulation *5*:609, 1952.
77. Helfant, R. H., Vokonas, P. S., and Gorlin, R.: Functional importance of human coronary collateral circulation. N. Engl. J. Med. *284*:1277, 1971.
78. Carroll, R. J., Verani, M. S., and Falsetti, H. L.: The effect of collateral circulation on segmental left ventricular contraction. Circulation *50*:709, 1974.
79. Levin, D. C.: Pathways and functional significance of the coronary collateral circulation. Circulation *50*:831, 1974.
80. Hamby, R. I., Aintablian, A., and Schwartz, A.: Reappraisal of the functional significance of the coronary collateral circulation. Am. J. Cardiol. *38*:304, 1976.
81. Carlton, R. A., and Boyd, T.: Traumatic laceration of the anterior descending coronary artery treated by ligation without myocardial infarction: Report of a case with review of the literature. Am. Heart J. *56*:136, 1958.
82. Gold, H. K., Leinbach, R. C., and Maroko, P. R.: Propranolol-induced reduction of signs of ischemic injury during acute myocardial infarction. Am. J. Cardiol. *38*:689, 1976.
83. Wackers, F. J. T., Lie, K. I., Sokole, E. B., Res, J., Schoot, J. B. V. D., and Durrer, D.: Prevalence of right ventricular involvement in inferior wall infarction assessed with myocardial imaging with thallium-201 and technetium-99m pyrophosphate. Am. J. Cardiol. *42*:358, 1978.
84. Isner, J. M., and Roberts, W. C.: Right ventricular infarction complicating left ventricular infarction secondary to coronary heart disease. Frequency, location, associated findings and significance from analysis of 236 necropsy patients with acute or healed myocardial infarction. Am. J. Cardiol. *42*:885, 1978.
85. Nixon, J. V.: Right ventricular myocardial infarction. Arch. Intern. Med. *142*: 945, 1982.
85a. Haupt, H. M., Hutchins, G. M., and Moore, G. W.: Right ventricular infarction: Role of the moderator band artery in determining infarct size. Circulation *67*:1268, 1983.
86. Rackley, C. E., Russell, R. O., Jr., Mantle, J. A., Rogers, W. J., Papapietro, S. E., and Schwartz, K. M.: Right ventricular infarction and function. Am. Heart J. *101*:215, 1981.
87. Wade, W. G.: The pathogenesis of infarction of the right ventricle. Br. Heart J. *21*:545, 1957.
88. Silverman, B. D., Carabajal, N. R., Chorches, M. A., and Taranto, A. I.: Tricuspid regurgitation and acute myocardial infarction. Arch. Intern. Med. *142*: 1394, 1982.
89. Lloyd, E. A., Gersh, B. J., and Kennelly, B. M.: Hemodynamic spectrum of dominant right ventricular infarction. Am. J. Cardiol. *48*:1016, 1981.
89a. Lopez-Sendon, J., Garcia-Fernandez, M. A., Coma-Canella, I., Yanguela, M. M., and Banuelos, F.: Segmental right ventricular function after acute myocardial infarction: Two-dimensional echocardiographic study in 63 patients. Am. J. Cardiol. *51*:390, 1983.
90. Cushing, E. H., Feil, H. S., Stanton, E. J., and Wartman, W. B.: Infarction of the cardiac auricles (atria): Clinical, pathological and experimental studies. Br. Heart J. *4*:17, 1942.
91. Wartman, W. B., and Hellerstein, H. K.: The incidence of heart disease in 2000 consecutive autopsies. Ann. Intern. Med. *28*:41, 1948.
92. Lowe, T. E., and Wartman, W. B.: Myocardial infarction. Br. Heart J. *6*:115, 183, 1944.
93. London, R. E., and London, S. B.: Rupture of the heart. A critical analysis of 47 consecutive autopsy cases. Circulation *31*:202, 1965.
94. Björck, G., Mogensen, L., Nyquist, O., Orinius, E., and Sjögren, A.: Studies of myocardial rupture with cardiac tamponade in acute myocardial infarction. Chest *61*:4, 1972.
95. Kassis, E., Vogelsang, M., and Lyngborg, K.: Cardiac rupture complicating myocardial infarction. A study concerning early diagnosis and possible management. Dan. Med. Bull. *48*:164, 1981.
96. Edmondson, H. A., and Hoxie, H. J.: Hypertension and cardiac rupture: Clinical and pathological study of 72 cases, in 13 of which rupture of the interventricular septum occurred. Am. Heart J. *24*:719, 1942.
97. Schuster, E. H., and Bulkley, B. H.: Expansion of transmural myocardial infarction: A pathophysiologic factor in cardiac rupture. Circulation *60*:1532, 1979.
98. Vlodaver, Z., Coe, J. L., and Edwards, J. E.: True and false left ventricular aneurysms. Circulation *51*:567, 1975.
99. Vlodaver, Z., and Edwards, J. E.: Rupture of ventricular septum or papillary muscle complicating myocardial infarction. Circulation *55*:815, 1977.
100. Radford, M. J., Johnson, R. A., Daggett, W. M., Fallon, J. T., Buckley, M. J., Gold, H. K., and Leinbach, R. C.: Ventricular septal rupture: A review of clinical and physiologic features and an analysis of survival. Circulation *64*: 545, 1981.
101. Matsui, K., Kay, J. H., Mendez, M., Zubiate, P., Vanstrom, N., and Yokoyama, T.: Ventricular septal rupture secondary to myocardial infarction. Clinical approach and surgical results. J.A.M.A. *245*:1537, 1981.
101a. Nishimura, R. A., Schaff, H. V., Shub, C., Gersh, B. J., Edwards, W. D., and Tajik, A.: Papillary muscle rupture complicating acute myocardial infarction: Analysis of 17 patients. Am. J. Cardiol. *51*:373, 1983.
102. Roberts, W. C., and Cohen, L. D.: Left ventricular papillary muscles. Description of the normal and a survey of conditions causing them to be abnormal. Circulation *46*:138, 1972.
103. Roberts, W. C., and Perloff, J. K.: Mitral valvular disease—A clinicopathologic survey of the conditions causing the mitral valve to function abnormally. Ann. Intern. Med. *77*:939, 1972.
104. Wei, J. Y., Hutchins, G. M., and Bulkley, B. H.: Papillary muscle rupture in fatal acute myocardial infarction. Ann. Intern. Med. *90*:149, 1979.
105. Abrams, D. L., Edelist, A., Luria, M. H., and Miller, A. J.: Ventricular aneurysm: A reappraisal based on a study of 65 consecutive autopsied cases. Circulation *27*:164, 1963.
106. Schlicter, J., Hellerstein, H. K., and Katz, L. N.: Aneurysm of the heart: A correlative study of one hundred and two proved cases. Medicine *33*:43, 1954.
107. Eaton, L. W., and Bulkley, B. H.: Expansion of acute myocardial infarction: Its relationship to infarct morphology in a canine model. Circ. Res. *49*:80, 1981.
108. Swan, H. J. C., Forrester, J. S., Diamond, G., Chatterjee, K., and Parmley, W. W.: Hemodynamic spectrum of myocardial infarction and cardiogenic shock. Circulation *45*:1097, 1972.
109. Graber, J. D., Oakley, C. M., Pickering, J. F., Goodwin, J. F., Raphael, M. J., and Steiner, R. E.: Ventricular aneurysm, an appraisal of diagnosis and surgical therapy. Br. Heart J. *34*:830, 1972.
110. Asinger, R. W., Mikell, F. L., Elsperger, J., and Hodges, M.: Incidence of left ventricular thrombosis after acute transmural myocardial infarction. Serial evaluation of two-dimensional echocardiography. N. Engl. J. Med. *305*:297, 1981.
111. Page, D. L., Caulfield, J. B., Kastor, J. A., DeSanctis, R. W., and Sanders, C. A.: Myocardial changes associated with cardiogenic shock. N. Engl. J. Med. *285*:133, 1971.
112. Alonso, D. R., Scheidt, S., Post, M., and Killip, T.: Pathophysiology of cardiogenic shock; quantification of myocardial necrosis, clinical, pathologic and electrocardiographic correlation. Circulation *48*:588, 1973.
112a. Resnekov, L.: Cardiogenic shock. Chest *83*:893, 1983.
113. Fraker, T. D., Jr., Wagner, G. S., and Rosati, R. A.: Extension of myocardial infarction: Incidence and prognosis. Circulation *60*:1126, 1979.
114. Gutovitz, A. L., Sobel, B. E., and Roberts, R.: Progressive nature of myocardial injury in selected patients with cardiogenic shock. Am. J. Cardiol. *41*:469, 1978.
115. Wackers, F. J., Lie, K. I., Becker, A. E., Durrer, D., and Wellens, H. J. J.: Coronary artery disease in patients dying from cardiogenic shock or congestive heart failure in the setting of acute myocardial infarction. Br. Heart J. *38*:906, 1976.
115a. Visser, C. A., Kan, G., Lie, K. I., and Durrer, D.: Incidence and one-year follow-up of left ventricular thrombus following acute myocardial infarction: An echocardiographic study of 96 patients. J. Am. coll. Cardiol. *1*:648, 1983.
116. Hellerstein, H. K., and Martin, J. W.: Incidence of thrombo-embolic lesions accompanying myocardial infarction. Am. Heart J. *33*:443, 1947.
117. Davies, M. J., Woolf, N., and Robertson, W. B.: Pathology of acute myocardial infarction with particular reference to occlusive coronary thrombi. Br. Heart J. *38*:659, 1976.
118. Eppinger, E. C., and Kennedy, J. A.: The cause of death in coronary thrombo-

sis, with special reference to pulmonary embolism. Am. J. Med. Sci. *195*:104, 1938.
119. Blau, N., Shen, B. A., Pittman, D. E., and Joyner, C. E.: Massive hemopericardium in a patient with post-myocardial infarction syndrome. Chest *71*:549, 1977.
120. Dressler, W.: The post-myocardial infarction syndrome: A report of forty-four cases. Arch. Intern. Med. *103*:28, 1959.
121. Lichstein, E., Arsura, E., Hollander, G., Greengart, A., and Sanders, M.: Current incidence of postmyocardial infarction (Dressler's) syndrome. Am. J. Cardiol. *50*:1269, 1982.
122. Lichstein, E., Lin, H. M., and Gupta, P.: Pericarditis complicating acute myocardial infarction: Incidence of complications and significance of electrocardiogram on admission. Am. Heart J. *87*:246, 1974.
123. Soloff, L. A.: Pericardial cellular response during the post-myocardial infarction syndrome. Am. Heart J. *82*:812, 1971.
124. McCabe, J. C., Ebert, P. A., Engle, M. A., and Zabriskie, J. B.: Circulating heart-reactive antibodies in the postpericardiotomy syndrome. J. Surg. Res. *14*:158, 1973.
124a. Spann, J. F.: Changing concepts of pathophysiology, prognosis and therapy in acute myocardial infarction. Am. J. Med. *74*:877, 1983.

PATHOPHYSIOLOGY

125. Pfeffer, M. A., Pfeffer, J. M., Fishbein, M. C., Fletcher, P. J., Spadaro, J., Kloner, R. A., and Braunwald, E.: Myocardial infarct size and ventricular function in rats. Circ. Res. *44*:503, 1979.
125a. Slutsky, R. A., Mattrey, R. F., Long, S. A., and Higgins, C. B.: In vivo estimation of myocardial infarct size and left ventricular function by prospectively gated computerized transmission tomography. Circulation *67*:759, 1983.
126. Herman, M. V., Heinle, R. A., Klein, M. D., and Gorlin, R.: Localized disorders in myocardial contraction. N. Engl. J. Med. *227*:222, 1967.
127. Forrester, J. S., Wyatt, H. L., DaLuz, P. L., Tyberg, J. V., Diamond, G. A., and Swan, H. J. C.: Functional significance of regional ischemic contraction abnormalities. Circulation *54*:64, 1976.
128. Diamond, G., and Forrester, J. S.: Effect of coronary artery disease and acute myocardial infarction on left ventricular compliance in man. Circulation *45*:11, 1972.
129. Rackley, C. E., Russell, R. O., Jr., Mantle, J. A., and Rogers, W. J.: Modern approach to the patient with acute myocardial infarction. Curr. Prob. Cardiol. *1*:49, 1977.
130. Klein, M. D., Herman, M. V., and Gorlin, R. G.: A hemodynamic study of left ventricular aneurysm. Circulation *35*:614, 1967.
131. Wynne, J., Sayres, M., Maddox, D. E., Idoine, J., Alpert, J. S., Neill, J., and Holman, B. L.: Regional left ventricular function in acute myocardial infarction: Evaluation with quantitative radionuclide ventriculography. Am. J. Cardiol. *45*:203, 1980.
132. Weiss, J. L., Bulkley, B. H., Hutchins, G. M., and Mason, S. J.: Two-dimensional echocardiographic recognition of myocardial injury in man: Comparison with postmortem studies. Circulation *63*:401, 1981.
133. Forrester, J. S., Diamond, G., Parmley, W., and Swan, H. J. C.: Early increase in left ventricular compliance after myocardial infarction. J. Clin. Invest. *51*:598, 1972.
134. Pirzada, F. A., Ekong, E. A., Vokonas, P. S., Apstein, C. S., and Hood, W. B., Jr.: Experimental myocardial infarction. XIII. Sequential changes in left ventricular pressure-length relationships in the acute phase. Circulation *53*:970, 1976.
135. Smith, M., Ratshin, R. A., Harrel, F. E., Jr., Russell, R. O., Jr., and Rackley, C. E.: Early sequential changes in left ventricular dimensions and filling pressure in patients after myocardial infarction. Am. J. Cardiol. *33*:363, 1974.
136. Ratshin, R. A., Rackley, C. E., and Russell, R. O., Jr.: Hemodynamic evaluation of left ventricular function in shock complicating myocardial infarction. Circulation *45*:127, 1972.
137. Eaton, L. W., and Bulkley, B. H.: Expansion of acute myocardial infarction. Its relationship to infarct morphology in a canine model. Circ. Res. *49*:80, 1981.
138. Erlebacher, J. A., Weiss, J. L., Eaton, L. W., Kallman, C., Weisfeldt, M. L., and Bulkley, B. H.: Late effects of acute infarct dilation on heart size: A two-dimensional echocardiographic study. Am. J. Cardiol. *49*:1120, 1982.
139. Rude, R. E., Muller, J. E., and Braunwald, E.: Efforts to limit the size of myocardial infarcts. Ann. Intern. Med. *95*:736, 1981.
140. Forrester, J. S., Diamond, G., Chatterjee, K., and Swan, H. J. C.: Medical therapy of acute myocardial infarction by application of hemodynamic subsets. N. Engl. J. Med. *295*:1356, 1404, 1976.
141. Russell, R. O., Jr., Mantle, J. A., Rogers, W. J., and Rackley, C. E.: Current status of hemodynamic monitoring: Indications, diagnosis and complications. *In* Rackley, C. E. (ed.): Critical Care Medicine. Cardiovascular Clinics. Philadelphia, F. A. Davis, 1981, pp. 1–14.
141a. Rabinowitz, B., Elazar, E., and Neufeld, H. N.: A hemodynamic and autonomic profile of patients belonging to the hyperkinetic subset of acute myocardial infarction. J. Am. Coll. Cardiol. *1*:649, 1983.
141b. Chou, T-C., Fowler, N. O., Gabel, M., van der Bel-Kahn, J., and Feltner, E. J.: Electrocardiographic and hemodynamic changes in experimental right ventricular infarction. Circulation *67*:1258, 1983.
141c. Baigrie, R. S., Haq, A., Morgan, C. D., Rakowski, H., Drobac, M., and McLaughlin, P.: The spectrum of right ventricular involvement in inferior wall myocardial infarction: A clinical, hemodynamic and noninvasive study. J. Am. Coll. Cardiol. *1*:1396, 1983.
142. Carabello, B., Cohn, P. F., and Alpert, J. S.: Hemodynamic monitoring in patients with hypotension after myocardial infarction. Chest *74*:5, 1978.
143. Coma-Canella, I., Lopez-Sendon, J., and Gamallo, C.: Low output syndrome in right ventricular infarction. Am. Heart J. *98*:613, 1979.
144. Haffajee, C. I., Love, J., Gore, J. M., and Alpert, J. S.: Reversibility of shock by atrial or atrioventricular sequential pacing in right ventricular infarction. Am. J. Cardiol. *49*:1025, 1982.
145. Marmor, A., Geltman, E. M., Biello, D. R., Sobel, B. E., Siegel, B. S., and Roberts, R.: Functional response to the right ventricle to myocardial infarction: Dependence on the site of left ventricular infarction. Circulation *64*:1005, 1981.
146. Braunwald, E.: Regulation of the circulation. N. Engl. J. Med. *290*:1124, 1420, 1974.
147 Biddle, T. L., Yu, P. N., Hodges, M., Chance, J. R., Ehrlich, D. A., Kronenberg, M. W., and Roberts, D. L.: Hypoxemia and lung water in acute myocardial infarction. Am. Heart J. *92*:692, 1976.
148. Biddle, T. L., Khanna, P. K., Yu, P. N., Hodges, M., and Shah, P. M.: Lung water in patients with acute myocardial infarction. Circulation *49*:115, 1974.
149. Lichtman, M. A., Cohen, J., Young, J. A., Whitbeck, A. A., and Murphy, M.: The relationships between arterial oxygen flow rate, oxygen binding by hemoglobin, and oxygen utilization after myocardial infarction. J. Clin. Invest. *54*:501, 1974.
150. DaLuz, P. L., Cavanilles, J. M., Michaels, S., Weill, M. H., and Shubin, H.: Oxygen delivery, anoxic metabolism and hemoglobin-oxygen affinity (P_{50}) in patients with acute myocardial infarction and shock. Am. J. Cardiol. *36*:148, 1975.
151. Hales, C. A., and Kazemi, H.: Small-airways function in myocardial infarction. N. Engl. J. Med. *290*:761, 1974.
152. Kazemi, H., Parsons, E. F., Valenca, L. M., and Strieder, D. J.: Distribution of pulmonary blood flow after myocardial ischemia and infarction. Circulation *41*:1025, 1970.
153. Datey, K. K., and Nanda, N. C.: Hyperglycemia after acute myocardial infarction. N. Engl. J. Med. *276*:262, 1976.
154. Vetter, N. J., Adams, W., Strange, R. C., and Oliver, M. F.: Initial metabolic and hormonal response to acute myocardial infarction. Lancet *1*:284, 1974.
155. Bertel, O., Buhler, F. R., Baitsch, G., Ritz, R., and Burkart, F.: Plasma adrenaline and noradrenaline in patients with acute myocardial infarction. Relationship to ventricular arrhythmias in varying severity. Chest *82*:64, 1982.
156. Taylor, S. H., Majid, P. A., Saxton, C., and Sharma, B.: Insulin secretion in heart failure. Am. Heart J. *83*:281, 1972.
157. Taylor, S. H., Saxton, C., Majid, P. A., Dykes, J. R. W., Ghosh, P., and Stoker, J. B.: Insulin secretion following myocardial infarction with particular respect to pathogenesis of cardiogenic shock. Lancet *2*:1373, 1969.
158. Ceremuzynski, L.: Hormonal and metabolic reactions evoked by acute myocardial infarction. Circ. Res. *48*:767, 1981.
159. Jefferson, L. S., Rannels, D. E., Munger, B. L., and Morgan, H. E.: Insulin in the regulation of protein turnover in heart and skeletal muscle. Fed. Proc. *33*:1098, 1974.
160. Opie, L. H.: Metabolism of free fatty acids, glucose, and catecholamines in acute myocardial infarction: Relation to myocardial ischemia and infarct size. Am. J. Cardiol. *36*:938, 1975.
161. Taggart, P., and Carruthers, M.: Endogenous hyperlipidemia induced by emotional stress of racing driving. Lancet *1*:363, 1971.
162. Valori, C., Thomas, M., and Shillingford, J.: Free noradrenaline and adrenaline excretion in relation to clinical syndromes following myocardial infarction. Am. J. Cardiol. *20*:605, 1969.
163. Gupta, D. K., Young, R., Jewitt, D. E., Hartog, M., and Opie, L. H.: Increased plasma free fatty acids and their significance in patients with acute myocardial infarction. Lancet *2*:1209, 1969.
164. Jequier, E., and Perret, C.: Urinary excretion of catecholamines and their main metabolites after myocardial infarction: Relationship to the clinical syndrome. Eur. J. Clin. Invest. *1*:77, 1970.
165. Logan, R. W., and Murdoch, W. R.: Blood levels of hydrocortisone, transaminases and cholesterol after myocardial infarction. Lancet *2*:521, 1966.
166. Baily, R. R., Abernethy, M. H., and Beaven, D. W.: Adrenocortical response to the stress of an acute myocardial infarction. Lancet *1*:970, 1976.
167. Steele, P., Rainwater, J., and Vogel, R.: Abnormal platelet survival time in men with myocardial infarction and normal coronary arteriogram. Am. J. Cardiol. *41*:60, 1978.
168. Laursen, B., and Gormsen, J.: Spontaneous fibrinolysis demonstrated by immunological technique. Thromb. Diath. Haemorrh. *17*:42, 1967.
169. Handin, R. I., McDonough, M., and Lesch, M.: Elevation of platelet factor 4 in acute myocardial infarction: Measurement by radioimmunoassay. J. Lab. Clin. Med. *91*:340, 1978.
170. Rickman, F. D., Handin, R., Howe, J. P., Alpert, J. S., Dexter, L., and Dalen, J. E.: Fibrin split products in acute pulmonary embolism. Ann. Intern. Med. *79*:664, 1973.
171. Jan, K. M., Chien, S., and Bigger, J. T., Jr.: Observation on blood viscosity changes after acute myocardial infarction. Circulation *51*:1079, 1972.
172. Hershberg, P. I., Wells, R. E., and McGandy, R. B.: Hematocrit and prognosis in patients with acute myocardial infarction. J.A.M.A. *219*:855, 1972.

CLINICAL FEATURES

173. Phipps, C.: Contributory causes of coronary thrombosis. J.A.M.A. *106*:761, 1936.
174. Master, A. M., Dack, S., and Jaffe, H. L.: Factors and events associated with onset of coronary artery thrombosis. J.A.M.A. *109*:546, 1937.
175. Smith, C., Sauls, H. C., and Ballew, J.: Coronary occlusion: A clinical study of 100 patients. Ann. Intern. Med. *17*:681, 1942.
176. French, A. J., and Dock, W.: Fatal coronary arteriosclerosis in young soldiers. J.A.M.A. *124*:1233, 1944.
177. Fitzhugh, G., and Hamilton, B. E.: Coronary occlusion and fatal angina pectoris: Study of the immediate causes and their prevention. J.A.M.A. *100*:475, 1933.
178. Knapp, R. B., Topkins, M. J., and Artusio, J. F., Jr.: The cerebrovascular accident and coronary occlusion in anesthesia. J.A.M.A. *182*:332, 1962.
179. Goldfischer, J. D.: Acute myocardial infarction secondary to ergot therapy. N. Engl. J. Med. *262*:860, 1960.
180. Roussak, N. J.: Myocardial infarction during serum sickness. Br. Heart J. *16*: 218, 1954.
181. Levine, H. D.: Acute myocardial infarction following wasp sting. Report of two cases and critical survey of the literature. Am. Heart J. *91*:365, 1976.
182. Lange, R. L., Reid, M. S., Tresch, D. D., Keelan, M. H., Bernhard, V. M., and Coolidge, G.: Nonatheromatous ischemic heart disease following withdrawal from chronic industrial nitroglycerin exposure. Circulation *46*:666, 1972.
183. Maseri, A., L'Abbate, A., Baroldi, G., Chierchia, S., Marzilli, M., Ballestra, A. M., Severi, S., Parodi, O., Biagini, A., Distante, A., and Pesola, A.: Coronary vasospasm as a possible cause of myocardial infarction. A conclusion derived from the study of "preinfarction" angina. N. Engl. J. Med. *299*:1271, 1978.
184. Jenkins, C. D.: Recent evidence supporting psychologic and social risk factors for coronary disease. N. Engl. J. Med. *294*:987, 1033, 1976.
185. Rahe, R. H., Romo, M., Bennett, L., and Siltanen, P.: Recent life changes, myocardial infarction, and abrupt coronary death. Arch. Intern. Med. *133*: 221, 1974.
186. Norris, N. M.: Myocardial Infarction. Edinburgh, Churchill Livingstone, 1982, 322 pp.
187. Alonzo, A. M., Simon, A. B., and Feinleib, M.: Prodromata of myocardial infarction and sudden death. Circulation *52*:1056, 1975.
188. Malliani, A., and Lombardi, F.: Consideration of the fundamental mechanisms eliciting cardiac pain. Am. Heart J. *103*:575, 1982.
189. Ikram, H., Orchard, R. T., and Read, S. E. C.: Intractable hiccupping in acute myocardial infarction. Br. Med. J. *2*:504, 1971.
190. Uretsky, B. F., Farquhar, D. S., Borezin, A., and Hood, W. B.: Symptomatic myocardial infarction without chest pain: Prevalence and clinical course. Am. J. Cardiol. *40*:498, 1977.
191. Margolis, J. R., Kannel, W. B., Feinleib, M., Dawber, T. R., and McNamara, P. M.: Clinical features of unrecognized myocardial infarction—Silent and symptomatic. Eighteen year follow-up: The Framingham Study. Am. J. Cardiol. *32*:1, 1973.
192. Sullivan, W., Vlodaver, Z., Tuna, N., Long, L., and Edward, J. E.: Correlation of electrocardiographic and pathologic findings in healed myocardial infarction. Am. J. Cardiol. *42*:724, 1978.
193. Bean, W. B.: Masquerade of myocardial infarction. Lancet *1*:1044, 1977.
194. Stone, P., and Muller, J. E.: Nifedipine therapy for recurrent ischemic pain following myocardial infarction. Clin. Cardiol. *5*:223, 1982.
195. Moran, T. J., French, W. J., Abrams, H. F., and Criley, J. M.: Post–myocardial infarction angina and coronary spasm. Am. J. Cardiol. *50*:197, 1982.
196. Koiwaya, Y., Torii, S., Takeshita, A., Nakagaki, O., and Nakamura, M.: Postinfarction angina caused by coronary arterial spasm. Circulation *65*:275, 1982.
197. Thoren, P. N.: Activation of left ventricular receptors with nonmedullated vagal afferent fibers during occlusion of a coronary artery in the cat. Am. J. Cardiol. *37*:1046, 1976.
198. Chadda, K. D., Lichstein, E., Gupta, P. K., and Choy, R.: Bradycardia-hypotension syndrome in acute myocardial infarction. Reappraisal of the overdrive effects of atropine. Am. J. Med. *59*:158, 1975.
199. Chizner, M. A.: Bedside diagnosis of the acute myocardial infarction and its complications. Curr. Probl. Cardiol. *7*:1, 1982.
200. Renner, W. F., and Renner, G. W.: The quality of resonance of the first heart sound after myocardial infarction: Clinical significance. Circulation *59*:1144, 1979.
201. Stein, P. D., Sabbah, H. N., and Barr, I.: Intensity of heart sounds in the evaluation of patients following myocardial infarction. Chest *75*:679, 1979.
202. Riley, C. P., Russell, R. O., Jr., and Rackley, C. E.: Left ventricular gallop sound and acute myocardial infarction. Am. Heart J. *86*:598, 1973.
203. Sawaya, J. I., Mujais, S. K., and Armenian, H. K.: Early diagnosis of pericarditis in acute myocardial infarction. Am. Heart J. *100*:144, 1980.
204. Thompson, P. L., and Robinson, J. S.: Stroke after acute myocardial infarction: Relation to infarct size. Br. Med. J. *2*:457, 1978.
205. Sobel, B. E., and Shell, W. E.: Serum enzyme determinations in the diagnosis and assessment of myocardial infarction. Circulation *45*:471, 1972.
206. Hearse, D. J.: Myocardial enzyme leakage. J. Mol. Med. *2*:185, 1977.
207. Pasyk, S., Bloor, C. M., Khouri, E. M., and Gregg, D. E.: Systemic and coronary effects of coronary artery occlusion in the unanesthetized dog. Am. J. Physiol. *220*:646, 1971.
208. Shell, W. E., Kjekshus, J. K., and Sobel, B. E.: Quantitative assessment of the extent of myocardial infarction in the conscious dog by means of analysis of serial changes in serum creatine phosphokinase activity. J. Clin. Invest. *50*: 2614, 1971.
209. Agress, C. M., and Kin, J. H. C.: Evaluation of enzyme tests in the diagnosis of heart disease. Am. J. Cardiol. *6*:641, 1960.
210. Vasudevan, G., Mercer, D. W., and Varat, M. A.: Lactic dehydrogenase isoenzyme determination in the diagnosis of acute myocardial infarction. Circulation *57*:1055, 1978.
211. Weidner, N.: Laboratory diagnosis of acute myocardial infarct. Usefulness of determination of lactate dehydrogenase (LDH)–1 level and the ratio of LDH–1 to total LDH. Arch. Pathol. Lab. Med. *106*:375, 1982.
212. Goldberg, D. M., and Windfield, D. A.: Diagnostic accuracy of serum enzyme assays for myocardial infarction in a general hospital population. Br. Heart J. *34*:597, 1972.
213. Roberts, R., and Sobel, B. E.: Isoenzymes of creatine phosphokinase and diagnosis of myocardial infarction. Ann. Intern. Med. *79*:741, 1973.
214. Tsung, S. H.: Several conditions causing elevation of serum CK-MB and CK-BB. Am. J. Clin. Pathol. *75*:711, 1981.
215. Roberts, R., Gowda, K. S., Ludbrook, P. A., and Sobel, B. E.: Specificity of elevated serum MB creatine phosphokinase activity in the diagnosis of acute myocardial infarction. Am. J. Cardiol. *36*:433, 1975.
216. Roberts, R., and Sobel, B. E.: Creatine kinase isoenzymes in the assessment of heart disease. Am. Heart J. *95*:521, 1978.
217. Roberts, R., Sobel, B. E., and Parker, C. W.: Radioimmunoassay for creatine kinase isoenzymes. Science *194*:855, 1976.
218. Alderman, E. L., Matlof, H. J., Shumway, N. E., and Harrison, D. C.: Evaluation of enzyme testing for the detection of myocardial infarction following direct coronary surgery. Circulation *48*:135, 1973.
219. Klein, M. S., Colemen, R. E., Weldon, C. S., Sobel, B. E., and Robert, R.: Concordance of electrocardiographic and scintigraphic criteria of myocardial injury after cardiac surgery. J. Thorac. Cardiovasc. Surg. *71*:934, 1976.
220. Roberts, R., Sobel, B. E., and Ludbrook, P. A.: Determination of the origin of elevated plasma CPK after cardiac catheterization. Cathet. Cardiovasc. Diagn. *2*:239, 1976.
221. Heller, G. V., Blaustein, A. S., and Wei, J. Y.: Implications of increased myocardial isoenzyme level in the presence of normal serum creatine kinase activity. Am. J. Cardiol. *51*:24, 1983.
221a. Smith, J. L., Ambos, D., Gold, H. K., Muller, J. E., Poole, W. K., Raabe, D. S., Jr., Rude, R. E., Passamani, E., Braunwald, E., Sobel, B. E., Roberts, R., and the MILIS Study Group. Am. J. Cardiol. *51*:1294, 1983.
222. Grande, P., Hansen, B. F., Christiansen, C., and Naestoft, J.: Estimation of acute myocardial infarct size in man by serum CK-MB measurements. Circulation *65*:756, 1982.
223. Hori, M., Inoue, M., Fukui, S., Shimazu, T., Mishima, M., Ohgitani, N., Minamino, T., and Abe, H.: Correlation of ejection fraction and infarct size estimated from the total CK released in patients with acute myocardial infarction. Br. Heart J. *41*:433, 1979.
224. Geltman, E. M., Ehsani, A. A., Campbell, M. K., Schechtman, K., Roberts, R., and Sobel, B. E.: The influence of location and extent of myocardial infarction on long-term ventricular dysrhythmia and mortality. Circulation *60*:805, 1979.
225. Goldberger, E., Alesio, J., and Woll, F.: The significance of hyperglycemia in myocardial infarction. N.Y. State Med. J. *45*:391, 1945.
226. Rahe, R. H., Rubin, R. T., Arthur, R. J., and Clark, B. R.: Serum uric acid and cholesterol variability. J.A.M.A. *206*:2875, 1973.
227. Tan, M. H., and Wilmshurst, E. G., Gleason, R. E., and Soeldner, J. S.: Effect of posture on serum lipids. N. Engl. J. Med. *289*:416, 1973.
228. Kagen, L., Scheidt, S., and Butt, A.: Serum myoglobin in myocardial infarction: The "staccato phenomenon." Is acute myocardial infarction in man an intermittent event? Am. J. Med. *62*:86, 1977.
229. Vallee, B. L.: The time course of serum copper concentrations of patients with myocardial infarction. Metabolism *1*:420, 1952.
230. Sunderman, F. W., Jr., Nomoto, S., Pradhan, A. M., Levine, H., Bernstein, S. H., and Hirsch, R.: Increased concentration of serum nickel after acute myocardial infarction. N. Engl. J. Med. *283*:896, 1970.
231. Wacker, W. E. C., Ulmer, D. D., and Vallee, B. L.: Metalloenzymes and myocardial infarction. II. Malic and lactic dehydrogenase activities and zinc concentrations in serum. N. Engl. J. Med. *255*:449, 1956.
232. Fitzsimons, E. J., and Kaplan, K.: Rapid drop in serum iron concentration in myocardial infarction. Am. J. Clin. Pathol. *73*:552, 1980.
233. Rector, W. G., Jr., DeWood, M. A., Williams, R. V., and Sullivan, J. F.: Serum magnesium and copper levels in myocardial infarction. Am. J. Med. Sci. *281*:25, 1981.
234. Eastham, R. D., and Morgan, E. H.: Plasma-fibrinogen levels in coronary-artery disease. Lancet *2*:1196, 1963.
235. Savage, R. M., Wagner, G. S., Ideker, R. E., Podolsky, S. A., and Hackel, D. B.: Correlation of postmortem anatomic findings with electrocardiographic changes in patients with myocardial infarction. Circulation *55*:279, 1977.
236. Cooksey, J. D., Dunn, M., and Massie, E.: Clinical Vectorcardiography and Electrocardiography. 2nd Ed. Chicago, Year Book Medical Publishers, 1977, p. 361.

237. Haiat, R., Worthington, F. X., Castellanos, A., and Lemberg, L.: Unusual normalization of the electrocardiogram on the 6th day of myocardial infarction. J. Electrocardiol. *4*:363, 1971.
238. Candell-Riera, J., Figueras, J., Valle, V., Alvarez, A., Gutierrez, L., Cortadellas, J., Cinca, J., Salas, A., and Rius, J.: Right ventricular infarction: Relationships between ST segment elevation in V_{4R} and hemodynamic, scintigraphic, and echocardiographic findings in patients with acute inferior myocardial infarction. Am. Heart J. *101*:281, 1981.
239. Chou, T., Van Der Bel-Kahn, J., Allen, J., Brockmeier, L., and Fowler, N.O.: Electrocardiographic diagnosis of right ventricular infarction. Am. J. Med. *70*: 1175, 1981.
240. Lieu, C. K., Greenspan, G., and Piccirillo, R. T.: Atrial infarction of the heart. Circulation *23*:331, 1961.
241. Silvertssen, E., Hoel, B., Bay, G., and Jorgensen, L.: Electrocardiographic atrial complex and acute atrial myocardial infarction. Am. J. Cardiol. *31*:450, 1973.
242. Stein, P. D., and Simon, A. P.: Vectorcardiographic diagnosis of diaphragmatic myocardial infarction. Am. J. Cardiol. *38*:568, 1976.
243. Howard, P. F., Benchimol, A., Desser, K. B., Reich, F. D., and Graves, C.: Correlation of electrocardiogram and vectorcardiogram with coronary occlusion and myocardial contraction abnormality. Am. J. Cardiol. *38*:582, 1976.
244. Levine, H. D., Young, E., and Williams, R. A.: Electrocardiogram and vectorcardiogram in myocardial infarction. Circulation *45*:457, 1972.
245. Yu, P. N., Fox, S. M., Imboden, C. A., Jr., and Killip, T.: Coronary care unit. I. A specialized intensive care unit for acute myocardial infarction. Mod. Concepts Cardiovasc. Dis. *34*:23, 1965.
246. Meltzer, L. E., and Cohen, H. E.: The incidence of arrhythmias associated with acute myocardial infarction. *In* Meltzer, L. E., and Dunning, A. J. (eds.): Textbook of Coronary Care. Philadelphia, Charles Press, 1972.
247. Pantridge, J. F., and Adgey, A. A. J.: Pre-hospital coronary care. The mobile coronary care unit. Am. J. Cardiol. *24*:666, 1969.
247a. Julian, D. G., Valentine, P. A., and Miller, G. G.: Disturbances of rate, rhythm and conduction in acute myocardial infarction. Am. J. Med. *37*:915, 1964.
248. Hinkel, L. E., Jr., Carver, S. T., and Stevens, M.: The frequency of asymptomatic disturbances of cardiac rhythm and conduction in middle-aged men. Am. J. Cardiol. *24*:629, 1969.
249. Adgey, A. A. J., Alley, J. D., Geddes, J. S., James, R. G. G., Webb, S. W., and Zaidi, S. A.: Acute phase of myocardial infarction. Lancet *2*:501, 1971.
250. Graner, L. E., Gershen, B. J., Orlando, M. M., and Epstein, S. E.: Bradycardia and its complications in the pre-hospital phase of acute myocardial infarction. Am. J. Cardiol. *32*:607, 1973.
251. Zipes, D. P.: The clinical significance of bradycardic rhythms in acute myocardial infarction. Am. J. Cardiol. *24*:814, 1969.
251a. Mark, A. L.: The Bezold-Jarisch reflex revisited: Clinical implications of inhibitory reflezes originating in the heart. J. Am. Coll. Cardiol. *1*:90, 1983.
252. Wei, J. Y., Markis, J. E., Malagold, M., and Braunwald, E.: Cardiovascular reflexes stimulated by reperfusion of ischemic myocardium in acute myocardial infarction. Circulation *67*:796, 1983.
253. Meltzer, L. E., and Kitchell, J. B.: The incidence of arrhythmias associated with acute myocardial infarction. Prog. Cardiovasc. Dis. *9*:50, 1966.
254. DeSanctis, R. W., Block, P., and Hutter, A. M.: Tachyarrhythmias in myocardial infarction. Circulation *45*:681, 1972.
255. Jewitt, D. E., Balcon, R., Raftery, E. B., and Oram, S.: Incidence and management of supraventricular arrhythmias after acute myocardial infarction. Lancet *2*:734, 1967.
256. Rothfeld, E. L., Parsonnet, J., McGorman, W., and Linden, S.: Harbingers of paroxysmal ventricular tachycardia in acute myocardial infarction. Chest *71*: 142, 1977.
257. El-Sherif, N., Gann, D., and Sung, R. J.: Initiation of ventricular fibrillation by supraventricular beats in patients with acute myocardial infarction. (Abstr.). Circulation *58*(Suppl. II):195, 1978.
258. James, T. N.: Myocardial infarction and atrial arrhythmias. Circulation *24*: 761, 1961.
259. Konecke, L. L., and Knoebel, S. B.: Nonparoxysmal junctional tachycardia complicating acute myocardial infarction. Circulation *45*:367, 1972.
260. Lown, B., Fakhro, A., Hood, W. B., and Thorn, G. W.: The coronary care unit—New perspectives and directions. J.A.M.A. *199*:188, 1967.
261. Julian, D. T., Valentine, P. Z., and Miller, G. G.: Disturbances of rate, rhythm and conduction in acute myocardial infarction. A prospective study of 100 consecutive unselected patients with the aid of electrocardiographic monitoring. Am. J. Med. *37*:915, 1964.
262. Lie, K. J., Wellens, H. J. J., Dorsnar, E., and Durrer, D.: Observations on patients with primary ventricular fibrillation complicating acute myocardial infarction. Circulation *52*:755, 1975.
263. El-Sherif, N., Myerburg, R. J., Scherlag, B. J., Befeler, B., Aranda, J. M., Castellanos, A., and Lazzara, R.: Electrocardiographic antecedents of primary ventricular fibrillation. Value of the R-on-T phenomenon in myocardial infarction. Br. Heart J. *38*:415, 1976.
264. Lawrie, D. M., Higgins, M. R., Godman, M. J., Julian, D. G., and Donald, K. W.: Ventricular fibrillation complicating acute myocardial infarction. Lancet *2*:523, 1968.
265. Williams, D. O., Scherlag, B. J., Hope, R. R., El-Sherif, N., and Lazzara, R.: The pathophysiology of malignant ventricular arrhythmias during acute myocardial ischemia. Circulation *50*:1163, 1974.
266. El-Sherif, N., Scherlag, B. J., and Lazzara, R.: Electrode catheter recordings during malignant ventricular arrhythmias following experimental acute myocardial ischemia. Evidence for reentry due to conduction delay and block in ischemic myocardium. Circulation *51*:1003, 1975.
267. DeSoyza, N., Meacham, D., Murphy, M. L., Kane, J. J., Doherty, J. E., and Bissett, J. K.: Evaluation of warning arrhythmias before paroxysmal ventricular tachycardia during acute myocardial infarction in man. Circulation *60*:814, 1979.
268. Roberts, R., Ambos, H. D., Loh, C. W., and Sobel, B. E.: Initiation of repetitive ventricular depolarizations by relatively late premature complexes in patients with acute myocardial infarction. Am. J. Cardiol. *41*:678, 1978.
269. Campbell, R. W. F., Murray, A., and Julian, D. G.: Relation of ventricular arrhythmias to ventricular fibrillation. Br. Heart J. *43*:109, 1980.
270. Wenger, T. L., Bigger, J. T., Jr., and Merrill, G. S.: Ventricular arrhythmias in the late hospital phase of acute myocardial infarction. Circulation *52*:110, 1975.
271. Schulze, R. A., Rouleau, J., Rigo, P., Bowers, S., Strauss, H. W., and Pitt, B.: Ventricular arrhythmias in the late phase of acute myocardial infarction: Relation to left ventricular function detected by gated cardiac blood pool scanning. Circulation *52*:1006, 1975.
272. Oliver, G. C., Nolle, F. M., and Tiefenbrunn, J.: Ventricular arrhythmias associated with sudden death in survivors of acute myocardial infarction. Am. J. Cardiol. *33*:160, 1974.
273. Moss, A. J., De Camilla, J. J., Davis, H. P., and Bayer, L.: Clinical significance of ventricular ectopic beats in the early post-hospital phase of myocardial infarction. Am. J. Cardiol. *39*:635, 1977.
274. Anderson, K. P., De Camilla, J., and Moss, A. J.: Clinical significance of ventricular tachycardia (three beats or longer) detected during ambulatory monitoring after myocardial infarction. Circulation *57*:890, 1978.
275. Bigger, J. T., Jr., Weld, F. M., and Rolnitzky, L. M.: Prevalence, characteristics and significance of ventricular tachycardia (three or more complexes) detected with ambulatory electrocardiographic recording in the late hospital phase of acute myocardial infarction. Am. J. Cardiol. *48*:815, 1981.
276. DeSoyza, N., Bissett, J. K., Kane, J. J., Murphy, M. L., and Doherty, J. E.: Association of accelerated idioventricular rhythm and paroxysmal ventricular tachycardia in acute myocardial infarction. Am. J. Cardiol. *34*:667, 1974.
277. Sclarovsky, S., Strasberg, B., Martonovich, G., and Agmon, J.: Ventricular rhythms with intermediate rates in acute myocardial infarction. Chest *74*:180, 1978.
278. Lichstein, E., Ribas-Meneclier, C., Gupta, P. K., and Chadda, K. D.: Incidence and description of accelerated idioventricular rhythm complicating acute myocardial infarction. Am. J. Med. *58*:192, 1975.
279. Lie, K. I., Liem, K. L., Schuilenburg, R. M., David, G. K., and Durrer, D.: Early identification of patients developing late in-hospital ventricular fibrillation after discharge from the coronary care unit. Am. J. Cardiol. *41*:674, 1978.
280. Shillingford, J., and Thomas, M.: Hemodynamic effects of acute myocardial infarction in man. Prog. Cardiovasc. Dis. *9*:571, 1967.
281. Lassers, B. E., Anderton, J. L., George, M., Muir, A. L., and Julian, D. G.: Hemodynamic effects of artificial pacing in complete heart block complicating acute myocardial infarction. Circulation *38*:308, 1968.
282. Ruskin, J., McHale, P. A., Harley, A., and Greenfield, J. C., Jr.: Pressure-flow studies in man; effects of atrial systole on left ventricular function. J. Clin. Invest. *49*:472, 1970.
283. Rahimtoola, S. H., Ehsani, A., Sinno, M. Z., Loeb, H. S., Rosen, K. M., and Gunnar, R. M.: Left atrial transport function in myocardial infarction; Importance of its booster function. Am. J. Med. *59*:686, 1975.
284. Damato, A. N., and Lau, S. H.: Clinical value of the electrogram of the conduction system. Prog. Cardiovasc. Dis. *13*:119, 1970.
285. Johansson, B. W.: Atrioventricular and bundle branch block in acute myocardial infarction. Natural history and prognosis. *In* Meltzer, L. E., and Dunning. A. J. (eds.): Textbook of Coronary Care. Philadelphia, Charles Press, 1972, p. 328.
286. Rotman, M., Wagner, G. S., and Wallace, A. G. P.: Bradyarrhythmias in acute myocardial infarction. Circulation *45*:703, 1972.
287. Friedberg, C. K., Cohen, H., and Donoso, E.: Advanced heart block as a complication of acute myocardial infarction. Role of pacemaker therapy. Prog. Cardiovasc. Dis. *10*:466, 1968.
288. Beregovich, J., Fenig, S., and Lassers, J.: Management of acute myocardial infarction complicated by advanced atrioventricular block: Role of artificial pacing. Am. J. Cardiol. *23*:54, 1969.
289. Lassers, B. W., and Julian, D. G.: Artificial pacing in management of complete heart block complicating myocardial infarction. Br. Med. J. *2*:142, 1968.
290. Chatterjee, K., Harris, A., and Leatham, A.: The risk of pacing after infarction, and current recommendation. Lancet *2*:1061, 1969.
291. Kostuk, W. J., and Beanland, D. S.: Complete heart block associated with acute myocardial infarction. Am. J. Cardiol. *26*:380, 1970.
292. Biddle, T. L., Ehrich, D. A., Hu, P. N., and Hodges, M.: Relation of heart block and left ventricular dysfunction in acute myocardial infarction. Am. J. Cardiol. *39*:961, 1977.
293. Hindman, M. C., Wagner, G. S., Jaro, M., Atkins, J. M., Scheinman, M. M., DeSanctis, R. W., Hutter, A. H., Yeatman, L., Rubenfire, M., Pujure, C., Rubvin, M., and Morris, J. J.: The clinical significance of bundle branch block complicating acute myocardial infarction. I. Clinical characteristics, hospital mortality and one-year follow-up. Circulation *58*:679, 1978.
294. Lie, K. I., Wellens, H. J., and Schuilenburg, R. M.: Bundle branch block and

acute myocardial infarction. *In* Wellens, H. J. J., Lie, K. I., and Janse, M. J. (eds.): The Conduction System of the Heart: Structure, Function and Clinical Implications. Philadelphia, Lea and Febiger, 1976, pp. 662–672.
295. Mullins, C. B., and Atkins, J. M.: Prognoses and management of ventricular conduction blocks in acute myocardial infarction. Mod. Concepts Cardiovasc. Dis. *45*:129, 1976.
296. Scheinman, M. M., and Gonzalez, R. P.: Fascicular block and acute myocardial infarction. J.A.M.A. *244*:2646, 1980.
297. Atkins, J. M., Leshin, S. J., Blomquist, G., and Mullins, C. B.: Ventricular conduction blocks and sudden death in acute myocardial infarction. N. Engl. J. Med. *288*:281, 1973.
298. Godman, M. J., Lassers, B. W., and Julian, D. G.: Complete bundle branch block complicating acute myocardial infarction. N. Engl. J. Med. *282*:237, 1970.
299. Kostuk, W., Barr, J. W., Simon, A. L., and Ross, J., Jr.: Correlations between the chest film and hemodynamics in acute myocardial infarction. Circulation *48*:624, 1973.
300. McHugh, T. J., Forrester, J. S., Adler, L., Zion, D., and Swan, H. J. C.: Pulmonary vascular congestion in acute myocardial infarction: Hemodynamic and radiologic correlations. Ann. Intern. Med. *79*:29, 1972.
301. Timmis, A. D., Fowler, M. B., Burwood, R. J., Gishen, P., Vincent, R., and Chamberlain, D. A.: Pulmonary oedema without critical increase in left atrial pressure in acute myocardial infarction. Br. Med. J. *283*:636, 1981.
302. Field, B. J., Russell, R. O., Jr., Moraski, R. E., Soto, B., Hood, W. P., Jr., Burdenshaw, J. A., Smith, M., Maurer, B. J., and Rackley, C. E.: Left ventricular size and function and heart size in the year following myocardial infarction. Circulation *50*:331, 1974.
303. Brattler, A., Karliner, J. S., Higgins, C. B., Slutsky, R., Gilpin, E. A., Froelicher, V. F., and Ross, J., Jr.: The initial chest x-ray in acute myocardial infarction. Prediction of early and late mortality and survival. Circulation *61*: 1004, 1980.
304. Gibson, R. S., Taylor, G. J., Watson, D. D., Stebbins, P. T., Martin, R. P., Crampton, R. S., and Beller, G. A.: Predicting the extent and location of coronary artery disease during the early postinfarction period by quantitative thallium-201 scintigraphy. Am. J. Cardiol. *47*:1010, 1981.
305. Willerson, J. T., Parkey, R. W., Lewis, S. E., Bonte, F. J., and Buja, L. M.: Hot-spot imaging for patients with acute myocardial infarction. J. Cardiovasc. Med. 7:291, 1982.
306. Geltman, E. M., Biello, D., Welch, M. J., Ter-Pogossian, M. M., Roberts, R., and Sobel, B. E.: Characterization of nontransmural myocardial infarction by positron-emission tomography. Circulation *65*:747, 1982.
306a. Lindvall, K., Erhardt, L., and Sjogren, A.: Serial M-mode echocardiographic mapping in myocardial infarction: A quantitative evaluation of left ventricular wall motion abnormalities. Clin. Cardiol. *6*:220, 1983.
307. Teichholz, L. E., Kreulen, T., Herman, M. V., and Gorlin, R.: Problems in echocardiographic volume determinations; echocardiographic-angiographic correlations in the presence or absence of asynergy. Am. J. Cardiol. *37*:7, 1976.
308. Corya, B. C., Rasmussen, S., Knoebel, S. B., and Feigenbaum, H.: Echocardiography in acute myocardial infarction. Am. J. Cardiol. *36*:1, 1975.
309. Nieminen, M., and Heikkilä, J.: Echoventriculography in acute myocardial infarction. II. Monitoring of left ventricular performance. Br. Heart J. *38*:271, 1976.
310. Fletcher, P. J., Berning, J., Wynne, J., Ostriker, G., Sayres, M., Holman, B. L., and Alpert, J. S.: Prospective evaluation of M-mode echocardiography in acute myocardial infarction: Comparison of gated radionuclide ventriculography. Br. Heart J.
311. Feigenbaum, H., Corya, B. C., Dillon, J. C., Weyman, A. E., Rasmussen, S., Black, M. J., and Chang, S.: Role of echocardiography in patients with coronary artery disease. Am. J. Cardiol. *37*:775, 1976.
312. Chandraratna, P. A. N., Balachandran, P. K., Shah, P. M., and Hodges, M.: Echocardiographic observation on ventricular septal rupture complicating acute myocardial infarction. Circulation *51*:506, 1975.
313. DeJoseph, R. L., Seides, S. F., Lindner, A., and Damato, A. N.: Echocardiographic findings of ventricular septal rupture in acute myocardial infarction. Am. J. Cardiol. *36*:346, 1975.
314. Sharpe, D. N., Botvinick, E. H., Shames, D. M., Schiller, N. B., Massie, B. M., Chatterjee, D., and Parmley, W. W.: The noninvasive diagnosis of right ventricular infarction. Circulation *57*:483, 1978.
315. Heger, J. J., Weyman, A. E., Wann, L. S., Dillon, J. C., and Feigenbaum, H.: Cross-sectional echocardiography in acute myocardial infarction: Detection and localization of regional left ventricular asynergy. Circulation *60*:531, 1979.
316. Visser, C. A., Lie, K. I., Becker, A. E., and Durrer, D.: Apex two-dimensional echocardiography. Alternative approach to quantification of acute myocardial infarction. Br. Heart J. *47*:461, 1982.
317. Gibson, R. S., Bishop, H. L., Stamm, R. B., Crampton, R. S., Beller, G. A., and Martin, R. P.: Value of early two dimensional echocardiography in patients with acute myocardial infarction. Am. J. Cardiol. *49*:1110, 1982.
318. Richards, K. L., Hoekenga, D. E., Leach, J. K., and Blaustein, J. C.: Dopplercardiographic diagnosis of interventricular septal rupture. Chest *76*: 101, 1979.
319. Bishop, H. L., Gibson, R. S., Stamm, R. B., Beller, G. A., and Martin, R. P.: Role of two-dimensional echocardiography in the evaluation of patients with ventricular septal rupture postmyocardial infarction. Am. Heart J. *102*:965, 1981.
320. Donaldson, R. M., and Ballester, M.: Echocardiographic visualization of the anatomic causes of mitral regurgitation resulting from myocardial infarction. Postgrad. Med. J. *58*:257, 1982.
321. Morganroth, J., Parisi, A., and Pohost, G. M. (eds.): Noninvasive Cardiac Imaging. Chicago, Year Book Medical Publishers, 1983, p. 203.
322. Hamosh, P., Cohn, J. N., Engleman, K., Broder, M. I., and Freis, E. D.: Systolic time intervals and left ventricular function in acute myocardial infarction. Circulation *45*:375, 1972.
323. Inoue, K., Young, G. M., Brievson, A. L., Smulyan, H., and Eich, R. H.: Isometric contraction period of the left ventricle in acute myocardial infarction. Circulation *42*:79, 1970.
324. Parker, M. E., and Just, H. G.: Systolic time intervals in coronary artery disease as indices of left ventricular function: Fact or fancy? Br. Heart J. *36*:368, 1974.
325. Brubakk, O., and Overskeid, K.: Systolic time intervals in acute myocardial infarction. Acta Med. Scand. *199*:33, 1976.
326. Khan, A. H., and Haywood, L. J.: Value of serial apexcardiograms during and after myocardial infarction. Chest *70*:367, 1976.
327. Swan, H. J. C., Ganz, W., Forrester, J. S., Marcus, H., Diamond, G., and Chonette, D.: Catheterization of the heart in man with use of a flow-directed balloon-tipped catheter. N. Engl. J. Med. *283*:447, 1970.
328. Russell, R. O., Jr., Rackley, C. E., Pombo, J., Hunt, D., Potanin, C., and Dodge, H. T.: Effects of increasing left ventricular filling pressure in patients with acute myocardial infarction. J. Clin. Invest. *49*:1539, 1970.
329. Crexells, C., Chatterjee, K., Forrester, J. S., Dikshit, K., and Swan, H. J. C.: Optimal level of filling pressure in the left side of the heart in acute myocardial infarction. N. Engl. J. Med. *289*:1263, 1973.
330. Raphael, L. D., Mantle, J. A., Moraski, R. E., Rogers, W. J., Russell, R. O., Jr., and Rackley, C. E.: Quantitative assessment of ventricular performance in unstable ischemic heart disease by dextran function curves. Circulation *55*:858, 1977.
331. Weisel, R. D., Berger, R. L., and Hechtman, H. B.: Measurement of cardiac output by thermodilution. N. Engl. J. Med. *292*:682, 1975.
332. Rahimtoola, S. H., Loeb, H. S., Ehsani, A., Sinno, Z., Chuquimia, R., Lal, R., Rosen, K. M., and Gunnar, R. M.: Relationship of pulmonary artery to left ventricular diastolic pressures in acute myocardial infarction. Circulation *46*: 283, 1972. .
333. Fuchs, R. M., Heuser, R.R., Yin, F. C. P., Brinker, J. A.: Limitations of pulmonary wedge V waves in diagnosing mitral regurgitation. Am. J. Cardio. *49*: 849, 1982.
334. Gewirtz, H., Gold, H. K., Fallon, J. T., Pasternak, R. C., and Leinbach, R. C.: Role of right ventricular infarction in cardiogenic shock associated with inferior myocardial infarction. Br. Heart J. *42*:719, 1979.
335. Meister, S. G., and Helfant, R. H.: Rapid bedside differentiation of ruptured interventricular septum from acute mitral insufficiency. N. Engl. J. Med. *287*: 1024, 1972.
336. Rigaud, M., Rocha, P., Boschat, J., Favcot, J. C., Bardet, J., and Bourdarias, J. P.: Regional left ventricular function assessed by contrast angiography in acute myocardial infarction. Circulation *60*:130, 1979.
337. Stewart, D. K., Hamilton, G. W., Murray, J. A., and Kennedy, J. W.: Left ventricular function and coronary artery anatomy before and after myocardial infarction: A study of six cases. Circulation *49*:47, 1974.
338. Baxley, W. A., Jones, W. B., and Dodge, H. T.: Left ventricular anatomical and functional abnormalities in chronic postinfarction heart failure. Ann. Intern. Med. *74*:499, 1971.
339. Moraski, R. E., Russell, R. O., Jr., Smith, M., and Rackley, C. E.: Left ventricular function in patients with and without myocardial infarction and one, two, or three vessel coronary artery disease. Am. J. Cardiol. *35*:1, 1975.
340. Bertrand, M. E., Rousseau, M. F., Lablanche, J. M., Carre, A. G., and Lekieffre, J. P.: Cineangiographic assessment of left ventricular function in the acute phase of transmural myocardial infarction. Am. J. Cardiol. *43*:472, 1979.
341. Ratshin, R. A., Rackley, C. E., and Russell, R. O., Jr.: Hemodynamic evaluation of left ventricular function in shock complicating myocardial infarction. Circulation *45*:127, 1972.
341a. Rapaport, E., and Remedios, P.: The high risk patient after recovery from myocardial infarction: Recognition and management. J. Am. Coll. Cardiol. *1*:391, 1983.
341b. Coll, S., Castaner, A., Sanz, G., Roig, E., Magrina, J., Navarro-Lopez, F., and Betriu, A.: Prevalence and prognosis after a first nontransmural myocardial infarction. Am. J. Cardiol. *51*:1584, 1983.
341c. Madsen, E. B., Hougaard, P., and Gilpin, E.: Dynamic evaluation of prognosis from time-dependent variables in acute myocardial infarction. Am. J. Cardiol. *51*:1579, 1983.
342. Killip, T., and Kimball, J. I.: Treatment of myocardial infarction in a coronary care unit. A two year experience with 250 patients. Am. J. Cardiol. *20*:457, 1967.
343. Peel, A. A. F., Semple, T., Wang, I., Lancaster, W. M., and Dall, J. L. G.: A coronary prognostic index for grading the severity of infarction. Br. Heart J. *24*:745, 1962.
344. Norris, R. M., Brandt, P. W. T., Caughey, D. E., Lee, A. J., and Scott, P. J.: A new coronary prognostic index. Lancet *1*:274, 1969.
344a. Buda, A. J., Macdonald, I. L., Dubbin, J. D., Orr, S. A., and Strauss, H. D.: Myocardial infarct extension: Prevalence, clinical significance, and problems in diagnosis. Am. Heart J. *105*:744, 1983.
345. Strauss, H. D.: Myocardial infarction extension: Clinical significance. Primary Cardiol. *8*:14, 1982.

346. Baker, J. T., Bramlet, D. A., Lester, R. M., Harrison, D. G., Roe, C. R., and Cobb, F. R.: Myocardial infarct extension: Incidence and relationship to survival. Circulation *65*:918, 1982.
347. Marmor, A., Geltman, E. M., Schechtman, K., Sobel, B. E., and Roberts, R.: Recurrent myocardial infarction: Clinical predictors and prognostic implications. Circulation *66*:415, 1982.
348. Marmor, A., Sobel, B. E., and Roberts, E.: Factors presaging early recurrent myocardial infarction ("extension"). Am. J. Cardiol. *48*:603, 1981.
349. Verdouw, P. D., Hagemeijer, F., van Dorp, W. G., van der Vorm, A., and Hugenholtz, P. G.: Short-term survival after acute myocardial infarction predicted by hemodynamic parameters. Circulation *52*:413, 1975.
350. Sanford, C. F., Corbett, J., Nicod, P., Curry, G. L., Lewis, S. E., Dehmer, G. J., Anderson, A., Moses, B., and Willerson, J. T.: Value of radionuclide ventriculography in the immediate characterization of patients with acute myocardial infarction. Am. J. Cardiol. *49*:637, 1982.
351. Miller, D. H., and Borer, J. S.: Exercise testing early after myocardial infarction. Risks and benefits. Am. J. Med. *72*:427, 1982.
351a. Becker, L. C., Silverman, K. J., Bulkley, B. H., Kallman, C. H., Mellits, E. D., and Weisfeldt, M.: Comparison of early thallium-201 scintigraphy and gated blood pool imaging for predicting mortality in patients with acute myocardial infarction. Circulation *67*:1272, 1983.
352. Holman, B. L., Chisholm, R. J., and Braunwald, E.: The prognostic implications of acute myocardial infarct scintigraphy with ^{99m}Tc-pyrophosphate. Circulation *57*:320, 1978.
353. Nasmith, J., Marpole, D., Rahal, D., Homan, J., Stewart, S., and Sniderman, A.: Clinical outcomes after inferior myocardial infarction. Ann. Intern. Med. *96*:22, 1982.
354. Gibson, R. S., Crampton, R. S., Watson, D. D., Taylor, G. J., Carabello, B. A., Holt, N. D., and Beller, G. A.: Precordial ST segment depression during acute inferior myocardial infarction: Clinical, scintigraphic and angiographic correlations. Circulation *66*:732, 1982.
355. Salcedo, J. R., Baird, M. G., Chambers, R. J., and Beanlands, D. S.: Significance of reciprocal S-T segment depression in anterior precordial leads in acute inferior myocardial infarction: Concomitant left anterior descending coronary artery disease? Am. J. Cardiol. *48*:1003, 1981.
355a. Ong, L., Valdellon, B., Coromilas, J., Brody, R., Reiser, P., and Morrison, J.: Precordial S-T segment depression in inferior myocardial infarction. Evaluation by quantitative thallium-201 scintigraphy and technetium-99m ventriculography. Am. J. Cardiol. *51*:734, 1983.
356. Schuster, E. H., and Bulkley, B. H.: Early post-infarction angina. Ischemia at a distance and ischemia in the infarct zone. N. Engl. J. Med. *305*:1101, 1981.
357. Edson, J. N.: Subendocardial myocardial infarction. Am. Heart J. *60*:323, 1960.
358. Erikssen, J., Muller, C., and Anderssen, J. N.: Atypical case histories and electrocardiograms in myocardial infarction. Acta Med. Scand. *188*:95, 1970.
359. Friedberg, C. K.: Symposium: Myocardial infarction 1972. Part 1. Introduction. Circulation *45*:179, 1972.
360. Hutter, A. M., Jr., DeSanctis, R. W., Flynn, T., and Yeatman, L. A.: Nontransmural myocardial infarction: A comparison of hospital and late clinical course of patients with that of matched patients with transmural anterior and transmural inferior myocardial infarction. Am. J. Cardiol. *48*:595, 1981.
361. Madias, J. E., Chahine, R. A., Gorlin, R., and Blacklow, D. J.: A comparison of transmural and nontransmural acute myocardial infarction. Circulation *49*: 498, 1974.
361a. Phibbs, B.: "Transmural" versus "Subendocardial" myocardial infarction: An electrocardiographic myth. J. Am. Coll. Cardiol. *1*:561, 1983.
362. Rigo, R., Murray, M., Taylor, D. R., Weisfeldt, M. L., Strauss, H. W., and Pitt, B.: Hemodynamic and prognostic findings in patients with transmural and nontransmural infarction. Circulation *51*:1064, 1975.
363. Madias, J. E., and Gorlin, R.: They myth of "mild" myocardial infarction. Ann. Intern. Med. *86*:347, 1977.
364. Madigan, N. P., Rutherford, B. D., and Frye, R. L.: The clinical course, early prognosis and coronary anatomy of subendocardial infarction. Am. J. Med. *60*: 634, 1976.
364a. DeFeyter, P. J., van Eenige, M. J., Dighton, D. H., and Roos, J. P.: Exercise testing early after myocardial infarction. Chest *83*:853, 1983.
365. Fuller, C. M., Raizner, A. E., Verani, M., Nahormek, P. A., Chahine, R. A., McEntee, C. W., and Miller, R. R.: Early post–myocardial infarction treadmill stress testing. Ann. Intern. Med. *94*:734, 1981.
365a. Nair, R., Allan, K., Reg, N., Baird, M. G., Beanlands, D. S., and Higginson, L. A.: A comparison of clinical and treadmill predictors of prognosis following acute myocardial infarction. J. Am. Coll. Cardiol. *1*:717, 1983.
365b. Gibson, R. S., Watson, D. D., Crampton, R. S., Beller, G. A.: Prospective comparison of submaximal exercise TL-201 scintigraphy 2 weeks after and symptom-limited maximal testing 3 months after myocardial infarction. J. Am. Coll. Cardiol. *1*:654, 1983.
366. Corbett, J. R., Dehmer, G. J., Lewis, S. E., Woodward, W., Henderson, E., Parkey, R. W., Blomqvist, C. G., and Willerson, J. T.: The prognostic value of submaximal exercise testing with radionuclide ventriculography before hospital discharge in patients with recent myocardial infarction. Circulation *64*:535, 1981.
366a. Hung,. J., Goris, M. L., Nash, E., Kraemer, H. C., and DeBusk, R. F.: The comparative prognostic value of standard treadmill testing, rest and exercise thallium myocardial perfusion scintigraphy and radionuclide ventriculography 3 weeks after myocardial infarction. J. Am. Coll. Cardiol. *1*:654, 1983.
367. Sanz, G., Castaner, A., Betriu, A., Magrina, J., Roig, E., Coll, S., Pare, J. C., and Navarro-Lopez, F.: Determinants of prognosis in survivors of myocardial infarction. A prospective clinical angiographic study. N. Engl. J. Med. *306*: 1065, 1982.
368. Borer, J. S., Rosing, D. R., Miller, R. H., Stark, R. M., Kent, K. M., Bacharach, S. L., Green, M. V., Lake, C. R., Cohen, H., Holmes, D., Donohue, D., Baker, W., and Epstein, S. E.: Natural history of left ventricular function during 1 year after acute myocardial infarction: Comparison with clinical, electrocardiographic and biochemical determinations. Am. J. Cardiol. *46*:1, 1980.
369. Mukharji, J., Rude, R., Gustafson, N., Poole, K., Passamani, E., Thomas, L. J., Jr., Strauss, H. W., Muller, J. E., Roberts, R., Raabe, D. S., Jr., Braunwald, E., Willerson, J. T., and cooperating investigators, MILIS: Late sudden death following myocardial infarction: Interdependence of risk factors. J. Am. Coll. Cardiol. *1*:585, 1983.
370. Moss, A. J., Bigger, J. T., Case, R. B., Gillespie, J., Goldstein, R., Greenberg, H., Krone, R., Marcus, F. I., Odoroff, C. L., and Oliver, G. C.: Risk stratification and prognostication after myocardial infarction. J. Am. Coll. Cardiol. *1*:716, 1983.

38 THE MANAGEMENT OF ACUTE MYOCARDIAL INFARCTION

by Burton E. Sobel, M.D., and Eugene Braunwald, M.D.

More than 60 per cent of the deaths associated with acute myocardial infarction (AMI) occur within one hour of the event and are attributable to malignant arrhythmias, usually ventricular fibrillation. This manifestation of ischemic heart disease is discussed in Chapter 23. Despite the importance of sudden death, more than 500,000 patients are hospitalized annually in the United States for AMI.[1] The pathological, physiological, and clinical features of this condition are presented in Chapter 37, while its management is considered here.

Careful monitoring of cardiac rhythm and the prompt treatment of arrhythmias have reduced sharply the incidence of in-hospital deaths from AMI.[2] Accordingly, most deaths among patients with this condition who reach the hospital are now attributable to left ventricular failure and shock and occur within the three or four days after the onset of infarction.[3] Only a minority of in-hospital deaths now result from intractable arrhythmias, and most of these occur in settings where monitoring and/or treatment is inadequate or are secondary to extensive infarction and left ventricular failure.[2,4–6]

Prior to the advent of coronary care units, treatment of AMI was directed almost exclusively toward allowing healing of the infarct, preventing cardiac rupture and other complications such as pulmonary and systemic embolism, and sustaining arterial pressure and urine output. Subsequently, the major emphasis of therapeutic strategy was on the prevention and aggressive treatment of arrhythmias. The concept that infarct size is an important determinant of prognosis (Fig. 37–8, p. 1271) and that its ultimate extent might be modified favorably by early implementation of selected physiological and pharmacological interventions has directed attention to protection of jeopardized myocardium by restoring perfusion to ischemic tissue or by a variety of pharmacological interventions.[7,8] However, as discussed later, the ultimate clinical benefits of this approach have yet to be realized. The treatment of AMI is discussed under five headings:

1. General measures
2. Treatment and prophylaxis of arrhythmias
3. Treatment of hemodynamic disturbances
4. Minimization of infarct size
5. Convalescence

GENERAL MEASURES

MOBILE CORONARY CARE UNITS. It is now well established that most deaths associated with AMI occur within the first hour after its onset and that death is usually due to ventricular fibrillation (Chap. 23).[9,10] Accordingly, the importance of the immediate implementation of definitive resuscitative efforts and of rapidly transporting the patient to a hospital cannot be overemphasized. Well-equipped ambulances, staffed by personnel trained in the care of the infarct victim, allow definitive therapy to commence while the patient is being transported to the hospital.[11,12] These specially equipped and staffed ambulances have been termed mobile coronary care units; to be used effectively, they must be placed strategically within a community and excellent radio-communication systems must be available. They should be equipped with a battery-operated monitoring oscilloscope and direct writing electrocardiograph; a battery-operated DC defibrillator; oxygen, endotracheal tubes, and suction apparatus; and commonly used cardiovascular drugs. A radiotelemetry system that allows transmission of the electrocardiogram to the hospital is desirable but not essential.

The effectiveness of these systems in Belfast, Ireland,[11] Seattle, Washington,[13] and Columbus, Ohio[14] has been amply documented. The rapid initiation of prehospital cardiopulmonary resuscitation facilitated by mobile coronary care units and trained paramedical personnel results in initially successful resuscitation in approximately two thirds of patients. It has been demonstrated that the frequency of death during transportation can be diminished from 22 to 9 per cent when defibrillation equipment and trained paramedical personnel are available.[15] In addition to prompt defibrillation, the efficacy of prehospital care appears to depend on several factors, including early relief of pain with its deleterious physiological sequelae, the reduction of excessive activity of the autonomic nervous system, and abolition of prelethal arrhythmias, such as ventricular tachycardia.

CORONARY CARE UNITS. During the past two decades the mortality of patients with AMI treated in coronary care units has declined significantly from what it had been before the introduction of these units.[4] Reduction in mortality has resulted almost entirely from the elimination of primary arrhythmias as a cause of death.[2] Most instances of this arrhythmia occur *before* the patient reaches the hospital, and only about 5 per cent of patients develop a primary ventricular arrhythmia *after* they reach the hospital, an average of five to six hours after the onset of the attack in most series. Deaths from primary ventricular fibrillation have been prevented because the coronary care unit allows continuous monitoring of cardiac rhythm by highly trained nurses with the authority to administer immediate treatment and prophylaxis of arrhythmias in the absence of physicians, and because of the specialized equipment (defibrillators, pacemakers) and drugs available for instantaneous use.[16] Although all these benefits can certainly be achieved for patients scattered throughout the hospital, the clustering of patients with AMI has greatly improved the efficient use of the trained personnel, facilities, and equipment. In recent years, with increasing emphasis on hemodynamic monitoring and treatment of the serious complications of AMI with such modalities as afterload reduction and intra-aortic balloon counterpulsation, the coronary care unit has assumed even greater importance.

At the same time, the value of coronary care units for patients with *uncomplicated AMI* has been questioned and restudied.[17] In one widely publicized randomized trial, patients with suspected infarction were evaluated initially at home; after a two-hour observation interval they were divided at random into home-management and hospital-management groups.[18] Although the six-week mortality rate among patients with infarction in the two groups was similar (13 per cent and 11 per cent, respectively), such low overall mortality rates make detection of small although real differences difficult. Furthermore, approximately one fourth of the patients with significant electrophysiological or hemodynamic complications were excluded. Thus, hospital care was provided for all high-risk patients. Furthermore, under the general conditions of medical practice in the United States, it is difficult to provide the same immediate intensive care at home for all patients with suspected infarction that was made available in this study. Since prediction of the occurrence of early complications is imperfect, we believe that the observation and prompt treatment possible in a well-staffed coronary care unit continue to justify the reliance placed upon this setting as the primary one for early management of patients with suspected or confirmed AMI. Patient delay in seeking medical attention and the medical system's delay in responding reduce the potential impact of the coronary care unit because the patients do not reach the unit until the maximum danger has passed. Therefore, education of the public, of patients at high risk of AMI, and those members of the medical profession involved in responding to the initial complaints of these patients is likely to be rewarded by further reductions of mortality.[17,19]

INTERMEDIATE CORONARY CARE UNITS. Since the hazard of *primary* ventricular fibrillation is essentially over in 24 to 36 hours, there is little need for patients with entirely *uncomplicated* infarcts to remain in a coronary care unit for more than two days. Obviously, patients with complicated infarcts, particularly those with arrhythmias and pump failure, require continued care in such a unit. There is an increased risk of ventricular tachycardia and ventricular fibrillation in the late MI period, and an increased vulnerability to ventricular fibrillation is responsible for these arrhythmias four to ten days after AMI, accounting for between 10 and 30 per cent of total hospital deaths.[20,21] In view of this significant in-hospital mortality after discharge from the coronary care unit, continued surveillance in intermediate coronary care units (also called "step-down units") is justifiable.

Risk factors for sudden death in the hospital *after* discharge from the coronary care unit include intraventricular conduction defects,[22] sinus tachycardia persisting for more than two days, and extensive anterior infarction, as well as episodes of ventricular fibrillation and of atrial flutter or fibrillation occurring while the patient is in the coronary care unit, and, possibly, marked electrocardiographic ST-segment abnormalities induced by low levels of activity.[23] Although not established with certainty, it is suspected that substantial reduction in the late hospital death rate can be achieved with the use of intermediate coronary care units, which permit prolonged continuous monitoring of the electrocardiogram and prompt, effective treatment of ventricular fibrillation and other serious arrhythmias.[2,4,10,22] The availability of these units may be useful also in helping to identify those patients who remain free from complications for a minimum of one week, since early discharge from the hospital appears to be feasible for this subset.[24,25] An additional potential advantage is facilitation of patient education in a group setting with formal lectures and videotape programs.

ANALGESIA. The alleviation or reduction of pain is a critical factor in the care of patients with AMI. Although a wide variety of agents has been used to treat the pain associated with MI, including meperidine, pentazocine, and morphine, the latter agent remains the drug of choice except in patients with well-documented morphine hypersensitivity. Four to 8 mg should be administered intravenously and doses of 2 to 8 mg repeated at intervals of 5 to 15 minutes until the pain is relieved or evident toxicity—i.e., hypotension, depression of respiration, or severe vomiting—precludes further administration of the drug. In some patients, remarkably large cumulative doses of morphine (2 to 3 mg/kg) may be required and are usually tolerated.

The reduction of anxiety resulting from morphine diminishes the patient's restlessness and the activity of the autonomic nervous system, with a consequent reduction of the heart's metabolic demands. The beneficial effect of morphine in patients with pulmonary edema is unequivocal (p. 571) and may relate to several factors, including peripheral arterial and venous dilatation (particularly among patients with excessive sympathoadrenal activity), reduction of the work of breathing, and slowing of heart rate secondary to combined withdrawal of sympathetic tone and augmentation of vagal tone.[26]

Hypotension following the administration of morphine can be minimized by maintaining the patient in a supine position and elevating the lower extremities if systolic arterial pressure declines below 100 mm Hg. Obviously, such positioning is undesirable in the presence of pulmonary edema, but morphine rarely produces hypotension under these circumstances. The concomitant administration of atropine in doses of 0.5 to 1.5 mg intravenously may be helpful in reducing the excessive vagomimetic effects of morphine, particularly when hypotension and bradycardia are present before it is administered. Respiratory depression is an unusual complication of morphine in the presence of severe pain or pulmonary edema, but as the patient's cardiovascular status improves, impairment of ventilation may supervene and should be watched for. It can be treated with Narcan, in doses of 0.4 mg intravenously at 5-minute intervals to a maximum of 1.2 mg. Nausea and vomiting may be troublesome side effects following large doses of morphine and may be treated with a phenothiazine in order to avoid the marked stress on the circulation resulting from emesis.

Other analgesics such as meperidine are less effective than is morphine but equally likely to produce side effects and prone to augment ventricular rate. Inhalation of *nitrous oxide*, in concentrations of from 20 to 50 per cent, combined with oxygen, has been utilized widely in Europe and with increasing frequency in the United States. It frequently provides effective analgesia, particularly in patients with relatively mild pain[27,28] and in those having recurrent prolonged episodes of pain. Nitrous oxide appears to influence myocardial oxygen demands favorably, since its sedative action diminishes the patient's total metabolic needs. It does not depress left ventricular function or produce significant hemodynamic changes or adverse reactions.

OXYGENATION. Hypoxemia is common in patients with AMI and is usually secondary to ventilation-perfusion abnormalities[29] (pp. 1276 and 1787), which are sequelae of left ventricular failure; patchy pneumonia and intrinsic pulmonary disease are additional causes of hypoxemia. It is common practice to treat all patients hospitalized with AMI with oxygen for 24 to 48 hours, based on the very common occurrence of arterial hypoxemia and both experimental[30] and clinical[31] evidence that increased oxygen in the inspired air protects ischemic myocardium. However, augmentation of the fraction of oxygen in the inspired air does not elevate oxygen delivery significantly in patients who are not hypoxemic. Furthermore, it may increase systemic vascular resistance and arterial pressure and thereby lower cardiac output slightly.

In view of these considerations, arterial oxygen tension should be measured at the time of the patient's admission to the coronary care unit; oxygen therapy may be omitted if it is normal. On the other hand, oxygen should be administered to patients with AMI when arterial hypoxemia is clinically evident or can be documented.[32] In these patients, serial arterial blood gas measurements may be employed to follow the efficacy of oxygen therapy. Although patients with AMI may exhibit a reduction in precordial ST-segment elevation during 100 per cent oxygen breathing, no long-term effect on survival or on the development of complications has been documented.[31]

In general, the delivery of 2 to 4 L/min of 100 per cent oxygen by mask or nasal prongs for two to three days is satisfactory for most patients with mild hypoxemia. If arterial oxygenation is still depressed on this regimen, the flow rate may have to be increased. In patients with pulmonary edema, endotracheal intubation and controlled ventilation at a positive pressure may be necessary. Although hyperbaric oxygen has been evaluated in experimental animals[33] and in patients[34] with AMI, routine implementation of this intervention in the conventional clinical setting is impractical, and no long-term benefit has been established. Alternative approaches designed to facilitate delivery of oxygen to ischemic myocardium, such as intravenous administration of fluorocarbon preparations, capable of enhancing oxygen-carrying capacity and reducing viscosity of the circulating blood, although promising in animal experiments, have not yet been evaluated clinically.

PHYSICAL ACTIVITY. In the absence of all complications, patients with AMI need not be confined to bed for more than 24 to 36 hours and may use a bedside commode from the time of admission. They may sit in a chair for two half-hour periods on the second and for two one-hour periods on the third day. If arrhythmia, heart failure, and other significant complications have not occurred or if they are controlled, the patient may be transferred out of the coronary care unit after three days. Monitoring for an additional two days in an intermediate care unit is desirable. A nurse should help wash the patient during the first five days. If the convalescence continues uneventfully, limited ambulation within the room can be begun on the fourth or fifth day. Activity can then increase progressively, and a shower may be allowed on the ninth or tenth day.

Hospitalization and enforced bed rest for any illness may lead to complications, particularly in elderly patients, such as constipation, decubitus ulcers, excessive resorption of bone with formation of renal calculi, atelectasis, thrombophlebitis, pulmonary emboli, urinary retention, mild anemia due to repetitive blood sampling for diagnostic tests, impaired oral intake of fluids, bleeding from the gastrointestinal tract due to stress ulcers, and deconditioning of cardiovascular reflex responses to postural changes. Because of the precarious status of the heart recovering from AMI, avoidance of such complications is of primary importance. For example, constipation may lead to straining, transitory reduction of venous return and diminution of cardiac output, impaired coronary perfusion, and ventricular arrhythmias, occasionally culminating in ventricular fibrillation. Early implementation of a bed-chair regimen appears to be useful in avoiding many of the difficulties encountered previously among patients confined to bed for several weeks.

Other general measures include (1) A liquid diet for 24 hours, because of the risk of nausea and vomiting or cardiac arrest early after infarction and the need to reduce the risk of aspiration. This should be followed by a 1500 calorie soft diet, with no added salt, divided into multiple small feedings for several days. Then, in the absence of heart failure, a regular diet, low in cholesterol and saturated fats, is appropriate. Caffeine-rich beverages should be avoided because of their possible arrhythmogenic effects. (2) Dioctyl sodium sulfosuccinate, 100 mg daily, or another stool softener should be used to prevent constipation and straining. (3) The emotional impact of an AMI and of hospitalization in a coronary care unit (p. 1829) should be offset by thoughtful explanations of the nature of the illness, the function of the equipment, and the purpose of the procedures. A deliberate effort should be made to maintain the atmosphere in the coronary care unit as quiet and restful as possible. Diazepam, 2 to 5 mg orally four times a day, is useful to allay the anxiety that is so common in this setting. Flurazepam, 15 to 30 mg, or an equivalent narcotic may be given for sleep. (4) Derangements potentially contributing to arrhythmias, such as hypoxemia, hypovolemia, disturbances of acid-base balance or of electrolytes, and digitalis toxicity should be identified and corrected. (5) The treatment of post–myocardial infarction pericarditis and Dressler's syndrome are discussed on pp. 1505 and 1514.

ANTICOAGULANTS. There are at least three theoretical reasons for anticipating that anticoagulants might be beneficial in the management of AMI: (1) Since the coronary occlusion responsible for the AMI is often a thrombus (p. 1265), anticoagulants might be expected to halt or slow progression and to prevent the development of new thrombi elsewhere in the coronary arterial tree (2) Anticoagulants might be expected to diminish the formation of mural thrombi (p. 1271) and resultant systemic embolization (3) Anticoagulants might be expected to reduce the incidence of venous thrombosis and pulmonary embolization.

Despite several decades of evaluation, the results of the treatment of AMI with anticoagulants are inconclusive. However, sporadic reports continue to appear of the favorable effects of anticoagulants on mortality among patients hospitalized with AMI.[36–39] Salutary effects on the underlying coronary disease, progression, or recurrence of infarction have not been clearly demonstrated with conventional anticoagulant drugs, yet it is clear that they decrease the incidence of cerebral emboli resulting from mural thrombi from approximately 10 to 4 per cent.[40] In addition, the administration of heparin in doses sufficient to influence activation of Factor X without affecting conventional laboratory tests of the coagulation system substantially diminish the incidence of deep vein thrombosis[41] and thereby reduce the incidence of pulmonary emboli. It appears advisable, therefore, to administer minidose heparin (5000 units subcutaneously) every 8 to 12 hours in the absence of specific contraindications.[42–44] The drug should be continued until two to three days prior to hospital discharge, although it is recognized that in patients with uncomplicated AMI's, there is no evidence that it reduces mortality.

In patients with high risk of embolism (e.g., those with ventricular aneurysm, marked obesity, cardiogenic shock, low output state, present or past thrombophlebitis, arterial or pulmonary embolism), there is evidence that in the absence of contraindications, anticoagulant treatment does exert a favorable effect on survival, and full-dose anticoagulation with heparin is indicated (e.g., intravenous administration of 15,000 units, followed by continuous infusion of 1000 units per hour) to maintain the clotting time and partial thromboplastin time at 1.5 to 2.5 times normal. After five to seven days of therapy, prothrombinopenic drugs or continued administration of subcutaneous, adjusted doses of heparin may be employed if conditions exist which suggest that venous thrombosis and embolism are likely to recur. These include continued or worsening heart failure, persistent thrombophlebitis, or the need for prolonged bed rest.

The long-term benefit of anticoagulants *following hospital discharge* is especially controversial. In one well-designed clinical trial on survivors of AMI exceeding 60 years of age, intensive and stable anticoagulant therapy reduced the risk of recurrent infarction and of cardiac death.[45] If these findings are confirmed, it will be essential to reconsider our present policy which limits the use of chronic anticoagulants to patients in the post-hospital phase to those with specific indications, including thrombophlebitis, a history of pulmonary or systemic embolism, evidence of a mural thrombus in the left ventricle on two-dimensional echocardiography (Fig. 5–68, p. 127), and severe heart failure. The role, if any, of sulfinpyrazone, aspirin, dipyridamole, and other antiplatelet agents in both the acute and the chronic convalescent phases of MI is unsettled and controversial at this time.

TREATMENT AND PROPHYLAXIS OF ARRHYTHMIAS

The electrophysiological mechanisms responsible for arrhythmias in patients with AMI are discussed on pp. 619 to 629. The incidence and consequences of arrhythmias and atrioventricular and intraventricular conduction defects in these patients are presented on p. 1284, the action of antiarrhythmic drugs on p. 653, and the role of cardiac pacing and of electric cardioversion on p. 669.

Arrhythmias occurring in patients with AMI require vigorous treatment when they impair hemodynamics, compromise myocardial viability by augmenting myocardial oxygen requirements, or predispose to malignant ventricular arrhythmias, i.e., ventricular tachycardia, ventricular fibrillation, or asystole.[46] There is evidence that both the diminished threshold to ventricular fibrillation[5] and the incidence of malignant ventricular arrhythmias associated with infarction[47–49] are affected by the extent of the underlying infarction.

When patients are seen early during the course of MI they almost invariably exhibit evidence of increased activity of the autonomic nervous system. Sinus bradycardia, sometimes associated with AV block, often reflecting augmented vagal activity, is particularly common in patients with inferoposterior infarction and is often accompanied by hypotension. Hypotension, regardless of cause, is hazardous in patients with AMI, since it impairs perfusion of marginally ischemic zones, intensifies ischemia, and may initiate or perpetuate the vicious circle illustrated in Figure 37–8, p. 1271.

Bradyarrhythmias and Conduction Defects

SINUS BRADYCARDIA (see also p. 1284). The cause of the vagotonia and resultant bradycardia and hypotension that often accompany AMI, particularly in patients with inferior and posterior infarcts, is not entirely clear. One factor appears to be stimulation of cardiac vagal afferent receptors[50] (which are more common in the inferoposterior than the anterior or lateral portions of the left ventricle), with resulting efferent cholinergic stimulation of the heart. In the first four to six hours following infarction, if the sinus rate is slow (under 60/min), administration of intravenous atropine in aliquots of 0.3 to 0.6 mg every 3 to 10 minutes (with a total dose not exceeding 2 mg) to bring heart rate up to approximately 60/min often abolishes premature ventricular beats commonly associated with sinus bradycardia.[51–54] Atropine often contributes to restoration of arterial pressure[9] and hence coronary perfusion. These favorable effects are frequently accompanied by regression of ST-segment elevation (Fig. 38–1). Elevation of the lower extremities will also often elevate arterial pressure by redistributing blood from the systemic venous bed to the thorax, thereby augmenting ventricular preload, cardiac output, and arterial pressure.

Sinus bradycardia occurring more than six hours after the onset of the AMI is often transitory, is caused by sinus node dysfunction or atrial ischemia rather than vagal hyperactivity, is usually not accompanied by hypotension, and does not usually predispose to ventricular arrhythmias. Treatment is not required unless ventricular performance is compromised or administration of propranolol or high doses of antiarrhythmic drugs, which may slow the sinus rate further, is planned. When atropine is ineffective and the patient is symptomatic and/or hypotensive, electrical pacing is indicated. In patients with depressed ventricular performance, who require the "atrial kick," atrial pacing or atrioventricular sequential pacing is superior to simple ventricular pacing.[55]

ATRIOVENTRICULAR BLOCK (see also pp. 730 and 1287). *First degree AV block* generally does not require specific treatment. However, if digitalis intoxication is sus-

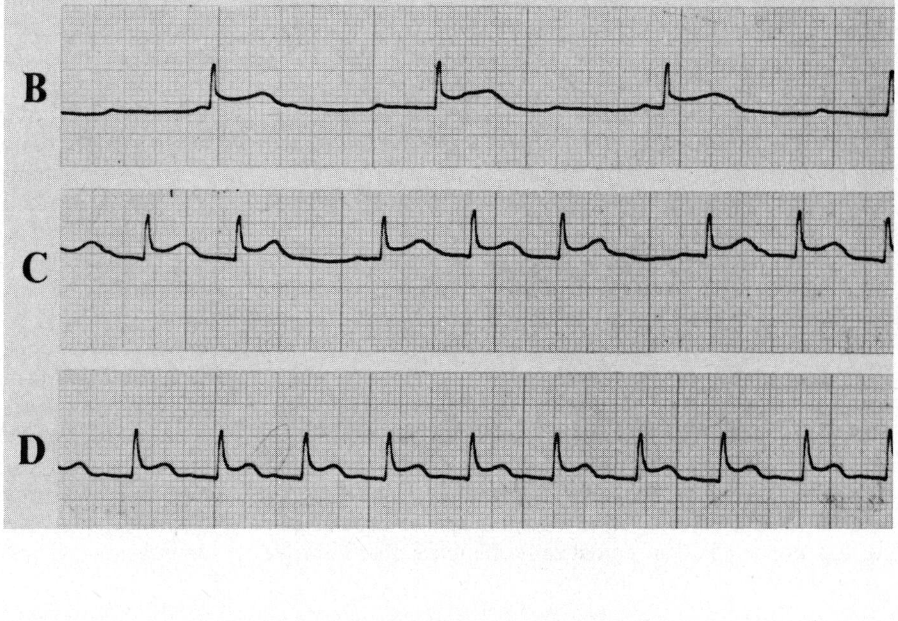

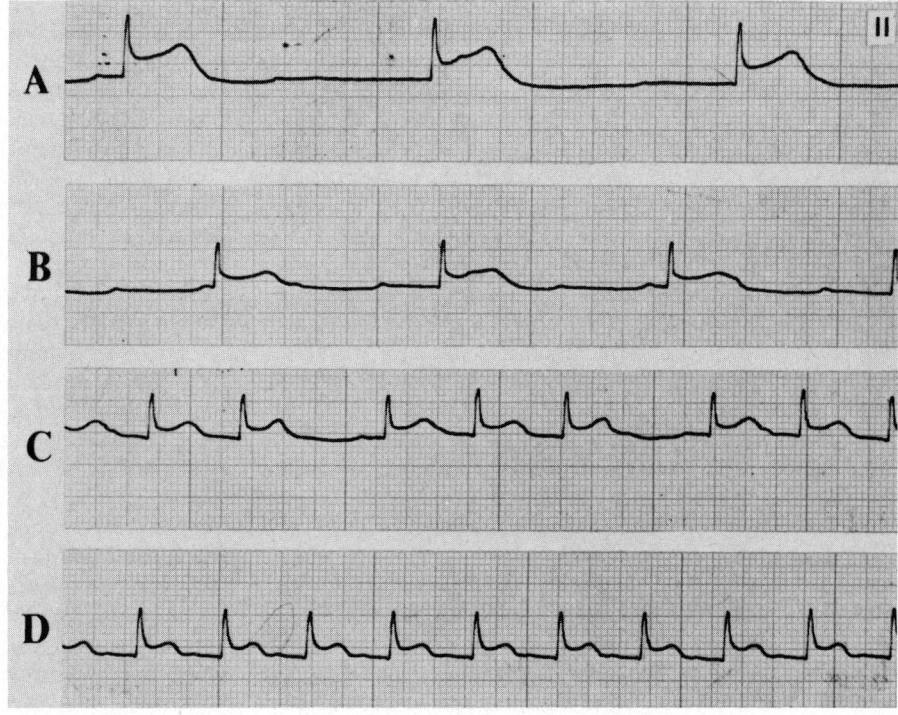

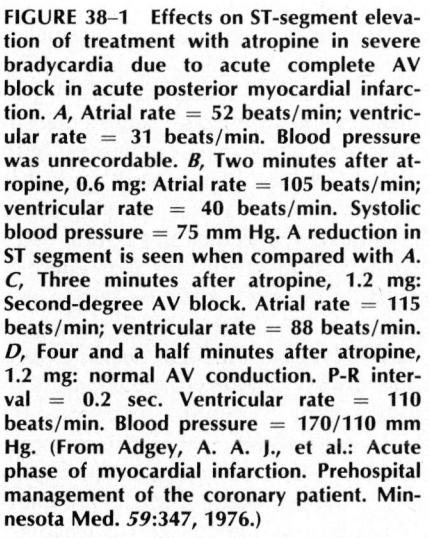

FIGURE 38–1 Effects on ST-segment elevation of treatment with atropine in severe bradycardia due to acute complete AV block in acute posterior myocardial infarction. *A,* Atrial rate = 52 beats/min; ventricular rate = 31 beats/min. Blood pressure was unrecordable. *B,* Two minutes after atropine, 0.6 mg: Atrial rate = 105 beats/min; ventricular rate = 40 beats/min. Systolic blood pressure = 75 mm Hg. A reduction in ST segment is seen when compared with *A. C,* Three minutes after atropine, 1.2 mg: Second-degree AV block. Atrial rate = 115 beats/min; ventricular rate = 88 beats/min. *D,* Four and a half minutes after atropine, 1.2 mg: normal AV conduction. P-R interval = 0.2 sec. Ventricular rate = 110 beats/min. Blood pressure = 170/110 mm Hg. (From Adgey, A. A. J., et al.: Acute phase of myocardial infarction. Prehospital management of the coronary patient. Minnesota Med. *59*:347, 1976.)

pected as the etiology, this drug should be discontinued. If the block is a manifestation of excessive vagotonia and is associated with sinus bradycardia and hypotension, administration of atropine, as outlined above, may be helpful. In all circumstances, careful surveillance is important in view of the possibility of progression to higher degrees of block.[56]

Specific therapy also is not required in patients with *second-degree AV block of the Mobitz type I* variety (Wenckebach), when the average ventricular rate is adequate and ventricular irritability, heart failure, or bundle branch block are absent. However, if these complications develop of if the ventricular rate falls below 60/min, immediate treatment with a temporary transvenous pacemaker is indicated. *Mobitz type II second-degree AV block* (p. 731) is relatively rare in AMI, but because of its potential for progression to complete heart block, it should be treated with a demand transvenous pacemaker with the rate set at approximately 60/min.[57]

Definitive data are not available concerning the importance of *complete AV block* as an *independent* risk factor for mortality and whether temporary transvenous pacing per se improves survival of patients with AMI. Some contend that ventricular pacing is useless when employed to correct complete AV block in patients with *anterior* infarction in view of the poor prognosis in this group regardless of therapy and therefore that ventricular pacing should be initiated only for complete AV block in association with inferior infarction and only when hemodynamic impairment is present. We believe, however, that ventricular or atrioventricular sequential pacing is indicated in essentially *all* patients with AMI with complete AV block. Pacing is likely to protect against transient hypotension with its attendant risks of extending infarction and precipitating malignant ventricular arrhythmias. Also, pacing protects against asystole, a particular hazard in patients with anterior infarction and infranodal block. Improved survival with pacing probably occurs in only a small fraction of patients with complete AV block and anterior wall infarcts, since the extensive destruction of the myocardium that almost invariably accompanies this condition results in a very high mortality rate, even in paced patients. Therefore, a large series of patients would be required to demonstrate the small reduction of mortality that might be achieved by pacing. The absence of data supporting such an effect, however, by no means excludes the possibility that it may be present. While it is generally agreed that pacing is indicated in patients with *inferior* wall infarction and complete AV block, it is of particular importance if the ventricular rate is very slow (<45 beats/min), if ventricular irritability is present, or if pump failure develops; atropine is of little value in these patients.

INTRAVENTRICULAR BLOCK. Complete bundle branch block (either left or right), the combination of right bundle branch block and left anterior divisional (fascicular) block, or any of the various forms of trifascicular block are more often associated with anterior than inferoposterior infarction. The poor prognosis associated with these intraventricular conduction defects is probably related more to the extent of infarction than to the direct consequences of the block itself.[57,58] Although, just as is the case for complete AV block, transvenous ventricular pacing has not resulted in statistically demonstrable improvement in prognosis among patients with AMI who develop intraventricular conduction defects, we believe that pacing is advisable in patients at high risk of developing complete AV block. This includes patients with *new* bilateral bundle branch block, i.e., right bundle branch block with left anterior or posterior divisional block and alternating right and left bundle branch block; first degree AV block adds to this risk. Isolated new block in only one of the three fascicles poses somewhat less risk; these patients can have a prophylactic pacemaker inserted or may be monitored closely and insertion of a pacemaker deferred unless conduction in a second fascicle becomes impaired or the P-R interval becomes prolonged. In our opinion, failure to demonstrate improved prognosis statistically does not belie the potential value of pacemaker therapy; it probably reflects the overriding impact on mortality of the extensive infarction responsible for the development of the conduction abnormality and the large number of patients required to permit statistical documentation of reduction of mortality. The presence of an intraventricular conduction defect *antedating* the AMI does not appear to predispose the patient to the development of complete AV block, and prophylactic pacing is not ordinarily indicated.

The question of permanent pacing in survivors of AMI associated with conduction defects is still controversial.[58-62] Patients with inferior infarction with *transient* Type II second-degree block or complete AV block without an associated intraventricular conduction defect do not appear to require permanent pacing. Some contend that prophylactic pacing makes little difference in the long-term survival of patients with AMI and bundle branch block complicated by transient high-degree block.[59] On the other hand, in a retrospective multicenter study, survivors of AMI and bundle branch block who experienced transient high-degree (Mobitz Type II second-degree, or third-degree) block had a high incidence of recurrent high-degree AV block and sudden death, and this incidence was reduced by insertion of a permanent demand pacemaker.[61-63] Thus, these findings suggest a role for prophylactic permanent pacing in patients with AMI and bundle branch block with transient high-degree atrioventricular block.

The question of the advisability of permanent pacemaker insertions is complicated by the fact that not all sudden deaths in this population are due to recurrent high-degree block. A high incidence of late in-hospital ventricular fibrillation occurs in coronary care unit survivors with anteroseptal myocardial infarction complicated by either right or left bundle branch block,[21] and if the propensity for this arrhythmia continued, ventricular fibrillation rather than asystole due to failure of atrioventricular conduction and of the infranodal pacemaker could be responsible for late sudden death.

VENTRICULAR ASYSTOLE. Sudden death associated with AMI is almost always due to ventricular fibrillation. Appearance of apparent ventricular asystole on oscilloscopic displays of continuously recorded electrocardiograms may be misleading, since the mechanism may in fact be fine ventricular fibrillation. Because of the predominance of ventricular fibrillation as the cause of cardiac arrest in this setting, initial therapy should include electrical countershock, even if definitive electrocardiographic documentation of this arrhythmia is not available. In the rare instance in which asystole can be documented to be the responsible electrophysiological disturbance, immediate transthoracic pacing (or stimulation with a transvenous pacemaker if one is already in place) is indicated.

Supraventricular Tachyarrhythmias and Premature Beats

Activation of receptors within atrial and ventricular myocardium by necrotic tissue may cause enhanced efferent sympathetic activity, increased concentrations of circulating catecholamines, and local release of catecholamines from nerve endings within the heart.[64] The latter may also result from direct ischemic damage of adrenergic neurons. In addition, ischemic myocardium may be hyperreactive to the arrhythmogenic effects of norepinephrine,[65,66] which may vary strikingly in concentration in different portions of the ischemic heart.[67] Sympathetic stimulation of the heart may also enhance the automaticity of ischemic Purkinje fibers. Furthermore, catecholamines facilitate propagation of slow current responses mediated by calcium (p. 624), and stimulation of ischemic myocardium by catecholamines may exacerbate arrhythmias dependent on such currents.[65,68,69] Cardiac catecholamine depletion induced by mediastinal ablation[70] or reduction of adrenergic stimulation by pharmacological means[6] protects against ventricular arrhythmias in experimental animals. Thus, although ventricular premature beats in patients with MI can usually be suppressed by administration of antiarrhythmic agents such as lidocaine, beta-adrenergic blocking agents may also be helpful in the treatment of ventricular arrhythmias, particularly when the latter are associated with other signs of heightened adrenergic activity such as sinus tachycardia.

Tachyarrhythmias of any origin may be deleterious, since they increase myocardial oxygen requirements, limit the time available for coronary perfusion and ventricular filling during diastole, and compromise cardiac output. Even electrophysiologically mild disturbances may have grave import in patients with AMI. For example, while atrial transport plays only a modest role in sustaining stroke volume in patients with normal hearts, cardiac output may be remarkably dependent upon maintenance of a properly timed atrial contraction in patients with AMI (Fig. 37–14, p. 1286). Therefore, aggressive management is indicated when hemodynamics are compromised by arrhythmias that disturb the sequence of atrial and ventricular contractions, such as wandering atrial pacemaker, AV junctional escape rhythms, frequent premature atrial contractions, accelerated idioventricular rhythm, and atrial fibrillation or flutter, even when the ventricular response is not excessively rapid, as well as when more serious derangements such as paroxysmal supraventricular tachycardia, AV dissociation with nodal tachycardia, and high degrees of AV block are present. The treatment of tachyarrhythmias involves not only the use of antiarrhythmic drugs but also correction of abnormalities of plasma electrolyte concentrations, acid-base balance disturbances, hypoxemia, and anemia. In addition, it is essential to treat pericarditis, pulmonary emboli, and pneumonia or other infections, which may give rise to sinus tachycardia or other supraventricular tachyarrhythmias.

SINUS TACHYCARDIA. This arrhythmia occurs in approximately one third of patients with AMI and may be associated with transient hypertension or hypotension and augmented sympathetic activity.[64,71] Sinus tachycardia may result from pain and fright or may be the only overt evidence of pump failure; it may result from associated infection or pulmonary embolism, pericarditis, hypovolemia, or fever. The etiology should be sought and appropriate treatment instituted, e.g., analgesics for pain, diuretics for heart failure, oxygen, beta blockers and nitroglycerin for ischemia, and aspirin for pericarditis.[72]

Administration of beta-adrenergic blocking agents, in the dosage and manner described on p. 1320, may be helpful in the treatment of sinus tachycardia, particularly when this arrhythmia is a manifestation of a hyperdynamic circulation, which is seen particularly in young patients with an initial MI without extensive cardiac damage (p. 1274). However, beta blockade is contraindicated in patients in whom the sinus tachycardia is a manifestation of pump failure, as reflected in a systolic arterial pressure below 100 mm Hg, rales involving more than one third of the lung fields, a pulmonary capillary wedge pressure exceeding 20 to 25 mm Hg, or a cardiac index below approximately 2.5 $L/min/m^2$.

ATRIAL FLUTTER AND FIBRILLATION (see pp. 626 and 1285). Both of these arrhythmias are more common during the first 24 hours after infarction than subsequently and are associated with increased mortality, particularly in patients with anterior wall infarction. However, because they are more common in patients with clinical and hemodynamic manifestations of extensive infarction and a poor prognosis, their *independent* contributions to increased mortality are not clear. Unfortunately, their management is complicated by frequent recurrence, particularly when they result from left atrial dilatation secondary to left ventricular failure.

Management of atrial flutter and fibrillation in patients with AMI is usually similar to their management in other settings (pp. 698 and 700). However, because of the possibility that a rapid ventricular rate can increase infarct size and because of the important role played by atrial contraction in the support of cardiac output in patients with AMI (Fig. 37–14, p. 1286), treatment must be prompt, especially when the ventricular rate exceeds 100/min. *Digitalis glycosides* are the principal agents used to slow the ventricular response. Digitalis may be supplemented by small intravenous doses of a beta blocker which also prolongs the AV nodal refractory period: 1 to 4 mg of propranolol in divided doses is often quite effective in reducing the ventricular rate and is well tolerated even in patients with mild heart failure and a rapid ventricular rate. Reduction of the rate of ventricular response to atrial fibrillation may be achieved also with verapamil administered intravenously[73] via bolus injections of 60 to 120 $\mu g/kg$, followed by a continuous infusion of 2.5 to 5.0 $\mu g/kg/min$, although caution must be exercised to avoid systemic arterial hypotension. On the other hand, when hemodynamic decompensation is prominent, electrical cardioversion with anterior and laterally placed paddles[74] employing low-energy, 5 to 20 watt-second discharges is indicated. An additional important option for the treatment of atrial flutter is the use of rapid atrial stimulation via a transvenous intraatrial electrode (p. 672); in contrast to DC cardioversion, this technique can be employed in the presence of possible digitalis intoxication, is less prone than DC countershock to elicit bradycardia after conversion to sinus rhythm, provides control of ventricular rate via atrial or ventricular pacing should this be necessary, and can be reapplied with less difficulty than cardioversion, should the patient experience recurrent atrial flutter. Following restoration of sinus rhythm, attention should be directed to the management of the underlying cause, usually heart failure, and to the prevention of recurrences, with antiarrhythmic agents such as quinidine.[75] Patients with recurrent episodes should be treated with oral anticoagulants.

OTHER ATRIAL ARRHYTHMIAS. *Premature atrial contractions* require no specific therapy. However, since they often herald more serious forms of atrial tachyarrhythmias, they merit attention. As is the case for patients with atrial flutter and fibrillation, premature atrial contractions may indicate atrial dilatation or excessive autonomic stimulation and they often reflect the presence of overt or occult heart failure; therefore they may respond to treatment of this condition. *Wandering atrial pacemaker* and *AV junctional rhythm* are important in patients with AMI because, as indicated above, the loss of atrial transport function may be tolerated poorly. Transvenous sequential atrioventricular pacing may be required to facilitate ventricular performance and maintain adequate peripheral perfusion.

Aggressive management is indicated for *paroxysmal supraventricular tachycardia* due to reentry involving the AV node (p. 626 and 707) because of the very rapid ventricular rate and its potentially adverse effects in patients with AMI. Augmentation of vagal tone by manual carotid sinus stimulation or intravenous administration of 10 mg of edrophonium (Tensilon) may restore sinus rhythm. Alpha-adrenergic agonists to increase arterial pressure and activate carotid sinus baroreceptors, an acceptable form of therapy for paroxysmal supraventricular tachycardia under other circumstances, are hazardous in patients with AMI, and intravenous verapamil is preferable.[73,76] Although digitalis glycosides may be useful in augmenting vagal tone, thereby terminating the arrhythmia, their effect is often delayed. Accordingly, low-energy DC countershock or rapid atrial stimulation via a transvenous intra-atrial electrode should be utilized just as for atrial flutter, particularly if hemodynamic decompensation occurs or if the rhythm is refractory to conventional measures. *Paroxysmal atrial tachycardia with AV block* (p. 701) may be a manifestation of digitalis intoxication and should be treated by withholding this drug and instituting potassium therapy, when it is accompanied by hypokalemia.

Ventricular Arrhythmias

VENTRICULAR PREMATURE CONTRACTIONS (see also pp. 719 and 1285). The suppression of ventricular premature contractions is based on the concept that in the face of myocardial ischemia the threshold for ventricular fibrillation is reduced and otherwise innocuous ventricular premature contractions may trigger ventricular fibrillation. While frequent ventricular premature contractions in the setting of ischemia are often used as a marker of the heart's propensity to fibrillate, successful suppression of ventricular premature contractions provides no assurance that ventricular fibrillation will not occur. Indeed, in more than half of the patients with AMI developing ventricular fibrillation, there are no premonitory ventricular premature contractions (p. 1286).[78] Furthermore, a large number of randomized trials have compared the routine administration of several potent antiarrhythmic drugs —lidocaine, quinidine, procainamide, and disopyramide, as well as beta-adrenergic blocking agents—against placebo. All of these agents reduced the frequency of ventricular premature contractions, and in the case of lidocaine, routine administration lowered the incidence of ventricular fibrillation.[79–81] None of the agents administered in this fashion, however, reduced mortality.[82]

Despite the results of these large trials and despite the complexity of the relationship between ventricular premature contractions and ventricular fibrillation, we favor the prophylactic administration of antiarrhythmic drugs in selected patients. This position is based partly on the concept that the abolition or reduction of ventricular premature contractions serves as a useful end-point that reflects an adequate overall pharmacological effect. Thus, when an appropriately selected agent is administered in sufficiently high doses, it can reduce the incidence of ventricular fibrillation even though its antifibrillatory activity can be monitored only indirectly, i.e., by reducing the incidence of ventricular premature contractions. It seems eminently desirable to reduce the incidence of ventricular fibrillation; although this potentially lethal arrhythmia may be treated effectively in centers where clinical trials on patients with AMI are being carried out, which usually have well-staffed and equipped coronary care units, this does not guarantee similar results in different settings.

Frequent ventricular premature contractions occurring very soon after the onset of MI, particularly during the first hour, may depend primarily on reentry rather than on increased automaticity.[81a] At this time, lidocaine, which impairs conduction in ventricular myocardium and diminishes automaticity, may be somewhat less effective than it is later.[82] When, at the very inception of an infarction, ventricular premature contractions are encountered in the presence of sinus tachycardia, augmented sympathoadrenal stimulation is often a contributing factor, and beta-adrenergic blockade is usually effective. Indeed, the effectiveness of beta-adrenergic blocking drugs under these circumstances may, in fact, play a role in the reduction in sudden deaths reported in patients who have recovered from AMI and are at high risk of recurrence.[83,84] The dose and mode of administration as well as the contraindications to beta-blockade are discussed on p. 1320.

In the absence of specific, correctable factors, such as sympathoadrenal hyperactivity with tachycardia, lidocaine should be administered to patients with AMI and frequent ventricular premature contractions (>6/min), multiform premature contractions and extrasystoles occurring in pairs or salvos, and early premature contractions (R on T), even though it is acknowledged that it may not be appropriate to consider these to be "warning arrhythmias." We favor the prophylactic administration of lidocaine, as described below, particularly in patients with AMI at high risk of developing ventricular fibrillation. This includes younger patients (< 50 years) without a prior history of heart failure or AMI and who present within the first six hours of infarction. Older patients (> 70 years) who are seen more than six hours after the onset of the MI are less likely to develop ventricular fibrillation and are at higher risk of developing lidocaine toxicity and should probably not receive prophylaxis routinely. The management of other patients must be individualized. The setting in which the patient is treated must also be considered. Obviously, the risk to life of ventricular fibrillation is greater at home or on a general hospital floor than in an expertly and fully staffed and equipped coronary care unit.

The pharmacology and pharmacokinetics of lidocaine are discussed on p. 653. With regimens depending on continuous infusion alone, therapeutic blood levels (1.5 to 5 μg/ml) are reached only after several hours because of the short half-life of the drug. Therefore, a loading dose of 100 mg or 1 mg/kg should be given intravenously as a bolus injection at the time of admission or during the patient's transportation to the hospital, followed in 5 to 10 minutes by an injection of 0.5 mg/kg. An intravenous infusion should be started concomitantly; a dose of 50 μg/kg/min in patients without heart failure and of 20 μg/kg/min in patients with heart failure is advised.[85] Intramuscular injections into the deltoid or gluteal muscles with conventional syringes and needles do not achieve therapeutic concentrations as promptly as those following intravenous injection.

The maintenance dose of lidocaine should be adjusted within the range of 1 to 4 mg/min to reduce sharply or abolish premature ventricular contractions. It should be recognized that the metabolism of lidocaine is slowed not only in patients with heart failure but also in those with diminution of hepatic blood flow due to effects of pharmacological agents such as propranolol.[86] Therefore, careful titration is needed to avoid toxicity, manifested primarily by central nervous system hyperactivity, as well as by depression of intraventricular and atrioventricular conduction and cardiac contractility (p. 656). Saturation of an extravascular pool normally occurs after a continuous infusion of approximately three hours, at which time blood levels will increase despite maintenance of a constant infusion rate.[87] At this time, it may be desirable to reduce the rate of administration by about 25 per cent.

This regimen is effective in suppressing ventricular premature contractions in approximately 75 per cent of patients seen within the first hour after the onset of ischemia;[9] it is effective in an even higher percentage—80 to 90 per cent—of patients seen later after the onset of ischemia, perhaps because enhanced automaticity becomes a progressively more important factor in the etiology of ventricular premature contractions with the passage of time from the onset of infarction and because of the particular effectiveness of the drug for arrhythmias on this basis.[88–91] Lidocaine has been shown to abolish reentrant ventricular arrhythmias in the late myocardial infarction phase by further depression and block of conduction in the reentrant pathway.[92]

When ventricular premature contractions compromise hemodynamics and persist despite administration of lidocaine, administration of *procainamide* intravenously in bolus doses of approximately 1 to 2 mg/kg intravenously over intervals of 5 minutes to a cumulative dose of approximately 1000 mg, followed by maintenance therapy with an intravenous infusion (20 to 80 μg/kg/min), may be effective.

Ventricular premature contractions that are unresponsive to lidocaine and procainamide in approximately the first six hours following AMI, particularly in the presence of sinus tachycardia, may be responsive to beta-adrenergic blocking agents. Newer investigational antiarrhythmic agents with actions resembling those of procainamide, such as acetyl procainamide,[93] aprindine,[76] and encainide[77] (p. 667), may be given to patients unresponsive to lidocaine and/or procainamide. Efficacy of these agents is noted in some patients with AMI and frequent ventricular premature contractions refractory to therapy with conventionally available agents.

Although *phenytoin* (Dilantin) (p. 661) (50 to 100 mg intravenously at 5 to 10 minute intervals to a total of 1000 mg) may diminish ventricular arrhythmia by decreasing the rate of phase IV depolarization, suppressing efferent cardiac sympathetic stimulation,[94] and further depressing and blocking conduction in ischemia-induced reentrant pathways,[95] it does not confer protection against ventricular fibrillation either in the first few hours[96] or later in the course of AMI. On the other hand, this drug may be effective when ventricular arrhythmias are initiated or potentiated by digitalis intoxication.

If ventricular premature contractions recur following initial intravenous treatment, oral administration of conventional antiarrhythmic agents is justified, including quinidine, procainamide, disopyramide, phenytoin, and propranolol, selected on the basis of the criteria outlined above and described in Chapter 20.

ACCELERATED IDIOVENTRICULAR RHYTHM (see also pp. 724 and 1286). The need for treatment of this arrhythmia with rates in the range of 60 to 100 beats/min remains controversial. Since these rhythms may deteriorate into ventricular tachycardia and since they may compromise cardiac function because of impairment of the physiological sequential relationship between atrial and ventricular contraction, it may be prudent to treat them by accelerating the sinus rate with atropine or atrial pacing or by suppressing the ventricular pacemaker with the administration of lidocaine intravenously. However, there is no definitive evidence that this arrhythmia, when left untreated, increases the incidence of either ventricular fibrillation or mortality.[10]

VENTRICULAR TACHYCARDIA (see also pp. 721 and 1286). Rapid abolition of this arrhythmia in patients with AMI is mandatory because of its deleterious effect on pump function and because it frequently deteriorates into ventricular fibrillation. When the ventricular rate is rapid (> 150/min) and/or there is a decline in arterial pressure, a single attempt at "thump version," i.e., striking a sharp blow to the precordium, is indicated (Fig. 38–2). If this maneuver is unsuccessful, it should be followed immediately by synchronized DC countershock, with the use of relatively low energies, i.e., 10 to 25 watts. When the ventricular rate is very rapid and synchronization is not possible, a defibrillatory impulse of 100 to 200 watt-seconds should be delivered. When the ventricular rate is slower than approximately 150/min and the arrhythmia is

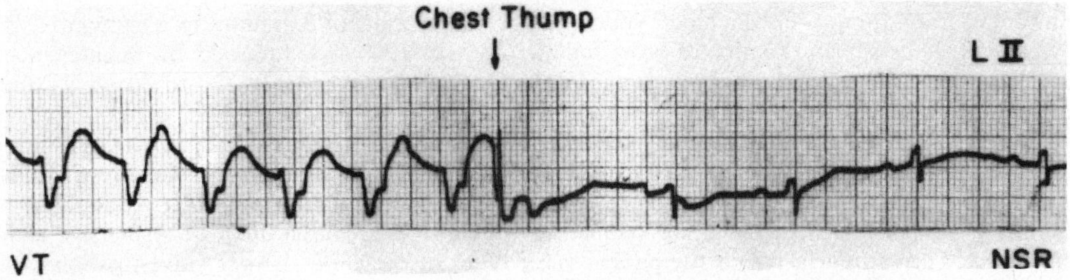

FIGURE 38–2 An example of reversion of ventricular tachycardia by a precordial thump. (Reproduced with permission from Pennington, J. E. Taylor, J., and Lown, B.: Chest thump for reverting ventricular tachycardia. N. Engl. J. Med. *283*:1192, 1970.)

well tolerated hemodynamically, a brief (15 to 20 min) trial of treatment with lidocaine or procainamide, using the loading doses described above, is in order. After reversion to sinus rhythm, every effort should be made to correct underlying abnormalities such as hypoxia, hypotension, acid-base or electrolyte disturbances, and digitalis excess. If these measures are unsuccessful, an infusion of bretylium tosylate (1–2 mg/min) may be tried. Recurrent or refractory ventricular tachycardia may respond to aneurysm resection, encircling endocardial ventriculotomy, or endocardial resection with or without coronary artery bypass grafting; these surgical procedures are generally reserved for use until after the acute phase.[97–99]

VENTRICULAR FIBRILLATION (see also pp. 728 and 1286). Several forms of ventricular fibrillation associated with acute ischemic episodes can be distinguished. Two forms are associated with the syndrome of sudden cardiac death among ambulatory patients (Chap. 23): (1) In the first, the majority of survivors do not evolve AMI, although they usually have serious coronary artery disease. Therefore this form, although a manifestation of acute myocardial ischemia, should not be classified as one associated with AMI. (2) The second form is seen among survivors of resuscitation from sudden out-of-hospital ventricular fibrillation and occurs within minutes or a very few hours after the onset of other symptoms of ischemia such as pain. Patients evolve an MI, and in them the arrhythmia may well be identical to another form, generally called (3) *primary ventricular fibrillation.* This form occurs usually during the first 24 hours (most commonly during the first six to eight hours) in the course of AMI in the absence of cardiac failure or shock, and accounts for approximately 80 per cent of in-hospital episodes of ventricular fibrillation. (4) The fourth form, *secondary ventricular fibrillation,* occurs most commonly between 12 hours and four days after infarction, and is accompanied by and is probably a consequence of heart failure, hypotension, cardiogenic shock, or all three. (5) The fifth form, termed *late in-hospital ventricular fibrillation,* usually occurs after the third or fourth day—often after discharge from the coronary care unit but prior to hospital discharge. It is the risk of developing this form of ventricular fibrillation that has served as a stimulus to the development of intermediate coronary care (step-down) units (p. 1302). Patients may have heart failure but are rarely in cardiogenic shock. Patients with intraventricular conduction defects, extensive anterior wall infarction, persistent sinus tachycardia, as well as atrial flutter or fibrillation early in their course, are at higher risk of suffering late in-hospital ventricular fibrillation than patients without these features. Thus, this form of ventricular fibrillation merges with the first form, i.e., that responsible for sudden death after hospital discharge in patients with healed infarcts.

Procainamide,[100] lidocaine,[101] and the beta-adrenergic blocker, metoprolal,[101a] administered prophylactically have all been reported to reduce the incidence of ventricular fibrillation in hospitalized patients.[88,102,103] However, they may not reduce overall mortality substantially because treatment of this arrhythmia is so successful in an effectively staffed coronary care unit. Despite the potentially lethal nature of primary ventricular fibrillation, the bulk of evidence (with one exception[104]) suggests that when it is treated promptly with electrical countershock, ventricular fibrillation does not affect prognosis adversely, either in the hospital or following discharge. On the other hand, secondary ventricular fibrillation occurring in association with marked left ventricular failure or hypotension entails a dire prognosis, with only 20 to 25 per cent of patients surviving hospitalization;[10] the prognosis is intermediate in so-called late in-hospital ventricular fibrillation.[2] In the latter two forms it is the impairment of cardiac function consequent to the loss of contracting myocardium rather than the arrhythmia *per se* which is responsible for the poor prognosis.

The treatment of ventricular fibrillation, described in detail on p. 729, is *electrical countershock,* implemented as rapidly as possible. The likelihood of successful restoration of an effective cardiac rhythm declines rapidly with time after the onset of uncorrected ventricular fibrillation. Irreversible brain damage may occur within 1 to 2 minutes, particularly in elderly patients. Despite the superficial appeal of "thump version," which may sometimes terminate ventricular tachycardia (as opposed to fibrillation), no time should be lost before treating patients with ventricular fibrillation with electrical countershock.

Prompt electrical countershock generally interrupts fibrillation and restores an effective cardiac rhythm in patients under direct medical observation in the coronary care unit. When ventricular fibrillation occurs outside of an intensive care unit, resuscitative efforts are much less likely to be successful, primarily because the time interval between the onset of the episode and institution of definitive therapy tends to be prolonged. Since closed-chest cardiopulmonary resuscitation with external cardiac compression provides only a marginal cardiac output even under optimal circumstances, countershock should be implemented as soon as possible after the detection of ventricular fibrillation rather than deferred under the mistaken impression that adequate circulatory and respiratory support can be maintained in the interim. Failure of electrical countershock to restore an effective cardiac rhythm is due almost always to rapidly recurrent ventricular tachycardia or ventricular fibrillation, to electromechanical dissociation, or, very rarely, to electrical asystole.

Ventricular fibrillation often recurs rapidly and repeatedly when the metabolic milieu of the heart has been compromised by severe or prolonged hypoxemia, acidosis, or electrolyte abnormalities. Under these conditions, continued cardiopulmonary resuscitation, prompt implementation of pharmacological and ventilatory maneuvers designed to correct these abnormalities, treatment with antiarrhythmic agents such as lidocaine, and rapidly repeated attempts with electrical countershock may be effective. Even though repeated shocks with excessive energy may damage the myocardium[105-107] and elicit arrhythmias,[108] speed is essential and prompt efforts with high-intensity shocks (generally 300-400 watts initially) are justified. When ventricular fibrillation persists without documented interruption by electrical countershock, the intracardiac administration of epinephrine (up to 10 ml of a 1:10,000 concentration) or calcium gluconate (up to 15 ml of 10 per cent calcium gluconate) may facilitate success in a subsequent attempt. Conversion of fine to coarse ventricular fibrillation by either or both of these drugs may augur well for subsequent successful defibrillation.

Successful interruption of ventricular fibrillation or prevention of refractory recurrent episodes may be facilitated by administration of *bretylium tosylate,* 5 mg/kg I.V., repeated 20 minutes later if necessary (p. 663).[109] When synchronous cardiac electrical activity is restored by countershock, but contraction is ineffective, i.e., during electromechanical dissociation—the usual underlying cause is very extensive myocardial ischemia, or necrosis, or rupture of the ventricular free wall or septum. If rupture has not occurred, intracardiac administration of calcium gluconate or epinephrine may facilitate restoration of an effective heart beat. Another antifibrillatory agent is amiodarone (p. 666) (investigational in the United States). It has a slow onset of action, and therefore its principal role may prove to be in the *prevention* rather than treatment of ventricular fibrillation. Despite the unequivocal antiarrhythmic efficacy of this agent[110] and its potential value in limiting infarct size,[111] ocular, cutaneous, endocrine, and pulmonary toxicities may preclude its widespread clinical use.

TREATMENT OF HEMODYNAMIC DISTURBANCES

As indicated on p. 1274, hemodynamic assessment of patients with AMI has delineated several subsets with characteristic hemodynamic profiles. A convenient classification is (1) normal hemodynamics, (2) hyperdynamic circulatory state, (3) hypovolemic hypotension, (4) left ventricular failure, and (5) cardiogenic shock.[112-114] As indicated in Table 38–1, therapy designed to maintain ventricular performance, support hemodynamics, and protect jeopardized myocardium should be selected with consideration of the class of each patient. This classification can be achieved most readily by means of hemodynamic monitoring.

HYPOTENSION IN THE PREHOSPITAL PHASE. During the *prehospital phase of AMI,* invasive hemodynamic monitoring is usually not practical, and during this period, therapy should be guided by frequent clinical assessment and measurement of arterial pressure by the cuff method, with the recognition that intense vasoconstriction can provide a falsely low pressure measured by this method. Hypotension associated with bradycardia often reflects excessive vagotonia, which may be responsive to atropine and elevation of the lower extremities. Relative or absolute hypovolemia is often present when hypotension occurs with a normal or rapid heart rate, particularly among patients receiving diuretics just prior to the occurrence of infarction. Marked diaphoresis, reduction of fluid intake, or vomiting during the period preceding and accompanying the onset of AMI may all contribute to the development of hypovolemia. Even if the effective vascular volume is normal, *relative* hypovolemia may be present, since ventricular compliance is reduced in AMI (p. 1247) and a left

TABLE 38–1 POTENTIALLY USEFUL THERAPEUTIC INTERVENTIONS IN HEMODYNAMIC CATEGORIES OF PATIENTS WITH ACUTE MYOCARDIAL INFARCTION*

Hemodynamic Category	P_a†	$\overline{PA}_o$‡	CI§	Suggested Intervention	Remarks
Normal	≤15	≤12	2.7–3.5	None	β-blockade may be beneficial
Hyperdynamic state	≤15	≤12	≥3.0	β-adrenergic blockage	Tachycardia is a hallmark of subset
Hypotension or shock secondary to hypovolemia	≤15	≤9	≤2.7	Repletion of vascular volume	Reclassification may be necessary after PA_o is increased to range of 14 to 18 mm Hg
LV failure					
Mild	≥22	≥18–≤22	≤2.5	Diuretics	Dyspnea, hypoxemia, or mild pulmonary vascular congestion
Severe	≥25	≥22	≤1.8	Vasodilators + diuretics	Pulmonary vascular congestion and pulmonary edema; cardiac glycosides; positive pressure ventilation and/or circulatory assist may be useful
Cardiogenic hypotension or shock	≥22	≥18	≤1.8	Circulatory assist	Sympathomimetic agents with positive inotropic effects such as dopamine or dobutamine may be useful

*Modified from references 3, 112, and 113.
†P_a, mean pulmonary artery pressure in mm Hg.
‡$\overline{PA}_o$, mean pulmonary artery occlusive pressure in mm Hg.
§CI, cardiac index in liters/minute/m².

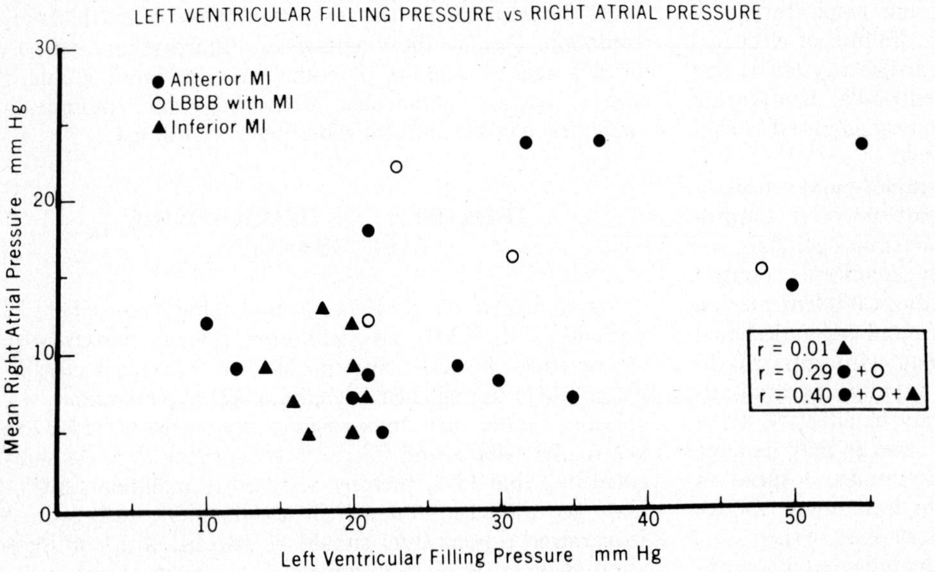

FIGURE 38–3 Comparison between left ventricular filling pressure and right atrial pressure in patients with acute myocardial infarction did not reveal a significant relationship. (From Rackley, C. E., et al.: Recognition of acute myocardial infarction. *In* Rackley, C. E., and Russell, R. O., Jr. (eds.): Coronary Artery Disease: Recognition and Management. Mt. Kisco, N.Y., Futura Publishing Co., 1979, p. 315.)

ventricular filling pressure as high as 20 to 24 mm Hg may be needed to provide an optimal preload.

In the absence of rales involving more than one third of the lung fields, the reverse Trendelenburg position should be assumed and in patients with sinus bradycardia, atropine should be administered (p. 690). If these measures do not correct the hypotension, crystalloid solutions should be administered intravenously, beginning with a bolus of 100 ml followed by 50-ml increments every five minutes. The patient should be carefully observed and the infusion stopped when the systolic pressure returns to approximately 100 mm Hg, if the patient becomes dyspneic or if pulmonary rales develop or increase. Because of the poor correlation between left ventricular filling pressure and mean right atrial pressure (Fig. 38–3), assessment of systemic venous pressure is of limited value as a guide to fluid therapy. Administration of cardiotonic agents (see below) is indicated during the prehospital phase if systemic arterial hypotension persists and is refractory to correction of hypovolemia and excessive vagotonia.

In the absence of invasive hemodynamic monitoring, assessment of peripheral vascular resistance must be based on clinical observations. If cutaneous vasoconstriction is present, therapy with dobutamine, which stimulates cardiac contractility without unduly accelerating heart rate and which does not increase the impedance to ventricular outflow, may be helpful (p. 543). In hypotensive patients with AMI, when there is clinical evidence of vasodilatation, an uncommon circumstance, norepinephrine is preferable.

INDICATIONS FOR INVASIVE HEMODYNAMIC MONITORING. Hemodynamic assessment becomes possible once the patient reaches the hospital. An estimation of the presence or absence of gross abnormalities in cardiac index and left ventricular filling pressure can be made on the basis of clinical examination in approximately 80 per cent of patients. Additional insights can sometimes be obtained with the use of noninvasive methods such as echocardiography to estimate the left atrial pressure, based on the timing of mitral valve closure and the interval from aortic valve closure to mitral valve opening.[115] Echocardiography can also demonstrate the presence of right ventricular dilatation in patients with right ventricular infarcts (Fig. 37–15, p. 1289). However, severe depression of cardiac index and/or elevation of left ventricular filling pressure may be unsuspected in as many as 15 per cent of patients when estimates are based exclusively on clinical criteria.[116]

In patients with *clinically uncomplicated AMI,* invasive hemodynamic monitoring is generally not necessary, since the status of the circulation can be assessed by careful clinical evaluation. This ordinarily consists of monitoring of heart rate and rhythm, measurement of systemic arterial pressure by cuff, obtaining chest roentgenograms to detect heart failure, careful and repeated auscultation of the lung fields for pulmonary congestion, measurement of urine flow, examination of the skin and mucous membranes for evidence of the adequacy of perfusion, and arterial sampling for pO_2, pCO_2, and pH when hypoxemia or metabolic acidosis is suspected.

Invasive monitoring ordinarily consists of inserting an arterial line for the continuous measurement of arterial pressure, and a balloon flotation catheter for measurement of pulmonary artery, pulmonary artery occlusive (equivalent to pulmonary wedge) and right atrial pressures, and cardiac output by thermodilution (p. 290); in patients with hypotension, a Foley catheter provides accurate and continuous measurement of urine output.

The importance of invasive hemodynamic monitoring[116] is based on the following principal factors:

1. The difficulty of interpreting clinical and radiographic findings of pulmonary congestion because of phase lags, such as those occurring after diuretic therapy.

2. The need for identifying noncardiac causes of arterial hypotension, particularly hypovolemia.

3. Possible contributions of reduced ventricular compliance to impaired hemodynamics, requiring judicious adjustment of intravascular volume to optimize left ventricular filling pressure.

4. Difficulty in assessing the severity and sometimes even the presence of lesions such as mitral regurgitation

and ventricular septal defect when the cardiac output or the systemic pressures are depressed.

5. Establishing a baseline of hemodynamic measurements and guiding therapy in patients with clinically apparent pulmonary edema or cardiogenic shock.

6. The underestimation of systemic arterial pressure by the cuff method in patients with intense vasoconstriction (p. 22).

Therefore, we believe the following to be indications for invasive hemodynamic monitoring in patients with AMI: (1) hypotension unresponsive to simple measures, such as elevation of the lower extremities and the administration of atropine in patients with accompanying bradycardia; (2) moderate or severe left ventricular failure, manifested by persistent or excessive dyspnea, rales, or radiographic evidence of pulmonary vascular congestion, pulmonary edema, or cardiomegaly; (3) unexplained or refractory sinus tachycardia or other tachyarrhythmias; (4) unexplained or severe cyanosis, hypoxemia, tachypnea, diaphoresis, or acidosis; and (5) clinical signs suggestive of mitral regurgitation, ventricular septal defect, or pericardial effusion.

HYPERDYNAMIC STATE. When infarction is not complicated by hemodynamic impairment, no therapy other than general supportive measures and treatment of arrhythmias is necessary. However, if the hemodynamic profile is of the hyperdynamic state, i.e., elevation of sinus rate, arterial pressure, and cardiac index, occurring singly or together in the presence of a normal or low left ventricular filling pressure, and if other causes of tachycardia such as fever, infection, and pericarditis can be excluded, treatment with beta-adrenergic blocking agents is indicated. The rationale, dose, and mode of administration are discussed on p. 1320.

HYPOVOLEMIC HYPOTENSION. Recognition of hypovolemia is of particular importance in hypotensive patients with AMI, because improvement in circulatory dynamics is so readily and safely achieved by augmentation of vascular volume. Since hypovolemia is often occult, it is frequently overlooked in the absence of invasive hemodynamic monitoring. It may be absolute, with low left ventricular filling pressure (<8 mm Hg), or relative, with normal (8 to 12 mm Hg) or even modestly increased (13 to 18 mm Hg) left ventricular filling pressures. Because of the reduction of left ventricular compliance that occurs with acute ischemia and infarction (p. 1246), left ventricular filling pressures between 13 and 18 mm Hg, while above the upper limits of normal, may be suboptimal.

Exclusion of hypovolemia as the cause of hypotension requires documentation of a reduced cardiac output despite left ventricular filling pressure of more than approximately 17 mm Hg. If, in a hypotensive patient, the pulmonary capillary wedge pressure (ordinarily measured as the pulmonary artery occlusive pressure) is below this level, fluid challenge should be carried out with sequential 50-ml intravenous bolus infusions[117] and serial assessments should be made of pulmonary capillary wedge pressure and cardiac output. Elevation of pulmonary capillary wedge pressure to between 18 and 24 mm Hg reflects the achievement of a left ventricular filling pressure associated with an optimal cardiac output (Fig. 38–4). If hypovolemia is documented, the fluid replaced should resemble the fluid lost. Thus, when a low hematocrit complicates AMI, infusion of whole blood is the treatment of choice. On the other hand, crystalloid or colloid solutions should be administered when the hematocrit is normal or elevated.

Hypotension Due to Right Ventricular Infarction. Hypotension caused by right ventricular infarction may be confused with that caused by hypovolemia, because both are associated with a low, normal, or minimally elevated left ventricular filling pressure. However, hypotension secondary to right ventricular infarction (which is frequently associated with inferior left ventricular infarction) is generally recognizable from discordant elevation of right compared to left ventricular filling pressure, diminution of right ventricular ejection fraction by radionuclide ventriculography,[118,119] and right ventricular dilatation on echocardiography (Fig. 37–15, p. 1289). The hypotension associated with right ventricular infarction often responds to the vigorous administration of fluid, and positive inotropic agents such as dobutamine;[118–120] the treatment of cardiogenic shock associated with right ventricular infarction is discussed on p. 1317).

Treatment of Left Ventricular Failure

The treatment of left ventricular failure with AMI requires meticulous attention to ventilation, since hypoxemia can impair the function of ischemic tissue at the margin of

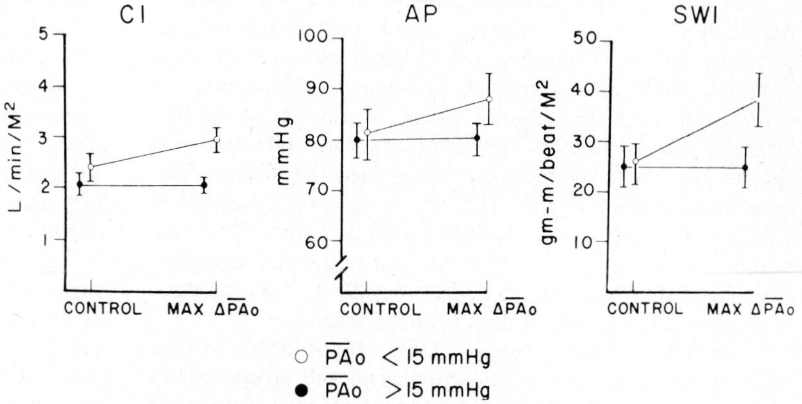

FIGURE 38–4 Effects of augmentation of vascular volume on ventricular function in patients with AMI who were categorized according to levels of pulmonary artery occlusive ($\overline{PAo}$) pressure (pulmonary capillary wedge pressure) as soon as possible after hospitalization. Vascular volume was augmented by infusion with dextran or hypertonic glucose solutions. As can be seen, among patients with high initial $\overline{PAo}$ pressure, cardiac index (CI) and mean aortic pressure ($\overline{AP}$) did not increase as a result of volume expansion, nor did the stroke work index (SWI) rise. On the other hand, in patients in whom initial values of $\overline{PAo}$ were not elevated substantially above the normal range, expansion of plasma volume led to an increase in cardiac index, elevation of mean aortic pressure, and an increased stroke work index—all compatible with improved ventricular performance achieved by the induction of more favorable loading conditions. Results expressed comprise mean values ± SE. (Reprinted by permission from Crexells, C., et al.: Optimal level of filling pressure in the left side of the heart in acute myocardial infarction. N. Engl. J. Med. *289*:1264, 1973.)

the infarct and thereby initiate the vicious circle, ultimately leading to the patient's demise (Fig. 37–8, p. 1271). The combination of pulmonary vascular congestion (or when it is severe, pulmonary edema), reduced pulmonary compliance, and the respiratory depression that may be associated with excessive doses of analgesics conspires to impair ventilatory function and arterial oxygenation (pp. 1276 and 1786). When arterial oxygen tension cannot be maintained above 60 to 70 mm Hg despite inhalation of 100 per cent oxygen delivered at 8 L/min by mask and the adequate use of bronchodilators, endotracheal intubation, assisted ventilation, and positive pressure should be considered. The improvement of arterial oxygenation and hence myocardial oxygen supply may help to restore ventricular performance. Invasive hemodynamic monitoring is necessary to guide therapy under these circumstances, since positive end-expiratory pressure may diminish systemic venous return and reduce effective left ventricular filling pressure.

When wheezing complicates pulmonary congestion, bronchodilators that act primarily on beta-2 adrenergic receptors, such as isoetharine or metaproterenol, given as aerosols, or terbutaline, which can be administered subcutaneously or orally, are more desirable than conventional bronchodilators, such as isoproterenol or epinephrine, whose primary effects are on beta-1 receptors.

Although positive inotropic agents may be useful, they do *not* represent the *initial* therapy of choice in patients with AMI. Instead, heart failure in this setting is managed most effectively first by reduction of blood volume and ventricular preload, and, if possible, by lowering afterload.

DIURETICS (also see p. 527). Mild heart failure in patients with AMI frequently responds well to diuretics such as furosemide, administered intravenously in doses of 40 mg, repeated at 3- to 4-hour intervals if necessary. The resultant reduction of pulmonary capillary pressure reduces dyspnea, and the lowering of left ventricular wall tension that accompanies the reduction of left ventricular diastolic volume diminishes myocardial oxygen requirements and may lead to improvement of contractility and augmentation of the ejection fraction, stroke volume, and cardiac output. The reduction of elevated left ventricular filling pressure may also enhance myocardial oxygen delivery by diminishing the impedance to coronary perfusion attributable to elevated ventricular wall tension (p. 1239). It may also improve arterial oxygenation by reducing pulmonary vascular congestion.

The intravenous administration of furosemide reduces pulmonary vascular congestion and pulmonary venous pressure within 15 minutes, before renal excretion of sodium and water have occurred; presumably this action results from a direct dilating effect of this drug on the systemic arterial bed (p. 527). It is important not to "overshoot" the mark by reducing left ventricular filling pressure much below 18 mm Hg, the lower range associated with optimal left ventricular performance, since this may reduce cardiac output further and cause arterial hypotension. Excessive diuresis may also result in hypokalemia, with its attendant risk of digitalis intoxication.

VASODILATORS (see p. 534). Myocardial oxygen requirements depend on left ventricular wall stress, which in turn is proportional to the product of peak developed left ventricular pressure, volume, and wall thickness (p. 1535). Vasodilator therapy is not recommended in patients with uncomplicated AMI, but is useful in patients whose MI is complicated by heart failure unresponsive to treatment with diuretics, hypertension, mitral regurgitation, or ventricular septal defect. In these patients, treatment with vasodilator agents increases stroke volume and reduces myocardial oxygen consumption. The necessity for hemodynamic monitoring of systemic arterial and pulmonary capillary wedge (or at least pulmonary artery) pressure of cardiac output in patients treated with these agents must be emphasized, since improvement of cardiac performance and energetics requires three simultaneous effects: (1) reduction of impedance to ventricular ejection; (2) avoidance of excessive systemic arterial hypotension in order to maintain effective coronary perfusion pressure; and (3) avoidance of excessive reduction of ventricular filling pressure with consequent diminution of cardiac output. In general, pulmonary capillary wedge pressure should be maintained at approximately 20 mm Hg and arterial diastolic blood pressure above 60 mm Hg in patients who were normotensive prior to the development of the AMI.

Appropriate doses of vasodilators generally enhance stroke volume and cardiac output, reduce left ventricular filling pressure and volume and calculated systemic vascular resistance, without causing serious reflex tachycardia. While available data are not conclusive and do not apply to all subsets of patients with AMI, at least one vasodilator, nitroglycerin, when given early in the course of AMI, has been reported also to protect ischemic myocardium and limit infarct size (p. 1322). Excessive doses of vasodilators may decrease cardiac output by reducing preload and left ventricular filling pressure below optimal levels or may decrease coronary perfusion by excessive depression of systemic arterial pressure. Compromise of coronary perfusion, in turn, may impair ventricular performance further, extend infarction, and give rise to lethal arrhythmias.

Vasodilator therapy is particularly useful when AMI is complicated by mitral regurgitation or rupture of the ventricular septum. In such patients, vasodilators alone or in combination with intra-aortic balloon counterpulsation can sometimes serve as a "holding maneuver" and provide hemodynamic stabilization to permit definitive catheterization and angiographic studies to be carried out and to prepare the patient for early surgical intervention. Because of the precarious state of patients with complicated infarcts and the need for meticulous adjustment of dosage, therapy is best initiated with agents that can be administered intravenously and that have a short duration of action, such as nitroprusside,[121–124] trimethaphan,[125] nitroglycerin,[126–133] isosorbide dinitrate,[134] or phentolamine.[135,136] After initial stabilization, oral medication with hydralazine;[137,138] long-acting nitrates given by mouth, sublingually, by ointment or transdermally;[139,140] prazosin;[141] calcium antagonists such as nifedipine;[142] and angiotensin-converting enzyme inhibitors such as captopril[143] may be useful.

There has been more experience with the intravenous infusion of *nitroprusside* in patients with AMI than with other vasodilators. It is generally given initially in doses of 0.5 μg/kg/min[145,146] and may be gradually and progressively increased up to 50 μg/kg/min. While increasing cardiac output in patients with AMI and left ventricular failure (Fig. 38–5),[147] nitroprusside diminishes arteriolar resistance

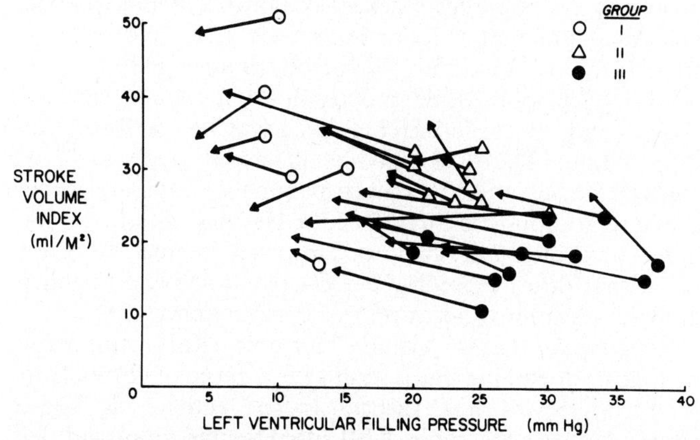

FIGURE 38–5 Hemodynamic responses to nitroprusside infusion in patients with acute myocardial infarction. Patients in Groups II and III with elevated left ventricular filling pressures (20 mm Hg or more) tend to respond to the vasodilator with an increase in the stroke volume and a marked drop in the filling pressure, whereas patients with left ventricular filling pressures below 15 mm Hg (Group I) show a reduction in the stroke volume and tend to have less marked decreases in filling pressures during nitroprusside infusion. Group III patients had stroke work indices below 20 g-m/m². (Reproduced with permission from Chatterjee, K., and Parmley, W. W.: The role of vasodilator therapy in heart failure. Prog. Cardiovasc. Dis. *19*:301, 1977.)

and impedance to left ventricular ejection, pulmonary capillary wedge pressure, myocardial oxygen requirements, and sometimes the frequency of ventricular premature contractions. With optimization of dose, improved segmental ventricular function of zones of apparent infarction has been observed.[124] Nitroprusside may augment cardiac output even in patients with cardiogenic shock, if arterial diastolic and coronary perfusion pressure are maintained by concomitant intra-aortic balloon counterpulsation.

Nitroglycerin has been shown in animal experiments to be less likely than nitroprusside to produce a "coronary steal," i.e., to divert blood flow from the ischemic to the nonischemic zone,[127] and therefore when it (or isosorbide dinitrate, which has a similar action[134]) is used intravenously it may be a particularly useful vasodilator in patients with AMI.[128] Ten to 15 μg/min is infused and the dose is increased by 5 μg/min every five minutes until the desired effect (improvement of hemodynamics or relief of ischemic chest pain) or a decline in systolic arterial pressure to 90 mm Hg, or by more than 15 mm Hg, has occurred. Since nitroglycerin adheres to polyvinyl chloride, this drug should be administered through specially available kits. Although both nitroglycerin and nitroprusside lower systemic arterial pressure, systemic vascular resistance, and the heart rate–systolic blood pressure product, the reduction of left ventricular filling pressure is more prominent with nitroglycerin because of its relatively greater effect than nitroprusside on venous capacitance vessels. Nevertheless, in patients with severe left ventricular failure, cardiac output often increases despite the reduction in left ventricular filling pressure produced by nitroglycerin.

Favorable effects on ventricular performance and jeopardized ischemic myocardium in patients with AMI have been obtained with *phentolamine* (at doses of 0.1 to 2.0 mg/min), an alpha-adrenergic blocking agent whose predominant effects are on arteriolar resistance vessels;[135,136] unfortunately, this agent is extremely expensive and causes tachycardia. Reduction of ventricular afterload with intravenous infusions of a ganglionic blocking agent, *trimethaphan*, in doses of 100 to 1000 μg/min in patients with AMI, associated with acute or chronic hypertension has been shown to protect ischemic myocardium and to reduce infarct size and early mortality in hypertensive patients with AMI.[125] This agent is less likely to produce reflex tachycardia than are directly acting vasodilators because of its inhibitory effects on sympathetic ganglia and therefore on baroreceptor-mediated reflexes.

The use of oral vasodilators in the treatment of chronic congestive heart failure is discussed on pp. 534 to 541. Here we focus on their use in the patients with AMI, which is generally begun after their condition has been stabilized with an intravenous agent.

Hydralazine (p. 538) (10 to 100 mg four times a day) is an orally effective vasodilator acting directly on arterioles. Although useful as an afterload-reducing agent in patients with chronic heart failure, it may be hazardous in patients in the first few days following AMI because of the tachycardia it sometimes induces owing to reflex stimulation. Furthermore, some[148,149] but not all[150,151] investigators have reported the development of pharmacological or physiological tolerance with prolonged use.

Prazosin (p. 539) (0.5 mg. with gradual increments to a maximum of 10 mg, three times daily), an orally active adrenergic-blocking agent, improves cardiac function in patients with chronic congestive heart failure.[141] Although it has not been evaluated extensively in the treatment of AMI, its unique pharmacological properties, compared with those of other alpha-adrenergic receptor antagonists, appear promising. In contrast to other alpha-receptor blocking agents, prazosin does not inhibit presynaptic sites, i.e., so-called alpha-2 receptors (Fig. 27–9, p. 914). Accordingly, negative feedback on presynaptic receptors by norepinephrine released from the nerve endings remains intact. This may account for the absence of tachycardia after administration of the drug, which should make it particularly useful in patients with AMI. Prazosin, like nitroprusside, affects both arteriolar and venous tone; effects persist for up to six hours after an oral dose.

Captopril (p. 539) (25 to 100 mg three times daily)[151] elicits sustained increases in cardiac index and diminution of left ventricular filling pressure, even among patients with congestive heart failure complicated by impaired renal function. Its inhibition of formation of angiotensin II results in retention of potassium due to decreased aldosterone levels, and hence it should be used with caution with potassium-sparing diuretics such as spironolactone, triamterene, or amiloride. It may potentiate the hypotensive effects of other agents such as thiazide or "loop" diuretics, which should therefore be used judiciously and sometimes at reduced dosage if employed concomitantly. Rare toxic effects on the hematopoietic system or on glomerular functional integrity and proteinuria are generally seen only with high doses. Captopril has not been evaluated extensively in patients with AMI, but it is of interest that it has been shown, in experimental studies, to reduce infarct size in dogs with coronary occlusion.[152]

Digitalis (see p. 508). Although digitalis increases contractility and the oxygen consumption of normal hearts, when heart failure is present the diminution of heart size and wall tension frequently results in a net reduction of myocardial oxygen requirements.[153] In animal experiments acetylstrophanthidin fails to improve ventricular performance immediately following experimental coronary occlusion, but salutary effects are elicited when it is administered several days later.[154] The absence of early beneficial effects may be due to the inability of ischemic tissue to respond to digitalis, the already maximal stimulation of contractility of the normal heart by circulating and neuronally released catecholamines, or the dissipation of the force of contraction of normal myocardium into dyskinetic areas. In experimental animals without congestive heart failure who are subjected to coronary occlusion, digitalis increases the distribution and severity of ischemia, presumably by stimulating oxygen requirements,[155] although it augments blood flow to ischemic zones in conscious dogs.[156] Digitalis reduces the severity of ischemia occurring in the presence of experimentally induced congestive heart failure,[157] presumably because of the reduction in myocardial oxygen requirements.

Although the issue is still controversial, arrhythmias may be increased by digitalis glycosides when they are given to patients in the first few hours after the onset of MI, particularly in the presence of hypokalemia. Also, undesirable peripheral systemic and coronary vasoconstriction may result from the rapid intravenous administration of these agents.[158]

Administration of digitalis to patients hospitalized with AMI should generally be reserved for the management of supraventricular tachyarrhythmias such as atrial flutter and fibrillation and of heart failure that persists despite treatment with diuretics. Digitalis causes modest improvement of cardiac performance in patients with mild heart failure (Killip Class II).[159,160] There is no indication for its use as an inotropic agent in patients without clinical evidence of left ventricular dysfunction (Killip Class I), and it is too weak an inotropic agent to be relied upon as the principal cardiac stimulant in patients in overt pulmonary edema or cardiogenic shock (Classes III or IV). It may, however, be useful as a supplement to vasodilator agents and in the treatment of persistent or recurrent left ventricular failure. Cardiac glycosides appear to become progressively more effective in the treatment of heart failure as the interval from the acute events lengthens; i.e., they are more effective in the treatment of chronic than of acute heart failure secondary to ischemic heart disease. However, the possibility that continued administration of digitalis might contribute to late mortality in the two years following AMI has been raised[161] and debated.[162] The possible long-term hazards of digitalis administration must be clarified before a definitive recommendation about its use in the convalescent phase can be made. At this time, it would appear to be indicated only if there is overt heart failure and/or supraventricular tachyarrhythmias, but it is of interest that it has been shown, in experimental studies, to reduce the area of infarct size in dogs with coronary occlusion and heart failure.[166]

BETA-ADRENERGIC AGONISTS (see also p. 542). When left ventricular failure is severe, as manifested by marked reduction of cardiac index (<2 L/min/m^2), and pulmonary capillary wedge pressure is at optimal (18 to 24 mm Hg) or excessive (>24 mm Hg) levels despite therapy with diuretics, beta-adrenergic agonists are indicated. Although isoproterenol is a potent cardiac stimulant and improves ventricular performance, it also causes tachycardia and augments myocardial oxygen consumption and lactate production;[163] in addition, it reduces coronary perfusion pressure by causing systemic vasodilation and increases the extent of experimentally induced infarction in animals.[155,164] Norepinephrine and metaraminol also increase myocardial oxygen consumption because of their peripheral vasoconstrictor as well as positive inotropic actions.

Dopamine and dobutamine, which are relatively cardioselective and stimulate beta-1 receptors, exert predominantly positive inotropic effects (p. 418) and may be particularly useful in patients with AMI and reduced cardiac output, increased left ventricular filling pressure, pulmonary vascular congestion, and hypotension.[164a] Fortunately, the potentially deleterious alpha-adrenergic vasoconstrictor effects exerted by *dopamine* occur only at higher doses than those required to increase contractility. Its vasodilating actions on renal and splanchnic vessels and its positive inotropic effects generally improve hemodynamics and renal function.[165] In patients with AMI and left ventricular failure, this drug should be administered at a dose of 3 μg/kg/min, while monitoring pulmonary capillary wedge and systemic arterial pressures as well as cardiac output. The dose may be increased stepwise to 20 μg/kg/min, in order to reduce pulmonary capillary wedge pressure to approximately 20 mm Hg and elevate cardiac index to exceed 2 L/min/m^2. However, it must be recognized that doses exceeding 5 μg/kg/min activate peripheral alpha receptors and cause vasoconstriction.

Dobutamine has a positive inotropic effect comparable to that of dopamine but a slightly less positive chronotropic effect,[166] with less vasoconstrictor activity at higher doses. In patients with AMI dobutamine improves left ventricular performance without augmenting enzymatically estimated infarct size.[167–169,169a] It may be administered in a starting dose of 2.5 μg/kg/min and increased stepwise to a maximum of 30 μg/kg/min. Both dopamine and dobutamine must be given carefully and with constant monitoring of the electrocardiogram, systemic arterial pressure, pulmonary artery or pulmonary artery occlusive pressure, and, if possible, frequent measurements of cardiac output. The dose must be reduced if systolic pressure exceeds 130 to 140 mm Hg, heart rate exceeds 100 to 110 beats/min, or supraventricular or ventricular tachyarrhythmias are precipitated.

TREATMENT OF CARDIOGENIC SHOCK

(see also p. 593)

Massive AMI may produce global impairment of left ventricular function which is so profound that cardiogenic shock supervenes. The etiology, pathophysiology, and clinical picture of this syndrome are considered in detail on pp. 591 and 1270. Cardiogenic shock is characterized by marked hypotension with systolic arterial pressure less than 80 mm Hg and a marked reduction of cardiac index (generally < 1.8 L/min/m^2) in the face of elevated left ventricular filling pressure (pulmonary capillary wedge pressure > 18 mm Hg).[169b] Spurious estimates of left ventricular filling pressure based on measurements of the pulmonary artery occlusive pressure can occur in the presence of marked mitral regurgitation, in which the tall *v* wave in the left atrial (and pulmonary artery occlusive) pressure tracing elevates the mean pressure above left ventricular end-diastolic pressure. Accordingly, mitral regurgitation and other mechanical lesions such as ventricular septal defect, ventricular aneurysm, and pseudoaneurysm must be excluded before the diagnosis of cardiogenic shock due to global impairment of left ventricular function can be established. These potentially catastrophic mechanical complications should be suspected in any patient with AMI in whom circulatory collapse occurs. Immediate hemodynamic and angiographic evaluations are necessary if these complications are likely to be responsible for the impairment of left ventricular performance, since primary therapy of such lesions usually requires immediate operative treatment with intervening support of the circulation by intra-aortic balloon counterpulsation.

Cardiotonic agents, particularly dopamine and dobutamine, are employed extensively in the treatment of cardiogenic shock owing to global impairment of left ventricular function.[170] While these drugs can improve hemodynamics in the absence of the above-mentioned mechanical complications, unfortunately they do not appear to affect mortality significantly. Similarly, vasodilators have been utilized in an effort to elevate cardiac output and to reduce left ventricular filling pressure. However, by lowering the already markedly reduced coronary perfusion pressure, myocardial perfusion can be compromised further, accelerating the vicious circle illustrated in Figure 37–8 p. 1271. Vasodilators may nonetheless be employed in conjunction with intra-aortic balloon counterpulsation and/or inotropic agents in an effort to increase cardiac output while sustaining or elevating coronary perfusion pressure.

The systemic vascular resistance is usually elevated in patients with cardiogenic shock, but occasionally resistance is normal, and in some instances vasodilation actually predominates. When systemic vascular resistance is *not* elevated in patients with cardiogenic shock, norepinephrine (in doses ranging from 2 to 10 μg/min), which has both alpha- and beta-adrenergic agonist properties, is often employed to increase diastolic arterial pressure, maintain coronary perfusion, and improve contractility, but, again, there is no definitive evidence that ultimate outcome is affected by this drug.[163,171] Norepinephrine should be used only when other means, including balloon counterpulsation, fail to maintain systemic arterial diastolic pressure above 50 to 60 mm Hg in a previously normotensive patient. The use of alpha-adrenergic agents such as phenylephrine or methoxamine is contraindicated in patients with cardiogenic shock.

INTRAAORTIC BALLOON COUNTERPULSATION. The implementation, underlying principles, and physiological consequences of this procedure in patients with cardiogenic shock are discussed on p. 593 and illustrated in Figure 18–10. This form of circulatory assistance augments diastolic aortic pressure and thereby facilitates coronary perfusion; it reduces left ventricular afterload and thereby reduces myocardial oxygen consumption;[172,173] as a consequence anaerobic metabolism[174] and myocardial ischemia are diminished. Favorable effects are sometimes reflected in prompt resolution of electrocardiographic signs of ischemia (Fig. 38–6).

Intraaortic balloon counterpulsation is utilized in the treatment of AMI in three groups of patients: (1) those who are hemodynamically unstable and in whom support of the circulation is required for the performance of diagnostic studies which are carried out to assess lesions that are potentially correctable surgically; (2) in cardiogenic shock that is unresponsive to medical management; and (3) in the presence of persistent ischemic pain that is unresponsive to treatment with inhalation of 100 per cent oxygen, beta-adrenergic blockade, nitrates, and calcium channel blocking agents during the postinfarction state. Unfortunately, among patients with cardiogenic shock, improvement is often only temporary, and "balloon dependence" is common.[175,176] Patients with cardiogenic shock treated with this modality can be successfully weaned from the supporting system only occasionally, and counterpulsation alone does not improve overall mortality, either in patients with or those without a surgically remediable mechanical lesion.[177,178] However, it may be life-saving in allowing the patient to tolerate catheterization and coronary arteriography and to be brought to the operating room for definitive treatment without irreversible organ damage. It is possible that left ventricular bypass, a technique that reduces left ventricular oxygen demands more drastically (p. 548), may ultimately prove to be more effective in improving survival in patients with cardiogenic shock than intraaortic balloon counterpulsation;[179] however, at the present time it is still experimental.

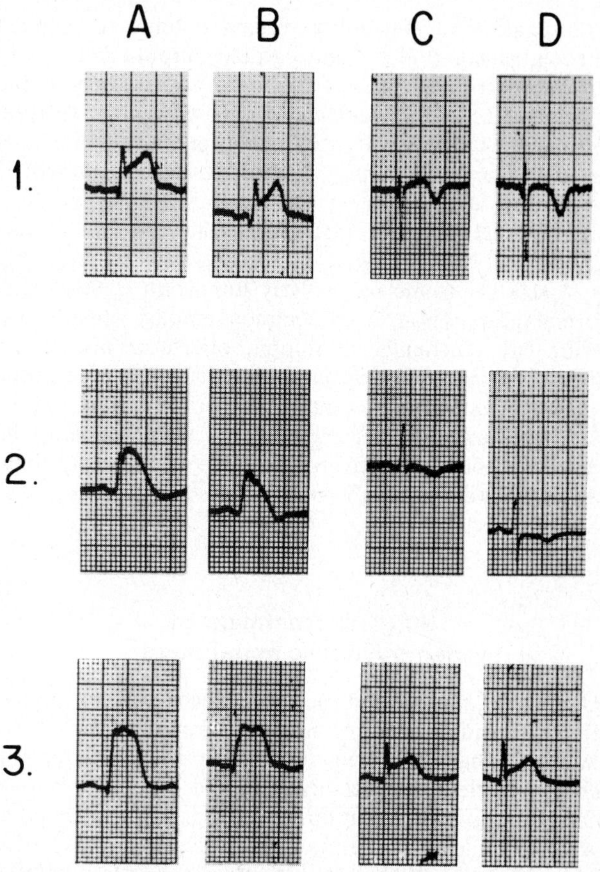

FIGURE 38–6 Precordial lead showing maximal ST-segment elevation in patients with acute myocardial infarction 1 hour before intraaortic balloon pumping (IABP) (column A), immediately before IABP (column B), 30 minutes after commencing IABP (column C), and 1 hour after IABP had begun (column D). The fall in ST-segment elevation in these leads during the hour before IABP was 26 per cent, compared with 84 per cent during the post-IABP hour. In all cases the ST response was greatest during the first 30 minutes of treatment. (Modified from Leinbach, R. C., et al.: Early intraaortic balloon pumping for anterior myocardial infarction without shock. Circulation *58*:204, 1978, by permission of the American Heart Association, Inc.)

Noninvasive approaches to circulatory assistance have been developed, such as external devices that apply pressure to the lower extremities during diastole, thereby promoting increased runoff during systole. However, this form of therapy likewise does not alter outcome decisively; its hemodynamic effects are, in fact, less than those of intraaortic counterpulsation.[180]

RIGHT VENTRICULAR INFARCTION (see also p. 1274). Unlike cardiogenic shock due solely or predominantly to left ventricular involvement, hemodynamics may be improved in patients with right ventricular infarction by a combination of expanding plasma volume to augment right ventricular preload and cardiac output, and the administration of arterial vasodilators. These drugs reduce the impedance to left ventricular outflow and in turn left ventricular diastolic, left atrial, and pulmonary (arterial) pressures, thereby lowering the impedance to right ventricular outflow and enhancing right ventricular output. A remarkably high survival rate of 60 per cent, albeit in a small series, makes recognition and vigorous medical therapy of this syndrome particularly important.[120] Since right ventricular infarction is so common among patients with inferior left ventricular infarction, otherwise unexplained systemic arterial hypotension or diminished cardiac output in such patients should lead to the prompt consideration of this diagnosis. Replacement of the tricuspid valve has been carried out in the treatment of severe tricuspid regurgitation secondary to right ventricular infarction.[181]

Surgical Treatment of Hemodynamic Impairment

Operative intervention is most successful in patients with AMI and circulatory collapse when a surgically correctable mechanical lesion can be identified and repaired, such as ventricular septal defect,[182,183] acute mitral regurgitation resulting from rupture of the head of a papillary muscle or of chordae tendineae, aneurysm, or pseudoaneurysm (p. 1270).[184] In such patients the circulation should at first be supported by intraaortic balloon pulsation and a positive inotropic agent such as dopamine or dobutamine in combination with a vasodilator unless the patient is hypotensive. Operation should not be delayed in patients with a correctable lesion who require pharmacologic and/or mechanical (counterpulsation) support (Fig. 38–7).[182,185,186] Such patients frequently develop a serious complication—infection, adult respiratory distress syndrome, extension of the infarct, renal failure, etc.—if operation is delayed. On the other hand, when the hemodynamic status of a patient with one of these mechanical lesions complicating an AMI remains stable after the patient has been weaned off pharmacologic and/or mechanical support, it may be desirable to postpone operation for two to four weeks to allow some healing of the infarct to occur.

Some favorable results have been reported from early revascularization and infarctectomy in patients who have cardiogenic shock due to ventricular failure without mechanical complications and who are unresponsive to all other measures.[187,188] However, this approach has not received widespread acceptance because of the high mortality rate, and the difficulties involved in selecting the proper time for operation—after it has become clear that the patient is in cardiogenic shock despite optimal medical management, yet before a critical quantity of myocardium has become irreversibly damaged.

Although cardiac rupture (p. 1268) is generally immediately fatal pericardiocentesis to abort cardiac tamponade, followed immediately by resection of the necrotic and ruptured myocardium with primary reconstruction, has on rare occasion been lifesaving.[188,189]

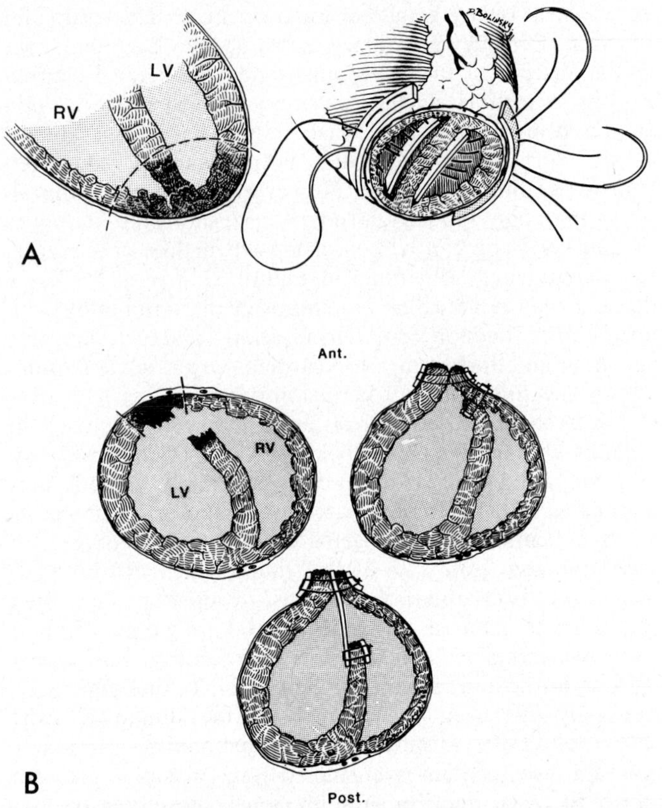

FIGURE 38–7 *A*, Closure of apical ventricular septal rupture. The infarcted apex is resected, and the remaining viable myocardium of the septum and the left and right ventricular free walls are buttressed together using Teflon felt inside and outside the ventricle. LV = left ventricle; RV = right ventricle. *B*, Closure of a ventricular septal rupture with an extensive anterior infarct. The septum is reconstructed with a heavy Dacron patch that is sewn to the base of remaining septum using Teflon bolsters on both sides. The free edge of the patch is then brought out and the left and right ventricular free walls are attached to it, as shown in *C*. Ant. = anterior; LV = left ventricle; Post = posterior; RV = right ventricle. (Reproduced with permission from Kopf, G. S., Meshkov, A., Laks, H., Hammond, G. L., and Geha, A. S.: Changing patterns in the surgical management of ventricular septal rupture after myocardial infarction. Am. J. Surg. *143*:465, 1982.)

LIMITATION OF INFARCT SIZE

As already noted, infarct size is an important determinant of prognosis in patients with AMI. Patients who succumb from cardiogenic shock exhibit massive infarcts,[191,192] and early impairment of ventricular function, presaging a poor prognosis, is correlated with extensive infarcts.[192–196] Survivors with large infarcts frequently exhibit late impairment of ventricular function, and the long-term mortality rate is higher than that for survivors with small infarcts (Fig. 38–8), who tend not to develop cardiac decompensation.[49,193,194,197–201] The influence of infarct size on mortality is most apparent during the patient's hospital course and in the first few months after infarction. The hospital mortality of patients with large infarcts, as estimated by technetium pyrophosphate scanning, is several-fold greater than it is in patients with small infarcts (Fig. 11–24, p. 387).[201] However, the importance of infarct size declines

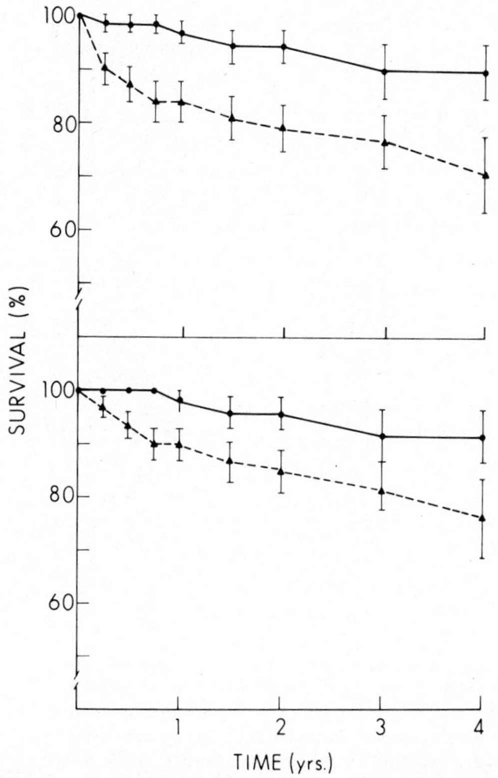

FIGURE 38–8 The influence of the extent of initial myocardial infarction on survival. Survival is shown after initial myocardial infarction in a total of 173 patients with infarct size index (expressed in terms of CK-gram-equivalents/m²) of <15 (solid line) vs. ≥15 (interrupted line). Brackets indicate standard errors. The upper panel depicts survival curves for all patients who survived for at least 24 hours after the onset of an initial myocardial infarction. The lower panel depicts curves for those patients who survived at least 21 days after infarction. In both groups, survival was significantly greater for patients with small compared to large infarcts ($p < 0.05$). (From Geltman, E. M., et al.: The influence of location and extent of myocardial infarction on long-term ventricular dysrhythmia and mortality. Circulation *60*:805, 1979, by permission of the American Heart Association, Inc.)

somewhat with time after the initial episode;[49] after recovery from an AMI it is the quantity of remaining myocardium whose viability is threatened because it is perfused by obstructed coronary vessels (p. 340) that becomes critical to the prognosis.

THE DYNAMIC NATURE OF INFARCTION. AMI is a dynamic process that often does not occur instantaneously but sometimes evolves relatively slowly (Fig. 37–7, p. 1271). As has been pointed out (p. 1256), in experimental animals the fate of jeopardized, ischemic tissue may be affected favorably by interventions that restore perfusion, reduce myocardial oxygen requirements, inhibit accumulation or facilitate washout of noxious metabolites, augment the availability of substrate for anaerobic metabolism,[7,8,155,202–204] or blunt the effects of mediators of injury such as calcium (Fig. 36–16, p. 1253),[205,206] metabolites, and constituents of cell membranes.[207,208]

The perfusion of the myocardium associated with AMI appears to be reduced maximally immediately following coronary occlusion. In experimental animals, increases in blood flow to the peripheral portions of the ischemic zones become evident within 24 hours of acute coronary occlusion,[209,210] suggesting that dynamic factors contribute to the early limitation of perfusion; these may include release of catecholamines as a consequence of ischemia of adrenergic neurons, as well as the efflux of potassium from injured myocardial cells.[211] Spasm of coronary vessels has been implicated not only in Prinzmetal's variant angina (p. 1360) but also in association with MI induced by atherosclerosis,[212–215] as well as in patients experiencing postinfarction angina at rest.[216,217]

Relatively prompt, *partial* restoration of reduced blood flow to the ischemic zone may result from spontaneous thrombolysis, from relief of coronary spasm, or from improved systemic hemodynamics; the latter includes augmented coronary perfusion pressure and reduced left ventricular end-diastolic pressure. Subsequently, perfusion may be enhanced by the development of collateral circulation.[218] The prompt implementation of measures designed to protect ischemic myocardium and support myocardial perfusion may provide sufficient time for the development of anatomical and physiological compensatory mechanisms that limit the ultimate extent of infarction.

AMI in hospitalized patients may be complicated by extension of infarction or early reinfarction (p. 1292). Depending on the criteria utilized for detection, the incidence of these complications ranges from 8 to 30 per cent.[219–221] It is possible that interventions designed to protect ischemic myocardium during the initial event may also reduce the incidence of extension of infarction or early reinfarction. On the other hand, it has been suggested that preservation of ischemic myocardium could lead to persistent survival of cells in regions subjected to repetitive episodes of severe ischemia, leading to the development of arrhythmias. The relatively poor late prognosis of patients with subendocardial infarction[222,223] and the very high risk of sudden death among patients with serious coronary artery disease but without MI who are successfully resuscitated from ventricular fibrillation[13] (Chap. 23) are consistent with this possibility. However, despite these hazards, there is no evidence that the implementation of interventions designed to protect ischemic myocardium results in any late deleterious effects. Furthermore, it has been reported that preservation of ischemic myocardium by trimethaphan in hypertensive patients with evolving infarction,[125] by intravenous nitroglycerin in normotensive patients,[132] and by the early administration of beta-adrenergic blocking agents[224–226] is actually associated with a reduced rather than an increased mortality.

Proof of the clinical efficacy of specific interventions has been difficult to acquire, in part because of the wide variations in the size of infarcts and their rate of evolution, in part because of the difficulties involved in measuring infarct size, and in part because it is difficult to predict what the size of any given infarction would have been had the intervention under study not been administered. In addition, since many patients usually reach the hospital five hours or even later after the onset of ischemia, it may be too late in these patients to salvage substantial quantities of ischemic myocardium in the first place. In addition, from a statistical point of view, detection of a 15 per cent difference in an estimate of infarct size would require anal-

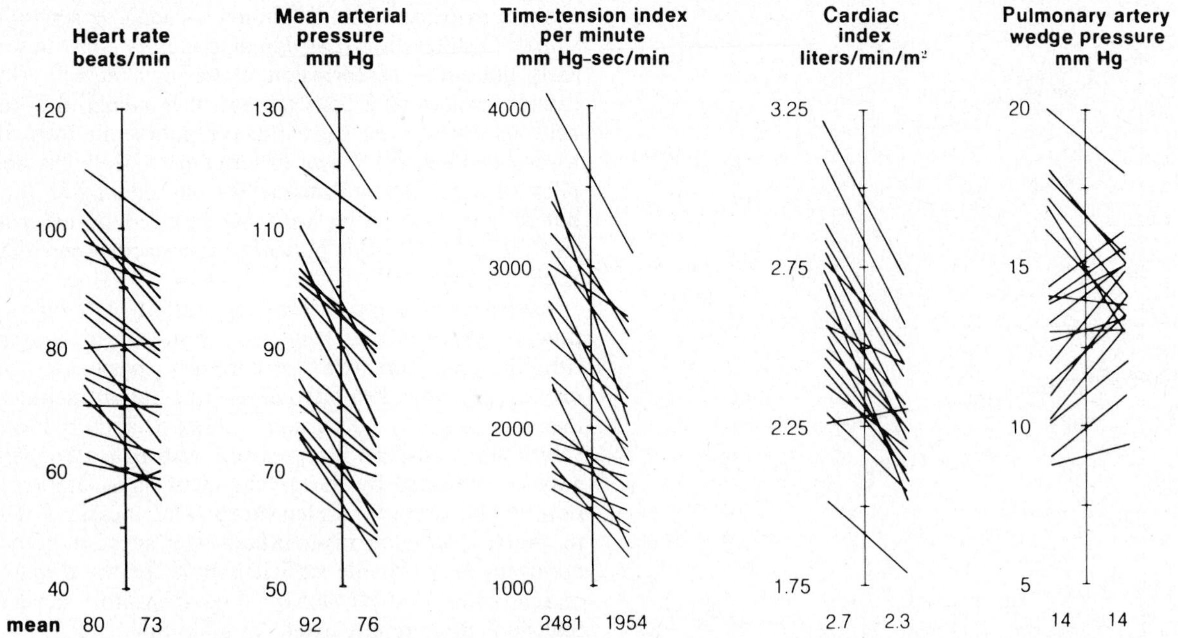

FIGURE 38–9 Hemodynamic effects of propranolol in patients with acute myocardial infarction. Control values are shown to the left of each scale and results after propranolol to the right. Heart rate, mean arterial pressure, and time-tension index are uniformly decreased after propranolol, and cardiac index is decreased in all but one patient. The response of pulmonary artery wedge pressure, however, is variable; in 6 patients with pressures above 15 mm Hg before treatment, propranolol produced a substantial reduction, whereas in the remaining patients, pressure was slightly increased. (From Mueller, H. S., et al.: How, when and why to use propranolol in acute MI. Cardiovasc. Med. *2*:321, 1977.)

ysis of the results in as many as 3000 patients initially entering a prospective study of the effects of treatment according to a rigorous protocol. With mortality as an endpoint, detection of a significant difference attributable to an intervention would require study of an even larger number of patients. Despite the difficulties in the unequivocal demonstration of efficacy of interventions designed to limit infarct size, we believe that therapeutic nihilism is not justified. By analogy, the well-documented high mortality in essential hypertension and the potential benefits of antihypertensive drugs led to their extensive and effective utilization long before improved survival with treatment was demonstrated unequivocally.

BETA-ADRENERGIC BLOCKADE. Beta blockers decrease cardiac index, stroke index, heart rate, blood pressure, and tension-time index (Fig. 38–9). The net effect of these drugs is a reduction in myocardial oxygen consumption per minute and per beat, in the setting of increased concentrations of circulating catecholamines and sympathetic nerve stimulation associated with AMI.[226] Favorable effects of beta-adrenergic blockade on the balance of myocardial oxygen supply and demand are reflected in the reduction of myocardial lactate production[227–229] and the diminution of ventricular arrhythmias.[230] Since beta-adrenergic blockade diminishes circulating levels of free fatty acids by antagonizing the lipolytic effects of catecholamines, and since elevated levels of fatty acids augment myocardial oxygen consumption and probably increase the incidence of arrhythmias, these metabolic actions of beta-blocking agents may be beneficial to the ischemic heart.[228,229]

Objective evidence of beneficial effects of beta-blockers in acute myocardial ischemia in patients has been reported by several investigators using various modifications of the precordial ST-segment mapping technique (Fig. 38–10).[231–234] Gold et al.[231] found that the likelihood of a beneficial clinical and electrocardiographic response increased in the presence of residual antegrade or collateral blood flow to the infarct zone, as determined by coronary arteriography. Waagstein and Hjalmarson[235] demonstrated, in a double-blind controlled study, that each of three cardioselective beta blockers decreased ST-segment elevations in transmural infarction and reduced ischemic chest pain in patients with transmural and nontransmural infarction; no diminution of ST-segment elevation occurred with the administration of saline or an analgesic. In addition, intravenous pindolol, a beta blocker with some intrinsic sympathomimetic activity, has been shown to reduce ST-segment elevation, relieve ischemic pain, and improve regional wall motion in patients with transmural AMI.[236]

However, just as is the case in the experimental situations (p. 1256), not all clinical trials of beta blockers in AMI have reported salutary effects. Thus, practolol (oral or intravenous followed by oral) begun early during the course of AMI did not result in major differences in the clinical course, although there was a lower mortality in the subgroup of practolol-treated patients who had tachycardia at the time of entry into the study.[237]

Studies of the effect of beta blockade on indexes of infarct size in patients are limited. Peter et al.[238] reported the results of a randomized trial of propranolol (0.1 mg/kg intravenously, followed by 320 mg orally over the next 27 hours). The patients treated *within four hours of onset of symptoms* of uncomplicated MI had significantly lower peak serum creatine kinase levels and less cumulative creatine kinase release into plasma than did patients without specific therapy (Figure 38–11). The same group[239] also found that patients with suspected MI, treated with propranolol within four hours of the onset of symptoms, had a significantly lower incidence of infarction, as indicated by electrocardiographic changes and serum creatine kinase elevation, suggesting that threatened infarction might actually be prevented by early beta blockade. Similarly, Yusuf et al. have reported that intravenous atenolol, given a median of four hours following symptoms of AMI, decreased the incidence of AMI, MB creatine kinase release, electrocardiographic evolution of infarction,[240] and the severity of ischemic pain.[241] Two randomized double-blind controlled studies with beta blockade carried out in the acute phase of infarction have indi-

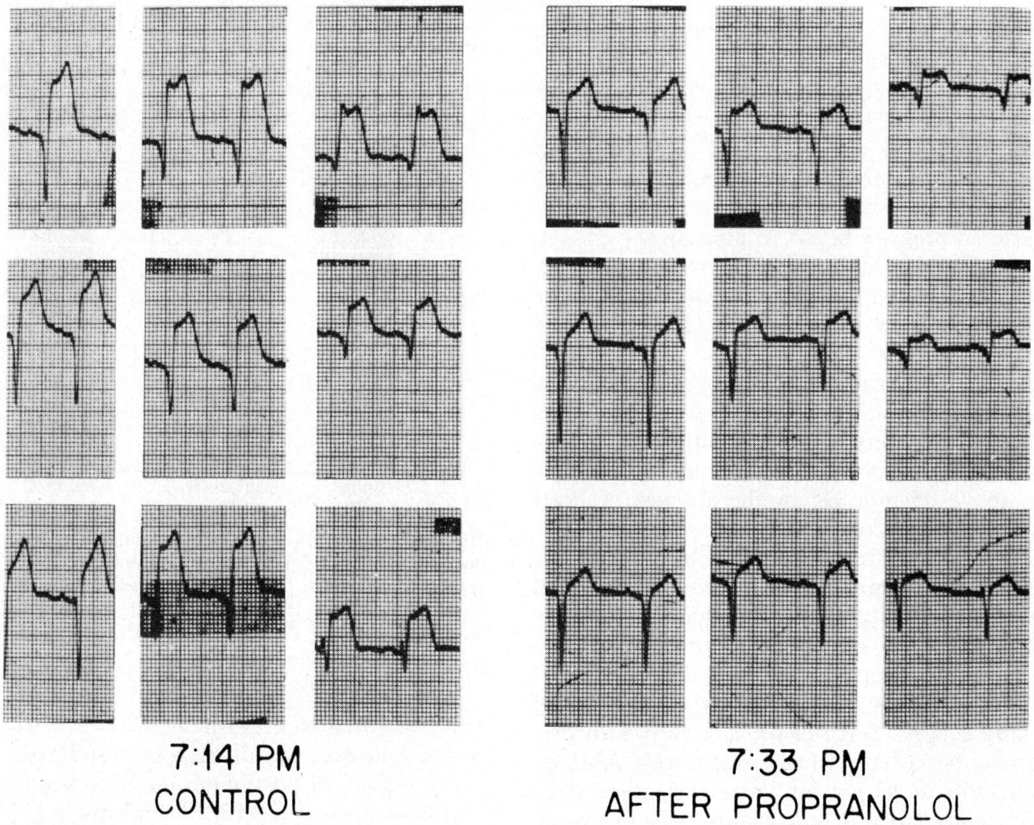

FIGURE 38–10 The effect of propranolol in the reduction of ST-segment elevation in a patient with acute myocardial infarction. The nine leads, depicted from the V_1, V_3, and V_5 positions, and the corresponding sites are one intercostal space above and below the standard positions. Note the marked reduction in ST-segment elevations after propranolol administration. (From Gold, H. K., et al.: Propranolol-induced reduction of signs of ischemic injury during acute myocardial infarction. Am. J. Cardiol. *38*:689, 1976.)

cated that such therapy can limit enzymatically estimated infarct size. One involved alprenolol[242] and the other the cardioselective beta-blocker metoprolol.[242a] In both of these investigations, beta-blocker therapy was initiated early in the course of infarction and was then maintained.

Although the precise indications for beta blockade in AMI are controversial, on the basis of available information, patients with the hyperdynamic state (sinus tachycardia, hypertension, no evidence of heart failure) as well as patients seen in the first four hours who will not be subjected to thrombolytic therapy would appear to be the best candidates; in addition, unless there are contraindications, beta blockade should probably be continued in patients who develop an AMI while receiving one of these agents. In addition, propranolol is indicated in patients in whom infarction is complicated by persistent or recurrent ischemic pain, progressive or repetitive serum enzyme elevations suggestive of infarct extension, or tachyarrhythmias refractory to lidocaine and procainamide early after the onset of infarction. On the other hand, it is unlikely that beta blockade (or any intervention) can reduce infarct size significantly if it is applied much later than six hours after the onset of the event, because by this time, the ultimate size of the infarct has been established in many patients.

In patients who have not received beta blockers in the preceding 24 hours, propranolol may be administered in initial amounts of 0.1 mg/kg intravenously, divided into three equal doses given at 5-minute intervals. During this period, heart rate and arterial pressure should be determined, either through an indwelling arterial catheter or by the cuff method, and an electrocardiographic strip should be recorded after each injection. Intravenous propranolol

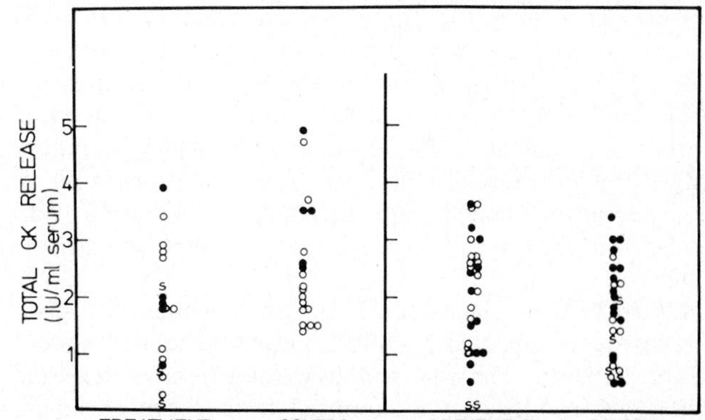

FIGURE 38–11 Effect of propranolol on total CK release after infarction as a function of the time of onset of myocardial infarction. Total calculated CK appearance in treated and control patients entering the trial, less than 4 hours (*left*) or more than 4 hours (*right*) after the onset of infarction. Solid circles indicate patients with anterior infarction and open circles indicate those with inferior infarction. Total CK appearance was 30 per cent less ($p < 0.025$) in patients treated within 4 hours of the onset than in control patients. No significant improvement occurred in patients treated more than 4 hours after the onset. (From Peter, T., et al.: Reduction of enzyme levels by propranolol after acute myocardial infarction. Circulation *57*:1091, 1978, by permission of the American Heart Association, Inc.)

should *not* be administered or its administration should be halted if any of the following events occur:

1. Second- or third-degree AV block or lengthening of the P-R interval beyond 0.24 sec.
2. Rales extending more than one third of the way up the lung fields, or wheezes detected on auscultation.
3. Ventricular rate below 50 per minute.
4. Systolic arterial pressure below 95 mm Hg.
5. Pulmonary artery wedge pressure above 24 mm Hg. (While it is useful, it is by no means necessary to monitor this pressure in patients in whom a beta blocker will be administered.)

The intravenous administration of propranolol is followed one hour later by oral propranolol given in a dose, generally 20 to 80 mg every six hours, adjusted to keep the heart rate between 50 and 65 beats/min and the systolic pressure above 95 mm Hg in the absence of heart failure, wheezing, or advanced AV block.

With the availability of cardioselective beta-adrenergic blocking agents such as alprenolol and metoprolol, and the favorable effects of alprenolol,[243] timolol,[83] metoprolol,[225] and propranolol[84] in double-blind, prospective, *secondary prevention* trials, it appears likely that the beneficial effects of all of these agents are attributable to their beta-1 receptor blocking actions. Some of the alternatives to propranolol that may be beneficial for patients with AMI include alprenolol (40 to 50 mg intravenously followed by 100 to 200 mg orally twice daily), metoprolol (15 mg intravenously followed by 100 mg orally twice daily), and timolol (10 mg orally twice daily). As experience with other available beta-blocking agents such atenolol, nadolol, and pindolol increases, their use in the setting of AMI will undoubtedly be evaluated and clarified as well.

Although antagonism of sympathetic stimulation to the heart might be expected to exacerbate pulmonary edema in patients with occult heart failure, only directionally inconsistent and small changes in pulmonary capillary wedge pressure occur when the drug is used in patients with AMI (Fig. 38–9); in patients with pulmonary capillary pressures below 25 mm Hg, propranolol may elevate the pressure but usually not to excess of this level.[227,228] In an equal number of patients, the elevated pulmonary capillary wedge pressure actually declines, presumably because of the lessening of ischemia and the resultant increase in ventricular compliance and improvement of ventricular performance.

NITRATES (see also p. 1256). Intravenous nitroglycerin has been reported to affect measurements of infarct size in patients. Derrida and associates[243] have reported preliminary results of a randomized trial of prolonged nitroglycerin infusion in patients with AMI. ECG mapping showed a greater reduction in ST-segment elevations after the start of nitroglycerin therapy and less R-wave fall at initially ischemic sites in the nitroglycerin-treated group. Furthermore, in patients with heart failure, mortality and serious ventricular arrhythmias appeared to be reduced in the nitroglycerin-treated group. Bussmann and associates[244] have also reported on a prospective, randomized trial of intravenous nitroglycerin in patients with AMI. Findings included significantly lower values of peak serum CK, lower rates of CK release, and smaller calculated infarct sizes in nitroglycerin-treated patients (Fig. 38–12). Becker and colleagues[245,246] have shown in a prospective, randomized trial that treatment with intravenous nitroglycerin for 48 hours followed by nitroglycerin ointment therapy for 72 hours enhanced postinfarction improvement of myocardial perfusion measured with ^{201}Tl scintigraphy; there is preliminary evidence from the same trial that nitroglycerin reduces the frequency of infarct extension and late ventricular arrhythmias.[247] Kim and Williams have reported that large and frequent doses of nitroglycerin used in the first four hours after the onset of the infarct limited the electrocardiographic signs of myocardial necrosis,[248] a finding consistent with that of other workers using intravenous nitroglycerin.[245,249,250]

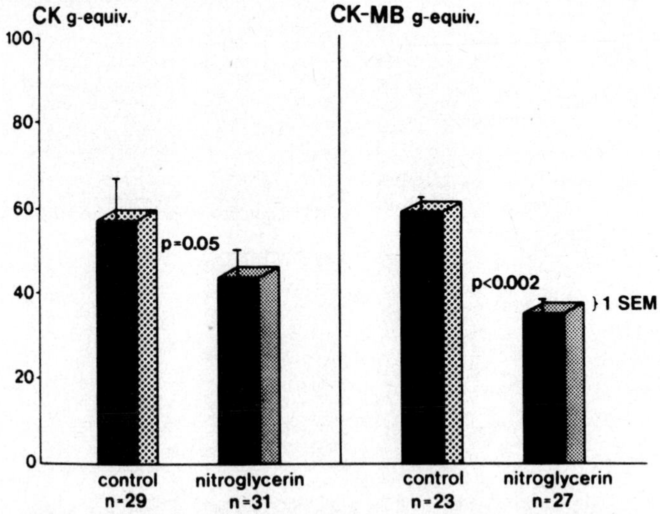

FIGURE 38–12 CK and CK-MB infarct size were significantly reduced in nitroglycerin-treated patients (n = 31) compared with untreated controls (n = 29). (Reproduced with permission from Bussmann, W. D., Passek, D., Seidel, W., and Kaltenbach, M.: Reduction of CK and CK-MB indexes of infarct size by intravenous nitroglycerin. Circulation *63*:615, 1981.)

In experimental animals, nitrates elicit small reductions in total coronary vascular resistance with improvement in the ratio of endocardial to epicardial flow in ischemic myocardium. Myocardial lactate production declines, reflecting diminished myocardial dependence on anaerobic metabolism. However, beneficial effects on coronary blood flow are blunted by the systemic hypotension and reflex tachycardia that are sometimes induced. In contrast to agents such as nitroprusside, nitroglycerin does not appear to produce a "coronary steal."[127] In dogs subjected to coronary occlusion, nitroglycerin reduces the incidence of spontaneous ventricular fibrillation, increases the threshold to induced fibrillation, and diminishes ST-segment elevation.[250] When systemic arterial hypotension and reflex tachycardia are prevented by the concomitant administration of methoxamine or phenylephrine, there is a marked reduction of ST-segment elevation accompanied by a reduction in experimental infarct size.[130]

In patients with AMI, the administration of nitroglycerin and other nitrates such as isosorbide dinitrate diminishes pulmonary capillary wedge pressure and systemic arterial pressure as well as left ventricular end-systolic and end-diastolic volumes. It also reduces ventricular asynergy, to the extent that the local impairment of the left ventricular function is due to reversibly injured, depressed myocardium rather than to zones of completed infarction or scar.[252]

As is true in experimental animals, the administration of nitroglycerin to patients with AMI depends on the existing hemodynamics. When systemic arterial and pulmonary capillary wedge pressures are normal or low prior to the administration of nitroglycerin, reflex tachycardia may result from the further reduction of ventricular filling and arterial pressures; nitroglycerin is probably contraindicated under these circumstances, although the administration of an alpha-adrenergic agonist such as methoxamine (5 mg intravenously or 10 to 15 mg intramuscularly) to augment systemic arterial resistance may be helpful.[130]

Intravenous nitroglycerin can be administered safely to patients with evolving MI as long as the dose is titrated carefully to avoid induction of reflex tachycardia or systemic arterial hypotension (systolic blood pressure $\leq$ 95 mm Hg).[254,255] One useful regimen employs an initial infusion rate of 10 μg/min with stepwise increases of 10 μg/min. Alternatively, it may be administered sublingually at doses of 0.3 to 0.6 mg. This route may be more hazardous, since the rate of absorption is difficult to control and arterial pressure may decline precipitously. Nitroglycerin is often useful for the relief of persistent pain and as a vasodilator in patients with infarction associated with left ventricular failure.

OTHER POTENTIALLY USEFUL APPROACHES TO PROTECTION OF ISCHEMIC MYOCARDIUM

The experimental observations indicating the potential usefulness of the agents described below are summarized on pp. 1255 to 1257.

Hyaluronidase. In several small prospective randomized trials, hyaluronidase diminished development of Q waves or loss of R waves in electrocardiographic sites initially exhibiting ST-segment elevation,[256-258] suggesting that ischemic myocardium was protected and that the evolution of infarction in jeopardized zones was limited. In other studies, it was associated with a small reduction in mortality.[259] It is ordinarily administered intravenously in doses of 500 NF units per kg every 6 hours for 48 hours. An advantage of this agent is the absence of any detectable hemodynamic action and the lack of adverse effects except for rare allergic reactions. It is undergoing further clinical trials.

Glucose-Insulin-Potassium. Administration of a solution of glucose-insulin-potassium (300 gm of glucose, 50 units of insulin, and 80 mEq of KCl in 1000 ml of H_2O administered at a rate of 1.5 ml/kg/hr) lowers the concentration of plasma free fatty acids and improves ventricular performance, as reflected in systolic arterial pressure, cardiac output, and stroke work at any level of left ventricular filling pressure (Fig. 14–3, p. 470)[260,261]; also the frequency of ventricular premature beats decreases.[262,263] In a nonrandomized study, mortality appeared to be reduced,[264,265] hemodynamics improved, global ejection fraction increased, and asynergy in the ischemic zone and pulmonary artery diastolic pressure reduced.[266,266a] However, no definitive effect on enzymatically estimated infarct size or long-term mortality has been described in a prospective, controlled, randomized trial.

Corticosteroids. Administration of a single large dose of methylprednisolone has been reported to decrease infarct size, estimated enzymatically.[267] However, the control and treated groups were not strictly comparable with respect to the apparent extent of infarction prior to the administration of the drug. In contrast to these favorable effects, in another study infarct size estimated enzymatically appeared to be *increased* by multiple doses of methylprednisolone.[268] Administration of the drug has led to persistent elevation of plasma MB-CK and the suspicion of an excessively high incidence of ventricular rupture, as well as an increase in mortality, perhaps because administration of corticosteroids inhibits healing of the infarct.[269-271] Accordingly, administration of multiple high doses of corticosteroids beginning several hours after the onset of ischemic injury appears to be deleterious rather than beneficial. However, on the basis of recent experimental work, it is possible that a single large dose of a glucocorticosteroid may reduce infarct size without interfering with myocardial healing.[272]

Intraaortic Balloon Counterpulsation. From a theoretical standpoint, intra aortic or external[273] balloon counterpulsation might be expected to limit infarct size for several reasons. In experimental animals, intra aortic balloon counterpulsation decreases afterload and myocardial oxygen consumption,[274] decreases preload, increases coronary blood flow, and improves cardiac performance.[173] When intraaortic balloon counterpulsation is carried out in experimental animals immediately after coronary occlusion, ischemic myocardium appears to be protected, based on analysis of ST-segment elevations, myocardial CK depletion, and histological and histochemical criteria of necrosis.[275-277] No definitive information is available indicating that intraaortic balloon counterpulsation alters the prognosis in patients with relatively uncomplicated infarction. Leinbach et al., however, have reported an immediate, persistent fall in ST-segment elevation. This occurred in patients with anterior MI who had preservation of precordial R waves and good ventricular function,[278] in whom the left anterior descending coronary artery was not totally occluded and who underwent intra-aortic balloon pumping within six hours.

REPERFUSION

When carried out within the first several hours after coronary occlusion, reperfusion improves hemodynamics and decreases infarct size, as assessed by epicardial ST-segment recordings, precordial QRS maps, myocardial CK depletion, positron emission tomography and morphology, in several species of experimental animals;[279-287] the extent of protection appears to be directly related to the rapidity with which reperfusion is implemented after the onset of coronary occlusion.[288] Potentially deleterious effects that may accompany reperfusion in experimental animals include myocardial hemorrhage[280,289] and ventricular fibrillation,[280-282] complications that may be particularly prominent when sufficient time (i.e., more than four or five hours) has elapsed after coronary occlusion such that microvascular integrity has become compromised.[282,284] Fortunately, it appears that hemorrhage occurs into tissue that is either already necrotic or destined to become so; therefore, reperfusion does not appear to *extend* infarction.[286]

SURGICAL REPERFUSION. Recent modifications of surgical technique and extensive improvements in intraoperative myocardial preservation with cardioplegia and hypothermia have allowed surgical reperfusion to be carried out at a very low mortality—approximately 2 per cent, in selected centers. This has kindled enthusiasm for emergency coronary revascularization as a possible therapy to protect jeopardized myocardium in patients undergoing AMI.[290-294] As appears to be the case for all methods designed to limit infarct size, this therapy can be successful only if it is applied within the first four or five hours of the onset of the acute event. It is logistically very difficult in the usual patient who develops an AMI outside of the hospital, to bring the patient to the hospital, carry out a clinical evaluation, outline the coronary anatomy by arteriography, assemble the surgical team, commence operation, and place the patient on cardiopulmonary bypass in less than four hours after the onset of the event. It is therefore unlikely that surgical reperfusion can or will be widely applied on a regular basis in the treatment of AMI. Indeed, operation is *contraindicated* in patients with uncomplicated transmural infarcts more than six hours after the onset of the event.

However, in some patients with AMI, including some with cardiogenic shock, infarction appears to occur in a stuttering fashion over an interval of several days.[295] Theoretically, revascularization carried out more than six hours after the onset of the event might be of benefit in this group, but this has yet to be established. Also, coronary bypass surgery can be carried out promptly in patients who appear to develop infarction in the course of cardiac catheterization, coronary arteriography, and transluminal coronary angioplasty,[296-298] as well as in patients whose coronary anatomy has been recently assessed by coronary arteriography and who develop an infarction in the hospital while awaiting operation. In these selected groups of patients, coronary artery bypass surgery is likely to be effective in limiting myocardial infarct size, since it can be carried out before irreversible myocardial damage has occurred. At the same time, bypass of non–infarct-related coronary obstructions can be expected to exert additional benefit. It must be appreciated, however, that definitive diagnostic criteria, such as elevations of plasma enzyme activity indicative of infarction, do not evolve instantaneously, and the decision to intervene surgically must often be implemented on the basis of clinical suspicion and at a time when the diagnosis of infarction cannot be established with certainty. These circumstances make objective evaluation of this form of therapy difficult.

INTRACORONARY THROMBOLYSIS. The appreciation that coronary thrombosis is often responsible for the initiation and/or the perpetuation of infarction (p. 1265) and the discovery that intracoronary administration of thrombolytic agents restores angiographic patency to coronary vessels in a majority of cases[300,301] have sparked interest in the potential value of clot lysis in salvaging jeopardized tissue and limiting the extent of injury sustained in patients evolving MI.

On the basis of experience gathered in several laboratories,[302–306] it now appears that:

1. Coronary arteriography can be carried out safely by a skilled and experienced team in patients presenting within the first four hours of what appears, on clinical grounds, to be an AMI with electrocardiographic evidence of early infarction, i.e., ST-segment elevation and early changes in the QRS complex.

2. A total occlusion that appears on coronary arteriography to be produced by a thrombus will be found in the infarct-related artery in approximately 95 per cent of such patients.

3. The direct intracoronary injection of nitroglycerin will relieve the obstruction in only a very small minority of such patients, i.e., less than 5 per cent.

4. Intracoronary infusion of streptokinase, according to the technique outlined on p. 336, will lyse the clot in 70 to 80 per cent of patients; large bolus doses of streptokinase (approximately 1.0 million units) administered intravenously will be successful in lysing clots in approximately 50 per cent (Fig. 38–13).

5. At least a portion of the successfully reperfused myocardium will show evidence of viability, as reflected in the uptake and concentration of Thallium-201 in previously unperfused areas (Fig. 38–14), or restoration of wall motion in previously akinetic segments, in approximately two thirds of patients treated within four hours.[306a,306b]

6. When carried out by experienced groups, the procedure is associated with a small risk of serious bleeding; reperfusion ventricular tachyarrhythmias are common[307] but can usually be controlled by lidocaine or DC cardioversion; therefore coronary thrombolysis is associated with a low mortality.

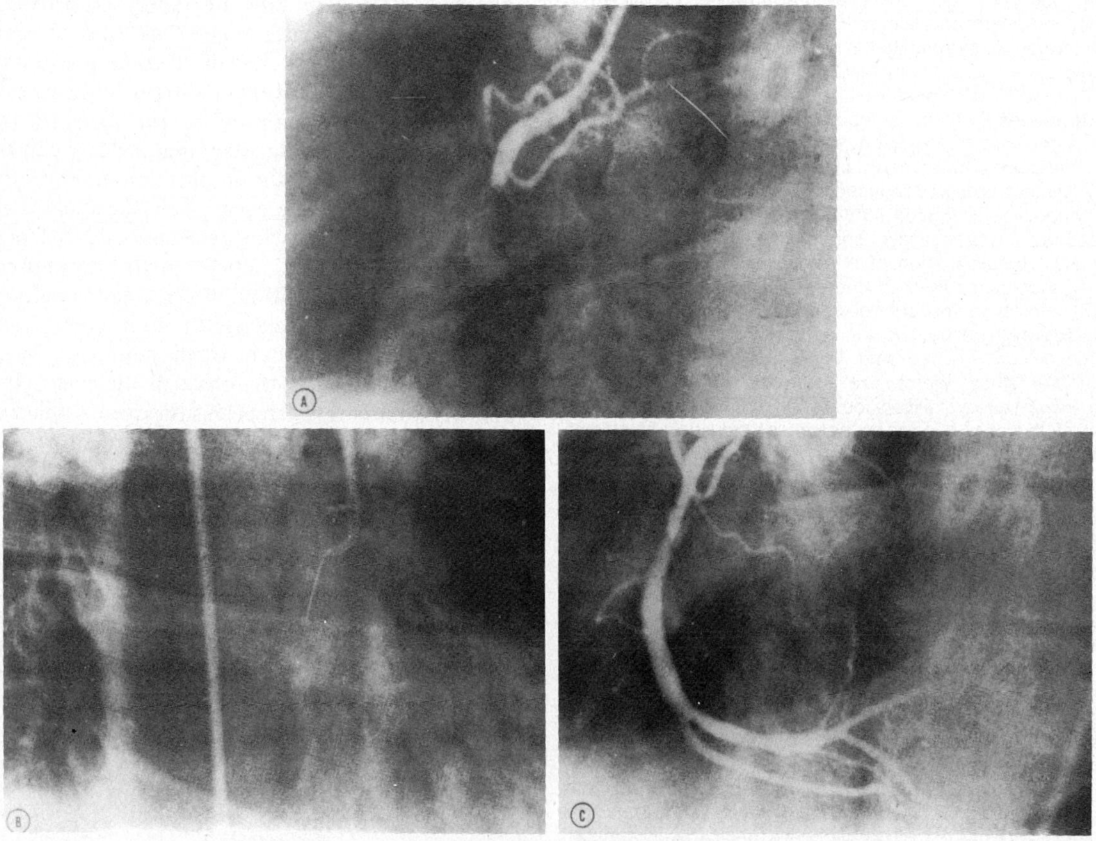

FIGURE 38–13 *A*, Complete occlusion of the right coronary artery in a 38-year-old male patient with evolving inferoposterolateral myocardial infarction. *B*, Infusion catheter advanced to site of occlusion. *C*, The artery was patent after 20 minutes of Thrombolysin infusion at a rate of 4,000 IU/min. The arteriogram was taken after an additional infusion of Thrombolysin, 120,000 IU in 60 minutes, which further improved patency. (Reproduced with permission from Ganz, W., Buchbinder, N., Marcus, H., Mondkar, A., Maddahi, J., Charuzi, Y., O'Connor, L., Shell, W., Fishbein, M. C., Kass, R., Miyamoto, A., and Swan, H. J. C.: Intracoronary thrombolysis in evolving myocardial infarction. Am. Heart J. *101*:4, 1981.)

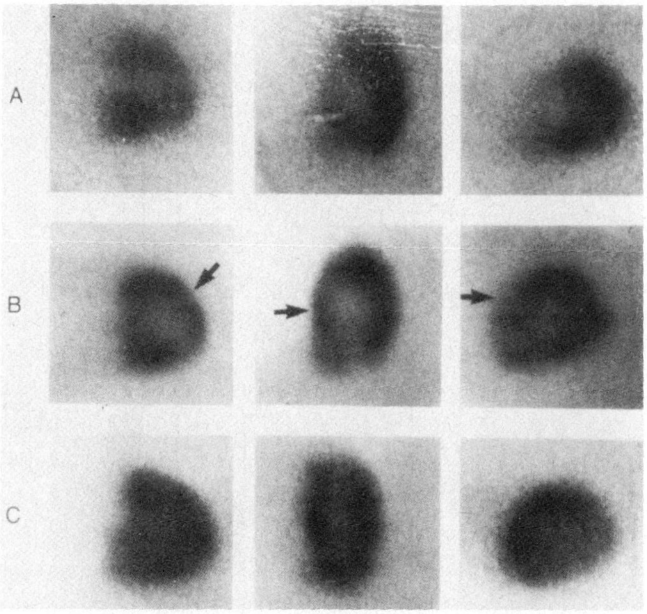

FIGURE 38–14 Intracoronary thallium-201 scintiscans performed in a patient before thrombolysis (*A*), immediately after thrombolysis (*B*), and three months after thrombolysis (*C*). There was a recanalization of the totally obstructed left anterior descending coronary artery. Views, from left to right, are the anterior, modified left anterior oblique, and 70-degree left anterior oblique. Panel *B* shows an increase in perfusion to the anteroseptal region (arrows). In Panel B in the modified left anterior oblique view at seven o'clock, there is an area of improved perfusion, which enhances a persistent filling defect present in the same view in Panel *A* at six o'clock. There is persistence of perfusion of the anteroseptal region at three months after thrombolysis (Panel *C*). (Reproduced with permission from Markis, J. E., Malagold, M., Parker, J. A., Silverman, K. J., Barry, W. H., Als, A. V., Paulin, S., Grossman, W., and Braunwald, E.: Myocardial salvage after intracoronary thrombolysis with streptokinase in acute myocardial infarction. N. Engl. J. Med. *305*:777, 1981.)

Despite the promise of this approach, its ultimate utility remains to be proven because of several unresolved issues.[308,308a] These include (1) difficulty in interpreting the significance of accelerated electrocardiographic changes and the appearance of enzymes in plasma; (2) problems in determining the presence of infarction definitively when thrombolysis is initiated early; (3) problems in interpreting an enhanced ejection fraction or wall motion following thrombolysis, which does not always portend myocardial salvage (the role of augmented sympathetic stimulation and of arterial pressure reduction due to the hypotensive effect of streptokinase infusion in improving myocardial wall remain to be established); (4) the potentially deleterious effects of reperfusion injury when lysis is induced late; (5) lack of proof, at this time, that survival is enhanced; and (6) lack of knowing the optimal manner of treatment following successful reperfusion (i.e., coronary artery bypass grafting,[309,309a] percutaneous transluminal angioplasty,[310,310a] or medical therapy with streptokinase or with clot-selective activators of the fibrinolytic system that do not induce a systemic lytic state. Thus, despite its distinct promise as a technique to limit infarct size, coronary thrombolysis remains an investigational modality at the time of this writing. The possibility that large doses of intravenous streptokinase may also lyse intracoronary thrombi is also under intense investigation.[310b]

IMPLICATIONS OF THE CONCEPT OF INFARCT SIZE LIMITATION FOR ROUTINE MANAGEMENT OF AMI

The recognition that the ultimate size of an MI does not depend solely on the pathological anatomy of the coronary vascular bed, but also on a variety of physiological variables, suggests emphasis on a number of principles in the management of AMI. These principles can and should be applied in routine care despite the fact that the clinical efficacy of the specific interventions described above has not yet been definitively established. First, and of greatest importance, it is mandatory to maintain an optimal balance between myocardial oxygen supply and demand so that as much of the jeopardized zone of the myocardium surrounding the most profoundly ischemic zones of the infarct can be salvaged. Myocardial oxygen consumption is minimized by maintaining the patient at rest, physically and emotionally, and by utilizing mild sedation and a quiet atmosphere that may lower heart rate, a major determinant of myocardial oxygen consumption. If the patient was receiving a beta-adrenergic blocking agent at the time the clinical manifestations of the infarct commenced, the drug should not be discontinued unless a specific contraindication develops, such as left ventricular failure or a bradyarrhythmia. Marked sinus bradycardia (heart rate less than approximately 50 beats/min) and the frequently coexisting hypotension should be treated with postural maneuvers (the reverse Trendelenburg position) to increase central blood volume and atropine or electrical pacing, but not with isoproterenol. On the other hand, the *routine* administration of atropine, with the resultant increase in heart rate, to patients without serious bradycardia is contraindicated. All forms of tachyarrhythmias require prompt and direct treatment, since they increase myocardial oxygen needs.

Diuretics are the first line of drugs indicated in the treatment of heart failure. If insufficient, vasodilators should be added,[255] unless the patient is already hypotensive. Inotropic agents such as the digitalis glycosides and cardioactive sympathomimetics should be added only if there is evidence of persistent ventricular failure despite diuretics and vasodilators; these agents should not be given prophylactically. Of the various sympathomimetic amines available, isoproterenol with its chronotropic and vasodilator effects is the most hazardous. Dobutamine, or small doses of dopamine, which has less effect on heart rate and systemic vascular resistance than do norepinephrine, epinephrine or isoproterenol is the drug of choice when cardiac contractility *must* be augmented.

Particular attention must be paid to preserving arterial oxygenation in patients with hypoxemia, such as occurs in patients with chronic pulmonary disease, pneumonia, or left ventricular failure. Oxygen-enriched air should be administered to patients with hypoxemia, and bronchodilators and expectorants should be used when indicated. Severe anemia, which can also extend the area of ischemic injury, should be corrected by the cautious administration of packed red cells, accompanied by a diuretic if there is any evidence of left ventricular failure. Associated conditions, particularly infections and the accompanying tachycardia, fever, and elevated myocardial oxygen needs, require immediate attention.

Systolic arterial pressure should not be allowed to deviate by more than approximately 25 to 30 mm Hg from the patient's usual level. In regard to the effect of changes in arterial pressure on myocardial injury, it is likely that each patient has an optimum level of arterial pressure. As coronary perfusion pressure deviates from this level, the unfavorable balance between oxygen supply (which is related to coronary perfusion pressure) and myocardial oxygen demand (which is related to ventricular wall tension) that ensues will increase the extent of ischemic injury.

Rather than simply maintaining the patient's vital signs, the physician's attention should be directed toward preserving the myocardium as well as maintaining perfusion of peripheral organs. However, these two objectives may sometimes conflict. In the first four to six hours following the onset of the clinical event, when the ultimate size of the infarct has not yet been established, myocardial preservation should ordinarily be given the highest priority. This may mean foregoing the stimulation of cardiac contractility by inotropic agents. Later, once the size of the infarct is fixed and if heart failure supervenes, it may be appropriate to stimulate the heart with positive inotropic agents, i.e., to employ an intervention that might have increased infarct size if given at an earlier time.

In some patients, particularly those with cardiogenic shock, tissue damage occurs in a "stuttering" manner with persistent release of CK into the blood stream (Fig. 38–15) rather than abruptly, a condition that might more properly be termed *subacute infarction*.[49,192] This concept of the dynamic nature of the infarct process as well as the observa-

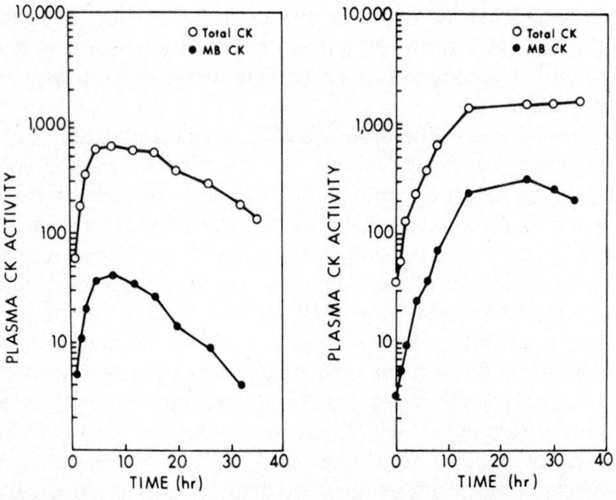

FIGURE 38–15 Plasma CK time-activity curves in a patient with uncomplicated acute myocardial infarction (*left*) and one with acute myocardial infarction associated with cardiogenic shock (*right*). As shown on the left, hemodynamically uncomplicated acute myocardial infarction is characterized by a relatively early occurrence of peak total and MB-CK activity, with a gradual subsequent smooth decline. On the other hand, as shown on the right, myocardial infarction associated with cardiogenic shock is characterized by a more prolonged interval prior to occurrence of peak enzyme activity in blood, indicative of persistent release of enzyme reflecting progressive damage of myocardium. Total CK activity may remain elevated in patients with myocardial infarction because of extracardiac release of enzyme, but the sustained elevation of MB-CK activity accompanying cardiogenic shock, as evident in the example shown on the right, is attributable to continuing cardiac damage. (From Gutovitz, A. L., et al.: The progressive nature of myocardial injury in selected patients with cardiogenic shock. Am. J. Cardiol. *41*:469, 1978.)

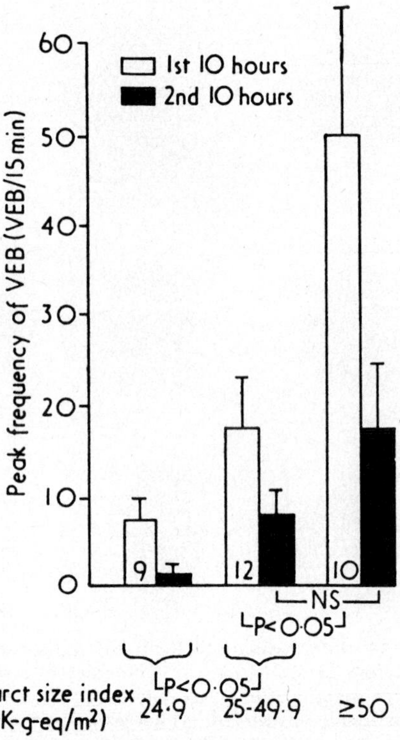

FIGURE 38–16 Dependence of ventricular ectopic activity, expressed as ventricular ectopic beats (VEB's), during the first 20 hours after admission in patients with acute myocardial infarction. Patients were divided into three groups according to infarct size index, expressed in terms of CPK-gram-equivalents/m². VEB frequency was greater in patients with larger infarcts during the first 10 hours after admission, as shown by the clear bars. A similar trend was evident during the second 10 hours after admission, as shown by the solid bars, although the overall frequency of VEB's was less during this interval compared with the first 10 hours after admission. Results expressed are means ±SE. (From Roberts, R., et al.: Relation between infarct size and ventricular arrhythmia. Br. Heart J. *37*:1169, 1975.)

tion that the incidence of ventricular ectopic activity in both the early (Fig. 38–16) and late (Table 38–2) post-infarct periods greatly expands the horizon for what can *potentially* be accomplished by techniques to limit myocardial necrosis.

However, it must be acknowledged that *definitive* proof that substantial quantities of tissue can be salvaged and that prognosis can thereby be improved is not yet available, despite (1) the inherent logic in attempting to reduce infarct size; (2) the availability of a wide variety of interventions that are effective in experimental animals; (3) the ability to apply these techniques with reasonable safety in patients; and (4) the results of an increasing number of trials in patients with encouraging results.

CONVALESCENCE

The time of discharge from the hospital is variable. It may be as early as one week after admission for patients who experience no complications, who can be followed readily at home, and for whom the family setting is conducive to convalescence.[311,312] Most complications that would preclude early discharge occur within the first day or two of admission and therefore, patients suitable for early dis-

TABLE 38–2 RELATION BETWEEN VENTRICULAR ECTOPIC ACTIVITY AND INFARCT SIZE LATE AFTER INFARCTION

LOCATION OF INFARCTION	ln PVC's/24 HR	
Transmural		
All patients	4.17(66)	
ISI < 15	2.93(20)	(P <0.005)
ISI ≥ 15	4.71(46)	
Inferior (Transmural)		
All patients	4.52(40)	
ISI < 15	3.81(14)	(P = N.S.)
ISI ≥ 15	4.90(26)	
Anterior (Transmural)		
All patients	3.64(26)	
ISI < 15	0.88(6)	(P < 0.001)
ISI ≥ 15	4.47(20)	
Subendocardial		
All patients	3.64(15)	
ISI < 15	2.48(11)	(P < 0.02)
ISI ≥ 15	6.81(4)	

The significance of relationships between infarct location, infarct size index (ISI) expressed as CK-gram-equivalents, and the frequency of premature ventricular complexes (PVC's). Numbers in parentheses indicate the number of patients sustaining an initial infarction occurring at the locus specified, with follow-up obtained from 3 to 38 months after infarction. Results are expressed as the natural logarithm (ln) of PVC frequency because the statistical distribution of PVC's is not normal but the distribution of ln PVC's is. (Reproduced with permission from Geltman, E. M., et al.: The influence of location and extent of myocardial infarction on long-term ventricular dysrhythmia and mortality. Circulation *60*:805, 1979, by permission of the American Heart Association, Inc.)

charge can be identified very early during the hospitalization.[312] Ordinarily, discharge of patients without complications is deferred until 10 to 12 days following infarction, at a time when the patient has become fully ambulatory. For patients who have experienced a complication, discharge is deferred until their condition has been stable for several days and it is clear that they are responding appropriately to necessary medications such as antiarrhythmic agents, vasodilators, or positive inotropic agents.

Before discharge from the hospital, the patient should receive detailed instruction concerning physical activity. Initially, this should consist of being ambulatory at home but avoiding isometric activity such as lifting; several rest periods should be taken daily. In addition, the patient should be given fresh nitroglycerin tablets and instructed in their use. As convalescence progresses, graded resumption of activity should be encouraged. Many approaches have been utilized, ranging from formal rigid guidelines to general advice advocating moderation and avoidance of any activity that evokes symptoms. There is some evidence that behavior alteration is possible after recovery from MI and that this may improve prognosis.[313,313a] The physical and psychological rehabilitation of patients convalescing from AMI are discussed in Chapters 40 and 57.

The concept of *secondary prevention* of reinfarction and death after recovery from an AMI has been actively investigated during the past two decades. Until quite recently, however, nearly all efforts at demonstrating secondary prevention had failed. Thus, studies of antiplatelet agents (aspirin, sulfinpyrazone[314]), lipid-lowering drugs, antiarrhythmic agents, anticoagulants, and even beta blockers had not provided undisputed proof of improvement of long-term survival following myocardial infarction. However, large trials with three beta blockers—timolol,[83] propranolol,[84] and metoprolol[225]—have demonstrated that these drugs do improve survival in a wide spectrum of postinfarction patients and also reduce the incidence of sudden death and reinfarction.

While the exact mechanism of this beneficial effect is unknown, it appears to be due to a "class" effect, i.e., it is secondary to beta blockade, since neither cardioselectivity, intrinsic sympathomimetic activity, or membrane stabilizing activity appear to be requisite. The reduction in mortality is seen in all age groups, for all types of infarction, and in all risk groups. Therefore, based on currently available evidence, patients without contraindication to beta blockade (asthma, congestive heart failure, bradyarrhythmias) should have prophylactic treatment with beta blockers initiated between one and four weeks after AMI. The dosage should be sufficient to blunt the heart rate response to exercise, and therapy should be continued for at least two years. The effectiveness of secondary prevention with other agents, including calcium-channel blockers, antiplatelet agents, anticoagulants, lipid lowering drugs, antiarrhythmics, prostacyclin analogs, and thromboxane synthetase inhibitors, requires further investigation.

In addition to exercise testing in the early convalescent phase (p. 1386), in many centers cardiac catheterization and angiography are being carried out more or less routinely in most survivors of AMI, regardless of whether or not they are symptomatic. Similar anatomical findings have been observed independent of the patient's postinfarction course; approximately one third of patients each have serious obstruction in one, two, and three vessels, while 10 per cent have left main coronary artery disease.[315] Two thirds of the patients have residual viable myocardium that is seriously jeopardized because it is perfused by critically narrowed vessels.[316] These provocative findings have raised the question of whether or not it is advisable to carry out coronary arteriography routinely in survivors of AMI in order to detect patients who might benefit from coronary artery bypass grafting. Insufficient information is available to take a firm position on this question,[317] but since it is possible to identify high-risk patients from their clinical course, combined with noninvasive exercise testing, including myocardial perfusion scintigraphy[318–320] (p. 374) as well as ambulatory electrocardiography,[320a,320b] it seems reasonable at this time to limit these invasive studies to such high-risk patients, as well as to those who have significant postinfarct angina, despite a good medical regimen, including a calcium-channel blocker.[321]

References

1. Hillis, L. D., and Braunwald, E.: Myocardial ischemia. N. Engl. J. Med. *296*: 971, 1034, 1093, 1977.
2. Norris, R. M.: Myocardial Infarction. Edinburgh, Churchill Livingstone, 1982.
3. Gillespie, T. A., and Sobel, B. E.: A rationale for therapy of acute myocardial infarction: Limitation of infarct size. Adv. Intern. Med. *22*:319, 1976.
4. Karliner, J. S., and Gregoratos, G.: Coronary Care. Edinburgh, Churchill Livingstone, 1981.
5. Bloor, C. M., Ehsani, A., White, F. C., and Sobel, B. E.: Ventricular fibrillation threshold in acute myocardial infarction and its relation to myocardial infarct size. Cardiovasc. Res. *9*:468, 1975.
6. Spann, J. F.: Changing concepts of pathophysiology, prognosis, and therapy in acute myocardial infarction. Am. J. Med. *74*:877, 1983.
7. Rude, R. E., Muller, J. E., and Braunwald, E.: Efforts to limit the size of myocardial infarcts. Ann. Intern. Med. *95*:736, 1981.
8. Lange, L. G., and Sobel, B. E.: Pharmacological salvage of myocardium. Ann. Rev. Pharmacol. Toxicol. *22*:115, 1982.
9. Pantridge, J. F., Webb, S. W., Adgey, A. A. J., and Geddes, J. S.: The first hour after the onset of acute myocardial infarction. *In* Yu, P. N., and

Goodwin, J. F. (eds.): Progress in Cardiology.Philadelphia, Lea and Febiger, 1974, p. 173.
10. Bigger, J. T., Jr., Dresdale, R. J., and Heissenbuttel, R. H., Weld, F. M., and Wit, A. L.: Ventricular arrhythmias in ischemic heart disease: Mechanism, prevalence, significance, and management. Prog. Cardiovasc. Dis. *19*:255, 1977.
11. Pantridge, J. R., and Geddes, J. S.: Diseases of the cardiovascular system. Management of acute myocardial infarction. Br. Med. J. *2*:168, 1976.
12. Adgey, A. A. J., Clements, I. P., Mulholland, H. C., Wilson, C., and Webb, S. W.: Acute phase of myocardial infarction. Prehospital management of the coronary patient. Minnesota Med. *59*:347, 1976.
13. Cobb, L. A., Baum, R. S., Alvarez, H., III, and Schaffer, W. A.: Resuscitation from out-of-hospital ventricular fibrillation: 4 years' follow-up. Circulation *51–52* (Suppl. III):223, 1975.
14. Lewis, R. P., Lanese, R. R., Stang, J. M., Chirikos, T. N., Keller, M. D., and Warren, J. V.: Reduction of mortality from prehospital myocardial infarction by prudent patient activation of mobile coronary care system. Am. Heart J. *103*:123, 1982.
15. Crampton, R. S., Aldrich, F. R., Gascho, J. A., Miles, J. R., Jr., and Stillerman, R.: Reduction of prehospital, ambulance and community coronary death rates by the community-wide emergency cardiac care system. Am. J. Med. *58*:151, 1975.
16. Goldman, L.: Coronary care units: A perspective on their epidemiologic impact. Int. J. Cardiol., *2*:284, 1982.
17. Morris, A. L., Nernberg, V., Roos, N. P., Henteleff, P., and Ross, L., Jr.: Acute myocardial infarction: Survey of urban and rural hospital mortality. Am. Heart J. *105*:44, 1983.
18. Hill, J. D., Hampton, J. R., and Mitchell, J. R. A.: A randomized trial of home-versus-hospital management for patients with suspected myocardial infarction. Lancet *1*:837, 1978.
19. Rowley, J. M., Hill, J. D., Hampton, J. R., and Mitchell, J. R. A.: Early reporting of myocardial infarction: Impact of an experiment in patient education. Br. Med. J. *284*:1741, 1982.
20. Graboys, T. B.: In-hospital sudden death after coronary care unit discharge: A high-risk profile. Arch. Intern. Med. *135*:512, 1975.
21. Wilson, C., and Adgey, A. A. J.: Survival of patients with late ventricular fibrillation after acute myocardial infarction. Lancet *2*:214, 1974.
22. Lie, K. I., Liem, K. L., Schuilenburg, R. M., David, G. K., and Durrer, B.: Early identification of patients developing late in-hospital ventricular fibrillation after discharge from the Coronary Care Unit. Am. J. Cardiol. *41*: 674, 1978.
23. Starling, M. R., Crawford, M. H., Kennedy, G. T., and O'Rourke, R. A.: Treadmill exercise tests predischarge and six week post-myocardial infarction todetect abnormalities of known prognostic value. Ann. Intern. Med. *94*:721, 1981.
24. McNeer, J. F., Wagner, G. S., Ginsburg, P. B., Wallace, A. G., McCants, C. B., Conley, M. J., and Rosati, R. A.: Hospital discharge one week after acute myocardial infarction. N. Engl. J. Med. *298*:229, 1978.
25. Severance, H. W., Jr., Morris, K. G., and Wagner, G. S.: Criteria for early discharge after acute myocardial infarction. Validation in a community hospital. Arch. Intern. Med. *142*:39, 1982.
26. Zelis, R., Mansour, E. J., Capone, R. J., and Mason, D. T.: The cardiovascular effects of morphine: The peripheral capacitance and resistance vessels in human subjects. J. Clin. Invest. *54*:1247, 1974.
27. Wynne, J., Mann, T., Alpert, J. S., and Grossman, W.: Beneficial effects of nitrous oxide in patients with ischemic heart disease. Circulation *55–56* (Suppl. III):18, 1977 (Abstr.).
28. Thompson, P. L., and Lown, B.: Nitrous oxide as an analgesic in acute myocardial infarction. J.A.M.A. *235*:924, 1976.
29. Fillmore, S. J., Shapiro, M., and Killip, T.: Arterial oxygen tension in acute myocardial infarction. Serial analysis of clinical state and blood gas changes. Am. Heart J. *79*:620, 1970.
30. Maroko, P. R., Radvany, P., Braunwald, E., and Hale, S. L.: Reduction of infarct size by oxygen inhalation following acute coronary occlusion. Circulation *52*:360, 1975.
31. Madias, J. E., and Hood, W. B., Jr.: Reduction of precordial ST-segment elevation in patients with anterior myocardial infarction by oxygen breathing. Circulation *53*(Suppl. I):198, 1976.
32. Singer, M. M., Wright, F., Stanley, L. K., Roe, B. B., and Hamilton, W. K.: Oxygen toxicity in man: A prospective study in patients after open-heart surgery. N. Engl. J. Med. *283*:1473, 1970.
33. Mogelson, S., Davidson, J., Sobel, B. E., and Roberts, R.: The effect of hyperbaric oxygen on infarct size in the conscious animal. Eur. J. Cardiol. *12*: 135, 1980.
34. Meijne, N. G.: Hyperbaric Oxygen and Its Clinical Value: With Special Emphasis on Biochemical and Cardiovascular Aspects. Springfield, Ill., Charles C Thomas, 1970.
35. Glogar, D. H., Kloner, R. A., Muller, J., DeBoer, L. W. V., Braunwald, E., and Clark, L. C., Jr.: Fluorocarbons reduce myocardial ischemic damage after coronary occlusion. Science *211*:1439, 1981.
36. Modan, B., Shani, M., Schor, S., and Modan, M.: Reduction of hospital mortality from acute myocardial infarction by anticoagulant therapy. N. Engl. J. Med. *292*:1359, 1975.
37. Wessler, S.: Antithrombotic agents are indicated in the therapy of acute myocardial infarction. Cardiovasc. Clin. *8*:131, 1977.
38. Tonaschia, J., Gordis, L., and Schmerler, H.: Retrospective evidence favoring use of anticoagulants for myocardial infarctions. N. Engl. J. Med. *292*:1362, 1975.
39. Horwitz, R. I., and Feinstein, A. R.: The application of therapeutic trial principles to improve the design of epidemiologic research: A case-control study suggesting that anticoagulants reduce mortality in patients with myocardial infarction. J. Chron. Dis. *34*:575, 1981.
40. Anticoagulants in acute myocardial infarction: Results of a cooperative clinical trial. J.A.M.A. *225*:724, 1973.
41. Wray, R., Maurer, B., and Shillingford, J.: Prophylactic anticoagulant therapy in the prevention of calf-vein thrombosis after myocardial infarction. N. Engl. J. Med. *288*:815, 1973.
42. Rosenberg, R. D.: Actions and interactions of antithrombin and heparin. N. Engl. J. Med. *292*:146, 1975.
43. Hull, R., Delmore, T., Carter, C., Hirsh, J., Genton, E., Gent, M., Turpie, G., and McLaughlin, D.: Adjusted subcutaneous heparin versus warfarin sodium in the long-term treatment of venous thrombosis. N. Engl. J. Med. *306*:189, 1982.
44. Pitt, A., Anderson, S. T., Habersberger, P. G., and Rosengarten, D. S.: Low dose heparin in the prevention of deep vein thromboses in patients with acute myocardial infarction. Am. Heart J. *99*:574, 1980.
45. A double-blind trial to assess long-term oral anticoagulant therapy in elderly patients with myocardial infarction. Report of the sixty-plus reinfarction study research group. Lancet *2*:989, 1980.
46. Corday, E., and Corday, S. R.: Advances in clinical management of acute myocardial infarction in the past 25 years. J. Am. Coll. Cardiol. *1*:126, 1983.
47. Cox, J. R., Jr., Roberts, R., Ambos, H. D., Oliver, G. C., and Sobel, B. E.: Relations between enzymatically estimated myocardial infarct size and early ventricular dysrhythmia. Circulation *53*(Suppl. I):150, 1976.
48. Roberts, R., Husain, A., Ambos, H. D., Oliver, G. C., Cox, J., Jr., and Sobel, B. E.: Relation between infarct size and ventricular arrhythmia. Br. Heart J. *37*: 1169, 1975.
49. Geltman, E. M., Ehsani, A. A., Campbell, M. K., Schechtman, K., Roberts, R., and Sobel, B. E.: The influence of location and extent of myocardial infarction on long-term ventricular dysrhythmia and mortality. Circulation *60*:805, 1979.
50. Thorén, P. N.: Activation of left ventricular receptors with nonmedullated vagal afferent fibers during occlusion of a coronary artery in the cat. Am. J. Cardiol. *37*:1046, 1976.
51. Adgey, A. A. J., Geddes, J. S., Mulholland, H. C., Keegan, D. A. J., and Pantridge, J. F.: Incidence, significance, and management of early bradyarrhythmia complicating acute myocardial infarction. Lancet *2*:1097, 1968.
52. Han, J.: Mechanisms of ventricular arrhythmias associated with myocardial infarction. Am. J. Cardiol. *24*:800, 1969.
53. Chadda, K. D., Lichstein, E., Gupta, P. K., and Choy, R.: Bradycardia-hypotension syndrome in acute myocardial infarction: Reappraisal of the overdrive effects of atropin. Am. J. Med. *59*:158, 1975.
54. Warren, J. V., and Lewis, R. P.: Beneficial effects of atropine in the pre-hospital phase of coronary care. Am. J. Cardiol. *37*:68, 1976.
55. Topol, E. J., Goldschlager, N., Ports, T. A., DiCarlo, L. A., Jr., Schiller, N. B., Botvinick, E. H., and Chatterjee, K.: Hemodynamic benefit of atrial pacing in right ventricular myocardial infarction. Ann. Intern. Med. *96*:594, 1982.
56. Norris, R. M., and Mercer, C. J.: Significance of idioventricular rhythms in acute myocardial infarction. Prog. Cardiovasc. Dis. *16*:455, 1974.
57. Haft, J. I.: Clinical implications of atrioventricular and intraventricular conduction abnormalities. II. Acute myocardial infarction. *In* Rios, J. C. (ed.): Clinical-Electrocardiographic Correlations. Philadelphia, F. A. Davis Co., 1977, p. 65.
58. Ritter, W. S., Atkins, J. M., Blomqvist, C. G., and Mullins, C. B.: Permanent pacing in patients with transient trifascicular block during acute myocardial infarction. Am. J. Cardiol. *38*:205, 1976.
59. Ginks, W. R., Sutton, R., Oh, W., and Leatham, A.: Long-term prognosis after acute inferior infarction with atrioventricular block. Br. Heart J. *39*:186, 1977.
60. Waters, D. D., and Mizgala, H. F.: Long-term prognoses of patients with incomplete bundle branch block complicating acute myocardial infarction. Am. J. Cardiol. *34*:1, 1974.
61. Hindman, M. C., Wagner, G. S., JaRo, M., Atkins, J. M., Scheinman, M. M., DeSanctis, R. W., Hutter, A. H., Jr., Yeatman, L., Rubenfire, M., Pujura, C., Rubin, M., and Morris, J. J.: The clinical significance of bundle branch block complicating acute myocardial infarction. I. Clinical characteristics, hospital mortality, and one-year followup. Circulation *58*:679, 1978.
62. Hindman, M. C., Wagner, G. S., JaRo, M., Atkins, J. M., Scheinman, M. M., DeSanctis, R. W., Hutter, A. H., Jr., Yeatman, L., Rubenfire, M., Pujura, C., Rubin, M., and Morris, J. J.: The clinical significance of bundle branch block complicating acute myocardial infarction. 2. Indications for temporary and permanent pacemaker insertion. Circulation *58*:689, 1978.
63. Hindman, M. C., and Wagner, G. S.: Bundle branch block during acute myocardial infarction. Primary Cardiol. *6*:73, 1980.
64. Malliani, A., Schwartz, P. J., and Zanchetti, A.: A sympathetic reflex elicited by experimental coronary occlusion. Am. J. Physiol. *217*:703, 1969.
65. Corr, P. B., and Gillis, R. A.: Autonomic neural influences on the dysrhythmias resulting from myocardial infarction. Circ. Res. *43*:1, 1978.
66. Harris, A. S., Otero, H., and Bocage, A. J.: The induction of arrhythmias by sympathetic activity before and after occlusion of a coronary artery in the canine heart. J. Electrocardiol. *4*:34, 1971.

67. Han, J., and Moe, G. K.: Nonuniform recovery of excitability in ventricular muscle. Circ. Res. *14*:44, 1964.
68. Cranefield, P. F.: The Conduction of the Cardiac Impulse: The Slow Response and Cardiac Arrhythmias. Mount Kisco, N.Y., Futura Publishing Company, 1975.
69. Wit, A. L., Hoffman, B. F., and Rosen, M. R.: Electrophysiology and pharmacology of cardiac arrhythmias. IX. Cardiac electrophysiologic effects of beta adrenergic receptor stimulation and blockade. Part A. Am. Heart J. *90*: 521, 1975.
70. Ebert, P. A., Venderbeek, R. B., Allgood, R. J., and Sabiston, D. C., Jr.: Effect of chronic cardiac denervation on arrhythmias after coronary artery ligation. Cardiovasc. Res. *4*:141, 1970.
71. Peterson, D. F., and Brown, A. M.: Pressor reflexes produced by stimulation of afferent fibers in the cardiac sympathetic nerves of the cat. Circ. Res. *28*: 605, 1971.
72. Berman, J., Haffajee, C. I., and Alpert, J. S.: Therapy of symptomatic pericarditis after myocardial infarction: Retrospective and prospective studies of aspirin, indomethacin, prednisone, and spontaneous resolution. Am. Heart J. *101*: 750, 1981.
73. Krikler, D. M., and Rowland, E.: The role of calcium-ion antagonists in cardiac arrhythmias. *In* Fleckenstein, A., and Roskamm, G. (eds.): Calcium Antagonismus. Berlin, Springer-Verlag, 1980, p. 55.
74. Kerber, R. E., Jensen, S. R., Grayzel, J., Kennedy, J., and Hoyt, R.: Elective cardioversion: Influence of paddle-electrode location and size on success rates and energyrequirements. N. Engl. J. Med. *305*:658, 1981.
75. Pantridge, J. F.: Emergency treatment of cardiac arrhythmias in myocardial infarction. *In* Scott, D. B., and Julian, D. G. (eds.): Lidocaine in the Treatment of Ventricular Arrhythmias. Edinburgh, E. & S. Livingstone, 1971, p. 77.
76. Zipes, D. P., and Troup, P. J.: New antiarrhythmic agents: Amiodarone, aprindine, disopyramide, ethmozin, mexiletine, tocainide, verapamil. Am. J. Cardiol. *41*:1005, 1978.
77. Abitbol, H., Califano, J. E., Abate, C., Beilis, P., and Castanellos, H.: Use of flecainide acetate in the treatment of premature ventricular contractions. Am. Heart J. *105*:227, 1983.
78. Dhurandher, R. W., MacMillan, R. L., and Brown, K. W. G.: Primary ventricular fibrillation complicating acute myocardial infarction. Am. J. Cardiol. *27*:347, 1971.
79. Lie, K. I., Wellens, H. J., and Van Capelli, F. J.: Lidocaine in the prevention of primary ventricular fibrillation. A double blind randomized study of 212 consecutive patients. N. Engl. J. Med. *291*:1324, 1974.
80. Routledge, P. A., Stargel, W. W., Barchowsky, A., Wagner, G. S., and Shand, D. G.: Control of lidocaine therapy: New perspectives. Therap. Drug Monitoring *4*:265, 1982.
81. DeSilva, R. E., Hennekens, C. H., Lown, B., and Casscells, S. W.: Lidocaine prophylaxis in acute myocardial infarction: An evaluation of methodology. Lancet *1*:855, 1981.
81a. Mehra, R., Zeiler, R. H., Gough, W. B. and El-Sherif, N.: Reentrant ventricular arrhythmias in the later myocardial infarction period. 9. Electrophysiologic-anatomic correlation of reentrant circuits. Circulation *67*:11, 1983.
82. May, G. S., Furberg, C. D., Eberlein, K. A., and Geraci, B. J.: Secondary prevention after myocardial infarction. A review of short-term acute phase trials. Prog. Cardiovasc. Dis. *25*:335, 1983.
83. The Norwegian Multicenter Study Group: Timolol-induced reduction in mortality and reinfarction in patients surviving acute myocardial infarction. N. Engl. J. Med. *304*:801, 1981.
84. The Beta-Blocker Heart Attack Trial. Beta Blocker Heart Attack Study Group. J.A.M.A. *246*:2073, 1981.
85. Lopez, L. M., Mehta, J. L., Robinson, J. D., and Roberts, R. J.: Optimal lidocaine dosing in patients with myocardial infarction. Therap. Drug. Monitoring *4*:271, 1982.
86. Prescott, L. F., Adjepon-Yamoah, K. K., and Talbot, R. G.: Impaired lignocaine metabolism in patients with myocardial infarction and cardiac failure. Br. Med. J. *1*:939, 1976.
87. LeLorier, J., Grenon, D., Latour, Y., Caille, G., Dumont, G., Brosseau, A., and Solignac, A.: Pharmacokinetics of lidocaine after prolonged intravenous infusions in uncomplicated myocardial infarction. Ann. Intern. Med. *87*:700, 1977.
88. Corr, P. B., and Sobel, B. E.: Mechanisms contributing to dysrhythmias induced by ischemia and their therapeutic implications. Adv. Cardiol. *22*:110, 1978.
89. Chopra, M. P., Portal, R. W., and Aber, C. P.: Lignocaine therapy after acute myocardial infarction. Br. Med. J. *1*:213, 1969.
90. Lown, B., and Vassaux, C.: Lidocaine in acute myocardial infarction. Am. Heart J. *76*:586, 1968.
91. Fehmers, M. C. O., and Dunning, A. J.: Intramuscularly and orally administered lidocaine in the treatment of ventricular arrhythmias in acute myocardial infarction. Am. J. Cardiol. *29*:514, 1972.
92. El-Sherif, N., Scherlag, B. J., Lazzara, R., and Hope, R. R.: Reentrant ventricular arrhythmias in the late myocardial infarction period. 4. Mechanism of action of lidocaine. Circulation *56*:395, 1977.
93. Kluger, J., Drayer, D. E., Reidenberg, M. M., and Lahita, R.: Acetylprocainamide therapy in patients with previous procainamide-induced lupus syndrome. Ann. Intern. Med. *95*:18, 1981.
94. Gillis, R. A., McClellan, J. R., Sauer, T. S.,and Standaert, F. G.: Depression of cardiac sympathetic nerve activity by diphenylhydantoin. J. Pharmacol. Exp. Ther. *179*:599, 1971.
95. El-Sherif, N., and Lazzara, R.: Reentrant ventricular arrhythmias in the late myocardial infarction period. 5. Mechanism of action of diphenylhydantoin. Circulation *57*:405, 1978.
96. Lown, B., and Wolf, M.: Approaches to sudden death from coronary heart disease. Circulation *44*:130, 1971.
97. Wald, R. W., Waxman, M. B., Corey, P. N., Gunstensen, J., and Goldman, B. S.: Management of intractable ventricular tachyarrhythmias after myocardial infarction. Am. J. Cardiol. *44*:329, 1979.
98. Guiraudon, G., Fontaine, G., Frank, R., Escande, G., Etievent, P., and Cabrol, C.: Encircling endocardial ventriculotomy: A new surgical treatment for life-threatening ventricular tachycardias resistant to medical treatment following myocardial infarction. Ann. Thorac. Surg. *26*:438, 1978.
99. Josephson, M. E., Harken, A. H., and Horowitz, L. N.: Endocardial excision: A new surgical technique for the treatment of recurrent ventricular tachycardia. Circulation *60*:1430, 1979.
100. Wyman, M. G., and Hammersmith, L.: Comprehensive treatment plan for the prevention of primary ventricular fibrillation in acute myocardial infarction. Am. J. Cardiol. *33*:661, 1974.
101. Lie, K. I., Wellens, H. J., van Capelle, F. J., and Durrer, D.: Lidocaine in the prevention of primary ventricular fibrillation: A double-blind, randomized study of 212 consecutive patients. N. Engl. J. Med. *291*:1324, 1974.
101a. Ryden, L., Ariniego, R., Arnman, K., Herlitz, J., Hjalmarson, A., Holmberg, S., Reyes, C., Smedgard, P., Svedberg, K., Vedin, A., Waagstein, F., Waldenstrom, A., Wilhelmsson, C., Wedel, H., and Yamamoto, M.: A double-blind trial of metoprolol in acute myocardial infarction. Effects on ventricular tachyarrhythmias. N. Engl. J. Med. *308*:614, 1983.
102. Engler, R. L., and LeWinter, M. M.: Ventricular arrhythmias: Diagnosis, treatment and prognosis. *In* Karliner, J. (ed.): Coronary Care. Edinburgh, Churchill Livingstone, 1981, pp. 367–390.
103. Jewitt, D. E., Kishon, Y., and Thomas, M.: Lignocaine in the management of arrhythmias after acute myocardial infarction. Lancet *1*:266, 1968.
104. Conley, M. J., McNeer, J. F., Lee, K. L., Wagner, G. S., and Rosati, R. A.: Cardiac arrest complicating acute myocardial infarction. Predictability and prognosis. Am. J. Cardiol. *39*:7, 1977.
105. Davis, J. S., Lie, J. T., Bentinck, D. C., Titus, J. L., Tacker, W. A., and Geddes, L. A.: Cardiac damage due to electric current and energy: Light microscopic and ultrastructural observations of acute and delayed myocardial cellular injuries. *In* Proceedings, Cardiac Defibrillation Conference, Purdue University, W. Lafayette, Ind., 1975.
106. Van Vleet, J. F., Tacker, W. A., Jr., Geddes, L. A., and Ferrans, V. J.: Acute cardiac damage in dogs given multiple transthoracic shocks with a trapezoidal wave-form defibrillator. Am. J. Vet. Res. *38*:617, 1977.
107. Ehsani, A., Ewy, G. A., and Sobel, B. E.: Effects of electrical countershock on serum creatine phosphokinase (CPK) isoenzyme activity. Am. J. Cardiol. *37*: 12, 1976.
108. Abboud, F. M., Pansegrau, D. G., and Mark, A. L.: Autonomic responses to ventricular defibrillation. *In* Proceedings, Cardiac Defibrillation Conference, Purdue University, W. Lafayette, Ind., 1975.
109. Heissenbuttel, R. H., and Bigger, J. T., Jr.: Bretylium tosylate, a newly available antiarrhythmic drug for ventricular arrhythmias. Ann. Intern. Med. *91*: 229, 1979.
110. Kaski, J. C., Girotti, L. A., Messuti, H., Rutitzky, B., and Rosenbaum, M. B.: Long-term management of sustained, recurrent symptomatic ventricular tachycardia with amiodarone. Circulation *64*:273, 1981.
111. DeBoer, L. W. V., Nosta, J. J., Kloner, R. A., and Braunwald, E.: Studies of amiodarone during experimental myocardial infarction: Beneficial effects on hemodynamics and infarct size. Circulation *65*:508, 1982.
112. Forrester, J. S., Diamond, G., Chatterjee, K., and Swan, H. J. C.: Medical therapy of acute myocardial infarction by application of hemodynamic subsets (First of Two Parts). N. Engl. J. Med. *295*:1356, 1976.
113. Forrester, J. S., Diamond, G., Chatterjee, K., and Swan, H. J. C.: Medical therapy of acute myocardial infarction by application of hemodynamic subsets (Second of Two Parts). N. Engl. J. Med. *295*:1404, 1976.
114. Klein, M. S., and Sobel, B. E.: Medical management of myocardial infarction. Ann. Rev. Med. *27*:89, 1976.
115. Askenazi, J., Koenigsberg, D. I., Ziegler, J. H., and Lesch, M.: Echocardiographic estimates of pulmonary artery wedge pressure. N. Engl. J. Med. *305*:1566, 1981.
116. Russell, R. O., Jr., Mantle, J. A., Rogers, W. J., and Rackley, C. E.: Current status of hemodynamic monitoring: Indications, diagnosis and complications. *In* Rackley, C. E. (ed.): Critical Care Medicine, Cardiovascular Clinics. Philadelphia, F. A. Davis, 1981, pp. 1–14.
117. Russell, R. O., Jr., Rackley, C. E., Pambo, J., Hunt, D., Potanin, C., and Dodge, H. T.: Effects of increasing left ventricular filling pressure in patients with acute myocardial infarction. J. Clin. Invest. *49*:1539, 1970.
118. Strauss, H. D., Sobel, B. E., and Roberts, R.: The influence of occult right ventricular infarction on enzymatically estimated infarct size, hemodynamics and prognosis. Circulation *62*:503, 1980.
119. Marmor, A., Geltman, E. M., Biello, D. R., Sobel, B. E., Siegel, B. A., and Roberts, R.: Functional response of the right ventricle to myocardial infarction: Dependence on the site of left ventricular infarction. Circulation *64*: 1005, 1981.
120. Lorell, B., Leinbach, R. C., Pohost, G. M., Gold, H. K., Dinsmore, R. E.,

Hutter, A. M., Jr., Pastore, J. O., and DeSanctis, R. W.: Right ventricular infarction. Clinical diagnosis and differentiation from cardiac tamponade and pericardial constriction. Am. J. Cardiol. *43*:465, 1979.

121. Durrer, J. D., Lie, K. I., VanCapelle, F. J. L., and Durrer, D.: Effect of sodium nitroprusside on mortality in acute myocardial infarction. N. Engl. J. Med. *306*:1121, 1982.

122. Cohn, J. N., Franciosa, J. A., Francis, G. S., Archibald, D., Tristani, F., Fletcher, R., Montero, A., Cintron, G., Clarke, J., Hager, D., Saunders, R., Cobb, F., Smith, R., Hoeb, H., and Settle, H.: Effect of short-term infusion on sodium nitroprusside in mortality rate in acute myocardial infarction complicated by left ventricular failure. Results of a Veterans Administration Cooperative study. N. Engl. J. Med. *306*:1129, 1982.

123. Passamani, E. R.: Nitroprusside in myocardial infarction. N. Engl. J. Med. *306*:1168, 1982.

124. Bodenheimer, M. M., Ramanathan, K., Banka, V. S., and Helfant, R. H.: Effect of progressive pressure reduction with nitroprusside on acute myocardial infarction in humans: Determination of optimal afterload. Ann. Intern. Med. *94*:435, 1981.

125. Shell, W. E., and Sobel, B. E.: Protection of jeopardized ischemic myocardium by reduction of ventricular afterload. N. Engl. J. Med. *291*:481, 1974.

126. Flaherty, J. T., Reid, P. R., Kelly, D. T., Taylor, D. R., Weisfeldt, M. L., and Pitt, B.: Intravenous nitroglycerin in acute myocardial infarction. Circulation *51*:132, 1975.

127. Chiariello, M., Gold, H. K., Leinbach, R. C., Davis, M. A., and Maroko, P. R.: Comparison between the effects of nitroprusside and nitroglycerin on ischemic injury during acute myocardial infarction. Circulation *54*:766, 1976.

128. Flaherty, J. T.: Intravenous nitroglycerin. Johns Hopkins Med. J. *151*:36, 1982.

129. Bussmann, W. D., Barthe, G., Klepzig, H., Jr., and Kaltenbach, M.: Controlled study of intravenous nitroglycerin treatment for two days in patients with recent myocardial infarction. Clin. Cardiol. *3*:399, 1980.

130. Borer, J. S., Redwood, D. R., Levitt, B., Cagin, N., Bianchi, C., Vallin, H., and Epstein, S. E.: Reduction in myocardial ischemia with nitroglycerin or nitroglycerin plus phenylephrine administered during acute myocardial infarction. N. Engl. J. Med. *293*:1008, 1975.

131. Come, P. C., Flaherty, J. T., Baird, M. G., Rouleau, J. R., Weisfeldt, M. L., Greene, H. L., Becker, L., and Pitt, B.: Reversal by phenylephrine of the beneficial effects of intravenous nitroglycerin in patients with acute myocardial infarction. N. Engl. J. Med. *293*:1004, 1975.

132. Derrida, J. P., Sal, R., and Chiche, P.: Nitroglycerin infusion in acute myocardial infarction. N. Engl. J. Med. *297*:336, 1977.

133. Awan, N. A., Amsterdam, E. A., Zakuddin, V., DeMaria, A. N., Miller, R. R., and Mason, D. T.: Reduction of ischemic injury by sublingual nitroglycerin in patients with acute myocardial infarction. Circulation *54*:761, 1976.

134. Rabinowitz, B., Tamari, I., Elazar, E., and Neufeld, H. N.: Intravenous isosorbide dinitrate in patients with refractory pump failure and acute myocardial infarction. Circulation *65*:771, 1982.

135. Kelly, D. T., Delgado, C. E., Taylor, D. R., Pitt, B., and Ross, R. S.: Use of phentolamine in acute myocardial infarction associated with hypertension and left ventricular failure. Circulation *47*:729, 1973.

136. Chatterjee, K., Parmley, W. W., Ganz, W., Forrester, J., Walinsky, P., Crexells, C., and Swan, H. J. C.: Hemodynamic and metabolic responses to vasodilator therapy in acute myocardial infarction. Circulation *48*:1183, 1973.

137. Franciosa, J. A., Pierpont, G., and Cohn, J. N.: Hemodynamic improvement after oral hydralazine in left ventricular failure. Ann. Intern. Med. *86*:388, 1977.

138. Chatterjee, K., Parmley, W. W., Massie, B., Greenberg, B., Werner, J., Klausner, S., and Norman, A.: Oral hydralazine therapy for chronic refractory heart failure. Circulation *54*:879, 1976.

139. Franciosa, J. A., Mikulic, E., Cohn, J. N., Jose, E., and Fabie, A.: Hemodynamic effects of orally administered isosorbide dinitrate in patients with congestive heart failure. Circulation *50*:1020, 1974.

140. Gold, H. K., Leinbach, R. C., and Sanders, C. A.: Use of sublingual nitroglycerin in congestive failure following acute myocardial infarction. Circulation *46*:839, 1972.

141. Magorien, R. D., Triffon, D. W., Desch, C. E., Bay, W. H., Unverferth, D. V., and Leier, C. V.: Prazosin and hydralazine in congestive heart failure. Ann. Intern. Med. *95*:5, 1981.

142. Cohen, R. A., Shepherd, J. T., and Vanhoutte, P. M.: Prejunctional and postjunctional actions of endogenous norepinephrine at the sympathetic neuroeffector junction in canine coronary arteries. Circ. Res. *52*:16, 1983.

143. Jaffe, A. S., Henry, P. D., Vacek, J. L., Sobel, B. E., and Roberts, R.: Administration of nifedipine to patients with acute myocardial infarction. *In* Vogel, J. H. K. (ed.): Cardiovascular Medicine 1982. New York, Raven Press, 1982, p. 91.

144. Cohn, J. N.: Editorial—Progress in vasodilator therapy for heart failure. N. Engl. J. Med. *302*:1414, 1980.

145. Kötter, V., Von Leitner, E. R., Wunderlich, J., and Schröder, R.: Comparison of haemodynamic effects of phentolamine, sodium nitroprusside, and glyceryl trinitrate in acute myocardial infarction. Br. Heart J. *39*:1196, 1977.

146. Franciosa, J. A., Guiha, N. H., Limas, C. J., Rodriguera, E., and Cohn, J. N.: Improved left ventricular function during nitroprusside infusion in acute myocardial infarction. Lancet *1*:650, 1972.

147. Hockings, B. E. F., Cope, G. D., Clarke, G. M., and Taylor, R. R.: Randomized controlled trial of vasodilator therapy after myocardial infarction. Am. J. Cardiol. *48*:345, 1981.

148. Packer, M., Meller, J., Medina, N., Yushak, M., and Gorlin, R.: Hemodynamic characterization of tolerance to long-term hydralazine therapy in severe chronic heart failure. N. Engl. J. Med. *306*:57, 1982.

149. Colucci, W. S., Williams, G. H., Alexander, R. W., and Braunwald, E.: Mechanisms and implications of vasodilator tolerance in the treatment of congestive heart failure. Am. J. Med. *71*:89, 1981.

150. Chatterjee, K., Ports, T. A., Brundage, B. H., Massie, B., Holly, A. N., and Parmley, W. W.: Oral hydralazine in chronic heart failure: Sustained beneficial hemodynamic effects. Ann. Intern. Med. *92*:600, 1980.

151. Dzau, V. J., Colucci, W. S., Williams, G. H., Curfman, G., Meggs, L., and Hollenberg, N. K.: Sustained effectiveness of converting-enzyme inhibition in patients with severe congestive heart failure. N. Engl. J. Med. *302*:1373, 1980.

152. Ertl, G., Kloner, R. A., Alexander, R. W., and Braunwald, E.: Limitation of experimental infarct size by angiotensin-converting enzyme inhibitor. Circulation *65*:40, 1982.

153. Covell, J. W., Braunwald, E., Ross, J., Jr., and Sonnenblick, E. H.: Studies on digitalis XVI. Effects on myocardial oxygen consumption. J. Clin. Invest. *45*: 1535, 1966.

154. Kumar, R., Hood, W. B., Jr., Joison, J., Gilmour, D. P., Norman, J. C., and Abelmann, W. H.: Experimental myocardial infarction. VI. Efficacy and toxicity of digitalis in acute and healing phase in intact conscious dog. J. Clin. Invest. *49*:358, 1970.

155. Maroko, P.R., Kjekshus, J. K., Sobel, B. E., Watanabe, T., Covell, J. W., Ross, J., Jr., and Braunwald, E.: Factors influencing infarct size following experimental coronary artery occlusions. Circulation *43*:67, 1971.

156. Vatner, S. F., Baig, H., Manders, W. T., and Murray, P. A.: Effects of a cardiac glycoside on regional function, blood flow, and electrograms in conscious dogs with myocardial ischemia. Circ. Res. *43*:413, 1978.

157. Watanabe, T., Covell, J. W., Maroko, P. R., Braunwald, E., and Ross, J., Jr.: The effects of increased arterial pressure and positive inotropic agents on the severity of myocardial ischemia in the acutely depressed heart. Am. J. Cardiol. *30*:371, 1972.

158. Ross, J., Jr., Waldhausen, J. S., and Braunwald, E.: Studies on digitalis. I. Direct effects on peripheral vascular resistance. J. Clin. Invest. *39*:930, 1960.

159. Morrison, J., Coromilas, J., Robbins, M., Ong, L., Eisenberg, S., Stechel, R., Zema, M., Reiser, P., and Scherr, L.: Digitalis and myocardial infarction in man. Circulation *62*:8, 1980.

160. Marcus, F. I.: Editorial—Use of digitalis in acute myocardial infarction. Circulation *62*:17, 1980.

161. Moss, A. J., Davis, H. T., Conard, D. L., DeCamilla, J. J., and Odoroff, C. L.: Digitalis-associated cardiac mortality after myocardial infarction. Circulation *64*:1150, 1981.

162. Ryan, T. J., McCabe, C. H., Bailey, D., Papapietro, S. E., Fisher, L. D., Mock, M., and Killip, T.: The effect of digitalis on survival in high risk patients (CASS). Circulation *64* (Suppl. 4): 43, 1981.

163. Mueller, H., Ayres, S. M., Giannelli, S., Jr., Conklin, E. F., Mazzara, J. T., and Grace, W. J.: Effect of isoproterenol, 1-norepinephrine, and intra-aortic counterpulsation on hemodynamics and myocardial metabolism in shock following acute myocardial infarction. Circulation *45*:335, 1972.

164. Shell, W. E., and Sobel, B. E.: Deleterious effects of increased heart rate on infarct size in the conscious dog. Am. J. Cardiol. *31*:474, 1973.

164a. Ichard, C., Ricome, J. L., Rimailho, A., Bottineau, G., and Auzepy, P.: Combined hemodynamic effects of dopamine and dobutamine in cardiogenic shock. Circulation *67*:620, 1983.

165. Holzer, J., Karliner, J. S., O'Rourke, R. A., Pitt, W., and Ross, J., Jr.: Effectiveness of dopamine in patients with cardiogenic shock. Am. J. Cardiol. *32* :79, 1973.

166. Tuttle, R. R., and Mills, J.: Development of a new catecholamine to selectively increase cardiac contractility. Circ. Res. *36*:185, 1975.

167. Gillespie, T. A., Ambos, H. D., Sobel, B. E., and Roberts, R.: Effects of dobutamine in patients with acute myocardial infarction. Am. J. Cardiol. *39*: 588, 1977.

168. Keung, E. C. H., Siskind, S. J., Sonnenblick, E. H., Ribner, H. S., Schwartz, W. J., and LeJemtel, T. H.: Dobutamine therapy in acute myocardial infarction. J.A.M.A. *245*:144, 1981.

169. Goldstein, R. A., Passamani, E. R., and Roberts, E.: Comparison of digoxin and dobutamine in patients with acute infarction and cardiac failure. N. Engl. J. Med. *303*:846, 1980.

169a. Maekawa, K., Liang, C-S., and Hood, W. B., Jr.: Comparison of dobutamine and dopamine in acute myocardial infarction. Effects of systemic hemodynamics, plasma catecholamines, blood flows and infarct size. Circulation *67*:750, 1983.

169b. Resnevkov, L.: Cardiogenic shock. Chest *83*:893, 1983.

170. Gunnar, R. M., and Loeb, H. S.: Shock in acute myocardial infarction: Evolution of physiologic therapy. J. Am. Coll. Cardiol. *1*:154, 1983.

171. Mueller, H., Ayres, S. M., Gregory, J. J., Gianelli, S., Jr., and Grace, W. J.: Hemodynamics, coronary blood flow, and myocardial metabolism in coronary shock; Response to L-norepinephrine and isoproterenol. J. Clin. Invest. *49*: 1885, 1970.

172. Mueller, H., Ayres, S. M., Conklin, E. F., Giannelli, S., Jr., Mazzara, J. T., Grace, W. T., and Nealon, T. F., Jr.: The effects of intra-aortic counterpulsation on cardiac performance and metabolism in shock associated with acute myocardial infarction. J. Clin. Invest. *50*:1885, 1971.

173. Saini, V. K., Hood, W. B., Jr., Hechtman, H. B., and Berger, R. L.: Nutrient myocardial blood flow in experimental myocardial ischemia. Circulation *52*: 1086, 1975.

174. Gold, H. K., Leinbach, R. C., Mundth, E. D., Sanders, C. A., and Buckley,

M. J.: Reversal of myocardial ischemia complicating acute infarction by intra-aorta balloon pumping (IABP). Circulation *45–46*(Suppl. II):22, 1972.
175. DeLaria, G. A., Johansen, K. H., Sobel, B. E., Sybers, H. D., and Bernstein, E. F.: Delayed evolution of myocardial ischemic injury after intra-aortic balloon counterpulsation. Circulation *50*(Suppl. II):242, 1974.
176. Johnson, S. A., Scanlon, P. J., Loeb, H. S., Moran, J. M., Pifarre, R., and Gunnar, R. M.: Treatment of cardiogenic shock in myocardial infarction by intraaortic balloon counterpulsation and surgery. Am. J. Med. *62*:687, 1977.
177. O'Rourke, M. F., Norris, R. M., Campbell, T. J., Chang, V. P., and Sammel, N. L.: Randomized controlled trial of intra-aortic balloon counterpulsation in early myocardial infarction with acute heart failure. Am. J. Cardiol. *47*:815, 1981.
178. Bitran, D., Hasin, Y., Weiss, A., Shefer, A., Freiman, I., Shimon, D., and Gotsman, M. S.: Intra-aortic balloon counterpulsation in acute myocardial infarction. Israel J. Med. Sci. *18*:215, 1982.
179. Pae, W. E., Jr., and Pierce, W. S.: Temporary left ventricular assistance in acute myocardial infarction and cardiogenic shock. Rationale and criteria for utilization. Chest *79*:692, 1981.
180. Gowda, S. K., Gillespie, T. A., Byrne, J. D., Ambos, H. D., Sobel, B. E., and Roberts, R.: Effects of external counterpulsation on enzymatically estimated infarct size and ventricular arrhythmia. Br. Heart J. *40*:308, 1978.
181. Korr, K. S., Lewvinson, H., Bough, E. W., Gheorghiade, M., Stone, J., McEnany, T., and Shulman, R. S.: Tricuspid valve replacement for cardiogenic shock after acute right ventricular infarction. J.A.M.A. *244*:1958, 1980.
182. Kopf, G. S., Meshkov, A., Laks, H., Hammond, G. L., and Beha, A. S.: Changing patterns in the surgical management of ventricular septal rupture after myocardial infarction. Am. J. Surg. *143*:465, 1982.
183. Montoya, A., McKeever, L., Scanlon, P., Sullivan, H. J., Gunnar, R. M., and Pifarre, R.: Early repair of ventricular septal rupture after infarction. Am. J. Cardiol. *45*:345, 1980.
184. Catherwood, E., Mintz, G. S., Kotler, M. N., Parry, W. R., and Segal, B. L.: Two-dimensional echocardiographic recognition of left ventricular pseudoaneurysm. Circulation *62*:294, 1980.
185. Miller, D. C., and Stinson, E. B.: Surgical management of acute mechanical defects secondary to myocardial infarction. Am. J. Surg. *141*:677, 1981.
186. Thomas, C. S., Jr., Alford, W. C., Jr., Burrus, G. R., Glassford, D. M., Jr., and Stoney, W. S.: Urgent operation for acquired ventricular septal defect. Ann. Surg. *195*:706, 1982.
187. Mundth, E. D.: Surgical treatment of cardiogenic shock and of acute mechanical complications following myocardial infarction. Cardiovasc. Clin. *8*:241, 1977.
188. Johnson, S. A., Scanlon, P. J., and Loeb, H. S.: Treatment of cardiogenic shock in myocardial infarction by intraaortic balloon counterpulsation and surgery. Am. J. Med. *62*:687, 1977.
189. Eisenmann, B., Bareiss, P., Pacifico, A. D., Jeanblanc, B., Kretz, J. G., Baehret, B., Warter, J., and Kieny, R.: Anatomic, clinical and therapeutic features of acute cardiac rupture. J. Thorac. Cardiovasc. Surg. *76*:78, 1978.
190. Russell, R. O., Jr., Turner, J. D., Rogers, W. J., Mantle, J. A., and Rackley, C. E.: Mortality reduction after acute myocardial infarction in a myocardial infarction research unit. Clin. Res. *26*:752A, 1978.
191. Page, D. L., Caulfield, J. B., Kastor, J. A., DeSanctis, R. W., and Sanders, C. A.: Myocardial changes associated with cardiogenic shock. N. Engl. J. Med. *285*:133, 1971.
192. Gutovitz, A. L., Sobel, B. E., and Roberts, R.: Progressive nature of myocardial injury in selected patients with cardiogenic shock. Am. J. Cardiol. *41*:469, 1978.
193. Kostuk, W. J., Ehsani, A. A., Karliner, J. S., Ashburn, W. L., Peterson, K. L., Ross, J., Jr., and Sobel, B. E.: Left ventricular performance, after myocardial infarction assessed by radioisotope angiocardiography. Circulation *47*:242, 1973.
194. Rogers, W. J., McDaniel, H. G., Smith, L. R., Mantle, J. A., Russell, R. O., Jr., and Rackley, C. E.: Correlation of angiographic estimates of myocardial infarct size and accumulated release of creatine kinase MB isoenzyme in man. Circulation *56*:199, 1977.
195. Peel, A. A. F., Semple, T., Wang, I., Lancaster, W. M., and Dall, J. L. G.: A coronary prognostic index for grading the severity of infarction. Br. Heart J. *24*:745, 1962.
196. Norris, R. M., Brandt, P. W. T., and Lee, A. J.: Mortality in a coronary-care unit analysed by a new coronary prognostic index. Lancet *1*:278, 1969.
197. Sobel, B. E., Bresnahan, G. F., Shell, W. E., and Yoder, R. D.: Estimation of infarct size in man and its relation to prognosis. Circulation *46*:640, 1972.
198. Shell, W. E., and Sobel, B. E.: Biochemical markers of ischemic injury. Circulation *53*(Suppl. I):98, 1976.
199. Bleifield, W., Mathey, D., Hanrath, P., Buss, H., and Effert, S.: Infarct size estimated from serial serum creatine phosphokinase in relation to left ventricular hemodynamics. Circulation *55*:303, 1977.
200. Mathey, D., Bleifield, W., Hanrath, P., and Effert, S.: Attempt to quantitate relation between cardiac function and infarct size in acute myocardial infarction. Br. Heart J. *36*:271, 1974.
201. Holman, B. L., Chisholm, R. J., and Braunwald, E.: The prognostic implications of acute myocardial infarct scintigraphy with ^{99}m Tc-pyrophosphate. Circulation *57*:320, 1978.
202. Sobel, B. E., and Shell, W. E.: Jeopardized, blighted and necrotic myocardium. Circulation *47*:215, 1973.
203. Braunwald, E., and Maroko, P. R.: The reduction of infarct size—an idea whose time (for testing) has come. Circulation *50*:206, 1974.
204. Braunwald, E., and Maroko, P. R.: Limitation of infarct size. Curr. Probl. Cardiol. *3*:1, 1978.
205. Christlieb, I. Y., Clark, R. E., and Sobel, B. E.: Three-hour preservation of the hypothermic globally ischemic heart with nifedipine. Surgery *90*:947, 1981.
206. Snyder, D. W., and Sobel, B. E.: Treatment of ischemic heart disease: Clinical therapy of ischemic heart disease. *In* Rosen, M., and Hoffman, B. (eds.): Medical Management of Ischemic Heart Disease. The Hague, The Netherlands, Martinus Nijhoff Publishers, in press.
207. Corr, P. B., Snyder, D. W., Lee, B. I., Gross, R. W., Keim, C. R., and Sobel, B. E.: Pathophysiological concentrations of lysophosphatides and the slow response. Am. J. Physiol., *12:187, 1982.*
208. Gross, R. W., Corr, P. B., Lee, B. I., Saffitz, J. E., Crafford, W. A., Jr., and Sobel, B. E.: Incorporation of radiolabeled lysophosphatidyl choline into canine Purkinje fibers and ventricular muscle: Electrophysiological, biochemical and autoradiographic correlations. Circ. Res., *51*:27, 1982.
209. Schaper, W., and Pasyk, S.: Influence of collateral flow on the ischemic tolerance of the heart following acute and subacute coronary occlusion. Circulation *53*(Suppl. I):57, 1976.
210. Bishop, S. P., White, F. C., and Bloor, C. M.: Regional myocardial blood flow during acute myocardial infarction in the conscious dog. Circ. Res. *38*:429, 1976.
211. Borda, L., Shuchleib, R., and Henry, P. D.: Effects of potassium on isolated canine coronary arteries. Circ. Res. *41*:778, 1977.
212. Oliva, P. B., and Breckinridge, J. C.: Arteriographic evidence of coronary arterial spasm in acute myocardial infarction. Circulation *56*:366, 1977.
213. Braunwald, E.: Coronary artery spasm as a cause of myocardial ischemia. J. Lab Clin. Med. *97*:299, 1981.
214. Maseri, A., L'Abbate, A., Baroldi, G., Chierchia, S., Marzilli, M., Ballestra, A. M., Severi, S., Parodi, O., Biagini, A., Distante, A., and Pesola, A.: Coronary vasospasm as a possible cause of myocardial infarction. N. Engl. J. Med. *299*: 1271, 1978.
215. Henry, P. D., and Yokoyama, M.: Supersensitivity of atherosclerotic rabbit aorta to ergonovine: Mediation by aserotonergic mechanism. J. Clin. Invest. *66*: 306, 1980.
216. Moran, T. J., French, W. J., Abrams, H. F., and Criley, J. M.: Post-myocardial infarction angina and coronary spasm. Am. J. Cardiol. *50*:192, 1982.
217. Koiwaya, Y., Torii, S., Takeshita, A., Nakagaki, O., and Nakamura, M.: Postinfarction angina caused by coronary arterial spasm. Circulation *65*:275, 1982.
218. Williams, D. O., Amsterdam, E. A., Miller, R. R., and Mason, D. T.: Functional significance of coronary collateral vessels in patients with acute myocardial infarction: Relation to pump performance, cardiogenic shock and survival. Am. J. Cardiol. *37*:345, 1976.
219. Strauss, H. D.: Myocardial infarction extension: Clinical significance. Primary Cardiol. *8*:14, 1982.
220. Baker, J. T., Bramlet, D. A., Lester, R. M., Harrison, D. C., Roe, C. R., and Cobb, F. R.: Myocardial infarct extension: Incidence and relationship to survival. Circulation *65*:918, 1982.
221. Marmor, A., Sobel, B. E., and Roberts, R.: Factors presaging early recurrent myocardial infarction ("extension"). Am. J. Cardiol. *48*:603, 1981.
222. Cannom, D. S., Levy, W., and Cohen, L. S.: The short- and long-term prognosis of patients with transmural and nontransmural myocardial infarction. Am. J. Med. *61*:452, 1976.
223. Hutter, A. M., Jr., DeSanctis, R. W., Flynn, T., and Yeatman, L. A.: Nontransmural myocardial infarction. A comparison of hospital and late clinical course of patients with that of matched patients with transmural anterior and transmural inferior myocardial infarction. Am. J. Cardiol. *48*:595, 1981.
224. Yusuf, S., Ramsdale, E., Peto, R., Furse, L., Bennet, D., Bray, C., and Sleight, P.: Early intravenous atenolol treatment in suspected acute myocardial infarction. Preliminary report of a randomized trial. Lancet *2*:73, 1980.
225. Lange, R., Kloner, R. A., and Braunwald, E.: First ultra-short-acting beta-adrenergic blocking agent: Its effect on size and segmental wall dynamics of reperfused myocardial infarcts in dogs. Am. J. Cardiol. *51*:1759, 1983.
226. Braunwald, E., Muller, J. E., Kloner, R. A., and Maroko, P. R.: Role of beta-adrenergic blockade in the therapy of patients with myocardial infarction. Am. J. Med. *74*:113, 1983.
227. Mueller, H. S., Ayres, S. M., Religa, A., and Evans, R. G.: Propranolol in the treatment of acute myocardial infarction: Effect on myocardial oxygenation and hemodynamics. Circulation *49*:1078, 1974.
228. Mueller, H. S., and Ayres, S. M.: The role of propranolol in the treatment of acute myocardial infarction. Prog. Cardiovasc. Dis. *19*:405, 1977.
229. Opie, L. H.: Metabolism of free fatty acids, glucose and catecholamines in acute myocardial infarction: Relation to myocardial ischemia and infarct size. Am. J. Cardiol. *36*:938, 1975.
230. Ahumada, G. G., Karlsberg, R. P., Jaffe, A. S., Ambos, H. D., Sobel, B. E., and Roberts, R.: Reduction of early ventricular arrhythmia by acebutolol in patients with acute myocardial infarction. Br. Heart J. *41*:654, 1979.
231. Gold, H. K., Leinbach, C., and Maroko, P. R.: Propranolol-induced reduction of signs of ischemic injury during acute myocardial infarction. Am. J. Cardiol. *38*:689, 1976.
232. Libby, P., Maroko, P. R., Covell, J. W., Malloch, C. I., Ross, J., Jr., and Braunwald, E.: Effect of practolol on the extent of myocardial ischemic injury after experimental coronary occlusion and its effect on ventricular function in the normal and ischemic heart. Cardiovasc. Res. *7*:167, 1973.
233. Muller, J. E., Maroko, P. R., and Braunwald, E.: Precordial electrocardio-

graphic mapping: A technique to assess the efficacy of interventions designed to limit infarct size. Circulation *57*:1, 1978.

234. Pelides, L. J., Reid, D. S., Thomas, M., and Shillingford, J. P.: Inhibition by beta-blockade of the ST segment elevation after acute myocardial infarction in man. Cardiovasc. Res. *2*:295, 1972.

235. Waagstein, F., and Hjalmarson, A. C.: Effect of cardioselective beta blockade on heart function and chest pain in acute myocardial infarction. Acta Med. Scand. *587*(Suppl.):201, 1975.

236. Heikkila, J., and Nieminen, M. S.: Failure of methylprednisolone to protect acutely ischemic myocardium: A contrast with subsequent beta-adrenergic blockade in man. Chest *73*:577, 1978.

237. Barber, J. M., Boyle, D. M., Chaturvedi, N. C., Singh, N., and Walsh, M. J.: Practolol in acute myocardial infarction. Acta Med. Scand. *587*(Suppl.):213, 1976.

238. Peter, T., Norris, R. M., and Clarke, E. D.: Reduction of enzyme levels by propranolol after acute myocardial infarction. Circulation *57*:1091, 1978.

239. Norris, R. M., Clarke, E. D., Sammel, N. L., Smith, W. M., and Williams, B.: Protective effect of propranolol in threatened myocardial infarction. Lancet *2*: 907, 1978.

240. Yusuf, S., Sleight, P., Rossi, P., Ramsdale, D., Peto, R., Furze, L., Sterry, H., Pearson, M., Motwani, R., Parish, S., Gray, R., Bennett, D., and Bray, C.: Reduction in infarct size, arrhythmias and chest pain by early intravenous beta blockade in suspected acute myocardial infarction. Circulation *67*:12, 1983.

240a. Yusuf, S., Ramsdale, D., Rossi, P., Peto, R., Pearson, M., Sterry, H., Furse, L., Motwani, R., Parish, S., Gray, R., Bennett, D., Bray, C., and Sleight, P.: Reduction in infarct size, morbidity and short term mortality by early intravenous beta blockade. J. Am. Coll. Cardiol. *1*:676, 1983.

241. Ramsdale, D. R., Faragher, E. B., Bennett, D. H., Bray, C. L., Ward, C., Cruickshank, J. M., Yusuf, S., and Sleight, P.: Ischemic pain relief in patients with acute myocardial infarction by intravenous atenolol. Am. Heart J. *103*: 459, 1982.

242. Jurgensen, H. J., Frederiksen, J., Hansen, D. A., and Pedersen-Bjorgaard, D.: Limitation of myocardial infarct size in patients less than 66 years treated with alprenolol. Br. Heart J. *45*:583, 1981.

242a. Hjalmarson, A., Herlitz, J., Holmberg, S., Ryden, L., Swedberg, K., Vedin, A., Waagstein, F., Waldenstrom, A., Waldenstrom, J., Wedel, H., Wilhelmsen, L., and Wilhelmsson, C.: The Goteborg metoprolol trial. Effects on mortality and morbidity in acute myocardial infarction. Circulation *67*:26, 1983.

243. Andersen, M. P., Fredriksen, J., and Jurgensen, H. J.: Effect of alprenolol on mortality among patients with definite or suspected acute myocardial infarction: Preliminary results. Lancet *2*:865, 1979.

244. Bussman, W. D., Passek, D., Seidel, W., and Kaltenbach, M.: Reduction of CK and CK-MB indexes of infarct size by intravenous nitroglycerin. Circulation *63*:615, 1981.

245. Becker, L. C., Bulkley, B. J., and Pitt, B.: Enhanced reduction of thallium-201 defects in acute myocardial infarction by nitroglycerin treatment: Initial results of a prospective randomized trial. Clin. Res. *26*:219A, 1978 (abst.).

246. Becker, L. C., Fortuin, N. J., and Pitt, B.: Effect of ischemia and antianginal drugs on the distribution of radioactive microspheres in the canine left ventricle. Circ. Res. *28*:263, 1971.

247. Flaherty, J. T., Becker, L. C., and Weisfeldt, M. L.: Results of a prospective randomized clinical trial of intravenous nitroglycerin in acute myocardial infarction. Circulation *62*(Suppl. 3):82, 1980 (abst.).

248. Kim, Y. I., and Williams, J. F., Jr.: Large dose sublingual nitroglycerin in myocardial infarction: Relief of chest pain and reduction of Q wave randomized prospective study. Circulation *64*(Suppl. 4):195, 1981.

249. Gold, H. K., Chiariello, M., Leinbach, R. C., Davis, M. A., and Maroko, P. R.: Deleterious effects of nitroprusside on myocardial injury during acute myocardial infarction. Herz *1*:161, 1976.

250. Jaffe, A. S., Geltman, E. M., Tiefenbrunn, A. J., Ambos, H. D., Snyder, D., Dukuyama, O., Bauwens, D., Sobel, B. E., and Roberts, R.: Reduction of the extent of inferior myocardial infarction with intravenous nitroglycerin: A randomized prospective study. Circulation *64*(Suppl. 4):195, 1981.

251. Borer, J. S., Kent, K. M., Goldstein, R. E., and Epstein, S. E.: Nitroglycerin-induced reduction in the incidence of spontaneous ventricular fibrillation during coronary occlusion in dogs. Am. J. Cardiol. *33*:517, 1974.

252. Shah, R., Bodenheimer, M. M., Banka, V. S., and Helfant, R. H.: Nitroglycerin and ventricular performance: Differential effect in the presence of reversible and irreversible asynergy. Chest *70*:473, 1976.

253. Myers, R. W., Scherer, J. L., Goldstein, R. A., Goldstein, R. E., Kent, K. M., and Epstein, S. E.: Effects of nitroglycerin and nitroglycerin-methoxamine during acute myocardial ischemia in dogs with pre-existing multivessel coronary occlusive disease. Circulation *51*:632, 1975.

254. Hill, N. S., Antman, E. M., Green, L. H., and Alpert, J. S.: Intravenous nitroglycerin. A review of pharmacology, indications, therapeutic effects and complications. Chest *79*:69, 1981.

255. Chatterjee, K., and Parmley, W. W.: Vasodilator therapy for acute myocardial infarction and chronic congestive heart failure. J. Am. Coll. Cardiol. *1*:133, 1983.

256. Maroko, P. R., Hillis, L. D., Muller, J. E., Tavazzi, L., Heyndrickx, G. R., Ray, M., Chiariello, M., Distante, A., Askenazi, J., Salerno, J., Carpentier, J., Reshetnaya, N. I., Radvany, P., Libby, P., Raabe, D. S., Chazov, E. I., Bobba, P., and Braunwald, E.: Favorable effects of hyaluronidase on electrocardiographic evidence of necrosis in patients with acute myocardial infarction. N. Engl. J. Med. *296*:898, 1977.

257. Saltissi, S., Coltart, D. J., Robinson, P. S., Webb-Peploe, M. M., and Croft, D. N: Effects of early administration of a highly purified hyaluronidase preparation (GL enzyme) on myocardial infarct size. Lancet *1*:867, 1982.

258. Henderson, A., Campbell, R. W. F., and Julian, D. G.: Effect of a highly purified hyaluronidase preparation (GL enzyme) on electrocardiographic changes in acute myocardial infarction. Lancet *1*:874, 1982.

259. Flint, E. J., Cadigan, P. J., DeGiovanni, J., Lamb, P., and Pentecost, B. L.: Effect of GL enzyme (a highly purified form of hyaluronidase) on mortality after myocardial infarction. Lancet *1*:871, 1982.

260. Rackley, C. E., Russell, R. O., Jr., Rogers, W. J., and Mantle, J. A.: Glucose-insulin-potassium infusion in acute myocardial infarction: Review of clinical experience. Postgrad. Med. *65*:93, 1979.

261. Mantle, J. A., Rogers, W. J., McDaniel, H. G., Holmes, R. A., Russell, R. O., Jr., and Rackley, C. E.: Metabolic support of mechanical performance in myocardial infarction in man—a randomized clinical trial of glucose-insulin-potassium. Am. J. Cardiol. *43*:395, 1979.

262. Rogers, W. J., Russel, R. O., Jr., McDaniel, H. G., and Rackley, C. E.: Acute effects of glucose-insulin-potassium infusion on myocardial substrates, coronary blood flow and oxygen consumption in man. Am. J. Cardiol. *40*:421, 1977.

263. Rogers, W. J., Segall, P. H., McDaniel, H. G., Mantle, J. A., Russell, R. O., Jr., and Rackley, C. E.: Prospective randomized trial of glucose-insulin-potassium in acute myocardial infarction. Am. J. Cardiol. *43*:801, 1979.

264. Russell, R. O., Jr., Rogers, W. J., Mantle, J. A., McDaniel, H. G., and Rackley, C. E.: Glucose-insulin-potassium, free fatty acids and acute myocardial infarction in man. Circulation *53* (Suppl. I):I–207, 1975.

265. Heng, M. K., Norris, R. M., Singh, B. N., and Barratt-Boyes, C.: Effects of glucose and glucose-insulin-potassium on haemodynamics and enzyme release after acute myocardial infarction. Br. Heart J. *39*:748, 1977.

266. Whitlow, P. L., Rogers, W. J., Smith, L. R., McDaniel, H. G., Papapietro, S. E., Mantle, J. A., Logic, J. R., Russell, R. O., Jr., and Rackley, C. E.: Enhancement of left ventricular function by glucose-insulin-potassium infusion in acute myocardial infarction. Am. J. Cardiol. *49*:811, 1982.

266a. Rogers, W. J., McDaniel, H. G., Mantle, J. A., and Rackley, C. E.: Prospective randomized trial of glucose-insulin-potassium in acute myocardial infarction: Effects on hemodynamics, short- and long-term survival. J. Am. Coll. Cardiol. *1*:628, 1983.

267. Morrison, J., Reduto, L., Pizzarello, R., Geller, K., Maley, T., and Gulotta, S.: Modification of myocardial injury in man by corticosteroid administration. Circulation *53* (Suppl. I):200, 1976.

268. Roberts, R., DeMello, V., and Sobel, B. E.: Deleterious effects of methylprednisolone in patients with myocardial infarction. Circulation *53* (Suppl. I):204, 1976.

269. Bulkley, B. H., and Roberts, W. C.: Steroid therapy during acute myocardial infarction: A cause of delayed healing and of ventricular aneurysm. Am. J. Med. *56*:244, 1974.

270. Kloner, R. A., Fishbein, M. C., Lew, H., Maroko, P. R., and Braunwald, E.: Mummification of the infarcted myocardium by high dose corticosteroids. Circulation *57*:56, 1978.

271. Maclean, D., Maroko, P. R., Fishbein, M. C., and Braunwald, E.: Effects of corticosteroids on myocardial infarct size and healing following experimental coronary occlusion. Am. J. Cardiol. *39*:280, 1977.

272. Hammerman, H., Kloner, R. A., Hale, S. L., Schoen, F. J., and Braunwald, E.: Is scar thinning and LV topographic alterations induced by anti-inflammatory agent of functional significance? Clin. Res., in press.

273. Amsterdam, E. A., et al.: Clinical assessment of external pressure circulatory assist in acute myocardial infarction. Report of a cooperative clinical trial. Am. J. Cardiol. 45:349, 1980.

274. Powell, W. J., Jr., Daggett, W. M., Magro, A. E., Bianco, J. A., Buckley, M. J., Sanders, C. A., Kantrowitz, A. R., and Austen, W. G.: Effects of intra-aortic balloon counterpulsation on cardiac performance, oxygen consumption, and coronary blood flow in dogs. Circ. Res. *26*:753, 1970.

275. Maroko, P. R., Bernstein, E. F., Libby, P., DeLaria, G. A., Covell, J. W., Ross, J., Jr., and Braunwald, E.: Effects of intraaortic balloon counterpulsation on the severity of myocardial ischemic injury following acute coronary occlusion: Counterpulsation and myocardial injury. Circulation *45*: 1150, 1972.

276. Nachlas, M. M., and Siedband, M. P.: The influence of diastolic augmentation on infarctsize following coronary artery ligation. J. Thorac. Cardiovasc. Surg. *53*:698, 1967.

277. Sugg, W. L., Webb, W. R., and Ecker, R. R.: Reduction of extent of myocardial infarction by counterpulsation. Ann. Thorac. Surg. *7*:310, 1969.

278. Leinbach, R. C., Gold, H. K., Harper, R. W., Buckley, M. J., and Austen, W. G.: Early intraaortic balloon pumping for anterior myocardial infarction without shock. Circulation *58*:204, 1978.

279. Ginks, W. R., Sybers, H. D., Maroko, P. R., Covell, J. W., Sobel, B. E., and Ross, J., Jr.: Coronary artery reperfusion: II. Reduction of myocardial infarct size at 1 week after the coronary occlusion. J. Clin. Invest. *51*:2717, 1972.

280. Lang, T., Corday, E., Gold, H., Meerbaum, S., Rubins, S., Costantini, C., Hirose, S., Osher, J., and Rosen, V.: Consequences of reperfusion after coronary occlusion: Effects on hemodynamic and regional myocardial metabolic function. Am. J. Cardiol. *33*:69, 1974.

281. Smith, G. T., Soeter, J. R., Haston, H. H., and McNamara, J. J.: Coronary reperfusion in primates: Serial electrocardiographic and histologic assessment. J. Clin. Invest. *54*:1420, 1974.

282. Symes, J. F., Arnold, I. M. F., and Blundell, P. E.: Early revascularization of the acute myocardial infarction: The critical time factor. Can. Med. Assoc. J. *107*:636, 1972.

283. Kloner, R. A., Fishbein, M. C., Cotran, R. S., Braunwald, E., and Maroko, P. R.: The effect of propranolol on microvascular injury in acute myocardial ischemia. Circulation *55*:872, 1977.

284. Deloche, A., Fabiani, J. N., Camilleri, J. P., Relland, J., Joseph, D., Carpentier, A., and Dubost, C.: The effect of coronary artery reperfusion on the extent of myocardial infarction. Am. Heart J. *93*:358, 1977.
285. Kloner, R. A., Rude, R. E., Carlson, N., Maroko, P. R., DeBoer, L. W. V., and Braunwald, E.: Ultrastructural evidence of microvascular damage and myocardial cell injury after coronary artery occlusion: Which comes first? Circulation *62*:945, 1980.
286. Kloner, R. A., Ellis, S. G., Lange, R., and Braunwald, E.: Studies of experimental coronary artery reperfusion: Effects on infarct size, myocardial function, biochemistry, ultrastructure and microvascular damage. Circulation, in press.
287. Bergmann, S. R., Lerch, R. A., Fox, K. A. A., Ludbrook, P. A., Welch, M. J., Ter-Pogossian, M. M., and Sobel, B. E.: The temporal dependence of beneficial effects of coronary thrombolysis characterized by positron tomography. Am. J. Med., *73*:573, 1982.
288. Reimer, K. A., and Jennings, R. B.: The wavefront phenomenon of myocardial ischemic cell death. II. Transmural progression of necrosis within the framework of ischemic bed size (myocardium at risk) and collateral flow. Lab. Invest. *40*:633, 1979.
289. Bresnahan, G. F., Roberts, R., Shell, W. E., Ross, J., Jr., and Sobel, B. E.: Deleterious effects due to hemorrhage after myocardial reperfusion. Am. J. Cardiol. *33*:82, 1974.
290. Hammermeister, K. E.: The effect of coronary bypass surgery on survival. Prog. Cardiovasc. Dis. *25*:297, 1983.
291. Phillips, S. J., Kongtahworn, C., Zeff, R. H., Benson, M., Iannone, L., Brown, T., and Gordon, D. F.: Emergency coronary artery revascularization: A possible therapy for acute myocardial infarction. Circulation *60*:241, 1979.
292. McIntosh, H. D., and Buccino, R. A.: Editorial—Emergency coronary artery revascularization of patients with acute myocardial infarction. You can . . . but should you? Circulation *60*:247, 1979.
293. Bery, R., Jr., Selinger, S. L., and Leonard, J. J.: Immediate coronary artery bypass for acute evolving myocardial infarction. J. Thorac. Cardiovasc. Surg. *81*:493, 1981.
294. DeWood, M. A., Spores, J., Notske, R. N., Lang, H. T., Shields, J. P., Simpson, C. S., Rudy, L. W., and Grunwald, R.: Medical and surgical management of myocardial infarction. Am. J. Cardiol. *44*:1356, 1979.
294a. DeWood, M. A., Heit, J., Spores, J., Berg, R., Jr., Selinger, S. L., Rudy, L. W., Hensley, G. R., and Shields, J. P.: Anterior transmural myocardial infarction: Effects of surgical coronary reperfusion on global and regional left ventricular function. J. Am. Coll. Cardiol. *1*:1223, 1983.
295. Kagen, L., Scheidt, S., and Butt, A.: Serum myoglobin in myocardial infarction: The "staccato phenomenon": Is acute myocardial infarction in man an intermittent event? Am. J. Med. *62*:86, 1977.
296. Loop, F. D., Cheanvechai, C., Sheldon, W. C., Taylor, P. C., and Effler, D. B.: Early myocardial revascularization during acute myocardial infarction. Chest *66*:478, 1974.
297. Gruntzig, A. R., Senning, A., and Siegenthaler, W. E.: Nonoperative dilatation of coronary artery stenosis. N. Engl. J. Med. *301*:61, 1979.
298. Kent, K. M., Bonow, R. O., Rosing, D. R., Ewels, C. J., Lipson, L. C., McIntosh, C. L., Bacharach, S., Green, M., and Epstein, S. E.: Improved myocardial function during exercise after successful percutaneous transluminal coronary angioplasty. N. Engl. J. Med. *306*:441, 1982.
299. DeWood, M. A., Spores, J., Notske, R., Mouser, L. T., Burroughs, R., Golden, M. S., and Lang, H. T.: Prevalence of total coronary occlusion during the early hours of transmural myocardial infarction. N. Engl. J. Med. *303*:897, 1980.
300. Rentrop, P., Blanke, H., Marsch, K. R., Kaiser, H., Kostering, H., and Leitz, K.: Selective intracoronary thrombolysis in acute myocardial infarction and unstable angina pectoris. Circulation *63*:307, 1981.
301. Ganz, W., Buchbinder, N., Marcus, H., Mondkar, A., Maddahi, J., Charuzi, Y., O'Conner, L., Shell, W., Fishbein, M. C., Cass, R., Miyamoto, A., and Swan, H. J. C.: Intracoronary thrombolysis in evolving myocardial infarction. Am. Heart J. *101*:4, 1981.
301a. Schroder, R., Biamino, G., Leitner, E-R. V., Linderer, T., Bruggemann, T., Heitz, J., Vohringer, H-F., and Wegscheider, K.: Intravenous short-term infusion of streptokinase in acute myocardial infarction. Circulation *67*:536, 1983.
301b. Feit, F., and Rentrop, K. P.: Thrombolytic therapy in acute myocardial infarction. Cardiovasc. Rev. Rep. *4*:426, 1983.
302. Markis, J. E., Malagold, M., Parker, J. A., Silverman, K. J., Barry, W. H., Als, A. V., Paulin, S., Grossman, W., and Braunwald, E.: Myocardial salvage after intracoronary thrombolysis with streptokinase in acute myocardial infarction: Assessment of intracoronary thallium-201. N. Engl. J. Med. *305*:777, 1981.
303. Mathey, D. G., Kuck, K-H., Tilsner, V., Krebber, H-J., and Bleifeld, W.: Nonsurgical coronary artery recanalization in acute transmural myocardial infarction. Circulation *63*:489, 1981.
304. Ganz, W., Geft, I., Maddahi, J., Berman, D., Charuzi, Y., Shah, P. K., and Swan, H. J. C.: Nonsurgical reperfusion in evolving myocardiol infarction. J. Am. Coll. Cardiol. *1*:1247, 1983.
305. Anderson, J. L., Marshall, H. W., Bray, B. E., Lutz, J. R., Frederick, P. R., Yanowitz, F. G., Datz, F. L., Klausner, S. C., and Hagan, A. D.: A randomized trial of intracoronary streptokinase in the treatment of acute myocardial infarction. N. Engl. J. Med. *308*:1312, 1983.
306. Maddahi, J., Ganz, W., Ninomiya, K., Hashida, J., Fishbein, M. C., Mondkar, A., Buchbinder, N., Marcus, H., Geft, I., Shah, P. K., Rozanski, A., Swan, H. J. C., and Berman, D. S.: Myocardial salvage by intracoronary thrombolysis in evolving acute myocardial infarction. Evaluation using intracoronary injection of thallium-201. Am. Heart J. *102*:664, 1981.
306a. Blanke, H., Schicha, H., Kaiser, H., Karsch, K. R., and Rentrop, K. P.: Long-term left ventricular function after intracoronary streptokinase therapy. J. Am Coll. Cardiol. *1*:579, 1983.
306b. Schwarz, F., Faure, A., Katus, H., VonOlshausen, K., Hofmann, M., Schuler, G., Manthey, J., and Kubler, W.: Intracoronary thrombolysis in acute myocardial infarction: An attempt to quantitate its effects by comparison of enzymatic estimate of myocardial necrosis with left ventricular ejection fraction. Am. J. Cardiol. *51*:1573, 1983.
307. Fujimoto, T., Peter, T., Hamamoto, H., and Mandel, W. J.: Electrophysiologic observations on ventricular tachyarrhythmias following reperfusion. Am. Heart J. *105*:201, 1983.
308. Sobel, B. E., and Bergmann, S. R.: Coronary thrombolysis: Some unresolved issues. Am. J. Med. *72*:1, 1982.
308a. Khaja, F., Walton, J. A., Jr., Brymer, J. F., Lo, E., Osterberger, L., O'Neill, W. W., Colfer, H. T., Weiss, R., Lee, T., Kurian, T., Goldberg, A. D., Pitt, B., and Goldstein, S.: Intracoronary fibrinolytic therapy in acute myocardial infarction. Report of a prospective randomized trial. N. Engl. J. Med. *308*:1305, 1983.
309. Krebber, H. J., Mathey, D., Kuck, K. J., Kalmar, P., and Rodewald, G.: Management of evolving myocardial infarction by intracoronary thrombolysis and subsequent aorta-coronary bypass. J. Thorac. Cardiovasc. Surg. *83*:186, 1982.
309a. Lolley, D. M., Fulton, R., Hamman, J., Reader, G. S., Johnson, J. L., Clarke, J. A., Sheth, M. K., and Hearne, M. J.: Early coronary artery surgery after intracoronary streptokinase thrombolytic therapy. J. Am. Coll. Cardiol. *1*:632, 1983.
310. Meyer, J., Merx, W., Dorr, R., Lambertz, H., Bethge, C., and Effert, S.: Successful treatment of acute myocardial infarction shock by combined percutaneous transluminal coronary recanalization (PTCR) and percutaneous transluminal coronary angioplasty (PTCA) Am. Heart J. *103*:132, 1982.
310a. Papapietro, S. E., MacLean, W. A. H., Stanley, A. W. H., Jr., Cooper, T. B., Hess, R. G., Siler, W., and Geer, D. A.: Percutaneous transluminal coronary angioplasty in acute myocardial infarction. J. Am. Coll. Cardiol. *1*:580, 1983.
310b. Schroder, R.: Systemic versus intracoronary streptokinase infusion in the treatment of acute myocardial infarction. J. Am. Coll. Cardiol. *1*:1254, 1983.
311. Ahlmark, G., Ahlberg, G., Saetre, H., Haglund, I., and Korsgren, M.: A controlled study of early discharge after uncomplicated myocardial infarction. Acta Med. Scand. *206*:87, 1979.
312. Lau, Y. K., Smith, J., Morrison, S. L., and Chamberlain, D. A.: Policy for early discharge after acute myocardial infarction. Br. Med. J. *281*:1489, 1980.
313. Friedman, M., Thoresen, C. E., Gill, J. J., Ulmer, D., Thompson, L., Powell, L., Price, V., Elek, S. R., Rabin, D. D., Breall, W. S., Piaget, G., Dixon, T., Bourg, E., Levy, R. A., and Tasto, D. L.: Feasibility of altering type A behavior pattern after myocardial infarction. Recurrent coronary prevention project study: Methods, baseline results and preliminary findings. Circulation *66*:83, 1982.
313a. Ewart, C. K., Taylor, C. B., Reese, L., and Debusk, R. F.: Effects of early postinfarction exercise testing on self perception and subsequent physical activity. J. Am. Coll. Cardiol. *1*:662, 1983.
314. Hood, W. B., Jr.: More on sulfinpyrazone after myocardial infarction. N. Engl. J. Med. *306*:988, 1982.
315. Rackley, C. E., Russell, R. O., Mantle, J. A., Rogers, W. J., and Papapietro, S. E.: Modern approach to myocardial infarction: Determination of prognosis and therapy. Am. Heart J. *101*:75, 1981.
316. Turner, J. D., Schwartz, K. M., Logic, J. R., Sheffield, L. T., Rensal, S., Roitman, D. I., Mantle, J. A., Russell, R. O., Rackley, C. E., and Rogers, W. J.: Detection of residual jeopardized myocardium three weeks after myocardial infarction by exercise testing with thallium 201 myocardial scintigraphy. Circulation *61*:729, 1980.
317. Forrester, J. S.: Do you routinely recommend coronary angiography after uncomplicated MI? J. Cardiovasc. Med. *6*:393, 1981.
318. Willerson, J. T., and Buja, L. M.: Cause and course of acute myocardial infarction. Am. J. Med. *69*:903, 1980.
319. Miller, D. H., and Borer, J. S.: Exercise testing early after myocardial infarction. Risks and benefits. Am. J. Med. *72*:427, 1982.
320. Fuller, C. M., Raizner, A. E., Verani, M. S., Nahormek, P. A., Chahine, R. A., McEntee, C. W., and Miller, R. R.: Early post-myocardial infarction treadmill stress testing. Ann. Intern. Med. *94*:734, 1981.
320a. Rapaport, E., and Remedios, P.: The high risk patient after recovery from myocardial infarction: Recognition and management. J. Am. Coll. Cardiol. *1*:391, 1983.
320b. Mukharji, J., Rude, R., Gustafson, N., Poole, K., Passamani, E., Thomas, L. J., Jr., Strauss, H. W., Muller, J. E., Roberts, R., Raabe, D. S., Jr., Braunwald, E., Willerson, J. T., and cooperating investigators, MILIS: Late sudden death following myocardial infarction: Interdependence of risk factors. J. Am. Coll. Cardiol. *1*:585, 1983
321. Stone, P. H., and Muller, J. E.: Nifedipine therapy for recurrent ischemic pain following myocardial infarction. Clin. Cardiol. *5*:223, 1982.

39 CHRONIC ISCHEMIC HEART DISEASE

by Peter F. Cohn, M.D., and Eugene Braunwald, M.D.

Chronic ischemic heart disease is most commonly due to obstruction of the coronary arteries, which in turn usually results from atherosclerosis, a condition described in Chapter 34. The importance of ischemic heart disease in contemporary society is attested to by the almost epidemic number of persons afflicted—especially when this number is compared with the anecdotal reports of its occurrence in the medical literature prior to this century. Coronary artery disease causes more deaths, disability, and economic loss in industrialized nations than any other group of diseases. In the United States arteriosclerosis is responsible for nearly half of all deaths: almost one million annually. Each year, 200,000 Americans under the age of 65 years die with what has been called *premature* ischemic heart disease and another two million people are afflicted with it. In addition to enormous personal and family suffering, it has been estimated that these diseases cost the United States more than $50 billion in health expenditures and lost productivity.

HISTORICAL PERSPECTIVES

To appreciate this disease entity, some historical perspective is useful. Angina pectoris serves as a useful example, since it is the most common clinical presentation of chronic ischemic heart disease. The term was first used by Dr. William Heberden in a report published in 1772.[1] Unlike the word "dolor," which means pain, the word "angina" was intended to indicate a sense of *strangling.* Heberden noted that fear of death ("angor animi") often accompanies this sensation in the chest (or rather, observed with this symptom complex, episodes of discomfort in the "breast"). Heberden's description of angina is as accurate today as it was more than two centuries ago: "There is a disorder of the breast, marked with strong and peculiar symptoms considerable for the kind of danger belonging to it, and not extremely rare, of which I do not recollect any mention among medical authors. The seat of it, and sense of strangling and anxiety, with which it is attended, may make it not improperly be called angina pectoris. Those, who are afflicted with it, are seized while they are walking and most particularly when they walk soon after eating, with a painful and most disagreeable sensation in the breast, which seems as if it would take their life away, if it were to increase or to continue; the moment they stand still, all this uneasiness vanishes."

The pathophysiological mechanism of angina pectoris as being related to an imbalance between myocardial oxygen supply and demand was first appreciated in 1799 by C.H. Parry: "The rigidity of the coronary arteries may act, proportionately to the extent of the ossification, as a mechanical impediment to the free motion of the heart; and though a quantity of blood may circulate through these arteries, sufficient to nourish the heart, yet there may probably be less than what is requisite for ready and vigorous action. Hence, though a heart so diseased may be fit for the purposes of common circulation, during a state of bodily and mental tranquility, and of health otherwise good, yet when any unusual exertion is required, its powers may fail, under the new and extraordinary demand."[2]

An indirect commentary on the incidence of coronary atherosclerosis is provided by the medical literature dealing with angina. Following Heberden's original account of angina pectoris, few reports dealt with this syndrome before the beginning of the 20th century. For example, in a textbook of medicine by Austin Flint published in 1866,[3] only two pages were devoted to angina pectoris. There appears to have been far less coronary artery disease 100 years ago than now, for it seems hard to believe that it could have escaped attention if acute myocardial infarction and sudden death occurred with any frequency in young and middle-aged men. In the mid-19th century, renewed interest in angina pectoris was stimulated by Brunton's report on the use of amyl nitrate for the treatment of angina pectoris,[4] yet when William Osler published his textbook of medicine in 1892,[5] he still referred to angina as a rare condition. Osler believed that complete obliteration of a coronary artery, if produced suddenly, was usually fatal. Although he recognized different gradations of anginal pain,[6] nonfatal acute myocardial infarction as a separate entity was appreciated for the first time with the reports of Obraztov and Strazhesko in Russia in 1910[7] and of Herrick in the United States in 1912.[8]

The work of these clinical pioneers did not receive much attention initially, possibly because the condition was not yet common enough for physicians to appreciate its importance. This may be due to the fact that even in the early 20th century, the large hospitals of the country were "reserved" for the indigent, who were often malnourished; the more affluent private patients in whom the incidence of ischemic heart disease was greater, were seen at home. P. D. White became interested in coronary artery disease early in the 20th century; however, while in medical school and as an intern and resident in Boston, he stated that he received no instruction or experience that helped him recognize this condition. In 1968, he reviewed the hospital records of 800 patients who had been under his care as an intern at the Massachusetts General Hospital in 1912–1913.[9] Of 700 men, mainly between the ages of 20 and 60 years, only eight were diagnosed as having angina pectoris; three had syphilitic aortitis as the cause of their pain, and one had rheumatic aortic regurgitation. Thus, it appears that symptomatic ischemic heart disease was quite uncommon at the Massachusetts General Hospital at the beginning of the 20th century. In the early 1920's, ischemic heart disease aroused more interest, and there were increasing reports of its occurrence. Wearn, at the Peter Bent Brigham Hospital, described a premonitory chest pain syndrome before the actual myocardial infarction occurred —a forerunner of the syndrome currently named unstable angina.[10]

With the development of cardiology as a specialty, interest in coronary artery disease grew rapidly. The diagnostic value of the electrocardiogram became appreciated, as did the importance of electrocardiographic abnormalities occasioned by exercise. Perhaps the most important next step in understanding the pathophysiology of chronic ischemic heart disease was the clinical-pathological correlation described by Blumgart, Schlesinger, and Zoll at Boston's Beth Israel Hospital.[11] Their studies were particularly important because they demonstrated the different histopathological findings in patients with angina pectoris and myocardial infarction, and they stressed the importance of the collateral circulation. Two decades after the work of Blumgart and associates the modern era of study of coronary artery disease began with the introduction of coronary arteriography by Sones in 1959,[12] allowing the evaluation of coronary anatomy in vivo.

There is no uniform presenting syndrome for chronic ischemic heart disease. Although chest discomfort is usually the predominant symptom in chronic (stable), unstable, or variant angina and acute myocardial infarction, syndromes of ischemic heart disease also occur in which ischemic chest discomfort is absent or not prominent. These include asymptomatic myocardial ischemia, cardiac arrhythmias, and congestive heart failure. Myocardial ischemia may also occur in the absence of coronary atherosclerosis (as in aortic valve disease, hypertrophic cardiomyopathy, and syphilitic aortitis), and coronary artery disease may occur together with these other forms of heart disease. Finally, the various syndromes characteristic of ischemic heart disease may complicate noncardiac disease, e.g., coronary artery disease may occur in patients with chronic renal failure requiring dialysis.

CHRONIC (STABLE) ANGINA PECTORIS

CLINICAL MANIFESTATIONS

CHARACTERISTICS OF ANGINA (see also p. 5). Heberden's initial description of the chest discomfort as conveying a sense of "strangling and anxiety" is still remarkably pertinent today, although adjectives used to describe this distress now include "viselike," "constricting," "suffocating," "crushing," "heavy," and "squeezing." In other patients, the quality of the sensation is even more vague and may be described as a mild pressure-like discomfort or an uncomfortable numb sensation. The site of the discomfort is usually retrosternal, but radiation is common and usually occurs down the ulnar surface of the left arm; commonly, the right arm and the outer surfaces of both arms are also involved.[13] Sampson and Cheitlin have documented the large number of regions that can be sites of radiation, with neck, jaw, and throat pain observed most commonly.[14] Headache is uncommon,[15] and discomfort below the epigastrium due to angina is rare. Anginal "equivalents" (i.e., symptoms of myocardial ischemia other than angina) such as breathlessness, faintness, fatigue, and belching have also been reported.

The etiology of the discomfort is complex and not fully understood.[16] For example, the specific substance that actually stimulates sympathetic afferents and begins the series of interactions that culminate in chest discomfort has not been identified.[17] Some evidence favors agents that are released from cells as a result of transient ischemia, such as bradykinin, histamine, or serotonin.[18] Acidosis or elevated potassium concentration in the involved tissues may trigger release of these substances to which the sensory end-plates of the intracardiac sympathetic nerves appear to be particularly sensitive. The end-plates are the receptors of a network of unmyelinated nerves that lie between cardiac muscle fibers and that are also found around coronary vessels, travel to the cardiac plexus, and then ascend to the sympathetic ganglia (C7-T4). Impulses are transmitted to corresponding spinal ganglia, then via the spinal cord to the thalamus, and finally to the cerebral cortex.

The discomfort of myocardial ischemia is perceived in various regions of the chest because it is "referred" to the corresponding peripheral dermatomes that supply afferent nerves to the same segment of the spinal cord as the heart. A plausible explanation is that a common pool of secondary neurons can be stimulated by somatic and visceral afferent impulses.[19] If visceral stimuli are excessive, the nearby intermediate neurons that are receptors for somatic impulses may be excited, and the discomfort will then be perceived as being cutaneous in origin. Thus, pain impulses can be referred to the medial aspects of the arm via common connections to the brachial plexus and can be referred to the neck via connections with the cervical roots.

It is not clear why some patients with clear-cut evidence of ischemic heart disease experience no chest discomfort; diabetics, in particular, appear to have a higher frequency of "silent" ischemia, presumably because of autonomic denervation. In some patients chest pain disappears after a myocardial infarction, even though other evidence of paroxysmal ischemia, such as ST-segment depression, may persist. It is postulated that in these patients the nerve endings may have been damaged as a result of the infarction. Finally, patients with reproducible evidence of myocardial ischemia may or may not experience chest pain with each of the various episodes. Ambulatory electrocardiography has revealed that the majority of patients with angina also experience numerous episodes of silent ischemia, i.e., ST-segment and T-wave changes, identical to those occurring during typical angina but unaccompanied by chest discomfort; the frequency of these episodes is reduced by treatment with beta blockers and calcium-channel blockers, supporting the contention that they represent instances of myocardial ischemia.

The fact that the discomfort of angina is not uniform and that other entities can mimic it often makes the differential diagnosis of chest pain difficult[13,17,20] (Table 1–1, p. 5). Differentiating the discomfort resulting from these noncardiac disorders from angina pectoris is usually possible when the *quality* of the pain and its *duration, precipitating factors,* and *associated symptoms* are taken into consideration (Table 39–1).[14] Thus, the *typical* anginal episode usually begins gradually and reaches maximum intensity over a period of minutes before dissipating—usually as a result of cessation of the activity that precipitated it. One should consider *noncoronary* causes in patients with sharp, stabbing, or burning chest pain that comes and goes in a matter of seconds or with a dull, continuous ache in the chest. Similarly, changes in posture do not usually affect the discomfort of myocardial ischemia, and this maneuver helps to distinguish angina from pericardial disease or hiatus hernia. In typical angina, the pain is related to an increase in myocardial oxygen demands, most commonly brought about by physical activity; the *rate* at which a task is carried out is important. Hurrying is particularly likely to precipitate angina, as are efforts involving motion of the hands over the head. Emotion or eating, particularly when combined with physical activity, commonly causes angina, as do a variety of other factors, including the excessive metabolic demands imposed by chills and fever, thyrotoxicosis, tachycardia from any cause, severe anemia, and hypoglycemia. In all these conditions, underlying fixed coronary artery obstruction in the form of atheromatous disease is usually present, and the other factors (e.g., exercise, fever) increase the activity of the heart, stimulate myocardial oxygen needs in the presence of a fixed and limited oxygen supply, and thus precipitate ischemia and chest discomfort.

There is increasing evidence, however, that angina may also be caused by transient reductions of oxygen supply as a consequence of *coronary vasoconstriction.*[21–24,24a,24b] As pointed out on page 1241, the coronary arterial bed is well innervated and a variety of stimuli alter coronary tone. There is a reciprocal relation between the severity of dynamic and organic obstruction required to cause myocardial ischemia. Thus, in persons with no organic lesions, only severe dynamic obstruction—as occurs in the coronary spasm of Prinzmetal's angina—can cause myocardial ischemia and resultant angina. On the other hand, in patients with severe, although subcritical, fixed obstruction to coronary flow, only a minor increase in dynamic obstruction is necessary to cause blood flow to fall below a critical level and cause myocardial ischemia (Fig. 39–1).

FIXED- VS. VARIABLE-THRESHOLD ANGINA. The variability of the threshold for angina differs among patients. In patients with *fixed-threshold angina,* with few if any dynamic (vasoconstrictive) components, the level of physical activity, a reflection of myocardial oxygen consumption, required to precipitate angina is relatively constant. Characteristically, these patients can predict with

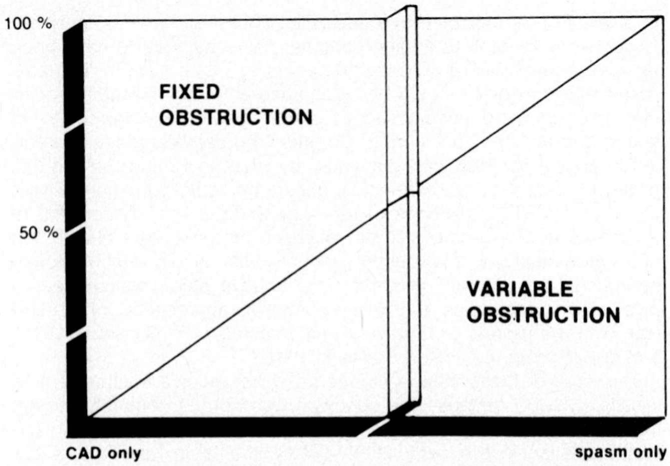

FIGURE 39–1 Different mixtures of fixed and variable obstruction may produce myocardial ischemia. The vertical bar represents a patient in whom both spasm (variable obstruction) and fixed obstruction play significant roles in occluding a coronary artery. This variable mixture of spasm and fixed obstruction may be present not only in Prinzmetal's angina but in classic angina and acute myocardial infarction as well. (From Muller, J. E.: Prinzmetal's angina: A model for the role of spasm in ischemic heart disease. J. Cardiovasc. Med. *5*:19, 1980.)

TABLE 39–1 CHARACTERISTICS OF ANGINA PECTORIS

Quality	
	Sensation of pressure or heavy weight on the chest
	Burning sensation
	Feeling of tightness
	Shortness of breath with feeling of constriction about the larynx or upper trachea
	Visceral quality (deep, heavy, squeezing, aching)
	Gradual increase in intensity followed by gradual fading away
Location	
	Over the sternum or very near to it
	Anywhere between epigastrium and pharynx
	Occasionally limited to left shoulder and left arm
	Rarely limited to right arm
	Limited to lower jaw
	Lower cervical or upper thoracic spine
	Left interscapular or suprascapular area
Duration	
	0.5 to 30 minutes
Precipitating Factors	
	Relationship to exercise
	Effort which involves use of arms above the head
	Cold environment
	Walking against the wind
	Walking after a large meal
	Emotional factors involved with physical exercise
	Fright, anger
	Coitus
Nitroglycerin Relief	
	Relief of pain occurring within 45 seconds to 5 minutes of taking nitroglycerin
Radiation	
	Medial aspect of left arm
	Left shoulder
	Jaw
	Occasionally right arm

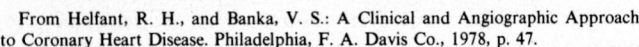

From Helfant, R. H., and Banka, V. S.: A Clinical and Angiographic Approach to Coronary Heart Disease. Philadelphia, F. A. Davis Co., 1978, p. 47.

precision the amount of physical activity that causes angina, e.g., walking up exactly two and a half flights of stairs. When these patients are tested on a treadmill or bicycle, the pressure-rate product that elicits angina and/or electrocardiographic evidence of ischemia is fixed or almost so. Patients with *variable-threshold angina,* who may or may not have a fixed obstructive lesion but in whom dynamic obstruction caused by vasoconstriction plays an important role in causing myocardial ischemia, typically have "good days," when they are capable of substantial physical activity, and "bad days," when even minimal activity can cause clinical and/or electrocardiographic evidence of myocardial ischemia or when angina occurs at rest. Often, even in the course of a single day, they may be capable of substantial physical activity at one time, while at another time minimal activity will result in angina. Patients with variable-threshold angina typically complain occasionally of angina at rest, nocturnal angina, and angina precipitated by the cold, emotion, and meals. It is presumed that coronary vasoconstriction is responsible for or contributes to the development of angina under all these circumstances. The anginal threshold tends to be lower in the morning than in the afternoon, correlating with the angiographic finding of smaller coronary arterial lumina at that time of day.[25] Many patients fall between these two extremes (Fig. 39–1), i.e., their anginal threshold is moderately variable; the term *mixed angina* is suggested to describe this large group.

Changes in the blood pressure–heart rate product (the double product) provide a rough approximation of myocardial oxygen requirements (p. 1238). In patients with effort-induced fixed-threshold angina, the threshold at which ischemia develops (as reflected in angina and ST-segment depression) is a function of myocardial oxygen requirement. In patients with (relatively) fixed-threshold angina, the time and effort required for the development of angina during treadmill exercise is relatively predictable and reproducible; it is probable that as the performance of the ventricle (and therefore its oxygen consumption) increases, a point is reached at which myocardial perfusion distal to a major coronary arterial obstruction can no longer increase, and ischemia ensues.

Observations in patients experiencing angina under circumstances other than exercise help to explain the pathophysiological bases of angina. For example, some patients with ischemic heart disease characteristically experience angina on exposure to *cold weather* or *during or after meals.* A cold environment has been shown to increase peripheral resistance at rest and during exercise.[26] The rise in arterial pressure, by augmenting myocardial oxygen requirements, lowers the threshold for the development of angina. An alternative, or additional, explanation is the development of coronary spasm.[27,28] The reduction in exercise capacity during or after meals has been explained by a more rapid rise in heart rate and blood pressure compared to preprandial values,[29] but the postprandial increase in myocardial oxygen needs may not be sufficient to explain the development of ischemia, and a dynamic component, i.e., coronary vasoconstriction, may also be involved.[30] Similarly, during angina induced by *emotional stress,* heart rate and blood pressure and therefore myocardial oxygen needs rise but usually not to the level required to produce angina during exercise. Therefore, a dynamic component probably plays a role as well.[31]

Relief of anginal discomfort is usually afforded by rest (not by "walking through") and by sublingual nitroglycerin; indeed, the response to the drug is often a useful diagnostic tool.[32] A longer delay before relief is obtained, i.e., more than 5 to 10 minutes, suggests that the pain is not ischemic in origin. As described by Levine, carotid sinus pressure can also often bring about rapid alleviation of discomfort.[33]

In *atypical angina* the precipitating factors may be similar, but the quality of the discomfort is different (sharp and stabbing, for example); or, if the quality of the discomfort is angina-like, the precipitating causes are unusual, such as varying body positions; or the discomfort may be typical in quality and occur only at rest but may not be accompanied by characteristic ST-segment changes. *Nonanginal chest pain* has neither the quality of typical angina nor its usual precipitating causes.

CLINICAL-PATHOLOGICAL CORRELATIONS OF ANGINA. The prevalence of coronary artery disease in subsets of patients with typical angina, atypical angina, and nonanginal chest pain has been estimated by Diamond and Forrester to be about 90 per cent, 50 per cent, and 16 per cent, respectively, while the prevalence of coronary artery disease in asymptomatic adults of comparable age is estimated to be 3 to 4 per cent.[34] Pasternak et al. reported that among 3242 patients in whom coronary angiograms were obtained for chest pain, 175 (5.4%) had essentially normal coronary vessels. Of the latter, about one-third had chest pain typical of angina and in two-thirds it was atypical.[35] There is a suggestion from a number of reports[36–39] that on the whole the clinical manifestations of ischemia may be more severe in patients with multivessel than single-vessel disease, but in any individual patient the nature of the underlying disease cannot be predicted from the severity, nature, duration, or quality of the discomfort. Perhaps the best examples of this lack of clinical-pathological correlation are two groups of patients who are relatively common: those with advanced obstructive disease and so-called "silent ischemia"[40–42] (p. 1362) and those with Prinzmetal's angina (p. 1360). For comparable degrees of obstructive coronary artery disease, as defined arteriographically, asymptomatic or minimally symptomatic patients have a better prognosis than do those with severe angina.[42] When infarction (without angina) is the first manifestation of ischemic heart disease, it is usually associated with single-vessel disease; when angina occurs before and/or after infarction, two- or three-vessel disease is usually present.[43]

Differential Diagnosis of Chest Pain
(Table 1–1, p. 5)

The differentiation of various disorders from coronary artery disease is challenging because the severity of the chest pain and the seriousness of the underlying disorder are not necessarily related. Compounding the difficulty in differential diagnosis is the common myth that pain in the left arm or left side of the chest is an ominous sign signifying the presence of coronary artery disease. A host of disorders can cause these types of discomfort.[20] *Esophagitis* can produce discomfort that can mimic that of myocardial ischemia because it is usually substernal in location and may have a "burning" component. Because there is usually an element of esophageal spasm, discomfort is often relieved by nitroglycerin or, unlike angina, by milk or antacids as well. Acid infusion studies, radiological studies, and esophagoscopy are helpful in confirming the diagnosis of this disorder.[44] Gastric reflux is often associated with *hiatus hernia,* which can also be diagnosed radiographically; postprandial distress is most marked in the recumbent position, and this feature helps to differentiate it from angina pectoris.[45] Distention of the splenic flexure of the colon can mimic anginal pain, but, unlike angina, relief of symptoms often follows a bowel movement. The major *musculoskeletal disorders* that can mimic angina include subacromial bursitis and costochondritis.[46] Cervical radiculitis may occur as a constant ache, often resulting in a sensory deficit. The pain may be related to motion of the neck, just as motion of the shoulder triggers attacks of pain that are due to *bursitis.* The full-blown *Tietze syndrome,* i.e., painful swelling of the costochondral junctions, is uncommon, whereas costochondritis causing tenderness of the costochondral joints is relatively common[47]; pain on palpation of these joints is a useful clinical sign. Physical examination may also detect pain brought about by movement of an arthritic shoulder, a calcified shoulder tendon, and the like. Occasionally, pain mimicking angina can be due to compression of the brachial plexus by a cervical rib.

Other cardiovascular diseases may also mimic angina pectoris. In addition to *aortic dissection,* which usually is characterized by sharp, intense, retrosternal pain with radiation to the back (p. 1550), *pulmonary hypertension* may also be a problem in differential diagnosis (p. 840). The discomfort produced by the latter is generally precordial and, although often precipitated by exertion, is usually more persistent than angina. Pulmonary hypertension must be severe to cause chest pain and may be readily recognized by the findings of right ventricular hypertrophy on physical examination and electrocardiography. The discomfort that is perhaps most difficult to differentiate from angina is that produced by *acute pericarditis* (p. 1474), which is usually relieved by sitting up and leaning forward and is intensified by the supine posture. A friction rub often helps to confirm the diagnosis.

In many of the disorders just mentioned, angina pectoris can usually be excluded by a careful history and physical examination. Brief episodes of sharp, stabbing pain or continual dull aches of a burning or boring quality commonly observed with gastrointestinal disorders are not characteristic of angina, nor is the response to antacids or eating. On the other hand, the major point in differentiating between angina and musculoskeletal disorders usually relates to an abnormality found on physical examination, with tenderness either on palpation or on movement of the affected part. It must be stressed, however, that ischemic heart disease can and frequently does *coexist* with any of these other disorders and that occasionally noncardiac disease can trigger a true anginal attack in a patient with coronary artery disease. For example, the sympathoadrenal discharge that accompanies biliary colic may increase heart rate and blood pressure and thereby increase myocardial oxygen requirements, so that myocardial ischemia may develop in a patient with obstructive coronary artery disease.

Chest Pain with Normal Coronary Arteriogram

The syndrome of angina or angina-like chest pain with a normal coronary arteriogram is an important clinical entity to be differentiated from classic ischemic heart disease caused by coronary atherosclerosis.[35,48–55] In this condition, the prognosis is usually excellent—contrasted with that in patients with coronary atherosclerosis—and hence its recognition is of critical importance. Patients with chest pain who have normal coronary arteries may constitute as many as 20 per cent of individuals undergoing coronary arteriography because of the strong suspicion of angina. The etiology of the syndrome is unknown. True myocardial ischemia, reflected in the production of lactate by the myocardium during exercise or pacing, is present in only a small fraction of these patients. However, in one study, the increase in coronary blood flow following dipyridamole, a potent coronary vasodilator, was found to be reduced, and this inability to augment coronary blood flow was associated with a decline of left ventricular function during exercise; presumably an abnormality of the small arteries was responsible for the angina and ischemia.[54] Some patients with angina and normal coronary arteries are found on extensive investigation to have a cardiomyopathy—either hypertrophic or congestive—and in these cases reduced perfusion, especially of the subendocardium, may be responsible for myocardial ischemia and resultant angina.[55] Herman et al. discussed some of the theories proffered for this syndrome; an abnormal oxyhemoglobin dissociation curve, misinterpretation of arteriography, occult cardiomyopathy, and psychomotor factors.[51] Patients with psychogenic chest pain, neurocirculatory asthenia, and Da Costa's syndrome (p. 6) also fall into this category. These patients are not considered to have coronary spasm because of the absence of a typical response to ergonovine (p. 1361); they rarely develop acute myocardial infarction, but if they do, their long-term prognosis tends to be favorable because they do not have diffuse coronary artery disease. The syndrome of angina or angina-like chest pain occurs more frequently in women, while obstructive coronary artery disease is far more common in men. Fewer than half the patients with chest pain with normal coronary arteriograms have typical angina; the majority have a variety of forms of atypical chest pain.

Abnormal physical findings such as precordial bulges, gallop sounds, and murmurs of mitral regurgitation are uncommon. The resting electrocardiogram may be normal, but nonspecific ST-T abnormalities are often observed. A minority, approximately 20 per cent of the patients with chest pain and normal coronary arteriograms, have positive exercise tests. Left ventricular function is usually normal at rest and after pacing,[56–58] unlike the situation in obstructive coronary artery disease in which function is or becomes impaired during stress. However, a small number of these patients exhibit lactate production and electrocardiographic changes (ST-segment depression) during stress, signifying ischemia, for as yet unexplained reasons. Myocardial perfusion studies have not shown any consistent pattern of abnormal myocardial blood flow,[59,60] although coronary vasodilator reserve may be impaired.[52,54] *Management* of patients with this syndrome is focused on the explanation of the relatively benign nature of the condition to the patient, psychological counseling, and analgesics to provide pain relief. However, many of these patients continue to remain disabled with chest discomfort despite these measures.[51]

Physical Examination of the Patient with Chronic Stable Angina

General physical examination of the patient with chronic ischemic heart disease and angina pectoris may be entirely normal or may reveal the presence of risk factors for the development of coronary atherosclerosis. Thus, the blood pressure either may be chronically elevated or may rise acutely (along with the heart rate) during an anginal attack.[61,62] The general examination may also reveal xanthomas suggestive of hypercholesterolemia (p. 17); arcus senilis in patients under 50 years of age also suggests this metabolic abnormality, but this sign is less significant in older persons. Precordial tenderness is uncommon in angina, and the presence of costosternal tenderness suggests that angina is not responsible for the chest discomfort. An interesting finding is the diagonal earlobe crease, reportedly more prevalent in patients with coronary artery disease[63]; however, the interpretation of this sign is controversial.[64] Retinal arteriolar changes are common in patients with coronary artery disease, even in those without diabetes mellitus or hypertension; an abnormal light reflex is the most sensitive sign, while abnormal vessel tortuosity and decreased caliber are less sensitive but more specific signs.[65]

The *cardiac examination,* long considered of little help in the diagnosis of chronic coronary artery disease, especially in patients with only a history of angina pectoris, actually may supply useful clues to both the diagnosis of ischemic heart disease and the functional state of the myocardium. First, the presence of murmurs of hypertrophic obstructive cardiomyopathy or aortic valve disease suggests that the ischemic chest pain may be due to conditions other than, or in addition to, coronary artery disease. Second, certain findings suggest ischemia as the basis for the chest pain if other obvious cardiac diseases are absent. A prime example is the presence of a third or a loud fourth heart sound,[66,67] and the presence of prominent early diastolic or presystolic filling waves on the apexcardiogram. Although these are common findings in patients with angina at rest,[66] their frequency is increased during handgrip exercise,[68] even if the latter does not precipitate angina pectoris. These sounds and pulsations are related to the functional state of the left ventricle, particularly its pressure and compliance during diastole (p. 50)[66–69]; their absence does not exclude significant coronary atherosclerosis but instead suggests the absence of left ventricular dysfunction. Although the specificity of the fourth heart sound as a finding diagnostic of cardiac disease has been questioned, since it is heard in many apparently normal subjects over 45 years of age,[70,71] we agree with Tavel[72] that a clear, loud fourth heart sound accompanied by a palpable presystolic wave is an abnormal finding. It is not specific for ischemic heart disease but may also be elicited in other conditions associated with left ventricular hypertrophy, like aortic stenosis and hypertension, in which left ventricular compliance is reduced. Paradoxical splitting of the second heart sound may occur transiently during an anginal attack. It appears to be related to asynergy and prolongation of left ventricular contraction. Abnormal left ventricular function may also be documented by abnormalities in systolic time intervals, i.e., prolongation of the preejection period (PEP), shortening of the systolic ejection period (SEP), and an increase in PEP/SEP (p. 55).

When patients with ischemic heart disease lie in the left lateral recumbent position, dyskinetic bulges at the apex may be palpated or recorded by means of apexcardiography (p. 62); the bulges correspond to dyskinetic areas and often complement the auscultatory findings of diastolic filling sounds. Transient or persistent apical systolic murmurs are quite common and have been attributed to papillary muscle dysfunction secondary to myocardial ischemia.[67] They are more prevalent in patients with extensive coronary artery disease, especially those with prior myocardial infarction and left ventricular dysfunction. The systolic murmur may assume a variety of configurations (early, late, or holosystolic) and may be accentuated by exertion or during angina. A midsystolic click, often followed by a late systolic murmur characteristic of mitral valve prolapse produced by papillary muscle dysfunction (p. 1076), also occurs in patients with coronary artery disease.[73] A diastolic murmur or a continuous murmur is a rare finding and has been attributed to turbulent flow across a proximal coronary artery stenosis.[74]

ELECTROCARDIOGRAM. The resting electrocardiogram is normal in one-fourth to one-half of patients with chronic stable angina pectoris, depending on the incidence of previous myocardial infarction in the particular series of patients.[75] Patients with normal tracings may have severe angina, but they usually have not previously suffered large infarctions. When the electrocardiogram is abnormal, the most common findings are nonspecific ST-T changes with or without evidence of prior transmural infarction; however, a variety of conduction disturbances, most frequently left bundle branch block and left anterior divisional block, have also been reported. However, these are nonspecific signs and occur in many conditions other than ischemic heart disease. A variety of arrhythmias, especially ventricular premature beats, may be present, but they too are nonspecific. P-wave abnormalities indicative of left atrial enlargement are frequently associated with impairment of left ventricular contractility. Q waves are specific although insensitive indicators of abnormal wall motion. Correlation between the electrocardiographic pattern of myocardial infarction and total obstruction of the coronary artery perfusing that segment of the ventricle is excellent.[76]

NONINVASIVE STRESS TESTING

The contemporary approach to the use of noninvasive stress testing in the diagnosis and evaluation of patients with known or suspected ischemic heart disease has been well summarized by Gibson and Beller.[77] For appropriate application of noninvasive tests, it is important to consider Bayes theorem (p. 273), which states that while the reliability of any test is defined by its sensitivity and specificity,* its predictability depends on the prevalence of the disease in the population under study (Fig. 39–2). In interpreting the results of stress tests for the diagnosis of

*For definition of these terms; see page 273.

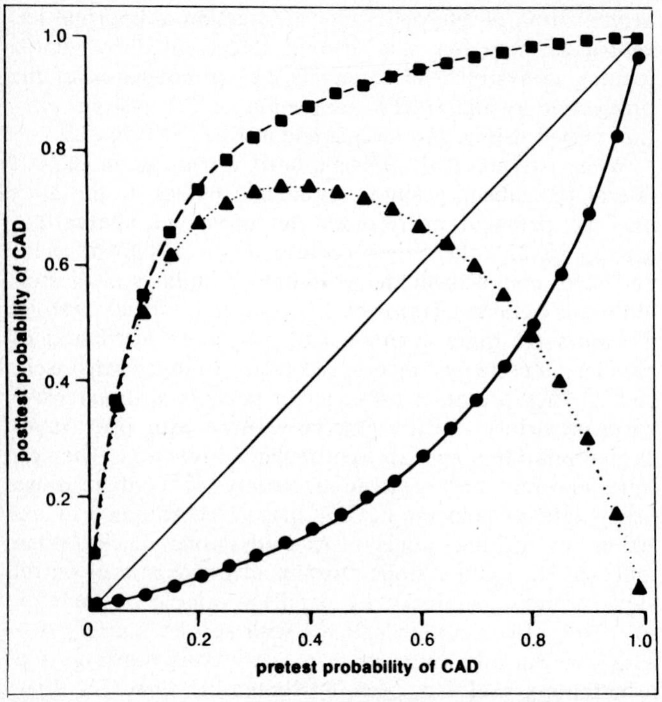

FIGURE 39–2 Pre- and posttest probability of CAD for abnormal and normal results of exercise-redistribution thallium-201 scintigraphy. The curve describing the difference between posttest probability of a normal and abnormal test result indicates the range of disease prevalence for which ^{201}Tl at exercise and redistribution discriminates most effectively between the presence and absence of disease. ^{201}Tl stress scintigraphy is most useful when the pretest prevalence of CAD is 20 to 60 per cent. *Example*: In a patient with a pretest probability of CAD of 60 per cent, a positive ^{201}Tl stress test increases the probability of CAD to about 95 per cent, but a negative test decreases it to about 25 per cent. On the other hand, at a very high or very low pretest probability of disease, not much will be gained by either a positive or a negative test result. ■ = abnormal; ▲ = posttest probability difference; ● = normal. (From Hamilton, G. W., et al.: Semin. Nucl. Med. *8*:358, 1978.)

ischemic heart disease, it is vital to consider the patient population being studied, i.e., the estimated prevalence of the disease *prior* to testing. Thus, if the pretest likelihood of the patient having coronary artery disease is low (less than 15 per cent), as occurs in asymptomatic persons or patients with so-called nonanginal chest pain, a normal result on any of the three commonly employed noninvasive tests (exercise electrocardiography, stress myocardial perfusion scintigraphy, and stress radionuclide angiography) may be used to exclude coronary disease. However, when a positive test in these individuals is a false-positive response, as often occurs, a second noninvasive test is indicated; if it too is positive, coronary artery disease is likely. On the other hand, when the pretest likelihood of disease is high, approximately 85 per cent, as in patients with typical angina pectoris, a positive test is helpful in that it confirms the disease and often provides an indication of its severity.[77] An unexpected negative result does not exclude the diagnosis of coronary disease; under these circumstances, a second or third noninvasive test would be of value, since it might identify the first test as being falsely negative. On the other hand, if the second test is also negative, reevaluation of the patient is clearly in order. Maximal benefit from noninvasive diagnostic testing is obtained when the pretest likelihood for disease is approximately 50 per cent, as in patients with atypical angina pectoris. In them, a positive test raises the likelihood of significant coronary artery disease to approximately 85 per cent and a negative test reduces it to 15 per cent.

EXERCISE ELECTROCARDIOGRAPHY (p. 267). The recording of an electrocardiogram during and after exercise, especially if angina is precipitated, can be a valuable adjunct in the evaluation of patients suspected of having ischemic heart disease[78,79]; this important technique is the subject of Chapter 8. The degree of ST-segment depression has been combined with the configuration, time of onset, and persistence of depression during treadmill testing to increase the sensitivity and specificity of the test.[80] Early onset of ST-segment depression, its long persistence following exercise, and most importantly its shape, i.e., the slope of the segment (Fig. 39–3), are all strongly associated with extensive coronary artery disease (Table 39–2). Increases in R-wave height with exercise in one or more leads, possibly reflecting an increase in left ventricular volume, are often associated with coronary artery disease and left ventricular dysfunction.[81]

There is increasing interest in *nonelectrocardiographic findings* during exercise testing as indicators of severe coronary artery disease. In particular, attention has been called to the development of hypotension as important in predicting the presence of coronary artery disease.[82,83] Multifactorial approaches are being utilized[84–86] that include both electrocardiographic and nonelectrocardiographic measurements, such as the duration of the test and the heart rate response, to improve the accuracy of the exercise test. The occurrence of chest pain early during the test has been correlated with increased risk of future myocardial infarction and coronary death[87] and appears to be an-

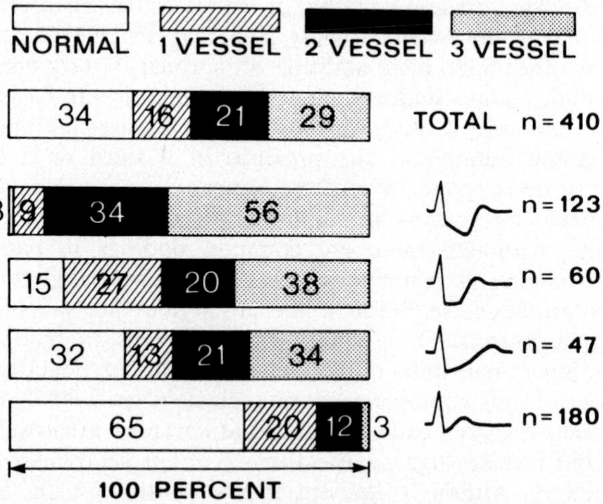

FIGURE 39–3 Relation between the type of ST-segment response in an exercise test and the extent of coronary artery disease. All numbers represent percentages. The total study population is represented at the top. Downsloping ST segments are highly specific for coronary disease, with only one false-positive response (0.8 per cent) encountered; most patients with this response (90 per cent) have double- and triple-vessel involvement. Neither the horizontal nor the slowly upsloping ST segments aid in identifying severe disease. A small percentage (15 per cent) of patients with entirely normal treadmill tests have double- and triple-vessel disease. (From Goldschlager, N., et al.: Treadmill stress tests as indicators of presence and severity of coronary artery disease. Ann. Intern. Med. *85*: 277, 1976.)

TABLE 39–2 CAUSES OF FALSE-POSITIVE EXERCISE ST-SEGMENT RESPONSE

1. Abnormality in baseline ECG at rest due to digitalis, left ventricular hypertrophy, Wolff-Parkinson-White syndrome and other preexcitation variants, hypokalemia, bundle branch block, or vasoregulatory asthenia.
2. Failure before exercise to exclude hyperventilation-induced ST abnormality, recent food intake, or anemia.
3. ECG baseline instability during test simulating ST-segment displacement.
4. Sudden excessive exercise with excessive double product.
5. Various cardiac disorders, such as valvular or congenital heart disease, cardiomyopathy, mitral valve prolapse syndrome, hypertension, hypertrophic obstructive cardiomyopathy, and pericardial disorders.

Exercise Test Variables Associated with Multivessel Coronary Artery Disease and Increased Risk for Subsequent Myocardial Infarction or Sudden Death

ST-segment response:
1. 2 mm or more horizontal or downsloping ST-segment depression at heart rate ≤ 130 beats/min.
2. Postexercise ST-segment depression persisting ≥ 5 min.

Systolic blood pressure response to progressive exercise:
1. Flat response (< 10 mm Hg rise for 2 stages).
2. Sustained decrease of ≥ 10 mm Hg.

Exercise capacity:
1. Inability to complete stage II of Bruce protocol or equivalent.
2. Maximal heart rate < 70 per cent of age-predicted maximum.

Frequent or complex ventricular arrhythmias at low heart rate.

From Gibson, R. S., and Beller, G. A.: Should exercise electrocardiographic testing be replaced by radioisotope methods? *In* Rahimtoola, S. H. (ed.): Controversies in Coronary Artery Disease. Philadelphia, F. A. Davis Co., 1983, p. 1–31.

other useful diagnostic feature. In patients with coronary arteriographically proven ischemic heart disease, survival correlated directly with the duration of exercise that the patient could tolerate[79] and with the time during the test at which ST-segment depression occurred (Figs. 8–11, p. 274, and 8–12, p. 275).

The exercise test is also useful for exposing ventricular ectopic activity[88] but is less sensitive in this regard than is *ambulatory electrocardiographic monitoring* for 24 hours.[89] Patients with the more severe forms of coronary artery disease and abnormal left ventricular function have been shown to have a greater prevalence of exercise-induced arrhythmias.[90,91] Ambulatory electrocardiographic monitoring can also document the presence of ischemia in patients with coronary artery disease, with a good correlation between ST-segment depression occurring during normal activity and severe arteriographic abnormalities having been reported[92]; pain often does not accompany the ST-segment depression.[93] However, false-positive responses in patients free of coronary artery disease limit the usefulness of ambulatory 24-hour monitoring.[94]

In 16 studies summarized by Gibson and Beller in which results of exercise electrocardiography and coronary arteriography were compared, the overall sensitivity of the former test averaged 64 per cent and the specificity 89 per cent.[77] The extent of coronary artery disease affects the sensitivity of the test, i.e., the test is substantially more sensitive as the number of involved coronary vessels increases, rising from 44 per cent in patients with one-vessel disease to 85 per cent in patients with three-vessel and left main coronary artery disease. Thus, in view of the relatively low sensitivity of the test, a negative result does not rule out ischemic heart disease; however, it does make three-vessel or left main disease much less likely. Conversely, an adequate maximum exercise test, one achieving more than 85 per cent of the predicted maximal heart rate, is unlikely to miss significant three-vessel or left main coronary artery disease. In normal asymptomatic persons, the incidence of false-positive exercise electrocardiograms is relatively high, approximately 40 per cent. Although the test is not very helpful for evaluating individual asymptomatic individuals, it is of great value in epidemiological studies, since *groups* of asymptomatic and apparently normal persons with a positive test are at much higher risk of developing overt coronary disease in the future than are those with negative tests.

A major limitation of the sensitivity of the exercise electrocardiogram is that it cannot be interpreted in many patients, including patients who are incapable of reaching the level of exercise required for near-maximal effort (85 per cent or more of maximal predicted heart rate), particularly those on propranolol or those who develop fatigue, leg cramps, or dyspnea, and patients with abnormalities in the baseline electrocardiogram, including those on digitalis (Table 39–2). The findings on exercise electrocardiograms in patients with multivessel coronary artery disease and those at high risk for subsequent myocardial infarctions and sudden death are shown in Table 39–2.

STRESS THALLIUM-201 MYOCARDIAL PERFUSION IMAGING (p. 369). In this technique, the radionuclide is injected at peak exercise and the image is obtained several minutes later when the patient is at rest; it demonstrates the regional perfusion pattern that existed during the stress of exercise. Defects represent either areas of stress-induced impairment of blood flow or infarction. If a delayed image is obtained 2 to 3 hours later and the initial defect persists, it is probably due to an infarction. On the other hand, if it exhibits delayed uptake, it represents an area of ischemic, transiently hypoperfused but viable myocardium.

In a summary of 22 published studies involving more than 2000 patients, the stress thallium-201 scintigram was usually superior to the exercise electrocardiogram, with a sensitivity of 83 per cent (compared with 73 per cent for the electrocardiogram) and a specificity of 90 per cent (compared with 82 per cent).[77,95] In patients with single-vessel coronary artery disease, the sensitivity of the electrocardiographic exercise test is particularly low, but this is not the case for thallium scintigraphy. Thallium defects in two or three vascular segments correctly predict multivessel disease in approximately 75 per cent of patients. Failure of normal redistribution into a defect is usually associated with wall motion abnormalities and with irreversible asynergy after a premature ventricular contraction on ventriculography, while asynergic segments at rest with redistribution on postexercise scintigrams usually show transient reversibility of the wall motion defect as well.[96] Patients with multiple defects of the redistribution type, with abnormal lung uptake during exercise-induced ischemia, reflecting a sudden rise in left ventricular diastolic pressure,[97,97a] are at particularly high risk for subsequent ischemic events. The thallium-perfusion defect can also be used to predict the ejection fraction[98] and the potential reversibility of perfusion abnormalities following surgical treatment.[99]

EXERCISE RADIONUCLIDE ANGIOGRAPHY (p. 365). In this test, measurements of ejection fraction and of regional wall motion are obtained both at rest and at increasing workloads.[100,100a,100b,100c] In a summary of 12 published studies comprising 771 patients, Gibson and Beller reported that the radionuclide angiogram had both sensitivity and specificity of approximately 90 per cent when both failure of a rise in ejection fraction and presence of a new regional wall motion abnormality were required for the test to be deemed positive.[77] (It is important to include exercise-induced regional wall motion abnormalities in order to define a positive exercise radionuclide angiogram, since the ejection fraction may fail to rise in patients with conditions other than ischemic heart disease, including cardiomyopathies, valvular heart disease, or hypertension, and in normal individuals receiving propranolol.)

The greater sensitivity of the two radionuclide techniques, i.e., exercise radionuclide angiography and stress thallium perfusion scintigraphy, compared to exercise electrocardiography, is probably related to the fact that abnormalities of perfusion and left ventricular contraction occur at a lower ischemic threshold than does exercise-induced ST-segment depression. Both radionuclide techniques are superior to exercise electrocardiography primarily because they allow evaluation of patients with electrocardiographic abnormalities at rest and of those who are unable to achieve adequate levels of exercise (Table 39–2).[100]

The sensitivity and specificity of both radionuclide techniques have been found to be similar in seven studies, comprising a total of 391 patients.[77] There is no consensus as to which of the two tests should be carried out first. We prefer to obtain the stress thallium-201 scintigram initially, since exercise radionuclide angiography can usually be performed on the same day after myocardial perfusion scintigraphy if the need arises, whereas the converse is not possible.

CLINICAL APPLICATION OF NONINVASIVE TESTS. In asymptomatic persons or in those with nonanginal chest pain who are being screened or evaluated for coronary artery disease, i.e., patients in whom the pretest likelihood of coronary disease is low (less than 15 per cent), a negative exercise electrocardiogram generally provides sufficient information to confirm the absence of ischemic heart disease; a positive test result should be followed by a thallium perfusion scan. When both of these tests are abnormal, the likelihood of significant coronary artery disease exceeds 80 per cent; however, if there is a discrepancy in the results of the two tests, either coronary arteriography or radionuclide angiography (and arteriography if the result is positive) is in order.

In patients with *atypical angina,* if two noninvasive tests are abnormal, the likelihood of coronary artery disease exceeds 95 per cent; if both tests are normal, this likelihood falls below 5 per cent. Results of noninvasive stress tests are independent of each other, and whenever they are discordant, a third noninvasive test will often be helpful. Also, when test results are discordant, they should be evaluated in the light of the level of exercise achieved as well as the degree of positivity (e.g., the presence of accompanying symptoms, the depth of the ST-segment response, the heart rate at which it occurred, and the persistence of the ST-segment response on the stress electrocardiogram; the size and number of perfusion defects on the stress perfusion scintigram; and the magnitude of the exercise-induced change in ejection fraction and regional wall motion disorder on the exercise radionuclide angiogram). Thus, a patient with a normal exercise electrocardiogram who develops multiple large perfusion defects on a thallium-201 scintigram (accompanied by chest pain at a heart rate of 160 beats/min) is more likely to have ischemic heart disease than one who has a normal exercise electrocardiogram and develops a single small perfusion defect without chest pain at a heart rate of 195 beats/min.

In patients with *typical angina* (i.e., those with a high pretest likelihood of disease) noninvasive testing is most valuable for establishing the extent and severity of underlying coronary artery disease. The development of exertional hypotension, marked or prolonged ST-segment depression at low work levels and/or heart rate, striking decreases in ejection fraction and wall motion, and large or multiple defects on the exercise thallium scintigram all point to severe multivessel disease in patients at high risk of subsequent coronary events, including sudden death.[101]

OTHER LABORATORY TESTS

In patients with angina pectoris, the *echocardiogram* may show abnormalities of motion of the septum and posterior wall, corresponding to obstruction of the left anterior descending and right or left circumflex coronary arteries, respectively (Fig. 5–64, p. 125).[102,103] These abnormalities are particularly marked in patients who have had a myocardial infarction in those regions. However, the areas of the ventricle that can be imaged by the conventional M-mode echocardiogram are limited; the apex and inferior and lateral walls of the left ventricle are usually missed. Larger sections of the ventricle can be visualized by two-dimensional echocardiography (p. 93),[104] and this technique is of substantial value for defining noninvasively those areas of the left ventricle which show abnormal wall motion and for assessing left ventricular function (Fig. 5–65, p. 126). Serial tracings often reveal disorders of wall motion as ischemia waxes or wanes. Two-dimensional echocardiography is also useful for defining obstructive lesions of the left main coronary artery.[105]

Serum levels of cardiac enzymes are normal in angina pectoris and serve to differentiate these patients from those with acute myocardial infarction. One of the striking features of chronic ischemic heart disease in relatively young persons is the frequency with which certain metabolic abnormalities are detected. Since *hyperlipidemia* and *carbohydrate intolerance* are recognized as risk factors for the development of ischemic heart disease, this finding is not unexpected, and the prevalence of these abnormalities, particularly in patients under the age of 50 years, is impressive (Chap. 35). Two studies found that over 90 per cent of patients under the age of 50 years with angiographically proven ischemic heart disease had either carbohydrate intolerance or Type II or IV hyperlipoproteinemia.[106,107]

The *chest roentgenogram* is usually within normal limits in patients with chronic ischemic heart disease. However, coronary artery calcification detected fluoroscopically may be more diagnostic of coronary artery disease than was once thought, especially in young people.[108,109] More than 90 per cent of patients with coronary artery calcification were found to have critical coronary artery obstruction;

however, coronary calcification on fluoroscopy is not a very sensitive test, since it is found in only 40 per cent of patients with angiographically documented coronary artery disease.[108] When fluoroscopic evidence of coronary calcification is present in combination with a positive exercise test, the probability of finding coronary artery disease on subsequent coronary angiography is very high.[34]

CATHETERIZATION, ANGIOGRAPHY, AND CORONARY ARTERIOGRAPHY

Although the clinical examination and noninvasive techniques described above are valuable, the definitive diagnosis of coronary artery disease and a precise assessment of its anatomical severity and its effects on cardiac performance and myocardial metabolism require cardiac catheterization (Chap. 9), left ventricular angiography (Chap. 6), and coronary arteriography (Chap. 10). Among patients with chronic stable angina pectoris, coronary arteriography usually reveals relatively equal distribution (approximately 25 per cent each) of one-, two-, and three-vessel disease; about 5 to 10 per cent of patients have obstruction of the left main coronary artery, and in approximately 15 per cent no critical obstruction is detectable (p. 1338). Total occlusion of at least one major coronary artery is more common in patients with chronic angina who have had prior infarctions than in those without infarction.[43]

Coronary artery ectasia, i.e., aneurysmal dilatation, is present in approximately 5 per cent of patients with ischemic heart disease. This angiographic lesion does not appear to affect either survival or the incidence of myocardial infarction; it is considered to be a variant of coronary atherosclerosis rather than a distinct clinical entity.[110] *Coronary collaterals* are observed only when there is 50 to 75 per cent stenosis* of a coronary artery, but in 15 to 20 per cent of patients with this degree of stenosis, no collaterals are visible.[111] The functional significance of collateral vessels is unclear (p. 1267).[112,113] When they are well developed, coronary collaterals may be adequate to protect against resting ischemia but may fail to meet the increased needs of exercise and therefore may not reduce the frequency or severity of angina. Also, patients with abundant collaterals appear to suffer smaller myocardial infarctions.[114,115] On the basis of canine experiments, it is not clear whether or not exercise alters the development of collaterals.[116,117]

Diastolic ventricular performance, as reflected in the early diastolic ventricular filling rate, is abnormally reduced at rest in many patients with chronic stable angina, even when systolic performance, as reflected in the ejection fraction, is normal. Diastolic filling becomes even more abnormal during exercise.[118]

The frequency of abnormal elevations of left ventricular end-diastolic pressure and of reduced cardiac output increases with the number of vessels exhibiting critical narrowing and with the number of prior infarctions,[119] but there is a great deal of overlap among individual patients[120] so that the severity of coronary arterial or left ventricular disease cannot be predicted from this measurement. The left ventricular end-diastolic pressure may be elevated because of reduced ventricular compliance, left ventricular failure, or a combination of these two processes[121–123]; both reduced compliance and left ventricular failure may occur as a consequence of acute ischemia and chronic scar formation. The elevation of left ventricular diastolic pressure has its clinical correlate in the presence of diastolic (third and fourth) heart sounds.

In the resting state, i.e., in the absence of active or recent ischemia, hemodynamic abnormalities in patients with chronic stable angina usually reflect the presence of prior myocardial infarction, but in many patients with normal hemodynamics in the basal state, abnormalities of left ventricular function can be elicited by dynamic or static exercise.[124,125] Elevations of left ventricular end-diastolic pressure usually occur *before* the patient complains of chest discomfort and before there is electrocardiographic ST-segment depression.

Pacing-induced and post-pacing angina can also be observed in the catheterization laboratory (Fig. 39–4, p. 1344). This form of stress testing is especially useful for combined hemodynamic-metabolic-ventriculographic studies[126] because quantitative left ventricular angiography and myocardial lactate metabolism can be studied during or immediately after pacing, uncomplicated by an elevation of systemic arterial lactate levels, as occurs in dynamic exercise. When atrial pacing to induce ischemia is carried out in patients with chronic angina secondary to chronic obstructive coronary artery disease, elevations in ventricular end-diastolic pressure occur frequently and usually in association with the development of typical anginal discomfort at a reproducible heart rate–blood pressure product.[126,127] Impaired ventricular relaxation and increased regional myocardial stiffness have also been demonstrated during pacing-induced ischemia[128] and may be one component of the altered diastolic properties of the ischemic ventricle (p. 1246).

Abnormalities of left ventricular wall motion on biplane left ventriculography (asynergy) occur in approximately two-thirds of patients with ischemic heart disease and chronic stable angina pectoris, often in conjunction with abnormal hemodynamic findings (Fig. 10–48, p. 339).[129] Asynergy in the basal state is usually due to necrotic tissue, reflecting prior infarction, and there is a good correlation between electrocardiographic evidence of infarction (Q waves) and corresponding regional asynergy.[130,131] In many other patients with chronic ischemic heart disease, areas of abnormal wall motion are apparent only after ischemia is induced acutely—as with atrial pacing[132] or with exercise[133] —and the asynergy is "reversible," that is, it reverts to normal when the ischemic episode ceases.

The potential reversibility of localized asynergy evident on the basal ventriculogram has become the center of intensive investigation using several approaches. The purpose of these studies has been to devise techniques to distinguish between areas that are irreversibly damaged as a result of infarction and those that are "stunned,"[134] i.e., reversibly ischemic, even in the absence of angina or acute electrocardiographic changes. Techniques to identify the latter areas, i.e., to study the "contractile reserve" of the left ventricle, make use of inotropic stimulation (epinephrine and postextrasystolic potentiation[135] as well as preload reduction with nitroglycerin[135,136]). A reversibly damaged portion of the left ventricle begins to contract normally

*Unless otherwise noted, "per cent stenosis" refers to reduction of luminal diameter.

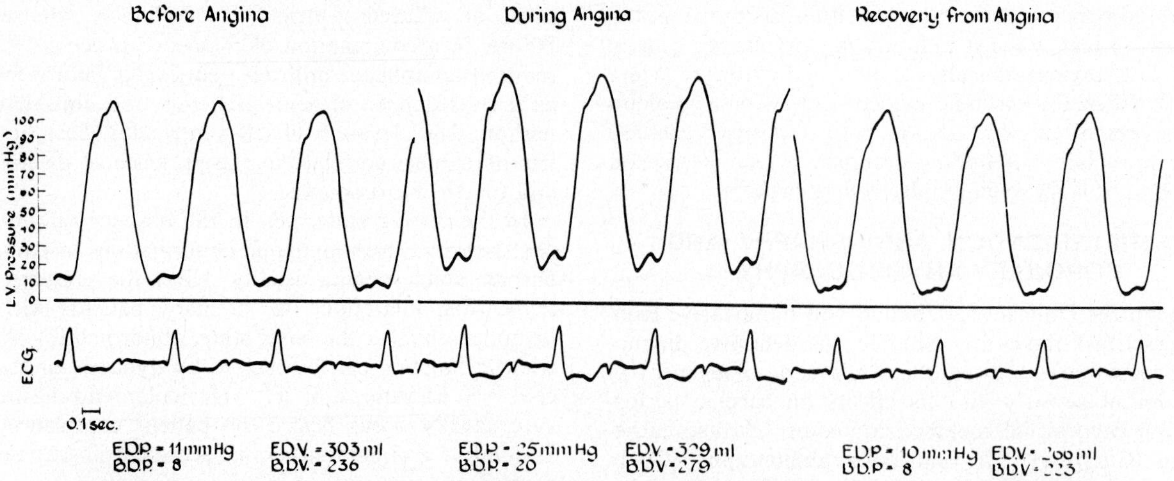

FIGURE 39–4 Records demonstrating changes in left ventricular pressure and an electrocardiographic tracing of a patient before angina, during angina, and after recovery from angina. Angina was produced by a brief period of atrial pacing at 140 beats/min, and the heart rate was maintained at approximately 95 beats/min during pressure recording. The beginning- and end-diastolic pressure (BDP and EDP, respectively) and corresponding ventricular volumes (BDV and EDV, respectively) are noted below each condition. (From Barry, W. H., et al.: Changes in diastolic stiffness and tone of the left ventricle during angina pectoris. Circulation *49*:255, 1974, by permission of the American Heart Association, Inc.)

when these interventions are applied, while irreversibly damaged myocardium does not. Histopathological studies performed on myocardial biopsy specimens obtained at the time of coronary artery bypass operations have demonstrated that those segments which exhibit reversible asynergy at angiography are made up predominantly of histologically normal myocardium, while the nonresponsive segments exhibit marked muscle loss and replacement by fibrous tissue.[137] The more responsive areas are usually better perfused, either by the native coronary artery or by collateral vessels, and are associated with a lower frequency of Q waves on the electrocardiogram.[138] The most severe aspect of left ventricular asynergy is the well-demarcated aneurysm, which not only exhibits contractile failure but also is unable to resist expansion during ventricular systole; in other words, it exhibits dyskinesis (paradoxical pulsation).

In addition to demonstrating areas of asynergy, left ventriculography may also show mitral valve prolapse (p. 1093), which occurs in 20 to 25 per cent of patients with obstructive coronary artery disease[139,140] and probably results from impaired contractility of the ventricular myocardium and papillary muscles.

Abnormal myocardial metabolism has also been documented by means of cardiac catheterization in patients with chronic stable angina. With a catheter in place in the coronary sinus, coronary arteriovenous lactate measurements are obtained at rest and after suitable stresses, such as the infusion of isoproterenol[141] or pacing.[142] Since lactate is a byproduct of anaerobic glycolysis, its production by the heart and subsequent appearance in coronary sinus blood is a sign of myocardial ischemia. When combined with coronary arteriography, this technique may be helpful in localizing significant coronary obstructive lesions and myocardial ischemia.[141]

MYOCARDIAL PERFUSION STUDIES. Several techniques based on washout of radioactive inert gases from the myocardium following injection into the coronary arteries can be used to measure regional myocardial blood flow, as described on page 377. Using these techniques, Cannon et al. have shown reductions in the perfusion of areas of myocardium subserved by totally obstructed coronary arteries compared with areas that are normally perfused. Less striking differences were observed with lesions compromising the lumen by 50 to 90 per cent.[143,144] Coronary blood flow measured by the regional xenon-133 technique has also been shown to be diminished in areas of abnormal ventricular wall motion, both at sites of previous infarction[145] and in noninfarcted regions.[146] This reduction in blood flow can be caused by coronary arterial stenosis or the reduced myocardial oxygen requirements of a noncontracting region or both. Whether any given area with low flow measured by this technique is contracting poorly because of reversible ischemia or is irreversibly damaged by scar formation is unclear, but there is evidence, obtained by means of postextrasystolic potentiation, that in regions with blood flow $\leq$ 50 ml/min/100 g in the basal state, the myocardium usually lacks contractile reserve and is probably irreversibly injured.[147] Atrial pacing has also been used with the xenon-133 technique to accentuate the differences between regions that are normally and poorly perfused in the basal state.[148] Regional myocardial blood flow can also be assessed noninvasively by myocardial perfusion scintigraphy, described in detail on page 369.[149]

MEDICAL MANAGEMENT

The medical management of ischemic heart disease involves four aspects: (1) correction of specific coronary risk factors, discussed in Chapter 35; (2) general and nonpharmacological methods, with particular attention toward adjustment of the patient's lifestyle;[150] (3) various specific medications used to treat angina; and (4) percutaneous transluminal angioplasty.

General Treatment

Fever, anemia, thyrotoxicosis, infection, tachycardia, hypoxemia, and certain drugs used to treat noncardiac diseases (such as amphetamines and isoproterenol mists) all increase myocardial oxygen needs and may precipitate or intensify angina. It is generally appreciated that cigarette smoking, the inhalation of smog, and ascent to high altitudes all lower the threshold for angina. It is less well known that breathing smoke-filled air from *other* people's cigarettes, i.e., passive smoking, may also aggravate angina.[151] These drugs and conditions should be eliminated. Congestive heart failure, by causing cardiac dilatation and cardiac tachyarrhythmias, can increase myocardial oxygen needs, and their treatment, as outlined in Chapters 16 and 21, will frequently diminish the frequency and severity of angina.

Other general measures include the treatment of hypertension (Chap. 27), which not only is a risk factor for the progression of atherosclerosis but also augments myocardial oxygen requirements. Attainment of an ideal weight is particularly important in the obese patient, since weight reduction raises the threshold for the development of angina pectoris.

Effective communication with both the patient and the family is essential. The psychosocial issues faced by the patient who develops chronic stable angina are similar to, though usually less intense than, those experienced by the patient with an acute myocardial infarction, discussed on page 1828. Many patients have an unrealistically gloomy perception of their prognosis; they should be offered a realistic appraisal, together with an understandable explanation of the pertinent clinical features of the disease. The advantages to the patient of having an effective anginal "warning system"[40] to prevent damage to the heart should be stressed. The role of personality type as an independent risk factor for coronary artery disease is discussed on pp. 1826 to 1828; some evidence indicates that counseling efforts to reduce the features of the "Type A" personality may improve prognosis in patients following myocardial infarction.[152] An important aspect of the physician's role is to counsel patients in the kind of work they can do, in their leisure activities, eating habits, vacation plans, and the like. It is desirable, if possible, to consult with the closest member(s) of the family, both to insure an accurate and full assessment of the patient's activities and to inform the family of what can be expected in the course of the patient's disease.

Certain changes in life style may be helpful, such as modifying strenuous activities if they constantly and repeatedly produce angina. These changes may be minor in many instances. For example, golfing could be modified to include use of a golfcart instead of walking. Many activities, such as shopping or climbing stairs, need not be discontinued. Often, it is merely necessary to perform them more slowly or to pause for brief periods of rest. The patient with chronic stable angina should avoid excessive fatigue and exhaustion; one or two regular rest periods during each day are often helpful. While it is desirable to minimize the number of bouts of angina, an occasional episode is not to be feared. The vast majority of patients with chronic stable angina should not be treated like invalids. Often, the propensity for angina actually declines,[153] perhaps as a result of the development of collaterals or because of training effects, discussed later; indeed, unless patients occasionally reach their anginal thresholds, they may not appreciate the extent of their exercise capacity.

Eliminating or reducing the factors that precipitate anginal episodes is of obvious importance. Each patient learns what his usual threshold is by trial and error. Since many anginal episodes are precipitated by increases in the mechanical activity of the heart (due to increases in heart rate and blood pressure), the patient should avoid *sudden* bursts of activity, particularly after long periods of rest. Thus, morning activities such as showering, shaving, and dressing should be done at a slower pace, and at certain times, prophylactic nitroglycerin is extremely useful (discussed below). The stress of sexual intercourse is ordinarily approximately equal to that of climbing one flight of stairs at a normal pace or of any activity that induces a heart rate of approximately 120 beats/min. With proper precautions, i.e., commencing more than 2 hours postprandially and taking an additional dose of propranolol one hour before and nitroglycerin 15 minutes before, the majority of patients with chronic stable angina are able to continue a satisfactory sexual life.

Just as there is a role for exercise in the management of coronary artery disease, so is there a role for rest, especially in situations in which angina has become frequent or severe. Marked restriction of activity or even complete bed rest, in addition to drug therapy, may be necessary to control symptoms. In less critical situations, merely reducing the amount of time spent working or increasing the rest periods will have a beneficial effect. For example, a long lunch break including a short nap may be beneficial. It may be necessary for the patient to use a face mask or scarf to cover the mouth or nose in cold weather. A hot, humid environment may also precipitate angina, and air conditioning may be a necessity rather than a luxury for patients with ischemic heart disease. Large meals can have a similar effect if they are followed by exertion. An effort should be made to minimize emotional outbursts, since they too increase myocardial oxygen requirements and sometimes induce coronary vasoconstriction. Occasionally antianxiety drugs or sedation may be useful.

Exercise (see also Chapter 40). There is a growing interest in the use of *physical exercise,* either in prevention of ischemic heart disease or in the reduction of complications once clinical manifestations occur. Despite observations that physical training has a beneficial effect on cardiac performance,[154] the relationship between physical activity and the development of coronary artery disease is unclear. Whether the widespread adoption of regular dynamic exercise (jogging, swimming, walking, bicycling) influences the development or rate of progression of coronary artery disease remains to be determined. Although the question of whether or not regular exercise accelerates the development of collateral vessels is still unsettled,[116,117] exercise does have a place, not only in the rehabilitation of individuals recovering from myocardial infarction, but in the management of patients with chronic angina as well.

The *conditioning effect of exercise* on skeletal muscle allows the patient to expend a greater physical effort at any level of total body oxygen consumption, and the conditioning effect of exercise on the heart, by decreasing the

TABLE 39–3 DOSAGE AND ACTIONS OF NITROGLYCERIN FOR ANGINAL THERAPY

NAME		EFFECTS°		DOSAGE						SIDE EFFECTS
Nonproprietary	*Proprietary*	*Physiologic*	*Therapeutic*	*Beginning*	*Average*	*Maximal*	*Formulation*	*Route*	*Supplied*	
Glyceryl trinitrate (nitroglycerin)	Nitrostat	Relaxes vascular smooth muscle	Decreases venous return	0.3 mg	0.6 mg	As needed	Sublingual tablets	SL	0.3, 0.4, and 0.6 mg	Headache Flushing Tachycardia
	Nitrobid	Dilates arterioles	Decreases blood pressure	2.5 mg bid	2.5 mg tid; 6.5 mg bid	6.5 mg tid	Sustained-release capsules	PO	2.5 and 6.5 mg	Dizziness Postural hypotension
	Nitroglyn	Reduces peripheral vascular resistance	Decreases net myocardial oxygen consumption	1.3 mg bid	1.3 mg tid; 6.5 mg bid	6.5 mg tid	Sustained-action tablets	PO	1.3, 2.6, and 6.5 mg	
	Nitrospan	Reduces mean arterial pressure		2.5 mg before breakfast and at hour of sleep			Sustained-release microdialysis cells	PO	2.5 mg	
	Nitro-SA	Reflex tachycardia		2.5 mg bid	2.5 mg bid	2.5 mg tid	Sustained-release capsules	PO	2.5 mg	
	Nitrong				2.6 mg tid		Controlled release tablets	PO	2.6 mg	
	Nitrol ointment			1 to 2 inches hs	2 inches hs	6 inches hs	Lanolin, petrolatum	Topically	1- and 2-oz tubes 2% TNG	

°These effects refer to all formulations of nitroglycerin.
Reproduced with permission from Wolfson, S., and Costin, J. C.: Medical therapy in angina pectoris. *In* Donoso, E., and Gorlin, R. (eds.): Angina Pectoris. Vol. III. New York, Stratton Intercontinental Medical Book Corp., 1977, p. 121.

to cause angina.[192,193] Used for this purpose, it may prevent anginal attacks for 30 to 45 minutes. Nitroglycerin tablets tend to lose their potency, especially if exposed to light, and should therefore be kept in dark containers. Adverse reactions are common and include headache, flushing, and hypotension. The last is only rarely severe but can be potentially dangerous if the chest pain is due to a myocardial infarction rather than angina and arterial pressure had already declined because of pump failure and/or a vagal reaction or hypovolemia. In addition, the partial pressure of oxygen in arterial blood may fall after nitroglycerin administration because of an increasing ventilation-perfusion imbalance owing to impairment of the lung's ability to vasoconstrict in areas of alveolar hypoxia and thereby redirect perfusion to less hypoxic tissue.[194] Methemoglobinemia is a rare complication of very large doses of nitrates (p. 1694).

Other nitrate preparations are available in sublingual, buccal, oral, and ointment form (Table 39–4). Isosorbide dinitrate and other long-acting preparations are available in 2.5- and 5.0-mg sublingual tablets, a 10-mg buccal (chewable) form, and 5-, 10-, and 20-mg tablets for oral use as well as in 40-mg "sustained-release" capsules. Since orally administered nitrates undergo rapid hepatic metabolism,[195] large doses (5 mg nitroglycerin and 20 mg isosorbide dinitrate or pentaerythritol tetranitrate) may be required. Oral nitrates are not very potent agents but they can raise the threshold of activity required for the development of angina and reduce the incidence of anginal attacks and the need for sublingual nitroglycerin.[196,197] They do not appear to cause tolerance to sublingual nitroglycerin.[198] Thadani et al. have reported that isosorbide dinitrate should be administered as frequently as every 2 to 3 hours for a continued beneficial effect.[199]

Topical Nitroglycerin. *Nitroglycerin ointment* (15 mg/inch) is efficacious when applied (most commonly to the chest) in strips of 0.5 to 2.0 inches. This form of the drug is particularly useful in patients with severe angina who are confined to bed and chair; since it is effective for 4 to 6 hours, it may also be used prophylactically after retiring by patients with nocturnal angina. While ordinary nitroglycerin ointment is not suitable for ambulatory patients, *sustained-release transdermal preparations* offer an alternative. A nitroglycerin-impregnated polymer is bonded to an adhesive bandage that should be applied to a site free of hair. Physically, these products resemble a "Band-Aid"; the drug is delivered at the inner surface, the outer layer is impermeable, and the entire unit is attached to the skin by an adhesive. The rate of delivery of the drug is determined by several means in different preparations, including a semipermeable membrane placed between the drug reservoir and the skin.[200] The dose depends on the size of the unit (5 to 30 cm^2) which releases 25 to 154 mg nitroglycerin over a 24-hour period. Clinical efficacy over a 24-hour period has been established.[201] Therapeutic plasma levels are achieved within 30 to 60 minutes of application and are maintained for at least 30 minutes after removal of the patch. Thus, transdermal delivery devices, suitable for

TABLE 39–4 DOSAGE AND ACTIONS OF LONG-ACTING NITRATES FOR ANGINAL THERAPY

NAME		EFFECTS°		DOSAGE						SIDE EFFECTS
Nonproprietary	*Proprietary*	*Physiologic*	*Therapeutic*	*Beginning*	*Usual*	*Maximal*	*Formulation*	*Route*	*Supplied*	
Isosorbide dinitrate	Isordil and Sorbitrate	Relaxes vascular smooth muscle	Decreases venous return	5 mg q 2–3 hr	5 to 10 mg q 3 hr	20 mg	Sublingual† tablets	SL	2.5, 5, 10, 20 mg	Headache Flushing Tachycardia Dizziness
				5 mg qid or 40 mg bid	5 to 30 mg qid or 40 mg bid	30 mg qid or 40 mg tid	Tablets and capsules	PO	5 and 10 mg	
Pentaerythritol tetranitrate	Peritrate	Dilates arterioles; reduces peripheral vascular resistance	Decreases blood pressure; decreases net myocardial oxygen consumption	10 mg qid	10 to 20 mg qid or 80 mg bid	60 mg q 4 hr	Oral†	PO	10 and 20 mg	Postural hypotension
Erythrityl tetranitrate	Cardilate	Reflex tachycardia		5 mg qid	5 to 15 mg qid	45 mg q 2 hr	Oral, sublingual, and chewable tablets	SL or PO	5, 10, 15 mg; 10-mg chewable	Possibly causes tachyphylaxis to nitroglycerin with prolonged use

°These effects refer to all long-acting nitrates.
†Also available as "sustained-action" tablets; efficacy not well documented.
Reproduced with permission from Wolfson, S., and Costin, J. C.: Medical therapy in angina pectoris. *In* Donoso, E., and Gorlin, R. (eds.): Angina Pectoris. Vol. III. New York, Stratton Intercontinental Medical Book Corp., 1977, p. 121.

once-a-day application in ambulatory patients, may prove to be a more convenient way to deliver the time-honored drug. Absorption through the skin by ointment or the transdermal route is advantageous, since it reaches target organs without being inactivated by the liver. Allergic contact dermatitis is occasionally associated with topical nitroglycerin.

Although chronic administration of nitrates does not usually induce clinically important tolerance or cross-tolerance to nitroglycerin, the lowest effective dosage of long-acting nitrates should be employed, since the development of tolerance to large doses does occasionally occur.[192] Because of the suggestion of nitrate dependence, nitrate therapy should be carefully withdrawn. Indeed, in individuals exposed to industrial doses of nitroglycerin, nitrate tolerance, nitrate dependence, and withdrawal symptoms may cause serious problems.[202]

The chronic combined administration of nitrates and beta-adrenergic blockers reduces the frequency of anginal episodes. Some investigators have reported an additive effect of the two drugs in increasing exercise tolerance.[203] Certainly, beta blockers have the desirable effect of blocking the reflex tachycardia that may accompany nitrate-induced hypotension.[204]

Beta-Adrenergic Blocking Agents

These drugs constitute a cornerstone of therapy for effort-induced, chronic stable angina.[205] A number of randomized, double-blind studies have shown that beta-adrenergic blockers, in doses that are generally well tolerated, reduce the frequency of anginal episodes and raise the anginal threshold.[206,207,207a] This action is dependent on their ability to cause competitive inhibition of the effects of neuronally released and circulating catecholamines on beta-adrenergic receptors (p. 418).[208] In this manner, these drugs attenuate the cardiac responses to adrenergic stimulation (chiefly increases in heart rate and contractility). Thus, beta blockers reduce myocardial oxygen demands primarily during activity or excitement when surges of increased sympathetic activity occur. Effects on heart rate and myocardial contractility at rest are less profound because of the lower adrenergic drive to the heart in the basal state. Beta-adrenergic blockers also lower myocardial oxygen needs by reducing arterial pressure and they are extremely useful antihypertensive agents (p. 916).

For optimal results, the dose of beta blocker should be carefully titrated. It is useful to start with 80 mg of propranolol daily (20 mg four times a day), or comparable doses of one of the other beta blockers, in an effort to reduce resting heart rates to 50 to 60 beats/min and to cause less than a 20-beat/min increase with modest exercise (e.g., climbing one flight of stairs). The usual dosage of propranolol ranges from 80 to 320 mg/day, but some patients require (and tolerate) doses as high as 1000 mg daily. Serum levels of 30 ng/ml are usually required to achieve a 25 per cent or greater reduction in the frequency of angina.[209,210]

Adverse Reactions. Beta blocking drugs may induce fatigue, mental depression, gastrointestinal upset, intensification of insulin-induced hypoglycemia, cutaneous reactions, bronchoconstriction, and heart block.[211,212] In patients who already have impaired left ventricular function, congestive heart failure may ensue or may be intensified, an effect that can be counteracted by the use of digitalis or diuretics. Beta blockers should *not* be used in patients with bradyarrhythmias of any kind unless a pacemaker is in place.

TABLE 39–5 PHARMACOKINETICS AND PHARMACOLOGY OF SOME BETA-ADRENERGIC BLOCKERS

	DRUG					
	Atenolol	*Metoprolol*	*Nadolol*	*Pindolol*	*Propranolol*	*Timolol*
Extent of absorption (%)	≃50	>95	≃30	>90	90	>90
Extent of bioavailability (% of dose)	≃40	≃50	≃30	≃90	≃30	75
Beta-blocking plasma concentration	0.2 to 0.5 μg/ml	50 to 100 ng/ml	50 to 100 ng/ml	50 to 100 ng/ml	50 to 100 ng/ml	5 to 10 ng/ml
Protein binding (%)	<5	12	≃30	57	93	≃10
Lipophilicity*	Low	Moderate	Low	Moderate	High	Low
Elimination half-life (hr)	6 to 9	3 to 4	14 to 25	3 to 4	3.5 to 6.0	3 to 4
Urinary recovery of unchanged drug (% of dose)	≃40	≃3	70	≃40	<1	≃20
Total urinary recovery (% of dose)	>95	>95	70	>90	>90	65
Drug accumulation in renal disease	Yes	No	Yes	No	No	No
Predominant route of elimination†	RE (mostly unchanged)	HM	RE	RE (≃40% unchanged) and HM	HM	RE (≃20% unchanged) and HM
Active metabolites	No	No	No	No	Yes	No
β_1-blocker potency ratio (propranolol = 1)	1.0	1.0	1.0	6.0	1.0	6.0
Relative β_1 sensitivity	+	+	0	0	0	0
Intrinsic sympathetic activity	0	0	0	+	0	0
Membrane-stabilizing activity	0	0	0	+	++	0
Usual maintenance dose	50 to 100 mg/qd	50 to 100 mg/qid	40 to 80 mg/qd	5 to 20 mg/tid	60 mg/qid	20 mg/bid

*Determined by the distribution ratio between octanol and water.
†RE = renal excretion; HM = hepatic metabolism.

Modified from Frishman, W. H.: Beta-adrenoceptor antagonists: New drugs and new indications. N. Engl. J. Med. *305*:500, 1981.

Sudden withdrawal of the drug in ambulatory patients has been reported to result in acute ischemic episodes.[213] There are several possible mechanisms for this "rebound" phenomenon; since the drug prevents or reduces the frequency of angina, patients increase their activities to a level that previously would have resulted in chest pain. When the drug is discontinued, they maintain their higher levels of activity but without the drug's protective effects. Since the greatest clinical benefit occurs in patients who were previously most disabled, the rebound effects might be expected to be most marked in those patients readily prone to myocardial ischemia. Other possible mechanisms involve the unmasking of the underlying coronary obstruction that has progressed during the course of drug administration, the elevation of arterial pressure, and an increase in the number of adrenergic beta receptors ("up-regulation").[214] The rebound phenomenon is much less marked in hospitalized patients, suggesting that the higher "set" of activity level is the major mechanism.

Blockade of noncardiac (i.e., beta$_2$) receptors inhibits catecholamine-induced glycogenolysis and the vasodilating effects of catecholamines in peripheral blood vessels. Therefore, noncardioselective beta blockers may impair the defense of insulin-induced hypoglycemia, may precipitate episodes of Raynaud's phenomenon, and may cause uncomfortable coldness of the distal extremities. Blockade of vasodilatory. (beta$_2$) receptors by noncardioselective beta blockers, such as propranolol, leaves the constrictor (alpha-adrenergic) receptors unopposed and thereby enhances vasoconstriction. Indeed, Kern et al. have shown in patients with chronic obstructive coronary artery disease that the coronary vasoconstriction that normally occurs during the cold pressor test is intensified by beta-adrenergic blockade with propranolol.[215] Propranolol prolongs episodes of myocardial ischemia in patients with Prinzmetal's angina[216] and is ordinarily contraindicated in this condition (p. 1360).

Six beta blockers are currently available in the United States (Table 39–5). They appear to be equally effective in the treatment of angina pectoris, but their differences in membrane-stabilizing properties, lipo- or hydrophilicity, cardioselectivity, and intrinsic sympathomimetic activity affect the other actions of these compounds. The hydrophilic beta blockers, i.e., atenolol and nadolol, are not as readily absorbed from the gastrointestinal tract as are the more lipophilic agents.[217] On the other hand, they are not as extensively metabolized and have relatively long plasma half-lives. Hydrophilic beta blockers tend not to penetrate into the central nervous system and therefore appear to be associated with less mental depression and sleep disturbances. Bronchoconstriction results from blockade of beta$_2$ receptors in the tracheobronchial tree; as a consequence, asthma and chronic obstructive lung disease are contraindications to the use of these agents. Since cardioselectivity is only relative, the use of such drugs (metoprolol and atenolol) in doses sufficient to prevent angina may still cause bronchoconstriction in susceptible patients.

One group of beta blockers with so-called intrinsic stimulating activity (ISA) cause not only blockade but also stimulation of beta receptors. Pindolol, a beta blocker with partial agonist activity, causes little if any slowing of heart rate, depression of atrioventricular (AV) conduction, and depression of contractility at rest but still blocks the effects of exercise on these parameters. Its partial agonist activity also induces bronchodilatation.[218–220] Accordingly, there is at least some theoretical advantage to using this beta blocker in patients with sinus bradycardia, AV block, left ventricular dysfunction and bronchospasm. However, additional clinical evidence is required to support these theoretical advantages.[207]

Calcium-Channel Blockers

The critical role played by calcium ions in the normal contraction of cardiac and vascular smooth muscle is discussed on page 413 and in myocardial ischemia on page 1253. Calcium-channel blocking agents have been found to be effective in the treatment of chronic stable angina, either alone or in combination with beta-adrenergic blockers and nitrates.[221,222,222a,222b,222c,222d] Three calcium-channel blocking agents—nifedipine, verapamil, and diltiazem—are now available in the United States. All three agents are effective in causing relaxation of vascular smooth muscle, in both the systemic arterial and the coronary arterial beds.

Nifedipine is the most potent vasodilator of the three. Although in vitro its actions on the myocardium and specialized cardiac tissue (i.e., the sinoatrial and AV nodes) are similar to those of the other agents, the concentration required to reproduce this effect is not reached in vivo because of its powerful vasodilating effects. Therefore, nifedipine's beneficial effects in the treatment of angina result from its capacity to reduce myocardial oxygen needs consequent to afterload reduction and to increase coronary blood flow consequent to its dilating action on the coronary vascular bed. Nifedipine decreases left ventricular afterload, while ejection fraction, velocity of circumferential fiber shortening, heart rate, and cardiac index all show slight reflex increases. In patients with elevated left ventricular end-diastolic volumes and pressures, nifedipine reduces ventricular end-diastolic pressure and left ventricular end-diastolic and end-systolic volumes and enhances ejection fraction more than it does in patients with normal baseline left ventricular function (Fig. 39–8 and Table 39–6).[223]

Side effects include headache, dizziness, flushing, nausea, and leg edema not related to heart failure. In a small number of patients, a paradoxical increase in myocardial ischemia may occur, presumably resulting from excessive lowering of arterial pressure and reflex tachycardia; cardiac depression is very rarely seen. The dose is 10 mg orally every 8 (or 6) hours increased to 20 mg every 8 (or 6) hours, guided by blood pressure response; 160 mg daily is considered to be the maximum dose.

Verapamil appears to decrease myocardial oxygen demand without any change in the anginal threshold (i.e., in the rate-pressure product) at the onset of angina, suggesting that increased oxygen delivery is not a principal mechanism of action.[224,225,225a] Charlap and Frishman[226] have summarized nine trials comparing verapamil with beta blockade (usually propranolol) in the treatment of effort-related angina. The two drugs were found to be comparable, both producing dose-dependent reductions in the frequency of anginal attacks (Fig. 39–9). In a comparison of propranolol, 480 mg/day, and verapamil, 320 mg/day, Leon et al. found verapamil to be superior.[227] Left ventricular diastolic filling is enhanced by verapamil in patients

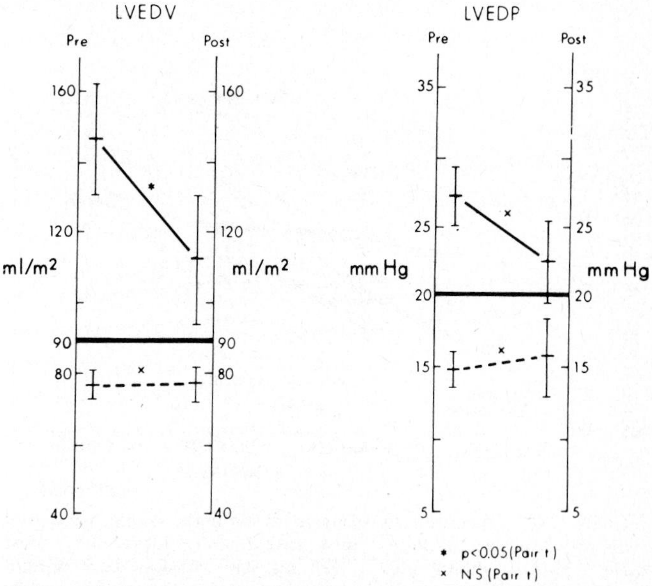

FIGURE 39–8 Left ventricular end-diastolic volume (LVEDV) and end-diastolic pressure (LVEDP) before and after nifedipine. Average EDV declined significantly in group 2 patients, in whom baseline LVEDV exceeded 90 ml/m², but was unchanged in group 1 patients, in whom initial LVEDV was normal. Average LVEDP declined in group 2 patients but did not change significantly in those in group 1. (From Ludbrook, P. A., et al.: Acute hemodynamic responses to sublingual nifedipine: Dependence on left ventricular function. Circulation *65*:489, 1982, by permission of the American Heart Association, Inc.)

with chronic stable angina both at rest and during exercise, but beta blockade does not have this effect.[227] The dose is *80* to *120* mg, *three or four times daily* (Table 39–7).

Diltiazem's actions are similar to those of verapamil—lowering arterial pressure at rest and during exertion and increasing the workload required to produce myocardial ischemia—but there is also some evidence that the drug may increase myocardial oxygen delivery.[228] Its action on the coronary vasculature is relatively selective, and this may explain the remarkably low incidence of adverse effects that have been reported. Like verapamil, diltiazem should be used only with great caution in patients with sick sinus syndrome and advanced degrees of AV block and left ventricular dysfunction. The dose is 30 to 60 mg four times daily.[229,229a]

Verapamil and diltiazem in doses used clinically not only cause systemic coronary vascular dilatation but also inhibit calcium influx into the myocardial and specialized cardiac cells, sometimes causing slowing of heart rate and AV conduction and impairing myocardial contractility.

TABLE 39–6 COMPARISON OF DRUG EFFECTS ON GLOBAL AND REGIONAL LEFT VENTRICULAR FUNCTION DURING EXERCISE (VS. CONTROL)

	Global LV Function								Regional LV Function		
	HR	*SBP*	*DBP*	*PAPD*	*CI*	*TVR*	*EF*	*EDVI*	*NL*	*ISCH*	*SCAR*
Nitroglycerin	(↑)	—	(↓)	↓	—	—	(↑)	(↓)	—	↑	—
Nifedipine	↑	↓	↓	↓	↑	↓	(↑)	—	—	↑	—
Metoprolol	↓	↓	—	↑	(↓)	↑	—	—	↓	(↑)	—

Significant group differences are represented by different symbols: arrows indicate changes vs. control; arrows in parentheses indicate changes that are significant by single comparison but not by multiple group comparison.

Abbreviations: LV = left ventricular; HR = heart rate; SBP = systolic blood pressure; DBP = diastolic blood pressure; PAPD = pulmonary artery diastolic pressure; CI = cardiac index; TVR = total vascular resistance; EF = ejection fraction; EDVI = end-diastolic volume index; NL = normal segment; ISCH = ischemic segment; SCAR = scar segment; ↑ = increase; ↓ = decrease; — = no significant change vs. control.

From Pfisterer, M., et al.: Comparative effects of nitroglycerin, nifedipine and metoprolol on regional left ventricular function in patients with one-vessel coronary disease. Circulation *67*: 291, 1983.

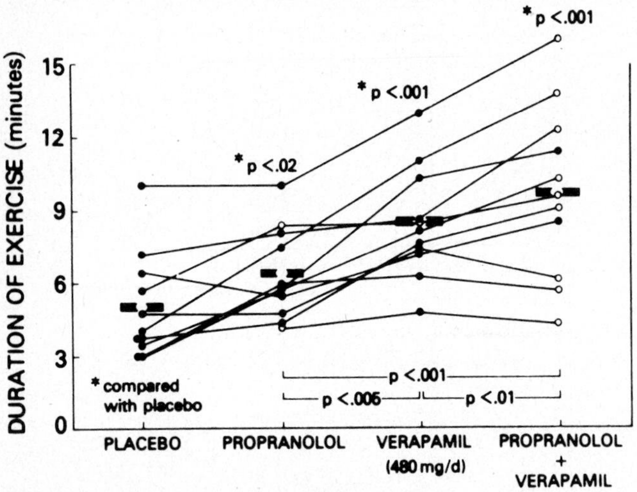

FIGURE 39–9 Duration of exercise in patients taking verapamil (480 mg/day), propranolol ("best dose"), and propranolol ("best dose") plus verapamil (407 ± 25 mg/day). Broken bars denote mean exercise time, closed circles represent exercise terminated by angina, and open circles represent exercise limited by fatigue or shortness of breath. (From Leon, M. B., et al.: Clinical efficacy of verapamil alone and combined with propranolol in treating patients with chronic stable angina pectoris. Am. J. Cardiol. *48*:131, 1981.)

The principal side effects of these three calcium-channel blockers are contrasted with those of beta blockers and nitrates in Table 39–8. The major side effects of nifedipine are hypotension, flushing, and headache. The drug lowers arterial pressure and may produce a mild reflex tachycardia and augmentation of myocardial contractility. On the other hand, verapamil and diltiazem, by blocking the influx of calcium ions into cardiac tissue, cause a depression of cardiac contractility and a slowing of heart rate and of AV conduction. Therefore, nifedipine is contraindicated in patients who are already hypotensive,[230] while verapamil and diltiazem should probably not be administered to patients with left ventricular dysfunction, sinus bradycardia, sick sinus syndrome, and AV block, particularly if they are already receiving a beta-adrenergic blocker that can exert similar deleterious effects. In such patients, nifedipine is the calcium-channel blocker of choice, since it has less negative effects on myocardial contractility or on the specialized automatic or conduction system than does verapamil or diltiazem.

RELATIVE ADVANTAGES OF BETA BLOCKERS AND CALCIUM ANTAGONISTS. There is some controversy at the present time about whether a calcium-channel blocking agent or a beta blocker should be employed first in the treatment of chronic stable angina if more than an occasional sublingual nitroglycerin tablet is required. As indicated in the foregoing discussion, both classes of agents appear to be about equally effective. Chronic administration of beta-adrenergic blockers has been found to prolong life in patients after acute myocardial infarction,[231,232] but this has not yet been demonstrated for calcium-channel blockers. Since many patients with chronic stable angina either have suffered a myocardial infarction or have a similar pathophysiological process, not only might they benefit from the symptomatic relief provided by beta-adrenergic blockade, but conceivably these agents may also improve survival and diminish mortality in patients with chronic stable angina. On the other hand, a number of conditions, such as moderate to severe left ventricular failure, sinus bradycardia, sick sinus syndrome, and advanced AV block as well as obstructive lung disease, are contraindications to beta blockade, and in such patients nifedipine is preferable. Hypertensive patients do well with both beta blockers and calcium-channel blockers, since both agents have antihypertensive effects.

One logical way to make a choice between a calcium antagonist and a beta blocker is to take a detailed history and determine whether the patient's anginal threshold is fixed or variable, as discussed on page 1336. When it is relatively fixed, it may be presumed that myocardial ischemia is caused primarily by an increase in myocardial oxygen needs during exercise in the face of a fixed supply, and a beta blocker would be considered the agent of choice; conversely, in patients with variable-threshold angina, in whom a reduction of myocardial blood supply caused by coronary vasospasm plays a role in the development of ischemia and angina, a calcium-channel blocking agent may be preferable to a beta blocker.

COMBINATION THERAPY. In patients with more severe angina, a combination of a beta-adrenergic blocker, a calcium antagonist, and long-acting nitrates may be employed. The hemodynamic spectrum of action of nitroglycerin, calcium antagonists, and beta blockers is sufficiently different to suggest that combination therapy might be useful (Table 39–6).[233] Indeed, a number of studies[234–239] have shown that the combination of a beta blocker and a calcium-channel blocker is superior to either drug alone (Fig. 39–9). While combined blockade of calcium entry and beta-adrenergic receptors is usually well tolerated, this combination should be approached with caution, since it can occasionally produce severe left ventricular dysfunction.[240,241] It is often possible to use low doses of each agent, so that the adverse effects of each drug are diminished.

In patients with angina severe enough to require combination therapy but without specific contraindications to any antianginal agents, the combination of a beta blocker

TABLE 39–7 CLINICAL PHARMACOKINETICS OF MAJOR CALCIUM ANTAGONISTS

Agent	Usual Adult dose	Absorption	Onset of Action	Peak Effect	Plasma Half-life
Verapamil	IV: 0.075 to 0.15 mg/kg	—	≈2 min	3 to 5 min	<1/2 hr
	Oral: 80 to 120 mg tid or qid	90%	2 hr	3 to 4 hr	3 to 7 hr*
Nifedipine	SL: 10 to 30 mg tid or qid	90%	<3 min	Not available	
	Oral: 10 to 30 mg tid or qid	90%	<20 min	1 to 2 hr	4 hr
Diltiazem	IV: 0.075 to 0.15 mg/kg	—		Not available	
	Oral: 30 to 90 mg tid or qid	90%	<15 min	30 min	4 hr

IV = intravenous; SL = sublingual.
*Single dose; may be lengthened to 4.5 to 12 hours after 6 to 10 consecutive oral doses.
From Singh, B. N.: Clinical pharmacology of calcium antagonist drugs. Cornell Postgraduate Course on Calcium Antagonists. New York, Medcom, Inc., 1982, p. 5.

TABLE 39–8 SIDE EFFECTS OF ANTIANGINAL DRUGS*

	Hypotension Flushing, Headache	Left Ventricular Dysfunction	Decreased Heart Rate Atrio-ventricular Block†	Gastro-intestinal Symptoms	Broncho-constriction‡
Beta blockers	0	++	+++	+	+++
Nitrates	+++	0	0	0	0
Diltiazem	+	+	+	0	0
Nifedipine	+++	0	0	0	0
Verapamil	+	+	++	++	0

*0 = absent; + = mild; ++ = moderate; +++ sometimes severe.
†In patients with sick sinus node syndrome or conduction system disease.
‡In patients with obstructive lung disease.
From Braunwald, E.: Mechanism of action of calcium channel blocking agents. N. Engl. J. Med. *307*:1618, 1982.

and nifedipine or of verapamil or diltiazem with a long-acting nitrate is appropriate. As already stated, since beta blockers and both verapamil and diltiazem exert negative inotropic effects and depress cardiac automaticity and conduction, this combination may be hazardous in patients who already have left ventricular dysfunction and in those with impaired function of the sinoatrial or AV nodes. The combination of nifedipine and nitrates may also be less than ideal, since both agents are potent vasodilators. In practice, antianginal drugs are begun in low doses and are gradually raised to tolerance. If the patient's lifestyle is limited by persistent angina despite all the aforementioned measures, and if there are no contraindications, surgical treatment should be considered.

OTHER ANTIANGINAL THERAPIES. Anticoagulant therapy with coumarin derivatives is no longer recommended for patients with chronic stable angina without other factors predisposing to venous thrombosis. Its use in the postmyocardial infarction state is discussed on page 1304. Whether treatment with sulfinpyrazone and other drugs that impair platelet function is of value is not yet clear.[242]

Percutaneous Transluminal Angioplasty (PTCA)

This technique consists of introducing a catheter incorporating a balloon under local anesthesia across a stenotic segment in a coronary artery and relieving the stenosis by inflating the balloon (Fig. 9–12, p. 298).[243,243a,243b,243c] Morphological studies have shown that this procedure, when successful, disrupts the intima and splits the atherosclerotic plaque.[244] The most appropriate candidates for this procedure are patients with (1) stable angina refractory to medical therapy and severe enough to warrant surgical revascularization; (2) a relatively proximal stenosis in one of the three major coronary arteries; and (3) a discrete stenosis, less than 1 cm in length, that is readily accessible.[245] Patients with left main coronary artery disease are *not* good candidates, and the role of this procedure in patients with multivessel disease is not yet clear.[245a,245b] Approximately 10 per cent of patients who are candidates for coronary artery bypass grafting are candidates for angioplasty.

Depending on the skill and experience of the operator, PTCA is successful in dilating the stenosis in 60 to 80 per cent of cases.[245–247] In these patients, angina is usually relieved and left ventricular function improves, as reflected in an elevation of the ventricular ejection fraction during exercise.[246,248] Coronary occlusion occurs in about 5 per cent of patients, and in these, myocardial infarction can sometimes be averted or limited by immediate coronary artery bypass grafting. Accordingly, a cardiac surgical team must be available on standby for treatment of this complication. Mortality rate changes from 0.5 to 1.0 per cent.[245,247] In about 20 per cent of the patients in whom the procedure is initially successful, stenosis recurs, usually during the first 6 months.[247a] In about two-thirds of these patients, a second angioplasty will be successful, with symptomatic improvement for more than one year.[247b] Exercise electrocardiography and ^{201}thallium perfusion imaging are helpful in following patients after angioplasty;[248a, 248b] recurrence of symptoms and abnormal findings on these noninvasive tests are useful in determining when arteriography should be repeated.[249,250]

Successful vaporization of atherosclerotic plaques and intracoronary thrombi using an argon laser passed through a fiberoptic catheter (i.e., transluminal laser coronary angioplasty) has been reported in a variety of animal and human necropsy models.[251,252,252a,252b,252c] This technique, like percutaneous transluminal coronary angioplasty, appears to be promising for the treatment of chronic stable angina in selected patients. Balloon angioplasty has also been employed successfully in the course of surgical revascularization to improve perfusion of vessels that cannot be reached by grafts.[253,254]

Guidelines for Medical Treatment of Chronic (Stable) Angina

Risk factor modification is most important in younger patients with chronic stable angina (under age 50). This is most easily accomplished by cessation of cigarette smoking and treatment of hypertension. What effect reduction of serum cholesterol levels will have on regression of atheromas is unclear, but it is unlikely to be significant unless a means is found to produce a radical reduction of markedly elevated serum cholesterol. Perhaps currently available methods of diet and drug therapy may slow the progression of the disease. Similarly, the relationship between maintenance of blood sugar within the normal range in diabetics and preventing vascular disease is far from settled.

In mild chronic stable angina, drug therapy may be limited to sublingual nitroglycerin on an "as necessary" basis if pain episodes are relatively infrequent (once or twice a week). It should also be used prophylactically in situations known to precipitate angina. If nitroglycerin is required on

like pain despite normal coronary arteriograms, discussed on page 1338. Myocardial ischemia not caused by coronary atherosclerosis can also result from embolism, as in infective endocarditis (Chap. 33); mitral valve prolapse (p. 1089); prosthetic valve thrombosis; primary tumors of the heart (Chap. 42); calcific emboli from calcified aortic valves; especially during operation; mural thrombi in patients with cardiomyopathy and myocardial infarction; and aortitis (lues, arteritis) (Chap. 45).

An interesting nonatherosclerotic ischemic syndrome has been described in workers in the nitrate industry who apparently experience nitrate withdrawal symptoms on weekends, presumed to be secondary to coronary spasm when there is no counterstimulation to the vasoconstriction that they undergo as an adaptation to the vasodilating actions of the high concentrations of nitrates to which they are exposed.[422]

SURGICAL MANAGEMENT OF ISCHEMIC HEART DISEASE

HISTORICAL PERSPECTIVE

Numerous operations have been proposed for the treatment of coronary artery disease. The earliest was cardiac denervation, consisting of excision of cardiac fibers. Although many patients reported relief of angina, this procedure did not gain wide acceptance. Procedures to revascularize the myocardium have included suturing the omentum directly to the epicardium,[423] obstruction of coronary venous outflow,[424] application of irritants to the epicardium in the hope that new blood vessels would form, and ligation of the distal internal mammary artery in order to increase blood flow through the pericardial branches.[425] These approaches were of little value because they did not take into account the magnitude of the blood flow deficit nor the fact that the major site of diminished perfusion was in the deep rather than superficial layers of the myocardium.[426]

In 1964, Vineberg and Walter reported on the generally favorable clinical course of 140 patients in whom the more physiologic operation (carried out over the preceding 13 years) of implantation of a systemic (internal mammary) artery deep into the myocardium, beyond the area of obstruction, resulted in the formation of new blood vessels that communicated with the distal branches of the obstructed coronary artery.[427] A beneficial effect on myocardial lactate metabolism as well as on myocardial blood flow was demonstrated in some patients.[428] Patency of the implants to the preexisting coronary circulation was demonstrated on selective arteriography in about half the cases. Although sustained relief of angina and reductions in mortality or in the rate of recurrent myocardial infarction, compared with medically treated patients, were never clearly demonstrated,[426,429] there is little doubt that in individual patients an internal mammary artery implant can act as the crucial source of blood to an otherwise severely underperfused region. In most patients, however, blood flow through the grafts is simply too low for adequate revascularization.[430]

Cardiovascular surgeons at the Cleveland Clinic then introduced or popularized several surgical procedures that directly involved the coronary arteries, including "roofing over" an atheromatous plaque with a pericardial patch graft, resecting the obstructed portion of the coronary artery and interposing a venous graft, and/or endarterectomy,[431,432] but none of these operations was shown to provide sustained benefit and all were often associated with a high operative mortality rate. A major advance took place in 1964, when DeBakey and colleagues anastomosed portions of an autologous saphenous vein proximally to the aorta and distally to the diseased coronary artery beyond the obstruction.[433] The internal mammary artery was then used for the same purpose.[434] These procedures were soon found to be qualitatively superior to the earlier operations because they were capable of delivering substantial quantities of blood to previously ischemic myocardium, providing marked and sustained relief of angina pectoris in most patients. These direct revascularization procedures are now being used widely on more than 100,000 patients per year in the United States. Thus, aortocoronary bypass grafting not only has become the most widely applied cardiac operation but is now one of the most frequently practiced of all major surgical procedures.

OPERATIVE PROCEDURE

(See also Chapter 55)

Beta-adrenergic blockers, nitrates, and calcium-channel blockers are continued until surgery, and anesthesia is employed to maintain a normal rate-pressure product during induction. Most surgeons employ coronary revascularization, carried out with the aid of cardiopulmonary bypass at moderate hypothermia (24° to 32° C) and hemodilution. A motionless heart is achieved by continuous aortic cross-clamping with profound cardiac hypothermia and cardioplegia with cold potassium solution.[435] The vein grafts are inverted so that the distal end of the vein is placed proximally as an end-to-side anastomosis on the aorta (Fig. 39–18). The distal end of the vein is then placed as an end-to-side anastomosis on the coronary artery (Fig. 39–19); side-to-side anastomoses permit revascularization of several coronary artery branches with a single saphenous vein graft. In order to avoid obstruction of the graft by thrombotic occlusion or kinking, care must be exercised in the physical handling of the veins used as bypass grafts as well as in the positioning and arching of the vessels as they exit from the aorta and at-

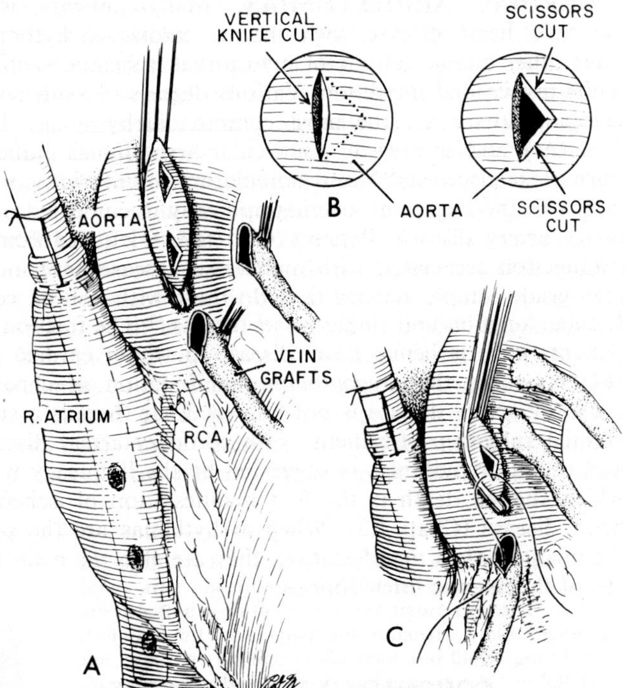

FIGURE 39–18 The aorticovenous anastomosis. *A* shows the direction of the anastomotic site for left-sided grafts; *B* shows details of aortic orifices; *C* shows the direction of right coronary artery (RCA) grafts. (From Cohn, L. H.: Surgical techniques of emergency coronary revascularization. *In* Cohn, L. H. (ed.): The Treatment of Acute Myocardial Ischemia: An Integrated Medical-Surgical Approach. Mt. Kisco, N.Y., Futura Publishing Co., 1979, p. 87.)

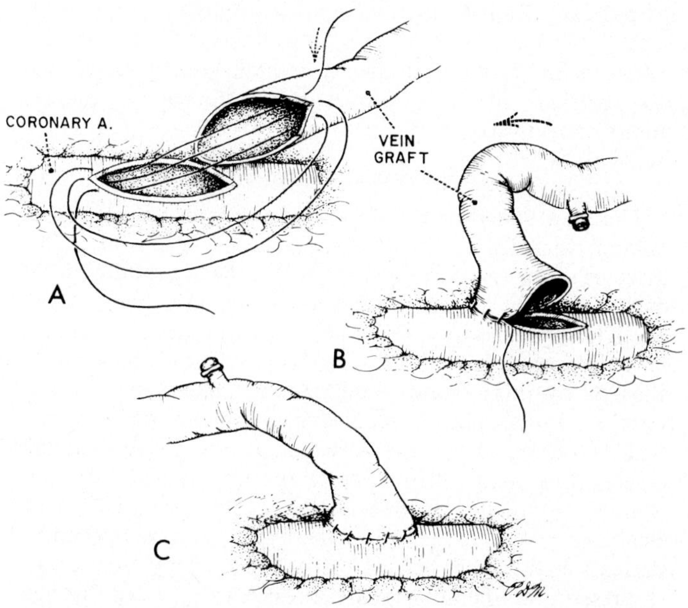

FIGURE 39–19 The venocoronary anastomosis to the proximal portion of the arteriotomy. (From Cohn, L. H.: Surgical techniques of emergency coronary revascularization. *In* Cohn, L. H. (ed.): The Treatment of Acute Myocardial Ischemia: An Integrated Medical-Surgical Approach. Mt. Kisco, N.Y., Futura Publishing Co., 1979, p. 87.)

tach to a coronary artery. Revascularization should include bypass of all major arterial segments with greater than 50 per cent stenosis of the luminal diameter.[436,437,437a]

Internal mammary artery bypass grafts may have certain advantages over vein grafts. The size of the internal mammary artery is similar to that of the native coronary vessel, and there is apparently little tendency for this graft to develop fibrous intimal hyperplasia, which may account for its reported higher patency rate.[434] However, because of its smaller internal diameter, it delivers less blood than do saphenous vein bypass grafts[438] and is also of limited value for revascularization of the posterior surface of the heart, because it is often too short to be used for more distal anastomoses. In general, internal mammary artery grafting also requires a longer time to perform and is therefore less desirable than saphenous vein grafting for emergency procedures. It is best suited for those patients in whom saphenous veins are not available because of prior bypass surgery or venous stripping of the leg for varicosities. Comparison of the efficacy of artery versus vein techniques must await followup results.

PATIENT SELECTION FOR CORONARY ARTERY SURGERY

To undergo coronary artery bypass grafting, patients must usually meet certain clinical, coronary arteriographic, and hemodynamic criteria.[439]

CLINICAL FACTORS

Chronic Stable Angina. We still agree with the Report of the Inter-Society Commission for Heart Disease Resources, presented in 1972, that the most widely accepted indication for coronary artery bypass surgery in stable angina is significant disability from moderate to severe angina pectoris, despite optimal medical care.[440] The threshold for "significant" disability varies widely among patients. Obviously, it differs for a relatively young man (under age 45) who is dependent on heavy physical work for his livelihood and an older woman (over age 75) who is sedentary and retired. In general, however, we would define "significant" disability as one that clearly interferes with the patient's desired lifestyle. Although this disability usually results from the coronary artery disease itself, it may be related to the side effects of the medications required to control the discomfort of myocardial ischemia. Angina pectoris can be controlled in most patients but sometimes only with excessive doses of antianginal agents. Optimal medical care, as described earlier (p. 1345), involves achievement of optimal weight; treatment of associated illnesses that can intensify myocardial ischemia, such as thyrotoxicosis or anemia; control of blood pressure, arrhythmias, and metabolic abnormalities such as carbohydrate intolerance and hyperlipidemias; abstinence from smoking; and most importantly, medication with beta blockers as well as short- and long-acting nitrates and calcium-channel blockers.

In published reports in the early 1970's, the majority of patients selected for operation were, in fact, in functional Classes III and IV.[441,442] However, with the reduction in perioperative mortality, a trend toward operating on less symptomatic or intensively treated patients has been noted. Other clinical factors considered in the selection of patients with arteriographically proven coronary obstructive disease include an increased concern for younger patients with coronary disease and evidence of previous myocardial infarction, even in patients with few symptoms. In many centers, the average age at operation is approximately 50 years, and more than half these patients have suffered previous myocardial infarction.[442]

Unstable Angina. The indications for operation in patients with unstable angina are more clear-cut than are those for stable angina and are discussed on page 1358. Initial medical management with bed rest, sedation, nitrates, beta blockade, and, if necessary, intraaortic balloon counterpulsation is the treatment of choice; *emergency* surgery is recommended only when this therapy fails to stabilize the patient. Patients with left main coronary artery disease should be operated upon on an urgent basis. In patients with coronary artery anatomy suitable for bypass who have been successfully treated medically, we recommend that operation be carried out 1 to 2 weeks after symptoms subside, generally during the same hospital stay. These patients could also return home, gradually increase activity, and maintain therapy with beta-adrenergic blockade, calcium-channel blocking agents, and nitrates; operation would be deferred until the patient developed either a second episode of unstable angina or sufficiently disabling chronic stable angina to satisfy the surgical requirements for the condition, as described above. It has been our experience that many patients with unstable angina will present one of these two indications within 6 months of discharge from the hospital, and the relatively high incidence of surgical treatment in the patients selected at random for medical therapy in the National Cooperative

Study confirms this.[287,443] It is for this reason and because of the relatively low risk of operation in the hands of a skilled surgical team and the excellent symptomatic results that we recommend early operation, i.e., prior to hospital discharge for the majority of patients with unstable angina. However, a number of randomized studies in addition to the National Cooperative Study have shown no advantage to urgent operation in this condition, and it must be acknowledged that firm data are lacking on the comparative advisability of early operation as opposed to the conservative course of postponing the procedure until required by the development of symptoms despite optimal medical management.

It is generally agreed that (1) patients with unstable angina treated surgically within the first 24 hours of presenting to the hospital have higher mortality and periinfarction rates than those operated upon later[444]; (2) the survival of patients operated upon early (1 to 2 weeks) after hospital admission is similar to that of medically treated patients; (3) surgically treated patients do better symptomatically than those treated medically; and (4) many medically treated patients ultimately require operation because of the recurrence of unstable angina or the development of severe chronic stable angina.

Prinzmetal's Angina. Although coronary artery bypass grafting is generally successful in relieving the pain of chronic stable angina pectoris, it is of little if any value in patients with *Prinzmetal's variant angina* without organic obstructive coronary artery disease. Since episodes of coronary artery spasm continue after operation, blood flow may be reduced sufficiently to cause thrombosis if spasm occurs in the area of insertion of the anastomosis of the graft into the native coronary artery. Patients with coronary artery spasm superimposed on obstructive arteriosclerotic coronary artery disease may fare better with coronary artery bypass than those in whom spasm occurs in unobstructed coronary arteries. Although some patients with variant angina clearly derive benefit from the bypass operation,[373] their response generally is inferior to that of patients with typical angina pectoris.

Heart Failure and Myocardial Infarction. In the absence of severe angina, patients with *heart failure* secondary to diffuse coronary artery disease (i.e., patients with ischemic cardiomyopathy) are not good candidates for coronary revascularization, since the mortality rate is higher than in patients with well-preserved left ventricular function.[445,446] However, there is some evidence that in patients in whom left ventricular dysfunction is due to chronically ischemic but not irreversibly damaged fibrotic tissue, surgical revascularization can improve left ventricular function[447,448] and perhaps survival as well.[449,450] Patients with heart failure should be studied carefully to exclude a mechanical lesion, such as mitral regurgitation or a ventricular aneurysm, which is usually amenable to surgical treatment.

Indications for coronary revascularization in patients with *acute myocardial infarction* or *cardiogenic shock* and *intractable ventricular arrhythmias* are discussed elsewhere (p. 1318). The number of patients with these manifestations of coronary artery disease subjected to these procedures has been relatively small, and suitable control series are not available. Although favorable results have been reported in patients with acute myocardial infarction both with [451–453] and without[454–456] cardiogenic shock, appropriate comparisons with nonsurgically treated patients have not been carried out, and the question of clinical benefits remains unresolved.

ARTERIOGRAPHIC FACTORS

The view stated in the Report of the Inter-Society Commission for Heart Disease Resources in 1972 still holds: there is "general agreement that the best candidates for bypass surgery are those with severe (greater than 75 per cent) luminal diameter obstructions in proximal segments of major branches of the coronary arteries," as demonstrated by high-quality angiograms taken in multiple views.[440] Intraoperative studies have shown that arteries with less than 50 per cent obstruction often have minimal, if any, pressure gradients across the lesions and little difference in blood flow through the artery, as measured by clearance of xenon-133, when the bypass graft is opened.[457] Patients with higher-grade obstructions usually have greater pressure gradients across the lesions, and flow through the artery could be shown to increase significantly when the bypass graft is opened.

The state of the distal vasculature is equally important. This can be evaluated directly by an angiographic assessment and indirectly by flow measurements. In one series of 154 venous grafts studied 2 months and 1 year after operation, it was concluded that late patency of the grafts was related to coronary arterial runoff, as determined by the diameter of the coronary artery into which the graft was inserted, the size of the distal vascular bed, and, to a lesser degree, the severity of coronary atherosclerosis distal to the site of insertion of the graft.[458] The highest graft patency rates were found when the lumina of the vessels distal to the graft insertion were greater than 1.5 mm in diameter, perfused a large peripheral vascular bed, and were free of atheromas occluding more than 25 per cent of the vessel lumen. Vessel diameters measured at coronary arteriography correlated satisfactorily with those obtained at operation.[459] The most accurate appraisal of the vascular bed distal to the principal obstruction can be made when the vessels fill in an antegrade manner. Assessment is less accurate when there is total proximal occlusion and distal filling occurs through adequate collaterals. In many such instances, the vessels are actually larger than the arteriogram suggests. Whenever there is any question about the ability of a vessel to accept a graft, the surgeon should attempt the anastomosis (consistent with patient safety, of course), since subjective improvement clearly depends on the completeness of revascularization.[460,461]

Flow rates through saphenous vein grafts measured at the time of operation average nearly 70 ml/min; those in which the flow is less than 45 ml/min—and especially less than 25 ml/min—are frequently associated with graft closure, whereas closure is less common at flow rates exceeding 45 ml/min.[462,463] The possible causes for reduced flow include subcritical obstruction of a proximal coronary artery; a technically poor anastomosis, with narrowing of the lumen due to kinking of the vessel or pinching at the site of the anastomosis; and a small myocardial mass perfused by the graft, which may in turn be due to diseased distal vasculature.

Ventricular Function. The relation between the presence of clinical evidence of congestive heart failure, hemodynamic evidence of left ventricular dysfunction, extensive wall motion disorders on left ventricular angiography, and poor surgical outcome is now well appreciated.[463–466] Clinical descriptors such as a history of heart failure, pulmonary rales, previous need of a diuretic or digitalis, and a cardiothoracic ratio of 0.50 or more are all associated with a significantly higher operative risk. In the Collaborative Study in Coronary Artery Surgery (CASS), the operative mortality was 1.9 per cent in patients with ejection fractions of 50 per cent or more and 6.7 per cent in those with ejection fractions below 19 per cent; these rates were 1.7 per cent in those with normal or minimally impaired wall motion and 9.1 per cent in those with greatly impaired wall motion.[467]

In estimating ejection fraction and wall motion in patients with coronary artery disease, it is important to analyze ventricular wall motion in the basal state as well as after inotropic stimulation or afterload reduction, in order to show enhancement of otherwise depressed wall motion.[135–137] As noted earlier, "contractile reserve" is the term used to describe the ability of ventricular wall segments that contract abnormally in the basal state to exhibit augmented contractility, often with an increase in overall ejection fraction, in response to a suitable stimulus.[468]

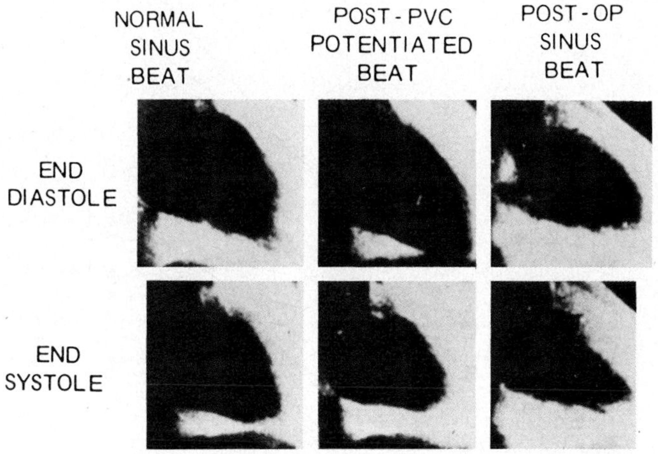

	PRE-OP NSB	PRE-OP p̄PVC	POST-OP
EDVI	138	151	156
ESVI	88	83	55
SVI	50	68	101
EF	36%	45%	65%

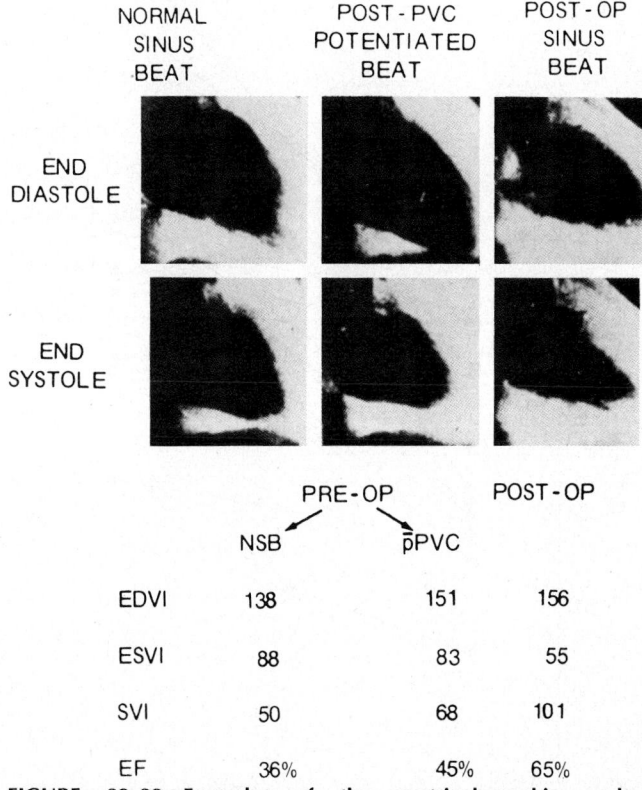

FIGURE 39–20 Examples of the ventriculographic analysis performed to evaluate the effects of an inotropic stimulus, including some of the calculations made. PVC = premature ventricular contraction; PRE-OP = preoperative; POST-OP = postoperative; NSB = normal sinus beat; pPVC = after premature ventricular contraction; EDVI = end-diastolic volume index (ml/m²); ESVI = end-systolic volume index (ml/m²); SVI = stroke volume index (ml/m²); EF = ejection fraction. (From Popio, K. A., et al.: Post extrasystolic potentiation as a predictor of potential myocardial viability. Am. J. Cardiol. *39*:944, 1977.)

Zones of the myocardium responding to inotropic stimulation or to a decrease in afterload may improve functionally after revascularization (Fig. 39–20).[469] The demonstration of augmentation of contractility acutely and similar improvement after revascularization are related to the finding that many hypokinetic (and even akinetic) areas of the ventricular wall are composed either of ischemic, though viable, muscle or of a mixture of the latter and fibrous scar; the viable muscle is capable of responding to stimulation and, after operation, to improved perfusion.[137] In contrast, necrotic tissue obviously cannot be stimulated to contract by any pharmacological or hemodynamic intervention nor by improved perfusion. In patients with poor left ventricular function and poor contractile reserve (less than 0.10 increase in ejection fraction with inotropic stimulation), perioperative mortality is higher and long-term survival is poorer than in patients with equally depressed left ventricular function but with normal contractile reserve.[468–470]

Although, as stated above, the risk of operation is higher in patients with depressed left ventricular function, many such patients will nonetheless experience striking relief of anginal discomfort, and symptoms of heart failure may diminish somewhat after coronary bypass grafting. Therefore, we generally recommend surgical treatment for patients with heart failure and disabling angina, recognizing the higher risks involved.

RESULTS

OPERATIVE MORTALITY. Operative mortality for the treatment of stable and unstable angina pectoris has been declining steadily. In the CASS, the overall mortality for 6630 patients operated upon between 1975 and 1978 was 2.3 per cent. In addition to being affected by left ventricular function, as described above, mortality increased with age (0 in patients under 30 years to 7.9 per cent in those over 70 years). It was higher in women than in men, varied with the number of vessels involved, and was highest in patients with left main coronary artery stenosis. Operative mortality was 1.7 per cent for elective surgery, 3.5 per cent for urgent surgery, and 10.8 per cent for emergency surgery.[467] Additional cardiac surgical procedures raised the risk to 8 per cent in patients undergoing resection or plication of aneurysm and to 24 per cent in patients undergoing mitral valve replacement.

As with other operations, the risks depend on the patient's general medical status and the presence of associated conditions, such as pulmonary or renal disease. It must be recognized that the surgical results reported in the literature are usually the best in the field and may be substantially superior to those in the institution where the patient under consideration is going to receive surgical care. Thus, operative mortality among the 15 participating centers ranged from 0.3 to 6.4 per cent, emphasizing that the experience and skill of the team (surgeons, anesthesiologists, and cardiologists) play decisive roles in determining the outcome. The presence of risk factors for coronary artery disease and a previous myocardial infarction did not appear to affect operative mortality. Kuchoukos et al. have emphasized that improved perioperative management, including anesthetic techniques, intraoperative protection of the myocardium, and preoperative stabilization of patients, have all played important roles in the steady decline of operative mortality.[436] In patients with active ischemia or extremely poor left ventricular function, operative mortality may be reduced when the intraaortic balloon is used to support the circulation during the perioperative period. Finally, the physician considering referral of a particular patient for surgical treatment must fully appreciate the recent results obtained by the surgical group selected.

LATE SURVIVAL. Lack of controlled studies in most series makes evaluation of the effect of surgical treatment of survival difficult. In large series, 4-year mortality rates range from 9 to 18 per cent.[471,472] Although operative mortality is also considered in these analyses, survival figures must be evaluated with the realization that, in general, operated patients have been preselected for good left ventricular function. Left ventricular function, reflected in the ejection fraction[473] and the qualitative assessment of left ventricular contraction,[474] influences late postoperative survival. The presence of associated peripheral vascular disease signifying diffuse atherosclerosis, cigarette smoking, hypertension, and hypercholesterolemia all correlate with an increased likelihood of late death.[475]

SYMPTOMATIC RESULTS. Between 70 and 95 per cent of patients with chronic stable angina operated upon report relief of anginal symptoms and reduction of nitroglycerin and propranolol use[429,475a]; 33 to 55 per cent of patients become totally asymptomatic, while symptoms increase in approximately 5 per cent.[474] In many reports, this improvement in symptoms is a subjective impression and open to criticism in view of the profound placebo effect of a thoracotomy. However, unlike a placebo effect, which is usually transient, the improvement persists, and the results of exercise testing carried out pre- and postoperatively often substantiate the belief that true clinical benefit has been achieved. Techniques that combine pre- and postoperative myocardial imaging with thallium-201 often indicate that the improved symptomatic state results from improved regional myocardial perfusion via patent grafts.[476] In general, the clinical benefits of the operation can be related to graft patency and completeness of revascularization.[441,472] Return of angina with graft closure implies that a placebo effect is not of major importance with this kind of surgery. However, recurrence of symptoms, which occurs at an annual rate of 3.5 per cent is related to obstruction of vein grafts in one-fourth of patients, to progression of atherosclerosis in native ungrafted vessels in half the patients, and to both in the remaining one-fourth.[474,447] However, despite the salutary clinical results, the employment rate among these patients shows little tendency to rise postoperatively.[478,479]

VENTRICULAR FUNCTION. Determining whether or not coronary revascularization improves left ventricular function is complicated by the occasional occurrence of perioperative myocardial infarction, progression of disease in the native coronary arteries, and closure of bypass grafts. Improvement in function, no change, and worsening have been reported to varying degrees.[480,481] Improvement in symptoms of cardiac failure is also variable. In most patients in whom pre- and postoperative comparisons were made at rest, the cardiac output, stroke volume, left ventricular end-diastolic pressure and volume, and ejection fraction show no significant change for the group as a whole, although in individual patients there may be substantial changes in either direction. On the other hand, an improvement in left ventricular function during exercise can often be demonstrated by means of radionuclide cine ventriculography (Fig. 39–21).[475] In addition, if motion of left ventricular wall segments improved with nitroglycerin, they will usually improve with coronary bypass grafting, as will some persistent deficits on thallium perfusion scans.[472] Coronary artery bypass grafting has also been shown to reverse exertional hypotension, a manifestation of acute left ventricular dysfunction caused by widespread ischemia. Thus, in most cases, failure to demonstrate that surgery leads to improvement in the resting state suggests that the reperfused myocardium is not ischemic at rest; rather, it is the stress-induced depression of left ventricular function that can be improved by revascularization.

PERIOPERATIVE COMPLICATIONS. The rate of perioperative *myocardial infarction* that has been reported to be associated with elective coronary revascularization is approximately 5 per cent.[436,481,482] The most accurate method for diagnosing this complication relies on electrocardiographic evidence of new and persistant Q waves combined with marked elevation of cardiac enzymes, especially the

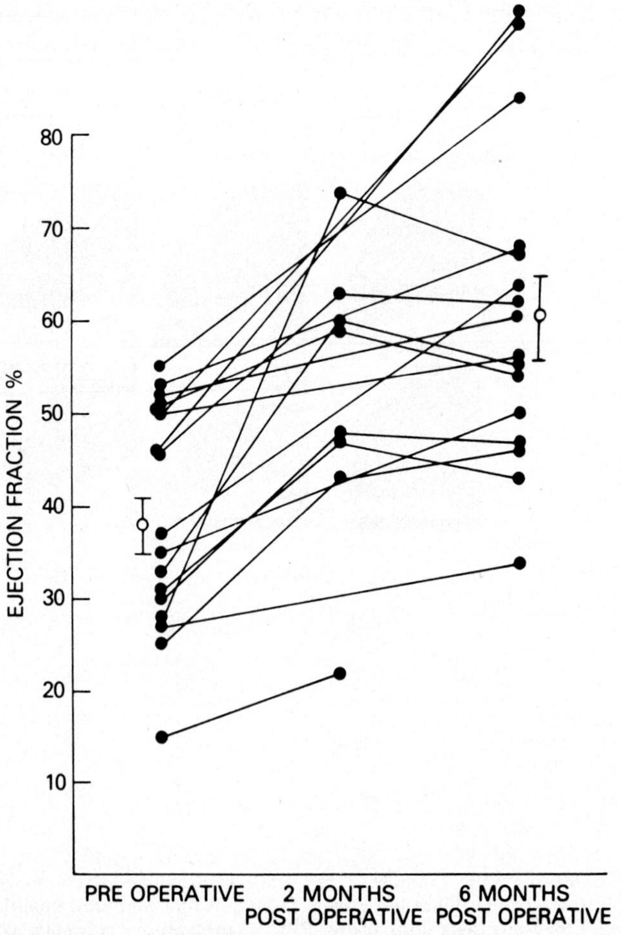

FIGURE 39–21 Radionuclide ejection fraction during exercise in 17 of 23 patients who showed improvement after operation. All 17 patients improved symptomatically (12 were entirely asymptomatic). By contrast, in the six patients with unchanged or decreased ejection fraction (not shown in figure), four had unchanged symptoms. (From Kent, K. M., et al.: Effects of coronary-artery bypass on global and regional left ventricular function during exercise. N. Engl. J. Med. *298*:1434, 1978.)

CK-MB fraction, and positive postoperative pyrophosphate scans.[483] The incidence of perioperative infarction is usually related to obstruction of a graft and correlates with the number of bypass grafts. Therefore, meticulous attention to anastomosis of the graft to the coronary artery is vital.[482] Although the loss of viable myocardium is obviously undesirable, in most patients the perioperative infarcts are small.

The development of *hypertension*[484] represents another postoperative problem peculiar to direct coronary revascularization. This complication, which may occur in up to one-third of all patients, can lead to fatal hemorrhage, cardiac failure, and arrhythmias. The mechanism responsible for the hypertension is unclear, but it may be related to increased levels of circulating catecholamines and renin. Intravenous sodium nitroprusside is effective for short-term management until appropriate oral antihypertensive agents, such as alpha-methyldopa, can be started.

GRAFT PATENCY RATE AND CHANGES IN THE NATIVE CIRCULATION. Overall, vein graft patency rates 6 to 12 months after operation range from 75 to 87 per cent[472]; since most patients receive multiple grafts, a larger percentage of patients, 84 to 95 per cent, have at least one patent graft.[429] Perhaps the most important single factor influencing graft patency is the flow rate through the graft, which in turn is a function of the severity of the obstruction in the native vessel proximal to the graft, the capacity of the distal arterial bed to accept the flow, and the technical adequacy of the operation; kinking or angulation of the graft, which diminishes flow rate, is particularly hazardous.[472a] Graft occlusion occurring within 6 to 12 months of operation is usually due to thrombosis; approximately half the occlusions occur within the first month after surgery.[472] Vein grafts may also undergo fibrous intimal, medial, and adventitial proliferation (Fig. 39–22) as well as atherosclerosis-like changes (Fig. 39–23),[485,486] and these morphological changes may represent a major cause of late graft closure,[487] which is approximately 2 per cent per year after the first year.[477,488] In a larger number of patients, particularly those with hyperlipidemia, progressive narrowing of the graft without total occlusion occurs.[485]

Contrast-enhanced computed tomography[489,490] represents a useful, relatively noninvasive way to assess patency of saphenous vein grafts (p. 191). In one prospective, randomized, double-blind trial, the effects of two platelet inhibitors on early postoperative vein graft patency were studied. Dipyridamole, begun 2 days before operation, and aspirin, begun 7 hours after operation, markedly reduced graft occlusion during a 4-month period.[491] Sulfinpyrazone has also been reported to reduce the incidence of early closure in grafts with flow rates exceeding 30 ml/min.[492]

Progression of atherosclerosis in the native coronary circulation may also contribute to poor clinical results. The tendency for proximal lesions to progress to complete stenosis is greater in operated than nonoperated vessels, but this is of little importance if the graft is patent; progression of disease distal to the graft can be expected to have more serious side effects. At an average followup of one

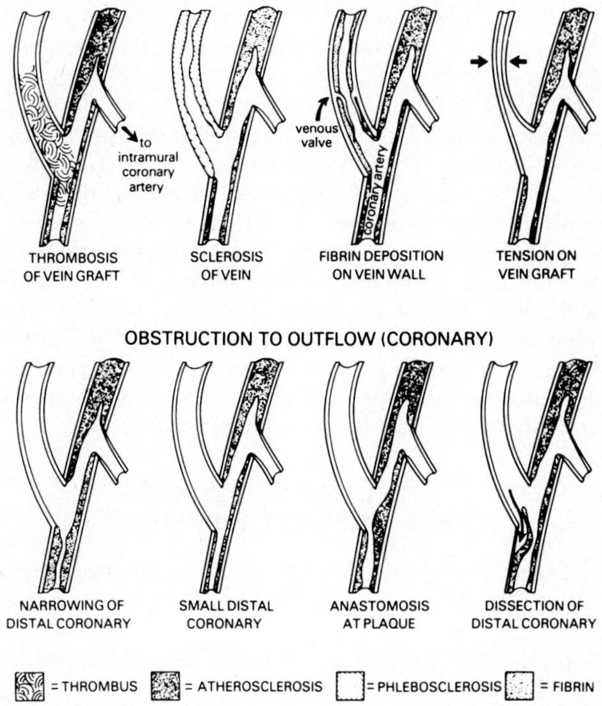

FIGURE 39–22 Anatomical and technical factors that can produce obstruction of a vein graft (top) and of arterial outflow (bottom). (From Spray, T. L., and Roberts, W. C.: Morphologic observations in biologic conduits between aorta and coronary artery. *In* Rahimtoola, S. (ed.): Coronary Bypass Surgery. Philadelphia, F. A. Davis, 1977, p. 11.)

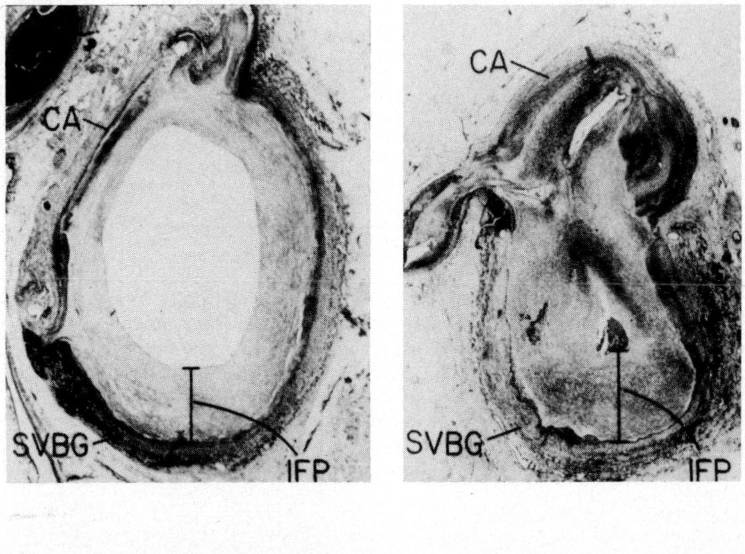

FIGURE 39–23 Postmortem histological sections through coronary artery (CA) anastomosis sites of saphenous vein bypass grafts (SVBG) show extensive fibrous tissue proliferation in the grafts' intimal layers. In the graft at left, the circumferential intimal fibrous plaque (IFP) developed in 5 months. In the graft at right, the process resulted in greater than 90 per cent stenosis 8 months after implantation. With time, such fibrous plaques may become infiltrated with lipids and calcium and increasingly resemble atherosclerotic plaques. (From Bulkley, B. H.: Why coronary bypass grafts fail: Early and late pathologic changes. J. Cardiovasc. Med. *5*:1025, 1980.)

year, the frequency of distal progression ranged from 27 to 35 per cent in two studies.[493,494] However, based on 5- to 7-year followup, grafting does not appear to accelerate distal progression.[495]

REOPERATION. Reoperation is indicated in patients with minimal relief of angina after the initial procedure or with recurrence of this symptom due to graft closure or progression of disease in unoperated arteries and in whom the distal vasculature and state of left ventricular function are still adequate for surgery. The procedure can be carried out with a relatively low mortality, only slightly higher than that for the initial procedure; relief of angina occurs in about two-thirds of the patients.[496,497] Reoperation tends to be more successful in relieving angina when it is performed in patients with new lesions in unoperated vessels than when carried out for graft occlusion.

EFFECT OF SURGICAL TREATMENT ON SURVIVAL

The question of whether or not coronary artery bypass grafting affects long-term survival is one of the most pressing questions in cardiology and can be answered only by a comparison of medically and surgically treated patients. This can be accomplished by the use of randomized trials as well as by comparing the outcome in suitably matched patients treated medically and surgically. There is general agreement that surgical treatment improves survival in patients with *left main coronary artery obstruction*[498–501] (Fig. 39–24). The greatest difference occurred in patients with associated disease of the right coronary artery and some degree of left ventricular dysfunction.

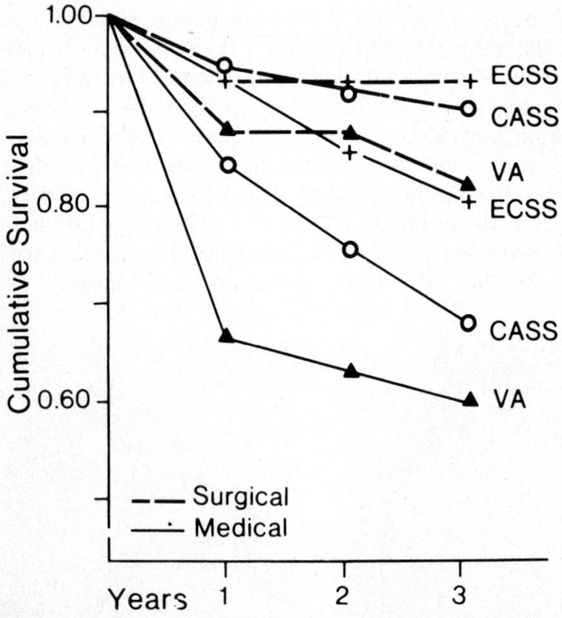

FIGURE 39–24 Cumulative 3-year survival rates of medically treated patients with left main coronary artery disease in three studies: Collaborative Study in Coronary Artery Surgery (CASS), the European Study (ECSS), and the Veterans Administration (VA) Study. (From Chaitman, B. R., et al.: Effect of coronary bypass surgery on survival patterns in subsets of patients with left main coronary artery disease. Am. J. Cardiol. *48*:765, 1981.)

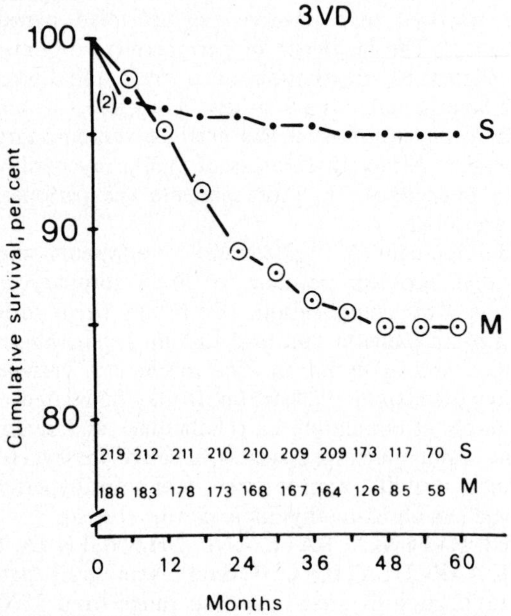

FIGURE 39–25 Cumulative survival curves for patients with three-vessel disease from the European Coronary Surgery Study. M = medical group; S = surgical group. Numbers along the bottom represent patients at risk at the beginning of each 6-month period. Numbers within parentheses indicate preoperative deaths in the surgical group. (From Varnauskas, E.: Prospective randomized study of coronary artery bypass surgery in stable angina pectoris. Lancet *2*: 491, 1980.)

Randomized trials in patients with chronic stable angina have shown that surgical treatment also prolongs life in patients with three-vessel disease (Fig. 39–25).[498,502] Among patients with two-vessel disease, those with proximal left anterior descending obstruction appeared to do better after surgery while other patients with two-vessel disease showed no change.[445] In one trial, surgical treatment has also been shown to improve longevity in patients at high risk, defined by four noninvasively determined characteristics: New York Heart Association Class III or IV, a history of hypertension, a history of prior myocardial infarction, and ST-segment depression on the resting electrocardiogram[503]; however, surgery did not have this effect in "low risk" patients. There is no evidence that surgical treatment improves survival in patients with any form of single-vessel disease, including isolated proximal left anterior descending coronary artery obstruction.[445] Asymptomatic or mildly symptomatic patients appear to have better prognoses than do seriously symptomatic patients,[389] and surgery appears to improve prognosis only in that subgroup of asymptomatic or mildly symptomatic patients who have three-vessel disease with some impairment of left ventricular function.[445] On the other hand, there is no evidence that surgery improves survival in asymptomatic survivors of two or three myocardial infarctions with multivessel disease.[450] Whether coronary surgery improves the prognosis of survivors of out-of-hospital ventricular fibrillation is unsettled, but based on some theoretical reasons and a few observations it may do so.[504]

INDICATIONS FOR SURGICAL TREATMENT (Table 39–10). Surgical treatment for chronic stable angina must be individualized. All patients in whom medical treatment has failed and who have persistent angina are

TABLE 39–10 CORONARY BYPASS SURGERY FOR ANGINA

Prolongs life
1. In LMCAD, particularly if LV function is moderately impaired
2. In three-vessel disease
3. In angina and ST depression on resting ECG + at least two of the following:
   NYHA Class III or IV
   History of myocardial infarction
   History of systemic hypertension *or* all three of the above with ECG changes

Symptomatic improvement

1.	50 to 70% asymptomatic	(0 to 9% with medical therapy)
2.	85 to 90% improved	(50% with medical therapy)
3.	81% no angina at rest	(65% with medical therapy)
4.	82% no unstable angina	(55% with medical therapy)
5.	75% no nitroglycerin	(36% with medical therapy)
6.	87% no propranolol	(33% with medical therapy)
7.	50% event-free course up to 7 years	(12% with medical therapy)

Risks
1. Operative mortality*
   a. 1.3%; varies from 0 to 3.5% in various subgroups:

Extext of CAD	*All patients*	*Normal LV function*	*Abnormal LV function*
One-vessel disease	0.5%	0.0%	1.7%
Two-vessel disease	0.8%	1.5%	0.0%
Three-vessel disease	1.5%	0.7%	2.1%
LMCAD	2.5%	0.0%	3.5%

   b. LV function: Normal 0.7%
      Abnormal 1.8%

   c. Age
      <45 years 0.0%
      45 to 65 years 1.3%
      >65 years 2.0%
2. Perioperative myocardial infarction ≤ 10% (may be as low as 2.5%)
3. Vein graft occlusion rate 10 to 15% (depends on state and location of grafted coronary artery; vein graft patency is 92% for LAD, 80% for RCA, and 70% for OM).
4. No patent grafts — 0 to 10% (depending on the number of grafts inserted)
5. No relief of pain — 5 to 10% (50% with medical therapy)
6. Angina worse — 6% (12% with medical therapy)
7. Recurrence of angina — 2 to 4% per year

Late survival
1. At 4 years 92.5% (91 to 94% is the 95% confidence interval)
2. Four-year survival in various subgroups:

   a.

Extent of CAD	*All patients*	*Normal LV function*	*Abnormal LV function*
One-vessel disease	97%	98%	94%
Two-vessel disease	95%	92%	97%
Three-vessel disease	90%	94%	87%
LMCAD	95%	97%	94%

   b. LV function: Normal 95%
      Abnormal 90%

   c. Age
      <45 years 98%
      45 to 65 years 93%
      ≥66 years 84%

*A 0% operative mortality means the operative mortality is very low but will not necessarily be 0% as more patients are operated.
Abbreviations: LMCAD = left main coronary artery disease; NYHA = New York Heart Association; LV = left ventricular; CAD = coronary artery disease; LAD = left anterior descending coronary artery; RCA = right coronary artery; OM = obtuse marginal coronary artery.
From Rahimtoola, S. H.: Coronary bypass surgery for chronic angina—A Perspective. Circulation *65*:225, 1982.

usually candidates for operation (or angioplasty). Patients with single-vessel disease are operated upon only to improve symptoms, not to prolong survival. Patients with left main coronary artery disease, with three-vessel coronary artery disease, and with two-vessel disease involving the proximal left anterior descending coronary artery who are moderately or severely symptomatic (but not necessarily medical failures) are ordinarily referred for surgery, unless there are specific contraindications.

The multicenter National Cooperative Study to Compare Medical and Surgical Therapy of Unstable Angina Pectoris evaluated 288 patients between 1972 and 1976.[286,443] One randomly selected group received intensive pharmacological treatment with nitrates and propranolol and another underwent emergency coronary revascularization. The surgical group had a higher early myocardial infarction rate and significantly improved long-term quality of life, compared with the medically treated group; almost half the latter eventually required surgical treatment. The finding of greater symptomatic relief with operation but without increased longevity has also been reported from smaller randomized series.[445] A major conclusion from these studies is that immediate bypass surgery can be reserved for patients with unstable angina who have signifi-

191. Hood, W. P., Jr., Amende, I., Simon, R., and Lichtlen, P. R.: The effects of intracoronary nitroglycerin on left ventricular and diastolic function in man. Circulation 61:1098, 1980.
192. Abrams, J.: Nitroglycerin and long-acting nitrates. N. Engl. J. Med. 302:1234, 1980.
193. Alpert, J. S.: Toward the more effective use of nitroglycerin. J. Cardiovasc. Med. 7:598, 1982.
194. Hales, C. A., and Westphal, D.: Hypoxemia following the administration of sublingual nitroglycerin. Am. J. Med. 65:911, 1978.
195. Needleman, P., Lang, S., and Johnson, E. M., Jr.: Organic nitrates: Relationship between biotransformation and rational angina pectoris therapy. J. Pharmacol. Exp. Ther. 181:489, 1972.
196. Glancy, D. L., Richter, M. A., Ellis, E. V., and Johnson, W.: Effect of swallowed isosorbide dinitrate on blood pressure, heart rate and exercise capacity in patients with coronary artery disease. Am. J. Med. 62:39, 1977.
197. Markis, J. E., Gorlin, R., Mills, R. M., Williams, R. A., Schweitzer, P., and Ransil, B. J.: Sustained effect of orally administered isosorbide dinitrate on exercise performance of patients with angina pectoris. Am. J. Cardiol. 43:265, 1979.
198. Lee, G., Mason, O. T., and DeMaria, A. N.: Effects of long-term oral administration of isosorbide dinitrate on the antianginal response to nitroglycerin. Am. J. Cardiol. 41:82, 1978.
199. Thadani, U., Fung, H. L., Darke, A. C., and Parker, J. O.: Oral isosorbide dinitrate in angina pectoris: Comparison of duration of action and dose-response relation during acute and sustained therapy. Am. J. Cardiol. 49:411, 1982.
200. Transdermal delivery systems for nitroglycerin. Med. Lett. 24:35, 1982.
201. Thompson, R. H.: The clinical use of transdermal delivery devices with nitroglycerin. Cardiovasc. Rev. Rep. 4:91, 1983.
202. Abrams, J.: Nitrate tolerance and dependence. Am. Heart J. 99:113, 1980.
203. Bassan, M. M., and Weiler-Ravell, D.: The additive antianginal action of oral isosorbide dinitrate in patients receiving propranolol. Magnitude and duration of effect. Chest 83:233, 1983.
204. Epstein, S. E., and Braunwald, E.: Inhibition of the adrenergic nervous system in the treatment of angina pectoris. Med. Clin. North Am. 52:1031, 1968.
205. Braunwald, E. (ed.): Beta-Adrenergic Blockade—A New Era in Cardiovascular Medicine. New York, Excerpta Medica, 1978, 309 pp.
206. Miller, R. R., Olson, H. G., and Pratt, C. M.: Efficacy of beta-adrenergic blockade in coronary heart disease: Propranolol in angina pectoris. Clin. Pharmacol. Ther. 18:598, 1975.
207. Manyari, D. E., Kostuk, W. J., Carruthers, G., Johnston, D. J., and Purves, P.: Pindolol and propranolol inpatients with angina pectoris and normal or near-normal ventricular function. Lack of influence of intrinsic sympathomimetic activity on global and segmental left ventricular function assessed by radionuclide ventriculography. Am. J. Cardiol. 51:427, 1983.
207a. Harris, F. J., Low, R. I., Palmer, L., Amsterdam, E. A., and Mason, D. T.: Antianginal efficacy and improved exercise performance with timolol. Twice-daily beta blockade in ischemic heart disease. Am. J. Cardiol. 51:13, 1983.
208. Watanabe, A. G.: Recent advances in knowledge about beta-adrenergic receptors: Application to clinical cardiology. J. Am. Coll. Cardiol. 1:82, 1983.
209. Alderman, E. L., Davies, R. O., Crowley, J. J., Lopes, M. G., Brooker, J. Z., Friedman, J. P., Graham, A. F., Matlof, H. J., and Harrison, D. C.: Dose response effectiveness of propranolol for the treatment of angina pectoris. Circulation 51:964, 1975.
210. Pine, M., Favrot, L., Smith, S., McDonald, K., and Chidsey, C. A.: Correlation of plasma propranolol concentration with therapeutic response in patients with angina pectoris. Circulation 52:886, 1975.
211. Parmley, W. W.: Beta blockers in coronary artery disease. Cardiovasc. Rev. Rep. 2:655, 1981.
212. Koch-Weser, J.: Beta-adrenoceptor antagonists: New drugs and new indications. N. Engl. J. Med. 305:500, 1981.
213. Miller, R. R., Olson, H. G., Amsterdam, E. A., and Mason, D. T.: Propranolol withdrawal rebound phenomenon. Exacerbation of coronary events after abrupt cessation of antianginal therapy. N. Engl. J. Med. 293:416, 1975.
214. Aarons, R. D., and Molinoff, P. B.: Changes in the density of beta adrenergic receptors in rat lymphocytes, heart and lung after chronic treatment with propranolol. J. Pharmacol. Exp. Ther. 221:439, 1982.
215. Kern, M. J., Ganz, P., Horowitz, J. D., Gaspar, J., Barry, W. H., Lorell, B. H., Grossman, W., and Mudge, G. H., Jr.: Potentiation of coronary vasoconstriction by beta-adrenergic blockade. Circulation 67:1178, 1983.
216. Robertson, R. M., Wood, A. J. J., Vaughn, W. K., and Robertson, D.: Exacerbation of vasotonic angina pectoris by propranolol. Circulation 65:281, 1982.
217. Cruickshank, J. M.: The clinical importance of cardioselectivity and lipophilicity in beta blockers. Am. Heart J. 100:160, 1980.
218. Frishman, W. H., and Kostis, J.: The significance of intrinsic sympathomimetic activity in beta-adrenoceptor blocking drugs. Cardiovasc. Rev. Rep. 3:503, 1982.
219. Kostis, J. B., Frishman, W., Hosler, M. H., Thorsen, N. L., Gonasun, L., and Weinstein, J.: Treatment of angina pectoris with pindolol: The significance of intrinsic sympathomimetic activity of beta blockers. Am. Heart J. 104:496, 1982.
220. Cannon, R. E., Slavin, R. G., and Gonasun, L. M.: The effect on asthma of a new beta blocker, pindolol. Am. Heart J. 104:438, 1982.
221. Krikler, D. M., and Rowland, E.: Clinical value of calcium antagonists in treatment of cardiovascular disorders. J. Am. Coll. Cardiol. 1:355, 1983.
222. Fleckenstein, A.: Calcium Antagonist in Heart and Smooth Muscle. New York, John Wiley and Sons, 1983.
222a. Sherman, G., and Liang, C-S.: Nifedipine in chronic stable angina: A double-blind placebo-controlled crossover trial. Am. J. Cardiol. 51:706, 1983.
222b. Stone, P. H., Turi, Z., Muller, J. E., Geltman, E., Jaffe, A., and Braunwald, E.: Experience with nifedipine in 845 patients with refractory angina pectoris. J. Am. Coll. Cardiol. 1:596, 1983.
222c. Subramanian, B.: Long-term therapy of angina with calcium antagonists. Cardiovasc. Rev. Rep. 4:493, 1983.
222d. Subramanian, V. B., Khurmi, N. S., Bowles, M. J., O'Hara, M., and Raftery, E. B.: Objective evaluation of three dose levels of diltiazem in patients with chronic stable angina. J. Am. Coll. Cardiol. 1:1144, 1983.
223. Ludbrook, P. A., Tiefenbrunn, A. J., Reed, F. R., and Sobel, B. E.: Acute hemodynamic responses to sublingual nifedipine: Dependence on left ventricular function. Circulation 65:489, 1982.
224. Klein, H. O., Ninio, R., Oren, V., Lang, R., Sareli, P., DiSegni, E., David, D., Guerrero, J., and Kaplinsky, E.: The acute hemodynamic effects of intravenous verapamil in coronary artery disease. Assessment by equilibrium-gated radionuclide ventriculography. Circulation 67:101, 1983.
225. Rouleau, J., Chatterjee, K., Ports, T. A., Doyle, M. B., Hiramatsu, B., and Parmley, W. W.: Mechanism of relief of pacing-induced angina with oral verapamil: Reduced oxygen demand. Circulation 67:94, 1983.
225a. Chew, C. Y. C., Brown, B. G., Singh, B. N., Wong, M. M., Pierce, C., and Petersen, R.: Effects of verapamil on coronary hemodynamic function and vasomobility relative to its mechanism of antianginal action. Am. J. Cardiol. 51:699, 1983.
226. Charlap, S., and Frishman, W. H.: Comparative effects of verapamil and beta blockers in the therapy for patients with stable angina pectoris. Cardiovasc. Rev. Rep. 4:66, 1983.
227. Leon, M. B., Rosing, D. R., Bonow, R. O., Lipson, L. C., and Epstein, S. E.: Clincial efficacy of verapamil alone and combined with propranolol in treating patients with chronic stable angina pectoris. Am. J. Cardiol. 48:131, 1981.
228. Wagniart, P., Ferguson, R. J., Chaitman, B. R., Achard F., Benacerraf, A., Delanguenhagen, B., Morin, B., Pasternac, A., and Bourassa, M. G.: Increased exercise tolerance and reduced electrocardiographic ischemia with diltiazem in patients with stable angina pectoris. Circulation 66:23, 1982.
229. Schroeder, J. S., McAuley, B., and Ginsburg, R.: Diltiazem: A clinical and pharmacologic profile. J. Cardiovasc. Med. 8:41, 1983.
229a. Smith, M. S., Verghese, C. P., Shand, D. G., and Pritchett, E. L. C.: Pharmacokinetic and pharmacodynamic effects of diltiazem. Am. J. Cardiol. 51:1369, 1983.
230. Marra, S., Paolillo, V., Baduini, G., Spadaccini, F., and Angelino, P. F.: Acute effects of chewable nifedipine on hemodynamic responses to upright exercise in patients with prior myocardial infarction and effort angina. Chest 83:50, 1983.
231. Furberg, C. D., Friedewald, W. T., and Eberlein, K. A. (eds.): Proceedings of the workshop on implications of recent beta-blocker trials for post-myocardial infarction patients. Circulation 67:1–111, 1983.
232. Turi, Z. G., and Braunwald, E.: The use of beta blockers after myocardial infarction. JAMA 249:2512, 1983.
233. Pfisterer, M., Glaus, L., and Burkart, F.: Comparative effects of nitroglycerin, nifedipine and metoprolol on regional left ventricular function in patients with one-vessel coronary disease. Circulation 67:291, 1983.
234. Johnson, S. M., Mauritson, D. R., Corbett, J. R., Woodward, W., Willerson, J. T., and Hillis, L. D.: Double-blind, randomized, placebo-controlled comparison of propranolol and verapamil in the treatment of patients with stable angina pectoris. Am. J. Med. 71:443, 1981.
235. Braunwald, E.: Mechanism of action of calcium-channel-blocking agents. N. Engl. J. Med. 307:1618, 1983.
236. Dargie, H. J., Lynch, P. G., Krikler, D. M., Harris, L., and Krikler, S.: Nifedipine and propranolol: A beneficial drug interaction. Am. J. Med. 71: 676, 1981.
237. Pfisterer, M., Muller-Brand, J., and Burkart, F.: Combined acebutolol/nifedipine therapy in patients with chronic coronary artery disease: Additional improvement of ischemia-induced left ventricular dysfunction. Am. J. Cardiol. 49:1259, 1982.
238. Bassan, M., Weiler-Ravell, D., and Shalev, O.: The additive antianginal action of oral nifedipine in patients receiving propranolol. Magnitude and duration of effect. Circulation 66:710, 1982
239. Winniford, M. D., Huxley, R. L., and Hillis, L. D.: Randomized, double-blind comparison of propranolol alone and a propranolol-verpamil combination in patients with severe angina of effort. J. Am. Coll. Cardiol. 1:492, 1983.
239a. Johnston, D. L., Gebhart, V., Lesoway, R., and Kostuk, W. J.: Hemodynamic evaluation of verapamil and propranolol alone and in combination: Assessment of radionuclide ventriculography. J. Am. Coll. Cardiol. 1:679, 1983.
239b. Lessem, J.: Combined therapy with verapamil and atenolol in chronic stable angina. J. Am. Coll. Cardiol. 1:596, 1983.
240. Packer, M., Meller, J., Medina, N., Yushak, M., Smith, H., Holt, J., Guererro, J., Todd, G. D., McAllister, R. G., Jr., and Gorlin, R.: Hemodynamic consequences of combined beta-adrenergic and slow calcium channel blockade in man. Circulation 65:660, 1982.
241. Kieval, J., Kirsten, E. B., Kessler, K. M., Mallon, S. M., and Myerburg, R. J.: The effects of intravenous verapamil on hemodynamic status of patients with coronary artery disease receiving propranolol. Circulation 65:653, 1982.
242. Hood, W. B., Jr.: More on sulfinpyrazone after myocardial infarction (Editorial). N. Engl. J. Med. 306:988, 1982.
243. Grüntzig, A. R., and Meier, B.: Percutaneous transluminal coronary angioplasty. The first five years and the future. Intern. J. Cardiol. 2:319, 1983.
243a. Dorros, G., Cowley, M. J., Simpson, J., Bentivoglio, L. G., Block, P. C., Bourassa, M., Detre, K., Goselin, A. J., Gruntzig, A. R., Kelsey, S. F., Kent, K. M., Mock, M. B., Mulin, S. M., Myuler, R. K., Passamani, E. R., Stertzer, S. H., and Williams, D. O.: Percutaneous transluminal coronary angioplasty: Report of complications from the National Heart, Lung and Blood Institute PTCA registry. Circulation 67:723, 1983.
243b. Holmes, D. R., Jr., Vlietstra, R. E., Mock, M. B., Reeder, G. S., Smith, H. C., Bove, A. A., Bresnahan, J. F., Piehler, J. M., Schaff, H. V., and Orszulak,

T. A.: Angiographic changes produced by percutaneous transluminal coronary angioplasty. Am. J. Cardiol. *51*:676, 1983.

243c. Meier, B., Hollman, J., and Gruentzig, A. R.: Percutaneous transluminal coronary angioplasty. Circulation *67*:1155, 1983.

244. Block, P. C., Myler, R. K., Stertzer, S., and Fallon, J. T.: Morphology after transluminal angioplasty in human beings. N. Engl. J. Med. *305*:382, 1981.

245. Meier, B., Grüntzig, A. R., Hollman, J., Ischinger, T., and Bradford, J. M.: Does length or eccentricity of coronary stenoses influence the outcome of transluminal dilatation? Circulation *67*:497, 1983.

245a. Vlietstra, R. E., Holmes, D. R., Jr., Mock, M. B., Smith, H. C., Reeder, G. S., Bresnahan, J. F., Bove, A. A., and Piehler, J. M.: Balloon angioplasty in multivessel coronary disease: Mayo Clinic experience. J. Am. Coll. Cardiol. *1*: 656, 1983.

245b. Williams, D. O., Kurzrok, S., Riley, R., Singh, A., and Most, A.: Partial revascularization by single vessel coronary angioplasty: Efficacious therapy of multivessel coronary artery disease. J. Am. Coll. Cardiol. *1*:655, 1983.

246. Kent, K. M., Bonow, R. O., Rosing, D. R., Ewels, C. J., Lipson, L. C., McIntosh, C. L., Bacharach, S., Green, M., and Epstein, S. E.: Improved myocardial function during exercise after successful percutaneous transluminal coronary angioplasty. N. Engl. J. Med. *306*:441, 1982.

247. Kent, K. M., Bentivoglio, L. G., Block, P. C., Cowley, M. J., Dorros, G., Gosselin, A. J., Grüntzig, A., Myler, R. K., Simpson, J., Stertzer, S. H., Williams, D. O., Fisher, L., Gillespie, M. J., Detre, K., Kelsey, S., Mullin, S. M., and Mock, M. B.: Percutaneous transluminal coronary angioplasty: Report from the registry of the National Heart, Lung, and Blood Institute, Am. J. Cardiol. *49*:2011, 1982.

247a. Hollman, J., Gruentzig, A., Meier, B., Bradford, J., and Galan, K.: Factors affecting recurrence after successful coronary angioplasty. J. Am. Coll. Cardiol. *1*:644, 1983.

247b. Williams, D. O., Gruntzig, A., Kent, K., Detre, K., Kelsey, C., Shalloner, K., and members of the Executive Committee, NHLBI: Role of repeated percutaneous transluminal coronary angioplasty (PTCA) for coronary restenosis: A report of the NHLBI PTCA registry. J. Am. Coll. Cardiol. *1*:644, 1983.

248. Sigwart, U., Grbic, M., Essinger, A., Bischof-Delaloye, A., Sadeghi, H., and Rivier, J.-L.: Improvement of left ventricular function after percutaneous transluminal coronary angioplasty. Am. J. Cardiol. *49*:651, 1982.

248a. Williams, D., Singh, A., and Most, A.: Sustained efficacy of coronary angioplasty documented by stress testing at one year. J. Am. Coll. Cardiol. *1*:724, 1983.

249. Hirzel, H. O., Nuesch, K., Grüntzig, A. R., and Leutolf, U. M.: Short- and long-term changes in myocardial perfusion after percutaneous transluminal coronary angioplasty assessed by thallium-201 exercise scintigraphy. Circulation *63*:1001, 1981.

250. Scholl, J. M., Chaitman, B. R., David, P. R., Dupras, G., Bevers, G., Val, P. G., Crepeau, J., Lesperance, J., and Bourassa, M. G.: Exercise electrocardiography and myocardial scintigraphy in the serial evaluation of the results of percutaneous transluminal coronary angioplasty. Circulation *66*:380, 1982.

251. Choy, D. S. J., Stertzer, S., Rotterdam, H. Z., Sharrock, N., and Kaminow, I. P.: Transluminal laser catheter angioplasty. Am. J. Cardiol. *50*:1206, 1982.

252. Choy, D. S. J., Stertzer, S. H., Rotterdam, H. Z., and Bruno M. S.: Laser coronary angioplasty: Experience with 9 cadaver hearts. Am. J. Cardiol. *50*:1209, 1982.

252a. Lee, G., Ikeda, R., Herman, I., Dwyer, R. M., Bass, M., Hussein, H., Kozina, J., and Mason, D. T.: The qualitative effects of laser irradiation on human arteriosclerotic disease. Am. Heart J. *105*:885, 1983.

252b. Choy, D. S., Stertzer, H., Quilici, P., Wallsh, E., Bruno, M. S., Loubeau, J-M., Kaminow, I., and Rotterdam, H.: Argon laser angioplasty in cadaver and animal models. J. Am. Coll. Cardiol. *1*:690, 1983.

252c. Gessman, L. J., Reno, C. W., and Hastie, R.: Model for testing coronary angioplasty by laser catheter. J. Am. Coll. Cardiol. *1*:690, 1983.

253. Mills, N. L., and Doyle, D. P.: Does operative transluminal angioplasty extend the limits of coronary artery bypass surgery? A preliminary report. Circulation *66*(Suppl. 1):26, 1982.

254. Jones, E. L., and King, S. B.: Intraoperative angioplasty in the treatment of coronary artery disease. J. Am. Coll. Cardiol. *1*:970, 1983.

255. Kannel, W. B., and Feinleib, M.: Natural history of angina pectoris in the Framingham study: Progress and survival. Am. J. Cardiol. *29*:154, 1972.

256. Frank, C. W., Weinblatt, W., and Shapiro, S.: Angina pectoris in men: Prognostic significance of related medical factors. Circulation *47*:509, 1973.

257. Vedin, A., Wilhelmsson, C., Elmfeldt, D., Save-Soderbergh, J., Tibblin, G., and Wilhelmsen, L.: Death and non-fatal reinfarctions during two years' follow-up after myocardial infarction. Acta Med. Scand. *198*:353, 1975.

258. Graham, I., Mulcahy, R., Hickey, N., O'Neill, W., and Daly, L.: Natural history of coronary heart disease: A study of 586 men surviving an initial acute attack. Am. Heart J. *105*:249, 1983.

259. Frank, C. W., Weinblatt, E., Shapiro, S., and Sager, R. V.: Prognosis of men with coronary heart disease as related to blood pressure. Circulation *38*:432, 1968.

260. Gorlin, R.: Natural history of coronary heart disease. *In* Gorlin, R.: Coronary Artery Disease. Philadelphia, W. B. Saunders Co., 1976, p. 195.

261. Spain, D. M., and Bradess, V. A.: Sudden death from coronary heart disease: Survival time, frequency of thrombi and cigarette smoking. Chest *58*:107, 1970.

262. Blackburn, H.: The prognostic importance of the electrocardiogram after myocardial infarction: Experience in the coronary drug project. Ann. Intern. Med. *77*:677, 1972.

263. Kotler, M. N., Tabatznik, B., Mower, M. M., and Tominaga, S.: Prognostic significance of ventricular ectopic beats with respect to sudden death in the late postinfarction period. Circulation *47*:959, 1973.

264. Kannel, W. B., Boyle, J. T., McNamara, P., Quickenton, P., and Gordon, T.: Precursors of sudden coronary death: Factors related to the incidence of sudden death. Circulation *51*:606, 1975.

265. Reeves, T. J., Oberman, A., Jones, W. B., and Sheffield, L. T.: Natural history of angina pectoris. Am. J. Cardiol. *33*:423, 1974.

266. Califf, R. M., Tomabechi, Y., Lee, K. L., Phillips, H., Pryor, D. B., Harrell, F. E., Jr., Harris, P. J., Peter, R. H., Behar, V. S., Kong, Y., and Rosati, R. A.: Outcome in one-vessel coronary artery disease. Circulation *67*:283, 1983.

267. Burggraf, G. W., and Parker, J. O.: Prognosis in coronary artery disease—angiographic, hemodynamic and clinical factors. Circulation *51*:146, 1975.

268. Humphries, J. O., Kuller, L., Ross, R. S., Friesinger, G. C., and Page, E. E.: Natural history of ischemic heart disease in relation to arteriographic findings. Circulation *49*:489, 1974.

269. Oberman, A., Jones, W. B., and Riley, C. P.: Natural history of coronary artery disease. Bull. N.Y. Acad. Med. *48*:1109, 1972.

270. Harris, P. J., Behar, V. S., Conley, M. J., Harrell, F. E., Jr., Lee, K. L., Peter, R. H., Kong, Y., and Rosati, R. A.: The prognostic significance of 50 per cent coronary stenosis in medically treated patients with coronary artery disease. Circulation *62*:240, 1980.

271. Kent, K. M., Rosing, D. R., Ewels, C. J., Lipson, L., Bonow, R., and Epstein, S. E.: Prognosis of asymptomatic or mildly symptomatic patients with coronary artery disease. Am. J. Cardiol. *49*:1823, 1982.

272. Proudfit, W. L., Bruschke, A. V., and Sones, F. M., Jr.: Natural history of obstructive coronary artery disease: Ten-year study of 601 nonsurgical cases. Progr. Cardiovasc. Dis. *22*:53, 1978.

273. Bruschke, A. V., Proudfit, W. L., and Sones, F. M., Jr.: Progress study of 490 consecutive nonsurgical cases of coronary disease followed 5–9 years. II. Ventriculographic and other correlations. Circulation *47*:1154, 1973.

274. Gross, H., Vaid, A. K., and Cohen, M. K.: Prognosis in patients rejected for coronary revascularization surgery. Am. J. Med. *64*:9, 1978.

275. Nelson, G. R., Cohn, P. F., and Gorlin, R.: Prognosis in medically treated coronary artery disease. The value of the ejection fraction compared with other measurements. Circulation *52*:408, 1975.

276. Harlan, W. R., Oberman, A., Grimm, R., and Rosati, R. A.: Chronic congestive heart failure in coronary artery disease: Clinical criteria, Ann. Intern. Med. *86*:133, 1977.

277. Bruschke, A. V., Proudfit, W. L., and Sones, F. M., Jr.: Progress study of 490 consecutive nonsurgical cases of coronary disease followed 5–9 years. I. Arteriographic correlations. Circulation *47*:1147, 1973.

278. Conti, C. R., Selby, J. H., and Christie, L. G.: Left main coronary artery stenosis: Clinical spectrum, pathophysiology and management. Progr. Cardiovasc. Dis. *22*:73, 1979.

278a. Takaro, T., Peduzzi, P., Detre, K. M., Hultgren, H. N., Murphy, M. L., Bel-Kahn, J., Thomsen, J., and Meadows, W. R.: Survival in subgroups of patients with left main coronary artery disease. Veterans Administration Cooperative Study of Surgery for Coronary Arterial Occlusive Disease. Circulation *66*:14, 1982.

279. Bemis, C. E., Gorlin, R., Kemp, H. G., and Herman, M. V.: The progression of coronary obstructive disease. A clinical arteriographic study. Circulation *47*: 455, 1973.

280. Kramer, J. R., Matsuda, Y., Mulligan, J. C., Aronow, M., and Proudfit, W. L.: Progression of coronary atherosclerosis. Circulation *63*:519, 1981.

281. Bruschke, A. V. G., Wijers, T. S., Kolsters, W., and Landmann, J.: The anatomic evolution of coronary artery disease demonstrated by coronary arteriography in 256 nonoperated patients. Circulation *63*:527, 1981.

281a. Hansteen, V., Moinichen, E., Lorenstsen, E., Andersen, A., Strom, O., Soiland, K., Dyrbekk, D., Refsum, A.-M., Tromsdal, A., Knudsen, K., Eika, C., Bakken, J., Jr., Smith, P., and Hoff, P. I.: One year's treatment with propranolol after myocardial infarction: Preliminary report of Norwegian multicentre trial. Br. Med. J. *284*:155, 1982.

UNSTABLE ANGINA

282. Adelman, A. G., and Goldman, B. S. (Eds.): Unstable Angina. Recognition and Management. Littleton, Col., 1981, PSG Publishing Co., Inc.

283. Fowler, N. O.: Preinfarction angina. Circulation *44*:775, 1971.

284. Willerson, J. T., Hillis, L. D., and Buja, L. M.: Ischemic Heart Disease. New York, Raven Press, 1982.

285. Robbins, S. L.: Clinicopathologic correlations in coronary atherosclerosis. Four hundred and thirty patients studied with postmortem coronary angiography. Circulation *27*:170, 1963.

286. Fulton, M., Lutz, W., Donald, K. W., Kirby, B. J., Duncan, B., Morrison, S. L., Kerr, F., Julian, D. G., and Oliver, M. F.: Natural history of unstable angina. Lancet *1*:860, 1972.

287. Report of the Unstable Angina Pectoris Study Group: Unstable angina pectoris: National Cooperative Group to Compare Medical and Surgical Therapy. II. In-hospital experience and initial follow-up results in patients with one, two, and three vessel disease. Am. J. Cardiol. *42*:839, 1978.

288. Gazes, P. C., Mobley, E. M., Jr., Faris, H. M., Jr., Duncan, R. C., and Humphries, G. B.: Preinfarctional (stable) angina—a prospective study; Ten year follow-up. Prognostic significance of electrocardiographic changes. Circulation *48*:331, 1973.

289. Victor, M. F., Likoff, M. J., Mintz, G. S., and Likoff, W.: Unstable angina pectoris of new onset: A prospective clinical and arteriographic study of 75 patients. Am. J. Cardiol. *47*:228, 1981.

290. Fischl, S., Gorlin, R., and Herman, M. V.: The intermediate coronary syndrome: Clinical, angiographic and therapeutic aspects. N. Engl. J. Med. *288*: 1193, 1973.

291. Plotnick, G. D., and Conti, C. R.: Transient ST-segment elevation in unstable angina. Clinical and hemodynamic significance. Circulation *51*:1015, 1975.
292. Bodenheimer, M. M., Banka, V. S., Trout, R. G., Hermann, G. A., Pasdar, H., and Helfant, R. H.: Pathophysiologic significance of ST and T wave abnormalities in patients with the intermediate coronary syndrome. Am. J. Cardiol. *39*:153, 1977.
293. Rackley, C. E., Russell, R. O., Jr., Rogers, W. J., Mantle, J. A., and Papapietro, S. E.: Unstable angina pectoris: Is it time to change our approach? Am. Heart J. *103*:154, 1982.
294. Alison, H. W., Russel, R. O., Jr., Mantle, J. A., Kouchoukos, N. T., and Rackley, C. E.: Coronary anatomy and arteriography in patients with unstable angina pectoris. Am. J. Cardiol. *41*:204, 1978.
295. Roberts, W. C., and Virmani, Z.: Quantitation of coronary arterial narrowing in clinically isolated unstable angina pectoris: An analysis of 22 necropsy patients. Am. J. Med. *67*:792, 1979.
296. Parker, F. B., Jr., Neville, J. F., Jr., Hanson, E. C., and Webb, W. R.: Retrograde and antegrade pressures and flows in preinfarction syndrome. Circulation *50*(Suppl. 11):122, 1974.
297. Sharma, B., Hodges, M., Asinger, R. W., Goodwin, J. F., and Francis, G. S.: Left ventricular function during spontaneous angina pectoris: Effect of sublingual nitroglycerin. Am. J. Cardiol. *46*:34, 1980.
298. Roughgarden, J. W.: Circulatory changes associated with spontaneous angina pectoris. Am. J. Med. *41*:947, 1966.
299. Cannom, D. S., Harrison, D. C., and Schroeder, J. S.: Hemodynamic observations in patients with unstable angina pectoris. Am. J. Cardiol. *33*:17, 1974.
300. Maseri, A.: Variant angina and coronary vasospasm: Clues to a broader understanding of angina pectoris. Cardiovasc. Med. *4*:647, 1979.
301. Chierchia, S., Brunelli, C., Simonetti, I., Lazzari, M., and Maseri, A.: Sequence of events in angina at rest: Primary reduction in coronary flow. Circulation *61*: 759, 1980.
302. Holmes, D. R., Jr., Hartzler, G. O., Smith, H. C., and Fuster, V.: Coronary artery thrombosis in patients with unstable angina. Br. Heart J. *45*:411, 1981.
303. Neill, W. A., Wharton, T. P., Jr., Fluri-Lundeen, J., and Cohen, I. S.: Acute coronary insufficiency—Coronary occlusion after intermittent ischemic attacks. N. Engl. J. Med. *302*:1157, 1980.
304. Specchia, G., de Servi, S., Falcone, C., Bramucci, E., Angoli, L., Mussini, A., Marioni, G. P., Montemartini, C., and Bobba, P.: Coronary arterial spasm as a cause of exercise-induced ST-segment elevation in patients with variant angina. Circulation *59*:948, 1979.
305. Biagini, A., Mazzei, M. G., Carpeggiani, C., Testa, R., Antonelli, R., Michelassi, C., L'Abbate, A., and Maseri, A.: Vasospastic ischemic mechanism of frequent asymptomatic transient ST-T changes during continuous electrocardiographic monitoring in selected unstable angina patients. Am. Heart J. *103*:13, 1982.
306. Johnson, S. M., Mauritson, D. R., Winniford, M. D., Willerson, J. T., Firth, B. G., Cary, J. R., and Hillis, L. D.: Continuous electrocardiographic monitoring in patients with unstable angina pectoris: Identification of high-risk subgroup with severe coronary disease, variant angina, and/or impaired early prognosis. Am. Heart J. *103*:4, 1982.
307. Donsky, M. S., Curry, G. C., Parkey, R. W., Meyer, S. L., Bonte, F. J., Platt, M. R., and Willerson, J. T.: Unstable angina pectoris. Clinical, angiographic, and myocardial scintigraphic observations. Br. Heart J. *38*:257, 1976.
308. Uthurralt, N., Davies, G. J., Parodi, O., Bencivelli, W., and Maseri, A.: Comparative study of myocardial ischemia during angina at rest and on exertion using thallium-201 scintigraphy. Am. J. Cardiol. *48*:410, 1981.
309. Nixon, J. V., Brown, C. N., and Smitherman, T. C.: Identification of transient and persistent segmental wall motion abnormalities in patients with unstable angina by two-dimensional echocardiography. Circulation *65*:1497, 1982.
310. Conti, R., Brawley, R., Pitt, B., and Ross, R.: Unstable angina: Morbidity and mortality in 57 consecutive patients evaluated angiographically. Am. J. Cardiol. *32*:745, 1973.
311. Scanlon, P. J., Nemickas, R., Moran, J. F., Talano, J. V., Amirparviz, F., and Pifane, R.: Accelerated angina pectoris. Clinical, hemodynamic, arteriographic and therapeutic experience in 85 patients. Circulation *47*:19, 1973.
312. Weintraub, R. M., Aroesty, J. M., Paulin, S., Levine, F. H., Markis, J. E., LaRaia, P. J., Cohen, S. I., and Kurland, G. S.: Medically refractory unstable angina pectoris. I. Long-term follow-up of patients undergoing intraaortic balloon counterpulsation and operation. Am. J. Cardiol. *43*:877, 1979.
313. Levine, F. H., Gold, H. K., Leinbach, R. C., Daggett, W. M., Austen, W. G., and Buckley, M. J.: Management of acute myocardial ischemia with intraaortic balloon pumping and coronary bypass surgery. Circulation *58*(Suppl. 1):69, 1978.
314. Conti, C. R.: Treatment of unstable angina: A model for step therapy. Cardiovasc. Rev. Rep. *3*:1306, 1982.
315. Cohn, P. F., and Cohn, L. H.: Medical/surgical treatment of unstable angina. *In* Cohn, L. H. (ed.): The Treatment of Acute Myocardial Ischemia: An Integrated Medical-Surgical Approach, Mt. Kisco, N.Y., Futura Publishing Co., 1979, p. 105.
316. Mohr, R., Smolinsky, A., and Goor, D. A.: Treatment of nocturnal angina with 10° reverse Trendelenburg bed position. Lancet *1*:1325, 1982.
317. Curfman, G. D., Heinsimer, J. A., Lozner, E. C., and Fung, H.: Intravenous nitroglycerin in the treatment of spontaneous angina pectoria: A prospective, randomized trial. Circulation *67*:276, 1983.
317a. Kaplan, K., Davison, R., Parker, M., Przybylek, J., Teagarden, J. R., and Lesch, M.: Intravenous nitroglycerin for the treatment of angina at rest unresponsive to standard nitrate therapy. Am. J. Cardiol. *51*:694, 1983.
318. Mehta, J., Pepine, C. J., Day, M., Guerrero, J. R., and Conti, C. R.: Short-term efficacy of oral verapamil in rest angina. A double-blind placebo controlled trial in CCU patients. Am. J. Med. *71*:977, 1981.
319. Moses, J. W., Wertheimer, J. H., Bodenheimer, M. M., Banka, V. S., Feldman, M., and Helfant, R. H.: Efficacy of nifedipine in rest angina refractory to propranolol and nitrates in patients with obstructive coronary artery disease. Ann. Intern. Med. *94*:425, 1981.
320. Gerstenblith, G., Ouyang, P., Achuff, S. C., Bulkley, B. H., Becker, L. C., Mellits, E. D., Baughman, K. L., Weiss, J. L., Flaherty, J. T., Kallman, C. H., Llewellyn, M., and Weisfeldt, M. L.: Nifedipine in unstable angina: A double-blind, randomized trial. N. Engl. J. Med. *306*:885, 1982.
320a. Robertson, R. M., Robertson, D., Davison, R., Kaplan, K., Haywood, L. J., Goldstein, S., Lee, T. G., Mehta, J., Conti, C. R., Simpson, R. J., and Singh, B.: Angina at rest: A double-blind, placebo-controlled, multicenter study of oral verapamil. J. Am. Coll. Cardiol. *1*:595, 1983.
321. Williams, D. O., Riley, R. S., Singh, A. K., Gewirtz, H., and Most, A. S.: Evaluation of the role of coronary angioplasty in patients with unstable angina pectoris. Am. Heart J. *102*:1, 1981.
322. Meyer, J., Schmidtz, H., Erbel, R., Kiesslich, T., Bocker-Josephs, B., Krebs, W., Braun, P. C., Bardos, P., Minale, C., Messmer, B. J., and Effert, S.: Treatment of unstable angina pectoris with percutaneous transluminal coronary angioplasty (PTCA). Cath. Cardiovasc. Diagn. *7*:361, 1981.
323. Hirsh, P. D., Hillis, L. D., Campbell, W. B., Firth, B. G., and Willerson, J. T.: Release of prostaglandins and thromboxane into the coronary circulation in patients with ischemic heart disease. N. Engl. J. Med. *304*:685, 1981.
324. Smitherman, T. C., Milam, M., Woo, J., Willerson, J. T., and Frenkel, L. P.: Elevated beta thromboglobulin in peripheral venous blood of patients with acute myocardial ischemia: Direct evidence for enhanced platelet reactivity in vivo. Am. J. Cardiol. *48*:395, 1981.
325. Tolts, J. D., Crowell, E. B., and Rowe, G. G.: Platelet aggregation in partially obstructed vessels and its elimination with aspirin. Circulation *54*:365, 1976.
326. Lewis, H. D., Davis, J. W., Archibald, D. G., Steinke, W. E., Smitherman, T. C., Doherty, J. E., LeWinter, M. M., Linares, E. Pouget, J. M., Sabharwal, S. C., Chesler, E., and DeMots, H.: Protective effects of 324 mg. aspirin daily in men with unstable angina: Results of a VA Cooperative Study. Circulation *66* (Part II):17, 1982 (Abstr.).
327. Krauss, K. R., Hutter, A. M., and DeSanctis, R. W.: Acute coronary insufficiency: Course and follow-up. Circulation *45*(Suppl. 1):66, 1972.
328. Schroeder, J. S., Lamb, I. H., and Hu, M.: Do patients in whom myocardial infarction has been ruled out have a better prognosis after hospitalization than those surviving infarction? N. Engl. J. Med. *303*:1, 1980.
329. Solomon, H. A., Edwards, A. L., and Killip, T.: Prodromata in acute myocardial infarction. Circulation *40*:463, 1969.

VARIANT ANGINA

330. Prinzmetal, M., Kennamer, R., Merliss, R., Wada, T., and Bor, N.: A variant form of angina pectoris. Am. J. Med. *27*:375, 1959.
331. Stein, J. H., Ambrose, J. A., King, B. D., and Herman, M. V.: An integrated approach to the recognition and treatment of variant angina. Cardiovasc. Rev. Rep. *3*:1297, 1982.
332. Weiner, L., Kasparian, H., Duca, P. R., Walinsky, P., Gottlieb, R.S., Hanckel, F., and Brest, A. N.: Spectrum of coronary arterial spasm. Clinical angiographic and myocardial metabolic experience in 29 cases. Am. J. Cardiol. *38*: 945, 1976.
333. Yasue, H., Omote, S., Takizawa, A., Nagao, M., Miwa, K., and Tanaka, S.: Cardiac variations of exercise capacity in patients with Prinzmetal's variant angina: Role of exercise-induced coronary arterial spasm. Circulation *59*:938, 1979.
334. Weiner, D. A., Schick, E. C., Jr., Hood, W. B., Jr., and Ryan, T. J.: ST-segment elevation during recovery from exercise. Chest *74*:133, 1978.
335. Oliva, P. B., Potts, D. E., and Pluss, R. G.: Coronary arterial spasm in Prinzmetal angina. Documentation by coronary arteriography. N. Engl. J. Med. *288*:745, 1973.
336. Dhurandhar, R. W., Watt, D. L., Silber, M. D., Trimble, A. S., and Adelman, A. G.: Prinzmetal's variant form of angina with arteriographic evidence of coronary arterial spasm. Am. J. Cardiol. *30*:902, 1972.
337. Higgins, C. B., Wexler, L., Silverman, J. F., and Schroeder, J. S.: Clinical and arteriographic features of Prinzmetal's variant angina: Documentation of etiology factors. Am. J. Cardiol. *37*:831, 1976.
338. Berman, N. D., McLaughlin, P. R., Huckell, V. F., Mahon, W. A., Morch, J. E., and Adelman, A. G.: Prinzmetal's angina with coronary artery spasm. Angiographic, pharmacologic, metabolic and radionuclide perfusion studies. Am. J. Med. *60*:727, 1976.
339. Freedman, B., Dunn, R. F., Richmond, D. R., and Kelly, D. T.: Coronary artery spasm during exercise: Treatment with verapamil. Circulation *64*:68, 1981.
340. Waters, D D., Theroux, P., Crittin, J., Dauwe, F., and Mizgala, H. F.: Previously undiagnosed variant angina as a cause of chest pain after coronary artery bypass surgery. Circulation *61*:1159, 1980.
341. Miller, D., Waters, D. D., Warnica, W., Szlachcic, J., Kreeft, J., and Theroux, P.: Is variant angina the coronary manifestation of a generalized vasospastic disorder? N. Engl. J. Med. *304*:763, 1981.
342. Antman, E., Muller, J., Goldberg, S., MacAlpin, R., Rubenfire, M., Tabatznik, B., Liang, C., Heupler, F., Achuff, S., Reichek, N., Geltman, E., Kerin, N. Z., Neff, R. K., and Braunwald, E.: Nifedipine therapy for coronary-artery spasm. Experience in 127 patients. N. Engl. J. Med. *302*:1269 1980.
343. Kerin, N. Z., Rubenfire, M., Naini, M., Wajszczuk, W. J., Pamatmat, A., and

Cascade, P. N.: Arrhythmias in variant angina pectoris: Relationship of arrhythmias to ST-segment elevation and R-wave changes. Circulation *60*:1343, 1979.
344. Sheehan, F. H., and Epstein, S. E.: Determinants of arrhythmic death due to coronary spasm: Effect of preexisting coronary artery stenosis on the incidence of reperfusion arrhythmia. Circulation *65*:259, 1982.
345. Kerin, N. Z., Rubenfire, M., Naini, M., Wajszezuk, W. J., Pamatmat, A., and Cascade, P. N.: Arrhythmias in variant angina pectoris. Relationship or arrhythmias to ST-segment elevation and R-wave changes. Circulation *60*:1343, 1979.
346. Biagini, A., Mazzei, M. G., Carpeggiani, C., Buzzigoli, G., Zucchelli, G., Parodi, O., L'Abbate, A., and Maseri, A.: Myocardial cell damage during attacks of vasospastic angina in the absence of persistent electrocardiographic changes. Clin. Cardiol. *4*:315, 1981.
347. Meller, J., Conde, C. A., Donoso, E., and Dack, S.: Transient Q waves in Prinzmetal's angina. Am. J. Cardiol. *35*:691, 1975.
348. Guazzi, M., Polese, A., Fiorentini, C., Magrini, F., and Bartorelli, C.: Left ventricular performance and related hemodynamic changes in Prinzmetal's variant angina pectoris. Br. Heart J. *33*:84, 1971.
349. Gaasch, W. H., Adyantha, A. V., Wang, V. H., Pickering, E., Quinons, M. A., and Alexander, J. K.: Prinzmetal's variant angina: Hemodynamic and angiographic observations during pain. Am. J. Cardiol. *35*:683, 1977.
350. Muller, J. E.: Prinzmetal's angina—A model for the role of spasm in ischemic heart disease. J. Cardiovasc. Med. *5*:19, 1980.
351. Selzer, A., Langston, M., Ruggeroli, C., and Cohn, K.: Clinical syndrome of variant angina with normal coronary arteriogram. N. Engl. J. Med. *295*:1343, 1976.
352. Cipriano, P. R., Koch, F. H., Rosenthal, S. J., and Schroeder, J. S.: Clinical course of patients following the demonstration of coronary artery spasm by angiography. Am. Heart J. *101*:127, 1981.
353. Waters, D. D., Theroux, P., Szlachcic, J., and Dauwe, F.: Provocative testing with ergonovine to assess the efficacy of treatment with nifedipine, diltiazem and verapamil in variant angina. Am. J. Cardiol. *48*:123, 1981.
354. Curry, R. C., Jr., Pepine, C. J., Sabom, M. B., Feldman, R. L., Christie, L. G., and Conti, C. R.: Effects of ergonovine in patients with and without coronary artery disease. Circulation *56*:803, 1977.
354a. Winniford, M. D., Johnson, S. M., Mauritson, D. R., and Hillis, L. D.: Ergonovine provocation to assess efficacy of long-term therapy with calcium antagonists in Prinzmetal's variant angina. Am. J. Cardiol. *51*:684, 1983.
355. Waters, D. D., Szlachcic, J., Theroux, P., Dauwe, F., and Mizgala, H. F.: Ergonovine testing to detect spontaneous remissions of variant angina during long-term treatment with calcium antagonist drugs. Am. J. Cardiol. *47*:179, 1981.
356. Ginsburg, R., Lamb, I. H., Bristow, M. R., Schroeder, J. S., and Harrison, D. C.: Application and safety of outpatient ergonovine testing in accurately detecting coronary spasm in patients with possible variant angina. Am. Heart J. *102*:698, 1981.
357. Waters, D. D., Theroux, P., Szlachcic, J., Dauwe, F., Crittin, J., Bonan, R., and Mizgala, H. F.: Ergonovine testing in a coronary care unit. Am. J. Cardiol. *46*:922, 1980.
358. Buxton, A., Goldberg, S., Hirshfeld, J. W., Wilson, J., Mann, T., Williams, O., Overlie, P., and Oliva, P.: Refractory ergonovine-induced coronary vasospasm: Importance of intracoronary nitroglycerin. Am. J. Cardiol. *46*:329, 1980.
359. Heupler, F. A., Jr.: Provocative testing for coronary arterial spasm: Risk, method and rationale. Am. J. Cardiol. *46*:335, 1980.
360. Yasue, H., Touyama, M., Shimamoto, M., Kato, H., Tanaka, S., and Akiyama, F.: Role of autonomic nervous system in the pathogenesis of Prinzmetal's variant form of angina. Circulation *50*:534, 1974.
361. Ginsburg, R., Bristow, M. R., Kantrowitz, N., Baim, D. S., and Harrison, D. C.: Histamine provocation of clinical coronary artery spasm: Implications concerning pathogenesis of variant angina pectoris. Am. Heart J. *102*:819, 1981.
362. Waters, D. D., Szlachcic, J., Bonan, R., Miller, D. D., Dauwe, F., and Theroux, P.: Comparative sensitivity of exercise, cold pressor and ergonovine testing in provoking attacks of variant angina in patients with active disease. Circulation *67*:310, 1983.
363. Maseri, A., Parodi, O., Severi, S., and Pesola, A.: Transient transmural reduction of myocardial blood flow, demonstrated by thallium-201 scintigraphy, as a cause of variant angina. Circulation *54*:280, 1976.
364. McLaughlin, P. R., Doherty, P. W., Martin, P. R., Goris, M. L., and Harrison, D. L.: Myocardial imaging in a patient with reproducible variant angina. Am. J. Cardiol. *39*:129, 1977.
365. Ricci, D. R., Orlick, A. E., Doherty, P. W., Cipriano, P. R., and Harrison, D. R.: Reduction of coronary blood flow during coronary artery spasm occurring spontaneously and after provocation by ergonovine maleate. Circulation *57*: 392, 1978.
366. Ginsburg, R., Lamb, I. H., Schroeder, J. S., Hu, M., and Harrison, D. C.: Randomized double-blind comparison of nifedipine and isosorbide dinitrate therapy in variant angina pectoris due to coronary artery spasm. Am. Heart J. *103*:44, 1982.
367. Schroeder, J. S., Lamb, I. H., Bristow, M. R., Ginsburg, R., Hung, J., and McAuley, B. J: Prevention of cardiovascular events in variant angina by long-term diltiazem therapy. J. Am. Coll. Cardiol. *1*:1507, 1983.
368. Braunwald, E.: Coronary artery spasm as a cause of myocardial ischemia. J. Lab. Clin. Med. *97*:299, 1981.
369. Gunther, S., Muller, J. E., Mudge, G. H., Jr., and Grossman, W.: Therapy of coronary vasoconstriction in patients with coronary artery disease. Am. J. Cardiol. *47*:157, 1981.
370. Colucci, W. S.: Alpha-adrenergic receptor blockade with prazosin. Consideration of hypertension, heart failure and potential new applications. Ann. Intern. Med. *97*:67, 1982.
371. Tzivoni, D., Keren, A., Benhorin, J., Gottlieb, S., Atlas, D., and Stern, S.: Prazosin therapy for refractory variant angina. Am. Heart J. *105*:262, 1983.
372. Miwa, K., Kambara, H., and Kawai, C.: Effect of aspirin in large doses on attacks of variant angina. Am. Heart J. *105*:351, 1983.
373. Schick, E. C., Jr., Davis, Z., Lavery, R. M., McCormick, J. R., Fay, M., and Berger, R. L.: Surgical therapy for Prinzmetal's variant angina. Ann. Thorac. Surg. *33*:359, 1982.
374. Waters, D. D., Szlachcic, J., Miller, D., and Theroux, P.: Clinical characteristics of patients with variant angina complicated by myocardial infarction or death within 1 month. Am. J. Cardiol. *49*:658, 1982.
375. Brunelli, C., Lazzari, M., Simonetti, I., L'Abbate, A., and Maseri, A.: Variable threshold of exertional angina: A clue to a vasopastic component. Eur. Heart J. *2*:155, 1981.
376. Ahmad, M., Dubiel, J. P., and Haibach, H.: Cold pressor thallium-201 myocardial scintigraphy in the diagnosis of coronary artery disease. Am. J. Cardiol. *50*:1253, 1982.
377. Mueller, H. S., Rao, P. S., Rao, P. B., Gory, D. J., Mudd, J. G., and Ayres, S. M.: Enhanced transcardiac l-norepinephrine response during cold pressor test in obstructive coronary artery disease. Am. J. Cardiol. *50*:1223, 1982.
378. Bertrand, M. E., LaBlanche, J. M., Tilmant, R. Y., Thieuleux, F. A., Delforge, M. R., Carre, A. G., Asseman, P., Berzin, B., Libersa, C., and Laurent, J. M.: Frequency of provoked coronary arterial spasm in 1089 consecutive patients undergoing coronary arteriography. Circulation *65*:1299, 1982.
379. Koiwaya, Y., Nakamura, M., Mitsutake, A., Tanaka, S., and Takeshita, A.: Increased exercise tolerance after oral diltiazem, a calcium antagonist, in angina pectoris. Am. Heart J. *101*:143, 1981.
380. Pine, M. B., Citron, P. D., Bailly D. J., Butman, S., Plasencia, G. O., Landa, D. W., and Wong, R. K.: Verapamil versus placebo in relieving stable angina pectoris. Circulation *65*:17, 1982.

ISCHEMIC HEART DISEASE IN WHICH DISCOMFORT IS NOT THE DOMINANT SYMPTOM

381. Kannel, W. B., Doyle, J. T., McNamara, P. M., Quickenton, P., and Gordon, T.: Precursors of sudden coronary death. Factors related to the incidence of sudden death. Circulation *51*:606, 1975.
382. Master, A. M., and Geller, A. M.: The extent of completely asymptomatic coronary artery disease. Am. J. Cardiol. *23*:173, 1969.
383. Cohn, P. F.: Severe asymptomatic coronary artery disease. A diagnostic, prognostic and therapeutic puzzle. Am. J. Med. *62*:565, 1977.
384. Froelicher, V. F., Yanowitz, F. G., Thompson, A. J., and Lancaster, M. C.: The correlation of coronary angiography and the electrocardiographic response to maximal threadmill testing in 76 asymptomatic men. Circulation *48*:597, 1973.
385. Borer, J. S., Brensike, J. D., Redwood, D. R., Itscoitz, S. B., Passamanin, E. R., Stone, N. J., Richardson, J. M., Levy, R. I., and Epstein, S. E.: Limitations of electrocardiographic response to exercise in predicting coronary artery disease. N. Engl. J. Med. *293*:367, 1975.
386. Erikssen, J., Enge, I., Forfang, K., and Storstein, O.: False positive diagnostic tests and coronary angiographic findings in 105 presumably healthy males. Circulation *54*:371, 1976.
387. O'Rourke, R. A., and Ross, J. R., Jr.: Ambulatory electrocardiographic monitoring to detect ischemic heart disease. Ann. Intern. Med. *81*:696, 1974.
388. Stern, S., and Tzivoni, D.: Early detection of silent ischemic heart disease by 24-hour electrocardiographic monitoring of active subjects. Br. Heart J. *36*: 481, 1976.
389. Cohn, P. F., Prognosis and treatment of asymptomatic coronary artery disease. J. Am. Coll. Cardiol. *1*:959, 1983.
390. Gorlin, R., Klein, M. D., and Sullivan, J. M.: Prospective correlative study of ventricular aneurysm. Mechanistic concept and clinical recognition. Am. J. Med. *42*:512, 1967.
391. Parmley, W. W., Chuck, L., Kivowitz, C., Matloff, J. M., and Swan, H. J. C.: In vitro length-tension relations of human ventricular aneurysms. Relation of stiffness to mechanical disadvantage. Am. J. Cardiol. *32*:889, 1973.
392. Erikson, U., Hallen, A., Helmius, G., and Sawada, S.: On the pathophysiology of left ventricular aneurysm. An analysis by cineangiography and videodensitometry. Fortschr. Röntgenstr. *137*:85, 1982.
393. Esente, P., Gensini, G. G.: Huntington, P. P., Kelly, A. E., and Black, A.: Left ventricular aneurysm without coronary arterial obstruction or occlusion. Am. J. Cardiol. *34*:658, 1974.
394. Cabin, H. S., and Roberts, W. C.: Left ventricular aneurysm, intraaneurysmal thrombus and systemic embolus in coronary heart disease. Chest *77*:586, 1980.
395. Stratton, J. R., Lighty, G. W., Jr., Pearlman, A. S., and Ritchie, J. L.: Detection of left ventricular thrombus by two-dimensional echocardiography: Sensitivity, specificity, and causes of uncertainty. Circulation *66*:156, 1982.
396. Froehlich, R. T., Falsetti, H. L., Doty, D. B., and Marcus, M.: Recognizing and treating left ventricular aneurysm. J. Cardiovasc. Med. *6*:465, 1981.
397. van Meurs-van Woezik, H., Meltzer, R. S., van den Brand, M., Essed, C. E., Michels, R. H. M., and Roelandt, J.: Superiority of echocardiography over angiocardiography in diagnosing a left ventricular thrombus. Chest *80*:321, 1981.
398. Ezekowitz, M. D., Leonard, J. C., Smith, E. O., Allen, E. W., and Taylor, F. B.: Identification of left ventricular thrombi in man using indium-111–labeled autologous platelets. A preliminary report. Circulation *63*:803, 1981.
399. Rigo, P., Murray, M., Strauss, H. W., and Pitt, B.: Scintiphotographic evalua-

tion of patients with suspected left ventricular aneurysm. Circulation *50*:985, 1974.
400. Parisi, A. F., Moynihan, P. F., Ray, B. J., and Pietro, D. A.: Two-dimensional echocardiography. J. Cardiovasc. Med. *5*:39, 1980.
401. Burch, G. E., DePasquale, N. P., and Phillips, J. H.: The syndrome of papillary muscle dysfunction. Am. Heart J. *75*:399, 1968.
402. Balu, V., Hershowitz, S., Zaki Masud, A. R., Bhayana, J. N., and Dean, D. C.: Mitral regurgitation in coronary artery disease. Chest *81*:550, 1982.
403. Gahl, K., Sutton, R., Pearson, M., Caspari, P., Lairet, A., and McDonald, L.: Mitral regurgitation in coronary heart disease. Br. Heart J. *39*:13, 1977.
404. Shelburne, J. C., Rubinstein, D., and Gorlin, R.: A reappraisal of papillary muscle dysfunction. Correlative, clinical and angiographic study. Am. J. Med. *46*:862, 1969.
405. Burch, G. E., Giles, T. D., and Colcolough, H. L.: Ischemic cardiomyopathy. Am. Heart J. *79*:291, 1970.
406. Yatteau, R. F., Peter, R. H., Behar, V. S., Bartel, A. G., Rosati, R. A., and Kong, Y.: Ischemic cardiomyopathy: The myopathy of coronary artery disease. Natural history and results of medical versus surgical treatment. Am. J. Cardiol. *34*:520, 1974.
407. Dash, H., Johnson, R. A., Dinsmore, R. E., and Harthorne, J. W.: Cardiomyopathic syndrome due to coronary artery disease. I. Relation to angiographic extent of coronary disease and to remote myocardial infarction. Br. Heart J. *39*:733, 1977.
408. Calvert, A., Lown, B., and Gorlin, R.: Ventricular premature beats and anatomically defined coronary heart disease. Am. J. Cardiol. *39*:4, 1977.
409. Levine, S. A., and Kauvar, A. J.: Association of angina pectoris or thrombosis with mitral stenosis. J. Mt. Sinai Hosp. *8*:754, 1942.
410. Gardner, F. E., and White, P. D.: Coronary occlusion and myocardial infarction associated with chronic rheumatic heart disease. Ann. Intern. Med. *31*: 1003, 1949.
411. Befeler, B., Kamen, A. R., and MacLeod, M. B.: Coronary artery disease and left ventricular function in mitral stenosis. Chest *57*:435, 1970.
412. Basta, L. L., Raines, D., Najjar, S., and Kioschos, J. M.: Clinical, haemodynamic, and coronary angiographic correlates of angina pectoris in patients with severe aortic valve disease. Br. Heart J. *37*:150, 1975.
413. Graboys, T. B., and Cohn, P. F.: The prevalence of angina pectoris and abnormal coronary arteriograms in severe aortic valvular disease. Am. Heart J. *93*: 683, 1977.
414. Hakki, A., Kimbiris, D., Iskanadrian, A. S., Segal, B. L., Mintz, G. S., and Bemis, C. E.: Angina pectoris and coronary artery disease in patients with severe aortic valvular disease. Am. Heart J. *100*:441, 1980.
415. Hancock, E. W.: Clinical assessment of coronary artery disease in patients with aortic stenosis. Am. J. Cardiol. *35*:142, 1975.
416. Harris, C. N., Kaplan, M. A., Parker, D. P., Dunne, E. F., Cowell, H. S., and Ellestad, M. H.: Aortic stenosis, angina, and coronary artery disease-interrelations. Br. Heart J. *37*:656, 1975.
417. Bagdade, J. D.: Atherosclerosis in patients undergoing maintenance hemodialysis. Kidney Int. (Suppl.)(3):370, 1975.
418. Gurland, H. J., Brunner, F. P., Dehn, H., Harlen, H., Parsons, F. M., and Scharer, K.: Combined report on regular dialysis and transplantation in Europe. Proc. Eur. Dial. Transpl. Assoc. *10*:17, 1973.
419. Lowrie, E. G., Lazarus, J. M., Mocelin, A. J., Bailey, G. L., Hampers, C. L., Wilson, R. E., and Merrill, J. P.: Survival of patients undergoing chronic hemodialysis and renal transplantation. N. Engl. J. Med. *288*:863, 1973.
420. Lindner, A., Charra, B., Sherrard, D. J., and Scribner, B. H.: Accelerated atherosclerosis in prolonged maintenance dialysis. N. Engl. J. Med. *290*:697, 1974.
421. Oakley, C. M.: Non-atheromatous ischemic heart disease. Postgrad. Med. J. *52*: 438, 1976.
422. Lange, R. L., Reid, M. S., Tresch, D. D., Keelan, M. H., Bernhard, J. M., and Coolidge, G.: Nonatheromatous ischemic heart disease following withdrawal from chronic industrial nitroglycerin exposure. Circulation *46*:666, 1972.

SURGICAL TREATMENT

423. O'Shaughnessy, L.: Surgical treatment of cardiac ischemia. Lancet *1*:185, 1937.
424. McAllister, F. F., Leighninger, D., and Beck, C. S.: Revascularization of the heart by graft of systemic artery into coronary sinus. J.A.M.A. *137*:436, 1948.
425. Glover, R. P., Davila, J. C., Kyle, R. H., Beard, J. C., Jr., Trout, R. G., and Kitchell, J. R.: Ligation of the internal mammary arteries as a means of increasing blood supply to the myocardium. J. Thorac. Surg. *34*:661, 1957.
426. Gorlin, R.: Revascularization of the myocardium. *In* Gorlin, R.: Coronary Artery Disease. Philadelphia, W. B. Saunders Co., 1976, p. 263.
427. Vineberg, A., and Walker, J.: The surgical treatment of coronary artery heart disease by internal mammary artery implantation: Report of 140 cases followed up to thirteen years. Dis. Chest. *45*:190, 1964.
428. Gorlin, R., and Taylor, W. J.: Myocardial revascularization with internal mammary artery implantation: Current status. J.A.M.A. *207*:907, 1969.
429. Mundth, E. D., and Austen, W. G.: Surgical measures for coronary heart disease. N. Engl. J. Med. *293*:13, 1975.
430. Participants of the Veterans Administration Coronary Bypass Surgery Cooperative Study Group: Long-term results of internal mammary artery implantation for coronary artery disease: A controlled trial. Ann. Thorac. Surg. *29*: 234, 1980.
431. Favalora, R.: Direct and indirect coronary surgery. Circulation *46*:1197, 1972.
432. Effler, D. B.: Myocardial revascularization surgery since 1945. Its evolution and impact. J. Thorac. Cardiovasc. Surg. *72*:823, 1976.
433. DeBakey, M. Garrett, H. E., and Dennis, E. W.: Aorto-coronary bypass with saphenous vein graft. Seven-year follow-up. J.A.M.A. *223*:792, 1973.
434. Green, G. E.: Internal mammary artery to coronary artery anastomosis: Three year experience with 165 patients. Ann. Thorac. Surg. *14*:260, 1972.
435. Loop, F. D., Sheldon, W. C., Lytle, B. W., Cosgrove, D. M., III, and Proudfit, W. L.: The efficacy of coronary artery surgery. Am. Heart J. *101*:86, 1981.
436. Kouchoukos, N. T., Oberman, A., Kirklin, J. W., Russell, R. O., Jr., Karp, R. B., Pacifico, A. D., and Zorn, G. L.: Coronary bypass surgery: Analysis of factors affecting hospital mortality. Circulation *62*(Suppl. I):84, 1980.
437. Frye, R. L., and Frommer, P. L. (eds.): Consensus Development Conference on Coronary Bypass Surgery. Medical and scientific aspects. Circulation *65* (Suppl. II):1–129, 1982.
437a. Jones, E. L., Carver, J. M., Guyton, R. P., Bone, D. K., Hatcher, C. R., Jr., and Riechwalt, N.: Importance of complete revascularization in performance of the coronary bypass operation. Am. J. Cardiol. *51*:7, 1983.
438. Dobrin, P., Canfield, T., Moran, J., Sullivan, H., and Pifarre, R.: Coronary artery bypass. The physiological basis for differences in flow with internal mammary artery and saphenous vein grafts. J. Thorac. Cardiovasc. Surg. *74*:445, 1977.
439. Cohn, P. F.: Clinical angiographic, and hemodynamic factors influencing selection of patients for coronary artery bypass surgery. Progr. Cardiovasc. Dis. *18*: 223, 1975.
440. Report of Inter-Society Commission for Heart Disease Resources: Optimal resources for coronary artery surgery. Circulation *46*:A-325, 1972.
441. Alderman, E. L., Matlof, H. J., Wexler, L., Shumway, N. E., and Harrison, D. C.: Results of direct coronary artery surgery for the treatment of angina pectoris. N. Engl. J. Med. *388*:535, 1973.
442. McNeer, J. F., Starmer, C. F., Bartel, A. G., Behar, V. S., Kong, Y., Peter, R. H., and Rosati, R. A.: The nature of treatment selection in coronary artery disease. Experience with medical and surgical treatment of a chronic disease. Circulation *49*:606, 1974.
443. Report of the Unstable Angina Pectoris Study Group: Unstable angina pectoris: National Cooperative Group to Compare Medical and Surgical Therapy. I. Report of protocol and patient population. Am. J. Cardiol. *37*:896, 1976.
444. Scanlon, P. J.: The intermediate coronary syndrome. Progr. Cardiovasc. Dis. *23*:351, 1981.
445. Hammermeister, K. E.: The effect of coronary bypass surgery on survival. Progr. Cardiovasc. Dis. *15*:297, 1983.
446. Tyers, G. F. O., Williams, D. R., and Babb, J. D.: The changing status of ejection fraction as a predictor of early mortality following surgery for acquired heart disease. Chest *71*:371, 1977.
447. Rozanski, A., Berman, D. S., Gray, R., Levy, R., Raymond, M., Maddahi, J., Pantaleo, N., Waxman, A. D., Swan, H. J. C., and Matloff, J.: Use of thallium-201 redistribution scintigraphy in the preoperative differentiation of reversible and nonreversible myocardial asynergy. Circulation *64*:936, 1981.
448. Rozanski, A., Berman, D., Gray, R., Diamond, G., Raymond, J., Prause, J., Maddahi, J., Swan, H. J. C., and Matloff, J.: Preoperative prediction of reversible myocardial asynergy by postexercise radionuclide ventriculography. N. Engl. J. Med. *307*:212, 1982.
449. Manley, J. C., King, J. F., and Zeft, H. J.: The "bad" left ventricle. Results of coronary surgery and effect on late survival. J. Thorac. Cardiovasc. Surg. *72*: 841, 1976.
450. Norris, R. M., Agnew, T. M., and Brandt, P. W. T.: Coronary surgery after recurrent myocardial infarction: Progress of a trial comparing surgical with nonsurgical management for asymptomatic patients with advanced coronary disease. Circulation *63*:785, 1981.
451. Faulkner, S. L., Stoney, W. S., and Alford, W. C.: Ischemic cardiomyopathy: Medical versus surgical treatment. J. Thorac. Cardiovasc. Surg. *74*:77, 1977.
452. Leinbach, R. C., Gold, H. K., and Dinsmore, R. E.: The role of angiography in cardiogenic shock. Circulation *48*(Suppl. III):95, 1976.
453. Johnson, S. A., Scanlon, P. J., and Loeb, H. S.: Treatment of cardiogenic shock in myocardial infarction by intraaortic balloon counterpulsation and surgery. Am. J. Med. *62*:687, 1977.
454. Berg, R., Jr., Selinger, S. L., and Leonard, J. J.: Immediate coronary artery bypass for acute evolving myocardial infarction. J. Thorac. Cardiovasc. Surg. *81*:493, 1981.
455. Phillips, S. J., Kongtahworn, C., and Zeff, R. H.: Emergency coronary artery revascularization: A possible therapy for acute myocardial infarction. Circulation *60*:241, 1979.
456. Selinger, S. L., Berg, R., Jr., and Leonard, J. J.: Surgical treatment of acute evolving anterior myocardial infarction. Circulation *64*(Suppl. II):28, 1981.
457. Smith, S. C., Jr., Gorlin, R., Herman, M. V., Taylor, W. J., and Collins, J. J., Jr.: Myocardial blood flow in man. Effect of coronary collateral circulation and coronary artery bypass surgery. J. Clin. Invest. *51*:2556, 1972.
458. Lesperance, J., Bourassa, M. G., Biron, P., Campeau, L., and Saltiel, J.: Aorta to coronary artery saphenous vein grafts. Preoperative angiographic criteria for successful surgery. Am. J. Cardiol. *30*:459, 1972.
459. Rosch, J., Dotter, C. T., Antonovic, R., Bonchek, L., and Starr, A.: Angiographic appraisal of distal vessel suitability for aortocoronary bypass graft surgery. Circulation *48*:202, 1973.
460. Cukingnan, R. A., Carey, J. S., Wittig, J. H., and Brown, B. G.: Influence of complete coronary revascularization on relief of angina. J. Thorac. Cardiovasc. Surg. *79*:188, 1980.
461. Murphy, E. S., and Kloster, F. E.: Coronary bypass surgery: What are the indications? J. Cardiovasc. Med. *8*:57, 1983.
462. Walker, J. A., Friedberg, H. D., Flemma, R. J., and Johnson, W. D.: Determinants of angiographic patency of aortocoronary vein bypass grafts. Circulation *45, 46*(Suppl. 1):86, 1972.
463. Grondin, C. M., Lapage, G., Castoguay, Y. R., Meere, C., and Grondin, P.:

Aorto-coronary bypass graft. Initial blood flow through the graft, and early postoperative patency. Circulation *44*:815, 1971.
464. Spencer, F. C., Green, G. E., Tice, D. A., Wallsh, E., Mills, N. L., and Glassman, E.: Coronary artery bypass grafts for congestive heart failure. A report of experiences with 40 patients. J. Thorac. Cardiovasc. Surg. *62*:529, 1971.
465. Kouchoukos, N. T., Doty, D. B., Buettner, L. E., and Kirklin, J. W.: Treatment of postinfarction cardiac failure by myocardial excision and revascularization. Circulation *45*(Suppl. 1):72, 1972.
466. Loop, F. D., Brettoni, J. N., Pichard, A., Siegel, W., Razani, M., and Effler, D. B.: Selection of the candidate for myocardial revascularization. A profile of high risk based on multivariate analysis. J. Thorac. Cardiovasc. Surg. *69*:40, 1975.
467. Kennedy, J. W., Kaiser, G. C., Fisher, L. D., Fritz, J. K., Myers, W., Mudd, J. G., and Ryan, T. J.: Clinical and angiographic predictors of operative mortality from the collaborative study in coronary artery surgery (CASS). Circulation *63*:793, 1981.
468. Cohn, P. F., Gorlin, R., Herman, M. V., Sonnenblick, E. H., Horn, H. R., Cohn, L. H., and Collins, J. J., Jr.: Relation between contractile reserve and prognosis in patients with coronary artery disease and a depressed ejection fraction. Circulation *51*:414, 1975.
469. Popio, K. A., Gorlin, R., Bechtel, D. L., and Levine, J. A.: Post extrasystolic potentiation as a predictor of potential myocardial viability. Am. J. Cardiol. *39*: 944, 1977.
470. Nesto, R. W., Cohn, L. H., Collins, J. J., Jr., Wynne, J., Holman, L., and Cohn, P. F.: Inotropic contractile reserve: A useful predictor of increased 5-year survival and improved postoperative left ventricular function in patients with coronary artery disease and reduced ejection fraction. Am. J. Cardiol. *50*: 39, 1982.
471. Starek, P. J. K.: Effects of coronary artery surgery and early and late survival. Cardiovasc. Rev. Rep. *4*:551, 1983.
472. Rahimtoola, S. H.: Coronary bypass surgery for chronic angina — 1981: A perspective. Circulation *65*:225, 1982.
472a. Waller, B. F., and Roberts, W. C.: Severe coronary narrowing at the site of or distal to the bypass graft anastomosis — the most important cause of early and late graft closure: analysis of 102 necropsy patients (108 arteries and 185 grafts) having an isolated aorto-coronary bypass operation. J. Am. Coll. Cardiol. *1*:719, 1983.
473. Solignac, A., Gueret, P., and Bourassa, M. G.: Influence of left ventricular function on survival 3 to 4 years after aortocoronary bypass. Eur. J. Cardiol. *2*: 421, 1975.
474. Hacker, R. W., Torka, M., and von der Emde, J.: Influence of preoperative variables upon the results of coronary artery bypass surgery. Cardiovascular Diseases, Bull Texas Heart Institute *7*:20, 1980.
475. Barboriak, J. J., Rimm, A. A., and Anderson, A. J.: Risk factors and mortality in patients with aortocoronary vein bypass operations. Cardiology *63*:237, 1978.
475a. Frick, M. H., Harjola, P-T., and Valle, M.: Persistent improvement after coronary bypass surgery: Ergometric and angiographic correlations at 5 years. Circulation *67*:491, 1983.
476. Greenberg, B. H., Hart, R., Botvinick, E. H., Werner, J. A., Brundage, B. H., Shames, P. M., Chatterjee, K., and Parmley, W. W.: Thallium-201 myocardial perfusion scintigraphy to evaluate patients after coronary bypass surgery. Am. J. Cardiol. *42*:167, 1978.
477. Seides, S. F., Borer, J. S., Kent, K. M., Rosing, D. R., McIntosh, C. L., and Epstein, S. E.: Long-term anatomic fate of coronary-artery bypass grafts and functional status of patients five years after operation. N. Engl. J. Med. *298*: 1213, 1978.
478. Johnson, W. D., Kayser, K. L. Pedraza, P. M., and Shore, R. T.: Employment patterns in males before and after myocardial revascularization surgery. A study of 2229 consecutive male patients followed for as long as 10 years. Circulation *65*:1086, 1982.
479. Danchin, N., David, P., Bourassa, M. G., Robert, P., and Chaitman, B. R.: Factors predicting working status after aortocoronary bypass surgery. Canad. Med. Assoc. J. *126*:255, 1982.
480. Freeman, M. R., Gray, R. J., Berman, D. S., Maddahi, J., Raymond, M. J., Forrester, J. S., and Matloff, J. M.: Improvement in global and segmental left ventricular function after coronary bypass surgery. Circulation *64*:II-34, 1981.
481. Hammermeister, K. E., Kennedy, J. W., Hamilton, G. W., Stewart, D. K., Gould, K. L., Lipscomb, K., and Murray, J. A.: Aortocoronary saphenous vein bypass. Failure of successful grafting to improve resting left ventricular function in chronic angina. N. Engl. J. Med. *290*:186, 1974.
482. Burton, J. R., FitzGibbon, G. M., Keon, W. J., and Leach, A. J.: Perioperative myocardial infarction complicating coronary bypass. Clinical and angiographic correlations and prognosis. J. Thorac. Cardiovasc. Surg. *82*:758, 1981.
483. Righetti, A., Crawford, M. H., O'Rourke, R. A., Hardason, T., Schelbert, H., Daily, P. O., De Luca, M., Ashburn, W., and Ross, J., Jr.: Detection of perioperative myocardial change after coronary artery bypass surgery. Circulation *55*:173, 1977.
484. Roberts, A. J., Subramanian, V. A., Herman, S. D., Case, D. B., Johnson, G. A., Jr., and Gay, W. A., Jr.: Systemic hypertension associated with coronary artery bypass surgery. J. Thorac. Cardiovasc. Surg. *74*:846, 1977.
485. Palac, R. T., Meadows, W. R., Hwang, M. H., Loeb, H. S., Pifarre, R., and Gunnar, R. M.: Risk factors related to progressive narrowing of aortocoronary vein grafts studied 1 and 5 years after surgery. Circulation *66*(Suppl. I):40, 1982.
486. Bulkley, B. H.: Why coronary bypass grafts fail: Early and late pathologic changes. J. Cardiovasc. Med. *5*:1025, 1980.
487. Spray, T. L., and Roberts, W. C.: Changes in saphenous veins used as aortocoronary bypass grafts. Am. Heart J. *94*:500, 1977.
488. Campeau, L., Lesperance, J., Corbara, F., Hermann, J., Grondin, C. M., and Bourassa, M. G.: Aortocoronary saphenous vein bypass graft changes 5 to 7 years after surgery. Circulation *58*(Suppl.):170, 1978.
489. Albrechtsson, U. J., Stahl, E., and Tylen, U.: Evaluation of coronary artery bypass graft patency with computed tomography. J. Computer Asst. Tomog. *5*: 822, 1981.
490. Ullyot, D. J., Turley, K., McKay, C. R., Brundage, B. H., Lipton, M. J., and Ebert, P. A.: Assessment of saphenous vein graft patency by contrast-enhanced computed tomography. J. Thorac. Cardiovasc. Surg. *83*:512, 1982.
491. Chesebro, J. H., Clements, I. P., Fuster, V., Elveback, L. R., Smith, H. C., Bardsley, W. T., Frye, R. L., Holmes, D. R., Jr., Vlietstra, R. E., Pluth, J. R., Wallace, R. B., Puga, F. J., Orszulak, T. A., Piehler, J. M., Schaff, H. V., and Danielson, G. K.: A platelet-inhibitor drug trial in coronary artery bypass operations. Benefit of perioperative dipyridamole and aspirin therapy on early postoperative vein graft patency. N. Engl. J. Med. *307*:73, 1982.
492. Baur, H. R., VanTassel, R. A., Pierach, C. A., and Gobel, F. L.: Effects of sulfinpyrazone on early graft closure after myocardial revascularization. Am. J. Cardiol. *49*:420, 1982.
493. Griffith, L. S. C., Achuff, S. C., Conti, C. R., Humphries, J. O., Brawley, R. K., Gott, V. L., and Ross, R. S.: Changes in intrinsic coronary circulation and segmental ventricular motion after saphenous-vein coronary bypass graft surgery. N. Engl. J. Med. *288*:589, 1973.
494. Levine, J. A., Bechtel, D. J., Gorlin, R., Cohn, P. F., Herman, M. V., Cohn, L. H., and Collins, J. J., Jr.: Coronary artery anatomy before and after direct revascularization surgery: Clinical and cinearteriographic studies in 67 selected patients. Am. Heart J. *89*:561, 1975.
495. Palac, R. T., Hwang, M. H., Meadows, W. R., Croke, R. P., Pifarre, R., Loeb, H. S., and Gunnar, R. M.: Progression of coronary artery disease in medically and surgically treated patients 5 years after randomization. Circulation *64*:II-17, 1981.
496. Shark, W. M., and Kass, R. M.: Repeat myocardial revascularization in coronary disease therapy: Consideration of primary bypass failure and success of second graft surgery. Am. Heart J. *102*:303, 1981.
497. Loop, F. D.: Is there a role for repeat coronary bypass surgery? J. Cardiovasc. Med. *6*:233, 1981.
498. European Coronary Surgery Study Group: Prospective randomized study of coronary artery bypass surgery in stable angina pectoris. Lancet *2*:491, 1980.
499. Chaitman, B. P., Fisher, L. D., and Bourassa, M. G.: Effect of coronary bypass surgery on survival patterns in subsets of patients with left main coronary artery disease. Report of the Collaborative Study in Coronary Artery Surgery (CASS). Am. J. Cardiol. *48*:765, 1981.
500. Takaro, T., Hultgren, H. N., and Lipton, M. J.: The VA Cooperative Randomized Study of surgery for coronary arterial occlusive disease. II. Subgroup with significant left main lesions. Circulation *54*(Suppl. III):107, 1976.
501. Oberman, A., Harrell, R. R., and Russel, R. O.: Surgical versus medical treatment in disease of the left main coronary artery. Lancet *2*:591, 1976.
502. Takaro, T., Hultgren, H. N., Detre, K. M., and Peduzzi, P.: The Veterans Administration Cooperative Study of Stable Angina: Current status. Circulation *65*(Part II):60, 1982.
503. Detre, K., Peduzzi, P., Murphy, M., Hultgren, H., Thomsen, J., Oberman, A., and Takaro, T.: Effect of bypass surgery on survival in patients in low- and high-risk subgroups delineated by the use of simple clinical variables. Circulation *63*:1329, 1981.
504. Myerburg, R. J., Ghahramani, A., and Mallon, S. M.: Coronary revascularization in patients surviving unexpected ventricular fibrillation. Circulation *52*(Suppl. III):219, 1975.
505. Cooperman, M., Stinson, E. B., Griepp, R. B., and Shumway, N. E.: Survival and function after left ventricular aneurysmectomy. J. Thorac. Cardiovasc. Surg. *69*:321, 1975.
506. Watson, L. E., Dickhaus, D. W., and Martin, R. H.: Left ventricular aneurysm. Preoperative hemodynamics, chamber volume, and results of aneurysmectomy. Circulation *52*:868, 1975.
506a. Cohen, M., Packer, M., and Gorlin, R.: Indication for left ventricular aneurysmectomy. Circulation *67*:717, 1983.
507. Lee, D. C., Johnson, R. A., Boucher, C. A., Wexler, L. F., and McEnany, M. T.: Angiographic predictors of survival following left ventricular aneurysmectomy. Circulation *56*(Suppl. II):12, 1977.
508. Liedtke, A. J., Hughes, H. C., and Zelis, R.: Functional reductions in left ventricular volume. Minimum chamber size consonant with effective hemodynamic performance. J. Thorac. Cardiovasc. Surg. *71*:195, 1976.
509. Stephens, J. D., Dymond, D. S., Stone, D. L., Rees, G. M., and Spurrell, R. A. J.: Left ventricular aneurysm and congestive heart failure: Value of exercise stress and isosorbide dinitrate in predicting hemodynamic results of aneurysmectomy. Am. J. Cardiol. *45*:932, 1980.
510. Froehlich, R. T., Falsetti, H. L., Doty, D. B., and Marcus, M. L.: Prospective study of surgery for left ventricular aneurysm. Am. J. Cardiol. *45*:923, 1980.
511. Aranda, J. M., Befeler, B., Thurer, R., Vargas, A., El-Sherif, W., and Lazana, R.: Long-term clinical and hemodynamic studies after ventricular aneurysmectomy and aorto-coronary bypass. J. Thorac. Cardiovasc. Surg. *73*:772, 1977.
512. Barnes, R. W., Liebman, P. R., Marszalek, P. B., Kirk, C. L., and Goldman, M. H.: The natural history of asymptomatic carotid disease in patients undergoing cardiovascular surgery. Surgery *90*:1075, 1981.
513. Mannick, J. A.: Editorial — Combined carotid and coronary surgery. J. Cardiovasc. Med. (*in press*).

40 REHABILITATION OF PATIENTS WITH CORONARY ARTERY DISEASE

by Albert Oberman, M.D., M.P.H.

Cardiovascular rehabilitation aims to improve and extend the quality of life for the cardiac patient by allowing him to function at the highest level compatible with the extent of his disease. A comprehensive program emphasizes physical fitness, intervention measures to retard the underlying disease process, and psychosocial adaptations. The ultimate goal of these activities is to enable the cardiac patient, largely by his own efforts, to regain his pre-illness capabilities or make the adjustments necessary for an active, productive life. Historically, cardiac rehabilitation has evolved from the techniques and principles developed from the long-term care of survivors of myocardial infarction.[1,2] Nevertheless, these same techniques can be applied to patients with other cardiac problems, including those who have had bypass grafting,[3] heart valve surgery,[4] and even cardiac transplantation.[5]

Cardiac rehabilitation is justified by the profound influence of cardiovascular disease on health and its overall costs, currently estimated for the U.S. at over $50 billion per annum.[6] The primary focus for cardiac rehabilitation has been coronary artery disease because of its high prevalence and adverse influence on disability and mortality. Coronary artery disease, the most prominent cause of premature disability in the American labor force, continues to be the leading cause of death among adults at all ages. In addition, the indirect health care costs for coronary artery disease are more than three times the direct costs, with lost income, lower productivity, disability, insurance expenses, and workman's compensation exceeding $20 billion, in comparison to the $5.5 billion spent directly for medical care.

Many patients remain incapacitated unnecessarily. They fail to return to ordinary activities owing to an overly restrictive approach in their management, even though coronary registries indicate the maximal physical capacity for patients after infarction is only 10 per cent less than healthy men of the same age.[7] Despite therapeutic advances, physicians have estimated declines in return to work since 1970 for patients with uncomplicated myocardial infarction;[8] in 1970, 85 to 89 per cent of previously employed patients less than 55 years of age returned to work, whereas only 79 to 84 per cent did so in 1979. Many do not work because of problems related to physical deconditioning, inappropriate medical advice, and psychological maladaptations rather than actual physical limitations.[9,10] Debusk and Davidson[11] determined on the basis of myocardial infarction alone that as many as 150,000 patients aged 35 to 65 and employed outside the home have special needs because of physical, psychosocial, and related vocational disabilities. Those patients afflicted with angina or valvular heart disease or those undergoing cardiac surgery add to this burden.

The magnitude of the problem plus the anticipated tendency toward an older work force in the next decade strongly point out the need for rehabilitation services.[12] The vast majority of cardiac patients, even those with complex medical, psychological, and vocational problems, referred to special work evaluation units can return to nearly normal levels of work and leisure activities.[11] However, it should be emphasized that return to work is but one of several potential benefits arising from successful rehabilitation efforts. Other outcome measures useful in assessing the value of a cardiac rehabilitation program include improvement in functional capacity, favorable physiological adaptations, symptomatic relief, lessened anxiety and depression, and the preservation of the patient's role in family and societal activities. Less certain is whether a comprehensive rehabilitation program with an exercise component can retard atherosclerosis, protect against further cardiac complications, and prolong life.

EXERCISE PROGRAM

RATIONALE. Exercise, a key element in the rehabilitative process, leads to various training adaptations, alleviating both the physiological and the psychological disorders brought about by cardiac disease.

Musculoskeletal Disability. Prolonged immobilization causes negative nitrogen and protein balance and decreases skeletal muscle mass, contractile strength, and efficiency.[13] After hospitalization, the cardiac patient experiences degeneration of the skeletal muscles and general deconditioning as a result of the prolonged bed rest. Perhaps the ideal candidate for an exercise program to relieve musculoskeletal disabilities is the patient who has had cardiac surgery, which has involved (1) restriction of activities prior to the operation as well as afterward, (2) manipulation of the sternum and chest wall, (3) immobilization in awkward positions during the operation, and (4) edema and paresthesias at the site of saphenous vein extraction after bypass grafting. Musculoskeletal problems also affect the morale of the patient and, if not managed properly, become sources of chronic disability. An appropriate conditioning routine allows a return to daily activities by restoring strength, flexibility, muscle coordination, and joint mobility.

Functional Capacity. Exercise involving large muscle groups at sufficient intensity and duration improves oxygen transport within the circulatory system and oxidative metabolic capacity of skeletal muscles, thus enhancing physical capacity for work and leisure time activities. The circulatory demands depend primarily on the relative workload, the proportion of maximal oxygen uptake required. Multiple studies have demonstrated that properly designed physical training programs increase maximal oxygen uptake and lower the relative aerobic requirements at submaximal workloads, lessening the metabolic and circulatory demands for most coronary patients, even those with impaired left ventricular function.[14–17] The percentage increase in maximal oxygen uptake depends on several factors; however, those patients initially with low capacity but *without* left ventricular dysfunction tend to show the greatest improvement. Those previously symptomatic with ordinary activities now may exert themselves at the same level without distress because the effort required represents a lesser percentage of maximal capacity. Ordinarily, the threshold for symptoms becomes manifest at about 75 per cent of functional capacity so that any exertion less than this threshold should not trouble patients.[18] Thus, even a *modest* increment in physical capacity may permit a *marked* improvement in the quality of life by allowing stair climbing, shopping, and other common activities. A patient unable to walk at 4 mph who increases his oxygen capacity from 20 ml/kg-min to 30 ml/kg-min after training should be able to walk comfortably at this same rate and conduct activities previously causing symptoms (Fig. 40–1). Not infrequently, patients are limited by leg fatigue or intermittent claudication. Though data are sparse, training appears to increase walking distance over a period of 3 or more months when conducted to the point of leg intolerance.[19,20]

Psychological Changes. Low-level exercise appears sufficient to stimulate positive psychosocial changes among men who have had myocardial infarctions.[21] Physical conditioning provides the means for allaying anxiety and preventing the onset and progression of depression, two major disorders encountered in cardiac patients. In contrast to the many restrictions imposed, exercise offers a positive and constructive approach by encouraging new activities and dispelling those fears associated with tasks requiring physical exertion. Such improvement in physical capacity encourages the patient to see himself in the context of previous health rather than as a cardiac cripple, strengthening feelings of well-being, self-esteem and self-confidence.[9,10,18] Psychological studies demonstrate that patients who exercise and become physically fit reduce their level of anxiety and suffer less depression and consequently are better able to tolerate life's stresses.[18,22]

Assessment for Exercise

Appropriate clinical evaluation and exercise testing allow selection of patients most likely to benefit from training programs and maximize compliance. The physician must determine whether the patient has any medical conditions that might preclude vigorous activity or influence the response to exercise. Quantification and prescription of exercise patterns for such a program can best be made by multistage exercise testing. However, a number of factors outside the exercise testing laboratory can also influence the patient's response to training: adverse environmental conditions (temperature, altitude, and air pollutants), prolonged exercise, competitive activities, noncompliance to the exercise regimen, and changes in health status. Careful observation of the patient in training through monitored exercise sessions for a period of at least 2 to 6

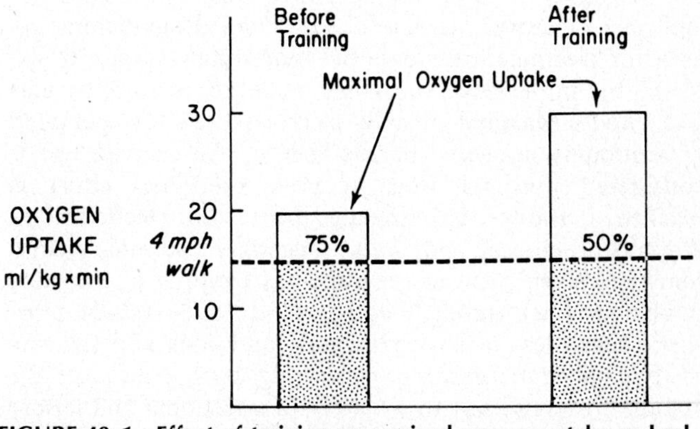

FIGURE 40–1 Effect of training on maximal oxygen uptake and relative oxygen cost (per cent $VO_2max = VO_2/VO_2max$) of walking at 4 mph on a level grade. (From Dehn, M. M., Pansegrau, D. G., and Mitchell, J. H.: Exercise training after acute myocardial infarction. *In* Wenger, N. K. (ed.): Exercise and the Heart. Philadelphia, F. A. Davis Co., 1978, pp. 117–132.)

weeks prior to more intense activities necessary for training adaptation allows more precise recommendations for long-term exercise.

CLINICAL EVALUATION. There are few absolute contraindications to exercise, but any acute illness, poorly controlled systemic disease, or unstable condition carries an unacceptable risk with exertion beyond that required for sedentary activities or more than several times basal metabolic needs. Cardiovascular contraindications to exercise requiring special consideration include (1) acute myocardial infarction, (2) unstable angina pectoris, (3) arrhythmias (ventricular tachycardia or any rhythm significantly compromising cardiac function), (4) congestive heart failure, (5) severe aortic stenosis or left ventricular outflow tract obstruction, (6) aortic dissection, (7) cardiomyopathy or myocarditis within the past year, (8) thrombophlebitis, and (9) recent embolism. Complete lists of possible contraindications and precautions for exercise are reviewed in recent publications.[23-27] Patients with diabetes, obstructive lung disease, renal disease, hernia, anemia, orthopedic disabilities, or other chronic illnesses deserve special attention but such disorders rarely constitute absolute contraindications. Drugs frequently alter the exercise response and cannot be ignored in establishing training guidelines but do not necessarily preclude training effects.[26,28,29] Agents such as beta blockers or antisympathetic drugs limit the heart rate response, whereas "cold" remedies and "mood elevators" exaggerate the sympathetic response to exercise and may predispose to dysrhythmias. Individuals on anticoagulants must be carefully watched to avoid local trauma and possible bleeding; insulin requirements for diabetics may decrease considerably with exercise. Digitalis, diuretics, tranquilizers, and antihypertensives augment ST-segment depression, whereas drug-induced hypokalemia can alter exercise tolerance.[24,26,30]

EXERCISE TESTING (see Chap. 8). Although a variety of protocols can be used for exercise testing, the procedures should be conducted in a standard fashion in order to compare data at different points in time between patients and longitudinally in the same patient. Submaximal exercise tests can be used, but it must be realized that age-predicted heart rates do not always apply to patients with symptomatic coronary disease. Maximal heart rate can be highly variable among individuals of the same sex and age; moreover, cardiac diseases and drugs commonly used for treatment attenuate the heart rate response to exercise by influencing the sinus node or atrioventricular (AV) node. Maximal capacity cannot be reliably estimated or accurately measured in this fashion. An exercise test is considered maximal when a peak exertional effort is reached or the test is terminated because of electrocardiographic or clinical endpoints. Generally, ischemic symptoms and signs occur at the same heart rate or at the same double product (product of heart rate and systolic pressure), regardless of environmental conditions and the mix of dynamic-static exercise, permitting extrapolation of the standard exercise test to a variety of vocational and leisure tasks.[11,31]

The multistage exercise test defines the patient's functional capacity; provokes heart rate, blood pressure, and electrocardiographic abnormalities not apparent at rest; furnishes prognostic information; and provides baseline data for evaluating progress. Opinions vary regarding the importance of exercise-induced premature ventricular contractions (PVC's) compared with those occurring at rest but decreasing with exercise.[32,33] Neither exercise testing nor prolonged ambulatory monitoring for PVC's has clarified the significance of such dysrhythmias for patients entering an exercise program.[32-34] However, recent data indicate a characteristic and reproducible relationship between PVC frequency and heart rate over the range of heart rates encountered during routine activities.[35]

The test situation can be used to great advantage in observing the patient during exercise for symptoms, signs, and general appearances and for teaching him how to judge his own performance. The Borg Scale is a technique for quantifying perceived exertion by having the patient rate the workload on a scale from 6 to 20.[36] Each odd number of 15 grade categories is characterized by appropriate descriptors, ranging from very, very light (7 rating) to very, very hard (19 rating). Such ratings can be used for assessing the patient's work tolerance and as an educational tool by which the patient can estimate whether he is achieving his training level independent of heart rate measurement.

Exercise Training

To be worthwhile, exercise must tax the cardiorespiratory system; yet the musculoskeletal and cardiovascular hazards to unfit middle-aged adults with coronary disease who undertake strenuous exercise cannot be overemphasized. The likelihood of such problems depends in large part on age, athletic abilities, prior inactivity, extent of coronary atherosclerosis, left ventricular dysfunction, and general health. Although these immutable variables can increase the risk of complications, an exercise program can be conducted in a fashion that will minimize any potential hazards. Regular exercise, even of high intensity, is safe for cardiac patients if they follow an individualized but well-structured program. The primary determinants of the magnitude of the adaptive response to such a program involve the intensity, frequency, and duration of the exercise session and the type of exercise.

INTENSITY. This appears to be the single most important determinant in achieving the desired training effects. The cardiac patient should train at 50 to 75 per cent of his maximal oxygen uptake, although a relative load of 40 per cent has sufficed in some instances.[14,23-27,37-39] As with normal subjects, the degree of improvement tends to be inversely proportional to the pretraining capacity for patients with coronary disease.[14] Because of the high linear correlation between oxygen uptake and heart rate at submaximal workloads, the heart rate may be substituted for the more difficult measurement of oxygen consumption. Available tables for predicting maximal heart rate by age cannot be used for this purpose. These predicted heart rates represent the average values for "normal" persons not on medication and therefore can be misleading and can negate the purpose of the individual prescription. Cardiac patients should have a target that takes into consideration symptoms and signs, so that the training intensity never exceeds the point at which ischemia becomes manifest. By actually testing the patient, the monitoring physician can take into account aberrant heart rate responses due to intrinsic cardiac disease or medications such as beta blockers. The usual effects of training are observed in patients on beta blockers, and the exercise heart rate, although lower than that in patients not receiving these drugs, remains a useful guide to their evaluation throughout a physicial training program.[28,29]

Ample data indicate that a training heart rate at 70 to 85 per cent of maximal capacity corresponds to the levels of maximal oxygen uptake (57 to 78 per cent) required for training (Fig. 40–2).[14–16,26,27,37–39] Another approach for estimating the target heart rate is to add 60 to 70 per cent of the difference between resting heart rate and maximal heart rate attained to the resting heart rate.[36–39] This technique takes the variability of the resting heart rate into account and generally gives a slightly higher target heart rate. The relationship of per cent maximal heart rate and per cent maximal oxygen uptake remains consistent for persons of all ages in the presence or absence of coronary disease and at all levels of training.[37] In practice, the target heart rate determined by either procedure applies to all training activities for the patient under usual environmental conditions.

Besides oxygen consumption and heart rate, the dosage intensity may be prescribed in METS. A MET is a unit of energy that approximates the amount of oxygen required under basal conditions at rest and is 3.5 ml/kg-min. Published tables[39,40] transform METS into energy requirements for common activities at work and home (Table 40–1). METS can be used only as a crude index because differences in individual energy expenditure vary according to environmental factors, physical condition, skills, and motivation. Yet the MET is recommended for translation into exercise programs, since it is easily understood by both the patient and the physician, can be applied to various tasks, and can be monitored by heart rate response. The average 40-year-old male in the U.S. can function at 10 METS at his maximum capacity; therefore, the concept of 1 MET as the energy cost of sitting provides a scale of 1 to 10 for applying physical activity components to the functional capacity of the average adult man.[24]

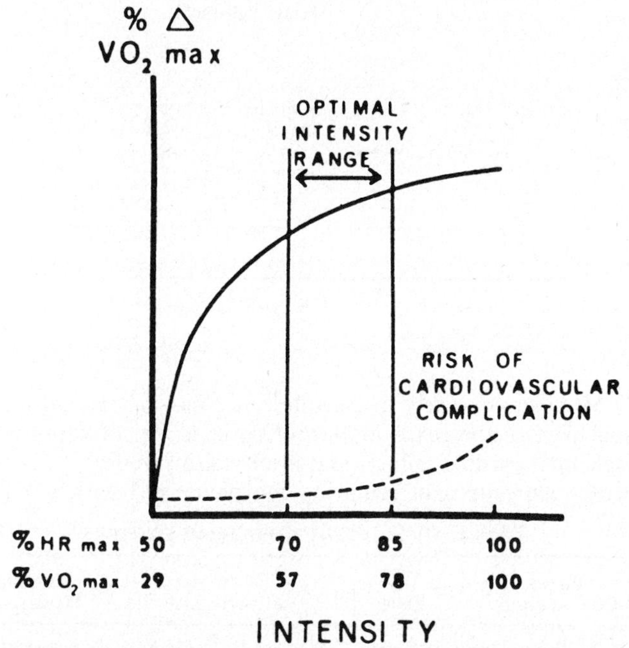

FIGURE 40–2 Relationship between per cent gain in aerobic capacity (ΔVO_2max) and intensity of exercise expressed as per cent of maximal heart rate (HR max) or per cent of VO_2max. The optimal intensity range is 70 to 85 per cent of HR max equivalent to 57 to 78 per cent VO_2max. As the intensity of exercise exceeds 85 per cent of HR max, the relative risks of arrhythmias, angina pectoris, and other ischemic manifestations increase abruptly, whereas the improvement in aerobic capacity levels off. (Adapted from Hellerstein, H. K., and Franklin, B. A.: Exercise testing and prescription. *In* Wenger, N. K., and Hellerstein, H. K. (eds.): Rehabilitation of the Coronary Patient. New York, John Wiley and Sons, 1978, pp. 149–202.)

DURATION. Although training adaptations can occur with brief sessions at high intensity, this is not advisable from the standpoint of safety. In addition, the logistics of getting to and from supervised sessions make a 30- to 45-minute exercise session more practical. However, frequent brief sessions may be necessary for those individuals unable to tolerate 30 minutes of moderate intensity (70 to 80 per cent or lower of maximal capacity). Training effects may be noted as soon as 2 weeks or as late as 6 weeks after starting but can be highly variable among individuals, depending upon initial functional capacity, health status, and response to specific activities.[37]

FREQUENCY OF TRAINING. To improve cardiovascular fitness, the exercise program should be performed at least 3 days a week, preferably nonconsecutively to avoid musculoskeletal stress. Maintenance programs of 2 to 3 days per week suffice to retain exercise adaptations. Frequency of training appears to be less important than either intensity or duration.

TYPE OF EXERCISE. The mode of exercise should be dynamic (isotonic) activities involving large muscle groups, designed to overload the oxygen transport system of the body, such as walking, jogging, swimming, and bicycling. Swimming, an ideal exercise from the standpoint of involving large muscle groups in the arms and legs, also provides relief for weight-bearing joints but has a high relative energy cost and can mask ischemic symptoms.[41,42] Recent studies suggest no difference between combined dynamic-static exercise compared with dynamic exercise alone at peak loads in causing induced ischemia, left ventricular dysfunction, or ventricular arrhythmias.[31,43] Adaptive training responses are peculiar to the muscle group exercised so that the patient's occupational and leisure time activities should be considered in order to establish appropriate exercises.[14–16] Most rehabilitation programs incorporate interval training techniques, a series of repeated bouts of exercise alternated with periods of relief during the exercise session. For most situations, such intermittent exercise offers several advantages over continuous training techniques: (1) The patient will be able to achieve higher intensity levels with less probability of leg fatigue by virtue of the rest periods; (2) it allows more diverse activities; (3) changing modes of exercise permit different muscle groups to be stressed; and (4) ischemic signs can be monitored more carefully during the recovery intervals.

Phases of Rehabilitation

The exercise program is divided into three phases: (1) early convalescence during hospitalization; (2) intermediate convalescence, the transition period between hospital and resumption of ordinary activities; and (3) the long-term program for maintenance of health (Table 40–2). Although guidelines for exercise remain the same throughout these

TABLE 40–1 APPROXIMATE ENERGY REQUIREMENTS FOR SELECTED ACTIVITIES

Energy Category	Self-Care or Home	Occupational	Recreational	Physical Conditioning
Very Light < 3 METS < 10 ml/kg-min < 4 kcal	Washing, shaving, dressing Desk work, writing Washing dishes Driving auto	Sitting (clerical, assembling) Standing (store clerk, bartender) Driving truck Janitorial work	Playing cards Horseshoes Bait casting Billiards Sewing, knitting Golf (cart)	Walking (level at 2 mph) Stationary bicycle (very low resistance) Very light calisthenics
Light 3–5 METS 11–18 ml/kg-min 4–6 kcal	Cleaning windows Raking leaves Weeding Power lawn mowing Waxing floors (slowly) Painting Carrying objects (15–30 lb)	Stocking shelves (light objects) Light welding Light carpentry Machine assembly Auto repair Paperhanging	Dancing (social and square) Golf (walking) Sailing Horseback riding Volleyball (6 man) Tennis (doubles)	Walking (3–4 mph) Level bicycling (6–8 mph) Light calisthenics
Moderate 5–7 METS 18–25 ml/kg-min 6–8 kcal	Easy digging in garden Level hand lawn mowing Climbing stairs (slowly) Carrying objects (30–60 lb) Splitting wood	Carpentry (exterior home building) Shoveling dirt Pneumatic tools	Light backpacking Tennis (singles) Water skiing Skating (ice and roller) Horseback riding (gallop)	Walking (4.5–5 mph) Bicycling (9–10 mph) Swimming (breast stroke)
Heavy 7–9 METS 25–32 ml/kg-min 8–10 kcal	Sawing wood Heavy shoveling Climbing stairs (moderate speed) Carrying objects (60–90 lb)	Tending furnace Digging ditches Pick and shovel	Canoeing Mountain climbing Touch football Paddleball	Jog (5 mph) Swim (crawl stroke) Rowing machine Bicycling (12 mph) Heavy calisthenics
Very Heavy > 9 METS > 32 ml/kg-min > 10 kcal	Carrying loads upstairs Carrying objects (> 90 lb) Climbing stairs (quickly) Shoveling heavy snow	Lumber jack Heavy laborer	Handball Squash Ski touring over hills	Running (≥ 6 mph Bicycle (≥ 13 mph or up steep hill) Rope jumping

Adapted from Haskell, W. L.: Design and implementation of cardiac conditioning programs. *In* Wenger, N. K., and Hellerstein, H. (eds.): Rehabilitation of the Coronary Patient. New York, John Wiley and Sons, 1978, pp. 203–241.

program phases, the objectives and methods differ somewhat in each.

PHASE ONE—IN HOSPITAL. Traditionally, 6 to 8 weeks of absolute bed rest was the rule for patients sustaining a myocardial infarction, although as early as the 1940's, Dr. Tinsley Harrison questioned the wisdom of undue restriction.[44] Deleterious effects of such mobilization include a decrement of 20 per cent or more in physical work capacity, hypovolemia, depression of pulmonary ventilation, and muscle degeneration.[13] Controversy surrounded early mobilization after infarction until a series of investigations, progressing from a "chair regimen"[45] to rapid mobilization, demonstrated the safety and efficacy of such activities for selected patients.[13,46–53] Coronary artery bypass grafting creates a situation not unlike that after myocardial infarction, in which carefully supervised activity programs during hospitalization result in shortened hospital stays, with no greater immediate risk than prolonged bed rest.[54]

Mobilization early in convalescence has become an integral part of the rehabilitation of patients free of continued ischemia, cardiac failure, and electrical instability. Patients with recurrent pain requiring morphine and with a CK-

TABLE 40–2 EXERCISE PROGRAM SCHEDULE

Phase of Convalescence*	Time	Activities	Average Workload
Early	1–3 weeks	Self care activities, low-level calisthenics, walking	2–4 METS
Intermediate	4–12 weeks	Moderate-level calisthenics, walking, structured endurance training	5–7 METS
Long-term	12 + weeks	High-level calisthenics, high-level endurance training	7 + METS

*Following myocardial infarction or coronary artery bypass surgery.

MB persisting for 72 hours or longer representing possible extension of the infarction[55] must be approached more cautiously. Most data reveal no immediate adverse effects of early mobilization and discharge,[56] but one randomized controlled trial noted an unexplained lower mortality during the second and third years of follow-up in the late mobilization group.[52] Although in-hospital exercise improved functional status at the time of discharge and led to an earlier and more complete return to work in some studies,[56] Sivarajan and colleagues[57] were unable to detect any significant beneficial or deleterious efforts of an early in-hospital exercise program combined with early evaluation and discharge. Another study showed significant functional improvement from early low-intensity exercises but only in a small subgroup able to exercise without evidence of ischemia.[58]

Early exercise testing (see also pp. 1293 and 1327) is useful for rehabilitation assessment in patients without congestive heart failure, severe arrhythmias, orthopedic complications, or other severe disabilities.[59–61,61a] Testing may merely involve monitoring the patient as he walks in a hospital corridor, with observation for angina, dyspnea, new murmurs, gallops, abnormalities of heart rate or blood pressure, and electrocardiographic changes. Of more value is a low-level testing protocol[11,60,62] to detect the threshold for adverse symptoms or signs, to judge whether a patient can tolerate self-care activities at home, and to provide prognostic information.[62a] The safety of early testing appears to be more related to the severity of disease than to the length of the interval following infarction or to details of the test protocol.

As early as the first few days after infarction, patients without complications can be started on self-care activities limited to several METS (Fig. 40–3). This modest exertional level rarely increases the heart rate more than 10 beats/min and permits the patient to feed himself, wash his hands and face, shave, and use the bedside commode with assistance. Activities as minimal as getting up and sitting in a chair several times daily, suggested by Levine and Lown years ago,[45] prevent orthostatic intolerance from protracted bed rest.[63] Programmed and progressive self-care activities allow patients to maintain the expectation of an independent life style. Calisthenics, valuable for flexibility, strength, and even endurance, may be started in conjunction with a walking program. Specific exercises to increase the strength of the pectoral muscles have been developed for the postoperative patient.[3] Isometric exercises are avoided because of the presumed excessive myocardial oxygen consumption and dysrhythmias imposed by the predominantly "pressure" workload, though recent studies question this concept.[31,43] Physical activities should be carried out under the supervision of the nursing staff with frequent reassessment of symptoms and signs during the early exercise sessions; just prior to discharge, physical activity should be monitored for abnormal responses to exercise. If problems occur, the level of activities should be either reduced or discontinued temporarily until the patient can resume progressive exercise safely.

PHASE TWO—INTERMEDIATE CONVALESCENCE. At the time of discharge from the hospital, the patient should be able to perform activities at peak levels of 3.5 to 4.0 METS for short durations corresponding to usual activities at home.[64] During initial days at home, patients continue the activities started at the hospital—dynamic warm-up exercises followed by walking at a graduated distance and pace. After the initial post-hospitalization examination, further advice about exercise can be given to those ready. During this period, the patient is asked first to walk at least a half mile in 10 minutes, then a mile in 20 minutes, subsequently decreasing the time to 15 minutes by increasing the speed. Provided there are no contraindications, the walking program is accelerated, first in distance and then in pace. Generally, if the duration can be doubled at a given intensity without producing symptoms or excessive heart rate response, the next higher level of intensity may be undertaken.[25] Next the walk is lengthened to 2 miles daily, with the speed maintained at 4 mph or the distance covered in 30 minutes. If a patient can maintain the pace, the distance can be increased to 3 or 4 miles per day at his physician's discretion. Not all patients can achieve this goal, but almost all can obtain great satisfaction in the attempt.

At 6 to 8 weeks after hospitalization, the emphasis shifts toward *dynamic exercises* to improve cardiopulmonary function. At this point, patients must be carefully reevaluated to determine possible adverse reactions to exercise or conditions requiring special precautions with more vigorous exertion. Some examples include prolonged fatigue, worsening angina or congestive failure, dysrhythmias, signs of cerebral dysfunction, development of orthopedic problems, electrocardiographic changes, or altered drug regimens. Recommendations for exercise should be made with the same care as for any other prescription. An inappropriately high intensity of exercise can lead to clinical events, orthopedic problems, and generally poor compliance, whereas homeopathic doses nullify any likely improvement and discourage patients from resuming ordinary activities. An appropriate prescription requires a maximal or symptom-sign–limited exercise test. In addition to the objective measurements of work capacity during the test, the patient's subjective estimate of exertion (Borg Scale) can be helpful in formulating the exercise prescription and in monitoring training effects.[36] At this stage of convalescence, the exercise prescription recommended for endurance training is based on the lower boundary of the target range, or about 60 per cent of the patient's maximal oxygen uptake, corresponding to 70 to 75 per cent of the maximal heart rate, achieved on the exercise test. For example, if the maximal heart rate achieved before termination of the exercise test is 160 beats/min, the target heart rate will be 75 per cent of 160 ($160 \times 0.75 = 120$ beats per minutes. With interval (intermittent) exercise, the changing energy demands may result in heart rates varying by about 10 per cent from the prescribed target heart rate. However, the heart rate should average out to the prescribed level over the total duration of the training session. Patients able to perform at levels of 5 METS or more should exercise at least three times per week, preferably on alternate days to avoid excessive bone-joint stress. The duration of the exercise may range from 20 to 30 minutes during the first few weeks of conditioning, after which the duration can be increased to as much as 45 minutes. Duration can be set empirically for those patients with functional capacities below 5 METS and can be adjusted thereafter, depending on the individual response to exercise. The frequency of exercise should be prescribed for

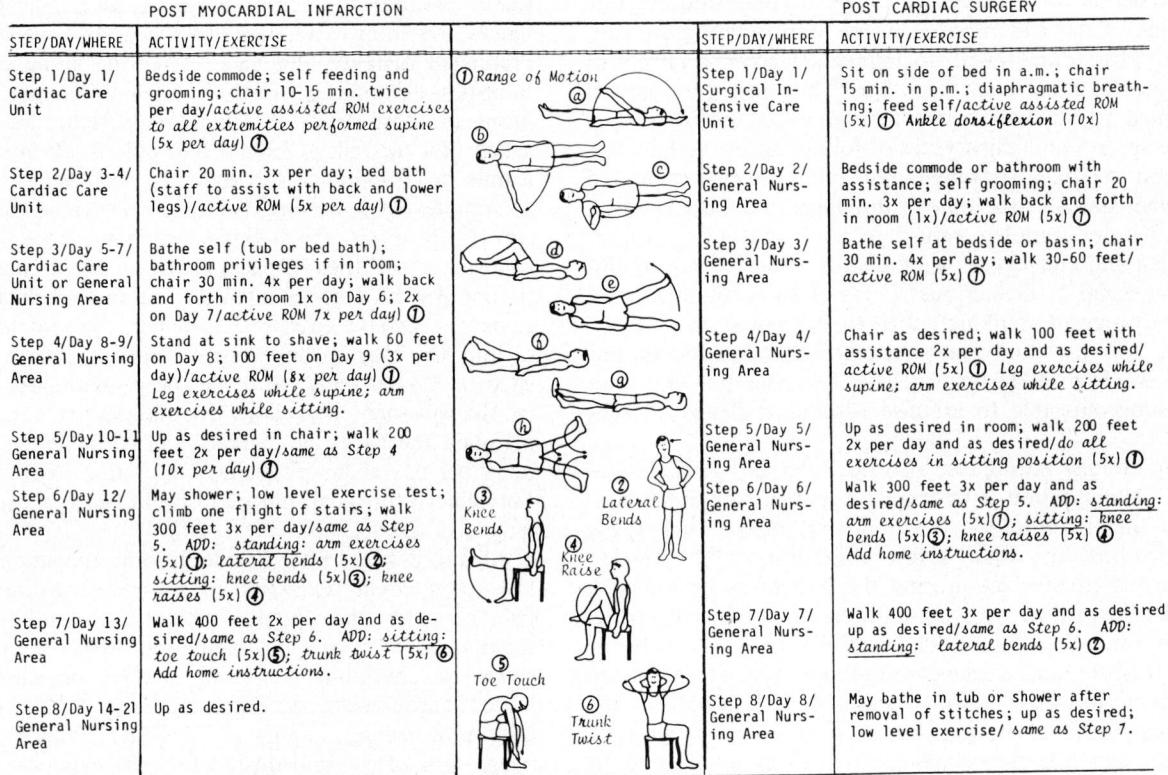

POST MYOCARDIAL INFARCTION

STEP/DAY/WHERE	ACTIVITY/EXERCISE
Step 1/Day 1/ Cardiac Care Unit	Bedside commode; self feeding and grooming; chair 10-15 min. twice per day/*active assisted ROM exercises to all extremities performed supine (5x per day)* ①
Step 2/Day 3-4/ Cardiac Care Unit	Chair 20 min. 3x per day; bed bath (staff to assist with back and lower legs)/*active ROM (5x per day)* ①
Step 3/Day 5-7/ Cardiac Care Unit or General Nursing Area	Bathe self (tub or bed bath); bathroom privileges if in room; chair 30 min. 4x per day; walk back and forth in room 1x on Day 6; 2x on Day 7/*active ROM 7x per day)* ①
Step 4/Day 8-9/ General Nursing Area	Stand at sink to shave; walk 60 feet on Day 8; 100 feet on Day 9 (3x per day)/*active ROM (8x per day)* ① *Leg exercises while supine; arm exercises while sitting.*
Step 5/Day 10-11 General Nursing Area	Up as desired in chair; walk 200 feet 2x per day/*same as Step 4 (10x per day)* ①
Step 6/Day 12/ General Nursing Area	May shower; low level exercise test; climb one flight of stairs; walk 300 feet 3x per day/*same as Step 5. ADD: standing: arm exercises (5x)①; lateral bends (5x)②; sitting: knee bends (5x)③; knee raises (5x)* ④
Step 7/Day 13/ General Nursing Area	Walk 400 feet 2x per day and as desired/*same as Step 6. ADD: sitting: toe touch (5x)⑤; trunk twist (5x)* ⑥ *Add home instructions.*
Step 8/Day 14-21 General Nursing Area	Up as desired.

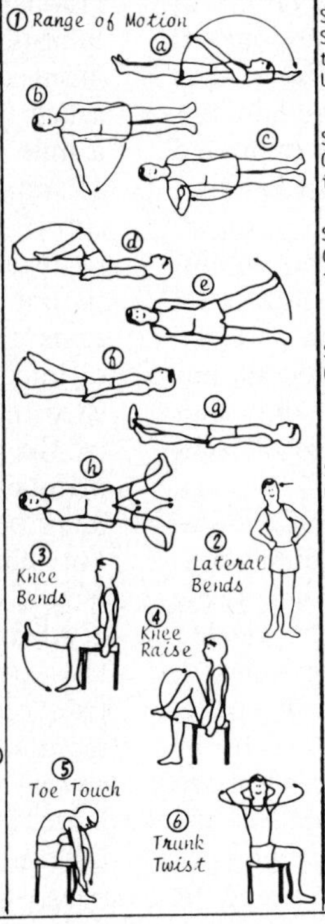

POST CARDIAC SURGERY

STEP/DAY/WHERE	ACTIVITY/EXERCISE
Step 1/Day 1/ Surgical Intensive Care Unit	Sit on side of bed in a.m.; chair 15 min. in p.m.; diaphragmatic breathing; feed self/*active assisted ROM* (5x) ① ***Ankle dorsiflexion*** (10x)
Step 2/Day 2/ General Nursing Area	Bedside commode or bathroom with assistance; self grooming; chair 20 min. 3x per day; walk back and forth in room (1x)/*active ROM* (5x) ①
Step 3/Day 3/ General Nursing Area	Bathe self at bedside or basin; chair 30 min. 4x per day; walk 30-60 feet/ *active ROM* (5x) ①
Step 4/Day 4/ General Nursing Area	Chair as desired; walk 100 feet with assistance 2x per day and as desired/ *active ROM* (5x) ① *Leg exercises while supine; arm exercises while sitting.*
Step 5/Day 5/ General Nursing Area	Up as desired in room; walk 200 feet 2x per day and as desired/*do all exercises in sitting position* (5x) ①
Step 6/Day 6/ General Nursing Area	Walk 300 feet 3x per day and as desired/*same as Step 5. ADD: standing: arm exercises* (5x)①; *sitting: knee bends* (5x)③; *knee raises* (5x) ④ *Add home instructions.*
Step 7/Day 7/ General Nursing Area	Walk 400 feet 3x per day and as desired; up as desired/*same as Step 6. ADD: standing: lateral bends* (5x) ②
Step 8/Day 8/ General Nursing Area	May bathe in tub or shower after removal of stitches; up as desired; low level exercise/ *same as Step 7.*

FIGURE 40–3 Inpatient activity schedule. Exercise instructions:
1. Range of motion (ROM):
a. With elbow straight, lift arm straight over head and return to side. Relax and repeat with opposite arm.
b. With elbow straight, lift arm away from body and over head, and then return to side. Relax and repeat with opposite arm.
c. With arm straight down by side, bend elbow and touch shoulder with fingertips. Relax and repeat with opposite arm.
d. Raise knee toward chest and return to starting position. Relax and repeat with opposite leg.
e. With leg straight, move leg out to side of body and return to starting position. Relax and repeat with opposite leg.
f. Straight leg raise.
g. Make circular patterns with both feet. Relax and repeat.
h. Roll legs in and out simultaneously. Relax and repeat.
2. Lateral bends: standing erect, bend trunk laterally to left then to right. Relax and repeat.
3. Knee bends: sitting erect, straighten and bend knees alternately. Relax and repeat.
4. Knee raise: sitting erect, raise knees toward the chest alternately. Relax and repeat.
5. Toe touch: sitting erect, bend trunk forward trying to touch toes with fingertips. Relax and repeat.
6. Trunk twist: sitting erect, twist trunk to left and then to right. Relax and repeat.
(Adapted from Georgia Baptist Medical Center, Cardiac Rehabilitation Unit, Atlanta, Georgia.)

three to five periods per week. Daily sessions for persons with capacities between 3 and 5 METS may be advisable, and for patients with functional capacities less than 3 METS, sessions of 5 minutes several times daily.[26] Within these guidelines, the exercise prescription for most patients will result in training adaptations without undue fatigue or hazard.

Group activities at an exercise facility offer certain advantages—trained personnel, established emergency routines, and motivation by other participants.[65] A model training session might proceed as follows: After 5 minutes of warm-up calisthenics, the patient exercises at the target rate set at about 75 per cent of the maximal heart rate achieved on the prior exercise test. Useful training devices include the treadmill, stationary bicycle, steps, rowing machine, arm ergometer, and arm wheel. On each device, the patient reaches his target rate within a minute or two and maintains this heart rate within 10 beats/min for the remainder of the 4-minute exercise period. After the fourth minute, there is a 2-minute recovery period before the patient moves to the next exercise station, with the patient alternating between arm and leg device stations. In this way the patient achieves a larger overall workload before the onset of fatigue or symptoms. After six exercise periods, or a total of 24 minutes of exercise, the patient walks around the room for a 5-minute cool-down period. Most patients are ready to begin their own long-term program after 6 to 12 of these supervised exercise sessions.

PHASE THREE—LONG-TERM PROGRAM. The long-term program is designed to retain training adaptations and stimulate further progress. The need for supervision is critical during the transition to more vigorous exertion with less structured routines, yet economic and other concerns necessitate the judicious use of unsupervised exercise programs for coronary patients.[66–69] Except for those patients benefiting from low-level activities such as walking, it is best to delay an unsupervised program. Patients may proceed to an unsupervised maintenance program after thorough evaluation on the basis of (1) a stable health status, (2) relatively low risk for subsequent cardiac events, (3) functional performance of at least 8 METS or more, and (4) a full understanding of the principles of exercise training and the disease process.[23,26]

Recreational activities equivalent to the peak energy requirements of the previous exercise test can be introduced in the absence of possible hazards, such as adverse environmental conditions, intensive competition, or marked emotional involvement. Sports and games vary in promoting the components of fitness—endurance, strength, and flexibility—and should be selected accordingly. A typical long-term exercise session for a patient attaining a maximal heart rate of 140 beats/min and 6 METS on the exercise test before developing angina would consist of the following components: (1) warm-up exercises for 5 minutes; (2) endurance training consisting of 20 to 30 minutes of walking, jogging, or cycling, at the target exertional level (85 per cent of maximal capacity, which is about 120 beats/min, or 5 METS); (3) a 5-minute cool-down period; (4) a 5-minute warm-up period; (5) a 20- to 30-minute recreational period; and (6) a final cool-down 5-minute walk (Fig. 40–4). The allotted time for structured endurance and recreational activities depends on individual preference, capabilities, and facilities. Heart rate estimates are more difficult to make with recreational activities, and the patient's subjective feelings of exertion (Borg Scale) become more important.[36] As the patient adapts to the training routine, the heart rate for a given exertional task will decrease, allowing progressive increments in the workload. Periodic evaluation will aid in adjusting the exercise prescription and in assessing progress. Recent publications review in detail exercise prescriptions, appropriate physical activities, and topics pertinent to cardiac rehabilitation programs.[70]

SECONDARY PREVENTION

Once manifest, coronary heart disease increases susceptibility to infarction, congestive failure, stroke, and premature death.[71] New rehabilitation studies document the importance of intervention programs in reducing the sequellae of coronary disease, prolonging life, and having a positive effect on life style.[72–76,76a] In addition to physical training, a rehabilitation program should incorporate risk factor intervention as well as clinical measures likely to alter the progression of disease and improve the long-term prognosis. Several clinical trials (p. 1352)[77,77a,77b,77c,77d,78] have now demonstrated that beta-blocking drugs can substantially reduce the rate of death during the first 2 years after myocardial infarction. Whether other kinds of coronary artery disease patients can benefit from these agents, the best time to initiate treatment, and the duration of therapy required for optimal benefits remain unknown. Recent reviews[79–81] corroborate the value of coronary artery bypass grafting in affecting the quality of life by relieving symptoms in 80 to 90 per cent of patients with angina, by increasing functional capacity, by reducing the number of cardiac related events, and by prolonging survival in patients with substantial stenosis of the left main coronary artery or "three-vessel" disease (p. 1372). These findings emphasize the importance of optimal clinical management in the rehabilitation process for selected categories of patients.

Risk Factor Modification (See Chap. 35)

The prognosis after myocardial infarction as well as the development of coronary artery disease is associated with major risk factors.[71,82–84] Patients should be advised to discontinue all forms of smoking, even filtered cigarettes,[85] as

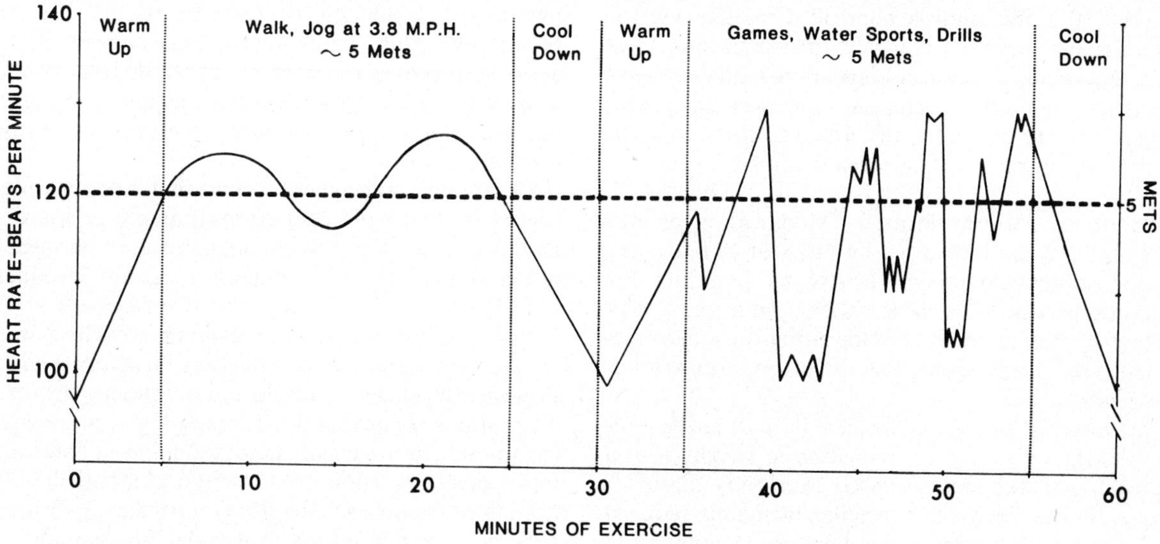

FIGURE 40–4 Long-term exercise program. The example is for the hypothetical patient who completed Stage 6 of the prior exercise test, attaining a maximum heart rate of 140 beats/min before developing angina. The program contains variable amounts of recreational activities in addition to the basic endurance exercises to maintain the patient's interest. The actual heart rate tends to fluctuate about the desired target level and is more difficult to approximate with recreational activities. With adequate supervision, the heart rate can be maintained within 10 beats of the prescribed target rate for most of the session. (From Oberman, A., and Kouchoukos, N. T.: Role of exercise after coronary artery surgery. *In* Wenger, N. K. (ed.): Exercise and the Heart. Philadelphia, F. A. Davis Co., 1978, pp. 155–172.)

early in the course of the disease as possible. Among coronary patients, ex-smokers have only one-half the subsequent mortality of those who continue to smoke;[71] in the Coronary Artery Surgery Study registry, 5-year survival was significantly less for those who continued to smoke.[86] Weight reduction favorably modifies cholesterol levels, blood pressure, glucose tolerance, and other metabolic factors associated with atherosclerotic disease.[71,87] Persuasive evidence exists that an elevated serum cholesterol level, especially with a low proportion of high-density lipoprotein cholesterol,[88] accelerates the progression of atherosclerosis and its complications,[84,89,90] yet data from the controlled trials justifying reduction of plasma lipids by means of drugs are not encouraging.[72,91]

One must extrapolate from the studies on the efficacy of antihypertensive treatment for the general population[92] and the anticipated greater myocardial oxygen costs in hypertension to justify treating hypertension in patients with coronary artery disease. Lowering elevated blood pressure in patients with coronary artery disease should diminish symptoms, enhance left ventricular function, and retard progression of disease, but no documentation from controlled trials among such populations is available. The situation is complicated by hemodynamic changes resulting from the myocardial infarction itself. In the Framingham experience, a decrease in blood pressure at 1 year after infarction adversely affected mortality;[71] however, by excluding those patients who had sustained a fall in blood pressure post infarction, the usual direct relationship between blood pressure and mortality was found. For the long-term management of coronary patients, optimal blood pressure levels have yet to be determined.

Exercise

In the past 10 years, multiple controlled randomized trials of exercise for survivors of myocardial infarction have supported the value of physical activity in reducing long-term mortality.[72] Possible mechanisms for secondary prevention involve retardation of the atherosclerotic process or protection against the occurrence of clinical manifestations.

Retardation of Atherosclerosis. Modification of atherogenic traits that are influenced by physical activity may improve the subsequent clinical course by retarding the atherosclerotic process. For those patients undergoing coronary artery bypass grafting, the prevention of atherosclerosis in the vein grafts themselves is an important long-term concern.[93]

Some atherogenic factors influenced by a training program include the following: (1) reduction in weight with a constant caloric intake and increased lean body mass;[94–96] (2) changes in the lipoprotein profile, including reduced levels of serum triglycerides and an increased amount of cholesterol carried by high-density lipoproteins,[94–98] but no clear concensus exists regarding the relationship of total cholesterol concentration to habitual exercise;[99] (3) increased cellular sensitivity to insulin, resulting in improved glucose tolerance;[95,100] (4) minimal blood pressure changes but generally a lowered resting diastolic blood pressure with a decrease in mean blood pressure during submaximal exercise;[15,16,96,101] (5) stimulation of desirable health habits, including modification of Type A behavior (p. 1826);[102,103] (6) decreased platelet adhesiveness and enhanced fibrinolysis;[104,105] (7) and a lessened adrenergic response to stress.[96,101,106]

Yet it is unlikely that coronary patients in a supervised exercise program not using additional intervention modalities will exhibit marked improvement in major risk factors.[107,108] Insufficient training adaptations due to poor compliance and the inability to attain the levels of exertion or the duration necessary for major changes in risk factors have been offered as explanations.[98,102,107–109] Alternatively, it is possible that exercise might act indirectly by blocking the effect of major risk factors. For example, training adaptations lower heart rate and blood pressure at submaximal work levels, accelerate carbon monoxide metabolism, and diminish platelet aggregation; any or all of these metabolic changes might counter the adverse effects of smoking.[107]

Protection Against Clinical Manifestations of Coronary Artery Disease. Properly executed physical training programs generally increase exercise tolerance by at least 20 per cent in most patients with coronary artery disease[15,25,110] and in some instances allow coronary patients to reach a degree of fitness seldom attained even by healthy individuals—that required for marathon races.[111–113] Training adaptations result in relative bradycardia at submaximal levels of exercise but induce little change in stroke volume. The increased maximum oxygen uptake depends primarily upon enhanced peripheral extraction of oxygen by redistribution of blood to working skeletal muscles and local adaptive changes in the skeletal muscle's capacity for aerobic metabolism.[15,16] Such training effects reduce cardiac work in proportion to total body work and enable an individual to respond to exertion without taxing the circulation and compromising myocardial oxygen needs.[14] Myocardial oxygen consumption, as estimated indirectly, is less for a given task owing to a systematic decrease in exercise heart rate and blood pressure.[101] More recent data suggest that training actually improves myocardial oxygen delivery or utilization, leading to an increased exercise tolerance and higher values for heart rate and systolic blood pressure before myocardial ischemia develops.[110,115–117]

Ehsani and colleagues[115] found that patients able to exercise at 65 to 85 per cent of maximum $\dot{V}O_2$ for 1 hour per day, 4 or 5 days per week, achieved a 38 per cent increase in maximum $\dot{V}O_2$ and increased the double product threshold. The extent of ST-segment displacement at the same double product and at the maximum workload was less after training, implying a reduction in myocardial ischemia. Presumably, skeletal muscle and autonomic nervous system adaptations occur rapidly, bringing about increased exercise capabilities, but cardiac adaptations occur later, only with more intense exertion over a period of months.[118,119] In addition, improvement in exercise performance[120–122] has been attributed to enhanced left ventricular function and increased stroke volume with prolonged, intensive exercise training. Failure to improve ventricular function during rest and exercise may be due to insufficient training levels.[118,119] Indirect evidence for favorable cardiovascular changes includes reversion of aberrant ballistocardiographic waveforms,[123] fewer electrocardiographic abnormalities,[124,125] and less ventricular ectopic activity[83,101] in men participating in vigorous exercise. Still uncertain is the degree to which the consequences of a myocardial infarct can be corrected or compensated for by an exercise program.

Experimental data from animals with surgically induced coronary artery lesions subjected to physical training suggest cardiovascular adaptations that might diminish myocardial ischemia: (1) improved myocardial function and metabolism and (2) augumented myocardial perfusion, possibly resulting from increased coronary vasculature, capillary to myocardial fiber ratio, and collateral circulation.[124,126] Monkeys fed an atherogenic diet and then exercised demonstrated larger coronary arteries and less surface area involved with atherosclerotic plaques than did sedentary controls, suggesting that exercise may prevent coronary artery disease in primates by augmenting the coronary vascular bed.[127] Nevertheless, studies of physical activity in patients with coronary artery disease have not demonstrated expanded collateral circulation,[116,126,128–130] but evaluation during exercise or more sensitive methods for determining myocardial perfusion might be needed.

Over the last decade a growing series of randomized trials[131–135] have demonstrated a differential mortality among survivors of myocardial infarction randomized to a physical training program compared with those in a "control" group (Table 40–3). These studies were based on supervised training programs consisting of two to four sessions per week lasting 20 to 60 minutes each. Despite major problems in adherence to the exercise regimen, all the trials but one showed reductions in mortality ranging from 20.6 to 37.0 per cent for the exercise group. Little effect on the incidence of reinfarction was noted. However, such trials were inadequate to test the hypothesis that exercise reduces overall mortality, as they were not designed with this as the primary outcome. The National Exercise and Heart Disease Project showed a substantial, but nonsignificant, 37 per cent reduction in total mortality, primarily due to fewer deaths from recurrent myocardial infarction.[135] The benefits of exercise were greatest in those patients whose physical capacity exceeded 7 METS, in cigarette smokers, and in those whose systolic blood pressure response to exercise testing exceeded 140 mm Hg. These data support an assumption of substantial benefit from supervised exercise among survivors of a myocardial infarction. Pooling of the results from these five comparable studies is consistent with a 19 per cent reduction ($p < 0.05$) in total mortality in the exercise intervention group.[72] In any event, these trials conclusively demonstrated that there was no additional hazard from supervised exercise among postinfarction patients. Haskell surveyed 30 rehabilitation programs in the U.S. and Canada treating 13,570 patients during the period evaluated and found the rate for all complications was 1 per 25,715 patient-hours and the fatal complication rate was 1 fatality per 116,402 patient-hours of participation.[136]

Comprehensive Rehabilitation Programs

There is now long-term information on several comprehensive Scandinavian rehabilitation intervention programs. In these studies a multidisciplinary rehabilitation team emphasized exercise, health education (advice on smoking cessation, diet, and stress reduction), and pharmacological management. Intervention included individual and group counseling with involvement of the spouses and specific informational material supplemented by audiovisual techniques. In the North Karelia Study,[73,74] 1300 patients with an acute myocardial infarction under the age of 65 participated in a special program for rehabilitation and secondary prevention from 1973 to 1977; these participants experienced a reduction in the incidence of recurrent infarction and new vocational invalidity pensions. A collaborative study from two Finnish centers assessed the effects of comprehensive rehabilitation on morbidity and mortality as well as on return to work and various other outcomes.[75] In this program, beginning 2 weeks after hospital discharge, the cumulative coronary mortality was 18.6 per cent in the intervention group and 29.4 per cent in the control group at the 3-year follow-up with differences due mainly to reduced numbers of sudden deaths following infarction. In a special clinic in Göteborg, there was a significant reduction in nonfatal reinfarction and new coronary events after 2 years of attendance.[76] New coronary rates were reduced by 50 per cent despite comparable values for initial risk factors between the intervention and reference group; total mortality was not changed significantly by intervention.

Substantial opportunities exist for secondary prevention

TABLE 40–3 SECONDARY PREVENTION WITH PHYSICAL TRAINING (PREVIOUS RANDOMIZED CONTROLLED TRIALS)

Trial	N	Intervention	Follow-up (months)	Mortality (%) Control	Mortality (%) Intervention	Effectiveness (%)*
Sweden (1968–72)	315	Supervised exercise, 3×/week	48	22.3	17.7	20.6
Finland (1969–72)	298	Supervised exercise, 2–3×/week	12	21.9	17.1	21.9
Finland (1969–72)	380	Daily home exercise	29	14.0	10.0	28.6
Canada (1972–78)	733	Partially supervised exercise, 2–4×/week	48	7.3	9.5	−30.0
United States (1974–79)	651	Supervised exercise, 3×/week	36	7.3	4.6	37.0

$$\text{*Effectiveness} = \frac{\text{control mortality} - \text{intervention mortality}}{\text{control mortality}} \times 100$$

among patients with coronary artery disease based on recent pharmacological and surgical trials.[77–80] Other promising interventions, especially exercise, require further testing in selected subgroups most likely to derive benefits from the regimen and in adequate numbers to test definitively the hypothesis that the intervention will reduce mortality.

PSYCHOSOCIAL CONCERNS

(See also Chap. 57)

During recovery, the patient and his family are forced to make a number of social and psychological adjustments. The emotional problems of the patient, from the onset of pain, through the period of hospitalization, and until he resumes ordinary activities, have been well described.[9,10,137–139] Post–myocardial infarction depression and anxiety are almost universal and can lead to permanent psychological problems unless they are anticipated and counteracted by appropriate counseling.[7] Fear of death, reinfarction, or inability to resume former living patterns is common[140] and should be amenable to rehabilitation. The patient's perception of his physical handicap is greatly influenced by his emotional state; not surprisingly, disability varies markedly at comparable levels of disease.

Impairment of personality and psychological functioning has been observed in a number of studies after open-heart surgery and specifically after coronary artery bypass procedures. Heller and coworkers[141] have reported that despite physical improvement after surgery, psychological problems remain a major barrier to rehabilitation in approximately one-third of patients. Even 1 year after operation, these patients were more passive, anxious, and depressed, and experienced increased somatic preoccupation, loss of self-esteem, and impaired sexual and marital functioning. Asymptomatic patients after operation are uncertain about their limitations and are fearful of precipitating pain, whereas those with continued symptoms or problems become discouraged and depressed. The patient's perception of his health status is probably as important as his actual functional capacity in determining the extent of disability after operation.[142]

Although the hospital setting provides an appropriate environment for motivating the patient to adapt to a healthier life style, the anxiety, fatigue, and acuteness of the situation limit educational opportunities. After the patient has left the hospital and resumed home activities, a more detailed educational program is possible. At this time explanation of the illness, the natural history of the disease, and the possibilities for long-term management should be addressed. An assortment of recent instructional materials and books can be used advantageously.[70,143–150] Involving the patient in planning for recovery, by teaching self-monitoring responses to physical activities and identifying areas in which he can make decisions for his own care, helps to encourage adherence to the medical regimen. Group discussions are especially helpful for both the patients and their families at various stages in the rehabilitation program. At all stages of convalescence, the spouse must be involved. Typically, the spouse has guilt feelings and is unable to express his or her own inadequacies in dealing with the situation; the spouse's anxiety and uncertainty may be as great as the patient's.[10,139] The spouse finds it difficult to help the patient while allowing him or her to be independent and resume activities. As a result of these conflicts and the major changes in life-long roles, marital tensions increase.

Resumption of sexual activity may be important in the marital relationship during these stressful readjustment periods. A common misconception is that sexual intercourse may be too strenuous for patients with coronary artery disease, yet the average rate of peak sexual activity is less than 120 beats/min and exertional requirements are no more than those of walking up one or two flights of stairs or taking a brisk walk for several blocks (p. 1832).[151–153] Family counseling should include discussion of life style adjustments to be anticipated during convalescence and the harm of unnecessary restriction. Although some patients profit from formal support and intervention, it is best that patients and their families assume responsibility for their rehabilitation and deal with the emotional aspects of their illness. Medical practitioners must recognize the importance of informal counseling and social support mechanisms for effecting optimal long-term recovery from cardiac disease.[154]

Early identification of those patients likely to have special psychological problems can speed recovery because few patients will express their fears or difficulties to the physician. In one controlled study, psychotherapy initiated during the hospitalization period resulted in fewer days in the intensive care unit with fewer medical and psychological problems.[155] Cay[137] has summarized the methods of treatment as informing the patient of the natural history of the disease, explaining the rationale of treatment, reassuring and encouraging him, giving practical help with concrete problems, nondirective guidance, drug therapy, and gradually increasing physical exercise. Patients and their families should be informed about community resources, including counseling services, home care agencies and services, vocational rehabilitation facilities, and coronary clubs. Group sessions allow patients to exchange information, gain social group support, express their feelings, and share common problems and solutions. Controlled studies of group psychotherapy in a variety of settings indicate its value.[156–158] Friedman and coworkers[159] found the infarction rate and cardiovascular mortality to be significantly lower in postinfarction patients who received both behavioral counseling to diminish Type A behavior and cardiological advice compared to the control subjects. Other management techniques involve medication, relaxation techniques, and follow-up counseling.[160] The marked psychological improvements may be the most striking aspect of a comprehensive rehabilitation program and may do much to restore overall performance and to enable the patient to return to as normal an active life as possible.

EMPLOYABILITY

Many consider the return to work to be *the* goal of cardiac rehabilitation. Actually, work outcomes can be viewed from several perspectives: the time required for resumption of usual work activities, current occupational activities compared with the patient's usual profession, the number of hours worked per week, or work capabilities. Currently, about 80 to 85 per cent of patients with an uncomplicated post-hospitalization course can return to their former jobs within 3 months of infarction;[8,64,161] about 65 per cent return to gainful employment post–coronary artery bypass grafting,[142] compared with an anticipated loss of 4 per cent per year in the general population in this age group.[162] Physiological improvements suffice in many instances to bring patients back to work, but other patients require additional motivation and reassurance from their physician and their families. Nonmedical factors appear paramount; the presence or absence of angina pectoris has limited impact on the percentage of patients returning to work after infarction,[163,164] although alleviation of postoperative symptoms plays a role in some studies.[142,162,164] Patients with more extensive coronary artery disease may delay their return to work, but the proportion returning to work is not substantially different from those with less disease; little correlation exists between employability and the severity or distribution of coronary artery disease.[142,165]

What does seem to be important in determining whether individuals will return to work is their ability to work *prior* to an infarction or cardiac operation. Individuals previously unemployed or retired rarely seek employment after medical treatment.[163] In fact, "doctor's advice" has been cited as another major reason for not working after myocardial infarction and coronary artery bypass grafting.[162,166] A number of factors have proved useful in determining whether a patient will return to work: employment and occupational type at admission to hospital, work history, nonwork income, availability to the previous job, perception of health, educational level, family and social stability, and psychological factors.[142,167] Cardiac rehabilitation has significantly helped in returning to employment men otherwise at high risk of remaining unemployed.[167]

In certain occupations—airplane pilots, truck drivers, and other positions where health is critical to the public welfare—resumption of previous activities is precluded. Other barriers to work rehabilitation include noncardiac disabilities, unsatisfactory work records, low occupational skills, unavailability of jobs, workmen's compensation and related legal decisions, and a variety of societal factors.[168] The misconception that myocardial infarction patients are not capable of hard physical work has led firms to reject cardiac patients from industrial positions, even though fewer than 10 per cent of occupational tasks are considered "heavy."[11] A useful publication for disability evaluation for cardiac disease is the American Medical Association's *Guide to the Evaluation of Permanent Impairment.*[169] Historically, determination of fitness to work has been established by work evaluation units. Although nonmedical factors greatly influence individual decisions on return to work, valuable information about prognosis and physical work capacity can be clarified by special evaluation techniques, especially exercise testing. If a patient exhibits no cardiovascular abnormalities under the physical stress of symptom-limited treadmill exercise testing, the probability is high that he will not encounter these abnormalities during ordinary working conditions.

DeBusk and Davidson[11] believe that short-term observation of the cardiovascular response during treadmill exercise testing is adequate to assess work potential, thus eliminating the need for simulation of the patient's occupational tasks. The job can be tailored to achievement on the exercise test using the maximal workload, heart rate, blood pressure response, and ischemic changes as guidelines for work activities. Ambulatory electrocardiograms or monitoring may be of value in special circumstances, but generally these more cumbersome methods are not necessary. The mean oxygen transport capacity for patients after a myocardial infarction ranges from 7 to 9 METS.[65,161] Such patients should be able to work easily at usual sedentary job requirements throughout the 8-hour day at an *average* level of 30 percent capacity,[24,170] or roughly 3 METS (Table 40–1). For those jobs involving strenuous activity, exertion tends to be of short duration, so that myocardial work is less than that during longer steady-state efforts. If the peak exertion required is brief, with the usual rest periods interspersed, even individuals with low physical work capacity can reach surprisingly high work levels before developing symptoms or signs of ischemia. However, both peak loads and average work requirements must be considered in evaluating work opportunities. The physician must understand the occupational requirements of patients and help them return to gainful employment.[12,162,171,172] Medical practitioners can work with employers to establish a satisfactory work environment perceived by the patients as nonthreatening to their health by recommending temporary limited-duty jobs, alternative job assignments, and job transfers that do not involve severe physiological or psychological stress.

Much remains to be done to identify and remove potential impediments to work for individuals with a standard of living or work ethic incompatible with early retirement. Delay in return to work or threatened loss of jobs poses major problems for them and society. Competition for jobs by younger individuals should be eliminated by the forthcoming shortage of younger workers during the next decade as the population ages. Such developments are likely to exaggerate the cost of failing to return to work cardiac patients capable of productive employment, as the rising cost of social services may well extend our working lifetimes past the current customary retirement age of 65.[12]

References

1. Hellerstein, H. K.: Cardiac rehabilitation: A retrospective view. *In* Pollock, M. L., and Schmidt, D. H. (eds.): Heart Disease Rehabilitation. Boston, Houghton Mifflin, 1979, pp. 509–520.
2. Kellerman, J.: Rehabilitation of patients with coronary heart disease. Prog. Cardiovasc. Dis. *17*:303, 1975.
3. Oberman, A., and Kouchoukos, N. T.: Role of exercise after coronary artery surgery. *In* Wenger, N. K. (Ed.): Exercise and the Heart. Philadelphia, F. A. Davis Co., 1978, pp. 155–172.
4. Newell, J. P., Kappagoda, C. T., Stoker, J. B., Deverall, P. B., Watson, D. A., and Linden, R. J.: Physical training after heart valve replacement. Br. Heart J. *44*:638, 1980.
5. Hassell, L. A., Fowles, R. E., and Stinson, E. B.: Patients with congestive cardiomyopathy as cardiac transplant recipients. Am. J. Cardiol. *47*:1205, 1981.
6. Arteriosclerosis 1981: Report of the Working Group on Arteriosclerosis for the National Heart, Lung, and Blood Institute, Vol. 2, June, 1981.
7. Sanne, H.: Selection of patients for cardiac rehabilitation. *In* James, W. E., and Amsterdam, E. A. (eds.): Coronary Heart Disease, Exercise Testing and Cardiac Rehabilitation. New York, Symposia Specialists, 1977, pp. 247–257.
8. Wenger, N. K., Hellerstein, H. K., and Blackburn, H.: Physician practice in the management of patients with uncomplicated myocardial infarction: Changes in the past decade. Circulation *65*:421, 1982.
9. Eliot, R. S.: Stress and the Major Cardiovascular Disorders. New York, Futura Publishing Co., 1979.
10. Croog, S. H., and Levine, S.: The Heart Patient Recovers. New York, Human Sciences Press, 1977.
11. DeBusk, R. F., and Davidson, D. M.: The work evaluation of the cardiac patient. J. Occup. Med. *22*:715, 1980.

12. Oberman, A., and Finklea, J. F.: Return to work after coronary artery bypass grafting. Ann. Thorac. Surg. *34*:353, 1982.
13. Wenger, N.: Research related to rehabilitation. Circulation *60*:1636, 1979.
14. Blomqvist, C. G., and Lewis, S. F.: Physiological effects of training: General circulatory adjustments. *In* Cohen, L. S., Mock, M. B., and Ringqvist, I. (eds.): Physical Conditioning and Cardiovascular Rehabilitation. New York, John Wiley and Sons, 1981, pp. 57–76.
15. Clausen, J. P.: Circulatory adjustments to dynamic exercise and effect of physical training in normal subjects and in patients with coronary artery disease. Prog. Cardiovasc. Dis. *18*:459, 1976.
16. Scheuer, J., and Tipton, C. M.: Cardiovascular adaptations to physical training. Ann. Rev. Physiol. *39*:221, 1977.
17. Conn, E. H., Williams, R. S., and Wallace, A. G.: Exercise responses before and after physical conditioning in patients with severely depressed left ventricular function. Am. J. Cardiol. *49*:296, 1982.
18. Report of the Task Force on Cardiovascular Rehabilitation of the National Heart and Lung Institute: Needs and Opportunities for Rehabilitating the Coronary Heart Disease Patient. Washington, D.C., DHEW Publication No. (NIH) 75–750, 1974.
19. Jonason, A., Jonzon, B., Ringqvist, I., and Omar-Rydbert, A.: Effect of physical training on different categories of patients with intermittent claudication. Acta Med. Scand. *206*:253, 1979.
20. Saltin, B.: Physical training in patients with intermittent claudication. *In* Cohen, L. S., Mock, M. B., and Ringqvist, I. (eds.): Physical Conditioning and Cardiovascular Rehabilitation. New York, John Wiley and Sons, 1981, pp. 181–196.
21. Stern, M. J., and Cleary, P.: National Exercise and Heart Disease Project: Psychosocial changes observed during a low-level exercise program. Arch. Intern. Med. *141*:1463, 1981.
22. Hackett, T. P., and Cassem, N. H.: Psychological aspects of rehabilitation after myocardial infarction factors related to exercise. *In* Wenger, N. K., and Hellerstein, H. K. (eds.): Rehabilitation of the Coronary Patient. New York, John Wiley and Sons, 1978, pp. 243–253.
23. Council on Scientific Affairs: Physician-supervised exercise programs in rehabilitation of patients with coronary heart disease. J.A.M.A. *245*:1463, 1981.
24. American Heart Association: The Exercise Standards Book. Circulation *59*:421A, 1979.
25. The Committee on Exercise: Exercise Testing and Training of Individuals with Heart Disease or at High Risk for its Development: A Handbook for Physicians. Dallas, American Heart Association, 1975.
26. American College of Sports Medicine: Guidelines for Graded Exercise Testing and Exercise Prescription. Philadelphia, Lea and Febiger, 1980.
27. Pollock, M. L., Ward, A., and Foster, C.: Exercise prescription for rehabilitation of the cardiac patient. *In* Pollock, M. L., and Schmidt, D. H. (eds.): Heart Disease Rehabilitation. Boston, Houghton Mifflin, 1979, pp. 413–445.
28. Pratt, C. M., Welton, D. E., Squires, W. G., Kirgy, T. E., Hartung, G. H., and Miller, R. R.: Demonstration of training effect during chronic beta-adrenergic blockade in patients with coronary artery disease. Circulation *64*:1125, 1981.
29. Vanhees, L., Fagard, R., and Amery, A.: Influence of beta adrenergic blockage on effects of physical training in patients with ischaemic heart disease. Br. Heart J. *48*:33, 1982.
30. Myocardial infarction, exercise and prognosis. Lancet *1*:78, 1980.
31. Hung, J., McKillip, J., Savin, W., Magder, S., Kraus, R., Houston, N., Goris, M., Haskell, W., and DeBusk, R.: Comparison of cardiovascular response to combined static-dynamic effort, postprandial dynamic effort and dynamic effort alone in patients with chronic ischemic heart disease. Circulation *65*:1411, 1982.
32. Viitasalo, M. T., Kala, R., Eisalo, A., and Halonen, A.: Ventricular arrhythmias during exercise testing, jogging, and sedentary life. Chest *76*:21, 1979.
33. McKinnis, R. A., Burks, H., Lee, K. L., Harrell, F. E., Behar, V. S., Pryor, V. S., Pryor, D. B., Wagner, G. S., and Rosati, R. A.: Prognostic implications of ventricular arrhythmias during 24 hour ambulatory monitoring in patients undergoing cardiac catheterization for coronary artery disease. Am. J. Cardiol. *50*:23, 1982.
34. Simoons, M., Lap, C., and Pool, J.: Heart rate levels and ventricular ectopic activity during cardiac rehabilitation. Am. Heart J. *100*:9, 1980.
35. Winkle, R. A.: The relationship between ventricular ectopic beat frequency and heart rate. Circulation *66*:439, 1982.
36. Borg, G. A.: Psychophysical bases of perceived exertion. Med. Sci. Sports Exercise *14*:377, 1982.
37. Wilson, P. K., Fardy, P. S., and Froelicher, V. F.: Cardiac Rehabilitation, Adult Fitness, and Exercise Testing. Philadelphia, Lea and Febiger, 1981, pp. 333–351.
38. Hellerstein, H. K., and Franklin, B. A.: Exercise testing and prescription. *In* Wenger, N. K., and Hellerstein, H. K. (eds.): Rehabilitation of the Coronary Patient. New York, John Wiley and Sons, 1978, pp. 149–202.
39. Haskell, W. L.: Design and implementation of cardiac conditioning programs. *In* Wenger, N. K., and Hellerstein, H. K. (eds.): Rehabilitation of the Coronary Patient. New York, John Wiley and Sons, 1978, pp. 203–241.
40. Fox, S. M., Naughton, J. P., and Gorman, P. A.: Physical activity and cardiovascular health: III. The exercise prescription: frequency and type of activity. Mod. Concepts Cardiovasc. Dis. *41*:25, 1972.
41. Magder, S., Linnarsson, D., and Gullstrand, L.: The effect of swimming on patients with ischemic heart disease. Circulation *63*:979, 1981.
42. Fletcher, G. F., Cantwell, J. D., and Watt, E. W.: Oxygen consumption and hemodynamic response of exercises used in training of patients with recent myocardial infarction. Circulation *60*:140, 1979.
43. Ferguson, R. J., Cote, P., Bourassa, M. G., and Corbara, F.: Coronary blood flow during isometric and dynamic exercise in angina pectoris patients. J. Cardiac Rehabil. *1*:21, 1981.
44. Harrison, T. R.: Abuse of rest as a therapeutic measure for patients with cardiovascular disease. J.A.M.A. *125*:1075, 1944.
45. Levine, S. A., and Lown, B.: "Armchair" treatment of acute coronary thrombosis. J.A.M.A. *148*:1365, 1952.
46. Harpur, J., Kellett, R. J., Conner, W. T., Galbraith, H. J. B., Hamilton, M., Murray, J. J., Swallow, J. H., and Rose, G. A.: Controlled trial of early mobilization and discharge from hospital in uncomplicated myocardial infarction. Lancet *2*:1331, 1971.
47. Lamers, H. J., Drost, W. S. J., Kroon, B. J. M., van Es, L. A., Meilink-Holdemaker, L. J., and Birkenhager, L. H.: Early mobilization after myocardial infarction.: A controlled study. Br. Med. J. *1*:277, 1973.
48. Boyle, J. A., and Lorimer, A. R.: Early mobilisation after uncomplicated myocardial infarction. Prospective study of 538 patients. Lancet *2*:346, 1973.
49. Hayes, M. J., Morris, G. K., and Hampton, J. R.: Comparison of mobilization after two and nine days in uncomplicated myocardial infarction. Br. Med. J. *3*:10, 1974.
50. Thornley, P. E., and Turner, R. W. D.: Rapid mobilisation after acute myocardial infarction; first step in rehabilitation and secondary prevention. Br. Heart J. *39*:471, 1977.
51. Lindvall, K., Erhardt, L. R., Lundman, T., Rehnqvist, N., and Sjögren, A.: Early mobilization and discharge of patients with acute myocardial infarction. A prospective study using risk indicators and early exercise tests. Acta Med. Scand. *206*:169, 1979.
52. West, R. R., and Henderson, A. H.: Randomized multicentre trial of early mobilisation after uncomplicated myocardial infarction. Br. Heart J. *42*:381, 1979.
53. Block, A., Maeder, J. P., Haissly, J. C., Felix, J., and Blackburn, H.: Early mobilization after myocardial infarction: A controlled study. Am. J. Cardiol. *34*:152, 1974.
54. Silvidi, G. E., Squires, R. W., Pollock, M. L., and Foster, C.: Hemodynamic responses and medical problems associated with early exercise and ambulation in coronary artery bypass graft surgery patients. J. Cardiac Rehab. *2*:355–362, 1982.
55. Baker, J. T., Bramlet, D. A., Lester, R. M., Harrison, D. G., Roe, C. R., and Cobb, F. R.: Myocardial infarct extension: Incidence and relationship to survival. Circulation *65*:918, 1982.
56. Wenger, N. K.: Rehabilitation of the coronary patient: Scope of the problem and responsibility of the primary care physician. Cardiovasc. Rev. Rep. *12*: 1249, 1981.
57. Sivarajan, E. S., Bruce, R. A., Almes, M. J., Green, B., Belanger, L., Lindskog, B. D., Newton, K. M., and Mansfield, L. W.: In-hospital exercise after myocardial infarction does not improve treadmill performance. N. Engl. J. Med. *305*:358, 1981.
58. DeBusk, R. F., Houston, N., Haskell, W., Fry, G., and Parker, M.: Exercise training soon after myocardial infarction. Am. J. Cardiol. *44*:1225, 1979.
59. Vaisrub, S.: Editorial: Exercise tests after myocardial infarction. J.A.M.A. *243*:261, 1980.
60. Jelinek, M. V., Ziffer, R. W., McDonald, D. G., Wasir, H., and Hale, S. G.: Early exercise testing and mobilization after myocardial infarction. Med. J. Aust. *29*:589, 1977.
61. Theroux, P., Waters, D. D., Halphen, C., Debaisieux, J. C., and Mizgala, H. F.: Prognostic value of exercise testing soon after myocardial infarction. N. Engl. J. Med. *301*:341, 1979.
61a. Ewart C. K., Taylor, B., Reese, L., and DeBusk, R. F.: Effects of early postinfarction exercise testing on self perception and subsequent physical activity. J. Am. Coll. Cardiol. *1*:662, 1983.
62. Bruce, R. A.: Exercise tests. *In* Cohen, L. S., Mock, M. B., and Ringqvist, I., (eds.): Physician Conditioning and Cardiovascular Rehabilitation. New York, John Wiley and Sons, 1981, pp. 3–22.
62a. Ewart, C. K., Taylor, C. B., Reese, L. B., and DeBusk, R. F.: Effects of early postmyocardial infarction exercise testing on self-perception and subsequent physical activity. Am. J. Cardiol. *51*:1076, 1983.
63. Hung, J., Criley, J. M., and Corne, R. A.: Effects of bedrest and deconditioning on exercise ventricular function in middle-aged men. American College of Cardiology Extended Learning Tape, Vol. 13, No. 11, November, 1981.
64. Acker, J. E., Jr.: Medical benefits and concerns in cardiac rehabilitation. *In* Pollock, M. L., and Schmidt, D. H. (eds.): Heart Disease and Rehabilitation. Boston, Houghton Mifflin Professional Publishers, 1979, pp. 654–662.
65. Naughton, J.: The National Exercise and Heart Disease Project: Development, Recruitment, and Implementation. *In* Wenger, N. K. (ed.): Exercise and the Heart. Philadelphia, F. A. Davis Co., 1978.
66. Williams, R. S., Miller, H., Koisch, F. P., Ribisl, P. and Graden, H.: Guidelines for unsupervised exercise in patients with ischemic heart disease. J. Cardiac Rehabil. *1*:213, 1981.
67. Pyfer, H. R.: Guidelines for unsupervised exercise in patients with ischemic heart disease, Commentary 1. J. Cardiac Rehabil. *1*:217, 1981.
68. Oberman, A.: Guidelines for unsupervised exercise in patients with ischemic heart disease, Commentary 2. J. Cardiac Rehabil. *1*:218, 1981.

69. Kavanagh, T., and Shephard, R. J.: Exercise for postcoronary patients: An assessment of infrequent supervision. Arch. Phys. Med. Rehabil. *61*:114, 1980.
70. Oberman, A.: Cardiac rehabilitation, key references. Circulation *62*:909, 1980.
71. Kannel, W. B.: Prospects for risk factor modification to reduce risk of reinfarction and premature death. J. Cardiac Rehabil. *1*:63, 1982.
72. May, G. S., Eberlein, K. A., Furberg, C. D., Passamani, E. R., and DeMets, D. L.: Secondary prevention after myocardial infarction: A review of long-term trials. Prog. Cardiovasc. Dis. *24*:331, 1982.
73. Salonen, J. T., and Puska, P.: A community programme for rehabilitation and secondary prevention for patients with acute myocardial infarction as part of a comprehensive community programme for control of cardiovascular disease (North Karelia Project). Scand. J. Rehabil. Med. *12*:33, 1980.
74. Puska, P., Tuomilehto, J., Salonen, J. T., et al.: Community control of cardiovascular disease: Evaluation of a comprehensive community programme for control of cardiovascular diseases in 1972–77 in North Karelia, Finland. Geneva, WHO Monograph Series, 1981.
75. Kallio, V., Hamalainen, H., Hakkila, J., and Luurila, O. J.: Reduction in sudden deaths by a multifactorial intervention programme after acute myocardial infarction. Lancet *2*:1091, 1979.
76. Vedin, A., Wilhemsson, C., Tibblin, G., and Wilhelmsen, L.: The post-infarction clinic in Göteborg, Sweden. A controlled trial of a therapeutic organization. Acta Med. Scand. *200*:453, 1976.
76a. Vermeulen, A., Lie, K. I., and Durrer, D.: Effects of cardiac rehabilitation after myocardial infarction: Changes in coronary risk factors and long-term prognosis. Am. Heart J. *105*:798, 1983.
77. The Norwegian Multicenter Study Group: Timolol-induced reduction in mortality and reinfarction in patients surviving acute myocardial infarction. N. Engl. J. Med. *304*:801, 1981.
77a. Hansteen, V.: Beta blockade after myocardial infarction: The Norwegian propranolol study in high-risk patients. Circulation *67* (Suppl. 1):57, 1983.
77b. Goldstein, S.: Propranolol therapy in patients with acute myocardial infarction: The beta-blocker heart attack trial. Circulation *67* (Suppl. 1):53, 1983.
77c. Turi, Z. G., and Braunwald, E.: The use of beta blockers after myocardial infarction. JAMA *249*:2512, 1983.
77d. Furberg, C. D., Friedewald, W. T., and Eberlein, K. A. (eds.): Proceedings of the workshop on implications of recent beta-blocker trials for post-myocardial infarction patients. Circulation *67*:1–111, 1983.
78. β-Blocker Heart Attack Trial Research Group: A randomized trial of propranolol in patients with acute myocardial infarction. I. Mortality Results. J.A.M.A. *247*:1707, 1982.
79. National Institutes Of Health Consensus Development Conference Statement on Coronary Bypass Surgery. Scientific and Clinical Aspects. Circulation *65* (Suppl. II):126, 1982.
80. Rahimtoola, S. H.: Coronary bypass surgery for chronic angina—1981: a perspective. Circulation *65*:225, 1982.
81. Ross, J. K., Monro, J. L., Diwell, A. E., Mackean, J. M., Marsh, J., and Barjer, D. H. P.: The quality of life after cardiac surgery. Br. Med. J. *282*:451, 1981.
82. Kannel, W. B., Doyle, J. T., and Ostfeld, A. M.: American Heart Association Committee Report: Risk factors and coronary disease. Circulation *62*:449A, 1980.
83. Oberman, A.: Natural history of coronary artery disease. *In* Racklay, C. E., and Russell, R. O. (eds.): Coronary Artery Disease: Recognition and Management. New York, Futura Publishing Co., 1979, pp. 1–30.
84. Schlant, R. C., Forman, S., Stamler, J., and Canner, P. L.: The natural history of coronary heart disease: Prognostic factors after recovery from myocardial infarction in 2789 men. The five-year findings of the Coronary Drug Project. Circulation *66*:401, 1982.
85. Castelli, W. P., Dawber, T. R., Feinleib, M., Garrison, R. J., McNamara, P. M., and Kannel, W. B.: The filter cigarette and coronary heart disease: The Framingham Study. Lancet *2*:109, 1981.
86. Vliestra, R. E., Kronmal, R. A., and Oberman, A.: Stopping smoking improves survival in patients with angiographically proven coronary artery disease (Abstr.). Am. J. Cardiol. *49*:984, 1982.
87. Ashley, F. W., Jr., and Kannel, W. B.: Relation of weight change to changes in atherogenic traits: The Framingham Study. J. Chron. Dis. *27*:103, 1974.
88. Castelli, W. P., Doyle, J. T., Gordon, T., Hames, C. G., Hjortland, M. C., Hulley, S. B., Kagan, A., and Zukel, W. J.: HDL-cholesterol and other lipids in coronary heart disease. The cooperative lipoprotein phenotyping study. Circulation *55*:767, 1977.
89. Joint Recommendations by the International Society and Federation of Cardiology Scientific Councils on Arteriosclerosis, Epidemiology and Prevention, and Rehabilitation. Br. Med. J. *282*:894, 1981.
90. Rationale of the diet-heart statement of the American Heart Association: Report of the AHA Nutrition Committee. Arteriosclerosis *4*:177, 1982.
91. Oliver, M. F.: Serum cholesterol—the knave of hearts and the joker. Lancet *2*:1090, 1981.
92. Hypertension Detection and Follow-Up Cooperative Group: Five-year findings of the Hypertension Detection and Follow-Up Program: I. Reduction in mortality of persons with high blood pressure, including mild hypertension. J.A.M.A. *242*:2562, 1979.
93. Bukley, B. H., and Hutchins, G. M.: Accelerated "atherosclerosis": A morphologic study of 97 saphenous vein coronary artery bypass grafts. Circulation *55*:163, 1977.
94. Hartung, G. H., Squires, W. G., and Gotto, A. M.: Effect of exercise training on plasma high-density lipoprotein cholesterol in coronary disease patients. Am. Heart J. *101*:181, 1981.
95. Bjorntorp, P., Berchtold, P., Grimby, G., Lindholm, B., Sanne, H., Tibblin, G., and Wilhelmsen, L.: Effects of physical training on glucose tolerance, plasma insulin after lipids and on body composition in men after myocardial infarction. Acta Med. Scand. *192*:439, 1972.
96. Fletcher, G. F., and Cantwell, J. D.: Exercise and Coronary Heart Disease. Springfield, Ill., Charles C Thomas, 1974, pp. 31–45.
97. Ballantyne, F. C., Clark, R. S., Simpson, H. S., and Ballantyne, D.: The effect of modern physical exercise on the plasma lipoprotein subfractions of male survivors of myocardial infarction. Circulation *65*:913, 1982.
98. Berg, A., Keul, J., Ringwald, G., Stippig, J., and Deus, B.: Serum lipoprotein cholesterol in sedentary and trained male patients with coronary heart disease. Clin. Cardiol. *4*:233, 1981.
99. Haskell, W. L.: Influence of habitual physical activity on blood lipids and lipoproteins. *In* Cohen, L. S., Mock, M. B., and Ringqvist, I. (eds.): Physical Conditioning and Cardiovascular Rehabilitation. New York, John Wiley and Sons, 1981, pp. 87–102.
100. Pedersen, O., Beck-Nielsen, H., and Heding, L.: Increased insulin receptors after exercise in patients with insulin-dependent diabetes mellitus. N. Engl. J. Med. *302*:886, 1980.
101. Haskell, W. L.: Mechanisms by which physical activity may enhance the clinical status of cardiac patients. *In* Pollock, M. L., and Schmidt, D. (eds.): Heart Disease and Rehabilitation. Boston, Mass., Houghton Mifflin Professional Publishers, 1979, pp. 276–296.
102. Stern, M. J., and Cleary, P.: Long-term psychosocial outcome. Arch. Intern. Med. *152*:1093, 1982.
103. Blumenthal, J. A., Williams, S., Williams, R. B., and Wallace, A. G.: Effects of exercise on the type A (coronary prone) behavior pattern. Psychosom. Med. *42*:289, 1980.
104. Epstein, S. E., Rosing, D. R., and Brakman, P.: Impaired fibrinolytic response to exercise in patients with type IV hyperlipoproteinemia. Lancet *2*:631, 1970.
105. Williams, R. S., Logue, E. E., and Lewis, J. L.: Physical conditioning augments the fibrinolytic response to venous occlusion in healthy adults. N. Engl. J. Med. *302*:987, 1980.
106. Fox, S. M., Naughton, J. P., and Gorman, P. A.: Physical activity and cardiovascular health (Part I). Mod. Concepts Cardiovasc. Dis. *41*:17, 1972.
107. Oberman, A., Cleary, P., LaRosa, J. C., Hellerstein, H. K., and Naughton, J.: Changes in risk factors among long-term exercise rehabilitation program participants. Adv. Cardiol. *31*, 1983.
108. Shephard, R. J.: Cardiac rehabilitation in prospect. *In* Pollock, M. L., and Schmidt, D. H. (eds.): Heart Disease and Rehabilitation. Boston, Houghton Mifflin Professional Publishers, 1979, pp. 521–547.
109. Williams, P. T., Wood, P. D., Haskell, W. L., and Vranizan, K.: The effect of running mileage and duration on plasma lipoprotein levels. J.A.M.A. *247*:2674, 1982.
110. Redwood, D. R., Rosing, D. R., and Epstein, S. E.: Circulatory and symptomatic effects of physical training in patients with coronary-artery disease and angina pectoris. N. Engl. J. Med. *286*:959, 1972.
111. Dressendorfer, R. H., and Scaff, J. H.: Cardiorespiratory responses to marathon running in cardiac patients. Med. Sci. Sports *7*:71, 1975.
112. Kavanagh, T., Shephard, R. H., and Pandit, V.: Marathon running after myocardial infarction. J.A.M.A. *229*:1602, 1974.
113. Kavanagh, T., Shephard, R. J., and Kennedy, J.: Characteristics of postcoronary marathon runners. *In* Milvy, P. (ed.): The Marathon: Physiological, Medical, Epidemiological, and Psychological Studies. New York, New York Academy of Sciences, 1977, pp. 455–515.
114. Gobel, F. L., Nordstrom, L. A., Nelson, R. R., Jorgensen, C. R., and Wang, Y.: The rate-pressure product as an index of myocardial oxygen consumption during exercise in patients with angina pectoris. Circulation *57*:549, 1978.
115. Ehsani, A. A., Heath, G. W., Hagberg, J. M., Sobel, B. E., and Holloszy, J. O.: Effects of 12 months of intense exercise training on ischemic ST-segment depression in patients with coronary artery disease. Circulation *64*:1116, 1981.
116. Sim, D. N., and Neill, W. A.: Investigation of the physiological basis for increased exercise threshold for angina pectoris after physical conditioning. J. Clin. Invest. *54*:763, 1974.
117. Detry, J. M., and Bruce, R. A.: Effects of physical training on exertional ST segment depression in coronary heart disease. Circulation *44*:390, 1971.
118. Ehsani, A. A., Martin, W. H., Heath, G., and Coyle, E. F.: Cardiac effects of prolonged and intense exercise training in patients with coronary artery disease. Am. J. Cardiol. *50*:246, 1982.
119. Paterson, D. H., Shephard, R. J., Cunningham, D., Jones, N. L., and Andrew, G.: Effects of physical training on cardiovascular function following myocardial infarction. J. Appl. Physiol. *47*:482, 1979.
120. Cobb, F. R., Williams, R. S., McEwan, P., Jones, R. H., Coleman, R. E., and Wallace, A. G.: Effects of exercise training on ventricular function in patients with recent myocardial infarction. Circulation *66*:100, 1982.
121. DeMaria, A. N., Neumann, A., Lee, G., Fowler, W., and Mason, D. T.: Alterations in ventricular mass and performance induced by exercise training in man evaluated by echocardiography. Circulation *57*:237, 1978.
122. Jensen, D., Atwood, J. E., Froelicher, V., McKirnam, M. D., Battler, A., Ashburn, W., and Ross, J.: Improvement in ventricular function during exercise studied with radionuclide ventriculography after cardiac rehabilitation. Am. J. Cardiol. *46*:770, 1980.
123. Holloszy, J. O., Skinner, J. S., Barry, A. J., et al.: Effect of physical condition-

ing on cardiovascular function—a ballistocardiographic study. Am. J. Cardiol. *14*:761, 1964.
124. Froelicher, V. F., and Brown, P.: Exercise and coronary heart disease. J. Cardiac Rehabil. *1*:277, 1981.
125. Epstein, L., Miller, G. J., Stitt, F. W., and Morris, J. N.: Vigorous exercise in leisure time, coronary risk factors, and resting electrocardiogram in middle-aged male civil servants. Br. Heart J. *38*:403, 1976.
126. Scheuer, J.: Effects of physical training on myocardial vascularity and perfusion. Circulation *66*:491, 1982.
127. Kramsch, D. M., Aspen, A. J., Abramowitz, B. M., Kreimendahl, T., and Hood, W. B.: Reduction of coronary atherosclerosis by moderate conditioning exercise in monkeys on an atherogenic diet. N. Engl. J. Med. *305*:1483, 1981.
128. Kennedy, C. C., Spiekerman, R. E., Lindsay, M. I., et al.: One-year graduated exercise program for men with angina pectoris. Mayo Clin. Proc. *51*:231, 1976.
129. Ferguson, R. J., Petitclerc, R., Choquette, G., et al.: Effect of physical training on treadmill exercise capacity, collateral circulation and progression of coronary disease. Am. J. Cardiol. *134*:764, 1974.
130. Nolewajka, A. J., Kostuk, W. J., Rechnitzer, P. A., and Cunningham, D. A.: Exercise and human collateralization: An angiographic scintigraphic assessment. Circulation *60*:114, 1979.
131. Wilhelmsen, L., Sanne, H., Elmfeldt, D., Grimby, G., Tibblin, G., and Wedel, H.: A controlled trial of physical training after myocardial infarction. Prev. Med. *4*:491, 1975.
132. Kentala, E.: Physical fitness and feasibility of physical rehabilitation after myocardial infarction in men of working age. Ann. Clin. Res. *4*(Suppl. 9):1, 1972.
133. Palatsi, I.: Feasibility of physical training after myocardial infarction and its effect on return to work, morbidity and mortality. Acta Med. Scand. (Suppl.):599, 1976.
134. Shephard, R. J.: Evaluation of earlier studies: Canada. *In* Cohen, L. S., Mock, M. B., and Ringqvist, I. (eds.): Physical Conditioning and Cardiovascular Rehabilitation. New York, John Wiley and Sons, 1981, pp. 271–288.
135. Shaw, L. W.: Effects of a prescribed supervised exercise program on mortality and cardiovascular morbidity in patients after a myocardial infarction. Am. J. Cardiol. *48*:39, 1981.
136. Haskell, W. L.: Cardiovascular complications during exercise training of cardiac patients. Circulation *57*:920, 1974.
137. Cay, E. L.: Psychological approach in patient after a myocardial infarction. Adv. Cardiol. *24*:120, 1978.
138. Stern, M. J., and Pascale, L.: Psychosocial adaptation post myocardial infarction: The spouse's dilemma. J. Psychosom. Res. *23*:83, 1979.
139. Davidson, D. M.: The family and cardiac rehabilitation. J. Fam. Pract. *8*:253, 1979.
140. International Society of Cardiology, Scientific Council on Rehabilitation of Cardiac Patients: Myocardial Infarction: How to Prevent, How to Rehabilitate, Mannheim, West Germany, Boehringer, 1973.
141. Heller, S. S., Frank, K. A., Kornfeld, D. S., et al.: Psychological outcome following open-heart surgery. Arch. Intern. Med. *5*:67, 1974.
142. Oberman, A., Wayne, J. B., Kouchoukos, N. T., Charles, E. D., Russell, R. O., and Rogers, W. J.: Employment status after coronary artery bypass surgery. Circulation *65*(Suppl. II):115, 1982.
143. Alpert, J. S.: The Heart Attack Handbook: A Common Sense Guide to Treatment, Recovery and Prevention. Boston, Little Brown and Co., 1978.
144. Farquhar, J. W.: The American Way of Life Need Not be Hazardous to Your Health. New York, W. W. Norton, 1978.
145. Halhuber, M. J.: Health education in cardiac rehabilitation. Adv. Cardiol. *24*:146, 1978.
146. Brammell, H. L., McDaniel, J. W., Niccoli, S. A., Darnell, R., and Roberson, D. R.: Cardiac Rehabilitation: A Handbook for Vocational Rehabilitation Counselors. Denver, University of Colorado Medical Center, Webb-Waring Lung Institute, 1979.
147. Cohn, K., Duke, D., and Madrid, J. A.: Coming Back: A guide to recovering from heart attack and living confidently with coronary disease. Reading, Mass., Addison-Wesley Publishing Co., 1979.
148. Zohman, L. R., Kattus, A. A., and Softness, D. G.: The Cardiologists' Guide to Fitness and Health Through Exercise. New York, Simon and Schuster, 1979.
149. American Medical Association: Book of Heart Care. New York, Random House, 1982.
150. An Active Partnership for the Health of Your Heart. Audiovisual modules. Santa Clara, Cal., American Heart Association, 1976.
151. Kavanagh, T., and Shephard, R. J.: Sexual activity after myocardial infarction. Can. Med. Assoc. J. *116*:1250, 1977.
152. Hellerstein, H. K., and Friedman, E. H.: Sexual activity and the postcoronary patient. Med. Aspects Hum. Sex. *3*:70, 1973.
153. McLane, M., Krop, H., and Mehta, J.: Psychosexual adjustment and counseling after myocardial infarction. Ann. Intern. Med. *92*:514, 1980.
154. Smith, R. T.: The role of social resources in cardiac rehabilitation. *In* Cohen, L. S., Mock, M. B., Ringqvist, I. (eds.): Physical Conditioning and Cardiovascular Rehabilitation. New York, John Wiley and Sons, 1981, pp. 221–232.
155. Gruen, W.: Effects of brief psychotherapy during the hospitalization period on the recovery process in heart attacks. J. Consult. Clin. Psychol. *43*:223, 1975.
156. Hackett, T. P.: The use of groups in the rehabilitation of the postcoronary patient. Adv. Cardiol. *24*:127, 1978.
157. Munford, E., Schlesinger, H. J., and Glass, G. V.: The effects of psychological intervention on recovery from surgery and heart attacks: An analysis of the literature. Am. J. Pub. Health *72*:141, 1982.
158. Rahe, R. H., Ward, H. W., and Hayes, V.: Brief group therapy in myocardial infarction rehabilitation; three- to four-year follow-up of a controlled trial. Psychosom. Med. *41*:229, 1979.
159. Friedman, M., Thoresen, C. E., Gill, J. J., Ulmer, D., Thompson, L., Powell, L., Price, V., Elek, S. R., Rabin, D. D., Breall, W. S., Piaget, G., Dixon, T., Bourg, E., Levy, R. A., and Tasto, D. L.: Feasibility of altering type A behavior pattern after myocardial infarction. Circulation *66*:83, 1982.
160. Hackett, T. P., and Rosenbaum, J. F.: Emotion, psychiatric disorders, and the heart. *In* Braunwald, E. (ed.): Heart Disease: A Textbook of Cardiovascular Medicine. Philadelphia, W. B. Saunders Co., 1984, pp. 1826–1844.
161. Muir, J. R.: The rehabilitation of cardiac patients. Proc. R. Soc. Med. *70*:655, 1977.
162. Johnson, W. D., Kayser, K. L., Pedraza, P. M., and Shore, R. T.: Employment patterns in males before and after myocardial revascularization surgery. A study of 229 consecutive male patients followed for as long as 10 years. Circulation *65*:1086, 1982.
163. Davidson, D. M., Taylor, C. B., and DeBusk, R. F.: Factors influencing return to work after myocardial infarction or coronary artery bypass surgery. J. Cardiac Rehabil. *10*:1, 1979.
164. Guvendik, L., Rahan, M., and Yacoub, M.: Symptomatic status and pattern of employment during a five year period following myocardial revascularization for angina. Ann. Thorac. Surg. *34*:383, 1982.
165. Nitter-Hauge, S., Noreik, K., Simonsen, S., Storstein, O., Bjorbaek, T., and Steen, A.: Studies of correlation between progression of coronary artery disease, as assessed by coronary arteriography, left ventricular end-diastolic pressure, ejection fraction, and employability. Br. Heart J. *39*:884, 1977.
166. Oberman, A., and Kouchoukos, N.: Working status of patients following coronary bypass surgery. Am. Heart J. *98*:132, 1979.
167. Schiller, E., and Baker, J.: Return to work after a myocardial infarction; evaluation of planned rehabilitation and of a predictive rating scale. Med. J. Austr. *1*:859, 1976.
168. American Heart Association: Report of the Committee on Stress, Strain and Heart Disease. Dallas, Texas, News from the AHA, 825A–835A, 1976.
169. American Medical Association, Committee on Rating of Mental and Physical Impairment: Guides to the evaluation of permanent impairment. Monroe, Wisconsin, 1977.
170. Astrand, P. O., and Rodahl, K.: Textbook of Work Physiology: Physiological Bases of Exercise. 2nd ed. New York, McGraw-Hill Book Co., 1977.
171. Liddle, H. V., Jenson, R., and Clayton, P. D.: The rehabilitation of coronary surgical patients. Ann. Thorac. Surg. *34*:374, 1982.
172. Horgan, J. H., Teo, K. K., Murren, K. M., and O'Riodan, J. M.: The response to exercise training and vocational counseling in post myocardial infarction and coronary artery bypass surgery patients. Ir. Med. J. *73*:444, 1980.

41

THE CARDIOMYOPATHIES AND MYOCARDITIDES

by Joshua Wynne, M.D., and Eugene Braunwald, M.D.

CLASSIFICATION

The cardiomyopathies are diseases involving the heart muscle itself.[1–3] They are unique in that they are not the result of ischemic,* hypertensive, congenital, valvular, or pericardial diseases (Table 41–1). While exclusion of these etiological factors is necessary for the diagnosis of cardiomyopathy, this form of heart disease is often sufficiently distinctive—both clinically and hemodynamically—to allow a positive diagnosis to be made.[4] With increasing awareness of this condition by clinicians, along with improvements in diagnostic techniques, cardiomyopathy is being recognized as a major cause of morbidity and mortality. In some areas of the world, it accounts for 30 per cent or more of all deaths due to heart disease.[5]

A variety of schemes have been proposed for classifying the cardiomyopathies.[2,3,5–8] Most useful from a clinical standpoint is a *functional* classification that emphasizes common pathophysiological abnormalities. Three basic categories of functional impairment have been described (Table 41–2): (1) *dilated* (formerly called congestive), characterized by ventricular dilatation, contractile dysfunction, and often symptoms of congestive heart failure; (2) *hypertrophic*, recognized by inappropriate left ventricular hypertrophy, often with asymmetrical involvement of the septum, with preserved or enhanced contractile function; and (3) *restrictive*, marked by endocardial scarring of the ventricle, with impairment of diastolic filling. The distinctions between these three functional categories are not absolute, and there is often overlap; in particular, patients with hypertrophic cardiomyopathy also have increased wall stiffness (as a consequence of the myocardial hypertrophy) and thus present some of the features of a restrictive cardiomyopathy.[9] Table 41–3 shows the echocardiographic characteristics of the three types of cardiomyopathies. We believe it is useful to divide the cardiomyopathies into primary and secondary forms. *Primary cardiomyopathies* are conditions in which: (1) the basic pathological process involves the myocardium rather than the valves or other cardiac structures, and (2) the cause of the heart disease is unknown and not part of a disorder affecting other organs. *Secondary cardiomyopathies* are conditions in which the cause of the myocardial abnormality is known or in which the cardiomyopathy is one manifestation of a systemic disease process, such as sarcoid.

ENDOMYOCARDIAL BIOPSY. Evaluation of the patient suspected of suffering from a cardiomyopathy has been facilitated by the use of endomyocardial biopsy (p. 297). Using a flexible bioptome, the clinician may obtain a tissue sample from the right or left ventricle via a transvenous or transarterial approach. Endomyocardial biopsy results in a small tissue sample (average size <1 mm^3),[10] and five or more biopsies are often required to be certain of a given histological finding, since pronounced topographic variations may be found within the myocardium.[11] It remains controversial as to which patients with cardiomyopathy should be subjected to biopsy, but there is general agreement that biopsy may be of benefit in certain specific situations (Table 41–4). Although on occasion endomyocardial biopsy may identify a specific etiological agent in an individual patient with cardiac disease of uncertain cause (Table 41–5 and Fig. 41–1), the clinical utility of routine biopsy in cardiomyopathy remains uncertain.[10,11] While diagnostic abnormalities may be detected in the hypertrophic and restrictive cardiomyopathies, no definitive pattern has been found in dilated cardiomyopathy.[10]

DILATED CARDIOMYOPATHY

IDIOPATHIC DILATED CARDIOMYOPATHY

Dilated cardiomyopathy is a syndrome characterized by cardiac enlargement and often by the development of congestive heart failure. Formerly called congestive cardiomyopathy, the term *dilated cardiomyopathy* is now preferred, since the earliest abnormality is ventricular enlargement and systolic contractile dysfunction, with congestive heart failure often (but not invariably) developing later. It is characterized principally by impaired systolic pump function,[9,12] and both the end-diastolic and end-systolic volumes are increased. Ventricular wall thickness may be normal, increased, or decreased, and left ventricular filling pressure is usually elevated as a consequence of the poorly contractile left ventricle,[13] although decreased left ventricular compliance may contribute to the elevated filling pressures.[14]

Although the etiology is not definable in many cases, the dilated cardiomyopathies probably represent a final common pathway that is the end result of myocardial damage produced by a variety of toxic, metabolic, or infectious agents.[12,13] Alcohol, for example, may lead to severe

*The term *ischemic cardiomyopathy* refers to the condition in which ischemic heart disease causes diffuse fibrosis or multiple infarctions and leads to heart failure with left ventricular dilatation; it may or may not be associated with angina pectoris (p. 1363).

TABLE 41–1 IMPORTANT CAUSES OF CARDIOMYOPATHY AND MYOCARDITIS

1. Inflammatory
   a. Infective
      Viral
      Rickettsial
      Bacterial
      Mycobacterial
      Spirochetal
      Fungal
      Parasitic
   b. Noninfective
      Collagen diseases
2. Metabolic
   a. Nutritional
      Thiamine
      Kwashiorkor
      Pellagra
      Scurvy
      Hypervitaminosis D
      Obesity
   b. Endocrine
      Acromegaly
      Thyrotoxicosis
      Myxedema
      Uremia
      Cushing's disease
      Pheochromocytoma
      Diabetes mellitus
   c. Altered metabolism
      Gout
      Oxalosis
      Porphyria
   d. Electrolyte imbalance
3. Toxic
   a. Cobalt
   b. Alcohol
   c. Bleomycin
   d. Adriamycin
   e. Phenothiazines
   f. Antimony compounds
   g. Carbon monoxide
   h. Lead
   i. Emetine and dehydroemetine
   j. Chloroquine
   k. Lithium
   l. Cyclophosphamide
   m. Hydrocarbons
   n. Catecholamines
   o. Phosphorus
   p. Mercury
   q. Insect stings
   r. Snake bites
   s. Paracetamol
   t. Reserpine
   u. Corticosteroids
4. Infiltrative
   a. Amyloidosis
   b. Hemochromatosis
   c. Neoplastic
   d. Glycogen storage disorders
   e. Sarcoidosis
   f. Mucopolysaccharidosis
   g. Fabry's disease
   h. Whipple's disease
   i. Gaucher's disease
5. Fibroplastic
   a. Endomyocardial fibrosis
   b. Endocardial fibroelastosis
   c. Löffler's fibroplastic endocarditis
   d. Becker's disease
   e. Carcinoid
6. Hematological
   a. Sickle cell anemia
   b. Polycythemia vera
   c. Thrombotic thrombocytopenic purpura
   d. Leukemia
7. Hypersensitivity
   a. Methyldopa
   b. Penicillin
   c. Sulfonamides
   d. Tetracycline
   e. Phenindione
   f. Phenylbutazone
   g. Antituberculous drugs
   h. Giant cell myocarditis
   i. Cardiac transplant rejection
8. Genetic
   a. Hypertrophic cardiomyopathy
      With gradient
      Without gradient
   b. Neuromuscular
      Duchenne's muscular dystrophy
      Facioscapulohumeral muscular dystrophy
      Limb-girdle dystrophy of Erb
      Myotonia dystrophica
      Friedreich's ataxia
9. Miscellaneous acquired
   a. Postpartum cardiomyopathy
   b. Obesity
10. Idiopathic
   a. Idiopathic dilated cardiomyopathy
   b. Idiopathic restrictive cardiomyopathy
   c. Idiopathic hypertrophic cardiomyopathy
11. Physical agents
   a. Heat stroke
   b. Hypothermia
   c. Radiation

cardiac dysfunction and congestive heart failure and present clinical, hemodynamic, and pathological findings identical to those present in idiopathic dilated cardiomyopathy, which, in the final analysis, is a diagnosis of exclusion. The course of idiopathic dilated cardiomyopathy is usually one of progressive deterioration[8a]; the majority of patients succumb within four years after the onset of symptoms,[9] although a minority improve, with a reduction in cardiac size and longer survival.[15] Age greater than 55 years, a cardiothoracic ratio greater than 0.55, and a cardiac index less than 3.0 liters/min/m^2 each identifies patients with a greater than 85 per cent mortality (Fig. 41–2).[15]

PATHOLOGY. *Postmortem examination* discloses enlargement and dilatation of all four chambers; the ventricles are more dilated than the atria. While the thickness of the ventricular wall is increased in some cases, the degree of hypertrophy is often inadequate for the severe dilatation present.[16] The development of left ventricular hypertrophy may have a protective or beneficial role in dilated cardiomyopathy, since it may serve to reduce systolic wall stress and protect against further cavity dilatation.[17] In patients with equivalent degrees of chamber enlargement, survival is longer in those with a greater degree of left ventricular hypertrophy.[17] The cardiac valves are intrinsically normal, and intracavitary thrombi, particularly in the ventricular apex, are common.[9,16] A nonspecific form of endocardial thickening that underlies the ventricular thrombi is often observed.[16,18] The coronary arteries are usually normal.[18]

Histological examination reveals extensive areas of interstitial and perivascular fibrosis, occasionally associated with calcification, within the walls of the ventricles.[16,19] Small areas of necrosis and cellular infiltrate are seen on occasion, but these are not prominent features.[18] Quantitative analysis of myocardial samples has shown a reduction in the number of neurons in dilated cardiomyopathy, but the significance of this finding is unclear at present.[20] Cardiac biopsy specimens obtained during life by a transvenous or transthoracic approach demonstrate a variety of

TABLE 41–2 FUNCTIONAL CLASSIFICATION OF THE CARDIOMYOPATHIES

	Dilated	Restrictive	Hypertrophic
Symptoms	Congestive heart failure, particularly left-sided Fatigue and weakness Systemic or pulmonary emboli	Dyspnea, fatigue Right-sided congestive heart failure Signs and symptoms of systemic disease: amyloidosis, iron storage disease, etc.	Dyspnea, angina pectoris Fatigue, syncope, palpitations
Physical Examination	Moderate to severe cardiomegaly; S_3 and S_4 Atrioventricular valve regurgitation, especially mitral	Mild to moderate cardiomegaly; S_3 or S_4 Atrioventricular valve regurgitation; inspiratory increase in venous pressure (Kussmaul's sign)	Mild cardiomegaly Apical systolic thrill and heave; brisk carotid upstroke S_4 common Systolic murmur that increases with Valsalva maneuver
Chest Roentgenogram	Moderate to marked cardiac enlargement, especially left ventricular Pulmonary venous hypertension	Mild cardiac enlargement Pulmonary venous hypertension	Mild to moderate cardiac enlargement Left atrial enlargement
Electrocardiogram	Sinus tachycardia Atrial and ventricular arrhythmias ST-segment and T-wave abnormalities Intraventricular conduction defects	Low voltage Intraventricular conduction defects AV conduction defects	Left ventricular hypertrophy ST-segment and T-wave abnormalities Abnormal Q waves Atrial and ventricular arrhythmias
Echocardiogram	Left ventricular dilatation and dysfunction Abnormal diastolic mitral valve motion secondary to abnormal compliance and filling pressures	Increased left ventricular wall thickness and mass Small or normal-sized left ventricular cavity Normal systolic function Pericardial effusion	Asymmetrical septal hypertrophy (ASH) Narrow left ventricular outflow tract Systolic anterior motion (SAM) of the mitral valve Small or normal-sized left ventricle
Radionuclide Studies	Left ventricular dilatation and dysfunction (RVG)	Infiltration of myocardium (^{201}Tl) Small or normal-sized left ventricle (RVG) Normal systolic function (RVG)	Small or normal-sized left ventricle (RVG) Vigorous systolic function (RVG) Asymmetrical septal hypertrophy (RVG or ^{201}Tl)
Cardiac Catheterization	Left ventricular enlargement and dysfunction Mitral and/or tricuspid regurgitation Elevated left- and often right-sided filling pressures Diminished cardiac output	Diminished left ventricular compliance "Square root sign" in ventricular pressure recordings Preserved systolic function Elevated left- and right-sided filling pressures	Diminished left ventricular compliance Mitral regurgitation Vigorous systolic function Dynamic left ventricular outflow gradient

RVG = Radionuclide ventriculogram; ^{201}Tl = thallium-201

abnormalities, including interstitial fibrosis, cellular hypertrophy, and myocardial cell degeneration.[19,20a] The mitochondria of myocytes are frequently abnormal, with swelling and loss of cristae, but specific and diagnostic electron microscopic findings are lacking.[19] Both left and right ventricular tissues possess reduced activities of mitochondrial enzymes, with elevated levels of lactate dehydrogenase.[21] These abnormalities of mitochondrial function are not unexpected in view of the known ultrastructural abnormalities of the mitochondria, and it is thought that the elevated levels of lactate dehydrogenase result from enhanced anaerobic glycolysis due to mitochondrial dysfunction.[21] No viruses or other etiological agents have been identified with any regularity in tissue from patients with dilated cardiomyopathy. Particularly disappointing has been the failure to identify any immunological, histochemical, morphological, ultrastructural, or microbiological markers that might be used to establish the diagnosis of idiopathic dilated cardiomyopathy or to clarify its cause. Because there are no specific morphological features that characterize the dilated cardiomyopathies, it is not surprising that endomyocardial biopsy is not widely used for diagnosis of this condition. However, biopsy may be useful in *excluding* other conditions, such as endomyocardial fi-

TABLE 41–3 ECHOCARDIOGRAPHIC FINDINGS IN THREE TYPES OF CARDIOMYOPATHY

	Dilated	Hypertrophic	Restrictive
LV cavity	++	– or N	N
LV wall thickness	N	+	+
LV contractility	–	+ or N	N or –

LV = left ventricular; – = decreased; N = normal; + = increased.

From DeMaria, A. N., Bommer, W., Lee, G., and Mason, D. T.: Value and limitations of two dimensional echocardiography in assessment of cardiomyopathy. Am. J. Cardiol. *46*:1225, 1980.

TABLE 41–4 COMMON INDICATIONS FOR ENDOMYOCARDIAL BIOPSY

1. To differentiate restrictive from constrictive disease.
2. To evaluate cardiac involvement in systemic disease.
3. To evaluate myocarditis.
4. To detect cardiotoxicity due to cardiotoxic agents.
5. To evaluate cardiac transplant rejection.
6. To evaluate cardiac tumors.

TABLE 41–5 SPECIFIC PATHOLOGICAL ENTITIES DETECTED BY ENDOMYOCARDIAL BIOPSY

1. Cardiac transplant rejection
2. Myocarditis
3. Adriamycin cardiotoxicity
4. Amyloidosis
5. Sarcoidosis
6. Hemochromatosis
7. Endocardial fibroelastosis
8. Endomyocardial fibrosis
9. Carcinoid
10. Glycogen storage disease
11. Cardiac tumor
12. Fabry's disease

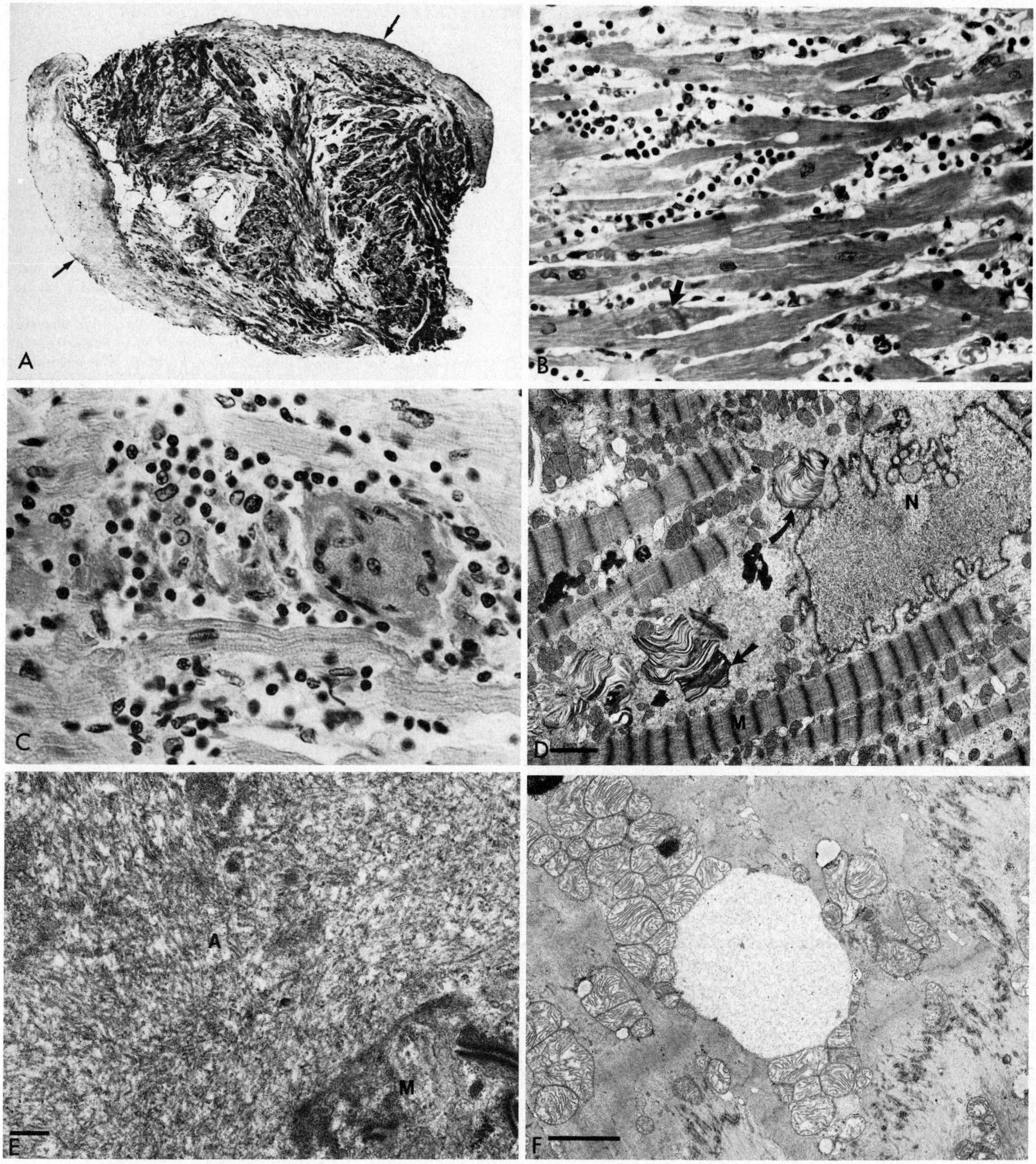

FIGURE 41–1 Representative examples of findings by endomyocardial biopsy. *A,* Low-power view of an entire transvenous right ventricular endomyocardial biopsy specimen. The endocardial surface is indicated by arrows. (Hematoxylin and eosin stain; original magnification × 90.) *B,* Inflammatory myocarditis with moderate, predominantly lymphocytic interstitial infiltrate throughout the myocardium. Focal myocardial cell necrosis is indicated by the arrow. (Hematoxylin and eosin stain; original magnification × 550.) *C,* Typical myocardial lesion in giant cell myocarditis with foci of mixed inflammatory infiltrate and multinucleated giant cells. (Hematoxylin and eosin stain; original magnification × 550.) *D,* Endomyocardial biopsy in patient with Fabry's disease. Transmission electron micrograph of cardiac muscle cell showing nucleus (N), myofibrils (M), and cytoplasmic inclusions (arrows) characteristic of Fabry's disease. (Original magnification × 3000. Bar at lower left-hand corner = 2 μm.) *E,* Cardiac amyloidosis revealed by endomyocardial biopsy. A very high magnification transmission electron photomicrograph (× 50,000) shows finely fibrillar amyloid material (A) in the interstitium surrounding individual myocytes. A portion of one myocyte is seen (M). (Bar at lower left = 0.1 μm.) *F,* Electron micrograph of endomyocardial biopsy specimen from a patient with adriamycin cardiotoxicity. The myocyte shown demonstrates swelling of the sarcoplasmic reticulum and diffuse myofibrillar loss. (Original magnification × 4500. Bar at lower left = 2 μm.) (Courtesy of Dr. Frederick J. Schoen, Department of Pathology, Brigham and Women's Hospital.)

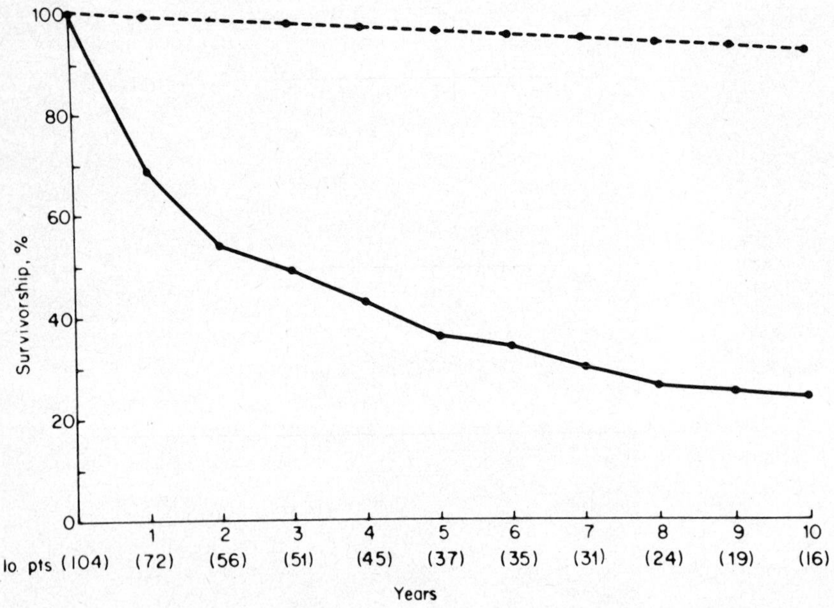

FIGURE 41–2 Observed survival plotted against time in years in 104 patients (pts.) with the diagnosis of idiopathic dilated cardiomyopathy (solid line). The dashed line represents the control expected survival, on the basis of age and sex distribution, according to the death rates of the Minnesota 1970 White Population Life Table. The number of living patients under observation at each followup interval is indicated in parentheses. (From Fuster, V., et al.: The natural history of idiopathic dilated cardiomyopathy. Am. J. Cardiol. *47*:525, 1981.)

brosis, myocarditis, and infiltrative diseases of the myocardium.[22] Also, by using a semiquantitative grading scale of the severity of histological changes in biopsy specimens, it may be possible to separate patients into groups with a poor prognosis (0 per cent survival at 4 years) and a better prognosis (better than 50 per cent 4-year survival), although there is disagreement on this point.[11,23]

ETIOLOGY. It is likely that primary dilated cardiomyopathy is a common expression of myocardial damage that has been produced by a variety of myocardial insults.[24] While the cause or causes remain unclear, at least four conditions, if not etiologically linked, appear to lower the threshold for the development of cardiomyopathy, and it is possible that in some cases a combination of factors results in severe myocardial damage.[24] Alcohol, pregnancy (see Chap. 53), systemic hypertension (see Chap. 26), and a variety of infections (pp. 1432 to 1442) may each be associated with myocardial dysfunction and congestive failure and are important causes of secondary dilated cardiomyopathy. Other causes include selenium deficiency and a variety of toxic agents, including cyclophosphamide (p. 1692) and adriamycin (p. 1690).

The possible progression of infective, particularly viral, myocarditis to cardiomyopathy has engendered the greatest speculation as a possible cause of "idiopathic" dilated cardiomyopathy.[24,25] While this hypothesis is inviting, it remains largely unsupported; there have been few observations of a transition from myocarditis to dilated cardiomyopathy and almost no evidence to suggest prior viral infections in patients with unequivocal cardiomyopathy.[26] However, there are patients who present with the clinical features of a dilated cardiomyopathy in which the apparent cause of the left ventricular enlargement and contractile dysfunction is an inflammatory myocarditis, possibly postviral (see p. 1433). Unlike the histological features of dilated cardiomyopathy, this form of myocarditis is characterized by a prominent round cell infiltrate. Identification of such patients requires endomyocardial biopsy, although myocardial uptake of the radionuclide gallium-67 may provide a noninvasive means of selecting patients for biopsy.[28,28a]

A variety of other possible causes has been proposed, again with little supportive evidence. Thus, endocrine and immunological abnormalities[27] as well as the effects of chemical or physical toxins have been suggested as possible etiological factors. Heart muscle from patients with dilated cardiomyopathy has been shown to bind immunoglobulins preferentially, and circulating antimyocardial antibodies may be demonstrated in many patients, although the significance and reproducibility of these findings remain unclear.[29,30] The observation that circulating lymphocytes of patients with idiopathic dilated cardiomyopathy demonstrate defective suppressor cell function in vitro is intriguing, but its significance, too, is not clear nor have the findings been completely reproducible.[31,32] It has been suggested that microvascular hyperreactivity (spasm) may lead to myocellular necrosis and scarring, with resultant heart failure, although this hypothesis remains speculative.[33]

In contrast to hypertrophic cardiomyopathy, in which familial transmission is quite common, in dilated cardiomyopathy it is rare. Occasional instances have been reported, and a genetic abnormality may be implicated in a small fraction of patients with dilated cardiomyopathy.[34–36]

Clinical Manifestations

Symptoms usually develop gradually in patients with dilated cardiomyopathy. Some patients may be asymptomatic yet have left ventricular dilatation for months or even years.[37,38] An unrecognized illness may result in left ventricular dilatation, which is clinically recognized only years later when symptoms develop or when routine chest roentgenography demonstrates cardiomegaly.[37] Although patients of any age may be affected, the disease is most common in middle age[37,39] and is more frequent in men than in women.[40]

The most striking symptoms are those of left ventricular failure. Dyspnea on exertion and, in more severe cases, orthopnea, paroxysmal nocturnal dyspnea, and dyspnea at rest are prominent.[38] Fatigue and weakness due to diminished cardiac output are common. Peripheral edema, hepatomegaly, and ascites are late and ominous signs. Vague chest pain is not uncommon, although angina pectoris is unusual and suggests the presence of coronary artery disease rather than dilated cardiomyopathy. In some patients there appears to be a reduction in myocardial perfusion despite normal coronary arteries, suggesting that subendocardial ischemia may play a role in the genesis of chest pain.[41] Chest pain secondary to pulmonary embolism and abdominal pain secondary to congestive hepatomegaly are frequent in the late stages of the illness.

Physical examination reveals variable degrees of cardiac enlargement and findings of congestive heart failure. The systolic blood pressure is usually normal or low, and the pulse pressure is narrow, reflecting a diminished stroke volume. The arterial pulse is of low amplitude and volume. Pulsus alternans (p. 25) is common when severe left ventricular failure is present. The jugular veins are frequently distended. Prominent *a* and *v* waves are visible—the latter a late manifestation of the presence of tricuspid valvular regurgitation. The liver may be engorged and pulsatile. Peripheral edema and ascites may be present.

The precordium usually reveals left and, occasionally, right ventricular impulses, but the heaves are not sustained, as they are in patients with considerable ventricular hypertrophy (p. 27). The apical impulse is usually displaced laterally, reflecting left ventricular dilatation. A presystolic *a* wave may be palpable. The second heart sound is usually normally split, although paradoxical splitting (p. 47) may be detected in the presence of left bundle branch block, an electrocardiographic finding which is not unusual in dilated cardiomyopathy. The pulmonary component of the second heart sound may be accentuated, and the splitting may be narrow if pulmonary hypertension is present.[42] Presystolic gallop sounds (S_4) often precede the development of overt congestive heart failure. Ventricular gallops (S_3) are the rule once cardiac decompensation occurs, and a summation gallop is often heard when there is tachycardia. Systolic murmurs are common and are usually due to mitral or, less commonly, tricuspid valvular regurgitation. Atrioventricular valvular regurgitation results from ventricular dilatation and resultant distortion of the geometry of the subvalvar apparatus.[43] Gallop sounds and regurgitant murmurs can often be elicited or intensified by isometric handgrip exercise[42] with its attendant enhancement of systemic vascular resistance and impedance to left ventricular outflow. Systemic emboli resulting from dislodgment of intracardiac thrombi from the left atrium and ventricle[38,42] and pulmonary emboli that originate in the venous system of the legs are common late complications.

NONINVASIVE EXAMINATION. The *chest roentgenogram* usually reveals left ventricular enlargement, although generalized cardiomegaly is often seen. Left ventricular failure may result in signs of pulmonary venous hypertension (i.e., pulmonary vascular redistribution) as well as interstitial and even alveolar edema (p. 173). Pleural effusions may be present, and the azygos vein and superior vena cava may be dilated when right heart failure supervenes. The *electrocardiogram* often shows sinus tachycardia when heart failure is present. The entire spectrum of atrial and ventricular tachyarrhythmias and atrioventricular conduction disturbances may be seen. Indeed, arrhythmias are second in frequency only to heart failure as clinical manifestations of congestive cardiomyopathy.[38,38a] A variety of intraventricular conduction defects is common, and Q waves may be present when there is extensive left ventricular fibrosis without discrete myocardial infarction;[37] ST-segment and T-wave abnormalities are common.

Systolic time intervals (p. 54) are usually abnormal in dilated cardiomyopathy and are useful in estimating and following the severity of left ventricular dysfunction in patients with this condition. The left ventricular ejection time (LVET) is reduced, the preejection period (PEP) is prolonged, and the ratio of the PEP/LVET exceeds the upper limits of normal, i.e., 0.43.[44]

Both M-mode and two-dimensional *echocardiography* are useful in assessing the degree of impairment of left ventricular function and for excluding concomitant valvular or pericardial disease (Chap 5). In addition to examination of all four cardiac valves for evidence of structural or functional abnormalities, the size of the ventricular cavity may be assessed, the thickness of the left and right ventricular walls evaluated, and an estimate made of ventricular function.[45] Left ventricular enlargement, with increased end-diastolic and end-systolic volumes, and reduced ejection fraction and fractional shortening are characteristically found. Mitral valve motion may be abnormal and may reflect the effects of diminished left ventricular compliance and elevated end-diastolic pressure. Right ventricular enlargement occurs late in the stage of the illness. A pericardial effusion may sometimes by demonstrated. *Thallium-201 imaging* at rest and with exercise is of limited value in distinguishing left ventricular enlargement due to dilated cardiomyopathy from that due to coronary artery disease unless a large defect indicative of a myocardial infarction is seen.[46]

Radionuclide ventriculography, like echocardiography, reveals elevated end-diastolic and end-systolic left ventricular volumes, reduced ejection fractions in both ventricles and wall-motion abnormalities.[46a] This technique is helpful both in the assessment of ventricular function and in evaluating the response to therapy.[47] In many cases, however, it is not necessary to carry out serial batteries of noninvasive tests in order to follow patients with dilated cardiomyopathy and evaluate their response to treatment. This is true particularly when the studies are performed only with the patient at rest, since clinical symptoms correlate best with exercise capacity, which in turn bears only a general relationship to resting ventricular performance.[48]

To identify potentially reversible secondary causes of dilated cardiomyopathy, several basic screening tests are often indicated, including determinations of serum phosphorus (hypophosphatemia), serum calcium (hypocalcemia), serum creatinine and urea nitrogen (uremia), and serum iron (hemochromatosis).[49]

CARDIAC CATHETERIZATION AND ANGIOCARDIOGRAPHY. The left ventricular end-diastolic, left atrial, and pulmonary artery wedge pressures are usually elevated. Modest degrees of pulmonary arterial hypertension are common.[42] Advanced cases may demonstrate right ventricular dilatation and failure as well, with resultant elevation of the right ventricular end-diastolic, right atrial, and central venous pressures. However, the end-diastolic pressure in the left ventricle usually exceeds that in the right by at least 5 mm Hg. Cardiac output is reduced,[50] often markedly.

Left ventriculography demonstrates enlargement of this chamber with diffuse reduction in wall motion.[9,42] The ejection fraction is decreased and the end-systolic volume is increased as a result of the impairment of left ventricular contractility. Sometimes left ventricular thrombi may be visualized within the left ventricle as intracavitary filling defects. Mild mitral regurgitation is often present.[42] On occasion, it may be difficult to distinguish left ventricular dilatation secondary to severe mitral regurgitation from a dilated cardiomyopathy with secondary mitral regurgitation. The left ventricular wall may be thickened, but this is usually not a prominent finding.[9]

Coronary arteriography usually reveals normal vessels.[50] This technique may be of particular value in patients with abnormal Q waves on the electrocardiogram, since such a pattern may be due to myocardial infarction as a result of obstructive coronary artery disease or, alternatively, extensive myocardial fibrosis secondary to severe dilated cardiomyopathy in the absence of coronary artery obstruction.

Treatment

Since the cause of idiopathic dilated cardiomyopathy is unknown, specific therapy is not possible. Treatment, therefore, is on the same basis as that for heart failure, discussed in detail in Chapter 16. Physical, dietary, pharmacological, mechanical, and surgical interventions may help to control symptoms,[51] although their role in prolonging life has not been established.

Patients with moderately severe left ventricular failure may be comfortable at rest but may develop severe symptoms with exercise, when they are unable to increase their cardiac output commensurately. It is reasonable to restrict activity for these patients to avoid precipitation of unwanted and poorly tolerated symptoms (Fig. 16–1, p. 504). Marked curtailment of exercise in the form of prolonged bed rest may result not only in improvement of symptoms but also in a reduction in heart size and an improvement in prognosis.[16] However, many patients are unable psychologically to tolerate strict bed rest, and the efficacy of immobilization per se has not been documented.[12,52] Perhaps prolonged bed rest in the hospital is helpful by ensuring a nutritious diet and removal of a toxin (e.g., alcohol). A reasonable compromise can usually be achieved in reducing activity without totally incapacitating the patient.[52] It has been suggested that in patients with heart failure due to dilated cardiomyopathy a beneficial effect may be seen with beta-adrenergic blockade[53,53a] along with deterioration on withdrawal of therapy.[54] The mechanism of improvement is said to be protection against the increased sympathetic nervous activity that may accompany heart failure. The results have not been confirmed in adequately controlled trials, and at this final the use of beta-adrenergic blockade in dilated cardiomyopathy should be considered speculative, experimental, and potentially dangerous.[55,55a] Prolonged improvement in clinical status and left ventricular function has been noted following a 3-day infusion of the synthetic catecholamine dobutamine.[56] Further trials should clarify the role of these experimental approaches in patients with dilated cardiomyopathy.

Antiarrhythmic agents should be used to treat symptomatic or serious arrhythmias. Because of the adverse effects of most available agents, many of which depress myocardial contractility (Chap. 20), treatment should be individualized, with both efficacy and toxicity carefully monitored. Because of the frequency and hazards of embolization,[56a] patients with dilated cardiomyopathy and heart failure should be treated with anticoagulants, even without direct evidence of thrombus formation if there are no specific contraindications to these agents.[14,38,52] Corticosteroids appear to have no place in the treatment of chronic idiopathic dilated cardiomyopathy.

Surgical replacement of regurgitant valves has been attempted rarely in patients with progressive atrioventricular valvular regurgitation (almost always mitral) which appeared to result in progressive cardiac enlargement and failure. The results of operation are often less than satisfactory because of the degree of preexisting cardiac dysfunction and damage. In appropriate patients, cardiac transplantation may be an alternative (p. 547),[57] with a 3-year survival rate of nearly 70 per cent compared with less than 5 per cent in nontransplanted patients.[58] The enormous emotional and economic investments required for carrying out this procedure must be appreciated, however.

ALCOHOLIC CARDIOMYOPATHY

Excessive consumption of alcohol is the major cause of secondary, non-ischemic dilated cardiomyopathy in the Western world,[59] resulting in cardiomegaly and low cardiac output. It is estimated that two-thirds of the adult population use alcohol to some extent, and greater than 10 per cent are heavy users. Therefore, it is not surprising that alcoholic cardiomyopathy is a major problem. Ceasing alcohol consumption may halt the progression or even reverse alcoholic cardiomyopathy,[60] which, unlike idiopathic or primary dilated cardiomyopathy, is usually marked by progressive deterioration.

The consumption of alcohol may result in myocardial damage by three basic mechanisms: (1) direct toxic effects; (2) nutritional effects, most commonly in association with thiamine deficiency, which leads to beriberi heart disease (p. 814); and (3) rarely, toxic effects due to additives in the alcoholic beverage (cobalt)[61] (p. 1408). There had been considerable speculation that alcohol caused myocardial damage only through dietary deficiencies, but it is now clear that alcoholic cardiomyopathy occurs in the absence of nutritional deficiencies.[59]

Typical Oriental beriberi is distinguished from alcoholic cardiomyopathy by the presence of high output failure in the former (p. 817); peripheral vasodilatation is prominent, with increased venous return and resultant high cardiac output.[62] This condition responds to thiamine administration, often in a dramatic fashion.[63] The existence of a variant of beriberi heart disease, termed Occidental beriberi, has been proposed; in contrast to the high output state in Oriental beriberi, Occidental beriberi heart disease is marked by cardiac dilatation, congestive failure, and diminished cardiac output without peripheral vasodilatation, increased venous return, or elevated cardiac output.[64] Because it occurs almost exclusively in alcoholic patients, is not usually observed in individuals with solely a dietary thiamine deficiency, does not respond well to thiamine administration, and is otherwise identical clinically to alcoholic cardiomyopathy, Occidental beriberi heart disease in fact is probably the same as alcoholic cardiomyopathy.[39]

Alcohol results in acute as well as chronic depression of myocardial contractility[65] and may produce demonstrable cardiac dysfunction even when ingested by normal individuals in quantities consumed in social drinking.[66] When conscious, chronically instrumented, but otherwise healthy dogs are given intravenous infusions of ethanol to produce blood levels well below the usual legal human limit for the operation of motor vehicles (150 mg/dl), cardiac dilatation and systolic dysfunction occur, with a fall in cardiac output and the maximum dP/dt.[67] The acute hemodynamic effects of alcohol appear to depend on its blood levels, since ventricular dysfunction following acute ethanol ingestion may be reversed within 15 to 30 minutes of hemodialysis.[68] Prior exposure to alcohol appears to modulate the hemodynamic response to acute challenge with alcohol. Larger doses of alcohol are required to produce cardiac dysfunction in chronic alcoholic patients without obvious heart disease than in normal subjects. On the other hand, the alcoholic person with clinically evident cardiac dysfunction appears to be more susceptible to the deleterious effects of alcohol than normal.[68]

The mechanism of the cardiac depression produced by alcohol remains unclear, and a direct causal relationship between alcohol and the development of cardiomyopathy has not been proved.[66] In acute studies, alcohol and its metabolite acetaldehyde have been shown to interfere with a number of cellular functions that involve the transport and binding of calcium, mitochondrial respiration, myocardial lipid metabolism, myocardial protein synthesis, and myofibrillar ATPase.[59,69,70,70a] Alcohol results in loss of potassium ions from myocardial cells, along with diminished uptake of free fatty acids but enhanced myocardial extraction of triglyceride.[71] The major unanswered question is how these metabolic effects result in persistent myocardial injury. It is possible that factors such as magnesium deficiency or the presence of a separate toxic compound associated with the alcohol may be involved in the production of alcoholic cardiomyopathy.[66]

Several studies in experimental animals and in chronic alcoholic patients admitted to the hospital have demonstrated cardiac dysfunction even when adequate nutrition was ensured.[60] Chronic experimental studies in a well-nourished alcoholic person given 12 to 16 ounces of whiskey per day for several months demonstrated the gradual development of heart failure. Without specific therapy, the features of congestive failure resolved within several weeks following the cessation of alcohol intake[71] (Fig. 41–3).

PATHOLOGY. The gross and microscopic pathological findings are nonspecific and similar to those observed in idiopathic dilated cardiomyopathy.[19,39] Edema of the vascular wall and perivascular fibrosis of the intramyocardial coronary arteries has been observed,[72,73] and it has been suggested that the myocardial damage in alcoholic cardiomyopathy may be the result of ischemia produced by disease of the small intramural coronary arteries.[73] Alcohol, even in small amounts, may result in alterations of mitochondrial structure.[74,75]

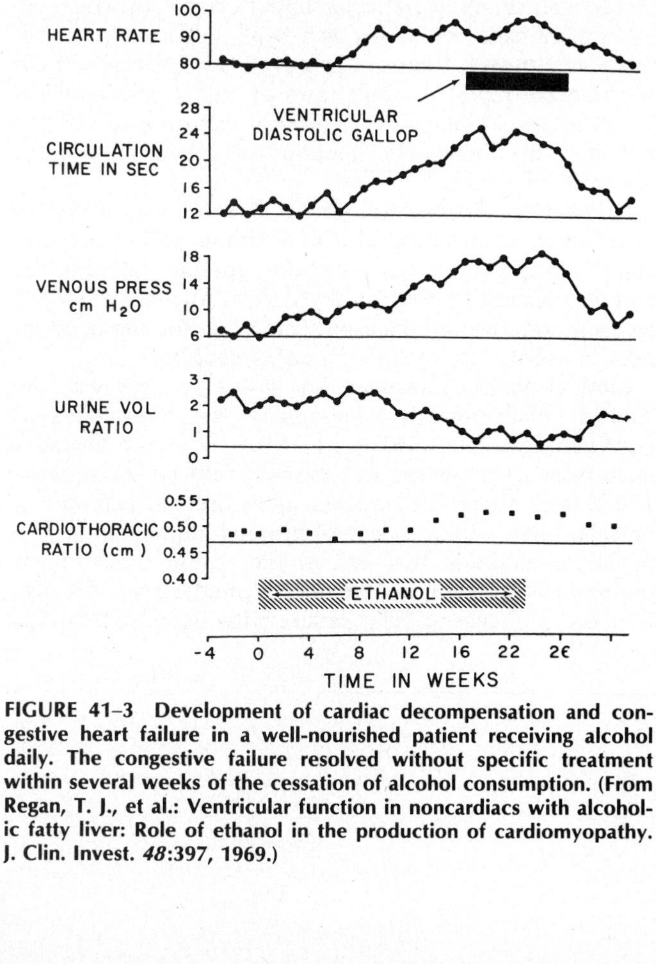

FIGURE 41–3 Development of cardiac decompensation and congestive heart failure in a well-nourished patient receiving alcohol daily. The congestive failure resolved without specific treatment within several weeks of the cessation of alcohol consumption. (From Regan, T. J., et al.: Ventricular function in noncardiacs with alcoholic fatty liver: Role of ethanol in the production of cardiomyopathy. J. Clin. Invest. *48*:397, 1969.)

CLINICAL MANIFESTATIONS

Alcoholic cardiomyopathy is most commonly seen in males 30 to 55 years of age who have been heavy consumers of whiskey, wine, or beer, usually for more than 10 years.[60,68,76,77] The male predominance appears to be largely the result of the higher frequency of alcoholism in this sex, although noninvasive testing of cardiac function in male and female alcoholic patients suggests that cardiac dysfunction is more likely in men than in women.[78] While alcoholic cardiomyopathy may be observed in the homeless, malnourished, "skid row" alcoholic man who is a candidate for and may often suffer from alcoholic cirrhosis, many patients are well-nourished individuals in the middle and even upper socioeconomic brackets without liver disease or peripheral neuropathy.[39,60,68,79] Therefore, unless a high index of suspicion is maintained, it may be easy to miss a history of alcohol abuse. Persistent questioning of the patient and particularly the relatives of patients with unexplained cardiomegaly or cardiomyopathy is often required to elicit a history of alcoholism.

It is frequently possible to demonstrate mild depression of cardiac function in chronic alcoholics even before cardiac dysfunction becomes clinically manifest.[68,80,81] Abnormalities of both systolic function (reduced ejection fraction) and diastolic function (increased myocardial wall stiffness) have been demonstrated in alcoholic patients without cardiac symptoms by a variety of invasive and noninvasive techniques.[68,80,81] Two basic patterns have been observed: (1) left ventricular dilatation with impaired systolic function and (2) left ventricular hypertrophy with diminished compliance and normal or increased contractile performance; left ventricular size is most substantially increased.[82–84] The development of symptoms may be insidious, although some patients present acute and florid left-sided congestive heart failure.[76] A paroxysm of atrial fibrillation is a relatively frequent initial presenting finding.[79] More advanced cases present findings of biventricular failure, with left ventricular dysfunction usually dominating.[39,76,79] Dyspnea, orthopnea, and paroxysmal nocturnal dyspnea are frequently observed.[79] Palpitations and syncope due to cardiac arrhythmias, usually supraventricular, are occasionally present.[76] Angina pectoris does not occur unless there is concomitant coronary artery disease or aortic stenosis.

Physical examination usually reveals a narrow pulse pressure, often with an elevated diastolic pressure secondary to excessive peripheral vasoconstriction.[39,76,79] There is cardiomegaly, and protodiastolic (S_3) and presystolic (S_4) gallop sounds are common. An apical systolic murmur of mitral regurgitation due to papillary muscle dysfunction is often found.[79] The severity of right heart failure varies, but jugular venous distention and peripheral edema are common.

LABORATORY EXAMINATION. The *chest roentgenogram* demonstrates cardiac enlargement, pulmonary congestion, and pulmonary venous hypertension. Pleural effusions are often seen. *Electrocardiographic abnormalities* are common and are frequently the only indication of alcoholic heart disease during the preclinical phase. Alcoholic patients without other evidence of heart disease often are seen after developing palpitations, chest discomfort, or syncope typically following a binge of alcohol consumption on a weekend, particularly during the year-end holiday season.[85] This is dubbed the "holiday heart syndrome." The most common arrhythmia observed is atrial fibrillation, followed by atrial flutter and frequent ventricular premature contractions.[85,86] Hypokalemia may play a role in the genesis of some of these arrhythmias. Supraventricular arrhythmias are also frequently observed in patients with overt alcoholic cardiomyopathy. Sudden, unexpected death is not uncommon in young adult alcoholics, and it is likely that ventricular fibrillation is responsible.[68] On the other hand, arrhythmias often cease in patients who abstain from alcohol.[85]

Atrioventricular conduction disturbances (most commonly first-degree heart block), bundle branch block, and left ventricular hypertrophy[79,87] are common electrocardiographic findings. Prolongation of the Q-T interval is noted frequently.[84] ST-segment and T-wave changes are often restored to normal within several days after cessation of alcohol consumption.[88] Q waves, presumably reflecting myocardial fibrosis, are usually not prominent.[76]

The hemodynamic findings observed at cardiac catheterization and the assessment of left ventricular function by noninvasive methods (echocardiography, isotope angiography, and systolic time intervals) resemble those found in idiopathic dilated cardiomyopathy.

The *natural history* of alcoholic cardiomyopathy depends on the drinking habits of the patient. Total abstinence in the earlier stages of the disease frequently leads to resolution of the manifestation of congestive heart failure and a return of heart size to normal.[77,79,89,90] Continued alcohol consumption leads to further myocardial damage and fibrosis, and the congestive heart failure becomes increasingly refractory to treatment, resulting eventually in the demise of the patient.[79] Death may also be due to arrhythmia, heart block, and systemic or pulmonary embolism.[39, 79]

TREATMENT. The key to the long-term treatment of alcoholic cardiomyopathy is *complete abstinence*, as early in the course of the disease as possible. The prognosis in patients who continue to drink, particularly if they have been symptomatic for a long period, is poor. In one study, 80 per cent of such patients died within a 3-year period.[77] In the overall population of patients with alcoholic cardiomyopathy, between 40 and 50 per cent succumb within a 3- to 6-year period.[77,89] Prolonged bed rest is also thought to result in functional improvement,[89] although its major benefit may simply be the decreased alcohol consumption.

The management of acute episodes of congestive heart failure is similar to that of idiopathic dilated cardiomyopathy. For patients with severe congestive heart failure, it is probably prudent to administer thiamine on the remote chance that beriberi may be contributing to the heart failure.

COBALT CARDIOMYOPATHY

A previously unrecognized syndrome of fulminating congestive heart failure appeared in 1966, first in Quebec City, Canada, and subsequently in Omaha, Nebraska; Minneapolis, Minnesota; and Belgium.[61] The disease was found in people who drank a particular brand of beer to which cobalt sulfate had been added as a foam stabilizer. After cobalt was removed from the process, no more cases of the disease were reported. Rare cases of cobalt cardiomyopathy have been found after industrial exposure to cobalt[91] and after the therapeutic ingestion of cobalt salts in the treatment of anemia.[92]

Pathological findings are those of a dilated, hypertrophied heart, often surrounded by a sizable pericardial effusion.[39] Microscopic examination reveals myofibrillar hyaline necrosis as well as myocardial vacuolization and degeneration. The mechanism responsible for the development of cobalt cardiotoxicity remains unclear.

Clinical Manifestations. The typical patient who developed cobalt-beer cardiomyopathy was a middle-aged man who had consumed large quantities of the contaminated beer.[61] The disease was characterized by severe heart failure, with death occurring in more than 40 per cent of patients, often within 3 days of hospital admission.[39,61] The typical presentation was that of the abrupt onset of left followed by right heart failure. Hemodynamic findings were those of biventricular failure with depressed cardiac output.[61]

HYPERTROPHIC CARDIOMYOPATHY

DEFINITIONS. The gross pathological features of hypertrophic obstructive cardiomyopathy (HOCM) were first systematically described in 1958.[93] The characteristic finding is pronounced myocardial hypertrophy, particularly involving the interventricular septum of a nondilated left ventricle. A distinctive clinical feature was soon recognized in many patients with hypertrophic cardiomyopathy: a dynamic pressure gradient in the subaortic area, evanescent in some patients, which divides the left ventricle into a high-pressure apical region and a lower-pressure subaortic region.[94] Hence the term *idiopathic hypertrophic subaortic stenosis* (*IHSS*) was suggested, although subsequent findings have indicated that many patients do not, in fact, ever have obstruction to left ventricular outflow, and thus *hypertrophic cardiomyopathy* is a more appropriate and inclusive way to describe the disease.

Much of the initial investigation in this disease was stimulated by the unique dynamic pressure gradient.[94] Unlike the constant gradient produced by fixed orifice obstruction (as in patients with valvular aortic stenosis or a discrete subaortic membrane), the gradient in HOCM often demonstrates wide fluctuations and in some patients varies between absent and severe. Other patients do not have gradients at rest, but these can be provoked by a variety of physiological or pharmacological interventions (Table 41–6).

Because of the unique obstructive features in hypertrophic cardiomyopathy, the names used to designate this disorder emphasized this characteristic. In the United States, the disease was called idiopathic hypertrophic subaortic stenosis (IHSS) and in Canada *muscular subaortic stenosis.* Investigations over the last 20 years have helped clarify the etiological, clinical, and pathological features of hypertrophic cardiomyopathy, but as a result of the rapid growth in the field, the disorder has been referred to by a bewildering array of more than 50 names![95–97] As we now understand the disease, many of the terms used to designate it are in reality merely *features* of the disease that may be seen in a greater or lesser percentage of afflicted patients.

The older terms, such as IHSS, which emphasized the obstructive features of the disease, have fallen into disfavor, since it is now clear that many and perhaps most patients do not in fact demonstrate an intraventricular pressure gradient. The most characteristic pathophysiological abnormality is not systolic but rather *diastolic* dysfunction.[24] Thus, hypertrophic cardiomyopathy is characterized by abnormal stiffness of the left ventricle during diastole, with resultant impaired ventricular filling. This abnormality in diastolic relaxation results in elevation of the left ventricular end-diastolic pressure. The elevated left ventricular filling pressure is associated with elevated left atrial, pulmonary venous, and pulmonary capillary pressures, causing dyspnea—the most common symptom in hypertrophic cardiomyopathy, despite typically *hypercontractile* left ventricular function. The disease appears to be genetically transmitted as an autosomal dominant trait with a high degree of penetrance in most patients, although sporadic cases occur, some of which may represent new mutations.[98] As might be expected with such a mode of inheritance, evidence of the disease is found in almost half the first-degree relatives of a patient with hypertrophic cardiomyopathy; in many of the relatives the disease is milder than in the propositus, the degree of hypertrophy is less, and outflow gradients are usually lacking. Symptoms are often absent, and the disease may be detected only by echocardiography.[98]

TABLE 41–6 EFFECTS OF INTERVENTIONS ON OUTFLOW GRADIENT AND SYSTOLIC MURMUR IN HOCM

	CONTRACTILITY	PRELOAD	AFTERLOAD
Increase in Gradient and Murmur			
Valsalva maneuver (during strain)	—	↓	↓
Standing	—	↓	—
Postextrasystole	↑	↑	—
Isoproterenol	↑	↓	↓
Digitalis	↑	↓	—
Amyl nitrite	— then ↑	↓ then ↑	↓
Nitroglycerin	—	↓	↓
Exercise	↑	↑	↑
Tachycardia	↑	↓	—
Hypovolemia	↑	↓	↓
Decrease in Gradient and Murmur			
Mueller maneuver	—	↑	↑
Valsalva overshoot	—	↑	↑
Squatting	—	↑	↑
Alpha-adrenergic stimulation (phenylephrine)	—	—	↑
Beta-adrenergic blockade	↓	↑	—
General anesthesia	↓	—	—
Isometric handgrip	—	—	↑

↑ = increase; ↓ = decrease; — = no major change.

PATHOLOGY

Gross examination of the heart discloses a marked increase in myocardial mass, and the ventricular cavities are small (Fig. 41–4). The atria are dilated and often hypertrophied,[99] reflecting the high resistance to filling of the ventricles and the effects of atrioventricular valve regurgitation (Table 41–7). The pattern of hypertrophy of the left ventricle, at least in certain population groups, is distinctive and differs from that seen with secondary hypertrophy (as in systemic hypertension or discrete obstruction to left ventricular outflow, i.e., subaortic, valvular, or supravalvular aortic stenosis) in that it is commonly associated with disproportionate involvement of the interventricular septum compared with the free wall of the left ventricle (Fig. 41–4). In both normal subjects as well as patients with left ventricular hypertrophy without HOCM, the ratio of the thickness of the interventricular septum to that of the left ventricular free wall has been shown at autopsy and by echocardiography to be around 1.0 and nearly always less than 1.3. However, this ratio usually exceeds 1.3 in HOCM. Asymmetrical septal hypertrophy (ASH) was at one time felt to be pathognomonic of HOCM, but modifications of this concept have been required.[100–111] Thus, it is now recognized that concentric left ventricular hypertrophy, with symmetrical thickening of the left ventricle, involving the septum and free wall equally, may oc-

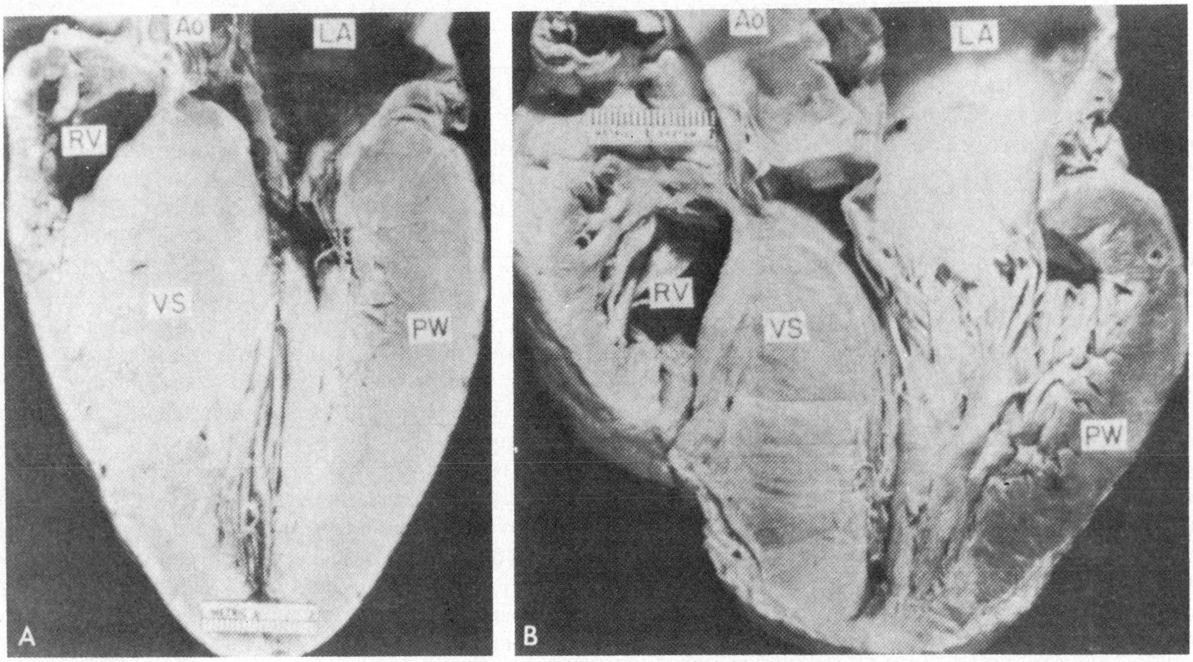

FIGURE 41–4 Two hearts showing hypertrophic cardiomyopathy, one with obstruction (*A*) and one without (*B*). The ventricular septum is markedly thickened in both, but the posterior wall is thickened only in the patient in *A*. Ao = aorta, LA = left atrium, RV = right ventricle, VS = ventricular septum, PW = posterior left ventricular wall. (From Henry, W. L., et al.: Differences in the distribution of myocardial abnormalities in patients with obstructive and nonobstructive asymmetric septal hypertrophy (ASH). Echocardiographic and gross anatomic findings. Circulation *50*:447, 1974, by permission of the American Heart Association, Inc.)

casionally be seen in patients with the genetically transmitted as well as the sporadic forms of hypertrophic cardiomyopathy.[101,102] Even in the majority of patients who manifest ASH the hypertrophy often extends beyond the septum to involve portions of the anterolateral left ventricular wall.[112] In some patients with hypertrophic cardiomyopathy there is substantial hypertrophy in unusual locations, such as the posterior portion of the septum; this may result in diagnostic confusion, since the hypertrophy may not be detectable by M-mode echocardiography but only by two-dimensional echocardiography.[113,113a]

Two types of an unusual form of hypertrophic cardiomyopathy localized to the *apical* portion of the left ventricle have been noted. One form, described in Japanese patients, imparts a characteristic spadelike configuration to the left ventricular chamber on two-dimensional echocardiographic or contrast ventriculographic study. Patients with apical hypertrophy of this type may demonstrate giant negative T waves in the precordial electrocardiographic leads, but they typically do not demonstrate pressure gradients.[114] The other form demonstrates a small, poorly contractile apical segment that communicates with the subaortic area through a markedly narrowed midventricular channel. In this form of apical hypertrophic cardiomyopathy the T waves are not deeply inverted, and an intraventricular pressure gradient may be found.[115] Disproportionate septal hypertrophy may be found in patients with a variety of acquired or congenital lesions in the absence of hypertrophic cardiomyopathy.[103–110] Thus, ASH is a normal finding during fetal life, in neonates, and in infants but normally disappears by the age of 1 or 2 years.[109,116] Conditions resulting in right ventricular pressure overload and thus right ventricular hypertrophy, such as pulmonic stenosis or primary pulmonary hypertension, often result in thickening of the interventricular septum, without affecting the free wall of the left ventricle.[108,109] Abnormal thickness of the septum relative to that of the free wall may also occur in coronary artery disease, presumably when infarction leads to fibrosis and thinning of the free wall of the left ventricle, while the noninfarcted septum exhibits compensatory hypertrophy.[117,118] Other conditions that may present similar patterns of disproportionate septal hypertrophy include lentiginosis, Turner's syndrome, acromegaly, hyperthyroidism, and Friedreich's ataxia, and HOCM may develop after aortic valve replacement.[119,119a] Athletes, weight lifters, and infants of diabetic mothers may demonstrate similar patterns. Rarely, apparent left ventricular hypertrophy is due to infiltration of the septum by tumor,[120,121] Pompe's disease,[122] or Fabry's disease.[123] To differentiate the various causes of septal–free wall disproportion, the term *disproportionate septal thickening* (DST) has been used to indicate the secondary form, while ASH is often reserved for the primary form found in HOCM. The degree of thickening of the interventricular septum ap-

TABLE 41–7 PATHOLOGICAL FINDINGS IN HYPERTROPHIC CARDIOMYOPATHY

Finding	Frequency (%)
Asymmetrical septal hypertrophy	95
Small or normal-sized ventricular cavities	95
Mural plaque in left ventricular outflow tract	75
Thickened mitral valve	75
Dilated atria	100
Abnormal intramural coronary arteries	50
Disarray of ventricular septal myocardial fibers	95

Data from Roberts, W. C., and Ferrans, V. J.: Pathologic anatomy of the cardiomyopathies. Idiopathic dilated and hypertrophic types, infiltrative types and endomyocardial disease with and without eosinophilia. Hum. Pathol. 6:287, 1975.

pears to be unrelated to the presence or absence of a pressure gradient.[99] However, patients who have had a left ventricular outflow gradient during life demonstrate secondary hypertrophy of the posterobasal wall, including the area immediately behind the posterior leaflet of the mitral valve and below the mitral annulus.[124] While hypertrophied, bizarrely shaped, and abnormally arranged myocardial cells are commonly present in the septum (Fig. 41–4), such abnormalities may be less common in the free wall,[125] although these findings are controversial.[119] The gross and histological appearance in the free wall resembles that seen in valvular aortic stenosis, suggesting that these changes are secondary to the high ventricular pressure caused by the pressure gradient. In patients *without* a gradient, portions of the free wall are hypertrophied and extensively involved by bizarre and disorganized myocardial fibers identical to those found in the septum, suggesting a diffuse myopathic process.[124,126]

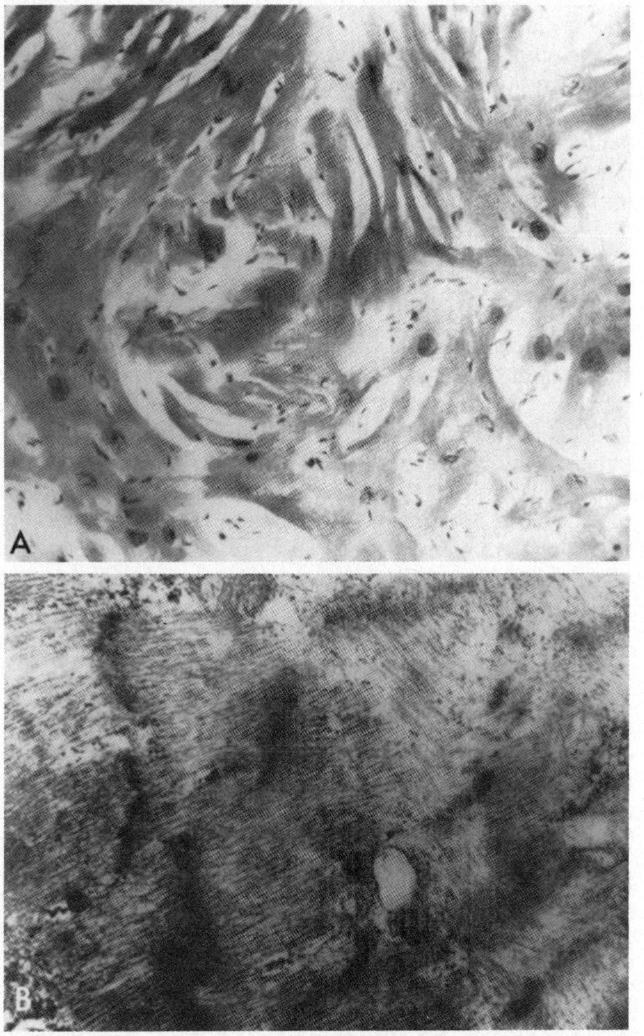

FIGURE 41–5 *A*, Photomicrograph of myocardium from the septal region in a patient firmly diagnosed clinically as suffering from hypertrophic cardiomyopathy. Extensive disarray of myocardial fibers and attempts at whorl formation are present. In addition, severe hypertrophy and an increase in collagen tissue, interrupting muscle bundles, can be seen. Nuclear changes are not prominent, and perinuclear halos are absent. Although not all diagnostic criteria are seen here, the combination of changes present characterizes this condition. (Hematoxylin and eosin stain; original magnification × 650.) *B*, Electron micrograph showing disarray of myocardial fibrils and widening of Z bands. (Lead citrate and uranyl acetate; original magnification × 38,400.) (From Olsen, E. G. J.: The pathology of idiopathic hypertrophic subaortic stenosis (hypertrophic cardiomyopathy): A critical review. Am. Heart J. *100*:553, 1980.)

A "contact lesion" in the form of a mural plaque on the endocardium of the left ventricular outflow tract is frequently found in patients with marked gradients at rest[99] (Table 41–7). This fibrous thickening appears to result from the trauma of the anterior mitral valve leaflet apposing the septum during systole. The thickening of the mitral valve that is often seen[99] is probably explained on a similar basis.

The bizarre form of myocardial fiber hypertrophy that results in myocardial fiber disarray is a prominent feature of HOCM[118] (Fig. 41–5). The disorganization and disarray seen in the septum is not confined to the muscle cell bundles but involves the myofibrils and myofilaments within individual cells as well[127,128] (Fig. 41–5). The myocardial cells are wider and shorter than in other conditions, but they often have bizarre shapes.[124,128] Foci of disorganized cells are often interspersed between areas of hypertrophied but otherwise normal-appearing muscle cells.[124] Similar cellular disorganization is found in a spontaneously occurring primary myocardial disease of dogs and cats.[129] While initially considered specific for HOCM, it is now recognized that abnormally arranged cardiac muscle cells in the septum may be found not only in a variety of disease states, including concentric left ventricular hypertrophy secondary to pressure overload, coronary artery disease, congenital heart disease, and cor pulmonale, but in normal hearts as well.[129a] However, there appears to be a quantitative relationship between the extent of cellular disarray and the underlying disease process, since the disorganization of myocardial fibers is far greater in HOCM than in other disorders.[127] There is a suggestion that the greater the extent of cellular disorganization, the worse the clinical outcome.[126] However, a somewhat surprising finding is that there is little correlation between the extent of cellular disorganization in surgically excised septectomy samples in patients with HOCM and the amount observed at subsequent necropsy.[130]

ETIOLOGY

The cause of the myocardial hypertrophy in HOCM remains unclear. While there are persuasive data that in most patients the disease is inherited,[113a] and in some instances linked to the HLA system,[130a] the basic defect is unknown. The disorganized myocardial fibers may be the result of mechanical stresses within the septum, since myocardial disarray is also seen frequently in other conditions characterized by excessive systolic pressure.[131,132] It has been suggested that the genetic defect in HOCM results in a catenoid shape and configuration of the septum that is concave to the left in the transverse plane but concave to the right in the apex-to-base plane. This abnormal configuration of the septum leads to prominent isometric contraction which might result in fiber disarray.[133] The reverse argument has also been made that the isometric contraction inherent in malaligned cells itself stimulates hypertrophy.[134]

Other suggested etiologies of HOCM include (1) abnormal sympathetic stimulation because of excessive production of or heightened responsiveness of the heart to circulating catecholamines[24,134]; (2) abnormal intramural coronary arteries that lead to myocardial ischemia, with resultant fibrosis and abnormal compensatory hypertrophy[135]; (3) abnormal rapid atrioventricular conduction that leads to asynchronous ventricular contraction resulting in abnormal myocardial hypertrophy[135]; (4) a primary abnormality of collagen that may lead to an abnormal and disorganized fibrous skeleton which, with the development of hypertrophy, leads to myocardial cellular disorganization and disarray[135]; and (5) subendocardial ischemia that depletes the energy stores essential for the sequestration of calcium during diastole, resulting in persistent interaction of the contractile elements during diastole and attendant increased diastolic stiffness.[136]

PATHOPHYSIOLOGY

Since the initial descriptions of hypertrophic cardiomyopathy, the feature that has attracted the greatest attention and has been the source of considerable controversy is the dynamic pressure gradient (Fig. 41–6). While this pressure gradient was initially felt to be due to a muscular sphincter action in the subaortic region, it appears to be related to further narrowing of an already smalltract (narrowed by the prominent septal hypertrophy and possibly abnormal location of the mitral valve) by systolic anterior motion (SAM) of the mitral valve against the septum. Even the view that the pressure gradient in HOCM is the result of mechanical obstruction as a consequence of SAM may require modification. The generation of a pressure gradient due to subaortic obstruction would imply that left ventricular ejection is slowed or impeded at some point during systole. Yet characteristic features of HOCM are rapid ventricular emptying and high ejection fractions. Hemodynamic studies have shown that the majority of flow (at least 80 per cent) is unusually rapid in hypertrophic cardiomyopathy and is completed earlier in systole than normal, regardless of whether gradients are absent, provocable, or present.[137] Since the total duration of systole is prolonged only in patients with gradients,[137] it is likely that a small residual amount of blood is in fact impeded in its ejection from the left ventricle as a consequence of dynamic obstruction.

CLINICAL MANIFESTATIONS

Symptoms. Although symptomatic HOCM is most commonly a disease of young adulthood (the average age of presentation is 26 years[138]), one-third of symptomatic patients coming to cardiac catheterization are over the age of 60 years.[139] The condition has been observed at necropsy in stillborns and both clinically and pathologically in octogenarians.[139–144] The importance of recognizing this disorder in children at the earliest possible time is highlighted by the high mortality rate; death is often sudden and unexpected. Since syncope and sudden death have been associated with competitive sports and severe exertion in patients with hypertrophic cardiomyopathy, these activities should be proscribed. A particularly high index of suspicion of this condition must be maintained to make the clinical diagnosis in the elderly, since their symptoms may easily be confused with those of coronary artery or aortic valve disease.[139,144] No sex predilection is apparent[145] although females are more likely to be severely disabled and may initially present at a younger age than males.[146]

The clinical picture varies considerably, ranging from the asymptomatic relative of a patient with recognized HOCM who has ASH on echocardiogram but no other manifestation of the illness to the patient with incapacitating symptoms.[138] Most patients with HOCM are asymptomatic and consist of the relatives of patients with known disease. Unfortunately, the first clinical manifestation of the disease in asymptomatic individuals may be sudden death (Fig. 41–7).[147]

The most common symptom is *dyspnea*,[138] which is largely a consequence of the elevated left ventricular diastolic (and therefore left atrial and pulmonary venous) pressure, which results largely from impaired ventricular filling and increased wall stiffness secondary to ventricular hypertrophy.[148] Angina pectoris, fatigue, and syncope are also common.[138,148] Palpitations, paroxysmal nocturnal dyspnea, overt congestive heart failure, and dizziness are found less frequently,[138] although marked congestive heart failure culminating in death may be seen in infants with hypertrophic cardiomyopathy.[149] Exertion tends to exacerbate many of the symptoms. A variety of mechanisms may contribute to the production of angina pectoris. It is at least in part the result of an imbalance between oxygen supply and demand as a consequence of the greatly increased myocardial mass.[150] Transmural infarction may occur in the absence of narrowing in the extramural coronary arteries.[151] Narrowing of the small coronary arteries may contribute to myocardial ischemia,[135] and a few patients with hypertrophic cardiomyopathy may also have atheromatous obstructive coronary artery disease. Impaired diastolic relaxation may produce subendocardial

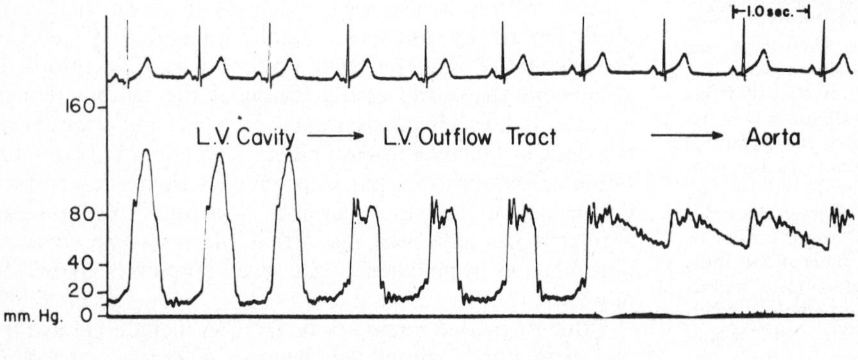

FIGURE 41–6 Pressure tracing recorded as retrograde aortic catheter was withdrawn from the left ventricular (LV) cavity through the left ventricular outflow tract and into the ascending aorta. Note that the pressure gradient occurs within the left ventricle. There is a notch on the left ventricular pressure pulse at approximately 100 mm Hg, the value of the peak systolic pressure distal to the obstruction. In the left ventricular outflow tract the pressure pulse exhibits a midsystolic dip and a secondary elevation late in systole. A similar contour is present during systole in the aortic pressure pulse. (From Braunwald, E., et al.: Idiopathic hypertrophic subaortic stenosis. Circulation *30*(Suppl. IV):67, 1964, by permission of the American Heart Association, Inc.)

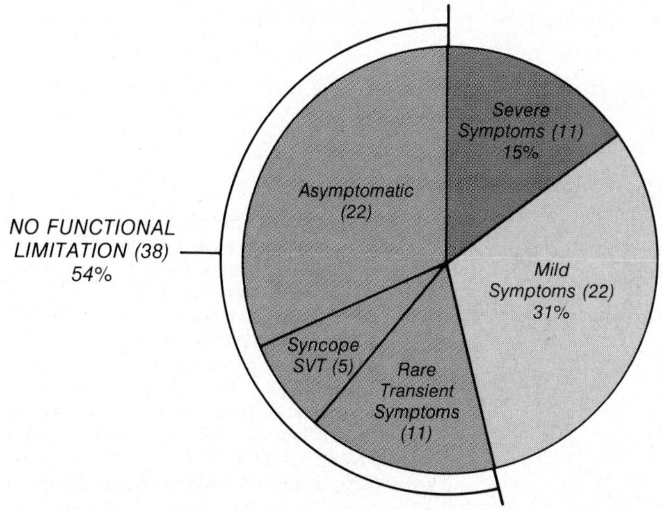

FIGURE 41–7 Functional state before sudden death or cardiac arrest in 71 patients with hypertrophic cardiomyopathy. SVT = supraventricular tachycardia. (From Maron, B. J., et al.: Sudden death in hypertrophic cardiomyopathy: A profile of 78 patients. Circulation *65*:1388, 1982, by permission of the American Heart Association, Inc.)

ischemia as a result of prolonged maintenance of wall tension with a concomitant slower-than-normal decrease in the impedance to coronary blood flow. As in patients with valvular aortic stenosis, syncope may result from an inability to increase cardiac output with exertion or from cardiac arrhythmias (p. 1099).[152] Near-syncopal ("graying out") spells that occur in the erect posture and that can be relieved by immediately lying down are common. However, in contrast to valvular aortic stenosis, syncope or near-syncope may not be an ominous finding in hypertrophic cardiomyopathy; some patients have a history of such episodes dating back many years without deterioration in the condition.[138]

Physical Examination. This may be normal in asymptomatic patients without gradients, save for a left ventricular lift and a loud fourth heart sound, but there are usually prominent findings in patients with a pressure gradient in the left ventricular outflow tract. The apical precordial impulse is often displaced laterally and is usually abnormally forceful and enlarged.[138,145] Because of decreased left ventricular compliance, a prominent presystolic apical impulse which results from forceful atrial systole is often present.[148] This may result in a double apical impulse as a result of the prominent *a* wave. A more characteristic but less frequently recognized abnormality is a triple apical beat, the third impulse being a late systolic bulge that occurs when the heart is nearly empty and is performing near-isometric contraction. These findings may be readily recorded by apexcardiography (Fig. 41–8).

A systolic thrill is commonly present, is most frequently palpable at the apex or along the lower left sternal border,[146] and bears only a rough relationship to the severity of the pressure gradient.[138,146] The jugular venous pulse usually demonstrates a prominent *a* wave, reflecting diminished right ventricular compliance secondary to the massive hypertrophy of the ventricular septum. The carotid pulse typically rises briskly and then declines in midsystole as the gradient develops, followed by a secondary rise. This may be well appreciated on physical examination and can be demonstrated more clearly by means of indirect pulse tracings (Figs. 41–8 and 41–9).

The first heart sound is normal and is often preceded by a fourth heart sound[138,146] that corresponds to the apical presystolic impulse.[145] The second heart sound is usually normally split. In some patients, however, it is narrowly split and in others, particularly those with severe outflow gradients, paradoxical splitting may be noted.[138,146] A third heart sound is common but does not have the same ominous significance as in patients with valvular aortic stenosis. Systolic ejection sounds are rare.[138] The auscultatory hallmark of HOCM is a systolic murmur (Fig. 41–8), which is typically harsh and crescendo-decrescendo in configuration; it often begins well after the first heart sound and is best heard between the apex and the left sternal border. It often radiates well to the lower sternal border, the axillae, and base of the heart but not into the neck vessels.[138,148] The murmur is often more holosystolic and blowing at the apex and in the axillae (probably due to mitral regurgitation) and midsystolic and harsher along the lower sternal border (due to flow across the outflow tract).[146,148]

The murmur is labile in intensity and duration, and a variety of maneuvers may be utilized to augment or suppress it (Table 41–6, p. 1409). The systolic murmur is due both to turbulence as the blood passes through the narrowed left ventricular outflow tract and to mitral regurgitation, which is invariably found when obstruction is present.[148] A diastolic rumbling murmur,[139] reflecting increased transmitral flow, may occur in patients with marked mitral regurgitation. The murmur of aortic regur-

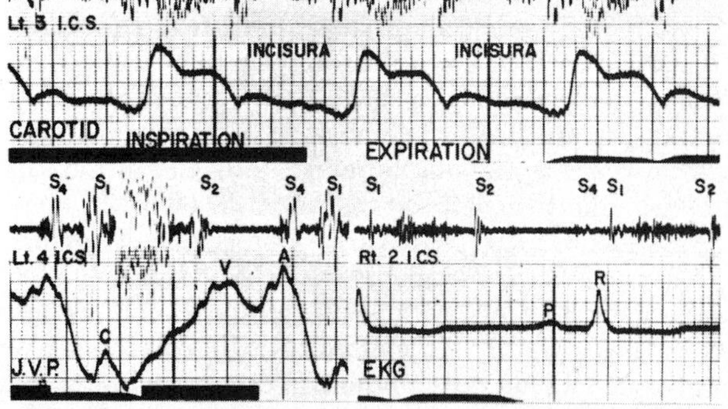

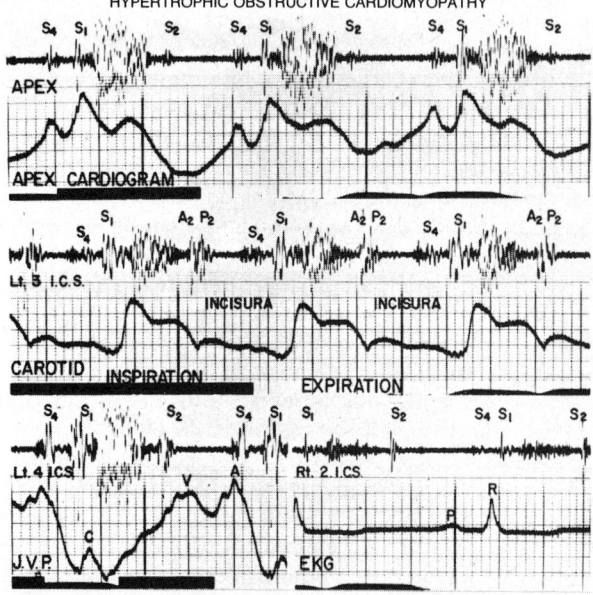

FIGURE 41–8 Phonocardiogram recorded at the apex, the third left intercostal space (Lt. 3 I.C.S.), the fourth left intercostal space (Lt. 4 I.C.S.), and the second right intercostal space (Rt. 2 I.C.S.). S_1 = first heart sound, S_2 = second heart sound, S_4 = fourth heart sound, J.V.P. = jugular venous pulse. Note the prominent S_4 and the presystolic expansion of the apexcardiogram, the prominent *a* wave of the J.V.P., and the rapid upstroke of the indirect carotid arterial pulse. The apexcardiogram exhibits early systolic collapse followed by late systolic expansion. The diamond-shaped midsystolic murmur is recorded best at the apex and is less prominent along the second right intercostal space. (From Braunwald, E., et al.: Idiopathic hypertrophic subaortic stenosis. Circulation *30*(Suppl. IV):14, 1964, by permission of the American Heart Association, Inc.)

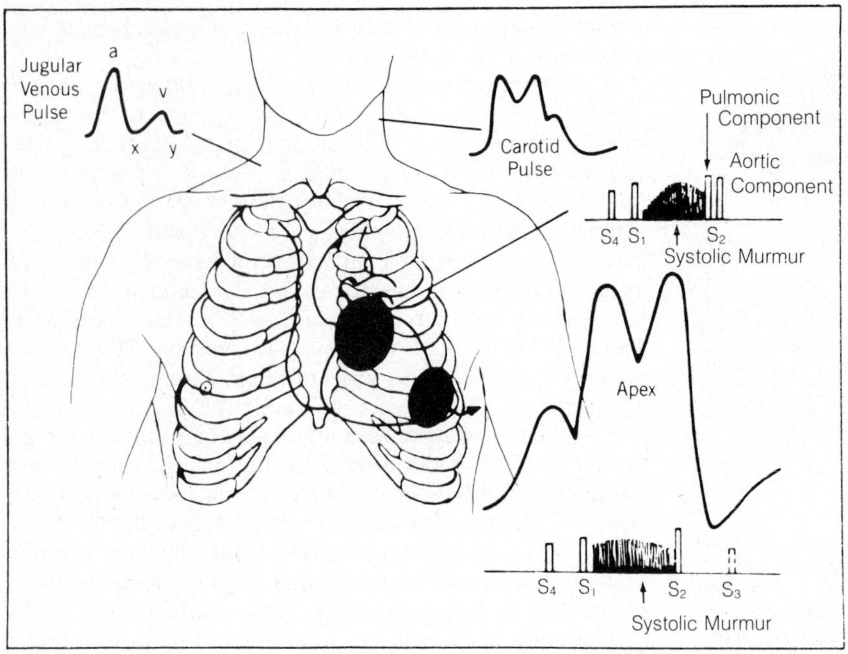

FIGURE 41–9 Salient physical signs of hypertrophic obstructive cardiomyopathy. Jugular venous pulse shows prominent *a* wave. Carotid pulse shows rapid rise and bifid pulse. Left ventricular apex shows prominent *a* wave and bifid systolic impulse. Auscultatory features are schematized. S_4 = fourth heart sound; S_1 = first heart sound; S_3 = third heart sound. (From Shah, P. M.: Newer concepts in hypertrophic obstructive cardiomyopathy II. J.A.M.A. *242*:1771, 1979. Copyright 1979, American Medical Association.)

gitation is observed only rarely in patients with HOCM, although it may develop after surgery to correct the outflow gradient[138,146] or following bacterial endocarditis.[153]

It is important to know the features of physical examination that permit differentiation of HOCM from fixed orifice obstruction, most commonly due to valvular aortic stenosis (Table 32–10, p. 1100). The character of the carotid pulse is the most useful feature in this regard. Because there is obstruction to left ventricular emptying from the beginning of systole with fixed valvular stenosis, the carotid upstroke is slowed and of low amplitude (pulsus parvus et tardus) (Fig. 3–22, p. 56, and Fig. 4–4, p. 70). With HOCM, initial ejection of blood from the left ventricle is unimpeded, and therefore the arterial upstroke is brisk. Other features that may be helpful but are of considerably less significance are the location of the murmur (it radiates along the carotid arteries in valvular aortic stenosis but not in HOCM), an ejection sound (present in patients with valvular aortic stenosis in the absence of calcification of the aortic valve and absent in HOCM), and the location of the systolic thrill (most prominent in the second right intercostal space in valvular aortic stenosis and in the fourth interspace along the left sternal border in HOCM).

ELECTROCARDIOGRAM. This is usually abnormal in hypertrophic cardiomyopathy and invariably so in symptomatic patients with left ventricular outflow gradients[153a] (Fig. 41–10). Normal electrocardiograms are seen in only one-fourth of asymptomatic patients without gradients.[138,154] The most common abnormalities are ST-segment and T-wave abnormalities, followed by evidence of left ventricular hypertrophy, with QRS complexes that are tallest in the midprecordial leads.[154,155,155a] There may be progressive electrocardiographic evidence of hypertrophy over time.[155b] Prominent, abnormal Q waves are relatively common, occurring in 20 to 50 percent of patients.[146,148] The Q-wave abnormalities often involve the inferior (II, III, aV_f) and/or lateral (V_4–V_6) leads (Fig. 41–10). They appear to be due to depolarization of myopathic cells in the septum that have abnormal electrophysiological properties.[156] A variety of other electrocardiographic abnormalities may occur, including abnormal electrical axis (usually left-axis deviation) and P-wave abnormalities (usually left atrial enlargement). Accessory atrioventricular pathways have been found in hypertrophic cardiomyopathy, although they appear to be rare. A short P-R interval followed by slurring of a tall R wave with normal QRS duration is a relatively frequent finding;[138] in many cases this appears to be unassociated with evidence of preexcitation.[157] Clinically significant abnormalities of AV conduction are unusual, but disturbances of AV nodal electrophysiology are surprisingly common in the small number of patients who have undergone electrophysiological study.[158,159] The electrophysiological abnormalities may be subtle manifestations of the fibrotic and cystic changes that have been found at necropsy in the conducting system of patients with HOCM.[160]

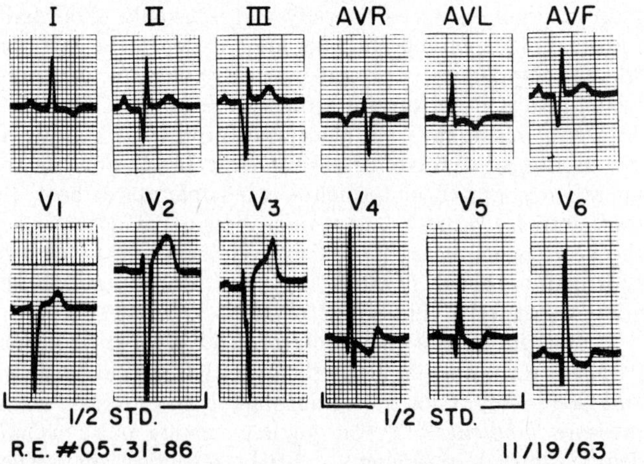

FIGURE 41–10 Electrocardiogram showing abnormal Q waves in leads II, III, aV_F, V_5, and V_6 in a patient with HOCM. Precordial leads exhibit the voltage criteria for left ventricular hypertrophy. (From Braunwald, E., et al.: Idiopathic hypertrophic subaortic stenosis. Circulation *30*(Suppl. IV):26, 1964, by permission of the American Heart Association, Inc.)

Although a hemodynamic mechanism may play a role in the demise of patients with hypertrophic cardiomyopathy, many and perhaps most deaths, particularly those that are known to have been sudden, are probably due to an arrhythmia. Because of the systolic and diastolic abnormalities in this disorder, rhythm disturbances are less well tolerated.

Ventricular arrhythmias are common in patients with hypertrophic cardiomyopathy, occurring in over three-fourths of patients undergoing continuous ambulatory electrocardiographic monitoring.[161,162] Ventricular tachycardia is found in about one-fourth of the patients studied, and in some it is a harbinger of subsequent sudden death.[161,162a] A similar spectrum of arrhythmias may be detected in those asymptomatic relatives of patients with hypertrophic cardiomyopathy who themselves have the disease (often undiagnosed).[163] Treadmill testing may expose arrhythmias that are not present at rest, although continuous ambulatory monitoring is superior in detecting repetitive ventricular tachyarrhythmias.[162,164] Supraventricular tachycardia may be found in one-fourth of patients.[165] Atrial fibrillation occurs in 5 to 10 per cent of patients, and the resultant loss of the atrial contribution to the filling of a hypertrophied, stiff ventricle may result in marked clinical deterioration—as a consequence of a reduction in cardiac output or elevation of the left atrial pressure or both.[146,148]

CHEST ROENTGENOGRAM. The findings on radiographic examination are variable; heart size, principally the left ventricle, may range from normal to markedly enlarged, but there is little correlation between heart size and the severity of the outflow tract gradient. Left atrial enlargement is frequently observed, especially when significant mitral regurgitation is present.[138,145,148] Aortic root enlargement and valvular calcification are not seen unless associated diseases are present, although calcification of the mitral annulus is common in HOCM.[166]

ECHOCARDIOGRAPHY (see also p. 128). Because echocardiography combines the attributes of high resolution and no known risk, it has been widely utilized in the evaluation of hypertrophic cardiomyopathy,[100,167–169] (Fig. 41–11, Fig. 5–36, p. 108, and Figs. 5–69 to 5–71, pp. 128 and 129). It is useful in the study of patients with suspected hypertrophic cardiomyopathy and also in the screening of relatives of patients with documented HOCM. The echocardiogram is of value in identifying and quantifying morphological (e.g., asymmetrical septal hypertrophy) as well as functional features (e.g., hypercontractile left ventricle).

The cardinal echocardiographic feature of hypertrophic cardiomyopathy is left ventricular hypertrophy. Maximal hypertrophy of the septum often occurs midway between the base and apex of the left ventricle. The finding of a thickened septum that is 1.3 or more times the thickness of the posterior wall when measured in diastole just prior to atrial systole has been the time-honored criterion for the diagnosis of asymmetrical septal hypertrophy (ASH).[100,170] The septum not only is relatively thicker than the posterior wall but is typically at least 15 mm in thickness (normal $\leq$ 11 mm). Approximately half the first-degree relatives of patients with hypertrophic cardiomyopathy will have such an abnormal septal/free wall ratio, despite the fact that they are often asymptomatic, have normal physical examinations, and are often unaware of any cardiac disease.[94] In patients with concentric left ventricular hypertrophy (due to systemic hypertension or aortic valve disease, for example), the septal/free wall ratio will often be close to 1:1,[171] although it has been reported on the basis of M-mode echocardiograms that many such patients will have ASH.[172,173] The use of a septal/free wall ratio of 1.5:1 may be more specific for hypertrophic cardiomyopathy, although some patients with HOCM will not be identified.[174]

M-mode echocardiography will not always provide accurate measurements of true septal thickness, however. In many cases in which the M-mode echocardiogram falsely suggests ASH, the finding is due to oblique imaging of an acutely anteriorly angled interventricular septum.[175] Two-dimensional echocardiography should be used to clarify septal orientation and thickness in such questionable or equivocal cases, although optimally it should be part of the routine examination of all patients with hypertrophic cardiomyopathy. Two-dimensional echocardiography is also useful for identifying patients with localized hypertrophy in unusual locations not accessible to the M-mode beam such as the posterior or apical septum, the anterior or lateral left ventricular free wall,[113] and the apex.[114,115] An unusual echocardiographic pattern consisting of a ground-glass appearance has been noted in portions of the hypertrophied myocardium in HOCM. It has been speculated

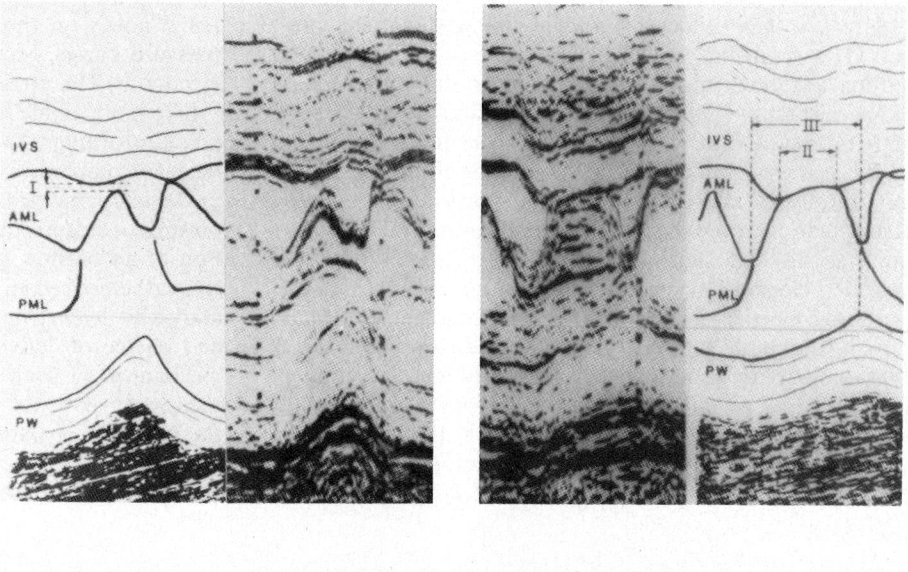

FIGURE 41–11 Determination of degree of systolic anterior motion of mitral valve. *Left,* Echocardiogram and line diagram from a patient with moderate systolic anterior motion. *Right* , A patient with severe systolic anterior motion. PML = posterior mitral leaflet; AML = anterior mitral leaflet; IVS = interventricular septum; PW = posterior left ventricular wall. (From Gilbert, B. W., et al.: Hypertrophic cardiomyopathy: Subclassification by M mode echocardiography. Am. J. Cardiol. *45*:861, 1980.)

that this pattern may be related to the abnormal cellular architecture and myocardial fibrosis that has been noted in pathological studies.[95] Two-dimensional echocardiograms in HOCM have suggested, in concordance with autopsy specimens, that the interventricular septum is configured in the shape of a catenoid, i.e., a curved surface with net zero curvature at all points.[176]

A second echocardiographic feature often found in hypertrophic cardiomyopathy in addition to ASH is narrowing of the left ventricular outflow tract, which is formed by the interventricular septum anteriorly and the anterior leaflet of the mitral valve posteriorly. The mitral valve apparatus is positioned abnormally close to the septum,[167] possibly the result of the posterior bulging of the septum. When hypertrophic cardiomyopathy is associated with a pressure gradient, there is abnormal systolic anterior motion (SAM) of the anterior leaflet of the mitral valve (Fig. 41–11).[167] Although the role of SAM in *producing* the gradient is controversial, there is a close relationship between the degree of SAM and the size of the outflow gradient.[177,178] Prolonged interventricular septal contact of the mitral apparatus is limited to hypertrophic cardiomyopathy with resting pressure gradients,[179] and there is a close temporal relationship between the onset of the pressure gradient and the onset of septal apposition of the mitral apparatus.[180]

Three explanations have been offered for SAM: (1) the mitral valve is *pulled* against the septum by contraction of the papillary muscles, because of the abnormal location and orientation of these muscles resulting from septal hypertrophy; (2) the mitral valve is *pushed* against the septum because of its abnormal position in the outflow tract;[181] (3) the mitral valve is drawn toward the septum because of the lower pressure that occurs as blood is ejected at a high velocity through a narrowed outflow tract (Venturi effect).[148] However, contrary to initial reports, SAM of the mitral valve and dynamic left ventricular gradients are not pathognomonic of HOCM but may be found in a variety of other conditions,[101,102] including hypercontractile states, left ventricular hypertrophy, transposition of the great arteries, and infiltration of the septum.[101,102,182–185] In many cases in conditions other than HOCM, SAM is due to buckling of the chordae tendineae rather than to movement of the anterior mitral valve leaflet as occurs in HOCM (although the chordae tendineae and papillary muscles may contribute to SAM in HOCM).[186]

Several other echocardiographic findings may be present: (1) a small left ventricular cavity;[187] (2) reduced septal motion and thickening during systole (presumably because of the disarray of the myofibrillar architecture and abnormal contractile function);[167] (3) normal or increased motion of the posterior wall; (4) a reduced rate of closure of the mitral valve in mid-diastole secondary to a decrease in left ventricular compliance[187] or abnormal transmitral flow during diastole;[188] (5) mitral valve prolapse;[189] and (6) partial systolic closure or, more commonly, coarse systolic fluttering of the aortic valve related to turbulent blood flow in the outflow tract.[190] The echocardiographic findings that accompany a left ventricular outflow tract gradient (SAM and aortic valve partial closure) may be quite labile, and provocative measures such as the Valsalva maneuver or pharmacologically induced vasodilatation with amyl nitrite (Fig. 3–23, p. 56), stimulation of contractility with isoproterenol, or an induced premature ventricular contraction may be required to precipitate the findings.[178]

Abnormalities of diastolic function may be shown by echocardiography in many patients with hypertrophic cardiomyopathy, independent of the presence or absence of a systolic pressure gradient. The isovolumetric relaxation time, measured from aortic valve closure to mitral valve opening, is frequently prolonged and the peak velocity of left ventricular filling is reduced.[191,192] Because the septum is typically hypokinetic, the rate of left ventricular filling is determined primarily by the rate of free wall thinning.[191]

RADIONUCLIDE SCANNING TECHNIQUES. These techniques are gaining popularity in the detection of hypertrophic cardiomyopathy. Thallium-201 myocardial imaging permits direct determination of the relative thicknesses of the septum and free wall and may be of particular value when technical constraints limit the reliability of echocardiographic evaluation in a given patient with presumed HOCM.[193] The utility of rest and exercise thallium-201 scintigraphy in identifying patients with hypertrophic cardiomyopathy whose angina pectoris is due to obstructive epicardial coronary artery disease is controversial;[194,195] at least in some patients, thallium-201 defects suggestive of regional myocardial ischemia are found despite angiographically normal coronary arteries.[194] Gated radionuclide ventriculography with blood pool labeling permits the evaluation of not only the size but also the motion of the septum and left ventricle.[196] Disproportionate upper septal thickening is a distinctive scintigraphic feature that may be seen in the steep left anterior oblique view.[196] As with the echocardiogram, abnormal diastolic filling of the ventricle has been observed in patients with hypertrophic cardiomyopathy (both with and without gradients) by computer analysis of the blood pool scan.[197]

Hemodynamics

Cardiac catheterization discloses diminished diastolic left ventricular compliance and a pressure gradient within the body of the left ventricle, which is separated from a subaortic chamber by the thickened septum and the anterior leaflet of the mitral valve that abuts the septum (Figs. 41–6 and 41–12). The pressure gradient may be quite labile and may vary between 0 and 175 mm Hg. There is often a notch on the ascending limb of the left ventricular pressure curve, occurring at the onset of left ventricular ejection.[138] The arterial pressure tracing may demonstrate a "spike and dome" configuration similar to the carotid pulse recording. As a consequence of diminished left ventricular compliance, the mean and particularly the *a* wave in the left atrial pressure pulse and the left ventricular end-diastolic pressures are usually elevated.[138] Artifact stimulation of an outflow gradient may occur if the left ventricular catheter becomes entrapped in the trabeculae of a markedly hypertrophied left ventricle.[148] Proper technique and choice of catheters with side holes should clarify the mechanism of such gradients. Cardiac output may be depressed in patients with longstanding severe gradients. In the majority of patients it is normal; occasionally it is elevated.

Hemodynamic abnormalities in hypertrophic cardiomy-

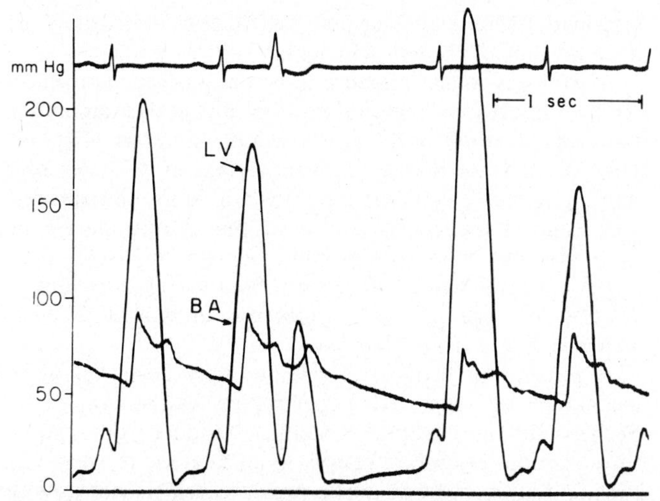

FIGURE 41–12 Simultaneous pressures recorded in the left ventricle (LV) and brachial artery (BA) in a patient with HOCM. During the postpremature contraction beat, the pulse pressure in the brachial artery is less than in the control beats. (From Braunwald, E., et al.: Idiopathic hypertrophic subaortic stenosis. Circulation *30*(Suppl. IV):78, 1964, by permission of the American Heart Association, Inc.)

opathy are not limited to the left heart. Approximately one-fourth of patients demonstrate pulmonary hypertension, which is usually mild but occasionally may be moderate to severe. This may be due to elevated mean left atrial pressures. A pressure gradient in the right ventricular outflow tract is seen in approximately 15 per cent of patients who have obstruction to left ventricular outflow[138,146] and appears to result from muscular contraction of the infundibulum. Right atrial and right ventricular end-diastolic pressures may be slightly elevated.

Angiocardiography. Left ventriculography shows a hypertrophied ventricle in which the anterior leaflet of the mitral valve moves anteriorly during systole and encroaches upon the outflow tract (Fig. 41–13). Associated with this motion of the leaflet is mitral regurgitation, which appears to be a constant finding in patients with gradients.[148] The left ventricular cavity is often small, and systolic ejection is typically vigorous, resulting in virtual obliteration of the cavity at end systole, although reduced afterload (end-systolic wall stress) may be related to the apparent hypercontractile state.[198,199] The papillary muscles are often prominent and may fill the left ventricular cavity in late systole. In some cases, the hypertrophy of the papillary muscles and midventricular myocardium may result in true muscular stenosis owing to a sphincter mechanism.[200]

It is often helpful to supplement angiographic evaluation of the left ventricle with simultaneous right ventriculography in a cranially angulated LAO projection in order to obtain optimal visualization of the size, shape, and configuration of the interventricular septum[201] (Fig. 41–14). The hypertrophy appears maximal in the lower portion of the

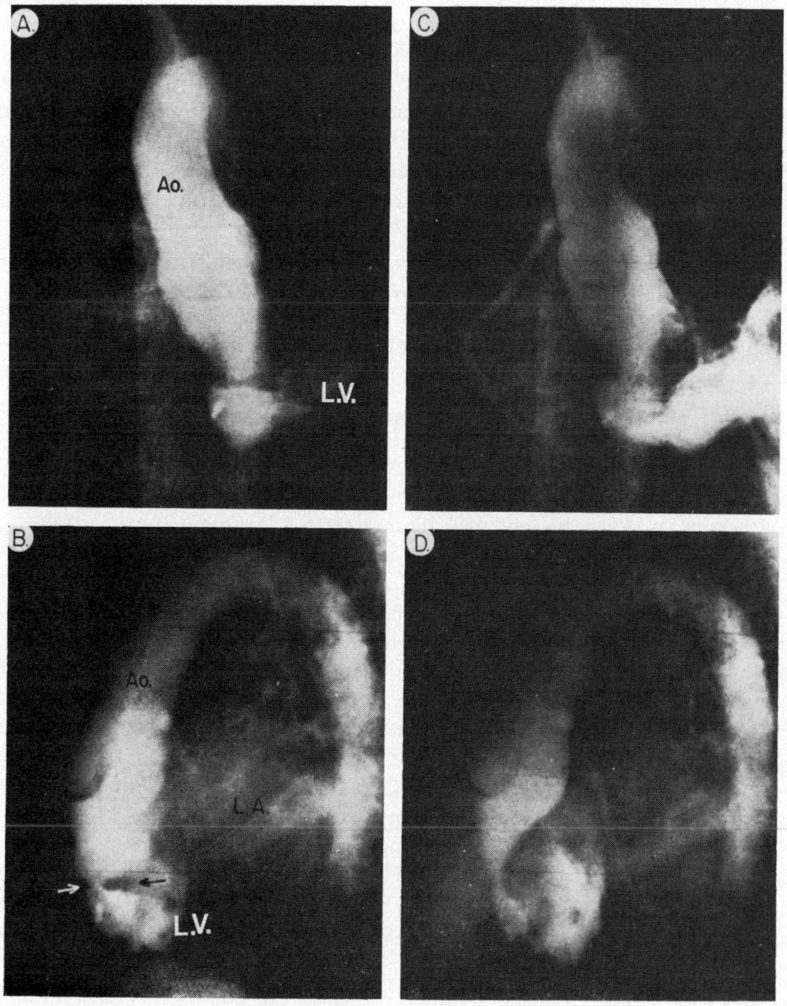

FIGURE 41–13 Angiograms showing obstruction in a patient with familial HOCM. Films were obtained during selective left ventricular angiography, in the frontal (*A* and *C*) and lateral (*B* and *D*) projections. During systole (*A* and *B*), a linear area of narrowing is apparent (arrows), which lies at the point where the hypertrophied septum impinges on the closed anterior leaflet of the mitral valve. Films exposed in diastole (*C* and *D*) also reveal the site of the mitral valve leaflet. Ao. = aorta, L.A. = left atrium, L.V. = left ventricle. (From Ross, J., Jr., Braunwald, E., Gault, J. H., Mason, D. T., and Morrow, A. G.: The mechanism of the intraventricular pressure gradient in idiopathic hypertrophic subaortic stenosis. Circulation *34*:558, 1966, by permission of the American Heart Association, Inc.)

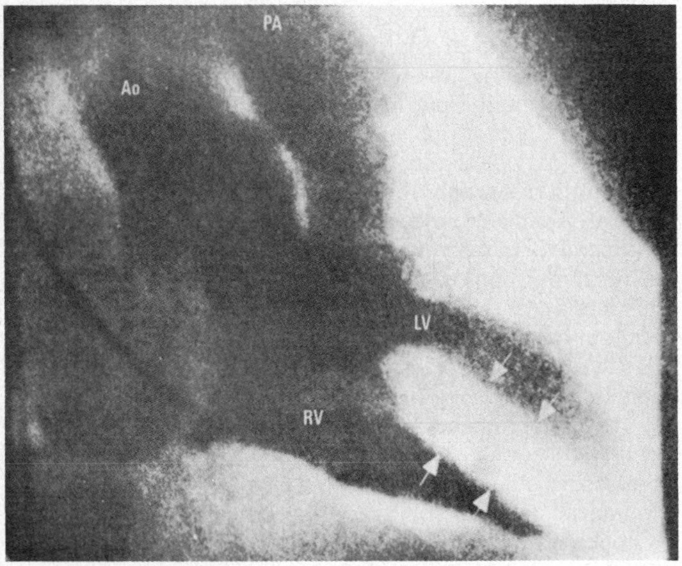

FIGURE 41–14 Right anterior oblique angiocardiogram showing HOCM. Selected systolic cine frame with simultaneous injection of contrast media into both right (RV) and left (LV) ventricles demonstrates the massive hypertrophy of the interventricular septum (arrows). The aorta (Ao) and pulmonary artery (PA) are simultaneously opacified. (From Van Houten, F. X., et al.: Radiology of valvular heart disease. *In* Sonnenblick, E. H., and Lesch, M. (eds.): Valvular Heart Disease. New York, 1974, p. 42, by permission of Grune and Stratton.)

septum, giving it a characteristic triangular appearance.[202] The left septal surface either is flat or bulges into the left ventricular cavity at its mid or lower portion, in contrast to the normal findings of the septum curving toward the right ventricle.[201]

In patients over 45 years of age, coronary artery obstructive disease is rather common, although the symptoms of ischemic pain are indistinguishable from those of patients with normal coronary angiograms and hypertrophic cardiomyopathy.[203] The left anterior descending[204] and septal perforator coronary arteries may demonstrate phasic narrowing during systole in the absence of fixed obstructive lesions.[205]

LABILITY OF GRADIENT

A feature characteristic of HOCM already referred to is the variability and lability of the left ventricular outflow gradient. A given patient may demonstrate a large outflow gradient on one occasion but have none at another time. In some patients without a resting gradient, it may be temporarily provoked.[178,206] Three basic mechanisms are involved in the production of dynamic gradients, all of which act by reducing ventricular volume and presumably accentuate the apposition of the anterior mitral leaflet against the septum: (1) increased contractility, (2) decreased preload, and (3) decreased afterload.[138,206] In a minority of patients with HOCM, the gradient is midventricular[200] and may be intensified by increased contractility, which exerts a direct muscular sphincteric action. The stimuli that provoke or intensify left ventricular outflow tract gradients in HOCM generally improve myocardial performance in normal subjects and in patients with most forms of heart disease[145] (Fig. 41–15). Conversely, reductions in contractility or increases in preload or afterload, which increase left ventricular dimensions, reduce or abolish the left ventricular outflow gradient.

Alterations in the magnitude of the gradient are reflected by changes in the findings on physical examination, noninvasive tests, and catheterization findings (Fig. 41–16). An increase in the gradient results in a louder murmur, a longer ejection period with a more characteristic spike and dome configuration in the carotid pulse, and more flagrant echocardiographic evidence of SAM of the anterior mitral leaflet. *It is this dynamic characteristic of HOCM that distinguishes it from the discrete forms of obstruction to ventricular outflow.*

A number of bedside procedures may be useful in the evaluation of suspected hypertrophic cardiomyopathy.[207] Perhaps the most helpful is sudden standing from a squatting position. Squatting results in an increase in venous return and an increase in aortic pressure, which increases the ventricular volume, diminishing the gradient and decreasing the intensity of the murmur. Sudden standing has the opposite effects and results in accentuation of the gradient and the murmur. The Valsalva maneuver is another useful bedside technique for eliciting or exacerbating the gradient, (Table 41–6 and Fig. 41–16). Following a transient increase in arterial pressure that usually lasts for four or five cardiac cycles after the onset of the strain coincident with an increase in heart rate, the arterial systolic and pulse pressures and ventricular volume decline, and the gradient (and murmur) increase. Following release of the strain, there is a compensatory overshoot of arterial pressure and venous return and cardiac slowing, all of which increase ventricular volume and reduce the magnitude of the gradient and the murmur.[207] In occasional patients, there may be paradoxical attenuation of the systolic murmur despite an increase in the pressure gradient.[208] The Mueller maneuver, i.e., deep inspiration against a closed glottis (the opposite of the Valsalva maneuver), results in the *lessening* of dynamic obstruction to left ventricular outflow.[209] Inhalation of amyl nitrite also intensifies the murmur and the abnormality of the arterial pulse (Fig. 3–23, p. 56).

One of the most potent stimuli for enhancing the gradient is *postextrasystolic potentiation* (p. 437), which may occur following a spontaneous premature contraction or be induced by mechanical stimulation with a catheter or an external precordial mechanical stimulator.[145,178] The resultant increase in contractility in the beat following the extrasystole is so marked that it outweighs the otherwise salutary effect of increased ventricular filling caused by the compensatory pause and produces an increase in the gradient and murmur. A characteristic change often occurs in the directly recorded arterial pressure tracing, which, in addition to displaying a more marked spike and dome configuration, exhibits a pulse pressure that fails to increase as expected or actually decreases (Fig. 41–12). This is one of the most reliable signs of dynamic obstruction of the left ventricular outflow tract.[210]

Digitalis glycosides and the beta-adrenergic agonist isoproterenol result in an increase in the gradient, since they increase myocardial contractility, while nitroglycerin and amyl nitrite exaggerate the gradient by decreasing arterial pressure and ventricular volume.[138,145] Hypovolemia (as a result of hemorrhage or overly aggressive diuresis) may also provoke overt obstruction to left ventricular outflow.

FIGURE 41–15 *Top,* Simultaneous pressures recorded in the left ventricle (L.V.) and brachial artery (B.A.) before and immediately after the injection of 2 μg of isoproterenol. The broken lines indicate the fall in the brachial artery pressure and the simultaneous elevation of the left ventricular systolic pressure. (From Braunwald, E., et al.: Idiopathic hypertrophic subaortic stenosis. Circulation *30*(Suppl. IV):87, 1964, by permission of the American Heart Association, Inc.)
Bottom, Effects of 2 mg of methoxamine in a patient with HOCM. *A,* Simultaneous left ventricular (LV) and brachial artery (BA) pressure pulses prior to the injection, showing a large pressure gradient. *B,* Continuous recording at a slow paper speed immediately after the injection, as the gradient gradually disappeared. *C,* Absence of a pressure gradient during the full effect of methoxamine. Note also that as the gradient disappeared, the brachial arterial pressure pulse became more normal and less characteristic of HOCM than it was prior to methoxamine administration (*A*). (From Braunwald, E., et al.: Idiopathic hypertrophic subaortic stenosis. Circulation *30*(Suppl. IV):91, 1964, by permission of the American Heart Association, Inc.)

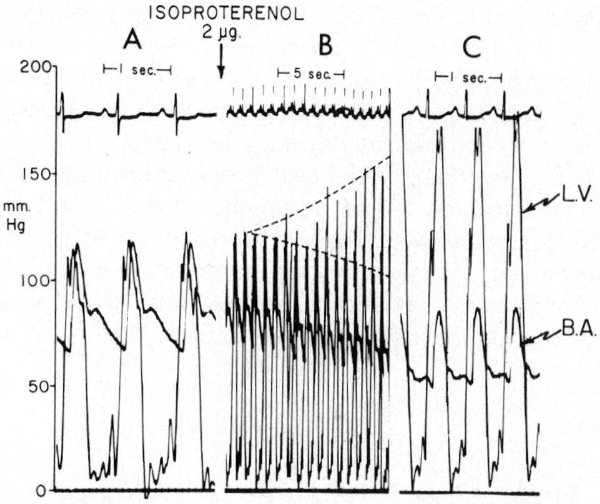

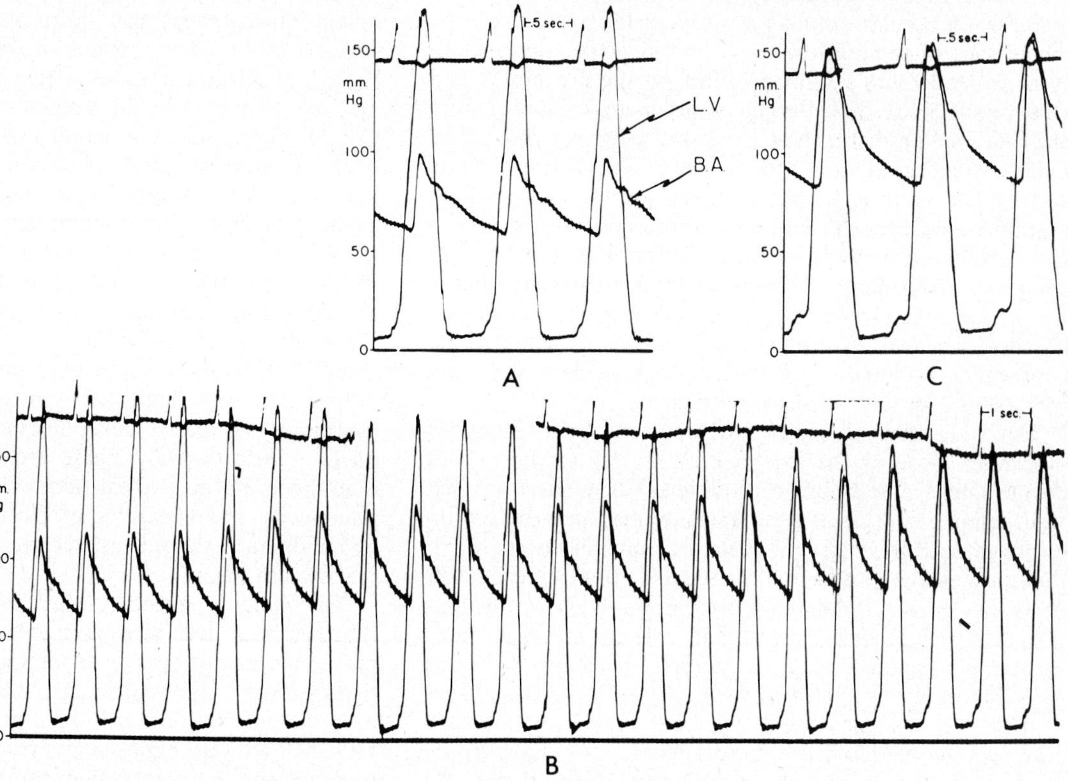

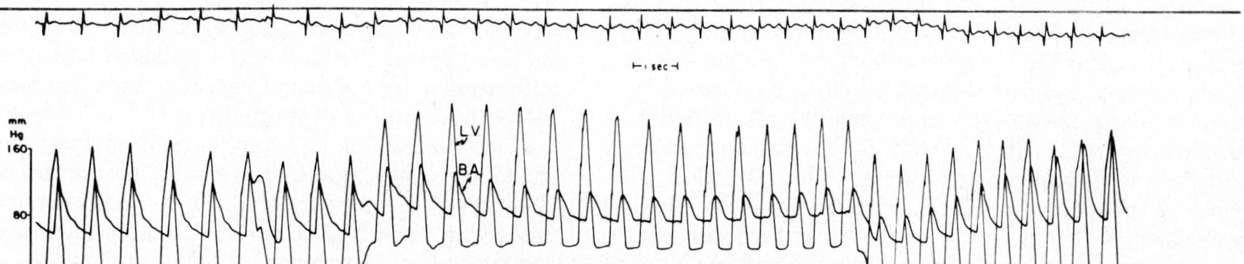

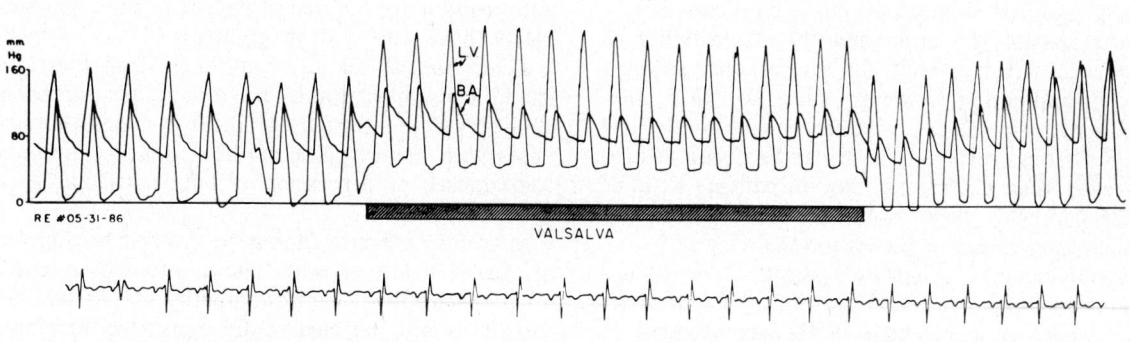

FIGURE 41–16 Effect of the Valsalva maneuver on simultaneous pressures recorded in the left ventricle (LV) and brachial artery (BA) of a patient with HOCM. Note that during the Valsalva maneuver a striking increase in the pressure gradient occurs, which diminishes following release of the Valsalva maneuver. (From Braunwald, E., et al.: Idiopathic hypertrophic subaortic stenosis. Circulation *30*(Suppl. IV):100, 1964, by permission of the American Heart Association, Inc.)

The intensity of the murmur and the left ventricular outflow gradient may be decreased by beta-adrenergic blockade, although the effect is often not dramatic and is of most hemodynamic benefit in protecting against the *increase* in the gradient that may be provoked by exercise. It has also been suggested that propranolol may exert a beneficial effect on diastolic compliance and result in an improvement in myocardial distensibility.[211] In most patients the severity of mitral regurgitation and the intensity of the apical blowing regurgitant murmur vary with the degree of obstruction of left ventricular outflow.[148,207]

TREATMENT

Interventions that decrease ventricular contractility or increase ventricular volume, systemic arterial pressure, the dimensions of the outflow tract, or ventricular distensibility in general exert a salutary effect on the symptoms and vice versa. Since digitalis glycosides increase contractility and thus the gradient, these drugs are generally proscribed unless atrial fibrillation with a very rapid ventricular rate and/or left ventricular dilatation and dysfunction without a gradient are present. Similarly, nitrates and beta-adrenergic stimulants are best avoided. Dyspnea is a prominent symptom in patients with hypertrophic cardiomyopathy but is not usually due to systolic dysfunction, and diuretics should be used sparingly, if at all, since reduction of intravascular volume may reduce ventricular size and increase the systolic pressure gradient.

The mainstay of medical therapy is beta-adrenergic blockade; most of the experience to date has been with propranolol. In addition to possible salutary effects on left ventricular compliance, beta blockade may prevent the increase in outflow obstruction that accompanies exercise, although resting gradients are largely unchanged.[9,212] It decreases the determinants of myocardial oxygen consumption and thus angina pectoris, and perhaps exerts an antiarrhythmic action.[9] Angina pectoris generally responds more favorably to treatment with a beta blocker than does dyspnea.[9] It has also been suggested that beta blockade may prevent sudden death, but its efficacy for this purpose has not been established.[9] Propranolol also blunts the chronotropic response, thus limiting the demand for increased myocardial oxygen delivery.[144a] Beta-adrenergic blockade may also have a beneficial effect on diastolic ventricular filling possibly by improving the distensibility of the left ventricle.[214] The overall clinical response to beta blockade is disappointing, however, since less than one-third of patients experience sustained symptomatic improvement.[131,215] It is reasonable to try large doses of propranolol (greater than 320 mg per day) in patients without contraindications who have not experienced adequate symptomatic improvement with conventional doses.[216]

The calcium-channel blocking agents, principally verapamil and nifedipine, are an increasingly popular alternative to beta-adrenergic blockade in the management of hypertrophic cardiomyopathy. Both the hypercontractile systolic function and the abnormalities of diastolic filling may be related to abnormal calcium kinetics, and drugs that block the inward transport of calcium across the myocardial cell membrane may be able to rectify both abnormalities.

Verapamil has been the most widely studied calcium-channel blocking agent in this condition. Its use was suggested, at least in part, by the observation that it produces a protective and beneficial effect in the hereditary cardiomyopathy of the Syrian hamster, a condition marked by intracellular calcium overload, in which propranolol is ineffective.[217] Although the vasodilator effects of verapamil should not be helpful in HOCM, it appears that by depressing myocardial contractility, verapamil can decrease the left ventricular outflow gradient when given intravenously or orally.[218–220,220a] Perhaps more important from a symptomatic point of view, verapamil improves diastolic filling in hypertrophic cardiomyopathy.[197,221,221a] While variable clinical responses have been reported with verapamil, some patients show increased exercise capacity and an improved symptomatic status.[220] Sustained symptomatic improvement has been noted with the long-term administration of verapamil in ambulatory patients,[222] although important adverse effects, including sudden death, may be seen in a small fraction of patients so treated.[223] Complications with verapamil include suppression of sinus node automaticity and inhibition of atrioventricular conduction, vasodilatation, and negative inotropic effects. These side effects may culminate in hypotension, pulmonary edema, and death; there is a suggestion that antiarrhythmic agents, especially quinidine, may exacerbate the deleterious hemodynamic effects of verapamil.[223] Because of these adverse effects, it has been suggested that verapamil should not be used, or be used only with extreme caution, in patients with high left ventricular filling pressure or symptoms of paroxysmal nocturnal dyspnea or orthopnea.[223] Unfortunately, these are usually precisely the patients who are in greatest need of therapy. In addition, patients with abnormalities of electrical impulse generation or conduction should not receive verapamil unless a pacemaker is in place.

Nifedipine is another calcium-channel blocking agent that has been used in hypertrophic cardiomyopathy, and it may have advantages over verapamil, since it causes less depression of atrioventricular conduction, although it is a more potent vasodilator.[136] It improves diastolic function in HOCM without depressing systolic function, apparently by increasing left ventricular compliance.[136] Nifedipine may also improve the chest pain associated with hypertrophic cardiomyopathy.[224] Combined administration of nifedipine and propranolol may be of benefit in some patients, particularly those with outflow gradients.[225]

Disopyramide, an antiarrhythmic drug that alters calcium kinetics, has produced symptomatic improvement and abolition of the pressure gradient in a small number of patients with hypertrophic cardiomyopathy, presumably as a consequence of depression of left ventricular systolic performance.[226]

Strenuous exercise should be avoided because of the risk of sudden death; it is the major cause of a fatal outcome in hypertrophic cardiomyopathy.[215] Atrial fibrillation should usually be electrically converted to sinus rhythm without delay because of the often catastrophic hemodynamic consequences of the loss of the atrial contribution to ventricular filling in this disorder. Infective endocarditis may occur in as many as 9 per cent of patients,[146,227,228] and antibiotic prophylaxis is indicated.[229] The infection usually occurs on the aortic valve or mitral apparatus, on the endocardium, or at the site of the contact lesion on the septum; thus, chronic endocardial trauma may provide a nidus for subsequent infection.[228] Anticoagulants should be given to patients with chronic atrial fibrillation when no contraindication exists.

Surgical Treatment

A variety of surgical procedures aimed at reducing the outflow gradient have been developed and are most commonly utilized in the markedly symptomatic patient who has not responded well to medical management. The most popular operation for HOCM consists of excising a portion of the hypertrophied septum (Fig. 41–17). A transaortic approach with septal myotomy-myectomy[230,231] is probably the most widely utilized procedure, although left transventricular[232] as well as combined transaortic and left ventricular approaches[233] have also been employed successfully. Operation often relieves the obstruction as well as the mitral regurgitation, although even when performed by surgeons experienced with this procedure, operative mortality is in the range of 5 to 10 per cent.[9,131,234–236] Even patients over the age of 65 years have undergone successful surgery, with benefits and risks comparable to those of younger adults.[237] Since symptoms are not closely correlated with the presence or magnitude of the pressure gradient, it is possible that the operation produces beneficial effects aside from the reduction in outflow gradient. Although replacement of the mitral valve has been advocated,[238] myotomy-myectomy alone is usually adequate and remains the surgical procedure of choice.[207,234,238a] Surgery results in improved exercise capacity with an increase in the peak exercise cardiac output.[239] Furthermore, septal myotomy-myectomy does not produce important impairment of global left ventricular function at rest or during exercise.[240]

Natural History

The clinical course in hypertrophic cardiomyopathy is varied, although in most patients symptoms remain stable or even improve over a period of 5 to 10 years.[146,215] The

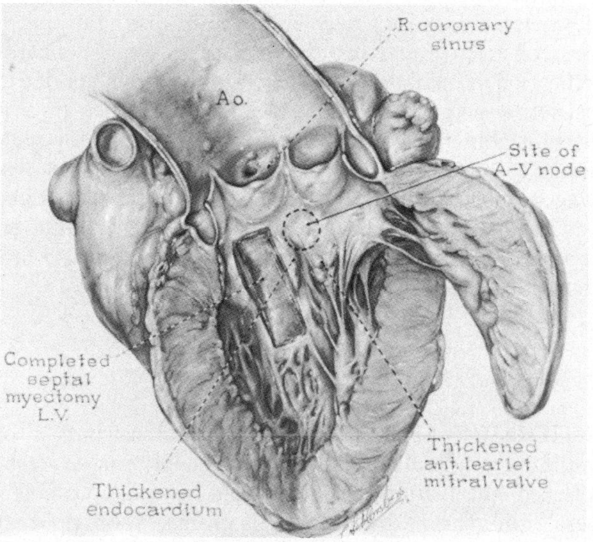

FIGURE 41–17 Appearance of the left ventricle after septal myotomy-myectomy. Ao = aorta. (From Morrow, A. G.: Hypertrophic subaortic stenosis. Operative methods utilized to relieve left ventricular outflow obstruction. J. Thorac. Cardiovasc. Surg. *76*:423, 1978.)

annual attrition is about 4 per cent a year, and clinical deterioration (aside from sudden death) is usually slow. Although symptoms are unrelated to the severity or even the presence of a gradient, the percentage of severely symptomatic patients does increase with age.[24,146,215] The onset of atrial fibrillation usually leads to a striking increase in symptoms, and prompt cardioversion is usually indicated.[24] Pregnancy appears to be well tolerated.[241,242]

Progression of HOCM to left ventricular dilatation and dysfunction without a gradient, i.e., dilated cardiomyopathy, is an interesting, serious, but unusual occurrence.[215,243] It usually takes place either after prior surgical resection of the septum[243,244] or as a consequence of myocardial infarction.[150,245] In patients with infarction, the extramural coronary arteries may be normal. Extensive areas of the myocardium may be scarred, resulting in left ventricular dilatation.[150]

Death is usually sudden in HOCM and may occur in previously asymptomatic patients, in individuals who were unaware they had the disease, or in patients with an otherwise stable course.[24,146,215,246,247] Paradoxically, younger patients, those without functional limitation, and those with mild or no gradients appear to be at particular risk of sudden death.[147,248] There is a subgroup of patients with hypertrophic cardiomyopathy in whose families premature death is unusually frequent.[247] Even individuals without such "malignant" family histories are at risk of sudden death. No specific clinical feature (other than a family history of sudden death due to hypertrophic cardiomyopathy and young age) appears to identify patients at risk of sudden death,[248] although it has been suggested that a history of syncope and severe dyspnea may be more common in patients at risk of sudden death.[249] Sudden death often occurs during exercise, and strenuous exertion should probably be proscribed in all patients with HOCM whether or not symptoms are prominent, although the risk of sudden death appears to decrease above the age of 40 years.[147,248] Unsuspected hypertrophic cardiomyopathy is the most common abnormality found at autopsy in young competitive athletes who die suddenly.[250]

It is presumed, but not established, that sudden death is due to a ventricular arrhythmia, although atrial arrhythmias may play a role in sensitizing the heart so that ventricular arrhythmias appear subsequently.[147] The protective effect of beta-adrenergic blockade, calcium-channel blockade, or antiarrhythmic agents in preventing sudden death has still not been established. Amiodarone is effective in suppressing repetitive ventricular tachyarrhythmias in hypertrophic cardiomyopathy, although whether this will translate into improved survival remains to be seen.[251]

The risk of sudden death appears to be reduced in patients surviving left ventricular myotomy-myectomy. A small number of patients with outflow gradients, minimal or absent symptoms, and prior cardiac arrest have undergone prophylactic surgery with encouraging short-term results, although whether surgery itself prevents repeat cardiac arrest is unclear, since these patients ordinarily receive antiarrhythmic agents after surgery.[252] Because an effective therapeutic strategy—either medical or surgical—has yet to demonstrate efficacy in preventing sudden death in hypertrophic cardiomyopathy, the results of ongoing investigative efforts are eagerly awaited, particularly those employing a variety of antiarrhythmic agents.[251]

RESTRICTIVE AND INFILTRATIVE CARDIOMYOPATHIES

Of the three major functional categories of the cardiomyopathies (dilated, hypertrophic, and restrictive), the restrictive are the least common in Western countries.[37] The hallmark of the restrictive cardiomyopathies is abnormal diastolic function; the ventricular walls are excessively rigid and impede ventricular filling. Contractile function, on the other hand, is relatively unimpaired, with normal systolic emptying of the ventricles. Thus, restrictive cardiomyopathy bears some functional resemblance to constrictive pericarditis, which is also characterized by normal or near-normal systolic function but abnormal ventricular filling[253] (p. 1490).

A variety of specific pathological processes may result in restrictive cardiomyopathy, although the cause often remains unknown. Myocardial fibrosis, hypertrophy, or infiltration is usually responsible for the abnormal diastolic behavior. Myocardial involvement with amyloid is a common cause of secondary restrictive cardiomyopathy, although restriction is also seen in hemochromatosis, glycogen deposition, endomyocardial fibrosis, and, less commonly, fibroelastosis, the eosinophilias, neoplastic infiltration, pseudoxanthoma elasticum, and myocardial fibrosis of diverse etiologies.[4,37,42,254,255]

In a minority of cases, no specific etiology is apparent. Some patients may manifest all the features of a restrictive cardiomyopathy and exhibit the pathological findings of left ventricular hypertrophy and fibrosis;[12] certainly ventricular hypertrophy can cause diminished ventricular compliance (Fig. 12–23, p. 428 and p. 454). It has been suggested that myocardial fibrosis of any cause may result in restrictive physiology when it is sufficiently severe.[254] Rare patients may present with findings of restrictive physiology but without fibrosis, infiltration, or other pathological findings demonstrable in the heart. It has been suggested that a defect in myocardial relaxation is present in these patients.[254]

To be useful as a clinical descriptor, the term "restrictive cardiomyopathy" must be limited to those patients who are characterized *primarily* by abnormal cardiac stiffness, rather than used to describe patients who have abnormal ventricular filling dynamics associated with impaired ventricular systolic function.[256] Thus, while the hearts of patients with grossly dilated, hypocontractile left ventricles (dilated cardiomyopathy) may well have abnormal diastolic properties, their *primary* abnormality is impairment of systolic function, leading to left ventricular enlargement and, often, asynergic contraction. Similarly, it is clear that while the diastolic properties of the heart are frequently, perhaps universally, abnormal in hypertrophic cardiomyopathy, the hallmark of this condition, by definition, is ventricular hypertrophy.

HEMODYNAMICS. The clinical and hemodynamic features of restrictive heart disease simulate those of chronic constrictive pericarditis,[4,253,256] and endomyocardial biopsy may be particularly useful in this setting. Exploratory thoracotomy may be required on rare occasions.[256] The characteristic hemodynamic feature in both conditions occurs in the ventricular pressure recording, which shows a deep and rapid early decline in ventricular pressure at the onset of diastole, with a rapid rise to a plateau in early diastole. This dip and plateau has been termed the "square root" sign[257] (Fig. 43–16, p. 1490) and is manifested in the atrial pressure tracing as a prominent *y* descent followed by a rapid rise and plateau. The *x* descent may also be rapid, and the combination results in the characteristic M or W waveform in the atrial pressure tracing. The *a* wave is prominent and often is of the same amplitude as the *v* wave.[4,258] Both systemic and pulmonary venous pressures are elevated, although patients with restrictive heart disease typically have higher left than right ventricular filling pressures, and this difference is accentuated by exercise.[256] In this respect they differ from patients with constrictive pericarditis, in whom diastolic pressures are similar in both ventricles. The pulmonary artery systolic pressure is usually greater than 50 mm Hg in patients with restrictive cardiomyopathy but is lower in constrictive pericarditis.[253,258] Furthermore, the plateau of the right ventricular diastolic pressure is usually at least one-third of the peak right ventricular systolic pressure in patients with constrictive pericarditis, while it is frequently less in restrictive cardiomyopathy.[253]

CLINICAL MANIFESTATIONS. Exercise intolerance is frequent because of the inability of patients with restrictive cardiomyopathy to increase their cardiac output by tachycardia without further compromising ventricular filling.[37] Weakness and dyspnea are often prominent.[256] Chest pain may be prominent in a small fraction of patients but is usually absent. Particularly in advanced cases, an elevated central venous pressure, with peripheral edema, enlarged liver, ascites, and anasarca may be present.[4,256] *Physical examination* may reveal jugular venous distention; an S_3, S_4, or both; and, occasionally, systolic murmurs reflecting atrioventricular valvular regurgitation.[4,256] An inspiratory increase in venous pressure (Kussmaul sign) may be seen.[4] However, in contrast to constrictive pericarditis, the apex impulse is usually palpable, and the apexcardiogram demonstrates a prominent rapid filling wave in restrictive cardiomyopathy.

Various ancillary laboratory findings in addition to endomyocardial biopsy may be useful in distinguishing between constrictive and restrictive disease. While pericardial calcification is neither absolutely sensitive nor specific for constrictive pericarditis[256] (p. 1492), its presence in a patient in whom the differential diagnosis rests between restrictive cardiomyopathy and constrictive pericarditis lends strong support to the latter diagnosis. The echocardiogram may demonstrate thickening of the left ventricular wall and an increase of left ventricular mass in patients with infiltrative disease causing restrictive cardiomyopathy.[259]

AMYLOIDOSIS

ETIOLOGY AND TYPES. Amyloidosis is a disease complex that results from deposition of unique twisted β-pleated sheet fibrils formed from various proteins by several different pathogenic mechanisms.[260] Amyloid may be found in almost any organ, but clinically evident disease does not appear unless there is extensive infiltration. Several different types of amyloid fibrils have been described; the two most common are those composed of immunoglobulin light chains (designated AL) and those composed of a nonimmunoglobulin protein (designated AA).[260–262]

Amyloidosis presents in one of three clinicopathological forms: (1) acquired systemic amyloidosis, (2) organ-limited amyloidosis, and (3) localized deposition. Three forms of acquired systemic amyloidosis are seen: (a) associated with an immunocyte dyscrasia (e.g., multiple myeloma), (b) reactive (e.g., due to chronic infectious or inflammatory conditions), and (c) heredofamilial. Three different forms of familial involvement are recognized, depending upon the principal organ system involved: nephropathic, neuropathic, and cardiopathic.[263] Organ-limited amyloidosis may involve several organ systems, including the heart, and is more common with aging, thus the designation *senile* amyloidosis.

Senile amyloidosis is becoming increasingly common as the average age of the population increases. Indeed, involvement of the heart by senile amyloidosis may be found in more than 10 per cent of routinely autopsied individuals over the age of 75 years, and the prevalence and severity of involvement increases with advancing age. The fibrillar protein is unlike that found in other forms of amyloidosis. Small deposits of amyloid may often be found in the pulmonary vessels or the vessels of other organs as well.[264]

Cardiac Amyloidosis

Involvement of the heart is a common finding and is the most frequent cause of death in amyloidosis associated with an immunocyte dyscrasia.[265] In reactive amyloidosis, on the other hand, clinically significant cardiac involvement is uncommon;[260,261] the myocardial deposits are typically small and perivascular and usually do not result in significant myocardial dysfunction.[266] Familial amyloidosis is only occasionally associated with overt cardiac involvement; the clinical course is usually dominated by neurological or renal dysfunction, particularly in familial Mediterranean fever, in which death at an early age from renal failure is common.[263] Cardiac involvement in senile amyloidosis varies from small atrial deposits that do not result in functional impairment to extensive ventricular involvement with resultant cardiac failure.[267]

Cardiac amyloidosis occurs more commonly in men than in women (except for the senile form), and it is rare before the age of 40 years.[261,267–269] Even in the familial form, the onset of clinical cardiac disease usually does not occur before the age of 35 years and generally occurs much later in life.[263]

PATHOLOGY. The pathological findings often include mild cardiac enlargement, usually without significant ventricular dilatation. The walls of both ventricles are typically firm, rubbery, noncompliant, and thickened.[268] Amyloid is present between the myocardial fibers, with extensive deposition in the papillary muscles occurring commonly.[269a] Serial sections of the sinoatrial and atrioventricular nodes and the bundle branches may disclose amyloid deposits,[268] but fibrosis of these structures is perhaps more common.[270] In addition, endocardial involvement of the atria and ventricles is frequent, often associated with overlying thrombi. The pericardium may contain focal deposits of amyloid as

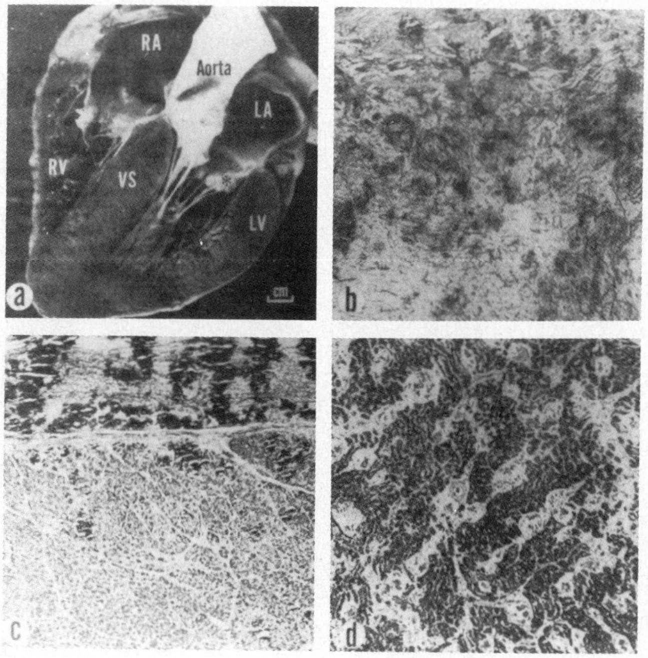

FIGURE 41–18 *a*, Gross appearance of unfixed heart in generalized cardiac amyloidosis. Note hypertrophied left ventricle (LV), right ventricle (RV), and ventricular septum (VS); rigid left atrium (LA) and right atrium (RA); and nodular thickening of mitral valve (*). *b*, Photomicrograph of mitral valve with extensive amyloid deposits (dark-staining patches) (× 64). *c*, Photomicrograph of left atrial wall. Note concentration of amyloid deposits in endocardium (dark-staining patches in upper part) (× 64). *d*, Photomicrograph of ventricular myocardium with diffuse amyloid deposits in interstitium and small blood vessels (pale-staining areas) surrounding irregular islands of muscle fibers (dark-staining areas) (× 64). (From Lie, J. T.: Amyloidosis and amyloid heart disease. Primary Cardiol. *8*:75, 1982.)

well. Amyloidosis often results in focal thickening or deposits on the cardiac valves, but these abnormalities do not appear to interfere with valvular function. The intramural coronary arteries and veins frequently contain amyloid deposits in the media and adventitia, occasionally compromising the lumina of the vessels,[270a] with attendant localized areas of ischemic necrosis that may produce intractable congestive heart failure (Fig. 41–19).[268,271]

CLINICAL MANIFESTATIONS. Involvement of the cardiovascular system by amyloidosis occurs in one of four general patterns:

1. The most common is congestive heart failure due to systolic dysfunction, which occurs in half or more patients.[265,268] Hemodynamic evidence of restriction of ventricular filling may not be prominent in these patients. The course of this form of the disease is often one of gradual progression, usually poorly responsive to treatment. The progress is usually rapid, with death due to cardiac failure generally occurring between 4 months and 2 years after the onset of symptoms.[261,265,268] Cardiomegaly is often demonstrated on chest roentgenography, although massive cardiac enlargement is uncommon. Angina pectoris occurs in one-third of the patients, often reflecting amyloid involvement of the coronary arteries.[268]

2. A second presentation of cardiac amyloidosis is that of a restrictive cardiomyopathy.[272] Right-sided findings dominate the clinical presentation, with peripheral edema a prominent finding while paroxysmal nocturnal dyspnea and orthopnea are absent. The amyloid infiltration of the

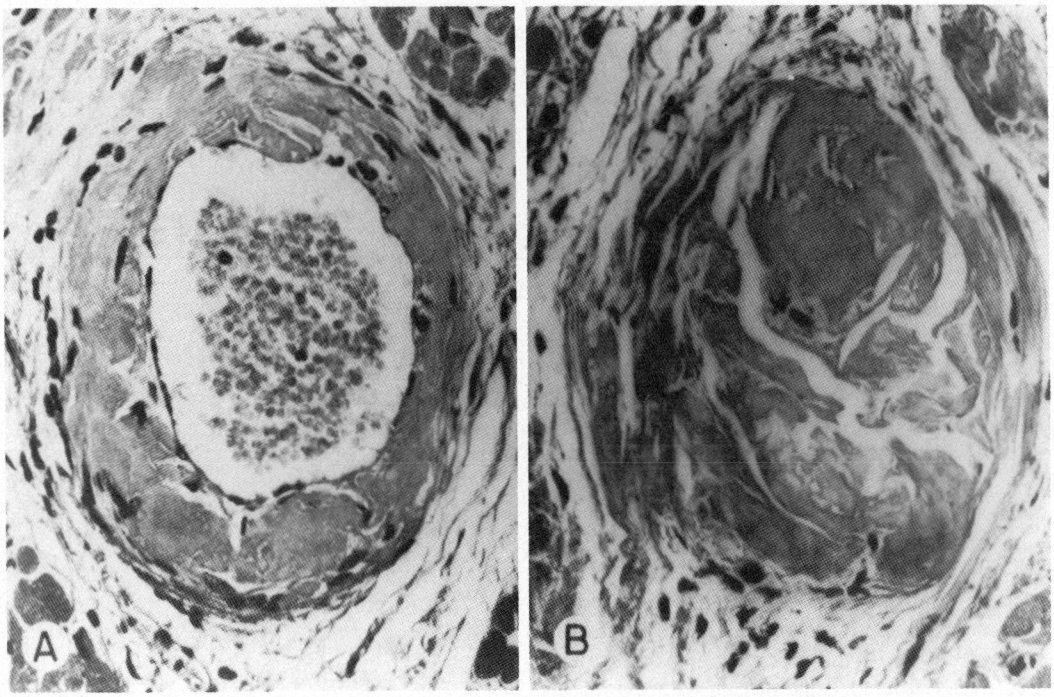

FIGURE 41–19 **Amyloidosis of intramyocardial arteries.** ***A,*** **Extensive medial deposition of amyloid with preservation of the vascular lumen.** ***B,*** **Complete loss of luminal patency as a result of the amyloid. (Hematoxylin and eosin stain; × 400, reduced by 28 per cent.) (From Smith, R. R. L., and Hutchins, G. M.: Ischemic heart disease secondary to amyloidosis of intramyocardial arteries. Am. J. Cardiol.** ***44*****:413, 1979.)**

myocardium results in increased stiffness of the myocardium, producing the characteristic diastolic dip and plateau (square root sign) in the ventricular pressure pulse.[256] In contrast to the accelerated early left ventricular diastolic filling found in constrictive pericarditis, cardiac amyloidosis is marked by an impaired rate of early diastolic filling, as a consequence of the stiffness of the ventricle[273] (Fig. 43–21, p. 1494).

3. An abnormality of cardiac impulse formation and conduction is a third mode of presentation and may result in arrhythmias and conduction disturbances, which are common in cardiac amyloidosis. One-third or more of patients with primary amyloidosis may experience lightheadedness or syncope.[261,265] Sudden death, presumably arrhythmic in origin, is relatively common.[272]

4. Orthostatic hypotension is the fourth mode of presentation. Although most likely due to amyloid infiltration of the autonomic nervous system or of blood vessels (p. 930), amyloid deposition in the heart and adrenals may contribute to this manifestation.[274] Hypovolemia as a result of the nephrotic syndrome secondary to renal amyloidosis may aggravate the postural hypotension.

Physical examination often reveals findings of congestive heart failure,[268] with systolic murmurs due to atrioventricular valvular regurgitation. Particularly in patients with restrictive cardiomyopathy, jugular venous distention, a protodiastolic gallop, hepatomegaly, peripheral edema, and a narrow pulse pressure are present.[274]

The *chest roentgenogram* usually shows cardiomegaly in patients with the clinical and hemodynamic picture of congestive cardiomyopathy, although heart size may be normal in patients with the restrictive form. Pulmonary congestion may be prominent in patients with congestive heart failure. Pleural effusions are common. *The electrocardiogram* is frequently abnormal;[268] the most characteristic feature is diffusely diminished voltage, occurring in approximately half the patients. Myocardial infarction is often simulated because of small or absent R waves in right precordial leads or, less frequently, by Q waves in the inferior leads. Left-axis deviation is seen in more than half the patients. Arrhythmias are common, particularly atrial fibrillation, which has been reported in 20 per cent of the patients. Various forms of AV conduction defects are often seen and have been found in one-third of patients with cardiac amyloidosis. Abnormalities of AV conduction appear to be particularly common in familial amyloidosis with polyneuropathy.[275] Sinus node involvement is common, and the clinical and electrocardiographic features of the sick sinus syndrome may be present (p. 693).[276] Patients with cardiac amyloidosis appear to be particularly sensitive to digitalis preparations, and the use of ordinary doses of digitalis glycosides may lead to serious arrhythmias.

Echocardiography (Fig. 5–73, p. 130) most commonly reveals increased thickness of the walls of the ventricles and an increased left ventricular mass.[259,272,277,278] The left ventricular cavity is usually normal or small in size, and wall excursions are often reduced.[259,272,277] A pericardial effusion is common, but rarely results in tamponade.[279] The appearance of the thickened cardiac walls is often distinctive on two-dimensional echocardiography, demonstrating a granular sparkling texture, presumably due to the amyloid deposit.[280] Echocardiographic demonstration of thick left ventricular walls with concomitant low voltage on the electrocardiogram appears to distinguish cardiac amyloidosis from pericardial disease or left ventricular hypertrophy, and this distinctive voltage/mass ratio is characteristic of myocardial infiltration by the amyloid fibrils.[281] Computer-assisted analysis of echocardiograms in amyloidosis has shown reduced ventricular distensibility and impaired diastolic filling.[282]

DIAGNOSIS. Whereas two or three decades ago the clinical diagnosis of systemic amyloidosis was made correctly antemortem only 25 per cent of the time, with more recent clinical awareness of the disease and the utilization of *biopsy techniques* the diagnosis is now made antemortem in almost 80 per cent of cases.[265,274] Rectal biopsy has been the single most useful diagnostic procedure, combining the attributes of relative ease of performance, sensitivity, and safety.[265] Biopsy of gingiva, bone marrow, liver, kidney, and various other tissues has also been employed. Endomyocardial biopsy of the right[283,284] or left ventricles[285] may be helpful in establishing the diagnosis of cardiac amyloidosis.

TREATMENT. The treatment of cardiac amyloidosis is generally ineffective, since there is no way to halt the progression of the underlying disease,[261] although several experimental trials are under way. Digitalis glycosides should be used with caution because patients with cardiac amyloidosis appear to be particularly sensitive to digitalis preparations, and the use of ordinary doses may lead to serious arrhythmias; this may relate to selective binding of digoxin to amyloid fibrils in the myocardium.[286] Insertion of a permanent pacemaker may be beneficial in patients with symptomatic conducting system disease.

INHERITED INFILTRATIVE DISORDERS CAUSING CARDIOMYOPATHY

The inherited disorders of Fabry's disease and Gaucher's disease are associated with the abnormal intramyocardial accumulation of a metabolic product. Such myocardial involvement results primarily in abnormal systolic contractile performance. However, the accumulation of the metabolic product in the myocardium may also impair the filling of the ventricles, thereby adding a restrictive component.

FABRY'S DISEASE. Fabry's disease (angiokeratoma corporis diffusum universale) is an X-linked disorder of glycosphingolipid metabolism due to a deficiency of the enzyme ceramide trihexosidase. It is characterized by an intracellular accumulation of a neutral glycolipid, with prominent involvement of the skin and kidneys as well as the myocardium. *Histological examination* often reveals widespread involvement of the myocardium, vascular endothelium, conducting tissues, and valves—particularly the mitral valve.[287,288] The major clinical manifestations of the disease result from the accumulation of the glycolipid substrate in endothelial cells, with eventual occlusion of small arterioles.[289] The accumulation of the glycolipid occurs in the lysosomes of the cardiac tissues and is responsible for the multiple cardiovascular manifestations of Fabry's disease.[287] Symptomatic cardiovascular involvement occurs eventually in most affected males, while female carriers are usually asymptomatic or only minimally symptomatic.[287] Systemic hypertension, myocardial ischemia or infarction, and congestive heart failure are common clinical manifestations.[287] Electrocardiographic abnormalities include left ventricular hypertrophy, P-wave abnormalities, conduction defects, and arrhythmias.[290] The echocardiogram usually reveals increased left ventricular wall thickness, presumably the result of glycolipid deposition.[289]

GAUCHER'S DISEASE. Gaucher's disease is an uncommon, inherited disorder of glycosyl ceramide metabolism. It is secondary to a deficiency of the enzyme beta-glucosidase and results in accumulation of cerebrosides in the spleen, liver, bone marrow, lymph nodes, brain, and myocardium. Diffuse interstitial infiltration of the left ventricle by cells laden with cerebroside occurs in Gaucher's disease, associated with reduced left ventricular compliance and cardiac output. Clinical evidence of cardiac involvement is uncommon, but when present it is characterized by left ventricular dysfunction.[291]

Hemochromatosis and Hemosiderosis

(See also p. 1682)

Hemochromatosis is characterized by excessive deposition of iron in a variety of parenchymal tissues (heart, liver, gonads, and pancreas). It may occur (1) as a familial or idiopathic disorder, (2) in association with a defect in hemoglobin synthesis resulting in ineffective erythropoiesis, (3) in chronic liver disease, and (4) with excessive oral intake of iron over many years. While patients who have iron deposits in the myocardium virtually always have deposits in other organs (e.g., liver, spleen, pancreas, bone marrow), the severity of myocardial involvement varies widely and parallels only roughly that in other organs.[292]

The *pathological findings* (Fig. 49–7, p. 1683) are a dilated heart with thickened ventricular walls. Myocardial iron deposits, often grossly visible, are most common in the subepicardial region, followed by the subendocardial region and papillary muscles, and are least common in the midmyocardial wall. They are more extensive in ventricular than atrial myocardium.[292] Iron deposits in myocardial cells are typically perinuclear in location initially but eventually occupy much of the fiber. Involvement of the cardiac conducting system is limited, compared with the relatively heavy infiltration of contracting cells.[293] Myocardial degeneration and fibrosis may also occur.

The severity of myocardial dysfunction is proportional to the amount of iron present in the myocardium.[293] Extensive deposits of cardiac iron (particularly those grossly visible at postmortem examination) are invariably associated with cardiac dysfunction—usually chronic congestive heart failure, which is often the cause of death. Extensive cardiac deposits usually occur in patients who receive more than 100 blood transfusions (unless there is associated iron loss due to bleeding).[292]

The *clinical manifestations* vary widely, depending on the extent of myocardial involvement. Some patients remain asymptomatic despite echocardiographic evidence of myocardial infiltration, which is expressed as an increase in left ventricular wall thickness.[259,293] Symptomatic cardiac involvement is usually associated with electrocardiographic abnormalities, including ST-segment and T-wave changes, as well as supraventricular arrhythmias; these electrocardiographic changes correlate with the degree of iron deposits in the heart.[292] Atrioventricular conduction disturbances and ventricular arrhythmias are uncommon.

Severe iron storage disease involving the heart usually produces a dilated and rarely a restrictive cardiomyopathy, characterized by exertional dyspnea, orthopnea, peripheral edema, and protodiastolic gallop sounds. The diagnosis is aided by finding elevated plasma iron levels (180 to 300 μg/dl; normal = 50 to 150), a normal or low total iron-binding capacity (200 to 300 μg/dl; normal = 250 to 370), and markedly elevated values for saturation of transferrin (80 to 100 per cent; normal = 22 to 46 per cent), serum ferritin (900 to 6000 ng/ml; normal = 3 to 180), urinary iron (9 to 23 mg/24 hr; normal = 0 to 2), and liver iron (600 to 1800 μg/100 mg dry wt; normal = 30 to 140).[294] Cardiac failure is usually progressive and largely refractory to therapy,[292] although repeated phlebotomies or the use of the chelating agent desferrioxamine may be beneficial.[295,296] (See further discussion of the treatment of iron storage disease on p. 1684.)

SARCOIDOSIS

Sarcoidosis is a granulomatous disorder of unknown etiology, characterized by multisystem involvement. Infiltration of the lungs, reticuloendothelial system, and skin usually dominates the clinical picture, but virtually any tissue may be affected. The most important manifestation results from pulmonary involvement. This often leads to diffuse fibrosis which may result in fatal right heart failure[297] (p. 1595). Primary cardiac involvement is not often recognized clinically, although it may be demonstrated at autopsy in 20 to 30 per cent of cases of sarcoid, most of which demonstrate generalized sarcoidosis.[298,299] Clinical manifestations of sarcoid heart disease are present in less than 5 per cent of patients, although myocardial involvement may result in heart block, congestive heart failure, and sudden death.[300,301] Myocardial sarcoidosis may have restrictive as well as congestive features, since cardiac infiltration by sarcoid granulomas results not only in increased stiffness of the ventricular wall but diminished systolic contractile function as well. Myocardial sarcoidosis typically affects young or middle-aged adults (mean age, 40 years) of either sex; there is usually evidence of generalized sarcoidosis.[297,302]

PATHOLOGY. The typical pathological feature of sarcoidosis is the presence of noncaseating granulomas,[303,304] which occur in many organs.[305] They infiltrate the myocardium and may eventually become fibrotic scars[306] (Fig. 41–20). The granulomas may involve any region of the heart, although the left ventricular free wall and the interventricular septum are the most common sites, and extensive granulomas and scar tissue in the cephalad portion of the interventricular septum is a constant finding in patients with abnormalities of the conduction system.[300,302] Occasional patients may have preferential and extensive involvement of the septum with minimal disease elsewhere in the heart.[307] Transmural involvement is common,[302] and large portions of the ventricular wall may be replaced by sarcoid tissue, which may lead to aneurysm formation. Even apparently uninvolved myocardium may demonstrate extensive mitochondrial damage upon examination by electron microscopy.[308] While involvement of small coronary artery branches may be found in sarcoidosis, the pathophysiological importance of this observation remains unclear.[309]

CLINICAL MANIFESTATIONS. Death was sudden in two-thirds of the patients in a large autopsy study of sarcoidosis of the heart; indeed, sudden death is the most common manifestation of cardiac sarcoidosis.[302] Many of the patients experienced antecedent arrhythmias or complete AV block.[302,309–312] Conduction disturbance is the most frequent clinical indication of myocardial sarcoid in nonfatal cases.[298] Syncope is common and may reflect paroxysmal arrhythmias or conduction disturbances.[307,313] Atrial and ventricular arrhythmias, especially ventricular tachycardia, are observed frequently.[301,302,314,315] Congestive heart failure is the other major manifestation of myocardial involvement. While cor pulmonale accounts for some of the symptoms of heart failure, many symptoms are caused by direct myocardial involvement by granulomas and scar tissue, and the patients show the clinical features of restrictive or dilated cardiomyopathy.[302,311,312,316] Symptoms of myocardial sarcoid may be present for variable lengths of time, with survival for up to 15 years reported.[300] However, the disease often progresses rapidly to death, and in the majority of patients the interval from the onset of the cardiac symptoms to death is less than 2 years.[302]

Cardiac dysfunction is often severe and progressive and

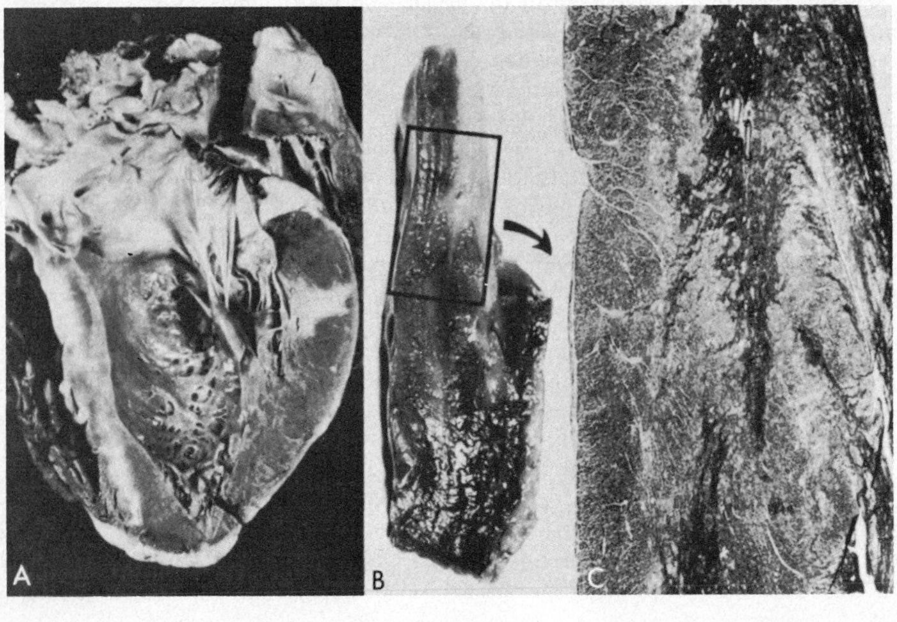

FIGURE 41–20 ***A,*** **Cardiac sarcoidosis, with hypertrophied and dilated left ventricle, diffuse fibrosis of the interventricular septum, and a focal discrete scar in the free left ventricular wall.** ***B,*** **Fibrosis in the region of interventricular septum.** ***C,*** **Histological section from the area delineated in** ***B,*** **demonstrating the darker staining fibrosed areas. (Original magnification × 5.) (From Lie, J. T., et al.: Sudden death from cardiac sarcoidosis with involvement of conduction system. Am. J. Med. Sci.** ***267*****:123, 1974.)**

usually refractory to therapy.[298] Occasionally, patients with extensive involvement develop overt left ventricular aneurysms.[301,302,317] Pericardial effusions and valvular involvement sometimes occur.[304,310] Calcification of the mitral valve annulus, probably reflecting the effects of the hypercalcemia that may accompany sarcoidosis, is sometimes found.[302]

The *physical examination* may reveal findings of extracardiac sarcoid or may be totally normal. Cardiac murmurs are common, usually reflecting mitral regurgitation.[298,302] This appears to be more the result of left ventricular dilatation or infiltration than of direct sarcoid involvement of the papillary muscles.[302]

The *electrocardiogram* is frequently abnormal in patients with known sarcoid and most commonly demonstrates T-wave abnormalities.[318] Sarcoidosis appears to have an affinity for involvement of the AV junction and bundle of His, and thus varying degrees of AV block are common.[298,302,309,311,319] With extensive myocardial involvement, pathological Q waves may appear and simulate myocardial infarction.[301,307]

DIAGNOSIS. In many cases the diagnosis may be suspected in patients with bilateral hilar lymphadenopathy on chest roentgenogram in whom there is clinical or electrocardiographic evidence of myocardial disease. Some patients may have myocardial involvement without other overt systemic indications of disease. In this situation, percutaneous endomyocardial biopsy may be particularly useful.[320] Myocardial imaging with thallium-201 may also be helpful in demonstrating segmental filling defects representing areas of infiltration of the myocardium[321] and may indicate myocardial involvement in more than one-third of patients with sarcoid but without clinical evidence of cardiac involvement.[322] Imaging may also indicate the presence of right ventricular hypertrophy in patients with right ventricular overload due to pulmonary fibrosis and pulmonary hypertension. Myocardial uptake of technetium pyrophosphate and gallium in myocardial sarcoidosis has also been reported.[322a]

TREATMENT. The treatment of myocardial sarcoidosis is difficult. Arrhythmias are often refractory to antiarrhythmic drugs, although quinidine with or without propranolol is sometimes efficacious.[300,323,324] Permanent pacing may be helpful,[300,309,324] and since sudden death is so common in sarcoid, it should be applied in all patients with advanced heart block.[324]

The evaluation of the response of sarcoidosis to therapy is made even more difficult by the occasional spontaneous improvement in conduction that may occur.[300] While the matter is not settled, it appears that corticosteroids may be of some benefit in treating the conduction disturbances, arrhythmias, and myocardial dysfunction of sarcoidosis.[300,325,326] Since the risk of the sudden death appears to be greatest in patients with extensive myocardial involvement, it is reasonable to attempt to halt the progression of the disease with steroids before irreversible fibrosis occurs.[299,319] Some evidence suggests that steroids may result in the healing of granulomas, although formation of a ventricular aneurysm may be a possible side effect.[302]

Whipple's Disease

Intestinal lipodystrophy, or Whipple's disease, may be associated with myocardial involvement, and PAS-positive macrophages may be found in the myocardium, pericardium, and heart valves of patients with this disorder.[327] Electron microscopy has demonstrated rod-shaped structures in the myocardium similar to those found in the small intestine, and it has been suggested that they are the causative agent of the myocardial abnormalities. There is often an associated inflammatory infiltrate and foci of fibrosis. The valvular fibrosis may be severe enough to result in malfunction. While asymptomatic, nonspecific electrocardiographic changes are most common, systolic murmurs, pericarditis, and even overt congestive heart failure may occur.[327]

BECKER'S DISEASE

Becker's disease (also called African cardiomyopathy) is an uncommon condition of obscure etiology that occurs most commonly in South Africa. It is characterized by cardiac dilatation without hypertrophy and by fibrosis of the papillary muscles, subendocardium, and endocardium; it is associated with pericardial effusion, myocardial necrosis, and mural thrombosis.[328,329] The disease appears to progress from an acute edematous serous myocarditis marked by fibrinoid necrosis to a chronic stage with endocardial necrosis and fibrosis, mural thrombosis, and organization leading to endocardial sclerosis.

At necropsy, the heart is dilated but not hypertrophied; a pericardial effusion is often present. White patches of endocardial thickening, composed of fibroelastic tissue, typically involve the apex, the papillary muscles, atria, and the outflow portion of the interventricular septum.[329] A thin fibrin layer usually covers the endocardium, but the cardiac valves are uninvolved. Mural thrombi are a ubiquitous finding, occurring most commonly in the left ventricle, followed in frequency by the left atrium, right atrium, and, rarely, the right ventricle.[328] There is marked interstitial edema of the myocardium, with a serous myocarditis and degenerated and necrotic muscle fibers. Perivascular fibrosis may be prominent. The aorta and its vasa vasorum may show focal nodular swellings and fibrinoid necrosis, and giant cells may be found within the intima of the pulmonary artery.[328,329]

ETIOLOGY. Although nutritional, toxic, hypersensitivity, and infectious causes of the disease have been suggested, the actual mechanism remains obscure. It is intriguing that patients at risk of developing Becker's disease appear to ingest a diet deficient in tryptophan[330] and that rats fed a similar diet for long periods of time develop cardiac lesions similar to those found in humans.[331] Jamaican cardiomyopathy[332] may represent the same or a closely related pathological process.

CLINICAL MANIFESTATIONS. The disease occurs in all ages and in all races in South Africa. It may present as congestive heart failure, which may be acute and rapidly progressive, with death occurring within 6 months, or may be chronic, with survival for up to three years.[329] Patients may show an acute illness marked by fever; leukocytosis (without eosinophilia); multiple emboli with infarction of the lungs, spleen, kidneys, or brain; and progressive congestive heart failure.[328,329] Dyspnea is an almost ubiquitous symptom, often associated with cough, peripheral edema, chest pain, and hemoptysis.[328] *Physical examination* reveals jugular venous distention, tachycardia, pulmonary congestion, edema, cardiomegaly, gallop rhythm, and a systolic murmur of atrioventricular valvular regurgitation.[329]

Chest roentgenography reveals an enlarged cardiac silhouette due to both cardiomegaly and pericardial effusion.[328] Findings typical of pulmonary congestion are common. The *electrocardiogram* is virtually always abnormal, principally with ST-segment and T-wave abnormalities.

ENDOMYOCARDIAL FIBROSIS

Endomyocardial fibrosis is a disease of unknown etiology that occurs most commonly in the residents of tropical and subtropical Africa, particularly Uganda and Nigeria. It is typified by fibrous endocardial lesions of the inflow portion of the right or left ventricle or both and often involves the atrioventricular valves, resulting in regurgitation. It is a relatively frequent cause of heart failure and death in equatorial Africa, accounting for 15 to 25 per cent of deaths due to heart disease.[329,333,334]

While most prominent in Africa, it is also found in tropical and subtropical regions in the rest of the world, including India, Brazil, Colombia, and Ceylon.[335–338] It is most common in specific ethnic groups, notably the Rwanda tribe in Uganda[339] and in people of low socioeconomic status.[334] The disease is equally frequent in both sexes, and, although most common in children and young adults, its reported age range is from 4 to 70 years of age.[329] It is most common in blacks, but cases have been reported occasionally in Caucasians in temperate climates who previously resided in tropical areas.[338]

PATHOLOGY. A pericardial effusion, which may be quite large, may be present. The heart is normal in size or slightly enlarged, but massive cardiomegaly does not occur.[337] Hypertrophy is typically absent. The right atrium is often dilated, and in patients with severe right ventricular involvement there may be massive enlargement of this chamber. Indentation of the right border of the heart above the apex as a result of apical scarring may occur. The right ventricular outflow tract is often dilated above this indentation.[339]

Combined right and left ventricular disease occurs in about half the cases, with pure left ventricular involvement occurring in 40 per cent and pure right ventricular involvement in the remaining 10 per cent of patients who are examined post mortem.[337] When affected, the right ventricle exhibits extensive, dense, fibrous thickening of the inflow tract and apex, with involvement of the papillary muscles and chordae tendineae. Involvement of the right ventricle may lead to obliteration of the apex, with a mass of thrombus and fibrous tissue filling the cavity.[329,337] The tricuspid valve is often pulled down and distorted by the fibrous process involving the supporting structures.[329] Right atrial thrombi occur commonly.[337,339] Left ventricular involvement is similar, with fibrosis extending from the apex up the inflow portion of the left ventricle to the posterior mitral valve leaflet. The anterior leaflet of the mitral valve and the outflow portion of the left ventricle are usually spared.[337] Thrombi may overlie the endocardial lesions, but obliteration of the left ventricular cavity does not occur.

Microscopically, the involved endocardium demonstrates a thick layer of hyalinized fibrous tissue on top of a layer of collagen fibers;[329] foci of calcification may be present,[340] and thrombus may cover the outer layer of fibrous tissue. Septa composed of fibrous and granulation tissue extend for variable distances into the myocardium.[329,340] The myocardial fibers may show degeneration, particularly in areas adjacent to the fibrous plaques.[339] Interstitial edema is often present, but there is no cellular infiltration.[329] Small patches of fibroelastosis may occur in both ventricular outflow tracts beneath the semilunar valves but are felt to be a secondary phenomenon due to local trauma rather than a result of the basic pathological process.[329] The coronary arteries and great vessels are uninvolved, as is the remainder of the body.

ETIOLOGY. A variety of causes of endomyocardial fibrosis have been suggested, but the true etiology remains unclear. Perhaps the most intriguing hypothesis involves the role of diet. Patients in whom the disease occurs often consume large quantities of bananas, which have a high serotonin content, and an analogy has been drawn between the fibrotic cardiac lesions seen in carcinoid heart disease (p. 1431) and those in endomyocardial fibrosis.[337] However, it is now generally accepted that neither malnutrition nor massive consumption of plantains is the critical variable that causes this disease.[341] Other hypotheses incriminate infection with viruses, streptococci, filaria, or infestation with *Loa loa.*[337,341] It has also been suggested that endomyocardial fibrosis may represent an immunological response to streptococcal infection in individuals who are particularly susceptible to malaria, although the nature of the relationship remains unclear. Whatever the nature of the inciting agent, it appears that endomyocardial fibrosis is one part of a spectrum of a disease process that includes Löffler's endocarditis[342] (p. 1430).

CLINICAL MANIFESTATIONS. Endomyocardial fibrosis may involve both ventricles or either ventricle selectively; left-sided involvement results in symptoms of pulmonary congestion, while predominant right-sided disease may present features of a restrictive cardiomyopathy and therefore simulate constrictive pericarditis. Frequently, the disease is discovered as an incidental finding at necropsy.[337] There is often regurgitation of one or both atrioventricular valves. The onset of the disease is usually insidious, but it is sometimes ushered in by an acute febrile illness.[329,336,337,339] Patients present symptoms of cardiac decompensation, including dyspnea, cough, tender hepatomegaly, ascites, edema, and palpitations.[343] Rarely, the disease appears to stabilize, and survival for up to 12 years has been observed, but it is usually relentlessly progressive, with poor response to treatment.[329,339] Progressive heart failure is the rule. In contrast to Becker's disease, pulmonary or systemic embolization is uncommon.[329] Death is due to progressive myocardial failure, often associated with pulmonary congestion, infection, or infarction.[343] The most important immediate cause of death is sudden, unexpected cardiovascular collapse, presumably arrhythmic in origin.[343] Patients with prominent involvement of the right side of the heart appear to survive longer than those with principally left-sided involvement.[343]

Right Ventricular Endomyocardial Fibrosis. Pure or predominant right ventricular involvement is characterized by fibrous obliteration of the right ventricular apex that diminishes the capacity of this chamber.[337] The fibrosis often extends to the supporting apparatus of the tricuspid valve, resulting in tricuspid regurgitation. Therefore, clinical manifestations in patients with right-sided involvement include an elevated jugular venous pressure, a prominent *v* wave, and a rapid *y* descent. A rapid subsequent ascent is often observed.[337,339] A protodiastolic gallop sound may be heard along the lower sternal border, reflecting right ventricular dysfunction. The liver is usually large and pulsatile, and ascites, splenomegaly, and peripheral edema are common.[339] Although cyanosis and clubbing of the digits may be seen, the cause is unclear.[336] Pulmonary congestion is not present in the absence of left-sided involvement, and the pulmonary artery and pulmonary capillary wedge pressures are normal. A pericardial effusion, which is sometimes quite large, may be present.[337] The right atrium is often enlarged, sometimes massively so.[335,336,339]

The *electrocardiogram* is usually abnormal, with diminished QRS voltage (probably resulting from the presence of a pericardial effusion), ST-segment and T-wave abnormalities, and findings of right atrial enlargement.[336,337,339] Occasionally, atrial fibrillation occurs.[337,339] The *chest roentgenogram* demonstrates cardiac enlargement, usually with gross prominence of the right atrium and a pericardial effusion. Calcification in the region of the right ventricular apex may be found.[337,339] The pulmonary vasculature is typically normal.[336] At *angiography* the right ventricular apex is characteristically not visualized because of obliteration by the fibrous endocardium,[336,337] but tricuspid regurgitation, right atrial enlargement, and filling defects in the right atrium due to intraatrial thrombi are sometimes seen.[336]

Left Ventricular Endomyocardial Fibrosis. Predominant *left-sided* involvement results in a different clinical picture. The endomyocardial fibrosis involves the apex of the ventricle and usually the chordae tendineae of the posterior mitral valve leaflet as well,[337] leading to mitral regurgitation.[339] The murmur may be confined to late systole, as is characteristic of the papillary muscle dysfunction type of murmurs, or it may be pansystolic.[337,339] Findings of pulmonary hypertension may be prominent, with a closely split second heart sound and an accentuated pulmonary component, right ventricular hypertrophy with a parasternal lift, a palpable pulmonary artery impulse, and, occasionally, the murmur of functional pulmonary regurgitation. A protodiastolic gallop is commonly heard.[337,339]

The *electrocardiogram* usually shows T-wave abnormalities and diminished QRS voltage. There may be findings of left atrial and right ventricular enlargement. Occasionally, atrial fibrillation is present.[337,339] *Cardiac catheterization* usually reveals pulmonary hypertension, with elevated left ventricular filling pressures and a reduced cardiac index. The left ventriculogram usually shows extensive left ventricular asynergy and mitral regurgitation.[335] A filling defect due to an intracavitary thrombus within the ventricle may be seen on occasion.

Biventricular Endomyocardial Fibrosis. This form of endomyocardial fibrosis occurs more frequently than either isolated right- or left-sided disease. If there is more than minimal right ventricular involvement, severe pulmonary hypertension does not occur, and the right-sided findings dominate the clinical presentation.[337] The typical patient with biventricular involvement may have the features of right ventricular endomyocardial fibrosis, as described above, with only a mitral regurgitant murmur to suggest left ventricular involvement.[337] Rarely, in patients with biventricular involvement, the left-sided features dominate the clinical picture.[339] Systemic embolization may occur in up to 15 per cent of patients; infective endocarditis is even less frequent and is found in less than 2 per cent.[337]

DIAGNOSIS. This is based on the presence of the typical clinical features in an individual from the appropriate geographical area. Eosinophilia is usually not a prominent feature and, when present, may reflect associated parasitic infestation.[339] The *chest roentgenogram* usually shows mild cardiomegaly and sometimes intracardiac calcification. Right ventricular involvement often results in characteristic findings on *echocardiography,* including right ventricular dilatation, abnormal septal motion, and thickening of the ventricular wall.[344,344a] *Endomyocardial biopsy* may occasionally be helpful in establishing the diagnosis.[338] However, this risks dislodging a mural thrombus, with resultant embolization. In addition, because the disease is often focal, the biopsy may miss the pathological process, particularly if a right ventricular biopsy is performed in a patient with isolated left-sided disease.[338] The typical findings at *cardiac catheterization*[334,335,337,337a] (impairment of ventricular filling, diminished ventricular stroke volume due to partial obliteration of the ventricular apex as well as atrioventricular valve regurgitation, and systolic dysfunction) are helpful but not specific for this condition.

TREATMENT. The treatment of endomyocardial fibrosis is often difficult. Digitalis glycosides may be helpful in controlling the ventricular rate in patients with atrial fibrillation, but the response of congestive symptoms is disappointing. Diuretics are not particularly helpful in the treatment of ascites.[337] Insertion of a subcutaneous pericardioperitoneal shunt may be of some benefit in patients with massive recurrent pericardial effusion.[345] Operative excision of the fibrotic endocardium and replacement of the mitral

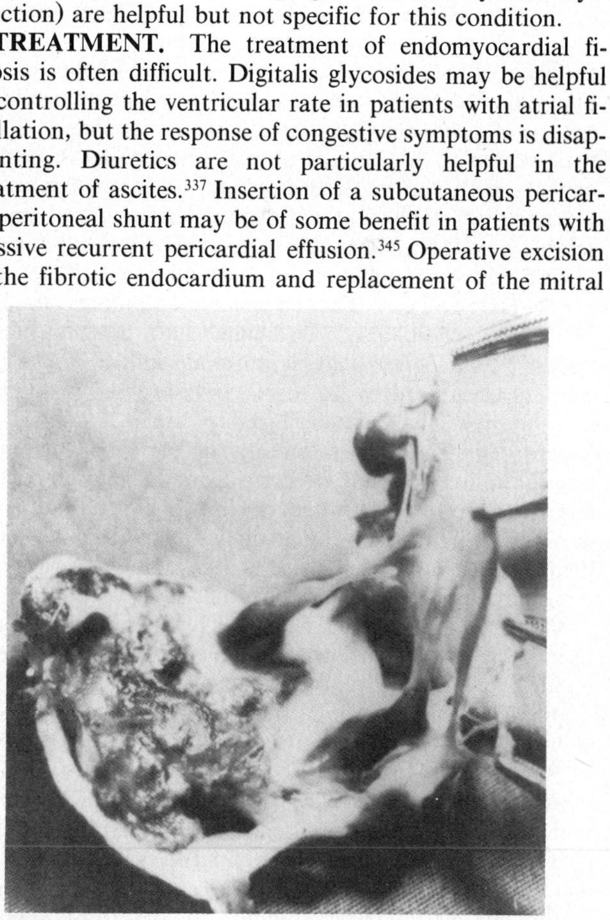

FIGURE 41–21 Appearance of the excised left ventricular endocardium and mitral valve. (From Moraes, C. R., et al.: Endomyocardial fibrosis: Report of 6 patients and review of the surgical literature. Ann. Thorac. Surg. *29*:243, 1980.)

or tricuspid valves has led to substantial symptomatic improvement (Fig. 41–21).[334,337a,346–348,348a,348b] Postoperative catheterization has also provided objective evidence of hemodynamic improvement with a reduction in ventricular filling pressures and an increase in cardiac output.[334,346] Although only a limited number of patients have undergone operation, this approach appears to be a promising alternative to medical treatment, which is often disappointing,[349] although operative mortality may be as high as 20 per cent.[350]

Löffler's Endocarditis (Hypereosinophilic Syndrome)

A variety of disease states are marked by prolonged and profound eosinophilia associated with localized or widespread eosinophilic infiltrates.[351,352] Cardiac involvement is the rule, occurring in more than 95 per cent of such patients.[352] The characteristic cardiac lesion is dense endocardial fibrosis with superimposed thrombus. Three general causes of the so-called hypereosinophilic syndrome (i.e., profound eosinophilia with tissue involvement) have been suggested: (1) leukemia; (2) reactive—that is, secondary to polyarteritis nodosa, Hodgkin's disease, tumors, parasitic infestation, asthma, or drug reaction; and (3) idiopathic. The last is the most common.[353,354]

One of the major unanswered questions in Löffler's endocarditis is the relation between the eosinophilia and the mechanism of the cardiac damage. It has been suggested that marked eosinophilia occurs in response to profound antigenic stimulation of unknown cause.[337] It appears that the cardiac damage itself may be the result of prolonged release of products from circulating eosinophils.[355] It has been proposed that, unlike normal eosinophils, those from patients with the hypereosinophilic syndrome possess receptors that result in their degranulation in response to soluble bloodborne substances, and this degranulation may in turn release unknown cardiotoxic substances.[355]

PATHOLOGY. The pathological findings in Löffler's endocarditis may be divided into three sequential stages.[340,353] The *first stage* is an acute inflammatory infiltrate, characterized by an eosinophilic myocarditis particularly prominent in the inner layers of the myocardium.[340,353] Myocardial necrosis and arteritis of the small intramural arterioles are common. Mural thrombi may be superimposed over the thickened but intact endocardium. The duration of illness from onset of symptoms to death in patients who demonstrate these acute findings averages less than 2 months.[340]

The *second stage* is characterized by thrombus formation over a thickened myocardium which is infiltrated by eosinophils,[340] while the *third stage* is one of fibrosis, with a prominent layer of hyaline fibrous tissue in the thickened endocardium. Mural thrombi are almost always present[353] in this stage of the disease. Arteritis and the eosinophilic infiltrate present in the earlier stages are now scanty or absent. The fibrotic lesions are located primarily in the inflow tract and apex of the ventricles, with frequent involvement of the papillary muscles and chordae tendineae.[353] The pathological findings in the third stage of Löffler's endocarditis are identical to those in endomyocardial fibrosis[340] (p. 1428), and there are no reliable gross or histological features to distinguish the two diseases.

The *hypereosinophilic syndrome* is characterized by the combination of a persistent eosinophilia, i.e., ≥ 1500 eosinophils/mm^3 for at least 6 months or until death, and evidence of organ involvement. A variety of organs are frequently involved besides the heart, including the lungs, bone marrow, and brain. Renal, gastrointestinal, dermatological, and hepatic involvement is observed less frequently.[337] The majority of patients are Caucasian men living in temperate climates.[353] The disease is primarily one of middle age, and, although any age group may be involved, children are least often affected.

CLINICAL MANIFESTATIONS. The principal clinical features include weight loss, fever, cough, skin rash, and congestive heart failure. Overt cardiac dysfunction occurs in more than half the patients with cardiac involvement and may be either right- or left-sided.[352] Cardiomegaly, often without overt symptoms of congestive heart failure, may be present, and the murmur of mitral regurgitation is common. Systemic embolism is frequent and may lead to neurological and renal dysfunction.[353,356] Once the disease becomes clinically evident, survival is usually brief, averaging nine months, although a minority of patients survive for four years or more. More recent reports have suggested a more benign course, with average survivals exceeding five years;[352] the reason for this apparent improvement in prognosis is unclear but may be related to improvement in therapy.[357] Death is usually due to congestive heart failure, often with associated renal, hepatic, or respiratory dysfunction.

LABORATORY EXAMINATION. A variety of abnormalities of the blood may be seen in addition to the eosinophilia. The erythrocyte sedimentation rate is frequently elevated, and occasionally patients have abnormal or depressed leukocyte alkaline phosphatase levels and chromosomal abnormalities (including the Philadelphia [Ph^1] chromosome).[352]

The *chest roentgenogram* may reveal cardiomegaly and pulmonary congestion or, less commonly, pulmonary infiltrates. The *electrocardiogram* most commonly shows nonspecific ST-segment and T-wave abnormalities. Left ventricular hypertrophy, arrhythmias, and conduction defects, particularly right bundle branch block, may also be present.[352,358]

The *echocardiogram* commonly demonstrates thickening of the right and left ventricular walls with an increase of the left ventricular mass.[359] Localized thickening of the posterobasal left ventricular wall may lead to mitral regurgitation.[359a] Enlargement of the left atrium and right and/or left ventricles may be seen; abnormal mitral valve motion reflecting diminished left ventricular compliance and pericardial effusions are found in one-fourth to one-third of patients.[357]

The *hemodynamic consequences* of the dense endocardial scarring seen in Löffler's endocarditis are those of a restrictive cardiomyopathy as described above (p. 1422) with abnormal diastolic filling due to increased stiffness of the ventricles and a reduction in the size of the ventricular cavity by organized thrombus. Systolic performance is also impaired and atrioventricular valvular regurgitation may occur because of involvement of the supporting apparatus of the mitral or tricuspid valves.[360] In rare cases the mitral and tricuspid valves themselves may become fibrotic, and stenosis may result.[360] *Cardiac catheterization* reveals markedly elevated ventricular filling pressures, and there may be evidence of tricuspid or mitral regurgitation. On angiography, contraction of the ventricles, particularly the right ventricle, is often asynergic.[351,356] Occasionally, verrucous deposits and friable vegetations on the valves are noted on angiography.[353]

TREATMENT. Therapy is generally unsatisfactory.[351] Digitalis is usually ineffective, and the congestive failure is inexorable.[361] Short-lived improvement after steroid therapy has been reported, but sustained efficacy has not been demonstrated.[351,352,361] Eosinophilia may be diminished by treatment with hydroxyurea and vincristine, a wide range of other myelo- and immunosuppressive agents, antihistamines, radiation, splenectomy, and antiparasitic drugs, but whether this results in any change in the natural history of the disease is not clear. A rare patient has undergone surgical removal of the fibrotic endocardial tissue and has shown clinical improvement.[362,363]

RELATION BETWEEN ENDOMYOCARDIAL FIBROSIS AND LÖFFLER'S ENDOCARDITIS. There are both important similarities and differences between endomyocardial fibrosis and Löffler's endocarditis. The similarities in the histological and the gross anatomical findings as well as the clinical and hemodynamic manifestations of advanced Löffler's endocarditis and endomyocardial fibrosis have led to the suggestion that they are related entities.[353,364]

In fact, a continuum has been suggested from tropical eosinophilia to Löffler's endocarditis to, finally, endomyocardial fibrosis.[364] According to this formulation, endocardial fibrosis may be the final expression of damage initially mediated through eosinophils, and endomyocardial fibrosis may be a late form of Löffler's endocarditis.[353] It may be that eosinophilia occurs early in the course of endomyocardial fibrosis, perhaps resulting from parasitic infection, only to disappear later.[365] A number of important differences between the two diseases should be borne in mind. They occur in different geographical areas and age groups. Endomyocardial fibrosis is associated with less thrombus formation than is Löffler's endocarditis, while Löffler's endocarditis may be associated with a generalized arteritis not found in endomyocardial fibrosis.[364] Despite these differences, we favor the view that endomyocardial fibrosis may, at least in some instances, be a later, "burned-out" phase of Löffler's endocarditis that is no longer associated with eosinophilia.[364]

Endocardial Fibroelastosis (See page 1049)

Carcinoid Heart Disease

Etiology and Pathology. The carcinoid syndrome is caused by a metastasizing carcinoid tumor and is characterized by cutaneous flushing, diarrhea, bronchoconstriction, and endocardial plaques composed of a unique type of fibrous tissue.[366] The vasomotor, bronchoconstrictor, and cardiac manifestations are undoubtedly related to circulating humoral substances secreted by the tumor.[367] The diarrhea is probably caused by serotonin, which is secreted in large amounts by carcinoid tumors, while the dermal flushes and bronchospasm appear to be related to the release of kinin peptides. Virtually all patients develop diarrhea and flushing, while cardiac abnormalities occur in over half the patients and bronchospasm in one third.[366,368]

Sixty to 90 per cent of tumors arise in the appendix, while the rest originate in the ileum, stomach, duodenum, or other areas of the gastrointestinal tract.[369] Only the carcinoid tumors of the ileum tend to metastasize, with involvement of the regional lymph nodes and liver. Also, only carcinoid tumors that invade the liver result in carcinoid heart disease.[370] The cardiac lesions may be related to large circulating quantities of serotonin (5-hydroxytryptamine) or other substances secreted by the tumor, which are usually inactivated by the liver, lungs, and brain.[369] Hepatic metastases apparently allow large quantities of tumor products to reach the heart without being inactivated by the liver.[369,371] Left-sided cardiac involvement is rare in the carcinoid syndrome, probably because of the inactivation of the offending humoral substance(s) by the lungs, although left-sided lesions may occur in the presence of an intracardiac communication that allows right-to-left shunting, thus avoiding the pulmonary circulation.[370]

The characteristic lesions are fibrous plaques that involve the tricuspid and pulmonic valves, the endocardium of the cardiac chambers, and the intima of the venae cavae, pulmonary artery, and coronary sinus (Fig. 41–22).[366,367,370] The fibrous tissue in the plaques results in distortion of the valves, leading to pulmonic stenosis and tricuspid regurgitation (p. 1117).[367] Histologically, the plaques consist of deposits of fibrous tissue located superficially on the endocardium with little or no extension into the underlying layers.[367] Ultrastructural studies have demonstrated that the plaques are composed of smooth muscle cells embedded in a stroma rich in acid mucopolysaccharides and collagen.[366] The plaques may form as a result of healing of a superficial endocardial injury, which is produced by a compound secreted by or derived from the tumor.[366]

Clinical Manifestations. *Physical examination* usually reveals a systolic murmur along the left upper sternal border, produced by valvular pulmonic stenosis, tricuspid regurgitation, or both. A right ventricular heave and systolic thrill are often present.[370]

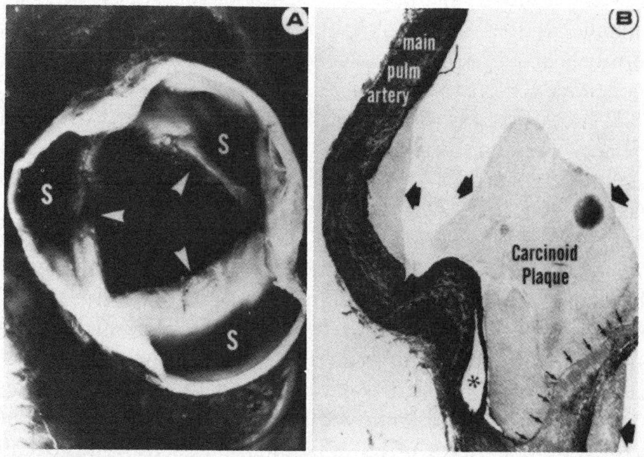

FIGURE 41–22 *A,* Gross photograph of deformed pulmonic valve with fixed, stenotic, triangular-shaped orifice (arrowheads) and sinuses (S) accentuated by thickened, retracted valve cusps. *B,* Photomicrograph of pulmonic valve cusp with a large carcinoid plaque (broad arrows) on the arterial surface (outlined by small arrows) and a smaller plaque on the ventricular surface of the valve cusp. A small plaque is also present on the intima of the buckled pulmonary artery. Empty space in pulmonary artery wall (*) is a section-preparation artifact. (Elastic Van Gieson's stain; × 16.) (From Lie, J. T.: Carcinoid tumors, carcinoid syndrome, and carcinoid heart disease. Primary Cardiol. *8*:163, 1982.)

The *chest roentgenogram* may reveal enlargement of the heart, although the pulmonary artery trunk is typically of normal size, without evidence of poststenotic dilatation. No specific *electrocardiographic pattern* is diagnostic of carcinoid heart disease, although low voltage is often present. Evidence of right atrial enlargement may be seen on occasion, but electrocardiographic evidence of right ventricular hypertrophy is usually lacking. Nonspecific ST-segment and T-wave abnormalities and right bundle branch block have also been reported.[370] *Echocardiography* may reveal evidence of tricuspid or pulmonary valve thickening.[371a]

The *hemodynamic findings* most commonly encountered are those of tricuspid regurgitation and pulmonic stenosis. Some patients with the carcinoid syndrome appear to be in a profound hyperkinetic state, which may lead to high-output heart failure[372] (p. 820). Cardiac catheterization appears to be hazardous in patients with the malignant carcinoid syndrome, and several deaths have been reported.[370,373]

Treatment. Treatment of patients with mild congestive heart failure consists of digitalis and diuretics.[367] Some of the vasomotor symptoms may be controlled with alpha-adrenergic blockers and serotonin antagonists.[367] Surgical replacement of the tricuspid valve and pulmonic valvotomy may be beneficial in severely symptomatic patients with serious valvular dysfunction and may permit prolonged survival.[369]

Obesity Heart Disease (See page 1741)

Diabetic Cardiomyopathy (See page 1738)

MYOCARDITIS

When the heart is involved in an inflammatory process, often caused by an infectious agent, myocarditis is said to be present. The inflammation may involve the myocytes, interstitium, vascular elements, and/or pericardium; involvement of the latter structure is discussed in Chapter 43.

Myocarditis is a common cause of acute congestive cardiomyopathy and has been described during and following a wide variety of viral, rickettsial, bacterial, protozoal, and metazoal diseases; indeed, virtually any infectious agent may produce cardiac inflammation. Infectious agents cause myocardial damage by three basic mechanisms: (1) invasion of the myocardium, e.g., by echovirus[374]; (2) production of a myocardial toxin, e.g., diphtheria[375]; and (3) autoimmunity, as occurs in acute rheumatic fever[376] and systemic lupus erythematosus (p. 1660). Myocarditis may also be caused by radiation and other physical agents, chemicals (e.g., lead), pharmacological agents (e.g., adriamycin, p. 1690), and metabolic disorders (e.g., uremia, p. 1760), as is discussed later in this chapter. In an unknown number of patients, acute myocarditis becomes chronic dilated cardiomyopathy. Conversely, an unknown number of cases of chronic dilated cardiomyopathy commence as acute myocarditis.

Myocarditis may be an acute or a chronic process. In North America, viruses are the most common agents producing myocarditis, while in South America, Chagas' disease (produced by *Trypanosoma cruzi*) is far more common. The identification of the specific etiological agent responsible for infectious myocarditis usually rests on the associated extracardiac findings, since the cardiovascular signs and symptoms are often nonspecific. The histological findings vary, depending on the stage of the disease, the mechanism of myocardial damage, and the specific etiological agent. Myocardial involvement may be focal or diffuse, but the myocardial lesions are generally randomly distributed in the heart, and thus the clinical consequences depend to a large extent on the size and number of the lesions. However, a single small lesion may have profound consequences if it is located within the cardiac conducting system.[377] The histological findings are usually nonspecific (except for some parasitic and granulomatous forms of myocarditis), and, with the exception of adriamycin cardiotoxicity,[378] myocardial biopsy is usually not rewarding in elucidating the etiology.

INFECTIOUS MYOCARDITIS

Clinical Manifestations

The clinical expression of myocarditis ranges from the asymptomatic state secondary to focal inflammation to fulminant fatal congestive heart failure due to diffuse myocarditis. An initial episode of viral myocarditis, perhaps unrecognized and forgotten, may be the initial event that eventually culminates in an "idiopathic" dilated cardiomyopathy (Fig. 41–23).[379] In support of this view is the observation in experimental animals that structural and functional myocardial alterations following viral myocarditis may persist well beyond the stage of viral replication and myocardial inflammatory response.[380]

While transient electrocardiographic abnormalities suggesting myocardial involvement are noted in many patients with infectious diseases,[381,382] most patients do not have other clinical manifestations of myocarditis. It is postulated that these electrocardiographic changes reflect subclinical myocardial involvement. That frequent but unrecognized myocardial involvement occurs with systemic infections is supported by histological evidence of myocarditis in 4 to 10 per cent of routine postmortem examinations.[383–387] Some degree of myocardial involvement, often subepicardial in location, also frequently occurs in patients with acute pericarditis.[388,389]

Since myocardial involvement is subclinical in most acute infectious diseases, the majority of patients have no specific complaints referable to the cardiovascular system;

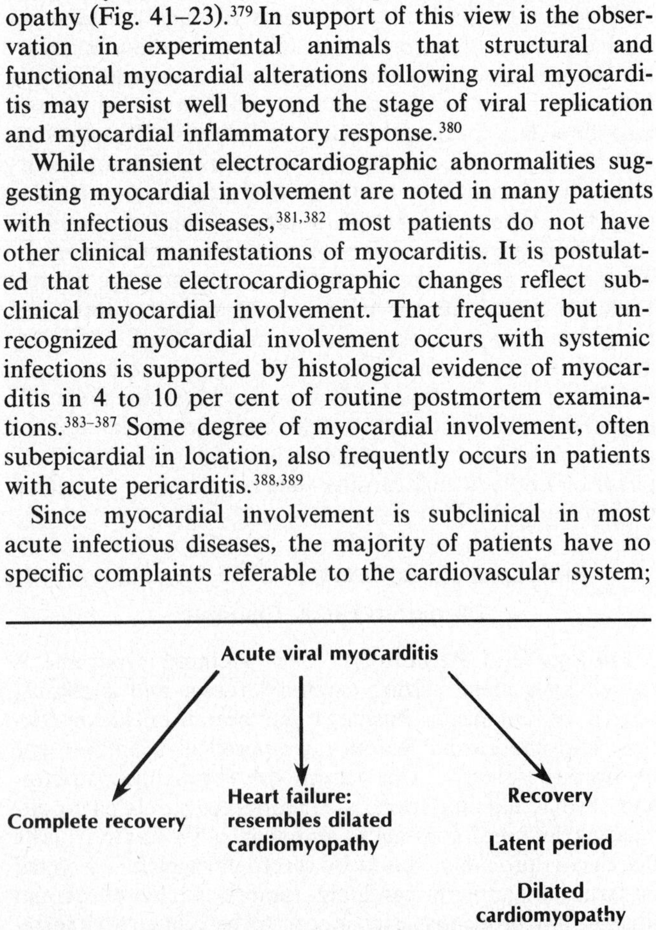

FIGURE 41–23 Viral myocarditis and cardiomyopathy. (From Goodwin, J. F.: The frontiers of cardiomyopathy. Br. Heart J. *48*:1, 1982.)

the presence of myocarditis is often inferred from the ST-segment and T-wave changes on the electrocardiogram.[383] From a clinical viewpoint, myocardial involvement is associated with nonspecific symptoms, including fatigue, dyspnea, palpitations, and precordial discomfort. Chest pain usually reflects associated pericarditis,[389] but precordial discomfort suggestive of myocardial ischemia is occasionally observed.[390]

On *physical examination,* tachycardia is usual and may be out of proportion to the temperature elevation.[385,391] The first heart sound is often muffled, and a protodiastolic gallop may be present. A transient apical systolic murmur may appear, but diastolic murmurs are rare.[381,384] Clinical evidence of congestive heart failure occurs only in the more severe cases.[381,383,385,390] Pulsus alternans is rare and is limited to patients with fulminant disease.[384] The heart is usually normal in size in the clinically silent cases, but it may be dilated in patients with congestive heart failure.[384] Pulmonary and systemic emboli may occur.[389,391]

As already indicated, *electrocardiographic* abnormalities are usually transient and occur far more frequently than does clinical myocardial involvement.[392] The most common changes are abnormalities of the ST segment and T wave, but atrial and in particular ventricular arrhythmias, atrioventricular (AV) and intraventricular conduction defects, and, rarely, Q waves may be seen.[379,393,394] Complete AV block is usually transient and resolves without sequelae, but it is occasionally a cause of sudden death in patients with myocarditis. On *radiological examination,* heart size may range from normal to markedly enlarged, and pulmonary congestion may be present in patients with fulminant disease. *Radionuclide scanning* after the administration of gallium-67 or technetium-99m pyrophosphate may identify inflammatory and necrotic changes characteristic of myocarditis.[396,397]

The *diagnosis* is often predicated on the identification of the associated systemic illness and its characteristic features. The diagnosis of viral myocarditis is supported by the identification of the virus in stool, throat washings, blood, myocardium, feces, or pericardial fluid, or by a distinct (usually fourfold) increase in virus neutralizing antibody, complement-fixation, or hemagglutination inhibition titers.[379] Even in fatal cases, isolation of virus from the myocardium at necropsy is difficult and is accomplished with regularity only with the Coxsackie, echo-, and poliomyelitis viruses.[380]

Most patients recover completely. The myocarditis frequently is clinically silent, and suspected only because of electrocardiographic changes.[394,398] However, some asymptomatic patients with prior myocarditis have left ventricular dysfunction that is not apparent clinically but may be demonstrated by exercise radionuclide ventriculography.[399] Some patients, most commonly infants and children, may succumb to the acute process. An unknown number of patients, probably a minority, develop chronic myocarditis, which may eventually culminate in "idiopathic" dilated cardiomyopathy.[392,400]

Pathology. Patients dying of or with myocarditis demonstrate a wide spectrum of gross and histological pathological changes, reflecting the range of disease seen clinically. Grossly, the hearts may be normal, dilated, hypertrophied, or flabby. An interstitial inflammatory reaction is usually observed and myocytolysis and necrosis may be seen.[401] Routine histological examination of the heart rarely provides a specific diagnosis, although in some instances electron microscopic and immunofluorescent techniques may allow elucidation of a specific etiology.

Treatment. Therapy is often supportive and is usually directed at the more prominent systemic manifestations of the disease. The demonstration of a particular predilection for involvement of the AV conducting system in some forms of myocarditis[402] suggests that patients with suspected myocarditis should be observed closely for any evidence of conduction abnormality. Since hypoxia and exercise intensify the damage from myocarditis in experimental animals, adequate oxygenation and rest are indicated.[403,404] Congestive heart failure responds to routine management, including digitalization and diuresis, although patients with myocarditis appear to be particularly sensitive to digitalis, and toxicity should be watched for.[389] Significant arrhythmias should be treated with antiarrhythmic agents, although beta-adrenergic blockers are probably best avoided in view of their negative inotropic action. The use of corticosteroids is controversial, but they are proscribed in acute viral myocarditis, since increased tissue necrosis and viral replication have been demonstrated following their use.[404] In some patients with rapidly progressive congestive heart failure of no identifiable cause, an inflammatory myocarditis may be demonstrable by right ventricular endomyocardial biopsy. A small number of patients have responded favorably to treatment with immunosuppressive agents, usually prednisone and azathioprine.[404a] Serial endomycardial biopsies have confirmed the resolution of the inflammatory infiltrate with treatment.[405] Prolonged bed rest has been advocated, but its utility in preventing long-term sequelae has not been established.[401]

It is hoped that effective antiviral agents for treating viral myocarditis will be developed. It may also be possible, in the future, to treat patients with myocarditis with agents that stimulate production of interferon, since this substance affords protection against the effects of viral myocarditis, at least in experimental animals.[406] Antibiotics may also be employed with benefit in infections caused by atypical pneumonia and psittacosis.

Viral Myocarditis*

Systemic infection with numerous viruses may be associated with clinical evidence of myocarditis[407] (Table 41–8). The myocarditis characteristically presents after a lag period of several weeks following the initial systemic infection, suggesting involvement of an immunological mechanism.[392] In animals, a variety of factors appears to enhance susceptibility to myocardial damage, including radiation, malnutrition, steroids, exercise, and previous myocardial injury.[400] Viral myocarditis may be particularly virulent in infants and in pregnant women.[404]

Coxsackie Virus. Both Coxsackie A and B viruses may produce myocarditis, although infection with Coxsackie B is more common,[400] and this agent is the most frequent cause of viral myocarditis.[393] The myocardium appears to be particularly susceptible to the effects of this virus because of the apparent affinity of myocardial membrane receptors for the viral particles.[404] Necropsy often demonstrates a

*Myocarditis secondary to psittacosis and *Mycoplasma pneumoniae* is described later in this chapter.

TABLE 41–8 PRINCIPAL VIRAL CAUSES OF MYOCARDITIS

Coxsackie (Groups A and B)
Echovirus
Adenovirus
Influenza
Varicella
Poliomyelitis
Mumps
Rabies
Viral hepatitis
Infectious mononucleosis
Cytomegalovirus
Arbovirus (Groups A and B)
Variola and vaccinia
Viral encephalitis
Yellow fever
Herpes simplex

pericardial effusion, pericarditis, cardiac enlargement, and a predominantly mononuclear inflammatory infiltrate, with necrosis of the atrial and ventricular myocardium.[39,408] In some cases, focal myocardial necrosis simulating myocardial infarction is seen, despite normal coronary arteries.[409]

Although most infections are probably subclinical,[410,411] Coxsackie myocarditis appears to be particularly virulent in the neonate. In most infections in adults, the other clinical manifestations of viral involvement, such as pleurodynia, myalgia, upper respiratory tract symptoms, and arthralgias, predominate. Severe cases in the adult are characterized by myopericardial involvement with pleuritic or pericarditic chest pain, palpitations, and fever. Many patients with overt myocardial involvement develop congestive heart failure with cardiomegaly and pulmonary edema.

The *electrocardiogram* is virtually always abnormal, with ST-segment and T-wave changes and arrhythmias, often ventricular in origin; AV conduction disturbances are common.[412] Blood levels of myocardial enzymes (serum glutamic oxaloacetic transaminase, creatine kinase) may be normal or elevated, reflecting the absence or presence of variable degrees of myocardial necrosis.[413]

Most patients recover completely within weeks, although it may require months for the electrocardiogram to return to normal.[414] Rarely, Coxsackie myocarditis is fatal in adults. Some patients become symptomatic following resolution of the infection, and they may present years later with dilated cardiomyopathy.[412] Occasionally, patients appear to recover completely only to develop symptoms subsequently.[415,416]

Treatment is symptomatic, and despite occasional postmortem evidence of intracardiac thrombi, anticoagulation should probably be avoided because of the risk of a hemorrhagic pericardial effusion.[412] Bed rest is indicated during the acute course of myocarditis, but there is no convincing evidence that a period of prolonged rest after apparent resolution of the acute process is useful.[417] Heart failure and cardiac arrhythmias are treated in the usual fashion.

Echovirus. Closely akin to the Coxsackie virus, the echoviruses may also be associated with myopericarditis, often during the course of an acute, pleurodynia-like illness,[418,419] although clinically apparent myocardial involvement during the course of an echovirus infection is rare.[401] Ventricular arrhythmias, complete AV block, and transient, nonspecific electrocardiographic changes have been reported.[420]

Adenovirus. Myocarditis is rare in adenovirus infection. Postmortem findings include dilated right and left ventricles, with a mononuclear infiltrate with fragmentation of the myocardial fibers.[421]

Influenza. Cardiovascular involvement may play an important role in patients with influenza, since one-third of fatal cases have evidence of active myocarditis.[422] Postmortem findings in fatal cases include biventricular dilatation, with evidence of subendocardial and subepicardial petechiae and hemorrhage. A mononuclear inflammation is prominent, especially in perivascular areas. Occasional fibrinoid necroses of the myocardial arterioles may be seen.[423] The earliest histological abnormalities include petechial hemorrhages and loss of myofibrillar striations. Then, fragmentation of the myocardial fibers becomes marked, and there is interstitial edema and hemorrhage.[422]

Cardiac involvement typically occurs within 1 to 2 weeks of the onset of the illness and may be severe, sometimes contributing to mortality.[423,424] The *clinical manifestations* include dyspnea, palpitations, anginal chest pain, arrhythmia, and heart failure[425]; there is often concomitant involvement of the pericardium. Sinus tachycardia or, less commonly, sinus bradycardia may be seen. The *electrocardiogram* may show transient ST-segment and T-wave abnormalities, conduction defects, and even complete AV block.[422] Sudden death is common and may be associated with massive hemorrhagic pulmonary edema due to viral involvement of the lungs.[422]

Varicella. Clinical myocarditis is a rare finding in varicella. Occasionally a patient may develop overt evidence of myocarditis with congestive heart failure.[426] Histological findings include rare but characteristic intranuclear inclusion bodies within the myocardial cells, along with interstitial edema, cellular infiltrates, and myonecrosis.[427] The electrocardiogram may show conduction abnormalities, and sudden death occurs rarely.[428]

Poliomyelitis. Myocarditis is a frequent finding in fatal cases of poliomyelitis, particularly during epidemics,[429] occurring in half or more of all patients dying with this disease. While myocardial involvement is usually focal and minimal in extent, some patients with bulbar disease succumb early in the course of the illness, often with cardiovascular collapse.[429,430] These patients all have viral infection of the medulla and severe systemic vasoconstriction that leads to pulmonary edema. Myocarditis appears to contribute to the heart failure.[429] The *electrocardiogram* is frequently abnormal, with ST-segment and T-wave abnormalities, prolongation of the P-R and Q-T intervals,[431] extrasystoles, tachycardia, and atrial fibrillation.[382] *Treatment* is symptomatic, with aggressive support of pulmonary function; tracheostomy and prolonged mechanical ventilatory support may be required. Fortunately, this disease has been largely eliminated by immunization.

Mumps. Myocardial involvement during the course of mumps is a rare phenomenon, occurring in less than 10 per cent of adults infected with this virus, and even less frequently in children.[432] The hearts of only a few patients with mumps have come to postmortem examination and they have been found to be both dilated and hypertrophied. Histologically, there is diffuse interstitial fibrosis, with infiltration of mononuclear cells and areas of focal necrosis.[433]

Cardiac involvement is usually unrecognized clinically, and the diagnosis of myocarditis is based on nonspecific electrocardiographic changes.[434] Transient ST-segment and T-wave abnormalities are most common, but extrasystoles and AV conduction block may occur; in a rare case, persistent complete heart block requires insertion of a permanent pacemaker.[435] Myocarditis generally occurs in the first week of illness and is transient, in most cases resolving within several weeks.[382,434] A few patients develop precordial chest pain, dyspnea, palpitations, and fatigue; cardiomegaly and congestive heart failure occur on occasion.[433] Tachycardia, a transient apical systolic murmur, and protodiastolic gallop may be present.[434]

Viral Hepatitis. The characteristic *pathological changes* in the myocardium associated with viral hepatitis are minute foci of necrosis of isolated muscle bundles, often surrounded by lymphocytes, and a diffuse serous inflammation.[436] The ventricles may be dilated, with petechial hemorrhages.[437] Hemorrhage into the interventricular septum involving the area of the conduction system is a conspicuous finding,[436,437] and electrocardiographic surveillance for evidence of conduction defects may be warranted in patients with clinical evidence of myocarditis during the course of viral hepatitis.

Electrocardiographic changes, including bradycardia, ventricular premature beats, and ST-segment and T-wave changes, may be seen during the course of hepatitis.[401,436,438] These abnormalities are usually transient and asymptomatic, although congestive heart failure, cardiomegaly, and sudden death have been reported.[437] Patients may present dyspnea, palpitations, and an anginal type of chest pain. Symptomatic myocarditis is generally observed during the first to third week of the disease.[438]

Infectious Mononucleosis. Examination of the hearts of patients with the myocarditis associated with infectious mononucleosis may reveal atypical lymphocytes within the myocardium, along with focal myocardial infiltrates and necrosis.[439] *Electrocardiographic changes* associated with infectious mononucleosis are common, although symptomatic cardiac involvement is only rarely observed.[439–441] ST-segment and T-wave changes may be observed, along with varying degrees of AV block. Ventricular arrhythmias occur rarely but may be fatal. Symptomatic patients may demonstrate a pericardial friction rub, an apical systolic murmur, and evidence of congestive heart failure.[439] Most patients follow an uncomplicated and nonfatal clinical course.[442]

Rubella and Rubeola. Congenital cardiovascular lesions may develop in the offspring when *rubella* is contracted by the mother during the first trimester of pregnancy, with persistent ductus arteriosus and pulmonary artery maldevelopment as prominent anomalies (p. 942). Abnormalities of the conduction system have been reported in postnatal rubella, but myocarditis does not appear to occur.[443]

In *rubeola,* transient electrocardiographic abnormalities,[444,445] including prolongation of the P-R interval, ST-segment and T-wave changes, AV conduction abnormalities, and ventricular tachycardia, have been reported.[381,444,445] The electrocardiographic changes are usually transient. Congestive heart failure occurs on rare occasions, and its appearance is a poor prognostic sign, often indicating a fatal outcome.[382] Histological examination of the heart in fatal cases has revealed evidence of myocarditis characterized predominantly by a perivascular lymphocytic infiltrate.[445]

Cytomegalovirus. Unrecognized infection with cytomegalovirus (CMV) is extremely common in childhood, and the majority of the adult population have antibodies to CMV.[446,447] Primary infection after the age of 35 years is uncommon, and generalized infection usually occurs only in immunosuppressed patients with neoplastic disease. The cardiovascular manifestations in adults are generally limited to asymptomatic and transient electrocardiographic changes. Symptomatic cardiac involvement is rare, although a hemorrhagic pericardial effusion may occur.[448] While fatalities are unusual, when they do occur histological examination of the heart may reveal focal lymphocytic infiltration and fibrosis.[448]

Arbovirus. Infections due to group A arbovirus (e.g., chikungunya) and group B arbovirus (e.g., dengue) often result in symptomatic cardiac involvement. In addition to symptoms due to systemic involvement (fever, headache, sweating), chest pain, dyspnea, palpitations, fatigue, dizziness, and paroxysmal nocturnal dyspnea are often prominent features. A protodiastolic gallop, apical systolic murmur, and cardiomegaly are common.[449–451] The latter often persists after the acute illness has resolved. The *electrocardiogram* is virtually always abnormal in patients with myocardial involvement, and ST segment and T wave abnormalities, sinus tachycardia, sinus bradycardia, conduction disturbances, and arrhythmias are found.[451] Atrial fibrillation, atrial premature depolarizations, and ventricular premature depolarizations are also seen. Sudden death may occur, most often due to ventricular arrhythmias or embolization.[449] Complete recovery is unusual, and most patients have persistent cardiomegaly and abnormalities of the electrocardiogram.[449,451]

Variola and Vaccinia. Cardiac involvement following smallpox is rare, although several cases of myocarditis associated with acute cardiac failure and death have been reported.[452] Myocarditis with pericardial effusion and congestive heart failure has also been observed as a complication of smallpox vaccination;[453] an immunological mechanism has been suggested and dramatic responses to steroids have been reported. The histological changes include a mixed mononuclear infiltrate, with interstitial edema and occasional degenerating or necrotic muscle bundles.[454]

Yellow Fever. Myocardial changes are occasionally seen in fatal cases of yellow fever, with petechial hemorrhages of the endocardial and epicardial surfaces, foci of myocardial necrosis, and cellular infiltration.[455]

Respiratory Syncytial Virus. Although respiratory syncytial virus is an important cause of respiratory disease, particularly in children, it rarely results in cardiac involvement.[456] Several patients have developed clinical congestive heart failure after an infection with this virus, with symptoms appearing several days after the initial respiratory manifestations[456,457] (Fig. 41–24). Complete heart block is a prominent feature, although cardiomegaly, ventricular arrhythmias, and cardiac decompensation may also be noted.

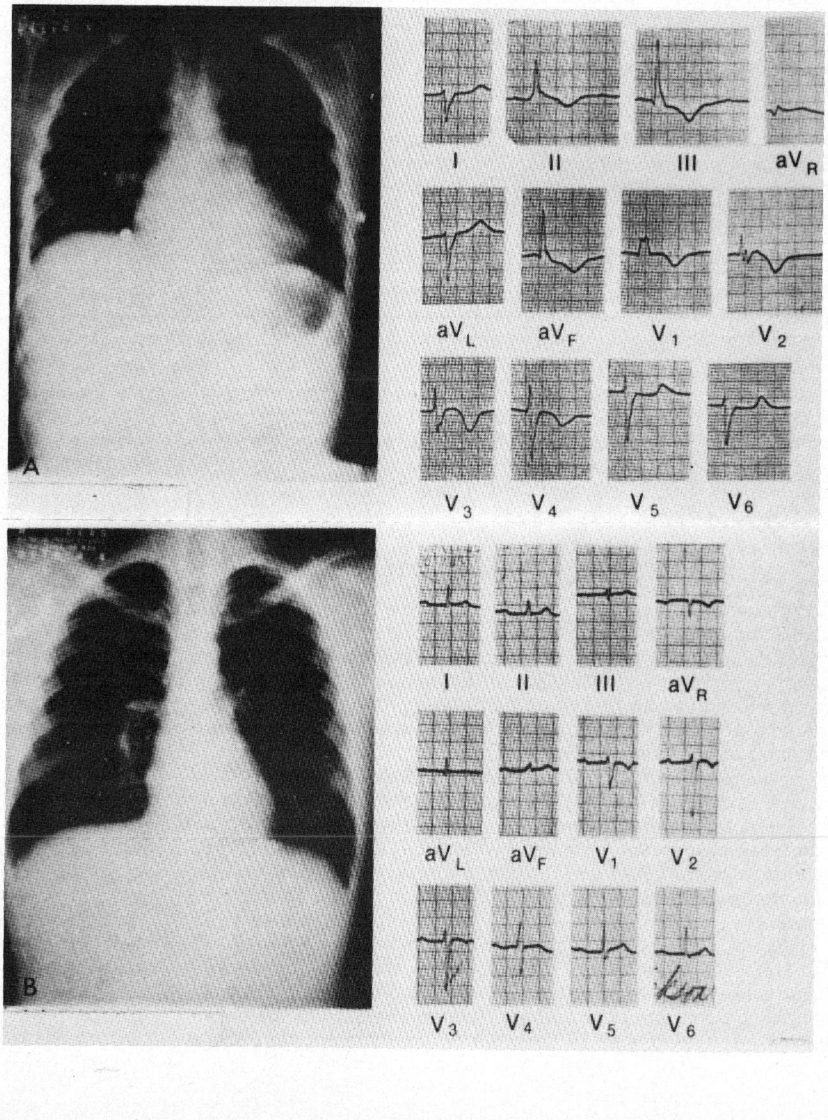

FIGURE 41–24 Recovery from myocardial involvement with respiratory syncytial virus. *A,* On admission, there is generalized cardiomegaly, prominence of the hilar vessels, and a pacing catheter within the right ventricle. The electrocardiogram demonstrates complete heart block with an idioventricular rhythm. *B,* One month later, following clinical recovery, the chest roentgenogram is normal, and the electrocardiogram is normal except for first-degree heart block. (From Giles, T. D., and Gond, R. S.: Respiratory syncytial virus and heart disease. A report of two cases. J.A.M.A. *236*:1128, 1976. Copyright 1976, American Medical Association.)

Mycoplasma pneumoniae. Electrocardiographic abnormalities are common during the course of atypical pneumonia, occurring in up to one-third of patients.[458] Nonspecific ST-segment and T-wave abnormalities are most common, particularly involving the right-sided precordial leads, but first-degree AV block is occasionally seen.[382,458] The electrocardiographic findings usually resolve within 1 to 2 weeks. Pericarditis may be a prominent finding, and congestive heart failure is occasionally seen.[459,460] A protodiastolic gallop and pericardial friction rub may be noted in occasional cases.[382] No specific treatment for the cardiovascular involvement is usually indicated. Complete recovery is the rule in most patients.[459]

Psittacosis. Myocarditis complicating psittacosis is a relatively common occurrence and is characterized by congestive heart failure and acute pericarditis.[461,462] *Pathological changes* include a fibrinous pericarditis, subendocardial hemorrhages, and interstitial edema, with lymphocytic and plasma cell infiltrates. Fatty degeneration or cloudy swelling of the muscle fibers may be seen. Fever, chest pain, electrocardiographic changes, cardiomegaly, systemic emboli, tachycardia, and hypotension may occur. While most patients recover completely, fatalities have been reported in a small fraction.[461] The systemic infection may be treated effectively with tetracycline, but the effect of the antibiotic on the myocardium is unknown.

Rickettsial Myocarditis

The rickettsial diseases are frequently associated with evidence of myocardial involvement. Transient ST-segment and T-wave alterations in particular are observed commonly.[463] The circulatory collapse that may accompany these diseases is largely a manifestation of abnormalities of the peripheral vascular bed, but a myocardial component may also be present. The basic histopathological process is a vasculitis, with a periarterial interstitial infiltrate.[464]

Scrub Typhus. Myocarditis is common during the course of scrub typhus (tsutsugamushi disease, caused by *R. tsutsugamushi*). The histological findings are those of a focal panvasculitis involving the small blood vessels. Myocardial necrosis is unusual, but hemorrhage into the heart and subepicardial petechiae may occur. Clinical evidence of myocardial involvement typically is not severe and is usually not associated with residual cardiac damage.[465,466] The electrocardiogram may show nonspecific ST-segment and T-wave abnormalities, as well as first-degree AV block. A protodiastolic gallop and apical systolic murmur suggestive of mitral regurgitation are occasionally found.

Rocky Mountain Spotted Fever. Clinical evidence of myocarditis is *not* usually a prominent feature of Rocky Mountain spotted fever (caused by *R. rickettsii*), although the heart is involved in the multisystem damage that occurs as the result of a widespread vasculitis.[467,468]

Q Fever. Endocarditis is the most common cardiac manifestation of infection with *R. burnettii* (Q fever). Myocarditis is not a prominent feature, although dyspnea and chest pain, perhaps reflecting associated pericarditis, occur frequently.[469] The electrocardiogram may demonstrate transient ST-segment and T-wave changes as well as paroxysmal ventricular arrhythmias.[469,470]

Bacterial Myocarditis

Diphtheria. Myocardial involvement is one of the most serious complications of diphtheria[471] and occurs in at least one fourth of cases. Indeed, myocardial involvement is the most common cause of death in this infection.[472] Cardiac damage is due to the liberation by the diphtheria bacillus of a toxin that inhibits protein synthesis by interfering with the transfer of amino acids from soluble RNA to polypeptide chains under construction.[473]

Pathological findings include a flabby and dilated heart with a myocardium that has a "streaky" appearance. Microscopic examination reveals characteristic fatty infiltration of the myocytes, often with an interstitial inflammatory infiltrate, myocytolysis, and hyaline necrosis of muscle fibers.[382] With time, fibrosis and hypertrophy of the remaining myocardial cells develop. The conduction system is often involved.

Typically, *clinical signs* of cardiac dysfunction appear at the end of the first week of the illness.[471] Cardiomegaly and severe congestive heart failure are often present.[382] A protodiastolic gallop and pulmonary congestion may be prominent features. Elevation of the serum transaminase levels may be seen; a high level is associated with a poor prognosis.[471] Sudden circulatory failure and death may occur.[382] Many patients develop ST-segment and T-wave abnormalities, but atrial and ventricular arrhythmias, bundle branch block, and various grades of AV conduction defects may also occur.[474] Persistently abnormal electrocardiograms are common following diphtheritic myocarditis, as are cardiomegaly and symptoms of reduced cardiac reserve.[382] Some patients recover fully.[471]

Because of the serious effects of the toxin on the myocardium, antitoxin should be administered as rapidly as possible. Antibiotic therapy is of less urgency. General supportive measures are indicated. Overt congestive heart failure may be resistant to therapy with cardiac glycosides. The development of complete AV block is a serious complication, but it may be amenable to treatment with a transvenous pacemaker.[475]

Salmonella. Symptomatic myocardial involvement during salmonella infections is rare, although electrocardiographic abnormalities are often seen, suggesting subclinical myocarditis. *Postmortem findings* in salmonella myocarditis may reveal a shaggy, fibrinous pericarditis and, in some cases, evidence of endocarditis.[476,477] Myocardial petechiae and hemorrhagic necrosis may occur, with evidence of biventricular dilatation. A polymorphonuclear leukocytic infiltrate with evidence of coronary arteritis may be found.[478] The arteritis may lead to thrombosis, infarction, and death. Other cardiovascular complications include infected mural thrombi, occasionally resulting in pulmonary and systemic emboli, and mycotic aneurysms.[476] Myocardial abscesses often develop and may rupture, producing fatal cardiac tamponade.[476] Myocarditis with congestive heart failure occurs most commonly in children who are severely ill with salmonellosis, and it is associated with a high mortality.[479] When myocarditis occurs, it often develops rapidly, with evidence of biventricular failure, tachycardia, a protodiastolic gallop, an apical systolic murmur of mitral regurgitation, and peripheral edema.[480]

Electrocardiographic abnormalities include ST-segment and T-wave changes, and prolonged P-R or Q-T intervals. These electrocardiographic changes typically appear in the second week of illness and usually resolve completely within a week.[480,481]

Tuberculosis. Tuberculous involvement of the myocardium is rare, particularly since the introduction of drugs effective against tuberculosis.[482] Children are more susceptible than adults to myocardial involvement.[483] Cardiac involvement may occur by direct extension from tuberculous hilar lymph nodes (probably the most common); lymphatic spread; and hematogenous spread.[484,485]

Miliary involvement of the heart is most common in children and occurs in 15 to 50 per cent of cases of miliary tuberculosis. The nodular and diffuse varieties are more common in adults.[483] The pericardium is typically free of tuberculous involvement in miliary tuberculosis, while the right side of the heart and interventricular septum are most commonly involved. *Nodular* myocardial involvement is the most common type of myocarditis in adults. Tuberculomas are isolated or multiple, rounded, circumscribed, firm nodules 2 to 70 mm in diameter.[486] The cardiac involvement may lead to compression of cardiac chambers with resulting functional abnormalities.[483] *Diffuse* infiltrating myocardial tuberculosis is the least common form of myocardial tuberculosis.[483] The myocardial involvement may lead to formation of a tuberculous aneurysm, and rupture with cardiac tamponade and death has been reported.[487] Infiltrative involvement of the heart appears to be predominantly right-sided, particularly the right atrium.[485,488] Most cases of myocardial tuberculosis are clinically silent and are diagnosed only at postmortem examination.[482,488] On rare occasions, tuberculous involvement of the myocardium may lead to arrhythmias, including atrial fibrillation and ventricular tachycardia, complete AV block, and congestive heart failure.

Streptococcus. The most common detected cardiac finding following beta-hemolytic streptococcal infection is acute rheumatic fever, which is discussed in detail in Chapter 48.

Direct infection of the heart by the streptococcus produces a myocarditis that is distinct from acute rheumatic carditis. It is characterized by an interstitial infiltrate composed of mononuclear cells with occasional polymorphonuclear leukocytes; the infiltrate may be focal or diffuse and may be localized to the subendocardial or perivascular region. There may be small areas of myocardial necrosis,[489] and direct bacterial invasion of the myocardium can sometimes be detected. *Electrocardiographic abnormalities*, including prolongation of the P-R and Q-T intervals, occur frequently;[382] while these abnormalities are rarely associated with other clinical manifestations of myocardial involvement, sudden death, conduction disturbances, and arrhythmias may occur.[490]

Meningococcus. Myocardial involvement is common during the course of meningococcal infections, particularly in men with fatal meningococcal infections.[491] *Pathological findings* include hemorrhagic myocardial lesions, occasionally associated with intracellular organisms. An interstitial myocarditis composed of lymphocytes, plasma cells, and polymorphonuclear leukocytes is often observed, occasionally with muscle necrosis.[393, 491] Fulminating meningococcemia associated with the Waterhouse-Friderichsen syndrome may exhibit focal muscle necrosis, severe fatty change, and cloudy swelling of the myocytes.[492]

Meningococcal myocarditis may result in congestive heart failure, which may be fatal, as well as in pericardial effusion.[493] Death may also occur suddenly and be associated with involvement of the AV node.[393] It is advisable to monitor the rhythm of patients with meningococcemia. In milder cases, transient electrocardiographic abnormalities, principally ST-segment and T-wave changes, are often seen and may resolve completely with time.[493]

Clostridia. Cardiac involvement is common in patients with clostridial infections with multiple organ involvement[494]; the myocardial damage results from the toxin elaborated by the bacteria. The *pathological findings* are distinctive, with gas bubbles usually present in the myocardium. Areas of degenerated muscle fibers are apparent, but an inflammatory infiltrate is usually absent.[494] *C. perfringens* may cause myocardial abscess formation with myocardial perforation and resultant purulent pericarditis.[495]

Bacterial Endocarditis. Myocardial infection is frequently observed as a consequence of infective endocarditis (Chap. 33).

Legionnaire's Disease. Although pneumonia, rhabdomyolysis, renal failure, and hepatic as well as central nervous system involvement are common with *Legionella pneumophila*, overt cardiac involvement is not. Occasional electrocardiograpic changes may be noted, consisting primarily of ST-segment and T-wave abnormalities. Rarely, myocarditis with evidence of myocardial necrosis and congestive heart failure may be seen.[496]

Spirochetal Infections

Syphilis. Aortitis is the most common manifestation of luetic involvement of the cardiovascular system. Aortic regurgitation and coronary ostial narrowing are associated findings (p. 1562). Syphilitic involvement of the myocardium itself in the form of gumma formation is rare and is usually unsuspected clinically. Involvement of the interventricular septum may result in damage to the conducting system and AV block.[497] Gummae may also impinge on the heart valves and interfere with their function.[498] While congenital syphilis may lead to a diffuse myocarditis,[499] the existence of this in adults is disputed.[500]

Leptospirosis [Weil's Disease]. Cardiac involvement is common in leptospirosis. The *pathological findings* include petechiae or larger foci of hemorrhage, often located in the epicardium.[501] An interstitial myocardial infiltration, often subendocardial in location, may occur, with involvement of the papillary muscles.[501] Involvement of the AV conduction system may be a prominent feature. The most common manifestations of cardiac involvement are ST-segment and T-wave changes; atrial and ventricular arrhythmias, sinus bradycardia, and conduction defects may occur.[502,503] Cardiomegaly, pulmonary congestion, a protodiastolic gallop, pericarditis, and symptoms of congestive heart failure occur rarely.[502]

Relapsing Fever. Many infections are currently observed in Ethiopia. During pandemics, mortality may be particularly high, reaching 70 per cent. Cardiac involvement is a common complication and is often implicated as a cause of death. AV conduction defects occur frequently and may be responsible for sudden death, although tachyarrhythmias have also been implicated.[504] Numerous petechiae are observed with a diffuse histiocytic interstitial infiltrate, particularly around small arterioles in the left ventricle.

Fungal Infections

Systemic fungal infections often occur in individuals with reduced resistance to infection, who are frequently patients with malignant disease and/or those receiving chemotherapy, steroids, radiation, or immunosuppressive therapy.

Aspergillosis. Myocardial involvement is not uncommon in generalized aspergillosis. On *pathological examination*, myocardial necrosis and infarction caused by thrombosis of vessels that contain fungal mycelia are commonly seen. The fungus often extends beyond the vessel walls and invades the surrounding necrotic myocardium.[505] The electrocardiogram may be normal in the face of significant myocardial damage but T-wave changes may be present.[506] The *diagnosis* of aspergillus infection is often difficult. Identification of aspergillus through open lung biopsy, aspiration lung biopsy, transtracheal aspiration, or bronchial brush technique is usually successful. Early institution of prolonged therapy with amphotericin B may result in significant improvement.[505]

Actinomycosis. Myocarditis is a rare complication of actinomycotic infection, occurring in less than 2 per cent of patients.[507] However, cardiac involvement is quite serious when it does occur. Involvement of the heart most commonly is the result of direct extension of disease within the thorax.[507] Initially the pericardium is invaded, with eventual obliteration of the pericardial space.[508] The myocardium is commonly involved by extension of the pericardial process. Myocardial seeding is less common. The myocardial lesion is a suppurative, necrotizing abscess containing the organism, surrounded by granulation tissue.[508] Both right- and left-sided failure are common manifestations.[508] A pericardial rub may be heard, sometimes associated with clinical evidence of a pericardial effusion. Arrhythmias occur infrequently.[507]

Blastomycosis. Blastomycosis involves the myocardium by spread from mediastinal lymph nodes, by hematogenous miliary seeding,[509,510] and most frequently by direct extension from the pericardium. *Pathological findings* include cardiac dilatation without hypertrophy but with caseation and tubercle formation. Thrombi may form above the endocardial lesions. Dyspnea, cyanosis, and peripheral edema may be prominent. Tachycardia and a systolic murmur are often present.[510]

Cryptococcosis. Cryptococcal infection of the myocardium occurs most commonly in patients with disseminated malignancy.[511] *Pathological examination* may show cardiac dilatation, with epithelial granulomas and giant cells and variable degrees of fibrosis.[512] Congestive heart failure occurs[512]; pulmonary congestion and muffled heart sounds may be found on physical examination, and cardiomegaly on the chest roentgenogram. The *electrocardiogram* may show first-degree AV block and T-wave inversions; ventricular arrhythmias have been observed.

Candidiasis. Disseminated monilial infections are common opportunistic infections, particularly in the compromised host.[513] Endocardi-

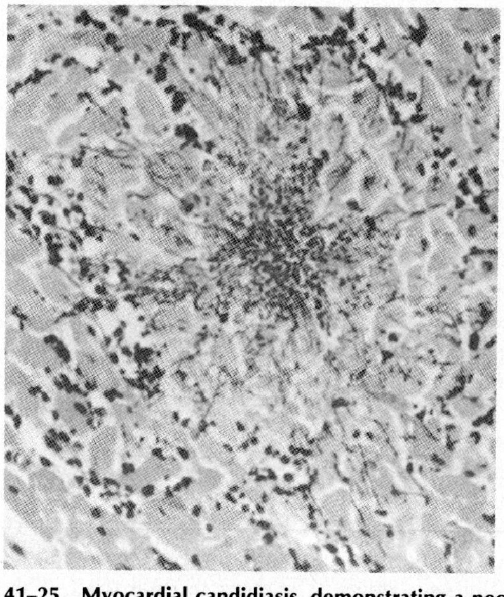

FIGURE 41-25 Myocardial candidiasis, demonstrating a necrotizing myocarditis with a surrounding inflammatory infiltrate. Fungal growth is apparent in the center of the figure. (Original magnification × 360.) (From Brooks, S. E. H., and Young, E. G.: Clinicopathologic observations on systemic moniliasis: A case report and review of the literature. Arch. Pathol. *73*:383, 1962. Copyright 1962, American Medical Association.)

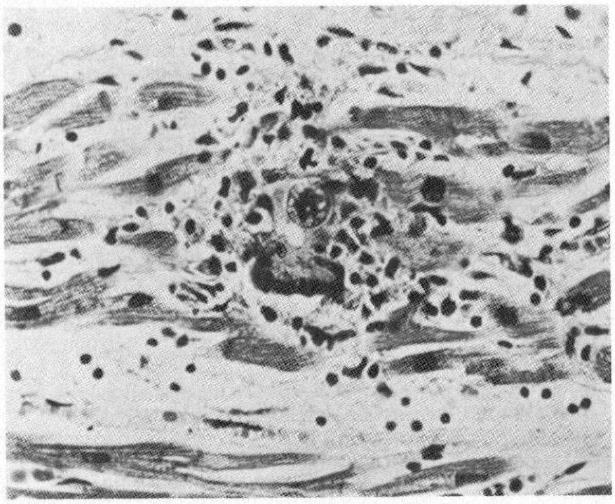

FIGURE 41–26 Disseminated coccidioidomycosis with myocardial involvement. There is a coccidioidal granuloma with evidence of necrosis, multinucleated giant cells, mononuclear cells, lymphocytes, and a coccidioidal spherule. (From Reingold, I. M.: Myocardial lesions in disseminated coccidioidomycosis. Am. J. Clin. Pathol. *20*: 1044, 1950.)

tis is the most frequent manifestation of cardiac involvement (p. 1170), although abscesses of the myocardium may occur as associated or independent findings. Complete heart block may be caused by microabscesses of the conduction system. Pseudohyphae and yeast forms are often found, and multiple foci in the myocardium are usually present.[514] The abscesses are composed of tubercles, with pseudohyphae in the center of the lesions and surrounding yeast forms; there may be polymorphonuclear leukocytes in the periphery of the lesion[514] (Fig. 41–25).

Coccidioidomycosis. Involvement of the heart is seen on occasion in patients with generalized coccidioidomycosis. The hearts may be grossly normal, although epicardial lesions with resultant pericarditis are frequent,[515] and progression to constrictive pericarditis may occur[516] (p. 1502). A nonspecific, focal, interstitial, and perivascular cellular infiltrate with associated muscle fiber degeneration and interstitial edema is commonly found, although granulomas containing fungi are also seen sometimes[515] (Fig. 41–26).

Histoplasmosis. Cardiac involvement in histoplasmosis is rare and usually is in the form of endocarditis (Chap. 33).[517] Pericarditis with effusion may also occur (p. 1502) and superior vena caval obstruction has been observed.[518] Myocardial involvement occurs less frequently, although atrial arrhythmias and T-wave abnormalities have been reported.[518]

Protozoal Myocarditis

TRYPANOSOMIASIS (CHAGAS' DISEASE)

Chagas' disease is caused by the protozoan *Trypanosoma cruzi.* The major cardiovascular manifestation is an extensive myocarditis that typically becomes evident years after the initial infection. The disease is prevalent in Central and South America, particularly in Brazil, Argentina, and Chile, where it is a major public health problem. More than 10 million people in South America may be afflicted.[519]

The natural history of Chagas' disease is characterized by three phases: acute, latent, and chronic. During the *acute phase,* the disease is transmitted to humans through the bite of a reduviid bug (subfamily *Triatominae*), which harbors the parasite in its gastrointestinal tract. This insect acquires the disease from feeding on infected animals, including the armadillo, raccoon, opossum, and skunk as well as domestic dogs and cats. The reduviid bug, popularly known in Argentina as "vinchuca," meaning "to let oneself drop," lives in the walls and roofs of houses and, during nocturnal feeding, drops from the ceiling onto the sleeping person below.[520] The bug then often bites the person around the eyes, and infection of the human host occurs when the trypanosomes in the animal's feces gain entry through abraded skin or through the conjunctivae. Occasionally, this results in unilateral periorbital edema and swelling of the eyelid, termed *Romaña's sign,* while entry through the skin may result in a lesion called a *chagoma.* Transmission may also occur through blood transfusions as well as congenitally.

ACUTE TRYPANOSOMIASIS. Following inoculation, the protozoa multiply and then migrate widely throughout the body. In a minority of cases an acute illness occurs, although inapparent acute infections are more common.[520,521] There appears to be a depression of T-cell function in those with inapparent acute infections, while those with evident acute disease have normal T-cell function.[521]

Pathological examination during the acute phase often reveals parasites in the cardiac fibers with a marked cellular infiltrate, particularly around cardiac cells that have ruptured and released the parasites. The cellular infiltrate is typically milder around intact muscle fibers harboring parasites. Degeneration of the myocardial fibers may occur. Involvement may extend into the endocardium, resulting in thrombus formation, and into the epicardium, resulting in pericardial effusion.[522] The pathogenesis of the myocardial lesions of acute Chagas' disease appears to relate in large part to immune lysis by antibody and cell-mediated immunity directed against antigens released from *T. cruzi*–infected cells, which become adsorbed onto the surface of infected and noninfected host cells.[523–525]

Clinical Manifestations. These include fever, muscle pains, sweating, hepatosplenomegaly, myocarditis, and, occasionally, meningoencephalitis.[520] The congestive heart failure is characterized by tachycardia, a protodiastolic gallop, arrhythmias, pulmonary congestion, and peripheral edema. Most patients recover, and their symptoms resolve over several months. Occasionally, patients develop fulminant necrotizing panmyocarditis, often with electrocardiographic evidence of right bundle branch block and findings suggesting extensive myocardial necrosis.[520] Young children most commonly develop clinical acute disease and generally are the most seriously ill.

CHRONIC TRYPANOSOMIASIS. The disease then enters a *latent phase,* not to reappear for 10 to 30 years. At an average of 20 years after the initial (and usually unrecognized) infestation, approximately 30 per cent of infected individuals develop findings of *chronic Chagas' disease,* characterized by cardiomegaly, congestive heart failure, arrhythmias, and right bundle branch block (Fig. 41–27). In this stage, cardiac dilatation typically involves all the cardiac chambers, although right-sided enlargement may predominate.[526] The right ventricle may exhibit increased compliance, dilatation and inflammation, with areas of necrosis.

The pathogenesis of chronic chagasic cardiomyopathy is becoming clearer. The central paradox in this disorder is the negative correlation between the severity of disease and the level of parasitemia.[524] It is not unusual to be unable to detect parasites in patients dying of Chagas' disease.[527] An autoimmune mechanism is thus suggested. It appears (at least in an animal model) that self-reactive cytotoxic T

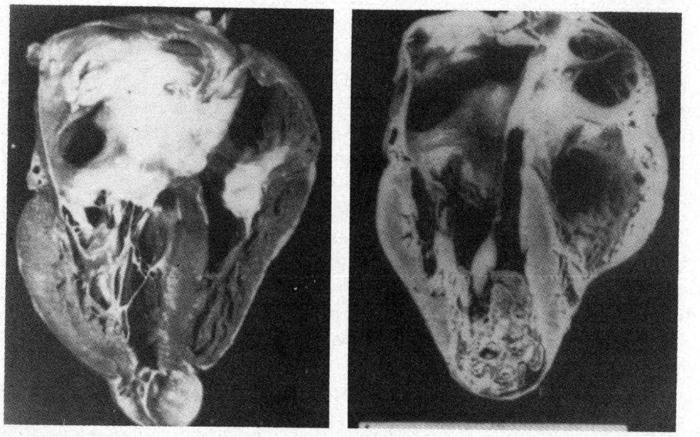

FIGURE 41–27 ***Left,*** **Chagas' heart disease with apical aneurysm.** ***Right,*** **Thrombosis of the apical aneurysm. (From Oliveira, J. S. M., et al.: Apical aneurysm of Chagas' heart disease. Br. Heart J.** ***46*****: 432, 1981.)**

lymphocytes develop following the initial infection, and these lymphocytes are able to lyse normal host cells in the absence of parasite antigens.[523] It is thought that the acute phase results in the release from parasite-modified host cells of self components that are immunogenic.

Pathology. Nerves and autonomic ganglia are frequently abnormal; megaesophagus and megacolon may occur; less commonly, there is dilatation of the stomach, duodenum, ureter, and bronchi.[528] Different strains of *T. cruzi* may account for the geographic differences in the expression of Chagas' disease; in Brazil, megaesophagus and megacolon are uncommon, but these conditions are usual in Venezuela.[529] Lesions of the cardiac nerves are routinely found in patients with chronic Chagas' disease.[526] Pathological cardiac findings include cardiac enlargement with dilatation and hypertrophy of all cardiac chambers.[520,526,528] The left ventricular apex is often thin and bulging, resembling an aneurysm[530] (Fig. 41–27). Thrombus formation is frequent and may fill much of the apex; the right atrium also frequently contains thrombus.[528]

The microscopic findings are principally those of extensive fibrosis, particularly of the left ventricle.[531] A chronic cellular infiltrate composed of lymphocytes, plasma cells, and macrophages is often present[528,531] (Fig. 41–28). In rare cases, granulomatous lesions or an arteritis is apparent.[528] Preferential involvement of the right bundle branch and the anterior fascicle of the left bundle branch by inflammatory and fibrotic changes explains the frequent occurrence of right bundle branch and left anterior fascicular block.[532] Parasites may be identified in one-fourth of patients[526]; the frequency with which they are found depends upon the diligence of the search for them.

Clinical Manifestations. Chronic progressive heart failure, often predominantly right-sided, is the rule. Thus, while pulmonary congestion is occasionally noted, the usual findings generally include fatigue due to diminished cardiac output, peripheral edema, ascites, and hepatic congestion.[520] Tricuspid regurgitation is often present, particularly in patients with severe right-sided heart failure, although mitral regurgitation is frequently present as well.[528] The second heart sound is widely split, often with an accentuated pulmonic component,[520] reflecting the combined effects of right bundle branch block and pulmonary hypertension.

The *chest roentgenogram* often demonstrates severe cardiomegaly, with or without pulmonary venous hypertension.[528] *Electrocardiographic abnormalities* are the rule, with right bundle branch block and left anterior hemiblock being the most common changes in patients with chronic Chagas' disease[520,528,528a] (Fig. 41–29). Left bundle branch block is uncommon. ST-segment and T-wave abnormalities are common,[520] while Q waves involving the inferior leads,[528] P-wave abnormalities, and AV block are occasionally seen.[522] Early in the disease, the electrocardiogram may be normal or nearly so. Administration of the antiarrhythmic agent ajmaline may precipitate the appearance of electrocardiographic abnormalities and thus identify patients with as yet clinically silent cardiac involvement.[533,534a]

Ventricular arrhythmias are a prominent feature of chronic Chagas' disease. Frequent ventricular premature depolarizations, often with multiple morphologies, are seen often, and bouts of ventricular tachycardia may occur. Ventricular arrhythmias are particularly common during and following exercise, occurring in the majority of patients subjected to stress electrocardiographic testing.[528] Syncope and sudden death due to ventricular fibrillation are a constant threat and may develop even before cardiomegaly or heart failure.[520] Sinus bradycardia may also be seen, even in patients with severe heart failure when a tachycardia would be expected.[520,526] Atrial arrhythmias, including atrial fibrillation, may also occur. Thromboembolic phenomena are a frequent complication.[528]

The *echocardiographic findings* in some are those of a dilated cardiomyopathy (Fig. 5–72, p. 130), with dilatation, increased end-diastolic and end-systolic volumes, reduced fractional systolic shortening of the left ventricle, and ejection fraction, often with enlargement of the left atrium and right ventricle.[528] In the majority of patients, the echocardiographic appearance is distinctive, with left ventricular posterior wall hypokinesis and relatively preserved interventricular septal motion; an apical aneurysm is often seen on two-dimensional echocardiography.[519]

Left ventricular cineangiography in advanced cases shows a dilated, hypokinetic left ventricle with a large apical aneurysm containing intracavitary thrombus, often with evidence of mitral regurgitation (Fig. 41–27). Mild

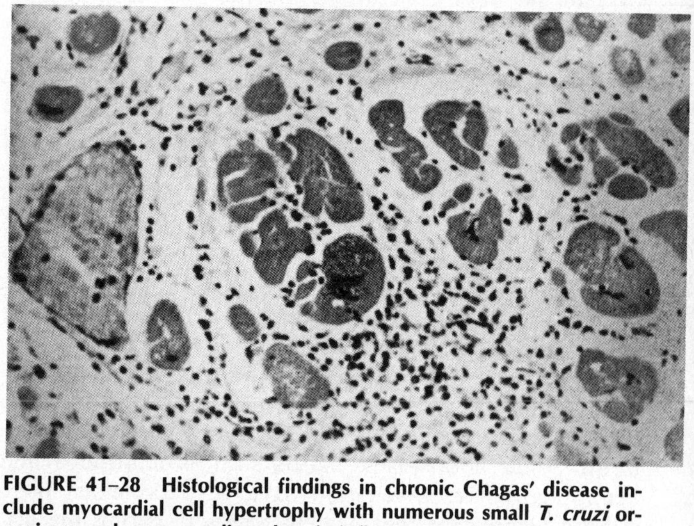

FIGURE 41–28 Histological findings in chronic Chagas' disease include myocardial cell hypertrophy with numerous small ***T. cruzi*** **organisms and a surrounding chronic inflammatory infiltrate. (Original magnification × 400.) (From Puigbo, J. J., et al.: Diagnosis of Chagas' cardiomyopathy. Noninvasive techniques. Postgrad. Med. J.** ***53*****: 527, 1977.)**

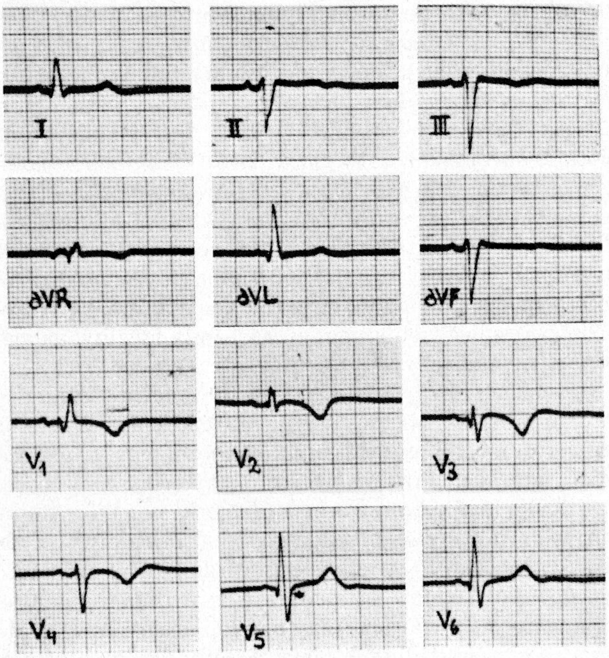

FIGURE 41–29 Electrocardiogram typical of chronic Chagas' disease, demonstrating left anterior hemiblock, right bundle branch block, and T-wave changes. (From Rosenbaum, M. B.: Chagasic myocardiopathy. Progr. Cardiovasc. Dis. *7*:199, 1964, by permission of Grune and Stratton.)

asynergy in the anteroapical region may be seen in some patients despite the absence of clinical, radiological or electrocardiographic evidence of cardiac involvement.[534,534a]

The *complement-fixation* test (Machado-Guerreiro test) is useful in diagnosis; it has a sensitivity of greater than 90 per cent, with a specificity of 99 per cent[520] for the identification of chronic Chagas' disease. Also used in diagnosis are the indirect immunofluorescent antibody, the enzyme-linked immunosorbent assay (ELISA), and the hemagglutination tests.[535,536] Another test that is occasionally useful is the detection of parasites in the blood of patients with chronic Chagas' disease (which occurs in 30 to 40 per cent of cases) by means of *xenodiagnosis.* The patient is bitten by reduviid bugs bred in the laboratory; the subsequent identification of parasites in the intestine of the insect is proof of infection in the human host.[520]

Diagnosis. Three forms of evidence should be available to establish a diagnosis of chronic Chagas' cardiomyopathy: (1) *epidemiological evidence*—the patient should be from a geographical area where the vectors are available and the disease occurs; (2) *clinical evidence*—the patient should have findings of a dilated cardiomyopathy with arrhythmias or conduction abnormalities, without evidence of intrinsic valvular, pericardial, coronary, or congenital disease; (3) *laboratory evidence*—the serological or xenodiagnostic test should be positive.[520]

Treatment. The management of Chagas' disease remains difficult; once cardiac decompensation develops, there is usually a rapid and inexorable progression to death. While antiparasitic agents such as nifurtimox and benzimidazole are effective in reducing parasitemia, there is no evidence that they are efficacious in curing the disease.[537] A more promising avenue of approach appears to be immunoprophylaxis, although a clinically useful vaccine is not yet available.[524]

African Trypanosomiasis. African sleeping sickness, due to *Trypanosoma gambiense* or *T. rhodesiense,* may be associated with myocardial abnormalities, although they are usually of less functional significance than in so-called American trypanosomiasis (Chagas' disease).[538] *T. rhodesiense*, in particular, may lead to cardiac failure, although the central nervous system findings (excessive somnolence) usually dominate the clinical picture.

Pathological examination uniformly reveals pericardial fluid. The heart is not as greatly dilated and hypertrophied as it is in Chagas' disease and may appear grossly to be normal. There is often epicardial thickening with a cellular exudate composed of lymphocytes, plasma cells, and histiocytes.[539] The myocardium typically displays a diffuse interstitial infiltrate, often with zones of patchy fibrosis and interstitial edema.[539,540]

Nonspecific *electrocardiographic changes*, usually T-wave abnormalities and prolongation of the Q-T interval,[538] are often observed. Unlike Chagas' disease, arrhythmias and conduction disturbances are usually not prominent features and the arterial pressure is usually normal. Some of the patients have asymptomatic cardiomegaly, although both pulmonary congestion and peripheral edema have been reported.

Toxoplasmosis. *Toxoplasma* infections are caused by an obligate intracellular parasite (*T. gondii*); both congenital and acquired forms may occur. Symptomatic, acquired, toxoplasmic infections occur most commonly in patients with malignant diseases who are being treated with corticosteroids, chemotherapy, radiation, or immunosuppressive drugs.[541] *Pathological findings* include cardiac enlargement and hypertrophy, with occasional endocardial thrombi.[542] Petechial hemorrhages, an inflammatory infiltrate with variable degrees of edema and degeneration of the muscle bundles, and pericardial effusion are often present.

Most adult cases are asymptomatic, but *Toxoplasma* infections may produce a severe, fatal disease with multisystem involvement.[541] Toxoplasmic myocarditis, often with pericarditis, may occur as an isolated disease process or as part of a multisystem disseminated disease. Manifestations may include arrhythmia (atrial and ventricular), AV block, pericarditis, and heart failure.[543] Large pericardial effusions may be seen on occasion.[544] Palpitations, tachycardia, chest discomfort, fatigue, pulmonary congestion, and peripheral edema may be prominent symptoms. *Physical examination* usually reveals cardiomegaly, congestive heart failure, gallop rhythm, systolic murmurs, and hypotension. The *electrocardiogram* may show a variety of abnormalities, including atrial and ventricular arrhythmias, bundle branch block or hypertrophy patterns, or AV conduction defects.[541,542,545] When the myocardial involvement is one manifestation of disseminated disease, the antibody titers are typically quite high or rise rapidly. On the other hand, isolated myocarditis may be associated with low and nondiagnostic titers.

Treatment is with a combination of pyrimethamine and triple sulfonamides, but the response to therapy is variable.[541,545] Corticosteroids may be helpful in treating arrhythmias or conduction defects.

Malaria. While myocardial changes may be demonstrated during the course of malaria, particularly with *Plasmodium falciparum*, clinical findings to indicate cardiac involvement are rare. The heart generally demonstrates few gross abnormalities. The principal findings are histological. The capillaries are often filled and even distended with an accumulation of parasites, sometimes totally occluding the lumen of the vessels. Thrombosis of the capillaries and ischemic myocardial changes may be seen.[546,547] Focal myocardial damage may be present, along with an interstitial infiltrate composed of lymphocytes, plasma cells, and macrophages. In rare cases, cardiac failure may contribute to or even cause death,[548] although it has not been demonstrated that chronic heart disease results from malaria. Slight ST-segment and T-wave changes on the electrocardiogram may be the only clinical indications of myocarditis.[549]

Metazoal Myocardial Disease

Schistosomiasis. Schistosomiasis is a major public health problem, with an infection rate as high as 85 per cent in heavily endemic areas, such as the Nile River basin in Africa and the Yangtze River basin in the Orient. Its principal cardiac effect is right heart overload secondary to pulmonary hypertension. Embolization of the schistosomal ova to the pulmonary vasculature results in an allergic pulmonary arteritis and a paravascular granulomatous reaction, which results in pulmonary hypertension. Right ventricular hypertrophy and right heart failure with chronic cor pulmonale occur typically in young adults.[550,551]

Direct myocardial involvement, on the other hand, is quite infrequent.[552] Myocardial invasion by the ova may result in an inflammatory myocarditis, with a perivasculitis composed principally of mononuclear cells and eosinophils.[552] It has also been proposed that a myocarditis may occur in the absence of direct invasion by the parasite, and a toxic or allergic etiology has been postulated.[553]

Heterophyiasis. This condition results from infestation by several intestinal flukes and is common, particularly in the Far East. The heart may become involved, presumably by hematogenous spread. The heart may be slightly dilated, particularly the right side, with prominent subepicardial hemorrhages. Chronic congestive heart failure is present for some time and may eventually culminate in the patient's demise.[553,554]

Cysticercosis. Cardiac involvement with *Cysticercus cellulosae*, the larval form of *Taenia solium*, is occasionally seen following a disseminated systemic infection. While electrocardiographic changes, including P- and T-wave abnormalities, as well as congestive heart failure have been reported, most cases of cardiac involvement are not apparent clinically.[555-557]

Echinococcus (Hydatid Cyst). *Echinococcus* is endemic in many sheep-raising areas of the world, particularly Argentina, Uruguay, New Zealand, Greece, North Africa, and Iceland, but cardiac involvement in hydatid disease is uncommon, occurring in less than 2 per cent of cases.[558] The usual host of *Echinococcus granulosus* is the dog, but human beings may serve as intermediate hosts (rather than the sheep, the usual intermediate host) if they accidentally ingest ova from contaminated dog feces. The parasites leave the intestine and enter the portal circulation, where the majority are trapped by the liver. Some of the parasites may escape the hepatic and pulmonary bed and become trapped in the myocardium.[559] Once in the myocardium, the parasite grows and a cyst is formed, which may range from a few millimeters to many centimeters in diameter; most exceed 5 centimeters.[560]

The left ventricle is the most common site of cardiac involvement, presumably because of its richer coronary circulation.[560-563] Involvement of the interventricular septum and right ventricle may also occur.[39,564-566] A myocardial cyst may degenerate and calcify, develop daughter cysts, or rupture. Rupture of the cyst is the most dreaded complication; rupture into the pericardium may result in acute pericarditis, which may progress to chronic constrictive pericarditis. Rupture into the cardiac chambers may result in systemic or pulmonary emboli. The liberation of hydatid fluid into the circulation may produce profound, fatal circulatory collapse due to an anaphylactic reaction to the protein constituents of the fluid.

Most patients with cardiac involvement are in the second to fourth decades, and men predominate.[560-562] The diagnosis may be made from the *chest roentgenogram*, which typically shows an abnormal cardiac silhouette with a distinct bulge of the cardiac border.[558,559,561] Expansion of the cyst may result in myocardial compression and damage, sometimes resulting in angina pectoris and electrocardiographic abnormalities.[565] The *electrocardiogram* often reflects the location of the cyst; T-wave changes and loss of QRS voltage may occur with left ventricular involvement, while AV conduction defects or right bundle branch block may be seen with involvement of the interventricular septum. P-wave abnormalities occur in the rare cases of atrial involvement. Arrhythmias are occasionally seen as well.[559] Chest pain is usually due to rupture of the cyst into the pericardial space wth resultant pericarditis.[558] Protrusion of a cyst from the interventricular septum into the right ventricular outflow tract may result in partial obstruction.[558,562,566]

Diagnosis of an echinococcal cyst of the heart is a relatively simple matter if there is evidence of cysts in other organs, particularly the liver and lung.[553,558] Unfortunately, the cardiac cyst is often an isolated, solitary finding. The *chest roentgenogram* frequently shows a calcified lobular mass adjacent to the left ventricle,[562] and fluoroscopy and tomography may furnish additional details regarding location, size, shape, and degree of cyst calcification. Two-dimensional echocardiography may prove useful in the early detection of cardiac involvement.[567] Definitive diagnosis is provided by cardiac catheterization and angiography.[558,559,562] Left ventricular angiography may be particularly helpful in differentiating a cyst from a ventricular aneurysm.[563] Coronary arteriography may be useful in defining the extent of the cyst by its displacement of the coronary vasculature.[559] Hemodynamic measurements may demonstrate a gradient between the right ventricle and pulmonary artery in patients with obstruction to right ventricular outflow.

Eosinophilia, present in some patients, is a useful adjunctive finding. The Casoni skin test is not very helpful because both false-positive and false-negative results occur. Serological tests, including hemagglutination and complement-fixation, are more useful.[559]

Until recently, *treatment* for hydatid disease was limited to surgical excision.[558,559] Recent experience suggests that the benzimidazole derivative mebendazole may be an effective agent in the medical management of this disease.[568] Because of the significant risk of rupture of the cyst and its attendant serious and sometimes fatal consequences, surgical excision is generally recommended for asymptomatic patients.[562] The surgical results have been favorable, with complete recovery in many cases.[562]

Visceral Larva Migrans. People are occasional accidental hosts of the roundworm infestations of dogs due to *Toxocara canis*. Most cases occur in children one to three years of age.[569] Myocarditis may occur in association with invasion of the myocardium by larvae. The myocardial lesions include granulomas or extensive inflammatory infiltrates with foci of muscle necrosis.[570] Congestive failure and death may occur, although complete recovery following the use of corticosteroids has been reported.[569,570]

TRICHINOSIS. Infestation with *Trichinella spiralis* is the most common human helminthic disease, and evidence of involvement may be found in almost 1 per cent of routine autopsies.[571] Unlike some parasitic diseases with cardiac involvement, myocarditis plays a prominent role in trichinosis and is in fact responsible for the majority of fatalities.[572] The mortality of acute trichinosis is reported to be approximately 5 per cent. Less frequently, death is due to pulmonary embolism secondary to venous thrombosis as well as encephalitis.[572]

Although the parasite frequently invades the heart, it does not usually encyst there, and it is rare to find larvae or larval fragments in the myocardium.[573] Nonetheless, *pathological findings* at postmortem examination may be impressive. The heart may be dilated and flabby and a pericardial effusion may be present. A prominent focal infiltrate composed of lymphocytes and eosinophils, with interstitial edema, hyperemia, and scattered hemorrhages, is commonly found.[553,571-573] Areas of muscle degeneration and necrosis are present. The lesions may be due to toxic effects of the products produced in the course of the host reaction.

The *clinical manifestations*, congestive heart failure and chest pain, usually appear around the third week of the disease, when the general constitutional symptoms are abating.[571,574] Often, the cardiac symptoms are mild or absent or are overshadowed by other symptoms. Physical examination may be normal, or there may be gross cardiomegaly with severe congestive heart failure.[573,575,576] Sudden death may occur, usually in the fourth to eighth week of the illness.[553,574]

Electrocardiographic abnormalities may be detected in one-fourth of patients with trichinosis[573] and parallel the time course of clinical cardiac involvement, initially appearing in the second or third week and usually resolving by the seventh week of the illness.[571,576] The most common electrocardiographic abnormalities are T-wave changes, followed by prolongation of the QRS complex, diminished QRS voltage, first-degree AV block,[576] and ventricular arrhythmias.[575] The electrocardiographic changes usually resolve completely.

The definitive *diagnosis* is based on the demonstration of

larval forms in tissue biopsy samples, usually of the gastrocnemius muscle. Eosinophilia, when present, is a supportive finding.[553] The skin test is usually but not invariably positive. Treatment is with corticosteroids; dramatic improvement in cardiac function has been reported following their use.[571,575] Recovery from myocarditis may occur without residual cardiac damage.

NONINFECTIOUS MYOCARDIAL DAMAGE

A wide variety of stimuli other than those produced by infection may act on the heart and damage the myocardium.[577,578] In some cases, the damage is acute, transient, and associated with evidence of myocardial inflammation (myocarditis). Other agents that damage the myocardium may lead to chronic changes with resulting histological evidence of fibrosis and a clinical picture of a dilated cardiomyopathy. Furthermore, many offending stimuli may be associated with both acute and chronic phases (e.g., alcohol, adriamycin). The response often is related to the dose and rate of exposure.

Numerous chemicals and drugs (both industrial and therapeutic) may lead to cardiac damage and dysfunction. Several physical agents (e.g., radiation and excessive heat) may also result in myocardial damage. Furthermore, myocardial involvement may be evident in a variety of systemic diseases, which are described in Part IV of this book.

Toxic, Chemical, and Drug Effects

Tricyclic Antidepressants (see also p. 1839). Although sudden death, disturbances in rhythm, and abnormalities of AV conduction may be seen with the tricyclic antidepressants, important depression of left ventricular function is usually not seen, even in patients with preexisting heart disease.[579] Postural hypotension may be exacerbated, however.

Phenothiazines (see also p. 1840). The phenothiazines may be associated with a variety of cardiac disturbances, including electrocardiographic changes, atrial and ventricular arrhythmias, and sudden death.[580-582] Of the most commonly used agents, evidence of cardiac involvement is most common with thioridazine (Mellaril), less common with chlorpromazine (Thorazine), and least common with trifluoperazine (Stelazine). The cardiac effects are largely dose-dependent. Electrocardiographic abnormalities may be seen with as little as 200 milligrams of thioridazine per day and consist of lengthening of the Q-T interval and T-wave changes.[583] Higher doses may lead to frank T-wave inversion and increase in the amplitude of the U wave.[580] Changes in the P wave, QRS complex, and ST segment are usually absent.

The phenothiazines appear to have a quinidine-like effect, except that they do not prolong the duration of the QRS complex.[583] Although the phenothiazines may lead to ventricular arrhythmias, they also apparently suppress atrial and ventricular ectopic beats, at least in experimental animals.[584] The electrocardiographic abnormalities and arrhythmias resolve with discontinuation of the drug, usually within 48 hours.[585] Ventricular irritability apparently is caused by the facilitation of reentry by the phenothiazines.

Pathological changes in the hearts of patients who have received psychotropic drugs and who have died suddenly include the deposition of acid mucopolysaccharide between muscle bundles in periarteriolar regions as well as the conduction system, with myofibrillar degeneration, and endothelial proliferation in the smaller blood vessels. A variety of explanations have been invoked for the cardiac damage, including direct toxic effects of the phenothiazines on the myocardium, stimulation of higher autonomic centers, and changes in circulating or myocardial levels of catecholamines.[586]

Emetine. Cardiovascular changes are common with the use of emetine, a drug often employed in the treatment of amebiasis and schistosomiasis.[587] Myocardial lesions may be observed in some but not all patients at autopsy, and similar cardiac damage is noted in experimental animals given emetine.[580,587,588] The myocardial lesions consist of myofibrillar degeneration and necrosis, with an interstitial infiltrate of mononuclear cells and histiocytes. Emetine appears to inhibit oxidative phosphorylation and results in reversible damage to the mitochondria.[587,589] However, the observation that potassium administration often results in normalization of the T waves suggests that the electrocardiographic changes are due to transient intracellular ionic shifts.[588,590]

The *electrocardiogram* most commonly shows reduced T-wave amplitude or inversion. Prolongation of the Q-T interval and ST-segment shifts may also be seen, although abnormalities of the P wave, P-R segment, and QRS complex are infrequent. The electrocardiographic changes usually resolve within weeks or months after cessation of treatment. Sinus tachycardia and hypotension may also be seen, although clinical evidence of myocardial toxicity is usually lacking.[588] Only rare fatalities have been reported. *Dehydroemetine* results in electrocardiographic abnormalities similar to those of emetine, but they are less prominent and of shorter duration.[588]

Emetine and dehydroemetine therapy should be discontinued upon appearance of clinical evidence of cardiac toxicity, but treatment may be continued cautiously if electrocardiographic changes are the only manifestation. Potassium supplementation may be employed so long as the serum potassium level is closely monitored.

Chloroquine. This drug has been widely used in the prophylaxis and treatment of a variety of parasitic diseases and has potent toxic cardiac effects, which appear to be related to its ability to inhibit cellular respiration by blocking the Krebs cycle.[591] It is a myocardial depressant in large doses, although routine doses are not usually associated with clinical evidence of cardiac dysfunction.[590,591] Electrocardiographic changes occur routinely and are similar to those seen with emetine, although they are less pronounced and of shorter duration. In toxic doses, chloroquine may result in depressed cardiac output, bradycardia, arrhythmias, heart block, and death.[591]

Antimony Compounds. Various antimony compounds, such as stibophen and tartar emetic, have been widely used in the treatment of schistosomiasis; less toxic agents are now becoming available. The antimony compounds are associated with electrocardiographic changes in almost all patients. Typical *electrocardiographic changes* include prolongation of the Q-T interval with flattening or inversion of T waves. ST-segment shifts and P-wave changes may be seen, although the QRS complex usually demonstrates no abnormality.[580] Most patients do not demonstrate cardiac findings, although chest pain, bradycardia, hypotension, ventricular arrhythmias (including paroxysmal ventricular tachycardia), and sudden death may occur.[592]

Lithium (see also p. 1841). Lithium carbonate, used in the treatment of manic-depressive disorders, is associated with T-wave changes in one-fourth or more of patients who receive the drug. Clinical evidence of myocardial involvement is usually lacking, although intoxication with lithium may be associated with ventricular arrhythmias, symptomatic sinus node abnormalities, atrioventricular conduction disturbances, and death.[593-595] In fatal lithium toxicity, the heart is dilated and there is evidence of myofibrillar degeneration associated with a lymphocytic interstitial infiltrate and fibrosis.[595]

Hydrocarbons. Ingestion of hydrocarbons may result in fragmentation and vacuolization of the muscle fibers with loss of cross-striations.[596] Electrocardiographic changes, arrhythmias, and cardiomegaly may occur. Involvement of the central nervous, renal, hepatic, and pulmonary systems may dominate the clinical presentation and obscure the myocardial damage, which may well contribute to the mortality of hydrocarbon ingestion.[596] The electrocardiographic changes include ST-segment and T-wave abnormalities, although patterns suggesting acute myocardial injury have been noted.[597]

The *fluorinated hydrocarbons*, commonly used as aerosol propellants, appear to be cardiac toxins, contrary to their reputation of being inert. In animal preparations, at least, the aerosol propellants cause ventricular tachyarrhythmias, depress myocardial contractility, and lower systemic vascular resistance and arterial pressure.[598] These cardiovascular effects may be involved in the sudden deaths seen in individuals who abuse aerosols for their psychotropic effect.

Catecholamines. Myocarditis is frequently observed in conjunction with pheochromocytoma, and the myocardial damage has been attributed to high levels of circulating catecholamines[599,600] (p. 1734). Similar changes have been demonstrated in experimental animals treated with prolonged infusions of L-norepinephrine. Catecholamines may produce an acute myocarditis, with focal myocardial necrosis, inflammation, epicardial hemorrhages, tachycardia, and arrhythmias.[601] Phenylpropanolamine, a sympathomimetic amine used in decongestants and appetite suppressants, may result in similar findings.[602]

A variety of mechanisms have been suggested. A direct toxic effect may be involved, or the damage may be secondary to relative tissue hypoxia because of heightened metabolic demands. Alternatively, the damage may result from changes in autonomic tone or enhanced lipid mobility induced by epinephrine.[603] Aspirin and dipyridamole appear to offer some protection against experimental myocardial necrosis by catecholamines, suggesting that platelet aggregation plays a major role. It has been suggested that the rare development of a myocardial infarction after prolonged stress may result from intravascular platelet thrombosis induced by catecholamines, which may lead to occlusion of a coronary artery previously narrowed by an atheroma.[603]

Lead. The prominent features in lead poisoning generally center on the gastrointestinal and central nervous systems. However, myocardial involvement may contribute to or be the principal cause of death in some cases.[577,604] Reported pathological changes include cloudy swelling of the myofibers, with interstitial fibrosis and edema but without much of a cellular infiltrate. Electrocardiographic changes, chest pain, atrioventricular conduction defects, and overt congestive heart failure may occur.[605] The electrocardiographic and myocardial changes appear to be reversible.

Carbon Monoxide. Both acute and chronic carbon monoxide toxicity are common. While central nervous system findings usually dominate the clinical presentation, significant and occasionally fatal cardiac abnormalities are often present. Because carbon monoxide has a higher affinity for hemoglobin than does oxygen, insufficient oxygen is transported to the tissues.[606] Thus, the cardiac toxicity is the result of myocardial hypoxia, but a direct toxic effect of the gas on myocardial mitochondria may also play a role.[607] The *histological features* include focal areas of necrosis, most marked in the subendocardium. Focal perivascular infiltrates and punctate hemorrhages are also seen.[606] The *electrocardiographic changes* in survivors are transient.[606] Administration of 100 per cent oxygen, bed rest, and surveillance for serious rhythm or conduction abnormalities will usually permit rapid recovery.[606]

Cardiac involvement may appear promptly after exposure or it may be delayed for up to several days. Palpitations, sinus tachycardia, and various arrhythmias, including ventricular extrasystoles and atrial fibrillation, are common.[606,608] Bradycardia and AV block may occur in more severe cases. In patients with ischemic heart disease, angina pectoris and myocardial infarction may be precipitated. Electrocardiographic ST-segment and T-wave abnormalities are quite common. Transient left ventricular wall motion abnormalities may be present.[609]

Mercury. Electrocardiographic abnormalities, principally ST-segment depression, T-wave changes, and prolongation of the Q-T interval, are common findings in mercury poisoning. However, no specific cardiac symptoms occur.[610]

Phosphorus. Ingestion of phosphorus leads to death in 30 to 50 per cent of individuals, with most deaths occurring within 36 hours.[611] The heart is dilated, with diffuse interstitial edema but without a cellular infiltrate. Electrocardiographic abnormalities occur in the majority of patients and consist of ST-segment and T-wave abnormalities, prolongation of the QRS complex and Q-T interval, and atrial arrhythmias.[611,612] Prominent clinical features include severe biventricular depression of contractile function, peripheral vasodilatation, and marked hypotension.

Hypocalcemia. In rare patients with chronic hypocalcemia (often due to hypoparathyroidism), congestive heart failure may occur and resolve only when the serum calcium level is raised.[613,614]

Selenium Deficiency. Dietary deficiency of the trace element selenium appears to be one of the principal factors responsible for a form of dilated cardiomyopathy endemic to certain rural areas in China that are deficient in selenium.[615] Termed *Keshan disease*, it affects mainly children and young women and can be prevented by the prophylactic administration of sodium selenite tablets.[616] A similar cardiomyopathy may be found in Occidentals subjected to prolonged parenteral hyperalimentation.[617]

Scorpion Sting. The venom of the scorpion is mainly neurotoxic, but cardiac findings may be prominent and even fatal, particularly in children.[577,618] Hearts are normal on gross examination with prominent microscopic changes usually but not invariably present, particularly in the subendocardial regions and papillary muscles.[618,619] Degeneration and necrosis of muscle fibers are noted, with interstitial edema and a mononuclear infiltrate. The histological features of scorpion sting suggest high levels of circulating catecholamines[618-620] and are similar to those seen with experimental catecholamine infusion and in pheochromocytoma (p. 1734). The parasympathetic system appears to be stimulated as well.[621]

The *electrocardiogram* often initially shows tall peaked T waves that progress to inversions and ST-segment shifts. Q waves may appear, and the Q-T interval is usually prolonged. Atrial, junctional, and ventricular arrhythmias may occur. Tachycardia, hypertension, anxiety, diaphoresis, and pulmonary edema—findings resembling those of a massive catecholamine effect—are striking in many patients.[618-620] A smaller number of patients are seen in shock with peripheral vascular collapse. Most deaths are due to pulmonary edema, presumably the result of left ventricular dysfunction. Occasionally, sudden and unexpected deaths occur in a smaller percentage of patients, presumably as a consequence of arrhythmias. Adrenergic blocking agents may be useful in the management of the cardiovascular manifestation of scorpion stings.[618]

Wasp and Spider Stings. Stings by the vespine wasps may lead to hypotension, circulatory collapse, and cyanosis,[622] manifestations of anaphylaxis. Occasional patients may have chest pain and clinical findings compatible with acute myocardial infarction. The mechanism of myocardial damage is unclear; perhaps it merely reflects necrosis from profound hypotension, although a direct toxic effect on the myocardium or an indirect effect on the coronary arteries may be involved.

Cardiovascular collapse may also appear after stings due to the "black widow" spider (*Latrodectus mactans*). Atrial arrhythmias, labile blood pressure, and increased urinary levels of vanillylmandelic acid suggest that the stings may result in increased catecholamine levels.[623]

Snake Bite. Cardiac complications are usually not prominent features of snake bites, and the clinical picture is usually dominated by the neurological, hematological, and vascular damage produced by the snakebite toxin.[624] Myocardial involvement is seen on occasion and may rarely contribute to morbidity and mortality.[577] T-wave abnormalities are the most common manifestation of myocardial involvement, although ST-segment depression and QRS prolongation may also be seen. The electrocardiographic changes are usually transient, but when persistent they are attributed to direct myocardial damage due to the toxin.[625] Death may occur from circulatory collapse in adder bites, and myocardial infarction due to hypotension and coronary artery thrombosis has been reported.[626]

Arsenic. Arsenicals are currently utilized in pesticides. Myocardial involvement may be seen in both acute and chronic poisoning; the heart may be dilated, with accumulation of pericardial fluid.[627] Multiple focal and confluent areas of subepicardial and subendocardial hemorrhage are characteristic findings.[627,628] The myocardium is usually abnormal, with evidence of a perivascular mononuclear infiltrate.

Clinically unrecognized, toxic, interstitial myocarditis[629] is reflected in T-wave inversions and ST-segment depressions, along with prolongation of the Q-T interval. The electrocardiographic changes usually revert to normal within two to four weeks. The electrocardiographic abnormalities appear to resolve more rapidly when BAL (British antilewisite, dimercaprol) is utilized in therapy.[630] Death is often due to acute renal failure, although circulatory collapse may occur.[627,628]

Industrial exposure to *arsine gas* is often rapidly fatal, with deaths due to myocardial failure and uremia.[631] The principal toxic effect of arsine is on the red blood cells, with the production of massive hemolysis. Cardiac dilatation is typically present at postmortem examination. Myocardial edema with subepicardial hemorrhage, fibrosis, cloudy swelling, and fragmentation of muscle fibers with a minimal cellular infiltrate constitute the principal histological findings. T-wave changes are common. Death from pulmonary edema usually occurs within two days of exposure.

Cyclophosphamide (see also p. 1692). High doses of cyclophosphamide (greater than 45 mg/kg/24 hr) have been associated with electrocardiographic changes, congestive heart failure, and death from a hemorrhagic myocarditis.[632,633] In the majority of patients treated a reversible decrease in QRS voltage and systolic function is seen, often asymptomatic, although more than 20 per cent may succumb owing to myopericarditis.[634] The hearts are dilated, with subepicardial and subendocardial ecchymoses, and the left ventricle is thickened.[634] The myocardial damage appears to result from direct endothelial damage and resultant fibrin microthrombi in the capillaries. Myopericarditis may occur within the first two weeks of the initiation of therapy, with development of dyspnea, tachycardia, orthopnea, hypotension, fluid retention, and decreased QRS voltage.[632]

Paracetamol. Paracetamol, a phenacetin metabolite, may result in massive liver necrosis. On occasion it also results in fatty degeneration and focal necrosis of the myocardium, typically on the second to fourth day after an overdose.[635]

Thyroid Hormone. Rare cases of sudden death have been seen with thyroid hormone abuse, and pathological examination has revealed evidence of myocarditis with focal leukocytic infiltration and fibrosis.[636]

Miconazole. Anaphylaxis and cardiac arrest may be seen in patients with hematological malignancies treated with the antifungal agent miconazole.[637] The mechanism of apparent cardiotoxicity is unclear.

Disopyramide (see also p. 659). The antiarrhythmic agent disopyramide may lead to depression of left ventricular function when given either intravenously or orally, although this effect usually is seen only in patients with preexisting left ventricular dysfunction.[638] In addition to an exacerbation of congestive failure, disopyramide may also precipitate profound cardiovascular collapse and death.[639]

5-Fluoro-uracil. This antineoplastic agent has rarely been associated with cardiotoxicity manifested by chest pain, electrocardiographic changes, and arrhythmia. Swelling of myocardial fibers has been demonstrated in an animal preparation.[640]

Daunorubicin and Adriamycin (see page 1690 to 1692).

Hypersensitivity

Hypersensitivity to a variety of agents may result in allergic reactions that involve the myocardium.[641] In addition to anaphylaxis and serum sickness, allergies to a variety of drugs or other sensitizers may lead to an allergic myocarditis, characterized by eosinophilia, and a perivascular infiltration of the myocardium by eosinophils, multinucleated giant cells, and leukocytes.

Methyldopa. This drug is widely used in the treatment of hypertension (p. 915). Although hepatitis is the most frequently encountered serious adverse reaction, sudden and unexpected death has been reported in a number of patients found at necropsy to have had an unsuspected myocarditis.[578] The *histological findings* have the characteristics of an allergic myocarditis, showing an interstitial inflammatory infiltrate with abundant eosinophils, a vasculitis, and focal myocardial necrosis.[642]

Penicillin. Allergic reactions to penicillin are fairly common, but myocardial involvement is rare.[577,578] *Histological findings* consist of a perivascular and interstitial infiltrate composed of eosinophils, plasma cells, lymphocytes, and histiocytes.[643] Both myocardial infarction and pericarditis may occur and account for some of the electrocardiographic changes.[644] Transient electrocardiographic changes may be the only manifestation of cardiac involvement, with bradycardia, ST-segment elevation, and T-wave inversion.

Sulfonamides. Sulfonamides may result in myocardial damage owing to a hypersensitivity vasculitis as well as a myocarditis.[645] Fatal cases usually demonstrate an eosinophilic myocarditis, sometimes with granulomas.[646] While usually clinically silent, severe and even fatal congestive heart failure may occur.[647] Electrocardiographic changes are usually absent, but nonspecific ST-segment and T-wave abnormalities may be seen.[580,647]

Tetracycline. Allergic reactions to antibiotics of the tetracycline class include fever, tachycardia, and first-degree AV block. Postmortem findings include cardiac dilatation, fibrinoid muscle cell degeneration, and a diffuse interstitial and perivascular infiltrate.[577,578,648]

Phenindione. Marked congestive heart failure with cardiomegaly and pulmonary edema has been reported following the use of phenindione. The electrocardiogram may show sinus tachycardia, low QRS voltage, and T-wave inversion.[578,649]

Phenylbutazone. Myocarditis is an uncommon complication[578] but is characterized by dyspnea, chest pain, hypotension, and extensive ST-segment elevations.[650] Pericardial effusions with a prominent perivascular infiltrate may be seen in the myocardium.[651]

Antituberculous Drugs. Most reactions to antituberculous drugs consist of a fever, rash, or both, but serious and fatal cardiac reactions may occur. *Paraaminosalicylic acid* may lead to the development of interstitial edema, acute inflammatory infiltrate, refractory congestive heart failure, hypotension, and ventricular irritability.[652] It is commonly associated with transient arrhythmias or cardiac dilatation.[653]

Streptomycin has been implicated as a rare cause of myocarditis. Pathological findings may include cardiac dilatation, myocarditis with necrosis, hemorrhage, and a fibrinous pericardial effusion.[654] Clinically, it may be associated with chest pain, dyspnea, fever, and rash, followed by collapse and death.

Lyme Carditis. Lyme disease is a process of uncertain etiology that appears to be transmitted by the tick *Ixodes dammini.* The disease is found only in areas of tick distribution, the majority of cases emanating from the northeastern coast of the United States.[655] Lyme disease usually begins during the summer months with a characteristic skin rash (erythema chronicum migrans), followed in days to months by neurological, joint, or cardiac involvement.[656] It is thought that the tick bite transmits an infectious agent that produces the initial skin eruption. The later manifestations, including carditis, appear to be immune-mediated, perhaps related to circulating immune complexes.[657]

About 10 per cent of patients with Lyme disease develop evidence of cardiac involvement, the most common manifestation being variable degrees of AV block. Syncope due to complete heart block is frequent with cardiac involvement, as are diffuse ST-segment and T-wave abnormalities.[657] Transient asymptomatic left ventricular dysfunction may be detected by radionuclide ventriculography in as many as one-third of patients, although cardiomegaly or symptoms of congestive heart failure are rare.[657]

The value of specific therapy in Lyme carditis remains uncertain. Although the skin eruption responds to penicillin or tetracycline, a beneficial effect of antibiotics on the carditis is unestablished.[657] Advanced AV block is usually treated with salicylates or prednisone, although patients with the most severe involvement (meningoencephalitis, complete AV block for longer than one week, or cardiomegaly) are treated routinely with corticosteroids. Temporary transvenous pacing may be required for up to a week in patients with complete heart block.[657]

Giant Cell Myocarditis. Giant cell myocarditis is a rare disease of unknown etiology characterized by the presence of multinucleated giant cells in the myocardium. Variously called acute isolated myocarditis and granulomatous myocarditis, this condition is typically a rapidly fatal disease of young to middle-aged adults.[658,659] *Pathological findings* are usually impressive. The ventricles are dilated, and when death is not sudden, mural thrombi may be present. A serpiginous area of myocardial necrosis may be seen involving the right as well as the left ventricle.[659] Multinucleated giant cells are found, particularly at the margins of the areas of myocardial necrosis. An extensive inflammatory infiltrate is present within the necrotic areas, composed of eosinophils, histiocytes, and other cells[658,659]; fibrosis is absent.[658]

Although giant cell myocarditis appears to be associated with thymoma, systemic lupus erythematosus, and thyrotoxicosis,[659,660] the cause of the disease remains obscure. In many ways the clinical features suggest a viral myocarditis except for the rapid and virulent course. However, despite careful investigation there has been no serological or bacteriological evidence of an infectious etiology.[658,661] Sarcoid, syphilis, and tuberculosis have all been proposed as possible causes, although these usually present distinctive histological features.[659] It has also been suggested that the cause is an autoimmune reaction,[662] although little evidence aside from the histological findings supports this view.

Both sexes are equally affected; the onset is typically rapid, with dyspnea, chest pain, orthopnea, and hypotension.[658,659,661] Fever is usually present with electrocardiographic evidence of widespread myocardial involvement. Sinus tachycardia, left bundle branch block, atrial and ventricular arrhythmias, complete heart block, and findings suggesting acute myocardial necrosis may be seen. Overt congestive heart failure and sudden death may occur.

Rejection of the Transplanted Heart. The major barrier to wider application of cardiac transplantation remains the problem of immunologically mediated injury as a result of rejection[663] (p. 547). Acute rejection is most frequent in the first three months after transplantation, occurring on the average of once per 21 patient-days. Among long-term survivors, on the other hand, episodes of acute rejection occur only once every 325 patient-days.

In the immediate postoperative period, immunosuppression is accomplished with high-dose prednisone, azathioprine, Cyclosporin A, and antithymocyte globulin.[57] The findings in rejection may be clinically subtle, and often the only indication is a decline in the QRS voltage presumably secondary to myocardial edema secondary to the rejection process. ST-segment and T-wave changes are also common.[57,664] Less commonly, atrial or ventricular arrhythmias appear. Mild rejection episodes are marked only by these electrocardiographic findings, and there is no reduction of cardiac reserve. A diastolic sound (usually an S_3, occasionally an S_4) is often present. An increase in thickness of the left ventricular wall is often detectable by echocardiography,[664] presumably the result of myocardial edema. Severe rejection is categorized by clinical evidence of diminished cardiac performance at rest, with hypotension, weakness, and congestive heart failure.[57,664]

The presence and severity of rejection can be evaluated by percutaneous right ventricular endomyocardial biopsy (Fig. 41-30).[665-667] A biopsy specimen is usually obtained as a baseline shortly after transplantation and the procedure repeated during suspected rejection episodes.[663] During rejection, the myocardium becomes dark and edematous. Interstitial edema, hemorrhage and myocyte degeneration and necrosis appear. Changes in the microvasculature are present, with swelling of endothelial cells and perivascular infiltration of mononuclear cells.[667] The clinical manifestation of these pathological changes is diminished ventricular compliance, resulting in restriction to myocardial filling.[664]

Treatment of early acute rejection by intensive immunosuppression is usually successful, although a significant number of infections and other serious complications occur as a result of the immunosuppression.[664] Late chronic rejection is felt to be responsible for the accelerated development of atherosclerosis in the coronary arteries of the transplanted heart.[57,668] The use of warfarin and dipyridamole as well as of diets low in cholesterol and saturated fats has reduced the incidence to approximately 20 per cent.[669]

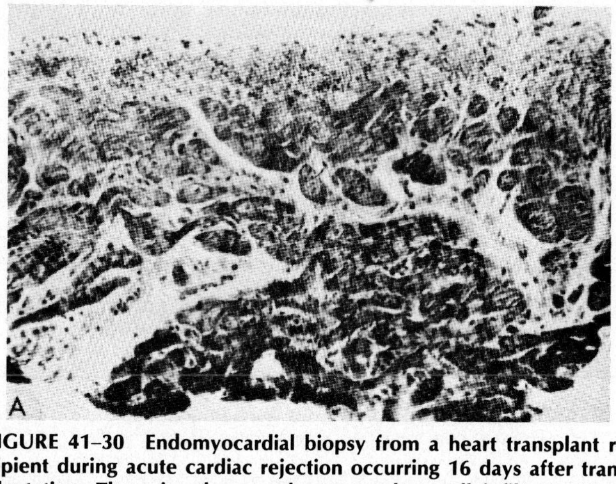

FIGURE 41-30 Endomyocardial biopsy from a heart transplant recipient during acute cardiac rejection occurring 16 days after transplantation. There is edema and mononuclear cell infiltrate. (From Caves, P., et al.: Transvenous endomyocardial biopsy—application of a method for diagnosing heart disease. Postgrad. Med. J. *57*:286, 1975.)

Physical Agents

Heat Stroke. This condition results from failure of the thermoregulatory center following exposure to high ambient temperature and is manifested principally by hyperpyrexia and central nervous system dysfunction. However, cardiovascular abnormalities are common. *Pathological changes* include dilatation of the right side of the heart, particularly the right atrium. Hemorrhages of the subendocardium and the subepicardium are frequently seen at necropsy and often involve the interventricular septum and posterior wall of the left ventricle. Histological findings include degeneration and necrosis of muscle fibers as well as interstitial edema.[670,671] Possible factors responsible for myocardial damage include direct thermal injury, myocardial hypoxia secondary to circulatory collapse, decreased coronary blood flow, and metabolic abnormalities resulting from widespread injury to other organs.[670] Hypotension and circulatory collapse may occur.

Sinus tachycardia is invariably present, while atrial and ventricular arrhythmias are usually absent. Transient prolongation of the Q-T interval may be seen, along with ST-segment and T-wave abnormalities. It may take up to several months for these repolarization abnormalities to resolve.[670] P-wave abnormalities may occur, but abnormalities of the QRS complex or of atrioventricular conduction are not usually seen. Serum enzyme levels may be elevated and may reflect myocardial damage, at least in part.

Hypothermia. Low temperature may also result in myocardial damage. Cardiac dilatation may occur with epicardial petechiae and subendocardial hemorrhages.[672] Microinfarcts are present in the ventricular myocardium, and fatty changes are common.[673] The lesions are not due to the low temperature per se but appear to be the result of the circulatory collapse, hemoconcentration, capillary sludging, and depressed cellular metabolism that accompany hypothermia.

Radiation. A variety of acute and chronic cardiac complications may result from the employment of ionizing radiation during radiotherapy or, less commonly, after radiation accidents. While the heart is one of the organs most resistant to the effects of radiation, damage to the pericardium (p. 1509), myocardium, and endocardium may occur.[674,675,675a,675b] Although radiation probably results in some degree of tissue damage in all patients,[676] clinical evidence of cardiac involvement occurs in approximately 5 per cent of patients with Hodgkin's disease or breast carcinoma treated with 4000 to 5000 rads to the chest.[677,678] Radiation-induced cardiac damage is related to the dose of radiation, the mass of heart irradiated, and the dose schedule of the radiation.

Acute cardiac damage has been studied in experimental animals, and it appears that the findings are similar in humans.[678] The initial changes are those of a pancarditis, with an exudative infiltrate of the pericardium, epicardium, myocardium, and endocardium, often with inflammation of the smaller arteries. The acute changes resolve within 48 hours, to be followed by a latent period in which there are no important pathological findings. The late cardiac damage following irradiation appears to result from a long-lasting injury of the capillary endothelial cells, which leads to cell death, capillary rupture, and microthrombi. Because of this damage to the microvasculature, ischemia results and is followed by myocardial fibrosis.[678] In addition to microvascular damage, the major epicardial coronary arteries may become narrowed.[675,679]

Only an occasional patient manifests acute cardiac abnormality clinically with radiation therapy; typically this consists of acute pericarditis. The more common clinical expressions of radiation heart disease occur months or years after the exposure. The pericardium is the most common site of clinical involvement, with findings of chronic pericardial effusion or pericardial constriction.[678] Myocardial damage occurs less frequently[678a, 678b] and is characterized by myocardial fibrosis with or without endocardial fibrosis or fibroelastosis.[678]

Electrocardiographic abnormalities may be the only clinical indication of cardiac involvement, although patients with myocardial fibrosis may develop intractable congestive heart failure.[674,678] It appears that radiation and cancer chemotherapeutic agents may act synergistically in producing myocardial damage and that withdrawal of corticosteroids may activate previously subclinical radiation injury.[677] In experimental animals, corticosteroids and nonsteroidal antiinflammatory agents, if given early, retard the development of radiation-induced heart disease.[680]

References

1. Shabetai, R.: Cardiomyopathy: How far have we come in 25 years, how far yet to go? J. Am. Coll. Cardiol. *1*:252, 1983.
2. Brigden, W.: Uncommon myocardial diseases: The non-coronary cardiomyopathies. Lancet *2*:1179, 1957.
3. Report of the WHO/ISFC task force on the definition and classification of cardiomyopathies. Br. Heart J. *44*:672, 1980.
4. Goodwin, J. F.: The frontiers of cardiomyopathy. Br. Heart J. *48*:1, 1982.
5. Burch, G. E., and DePasquale, N. P.: Recognition and prevention of cardiomyopathy. Subcommittee on Cardiomyopathy. Circulation *42*:A-47, 1970.
6. Carlisle, R.: A classification for the cardiomyopathies. Am. J. Cardiol. *28*:242, 1971.
7. Fejfar, Z.: Definition and classification of the cardiomyopathies. Pathol. Microbiol. *35*:17, 1970.
8. Olsen, E. G. J.: The pathology of cardiomyopathies. A critical analysis. Am. Heart J. *98*:385, 1979.

8a. Franciosa, J. A., Wilen, M., Ziesche, S., and Cohn, J. N.: Survival in men with severe chronic left ventricular failure due to either coronary heart disease or idiopathic dilated cardiomyopathy. Am. J. Cardiol. *51*:831, 1983.

9. Goodwin, J. F.: Congestive and hypertrophic cardiomyopathies. A decade of study. Lancet *1*:731, 1970.
10. Baandrup, U., and Olsen, E. G. J.: Critical analysis of endomyocardial biopsies from patients suspected of having cardiomyopathy. I. Morphological and morphometric aspects. Br. Heart J. *45*:475, 1981.

DILATED CARDIOMYOPATHY

11. Baandrup, U., Florio, R. A., Rehahn, M., Richardson, P. J., and Olsen, E. G. J.: Critical analysis of endomyocardial biopsies from patients suspected of having cardiomyopathy. II. Comparison of histology and clinical/hemodynamic information. Br. Heart J. *45*:487, 1981.
12. Ziady, G. M., Oakley, C. M., Raphael, M. J., and Goodwin, J. F.: Primary restrictive cardiomyopathy. Br. Heart J. *37*:556, 1975.
13. Adelman, A. G., Wigle, E. D., Felderhof, C. H., Corrigal, D. M., and Gilbert, B. W.: Current concepts of primary cardiomyopathy. Cardiovasc. Med. *2*:495, 1977.
14. Grossman, W., McLaurin, L. P., and Rolett, E. L.: Alterations in left ventricular relaxation and diastolic compliance in congestive cardiomyopathy. Cardiovasc. Res. *13*:514, 1979.
15. Fuster, V., Gersh, B. J., Giuliani, E. R., Tajik, A. J., Brandenburg, R. O., and Grye, R. L.: The natural history of idiopathic dilated cardiomyopathy. Am. J. Cardiol. *47*:525, 1981.
16. McDonald, C. D., Burch, G. E., and Walsh, J. J.: Prolonged bed rest in the treatment of idiopathic cardiomyopathy. Am. J. Med. *52*:41, 1972.
17. Benjamin, I. J., Schuster, E. H., and Bulkley, B. H.: Cardiac hypertrophy in idiopathic dilated congestive cardiomyopathy: A clinicopathologic study. Circulation *64*:442, 1981.
18. Olsen, E. G. J.: Pathological recognition of cardiomyopathy. Postgrad. Med. J. *51*:277, 1975.
19. Roberts, W. C., and Ferrans, V. J.: Morphologic observations in the cardiomyopathies. *In* Fowler, N. O. (ed.): Myocardial Diseases. New York, Grune and Stratton, 1973, p. 59.
20. Amorim, D. S., and Olsen, E. G. J.: Assessment of heart neurons in dilated (congestive) cardiomyopathy. Br. Heart J. *47*:11, 1982.

20a. Schwarz, F., Mall, G., Zebe, H., Blickle, J., Derks, H., Manthey, J., and Kübler, W.: Quantitative morphologic findings of the myocardium in idiopathic dilated cardiomyopathy. Am. J. Cardiol. *51*:501, 1983.

21. Peters, T. J., Wells, G., Oakley, C. M., Brooksby, I. A. B., Jenkins, B. S., Webb-Peploe, M. M., and Coltart, D. J.: Enzymatic analysis of endocardial biopsy specimens from patients with cardiomyopathies. Br. Heart J. *39*:1333, 1977.
22. Olsen, E. G. J.: Endomyocardial biopsy. Br. Heart J. *40*:95, 1978.
23. Kuhn, H., Breithardt, G., Knieriem, H-J., Köhler, E., Lösse, B., Seipel, L., and Loogen, F.: Prognosis and possible presymptomatic manifestations of congestive cardiomyopathy (COCM). Postgrad. Med. J. *54*:451, 1978.
24. Matsumori, A., and Kawai, C.: An animal model of congestive (dilated) cardiomyopathy: Dilatation and hypertrophy of the heart in the chronic stage in DBA/2 mice with myocarditis caused by encephalomyocarditis virus. Circulation *66*:355, 1982.
25. Cambridge, G., MacArthur, C. G. C., Waterson, A. P., Goodwin, J. F., and Oakley, C. M.: Antibodies to Coxsackie B viruses in congestive cardiomyopathy. Br. Heart J. *41*:692, 1979.
26. Brooksby, I. A. B., Coltart, D. J., and Webb-Peploe, M. M.: Progress in endomyocardial biopsy. Mod. Concepts Cardiovasc. Dis. *44*:65, 1975.
27. Jacobs, B., Matsuda, Y., Deodhar, S., and Shirey, E.: Cell-mediated cytotoxicity to cardiac cells of lymphocytes from patients with primary myocardial disease. Am. J. Clin. Pathol. *72*:1, 1979.
28. O'Connell, J. B., Robinson, J. A., Henkin, R. E., and Gunnar, R. M.: Immunosuppressive therapy in patients with congestive cardiomyopathy and myocardial uptake of gallium-67. Circulation *64*:780, 1981.

28a. O'Connell, J. B., Fowles, R. E., Robinson, J. A., Subramanian, R., and Gunnar, R. M.: A possible role for myocarditis in the pathogenesis of familial dilated cardiomyopathy. J. Am. Coll. Cardiol. *1*:584, 1983.

29. Eckstein, R., Mempel, W., and Bolte, H.-D.: Reduced suppressor cell activity in congestive cardiomyopathy and in myocarditis. Circulation *65*:1224, 1982.
30. Trueman, T., Thompson, R. A., Cummins, P., and Littler, W. A.: Heart antibodies in cardiomyopathies. Br. Heart J. *46*:296, 1981.
31. Fowles, R. E., Bieber, C. P., and Stinson, E. B.: Defective *in vitro* suppressor cell function in idiopathic cardiomyopathy. Circulation *59*:483, 1979.
32. Anderson, J. L., Greenwood, J. H., and Kawanishi, H.: Evaluation of suppressor immune regulatory function in idiopathic congestive cardiomyopathy and rheumatic heart disease. Br. Heart J. *46*:410, 1981.
33. Factor S. M., and Sonnenblick E. H.: Hypothesis: Is congestive cardiomyopathy caused by hyperactive myocardial microcirculation (microvascular spasm)? (Editorial) Am. J. Cardiol. *50*:1149, 1982.
34. Ross, R. S., Bulkley, B. H., Hutchins, G. M., Harshley, J. S., Jones, R. A., Kraus, H., Liebman, J., Thorne, C. M., Weinberg, S. B., Weech, A. A., and Weech, A. A., Jr.: Idiopathic familial myocardiopathy in three generations: A clinical and pathologic study. Am. Heart J. *96*:170, 1978.
35. Hartveit, F., Moehle, B. O., and Pihl, T.: A family with congestive cardiomyopathy. Cardiology *68*:193, 1981.
36. Sacks, H. N., Crawley, I. S., Ward, J. A., and Fine, R. M.: Familial cardiomyopathy, hypogonadism and collagenoma. Ann. Intern. Med. *93*:813, 1980.
37. Oakley, C. M.: Clinical recognition of the cardiomyopathies. Circ. Res. *34/35* (Suppl. II):11, 1974.
38. Segal, J. P., Harvey, W. P., and Stapleton, J. F.: Clinical features and natural history of cardiomyopathy. *In* Fowler, N. O. (ed.): Myocardial Diseases. New York, Grune and Stratton, 1973, p. 37.

38a. Huang, S. K., Messer, J. V., and Denes, P.: Significance of ventricular tachycardia in idiopathic dilated cardiomyopathy: Observations in 35 patients. Am. J. Cardiol. *51*:507, 1983.

39. McKinney, B.: Pathology of the cardiomyopathies. London, Butterworths, 1974.
40. Torp, A.: Incidence of congestive cardiomyopathy. Postgrad. Med. J. *54*:435, 1978.
41. Pasternac, A., Noble, J., Streulens, Y., Elie, R., Henschke, C., and Bourassa, M. G.: Pathophysiology of chest pain in patients with cardiomyopathies and normal coronary arteries. Circulation *65*:778, 1982.
42. Schlant, R. C.: Physiology of idiopathic cardiomyopathies. *In* Burch, G. E. (ed.): Cardiomyopathy. (Cardiovascular Clinics Series.) Philadelphia, F. A. Davis Co., 1972, p. 62.
43. Phillips, J. H., Burch, G. E., and DePasquale, N. P.: The syndrome of papillary muscle dysfunction. Its clinical recognition. Ann. Intern. Med. *59*:508, 1963.
44. Weissler, A. M.: Current concepts in cardiology. Systolic-time intervals. N. Engl. J. Med. *296*:321, 1977.
45. Marsh, J. D., Green, L. H., Wynne, J., Cohn, P. F., and Grossman, W.: Left ventricular end-systolic pressure—dimension and stress-length relations in normal human subjects. Am. J. Cardiol. *44*:1311, 1979.
46. Saltissi, S., Hockings, B., Croft, D. N., and Webb-Peploe, M. M.: Thallium-201 myocardial imaging in patients with dilated and ischemic cardiomyopathy. Br. Heart J. *46*:290, 1981.

46a. Greenberg, J., Boucher, C. A., Okada, R. D., Murphy, J. H., Palacios, I., Pohost, G. M., and Strauss, H. W.: Incidence of regional wall motion abnormalities in primary congestive cardiomyopathy. J. Am. Coll. Cardiol. *1*:723, 1983.

47. Colucci, W., Wynne, J., Holman, B. L., and Braunwald, E.: Chronic therapy of heart failure with prazosin: A randomized double-blind trial. Am. J. Cardiol. *45*:337, 1980.
48. Engler, R., Ray, R., Higgins, C. B., McNally, C., Buxton, W. H., Bhargava, V., and Shabetai, R.: Clinical assessment and follow-up of functional capacity in patients with chronic congestive cardiomyopathy. Am. J. Cardiol. *49*:1832, 1982.
49. Johnson, R. A., and Palacios, I.: Dilated cardiomyopathy of the adult. N. Engl. J. Med. *307*:1051 and 1119, 1982.
50. Kawai, C., and Takatsu, T.: Clinical and experimental studies on cardiomyopathy. N. Engl. J. Med. *293*:592, 1975.
51. Pierpont, G. L., Cohn, J. N., and Franciosa, J. A.: Congestive cardiomyopathy: Pathophysiology and response to therapy. Arch. Intern. Med. *138*:1847, 1978.
52. Abelmann, W. H.: Treatment of congestive cardiomyopathy. Postgrad. Med. J. *54*:477, 1978.
53. Swedberg, K., Hjalmarson, A., Waagstein, F., and Wallentin, I.: Beneficial effects of long-term beta-blockade in congestive cardiomyopathy. Br. Heart J. *44*: 117, 1980.

53a. Waagstein, F., Hjalmarson, A., Swedeberg, K., and Wallentin, C.: Beta-blockers in dilated cardiomyopathies: They work. Europ. Heart J. *4* (Suppl. A):173, 1983.

54. Swedberg, K., Hjalmarson, A., Waagstein, F., and Wallentin, I.: Adverse effects of beta-blockade withdrawal in patients with congestive cardiomyopathy. Br. Heart J. *44*:134, 1980.
55. Ikram, H., and Fitzpatrick, D.: Double-blind trial of chronic oral beta blockade in congestive cardiomyopathy. Lancet *2*:490, 1981.

55a. Ikram, H., and Fitzpatrick, M. A.: Beta blockade for dilated cardiomyopathy: The evidence against therapeutic benefit. Europ. Heart J. *4* (Suppl. A):179, 1983.

56. Unverferth, D. V., Magorien, R. D., Lewis, R. P., and Leier, C. V.: Long-term benefit of dobutamine in patients with congestive cardiomyopathy. Am. Heart J. *100*:622, 1980.

56a. Lapeyre, A. C., Steele, P. M., Kazmier, F. J., Chesebro, J. H., Vlietstra, R. e., and Fuster, V.: Low incidence of systemic embolism in left ventricular aneurysm—A comparison with idiopathic dilated cardiomyopathy. J. Am. Coll. Cardiol. *1*:704, 1983.

57. Schroeder, J. S.: Current status of cardiac transplantation, 1978. J.A.M.A. *241*: 2069, 1979.
58. Hassell, L. A., Fowles, R. E., and Stinson, E. B.: Patients with congestive cardiomyopathy as cardiac transplant recipients: Indications for and results of cardiac transplantation and comparison with patients with coronary artery disease. Am. J. Cardiol. *47*:1205, 1981.
59. Rubin, E.: Alcoholic myopathy in heart and skeletal muscle. N. Engl. J. Med. *301*:28, 1979.
60. Regan, T. J., Haider, B., Ahmed, S. S., Lyons, M. M., Oldewurtel, H. A., and Ettinger, P. O.: Whiskey and the heart. Cardiovasc. Med. *2*:165, 1977.
61. Alexander, C. S.: Cobalt-beer cardiomyopathy. A clinical and pathological study of twenty-eight cases. Am. J. Med. *53*:395, 1972.
62. Albarian, M., Yankopoulos, N. A., and Abelmann, W. H.: Hemodynamic studies in beriberi heart disease. Am. J. Med. *41*:197, 1966.
63. Jeffrey, F. E., and Abelmann, W. H.: Recovery from proved Shoshin beriberi. Am. J. Med. *50*:123, 1971.
64. Weiss, S.: Occidental beriberi with cardiovascular manifestations. Its relation to thiamine deficiency. J.A.M.A. *115*:832, 1940.
65. Segel, L. D., Rendig, S. V., and Mason, D. T.: Left ventricular dysfunction of isolated working rat hearts after chronic alcohol consumption. Cardiovasc. Res. *13*:136, 1979.
66. Friedman, H. S., and Lieber, C. S.: Cardiotoxicity of alcohol. Cardiovasc. Med. *2*:111, 1977.
67. Horwitz, L. D., and Atkins, J. M.: Acute effects of ethanol on left ventricular performance. Circulation *49*:124, 1974.
68. Regan, T. J., Ettinger, P. O., Lyons, M. M., Moschos, C. B., and Weisse, A. B.: Ethyl alcohol as a cardiac risk factor. Cur. Probl. Cardiol. *2*:1, 1977.
69. Bing, R. J.: Cardiac metabolism: Its contribution to alcoholic heart disease and myocardial failure. Circulation *58*:965, 1978.
70. Rubin, E.: Alcoholic myopathy in heart and skeletal muscle. N. Engl. J. Med. *301*:28, 1979.

70a. Lange, L. G., and Sobel, B. E.: Impaired cardiac mitochondrial function induced by specific metabolites of ethanol: Fatty acid ethyl esters. J. Am. Coll. Cardiol. *667*:1983.

71. Regan, T. J., Levinson, G. E., Oldewurtel, H. A., Frank, M. J., Weisse, A. B., and Moschos, C. B.: Ventricular function in noncardiacs with alcoholic fatty liver: Role of ethanol in the production of cardiomyopathy, J. Clin. Invest. *48*: 397, 1969.
72. Burch, G. E., and Giles, T. D.: The small coronary arteries in alcoholic cardiomyopathy. Am. Heart J. *94*:471, 1977.
73. Factor, S. M.: Intramyocardial small-vessel disease in chronic alcoholism. Am. Heart J. *92*:561, 1976.
74. Klein, H., and Harmjanz, D.: Effect of ethanol infusion on the ultrastructure of human myocardium. Postgrad. Med. J. *51*:325, 1975.
75. Weisharr, R., Sarma, J. S. M., Maruyama, Y., Fischer, R., Bertuglia, S., and Bing, R. J.: Reversibility of mitochondrial and contractile changes in the myocardium after cessation of prolonged ethanol intake. Am. J. Cardiol. *40*:556, 1977.
76. Bridgen, W.: Alcoholic cardiomyopathy. *In* Burch, G. E. (ed.): Cardiomyopathy. (Cardiovascular Clinics Series.) Philadelphia, F. A. Davis Co., 1972, p. 188.
77. Demakis, J. G., Proskey, A., Rahimtoola, S. H., Jamil, M., Sutton, G. C., Rosen, K. M., Gunnar, R. M., and Tobin, J. R., Jr.: The natural course of alcholic cardiomyopathy. Ann. Intern. Med. *80*:293, 1974.
78. Wu, C. F., Sudhaker, M., Jaferi, G., Ahmed, S. S., and Regan, T. J.: Preclinical cardiomyopathy in chronic alcoholics: A sex difference. Am. Heart J. *91*: 291, 1976.
79. Burch, G. E., and DePasquale, N. P.: Alcoholic cardiomyopathy. Am. J. Cardiol. *23*:723, 1969.
80. Spodick, D. H., Pigott, V. M., and Chirife, R.: Preclinical cardiac malfunction in chronic alcoholism. N. Engl. J. Med. *287*:677, 1972.
81. Levi, G. F., Quadri, A., Ratti, S., and Basagni, M.: Preclinical abnormality of left ventricular function in chronic alcoholics. Br. Heart J. *39*:35, 1977.
82. Mathews, E. C., Gardin, J. M., Henry, W. L., Del Negro, A. A., Fletcher, R. D., Snow, J. A., and Epstein, S. E.: Echocardiographic abnormalities in chronic alcoholics with and without overt congestive heart failure. Am. J. Cardiol. *47*:570, 1981.
83. Askanas, A., Udoshi, M., and Sadjadi, S. A.: The heart in chronic alcoholism. A noninvasive study. Am. Heart J. *99*:9, 1980.
84. Kino, M., Imamitchi, H., Morigutchi, M., Kawamura, K., and Takatsu, T.: Cardiovascular status in asymptomatic alcoholics, with reference to the level of ethanol consumption. Br. Heart J. *46*:545, 1981.
85. Ettinger, P. O., Wu, C. F., De La Cruze, C., Jr., Weisse, A. B., Ahmed, S. S., and Regan, T. J.: Arrhythmias and the "holiday heart": Alcohol-associated cardiac rhythm disorders. Am. Heart J. *95*:555, 1978.
86. Greenspan, A. J., and Schaal, S. F.: The "holiday heart": Electrophysiologic studies of alcohol effects in alcoholics. Ann. Intern. Med. *98*:135, 1983.
87. Bashour, T. T., Fahdul, H., and Cheng, T. O.: Electrocardiographic abnormalities in alcoholic cardiomyopathy. A study of 65 patients. Chest *68*:24, 1975.
88. Lacour, F., Sr., and Suire, E. M.: The diagnosis of alcohol cardiomyopathies. J. La. State Med. Soc. *130*:159, 1978.
89. McDonald, C. D., Burch, G. E., and Walsh, J. J.: Alcoholic cardiomyopathy managed with prolonged bed rest. Ann. Intern. Med. *74*:681, 1971.
90. Schwartz, L., Sample, K. A., and Wigle, E. D.: Severe alcoholic cardiomyopathy reversed with abstention from alcohol. Am. J. Cardiol. *36*:963, 1975.
91. Barborik, M., and Dusek, J.: Cardiomyopathy accompanying industrial cobalt exposure. Br. Heart J. *34*:113, 1972.
92. Manifold, I. H., Platts, M. M., and Kennedy, A.: Cobalt cardiomyopathy in a patient on maintenance haemodialysis. Br. Med. J. *2*:1609, 1978.

HYPERTROPHIC CARDIOMYOPATHY

93. Teare, R. D.: Asymmetrical hypertrophy of the heart in young adults. Brit. Heart J. *20*:1, 1958.
94. Morrow, A. G., and Braunwald, E.: Functional aortic stenosis: A malformation characterized by resistance to left ventricular outflow without anatomic obstruction. Circulation *20*:181, 1959.
95. Martin, R. P., Rakowski, H., French, J., and Popp, R. L.: Idiopathic hypertrophic subaortic stenosis viewed by wide-angle, phased-array echocardiography. Circulation *59*:1206, 1979.
96. Maron, B. J., and Epstein, S. E.: Hypertrophic cardiomyopathy: Recent observations regarding the specificity of three hallmarks of the disease: asymmetric septal hypertrophy, septal disorganization and systolic anterior motion of the anterior mitral leaflet. Am. J. Cardiol. *45*:141, 1980.
97. Doi, Y. L., McKenna, W. J., Gehrke, J., Oakley, C. M., and Goodwin, J. F.: M-mode echocardiography in hypertrophic cardiomyopathy: Diagnostic criteria and prediction of obstruction. Am. J. Cardiol. *45*:6, 1980.
98. Clark, C. E., Henry, W. L., and Epstein, S. E.: Familial prevalence and genetic transmission of idiopathic hypertrophic subaortic stenosis. N. Engl. J. Med. *289*:709, 1973.
99. Roberts, W. C., and Ferrans, V. J.: Pathologic anatomy of the cardiomyopathies. Idiopathic dilated and hypertrophic types, infiltrative types and endomyocardial disease with and without eosinophilia. Hum. Pathol. *6*:287, 1975.
100. Epstein, S. E., Henry, W. L., Clark, C. E., Roberts, W. C., Maron, B. J., Ferrans, V. J., Redwood, D. R., and Morrow, A. G.: Asymmetric septal hypertrophy. Ann. Intern. Med. *81*:650, 1974.
101. Maron, B. J., Gottdiener, J. S., Roberts, W. C., Henry, W. L., Savage, D. D., and Epstein, S. E.: Left ventricular outflow tract obstruction due to systolic anterior motion of the anterior mitral leaflet in patients with concentric left ventricular hypertrophy. Circulation *57*:527, 1978.
102. Come, P. C., Bulkley, B. H., Goodman, Z. D., Hutchins, G. M., Pitt, B., and Fortuin, N. J.: Hypercontractile cardiac states simulating hypertrophic cardiomyopathy. Circulation *55*:901, 1977.
103. Buxton, A. E., Morganroth, J., Josephson, M. E., Perloff, J. K., and Shelborne, J. C.: Isolated dextroversion of the heart with asymmetric septal hypertrophy. Am. Heart J. *92*:785, 1976.
104. Sommerville, J., and Becu, L.: Congenital heart disease associated with hypertrophic cardiomyopathy. Johns Hopkins Med. J. *140*:151, 1977.
105. Maron, B. J., Gottdiener, J. S., Roberts, W. C., Hammer, W. J., and Epstein, S. E.: Nongenetically transmitted disproportionate ventricular septal thickening associated with left ventricular outflow obstruction. Br. Heart J. *41*:345, 1979.
106. Sommerville, J., and Becu, L.: Congenital heart disease associated with hypertrophic cardiomyopathy. Br. Heart J. *40*:1034, 1978.
107. Abbasi, A., Slaughter, J. C., and Allen, M. W.: Asymmetrical septal hypertrophy in patients with long-term hemodialysis. Chest *74*:548, 1978.
108. Maron, B. J., Clark, C. E., Henry, W. L., Fukuda, T., Edwards, J. E., Mathews, E. C., Jr., Redwood, D. R., and Epstein, S. E.: Prevalence and characteristics of disproportionate ventricular septal thickening in patients with acquired or congenital heart disease. Echocardiographic and morphologic findings. Circulation *55*:489, 1977.
109. Larter, W. E., Allen, H. D., Sahn, D. J., and Goldberg, S. J.: The asymmetrically hypertrophied septum. Further differentiation of its causes. Circulation *53*: 19, 1976.
110. Stern, A., Kessler, K. M., Hammer, W. J., Kreulen, T., and Spann, J. F.: Septal-free wall disproportion in inferior infarction: The echocardiographic differentiation from hypertrophic cardiomyopathy. Circulation *58*:700, 1978.
111. Raj, M. V. J., Srinivas, V., Graham, I. M., and Evans, D. W.: Coexistence of asymmetric septal hypertrophy and aortic valve disease in adults. Thorax *34*: 91, 1979.
112. Maron, B. J., Gottdiener, J. S., and Epstein, S. E.: Patterns and significance of distribution of left ventricular hypertrophy in hypertrophic cardiomyopathy: A wide-angle two-dimensional echocardiographic study of 125 patients. Am. J. Cardiol. *48*:418, 1981.
113. Maron, B.J., Gottdiener, J. S., Bonow, R. O., and Epstein, S. E.: Hypertrophic cardiomyopathy with unusual locations of left ventricular hypertrophy undetectable by M-mode echocardiography: Identification by wide-angle two-dimensional echocardiography. Circulation *63*:409, 1981.

113a. Ciro, E., Nichols, P. F., III, and Maron, B. J.: Heterogeneous morphologic expression of genetically transmitted hypertrophic cardiomyopathy. Circulation *67*:1227, 1983.

114. Yamaguchi, H., Ishimura, T., Nishiyama, S., Nagasaki, F., Nakanishi, S., Takatsu, F., Nishijo, T., Umeda, T., and Machii, K.: Hypertrophic nonobstructive cardiomyopathy with giant negative T waves (apical hypertrophy): Ventriculographic and echocardiographic features in 30 patients. Am. J. Cardiol. *44*:401, 1979.
115. Maron, B. J., Bonow, R. O., Seshagiri, T. N. R., Roberts, W. C., and Epstein, S. E.: Hypertrophic cardiomyopathy with ventricular septal hypertrophy localized to the apical region of the left ventricle (apical hypertrophic cardiomyopathy). Am. J. Cardiol. *49*:1838, 1982.

116. Bulkley, B. H., Weisfeldt, M. L., and Hutchins, G. M.: Asymmetric septal hypertrophy and myocardial fiber disarray. Features of normal, developing and malformed hearts. Circulation *56*:292, 1977.
117. Rassmussen, S., Corya, B. C., Feigenbaum, H., and Knoebel, S. B.: Detection of myocardial scar tissue by M-mode echocardiography. Circulation *57*:230, 1978.
118. Maron, B. J., Savage, D. D., Clark, C. E., Henry, W. L., Vlodaver, Z., Edwards, J. E., and Epstein, S. E.: Prevalence and characteristics of disproportionate ventricular septal thickening in patients with coronary artery disease. Circulation *57*:250, 1978.
119. Olsen, E. G. J.: The pathology of idiopathic hypertrophic subaortic stenosis (hypertrophic cardiomyopathy). A critical review. Am. Heart J. *100*:553, 1980.
119a. Thompson, R., Ahmed, M., Pridie, R., and Yacoub, M.: Hypertrophic cardiomyopathy after aortic valve replacement. Am. J. Cardiol. *45*:33, 1980.
120. Isner, J. M., Falcone, M. W., Virmani, R., and Roberts, W. C.: Cardiac sarcoma causing "ASH" and simulating coronary heart disease. Am. J. Med. *66*: 1025, 1979.
121. Cabin, H. S., Costello, R. M., Vasudevan, G., Maron, B. J., and Roberts, W. C.: Cardiac lymphoma mimicking hypertrophic cardiomyopathy. Am. Heart J. *102*:466, 1981.
122. Bulkley, B. H., and Hutchins, G. M.: Pompe's disease presenting as hypertrophic myocardiopathy with Wolff-Parkinson-White syndrome. Am. Heart J. *96*: 246, 1978.
123. Colucci, W. S., Lorell, B. H., Schoen, F. J., Warhol, M. J., and Grossman, W.: Hypertrophic obstructive cardiomyopathy due to Fabry's disease. N. Engl. J. Med. *307*:926, 1982.
124. Henry, W. L., Clark, C. E., Roberts, W. C., Morrow, A. G., and Epstein, S. E.: Differences in the distribution of myocardial abnormalities in patients with obstructive and nonobstructive asymmetric septal hypertrophy (ASH). Echocardiographic and gross anatomic findings. Circulation *50*:447, 1974.
125. Maron, B. J., Ferrans, V. J., Henry, W. L., Clark, C. E., Redwood, D. R., Roberts, W. C., Morrow, A. G., and Epstein, S. E.: Differences in distribution of myocardial abnormalities in patients with obstructive and nonobstructive asymmetric septal hypertrophy (ASH). Light and electron microscopic findings. Circulation *50*:436, 1974.
126. Maron, B. J., Anan, T. J., and Roberts, W. C.: Quantitative analysis of the distribution of cardiac muscle cell disorganization in the left ventricular free wall of patients with hypertrophic cardiomyopathy. Circulation *63*:882, 1981.
127. Maron, B. J., and Roberts, W. C.: Quantitative analysis of cardiac muscle cell disorganization in the ventricular septum of patients with hypertrophic cardiomyopathy. Circulation *59*:689, 1979.
128. Ferrans, V. J., Morrow, A. G., and Roberts, W. C.: Myocardial ultrastructure in idiopathic hypertrophic subaortic stenosis. A study of operatively excised left ventricular outflow tract muscle in 14 patients. Circulation *45*:769, 1972.
129. Maron, B. J., and Roberts, W. C.: Hypertrophic cardiomyopathy and cardiac muscle cell disorganization revisited: Relation between the two and significance. Am. Heart J. *102*:95, 1981.
129a. Wigle, E. D., and Silver, M. D.: Editorial: Myocardial fiber disarray and ventricular septal hypertrophy in asymmetrical hypertrophy of the heart. Circulation *58*:398, 1978.
130. Isner, J. M., Maron, B. J., and Roberts, W. C.: Comparison of amount of myocardial cell disorganization in operatively excised septectomy specimens with amount observed at necropsy in 18 patients with hypertrophic cardiomyopathy. Am. J. Cardiol. *46*:42, 1980.
130a. Kishimoto, C., Kaburagi, T., Takayama, S., Yokoyama, S., Hanyu, I., Takatsu, Y., and Tomimoto, K.: Two forms of hypertrophic cardiomyopathy distinguished by inheritance of HLA haplotypes and left ventricular outflow tract obstruction. Am. Heart J. *105*:988, 1983.
131. Shah, P. M.: Idiopathic hypertrophic subaortic stenosis (hypertrophic obstructive cardiomyopathy). Changing concepts — 1975. Chest *68*:814, 1975.
132. Hamby, R. I., Roberts, G. S., and Meron, J. M.: Hypertension and hypertrophic subaortic stenosis. Am. J. Med. *51*:474, 1971.
133. Hutchins, G. M., and Bulkley, B. H.: Catenoid shape of the interventricular septum: Possible cause of idiopathic hypertrophic subaortic stenosis. Circulation *58*:392, 1978.
134. Perloff, J. K.: Pathogenesis of hypertrophic cardiomyopathy: Hypothesis and speculation. Am. Heart J. *101*:219, 1981.
135. James, T. N., and Marshall, T. K.: De Subitaneis Mortibus. XII. Asymmetrical hypertrophy of the heart. Circulation *51*:1149, 1975.
136. Lorell, B. H., Paulus, W. J., Grossman, W., Wynne, J., and Cohn, P. F.: Modification of abnormal left ventricular diastolic properties by nifedipine in patients with hypertrophic cardiomyopathy. Circulation *65*:499, 1982.
137. Murgo, J. P., Alter, B. R., Dorethy, J. F., Altobelli, S. A., and McGrawahan, G. M., Jr.: Dynamics of left ventricular ejection in obstructive and nonobstructive hypertrophic cardiomyopathy. J. Clin. Invest. *66*:1369, 1980.
138. Braunwald, E., Lambrew, C. T., Rockoff, S. D., Ross, J., Jr., and Morrow, A. G.: Idiopathic hypertrophic subaortic stenosis. Circulation *29/30* (Suppl. IV):1, 1964.
139. Whiting, R. B., Powell, W. J., Jr., Dinsmore, R. E., and Sanders, C. A.: Idiopathic hypertrophic subaortic stenosis stenosis in the elderly. N. Engl. J. Med. *285*:196, 1971.
140. Neufeld, H. N., Ongley, P. A., and Edwards, J. E.: Combined congenital subaortic stenosis and infundibular pulmonary stenosis. Br. Heart. J. *22*:686, 1960.
141. Maron, B. J., Edwards, J. E., Henry, W. L., Clark, C. E., Bingle, G. J., and Epstein, S. E.: Asymmetric septal hypertrophy (ASH) in infancy. Circulation *50*:809, 1974.
142. Fiddler, G. I., Tajik, A. J., Weidman, W. H., McGoon, D. C., Ritter, D. G., and Guiliani, E. R.: Idiopathic hypertrophic subaortic stenosis in the young. Am. J. Cardiol. *42*:793, 1978.
143. Hamby, R. I., and Aintablian, A.: Hypertrophic subaortic stenosis is not rare in the eighth decade. Geriatrics *31*:71, 1976.
144. Krasnow, N., and Stein, R. A.: Hypertrophic cardiomyopathy in the aged. Am. Heart J. *96*:326, 1978.
145. Spodick, D. H.: Hypertrophic obstructive cardiomyopathy of the left ventricle (idiopathic hypertrophic subaortic stenosis). *In* Burch, G. E. (ed.): Cardiomyopathy. (Cardiovascular Clinics Series.) Philadelphia, F. A. Davis Co., 1972, p. 133.
146. Frank, S., and Braunwald, E.: Idiopathic hypertrophic subaortic stenosis. Clinical analysis of 126 patients with emphasis on the natural history. Circulation *37*:759, 1968.
147. Maron, B. J., Roberts, W. C., Edwards, J. E., McAllister, H. U., Jr., Foley, D. D., and Epstein, S. E.: Sudden death in patients with hypertrophic cardiomyopathy: Characterization of 26 patients without functional limitation. Am. J. Cardiol. *41*:803, 1978.
148. Wigle, E. D., Felderhof, C. H., Silver, M. D., and Adelman, A. G.: Hypertrophic obstructive cardiomyopathy (muscular or hypertrophic subaortic stenosis). *In* Fowler, N. O. (ed.): Myocardial Diseases. New York, Grune and Stratton, 1973, p. 297.
149. Maron, B. J., Tajik, A. J., Ruttenberg, H. D., Graham, T. P., Atwood, G. F., Victorica, B. E., Lie, J. T., and Roberts, W. C.: Hypertrophic cardiomyopathy in infants: Clinical features and natural history. Circulation *65*:7, 1982.
150. Sutton, M. G. St. J., Tajik, A. J., Smith, H. C., and Ritman, E. L.: Angina in idiopathic hypertropic subaortic stenosis. A clinical correlation of regional left ventricular dysfunction: A videometric and echocardiographic study. Circulation *61*:561, 1980.
151. Maron, B. J., Epstein, S. E., and Roberts, W. C.: Hypertrophic cardiomyopathy and transmural myocardial infarction without significant atherosclerosis of the extramural coronary arteries. Am. J. Cardiol. *43*:1086, 1979.
152. McKenna, W., Harris, L., and Deanfield, J.: Syncope in hypertrophic cardiomyopathy. Br. Heart J. *47*:117, 1982.
153. Wiener, M. W., Vondoenhoff, L. J., and Cohen, J.: Aortic regurgitation first appearing 12 years after successful septal myectomy for hypertrophic obstructive cardiomyopathy. Am. J. Med. *72*:157, 1982.
153a. Henderson, M. A., Ruddy, T. D., Makowski, H., and Wigle, E. D.: Left ventricular hypertrophy by ECG in hypertrophic cardiomyopathy. J. Am. Coll. Cardiol. *1*:693, 1983.
154. Savage, D. D., Seides, S. F., Clark, C. E., Henry, W. L., Maron, B. J., Robinson, F. C., and Epstein, S. E.: Electrocardiographic findings in patients with obstructive and nonobstructive hypertrophic cardiomyopathy. Circulation *58*: 402, 1978.
155. Chen, C-H., Nobuyoshi, M., and Kawai, C.: ECG pattern of left ventricular hypertrophy in nonobstructive hypertrophic cardiomyopathy: The significance of the mid-precordial changes. Am. Heart J. *97*:687, 1979.
155a. Maron, B. J., Wolfson, J. K., Ciro, E., and Spirito, P.: Relation of electrocardiographic abnormalities and patterns of left ventricular hypertrophy identified by 2-dimensional echocardiography in patients with hypertrophic cardiomyopathy. Am. J. Cardiol. *51*:189, 1983.
155b. McKenna, W. J., Borggrefe, M., England, D., Deanfield, J., Oakley, C. M., and Goodwin, J. F.: The natural history of left ventricular hypertrophy in hypertrophic cardiomyopathy: An electrocardiographic study. Circulation *66*: 1233, 1982.
156. Cosio, F. G., Moro, C., Alonso, M., de la Calzada, C. S., and Llovet, A.: The Q waves of hypertrophic cardiomyopathy: An electrophysiologic study. N. Engl. J. Med. *302*:96, 1980.
157. Krikler, D. M., Davies, M. J., Rowland, E., Goodwin, J. F., Evans, R. C., and Shaw, D. B.: Sudden death in hypertrophic cardiomyopathy: Associated accessory atrioventricular pathways. Br. Med. J. *43*:245, 1980.
158. Ingham, R. E., Mason, J. W., Rossen, R. M., Goodman, D. J., and Harrison, D. C.: Electrophysiologic findings in patients with idiopathic hypertrophic subaortic stenosis. Am. J. Cardiol. *41*:811, 1978.
159. Spilkin, S., Mitha, A. S., Matisonn, R. E., and Chesler, E.: Complete heart block in a case of idiopathic hypertrophic subaortic stenosis. Noninvasive correlates with the timing of atrial systole. Circulation *55*:418, 1977.
160. Bharati, S., McAnulty, J. H., Lev, M., and Rahimtoola, S. H.: Idiopathic hypertrophic subaortic stenosis with split His bundle potentials: Electrophysiologic and pathologic correlations. Circulation *62*:1373, 1980.
161. McKenna, W. J., Chetty, S., Oakley, C. M., and Goodwin, J. F.: Arrhythmia in hypertrophic cardiomyopathy: Exercise electrocardiographic and 48 hour ambulatory electrocardiographic assessment with and without beta adrenergic blocking therapy. Am. J. Cardiol. *45*:1, 1980.
162. Savage, D. D., Seides, S. F., Maron, B. J., Myers, D. J., and Epstein, S. E.: Prevalence of arrhythmias during 24-hour electrocardiographic monitoring and exercise testing in patients with obstructive and nonobstructive hypertrophic cardiomyopathy. Circulation *59*:866, 1979.
162a. Anderson, K. P., Stinson E. B., Derby, G. C., Oyer, P. E., and Mason, J. W.: Vulnerability of patients with obstructive hypertrophic cardiomyopathy to ventricular arrhythmia induction in the operating room. Analysis of 17 patients. Am. J. Cardiol. *51*:811, 1983.
163. Bjarnason, I., Hardarson, T., and Jonsson, S.: Cardiac arrhythmias in hypertrophic cardiomyopathy. Br. Heart J. *48*:198, 1982.
164. Ingham, R. E., Rossen, R. M., Goodman, D. T., and Harrison, D. C.: Treadmill arrhythmias in patients with idiopathic hypertrophic subaortic stenosis. Chest *68*:759, 1975.

165. McKenna, W. J., England, D., Doi, Y. L., Deanfield, J. E., Oakley, C., and Goodwin, J. F.: Arrhythmia in hypertrophic cardiomyopathy. I. Influence on prognosis. Br. Heart J. *46*:168, 1981.
166. Kronzon, I., and Glassman, E.: Mitral ring calcification in idiopathic hypertrophic subaortic stenosis. Am. J. Cardiol. *42*:60, 1978.
167. Shah, P. M., and Sylvester, L. J.: Echocardiography in the diagnosis of hypertrophic obstructive cardiomyopathy. Am. J. Med. *62*:830, 1977.
168. Schapira, J. N., Stemple, D. R., Martin, R. P., Rakowski, H., Stinson, E. B., and Popp, R. L.: Single and two-dimensional echocardiographic visualization of the effects of septal myectomy in idiopathic hypertrophic subaortic stenosis. Circulation *58*:850, 1978.
169. Weyman, A. E., Feigenbaum, H., Hurwitz, R. A., Girod, D. A., Dillon, J. C., and Chang, S.: Localization of left ventricular outflow obstruction by cross-sectional echocardiography. Am. J. Med. *60*:33, 1976.
170. Maron, B. J., Henry, W. L., and Epstein, S. E.: Pathophysiology of asymmetric septal hypertrophy. Ann. Radiol. *20*:359, 1977.
171. Abbasi, A. S., MacAlpin, R. N., Eber, L. M., and Pearce, M. L.: Left ventricular hypertrophy diagnosed by echocardiography. N. Engl. J. Med. *289*:118, 1973.
172. Wei, J. Y., Weiss, J. L., and Bulkley, B. H.: The heterogeneity of hypertrophic cardiomyopathy: An autopsy and one-dimensional echocardiographic study. Am. J. Cardiol. *45*:24, 1980.
173. Doi, Y. L., Deanfield, J. E., McKenna, W. J., Dargie, H. J., Oakley, C. M., and Goodwin, J. F.: Echocardiographic differentiation of hypertensive heart disease and hypertrophic cardiomyopathy. Br. Heart J. *44*:395, 1980.
174. Kansal, S., Roitman, D., and Sheffield, L. T.: Interventricular septal thickness and left ventricular hypertrophy. An echocardiographic study. Circulation *60*: 1058, 1979.
175. Fowles, R. E., Martin, R. P., and Popp, R. L.: Apparent asymmetric septal hypertrophy due to angled interventricular septum. Am. J. Cardiol. *46*:386, 1980.
176. Silverman, K. J., Hutchins, G. M., Weiss, J. L., and Moore, G. W.: Catenoid shape of the interventricular septum in idiopathic hypertrophic subaortic stenosis: Two-dimensional echocardiographic confirmation. Am. J. Cardiol. *49*: 27, 1982.
177. Henry, W. L., Clark, C. E., Glancy, L., and Epstein, S. E.: Echocardiographic measurement of the left ventricular outflow gradient in idiopathic hypertrophic subaortic stenosis. N. Engl. J. Med. *288*:989, 1973.
178. Angoff, G. H., Wistran, D., Sloss, L. J., Markis, J. E., Come, P. C., Zoll, P. M., and Cohn, P. F.: Value of a noninvasively induced ventricular extrasystole during echocardiographic and phonocardiographic assessment of patients with idiopathic hypertrophic subaortic stenosis. Am. J. Cardiol. *42*:919, 1978.
179. Gilbert, B. W., Pollick, C., Adelman, A. G., and Wigle, E. D.: Hypertrophic cardiomyopathy: Subclassification by M mode echocardiography. Am. J. Cardiol. *45*:861, 1980.
180. Pollick, C., Morgan, C. D., Gilbert, B. W., Rakowski, H., and Wigle, E. D.: Muscular subaortic stenosis: The temporal relationship between systolic anterior motion of the anterior mitral leaflet and the pressure gradient. Circulation *66*:1087, 1982.
181. Henry, W. L., Clark, C. E., Griffith, J. M., and Epstein, S. E.: Mechanism of left ventricular outflow obstruction in patients with obstructive asymmetric septal hypertrophy (idiopathic hypertrophic subaortic stenosis). Am. J. Cardiol. *35*:337, 1975.
182. Awdeh, N., Ervin, S., Young, J. M., and Nunn, S.: Systolic anterior motion of the mitral valve caused by sarcoid involving the septum. South Med. J. *71*: 969, 1978.
183. Rees, A., Elbl, F., Minhas, K., and Solinger, R.: Echocardiographic evidence of outflow tract obstruction in Pompe's disease (glycogen storage disease of the heart). Am. J. Cardiol. *37*:1103, 1976.
184. Crawford, M.H., Groves, B. M., and Horwitz, L. D.: Dynamic left ventricular outflow tract obstruction and systolic anterior motion of the mitral valve in the absence of asymmetric septal hypertrophy. Am. J. Med. *65*:703, 1978.
185. Maron, B. J., Gottdiener, J. S., and Perry, L. W.: Specificity of systolic anterior motion of anterior mitral leaflet for hypertrophic cardiomyopathy: Prevalence in large population of patients with other cardiac diseases. Br. Heart J. *45*:206, 1981.
186. Gardin, J. M., Talano, J. V., Stephanides, L., Fizzano, J., and Lesch, M.: Systolic anterior motion in the absence of asymmetric septal hypertrophy: A buckling phenomenon of the chordae tendineae. Circulation *63*:181, 1981.
187. Feizi, O., and Emmanuel, R.: Echocardiographic spectrum of hypertrophic cardiomyopathy. Br. Heart J. *37*:1286, 1975.
188. Venco, A., Recusani, F., and Sgalambro, A.: Diastolic movement of mitral valve in hypertrophic cardiomyopathy: An echocardiographic study. Br. Heart J. *43*:159, 1980.
189. Chandraratna, P. A. N., Tolentino, A. O., Mutricumarana, W., and Lomez, A. L.: Echocardiographic observations on the association between mitral valve prolapse and asymmetric septal hypertrophy. Circulation *55*:622, 1977.
190. Sabbah, H. N., Alam, M., Anbe, D. T., and Stein, P. D.: Mid-systolic closure of the aortic valve in hypertrophic obstructive cardiomyopathy: A pressure-related phenomenon induced by turbulent blood flow. Cath. Cardiovasc. Diag. *6*: 397, 1980.
191. St. John Sutton, M. G., Tajik, A. J., Gibson, D. G., Brown, D. J., Seward, J. B., and Giuliani, E. R.: Echocardiographic assessment of left ventricular filling and septal and posterior wall dynamics in idiopathic hypertrophic subaortic stenosis. Circulation *57*:512, 1978.
192. Hanrath, P., Mathey, D. G., Siegert, R., and Bleifeld, W.: Left ventricular relaxation and filling pattern in different forms of left ventricular hypertrophy: An echocardiographic study. Am. J. Cardiol. *45*:15, 1980.
193. Bulkley, B. H., Rouleau, J., Strauss, H. W., and Pitt, B.: Idiopathic hypertrophic subaortic stenosis: Detection by thallium-201 myocardial perfusion imaging. N. Engl. J. Med. *293*:1113, 1975.
194. Pitcher, D., Wainwright, R., Maisey, M., Curry, P., and Sowton, E.: Assessment of chest pain in hypertrophic cardiomyopathy using exercise thallium-201 myocardial scintigraphy. Br. Heart J. *44*:650, 1980.
195. Rubin, K. A., Morrison, J., Padnick, M. B., Binder, A. J., Chiaramida, S., Margouleff, D., Padmanabhan, V. T., and Gulotta, S. J.: Idiopathic hypertrophic subaortic stenosis: Evaluation of anginal symptoms with thallium-201 myocardial imaging. Am. J. Cardiol. *44*:1040, 1979.
196. Pohost, G. M., Vignola, P. A., McKusick, K. E., Block, P. C., Myers, G. S., Walker, H. J., Copen, D. L., and Dinsmore, R. E.: Hypertrophic cardiomyopathy. Evaluation by gated cardiac blood pool scanning. Circulation *55*:92, 1977.
197. Bonow, R. O., Rosing, D. R., Bacharach, S. L., Green, M. V., Kent, K. M., Lipson, L. C., Maron, B. J., Leon, M. B., and Epstein, S. E.: Effects of verapamil on left ventricular systolic function and diastolic filling in patients with hypertrophic cardiomyopathy. Circulation *64*:787, 1981.
198. Raizner, A. E., Chahine, R. A., Ishimon, T., and Audek, M.: Clinical correlates of left ventricular cavity obliteration. Am. J. Cardiol. *40*:303, 1977.
199. Hirota, Y., Furubayashi, K., Kaku, K., Shimizu, G., Kino, M., Kawamura, K., and Takatsu, T.: Hypertrophic nonobstructive cardiomyopathy: A precise assessment of hemodynamic characteristics and clinical implications. Am. J. Cardiol. *50*:990, 1982.
200. Falicov, R. E., and Resnekov, L.: Mid ventricular obstruction in hypertrophic obstructive cardiomyopathy. New diagnostic and therapeutic challenge. Br. Heart J. *39*:701, 1977.
201. Redwood, D. R., Scherer, J. L., and Epstein, S. E.: Biventricular cineangiography in the evaluation of patients with asymmetric septal hypertrophy. Circulation *49*:1116, 1974.
202. Delius, W., Wirtzfeld, A., Schinz, A., Mathes, P., Sebening, H., and Blomer, H.: Evaluation of the ventricular septum by biventricular cineangiography in congestive and hypertrophic cardiomyopathies. Ann. Radiol. *21*:463, 1978.
203. Walston, A., II, and Behar, V. S.: Spectrum of coronary artery disease in idiopathic hypertrophic subaortic stenosis. Am. J. Cardiol. *38*:12, 1976.
204. Brugada, P., Bär, F. W. H. M., de Zwaan, C., Roy, D., Green, M., and Wellens, H. J. J.: "Sawfish" systolic narrowing of the left anterior descending coronary artery: An angiographic sign of hypertrophic cardiomyopathy. Circulation *66*:800, 1982.
205. Pichard, A. D., Meller, J., Teichholz, L. E., Lipnik, S., Gorlin, R., and Herman, M. V.: Septal perforator compression (narrowing) in idiopathic hypertrophic subaortic stenosis. Am. J. Cardiol. *40*:310, 1977.
206. Glancy, D. L., Shephard, R. L., Beiser, G. D., and Epstein, S. E.: The dynamic nature of left ventricular outflow obstruction in idiopathic hypertrophic subaortic stenosis. Ann. Intern. Med. *75*:589, 1971.
207. Delman, A. J., and Stein, E.: Dynamic Auscultation and Phonocardiography. Philadelphia, W. B. Saunders Co., 1979, p. 825.
208. Stefadouros, M. A., Mucha, E., and Frank, M. J.: Paradoxic response of the murmur of idiopathic hypertrophic subaortic stenosis to the Valsalva maneuver. Am. J. Cardiol. *37*:89, 1976.
209. Bartall, H., Amber, S., Desser, K. B., and Benchimol, A.: Normalization of the external carotid pulse tracing of hypertrophic subaortic stenosis during Müller's maneuver. Chest *74*:77, 1978.
210. Brockenbrough, E. C., Braunwald, E., and Morrow, A. G.: A hemodynamic technic for the detection of hypertrophic subaortic stenosis. Circulation *23*: 189, 1961.
211. Saenz de la Calzada, C., Ziady, G. M., Hardarson, T., Curiel, R., and Goodwin, J. F.: Effect of acute administration of propranolol on ventricular function in hypertrophic obstructive cardiomyopathy measured by noninvasive techniques. Br. Heart J. *38*:798, 1976.
212. Cohen, L. S., and Braunwald, E.: Amelioration of angina pectoris in idiopathic hypertrophic subaortic stenosis with beta-adrenergic blockade. Circulation *35*: 847, 1967.
213. Thompson, D. S., Haqvi, N., Juul, S. M., Swanton, R. H., Coltart, D. J., Jenkins, D. S., and Webb-Peploe, M. M.: Effects of propranolol on myocardial oxygen consumption, substrate extraction and haemodynamics in hypertrophic cardiomyopathy. Br. Heart J. *44*:488, 1980.
214. Alvares, R. F., and Goodwin, J. F.: Noninvasive assessment of diastolic function in hypertrophic cardiomyopathy on and off beta adrenergic blocking drugs. Br. Heart J. *48*:204, 1982.
215. Shah, P. M., Adelman, A. G., Wigle, E. D., Gobel, F. L., Burchell, H. B., Hardarson, T., Curill, R., de al Calzada, C., Oakley, C. M., and Goodwin, J. F.: The natural (and unnatural) history of hypertrophic obstructive cardiomyopathy. Circ. Res. *34/35* (Suppl. II):11, 1974.
216. Canedo, M. I., Frank, M. J., and Abdulla, A. M.: Rhythm disturbances in hypertrophic cardiomyopathy: Prevalence, relation to symptoms and management. Am. J. Cardiol. *45*:848, 1980.
217. Rouleau, J.-L., Chuck, L. H. S., Hollosi, G., Kidd, P., Sievers, R. E., Wikman-Coffelt, J., and Parmley, W. W.: Verapamil preserves myocardial contractility in the hereditary cardiomyopathy of the Syrian hamster. Circ. Res. *50*: 405, 1982.
218. Kaltenbach, M., Hopf, R., Kober, G., Bussmann, W.-D., Keller, M., and Petersen, Y.: Treatment of hypertrophic obstructive cardiomyopathy with verapamil. Br. Heart J. *42*:35, 1979.
219. Rosing, D. R., Kent, K. M., Borer, J. S., Seides, S. F., Maron, B. J., and Epstein, S. E.: Verapamil therapy: A new approach to the pharmacologic treatment of hypertrophic cardiomyopathy. I. Hemodynamic effects. Circulation *60*: 1201, 1979.

220. Rosing, D. R., Kent, K. M., Maron, B. J., and Epstein, S. E.: Verapamil therapy: A new approach to the pharmacologic treatment of hypertrophic cardiomyopathy. II. Effects on exercise capacity and symptomatic status. Circulation *60*:1208, 1979.

220a. Spicer, R. L., Rocchini, A. P., Crowley, D. C. Vasiliades, J., and Rosenthal, A.: Hemodynamic effects of verapamil in children and adolescents with hypertrophic cardiomyopathy. Circulation *67*:413, 1983.

221. Hanrath, P., Mathey, D. G., Kremer, P., Sonntag, F., and Bleifeld, W.: Effect of verapamil on left ventricular isovolumic relaxation time and regional left ventricular filling in hypertrophic cardiomyopathy. Am. J. Cardiol. *45*:1258, 1980.

221a. Bonow, R. O., Frederick, T. M., Bacharach, S. L., Green, M. V., Goose, P. W., and Rosing, D. R.: Atrial systole and left ventricular filling in patients with hypertrophic cardiomyopathy: Effect of verapamil. J. Am. Coll. Cardiol. *1*: 738, 1983.

222. Rosing, D. R., Condit, J. R., Maron, B. J., Kent, K. M., Leon, M. B., Bonow, R. O., Lipson, L. C., and Epstein, S. E.: Verapamil therapy: A new approach to the pharmacologic treatment of hypertrophic cardiomyopathy. III. Effects of long-term administration. Am. J. Cardiol. *48*:545, 1981.

223. Epstein, S. E., and Rosing, D. R.: Verapamil: Its potential for causing serious complications in patients with hypertrophic cardiomyopathy. Circulation *64*: 437, 1981.

224. Koide, T., Kakihana, M., Takabatake, Y., Iizuka, M., Uchida, Y., Ozeki, K., Morooka, S., Kato, A., Tanaka, S., Oya, T., Momomura, S., and Murao, S.: Long term clinical effects of calcium inhibitors in hypertrophic cardiomyopathy compared to the effect of beta-blocking agents. Jap. Heart J. *22*:87, 1981.

225. Landmark, K., Sire, S., Thaulow, E., Amlie, J. P., and Nitter-Hauge, S.: Haemodynamic effects of nifedipine and propranolol in patients with hypertrophic obstructive cardiomyopathy. Br. Heart J. *48*:19, 1982.

226. Pollick, C.: Muscular subaortic stenosis. Hemodynamic and clinical improvement after disopyramide. N. Engl. J. Med. *307*:997, 1982.

227. Adelman, A. G., Wigle, E. D., Ranganathan, N., Webb, G. D., Kidd, B. S. L., Bigelow, W. G., and Silver, M. D.: The clinical course in muscular subaortic stenosis. A retrospective and prospective study of 60 hemodynamically proven cases. Ann. Intern. Med. *77*:515, 1972.

228. LeJemtel, T. H., Factor, S. M., Koenigsberg, M., O'Reilly, M., Frater, R., and Sonnenblick, E. H.: Mural vegetations at the site of endocardial trauma in infective endocarditis complicating idiopathic hypertrophic subaortic stenosis. Am. J. Cardiol. *44*:569, 1979.

229. Chagnac, A., Rudniki, C., Loebel, H., and Zahavi, I.: Infectious endocarditis in idiopathic hypertrophic subaortic stenosis: Report of three cases and review of the literature. Chest *81*:346, 1982.

230. Morrow, A. G.: Hypertrophic subaortic stenosis. Operative methods utilized to relieve left ventricular outflow obstruction. J. Thorac. Cardiovasc. Surg. *76*: 423, 1978.

231. Maron, B. J., Koch, J.-P., Kent, K. M., Epstein, S. E., and Morrow, A. G.: Results of surgery for idiopathic subaortic stenosis. J. Cardiovasc. Med. *5*:145, 1980.

232. Senning, A.: Transventricular relief of idiopathic hypertrophic subaortic stenosis. J. Cardiovasc. Surg. *17*:371, 1976.

233. Agnew, T. M., Barratt-Boyes, B. G., Brandt, P. W. T., Roche, A. H. G., Lowe, J. B., and O'Brien, K. P.: Surgical resection in idiopathic hypertrophic subaortic stenosis with a combined approach through aorta and left ventricle. J. Thorac. Cardiovasc. Surg. *74*:307, 1977.

234. Roberts, W. C.: Operative treatment of hypertrophic obstructive cardiomyopathy. The case against mitral valve replacement. Am. J. Cardiol. *32*:377, 1973.

235. Maron, B. J., Merrill, W. H., Freier, P. A., Kent, K. M., Epstein, S. E., and Morrow, A. G.: Long-term clinical course and symptomatic status of patients after operation for hypertrophic subaortic stenosis. Circulation *57*:1205, 1978.

236. Tajik, A. J., Giuliani, E. R., Weidman, W. H., Brandenburg, R. O., and McGoon, D. C.: Idiopathic hypertrophic subaortic stenosis. Long-term surgical followup. Am. J. Cardiol. *34*:815, 1974.

237. Koch, J.-P., Maron, B. J., Epstein, S. E., and Morrow, A. G.: Results of operation for obstructive hypertrophic cardiomyopathy in the elderly: Septal myotomy and myectomy in 20 patients 65 years of age or older. Am. J. Cardiol. *46*:963, 1980.

238. Cooley, D. A., Leachman, R. D., and Wukasch, D. C.: Diffuse muscular subaortic stenosis: Surgical management. Am. J. Cardiol. *31*:1, 1973.

238a. Beahrs, M. M., Tajik, A. J., Seward, J. B., Giuliani, E. R., and McGoon, D. C.: Hypertrophic obstructive cardiomyopathy: Ten- to 21-year followup after partial septal myectomy. Am. J. Cardiol. *51*:1160, 1983.

239. Redwood, D. R., Goldstein, R. E., Hirshfeld, J., Borer, J. S., Morganroth, J., Morrow, A. G., and Epstein, S. E.: Exercise performance after septal myotomy and myectomy in patients with obstructive cardiomyopathy. Am. J. Cardiol. *44*:215, 1979.

240. Borer, J. S., Bacharach, S. L., Green, M. V., Kent, K. M., Rosing, D. R., Seides, S. F., Morrow, A. G., and Epstein, S. E.: Effect of septal myotomy and myectomy on left ventricular systolic function at rest and during exercise in patients with IHSS. Circulation *60*(Suppl. I):I–82, 1979.

241. Kolibash, A. J., Ruiz, D. E., and Lewis, R. P.: Idiopathic hypertrophic subaortic stenosis in pregnancy. Ann. Intern. Med. *82*:791, 1975.

242. Oakley, G. D. G., McGarry, K., Limb, D. G., and Oakley, C. M.: Management of pregnancy in patients with hypertrophic cardiomyopathy. Br. Med. J. *1*:1749, 1979.

243. Beder, S. D., Gutgesell, H. P., Mullins, C. E., and McNamara, D. G.,: Progression from hypertrophic obstructive cardiomyopathy to congestive cardiomyopathy in a child. Am. Heart J. *104*:155, 1982.

244. ten Cate, F. J., and Roelandt, J.: Progression of left ventricular dilatation in patients with hypertrophic obstructive cardiomyopathy. Am. Heart J. *97*:762, 1979.

245. Waller, B. F., Maron, B. J., Epstein, S. E., and Roberts, W. C.: Transmural myocardial infarction in hypertrophic cardiomyopathy: A cause of conversion from left ventricular asymmetry to symmetry and from normal-sized to dilated left ventricular cavity. Chest *79*:461, 1981.

246. Powell, W. J., Jr., Whiting, R. B., Dinsmore, R. E., and Sanders, C. A.: Symptomatic prognosis in patients with idiopathic hypertrophic subaortic stenosis (IHSS). Am. J. Med. *55*:15, 1973.

247. Maron, B. J., Lipson, L. C., Roberts, W. C., Savage, D. D., and Epstein, S. E.: "Malignant" hypertrophic cardiomyopathy: Identification of a subgroup of families with unusually frequent premature deaths. Am. J. Cardiol. *41*:1133, 1978.

248. Baron, B. J., Roberts, W. C., Epstein, S. E.: Sudden death in hypertrophic cardiomyopathy: A profile of 78 patients. Circulation *65*:1388, 1982.

249. McKenna, W., Deanfield, J., Faruqui, A., England, D., Oakley, C., and Goodwin, J.: Prognosis in hypertrophic cardiomyopathy: Role of age and clinical, electrocardiographic and hemodynamic features. Am. J. Cardiol. *47*:532, 1981.

250. Maron, B. J., Roberts, W. C., McAllister, H. A., Rosing, D. R., and Epstein, S. E.: Sudden death in young athletes. Circulation *62*:218, 1980.

251. McKenna, W. J., Harris, L., Perez, G., Krikler, D. M., Oakley, C., and Goodwin, J. F.: Arrhythmia in hypertrophic cardiomyopathy. II. Comparison of amiodarone and verapamil in treatment. Br. Heart J. *46*:173, 1981.

252. Morrow, A. G., Koch, J.-P., Maron, B. J., Kent, K. M., and Epstein, S. E.: Left ventricular myotomy and myectomy in patients with obstructive hypertrophic cardiomyopathy and previous cardiac arrest. Am. J. Cardiol. *46*:313, 1980.

RESTRICTIVE AND INFILTRATIVE CARDIOMYOPATHIES

253. Hirschmann, J. V.: Pericardial constriction. Am. Heart J. *96*:110, 1978.

254. Benotti, J. R., Grossman, W., and Cohn, P. F.: The clinical profile of restrictive cardiomyopathy. Circulation *61*:1206, 1980.

255. Navarro-Lopez, F., Llorian, A., Ferrer-Roca, O., Betriu, A., and Sanz, G.: Restrictive cardiomyopathy in pseudoxanthoma elasticum. Chest *78*:113, 1980.

256. Meaney, E., Shabetai, R., Bhargana, V., Shearer, M., Weidner, C., Mangiardi, L. M., Smalling, R., and Peterson, K.: Cardiac amyloidosis, constrictive pericarditis and restrictive cardiomyopathy. Am. J. Cardiol. *38*:547, 1976.

257. Hansen, A. T., Eskildsen, P., and Gotzsche, H.: Pressure curves from the right auricle and the right ventricle in chronic constrictive pericarditis. Circulation *3*: 881, 1951.

258. Shabetai, R.: Profiles in constrictive pericarditis, cardiac tamponade and restrictive cardiomyopathy. *In* Grossman, W. (ed.): Cardiac Catheterization and Angiography. Philadelphia, Lea and Febiger, 1974, p. 304.

259. Borer, J. S., Henry, W. L., and Epstein, S. E.: Echocardiographic observations in patients with systemic infiltrative disease involving the heart. Am. J. Cardiol. *39*:184, 1977.

260. Glenner, G. C.: Amyloid deposits and amyloidosis: The β-fibrilloses. N. Engl. J. Med. *302*:1283 and 1333, 1980.

261. Kyle, R. A., and Baynd, E. D.: Amyloidosis: Review of 236 cases. Medicine *54*:271, 1975.

262. Pear, B. L.: Big heart, tongue, and kidneys—stiff intestines: The roentgenographic diagnosis of amyloidosis. J.A.M.A. *241*:58, 1979.

263. Gafni, J., Sohar, E., and Heller, H.: The inherited amyloidoses. Their clinical and theoretical significance. Lancet *1*:71, 1964.

264. Westermark, P., Natvig, J. B., and Johansson, B.: Characterization of an amyloid fibril protein from senile cardiac amyloid. J. Exp. Med. *146*:631, 1977.

265. Barth, W. F.: Amyloidosis: Review of cardiac and renal manifestations. Med. Ann. D.C. *36*:228, 266, 1967.

266. Dahlin, D. C.: Classification and general aspects of amyloidosis. Med. Clin. North Am. *34*:1107, 1950.

267. Hodkinson, H. M., and Pomerance, A.: The clinical significance of senile cardiac amyloidosis: A prospective clinicopathological study. Q. J. Med. *46*:381, 1977.

268. Buja, L. M., Khoi, N. B., and Roberts, W. C.: Clinically significant cardiac amyloidosis. Am. J. Cardiol. *26*:394, 1970.

269. Pomerance, A.: Senile cardiac amyloidosis. Br. Heart J. *27*:711, 1965.

269a. Maule, W. F., and Martin, R. H.: Primary cardiac amyloidosis: An angiographic clue to early diagnosis. Ann. Intern. Med. *98*:177, 1983.

270. Ridolfi, R. L., Bulkley, B. H., and Hutchins, G. M.: The conduction system in cardiac amyloidosis. Clinical and pathologic features of 23 patients. Am. J. Med. *62*:677, 1977.

270a. Saffitz, J. E., Sazama, K., and Roberts, W. C.: Amyloidosis limited to small arteries causing angina pectoris and sudden death. Am. J. Cardiol. *51*:1234, 1983.

271. Smith, R. R. L., and Hutchins, G. M.: Ischemic heart disease secondary to amyloidosis of intramyocardial arteries. Am. J. Cardiol. *44*:413, 1979.

272. Chew, C., Ziady, G. M., Raphael, M. J., and Oakley, C. M.: The functional defect in amyloid heart disease: The "stiff heart" syndrome. Am. J. Cardiol. *36*: 438, 1975.

273. Tyberg, T. I., Goodyer, A. V., Hurst, V. W., III, Alexander, J., and Langou, R. A.: Left ventricular filling in differentiating restrictive amyloid cardiomyopathy and constrictive pericarditis. Am. J. Cardiol. *47*:791, 1981.

274. Garcia, R., and Saleh, S. M.: Amyloidosis. Cardiovascular manifestations in five illustrative cases. Arch. Intern. Med. *121*:259, 1968.
275. Olofsson, B. O., Andersson, R., and Furberg, B.: Atrioventricular and intraventricular conduction in familial amyloidosis with polyneuropathy. Acta Med. Scand. *208*:77, 1980.
276. Gray, L. W., Duca, P. R., and Chung, E. K.: Sick sinus syndrome due to cardiac amyloidosis. Cardiology *63*:212, 1978.
277. Giles, T. D., Leon-Galindo, J., and Burch, G. E.: Echocardiographic findings in amyloid cardiomyopathy. South. Med. J. *71*:1393, 1978.
278. Child, J. S., Krivokapich, J., and Abbasi, A. S.: Increased right ventricular wall thickness on echocardiography in amyloid infiltrative cardiomyopathy. Am. J. Cardiol. *44*:1391, 1979.
279. Brodarick, S., Paine, R., Higa, E., and Carmichael, K. A.: Pericardial tamponade, a new complication of amyloid heart disease. Am. J. Med. *73*:133, 1982.
280. Siqueira-Filho, A. G., Cunha, C. L. P., Tajik, A. J., Seward, J. B., Schattenberg, T. T., and Giuliani, E. R.: M-mode and two-dimensional echocardiographic features in cardiac amyloidosis. Circulation *63*:188, 1981.
281. Carroll, J. D., Gaasch, W. H., and McAdam, K. P. W. J.: Amyloid cardiomyopathy: Characterization by a distinctive voltage/mass relation. Am. J. Cardiol. *49*:9, 1982.
282. St. John Sutton, M. D., Reicheck, N., Kastor, J. A., and Giuliani, E. R.: Computerized M-mode echocardiographic analysis of left ventricular dysfunction in cardiac amyloid. Circulation *66*:790, 1982.
283. Schroeder, J. S., Billigham, M. E., and Rider, A. K.: Cardiac amyloidosis. Diagnosis by transvenous endomyocardial biopsy. Am. J. Med. *59*:269, 1975.
284. Hedner, P., Rausing, A., Steen, K., and Torp, A.: Diagnosis of cardiac amyloidosis by myocardial biopsy. Acta Med. Scand. *198*:525, 1975.
285. Chan, W., and Ikram, H.: Primary amyloidosis with cardiac involvement diagnosed by left ventricular endomyocardial biopsy. Aust. N.Z. J. Med. *7*:427, 1977.
286. Rubinow, A., Skinner, M., and Cohen, A. S.: Digoxin sensitivity in amyloid cardiomyopathy. Circulation *63*:1285, 1981.
287. Desnick, R. J., Blieden, L. C., Sharp, H. L., Hofschire, P. J., and Moller, J. H.: Cardiac valvular anomalies in Fabry disease. Clinical, morphologic and biochemical studies. Circulation *54*:818, 1976.
288. Becker, A. E., Schoorl, R., Balk, A. G., and van der Heide, R. M.: Cardiac manifestations of Fabry's disease. Report of a case with mitral insufficiency and electrocardiographic evidence of myocardial infarction. Am. J. Cardiol. *36*: 829, 1975.
289. Bass, J. L., Shrivastava, S., Grabowski, G. A., Desnick, R. J., and Moller, J. H.: The M-mode echocardiogram in Fabry's disease. Am. Heart J. *100*:807, 1980.
290. Mehta, J., Tuna, N., Moller, J. H., and Desnick, R. J.: Electrocardiographic and vectorcardiographic abnormalities in Fabry's disease. Am. Heart J. *93*: 699, 1977.
291. Smith, R. R. L., Hutchins, G. M., Sack, G. H., and Ridolfi, R. L.: Unusual cardiac, renal and pulmonary involvement in Gaucher's disease. Interstitial glucocerebroside accumulation, pulmonary hypertension, and fatal bone marrow embolization. Am. J. Med. *65*:352, 1978.
292. Buja, L. M., and Roberts, W. C.: Iron in the heart. Etiology and clinical significance. Am. J. Med. *51*:209, 1971.
293. Arnett, E. N., Nienhuis, A. W., Henry, W. L., Ferrans, V. J., Redwood, D. R., and Roberts, W. C.: Massive myocardial hemosiderosis: A structure-function conference at the National Heart and Lung Institute. Am. Heart J. *90*: 777, 1975.
294. Cartwright, G. E.: Hemochromatosis. *In* Thorn, G. W., Adams, R. D., Braunwald, E., Isselbacher, K. J., and Petersdorf, R. G. (eds.): Harrison's Principles of Internal Medicine. New York, McGraw-Hill, 1977, p. 652.
295. Cutler, D. J., Isner, J. M., Bracey, A. W., Hufnagel, C. A., Conrad, P. W., Roberts, W. C., Kerwin, D. M., and Weintraub, A. M.: Hemochromatosis heart disease: An unemphasized cause of potentially reversible restrictive cardiomyopathy. Am. J. Med. *69*:923, 1980.
296. Short, E. M., Winkle, R. A., and Billingham, M. E.: Myocardial involvement in idiopathic hemochromatosis. Morphologic and clinical improvement following venesection. Am. J. Med. *70*:1275, 1981.
297. Editorial: Sarcoid heart disease. Br. Med. J. *4*:627, 1972.
298. Gozo, E. G., Jr., Cosnow, I., Cohen, H. C., and Okun, L.: The heart in sarcoidosis. Chest *60*:379, 1971.
299. Silverman, K. J., Hutchins, G. M., and Bulkley, B. H.: Cardiac sarcoid: A clinicopathologic study of 84 unselected patients with systemic sarcoidosis. Circulation *58*:1204, 1978.
300. Lie, J. T., Hunt, D., and Valentine, P. A.: Sudden death from cardiac sarcoidosis with involvement of conduction system. Am. J. Med. Sci. *267*:123, 1974.
301. Lull, R. J., Dunn, B. E., Gregoratos, G., Cox, W. A., and Fisher, G. W.: Ventricular aneurysm due to cardiac sarcoidosis with surgical cure of refractory ventricular tachycardia. Am. J. Cardiol. *30*:282, 1972.
302. Roberts, W. C., McAllister, H. A., and Ferrans, V. J.: Sarcoidosis of the heart. A clinicopathologic study of 35 necropsy patients (Group I) and review of 78 previously described necropsy patients (Group II). Am. J. Cardiol. *63*:86, 1977.
303. Fawcett, F. J., and Goldberg, M. J.: Heart block resulting from myocardial sarcoidosis. Br. Heart J. *36*:220, 1974.
304. Porter, G. H.: Sarcoid heart disease. N. Engl. J. Med. *263*:1350, 1960.
305. Ghosh, P., Fleming, H. A., Gresham, G. A., and Stonin, P. G. I.: Myocardial sarcoidosis. Br. Heart J. *34*:769, 1972.
306. Bulkley, B. H., and Hutchins, G. M.: Sarcoidosis, myocarditis and sudden death. Primary Cardiology July/Aug:38, 1977.
307. Phinney, A. O., Jr.: Sarcoid of the myocardial septum with complete heart block: Report of two cases. Am. Heart J. *62*:270, 1961.
308. Ferrans, V. J., Hibbs, R. G., Block, W. C., Walsh, J. J., and Burch, G. E.: Myocardial degeneration in cardiac sarcoidosis: Histochemical and electron microscopic studies. Am. Heart J. *69*:159, 1965.
309. James, T. N.: De Subitaneis Mortibus. XXV. Sarcoid heart disease. Circulation *56*:320, 1977.
310. Shiff, A. D., Blatt, C. J., and Colp, C.: Recurrent pericardial effusion secondary to sarcoidosis of the pericardium. A biopsy-proved case. N. Engl. J. Med. *281*:141, 1969.
311. McTaggart, D. R.: Sarcoidosis with cardiac involvement. Med. J. Aust. *2*:689, 1973.
312. Fleming, H. A.: Sarcoid heart disease. Br. Heart J. *36*:54, 1974.
313. Abeler, V.: Sarcoidosis of the cardiac conducting system. Am. Heart J. *97*:701, 1979.
314. Walsh, M. J.: Systemic sarcoidosis with refractory ventricular tachycardia and heart failure. Br. Heart J. *40*:931, 1978.
315. Serwer, G. A., Edwards, S. B., Benson, W., Jr., Anderson, P. A. W., and Spack, M.: Ventricular tachycardia due to cardiac sarcoidosis in a child. Pediatrics *62*:322, 1978.
316. Miller, A., Jackler, I., and Chuang, M.: Onset of sarcoidosis with left ventricular failure and multisystem involvement. Chest *70*:302, 1976.
317. Ahmed, S. S., Rozefort, R., Taclob, L. T., and Brancato, R. W.: Development of ventricular aneurysm in cardiac sarcoidosis. Angiology *28*:323, 1977.
318. Stein, E., Jackler, I., Stimmel, B., Stein, W., and Siltzbach, L. E.: Asymptomatic electrocardiographic alterations in sarcoidosis. Am. Heart J. *86*:474, 1973.
319. Strauss, G. S., Lawton, B. R., Wenzel, F. J., and Ray, J. F., III: Detection of covert myocardial sarcoidosis by scalene node biopsy. Chest *69*:790, 1976.
320. Lorell, B., Alderman, E. L., and Mason, J. W.: Cardiac sarcoidosis. Diagnosis with endomyocardial biopsy and treatment with corticosteroids. Am. J. Cardiol. *42*:143, 1978.
321. Bulkley, B. H., Rouleau, J. R., Whitaker, J. Q., Strauss, H. W., and Pitt, B.: The use of ^{201}thallium for myocardial perfusion imaging in sarcoid heart disease. Chest *72*:27, 1977.
322. Kinney, E. L., Jackson, G. L., Reeves, W. C., and Zelis, R.: Thallium-scan myocardial defects and echocardiographic abnormalities in patients with sarcoidosis without clinical cardiac dysfunction. An analysis of 44 patients. Am. J. Med. *68*:497, 1980.
323. Stein, E., Stimmel, B., and Siltzbach, L. E.: Clinical course of cardiac sarcoidosis. Ann. N.Y. Acad. Sci. *278*:470, 1976.
324. Duvernoy, W. F. C., and Garcia, R.: Sarcoidosis of the heart presenting with ventricular tachycardia and atrioventricular block. Am. J. Cardiol. *28*:348,1971.
325. Friedman, H. S., Parikh, N. K., Chandler, N., and Calderon, J.: Sarcoidosis with incomplete bilateral bundle branch block pattern disappearing following steroid therapy. An electrophysiological study. Eur. J. Cardiol. *4*:141, 1976.
326. Bashour, F. A., McConnell, J., Skinner, W., and Hanson, M.: Myocardial sarcoidosis. Dis. Chest *53*:413, 1968.
327. McAllister, H. A., and Fenoglio, J. J.: Cardiac involvement in Whipple's disease. Circulation *52*:152, 1975.
328. Becker, B. J. P., Chatgidakis, C. B., and Van Lingen, B.: Cardiovascular collagenosis with parietal endocardial thrombosis. A clinicopathological study of forty cases. Circulation *7*:345, 1953.
329. Davies, J. N. P., and Coles, R. M.: Some considerations regarding obscure disease affecting the mural endocardium. Am. Heart J. *59*:606, 1960.
330. Reid, J. V. O., and Berjak, P.: Tryptophan and serotonin levels in patients with or susceptible to African cardiomyopathy. Am. Heart J. *74*:337, 1967.
331. Reid, J. V. O., and Berjak, P.: Dietary production of myocardial fibrosis in the rat. Am. Heart J. *71*:240, 1966.
332. Hill, K. R., Still, W. J. S., and McKinney, B.: Jamaican cardiomyopathy. Br. Heart J. *29*:594, 1967.
333. Brink, A. J., and Lewis, C. M.: Coronary blood flow, energetics, and myocardial metabolism in idiopathic mural endomyocardiopathy. Am. Heart J. *73*: 339, 1967.
334. Lepley, D., Jr., Aris, A., Korns, M. E., Walker, J. A., and D'Cunha, R. M.: Endomyocardial fibrosis. A surgical approach. Ann. Thorac. Surg. *18*:626, 1974.
335. Vijayaraghavan, G., Cherian, G., Krishnaswami, S., and Sukumar, I. P.: Left ventricular endomyocardial fibrosis in India. Br. Heart J. *39*:563, 1977.
336. Guimaraes, A. C., Esteves, J. P., Filho, A. S., and Macedo, V.: Clinical aspects of endomyocardial fibrosis in Bahia, Brazil. Am. Heart J. *81*:7, 1971.
337. Shaper, A. G., Hutt, M. S. R., Edington, G. M., Somers, K., and Fowler, J. M.: Endomyocardial fibrosis. Cardiologia *52*:20, 1968.
337a. Cherian, G., Vijayaraghavan, G., Krishnaswami, S., Sukumar, I. P., John, S., Jairaj, P. S., and Bhaktaviziam, A.: Endomyocardial fibrosis: Report on the hemodynamic data in 29 patients and review of the results of surgery. Am. Heart J. *105*:659, 1983.
338. Beck, W., and Schrire, V.: Endomyocardial fibrosis in Caucasians previously resident in tropical Africa. Br. Heart J. *34*:915, 1972.
339. Connor, D. H., Somers, K., Hutt, M. S. R., Manion, W. C., and D'Arbela, P. G.: Endomyocardial fibrosis in Uganda (Davies disease): Part I. An epidemiologic, clinical and pathologic study. Am. Heart J. *74*:687; *75*:107, 1968.
340. Olsen, E. G.: Endomyocardial fibrosis and Löffler's endocarditis parietalis fibroplastica. Postgrad. Med. J. *53*:538, 1977.

341. Carlisle, R., Ogunba, E. D., McFarlane, H., Onayemi, D. A., and Oyeleye, V. O.: Immunoglobulins and antibody to *Loa loa* in Nigerians with endomyocardial fibrosis and other heart disease. Br. Heart J. *34*:678, 1972.
342. Roberts, W. C., Liegler, D. G., and Carbone, P. P.: Endomyocardial disease and eosinophilia: A clinical and pathologic spectrum. Am. J. Med. *46*:28, 1969.
343. D'Arbela, P. G., Mutazindwa, T., Patel, A. K., and Somers, K.: Survival after first presentation with endomyocardial fibrosis. Br. Heart J. *34*:403, 1972.
344. George, B. O., Talabi, A. I., Gaba, F. E., and Adeniyi, D. S.: Echocardiography in the diagnosis of right ventricular endomyocardial fibrosis. Postgrad. Med. J. *58*:467, 1982.
344a. Acquatella, H., Schiller, N. B., Puigbo, J. J., Gomez-Mancebo, J. R., Suarez, C., and Acquatella, G.: Value of two-dimensional echocardiography in endomyocardial disease with and without eosinophilia. A clinical and pathologic study. Circulation *67*:1219, 1983.
345. Adebonojo, S. A., and Jaiyesimi, F.: Pericardioperitoneal shunt for massive recurrent pericardial effusion in patients with endomyocardial fibrosis. Int. Surg. *62*:349, 1977.
346. Hess, O. M., Turina, M., Senning, A., Goebel, N. H., Scholer, Y., and Krayenbuehl, H. P.: Pre- and postoperative findings in patients with endomyocardial fibrosis. Br. Heart J. *40*:406, 1978.
347. Sheikhzadeh, A. H., Tarbiat, S., Nazarian, I., Aryanpur, I., and Sening. Å.: Constrictive endocarditis: Report of a case with successful surgery. Br. Heart J. *42*:224, 1979.
348. Goebel, N., Gander, M. P., and Hess, O. M.: Angiographic aspects of endomyocardial fibrosis. Ann. Radiol. *21*:475, 1978.
348a. Cherian, K. M., John, T. A., and Abraham, K. A.: Endomyocardial fibrosis: Clinical profile and role of surgery in management. Am. Heart J. *105*:706, 1983.
348b. Gonzalez-Lavin, L., Friedman, J. P., Hecker, S. P., and McFadden, P. M.: Endomyocardial fibrosis: Diagnosis and treatment. Am. Heart J. *105*:699, 1983.
349. Dubost, C., Prigent, C., Gerbaux, A., Maurice, P., Passelecq, J., Rulliere, R., Carpentier, A., and Deloche, A.: Surgical treatment of constrictive fibrous endocarditis. J. Thorac. Cardiovasc. Surg. *82*:585, 1981.
350. Metras, D., Coulibaly, A. O., Chauvet, J., Ekra, A., Longechaud, A., and Bertrand, E.: Endomyocardial fibrosis. J. Thorac. Cardiovasc. Surg. *83*:52, 1982.
351. Hall, S. W., Jr., Theologides, A., From, A. H. L., Gobel, F. L., Fortuny, I. E., Lawrence, C. J., and Edwards, J. E.: Hypereosinophilic syndrome with biventricular involvement. Circulation *55*:217, 1977.
352. Chusid, M. J., Dale, D. C., West, B. C., and Wolff, S. M.: The hypereosinophilic syndrome: Analysis of fourteen cases with review of the literature. Medicine *51*:1, 1975.
353. Brockington, I. F., and Olsen, E. G. J.: Löffler's endocarditis and Davies' endomyocardial fibrosis. Am. Heart J. *85*:308, 1973.
354. Brink, A. J., and Weber, W. H.: Fibroplastic parietal endocarditis with eosinophilia: Löffler's endocarditis. Am. J. Med. *34*:52, 1963.
355. Spry, C. J. F., and Tai, P. C.: Studies on blood eosinophils. II. Patients with Löffler's cardiomyopathy. Clin. Exp. Immunol. *24*:423, 1976.
356. Bell, J. A., Jenkins, B. S., and Webb-Peploe, M. M.: Clinical, haemodynamic, and angiographic findings in Löffler's eosinophilic endocarditis. Br. Heart J. *38*: 541, 1976.
357. Parrillo, J. E., Borer, J. S., Henry, W. L., Wolff, S. M., and Fauci, A. S.: The cardiovascular manifestations of the hypereosinophilic syndrome. Prospective study of 26 patients, with review of the literature. Am. J. Med. *67*:573, 1979.
358. Raizner, A. E., Silverman, M. E., and Waters, W. C., III: Conduction disturbances and pacemaker failure in Löffler's endomyocarditis. Am. J. Med. *53*: 343, 1972.
359. Rodger, J. C., Irvine, K. G., and Lerski, R. A.: Echocardiography in Löffler's endocarditis. Br. Heart J. *46*:110, 1981.
359a. Gottdiener, J. S., Maron, B. J., Schooley, R. T., Harley, J. B., Roberts, W. C., and Fauci, A. S.: Two dimensional echocardiographic assessment of the idiopathic hypereosinophilic syndrome. Anatomic basis of mitral regurgitation and peripheral embolization. Circulation *67*:572, 1983.
360. Weyman, A. E., Rankin, R., and King, H.: Löffler's endocarditis presenting as mitral and tricuspid stenosis. Am. J. Cardiol. *40*:438, 1977.
361. Scott, M. E., and Bruce, J. H.: Löffler's endocarditis. Brit. Heart J. *37*:534, 1975.
362. Fournial, G., Schlanger, R., Berthoumieu, F., Pris, J., Marco, J., and Eschapasse, H.: Surgery for cardiac complications caused by endocardial mural fibrin deposits in a hypereosinophilic syndrome. Circulation *65*:1010, 1982.
363. Cohen, J., Davies, J., Goodwin, J. F., and Spry, C. J. F.: Arrhythmias in patients with hypereosinophilia: A comparison of patients with and without Löffler's endomyocardial disease. Postgrad. Med. J. *56*:828, 1980.
364. Oakley, C. M., and Olsen, E. G. J.: Eosinophilia and heart disease. Brit. Heart J. *39*:233, 1977.
365. Andy, J. J., Bishara, F. F., and Soyinka, O. O.: Relation of severe eosinophilia and microfilariasis to chronic African endomyocardial fibrosis. Br. Heart J. *45*: 672, 1981.
366. Ferrans, V. J., and Roberts, W. C.: The carcinoid endocardial plaque. An ultrastructural study. Hum. Pathol. 7:387, 1976.
367. Grahame-Smith, D. G.: The carcinoid syndrome. Am. J. Cardiol. *21*:376, 1968.
368. Grahame-Smith, D. G.: The carcinoid syndrome. *In* Bondy, P. K., and Rosenberg, L. E. (eds.): Metabolic Control and Disease. 9th ed. Philadelphia, W. B. Saunders Co., 1980, p. 1703.
369. Hendel, N., Leckie, B., and Richards, J.: Carcinoid heart disease: Eight-year survival following tricuspid valve replacement and pulmonary valvotomy. Ann. Thorac. Surg. *30*:391, 1980.
370. Roberts, W. C., and Sjoerdsma, A.: The cardiac disease associated with the carcinoid syndrome (carcinoid heart disease). Am. J. Med. *36*:5, 1969.
371. Stephan, E., and deWit J.: Carcinoid heart disease from primary carcinoid tumour of the ovary. Haemodynamic and cine coronary angiocardiographic study after operation. Br. Heart J. *36*:613, 1974.
371a. Howard, R. J., Drobac, M., Rider, W. D., Keane, T. T., Finlayson, J., Silver, M. D., Wigle, E. D., and Rakowski, H.: Carcinoid heart disease: Diagnosis by two-dimensional echocardiography. Circulation *66*:1059, 1982.
372. Schwaber, J. R., and Lukas, D. S.: Hyperkinemia and cardiac failure in the carcinoid syndrome. Am. J. Med. *32*:846, 1962.
373. Biörck, G., Axen, O., and Thorson, A.: Unusual cyanosis in a boy with congenital pulmonary stenosis and tricuspid insufficiency. Fatal outcome after angiocardiography. Am. Heart J. *44*:143, 1952.

MYOCARDITIS

374. Monif, G. R. G., Lee, C. W., and Hsiung, G. D.: Isolated myocarditis with recovery of ECHO type 9 virus from the myocardium. N. Engl. J. Med. *277*: 1353, 1967.
375. Morales, A. R., Vichitbandha, P., Chandruang, P., Evans, H., and Bourgeois, C. H.: Pathologic features of cardiac conduction disturbances in diphtheritic myocarditis. Arch. Pathol. *91*:1, 1971.
376. Kaplan, M. H., and Meyeserian, M.: An immunological cross-reaction between Group-A streptococcal cells and human heart tissue. Lancet *1*:706, 1962.
377. James, T. N., Schlant, R. C., and Marshall, T. K.: De Subitaneis Mortibus. XXIX. Randomly distributed focal myocardial lesions causing destruction in the His bundle or a narrow origin left bundle branch. Circulation *57*:816, 1978.
378. Friedman, M. A., Bozdeck, M. J., Billingham, M. E., and Rider, A. K.: Daunorubicin cardiotoxicity. Serial endomyocardial biopsies and systolic time intervals. J.A.M.A. *240*:1603, 1978.
379. Ablemann, W. H.: Viral myocarditis and its sequelae, Annu. Rev. Med. *24*: 145, 1973.
380. Adesanya, C. O.: Heart muscle performance after experimental viral myocarditis. J. Clin. Invest. *57*:569, 1976.
381. Fine, I., Brainerd, H., and Sokolow, M.: Myocarditis in acute infectious diseases: A clinical and electrocardiographic study. Circulation *2*:859, 1950.
382. Weinstein L.: Cardiovascular manifestations in some of the common infectious diseases. Mod. Concepts Cardiovasc. Dis. *23*:229, 1954.
383. Abelmann, W. H.: Myocarditis. N. Engl. J. Med. *275*:832, 944, 1966.
384. De La Chapelle, C. E., and Kossmann, C. E.: Myocarditis. Circulation *10*:747, 1954.
385. Saphir, O., Wile, S. A., and Reingold, J. M.: Myocarditis in children. Am. J. Dis. Child. *67*:294, 1944.
386. Saphir, O.: Myocarditis: A general review with an analysis of two hundred and forty cases. Arch. Pathol. *32*:1000, 1941; *33*:88, 1942.
387. Stevens, P. J., and Underwood Ground, K. E.: Occurrence and significance of myocarditis in trauma. Aerospace Med. *41*:776, 1970.
388. Pankey, G. A.: Effect of viruses on the cardiovascular system. Am. J. Med. Sci. *250*:103, 1965.
389. Woodward, T. E., Togo, Y., Lee, Y-C., and Hornick, R. B.: Specific microbial infections of the myocardium and pericardium. A study of 82 patients. Arch. Intern. Med. *120*:270, 1967.
390. Gore, I., and Saphir, O.: Myocarditis: A classification of 1402 cases. Am. Heart J. *34*:827, 1947.
391. Editorial: Non-rheumatic myopericarditis. Br. Med. J., *2*:544, 1971.
392. Sanders, V.: Viral myocarditis. Am. Heart J. *66*:707, 1963.
393. Robboy, S. J.: Atrioventricular-node inflammation. Mechanisms of sudden death in protracted meningococcemia. N. Engl. J. Med. *286*:1091, 1972.
394. Gerzen, P., Granath, A., Holmgren, B., and Zetterquist, S.: Acute myocarditis. A followup study. Br. Heart J. *34*:575, 1972.
395. Lim, C. H., Toh, C. C. S., Chia, B-L., and Low, L-P.: Stokes-Adams attacks due to acute nonspecific myocarditis. Am. Heart J. *90*:172, 1975.
396. Reeves, W. C., Jackson, G. L., Flickinger, F. W., Divee, H. G., Schwiter, E. J., Werner, J., Whitesell, L., Bidde, M. A., Copenhover, G., Shaikh, B. S., and Zelis, R.: Radionuclide imaging of experimental myocarditis. Circulation *63*: 640, 1981.
397. Matsumori, A., Kadota, K., and Kawai, C.: Technetium-99m pyrophosphate uptake in experimental viral perimyocarditis. Sequential study of myocardial uptake and pathologic correlates. Circulation *61*:802, 1980.
398. Bengtsson, E., and Lamberger, B.: Five-year followup study of cases suggestive of acute myocarditis. Am. Heart J. *72*:751, 1966.
399. Das, S. K., Brady, T. J., Thrall, J. H., and Pitt, B.: Cardiac function in patients with prior myocarditis. J. Nucl. Med. *21*:689, 1980.
400. Burch, G. E., and Giles, T. D.: The role of viruses in the production of heart disease. Am. J. Cardiol. *29*:231, 1972.
401. Abelmann, W. H.: Clinical aspects of viral cardiomyopathy. *In* Fowler, N. O. (ed.): Myocardial Diseases. New York, Grune and Stratton, 1973, p. 253.
402. Wenger, N. K.: Infectious myocarditis. *In* Burch, G. E. (ed.): Cardiomyopathy. (Cardiovascular Clinics Series.) Philadelphia, F. A. Davis Co., 1972, p. 168.
403. Pearce, J. H.: Heart disease and filtrable virus. Circulation *21*:448, 1960.

404. Lerner, A. M.: Coxsackie virus myocardiopathy. J. Infect. Dis. *120*:496, 1969.
404a. Fenoglio, J. J., Ursell, P. C., Kellogg, C. F., Drusin, R. E., and Weiss, M. B.: Diagnosis and classification of myocarditis by endomyocardial biopsy. N. Engl. J. Med. *308*:12, 1983.
405. Mason J. W., Billingham, M. E., and Ricci, D. R.: Treatment of acute inflammatory myocarditis assisted by endomyocardial biopsy. Am. J. Cardiol. *45*: 1037, 1980.
406. Norris, D., and Loh, P. C.: Coxsackie virus myocarditis: Prophylaxis and therapy with an interferon stimulator. Proc. Soc. Exp. Biol. Med. *142*:133, 1973.
407. Levine, H. D.: Virus myocarditis: A critique of the literature from clinical, electrocardiographic, and pathologic standpoints. Am. J. Med. Sci. *277*:132, 1979.
408. Price, R. A., Garcia, J. H., and Rightsel, W. A.: Choriomeningitis and myocarditis in an adolescent with isolation of Coxsackie B-5 virus. Am. J. Clin. Pathol. *53*:825, 1970.
409. Desa'Neto, A., Bullington, D., Bullington, R. H., Desser, K. B., and Benchimol, A.: Coxsackie B5 heart disease. Demonstration of inferolateral wall myocardial necrosis. Am. J. Med. *68*:295, 1980.
410. Grist, N. R., and Bell, E. J.: Coxsackie viruses and the heart. Am. Heart J. *77*: 295, 1969.
411. Ray, C. G., Portman, J. N., Stamm, S. J., and Hickman, R. O.: Hemolytic-uremic syndrome and myocarditis. Association with coxsackievirus B infection. Am. J. Dis. Child. *122*:418, 1970.
412. Smith, W. G.: Coxsackie B myopericarditis in adults. Am. Heart J. *80*:34, 1970.
413. Hirschman, S. F., and Hammer, G. S.: Coxsackie virus myopericarditis. A microbiological and clinical review. Am. J. Cardiol. *34*:224, 1974.
414. Sainani, G. S., Dekate, M. P., and Rao, C. P.: Heart disease caused by Coxsackie virus B infection. Br. Heart J. *37*:819, 1975.
415. Rose, H. D.: Recurrent illness following acute Coxsackie B-4 myocarditis. Am. J. Med. *54*:544, 1973.
416. Burch, G. E., and Colcolough, H. L.: Progressive Coxsackie viral pericarditis and nephritis. Ann. Intern Med. *71*:963, 1969.
417. Editorial: Acute myocarditis and its sequelae. Br. Med. J. *3*:783, 1972.
418. Bell, E. J., and Grist, N. R.: Echoviruses, carditis and acute pleurodynia. Am. Heart J. *82*:133, 1971.
419. Bell, E. J., and Grist, N. R.: Echovirus, carditis and actue pleurodynia. Lancet *1*:326, 1970.
420. Schleissner, L. A., Fiala, M., Imagawa, D. T., and Casaburi, R.: Application of systolic time intervals to acute cardiomyopathy with echovirus 2. Chest *69*: 563, 1976.
421. Henson, D., and Nufson, M. A.: Myocarditis and pneumonitis with type 21 adenovirus infection. Association with fatal myocarditis and pneumonitis. Am. J. Dis. Child *121*:334, 1971.
422. Verel, D., Warrack, A. J. N., Potter, C. W., Ward, C., and Rickards, D. F.: Observations on the A_2 England influenza epidemic: A clinicopathological study. Am. Heart J. *92*:290, 1976.
423. Oseasohn, R., Adelson, L., and Kaji, M.: Clinicopathological study of thirty-three fatal cases of Asian influenza. N. Engl. J. Med. *260*:509, 1959.
424. Coltman, C. A., Jr.: Influenza myocarditis: Report of a case with observations on serum glutamic oxaloacetic transaminase. J.A.M.A. *180*:204, 1962.
425. Adams, C. W.: Postviral myopericarditis associated with the influenza virus. Am. J. Cardiol. *4*:56, 1959.
426. Moore, C. M., Henry, J., Benzing, G., III, and Kaplan, S.: Varicella myocarditis. Am. J. Dis. Child *118*:899, 1969.
427. Hackel, D. B.: Myocarditis in association with varicella. Am. J. Pathol. *29*: 369, 1953.
428. Morales, A. R., Adelman, S., and Fine, G.: Varicella myocarditis: A case of sudden death. Arch. Pathol. *91*:29, 1971.
429. Hildes, J. A., Schaberg, A., and Alcock, A. J. W.: Cardiovascular collapse in acute poliomyelitis. Circulation *12*:986, 1955.
430. Teloth, H. A.: Myocarditis in poliomyelitis. Arch. Pathol. *55*:408, 1953.
431. Weinstein, L., and Shelokov, A.: Cardiovascular manifestations of acute poliomyelitis. N. Engl. J. Med. *244*:281, 1951.
432. Mohammed, I., and Carlisle, R.: Cardiac and renal involvement in mumps. West Afr. Med. J.: *20*:367, 1971.
433. Roberts, W. C., and Fox, S. M., III: Mumps of the heart: Clinical and pathologic features. Circulation *32*:342, 1965.
434. Bengtsson, E., and Orndahl, G.: Complications of mumps with special reference to the incidence of myocarditis. Acta Med. Scand. *149*:381, 1954.
435. Arita, M., Ueno, Y., and Masuyama, Y.: Complete heart block in mumps myocarditis. Br. Heart J. *46*:342, 1981.
436. Saphir, O., Amromin, G. D., and Yokoo, H.: Myocarditis in viral (epidemic) hepatitis. Am. J. Med. Sci. *231*:168, 1956.
437. Bell, H.: Cardiac manifestations of viral hepatitis. J.A.M.A. *218*:387, 1971.
438. Nagaratnam, N., deSilva, D. P. K. M., and Gunawardene, K. R. W.: Myocardial involvement in infectious hepatitis. Postgrad. Med. J. *47*:785, 1971.
439. Webster, B. H.: Cardiac complications of infectious mononucleosis: A review of the literature and report of five cases. Am. J. Med. Sci. *234*:62, 1957.
440. Frishman, W., Kraus, M. E., Zabkar, J., Brooks, V., Alonso, D., and Dixon, L. M.: Infectious mononucleosis and fatal myocarditis. Chest *72*:535, 1977.
441. Miller, R., Ward, C., Amsterdam, E., Mason, D. T., and Zelis, R.: Focal mononucleosis myocarditis simulating myocardial infarction. Chest *63*:102, 1973.
442. Hudgins, J. M.: Infectious mononucleosis complicated by myocarditis and pericarditis. J.A.M.A. *235*:2626, 1976.
443. Goldfinger, D., Schreiber, W., and Wosika, P. H.: Permanent heart block following German measles. Am. J. Med. *2*:320, 1947.
444. Goldfield, M., Bayer, N. H., and Weinstein, L.: Electrocardiographic changes during the course of measles. J. Pediatr. *46*:30, 1955.
445. Degen, J. A.: Visceral pathology in measles: A clinico-pathologic study of 100 cases. Am. J. Med. Sci. *194*:104, 1937.
446. Wilson, R. S., Morris, T. H., and Rossell Rees, J.: Cytomegalovirus myocarditis. Br. Heart J. *34*:865, 1972.
447. Wink, K., and Schmitz, H.: Cytomegalovirus myocarditis. Am. Heart J. *100*: 667, 1980.
448. Tuila, E., and Leinikki, P.: Fatal cytomegalovirus infection in a previously healthy boy with myocarditis and consumption coagulopathy as presenting signs. Scand. J. Infect. Dis. *4*:57, 1972.
449. Obeyesekere, I., and Herman, Y.: Arbovirus heart disease: Myocarditis and cardiomyopathy following dengue and chikungunya fever—a follow-up study. Am. Heart J. *85*:186, 1973.
450. Nagaratham, N., Siripala, K., and deSilva, N.: Arbovirus (dengue type) as a cause of acute myocarditis and pericarditis. Br. Heart J. *35*:204, 1973.
451. Obeyesekere, I., and Herman, Y.: Myocarditis and cardiomyopathy after arbovirus infections (dengue and chikungunya fever). Br. Heart J. *34*:821, 1972.
452. Anderson T., Foulis, M. A., Grist, N. R., and Landsman, J. B.: Clinical and laboratory observations in a smallpox outbreak. Lancet *1*:1248, 1951.
453. Matthews, A. W., and Griffiths, I. D.: Post-vaccinal pericarditis and myocarditis. Br. Heart J. *36*:1043, 1974.
454. Finlay-Jones, L. R.: Fatal myocarditis after vaccinations for smallpox. N. Engl. J. Med. *270*:41, 1964.
455. Connell, D. E.: Myocardial degeneration in yellow fever. Am. J. Pathol. *4*:431, 1928.
456. Gills, T. D., and Gohd, R. S.: Respiratory syncytial virus and heart disease. A report of two cases. J.A.M.A. *236*:1128, 1976.
457. Bairan, A. C., Cherry, J. D., Fagan, L. F., and Coff, J. E., Jr.: Complete heart block and respiratory syncytial virus infection. Am. J. Dis. Child. *127*:264, 1974.
458. Lewes, D., Rainsford, D. J., and Lane, W. F.: Symptomless myocarditis and myalgia in viral and *Mycoplasma pneumoniae* infections. Br. Heart J. *36*:924, 1974.
459. Sands, M. J., Jr., Satz, J. E., Turner, W. E., and Soloff, L. A.: Pericarditis and perimyocarditis associated with active *Mycoplasma pneumoniae* infection. Ann. Intern. Med. *86*:544, 1977.
460. Pickens, S., and Catterall, J. R.: Disseminated intravascular coagulation and myocarditis associated with *Mycoplasma pneumoniae* infection. Br. Med. J. *1*: 1526, 1978.
461. Dymock, I. W., Lawson, J. M., MacLennan, W. J., and Ross, C. A. C.: Myocarditis associated with psittacosis. Br. J. Clin. Pract. *25*:240, 1971.
462. Sutton, G. C., Morrissey, R. A., Tobin, J. R., Jr., and Anderson, T. V.: Pericardial and myocardial disease associated with serologic evidence of infection by agents of the psittacosis-lymphogranuloma venereum group (Chlamydiaceae). Circulation *36*:830, 1967.
463. Woodward, I. E., McCrumb, F. R., Jr., Carey, I. N., and Tago, Y.: Viral and rickettsial causes of cardiac disease including the Coxsackie virus etiology of pericarditis and myocarditis. Ann. Intern. Med. *53*:1130, 1960.
464. Allen, A. C., and Spitz, S.: A comparative study of the pathology of scrub typhus (tsutsugamushi disease) and other rickettsial diseases. Am. J. Pathol. *21*: 603, 1945.
465. Ognibane, A. J., O'Leary, D. S., Czarnocki, S. W., Flannery, E. P., and Grove, R. B.: Myocarditis and disseminated intravascular coagulation in scrub typhus. Am. J. Med. Sci. *262*:233, 1971.
466. Levine, H. D.: Pathologic study of thirty-one cases of scrub typhus fever with special reference to the cardiovascular system. Am. Heart J. *31*:314, 1946.
467. Bradford, W. D., and Hackel, D. B.: Myocardial involvement in Rocky Mountain spotted fever. Arch. Pathol. Lab. Med. *102*:357, 1978.
468. Hand, W. L., Miller, J. B., Reinary, J. A., and Sanford, J. P.: Rocky Mountain spotted fever: A vascular disease. Arch. Intern. Med. *125*:879, 1970.
469. Sheridan, P., MacCraig, J. N., and Hart, R. J. C.: Myocarditis complicating Q fever. Br. Med. J. *2*:155, 1974.
470. Barraclough, D., and Popert, A. J.: Q fever presenting with paroxysmal ventricular tachycardia. Br. Med. J. *2*:423, 1975.
471. Taheinia, A. C.: Electrocardiographic abnormalities and serum transaminase levels in diphtheritic myocarditis. J. Pediatr. *75*:1008, 1969.
472. Riley, H. D., Jr., and Weaver, T. S.: Cardiovascular and nervous system complications of diphtheria. Am. Pract. *3*:536, 1952.
473. Collier, R. J., and Pappenheimer, A. M.: Studies on the mode of action of diphtheria toxin. J. Exp. Med. *120*:1007; 1018, 1964.
474. Ledbetter, M. K., Cannon, A. B., and Costa, A. F.: The electrocardiogram in diphtheritic myocarditis. Am. Heart. J. *68*:599, 1964.
475. Matisonn, R. E.: Successful electrical pacing for complete heart block complicating diphtheritic myocarditis. Br. Heart J. *38*:423, 1976.
476. Sanders, V., and Misanik, L. F.: Salmonella myocarditis: Report of a case with ventricular rupture. Am. Heart J. *68*:682, 1964.
477. Hennigar, G. R., Thabet, R., Bundy, W. C., and Sutton, L. E.: Salmonellosis complicated by pancarditis. J. Pediatr. *43*:524, 1953.
478. Shilkin, K. B.: *Salmonella typhimurium* pancarditis. Postgrad. Med. J. *45*:40, 1969.
479. Le-Van-Diem, A. K.: Typhoid fever with myocarditis. Am. J. Trop. Med. Hyg. *23*:218, 1974.
480. Mainzer, F.: Electrocardiographic study of typhoid myocarditis. Br. Heart J. *9*: 145, 1947.

481. Thiruvengadam, K. V., Shetty, M. R., and Mallick, M. A.: Myocarditis in enteric fever. J. Indian Med. Assoc. *48*:115, 1967.
482. Kinare, S. G., and Deshmulh, M. M.: Complete atrioventricular block due to myocardial tuberculosis. Arch. Pathol. *88*:684, 1969.
483. Auerbach, O., and Guggenheim, A.: Tuberculosis of the myocardium: A review of the literature and a report of six new cases. Q. Bull. Sea View Hosp. *2*: 264, 1937.
484. Horn, H., and Saphir, O.: The involvement of the myocardium in tuberculosis. A review of the literature and report of 3 cases. Am. Rev. Tuberc. *32*:492, 1935.
485. Rosenbaum, H., and Linn, H. J.: Tuberculosis of myocardium. Am. J. Clin. Pathol. *18*:162, 1948.
486. Claiborne, T. S.: Caseating granuloma of the heart. Am. J. Cardiol. *33*:920, 1974.
487. Jones, K. P., and Tilden, I. L.: Tuberculous myocardial aneurysm, with rupture and sudden death from tamponade: Review of the literature and report of a case. Hawaii Med. J. *1*:295, 1942.
488. Rawls, W. J., Shuford, W. H., Kogan, W. D., Hurst, J. W., and Schlant, R. C.: Right ventricular outflow tract obstruction produced by a myocardial abscess in a patient with tuberculosis. Am. J. Cardiol. *21*:738, 1968.
489. Gore, I.: Myocarditis in infectious diseases. Am. Pract. *1*:292, 1947.
490. Brody, A., and Smith, L. W.: Visceral pathology in scarlet fever and related streptococcal infections. Am. J. Pathol. *12*:373, 1936.
491. Hardman, J. M., and Earle, K. M.: Myocarditis in 200 fatal meningococcal infections. Arch. Pathol. *87*:318, 1969.
492. d'Agati, V., and Marangoni, B. A.: The Waterhouse-Friderichsen syndrome. N. Engl. J. Med. *232*:1, 1945.
493. Denmark, I. C., and Knight, E. L.: Cardiovascular and coagulation complications of Group C meningococcal disease. Arch. Intern. Med. *127*:238, 1971.
494. Roberts, W. C., and Beard, G. W.: Gas gangrene of the heart in clostridial septicemia. Am. Heart J. *74*:482, 1967.
495. Guneratre, P.: Gas gangrene (abscess) of heart. N.Y. State J. Med. *75*:1766, 1975.
496. Gross, D., Willens, H., and Zeldis, S. M.: Myocarditis in Legionnaire's disease. Chest 79:232, 1981.
497. Doscia, J. L., Fisco, J. M., and Brace, W. T.: Complete heart block due to a solitary gumma. Am. J. Cardiol. *13*:553, 1964.
498. Spain, D. M., and Johannsen, M. W.: Three cases of localized gummatous myocarditis. Am. Heart J. *241*:689, 1942.
499. Boss, J. H., Liftkowtiz, M., and Freud, M.: Unusual manifestations of syphilitic cardiovascular disease. Ann. Intern. Med. *55*:824, 1961.
500. Saphir, O.: Syphilitic myocarditis. Arch. Pathol. *13*:266, 1932.
501. Arean, V. M.: Leptospiral myocarditis. Lab. Invest. *6*:462, 1957.
502. Edwards, G. A., and Damm, B. M.: Human leptospirosis. Medicine *39*:117, 1960.
503. Sodeman, W. A., and Kellough, J. H.: The cardiac manifestations of Weil's disease. Am. J. Trop. Med. *31*:479, 1957.
504. Judge, D. M., Samuel, I., Perine, P. L., Vukotic, D., and Ababa, A.: Louse-borne relapsing fever in man. Arch. Pathol. *97*:136, 1974.
505. Williams, A. H.: Aspergillus myocarditis. Am. J. Clin. Pathol. *61*:247, 1974.
506. Cade, J. F.: Pulmonary aspergillosis with myocarditis. Med. J. Aust. *1*:581, 1966.
507. Zoeckler, S. J.: Cardiac actinomycosis: A case report and survey of the literature. Circulation *3*:854, 1951.
508. Edwards, A. C.: Actinomycosis in children: A review of the literature and report of cases. Am. J. Dis. Child. *41*:1419, 1931.
509. Martin, D. S., and Smith, D. T.: Blastomycosis (American blastomycosis, Gilchrist's disease). I. A review of the literature. Am. Rev. Tuberc. *39*:275, 1939.
510. Baker, R. D., and Brian, E. W.: Blastomycosis of the heart: Report of two cases. Am. J. Pathol. *13*:139, 1937.
511. Hutter, R. V. P., and Collins, H. S.: The appearance of opportunistic fungus infections in a cancer hospital. Lab. Invest. *11*:1035, 1962.
512. Jones, I., Nassau, E., and Smith, P.: Cryptococcosis of the heart. Br. Heart J. *27*:462, 1965.
513. Van Kirk, J. E., Simon, A. B., and Armstrong, U. R.: Candida myocarditis causing complete atrioventricular block. J.A.M.A. *227*:931, 1974.
514. Brooks, S. E. H., and Young, E. G.: Clinicopathologic observations on systemic moniliasis: A case report and review of the literature. Arch. Pathol. *73*:383, 1962.
515. Reingold, I. M.: Myocardial lesions in disseminated coccidioidomycosis. Am. J. Clin. Pathol. *20*:1044, 1950.
516. Larson, R., and Schert, R. E.: Coccidioidal pericarditis. Circulation *7*:211, 1953.
517. Merchant, R. K., Louria, D. B., Geisler, P. H., Edgcomb, J. H., and Utz, S. P.: Fungal endocarditis. Review of the literature and report of three cases. Ann. Intern. Med. *48*:242, 1958.
518. Owen, G. E., Scherr, W. N., and Segre, E. J.: Histoplasmosis involving the heart and great vessels. Am. J. Med. *32*:552, 1962.
519. Acquatella, H., Schiller, N. B., Puigbo, J. J., Giordano, H., Suarez, J. A., Casal, H., Arreaza, N., Valecillos, R., and Hirschhaut, E.: M-mode and two-dimensional echocardiography in chronic Chagas' heart disease. A clinical and pathologic study. Circulation *62*:787, 1980.
520. Rosenbaum, M. B.: Chagasic myocardiopathy. Progr. Cardiovasc. Dis. *7*:199, 1964.
521. Teixeira, A. R. L., Teixeira, G., Macedo, V., and Prata, A.: Acquired cell-mediated immunodepression in acute Chagas' disease. J. Clin. Invest. *62*:1132, 1978.
522. Winslow, D. J., and Chaffee, E. F.: Preliminary investigations in Chagas disease. Milit. Med. *130*:826, 1965.
523. Ribeiro Dos Santos, R., and Hudson, L.: *Trypanosoma cruzi*: Immunological consequences of parasite modification of host cells. Clin. Exp. Immunol. *40*:36, 1980.
524. Editorial: Chagas' disease: Potential for immunoprophylaxis. Lancet *1*:466, 1980.
525. Ribeiro Dos Santos, R., and Hudson, L.: *Trypanosoma cruzi*: Binding of parasite antigens to mammalian cell membranes. Parasite Immunol. *2*:1, 1980.
526. Mott, K. E., and Hagstrom, J. W. C.: The pathologic lesions of the cardiac autonomic nervous system in chronic Chagas' myocarditis. Circulation *31*:273, 1965.
527. Teixeira, A. R. L.: Chagas' disease: Trends in immunological research and prospects for immunoprophylaxis. Bull. WHO *57*:697, 1979.
528. Puigbó, J. J., Valecillos, R., Hirschhault, E, Giordano, H., Boccalandro, I., Suarez, C., and Aparicio, J. M.: Diagnosis of Chagas' cardiomyopathy. Non-invasive techniques. Postgrad. Med. *53*:527, 1977.
528a. Maguire, J. H., Mott, K. E., Lehman, J. S., Hoff, R.., Muniz, T. M, Guimãraes, A. C., Sherlock, I., and Morrow, R. H. : Relationship of electrocardiographic abnormalities and seropositivity to Trypanosoma cruzi within a rural community in Northeast Brazil. Am. Heart J. *105*:287, 1983.
529. Miles, M. A., Cedillos, R. A., Povoa, M. M., De Souza, A. A., Prata, A., and Macedo, V.: Do radically dissimilar *Trypanosoma cruzi* strains (zymodemes) cause Venezuelan and Brazilian forms of Chagas' disease? Lancet *1*:1338, 1981.
530. Oliveira, J. S. M., Oliveira, J. A. M., Frederigue, V., Jr., and Filho, E. C. L.: Apical aneurysm of Chagas' heart disease. Br. Heart J. *46*:432, 1981.
531. Laranja, F. S., Dias, E., Nobrega, G., and Miranda, A.: Chagas' disease: A clinical, epidemiologic, and pathologic study. Circulation *14*:1035, 1956.
532. Andrade, Z. A., Andrade, S. G., Oliveira, G. B., and Alonso, D. R.: Histopathology of the conducting tissue of the heart in Chagas' myocarditis. Am. Heart J. *95*:316, 1978.
533. Chiale, P. A., Przybylski, J., Laino, R. A., Halpern, M. S., Sanchez, R. A., Gafrieli, A., Elizari, M. V., and Rosenbaum, M. B.: Electrocardiographic changes evoked by ajmaline in chronic Chagas' disease without manifest myocarditis. Am. J. Cardiol. *49*:14, 1982.
534. Carrasco, H. A., Barboza, J. S., Inglessis, G., Fuenmayor, A., and Molina, C.: Left ventricular cineangiography in Chagas' disease: Detection of early myocardial damage. Am. Heart J. *104*:595, 1982.
535. Araujo, F., Chiari, E., and Dias, J. C. P.: Demonstration of *Trypanosoma cruzi* antigen in serum from patients with Chagas' disease. Lancet *1*:246, 1981.
536. Mott, K. E., Lehman, J. S., Jr., Hoff, R., Morrow, R. H., Muniz, T. M., Sherlock, I., Draper, C. C., Pugliese, C., and Guimaraes, A.: The epidemiology and household distribution of seroreactivity to *Trypanosoma cruzi* in a rural community in northeast Brazil. Am. J. Trop. Med. Hyg. *25*:552, 1976.
537. Brener, Z., and Andrade, Z. A. (eds.): *Trypanosoma cruzi* e Doenca de Chagas. Rio de Janeiro, Guanabara Koogan, 1979, p. 362.
538. Francis, T. I.: Visceral complications of Gambian trypanosomiasis in a nigerian. Trans. R. Soc. Trop. Med. Hyg. *66*:140, 1972.
539. deRaadt, P., and Koten, J. W.: Myocarditis in rhodesiense trypanosomiasis. East Afr. Med. J. *45*:128, 1968.
540. Poltera, A. A., Cox, N., and Owor, R.: Pancarditis affecting the conducting system and all valves in human African trypanosomiasis. Br. Heart J. *38*:827, 1976.
541. Theologides, A., and Kennedy, B. J.: Toxoplasmic myocarditis and pericarditis (editorial). Am. J. Med. *47*:169, 1969.
542. Van der Horst, R., Kleverman, P., Schonland, M., and Gotsman, M.: Fatal myocardial necrosis probably due to toxoplasma myocarditis. S. Afr. Med. J. *46*:949, 1972.
543. Leak, D., and Meghji, M.: Toxoplasmic infection in cardiac disease. Am. J. Cardiol. *43*:841, 1979.
544. Sagrista-Sauleda, J., Permanyer-Miralda, G., Juste-Sanchez, C., de Buen-Sanchez, M. L., Pujadas-Capmany, R., Arcalis-Arce, L., and Soler-Soler, J.: Huge chronic pericardial effusion caused by *Toxoplasma gondii*. Circulation *66*: 895, 1982.
545. Mary, A. S., and Hamilton, M.: Ventricular tachycardia in a patient with toxoplasmosis. Br. Heart J. *35*:349, 1973.
546. Rojas, R. A., and Deza, D.: Cardiac changes in malarial patients. Am. Heart J. *33*:702, 1947.
547. Merkel, W. C.: *Plasmodium falciparum* malaria: The coronary and myocardial lesions observed at autopsy in two cases of acute fulminating *Plasmodium falciparum* infection. Arch. Pathol. *41*:290, 1946.
548. Herrera, J. M.: Cardiac lesions in vivax malaria: Study of a case with coronary and myocardial damage. Arch. Inst. Cardiol. Mex. *30*:26, 1960.
549. Simonson, E., and Keys, A.: Experimental malaria in man. III. The changes in the electrocardiogram. J. Clin. Invest. *29*:68, 1950.
550. Wessel, H. U., Sommers, H. M., Cugell, D. W., and Paul, M. H.: Variants of cardiopulmonary manifestations of Manson's schistosomiasis: Report of two cases. Ann. Intern Med. *62*:757, 1965.
551. Bedford, D. E., Aidaros, S. M., and Girgis, B.: Bilharzial heart disease in Egypt: Cor pulmonale due to bilharzial pulmonary endarteritis. Br. Heart J. *8*: 87, 1946.
552. Zahawi, S., and Shukri, N.: Histopathology of fatal myocarditis due to ectopic schistosomiasis. Trans. R. Soc. Trop. Med. Hyg. *50*:166, 1956.
553. Kean, B. H., and Breslou, R. C.: Parasites of the Human Heart. New York, Grune and Stratton, 1964.

554. Africa, C. M., Garcia, E. Y., and DeLeon, W.: Intestinal heterophyiasis with cardiac involvement. A contribution to the etiology of heart failure. J. Philipp. Isl. Med. Assoc. *15*:358, 1935.
555. Helimsky, A. M.: Cysticercosis of the brain, heart and skeletal muscles. Med. Parazitol. (Mosk.) *31*:610, 1962.
556. Goldsmid, J. M.: Two unusual cases of cysticercosis in man in Rhodesia. J. Helminthol. *40*:331, 1966.
557. Ibarra-Perez, C., Fernandez-Diez, J., and Rodriguez-Trujillo, F.: Myocardial cysticercosis: Report of two cases with coexisting heart disease. South. Med. J. *65*:484, 1972.
558. Murphy, T. E., Kean, B. H., Venturine, A., and Lillekei, C. W.: Echinococcus cyst of the left ventricle: Report of a case with review of the pertinent literature. J. Thorac. Cardiovasc. Surg. *61*:443, 1970.
559. Dodek, A., DeMots, H., Antonomic, J. A., and Hodam, R. P.: Echinococcus of the heart. Am. J. Cardiol. *30*:293, 1972.
560. DiBello, R., Urioste, H. A., and Rubio, R.: Hydatid cysts of the ventricular septum of the heart: A study based on two personal cases and forty-one observations in the literature. Am. J. Cardiol. *14*:237, 1964.
561. Dighiero, J., Canabal, E. J., Aguirre, C. V., Hazan, J., and Horjales, J. O.: Echinococcus disease of the heart. Circulation *17*:127, 1958.
562. Heilbrunn, A., Kittle, C. F., and Dunn, M.: Surgical management of echinococcal cysts of the heart and pericardium. Circulation *27*:219, 1963.
563. Gibson, D. S.: Cardiac hydatid cysts. Thorax *19*:151, 1964.
564. Artucio, H., Roglia, J. L., DiBello, R., Dubra, J., Gorlero, A., Polero, J., and Urioste, H. A.: Hydatid cyst of the interventricular septum of the heart with rupture into the right ventricle. J. Thorac. Cardiovasc. Surg. *44*:110, 1962.
565. De Los Arcos, E., Madurga, M. P., Leon, J. P., Martinez, J. L., and Urquira, M.: Hydatid cyst of the interventricular septum causing left anterior hemiblock. Br. Heart J. *33*:623, 1971.
566. Naaman, Y. D., Samarrai, A. A. R., and al-Omeri, M. M.: Hydatid disease of the heart. A report of four cases. J. Cardiovasc. Surg. *14*:95, 1973.
567. Oliver, J. M., Benito, L. P., Ferrufino, O., Sotillo, J. F., and Nunez, L.: Cardiac hydatid cysts diagnosed by two-dimensional echocardiography. Am. Heart J. *104*:164, 1982.
568. Editorial: Medical treatment of hydatid disease. Br. Med. J. *2*:563, 1979.
569. Becroft, D. M. O.: Infection by the dog roundworm *Toxocara canis* and fatal myocarditis. N. Engl. J. Med. *63*:729, 1964.
570. Friedman, S., and Hervada, A. R.: Severe myocarditis with recovery in a child with visceral larva migrans. J. Pediatr. *56*:91, 1960.
571. Barr, R.: Human trichinosis: Report of four cases, with emphasis on central nervous system involvement, and a survey of 500 consecutive autopsies at the Ottawa Civic Hospital. Can. Med. Assoc. J. *95*:912, 1966.
572. Edwards, J. L., Hood, C. I., and Laite, H. B.: Studies on the pathogenesis of cardiac and cerebral lesions of experimental trichinosis in rabbits. Am. J. Pathol. *40*:711, 1962.
573. Chase, G. O.: Death due to eosinophilic myocarditis related to trichinosis. J.A.M.A. *165*:1826, 1957.
574. Grey, D. F., Morse, B. S., and Phillips, W. F.: Trichinosis with neurologic and cardiac involvement: Review of the literature and report of three cases. Ann. Intern. Med. *57*:230, 1962.
575. Segar, L. F., Kashtan, H. A., and Miller, P. B.: Trichinosis with myocarditis. Report of a case treated with ACTH. N. Engl. J. Med. *252*:397, 1955.
576. Solarz, S. D.: An electrocardiographic study of one hundred and fourteen consecutive cases of trichinosis. Am. Heart J. *34*:230, 1947.
577. Van Stee, E. W. (ed.): Cardiovascular Toxicology. New York, Raven Press, 1982, 388 pp.
578. Bristow, M. R. (ed.): Drug-Induced Heart Disease. Amsterdam, Elsevier Press, 1980, 476 pp.
579. Veith, R. C., Raskind, M. A., Caldwell, J. H., Barnes, R. F., Gumbrecht, G., and Ritchie, J. L.: Cardiovascular effects of tricyclic antidepressants in depressed patients with chronic heart disease. N. Engl. J. Med. *306*:954, 1982.
580. Surawicz, B., and Lasseter, K. C.: Effect of drugs on the electrocardiogram. Prog. Cardiovasc. Dis. *13*:26, 1970.
581. Fletcher, G. F., Kazamias, T. M., and Wenger, N. K.: Cardiotoxic effect of mellaril: Conduction disturbances and supraventricular arrhythmias. Am. Heart J. *78*:135, 1969.
582. Fowler, N. O., McCall, D., Chou, T. C., Holmes, J. C., and Hanenson, I. B.: Electrocardiographic changes and cardiac arrhythmias in patients receiving psychotropic drugs. Am. J. Cardiol. *37*:223, 1976.
583. Kelley, H. G., Fay, J. E., and Laverty, S. G.: Thioridazine hydrochloride (Mellaril): Its effect on the electrocardiogram and a report of two fatalities with electrocardiographic abnormalities. Can. Med. Assoc. J. *89*:546, 1963.
584. Madan, B. R., and Pendse, V. K.: Antiarrhythmic activity of thioridazine hydrochloride (Mellaril). Am. J. Cardiol. *11*:78, 1963.
585. Burda, D. C.: Electrocardiographic abnormalities induced by thioridazine (Mellaril). Am. Heart J. *76*:153, 1968.
586. Raisfeld, I. H.: Cardiovascular complications of antidepressant therapy. Interactions at the adrenergic neuron. Am. Heart J. *83*:129, 1972.
587. Pearce, M. B., Bullock, R. T., and Murphy, M. L.: Selective damage of mitochondria due to emetine hydrochloride. Arch. Pathol. *91*:8, 1971.
588. Dempsy, J. J., and Salem, H. H.: An enzymatic electrocardiographic study on toxicity of dehydroemetine. Br. Heart J. *28*:505, 1966.
589. Murphy, M. L., Bullock, R. T., and Pearce, M. B.: The correlation of metabolic and ultrastructural changes in emetine myocardial toxicity. Am. Heart J. *87*: 105, 1974.
590. Sanghri, L. M., and Mathur, B. B.: Electrocardiogram after chloroquine and emetine. Circulation *32*:281, 1965.
591. Michael, T. A. D., and Arivazzadek, S.: The effects of acute chloroquine poisoning with special reference to the heart. Am. Heart J. *79*:831, 1970.
592. Honey, M.: The effects of sodium antimony tartrate on the myocardium. Br. Heart J. *22*:601, 1960.
593. Wellens, H. J., Cats, V. M., and Duren, D. R.: Symptomatic sinus node abnormalities following lithium carbonate therapy. Am. J. Med. *59*:285, 1975.
594. Tilkian, A., Schroeder, J. S., Kao, J., and Hultgren, H.: Effect of lithium on cardiovascular performance: Report on extended ambulatory monitoring and exercise testing before and during lithium therapy. Am. J. Cardiol. *38*:701, 1976.
595. Tseng, H. C.: Interstitial myocarditis probably related to lithium carbonate intoxication. Arch. Pathol. *92*:444, 1971.
596. James, F. W., Kaplan, S., and Benzing, G., III: Cardiac complications following hydrocarbon ingestion. Am. J. Dis. Child *121*:431, 1971.
597. Steiner, M. H.: Syndromes of kerosene poisoning in children. Am. J. Dis. Child. *74*:32, 1947.
598. Harris, W. S.: Toxic effects of aerosol propellants on the heart. Arch. Intern. Med. *131*:162, 1973.
599. Bagnell, W. E., Salway, S. G., and Jackson, E. W.: Phaeochromocytoma with myocarditis managed with *l*-methyl-*p*-tyrosine. Postgrad. Med. J. *52*:653, 1976.
600. Van Vliet, P. D., Burchell, H. B., and Titus, J. L.: Focal myocarditis associated with pheochromocytomas. N. Engl. J. Med. *274*:1102, 1966.
601. Szakacs, J. E., and Mehlman, B.: Pathologic changes induced by *l*-norepinephrine: Quantitative aspects. Am. J. Cardiol. *5*:619, 1960.
602. Pentel, P. R., Mikell, F. L., and Zavoral, J. H.: Myocardial injury after phenylpropanolamine ingestion. Br. Heart J. *47*:51, 1982.
603. Haft, J. I., Gershengorn, K., Kranz, P. D., and Oestreicher, R.: Protection against epinephrine-induced myocardial necrosis by drugs that inhibit platelet aggregation. Am. J. Cardiol. *30*:838, 1972.
604. Kline, T. S.: Myocardial changes in lead poisoning. Am. J. Dis. Child. *99*:48, 1960.
605. Freeman, R.: Reversible myocarditis due to chronic lead poisoning in childhood. Arch. Dis. Child. *40*:389, 1965.
606. Anderson, R. F., Allensenarth, D. C., and DeGroot, W. J.: Myocardial toxicity from carbon monoxide poisoning. Ann. Intern. Med. *67*:1172, 1967.
607. Hayes, J. M., and Hall, G. V.: The myocardial toxicity of carbon monoxide. Med. J. Aust. *1*:865, 1964.
608. Shafer, N., Smilay, M. G., and MacMillan, F. P.: Primary myocardial disease in man resulting from acute carbon monoxide poisoning. Am. J. Med. *38*:316, 1965.
609. Corya, B. C., Black, M. J., and McHenry, P. L.: Echocardiographic findings after acute carbon monoxide poisoning. Br. Heart J. *38*:712, 1976.
610. Dahhan, S. S., and Orfaly, H.: Electrocardiographic changes in mercury poisoning. Am. J. Cardiol. *14*:178, 1964.
611. Talley, R. C., Tinhart, J. W., Trevino, A. J., Moore, C., and Beller, B. M.: Acute elemental phosphorus poisoning in man: Cardiovascular toxicity. Am. Heart J. *84*:139, 1972.
612. Diaz-Rivera, R. S., Ramos-Morales, R., Garcia-Palmieri, M. R., and Ramirez, E. A.: The electrocardiographic changes in acute phosphorus poisoning in man. Am. J. Med. Sci. *241*:758, 1961.
613. Connor, T. B., Rosen, B. L., Blaustein, M. P., Applefeld, M. M., and Doyle, L. A.: Hypocalcemia precipitating congestive heart failure. N. Engl. J. Med. *307*:869, 1982.
614. Giles, T. D., Iteld, B. J., and Rives, K. L.: The cardiomyopathy of hypoparathyroidism. Chest *79*:225, 1981.
615. Editorial: Selenium in the heart of China. Lancet *2*:889, 1979.
616. Keshan Disease Research Group of the Chinese Academy of Medical Sciences: Observations on the effect of sodium selenite in prevention of Keshan disease. Chin. Med. J. (Engl.) *92*:471, 1979.
617. Johnson, R. A., Baker, S. S., Fallon, J. T., Maynard, E. P., III, Ruskin, J. N., Wen, A., Ge, K., and Cohen, H. J.: An occidental case of cardiomyopathy and selenium deficiency. N. Engl. J. Med. *304*:1210, 1981.
618. Gueron, M., and Yarom, R.: Cardiovascular complications of severe scorpion sting: Clinicopathologic correlations. Chest *57*:156, 1970.
619. Gueron, M., Stern, J., and Cohen, W.: Severe myocardial damage and heart failure in scorpion sting: Report of five cases. Am. J. Cardiol. *19*:719, 1967.
620. Bisarya, B. N., Vasavada, J. P., Bhatt, A., Nair, P. N. R., and Sharma, V. R.: Hemiplegia and myocarditis following scorpion bite (a case report). Indian Heart J. *29*:97, 1977.
621. Gueron, M., Adolph, R. J., Grupp, I. L., Gabel, M., Grupp, G., and Fowler, N. O.: Hemodynamic and myocardial consequences of scorpion venom. Am. J. Cardial. *45*:979, 1980.
622. Levine, H. D.: Acute myocardial infarction following wasp sting: Report of two cases and critical survey of the literature. Am. Heart J. *91*:365, 1976.
623. Weitzman, S., Margulis, G., and Lehmann, E.: Uncommon cardiovascular manifestations and high catecholamine levels due to "black widow" bite. Am. Heart J. *93*:89, 1977.
624. Reid, H. A.: Snakebite in the tropics. Br. Med. J. *3*:359, 1968.
625. Reid, H. A., Thean, P. C., Chan, K. E., and Baharom, A. R.: Clinical effects of bites by Malayan viper (*Ancistrodon rhodostoma*). Lancet *1*:617, 1963.
626. Chadha, J. S., Ashby, D. W., and Brown, J. O.: Abnormal electrocardiogram after adder bite. Br. Heart J. *30*:138, 1968.
627. Weinberg, S. L.: The electrocardiogram in acute arsenic poisoning. Am. Heart J. *60*:971, 1960.
628. Barry, K. G., and Herndon, E. G., Jr.: Electrocardiographic changes associated with acute arsenic poisoning. Med. Ann. D.C. *31*:25, 1962.
629. Wenzel, D. G.: Drug-induced cardiomyopathies. J. Pharm. Sci. *56*:1209, 1967.

630. Glazener, F. S., Ellis, J. G., and Johnson, P. K.: Electrocardiographic findings with arsenic poisoning. Calif. Med. *109*:158, 1968.
631. McKinstry, W. J., and Hicks, V. M.: Emergency-arsine poisoning. Arch. Intern. Med. *100*:34, 1957.
632. Appelbaum, F., Strauchen, J. A., and Graw, R. G., Jr.: Acute lethal carditis caused by high-dose combination chemotherapy. A unique clinical and pathological entity. Lancet *1*:58, 1976.
633. O'Connell, T. X., and Berenbaum, M. C.: Myocardial and pulmonary effects of high doses of cyclophosphamide and isophosphamide. Cancer Res. *34*:1586, 1974.
634. Gottdiener, J. S., Appelbaum, F. R., Ferrans, V. J., Deisseroth, A., and Ziegler, J.: Cardiotoxicity associated with high-dose cyclophosphamide therapy. Arch. Intern. Med. *141*:758, 1981.
635. Sanerkin, N. G.: Acute myocardial necrosis in paracetamol poisoning. Br. Med. J. *3*:478, 1971.
636. Bhasin, S., Wallace, W., Lawrence, J. B., and Lesch, M.: Sudden death associated with thyroid hormone abuse. Am. J. Med. *71*:887, 1981.
637. Fainstein, V., and Bodey, G. P.: Cardiorespiratory toxicity due to miconazole. Ann. Intern. Med. *93*:432, 1980.
638. Kowey, P. R., Friedman, P. L., Podrid, P. J., Zielonka, J., Lown, B., Wynne, J., and Holman, B. L.: Use of radionuclide ventriculography for assessment of changes in myocardial performance by disopyramide phosphate. Am. Heart J. *104*:769, 1982.
639. Morady, F., Scheinman, M. M., and Desai, J.: Disopyramide. Ann. Intern. Med. *96*:337, 1982.
640. Vorobiof, D. A.: Cardiotoxicity of 5-fluoro-uracil. A case report. South Africa Med. J. *61*:634, 1982.
641. Harkavy, J.: Cardiac manifestations due to hypersensitivity. Ann. Allergy *28*: 242, 1970.
642. Mullick, F. G., and McAllister, H. A.: Myocarditis associated with methyldopa therapy. J.A.M.A. *237*:1699, 1977.
643. Plafker, J.: Penicillin-related nephritis and myocarditis: A case report. South. Med. J. *64*:852, 1971.
644. Schoenivetter, A. H., and Silber, E. N.: Penicillin hypersensitivity, acute pericarditis, and eosinophilia. J.A.M.A. *191*:672, 1965.
645. Simon, M. A.: Pathologic lesions following the administration of sulfonamide drugs. Am. J. Med. Sci. *205*:439, 1943.
646. Blanchard, A. J., and Mertens, G. A.: Hypersensitivity myocarditis occurring with sulphamethoxypridazine therapy. Can. Med. Assoc. J. *79*:627, 1958.
647. MacSearraegh, E. T. M., and Patel, I. C. M.: Cardiomyopathy as a complication of sulphonamide therapy. Br. Med. J. *3*:33, 1968.
648. Kline, L. K., Kline, T. S., and Saphir, O.: Myocarditis in senescence. Am. Heart J. *65*:446, 1963.
649. Kerwin, A. J.: Fatal myocarditis due to sensitivity to phenindione. Can. Med. Assoc. J. *90*:1418, 1964.
650. Hodge, P. R., and Lawrence, J. R.: Two cases of myocarditis associated with phenylbutazone therapy. Med. J. Aust. *1*:640, 1957.
651. Edelstein, J. M.: Butazolidin angiitis and periangiitis simulating Aschoff nodule. Am. Heart J. *69*:573, 1965.
652. Barrett, D. A., II, Dalldorf, F. G., Barnwell, W. H., II, and Hudson, R. P.: Allergic giant cell myocarditis complicating tuberculosis chemotherapy. Arch. Pathol. *91*:201, 1971.
653. Hubaytar, R. T., and Simpson, D. G.: Atrial fibrillation due to hypersensitivity due to para-aminosalicylic acid. Am. Rev. Respir. Dis. *86*:720, 1962.
654. Chatterjee, S. S., and Thakre, M. W.: Fiedler's myocarditis; Report of a fatal case following intramuscular injection of streptomycin. Tubercle *39*:240, 1958.
655. Schrock, C. G.: Lyme disease: Additional evidence of widespread distribution. Recognition of a tick-borne dermatitis-encephalitis-arthritis syndrome in an area of known Ixodes tick distribution. Am. J. Med. *72*:700, 1982.
656. Steere, A. C., Malawista, S. E., Newman, J. H., Spiebler, P. N., and Bartenhagen, N. H.: Antibiotic therapy in Lyme disease. Ann. Intern. Med. *93*: 1, 1980.
657. Steere, A. C., Batsford, W. P., Weinberg, M., Alexander, J., Berger, H. J., Wolfson, S., and Malawista, S. E.: Lyme carditis: Cardiac abnormalities of Lyme disease. Ann. Intern. Med. *93*:8, 1980.
658. Peison, B., and Lowenstein, E. C.: Giant-cell myocarditis. N.Y. State J. Med. *73*:2259, 1973.
659. Davies, M. J., Pomerance, A., and Teare, R. D.: Idiopathic giant cell myocarditis—a distinctive clinicopathological entity. Br. Heart J. *37*:192, 1975.
660. Pyun, K. S., Kim, Y. H., Katzenstein, R. E., and Kikkawn, Y.: Giant cell myocarditis. Light and electron microscopic study. Arch. Pathol. *90*:181, 1970.
661. Nakahara, K.: Giant cell myocarditis. Hawaii Med. J. *34*:56, 1975.
662. Dragatakis, L. M., Klassen, J., Hüttner, I., Fraser, D. G., Poirier, N. L., and Klassen, G. A.: Autoimmune myocarditis: A clinical entity. Canad. Med. Assoc. J. *120*:317, 1979.
663. Graham, A. F., Rider, A. K., Caves, P. K., Stinson, E. B., Harrison, D. C., and Schroeder, J. S.: Acute rejection in the long-term cardiac transplant survival. Clinical diagnosis, treatment and significance. Circulation *49*:361, 1974.
664. Gripp, R. B., Stinson, E. B., Dong, E., Jr., Clark, D. A., and Shumway, N. E.: Acute rejection of the allografted human heart. Diagnosis and treatment. Ann. Thorac. Surg. *12*:113, 1971.
665. Caves, P. K., Stinson, E. B., Billingham, M. E., Rider, A. K., and Shumway, N. E.: Diagnosis of human cardiac allograft rejection by serial cardiac biopsy. J. Thorac. Cardiovasc. Surg. *66*:461, 1973.
666. Caves, P. K., Stinson, E. B., Graham, A. F., Billingham, M. E., Grehl, T. M., and Shumway, N. E.: Percutaneous transvenous endomyocardial biopsy. J.A.M.A. *225*:288, 1973.
667. Bieber, C. P., Stinson, E. B., Shumway, N. E., Payne, R., and Kosek, J.: Cardiac transplantation in man. VII. Cardiac allograft pathology. Circulation *41*: 753, 1970.
668. Thomson, J. G.: Production of severe atheroma in a transplanted human heart. Lancet *2*:1088, 1969.
669. Griepp, R. B., Stinson, E. B., Bieher, C. P., Reitz, B. A., Copeland, J. G., Oyer, P. E., and Shumway, N. E.: Control of graft arteriosclerosis in human heart transplant recipients. Surgery *81*:262, 1977.
670. Kew, M. C., Tucker, R. B. K., Bersohn, I., and Seftel, H. C.: The heart in heatstroke. Am. Heart J. *77*:324, 1969.
671. Malamud, N., Haymaker, W., and Luster, R. F.: Heatstroke: A clinicopathological study of 125 fatal cases. Milit. Surg. *99*:397, 1946.
672. Duguid, H., Simpson, R. G., and Stowers, R. G.: Accidental hypothermia. Lancet *2*:1213, 1961.
673. Read, A. E., Ainslie-Smith, D., Gough, K. R., and Holmes, R.: Pancreatitis and accidental hypothermia. Lancet *2*:1219, 1961.
674. Biran, S., Hochmann, A., and Stern, S.: Therapeutic irradiation of the chest and electrocardiographic changes. Clin. Radiol. *20*:433, 1969.
675. McReynolds, R. A., Gold, G. L., and Roberts, W. C.: Coronary heart disease after mediastinal irradiation for Hodgkin's disease. Am. J. Med. *60*:39, 1976.
675a. Applefeld, M. M., and Wiernik, P. H.: Cardiac disease after radiation therapy for Hodgkin's disease: Analysis of 48 patients. Am. J. Cardiol. *51*:1679, 1983.
675b. Totterman, K. J., Pesonen, E., and Siltanen, P.: Radiation-related chronic heart disease. Chest *83*:875, 1983.
676. Arom, K. V., Bishop, V. S., Grover, F. L., and Trinkle, J. K.: Effect of therapeutic-dose irradiation of left ventricular function in conscious dogs. Ann. Thorac. Surg. *28*:166, 1979.
677. Weinstein, P., Greenwald, E. S., and Grossman, J.: Unusual cardiac reaction to chemotherapy following mediastinal irradiation in a patient with Hodgkin's disease. Am. J. Med. *60*:152, 1976.
678. Stewart, J. R., and Fajardo, C. F.: Radiation-induced heart disease. Clinical and experimental aspects. Radiol. Clin. North Am. *9*:511, 1971.
678a. Gottdiener, J. S. Katin, M. J., Borer, J. S., Bacharach, S. L., and Green, M. V.: Late cardiac effects of therepeutic mediastinal irradiation. Assessment by echocardiography and radionuclide ventriculography. N. Engl. J. Med. *308*: 569, 1983.
678b. Burns, R. J., Bar-Shlomo, B-Z., Druck, M. N., Herman, J. G., Gilbert, B. W., Perrault, D. J., and McLaughlin, P. R.: Detection of radiation cardiomyopathy by gated radionuclide angiography. Am. J. Med. *74*:297, 1983.
679. Brosius, F. C., III, Waller, B. F., and Roberts, W. C.: Radiation heart disease: Analysis of 16 young (aged 15 to 33 years) necropsy patients who received over 3,500 rads to the heart. Am. J. Med. *70*:519, 1981.
680. Reeves, W. C., Cunningham, D., Schwiter, E. J., Abt, A. Skarlatos, S., Wood, M. A., and Whitesell, L.: Myocardial hydroxyproline reduced by early administration of methylprednisolone or ibuprofen to rabbits with radiation-induced heart disease. Circulation *65*:924, 1982.

42 PRIMARY TUMORS OF THE HEART

by Wilson S. Colucci, M.D., and Eugene Braunwald, M.D.

"A diagnosis is easy as long as you think of it."
SOMA WEISS

The incidence of primary tumors of the heart* in autopsy series ranges from 0.0017 to 0.28 per cent.[1-5] Thus, these tumors are far less common than metastatic tumors to the heart.[6] The diagnosis is further complicated by an extraordinary variety of nonspecific clinical signs and symptoms that are capable of masquerading as many other more common cardiovascular and systemic diseases (Table 42–1). Prior to the advent of modern cardiopulmonary bypass surgical techniques, the correct antemortem diagnosis of an intracardiac tumor was largely academic, since effective therapy was not possible. However, now that many cardiac tumors are curable by operation, it is critically important to establish this diagnosis whenever possible. During the last decade, major advances in noninvasive cardiovascular diagnostic techniques have greatly facilitated this task, and it is now possible safely and readily to screen patients suspected of having a cardiac tumor, in many cases arriving at a definitive diagnosis preoperatively. Nevertheless, a high index of suspicion remains the most important element in diagnosing a cardiac tumor.

HISTORICAL PERSPECTIVE

Although primary tumors of the heart have been recognized since at least as early as the sixteenth century,[6a] a correct antemortem diagnosis was not recorded until 1934.[7] The modern era of diagnosis began with the development of angiography, which permitted the visualization of cardiac tumors during life, and, in 1952, Goldberg et al. reported the first angiographic diagnosis of a left atrial myxoma.[8]

Before the development of modern open heart surgical techniques, there were only rare reports of the successful removal of cardiac tumors, most on the epicardial surface.[9,10] Prior to the use of cardiopulmonary bypass, most attempts to remove intracardiac were unsuccessful.[11] In 1954, Crafoord performed the first successful excision of an intracardiac tumor, a left atrial myxoma, utilizing total cardiopulmonary bypass under direct vision.[12] The successful surgical excision of a wide variety of cardiac tumors is now possible, and in many instances a complete cure has been achieved.[11,13-17]

Advances in the field of noninvasive cardiovascular diagnosis have had a major impact on the ability of physicians to recognize correctly cardiac tumors antemortem. A cardiac tumor was first demonstrated by M-mode echocardiography in 1959,[18] and, subsequently, echocardiography has become the cornerstone of the noninvasive diagnosis of cardiac tumors. Cross-sectional echocardiography has proved to be extremely useful and, in most situations, superior to M-mode echocardiography[18-24]. Radionuclide gated blood pool scanning[25-27] and computed tomography[28-32] have also been shown to be of value in the diagnosis of cardiac tumors. Thus, during the past quarter century it has become possible to diagnose and successfully treat the majority of primary cardiac tumors. An appreciation of the clinical features, therefore, is now of far greater importance than heretofore.

CLINICAL PRESENTATION (Table 42–1)

SYSTEMIC FINDINGS. Cardiac tumors can produce a broad array of systemic (i.e., noncardiac) findings, including fever, cachexia, malaise, arthralgias, Raynaud's phenomenon, rash, clubbing, and episodic bizarre behavior,[33-37] as well as systemic and pulmonary emboli. A variety

*Tumors arising elsewhere in the body and metastasizing to the pericardium and heart are discussed in Chapter 43 (Diseases of the Pericardium) and Chapter 49 (Hematologic-Oncologic Disorders and Heart Disease).

TABLE 42–1 CLINICAL PRESENTATIONS OF CARDIAC TUMORS

Cardiovascular Signs and Symptoms
1. Chest pain
2. Syncope
3. Congestive heart failure (left and/or right heart)
4. Valvular stenosis and/or insufficiency
5. Constrictive pericarditis
6. Pericardial effusion or tamponade
7. Arrhythmias
8. Conduction blocks
9. Intracardiac shunts
Systemic Signs and Symptoms
1. Systemic embolization
2. Pulmonary embolization and pulmonary hypertension
3. Fever
4. Cachexia and malaise
5. Arthralgia
6. Rash
7. Clubbing
8. Raynaud's phenomenon
9. Hypergammaglobulinemia
10. Anemia or polycythemia
11. Thrombocytosis or thrombocytopenia
12. Leukocytosis

of laboratory findings have been reported, including hypergammaglobulinemia, an elevated erythrocyte sedimentation rate, thrombocytosis, thrombocytopenia, polycythemia, leukocytosis, and anemia.[33–35,38–40] The mechanism by which cardiac tumors cause these systemic manifestations is not known with certainty, but it has been attributed to secretory products of the tumor or to tumor necrosis.[33,34,41] An immunological basis for the systemic manifestations is suggested by the finding of an increased titer of antimyocardial antibodies in a patient with a myxoma and a fall in the titer following surgical removal of the tumor.[42] A case of multiple myeloma has been attributed to continuous immunological stimulation by a left atrial myxoma.[43] Because the cardiac findings are nonspecific and may be subtle or absent, it is not unusual for these systemic findings to lead to a diagnosis of collagen vascular disease, infection, or noncardiac malignancy.[44–46] Rarely, myxomas may be superinfected by bacteria or fungi.[47]

EMBOLIC PHENOMENA. The embolization of tumor fragments or of thrombi from the surface of a tumor is a frequent and often dramatic clinical occurrence.[48–55] Although myxomas are the source of most tumor emboli because of the combination of their friable consistency and intracavitary location, other types of cardiac tumors occasionally may embolize.

The distribution of tumor emboli depends upon the location of the tumor and the presence or absence of intracardiac shunts. Left-sided tumors embolize to the systemic circulation, resulting in infarction and hemorrhage of viscera, including the heart, as well as peripheral limb ischemia and vascular aneurysms.[35,48–57] The diagnosis of an intracardiac tumor may be made after histological examination of systemic embolic material,[48,51,56] and, therefore, it is of critical importance to make every effort to recover and examine embolic material. In some cases, particularly when petechiae are present, biopsy of skin or muscle[35] may demonstrate intravascular tumor emboli.

Multiple systemic emboli may mimic systemic vasculitis[35,44,46] or infective endocarditis,[45,52] especially when associated with other manifestations of a systemic illness such as fever, weight loss, arthralgias, elevated erythrocyte sedimentation rate, and elevated serum gamma globulins. The finding at angiography of multiple vascular aneurysms secondary to tumor emboli in the cerebral, renal, femoral, and coronary arteries may lead to the diagnosis of polyarteritis nodosa.[53] The neurological consequences of embolization include transient ischemic attacks, seizures, syncope, and cerebral, cerebellar, brain stem, spinal cord or retinal infarction.[54,55,58] The neurological event may occasionally be the first or only clinical manifestation of a cardiac tumor. An embolic stroke in a young person without evidence of cerebrovascular disease, particularly in the presence of sinus rhythm, should raise the possibility of intracardiac myxoma, as well as infective endocarditis (p. 1155) and prolapse of the mitral valve (p. 1094).

Right-sided cardiac tumors, and left-sided cardiac tumors proximal to left-to-right intracardiac shunts, may result in pulmonary emboli.[59–61] Indeed, serious pulmonary hypertension and secondary cor pulmonale due to chronic recurrent pulmonary emboli from a right atrial myxoma have been noted.[60] Clinically, the findings may be indistinguishable from pulmonary emboli secondary to venous thromboembolism (p. 1582). Although the findings on chest roentgenogram are relatively nonspecific,[61] perfusion lung scanning in such patients (pp. 390 and 1586) may be atypical of pulmonary embolism in two respects: (1) The tumor-produced perfusion defects may remain static for long periods of time, as opposed to typical pulmonary embolic disease in which the defects usually resolve over the course of a few weeks; and (2) there may be complete absence of flow to one lung in the presence of completely normal perfusion of the opposite lung, a pattern unusual with typical pulmonary emboli.[61,62]

Cardiac Manifestations

The specific signs and symptoms produced by tumors are more closely related to their precise anatomical location than to their histological types.[63] Thus, it is useful to consider the constellation of findings which is typical of each location. The presentation of *pericardial tumors* is considered on pages 1507 to 1509 and will not be discussed here except to point out that primary tumors of the myocardium and endocardium may extend into the pericardial space and produce many of the clinical manifestations of pericardial tumors, including hemorrhagic pericardial effusion and compression of the heart by the effusion or the tumor itself.

MYOCARDIAL TUMORS. When clinically apparent, myocardial tumors most commonly result in disturbances of conduction or rhythm,[63–66] the precise nature of which is determined by the location of the tumor. Thus, tumors in the area of the atrioventricular node, typically angiomas and mesotheliomas, may produce atrioventricular (AV) conduction disturbances, including complete heart block and asystole, and can lead to sudden death.[64,65] A wide variety of arrhythmias may be produced, including atrial fibrillation or flutter, paroxysmal atrial tachycardia with or without block, nodal rhythm, ventricular premature beats, ventricular tachycardia, and ventricular fibrillation.[63] Intramural tumors may also produce symptoms by virtue of their size and location. Impairment of ventricular performance may simulate congestive, restrictive, or hypertrophic cardiomyopathy (Chap. 41).[67,68] Myocardial rupture rarely may result from tumor infiltration of the myocardial wall.

LEFT ATRIAL TUMORS. Mobile, predunculated, left atrial tumors may prolapse to variable degrees into the mitral valve orifice, resulting in obstruction to atrioventricular blood flow and, frequently, mitral regurgitation. The resultant signs and symptoms often mimic those of mitral valve disease[60] (Chap. 32) and include dyspnea, orthopnea, paroxysmal nocturnal dyspnea, acute pulmonary edema, cough, hemoptysis, chest pain, peripheral edema, and fatigue. However, weight loss, pallor, syncope, and sudden death—manifestations uncommon for mitral valve disease—also occur.[63] It is not unusual for the symptoms to be sudden in onset, intermittent, and related to the patient's body position.[52,63] Although the majority of symptoms produced by left atrial tumors are nonspecific, the occurrence of paroxysmal symptoms that arise characteristically in a particular body position and are out of proportion to the clinical findings should raise the possibility of a left atrial tumor.

Physical examination may disclose signs of pulmonary congestion, an S_4, a loud S_1 which is often widely split, a holosystolic murmur which is loudest at the apex and resembles mitral regurgitation, and a diastolic murmur resulting from the obstruction to flow through the mitral orifice produced by the tumor. In many cases an early diastolic sound, termed a tumor "plop," can be identified (Fig. 42–1). It is thought to be produced as the tumor strikes the endocardial wall or as its excursion is abruptly halted[70] (Fig. 3–15, p. 50). Although in most cases the tumor "plop" occurs later than the opening snap of the mitral valve and earlier than the S_3, it is not surprising that this sound is frequently confused with the opening snap or the S_3.

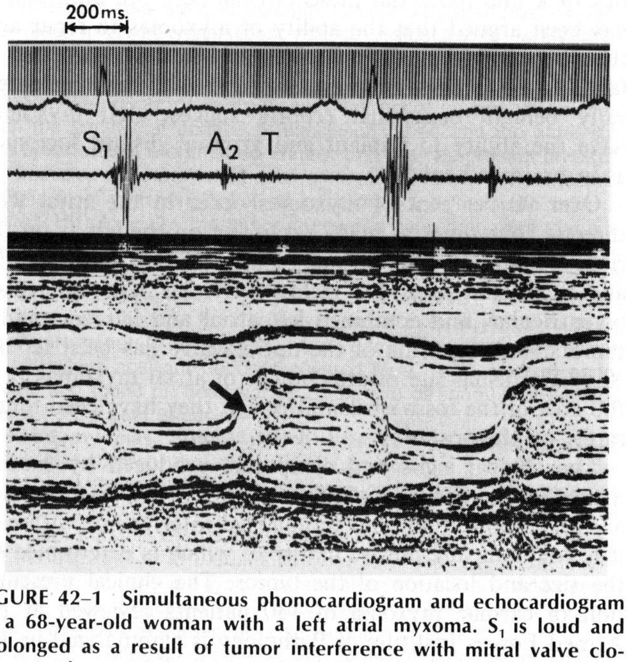

FIGURE 42–1 Simultaneous phonocardiogram and echocardiogram of a 68-year-old woman with a left atrial myxoma. S_1 is loud and prolonged as a result of tumor interference with mitral valve closure. A characteristic tumor "plop" (T) occurs approximately 100 msec after A_2 and corresponds with movement of the tumor into the mitral valve orifice (arrow) on the echocardiogram. (Courtesy of L.J. Sloss, M.D., Brigham and Women's Hospital, Boston.)

RIGHT ATRIAL TUMORS. Right atrial tumors frequently produce symptoms of right heart failure, including fatigue, peripheral edema, ascites, hepatomegaly, and prominent *a* waves in the jugular venous pulse.[52,71] The average time interval from the symptomatic presentation to the correct diagnosis of right atrial tumor is 3 years.[72] The development of right heart failure may be rapidly progressive and is often associated with new systolic or diastolic murmurs or both.[61,73] The murmurs are generally the result of tumor obstruction to tricuspid valve flow, or of tricuspid regurgitation caused by tumor interference with valve closure or valve destruction as a result of trauma by the tumor.[74] It is not surprising that right atrial tumors have been misdiagnosed as Ebstein's anomaly of the tricuspid valve, constrictive pericarditis, tricuspid stenosis, carcinoid syndrome, superior vena caval syndrome, and cardiomyopathy.[52] Pulmonary embolism and pulmonary hypertension occur and may simulate classic thromboembolic disease.[60–62] Right atrial hypertension may cause right-to-left shunting through a patent foramen ovale, with systemic hypoxia, cyanosis, clubbing, and polycythemia.[61,62,71]

Physical examination may reveal peripheral edema, superior vena caval syndrome, hepatomegaly, and ascites. An early diastolic rumbling murmur, alone or in combination with a holosystolic murmur secondary to tricuspid regurgitation, may be heard and may demonstrate respiratory or positional variation.[52] Because of the rarity of isolated rheumatic tricuspid valvular disease, the lack of other valvular findings should raise the question of a right atrial tumor.[71] A protodiastolic tumor plop has been described and is thought to be similar in etiology to that produced by the left atrial tumor.[74a] The jugular venous pressure may be elevated, and a prominent *a* wave and steep *y* descent have been described.[75]

RIGHT VENTRICULAR TUMORS. Right ventricular tumors often present with right heart failure as a result of obstruction to right ventricular filling or outflow. Clinical manifestations include peripheral edema, hepatomegaly, ascites, shortness of breath, syncope, and sudden death.[76]

A systolic ejection murmur at the left sternal border is usually found on physical examination.[77] A presystolic murmur[78] and a diastolic rumble[63] have been noted and are thought to be due to obstruction of the tricuspid valve. An S_3 may be audible, and a low-pitched diastolic sound that coincides with the maximal anterior excursion of the tumor has been ascribed either to tumor or to late closure of the pulmonary valve.[76] P_2 is often delayed, and its intensity may be normal, decreased, or increased. Tumor emboli to the pulmonary arteries may result in pulmonary hypertension, and the presence of tumor in the pulmonic valve orifice may lead to pulmonary regurgitation. The jugular veins are frequently distended with a prominent *a* wave and may demonstrate a Kussmaul's sign (p. 21).[78]

The cardiac findings often lead to a diagnosis of pulmonic stenosis, restrictive cardiomyopathy, or tricuspid regurgitation.[77,79] Whereas pulmonic stenosis is often asymptomatic and slowly progressive, the symptoms of right ventricular tumors are often rapidly progressive, and there is no poststenotic dilatation or systolic ejection click.

LEFT VENTRICULAR TUMORS. When left ventricular tumors are predominantly intramural in location, they are often asymptomatic, or they may present as conduction disturbances, arrhythmias, or interference with

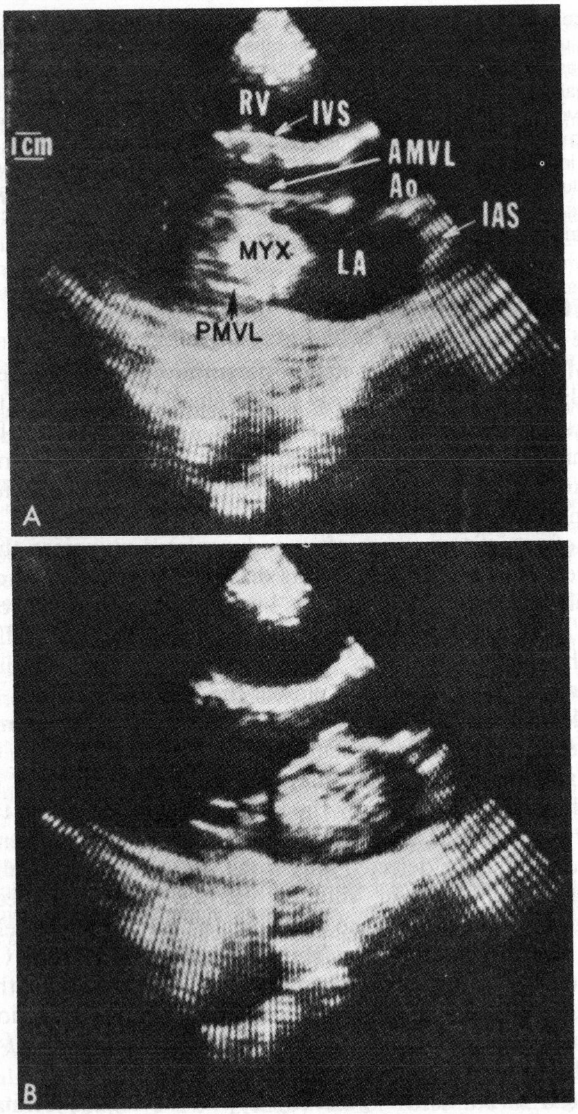

FIGURE 42–2 Two-dimensional sagittal echocardiogram, showing highly mobile tumor, 3 × 4 cm, prolapsing well into the left ventricle during diastole (*A*, top) and returning to left atrium (LA) during systole (*B*, bottom). Note normal-appearing echoes of mitral valve. RV = right ventricle; IVS = interventricular septum; AMVL = anterior mitral valvular leaflet; Ao = aorta; IAS = interatrial septum; MYX = myxoma; and PMVL = posterior mitral valvular leaflet. (From Lappe, D.L., et al.: Two-dimensional echocardiographic diagnosis of left atrial myxoma. Chest *74*:55, 1978.)

mobility.[19] In addition, the cross-sectional method is more sensitive than the M-mode for the detection of small tumors[19] and is especially useful in the detection of left ventricular tumors and tumors that do not prolapse through the mitral or tricuspid valve orifices. Phased-array techniques may facilitate the differentiation between left atrial thrombus and myxoma, because the former typically produces a layered appearance and is generally situated in the posterior portion of the atrium, whereas the latter is often mottled in appearance[150] and rarely occurs in the posterior portion of the atrium. In some atrial myxomas, areas of echolucency may be seen within the tumor mass, corresponding to areas of hemorrhage within the tumor.[151] Since these areas of echolucency are not found in thrombotic or infective lesions, this finding may be of value in the differential diagnosis of an intraatrial mass.

Radionuclide Imaging (Fig. 42–3). Gated blood pool scanning has been used to identify atrial, ventricular, and intramuscular tumors.[25–27,152,153] Radionuclide ventriculography generally has a lower rate of resolution than does echocardiography or contrast injection angiography and therefore may be less sensitive for the detection of small filling defects. However, radionuclide ventriculography may provide clear visualization of filling defects in some cases when other methods are nondiagnostic, particularly in the case of ventricular or intramural tumors.[25,26] In some cases, gated blood pool scanning may provide more detailed information regarding myocardial geometry and tumor size and location than that obtained by echocardiography.[25] Mobile left atrial tumors may be seen to prolapse into the left ventricle during diastole.[25] Thus, gated blood pool scanning may, in some cases, provide information complementary to that obtained by echocardiography.[25–27]

Computed Tomography (p. 189). Computed tomography of the heart has been used in several cases to demonstrate cardiac tumors[28–32] (Fig. 42–4). Although more experience will be necessary in order to establish its role, certain advantages and disadvantages are already apparent. The former include a high degree of tissue discrimination, which may allow definition of the degree of intramural tumor extension; evaluation of the extracardiac structures; and the ability to construct images in any plane. Disadvantages include poor resolution consequent to movement and long exposure times, and patient exposure to contrast agents and radiation.[29] At present, computed tomography appears to be most useful in the evaluation of suspected malignant tumors in order to determine the degree of myocardial invasion and the involvement of pericardial and extracardiac structures.

Other Noninvasive Methods. Cardiac tumors cannot be diagnosed by phonocardiography, apex cardiography, or jugular venous or carotid pulse analysis. However, when valvular or myocardial disease is suspected on clinical grounds, certain atypical findings may raise the ques tion of cardiac tumor. The intensity of the systolic or diastolic murmur caused by a left atrial myxoma is often exquisitely sensitive to positional change, a finding atypical of valvular heart disease.[63] The first heart sound may be delayed as a consequence of an elevated left atrial pressure, as in mitral stenosis (p. 1068) It is often intense and widely split, and an early systolic sound may occur, representing tumor movement toward the atrium during systole.[154] In addition, a tumor "plop" may be present about 100 msec after the second heart sound, which appears to result from the sudden tensing

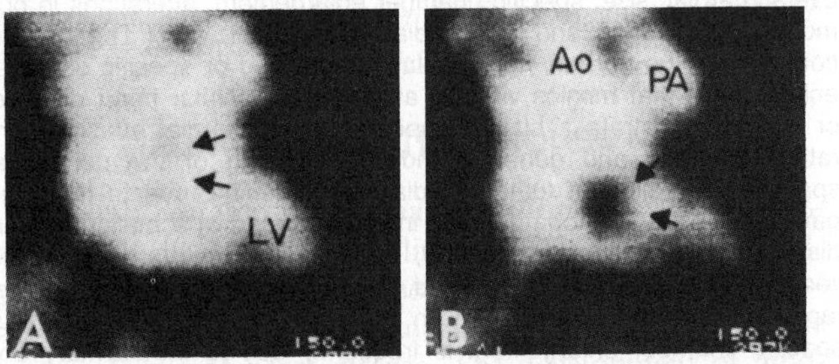

FIGURE 42–3 Gated blood pool scan of a patient with a left atrial myxoma. During systole (*A*) the tumor is faintly visualized in the left atrium (arrows). However, during diastole (*B*) the tumor is clearly seen as a filling defect in the left ventricle (arrows). Ao = aorta; PA = pulmonary artery; LV = left ventricle. (From Pohost, G.M., et al.: Detection of left atrial myxoma by gated radionuclide cardiac imaging. Circulation *55*:88, 1977, by permission of the American Heart Association, Inc.)

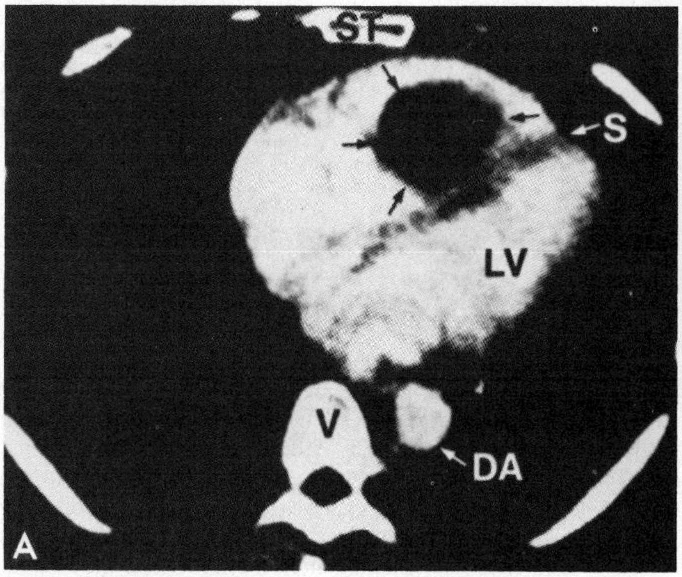

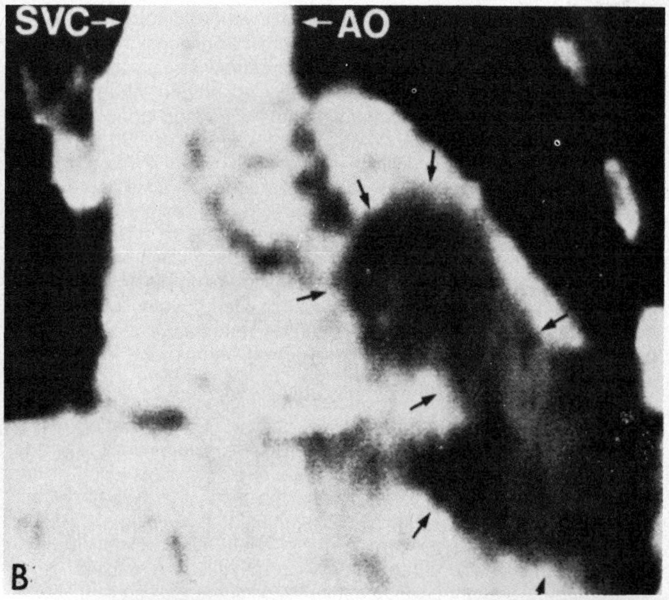

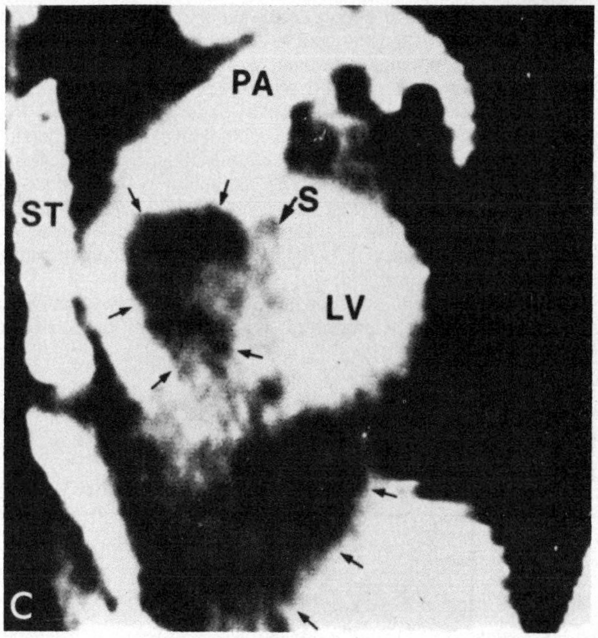

FIGURE 42–4 *A,* Transverse computed tomographic (CT) scan through the right and left ventricles (RV and LV) during IV infusion of 76 per cent diatrizoate of a patient with a cardiac liposarcoma. The patient's right side is projected at the left side of the illustration, as in a conventional radiograph of the chest. The sternum (ST) and vertebral body (V) are marked for orientation. Contrast fills the ventricles and descending aorta (DA). The large, low-density tumor (arrows) occupies the cavity of the right ventricle and lies alongside the interventricular septum (S). *B,* Reformatted CT image made from contiguous transverse CT slices taken during contrast infusion. The plane of reformatting passes through the RV, corresponding to the right anterior oblique projection of an angiocardiogram. The low-density tumor (arrows) forms a pedunculated mass in the cavity of the RV with invasion through the myocardium of the apex of the RV into the pericardial sac. The lowermost arrows indicate the intrapericardial component of the tumor. SVC = superior vena cava; AO = ascending aorta. *C,* Reformatted CT image made from contiguous transverse CT slices taken during contrast infusion. The plane of reformatting passes through both ventricles, corresponding to the left anterior oblique projection of an angiocardiogram, but the plane is also angled along the axis extending from the right ventricular apex to the outflow tract, roughly corresponding to a half-axial projection. The pedunculated, low-density tumor (arrows) is again visualized in the right ventricular cavity and extending through the apex into the pericardial sac (lowermost arrows). ST = sternum; PA = pulmonary artery; S = interventricular septum; LV = left ventricular cavity. (Reproduced with permission from Godwin, J.D., et al.: Computed tomography: A new method for diagnosing tumor of the heart. Circulation *63*:448, 1981.)

of the tumor stalk as it prolapses into the left ventricle during diastole or from the tumor striking the myocardium[63,70] (Figs. 42–1 and 3–15, p. 50). The tumor "plop" *precedes* the end of the rapidly filling wave of the apex cardiogram and can thereby be differentiated from an S_3; as noted, it usually occurs later than an opening snap. Systolic time intervals are usually consistent with a reduced stroke volume (p. 54). The apexcardiography often shows a deep notch on the upstroke which occurs at the time of extrusion of the tumor through the mitral valve in early systole.

Right atrial tumors may also result in a widely split first heart sound and an early systolic sound. The second heart sound may be paradoxically split as a result of early pulmonic valve closure.[155] A tumor "plop" and systolic and diastolic murmurs which are increased by inspiration may also occur with right atrial tumors.[154] The jugular venous pulse tracing may reflect obstruction of the tricuspid orifice, demonstrating an accentuated *a* wave, attenuation of the *x* descent, or an early, broad *v* wave.[154]

ANGIOGRAPHY

Cardiac catheterization and selective angiocardiography are not necessary in all cases of cardiac tumors, since, as discussed above, in many cases adequate preoperative information may be obtained by echocardiography, gated blood pool scanning, and/or computed tomography. However, several circumstances exist in which the risk of cardiac catheterization is outweighed by the supplemental information it may provide. These situations include cases in which (1) noninvasive evaluation has not been fully adequate in defining tumor location or attachment; (2) all four cardiac chambers have not been adequately visualized noninvasively; (3) a malignant cardiac tumor is considered likely; or (4) other cardiac lesions may coexist with a cardiac tumor and possibly dictate a different surgical approach. For instance, when a malignant cardiac tumor is suspected, cardiac angiography may provide valuable information regarding the degree of myocardial, vascular, and/or pericardial invasion. Likewise, in certain cases, such as the presence of pulmonary hypertension or the coexistence of significant valvular or coronary artery lesions, cardiac catheterization and angiography may provide information that significantly affects the surgical approach.

The major angiographic findings in patients with cardiac tumors include (1) compression or displacement of cardiac chambers or large vessels, (2) deformity of cardiac chambers, (3) intracavitary filling defects, (4) marked variations in myocardial thickness, (5) pericardial effusion, and (6) local alterations in wall motion.[137,138] Displacement of the cardiac chambers or the great vessels without deformation of the internal contour may be observed in both benign and malignant tumors, whereas deformation of a cardiac chamber usually indicates an infiltrating malignant lesion.[138] The most frequent angiographic findings are intracavitary filling defects, which may be either fixed or mobile. Fixed defects may be lobulated or appear as a coarse nodularity of the myocardium often difficult to distinguish from a mural thrombus. Such defects may reflect endocardial tumors with broad attachments or intramural tumors with intracavitary extension. Mobile intracavitary defects are usually pedunculated tumors, typically myxomas, although the stalk may be difficult to visualize. Such tumors may prolapse into the atrioventricular valve orifice during diastole (Fig. 42–5) or, in the case of ventricular tumors, into the left ventricular outflow tract during systole. An atrial ball thrombus may mimic a pedunculated tumor but is more likely to be associated with clot in the atrial appendage.

A localized increase in myocardial wall thickness, especially when accompanied by a pericardial effusion, suggests an infiltrating malignant tumor. It is often difficult to differentiate myocardial thickening from pericardial effusion, but this may be aided by observation of the thickness of the right atrial wall. Since the right atrial wall is seldom infiltrated by tumor, the finding of right atrial thickening to greater than 5 mm suggests a pericardial effusion.[138] In myocardial infiltration, localized areas of disordered wall motion may also be noted by cineangiography. Coronary arteriography may in some cases allow visualization of the vascular supply of the tumor, thus demarcating the extent of tumor invasion, the source of its blood supply, and its relation to the coronary arteries. However, the vascular pattern of cardiac tumors has not proved to be a useful sign of malignancy.[138]

False-negative angiographic studies generally occur when the diagnosis is not suspected prior to catheterization.[23,142] False-positive studies are most often the result of thrombus, but may also be produced by many entities: such as streaming of nonopaque venous blood, a hematoma in the atrial septum, an aneurysm of the muscular or membranous ventricular septum, Bernheim syndrome, congenital septal dysplasia, and hydatid cysts of the interventricular septum.[138,156]

The major risk of angiography is peripheral embolization due to dislodgement of a fragment of tumor or of an associated thrombus.[138,157] Therefore, the thorough evaluation of all cardiac chambers by *noninvasive* methods prior to catheterization is to be recommended in patients suspected of having cardiac tumors so that contrast material can be injected into the chamber proximal (upstream) to the location of the tumor.[138] The transseptal approach to the left atrium (p. 283) is particularly hazardous because of the frequent occurrence of left atrial myxomas in the region of the fossa ovalis.

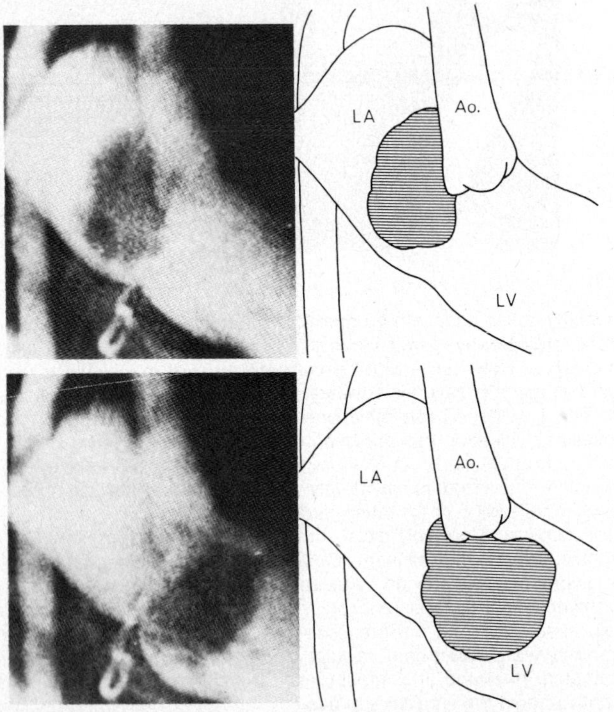

FIGURE 42–5 Cineangiogram of a patient with left atrial myxoma. The tumor appears as a filling defect in the left atrium during systole (upper panel) and prolapses into the left ventricle during diastole (lower panel). LA = left atrium; Ao. = aorta; LV = left ventricle. (From Selzer, A., et al.: Protean clinical manifestations of primary tumors of the heart. Am. J. Med. *52*:9, 1972.)

TREATMENT AND PROGNOSIS

BENIGN TUMORS. Operative excision is the treatment of choice for most benign cardiac tumors and in many cases results in a complete cure.[4,11,13,14,17] Although many tumors are histologically benign, all cardiac tumors are potentially lethal as a result of intracavitary or valvular obstruction, peripheral embolization, and disturbances of rhythm or conduction. Unfortunately, it is not unusual for patients to die or experience a major complication while awaiting operation, and therefore it is mandatory to carry out the operation promptly after the diagnosis has been established.

Although some epicardial tumors may be removed without the aid of extracorporeal circulation, most mural and intracavitary tumors must be excised under direct vision, with use of the heart-lung machine.[11] Closed approaches, although occasionally used in the past,[158] are not now recommended because of increased risk of dislodging tumor fragments. In addition, excision cannot be as complete, and adequate inspection of the other cardiac chambers for additional tumors is not possible.

The dislodgement of tumor fragments constitutes a major risk of operation and may result in peripheral emboli or the dispersion of micrometastases, which may seed peripherally. To reduce this risk, manipulation of the heart prior to cardiopulmonary bypass should be minimized. Some surgeons recommend that venous cannulation for cardiopulmonary bypass be performed via the femoral or azygous veins rather than through the right atrium in order to avoid dislodging an unsuspected right atrial tumor.[121] In addition, the tumor should be removed en bloc when possible, and the chamber then irrigated well with saline.

Atrial Myxomas. Numerous reports document complete cure of left and right atrial myxomas with follow-up periods of 10 to 15 years.[4,11,16,17] However, in about 1 to 5 per cent of cases, a recurrence or second cardiac myxoma has been reported following resection of the initial myxoma.[159] Possible etiologies of the second tumor include incomplete excision of the original tumor with regrowth, growth from a second "pretumorous" focus, or intracardiac implantation from the original tumor.[159] Because of the first two possibilities, some surgeons advocate excision of the entire region of the fossa ovalis and repair of the resultant atrial septal defect in order to remove presumably high concentrations of "pretumor" cells thought to be located in that region.[160,161] Other surgeons have reported equally successful long-term recurrence-free periods with simple excision of the tumor and a small rim at the base.[13,16] Regardless of the extent of tumor resection performed, such patients should receive periodic long-term follow-up by cross-sectional echocardiography.

Other Benign Tumors. Although the majority of operations for cardiac tumors have been performed for atrial myxomas owing to their high frequency, successful excision has also been reported for ventricular myxomas, as well as most other types of benign cardiac tumor, including rhabdomyoma, hamartoma, fibroma, lipoma, hemangioma, and papillary fibroelastoma.[17,99,102,110,112,120,162–166] The major surgical considerations in excision of ventricular tumors include preservation of adequate ventricular myocardium, maintenance of proper atrioventricular valve function, and preservation of as much of the conduction system as possible. Often, however, papillary muscles, chordae tendineae, or the AV conduction system must be sacrificed during the resection of a tumor, thereby necessitating replacement of the atrioventricular valve, implantation of a pacemaker, or both.

MALIGNANT TUMORS. Operation is not an effective treatment for the great majority of primary malignant tumors of the heart because of the large mass of cardiac tissue involved or the presence of metastases. The major role for surgery in such cases is to establish a diagnosis in order to exclude the possibility of a curable benign tumor. Nevertheless, in some cases palliation of hemodynamic and/or constitutional symptoms and extension of life may be achieved by aggressive therapy. Survivals of from 1 to 3 years have been reported following partial resection, chemotherapy, radiation therapy, or various combinations of these modalities.[123,131,167–169] In some instances, localized recurrences have been eliminated by as many as five operations.[14,15] Some success in palliation of symptoms has been reported following the combination of chemotherapy and radiation therapy[170] and radiation therapy alone.[171] Lymphosarcoma of the heart frequently responds to chemotherapy, radiation therapy, or both.[172,173] Unfortunately, many other reports indicate a failure to alter the course of cardiac sarcomas despite various combinations of surgery, chemotherapy, and radiation therapy.

References

1. Straus, R., and Merliss, R.: Primary tumors of the heart. Arch. Pathol. *39*:74, 1945.
2. Fine, G.: Neoplasms of the pericardium and heart. *In* Gould, S. E. (ed.): Pathology of the Heart and Blood Vessels. Springfield, Ill., Charles C Thomas, 1968, p. 851.
3. Heath, D.: Pathology of cardiac tumors. Am. J. Cardiol. *21*:315, 1968.
4. McAllister, H. A., and Fenoglio, J. J.: Tumors of the cardiovascular system. *In* Atlas of Tumor Pathology. Washington, D. C., Armed Forces Institute of Pathology, 1978. Fasc. 15, 2nd series.
5. McAllister, H. A., Jr.: Primary tumors of the heart and pericardium. Pathol. Ann. *17*:325, 1979.
6. Fabian, J. T., and Rose, A. G.: Tumours of the heart. S. Afr. Med. J. *61*:71, 1982.

6a. Mahaim, I.: Les Tumeurs et les Polypes de Coeur: Étude Anatomo-Clinique. Paris, Masson, 1945.

7. Barnes, A. R., Beaver, D. C., and Snell, A. M.: Primary sarcoma of the heart: Report of a case with E. C. G. and pathological studies. Am. Heart J. *9*:480, 1934.
8. Goldberg, H. P., Glenn, F., Dotter, C. T., and Steinberg, I.: Myxoma of the left atrium. Diagnosis made during life with operative and postmortem findings. Circulation *6*:762, 1952.
9. Beck, C. S.: An intrapericardial teratoma and a tumor of the heart: Both removed operatively. Ann. Surg. *116*:161, 1942.
10. Maurer, E. R.: Successful removal of tumor of the heart. J. Thorac. Surg. *23*: 473, 1952.
11. Castaneda, A. R., and Varco, R. L., Tumors of the heart: Surgical considerations. Am. J. Cardiol. *21*:357, 1968.
12. Crafoord, C. L.: Case report. *In* Lam, C. R. (ed.): Proceedings, International Symposium on Cardiovascular Surgery. Philadelphia, W. B. Saunders Co., 1955, p. 202.
13. Melo, J., Ahmad, A., Chapman, R., Wood, J., and Starr, A.: Primary tumors of the heart: A rewarding challenge. Am. Surg. *45*:681, 1979.
14. Gabelman, C., Al-Sadir, J., Lamberti, J., Fozzard, H. A., Laufer, E., Replogle, R. L., and Myerowitz, P. D.: Surgical treatment of recurrent primary malignant tumor of the left atrium. J. Thorac. Cardiovasc. Surg. *77*:914, 1979.
15. Yashar, J., Witoszka, M., Savage, D. D., Klie, J., Dyckman, J., Yashar, J. J., Reddick, R. L., Watson, D. C., and McIntosh, C. L.: Primary osteogenic sarcoma of the heart. Ann. Thorac. Surg. *28*:594, 1979.
16. Silverman, N. A.: Primary cardiac tumors. Ann. Surg. *191*:127, 1980.
17. Houser, S., Forbes, N., and Stewart, S.: Rhabdomyoma of the heart: A diagnostic and therapeutic challenge. Ann. Thorac. Surg. *29*:373, 1980.
18. Effert, S., and Domanig, E.: The diagnosis of intra-atrial tumor and thrombi by the ultrasonic echo method. Ger. Med. Mon. *4*:1, 1959.
19. Lappe, D. L., Bulkley, G. H., and Weiss, J. L.: Two-dimensional echocardiographic diagnosis of left atrial myxoma. Chest *74*:55, 1978.
20. Lewis, B. S., Lewis, N., Popp, R. L., Weiss, A. T., Borman, J. B., and Gotsman, M. S.: Diagnostic value of cross-sectional echocardiography in left atrial myxoma. Isr. J. Med. Sci. *15*:426, 1979.
21. Come, P. C., Kurland, G. S., and Vine, H. S.: Two dimensional echocardiography in differentiating right atrial and tricuspid valve mass lesions. Am. J. Cardiol. *44*:1207, 1979.
22. Fye, W. B., and Molina, J. E.: Right atrial angiosarcoma: Echocardiographic diagnosis and surgical correction. Johns Hopkins Med. J. *147*:111, 1980.
23. Fowles, R. E., Miller, C., Egbert, B. M., Fitzgerald, J. W., and Popp, R. L.: Systemic embolization from a mitral valve papillary endocardial fibroma detected by two-dimensional echocardiography. Am. Heart J. *102*:128, 1981.
24. Tway, K. P., Shah, A. A., and Rahimtoola, S. H.: Multiple biatrial myxomas demonstrated by two-dimensional echocardiography. Am. J. Med. *71*:896, 1981.
25. Pohost, G. M., Pastore, J. O., McKusick, K. A., Chiotellis, P. N., Kapeliakis, G. Z., Myers, G. S., Dinsmore, R. E., and Block, P. C.: Detection of left atrial myxoma by gated radionuclide cardiac imaging. Circulation *55*:88, 1977.
26. Pitcher, D., Wainwright, R., Brennand-Roper, D., Deverall, P., Sowton, E., and Maisey, M.: Cardiac tumors: Non-invasive detection and assessment by gated blood pool radionuclide imaging. Br. Heart J. *44*:143, 1980.
27. Winzelberg, G. G., Rapoport, F., Boucher, C. A., Carey, R. W., McKusick, K. A., and Strauss, H. W.: Combined gated cardiac blood pool scintigraphy and ^{67}Ga-citrate scintigraphy for detection of cardiac lymphoproliferative disorders. Radiology *141*:191, 1981.
28. Huggins, T. J., Huggins, M. J., Schnapf, D. J., Brott, W. H., Sinnott, R. C., and Shawl, F. A.: Left atrial myxoma: Computed tomography as a diagnostic modality. J. Comput. Assist. Tomogr. *4*:253, 1980.
29. Godwin, J. D., Axel, L., Adams, J. R., Schiller, N. B., Simpson, P. C., Jr., and Gertz, E. W.: Computed tomography: A new method for diagnosing tumor of the heart. Circulation *63*:448, 1981.
30. Köhler, E., Bocker, K., Leuner, C., Jungblut, R., Schoppe, W., Nessler, L., Minami, K., and Loogen, F.: The diagnostic value of M-mode, two-dimensional echocardiography, and computed tomography in comparison to the results of cardiac catheterization in the diagnosis of tumors of the heart. Z. Kardiol. *70*:571, 1981.
31. Sutton, D., Al-Kutoubi, M. A., and Lipkin, D. P.: Left atrial myxoma diagnosed by computerized tomography. Br. J. Radiol. *55*:80, 1982.
32. Lackner, K., Heuser, L., Friedman, G., and Thurn, P.: Computerkardiotomographie bei Tumoren des linken Vorhofes. Forstchr. Roentgenstr. *129*:735, 1978.
33. Goodwin, J. F.: Symposium on cardiac tumors. The spectrum of cardiac tumors. Am. J. Cardiol. *21*:307, 1968.
34. MacGregor, G. A., and Cullen, R. A.: The syndrome of fever, anaemia and high sedimentation rate with an atrial myxoma. Br. Med. J. *5*:158, 1959.
35. Huston, K. A., Combs, J. J., Lie, J. T., and Giuliani, E. R.: Left atrial myxoma simulating peripheral vasculitis. Mayo Clin. Proc. *53*:752, 1978.
36. Caralis, D. G., Kennedy, H. L., Bailey, I., and Bulkley, B. H.: Primary right cardiac tumor. Chest *77*:100, 1980.
37. Willey, R. F., Mathews, M. B., and Walbaum, P. R.: An unusual case of large right atrial myxoma. Br. Heart J. *44*:108, 1980.
38. Firor, W. B., Aldridge, H. E., and Bigelow, W. G.: A follow-up study of three patients after removal of left atrial myxoma five to ten years previously. J. Thorac. Cardiovasc. Surg. *51*:515, 1966.
39. Levinson, J. P., and Kincaid, O. W.: Myxoma of the right atrium associated with polycythemia. N. Engl. J. Med. *264*:1187, 1961.
40. Vuopio, P., and Nikkila, E. A.: Hemolytic anemia and thrombocytopenia in a case of left atrial myxoma associated with mitral stenosis. Am. J. Cardiol. *17*: 585, 1966.
41. Boss, J. H., and Bechar, M.: Myxoma of the heart. Report based on four cases. Am. J. Cardiol. *3*:823, 1959.
42. Curry, H. L. F., Mathews, J. A., and Robinson, J.: Right atrial myxoma mimicking a rheumatic disorder. Br. Med. J. *1*:542, 1967.
43. Graham, S. L., and Sellers, A. L.: Atrial myxoma with multiple myeloma. Arch. Intern. Med. *139*:116, 1979.
44. Kaminsky, M. E., Ehlers, K. H., Engle, M. A., Klein, A. A., Levin, A. R., and Subramanian, V. A.: Atrial myxoma mimicking a collagen disorder. Chest *75*:93, 1979.
45. Rajpal, R. S., Leibsohn, J. A., Liekweg, W. G., Gross, C. M., Olinger, G. N., Rose, H. D., and Bamrah, V. S.: Infected left atrial myxoma with bacteremia simulating infective endocarditis. Arch. Intern. Med. *139*:1176, 1979.
46. Byrd, W. E., Matthews, O. P., and Hunt, R. E.: Left atrial myxoma presenting as a systemic vasculitis. Arth. Rheum. *23*:240, 1980.
47. Joseph, P., Himmelstein, D. U., Mahowald, J. M., and Stullman, W. S.: Atrial myxoma infected with Candida: First survival. Chest *78*:340, 1980.
48. Silverman, J., Olwin, J. S., and Graettinger, J. S.: Cardiac myxomas with systemic embolization. Circulation *26*:99, 1962.

43 PERICARDIAL DISEASE

by Beverly H. Lorell, M.D., and Eugene Braunwald, M.D.

HISTORICAL BACKGROUND[1,2]

In the ancient world knowledge of the pericardium was gained from anatomical observations of animal sacrifices and human corpses during war. Both Homer and Pliny wrote about the anatomical finding of "hairy hearts" in warriors who died on the battlefield. Hippocrates accurately described the normal pericardium as "a smooth mantle surrounding the heart and containing a small amount of fluid resembling urine." In the Dead Sea Scrolls (A.D. 1) the pericardium was referred to as "the foreskin of the heart." Galen (A.D. 131–201) named the pericardium and recognized its protective function.

In the 17th century, Riolan advocated the technique of pericardial aspiration for treating patients with large pericardial effusions, and William Harvey vividly demonstrated to King Charles that much of the visceral pericardium is pain-insensitive by palpating the beating heart of a young nobleman who had a large defect in the left chest. In the same century, the Cornish physiologist Richard Lower made remarkable observations about the physiology of constrictive pericarditis and cardiac tamponade: "Just as the heart labors when affected by disease within, so it does when oppressed from without by disease of its covering. So it happens when that same covering of the heart fills with an effusion and the walls are compressed with water on every side, so that they cannot dilate to receive the blood, then truly the pulse diminishes until at length it is suppressed by even more water, when syncope, and death itself follows. Just as the accumulation of too much water harms the heart, so too does trouble come when the heart and the pericardium become everywhere adherent. . . ."

Early in the 19th century, Morgagni described cardiac compression by hemopericardium and by pericardial calcification, noted that the apex beat was often absent in patients with extensive pericardial adhesion, and advocated pericardiocentesis via incision for treatment of pericardial tamponade. Corvisart and his student Laennec distinguished adhesive pericarditis from pericardial effusion by physical examination. Romero reported the first successful pericardiotomy to relieve pericardial effusion, and in 1840, Franz Schuh performed the first successful "blind" pericardiocentesis with a trocar to relieve cardiac tamponade. Norman Cheevers of Guy's Hospital in London astutely appreciated the physiology of constrictive pericarditis: "The principal cause of dangerous symptoms . . . appears to arise from the occurrence of gradual contraction in the layer of adhesive material which has been deposited around the heart, compressing its muscular tissue and embarrassing its systolic and diastolic movement, but more particularly the latter. The ventricles, having become diminished in capacity, make up for this loss by the rapidity of their contractions. . . ."

In the mid-1800's, Joseph Skoda reported the characteristic physical findings of constrictive pericarditis including the "diastolic heart beat" (pericardial knock), systolic precordial retraction, and sudden diastolic collapse of the cervical veins (prominent venous *y* descent). Kussmaul made the classic bedside observations of neck vein distention in compressive pericardial disorders and pulsus paradoxus, the hallmark of acute cardiac tamponade, which he described as paradoxical because the palpated pulse disappeared during inspiration even though the heart continued to beat. He also described the finding of an inspiratory increase in central venous pressure in constrictive pericarditis, now known as *Kussmaul's sign.* Early in the 20th century, the first pericardiectomy for constrictive pericarditis was performed by Hallopeau.

Even with the tremendous experimental advances made in this century toward understanding the physiology of the normal and diseased pericardium and appreciating the clinical picture of pericardial disease, Sir William Osler's caveat is still applicable: "Even with copious effusion, the onset and course may be so insidious that no suspicion of the true nature of the disease is aroused. . . . Perhaps no serious disease is so frequently overlooked by the practitioner. Postmortem experience shows how often pericarditis is not recognized or goes on to resolution and adhesion without attracting notice."

ANATOMY

The pericardium forms a strong flask-shaped sac with short tube-like extensions that enclose the origins of the aorta and its junction with the aortic arch, the pulmonary artery where it branches, the proximal pulmonary veins, and venae cavae. Fibrous tissue of the pericardium actually blends with adventitia of the great arteries to form very strong attachments. In addition, the pericardium has firm ligamentous attachments anteriorly to the sternum and xiphoid process, posteriorly to the vertebral column, and inferiorly to the diaphragm.[3]

The human pericardium receives its arterial blood supply from small branches of the aorta and internal mammary and musculophrenic arteries. The pericardium is innervated by the vagus, left recurrent laryngeal nerve, and esophageal plexus and also has rich sympathetic innervation from the stellate and first dorsal ganglia and the cardiac, aortic, and diaphragmatic plexuses. The phrenic nerves course over the pericardium en route to the diaphragm. The afferent nerves responsible for pain perception appear to be transmitted via the phrenic nerve entering the spinal cord at C4–C5.[3,4] It appears that the anterior parietal pericardium is pain-sensitive while the lateral and posterior parietal pericardial regions are not.

The pericardium is composed of a fibrous outer layer composed of collagen bundles and elastin fibers and an inner serous membrane composed of a single layer of mesothelial cells. The inner serous layer is intimately attached to the surface of the heart and epicardial fat to form the *visceral pericardium*, and this inner serous membrane reflects back on itself to line the outer fibrous layer to form the *parietal pericardium*. The pericardium has two major serosal tunnels: the transverse sinus, which lies posterior to the great arteries and anterior to the atria and superior vena cava, and the oblique sinus, which lies posterior to the left atrium so that the posterior left atrial wall is actually separated from the pericardial space. The fact that the oblique sinus is usually not fluid-filled in the presence of a pericardial effusion is clinically important in that it explains why an echo-free space denoting an effusion is often not detected behind the left atrium during echocardiography.

The serous visceral pericardium is attached to the parietal pericardium by delicate connective tissue with elastin fibers. The parietal pericardium is composed of collagen fibers interlaced with extensive elastic fibers, which are wavy during childhood and become progressively straighter with age, suggesting that young pericardia are more compliant than those of the elderly. Electron microscopy reveals that exuberant microvilli and long, single cilia project from the serous mesothelium composing the visceral pericardium and the inner lining of the parietal pericardium (Fig. 43–1).[5] The microvilli are believed to increase markedly the surface area available for fluid transport, and both microvilli and cilia provide a specialized surface to permit movement of the pericardial membranes over each other during each cardiac cycle and to permit the pericardium to accommodate changes in cardiac shape during contraction.

The human pericardium normally contains up to 50 ml of clear fluid.[6] The visceral pericardium is believed to be the source of normal pericardial fluid and of excessive fluid in disease states. Normal pericardial fluid appears to be an ultrafiltrate of plasma, since electrolytes are present in pericardial fluid in concentrations compatible with such an ultrafiltrate; protein concentrations are about one-third those of the plasma, and albumin is present in a higher ratio in pericardial fluid reflecting its lower molecular weight.[7] The membrane characteristics of the pericardium tend to favor fluid removal rather than accumulation,[8] which may be a safety factor preventing the development of cardiac tamponade. Current data suggest that drainage of the pericardial space occurs both by the thoracic duct via the parietal pericardium and by the right lymphatic duct via the right pleural space.

FUNCTIONS OF THE PERICARDIUM

The pericardium serves several membrane functions. Its ligamentous attachments help to fix the heart anatomically and prevent excessive motion with changes in body position. The pericardium also reduces friction between the heart and surrounding organs and provides a barrier against the extension of infection and malignancy from contiguous organs to the heart itself. The role of the pericardium in the regulation of the circulation is controversial, since congenital absence or surgical excision of the pericardium is *not* associated with overt disturbances of cardiac function. However, observations in both dogs and man indicate that the pericardium may play a role in (1) the distribution and equalization of hydrostatic forces on the heart, (2) the prevention of acute cardiac dilatation, and (3) diastolic coupling of the two ventricles[7a] (see later).

The normal pericardium is stiff, and the relationship between pressure within the pericardium and total intrapericardial volume, which is the sum of the volume of the heart itself and the reserve volume of the surrounding peri-

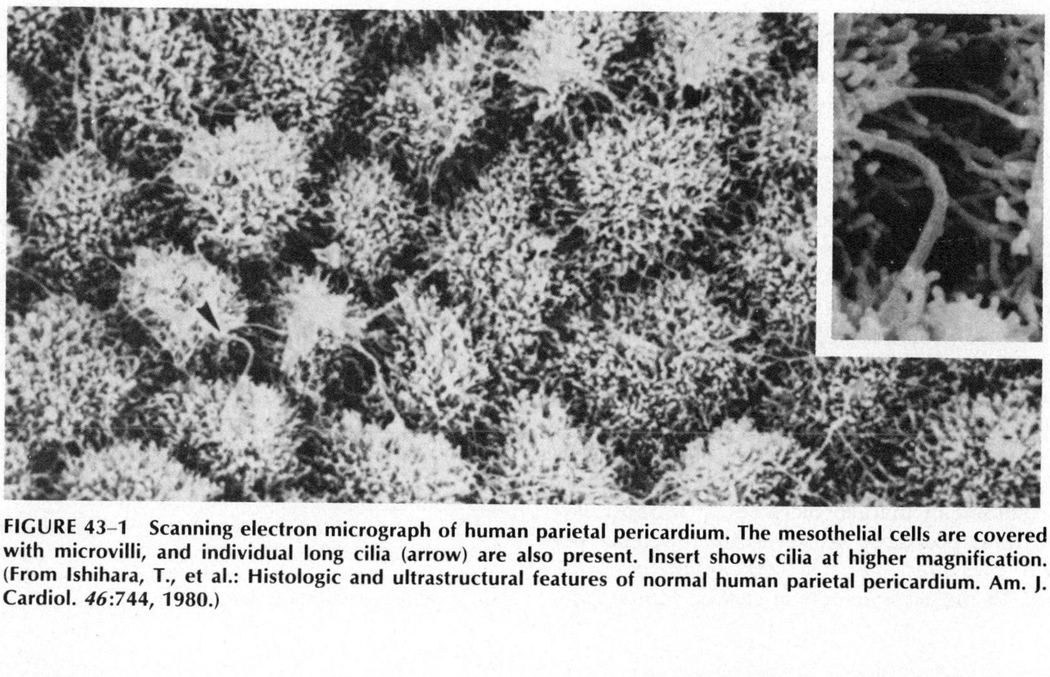

FIGURE 43–1 Scanning electron micrograph of human parietal pericardium. The mesothelial cells are covered with microvilli, and individual long cilia (arrow) are also present. Insert shows cilia at higher magnification. (From Ishihara, T., et al.: Histologic and ultrastructural features of normal human parietal pericardium. Am. J. Cardiol. *46*:744, 1980.)

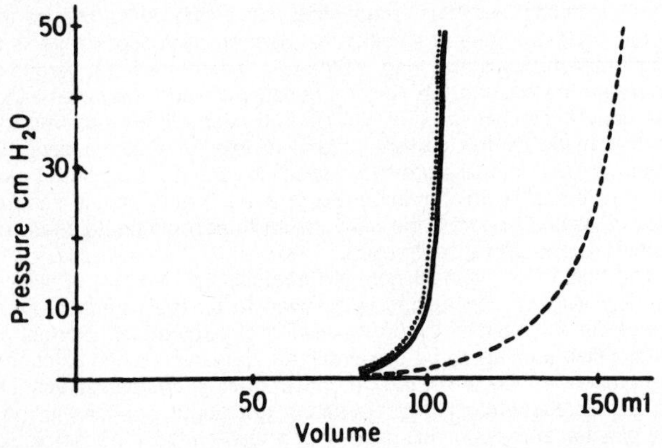

FIGURE 43–2 Pressure-volume curves before (left) and after (right) removal of the pericardium of an isolated dog heart. Solid line is pericardial volume, dotted line is heart volume within the pericardium, and dashed line is heart volume after removal of pericardium. Note that the curve at left is flat initially but becomes extremely steep as total volume within the pericardium increases. After removal of the pericardium (right curve), an increase in heart volume results in a lesser rise in pressure than with the pericardium intact. (From Hort, W.: Herzbentel and Herzgrosse. Arch. Kreislaufforsch. *44*:21, 1964.)

cardial sac, appears as a steep curve when plotted on a graph.[3] Thus, once the pericardium is filled, intrapericardial pressure rises sharply as volume is increased (Fig. 43–2). Normally, the pericardial sac is filled with a thin film of fluid distributed throughout the pericardial space in such a way that the pericardial reserve volume is not exceeded. This permits respiratory and postural changes in cardiac volume and total intrapericardial volume to occur without significant changes in intrapericardial pressure. Normally, pericardial pressure is equal to intrapleural pressure and varies from −5 to +5 cm H_2O during the respiratory cycle.[9] Pericardial pressure is transmitted uniformly throughout the fluid-filled intrapericardial space, thus minimizing the impact of gravitational or inertial forces on the circulation. This is analogous to the hydraulic function of cerebral spinal fluid relative to the cerebral circulation.[10]

Pericardial pressure is also a determinant of the *transmural distending pressure* of the cardiac chambers and contributes to the operation of the Frank-Starling mechanism in the beat-to-beat regulation of stroke volume. The transmural distending pressure of either ventricle is the difference between intracardiac and intrapericardial pressures and is independent of gravity. For example, when left ventricular end-diastolic pressure is +5 mm Hg and intrapericardial pressure is −2 mm Hg, relative to atmosphere, the actual ventricular distending pressure is $5 - (-2) = 7$ mm Hg. With the chest closed, the presence of equal transmural pressures at all levels of the heart relative to gravity helps to insure uniform diastolic fiber stretch and operation of the Frank-Starling mechanism.[11]

When the volume of the heart or other contents of the pericardial sac increase and exceed the elastic limits of the pericardium, during diastole the heart is shifted to the steep portion of the curve relating intrapericardial pressure and volume, resulting in marked increases in intrapericardial and intracardiac pressures. However, the difference between the two pressures, i.e., the *transmural pressure*, usually declines. In the extreme case of cardiac tamponade, in which both intrapericardial and intracardiac pressures are markedly increased, the transmural pressure distending the ventricles may fall precipitously, resulting in decreased ventricular diastolic volumes and preload. Conversely, when a reduction in elevated intracardiac volume occurs, intrapericardial pressure also falls, which promotes ventricular filling. This is exemplified by the changes in intrapericardial pressure and venous return that occur during ventricular ejection in every cardiac cycle. Ventricular ejection is accompanied by abrupt descent of the atrioventricular junction (the "base" of the heart) and a reduction in right atrial pressure, manifest by the *x* descent* in the right atrial pressure pulse as well as by a decline in intrapericardial pressure. These changes result in a surge of venous return during systole, particularly when ventricular and pericardial pressures are increased.[12] Brecher has shown that the acceleration of venous return during systolic ejection is diminished by opening of the pericardium.[13] These findings, taken together, indicate that changes in intrapericardial pressure modulate the regulation of stroke volume by ventricular preload, i.e., the Frank-Starling mechanism, particularly at higher ventricular and pericardial pressures.

Limitation of Cardiac Distention. The relatively nondistensible pericardium may help to limit acute distention of the heart.[14,15] This was appreciated as early as 1898 by Bernard, who used a pump to increase pressure in excised hearts with and without the pericardium and noted that hearts unsupported by the pericardium ruptured at lower pressures than did hearts with intact pericardia.[16] More recent studies in dogs have suggested that the pericardium may *restrain* left ventricular filling, so that ventricular volume is greater at any given ventricular pressure with the pericardium removed than with the pericardium intact.[17–20] In addition, acute changes in intracardiac and total intrapericardial volume result in an upward shift of the left ventricular pressure-volume relationship, which is in part mediated by the restraining effect of the pericardium.

Thus, Shirato and Shabetai demonstrated that acute volume loading with dextran in dogs with intact pericardia resulted in an upward shift in the left ventricular pressure–segment length relation, i.e., left ventricular pressure was higher at any given segment length while the reduction of venous return and cardiac volume by means of nitroprusside administration shifted the curves downward toward control levels (see Figure 12–24, p. 429).[21] This occurred because nitroprusside and other vasodilators that decrease right heart filling reduce the total volume occupied by the heart within the pericardial space and thus reduce the restraining of the left ventricle by the pericardium; in turn, this causes a downward shift of the left ventricular pressure-volume relation so that a given left ventricular volume is associated with a lower left ventricular diastolic pressure. After pericardiectomy, volume loading resulted in a rightward shift in the pressure–segment length relation[21a] and, after nitroprusside, a leftward shift along a single

*It is recognized that the descent in venous pressure after the *a* wave is usually termed the *x* descent and, after the *c* wave, the *x'* descent. In this chapter, the major systolic venous pressure descent after the *a* and *c* waves will be termed the *x* descent.

curve. When the effect of the pericardium was eliminated by plotting left ventricular *transmural pressure* versus segment length, the points during all interventions also fell along a single curve.

Refsum et al. investigated the role of the pericardium in the mechanism of shifts in the left ventricular pressure-volume relationship by infusing saline both intravenously and into the pericardial sac in closed-chest dogs in which intrapericardial and cardiac volumes were assessed by computed tomography.[22] Acute upward shifts in the left ventricular diastolic pressure-volume relationship during volume loading were due to elevations in intrapericardial pressure induced by increases in total intrapericardial volume.

A restraining effect of the pericardium has also been observed early in the course of chronic volume overloading induced by formation of arteriovenous shunts in dogs prior to enlargement of the pericardium by stretch or hypertrophy, but this restraining effect was not apparent in dogs studied late during the course of chronic volume overload.[23] This finding suggests that chronic left ventricular enlargement and hypertrophy are accompanied by compensatory hypertrophy or stretch of the pericardium and an increase in total intrapericardial volume.

These observations, taken together, suggest that shifts in the left ventricular intracavity pressure-volume relation following volume loading or vasodilator administration are largely due to changes in intrapericardial pressure. However, the pericardium does not affect *intrinsic* myocardial compliance[24] nor does it account for changes in the left ventricular diastolic pressure-volume relationship observed during ischemia.[25]

Ventricular Interdependence. The pericardium also contributes to *diastolic coupling* between the two ventricles, i.e., to ventricular interdependence. The distention of one ventricle alters the distensibility of the other, even in the absence of the pericardium.[26–29] This effect appears to be mediated in part by shared encircling muscle bands and by the interventricular septum, which tends to bulge into the left ventricle, causing a change in the shape of the left ventricle when the right ventricle is distended.[30–32] In the *absence* of the pericardium, large increases in right ventricular volume and pressure are required to cause an appreciable increase in left ventricular filling pressure (Fig. 43–3).[33,34] In contrast, the presence of an intact pericardium markedly accentuates the coupling between ventricular diastolic pressures.[35–39] When right ventricular volume and pressure are increased with the pericardium intact, right and left ventricular filling pressures are closely correlated and left ventricular volume is smaller than in the absence of the pericardium, when cardiac distensibility is primarily related to properties of the myocardium.[39] This effect of the pericardium on diastolic ventricular interaction is present at normal filling pressures and becomes of increasing importance at high right ventricular filling pressures.[33] The normal pericardium does not appear to contribute importantly to the interaction of the ventricles during systole.[40]

In *summary,* there is experimental evidence that the pericardium limits acute distention of the heart, mediates changes in the relationship between ventricular pressure and volume, and enhances the effect that distention of one ventricle has on the diastolic pressure-volume relations of the contralateral ventricle.

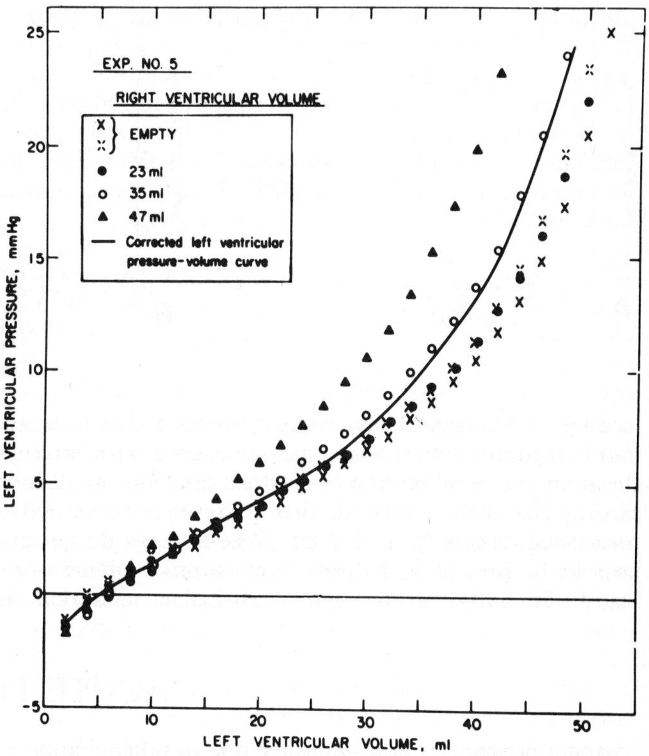

FIGURE 43–3 Left ventricular pressure-volume curves of the canine left ventricle without the pericardium obtained with the right ventricle empty and containing several different volumes. Increases in right ventricular volume result in a higher left ventricular pressure at the same left ventricular volume. This effect is most pronounced over the range of elevated left ventricular pressures and volumes. (From Taylor, R. R., et al.: Dependence of ventricular distensibility on filling of the opposite ventricle. Am. J. Physiol. *213*:711, 1967.)

Functions of the Pericardium in Man. Although one must be cautious in extrapolating the findings of animal experiments to the intact human heart, there is evidence in man that the restraining effects of the pericardium are clinically relevant. First, in humans after pericardiotomy, there is a downward shift of the left ventricular pressure-volume curve that is increasingly apparent as left ventricular volume increases.[41] In addition, angiotensin, nitroprusside, and nitroglycerin infusions, which alter intracardiac volume, cause acute shifts in the left ventricular diastolic pressure-volume relation[42–44] (Fig. 12–24, p. 429), an effect which probably depends on the presence of the pericardium. Ludbrook demonstrated in humans that the downward shift in the left ventricular pressure-volume curve that occurs during nitroglycerin administration is *not* observed with amyl nitrite, which alters aortic pressure but has no acute effect on intracardiac and intrapericardial volumes (Fig. 43–4).[45] After pericardiotomy and loss of the restraining effect of the pericardium, the human left ventricular pressure-volume curve is *not* altered by nitroprusside administration.[46] These observations indicate that the beneficial effects of interventions such as nitroprusside infusion, in which an augmentation of stroke volume may be observed at a lower ventricular filling pressure, are in part due to an alteration of apparent cardiac distensibility mediated by reducing the restraining effect of the pericardium.[47]

The pericardium may also provide a significant restraining effect on acute cardiac dilatation during acute volume

enlargement. Pericardiocentesis (p. 1486) is *not* indicated unless there is evidence of cardiac compression due to cardiac tamponade or unless analysis of pericardial fluid is essential to establish a diagnosis such as bacterial pericarditis.

CHRONIC PERICARDIAL EFFUSIONS

Chronic pericardial effusions persisting for more than six months may occur in any form of pericardial disease. Often they are surprisingly well tolerated, with no symptoms of cardiac compression, and are discovered when a routine chest roentgenogram discloses an unexpectedly large cardiac silhouette.[90] Chronic pericardial effusions are particularly likely to be found in patients with previous idiopathic or viral pericarditis, uremic pericarditis, and pericarditis secondary to myxedema or neoplasm. The management of chronic pericardial effusion depends in part on the etiology. Stable and apparently idiopathic effusions usually require no specific treatment except for avoidance of anticoagulants.[91] Chronic effusions secondary to tuberculosis, neoplasm, purulent infection, or hemorrhage into the pericardium may progress to cardiac tamponade or pericardial fibrosis, calcification, and constriction. As discussed on page 1505, large chronic effusions secondary to uremia may contribute to intermittent hypotension and instability during dialysis. When chronic pericardial effusion causes serious symptoms, a large subxiphoid pericardiotomy or total pericardiectomy may be warranted.[92,93] In the setting of chronic pericardial effusion, these surgical approaches allow evacuation of loculated fluid, fibrin, or thrombus and sampling of pericardial tissue for culture and histological examination.

PERICARDIAL EFFUSION WITH CARDIAC COMPRESSION: CARDIAC TAMPONADE

An increase in intrapericardial pressure secondary to fluid accumulation within the pericardial space results in cardiac tamponade, which is characterized by (1) an elevation of intracardiac pressures, (2) progressive limitation of ventricular diastolic filling, and (3) a reduction of stroke volume.

PATHOPHYSIOLOGY

As already noted, intrapericardial pressure is normally very close to intrapleural pressure and several mm Hg lower than right and left ventricular diastolic pressures. When the addition of fluid into the pericardial space causes intrapericardial pressure to rise to the level of the right atrial and right ventricular diastolic pressures, the transmural pressure distending these chambers declines to close to zero and cardiac tamponade occurs.[94] The rise of right atrial and intrapericardial pressures is less marked in the presence of hypovolemia, and therefore cardiac tamponade may be masked when hypovolemia is present (Fig. 43–8). Further accumulation of intrapericardial fluid causes both intrapericardial and right ventricular diastolic pressures to rise together to the level of left ventricular diastolic pressure, and subsequently, all three pressures rise together associated with a fall in systemic arterial pressure (Fig. 43–9). If left ventricular diastolic pressure is markedly elevated owing to preexisting left ventricular disease, cardiac tamponade occurs when right ventricular diastolic and pericardial pressures equalize but at a lower level than the left ventricular diastolic pressure.[95]

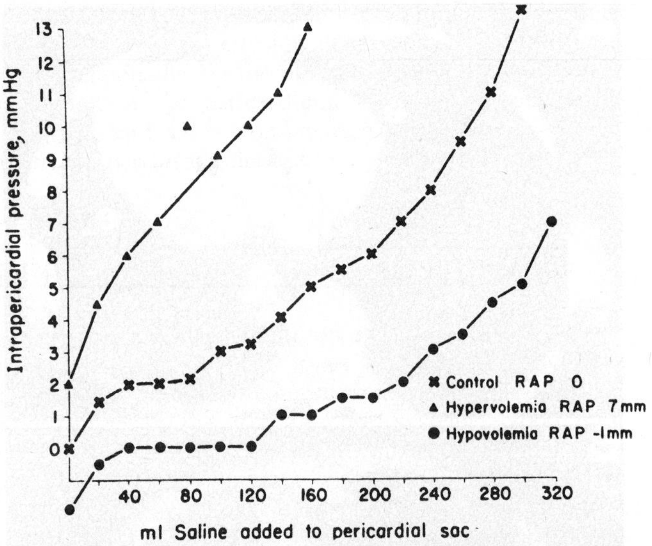

FIGURE 43–8 **Pericardial pressure-volume curves obtained by adding saline solution to the pericardial sac in closed-chest anesthetized dogs. The curve is steeper with hypervolemia and less steep with hypovolemia, compared with control, because the heart occupies a greater volume in the pericardial cavity with hypervolemia and a smaller volume with hypovolemia. (From Fowler, N. O.: Physiology of cardiac tamponade and pulsus paradoxus. II. Physiological, circulatory, and pharmacological responses in cardiac tamponade. Mod. Conc. Cardiovasc. Dis. *47*:116, 1978, by permission of the American Heart Association, Inc.)**

Equalization of intrapericardial and ventricular filling pressures results in markedly diminished diastolic volumes of both ventricles and a fall in stroke volume. These findings have been observed both in animals subjected to acute experimental tamponade and in humans with acute cardiac

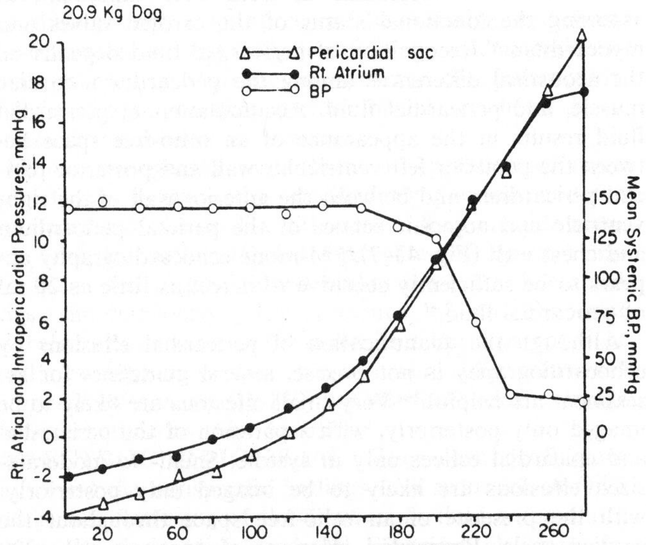

FIGURE 43–9 **Experimental cardiac tamponade produced by injection of saline into the pericardial sac of an anesthetized dog. As more than 160 ml is injected, right atrial and intrapericardial pressures rise sharply and equilibrate, and blood pressure (BP) falls abruptly. (From Fowler, N. O.: Physiology of cardiac tamponade and pulsus paradoxus. II. Physiological, circulatory, and pharmacological responses in cardiac tamponade. Mod. Conc. Cardiovasc. Dis. *47*: 115, 1978, by permission of the American Heart Association, Inc.)**

tamponade.[95–98] The reduction in stroke volume is initially compensated for by reflex increases in adrenergic tone; both tachycardia and increases in ejection fraction intially help to maintain forward cardiac output.[94,99] The importance of the adrenergic support of the heart is reflected in the finding that when beta-adrenergic blockade is carried out in cardiac tamponade, ejection fraction and stroke volume decline.[98] Systemic vascular resistance increases so that, at first, systemic arterial pressure is maintained at the expense of cardiac output. With severe cardiac tamponade, as cardiac output declines, compensatory mechanisms are no longer sufficient to maintain systemic arterial pressure, and perfusion of vital organs becomes impaired[99]; reduced coronary perfusion causes selective hypoperfusion of the subendocardium.[100,101] The addition of myocardial ischemia during cardiac tamponade could further compromise left ventricular stroke volume. In extreme cardiac tamponade, transmural diastolic ventricular pressures may actually be less than zero, suggesting that ventricular filling occurs by diastolic suction.[102] Sinus bradycardia, mediated by the cardiac depressor branches of the vagus nerve and by the nonvagal mechanism of sinoatrial node ischemia, may also occur during severe cardiac tamponade.[103,104] Profound bradycardia often occurs during severe hypotension and precedes the development of electrical-mechanical dissociation and death.[105]

Cardiac tamponade also alters the dynamics of systemic venous return and cardiac filling. Normally, one surge of systemic venous return occurs during ventricular ejection coincident with the systolic x descent of the venous pressure pulse, and a second surge occurs with the opening of the tricuspid valve in diastole, corresponding to the y descent. In cardiac tamponade, the heart is compressed throughout the cardiac cycle. During ejection, intracardiac volume transiently decreases, resulting in a transient fall in both intrapericardial and right atrial pressures, manifest as the x descent, which is accompanied by a surge of systemic venous return into the right atrium. However, in diastole, the total volume within the pericardial space remains elevated despite opening of the tricuspid valve; intrapericardial pressure remains elevated and equal to right atrial pressure so that transmural distending pressure is close to zero. As a result, the usual surge of systemic venous return during early diastole is abolished. These events are graphically reflected in the right atrial or systemic venous waveform in cardiac tamponade, in that the systolic x descent is prominent while the diastolic y descent is usually completely absent or attenuated (Fig. 43–10).

Pulsus Paradoxus. Inspiration and the transmission of negative intrathoracic pressure to the pericardial space further alter the dynamics of right and left ventricular filling and are responsible for *pulsus paradoxus*, the inspiratory fall of aortic systolic pressure greater than 10 mm Hg (Fig. 43–11).[106] The finding of weakening of the arterial pulse during inspiration was first recorded in 1854 by Vieordt in a description of purulent pericarditis and was subsequently described by Kussmaul in 1873 as the apparent paradox of the disappearance of the pulse during inspiration despite persistence of the heart beat. It should be emphasized that pulsus paradoxus is in fact an exaggeration of the normal inspiratory decline of left ventricular stroke volume by about 7 per cent and of systemic arterial pressure by 3 per cent.[107]

The complex mechanism of *pulsus paradoxus* in cardiac tamponade has been the subject of considerable controversy.[108] Experimental studies on the effects of inspiration in animals and man have helped to clarify this mechanism. Experiments in humans using radiopaque markers and electromagnetic flowmeters[109,110] have shown that inspiration is normally accompanied by an increase in diastolic dimensions of the right ventricle, a small decrease in left ventricular dimension, and increased velocity of flow from the venae cavae into the right atrium. Pulsus paradoxus in cardiac tamponade appears to result from an exaggeration of these normal findings. Measurement of intracardiac pressures and flow during experimental tamponade[111] and in man during cardiac tamponade[107,112] have demonstrated that inspiration is associated with falls in intrapericardial and right atrial pressures, which results in augmentation of flow from the venae cavae into the right atrium and right ventricle and augmentation of pulmonary artery flow and pulmonary artery systolic pressure. On the left side of the

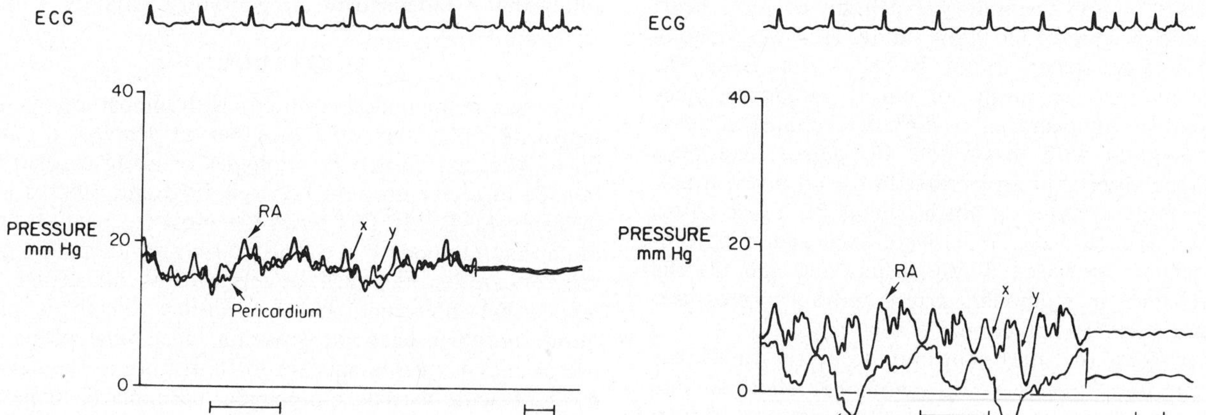

FIGURE 43–10 Right atrial (RA) and pericardial pressure measurements in a patient with cardiac tamponade. *Left panel,* Before pericardiocentesis, RA and pericardial pressures are elevated and equal, and the waveforms show the presence of the systolic x descent and near-absence of the diastolic y descent. *Right panel,* After removal of only 100 ml of pericardial fluid, and before pericardial pressure returns to zero, there is a reduction and separation of RA and pericardial pressures. Note that the RA waveform now shows a prominent diastolic y descent.

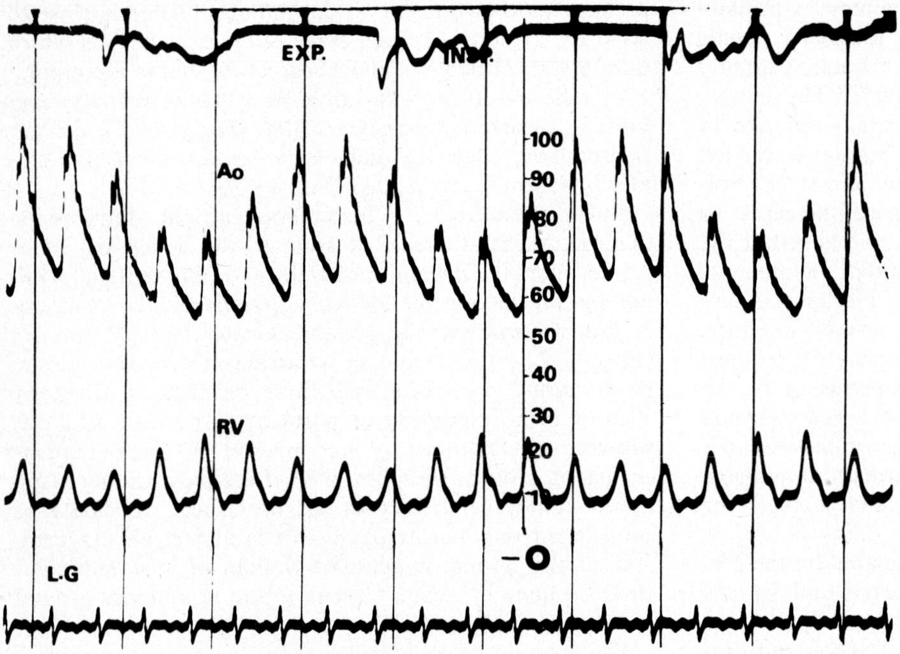

FIGURE 43–11 Recording of aortic (Ao) and right ventricular (RV) pressures in a patient with cardiac tamponade complicated by hypovolemia. *Pulsus paradoxus* is evident as a marked inspiratory decline in aortic systolic and pulse pressures during inspiration (INSP). RV pressure variation is out of phase with aortic pressure. Note that the RV waveform does *not* show a dip-and-plateau configuration. (From Shabetai, R., et al.: The hemodynamics of cardiac tamponade and constrictive pericarditis. Am. J. Cardiol. *26*:480, 1970.)

heart, left atrial and left ventricular diastolic pressures fall, accompanied by a fall in aortic flow and systolic arterial pressure.[107,113] The increase in venous return flow during inspiration results in a marked and exaggerated *increase in right ventricular dimensions* accompanied by a reduction in left ventricular dimensions and flattening and displacement of the septum toward the left ventricle.[114,115] *Thus, pulsus paradoxus in cardiac tamponade is critically dependent on the inspiratory augmentation of systemic venous return and right ventricular filling.*

Shabetai et al. demonstrated clearly that when experimental cardiac tamponade was induced in dogs, pulsus paradoxus did *not* develop when either the right heart was bypassed or right ventricular volume was strictly controlled.[111] These experiments also demonstrated that inspiratory pooling of blood within the lungs or traction on the heart by the diaphragm were *not* essential mechanisms of pulsus paradoxus in cardiac tamponade. Thus, these observations indicate that pulsus paradoxus in cardiac tamponade depends on the inspiratory expansion of right heart filling at the expense of left heart filling. However, competition for a "fixed space" within the pericardium is not the entire mechanism accounting for pulsus paradoxus, since (1) the sum of right and left ventricular volumes actually increases slightly with inspiration; (2) pulsus paradoxus occurs in the absence of an increase in the intrapericardial-pleural pressure gradient, which would be expected to occur if intrapericardial volume were fixed and right ventricular volume increased during inspiration; and (3) the cyclic variations in pulmonary artery and aortic pressures are not precisely 180 degrees out of phase.

Another factor that may contribute to pulsus paradoxus is an inspiratory increase in left ventricular afterload due to an inspiratory rise in transmural aortic pressure.[116] Furthermore, when left ventricular diastolic volume is markedly reduced, the left ventricle may be operating on the steep ascending limb of the Starling curve so that a small inspiratory reduction of left ventricular filling results in marked depression of left ventricular stroke volume and systolic pressure.[117,118] Pulsus paradoxus is occasionally observed in constrictive pericarditis and restrictive heart disease, and the latter mechanism may account for its presence in these disorders.

Pulsus paradoxus has also been observed in lung disease secondary to emphysema, bronchitis, asthma, acute airway obstruction secondary to tracheal compression, tension pneumothorax, and massive pulmonary embolism.[119–122] Under these circumstances, pulsus paradoxus is probably related both to the transmission of excessively negative intrathoracic pressure during inspiration to the aorta and to exaggerated right heart filling with an associated decrease in left heart filling during inspiration. Pulsus paradoxus may be absent in cardiac tamponade when underlying heart disease causes a marked elevation of left ventricular diastolic pressure so that the two ventricles are unequally compressed,[95] in atrial septal defect when the increase in systemic venous return during inspiration is shared between the two sides of the heart,[123] and in aortic regurgitation when there is a major component of left ventricular filling that is independent of respiratory variation.

ETIOLOGY

Cardiac tamponade may occur with almost any cause of pericarditis and may exist in either an acute or a chronic form. The distribution of etiologies of acute cardiac tamponade in a city hospital between 1963 and 1980 is noted in Table 43–4.[124] In this series the most frequent etiologies of cardiac tamponade were neoplasm and idiopathic or viral pericarditis, followed by pericarditis associated with myocardial infarction, invasive cardiac diagnostic procedures, purulent bacterial infection, and tuberculosis. The use of anticoagulants appears to contribute to the development of acute cardiac tamponade, particularly in patients with pericarditis due to acute myocardial infarction or after cardiac surgery.[124,125]

CLINICAL MANIFESTATIONS

The triad of (1) a decline in systemic arterial pressure; (2) elevation of systemic venous pressure; and (3) a small,

TABLE 43–4 COMMON ETIOLOGIES OF CARDIAC TAMPONADE

Disorder	%
Malignant disease	32
Idiopathic pericarditis	14
Uremia	9
Acute cardiac infarction (receiving heparin)	9
Diagnostic procedures with cardiac perforation	7.5
Bacterial	7.5
Tuberculosis	5
Radiation	4
Myxedema	4
Dissecting aortic aneurysm	4
Postpericardiotomy syndrome	2
Systemic lupus erythematosus	2
Cardiomyopathy (receiving anticoagulants)	2

Modified from Guberman, B. A., et al.: Cardiac tamponade in medical patients. Circulation *64*:633, 1981.

quiet heart was described by the thoracic surgeon Claude S. Beck in 1935.[126] These three features are typical of cardiac tamponade from intrapericardial hemorrhage due to penetrating heart wounds, aortic dissection, and intrapericardial rupture of an aortic or cardiac aneurysm. This syndrome develops when the pericardium is not enlarged or stretched, so that the addition of less than 200 ml of fluid or blood causes intrapericardial pressure to rise abruptly to above 20 to 30 mm Hg. In cases that are not immediately fatal, both cardiac output and arterial pressure fall, accompanied by tachycardia and tachypnea. The patient may be stuporous or agitated and restless, and the additional important finding of pulsus paradoxus may be difficult to appreciate when profound hypotension is present.

Jugular venous pressure is usually markedly elevated, with a typical waveform devoid of a diastolic *y* descent, but this may be difficult to appreciate at the bedside owing to the presence of tachypnea and the use of accessory respiratory muscles. Precordial heart activity is usually not palpable and heart sounds are distant or inaudible. Cold, clammy extremities and anuria may be present.

Cardiac tamponade is easily confused with other etiologies of shock, such as sepsis or internal hemorrhage. However, systemic venous pressure is not elevated in these conditions (Chap. 18). Therefore, a keen awareness of the possibility of acute cardiac tamponade is essential in patients with a history of accident, trauma, or an invasive cardiac procedure. Cardiac tamponade due to rupture of the heart from acute myocardial infarction may also be confused with cardiogenic shock due to myocardial failure per se, but in the latter condition severe left atrial hypertension with pulmonary edema as well as jugular venous distention are likely to be present. Cardiac tamponade may occasionally be confused with shock due to right ventricular infarction with jugular venous distention and clear lungs. However, the hemodynamics of right ventricular infarction are more like those of constrictive physiology than of tamponade (p. 1505).

Patients in whom cardiac tamponade develops slowly differ from those with cardiac tamponade due to cardiac penetration or rupture. In the setting of more slowly developing cardiac tamponade, patients usually appear acutely ill but not in extremis and the major complaint is usually dyspnea.[124,127] Chest pain of either a pleuritic or an oppressive nature may also be present. In patients with chronic development of tamponade, additional systemic symptoms may include weight loss, anorexia, and profound weakness.

The most common physical finding in a series of medical patients with cardiac tamponade was *jugular venous distention.*[124] In addition to absolute elevation of the systemic venous pressure, a characteristic waveform consisting of a prominent systolic *x* descent and absent diastolic *y* descent can often be appreciated at the bedside. Other common physical findings include tachypnea (80 per cent), tachycardia (77 per cent), pulsus paradoxus (77 per cent), pulsus paradoxus with total inspiratory disappearance of the brachial pulse and Korotkoff sounds (23 per cent), pericardial friction rub (29 per cent), hepatomegaly (55 per cent), and diminished heart sounds (34 per cent). It is noteworthy that systolic arterial hypotension, consisting of a systolic pressure less than 100 mm Hg, was present in a minority (36 per cent), and the majority of patients were alert, with warm extremities and preserved urine output.[124]

The finding of *pulsus paradoxus* is critical in making the diagnosis of cardiac tamponade, since most patients with slowly developing cardiac tamponade do not have the classic physical findings of a small, quiet heart and severe hypotension.[124,128] Pulsus paradoxus can be detected on physical examination as an inspiratory decrease in the amplitude of the palpated pulse in the femoral or carotid arteries. Total paradox, i.e., complete disappearance of the palpated pulse during inspiration, occurs during very severe cardiac tamponade or tamponade combined with hypovolemia. The magnitude of the paradoxical pulse can be accurately quantified by means of an intraarterial catheter but may be estimated by cuff sphygmomanometry. The cuff should be inflated 20 mm Hg above systolic pressure and slowly deflated until the Korotkoff sounds are heard only during expiration. The cuff should then be deflated to the point at which Korotkoff sounds are heard equally well in inspiration and expiration. The difference between these pressures is the estimated magnitude of pulsus paradoxus.

Other disorders with systemic venous distention, pulsus paradoxus, and clear lungs that can be confused with cardiac tamponade include obstructive pulmonary disease,[121,122] constrictive pericarditis, restrictive cardiomyopathy,[129] right ventricular infarction,[49] and massive pulmonary embolism.[119,120] Pulsus paradoxus is occasionally noted in shock, but jugular venous distention is usually absent.[130]

The clinical findings may be further modified in patients with so-called *low-pressure cardiac tamponade*[131] who are normotensive and in whom the physical examination is normal except for moderate elevation of jugular venous pressure to about 5 to 15 mm Hg. This syndrome represents an early stage in the development of cardiac tamponade in which accumulation of a pericardial effusion causes intrapericardial pressure to rise to a level of 5 to 15 mm Hg, with equilibration of intrapericardial and right heart diastolic filling pressures. Pericardiocentesis reduces intrapericardial pressure and the separation of right atrial and intrapericardial pressures. Low-pressure cardiac tamponade has been reported in patients with tuberculosis and neoplastic pericarditis and is often associated with severe dehydration.

CHEST ROENTGENOGRAM. There are no roentgenographic features diagnostic of cardiac tamponade. The heart may appear completely normal in size in cardiac tamponade that develops from acute hemopericardium due to cardiac rupture or laceration. On the other hand, if an effusion accumulates more slowly to more than 250 ml, the cardiac silhouette may be enlarged.[127] Other roentgenographic findings may include obscuring of vessels at the hilum, a globular or waterbottle configuration of the heart, clear lungs, and separation of epicardial and pericardial fat pads. These findings suggest the presence of a large pericardial effusion but supply no information about its hemodynamic significance.

ELECTROCARDIOGRAM. The electrocardiographic abnormalities seen in acute cardiac tamponade include those of acute pericarditis and pericardial effusion per se (p. 1476). The development of electrical alternans[132–135] is a more specific indicator of pericardial tamponade and reflects pendular swinging of the heart within the pericardial space (Fig. 43–12).[136–138] Electrical alternans may also occur in constrictive pericarditis, in tension pneumothorax, after myocardial infarction, and with severe cardiac muscle dysfunction. However, the appearance of electrical alternans in a patient with a known pericardial effusion is highly suggestive of cardiac tamponade—a finding that has been confirmed in experimental cardiac tamponade.[139] Electrical alternans of the QRS complex may occur in a 2:1 or 3:1 pattern. Alternans is usually limited to the QRS complex, but alternans of the P wave, QRS complex, and T wave may rarely occur and appears to be limited to extreme cardiac tamponade,[140] often in association with neoplastic or tuberculous effusion. Both the abnormal heart motion within the pericardial sac and electrical alternans disappear when pericardial fluid is aspirated.

ECHOCARDIOGRAM. In patients with jugular venous distention and the possibility of cardiac tamponade, echocardiography is extremely useful and should be performed prior to consideration of pericardiocentesis. In a rare patient who is in extremis from the extremely rapid development of cardiac tamponade, the physician may have to rely on the history and physical findings to make a judgment about the need for pericardiocentesis. If echocardiography is readily available and the patient with suspected cardiac tamponade is not moribund, obtaining an echocardiogram will increase the likelihood of diagnosing cardiac tamponade correctly. First, the echocardiogram helps to document the presence and magnitude of a pericardial effusion (Figs. 5–74, p. 131, and 5–75 and 5–76, p. 133), the absence of echocardiographic evidence of a pericardial effusion virtually excludes the diagnosis of cardiac tamponade (with the important exception of the postoperative cardiac surgery patient in whom loculated fluid or thrombus may cause cardiac compression). Second, the echocardiogram can rapidly differentiate cardiac tamponade from other causes of systemic venous hypertension and hypotension, including constrictive pericarditis, cardiac muscle dysfunction, and right ventricular infarction. The appearance of dense echoes in the pericardial space or extrinsic to the pericardium suggests the presence of material other than free fluid. Both massive extracardiac hematoma and extrinsic compression of the heart by tumor[141,142] can cause cardiac compression with the physiology of cardiac constriction or cardiac tamponade. When the echocardiogram excludes a pericardial effusion, inappropriate and potentially lethal attempts at pericardiocentesis or pericardiotomy can be avoided.

The echocardiogram can provide additional clues that a pericardial effusion is associated with cardiac tamponade. These important features include a gross reduction in the E-to-F slope and excursion of the anterior mitral valve leaflet,[115] early systolic notching of the anterior right ventricular wall, and sudden posterior motion of the interventricular septum during inspiration.[143] Acute cardiac tamponade has also been shown to be associated with right ventricular diastolic collapse[144] and an exaggerated inspiratory increase and expiratory decrease in right ventricular size.[144,145,145a] The echocardiographic findings of a pericardial effusion, a progressive fall in right ventricular dimensions during expiration, and an inspiratory increase in right ventricular dimensions suggest the diagnosis of cardiac tamponade. However, these changes are not specific,[146] and experimental studies indicate that a single echocardiogram cannot predict the presence or severity of cardiac tamponade.[147]

Radionuclide angiography can also detect right ventricu-

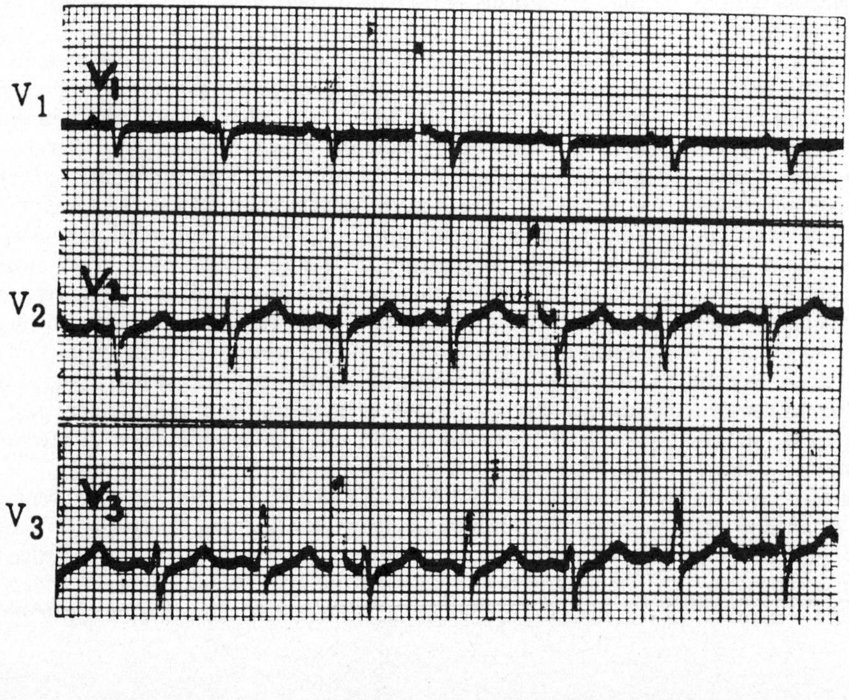

FIGURE 43–12 Electrical alternans (phasic alteration of the amplitude of the R wave) is present in a patient with pericardial effusion and cardiac tamponade. In lead V_3, the polarity of the QRS complex also alternates every other beat. (From Goldman, M. J.: Principles of Clinical Electrocardiography, 11th Edition. Los Altos, Lange Medical Publications, 1982, p. 305.)

lar and right atrial compression and compression of the superior vena cava as it enters the pericardium,[148] but these findings, while suggestive of cardiac tamponade, also lack sensitivity and specificity. Therefore it must be emphasized that cardiac tamponade is a clinical not an echocardiographic or a radionuclide diagnosis that is established definitively by documentation of the elevation and equilibration of intrapericardial and right atrial pressures and the reversal of these findings by evacuation of pericardial fluid.

CARDIAC CATHETERIZATION AND ANGIOGRAPHY

Cardiac catheterization is invaluable in establishing the hemodynamic importance of a pericardial effusion. Except in extreme emergencies, situations when the patient is moribund, we prefer to catheterize the right heart and pericardial space in conjunction with pericardiocentesis. Cardiac catheterization (1) provides absolute confirmation of the diagnosis of cardiac tamponade; (2) quantitates the magnitude of hemodynamic compromise; (3) guides pericardiocentesis by documenting that pericardial aspiration is associated with hemodynamic improvement; and (4) permits the detection of coexisting hemodynamic problems including left ventricular failure, right atrial hypertension due to tricuspid valve disease,[149] and effusive-constrictive pericarditis (p. 1496).

Cardiac catheterization typically demonstrates elevation of right atrial pressure with a characteristic prominent systolic x descent and a diminutive or absent y descent. When intrapericardial and right atrial pressures are recorded simultaneously, both are elevated and virtually identical (Fig. 43–10); both pressures fall during inspiration, and intrapericardial pressure may fall slightly below right atrial pressure during systolic ejection at the time of the x descent. If intrapericardial pressure is not elevated, and if right atrial and intrapericardial pressures are not virtually identical, the diagnosis of cardiac tamponade must be reconsidered.

Right ventricular diastolic pressure is elevated and equal to right atrial and intrapericardial pressures and lacks the dip-and-plateau configuration characteristic of constrictive pericarditis. Since right ventricular and pulmonary artery systolic pressures are equal to the pressure developed by the right ventricle plus the intrapericardial pressure, right ventricular and pulmonary artery systolic pressures are usually moderately elevated in the range of 35 to 50 mm Hg. It may be difficult to differentiate right ventricular and pulmonary artery waveforms without the use of fluoroscopy. In the case of severe cardiac compression, right ventricular systolic pressure may be reduced and only slightly higher than right ventricular diastolic pressure.

Usually, the pulmonary capillary wedge pressure and left ventricular diastolic pressure are elevated and equal to intrapericardial pressure when recorded simultaneously. However, in patients with severe underlying left ventricular dysfunction and marked elevation of the left ventricular diastolic pressure prior to the development of pericardial effusion, cardiac tamponade can be present when intrapericardial and right atrial pressures are equal but lower than left ventricular diastolic pressure.[95] Depending on the severity of cardiac compression, left ventricular systolic and aortic pressures may be normal or reduced.

Pulsus paradoxus can be easily documented by intraarterial catheterization and pressure measurement. Simultaneous recording of systemic arterial and right ventricular pressures shows that the inspiratory pressure variation is out of phase (Fig. 43–11). Stroke volume is usually markedly depressed. Cardiac output may be normal, owing to the compensatory effect of tachycardia, or it may be markedly reduced when cardiac tamponade is severe; systemic vascular resistance is usually elevated.

Angiographic studies are not essential if echocardiographic findings suggestive of cardiac tamponade were obtained prior to cardiac catheterization. Right atrial angiography usually demonstrates an abnormal concave appearance of the right atrial heart border and a water density extrinsic to the contrast-filled right atrium due to presence of the pericardial effusion.[150] In an otherwise normal heart, right and left ventricular end-diastolic volumes are usually reduced with normal or increased ejection fractions.

Aspiration of pericardial fluid results initially in the lowering of the identical intrapericardial, right atrial, right ventricular, and left ventricular diastolic pressures, followed by a fall of intrapericardial pressure below right atrial pressure and reappearance of the y descent in the right atrial waveform (Fig. 43–10). Further aspiration causes intrapericardial pressure to fall to a mean level of zero. Since the pressure-volume curve of the pericardium is steep, the initial aspiration of 50 to 100 ml of pericardial fluid usually leads to a striking reduction in intrapericardial pressure, a striking improvement in systemic arterial pressure and cardiac output, and abolition of pulsus paradoxus (Fig. 43–13).

If intrapericardial pressure falls to zero or becomes negative and right atrial pressure remains elevated, *effusive-*

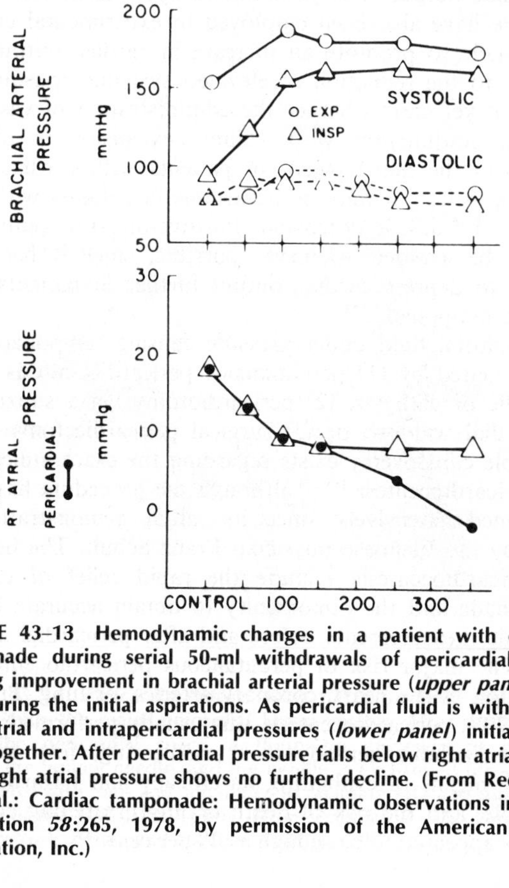

FIGURE 43–13 Hemodynamic changes in a patient with cardiac tamponade during serial 50-ml withdrawals of pericardial fluid. Striking improvement in brachial arterial pressure (*upper panel*) occurs during the initial aspirations. As pericardial fluid is withdrawn, right atrial and intrapericardial pressures (*lower panel*) initially decline together. After pericardial pressure falls below right atrial pressure, right atrial pressure shows no further decline. (From Reddy, P. S., et al.: Cardiac tamponade: Hemodynamic observations in man. Circulation *58*:265, 1978, by permission of the American Heart Association, Inc.)

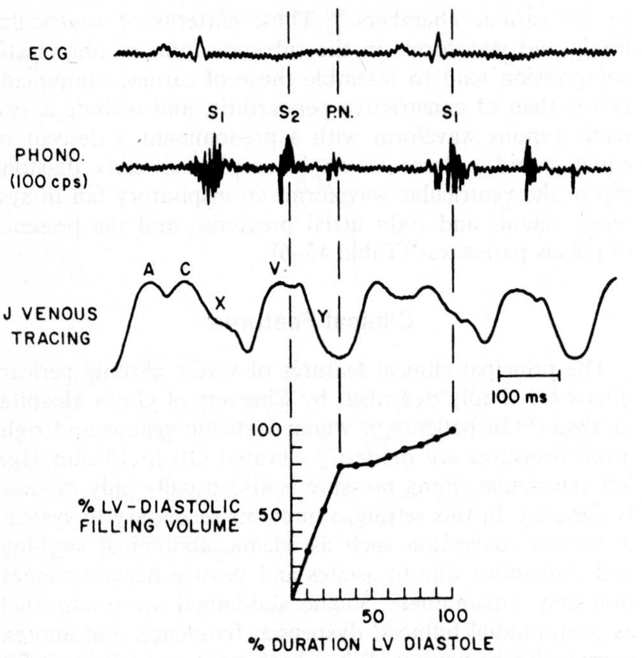

FIGURE 43–18 Electrocardiogram (ECG), phonocardiogram (PHONO), jugular venous pulse tracing, and left ventricular (LV) diastolic filling curve in a patient with constrictive pericarditis and pericardial knock (PN). The pericardial knock occurs simultaneously with the nadir of the diastolic *y* descent and sudden plateau of the LV filling curve. (From Tyberg, T. I., et al.: Genesis of pericardial knock in constrictive pericarditis. Am. J. Cardiol. *46*:570, 1980.)

tion and chronic constrictive pericarditis by neck vein examination at the bedside. The finding of Kussmaul's sign (an inspiratory increase in systemic venous pressure) is difficult to appreciate at the bedside and may be confused with exaggerated amplitude of the venous waves during inspiration.

The arterial pulse may be normal or show a diminished pulse pressure. Severe pulsus paradoxus is uncommon in rigid constrictive pericarditis and rarely exceeds 15 mm Hg unless pericardial fluid under pressure is also present. In some patients the precordium is quiet, while in others there is strikingly visible systolic retraction of the apical impulse. The most impressive abnormality during auscultation is the *diastolic pericardial knock* (see Figure 3–16, p. 51), an early diastolic sound that is often heard along the left sternal border in rigid constrictive pericarditis, infrequently heard in subacute constrictive pericarditis of the fibroelastic variety, and not heard in pure cardiac tamponade.[189] The pericardial knock usually occurs 0.09 to 0.12 second after A_2 and corresponds in timing to the sudden cessation of ventricular filling and the premature diastolic plateau of the diastolic ventricular volume curve (Fig. 43–18).[203,204] The pericardial knock tends to occur earlier and to have a higher acoustic frequency than the typical S_3 gallop sound, and therefore it may be confused with the opening snap of mitral stenosis. Widening of the aortic and pulmonic components of the second heart sound may occur in constrictive pericarditis. This is attributed to a fixed right ventricular stroke volume during inspiration due to pericardial compression as well as the presence of premature aortic valve closure due to a transitory inspiratory decrease in left ventricular stroke volume.[205]

Hepatomegaly is usually present and may be accompanied by ascites. Other evidence of hepatic dysfunction secondary to passive liver congestion and diminished cardiac output may include icterus, spider angiomas, and palmar erythema. In young patients with competent venous valves, edema of the extremities may be noticeably absent in the presence of marked abdominal distention. Older patients with longstanding constrictive pericarditis may have enormous ascites and massive swelling of the scrotum, thighs, and calves. In contrast, the upper torso and arms may show evidence of marked muscle wasting and cachexia.

CHEST ROENTGENOGRAM (See also page 176). The cardiac silhouette may be small, normal, or enlarged. Cardiac enlargement may be apparent due to coexisting pericardial effusion, the contribution of an enormously thickened pericardium, or preexisting cardiac chamber enlargement or hypertrophy. The right superior mediastinum may be prominent due to engorgement of the superior vena cava, and left atrial enlargement is common.[206] Extensive calcification of the pericardium is present in approximately half the patients and raises the possibility of a tubercular etiology. However, this finding is not specific for constrictive pericarditis in that a calcified pericardium is not necessarily a constricted one. Calcification of the pericardium is often detected on the lateral chest film in the atrioventricular groove or along the anterior and diaphragmatic surfaces of the right ventricle. Fluoroscopy may be helpful in distinguishing pericardial calcification from calcium within the wall of a myocardial aneurysm or thrombus or within the mitral or aortic valves, mitral annulus, or coronary arteries. Pleural effusions are present in the majority of patients.[207] Since left atrial pressure is commonly elevated to between 15 to 30 mm Hg, there may be evidence of redistribution of blood flow, while Kerley's B lines or infiltrates suggestive of frank pulmonary edema are rare (Table 43–7).

ELECTROCARDIOGRAM. Electrocardiographic findings include low QRS voltage, generalized T-wave inversion or flattening, and left atrial abnormalities suggestive of P mitrale (Fig. 43–19).[58,199] Atrial fibrillation occurs in less than half the patients with constrictive pericarditis and is thought to be related to longstanding elevation of atrial pressures and atrial enlargement. In a study of constrictive pericarditis in which postmortem specimens were available, Levine noted that atrioventricular block, intraventricular conduction defects, and pseudoinfarction patterns with deep wide Q waves seemed to be related to an extension of calcification into the myocardium and around the coronary arteries, compromising coronary blood flow.[197] An unusual pattern of right ventricular hypertrophy and right-axis deviation may be present in patients with dense pericardial scar overlying the right ventricular outflow tract.[208]

ECHOCARDIOGRAM (See also page 133). One distinct pattern of pericardial thickening in constrictive peri-

TABLE 43–7 RADIOLOGICAL FEATURES OF CONSTRICTIVE PERICARDITIS

Normal heart size	33%
Enlarged heart	67%
Calcified pericardium	43%
Pleural effusion	83%
Pulmonary venous congestion	86%
Left atrial enlargement	85%

Modified from Pulvaneswary, M., et al.: Constrictive pericarditis: Clinical, hemodynamic, and radiologic correlation. Australas. Radiol. *26*:53, 1982.

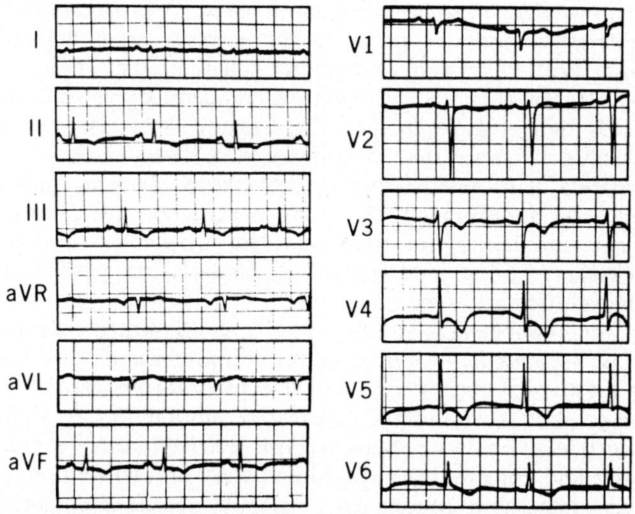

FIGURE 43–19 **Electrocardiogram of a patient with chronic constrictive pericarditis showing a wide notched P wave in lead II and diffuse T-wave inversion. (From Spodick, D. H.: Pathogenesis and clinical correlations of the electrocardiographic abnormalities of pericardial disease. Cardiovasc. Clin. *8*:201, 1977.)**

carditis consists of two parallel lines representing the visceral and parietal pericardia separated by a clear space of at least 1 mm; another consists of multiple dense echoes (Fig. 43–20).[209] In the absence of a pericardial effusion, it is sometimes difficult to differentiate a thickened pericardium from other causes of thickening of the left ventricular posterior wall, such as myocardial hypertrophy or infiltration. Extreme respiratory variation in the depth of the pulmonic valve *a* wave[210] and premature pulmonic valve opening secondary to a high right ventricular early diastolic pressure may be present,[211] but these changes are also seen in other disorders with high right ventricular early diastolic pressure, such as tricuspid and pulmonic regurgitation. Other echocardiographic abnormalities include reduced motion of the left ventricular posterior wall endocardium of less than 1 mm[212] and abnormal motion of the interventricular septum, evident as systolic flattening and abrupt posterior motion in early diastole, coinciding with the pericardial knock.[213,214] The abnormality in septal motion is not specific and may also occur in bundle branch block, volume overload, and aortic regurgitation in which rapid early diastolic left ventricular filling occurs. The abnormal pattern of rapid early diastolic filling seen in constrictive pericarditis may be reflected in an echocardiographic pattern of abrupt early diastolic posterior motion of the aortic root,[215] and the pattern of a rapid increase in left ventricular dimension in early diastole followed by no change in dimension in mid or late diastole.[216]

About 75 per cent of patients with constrictive pericarditis have at least one of the above findings.[217] The presence of pericardial thickening alone is not diagnostic of constrictive pericarditis, and the likelihood of this diagnosis increases if there is also evidence of an abnormal early rapid diastolic filling pattern and elevation of right ventricular diastolic pressure.

Two-dimensional echocardiography in constrictive pericarditis has been reported to show an immobile and dense appearance of the pericardium, bulging of the interventricular septum into the left ventricle during inspiration, prominent early diastolic filling, and dilatation of the hepatic veins and inferior vena cava.[218]

Other Laboratory Findings. Other abnormal laboratory findings may be present due to chronic elevation of right atrial pressure causing passive congestion of the liver, kidneys, and gastrointestinal tract. These include depressed serum albumin, elevated serum globulin, elevated conjugated and unconjugated serum bilirubin, and abnormal hepatocellular function tests. Protein-losing enteropathy may be evident from the presence of albumin in the stool, and lymphangiectasis on small bowel biopsy.[219,220] Elevated systemic venous pressure may also produce variable degrees of albuminuria as well as pronounced protein loss consistent with the nephrotic syndrome.[221,222] Nonspecific evidence of the presence of chronic disease such as a normocytic and normochromic anemia may be found.

Cardiac Catheterization and Angiography

Cardiac catheterization is useful in the assessment of patients suspected of having constrictive pericarditis (1) to document the presence of elevation and equilibration of diastolic filling pressures, (2) to assess the effects of constrictive pericarditis on stroke volume and cardiac output, (3) to evaluate myocardial systolic function, and (4) to assist in the difficult discrimination between constrictive pericarditis and restrictive cardiomyopathy.

Catheterization of both the right and left ventricles should be performed to permit the simultaneous recording of right and left heart filling pressures. Typical findings include the elevation and virtual identity (within 5 mm Hg) of right atrial, right ventricular diastolic, left atrial (pulmonary capillary wedge), and left ventricular diastolic

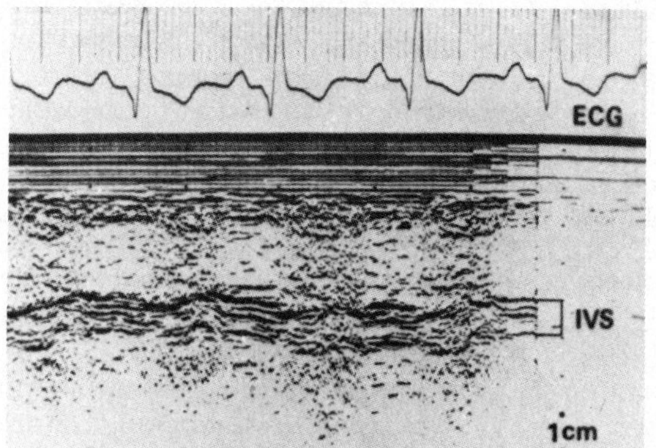

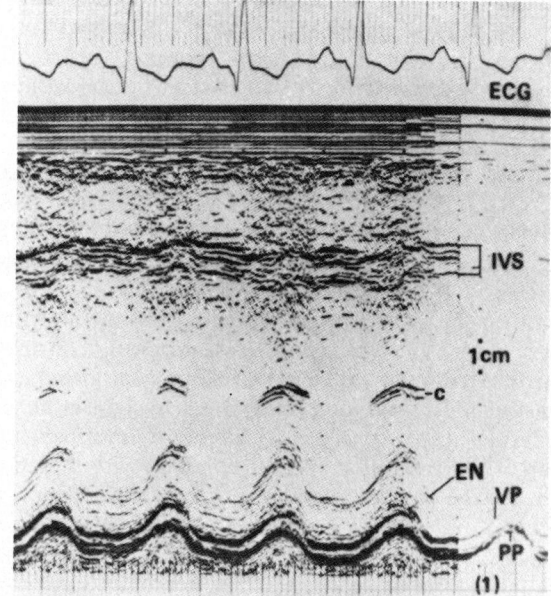

FIGURE 43–20 **Echocardiogram from a patient with constrictive pericarditis. Two intense parallel echoes, separated by a small clear space, can be seen posterior to the left ventricular endocardium (EN). At surgery or autopsy, this pattern is usually associated with dense adhesions between the parietal (PP) and visceral (VP) pericardium. ECG = electrocardiogram; IVS = interventricular septum. (From Schnittger, I., et al.: Echocardiography: Pericardial thickening and constrictive pericarditis. Am. J. Cardiol. *42*:388, 1978.)**

pressures. Right atrial pressure is characterized by a preserved systolic *x* descent, a prominent early diastolic *y* descent, and *a* and *v* waves that are small and equal in height and result in the typical "M" or "W" configurations. Both the right and left ventricular diastolic pressures show an early diastolic dip followed by a pressure plateau.[99,167,223] This sign may be obscured by the presence of tachycardia (Fig. 43–16). Care must be taken during pressure recording to use small displacement transducers and to avoid excessive use of connecting tubes or bubbles within the catheters and transducers. Right ventricular and pulmonary artery systolic pressures are usually modestly elevated, in the range of 35 to 40 mm Hg, and rarely exceed 60 mm Hg.

Careful recordings during respiration show that mean right atrial pressure fails to decrease normally or actually rises during inspiration. Since inspiration is associated with the transient pooling of blood within the pulmonary bed and a reduction in right ventricular afterload, inspiration causes a fall in pulmonary artery and right ventricular systolic pressures, pulmonary capillary wedge pressure, and left ventricular diastolic pressure. Because constrictive pericarditis is not associated with marked inspiratory swings in right ventricular filling, pulsus paradoxus is usually absent or less prominent than that observed in cardiac tamponade. Both cardiac output and stroke volume are low-normal or depressed.[167,224] When they are depressed, compensatory tachycardia and elevation of systemic vascular resistance may be found.

The *left ventricular angiogram* usually demonstrates that left ventricular end-systolic and end-diastolic volumes are normal or decreased. In the absence of myocardial fibrosis or inflammation, both isovolumetric and ejection phase indices of systolic function (Chap. 14) are normal.[223,225] Venous angiography may demonstrate superior vena caval dilatation and straightening of the right heart border[226]; pericardial thickening may be detectable. Coronary angiography may demonstrate that the coronary arteries are within the cardiac silhouette rather than on the surface of the heart,[227,228] and rarely diastolic pinching or external compression of the coronary arteries may be detected.[229]

HEMODYNAMIC DIFFERENTIATION AMONG CONSTRICTIVE PERICARDITIS, CARDIAC TAMPONADE, AND RESTRICTIVE CARDIOMYOPATHY. Although both constrictive pericarditis and tamponade are characterized by elevation and equilibration of right and left ventricular diastolic pressures, several hemodynamic features differ. In contrast to patients with constrictive pericarditis, patients with cardiac tamponade demonstrate (1) marked pulsus paradoxus, (2) a fall in right atrial pressure during inspiration, (3) elevation of intrapericardial pressure, (4) a right atrial pressure tracing with a predominant *x* descent and an attenuated or absent *y* descent, and (5) *lack* of a prominent dip-and-plateau pattern in the right and left ventricular pressure pulses.

The findings of cardiac catheterization help to differentiate some but not all patients with *constrictive pericarditis* from those with *restrictive cardiomyopathy* (p. 1422) due to amyloidosis, hemochromatosis, or other causes. In both conditions, right and left ventricular diastolic pressures are elevated, stroke volume and cardiac output are depressed, left ventricular end-diastolic volume is normal or decreased, and diastolic filling is impaired.[230] A diagnosis of restrictive cardiomyopathy is more likely when marked right ventricular systolic hypertension is present (pressure > 60 mm Hg), and left ventricular diastolic pressure exceeds right ventricular diastolic pressure at rest or during exercise by more than 5 mm Hg.[231,232] However, in some patients with restrictive cardiomyopathy, hemodynamics may be indistinguishable from constrictive pericarditis, with equilibration of right and left ventricular diastolic pressures and a predominant dip-and-plateau pattern in the ventricular waveforms.[167,232,233]

Angiographically, straightening of the right heart border may be present in both conditions, and thickening of the heart border may be detected due to either pericardial or myocardial thickening.[234] Decreased motion of the right ventricular free wall occurs in both restrictive cardiomyopathy and constrictive pericarditis, while normal motion of the crista supraventricularis is usually present in constrictive pericarditis but not in restrictive cardiomyopathy.[235]

The finding of a depressed left ventricular ejection fraction in the presence of a small heart has been suggested as a discriminating feature of restrictive cardiomyopathy.[234] However, the left ventricular ejection fraction may be normal in some patients with restrictive cardiomyopathy and, conversely, is occasionally reduced in patients with constrictive pericarditis.[232,233] Frame-by-frame analysis of left ventricular filling has been suggested as a method for distinguishing between constrictive pericarditis and restrictive cardiomyopathy.[236] In constrictive pericarditis, early diastolic filling tends to be excessively rapid in contrast to restrictive cardiomyopathy, in which early diastolic filling is slower than normal (Fig. 43–21).

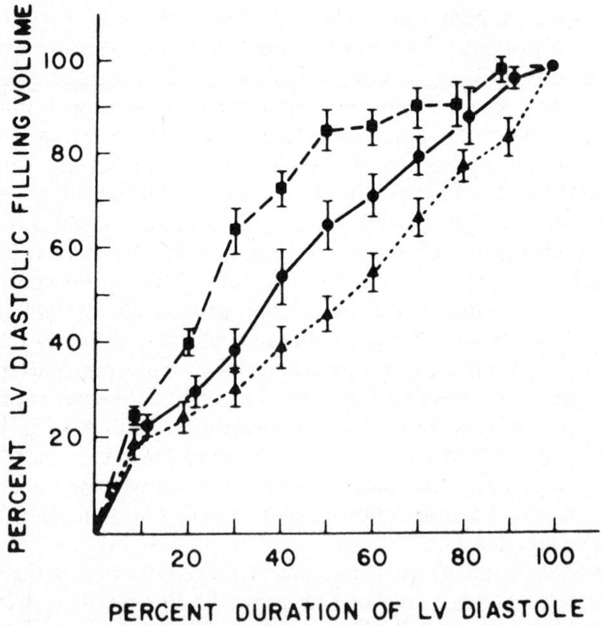

FIGURE 43–21 Composite left ventricular (LV) filling volume curves in normal subjects (solid line, circles), in patients with constrictive pericarditis (dashed line, solid squares), and in patients with restrictive amyloid cardiomyopathy (dotted line, triangles). Early left ventricular filling is exceedingly rapid in patients with constrictive pericarditis, whereas in patients with restrictive cardiomyopathy it is slower than normal. (From Tyberg, T. I., et al.: Left ventricular filling in differentiating restrictive amyloid cardiomyopathy and constrictive pericarditis. Am. J. Cardiol. *47*:791, 1981.)

Endomyocardial biopsy has also proved useful in documenting the presence of amyloidosis in patients in whom constrictive pericarditis and restrictive cardiomyopathy could not be differentiated at cardiac catheterization.[232] However, normal findings on endomyocardial biopsy do not exclude the presence of restrictive cardiomyopathy.[233] Furthermore, a pericardial effusion may rarely coexist with amyloid heart disease.[237,238] In a minority of patients, exploratory thoracotomy with careful examination of both pericardial and myocardial biopsy specimens is warranted to differentiate constrictive pericarditis, a condition that is usually treatable surgically, from restrictive cardiomyopathy, in which treatment is usually expectant.[238]

Diagnosis

Constrictive pericarditis should be suspected in patients with jugular venous distention, unexplained cardiac enlargement, hepatomegaly, systemic edema, or ascites.[202] It must be distinguished from superior vena caval obstruction, nephrotic syndrome, hepatic or intraabdominal disease due to malignancy, and other cardiac causes of right atrial hypertension including restrictive cardiomyopathy, tricuspid stenosis, tricuspid regurgitation, hypertrophic cardiomyopathy, and right atrial myxoma. Supportive, but nondiagnostic clinical features include a history of prior cardiothoracic trauma, acute pericarditis, or prior mediastinal irradiation; on physical examination there may be an early diastolic sound or knock in the absence of cardiac murmurs, and the heart is not massively enlarged. The roentgenogram may show pericardial calcification, and the echocardiogram reveals a thickened pericardium and abnormal diastolic filling patterns. The electrocardiogram may reveal notched P waves, atrial fibrillation, and low QRS voltage.

In the presence of findings suggestive of constrictive pericarditis, right and left heart catheterization with simultaneous pressure measurements should be performed to document the presence of constrictive physiology and to exclude other cardiac causes of right atrial hypertension. Diuresis should be avoided prior to catheterization, since hypovolemia may obscure both the characteristic abnormal waveforms and the elevation and equilibration of right and left heart filling pressures. In patients with a suggestive history but normal hemodynamics, a rapid saline volume challenge should be performed to exclude occult constrictive pericardial disease (p. 1496).

When pericardiocentesis is performed in the catheterization laboratory for cardiac tamponade, right and left heart filling pressures should be meticulously recorded after aspiration to exclude the presence of residual constrictive physiology due to effusive-constrictive pericarditis (p. 1496).

As discussed above, it may be extremely difficult to distinguish patients with constrictive pericarditis from those with restrictive physiology due to amyloidosis,[239–241] hemochromatosis,[242] endomyocardial fibrosis,[243] or eosinophilic endocarditis.[244,245] Both constrictive pericarditis and restrictive cardiomyopathy may show the electrocardiographic changes of atrial fibrillation, left atrial abnormalities, and diffuse low QRS voltage with T-wave flattening. The presence of atrioventricular block and conduction disturbances simulating myocardial infarction favors the diagnosis of restrictive cardiomyopathy. Echocardiography in some patients with restrictive cardiomyopathy may show abnormal thickening of the ventricular myocardium or a peculiar "sparkling" appearance when amyloidosis is present.[246–248] The simultaneous use of electrocardiography and echocardiography to demonstrate a reduction of the voltage/mass ratio has been described in patients with amyloid restrictive cardiomyopathy in whom diffuse low QRS voltage is associated with increased thickness of the left ventricular wall due to amyloid deposition.[249] As noted above, cardiac catheterization and angiography, often with endomyocardial biopsy, are usually helpful in discriminating constrictive pericarditis from restrictive cardiomyopathy in many patients, but, in a minority, an exploratory thoracotomy may be required.

Management

Constrictive pericarditis is a progressive disease without spontaneous reversal of either pericardial thickening or abnormal symptoms and hemodynamics. A minority of patients may survive for many years with modest jugular venous distention and peripheral edema that is controlled by the judicious use of diet and diuretics. The majority of patients who are symptomatic and come to medical attention, however, become progressively more disabled by weakness, ascites and peripheral edema and subsequently suffer the complications of severe cardiac cachexia. Treatment for constrictive pericarditis is complete resection of the pericardium.

Prior to 1971, surgical mortality from pericardiectomy performed for constrictive pericarditis ranged from 4 to 23 per cent.[250,251] Recent changes in technique have included the use of a median sternotomy, cardiopulmonary bypass to permit greater mobilization of the heart,[252] and performance of pericardiectomy earlier in the course of the disease prior to the appearance of cardiac cachexia and dense pericardial calcification. More recent series have cited an operative mortality of about 4 to 6 per cent,[253–255] and long-term improvement in hemodynamics and symptoms has been reported in about 75 per cent of patients who survive the operation.[253,255–265]

Pericardiectomy should probably not be attempted in patients with very early and mild disease whose symptoms can be completely controlled with the use of a mild diuretic or in very elderly patients with severe liver dysfunction, cachexia, densely calcified pericardium, and massive cardiac enlargement indicative of underlying myocardial damage.[258] Patients with known or suspected tubercular pericarditis should be treated with multidrug anti tuberculosis therapy for two to four weeks prior to operation; if the diagnosis is confirmed, these drugs should be continued for 6 to 12 months after pericardiectomy.

The most common surgical approach for pericardiectomy is via a median sternotomy with cardiopulmonary bypass to permit maximum mobilization of the heart and extensive resection of the pericardium. Complete removal of the parietal pericardium from the phrenic nerve to phrenic nerve is attempted, including freeing up of the atria and venae cavae if obvious constricting bands are present[252,253]; however, care must be taken to avoid laceration of the thin-walled atria and epicardial veins and arteries. If the heart fails to expand and pulsate more vigorously after removal of the parietal pericardium, the possibility of epicardial constriction and the need for visceral pericardiectomy must be considered by the surgeon.

Marked hemodynamic and symptomatic improvement is apparent in some patients immediately after operation. In others, symptomatic improvement and resolution of elevated jugular venous pressure and abnormal filling patterns may be delayed for weeks to months.[253,256,262,263] This delayed or inadequate response to pericardiectomy has been attributed to incomplete pericardial resection,[264] myocardial involvement by the calcified and fibrotic inflammatory process,[265] and epicardial sclerosis.[266]

EFFUSIVE-CONSTRICTIVE PERICARDITIS

Effusive-constrictive pericarditis is the condition of a tense pericardial effusion in the presence of visceral pericardial constriction.[267,268] The hallmark of this condition is continued elevation of right atrial pressure after the aspiration of pericardial fluid and restoration of intrapericardial pressure to zero. This entity may represent a stage in the development of classic constrictive pericarditis. The most common causes of effusive-constrictive pericarditis are the same as for chronic constrictive pericarditis (p. 1489) and include idiopathic or presumed viral pericarditis, tuberculosis, neoplastic infiltration of the pericardium, and mediastinal irradiation.[141,268] *Symptoms* are nonspecific and include atypical chest pain and a heavy sensation over the precordium; in advanced cases, exertional dyspnea may be present.

The *physical findings* usually resemble those of cardiac tamponade, including pulsus paradoxus, a normal or diminished pulse pressure, and jugular venous distention with a predominant *x* descent and an absent *y* descent. The chest roentgenogram usually shows cardiac enlargement consistent with the presence of a pericardial effusion, and the electrocardiogram may show nonspecific ST- and T-wave abnormalities or diffuse low QRS voltage. Both M-mode and wide-angle two-dimensional echocardiograms may show a pericardial effusion sandwiched between thickened pericardial membranes with fibrinous pericardial bands (Fig. 43–22).[269,270]

Although effusive-constrictive pericarditis can be suspected on clinical grounds, the diagnosis is made by recording right heart and intrapericardial pressures both before and after pericardiocentesis. Prior to pericardiocentesis, the physiology of cardiac tamponade may be present (p. 1480) with elevation and equilibration of intrapericardial, right atrial, right ventricular, and left ventricular diastolic pressures. The right atrial pressure tracing usually shows a prominent *x* descent and an inspiratory fall in right heart filling pressure. Pericardiocentesis with restoration of intrapericardial pressure to zero may reduce pulsus paradoxus and improve cardiac output, but it does not restore the hemodynamics entirely to normal. After pericardiocentesis, there is persistent elevation and equilibration of right atrial and right and left ventricular diastolic pressures. The waveforms convert to a pattern like that in constrictive pericarditis, with a prominent *y* descent in the right atrial pressure tracing, a dip-and-plateau pattern in the right ventricular pressure, and the absence of respiratory variation in right heart filling pressures (Fig. 43–23).

Pericardiocentesis may be useful in transiently improving systemic arterial pressure and cardiac output. However, persistent constriction after successful pericardiocentesis indicates the presence of a thickened, constrictive visceral pericardium and the need for further intervention. Treatment consists of total parietal and visceral pericardiectomy[271] and specific therapy for underlying malignancy or tuberculosis, if present.

Occult Constrictive Pericarditis

Bush and coworkers have described a variant of constrictive pericarditis characterized by the presence of significant pericardial disease without overt evidence of cardiac constriction on physical examination or during routine cardiac catheterization.[272,273] The majority of patients have a history of prior acute pericarditis; symptoms are nonspecific and include chronic disabling chest pain, fatigue, and dyspnea. In most patients, the chest roentgenogram reveals borderline cardiomegaly while pericardial calcification is infrequent. The electrocardiogram shows nonspecific ST- and T-wave abnormalities. The echocardiogram is normal in most patients and a minority show either a small pericardial effusion or a filling pattern suggestive of constrictive pericarditis.[272]

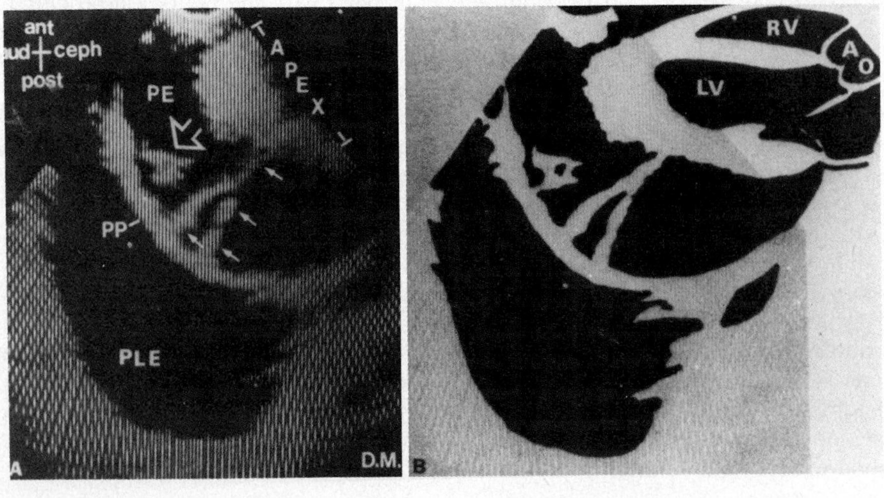

FIGURE 43–22 Two-dimensional echocardiogram (*A*) and schematic diagram (*B*) from a patient with postradiation pericarditis. Dense intrapericardial bands denoting pericardial adhesions (large and small arrows) are present within the pericardial effusion (PE). PP = parietal pericardium; PLE = pleural effusion; RV = right ventricle; AO = aorta; LV = left ventricle. (From Martin, R. P., et al.: Intrapericardial abnormalities in patients with pericardial effusion. Circulation *61*: 568, 1980, by permission of the American Heart Association, Inc.)

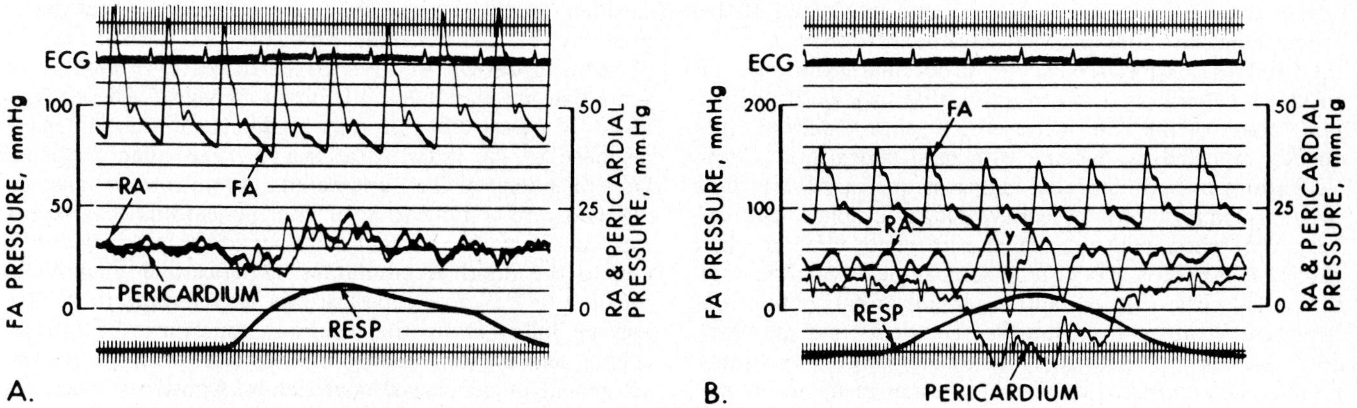

FIGURE 43–23 Femoral arterial (FA), right atrial (RA), and intrapericardial pressure tracings before (*A*) and after (*B*) pericardiocentesis in a patient with effusive-constrictive pericarditis. Before pericardiocentesis, right atrial and intrapericardial pressures are elevated and identical, and the *y* descent is absent from the right atrial waveform. After pericardiocentesis, mean intrapericardial pressure falls to zero, and the right atrial pressure remains elevated and develops a prominent diastolic *y* descent. (From Mann, T. et al.: Effusive-constrictive hemodynamic pattern due to neoplastic involvement of the pericardium. Am. J. Cardiol. *41*:781, 1978.)

Hemodynamics at rest are normal. However, the rapid infusion of 1,000 ml of prewarmed normal saline over 6 to 8 minutes transforms normal basal hemodynamics into a pattern of constrictive physiology, with elevation and equilibration of right and left ventricular diastolic pressures, the appearance of a prominent *y* descent in the right atrial pressure tracing, a dip-and-plateau pattern in the right ventricular pressure tracing, and loss of normal respiratory variation in the right atrial pressure pulse. These findings differ from those in normal subjects who usually experience no rise in filling pressures and from patients with myocardial disease in whom right and left ventricular diastolic pressures rise but fail to equilibrate after volume expansion. However, the sensitivity and specificity of volume challenge in the evaluation of patients with atypical chest pain and normal coronary arteries have not been well defined. In particular, the response of patients with atypical chest pain previously treated with beta-adrenergic blocking agents is not known. The likelihood that an abnormal response to volume challenge in patients with atypical chest pain reflects occult constrictive pericarditis is probably improved when there is also a history of remote pericarditis and an abnormal echocardiogram with evidence of pericardial thickening or pericardial effusion.

Total pericardiectomy has been reported in 12 patients with this diagnosis in whom there was histological confirmation of an abnormal pericardium and complete or near-complete resolution of symptoms postoperatively.[273] A few patients who have been restudied by volume challenge after operation no longer demonstrated equilibration of right and left heart filling pressures. It is not clear whether relief of chest pain after pericardiectomy was related to the relief of occult constrictive physiology per se or to relapsing pericarditis.

SPECIFIC FORMS OF PERICARDITIS

VIRAL PERICARDITIS

ETIOLOGY AND PATHOGENESIS. The viruses that most commonly cause acute pericarditis are Coxsackie virus group B and echovirus type 8.[274] Other viruses responsible for acute pericarditis include those which cause mumps, influenza, infectious mononucleosis, poliomyelitis, varicella, and hepatitis B.[275–278] Infectious mononucleosis may cause acute pericarditis with the complications of cardiac tamponade and constrictive pericarditis.[276] Varicella (chickenpox) may be associated with the complications of both severe viral pneumonia and acute pericarditis.[277] *Mycoplasma pneumoniae,* an important cause of adult nonbacterial pneumonia, also rarely causes myopericarditis.[279] There are no clinical features that distinguish acute viral pericarditis from idiopathic pericarditis, and it is likely that many cases of idiopathic pericarditis are due to unrecognized viral infections. The seasonal peak incidence of idiopathic pericarditis is in the spring and fall, which coincides with the increased incidence of enterovirus epidemics.

PATHOLOGY. Viral pericarditis causes inflammation of the visceral and parietal pericardial membranes, with infiltration first of polymorphonuclear leukocytes and then of lymphocytes around small vessels. Fibrin is deposited in the pericardial space, giving the pericardium a shaggy, reddened appearance. The underlying epicardium may also be involved by the inflammatory process. In some cases, the inflammation may result in a serous, serofibrinous, suppurative, or hemorrhagic effusion that may reach a volume of 200 ml, with a predominance of lymphocytes. Serous or serofibrinous effusions usually resolve completely by digestion of fibrin, or they may organize and obliterate the intrapericardial space. Depending on the volume, rate of accumulation, and thickness of the underlying pericardium, a pericardial effusion may result in subacute cardiac tamponade. Both echo and Coxsackie viruses may produce suppurative effusions that resolve by organization, formation of thick adhesions, calcification, and thickening of the pericardium, resulting in constrictive pericarditis.[181,280]

CLINICAL FINDINGS. A prodromal syndrome of an upper respiratory tract infection that may be described as a "cold" or the "flu" within the preceding weeks is frequently reported by patients with viral pericarditis. Clinical features of both viral and idiopathic pericarditis include chest discomfort, fever, pleurisy, cough, dyspnea, and fatigue. The chest pain associated with acute viral or idiopathic pericarditis may be excruciating, and lack of pericardial chest pain is unusual. A pericardial friction rub is present in up to three-fourths of patients and may last up to a week.[281-283] The chest roentgenogram demonstrates a pulmonary infiltrate or pleural effusion in up to 30 per cent of patients, and cardiac enlargement suggestive of a pericardial effusion is present in approximately half the patients.[284]

Viral or idiopathic pericarditis should be suspected in young or otherwise healthy adults with a characteristic prodromal illness and a syndrome of acute pericardial pain. It must be differentiated from pericarditis due to trauma, purulent pericardial infection, myocarditis, and systemic lupus erythematosus. In older patients, pericarditis due to rheumatoid disorders, myocardial infarction, tuberculosis, or neoplasm should be investigated before one presumes a viral etiology. The diagnosis of viral infection is strongly supported by the finding of a greater than fourfold rise in serial neutralizing antibody titers during the initial three weeks of illness.[282] It is rarely productive to attempt to isolate virus from blood, pericardial fluid, pleural fluid, or stool. Pericarditis due to infectious mononucleosis is suggested in the clinical setting of the young patient with high fever, adenopathy, sore throat, and positive heterophile test.

In a patient with a viral illness, the diagnosis of suspected pericarditis is confirmed clinically by the finding of a characteristic pericardial friction rub. Serial electrocardiographic changes of acute pericarditis (p. 1476) are not specific for the etiology of either viral or idiopathic pericarditis; however, the appearance of characteristic electrocardiographic changes may lead to the recognition of pericardial involvement in patients with a viral upper respiratory tract infection. Atrial arrhythmias and sinus tachycardia occur in about one-fourth of patients.[283] Echocardiographic documentation of a pericardial effusion is also evidence of pericardial inflammation in a patient with a viral upper respiratory tract infection and chest pain. Other laboratory findings suggestive of inflammation but not diagnostic of pericarditis include elevation of the sedimentation rate and leukocytosis. Cardiac isoenzymes may be abnormally elevated if there is extensive associated epicarditis or myocarditis.

Acute viral or idiopathic pericarditis is usually a short, dramatic, self-limited illness lasting 1 to 3 weeks. Important complications of acute viral or idiopathic pericarditis include (1) associated myocarditis, (2) recurrent pericarditis, (3) pericardial effusion with cardiac tamponade, and (4) the late development of constrictive pericarditis. Acute myocarditis, which may develop in association with pericarditis due to Coxsackie and echoviruses, may result in acute congestive heart failure, conduction disturbances, and cardiac enlargement that usually resolves completely or rarely leads to the development of a chronic congestive cardiomyopathy. Pericarditis may recur several weeks later in about 15 to 40 per cent of patients, and a small number of patients develop disabling recurrences over months to years that are extremely difficult to manage.[282] These recurrences of pericardial pain may be due to an immunological response to the initial viral injury rather than recurrent viral infections of the pericardium. Acute cardiac tamponade is a rare complication of viral pericarditis that occurs early in the course of acute viral or idiopathic pericarditis due to the rapid accumulation of pericardial fluid under pressure.[281,284,285] Acute pericarditis may appear to resolve and be followed by the insidious appearance of fatigue, edema, and ascites weeks to months later owing to the development of pericardial constriction. Constrictive pericarditis is a long-term complication that occurs in less than 10 per cent of patients with Coxsackie viral pericarditis.[280] Symptoms and abnormal hemodynamics resolve after surgical removal of the visceral as well as parietal pericardium.

MANAGEMENT. Treatment is directed against symptoms, with close observation for the development of cardiac tamponade or myocarditis early in the patient's course. For these reasons, most patients with an initial acute episode of pericarditis should be observed in the hospital. Bed or chair rest is warranted, and the avoidance of excessive motion and exercise helps to relieve pericardial pain and dyspnea. Pericardial pain and fever usually respond to nonsteroidal antiinflammatory agents and occasionally require steroids, as described on page 1477. Patients may be discharged from the hospital when fever and pericardial pain have disappeared and any pericardial effusion that was present has decreased in size. However, patients should be examined at regular intervals over the next few weeks to look for the complications of effusive-constrictive pericarditis and at longer intervals for the development of late constrictive pericarditis. Patients who develop tachyarrhythmias or acute conduction defects suggestive of myocardial involvement warrant close observation and electrocardiographic monitoring.

Recurrent pericarditis may require the reinstitution of antiinflammatory drug therapy with titration to the minimum dose needed to relieve symptoms, followed by gradual tapering of the drug over several weeks to months. Pericardiectomy is rarely needed for relief of severe recurrent pericardial pain in patients who cannot be weaned from steroids or other antiinflammatory drugs[286] or who have more than four recurrent attacks.

TUBERCULOUS PERICARDITIS

ETIOLOGY AND PATHOGENESIS. In industrialized nations, the incidence of tuberculous pericarditis has decreased within the past three decades as a result of effective chemotherapy and public health surveillance. The incidence of tuberculous pericarditis among patients with pulmonary tuberculosis ranges from about 1 to 8 per cent.[287] In earlier decades, tuberculous pericarditis was frequently seen in children and young adults,[288] but today it occurs predominantly in middle-aged and elderly males. The disease continues to be important in immunosuppressed patients and among the underprivileged, including South and

West African blacks, the black poor of the United States, and Asian and African immigrants.[287,289–292]

Tuberculous pericarditis usually develops by retrograde spread from peribronchial, peritracheal, or mediastinal lymph nodes or by early hematogenous spread from the primary tuberculous infection.[288,293,294] Less commonly, the pericardium is involved by the breakdown and contiguous spread of a necrotic tuberculous lesion in the lung, pleura, or spine or by hematogenous spread from distant secondary genitourinary or skeletal infections.[295]

PATHOLOGY. Tuberculous pericarditis usually begins with diffuse fibrin deposits, granuloma formation, and the presence of viable acid-fast bacilli.[294] A pericardial effusion then develops, which may be serous but more often contains some blood with a protein content exceeding 2.5 gm/dl. Although polymorphonuclear leukocytes are present early in the development of the effusion, they are later replaced by lymphocytes, monocytes, and plasma cells. Both complement-fixing antimyolemmal and antimyosin-type antibodies have been demonstrated in about 75 per cent of patients with *acute* tuberculous pericarditis in contrast to the much lower incidence in patients with viral pericarditis or constrictive pericarditis due to all types of tuberculosis, which suggests that cytolysis mediated by antimyolemmal antibodies may contribute to the development of exudative tuberculous pericarditis.[296] A tuberculous pericardial effusion usually develops very slowly and therefore does not cause hemodynamic complications; however, when it accumulates rapidly, even a small effusion may produce cardiac tamponade. As the effusion is absorbed, the pericardium thickens, granulomas proliferate, and a thick coat of fibrin is deposited on the parietal pericardium. At this stage, viable acid-fast bacilli may no longer be present, but caseation may develop and penetrate the myocardium. Finally, fibrous pericarditis develops as the granulomatous reaction is replaced by fibrous tissue and collagen. These changes are followed by the accumulation of cholesterol crystals and the development of pericardial calcification. Constrictive pericarditis develops in almost all patients with tuberculous pericarditis and in about half or less of the patients who receive antituberculosis chemotherapy.[297,298]

CLINICAL MANIFESTATIONS. Tuberculous pericarditis is usually detected clinically either in the effusive stage or late, i.e., after the development of constrictive pericarditis. It usually develops slowly, with nonspecific systemic symptoms such as low-grade fever, malaise, dyspnea, anorexia, weakness, and weight loss. Severe pericardial pain characteristic of viral and idiopathic pericarditis is uncommon in tuberculous pericarditis.[298] A large pericardial effusion usually causes dyspnea and a feeling of heaviness in the chest. Heavy sputum production, cough, and hemoptysis—clues to the presence of cavitary pulmonary tuberculosis—are usually absent.

Abnormalities on *physical examination* usually include fever, dyspnea, and a pericardial friction rub. If the complications of cardiac tamponade or effusive-constrictive pericarditis are present, the physical examination may reveal edema, jugular venous distention, pulsus paradoxus, distant heart sounds, hepatomegaly, and ascites. The *chest roentgenogram* usually shows an enlarged cardiac silhouette, and pleural effusions may be detected in about half the patients.[282] However, the apices and hila of the lung are usually normal, and pulmonary infiltrates or calcification is present in a minority of the patients. Tuberculous pericarditis may rarely present as a solitary mediastinal mass.[299]

DIAGNOSIS. Tuberculous pericarditis should be suspected in patients with fever and unexplained cardiomegaly, particularly those who are susceptible to tuberculosis, i.e., the underprivileged or immunosuppressed. It is noteworthy that tuberculous pericarditis may develop during chemotherapy for pulmonary tuberculosis.[300] In a minority of patients with pericarditis, a definitive diagnosis of a tuberculous origin may be made by culture or histological demonstration of tuberculosis outside the pericardium (sputum, gastric wash, pleural fluid, liver or bone marrow biopsy). A definitive diagnosis can be made by isolation of the bacillus from the pericardial fluid or pericardial biopsy. It is difficult to establish a definitive bacteriological diagnosis because of the low yield of the bacillus when pericardial fluid is examined by acid-fast stain on microscopy; failure of the bacillus to grow on appropriate media or in guinea pigs, even in patients with known tuberculous pericardial effusion; and the need to observe bacterial cultures for at least eight weeks. The probability of obtaining a definitive diagnosis is greatest if both pericardial fluid and a pericardial biopsy specimen are examined early in the effusive stage.[301] However, it must be emphasized that a negative pericardial biopsy does not exclude tuberculous pericarditis, since in some patients examination of the entire pericardium removed at pericardiectomy or autopsy is required to demonstrate clear-cut evidence of tuberculosis.[302,303]

It may be necessary to make a presumptive clinical diagnosis of tuberculous pericarditis in patients with a large pericardial effusion, a positive tuberculin skin test, and systemic symptoms such as weight loss and anorexia, even when examination of the pericardial fluid and biopsy does not reveal tuberculosis. In such patients, clinical improvement may occur after initiation of antituberculosis chemotherapy. A negative tuberculin skin test may be found in anergic patients. Making a presumptive clinical diagnosis of tuberculous pericarditis requires exquisite judgment, since, on the one hand, treatment should not be withheld from the seriously ill patient, while, on the other, it is not prudent to commit patients with nontuberculous effusions to a prolonged course of multiple-drug antituberculosis therapy.

MANAGEMENT. In the era before antituberculosis chemotherapy, tuberculous pericarditis was rapidly fatal, with a mortality rate greater than 80 per cent; the remaining patients had a protracted course of months to years with a frequently fatal outcome due to miliary tuberculosis or constrictive pericarditis. Since the introduction of early chemotherapy, mortality from acute tuberculous pericarditis has fallen to less than 50 per cent, but the effectiveness of antituberculosis chemotherapy in preventing the development of constrictive pericarditis is controversial.[290,297,298]

Treatment of tuberculous pericarditis includes hospitalization with bed rest and particular attention to findings on physical examination, electrocardiography, and echocardiography that suggest the development of an enlarging pericardial effusion and tamponade. Initial chemotherapy should usually consist of a three-drug regimen, ordinarily oral isoniazid, oral ethambutol, and intramuscular streptomycin. The use of corticosteroids has been advocated to reduce pericardial inflammation and enhance resorption of pericardial effusion, but there is no conclusive evidence that steroids reduce the risk of developing tuberculous constrictive pericarditis.[298,304] We believe that corticosteroids should be reserved for patients with recurrent large effusions or cardiac compression caused by granulation tissue who do not respond to antituberculosis drugs alone. In patients with documented cardiac tamponade or with a large pericardial effusion seen on echocardiogram, the effusion should be drained initially by percutaneous pericardiocentesis with continued catheter drainage. Pericardiectomy should be performed after two to four weeks of antituberculosis drug therapy if patients develop large recurrent effusions or cardiac compression due to effusive-constrictive disease or constrictive pericarditis.[287,290,304,305] Pericardiectomy should be performed early in the course in patients with clinical and hemodynamic evidence of cardiac compression, since mortality is high among patients who undergo pericardiectomy at the late stage of calcific pericardial constriction.

BACTERIAL (PURULENT) PERICARDITIS

Although the clinical spectrum of bacterial purulent pericarditis has changed over the past four decades, mortality remains high. Since the introduction of antibiotics in the 1940's, the incidence of bacterial pericarditis detected at autopsy has decreased.[306,307] Prior to 1943, purulent pericarditis occurred primarily in young, previously healthy males as a complication of pneumococcal pneumonia or empyema, and uncontrolled pleuropulmonary disease due to staphylococci or streptococci.[306] During the antibiotic era, there has been a decline in the incidence of pneumococcal and streptococcal pericarditis, although these organisms continue to cause life-threatening pericarditis.[307–309] The incidence of hospital-acquired penicillin-resistant staphylococcal pericarditis in post-thoracotomy patients has increased, and there is a widened spectrum of organisms responsible for bacterial pericarditis including the gram-negative bacilli (Proteus, *E. coli*, Pseudomonas, Klebsiella),[307] *Neisseria meningitidis*,[310–313] Salmonella species,[314,315] *Neisseria gonorrhoeae*,[316] *Hemophilus influenzae*,[317] *Pasteurella tularensis*,[318] *Streptococcus mitis*,[319] anaerobic organisms,[319] and other unusual pathogens.[320–323] Important predisposing factors for the development of purulent pericarditis include a preexisting sterile pericardial effusion[324] as well as immunodepression due to burns, immunotherapy, lymphoma, or leukemia.[319,325]

The routes of pericardial infection have also changed. Direct pulmonary extension of bacterial pneumonia or empyema now accounts for only about 20 per cent of cases of purulent pericarditis.[319] Today, purulent pericarditis tends to occur in adults via (1) contiguous spread from an early postoperative infection after thoracic surgery or trauma, (2) infection related to infective endocarditis, (3) extension from a subdiaphragmatic suppurative source, and (4) hematogenous spread during bacteremia. In patients with endocarditis, bacterial pericarditis is common and is detected in about 1 out of 8 patients with endocarditis studied at autopsy and in a higher percentage of those with staphylococcal endocarditis.[307] In such patients, bacterial pericarditis may develop by (1) extension from a valve ring abscess, (2) rupture of an aneurysm, (3) extension from a myocardial abscess, or (4) septic coronary embolus (Fig. 43–24). An infected myocardial infarction or aneurysm may also be a source for the development of purulent bacterial pericarditis.[307]

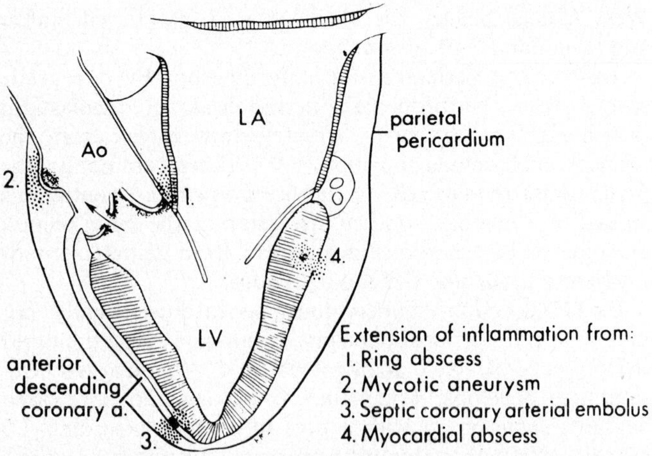

FIGURE 43–24 Schematic representation of the pathogenesis of pericarditis in infective endocarditis. Ao = aorta; LV = left ventricle; LA = left atrium. (From Roberts, W. C., and Spray, T. L.: Pericardial heart disease: A study of its causes, consequences, and morphologic features. *In* Spodick, D. H. (ed.): Pericardial Diseases. Philadelphia, F. A. Davis Co., 1976, p. 31.)

In *children*, bacterial pericarditis is second only to rheumatic fever as a cause of pericarditis[325]; the most common organisms include *Staphylococcus aureus* followed by *Hemophilus influenzae* and *Neisseria meningitidis*.[317,326–328] Pediatric illnesses associated with the development of bacterial pericarditis include pharyngitis, pneumonia, meningitis, otitis media, impetigo, endocarditis, and bacterial arthritis. The development of childhood bacterial pericarditis carries a high mortality of 36 to 70 per cent, depending on the organism and the risk of extremely rapid early development of constrictive pericarditis, which has also been reported in infants.[329–331] The high mortality rate in children appears to be markedly reduced by early diagnosis and combined treatment with parenteral antibiotics and open surgical pericardial drainage.[332,333]

PATHOLOGY. Bacterial pericarditis occurs most commonly by contiguous spread of an intrathoracic infection. In this setting, the initial lesion is an area of acute inflammation of the parietal pericardium adjacent to the thoracic source. Pericardial fluid may then accumulate and is clear at first, after which bacteria and fibrin appear; the late picture is of grossly purulent fluid with viable organisms, a high white blood cell count, and a low glucose content. Usually, bacterial pericarditis is frankly suppurative by the time it is detected clinically. The inflammation may result in organization and dense adhesions that cause obliteration of the pericardial space, thickening, and eventual calcification of the pericardium. In some patients, the inflammation may involve the adjacent sternum, pleura, and diaphragm with formation of dense adhesions between the parietal pericardium and contiguous structures.

CLINICAL FEATURES. Bacterial pericarditis is usually an acute fulminant illness of only a few days' duration. In one series,[319] the mean duration of symptoms prior to hospitalization was only three days. High fevers, shaking chills, night sweats, and dyspnea are common. In most patients the symptom of typical pericardial chest pain is absent. Tachycardia is present in nearly all patients, but a pericardial friction rub is present in less than half. In many cases, the pericarditis remains unsuspected because of the dominant presence of symptoms and signs related to an underlying known infection such as pneumonia or mediastinitis following complicated thoracic surgery or trauma. The appearance of new jugular venous distention and pulsus paradoxus may be the first evidence of pericardial involvement, and these ominous signs reflect the development of cardiac tamponade due to the acute accumulation of suppurative fluid under pressure.[319]

Laboratory findings usually include a leukocytosis with a marked leftward shift. The chest roentgenogram usually shows enlargement of the cardiac shadow and, less commonly, widening of the mediastinum. In the majority of cases, the roentgenogram shows evidence of underlying pneumonia, empyema, or mediastinitis without overt evidence of pericardial involvement. Electrocardiographic changes typically include ST-segment and T-wave changes characteristic of pericarditis in the majority of patients.[309,319] The appearance of electrical alternans suggests the presence of a massive suppurative effusion and raises the possibility of cardiac tamponade. In patients with suspected infective endocarditis, the appearance of a prolonged P-R interval, atrioventricular dissociation, or bundle branch block is strong evidence of extension of infection from the valve ring into the adjacent myocardium—an important predisposing factor for the development of pericarditis, especially in patients with staphylococcal endocarditis.[319]

Pericardial fluid usually shows polymorphonuclear leukocytosis and sometimes frank pus. Pericardial glucose levels are usually depressed and the protein content is elevated[319]; lactate dehydrogenase values may also be markedly elevated.

Purulent bacterial pericarditis should be suspected in a debilitated patient with unexplained high spiking fevers, dyspnea, markedly elevated white blood cell count, and an increase in the size of the cardiac silhouette on chest roentgenogram. The key to the diagnosis, which unfortunately is frequently not made before death, is a high index of suspicion. An echocardiogram should be promptly obtained to look for evidence of a new pericardial effusion and/or loculation of fluid with adhesions. The suspicion of purulent pericardial fluid is an indication to explore the pericardial space. This may be done by percutaneous pericardiocentesis *only* if there is echocardiographic evidence of a large anterior and posterior pericardial effusion that may be safely tapped or, preferably, by a generous subxiphoid pericardial window with thorough pericardial drainage.

Both pericardial fluid and pericardial tissue should be immediately studied by means of Gram-stained, acid-fast, and fungal smears by an experienced examiner. The fluid should then be cultured for aerobic and anaerobic bacteria with appropriate antibiotic sensitivity testing and for fungi and tuberculosis. Meticulous culturing for fungi as well as bacteria is important because of the increasing incidence of fungal pericarditis in patients who have received broad-spectrum antibiotics in the setting of immunosuppression or recent major surgery.[334] Pericardial fluid should also be examined for white blood cell count and differential, hematocrit, and glucose and protein content. Cultures of blood, sputum, and recent surgical wounds should also be obtained.

Despite the lower incidence of purulent bacterial pericarditis in the antibiotic era, overall survival continues to be extremely poor, averaging about 30 per cent in modern series.[306,319,335] The poor prognosis stems in large part from failure of clinical diagnosis before death. The high mortality from purulent pericarditis can be reduced substantially through the institution of both appropriate parenteral antibiotic therapy and early complete surgical drainage. The survival rate when the disease is recognized early and managed appropriately is about 50 per cent.[306,319,335] Early surgical drainage of the pericardium also helps to prevent the complication of constrictive pericarditis.

In patients treated only with antibiotics without pericardial drainage, the rapid unsuspected development of a large pericardial effusion may result in sudden cardiovascular collapse and death due to cardiac tamponade. In one series, cardiac tamponade developed acutely in 38 per cent of the patients with bacterial endocarditis, provided the initial clue to the presence of purulent pericarditis, and contributed to death in the majority.[319]

A special comment is warranted about pericarditis associated with *meningococcal* infection. The pericardium may become infected early during meningococcal sepsis (in the presence or absence of meningitis) causing purulent pericarditis with cardiac tamponade, with a natural history as described above.[312] In these cases, the pericardial fluid is frankly purulent and viable organisms can usually be isolated. In addition, sterile pericarditis may occur late in the convalescent period in association with arthritis, pleuritis, and ophthalmitis.[319,336,337] This syndrome appears to have an immunological etiology, does not require further antibiotic therapy if the primary infection has been adequately treated, and responds to antiinflammatory agents. A febrile, self-limited polyserositis with pericarditis has also been reported after 2 to 3 weeks of effective treatment of sepsis due to *Staphylococcus aureus.*[338] Acute self-limited pericarditis due to an allergic reaction to penicillin has been described; the presence of marked peripheral eosinophilia provides an important clue that pericarditis is a feature of the drug reaction rather than purulent bacterial pericarditis.[339]

MANAGEMENT. Results of Gram-staining of the pericardial fluid should be used in the selection of antibiotics for initial therapy. If the effusion is purulent but no organisms can be easily identified and tuberculosis is not considered likely, therapy should be initiated with both a semisynthetic antistaphylococcal antibiotic and an aminoglycoside. Dosage should be adjusted in the presence of renal or hepatic dysfunction. Depending on the results of the cultures of the pericardial fluid and blood, antibiotic therapy may then be modified. High concentrations of antibiotics can be achieved in pericardial fluid, so that instillation of antibiotics into the pericardial space is not warranted.[340] However, systemic antibiotics alone are inadequate treatment, and prompt and thorough surgical drainage of the pericardium is essential in almost all patients with bacterial pericarditis.[306,319] Pericardial aspiration of a large anterior and posterior effusion may be extremely helpful in making an initial bacteriological diagnosis and initiating therapy. However, purulent pericardial effusions are likely to recur. Therefore, open drainage, through creation of subxiphoid pericardial window, is usually adequate when the diagnosis is made early and when the pericardial fluid is thin and the pericardium minimally thickened. This procedure is also the preferred route of drainage in severely disabled patients, since it can be performed under local anesthesia and avoids the pleural cavities. In a patient with a thick purulent effusion and dense adhesions with loculation, extensive pericardiectomy is needed to achieve adequate drainage and to prevent late development of constrictive pericarditis.[307,341]

FUNGAL PERICARDITIS

ETIOLOGY AND PATHOPHYSIOLOGY. *Histoplasmosis* is the most common cause of fungal pericarditis.[282,342,343] This diagnosis should be considered in patients suspected of having tuberculous pericarditis who live in the Ohio or Mississippi River Valley or the Western Appalachians, where the fungus is endemic.[343–345] In these areas, histoplasmosis is acquired by inhalation of spores from soil contaminated by infected birds, bats, or chickens. Other fungal infections responsible for pericarditis include coccidioidomycosis, aspergillosis, blastomycosis, and those caused by *Candida albicans* and *Candida tropicalis*.[282,346–348] Coccidioidomycosis pericarditis occurs in patients who have inhaled chlamydospores from soil or dust in areas of the American Southwest, particularly the San Joaquin Valley, and Argentina, where it is endemic.[346,347] Groups at increased risk for the development of fungal pericarditis consequent to disseminated infection include patients addicted to the use of intravenous narcotics and patients who are immunosuppressed or who have received potent broad-spectrum antibiotics.[319,349]

Histoplasmosis pericarditis can develop by direct extension from infected hilar lymph nodes or by hematogenous dissemination from the primary pulmonary focus. The isolation of organisms from pericardial fluid is unusual, which suggests that either too few organisms are present for identification or the pericarditis represents a sterile immune reaction to histoplasmosis antigen in the pericardial space.[343,344] Pericarditis due to fungi other than histoplasmosis may occur as a complication of open heart surgery in adults and children,[350] owing to spread from contiguous infected lymph nodes or pulmonary lesions, or as a result of hematogenous dissemination in patients who are profoundly immunosuppressed with fungal sepsis.

PATHOLOGY. Pericardial fluid may accumulate extremely rapidly and to massive quantities in patients with histoplasmosis.[351] In cases of fungal pericarditis due to agents other than Histoplasma, exudative pericardial effusions tend to accumulate slowly, so that an effusion may be present for months. Fungal pericardial effusions occasionally become organized, with pericardial thickening and the development of a constricting, calcified pericardium.[352]

Histoplasmosis may cause infection of the myocardium and endocardium as well as of the pericardium.[351, 353] Similarly, aspergillosis and coccidioidomycosis may cause pericarditis in the context of pulmonary infection, endocarditis, and myocardial abscess. Therefore, cardiac decompensation in patients with fungal pericarditis may be due both to the presence of cardiac compression from a pericardial effusion or a constrictive pericardium and to an underlying myocardial infection.

CLINICAL FEATURES. Patients with histoplasmosis pericarditis usually develop the disease in the context of an asymptomatic or mild pneumonitis with benign self-limited dissemination to other organs or, rarely, in the setting of severe prolonged disseminated infection.[282,343,345] In the latter situation, disseminated histoplasmosis infection may be evident by fever, anemia, leukopenia, and the syndrome of pneumonitis progressing to pulmonary cavitation, massive hepatomegaly, meningitis, myocarditis, or endocarditis.[351] Marked variability in the severity of histoplasmosis infection is repeatedly observed among patients affected in the same outbreak, but severe disseminated infections are especially likely to occur in young infants and elderly males.

Coccidioidomycosis pericarditis does not occur in the brief self-limited influenza-like form of the infection but is instead a complication of the progressive disseminated form of coccidioidomycosis.[346,347] Blacks, Philippinos, and Chicanos appear to be especially vulnerable to the development of severe and progressive disseminated coccidioidomycosis. These patients are usually chronically ill and debilitated, with fever, weight loss, and the complications of pulmonary infiltrate progressing to cavitary disease with lymphadenopathy, osteomyelitis, and meningitis. In immunocompromised patients, the insidious appearance of symptoms of fungal pericarditis and underlying myocardial infection may initially be overlooked because attention is focused on symptoms related to underlying lymphoma, leukemia, or known valvular endocarditis. In these patients, nonspecific symptoms of fever, chest pain, dyspnea, and malaise may be falsely attributed to the underlying disease.

Physical findings suggestive of cardiac compression (jugular venous distention, hypotension, pulsus paradoxus) may be the first clues to the diagnosis of fungal pericarditis. The chest roentgenogram may show infiltrates, hilar adenopathy or cavitary lesions suggestive of pulmonary fungal infection, or a progressive increase in the size of the cardiac silhouette if a large pericardial effusion develops. However, there are no roentgenographic, electrocardiographic, or echocardiographic features characteristic of fungal pericarditis.

DIAGNOSIS. In patients with evidence of pericarditis, a presumptive clinical diagnosis of *histoplasmosis pericarditis* can be made on the basis of (1) exposure to soil in an endemic area, (2) an elevated complement-fixation titer, (3) a positive Histoplasma skin test, and (4) evidence of characteristic miliary calcifications in the spleen and lung. The Histoplasma skin test should always be performed *after* serological testing to avoid misinterpretation of the latter. Histoplasmosis pericarditis, which occurs in the setting of severe disseminated infection and massive lymphadenopathy, must be differentiated from sarcoidosis, tuberculosis, Hodgkin's disease, and brucellosis. Histological tissue examination and culture are important. In disseminated progressive histoplasmosis, the organism may be isolated from extrapericardial sites such as the bone marrow, exudate from ulcers, or sputum by inoculation on Sabouraud's medium or by guinea pig inoculation with subsequent subculture of the spleen. Histoplasmosis pericarditis may also occur in the absence of progressive disseminated infection. In this latter setting, cultures of pericardial fluid, bone marrow, and pleural fluid are likely to be sterile, and the diagnosis is made by a fourfold or greater rise in complement-fixation antibody titer.[343]

A presumptive diagnosis of *coccidioidomycosis pericarditis* is made in a patient with pericarditis by (1) a history of dust exposure in an endemic area in the American Southwest or South America, (2) a characteristic clinical picture of disseminated coccidioidomycosis involving the lungs and other organs, (3) the appearance of a positive serum precipitin test early in the infection followed by a rising positive complement-fixation antibody titer, and (4) microscopic evidence of the characteristic spherule in biopsy material or exudates. A definitive diagnosis is made by culture identification of the organism on Sabouraud's medium. Coccidioidin skin tests are often negative in the presence of progressive disseminated disease. If pericarditis due to other fungal organisms is suspected, appropriate complement-fixing antibody titers should be measured. Depending on the clinical setting it may be important to obtain pericardial fluid and a pericardial biopsy specimen. The microscopic finding of granulomas alone is nonspecific and may occur in tuberculosis, fungal and parasitic infections, and sarcoid involvement of the pericardium. Therefore, histological documentation of the characteristic appearance of the fungus and subsequent culture identification are important.

MANAGEMENT. Histoplasmosis may cause massive effusions with acute cardiac tamponade.[351,353] Although pericardial calcification and pericardial constriction have been reported in histoplasmosis pericarditis, these are uncommon.[352,354] Intravenous amphotericin B is required only for patients with histoplasmosis pericarditis and severe systemic disease. In nonhistoplasmosis fungal pericarditis, spontaneous remissions do *not* occur; infection progresses until the patient dies either of the underlying disease or of fungal pericardial and myocardial involvement. Drug therapy for pericarditis associated with disseminated coccidioidomycosis, aspergillosis, and blastomycosis consists of prolonged intravenous therapy with amphotericin B. The South American form of blastomycosis may require the addition of a sulfonamide. In many cases of nonhistoplasmosis fungal pericarditis, chronic pericardial fungal infection progresses to severe pericardial constriction or, less commonly, cardiac tamponade.[355] Therefore, depending on the patient's underlying medical condition, pericardiectomy is usually indicated. Intrapericardial instillation of antifungal agents has not proved helpful in these diseases. The marked toxicity associated with prolonged amphotericin B administration underscores the importance of making a definitive diagnosis after histological examination or culture. *Candida pericarditis* associated with fungal sepsis and disseminated infection is treated with amphotericin B, 5-fluorocytosine, and miconazole. Fungal pericarditis occurring in the presence of valvular fungal endocarditis should also be treated by valve replacement.

Pericarditis may also be caused by *Actinomyces israelii* and *Nocardia asteroides,* which are intermediate forms between fungi and bacteria,[356-359] and by parasitic infestations of amebiasis,[360-362] acquired toxoplasmosis,[363,364] and echinococcosis.[365-367] Very rare causes of parasitic pericarditis include dracunculosis,[368] cysticercosis, and filariasis.[369] These unusual pathogens rarely cause acute cardiac tamponade but may cause chronic constrictive pericarditis (Table 43–8).

PERICARDITIS FOLLOWING ACUTE MYOCARDIAL INFARCTION (See page 1279)

Pericarditis occurs commonly during the first few days after acute myocardial infarction. Although it is recognized clinically in approximately 10 to 15 per cent of patients with acute myocardial infarction, a much higher incidence is detected at autopsy.[370-372] Almost all patients with acute transmural myocardial infarction are found to have evidence of a localized fibrinous pericarditis overlying the infarction at autopsy. Pericarditis occurs following anterior, inferior, and lateral left ventricular infarction and in predominant right ventricular infarction as well. Other forms of pericardial involvement after myocardial infarction include acute pericardial hemorrhage secondary to cardiac rupture (p. 1268) and the late occurrence of Dressler's syndrome (p. 1513).

Pericarditis due to acute myocardial infarction usually involves the deposition of fibrin on the visceral and parietal pericardial surfaces overlying the region of transmural myocardial necrosis. Diffuse postinfarction pericarditis may resolve with the formation of delicate fibrinous adhesions within the pericardial space, obliteration of the pericardial space, or fibrotic pericardial thickening.

CLINICAL FEATURES. Pericarditis is recognized clinically by the appearance of a pericardial friction rub and pericardial chest pain within 12 hours to 10 days after acute myocardial infarction. In most patients with postinfarction pericarditis, a pericardial friction rub and pericardial chest pain appear within four days of infarction.[370,371,373] Appearance of a new friction rub more than 10 days after acute infarction probably represents the onset of Dressler's syndrome (p. 1513) or pericarditis complicating a second infarction. Detection of a pericardial friction rub is an important clue in the diagnosis of pericarditis in patients with postinfarction chest pain. Since pericardial friction rubs are notoriously evanescent, serial auscultatory evaluation of patients in various positions in a quiet room is important for detection. Pericardial rubs with a single systolic component heard near the apex may be confused with a new murmur of mitral regurgitation due to papillary muscle dysfunction or rupture. The pericardial friction rub of postinfarction pericarditis is not associated with any hemodynamic deterioration unless a pericardial effusion under pressure develops, causing cardiac tamponade.

Hemorrhagic cardiac tamponade has been reported in patients with postinfarction pericarditis in the absence of postinfarction rupture of the heart or leakage from a coronary artery.[374] Most, but not all, patients reported to have developed hemorrhagic cardiac tamponade in this context were receiving systemic anticoagulants.[375-378] These observations suggest that systemic anticoagulation contributes to the risk of bleeding into a pericardial effusion in patients with acute pericarditis complicating myocardial infarction.

The electrocardiographic ST-segment and T-wave changes typical of acute pericarditis may be difficult to recognize

TABLE 43–8 UNUSUAL INFECTIOUS CAUSES OF PERICARDITIS

Etiology	Route of Pericardial Involvement	Pathology	Diagnosis	Management
Fungi				
Actinomyces israelii	Extension from necrotic foci in mediastinum, lungs, or esophagus; hematogenous spread from necrotic mouth lesion.	1. Anaerobe; causes early mononuclear infiltrate that progresses to necrotic, suppurative lesion with granulomas. 2. May cause pericardial constriction.	1. Clinical evidence of underlying pulmonary or mediastinal infection. 2. Histological demonstration of filamentous acid-fast organisms with sulfur granules or, occasionally, a "ray fungus" colony on pericardial biopsy.	1. Fatal if untreated. 2. High-dose penicillin or tetracycline should be continued for several weeks after apparent cure. 3. Pericardiectomy for pericardial constriction or abscesses.
Nocardia asteroides	Extension from pulmonary focus in immunocompromised or debilitated patients.	1. Aerobe; pathology resembles tuberculosis with granulomas and caseation. 2. May cause pericardial constriction.	1. Histological demonstration of weakly acid-fast, branching filaments.	1. Sulfadiazine or combination of ampicillin and erythromycin. 2. Pericardiectomy for pericardial constriction.
Parasites				
Entamoeba histolytica	Rupture of hepatic abscess through diaphragm.	1. Noninfected serous effusion (20%). 2. Purulent effusion caused by cytolytic damage from parasite enzymes with secondary bacterial infection; pericardial abscesses may develop.	1. Histological demonstration of trophozoites in pericardial biopsy or fluid; "anchovy sauce" appearance of pericardial fluid. 2. Documentation of amebae in other organs *plus* improvement after therapeutic trial.	1. Metronidazole, 500 to 700 mg three times daily for 10 days. 2. Pericardial constriction or abscess requires pericardiectomy.
Toxoplasma gondii	1. Accidental cyst ingestion after exposure to infected animals or following organ transplantation or transfusion (rare). 2. Subsequent trophozoite invasion of nucleated cells.	1. Often involves both myocardium and pericardium. 2. Rupture of inflamed pericardial and epicardial blood vessels with subsequent formation of central necrotic zone with granuloma formation, fibrosis, and calcification.	1. Histological identification of intracellular toxoplasma on pericardial or lymph node biopsies or in spinal fluid. 2. Rising serum antibody titers of dye, complement fixation, or indirect hemagglutination tests.	1. Combination therapy with sulfonamide and 5-p-chlorophenyl-2,4-diamino-6-ethylpyrimidine (Daraprim).
Echinococcus granulosus	1. Ingestion of larvae of dog tapeworms that have passed from duodenum to portal veins as embryos and encyst in myocardium. 2. Pericardial cysts form after rupture of myocardial cysts.	1. Hydatid cysts containing clear fluid with surrounding fibrous shell of giant cells, eosinophils, and fibroblasts.	1. Histological demonstration of scolices in pericardial fluid with Ziehl-Neelsen stain. 2. Positive indirect hemagglutination test.	1. Surgical excision of pericardial cysts with sterilization of cyst contents prior to removal. 2. Indirect cyst aspiration should not be attempted due to risk of constrictive pericarditis following cyst spillage.

in patients with baseline alterations of the ST segment due to prior infarction. However, there are a few useful clues: (1) when pericarditis develops after myocardial infarction, the ST-segment vector may shift leftward and posteriorly from its original position; (2) ST-segment elevation tends to be higher when acute pericarditis complicates transmural myocardial infarction[371]; (3) the *new* appearance of diffuse transient ST-segment elevation or of P-R–segment depression 1 to 4 days after a localized myocardial infarction is suggestive of acute pericarditis; and (4) atrial tachyarrhythmias appear to be more common in patients with pericarditis following infarction.[379,380] However, the appearance of acute postinfarction pericarditis per se does not appear to affect adversely the mortality after acute infarction.[371,373,381]

Postinfarction pericarditis without cardiac compression must be differentiated from acute stress ulcer or gastritis, acute pulmonary embolus, hyperventilation, and, most importantly, recurrent myocardial ischemia. Pericardial pain usually has a typical sharp pleuritic character that becomes intensified in the supine position. In some patients, the pain may have a dull, aching quality and be mistaken for that of myocardial ischemia. Myocardial ischemic pain can usually be differentiated from the pain of postinfarction pericarditis by (1) obvious amelioration of the pain by nitroglycerin and (2) the appearance of new ST-segment and T-wave changes with reciprocal changes.

The development of cardiac tamponade in patients with myocardial infarction may be related to pericardial hemorrhage secondary to pericarditis or to myocardial rupture within the first three days after infarction. Both situations may be associated with cardiovascular collapse, severe hypotension, anuria, jugular venous distention, and an abrupt increase in heart size on the chest roentgenogram. Pericardiocentesis may successfully relieve hemorrhagic cardiac tamponade in patients with postinfarction pericarditis. Massive cardiac hemorrhage secondary to cardiac rupture is usually followed by the rapid development of electromechanical dissociation and death despite successful aspiration of the pericardial space, although survivors have been reported after subacute rupture.[382]

Acute cardiac tamponade secondary to postinfarction pericarditis must also be differentiated from cardiogenic shock without intrapericardial hemorrhage due to an acute ventricular septal defect or mitral regurgitation. The appearance of a new, loud systolic murmur points to an etiology of acute mitral regurgitation or ventricular septal defect, which can be confirmed by findings on echocardiography and cardiac catheterization. In the setting of an inferior myocardial infarction, the appearance of hypotension, pulsus paradoxus, and jugular venous distention may be related to massive right ventricular infarction rather than to cardiac tamponade.[49,50,383,384] Echocardiographic findings of right ventricular enlargement without a significant pericardial effusion, and catheterization findings suggestive of constrictive physiology (right atrial waveform with steep *y* descent) rather than cardiac tamponade (right atrial waveform with attenuated *y* descent) help to differentiate massive right ventricular infarction from cardiac tamponade and prevent inappropriate and possibly disastrous attempts at pericardiocentesis.

MANAGEMENT. Postinfarction pericarditis may produce mild symptoms that require no specific therapy or severe chest pain that persists for several days. If the pain is severe, aspirin or indomethacin will relieve pain within 48 hours in almost all patients.[385] A short course of prednisone may be required in patients whose pain does not improve after a 36-hour trial of nonsteroidal antiinflammatory agents.

There is experimental evidence that indomethacin may increase infarct size[386] and cause coronary vasoconstriction[387] and that indomethacin,[388] ibuprofen,[389] and multiple large doses of corticosteroids[390] interfere with the conversion of the myocardial infarct into a scar, so that marked thinning of the myocardial wall occurs. Although the clinical importance of these experimental findings is not clear, they suggest that steroids and nonsteroidal antiinflammatory drugs should be employed only with caution in patients with acute myocardial infarction. Fortunately, aspirin does not cause any of these adverse effects, and postinfarction pericarditis usually responds well to aspirin. Accordingly, we favor use of this drug.

UREMIC PERICARDITIS (See also page 1757)

ETIOLOGY. Pericarditis is a frequent and serious complication of chronic renal failure. Bright noted the presence of pericarditis in 8 per cent of autopsied patients with chronic renal failure reported in 1836 from Guy's Hospital.[391] Uremic pericarditis was detected in about half the patients with untreated chronic renal failure, although the incidence has decreased slightly in the dialysis era.[392,393]

The etiology of uremic pericarditis is unknown. Viral and bacterial causes have been proposed, but there is no consistent evidence to suggest an infectious origin in the majority of cases of uremic pericarditis.[394] Secondary infections of uremic pericardial effusions occur,[324] and it is unwise to assume that pericarditis in a patient with severe renal disease is simply related to uremia. Excess chronic exposure to toxic catabolic nitrogen metabolites has been suggested as the mechanism responsible for uremic pericarditis. This hypothesis is supported by the observations that uremic pericarditis is rare in patients with acute mild renal failure and that uremic pericarditis often improves with initiation of dialysis in previously untreated patients. However, there is no clear correlation between the development of pericarditis and the levels of blood urea nitrogen, and pericarditis can develop in patients undergoing regular dialysis with near-normal serum creatinine and electrolyte levels.[395,396] Pericarditis appears to be less common in patients undergoing peritoneal dialysis compared with hemodialysis, suggesting the role of an unknown toxin. It has also been proposed that pericarditis in dialysis patients may reflect an immunological response to substances introduced during dialysis. It is possible that etiological factors in nondialyzed patients differ from those in patients undergoing regular dialysis. In the latter group, systemic and regional heparinization during dialysis itself may exacerbate uremic pericarditis by promoting the tendency of vascular pericardial granulation tissue to bleed into the pericardial space.

Acute uremic pericarditis is characterized by the appearance of shaggy, hemorrhagic, fibrinous exudate on both parietal and visceral pericardial surfaces with little acute inflammatory cellular reaction (Fig. 43–25). In some patients, the vascular and friable pericardial surface may bleed, giving rise to hemorrhagic pericardial effusion. If

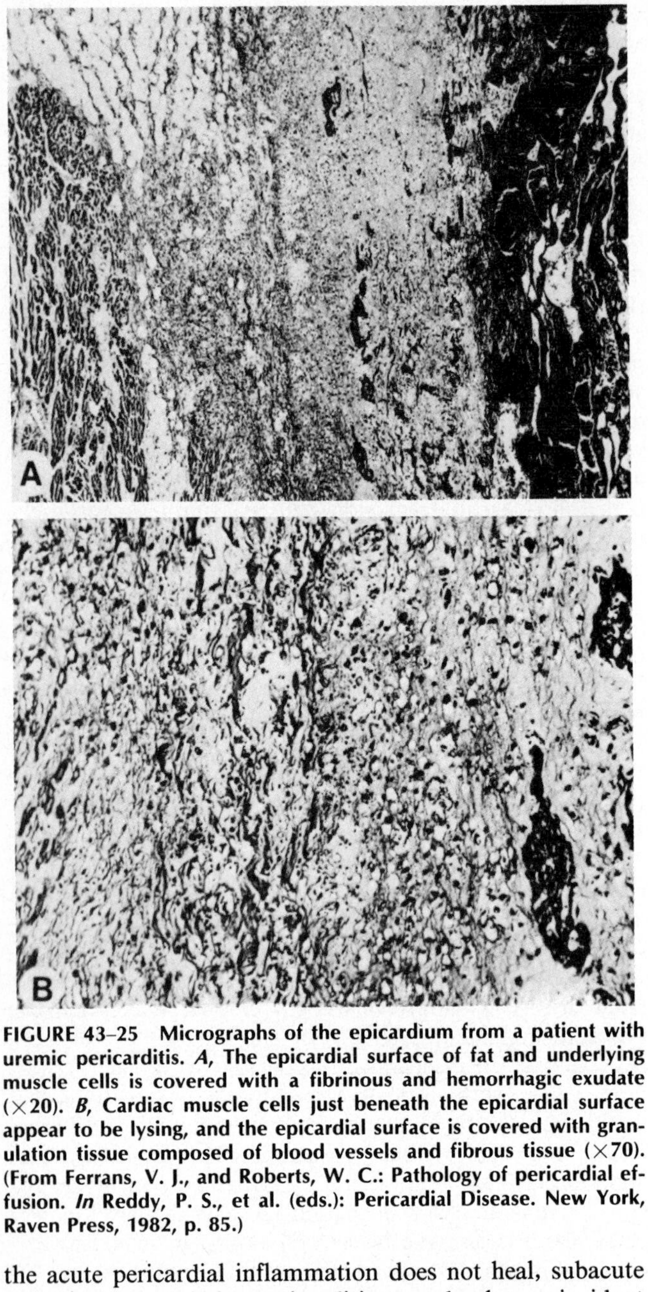

FIGURE 43-25 Micrographs of the epicardium from a patient with uremic pericarditis. *A*, The epicardial surface of fat and underlying muscle cells is covered with a fibrinous and hemorrhagic exudate (×20). *B*, Cardiac muscle cells just beneath the epicardial surface appear to be lysing, and the epicardial surface is covered with granulation tissue composed of blood vessels and fibrous tissue (×70). (From Ferrans, V. J., and Roberts, W. C.: Pathology of pericardial effusion. *In* Reddy, P. S., et al. (eds.): Pericardial Disease. New York, Raven Press, 1982, p. 85.)

the acute pericardial inflammation does not heal, subacute or chronic constrictive pericarditis may develop, coincident with organization of the effusion and formation of thick adhesions within the pericardial space. The pericardium may ultimately become very thick and fibrotic with an onion-peel appearance causing pericardial constriction, although extensive calcification is not common.[397]

CLINICAL FEATURES. The development of pericarditis in patients undergoing dialysis is of clinical importance, since it may (1) cause disability or life-threatening cardiac tamponade in patients who are otherwise well-compensated on dialysis, (2) compromise the status of patients who are candidates for renal transplantation, and (3) cause hemodynamic complications during routine dialysis. Uremic pericarditis with a large pericardial effusion may first come to clinical attention when an otherwise asymptomatic patient becomes hypotensive and confused upon fluid removal during ultrafiltration. This occurs because volume depletion may cause an abrupt fall in systemic blood pressure when ventricular filling is already compromised by the presence of a large, tense pericardial effusion. The patient's hemodynamic status may be further compromised if a large pericardial effusion coexists with uremic cardiomyopathy (p. 1760) so that a large left ventricular end-diastolic volume is needed to maintain stroke volume and cardiac output.

In addition, some patients develop symptoms of fever and substernal chest pain that is worse in the supine position and increases during inspiration. Patients with a large pericardial effusion may complain of dyspnea, the etiology of which may be difficult to differentiate from pulmonary venous congestion due to underlying myocardial dysfunction or cardiac compression.

The *physical examination* usually discloses tachycardia and a pericardial friction rub.[398] Patients with acute or subacute cardiac tamponade secondary to hemorrhagic effusion may have findings of jugular venous distention, pulsus paradoxus, and hypotension. In patients with a large pericardial effusion, increase in the size of the cardiac silhouette often develops on chest roentgenography, and this must be differentiated from changes in heart size due to myocardial dysfunction and chamber enlargement.

As in other forms of pericarditis, *echocardiography* is extremely useful in documenting the presence or absence of a pericardial effusion, estimating its size, and suggesting the presence of cardiac tamponade[399-401] as well as in detecting evidence of underlying myocardial dysfunction.

Before one makes a presumptive diagnosis of uremic pericarditis, other causes of pericardial effusion should be considered, including purulent pericarditis, neoplastic pericarditis, and pericarditis due to hypothyroidism. New, positive conversion of a tuberculin skin test in the context of the appearance of pericarditis and pericardial effusion should raise the suspicion of tuberculosis in the uremic patient. Cardiac catheterization is recommended in patients who are intolerant of dialysis and who develop dyspnea and hypotension owing to suspected cardiac tamponade. Prior to consideration of pericardiocentesis or pericardiectomy, it is important to document that these clinical findings are indeed related to the hemodynamics of cardiac tamponade (elevation and equilibration of right and left heart filling pressures) rather than to underlying congestive cardiomyopathy, ischemic heart disease, or excessively vigorous ultrafiltration. It must be remembered that pulsus paradoxus may be absent in uremic patients with cardiac tamponade and coexisting left ventricular failure and elevated left ventricular filling pressures.

In the past, uremic pericarditis was a terminal complication of untreated chronic renal failure and was almost uniformly fatal. Now, approximately one-third of dialyzed patients recover from uremic pericarditis without complication while about 20 per cent experience problems of hypotension and arrhythmias and fewer than 10 per cent experience the complications of tamponade and subacute chronic constrictive pericarditis.[396,397,399,402]

MANAGEMENT. Treatment of uremic pericarditis with a pericardial effusion is controversial, and multiple approaches have been advocated. However, the following principles have emerged: (1) no treatment is required for small, asymptomatic pericardial effusions that can be followed simply by serial echocardiography; and (2) large pericardial effusions in symptomatic patients may resolve after an increase in the frequency of dialysis,[399,403,404] but only half the patients recover with this therapy alone. Fever and a pericardial rub accompanied by a large pericardial effusion may markedly improve with intensification of dialysis combined with a nonsteroidal antiinflammatory drug such as indomethacin.[405–407] The addition of a corticosteroid may also promote an improvement in symptoms and regression of the pericardial effusion in patients who do not respond to dialysis alone, but the complications of long-term steroid administration limit its usefulness in the treatment of recurrent uremic pericarditis. Pericarditis tends to recur when antiinflammatory agents are discontinued, suggesting that these agents only suppress and do not cure the inflammatory process.

Pericardiocentesis followed by instillation of a nonresorbable steroid into the pericardial space has also been advocated,[408,409] but this procedure has been complicated by the development of purulent pericarditis.[410] There are reports of repetitive pericardiocenteses with low morbidity and mortality in uremic patients,[411] but other series have reported a substantial mortality as a consequence of pericardiocentesis.[412] The presence of a friable visceral pericardium increases the risk of cardiac trauma and intrapericardial hemorrhage in uremic pericarditis, and many patients are also compromised by the presence of left ventricular dysfunction. These considerations warrant special caution during the performance of pericardiocentesis in uremic patients and this procedure should probably be carried out only by experienced personnel in an optimal environment, with echocardiographic documentation that a large anterior and posterior effusion is present that can be safely aspirated.

Early pericardiectomy—total, subxiphoid, or limited—in uremic patients with a large pericardial effusion has been advocated to prevent the development of cardiac tamponade and constrictive pericarditis and to allow the procedure to be carried out at a time when the patient is clinically stable.[162,173,412–417] We feel that this approach is excessively aggressive, since many uremic patients with pericardial effusion respond well to medical therapy. Instead, we believe that pericardiectomy should be reserved for patients with pericardial constriction or recurrent cardiac tamponade resistant to antiinflammatory therapy and intensification of dialysis.

We recommend an increased frequency of dialysis combined with the use of a nonsteroidal antiinflammatory agent for the treatment of hemodynamically stable patients with uremic pericarditis. Patients who are hemodynamically unstable with hemodynamic evidence of cardiac tamponade and echocardiographic evidence of a large anterior and posterior effusion may be treated by percutaneous pericardiocentesis with continued catheter drainage of the pericardial sac for 24 to 48 hours. Subxiphoid pericardiotomy is advocated for patients with hemodynamic instability associated with recurrent pericardial effusions following pericardiocentesis or loculated pericardial effusions.

NEOPLASTIC PERICARDITIS

PATHOLOGY. At autopsy, the pericardium is involved in 5 to 10 per cent of patients with malignant neoplasm.[418–422] Lung cancer, breast cancer, leukemia, Hodgkin's disease, and non-Hodgkin's lymphoma account for about 80 per cent of reported cases of malignant pericarditis.[422–431] Other malignancies commonly reported to lead to pericardial involvement include gastrointestinal cancer, sarcomas, and melanoma.[432] Less common causes of malignant pericarditis include systemic mastocytosis, teratoma, and parotid carcinoma.[433–435] *Primary malignancies* of the pericardium are rare and include primarily mesothelioma and, less frequently, malignant fibrosarcoma, angiosarcoma, and benign and malignant teratomas.[436–440]

Metastatic involvement of the pericardium may cause an exudative pericardial effusion with tumor cells in the effusion, thickening and infiltration of the pericardium, and nodular tumor deposits.[441,442] Pericardial metastases *without* associated myocardial metastases are detected in about 75 per cent of cases of cardiac involvement.[431]

Neoplastic pericarditis may cause several syndromes of cardiac compression. Hemorrhagic effusion due to neoplastic infiltration of the pericardium may develop extremely rapidly, causing acute or subacute cardiac tamponade (Fig. 43–26). Pericardial involvement by tumors such as sarcomas, mesotheliomas, and melanomas can also produce a hemorrhagic effusion by erosion of the cardiac chamber or intrapericardial blood vessels, causing acute pericardial distention and abrupt fatal cardiac tamponade. Cardiac tamponade is occasionally the initial presentation of extracardiac malignancy and leukemia.[443–445] Cardiac compression may also occur as a consequence of the development of both a thickened pericardium and a pericardial effusion under pressure (effusive-constrictive pericarditis), or it may be caused by thickening of the pericardium produced by tumor encasement of the heart, causing the physiology of constrictive pericarditis.[141,142,446,447]

CLINICAL FEATURES. Neoplastic pericarditis is often totally asymptomatic and detected only as an incidental finding at autopsy. In other patients, it may cause severe symptoms or fatal complications. Thurber et al. reported that 29 per cent of 189 patients with pericardial metastases detected at autopsy had symptoms referable to the pericardium prior to death, but pericardial involvement was cor-

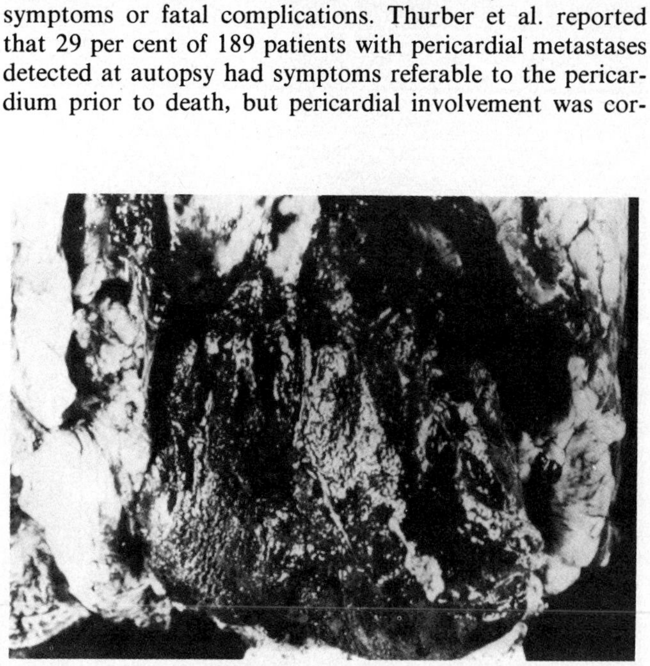

FIGURE 43–26 Gross pathologic specimen of malignant lymphoma metastatic to the heart. The lymphoma has diffusely infiltrated the pericardium and epicardium, resulting in a shaggy hemorrhagic exudate. A mixture of thrombus and blood was present within the pericardial space. (From Bloor, C. M.: Cardiac Pathology. Philadelphia, J. B. Lippincott Co., 1978.)

rectly diagnosed antemortem in only 8.5 per cent.[425] Among those patients with pericardial involvement, it was the direct cause of death in 36 per cent and a contributory factor in 49 per cent. In malignant pericarditis, dyspnea, cough, and chest pain occur frequently, while the physical findings of distant heart sounds and a pericardial friction rub are rarely detected. In many patients, symptoms resulting from pericardial involvement, such as dyspnea, hepatomegaly, and edema, may be incorrectly attributed to the underlying neoplasm, so that malignant pericarditis is not suspected until symptoms and signs of severe cardiac compression appear. Facial swelling, jugular venous distention, pulsus paradoxus, and cardiac tamponade relieved by pericardiocentesis occurred more frequently with neoplastic pericarditis than in patients with an underlying neoplasm and idiopathic or radiation-induced pericarditis.[448]

The *chest roentgenogram* is abnormal in more than 90 per cent of patients with malignant pericarditis and may show cardiac enlargement, mediastinal widening, a hilar mass, or, less commonly, an irregular nodular contour of the cardiac silhouette.[425,448] The *electrocardiogram* is usually abnormal but nonspecific, showing tachycardia, ST- and T-wave changes, low QRS voltage, and occasionally atrial fibrillation. Electrical alternans suggests the presence of a large malignant pericardial effusion under pressure.[449] Electrocardiographic findings rarely seen in pericarditis, such as atrioventricular conduction disturbances, suggest malignant invasion of the myocardium and conduction system.

DIAGNOSIS. The diagnosis of malignant pericarditis depends on both documentation of pericardial involvement and substantiation that pericarditis is due to neoplasm. Approximately half the patients with symptomatic pericarditis and neoplastic disease may have *nonmalignant* pericarditis due to prior radiation, idiopathic causes, infection, or an autoimmune disorder.[448] Many patients with advanced neoplastic disease are immunosuppressed as a consequence of their malignancy and/or therapy and are therefore at high risk for tubercular and fungal pericarditis. Acute pericarditis has also been reported as a complication of the intravenous administration of the chemotherapeutic agents adriamycin and daunorubicin.

Echocardiography often provides critical information about the presence and size of a pericardial effusion and the thickness and motion of the pericardium and may suggest the presence of abnormal diastolic filling of the heart due to cardiac compression. Two-dimensional echocardiography may be helpful in the detection of irregular undulating masses that protrude into the pericardial space and suggest the presence of pericardial metastases (Fig. 43–27).[450] Cardiac radionuclide scanning with gallium-67 citrate and technetium-99m pyrophosphate has also been used to detect malignant pericardial effusion,[451,452] but the specificity and sensitivity of these techniques are not established.

As in other forms of pericarditis, pericardiocentesis should be performed in conjunction with cardiac catheterization in patients with a large anterior and posterior pericardial effusion, documented by echocardiography, and suspected cardiac tamponade. Superior vena caval obstruction may coexist with malignant cardiac tamponade and contribute to the development of facial edema and jugular

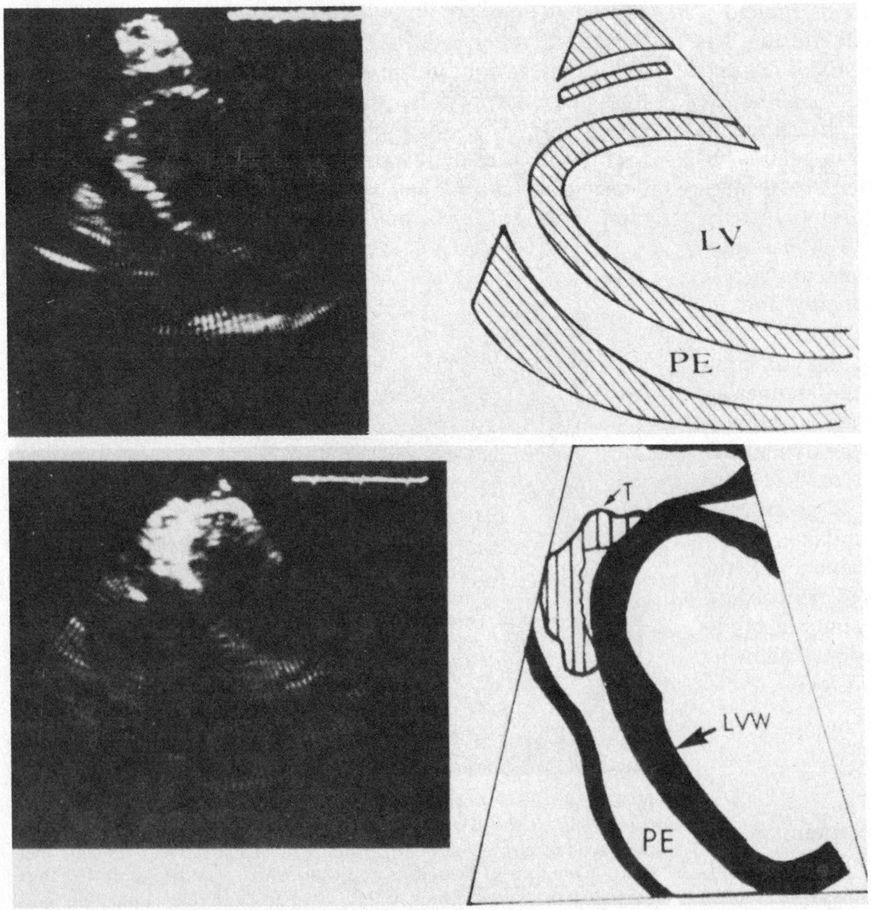

FIGURE 43–27 *Upper panel,* Cross-sectional echogram of an uncomplicated pericardial effusion showing a large clear space that denotes the pericardial effusion (PE) posterior to the left ventricle (LV). *Lower panel,* In contrast, the cross-sectional echogram from a patient with a malignant pericardial effusion shows irregular cauliflower-like masses (T) protruding into the pericardial effusion that represent bulky metastases. (From Chandraratna, P. A. N., et al.: Detection of pericardial metastases by cross-sectional echocardiography. Circulation *63*:167, 1981, by permission of the American Heart Association, Inc.)

venous distention and should be systematically excluded at cardiac catheterization in cancer patients.[156,448,453]

Pericardial fluid obtained at pericardiocentesis is serosanguineous or hemorrhagic in about two-thirds of patients and serous in the remainder. The appearance of the fluid does *not* differentiate between neoplastic, radiation, or idiopathic etiologies. Since treatment strategies differ, it is necessary to carry out a meticulous cytological examination of pericardial fluid in an attempt to differentiate malignant pericarditis from radiation-induced or idiopathic pericarditis. Cytological examination of pericardial fluid is diagnostic of a malignancy in about 85 per cent of cases of malignant pericarditis.[448,454,455] False-negative cytological diagnoses are uncommon in carcinomatous pericarditis but occur more commonly in involvement of the pericardium by lymphoma of mesothelioma.[156,448,456] In patients strongly suspected of neoplastic pericarditis, open pericardial biopsy may be required if the cytological examination of pericardial fluid is negative. If a sufficiently large biopsy specimen is obtained, open pericardial biopsy should provide a histological diagnosis in up to 90 per cent of cases.[454] However, false-negative diagnoses may occur if only a small tissue sample is obtained, and in critically ill patients open pericardial biopsy is not without risk.

In patients with echocardiographic evidence of a thickened pericardium and the physical findings of cardiac compression (jugular venous distention, edema, ascites, and hepatomegaly), cardiac catheterization is useful for documenting the presence of constrictive physiology before a decision is made to proceed with aggressive surgical intervention, i.e., extensive pericardiectomy.

Neoplastic pericarditis with cardiac compression must be differentiated from other causes of jugular venous distention, hepatomegaly, and peripheral edema in cancer patients. The most important of these are (1) underlying left ventricular dysfunction secondary to prior cardiac disease or adriamycin cardiac toxicity, (2) superior vena caval obstruction, (3) malignant hepatic involvement with portal hypertension, and (4) lymphangitic tumor spread in the lungs with secondary pulmonary hypertension.

NATURAL HISTORY. If cardiac tamponade can be avoided or successfully treated, the mere presence of neoplastic pericarditis does not imply that death is imminent. The reported *mean* survival of patients with neoplastic pericarditis ranges from 9 to 13 months.[457] In one series, a Kaplan-Meier analysis indicated a median survival of 4 months.[448] Long-term survival may be seen with neoplastic pericarditis and cardiac tamponade secondary to breast cancer.[458] In one series, 15 patients survived this complication for 1 to 2 years.[456]

MANAGEMENT. Decisions about the management of neoplastic pericardial effusion depend on the underlying condition of the patient, the presence or absence of clinical manifestations related to cardiac compression, and the prognosis and treatment options available for the specific histology and stage of the underlying malignancy. At one extreme are debilitated patients with end-stage malignant disease who have no promising treatment option for the underlying malignancy and a bleak prognosis. In this setting, diagnostic procedures should be as brief and painless as possible, and intervention should be directed toward alleviation of *symptoms* with the goal of improving the quality of the remaining days or weeks of life. In these patients, pericardiocentesis with catheter drainage is indicated for immediate relief of severe dyspnea, chest pain, or orthopnea. When the general prognosis of the patient is better, several more aggressive treatment options are available, the goals of which are (1) relief of cardiac tamponade, (2) prevention of recurrence of the malignant effusion, and (3) treatment or prevention of constrictive pericardial disease.[459]

In patients with asymptomatic pericardial effusion who have a treatment option of effective chemotherapy or hormonal therapy directed against the underlying malignancy, treatment with systemic agents alone can be attempted while progression of the effusion is observed by means of echocardiography. In patients with cardiac tamponade and large effusions secondary to neoplastic pericarditis, pericardiocentesis with catheter drainage in combination with systemic chemotherapy can be attempted.[156,448,460] If a symptomatic pericardial effusion recurs, more prolonged palliation can be attempted with a subxiphoid pericardiotomy.[461,462] This procedure has the disadvantage of being relatively ineffective when there is extensive tumor encasement of the heart, and pericardial windows may close secondary to the development of adhesions, thereby necessitating more extensive drainage procedures.

Another approach is the instillation of various chemotherapeutic agents or radioisotopes into the pericardial space following pericardiocentesis and catheter drainage. A successful response, i.e., reduction or disappearance of an effusion, is presumably related to sclerosis of the pericardial membranes and obliteration of the pericardial space. Control of recurrent malignant pericardial effusions has been reported with intrapericardial instillation of talc,[460] tetracycline,[463] and antineoplastic agents such as nitrogen mustard, thiotepa, 5-fluorouracil, and methotrexate.[457,459,464–468] Encouraging results have also been claimed after the intrapericardial instillation of radioactive phosphorus (^{32}P), yttrium (^{90}Y), and gold (^{198}Au).[468–471] Side effects of instillation of intrapericardial agents include chest pain, nausea, and fever.

External-beam radiation therapy is an important option for patients with radiosensitive tumors who have not yet received extensive mediastinal or cardiac radiation as a treatment modality.[472] Approximately half the patients with malignant pericarditis due to a variety of primary tumors have responded to this form of treatment.[459,472–475] In one series, malignant pericardial effusion improved significantly in 11 of 16 patients with breast cancer and two of seven patients with lung cancer following 2,500 to 3,000 rads of cardiac radiation, while six of seven patients with malignant pericarditis secondary to leukemia or lymphoma improved with lower doses of cardiac radiation.[474] Extensive surgical pericardiectomy is reserved for patients with symptoms of cardiac compression due to constrictive pericarditis or tumor encasement of the heart who otherwise have a good prognosis (one- to two-year survival) relative to the underlying malignancy.

RADIATION PERICARDITIS

ETIOLOGY. Radiation injury to the heart and pericardium is an important complication of megavoltage radiation therapy used in the treatment of breast carcinoma, Hodgkin's disease, and non-Hodgkin's lymphoma. It is estimated that a threshold dose of around 4,000 rads (1,500 rems) delivered to the heart is required to produce radiation injury to the pericardium.[459,476] In a series of 117 patients with carcinoma of the breast who received radiation therapy, the incidence of radiation-induced cardiac injury was 3.4 per cent,[459] while the incidence of radiation injury to the pericardium in 81 patients who underwent mantle irradiation for Hodgkin's disease was 29 per cent.[477] Pericardial injury may occur during the course of treatment or weeks to months later.[478–482] In one series, 92 per cent of cases presenting with pericardial effusions occurred within 12 months after completion of the course of radiation therapy.[477] However, it is now recognized that radiation pericarditis manifest as chronic pericardial effusion or constrictive pericarditis may become apparent *many years* after radiation therapy.[483–485] Currently employed radiotherapy techniques using subcarinal blocks that shield the heart have helped to decrease the risk of radiation-induced pericardial injury.[486]

PATHOLOGY. Acute radiation pericarditis is associated with fibrin deposition and pericardial fibrosis (Fig. 43–28). The acute inflammatory stage may be accompanied by a pericardial effusion that can be serous, serosanguineous, or hemorrhagic with a high protein and lymphocyte content.[487,488] The inflammation and initial effusion may resolve spontaneously, or the effusion may organize and progress to a stage of dense fibrinous adhesions with gradual obliteration of the pericardial space and thickening of the pericardium, causing a chronic pericardial effusion or a constricting pericardium. Radiation pericarditis is one of the most common causes of effusive-constrictive pericardial disease.[268] Radiation injury represents an important cause of constrictive pericarditis in children, in whom constrictive diseases are otherwise rare.[489]

It is important to recognize that radiation may also injure the heart itself, causing interstitial myocardial fibrosis, valvular thickening, and premature atherosclerosis of the epicardial coronary arteries.[487,490]

CLINICAL FEATURES. The acute form of pericarditis with postradiation pericardial effusion may be transient and asymptomatic, so that the mode of presentation is an increase in heart size seen on the chest roentgenogram. Other patients may present with a syndrome of acute pericarditis consisting of fever, pericardial pain, anorexia, malaise, a pericardial friction rub, and electrocardiographic abnormalities suggestive of this disease. Radiation-induced pericardial effusion may rarely produce fatal cardiac tamponade.[481] In the chronic form of pericardial injury, patients may present more than 20 years after radiation therapy with the insidious onset of fatigue, dyspnea, systemic edema, and jugular venous distention due to the development of constrictive pericarditis.[479,484,485,491,492] The clinical recognition and consequences of this delayed form of pericardial injury have become increasingly important as patients with breast cancer and Hodgkin's disease have prolonged survival and cures.

DIAGNOSIS. Radiation-induced pericarditis with a pericardial effusion is most often confused with pericarditis due to the underlying malignancy. However, patients with malignant pericardial effusion are more likely to present with massive effusions and cardiac tamponade, and cytological examination of pericardial fluid can identify a ma-

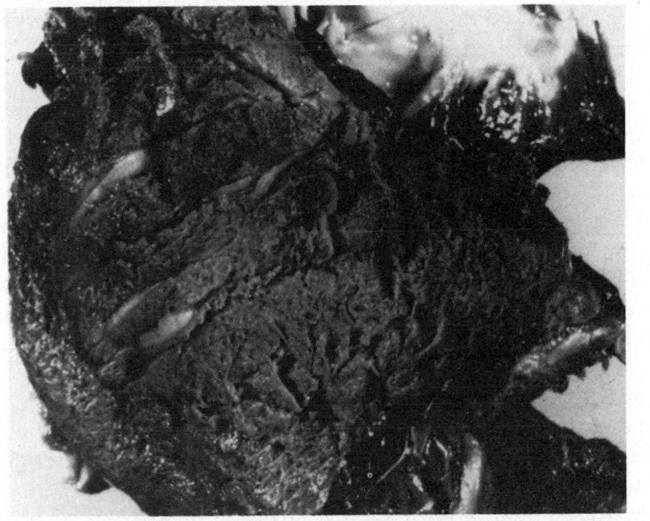

FIGURE 43–28 Gross pathologic specimen of a heart with radiation pericarditis that developed after radiation therapy for lung carcinoma. The surface of the heart is covered with a thick, shaggy, fibrinous pericarditis that was associated with a pericardial effusion. (From Bloor, C. M.: Cardiac Pathology. Philadelphia, J. B. Lippincott Co., 1978.)

lignant origin in about 85 per cent of cases.[448] In some patients, it may be extremely difficult to differentiate between these two entities without resorting to pericardial biopsy and histological examination of the pericardium. When symptoms referable to the pericardium occur years after apparently successful treatment of Hodgkin's disease or lymphoma, the pericarditis is much more likely to be related to radiation injury than to recurrent mediastinal malignancy.

MANAGEMENT. Patients in whom an asymptomatic pericardial effusion develops following radiation therapy may be followed by physical examination and serial echocardiography without the institution of specific therapy. Percutaneous pericardiocentesis should be limited to the treatment of cardiac tamponade or to drainage of a large pericardial effusion when cytological examination is required for management. Systemic corticosteroids may reduce chest pain and the size of the radiation-induced pericardial effusion, and in patients in whom purulent pericarditis is not suspected, a short course of corticosteroids is advised.[493,494] Sometimes pericarditis recurs after withdrawal of corticosteroids.[494,495] Pericardiectomy is required for that small number of symptomatic patients with large recurrent pericardial effusion, severe effusive-constrictive, or constrictive pericarditis. For some patients with constrictive pericarditis the outcome is reported to be excellent after pericardiectomy, while in others the outcome is poor due to persistent visceral pericardial constriction (epicarditis) or underlying myocardial injury.[496,497]

PERICARDITIS RELATED TO HYPERSENSITIVITY OR AUTOIMMUNITY

ACUTE RHEUMATIC FEVER (See also page 1646)

During the 19th century, acute rheumatic fever was believed to be the most common cause of pericarditis, and it was recognized that rheumatic pericarditis could occur independently of overt endocarditis.[498] The condition is now uncommon, but occasionally the development of a pericardial friction rub or effusion is the initial clue to the presence of rheumatic carditis.

Pathophysiology. Rheumatic pericarditis is characterized by fibrin deposition with localized or diffuse fibrous thickening of the pericardium. Osler reported that pericarditis could be accompanied by a fibrinous, serofibrinous, or purulent exudate.[498] The pericardial reaction may resolve spontaneously, and at autopsy there may be little evidence of prior pericardial inflammation in patients who die late from rheumatic heart disease. The development of chronic calcification and constrictive pericarditis, although reported, is very rare.[499]

Clinical Features. Rheumatic pericarditis usually occurs at the onset of the initial episode of acute rheumatic fever and may be asymptomatic or associated with typical pericardial pain and other symptoms of acute rheumatic fever, including fever, malaise, and arthralgias (p. 1648). When present, pericarditis often indicates an extensive pancarditis. The *diagnosis* of rheumatic pericarditis is based on the presence of pericardial chest pain, a pericardial friction rub, or echocardiographic evidence of a pericardial effusion in association with the usual serological and clinical criteria for acute rheumatic fever (p. 1649). In children, the onset of pericarditis, which is otherwise rare in this age group, should prompt a rigorous search for evidence of acute rheumatic fever. In the current era of antibiotic therapy and public hygiene in developed nations where acute rheumatic fever is no longer a common disease, acute rheumatic fever may not be recognized, and the combination of pericarditis, fever, arthralgias, and rash in a child or young adult may be mistaken for a viral exanthem, infectious endocarditis, juvenile rheumatoid arthritis, systemic lupus erythematosus, Henoch-Schönlein purpura, Crohn's disease, or sickle cell crisis.

Management. The treatment of rheumatic pericarditis is that of acute rheumatic fever and includes bed rest and penicillin as well as digoxin if myocardial failure is present. Chest pain associated with rheumatic pericarditis or arthralgias should be treated with aspirin, as described on page 1654. Rarely, corticosteroids are required. Small or moderate-sized pericardial effusions usually resolve spontaneously, and pericardiocentesis should not be performed solely for diagnostic reasons in a patient with documented acute rheumatic fever.

PERICARDITIS ASSOCIATED WITH SYSTEMIC LUPUS ERYTHEMATOSUS (See also page 1661)

Pericarditis usually occurs during flare-ups of disease activity in patients with systemic lupus erythematosus and is rare during quiescent phases of the disease. Pericarditis is detected clinically in about half these patients during the course of their disease, while the prevalence of pericarditis in autopsied patients is as high as 75 per cent.[500–502] The inflammatory process may cause fibrinous or effusive pericarditis with the rare occurrence of pathognomonic hematoxylin bodies in the visceral pericardium.[500] Pericardial fluid may be serous or grossly hemorrhagic with a high protein content, low glucose content, and white cell count below 10,000/mm^2 (composed primarily of polymorphonuclear leukocytes).[501] Pericardial fluid complement levels that are lower than normal serum values have been reported in patients with systemic lupus erythematosus, but caution must be used in interpreting this finding, since total hemolytic complement levels appear to be normally low in pericardial fluid.[501,503] Pericardial effusions may also contain lupus erythematosus cells and immune complexes.[504,505] Cardiac tamponade occurs in less than 10 per cent of patients with systemic lupus erythematosus and clinically recognized pericarditis, while the development of constrictive pericarditis has been reported but is extremely rare.[501,506] Pericarditis due to systemic lupus erythematosus may be accompanied by other cardiac lesions, including verrucous endocarditis,[507] inflammation and necrosis involving the conduction system, and coronary artery vasculitis (p. 1660).[508,509]

Clinical Features. Patients commonly complain of typical pericardial pain, dyspnea, and fever and present with a pericardial friction rub. Diffuse serositis including the presence of unilateral or bilateral pleuritis and pleural effusion is present in about one-fourth of patients.[501,510] The *chest roentgenogram* may show enlargement of the cardiac silhouette, pleural effusions, and parenchymal infiltrates. The roentgenographic findings of new cardiac enlargement and pulmonary venous hypertension due to a pericardial effusion under pressure must be differentiated from congestive heart failure secondary to myocardial dysfunction, a common problem in patients with systemic lupus erythematosus. *Electrocardiographic abnormalities* are those characteristic of acute pericarditis.

Pericarditis should be suspected when patients with systemic lupus erythematosus develop pleuritic chest pain, a pericardial rub, and an enlarging cardiac silhouette on the chest roentgenogram.[510] Since pericarditis usually occurs during periods of active disease, there is typically evidence of increased disease activity on blood tests for complement-fixation levels, antinuclear antibodies, lupus erythematosus cell preparations, and sedimentation rate. The *echocardiogram* may show evidence of a new pericardial effusion, confirming the presence of pericardial inflammation. Since many patients with systemic lupus erythematosus are treated with immunosuppressive corticosteroids and cytotoxic agents, a careful physical examination, blood cultures, and tuberculin skin test should be performed to search for evidence of purulent, fungal, or tuberculous pericarditis. Except when purulent pericarditis is strongly suspected, it is usually not necessary to confirm the clinical diagnosis of systemic lupus erythematosus pericarditis by performing pericardiocentesis. Systemic lupus erythematosus pericarditis can usually be distinguished from viral pericarditis by the absence of a prodromal upper respiratory infection and by the presence of other clinical findings suggestive of active systemic lupus erythematosus.

Management. In the majority of patients, pericarditis subsides when the systemic disease becomes inactive following treatment with corticosteroids or immunotherapy. The unusual complication of cardiac tamponade can ordinarily be treated with pericardiocentesis and usually does not require surgical intervention (i.e., a pericardial window or pericardiectomy). However, since the development of acute cardiac tamponade is unpredictable, patients with systemic lupus erythematosus pericarditis should be hospitalized and under close observation.

RHEUMATOID ARTHRITIS (See also page 1658)

Rheumatoid pericarditis was first described by Charcot, who observed pericardial fibrosis in four of nine autopsied patients.[511] Although pericarditis is detected at autopsy in up to 50 per cent of patients with rheumatoid arthritis, the clinical incidence of symptomatic pericarditis is less than 10 per cent.[501,512-514] Based on echocardiographic criteria for the presence of a pericardial effusion, pericarditis has been detected in 50 per cent of patients with chronic nodular rheumatoid arthritis, in 15 per cent of patients with typical non-nodular rheumatoid arthritis, and in no patients of comparable age with osteoarthritis.[515] Pericarditis tends to appear in patients with other evidence of severe rheumatoid arthritis, including extensive joint deformity, subcutaneous rheumatoid nodules, pneumonitis, and positive serum rheumatoid factor. The development of rheumatoid pericarditis, however, does not appear to correlate with the duration of the arthritis.[512] Rheumatoid pericarditis in adults can cause cardiac tamponade and has become recognized as an important cause of effusive-constrictive pericarditis and constrictive pericarditis.[268,512,516,517] In children with juvenile rheumatoid arthritis, pleuritis, pericarditis, and pneumonitis may occur without evidence of active joint involvement.[518-520]

Pathology. Typical pathological changes in the pericardium described at autopsy are those of nonspecific fibrous thickening of the visceral and parietal pericardium with adhesions and, occasionally, focal deposition of calcium and cholesterol. Rarely, small, necrotic granulomatous nodules are detected on the epicardial surface that are histologically identical to the subcutaneous rheumatoid nodule. Pericardial effusions associated with rheumatoid arthritis pericarditis are usually serous or hemorrhagic, with greater than 5 gm/dl of protein, glucose levels less than 45 mg/dl, and white blood cell counts ranging from 20,000 to 90,000/mm^3.[501,512] Pericardial effusion may also contain polymorphonuclear leukocytes with cytoplasmic inclusion bodies characteristic of rheumatoid arthritis. Gamma globulin complexes, positive latex-fixation titers, and low complement levels in the pericardial fluid have also been described.[521] Acute pericarditis may progress to cause diffusely constricting fibrotic pericarditis and can coexist with other cardiac lesions, including granulomatous aortic and mitral valve deformity causing chronic mitral or aortic insufficiency.

Clinical Features. Rheumatoid arthritis is often associated with fever, precordial chest pain, and dyspnea in association with a pericardial friction rub.[521] Pericarditis commonly coexists with an exacerbation of joint inflammation and pleuritis, manifest on the chest roentgenogram as a unilateral or bilateral pleural effusion in about 65 per cent of cases.[521] The electrocardiogram usually shows nonspecific ST-segment and T-wave changes. The presence of atrioventricular block in patients with rheumatoid pericarditis probably reflects rheumatoid myocardial involvement (p. 1660). On echocardiography a pericardial effusion is present in approximately half the patients with nodular rheumatoid arthritis. An effusion may be associated with echocardiographic evidence of mitral valve abnormalities in about 25 per cent of patients.[515,522,523]

Although rheumatoid pericarditis is usually self-limited and benign, cardiac tamponade may develop abruptly in 3 to 25 per cent of patients.[501,512,517] Cardiac tamponade occurs in both adult and juvenile rheumatoid arthritis[518,519,524] and has been reported as a complication of sudden steroid withdrawal.[525] An uncommon but major complication is the rapid onset of subacute constrictive or effusive-constrictive pericarditis.[512,516,517]

Management. Patients with symptomatic pericarditis may be treated with aspirin or other nonsteroidal antiinflammatory agents, as described on page 1477. Pericardiocentesis is indicated for relief of a large anterior-posterior effusion causing cardiac tamponade. Although some authors advocate treatment with corticosteroids,[521] there is no clear evidence that steroids alter the natural history of effusions or prevent the development of the complication of effusive-constrictive pericarditis.[512] In patients with documented effusive-constrictive or constrictive pericarditis, pericardiectomy can provide gratifying hemodynamic and symptomatic improvement.[512,516,517,526,527]

SCLERODERMA PERICARDITIS (See also page 1663)

Pericardial involvement is found at autopsy in about 50 per cent of patients with progressive systemic sclerosis (scleroderma), while pericarditis is detected clinically in about 10 per cent of patients.[501,528-530] While the pathogenesis of scleroderma pericarditis is unknown, it has been suggested that increased collagen formation by fibroblasts, in combination with tissue hypoxia, may result in aberrant collagen metabolism. Histological changes are nonspecific fibrotic pericardial thickening with adhesions and perivascular inflammatory cells. Pericardial effusion was detected by means of echocardiography in 41 per cent of patients with scleroderma, although it had been suspected clinically in only a minority of these.[531]

When present, the pericardial effusion is straw-colored and characterized by a protein content greater than 5 gm/dl, low cell count, and—in contrast to the characteristics of pericardial effusions in systemic lupus erythematosus and rheumatoid arthritis—the *absence* of autoantibodies, low complement levels, and immune complexes.[501] Pericardial involvement is often associated with sclerodermatous infiltration of the heart, causing a restrictive cardiomyopathy.[530]

Scleroderma pericardial disease may present as an acute syndrome resembling viral myocarditis, with fever, chest pain, a pericardial friction rub, and nonspecific electrocardiographic ST- and T-wave changes.[529] Other patients develop a chronic pericardial effusion with symptoms of right and left atrial hypertension, cardiomegaly and pleural effusions on the chest roentgenogram, and low QRS voltage on the electrocardiogram.[501]

There is no definitive treatment for scleroderma pericarditis. Patients with the syndrome of acute pericarditis may be treated with aspirin, as described on page 1477. Rarely, pericardial effusions with cardiac tamponade may develop, necessitating pericardiocentesis.[532] Patients with symptoms and hemodynamic abnormalities due to constrictive pericarditis may require pericardiectomy. It is especially important to perform cardiac catheterization in patients with scleroderma and suspected cardiac tamponade or constrictive pericarditis, since dyspnea and systemic venous hypertension may be related to sclerodermatous cardiac involvement or to pulmonary hypertension with right ventricular failure secondary to pulmonary fibrosis. The development of pericarditis in patients with scleroderma is ominous, since the five-year survival rate is about 25 per cent when isolated pericardial or other cardiac involvement is present and about 75 per cent in patients without heart, lung, or kidney involvement.[533]

PERICARDITIS IN OTHER CONNECTIVE TISSUE DISORDERS

Pericarditis may rarely develop in other connective tissue disorders, including mixed connective tissue disease, Sjögren's syndrome, dermatomyositis, ankylosing spondylitis, Reiter's syndrome, Wegener's granulomatosis, Felty's syndrome, and severe serum sickness.[501,534–536] Pericarditis associated with polyarteritis nodosa may occur in patients who are hepatitis B antigen–positive. It also occurs in disorders of possible autoimmune etiology, including temporal arteritis,[537] inflammatory bowel disease,[538–540] Kawasaki's disease,[541] Still's disease,[542] Whipple's disease,[543] Behçet's disease, and Henoch-Schönlein purpura.[501] Amyloidosis is well known as a cause of infiltrative restrictive myopathy, the hemodynamics of which may mimic constrictive pericarditis (p. 1488), but may also involve the pericardium and cause pericardial effusions.[237,238]

DRUG-RELATED PERICARDITIS

Pericarditis occurs in about 25 per cent of patients with procainamide-related and 2 per cent of those with hydralazine-related development of the systemic lupus erythematosus syndrome.[508,544] In these patients, pericarditis may occasionally be complicated by the development of cardiac tamponade or pericardial constriction.[545–547] Other drugs that may produce pericarditis in association with the drug-induced syndrome of systemic lupus erythematosus include reserpine, methyldopa, isoniazid, and diphenylhydantoin.[502,508,548]

Other drugs appear to produce pericarditis through separate mechanisms. Pericarditis has been reported as a complication of a hypersensitivity reaction with peripheral eosinophilia after administration of penicillin[339] and cromolyn sodium.[549] The mechanisms of drug-induced pericarditis following administration of 6-amino-9-D-psicofuranosylpurine[550] and minoxidil[551,552] are not understood. Pleural and pericardial effusions have also been reported in several patients after administration of dantrolene sodium.[553] Methysergide has been reported to cause constrictive pericarditis as part of a generalized process of mediastinal fibrosis.[554] The anthracycline neoplastic agents doxorubicin and daunorubicin may cause acute pericarditis as well as myocardial inflammation within the first three weeks of drug administration (p. 1690).[555]

Acute drug-related pericarditis usually resolves when the offending drug is discontinued, and improvement may be accelerated by the administration of corticosteroids. The rare development of chronic constrictive pericarditis may be treated by pericardiectomy.

POSTMYOCARDIAL INFARCTION (DRESSLER'S) SYNDROME

Dressler's syndrome is an acute illness with fever, pericarditis, and pleuritis, probably of autoimmune origin, that occurs weeks to months after an acute myocardial infarction.[556] In the majority of the 44 patients described by Dressler in 1959, pericarditis occurred between the 7th and 11th weeks after infarction.[557] Today, a distinction is usually made between simple acute pericarditis, which occurs during the first week after infarction (p. 1503), and Dressler's syndrome, which usually appears two to three weeks after infarction, with a range of one week to several months. Dressler estimated that this syndrome occurred in up to 4 per cent of patients after acute myocardial infarction[557]; however, a recent series from the same hospital indicates that the incidence of Dressler's syndrome has markedly decreased.[558]

The etiology of Dressler's syndrome is unknown. The association of symptoms and the appearance of antimyocardial antibodies has led to the hypothesis that an autoimmune mechanism, with or without a latent viral infection, is the etiology,[559,560] while some workers have concluded that the development of antimyocardial antibodies is not specific for the presence of Dressler's syndrome.[558,561] Leakage of blood into the pericardial space is another proposed mechanism, and the lower current incidence of the syndrome may reflect changing patterns of anticoagulant use in the postinfarction period.[558] It is likely that there are common factors in the pathogenesis of Dressler's syndrome and the postpericardiotomy syndrome (p. 1514), both of which have the following features: (1) an initial insult of endothelial cell injury and entry of blood into the pericardial space; (2) a delayed response after the initial insult, consisting of fever and inflammation of the pericardial surfaces; (3) development of antiheart antibodies; (4) a dramatic response to antiinflammatory agents; and (5) the common occurrence of relapses at intervals as long as two years after the initial episode.

Pathology. The histology of the pericardium usually reveals a nonspecific inflammation with fibrin deposition. In contrast to the acute pericarditis following myocardial infarction in which pericardial inflammation is often patchy, overlying the regions of infarction, the pericarditis in Dressler's syndrome is usually diffuse. A small to moderate-sized serous pericardial effusion may develop, but the incidence of this complication is not known.

Clinical Features. Patients characteristically present with severe malaise, fever, chest pain, and pleurisy.[557,562] The chest pain may be severe enough initially to cause both patient and physician to consider that it is caused by a second myocardial infarction. In other patients, the pain is characterized as a mild, vague discomfort or as pain localized to the substernal, precordial, neck, or back regions with a pleuritic or generalized aching quality. The pain may be severe and unremitting for days to weeks and is not relieved by nitroglycerin. Physical examination often discloses a pericardial friction rub and sometimes a pleural friction rub as well. The chest roentgenogram commonly reveals an enlarged cardiac silhouette secondary to pericardial effusion associated with pleural effusions[557] and, occasionally, transient pulmonary infiltrates. Pericardial effusions too small to be detected on the chest roentgenogram may be detected by echocardiography. Electrocardiographic abnormalities usually consist of serial ST-segment and T-wave changes strongly suggestive of acute pericarditis, but the electrocardiogram may not be helpful in patients with persistent repolarization abnormalities following infarction. Blood tests usually reveal the nonspecific findings of an increased erythrocyte sedimentation rate and peripheral leukocytosis. Tests for antimyocardial antibodies are often positive but are not specific and not widely available or established as a means of confirming the diagnosis.

Dressler's syndrome can usually be discriminated from recurrent myocardial infarction by (1) the characteristics of the chest pain, as described above; (2) the absence of new Q waves on the electrocardiogram; and (3) the absence of a marked rise in the CK-MB band. Small increases in cardiac enzyme levels may occur in pericarditis when the underlying epicardium is involved. Dressler's syndrome must also be distinguished from hemorrhagic pericarditis secondary to chronic systemic anticoagulation, pulmonary embolism and infarction, and progressive cardiac failure.

Management. A single episode of Dressler's syndrome is usually self-limited, but the syndrome does tend to recur. The initial episode usually warrants hospital admission and observation for the development of pericardial effusion or cardiac tamponade. Oral anticoagulants should be discontinued because of the risk of hemorrhage into a pericardial effusion. As in other patients with acute pericarditis, patients who are severely symptomatic with fever and chest pain usually benefit from treatment with aspirin or a nonsteroidal antiinflammatory agent. Therapeutic failure with these agents is an indication for a trial of corticosteroids, which should be tapered within four weeks followed by substitution with aspirin. Recurrent episodes of Dressler's syndrome may respond only to corticosteroids and occasionally require complete pericardiectomy for relief of intractable pericardial pain or prevention of recurrence.[563] Cardiac tamponade, although uncommon, has been reported[564] and can usually be managed with pericardiocentesis. Constrictive pericarditis is an extremely rare complication of Dressler's syndrome that may be relieved by pericardiectomy.[565,566]

POSTPERICARDIOTOMY SYNDROME

Etiology. Postpericardiotomy syndrome is identified by the appearance of fever, pericarditis, and pleuritis two to four weeks after a cardiac operation in which the pericardium has been opened and manipulated. This syndrome was first recognized in patients after mitral commissurotomy for rheumatic heart disease, and it was initially believed to represent a reactivation of rheumatic fever.[567] Subsequently it was appreciated that the syndrome could occur following cardiac operations in patients without rheumatic heart disease and that the common denominator appeared to be wide incision and manipulation of the pericardium.[568–570] An identical clinical syndrome has been reported following cardiac perforation by a catheter or transvenous pacemaker, blunt chest trauma, percutaneous diagnostic left ventricular puncture, and epicardial pacemaker implantation.[569] The incidence of postpericardiotomy syndrome following cardiac surgery ranges from 10 to 40 per cent in various series and averages about 30 per cent.[570–573] The observation of a 31 per cent incidence of postpericardiotomy syndrome in patients undergoing cardiac surgery for the Wolff-Parkinson-White syndrome clearly indicates that pericardial damage prior to surgery is *not* a prerequisite for development of the syndrome.[573] Furthermore, pericardial drainage techniques do not appear to affect the frequency of development of the syndrome after cardiac surgery.[574]

Analogous to Dressler's syndrome, the etiology of postpericardiotomy syndrome is hypothesized to be an autoimmune reaction directed against the epicardium in concert with a new or reactivated viral infection.[560,575] Studies by Engle and colleagues have demonstrated that antiheart antibodies appear in the serum of some patients who undergo pericardiotomy and that there is a positive correlation between the level of the titers and the incidence of the syndrome.[572,575] Approximately 70 per cent of patients with the postpericardiotomy syndrome and high antiheart antibody titers also develop a fourfold or higher rise in titer against one or more viral antigens, while in patients without the postpericardiotomy syndrome, a rise in viral titers occurs in only 8 per cent of those with negative antiheart antibody titers and in only 19 per cent of those with low levels of antiheart antibody titers[575]; these findings suggest that viral infection may be a triggering or permissive factor. The postpericardiotomy syndrome is rare in children under 2 years of age who undergo cardiac surgery, a finding that may be related to the short exposure time to viruses or to protective maternal antibodies transmitted via the placenta. The development of pleuritis and pleural effusions is believed to reflect involvement of the pleura adjacent to the inflamed pericardium; involvement of serous membranes distant from the heart is uncommon.

Pathology. There are no pathognomonic histological features of postpericardiotomy syndrome. The presence of blood in the pericardial space adjacent to an injured epicardium may result in the later development of pericardial adhesions, thickening of the pericardial membranes, and occasionally fibrinous obliteration of the pericardial space, causing pericardial constriction. Pericardial effusions in patients with postpericardiotomy syndrome may be straw-colored, serosanguineous, or frankly hemorrhagic, with a protein content higher than 4.5 gm/dl and a white blood cell count between 3,000 and 8,000/mm^3 (composed of both lymphocytes and granulocytes).[576]

Clinical Features. Patients typically develop an acute illness characterized by fever, malaise, and pleuritic chest pain that usually begins during the second or third postoperative week. In some cases, the fever may reflect a continuation of the more common problem of fever in the first week after operation. The chest pain is typical of acute pericarditis (p. 1474) and often has a pleuritic quality. The physician may not recognize the implication of the chest pain and may inappropriately ascribe it to the surgical incision or the presence of chest tubes. Nonspecific myalgias, arthralgias, and anorexia may also be present.

Physical examination often reveals a pericardial friction rub. It should be noted that the friction rub present in almost all patients during the first few days after cardiac surgery disappears in most patients who do not develop postpericardiotomy syndrome by the end of the first postoperative week. The chest roentgenogram demonstrates bilateral pleural effusions in about two-thirds of patients, pulmonary infiltrates in about one-tenth, and transient enlargement of the cardiac silhouette in half.[573] Electrocardiographic changes include nonspecific ST-segment and T-wave changes and a variety of episodic tachyarrhythmias.

Echocardiography is useful in monitoring the appearance and size of a pericardial effusion, which may be detected in about 40 per cent of patients with the postpericardiotomy syndrome.[577] Thus, the diagnosis of postpericardiotomy syndrome is made on clinical grounds based on recognition of the distinctive features of the syndrome in the postoperative patient. Other causes of postoperative fever, particularly infection, including the viral-induced postperfusion syndrome of atypical lymphocytosis, fever, and hepatosplenomegaly, must be excluded.[578]

Management. The postpericardiotomy syndrome is a self-limited but often prolonged and disabling illness. Fever and severe chest pain are usually relieved by aspirin or nonsteroidal antiinflammatory drugs. Corticosteroids should be reserved for patients in whom fever and chest pain are not relieved within 48 hours by other antiinflammatory agents. Recurrences tend to appear during the first six months after surgery and may occur in up to 50 per cent of patients.

Cardiac tamponade is an important and well-recognized complication of the postpericardiotomy syndrome.[576,579–582] In one large recently reported series of adult patients who survived cardiac surgery, almost 1 per cent developed cardiac tamponade an average of 49 days after surgery, in association with fever, a pericardial friction rub, and pericardial chest pain typical of the postpericardiotomy syndrome.[576] In contrast to the important role of anticoagulation in *early* postoperative bleeding after cardiac surgery, the use of anticoagulants did not appear to be a prerequisite for the development of cardiac tamponade in association with the postpericardiotomy syndrome. Patients at risk for the development of cardiac tamponade tend to have a large pericardial effusion (greater than 500 ml), detected by simple M-mode echocardiography. Cardiac tamponade can be managed conservatively by pericardiocentesis followed by the administration of antiinflammatory agents.[576] Patients with recurrent tamponade require pericardiectomy. Percutaneous pericardiocentesis should not be attempted in patients with echocardiographic evidence of only a posterior effusion, a loculated effusion, or an effusion with dense echoes suggesting the presence of both thrombus and free fluid. Constrictive pericarditis is a complication that may occur months to years after the postpericardiotomy syndrome.[583]

POSTOPERATIVE HEMOPERICARDIUM

Acute cardiac tamponade and pericardial constriction in the *absence* of typical features of the postpericardiotomy syndrome also occur secondary to hemopericardium following cardiac surgery and perforation of the heart during cardiac catheterization, pacemaker insertion, pericardiocentesis, and transthoracic cardiac puncture.[584–586] Although it is a form of traumatic pericarditis, it is included here because of its superficial similarities to the postpericardiotomy syndrome. In some patients, postoperative cardiac tamponade has been successfully managed with pericardiocentesis.[587] However, the development of early and late postoperative tamponade is usually due to the combination of free fluid and organizing thrombus, which requires open surgical drainage of the pericardial space. Localized compression of the left ventricle and right atrium has also been reported as a complication of postoperative cardiac tamponade.[588,589]

Constrictive pericarditis is being recognized increasingly as a complication of cardiac surgery and may occur in patients in whom the pericardium is left open but in situ.[590–594] In a recent review of 5,207 adults who underwent cardiac surgery, 0.2 per cent (11 patients) developed constrictive pericarditis documented by cardiac catheterization an average of 82 days after operation.[595] Important clinical features in these patients included dyspnea, jugular venous distention, pedal edema, and increased roentgenographic heart size, while echocardiographic evidence of pericardial thickening with a posterior pericardial effusion was detected in the majority. In this series, three patients responded to medical therapy with diuretics and antiinflammatory drugs, while the remainder improved after undergoing extensive pericardiectomy and were found to have hemorrhage-induced fibrosis of the pericardium, usually associated with a posterior organized hematoma.[595] Loculated hemorrhage in the posterior pericardial space in association with injury to the pericardium from local hypothermia and povidone-iodine irrigants is postulated to be the triggering stimulus in the development of pericardial inflammation and fibrosis.[592,595]

OTHER FORMS OF PERICARDIAL DISEASE

MYXEDEMA PERICARDIAL DISEASE

Myxedema is frequently associated with a myopathy; pericardial effusion also occurs in up to one-third of patients.[596–599] Since myxedematous patients frequently have ascites, pleural effusions, and uveal edema, it has been suggested that pericardial effusion may be related to a combination of sodium and water retention, slow lymphatic drainage, and increased capillary permeability with protein extravasation.[600] The pericardial fluid is usually clear or straw-colored, with elevated protein and cholesterol concentrations and few leukocytes or red blood cells. Pericardial fluid usually accumulates very slowly and may achieve volumes of 5 to 6 liters. Cholesterol crystals may also be present.[601] Occasionally, the pericardial effusion may resemble a viscous jelly rather than a clear fluid.

Myxedematous pericardial effusions usually do not cause symptoms. Often attention is called to the heart by the finding of marked cardiomegaly on a chest roentgenogram, and a large pericardial effusion is then detected on an echocardiogram.[596] The electrocardiogram often shows nonspecific abnormalities, including low QRS voltage and flattened or inverted T waves due to either myxedematous heart disease or pericardial effusion. The heart rate of myxedematous patients with pericardial effusion has been reported to be even slower than that of myxedematous patients without effusions.[596]

Myxedematous pericardial effusions tend to regress slowly and ultimately disappear over a period of months after patients have been treated with thyroid replacement and have returned to the euthyroid state.[596,599] Cardiac tamponade has been reported, but it is a rare complication.[601–605]

CHOLESTEROL PERICARDITIS

Cholesterol pericarditis results from pericardial injury associated with deposition of cholesterol crystals and a mononuclear cell inflammatory reaction consisting of foam cells, macrophages, and giant cells. The presence of cholesterol crystals in the pericardial space is believed to provoke a chronic inflammatory response that results in effusion and may ultimately lead to the development of constrictive pericarditis. A pericardial effusion that contains cholesterol crystals typically has a glittering "gold" appearance.[601] Cholesterol in the pericardial space may be derived from damaged or necrotic epicardial cells or lysed erythrocytes following hemopericardium.[606,607] The similarities in the lipid and cholesterol contents of pericardial fluid and serum in patients with cholesterol pericarditis suggest that simple transudation may explain the high cholesterol content in the pericardial space.

The management of patients with cholesterol pericarditis includes the detection and treatment of any underlying predisposing condition associated with the development of cholesterol pericarditis, such as tuberculous, rheumatoid, or myxedematous pericarditis or hypercholesterolemia. However, in the majority of cases, cholesterol pericarditis occurs in the absence of a clear underlying disease.[607] Cholesterol pericardial effusions are usually large, but since they develop slowly, they cause cardiac tamponade only occasionally. Pericardiectomy is indicated in the unlikely event of cardiac tamponade as well as in the treatment of massive cholesterol pericardial effusion, which may cause dyspnea and chest pain.[608] The development of constrictive pericarditis requiring pericardiectomy is rare.[609]

CHYLOPERICARDIUM

Chylopericardium consists of the accumulation of a chylous effusion in the pericardial space. Idiopathic chylopericardium is rare, and chylopericardium is usually associated with mechanical obstruction of the thoracic duct or its drainage into the left subclavian vein resulting from (1) surgical or traumatic rupture of the thoracic duct or (2) lymphatic blockage by neoplasms, tuberculosis, or lymphangiectasis.[610] Thoracic duct obstruction with failure of adequate collateral drainage then results in reflux of chyle through lymphatics draining the pericardium. Most patients with chylopericardium are asymptomatic and come to clinical attention when a large, slowly accumulating pericardial effusion is detected on chest roentgenogram or echocardiogram.[610,611] The presence of a connection between a damaged thoracic duct and the pericardial space can be established by lymphangiography[610] and computed tomography[612] as well as by the recovery of ingested Sudan III, a lipophilic dye, from pericardial aspirate.[610]

The pericardial fluid is usually milky white with a high cholesterol and triglyceride content, protein content greater than 3.5 gm/dl, and microscopic fat droplets.[610] Lymphopericardium, which is due to pericardial angiomas as part of a generalized lymphangiectasis, is characterized by clear pericardial fluid.

Cardiac tamponade is rare. The management of symptomatic chylopericardium consists of efforts to reduce the likelihood of recurrence. These include ingestion of a diet rich in medium-chain triglycerides[610] or, if this is unsuccessful, in ligation of the injured thoracic duct, if one is present, above the diaphragm, and parietal pericardiectomy to evacuate chylous fluid and prevent reaccumulation.[610]

TRAUMATIC PERICARDITIS

In addition to penetrating or nonpenetrating cardiac trauma (Chap. 44), other important causes of traumatic pericarditis include rupture of the esophagus into the pericardial space, which may occur from esophageal erosion secondary to esophageal carcinoma or sudden rupture of the esophageal contents into the pericardial space in Boerhaave's syndrome or as a complication of esophagogastrectomy. Traumatic pericarditis due to esophageal rupture is usually followed by intense erosive pericardial inflammation and infection secondary to the presence of bacteria and foreign bodies (food, salivary amylase, or stomach hydrochloric acid). Esophageal rupture or perforation may also be followed by the development of an esophagopericardial fistula.[613] All these disorders require immediate surgical intervention.[613,614] Pericarditis may also occur secondary to pancreatitis associated with a pericardial effusion with high amylase content and, rarely, the development of cardiac tamponade or a pancreatic-pericardial fistula.[615–617]

Pericardial trauma may also give rise to unusual traumatic syndromes, including cardiovascular collapse following herniation of the heart through a rent in the pericardium, mimicking congenital partial absence of the pericardium[618] with cardiac subluxation,[619] and intrapericardial diaphragmatic hernia.[620,621] Life-threatening cardiac herniation may also occur following radical left pneumonectomy with partial pericardial resection.[622] Herniation of the heart out of the pericardial sac can be diagnosed by thoracoscopy.[623] The rare problem of *traumatic pneumopericardium* may be caused by ulceration of the esophagus with fistula formation to the pericardium, puncture of the pericardium without cardiac laceration during sternal bone marrow aspiration, and artificial ventilation in newborns.[624]

A variety of other diseases have been reported in association with pericarditis (Table 43–9), but it is not clear whether the association is causal or coincidental.[625–632]

TABLE 43–9 DISORDERS OCCASIONALLY ASSOCIATED WITH PERICARDITIS

Atrial septal defects
Right atrial myxoma
Familial Mediterranean fever
Dego's disease
Gout
Gaucher's disease
Myeloid metaplasia
Silicosis
Scorpionfish (*Scorpaena buttuta*) sting
Pseudomyxoma peritonei

PERICARDIAL CYSTS

Pericardial cysts are uncommon and are typically located at the right costophrenic angle.[633] Unusual locations include the left costophrenic angle, hilum, and superior mediastinum at the level of the aortic arch. These anomalies, which come about through abnormal development of mesenchymal tissue during fetal life, are usually unilocular and filled with clear liquid, giving rise to the term "spring-water cysts."[634] Occasionally, the wall of the cyst calcifies.

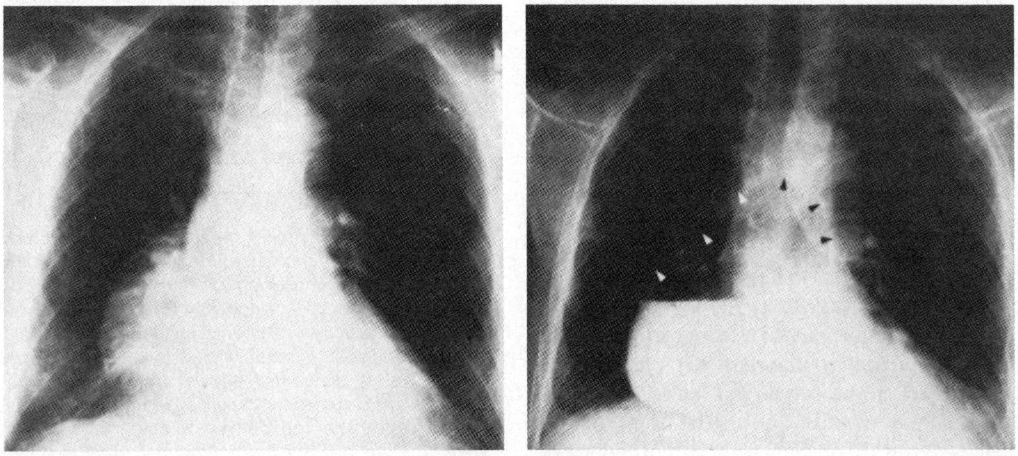

FIGURE 43–29 Chest roentgenogram in a patient with a benign pericardial cyst in a standard upright posteroanterior view. *Left panel,* Typical appearance of the cyst as a density at the lower right heart border. *Right panel,* Appearance after cyst puncture and instillation of contrast media and air. The superior portion of the cyst cavity (arrows) extends medially over the great vessels. (From Peterson, D. T., et al.: Pericardial cyst ten years after pericarditis. Chest *67*:719, 1975.)

Pericardial cysts usually do not give rise to symptoms or unusual findings on physical examination. Rarely, chest pain may occur owing to torsion of the cyst.[635] These lesions typically come to medical attention as an unsuspected finding on a chest roentgenogram and must be differentiated from other conditions such as solid tumors, cardiac aneurysms or pseudoaneurysms, and herniation of the omentum or liver through a diaphragmatic defect. In most cases, a cyst can be differentiated from solid tumor or aneurysm by two-dimensional echocardiography or computerized tomography.[636] When a suspected pericardial cyst is present in an unusual location, angiography may occasionally be needed to discriminate a cyst from an aneurysm or pseudoaneurysm. Pericardial cysts located at the right costophrenic angle can be accurately diagnosed and treated by percutaneous aspiration under fluoroscopic guidance (Fig. 43–29).[637] Because long-term followup studies have shown that asymptomatic patients do not develop symptoms or show progressive cyst enlargement, most patients should be managed conservatively, without surgical exploration.[638]

CONGENITAL ABSENCE AND DEFECTS OF THE PERICARDIUM

Congenital absence of the pericardium was first described anatomically by Realdus Columbus in 1559,[2] but its antemortem detection did not occur until 1959.[639] This anomaly usually involves a defect of the left-sided pericardium; total or partial absence of the right-sided pericardium is extremely rare.[640–642]

There is a 3:1 male-to-female predominance among patients with pericardial defects, and about 30 per cent have other congenital anomalies, including atrial septal defect, bicuspid aortic valve, bronchogenic cysts, or pulmonic sequestration.[643,644] Pocock has also suggested an association between congenital absence of the pericardium and mitral valve prolapse.[645]

Total absence of the pericardium is usually associated with no symptoms. Occasionally the patient may complain of chest discomfort and dyspnea. The more common condition of absence of the left pericardium may be associated with no symptoms or with nonexertional chest pain, dyspnea, palpitations, and recurrent pulmonary infections.[644] The etiology of these symptoms is unknown, but they may be related to torsion of the great vessels due to excess mobility of the heart or pleural-epicardial adhesions. The development of empyema, pericarditis, or pleurisy with effusion in these patients is attributed to loss of the anatomical barrier between the heart and the left lung. Absence of the left pericardium is also hypothesized to predispose to the development of post-traumatic mitral regurgitation and ventricular septal defect.[646]

Clinical features include widened splitting of the second heart sound, leftward displacement of the apical impulse, and a systolic murmur at the upper left sternal border that may be related to turbulent blood flow in an unusually mobile heart. Electrocardiographic abnormalities include right-axis deviation due to levoposition of the heart,[641,643] incomplete right bundle branch block, and clockwise displacement of the QRS transition zone of the precordial leads. Tall and peaked P waves in the right precordial leads have also been described.[647]

The standard posteroanterior view of the chest roentgenogram reveals marked leftward displacement of the cardiac silhouette (Fig. 43–30), prominence and clear demarcation of the main pulmonary artery, and interposition of radiolucent lung tissue between the aorta and main pulmonary artery or between the left hemidiaphragm and inferior cardiac border.[640,642] This anomaly must be differentiated from other conditions that cause prominence of the left hilum or pulmonary artery on the standard chest film, including pulmonic valve stenosis, atrial septal defect, idiopathic dilatation of the pulmonary artery, and hilar adenopathy.

M-mode echocardiographic changes in patients with complete absence of the left-sided pericardium are similar to those seen in right ventricular volume overload and include dilatation of the right ventricle and paradoxical anterior motion of the septum in systole.[648] Two-dimensional echocardiography has shown that the anterior movement of the septum toward the transducer in systole is an artifact related to cardiac rotation and exaggerated anterior displacement of the left ventricle.[649] Although the echocardiographic features are not diagnostic, echocardiography adds important supportive evidence to the diagnosis of congenital left-sided pericardial defect and helps to exclude other congenital anomalies, such as pulmonic valve stenosis or atrial septal defect, with which this condition may be confused. Radionuclide perfusion imaging can be used to confirm the diagnosis by the demonstration of a wedge of lung tissue between the heart and left hemidiaphragm[650]; computed tomography can also be used to detect absence of the left pericardium.[651]

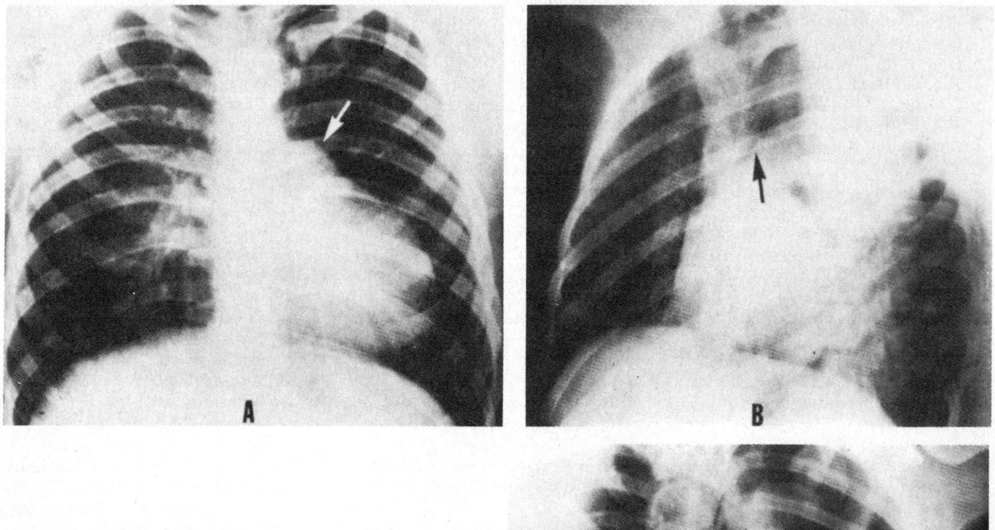

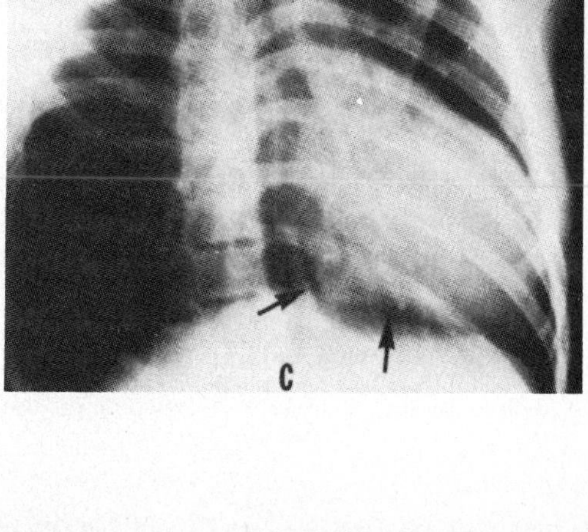

FIGURE 43–30 Chest roentgenograms in a patient with total absence of the left pericardium in posteroanterior (*A*), left anterior oblique (*B*), and right anterior oblique (*C*) views. The heart is shifted leftward, and the pulmonary artery segment is prominent (white arrow). There is a tongue of lung between the aorta and main pulmonary artery (*B*, black arrow) and between the left hemidiaphragm and inferior border of the heart (*C*, black arrows). (From Nassar, W. K., et al.: Congenital absence of left pericardium. Circulation *34*:100, 1966, by permission of the American Heart Association, Inc.)

Findings at cardiac catheterization are usually normal. Cardiac angiography with diagnostic left pneumothorax has been used in the past to outline the pericardium, but this procedure is hazardous and is now rarely needed to make the diagnosis of complete absence of the left pericardium if radiological and echocardiographic findings are compatible with the diagnosis. Cardiac catheterization with angiography is indicated only if there is a strong suspicion of associated congenital anomalies requiring surgical correction. Usually no specific therapy is required for management of complete absence of the left-sided pericardium.

Partial left-sided pericardial defects may be complicated by herniation of the left atrial appendage, atrium, or left ventricle through the defect, associated with chest pain, dizziness, syncope, and peripheral emboli.[641,649] Sudden death has been reported secondary to herniation and strangulation of the heart through the defect.[652] Radiological findings are less specific in partial left-sided defects than in complete absence of left pericardium. Pulmonary artery angiography with follow-through of contrast opacification to the left heart is probably the best method for definitively demonstrating herniation of the left atrium or left atrial appendage beyond the left heart border.[653]

The even rarer anomaly of *partial right-sided pericardial defect* may be associated with inspiratory right-sided chest pain secondary to herniation of the right atrium and right ventricle through the defect[654] or herniation of lung into the pericardial cavity.[655] The chest roentgenogram may show an unusual protuberance of the right heart border, and technetium-99m cardiac blood pool imaging may demonstrate that the abnormal contour of the right heart border fills simultaneously with the right atrium.[654] Right atrial angiography in the left anterior oblique projection is helpful in documenting herniation of the right atrium and right ventricle through the pericardial defect. Surgical treatment of partial left- or right-sided pericardial defects is usually indicated to relieve symptoms and prevent cardiac strangulation. The defect may be approached by excision of the atrial appendage, pericardioplasty, or extension of the defect.[641] Attempts to close a large defect may be unsuccessful owing to compression of the heart by the taut pericardium.[654]

References

1. Boyd, L. J., and Elias, H.: Contribution to diseases of the heart and pericardium. Historical introduction. Bull. N. Y. Med. Coll. *18*:1, 1955.
2. Spodick, D. H.: Medical history of the pericardium. The hairy hearts of hoary heroes. Am. J. Cardiol. *26*:447, 1970.
3. Holt, J. P.: The normal pericardium. Am. J. Cardiol. *26*:455, 1970.
4. Spodick, D. H.: Acute Pericarditis. New York, Grune and Stratton, 1959.
5. Ishihara, T., Ferrans, V. J., Jones, M., Boyce, S. W., Kawanami, O., and Roberts, W. C.: Histologic and ultrastructural features of normal human perietal pericardium. Am. J. Cardiol. *46*:744, 1980.
6. Roberts, W. C., and Spray, T. L.: Pericardial heart disease: A study of its causes, consequences and morphologic features. *In* Spodick, D. H. (ed.): Pericardial Diseases. Philadelphia, F. A. Davis, 1976, pp. 11–65.
7. Gibson, A. T., and Segal, M. B.: A study of the composition of pericardial fluid, with special reference to the probable mechanism of fluid formation. J. Physiol. (Lond.) *277*:367, 1978.

7a. Spodick, D. H.: The normal and diseased pericardium: Current concepts of pericardial physiology, diagnosis and treatment. J. Am. Coll. Cardiol. *1*:240, 1983.

8. Pegram, B. L., and Bishop, V. S.: An evaluation of the pericardial sac as a safety factor during tamponade. Cardiovasc. Res. *9*:715, 1975.
9. Morgan, B. C., Guntheroth, W. C., and Dillard, D. H.: The relationship of pericardial to pleural pressure during quiet respiration and cardiac tamponade. Circ. Res. *16*:493, 1965.
10. Avasthey, P., and Wood, E. H.: Intrathoracic and venous pressure relationships during responses to changes in body position. J. Appl. Physiol. *37*:166, 1974.
11. Holt, J. P.: Ventricular end-diastolic volume and transmural pressure. Cardiologia *50*:281, 1967.
12. Holt, J. P., Rhode, E. A., and Kines, H.: Pericardial and ventricular pressure. Cir. Res. *8*:1171, 1960.
13. Brecher, G. A.: Venous Return. New York, Grune and Stratton, 1956.
14. Kuno, Y.: The significance of the pericardium. J. Physiol. *50*:1, 1915.
15. Berglund, E., Sarnoff, S. J., and Isaacs, J. P.: Ventricular function—Role of the pericardium in regulation of cardiovascular hemodynamics. Circ. Res. *3*: 133, 1955.
16. Bernard, H. L.: The functions of the pericardium. J. Physiol. *22*:43, 1898.
17. Bartle, S. H., Hermann, H. J., Cavo, J. W., Moore, R. A., and Costenbader, J. M.: Effect of the pericardium on left ventricular volume and function in acute hypervolaemia. Cardiovasc. Res. *2*:284, 1968.
18. Spotnitz, H. M., and Kaiser, G. A.: The effect of the pericardium on pressure-volume relations in the canine left ventricle. J. Surg. Res. *11*:375, 1971.
19. Gibbon, J. H., Jr., and Churchill, E. D.: The mechanical influence of the pericardium upon cardiac function. J. Clin. Invest. *10*:405, 1931.
20. Stokland, O., Miller, M. M., Lekven, J., and Ilebekk, A.: The significance of the intact pericardium for cardiac performance in the dog. Circ. Res. *47*:27, 1980.
21. Shirato, K., Shabetai, R., Bhargave, V., Franklin, D., and Ross, J., Jr.: Alteration of the left ventricular diastolic pressure-segment length relation produced by the pericardium. Circulation *57*:1191, 1978.

21a. Crawford, H. H., Badke, F. R., and Amon, K. W.: Effect of the undisturbed pericardium on left ventricular size and performance during acute volume loading. Am. Heart J. *105*:267, 1983.

22. Refsum, H., Junemann, M., Lipton, M. J., Skioldebrand, C., Carlsson, E., and Tyberg, J. V.: Ventricular diastolic pressure-volume relations and the pericardium. Circulation *64*:997, 1981.
23. LeWinter, M. M., and Pavelec, R.: Influence of the pericardium on left ventricular end-diastolic pressure-segment relations during early and later stages of experimental chronic volume overload in dogs. Circ. Res. *50*:501, 1982.
24. Mirsky, I., and Rankin, J. S.: The effects of geometry, elasticity, and external pressures on the diastolic pressure-volume and stiffness-stress relations. How important is the pericardium? Circ. Res. *44*:601, 1979.
25. Serizawa, T., Carabello, B. A., and Grossman, W.: Effect of pacing induced ischemia on left ventricular diastolic pressure-volume relations in dogs with coronary stenoses. Circ. Res. *46*:430, 1980.
26. Taylor, R. R., Covell, J. W., Sonnenblick, E. H., and Ross, J., Jr.: Dependence of ventricular distensibility on filling of the opposite ventricle. Am. J. Physiol. *213*:711, 1967.
27. Laks, M. M., Garner, D., and Swan, H. J. C.: Volumes and compliances measured simultaneously in the right and left ventricles of the dog. Circ. Res. *20*: 565, 1967.
28. Elzinga, G., Van Grondelle, R., Westerhof, N., and Van Den Bos, G. C.: Ventricular interference. Am. J. Physiol. *226*:941, 1974.
29. Santamore, W. P., Lynch, P. R., Meier, G., Heckman, J., and Bove, A. A.: Myocardial interaction between the ventricles. J. Appl. Physiol. *41*:362, 1976.
30. Bemis, C. E., Serur, J. R., Borkenhagen, D., Sonnenblick, E. H., and Urschel, C. W.: Influence of right ventricular filling pressure on left ventricular pressure and dimension. Circ. Res. *34*:498, 1974.
31. Brinker, J. A., Weiss, J. L., Lappe, D. L., Rabson, J. L., Summer, W. R., Permutt, S., and Weisfeldt, M. L.: Leftward septal displacement during right ventricular loading in man. Circulation *61*:626, 1980.
32. Brenner, J. I., and Waugh, R. A.: Effect of phasic respiration on left ventricular dimension and performance in a normal population. Circulation *57*: 122, 1978.
33. Spadaro, J., Bing, O. H., Gaasch, W. H., and Weintraub, R. M.: Pericardial modulation of right and left ventricular diastolic interaction. Circ. Res. *48*: 233, 1981.
34. Lorell, B. H., Palacios, I., Daggett, W. M., Jacobs, M. L., Fowler, B. N., and Newell, J. B.: Right ventricular distention and left ventricular compliance. Am. J. Physiol. *240*:H87, 1981.
35. Janicki, J. S., and Weber, K. T.: The pericardium and ventricular interaction, distensibility, and function. Am. J. Physiol. *238*:H494, 1980.
36. Bove, A. A., and Santamore, W. P.: Ventricular interdependence. Progr. Cardiovasc. Dis. *23*:365, 1981.
37. Shirato, K., Kanazawa, M., Ishikawa, K., Nakajima, T., and Takishima, T.: The effect of the pericardium on the diastolic properties of the heart. Jpn. Circ. J. *46*:113, 1982.
38. Maruyama, Y., Ashikawa, K., Isoyama, S., Kanatsuke, H., Ino-Oka, E., and Takishima, T.: Mechanical interactions between four heart chambers with and without the pericardium in canine hearts. Circ. Res. *50*:86, 1982.
39. Glantz, S. A., Misbach, G. A., Moores, W. Y., Mathey, D. G., Levken, J., Stowe, D. F., Parmley, W. W., and Tyberg, J. V.: The pericardium substantially affects the left ventricular diastolic pressure-volume relationship in the dog. Circulation *42*:433, 1978.
40. Mangano, D. T.: The effect of the pericardium on ventricular systolic function in man. Circulation *61*:352, 1980.
41. Ringertz, H. G., Misbach, G. A., and Tyberg, J. V.: Effect of the normal pericardium on the left ventricular diastolic pressure-volume relationship. Acta Radiol. *22*:529, 1981.
42. Alderman, E. L., and Glantz, S. A.: Acute hemodynamic interventions shift the diastolic pressure-volume curve in man. Circulation *54*:662, 1976.
43. Brodie, B. R., Grossman, W., Mann, T., and McLaurin, L. P.: Effects of sodium nitroprusside on left ventricular diastolic pressure-volume relations. J. Clin. Invest. *59*:59, 1977.
44. Ludbrook, P. A., Byrne, J. D., Kurnik, P. B., and McKnight, R. C.: Influence of reduction of preload and afterload by nitroglycerin on left ventricular diastolic pressure-volume relations and relaxation in man. Circulation *56*:937, 1977.
45. Ludbrook, P. A., Byrne, J. D., and McKnight, R. C.: Influence of right ventricular hemodynamics on left ventricular diastolic pressure-volume relations in man. Circulation *59*:21, 1979.
46. Wong, C. Y., and Spotnitz, H. M.: Effect of nitroprusside on end-diastolic pressure-diameter relations of the human left ventricle after pericardiotomy. J. Thorac. Cardiovasc. Surg. *82*:350, 1981.
47. Ross, J., Jr.: Acute displacement of the diastolic pressure-volume curve of the left ventricle: Role of the pericardium and the right ventricle. Circulation *59*: 32, 1979.
48. Bartle, S. H., and Hermann, H. J.: Acute mitral regurgitation in man. Hemodynamic evidence and observations indicating an early role for the pericardium. Circulation *36*:839, 1967.

49. Lorell, B. H., Leinbach, R. C., Pohost, G. M., Gold, H. K., Dinsmore, R. E., Hutter, A. M., Jr., Pastore, J. O., and DeSanctis, R. W.: Right ventricular infarction. Am. J. Cardiol. *43*:465, 1979.
50. Goldstein, J. A., Vlahakes, G. H., Verrier, E. D., Schiller, N. B., Tyberg, J. V., Ports, T. A., Parmley, W. W., and Chatterjee, K.: The role of right ventricular systolic dysfunction and elevated intrapericardial pressure in the genesis of low output in experimental right ventricular infarction. Circulation *65*: 513, 1982.

ACUTE PERICARDITIS

51. Sodeman, W. A., and Smith, R. H.: A re-evaluation of the diagnostic criteria for acute pericarditis. Am. J. Med. Sci. *235*:672, 1958.
52. Dunn, M., and Rinkenberger, R. L.: Clinical aspects of acute pericarditis. Cardiovasc. Clin. *7-3*:131, 1976.
53. Markiewicz, W., Brik, A., Brook, G., Edoute, Y., Monakier, I., Markiewicz, Y.: Pericardial rub in pericardial effusion: Lack of correlation with amount of fluid. Chest *77*:643, 1980.
54. Spodick, D. H.: Pericardial rub: Prospective, multiple observer investigation of pericardial friction in 100 patients. Am. J. Cardiol. *35*:357, 1975.
55. Spodick, D. H.: Pathogenesis and clinical correlations of the electrocardiographic abnormalities of pericardial disease. Cardiovasc. Clin. *8-3*:201, 1977.
56. Hull, E.: The electrocardiogram in pericarditis. Am. J. Cardiol. *7*:21, 1961.
57. Spodick, D. H.: Diagnostic electrocardiographic sequences in acute pericarditis: Significance of PR segment and PR vector changes. Circulation *48*: 575, 1973.
58. Surawicz, B., and Lasseter, K. C.: Electrocardiogram in pericarditis. Am. J. Cardiol. *26*:471, 1970.
59. Spodick, D. H.: Acute pericarditis: ECG changes. Primary Cardiol. *8*:78, 1982.
60. Bruce, M. A., and Spodick, D. H.: Atypical electrocardiogram in acute pericarditis: Characteristics and prevalence. J. Electrocardiol. *13*:61, 1980.
61. Coffin, C. W., and Scarf, M.: Acute pericarditis simulating coronary artery occlusion. Am. Heart J. *32*:515, 1946.
61a. Wanner, W. R., Schaal, S. F., Bashore, T. M., Norton, V. J., Lewis, R. P., and Fulkerson, P. K.: Repolarization variant vs. acute pericarditis. A prospective electrocardiographic and echocardiographic evaluation. Chest *83*:180, 1983.
62. Spodick, D. H.: Differential characteristics of the electrocardiogram in early repolarization and acute pericarditis. N. Engl. J. Med. *295*:523, 1976.
63. Ginzton, L. E., and Laks, M. M.: The differential diagnosis of acute pericarditis. Circulation *65*:1004, 1982.
64. James, T. N.: Pericarditis and the sinus node. Arch. Intern. Med. *110*:305, 1962.
65. Dressler, N.: Sinus tachycardia complicating and outlasting pericarditis. Am. Heart J. *72*:422, 1966.
66. Olson, H. G., Lyons, K. P., Aronow, W. S., Kuperus, J., Orlando, J. R., and Waters, H. J.: Technetium-99m stannous pyrophosphate myocardial scintigrams in pericardial disease. Am. Heart J. *99*:459, 1980.
67. Kadota, K., Matsumori, A., Kambara, H., and Kawai, C.: Myocardial uptake of technetium-99m stannous pyrophosphate in experimental viral myopericarditis. J. Nucl. Med. *20*:1047, 1979.
68. Ahmad, M., and Dubiel, J. P.: Tc-99m pyrophosphate myocardial imaging in perimyocarditis. J. Nucl. Med. *22*:452, 1981.
69. Martin, P., Devriendt, J., Goffin, Y., and Verhas, M.: Gallium 67 scintigraphy in fibrinous pericarditis associated with bacterial endocarditis. Eur. J. Nucl. Med. *7*:192, 1982.
70. Taillefer, R., and Lemieux, R. J., Picard, D., and Dupras, G.: Gallium 67 imaging in pericarditis secondary to tuberculosis in histoplasmosis. Clin. Nucl. Med. *6*:413, 1981.
71. Schreiner, D. P., Krishnaswami, V., and Murphy, J. H.: Unsuspected purulent pericarditis detected by gallium-67 scanning: A case report. Clin. Nucl. Med. *6*: 411, 1981.
72. Tiefenbrunn, A. J., and Roberts, R.: Elevation of plasma MB creatine kinase and the development of new Q waves in association with pericarditis. Chest *77*: 438, 1980.
73. Marmor, A., Grenadir, E., Keidar, A., Edward, S., and Palant, A.: The MB fraction of creatine phosphokinase: An indicator of myocardial involvement in acute pericarditis. Arch. Intern. Med. *139*:819, 1979.
74. Hancock, E. W.: Management of pericardial disease. Mod. Conc. Cardiovasc. Dis. *48*:1, 1979.

PERICARDIAL EFFUSION

75. Steinberg, I.: Pericarditis with effusion: New observations with a note on Ewart's sign. Ann. Intern. Med. *49*:428, 1958.
76. Carsky, E. W., Mauceri, R. A., and Azimi, F.: The epicardial fat pad sign: Analysis of frontal and lateral chest radiographs in patients with pericardial effusion. Radiology *137*:303, 1980.
77. Dinsmore, R. E., Miller, A. R., Potsaid, M. S., and Shawdon, H. H.: Cineangiographic patterns in pericardial disease. Am. J. Roentgenol. *86*:425, 1966.
78. Mattsson, O.: Scintigraphy of pericardial effusion. Acta Radiol. Diag. *17*:737, 1976.
79. Wolverson, M. K., Grider, R. D., Sundaram, M., Heiberg, E., and Johnson, F.: Demonstration of unsuspected malignant disease of the pericardium by computed tomography. C. T. *4*:330, 1980.
80. Tomoda, H., Hoshiai, M., Furuya, H., Oeda, Y., Matsumoto, S., Tanabe, T., Tamachi, H., Sasamoto, H., Koide, S., Kuribayashi, S., and Matsuyama, S.: Evaluation of pericardial effusion with computed tomography. Am. Heart J. *99*:701, 1980.
81. Wong, B. Y. S., Lee, K. R., and MacArthur, R. I.: Diagnosis of pericardial effusion by computed tomography. Chest *81*:177, 1982.
82. Isner, J. M., Carter, B. L., Bankoff, M. S., Konstam, M. D., and Salem, D. N.: Computed tomography in the diagnosis of pericardial heart disease. Ann. Intern. Med. *97*:473, 1982.
83. Unverferth, D. V., Williams, T. E., and Fulkerson, P. K.: Electrocardiographic voltage in pericardial effusion. Chest *75*:157, 1979.
84. Allen, J. W., Harrison, E. D., Camp, J. C., Bursari, A., Turnier, E., and Lau, F. Y. K.: The role of serial echocardiography in the evaluation and differential diagnosis of pericardial disease. Am. Heart J. *93*:560, 1977.
85. Feigenbaum, H.: Echocardiographic diagnosis of pericardial effusion. Am. J. Cardiol. *26*:475, 1970.
86. Horowitz, M. S., Schultz, C. S., and Stinson, E. B.: Sensitivity and specificity of echocardiographic diagnosis of pericardial effusion. Circulation *50*:239, 1974.
86a. Parameswaran, R., and Goldberg, H.: Echocardiographic quantitation of pericardial effusion. Chest *83*:767, 1983.
87. Ratshin, R. A., Smith, M. K., and Hood, W. P., Jr.: Possible false positive diagnosis of pericardial effusion by echocardiography in the presence of large left atrium. Chest *65*:112, 1974.
88. Martin, R. P., Rakowski, H., French, J., and Popp, R. L.: Localization of pericardial effusion with wide angle phased array echocardiography. Am. J. Cardiol. *42*:904, 1978.
89. Friedman, M. J., Sahn, D. J., and Haber, K.: Two-dimensional echocardiography and B-mode ultrasonography for the diagnosis of loculated pericardial effusion. Circulation *60*:1644, 1979.
90. Brown, A. K.: Chronic idiopathic pericardial effusion. Br. Heart J. *28*:609, 1966.
91. Bedford, D. E.: Chronic effusive pericarditis. Br. Heart J. *26*:499, 1964.
92. Santos, G. H., and Frater, R. W. M.: The subxiphoid approach in the treatment of pericardial effusion. Ann. Thorac. Surg. *23*:467, 1977.
93. Hatcher, C. R., Jr., Logue, R. B., Logan, W. D., Jr., Symbas, R. B., Mansour, D. A., and Abbott, O. A.: Pericardiectomy for recurrent pericarditis. J. Thorac. Cardiovasc. Surg. *62*:371, 1971.
94. Fowler, N. O.: Physiology of cardiac tamponade and pulsus paradoxus. Physiological, circulatory, and pharmacologic responses in cardiac tamponade. Mod. Conc. Cardiovasc. Dis. *47*:115, 1978.
95. Reddy, P. S., Curtiss, E. I., O'Toole, J. D., and Shaver, J. A.: Cardiac tamponade: Hemodynamic observations in man. Circulation *58*:265, 1978.
96. Craig, R. J., Whalen, R. E., Behar, V. S., and McIntosh, H. D.: Pressure and volume changes of the left ventricle in acute pericardial tamponade. Am. J. Cardiol. *22*:65, 1968.
97. Shabetai, R., Mangiardi, L., Bhargava, V., Ross, J., Jr., and Higgins, C. B.: The pericardium and cardiac function. Progr. Cardiovasc. Dis. *22*:107, 1979.
98. Pegram, B. L., Kardon, M. B., and Bishop, V. S.: Changes in left ventricular internal diameter with increasing pericardial pressure. Cardiovasc. Res. *9*:707, 1975.
99. Shabetai, R., Fowler, N. O., and Guntheroth, W. G.: The hemodynamics of cardiac tamponade and constrictive pericarditis. Am. J. Cardiol. *26*:480, 1970.
100. Wechsler, A. S., Auerbach, B. J., Graham, T. C., and Sabiston, D. C.: Distribution of intramyocardial blood flow during pericardial tamponade: Correlation with microscopic anatomy and intrinsic myocardial contractility. J. Thorac. Cardiovasc. Surg. *68*:847, 1974.
101. Frank, M. J., Nadimi, M., Lesniak, L. J., Hilmi, K. I., and Levinson, G. E.: Effects of cardiac tamponade on myocardial performance, blood flow and metabolism. Am. J. Physiol. *220*:179, 1971.
102. Brecher, G. A.: Critical review of recent work on ventricular diastolic suction. Circ. Res. *6*:554, 1958.
103. Kostreva, D. R., Castaner, A., Pedersen, D. H., and Kampine, J. P.: Nonvagally mediated bradycardia during cardiac tamponade or severe hemorrhage. Cardiology *68*:65, 1981.
104. Castaner, A., Kostreva, D. R., and Kampine, J. P.: Changes in autonomic nerve activity during acute cardiac tamponade. Cardiology *66*:163, 1980.
105. Friedman, H. S., Gomes, J. A., Tardio, A. R., and Haft, J. I.: The electrocardiographic features of acute cardiac tamponade. Circulation *50*:260, 1974.
106. Fowler, N. O.: Cardiac Diagnosis and Treatment. 3rd ed. New York, Harper and Row, 1980, p. 981.
107. Ruskin, J., Bache, R. J., Rembert, J. C., and Greenfield, J. C., Jr.: Pressure-flow studies in man: Effect of respiration on left ventricular stroke volume. Circulation *48*:79, 1973.
108. Fowler, N. O.: Physiology of cardiac tamponade and pulsus paradoxus. I. Mechanisms of pulsus paradoxus in cardiac tamponade. Mod. Conc. Cardiovasc. Dis. *47*:109, 1978.
109. Goldblatt, A., Harrison, D. C., Glick, G., and Braunwald, E.: Studies on cardiac dimensions in intact, unanesthetized man. II. Effects of respiration. Circ. Res. *13*:448, 1963.
110. Wexler, L., Bergel, D. H., Gabe, I. T., Makin, G. S., and Mills, C. J.: Velocity of blood flow in normal human venae cavae. Circ. Res. *23*:349, 1968.
111. Shabetai, R., Fowler, N. O., Fenton, J. C., and Masangkay, M.: Pulsus paradoxus. J. Clin. Invest. *44*:1882, 1965.
112. Shabetai, R., Fowler, N. O., and Gueron, M.: The effects of respiration on aortic pressure and flow. Am. Heart J. *65*:525, 1963.
113. Gabe, I. T., Mason, D. T., Gault, J. H., Ross, J., Jr., Zelis, R., Mills, C. J.,

Braunwald, E., and Schillingford, J. P.: Effect of respiration on venous return and stroke volume in cardiac tamponade. Br. Heart J. *32*:592, 1970.
114. Settle, H. P., Adolph, R. J., Fowler, N. O., Engel, P., Agruss, N. S., and Levenson, N. I.: Echocardiographic study of cardiac tamponade. Circulation *56*:951, 1977.
115. D'Cruz, I. A., Cohen, H. C., Prabhu, R., and Glick, G.: Diagnosis of cardiac tamponade by echocardiography: Changes in mitral valve motion and ventricular dimensions, with special reference to paradoxical pulse. Circulation *52*:460, 1975.
116. McGregor, M.: Current concepts: Pulsus paradoxus. N. Engl. J. Med. *301*: 480, 1979.
117. Friedman, H. S., Sakurai, H., and Lajam, F.: Pulsus paradoxus: A manifestation of a marked reduction of left ventricular end-diastolic volume in cardiac tamponade. J. Thorac. Cardiovasc. Surg. *79*:74, 1980.
118. Robotham, J. L., and Mitzner, W.: A model of the effects of respiration on left ventricular performance. J. Appl. Physiol. *46*:411, 1979.
119. Burdine, J. A., and Wallace, J. M.: Pulsus paradoxus and Kussmaul's sign in massive pulmonary embolism. Am. J. Cardiol. *15*:413, 1965.
120. Cohen, S. I., Kupersmith, J., Aroesty, J., and Rowe, J. W.: Pulsus paradoxus and Kussmaul's sign in acute pulmonary embolism. Am. J. Cardiol. *32*:271, 1973.
121. Rebuck, A. S., and Pengelly, L. D.: Development of pulsus paradoxus in the presence of airways obstruction. N. Engl. J. Med. *288*:66, 1973.
122. Settle, H. P., Jr., Engel, P. J., Fowler, N. O., Allen, J. M., Vassollo, C. L., Hackworth, J. N., Adolph, R. J., and Eppert, D. C.: Echocardiographic study of the paradoxical arterial pulse in chronic obstructive lung disease. Circulation *62*:1297, 1980.
123. Winer, H. E., and Kronzon, I.: Absence of paradoxical pulse in patients with cardiac tamponade and atrial septal defects. Am. J. Cardiol. *44*:378, 1979.
124. Guberman, B. A., Fowler, N. O., Engel, P. J., Gueron, M., and Allen, J. M.: Cardiac tamponade in medical patients. Circulation *64*:633, 1981.
125. Hardesty, R. L., Thompson, M., Lerberg, D. B., Siewers, R. D., O'Toole, J. D., Salerni, R., and Bahnson, H. T.: Delayed postoperative cardiac tamponade: Diagnosis and management. Ann. Thorac. Surg. *26*:155, 1978.
126. Beck, C. S.: Two cardiac compression triads. J.A.M.A. *104*:714, 1935.
127. Symmes, J. C., and Berman, N. D.: Early recognition of cardiac tamponade. Canad. Med. Assoc. J. *116*:863, 1977.
128. Jacobs, W. R., and Talano, J. V.: Cardiomegaly and paradoxical pulse. Arch. Intern. Med. *138*:1125, 1978.
129. Hetzel, P. S., Wood, E. H., and Burchell, H. B.: Pressure pulses in the right side of the heart in a case of amyloid heart disease and in a case of idiopathic heart failure simulating constrictive pericarditis. Mayo Clin. Proc. *28*:107, 1953.
130. Cohn, J. N., Pinkerson, A. L., and Tristani, F. E.: Mechanism of pulsus paradoxus in clinical shock. J. Clin. Invest. *46*:1744, 1967.
131. Antman, E. M., Cargill, V., and Grossman, W.: Low-pressure cardiac tamponade. Ann. Intern. Med. *91*:403, 1979.
132. Niarchos, A. P.: Electrical alternans in cardiac tamponade. Thorax *30*:228, 1975.
133. McGregor, M., and Baskind, E.: Electrical alternans in pericardial effusion. Circulation *11*:837, 1955.
134. Bashour, F. A., and Cochran, P. W.: The association of electrical alternans with pericardial effusion. Dis. Chest *44*:146, 1963.
135. Littmann, D., and Spodick, D. H.: Total electrical alternation in pericardial disease. Circulation *17*:912, 1958.
136. Feigenbaum, H., Zaky, A., and Grabhorn, L. L.: Cardiac motion in patients with pericardial effusion. A study using reflected ultrasound. Circulation *34*: 611, 1966.
137. Usher, B. W., and Popp, R. L.: Electrical alternans: Mechanism in pericardial effusion. Am. Heart J. *83*:459, 1972.
138. Sbarbaro, J. A., and Brooks, H. L.: Pericardial effusion and electrical alternans: Echocardiographic assessment. Postgrad. Med. *63*:105, 1978.
139. Friedman, H. S., Lajam, F., Calderon, J., Zaman, Q., Marino, N. D., and Gomes, J. A.: Electrocardiographic features of experimental cardiac tamponade in closed-chest dogs. Eur. J. Cardiol. *6*:311, 1977.
140. Spodick, D. H.: Acute cardiac tamponade: Pathologic physiology, diagnosis and management. Progr. Cardiovasc. Dis. *10*:64, 1967.
141. Mann, T., Brodie, B. R., Grossman, W., and McLaurin, L.: Effusive-constrictive hemodynamic pattern due to neoplastic involvement of the pericardium. Am. J. Cardiol. *41*:781, 1978.
142. Wynne, J., Markis, J. E., and Grossman, W.: Extrinsic compression of the heart by tumor masquerading as cardiac tamponade. Cath. Cardiovasc. Diag. *4*:81, 1978.
143. Cosio, F. G., Martinez, J. P., Serrano, C. M., Calzada, C. S., and Alcaire, C. C.: Abnormal septal motion in cardiac tamponade with pulsus paradoxus. Echocardiographic and hemodynamic observations. Chest *71*:787, 1977.
144. Armstrong, W. F., Schilt, B. F., Helper, D. J., Dillon, J. C., and Feigenbaum, H.: Diastolic collapse of the right ventricle with cardiac tamponade: An echocardiographic study. Circulation *65*:1491, 1982.
145. Schiller, N. B., and Botvinick, E. H.: Right ventricular compression as a sign of cardiac tamponade: An analysis of echocardiographic ventricular dimensions and their clinical implications. Circulation *56*:774, 1977.
145a. Kronzon, I., Cohen, M. J., and Winer, H. E.: Contribution of echocardiography to the understanding of the pathophysiology of cardiac tamponade. J. Am. Coll. Cardiol. *1*:1180, 1983.
146. Winer, H., Kronzon, I., and Glassman, E.: Echocardiographic findings in severe paradoxical pulse due to pulmonary embolism. Am. J. Cardiol. *40*:808, 1977.
147. Martins, J. B., and Kerber, R. E.: Can cardiac tamponade be diagnosed by echocardiography? Circulation *60*:737, 1979.
148. Uren, R. F., McLaughlin, A. F., and Cormack, J.: Cardiac tamponade: Accurate diagnosis by radionuclide angiography. Aust. N. Z. J. Med. *10*:414, 1980.
149. Shabetai, R., Aravindakshan, V., Danielson, G., and Bryant, L.: Traumatic hemopericardium with tricuspid incompetence. J. Thorac. Cardiovasc. Surg. *57*: 294, 1969.
150. Spitz, H. B., and Holmes, J. C.: Right atrial contour in cardiac tamponade. Radiology *103*:69, 1972.
151. Fowler, N. O., and Holmes, J. C.: Hemodynamic effect of isoproterenol and norepinephrine in acute cardiac tamponade. J. Clin. Invest. *48*:502, 1969.
152. Gascho, J. A., Martins, J. B., Marcus, M. L., and Kerber, R. E.: Effects of volume expansion and vasodilators in acute pericardial tamponade. Am. J. Physiol. *240*:H49, 1981.
153. Moller, C. T., Schoonbee, C. G., and Rosendorff, C.: Hemodynamics of cardiac tamponade during various modes of ventilation. Br. J. Anaesth. *51*:409, 1979.
154. Kotte, J. H., and McGuire, J.: Pericardial paracentesis. Mod. Conc. Cardiovasc. Dis. *20*:102, 1951.
155. Kilpatrick, Z. M., and Chapman, C. B.: On pericardiocentesis. Am. J. Cardiol. *16*:722, 1965.
156. Krikorian, J. G., and Hancock, E. W.: Pericardiocentesis. Am. J. Med. *65*:808, 1978.
157. Wong, B., Murphy, J., Chang, C. J., Hassenein, K., and Dunn, M.: The risk of pericardiocentesis. Am. J. Cardiol. *44*:1110, 1979.
158. Kaiser, E., and Loewenneck, H.: Pericardial puncture. The most favorable anatomical approach. Münch. Med. Wschr. *123*:1697, 1981.
159. Heilerli, B., Anderes, U., and Follath, F.: Diagnosis and therapy of cardiac tamponade. An analysis of 50 patients. Schweiz. Med. Wschr. *111*:735, 1981.
159a. Callahan, J. A., Seward, J. B., Tajik, A. J., Holmes, D. R., Jr., Smith, H. C., Reeder, G.S., and Miller, F. A.: Enhanced safety of two-dimensional echocardiography-directed pericardiocentesis: A technique of choice. J. Am. Coll. Cardiol. *1*:738, 1983.
160. Aron, D. V., Richardson, J. D., Webb, G., Grover, F. L., and Trinkle, J. K.: Subxiphoid pericardial window in patients with suspected traumatic pericardial tamponade. Ann. Thorac. Surg. *23*:545, 1977.
161. Schepers, G. W. H.: Tuberculous pericarditis. Am. J. Cardiol. 9:248, 1962.
162. Morin, J. G., Mulder, D. S., and Long, R.: Pericardiectomy for uremic tamponade. Canad. J. Surg. *19*:109, 1976.
163. Gotsman, M. S., and Schrire, V.: Pericardiocentesis electrode needle. Br. Heart J. *28*:566, 1966.
164. Glancy, D. L., and Richter, M. A.: Catheter drainage of the pericardial space. Cath. Cardiovasc. Diag. *1*:311, 1975.
165. Lubell, D. K., and Glass, P.: Construction of a simplified pericardiocentesis electrode. Dis. Chest *41*:657, 1962.
166. Owens, W. C., Shaefer, R. A., and Rahimtoola, S. H.: Pericardiocentesis: Insertion of a pericardial catheter. Cath. Cardiovasc. Diag. *1*:317, 1975.
167. Shabetai, R., and Grossman, W.: Profiles in constrictive pericarditis, restrictive cardiomyopathy, and cardiac tamponade. *In* Grossman, W. (ed.): Cardiac Catheterization and Angiography. 2nd ed. Philadelphia, Lea and Febiger, 1980, pp. 358–376.
168. Wei, J. Y., Taylor, G. J., and Aschuff, S. C.: Recurrent cardiac tamponade and large pericardial effusion: Management with an indwelling pericardial catheter. Am. J. Cardiol. *42*:281, 1978.
169. Larrey, D. J.: New surgical procedure to open the pericardium and determine the cause of fluid in its cavity. Clin. Chirurg. *36*:393, 1829.
170. Alcan, K. E., Zabetakis, P. M., Marino, N. D., Franzone, A. J., Michelis, M. F., and Bruno, M. S.: Management of acute cardiac tamponade by subxiphoid pericardiotomy. J.A.M.A. *247*:1143, 1982.
171. Fontenelle, L. J., Cuello, L., and Dooley, B. N.: Subxiphoid pericardial window—A simple and safe method for diagnosing and treating acute and chronic pericardial effusions. J. Thorac. Cardiovasc. Surg. *62*:95, 1971.
172. Fredriksen, R. T., Cohen, L. S., and Mullins, C. B.: Pericardial windows or pericardiocentesis for pericardial effusions. Am. Heart J. *82*:158, 1971.
173. Ribot, S., Frankel, H. J., and Gielchinsky, I.: Treatment of uremic pericarditis. Clin. Nephrol. *27*:127, 1974.
174. Lajos, T. Z., Black, H. E., Cooper, R. G., and Wanka, J.: Pericardial decompression. Ann. Thorac. Surg. *19*:47, 1975.
175. Ibarra, P. C., and Gonzalez, R. L.: Diagnosis and treatment of pericarditis by the subxiphoid approach. Am. J. Surg. *44*:602, 1978.

CONSTRICTIVE PERICARDITIS

176. Agarwal, S., and Chopra, P.: Constrictive pericarditis: A histopathological study of 91 cases. Indian Heart J. *29*:278, 1977. Constrictive Pericarditis
177. Chesler, E., Matha, A. S., Matisonn, R. E., and Rogers, M. N. A.: Subpulmonic stenosis as a result of noncalcific pericarditis. Chest *69*:425, 1976.
178. McGaff, F. J., Haller, J. A., Jr., Leight, L., and Towery, B. T.: Subvalvular pulmonic stenosis due to constriction of the right ventricular outflow tract by a pericardial band. Am. J. Med. *34*:142, 1963.
179. Paul, O., Castleman, B., and White, P. D.: Chronic constrictive pericarditis: A study of 53 cases. Am. J. Med. Sci. *216*:361, 1948.
180. Andrews, G. W. S., Pickering, G. W., and Sellors, T. H.: The aetiology of con-

strictive pericarditis with special reference to tuberculous pericarditis, together with a note on polyserositis. Quart. J. Med. *17*:291, 1948.
181. Howard, E. J., and Maier, H.: Constrictive pericarditis following acute Coxsackie viral pericarditis. Am. Heart J. *75*:247, 1968.
182. Haycock, G. B., and Jordan, S. C.: Chronic pericardial constriction with effusion in childhood. Arch. Dis. Child. *54*:890, 1979.
183. Bonische, C. H., and Jaffe, J. P.: Spontaneous severe constrictive pericarditis in congenital afibrinogenemia: Mechanism, evaluation and successful surgical management. Am. Heart J. *101*:503, 1981.
184. Perheentupa, J., Autio, S., Leisti, S., Raitta, C., and Tuuteri, L.: Mulibrey nanism, and autosomal recessive syndrome with pericardial constriction. Lancet *2*:351, 1973.
185. Perheentupa, J., Autio, S., Leisti, S., and Raitta, C.: Mulibrey nanism: Dwarfism with muscle, liver, brain and eye involvement. Acta Pediat. Scand. (Suppl.) *206*:74, 1970.
186. Voorhees, M. L., Husson, G. S., and Blackman, M. S.: Growth failure with pericardial constriction. The syndrome of mulibrey nanism. Am. J. Dis. Child. *130*:1146, 1976.
187. Shabetai, R., Mangiardi, L., Bhargava, V., Ross, J., Jr., and Higgens, C. B.: The pericardium and cardiac function. Progr. Cardiovasc. Dis. *22*:107, 1979.
188. Moscovitz, H. L.: Pericardial constriction versus cardiac tamponade. Am. J. Cardiol. *26*:546, 1970.
189. Hancock, E. W.: Constrictive pericarditis: Modern view of diagnosis and management. J. Cardiovasc. Med. *41*:367, 1980.
190. Lewis, B. S., and Gotsman, M. S.: Left ventricular function in systole and diastole in constrictive pericarditis. Am. Heart J. *86*:23, 1973.
191. Armstrong, T. G., Lewis, B. S., and Gotsman, M. S.: Systolic time intervals in constrictive pericarditis and severe primary myocardial disease. Am. Heart J. *85*:6, 1973.
192. Khattri, H. N., Bidwei, P. S., Mahapatra, S. S., Sharma, J. K., and Wahi, P. L.: Systolic time intervals in constrictive pericarditis. Indian Heart J. *29*:70, 1977.
193. Gaasch, W. H., Peterson, K. L., and Shabetai, R.: Left ventricular function in chronic constrictive pericarditis. Am. J. Cardiol. *34*:107, 1974.
194. Harvey, R. M., Ferrer, M. I., Cathcart, R. T., Richards, D. W., and Cournand, A.: Mechanical and myocardial factors in chronic constrictive pericarditis. Circulation *8*:695, 1953.
195. Dines, D. E., Edwards, J. E., and Burchell, H. B.: Myocardial atrophy in constrictive pericarditis. Proc. Staff Meet. Mayo Clin. *33*:93, 1958.
196. Vogel, J. H. K., Horgan, J. A., and Strahl, C. L.: Ventricular function in chronic constrictive pericarditis: Observations on fiber shortening rate. Cardiol. Digest *6*:21, 1971.
197. Levine, H. D.: Myocardial fibrosis in constrictive pericarditis. Electrocardiographic and pathologic observations. Circulation *48*:1268, 1973.
198. Kesteloot, H., and Denef, B.: Value of reference tracings in diagnosis and assessment of constrictive epi- and pericarditis. Br. Heart J. *32*:675, 1970.
199. Wood, P.: Chronic constrictive pericarditis. Am. J. Cardiol. *7*:48, 1961.
200. Hancock, E. W.: On the elastic and rigid forms of constrictive pericarditis. Am. Heart J. *100*:917, 1980.
200a. Cheevers, N.: Observations on the disease of the orifice and valves of the aorta. Guy's Hosp. Rep. *7*:387, 1842.
201. Gimlette, T. M. D.: Constrictive pericarditis. Br. Heart J. *21*:9, 1959.
202. Hancock, E. W.: Constrictive pericarditis. Clinical clues to diagnosis. J.A.M.A. *232*:176, 1975.
203. Mounsey, P.: The early diastolic sound of constrictive pericarditis. Br. Heart J. *17*:143, 1955.
204. Tyberg, T. I., Goodyer, A. V. N., and Langou, R. A.: Genesis of pericardial knock in constrictive pericarditis. Am. J. Cardiol. *46*:570, 1980.
205. Beck, W., Shrire, V., and Vogelpoel, L.: Splitting of the second heart sound in constrictive pericarditis with observations on the mechanism of pulsus paradoxus. Am. Heart J. *64*:765, 1962.
206. Plus, G. E., Brower, A. J., and Clagett, O. T.: Chronic constrictive pericarditis: Roentgenologic findings in 35 surgically proved cases. Proc. Staff Meet. Mayo Clin. *32*:555, 1957.
207. Heinz, R., and Abrams, H. L.: Radiologic aspects of operable heart disease. IV. Appearances of constrictive pericarditis. Radiology *69*:54, 1957.
208. Chesler, E., Mitha, A. S., and Matisonn, R. E.: The ECG of constrictive pericarditis—Pattern resembling right ventricular hypertrophy. Am. Heart J. *91*:420, 1976.
209. Schnittger, I., Bowden, R. E., Abrams, J., and Popp, R. L.: Echocardiography: Pericardial thickening and constrictive pericarditis. Am. J. Cardiol. *42*:388, 1978.
210. Doi, Y. L., Sugiura, T., and Spodick, D. H.: Motion of pulmonic valve and constrictive pericarditis. Chest *80*:513, 1981.
211. Tanaka, C. N., Nishimoto, M., Takeuchi, K., Fukukawa, K., Kawai, S., and Oku, H.: Presystolic pulmonic valve opening in constrictive pericarditis. Jpn. Heart J. *20*:419, 1979.
212. Voekel, A. G., Pietro, D. A., Folland, E. D., Fisher, M. L., and Parisi, A. F.: Echocardiographic features of constrictive pericarditis. Circulation *58*:871,1978.
213. Gibson, T. C., Grossman, W., McLaurin, L. P., Moos, S., and Craige, E.: An echocardiographic study of the interventricular septum in constrictive pericarditis. Br. Heart J. *38*:738, 1976.
214. Candell-Riera, J., Garcia del Castillo, H., Permanyer-Miralda, G., and Soler-Soler, J.: Echocardiographic features of the interventricular septum in chronic constrictive pericarditis. Circulation *57*:1154, 1978.
215. Struck, B. L., Fitzgerald, J. W., and Lipton, M.: The posterior aortic wall echocardiogram: Its relationship to left atrial volume change. Circulation *54*:744, 1976.
216. Laurent, F., DeVernejoul, F., Galey, J. J., and Brun, P.: Echocardiography in the evaluation of constrictive pericarditis. Arch. Mal. Coeur *73*:85, 1980.
217. Chandraratna, P. A. N., Aronow, W. S., and Imaizumi, T.: Role of echocardiography in detecting the anatomic and physiologic abnormalities of constrictive pericarditis. Am. J. Med. Sci. *283*:141, 1982.
218. Lewis, B. S.: Real time two-dimensional echocardiography in constrictive pericarditis. Am. J. Cardiol. *49*:1789, 1982.
219. Plauth, W. H., Jr., Waldmann, T. A., Wochner, R. D., Braunwald, N. S., and Braunwald, E.: Protein-losing enteropathy secondary to constrictive pericarditis in childhood. Pediatrics *34*:636, 1964.
220. Wilkinson, P., Pinto, B., and Senior, J. R.: Reversible protein-losing enteropathy with intestinal lymphangiectasia, secondary to chronic constrictive pericarditis. N. Engl. J. Med. *273*:1178, 1965.
221. Pastor, B. H., and Cahn, M.: Reversible nephrotic syndrome resulting from constrictive pericarditis. N. Engl. J. Med. *262*:872, 1960.
222. Daugherty, G. W., Broadbent, J. C., and Brown, A. L., Jr.: Chronic constrictive pericarditis associated with the nephrotic syndrome: Report of case. Proc. Staff Meet. Mayo Clin. *37*:283, 1962.
223. Hansen, A. T., Eskildsen, P., and Gotzsche, H.: Pressure curves from the right auricle and the right ventricle in chronic constrictive pericarditis. Circulation *3*:881, 1951.
224. Conti, C. R., and Friesinger, G. C.: Chronic constrictive pericarditis, clinical and laboratory findings in 11 cases. Johns Hopkins Med. J. *120*:262, 1967.
225. Lewis, B. S., and Gotsman, M. S.: Left ventricular function in systole and diastole in constrictive pericarditis. Am. Heart J. *86*:23, 1973.
226. Figley, M. M., and Bagshaw, M. A.: Angiocardiographic aspects of constrictive pericarditis. Radiology *69*:46, 1957.
227. Ramsey, H. W., Sbar, S., Elliot, L. P., and Eliot, R. S.: The differential diagnosis of restrictive myocardiopathy and chronic constrictive pericarditis without calcification: Value of coronary arteriography. Am. J. Cardiol. *25*:635, 1970.
228. Alexander, J., Kelley, M. J., Cohen, L. S., and Langou, R. A.: The angiographic appearance of the coronary arteries in constrictive pericarditis. Radiology *131*:609, 1979.
229. Goldberg, E., Stein, J., Berger, M., and Berdoff, R. L.: Diastolic segmental coronary artery obliteration in constrictive pericarditis. Cath. Cardiovasc. Diag. *7*:197, 1981.
230. Shabetai, R., Fowler, N. O., and Fenton, J. C.: Restrictive cardiac disease. Pericarditis and the myocardiopathies. Am. Heart J. *69*:271, 1965.
231. Bhatia, M. D., Grover, D. N., and Roy, S. B.: Haemodynamic effects of exercise in patients with constrictive pericarditis before and after pericardiectomy. Indian Heart J. *29*:272, 1977.
232. Swanton, R. H., Brooksby, I. A. B., Davies, M. J., Coltart, D. J., Jenkins, B. S., and Webb-Peploe, M. M.: Systolic and diastolic ventricular function in cardiac amyloidosis. Studies in six cases diagnosed with endomyocardial biopsy. Am. J. Cardiol. *39*:658, 1977.
233. Benotti, J. R., Grossman, W., and Cohn, P. F.: Clinical profile of restrictive cardiomyopathy. Circulation *61*:1206, 1980.
234. Chew, C., Ziady, G., Raphael, M. J., and Oakley, C. M.: The functional defect in amyloid heart disease. Am. J. Cardiol. *36*:438, 1975.
235. Chang, L. W., and Grollman, J. H., Jr.: Angiographic differentiation of constrictive pericarditis and restrictive cardiomyopathy due to amyloidosis. Am. J. Radiol. *130*:451, 1978.
236. Tyberg, T. I., Goodyer, A. V. N., Hurst, V. W., Alexander, J., and Langou, R. A.: Left ventricular filling in differentiating restrictive amyloid cardiomyopathy and constrictive pericarditis. Am. J. Cardiol. *47*:791, 1981.
237. Broadarick, S., Paine, R. Higa, E., and Carmichael, K. A.: Pericardial tamponade—A new complication of amyloid heart disease. Am. J. Med. *73*:133, 1982.
238. Kern, M. J., Lorell, B. H., and Grossman, W.: Cardiac amyloidosis masquerading as constrictive pericarditis. Cath. Cardiovasc. Diag. *8*:629, 1982.
239. Gunnar, R. M., Dillon, R. F., Wallyn, R. J., and Elisberg, E. I.: The physiologic and clinical similarity between primary amyloid of the heart and constrictive pericarditis. Circulation *12*:827, 1955.
240. Hetzel, P. S., Wood, E. H., and Burchell, H. B.: Pressure pulses in the right side of the heart in a case of amyloid disease and in a case of idiopathic heart failure simulating constrictive pericarditis. Proc. Staff Meet. Mayo Clin. *28*:107, 1963.
241. Hoyningen-Huene, C. B. J.: Systemic amyloidosis presenting as constrictive pericarditis. A case studied with cardiac catheterization. Am. Heart J. *67*:290, 1964.
242. Wasserman, A. J., Richardson, D. W., Baird, C. L., and Wyso, E. M.: Cardiac hemochromatosis simulating constrictive pericarditis. Am. J. Med. *32*:316, 1962.
243. Clark, G. M., Valentine, E., and Blount, S. G.: Endocardial fibrosis simulating constrictive pericarditis. N. Engl. J. Med. *254*:349, 1956.
244. Brink, A. J., and Weber, H. W.: Fibroplastic parietal endocarditis with eosinophilia. Loeffler's endocarditis. Am. J. Med. *34*:52, 1963.
245. Parrillo, J. E., Borer, J. S., Henry, W. L., Wolff, S. M., and Fauci, A. S.: The cardiovascular manifestations of the hypereosinophilic syndrome. Am. J. Med. *67*:572, 1979.
246. Child, J. S., Levisman, J. A., Abbasi, A. S., and MacAlpin, R. N.: Echocardiographic manifestations of infiltrative cardiomyopathy. A report of seven cases due to amyloid. Chest *70*:726, 1976.

247. Borer, J. S., Henry, W. L., and Epstein, S. E.: Echocardiographic observations in patients with systemic infiltrative disease involving the heart. Am. J. Cardiol. *39*:184, 1977.
248. Child, J. S., Krivokapich, J., and Abbasi, A. S.: Increased right ventricular wall thickness on echocardiography in amyloid infiltrative cardiomyopathy. Am. J. Cardiol. *44*:1391, 1979.
249. Carroll, J. D., Gaasch, W. H., and McAdam, K. P. W. J.: Amyloid cardiomyopathy: Characterization by a distinctive voltage/mass ratio. Am. J. Cardiol. *49*:9, 1982.
250. Fowler, N. O.: [Chapter 48] *In* Cardiac Diagnosis and Treatment. 3rd ed. New York, Harper and Row, 1980, pp. 976–1009.
251. Cooley, J. C., Clagett, O. T., and Kirklin, J. W.: Surgical aspects of chronic constrictive pericarditis. A review of 72 operative cases. Ann. Surg. *147*:488, 1958.
252. Copeland, J. G., Stinson, E. B., Griepp, R. B., and Shumway, N. E.: Surgical treatment of chronic constrictive pericarditis using cardiopulmonary bypass. J. Thorac. Cardiovasc. Surg. *69*:236, 1975.
253. Somerville, W.: Constrictive pericarditis: With special reference to the change in natural history brought about by surgical intervention. Circulation *38* (Suppl. V):102, 1968.
254. Stalpaert, G., Suy, R., Daenen, W., and Nevelsteen, A.: Total pericardiectomy for chronic constrictive pericarditis. Acta Chir. Belg. *80*:277, 1981.
255. Wychulis, A. R., Connolly, D. C., and McGoon, D. C.: Surgical treatment of pericarditis. J. Thorac. Cardiovasc. Surg. *62*:608, 1971.
256. Collins, H. A., Woods, L. P., and Daniel, R. A., Jr.: Late results of pericardiectomy. Arch. Surg. *89*:921, 1964.
257. Fowler, N. O.: Constrictive pericarditis: New aspects. Am. J. Cardiol. *50*:1014, 1982.
258. Zucherman, J. F., Rubio, P. A., Guinn, G. A., and Korompai, F. L.: Rational use of operation in pericardial constriction. Int. Surg. *62*:204, 1977.
259. Kamaras, J., and Zaborszky, B.: Chronic constrictive pericarditis in children. Cor. Vasa. *23*:66, 1981.
260. Kloster, F. E., Crislip, R. L., Bristow, J. D., Herr, R. H., Ritzmann, L. W., and Griswold, H. E.: Hemodynamic studies following pericardiectomy for constrictive pericarditis. Circulation *32*:415, 1965.
261. Culliford, A. T., Lipton, M., and Spencer, F. C.: Operation for chronic constrictive pericarditis: Do the surgical approach and degree of pericardial resection influence the outcome significantly? Ann. Thorac. Surg. *29*:146, 1980.
262. Viola, A. R.: The influence of pericardiectomy on the hemodynamics of chronic constrictive pericarditis. Circulation *48*:1038, 1973.
263. Sawyer, C. G., Burwell, C. S., Dexter, L., Eppinger, E. C., Goodale, W. T., Gorlin, R., Harkin, D. E., and Haynes, F. W.: Chronic constrictive pericarditis. Further consideration of the pathologic physiology of the disease. Am. Heart J. *44*:207, 1952.
264. Chambliss, J. R., Jaruszewski, E. J., Brofman, B. L., Martin, J. F., and Feil, H.: Chronic cardiac compression (chronic constrictive pericarditis): A critical study of sixty-one operated cases with followup. Circulation *4*:816, 1951.
265. Dalton, J. C., Pearson, R. J., and White, P. D.: Constrictive pericarditis: A review and long-term followup of 78 cases. Ann. Intern. Med. *45*:445, 1956.
266. Walsh, T. J., Baughman, K. L., Gardner, T. J., and Bulkley, B. H.: Constrictive epicarditis as a cause of delayed or absent response to pericardiectomy. J. Thorac. Cardiovasc. Surg. *83*:126, 1982.
267. Spodick, D. H., and Kumar, S.: Subacute constrictive pericarditis with cardiac tamponade. Dis. Chest *54*:62, 1968.
268. Hancock, E. W.: Subacute effusive constrictive pericarditis. Circulation *43*:183, 1971.
269. Martin, R. P., Bowden, R., Filly, K., and Popp, R. L.: Intrapericardial abnormalities in patients with pericardial effusion. Circulation *61*:568, 1980.
270. Horowitz, M. S., Rossen, R., and Harrison, D. C.: Echocardiographic diagnosis of pericardial disease. Am. Heart J. *97*:420, 1979.
271. Rasaretnam, R., and Chanmugam, D.: Subacute effusive-constrictive pericarditis. Br. Heart J. *44*:44, 1980.
272. Bush, C. A., Stang, J. M., Wooley, C. G., and Kilman, J.: Occult constrictive pericardial disease. Diagnosis by rapid volume expansion and correction by pericardiectomy. Circulation *56*:924, 1977.
273. Kilman, J. W., Bush, C. A., Wooley, C. G., Stang, J. M., Teply, J., and Baba, N.: The changing spectrum of pericardiectomy for chronic pericarditis: Occult constrictive pericarditis. J. Thorac. Cardiovasc. Surg. *74*:668, 1977.

SPECIFIC FORMS OF PERICARDITIS

274. Brodie, H. R., and Marchessault, V.: Acute benign pericarditis caused by Coxsackie virus group B. N. Engl. J. Med. *262*:1278, 1960.
275. Kleinfeld, M., Milles, S., and Lidsky, M.: Mumps pericarditis: Review of the literature and report of a case. Am. Heart J. *55*:153, 1958.
276. Wilson, D. R., Lenkei, S. C., and Patterson, J. F.: Acute constrictive epicarditis following infectious mononucleosis. Circulation *23*:257, 1961.
277. Helmly, R. B., Smith, J. O., Jr., and Eisen, B.: Chickenpox with pneumonia and pericarditis. J.A.M.A. *186*:870, 1963.
278. Adler, R., Takahashi, M., and Wright, H. T., Jr.: Acute pericarditis associated with hepatitis B infection. Pediatrics *61*:716, 1978.
279. Ponka, A.: Carditis associated with *Mycoplasma pneumoniae* infection. Acta Med. Scand. *206*:77, 1979.
280. Cooper, D. K. C., and Sturridge, M. F.: Constrictive pericarditis following Coxsackie virus infection. Thorax *31*:472, 1976.
281. Brown, M.D.: Acute benign pericarditis. N. Engl. J. Med. *244*:666, 1951.
282. Fowler, N. O., and Manitsas, G. T.: Infectious pericarditis. Progr. Cardiovasc. Dis. *16*:323, 1973.
283. Bradley, E. C.: Acute benign pericarditis. Am. Heart J. *67*:121, 1964.
284. Connolly, D. C., and Burchell, H. B.: Pericarditis: A ten-year survey. Am. J. Cardiol. *7*:7, 1961.
285. Goodman, H. C.: Acute nonspecific pericarditis with cardiac tamponade: A fatal case associated with anticoagulant therapy. Ann. Intern. Med. *48*:406, 1958.
286. Blakemore, W. S., Zinsser, H. F., Kirby, C. K., Whitaker, W. B., and Johnson, J.: Pericardiectomy for relapsing pericarditis and chronic constrictive pericarditis. J. Thorac. Cardiovasc. Surg. *39*:26, 1960.
287. Larrieu, A. J., Tyers, G. F., Williams, E. H., and Derrick, J. R.: Recent experience with tuberculous pericarditis. Ann. Thorac. Surg. *29*:464, 1980.
288. Bellett, S., McMillan, T. M., and Gouley, G. A.: Tuberculous pericarditis: Clinical and pathological study based upon a series of 17 cases. Med. Clin. N. Am. *18*:201, 1934.
289. Roy, J. C., Gimei, Y., Condat, J. M., Lokrou, A., Ferrus, P., Soubeyrand, J., and Beda, B. Y.: Pericarditis in adults in Abidjan. Semin. Hop. Paris *57*:978, 1981.
290. Desai, H. N.: Tuberculous pericarditis: A review of 100 cases. S. Afr. Med. J. *55*:877, 1979.
291. Williams, I. M., and Hetzel, M. R.: Tuberculous pericarditis in South-West London: An increasing problem. Thorax *33*:816, 1978.
292. Gooi, H. C., and Smith, J. M.: Tuberculous pericarditis in Birmingham. Thorax *33*:94, 1978.
293. Bialock, A., and Levy, S. E.: Tuberculous pericarditis. J. Thorac. Surg. *7*:132, 1937.
294. Peel, A. A. F.: Tuberculous pericarditis. Br. Heart J. *10*:195, 1948.
295. Auerbach, O.: Pleural, peritoneal, and pericardial tuberculosis. Am. Rev. Tuberc. *61*:845, 1950.
296. Maisch, B., Maisch, S., and Kocksiek, K.: Immune reactions in tuberculous and chronic constrictive pericarditis. Am. J. Cardiol. *50*:1007, 1982.
297. Schrire, V.: Experience with pericarditis of Groote Schuur Hospital, Cape Town: An analysis of one hundred and sixty cases over a six-year period. S. Afr. Med. J. *33*:810, 1959.
298. Hageman, J. H., D'Esopo, N. D., and Glenn, W. W. L.: Tuberculosis of the pericardium: A long-term analysis of forty-four cases. N. Engl. J. Med. *270*:327, 1964.
299. Lesar, M. S., Orcutt, J., Wehunt, W. D., and Babcock, T. E.: Pericardial tuberculoma. An unusual cause of mediastinal mass. Radiology *138*:309, 1981.
300. Hirasing, R. A., and Van Bel, F.: Tuberculous pericarditis developing during chemotherapy. Eur. J. Resp. Dis. *63*:73, 1982.
301. Barr, J. F.: The use of pericardial biopsy in establishing etiologic diagnosis in acute pericarditis. Arch. Intern. Med. *96*:693, 1955.
302. Cheitlin, M. D., Serfos, L. J., Sbar, S. S., and Glosser, S. P.: Tuberculous pericarditis: Is limited pericardial biopsy sufficient for diagnosis: Am. Rev. Resp. Dis. *98*:287, 1968.
303. Deterling, R. A., Jr., and Humphreys, G. H.: Factors in the etiology of constrictive pericarditis. Circulation *12*:30, 1955.
304. Rooney, J. J., Crocco, J. A., and Lyons, H. A.: Tuberculous pericarditis. Ann. Intern. Med. *72*:73, 1970.
305. Ortbals, P. W., and Avioli, L. V.: Tuberculous pericarditis. Arch. Intern. Med. *139*:231, 1979.
306. Boyle, J. D., Pearce, M. L., and Guz, L. B.: Purulent pericarditis. Review of literature and report of eleven cases. Medicine *40*:119, 1961.
307. Klacsmann, P. B., Bulkley, B. H., and Hutchins, G. M.: The changed spectrum of purulent pericarditis. An 86 year autopsy experience in 200 patients. Am. J. Med. *63*:666, 1977.
308. Berk, S. L., Rice, P. A., Reynolds, C. A., and Finland, M.: Pneumococcal pericarditis: A persisting problem in contemporary diagnosis. Am. J. Med. *70*:247, 1981.
309. Kauffman, C. A., Watanakunakorn, C., and Phair, J. P.: Purulent pneumococcal pericarditis: A continuing problem in the antibiotic era. Am. J. Med. *54*:743, 1973.
310. Lukash, W. M.: Massive pericardial effusion due to meningococcic pericarditis. J.A.M.A. *185*:598, 1963.
311. Penny, J. L., Grace, W. J., and Kennedy, R. L.: Meningococci pericarditis. Am. J. Cardiol. *18*:281, 1966.
312. Herman, R. A., and Rubin, H. A.: Meningococcal pericarditis without meningitis presenting as tamponade. N. Engl. J. Med. *290*:143, 1974.
313. Rao, V. S., Rajashekaraian, K. L., Rice, T., Riaz, M., Towne, W., and Kallick, C. A.: Primary meningococcal pericarditis. South. Med. J. *73*:1276, 1980.
314. Levin, H. S., and Hosier, D. M.: Salmonella pericarditis. Report of a case and review of the literature. Ann. Intern. Med. *55*:817, 1961.
315. Theler, B. D., Noseda, G., Reiner, M., and Keller, H.: Pericarditis and myocarditis in salmonellosis. Schweiz. Med. Wschr. *110*:1394, 1980.
316. Vietzke, W. M.: Gonococcal arthritis with pericarditis. Arch. Intern. Med. *117*:270, 1966.
317. Benzing, G., III, and Kaplan, S.: Purulent pericarditis. Am. J. Dis. Child. *106*:289, 1963.
318. Meredith, H. C., Jr.: Tularemic pericarditis: A report of two cases, including one of constrictive pericarditis. Ann. Intern. Med. *32*:688, 1950.
319. Rubin, R. H., and Moellering, R. C., Jr.: Clinical, microbiologic, and therapeutic aspects of purulent pericarditis. Am. J. Med. *59*:68, 1975.

320. Callahan, D. L., Morriss, M. J., Kaplan, S. L., and Park, I.: Constrictive pericarditis due to *Streptococcus sanguis.* South. Med. J. *74*:377, 1981.
321. Hanson, G., and Engel, P. J.: Purulent pericarditis caused by beta-hemolytic group C streptococcus. Arch. Intern. Med. *414*:1351, 1981.
322. Lieber, I. H., Rensimer, E. R., and Ericsson, C. D.: Campylobacter pericarditis in hypothyroidism. Am. Heart J. *102*:462, 1981.
323. Rahman, M.: Bacteremia and pericarditis from Campylobacter infection. Br. J. Clin. Pract. *33*:131, 1979.
324. Solomon, C., Roberts, J. E., and Lisa, J. R.: The heart in uremia. Am. J. Pathol. *18*:729, 1942.
325. Nadas, A. S., and Levy, J. M.: Pericarditis in children. Am. J. Cardiol. *7*:109, 1961.
326. Feldman, W. E.: Bacterial etiology and mortality of purulent pericarditis in pediatric patients. Am. J. Dis. Child. *133*:164, 1979.
327. Leggiadro, R. J., and Balsam, D.: *Haemophilus influenzae* sepsis leading to pericarditis despite antimicrobial therapy. Johns Hopkins Med. J. *146*:133,1980.
328. Wyler, F., Knusli, D., Rutishauser, M., Stocker, F., Weber, J., and Real, F.: Pericarditis purulenta in children. Helv. Paediat. Acta *32*:135, 1977.
329. Jaiyesimi, F., Abioye, A. A., and Antia, A. U.: Infective pericarditis in Nigerian children. Arch. Dis. Child. *54*:384, 1979.
330. Chun, P. K., and Rocchini, A. P.: Occult constrictive pericarditis in infancy. Chest *78*:648, 1980.
331. Vogt, J., Rupprath, G., Divivie, E. R., Dahn, D., and Kunze, E.: Constrictive pericarditis in early infancy. Klin. Paediat. *192*:384, 1980.
332. Cheatham, J. E., Jr., Grantham, R. N., Peyton, M. D., Thompson, W. M., Luckstead, E. F., Razook, J. D., and Elkins, R. C.: *Hemophilus influenzae* purulent pericarditis in children: Diagnostic and therapeutic considerations. J. Thorac. Cardiovasc. Surg. *79*:933, 1980.
333. Stoobant, J., Leanage, R., Deanfield, J., and Taylor, J. F.: Acute infective pericarditis in infancy. Arch. Dis. Child. *57*:73, 1982.
334. Zimmerman, L. E.: Candida and Aspergillus endocarditis. Arch. Parthol. *50*: 591, 1950.
335. Gould, K., Barnett, J. A., and Sanford, J. P.: Purulent pericarditis in the antibiotic era. Arch. Intern. Med. *134*:923, 1974.
336. Morse, J. R., Oretsky, M. I., and Hudson, J. A. M.: Pericarditis as a complication of meningococcal meningitis. Ann. Intern. Med. *74*:212, 1971.
337. Pierce, H. I., and Cooper, E. B.: Meningococcal pericarditis: Clinical features and therapy in five patients. Arch. Intern. Med. *129*:918, 1972.
338. Miller, G. C., and Witham, A. C.: Delayed febrile pleuropericarditis after sepsis. Ann. Intern. Med. *79*:194, 1973.
339. Schoenwetter, A. H., and Silber, E. N.: Penicillin hypersensitivity, acute pericarditis and eosinophilia. J.A.M.A. *191*:136, 1965.
340. Tan, J. S., Holmes, J. C., Fowler, N. O., Manitsas, G. T., and Phair, J. P.: Antibiotic levels in pericardial fluid. J. Clin. Invest. *53*:7, 1974.
341. Das, P. B.: Staphylococcal pericarditis and its treatment by early pericardiectomy. Indian Heart J. *29*:90, 1977.
342. Saslaw, S., NorFleet, R. G., and Dapra, D. J.: Acute Histoplasma pericarditis. Arch. Intern. Med. *122*:162, 1968.
343. Picardi, J. L., Kauffman, C. A., Schwarz, J., Holmes, J. C., Phair, J. P., and Fowler, N. O.: Pericarditis caused by *Histoplasma capsulatum.* Am. J. Cardiol. *37*:82, 1976.
344. Young, E. J., Vainrub, B., and Musher, D. M.: Pericarditis due to histoplasmosis. J.A.M.A. *240*:1750, 1978.
345. Kirchner, S. G., Heller, R. M., Sell, S. J., and Altemeier, W. A. III: The radiological features of histoplasma pericarditis. Pediat. Radiol. *7*:7, 1978.
346. Larsen, R., and Scherb, R. E.: Coccidioidal pericarditis. Circulation *7*:211, 1953.
347. Chapman, M. G., and Kaplan, L.: Cardiac involvement in coccidioidomycosis. Am. J. Med. *23*:87, 1957.
348. Gronemyer, P. S., Weisfeld, A. S., and Sonnenwirth, A. C.: Purulent pericarditis complicating systemic infection with *Candida tropicalis.* Am. J. Clin. Pathol. *77*:471, 1982.
349. Walsh, T. J., and Bulkley, B. J.: Aspergillus pericarditis: Clinical and pathologic features in the immunocompromised patient. Cancer *49*:48, 1982.
350. Walsh, T. J., and Hutchins, G. M.: Postoperative Candida infections in children: Clinicopathologic study of continuing problem of diagnosis and therapy. J. Pediat. Surg. *15*:325, 1980.
351. Dix, J. H., and Gurkaynak, N.: Histoplasmosis with massive pericardial effusion and systemic involvement. J.A.M.A. *182*:687, 1962.
352. Kleger, H. L., and Fisher, E. R.: Fibrocalcific constrictive pericarditis due to *Histoplasma capsulatum.* N. Engl. J. Med. *267*:593, 1962.
353. Prager, R. L., Burney, D. P., Waterhouse, G., and Bender, H. W., Jr.: Pulmonary, mediastinal, and cardiac presentations of histoplasmosis. Ann. Thorac. Surg. *30*:385, 1980.
354. Wooley, C. F., and Hosier, D. M.: Constrictive pericarditis due to *Histoplasma capsulatum.* N. Engl. J. Med. *264*:1230, 1961.
355. Eng, R. J., Sen, P., Browne, K., and Louria, D. B.: Candida pericarditis. Am. J. Med. *70*:867, 1981.
356. Schlossberg, D., Franco-Jove, D., Woodward, C., and Shulman, C.: Pericarditis with effusion caused by *Actinomyces israelii.* Chest *69*:680, 1976.
357. Mohan, K., Dass, S. I., and Kemble, E. E.: Actinomycosis of the pericardium. J.A.M.A. *229*:321, 1974.
358. Causey, W. A., Arnell, P., and Brinker, J.: Systemic Nocardia infection. Chest *65*:360, 1974.
359. Susens, G. P., Al-Shamma, A., Rowe, J. C., Herbert, C. C., Bassis, M. L., and Coggs, G. C.: Purulent constrictive pericarditis caused by *Nocardia asteroides.* Ann. Intern. Med. *67*:1021, 1967.
360. Tyagi, S. K., Anand, I. S., Deodhar, S. D., and Datta, D. V.: A clinical study of amoebic pericarditis. J. Assoc. Physic. India *28*:515, 1980.
361. Bansal, B. C., and Gupta, D. S.: Amoebic pericarditis. Postgrad. Med. J. *47*: 678, 1971.
362. Kala, P. C., and Sharma, G. C.: Amoebic pericarditis treated by pericardiectomy. J. Indian Med. Assoc. *74*:194, 1980.
363. Sagrista-Sauleda, J., Permanyer-Miralda, G., Juste-Sanchez, C., De Buen-Sanchez, M. L., Pujadas-Capmany, R., Arcalis-Arce, L., and Soler-Soler, J.: Huge chronic pericardial effusion caused by *Toxoplasma gondii.* Circulation *66*: 895, 1982.
364. Feldman, H. A.: Medical progress: Toxoplasmosis. N. Engl. J. Med. *279*:1370, 1968.
365. Chens, W.: Hydatid cysts in the pericardium—A new case and review of the literature. J. Thorac. Cardiovasc. Surg. *30*:56, 1982.
366. Halliday, J. H., Jose, A. D., and Nicks, R.: Constrictive pericarditis following rupture of a ventricular hydatid cyst. Br. Heart J. *25*:821, 1963.
367. DiBello, R.: Cardiac echinococcosis. Late sudden death after surgical treatment. Chest *79*:110, 1981.
368. Kinare, S. G., Parulkar, G. B., and Sen, P. K.: Constrictive pericarditis resulting from dracunculosis. Br. Med. J. *1*:845, 1962.
369. Charon, A., and Sinha, K.: Constrictive pericarditis following filiariasis. Indian Heart J. *25*:213, 1973.
370. Thadani, U., Chopra, M. P., Aber, C. P., and Portal, R. W.: Pericarditis after acute myocardial infarction. Br. Med. J. *2*:135, 1971.
371. Lichstein, E. M., Lieu, H. M., and Gupta, P.: Pericarditis complicating acute myocardial infarction: Incidence of complications and significance of electrocardiogram on admission. Am. Heart J. *87*:246, 1974.
372. Stewart, C. F., and Turner, K. B.: A note on pericardial involvement in coronary thrombosis. Am. Heart J. *15*:232, 1938.
373. Khan, A. J.: Pericarditis of myocardial infarction: Review of the literature with case presentation. Am. Heart J. *90*:788, 1975.
374. Anderson, M. W., Christensen, N. A., and Edwards, J. E.: Hemopericardium complicating myocardial infarction in the absence of cardiac rupture. Arch. Intern. Med. *90*:634, 1952.
375. Aarseth, S., and Lange, H. F.: The influence of anticoagulant therapy on the occurrence of cardiac rupture and hemopericardium following heart infarction. I. A study of 89 cases of hemopericardium. Am. Heart J. *56*:250, 1958.
376. Lange, H. F., and Aarseth, S.: The influence of anticoagulant therapy on the occurrence of cardiac rupture and hemopericardium following heart infarction. II. A controlled study of a selected treated group based on 1,044 autopsies. Am. Heart J. *56*:257, 1958.
377. Miller, R. L.: Hemopericardium with use of oral anticoagulant therapy. J.A.M.A. *209*:1362, 1969.
378. Goldstein, R., and Wolff, L.: Hemorrhagic pericarditis in acute myocardial infarction treated with bishydroxycoumarin. J.A.M.A. *146*:616, 1951.
379. Liberthson, R. R., Salisbury, K. W., and Hutter, A. M., Jr.: Atrial tachyarrhythmias in acute myocardial infarction. Am. J. Med. *60*:956, 1976.
380. Liem, K. L., Durrer, D., and Lie, K. L.: Pericarditis in acute myocardial infarction. Lancet *2*:1004, 1975.
381. Sawaya, J. I., Mujais, S. K., and Armenian, H. K.: Early diagnosis of pericarditis in acute myocardial infarction. Am. Heart J. *100*:144, 1980.
382. Dvorak, K., and Cerny, J.: Long-term survival of subacute cardiac rupture with tamponade in acute myocardial infarction, without surgical intervention (the role of pericardiocentesis). Cor. Vasa. *21*:233, 1979.
383. Jensen, D. P., Goolsby, J. P., Jr., and Oliva, P. B.: Hemodynamic pattern resembling paricardial constriction after acute inferior myocardial infarction with right ventricular infarction. Am. J. Cardiol. *42*:858, 1978.
384. Butman, S., Olson, H. G., Aronow, W. S., and Lyons, K. P.: Remote right ventricular myocardial infarction mimicking chronic pericardial constriction. Am. Heart J. *103*:912, 1982.
385. Berman, J., Haffajee, C. I., and Alpert, J. S.: Therapy of symptomatic pericarditis after myocardial infarction: Retrospective and prospective studies of aspirin, indomethacin, prednisone, and spontaneous resolution. Am. Heart J. *101*: 750, 1981.
386. Jugdutt, B. I., Hutchins, G. M., Bulkley, B., Pitt, B., and Becker, L. C.: Effect of indomethacin on collateral blood flow and infarct size in the conscious dog. Circulation *59*:734, 1979.
387. Friedman, P. L., Brugada, P., Kuck, K. H., Bär, F. W. H. M., and Wellens, H. J. J.: Coronary vasoconstrictor effect of indomethacin in patients with coronary artery disease. N. Engl. J. Med. *305*:1171, 1981.
388. Hammerman, H., Kloner, R. A., Schoen, F. J., Brown, E. J., Hale, S., and Braunwald, E.: Indomethacin induced scar thinning following experimental myocardial infarction. Circulation *67*:1290, 1983.
389. Brown, E. J., Kloner, R. A., Schoen, F. J., Hammerman, H., Hale, S., and Braunwald, E.: Scar thinning due to ibuprofen administration following experimental myocardial infarction. Am. J. Cardiol. *51*:877, 1983.
390. Hammerman, H., Kloner, R. A., Schoen, F. J., Brown, E. J., Hale, S., and Braunwald, E.: Scar thinning due to indomethacin administration following experimental myocardial infarction. Clin. Res. *30*:547A, 1982.
391. Bright, R.: Tabular view of the morbid appearance in 100 cases connected with albuminous urine: With observations. Guy's Hosp. Rep. *1*:380, 1836.
392. Wacker, W., and Merrill, J. P.: Uremic pericarditis in acute and chronic renal failure. J.A.M.A. *156*:764, 1954.

393. Skov, P. E., Hansen, H. E., and Spencer, E. S.: Uremic pericarditis Acta Med. Scand. *186*:421, 1969.
394. Osanloo, E., Shalhoub, R. J., Cioffi, R. F., and Parker, R. H.: Viral pericarditis in patients receiving hemodialysis. Arch. Intern. Med. *139*:310, 1979.
395. Bailey, G. L., Hampers, C. L., and Merrill, J. P.: Reversible cardiomyopathy in uremia. Trans. Am. Soc. Artif. Intern. Organs *13*:263, 1967.
396. Shabetai, R.: Uremia, dialysis, and metabolic causes of pericardial disease. *In*: The Pericardium. New York, Grune and Stratton, 1981, pp. 385–389.
397. Lindsay, J., Jr., Crawley, I. S., and Callaway, G. M.: Chronic constrictive pericarditis following uremic hemopericardium. Am. Heart J. *79*:390, 1970.
398. Comty, C. M., Cohen, S. L., and Shapiro, F. L.: Pericarditis in chronic uremia and its sequels. Ann. Intern. Med. *75*:173, 1971.
399. Luft, L. C., Gilman, J. K., and Weyman, A. E.: Pericarditis in the patient with uremia: Clinical and echocardiographic evaluation. Nephron *25*:160, 1980.
400. D'Cruz, I. A., Bhatt, G. R., Cohen, H. C., and Glick, G.: Echocardiographic detection of cardiac involvement in patients with chronic renal failure. Arch. Intern. Med. *138*:720, 1978.
401. Goldstein, D. J., Nagar, C., Srivastava, N., Schacht, R. A., Ferris, F. Z., and Flowers, N. C.: Clinically silent pericardial effusions in patients on long-term hemodialysis. Chest *72*:744, 1977.
402. Morin, J. E., Hollomby, D., Gonda, A., Long, R., and Dobell, A. R. C.: Management of uremic pericarditis: A report of 11 patients with cardiac tamponade and a review of the literature. Ann. Thorac. Surg. *22*:588, 1976.
403. Alfrey, A. C., Goss, J. E., and Ogden, D. A.: Uremic hemopericardium. Am. J. Med. *45*:391, 1968.
404. Masson, J. F., Maes, M. L., and Zilberman, C.: Pericarditis in chronic renal insufficiency treated by periodic hemodialysis. Rev. Med. Intern. *2*:447, 1981.
405. Kwasnik, E. M., Koster, J. K., Lazarus, J. M., Sloss, L. J., Mee, R. B. B., Cohn, L. H., and Collins, J. J.: Conservative management of uremic pericardial effusions. J. Thorac. Cardiovasc. Surg. *76*:629, 1978.
406. Silverberg, S., Oreopoulos, D. G., Wise, D. J., Uden, D. E., Meindok, H., Jones, M., Rapaport, A., and deVeber, G. A.: Pericarditis in patients undergoing long-term hemodialysis and peritoneal dialysis. Am. J. Med. *63*:874,1977.
407. Minuth, A. M. W., Nottebohm, G. A., Eknoyan, G., and Suki, W. N.: Indomethacin treatment of pericarditis in chronic hemodialysis patients. Arch. Intern. Med. *135*:807, 1975.
408. Buselmeir, T. J., Simmons, R. L., Najarian, J. S., Mauer, S. M., Matas, A. J., and Kjellstrand, C. M.: Uremic pericardial effusion. Nephron *16*:371, 1976.
409. Fuller, T. J., Knochel, J. P., Brennan, J. P., Fetner, C. D., and White, M. G.: Reversal of intractable uremic pericarditis by triamcinolone hexacetonide. Arch. Intern. Med. *136*:979, 1976.
410. Feinroth, M. V., Goldstein, E. J., Josephson, A., and Friedman, E. A.: Infection complicating intrapericardial steroid instillation in uremic pericarditis. Clin. Nephrol. *15*:331, 1981.
411. Beaudry, C., Nakamoto, S., and Koloff, W. J.: Uremic pericarditis and cardiac tamponade in chronic renal failure. Ann. Intern. Med. *64*:990, 1966.
412. Singh, S., Newmark, K., Ishikasa, I., Mitra, S., and Berman, L. B.: Pericardiectomy in uremia. The treatment of choice for cardiac tamponade in chronic renal failure. J.A.M.A. *228*:1132, 1974.
413. Engelman, R. M., Levitsky, S., Konchigeri, H. N., Wyndham, C. R. C., Roper, K., and Kurtzman, N. A.: Total pericardiectomy for uremic pericarditis. World J. Surg. *1*:769, 1977.
414. Nickey, W. A., Chinitz, J. L., Flynn, J. J., Adam, A., Kim, K. E., Schwartz, A. B., Onesti, G., and Swartz, C. D.: Surgical correction of uremic constrictive pericarditis. Ann. Intern. Med. *75*:227, 1971.
415. Koopot, R., Zerefos, N. S., and Lavender, A. R.: Cardiac tamponade in uremic pericarditis: Surgical approach and management. Am. J. Cardiol. *32*:846, 1973.
416. Van Baestelaere, W., Verbanck, J., Verschuere, I., Ringoir, S., and Derom, F.: Surgical therapy of uremic pericarditis. Acta Chir. Belg. *80*:293, 1981.
417. Nevelsteen, A., Daenen, W., Suy, R., and Stalpaert, G.: Treatment by limited pericardiectomy. Acta Chir. Belg. *80*:299, 1981.
418. DeLoach, J. F., and Haynes, J. W.: Secondary tumors of the heart and pericardium. Arch. Intern. Med. *91*:224, 1953.
419. Roberts, W. C., Bodey, G. P., and Wertlake, P. T.: The heart in acute leukemia: A study of 420 autopsy cases. Am. J. Cardiol. *21*:388, 1968.
420. Hanfling, S. M.: Metastatic cancer to the heart. Circulation *22*:474, 1960.
421. Young, J. M., and Goldman, I. R.: Tumor metastases to the heart. Circulation *9*:220, 1954.
422. Roberts, W. C., Glancy, D. L., and DeVita, V. T.: Heart in malignant lymphoma (Hodgkin's disease, lymphosarcoma, reticulum cell sarcoma and mycosis fungoides): A study of 196 autopsy cases. Am. J. Cardiol. *22*:85, 1968.
423. Goudie, R. B.: Secondary tumors of the heart and pericardium. Br. Heart J. *17*: 183, 1955.
424. Gassman, H. S., Meadows, R., and Baker, L. A.: Metastatic tumors of the heart. Am. J. Med. *19*:357, 1955.
425. Thurber, D. L., Edwards, J. E., and Achor, R. W.: Secondary malignant tumors of the pericardium. Circulation *26*:228, 1962.
426. Cohen, G. U., Perry, T. M., and Evens, J. M.: Neoplastic invasion of the heart and pericardium. Ann. Intern. Med. *42*:1238, 1955.
427. Onuigbo, W. I. B.: The spread of lung cancer to the heart, pericardium, and great vessels. Jpn. Heart J. *15*:235, 1974.
428. Aymard, J. P., Voiriot, P., Witz, F., Colomb, J. N., Lederlin, P., Thibaut, G., Guerci, O., and Herbeuval, R.: Pericarditis as the presenting manifestation of acute monoblastic leukemia. Ann. Med. Intern. *131*:302, 1980.
429. Peterson, C. D., Robinson, W. A., and Kurnick, J. E.: Involvement of the heart and pericardium in the malignant lymphomas. Am. J. Med. Sci. *272*:161, 1976.
430. Jakob, H. G., and Zirkin, R. M.: Hodgkin's disease with involvement of the heart and pericardium. J.A.M.A. *73*:82, 1960.
431. Hagans, J. A.: Hodgkin's granuloma with pericardial effusion. Am. Heart J. *40*: 624, 1950.
432. Glancy, D. L., and Roberts, W. C.: The heart in malignant melanoma: A study of 70 autopsy cases. Am. J. Cardiol. *21*:555, 1968.
433. Thomas, D., Dragodanne, C., Frank, R., Prier, A., Chomette, G., and Grosgogeat, Y.: Systemic mastocytosis with myopericardial localization and atrioventricular block. Arch. Mal. Coeur *74*:215, 1981.
434. Arciniegas, E., Hakimi, M., Farooki, Z. Q., and Green, E. W.: Intrapericardial teratoma in infancy. J. Thorac. Cardiovasc. Surg. *79*:306, 1980.
435. Becker, S. N., Reza, M. J., Greenberg, S. H., and Stein, J. J.: Pericardial effusion secondary to mucoepidermoid carcinoma of the parotid gland. A report of an unusual case. Cancer *36*:1080, 1975.
436. Talib, S. H., Chawhan, R. N., Yadov, S. B., Hogade, P. R., and Talib, V. H.: Primary malignant mesothelioma of the pericardium. Indian Heart J. *30*:174, 1978.
437. Harveit, F., Brubakk, O., and Roksted, K.: Pericardial angiomatosis. Acta Med. Scand. *199*:519, 1976.
438. Poole-Wilson, P. A., Farnsworth, A., Braimbridge, M. V., and Pambakian, H.: Angiosarcoma of pericardium. Problems in diagnosis and management. Br. Heart J. *38*:240, 1976.
439. Das, P. B., Fletcher, A. G., and Deodhare, S. G.: Primary mesothelioma of the pericardium. Indian J. Chest Dis. Allied Sci. *18*:262, 1976.
440. Churg, A., Warnock, M. L., Bensch, K. G.: Malignant mesothelioma arising after direct application of asbestos and fiber glass to the pericardium. Am. Rev. Resp. Dis. *118*:419, 1978.
441. Nakayama, R., Yoneyama, T., and Takatani, O.: A study of metastatic tumors to the heart, pericardium, and great vessels. Incidences of metastases to the heart, pericardium and great vessels. Jpn. Heart J. *7*:227, 1966.
442. Kline, J. K.: Cardiac lymphatic involvement by metastatic tumor. Cancer *29*: 799, 1972.
443. Liepman, M. K., and Goodlerner, S.: Surgical management of pericardial tamponade as a presenting manifestation of acute leukemia. J. Surg. Oncol. *17*: 183, 1981.
444. Almagro, V. A., Caya, J. G., and Remeniuk, E.: Cardiac tamponade due to malignant pericardial effusion in breast cancer: A case report. Cancer *49*:1929, 1982.
445. Fraser, R. S., Viloria, J. B., and Wang, N. S.: Cardiac tamponade as a presentation of extracardiac malignancy. Cancer *45*:1697, 1980.
446. Donnelly, M. S., Weinberg, D. S., Skarin, A. T., and Levine, H. D.: Sick sinus syndrome with seroconstrictive pericarditis in malignant lymphoma involving the heart: A case report. Med. Pediat. Oncol. *9*:273, 1981.
447. Elguezabal, A., Farry, J. P., and Depace, N. L.: Massive metastatic cardiac tumor encasement with pericardial constriction. J. Med. Soc. N.J. *77*:820, 1980.
448. Posner, M. R., Cohen, G. I., and Skarin, A. T.: Pericardial disease in patients with cancer. Am. J. Med. *71*:407, 1981.
449. Usher, B. W., and Popp, R. L.: Electrical alternans: Mechanism in pericardial effusion. Am. Heart J. *83*:459, 1972.
450. Chandraratna, P. A. N., and Aronow, W. S.: Detection of pericardial metastases by cross-sectional echocardiography. Circulation *63*:197, 1981.
451. Simpson, A.J.: Malignant pericardial effusion diagnosed by combined ^{67}Ga-citrate and ^{99m}Tc-pertechnetate scintigraphy. Clin. Nucl. Med. *3*:445, 1978.
452. Quaife, M. A., Boschult, P., Baltaxe, H. A., Jr., and Dzindzio, B.: Myocardial accumulation of labelled phosphate in malignant pericardial effusion. J. Nucl. Med. *20*:392, 1979.
453. Comyn, D. J.: Cardiac tamponade with superior vena caval obstruction. S. Afr. Med. J. *54*:750, 1978.
454. Zipf, R. E., Jr., and Johnston, W. W.: The role of cytology in the evaluation of pericardial effusion. Chest *62*:593, 1972.
455. King, D. T., and Nieberg, R. K.: The use of cytology to evaluate pericardial effusions. Ann. Clin. Lab. Sci. *9*:18, 1979.
456. Yazdi, H. M., Hajdu, S. I., and Melamed, M. R.: Cytopathology of pericardial effusions. Acta Cytol. J. *24*:401, 1980.
457. Smith, F. E., Lane, M., and Hudgins, D. T.: Conservative management of malignant pericardial effusion. Cancer *33*:47, 1974.
458. Hirsch, D. M., Nydick, I., and Farrow, I. W.: Malignant pericardial effusion secondary to metastatic breast carcinoma: A case of long-term remission. Cancer *19*:1269, 1966.
459. Theologides, A.: Neoplastic cardiac tamponade. Semin. Oncol. *5*:181, 1978.
460. Flannery, E. P., Gregoratos, G., and Corder, M. P.: Pericardial effusion in patients with malignant diseases. Arch. Intern. Med. *135*:976, 1975.
461. Hankins, J. R., Satterfield, J. R., Aisner, J., Wiernik, P. H., and McLaughlin, J. S.: Pericardial window for malignant pericardial effusion. Ann. Thorac. Surg. *30*:465, 1980.
462. Hill, G. J., and Cohen, B. I.: Pleural pericardial window for palliation of cardiac tamponade due to cancer. Cancer *26*:81, 1970.
463. Davis, S., Sharma, S. M., Blumberg, E. D., and Kim, C. S.: Intrapericardial tetracycline for the management of cardiac tamponade secondary to malignant pericardial effusion. N. Engl. J. Med. *299*:1113, 1978.
464. Weisberger, A. S., Levine, B., and Storaasli, L. P.: Use of nitrogen mustard in treatment of serous effusions of neoplastic origin. J.A.M.A. *159*:1704, 1955.

465. Suhrland, L. G., and Weisberger, A. S.: Intracavitary 5-fluoruracil in malignant effusions. Arch. Intern. Med. *116*:431, 1965.
466. Weisberger, A. S.: Direct instillation of nitrogen mustard in the management of malignant effusions. N. Y. Acad. Sci. *68*:1091, 1958.
467. Terpenning, M., Orringer, M., Wheeler, R.: Intrapericardial nitrogen mustard with catheter drainage for the treatment of malignant effusions. Proc. Am. Assoc. Cancer Res. *20*:286, 1979.
468. Mauch, P. E.: Treatment of malignant pericardial effusions. *In* DeVita, V. T., Hellman, S., and Rosenberg, S. A. (eds.): Cancer. Principles and Practice of Oncology. Philadelphia, J. B. Lippincott Co., pp. 1571–1573.
469. Martini, N., Freiman, A. J., Watson, R. C., and Hilaris, B. S.: Intrapericardial instillation of radioactive chromic phosphate in malignant pericardial effusion. Am. J. Roentgenol. *128*:639, 1977.
470. O'Bryan, R. M., Talley, R. W., and Brennan, M. J.: Critical analysis of the control of malignant effusions with radioisotopes. Henry Ford Hosp. Med. J. *16*:3, 1968.
471. Clarke, T. H.: Radioactive colloidal gold Au^{198} in the treatment of neoplastic effusion. Northwest Med. Sch. Quart. Bull. *26*:98, 1952.
472. Bian, S., Brufman, G., Klein, E., and Hochman, A.: The management of pericardial effusion in cancer patients. Chest *71*:182, 1977.
473. Terry, L. N., and Kligerman, M. M.: Pericardial and myocardial involvement in lymphomas and leukemias—the role of radiotherapy. Cancer *25*:1003, 1970.
474. Cham, W. C., Freiman, A. H., and Carstens, P. H. B.: Radiation therapy of cardiac and pericardial metastases. Ther. Radiol. *114*:701, 1975.
475. Lokich, J. J.: The management of malignant pericardial effusion J.A.M.A. *224*: 1401, 1973.
476. Steward, J. R., Cohn, K. E., and Fajardo, L. F.: Radiation-induced heart diesease: A study of twenty-five patients. Radiology *89*:302, 1967.
477. Martin, R. G., Ruckdeschel, J. C., Chang, P., Byhardt, R., Bouchard, R. J., and Wiernik, P. H.: Radiation-related pericarditis. Am. J. Cardiol. *35*:216, 1975.
478. Cohn, K. E., Stewart, J. R., Fajardo, L. F., and Hancock, E. W.: Heart disease following radiation. Medicine *46*:281, 1967.
479. Muggia, F. M., and Cassileth, P. A.: Constrictive pericarditis following radiation therapy. Am. J. Med. *44*:116, 1968.
480. Masland, D. S., Rotz, C. T., Jr., and Harris, J. H.: Post-radiation pericarditis with chronic pericardial effusion. Ann. Intern. Med. *68*:97, 1968.
481. Ruckdeschel, J. C., Chang, P., Martin, R. G., Byhardt, R. W., O'Connell, M. J., Sutherland, J. C., and Wiernik, P. J.: Radiation-related pericardial effusions in patients with Hodgkin's disease. Medicine *54*:245, 1975.
482. DiMatteo, J., Vacheron, A., Heulin, A., Meeus, L., DiMatteo, G., Gilles, R., DeLage, F., and de Ratuld, A.: Cardiac complications of thoracic radiotherapy. Arch. Mal. Coeur. *71*:447, 1978.
483. Scott, D. L., and Thomas, R. D.: Late onset constrictive pericarditis after thoracic radiotherapy. Br. Med. J. *1*:341, 1978.
484. Applefeld, M. M., Slawson, R. G., Hall-Craigs, M., Green, D. C., Singleton, R. T., and Wiernik, P. H.: Delayed pericardial disease after radiotherapy. Am. J. Cardiol. *47*:210, 1981.
485. Haas, J.: Symptomatic constrictive pericarditis developing 45 years after radiation therapy to the mediastinum. Am. Heart J. *77*:89, 1969.
486. Carmel, R. J., and Kaplan, H. S.: Mantle irradiation in Hodgkin's disease. Cancer *37*:2813, 1976.
487. Fajardo, L. F., Stewart, J. R., and Cohn, K. E.: Morphology of radiation-induced heart disease. Arch. Pathol. *86*:512, 1968.
488. Glicksman, A. S., and Nickson, J. J.: Acute and late reactions to irradiation in the treatment of Hodgkin's disease. Arch. Intern. Med. *131*:369, 1973.
489. Greenwood, R. D., Rosenthal, A., Cassedy, R., Jaffe, N., and Nadas, A. S.: Constrictive pericarditis in childhood due to mediastinal irradiation. Circulation *50*:1033, 1974.
490. Brosius, F. C., Waller, B. F., and Roberts, W. C.: Radiation heart disease. Am. J. Med. *70*:519, 1981.
491. Steinberg, I.: Effusive-constrictive pericarditis: Two cases illustrating value of angiocardiography in diagnosis. Am. J. Cardiol. *19*:434, 1976.
492. Stroobandt, R., Knieriem, H. J., DeWolf, L., and Joosens, J. V.: Radiation-induced heart disease. Acta Cardiol. *30*:383, 1975.
493. Biran, S.: Corticosteroids in radiation-induced pericarditis. Chest *74*:96, 1978.
494. Keelan, M. H., and Rudders, R. A.: Successful treatment of radiation pericarditis with corticosteroids. Arch. Intern. Med. *134*:145, 1974.
495. Castellino, R. A., Gladstein, E., and Turbow, M. M.: Latent radiation injury of lungs or heart activated by steroid withdrawal. Ann. Intern. Med. *80*:593, 1974.
496. Morton, D. L., Kagan, A. R., Roberts, W. C., O'Brien, K. P., Holmes, E. C., and Adkins, P. C.: Pericardiectomy for radiation-induced pericarditis with effusion. Ann. Thorac. Surg. *8*:195, 1969.
497. Applefeld, M. M., Cole, J. F., Pollock, S. H., Sutton, F. J., Slawson, R. G., Singleton, R. T., and Wiernik, P. H.: The late appearance of chronic pericardial disease in patients treated by radiotherapy for Hodgkin's disease. Ann. Intern. Med. *94*:338, 1981.
498. Osler, W.: The Principles and Practice of Medicine. New York, D. Appleton and Company, 1892, p. 273.
499. Przybojewski, J. Z.: Rheumatic constrictive pericarditis. A case report and review of the literature. S. Afr. Med. J. *59*:682, 1981.
500. Bulkley, B. H., and Roberts, W. C.: The heart in systemic lupus erythematosus and the changes induced in it by corticosteroid therapy. Am. J. Med. *58*:243, 1975.
501. Cohen, A. S., and Canoso, J. J.: Pericarditis in the rheumatologic diseases. *In* Spodick, D. H. (ed.): Pericardial Diseases. Philadelphia, F. A. Davis Co., 1976, pp. 237–255.
502. Cohen, A. S., and Canoso, J. J.: Pericarditis in the rheumatologic diseases. Cardiovasc. Clin. *1*:237, 1976.
503. Kinney, E., Wynn, J., Hinton, D. M., Demers, S. L., O'Neill, M., Parr, G., Ward, S., and Zelis, R.: Pericardial-fluid complement. Normal values. Am. J. Clin. Pathol. *72*:972, 1979.
504. Quismorio, J. P., Jr.: Immune complexes in pericardial fluid in systemic lupus erythematosus. Arch. Intern. Med. *140*:112, 1980.
505. Jacobsen, E. J., and Reza, M. J.: Constrictive pericarditis in systemic lupus erythematosus. Demonstration of immunoglobulins in the pericardium. Arthritis Rheum. *21*:972, 1978.
506. Starkey, R. H., and Hahn, B. H.: Rapid development of constrictive pericarditis in a patient with systemic lupus erythematosus. Chest *63*:448, 1973.
507. Libman, E., and Sacks, B.: A hitherto undescribed form of valvular and mural endocarditis. Arch. Intern. Med. *33*:701, 1924.
508. Perlroth, M. G.: Connective tissue disease and the heart. J.A.M.A. *231*:410, 1975.
509. Homcy, C. J., Liberthson, R. R., Fallon, J. T., Gross, S., and Miller, L. M.: Ischemic heart disease in systemic lupus erythematosus in the young patient: Report of six cases. Am. J. Cardiol. *49*:478, 1982.
510. Collins, R. L., Turner, R. A., Nomeir, A. M., Hunt, R., Johnson, A. M., McLean, R. L., and Watts, L. E.: Cardiopulmonary manifestations of systemic lupus erythematosus. J. Rheumatol. *5*:299, 1978.
511. Charcot, J. M.: Clinical lecture on senile and chronic diseases. London, Sydenham Society, 1981, pp. 172–175.
512. Thadani, U., Iveson, J. M., and Wright, V.: Cardiac tamponade, constrictive pericarditis and pericardial resection in rheumatoid arthritis. Medicine *54*:261, 1975.
513. Gordon, D. A., Stein, J. N., and Broder, I.: Extra-articular features of rheumatoid arthritis: A systemic analysis of 127 cases. Am. J. Med. *54*:445, 1973.
514. Lebowitz, W. B.: The heart in rheumatoid arthritis (rheumatoid disease). A clinical and pathologic study of 22 cases. Ann. Intern. Med. *58*:102, 1963.
515. Kirk, J., and Cosh, J.: The pericarditis of rheumatoid arthritis. Quart. J. Med. *38*:397, 1969.
516. John, J. T., Jr., Hough, A., and Sergent, J. S.: Pericardial disease in rheumatoid arthritis. Am. J. Med. *66*:385, 1979.
517. Burney, D. P., Martin, C. E., Thomas, C. S., Fisher, R. D., and Bender, H. W., Jr.: Rheumatoid pericarditis. Clinical significance and operative management. J. Thorac. Cardiovasc. Surg. *77*:511, 1979.
518. Majeed, H. A., and Kvasnicka, J.: Juvenile rheumatoid arthritis with cardiac tamponade. Ann. Rheum. Dis. *37*:273, 1978.
519. Vukman, R. B., and Fay, G. J.: Juvenile rheumatoid arthritis with pericardial tamponade in an adult. Arch. Intern. Med. *141*:1078, 1981.
520. Yousefadeh, D. K., and Fishman, P. A.: The triad of pneumonitis, pleuritis, and pericarditis in juvenile rheumatoid arthritis. Pediat. Radiol. *8*:147, 1979.
521. Franco, A. E., Levine, H. D., and Hall, A. P.: Rheumatoid pericarditis. Ann. Intern. Med. *77*:837, 1972.
522. Parkash, R., Atassi, A., Poske, R., and Rosen, K. M.: Prevalence of pericardial effusion and mitral valve involvement in patients with rheumatoid arthritis without cardiac symptoms. N. Engl. J. Med. *289*:597, 1973.
523. Nomeir, A., Turner, R., and Watts, E.: Cardiac involvement in rheumatoid arthritis. Ann. Intern. Med. *79*:800, 1973.
524. Yancey, C. L., Doughty, R. A., Cohlan, B. A., and Athreya, B. H.: Pericarditis and cardiac tamponade in juvenile rheumatoid arthritis. Pediatrics *68*:369, 1981.
525. Mathew, P. K.: Pericardial tamponade secondary to sudden steroid withdrawal in chronic rheumatoid arthritis. Chest *75*:532, 1977.
526. Keith, T. A.: Chronic constrictive pericarditis in association with rheumatoid disease. Circulation *25*:477, 1962.
527. Kennedy, W. P. U, Partridge, R. E. H., and Matthews, M. B.: Rheumatoid pericarditis with cardiac failure treated by pericardiectomy. Br. Heart J. *28*: 602, 1966.
528. Nassar, W. K., Miskin, M. E., and Rosenbaum, D.: Pericardial and myocardial disease in progressive systemic sclerosis. Am. J. Cardiol. *22*:538, 1968.
529. McWhorter, J. E., and LeRoy, E. C.: Pericardial disease in scleroderma (systemic sclerosis). Am. J. Med. *57*:566, 1974.
530. Bulkley, B. H., Rjdolfi, R. T., Salyer, W. R., and Hutchins, G. M.: Myocardial lesions of progressive systemic sclerosis. Circulation *53*:483, 1976.
531. Smith, J. W., Clements, P. J., Levisman, J., Furst, D., and Foss, M.: Echocardiographic features of progressive systemic sclerosis. Am. J. Med. *66*: 28, 1979.
532. Uhl, G. S., and Kippes, G. M.: Pericardial tamponade in systemic sclerosis (schleroderma). Br. Heart J. *42*:345, 1979.
533. Medsger, T. A., Jr., Masi, A. T., and Rodnan, G. P.: Survival with systemic sclerosis (scleroderma). A life-table analysis of clinical and demographic factors in 309 patients. Ann. Intern. Med. *75*:369, 1971.
534. Csonka, G. W., and Oates, J. K.: Pericarditis and electrocardiographic changes in Reiter's syndrome. Br. Med. J. *1*:866, 1957.
535. Goldman, M. J., and Lau, F. Y. K.: Acute pericarditis associated with serum sickness. N. Engl. J. Med. *250*:278, 1954.
536. Shapiro, L., and Buckingham, R. B.: Septic rheumatoid pericarditis complicating Felty's syndrome. Arthritis Rheum. *24*:1435, 1981.
537. Dupond, J. L., and Leconte-des-Floris, R.: Temporal arteritis manifested as an acute febrile pericarditis. J.A.M.A. *247*:2371, 1982.

538. Dawes, P. T., and Atherton, S. T.: Coeliac disease presenting as recurrent pericarditis. Lancet *1*:1021, 1981.
539. Thompson, D. C., Lennard-Jones, J. E., Swarbrick, E. T., and Bown, R.: Pericarditis and inflammatory bowel disease. Quart. J. Med. *48*:93, 1979.
540. Becker, S. A., Wishnitzler, R., Botwin, S., Eliraz, A., and Bass, D. D.: Myopericarditis associated with inflammatory bowel disease. J. Clin. Gastroenterol. *3*:267, 1981.
541. Laane, B. F.: Infantile polyarteritis nodosa or mucocutaneous lymph node syndrome (Kawasaki disease). Arterities associated with aneurysm, thromboses and rupture of the coronary artery with cardiac tamponade. Tisddkr. Nor. Laegeforen. *101*:1583, 1981.
542. Desablens, B., Lesbre, J. P., Wattebled, R., Herve, M. A., Schurtz, C., DeLobel, J., and Messerschmitt, J.: Adult Still's disease with constrictive pericarditis. Sjögren's syndrome, and varied leucocytic abnormalities. Semin. Hop. Paris *56*:1163, 1980.
543. Vlietstra, R. E., Lie, J. T., Kuhl, W. E., Danielson, G. K., and Roberts, M. K.: Whipple's disease involving the pericardium: Pathologic confirmation during life. Aust. N. Z. J. Med. *8*:649, 1978.
544. Alarçon-Segovia, D.: Drug-induced lupus syndromes. Mayo Clin. Proc. *44*: 664, 1969.
545. Stein, H. B., Dodek, A., Lawson, L., and Rae, A.: Procainamide-induced lupus erythematosus: Report of a case with a large pericardial effusion and fluid analysis. J. Rheumatol. *6*:543, 1979.
546. Goldberg, M. J., Husain, M., Wajszczuk, W. J., and Rubenfire, M.: Procainamide-induced lupus erythematosus pericarditis encountered during coronary artery bypass surgery. Am. J. Med. *69*:159, 1980.
547. Carey, R. M., Coleman, M., and Feder, A.: Pericardial tamponade: A major manifestation of hydralazine-induced lupus syndrome. Am. J. Med. *54*:84, 1973.
548. Harrington, T. M., and Davis, D. E.: Systemic lupus-like syndrome induced by methyldopa therapy. Chest *79*:696, 1981.
549. Slater, E. E.: Cardiac tamponade and peripheral eosinophilia in a patient receiving cromolyn sodium. Chest *73*:878, 1978.
550. Yates, R. C., and Olson, K. B.: Drug-induced pericarditis. Report of three cases due to 6-amino-9-D-psicofuranosylpurine. N. Engl. J. Med. *265*:274, 1961.
551. Bennett, W. M.: Pericardial effusions associated with minoxidil. Lancet *2*:1356, 1977.
552. Houston, M. C., McChesney, J. A., and Chatterjee, K.: Pericardial effusion associated with minoxidil therapy. Arch. Intern. Med. *141*:69, 1981.
553. Petusevsky, M. L., Faling, L. J., Rocklin, R. E., Snider, G. L., Merliss, A. D., Moses, J. M., and Dorman, S. A.: Pleuropericardial reaction to treatment with Dantrolene. J.A.M.A. *242*:2772, 1979.
554. Meeran, M. K., Ahmed, A. H., Parsons, F. M., and Anderson, C. K.: Constrictive pericarditis due to methysergide therapy. S. Afr. Med. J. *50*:1595, 1976.
555. Bristow, M. R., Thompson, P. D., Martin, R. P., Mason, J. W., Billingham, M. E., Harrison, D. C.: Early anthracycline toxicity. Am. J. Med. *65*:823, 1978.
556. Dressler, W.: A postmyocardial infarction syndrome. Preliminary report of a complication resembling idiopathic recurrent benign pericarditis. J.A.M.A. *160*: 1379, 1956.
557. Dressler, W.: The post-myocardial infarction syndrome. A report of forty-four cases. Arch. Intern. Med. *103*:28, 1959.
558. Lichstein, E., Arsura, E., Hollander, G., Greengart, A., and Sanders, M.: Current incidence of post-myocardial infarction (Dressler's) syndrome. Am. J. Cardiol. *50*:1269, 1982.
559. Davies, A. M., and Gery, I.: The role of autoantibodies in heart disease. Am. Heart J. *60*:669, 1960.
560. Van der Geld, H.: Anti-heart antibodies in the post-pericardiotomy and the post-myocardial infarction syndrome. Lancet *2*:617, 1964.
561. Liem, K. L., ten Veen, J. H., Lie, K. I., Feltkamp, T. E. W., and Durrer, D.: Incidence and significance of heart muscle antibodies in patients with acute myocardial infarction and unstable angina. Acta Med. Scand. *206*:473, 1971.
562. Weiser, N. J., Kantor, M., and Russell, H. K.: Post-myocardial infarction syndrome. Circulation *20*:371, 1959.
563. Gibbons, J. A., and Vieweg, W. V.: Dressler's syndrome and angina pectoris relieved by surgery. Chest *77*:431, 1980.
564. Blau, N., Shen, B., and Pittman, D. E.: Massive hemopericardium in a patient with postmyocardial infarction syndrome. Chest *71*:4, 1977.
565. Goldhaber, S. Z., Lorell, B. H., and Green, L. H.: Constrictive pericarditis. A case requiring pericardiectomy following Dressler's postmyocardial infarction syndrome. J. Thorac. Cardiovasc. Surg. *81*:793, 1981.
566. Haiat, R., Desoutter, P., Stolitz, J. P., Chousterman, M., Cattan, P., and Gandjbakhch, I.: Constrictive pericarditis secondary to myocardial infarction. Arch. Mal. Coeur *74*:1349, 1981.
567. Soloff, L. A., Zatuchni, J., Janton, D. H., O'Neill, T. J. E., and Glover, R. P.: Reactivation of rheumatic fever following mitral commisurotomy. Circulation *8*:481, 1953.
568. Engle, M. A., and Ito, T.: The postpericardiotomy syndrome. Am. J. Cardiol. *7*:73, 1961.
569. Peters, R. W., Scheinman, M. M., Raskin, S., and Thomas, A. N.: Unusual complications of epicardial pacemakers. Am. J. Cardiol. *45*:1088, 1980.
570. Engle, M. A., Klein, A. A., Hepner, S., and Enlers, K. H.: The postpericardiotomy and similar syndromes. Cardiovasc. Clin. *7*:211, 1976.
571. Livelli, F. D., Jr., Johnson, R. A., McEnany, M. T., Sherman, E., Newell, J., Block, P. C., and DeSanctis, R. W.: Unexplained in-hospital fever following cardiac surgery: Natural history, relationship to postpericardiotomy syndrome and a prospective study of therapy with indomethacin versus placebo. Circulation *57*:968, 1978.
572. Engle, M. A., Gay, W. A., Jr., Kaminsky, M. E., Zabriskie, J. B., and Senterfit, L. B.: Postpericardiotomy syndrome then and now. Curr. Probl. Cardiol. *3*:1, 1978.
573. Kaminsky, M. E., Rodan, B. A., Osborne, D. R., Chen, J. T. T., Sealy, W. C., and Putman, C. E.: Postpericardiotomy syndrome. Am. J. Radiol. *138*:503, 1982.
574. DeSaulniers, D., Gervais, N., and Rouleau, J.: Does pericardial drainage decrease the frequency of the postpericardiotomy syndrome? Canad. J. Surg. *24*: 265, 1981.
575. Engle, M. A., Ehlers, K. H., O'Loughlin, J. E., Jr., Linday, L. A., and Fried, R.: The postpericardiotomy syndrome: Iatrogenic illness with immunologic and virologic components. *In* Engle, M. A. (ed.): Pediatric Cardiovascular Disease. Cardiovasc. Clin. 1981, pp. 381–391.
576. Ofori-Krakye, S. K., Tyberg, T. I., Geha, A. S., Hammond, G. L., Cohen, L. S., and Langou, R. A.: Late cardiac tamponade after open heart surgery: Incidence, role of anticoagulants in its pathogenesis and its relationship to the postpericardiotomy syndrome. Circulation *63*:1323, 1981.
577. Ikaheimo, M., and Takkunen, J.: Postpericardiotomy syndrome diagnosed by echocardiography. Scand. J. Thorac. Cardiovasc. Surg. *13*:305, 1979.
578. Wheeler, E. O., Turner, J. D., and Scannell, J. G.: Fever, splenomegaly, and atypical lymphocytes. A syndrome observed after cardiac surgery utilizing a pump oxygenator. N. Engl. J. Med. *266*:454, 1962.
579. Berger, R. L., Loveless, G., and Warner, O.: Delayed and latent postcardiotomy tamponade: Recognition and nonoperative treatment. Ann. Thorac. Surg. *12*:22, 1971.
580. McCabe, J. C., Engle, M. A., and Ebert, P. A.: Chronic pericardial effusion requiring pericardiectomy in the postpericardiotomy syndrome. J. Thorac. Cardiovasc. Surg. *67*:814, 1974.
581. King, T. E., Jr., Stelzner, T. J., and Sahn, S. A.: Cardiac tamponade complicating the postpericardiotomy syndrome. Chest *83*:500, 1983.
582. Herzog, D. B., Gilberg, E. M., and Levy, J. M.: Pericardial window complicated by acute congestive heart failure in a patient with chronic pericardial effusion. Pediatrics *57*:967, 1976.
583. Rice, E. P. L., Pifarre, R., and Montoya, A.: Constrictive pericarditis following cardiac surgery. Ann. Thorac. Surg. *31*:450, 1981.
584. Dane, T. E. B., and King, E. B.: Fatal cardiac tamponade and other mechanical complications of central venous catheters. Br. J. Surg. *62*:6, 1975.
585. Foster, C. J., Constrictive pericarditis complicating an endocardial pacemaker. Br. Heart J. *47*:497, 1982.
586. Schwartz, D. J., Thanavaro, S., Kleiger, R. E., Krone, R. J., Connors, J. P., and Oliver, G. C.: Epicardial pacemaker complicated by cardiac tamponade and constrictive pericarditis. Chest *76*:226, 1979.
587. Lindenau, K. F., Warnke, H., and Bergmann, U.: Cardiac tamponade following open heart surgery. Zentralbl. Chir. *104*:1345, 1979.
588. Jones, M. R., Vine, D. L., Attas, M., and Todd, E. P.: Late isolated left ventricular tamponade. J. Thorac. Cardiovasc. Surg. *77*:142, 1979.
589. Marx, P., Jaffe, C., Laks, H., and Wolfson, S.: Delayed post–cardiac-surgery tamponade producing localized right atrial compression. Cath. Cardiovasc. Diag. *7*:275, 1981.
590. Kanakis, C., Sheikh, A. I., and Rosen, K. M.: Constrictive pericardial disease following mitral valve replacement. Chest *79*:593, 1981.
591. Little, W. C., Primm, R. K., Karp, R. B., and Hood, W. P., Jr.: Clotted hemopericardium with the hemodynamic characteristics of constrictive pericarditis. Am. J. Cardiol. *45*:386, 1980.
592. Marsa, R., Mehta, S., Willis, N., and Bailey, L.: Constrictive pericarditis after myocardial revascularization: Report of three cases. Am. J. Cardiol. *44*:177, 1979.
593. Cohen, M. V., and Greenberg, M. A.: Constrictive pericarditis: Early and late complication of cardiac surgery. Am. J. Cardiol. *43*:657, 1979.
594. Brown, D. F., and Older, T.: Pericardial constriction as a late complication of coronary bypass surgery. J. Thorac. Cardiovasc. Surg. *74*:61, 1977.
595. Kutcher, M. A., King, S. B., Alimurung, B. N., Craver, J. M., and Logue, R. B.: Constrictive pericarditis as a complication of cardiac surgery: Recognition of an entity. Am. J. Cardiol. *50*:742, 1982.
596. Kerber, R. E., and Sherman, B.: Echocardiographic evaluation of pericardial effusion in myxedema. Incidence and biochemical and clinical correlations. Circulation *52*:823, 1975.
597. Kern, R. A., Soloff, L. A., Snope, W. J., and Bello, C. T.: Pericardial effusion: A constant, early, and major factor in the cardiac syndrome of hypothyroidism (myxedema heart). Am. J. Med. Sci. *217*:609, 1949.
598. Kurtzman, R. S., Chepey, J. J., and Otto, D. L.: Myxedema heart disease. Radiology *84*:624, 1965.
599. Hardisty, C. A., Naik, D. R., and Munro, D. S.: Pericardial effusion in hypothyroidism. Clin. Endocrinol. *13*:349, 1980.
600. Parving, H., Hansen, J. M., Nielsen, S. V., Rossing, N., Munck, O., and Lassen, N. A.: Mechanisms of edema formation in myxedema-increased protein extravasation and relatively slow lymphatic drainage. N. Engl. J. Med. *301*:460, 1981.
601. Davis, P. J., and Jacobson, S.: Myxedema with cardiac tamponade and pericardial effusion of "gold paint" appearance. Arch. Intern. Med. *120*:615, 1967.

602. Sharma, S. K., and Bordia, A.: Cardiac tamponade due to pericardial effusion in myxedema. Indian Heart J. *21*:210, 1969.
603. Das, S., Lieberman, A. N., and Schussler, G. C.: Prolonged persistence of a large pericardial effusion and hemodynamic evidence of cardiac tamponade during treatment of myxedema. Clin. Cardiol. *5*:459, 1982.
604. Singh, A., and Krishan, I.: Cardiac tamponade due to massive pericardial effusion in myxedema. Br. J. Med. Prac. *24*:347, 1970.
605. Spitzer, S., Adam, A., and Mason, D.: Myxedema complicated by pericardial tamponade. Penn. Med. *73*:33, 1970.
606. Brawley, R. K., Vasko, J. S., and Marrow, A. G.: Cholesterol pericarditis. Considerations of its pathogenesis and treatment. Am. J. Med. *41*:235, 1966.
607. Rosenbau, D. L., and Yu, P. N.: Idiopathic cholesterol pericarditis with effusion. Am. Heart J. *70*:515, 1965.
608. Ridenhouse, C. E., and Kiphart, R. J.: Idiopathic cholesterol pericarditis treated with pericardiectomy. Ann. Thorac. Surg. *4*:360, 1967.
609. Stanley, R. J., Subramanian, R., and Lie, J. T.: Cholesterol pericarditis terminating as constrictive calcific pericarditis. Follow-up study of patient with 40-year history of disease. Am. J. Cardiol. *46*:511, 1980.
610. Dunn, R. P.: Primary chylopericardium: A review of the literature and an illustrated case. Am. Heart J. *89*:369, 1975.
611. Pollard, W. M., Schuchmann, G. F., and Bowen, T. E.: Isolated chylopericardium after cardiac operations. J. Thorac. Cardiovasc. Surg. *81*:943, 1981.
612. Rankin, R. N., Raval, B., and Finley, R.: Primary chylopericardium: Combined lymphangiographic and CT diagnosis. J. Comput. Assist. Tomog. *4*: 869, 1980.
613. Shahian, D. M., and Kittle, C. F.: Successful management of esophagopericardial fistula complicating esophagogastrectomy. J. Thorac. Cardiovasc. Surg. *82*:83, 1981.
614. Hardy, G. J., Nicholson, D. M., Murphy, D. A., Johnstone, D. E., and Marrie, T. J.: Polymicrobial purulent pericarditis. Canad. J. Surg. *24*:80, 1981.
615. Mitchell, C. E.: Relapsing pancreatitis with recurrent pericardial and pleural effusions. Ann. Intern. Med. *60*:1047, 1964.
616. Davidson, E. D., Horney, J. T., and Salter, P. P.: Internal pancreatic fistula to the pericardium and pleura. Surgery *85*:478, 1979.
617. Withrington, R., and Collins, P.: Cardiac tamponade in acute pancreatitis. Thorax *35*:959, 1980.
618. King, J. B., and Sapsford, R. N.: Acute rupture of the pericardium with delayed dislocation of the heart: A case report. Injury 9:303, 1978.
619. Christides, C., Laskar, M., Kim, M., Grousseau-Renaudie, D., and Pouget, X.: Post-traumatic rupture of the pericardium with cardiac luxation associated with myocardial infarction and a rupture of the aortic isthmus. J. Chir. *118*: 505, 1981.
620. Meng, R. L., Straus, A., Milloy, F., Kittle, C. F., and Langston, H.: Intrapericardial diaphragmatic hernia in adults. Ann. Surg. *189*:359, 1979.
621. Larrieu, A. J., Weiner, I., Alexander, R., and Wolma, F. J.: Pericardiodiaphragmatic hernia. Am. J. Surg. *139*:436, 1980.
622. Hasse, J., Perruchoud, A., Wolff, G., and Gradel, E.: Right-to-left atrial shunt in cardiac dislocation following extensive pneumonectomy. Thorac. Cardiovasc. Surg. *27*:330, 1979.
623. Rodgers, B. M., Moulder, P. V., and Delaney, A.: Thoracoscopy: New method of early diagnosis of cardiac herniation. J. Thorac. Cardiovasc. Surg. *78*:623, 1979.
624. Schuhfried, G.: Pneumopericardium in newborns during artificial ventilation. Paediat. Paedol. *14*:135, 1979.
625. Semler, H. J., Brandenburg, R. O., and Kirklin, J. W.: Pericardial disease complicating congenital heart lesions. Ann. Intern. Med. *53*:494, 1960.
626. Yahini, J. H., Goor, D., Kraus, Y., Pauzner, Y. H. M., and Neufeld, H. N.: Atrial septal defect and constrictive pericarditis. Am. J. Cardiol. *17*:718, 1966.
627. Engle, M. A.: Cardiac involvement in Cooley's anemia. Ann. N.Y. Acad. Sci. *119*:694, 1964.
628. Zemer, D., Cabili, S., Revach, M., and Shahin, N.: Constrictive pericarditis in familial Mediterranean fever. Israel J. Med. Sci. *13*:55, 1977.
629. Frenkenfeld, R. H., Waters, C. H., and Steiner, R. C.: Bilateral myxomas of the heart. Ann. Intern. Med. *53*:827, 1960.
630. Pierce, R. N., and Walker-Smith, G. J.: Intrathoracic manifestations of Dego's disease (malignant atrophic papulosis). Chest *73*:79, 1978.
631. Paulley, J. W., Barlow, K. E., and Cutting, P. E. J.: Acute gouty pericarditis. Lancet *1*:21, 1963.
632. Abdun Nur, D., Marcus, C. S., and Russell, F. E.: Pericarditis associated with scorpionfish (*Scorpaena buttata*) sting. Toxicon *19*:579, 1981.
633. Feigin, D. S., Fenoglio, J. J., McAllister, H. A., and Madewell, J. E.: Pericardial cysts: A radiologic-pathologic correlation and review. Radiology *125*:15, 1977.
634. Maier, H. C.: Diverticulum of the pericardium: With observations on mode of development. Circulation *16*:1040, 1957.
635. Mabille, J. P., Pignon, L., Trigalou, D., and Viard, H.: Twisted pedunculated pleuro-pericardial cyst. J. Radiol. (Fr.) *61*:177, 1980.
636. Rogers, C. I., Seymour, E. Q., and Brock, J. G.: Atypical pericardial cyst location: The value of computed tomography. J. Comput. Assist. Tomog. *4*:683, 1980.
637. Klatte, E. C., and Yune, H. Y.: Diagnosis and treatment of pericardial cysts. Radiology *104*:541, 1972.
638. Unverferth, D. V., and Wooley, C. F.: The differential diagnosis of paracardiac lesions: Pericardial cysts. Cath. Cardiovasc. Diag. *5*:31, 1979.
639. Ellis, K., Leeds, N. E., and Himmelstein, A.: Congenital deficiencies in partial pericardium: Review of two new cases including successful diagnosis by plain roentgenography. Am. J. Roentgenol. *82*:125, 1959.
640. Glover, L. B., Barcia, A., and Reeves, T. J.: Congenital absence of the pericardium. Am. J. Roentgenol. *106*:542, 1969.
641. Nasser, W. K.: Congenital absence of the left pericardium. Am. J. Cardiol. *26*: 466, 1970.
642. Bor, I., and Kafke, V.: Aplasia of pericardium. J. Cardiovasc. Surg. *2*:389, 1961.
643. Morgan, J. R., Rogers, A. K., and Forker, A. D.: Congenital absence of the left pericardium. Ann. Intern. Med. *74*:370, 1971.
644. Pisano, D., Angeloni, J., Goldberg, H., and Nakhjavan, F. K.: Congenital absence of the pericardium: Report of a case. J. A.O.A. *80*:407, 1981.
645. Pocock, W. A., Lakier, J. B., and Benjamin, J. D.: Billowing mitral valve syndrome in association with absent left pericardium. S. Afr. Med. J. *52*:813, 1977.
646. Reginao, E., Speroni, F., Riccardi, M., Verunelli, F., and Eufrate, S.: Post-traumatic mitral regurgitation and ventricular septal defect in absence of left pericardium. Thorac. Cardiovasc. Surg. *28*:213, 1980.
647. Inoue, H., Fujii, J., Mashima, S., and Marao, S.: Pseudo right atrial overloading pattern in complete defect of the left pericardium. J. Electrocardiol. *14*:413, 1981.
648. Payvandi, M. N., and Kerber, R. E.: Echocardiography in congenital and acquired absence of the pericardium. An echocardiographic mimic of right ventricular volume overload. Circulation *53*:86, 1976.
649. Nicolosi, G. L., Borgioni, L., Alberti, E., Burelli, C., Maffesanti, M., Marino, P., Slavich, G., and Zanuttini, D.: M-mode and two-dimensional echocardiography in congenital absence of the pericardium. Chest *81*:610, 1982.
650. D'Altoria, R. A., and Caro, J. Y.: Congenital absence of the left pericardium detected by imaging of the lung: Case report. J. Nucl. Med. *18*:267, 1977.
651. Baim, R. S., MacDonald, I. L., Wise, D. J., and Lenkei, S. C.: Computed tomography of absent pericardium. Radiology *135*:127, 1980.
652. Saito, R., and Hotta, F.: Congenital pericardial defect associated with cardiac incarceration: Case report. Am. Heart J. *100*:866, 1980.
653. Rogge, J. D., Mishkin, M. E., and Genovese, P. D.: Congenital partial pericardial defect with herniation of the left atrial appendage. Ann. Intern. Med. *64*: 137, 1966.
654. Minocha, G. K., Falicov, R. E., and Nijensohn, E.: Partial right-sided congenital pericardial defect with herniation of the right atrium and right ventricle. Chest *76*:484, 1979.
655. Moene, R. J., Dekker, A., and van der Harten, H. J.: Congenital right-sided pericardial defect with herniation of part of the lung into the pericardial cavity. Am. J. Cardiol. *31*:519, 1973.

44 TRAUMATIC HEART DISEASE

by Peter F. Cohn, M.D., and Eugene Braunwald, M.D.

THE PROBLEM IN PERSPECTIVE

Unfortunately, traumatic heart disease is often regarded as an uncommon and even esoteric form of heart disease of interest primarily to physicians in the military service. That this is not the case is attested to by the statistics—violent injury accounts for the majority of deaths in persons under 40 years of age,[1] and among these victims cardiac trauma is one of the leading causes of death.[2,3] In recent years, reports of increasing traumatic heart disease in civilians may be attributed to the accelerating mechanization of contemporary life—whether on the farm, in the home, in industry, or on the roads. For example, it has been estimated that almost 20 per cent of over five million instances of bodily injury of at least moderate severity resulting from auto accidents are associated with cardiac trauma.[4] The increasing frequency of physical violence has resulted in a corresponding increase in the incidence of traumatic heart disease. Although all age groups and both sexes are susceptible to traumatic heart disease, *young adult males* are the most frequent victims, since they are more likely to have automobile and motorcycle accidents, incur injuries while performing heavy labor, and be involved in acts of physical violence.

There is, regrettably, no evidence that the frequency of these mishaps is declining or even approaching a plateau. At Boston City Hospital, for example, the annual incidence of penetrating wounds of the heart rose from 2.8 cases during the period from 1956 through 1964 to 8.0 cases from 1965 through 1976.[5] In addition, the incidence of medically related cardiac trauma is also rising, such as increased use of intravascular and intracardiac catheters leading to penetrating injuries of the heart and great vessels, and resuscitative cardiac massage causing a variety of nonpenetrating injuries of these organs.

The two principal, immediate consequences of cardiac injury are *exsanguinating hemorrhage* and *cardiac tamponade.* Effective treatment has resulted in an increasing number of immediate survivors, and later sequelae, including myocardial infarction, aneurysm, pseudoaneurysm, ventricular septal defect, valvular damage, recurrent pericarditis, and constrictive pericarditis, are becoming far more common. Serious cardiac trauma is frequently overlooked in patients with nonpenetrating injury, particularly when other structures such as the thoracic cage and lungs are obviously damaged. Such oversight can be tragic, because the lethal consequences of cardiac injury may suddenly emerge after the more superficial injuries have been attended to. Clearly, a much higher index of suspicion of this possibility is necessary if the increasing magnitude of this problem is to be halted and reversed.

NONPENETRATING CARDIAC INJURY

Nonpenetrating injuries result from the effects of external physical forces, but it is important to recognize that these forces need not be applied directly to the chest, since injuries to the heart and great vessels may also occur with trauma to other parts of the body. Parmley et al. have summarized the mechanisms of nonpenetrating injuries to the heart as follows: (1) direct force against the chest; (2) bidirectional force against the thorax; (3) indirect forces resulting in a marked increase in intravascular pressure, as from sudden compression in the abdomen and lower extremities; (4) decelerative forces; (5) blast forces; (6) concussive forces; and (7) combinations of the above.[6]

The most common cause of nonpenetrating injury in civilian life is probably that directly related to vehicular impact, either by direct compression, usually with the steering wheel squeezing the heart between the sternum and the spine, or by indirect compression.[7,8] Causes of nonpenetrating injuries other than automobile and motorcycle accidents include direct blows to the chest by any kind of blunt object or missile, such as a clenched fist or even various kinds of sporting equipment, as well as by the kicks of animals, falls, and cardiac resuscitative procedures. Fractures of the bony structures of the chest wall are *not* necessary accompaniments of cardiac injury in any of these situations. This point is of critical importance, since *the absence of such obvious injuries following trauma should by no means exclude the possibility of nonpenetrating injury to the heart.* The clinical manifestations may not be apparent for days or even weeks after the accident.[9]

Pathological findings following nonpenetrating cardiac injury usually include some degree of pericarditis, which may be associated with the late development of constriction. Changes in the heart itself range from minute ecchymotic areas in the subepicardium or subendocardium to transmural contusions with edematous, fragmented, or necrotic muscle fibers, surrounded at first by red blood cells and invaded soon thereafter by polymorphonuclear leukocytes. The external appearance of the heart may be misleading in the case of nonpenetrating injury, since large areas of intramural contusion,[10] including involvement of the interventricular septum, may not be apparent. In patients who survive the injury, healing is by scar formation resembling that following acute myocardial infarction, and post-traumatic aneurysms resembling postinfarction aneurysms may develop. The types of cardiac injury resulting from blunt (nonpenetrating) trauma are listed in Table 44–1, the most severe forms being rupture of the aortic or mitral valve and rupture of the interventricular septum or even of the free wall of a cardiac chamber. These injuries are frequently fatal, but fortunately they constitute only a small fraction of all nonpenetrating injuries (Table 44–2).

TABLE 44–1 TYPES OF CARDIAC INJURY FROM BLUNT TRAUMA

A. Myocardium
   1. Contusion
   2. Laceration
   3. Rupture
   4. Septal perforation
   5. Aneurysm, pseudoaneurysm
   6. Hemopericardium, tamponade
   7. Thrombosis, systemic embolism
B. Pericardium
   1. Pericarditis
   2. Postpericardiotomy syndrome
   3. Constrictive pericarditis
   4. Pericardial laceration
   5. Hemorrhage
   6. Cardiac herniation
C. Endocardial structures
   1. Rupture of papillary muscle
   2. Rupture of chordae tendineae
   3. Rupture of atrioventricular and semilunar valves
D. Coronary artery
   1. Thrombosis
   2. Laceration
   3. Fistula

From Jackson, D. H., and Murphy, G. W.: Nonpenetrating cardiac trauma. Mod. Conc. Cardiovasc. Dis. *45*:123, 1976, by permission of the American Heart Association, Inc.

Pericardium (See also p. 1480)

Injury to the pericardium in blunt trauma may range from contusion to laceration or rupture. Whether the pericardium tears or not, some degree of traumatic pericarditis is found at autopsy or operation in most patients sustaining severe blunt trauma of the chest, especially of the precordial area. Parmley et al. reported pericardial laceration or rupture in 249 of 546 autopsy cases of nonpenetrating trauma to the heart,[6] but it should be noted that this rarely occurs as an isolated lesion (Table 44–2) and is usually associated with cardiac contusion and even more serious cardiac injury. On the basis of a series of experiments in a canine model, in which 14 of 18 dogs receiving sublethal blunt chest trauma developed pericardial rents, DeMuth et al. suggested that a higher frequency of pericardial tears than is generally appreciated occurs in survivors of chest trauma.[11] Herniation of the heart or a portion of it through the defect may result from such injuries.[12] Clinically, a rent in the pericardium can occur as a consequence of blunt trauma, and delayed herniation of the heart through

TABLE 44–2 NONPENETRATING CARDIAC TRAUMA

Type and/or Site of Injury	Number of Cases	Cases Combined with Aortic Rupture	Total
Rupture	273	80	353
Right ventricle	56	10	66
Left ventricle	46	13	59
Right atrium	35	6	51
Left atrium	24	2	26
IV septum	25(20*)	7(4*)	30(24*)
IA septum	18(10*)	5(3*)	25(13*)
Multiple chamber ruptures	69	37	106
			128
Contusion/laceration	105	24	
Pericardial laceration	18	18	36
Hemopericardium	13	12	25
Valvular laceration/rupture	1(2†)	0(4†)	1(6†)
Aortic valve	1(1†)	0(2†)	1(3†)
Pulmonic valve	0(4†)	0	0(4†)
Tricuspid valve	0(8†)	0	0(8†)
Mitral valve	0(8†)	0(1†)	0(9†)
Mitral and tricuspid valves	0(1†)	0(1†)	0(2†)
Coronary artery laceration/rupture	0(7†)	1(2†)	1(9†)
Papillary muscle laceration/rupture	1(23†)	0	1(23†)
TOTAL	411	135	546

Numbers in parentheses indicate more significant associated cardiac injuries (tabulated in another column).
*Associated with other sites of cardiac rupture.
†Combined with cardiac rupture or other cardiac injury.
From Parmley, L. F., et al.: Nonpenetrating traumatic injury of the heart. Circulation *18*:371, 1958, by permission of the American Heart Association, Inc.

trauma, and delayed herniation of the heart through the rent may then acutely compromise circulatory function.[13]

CLINICAL FEATURES AND DIAGNOSIS. Clinically, traumatic pericarditis is manifested by the development of a typical pericardial friction rub and ST-T–wave changes on the electrocardiogram characteristic of pericarditis (p. 1475 and 1476). During and immediately following the acute episode, the major problem is not the pericarditis itself, but its most common complications, i.e., hemopericardium and resultant tamponade, discussed on p. 1480. Commonly, the patient is restless, with hypotension, oliguria or anuria, distant heart sounds, and pulsus paradoxus. There is usually diffuse low voltage on the electrocardiogram. Pericardial fluid on the echocardiogram (p. 1484) is a key finding.

TREATMENT AND PROGNOSIS. As a rule, uncomplicated pericarditis simply resolves. Tamponade, however, requires emergency operative treatment, as discussed below. Recurrent pericardial effusions sometimes associated with chest pain and fever, i.e., the so-called postcardiotomy syndrome, occur in a small number of patients. The etiology of this syndrome is not clear (p. 1514). Patients with recurrent effusions usually respond to aspirin or indomethacin, but occasionally glucocorticosteroids are necessary. Constrictive pericarditis occurs as a rare complication of traumatic pericarditis, with or without recurrent effusions.

Myocardium

Early experimental studies stressed the vulnerability of the heart to blunt trauma.[14] A method of producing a standard, graded, isolated injury to the myocardium through the intact chest wall of anesthetized dogs using a captive-bolt handgun or an air pressurized impactor with energy transferred through a metal disc has been described.[15–17] As the power was increased, the degree of injury became correspondingly more severe. The first level of energy produced only arrhythmias, intermediate levels produced varying degrees of hematoma associated with impairment of ventricular function, and the highest level of energy was nearly always fatal. An important and surprising finding was gross pathological change in the hearts of animals that showed no clinically apparent ill effects.

Since the consequences of nonpenetrating injury to the myocardium vary in intensity from mild contusion to cardiac rupture, it is not surprising that clinical manifestations also vary proportionately and that a high index of suspicion is often necessary for their recognition in all but the most obvious cases.[18] In patients with preexisting ischemic, valvular, or myopathic heart disease, the added insult of the myocardial trauma can be more serious than a comparable injury in a normal person.

CONTUSION

Myocardial contusion usually produces no significant symptoms and often goes unrecognized. At times, manifestations of the injury are masked by injury to the chest wall or other organs. The importance of a high index of suspicion of this complication is reflected in the experience at the Charity Hospital in New Orleans.[19] From 1963 to 1970, an average of two patients a year with cardiac contusion were admitted to the surgical service but, with increasing interest in and attention devoted to this problem, an average of eight patients per year were admitted from 1971 through 1973; in many of the latter patients, the diagnosis was not evident immediately but was established 48 hours after admission or even later. Most of the patients were young males involved in automobile accidents. Thus, as is the case with any condition, there is a higher frequency of diagnosis of cardiac contusion associated with increasing awareness of the lesion.

Clinical Features and Diagnosis. The most common symptom of myocardial contusion is precordial pain resembling that of myocardial infarction, but the pain from other sites of chest trauma can confuse the clinical picture.[20] As with myocardial infarction, nitroglycerin and related drugs have little effect in relieving the pain. The *electrocardiogram* probably represents one of the most helpful tools for recognizing this syndrome.[21–23] Either nonspecific ST-T abnormalities or the classic findings of pericarditis are the most common changes noted. Initially, electrocardiographic signs of deeper injury to the myocardium, i.e., pathological Q waves, may be dwarfed by pericardial inflammation; only as the latter subsides does injury to the myocardium become more evident. However, because the possibility of cardiac trauma is not considered, an electrocardiogram is often not recorded immediately on patients with chest injuries and the diagnosis may be missed. Just as in acute myocardial infarction, serial findings, i.e., Q waves and the subsidence of the ST-segment and T-wave abnormalities, are of critical importance.

Since *serum enzyme levels* may be elevated by trauma to noncardiac as well as to cardiac tissue, they too are of limited diagnostic value. With the increasing availability of reliable measurements of the MB band of creatine kinase (CK), the cardiospecific isoenzyme of creatine kinase (p. 1254), the presence or absence of cardiac necrosis can be better documented in patients with blunt trauma.[24] Indeed, with the electrocardiogram and CK-MB as screening tests, the detection of myocardial contusion has increased from 7 to 17 per cent of patients with blunt chest trauma presenting to the Henry Ford Hospital.[25]

Another potentially important diagnostic tool is *radionuclide imaging* (Chap. 11).[26] Myocardial perfusion is reduced in areas of myocardial contusion.[27] Chiu et al. have used technetium-labeled pyrophosphate to demonstrate images of positive uptake that were then correlated with postmortem angiograms showing extravasation of contrast material.[28] Images usually became negative 1 week after the trauma. Contused myocardium was found to concentrate ^{99m}Tc-pyrophosphate in quantities comparable to the level observed in ischemic injury.[29] Scanning following injection of radioactive thallium to detect areas of reduced perfusion and of labeled pyrophosphate to locate areas of recent necrosis may be expected to identify patients with myocardial damage following blunt trauma, to localize this damage, and to indicate the extent of the damage. Radionuclide ventriculography often shows a reduced ventricular ejection fraction in such patients.[30] These tests show changes similar to those observed in patients with acute myocardial infarction (Chap. 11).

A wide variety of *arrhythmias* is common with areas of extensive contusion,[31,32] and ventricular tachycardia that degenerates into ventricular fibrillation represents a frequent cause of death in these patients. The precise mechanism responsible for these arrhythmias has not been defined, but in the dog, increasing frequencies of ventricular premature beats were observed with increasing grades of trauma.[16] In addition, both atrioventricular and intraventricular conduction defects, as well as sinus node dysfunction, are seen.[33–35] In contrast to acute myocardial infarction, cardiac contusion rarely leads to severe heart failure unless severe damage to a valve or rupture of the interventricular septum has occurred. However, moderate impairment of right and/or left ventricular function, as reflected in depressed ejection fractions and ventricular function (myocardial performance) curves, is common.[30,36]

Treatment and Prognosis. Treatment of myocardial contusion has traditionally involved a 4- to 6-week period of bed rest with progressive ambulation thereafter.[7] However, in this era of progressively earlier ambulation for patients with myocardial infarction, a more aggressive approach appears to be reasonable. From the point of view of physical activity, we recommend treating these patients in a manner similar to those with acute myocardial infarction with comparable extent of myocardial damage (p. 1303). Treatment with anticoagulants is contraindicated, however, since it may precipitate or exacerbate intramyocardial or intrapericardial hemorrhage. Atrial fibrillation, when present, usually reverts to sinus rhythm spontaneously, but if it does not, digitalis glycosides may be used to slow the ventricular rate and may also cause reversion to sinus rhythm. Chest pain is best treated with analgesics.

The prognosis for complete or partial recovery is generally excellent, but these patients require careful follow-up, since late complications, ranging from ventricular arrhythmias to cardiac rupture, may occur. Coronary occlusion,[37] sinus of Valsalva–right atrial fistula,[38] and cardiac aneurysms[39] are occasional sequelae, and there is no agreement about whether or not surgical resection of the last-named is required.[40] It is our policy to use the presence of heart failure as an indication for operation of aneurysms analogous to that in patients with postinfarct aneurysms (p. 1374).

Although many analogies can be drawn between the cardiac necrosis caused by trauma and that caused by coronary artery disease, a number of critically important differences must be emphasized. Patients with acute myocardial infarction generally have diffuse, obstructive, gradually progressive coronary artery disease, are frequently middle-aged or elderly, and may have underlying heart disease such as that secondary to prolonged hypertension or diabetes mellitus; patients with traumatic myocardial contusion generally have normal coronary vessels and only a discrete area of myocardial damage;[41] most often, they are young and without underlying cardiovascular illness. Hence, the long-term prognosis in patients with myocardial necrosis secondary to trauma tends to be far better, *if they survive the acute episode.*

RUPTURE

There appear to be two mechanisms of cardiac rupture; (1) acute laceration due to compression of the heart by direct force, and (2) contusion and hemorrhage that proceed to necrosis, softening, and rupture several days following the trauma. Rupture of a cardiac chamber usually, but not always, results in immediate death. However, Bright and Beck reported that 30 of 152 patients with ventricular rupture survived 30 minutes or longer after the initial trauma.[14] It is this minority of patients that must be assessed and treated immediately in the emergency room setting.

Clinical Features and Diagnosis. In the patient who survives the first few minutes of cardiac rupture, the clinical picture of cardiac tamponade described above is common. Although ventricular rupture is far more common than is atrial rupture, the latter occurs particularly following automobile accidents.[42] Rupture of the interventricular septum should be suspected in patients who develop severe congestive heart failure immediately or within several days of the trauma, together with a new holosystolic murmur along the left sternal border; however, trauma to the mitral valve apparatus, which may present with a similar picture clinically, must be excluded. Based on a series of 546 autopsy cases of nonpenetrating injury to the heart, the incidence of rupture of the ventricular septum has been estimated by Parmley et al. to be a little more than 5 per cent, with a similar number of patients experiencing rupture of the atrial septum (Table 44–2).[6] These lesions may occur without other serious cardiac injuries, but occasionally other abnormalities are present, including valve cusp perforations and a variety of intracardiac shunts.[43,44] The predilection for perforation of the ventricular septum is highest at the apex, but any portion of the muscular septum may be involved, and multiple perforations are not uncommon. The diagnosis of ventricular septal defect and of damage to the mitral valve apparatus can be confirmed by means of catheterization, demonstration of an oxygen step-up in the right ventricle, and left ventricular angiography.[45]

Treatment and Prognosis. Patients with external rupture of the heart obviously require emergency operation if they are to have any chance of survival. Although surgery should not be postponed, pericardiocentesis and expansion of the intravascular volume can be carried out while the most rapid preparations possible for operation are undertaken. Successful surgical treatment of external cardiac rupture has been reported in a small number of cases.[4,46] In contrast, patients with rupture of the interventricular septum do not always require emergency operation. Indeed, many defects are small, with minimal left-to-right shunts, and may even heal spontaneously. If heart failure subsequently develops, as occurs in many patients, surgical correction should be carried out promptly and is often successful.[44]

COMPLICATIONS OF CARDIAC RESUSCITATION

In 1960, Kouwenhoven et al. described the technique of closed-chest (external) cardiac massage, and this technique quickly replaced open-chest massage in the management of cardiac arrest.[47] This procedure is generally thought to be safe and simple—so much so that it is included as part of the cardiopulmonary resuscitation technique taught to laymen. What is not sufficiently appreciated is that the procedure itself can often result in serious complications, which may go unrecognized because many of the patients

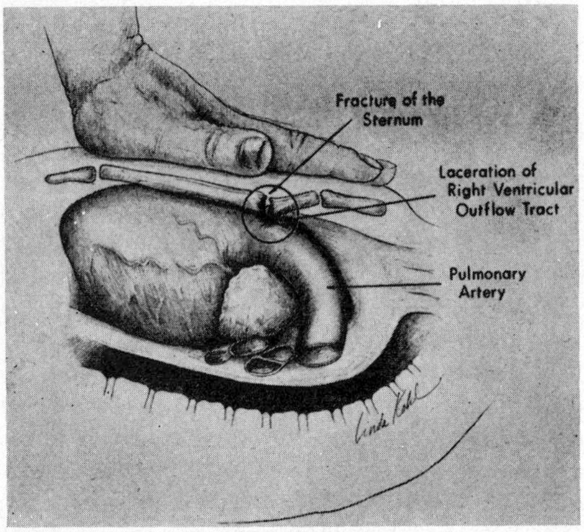

FIGURE 44–1 Schematic diagram showing the mechanism and site of laceration of the right ventricular outflow tract during external cardiac massage. (From Sethi, G.K., et al.: Complications of external cardiac massage. Report of a case of laceration of the right ventricular outflow tract. J. Cardiovasc. Surg. *18*:187, 1977.)

succumb to the cardiac arrest itself.[48] Even at postmortem examination, the complications may be improperly attributed to the underlying cardiac disease.

Rupture of the left ventricle is a more common complication of cardiac massage than rupture of the right ventricle (Figs. 44–1 and 44–2), but rupture of either chamber may occur and may be life-threatening if the patient survives the cardiac dysrhythmia that necessitated massage in the first place. In a series of autopsies on 60 patients in whom external cardiac massage had been carried out, Adelson observed four instances of laceration of the left ventricle and one each of the left atrium and cardiac vein.[49] Since in most instances external resuscitation is performed for patients with myocardial infarction, it may not always be clear whether the left ventricular rupture preceded or occurred as a consequence of the massage.

Rupture of right ventricular papillary muscles with acute tricuspid regurgitation has also been reported as a complication of closed-chest cardiac massage,[50] as has rupture of the atria[51] and aorta[52] and a variety of noncardiovascular traumatic lesions, such as fracture of the sternum, hemothorax, pneumothorax, and laceration of abdominal organs.[53] Because of the efficacy of cardiopulmonary resuscitation and its increasing use by paramedical personnel and laymen, an increasing number of such complications may be anticipated in the future. This increased incidence will be stemmed only by extensive and repeated educational programs for all individuals likely to employ this technique.

PENETRATING CARDIAC INJURY

Symbas has noted the long medical history of penetrating cardiac wounds, which have been recorded since the time of Hippocrates.[8] Up to the end of the nineteenth century, this type of wound was thought to be invariably fatal.[54]

Penetrating cardiac injuries occurring in civilian life are due to a variety of objects, such as bullets, knives, ice picks, and the like,[55,56] but they may also be due to the inward displacement of ribs or sternal fragments accompanying chest injuries. The chamber most commonly involved in this type of injury is the right ventricle because of its anterior position, followed, in descending order of frequency, by the left ventricle, the right atrium, and the left atrium.[57,58] However, penetrating wounds of the precordium are not the only types of wounds that may result in cardiac injury. Occasionally, wounds of other areas of the

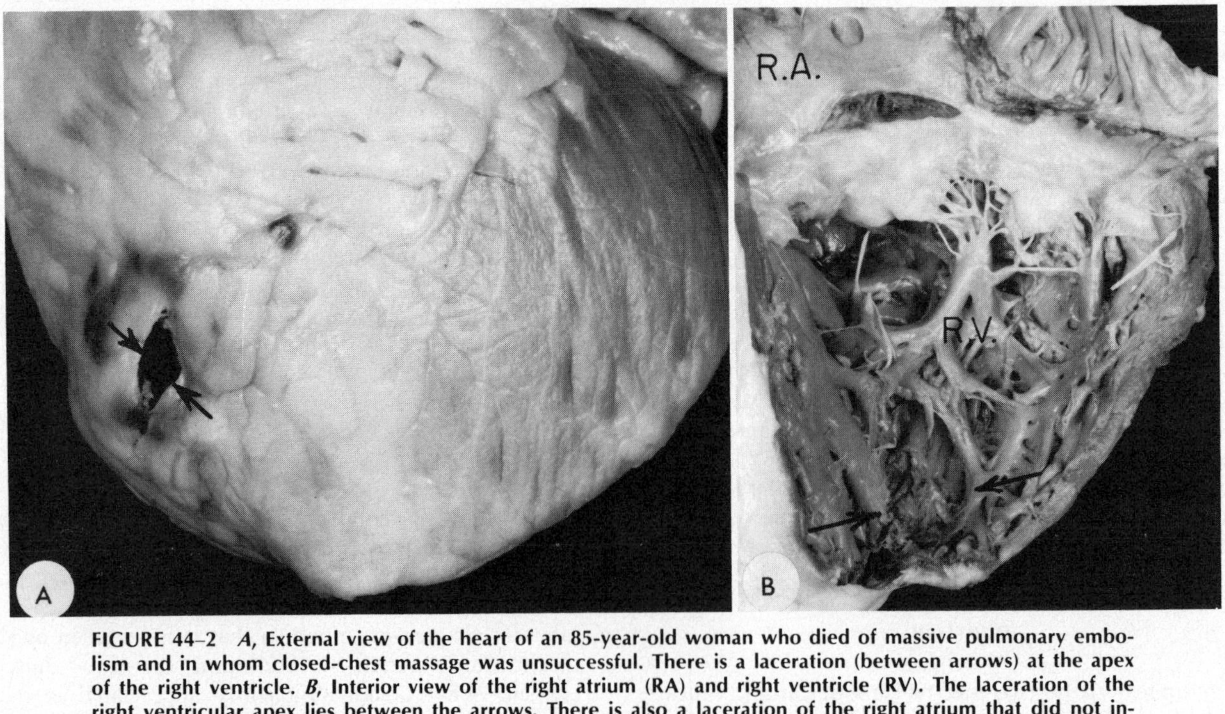

FIGURE 44–2 *A*, External view of the heart of an 85-year-old woman who died of massive pulmonary embolism and in whom closed-chest massage was unsuccessful. There is a laceration (between arrows) at the apex of the right ventricle. *B*, Interior view of the right atrium (RA) and right ventricle (RV). The laceration of the right ventricular apex lies between the arrows. There is also a laceration of the right atrium that did not involve the full thickness of the wall. (From Baldwin, J.J., and Edwards, J.E.: Rupture of right ventricle complicating closed chest massage. Circulation *53*:562, 1976, by permission of the American Heart Association, Inc.)

chest, as well as of the neck and upper abdomen, are associated with penetration of the heart. In addition, intravenous or intracardiac catheters may fracture and become impaled within the walls of a great vessel or cardiac chamber (Chap. 9).[59] Migration of an indwelling venous catheter into the pulmonary artery, which may ultimately lead to perforation of this vessel, is another complication that has increased in frequency with its widespread use in intensive care units.[60] Formerly, thoracotomy was necessary to remove these catheter fragments, but noninvasive snare devices are now available for this purpose.[61]

Perforation of the right ventricle with a transvenous pacing electrode is not uncommon, but tamponade is rare.[62] The postcardiotomy syndrome (p. 1514) however, may occur following such a perforation.[63] During cardiac catheterization, perforation of the thin-walled right atrium or outflow tract of the right ventricle has been reported.[64] Such patients usually require only careful observation, but when tamponade occurs, immediate drainage is mandatory.[65] Dissection of the aorta or arch vessels has been reported as a complication of retrograde arterial catheterization and occasionally is also severe enough to require operative intervention.[66]

Penetrating wounds of the heart often result in laceration of the pericardium, sometimes occurring alone but usually associated with laceration of the myocardium itself. One or more chambers but also the cardiac valves and their accessory structures, as well as the interventricular and interatrial septa, may be perforated. When laceration of the pericardium occurs as an isolated lesion, acute compromise of cardiac function resulting from herniation of the heart may be the presenting manifestation. Occasionally, low-velocity missiles may penetrate the cardiac chambers but may be retained within the myocardium.

The most common penetrating injuries resulting from physical violence are stab and gunshot wounds.[67] The former do not necessarily cause extensive cellular destruction adjacent to the wound; they resemble surgical incisions, and transmural wounds in the thick-walled left ventricle may actually seal quickly without disastrous consequences. In contrast, bullet wounds are associated with bleeding that is not usually self-limited and extensive cellular destruction in and adjacent to the path of the bullet. When a coronary artery is lacerated or perforated, myocardial infarction may ensue.

CLINICAL FEATURES AND DIAGNOSIS. The clinical picture of a penetrating wound of the heart depends on several factors, including the mechanism of injury (i.e., bullet, knife, ice pick), the size of the wound, and the precise location of the structures injured. Pericardial laceration occurring by itself is uncommon and of relatively little significance, unless infection supervenes. Rather, the injuries to underlying cardiac structures usually determine the clinical presentation, course, and choice of treatment. However, the *nature* of the pericardial wound is important, i.e., whether or not the wound is open and allows free drainage of intrapericardial blood. If the pericardium remains open and extravasated blood can pass freely into the pleural cavities or mediastinum, cardiac tamponade will not develop, at least initially, and the presenting signs and symptoms will be those of hemorrhage and hemothorax. On the other hand, if the pericardium does *not* permit free drainage, because its opening has been obliterated by a blood clot, adjacent lung tissue, or other structures, or because a flap develops in the pericardial rent, immediate exsanguination may be averted, but tamponade may occur minutes or hours later.[68] In some instances, blood accumulates both intra- and extrapericardially.

Whether the hemorrhage is intra- or extrapericardial, its severity can often be surmised from the clinical picture. Traumatic penetrating lesions of the heart are usually associated with injuries to the lungs and other organs, which may predominate at first; a high index of suspicion of cardiac penetration is necessary when patients are evaluated following thoracic or upper abdominal trauma. Though extensive injuries to the pericardium and underlying heart are usually immediately fatal or result in shock, delayed clinical manifestations of cardiac injury as a result of hemorrhage, infection, retained foreign bodies, or arrhythmias may become apparent after the other bodily injuries have been attended to. Failure to give serious consideration to the possibility that *cardiac* damage has occurred in a patient with obvious noncardiac trauma may lead to an unanticipated catastrophe.

Although echocardiography is extremely valuable in the recognition of pericardial effusion (p. 1478) and in the recognition of foreign bodies in the heart,[68a] it is not always readily available in an emergency setting. When agitation, cool and clammy skin, neck vein distention, pulsus paradoxus, and other classic findings of tamponade (considered earlier) are present, the diagnosis can be relatively simple; in patients without such typical findings, the clinical picture may be attributed to blood loss, especially since volume expansion can improve the hemodynamic state at least temporarily.[69] Fallah-Nejad et al. reported a series of 20 cases of penetrating cardiac injuries; the diagnosis was not immediately obvious in 10 patients in whom the signs of cardiac tamponade were either obscured or occurred late.[70] In several of these patients an initial salutary response to a volume load—with restoration of hemodynamics to apparently normal levels—was responsible for the failure to recognize the underlying cardiac injury. Whether or not pericardiocentesis should be performed as a diagnostic test is controversial. If nonclotting blood is obtained, the diagnosis of hemopericardium is confirmed, and the accompanying decompression may constitute effective, albeit temporary, initial treatment. If the pericardiocentesis is negative, however, cardiac tamponade cannot be ruled out. Since, as discussed below, the primary management in any event is thoracotomy, it seems to us pointless to waste valuable time with pericardial aspiration unless there is doubt regarding the diagnosis.

TREATMENT. Successful treatment of penetrating wounds by pericardial aspiration was reported several times during the nineteenth century. Nonetheless, until the first successful cardiorrhaphy,[54] there was great pessimism about survival following penetrating cardiac injury. Today, the definitive treatment of cardiac wounds *accompanied by severe hemorrhage* is immediate thoracotomy and cardiorrhaphy. Although multiple pericardiocenteses are no longer considered a substitute for thoracotomy in the treatment of cardiac wounds associated with cardiac tamponade, there may still be a role for pericardial aspiration *while preparing for operation* (Table 44–3). The availability

TABLE 44–3 MANAGEMENT OF PATIENTS WITH STAB WOUNDS TO THE HEART

1. Immediate pericardiocentesis
2. Placement of central venous pressure (CVP) catheter to withdraw blood and infuse fluids
3. Chest roentgenogram only if condition permits
4. Thoracotomy and repair of bleeding site
5. Wound closure with placement of pericardial drainage tubes
6. Postoperative antibotic therapy

From Harvey, J. C., and Pacifico, A. D.: Primary operative management: Method of choice for stab wounds to the heart. South. Med. J. *68*:149, 1975, by permission of the Southern Medical Journal.

in many hospitals of surgical teams and equipment for cardiopulmonary bypass has permitted the safe and effective repair of many penetrating injuries of the heart.

Lemos and associates described a 13-year experience with 121 patients undergoing surgical treatment of cardiac wounds in Brazil.[71] Gunshot wounds outnumbered stab wounds, nearly 72 per cent of the patients were in shock or "pre-shock," and 33 per cent had cardiac tamponade at the time of presentation to the hospital. Over 40 per cent of these patients were taken to the operating room within 30 minutes of arrival at the hospital, and an overall mortality of 26 per cent in patients with isolated cardiac wounds was reported. Harvey and Pacifico noted that there were no deaths among 24 patients with cardiac stab wounds who received primary operative management, but in contrast there were three deaths among 10 patients who were managed conservatively (including multiple pericardial aspirations).[72] Symbas et al. studied a series of 102 patients with bullet and stab wounds and concluded that immediate operation is the treatment of choice for tamponade.[73] Szentpetery and Lower concluded in their study of 30 consecutive patients with penetrating wounds that immediate operation is recommended for all penetrating injuries but that pericardiocentesis still has a role in the emergency relief of tamponade.[74]

Obviously, the decision for or against thoracotomy must depend, in part, on the setting in which the patient is encountered, the availability and skill of the surgical team, and facilities for cardiopulmonary bypass, all measured against the gravity of the clinical picture. Even in hospitals without the facilities for cardiopulmonary bypass, treatment of penetrating injuries of the heart may be very successful.[67,75] In 34 such patients, of whom 31 were in shock at the time of operation, there was no immediate mortality, although the late mortality was 23 per cent.

Occasionally, thoracotomy may be performed in moribund patients for whom general anesthesia is unnecessary. However, every effort must be made to maintain adequate ventilation. Administration of antibiotics and tetanus prophylaxis should also be instituted as routine measures. Operative treatment includes repair of the pericardium, myocardium, aorta, and valves as well as of any lacerations of the coronary arteries. At operation, the heart and great vessels should be thoroughly examined for the presence of multiple wounds. When the bullet has penetrated the anterior wall of the heart, the posterior wall should always be inspected for an exit wound before the chest is closed. Many victims of penetrating cardiac injury, young and otherwise in good health, can withstand relatively long periods of hypoperfusion without irreversible brain, renal, or cardiac damage. Therefore, one should err on the side of aggressive attempts at resuscitation in patients who arrive moribund in the operating room. Retained foreign bodies in the heart are less of a problem in civilian than in military injuries, because shootings in civilian life usually occur at short range and thus result in through-and-through wounds.

There is disagreement concerning whether or not retained foreign bodies should be removed. Certainly, if the projectile is accessible, it should be removed; otherwise, if small (less than 1 cm in diameter), it can probably be left in place,[76] although there is some risk of later infection, pain, aneurysm formation, or migration of the foreign body.[77,78] In addition, dealing with a patient who is preoccupied with the knowledge that he has a foreign body retained in or close to the heart may present some difficulty; indeed, anxiety can become excessive, impairing the patient's function more than the physical damage and, occasionally, becoming an indication for reoperation and extraction of the object. The serious consequences of a foreign body embolus from the left ventricle also encourages a more aggressive surgical policy toward foreign bodies lodged in that chamber than in the right ventricle. Foreign bodies embedded at strategic points in great vessels may erode the vessel and cause potentially severe hemorrhage or may embolize. As noted by Mattox et al. in a series of 28 patients with bullet emboli, complications are usually secondary to associated injuries rather than to removal of the bullets.[79]

Late complications of penetrating wounds of the heart are quite common and include post-traumatic pericarditis and infection as well as arrhythmias, ventricular septal defect, and ventricular aneurysm.

PROGNOSIS. The outlook following a penetrating wound depends, first and foremost, on the extent of the injury. Gunshot wounds of the heart are usually immediately fatal, with a slightly lower mortality for stab wounds; among the latter, knife wounds are more serious than are ice pick wounds. Wilson and Bassett have estimated that 80 to 90 per cent of patients with *stab* wounds who *reach* the hospital alive can be saved.[55] In addition, wounds that cause cardiac tamponade rather than massive extrapericardial hemorrhage are more likely to be successfully corrected. Patients who require 500 ml or less of blood preoperatively to maintain a satisfactory arterial pressure exhibited a mortality of 10 per cent, compared with those requiring more than 1000 ml, in whom mortality was much higher (36 per cent).[55] Salvage rates are lower in patients with penetrating wounds involving thin-walled structures such as the atria or the pulmonary artery (43 and 67 per cent, respectively), since they rarely seal off spontaneously, whereas injury to the ventricles is associated with distinctly higher survival (about 85 per cent). The state of consciousness and the extent of damage to the central nervous system, if any, at the time the patient presents to the hospital also affect prognosis; Wilson and Bassett reported that over half of those in coma succumbed compared with 11 per cent of conscious patients.[55] It is clear that delay in performing the initial thoracotomy also adversely influences the chances for survival.

Rupture of the interventricular septum is often a late complication of penetrating injury as it is with blunt inju-

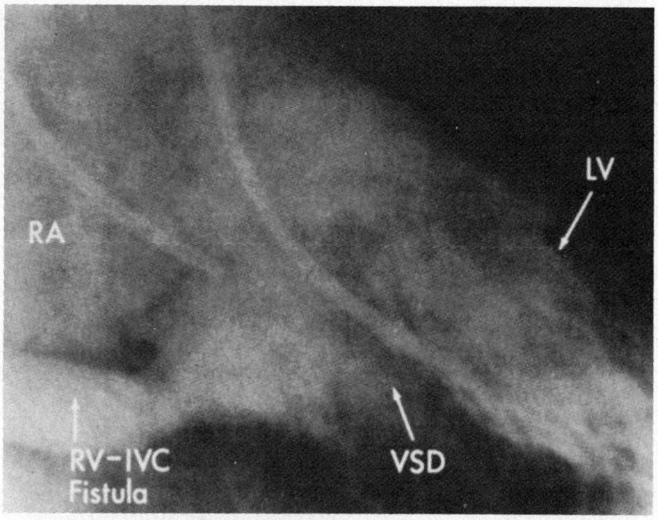

FIGURE 44–3 Angiocardiogram demonstrating ventricular septal defect (VSD) and right ventricular–inferior vena caval (RV-IVC) fistula in a 16-year-old boy who sustained a bullet wound to the chest 3 months earlier. At that time, emergency thoracotomy revealed only an entrance wound of the left ventricle (LV), which was sutured. Three months later, he was readmitted with severe congestive heart failure, and angiography was performed by injecting contrast media into the left ventricle. (From Rayner, A. V. S., et al.: Post-traumatic intracardiac shunts. Report of 2 cases and review of the literature. J. Thorac. Cardiovasc. Surg. *73*:728, 1977.)

ry (Fig. 44–3). Asfaw et al. described 12 patients with stab wounds who presented with cardiac tamponade and who had epicardial and pericardial wounds which were repaired at thoracotomy.[80] Days to years later, septal defects were diagnosed, but only four patients were symptomatic enough to warrant subsequent reoperation for closure of the defect.

INJURIES TO CARDIAC VALVES, PAPILLARY MUSCLES, AND CHORDAE TENDINEAE

Historically, reports of injuries to the cardiac valves and their accessory structures date back to the late nineteenth century. Patients with preexisting valvular heart disease may be at higher risk than those with normal valves for the development of valvular injury following blunt trauma. Parmley et al. reported a 9 per cent incidence of valvular injury in their report of 546 cases of nonpenetrating chest trauma (Table 44–2).[6] Damage to the aortic valve is by far the most common of these lesions (Fig. 44–4). (Parmley's series appears to be an exception in this regard). This is followed, in order, by damage to the mitral and tricuspid valves, presumably owing to the higher pressures generated by blunt trauma to the aorta, as noted by Jackson and Murphy.[4] The aortic valve is probably most vulnerable to damage early in diastole, when the ventricle and aorta are nearly full.[81] Damage to cardiac valves may also occur as a consequence of penetrating wounds of the heart, but, in contrast to the damage caused by nonpenetrating injury, these are rarely solitary lesions. Indeed, sustained damage of the aortic valve should be suspected in any patient without a history of heart disease who presents with a heart murmur after severe blunt trauma to the chest.

CLINICAL FEATURES AND DIAGNOSIS. New, loud, musical murmurs are characteristic of injury to the valves and their supporting structures. The combination of a high-pitched diastolic blowing murmur with a widened pulse pressure following blunt trauma to the chest suggests rupture of the *aortic valve.* The murmur and the hemodynamic consequences of the rupture may not appear for several days following the trauma. Aortic regurgitation may also occur transiently owing to perivalvular edema or hemorrhage.

Rupture of the *mitral valve* or of a papillary muscle appears to occur as a consequence of sudden obstruction to left ventricular outflow due to blunt injury in early diastole. It is usually associated with the development of precordial pain and a loud, harsh holosystolic murmur that radiates to the apex. Fulminant pulmonary edema quickly develops; those patients with lesser degrees of regurgitation due to torn leaflets or chordae tendineae may remain compensated for longer periods of time, although they may eventually show signs of decompensation.

Rupture of the *tricuspid valve* is rare[82,83] and more benign than mitral valve rupture, with symptoms ranging from fatigue to ascites and edema.[7] Physical findings can be striking, with prominent systolic venous pulsations, hepatic pulsations, and a typical holosystolic murmur with inspiratory accentuation. At cardiac catheterization, "ventricularization" of the atrial pressure, i.e., giant v waves in the right atrial pressure pulse, can be demonstrated. A valve damaged by trauma is flail, and this can be recognized by echocardiography, whereas left-heart catheterization and selective angiocardiography are most useful in assessing the severity and hemodynamic consequences of the injury.

TREATMENT AND PROGNOSIS. The prognosis depends largely on the severity of the regurgitation. Since the lesion usually develops suddenly, the ventricle does not have the opportunity to adapt to this burden, as it does in most forms of chronic valvular regurgitation. Obviously, the baseline condition of the ventricle prior to the trauma and the presence of other injuries occurring simultaneously affect the heart's ability to tolerate the insult. Before the

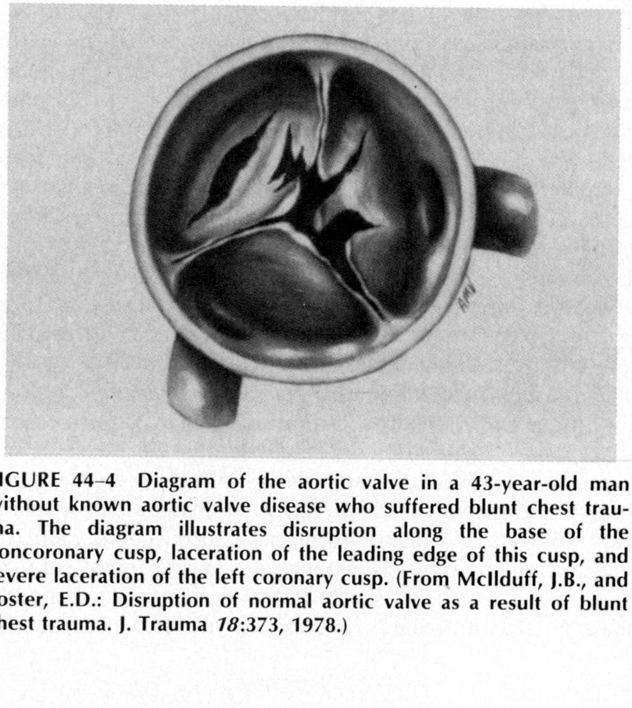

FIGURE 44–4 Diagram of the aortic valve in a 43-year-old man without known aortic valve disease who suffered blunt chest trauma. The diagram illustrates disruption along the base of the noncoronary cusp, laceration of the leading edge of this cusp, and severe laceration of the left coronary cusp. (From McIlduff, J.B., and Foster, E.D.: Disruption of normal aortic valve as a result of blunt chest trauma. J. Trauma *18*:373, 1978.)

development of cardiac surgery, a mean survival of 3½ years was reported in patients with traumatic aortic regurgitation.[84] Even in the current era when effective surgical treatment is possible, survival without the need for operation is not uncommon in patients with mild or moderate regurgitation. With severe left ventricular failure due to a ruptured mitral valve or papillary muscle, however, early surgery is mandatory, and, as in the case for the aortic valve,[85] replacement of the valve is usually preferred over valvuloplasty. It must be appreciated that the diagnosis of acute left ventricular failure may be difficult immediately after serious trauma, because fractured ribs and pulmonary contusions may be blamed for the shortness of breath and dyspnea. When left ventricular failure develops slowly or the lesion is not hemodynamically significant, as with lesser degrees of injury, medical therapy may suffice. Hemorrhage into a papillary muscle may cause late necrosis and delayed rupture, and these patients must be observed carefully.

Post-traumatic *tricuspid* regurgitation appears to have a more benign course, and many patients survive for long periods with supportive treatment. However, when failure does occur, valve replacement is the procedure of choice.

INJURIES TO THE CORONARY ARTERIES

Transmural myocardial infarctions have been reported following blunt trauma, but angiographic confirmation of coronary obstruction is rare, and, when found, its relationship to preexisting coronary atherosclerosis may be difficult to determine. When infarction occurs, it may not be clear whether it results directly from myocardial contusion, from trauma to a coronary artery, or from some combination of these two processes. In many cases of myocardial infarction, preexisting coronary artery disease has been present, and it is reasonable to postulate that the injury dislodges a plaque, which then obstructs the vessel completely.[86] However, it is also possible that a normal coronary artery becomes occluded, by either a traumatically induced intimal tear or hemorrhage. Indeed, coronary arteriography has provided strong evidence that myocardial infarction follows blunt chest trauma in previously asymptomatic persons with normal vessels except for complete obstruction of the vessel supplying the infarcted area (Fig. 44–5).[87,88] The complications of myocardial infarction —arrhythmias, pump failure, and late development of aneurysms—are similar when the lesion has an atherosclerotic basis, and treatment is similar as well. However, it may be anticipated that following survival from the initial episode, the long-term prognosis will be more favorable in patients with traumatic damage of a coronary artery, because the remaining vessels are usually normal.

Left ventricular *aneurysms* and *pseudoaneurysms* following injury to the coronary arteries can lead to rupture, cardiac failure, embolism, or arrhythmia. Operative intervention is indicated, particularly in the presence of a pseudoaneurysm, in which the myocardium has actually ruptured but in which a thrombus, fibrous tissue, and/or pericardium prevent exsanguination, since external rupture —an event which is usually fatal—is likely to occur ultimately if left untreated. Pseudoaneurysm can often be differentiated from true aneurysm by contrast or radionuclide angiography.

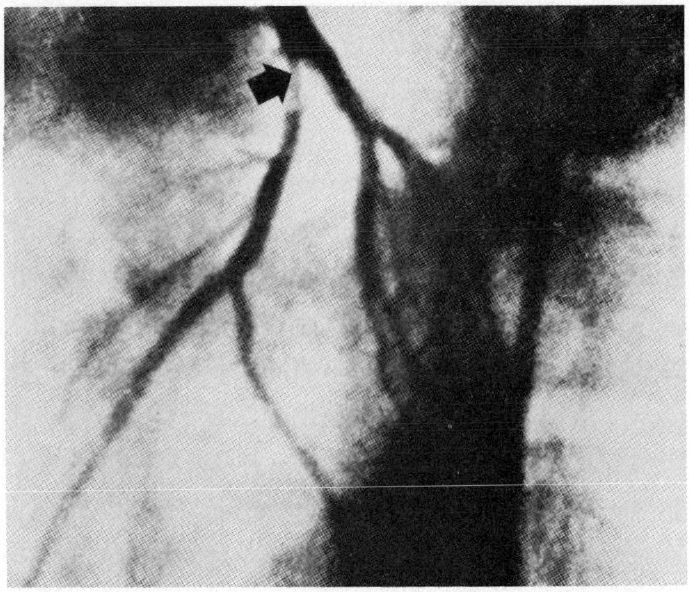

FIGURE 44–5 Left coronary arteriogram in the left anterior oblique position in a 26-year-old man who sustained an anterior wall myocardial infarction following blunt chest trauma. Arteriography performed 6 months later because of recurrent chest pain demonstrated an obstructive lesion in the left anterior descending artery (arrow). (From Jenkins, J.L., and Nishimura, A.: Coronary artery obstruction and myocardial infarction resulting from nonpenetrating chest trauma. Tex. Med. *71*:78, 1975.)

Formation of an *arteriovenous fistula* is an unusual complication of traumatic damage of a coronary artery.[89,90] Injury to the right coronary artery is more commonly followed by an arteriovenous fistula than is injury to the left. The venous side of the fistula may be the coronary sinus, the great cardiac vein, the right atrium, or the right ventricle; in the last instance, the fistula should be termed an "arteriocameral fistula." The murmur in traumatic coronary arteriovenous or arteriocameral fistula is usually loud, widely radiating, and continuous; the electrocardiogram frequently shows transmural myocardial infarction, and the roentgenogram exhibits cardiomegaly with increased pulmonary vascularity. In patients who do not undergo surgical repair, symptoms of congestive heart failure and chest pain are frequent.[91]

In 1969, Rea et al. reviewed 58 patients with *laceration of a coronary artery* due to penetrating injury and added 22 new cases.[92] The overall mortality ranged from 40 per cent with stab wounds to 67 per cent with gunshot wounds. Espada et al. reported nine patients with coronary artery lacerations among a series of 76 penetrating wounds of the heart, including seven patients with stab wounds and two with gunshot wounds.[93] As might be anticipated, the left anterior descending coronary artery is the vessel most commonly involved, and at operation, the treatment of choice is suture-ligation of the cut vessel with coronary artery bypass grafting if the lacerated vessel is large and the lesion is a proximal one. Angiography is not advised in the emergency setting, as it is with nonpenetrating trauma. However, postoperative angiography is useful in localizing the presence of possible residual injuries such as a coronary arteriocameral fistula.

INJURIES TO THE GREAT VESSELS

(See also pp. 1564–1566)

Rupture of the aorta is one of the most common traumatic lesions involving the heart or great vessels. The first case of rupture of the aorta due to *blunt* trauma was reported by Vesalius in 1557,[94] and its relative frequency is reflected in the finding that in one of every six automobile accident victims dying from blunt chest trauma the aorta is ruptured.[95] To a lesser extent, aortic rupture also occurs with falls from heights and other types of crushing injuries. Rupture occurs in the isthmus in 90 per cent of cases. Multiple tears may be present in some patients, and in others the edges of the torn aorta may be separated by several centimeters, producing a mediastinal hematoma or pseudoaneurysm.

It has been estimated that 10 to 20 per cent of patients with ruptured aorta live long enough to be treated successfully under ideal circumstances,[96] which include a high level of awareness of the possibility of aortic rupture in victims of automobile accidents as well as a well-coordinated team approach.[97] As with cardiac injury, rupture of the aorta may be overshadowed by injuries to other organs, and the diagnosis may be overlooked. Patients with aortic rupture often complain of pain in the back in addition to the chest, similar to that in patients with aortic dissection (p. 1550). If the expanding mediastinal hematoma or false aneurysm narrows the aortic lumen, or if the torn intima and media cause partial aortic obstruction, ischemia of the spinal cord and kidneys may ensue. A systolic murmur may be heard in the midscapular region, and widening of the superior mediastinum is visible on the chest roentgenogram (Fig. 44–6).[98]

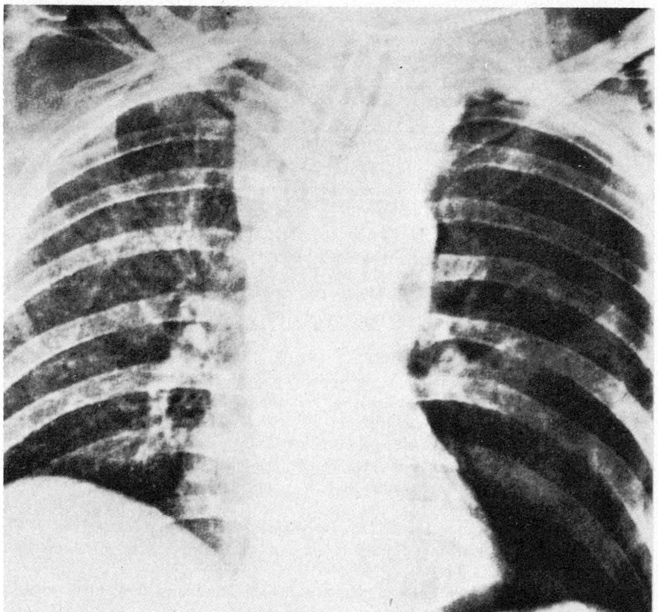

FIGURE 44–6 Chest x-ray demonstrating pronounced widening of the upper mediastinum, tracheal displacement, and left pneumothorax in a 35-year-old man who sustained traumatic rupture of the aorta as a result of an automobile accident. (From Puijlaert, C. B. A. J.: Roentgen diagnosis of traumatic rupture of the aorta. Radiologia Clin. *45*:217, 1976.)

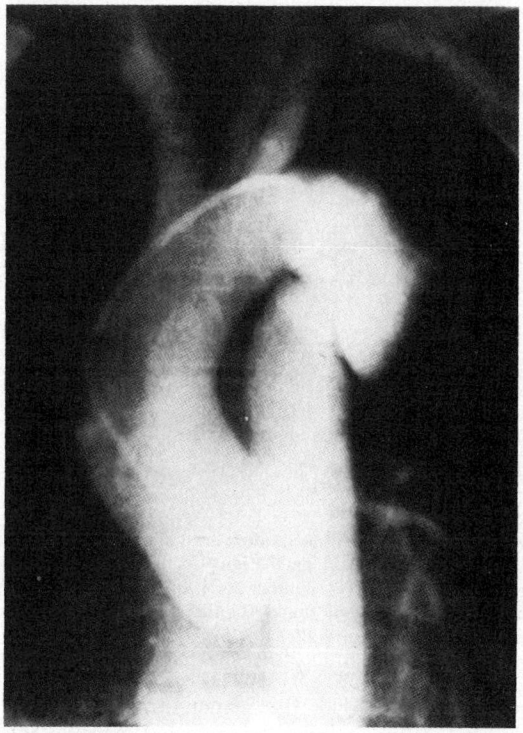

FIGURE 44–7 In a 27-year-old male, acute false and irregular aneurysm of the thoracic aorta just distal to the left subclavian artery. (Reproduced with permission from Andresen, J., and Axelsen, F.: Traumatic rupture of the thoracic aorta. Scand. J. Thorac. Cardiovasc. Surg. *14*:281, 1980.)

A diagnostic triad that occurs in well over half the cases of ruptured aorta consists of (1) increased arterial pressure and pulse amplitude in the upper extremities, (2) decreased pressure and pulse amplitude in the lower extremities, and (3) radiological evidence of widening of the superior mediastinum.[98,99] Chronic rupture of the aorta may be manifested by hoarseness, dysphagia, and cough. The diagnosis can be confirmed by aortography, which should be performed as soon as the nature of the injury is suspected. Aortography is essential for diagnosing and localizing the injury; the entire thoracic aorta and its branches should be visualized so as not to overlook a rupture occurring at an unusual site or multiple sites of rupture (Fig. 44–7).[100]

Penetrating trauma to the great vessels, which is usually the result of bullet or stab wounds, occurs most commonly in conjunction with cardiac wounds. Cardiac tamponade is a frequent complication of injury to the intrapericardial segment of one of the great vessels, but when it is extrapericardial, massive hemothorax is usually the presenting finding. The superior vena cava, trachea, or esophagus or some combination of these structures may be compressed if a large mediastinal hematoma forms as a result of bleeding. Injury to the innominate or carotid arteries may compress these vessels, with resultant neurological signs. An arteriovenous fistula may develop with symptoms of congestive heart failure accompanied by a systolic or, more commonly, a continuous murmur.[101] These fistulous connections may also involve the systemic and pulmonary vessels.[102]

Penetrating injury to the great vessels should be suspected in any patient in whom a projectile traverses the mediastinum and is suggested by radiological evidence of a

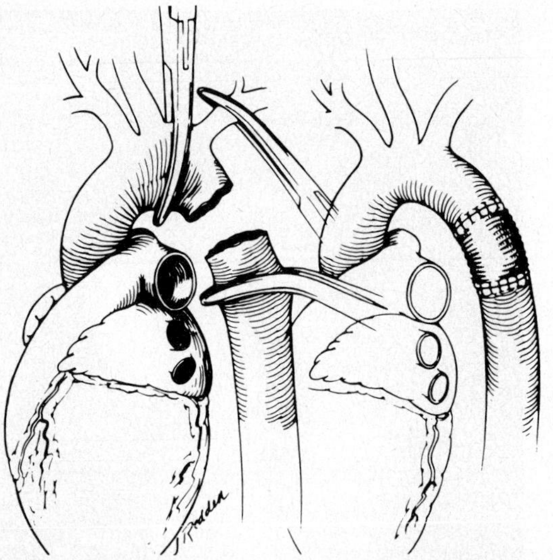

FIGURE 44–8 Method of obtaining vascular control (left) and attaching the woven Dacron graft (right) in patients with transections of the descending aorta secondary to blunt trauma. (From Pickard, L.R., et al.: Transection of the descending thoracic aorta secondary to blunt trauma. J. Trauma *17*:749, 1977.)

widened mediastinum. Aortography should be performed immediately, provided that emergency thoracotomy for shock or tamponade can be deferred briefly. Immediate operation, sometimes using a heparinized shunt between the ascending and descending aorta, should be carried out as soon as the diagnosis of thoracic aortic disruption has been established.[103] At the time of operation, the widest possible exposure is recommended. Pickard et al. described their experience with 22 patients with transection of the descending thoracic aorta secondary to blunt trauma who reached the hospital alive; five patients died shortly after admission, three died in the operating room, three died within 30 days of operation, and one died more than 1 year after the injury.[104] Ten patients were long-term survivors. A Dacron tube graft was utilized to bridge the defect in the majority of patients (Fig. 44–8). Similarly, 29 of 36 patients treated at the Grady Memorial Hospital from 1967 to 1972 for penetrating wounds of the great vessels recovered.[105]

In order to avoid the problem inherent in heparinization, i.e., bleeding from what are often multiple sites of trauma, tears of the descending thoracic aorta may often be repaired without cardiopulmonary bypass by simple aortic cross-clamping, as long as the cross-clamp time is restricted to less than 30 minutes.[106,107] An experienced surgeon can interpose a graft into the aorta with a total occlusion time ranging from 13 to 21 minutes, and ischemic injury to the spinal cord or kidneys should not occur. This technique may be aided by the intravenous administration of nitroprusside, which can maintain proximal aortic systolic pressure below 140 mm Hg.

Antiadrenergic agents such as guanethidine, reserpine, and propranolol, which have been utilized in the treatment of spontaneous dissection of the aorta (p. 1553), may also have a role in treatment of patients with aortic rupture if, for logistical reasons, operation must be deferred.

References

1. Committee on Trauma and Committee on Shock: Accidental death and disability: The neglected diseases of modern society. Washington, D.C., National Academy of Sciences, 1965, p. 5.
2. Cheitlin, M. D.: Cardiovascular trauma, part I (key references). Circulation *65*: 1529, 1982.
3. Cheitlin, M. D.: Cardiovascular trauma, part II (key references). Circulation *66*: 244, 1982.
4. Jackson, D. H., and Murphy, G. W.: Nonpenetrating cardiac trauma. Mod. Concepts Cardiovasc. Dis. *45*:123, 1976.
5. Sherman, M. M., Saini, V. K., Yarnoz, M. D., Ramp, J., Williams, L. F., and Berger, R. L.: Management of penetrating heart wounds. Am. J. Surg. *135*: 553, 1978.
6. Parmley, L. F., Manion, W. C., and Mattingly, T. W.: Nonpenetrating traumatic injury of the heart. Circulation *18*:371, 1958.
7. Liedtke, A. J., and DeMuth, W. E., Jr.: Nonpenetrating cardiac injuries: A collective review. Am. Heart J. *86*:687, 1973.
8. Symbas, P. N.: Cardiac trauma. Am. Heart J. *92*:387, 1976.
9. MacKintosh, A. F., and Fleming, H. A.: Cardiac damage presenting late after road accidents. Thorax *36*:811, 1981.
10. Allen, R. P., and Liedtke, A. J.: The role of coronary artery injury and perfusion in the development of cardiac contusion secondary to nonpenetrating chest trauma. J. Trauma *19*:153, 1979.
11. DeMuth, W. E., Lerner, E. H., and Liedtke, A. J.: Nonpenetrating injury of the heart: An experimental model. J. Trauma *13*:639, 1973.
12. Coats, R. R., Sakai, K., and Lam, C. R.: Extensive diaphragmatic rupture—Pericardial rupture from blunt trauma. J. Thorac. Cardiovasc. Surg. *17*:223, 1974.
13. King, J. B., and Sapsford, R. N.: Acute rupture of the pericardium with delayed dislocation of the heart: A case report. Injury *9*:303, 1978.
14. Bright, E. F., and Beck, C. S.: Nonpenetrating wounds of the heart: Clinical and experimental studies. Am. Heart J. *10*:293, 1935.
15. Anderson, A. E., and Doty, D. B.: Cardiac trauma: An experimental model of isolated myocardial contusion. J. Trauma *15*:237, 1975.
16. Lau, V.-K., Viano, D.C., and Doty, D. B.: Experimental cardiac trauma—Ballistics of a captive bolt pistol. J. Trauma *21*:39, 1982.
17. Stein, P. D., Sabbah, H. N., Viano, D. C., and Vostal, J. J.: Response of the heart to nonpenetrating cardiac trauma. J. Trauma *22*:364, 1982.
18. Gay, W.: Blunt trauma to the heart and great vessels. Surgery *91*:507, 1982.
19. Jones, J. W., Hewitt, R. L., and Drapanas, T.: Cardiac contusion: A capricious syndrome. Ann. Surg. *181*:567, 1975.
20. Saunders, C. R., and Doty, D. B.: Myocardial contusion Surg. Gynecol. Obstet. *144*:595, 1977.
21. Watson, J. H., and Bartholomae, W. M.: Cardiac injury due to nonpenetrating chest trauma. Ann. Intern. Med. *52*:871, 1960.
22. Potkin, R. T., Werner, J. A., Trobaugh, G. B., Chestnut, C. H., III, Carrico, C. J., Hallstrom, A., and Cobb, L. A.: Evaluation of noninvasive tests of cardiac damage in suspected cardiac contusion. Circulation *66*:627, 1982.
23. Katz, S., Gimmon, Z., and Appelbaum, A.: Cardiac contusion in the patient with multiple injuries. Injury *12*:180, 1980.
24. Lindsey, D., Navin, T. R., and Finley, P. R.: Transient elevation of serum activity of MB isoenzyme of creatine phosphokinase in drivers involved in automobile accidents. Chest *74*:15, 1978.
25. Torres-Mirabal, P., Gruenberg, J. C., Brown, R. S., and Obeid, F. N.: Spectrum of myocardial contusion. Am. Surg. *48*:383, 1982.
26. McConnell, B. J., McConnell, R. W., and Guiberteau, M. J.: Radionuclide imaging in blunt trauma. Radiol. Clin. North Am. *19*:37, 1981.
27. Ware, R. E., Martin, L. G., Tyras, D. H., Kourias, E., and Symbas, P. N.: Coronary arterial injection of radioactive albumin microspheres in diagnosis of experimental myocardial contusion. Surg. Forum *23*:138, 1972.
28. Chiu, C. L., Roelofs, J. D., Go, R. T., Doty, D. B., Rose, E. F., and Christie, J. H.: Coronary angiographic and scintigraphic findings in experimental cardiac contusion. Radiology *116*:679, 1975.
29. Downey, J., Chagrasulis, R., Fore, D., and Parmley, L.F.: Accumulation of technetium-99m stannous pyrophosphate in contused myocardium. J. Nucl. Med. *18*:1171, 1977.
30. Sutherland, G. R., Calvin, J. E., Driedger, A. A., Holliday, R. L., and Sibbald, W. J.: Anatomic and cardiopulmonary responses to trauma with associated blunt chest injury. J. Trauma *21*:1, 1981.
31. Bharati, S., Chervony, A., Gruhn, J., Rosen, K. M., and Lew, M.: Atrial arrhythmias related to trauma to the sinoatrial node. Chest *61*:331, 1972.
32. Fox, K. M., Rowland, E., Krikler, D. M., Bentall, H. H., and Goodwin, J. F.: Electrophysiological manifestations on nonpenetrating cardiac trauma. Br. Heart J. *43*:458, 1980.
33. Fox, K. M., Rowland, E., Krikler, D. M., Bentall, H. H., and Goodwin, J. F.: Electrophysiological manifestations of nonpenetrating cardiac trauma. Br. Heart J. *43*:458, 1980.
34. Brennan, J. A., Field, J. M., and Liedtke, A. J.: Reversible heart block following nonpenetrating chest trauma. J. Trauma *19*:784, 1979.
35. Bognolo, D. A., Rabow, F. I., Vijayanagar, R. R., and Eckstein, P. F.: Traumatic sinus node dysfunction. Ann. Emerg. Med. *11*:319, 1982.
36. Torres-Mirabal, P., Gruenberg, J. C., Talbert, J. G., and Brown, R. S.: Ventricular function in myocardial contusion: A preliminary study. Crit. Care Med. *10*:19, 1982.
37. Wainwright, R. J., Edwards, A. C., Maisey, M. N., and Sowton, E.: Early occlusion and late stricture of normal coronary arteries following blunt chest trauma. Chest *78*:796, 1980.
38. DeSa'Neto, A., Padnick, M. B., Desser, K. B., and Steinhoff, N. G.: Right sinus of valsalva–right atrial fistula secondary to nonpenetrating chest trauma. Circulation *60*:205, 1979
39. Rheuban, K. S., Tompkins, D. G., Nolan, S. P., Berger, B., Martin, R., and

Schneider, J. A.: Myocardial necrosis and ventricular aneurysm following closed chest injury in a child. J. Trauma *21*:170, 1981.
40. Candell, J., Valle, V., Payá, J., Cortadellas, J., Esplugas, E., and Rius, J.: Post-traumatic coronary occlusion and early left ventricular aneurysm. Am. Heart J. 97:509, 1979.
41. Allen, R. P., and Liedtke, A. J.: The role of coronary artery injury and perfusion in the development of cardiac contusion secondary to nonpenetrating chest trauma. J. Trauma *19*:153, 1979.
42. Smith, J. M., III, Grober, F. L., Marcos, J. J., Arom, K. V., and Trinkle, J. K.: Blunt traumatic rupture of the atria. J. Thorac. Cardiovasc. Surg. *71*:617, 1976.
43. Hines, G. L., Doyle, E., and Acinapura, A. J.: Post-traumatic ventricular septal defect, mitral insufficiency, and multiple coronary cameral fistulas. J. Trauma *17*:234, 1977.
44. Rayner, A. V. S., Fulton, R. L., Hess, P. J., and Daicoff, G. R.: Post-traumatic intracardiac shunts. Report of 2 cases and review of the literature. J. Thorac. Cardiovasc. Surg. *73*:728, 1977.
45. Pickard, L. R., Mattox, K. L., and Beall, A. C., Jr.: Ventricular septal defect from blunt chest injury. J. Trauma *20*:329, 1980.
46. Williams, J. B., Silver, D. G., and Laws, H. L: Successful management of heart rupture from blunt trauma. J. Trauma *21*:534, 1981.
47. Kouwenhoven, W. B., Jude, J. R., and Knickerbocker, G. G.: Closed chest cardiac massage. J.A.M.A. *173*:1064, 1966.
48. Bodily, K., and Fischer, R. P.: Aortic rupture and right ventricular rupture induced by closed chest cardiac massage. Minn. Med. *62*:225, 1979.
49. Adelson, L.: A clinicopathologic study of the anatomic changes in the heart resulting from cardiac massage. Surg. Gynecol. Obstet. *104*:513, 1957.
50. Gerry, J. L., Bulkley, B. H., and Hutchins, G. M.: Rupture of the papillary muscle of the tricuspid valve. A complication of cardiopulmonary resuscitation and a rare cause of tricuspid insufficiency. Am. J. Cardiol. *40*:825, 1977.
51. Wolfe, W. G., Dudley, A. W., Jr., and Wallace, A. G.: A pathological study of unsuccessful cardiac resuscitation. Arch. Surg. *96*:123, 1968.
52. Nelson, D. A., and Ashley, P. F.: Rupture of aorta during closed-chest cardiac massage. J.A.M.A. *193*:681, 1965.
53. Clark, D. T.: Complications following closed-chest massage. J.A.M.A. *181*: 337, 1962.
54. Rehn, L.: Ueber penetrirende Herzwunden und Herznaht. Arch. Klin. Chir. *55*: 315, 1897.
55. Wilson, R. F., and Bassett, J.S.: Penetrating wounds of the pericardium or its contents. J.A.M.A. *195*:513, 1966.
56. Symbas, P. N.: Chest trauma: What injury, what treatment approach? J. Cardiovasc. Med. *6*:989, 1981.
57. Jones, E. W., and Helmsworth, J.: Penetrating wounds of the heart. Thirty years' experience. Arch. Surg. *96*:671, 1968.
58. Fallahnejad, M., Kutty, A. C. K., and Wallace, H. W.: Secondary lesions of penetrating cardiac injuries. Ann. Surg. *191*:228, 1980.
59. Doering, R. B., Stemmer, E. A., and Connolly, J. E.: Complications of indwelling venous catheters with particular reference to catheter embolus. Am. J. Surg. *114*:259, 1967.
60. Bernhardt, L. C., Wegner, G. P., and Mendenhall, J. T.: Intravenous catheter embolization to the pulmonary artery. Chest *57*:329, 1970.
61. Bloomfield, D. A.: The nonsurgical retrieval of intracardiac foreign bodies—An international survey. Cathet. Cardiovasc. Diagn. *4*:1, 1978.
62. Escher, D. J. W.: Types of pacemakers and their complications. Circulation *47*: 1119, 1973.
63. Kaye, D., Frankl, D., and Arditi, L. I.: Probable postcardiotomy syndrome following implantation of a transvenous pacemaker. Report of the first case. Am. Heart J. *90*:627, 1975.
64. Gorlin, R.: Perforations and other cardiac complications. Chapter 6 in Cooperative Study on Cardiac Catheterization. Circulation *47* (Suppl. 3):36, 1968.
65. Morrow, A. G., Reis, R. L., and Ross, J., Jr.: Cardiac tamponade during cardiac catheterization. Management by immediate pericardiostomy and drainage. Am. Heart J. *77*:167, 1969.
66. Wellons, H. A., Jr., and Singh, R.: Acute dissecting aortic aneurysm resulting from retrograde brachial arterial catheterization. Successful operative intervention. Am. J. Cardiol. *33*:562, 1974.
67. Wilder, J. R., Dhar, N., Kudchadkar, A., and Kryger, S.: Penetration injury to the heart. J.A.M.A. *244*:2080, 1980.
68. Boyd, T. F., and Strieder, J. W.: Immediate surgery for traumatic heart disease. J. Thorac. Cardiovasc. Surg. *50*:305, 1965.
68a. Hassett, A., Moran, J., Sabiston, D. C., and Kisslo, J.: Use of echocardiography for the evaluation and management of penetrating missile wounds of the heart. J. Am. Coll. Cardiol. *1*:708, 1983.
69. Cooper, F. W., Jr., Stead, E. A., Jr., and Warren, J. V.: The beneficial effect of intravenous infusions in acute pericardial tamponade. Ann. Surg. *120*:822, 1944.
70. Fallah-Nejad, M., Wallace, H. W., Su, C. C., Kutty, A. C., and Blakemore, W. S.: Unusual manifestation of penetrating cardiac injuries. Arch. Surg. *11*: 1257, 1975.
71. Lemos, P. C. P., Akumura, M., Azeveda, A. C., DePaula, W., and Zerbini, E. J.: Cardiac wounds: Experience based on a series of 121 operated cases. J. Cardiovasc. Surg. *17*:1, 1976.
72. Harvey, J. C., and Pacifico, A. D.: Primary operative management. Method of choice for stab wounds to the heart. South. Med. J. *68*:149, 1975.
73. Symbas, P. N., Harlaftis, M. D., and Waldo, J. W.: Penetrating cardiac wounds: A comparison of different therapeutic methods. Ann. Surg. *183*:377, 1976.
74. Szentpetery, S., and Lower, R. R.: Changing concepts in the treatment of penetrating cardiac injuries. J. Trauma *17*:457, 1977.
75. Beach, P. M., Jr., Bognolo, D., and Hutchinson, J. E.: Penetrating cardiac trauma. Experience with 34 patients in a hospital without cardiopulmonary bypass capability. Am. J. Surg. *131*:411, 1976.
76. Bland, E. F., and Beebe, G. W.: Missiles in the heart. A twenty-five year follow-up report of World War II cases. N. Engl. J. Med. *274*:1039, 1966.
77. Moncada, R., Matuga, T., Unger, E., Freeark, R., and Pizarro, A.: Migratory trauma—cardiovascular foreign bodies. Circulation *57*:186, 1978.
78. Alsofrom, D. J., Marcus, N. H., Seigel, R. S., Talbot, W. A., Akl, B. F., Schiller, W. R., and Sklar, D. P.: Shotgun pellet embolization from the chest to the middle cerebral arteries. J. Trauma *22*:155, 1982.
79. Mattox, K. L., Beall, A. C., Jr., Ennix, C. L., and DeBakey, M. E.: Intravascular migratory bullets. Am. J. Surg. *137*:192, 1979.
80. Asfaw, I., Thoms, N. W., and Arfulu, A.: Interventricular septal defects from penetrating injuries of the heart. A report of 12 cases and review of the literature. J. Thorac. Cardiovasc. Surg. *69*:450, 1975.
81. Morritt, G. N., Taylor, N. C., Miller, H. C., and Walbaum, P. R.: Traumatic aortic regurgitation. J. R. Coll. Surg. (Edinb.) *24*:87, 1979.
82. Stephenson, L. W., MacVaugh, H., III, and Kastor, J. A.: Tricuspid valvular incompetence and rupture of the ventricular septum caused by nonpenetrating trauma. J. Thorac. Cardiovasc. Surg. *77*:768, 1979.
83. Watanabe, T., Katsume, H., Matsukubo, H., Furukawa, K., and Ijichi, H.: Ruptured chordae tendineae of the tricuspid valve due to nonpenetrating trauma. Chest *80*:751, 1981.
84. Howard, C. P.: Aortic insufficiency due to rupture by strain of a normal aortic valve. Can. Med. Assoc. J. *19*:12, 1928.
85. Kimbler, R. W., Stokes, J. P., and Barnhorst, D. A.: The surgical treatment of traumatic rupture of the aortic valve. Report of a case after blunt trauma. J. Trauma *17*:168, 1977.
86. Roberts, W. C., and Maron, B. J.: Sudden death while playing professional football. Am. Heart J. *102*:1061, 1981.
87. Pifarre, R., Grieco, J., Garibaldi, A., Sullivan, H. J., Montoya, A., and Bakhos, M.: Acute coronary artery occlusion secondary to blunt chest trauma. J. Thorac. Cardiovasc. Surg. *83*:122, 1982.
88. Vlay, S. C., Blumenthal, D. S., Shoback, D., Fehir, K., and Bulkley, B. H.: Delayed acute myocardial infarction after blunt chest trauma in a young woman. Am. Heart J. *100*:907, 1980.
89. Anderson, G. P., Adicoff, A., Motsay, G. J., Sako, Y., and Gobel, F. L.: Traumatic right coronary arterial–right atrial fistula. Am. J. Cardiol. *35*:439, 1975.
90. Alter, B. R., Wheeling, J. R., Martin, H. A., Margo, J. P., Treasure, R. L., and McGranahan, G. M., Jr.: Traumatic right coronary artery–right ventricular fistula with retained intramyocardial bullet. Am. J. Cardiol. *40*:815, 1971.
91. Snyder, J. S., Lindsay, J., Jr., Faris, J. V., and Glasser, S. P.: Traumatic coronary artery fistula. South. Med. J. *71*:649, 1978.
92. Rea, W. J., Sugg, W. L., Wilson, L. C., Webb, W. R., and Ecker, R. R.: Coronary artery lacerations: An analysis of 22 patients. Ann. Thorac. Surg. *7*: 518, 1969.
93. Espada, R., Whisennard, H. H., Mattox, K. L., and Beall, A. C., Jr.: Surgical management of penetrating injuries to the coronary arteries. Surgery *78*:755, 1975.
94. Symbas, P. N.: Great vessels injury. Am. Heart J. *93*:518, 1977.
95. Greendyke, R. M.: Traumatic rupture of the aorta. Special reference to automobile accidents. J.A.M.A. *195*:527, 1966.
96. Spencer, K. L., Guerin, P. F., Blake, H. A., and Bahnson, H. T.: A report of 15 patients with traumatic rupture of the aorta. J. Thorac. Cardiovasc. Surg. *41*:1, 1961.
97. Ayella, R. J., Hankins, J. R., Turney, S. Z., and Cowley, R. A.: Ruptured thoracic aorta due to blunt trauma. J. Trauma *17*:199, 1977.
98. Puijlaert, C. B. A. J.: Roentgen diagnosis of traumatic rupture of the aorta. Radiologia Clin. *45*:217, 1976.
99. Symbas, P. N., Tyras, D. H., Ware, R. E., and Hatcher, C. R., Jr.: Rupture of the aorta. A diagnostic triad. Ann. Thorac. Surg. *15*:405, 1973.
100. Kirsh, M. M., Orringer, M. B., Behrendt, D. M., Mills, L. J., Tashjian, J., and Sloan, H.: Management of unusual traumatic ruptures of the aorta. Surg. Gynecol. Obstet. *146*:365, 1978.
101. Norman, J. C., Weber, W. J., Wilson, W. S., and Sloan, H.: Post-traumatic fistula of the aorta, pulmonary artery and right ventricle. Ann. Surg. *161*: 357, 1965
102. Arom, K. V., and Lyons, G. W.: Traumatic pulmonary arteriovenous fistula. J. Thorac. Cardiovasc. Surg. *70*:918, 1975.
103. Akins, C. W., Buckley, M. J., Daggett, W., McIlduff, J. B., and Austen, W. G.: Acute traumatic disruption of the thoracic aorta: A ten-year experience. Ann. Thorac. Surg. *31*:305, 1981.
104. Pickard, L. R., Mattox, K. L., Espada, R., Beall, A. C., and DeBakey, M. E.: Transection of the descending thoracic aorta secondary to blunt trauma. J. Trauma *17*:749, 1977.
105. Symbas, P. N., Kourias, E., Tyras, D. H., and Hatcher, C. R., Jr.: Penetrating wounds of great vessels. Ann. Surg. *179*:757, 1974.
106. Vasko, J. S., Raess, D. H., Williams, T. E., Jr., Kakos, G. S., Kilman, J. W., Meckstroth, C. V., Cattaneo, S. M., and Klassen, K. P.: Nonpenetrating trauma to the thoracic aorta. Surgery *82*:400, 1977.
107. Turney, S. Z., Attar, S., Ayella, R., Cowley, R. A., and McLaughlin, J.: Traumatic rupture of the aorta. A five-year experience. J. Thorac. Cardiovasc. Surg. *72*:727, 1976.

45 DISEASES OF THE AORTA

by Eve E. Slater, M.D., and Roman W. De Sanctis, M.D.

THE NORMAL AORTA

Function. Appropriately called by the ancients "the greatest artery," the aorta is admirably suited for its job. This thin but large and remarkably tough vessel must absorb the impact of 2.5 to 3 billion heartbeats in the average lifetime of an individual, while over the same span carrying roughly 200,000,000 liters of blood to the periphery!

Arteries can be categorized as either "conductance" or "resistance" vessels. Conductance vessels are the conduits for blood, and the aorta is the epitome of a conductance vessel. It is composed of three layers: a thin inner tunica intima; a thick tunica media; and a rather thin outer layer, the tunica adventitia. The strength of the aorta resides in its media, which is composed of laminated but intertwining sheets of elastic tissue arranged in a spiral fashion to afford maximum strength. As thin as it is, the wall of the aorta can withstand the experimental pressure of thousands of millimeters of mercury without bursting. In contrast to the peripheral arteries, the aortic media contains very little smooth muscle, although there is a network of some smooth muscle and collagen between the elastic membranes. This tremendous accretion of elastic tissue in the aorta gives it not only great tensile strength but also elasticity, which serves a vital circulatory function. The aortic intima is a thin, delicate layer linked by endothelium and easily traumatized. The adventitia contains mainly collagen but also houses the important vasa vasorum and lymphatics, which nourish the aortic wall.

As ventricular systole develops, part of the force imparted by the contracting ventricle is converted into potential energy stored in the wall of the aorta as it is distended by the bolus of blood ejected into it. In diastole, this potential energy in the stretched aortic wall is transformed into kinetic energy as the resilient aorta decompresses, and the force that is created acts against the column of blood contained within the lumen. With a competent aortic valve proximally, the blood is thus further propelled distally into the arterial bed. The pulse wave itself with its milking effect is transmitted along the aorta to the periphery at a speed of about 5 meters per second. This is much faster than the velocity of the intraluminal blood, which travels only 40 to 50 cm per second. Thus, the aorta plays a major role in keeping the blood circulating after it is delivered into the aorta by the heart.

The systolic pressure developed within the aorta is a function of the volume of blood ejected into the aorta, the compliance or distensibility of the aorta, and the resistance to blood flow. The last is determined primarily by the tone in the peripheral muscular arteries and arterioles and to a slight extent by the inertia of the column of blood in the aorta when systole commences. The aorta and its arterial branches tend to stiffen with age, accounting for the increase in systolic blood pressure as people grow older.

In addition to its conductance and pumping functions, the aorta plays a role in the control of systemic vascular resistance and heart rate. Pressure-responsive receptors analogous to those in the carotid sinus lie in the ascending aorta and the aortic arch and send afferent signals to the vasomotor center in the brain stem by way of the vagus nerves. Raising the aortic pressure causes reflex reduction of vascular resistance and bradycardia, whereas lowering the pressure increases the heart rate.

Anatomic Considerations. The aorta consists of thoracic and abdominal portions. In turn, the thoracic aorta is composed of three segments: the ascending aorta, the aortic arch, and the descending thoracic aorta.

The *ascending aorta* in a normal adult is about 3 cm wide at its origin from the base of the heart and extends 5 to 6 cm cephalad to join the arch. Normally, the ascending aorta lies just to the right of the midline. Its proximal portion is within the pericardial cavity. Nearby structures include the pulmonary trunk in front and the left atrium, right pulmonary artery, and right main stem bronchus behind.

The *arch of the aorta* gives rise to all of the brachiocephalic vessels. It courses slightly leftward in front of the trachea and then proceeds dorsally and inferiorly above the left main stem bronchus to the left of the trachea and esophagus. The arch assumes almost a directly anteroposterior orientation in the superior mediastinum. Other closely related structures are the left phrenic and vagus nerves to the left of the arch; inferiorly lie the bifurcation of the pulmonary trunk and most of the left lung. The left recurrent laryngeal nerve also loops underneath it distally.

The *descending thoracic aorta* is the continuation of the aorta beyond the arch. It lies in the posterior mediastinum to the left of the vertebral column, gradually courses in front of the vertebral column as it descends, occupying a position behind the esophagus, and passes through the diaphragm, usually at the level of the 12th thoracic vertebra.

A small but important segment called the *aortic isthmus* is the point at which the arch and descending thoracic aorta join. This is where coarctations of the aorta are usually located, and it is also the point at which the mobile portion of the aorta—the ascending aorta and arch—becomes relatively fixed to the thorax by the pleural reflections, intercostal arteries, and left subclavian artery. The aorta is especially vulnerable to trauma at this point.

The *abdominal aorta* forms the continuation of the thoracic aorta, giving off the important splanchnic vessels and ending in the aortic bifurcation at the level of the 4th lumbar vertebra.

EXAMINATION OF THE AORTA

Unless the aorta is abnormally enlarged, the only location at which it can be palpated is in the abdomen. The ease with which it can be felt depends largely on the body habitus and on the pulse pressure; it is readily felt in thin individuals. It is quite sensitive to pressure. Auscultation usually is unrevealing in aortic diseases, except for occasional bruits at sites of narrowing of the aorta or its tributary branches. Diseases of the proximal ascending aorta sometimes involve the aortic valve, with resultant aortic regurgitation.

Chest roentgenography and fluoroscopy are valuable and simple procedures for assessing the aorta. Normally, the ascending aorta is not visible on the direct anteroposterior chest roentgenogram. The aortic arch is seen as the aortic "knob" or "knuckle" in the superior mediastinum just to the left of the vertebral column (Fig. 6–1, p. 147). The edge of the descending thoracic aorta can often be recognized to the left of the spine.

On the lateral chest roentgenogram, the proximal ascending aorta can be seen as an indistinct shadow in the middle mediastinum arising from the base of the heart. The ascending aorta and arch are best demonstrated in a left anterior oblique projection—a view that should always be included when disease of the thoracic aorta is suspected (Fig. 6–12, p. 155).

Calcification in the aortic knob is often present, particularly in older people and patients with hypertension. It has little significance. Arteriosclerosis often results in extensive aortic calcification. The location of aortic calcification is useful in the differential diagnosis of aortic disease. For example, syphilis usually causes calcification of the ascending aorta predominantly, whereas arteriosclerotic calcification is ordinarily densest in the arch and the descending thoracic and abdominal aorta. Aneurysms of the abdominal aorta can often be seen radiographically if they are calcified. A lateral film of the abdomen is the most useful view for demonstrating them.

Normally, the aorta tends to elongate and widen slightly with age, a process which is accelerated by hypertension. Aneurysms, of course, appear as localized dilations of the aorta. It is sometimes difficult to distinguish aneurysms from other mediastinal masses. In such cases fluoroscopy may be very helpful by showing the presence or absence of pulsations in the mass.

Angiographic study of the aorta has represented a signal advance in the evaluation of aortic diseases. Aneurysms, aortic dissections, and occlusive disease of the aorta and its arterial branches can usually be readily demonstrated by a contrast study (Fig. 45–7). There is expectation that with technical improvements in digital subtraction angiography, performed by venous injection of contrast material, adequate aortic definition will be possible while obviating the need for catheterization of the aorta.[1]

Ultrasonography has also provided an important adjunct to the diagnosis of aortic diseases. The presence or absence of an abdominal aortic aneurysm can be definitively established by this simple noninvasive technique. In particular, cross-sectional (2-D) echocardiography (p. 135) is extremely accurate in both diagnosing and sizing abdominal aortic aneurysms (Fig. 45–1) and can also provide valuable information about the location and size of aortic root aneurysms.[2–4]

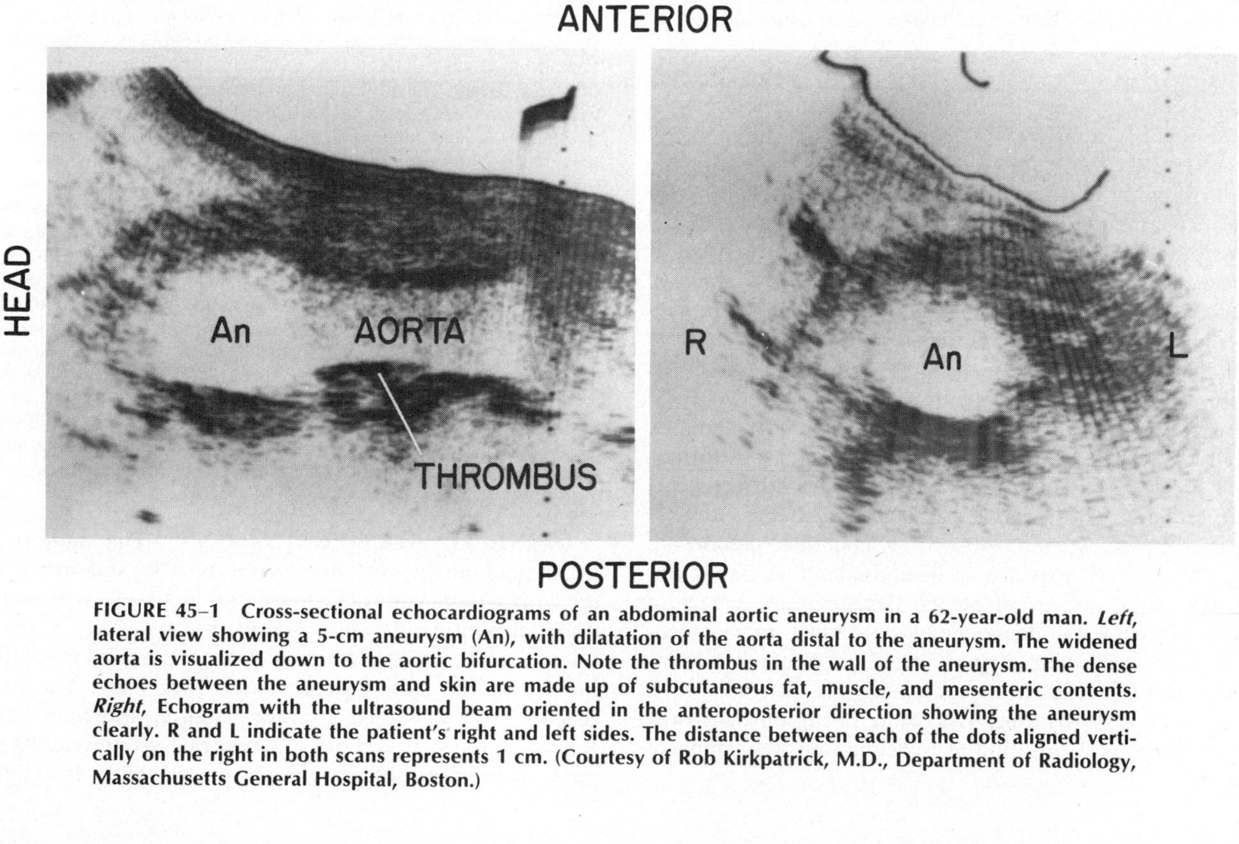

FIGURE 45–1 Cross-sectional echocardiograms of an abdominal aortic aneurysm in a 62-year-old man. *Left,* lateral view showing a 5-cm aneurysm (An), with dilatation of the aorta distal to the aneurysm. The widened aorta is visualized down to the aortic bifurcation. Note the thrombus in the wall of the aneurysm. The dense echoes between the aneurysm and skin are made up of subcutaneous fat, muscle, and mesenteric contents. *Right,* Echogram with the ultrasound beam oriented in the anteroposterior direction showing the aneurysm clearly. R and L indicate the patient's right and left sides. The distance between each of the dots aligned vertically on the right in both scans represents 1 cm. (Courtesy of Rob Kirkpatrick, M.D., Department of Radiology, Massachusetts General Hospital, Boston.)

Computed tomographic scanning of the body (CT scan), enhanced by intravenous injection of contrast material, is being used increasingly for noninvasive visualization of the aorta (see Fig. 45–4). CT scans are particularly useful for the diagnosis and sizing of thoracic and abdominal aortic aneurysms and for the diagnosis of aortic dissection and traumatic aneurysms of the aorta.[5,6,6a] In determining the size of abdominal aortic aneurysms, the CT scan is as accurate as ultrasonography, if not more so.

DISEASES OF THE AORTA

Pathogenesis

Although the pathogenesis of diseases of the aorta is discussed in several of the individual subsections, a brief commentary upon those factors which act adversely upon the aorta is appropriate at this point. Diseases of the aorta are either congenital or acquired. Congenital defects in turn are either gross anatomical abnormalities, such as coarctation, right aortic arch, anomalous arterial branches, double aortic arches, and so on, or histological disorders, such as degenerative abnormalities in the aortic wall that predispose to later problems, e.g., cystic medial degeneration in the Marfan syndrome and other inherited connective tissue disorders.

Acquired diseases of the aorta are primarily the result of degenerative changes in the aortic wall. Prominent among the factors which lead to this degeneration are aging, arteriosclerosis, hypertension, and specific infectious, inflammatory, or autoimmune diseases that involve the aorta focally or diffusely. Some of these processes may affect the aortic root, with resultant aortic regurgitation, or the major arterial branches arising from the aorta. Recently, the importance of the velocity at which blood is ejected from the left ventricle (dV/dt) as a major shearing stress on the aortic wall has also been emphasized as promoting aortic dissection.[8]

Arteriosclerosis is especially important in the pathogenesis of aortic aneurysms. There are several current theories, none mutually exclusive, to explain the development of atherosclerosis.[5] These are reviewed in Chapter 34.

Iwatsuki and colleagues have conducted a fascinating series of experiments: The initiation and maintenance of experimentally induced hypertension could be prevented or reversed by the inhibition of collagen cross linkage through administration of β-aminopropionitrile. This suggests that hypertension leads to structural aortic changes which, in turn, initiate an aortic response that serves to perpetuate the hypertensive syndrome.[9]

Indeed, hypertension itself may promote further damage, not only by injuring the endothelium or increasing formation of collagen but also by accelerating medial degeneration in patients with a molecular defect in their structural proteins, i.e., collagen or elastin—which then deteriorate more rapidly when exposed to hemodynamic stress. It appears that some degree of medial degeneration is part of the aging process, but these changes are much more extensive in individuals with hypertension.[10–12] Acute hypertension has also been shown experimentally to decrease blood flow into the vasa vasorum, thereby reducing nutrient flow into the media and resulting in ischemia and weakening of the wall.[13]

The only congenital gross anatomical disease considered in this chapter is pseudocoarctation. *Coarctation* is discussed on pages 887, 973, and 1038. All other conditions discussed either are acquired or result from congenital histological changes in the aortic wall.

ARTERIOSCLEROTIC AORTIC ANEURYSMS

Abdominal Aortic Aneurysms

Approximately three-quarters of all arteriosclerotic aortic aneurysms are confined to the abdominal aorta. Normally, in the adult, the aorta measures 2 cm in diameter at the level of the celiac axis, measures 1.8 cm just below the renal arteries, and continues to taper slightly to the iliac vessels. It is in the area between the renal arteries and the aortic bifurcation that most abdominal aneurysms occur. Clinically significant aneurysms measure 4 cm or more in diameter. (Charles De Gaulle, Albert Einstein, and Robert Frost all succumbed to ruptured abdominal aortic aneurysms.)

Etiology and Pathogenesis. Abdominal aortic aneurysms arise in some areas of dense atherosclerosis. The atherosclerotic process erodes the aortic wall, destroying the medial elastic elements. This causes weakening of the aortic wall and eventually leads to fusiform or, rarely, saccular dilatation of the abdominal aorta. As the aorta widens, tension in the wall of the aorta rises in accordance with Laplace law, which states that tension is proportional to the product of pressure and radius. Further widening results in greater tension, which in turn leads to acceleration in the rate of enlargement of the aneurysm. A vicious circle is thus established which produces dilatation that is often rapidly progressive. Hypertension may also contribute to the pathogenesis of these aneurysms.

Most abdominal aortic aneurysms arise just below the renal arteries and extend to, and sometimes involve, the aortic bifurcation. Only 2 to 5 per cent of abdominal aortic aneurysms are suprarenal, and these usually result from the distal extension of a thoracic aneurysm into the abdomen.[14] As aneurysms expand they may compress contiguous structures. Laminated thrombi frequently form in areas of stagnant flow within the aneurysm. Thrombotic and arteriosclerotic debris may embolize distally[15] (p. 1566) and compromise the circulation of tributary arteries. Finally, the aneurysm may rupture. Of those aneurysms which do rupture, 80 to 90 per cent rupture retroperitoneally, with a mean interval of 24 hours between rupture and death. The remainder rupture into the peritoneal cavity, causing rapid demise from exsanguination.[16]

CLINICAL MANIFESTATIONS. The majority of abdominal aneurysms are asymptomatic and are discovered on routine physical examination or on a routine abdominal roentgenogram.[17] Aneurysms may cause a sense of fullness in the epigastrium. If pain is present, it is usually located in the hypogastrium and lower back. The pain is usually steady, with a gnawing quality, and may last for hours or days at a time. In contrast to musculoskeletal back pain, it is not affected by movement, although patients may be more comfortable in certain positions, such as with the legs drawn up. Some astute asymptomatic patients may suspect an aneurysm by recognizing an abnormal pulsation of the aorta, as when lying down reading a book perched on the abdomen. Expansion and impending rupture are heralded by the development of pain, often of sudden onset, which is characteristically constant and severe and located in the back or lower abdomen, sometimes with radiation into groin, buttocks, or legs. Actual rupture is associated with the abrupt onset of catastrophic abdominal or back pain or both, hypotension, and usually shock. Pain is ordinarily particularly severe in the retroperitoneal area.[18,19]

Many aneurysms can be detected on physical examination, although even large aneurysms may be difficult or impossible to detect in obese individuals. When palpable, a pulsatile mass extending variably from between the xiphoid process to the umbilicus may be appreciated. Owing to difficulty in separating the abdominal aorta from surrounding structures by palpation, the size of an aneurysm tends to be overestimated in the physical examination. Moreover, it may sometimes be difficult to differentiate a tortuous, ectatic aorta from true aneurysmal dilatation. Aneurysms are often sensitive to palpation and may be quite tender if they are rapidly expanding or about to rupture. Aneurysms should always be palpated cautiously, particularly if they are tender.[20]

Associated occlusive arterial disease is sometimes present in the femoral pulses and pulses distally in the legs or feet. Bruits may be heard over the aneurysm or arising from the diseased arteries but are not requisite to the diagnosis. Rarely, an aneurysm may expand in such a way to occlude the inferior vena cava or one of the iliac veins, resulting in venous congestion and edema in one or both legs. Occasionally an arteriovenous fistula may be formed by spontaneous rupture into the inferior vena cava or iliac vein, and a syndrome of high-output cardiac failure results.

Patients who suffer rupture of an abdominal aortic aneurysm are critically ill. Hemorrhagic shock may ensue rapidly and is manifested by hypotension, vasoconstriction, skin mottling, diaphoresis, mental obtundation, and oliguria. Retroperitoneal hemorrhage may be signaled by hematomas in the flanks and groin. Rupture into the abdominal cavity may result in abdominal distention, whereas rupture into the duodenum presents as massive gastrointestinal hemorrhage.

DIAGNOSIS AND SIZING OF ANEURYSMS. Currently, aneurysms may be detected and their size estimated by six methods: (1) physical examination, (2) routine roentgenography, (3) abdominal cross-sectional echocardiography, (4) CT scan, (5) abdominal aortic angiography, and (6) digital subtraction angiography.

Brewster and colleagues have carefully compared the physical examination, routine roentgenography, two-dimensional echocardiography and aortic angiography for sizing abdominal aortic aneurysms.[21] Physical examination is clearly the least accurate. Lateral x-ray examination of the lumbar spine is inexpensive and reliably detects the outline of the aneurysm if its wall is calcified (Fig. 45–2). However, this is not the case in at least one-quarter of all patients with aneurysms; in them, therefore, the lesion cannot be visualized radiographically.[22]

Cross-sectional ultrasound is very accurate and is easily and atraumatically performed (Fig. 45–1). Refinements in ultrasonic techniques have permitted precise determination of the aortic adventitial border. Thus abdominal ultrasound is currently the simplest and best way to detect and size an abdominal aortic aneurysm.

Abdominal aortic angiography is less accurate in predicting size because the full width of an aneurysm may be masked by the presence of nonopacified mural thrombus (Fig. 45–3). Moreover, angiography carries with it a small but definite incidence of complications, including hematoma, localized dissection, infection, embolization, and renal

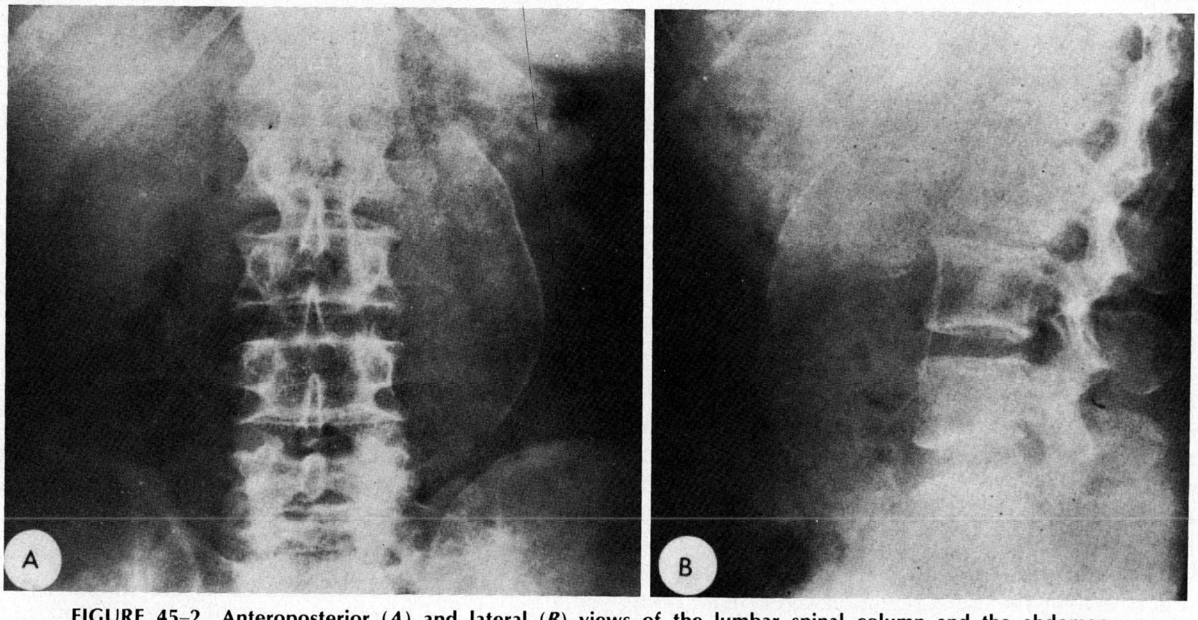

FIGURE 45–2 Anteroposterior (*A*) and lateral (*B*) views of the lumbar spinal column and the abdomen, disclosing a soft tissue mass with curvilinear calcification. (From Estes, J. E., Jr.: Abdominal aortic aneurysm: A study of one hundred and two cases. Circulation *2*:261, 1950, by permission of the American Heart Association, Inc.)

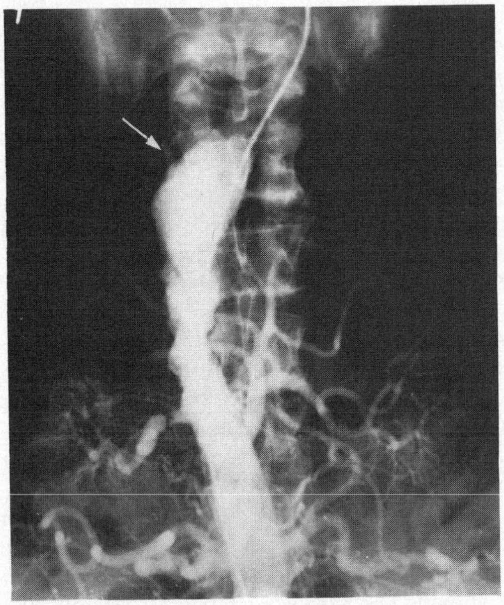

FIGURE 45–3 Abdominal aortogram showing an abdominal aortic aneurysm in a 64-year-old man. The aneurysm measures almost 6 cm in diameter and is wider than it appears because of a laminated thrombus in its wall. A faint rim of calcification outlining the left side of the aneurysm can be seen (arrow). The left renal artery is significantly narrowed. (Courtesy of Christos Athanasoulis, M.D., and Arthur Waltman, M.D., Section of Vascular Radiology, Massachusetts General Hospital, Boston.)

failure. Nevertheless, when angiography is performed in experienced hands, the morbidity from the procedure is minimal, and valuable information is often gleaned from it. Thus, in a survey of 190 patients, angiography of the aorta and distal circulation resulted in only minor complications in 2 per cent; averted an incorrect diagnosis in 11 per cent; revealed extension of the aneurysm above the renal arteries in 5 per cent; showed renal artery stenosis in 22 per cent and atypical renal arterial anatomy in 17 per cent; and delineated significant occlusive vascular disease in 48 per cent and associated aneurysms of the iliac, hypogastric, femoral, and popliteal vessels in 50 per cent.[23] Thus, aortography—if performed by experienced angiographers—is currently recommended for patients in whom there is any question of a correct diagnosis, for hypertensive patients with possible renal arterial disease, when the extent of the aneurysm is unclear, and for patients with suspected associated occlusive or aneurysmal diseases. In fact, at our institution, it is done routinely in most patients under consideration for surgery in order to facilitate perioperative management.

Current experience with CT scanning indicates that it may prove to be as useful as or even more accurate than ultrasound in the diagnosis and measurement of abdominal aortic aneurysms (see Fig. 45–4). CT scanning has additional advantages over ultrasound in that it provides information about the location of the renal arteries in relationship to the aneurysm; it may demonstrate retroperitoneal hemorrhage from an aneurysm; and it provides potentially useful information about other abdominal organs.[5,6] On the other hand, it does involve the use of radiation and is more costly and time-consuming than ultrasound.

Although experience with *digital subtraction angiography* (p. 191) is only now being accumulated, it is hoped that this technique will eventually yield information as detailed as that provided by aortography, while eliminating the need for intraarterial injection.

NATURAL HISTORY. There is a crucial relationship between the size of aneurysms and their natural history, which is why it is so important to determine their width. Half of all aneurysms greater than 6 cm in diameter rupture within 1 year, compared with 15 to 20 per cent of aneurysms less than 6 cm.[24] In a review of 24,000 consecutive autopsies, Darling et al. found that aneurysms 10 cm or larger had a 60 per cent incidence of rupture; those between 7 and 10 cm had a 45 per cent incidence of rupture; and those measuring 4 to 7 cm had a 25 per cent incidence of rupture.[25] The time course of rupture is hard to judge in such studies because so many patients succumb to complications of associated arteriosclerosis elsewhere, especially disease of the cerebrovascular and coronary arteries. However, Szilagyi et al. have computed mean survival for patients with aneurysms of less than 6 cm as 34.1 months, compared with 17.0 months for aneurysms greater than 6 cm.[24]

MANAGEMENT. At present, elective surgery is advised for all abdominal aortic aneurysms 6 cm in diameter or wider, assuming that surgical risks are not prohibitive because of other medical problems. Indeed, on the basis of Darling's studies, aneurysms as small as 4 cm should be resected in otherwise good surgical candidates. In poor-risk patients with aneurysms of 4 to 6 cm, close follow-up is advised with immediate surgery if the aneurysm is expanding or shows signs of impending rupture.

Surgery consists of resection of the aneurysm and insertion of a prosthesis, of which Dacron is the most widely

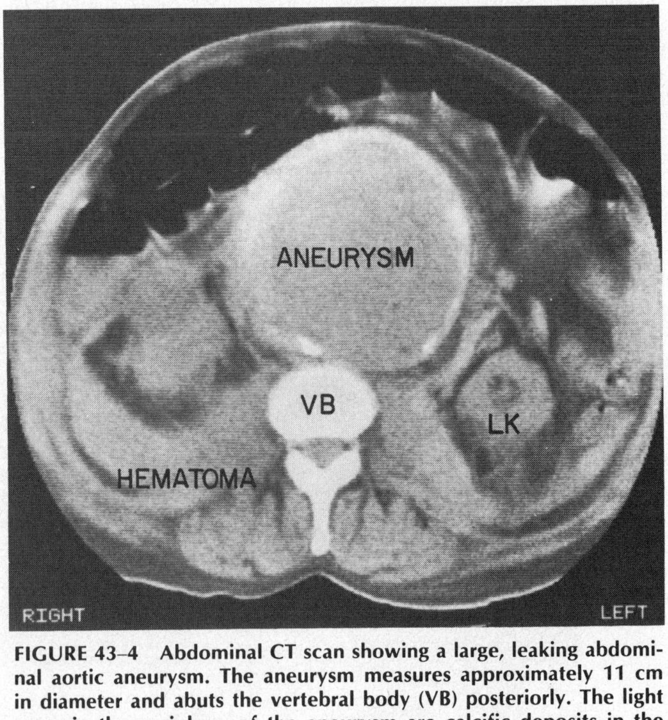

FIGURE 43–4 Abdominal CT scan showing a large, leaking abdominal aortic aneurysm. The aneurysm measures approximately 11 cm in diameter and abuts the vertebral body (VB) posteriorly. The light areas in the periphery of the aneurysm are calcific deposits in the aortic wall. The lower pole of the left kidney is identified (LK), and behind the right kidney is a retroperitoneal hematoma. (Courtesy of Dr. Jack Wittenberg, Department of Radiology, Massachusetts General Hospital, Boston.)

used at present.[26] Sometimes a simple tube graft is all that is necessary, although frequently the operation must be carried distally into one or both iliac vessels in order to excise the aneurysm completely. With large aneurysms, much of the wall of the aneurysm may be left in situ ("intrasaccular" approach of Creech). This reduces the need for extensive dissection, thereby decreasing aortic cross-clamping time, and has significantly diminished the problem of postoperative sexual dysfunction.

Expanding or ruptured abdominal aortic aneurysms are true surgical emergencies. In the case of rupture, patients can sometimes be stabilized by using a compression G-suit, a garment which may diminish the rate of bleeding by exerting counterforce externally against the abdomen. However, operation must be undertaken as soon as possible.[16]

Advances in perioperative management have improved survival rates in patients undergoing surgical resection of abdominal aortic aneurysms. Many of these patients have significant heart disease, and monitoring of the arterial blood pressure, cardiac output, cardiac filling pressures, and urine output may help enormously in their operative management.[27] These measurements provide a valuable guide to volume replacement. So-called "declamping shock" has been virtually eliminated by volume replacement guided by monitored pressures.[28] This term is applied to a syndrome characterized by marked hypotension upon release of the aortic cross clamp at the completion of surgery; the cause is believed to be pooling of blood in the dilated distal vascular bed and release of vasodepressor substances that have accumulated during surgery distal to the aortic clamp. The administration of mannitol and potent loop diuretics such as intravenous furosemide has reduced the frequency of postoperative renal failure.[29] The occurrence of renal failure postoperatively in patients with ruptured abdominal aortic aneurysms has correlated with very poor survival rates.[30] Autotransfusion has led to less frequent occurrence of hepatitis and fewer transfusion reactions.[31] Antibiotic coverage has reduced the frequency of infections. Hypothermia has been better controlled, and better understanding of the clotting system has improved management of hemostasis.[32]

Many patients with abdominal aortic aneurysms are heavy smokers and have serious chronic obstructive lung disease. Such patients have benefited greatly by improvements in postoperative respiratory care. Preoperative preparation of pulmonary patients is also important, and smokers should abstain from tobacco for at least 1 month in advance of surgery.[33]

If there is evidence of carotid artery disease in patients facing elective aneurysm resection, preoperative evaluation and surgery for critical carotid stenoses, if indicated, have resulted in fewer strokes. In occasional patients with severe coronary artery disease, it has proved wise to evaluate the coronary arterial tree angiographically and to perform coronary bypass surgery, if indicated, before subjecting the patient to aneurysm resection.[34] In cases of associated renal artery stenosis with renin-dependent hypertension or severe stenosis jeopardizing renal function, simultaneous renal artery reconstruction is often performed.[35]

OPERATIVE RISK. The risk of operation obviously depends on the general status of the patient and on whether or not the aneurysm has ruptured. Prompt recognition and immediate operation for patients with rupture have markedly improved survival rates. In low-risk patients, the mortality from the elective resection of abdominal aortic aneurysms should be 2 to 7 per cent. With expanding aneurysms, mortality is 5 to 15 per cent, and with rupture, mortality has reached a plateau at approximately 50 per cent, the major determinant of survival being the speed with which surgery is accomplished.[24,29,32,35–39]

Age and preexisting cardiac, pulmonary, cerebrovascular, and/or renal diseases all add to the risk of operation. Nevertheless, resection of nonruptured aneurysms in 63 octogenarian patients was accomplished with a 5 per cent overall mortality in an experienced center, contrasted with a 50 per cent mortality for unoperated-on patients; thus age per se should not be a definite contraindication for surgery in an otherwise healthy patient.[40]

An alternative to aneurysmectomy for very high-risk patients has been reported by Leather et al.[41] This group has combined thrombosis of the aortic aneurysm with right axillary to bilateral femoral artery bypass conduits. Thrombosis of the aneurysm usually followed the interruption of flow below the aortic bifurcation achieved by ligation of the iliac outflow vessels. If the aneurysm did not thrombose within 72 hours, the iliac outflow vessels responsible for continued patency were identified by angiography and were occluded by intraarterial injection of bucrylate. Although the perioperative and late mortality in these patients was high (6 deaths among 15 patients), the deaths were mostly related to associated diseases and not to the operative procedure itself.

The statistics showing better survival with elective resection of aneurysms are impressive. From several reports, the 5-year survival rate is only 5 to 10 per cent in patients with unexcised aneurysms larger than 6 cm, compared with over 50 per cent for those who undergo resection and 80 per cent for the age-matched "normal" population. *Late* survival is unaffected by whether the aneurysm was electively resected, acute, or ruptured.[39] With aneurysms smaller than 6 cm, the 5-year unoperated survival rate is about 50 per cent, as opposed to 60 to 70 per cent for those who undergo resection.[20,42–45]

COMPLICATIONS. The rate of late complications of aneurysmectomy has been reported as 8.5 per cent.[46] These complications include occlusion of the prosthesis (4 per cent), stenosis (0.6 per cent), false aneurysm formation (3 per cent), enteric fistula formation (1 per cent), and infection (3 per cent). Patients with graft occlusion usually have evidence of prior distal vascular disease which impedes aortic runoff. Occlusions occur mainly at the sites of anastomosis, and patients usually develop ischemic symptoms distal to the graft site. These stenoses may be increasingly amenable to correction by balloon catheter angioplasty (p. 297). False aneurysms may be caused by infection, but others arise spontaneously and are seen as expanding masses in the groin, abdomen, or lower back. Enteric fistulas are caused by rupture of the graft into the duodenum, resulting in gastrointestinal hemorrhage, and are associated with a high mortality. This complication can occur anywhere from 1 day to several years after operation, and the diagnosis must be suspected in any patient who has undergone abdominal aneurysmectomy and who presents with melena, hematemesis, hematochezia, or abdominal pain.[47] Recognition is obtained by gastrointestinal series, endoscopy, colonoscopy, or angiography. Infections most commonly are seen as a painful or tender groin mass, with or without a draining sinus. Recommended therapy involves administration of antibiotics, removal of the infected prosthetic material, and reestablishment of the circulation by an alternate route, usually axillofemoral bypass.

Attention has been called to the occasional occurrence of colonic ischemia following aneurysm surgery, caused by the necessary intraoperative sacrifice of the inferior mesenteric artery in patients with concomitantly diseased superior or mesenteric and hypogastric arteries, resulting in inadequate perfusion of the colon.[48,49] This complication is best avoided by paying careful attention to collateral blood flow to the colon, maintaining an inadequate blood pressure during surgery, and handling the distal colon carefully at the time of operation. If necessary, reimplantation of the inferior mesenteric artery can be performed if collateral circulation is inadequate.

THORACIC AORTIC ANEURYSMS

About one-quarter of all arteriosclerotic aneurysms involve the thoracic aorta.[50] Dilatation may occur anywhere along the thoracic aorta—that is, the ascending segment, the arch, or the descending portion; the latter two sites are the more common ones. This contrasts with luetic aneurysms, which are located predominantly in the ascending aorta. Sometimes the entire aorta is ectatic, with localized aneurysms at many sites in both the thoracic and the abdominal aorta. Aneurysms of the descending thoracic aorta not infrequently extend into the abdominal aorta, creating a thoracoabdominal aneurysm.

Pathogenesis. The pathogenesis of arteriosclerotic aneurysms is identical to that of those in the abdominal aorta. The arteriosclerotic process leads to weakening of the aortic wall, medial degeneration, and localized dilatation. Hypertension often coexists and contributes both to the undermining of the strength of the aortic wall and to expansion of the aneurysm. In the thorax, localized saccular aneurysms are somewhat more common than circumferential or fusiform aneurysms. The natural history of thoracic aneurysms differs somewhat from that of abdominal aortic aneurysms in that spontaneous rupture without warning is less common, because evidence of a growing thoracic aneurysm is usually afforded by symptoms caused by the compression of surrounding structures.[51]

CLINICAL MANIFESTATIONS. Thoracic aneurysms are very frequently associated with widespread atherosclerosis, particularly of the renal, cerebral, and cardiac arteries. In fact, the consequences of arterial obliterative disease in these other areas may dominate the clinical picture.

Symptoms and signs of thoracic aneurysms are related to their size and location and are caused primarily by their impingement upon adjacent structures. Thus, tracheal deviation, wheezing, cough, dyspnea, stridor, hemoptysis, recurrent pneumonitis, and intrapulmonary hemorrhage are the direct result of compression of the tracheobrachial tree and contiguous lung, especially the left main stem bronchus, by aneurysms of the descending thoracic aorta. Occasionally, an asymptomatic arch aneurysm will be visible or palpable rising above the suprasternal notch. Hoarseness may follow compression of the recurrent laryngeal nerve. Arch aneurysms sometimes produce a tracheal tug. Dysphagia arises from pressure against the nearby esophagus. The superior vena caval syndrome can develop as a consequence of obstruction of venous return from the superior vena cava or innominate veins.

Pain is due to compression and erosion of adjacent musculoskeletal structures. It is usually steady and boring—occasionally pulsating—and may be extremely severe. The sternum and right thoracic cage may be eroded by large aneurysms of the ascending aorta, and the vertebral column and posterior left ribs by descending thoracic aortic aneurysms. Visible and pulsatile masses are evident when aneurysms reach and begin to erode through the chest wall. Rupture of an aneurysm is heralded by the dramatic onset of excruciating pain, usually in the area where some pain had existed previously.

DIAGNOSIS. Most thoracic aortic aneurysms are readily visible on chest roentgenograms (Fig. 45–5), with fluoroscopy helping to differentiate an aneurysm from other types of mediastinal masses, such as neoplasms. However, some aneurysms are small, especially saccular aneurysms, which may rupture without having been visible on chest roentgenogram (Fig. 45–6).

Aortic angiography is clearly the definitive procedure for outlining an aneurysm, to make a diagnosis and to reveal the anatomical features of the aneurysm (Fig. 45–7). It should be performed in all patients under consideration for surgical repair. CT enhanced by the use of a contrast medium can be used to identify and size aneurysms of both the ascending and the descending thoracic aorta.[6,7] Alternatively, significant aneurysms of either the ascending or the descending thoracic aorta can be defined by cross-sectional echocardiography, but in the thoracic aorta, as contrasted with the abdominal aorta, this technique is not nearly so accurate as the CT scan, especially in the descending thoracic aorta.

NATURAL HISTORY. Data for the true natural history of arteriosclerotic thoracic aortic aneurysms are somewhat scanty, but, as with abdominal aneurysms, ultimate survival is related to the size of the aneurysms. Thoracic aneurysms greater than 6 or 7 cm in diameter are more prone to rupture than smaller ones.[51] Aneurysms that indicate expansion by producing symptoms of compression of surrounding structures are obviously diagnosed and treated earlier than aneurysms at silent sites. As noted, thoracic aneurysms are frequently associated with severe generalized arteriosclerosis, and many patients die of complications of arteriosclerosis before an aneurysm can rupture. When aneurysms do pursue a natural course, it has been found that symptomatic aneurysms are more prone to rupture than asymptomatic ones. In the study of Joyce et al. of 107 patients with thoracic aneurysms—73 per cent of which were arteriosclerotic—a 27 per cent 5-year survival rate for patients with symptomatic aneurysms was reported, as opposed to a 58 per cent 5-year survival rate for those without symptoms.[52] One-third of all deaths were attributed to aneurysm rupture, but over one-half of the mortality was caused by complications of arteriosclerosis unrelated to the aneurysm.

MANAGEMENT. Historically, surgical therapy once consisted of the introduction of long lengths of thrombogenic wire into an aneurysm, with the resultant thrombus

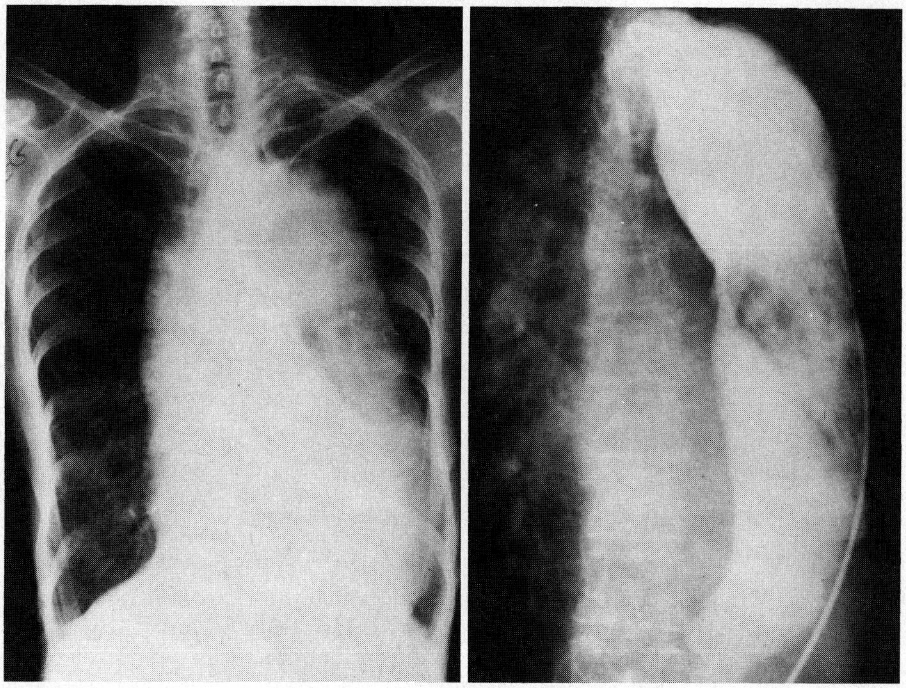

FIGURE 45–5 Large arteriosclerotic aneurysm of the descending thoracic aorta in a 69-year-old man. *Left,* Posteroanterior chest roentgenogram showing the widened aorta. *Right,* The aneurysm is outlined with contrast medium and originates just distal to the aortic arch, extending to the level of the diaphragm. (Courtesy of Robert Dinsmore, M.D., Chief of Cardiac Radiology, Massachusetts General Hospital, Boston.)

buttressing the wall of the aneurysm.[53] Direct wrapping of the aneurysm has also been tried. Currently, surgical excision is the procedure of choice whenever possible and is advised for aneurysms measuring 7 cm or more in diameter in the ascending and descending thoracic aorta. Clearly, even smaller aneurysms should be resected if they are producing symptoms. The aggressiveness with which surgical repair is undertaken depends greatly upon the general condition of the patient. The surgical procedure must be tailored to the specific aneurysm. Saccular aneurysms can sometimes be excised directly without resection of the aorta. Fusiform aneurysms in the ascending and descending thoracic aorta are best resected and replaced with a prosthetic tubular sleeve of appropriate size. Total cardiopulmonary bypass is necessary for the removal of ascending aortic aneurysms, and partial bypass to support the circulation distal to the aneurysm is often advisable in the resection of descending thoracic aortic aneurysms. A temporary shunt (Gott shunt) may be required from the proximal aorta to the aorta beyond the aneurysm to divert blood around the site of the aneurysm while it is being repaired.

Although fusiform aneurysms of the arch have been successfully excised surgically, the risks of operation in this area are high. Arch aneurysmectomy requires not only excision of the aneurysm but also reimplantation of all the brachiocephalic vessels. Perfusion by local cannulation of each of these important arteries is necessary while they are being reimplanted. Alternatively, resection of the aneurysm using profound hypothermia and circulatory arrest, a technique that is becoming increasingly favored by many surgical groups, has been employed successfully.[54,55]

Surgical results have improved considerably in recent years, with most major centers reporting an 80 to 85 per cent survival rate for the elective resection of ascending and descending thoracic aortic aneurysms.[56] Kidd et al. reported the results of operation in 83 patients with arteriosclerotic aneurysms of the ascending aorta operated upon between 1970 and 1975.[57] There was a 90 per cent early and an 84 per cent late survival rate. In a report on 82 patients with thoracoabdominal aneurysms, the survival rate was 94 per cent.[58]

Major complications of the operation are technical, especially hemorrhage from tearing of the diseased aorta. A

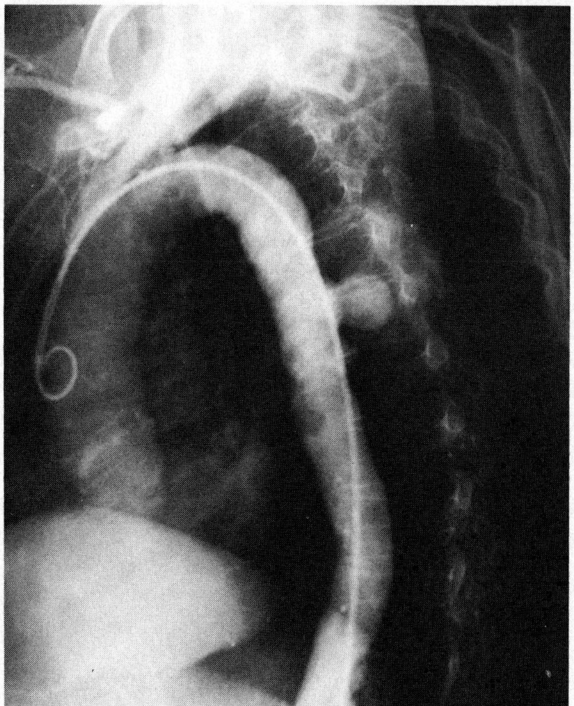

FIGURE 45–6 A localized saccular aneurysm in the descending thoracic aorta is clearly shown in the aortic angiogram of this 62-year-old man. The aneurysm had leaked, and a faint halo caused by the hematoma can be seen surrounding the aneurysm. The routine chest film appeared normal in this patient. (Courtesy of Christos Athanasoulis, M.D., and Arthur Waltman, M.D., Section of Vascular Radiology, Massachusetts General Hospital, Boston.)

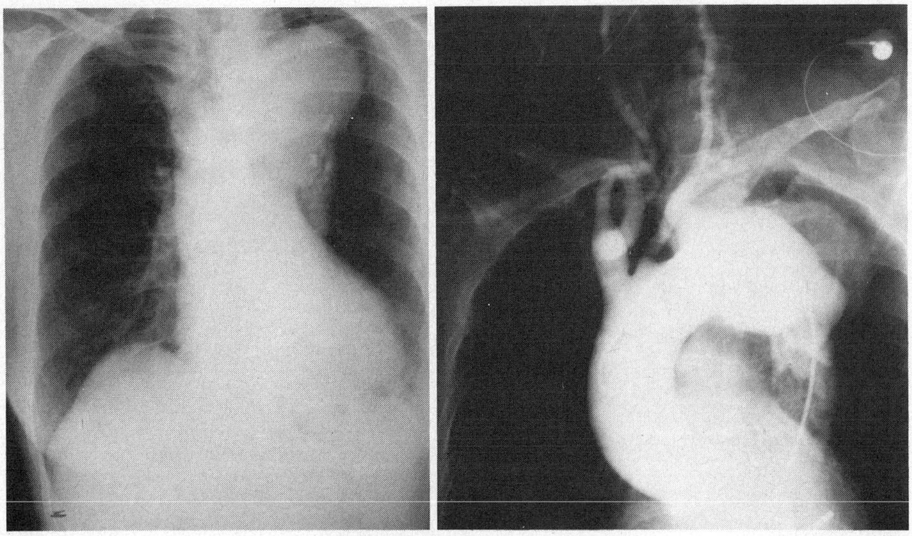

FIGURE 45–7 *Left,* Posteroanterior chest roentgenogram in a 66-year-old woman with an arteriosclerotic aneurysm of the descending thoracic aorta. *Right,* Aortographic appearance in the left oblique anterior projection. The aneurysm arises just at the site of origin of the left subclavian artery. Thrombus is evident in the outer wall of the aneurysm on the angiogram. (Courtesy of Christos Athanasoulis, M.D., and Arthur Waltman, M.D., Section of Vascular Radiology, Massachusetts General Hospital, Boston.)

catastrophic complication of resection of descending thoracic aortic aneurysms is paraplegia from the inadvertent interruption of the arterial blood supply to the spinal cord. This problem has been reduced considerably by maintaining distal aortic perfusion during surgery; by reducing the period of aortic cross clamping; by removal of minimal segments of aorta with the attendant intercostal arteries, especially in the areas of T7 through T9; and by prompt treatment of hypertension in the proximal aorta, which elevates cerebrospinal fluid pressure, thus reducing collateral blood flow to the spinal cord.[55,59–61] Complications of associated arteriosclerosis, such as myocardial infarction, cerebrovascular infarcts, and renal failure, often manifest themselves under the massive physiological stress of surgery.

Many patients with arteriosclerotic aneurysms are heavy smokers, and pulmonary complications are frequent. The left lung may be severely traumatized in resection of large aneurysms of the descending thoracic aorta, a complication which may seriously jeopardize the patient, particularly if there is underlying pulmonary disease.

Widespread aneurysmal dilatation of the aorta often precludes operation, although there are isolated reports of successful surgical replacement of essentially the entire diseased thoracic and abdominal aorta.[62] Associated diseases —especially pulmonary—make any operation impossible in still others. Although it seems logical to reduce blood pressure vigorously in patients with aneurysms and to reduce the velocity of ventricular ejection (p. 1553), the long-term impact of such therapy on retarding the expansion of aneurysms and improving survival is unknown.

AORTIC DISSECTION

Acute aortic dissection is a relatively common catastrophic illness and occurs at the rate of at least 2000 new cases per year in the United States.[63–65] Over the past two decades, great strides have been made in the diagnosis and the medical and surgical treatment of this highly lethal disease. It has been cogently pointed out that the term *dissecting hematoma* describes this entity more accurately than does the more widely used dissecting aneurysm. More recently, the simpler term *aortic dissection* has gained favor.

Aortic dissection is caused by the sudden development of a tear in the aortic intima, opening the way for a column of blood driven by the force of the arterial pressure to enter the aortic wall, destroying the media and stripping the intima from the adventitia for variable distances along the length of the aorta.[65a] It is uncertain whether the primary event in aortic dissection is rupture of the intima with secondary dissection into the media, or hemorrhage within a diseased media followed by disruption of the subjacent intima and subsequent propagation of the dissection through the intimal tear (Fig. 45–8). However, it is clear that occasional cases of extensive aortic dissection can occur without any identifiable intimal tear.

The manifestations of aortic dissection in any given patient are determined by the path taken by the dissecting hematoma as it progresses through the aorta. Thus, the circulation of any major artery arising from the aorta may be compromised; disruption of the support of the aortic valve by extension into the aortic root may cause aortic incompetence; and finally the dissecting column may rupture through the adventitia anywhere along the aorta, although the two most common sites of rupture are the pericardial space and the left pleural cavity.

CLASSIFICATION. Most schemata for classification of aortic dissection are based upon the fact that over 95 per cent of all dissections arise in one of two locations: (1) the ascending aorta within several centimeters of the aortic valve; and (2) the descending thoracic aorta, usually just beyond the origin of the left subclavian artery at the site of the ligamentum arteriosum.[64] The widely used classification of DeBakey et al. recognizes three groups (Fig. 45–9).[66] Types I and II both begin in the ascending aorta; Type I extends beyond the ascending aorta and arch, whereas Type II is confined to the ascending aorta. Type III originates in the descending thoracic aorta and usually propagates distally for a variable distance; more rarely, it extends retrograde into the arch and ascending aorta. An additional category, Type IV, has recently been proposed to include iatrogenic retrograde dissection due to intraarterial catheterization or cannulation.[67]

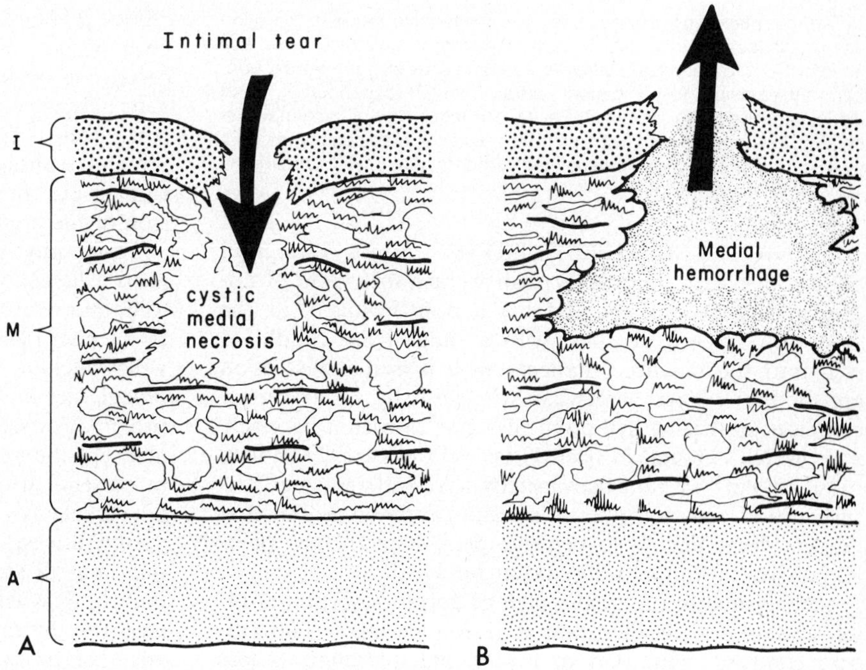

FIGURE 45-8 Proposed mechanisms of initiation of aortic dissection. In both cases, cystic medial necrosis is present. In *A*, an intimal tear is the initial event, allowing aortic blood to enter the media. In *B*, the primary event is hemorrhage into the media, with secondary rupture of the overlying intima. I = intima; M = media; A = adventitia.

Still another classification, based upon approach to therapy and proposed by Daily et al., delineates two types, A and B.[68] Type A includes all proximal dissections and those distal dissections that extend retrograde to the arch and ascending aorta; Type B refers to all other distal dissections without proximal extension.

Since the behavior and management of Types I and II dissections are similar, many investigators, including ourselves, have adopted a simple two-category classification into "proximal" (DeBakey Types I and II) and "distal" (DeBakey Type III) dissections.[69] "Ascending" and "descending" have also been used synonymously with "proximal" and "distal." Proximal dissections occur more frequently than distal dissections in a ratio of almost two to one in autopsy series. However, because proximal dissections are more rapidly lethal, many clinical series report larger numbers of patients with distal than proximal dissection.[69,70]

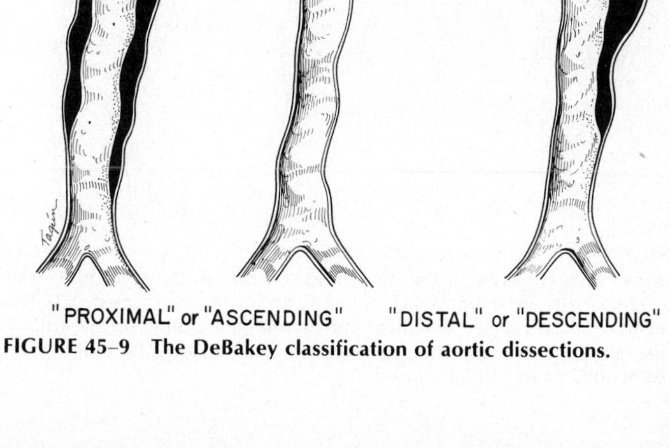

FIGURE 45-9 The DeBakey classification of aortic dissections.

Occasional other sites of origin are the aortic arch and the abdominal aorta. Furthermore, individual arteries may be the locus of isolated dissection, especially the coronary and carotid arteries.[71,72] The subject of aortic dissection has been discussed in several recent reviews.[63-65]

ETIOLOGY AND PATHOGENESIS. Degeneration of the aortic media is believed to be the pathological prerequisite for the development of aortic dissection.[64,65,65a] Usually, this consists of deterioration of the collagen and elastic tissue, often with cystic changes. This process, termed cystic medial necrosis or degeneration, most often is the result of chronic stress against the aortic wall, such as might occur with longstanding hypertension. Indeed, hypertension is an important contributing factor to aortic dissection and is found in well over half of all cases. It is especially prevalent with distal dissection.

Although some degree of medial degeneration has been shown to be part of the normal aging process in the aorta, these changes are qualitatively and quantitatively much greater in patients with aortic dissection.[11,12] Cystic medial degeneration is an intrinsic feature of the hereditary defects of connective tissue, especially the Marfan (p. 1665) and Ehler-Danlos (p. 1668) syndromes. Indeed, aortic dissection—especially proximal dissection—is a frequent and serious complication of Marfan (see p. 1556) syndrome. However, cystic medial degeneration and aortic dissection may occur in the absence of an associated phenotypic syndrome.[73] Certain congenital cardiovascular abnormalities, especially coarctation of the aorta and bicuspid aortic valves, seem to predispose to aortic dissection.[74,75] A combination of bicuspid aortic valve, cystic medial degeneration, and aortic root dissection in the absence of the Marfan syndrome has been described.[76]

An unexplained relationship exists between pregnancy and aortic dissection. About half of all aortic dissections in women under the age of 40 occur during pregnancy, usually in the last trimester. Isolated coronary artery dissection also usually occurs during pregnancy.

In older patients, dissections occasionally originate by way of perforation through an intimal atheromatous plaque. Trauma almost never causes a classic aortic dissection, although a localized tear in the region of the aortic isthmus is not uncommon following massive chest trauma.[77] Rarely, dissection of the aorta is a complication of other forms of vasculitis, including granulomatous arteritis (p. 1663).

Although strenuous physical exertion and emotional stress have been linked to aortic dissection, such a relationship is not usual. In a series of 124 cases of aortic dissection that we reviewed, we found such a history in only 14 per cent.[69]

The role played by chemicals toxic to connective tissue in the etiology of dissecting aneurysm in human beings is unknown. It is well known that the seeds of *Lathyrus odoratus* (sweet pea), which contain aminopropionitrile, cause cystic medial degeneration and dissecting aneurysm in rats.[78] We have encountered a proximal dissection in a young man with no other obvious predisposing factors who had a prolonged industrial exposure to dimethyl hydrazine, a connective tissue toxin.[69]

CLINICAL MANIFESTATIONS. Aortic dissection afflicts men more frequently than women in a ratio of approximately two to one and has a peak incidence in the sixth and seventh decades, with a range from childhood well into the nineties.[79] Patients with proximal dissection are on the average somewhat younger.[80] By far the most common presenting symptom of aortic dissection is *severe pain,* which is found in over 90 per cent of cases.[80a] In fact, those patients without pain usually have suffered some disturbance of consciousness as a result of the dissection that renders them unable to perceive pain. Nonetheless, painless dissection can and does occur rarely.[81]

Cataclysmic in onset, the pain of aortic dissection is often as severe at its inception as it ever becomes. This feature contrasts with that of myocardial infarction, where the pain usually has a crescendo-like onset. The pain of dissection may be all but unbearable, forcing the patient to writhe in agony or to pace restlessly in an attempt to gain some measure of relief. Several features of the pain may arouse suspicion of aortic dissection. The quality of the pain as described by the patient is often remarkably appropriate to the actual event. Adjectives such as "tearing," "ripping," and "stabbing" are frequently used. Another characteristic of the pain of aortic dissection is its tendency to migrate from the point of its origin to other sites, following the path of the dissecting hematoma as it extends through the aorta. Vasovagal manifestations, such as a drenching sweat, apprehension, nausea, vomiting, and faintness, are common at the outset.

The location of pain may be of some help in suggesting the site of origin.[69] Pain felt maximally in the anterior thorax is more frequent with proximal dissection, whereas pain that is most severe in the interscapular area is much more common with a distal site of origin. Although pain may be felt simultaneously in the anterior and posterior chest with both proximal and distal dissection, the *absence* of posterior interscapular pain strongly militates against a distal dissection, since over 90 per cent of patients with distal dissection report some back pain. Pain in the neck, throat, jaw, or teeth often occurs in dissections that involve the ascending aorta or arch.

Less common modes of presentation include congestive heart failure with or without associated chest pain, cerebrovascular accidents, syncope, paraplegia, and pulse loss with or without ischemic pain. Heart failure usually results from severe aortic regurgitation secondary to the dissection. The occurrence of syncope in aortic dissection may bear special significance. Syncope without focal neurological signs occurred in 6 of 124 patients in our series. In each case, there was evidence for rupture of the dissection into the pericardial cavity with cardiac tamponade.[69]

DIAGNOSIS. The diagnosis of aortic dissection can often be made with reasonable assurance from the *physical examination* alone. It has been noted that patients with aortic dissection may appear to be in shock; however, the blood pressure when measured is frequently elevated.[82] Over 50 per cent of patients with distal dissection are hypertensive on initial presentation. Hypotension usually results from cardiac tamponade; intrapleural or intraperitoneal rupture; or dissection of the brachiocephalic vessels resulting in "pseudohypotension," i.e., the inability to measure the blood pressure accurately because of occlusion of the brachial arteries.

Those physical findings most typically associated with aortic dissection, namely, pulse deficits, aortic regurgitation, and neurological manifestations, are more characteristic of proximal than distal dissection. Pulse abnormalities, which include the absence, diminution, or reduplication of pulses, occur in approximately one-half of patients with proximal dissection and, most commonly, involve the brachiocephalic vessels. Pulse deficits are much less common in patients with distal dissection and tend to involve the left subclavian and femoral arteries, although the femoral vessels are equally affected by the distal propagation of a proximal dissection. As depicted in Figure 45–10, pulses may be lost either by direct compression of the lumen of an artery by extension of the dissection into it or by blockade due to a flap of intima overlying the vessel orifice. Rarely, intimointimal intussusception may occur.[83] In either case, pulse deficits in aortic dissection may be transitory owing to decompression of the hematoma by distal reentry into the true lumen or by movement of the intimal flap away from the occluded orifice.

Aortic regurgitation is an important feature of proximal dissection and occurs in over 50 per cent in most series.[83a] When aortic regurgitation is present in patients with distal dissection, it most commonly antedates the dissection and results from preexisting dilatation of the aortic root due to severe hypertension or annuloaortic ectasia. The murmur of aortic regurgitation in aortic dissection often has a musical quality and may be heard better along the right than the left sternal border (p. 1111). It may wax and wane, the intensity varying directly with the height of the arterial blood pressure. Depending upon the severity of the regurgitation, other peripheral signs of aortic incompetence may be present, such as collapsing pulses and a wide pulse pressure. There are three mechanisms of aortic regurgitation in proximal dissection (Fig. 45–11): First, the dissec-

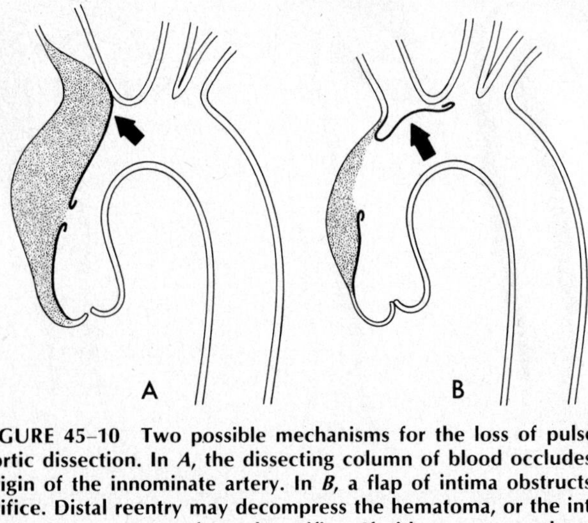

FIGURE 45–10 Two possible mechanisms for the loss of pulses in aortic dissection. In *A*, the dissecting column of blood occludes the origin of the innominate artery. In *B*, a flap of intima obstructs the orifice. Distal reentry may decompress the hematoma, or the intimal flap may move away from the orifice. If either occurs, pulses may be wholly or partially restored.

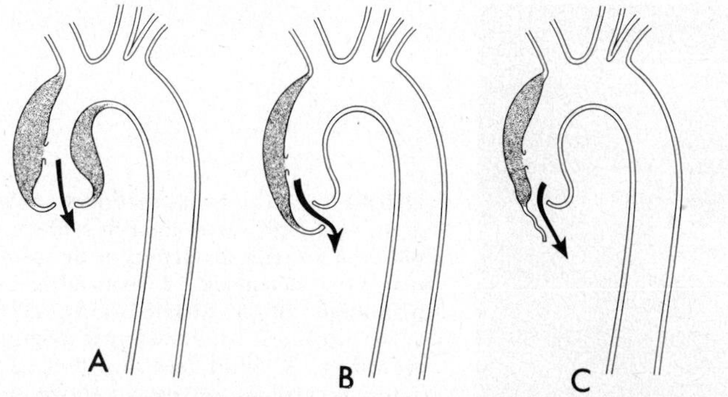

FIGURE 45–11 Mechanisms of aortic regurgitation in proximal dissecting aortic aneurysm. *A*, A circumferential tear pulls the annulus apart, preventing the leaflets from coapting. *B*, With asymmetrical dissection, pressure from the hematoma depresses one leaflet below the line of closure of the other. *C*, The annular support is disrupted, resulting in a flail aortic leaflet and aortic regurgitation.

tion may dilate the aortic root, widening the annulus so that aortic leaflets are unable to coapt in diastole; second, in an asymmetrical dissection, pressure from the dissecting hematoma may depress one leaflet below the line of closure of the others; and third, the annular support of the leaflets or the leaflets themselves may be torn so as to render the valve incompetent.

As noted, patients with proximal dissection sometimes have heart failure, which is almost always due to the sudden onset of severe aortic insufficiency. In rare cases, the congestive failure may be so severe as to mask the murmur and other usual signs of aortic regurgitation. In a few such patients whom we have encountered, the presence of disproportionately bounding pulses in the face of severe heart failure, coupled with a history highly suggestive of aortic dissection, served as a clue to the correct diagnosis.

Neurological deficits associated with aortic dissection include cerebrovascular accidents, ischemic peripheral neuropathy, ischemic paraparesis, and disturbances of consciousness.[84] Each of these is more common with proximal dissection, but deficits in the lower extremities are equally frequent in proximal and distal dissection.

Other occasionally encountered clinical manifestations of aortic dissection include pulsation of one of the sternoclavicular joints,[85] Horner's syndrome due to compression of the superior cervical sympathetic ganglion, vocal cord paralysis and hoarseness from pressure against the left recurrent laryngeal nerve, superior mediastinal syndrome from superior vena caval compression,[86] pulsating neck masses, tracheal or bronchial compression with bronchospasms,[64,87] hemorrhage into the tracheobronchial tree with hemoptysis,[88] hematemesis due to perforation into the esophagus,[89] heart block from retrograde burrowing of a dissection into the interatrial septum and thence down to the AV node,[90] and a continuous murmur due to rupture into the right atrium or ventricle.[91] Pleural effusions result from rupture of the dissection into one of the pleural spaces—usually the left—or simply from an exudative inflammatory reaction around the involved aorta. Additional complications may result from occlusion of important arteries by the dissection. Mesenteric infarction, renal infarction with severe renovascular hypertension, and myocardial infarction (seen in 1 to 2 per cent of patients with proximal dissection) are among the more serious occlusive events. Occasionally, high fever results presumably from the release of pyrogenic substances from the hematoma or from associated effusions.

Routine laboratory studies are not very helpful in making the diagnosis of aortic dissection. Anemia may develop from significant hemorrhage or sequestration of blood in the false channel. A mild to moderate polymorphonuclear leukocytosis (10,000 to 14,000/mm^3) is common. Lactic acid dehydrogenase (LDH) and bilirubin levels are sometimes elevated because of hemolysis of blood sequestered within the false lumen. Serum glutamic oxaloacetic transaminase (SGOT) and creatine phosphokinase (CPK or CPK-MB) values are usually normal. Disseminated intravascular coagulation has been reported rarely.[92] The electrocardiogram frequently shows left ventricular hypertrophy from preexistent hypertension and usually the absence of acute ischemic changes. The absence of electrocardiographic changes of myocardial ischemia or infarction in a patient with severe chest pain is a helpful point in differential diagnosis from myocardial infarction.

Diagnostic ultrasound (M-mode), in combination with cross-sectional (2-D) echocardiography, is helpful in the detection of a proximal dissection by revealing a widened aortic root, with delineation of the dissecting hematoma[93–95,95a] (Fig. 45–12). CT scan with contrast injection is quite accurate in defining both ascending and descending dissections, provided there is identification of a false lumen to distinguish the dissection from a fusiform aneurysm.[6,7,95–97,95a] Although 2-D echocardiography and CT clearly offer the advantage of noninvasive diagnosis,[95b] angiography is generally required to define the full extent of the dissection, to outline the relationship of the dissection to the major aortic branches, to evaluate aortic valve competency, and to identify the site of the intimal tear. Thus, these noninvasive techniques—especially the CT scan—may be most useful in the long-term follow-up of treated patients with aortic dissection, for evidence of localized aneurysm formation.[98,99] Chest roentgenogram and aortic angiography provide the most substantive laboratory means of initial and definitive diagnosis, respectively. Chest roentgenography almost always reveals an abnormally widened aortic contour.[100] A localized bulge may overlay the site of origin, and the aortic silhouette may be widened wherever the dissection extends. If the aortic knob is calcified, a greater than 1 cm separation of the intimal calcification from the adventitial border (the "calcium sign") is virtually pathognomonic of aortic dissection (Fig. 45–13). Tracheal deviation or a left pleural effusion may be seen. Comparison to previous films is most helpful. On the other hand, it is possible for extensive aortic dissection to occur without radiographic abnormalities.

Fluoroscopy of the aorta may suggest aortic dissection in that pulsations in the abnormally widened aorta are diminished or absent over an area of dissection. This contrasts with the exaggerated pulsations usually seen in a true aneurysm.

The single, most important study in the diagnosis of aortic dissection is *aortic angiography.* Although originally performed by injection of contrast material into the pulmonary artery with aortic opacification following the pulmonary venous phase, retrograde angiography is now the method of choice. The hazards of this approach have proved minimal, provided the catheter is carefully inserted

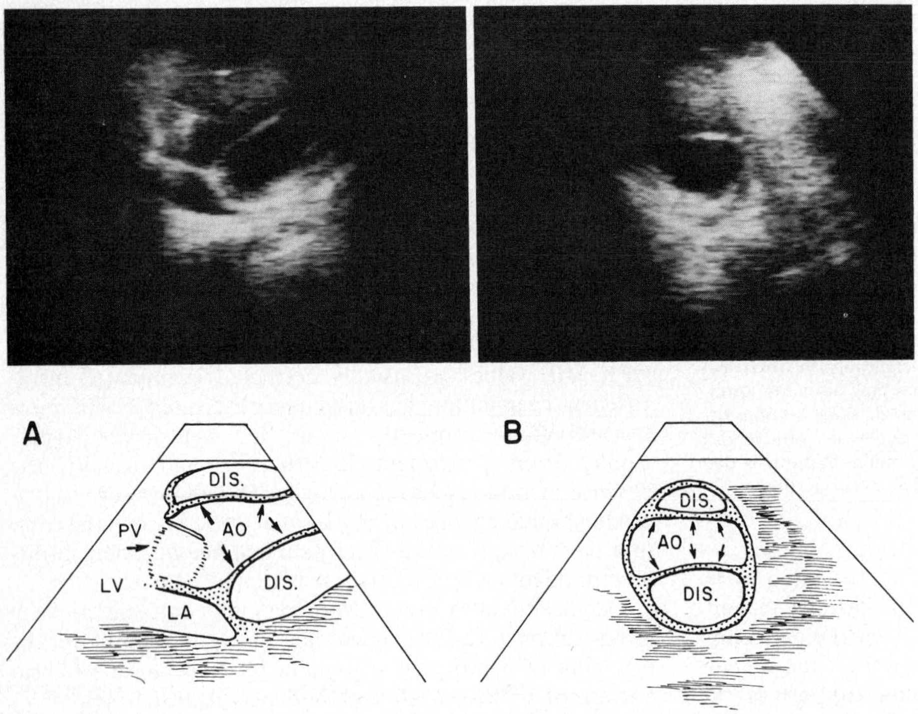

FIGURE 45–12 Cross-sectional echogram of the proximal aorta in a 63-year-old woman with dissection of the proximal aorta occurring 12 years after implantation of a Starr-Edwards aortic valve prosthesis. *A*, Parasternal long-axis recording. *B*, Short-axis recording. The actual recordings are shown above, and diagrammatic representations of the findings are pictured below. The echo-dense prosthetic valve (PV) is easily seen on the long-axis recording. Surrounding the aorta (AO) is the false channel of the dissection (DIS). (From Weyman, A. E.: Cross-sectional Echocardiography. Philadelphia, Lea and Febiger, 1982.)

and contrast material is not injected into the false channel. Aortic angiography has three objectives: (1) to establish a definite diagnosis, (2) to identify the site of origin of the dissection, and (3) to delineate the extent of the dissection and the distal circulation to vital organs (Fig. 45–14 and 45–15).

One additional feature to be assessed by angiography is the degree to which the false channel is opacified. There is evidence that the prognosis in medically treated patients is better in those with a nonopacified false channel, presumably an indication of thrombus formation in the channel which may serve to buttress the wall of the dissected aorta.[101] Although highly accurate, angiography is not without occasional pitfalls in the detection of aortic dissection. Failure of angiography to show a dissection can occur if there is faint opacification of the false lumen, unusual tearing of the intima, a very small and localized dissection, or equal simultaneous opacification of both channels.[102] Nevertheless, when properly performed and interpreted, angiography provides a definitive diagnosis in almost every case and is well tolerated by even critically ill patients.

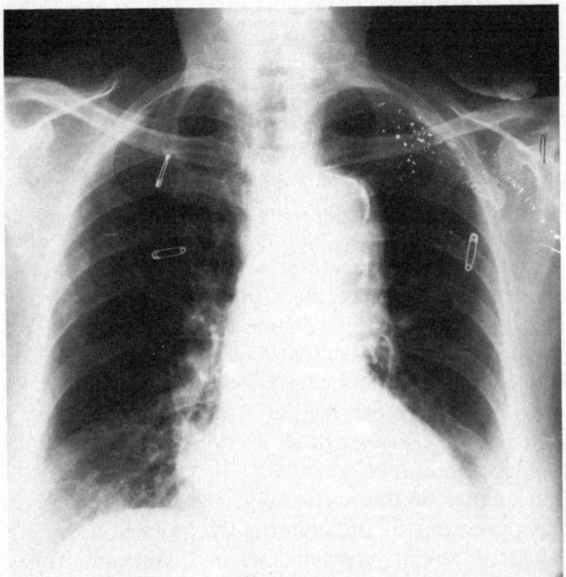

FIGURE 45–13 "Calcium sign" in distal dissection in an 80-year-old woman with longstanding hypertension. Note the marked separation of the calcification in the aortic knob and descending thoracic aorta from the outer wall of the aorta. This distance is normally no greater than 0.5 cm.

MANAGEMENT. Therapy for aortic dissection is directed at halting the progression of the dissecting hematoma, since fatal complications arise not from the intimal tear itself, but rather from the subsequent course taken by the dissection.[102a] Without treatment, aortic dissection is almost always fatal. In a collective review of long-term survival in untreated aortic dissection, more than one-quarter of all patients were dead within 24 hours, more than one-half died within the first week, more than three-quarters died within 1 month, and more than 90 per cent died within 1 year.[103]

The first surgical approach to aortic dissection was the so-called fenestration procedure by which the dissected aorta was incised and a distal communication was created between the true and false channels, thereby decompressing the false lumen.[104,105] Definitive surgical therapy was pioneered by DeBakey and colleagues in the early 1950's.[106] Its principles are to excise the intimal tear; to obliterate the false channel by oversewing aortic edges; to reconstitute the aorta with or without interposition of a synthetic graft; and to restore aortic valve competence by resuspension of the displaced aortic leaflets or by prosthetic valve replacement of the aortic valve in the case of proximal dissection.

In the midst of growing enthusiasm for surgical therapy.

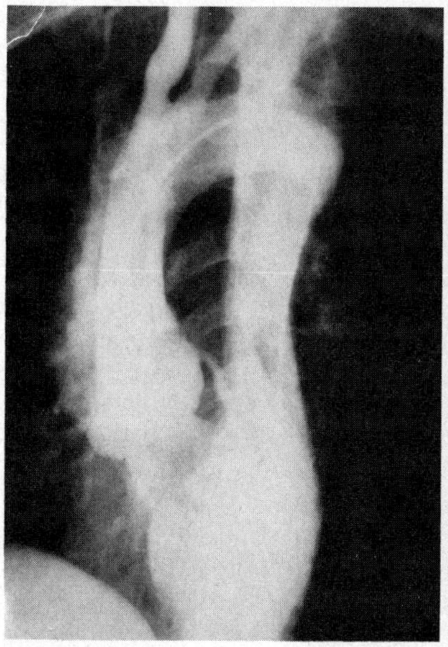
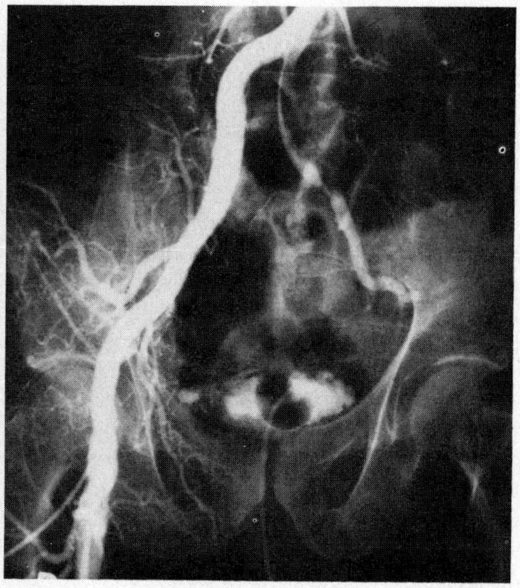

FIGURE 45-14 *Left,* Thoracic aortogram in the left anterior oblique projection showing a dissection beginning in the ascending aorta and spiraling through the aortic arch into the descending aorta. The false lumen can be faintly visualized. *Right,* Angiogram of the distal aorta showing virtual obstruction of the left iliac artery by the dissection. (Courtesy of Christos Athanasoulis, M.D., and Arthur Waltman, M.D., Section of Vascular Radiology, Massachusetts General Hospital, Boston.)

aggressive medical treatment of aortic dissection was first advocated by Wheat, Palmer, and collaborators.[107] They established two goals for pharmacological therapy: (1) reduction of the systolic blood pressure, and (2) diminution of the velocity of left ventricular ejection (dV/dt), which Prokop, Palmer, and Wheat consider a major stress acting upon the aortic wall that contributes to the genesis and propagation of aortic dissection.[8] Originally introduced for patients too ill to withstand surgery, medical therapy now forms the basis for the initial treatment of virtually all patients with aortic dissection prior to definitive diagnosis by angiography and serves as primary long-term therapy in a large additional subset of patients.

Early Emergency Treatment. All patients in whom there is a strong index of suspicion for aortic dissection should be immediately admitted to an intensive care unit, where blood pressure, cardiac rhythm, central venous pressure, urine output, and, when necessary, pulmonary wedge pressure and cardiac output can be monitored. Initial therapeutic goals are the elimination of pain and the reduction of systolic blood pressure to 100 to 120 mm Hg or to the lowest level commensurate with adequate vital organ (cardiac, renal, and cerebral) perfusion. Simultaneously, arterial dV/dt, which reflects the velocity of left ventricular ejection, should be reduced by beta-adrenergic blockade regardless of whether systolic hypertension or pain is present.

For acute reduction of arterial pressure, the potent vasodilator sodium nitroprusside is very effective, mixed as 50 to 100 mg in 500 ml of 5 per cent dextrose in water and infused initially at 25 to 50 μg/min, with dosages varying according to blood pressure response. Side effects include nausea, restlessness, somnolence, hypotension, and cyanide or thiocyanate toxicity, which can develop after more than 48 hours of continuous use (p. 537). Sodium nitroprusside alone can cause an increase in dV/dt, which can potentially contribute to propagation of the dissection.[108] Thus, adequate simultaneous beta-adrenergic blockade is essential when this drug is used.[107a]

If sodium nitroprusside is ineffective or poorly tolerated, the ganglionic blocking agent trimethaphan (Arfonad), mixed as 500 mg to 2.0 gm in 500 ml of 5 per cent glucose and water, is used. Initial infusion rate is 1 mg/min, titrating the dose against the blood pressure response, which is enhanced by the orthostatic maneuver of elevating the head of the bed. Limitations in the use of this powerful agent include severe hypotension, tachyphylaxis, somnolence, and sympathoplegia with urinary retention, constipation, ileus, and pupillary dilatation. In contrast with sodium nitroprusside, trimethaphan depresses dV/dt, which should provide a relative advantage in the treatment

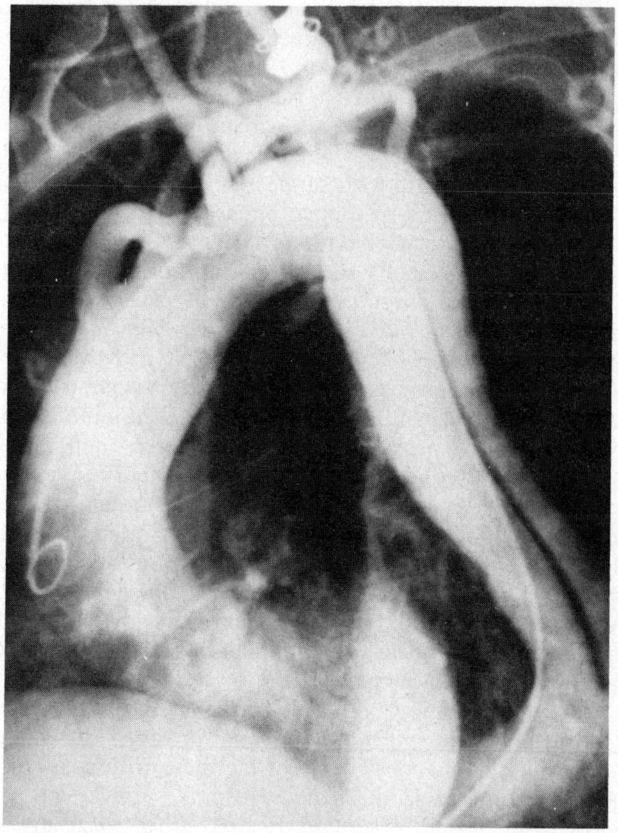

FIGURE 45-15 Left oblique anterior view of the aorta outlined angiographically showing a distal aortic dissection in a 63-year-old man. The true and false channels are clearly seen. The false channel is heavily opacified.

of aortic dissection. However, its unpleasant side effects and rapid tachyphylaxis have relegated this drug to a position of second choice in acute therapy in most centers.

To reduce dV/dt acutely, propranolol should be used in incremental doses of 1 mg intravenously every 5 minutes until there is evidence of satisfactory beta-adrenergic blockade, usually indicated by a pulse rate of 60 to 80 beats/min in the acute setting. A test dose of 0.5 mg intravenously is advised. Maximum initial total dose should not exceed 0.15 mg/kg. Further propranolol should be given intravenously every 4 to 6 hours in order to maintain adequate beta-adrenergic blockade, as reflected in heart rate, usually in dosages somewhat less than the initial amount, i.e., 2 to 6 mg. In chronic stable dissection, propranolol (or an alternative beta blocker) can be started orally, using 20 to 40 mg every 6 hours. Propranolol is contraindicated in the presence of bradycardia, asthma or heart failure. An alternative drug to reduce both blood pressure and dV/dt acutely is reserpine, 1 to 2 mg intramuscularly every 4 to 6 hours. Side effects of reserpine are drowsiness, depression, and peptic ulceration from the stimulation of hydrochloric acid secretion by the stomach. The latter risk can be minimized by concomitant administration of cimetidine, 300 mg intravenously or orally every 6 hours.

Once stabilized, the patient should undergo angiography for a definitive diagnosis. Angiography should be performed within 6 hours after admission, unless a life-threatening complication such as aortic rupture, free aortic regurgitation, cardiac tamponade, or compromise of a vital organ has supervened. If any of these potentially lethal problems arise, then surgery must be undertaken immediately, with angiography performed if possible while the operating room is being readied.

Definitive Subsequent Therapy. Despite minor variations from center to center, a remarkably consistent approach to definitive therapy of aortic dissection has evolved, based upon experience with surgical and medical treatment over the past decade. Although either medical or surgical therapy can be associated with an extremely successful outcome, it can be generally stated that *surgical results are superior to medical results in proximal dissection,* and, conversely, *medical therapy offers a relative advantage over surgery in most cases of uncomplicated distal dissection.*[109–114] These differences are based largely upon the disparate natural history of proximal and distal disease. Even minute progression of a proximal dissection poses potentially devastating consequences such as pulse loss, aortic regurgitation, neurological compromise, or cardiac tamponade. Thus, immediate surgical repair promises a better outcome. In contrast, patients with distal dissection are for the most part older and have a relatively increased incidence of advanced atherosclerotic or cardiopulmonary disease, thus rendering their surgical risks considerably higher. Medical therapy has proved to be quite effective in this group.

Recent studies report a hospital survival of approximately 60 per cent for patients with acute proximal dissection treated surgically and 80 per cent for those with acute distal dissection treated medically. Hospital survival for patients with chronic dissection treated either surgically—usually because of aortic insufficiency or an enlarging aneurysm—or medically is greater than 80 per cent.[113–116] The somewhat poorer results for surgically treated patients with acute dissection are mostly attributable to complications that have already occurred as a result of the dissection prior to the utilization of definitive therapy.[114] The definitely improved survival in patients with chronic dissection derives from this same principle, i.e., they have already selected themselves out as a group destined to do well because they have survived the initial high mortality that occurs within the first 2 weeks of onset of the dissection.[66,110,112–114] The results of long-term follow-up will be discussed below.

The generally advocated *indications for definitive surgical therapy* are summarized in Table 45–1. Note that occasional patients with proximal dissection who refuse surgery or for whom surgery is contraindicated by age or prior debilitating illness can be treated successfully by medical therapy. Moreover, both early and late medical therapy are usually required in *all* patients, including those treated surgically, to provide stabilization initially and to protect against redissection subsequently.

Surgical Therapy

Although the precise timing of surgery in patients without life-threatening complications is somewhat controversial, prompt repair is generally recommended to obviate even minute progression of the hematoma resulting in further complications. Surgical risk for all patients is obviously increased by age; associated diseases, especially pulmonary emphysema; aneurysm leakage; cardiac tamponade; shock; difficulty with blood pressure control; or vital organ compromise, in particular myocardial infarction or cerebrovascular accident.

As noted, the objectives of definitive surgical therapy are excision of the intimal tear and obliteration of entry into the false lumen by suturing together the edges of the dissected aorta proximally and distally. Aortic continuity is then reestablished either by joining the edges of the aorta directly, or, more commonly, by interposing a prosthetic sleeve graft between the two ends of the aorta (Fig. 45–16). Knowledge of the routes of perfusion of vital organs distal to the surgical site as determined by angiography may be of importance. For example, one or both renal arteries occasionally are found to be fed from the false lumen, in which case the false channel in the distal end of the surgically transected aorta might be left unclosed.[114a]

TABLE 45–1 INDICATIONS FOR DEFINITIVE SURGICAL AND MEDICAL THERAPY IN AORTIC DISSECTION

Surgical

1. Treatment of choice for proximal dissection.
2. Treatment for distal dissection complicated by the following:
   a. Progression with vital organ compromise.
   b. Rupture or impending rupture (saccular aneurysm formation).
   c. Aortic regurgitation.
   d. Inability to control pain or blood pressure medically.
   e. Retrograde extension into the ascending aorta.
   f. Marfan syndrome.

Medical

1. Treatment of choice for uncomplicated distal dissection.
2. Treatment for uncomplicated proximal dissection if the site of origin cannot be clearly identified.*
3. Treatment for stable, isolated arch dissection.
4. Treatment of choice for chronic dissection, i.e., uncomplicated dissection presenting 2 weeks or later after onset.

*Some authors advise surgical therapy for all proximal dissections, regardless of site of origin.[113]

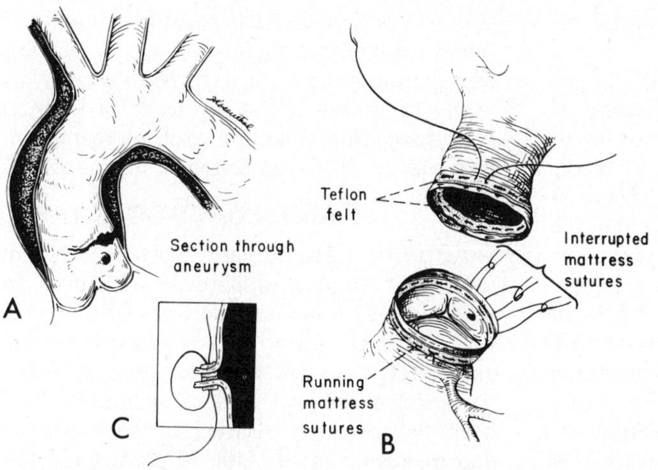

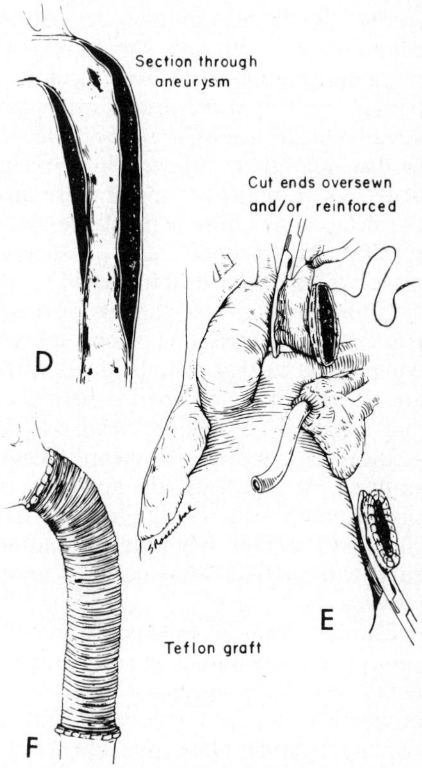

FIGURE 45–16 **Several steps in the surgical repair of a proximal (*A, B,* and *C*) and a distal (*D, E,* and *F*) aortic dissection. *A* and *D* show the dissections and the intimal tears. *B,* The aorta has been transected, and the ends of the aorta have been oversewn to obliterate the false lumen and have been buttressed with Teflon felt to prevent the sutures from tearing through the fragile tissue. *C,* The aortic ends are brought together in such a way that the Teflon is again used to reinforce the suture line between the two ends of the aorta or between the aorta and a sleeve graft, if such a graft is necessary for reconstitution of the aorta. *E* shows resection of a distal dissection, with a Teflon graft interposed in *F.* (*D, E,* and *F* reprinted by permission from Austen, W. G., and DeSanctis, R.: Surgical treatment of dissecting aneurysm of the thoracic aorta. N. Engl. J. Med. *272*:1314, 1965.)**

When aortic regurgitation complicates aortic dissection, simple decompression of the false channel may be all that is necessary to resuspend the leaflets and restore valvular competence. However, most surgeons have become increasingly aggressive about replacing the aortic valve with a prosthesis if it appears that even moderate aortic regurgitation will be present after the leaflets are decompressed, thus avoiding the high risk of having to replace the aortic valve with a second operation through a diseased aorta at some later date.

For repair of a proximal dissection, full cardiopulmonary bypass is necessary. On occasion, because of extensive dissection of the aorta, it may be difficult to find a safe site for placement of a perfusion cannula. In rare cases, we have had to abandon plans for surgical repair of a proximal dissection for this reason. In the repair of dissections of the descending thoracic aorta, support of the distal circulation may be necessary and can be achieved either by partial left heart bypass or by using a conduit which carries blood from the proximal to the distal aorta, circumventing the site of the dissection.

The actual operative procedure itself, in aortic dissection, is technically demanding. The wall of the diseased aorta is often friable, and the repair must be performed with meticulous care. The use of Teflon felt to buttress the wall and prevent sutures from tearing through the fragile aorta (Fig. 45–16*B*) has represented a significant technical advance. An alternate surgical approach consists of the wrapping of an unstable arch dissection with Dacron.[117] Bleeding, infection, and pulmonary or renal insufficiency constitute the most common early complications of surgical therapy. Spinal cord ischemia with resultant paraplegia due to inadvertent interruption of blood supply from the anterior spinal or intercostal arteries is a rare but dreaded consequence. Late complications include progressive aortic regurgitation if the aortic valve has not been replaced, localized aneurysm formation, and rarely, redissection at the original site of repair or at an independent secondary site.

Several innovative techniques for high-risk patients have been reported recently. One utilizes an intraluminal sutureless prosthesis for patients with friable thoracic aortic tissue.[118] The other, applied especially to distal, but also to proximal dissection, consists of bypassing the dissected aorta with a Dacron sleeve, ligating the aorta at the site of proximal extension of the dissection, and creating reversal of flow in the distal aorta to perfuse the major arterial branches arising from the dissected segment.[119] Both techniques have been used on only small numbers of patients, and long-term follow-up is lacking.

Medical Therapy. Indications for *definitive medical therapy* are summarized in Table 45–1. Clearly, operation must be performed if there is medical failure, for example, rupture or impending rupture, progression of the dissection with vital organ compromise, aortic regurgitation, or inability to control pain or blood pressure with drugs. Although we prefer medical therapy for low-risk patients with stable distal dissection, some centers advise surgery in this group as well.[113] Unfortunately, controlled studies of medically versus surgically treated patients with distal dissection and comparable surgical risks are lacking.

Although there is not unanimous agreement, medical therapy is still generally recommended for uncomplicated proximal dissection if the site of origin cannot be identified or isolated surgically. Similarly, because of the extreme difficulty of the operation involved with aortic arch dissections, medical therapy is usually advocated in those rare dissections which originate in the arch, with operative intervention reserved for serious complications that might occur on medical treatment.

Medical therapy is advocated for patients with chronic dissection, defined as a stable aortic dissection that has occurred 2 or more weeks prior to presentation, unless, of course, aortic regurgitation related to the dissection becomes hemodynamically significant.

Complications of medical therapy include severe hypotension related to the drugs, with possible precipitation of acute tubular necrosis, cerebrovascular accident, or myocardial infarction, although in a recent report of 52 medically treated patients none of these proved fatal.[114] Some of the drugs may cause somnolence and depression, and the specific side reactions and problems of each particular drug regimen must be anticipated.

Late follow-up of patients leaving the hospital with treated aortic dissection shows an actuarial survival rate comparable to that of individuals without dissection; there are no significant differences between patients with proximal vs. distal dissection, acute vs. chronic dissection, or medical vs. surgical treatment.[114] Thus, initially successful surgical or medical therapy for aortic dissection is sustained on long-term follow-up. Late complications include redissection, regurgitation, and localized saccular aneurysm formation; these occur in fewer than 3 per cent of patients.

Chronic medical therapy to control hypertension and continuous beta-adrenergic blockade is indicated for all patients who have sustained an aortic dissection, regardless of whether they have received definitive surgical or medical therapy. Systolic blood pressure should be controlled at or below a level of 130 to 140 mm Hg, or even lower if tolerated. Preferred agents are those with a negative inotropic as well as hypotensive effect, such as the beta blockers, methyldopa, clonidine, or reserpine, together with a diuretic. Hydralazine or minoxidil increases cardiac output and arterial dV/dt and should be used only in the presence of adequate beta-adrenergic blockade. There is at present insufficient experience using the converting enzyme inhibitors or calcium channel antagonists in aortic dissection to comment upon their use in the treatment of this disease.

Follow-up of patients who have sustained an aortic dissection should include careful and repeated physical examinations; periodic chest roentgenograms, CT scans, 2-D echocardiographic studies, or, where available, high-resolution digital subtraction angiography may also be useful in long-term follow-up for evidence of localized aortic aneurysm formation. The approach to therapy in patients with proximal or distal dissection is summarized in Table 45–2.

TABLE 45–2 APPROACH TO THE PATIENT WITH ACUTE AORTIC DISSECTION

Initial

1. Immediate monitoring and stabilization of vital signs, including pulse, blood pressure, cardiac rhythm, central venous pressure, urinary output, and, if necessary, pulmonary capillary wedge pressure.
2. Reduce systolic blood pressure to 100–120 mm Hg or lowest possible level commensurate with adequate organ perfusion. Use *nitroprusside*, 50–100 mg in 500 ml D_5W, infuse at 25–50 μg/min; or *trimethaphan*, 500 mg–2 gm in 500 ml D_5W, infuse at 1 mg/min and titrate against blood pressure response.
3. Institute beta blockade with propranolol, 1.0 mg IV over 5 min, and repeat until pulse ≤ 60 or to a total of 0.15 mg/kg. Repeat dose every 4–6 hours.
4. Once stable, proceed to definite diagnosis by angiography. Decide whether to use medical or surgical therapy.

Subsequent Definitive

1. *Proximal Dissection.* Surgery unless definite contraindication. (If associated with myocardial infarct or cerebrovascular accident, surgical results are poor.)
2. *Distal Dissection.* Medical unless:
   a. Rupture or impending rupture (large dilated and opacified false lumen and/or late development of a saccular aneurysm).
   b. Progression with vital organ compromise.
   c. Aortic regurgitation.

Note: Regardless of the type of dissection or ultimate therapy, medical therapy must be administered both initially and as long-term treatment to control blood pressure and arterial dV/dt and thus diminish the risk of hematoma progression or redissection.

ANNULOAORTIC ECTASIA

As aortic valve surgery evolved, it became clear that a significant number of patients with pure aortic regurgitation had this lesion on the basis of idiopathic dilatation of the proximal aorta and the aortic annulus. The term annuloaortic ectasia was first used by Ellis et al. in 1961 to describe this pathological condition.[120] The entity has been subsequently recognized with increasing frequency and makes up about 5 to 10 per cent of the population of patients who currently undergo aortic valve replacement for pure aortic regurgitation.

Etiology and Pathogenesis. The common pathological feature shared by patients with annuloaortic ectasia is that of severe changes of cystic medial necrosis in the wall of the afflicted aorta. Some degree of cystic medial necrosis with annuloaortic ectasia is found in virtually all cases of the Marfan syndrome.[121,122] In fact, it can be severe and is a frequent cause of death from fatal aortic rupture or dissection in Marfan syndrome (p. 1665). In most reported series of patients with annuloaortic ectasia, however, patients with classic Marfan syndrome have been excluded. Careful examination of patients with this condition usually reveals that about one-fourth to one-half have other stigmata of Marfan syndrome, indicating that many of these patients represent a forme fruste of that connective tissue disorder. In a clinicogenetic study of 18 patients with severe aortic regurgitation and dilatation of the ascending aorta but without other evidence of the Marfan syndrome except on pathological examination of the aorta, Emanuel et al. reported that 37.3 per cent of 126 first-degree relatives whom they examined had one or more stigmata of Marfan syndrome.[122a] Thus, it appears clear that many of these patients have primarily the aortic abnormalities of Marfan syndrome without the other manifestations of the disease. In summary, then, patients with annuloaortic ectasia appear to fall into three groups: (1) those with classic Marfan syndrome; (2) those with a forme fruste of the Marfan syndrome; and (3) those with cystic medial necrosis with no obvious underlying cause.

As the media degenerates, the aorta widens. The aortic root is involved, and the annulus dilates, carrying the aortic leaflets apart and eventually making it impossible for these edges to meet in diastole; aortic regurgitation ensues. The diseased aorta may dissect, and this may aggravate the aortic regurgitation.

CLINICAL MANIFESTATIONS. Men predominate over women in virtually all series by a ratio of anywhere between 2 and 8 to 1. Those patients without obvious Marfan syndrome usually are seen in the fourth, fifth, and sixth decades with progressively more severe aortic regurgitation. Patients with the classic Marfan syndrome or a forme fruste are generally younger. Some patients with annuloaortic ectasia experience sudden onset and rapid progression of symptoms, which may be due in part to severe aortic regurgitation secondary to aortic dissection. In the study of Lemon and White, recent aortic root dissection was found in 11 of 25 patients with annuloaortic ectasia who came to surgery.[123] All 11 of these patients had experienced chest pain before operation, although chest pain was also present in several patients with annuloaortic ectasia proven subsequently not to have had an aortic dissection.

The abnormal pulsation of the dilated aorta is sometimes palpable in the chest over the 2nd and 3rd right intercostal spaces, especially if the examination is done with

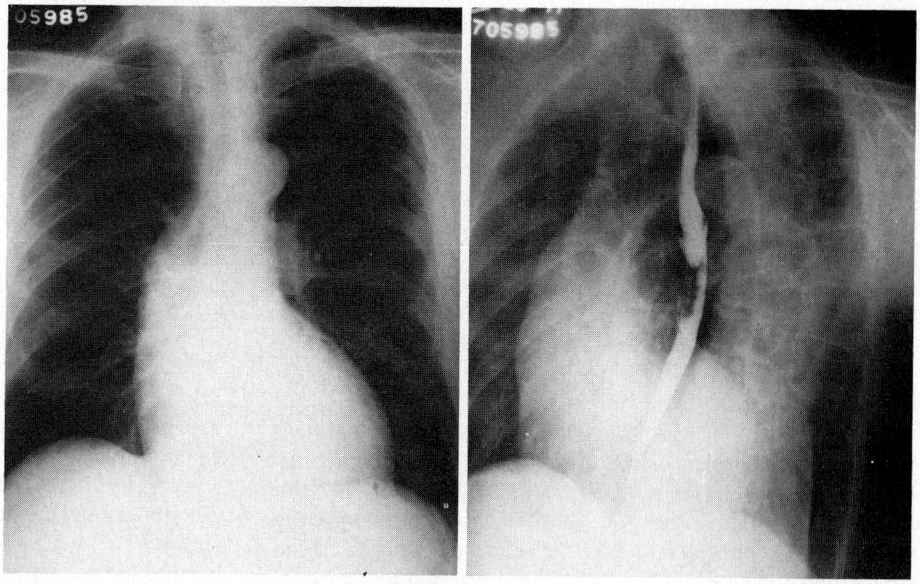

FIGURE 45–17 Posteroanterior (*left*) and left anterior oblique (*right*) chest roentgenograms in a 65-year-old man who had annuloaortic ectasia with severe aortic regurgitation that had developed over a 4-year period. Note the wide ascending aorta.

the patient sitting and in full expiration. We have also seen two patients with annuloaortic ectasia who had pulsation of the right sternoclavicular joint.

There is nothing especially unique to the signs and symptoms of aortic regurgitation in patients with annuloaortic ectasia as opposed to those who have aortic regurgitation from other causes, except for the greater intensity of the diastolic murmur to the right of the sternum in the former group and to the left in patients with a primary valvular abnormality. Lemon and White did find that the two features of an acute or subacute development of symptoms and the presence of chest pain were more frequently found in the group of patients with annuloaortic ectasia than in those with pure aortic valvular regurgitation, presumably on a rheumatic basis.[123] Features of the Marfan syndrome should be sought. They may be obvious, subtle, or absent.

The chest film usually shows a grossly dilated aortic root and ascending aorta (Fig. 45–17), with left ventricular enlargement proportionate to the severity of aortic regurgitation. Calcification in the aortic valve and dilated aorta is usually absent. Echocardiography or CT scan, in addition to showing classic features of aortic regurgitation (p. 115), demonstrates an abnormally widened aortic root. The huge aorta and the aortic regurgitation are easily demonstrated angiographically. Lemon and White identified three types of angiographic aortic enlargement: (1) "pear-shaped" enlargement (56 per cent) (Fig. 45–18); (2) diffuse symmetrical dilatation (27 per cent); and (3) dilatation limited to the sinuses of Valsalva (6 per cent).[123] In our own unpublished experience, aneurysmal dilatation of the sinuses of Valsalva is typically seen in those with Marfan syndrome. The mean maximal aortic diameter in Lemon and White's patients was 7.6 ± 2.7 cm and ranged from

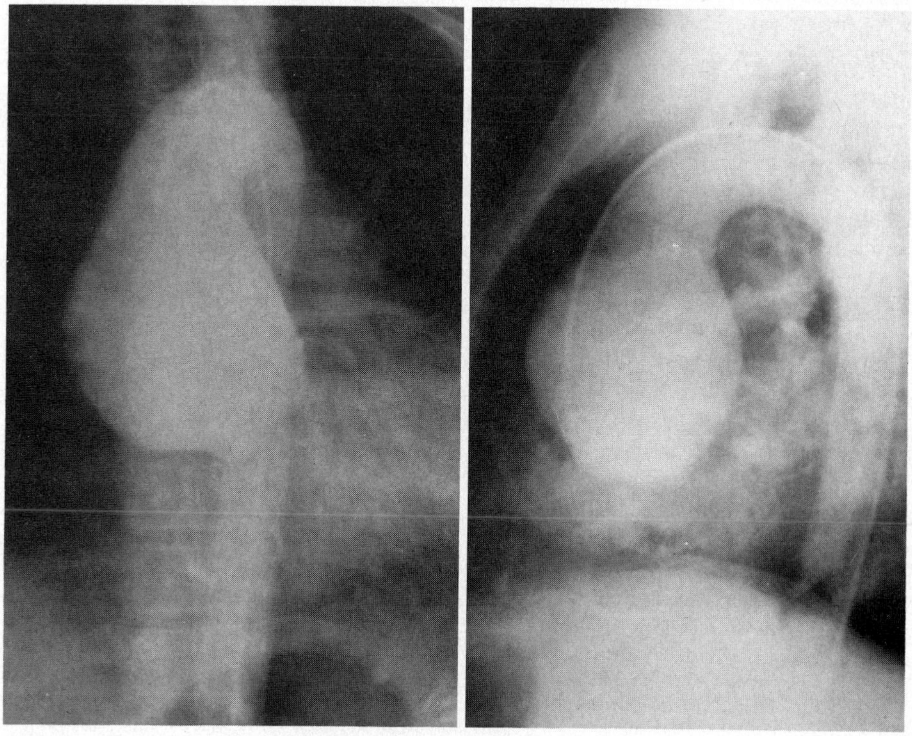

FIGURE 45–18 Anteroposterior (*left*) and lateral (*right*) aortogram in a man with annuloaortic ectasia. The bulbous, pear-shaped aortic root can be easily seen. The left ventricle is opacified consequent to aortic regurgitation. (Courtesy of Christos Athanasoulis, M.D., and Arthur Waltman, M.D., Section of Vascular Radiology, Massachusetts General Hospital, Boston.)

4.8 to 15 cm. This is two to five times the normal aortic diameter. Because dissections are characteristically small, circumscribed, and confined to the ascending aorta, they may not be easy to identify angiographically.

MANAGEMENT. Surgical correction using full cardiopulmonary bypass is usually undertaken for relief of the aortic regurgitation, when the latter is severe and responsible for symptoms of left ventricular failure or when the left ventricle or ascending aorta is increasing in size. However, in addition to replacing the aortic valve, resection of the aneurysmal aorta with insertion of a prosthetic (Dacron or Teflon) graft is generally required. Some surgeons advise sewing an artificial aortic valve to one end of a long prosthetic sleeve and suturing this in place from the aortic annulus at the end to the ascending aorta where it narrows beyond the aneurysm at the other. This reconstruction necessitates reimplantation of the coronary arteries. In fact, with aneurysmal sinuses of Valsalva, the coronary ostia may be carried cephalad by the enlarging sinuses, again necessitating ligation and reimplantation of the coronary arteries or the construction of saphenous vein bypass conduits from the aorta to the ligated coronary arteries. Because of the magnitude of the operation and the frequently friable tissues which make operation difficult, the risks of failure of aortic valve replacement and aneurysm resection are between 10 and 15 per cent in most centers; 5- and 10-year survival rates have been reported at 77 per cent and 57 per cent, respectively.[124] A recent report describing early and late survival for patients with the Marfan syndrome requiring aortic valve replacement and ascending aortic repair revealed no hospital mortality and a late survival rate of 61 per cent.[125] A tentative recommendation for elective repair of the aorta in patients with Marfan syndrome and aortic root diameter greater than 5.5 cm was made.[124]

Although postoperative results in survivors may be excellent, there is a disturbing occurrence of late sudden deaths, mostly from aortic dissection. However, death from progressive heart failure and sudden cardiac deaths also occur.

AORTIC ARTERITIS SYNDROMES

Takayasu's Arteritis

This peculiar arteritis was first noted in 1908 by the Japanese ophthalmologist Takayasu, who described a young woman with cataracts and unusual wreath-like arteriovenous anastoamoses surrounding the optic papillae[126] (Fig. 2–2*C*, p. 18). In discussing this case, Takayasu's colleagues called attention to two patients with similar ocular findings who also had absent radial pulses. Subsequently, this disease entity has been described by a variety of terms which reflect some of its many features, such as "aortic arch syndrome," "pulseless disease," "reversed coarctation," "occlusive thromboaortopathy," "young female arteritis," as well as Takayasu's arteritis.

DESCRIPTION, PATHOPHYSIOLOGY, AND ETIOLOGY. Although the majority of cases have been reported from Asia and Africa and most large series consist of Orientals, with a heavy predilection for women, this disease occurs worldwide.[127,128]

The basic pathological process is that of marked intimal proliferation and fibrosis and fibrous scarring and degeneration of the elastic fibers of the media, with round cell infiltration of variable intensity. However, fibrosis predominates over cellular reaction. The adventitia and intima become markedly thickened and vasa vasorum are destroyed. In its advanced cicatricial stage, the gross appearance of the aorta strikingly resembles the tree-barking of luetic aortitis. The proliferation process leads to obliterative luminal changes in the aorta and involved arteries. Localized aneurysm formation, poststenotic dilatation, and calcification in the aortic and arterial walls are late complications.[129,130] The process most often involves the arch of the aorta and its major branches, usually with changes that are most marked at the points of origin of the arteries from the aorta. It may present as multisegmental aortic disease with areas of normal wall between affected sites, diffuse involvement of the aorta, or predominantly disease of individual arteries arising from the aorta. The pulmonary arterial tree may also be affected.

Ueno et al. have subdivided the disease into three types, depending upon the sites of involvement (Fig. 45–19).[131] Type I involves primarily the aortic arch and its branches. Type II spares the aortic arch, involving the thoracoabdominal aorta and its branches; Type III combines features of both. More recently, Lupi-Herrera and colleagues have suggested a fourth category, Type IV, in which there is pulmonary arterial involvement.[128] In their series of 107 cases, the incidence of the various types was as follows: Type I, 8 per cent; Type II, 11 per cent; Type III, 65 per cent; and Type IV, 45 per cent (including several patients in the other groups).

A specific etiology for Takayasu's arteritis has not been forthcoming.[132] It has been linked to rheumatic fever, streptococcal infections, rheumatoid arthritis, and other collagen vascular diseases. Although giant cells are occasionally found in pathological specimens of vessels involved by the disease, the entity seems clearly distinct from giant cell arteritis, which affects predominantly patients over the age of 50 and involves mainly medium-sized muscular arteries. Although the aortic scarring of advanced Takayasu's arteritis resembles that of syphilis, nothing else suggests a causal relationship. Some investigators have reported a

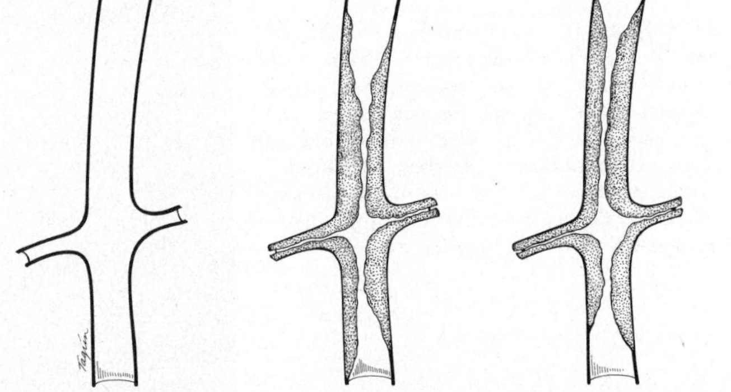

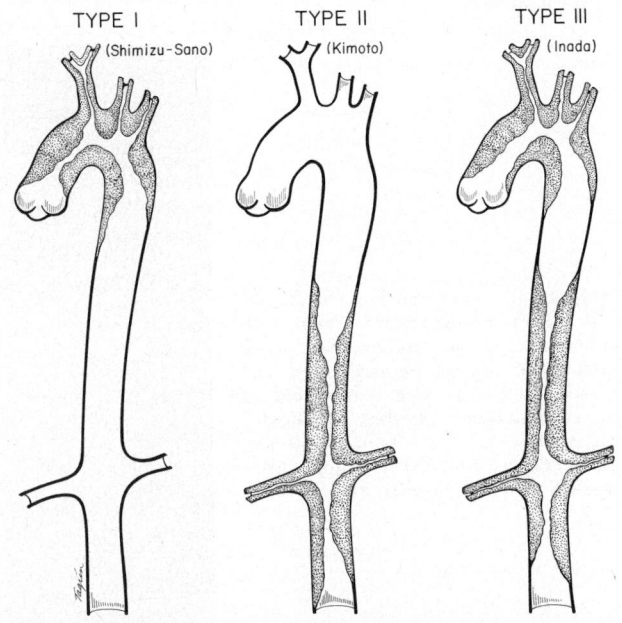

FIGURE 45–19 Types of Takayasu's arteritis. Type I involves primarily the aortic arch and brachiocephalic vessels. Type II affects the thoracoabdominal aorta and particularly the renal arteries. Type III combines features of both Types I and II. Types I and III may be complicated by aortic regurgitation. The eponyms for each type are noted.

strikingly higher incidence of tuberculin skin reactivity to both *Mycobacterium tuberculosis* and atypical mycobacteria in patients with Takayasu's arteritis compared with the general population, raising the possibility of a relationship to tuberculosis.[133] Although antiaortic antibodies have been detected in patients with this disease, their etiologic role is uncertain. Overall, the bulk of evidence favors an autoimmune etiology. It is likely that the arteritis represents the final common pathological expression of a number of different antigenic stimuli in susceptible patients. Recent evidence emphasizes an association between Takayasu's arteritis and certain HLA antigen subtypes.[134,135]

CLINICAL MANIFESTATIONS. The disease affects more women than men, in a ratio of 8.5 to 1. In as many as three-fourths of cases, onset is in the teenage years, although cases beginning in infancy or late middle age have been reported.[128,136,137] More than half the patients with this disease develop an initial systemic illness characterized by symptoms such as fever, anorexia, malaise, weight loss, night sweats, arthralgias, pleuritic pain, and fatigue. Localized pain and tenderness may be noted over affected arteries. This phase subsides, and these patients—as well as those who do not go through this so-called initial "systemic phase"—after a latent period of variable duration show symptoms and signs referable to the obliterative and inflammatory changes in the vessels. These late manifestations include diminished or absent pulses in 96 per cent, bruits in 94 per cent, hypertension in 74 per cent, and heart failure in 28 per cent.[128] The retinopathy originally described by Takayasu is seen in only about 25 per cent and is usually associated with carotid arterial involvement. The ocular process may lead to retinal detachment and loss of vision.

Patients with Types I and III manifest those findings which are considered to be most typical of this disease, namely "reversed" coarctation of the aorta with absent or diminished upper body pulses and barely detectable blood pressure in the arms, higher pressures in the lower extremities, bruits overlying diseased arteries, manifestations of ischemia at various affected sites, and syncope. Patients with Type II arteritis may have abdominal angina and claudication of the limbs but also tend to develop hypertension because of renal arterial involvement. In fact, hypertension is an extremely important complication of this disease, and it may be difficult to recognize because of the diminished pulsations in the arms. Hypertension appears to arise through several mechanisms, the two most important of which are hemodynamically significant coarctation of the aorta and renal artery stenosis. Decreased aortic capacitance and reduced baroreceptor reactivity may be contributory.[138,139]

Heart failure, when present, is usually seen in very young patients and appears to be a consequence of systemic hypertension. Rarely, aortic regurgitation can also contribute to congestive failure and is due to severe hypertension or to inflammation and scarring of the aortic valve by the inflammatory process.[140] The ostia and proximal segments of the coronary arteries can be affected, resulting in angina or myocardial infarction.[141,142] Rarely, aneurysms are palpable or arteriovenous fistulas occur.[137] Takayasu's arteritis may be a common cause of atypical coarctation syndromes in adults.[130,136,143,144] The frequent ab-

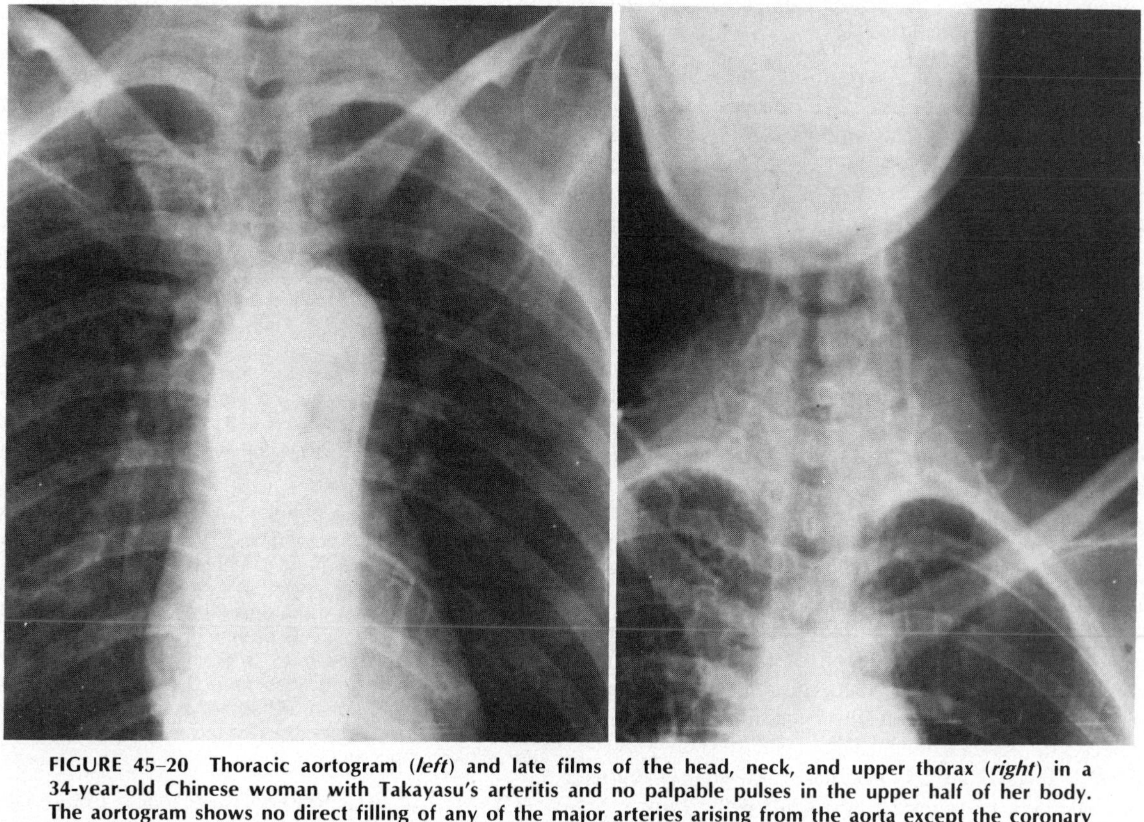

FIGURE 45-20 Thoracic aortogram (*left*) and late films of the head, neck, and upper thorax (*right*) in a 34-year-old Chinese woman with Takayasu's arteritis and no palpable pulses in the upper half of her body. The aortogram shows no direct filling of any of the major arteries arising from the aorta except the coronary arteries. In the delayed film (*right*) collateral channels faintly fill the carotid and vertebral systems.

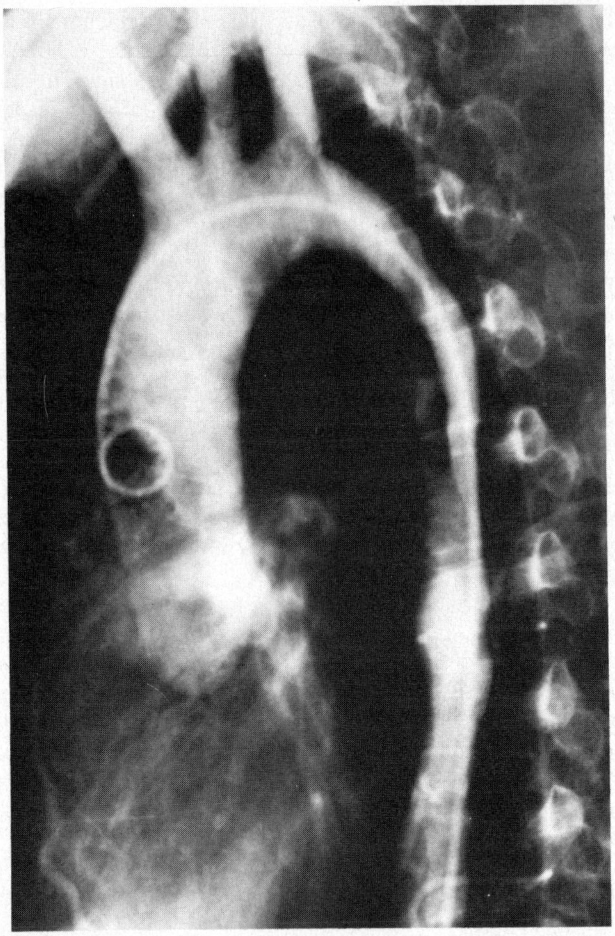

FIGURE 45–21 Aortogram in a 28-year-old Korean man with the clinical features of coarctation of the aorta that proved to be the result of Takayasu's arteritis. Note the typical "rat-tail" angiographic appearance of the descending thoracic aorta.

sence of antecedent systemic symptoms and the more equal sex distribution of this form of the disease have been stressed. It is also believed that Takayasu's arteritis may be responsible for some cases of what appear to be primary pulmonary hypertension.[145,146]

Laboratory abnormalities during the systemic phase are frequent.[133] The sedimentation rate is usually elevated, and a low-grade leukocytosis and mild anemia of chronic disease are common. These return toward normal when the systemic phase resolves. IgG values are almost invariably increased. Other serological abnormalities are common but not specific. These include elevated levels of C-reactive protein, increased antistreptolysin-O titers, and the occasional presence of rheumatoid factor and antinuclear antibodies.

Chest roentgenograms are usually unrevealing, although a rim of calcification is sometimes seen in the walls of the affected arteries. Arteriography reveals typical findings of an irregular intimal surface, with stenosis of the aorta or its tributary arteries, poststenotic dilatations, saccular aneurysms, and even complete occlusion of vessels (Fig. 45–20). Lande and Rossi have described the affected thoracic aorta as having a typical, narrowed, "rat tail" angiographic appearance (Fig. 45–21).[147]

TREATMENT AND PROGNOSIS. Adrenal corticosteroids are effective in relieving constitutional symptoms in patients with the systemic phase of the disease.[148] Fever, malaise, and fatigue are often dramatically relieved by steroids, and the sedimentation rate, which is a sensitive indicator of the activity of the disease, falls toward normal. There is also some evidence that corticosteroids may retard progression of arterial narrowing during the active stage of the disease. Anticoagulant drugs, including those of the warfarin family, and drugs that inhibit platelet function, such as aspirin and dipyridamole, are recommended both for treatment of transient ischemic symptoms and for prevention of progression of the disease. Their precise efficacy is not established. *Surgical treatment* of many different types may be needed to deal with late complications of Takayasu's arteritis.[149–151] These include endarterectomy, bypass of obstructed arteries (especially the renal arteries), resection of localized coarctations, excision of saccular aneurysms, and, rarely, aortic valve replacement.

The course of the disease is unpredictable, but slow progression over a period of months to years is usual. Morbidity and mortality depend upon the presence or absence of severe complications, which include retinopathy, secondary hypertension, aortic regurgitation, and aortic or arterial aneurysms. In one series, eventless survival over 7 years was 97 per cent in patients without major complications, compared with 59 per cent in patients with complications.[152] Heart failure and cerebrovascular accidents are common causes of death.

Giant Cell Arteritis

This disease of unknown cause is predominantly a disease of elderly people and characteristically involves medium-sized arteries. However, the aorta and its major branches are affected in about 15 per cent of cases.[153,154] The disease is also referred to as "granulomatous arteritis," "cranial" or "temporal" arteritis, and "arteritis of the aged." It is closely allied to a syndrome characterized by diffuse muscular aching and stiffness called polymyalgia rheumatica.

Pathophysiology and Etiology. The many names given this disease describe its important features. The characteristic pathological lesion that distinguishes it from other arteritis syndromes is granulomatous inflammation of the media of small- to medium-caliber arteries, about the size of the temporal artery, and especially vessels of the head and neck. In addition to the granulomas, an inflammatory infiltrate is usually found, composed largely of eosinophils, plasma cells, and other mononuclear elements. Endarteritis is not an important feature, but the mural involvement can lead to obstruction of the lumen of involved arteries. Rarely, the aortic wall may be weakened by the granulomatous process, leading to localized aneurysm formation, aortic annular dilatation, and aortic regurgitation. One of the more vivid examples of such aortic involvement by giant cell arteritis is the case report by Austen and Blennerhassett of a young black woman with an aortic aneurysm extending from the aortic valve to the origin of the innominate artery, with wide-open aortic regurgitation from annular dilatation.[155]

Involvement of the aorta and its major tributaries, when it occurs, may coexist with the more classic and prevalent syndromes of temporal arteritis and polymyalgia rheumatica, or, rarely, the aorta may serve as the primary target of this disease.

The etiology of giant cell arteritis is unknown, although the generalized systemic manifestations of the disease and its occasional apparent temporal relationship to prior immunization or a viral illness suggest a possible infectious or autoimmune origin.[156] Klein et al. point out that involvement of the aorta and larger arteries may often arise as corticosteroid therapy for the more classic forms of this disease is being tapered.[153]

CLINICAL MANIFESTATIONS. Giant cell arteritis typically affects patients over the age of 50 and occurs predominantly in women. The classic presentation is a triad of severe headache, marked malaise, and fever. Other severe constitutional symptoms are common and include anorexia, weight loss, lassitude, myalgias, and night sweats. Headaches are sometimes intense and almost unbearable. Headache typically occurs over involved arteries, usually the temporal arteries, but occasionally the occipital region. The area around the arteries is exquisitely sensitive to pressure, and complaints such as being unable to rest the head comfortably against a pillow are common. Claudication in the jaw muscles while chewing occurs in up to two-thirds of patients and is considered most suggestive of the diagnosis.[157] A serious complication that may occur anywhere in the course of the disease is the onset of blindness from involvement of the ophthalmic artery—blindness that is often irreversible. Visual symptoms ranging from blurring to diplopia and visual loss occur in 25 to 50 per cent of patients.[157] In its milder forms, patients may complain only of generalized muscular aches and pains and unusual fatigue, the syndrome of polymyalgia rheumatica. Blindness in these cases is uncommon.[157]

On rare occasions, consequences of involvement of the aorta or its major tributaries may be the first manifestations of the disease, although more typically, when such involvement occurs, it is part of the more generalized syndrome. However, when aortic or major branch disease is present, the symptoms are similar to those of Takayasu's arteritis and are the result of ischemia in the structures supplied by the involved arteries. Specifically, symptoms may include claudication of either upper or lower extremities, paresthesias, Raynaud's phenomenon, abdominal angina, coronary ischemia, transient cerebral ischemic attacks, and aortic arch and great vessel "steal" syndromes. More rarely, aortic aneurysms, aortic regurgitation, and aortic dissection may occur.[158] Interestingly, renal artery involvement is almost never seen, in contrast with Takayasu's arteritis.[153] Death can occur from aortic rupture or dissection.

On *physical examination*, fever is almost universal and patients appear toxic. Involved vessels are thickened and very tender. Indeed, an experienced examiner can often make the diagnosis of temporal arteritis with virtual certainty at the bedside simply by palpating an indurated, beaded, tender, temporal artery. Pulses may be lost, and bruits may occur over sites of arterial occlusion. Signs of aortic regurgitation are rarely present.

The *laboratory* may be helpful in making the diagnosis. A very high sedimentation rate is virtually a sine qua non for this disease and is a valuable guide to the activity of the process. A moderate normochromic, normocytic anemia is the rule. Acute phase reactants such as $alpha_2$ globulin are increased, and IgG levels also are often elevated.

The *diagnosis* is usually confirmed by biopsy of an involved artery, usually the temporal artery. In cases of larger vessel and aortic involvement, angiography may serve to differentiate arteritis from arteriosclerosis by the following features as described by Klein et al.: (1) long, smooth tapering stenosis alternating with segments of normal or even slightly increased diameter; (2) the absence of irregular ulcerated atheromatous plaques seen in profile; and (3) the more typical anatomical distribution of arteritis to include subclavian, axillary, and brachial arteries.[153]

MANAGEMENT. High-dose steroid therapy, e.g., 60 to 80 mg of prednisone per day, is recommended in all patients with granulomatous arteritis. The intent of therapy is not only to reverse the disease but also to prevent progression, especially in the ophthalmic arteries with resultant blindness. Using constitutional symptoms and the sedimentation rate as a guide, steroids usually can be reduced gradually, and the overall course is one of progressive improvement and eventual complete resolution. However, in many patients, the course of the disease may be protracted for months or years. Very rarely, surgical resection of an expanding aneurysm or replacement of a regurgitant aortic valve is necessary.[132,155,158,159]

Other Arteritis Syndromes

In addition to the aortic inflammation of Takayasu's and giant cell arteritis, isolated aortic regurgitation due to dilatation of the aortic valve ring with associated aortic root involvement may occur during the course of ankylosing spondylitis, psoriatic arthritis, arthritis associated with ulcerative colitis, relapsing polychondritis, and Reiter's syndrome.[160–164] Additionally, it is likely that aortic aneurysms rarely can complicate Behcet's syndrome.[165]

Reported instances of aortitis complicating each of these diseases is rare. For example, it is seen in 1 to 4 per cent of patients with ankylosing spondylitis (p. 1656), and only 15 well-described cases of Reiter's syndrome with aortic regurgitation have been documented (p. 1658). Nevertheless, the symptoms of aortic regurgitation and resultant heart failure may eventually dominate the clinical picture. In each case of arthritis-associated aortitis, the underlying arthritic disease is particularly fulminant and prolonged, and multiple extraarticular features are usually manifest.

Pathological features. These appear to be similar in each of the above diseases. In the early stages of inflammation there is marked dilatation of the aortic valve ring with patchy elastic tissue disruption, an active inflammatory cell infiltrate, and subendothelial fibrosis.[163] These changes are most marked in the aortic root. Later, the proximal ascending aorta develops a picture not unlike that of luetic aortitis, with intimal thickening, coarse, granular plaque formation, and characteristic obliterative endarteritis of the vasa vasorum. The aortic root dilates but usually without frank aneurysm formation. Early, the aortic valve cusps remain essentially normal and later become thickened and retracted, presumably as a result of the incompetence that arises from root dilatation.

The clinical features are those of aortic regurgitation and especially resemble those of annuloaortic ectasia. However, it is worth noting that the course of this disease is variable. Some patients evolve a rapidly progressive course of cardiac decompensation, whereas others have a more indolent and stable natural history. Thus the development of aortic regurgitation does not necessarily signify an irreversible downhill course. There is some evidence that the inflammation of the aortic root may be episodic; worsening of aortic regurgitation may also follow an intermittent course.

Paulus et al. make particular note of the seemingly high incidence of first-degree heart block in their patients with Reiter's syndrome.[163] This block was transient in two of their three patients, and, in one, it antedated the murmur of aortic regurgitation by 3 years. Heart block presumably results from inflammatory infiltrate in the area of the atrioventricular node and can progress to higher grade block. In fact, complete heart block can occur.

Treatment consists of that required for the underlying

arthritis or other disease. Aortic valve replacement should be performed when indicated, although special problems may be encountered in these patients. For example, pulmonary function is often impaired in ankylosing spondylitis as a result of rigidity of the thoracic spine and chest wall. In the rare patient with ulcerative colitis who requires aortic valve replacement, a porcine valve is recommended so that anticoagulation will be unnecessary. In contrast to annuloaortic ectasia, replacement of the ascending aorta itself is almost never necessary.

CARDIOVASCULAR SYPHILIS

Once accounting for between 5 and 10 per cent of all cardiovascular deaths, syphilitic disease of the heart and aorta has become a relative rarity in most major medical centers today owing to the aggressive treatment of lues in its early stages with effective antibiotics. However, the resurgence of syphilis over the past two decades makes it likely that a corresponding increase in the number of cases of cardiovascular syphilis will appear in the future.

Cardiovascular complications occur in approximately 10 to 12 per cent of cases of untreated lues.[166] The latent period may extend from 5 to 40 years after the initial spirochetal infection, with a usual time of 10 to 25 years.

Pathology. The consequences of lues are the direct results of spirochetal infection of the aortic media, thought to occur usually during the secondary phase of the disease, with subsequent inflammation and scarring of the aortic wall. Although the aorta may be invaded anywhere along its course, the most common location—and, in fact, the hallmark of the disease—is the ascending aorta. It is postulated that this area has a proclivity for syphilitic involvement because it is richer in lymphatics than any other portion of the aorta. The muscular and elastic tissues of the media are destroyed by the spirochetal invasion and resultant inflammatory process and are replaced by vascular fibrous tissue. There is an occlusive endarteritis of the vasa vasorum, with perivascular cuffing by plasma cells and lymphocytes.

The aortic wall becomes progressively weakened by the inflammatory process, and it may become calcified. Weakening of the wall leads to the development of aneurysmal dilatation. The overlying intima assumes a furrowed, wrinkled appearance covered with large plaques of a glistening, pearly material. This accounts for the "tree bark" appearance of the involved aorta that is characteristic, but not pathognomonic, of luetic aortitis.

The infection may extend into the aortic root, resulting in aortic regurgitation which is due to dilatation of the aortic annulus and separation of the aortic valve commissures. The support of the leaflets is undermined, and this combination of separation of the leaflets by widening of the annulus and undermining of the support of the cusps leads to progressively more severe aortic regurgitation. The leaflets are often floppy with curling of their edges, although this may be as much a consequence as a cause of the regurgitation. Often with aortic regurgitation there is an associated aneurysm, with calcification in the wall of the aneurysm and the annulus of the valve and base of the leaflets. An obliterative endarteritis may also obstruct the ostia of the two coronary arteries. Unfortunately, the scarring and injury from lues may progress long after the spirochetal organisms have been eradicated, accounting for what is so often a very long latent period before luetic aortitis becomes manifest.

There are four categories of syphilitic heart disease:[167] (1) uncomplicated syphilitic aortitis, (2) syphilitic aortic aneurysm, (3) syphilitic aortic valvulitis with aortic regurgitation, and (4) syphilitic coronary ostial stenosis. From autopsy studies, about one-third of patients with cardiovascular lues are "asymptomatic," meaning that they have postmortem pathological evidence of luetic involvement of the aortic wall without clinical manifestations. About half have a significant aortic aneurysm, and, of these, one-half to one-third have associated aortic regurgitation. Five to 10 per cent will have essentially pure aortic regurgitation, and 26 per cent will have significant luetic coronary ostial stenosis, often in association with aortic regurgitation or an aortic aneurysm, but occasionally as the only luetic manifestation.[167]

CLINICAL MANIFESTATIONS. Luetic aneurysms can arise anywhere along the aorta, but the most typical location is in the ascending aorta. They are usually saccular but may be fusiform. In the absence of aortic regurgitation, aneurysms may undergo significant enlargement without producing symptoms. Eventually, an aneurysm may expand enough to reach, compress, and even erode contiguous structures, particularly the sternum and anterior right thoracic cage in the case of aneurysms of the ascending aorta. A thrusting, pulsating mass may be seen and palpated. Although luetic aneurysms frequently rupture, they very rarely lead to aortic dissection.

Erosion of the bony structures of the chest wall causes pain at the site of involvement. Ascending aortic aneurysms and those involving the arch may produce a tracheal tug, stridor, and dysphagia. Aneurysms elsewhere may cause symptoms from compression of adjacent structures similar to those of any type of aneurysm located in the same area, such as hoarseness from compression of the left recurrent laryngeal nerve and cough from pressure against the left main stem bronchus in the case of aneurysms of the descending thoracic aorta. Compression of the main pulmonary artery, causing pulmonic stenosis, and rupture of syphilitic aneurysms into a pulmonary artery have been reported rarely.[168]

Although rare, luetic abdominal aortic aneurysms most commonly originate at the level of the 12th thoracic to the 2nd lumbar vertebrae, appearing before age 50, in contrast with arteriosclerotic aneurysms that tend to occur in older patients and are usually located below the level of the renal arteries.[169]

Luetic aortic regurgitation (p. 1106) tends to occur in older patients with luetic cardiovascular disease, presumably because of the longer duration of the disease in these individuals.[170] The earliest auscultatory sign of luetic aortic valve involvement is a tambour-like aortic closure sound. Because of the dilated aortic root, the murmur of luetic aortic regurgitation may be more prominent along the right sternal edge rather than the left, which is usually the case with rheumatic aortic regurgitation. The luetic aortic regurgitant murmur is often musical in quality. Rarely, eversion of one of the aortic cusps—especially the noncoronary leaflet—causes a spectacular, cooing diastolic murmur that is grade 5 or 6 in intensity, with a thrill. It may be heard intermittently and is often mistaken for a systolic murmur because of its loudness and honking quality.

Because there is often considerable calcification in the aortic annulus and stiffness of the base of the aortic leaflets, and because of the usually dilated proximal aorta, a loud systolic ejection murmur, sometimes with a thrill, is often present in luetic aortic valve disease in the absence of any significant aortic stenosis. Also, a loud, slapping, systolic ejection sound is sometimes caused by sudden distention of the dilated aorta by a large volume of blood in early systole.

A few clinical features of luetic aortic regurgitation may

be peculiar to it. Thus an associated aneurysm of the ascending aorta may be felt. Also, because of the concomitant coronary ostial stenosis, angina may be disproportionately severe for the degree of apparent aortic regurgitation. Atrial fibrillation, rare in other types of pure aortic regurgitation, is more frequent in luetic heart disease, perhaps again owing to the occasional occurrence of coronary ostial disease. Otherwise, the bounding pulses, wide pulse pressure, other signs of aortic diastolic runoff, and electrocardiographic evidence of left ventricular hypertrophy do not serve to distinguish luetic from other types of aortic regurgitation of equal severity.

DIAGNOSIS. Usually, there is a history of syphilis, and other manifestations of tertiary lues are found in 10 to 30 per cent of patients with cardiovascular syphilis. Fifteen to 30 per cent of patients have negative routine serological tests (Wasserman, Hinton, Kahn, Venereal Disease Research Laboratories [VDRL], and Kolmer) for syphilis.[171] On the other hand, serological tests directed against a specific treponema antigen, such as the *Treponema pallidum* immobilization (TPI) test or the fluorescent treponemal antibody absorption (FTA-ABS) test are almost invariably positive. The chest roentgenogram may afford extremely valuable clues to the diagnosis of luetic aortitis. The calcification in the ascending aorta proximal to the brachiocephalic vessels is almost always much more extensive than that elsewhere. This is in sharp contrast to arteriosclerosis.

Angiography may delineate the aneurysm (Fig. 45–22) and help to quantify the severity of aortic regurgitation. In patients suspected of having coronary ostial stenosis and in any patient with cardiovascular syphilis in whom surgical correction is contemplated, the coronary artery anatomy—and, particularly, the ostia—should be visualized by angiography if possible. Sometimes, the ostial lesion is so pronounced that it may prove to be impossible to enter the lumen of the affected artery with the catheter.

TREATMENT. All patients with syphilis, including cardiovascular syphilis, who are seen 1 year or more after the initial contact should be given a course of antibiotic therapy aimed at curing the spirochetal infection. Penicillin is still the most effective antibiotic and can be given by either of two schedules: (1) benzathine penicillin G, (Bicillin), 2.4 million units intramuscularly weekly for 3 weeks (total of 7.2 million units), or (2) aqueous procaine penicillin G, 600,000 units intramuscularly daily for 15 days. For patients allergic to penicillin, the recommended therapy is tetracycline, 500 mg orally four times daily for 30 days, or cephaloridine, 0.5 to 1.0 gm intramuscularly daily for 10 days. Although some suggest erythromycin, 500 mg orally four times daily for 30 days, as another alternative to penicillin, this regimen is generally considered to be less effective than the others. The effectiveness of treatment can be monitored by a decrease in VDRL titer, with the desired result being a fourfold reduction in titer in 12 to 24 months.[171,172]

Although a course of antibiotics is recommended in any previously untreated patient with cardiovascular syphilis, even those with a negative serology, there is no good evidence that such treatment reverses, or even halts, the progression of aortitis or aortic regurgitation. In cases of cardiovascular syphilis, cerebrospinal fluid examination should also be performed, and, if positive, this too should be followed to assure the adequacy of therapy. Since the efficacy of antibiotics other than penicillin against syphilis is not well studied beyond 1 year, close follow-up of patients treated with these alternative modes is recommended.

The indications for excision of the luetic aneurysms are similar to those for other thoracic aortic aneurysms (p. 1547): a diameter of 7 cm or larger or an aneurysm of any size that produces symptoms or is expanding rapidly. Since many luetic aneurysms are saccular, aneurysmorrhaphy is occasionally adequate. However, since ongoing aortitis and scarring are possible, it is probably wiser to replace as much as possible of the diseased aorta with a prosthetic graft. Prosthetic replacement of the aortic valve is indicated for significant aortic regurgitation, and the results are as good as in aortic regurgitation of other causes. Since the coronary artery disease of syphilis is usually ostial, a localized endarterectomy at the orifices of the coronary arteries may be possible.[173] If an adequate lumen cannot be obtained by endarterectomy, bypass conduits may be necessary.

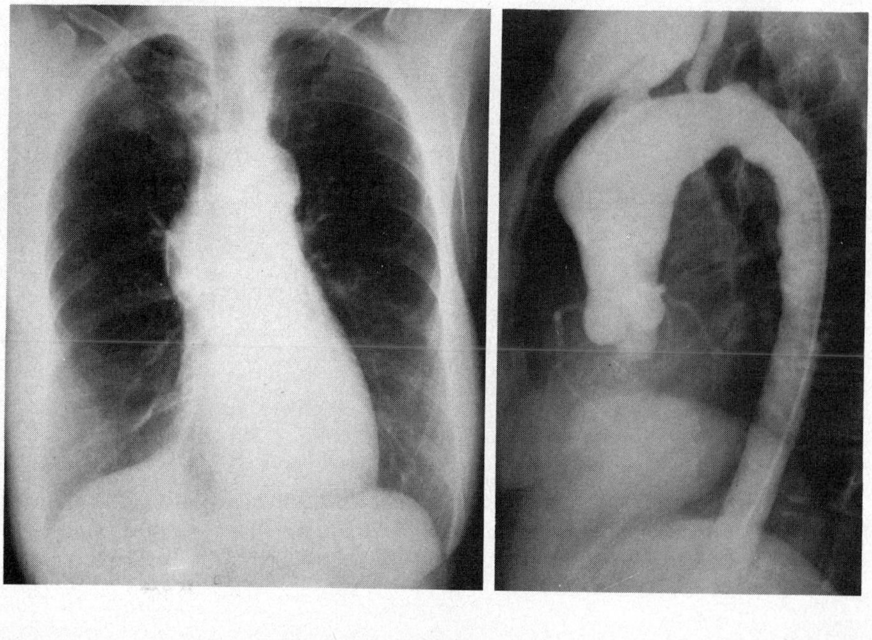

FIGURE 45–22 Films obtained from a 58-year-old woman with luetic aortitis. *Left,* Posteroanterior chest film showing an aneurysm of the ascending aorta with a faint rim of calcification. *Right,* Angiographic appearance of the aneurysm in the lateral view. (Courtesy of Christos Athanasoulis, M.D., and Arthur Waltman, M.D., Section of Vascular Radiology, Massachusetts General Hospital, Boston.)

PSEUDOCOARCTATION

Pseudocoarctation of the aorta is a rare condition resulting from elongation of the aortic arch, with redundancy and kinking of the aorta just distal to the origin of the left subclavian artery at the level of the ligamentum arteriosum.[174,175] Other terms used to describe this entity have included "mild coarctation," "atypical coarctation," or "subclinical coarctation."[176] Etiology is believed to be congenital, with a lack of compression and fusion of certain of the segments of the dorsal aortic root and fourth arch.[177] It is of interest that the incidence and distribution of associated cardiac anomalies parallel those seen in true coarctation. These anomalies include bicuspid aortic valve, sinus of Valsalva aneurysms, ventricular septal defect, and corrected transposition.[178]

Clinical Manifestations. The pressure gradient across the deformed area is usually trivial or absent. Thus, the clinical features of true coarctation—upper extremity hypertension, lower extremity hypotension, and the development of collateral arterial circulation—are absent. Physical findings are often those of the associated lesions, although a murmur is sometimes heard over the aortic kink in the interscapular area. With mild degrees of obstruction, blood pressure in the lower extremities may be slightly reduced, and there may be a subtle pulse lag between the radial and femoral arteries.

The entity can usually be recognized on chest roentgenography. The typical appearance is that of a double rounded density in the left superior mediastinum. Pitfalls in interpretation of the x-ray films are common. The upper density, though relatively translucent, represents the uppermost extension of redundant aorta and is often mistaken for tumor or aneurysm.[179] The lower density is the area of the aorta involved by poststenotic dilatation, and it is often misinterpreted as the aortic knob. Calcification may occur in the area of narrowing. Angiography confirms the diagnosis.

Significance. Problems may arise in pseudocoarctation from the formation of aneurysms by enlargement of the area either proximal or distal to the kink (Fig. 45–23). Associated aneurysms of the left subclavian artery have been reported.[180,181] Rarely, thrombus forms at the site of atheromatous degeneration and calcification in the kinked segment.[182] Complete thrombosis can produce a picture mimicking true coarctation, although collateral arterial circulation is notably absent.[182,183] Thrombus can also propagate directly into tributary vessels or embolize distally. The left subclavian artery is particularly vulnerable because of its proximity to the pseudocoarctation. Infection at the site of aortic narrowing is a rare problem.

Treatment. Therapy is necessary only for complications of pseudocoarctation. In the absence of complications, surgical resection is not indicated.[184] If a bruit or pressure gradient is present over an area of pseudocoarctation, antibiotic prophylaxis for endocarditis should be given before dental or surgical procedures.

AORTIC TRAUMA

(Also see p. 1537)

Blunt Trauma

Aortic injuries are associated with severe blunt trauma, and they are far from rare. In one autopsy series of fatal automobile accidents, rupture of the aorta was found in one-sixth of all victims.[185]

Etiology and Pathogenesis. Aortic trauma most commonly results from injuries associated with sudden high-speed deceleration upon impact, such as that resulting from motor vehicle accidents or severe falls.[185–188] The abrupt deceleration of the body as it crashes to a sudden stop creates enormous shearing forces which act maximally at those points where a highly mobile portion of the aorta joins a fixed segment. Less frequently, pressure or blast injuries may produce rupture of the aorta, believed to be caused by an acute increase in intraaortic pressure generated by the compression of blood contained within the aorta and further increased by the force imparted by cardiac systole.

Although the aorta may be torn anywhere along its length, the most frequent point of rupture, the site of 90 per cent of cases, is in the aortic isthmus at the site of insertion of the ligamentum arteriosum, just distal to the origin of the left subclavian artery. Here, the relatively mobile descending thoracic aorta sweeps dorsally to become fixed to the thoracic cage by the ligamentum arteriosum, the intercostal arteries, and the left subclavian artery. The injury may vary from a miniscule rent in the aortic wall to a complete circumferential transection of all three layers of the aorta. In the series of Parmley et al., 80 per cent of 296 cases of aortic trauma had a circumferential tear.[186] If the aorta is partially transected and the patient survives, a localized saccular aneurysm or pseudoaneurysm may develop subse-

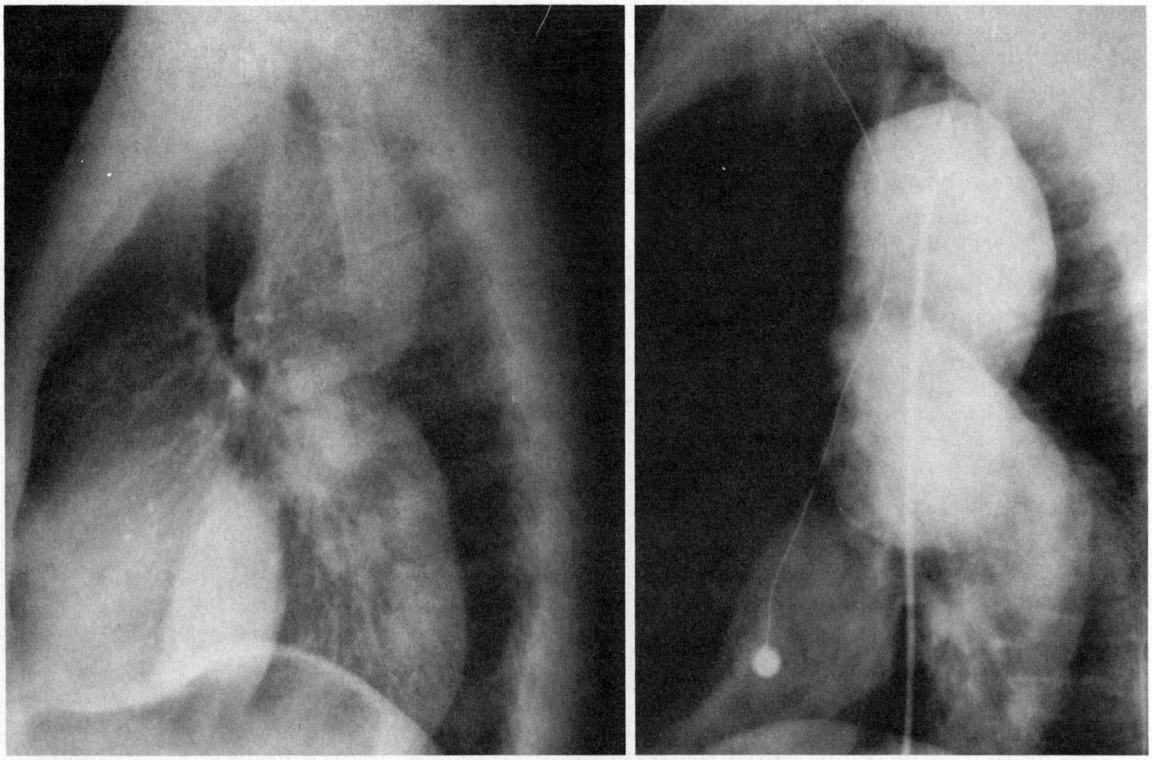

FIGURE 45–23 Pseudocoarctation of the aorta, with aneurysmal dilatation of the aorta proximal and distal to the point of narrowing. *Left,* Lateral chest roentgenogram. *Right,* The aorta is outlined with contrast material.

quently at the site of the tear. Pseudoaneurysms may also form between the two ends of a totally transected aorta.

In addition to the aortic isthmus, which is the locus of 90 per cent of all aortic injuries, other areas of injury include the supravalvular portion of the ascending aorta; the innominate artery, which may be avulsed from the aorta; the aortic arch; other portions of the descending thoracic aorta; the abdominal aorta; and combinations of these.

CLINICAL MANIFESTATIONS. The diagnosis of aortic trauma is often obscured by the presence of other serious injuries, such as central nervous system damage, visceral injury, and multiple systemic fractures. About two-thirds of patients with aortic rupture have clear-cut evidence of other thoracic trauma, such as chest or cardiac contusions, rib or vertebral fractures, pulmonary contusions, and hemorrhagic pleural effusions. The remaining one-third are surprisingly free of overt evidence of chest-wall injury.[187]

Few symptoms are directly attributable to the aortic trauma per se. Pressure from a localized hematoma can cause dyspnea and stridor from tracheal or bronchial compression, dysphagia from esophageal compression, or superior vena caval syndrome from caval compression. Although it is uncommon, the syndrome of so-called "acute coarctation" with upper extremity hypertension, reduced blood pressure in the lower extremities, a systolic murmur over the precordium or in the interscapular area, and a palpable radial-femoral pulse lag is virtually classic for the diagnosis.[189] An interscapular systolic bruit may be heard. Otherwise, the physical examination is quite unrevealing. Localized aneurysms developing in the aortic isthmus late after trauma may cause hoarseness, cough, and dysphagia from compression of the adjacent recurrent laryngeal nerve, bronchus, and esophagus.

DIAGNOSIS. Because the diagnosis is so frequently overshadowed by the presence of other severe injuries, rupture of the aorta is often overlooked. *A high index of suspicion is crucial, and evidence of aortic trauma should be sought in any patient with severe bodily injuries.* In the absence of classic physical findings, a common situation, the diagnosis is best suspected from the chest roentgenogram, which, if properly performed and interpreted, is abnormal in over 90 per cent of patients with traumatic aortic rupture; the most important radiologic abnormality is widening of the mediastinum.[190–192] Marsh and Sturm have delineated criteria for rupture of the aorta based upon a 40-degree anteroposterior supine chest film. The numbers on Figure 45–24 correspond to these criteria: (1) mediastinum measuring greater than 8 cm at the level of the aortic knob; (2) shift of trachea toward the right; (3) blurring of the normally sharp outline of the aorta; (4) obliteration of the medial aspect of the apex of the upper lobe of the left lung; (5) opacification of the clear space between the aorta and pulmonary artery; and (6) depression of the left main stem bronchus below 40 degrees.[193] Ayella et al. have emphasized the need for a true erect anteroposterior chest film, with the patient tilted a few degrees forward from the vertical axis to facilitate recognition of a widened mediastinum.[188] Additionally, the presence of a left apical cap due to mediastinal bleeding that extends into the left extrapleural apical space should prompt further search for traumatic aortic rupture.[194] CT with contrast injection may confirm the diagnosis and should be performed as expeditiously as possible in a stable patient who has sustained severe chest trauma.[7] Should the diagnosis remain in question or if the patient is unstable the threshold for performing angiography in suspected cases should be low (Fig. 45–25).

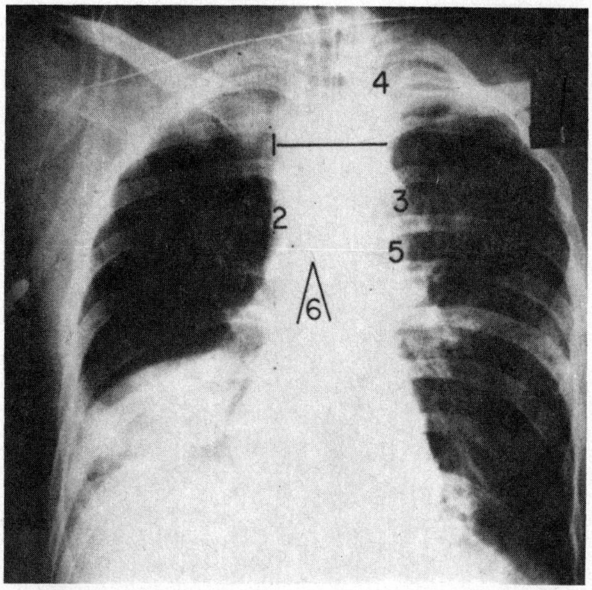

FIGURE 45–24 Aortic trauma. Roentgenographic characteristics of rupture of the proximal descending thoracic aorta in the supine anteroposterior projection (film-to-tube distance = 40 inches). See text for key to numbers. (From Marsh, D. G., and Sturm, J. T.: Traumatic aortic rupture: Roentgenographic indications for angiography. Ann. Thorac. Surg. *27*:337, 1976.)

COURSE AND PROGNOSIS. Approximately 80 per cent of patients with aortic rupture die instantly, although usually from other injuries, such as massive hemorrhage from other sites, trauma to other vital organs, or brain damage. Of those who survive the initial event, death often occurs from progressive hemorrhage at the site of the aortic tear within the first week. However, even with complete transection of the aorta, patients may be remarkably stable. About 2 to 5 per cent of patients with partial tears of the aorta go on to develop a localized aneurysm or pseudoaneurysm over a period of months or years, usually anterior to the aortic isthmus. This may either remain stable or ultimately expand. Such traumatic aneurysms frequently calcify or may become infected.[195,196]

TREATMENT. The treatment of aortic trauma is operative repair, which should be undertaken as soon as possible once the condition is recognized. Occasionally, other serious injuries make it necessary to delay operation in order to stabilize the patient, but even in the face of other severe trauma, surgery should be performed if there is evidence of progressive hemorrhage from the aorta. Rupture of the aorta is usually treated by resecting the torn segment of the aorta and inserting an interposed prosthetic graft into the two ends of the aorta. It may be necessary to support the distal circulation with a pump oxygenator or conduit bypass from the proximal to the distal aorta around the rupture in order to avoid ischemic damage to the spinal cord, abdominal viscera, and kidneys. Prompt recognition and operation for a ruptured aorta has resulted in survival of 75 to 80 per cent of patients with this injury who reach the hospital alive.[188]

In cases of localized saccular aneurysms developing late after trauma, surgical excision is advised if the patient is

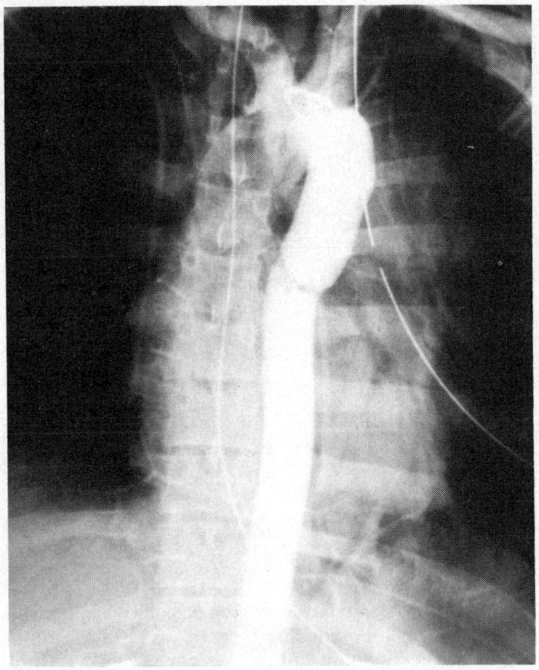

FIGURE 45-25 Thoracic aortogram in a 26-year-old man injured in a motor vehicle accident, showing traumatic transection of the aorta. The site of the tear can be clearly seen. (Courtesy of Robert Dinsmore, M.D., Massachusetts General Hospital, Boston.)

an otherwise reasonable operative candidate. The long-term follow-up of patients with such lesions indicates that about half of the aneurysms slowly expand and may even rupture. Surgery is curative and can be undertaken at a small risk (1 to 3 per cent).

Penetrating Trauma

Penetrating trauma of the aorta or any of its major arterial trunks is caused by puncture or laceration by missiles or knives, particularly bullet and stab wounds. Massive hemorrhage, often leading to rapidly fatal exsanguination, is common. The consequences of the trauma depend upon the site and severity of perforation. Thus, perforation of the aorta within the pericardial sac may lead to cardiac tamponade. Perforation of the aorta elsewhere may cause massive hemorrhage, with compression of surrounding structures by the hematoma, such as the vena cava, tracheobronchial tree, and esophagus. Occlusion of a lacerated artery itself or of adjacent vessels may occur, producing focal signs and symptoms such as loss of the right carotid and brachial pulses, with right hemispheric neurological signs in the case of occlusion of the innominate artery. Occasionally, simultaneous penetration of an adjacent artery and vein may cause an arteriovenous fistula, with a resultant continuous murmur, wide pulse pressure, and increased cardiac output.

MANAGEMENT. Immediate surgical repair should be undertaken in any patient suspected of having a penetrating wound of the aorta, i.e., one with a missile or stab wound of the chest associated with a wide mediastinum on roentgenogram. If the patient's condition allows it, emergency angiography can usually pinpoint the site of perforation. However, in most patients who survive to reach the hospital, immediate operation for closure of the wound and evacuation of the hematoma is necessary. Similarly, laceration or penetrating wounds of arteries require urgent surgical correction.

AORTIC THROMBOEMBOLIC DISEASE

Aortic Embolism

Between 10 and 25 per cent of peripheral arterial emboli affect the aortic bifurcation, resulting in what are termed "saddle emboli." At least 90 per cent of these emboli originate within the chambers of the left side of the heart; 5 per cent come from the aorta itself, usually from thrombus overlying an arteriosclerotic plaque; and the remainder came from undetermined sites.[197] Rarely, paradoxical systemic embolism from the venous circulation occurs through a patent foramen ovale or atrial septal defect. Conditions that predispose to peripheral embolism are myocardial infarction with mural thrombus, ventricular aneurysm, prosthetic valves, congestive cardiomyopathy, and atrial fibrillation, especially in patients with rheumatic mitral stenosis. So-called "marantic endocarditis" is occasionally encountered in chronically ill patients, especially those with malignant disease, and consists of sterile intracardiac thrombi that may dislodge and travel to distal sites. Other less frequent conditions that serve to cause arterial emboli are left atrial myxomas and acute and subacute bacterial endocarditis. Emboli in endocarditis are usually small, although large emboli are seen in acute bacterial endocarditis and fungal (*Candida*) endocarditis. An increased tendency to thromboembolism is encountered in women taking contraceptive pills and estrogens, in patients with malignant diseases, particularly carcinoma of the pancreas, and, rarely, in patients with antithrombin III deficiency.[198]

CLINICAL MANIFESTATIONS. Aortic bifurcation embolism is heralded by the sudden onset of excruciating pain in both legs. The pain usually extends distally from the midthigh area, but can also involve the buttocks, lumbosacral area, and perineum. Associated with the intense pain are numbness, symmetrical weakness, and paresthesias. Schatz and Stanley have summarized in alliteration this classic presentation as "*p*ain, *p*aralysis, *p*aresthesias, *p*ulselessness, and *p*allor."[199]

Examination reveals cold, pale extremities which are cyanotic and often exhibit a mottled, reticulated, reddish-blue appearance. These changes may progress to the blue-black color of gangrene, beginning first in the toes and extending proximally. Pulses are absent below the abdominal aorta. Initially sluggish, capillary filling is ultimately absent. Signs of ischemic neuropathy are present and include diminished or absent deep tendon reflexes, symmetrical weakness, and loss of all modalities of sensation, usually with demarcation at the level of the midthigh. If ischemia persists long enough, there may be myonecrosis with the release of products of muscle breakdown into the bloodstream, causing shock, hypotension, hyperkalemia, myoglobinuria, and acute tubular necrosis. Sepsis may add a serious further dimension to an already desperate problem. If perfusion is not reestablished within a few hours, death is almost inevitable.

The *differential diagnosis* includes acute aortic thrombosis from arteriosclerotic disease and dissecting aortic aneurysm. With thrombosis, there is usually a history of prior claudication, and an embolic source is lacking. With aortic dissection, a history of severe chest or back pain and an abnormal aortic contour on chest x-ray film usually provide distinguishing features.

The diagnosis is confirmed by angiography. However, most investigators advise prompt surgical intervention without angiography if the diagnosis is strongly suspected in order to avoid the loss of valuable time that could lead to irreversible ischemic damage to the limbs.

THERAPY. Most emboli can be removed by using Fogarty balloon-tipped catheters inserted through a transfemoral arterial approach under local anesthesia. In addition to retrieving the embolic material, passage of the Fogarty catheters into the distal arterial bed may result in the removal of any thrombus that may have formed as a result of the stagnant flow beyond the embolus. If the embolus cannot be retrieved with Fogarty catheters, removal by direct transabdominal aortotomy is necessary. Operative mortality ranges from 15 to 30 per cent, with death due to the underlying cardiac disease; limb salvage is estimated at 80 to 90 per cent in most series.[200] Anticoagulation with constant intravenous heparin is instituted upon completion of the operation and continued until therapeutic levels are achieved with one of the warfarin sodium family of drugs. Depending upon the clinical situation, long-term anticoagulant therapy using warfarin or antiplatelet agents may be required. Using the transfemoral approach, surgery can be carried out with a low mortality even in patients whose other disease makes them poor operative risks. Limbs are almost uniformly salvaged if operation is undertaken promptly. All embolic debris should be cultured and examined microscopically. Left atrial myxomas are sometimes first recognized by the pathological examination of embolic specimens.

Aortic Thrombosis

Rarely, primary thrombosis of the distal abdominal aorta may be seen as a result of atheromatous disease or in rare patients with deficiency in antithrombin III. In such patients, treatment is generally surgical, although an occasional case of successful balloon catheter dilation has been reported.[198,201]

Atheromatous Emboli

Embolism of atheromatous debris from the disruption of arteriosclerotic plaques in the aorta or its major arterial trunks has been noted with increasing frequency. Usually, such embolism takes the form of showers of microemboli, measuring between 150 and 600 μm in size, into small arterial branches—an entity that is also termed "cholesterol embolism." However, the obstruction of large arteries by embolic arteriosclerotic material may also occur. By far the most common cause of cholesterol embolism is surgery which involves the manipulation of an atherosclerotic aorta.[15] Thus, atheromatous embolism into the renal and splanchnic vascular beds is common after major abdominal vascular procedures, particularly the resection of abdominal aortic aneurysms. Embolism of atheromatous material also occurs as an occasional complication of intra-arterial cannulation, cardiac catheterization, and cardiopulmonary bypass. In addition to these iatrogenic causes, however, spontaneously occurring cholesterol embolism is encountered, particularly from the aorta into the femoral-popliteal system. Recent studies have suggested a causal relationship between cholesterol embolism and anticoagulant therapy, especially long-term anticoagulation with warfarin sodium–type drugs. Presumably, anticoagulation promotes hemorrhage into plaques, leading to their disruption, or prevents the formation of protective thrombus over ulcerated plaques. Finally, atheromatous embolism has followed blunt trauma to the aorta.[202]

CLINICAL MANIFESTATIONS. The consequences of cholesterol embolism depend upon the vascular bed involved as well as the extent to which the small arterial vessels are occluded. Two important complications of cholesterol embolism following abdominal aortic surgery are pancreatitis and renal failure from diffuse microinfarction of the pancreas and kidneys, respectively.[14,203] Renal failure may be severe and irreversible[204] (p. 1752). Occasionally, cholesterol embolism has been implicated as a cause of severe renovascular hypertension.[205] Gastrointestinal hemorrhage from microinfarction of abdominal viscera is also encountered.[206] Showers of atheromatous emboli may affect the cerebral circulation, producing either focal neurological defects or a diffuse encephalopathic picture. In such cases, shiny cholesterol particles are sometimes visible in the retinal arteries.[203]

Spontaneously occurring cholesterol embolism in the lower extremities is manifested by bilateral pain, livedo reticularis, and purpuric and ecchymotic lesions in the lower legs, feet, and toes. These manifestations may be paroxysmal as emboli intermittently dislodge from their sites of origin. Skin necrosis and ischemic gangrene are common, especially in the toes ("purple toe syndrome"). In the face of this clinical evidence of severe ischemia, arterial pulses are characteristically well preserved unless there is coincidental peripheral vascular disease.

The clinical picture may mimic that of a vasculitis or septic embolism from neisserial organisms—especially meningococcemia—or bacterial endocarditis. The absence of fever and other signs of systemic illness and the localized distribution of the lesions serve to distinguish cholesterol embolism from these other entities. The diagnosis has been made by muscle biopsy, which may show cholesterol particles in the arterioles.[204]

THERAPY. For the most part, there is no specific treatment for cholesterol microembolism. Careful attention to the prevention of necrosis and infection in the involved extremities is important. Although the amputation of gangrenous digits is occasionally necessary, the ultimate prognosis for recovery is quite good, unless embolism is frequent and recurrent. Pancreatitis often subsides, even though it may be severe. Renal failure may be irreversible.

The use of anticoagulants in the prevention of further embolism is controversial, with some investigators advocating that they be given and others contending that they promote further atheromatous emboli.[203,207] Overall, it appears that they are not of much value.

In instances of recurrent atheromatous embolism, it may be possible to pinpoint the source of the cholesterol particles by angiography and perform an endarterectomy or an excision of the involved segment with replacement with a prosthetic graft.

AORTIC BACTERIAL INFECTIONS

The term "infected aneurysm" has gradually replaced the original designation of "mycotic aneurysm" used by

Osler to define any localized dilation caused by sepsis in the wall of the aorta or any artery and thus to avoid confusion with infections of truly fungal origin. Infection can cause virtually any kind of aneurysmal dilatation, including fusiform, saccular, and false aneurysms. Rupture into the venous system may cause arteriovenous fistulas. Alternatively, infection may arise within preexisting arteriosclerotic aneurysms. Infected aortic aneurysms are rare, with only 1.2 cases per year recently being reported from a large general hospital.[208] Rarely, tuberculosis can infect the aorta, but, as of 1965, only 110 cases of tuberculous aortitis had been reported in the world's literature.[209]

Pathogenesis. Vascular infection may arise by any of three different mechanisms. First, septic emboli from bacterial endocarditis or diffuse bacteremia may infect normal or diseased tissue. This mechanism of infection has become less frequent owing to the widespread use of effective antibiotics for the control of septicemia. Second, there may be contiguous spread from adjacent abscesses, infected lymph nodes, empyema, and so on. This is the usual cause for tuberculous vascular involvement. Third, sepsis may be introduced directly from an external source, such as trauma, intravenous injections, or surgery. The incidence of this type of infection is increasing because of more frequent motor vehicle accidents, the widespread use of intravenous narcotics by drug addicts, and the performance of more intravascular procedures which may produce a portal for infection, such as cardiac catheterization and intraaortic balloon counterpulsation. With this type of sepsis, the peripheral arteries are obviously more frequently involved than the aorta per se.

Although virtually any organism may infect the arterial tree, certain bacteria seem to have a proclivity for this type of infection. In particular, this is true of the *Salmonella* group, which tends to infect arteriosclerotic aneurysms.

CLINICAL MANIFESTATIONS. Most patients with infected aortic aneurysms are febrile; the height of the fever depends upon the severity of infection, the organism, and the site of the infection. Extremely high fever and rigors are common. Symptoms may arise from localized expansion of an infected aneurysm, such as dysphagia from esophageal compression and pain in areas contiguous to the infected sac. If palpable, infected aneurysms are almost always tender. A tender and pulsatile mass in a febrile patient should be considered an infected aneurysm until proved otherwise. Jarrett et al. have suggested that infected aortic aneurysms can be differentiated from sterile ones by the presence of fever, relative preponderence in women, tenderness, lack of calcification, and a tendency for early vertebral erosion.[208] With tuberculous involvement, evidence is almost always seen on chest x-ray film.[210] This, coupled with a pulsating mass lesion, should elicit the correct diagnosis.

Sepsis in more peripheral arteries presents most commonly as fever with a palpable, painful, pulsating mass. Symptoms of compression of contiguous structures may also be present, such as arterial regurgitation or a neuropathy.[211] Small abscesses in the distribution of the artery are often seen in staphylococcal infections.

Leukocytosis, elevated sedimentation rate, and positive blood cultures are present in most cases. Commonly reported organisms are *Staphylococcus aureus* and *Salmonella* species; other gram-positive and gram-negative organisms, such as pneumococcus, *Pseudomonas*, and anaerobes, are found less frequently. Rarely, fungal infections with *Candida* or *Aspergillus* may occur. Localization of suspected infected aneurysms in a patient with sepsis can be aided by angiography. Valuable information can sometimes be obtained from ultrasound, gallium, and CT scans.

The natural history of infected aneurysms is that of progressive expansion, thinning of the aneurysm wall, and eventual rupture. Jarrett et al. found a more rapid progression in patients with gram-negative infections.[208]

THERAPY. Treatment is always surgical excision, combined with appropriate antibiotic or antituberculous chemotherapy. Wide excision of infected tissue is advised.[208,212] Usually a prosthetic tube graft must be inserted if the aorta or a major artery is involved. Early recognition and therapy clearly alter the outcome favorably.

AORTIC TUMORS

A review cites 21 cases of primary aortic tumors recorded in the world's literature.[213] Clearly secondary tumors can arise from direct extension and invasion from adjacent lung or abdominal neoplasms or from embolic spread. Histological types include fibrosarcoma (most commonly), fibromyxosarcoma, myxosarcoma, fibromyxoma, angiosarcoma, malignant fibrous histocytoma, and leiomyosarcoma.

In the 21 cases of primary aortic tumors, the age of the patients ranged from infancy to 70 years with a mean of 53 years; sex distribution was equal. Presentation in over half of the cases was pain with proximal hypertension due to the acquired coarctation, decreased femoral pulses, fever, claudication, and, occasionally, bruits. Diagnosis is made by the usual noninvasive or angiographic techniques, with the irregular appearance of the lumen and lack of enlargement of the outer diameter of the aorta being key features.

References

1. Buonocore, E., Meaney, T. F., Borkowski, G. P., Pavlicek, W., and Gallagher, J.: Digital subtraction angiography of the abdominal aorta and renal arteries. Radiology *139*:281, 1981.
2. Ferrucci, J. T., Jr.: Body ultrasonography. N. Engl. J. Med. *300*:538, 590, 1979.
3. DeMaria, A. N., Bommer, W., Neumann, A., Weinert, L., Bogren, H., and Mason, D. T.: Identification and localization of aneurysms of the ascending aorta by cross-sectional echocardiography. Circulation *59*:755, 1979.
4. Meyer, J. F., and Wall, H. N., Jr.: Ultrasonic evaluation of the aorta. *In* Lindsay, J., Jr., and Hurst, J. W. (eds.): The Aorta. New York, Grune and Stratton, 1979, p. 345.
5. Eriksson, I., Hemmingsson, A., and Lindgren, P. G.: Diagnosis of abdominal aortic aneurysms by aortography, computer tomography and ultrasound. Acta Radiol. [Diagn.] *21*:209, 1980.
6. Godwin, J. D., Herfkens, R. H., Skioldebrand, C. G., Federle, M. P., and Lipton, M. J.: Evaluation of dissections and aneurysms of the thoracic aorta by conventional and dynamic CT scanning. Radiology *136*:125, 1980.

6a. Moncada, R., Demos, T. C., and Churchill, R.: Detecting disease of the aorta by computed tomography. J. Cardiovasc. Med. *8*:186, 1983.

7. Egan, T. J., Neiman, H. L., Herman, R. J., Malave, S. R., and Sanders, J. H.: Computed tomography in the diagnosis of aortic aneurysm dissection of traumatic injury. Radiology *136*:141, 1980.
8. Prokop, E. K., Palmer, R. F., and Wheat, M. W., Jr.: Hydrodynamic forces in dissecting aneurysms. In vitro studies in a Tygon model and in dog aortas. Circ. Res. *27*:121, 1970.
9. Iwatsuki, K., Cardinale, G. J., Spector, S., and Udenfriend, S.: Reduction of blood pressure and vascular collagen in hypertensive rats by β-aminopropionitrile. Proc. Natl. Acad. Sci. USA *74*:360, 1977.
10. Saruk, M., and Eisenstein, R.: Aortic lesion in Marfan syndrome—The ultrastructure of cystic medial degeneration. Arch. Pathol. Lab. Med. *101*:74, 1977.
11. Schlatmann, T. J. M., and Becker, A. E.: Histologic changes in the normal aging aorta. Am. J. Cardiol. *39*:13, 1977.
12. Schlatmann, T. J. M., and Becker, A. E.: Pathogenesis of dissecting aneurysm of the aorta. Am. J. Cardiol. *39*:21, 1977.
13. Heistad, D. D., Marcus, M. L., Law, E. G., Armstrong, M. L., Ehrhardt, J. C., and Abboud, F. M.: Regulation of blood flow to the aortic media in dogs. J. Clin. Invest. *62*:133, 1978.
14. Crane, C.: Arteriosclerotic aneurysm of the abdominal aorta. Some pathologic and clinical correlations. N. Engl. J. Med. *253*:954, 1955.
15. Thurlbeck, W. M., and Castleman, B.: Atheromatous emboli to the kidneys after aortic surgery. N. Engl. J. Med. *257*:442, 1957.
16. Darling, R. C.: Ruptured arteriosclerotic abdominal aortic aneurysms. Am. J. Surg. *119*:397, 1970.
17. Weintraub, A. M., and Gomes, M. N.: Clinical manifestations of abdominal aortic aneurysm and thoracoabdominal aneurysm. *In* Lindsay, J., Jr., and Hurst, J. W. (eds.): The Aorta. New York, Grune and Stratton, 1979, p. 131.
18. Moore, H. D.: Abdominal aortic aneurysms. J. Cardiovasc. Surg. *17*:47, 1976.
19. McGregor, J. C.: Unoperated ruptured abdominal aortic aneurysms: A retro-

spective clinicopathologic study over a 10-year period. Br. J. Surg. *63*:113, 1976.
20. Hertzer, N. R., and Beven, E. G.: Abdominal aortic aneurysm. Postgrad. Med. *61*:72, 1977.
21. Brewster, D. C., Darling, R. C., Raines, J. K., Sarno, R., O'Donnell, T. F., Ezpeleta, M., and Athanasoulis, C.: Assessment of abdominal aortic aneurysm size. Circulation *56*:164, 1977.
22. Retief, P. J., and Loubser, J. S.: Diagnosis and treatment of abdominal aortic aneurysm. A report of 82 cases. S. Afr. Med. J. *56*:67, 1979.
23. Brewster, D. C., Retana, A., Waltman, A. C., and Darling, R. C.: Angiography in the management of aneurysms of the abdominal aorta. Its value and safety. N. Engl. J. Med. *292*:822, 1975.
24. Szilagyi, D. E., Smith, R. F., DeRusso, F. J., Elliott, J. P., and Sherrin, F. W.: Contribution of abdominal aortic aneurysmectomy to prolongation of life. Ann. Surg. *164*:678, 1966.
25. Darling, R. C., Messina, C. R., Brewster, D. C., and Ottinger, L. W.: Autopsy study of unoperated abdominal aortic aneurysms. The case for early resection. Circulation *56*(Suppl. II):161, 1977.
26. Linton, R. R.: Atlas of Vascular Surgery. Philadelphia, W. B. Saunders Co., 1973, pp. 266–269.
27. Attia, R. R., Murphy, J. D., Snider, M., Lappas, D. G., Darling, R. C., and Lowenstein, E.: Myocardial ischemia due to infrarenal aortic cross-clamping during aortic surgery in patients with severe coronary artery disease. Circulation *53*:961, 1976.
28. Bush, H. L., Jr., LoGerfo, F. W., Weisel, R. D., Mannick, J. A., and Hechtman, H. B.: Assessment of myocardial performance and optimal volume loading during elective abdominal aortic resection. Arch. Surg. *112*:1301, 1977.
29. Thompson, J. E., Hollier, L. H., Patman, R. D., and Persson, A. V.: Surgical management of abdominal aortic aneurysms: Factors influencing mortality and morbidity—A 20-year experience. Ann. Surg. *181*:654, 1975.
30. Cullen, D. J., Ferrara, L. C., Briggs, B. A., Walker, P. F., and Grehert, J.: Survival, hospitalization charges and follow-up results in critically ill patients. New Engl. J. Med. *294*:982, 1976.
31. Brener, B. J., Raines, J. K., and Darling, R. C.: Intraoperative autotransfusion in abdominal aortic resections. Arch. Surg. *107*:78, 1973.
32. Levin, P. M., Shore, E. H., Treiman, R. L., and Foran, R. F.: Ruptured abdominal aortic aneurysms. Surgical treatment. West. J. Med. *123*:431, 1975.
33. Spencer, F. C.: Diseases of great vessels. *In* Schwartz, S. I., and Shires, T.: Principles of Surgery. 3rd ed. New York, McGraw-Hill Book Co., 1979, p.883.
34. Young, A. E., and Couch, N. P.: Coronary artery disease and aortic aneurysm surgery. Lancet *1*:1005, 1977.
35. Brewster, D. C., Bluth, J., Darling, R. C., and Austen, W. G.: Combined aortic and renal artery reconstruction. Am. J. Surg. *131*:457, 1976.
36. Crawford, E. S., Saleh, S. A., Babb, J. W., III, Glaeser, D. H., Vaccaro, P. S., and Silvers, A.: Infrarenal abdominal aortic aneurysm: Factors influencing survival after operation performed over a 25-year period. Ann. Surg. *193*:699, 1981.
37. Ottinger, L. W.: Ruptured arteriosclerotic aneurysms of the abdominal aorta: Reducing mortality. J.A.M.A. *233*:147, 1975.
38. Darling, R. C., and Brewster, D. C.: Elective treatment of abdominal aortic aneurysms. World J. Surg. *4*:661, 1980.
39. Fielding, J. W. L., Black, J., Ashton, F., Slaney, G., and Campbell, D. J.: Diagnosis and management of 528 abdominal aortic aneurysms. Br. Med. J. *283*:355, 1981.
40. O'Donnell, T. F., Darling, R. C., and Linton, R. R.: Is 80 years too old for aneurysmectomy? Arch. Surg. *111*:1250, 1976.
41. Leather, R. P., Shah, D., Goldman, M., Rosenberg, M., and Karmody, A. M.: Nonresective treatment of abdominal aortic aneurysms. Use of acute thrombosis and axillofemoral bypass. Arch. Surg. *114*:1402, 1979.
42. Baker, A. G., and Roberts, B.: Long-term survival following abdominal aortic aneurysmectomy. J.A.M.A. *212*:445, 1970.
43. DeWeese, J. A., Blaisdell, F. W., and Foster, J. H.: Optimal resources for vascular surgery. Circulation *46*:305, 1972.
44. Hicks, G. L., Eastland, M. W., and DeWeese, J. A.: Survival improvement following aortic aneurysm resection. Ann. Surg. *181*:863, 1975.
45. Soreide, O., Lillestol, J., Christensen, O., Gromsgaard, L., Myhre, H. O., Solheim, K., and Trippestad, A.: Abdominal aortic aneurysms: Survival analysis of four hundred thirty-four patients. Surgery *91*:188, 1982.
46. Thompson, W. M., Johnsrude, I. S., Jackson, D. C., Older, R. A., and Wechsler, A. S.: Late complications of abdominal aortic reconstructive surgery: Roentgen evaluation. Ann. Surg. *185*:326, 1977.
47. Kierman, P. D., Pairolero, P. C., Hubert, J. P., Jr., Mucha, P., Jr., and Wallace, R. B.: Aortic graft–enteric fistula. Mayo Clin. Proc. *55*:731, 1980.
48. Ottinger, L. W., Darling, R. C., Nathan, M. J., and Linton, R. R.: Left colon ischemia complicating aorto-iliac reconstruction. Causes, diagnosis, management and prevention. Arch. Surg. *105*:841, 1972.
49. Ernst, C. B., Hagihara, P. F., Daugherty, M. E., Sachatello, C. R., and Griffen, W. O.: Ischemic colitis incidence following abdominal aortic reconstruction. A prospective study. Surgery *80*:417, 1976.
50. Lindsay, J., Jr.: Thoracic aneurysms. *In* Lindsay, J., Jr., and Hurst, J. W. (eds.): The Aorta. New York, Grune and Stratton, 1979, p. 121.
51. Crisler, C., and Bahnson, H. T.: Aneurysm of the aorta. Curr. Probl. Surg. 1–64, 1972.
52. Joyce, J. W., Fairbairn, J. F., Kincaid, O. W., and Juergens, J. L.: Aneurysms of the thoracic aorta—A clinical study with special reference to prognosis. Circulation *29*:176, 1964.
53. Altman, P., and Voorhees, A. B.: Aneurysm of the aorta treated by wiring. Case report of a 38-year survival. Ann. Surg. *184*:738, 1976.
54. Griepp, R. B., Stinson, E. B., Hollingsworth, J. F., and Buehler, D.: Prosthetic replacement of the aortic arch. J. Thorac. Cardiovasc. Surg. *70*:1051, 1975.
55. Culliford, A. T., Ayvaliotis, B., Shemin, R., Colvin, S. B., Isom, O. W., and Spencer, F. C.: Aneurysms of the ascending aorta and transverse arch: Surgical experience in 80 patients. J. Thorac. Cardiovasc. Surg. *83*:701, 1982.
56. Symbas, P. N.: Treatment of thoracic surgical aortic diseases. *In* Lindsay, J., Jr., and Hurst, J. W. (eds.): The Aorta. New York, Grune and Stratton, 1979, p. 259.
57. Kidd, J. N., Reul, G. J., Cooley, D. A., Sandiford, F. M., Kyger, E. R., and Wukasch, D. C.: Surgical treatment of aneurysms of the ascending aorta. Circulation *54*(Suppl. III):118, 1976.
58. Crawford, E. S., Snyder, D. M., Cho, G. C., and Roehm, J. O. F., Jr.: Progress in treatment of thoracabdominal and abdominal aortic aneurysms involving celiac, superior mesenteric, and renal Ann. Surg. *188*:404, 1978.
59. Crawford, E. S., and Rubio, P. A.: Reappraisal of adjuncts to avoid ischemia in the treatment of aneurysms of descending thoracic aorta. J. Thorac. Cardiovasc. Surg. *66*:693, 1973.
60. Wakabayashi, A., and Connolly, J. E.: Prevention of paraplegia associated with resection of extensive thoracic aneurysms. Arch. Surg. *111*:1186, 1976.
61. Stallone, R. J., Iverson, L. I. G., and Young, J. N.: Descending thoracic aortic aneurysm: A 10 year surgical experience. Am. J. Surg. *142*:106, 1981.
62. Mannick, J. A.: Surgical treatment of aneurysms of the abdominal and thoracic aorta. Prog. Cardiovasc. Dis. *16*:69, 1973.
63. Wheat, M. W., Jr.: Acute dissecting aneurysms of the aorta: Diagnosis and treatment—1979. Am. Heart J. *99*:373, 1980.
64. Roberts, W. C.: Aortic dissection: Anatomy, consequences, and causes. Am. Heart J. *101*:195, 1981.
65. Doroghazi, R. M., and Slater, E. E. (eds.): Aortic Dissection. New York, McGraw-Hill Book Co., 1983.
65a. Wheat, M. W., Jr.: Pathogenesis of aortic dissection. *In* Aortic Dissection. Doroghazi, R. M., and Slater, E. E. (eds.): New York, McGraw-Hill Book Company, 1983, p. 55.
66. DeBakey, M. E., Henly, W. S., Cooley, D. A., Morris, G. C., Jr., Crawford, E. S., and Beall, A. C.: Surgical management of dissecting aneurysms of the aorta. J. Thorac. Cardiovasc. Surg. *49*:130, 1965.
67. Sethi, G. K., Hughes, R. K., and Takaro, T.: Dissecting aortic aneurysms. Ann. Thorac. Surg. *18*:201, 1974.
68. Daily, P. O., Trueblood, H. W., Stinson, E. B., Wuerflein, R. D., and Shumway, N. E.: Management of acute aortic dissection. Ann. Thorac. Surg. *10*:237, 1970.
69. Slater, E. E., and DeSanctis, R. W.: The clinical recognition of dissecting aortic aneurysm. Am. J. Med. *60*:625, 1976.
70. Leonards, J. C., and Hasleton, P. S.: Dissecting aortic aneurysms: A clinicopathological study. Q. J. Med. *48*:55, 1979.
71. Bulkley, B. H., and Roberts, W. C.: Dissecting aneurysm (hematoma) limited to coronary artery. Am. J. Med. *55*:747, 1973.
72. Hochberg, F. H., Bean, C., Fisher, C. M., and Roberson, G. H.: Stroke in a 15-year-old girl secondary to terminal carotid dissection. Neurology *25*:725, 1975.
73. Loeppky, C. B., Alpert, M. A., Hamel, P. C., Martin, R. H., and Saab, S. B.: Extensive aortic dissection from combined-type cystic medial necrosis in a young man without predisposing factors. Chest *79*:116, 1981.
74. Fukuda, T., Tadavarthy, S. M., and Edwards, J. E.: Dissecting aneurysm of aorta complicating aortic valvular stenosis. Circulation *53*:169, 1976.
75. Gore, I., and Seiwert, V. J.: Dissecting aneurysm of the aorta: Pathologic aspects. Arch. Pathol. *53*:121, 1952.
76. McKusick, V. A., Logue, R. B., and Bahnson, H. T.: Association of aortic valvular disease and cystic medial necrosis of the ascending aorta; report of four instances. Circulation *16*:188, 1957.
77. Faraci, R. M., and Westcott, J. L.: Dissecting hematoma of the aorta secondary to blunt chest trauma. Diagn. Radiol. *123*:569, 1977.
78. Ponseti, I. V., and Baird, W. A.: Scoliosis and dissecting aneurysm of the aorta in rats fed with *Lathyrus odoratus* seeds. Am. J. Pathol. *28*:1059, 1952.
79. Fikar, C. R., Amrhein, J. A., Harris, J. P., and Lewis, E. R.: Dissecting aortic aneurysm in childhood and adolescence. Clin. Pediatr. *20*:578, 1981.
80. Hirst, A. E., Jr., Johns, V. J., Jr., and Kime, S. W., Jr.: Dissecting aneurysm of the aorta. A review of 505 cases. Medicine *37*:217, 1958.
80a. Slater, E. E.: Aortic dissection: Presentation and diagnosis. *In* Doroghazi, R. M., and Slater, E. E. (eds.): Aortic Dissection. New York, McGraw-Hill Book Company, 1983, p. 61.
81. Cohen, S., and Littman, D.: Painless dissecting aneurysm of the aorta. N. Engl. J. Med. *271*:143, 1964.
82. Lindsay, J., Jr., and Hurst, J. W.: Clinical features and prognosis in dissecting aneurysm of the aorta. A reappraisal. Circulation *35*:880, 1967.
83. Symbas, P. N., Kelly, T. F., Vlasis, S. E., Drucker, M. H., and Arensberg, D.: Intimo-intimal intussusception and other unusual manifestations of aortic dissection. J. Thorac. Cardiovasc. Surg. *79*:926, 1980.
83a. Hirst, A. E., and Gore, I.: The etiology and pathology of aortic regurgitation. *In* Doroghazi, R. M., and Slater, E. E. (eds.): Aortic Dissection. New York, McGraw Hill Book Company, 1983, p. 13.
84. Weisman, A. D., and Adams, R. D.: Neurological complications of dissecting aortic aneurysm. Brain *67*:69, 1944.
85. Logue, R. B., and Sikes, C.: New sign in dissecting aneurysm of the aorta. Pulsation of sternoclavicular joint. J.A.M.A. *148*:1209, 1952.

86. Riley, D. J., Liv, R. T., and Saxanoff, S.: Aortic dissection: A rare cause of the superior vena cava syndrome. J. Med. Soc. N. J. *78*:187, 1981.
87. Buja, M. L., Ali, N., and Roberts, W. C.: Stenosis of the right pulmonary artery: A complication of acute dissecting aneurysm of the ascending aorta. Am. Heart J. *83*:89, 1972.
88. McCarthy, C., Dickson, G. H., Besterman, E. M. M., Bromley, L. L., and Thompson, A. E.: Aortic dissection with rupture through ductus arteriosus into pulmonary artery. Br. Heart J. *34*:284, 1972.
89. Roth, J. A., and Parekh, M. A.: Dissecting aneurysms perforating the esophagus. N. Engl. J. Med. *299*:776, 1978.
90. Thiene, G., Rossi, L., and Becker, A. E.: The atrioventricular conduction system in dissecting aneurysm of the aorta. Am. Heart J. *98*:447, 1979.
91. Morris, A. L., and Barwinsky, J.: Unusual vascular complications of dissecting thoracic aortic aneurysm. Cardiovasc. Radiol. *1*:95, 1978.
92. ten Cate, J. W., Timmers, H., and Becker, A. E.: Coagulopathy in ruptured or dissecting aortic aneurysms. Am. J. Med. *59*:171, 1975.
93. Matsumoto, M., Matsuo, H., Ohara, T., Yoshioka, Y., and Abe, H.: A two-dimensional echoaortocardiographic approach to dissecting aneurysms of the aorta to prevent false positive diagnoses. Radiology *127*:491, 1978.
94. Victor, M. F., Mintz, G. S., Kotler, M. N., Wilson, A. R., and Segal, B. L.: Two dimensional echocardiographic diagnosis of aortic dissection. Am. J. Cardiol. *48*:1155, 1981.
95. Larde, D., Belloir, C., Vasile, N., Frija, J., and Ferrane, J.: Computed tomography of aortic dissection. Radiology *136*:147, 1980.
95a. Perez, J. E.: Noninvasive diagnosis: Computed tomography and ultrasound. *In* Doroghazi, R. M., and Slater, E. E. (eds.): Aortic Dissection. New York, McGraw-Hill Book Company, 1983, p. 133.
95b. Smith, D. C., and Jang, G. C.: Radiological diagnosis and aortic dissection. *In* Doroghazi, R. M., and Slater, E. E. (eds.): Aortic Dissection. New York, McGraw Hill-Book Company, 1983, p. 71.
96. Heiberg, E., Wolverson, M., Sundaram, M., Connors, J., and Susman, N.: CT findings in thoracic aortic dissection. Am. J. Radiol. *136*:13, 1981.
97. Moncada, R., Salinas, M., Churchill, R., Love, L., Reynes, C., Demos, T. C., Gunnar, R. M., and Pifarre, R.: Diagnosis of dissecting aortic aneurysm by computed tomography. Lancet *1*:238, 1981.
98. Turley, K., Ullyot, D. J., Godwin, J. D., Wilson, J. M., Lipton, M., Carlsson, E., and Ebert, P. A.: Repair of dissection of the thoracic aorta. Evaluation of false lumen utilizing computed tomography. J. Thorac. Cardiovasc. Surg. *81*:61, 1981.
99. Godwin, J. D., Turley, K., Herfkens, R. J., and Lipton, M. J.: Computed tomography for follow-up of chronic aortic dissections. Radiology *139*:655, 1981.
100. Earnest, F., IV, Muhm, J. R., and Sheedy, P. F., II: Roentgenographic findings in thoracic aortic dissection. Mayo Clin. Proc. *54*:43, 1979.
101. Dinsmore, R. E., Willerson, J. T.,, and Buckley, M. J.: Dissecting aneurysm of the aorta. Aortographic features affecting prognosis. Diagn. Radiol. *105*:567, 1972.
102. Shuford, W. H., Sybers, R. G., and Weens, H. S.: Problems of the aortographic diagnosis of dissecting aneurysms of the aorta. N. Engl. J. Med. *280*:225, 1969.
102a. Collins, J. J., Jr., Koster, J. K., Jr., Cohn, L. H., and VanDevanter, S. H.: Common aortic aneurysms: When to intervene. J. Cardiovas. Med. *8*:245, 1983.
103. Anagnostopoulos, C. E., Prabhakar, M. J. S., and Kittle, C. F.: Aortic dissections and dissecting aneurysms. Am. J. Cardiol. *30*:263, 1972.
104. Gurin, D., Bulmer, J. W., and Derby, R.: Dissecting aneurysms of the aorta. Diagnosis and operative relief of acute arterial obstructions due to this course. N.Y. State J. Med. *35*:1200, 1935.
105. Shaw, R. W.: Acute dissecting aortic aneurysms: Treatment by fenestration of the internal wall of the aneurysm. N. Engl. J. Med. *253*:331, 1955.
106. DeBakey, M. E., Cooley, D. A., and Creech, O., Jr.: Surgical considerations of dissecting aneurysm of the aorta. Ann. Surg. *142*:586, 1955.
107. Wheat, M. W., Jr., Palmer, R. F., Bartley, T. D., and Seelman, R. C.: Treatment of dissecting aneurysms of the aorta without surgery. J. Thorac. Cardiovasc. Surg. *50*:364, 1965.
107a. Wheat, M. W.: Intensive drug therapy. *In* Doroghazi, R. M., and Slater, E. E. (eds.): Aortic Dissection. New York, McGraw-Hill Book Company, 1983, p. 165.
108. Palmer, R. F., and Lasseter, K. C.: Nitroprusside and aortic dissecting aneurysm (letter). N. Engl. J. Med. *294*:1403, 1976.
109. Anagnostopoulos, C. E., Athanasuleas, C. L., Garrick, T. R., and Paulissian, R.: Acute Aortic Dissections. Baltimore, University Park Press, 1975.
110. Appelbaum, A., Karp, R. B., and Kirklin, J. W.: Ascending versus descending aortic dissections. Ann. Surg. *183*:296, 1976.
111. Reul, G. J., Jr., Cooley, D. A., Hallman, G. L., Reddy, S. B., Kyger, E. R., III, and Wukasch, D. C.: Dissecting aneurysm of the descending aorta—Improved surgical results in 91 patients. Arch. Surg. *110*:632, 1975.
112. Kidd, J. N., Reul, G. J., Jr., Cooley, D. A., Sandiford, F. M., Kyger, E. R., III, and Wukasch, D. C.: Surgical treatment of aneurysms of the ascending aorta. Cardiovasc. Surg *54*(Suppl.):118, 1976.
113. Miller, D. C., Stinson, E. B., Oyer, P. E., Rossiter, S. J., Reitz, B. A., Griepp, R. B., and Shumway, N. E.: The operative treatment of aortic dissections: Experience with 125 patients over a sixteen year period. J. Thorac. Cardiovasc. Surg. *78*:365, 1979.
114. Doroghazi, R. M., Slater, E. E., Austen, W. G., Buckley, M. J., and DeSanctis, R. W.: Long-term survival for 163 patients with treated aortic dissection. Am. J. Cardiol. (In press.)
114a. Miller, D. C.: Surgical management of aortic dissections: Indications, perioperative management and long-term results. *In* Doroghazi, R. M., and Slater, E. E. (eds.): Aortic Dissection. New York, McGraw-Hill Book Company, 1983, p. 193.
115. Vecht, R. J., Besterman, E. M. M., Bromley, L. L., Eastcott, H. H. G., and Kenyon, J. R.: Acute dissection of the aorta: Long-term review and management. Lancet *1*:110, 1980.
116. Cachera, J. P., Vouhe, P. R., Loisance, D. Y., Menu, P., Poulain, H., Bloch, G., Vasile, N., Aubry, P., and Galey, J. J.: Surgical management of acute dissections involving the ascending aorta. J. Thorac. Cardiovasc. Surg. *82*:576, 1981.
117. Kolff, J., Bates, R. J., Balderman, S. C., Shenkoya, K., and Anagnostopoulos, C. E.: Acute aortic arch dissection: Re-evaluation of the indications for medical and surgical therapy. Am. J. Cardiol. *39*:727, 1977.
118. Lemole, G. M., Strong, M. D., Spagna, P. M., and Karmilowicz, N. P.: Improved results for dissecting aneurysms: Intraluminal sutureless prosthesis. J. Thorac. Cardiovasc. Surg. *83*:249, 1982.
119. Carpentier, A., Deloche, A., Fabiani, J. N., Chauvaud, S., Relland, J., Nottin, R., Vouhe, P., Massoud, H., and Dubost, C.: New surgical approach to aortic dissection: Flow reversal and thromboexclusion. J. Thorac. Cardiovasc. Surg. *81*:659, 1981.
120. Ellis, P. R., Cooley, D. A., and DeBakey, M. E.: Clinical consideration and surgical treatment of annulo-aortic ectasia. J. Thorac. Cardiovasc. Surg. *42*:363, 1961.
121. Lindsay, J., Jr.: The Marfan syndrome and idiopathic cystic medial degeneration. *In* Lindsay, J., Jr., and Hurst, J. W. (eds.): The Aorta. New York, Grune and Stratton, 1979, p. 263.
122. Pyeritz, R. E., and McKusick, V. A.: The Marfan syndrome: Diagnosis and management. N. Engl. J. Med. *300*:772, 1979.
122a. Emanuel, R., Ng, R.A.L., Marcomichelakis, J., Moores, E. C., Jefferson, K. E., Macfaul, P. A., and Withers, R.: Formes frustes of Marfan's syndrome presenting with severe aortic regurgitation. Clinicogenetic study of 18 families. Br. Heart J. *39*:190, 1977.
123. Lemon, D. K., and White, C. W.: Anuloaortic ectasia: Angiographic, hemodynamic and clinical comparison with aortic valve insufficiency. Am. J. Cardiol. *41*:482, 1978.
124. Miller, D. C., Stinson, E. B., Oyer, P. E., Moreno-Cabral, R. J., Reitz, B. A., Rossiter, S. J., and Shumway, N. E.: Concomitant resection of ascending aortic aneurysm and replacement of the aortic valve. J. Thorac. Cardiovasc. Surg. *79*:388, 1980.
125. McDonald, G. R., Schaff, H. V., Pyeritz, R. E., McKusick, V. A., and Gott, V. L.: Surgical management of patients with the Marfan syndrome and dilatation of the ascending aorta. J. Thorac. Cardiovasc. Surg. *81*:180, 1981.
126. Takayasu, M.: Case with unusual changes of the central vessels in the retina. Acta Soc. Ophthalmol. Jap. *12*:554, 1908.
127. McKusick, V.: A form of vascular disease relatively frequent in the Orient. Am. Heart J. *63*:57, 1962.
128. Lupi-Herrera, E., Sanchez-Torres, G., Marcushamer, J., Mispireta, J., Horowitz, S., and Espino Vela, J.: Takayasu's arteritis. Clinical study of 107 cases. Am. Heart J. *93*:94, 1977.
129. Lande, A., and LaPorta, A.: Takayasu arteritis—An arteriographic-pathological correlation. Arch. Pathol. Lab. Med. *100*:437, 1976.
130. Lande, A.: Takayasu's arteritis and congenital coarctation of the descending thoracic and abdominal aorta. A critical review. Am. J. Roentgenol. *127*:227, 1976.
131. Ueno, A., Awane, G., and Wakahayachi, A.: Successfully operated obliterative brachiocephalic arteritis (Takayasu) associated with the elongated coarctation. Jap. Heart J. *8*:538, 1967.
132. Lande, A., Bard, R., Bole, P., and Guarnaccia, M.: Aortic arch syndrome (Takayasu's arteritis). Arteriographic and surgical considerations. J. Cardiovasc. Surg. *19*:507, 1978.
133. Nakao, K., Ikeda, M., Kimata, S., Nhtani, H., Miyahara, M., Ishimi, Z., Hashiba, K., Takeda, Y., Ozawa, T., Matsushita, S., and Kuramochi, M.: Takayasu's arteritis—Clinical report of eighty-four cases and immunological studies of seven cases. Circulation *35*:1141, 1967.
134. Numano, F., Isohisa, I., Maezawa, H., and Juji, T.: HL-A antigens in Takayasu's disease. Am. Heart J. *98*:153, 1979.
135. Volkman, D. J., Mann, D. L., and Fauci, A. S.: Association between Takayasu's arteritis and a B-cell alloantigen in North Americans. N. Engl. J. Med. *306*:464, 1982.
136. Inada, K., Shimizu, H., and Yokoyama, T.: Pulseless disease and atypical coarctation of the aorta with special reference to their genesis. Surgery *52*:133, 1962.
137. Gronemeyer, P. S., and deMello, D. E.: Takayasu's disease with aneurysm of right common iliac artery and iliocaval fistula in a young infant: Case report and review of the literature. Pediatrics *69*:626, 1982.
138. Swinton, N. W., and Cook, G. A.: Systolic hypertension and cardiac mortality of Takayasu's aortoarteritis. Angiology *27*:568, 1976.
139. Takishita, A., Tanaka, S., Orita, G., Kanaide, H., and Nakamura, M.: Baroflex sensitivity in patients with Takayasu's aortitis. Circulation *55*:803, 1977.
140. Akikusa, B., Kondo, Y., and Muraki, N.: Aortic insufficiency caused by Takayasu's arteritis without usual clinical features. Arch. Pathol. Lab. Med. *105*:650, 1981.
141. Pasternac, A., Lesperance, J., Grondin, P., and Cantin, M.: Primary arteritis in Takayasu's disease. A case studied by selective coronary arteriography. Am. J. Roentgenol. *128*:488, 1977.

142. Cipriano, P. R., Silverman, J. F., Perlroth, M. G., Griepp, R. B., and Wexler, L.: Coronary arterial narrowing in Takayasu's aortitis. Am. J. Cardiol. *39*:744, 1977.
143. Sen, P. K., Kinare, S. G., Engineer, S. D., and Parulkar, G. B.: The middle aortic syndrome. Br. Heart J. *25*:610, 1963.
144. Slater, E. E., and Fallon, J. T.: Upper extremity hypertension in a 28-year-old Korean man. Case Records of the Massachusetts General Hospital. N. Engl. J. Med. *299*:1002, 1978.
145. Lande, A., and Bard, R.: Takayasu's arteritis. An unrecognized cause of pulmonary hypertension. Angiology *27*:114, 1974.
146. Lupi, H. E., Sanchez, T. G., Horwitz, S., and Gutierrez, F. E.: Pulmonary artery involvement in Takayasu's arteritis. Chest *67*:69, 1975.
147. Lande, A., and Rossi, P.: The value of total aortography in the diagnosis of Takayasu's arteritis. Radiology *114*:287, 1975.
148. Bonventre, M. V.: Takayasu's disease revisited, N.Y. State J. Med. *74*:1960, 1974.
149. Sunamori, M., Hatano, R., Yokokawa, T., Tsukuura, T., Sakamoto, T., Suzuki, T., Murakami, T., Yokoawa, M., and Numano, F.: Aortitis syndrome due to Takayasu's disease. A guideline for the surgical indication. J. Cardiovasc. Surg. *17*:443, 1976.
150. Bloss, R. S., Duncan, J. M., Cooley, D. A., Leatherman, L. L., and Schnee, M. J.: Takayasu's arteritis: Surgical considerations. Ann. Thorac. Surg. *27*:574, 1979.
151. Hallett, J. W., Jr., Brewster, D. C., Darling, R. C., and O'Hara, P. J.: Coarctation of the abdominal aorta: Current options in surgical management. Ann. Surg. *191*:430, 1980.
152. Ishikawa, K.: Survival and morbidity after diagnosis of occlusive thromboaortopathy (Takayasu's disease). Am. J. Cardiol. *47*:1026, 1981.
153. Klein, R. G., Hunder, G. G., Stanson, A. W., and Sheps, S. G.: Large artery involvement in giant cell (temporal) arteritis. Ann. Intern. Med. *83*:806, 1975.
154. Hamrin, B.: Polymyalgia arteritica. Acta Med. Scand. (Suppl.)*533*:1, 1972
155. Austen, W. G., and Blennerhassett, M. B.: Giant cell aortitis causing an aneurysm of the ascending aorta and aortic regurgitation. N. Engl. J. Med. *272*:80, 1965.
156. Ghose, M. K., Shensa, S., and Lerner, P. I.: Arteritis of the aged (giant cell arteritis) and fever of unexplained origin. Am. J. Med. *60*:429, 1976.
157. Huston, K. A., and Hunder, G. G.: Giant cell (cranial) arteritis: A clinical review. Am. Heart J. *100*:99, 1980.
158. Salisbury, R. S., and Hazleman, B. L.: Successful treatment of dissecting aortic aneurysm due to giant cell arteritis. Ann. Rheum. Dis. *40*:507, 1981.
159. Soorae, A. S., McKeown, F., and Cleland, J.: Aortic valve replacement for severe aortic regurgitation caused by idiopathic giant cell aortitis. Thorax *35*:60, 1980.
160. Davidson, P., Bagenstoss, A. H., Slocumb, C. H., and Daugherty, G. W.: Cardiac and aortic lesions in rheumatoid spondylitis. Proc. Mayo Clin. *36*:427, 1963.
161. Zvaifler, N. J., and Weintraub, A. M.: Aortitis and aortic insufficiency in chronic rheumatic disorders. A reappraisal. Arthritis Rheum. *6*:241, 1963.
162. Pearson, C. M., Kroening, R., Verity, M. A., and Getzen, J. H.: Aortic insufficiency and aortic aneurysm in relapsing polychondritis. Trans. Assoc. Am. Phys. *80*:71, 1967.
163. Paulus, H. E., Pearson, C. M., and Pitts, W.: Aortic insufficiency in five patients with Reiter's syndrome. A detailed clinical and pathologic study. Am. J. Med. *53*:464, 1972.
164. Muna, W. F., Roller, D. H., Craft, J., Shaw, R. K., and Ross, A. M.: Psoriatic arthritis and aortic regurgitation. J.A.M.A. *244*:363, 1980.
165. Little, A. G., and Zarins, C. K.: Abdominal aortic aneurysm and Behçet's disease. Surgery *91*:359, 1982.
166. Kampmeier, R. H.: Manifestations of late syphilis. South. Med. Bull. *53*:17, 1965.
167. Heggtveit, H. A.: Syphilitic aortitis. A clinicopathologic autopsy study of 100 cases, 1950 to 1960. Circulation *29*:346, 1964.
168. Carter, C. H., Agostas, W. N., Sydenstricker, V. P.: Rupture of an aortic aneurysm into the pulmonary artery. A case report. Circulation *5*:449, 1952.
169. Kampmeier, R. H.: Aneurysm of the abdominal aorta. A study of 73 cases. Am. J. Med. Sci. *192*:97, 1936.
170. Prewitt, T. A.: Syphilitic aortic insufficiency. Its increased incidence in the elderly. J.A.M.A. *211*:637, 1970.
171. Sparling, A. F.: Diagnosis and treatment of syphilis. N. Engl. J. Med. *284*:642, 1971.
172. Centers for Disease Control: Syphilis Recommended Treatment Schedules, 1976. The Venereal Disease Control Advisory Committee. Ann. Intern. Med. *85*:94, 1976.
173. Beck, W., Barnard, C. N., and Schrire, V.: Syphilitic obstruction of coronary ostia successfully treated by endarterectomy. Br. Heart J. *27*:911, 1965.
174. Steinberg, I.: Anomalies (pseudocoarctation) of the arch of the aorta—Report of 8 new and review of 8 previously published cases. Am. J. Roentgenol. *88*:73, 1962.
175. Brinsfield, D. E., Shuford, W. M., Plauth, W. H., Jr., and Sybers, R. G.: Congenital anomalies of the aorta. *In* Lindsay, J., Jr., and Hurst, J. W. (eds.): The Aorta. New York, Grune and Stratton, 1979, p. 271.
176. Keller, H. I., and Cheitlin, M. D.: The occurrence of mild coarctation of the aorta (pseudocoarctation) and coarctation in one family. Am. Heart J. *70*:115, 1965.
177. Lavin, N., Mehta, S., Liberson, M., and Pouget, J. M.: Pseudocoarctation of the aorta. An unusual variant with coarctation. Am. J. Cardiol. *24*:584, 1969.
178. Lajos, T. Z., Meckstroth, C. V., Klassen, K. P., and Sherman, N. J.: Pseudocoarctation of the aorta. A variant or an entity? Chest *58*:571, 1970.
179. Griffen, J. F.: Congenital kinking of the aorta (pseudocoarctation). N. Engl. J. Med. *271*:726, 1964.
180. Turner, A. F., Swenson, B. E., Jacobson, G., and Kay, J. H.: Kinking or buckling of the aorta. Case report with complication of aneurysm formation. Am. J. Roentgenol. *97*:411, 1966.
181. Bahabozorgui, S., Bernstein, R. G., and Frater, R. W. M.: Pseudocoarctation of the aorta associated with aneurysm formation. Chest *60*:616, 1971.
182. Bland, E. F., and Castleman, B.: Vascular collapse in a woman with an unusual calcified ring in the aortic arch. N. Engl. J. Med. *280*:1466, 1969.
183. Steinberg, I.: Calcified and dilated ascending aorta due to atheromatous occlusive disease simulating coarctation of the aorta: A report of a case and theory of pathogenesis. Am. J. Roentgenol. *98*:840, 1966.
184. Prian, G. W., Kinard, S. A., Read, C. T., and Diethrich, E. B.: Pseudocoarctation: Diagnosis, etiology, natural history with emphasis on timing and technique of surgical correction. Vasc. Surg. *6*:198, 1972.
185. Greendyke, R. M.: Traumatic rupture of aorta: Special reference to automobile accidents. J.A.M.A. *195*:527, 1966.
186. Parmley, L. F., Mattingly, T. W., Manion, W. C., and Jahnke, E. J.: Nonpenetrating traumatic injury of the aorta. Circulation *17*:1086, 1958.
187. Fleming, A. W., and Green, D. C.: Traumatic aneurysms of the thoracic aorta: Report of 43 patients. Ann. Thorac. Surg. *18*:91, 1974.
188. Ayella, R. J., Hankins, J. R., Turney, S. Z., and Cowley, R. A.: Ruptured thoracic aorta due to blunt trauma. J. Trauma *17*:199, 1977.
189. Malm, J. R., and Deterling, R. A.: Traumatic aneurysm of the thoracic aorta simulating coarctation: A case report. J. Thorac. Cardiovasc. Surg. *40*:271, 1960.
190. Kirsh, M. M., Behrendt, D. M., Orringer, M. B., Gago, O., Gray, L. A., Mills, L. J., Walter, J. F., and Sloan, H.: The treatment of acute traumatic rupture of the aorta. A 10-year experience. Ann. Surg. *184*:308, 1976.
191. Bodily, K., Perry, J. F., Strate, R. G., and Fischer, R. P.: The salvageability of patients with post-traumatic rupture of the descending thoracic aorta in a primary trauma center. J. Trauma *17*:754, 1977.
192. Jang, G. C., Brody, W. R., and Dinsmore, R. E.: Radiologic diagnosis or aortic disease. *In* Lindsay, J., Jr., and Hurst, J. W. (eds.): The Aorta. New York, Grune and Stratton, 1979, p. 295.
193. Marsh, D. G., and Sturm, J. T.: Traumatic aortic rupture: Roentgenographic indications for angiography. Ann. Thorac. Surg. *21*:337, 1976.
194. Simeone, J. F., Deren, M. M., and Cagle, F.: The value of the left apical cap in the diagnosis of aortic rupture. Diagn. Radiol. *139*:35, 1981.
195. Bennett, D. E., and Cherry, J. K.: The natural history of traumatic aneurysms of the aorta. Surgery *61*:516, 1967.
196. Schwartz, M. L., Fisher, R., Sako, Y., Castaneda, A. R., Grage, T. B., and Nicoloff, D. M.: Post-traumatic aneurysms of the thoracic aorta. Surgery *78*:589, 1975.
197. Heiskell, C. A., and Conn, J., Jr.: Aortoarterial emboli. Am. J. Surg. *132*:4, 1976.
198. Shapiro, M. E., Rodvien, R., Bauer, K. A., and Salzman, E. W.: Acute aortic thrombosis in antithrombin III deficiency. J.A.M.A. *245*:1759, 1981.
199. Schatz, I. J., and Stanley, J. C.: Saddle embolus of the aorta. J.A.M.A. *235*: 1262, 1976.
200. Thompson, J. E., and Garrett, W. V.: Peripheral-arterial surgery. N. Engl. J. Med. *302*:491, 1980.
201. Tegtmeyer, C. J., Wellons, H. A., and Thompson, R. N.: Balloon dilation of the abdominal aorta. J.A.M.A. *244*:2636, 1980.
202. Hertzer, N. R.: Peripheral atheromatous embolization following blunt abdominal trauma. Surgery *82*:244, 1977.
203. Perdue, G. D., and Smith, R. B.: Atheromatous microemboli. Ann. Surg. *169*:954, 1969.
204. Carvajal, J. A., Anderson, R., Weiss, L., Grisiner, J., and Berman, R.: Atheroembolism. An etiologic factor in renal insufficiency, gastrointestinal hemorrhages and peripheral vascular diseases. Arch. Intern. Med. *119*:593, 1967.
205. Handler, F. P.: Clinical and pathologic significance of atheromatous embolization, with emphasis on an etiology of renal hypertension. Am. J. Med. *20*:366, 1956.
206. Anderson, W. R., Richards, A. M., and Weiss, L.: Hemorrhage and necrosis of the stomach and bowel due to atheroembolism. A correlative study of atheromatous emboli to the gastrointestinal tract in humans and experimental animals. Am. J. Clin. Pathol. *48*:30, 1967.
207. Moldveen-Geronimus, M., and Merriam, J. C.: Cholesterol embolization. From pathological curiosity to clinical entity. Circulation *35*:946, 1967.
208. Jarrett, F., Darling, R. C., Mundth, E. D., and Austen, W. G.: Experience with infected aneurysms of the abdominal aorta. Arch. Surg. *110*:1281, 1975.
209. Silbergleit, A., Arbulu, A., Defever, B. A., and Nedwicki, E. G.: Tuberculous aortitis. Surgical resection of ruptured abdominal false aneurysm. J.A.M.A. *193*:83, 1965.
210. Felson, B., Akers, P. V., Hall, G. S., Schreiber, J. T., Greene, R. E., and Pedrosa, C. S.: Mycotic tuberculous aneurysm of the thoracic aorta. J.A.M.A. *237*:1104, 1977.
211. Feinsod, F. M., Norfleet, R. G., and Hoehn, J. L.: Mycotic aneurysm of the external iliac artery. A triad of clinical signs facilitating early diagnosis. J.A.M.A. *238*:245, 1977.
212. Anderson, C. B., Butcher, H. R., and Ballinger, W. F.: Mycotic aneurysms. Arch. Surg. *109*:712, 1974.
213. Chen, K. T. K.: Primary malignant fibrous histiocytoma of the aorta. Cancer *48*:840, 1981.

46 COR PULMONALE AND PULMONARY THROMBOEMBOLISM

by E. Regis McFadden, Jr., M.D., and Eugene Braunwald, M.D.

According to the World Health Organization, the chronic form of cor pulmonale is composed of some combination of hypertrophy and dilatation of the right ventricle secondary to pulmonary hypertension; the latter is caused by disease of the pulmonary parenchyma and/or pulmonary vascular system between the origins of the main pulmonary artery and the entry of the pulmonary veins into the left atrium.[1] Acute cor pulmonale is defined as acute right heart strain or overload resulting from the pulmonary hypertension usually due to massive pulmonary embolism.[2] Cor pulmonale includes many disease states with diverse etiologies, pathophysiological mechanisms, and clinical characteristics which have in common only a disturbance of the pulmonary circulation. This chapter focuses on those conditions (with the exclusion of primary pulmonary hypertension, Chap. 25) which act directly on the pulmonary vessels, both acutely and chronically, and those which produce pulmonary hypertension by acting primarily on the gas-exchanging, neuromuscular, and ventilatory control functions of the respiratory system.

ANATOMICAL AND PATHOPHYSIOLOGICAL CORRELATES

Right Ventricular Anatomy

In the first 3 months of life in infants born at, or near, sea level, the right ventricle is larger and heavier and has a greater end-diastolic volume than the left.[3-7] With advancing age, the left ventricle becomes dominant, and in the adult, the right ventricular wall is relatively thin and has a crescentic configuration on cross section. However, in high-altitude dwellers, the situation is different. The degree of right ventricular preponderance, both at birth and for the first 3 months of life, is greater than that seen in low-altitude residents, and the normal regression in size is so delayed that the right ventricular enlargement can persist through the first decade.[6] In native adults living above 12,000 feet, 93 per cent of the hearts in a necropsy series showed some degree of right ventricular enlargement.[8] These morphological findings have a close relationship with the hemodynamic characteristics of individuals at high altitudes and can be related to the degree of pulmonary arterial hypertension.[9]

Several methods are used to ascertain the characteristics, presence, and severity of right ventricular hypertrophy; the two traditional methods involve the measurement of ventricular weight and wall thickness. Many investigators believe that wall thickness determinations are not sufficiently precise. Fulton et al. have provided weight criteria that are used widely.[10] In their technique, the right ventricle is dissected free, and the septum is weighed together with the left ventricle. Right ventricular weight can then be described in absolute terms or as a ratio of the left ventricle (LV) plus the septum (S), i.e., (LV + S)/RV. Using these criteria, a heart is considered normal only if the total ventricular weight is less than 250 gm, the free wall of the right ventricle weighs less than 65 gm, and the ratio of (LV + S)/RV is between 2.3:1 and 3.3:1. If left ventricular hypertrophy is also present, the ratio may be within normal limits or even raised. Using this method, Mitchell and colleagues found that the upper limits of normal (as defined by the mean plus 2 standard deviations) in men 40 or more years of age at death were 69 gm for the right ventricle and 203 gm for the left ventricle plus septum. These observers also noted that in their study right ventricular thickness was a relatively poor index of hypertrophy.[11]

Others have determined muscle fiber size morphometrically and found the distribution of myocardial fiber diameters to be uniform, with a distinct bell-shaped distribution noted for the right ventricle, left ventricle, and septum.[12] In cases of pure right ventricular hypertrophy, the distribution always shifted so that the mean diameter of the muscle fibers from the right ventricle exceeded that of the septum or normal left ventricle.

Right Ventricular Function

Because right ventricular hypertrophy occurs most commonly in association with longstanding elevations in pulmonary arterial pressures, an analogy has often been made between the left ventricle in systemic hypertension and the right ventricle in pulmonary hypertension. Since there is no fundamental difference in either the configuration or the pumping action of the two ventricles before birth, the differences that exist in the adult have been attributed to the flow resistance in the respective circulations.[13] As already noted, the normal adult right ventricle has thin walls and a crescent shape; its pumping action is akin to that of a bellows working in series with a low-pressure circuit, in contrast to the concentric contraction of the left ventricle. The right ventricle is more compliant,[14] and in comparison with the left it is better able to handle an increase in a volume than a pressure load. The evidence in support of this statement is derived in the main from animal data[15–18] (Fig. 46–1), which contrasts the effects of increasing preload and afterload on right and left ventricular function. In the left-hand panel, stroke volume is plotted as a function of various afterloads that were produced by actively constricting the main pulmonary artery and aorta in the dog.[15,16] Small increments in pulmonary artery pressure are associated with sharp decreases in right ventricular stroke volume. In contrast, the left ventricle, which normally works against high initial pressures, continues to maintain stroke volume despite substantial increases in systemic arterial pressure.

The right-hand portion of this figure demonstrates the effects of increasing preload. These ventricular function curves (Chap. 12) were obtained by volume infusions into the atria of dogs.[17,18] Note the marked differences in the respective ventricular stroke work that occur as right and left atrial pressures are increased. For a fourfold elevation in filling pressure (i.e., from 5 to 20 cm H_2O), the increase in left ventricular work was approximately five times that of the right.

In response to chronic pressure loads, significant changes develop in the configuration, mass, and functional characteristics of the right ventricle. The rate at which these occur in man and the magnitude of the pressures needed to produce them are unknown. However, animal studies indicate that alterations in structure and function can be quite rapid following experimental outflow tract obstruction. Spann et al. observed a 71 per cent increase in right ventricular weight in cats 2 days after the pulmonary artery was banded, and within a month weight had risen to 2.5 times the normal value.[19] This increase was not from an elevation in cardiac tissue water, since the wet to dry weight ratios were not significantly different from normal. It is doubtful that the response is as rapid in man.

The lumen of the main pulmonary artery can be reduced by 60 to 80 per cent before aortic pressure declines.[20–22] Because these experiments ignored the effects of neurohumoral compensations that support the systemic circulation, the impression has arisen that the acute right ventricular response is an abrupt, all-or-none event. However, as suggested in Figure 46–1, right ventricular decompensation is really a continuum.[15,18] At right ventricular systolic pressures of 60 to 80 mm Hg, right ventricular dilatation and failure occur with systemic hypotension and hypoperfusion.[23] The rate and/or absolute level of outflow tract obstruction at which these alterations develop can be greatly amplified or attenuated by respectively decreasing or increasing right coronary artery blood flow[23] (Fig. 46–2). The relative role played by changes in coronary blood flow in acute right heart failure secondary to massive thromboembolism in humans has yet to be determined.

Pulmonary Vascular Anatomy

Development. Embryologically, the primitive main pulmonary artery and its main right and left branches are derived from the aortic sac, whereas the peripheral pulmonary arteries arise from a network of vessels around the bronchial bud.[24] Each pulmonary artery forms a close relationship with a stem bronchus and provides an arterial partner for each new airway ramification. This branching pattern of airways and arteries is complete all the way out to the preacinar region by week 16 of intrauterine life, and further growth occurs only in dimensions.[25]

At birth the alveolar region is represented by primitive air sacs, and during early childhood the acini grow rapidly by budding new alveoli from respiratory bronchioli, alveolar ducts, and more distal air spaces.[26,27] New arteries and veins continue to develop up to the 18th month of life and then increase in size with further age.[26] These vessels follow the course of the alveoli and not the airway. By the age of

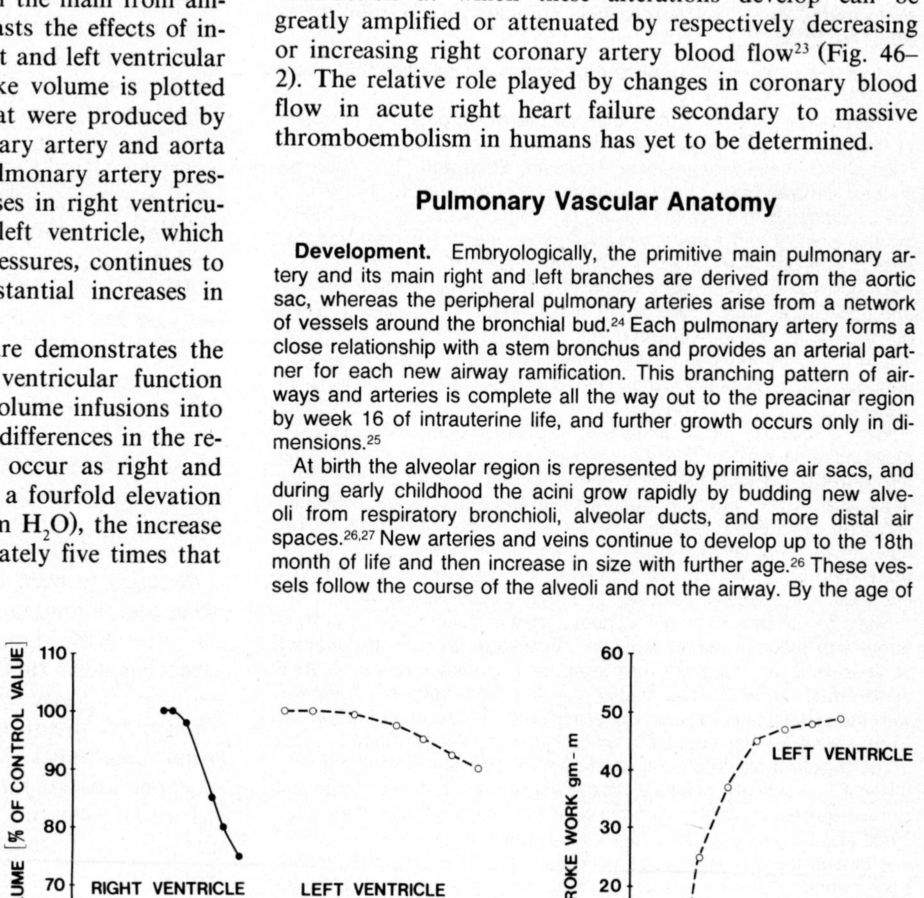

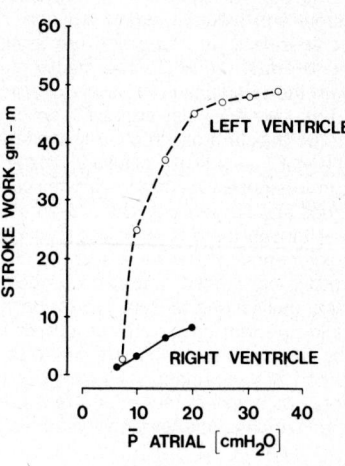

FIGURE 46–1 Effects of increasing preload and afterload on right and left ventricular function. The data in the left panel were obtained by constricting the main pulmonary artery and aorta in dogs. The right panel demonstrates the effect of increasing preloads.

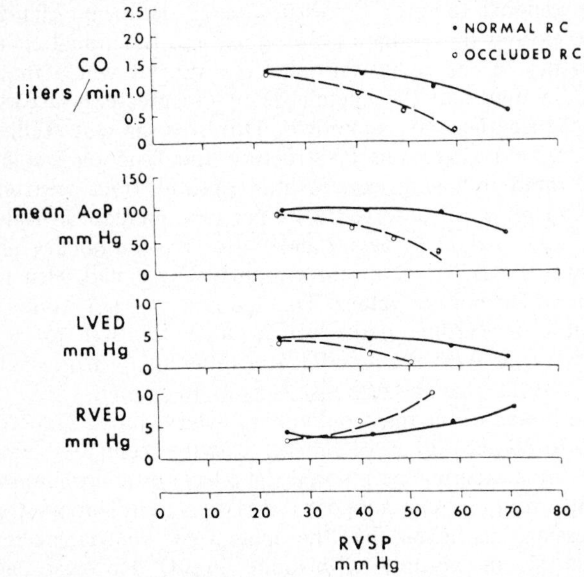

FIGURE 46–2 Hemodynamic responses to increasing levels of right ventricular systolic stress induced by incremental pulmonary artery obstruction before (solid lines) and after (broken lines) right coronary artery (RC) occlusion. CO = cardiac output; AoP = mean aortic pressure; LVED = left ventricular end-diastolic pressure; RVED = right ventricular end-diastolic pressure; RVSP = right ventricular systolic pressure. (From Brooks, H., et al.: Performance of the right ventricle under stress: Relation to right coronary flow. J. Clin. Invest. *50*:2176, 1971.)

8 years the number of alveoli and blood vessels reaches that of the adult.[26]

It has been traditionally held that the branching pattern and course of the airways and pulmonary arteries always parallel each other, at least within the alveolar region. However, Elliot and Reid have described an irregular branching pattern from the hilum to the level of the capillaries with so-called "axial" or "conventional" arteries following the airways and supernumerary arteries, which are side branches arising from the main arteries but without a corresponding airway.[28] Two types of supernumerary vessels have been recognized: aberrant and accessory. An *aberrant* artery arises independently of any airway but then joins one downstream and branches with it. An *accessory* artery branches independently of any airway and usually enters the periphery of a respiratory unit. The function of these vessels is unknown.

Wall Structure. In keeping with its embryological derivation, the main pulmonary artery and the first five generations are elastic in nature but less so than the aorta and major systemic arteries.[29] These vessels are over 3000 μm in diameter in the adult. In the axial pathway, the next three generations are said to be transitional.[30] They have fewer internal and external elastic laminae and range in size from 2000 to 3000 μm. The remainder of the artery is then divided into muscular, partially muscular, and nonmuscular segments.[31]

Muscular arteries have a continuous muscle coat limited by both internal and external elastic laminae. These arteries form the majority of vessels in the lung and are found in a diameter range of 30 to 2000 μm in the adult. The medial muscle coat is very thin compared with the arterioles in the systemic circulation. These vessels give way to partially muscular arteries in which the muscle is arranged in a spiral so that in cross section it appears as a crescent, with the rest of the wall being like a capillary. These vessels are between 30 to 250 μm in external diameter. Nonmuscular arteries are larger than capillaries and range from 30 to 75 μm in diameter in adults.

Although there is great variation in the sizes of arteries that accompany conducting airways such as lobar bronchi, those that follow the respiratory bronchi and alveolar ducts are muscular or partially so.[28-30] The implications for function of these observations are severalfold. It is known that gas exchange occurs in respiratory bronchi and alveolar ducts through the arteries that accompany these structures.[32] When this information is coupled with the fact that hypoxia acts directly to constrict muscular arteries,[32,33] it is apparent that this area of the lung has the propensity for active control of pulmonary blood flow. Further, since the spiral of muscle in the partially muscular arteries is directly contiguous with the muscle encircling the larger vessels, retrograde propagation of the hypoxic stimulus can occur in the intracellular pathways of the muscle syncytium,[34] and a wider and more severe response can develop.

Innervation. In further contrast to the peripheral circulation, it has proved difficult to demonstrate a nerve supply in the pulmonary circulation. Evidence suggests that although both adrenergic and cholinergic fibers are present, they are sparse in comparison with those of systemic vessels of similar size, and their distribution tends to be concentrated in the larger vessels at the hilum.[31,35]

In summary, the structure of the pulmonary circulation is in keeping with its hemodynamics. The thin-walled, sparsely innervated vessels which contain relatively small amounts of smooth muscle do not favor the development of marked vasomotor responses, and, indeed, vasoconstriction alone is not sufficient to overload the right ventricle to the point of producing acute cor pulmonale.[36] Consequently, mechanical occlusion of the pulmonary circulation can be inferred when there is acute cor pulmonale, and structural alterations in the pulmonary vascular bed must be present in the chronic form.

Physiology of the Pulmonary Circulation

(See also Chapter 25)

The physiology of the pulmonary circulation is unique from several standpoints. Most of this vascular bed is contained within the parenchyma of the lung, and thus the vessels are subjected to external distending and compressive forces which can act independently of any intrinsic properties of the vessels themselves. In addition, the pulmonary circulation is in series with a pump capable of developing only low pressures, yet it must accommodate the entire cardiac output under all states of physical activity. Consequently, it must adjust to wide variations in blood flow without much change in pressure so as not to overload the right ventricle. This section will deal with the pressure, flow, and volume relationships of the pulmonary circulation as they interrelate with the mechanical and gas-exchanging properties of the lungs.

PRESSURE-VOLUME RELATIONSHIPS. Historically, it has been thought that the pulmonary circulation is highly distensible and that the vessels dilate to accommodate increases in cardiac output and, in this manner, prevent an increase in pulmonary artery pressure in high-flow states.[37,38] However, actual measurements of the compliance of the pulmonary vessels have shown that this vascular bed is significantly stiffer than its systemic counterpart[39,40] (Fig. 46–3), and only small increments in blood volume can be accepted by the large pulmonary vessels.[41-44] It has subsequently been demonstrated that a major mechanism to accommodate increased blood volume is the recruitment of previously unperfused vessels.[39,45] Morphological evidence suggests that both recruitment and distention occur with an increase in pulmonary blood flow and that the transmural pressures to which the vessel is subjected are what determines which one predominates.[46] In superior portions of the lung where the vessels are collapsed or where alveolar pressure is greater than pulmonary venous pressure, recruitment appears to be the major mechanism. Distention is more important when pulmonary venous pressure is greater than alveolar pressure (see below).[31]

PRESSURE-FLOW RELATIONSHIPS. Evaluation of the pressure-flow relationships of the pulmonary circulation in normal humans at any fixed lung volume demonstrates a hyperbolic configuration in which large changes in pulmonary blood flow are associated with small eleva-

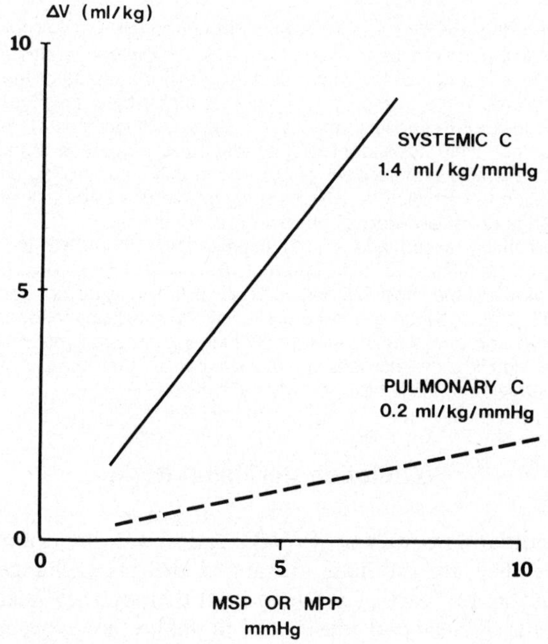

FIGURE 46–3 Comparison of compliances of pulmonary and systemic vascular beds. MSP = mean systemic pressure; MPP = mean pulmonary pressure; C = compliance; ΔV = change in volume. (Redrawn from Guyton, A. C.: Circulatory Physiology: Cardiac Output and Its Regulation. Philadelphia, W. B. Saunders Co., 1963.)

tions in pulmonary artery pressure (Fig. 46–4*A*). The net result is that as flow increases, pulmonary vascular resistance decreases (Fig. 46–4*B*).[36] Consequently, irrespective of whether distention or recruitment occurs, both mechanisms subserve the necessity of maintaining a low pressure circuit during situations of increased blood flow.

If one examines pulmonary vascular resistance as a function of lung volume, a U-shaped curve is found (Fig. 46–4*C*).[43] At the extremes of lung volume of full inflation and deflation, vascular resistance is high, and it reaches its nadir at about the resting end-expiratory position (i.e., at functional residual capacity). These findings can be explained by considering the geometry assumed by the alveolar and intrapulmonic but extraalveolar vessels in response to the transmural pressures to which they are exposed.

Because the pulmonary vessels are within the substance of the lung, their dimensions reflect the forces exerted upon them by the pulmonary parenchyma. At low lung volumes, the extraalveolar vessels tend to collapse because radial traction no longer supports them. Simultaneously, the alveolar vessels are pulled open by the increased recoil forces generated by the tendency of the alveoli to become smaller. As the lung is inflated to volumes above functional residual capacity, the larger vessels tend to be pulled open, but there is now a progressive increase in the resistance of the small vessels as they are squeezed and lengthened by enlarging alveoli. In addition to this deformation, alterations in alveolar pressure can also dynamically influence the lumens of small vessels. When alveolar pressure is positive, as it is during expiration or with the Valsalva maneuver, vessels are compressed. Alternatively, with negative pressure, as with inspiration or the Mueller maneuver, small vessels are subjected to a proportional distending pressure. With this information, it is relatively easy to appreciate that alveolar pressure can play a critical role in determining the distribution of pulmonary blood flow and, accordingly, gas exchange.

DETERMINANTS OF PULMONARY GAS EXCHANGE

Distribution of Pulmonary Blood Flow

In the normal upright human, blood flow per unit volume of lung steadily increases from the apex to the base, with flow at the apex being virtually nil.[47,48] This distribution is affected by changes of posture and by exercise. When a subject is in the supine position, apical blood flow increases but the basal flow remains virtually unchanged, with the result that the distribution from apex to base becomes almost uniform. In this posture, however, flow in the posterior or dependent regions exceeds that in the anterior parts. During mild exercise, flow to both the upper and the lower zones increases but more to the upper, so that flow becomes more evenly distributed.

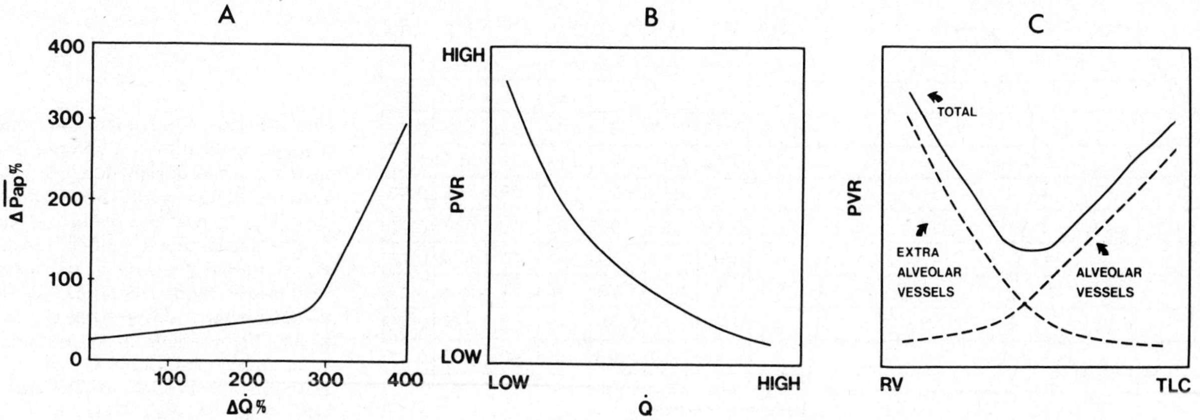

FIGURE 46–4 Some aspects of pulmonary vascular physiology. *A*, Pressure-flow relationship. *B*, Resistance-flow relationship. *C*, Pulmonary vascular resistance as a function of lung volume for the total system and for extraalveolar and alveolar vessels. $\Delta\overline{PAP}$ = per cent change of mean pulmonary artery pressure from control; ΔQ = per cent change in cardiac output; 100 = normal cardiac output; RV = residual volume; TLC = total lung capacity.

West and colleagues[47–50] and Permutt and Riley[51] have independently demonstrated that the pressure-flow relationships through the lung can be analogous to those of a "waterfall" or Starling resistor. The basic point of these studies is that the effective pressure drop in the pulmonary vasculature is not always the difference between inflow (pulmonary artery) and outflow (left atrial) pressures but often is between the inflow pressure and the closing pressure of small vessels downstream.

In normal human lungs pulmonary arterial and venous pressures both increase from superior to dependent regions because of hydrostatic effects resulting from gravity acting on the blood.[49–52] However, alveolar pressures remain essentially constant throughout the lung. Alveolar pressure exceeds venous pressure at a more dependent portion of the lung than does arterial pressure. This results in distribution of blood flow to three major areas (Fig. 17–4, p. 564). In the most superior area (zone I) no flow occurs because alveolar pressure exceeds pulmonary arterial pressure. Presumably, this is because thin-walled collapsible vessels are directly exposed to alveolar pressure. In humans, the pulmonary artery pressure is sufficiently high to bring blood to the apex of the lung so that no zone I is present under normal conditions. It can develop, however, if pulmonary artery pressure falls or if alveolar pressure is elevated, as it is in obstructive airway disease. In the middle zone (zone II), arterial pressure exceeds alveolar pressure, but the latter is greater than venous pressure. Here, flow through the capillaries is proportional to the difference between arterial and alveolar pressure. In the lowest zone, zone III, venous pressure exceeds alveolar pressure, the vessels are held open, and flow is determined in the usual way by the arterial-venous pressure difference. Hughes and associates[53] and West et al.[54] have also observed a small zone of reduced flow at the very base of the lung and have attributed this to a possible increase in the interstitial pressure as a consequence of the reduced expansion of the lung parenchyma in the lower zone. This has, therefore, been called zone IV. There is still some uncertainty about the cause of the reduced flow in this area, but the concept of reduction in flow caused by an increased interstitial pressure is almost certainly important in mitral stenosis and may be responsible for the reduction in basilar blood flow observed in that condition.

Distribution of Ventilation

The distribution of ventilation, like that of perfusion, decreases from base to apex in the normal lung, but the rate of change is only about one third that seen with blood flow[47] (Fig. 46–5). Here, too, gravity plays a role, and changes in posture have an influence. Thus, when normal subjects lie supine, the difference in ventilation between the anatomical upper and lower zones is abolished,[47] and in the inverted lung, the apex ventilates better than the base, so the normal pattern is reversed.

Evaluation of the relative rates of expansion of the upper and lower zones in the upright position reveals different patterns of distribution, depending upon the lung volume from which inspiration is initiated.[55–57] As a consequence of the effect of gravity and the shape of the pressure-volume curve of the lung, when a normal subject takes a breath from functional residual capacity (FRC), ventilation is preferentially distributed to the dependent lung zones. Since blood flow in the resting state is also preferentially distributed to this area, this matching of ventilation to perfusion in different body positions insures efficient gas exchange under a variety of physiological conditions.

If breathing takes place at lung volumes lower than FRC, the distribution of ventilation is quite different. Because of closure of dependent airways, the most inferior portions of the lung do not ventilate, and all of the inspired gas goes preferentially to the upper zones. The phenomenon of airway closure at low lung volumes has major physiological significance and can produce substantial alterations in ventilation-perfusion relationships and arterial hypoxia.[58,59]

Ventilation-perfusion Ratios

Ventilation-perfusion ($\dot{V}_A/\dot{Q}$) ratios are important because they are the determinants of the gas exchange that occurs in any part of the lung, and thereby they affect the overall efficiency of the lungs in taking up oxygen and eliminating carbon dioxide.[47,60–62] The partial pressure of oxygen in the alveolar gas (and therefore in the end-capillary blood) is set by a balance between the rate of removal by the blood and its rate of replenishment by ventilation. If ventilation is gradually reduced and perfusion maintained to an alveolus, oxygen tension falls and carbon dioxide tension rises. The limit is reached when the unit is not ventilated at all, and the pulmonary venous oxygen and carbon dioxide will be those of mixed venous blood. This is a $\dot{V}_A/\dot{Q}$ relationship of zero and corresponds to the situation in which there is a true anatomical pulmonary arteriovenous shunt, e.g., a pulmonary arteriovenous fistula or a functional one such as produced by atelectasis. By contrast, if perfusion to a normally ventilating alveolus is gradually reduced, the oxygen tension in the venous blood draining this alveolus rises and the partial pressure of carbon dioxide falls. The limit now occurs when the unit is unperfused. This is a $\dot{V}_A/\dot{Q}$ of infinity and is seen in situations in which blood supply is disrupted, such as by pulmonary emboli or other disease in which occlusion of the pulmonary arterial circulation occurs. Between these two

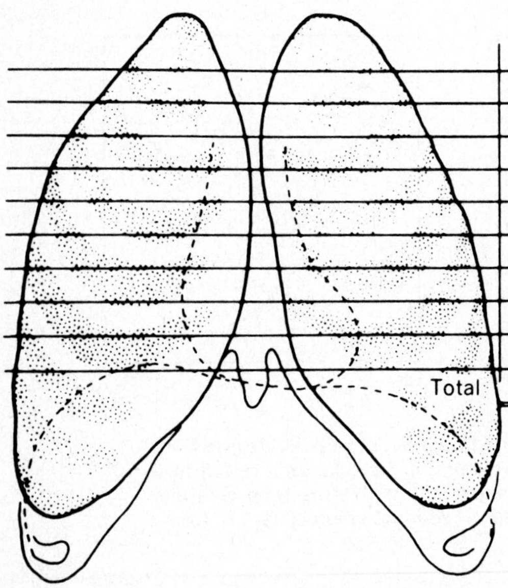

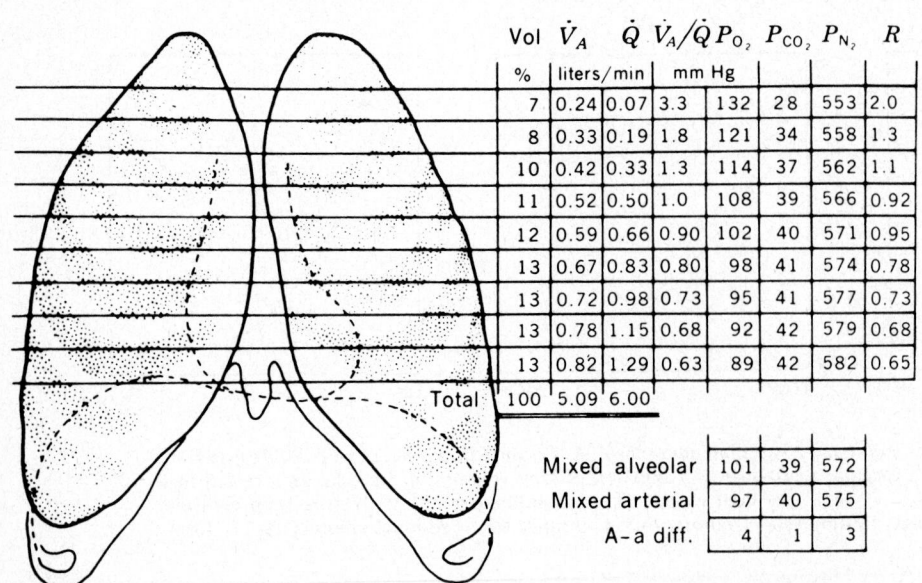

Vol	$\dot{V}_A$	$\dot{Q}$	$\dot{V}_A/\dot{Q}$	P_{O_2}	P_{CO_2}	P_{N_2}	R
%	liters/min			mm Hg			
7	0.24	0.07	3.3	132	28	553	2.0
8	0.33	0.19	1.8	121	34	558	1.3
10	0.42	0.33	1.3	114	37	562	1.1
11	0.52	0.50	1.0	108	39	566	0.92
12	0.59	0.66	0.90	102	40	571	0.95
13	0.67	0.83	0.80	98	41	574	0.78
13	0.72	0.98	0.73	95	41	577	0.73
13	0.78	1.15	0.68	92	42	579	0.68
13	0.82	1.29	0.63	89	42	582	0.65
Total 100	5.09	6.00					

	P_{O_2}	P_{CO_2}	P_{N_2}
Mixed alveolar	101	39	572
Mixed arterial	97	40	575
A-a diff.	4	1	3

FIGURE 46–5 Regional differences in alveolar ventilation ($\dot{V}_A$) and perfusion ($\dot{Q}$) in the normal upright lung. Vol = lung volume; $\dot{V}_A/\dot{Q}$= ventilation-perfusion ratios; P_{O_2} = partial pressure of oxygen; P_{CO_2} = partial pressure of carbon dioxide; P_{N_2} = partial pressure of nitrogen; R = respiratory exchange ratio; A-a diff. = alveolar-arterial differences. (From West, J. B.: Disturbances of respiratory function. *In* Petersdorf, R. G., et al. (eds.): Harrison's Principles of Internal Medicine. 10th ed. New York, McGraw-Hill Book Co., 1983.)

extreme examples, a wide range of $\dot{V}_A/\dot{Q}$ abnormalities is possible.

The alveoli hypoventilated in relation to their perfusion (i.e., low $\dot{V}_A/\dot{Q}$ ratio) cause hypoxemia, and their presence has the same effect as mixing venous and arterial blood. This is termed venous admixture or wasted blood and is evaluated clinically by determining the oxygen tension difference between ideal alveolar gas and arterial blood. Normally, venous admixture or "shunt effect" is only about 2 to 3 per cent of cardiac output,[63–65] but in severe disease it may rise to 30 per cent or more. The normal alveolar-arterial difference of oxygen (A-aDO_2) is 20 mm Hg or less.[63–65]

The alveoli which are hyperventilated in relation to their perfusion (i.e, high $\dot{V}_A/\dot{Q}$ ratio) mainly affect CO_2 elimination. They behave as if part of the inspired gas bypassed the alveoli, so this effect has been called "wasted ventilation" or an increase in "physiological dead space." It is evaluated by comparing mixed expired and arterial CO_2, using the Bohr equation. Normally the physiological dead space is less than 30 per cent of the tidal volume.[65,66] In severe lung disease it can rise to 50 per cent or more. Every pathological condition that directly affects the pulmonary parenchyma or its vascular bed results in mismatched ventilation and blood flow. Consequently, this abnormality is by far the most common cause of arterial hypoxemia in disease states. Both venous admixture and physiological dead space are typically increased in chronic obstructive and infiltrative lung diseases. In pulmonary thromboembolism an increase in dead space predominates.

In many pulmonary parenchymal diseases, blood supply to poorly ventilating areas tends to be reduced, so that the $\dot{V}_A/\dot{Q}$ ratios are not as low as they would otherwise be. One reason for this is that the local pathological process tends to disturb both ventilation and perfusion by its mechanical effects. Another is local hypoxic vasoconstriction, which shunts blood away from the involved alveoli.[32,33,67–69] In the case of thromboembolic phenomena, the regional decreases in CO_2 concentration that occur cause local increases in the resistance of small airways and thus reduce ventilation to the affected region.[70]

Other Causes of Abnormal Arterial Blood Gases

In addition to $\dot{V}_A/\dot{Q}$ inequalities, there are four other causes of arterial hypoxemia: (1) anatomical right-to-left intracardiac or intrapulmonary shunts (Chaps. 29 and 30); (2) reductions in the inspired concentration of O_2; (3) defects in the diffusion of O_2 from the alveolus to the blood; and (4) alveolar hypoventilation.

Although it was originally thought that measurements of the *diffusing capacity* of the lung for oxygen demonstrated a specific impairment in molecular O_2 transfer across a thickened membrane (i.e., alveolar capillary block),[71] it is now appreciated that single breath tests of diffusing capacity that employ carbon monoxide are profoundly influenced by three variables: (1) the surface area available for diffusion, (2) the volume of blood within the capillaries, and (3) the rate of combination of CO and hemoglobin.[72] Other factors, such as the molecular path for diffusion and the stratified heterogeneity of gas mixtures, also play a role.[73] In addition to the above, steady-state methods are also influenced by regional $\dot{V}_A/\dot{Q}$ relationships.[72] Thus, these techniques do not measure the thickness of the alveolar-capillary membrane, and in any disease associated with a loss of elastic recoil (loss of surface area through disruption of alveolar walls), marked $\dot{V}_A/\dot{Q}$ heterogeneities or loss of capillary bed will be associated with a reduced "diffusing capacity." Even so, the effect that this has on gas exchange is, at most, small.[74]

Alveolar hypoventilation is a condition in which insufficient gas exchange occurs to meet metabolic demands. It can result from many causes: severe $\dot{V}_A/\dot{Q}$ inequalities; reduced drive from the respiratory center so that the patient "will not breathe"; failure of the patient's respiratory system to act on the information sent from the central nervous system because of severe intrinsic pulmonary disease; or abnormalities of the neuromuscular apparatus of the chest wall or diaphragm.[75] In the latter cases the patient "cannot breathe." Regardless of cause, the cardinal features of the arterial blood are hypoxemia and hypercapnia, and both must be present to establish the diagnosis. The various diseases associated with alveolar hypoventilation and the mechanisms by which it comes about in each are discussed as examples of chronic cor pulmonale later in this chapter.

Effects of Alveolar Gas Tensions on the Pulmonary Circulation

The most potent stimulus for the development of pulmonary vasoconstriction is alveolar hypoxia.[31,33,67,68,76] Although acute vasoconstriction appears when the alveolar pO_2 is 60 mm Hg or lower, this response is found only in approximately two-thirds of normal subjects.[77] It is speculated that the subjects who respond to hypoxemia with pulmonary vasoconstriction are those who would be prone to develop chronic cor pulmonale if they developed a disease that interfered with effective alveolar ventilation.[78]

Acidosis also has been shown to produce significant increases in pulmonary vascular resistance as well as to act synergistically with hypoxia.[79] In contrast, an increase in arterial pCO_2 seems to exert no direct effect. Instead it seems to operate by way of the increase in hydrogen ion concentration that it induces. The interaction of hypoxia and acidemia is clinically important; these two conditions frequently coexist, and their interplay follows a predictable pattern (Fig. 46–6). At minor degrees of oxygen unsaturation, pulmonary artery pressure is relatively insensitive to hydrogen ion concentration, whereas it is extremely sensitive at high levels of unsaturation.[79] On the other hand, when the pH is high, the pressor effect of hypoxia is blunted.

Although the localization of the pulmonary vascular pressor response within the lung is still controversial, most studies indicate that it occurs in partially muscular arteries

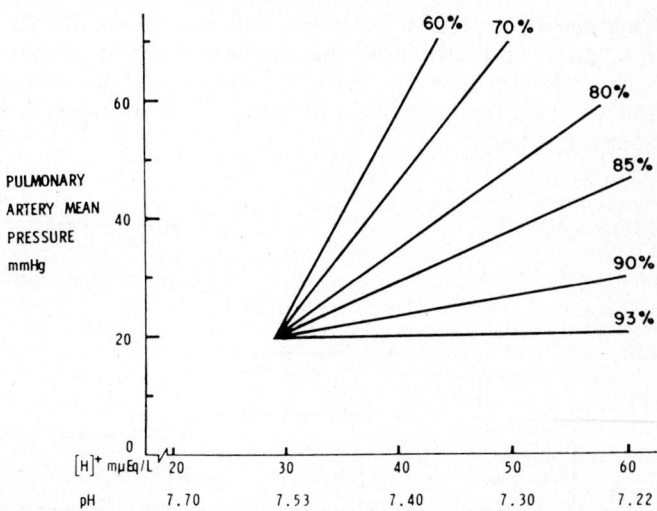

FIGURE 46–6 Relationship of arterial oxygen saturation and hydrogen ion concentration to pulmonary artery pressure. (From Enson, Y., et al.: The influence of hydrogen ion concentration and hypoxia on the pulmonary circulation. J. Clin. Invest. *43*:1146, 1964.)

less than 200 μm in diameter.[67,69,80,81] The mechanism by which hypoxia causes pulmonary arterial smooth muscle to constrict is unclear.[68]

However, the available information points toward two major alternatives: an indirect effect by which hypoxia might cause certain cells in the pulmonary parenchyma to release vasoactive substances (e.g., histamine from mast cells) or a direct effect of hypoxia on pulmonary arterial smooth muscle. Other influences may enhance hypoxic pulmonary vasoconstriction. For example, it is possible that extrapulmonic reflexes or the adrenergic neurotransmitter norepinephrine may augment the pressor response.

PULMONARY THROMBOEMBOLISM AND ACUTE COR PULMONALE

Incidence

It has been estimated that approximately 650,000 patients are afflicted annually with symptomatic pulmonary emboli.[82] Approximately one-fourth of these are fatal (Fig. 46–7). The incidence of pulmonary emboli in autopsy series has been reported to vary from 10 to 64 per cent.[83–86] This large range can be explained by the criteria used to establish the diagnosis and the patient populations studied. In unselected autopsies of adults with grossly visible thromboemboli as the endpoint, the usual figure quoted is around 10 per cent.[83,84] In older patients, particularly those with chronic lung or heart diseases or both, figures of 30 per cent or more are common.[85] However, when subtle pathological effects such as traces of emboli and healed residue are diligently sought in addition to visible thromboemboli, the incidence of pulmonary embolism reportedly can exceed 60 per cent.[86] A large fraction of these emboli, however, are of little clinical significance.

In contrast, the incidence of acute cor pulmonale, fatal pulmonary emboli, or a combination of the two is unknown. Estimates range from 0.1 to 1 per cent of all postsurgical patients.[87,88] Acute pulmonary embolism may be the most common form of acute lung disease among hospitalized patients[89] and, in some series, has been found to be the most common cause of sudden unexpected death in this population[90] (p. 776). Since the diagnosis was not suspected clinically in many of the above studies, the notion has arisen that pulmonary embolism is a very common, but clinically silent, disorder. Although this is undoubtedly true in populations who are chronically ill, bedridden, or postsurgical, the true prevalence of pulmonary embolism in a previously normal population is unknown; this condition may be grossly overdiagnosed in such individuals.[91]

Etiology

From both clinical and pathophysiological standpoints, the preponderant cause of acute cor pulmonale is the rapid obstruction of the pulmonary circulation by thrombi embolized from distant sources.[92] These may be massive and produce partial or complete occlusion of major arteries, or they may be extensive with multiple obstructions of small arterioles. By far the most common source of emboli is the deep veins of the legs,[93–95] and the incidence of lower extremity thrombosis among patients with thromboemboli ranges from 80 to 100 per cent.[96,97] It has been shown convincingly that when thrombi are present in the legs there will be clinical evidence of their presence in only about 50 per cent of cases.[95] Havig performed a complete dissection of the whole lower venous tree, including the plantar and iliac veins, in 80 per cent of the patients who died in a major hospital in Oslo and demonstrated that deep vein thrombosis may start independently at all levels of the venous tree but usually begins in the large venous sinuses of the calf and plantar muscles and in the valve pockets of the axial calf and thigh veins.[98] There is some suspicion that a clot formed in the thigh area is more prone to embolize than is one in a calf.[99]

Three factors are usually listed as fostering the development of venous thrombosis: stasis or slowing of blood in the extremities, damage to the vessel wall, and alterations in the coagulating mechanism of the blood.[92] Of these three, the last is the least well documented, and only a congenital deficiency of antithrombin III has been shown to correlate with excessive thrombotic risk.[100] By far the most common clinical problem is stasis, and it is encountered in many contexts, such as bed rest in the postoperative period and in the presence of congestive heart failure, as well as prolonged periods of sitting during ground or air travel.

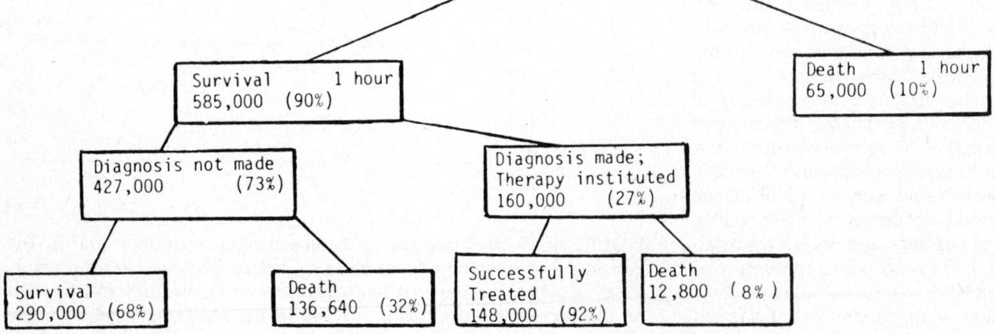

FIGURE 46–7 Diagrammatic representation showing estimated total annual incidence of patients with symptomatic pulmonary emboli in the United States (top box). The outcome in each category (number of patients and per cent) is shown in descending order from top to bottom. (Reproduced with permission from Bell, W. R., and Simon, T. L.: Am. Heart J. *103*: 239, 1982.)

Since the clinical signs and symptoms of venous thrombosis are frequently slight or absent, various laboratory approaches have been devised to facilitate the diagnosis.

Radiofibrinogen techniques rely upon the incorporation of labeled fibrinogen into the thrombus. Once this has occurred, the thrombus is detectable by surface counting. This technique has been used in two circumstances with slightly differing results. When employed *before* thrombus formation has occurred in high-risk groups of patients, it has proved to be a highly sensitive and reliable method of early detection and follow-up.[101,102] However, when used *after a* thrombus has formed, it will detect the presence of the clot only 60 to 80 per cent of the time.[103]

Impedance phlebography and Doppler ultrasound methods measure the speed with which blood leaves the legs. Both involve mechanical obstruction to venous outflow to induce a pooling of blood in the veins, followed by release and monitoring of the flow generated. Impedance phlebography relies upon calf resistance, whereas the Doppler method records frequency shifts in the ultrasound signal.[97,103] These techniques rarely produce false-positive results, but both have a significant incidence of false-negative results because they are relatively insensitive, requiring moderate to marked venous obstruction for best measurements.[92,97]

Although it is generally considered that the legs should be considered the source of an embolus in the absence of other clearly recognizable loci of thrombi, such as the right side of the heart or pelvic veins, it is important to recognize that emboli can also arise from axillary, hepatic portal, and renal veins.[104–106] Renal vein embolus is often associated with distinct symptom complexes characterized by evanescent pulmonary infiltrates in conjunction with the nephrotic syndrome. Other occlusive matter, such as amniotic fluid released during cesarean section or prolonged and difficult labor,[107] bone marrow particulates following trauma or cardiopulmonary resuscitation,[108] fat emboli following trauma,[109] air emboli or insufflation from open wounds in the neck or by intravenous introduction,[110] and tumor emboli[111] have also been implicated, on occasion, in the production of acute cor pulmonale. Still less common but quite dramatic forms of acute cor pulmonale have been encountered in massive pneumothorax, massive atelectasis, mediastinal emphysema, blast injuries, and, rarely, with rupture of an aortic aneurysm into the pulmonary artery.[112]

Pathophysiology

Since pulmonary embolism is a common disorder that has been intensively investigated, one would anticipate that it would be possible to describe its pathophysiology with great precision. Unfortunately, this is not the case, and a number of mechanisms have been proposed to explain the hemodynamic impact with its attendant cardiopulmonary and systemic sequelae.[92] Part of the reason for this is that in the past relatively little in the way of detailed investigation has been performed in acutely ill patients, and the cardiopulmonary alterations are often transient. Therefore, most concepts have been based upon acute, controlled animal studies. Here, too, difficulties have arisen because data have been derived from different species, and occlusions have been produced by ligatures or embolic material that has varied from inert beads and starch granules to clots formed in vivo.

ROLES OF VASCULAR OBSTRUCTION AND NEUROHUMORAL FACTORS. Obstruction of the pulmonary circulation is the sine qua non for the development of the acute, severe, pulmonary hypertension that occurs with emboli, but debate rages over whether it is the sole factor. Quantitatively, it has been recognized since early in this century that mechanical occlusion of 60 to 80 per cent of the lumen of the main pulmonary artery is necessary before the right ventricle dilates and fails.[15,113–115] Hyland and colleagues extended these observations by injecting polystyrene spheres, glass beads, or aged blood clots of precisely graded size into the right atria of dogs to occlude selectively the pulmonary arteries from lobar branches down to small precapillary vessels.[116] They found that irrespective of the material embolized, the majority of vessles at each level had to be obstructed before hypertension appeared. They therefore concluded that mechanical obstruction rather than vasoconstriction was the mechanism underlying the development of pulmonary hypertension. McIntyre and Sasahara reached similar conclusions in humans by observing a linear relationship between the extent of vascular obstruction, as measured during angiography, and mean pulmonary arterial pressure in patients free of cardiopulmonary disease prior to an embolic episode[117] (Fig. 46–8). However, this relationship did not exist in patients with heart or lung disease.[118]

Although mechanical obstruction is obviously quite important, this mechanism is irreconcilable with the observation that total occlusion of either the right or the left main pulmonary artery by a balloon is entirely innocuous in normal humans and produces only minor changes in pulmonary artery pressure.[70,119] Yet, in the study of McIntyre and Sasahara cited above, obstruction of 30 per cent of the

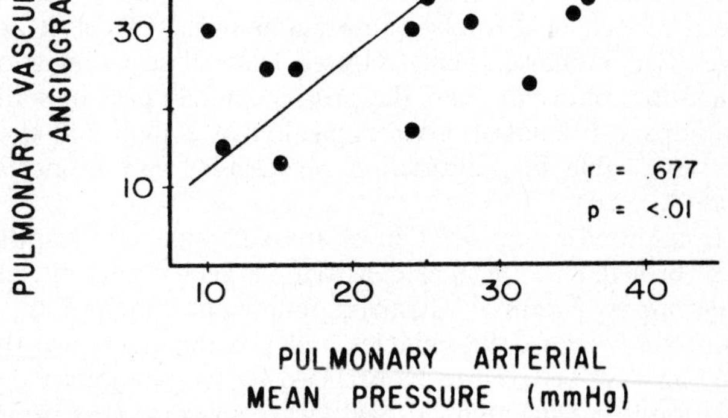

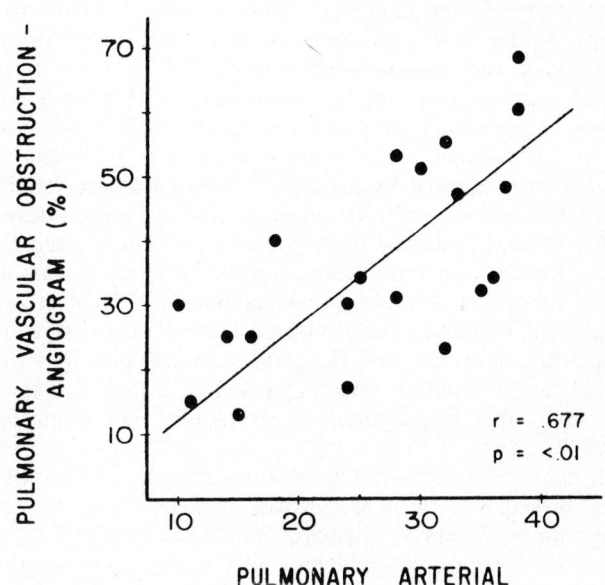

FIGURE 46–8 Relationship between percentage of angiographic obstruction and mean pulmonary artery pressure in patients free of cardiopulmonary disease prior to pulmonary embolization. (From McIntyre, K. M., and Sasahara, A. A.: Hemodynamic response to pulmonary embolism in patients free of prior cardiopulmonary disease. Am. J. Cardiol. *28*:228, 1971.)

pulmonary vasculature with emboli was associated with significant symptomatology, mean pulmonary artery pressures in excess of 30 mm Hg, and an elevation of total pulmonary resistance.[117] Consequently, since the full, acute syndrome occurs when much less than half of the vascular bed is occluded, *mechanical obstruction alone does not completely define the circulatory effects of embolization.*[117,118,120–124] Further, the mechanical theory does not readily explain the abnormalities that also occur in lung mechanics and gas exchange. Therefore, reflex neural and humoral factors must also be considered as participating in the genesis of the clinical picture.

Powerful evidence for humoral activity is derived from the work of Halmagyi et al.[125] In cross circulation experiments in sheep, these investigators demonstrated that pulmonary embolism induced in the donor simultaneously produced a rise in pulmonary artery pressure and a fall in lung compliance in both the donor and the recipient. The transmitted effects could be reversed in the recipient by interrupting the cross circulation and inflating the lung.

The injection of barium sulfate into the pulmonary circulation, in addition to increasing pulmonary vascular resistance,[126] constricts alveolar ducts and terminal bronchi with resultant marked decreases in pulmonary compliance.[127] These physiological effects are indistinguishable from those observed following pulmonary arterial infusions of collagen[128] or thrombin,[128] and it appears that the common denominator underlying these diverse agents is platelet aggregation with release of their potent vaso- and bronchoactive contents.[126,128–131] These observations have direct bearing on the pathogenesis of macroembolization.

Even though the precise pathophysiological sequence has not been worked out, morphological and pharmacological evidence suggests that in vivo autologous thromboemboli contain traces of thrombin and its precursors that cause aggregation of platelets on the embolus and release of their contents.[132] Emboli recovered from the lungs of dogs have been shown to have a coating of fibrin, leukocytes, and degranulated platelets that were not present at their site of formation in the limbs.[133] If platelet adhesion is prevented by platelet aging or washing the clot or by pretreatment with indomethacin,[131] or if thrombin formation is blocked by heparin,[132,134] the cardiopulmonary consequences of emboli are aborted. Similar findings occur if the products released from platelets are counteracted by administration of specific antagonists[129,134,135] or if emboli are produced in thrombocytopenic animals.[132] Thus, it appears that humoral agents released from platelets, such as histamine, serotonin, and the prostaglandins, pass into the pulmonary circulation after impaction of emboli and may be responsible for contraction of vascular and bronchial smooth muscle.

In addition to constriction of alveolar ducts and respiratory bronchioles, bronchoconstriction also occurs in airways up to 3 mm in diameter following embolization.[136] Since the terminal bronchioles and alveolar ducts are the only airways believed to be perfused by the pulmonary circulation,[137] constriction of these larger airways must be accomplished in some other way. It is possible that after release, the agents may diffuse locally, producing concentration gradients along the airway walls or in adjacent tissues. Alternatively, recirculation via the bronchial circulation could constrict airways. It is important to recognize, however, that local amplification of the biochemical response is also possible. For example, plasmin activated via the fibrinolytic pathway can initiate enzymatic reactions that can generate anaphylatoxins, which in turn can cause tissue mast cells to release their potent vasoactive and bronchoconstricting chemicals. This reaction would be expected to be intense but relatively short-lived, since the inhibitors of these compounds are also present or can be generated locally—a circumstance that also fits with the time course of the clinical sequelae of emboli.

It is apparent that the ingredients for severe, regional, and systemic effects are present. Bronchoconstriction and closure of distal lung units in embolized and nonembolized areas can produce wheezing and dyspnea as well as local ventilation-perfusion imbalances that can explain the *arterial hypoxemia* so commonly encountered in pulmonary embolism. *Hyperpnea* and *tachypnea* can also occur from summation of the stimuli of anxiety, systemic hypotension, reflex stimulation of lung afferents, and arterial hypoxemia if severe enough. The resulting hyperventilation gives rise to hypocapnia, which can aggravate airway smooth muscle contraction. All the effects need not be purely local, for at least one biological amine that figures prominently in the reaction (histamine) has been demonstrated to be a potent stimulant of vagal afferent discharges,[138] and it is likely that other agents released or generated may also activate vagal reflexes.[131]

HEMODYNAMIC RESPONSES. Because patients with pulmonary emboli are often so acutely ill, relatively few data on the human dynamics of this condition were available until recently. However, with publication of results of the second phase of the Urokinase–Pulmonary Embolism Trial,[124] it became possible to piece these voluminous data together with previous studies of smaller numbers of patients[117,118,123,139,140] to gain both general and specific insights.

In this national cooperative study,[124] complete hemodynamic measurements were obtained prior to treatment in 143 patients with angiographically proved thromboemboli. The most common abnormalities noted were arterial hypoxemia and right ventricular systolic pressures greater than 25 mm Hg. In decreasing order of frequency were elevations in total pulmonary resistance (>200 dynes-sec-cm^{-5}), right ventricular end-diastolic pressure (>6 mm Hg), mean pulmonary artery pressure (>20 mm Hg), and mean right atrial pressure (>6 mm Hg). Decreases in cardiac index (<2.7 liter/min/meter^2) paralleled the changes in mean right atrial pressure. Comparisons of the extent of the embolism with the hemodynamic response indicate that those patients with massive embolism (defined as obstruction of two or more lobar arteries) had more marked abnormalities (Fig. 46–9). In patients with massive obstruction, mean right atrial, right ventricular systolic and end-diastolic, and mean pulmonary artery pressures were all higher and cardiac index and arterial oxygen tensions were lower than in patients with submassive obstruction. However, despite the statistical significance of these findings, considerable overlap was seen in the values for individuals in the submassive and massive groups as well as in the normal range. In addition, this type of analysis did not take into consideration the state of cardiopulmonary function before the insult.

When the latter is taken into account, the most fre-

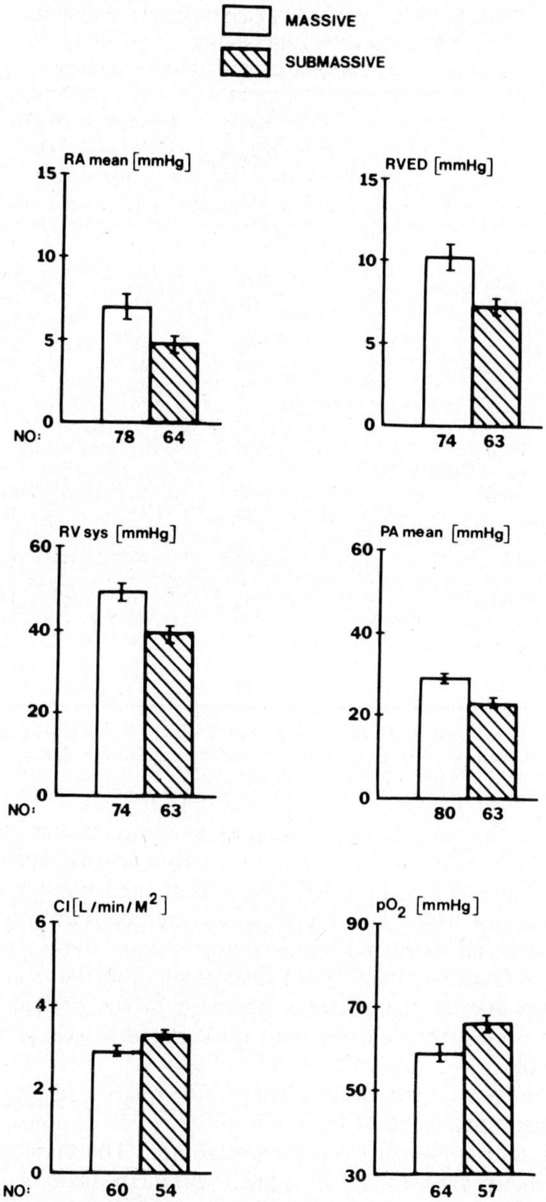

FIGURE 46–9 Cardiac hemodynamics following massive and submassive pulmonary emboli. The heights of the bars represent mean values, and the brackets are standard errors of the mean. The numbers below each graph indicate the size of the population studied. RA mean = right atrial mean pressure; RVED = right ventricular end-diastolic pressure; RV sys = right ventricular systolic pressure; PA mean = mean pulmonary artery pressure; CI = cardiac index; pO_2 = arterial oxygen tension. (Redrawn from National Cooperative Study: The urokinase pulmonary embolism trial. Circulation *47* (Suppl. II):1, 1973, by permission of the American Heart Association, Inc.)

quently observed postembolic abnormality in patients free of prior cardiac or pulmonary disease is *arterial hypoxemia.*[117,124,141] This usually occurs as the only manifestation of embolism when 25 per cent or less of the vasculature is obstructed.[117] Consequently, in the absence of other diseases that can produce hypoxemia, this finding is of great clinical value.[141]

A normal PaO_2 does not exclude the diagnosis.[87,124] In the urokinase trial, approximately 12 per cent of the patients had a PaO_2 of 80 mm Hg or more.[124] Use of the alveolar-arterial gradient for oxygen (A-aDO_2) is much more discriminatory, and, although no formal studies exist, it will probably always be abnormal in patients with significant pulmonary embolization. For example, if the PaO_2 were 85 mm Hg and the $PaCO_2$ were 30 mm Hg, with the patient breathing room air at sea level, the A-aDO_2 would be abnormally elevated to at least 28 mm Hg. This value can be calculated from an abbreviated version of the alveolar air equation:

$$PAO_2 = PIO_2 - \frac{PaCO_2}{RQ}$$

where PAO_2 = alveolar O_2 tension
PIO_2 = inspired O_2 tension (fractional concentration multiplied by the barometric pressure minus water vapor)
$PaCO_2$ = arterial CO_2 tension
RQ = respiratory quotient

In this case, PIO_2 is equal to 0.21 × (760 − 47), or 150 mm Hg. Since in practice RQ is tedious to measure, for clinical purposes one can assume a steady-state value of 0.8. This would be the lower limit if the patient were not retaining CO_2, because unsteady-state conditions other than this would tend to produce values of 1 or more and so further reduce the $PaCO_2$/RQ ratio. Thus,

$$PAO_2 = 150 - \frac{30}{0.8}$$

$$\begin{aligned} A\text{-}aDO_2 &= PAO_2 - PaO_2 \\ &= 113 - 85 \\ &= 28 \end{aligned}$$

If RQ were 1, then A-aDO_2 would be even more abnormal, i.e., 35 mm Hg. Thus, even though the absolute arterial oxygen tension is normal, gas exchange can still be abnormal.

The next most frequent derangement is *pulmonary hypertension.* It has been observed in approximately 70 per cent of the patients in several series[117,120,123,139] and can be expected to occur after 25 to 35 per cent of the vasculature has been obstructed in a previously normal vascular bed. A mean pulmonary artery pressure exceeding 40 mm Hg, even in the face of massive obstruction, seems to be the maximum pressureload that a previously normal right ventricle can generate.[117,123,139] Thus, pressures at such levels suggest massive obstruction, chronic recurrent embolization, or other causes of prior pulmonary artery hypertension.[117,118]

Elevation in right atrial mean pressure can be expected in approximately 50 per cent of cases, and it bears a direct relationship to the degree of pulmonary hypertension. In one study, right atrial mean pressure was always elevated whenever mean pulmonary artery pressure exceeded 30 mm Hg.[117] Thus, neck vein distention following a pulmonary embolus in a person without previous pulmonary hypertension signifies massive embolization.

In the absence of cardiac failure, the cardiac index is typically elevated in response to pulmonary emboli.[117,124,139] When depression of output occurs, it is virtually always in association with massive obstruction. It has been suggested that one of the mechanisms for cardiac depression is the mechanical compromise of right coronary artery blood flow.[23] However, this seems unlikely as there is now abundant evidence that perfusion of both coronary beds reflexly increases following pulmonary embolization.[142–145]

In patients with prior heart or lung disease, or both, the consequences of pulmonary emboli are markedly different. In general, for any degree of obstruction, the hemodynamic abnormalities are significantly greater than in previously normal individuals who suffer an embolus.[118] Mean pulmonary artery pressures of 40 mm Hg or more are common in this group, and elevations in right atrial pressures and depressions of cardiac index are the rule rather than the exception.[118,124] These patients are also more likely to develop acute left ventricular or global heart failure;[146] massive obstruction with survival is extremely uncommon.

Clinical Manifestations

SIGNS AND SYMPTOMS. The largest antemortem collection of the presenting signs and symptoms of patients with confirmed pulmonary emboli is summarized in Tables 46–1 and 46–2.[121,122] These 327 patients had been included in either the Urokinase–Pulmonary Embolism Trial[124] or the Urokinase-Streptokinase Embolism Trial,[121] and of them, 215 were free of preexisting cardiac or pulmonary disease prior to embolization[122] (Table 46–2). These data support the general clinical impression that no single symptom or combination of symptoms is diagnostic of pulmonary embolism.[89,118,147] Chest pain and dyspnea, found in over 85 per cent of the patients, were the most frequent symptoms. (In three-fourths of the group, the pain was pleuritic in nature.) Apprehension and cough were seen in 50 to 60 per cent of the patients. Hemoptysis, diaphoresis, and syncope were present in only a minority. When the extent of the embolization was examined in relation to symptoms, apprehension and syncope occurred with signficantly greater frequency in those with massive emboli, whereas pleuritic chest pain and hemoptysis were more common in patients with less extensive involvement. Quite similar patterns were noted in those without antecedent cardiopulmonary disease (Table 46–2). Dyspnea and cough tended to be prodromal, often noted by the patient as early as 5 or more days before the diagnosis was established. Chest pain tended to develop 3 to 4 days before definitive work-up, and the symptoms of apprehension, diaphoresis, and syncope were acute, usually occurring within 36 hours or less of presentation.

Tachypnea was the most common sign. Rales, an increased pulmonic component of the second heart sound, tachycardia, and fever were the next most frequent physical findings. Gallop rhythms, diaphoresis, and phlebitis

TABLE 46–1 INCIDENCE OF SYMPTOMS AND SIGNS IN 327 PATIENTS WITH THROMBOEMBOLISM

	Total Series n = 327 (%)	Massive Emboli n = 197 (%)	Submassive Emboli n = 130 (%)
Symptoms			
Chest pain	88	85	82
Dyspnea	84	85	82
Apprehension	59	65	50
Cough	53	53	52
Hemoptysis	30	23	40
Diaphoresis	27	29	23
Syncope	13	20	4
Signs			
Tachypnea (resp. > 16/min)	92	95	87
Rales	58	57	60
Increased pulmonic 2nd sound	53	58	45
Tachycardia (pulse > 100/min)	44	48	38
Fever (temp. > 37.8°C)	43	43	42
Gallop	34	39	25
Diaphoresis	36	42	27
Phlebitis	32	36	26
Edema	24	23	25
Murmur	23	27	16
Cyanosis	19	25	9

From Bell, W. R., et al.: The clinical features of submassive and massive pulmonary emboli. Am. J. Med. *62*:355, 1977.

TABLE 46–2 INCIDENCE OF SYMPTOMS AND SIGNS IN 214 PATIENTS WITH THROMBOEMBOLISM WITHOUT PREEXISTING CARDIAC OR PULMONARY DISEASE

	Total Series n = 214 (%)	Massive Emboli n = 145 (%)	Submassive Emboli n = 69 (%)
Symptoms			
Chest pain	74	67	85
Dyspnea	84	86	78
Apprehension	63	70	50
Cough	50	48	55
Hemoptysis	28	23	35
Diaphoresis	36	44	20
Syncope	13	17	4
Signs			
Tachypnea (resp. > 20/min)	85	87	81
Rales	56	55	56
Increased pulmonic 2nd sound	57	62	47
Tachycardia (pulse > 100/min)	58	66	42
Fever (temp. > 37.8°C)	50	50	51
Diaphoresis	36	44	20
Phlebitis	41	39	47
Cyanosis	18	24	3

From Stein, P. D., et al.: History and physical examination in acute pulmonary embolism in patients without preexisting cardiac or pulmonary disease. Am. J. Cardiol. *47*:218, 1981.

were each found in approximately one-third of the population, whereas edema, murmurs, and cyanosis were each noted in one-fourth or less. An accentuated pulmonic second sound, third and fourth heart sounds, murmurs, and cyanosis all occurred more frequently in those patients who had suffered massive rather than submassive embolization. Again, the patterns observed in the patients who were previously well mirrored those noted in this group as a whole.

The "classic triads" of hemoptysis, cough, and diaphoresis; hemoptysis, chest pain, and dyspnea; or dyspnea, chest pain, and apprehension were uncommon. The same lack of specificity was found in signs. Although tachypnea occurred in over 90 per cent of the population, its presence or absence, as that of hypoxemia, does not establish or eliminate the diagnosis. The combination of elevated heart rate, respiration, and temperature (Allen's sign) was present in only 23 per cent of patients. In the patients without preexisting heart or lung disease, the presenting symptoms were (1) pleuritic pain without hemoptysis (41 per cent); (2) pulmonary infarction with hemoptysis (25 per cent); (3) uncomplicated embolism with only dyspnea (10 per cent); and (4) circulatory collapse with shock (10 per cent) and syncope (9 per cent). Three per cent had nonpleuritic chest pain with dyspnea, and 0.5 per cent showed deep venous thrombosis with tachypnea. Thus, regardless of their varying degree of sensitivity, the symptoms and signs of pulmonary embolism are quite nonspecific.

With usual medical treatment, the clinical parameters clear progressively. Within a week after heparin therapy was initiated in the National Cooperative Trial,[124] the complaints of dyspnea, chest pain, and apprehension had cleared in 78, 74, and 85 per cent of the patients, respectively. However, cough resolved more slowly: 2 weeks after embolization, 48 per cent of the patients still had this complaint. Generally, the signs cleared more slowly than did the symptoms. Although diaphoresis disappeared in 83 per cent of the patients within 1 week, 62 and 63 per cent still had rales and an accentuated pulmonic component of the second heart sound, respectively.

In addition to the usual symptom complex associated with embolization, variant clinical expressions also occur. Thus, Israel and Goldstein[89] and Potts and Sahn[148] have described a total of 14 patients in whom abdominal pain was the predominant symptom. In 8 of the patients, these complaints were so severe that the correct diagnosis was delayed while attention was diverted to what appeared to be acute surgical abdomens. Another infrequent but perplexing manifestation is acute bronchospasm. Although many patients with recent emboli characteristically develop airway obstruction,[149] this is usually detectable only by appropriate pulmonary function tests. Occasionally, however, this airflow obstruction is so severe that acute wheezing develops, and the patient initially is thought to have bronchial asthma.[150–152] Pulmonary embolism may also masquerade as coronary insufficiency.[153]

ELECTROCARDIOGRAM (see also p. 212). Like the signs and symptoms of acute pulmonary embolization, the electrocardiographic alterations are highly variable and in the majority of instances are nondiagnostic[124,141,154–156] (Chap. 7). The types of changes observed in a large series of patients and their frequency distribution are summarized in Table 46–3.[124] In this study the pretreatment electrocardiograms were entirely normal in only 13 per cent of patients. Rhythm disturbances were present in 11 per cent, with premature ventricular beats the most common. Conduction disturbances were found in 65 per cent of the patients, ST-T changes in 64 per cent, and T-wave inversion in 40 per cent. The electrocardiographic manifestations of acute cor pulmonale ($S_1Q_3T_3$, complete or incomplete right bundle branch block, P-pulmonale, or right axis deviation) were uncommon. Patients with prior cardiopulmonary disease had a greater frequency of arrhythmias, conduction disturbances, and QRS changes, whereas patients with massive emboli had more QRS, ST-T segment, and T-wave changes. These findings are in general agreement with those of other investigations[141,154] and indicate that the electrocardiogram is not specific in pulmonary embolus and not particularly helpful in establishing the diagnosis. Moreover, it is insensitive to the rate of resolution of the emboli.

Even though the results of the studies described above are disappointing from a diagnostic standpoint, some data suggest that the hemodynamic variables are altered in a characteristic fashion (Figs. 7–16, p. 213, and 46–10) when the electrocardiogram is conclusive for, or suggestive of, acute right-heart strain in patients without cardiopulmonary disease prior to embolization. Such electrocardiograms were observed only when the mean pressures in the pulmonary artery and right atria exceeded 30 and 8 mm Hg, respectively; the total pulmonary resistance was greater than 500 dynes-sec-cm^{-5}; cardiac index was depressed; and the degree of pulmonary vascular obstruction exceeded 40 per cent.[154] Thus in the patients whose electrocardiograms were diagnostic of, or consistent with, right-heart strain, the clinical picture indicated that a cardiopulmonary catastrophe had occurred. Consequently, although the electrocardiogram can be of little value in arousing the clinical suspicion of pulmonary embolism per se, it may be useful in distinguishing between the two most frequent cardiopul-

TABLE 46–3 ELECTROCARDIOGRAPHIC ABNORMALITIES IN 131 PATIENTS WITH PULMONARY EMBOLISM

	PER CENT OF PATIENTS
Rhythm Disturbances	
Premature beats	11
Atrial	3
Ventricular	9
Atrial fibrillation	3
QRS Abnormalities	65
Right axis	5
Left axis	12
Incomplete right bundle branch block	5
Complete right bundle branch block	11
Right ventricular hypertrophy	5
$S_1 S_2 S_3$ pattern	9
$S_1 Q_3 T_3$ pattern	11
ST-T Abnormalities	64
T-wave inversion	40
ST-T segment depression	33
ST-T segment elevation	11

From National Cooperative Study: Urokinase–Pulmonary Embolism Trial. Circulation *47* (Suppl. II): 1, 1973, by permission of the American Heart Association, Inc.

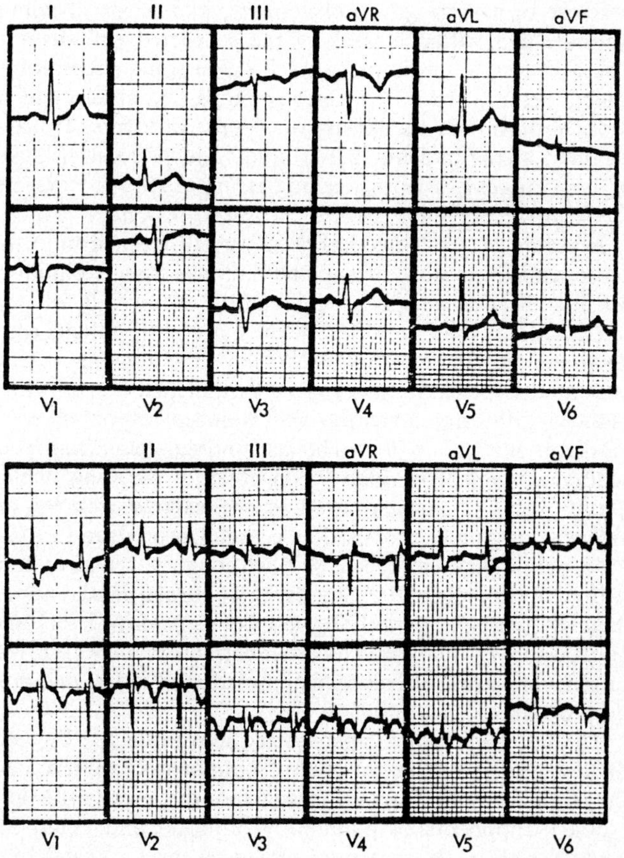

FIGURE 46–10 Normal (*top*) and postembolic (*bottom*) electrocardiograms in a 26-year-old patient who underwent arthrotomy of the knee. The bottom tracing shows the diagnostic features of acute right ventricular strain. Changes include acute development of a prominent S1, Q3 pattern with incomplete right bundle branch block, tachycardia (150 beats/min), and an axis shift from 0 to +30 degrees. (From McIntyre, K. M., et al.: Relation of the electrocardiogram to hemodynamic alterations in pulmonary embolism. Am. J. Cardiol. *30*:205, 1972.)

monary catastrophes: acute myocardial infarction and acute massive pulmonary embolism.

ABNORMALITIES IN RESPIRATORY FUNCTION. As described earlier in this chapter, acute pulmonary embolization in experimental animals has been shown to affect airways as well as blood vessels in both embolized and nonembolized areas. Consequently, both the mechanical and the gas-exchanging properties of the lungs are disturbed. Functionally, this produces tachypnea, hypoxemia, increased arterial-alveolar differences for oxygen and carbon dioxide, elevated physiological dead space, diminished lung compliance, increased airway resistance, and a fall in lung volume.[125–127,131,134,157–161] Many of these alterations in lung function result from closure of dependent airways and constriction of small bronchi, respiratory bronchioles, and alveolar ducts. The net effect is a disruption of normal ventilation-perfusion relationships so that gas exchange is impaired.

In humans, the acute effects of embolization per se are considerably less clear because the interpretation of the various functional abnormalities that have been described is limited by such factors as time of study and patient selection. For example, very few studies of mechanical lung function have been performed close in time to an embolic episode. Sasahara and colleagues reported reductions in vital capacity and forced expiratory volumes in 80 per cent or more of a large group of patients, two-thirds of whom were studied within a week of the suspected embolism.[149] These abnormalities improved acutely in some patients following heparin treatment, thereby suggesting an element of bronchospasm via the release of platelet products. However, most of the patients in this study had preexisting heart or lung disease or both, making it impossible to sort out the relative contributions of each disease process.

Alveolar gas exchange has been studied frequently in the acute embolic period, presumably because these techniques do not require extensive manipulation of severely ill persons, and the data are often directly useful in patient care. As in animal studies, a number of investigations have demonstrated hypoxemia, tachypnea, mismatched $\dot{V}_A/\dot{Q}$ ratios, reduced diffusing capacities, and widened arterial-alveolar gradients for CO_2.[149,162–168] The last finding stems from ventilation coming from high $\dot{V}_A/\dot{Q}$ areas of the lung, which dilutes the CO_2 concentration in the expired alveolar air and was originally proposed as a useful procedure to diagnose pulmonary embolism.[163,164] Although a sensitive test, it is time-dependent (i.e., apt to be abnormal in the immediate postembolic period and not hours or days later) and nonspecific in that any focal abnormality in $\dot{V}_A/\dot{Q}$ will produce it. Hence it has been superseded by other diagnostic procedures.

The fall in diffusing capacity has been explained by a reduction in the functional area of pulmonary capillaries by the embolization. Daum investigated the membrane and blood components of pulmonary diffusion and could account for all of the measured resistance to O_2 transfer by a reduction in capillary blood volume.[167] Thus, this is not an impairment of diffusion in the sense of an "alveolar capillary" block.

The chief mechanism at work in producing hypoxemia appears to be widespread regional inequalities in $\dot{V}_A/\dot{Q}$ ratios of various magnitudes that are scattered throughout the lungs. Wilson and coworkers have suggested that the immediate cause of hypoxemia in patients with no previous heart or lung disease is related to venous admixture but that the persistence of hypoxemia beyond the acute phase resulted from right-to-left shunting secondary to atelectasis.[168] The reason why the latter should develop is unknown, but some data indicate that surfactant formation (and hence alveolar stability) is reduced by temporarily interrupting pulmonary arterial supply to an area of the lung.[169]

The long-term effects of emboli on lung function in patients who were previously normal are frequently quite subtle at rest and consist of mild reductions in vital capacity, arterial oxygen tension, and diffusing capacities.[170] With exercise, wasted ("dead space") ventilation often increases abnormally or fails to fall if elevated initially, and hypoxemia worsens.[171,172] Because of these findings and the often vague clinical complaints associated with small embolic episodes, performance of detailed studies of gas exchange, both at rest and during physical exertion, in patients suspected of having occlusive pulmonary vascular disease can be quite rewarding in suggesting the diagnosis.

RADIOGRAPHIC ABNORMALITIES (see also Chap. 6). Before considering the roentgenographic manifestations of pulmonary thromboembolism, it must be noted that the majority of episodes confirmed by angiography show no abnormalities on plain chest radiographs.[173,174] When changes are present, however, they may be distinctive and can strongly suggest the diagnosis. The four manifestations of embolization *without infarction* are oligemia, change in vessel size, alterations in size and configuration of the heart, and loss of lung volume.

Loss of lung volume, as manifested, for example, by an elevated diaphragm, is the most common radiographic sign of pulmonary embolism. It has been observed in as many as 41 per cent of the patients in one large series.[124] In contrast, local pulmonary oligemia occurs infrequently and only with occlusion of large vessels. Although this finding has been confirmed as a valid sign of embolization,[175,176] it is seldom of sufficient degree to be convincing.[174,177] Oligemia is more often detected when a whole lung, or a major part of it, is deprived of its pulmonary arterial circulation (Fig. 46–11). In these circumstances, the unilateral oligemia contrasts markedly with the pleonemia of the other lung.[178] Generalized pulmonary oligemia is almost invariably the result of widespread obstruction of smaller pulmonary arteries from recurrent embolization. This finding is nearly always associated with the signs of pulmonary hypertension (see below). Enlargement of a major hilar artery is an important radiographic sign.[177,179–181] This is particularly valuable diagnostically when serial roentgenograms reveal progressive enlargement of the affected vessel[179] (Fig. 46–11). Equally important to the increase in size is the abrupt tapering of an occluded vessel (knuckle sign).[176] These alterations were found in 23 per cent of the patients in the National Cooperative Urokinase Trial, whereas focal oligemia was recorded in only 15 per cent.[124]

The postembolic cardiac changes consist of cardiac enlargement due to dilatation of the right ventricle, increase in size of the main pulmonary artery, and increase in the size and rapidity of tapering of the hilar vessels.[179] Dilatation of the azygous vein and of the superior vena cava, reflecting right-sided heart failure, may also be found. Cardiac changes are the least common roentgenographic

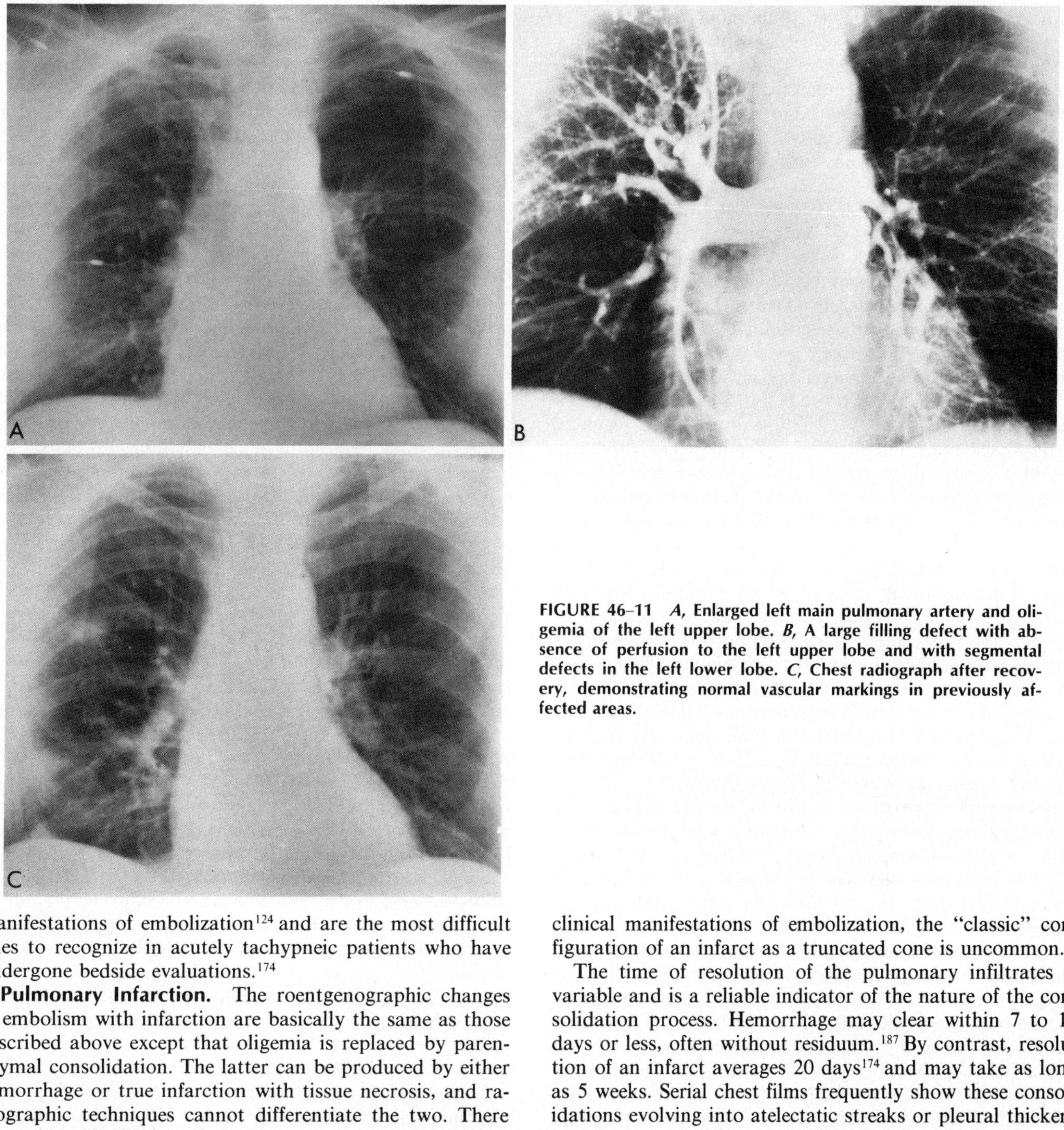

FIGURE 46–11 *A*, Enlarged left main pulmonary artery and oligemia of the left upper lobe. *B*, A large filling defect with absence of perfusion to the left upper lobe and with segmental defects in the left lower lobe. *C*, Chest radiograph after recovery, demonstrating normal vascular markings in previously affected areas.

manifestations of embolization[124] and are the most difficult ones to recognize in acutely tachypneic patients who have undergone bedside evaluations.[174]

Pulmonary Infarction. The roentgenographic changes in embolism with infarction are basically the same as those described above except that oligemia is replaced by parenchymal consolidation. The latter can be produced by either hemorrhage or true infarction with tissue necrosis, and radiographic techniques cannot differentiate the two. There is considerable difference of opinion about what percentage of emboli results in infarction of lung parenchyma, but postmortem findings indicate that as few as 10 to 15 per cent do so.[86,182] Infarction tends to occur in situations in which either the pulmonary venous drainage or the bronchial circulation has been compromised by a preexisting disease process, particularly congestive failure, malignancy, or chronic lung disease.[183–185] The reasons for this are not entirely clear, but it appears that after an embolus the viability of the pulmonary tissue is determined at least in part by the integrity of the bronchial circulation, the magnitude of the obstruction, and the site of the embolization.

The time interval between an embolic episode and the development of a radiographic density varies greatly. A pulmonary infiltrate may occur within 10 to 12 hours[175] or as late as a week after the occlusion.[175,186] As with the other clinical manifestations of embolization, the "classic" configuration of an infarct as a truncated cone is uncommon.

The time of resolution of the pulmonary infiltrates is variable and is a reliable indicator of the nature of the consolidation process. Hemorrhage may clear within 7 to 10 days or less, often without residuum.[187] By contrast, resolution of an infarct averages 20 days[174] and may take as long as 5 weeks. Serial chest films frequently show these consolidations evolving into atelectatic streaks or pleural thickening. Rarely, an infarcted area undergoes liquefaction and cavitation.[188–192] This can occur in the absence of sepsis or pulmonary infection and in extremely rare instances can result in the development of a bronchopleural fistula.[192] Pleural effusion is as common as parenchymal consolidation as a roentgenographic manifestation of thromboembolic disease, and usually indicates that infarction has occurred.[193] The amount of fluid varies. It is frequently small but on occasion may be abundant. It usually develops and absorbs synchronously with the infarction, though it may appear later and clear sooner.[174]

Diagnosis

As already indicated, the bedside diagnosis of pulmonary thromboembolism is unreliable because the clinical features of the disorder are varied and nonspecific. Szucs et al. assessed the sensitivity of certain laboratory tests in a prospective study of patients with angiographically documented acute pulmonary embolism.[141] Electrocardiographic evidence of right-heart strain occurred in 18 per cent; each had massive pulmonary embolism. Nonspecific chest roentgenographic abnormalities (infiltrates, effusion, or elevated diaphragm) occurred in 71 per cent. Lactic dehydrogenase was increased in 83 per cent of the patients, but serum glutamic oxaloacetic transaminase and bilirubin determinations were of little value. Arterial oxygen tensions, measured while the patient breathed room air, were decreased (≤ 80 mm Hg) in all patients. Thus, although diagnostic strategies of various accuracy have been proposed,[110,194] the most definitive procedures available are photoscanning and selective pulmonary angiography.

VENTILATION-PERFUSION SCINTIGRAPHY (also see pp. 388 to 392). The use of perfusion scanning in the assessment and diagnosis of pulmonary embolism was first described by Wagner and associates in 1964 and allows for determinations of the distribution of pulmonary blood flow in vessels as small as 50 μm.[195] Consequently, this procedure is very sensitive, but it lacks specificity. Although a normal scan provides convincing evidence for the absence of pulmonary emboli,[147,196] an abnormal scan can be ambiguous diagnostically because it can be produced by any condition that alters regional blood flow.[197] This is exemplified by a recent report of scan abnormalities in 88 per cent of 59 patients *without* angiographic demonstration of embolism.[198] The converse is even more disturbing. Bell and Simon observed 18 patients who were reported by scan to have a low probability of emboli, yet 10 had massive and 7 submassive emboli on angiography.[199]

Because of observations like these, various indices have been proposed to improve the scintigraphic definition of pulmonary embolism. The most common are (1) the size and distribution of perfusion abnormalities,[196,198] (2) the relationship between regional perfusion and ventilation,[199,200] (3) comparison of perfusion patterns after variable time intervals,[201,202] and (4) correlation with the conventional chest film.[197,198] Analysis of the relative value of the first three factors in patients with angiographically proved emboli indicates that a large perfusion defect and a $\dot{V}_A/\dot{Q}$ mismatch correlate strongly with pulmonary embolism.

McNeil et al.[192] and others[196,198] have found that lung or lobar defects on scan are likely to be the result of vascular obstruction. This is the so-called high-probability scan.[198] In this study, 80 per cent of lobar defects were associated with emboli, whereas segmental or subsegmental defects alone showed only a 30 per cent association. Thus, perfusion patterns per se are only fair discriminants. The addition of a ventilation scan (also discussed in Chapter 11) to look for $\dot{V}_A/\dot{Q}$ mismatches in the nonperfused area considerably strengthens the diagnostic capabilities.[197,198,200] In patients with multiple segmental and lobar perfusion defects and normal ventilation, the possibility of pulmonary embolism being shown by angiography is said to exceed 90 per cent.[203,204] A matched loss of perfusion and ventilation is not usually observed with embolization; thus, when found, it suggests other pathological processes such as chronic lung disease or heart failure. However, atelectasis, which may occur in embolization, with or without infarction, is associated with both abnormal ventilation and perfusion. In addition, it is doubtful whether a ventilation scan can exclude the diagnosis of pulmonary embolism in patients with obstructive airway disease or extensive parenchymal disease, since these diseases reduce the likelihood of finding a defect on a perfusion scan without an associated abnormality on the ventilation scan.

Sequential examinations reveal that scanning is most useful early in the disease. In the absence of recurrent emboli, the reliability of the scan diminishes rapidly as perfusion improves, finally returning to normal or to a pattern of diagnostic uncertainty.[139,197,201,202,205] Thus in the absence of other, quickly reversible, pathological conditions (asthma, pneumonia, congestive heart failure), a changing perfusion pattern suggests the presence of pulmonary embolus. Conversely, a fixed pattern is unlikely to represent embolic sequelae. A word of caution, however, in interpreting sequential scans is in order. Several observers[206,207] have described the appearance and disappearance of perfusion shifts in serial lung scans in angiographically patent vessels. Investigations failed to reveal new embolization, and it was concluded that the resolution of thromboemboli caused physiological redistribution of perfusion secondary to changes in relative impedance to flow in different areas of the lung.

A fourth way of increasing the specificity of the perfusion scan is to utilize the chest roentgenogram. The predictability of pulmonary embolism in high probability scans may be increased further if the chest film shows at least one of the following features of pulmonary embolism: infiltrate, pleural effusion, atelectasis, and elevated hemidiaphragm. If two features are present, the predictive value approaches 100 per cent.[197,198]

PULMONARY ANGIOGRAPHY. Selective pulmonary arteriography (the injection of contrast material into pulmonary artery branches which supply a segment or lobe) is considered to be the most specific test available for the detection of pulmonary embolism.[124,198,205,208,209] The absolute accuracy of pulmonary arteriography is difficult to assess, since small emboli may undergo rapid lysis[205] and an immediate postmortem examination is a rare event in humans. Unlike scanning procedures, which are maximally useful in detecting small emboli, angiography is seldom of value when the obstructed vessels are 2 mm or less in diameter.[177,205]

The most dependable roentgenographic signs are actual cut-offs (Fig. 46–11) or filling defects in the larger arteries or segmental vessels (Fig. 46–12).[176,177,198,208] Other findings that may suggest the diagnosis include local segmental hypovascularity; absent, diminished, or delayed arterial and venous flow; tortuous sequential vessels; alteration in the caliber of arteries proximal or distal to an embolus; and loss of volume of the affected lung segments.[176,177,198,208]

In their study of the criteria of the angiographic diagnosis of acute pulmonary embolism, Stein and colleagues emphasized the importance of evaluating the presence of other disease that might affect the pulmonary vasculature and thereby alter the angiographic pattern.[210] These observers noted that filling defects, vessel cut-offs, and pruning of the peripheral vessels occur only in pulmonary embolism. However, if oligemia and asymmetry of blood flow are used as the criteria, the possibility of false-positive diagnosis exists in that these abnormalities can be found in association with chronic lung disease or congestive heart

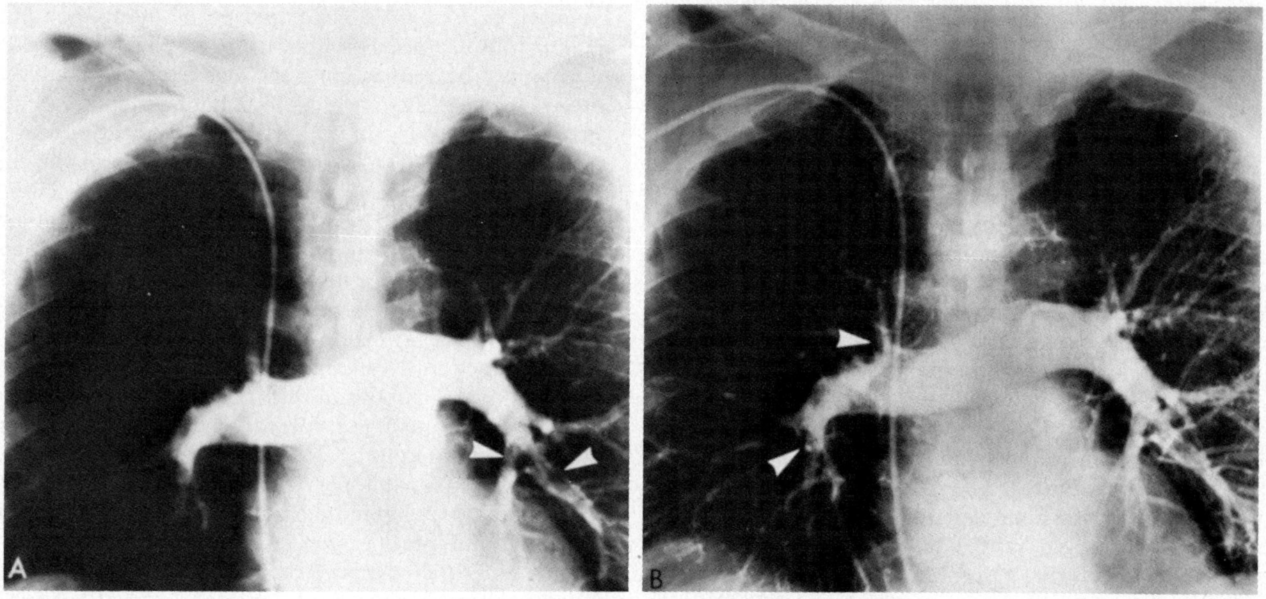

FIGURE 46–12 Multiple bilateral filling defects (arrows).

failure in the absence of intrinsic vascular occlusion.

Pulmonary arteriography in experienced hands is a relatively safe procedure. In five separate series involving almost 2600 patients, only six deaths related to pulmonary arteriography occurred; all of these occurred in patients with severe underlying embolic disease or pulmonary hypertension.[124,198,204,208,211] Nonfatal complications have been reported in approximately 4 per cent of patients.[208,211] Half of these related to the catheterization (cardiac perforation and arrhythmia) and the other half related to the contrast material (bronchospasm and anaphylaxis).

LABORATORY DIAGNOSIS. The triad of increased LDH, normal SGOT, and increased bilirubin has been reputed to be indicative of pulmonary embolism and infarction and useful in differentiation from myocardial infarction or pneumonia.[212] Subsequent investigation has not confirmed the original enthusiasm for its value, and several studies have found enzyme levels to be of little if any value in diagnosis.[124,141,213] As with other diagnostic procedures, variations in reported results may reflect different time intervals between the embolic episode and performance of the test, and different patient populations. Recently, interest has been generated in measurements of fibrin split products in patients with suspected embolism.[214] The data available thus far suggest that this test is sensitive, but its specificity needs further assessment.

Treatment (See Table 46–4)

The management of pulmonary embolism is determined importantly by the degree to which the circulation has been compromised.[215] Since most emboli resolve in time, the goals of treatment with the available agents are simple and twofold: to sustain life and to prevent recurrence. The studies of Barritt and Jordan[216] and others[217] have clearly

TABLE 46–4 TREATMENT REGIMENS IN PULMONARY EMBOLISM (PE)

1. Submassive PE	*2. Massive PE*	*3. Anticoagulants Contraindicated*
a. Heparin 70 μ/kg IV simultaneously with infusion of 20–25 μ/kg/hr IV regulated to keep APTT between 60–80 sec or Lee-White CT between 20–40 min for 7–10 days or b. Heparin, 55–70 μ/kg every 4 hr IV 7–10 days	a. Heparin 10,000 units IV simultaneously with infusion of 25 μ/kg/hr IV for 7–10 days regulated by laboratory test or b. Heparin, 7000–10,000 units every 4 hr IV for 24–48 hours followed by 55–75 μ/kg every 4 hours for 7–9 days or c. Streptokinase, 250,000 units IV for 30 minutes followed by 100,000 μ/hr for 24 hr; or urokinase, 4400 CTA μ/kg for 10 minutes followed by 4400 CTA μ/kg/hr for 12–24 hr. During thrombolytic therapy, the thrombin time should be 2–7× baseline. At completion of thrombolytic infusion when thrombin time is less than 2× baseline (3–4 hr later), start heparin therapy as in 2a or b.	Vena caval of ligation, umbrella or balloon, for life-threatening embolus; plication for other cases

Long-term therapy
a. Warfarin to keep prothrombin 8–25% activity, overlap 3–5 days with heparin and continue at least 12 weeks; further therapy guided by status of predisposing conditions

b. Heparin, 5000 units every 8–12 hr or subcutaneously for a minimum of 12 weeks

APTT = activated partial thromboplastin time; CT = clotting time. (Reproduced with permission from Bell, W. R., and Simon, T. L.: Am. Heart J. *103*:239, 1982.)

shown a significant reduction in mortality after pulmonary embolism, from approximately 25 to 5 per cent, among patients treated with anticoagulants. Therapy with heparin is adequate in most instances.[218]

In the absence of contraindications to anticoagulants, the current recommendation is 10,000 units of heparin intravenously in a single injection when pulmonary embolism is first suspected and diagnostic studies are not complete. After confirmation, heparin should be continued in amounts adequate to prevent platelet-thrombin interaction:[219,220] 5000 to 7500 units every 4 hours by intravenous administration, or, preferably, 1000 units per hour by constant infusion. Two controlled trials have shown continuous heparin therapy to be significantly safer from hemorrhagic complications,[221,222] but there is some suggestion that recurrent thromboembolism may be more prevalent with this approach.[223] The need for clotting time or partial thromboplastin time determinations to monitor the dose has been debated in the past; properly performed, these tests are helpful in reducing the incidence of hemorrhagic complications.[124] Heparin should be continued until the patient's cardiopulmonary status has stabilized and any evidence of venous thrombosis has resolved, which requires about 8 days.

Oral anticoagulants are usually instituted when the heparin is being tapered and the patient begins ambulation. No guidelines for duration of oral anticoagulation have been available, and most authorities recommend 3 to 6 months.[212] One randomized trial in which patients were treated for either 6 weeks or 6 months concluded that there was no benefit from oral anticoagulants administered for longer than 6 weeks in patients experiencing a single episode of phlebitis or pulmonary embolism or both.[224] In this study, the indications for therapy for 6 months were a past history of venous thromboembolism, a recurrent thrombotic tendency, or continuing predisposing cause. If the embolization is small and is the result of a specific predisposing factor that has subsequently resolved, anticoagulation, of course, may be discontinued sooner.

Although heparin is the cornerstone of therapy, it has the disadvantage of not being thrombolytic. The value of two thrombolytic agents, streptokinase and urokinase, has been extensively investigated. Urokinase has received most attention because it is not antigenic or pyrogenic, and its administration does not appear to require precise dosage or complex laboratory controls. The experience gained indicates that patients with acute pulmonary emboli who receive lytic therapy gain a short-lived advantage over those given heparin.[124,125] There is greater resolution of the emboli and hemodynamic improvement in the first 24 hours with thrombolytic therapy, particularly in patients with massive emboli, but this difference quickly disappears. Controlled trials have not shown any significant differences in mortality rates between the two therapeutic approaches. The available data suggest that thrombolytic therapy may prove valuable in treating patients with massive pulmonary embolism with hemodynamic compromise who were previously considered candidates for emergency pulmonary embolectomy.

Aside from pulmonary embolectomy, the surgical approaches to pulmonary embolism are also designed to prevent recurrent episodes. Accumulated experience has shown that either clipping or tying the inferior vena cava or interrupting flow with an "umbrella" directly below the renal veins is the procedure of choice (Fig. 46–13).[226-228] The patients most likely to need this therapy are those with contraindications to anticoagulants or those in whom recurrent emboli develop despite well-controlled anticoagulation.[219,227] As noted, the recognition of a recurrence during the acute phase of pulmonary embolism is a difficult clinical problem that requires angiography for confirmation; it can be hazardous to rely only on clinical findings or lung scans.[206,207] Even surgical procedures are not absolutely effective, and recurrences can occur[227,229] because sizable collateral channels develop through which embolization may recur with the passage of time and thrombi may form proximal to the site of caval manipulation.

Pulmonary embolectomy appears to be useful in very selective instances. The procedure requires cardiopulmonary bypass and carries with it a very high mortality, often exceeding 50 per cent.[230-232] Currently, indications for surgery are massive embolization with shock which fails to respond to vigorous medical therapy with isoproterenol, oxygen, and heparin.[220,233]

The most recent trend in the approach to pulmonary embolism is the prevention of its occurrence in high-risk

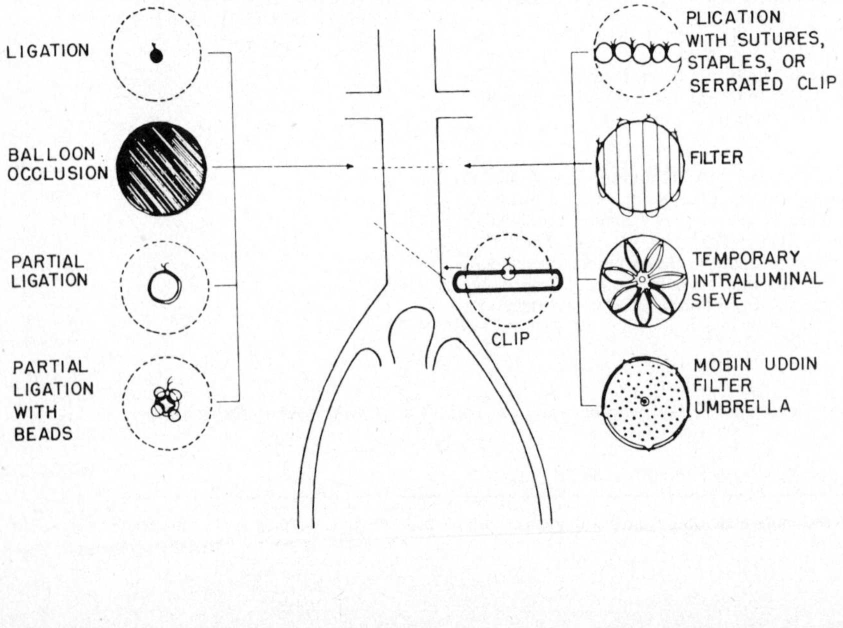

FIGURE 46–13 The various methods and devices used in the inferior vena cava to arrest emboli of lethal size. (From Gardner, A. M. N.: Inferior vena cava interruption in the prevention of fatal pulmonary embolism. Am. Heart J. *95*:679, 1978.)

groups. One of the most efficient ways of achieving this goal is to prevent the development of venous thrombosis in the lower extremities by early ambulation.[234] In those patients in whom this approach is not feasible, the classic study of Sevitt and Gallagher has clearly established the role of prophylactic anticoagulation as a useful alternative.[235] The most favored approach at present is to administer small doses of heparin (5000 units of high-potency heparin) every 12 hours to patients 40 years of age or older who are to undergo thoracoabdominal or gynecological surgery under general anesthesia. Data regarding prevention of deep venous thrombosis and pulmonary embolization in patients treated with this regimen are quite persuasive.[236,237] However, this approach does have limitations, and it has not been found to be very effective in patients with hip fracture or in those undergoing prostatic surgery.[238]

Prognosis

The natural history of pulmonary thromboembolism is not completely known. Available data indicate that considerably less than 10 per cent of all emboli are lethal in the acute phase,[88,182,239,240] and in those that are, 75 per cent of the deaths occur within 60 minutes of the onset of symptoms, with the remaining 25 per cent occurring within the next 48 hours.[241,242] Consequently, death in those who survive the acute insult long enough to be diagnosed and placed on therapy is a relatively rare event.[232,242]

Experimental studies in dogs have demonstrated that resolution of pulmonary vascular obstruction by fresh autologous blood clots begins within hours of embolism, and small emboli are lysed so rapidly that little or no evidence of their presence is detectable 5 to 13 days later, even with careful histological examination.[243] In humans, resolution appears to be slower. There is usually minimal angiographic and hemodynamic resolution of the vascular obstruction in the first 7 days following embolization, and complete clearing usually takes many weeks.[139] In one study in which serial lung scans were used, 15 per cent of patients showed complete resolution at 2 weeks, and 30 per cent required a month.[201] In the National Cooperative Urokinase Trial, lung scans had improved by only 50 per cent at 14 days, and prominent residual scan defects remained for 3 months.[124] In fact, 16 per cent of the patients had not completely cleared their defects in a year.

The factors that determine which patients will experience complete resolution and which will have persistent unresolved embolism have not been delineated. Similarly, the frequency of chronic cor pulmonale due to unresolved or recurrent embolism is not known. Paraskos and associates evaluated 50 patients with documented acute pulmonary embolism 1 to 7 years after the acute episode.[202] Their findings demonstrate that the vast majority of patients will return to their usual state of health and that unresolved embolism is an uncommon event. In this study, the most important factor influencing long-term survival was the presence of preexisting heart disease, especially left ventricular failure. The frequency of cor pulmonale or recurrent pulmonary embolism was less than 1 per cent. Thus the long-term prognosis in patients previously in good health appears to be quite good.

CHRONIC COR PULMONALE

Incidence

Because of its association with chronic lung disease, chronic cor pulmonale is believed to be a common type of heart disease.[1,76,244] Although precise figures on prevalence are lacking, it is possible to appreciate the potential magnitude of the problem by recognizing that chronic bronchitis and emphysema are its most common causes and that these two diseases result in approximately 30,000 deaths per year.[245] In one study in England, cor pulmonale was responsible for 30 to 40 per cent of all clinical cases of heart failure, of a total of 487 cases of cardiac disease,[246] and in the United States 10 to 30 per cent of hospital admissions for congestive heart failure are due to cor pulmonale.[247] Most patients are 45 years of age or older, and men are affected more frequently than women.

Etiology

There are many causes of cor pulmonale. Any disease that affects ventilatory mechanics, gas exchange, or the vascular bed either directly, through intrapulmonic events, or indirectly, via its effect on ventilatory control or the neuromuscular apparatus of respiration, may cause cor pulmonale. Since this is true of essentially all primary pulmonary disorders, the development of cor pulmonale simply indicates that the primary disease was sufficiently advanced to raise pulmonary artery pressure, cause right ventricular hypertrophy, and impair right ventricular function. Fortunately, most disorders affect too little of the lungs or are too circumscribed in their effects on gas exchange to initiate the train of events that leads to right ventricular hypertrophy and failure. A list of the various disease categories commonly associated with cor pulmonale, along with some specific examples of each process, is presented in Table 46–5.

Pathophysiology

Factors Contributing to the Development of Pulmonary Hypertension. The most important pathogenetic mechanisms that produce abnormalities in right ventricular structure and function are pulmonary hypertension and abnormal concentrations of blood gases that directly modify myocardial performance.[247a] As noted above (p. 1574), the normal pulmonary circulation is a low-resistance system with considerable reserve; therefore, substantial reductions in the size of the effective vascular bed must occur before pulmonary hypertension develops and becomes sustained. The pathogenetic sequence is unknown, and probably a number of mechanisms interact to produce pulmonary hypertension. Any theory regarding the development of cor pulmonale must take into account the effects

TABLE 46–5 DISEASE CATEGORIES ASSOCIATED WITH CHRONIC COR PULMONALE

Disorders of Pulmonary Parenchyma and Intrathoracic Airways
Chronic obstructive pulmonary disease
Chronic suppurative lung disease
Restrictive lung disease
Disorders of the Neuromuscular Apparatus and Chest Wall
Myopathic
Neurological
Thoracic deformity
Inadequate Ventilatory Drive
Obesity-hypoventilation syndromes
Primary alveolar hypoventilation
Sleep apnea syndromes (central)
Chronic mountain sickness
Upper Airway Obstruction
Pharyngeal-tracheal obstruction
Sleep apnea (obstructive)
Pulmonary Vascular Disorders
Multiple pulmonary emboli
Primary pulmonary hypertension
Miscellaneous

of the anatomical loss of vessels, i.e., anatomical restriction of the pulmonary vascular bed, pulmonary arteriolar constriction, increased blood viscosity, and increased blood flow, although their relative roles have not been clearly defined.[244]

It has long been thought that the essential pathology in chronic cor pulmonale is a *physical loss of vessels,* leading to a restricted vascular bed. Although it is certainly true that this mechanism contributes to the pulmonary hypertension seen in vascular occlusion resulting from multiple pulmonary emboli, aplasia, or extensive excision of lung tissue,[36,76,248] other factors also must be considered since emphysema, a disease in which alveolar vessels are widely destroyed, is typically associated with resting pulmonary hypertension and cor pulmonale only late in its course.[249,250] Thus, a decrease in the anatomical extent of the pulmonary vascular bed does not play a major role in the development of pulmonary hypertension unless the reduction is extreme. However, other processes (i.e., a constricted vascular bed) can *decrease the effective cross-sectional area without a loss of vessels.* The effective area can be reduced by arteriolar constriction secondary to alveolar hypoxemia and acidosis[32,33,67–70,76–80] and by the pathological changes responsible for pulmonary hypertension[251–254] (Chap. 25).

The potent vasoconstricting influence resulting from alveolar hypoxia (Fig. 46–14) is shared by the disease entities responsible for chronic cor pulmonale and listed in Table 46–5. The resulting pulmonary hypertension, when persistent, can make the vessels rigid and reduce their lumina by producing intimal thickening, inflammatory changes, and medial hypertrophy.[251–255]

Intimal thickening, regardless of its mechanism, often has a patchy distribution and is a frequent postmortem finding in patients beyond the age of 40 years who were free of pulmonary hypertension during life.[255] Therefore, the extent must be great to account for the perpetuation or worsening of pulmonary hypertension. The reversibility of this process is unknown, but when intimal thickening is produced by fibrosis, it is presumably permanent. Inflammatory changes vary from cellular infiltrates to fibrinoid necrosis and fibrosis. Most often these types of alterations are found in diffuse inflammatory lung lesions or with systemic illness with vasculitis; however, they have been noted secondary to pulmonary hypertension of any cause[252,255,256] (Chap. 25). Hypertrophy and hyperplasia of the smooth muscle in the media of the arterioles are regular findings in long-standing pulmonary hypertension and have been found to be reversible to some extent.[251–253]

An *increase in the viscosity of blood* has been shown experimentally to raise pulmonary vascular resistance[257] (p. 824). Viscosity is generally elevated as a result of chronic

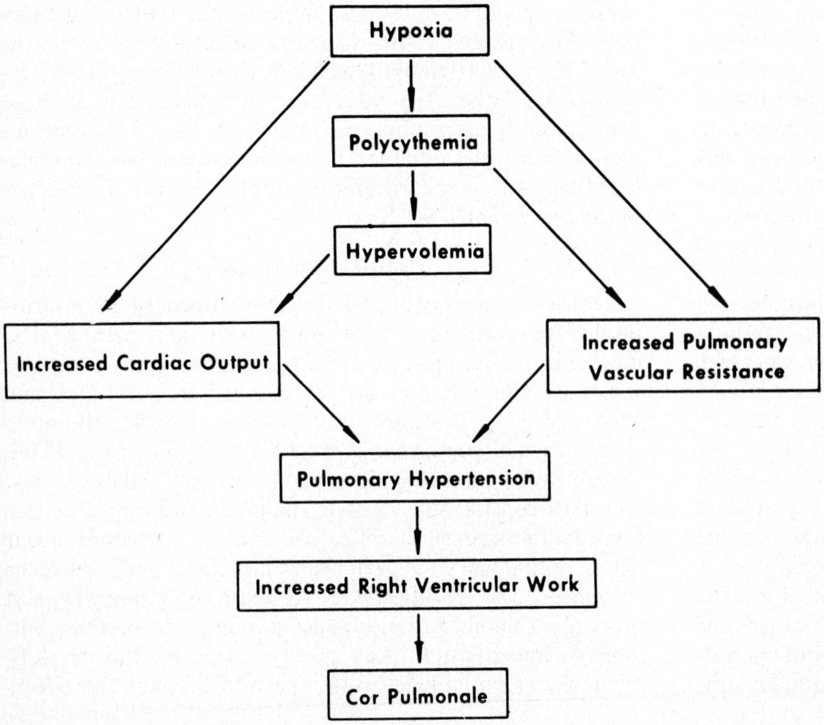

FIGURE 46–14 Schematic representation of the pathogenetic consequences of chronic hypoxia, regardless of cause, that culminate in cor pulmonale. (Reproduced with permission from Murray, J. F.: Respiration. In Pathophysiology—The Biological Principles of Disease. Smith, L. H., Jr., and Thier, S. O. (eds.): W. B. Saunders Co., Philadelphia, 1981, 1871 pp.)

hypoxemia stimulating red cell production through erythropoietin release. It represents an adaptation in that it provides the body with an increased oxygen-carrying capacity. However, the compensatory mechanism is useful only up to a point because the high hematocrit can interfere with blood flow in the capillaries and offset any potential benefits. The mechanism by which this occurs is complex. Blood is a non-Newtonian fluid, and its viscosity is an inverse function of shear rate, which varies with flow.[258] With high hematocrits the shear rates are low, and as the blood flow slows in the capillaries, viscosity increases even further, requiring a greater driving pressure. These considerations have served as the rationale for phlebotomy in selected patients with cor pulmonale.

The final factor that has been proposed as contributing to pulmonary hypertension is an *increase in pulmonary blood flow.* Extensive intimal hypertrophy and pathological medial necrosis have been created in the pulmonary circulation of animals by anastomosing a pulmonary artery either to the aorta or to one of its main branches.[259] Although studies demonstrate that bronchial artery–pulmonary vasculature collateral channels develop in chronic obstructive pulmonary disease,[260,261] these channels are seldom of quantitative significance except in the case of bronchiectasis.[261] As discussed below, increased cardiac outputs can raise pulmonary pressures in patients with both constricted and restricted vascular beds.

It is not clear how the above-described pathogenetic mechanisms interrelate in the development of pulmonary hypertension. It is easy to appreciate that the loss of vessels and diffuse constriction of the arterioles with its attendant pathological changes in their walls and lumina can combine to cause a reduction of the pulmonary vascular bed, which in turn causes an increase in pulmonary vascular resistance. However, these changes need not be manifest at rest as an elevated pulmonary artery pressure. As shown in Figure 46–4, the normal pulmonary vascular bed has the ability to accept large increases in flow without increasing pressure, probably through the recruitment of parallel vascular channels. In the case of a restricted vascular bed, this reserve is lost and the patients act as though they were starting at the bend of the normal pressure-flow relationship (Fig. 46–15).

Under these circumstances pressure can rise dramatically with exercise or any other condition that causes cardiac output to increase. With time and progression of the underlying disease as the secondary changes in the vessels develop, further reducing pulmonary vascular reserve, pulmonary artery pressure becomes elevated, even at rest. Now the pressure-flow relationship (Fig. 46–4*A*) is shifted upward and to the left as in a constricted bed, so that small increments in flow produce large increases in pressure over the entire range of cardiac outputs. It may be inferred that small increases in output are accompanied by large increases in work. Increases in viscosity and collateral blood flow worsen the situation by further increasing pulmonary artery pressure.

The data to support this general picture are derived from observations on the response to exercise of patients with chronic bronchitis (constricted vascular bed) and emphysema (restricted vascular bed).[262–264] In the former, pulmonary diffusing capacity *increases normally* with increases in cardiac output with exercise, and the work capacity of

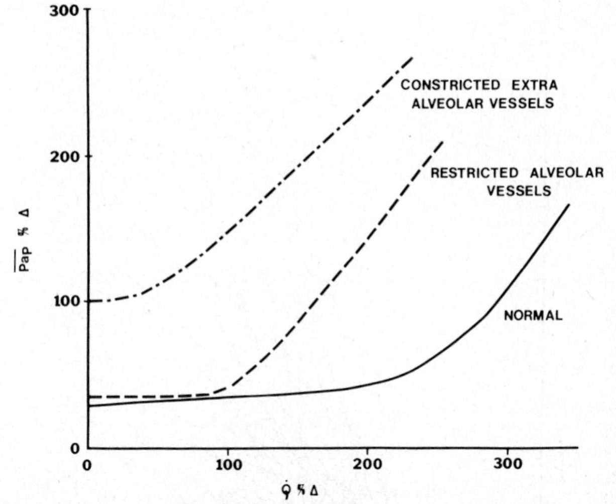

FIGURE 46–15 Pressure-flow relationship of normal, restricted, and constricted pulmonary vascular beds. The vertical axis indicates the percentage of change in mean pulmonary artery pressure ($\overline{PAP}$ % Δ), whereas the horizontal scale shows the percentage of change in cardiac output ($\dot{Q}$ % Δ). In both instances 100% = normal, basal level.

these patients is limited by their state of pulmonary mechanics and resulting gas exchange. It appears that the ability to dilate extraalveolar vessels normally and recruit alveolar vessels intact, although pulmonary artery pressure rises. Conversely, in patients with emphysema without resting pulmonary hypertension, diffusing capacity *does not increase normally* with exercise. The work capacity of these patients is limited by insufficient effective alveolar-capillary surface rather than by cardiac output or ventilation, and recruitment of alveolar vessels is severely curtailed.[262]

RIGHT VENTRICULAR DYNAMICS. The hemodynamic findings in cor pulmonale depend to some extent on the cause and duration of the underlying pathological process. Patients with relatively mild obstructive lung disease without severe hypoxemia generally have normal mean right atrial and right ventricular end-diastolic pressures, normal or low cardiac outputs, normal or slightly elevated pulmonary artery pressures, and slightly elevated pulmonary vascular resistances at rest.[264–272,272a,272b] Right ventricular ejection fractions, as determined by radionuclide techniques, tend to be normal.[270,271] With exercise, pulmonary artery pressure rises further, right ventricular stroke work increases (Fig. 46–16), and right ventricular ejection fractions fall.[270,271] Relating end-diastolic pressure to stroke work suggests that these patients operate on an extension of the normal right ventricular function curve.[269] This set of findings need not be accompanied by clinical or electrocardiographic evidence of right ventricular hypertrophy.[264] However, acute right ventricular failure can develop in these patients if respiratory failure is precipitated by a pulmonary infection.

Progression of the airway obstruction tends to accentuate these findings. As the ventilatory impairment worsens, the hemodynamic alterations follow suit. At the stage when severe chronic hypoxemia develops, usually in association with chronic hypercapnia, there is moderate pulmonary hypertension at rest, which becomes more severe during exercise in association with abnormal right ventricular filling pressures and function.[269–271] Cardiac output tends to be normal or slightly elevated at rest but increases little with exercise while air is being breathed; oxy-

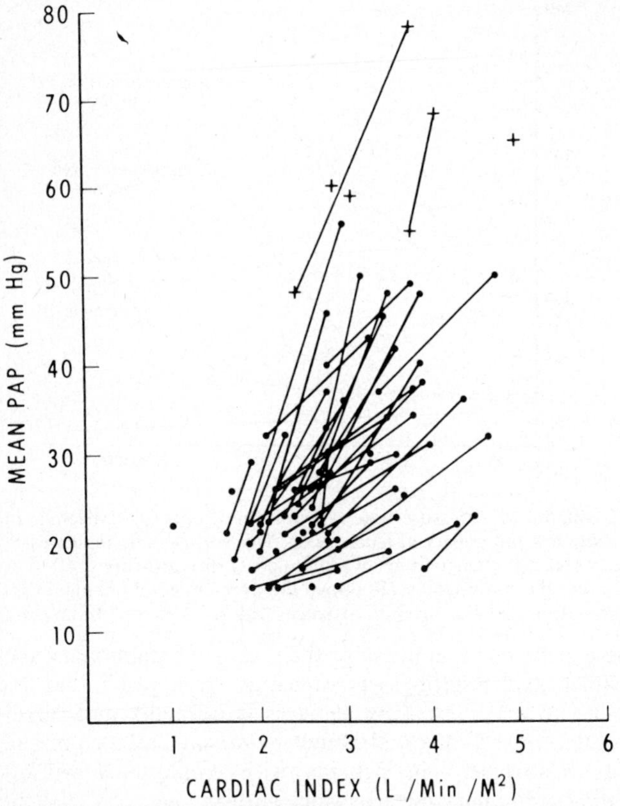

FIGURE 46–16 Relationship between mean pulmonary artery pressure (PAP) and cardiac index at rest and during exercise in patients with chronic obstructive lung disease. Crosses (+) indicate patients with arterial oxyhemoglobin saturation of less than 80 per cent. Resting and exercise values are connected by solid lines. (Reprinted with permission from Burrows, B., et al.: Patterns of cardiovascular dysfunction in chronic obstructive lung disease. N. Engl. J. Med. *286*: 912, 1972.)

gen administration, however, may improve the right ventricular ejection fraction.[271] Mean pulmonary artery pressures can reach levels of 60 to 80 mm Hg, and these patients are likely to show the clinical and electrocardiographic changes usually ascribed to cor pulmonale. Failure of the right ventricle is associated with an expanded circulating blood volume. However, in contrast to left ventricular failure, the pulmonary blood volume/total volume ratio remains essentially normal (approximately 1 to 10) even though red cell mass may be considerably increased.[273] Both circulating plasma volume and lung water increase,[273, 274] and both have been shown to decrease as pulmonary artery pressure is lowered with therapy.

LEFT VENTRICULAR DYNAMICS. Abnormally elevated pulmonary venous pressures, with or without overt left ventricular failure, invariably produce alterations in pulmonary mechanics and gas exchange, even in patients with normal lungs (Chapter 54). Consequently, left ventricular dysfunction could have deleterious effects in cor pulmonale. Controversy persists about whether the combined pulmonary–right ventricular pathologic condition in these patients produces the left ventricular disease, or whether the latter results from independent causes.

The view that disorders of the right ventricle may result in left ventricular disease has gained support from several sources. Animal experiments have shown that (1) right ventricular failure following banding of the pulmonary artery leads to similar morphological and biochemical changes in both cardiac chambers and to reduced contractility of the left ventricle,[275–277] (2) in both isolated hearts and intact animals alterations in right ventricular compliance or dimensions also change the mechanical properties of the left ventricle,[14,278,279] and (3) cattle with severe pulmonary hypertension at high altitude have increased left ventricular end-diastolic pressures.[280] Although these observations are provocative, their relevance to human disease is uncertain.

Autopsy studies have shown that left ventricular hypertrophy occurs in some patients with cor pulmonale,[281–283] and left ventricular dysfunction of varying degrees has been observed in vivo.[283–285] In all of these investigations, none of the usual etiologies of left ventricular disease were apparent. Thus, it appears that the structure and function of the left ventricle can become abnormal in association with the pathogenetic mechanisms underlying cor pulmonale. However, this is probably a very uncommon occurrence and the weight of current evidence indicates that cor pulmonale need not seriously affect left ventricular performance.[264,269,282,286–292] When abnormalities have been found, they could be explained either by a reduction in right ventricular stroke volume causing diminished left-sided filling or by independent disease processes such as coronary arteriosclerosis.[292] However, given the heterogeneity of the population with cor pulmonale and the variance of its natural history, the controversy will undoubtedly continue.[291]

Clinical Manifestations

As with other aspects of cor pulmonale, the clinical, radiological, therapeutic, and prognostic features are strongly influenced by the underlying disease process responsible for the pulmonary hypertension. For this reason, the subsequent presentation deals with many of these parameters as they specifically apply to the various disease categories listed in Table 46–5. Without doubt, the diseases that affect the pulmonary parenchyma, the intrathoracic airways, or both account for the vast majority of the cases of cor pulmonale. Within this category, the most common cause is chronic obstructive lung disease.

CHRONIC OBSTRUCTIVE PULMONARY DISEASE (COPD). COPD consists of chronic bronchitis, emphysema, and bronchial asthma. However, atopic asthma does *not* produce chronic cor pulmonale[250] and intrinsic, or nonatopic, asthma is often a variant of chronic bronchitis; in this chapter, COPD is used to denote chronic bronchitis and emphysema exclusively.

In most patients with COPD, chronic bronchitis and emphysema coexist, but cor pulmonale is restricted to those with functionally significant airway disease with or without emphysema.[250] This admixture has given rise to a great deal of confusion in terminology in the literature, and until the matter was sorted out by Burrows and colleagues[293] and Mitchell and Filley,[294] the terms bronchitis and emphysema were frequently considered to be synonymous. Additional observations uncovered fundamental differences in the clinical, physiological, and pathological features of the two conditions and laid the groundwork for a better understanding of these diseases.[75,262,293,295,296]

On the basis of this information, it is possible to think

TABLE 46–6 COMPARISON OF THE CLINICAL AND PHYSIOLOGICAL FEATURES OF EMPHYSEMA AND CHRONIC BRONCHITIS

	EMPHYSEMA	CHRONIC BRONCHITIS
Synonyms	Pink puffer Fighter	Blue bloater Nonfighter
Signs and Symptoms		
Cough and sputum	Scant	Marked
Dyspnea at rest	Marked	Usually absent
Recurrent chest infections	Unusual	Frequent
Cyanosis	No	Yes
Edema	No	Yes
Increased AP diameter of thorax	Marked	Mild
Hyperresonance to percussion	Marked	Mild
Pulmonary Gas Exchange		
Hematocrit	Normal	Elevated
P_aO_2	Slight reduction	Marked reduction
P_aCO_2	Low or normal	Elevated
Diffusing capacity	Markedly decreased	Normal or slightly reduced
Pulmonary Mechanics		
Expiratory flow rates	Reduced	Reduced
Elastic recoil	Markedly reduced	Normal or slightly reduced
Lung volumes	Marked hyperinflation	Mild hyperinflation
Pulmonary Circulation		
Pulmonary hypertension at rest	None or mild	Marked
with exercise	Moderate	Marked
Right heart failure	Terminal	Repeated

of COPD as a continuum, with chronic bronchitis at one extreme and emphysema at the other and the majority of patients having features of both conditions. The distinctions between the two groups are presented in Table 46–6. In the chronic bronchitis variety ("blue bloater," "nonfighter"), chronic cough with sputum production, frequently recurring chest infection, secondary erythrocytosis, and repeated bouts of right heart failure are common. Physiologically, the patients have hypoxemia and hypercapnia at rest, normal diffusing capacities, and elevated residual volumes, functional residual capacities, and airway resistances, with relatively normal values for total lung capacity and pulmonary compliance. Maximum flow rates and forced expiratory volumes are abnormally depressed. Chest radiographs show hyperinflated lungs, increased lung markings, and cardiomegaly.

The basic abnormality is widespread but regionally unequal airway obstruction that results in mismatched $\dot{V}_A/\dot{Q}$ relationships. In regions of low $\dot{V}_A/\dot{Q}$ ratios, pulmonary arterial constriction on the basis of hypoxia, hypercapnia, and/or acidosis occurs. With progression, net alveolar hypoventilation develops, the vascular bed becomes constricted, and resting pulmonary hypertension ensues.

In the emphysematous type ("pink puffer," "fighter"), dyspnea is the predominant symptom, and cough and sputum are considerably less prominent. Erythrocytosis is uncommon, and right heart failure tends to occur as a terminal event. In keeping with the hyperventilation, the alveolar-arterial gradient for oxygen is abnormally elevated, but arterial oxygen tension is usually normal or only slightly depressed; hypocapnia is common. Standard spirometric indices cannot differentiate this group from those with chronic bronchitis, as the degree of obstruction as measured by this technique is similar. However, the pink puffer has abnormally low diffusing capacities, enormous lung volumes, and very high values for pulmonary compliance. Roentgenograms of the chest reveal marked hyperinflation with flattened diaphragms, oligemia of the peripheral lung fields, and a small heart. With the onset of cor pulmonale, the prominence of the vascular markings increases, but right ventricular enlargement may be difficult to appreciate.

Although there is some airway disease in this condition, the primary pathological defect is widespread destruction of alveolar septa. As a result, the surface area for gas exchange is lost more or less in proportion to alveolar vessels, and arterial gas tensions can be reasonably well maintained for a period of time by increasing ventilation. However, the destruction of the parenchyma results in loss of lateral traction of small airways so that they narrow and collapse. Then the regional distribution of inspired air becomes more impaired, with resultant worsening of the abnormalities in $\dot{V}_A/\dot{Q}$ ratios. These patients initially have a restricted vascular bed, with normal pulmonary artery pressures at rest. As their disease process worsens with airway disease and further deterioration of gas exchange, secondary changes in the vasculature occur and resting pulmonary artery hypertension and cor pulmonale develop.

The *clinical manifestations* of cor pulmonale with heart failure are increasing dyspnea; episodes of paroxysmal cough, occasionally with syncope; and fluid retention with pitting edema and sometimes ascites. The distended neck veins exhibit prominent *a* and *v* waves and do not collapse with inspiration. Central cyanosis and an enlarged, tender liver are often present. Right ventricular hypertrophy is indicated by a palpable parasternal or subxiphoid heave. On auscultation, an S3 gallop, accentuated by inspiration, and a loud pulmonic second sound are frequently present. A holosystolic murmur along the lower left parasternal edge, accentuated by inspiration, usually indicates tricuspid regurgitation. These cardiac findings can be evanescent and can develop quickly when acute respiratory failure is superimposed on COPD. Examination of the lungs reveals diffuse inspiratory and expiratory rhonchi and wheezes. If acute respiratory failure is present in addition, papilledema, confusion, a hyperkinetic circulation, and asterixis may also be present.

Fundamental *treatment* of cor pulmonale in COPD is to relieve pulmonary hypertension by improving gas exchange.[297] This is accomplished by reducing bronchial smooth muscle constriction, promoting drainage of retained secretions, treating respiratory tract infections, and providing supplemental oxygen. The first two goals can be achieved simultaneously with the use of bronchodilators. In addition to relieving smooth muscle spasm, the sympathomimetics also increase mucociliary transport.[298] The net effect of these measures is the reduction of airway obstruction and the improvement of the regional distribution of inspired air and, through that, $\dot{V}_A/\dot{Q}$ relationships. Methylxanthines provide benefits above and beyond the usual bronchodilatation, for this class of compounds may produce favorable hemodynamic effects as well. In one study the intravenous administration of aminophylline in patients with cor pulmonale was shown to reduce mean pulmonary artery and right and left ventricular end-diastolic pressures significantly without inducing a change in the cardiac index,[299] and in another, right and left ventricular ejection fractions were increased.[300]

The beneficial effects of controlled oxygen therapy are well established in several circumstances. In acute respiratory failure, supplemental O_2 results in prompt and often dramatic improvement in pulmonary hemodynamics[264,265] (Fig. 46–17). In patients with progressive right ventricular hypertrophy or recurrent heart failure from cor pulmonale associated with severe hypoxemia ($PaO_2 < 50$ mm Hg) and severe pulmonary hypertension, marked improvement has been found when O_2 was administered for 15 or more hours per day.[301,302] However, a multicenter controlled trial showed that continuous O_2 for 24 hours a day provided the optimal therapy.[303] Such treatment appears to be safe, and some data suggest that it leads to prolonged survival.[304] However, if chronic O_2 therapy is being contemplated, it is *mandatory* to demonstrate that the supplemental O_2 does not result in worsening of alveolar hypoventilation with progressive hypercapnia.

The indications for the use of ancillary therapeutic measures such as phlebotomy, diuretics, and cardiac glycosides are considerably less clear. In the case of phlebotomy, most studies, including a recent double-blind investigation, have demonstrated an improvement in the subjective complaints related to vascular engorgement but no evidence of improvement in pulmonary gas exchange, mechanics, or hemodynamics.[305,306] Diuretics are commonly used for cor pulmonale with failure, and, although there is little question of their effectiveness in relieving fluid retention, there are scant data to demonstrate that they improve pulmonary hemodynamics or gas exchange in the absence of left ventricular decompensation. Nobel et al. reported an improvement in arterial blood gases with furosemide, but each of their four patients was given O_2 and other therapy concomitantly.[307] Attempts to reduce pulmonary artery pressures with vasodilators have led to conflicting results.[308,309]

The use of digitalis glycosides in patients with cor pulmonale is quite controversial. Digitalis apparently is effective in raising cardiac output in patients with cor pulmonale at rest but only at the expense of concomitant increases in pulmonary artery pressures. The subject has been reviewed, and the consensus is that there is no clear-cut evidence that cardiac glycosides are of substantial benefit unless left ventricular failure coexists.[310,311]

The *prognosis* of cor pulmonale in patients with COPD is difficult to state with certainty, for it is inextricably linked to the underlying disorder. When cor pulmonale de-

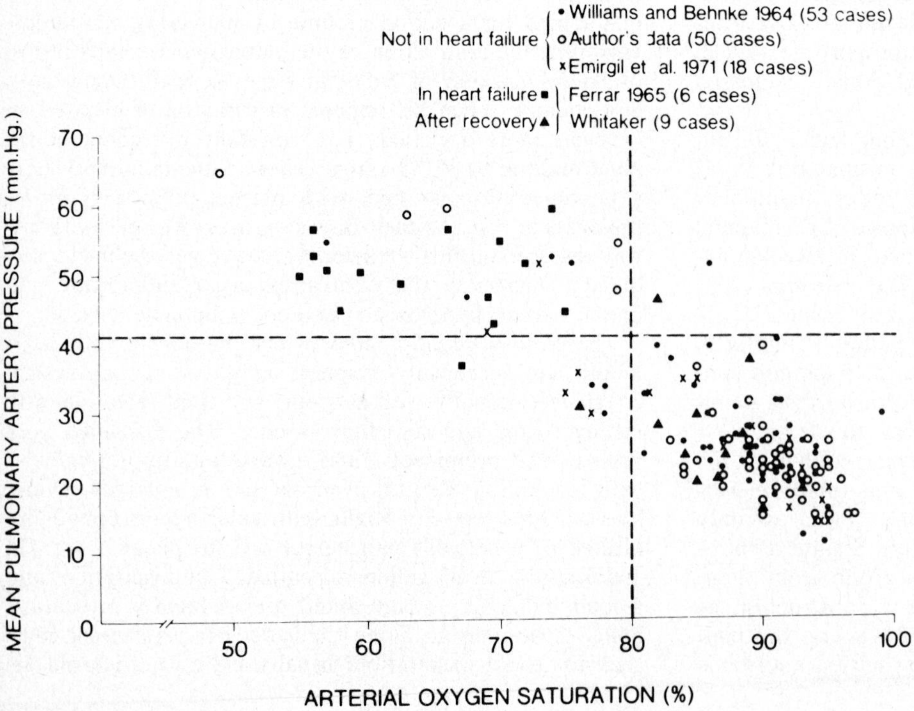

FIGURE 46–17 Relationship of resting mean pulmonary artery pressure to arterial oxygen saturation in 136 cases of chronic obstructive pulmonary disease. Solid squares represent data obtained in patients in heart failure; solid triangles, data from same subjects after recovery. The dashed lines are drawn at arbitrary points to indicate the relative risks of severe pulmonary hypertension (i.e., mean pulmonary artery pressure >40 mm Hg) in patients with arterial O_2 saturation values greater than, or less than, 80 per cent. (From Burrows, B.: Arterial oxygenation and pulmonary hemodynamics in patients with chronic airways obstruction. Proceedings of Conference on Scientific Basis of Respiratory Therapy. Am. Rev. Respir. Dis. *110*:64, 1974.)

velops in patients with emphysema, life expectancy is quite short, yet patients with bronchitis usually tolerate three to five such episodes before ultimately succumbing to their disease. Although long-term survival has been reported following the onset of cor pulmonale with heart failure, the 2- to 3-year survival rate ranges from 33 to 50 per cent,[312–315] but it may be improving with continuous O_2 therapy.

CHRONIC SUPPURATIVE PULMONARY DISEASE. The two prime examples of chronic suppurative disease associated with chronic cor pulmonale are bronchiectasis and cystic fibrosis.

Bronchiectasis. This chronic inflammatory disease is characterized clinically by cough and the production of copious amounts of purulent sputum and pathologically by cylindrical and saccular dilatation of airways.[316,317] In the majority of patients one can elicit a history of pneumonia developing as a complication of measles, pertussis, or some other contagious disease of childhood. It is thought that bacterial pneumonia and associated atelectasis are responsible for the destruction and dilatation of the bronchial walls. A small percentage of cases are associated with congenital defects such as Kartagener triad (p. 1618) and either congenital or acquired defects in immune mechanisms. Cor pulmonale develops in far-advanced cases in which destruction of lung tissue and fibrosis are extensive. The mechanism for pulmonary hypertension is believed to be capillary loss, hypoxia, and increased bronchial-pulmonary collateral blood flow. Formerly this was a relatively common affliction, but bronchiectasis has decreased considerably in incidence since the advent of the antibiotic era.

Cystic Fibrosis. This genetic defect is characterized by the secretion from exocrine glands of thick, tenacious mucus in which the mucopolysaccharide content is relatively insoluble and easily denatured. The lungs are involved to some extent in virtually all patients with the disease, and the thick mucus throughout the tracheobronchial tree partially or completely obstructs air passages, giving rise to focal atelectasis, pneumonia, bronchiectasis, and abscess formation.[318] Cor pulmonale is an important feature in the natural history, and it contributes to 70 per cent of the deaths.[319] An echocardiographic scoring system has been devised that provides a method for assessing the progression of the cardiac involvement in patients with cystic fibrosis and for evaluating prognosis.[320] Physiological studies have suggested that hypoxia is the principal stimulus to the production of pulmonary hypertension,[321] and pathological data have supported this by demonstrating that the thickening of the medial muscle layer is proportional to the degree of right ventricular hypertrophy.[322] In the past, the development of cardiac failure usually presaged death within a few months. In recent years, however, the prognosis has been improving, and a number of patients have survived for considerable periods.[323] These patients have been maintained on a vigorous, comprehensive, pulmonary care program with postural drainage, antibiotics, and bronchodilators.

RESTRICTIVE LUNG DISEASES. This category encompasses a multitude of diseases which have in common a loss of functioning pulmonary parenchyma with restriction of the pulmonary vascular bed. The latter results from a physical loss of vessels as well as from intrinsic abnormalities in the lumina and walls of those remaining. Essentially, five processes alone or in combination can produce this effect: (1) diffuse interstitial, (2) diffuse alveolar, (3) mixed alveolar-interstitial, (4) chest wall and pleural, and (5) extensive resection of lung tissue with disease in the residual parenchyma. Specific examples of the first three categories are sarcoidosis, radiation fibrosis, connective tissue disorders with primary or secondary lung involvement, fibrosing alveolitis, alveolar proteinosis, pneumoconiosis, and progressive massive fibrosis. The prototypes for the fourth and fifth categories are thoracoplasty for chronic tuberculosis and surgical resections for granulomatous disease or bronchiectasis.

Pulmonary parenchymal disease, especially when complicated by fibrosis of tissue and secondary vascular changes, can lead to severe pulmonary hypertension. As with the other conditions with a restricted vascular bed, the pulmonary hypertension is initially confined to circumstances in which the cardiac output is elevated. As the vascular bed becomes further restricted and the vessels stiffen, pulmonary hypertension persists at rest and intensifies with increased blood flow. As long as hypoxemia remains mild, pulmonary hypertension is modest, but cor pulmonale develops with respiratory failure. Fortunately, the sequence is not inevitable in most patients with these problems. If the pathological process stabilizes, as is often the case, the patient is left with modest pulmonary hypertension at rest, which is usually well tolerated.[76]

In these diseases, the lungs are stiff, with reduced volumes, and minute ventilations are high, with or without an elevated alveolar ventilation. Arterial O_2 and CO_2 tensions are usually moderately disturbed at rest, but severe hypoxemia may develop with exercise. The diffusing capacity is low and fails to increase normally as cardiac output is increased. In contrast to the chronic obstructive syndromes, a poor correlation exists between arterial blood gases and pulmonary artery pressure,[324] and there seems to be a parallel deterioration in pulmonary mechanics and hemodynamics.[325] As a general rule, when the vital capacity is greater than 80 per cent of normal, hemodynamics are normal. When vital capacity lies between 50 and 80 per cent, vascular resistance is increased and pulmonary artery pressure in the resting state is at the upper limits of normal. When vital capacity is below 50 per cent, pulmonary hypertension is present at rest. The role of hypoxic vasoconstriction in these patients has been difficult to clarify. Experimental evidence indicates that the ability of the pulmonary vasculature to respond to alveolar hypoxia is abnormal in diseased regions, so that when hypoxia does occur, blood is shifted toward the affected areas, thus worsening net gas exchange.[326] In any event, the development of severe hypoxemia and carbon dioxide retention heralds the onset of right ventricular failure, which is usually seen late in the course.

In keeping with the pathophysiology, the prominent symptoms of restrictive lung disease are tachypnea at rest and severe dyspnea on exertion. Fine inspiratory rales are found, along with the previously mentioned signs of pulmonary hypertension and right ventricular hypertrophy and/or failure. Early in the course of patients with pulmonary fibrosis, glucocorticoids or immunosuppressive drugs may be helpful if noninfectious inflammatory processes are believed present. In the late stages with extensive pulmonary fibrosis, these modalities are unsuccessful; all that can be offered is continuous O_2 therapy, diuretics, and cardiac glycosides. Although many of the diseases in this category progress slowly, once cor pulmonale develops the prognosis is grim.

DISORDERS OF THE NEUROMUSCULAR APPARATUS AND CHEST WALL. These disorders have in common the mechanical failure of the bellows apparatus, through weakness or paralysis of the respiratory muscles or through distortion of the geometry of the thorax. Several factors contribute to the development of cor pulmonale.

Failure of the Neuromuscular Apparatus. Respiratory muscle weakness can result from generalized diseases of muscles such as myopathic infiltrating diseases or muscular dystrophy, but it more commonly follows a neurological disorder, such as a cord lesion at or below the third cervical vertebra, amyotrophic lateral sclerosis, myasthenia gravis, poliomyelitis, Guillain-Barré syndrome, and so on.[327] In all of these diseases, the primary derangement is *generalized alveolar hypoventilation* from mechanical impedance to the movement of the rib cage, diaphragm, or both. The lungs and airways are usually not diseased, although they can become so with retained secretions and multiple aspirations. Although acute respiratory failure is common in these diseases, for cor pulmonale to develop in response to the hypoxic and hypercapneic stimuli the disorder must be chronic; consequently, this complication tends to be seen more often with cord lesions than with the other conditions just noted. Mechanical ventilatory support is the only treatment for the hypoventilation; a cuirass type of respirator is effective in these patients. Along with this, vigorous bronchial toilet facilitates the impaired handling of secretions that frequently coexists.

Bilateral diaphragmatic paralysis is an uncommon but insidious and frequently missed cause of cor pulmonale.[328] In the upright position ventilation is reasonably normal, but with assumption of the supine position gas exchange deteriorates. The diagnosis may be suspected in the patient with supine breathlessness, a disturbed sleep pattern, paradoxical (i.e., inward) motion of the abdomen on inspiration, and a low vital capacity in the erect position. Treatment consists of assisting ventilation during sleep. This can easily be accomplished under most circumstances with a rocking bed. When this is inadequate, electrical pacing of the diaphragm may be used.[329] Occasionally, diaphragmatic fatigue can contribute to the respiratory failure of COPD.[330]

Chest-Wall Disorders. The common congenital or acquired abnormalities that distort the geometry of the thoracic cage are kyphoscoliosis, pectus excavatum, pectus carinatum, and ankylosing spondylitis; only kyphoscoliosis is associated with cor pulmonale.[331] Kyphosis refers to any posterior angulation of the spine, and scoliosis consists of a lateral displacement with at least one compensatory curve in the opposite direction. Of these two processes, a kyphotic angle exceeding 100 degrees or an angle of scoliosis in excess of 120 degrees may be associated with cor pulmonale.[332] Such marked structural abnormalities of the thorax lead to abnormal positioning and functioning of the respiratory muscles, compression of the lung and pulmonary vasculature, and abnormal gas exchange.[332,333] In addition, it has been suggested that scoliosis interferes with the growth and development of alveoli and pulmonary arteries;[334] dyspnea is the major symptom of these disorders.

Therapy is directed toward avoiding complicating infections; episodes of acute respiratory failure are treated with mechanical ventilation. Surgical improvement of the thoracic deformity is not often associated with a commensurate change in cardiorespiratory function.[335]

INADEQUATE VENTILATORY DRIVE. The common denominator in this category is a depressed output from the respiratory center, with resultant generalized alveolar hypoventilation. Cor pulmonale is then the result of chronic hypoxemia and hypercapnia.

Obesity-Hypoventilation Syndrome. The association of extreme obesity with alveolar hypoventilation was originally made by Sir William Osler; Burwell et al. subsequently coined the term "pickwickian syndrome" to describe the combination of obesity, somnolence, plethora, and edema.[336] Despite many investigations, the pathogenesis of the hypoventilation in this syndrome remains obscure.[337] Excessive reduction of chest-wall compliance and muscle weakness secondary to obesity may account for part, but many extremely obese individuals with these defects do not hypoventilate. These patients may have abnormally low ventilatory responses to hypercapneic and anoxic stimulation, which improve with treatment.[338,339] Consequently, hyposensitivity of the respiratory center, whether acquired or preexistent, is probably a background factor.

The primary *treatment* of this disorder consists of weight reduction. The respiratory stimulant progesterone and its congeners have been shown to increase alveolar ventilation so that hypoxemia, hypercapnia, and cor pulmonale all improve substantially.[339,340] This may prove to be a useful adjunct until weight is reduced. If the respiratory and cardiac failure are life-threatening, ventilatory assistance may be required.

Some obese patients have periodic respirations, particularly during sleep. This sleep apnea syndrome is discussed next.

Sleep Apnea Syndromes. After the description of the Pickwickian syndrome, variant manifestations such as periodic respirations and hypersomnia were recognized, and it soon became apparent that many of the clinical and pathophysiological changes were secondary to abnormal respiratory patterns during sleep.[341] Three types of patterns have been recorded: (1) central apnea, in which airflow stops in conjunction with cessation of all respiratory muscle effort; (2) obstructive apnea, in which upper airway obstruction causes airflow to cease despite continuing or increasing efforts of the inspiratory muscles (the obstruction is believed to result from relaxation or discoordination of the buccal and pharyngeal muscles); and (3) mixed apnea, in which airflow and respiratory effort stop early in the episode, followed by a resumption of unsuccessful respiratory effort.[341,342] Irrespective of the mechanism, if the apneic periods are prolonged or repetitive, hypoventilation with hypoxemia, hypercapnia, and pulmonary hypertension develop, at first with sleep and then gradually when the patient is awake. Pulmonary capillary wedge pressures may also increase during periods of apnea.[343] The clinical symptomatology differs depending on the type, frequency, and intensity of the abnormal, sleep-related respiratory pattern.

The common clinical manifestations are loud snoring, abnormal behavior during sleep (somnambulism, tremors, or myoclonus), altered states of consciousness, nocturnal enuresis, morning headache, daytime hypersomnolence, and hypnagogic hallucinations. Most of these stem from the fact that the patient rarely reaches the deep stages of sleep because of hypoxic arousal and so is chronically sleep-deprived. The majority of patients with sleep apnea are *not obese* and ventilate normally when awake. Patients with obstructive apnea tend to have less severe hypoventilation and fewer hemodynamic abnormalities than patients with the other varieties. Treatment of central apnea consists of nocturnal diaphragmatic pacing;[329,344] tracheostomy is indicated in the obstructive variety.[345] If the latter type occurs in an obese patient, weight reduction may obviate the need for a permanent tracheal cannula. In the mixed group—those with combined central and obstructive etiologies—combined tracheostomy and diaphragmatic pacing are currently recommended.[344] Nocturnal O_2 therapy may be helpful in some patients by reducing the duration of the apneic periods and decreasing the related arrhythmias.[346]

Primary Alveolar Hypoventilation. Generalized alveolar hypoventilation in the absence of obesity or intrinsic disease of the lungs, chest wall, or neuromuscular apparatus has been ascribed to a failure of the autonomic control of ventilation. Most cases are acquired and are seen following encephalitis, brain stem surgery, meningitis, and the like, but congenital occurrence has been reported.[85,347] In this rare disease, the respiratory center does not respond to its chemical stimuli, and the patient has a flat or markedly depressed ventilatory–carbon dioxide response curve. However, an affected patient can improve alveolar ventilation and restore the arterial oxygen and carbon dioxide to normal by voluntary hyperventilation. This syndrome has been called *Ondine's curse.* The pathogenesis and treatment are similar to that outlined for other forms of generalized alveolar hypoventilation. An interesting therapeutic development is long-term pacing of the diaphragm by means of electrical stimulation of the phrenic nerves.[329]

Chronic Mountain Sickness. Some acclimatized residents of high altitudes suffer a transient loss of their adaptation after short stays at sea level and, upon return to altitude, develop acute pulmonary edema with circulatory and electrocardiographic changes similar to those seen in acute cor pulmonale[348] (p. 568). Some persons remaining at high altitude lose their acclimatization and develop signs and symptoms of generalized alveolar hypoventilation with chronic cor pulmonale. This syndrome is variously called *chronic mountain sickness, soroche,* or *Monge disease.*[349,350] The mechanism for the hypoventilation is unknown, but Severinghaus et al. have postulated that it is due to an adaptation or desensitization of the hypoxic chemoreceptors in the carotid body to chronic hypoxia.[351] The only treatment is removal of the patient to sea level, where pulmonary artery pressure falls acutely. With prolonged residence polycythemia disappears, and there is believed to be some involution of the structural changes of the pulmonary vessels.

UPPER AIRWAY OBSTRUCTION. Obstruction of the upper airways may be responsible for an inadequate ventilatory drive, global alveolar hypoventilation, and cor pulmonale. For the most part this occurs in children, especially black children, who have enlarged tonsils and adenoids.[352] Other causes include vascular ring (p. 1013), macroglossia, micrognathia, laryngotracheomalacia, laryngeal web, Crouzon disease, Hurler syndrome, and severe Pierre Robin syndrome,[353,354] but it can also develop with obstruction during sleep in both children and adults.[344] The mechanism for the hypoventilation is not at all clear. It has been suggested that an abnormally reactive pulmonary vascular bed, a defect in the central control of respiration, and an interference with normal sleep physiology, as in the sleep apnea syndrome, may play a part. There is little direct evidence for the first mechanism. However, it is known that ventilatory responsiveness to carbon dioxide is blunted in these patients and that it does not return to normal following therapy.[355]

The clinical features may mimic asthma, but more often the patients display somnolence, respiratory stridor, and recurrent respiratory tract infections. Treatment consists of surgical removal of the obstruction.

PULMONARY VASCULAR DISORDERS (see also Chap. 25). This category consists of diseases that primarily affect the pulmonary vasculature, with minimal or no parenchymal involvement. These diseases represent the most straightforward pathogenetic sequence in which pulmonary hypertension and right ventricular overloading are consequences of a progressive increase in pulmonary vascular resistance resulting from gradual obliteration of the blood vessels. In addition to their pathophysiology, these diseases also share in common the symptom of dyspnea and strikingly high pulmonary artery pressures, despite the fact that both vital capacity and pulmonary gas exchange may be only minimally impaired.[356] The latter is frequently of considerable diagnostic importance.

Multiple Pulmonary Emboli. Chronic thromboembolic disease occurs in two fashions. In the first, an obvious onset of the disease in the form of pleurisy or pulmonary infarction is followed by a protracted course characterized by step-wise impairment from acute attacks of dyspnea. In the second, patients tend to develop pulmonary hypertension and cor pulmonale slowly and silently without any antecedent gross pulmonic event.[248] Tachypnea, persisting during sleep, is an outstanding clinical feature of both varieties. Nonspecific symptoms such as tiredness, tachycardia, atypical chest pain, cough, and episodes of fever may also be part of the picture. Plain chest films may be of value in making the diagnosis if locally reduced vascular markings are found, but the diagnostic mainstay is pulmonary angiography. The prognosis is poor without early diagnosis. Treatment consists of preventing further embolization with anticoagulants or vena caval interruption or rarely by surgical evaluation of emboli in the pulmonary arterial bed.

Other Causes of Pulmonary Hypertension. *Schistosomiasis* is endemic in many parts of the world. Pulmonary hypertension is produced by ova emboli released by female worms lodged in pelvic or mesenteric veins.[357]

Sickle cell anemia can produce pulmonary hypertension through several mechanisms. The major one is extensive occlusion and microinfarction due to aggregation and sickling of the red blood cells in the pulmonary circulation (Chap. 49). Contributing factors are increased collateral blood flow and hyperviscosity.[358,359]

Pulmonary and/or systemic arteritis (Chap. 48) can be associated with the development of pulmonary hypertension. Most often this occurs in conjunction with collagen-vascular diseases such as scleroderma, lupus erythematosus, and rheumatoid arthritis. Usually there is pulmonary fibrosis in addition to the arteritis, but occasionally cor pulmonale can develop in its absence.[256]

Pulmonary venoocclusive disease is a rare disorder in which there is gradual obliteration of the pulmonary veins and venules (Chap. 25).[360] It tends to affect children and young adults, and its etiology is unknown. Chest radiographs show Kerley B lines and may help differentiate this disease from other entities like primary pulmonary hypertension and recurrent pulmonary emboli, but the diagnosis rests on lung biopsy.[361] The morphological picture shows narrowing and occlusion of small veins by organized thrombi. Nodular areas of congestion, interstitial fibrosis, and pneumonitis are regularly present as well. Anticoagulants do not seem to be of benefit, but successful treatment with immunosuppressive drugs has been reported.[362]

Electrocardiographic Findings (Table 46–7)

In the past, the use of the electrocardiogram to make the diagnosis of cor pulmonale has centered largely, if not exclusively, upon the demonstration of right ventricular hypertrophy. The classic criteria of a shift of the mean QRS axis to the right (right axis deviation greater than + 110 degrees), an R:S ratio in V_1 greater than 1, and an R:S ratio in V_6 of less than 1 were derived from patients with congenital heart disease[363,364] and have proved to be relatively poor criteria of cor pulmonale in patients with chronic obstructive lung disease.[365,366] The reason is that right ventricular hypertrophy per se is a late manifestation in these syndromes and occurs only after repeated dilatation of the ventricle.[156]

Kilcoyne and associates studied 200 patients with chronic obstructive lung disease and were able to demonstrate that when the arterial oxygen saturation fell below 85 per cent and mean pulmonary pressure was 25 mm Hg or greater, one or more of the following changes would develop in the electrocardiogram: (1) a rightward shift of the mean QRS axis of 30 degrees or more from its previous position; (2) inverted, biphasic, or flattened T waves in the right precordial leads; (3) depressed ST segments in leads II, III, and aV_f; and (4) incomplete or complete right bundle branch block.[366] With an increase in arterial saturation, these alterations disappeared. The T-wave changes in the right precordial leads and the axis shifts to the right occurred with only modest elevations of pulmonary artery pressure, but if these elevations became more severe, and if recurrences were frequent, then the rightward rotation of the QRS axis and the T-wave changes in the right precordial leads tended to become persistent. If pulmonary function were not improved, true right-axis deviation (a frontal plane axis greater than +90 degrees) and increased R-wave voltage in the right precordial leads developed. Once the latter occurred, the electrocardiogram was less likely to mirror any physiological variability, as reversion of the increased voltage to normal rarely occurred after improvement in arterial blood gases.

Other studies have suggested that clockwise rotation, right-axis deviation, a qR pattern in aV_r, and electrocardiographic evidence of right atrial enlargement, in that order, would also point to right ventricular hypertrophy in patients with chronic cor pulmonale (Chap. 7).[367] Occasionally in chronic obstructive lung disease the mean QRS axis may be directed posteriorly, superiorly, and to the right so that there is apparent left-axis deviation in the standard limb leads.[368] This pattern, along with low voltage, is most often associated with emphysema.[369]

Electrocardiographic features of prognostic importance in severe chronic bronchial obstruction have been outlined by Kok-Jensen.[370] In a study of 288 patients, survival was found to be very poor in patients with a QRS axis of +90 to +180 degrees and an amplitude of the P wave in lead II of 0.20 mV or more; only 37 and 42 per cent, respectively, of the patients with these changes were alive after 4 years.

TABLE 46–7 ELECTROCARDIOGRAPHIC CHANGES IN COR PULMONALE

ECG Criteria for Cor Pulmonale **without** *Obstructive Disease of the Airways**
1. Right-axis deviation with a mean QRS axis to the right of + 110°
2. R/S amplitude ratio in V_1 > 1
3. R/S amplitude ratio in V_6 < 1
4. Clockwise rotation of the electrical axis
5. P-pulmonale pattern
6. S_1Q_3 or $S_1S_2S_3$ pattern
7. Normal-voltage QRS
ECG Changes in Chronic Cor Pulmonale **with** *Obstructive Disease of the Airways†*
1. Isoelectric P waves in lead I or right-axis deviation of the P vector
2. P-pulmonale pattern (an increase in P-wave amplitude in II, III, aV_f)
3. Tendency for right-axis deviation of the QRS
4. R/S amplitude ratio in V_6 < 1
5. Low-voltage QRS
6. S_1Q_3 or $S_1S_2S_3$ pattern
7. Incomplete (and rarely complete) right bundle branch block
8. R/S amplitude ratio in V_1 > 1
9. Marked clockwise rotation of the electrical axis
10. Occasional large Q wave or QS in the inferior or midprecordial leads, suggesting healed myocardial infarction

*Any one of the first three criteria suffices to raise suspicion of right ventricular hypertrophy. The diagnosis becomes more certain if two or more of these findings are present (2 and 7). The last four criteria commonly occur in cor pulmonale secondary to primary alveolar hypoventilation interstitial disease of the lung, or pulmonary vascular disease.

†The first seven criteria are suggestive but nonspecific; the last three are more characteristic of cor pulmonale in obstructive disease of the airways.

Reproduced with permission from Holford, F. D.: The electrocardiogram in lung disease. *In* Fishman, A. P. (ed.): Pulmonary Diseases and Disorders. New York, McGraw-Hill, 1980, p. 140.

References

1. Chronic cor pulmonale: Report of an expert committee. Wld. Hlth. Org. Tech. Rep. Ser. *213*:1, 1961.
2. McGinn, S., and White, P. D.: Acute cor pulmonale resulting from pulmonary embolism, J.A.M.A. *104*:1473, 1935.
3. Lewis, T.: Observations upon ventricular hypertrophy with especial reference to preponderance of one or other chamber. Heart *5*:367, 1914.
4. Emery, J. L., and Mithal, A.: Weight of cardiac ventricles at and after birth. Br. Heart J. *23*:313, 1961.
5. Keen, E. N.: The post-natal development of the human cardiac ventricles. J. Anat. *89*:484, 1955.
6. Arias-Stella, J., and Recavarren, S.: Right ventricular hypertrophy in native children living at high altitude. Am. J. Pathol. *41*:55, 1962.
7. Mathew, R., Thilenius, O. G., and Arcilla, R. A.: Comparative response of right and left ventricles to volume overload. Am. J. Cardiol. *38*:239, 1976.
8. Recavarren, S., and Arias-Stella, J.: Right ventricular hypertrophy in people born and living at high altitudes. Br. Heart J. *26*:806, 1964.
9. Penaloza, D., Sime, F., Banchero, N., Gamboa, R., Cruz, J., and Martico-

Rena, E.: Pulmonary hypertension in healthy men born and living at high altitudes. Am. J. Cardiol. *11*:150, 1963.
10. Fulton, R. M., Hutchinson, E. C., and Jones, A. M.: Ventricular weight in cardiac hypertrophy. Br. Heart J. *14*:413, 1952.
11. Mitchell, R. S., Stanford, R. E., Silvers, G. W., and Dart, G.: The right ventricle in chronic airway obstruction: A clinicopathologic study. Am. Rev. Respir. Dis. *114*:147, 1976.
12. Ishikawa, S., Fattal, G. A., Popiewicz, J., and Wyatt, J. P.: Functional morphometry of myocardial fibers in cor pulmonale. Am. Rev. Respir. Dis. *105*:358, 1972.
13. Brecher, G. A., and Galletti, P. M.: Functional anatomy of cardiac pumping. *In* Hamilton, A. F., and Dow, P. (eds.): Handbook of Physiology; Circulation. Vol. II. Washington, D.C., American Physiological Society, 1963, p. 759.
14. Laks, M. M., Garner, D., and Swan, H. J. C.: Volumes and compliances measured simultaneously in the right and left ventricles of the dog. Circ. Res. *20*:565, 1967.
15. Abel, F. L., and Waldhausen, J. A.: Effects of alterations in pulmonary vascular resistance on right ventricular function. J. Thorac. Cardiovasc. Surg. *54*:886, 1967.
16. Abel, F. L.: Effects of alterations in peripheral resistance on left ventricular function. Proc. Soc. Exp. Biol. Med. *120*:52, 1965.
17. de V. Cotten, M., and Maling, H. M.: Relationships among stroke work, contractile force and fiber length during changes in ventricular function. Am. J. Physiol. *189*:580, 1957.
18. Sarnoff, S. J., and Berglund, E.: Ventricular function. I. Starling's law of the heart studied by means of simultaneous right and left ventricular function curves in the dog. Circulation *9*:706, 1954.
19. Spann, J. R., Buccino, R. A., Sonnenblick, E. H., and Braunwald, E. B.: Contractile state of cardiac muscle obtained from cats with experimentally produced ventricular hypertrophy and heart failure. Circ. Res. *21*:341, 1967.
20. Haggart, G. E., and Walker, A. M.: The physiology of pulmonary embolism as disclosed by quantitative occlusion of the pulmonary artery. Arch. Surg. *6*:764, 1923.
21. Gibbond, J. H., Hopkinson, M., and Churchill, E. D.: Changes in the circulation produced by gradual occlusion of the pulmonary artery. J. Clin. Invest. *11*:543, 1932.
22. Fineberg, M. H., and Wiggens, C. J.: Compensation and failure of the right ventricle. Am. Heart J. *11*:255, 1936.
23. Brooks, H., Kirk, E. S., Vokonas, P. S., Urschel, C. W., and Sonnenblick, E. H.: Performance of the right ventricle under stress: Relation to right coronary flow. J. Clin. Invest. *50*:2176, 1971.
24. Krahl, V. E.: Anatomy of the mammalian lung. *In* Fenn, O. W., and Rahn, H. (eds.): Handbook of Physiology; Respiration. Vol. I. Washington, D.C., American Physiological Society, 1964, p. 224.
25. Hislop, A., and Reid, L.: Intrapulmonary arterial development during fetal life—branching pattern and structure. J. Anat. *113*:35, 1972.
26. Davies, G. M., and Reid, L.: Growth of the alveoli and pulmonary arteries in childhood. Thorax *25*:669, 1975.
27. Boyden, E. A., and Tompsett, D. H.: The changing patterns in the developing lungs of infants. Acta Anat. *61*:164, 1965.
28. Elliott, F. M., and Reid, L.: Some new facts about the pulmonary artery and its branching pattern. Clin. Radiol. *16*:193, 1965.
29. Hislop, A., and Reid, L.: Pulmonary arterial development during childhood; Branching pattern and structure. Thorax *28*:129, 1973.
30. Reid, L.: Morphology of pulmonary circulation in health and disease. Kongr. Ber. Wiss. Tag. Norddtsch. Lung. Bronchialhk. *14*:333, 1975.
31. Fishman, A. P.: Regulation of the pulmonary circulation. *In* Fishman, A. P. (ed.): Pulmonary Diseases and Disorders. New York, McGraw-Hill Book Co., 1980, p. 397.
32. Staub, N. C., and Storey, W. F.: Relation between morphological and physiological events in lung using rapid freezing. J. Appl. Physiol. *17*:381, 1962.
33. von Euler, U. S., and Liljestrand, G.: Observations on the pulmonary arterial blood pressure in the cat. Acta Physiol. Scand. *12*:301, 1946.
34. Barr, L.: Smooth muscle as an electrical syncytium. *In* Fishman, A. P., and Hecht, H. H. (eds.): The Pulmonary Circulation and the Interstitial Space. Chicago, University of Chicago Press, 1969, p. 161.
35. Hebb, C.: Motor innervation of the pulmonary blood vessels of mammals. *In* Fishman, A. P., and Hecht, H. H. (eds.): The Pulmonary Circulation and the Interstitial Space. Chicago, University of Chicago Press, 1969, p. 195.
36. Fishman, A. P.: Dynamics of the pulmonary circulation. *In* Hamilton, W. F., and Dow, P. (eds.): Handbook of Physiology; Circulation. Vol. II, Washington, D. C., American Physiological Society, 1963, p. 1667.
37. Bard, P.: The pulmonary circulation and respiratory variations in the systemic circulation. *In* Bard, P. (ed.): Medical Physiology. St. Louis, Mosby, 1961, p. 231.
38. Brofman, B. L., Charms, B. L., Kohn, P. M., Elder, J., Newman, R., and Rizika, M.: Unilateral pulmonary artery occlusion in man. Control Studies. J. Thorac. Surg. *34*:206, 1957.
39. Guyton, A. C.: Circulatory Physiology: Cardiac Output and Its Regulation, Philadelphia, W. B. Saunders Co., 1963.
40. Maseri, A., Caldini, P., Howard, P., Joshi, R. C., Permutt, S., and Zierler, K. L.: Determinants of pulmonary vascular volume—recruitment versus distensibility. Circ. Res. *31*:218, 1972.
41. Lanari, A., and Agrest, A.: Pressure-volume relationship in the pulmonary vascular bed. Acta Physiol. Lat. Am. *4*:116, 1954.
42. Caro, C. G.: Extensibility of blood vessels in isolated rabbit lung. J. Physiol. (Lond.) *178*:193, 1965.
43. Howell, J. B. L., Permutt, S., Proctor, D. F., and Riley, R. L.: Effect of inflation of the lung on different parts of the pulmonary vascular bed. J. Appl. Physiol. *16*:71, 1961.
44. Engelberg, J., and DuBois, A. B.: Mechanics of pulmonary circulation in isolated rabbit lungs. Am. J. Physiol. *186*:401, 1959.
45. Maseri, A., Caldini, P., Permutt, S., and Zierler, K. L.: Pressure volume relationship in the pulmonary circulation. *In* Widimsky, J., Daum, S., and Herzog, H. (eds.): Progress in Respiration Research. Vol. 5. Basel, S. Karger, 1970, p. 53.
46. Glazier, J. B., Hughes, J. M. B., Maloney, J. E., and West, J. B.: Measurements of capillary dimensions and blood volume in rapidly frozen lungs. J. Appl. Physiol. *26*:65, 1969.
47. West, J. B.: Ventilation/Blood Flow and Gas Exchange. 2nd ed. Philadelphia, F. A. Davis Co., 1970.
48. West, J. B.: The use of radioactive materials in the study of lung function. *In* Fishman, A. P. (ed.): Pulmonary Diseases and Disorders. New York, McGraw-Hill Book Co., 1980, p. 378.
49. West, J. B., Dollery, C. T., and Nelmark, A.: Distribution of blood flow in isolated lungs: Relation to vascular and alveolar pressures. J. Appl. Physiol. *19*:713, 1964.
50. West, J. B., and Dollery, C. T.: Distribution of blood flow and the pressure-flow relations of the whole lung. J. Appl. Physiol. *20*:175, 1965.
51. Permutt, S., and Riley, R. L.: Hemodynamics of collapsible vessels with tone: The vascular waterfall. J. Appl. Physiol. *18*:924, 1963.
52. West, J. B., and Dollery, C. T.: Distribution of blood flow and ventilation-perfusion ratio in the lung, measured with radioactive CO_2. J. Appl. Physiol. *15*:405, 1960.
53. Hughes, J. M. B., Glazier, J. B., Maloney, J. E., and West, J. B.: Effect of interstitial pressure on pulmonary blood flow. Lancet *1*:192, 1967.
54. West, J. B., Dollery, C. J., and Heard, B. E.: Increased pulmonary vascular resistance in the dependent zone of the isolated dog lung caused by perivascular edema. Circ. Res. *17*:191, 1965.
55. Kaneko, K., Milic-Emili, J., Dolovich, M. B., Dawson, A., and Bates, D. V.: Regional distribution of ventilation and perfusion as a function of body position. J. Appl. Physiol. *16*:465, 1961.
56. Milic-Emili, J., Henderson, J. A. M., Dolovich, M. B., Trop, D., and Kaneko, K.: Regional distribution of inspired gas in the lung. J. Appl. Physiol. *21*:749, 1966.
57. Klocke, R. A.: Intrapulmonary distribution of air and blood. *In* Fishman, A. P. (ed.): Pulmonary Diseases and Disorders. New York, McGraw-Hill Book Co., 1980, p. 373.
58. LeBlanc, P., Ruff, F., and Milic-Emili, J.: Effect of age and body position on airway closure in man. J. Appl. Physiol. *28*:448, 1970.
59. Craig, D. B., Wahba, W. M., Don, H. F., Coutre, J. G., and Becklake, M. R.: Closing volume and its relationship to gas exchange in seated and supine position. J. Appl. Physiol. *31*:717, 1971.
60. Farhi, L. E.: Ventilation-perfusion relationship and its role in alveolar gas exchange. *In* Caro, C. (ed.): Recent Advances in Respiratory Physiology. London, W. H. Arnold, 1965.
61. Rahn, H., and Farhi, L. E.: Ventilation, perfusion, and gas exchange—the $\dot{V}a/\dot{Q}$ concept. *In* Fenn, W. O., and Rahn, H. (eds.): Handbook of Physiology: Respiration. Vol. 1. Washington, D.C., American Physiological Society, 1964, p. 735.
62. West, J. B.: Ventilation-perfusion inequality and overall gas exchange in computer models of the lung. Respir. Physiol. *7*:88, 1969.
63. Lenfant, C.: Measurements of ventilation-perfusion distribution with alveolar-arterial differences. J. Appl. Physiol. *18*:1090, 1963.
64. Filley, G. F., Gregorie, F., and Wright, G. W.: Alveolar and arterial oxygen tensions and the significance of the alveolar-arterial oxygen tension differences in normal man. J. Clin. Invest. *33*:517, 1954.
65. Raine, J. M., and Bishop, J. M.: A-a difference in O_2 tension and physiologic dead space in normal man. J. Appl. Physiol. *18*:284, 1963.
66. Severinghaus, J. W., and Stupfel, M.: Alveolar dead space as an index of distribution of blood flow in pulmonary capillaries. J. Appl. Physiol. *10*:335, 1957.
67. Fishman, A. P.: Respiratory gases in the regulation of the pulmonary circulation. Physiol. Rev. *41*:214, 1961.
68. Fishman, A. P.: Hypoxia and its effects on the pulmonary circulation. Circ. Res. *38*:221, 1976.
69. Bergofsky, E. H.: Mechanisms underlying vasomotor regulation of regional pulmonary blood flow in normal and disease states. Am. J. Med. *57*:378, 1974.
70. Swenson, E. W., Finley, T. N., and Guzman, S. V.: Unilateral hypoventilation in man during temporary occlusion of one pulmonary artery. J. Clin. Invest. *40*:828, 1961.
71. Austrian, R., McClement, J. H., Renzetti, A. D., Jr., Donald, K. W., Riley, R. L., and Cournand, A.: Clinical and physiologic features of some types of pulmonary diseases with impairment of alveolar-capillary diffusion. The syndrome of "alveolar-capillary block." Am. J. Med. *11*:667, 1951.
72. Bates, D. V., Macklem, P. T., and Christie, R. V.: Respiratory Function in Disease, 2nd Ed. Philadelphia, W. B. Saunders Co., 1971, p. 75.
73. Engel, L. A., and Macklem, P. T.: Gas mixing and distribution in the lung. *In* Widdicombe, J. G. (ed.): Respiratory Physiology II. International Review of Physiology, Vol. 14. Baltimore, University Park Press, 1977, p. 37.

74. Rahn, H., and Fenn, W. O.: A Graphical Analysis of the Respiratory Gas Exchange. Washington, D.C., American Physiological Society, 1962.
75. Sykes, M. K., McNicol, M. W., and Campbell, E. J. M.: Respiratory Failure. Oxford, Blackwell Scientific Publications, 1971, p. 56ff.
76. Fishman, A. P.: Cor pulmonale. Am. Rev. Respir. Dis. *114*:775, 1976.
77. Fowler, K. T., and Read, J.: Effect of alveolar hypoxia on zonal distribution of pulmonary blood flow. J. Appl. Physiol. *18*:244, 1963.
78. Lindsay, D. A., and Reed, J.: Pulmonary vascular responsiveness in the prognosis of chronic obstructive lung disease. Am. Rev. Respir. Dis. *105*:242, 1972.
79. Enson, Y., Guintini, C., Lewis, M. L., Morris, T. Q., Ferrer, I. M., and Harvey, R. M.: The influence of hydrogen ion concentration and hypoxia on the pulmonary circulation. J. Clin. Invest. *43*:1146, 1964.
80. Bergofsky, E. H., Haas, F., and Procelli, R. J.: Determination of the sensitive vascular sites from which hypoxia and hypercapnia elicit rises in pulmonary arterial pressure. Fed. Proc. *27*:1420, 1968.
81. Aviado, D. M.: The Lung Circulation. Vol. 1. London, Pergamon Press, 1965.

PULMONARY THROMBOEMBOLISM

82. Bell, W. R., and Simon, T. L.: Current status of pulmonary thromboembolic disease: Pathophysiology, diagnosis, prevention, and treatment. Am. Heart J. *103*:239, 1982.
83. Parker, B. M., and Smith, J. R.: Pulmonary embolism and infarction: Review of physiologic consequences of pulmonary arterial obstruction. Am. J. Med. *24*:402, 1958.
84. Allison, P. R., Dunnill, M. S., and Marshall, R.: Pulmonary embolism. Thorax *15*:273, 1960.
85. Moran, T.: Autopsy incidence of pulmonary embolism in coronary heart disease. Ann. Intern. Med. *32*:949, 1956.
86. Freiman, D. G., Suyemoto, J., and Wessler, S.: Frequency of pulmonary thromboembolism in man. N. Engl. J. Med. *272*:1278, 1965.
87. Dexter, L., and Dalen, J. E.: Pulmonary embolism and acute cor pulmonale. *In* Hurst, J. W. (ed.): The Heart. 4th ed. New York, McGraw-Hill Book Co., 1974, p. 1472.
88. Poe, N. D., Dore, E. K., Swanson, L. A., and Taplin, G. V.: Fatal pulmonary embolism. J. Nucl. Med. *10*:28, 1969.
89. Israel, H. L., and Goldstein, F.: The varied clinical manifestations of pulmonary embolism. Ann. Intern. Med. *47*:202, 1957.
90. McIntyre, K. M., and Levine, H. J.: Cardiac arrest and resuscitation. *In* Spitzer, S., Oaks, W. W., and Moyer, J. (eds.): Emergency Medical Management. New York, Grune and Stratton, 1971, p. 4.
91. Robin, E. D.: Overdiagnosis and overtreatment of pulmonary embolism: The Emperor may have no clothes. Ann. Intern. Med. *87*:775, 1977.
92. Fishman, A. P.: Pulmonary thromboembolism. Pathophysiology and clinical features. *In* Fishman, A. P. (ed.): Pulmonary Diseases and Disorders. New York, McGraw-Hill Book Co., 1980, p. 809.
93. Sevitt, S.: Venous thrombosis and pulmonary embolism. Am. J. Med. *33*:703, 1962.
94. Byrne, J. J., and O'Neil, E. E.: Fatal pulmonary emboli: A study of 130 autopsy proven fatal emboli. Am. J. Surg. *83*:47, 1952.
95. Kistner, R. L., Ball, J. J., Nordyke, R. A., and Freedman, G. G.: Incidence of pulmonary embolism in the course of thrombophlebitis of the lower extremities. Am. J. Surg. *124*:169, 1972.
96. Sharma, G. V. R. K., O'Connell, D. C., Wheeler, H. B., Belko, J. S., and Sasahara, A. A.: Deep venous thrombosis as a diagnosis clue to pulmonary embolism. Am. J. Cardiol. *33*:170, 1974.
97. Young, A. E., Henderson, B. A., Phillips, D. A., and Couch, N. P.: Impedance plethysmography: Its limitations as a substitute for phlebography. Cardiovasc. Radiol. *1*:233, 1978.
98. Havig, O.: Deep vein thrombosis and pulmonary embolism. Acta Chir. Scand. (Suppl.) *478*:1, 1977.
99. Moser, K. M., and LeMoine, J. R.: Is embolic risk conditioned by location of deep venous thrombosis? Ann. Intern. Med. *94*:439, 1981.
100. Rosenburg, R. D.: Hypercoagulability and Methods for Monitoring Anticoagulant Therapy. Washington, D.C., U.S. Department of Health, Education and Welfare, Publication No. (NIH) 76-866, 1976.
101. Kakkar, V. V., and Corrigan, T. P.: Detection of deep venous thrombosis: Survey and current states. Progn. Cardiovasc. Dis. *17*:207, 1974.
102. O'Brien, J. R.: Detection of thrombosis with ^{125}iodine-fibrinogen. Lancet *2*:396, 1970.
103. Moser, K. M., Branch, B. B., and Dolan, G. F.: Comparison of venography, impedance plethysmography and radiolabelled fibrinogen in clinically suspected deep venous thrombosis of the lower extremities. J.A.M.A. *237*:2195, 1977.
104. Falicov, R. E., Resnekov, L., and Petasnick, J.: Progressive pulmonary vascular obstruction and cor pulmonale due to repeated embolism from axillary vein thrombosis. Ann. Intern. Med. *73*:429, 1970.
105. Pollak, V. E., Kark, R. M., Pirani, C. L., Shafter, H. A., and Muehrcke, R. C.: Renal vein thrombosis and the nephrotic syndrome. Am. J. Med. *21*:496, 1956.
106. Senior, R. M., Britton, R. C., Turino, G. M., Wood, J. A., Langer, G. A., and Fishman, A. P.: Pulmonary hypertension associated with cirrhosis of the liver and with portacaval shunts. Circulation *38*:88, 1968.
107. Peterson, E. P., and Taylor, H. B.: Amniotic fluid embolism: An analysis of 40 cases. Obstet. Gynecol. *35*:787, 1970.
108. Rogel, S., Rosenmann, E., and Rachmilewitz, E. A.: Multiple pulmonary infarctions caused by bone marrow emboli. N. Engl. J. Med. *272*:732, 1965.
109. Dines, D. D., Linscheid, R. L., and Didier, E. P.: Fat embolism syndrome. Mayo Clin. Proc. *47*:237, 1972.
110. Deal, C. W., Fielden, B. P., and Monk, I.: Hemodynamic effects of pulmonary air embolism. J. Surg. Res. *11*:533, 1971.
111. Winterbauer, R. H., Elfenbein, I. B., and Ball, W. C., Jr.: Incidence and clinical significance of tumor embolization to the lungs. Am. J. Med. *45*:271, 1968.
112. Ingram, R. H., Jr.: Cor pulmonale with diseases affecting the pulmonary circulation. *In* Practice of Medicine. Vol. 6. Hagerstown, Md., Harper Medical, Harper and Row, 1971, p. 2.
113. Fineberg, M. H., and Wiggers, C. J.: Compensation and failure of the right ventricle. Am. Heart J. *11*:255, 1936.
114. Haggart, G. E., and Walker, A. M.: The physiology of pulmonary embolism as disclosed by quantitative occlusion of the pulmonary artery. Arch. Surg. *6*:764, 1923.
115. Gibbon, J. H., Hopkins, M., and Churchill, E. D.: Changes in the circulation produced by gradual occlusion of the pulmonary artery. J. Clin. Invest. *11*:543, 1932.
116. Hyland, J. W., Smith, G. T., McGuire, L. B., Harrison, D. C., Haynes, F. W., and Dexter, L.: Effect of selective embolization of various sized pulmonary arteries in dogs. Am. J. Physiol. *204*:619, 1963.
117. McIntyre, K. M., and Sasahara, A. A.: Hemodynamic response to pulmonary embolism in patients free of prior cardiopulmonary disease. Am. J. Cardiol. *28*:228, 1971.
118. McIntyre, K. M., Sasahara, A. A., and Sharma, G. V.: Pulmonary thromboembolism: Current concepts. Adv. Intern. Med. *18*:199, 1972.
119. Brandfonbrenner, M., Turino, G. M., Himmelstein, A., and Fishman, A. P.: Effects of occlusion of one pulmonary artery on pulmonary circulation in man. Fed. Proc. *17*:19, 1958.
120. McDonald, I. G., Hirsh, J., Hale, G. S., and O'Sullivan, E. F.: Major pulmonary embolism; A correlation of clinical findings, hemodynamics, pulmonary angiography, and pathological physiology. Br. Heart J. *34*:356, 1972.
121. Bell, W. R., Simon, T. L., and DeMets, D. L.: The clinical features of submassive and massive pulmonary emboli. Am. J. Med. *62*:355, 1977.
122. Stein, P. D., Willis, P. W., and DeMets, D. L.: History and physical examination in acute pulmonary embolism in patients without preexisting cardiac or pulmonary disease. Am. J. Cardiol. *47*:218, 1981.
123. Miller, G. A. H., and Sutton, G. C.: Acute massive pulmonary embolism. Clinical and haemodynamic findings in 23 patients studied by cardiac catheterization and pulmonary arteriography. Br. Heart J. *32*:518, 1970.
124. National Cooperative Study: The urokinase-pulmonary embolism trial. Circulation *47*(Suppl. II):1, 1973.
125. Halmagyi, D. F., Starzecki, B., and Horner, G. J.: Humoral transmission of cardiorespiratory changes in experimental lung embolism. Circ. Res. *14*:546, 1964.
126. Bo, G., Hognestad, J., and Vaage, J.: The role of blood platelets in pulmonary responses in microembolization with barium sulfate. Acta Physiol. Scand. *90*:244, 1974.
127. Nadel, J. A., Colebatch, H. J. H., and Olsen, C. R.: Location and mechanism of airway constriction after barium sulfate microembolism. J. Appl. Physiol. *19*:387, 1964.
128. Bo, G., and Hognestad, J.: Effects on the pulmonary circulation of suddenly induced intravascular aggregation of blood platelets. Acta Physiol. Scand. *85*:523, 1972.
129. Swendenborg, J.: Thrombin-induced vasoconstriction in the pulmonary circulation. Scand. J. Clin. Lab. Invest. *27*:321, 1971.
130. Stein, M., and Thomas, D. P.: Role of platelets in the acute pulmonary responses to endotoxin. J. Appl. Physiol. *23*:47, 1967.
131. Vaage, J.: Vagal reflexes in the bronchoconstriction occurring after induced intravascular platelet aggregation. Acta Physiol. Scand. *97*:94, 1976.
132. Thomas, D. P., Gurewich, V., and Ashford, T. P.: Platelet adherence to thromboemboli in relation to the pathogenesis and treatment of pulmonary embolism. N. Engl. J. Med. *274*:953, 1966.
133. Wessler, S., Reiner, L., Freiman, D. G., Reimer, S. M., and Lertzman, M.: Serum-induced thrombosis: Studies of its induction and evolution under controlled conditions *in vivo*. Circulation *20*:864, 1959.
134. Thomas, D., Stein, M., Tanabe, G., Rege, V., and Wessler, S.: Mechanism of bronchoconstriction produced by thromboemboli in dogs. Am. J. Physiol. *206*:1207, 1964.
135. Rosoff, C. B., Salzman, E. M., and Gurewich, V.: Reduction of the platelet serotonin and the response to pulmonary emboli. Surgery *70*:12, 1971.
136. Clarke, S. W., Graf, P. D., and Nadel, J. A.: *In vivo* visualization of small airway constriction after pulmonary microembolism in cats and dogs. J. Appl. Physiol. *29*:646, 1970.
137. Von Hayek, H.: The Human Lung. New York, Hafner, 1960.
138. Nadel, J. A.: Mechanisms of airway response to inhaled substances. Arch. Environ. Health *16*:171, 1968.
139. Dalen, J. E., Banas, J. S., Brooks, H. L., Evans, G. L., Paraskos, J. A., and Dexter, L.: Resolution rate of acute pulmonary embolism in man. N. Engl. J. Med. *280*:1194, 1969.
140. Tibbutt, D. A., Davies, J. A., Anderson, J. A., Fletcher, E. W. L., Hamill, J., Holt, J. M., Thomas, M. L., Lee, G. D. J., Miller, G. A. H., Sharp, A. A., and Sutton, G. C.: Compression by controlled clinical trial of streptokinase and heparin in the treatment of life-threatening pulmonary embolism. Br. Med. J. *1*:343, 1974.
141. Szucs, M. M., Brooks, H. L., Grossman, W., Banas, J. S., Meister, S. G., Dexter, L., and Dalen, J. E.: Diagnostic sensitivity of laboratory findings in acute pulmonary embolism. Ann. Intern. Med. *74*:161, 1971.

142. Stein, P. D., Alshabkhoun, S., Hawkins, H. F., Hyland, J. W., and Jarret, C. E.: Right coronary blood flow in acute pulmonary embolism. Am. Heart J. *77*:356, 1969.
143. Vatner, S. F., and Van Citters, R. L.: Effects of acute pulmonary embolism on coronary dynamics in the conscious dog. Am. Heart J. *83*:50, 1972.
144. Symbas, P., and Bonanno, J. A.: Coronary blood flow in acute experimental pulmonary embolization. J. Surg. Res. *10*:377, 1970.
145. Stein, P. D., Alshabkhoun, S., Hatem, C., Pur-Shahriari, A. A., Haynes, W., Harken, D. E., and Dexter, L.: Coronary artery blood flow in acute pulmonary embolism. Am. J. Cardiol. *21*:32, 1968.
146. Dexter, L.: Clinical aspects of pulmonary embolism and their relation to pathophysiology. Bull. Physio-Pathol. Respir. *6*:21, 1970.
147. Romhitt, D. W., Holmes, J. C., and Fowler, N. O.: Mimicry in pulmonary embolism. Geriatrics *27*:73, 1972.
148. Potts, D. E., and Sahn, S. A.: Abdominal manifestations of pulmonary embolism. J.A.M.A. *235*:2835, 1976.
149. Sasahara, A. A., Cannilla, J. E., Morse, R. L., Sidd, J. J., and Tremblay, G. M.: Clinical and physiologic studies in pulmonary thromboembolism. Am. J. Cardiol. *20*:10, 1967.
150. Windebank, W. J., Boyd, G., and Moran, F.: Pulmonary thromboembolism presenting as asthma. Br. Med. J.: *1*:90, 1973.
151. Webster, J. R., Saadeh, G. B., Eggum, P. R., and Suker, J. R.: Wheezing due to pulmonary embolism. Treatment with heparin. N. Engl. J. Med. *274*:931, 1966.
152. Olazabal, F., Roman-Irizarry, L. A., Oms, J. D., Conde, L., and Marchand, E. J.: Pulmonary emboli masquerading as asthma. N. Engl. J. Med. *278*:999, 1968.
153. Shaw, R. A., Schonfeld, S. A., and Whitcomb, M. E.: Pulmonary embolism presenting as coronary insufficiency. Arch. Intern. Med. *141*:651, 1981.
154. McIntyre, K. M., Sasahara, A. A., and Littman, D.: Relation of the electrocardiogram to hemodynamic alterations in pulmonary embolism. Am. J. Cardiol. *30*:205, 1972.
155. Webber, D. M., and Phillips, J. H.: A re-evaluation of electrocardiographic changes accompanying acute pulmonary embolism. J. Med. Sci. *251*:381, 1966.
156. Holford, F. D.: The electrocardiogram in lung diseases. *In* Fishman, A. P. (ed.): Pulmonary Diseases and Disorders. New York, McGraw-Hill Book Co., 1980, p. 139.
157. Levy, S. E., Stein, M., Totten, R. S., Bruderman, I., Wessler, S., and Robin, E. D.: Ventilation perfusion abnormalities in experimental pulmonary embolism. J. Clin. Invest. *44*:1699, 1965.
158. Julian, D. G., Travis, D. M., Robin, E. D., and Crump, C. H.: Effect of pulmonary artery occlusion upon end-tidal CO_2 tension. J. Appl. Physiol. *15*:87, 1960.
159. Fisher, S. R., Duranceau, A., Floyd, R. D., and Wolfe, W. G.: Comparative changes in ventilatory dead space following micro and massive pulmonary emboli. J. Surg. Res. *20*:195, 1976.
160. Levy, S. E., and Simmons, D. H.: Redistribution of alveolar ventilation following pulmonary thromboembolism in the dog. J. Appl. Physiol. *36*:60, 1974.
161. Levy, S. E., and Simmons, D. H.: Mechanism of arterial hypoxemia following pulmonary thromboembolism in dogs. J. Appl. Physiol. *39*:41, 1975.
162. Colp, C. R., and Williams, M. H., Jr.: Pulmonary functions following pulmonary embolization. Am. Rev. Respir. Dis. *85*:799, 1962.
163. Robin, E. D., Forkner, C. E., Bromberg, P. A., Croteau, J. R., and Travis, D. M.: Alveolar gas exchange in clinical pulmonary embolism. N. Engl. J. Med. *262*:283, 1960.
164. Robin, E. D., Julian, D. G., Travis, D. M., and Crump, C. H.: A physiologic approach to the diagnosis of acute pulmonary embolism. N. Engl. J. Med. *260*:586, 1959.
165. Bass, H., Heckscher, T., and Anthonisen, N. R.: Regional pulmonary gas exchange in patients with pulmonary embolism. Clin. Sci. *33*:355, 1967.
166. Stanek, V., Widimsky, J., and Jebavy, P.: Respiratory function in recurrent pulmonary embolism. Respiration *30*:223, 1973.
167. Daum, S.: The diffusing capacity of the lungs in pulmonary embolism. Respiration *26*:8, 1969.
168. Wilson, J. E., III, Pierce, A. K., Johnson, R. L., Jr., Winga, E. R., Harrell, W. R., Curry, G. C., and Mullins, C. B.: Hypoxemia in pulmonary embolism, a clinical study. J. Clin. Invest. *50*:481, 1971.
169. Morgan, T. E., and Edmunds, L. H., Jr.: Pulmonary artery occlusion. III. Biochemical alterations. J. Appl. Physiol. *22*:1012, 1967.
170. Kafer, E. R.: Respiratory function in pulmonary thromboembolic disease. Am. J. Med. *47*:904, 1969.
171. Jones, N. L., and Goodwin, J. F.: Respiratory function in pulmonary thromboembolic disorders. Br. Med. J. *1*:1089, 1965.
172. Nadel, J. A., Gold, W. M., and Burgess, S. H.: Early diagnosis of chronic pulmonary vascular obstruction. Value of pulmonary function tests. Am. J. Med. *44*:16, 1968.
173. Williams, J. R., and Wilcox, W. C.: Pulmonary embolism: Roentgenographic and angiographic considerations. Am. J. Roentgenol. *89*:333, 1963.
174. Figley, M. M., Gerdes, A. J., and Ricketts, H. J.: Radiographic aspects of pulmonary embolism. Semin. Roentgenol. *2*:389, 1967.
175. Fleischner, F. G.: Roentgenology of the pulmonary infarct. Semin. Roentgenol. *2*:61, 1967.
176. Lamas, R., and Swenson, E. W.: Diagnostic clues in pulmonary thromboembolism evaluated by angiographic and ventilation blood flow studies. Thorax *20*:327, 1965.
177. Weiner, S. N., Edelstein, J., and Charms, B. L.: Observations on pulmonary embolism and the pulmonary angiogram. Am. J. Roentgenol. *98*:859, 1966.
178. Fleischner, F. G.: Unilateral pulmonary embolism with increased compensatory circulation through the unoccluded lung: Roentgen observations. Radiology *73*:591, 1959.
179. Fleischner, F. G.: Pulmonary embolism. Clin. Radiol. *13*:169, 1962.
180. Chrispin, A. R., Goodwin, J. F., and Steiner, R.: The radiology of obliterative pulmonary hypertension and thromboembolism. Br. J. Radiol. *36*:705, 1963.
181. Teplick, J. G., Haskin, M. E., and Steinberg, S. B.: Changes in the main pulmonary artery segment following pulmonary embolism. Am. J. Roentgenol. *92*:557, 1964.
182. Smith, G. T., Dammin, G. J., and Dexter, L.: Postmortem arteriographic studies of the human lung in pulmonary embolization. J.A.M.A. *188*:143, 1964.
183. Dalen, J. E., Haffajee, C. I., Alpert, J. S., Howe, J. P., III, Ockene, I. S., and Paraskos, J. A.: Pulmonary embolism, pulmonary hemorrhage, and pulmonary infarction. N. Engl. J. Med. *296*:1431, 1977.
184. Tsao, M. S., Schraufnagel, D., and Wang, N.-S.: Pathogenesis of pulmonary Infarction. Am. J. Med. *72*:599, 1982.
185. Ellis, F. H., Jr., Grindlay, J. H., and Edwards, J. E.: The bronchial arteries. II. Their role in pulmonary embolism and infarction. Surgery *31*:167, 1952.
186. Stein, G. N., Chen, J. T., Goldstein, F., Israel, H. L., and Finkelstein, A.: The importance of chest roentgenography in the diagnosis of pulmonary embolism. Am. J. Roentgenol. *81*:255, 1959.
187. Castleman, B.: Pathologic observations on pulmonary infarction in man. *In* Sasahara, A. A., and Stein, M. (eds.): Pulmonary Embolic Disease. New York, Grune and Stratton, 1965, p. 86.
188. Vidal, E., LeVeen, H. H., Yarnoz, M., and Piccone, V. A., Jr.: Lung abscess secondary to pulmonary infarction. Ann. Thorac. Surg. *6*:557, 1971.
189. Scharf, J., Nahair, A. M., Munk, J., and Lichtig, C.: Aseptic cavitation in pulmonary infarction. Chest *59*:456, 1971.
190. Levin, L., and Kernohan, J. W.: Pulmonary abscess secondary to bland pulmonary infarction. Dis. Chest. *14*:218, 1948.
191. Chester, E. M., and Krause, G. R.: Lung abscess secondary to aseptic pulmonary infarction. Radiology *39*:647, 1942.
192. McFadden, E. R., Jr., and Luparello, F.: Bronchopleural fistula complicating massive pulmonary infarction. Thorax *24*:500, 1969.
193. Fraser, R. G., and Paré, J. A. P.: Diagnosis of Diseases of the Chest. Vol. 2. Philadelphia, W. B. Saunders Co., 1970.
194. McNeil, B. J.: A diagnostic strategy using ventilation-perfusion studies in patients suspect for pulmonary embolism. J. Nucl. Med. *17*:613, 1976.
195. Wagner, H. N., Jr., Sabiston, D. C., Jr., McAfee, J. G., Tow, D. E., and Stern, H. S.: Diagnosis of massive pulmonary embolism in man by radioisotope scanning. N. Engl. J. Med. *271*:377, 1964.
196. Gilday, D. L., Poulouse, K. P., and Deland, F. H.: Accuracy of detection of pulmonary embolism by lung scanning correlated with pulmonary angiography. Am. J. Roentgenol. Radium Ther. Nucl. Med. *115*:732, 1972.
197. McNeil, B. J., Holman, L., and Adelstein, S. J.: The scintigraphic definition of pulmonary embolism. J.A.M.A. *227*:753, 1974.
198. Moses, D. C., Silver, T. M., and Bookstein, J. J.: The complementary roles of chest radiography, lung scanning and selective pulmonary angiography in the diagnosis of pulmonary embolism. Circulation *49*:179, 1974.
199. Bell, W. R., and Simon, T. L.: A comparative analysis of pulmonary perfusion scans with pulmonary angiograms. Am. Heart J. *92*:700, 1976.
200. DeNardo, C. L., Goodwin, D. A., Ravasini, R., and Dietrich, P. A.: The ventilatory lung scan in the diagnosis of pulmonary embolism. N. Engl. J. Med. *282*:1334, 1970.
201. Tow, D. E., and Wagner, H. N., Jr.: Recovery of pulmonary arterial blood flow in patients with pulmonary embolism. N. Engl. J. Med. *276*:1053, 1967.
202. Paraskos, J. A., Aldestein, S. J., Smith, R. E., Rickman, F. D., Grossman, W., Dexter, L., and Dalen, J.: Late prognosis of acute pulmonary embolism. N. Engl. J. Med. *289*:55, 1973.
203. McNeil, B. J.: A diagnostic strategy using ventilation-perfusion studies in patients suspect for pulmonary embolism. J. Nucl. Med. *17*:613, 1976.
204. Cheely, R., McCartney, W. H., Perry, J. R., Delaney, D. J., Bustad, L., Wynia, V. H., and Griggs, T. R.: The role of non-invasive tests versus pulmonary angiography in the diagnosis of pulmonary embolism. Am. J. Med. *70*:17, 1981.
205. Moser, K. M., Harsanyi, P., Rius-Garriga, G., Guisan, M., Landis, G. A., and Miale, A.: Assessment of pulmonary photoscanning and angiography in experimental pulmonary embolism. Circulation *39*:663, 1969.
206. Isawa, T., Wasserman, K., and Taplin, G. V.: Variability of lung scans following pulmonary embolization. Am. Rev. Respir. Dis. *101*:207, 1970.
207. Moser, K. M., Longo, A. M., Ashburn, W. L., and Guisan, M.: Spurious scintiphotographic recurrence of pulmonary emboli. Am. J. Med. *55*:434, 1973.
208. Dalen, J. E., Brooks, H. C., Johnson, L. W., Meister, S. G., Szücs, M. M., Jr., and Dexter, L.: Pulmonary angiography in acute pulmonary embolism: Indications, techniques, and results in 367 patients. Am. Heart J. *81*:175, 1971.
209. Sasahara, A. A., Stein, M., Simon, M., and Littman, D.: Pulmonary angiography in the diagnosis of thromboembolic disease. N. Engl. J. Med. *270*:1075, 1964.
210. Stein, P. D., O'Connor, J. F., Dalen, J. E., Pur-Shahriari, A. A., Hoppin, F. G., Jr., Hammond, D. T., Haynes, F. W., Fleischner, F. G., and Dexter, L.: The angiographic diagnosis of acute pulmonary embolism: Evaluation of criteria. Am. Heart J. *73*:730, 1967.
211. Mills, S. R., Jackson, D. C., Older, R. A., Heaston, D. K., and Moore, R. V.: The incidence, etiologies, and avoidance of complications of pulmonary angiography in a large series. Diagn. Radiol. *136*:295, 1980.
212. Wacker, W. E., Rosenthal, M., Snodgrass, P. J., and Amador, E.: A triad for the diagnosis of pulmonary embolism and infarction. J.A.M.A. *178*:8, 1961.

213. Schonell, M. E., Crompton, G. K., Forshall, J. M., and Whitby, L. G.: Failure to differentiate pulmonary infarction from pneumonia by biochemical tests. Br. Med. J. *1*:1146, 1966.
214. Bynum, L., Crotty, C. M., and Wilson, J. E., III: Diagnostic value of tests of fibrin metabolism in patients predisposed to pulmonary embolism. Arch. Intern. Med. *139*:283, 1979.
215. Moser, K. L.: Pulmonary thromboembolism. *In* Petersdorf, P., et al. (eds.): Harrison's Principles of Internal Medicine. 10th ed. New York, McGraw-Hill Book Co., 1983, p. 1248.
216. Barritt, D. W., and Jordan, S. C.: Anticoagulant drugs in the treatment of pulmonary embolism. A controlled trial. Lancet *1*:1309, 1960.
217. Kernahan, R. J., and Todd, C.: Heparin therapy in thromboembolic disease. Lancet *1*:621, 1966.
218. Colman, R. W.: Prophylaxis and treatment of thromboembolism based on pathophysiology of clotting mechanisms. *In* Fishman, A. P. (ed.): Pulmonary Diseases and Disorders. New York, McGraw-Hill Book Co., 1980, p. 827.
219. Deykin, D.: Current status of anticoagulant therapy. Am. J. Med. *72*:659, 1982.
220. Sasahara, A. A.: Therapy for pulmonary embolism. J.A.M.A. *229*:1975, 1974.
221. Glazier, R. L., and Crowell, E. B.: Randomized prospective trial of continuous vs. intermittent heparin therapy. J.A.M.A. *236*:1365, 1976.
222. Salzman, E. W., Deykin, D., Mayer-Shapiro, R., and Rosenberg, R.: Management of heparin therapy: Controlled prospective trial. N. Engl. J. Med. *292*:1046, 1975.
223. Wilson, J. E., Bynum, L. J., and Parkey, R. W.: Heparin therapy in venous thromboembolism. Am. J. Med. *70*:808, 1981.
224. O'Sullivan, E. F.: Duration of anticoagulant therapy in venous thromboembolism. Med. J. Aust. *2*:1104, 1972.
225. Sharma, G. V. R. K., Cella, G., Parisi, A. F., and Sasahara, A. A.: Thrombolytic therapy. N. Engl. J. Med. *306*:1268, 1982.
226. Donaldson, M. C., Wirthlin, L. S., and Donaldson, G. A.: Thirty-year experience with surgical interruption of the inferior vena cava for prevention of pulmonary embolism. Ann. Surg. *191*:367, 1980.
227. Silver, D., and Sabiston, D. C.: The role of vena caval interruption in the management of pulmonary embolism. Surgery *77*:1, 1975.
228. Mobin-Uddin, K., Callard, G. M., Bolooki, H., Rubinson, R., Michie, D., and Jude, J. R.: Transvenous caval interruption with umbrella filter. N. Engl. J. Med. *286*:55, 1972.
229. Gurewich, U., Thomas, D. P., and Rabinov, K. R.: Pulmonary embolism after ligation of the inferior vena cava. N. Engl. J. Med. *274*:1350, 1966.
230. Cooley, D. A., and Beall, A. C.: Embolectomy for acute massive pulmonary embolism. Surg. Gynecol. Obstet. *126*:805, 1968.
231. Warren, R.: The current status of pulmonary embolectomy. *In* Sasahara, A. A., and Stein, M. (eds.): Pulmonary Embolic Disease. New York, Grune and Stratton, 1965, p. 283.
232. Alpert, J. S., Smith, R. E., Ockene, I. S., Askenazi, J., Dexter, L., and Dalen, J. E.: Treatment of massive pulmonary embolism: The role of pulmonary embolectomy. Am. Heart J. *89*:413, 1975.
233. McDonald, I. G., Hirsh, J., Hale, G. S., Cade, J. F., and McCarthy, R. A.: Isoproterenol in massive pulmonary embolism: Hemodynamic and clinical effects. Med. J. Aust. *2*:201, 1968.
234. Miller, R. R., Lies, J. E., Carretta, R. F., Wampold, D. B., DeNardo, G. L., Krans, J. F., Amsterdam, E. A., and Mason, D. T.: Prevention of lower extremity venous thrombosis by early mobilization. Confirmation in patients with acute myocardial infarction by ^{125}I-fibrinogen uptake and venography. Ann. Intern. Med. *84*:700, 1976.
235. Sevitt, S., and Gallagher, N. G.: Prevention of venous thrombosis and pulmonary embolism in injured patients. Lancet *2*:981, 1959.
236. Kakkar, U. V., Corrigan, T. P., and Fossard, D. P.: Prevention of fatal postoperative embolism by low dose heparin: An international multicenter trial. Lancet *2*:45, 1975.
237. Wessler, S., and Yin, E. T.: Theory and practice of minidose heparin in surgical patients: A status report. Circulation *47*:671, 1973.
238. Evarts, M., and Alfide, J.: Thromboembolism after total hip reconstruction: Failure of low doses of heparin in prevention. J.A.M.A. *225*:515, 1973.
239. Horowitz, R. E., and Tatter, D.: Lethal pulmonary embolism. *In* Sherry, S., Brinkhous, K. M., and Genton, E. (eds.): Thrombosis. Washington, D.C., National Academy of Sciences, 1961, p. 19.
240. Howe, M., Sevitt, S., and Thomas, D. P.: Venous Thrombosis and Pulmonary Embolism. Cambridge, Harvard University Press, 1970.
241. Donaldson, G. A., Williams, C., Scannell, J. G., and Shaw, R. S.: Reappraisal of application of the Trendelenburg operation to massive fatal embolism. N. Engl. J. Med. *268*:171, 1963.
242. Alpert, J. S., Smith, R., Carlson, J., Ockene, I. S., Dexter, L., and Dalen, J. E.: Mortality in patients treated for pulmonary embolism. J.A.M.A. *236*:1477, 1976.
243. Austin, J. H. M., Wilner, G. D., and Dominguez, C.: Natural history of pulmonary thromboemboli in dogs. Radiology *116*:519, 1975.

CHRONIC COR PULMONATE

244. Fishman, A. P.: Cor pulmonale. *In* Fishman, A. P. (ed.): Pulmonary Diseases and Disorders. New York, McGraw-Hill Book Co., 1980, p. 853.
245. Respiratory Disease. Task force report on prevention, control and education. Washington, D.C., U.S. Department of Health Education and Welfare, Public Health Service, National Institute of Health, 1977, p. 83.
246. Stuart-Harris, C. H., Twidle, R. H. S., and Clifton, M. A.: Hospital study of congestive heart failure with special reference to cor pulmonale. Br. Med. J. *2*:201, 1959.
247. Inter-Society Commission for Heart Disease Resources: Primary prevention of pulmonary heart disease. Circulation *41*:A-17, 1970.
247a. Berbel, L. N., and Miro, R. E.: Pulmonary hypertension in the pathogenesis of cor pulmonale. Cardiovasc. Rev. *4*:359, 1983.
248. Wilhelmsen, L., Selander, S., Sonderholm, B., Paulin, S., Varnauskas, E., and Werko, L.: Recurrent pulmonary embolism. Medicine *42*:335, 1963.
249. Hicken, P., Brewer, D., and Heath, D.: The relationship between the weight of the right ventricle of the heart and the internal surface area and number of alveoli in the human lung in emphysema. J. Pathol. Bacteriol. *92*:529, 1966.
250. Thurlbeck, W. M., Henderson, J. A., Fraser, R. G., and Bates, D. V.: Chronic obstructive lung disease. A comparison between clinical, roentgenologic, functional and morphologic criteria in chronic bronchitis, emphysema, asthma and bronchiectasis. Medicine *48*:81, 1970.
251. Edwards, J. E.: Pathology of chronic pulmonary hypertension. Pathol. Annu. *9*:1, 1974.
252. Wagenvoort, C. A., and Wagenvoort, N.: Hypoxic pulmonary vascular lesions in man at high altitude and in patients with chronic respiratory disease. Pathol. Microbiol. *39*:276, 1973.
253. Semmens, M., and Reid, L.: Pulmonary arterial muscularity and right ventricular hypertrophy in chronic bronchitis and emphysema. Br. J. Dis. Chest. *68*:253, 1974.
254. Oppenheimer, E. H., and Esterly, J. R.: Medial mucoid lesions of the pulmonary artery in cystic fibrosis, pulmonary hypertension, and other disorders. Lab. Invest. *30*:411, 1974.
255. Wagenvoort, C. A., Heath, D., and Edwards, J. E.: The Pathology of the Pulmonary Vasculature. Springfield, Ill., Charles C Thomas, 1964.
256. Clausen, K. P., and Geer, J. C.: Hypertensive pulmonary arteritis. Am. J. Dis. Child. *118*:718, 1969.
257. Roos, A.: Poiseuille's law and its limitation in vascular systems. *In* Grover, R. F. (ed.): Progress in Research in Emphysema and Chronic Bronchitis. Basel, Karger, 1963, p. 32.
258. Wells, R. E., and Merrill, E. W.: Influence of flow properties of blood upon viscosity hematocrit relationships. J. Clin. Invest. *41*:1591, 1962.
259. Saldana, M. A., Harley, R. A., Liebow, A. A., and Carrington, C. B.: Experimental extreme pulmonary hypertension and vascular disease in relation to polycythemia. Am. J. Pathol. *52*:935, 1968.
260. Balchum, O. J., Jung, R. C., Turner, A. F., and Jacobson, G.: Pulmonary artery to vein shunts in obstructive pulmonary disease. Am. J. Med. *43*:178, 1967.
261. Boushy, S. F., North, L. B., and Trice, J. A.: The bronchial arteries in chronic obstructive pulmonary disease. Am. J. Med. *46*:506, 1969.
262. Marcus, J. H., McLean, R. L., Duffell, G. M., and Ingram, R. H.: Exercise performance in relation to the pathophysiologic type of chronic obstructive pulmonary disease. Am. J. Med. *49*:14, 1970.
263. Harris, P., Segal, N., and Bishop, J. M.: The relation between pressure and flow in the pulmonary circulation in normal subjects and in patients with chronic bronchitis and mitral stenosis. Cardiovasc. Res. *2*:73, 1968.
264. Burrows, B., Kettel, L. J., Niden, A. H., Rabinowitz, M., and Diener, C. F.: Patterns of cardiovascular dysfunction in chronic obstructive lung disease. N. Engl. J. Med. *286*:912, 1972.
265. Whitaker, W.: Pulmonary hypertension in congestive heart failure complicating chronic lung disease. Q. J. Med. *23*:57, 1954.
266. Ferrer, M. I.: Disturbances in the circulation in patients with cor pulmonale. Bull. N.Y. Acad. Med. *41*:942, 1965.
267. Williams, J. F., and Behnke, R. H.: The effect of pulmonary emphysema upon cardiopulmonary hemodynamics at rest and during exercise. Ann. Intern. Med. *60*:824, 1964.
268. Emirgil, C., Sobol, B. J., Herbert, W. H., and Trout, K. W.: Routine pulmonary function studies as a key to the status of the lesser circulation in chronic obstructive pulmonary disease. Am. J. Med. *50*:191, 1971.
269. Khaja, F., and Parker, J. D.: Right and left ventricular performance in chronic obstructive lung disease. Am. Heart J. *82*:319, 1971.
270. Berger, H. S., Matthay, R. A., Loke, J., Marshall, R. C., Gottschalk, A., and Zaret, B. L.: Assessment of cardiac performance with quantitative radionuclide angiocardiography: Right ventricular ejection fraction with reference to findings in chronic obstructive pulmonary disease. Am. J. Cardiol. *41*:897, 1978.
271. Olvey, S. K., Redufo, L. A., Stevens, P. M., Deaton, W. J., and Miller, R. R.: First pass radionuclide assessment of right and left ventricular ejection fraction in chronic pulmonary disease. Effect of oxygen upon exercise response. Chest *78*:4, 1980.
272. Stein, P. D., Sabbah, H. N., Anbe, D. T., and Marzilli, M.: Performance of the failing and non-failing right ventricle of patients with pulmonary hypertension. Am. J. Cardiol. *44*:1050, 1979.
272a. Kawakami, Y., Kishi, F., Yamamoto, H., and Miyamoto, K.: Relation of oxygen delivery, mixed venous oxygenation and pulmonary hemodynamics to prognosis in chronic obstructive pulmonary disease. N. Engl. J. Med. *308*: 1045, 1983.
272b. Bergofsky, E. H.: Tissue oxygen delivery and cor pulmonale in chronic obstructive pulmonary disease. N. Engl. J. Med. *308*:1092, 1983.
273. Samet, P., Fritts, H. W., Jr., Fishman, A. P., and Cournand, A.: The blood volume in heart disease. Medicine *36*:211, 1957.
274. Turino, G. M., Edelman, N. H., Richards, E. C., and Fishman, A. P.: Extravascular lung water in cor pulmonale. Bull. Physiol. Pathol. Respir. *4*:47, 1968.
275. Chidsey, C. A., Kaiser, G. A., Sonnenblick, E. H., Spann, J. F., and Braun-

wald, E.: Cardiac norepinephrine stores in experimental heart failure in the dog. J. Clin. Invest. *43*:2386, 1964.
276. Chandler, B. M., Sonnenblick, E. H., Spann, J. F., Jr., and Pool, P. E.: Association of depressed myofibrillar adenosine triphosphatase and reduced contractility in experimental heart failure. Circ. Res. *21*:717, 1967.
277. Buccino, R. A., Harris, E., Spann, J. F., Jr., and Sonnenblick, E. H.: Response of myocardial connective tissues to development of experimental hypertrophy. Am. J. Physiol. *216*:425, 1969.
278. Kelly, D. T., Spotnitz, H. M., Beiser, G. D., Pierce, J. E., and Epstein, S. E.: Effects of chronic right ventricular volume and pressure loading on left ventricular performance. Circulation *44*:403, 1971.
279. Stool, E. W., Mullins, C. B., Leshin, S. J., and Mitchell, J. H.: Dimensional changes of the left ventricle during acute pulmonary arterial hypertension in dogs. Am. J. Cardiol. *33*:868, 1974.
280. Hecht, H. H., Kuida, H., and Tsagaris, T. J.: Brisket disease. IV. Impairment of left ventricular function in a form of cor pulmonale. Trans. Assoc. Am. Physicians *75*:263, 1962.
281. Fluck, D. C., Chandrasekar, R. G., and Gardner, F. U.: Left ventricular hypertrophy in chronic bronchitis. Br. Heart J. *28*:92, 1966.
282. Murphy, M. L., Adamson, J., and Hutcheson, F.: Left ventricular hypertrophy in patients with chronic bronchitis and emphysema. Ann. Intern. Med. *81*:307, 1974.
283. Rao, S. B., Cohn, K. E., Eldridge, F. L., and Hancock, E. W.: Left ventricular failure secondary to chronic pulmonary disease. Am. J. Med. *45*:229, 1968.
284. Jezek, V., and Schrijen, F.: Left ventricular function in chronic obstructive pulmonary disease with and without cardiac failure. Clin. Sci. Mol. Med. *45*:267, 1973.
285. Baum, G. L., Schwartz, A., Llamas, R., and Castillo, C.: Left ventricular function in chronic obstructive lung disease. N. Engl. J. Med. *285*:361, 1971.
286. Frank, M. J., Weisser, A. B., Moschos, C. B., and Levinson, G. E.: Left ventricular function, metabolism, and blood flow in chronic cor pulmonale. Circulation *48*:798, 1973.
287. Williams, J. F., Childress, R. H., Boyd, D. L., Higgs, L. M., and Behnke, R. H.: Left ventricular function in patients with chronic obstructive pulmonary disease. J. Clin. Invest. *47*:1143, 1968.
288. Unger, K., Shaw, D., Karliner, J. S., Crawford, M., O'Rourke, R. A., and Moser, K. M.: Evaluation of left ventricular performance in acutely ill patients with chronic obstructive lung disease. Chest *68*:135, 1975.
289. Steele, P., Ellis, J. H., Jr., Van Dyke, D., Sutton, F., Creagh, E., and Davies, H.: Left ventricular ejection fraction in severe chronic obstructive airways disease. Am. J. Med. *59*:21, 1975.
290. Christianson, L. C., Shah, A., and Fisher, V. J.: Quantitative left ventricular cineangiography in patients with chronic obstructive pulmonary disease. Am. J. Med. *66*:399, 1979.
291. Gabinski, C., Courty, G., Besse, P., and Castaing, R.: Left ventricular function in chronic obstructive lung disease. Bull. Eur. Physiopathol. Resp. *15*:755, 1979.
292. Slutsky, A., Hooper, W., Ackerman, W., Ashburn, W., Gerber, R., Moser, K., and Karliner, J.: Evaluation of left ventricular function in chronic pulmonary disease by exercise gated equilibrium radionuclide angiography. Am. Heart J. *101*:414, 1981.
293. Burrows, B., Fletcher, C. M., Heard, B. E., Jones, N. L., and Wootliff, S. S.: Emphysematous and bronchial types of chronic airways obstruction: Clinicopathological study of patients in London and Chicago. Lancet *1*:830, 1966.
294. Mitchell, R. S., and Filley, G. F.: Chronic obstructive bronchopulmonary disease. I. Clinical features. Am. Rev. Respir. Dis. *89*:360, 1964.
295. Mitchel, R. S., Vincent, T. N., and Filley, G. F.: Chronic obstructive bronchopulmonary disease. IV. The clinical and physiological differential of chronic bronchitis and emphysema. Am. J. Med. Sci. *247*:513, 1964.
296. Burrows, B., Strauss, R. H., and Niden, A. H.: Chronic obstructive lung disease. III. Interrelationships of pulmonary function data. Am. Rev. Respir. Dis. *91*:861, 1965.
297. Ingram, R.: Chronic bronchitis, emphysema, and chronic airways obstruction. *In* Petersdorf, R., et al. (eds.): Harrison's Principles of Internal Medicine. 10th ed. New York, McGraw-Hill Book Co., 1983, p. 1545.
298. Santa Cruz, R., Landa, J., Hirsch, J., and Sackner, M. A.: Tracheal mucous velocity in normal man and patients with obstructive lung disease: Effects of terbutaline. Am. Rev. Respir. Dis. *109*:458, 1974.
299. Parker, J. O., Kelkar, K., and West, R. S.: Hemodynamic effects of aminophylline in cor pulmonale. Circulation *33*:17, 1966.
300. Matthay, R. A., Berger, H. J., Locke, J., Gottschalk, A., and Zaret, B. L.: Effect of aminophylline upon right and left ventricular performance in chronic obstructive pulmonary disease. Noninvasive assessment by radionuclide angiocardiography. Am. J. Med. *65*:903, 1978.
301. Burrows, B.: Arterial oxygenation and pulmonary hemodynamics in patients with chronic airways obstruction. (Proceedings of Conference on the Scientific Basis of Respiratory Therapy.) Am. Rev. Respir. Dis. *110*:64, 1974.
302. Stark, R. D., Finnegan, P., and Bishop, J. M.: Daily requirements of oxygen to reverse pulmonary hypertension in patients with chronic bronchitis. Br. Med. J. *3*:724, 1972.
303. Nocturnal Oxygen Therapy Trial Group. Continuous or Nocturnal oxygen therapy in hypoxemic chronic obstructive lung disease. A clinical trial. Ann. Intern. Med. *93*:391, 1980.
304. Neff, T. A., and Petty, T. L.: Longterm oxygen therapy in chronic airway obstruction: Mortality in relationship to cor pulmonale, hypoxia, and hypercapnia. Ann. Intern. Med. *72*:621, 1970.
305. Dayton, L. M., McCullough, R. E., Scheinhorn, D. J., and Weil, J. V.: Symptomatic and pulmonary response to acute phlebotomy in secondary polycythemia. Chest *68*:785, 1975.
306. Rakita, L., Gillespie, D. G., and Sancetta, S. M.: The acute and chronic effects of phlebotomy on general hemodynamics and pulmonary function of patients with secondary polycythemia associated with pulmonary emphysema. Am. Heart J. *70*:466, 1965.
307. Nobel, M. I. M., Trenchard, D., and Guz, A.: The value of diuretics in respiratory failure. Lancet *2*:257, 1966.
308. Rubin, L. J., and Peter, R. H.: Hemodynamics at rest and during exercise after oral hydralazine in patients with cor pulmonale. Am. J. Cardiol. *47*:116, 1981.
309. Packer, M., Greenberg, B., Massiz, B., and Dash, H.: Deleterious effects of hydralazine in patients with pulmonary hypertension. N. Engl. J. Med. *306*:1326, 1982.
310. Green, L. H., and Smith, T. W.: The use of digitalis in patients with pulmonary disease. Ann. Intern. Med. *87*:459, 1977.
311. Mathur, P. N., Powles, A. C. P., Pugsley, S. O., McEwan, M. P., and Campbell, E. J. M.: Effect of digoxin on right ventricular function in severe chronic airway obstruction. Ann. Intern. Med. *95*:283, 1981.
312. Gottlieb, L. S., and Balchum, O. J.: Course of chronic obstructive pulmonary disease following first onset of respiratory failure. Chest *63*:5, 1973.
313. Stevens, P. M., Terplan, M., and Knowles, J. H.: Prognosis of cor pulmonale. N. Engl. J. Med. *269*:1289, 1963.
314. Burrows, B., and Earle, R. H.: Course and prognosis of chronic obstructive lung disease. A prospective study of 200 patients. N. Engl. J. Med. *280*:397, 1969.
315. Mitchell, R. S., Webb, N. C., and Filley, G. F.: Chronic obstructive lung disease. III. Factors influencing prognosis. Am. Rev. Respir. Dis. *89*:878, 1964.
316. Glauser, E. M., Cook, C. D., and Harris, C. B. C.: Bronchiectasis. A review of 187 cases in children with follow-up pulmonary function studies in 58. Acta Paediatr. Scand. (Suppl.)*165*:1, 1966.
317. Reid, L.: Reduction in bronchial subdivisions in bronchiectasis. Thorax *5*:233, 1950.
318. Schwachmann, H.: Cystic fibrosis. *In* Petersdorf, R., et al. (eds.): Harrison's Principles of Internal Medicine. 10th ed. New York, McGraw-Hill Book Co., 1983, p. 1542.
319. Royce, J. W.: Cor pulmonale in infancy and childhood. Report on 34 patients with special reference to the occurrence of pulmonary heart disease in cystic fibrosis of the pancreas. Pediatrics *8*:255, 1951.
320. Lester, L. A., Egge, A. C., Hubbard, V. S., Camerini-Otero, C. S., and Fink, R. J.: Echocardiography in cystic fibrosis: A proposed scoring system. J. Pediatr. *97*:742, 1980.
321. Goldring, R. M., Fishman, A. P., Turino, G. M., Cohen, H. I., Denning, C. R., and Anderson, D. H.: Pulmonary hypertension and cor pulmonale in cystic fibrosis of the pancreas. J. Pediatr. *65*:50, 1964.
322. Ryland, D., and Reed, L.: The pulmonary circulation in cystic fibrosis. Thorax *30*:285, 1975.
323. Wood, R. E., Boat, T. F., and Doershuk, C. F.: Cystic fibrosis: State of the art. Am. Rev. Respir. Dis. *113*:833, 1976.
324. Emirgil, C., Sobol, B. J., Herbert, W. H., and Trout, K.: The lesser circulation in pulmonary fibrosis secondary to sarcoidosis and its relationship to respiratory function. Chest *60*:371, 1971.
325. Enson, Y., Thomas, H. M., III, Bosken, C. H., Wood, J. A., LeRoy, E. C., Blanc, W. A., Wigger, H. J., and Harvey, R. M.: Pulmonary hypertension in interstitial lung disease: Relationship of vascular resistance to abnormal lung structure. Trans. Assoc. Am. Physicians *88*:248, 1975.
326. Irwin, R. S., Martinez-Gonzalez-Rio, J., Thomas, H. M., III, and Fritts, H. W., Jr.: The effect of granulomatous pulmonary disease in dogs on the response of the pulmonary circulation to hypoxia. J. Clin. Invest. *60*:1258, 1977.
327. Keltz, H.: The effect of respiratory muscle dysfunction on pulmonary function in patients with neuromuscular disease. Am. Rev. Respir. Dis. *91*:934, 1965.
328. Newsom Davis, J., Goldman, M., Loh, L., and Casson, M.: Diaphragm function and alveolar hypoventilation. Q. J. Med. *45*:87, 1976.
329. Glenn, W. W. L., Holcomb, W. C., Hogan, J., Matano, I., Gee, J. B. L., Motoyama, E. K., Kim, C. S., Poirier, R. S., and Forbes, G.: Diaphragm pacing by radiofrequency transmission in the treatment of chronic ventilatory insufficiency: Present status. J. Thorac. Cardiovasc. Surg. *66*:505, 1973.
330. Aubier, M., DeTroyer, A., Sampson, M., Macklem, P. T., and Roussos, C.: Aminophylline improves diaphragmatic contractility. N. Engl. J. Med. *305*:249, 1981.
331. Bergofsky, E. H.: Respiratory failure in disorders of the thoracic cage. Am. Rev. Respir. Dis. *119*:643, 1979.
332. Bergofsky, E. H., Turino, G. M., and Fishman, A. P.: Cardiorespiratory failure in kyphoscoliosis. Medicine *38*:263, 1959.
333. Bjure, J., Grimby, G., Kasalicky, J., Lindh, M., and Nachemson, A.: Respiratory impairment and airway closure in patients with untreated idiopathic scoliosis. Thorax *25*:451, 1970.
334. Davies, G., and Reid, L.: Effect of scoliosis on growth of alveoli and pulmonary arteries and on the right ventricle. Arch. Dis. Child. *46*:623, 1971.
335. Westgate, H. D., and Moe, J. H.: Pulmonary function in kyphoscoliosis before and after correction by the Harrington instrumentation method. J. Bone Joint Surg. *51*:935, 1969.
336. Burwell, C. S., Robin, E. D., Whaley, R. D., and Bickelman, A. G.: Extreme obesity associated with alveolar hypoventilation—A Pickwickian syndrome. Am. J. Med. *21*:811, 1956.
337. Rochester, D. F., and Enson, Y.: Current concepts in the pathogenesis of the obesity-hypoventilation syndrome. Am. J. Med. *57*:402, 1974.

338. Zwillich, C. W., Sutton, F. D., Pierson, D. J., Creagh, E. M., and Weil, J. V.: Decreased hypoxic ventilatory drive in the obesity-hypoventilation syndrome. Am. J. Med. *59*:343, 1975.
339. Lyons, H. A., and Huang, C. T.: Therapeutic use of progesterone in alveolar hypoventilation associated with obesity. Am. J. Med. *44*:881, 1968.
340. Sutton, F. D., Zwillich, C. W., Creagh, C. E., Pierson, D. J., and Weil, J. V.: Progesterone for outpatient treatment of pickwickian syndrome. Ann. Intern. Med. *83*:476, 1975.
341. Cherniack, N. S.: Respiratory dysrhythmias during sleep. N. Engl. J. Med. *305*:325, 1981.
342. Guilleminault, C., Tilkian, A., and Dement, W. C.: The sleep apnea syndrome. Annu. Rev. Med. *27*:465, 1976.
343. Buda, A. J., Schroeder, J. S., and Guilleminault, C.: Abnormalities of pulmonary wedge pressures in sleep-induced apnea. Int. J. Cardiol. *1*:67, 1981.
344. Glenn, W. W. L., Gee, J. B. L., Cole, D. R., Farmer, W. C., Shaw, R. K., and Beckman, C. B.: Combined central alveolar hypoventilation and upper airway obstruction. Treatment by tracheostomy and diaphragm pacing. Am. J. Med. *64*:50, 1978.
345. Walsh, R. E., Michaelson, E. D., Harkleroad, L. E., Zighelboim, A., and Sackner, M. A.: Upper airway obstruction in obese patients with sleep disturbance and somnolence. Ann. Intern. Med. *76*:185, 1972.
346. Martin, R. J., Sanders, M. H., Gray, B. A., and Pennock, B. E.: Acute and long-term ventilatory effects of hyperoxia in the adult sleep apnea syndrome. Am. Rev. Respir. Dis. *125*:175, 1982.
347. Mellins, R. B., Balfour, H. H., Jr., Turino, G. M., and Winters, R. W.: Failure of automatic control of ventilation (Ondine's curse). Medicine *49*:487, 1970.
348. Penaloza, D., and Sime, F.: Circulatory dynamics during high altitude pulmonary edema. Am. J. Cardiol. *23*:369, 1969.
349. Monge, C.: Chronic mountain sickness. Physiol. Rev. *23*:148, 1943.
350. Penoloza, D., and Sime, F.: Chronic cor pulmonale due to loss of altitude acclimatization (chronic mountain sickness). Am. J. Med. *50*:728, 1971.
351. Severinghaus, J. W., Bainton, C. R., and Carcelen, A.: Respiratory insensitivity to hypoxia in chronically hypoxic man. Respir. Physiol. *1*:308, 1966.
352. Bland, J. W., Edwards, F. K., and Brainsfield, D.: Pulmonary hypertension and congestive heart failure in children with chronic upper airway obstruction. New concepts and etiologic factors. Am. J. Cardiol. *23*:830, 1969.
353. Noonan, J. A.: Pulmonary heart disease. Pediatr. Clin. North Am. *18*:1255, 1971.
354. Johnson, G. M., and Todd, D. W.: Cor pulmonale in severe Pierre Robin syndrome. Pediatrics *65*:152, 1980.
355. Ingram, R. H., Jr., and Bishop, J. B.: Ventilatory response to carbon dioxide after removal of chronic upper airway obstruction. Am. Rev. Respir. Dis. *102*:645, 1970.
356. Williams, M. H., Jr., Adler, J. J., and Colp, C.: Pulmonary function studies as an aid in the differential diagnosis of pulmonary hypertension. Am. J. Med. *47*:378, 1969.
357. Obeyesekere, I., and Peiris, D.: Pulmonary hypertension and filariasis. Br. Heart J. *36*:676, 1974.
358. Moser, K. M., and Shea, J. G.: The relationship between pulmonary infarction, cor pulmonale, and the sickle states. Am. J. Med. *22*:561, 1957.
359. Heath, D., and Thompson, I. M.: Bronchopulmonary anastomoses in sickle cell anaemia. Thorax *24*:232, 1969.
360. Wagenvoort, C. A.: Pulmonary veno-occlusive disease. Chest *69*:82, 1976.
361. Scheibel, R. L., Dedeker, K. L., Gleason, D. F., Pliego, M., and Kieffer, S. A.: Radiographic and angiographic characteristics of pulmonary veno-occlusive disease. Radiology *103*:47, 1972.
362. Sanderson, J. E., Spiro, S. G., Hendry, A. T., and Turner-Warwick, M.: A case of pulmonary veno-occlusive disease responding to treatment with azathioprine. Thorax *32*:140, 1977.
363. Sokolow, M., and Lyon, T. P.: The ventricular complex in right ventricular hypertrophy as obtained by unipolar precordial and limb leads. Am. Heart J. *38*:273, 1949.
364. Goodwin, J. F., and Abdin, Z. N.: The cardiogram of congenital and acquired right ventricular hypertrophy. Br. Heart J. *21*:523, 1959.
365. Phillips, R.W.: The electrocardiogram in cor pulmonale secondary to pulmonary emphysema: A study of 18 cases proved by autopsy. Am. Heart J. *56*:352, 1958.
366. Kilcoyne, M. M., Davis, A. L., and Ferrer, M. I.: A dynamic electrocardiographic concept useful in the diagnosis of cor pulmonale. Circulation *42*:903, 1970.
367. Padmavati, S., and Raizada, V.: Electrocardiogram in chronic cor pulmonale. Br. Heart J. *34*:658, 1972.
368. Schaeffer, J. W., and Pryor, R.: Pseudo left axis deviation and the $S_1S_2S_3$ syndrome in chronic airway obstruction. Chest *71*:453, 1977.
369. Shmock, C. L., Pomerantz, B., Mitchell, R. S., Pryor, R., and Maisel, J. C.: The electrocardiogram in emphysema with and without airways obstruction. Chest *60*:328, 1971.
370. Kok-Jensen, A.: Simple electrocardiographic features of importance for prognosis in severe chronic bronchial obstruction. Scand. J. Respir. Dis. *56*:273, 1975.

PART IV

HEART DISEASE AND DISEASES OF OTHER ORGAN SYSTEMS

47 GENETICS AND CARDIOVASCULAR DISEASE

by Joseph L. Goldstein, M.D., and Michael S. Brown, M.D.

GENERAL PRINCIPLES OF CARDIOVASCULAR GENETICS

As with diseases affecting other body systems, genetic factors play a significant role in the pathogenesis of most diseases of the heart. In some disorders, such as the Marfan syndrome and familial hypercholesterolemia, the genetic effects are relatively clearly discernible and easy to analyze. In other diseases, such as most forms of congenital heart disease, the role of hereditary factors, although demonstrable, is less clear-cut, and the fundamental genetic mechanisms remain obscure.

In this chapter, we first review the general principles of hereditary disease as they apply to the major forms of heart disease. This is followed by a discussion of those disorders of the cardiovascular system for which a clear-cut genetic etiology has been demonstrated. In discussing a disorder, we have placed the major emphasis on the genetic aspects rather than on the clinical features, which are discussed elsewhere in this book.

MOLECULAR BASIS OF GENE EXPRESSION. All hereditary information is transmitted from parent to offspring through the inheritance of deoxyribonucleic acid (DNA). *DNA* is a linear polymer composed of purine and pyrimidine bases, the sequence of which ultimately determines the sequence of amino acids in every protein molecule made by the body. The four types of bases in DNA are arranged in groups of three, each group forming a code word or codon that signifies a particular amino acid. A *gene* represents the sequence of bases in DNA that codes for the amino acid sequence of a single polypeptide chain of a protein molecule.[1] The gene is the basic unit of heredity that is transmitted to each offspring during the formation of sperm and ova. The recent discovery that genes are not continuous sequences of DNA but consist of coding sequences (exons) interrupted by intervening sequences (introns) has led to a new view of gene expression that is beyond the scope of this chapter (for review, see reference 1).

It is estimated that the amount of DNA in the nucleus of each human cell is sufficient to code for several million genes. The genes are arranged in linear sequence organized into rod-shaped bodies called *chromosomes.* Each human cell contains 46 chromosomes, arranged in 23 pairs, one member of each pair having been derived from each of the individual's parents. Thus, each individual inherits two copies of each chromosome and hence two copies of each gene. The site at which a gene is located on a particular chromosome is termed the *genetic locus.* When a gene occupying a genetic locus exists in two or more different forms, these alternate forms of the gene are referred to as *alleles.*

A given gene always resides at a specified genetic locus on one particular chromosome. For example, the genetic locus for the human Rh blood group is on chromosome No. 1; at this chromosomal site in each individual there are two Rh genes, one on chromosome No. 1 derived from the mother and the other on chromosome No. 1 derived from the father. When both genes at the same genetic locus are identical, the individual is a *homozygote.* When the two genes differ (i.e., two alleles are present at the locus), the individual is a *heterozygote.* Each individual is homozygous at some loci and heterozygous at others.

Considerable progress has been made in recent years in delineating the human gene map. The chromosomal location of more than 350 genes is now known.[2]

MUTATION AS THE ORIGIN OF GENETIC DISEASE. A *mutation* is a stable, heritable alteration in DNA. Although the causes of mutation in human beings are largely unknown, a variety of environmental agents, such as radiation, viruses, and chemicals, are among the factors that are implicated.

Mutations can involve a visible alteration in the structure of a chromosome, such as a deletion or translocation of a portion of a chromosome, or they can involve a minute change in one of the purine or pyrimidine bases of a single gene. Most commonly, such "point" mutations consist of the substitution of one base for another, thus changing the meaning of the codon containing that base; hence, their designation as *missense mutations.* Of all of the human mutations so far elucidated, the vast majority involve such single-base changes. These missense mutations cause the substitution of one amino acid for another in the protein specified by the mutant gene. Such substitution can have little effect on the function of the protein, or it can totally eliminate all function. If the protein that is involved happens to be an enzyme, the loss of function may produce a metabolic disease.

CELLULAR MECHANISM BY WHICH MUTANT GENES PRODUCE DISEASES. Critical to the modern understanding of heredity is the concept that the only information transmitted from generation to generation is the sequence of bases in DNA and that these sequences, in turn, specify only the primary structure of RNA and protein molecules. All other chemical reactions within a cell—such as the synthesis of complex lipids and carbohydrates, the formation of membranes and other cellular organelles, the accumulation and partitioning of inorganic ions, and so on—occur as a secondary consequence of the action of specific proteins. Many of these proteins are enzymes that catalyze the biochemical conversion of one molecule into another. Others are structural proteins, such as collagen and elastin, and still others are regulatory proteins that dictate how much of each enzyme and each structural protein is to be made.

Since proteins are the cellular molecules the structures of which are encoded by genes, mutations in genes exert their deleterious effects by altering the structure of enzymes, structural proteins, or regulatory proteins. Thus, in a disease like Pompe disease (Type II glycogen storage disease), massive accumulation of glycogen in the heart is due not to a primary structural abnormality in the polysaccharide glycogen but to a structural abnormality in a protein, acid maltase, a lysosomal enzyme that is required to degrade glycogen.

GENETIC HETEROGENEITY. This exists when two or more mutations can produce a similar clinical syndrome. It is now believed that most, if not all, hereditary diseases, when carefully analyzed, will be shown to be genetically heterogeneous.[3]

Genetic heterogeneity may result from the existence of mutations at a single genetic locus (allelic mutations) or from mutations at different genetic loci (nonallelic mutations). In some cases of heterogeneity, not merely does the genetic locus differ but the mode of inheritance will also differ. For example, atrial septal defect can be inherited by an autosomal dominant mechanism in some families and by a multifactorial mechanism in other families.

CATEGORIES OF GENETIC DISORDERS AFFECTING THE CARDIOVASCULAR SYSTEM

Genetic diseases of the cardiovascular system, like all genetic disorders, generally fall into one of three categories:

1. *Chromosomal disorders* involve the lack, excess, or abnormal arrangement of one or more chromosomes, producing excessive or deficient genetic material and affecting many genes.
2. *Mendelian* or *single-gene disorders* are determined primarily by a single mutant gene that is transmitted to offspring in a predictable way. As a result, these disorders display simple (mendelian) inheritance patterns which can be classified into autosomal dominant, autosomal recessive, or X-linked types.
3. *Multifactorial disorders* are caused by an interaction of multiple genes and multiple exogenous or environmental factors. Although many of these multifactorial disorders, such as coronary artery disease (CAD) and most types of congenital heart disease, "run in families," the inheritance pattern is complex and unpredictable. In general, the risk to relatives is much less than that seen in the single-gene disorders. As discussed below, each of these three categories of genetic disease presents different problems with respect to causation, prevention, diagnosis, genetic counseling, and treatment.

Chromosomal Disorders

As noted, the number of chromosomes in normal individuals is 46, of which 44 represent the 22 pairs of *auto-*

somes and the other 2 are the *sex chromosomes.* Females have 2 X chromosomes (XX) and males have 1 X chromosome and 1 Y chromosome (XY). Each of the 22 pairs of autosomes and the 2 sex chromosomes can be identified microscopically on the basis of size, location of the centromere (which divides the chromosome into arms of equal or unequal length), and unique banding pattern (which is determined after treatment with special dyes and proteolytic enzymes).

Of the two most common chromosomal disorders causing heart disease, one results from an extra chromosome and the other results from a deficiency of one chromosome. Trisomy 21 (Down syndrome or mongolism) is characterized by the presence of three rather than two copies of chromosome 21, and the common form of Turner syndrome is characterized by the presence of one X chromosome rather than two X's or an X and a Y. The abnormality in both of these disorders appears to arise through *nondisjunction,* either during meiosis in one parent (i.e., in spermatogenesis or oogenesis) or in the first mitotic cleavage of the zygote. In meiotic nondisjunction, a pair of chromosomes does not separate normally so that both members of the pair (or none) pass into one gamete. When an additional copy of the chromosome is added during fertilization, three copies of the same chromosome (or only one) are in the new zygote instead of the pair found in normal persons.

The detected frequency of chromosomal aberrations among unselected newborn infants is 1 in 200 (0.5 per cent), whereas among first trimester spontaneous abortions the frequency of chromosomal defects is as high as 50 per cent. Thus, the vast majority of chromosomal abnormalities are lost in early fetal life. In most instances chromosomal disorders occur as new mutations; both parents are usually normal, and the risk of recurrence to relatives is usually low.

Single-gene Disorders

Disorders caused by the transmission of a single mutant gene show one of three simple (or mendelian) patterns of inheritance: (1) autosomal dominant, (2) autosomal recessive, or (3) X-linked. The distinction between "dominant" and "recessive" must be understood as one of convenience in pedigree analysis rather than as necessarily implying a fundamental difference in genetic mechanism. The term *dominant* implies that a mutation will be clinically manifest when an individual has a single dose of this mutation (or is *heterozygous* for it), whereas the term *recessive* implies that a double dose (or *homozygosity*) is required for clinical detection. Genes themselves are never dominant or recessive; their effects, however, produce clinical patterns that are classified as dominant or recessive.

The demonstration that a particular syndrome shows one of the three mendelian patterns of inheritance implies that its pathogenesis, no matter how complex, is due to an abnormality in a single protein molecule. For example, in the Marfan syndrome, all the clinical manifestations, which include such seemingly unrelated disturbances as ectopia lentis, scoliosis, arachnodactyly, and dissecting aneurysm, are the physiological consequences of a single abnormal protein that is encoded by a single abnormal gene. In many mendelian disorders, especially in those with dominant inheritance, it is not yet possible to demonstrate directly the protein that is primarily altered by the mutation. In such cases, only the distal physiological effects of the mutation are recognizable. Nevertheless, it is safe to assume that a single primary defect exists whenever a disease is transmitted by a single gene mechanism and that the various manifestations of the disease can all be related to the mutational event by a more or less complicated "pedigree of causes."

AUTOSOMAL DOMINANT DISORDERS. Dominant diseases are those manifest in the heterozygous state, i.e., when only one abnormal gene (*mutant allele*) is present and the corresponding partner allele on the homologous chromosome is normal. The gene responsible for an autosomal dominant disorder is located on 1 of the 22 autosomes; thus, both males and females can be affected. Since alleles segregate independently at meiosis, there is a one in two chance that the offspring of an affected heterozygote will inherit the mutant allele and, similarly, a one in two chance of his or her inheriting the normal allele.

The following features are characteristic of autosomal dominant inheritance: (1) Each affected individual has an affected parent (unless the condition arose by a new mutation in the individual or is mildly expressed in the affected parent); (2) an affected individual will bear, on the average, both normal and affected offspring in equal proportions; (3) normal children of an affected individual will have only normal offspring; (4) men and women are affected in equal proportion; (5) each sex is equally likely to transmit the condition to male and female offspring, with male-to-male transmission occurring; and (6) vertical transmission of the condition through successive generations occurs, especially when the trait does not impair reproductive capacity.

Although half the offspring of an individual with an autosomal dominant condition will inherit the disease, it is not necessarily true that each affected person must have an affected parent. In every autosomal dominant disease a certain proportion of affected persons owe the disorder to a new mutation rather than to an inherited mutation. The parent in whose germ cells the new mutation arose will be clinically normal. Likewise, the siblings of the affected individual will be normal, since the mutation will affect only a single germ cell. However, the affected individual will transmit the disease and half of his or her children will be affected.

The proportion of patients with dominant disorders who represent new mutations is inversely proportional to the effect of the disease on *biological fitness.* Biological fitness refers to the ability of an affected individual to produce children who survive to adult life and reproduce. In the extreme case, if a dominant mutation produces absolute infertility, then all observed cases would of necessity represent new mutations, and it would be impossible to prove the genetic transmission of the trait. In less severe disorders, as in the Marfan syndrome, the cardiac disease reduces biological fitness to about 85 per cent of normal, and the proportion of cases due to new mutations is about 15 per cent.

Before concluding that a dominant disorder in a given patient with unaffected parents is the result of a new mutation, two other considerations are important: (1) the possibility that the gene may be carried by one parent in whom the disease is of low expressivity (discussed below), and (2) the possibility that extramarital paternity may have occurred, which is found in about 3 to 5 per cent of randomly studied children in the United States.

Most autosomal dominant disorders show two characteristic features that are not usually seen in recessive syndromes: (1) *delayed age of onset,* and (2) *variability in clinical expression.* Delayed age of onset is seen in such disorders as myotonic dystrophy (p. 1708) and hypertrophic obstructive cardiomyopathy (p. 1409). These disorders typically do not become manifest clinically until adult life, even though the mutant gene is present from the time of conception. Variability in clinical expression is illustrated dramatically by the Holt-Oram syndrome (discussed below). Patients in the same family inheriting the same abnormal gene may manifest any one of the following: (1) atrial septal defect and a skeletal abnormality of the upper extremity, (2) only atrial septal defect, or (3) only a skeletal abnormality of the upper extremity. This diversity in clinical manifestations makes it difficult to recognize that each family member suffers from the same genetic abnormality.

Since dominant mutations involve a type of gene product that in a 50 per cent deficiency is capable of producing clinical symptoms in heterozygotes, the responsible mutations are likely to involve abnormalities in two classes of proteins: (1) those that regulate complex metabolic pathways, such as membrane receptors and rate-limiting enzymes in pathways under feedback control, and (2) key structural proteins, such as those involved in connective tissue formation. At present, however, the basic biochemical defects have been identified in only a handful of the known autosomal dominant disorders.

Examples of autosomal dominant disorders that involve the cardiovascular system include the Holt-Oram syndrome, the Noonan syndrome, the Marfan syndrome, hypertrophic obstructive cardiomyopathy, and familial hypercholesterolemia.

AUTOSOMAL RECESSIVE DISORDERS. Autosomal recessive conditions are clinically apparent only in the homozygous state, i.e., when both alleles at a particular genetic locus are mutant alleles. The gene responsible for an autosomal recessive disorder is located on 1 of the 22 autosomes; thus, both men and women can be affected.

The following features are characteristic of autosomal recessive inheritance: (1) the parents are clinically normal; (2) only siblings are affected and vertical transmission does not occur; and (3) men and women are affected in equal proportions.

The relative infrequency of recessive genes in the population and the requirement that two abnormal genes be present for clinical expression combine to create special conditions for autosomal recessive inheritance: (1) If a husband and a wife are both carriers for the same autosomal recessive gene, 25 per cent of the children will be normal, 50 per cent will be heterozygous carriers, and 25 per cent will be homozygous and affected with the disease; (2) if an affected individual marries a heterozygote (as may occur with consanguineous marriage), half the children will be affected, and a pedigree simulating dominant inheritance would result; (3) if two individuals with the same recessive disease marry, all of their children will be affected; and (4) the more infrequent the mutant gene in the population, the stronger the likelihood that affected individuals will be the product of consanguineous matings.

In general, consanguinity is an infrequent finding clinically in most families with recessive diseases in the United States. This is because the background rate for consanguinity in the general population is very low. Thus, in most of the United States (as opposed to areas with relative geographical isolation, such as northern Norway, Switzerland, and so on), a disorder must be extremely rare before it is associated with an important frequency of consanguinity. For example, consanguinity is expected in a large proportion of families having children with very rare disorders such as the Kartagener syndrome and mulibrey nanism.

The clinical picture in autosomal recessive disorders tends to be more uniform than that of dominant diseases, and onset often occurs early in life. As a general rule, recessive disorders are more commonly diagnosed in children, whereas dominant diseases are more frequently encountered in adults.

Inasmuch as only one of four children in a sibship is expected to be affected with a recessive disease, multiple cases in a family may not occur. This is especially true in a society in which small families are common. Consider, for example, 16 families in which both parents are heterozygous for the same recessive disorder. If each family has 2 children, 9 of the families will have no affected children, 6 will have 1 affected and 1 normal child, and only 1 of the 16 families will have 2 affected children. Thus, in the United States, physicians will usually see sporadic or isolated cases of a recessive disorder without an affected sibling to alert them to the possibility of a genetic etiology. Fortunately, because of the relatively uniform clinical picture of recessive disorders and because most can be diagnosed by biochemical tests, the correct diagnosis can usually be made even when no other members of a family are clinically affected.

The basic biochemical lesions underlying many autosomal recessive disorders have been identified. Of the three types of proteins in which mutations could occur (i.e., enzymes, structural proteins, and regulatory proteins), the most easy to study have been the enzymes. A mutation that destroys the catalytic activity of an enzyme generally does not impair the health of a heterozygote (i.e., an individual who has one mutant allele specifying a functionless enzyme and one normal allele on the partner chromosome specifying a normal enzyme). In this situation each cell in the body usually produces about 50 per cent of the normal number of active enzyme molecules. However, metabolic regulatory mechanisms avert any clinical consequences of this 50 per cent deficiency, and so heterozygotes are usually clinically normal. On the other hand, when an individual inherits functionless alleles at both loci specifying an enzyme, the reduction in enzyme activity is too great for any compensatory mechanism to overcome, and a disease results. Thus, heterozygotes for homocystinuria, in which patients have half the normal activity of cystathionine synthase, are clinically asymptomatic because the body compensates for the half-normal level of the enzyme by raising the homocystine concentration approximately twofold. Under these conditions a normal amount of homocystine can be metabolized and no symptoms occur. On the other hand, the homozygote for homocystinuria has such a severe reduction in cystathionine synthase activity that enormous levels accumulate within the blood and tissues, causing thrombotic events at a young age.

Examples of autosomal recessive disorders involving the heart include Pompe disease (pp. 1051 and 1622), the Kartagener syndrome (p. 1618), homocystinuria, and the Jervell and Lange-Nielsen syndrome (p. 1626).

X-LINKED DISORDERS. The genes responsible for one class of disorders are located on the X chromosome, and thus the clinical risk and severity of the disease are different for the two sexes. Since a woman has two X chromosomes, she may be either heterozygous or homozygous for the mutant gene, and the trait may therefore demonstrate either recessive or dominant expression. Men, on the other hand, have only one X chromosome, so they can be expected to display the full syndrome whenever they inherit the gene, regardless of whether the gene behaves as a recessive or as a dominant trait in a woman. Thus, the terms *X-linked dominant* or *X-linked recessive* refer only to the expression of the gene in women.

An important feature of all X-linked inheritance is the absence of male-to-male (i.e., father-to-son) transmission of the trait. This follows from the fact that a man must always contribute his Y chromosome to his sons; hence, he can never contribute his X chromosome. On the other hand, a man contributes his X chromosome to all of his daughters.

The characteristic features of X-linked recessive inheritance are as follows: (1) In contrast to the vertical transmission in dominant traits (parents and children affected) and the horizontal transmission in autosomal recessive traits (siblings affected), the pedigree pattern in X-linked recessive traits tends to be oblique because of the occurrence of the trait in the sons of normal carrier sisters of affected males (uncles and nephews affected); (2) male offspring of carrier women have a 50 per cent chance of being affected; (3) all female offspring of affected males are carriers; (4) affected males do not transmit the trait to any offspring; and (5) affected homozygous females occur only when an affected male marries a carrier female.

Examples of X-linked recessive disorders involving the heart include Duchenne muscular dystrophy (p. 1704), Fabry disease (p. 1425), and the Hunter syndrome.

Multifactorial Genetic Diseases

Most of the common diseases of the heart, such as coronary artery disease and congenital heart disease, have long been known to "run in families." They fit best into the category of *multifactorial genetic diseases.* The genetic element in these disorders rarely manifests itself in an all-or-none fashion as it does in the single-gene disorders and in chromosomal aberrations. Instead, the interaction of multiple genes with multiple environmental factors produces the familial aggregation.[4]

In the multifactorial genetic diseases, there is a *polygenic component* consisting of multiple genes that interact in a cumulative fashion. An individual inheriting the right combination of these genes passes beyond a "threshold of risk," at which point an *environmental component* determines whether or not and to what extent he or she is clinically affected. For another individual in the same family to express the same syndrome, he must inherit the same or a very similar combination of genes. Since the first-degree relatives of an affected individual (i.e., parents, siblings, and offspring) each share half his genes, they are all at increased risk of exhibiting the same polygenic syndrome. Second-degree relatives (uncles, aunts, and grandparents) share on the average one-fourth of an individual's genes $(1/2)^2$, and third-degree relatives (cousins) share one-eighth $(1/2)^3$. Thus, as the degree of relation becomes more distant, the likelihood of a relative inheriting the same combination of genes becomes less. Moreover, the chance of any relative inheriting the right combination of risk genes decreases as the number of genes required for the expression of a given trait increases.

Since the precise number of genes responsible for polygenic traits is unknown, one cannot calculate the precise risk of inheritance for a relative of an affected individual. Rather, one must rely on empirical risk figures (i.e., a direct tally of the proportion of affected relatives in previously reported families). In contrast to the single-gene disorders, in which 25 or 50 per cent of the first-degree relatives of an affected proband are at genetic risk, multifactorial genetic disorders generally affect no more than 5 to 10 per cent of first-degree relatives. Moreover, in contrast to mendelian traits, the recurrence risk of multifactorial conditions varies from family to family, and its estimation is significantly influenced by two factors: (1) the number of affected persons already present in the family, and (2) the severity of the disorder in the index case. The larger the number of affected relatives and the more severe their disease, the higher the risk to other relatives.

The hypothesis of a polygenic component in the inheritance of multifactorial diseases has been given a sound basis in recent years by the demonstration that at least one-third of all gene loci harbor different alleles that vary among individuals. Such a large degree of variation in normal genes, such as those that specify blood groups and the HLA system, undoubtedly provides the substratum for variations in genetic predisposition with which environmental factors can interact. Such variation among a normal gene is termed a *polymorphism.* An important observation of recent years has been the finding that certain alleles at the HLA loci predispose individuals to certain specific diseases. For example, if one inherits the B-27 allele at the HLA-B locus, one has a 120-fold greater chance for developing ankylosing spondylitis than an individual who lacks this allele. Ankylosing spondylitis remains a multifactorial disease, however, because its development clearly requires one or more other factors in addition to the B-27 allele. Thus, fewer than 15 per cent of people who inherit this allele develop this disease.

Multifactorial disorders are heterogeneous in the sense that the relative contribution of the polygenic factors ("risk genes") and environmental factors to the etiology will vary greatly from patient to patient. However, it is important to remember that among common phenotypes that are largely multifactorial, there will often be a small proportion in whom the phenotype is created by major mutant genes. For example, although coronary artery disease is usually of multifactorial etiology, about 5 per cent of subjects with premature myocardial infarctions are heterozygotes for familial hypercholesterolemia, a single-gene disorder that produces atherosclerosis in the absence of any other predisposing factor.[5] Similarly, in a small proportion of patients with other common cardiovascular diseases such as atrial septal defect, the condition is not multifactorial but determined by a single gene, as in the Holt-Oram syndrome.

GENE ACTION AND THE CARDIOVASCULAR SYSTEM

The existence of a gene affecting a specific cardiac function is frequently inferred from genetic analysis of pedigrees showing mendelian inheritance of a heart disorder. The function of the gene is deduced by analysis of the defect produced in family members who carry a mutant allele. Since at least 50 simply inherited disorders of the heart and vasculature are currently recognized (composing about 5 per cent of all mendelian disorders currently known to exist in humans),[6] there must be at least 50 genes and hence 50 protein molecules that affect cardiac function in a major way. Mutation of these genes produces cardiac dysfunction, which can be manifest clinically at several levels, including congenital cardiac malformations, derangement of the connective tissue elements of the heart and vascular system, cardiomyopathies, cardiac arrhythmias and conduction defects, pericarditis, cardiac tumors, and coronary artery disease. The nature of the proteins specified by these 50 critical genes is generally unknown.

The single-gene–determined disorders of the heart may potentially provide investigative models for unraveling the complexities of cardiovascular physiology and biochemistry. Most significant has been the use of the familial hypercholesterolemia syndrome to delineate a mechanism by which human cholesterol metabolism is regulated.[7] Inasmuch as several mendelian disorders that affect cardiac muscle structure (such as hypertrophic obstructive cardiomyopathy) are now recognized, it is predictable that the elucidation of the basic defect in each of them will provide biochemical information necessary to define the basis of human structural abnormalities, such as cardiac hypertrophy.

GENETIC COUNSELING IN CARDIOLOGY

THE FAMILY HISTORY

When caring for a patient with a possible genetic disorder involving the heart, the physician begins by taking a careful *family history* and by carrying out a *family evaluation.* The first step involves obtaining certain information on the *proband* or *index case* (i.e., the clinically affected person who has brought the family to attention) and on each of the patient's *first-degree relatives* (i.e., the parents, sibs, and offspring of the proband). This information includes the given name, surname, and maiden name; birth date or current age; age at death, whether an autopsy was performed, and cause of death; and presence of any disease or defect. Ideally, the family history should also include the name and address of the individuals' physicians and the hospitals to which they were admitted.

The second step includes asking six questions designed to survey the family for the presence of disease:

1. Is there any relative with an identical or similar trait?
2. Is there any relative with a trait that is absent in the proband but that is known to occur in some patients with the same disease? This question requires that the physician have some knowledge about the manifestations of the disease in question. For example, when obtaining the family history from a proband with dissecting aneurysm possibly caused by the Marfan syndrome, one should ask about the occurrence of eye abnormalities, cardiac abnormalities, and skeletal abnormalities in the proband's relatives.
3. Is there any relative with a trait that is recognized to be genetically determined? The purpose of this question is to ascertain the occurrence of hereditary disease in the family even though the patients may not consider themselves to be involved.
4. Is there any relative with an unusual disease, or has any relative died of a rare condition? The purpose of this question is to identify a condition that might be genetically determined though not recognized as such by the patient. In addition, this question may help to identify conditions in relatives that might be etiologically related to the patient's problem. For example, a patient with a cardiac tumor should be suspected of having underlying tuberous sclerosis if he or she has a brother with adenoma sebaceum and mental retardation, both of which can be manifestations of the tuberous sclerosis gene.
5. Is there any consanguinity in the family? Not only should this inquiry be made directly, but, in addition, one should ask whether common last names appear in the families of husband and wife. Consanguineous marriage may be the source of a rare autosomal recessive syndrome, such as Pompe disease, and sometimes its presence in the family may not be known by the proband.
6. What is the ethnic origin of the family? Persons of certain ethnic origins have an increased chance of certain genetic diseases. Mulibrey nanism (p. 1626) is one example of a familial heart disease that occurs with increased frequency in a specific ethnic group, the Finns.

The third step involves an examination of available family members, both those affected and those believed to be unaffected.

RETROSPECTIVE GENETIC COUNSELING

The prevention of hereditary cardiac diseases requires the identification of matings that are capable of producing defective offspring. These may be matings in which one of the two individuals is carrying a dominant or X-linked gene mutation or matings in which both individuals are carriers of a deleterious recessive gene. Such individuals are usually identified through an affected child or near relative, in which case retrospective genetic counseling can be provided.

When advising family members about the risk of transmitting a disorder that has already affected someone in the family, the first step is to be certain of the *correct diagnosis* —in particular, to make certain that the problem in question is really of genetic origin. This is especially important in cardiac disorders that may have both genetic and nongenetic causes. For example, some cases of patent ductus arteriosus are caused by a multifactorial genetic mechanism, whereas others are caused by rubella (p. 942).

Second, if the disease has a hereditary element, one must consider the possibility of *genetic heterogeneity*, a situation in which clinically similar genetic disorders show varying patterns of inheritance. For example, there are two types of atrial septal defect that resemble each other closely: a rare form showing autosomal dominant inheritance, as in the Holt-Oram syndrome (p. 1030 and 1616), and a common form having a multifactorial etiology.

To estimate the *recurrence risk*, one must consider what is known of the genetic mechanisms determining the relevant disorder. When more than one genetic mechanism exists, or when environmental factors can cause clinically indistinguishable traits, then the *relative probabilities* of the different mechanisms operating in the particular family are computed. For conditions determined by simple mendelian inheritance, there is no difficulty in predicting the probability of an offspring being affected, provided the genotypes of the parents can be recognized. Identification of the parental genotype is easiest for autosomal recessive and X-linked disorders, since the basic lesions in these two forms of mendelian inheritance usually involve simple enzyme deficiencies for which biochemical tests are now available.

Identification of the parental genotype is considerably more difficult for autosomal dominant disorders, since the basic defect is known for only a few. Thus, diagnosis of the heterozygote for a dominant disorder depends almost exclusively on the clinical evaluation and a careful pedigree analysis. In counseling a family in which one relative is affected with a dominant disorder, it is important that appropriate clinical examination of all first-degree relatives and appropriately selected distant relatives be carried out. If relatives appear unaffected, one must constantly consider the possibility that the clinical symptoms may be masked by *delayed age of onset* and *variability in expression.* When no relatives are affected, the possibility of a new dominant mutation must be entertained. The probability of a case of an autosomal dominant disorder being the result of a new mutation is inversely proportional to the reproductive fitness of the disorder.

In advising families about multifactorial genetic diseases in which the inheritance pattern is not clear-cut, such as premature coronary artery disease, the physician must resort to empirical risk estimates that have been derived from retrospectively assembled data (see Chap. 35).

Once the parental genotypes are determined, the genetic prognosis is usually presented in terms of probability that a given couple will produce an affected offspring. The physician providing genetic counseling must make certain that the couple understands not only the meaning of such absolute risk figures but also the severity of the disease and the variability in clinical expression. In other words, in dealing with a disorder such as the Noonan syndrome, it is important not only that the parents realize that they have a 50 per cent risk of producing a child with this disorder but also that they know that a certain proportion of patients with the disorder have severe disease, a certain proportion have mild disease, and so on. They should also have an understanding of the potential impact of the disease on their family. Thus, a disease that is lethal at birth might be classified by some as more "severe" than one that is lethal at age 16, but the latter is likely to have a much more profound impact on the family.

Although different families initially react in different ways to the same risk, most couples who seek genetic advice can be expected to take a responsible course of action that is based on the information quoted. Thus, the physician avoids giving direct advice to the couple concerning whether they "should" or "should not" have children. For serious genetic disease, it has been observed that when the recurrence risk is high, i.e., equal to or greater than 1 in 10, most parents are deterred from planning further children. When the risks are low, i.e., less than 1 in 10, most parents continue with additional pregnancies.[8]

PRENATAL DIAGNOSIS

The use of transabdominal amniocentesis permits diagnosis of certain genetic diseases at an early enough stage to terminate the pregnancy to prevent the birth of a defective child. This procedure allows high-risk couples the opportunity to have unaffected children, provided they are willing to have the pregnancy terminated in the event that an abnormal fetus is detected.[1,9]

TABLE 47–1 GENETIC DISORDERS AFFECTING THE HEART FOR WHICH PRENATAL DIAGNOSIS IS FEASIBLE

Disorder	Expression in Cultured Amniotic Fluid Cells	Detectable Abnormality
Down syndrome	Yes	Trisomy 21 or unbalanced 14/21 translocation by karyotype
Ellis–van Creveld syndrome	No	Visualization of bilateral polydactyly by fetoscopy
Duchenne muscular dystrophy	No	Decreased level of creatine phosphokinase (CPK) in fetal blood
Myotonic dystrophy	No	Gene for *myotonic dystrophy* closely linked with *secretor* gene, the product of which is present in amniotic fluid
Ehlers-Danlos, Type IV	Yes	Deficient synthesis of Type III collagen
Homocystinuria	Yes	Deficiency of cystathionine synthase
Pompe disease	Yes	Deficiency of lysosomal acid maltase
Homozygous familial hypercholesterolemia	Yes	Deficiency of receptors for low-density lipoprotein
Cholesteryl ester storage disease	Yes	Deficiency of lysosomal acid lipase
Fabry disease	Yes	Deficiency of α-galactosidase A
Mucopolysaccharidoses		
Type I-H, Hurler syndrome	Yes	Deficiency of α-L-iduronidase
Type I-S, Scheie syndrome	Yes	Deficiency of α-L-iduronidase
Type I-H/S, Hurler-Scheie compound	Yes	Deficiency of α-L-iduronidase
Type II, Hunter syndrome	Yes	Deficiency of sulfoiduronide sulfatase
Type IV, Morquio syndrome	Yes	Deficiency of *N*-acetylhexosamine sulfate sulfatase
Type VI, Maroteaux-Lamy syndrome	Yes	Deficiency of arylsulfatase B
Mucolipidosis, Type III	Yes	Deficiency of *N*-acetylglucosamine-1-phosphotransferase

Prenatal diagnosis usually requires obtaining amniotic fluid at week 16 of gestation, centrifuging the fluid to obtain fetal amniotic cells, and culturing the fetal cells in vitro. The culture process requires about 3 weeks. By this means the karyotype of the fetus can be determined to ascertain fetal sex and to detect various chromosomal aberrations, such as Down syndrome. Moreover, many inborn errors of metabolism can be detected by suitable assays of specific enzyme activities in the cultured fetal cells.

In addition to the use of amniotic cells for prenatal diagnosis, other methods, such as fetoscopy and radiology, can be employed. For example, the Ellis–van Creveld syndrome can be diagnosed in utero by visualization of bilateral polydactyly. Moreover, fetal blood sampling for measurement of the level of creatine phosphokinase (CPK) can be used in the prenatal diagnosis of muscular dystrophy. Table 47–1 lists those genetic disorders affecting the cardiovascular system for which prenatal diagnosis is currently feasible.

GENETICS OF SPECIFIC FORMS OF CARDIOVASCULAR DISEASE

CONGENITAL HEART DISEASES

(See also Chaps. 29 and 30)

Chromosomal Disorders

Approximately 5 per cent of all congenital heart malformations can be traced to a chromosomal aberration.[10] Virtually all cases of a congenital heart malformation associated with a chromosomal defect occur as part of a multiple malformation syndrome. Congenital heart disease is a characteristic feature of most chromosomal disorders, such as trisomy 13, trisomy 18, trisomy 21 (Down syndrome), deletion of the short arm of chromosome 4, deletion of the long arm of chromosome 13, deletion of the long arm of chromosome 18, and Turner syndrome (XO). A chromosomal syndrome that does *not* show an increased frequency of congenital heart disease is the Klinefelter syndrome (XXY). A discussion follows of the two chromosomal syndromes that most commonly cause congenital heart disease, Down syndrome and Turner syndrome.

DOWN SYNDROME. The trisomy 21 form of Down syndrome (mongolism) is the most common human chromosomal aberration, occurring in approximately 1 in every 600 neonates. Congenital heart disease, which is found in as many as 50 per cent of patients with this disorder, constitutes a major source of morbidity and mortality.[11–14]

The two most common cardiac lesions in Down syndrome are ventricular septal defect and endocardial cushion defect. Among patients with the complete form of endocardial cushion defect, those with Down syndrome account for about 50 per cent.[14] Secundum atrial septal defect, tetralogy of Fallot, and isolated patent ductus arteriosus are also observed in patients with Down syndrome. Transposition of the great arteries and coarctation of the aorta are rarely seen. Most patients having Down syndrome with congenital heart disease have a single lesion. However, as many as 30 per cent of those with heart disease may have multiple cardiac defects.[13]

The decision to repair surgically a congenital heart lesion in a patient with Down syndrome is often a complicated one. Factors to be considered include the seriousness of the defect; whether the patient is living at home or with relatives or is institutionalized; and the patient's degree of cooperation. Although it is generally believed that patients with Down syndrome are poor operative candidates because of their increased susceptibility to infections, recent surgical follow-up studies suggest that their postoperative mortality is no higher than that of a non–Down syndrome population with similar cardiac lesions.[11,15]

The most important factor in preventing the birth of a child with the trisomy 21 form of Down syndrome is maternal age. A marked increase in incidence occurs in children born to older mothers,[16,17] as shown in Table 47–2.

The recurrence risk to a couple who has had one child with the trisomy 21 form of Down syndrome is 2 per cent, i.e., there is a 1 in 50 chance that the next child will also have the trisomy 21 form of Down syndrome.[16] The recurrence risk is 2 per cent regardless of whether the mother is young (age 20) or old (age 45).[16] All women who are 36 years of age and older and all women who have had one child with trisomy 21 Down syndrome should have each of their subsequent pregnancies monitored by amniocentesis for a prenatal diagnosis.

The trisomy 21 aberration accounts for virtually all cases of Down syndrome born to women above age 30 and for 90 per cent of all cases born to women below age 30. The remaining 10 per cent of patients with Down syndrome born to women below age 30 have a translocation form. On karyotype analysis, such patients have the normal number of 46 chromosomes, including 2 normal chromosomes No. 21, 1 normal chromosome No. 14, and an unpaired large chromosome that represents an extra chromosome No. 21 that is joined to 1 chromosome No. 14. There are no clinical differences between children with the trisomy 21 form of Down syndrome and those with the translocation form.

Karyotypes of the parents of children with the translo-

TABLE 47–2 RISK OF HAVING A CHILD WITH DOWN SYNDROME AS A FUNCTION OF MATERNAL AGE

Maternal Age	Estimated Risk
$<$ 20 years	1 in 1800
20–29 years	1 in 1200
30–34 years	1 in 750
35–39 years	1 in 250
40–44 years	1 in 80
$\geq$ 45 years	1 in 25

cation form of Down syndrome exhibit one of the following:

1. In about 90 per cent of cases, both parents have normal karyotypes, so the translocation is assumed to have originated during gametogenesis, and the risk of recurrence is no more than 2 per cent to subsequent children.
2. In 10 per cent of cases one of the parents will have an abnormal karyotype consisting of 45 chromosomes with 1 normal chromosome No. 14, 1 normal chromosome No. 21, and a large chromosome that contains fused copies of both the 14 and 21 chromosomes.

About 5 to 20 per cent of the live-born offspring of an individual who is a "balanced" translocation carrier for the 14/21 chromosome will have Down syndrome, depending on whether the father (5 per cent) or the mother (20 per cent) carries the "balanced" translocation.[16] Other types of translocation occur, but these are much less frequent. Overall, the inherited translocation form of Down syndrome is extremely rare, especially compared with the trisomy 21 form of the disorder. Nevertheless, it is important to identify all such cases so that the pregnancies of all family members who are translocation carriers can be appropriately monitored by amniocentesis.

TURNER SYNDROME (see also p. 1038). Turner syndrome is characterized by the occurrence in a phenotypic female of the following clinical features: shortness of stature, amenorrhea due to gonadal dysgenesis, shield-shaped chest, pigmented nevi, webbing of the neck, cubitus valgus, shortening of metacarpals and metatarsals, renal abnormalities, and cardiovascular abnormalities. In about 60 per cent of patients with these clinical features, all the cells in the body will be deficient in one of the two X chromosomes (45,X form). The remaining 40 per cent of patients include individuals who have a mixture of cells, some of which show the 45,X karyotype and some of which show the normal karyotype (45,X/46,XX mosaicism), and individuals whose cells show structural abnormalities in one of the two X chromosomes (such as a single isochromosome X or a single ring X chromosome). Patients with the 45,X/46,XX form of Turner syndrome are often less severely clinically involved and may be nearly normal.

Most fetuses with the 45,X form of Turner syndrome die in utero and are aborted spontaneously. Recent studies indicate that the 45,X chromosomal abnormality occurs in as many as 5 per cent of all spontaneous abortions and in about 1 in 2500 female live births.[18]

Cardiovascular abnormalities occur in 35 to 50 per cent of all patients with the 45,X form of Turner syndrome.[19–22] Coarctation of the aorta is by far the most common abnormality that is encountered, accounting for 70 per cent of all cardiac anomalies. Other congenital malformations are occasionally seen, including bicuspid aortic valve, hypertrophic obstructive cardiomyopathy, ventricular septal defect, prolapse of the mitral valve, and dextrocardia.[19–23] Stenosis of the pulmonic valve is rarely, if ever, seen in Turner syndrome. This is in striking contrast to findings in the superficially similar Noonan syndrome, in which coarctation of the aorta is rarely encountered and stenosis of the pulmonic valve is the cardinal cardiac manifestation[22] (discussed below).

Patients with Turner syndrome caused by an isochromosome X or a ring X differ clinically from patients with the 45,X karyotype in that webbing of the neck and coarctation of the aorta are absent.[19,21] In patients with mosaic Turner syndrome, coarctation of the aorta occurs, but its frequency is considerably less than in the 45,X patients.

Adults with Turner syndrome are prone to systemic hypertension. This association between Turner syndrome and hypertension occurs in the absence of coarctation of the aorta and appears to be unrelated to the karyotypic abnormality.[19] The mechanism underlying the hypertension has not been defined.

Family studies have revealed a high frequency of both diabetes mellitus and thyroid autoantibodies in the chromosomally normal relatives of patients with Turner syndrome.[19] These findings have suggested that a genetic tendency to autoantibody formation in parents may predispose to the occurrence of chromosomal abnormalities in their offspring.

Elevated maternal age does not appear to predispose to offspring with Turner syndrome, unlike Down syndrome. Once a couple has had one child with Turner syndrome, the recurrence risk to subsequent offspring is virtually zero.

Single-gene Disorders

At least eight forms of congenital heart disease are now recognized to be caused by single-gene mutations. Together, these eight disorders account for about 5 per cent of all forms of congenital heart disease. In six of these disorders, the responsible mutation causes a multisystem syndrome of which congenital heart disease is only one component. Each of these mutations presumably disrupts the function of a single protein the action of which is necessary for several developmental events, including normal embryogenesis of the heart. Virtually nothing is known of how these mutant genes act at the molecular and cellular level.

The identification of any one of these eight single-gene disorders in a given individual enables the cardiologist to apply knowledge of the genetics of the syndrome to the identification of further cases in the same family and to provide genetic counseling to appropriate family members.

NOONAN SYNDROME (see also p. 986). The eponym Noonan syndrome describes a common clinical entity characterized by shortness of stature, mild mental retardation, a unique facial appearance (Fig. 47–1), webbing of the neck, cryptorchidism, renal anomalies, and congenital heart disease.[24–29] Skeletal deformities are also frequent, including scoliosis and pectus carinatum. Affected individuals superficially resemble patients with Turner syndrome in that shortness of stature, webbing of the neck, cubitus valgus, skeletal anomalies, renal abnormalities, and congenital heart disease are present in both disorders. Because of these clinical similarities, Noonan syndrome has frequently been referred to in the literature as male "Turner syndrome," "Turner phenotype with normal chromosomes," and XX and XY "Turner phenotype."[24–28]

However, several striking genetic and clinical differences between Noonan syndrome and Turner syndrome clearly separate these two disorders as distinct entities. (1) In contrast to Turner syndrome, in Noonan syndrome both males and females are affected and the karyotype in both

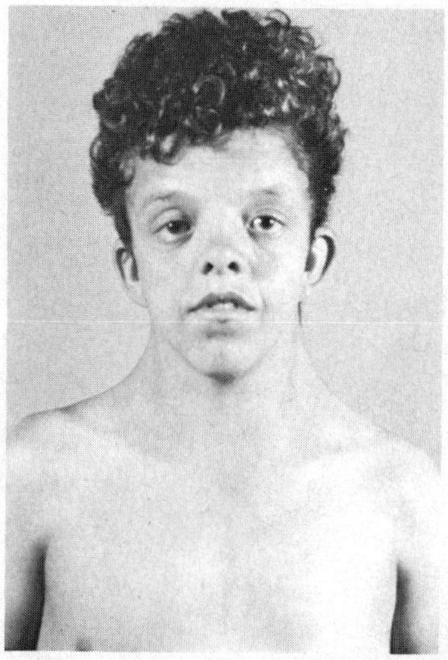

FIGURE 47–1 Eighteen-year-old boy with the Noonan syndrome. The facial abnormalities consist of curly hair, epicanthal folds, ptosis of eyelids, hypertelorism, strabismus, small chin, and low-set ears with abnormal auricles. Webbing of the neck is also evident.

males and females are affected and the karyotype in both sexes is normal;[24–28] (2) coarctation of the aorta, which rarely occurs in Noonan syndrome, is the most frequent cardiac lesion in Turner syndrome; conversely, *pulmonic stenosis*, which does not occur in Turner syndrome, is the most common cardiac lesion in Noonan syndrome;[23–31] and (3) Noonan syndrome is determined by a single mutant gene inherited as an autosomal dominant trait.[25,27,28,32–34]

Approximately 50 per cent of patients with Noonan syndrome have congenital heart disease.[29] The most common lesion is valvular pulmonary stenosis, occurring in about 60 per cent of those patients who have a congenital cardiac malformation. The stenotic pulmonic valve is frequently dysplastic. Characteristically, the annulus is of normal size, but the cusps are thickened and immobile.[23–31] The electrocardiogram is often different from the pattern usually seen in pulmonary valve stenosis: Left anterior hemiblock is common, and a deep S wave is frequently present in the precordial leads.[11,23]

Atrial septal defect and hypertrophic cardiomyopathy occur in about 20 per cent of patients with Noonan syndrome who have congenital heart disease. The cardiomyopathy frequently produces an eccentric hypertrophy of the left ventricle that can easily be missed during cardiac catherization limited to the right side of the heart.[35–38] Although the majority of patients show a single heart defect, some show a combination of pulmonary stenosis and either atrial septal defect or hypertrophic cardiomyopathy.

In addition to anomalies of the heart itself, abnormalities of the systemic arteries have been reported in patients with Noonan syndrome. These include fistulas of the coronary arteries, peripheral pulmonic stenosis, anomalous pulmonary venous septum, hemangiomas, peripheral lymphedema, and intestinal lymphangiectasis.[31]

Patients with Noonan syndrome undergoing cardiac surgery are particularly vulnerable to several complications: (1) technical difficulties because of the dysplastic nature of the pulmonic valve, sometimes necessitating total valve replacement—a formidable problem in infants and young children; (2) difficulty in establishing outflow drainage during total cardiopulmonary bypass because of the systemic venous anomalies; (3) increased risk of malignant hyperpyrexia during general anesthesia; and (4) development of persistent chylothorax because of pulmonary lymphangiectasis.[31]

The evidence for a genetic etiology of Noonan syndrome is provided by its occurrence in multiple siblings and in multiple generations of the same family. Family studies are consistent with autosomal dominant inheritance of a single mutant gene.[25,27,28,32–34] Figure 47–2 shows a pedigree of a family with Noonan syndrome: The mutant gene segregated through three generations, and one affected woman had affected children with two different husbands. As with most autosomal dominant traits, the Noonan syndrome gene shows a marked variation in its clinical expression; some affected individuals show only minor abnormalities (such as epicanthal folds and low-set ears), whereas others in the same family show the full syndrome with severe congenital heart disease.

Although male-to-male transmission of the mutant gene has been documented in several pedigrees,[32–34] most affected men, unlike affected women, show a deficiency in the number of offspring. This deficiency can be attributed to two factors: (1) Males appear to have a higher frequency of severe cardiac lesions than do females and therefore have less chance of surviving to reproductive age, and (2) about 75 per cent of affected males have bilateral cryptorchidism, whereas the affected females appear to have normal gonadal function.[24–34] This striking diminution in reproductive fitness in males with Noonan syndrome is consistent with the clinical observation that as many as 50 per cent of all cases of Noonan syndrome are sporadic cases. Such sporadic cases presumably represent new mutations.

It has been only fourteen years since Noonan syndrome was recognized as a distinct clinical and genetic entity separate from Turner syndrome. Nevertheless, in this short time more than 500 cases of Noonan syndrome have been reported. It has been estimated that the disorder may occur more frequently than 1 in 1000 persons in the population.[39] The basic defect underlying Noonan syndrome is

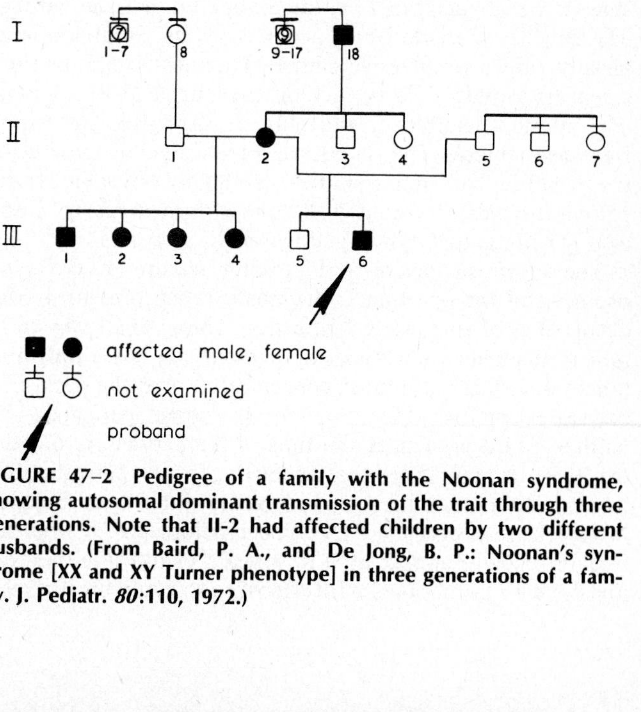

FIGURE 47–2 Pedigree of a family with the Noonan syndrome, showing autosomal dominant transmission of the trait through three generations. Note that II-2 had affected children by two different husbands. (From Baird, P. A., and De Jong, B. P.: Noonan's syndrome [XX and XY Turner phenotype] in three generations of a family. J. Pediatr. *80*:110, 1972.)

unknown. If it follows the pattern of other extremely common genetic diseases, it will ultimately be found to be genetically heterogeneous in that several different mutations will be able to cause a similar clinical syndrome.

In view of the high frequency of Noonan syndrome, the cardiologist should have a high index of suspicion of this disorder whenever a patient with congenital pulmonic stenosis is encountered. Attribution of this lesion to Noonan syndrome may be difficult, especially since 50 per cent of the cases may represent new mutations and thus exhibit a negative family history. The diagnosis is made even more difficult because many of the patients with documented Noonan syndrome have only mild facial abnormalities. Webbing of the neck and associated skeletal abnormalities may be absent. The invariant associated lesion is shortness of stature, so the physician should consider the presumptive diagnosis of Noonan syndrome whenever a patient with pulmonic stenosis and short stature is seen. In these cases, all first-degree relatives should be examined for the presence of mild facial abnormalities of the Noonan type as well as for occult cardiac lesions, especially pulmonic stenosis. The importance of making the diagnosis of Noonan syndrome lies in the ability of the physician to advise the patient that half of his or her children will be similarly affected.

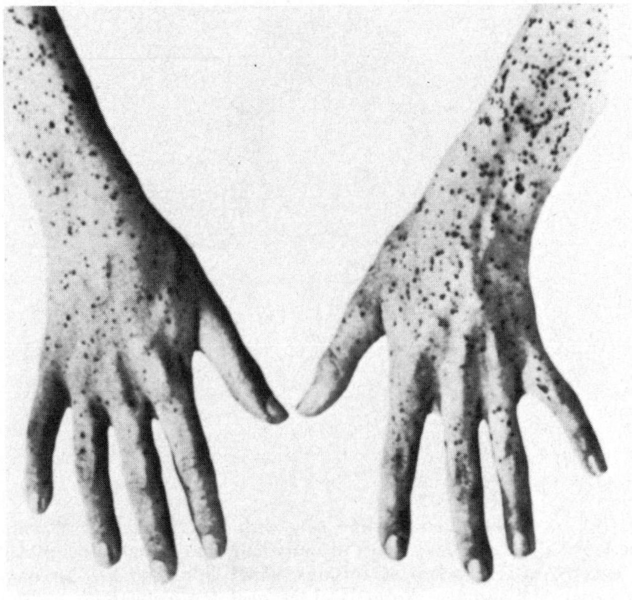

FIGURE 47–3 Skin of a 16-year-old boy with the LEOPARD syndrome covered with numerous deeply pigmented lentigines. (From Polani, P. E., and Moynahan, E. J.: Progressive carciomyopathic lentiginosis. Q. J. Med. *41*:205, 1972.)

LEOPARD SYNDROME. The LEOPARD syndrome is a rare, single gene–determined complex of congenital malformations affecting the cardiovascular system, the skin, the inner ear, and somatic and sexual development.[40–42] The cardinal features of the disorder are embodied in the mnemonic device LEOPARD: *L*, lentigenes; *E*, electrocardiographic conduction defects; *O*, ocular hypertelorism; *P*, pulmonic valve stenosis; *A*, abnormalities of genitals; *R*, retardation of growth, and *D*, deafness, sensorineural.[40]

Cardiac abnormalities, a common feature of the disorder, consist of anatomical malformations as well as electrocardiographic conduction defects. Stenosis of the pulmonic valve appears to be the most frequently encountered cardiac lesion. It may exist as an isolated anomaly, or it may be combined with aortic stenosis. Other cardiac defects that have been reported include endocardial fibroelastosis and hypertrophic cardiomyopathy.[40–44] The cardiac disease characteristically appears early in childhood and usually runs a progressive course. The most common electrocardiographic defects include prolonged P-R interval, left anterior hemiblock, widening of the QRS, and complete heart block. The functional significance of these electrocardiographic abnormalities is highly variable from patient to patient, being well tolerated in some or sufficiently serious to produce sudden death in others.

The most distinctive and striking feature of the syndrome, and the one that is diagnostic when present, is the occurrence of numerous lentigenes. These small (up to 5 mm in diameter), dark-brown spots, which spare only the mucosal surfaces, are most concentrated over the neck and upper extremities (Fig. 47–3). In some patients, the lentigenes are present at the time of birth, whereas in others they appear shortly after birth. In all patients, the number increases with age. Lentigenes differ from freckles in several respects: (1) They appear before age 5, whereas freckles usually appear at 6 to 8 years of age; (2) they do not increase in numbers with exposure to sunlight, whereas freckles do; and (3) microscopically, the quantity of melanocytes and the distribution of melanin in the pigmented and adjacent nonpigmented skin differ.[40]

The LEOPARD syndrome is inherited as an autosomal dominant trait. The clinical findings are highly variable from patient to patient, both within the same family as well as between affected individuals from different families. The most frequently encountered manifestations of the mutant gene are those relating to the cardiovascular system, occurring in at least 95 per cent of affected subjects. About 80 per cent have lentigenes. Deafness and abnormalities of genitals (hypospadias and undescended testes in the male) occur in about 20 per cent of patients.

The population frequency of the gene causing the LEOPARD syndrome is very low. Nothing is currently known about the relative proportion of cases arising from familial transmission of the mutant gene versus those arising from new mutations. Moreover, nothing is known regarding the biochemical action of the mutant gene.

HOLT-ORAM SYNDROME (see also p. 1030). Although atrial septal defect almost always occurs as a sporadic disorder, there are occasional families in which the pedigree pattern suggests the operation of a single mutant gene. The Holt-Oram syndrome and familial atrial septal defect with prolonged atrioventricular (AV) conduction are two examples of rare autosomal dominant disorders that are hidden among the more common sporadic cases of atrial septal defect.

The cardinal clinical manifestation of the Holt-Oram syndrome is the occurrence of an upper limb deformity in a patient with congenital heart disease.[45–50] Atrial septal defect of the secundum type is the most frequently encountered congenital heart malformation in affected individuals. This is usually accompanied by one or more electrocardiographic abnormalities, such as first-degree atrioventricular block, right bundle branch block, or bradycardia. Ventricular septal defect is the second most commonly encountered congenital heart lesion. Although virtually any form of congenital heart disease has been reported to occur in the syndrome, 70 per cent of affected individuals have either an atrial septal defect or a ventricular septal defect.

Many different upper limb deformities have been observed in association with the congenital heart disease in the Holt-Oram syndrome.[51] These limb deformities are typically bilateral but not necessarily symmetrical. If asymmetry is present, the skeletal lesions are usually more severe on the left side.[47] The most characteristic anomaly involves the thumbs. They may be absent, hypoplastic, triphalangeal, or finger-like. The last-named anomaly is referred to as "digitalization of the thumbs." The radius and the forearm are variably involved, the defects ranging in different patients from absent or hypoplastic radii to phocomelia.

Although deformities of the thumb are the best known features of the Holt-Oram syndrome, they do not occur in every case, nor are they pathognomonic.[51] Bilateral thumb abnormalities may also occur in the Diamond-Blackfan syndrome, in Fanconi anemia, or in thalidomide embryopathy. The most frequently encountered and specific upper limb abnormalities—namely, the presence of an abnormal scaphoid bone and/or accessory carpal bones—are detected on radiographs of the wrists. Various abnormalities also occur in the shoulder. The most common finding is a rotation of the scapula. Deformities of the humeral head and accessory ossicles around the shoulder have also been frequently noted.[51]

As in many dominantly inherited syndromes, individuals inheriting the Holt-Oram gene show varying degrees of clinical involvement. Intrafamilial variability appears to be as great as interfamilial variability.[52] The penetrance of the Holt-Oram gene is nearly 100 per cent, i.e., all individuals who inherit the gene manifest one or more clinical abnormalities, provided that appropriate studies, including wrist radiographs and electrocardiograms, are performed.[49] In about 60 per cent of cases, one of the parents is affected. The other 40 per cent of cases occur sporadically and apparently represent new mutations occurring in the germ cells of one of the parents.[47] Although the biochemical action of the mutant gene has not been defined, it presumably acts by disrupting a critical embryonic event common to the formation of the upper limbs and the heart.

The population frequency of the Holt-Oram syndrome has not been determined. However, the disorder is probably greatly underdiagnosed, with most cases being mistakenly considered as "garden-variety" atrial septal defects. The importance of separating the patient with the Holt-Oram syndrome from those cases of atrial septal defect that are not determined by a single-gene mechanism cannot be overemphasized. If the patient has Holt-Oram syndrome, then 50 per cent of the first-degree relatives (i.e., offspring, siblings, and parents) will be affected. In contrast, if a patient has a sporadic type of atrial septal defect, only about 3 per cent of the first-degree relatives would be affected. Thus, genetic counseling is quite different in these two situations.

FAMILIAL ATRIAL SEPTAL DEFECT WITH PROLONGED AV CONDUCTION. The syndrome of atrial septal defect with prolonged AV conduction represents a second example (the first being the Holt-Oram syndrome) of a single-gene–determined form of atrial septal defect. Pedigree studies of at least 20 large families leave little doubt about the autosomal dominant inheritance of this disorder.[53–56] The mutant gene shows a high degree of penetrance, and there is surprisingly little pleiotropy. That is, the mutant gene appears to cause only atrial septal defect and an abnormality of the AV conduction system. The latter is manifest clinically as either first- or second-degree heart block. Rarely, complete heart block occurs.

In the absence of a biochemical marker for the mutant gene, the diagnosis can be made only through careful clinical examination of family members of suspected cases. "Garden-variety" atrial septal defect can be excluded both by a family pedigree showing dominant inheritance and by electrocardiographic evidence of AV conduction block. The Holt-Oram syndrome can be ruled out by a normal clinical and radiological examination of the upper extremities.

ELLIS–VAN CREVELD SYNDROME. The Ellis–van Creveld syndrome constitutes a rare form of congenital heart disease that is inherited as an autosomal recessive trait. Affected individuals manifest abnormalities not only of the heart but also of the skeletal system, the nails, and the mouth.[57–59]

Congenital heart disease occurs in 50 to 60 per cent of patients and frequently causes deaths in infancy. The most common cardiac lesion involves the atrium, producing either a single atrium or a large atrial septal defect. The atrial lesion may occur alone, or it may be associated with another cardiac defect, such as aortic atresia, hypoplastic ascending aorta, or hypoplastic left ventricle.

The skeletal findings in the Ellis–van Creveld syndrome are characteristic. The patients have an abnormally small stature that is present from the time of birth. They exhibit a particularly striking shortening in the distal parts of the extremities. Bilateral polydactyly and fusion of the carpal bones are also present. Additional findings include the presence of hypoplastic nails and several oral abnormalities, including labiogingival adherences, accessory frenula, and hypodontia.

About half of affected individuals die in early infancy as a result of cardiorespiratory problems. The majority of survivors have normal intelligence. Eventual adult stature is in the range of 45 to 60 inches (115 to 150 cm).

Although the Ellis–van Creveld syndrome is an extremely rare disorder in the general population, it occurs with high frequency in certain isolated groups. As a result, the genetics of the disease have been well delineated.[58] The following observations support an autosomal recessive inheritance pattern: (1) The disorder occurs with equal frequency in males and females; (2) only siblings are affected in a given family; and (3) about one-third of all cases result from parental consanguinity. Most cases of the disorder in the United States occur in the Old Order Amish, an inbred religious isolate in Lancaster County, Pennsylvania, in which 13 per cent of the population carries the mutant gene.[58]

The underlying biochemical defect responsible for the Ellis–van Creveld syndrome has not yet been identified. Nonetheless, since affected individuals always manifest bilateral polydactyly of the hands, it is possible to make a prenatal diagnosis in pregnancies at risk by inspecting the fetus in utero, using fetoscopy to determine whether or not polydactyly is present.[60]

FAMILIAL SUPRAVALVULAR AORTIC STENOSIS (see also p. 981). Supravalvular aortic stenosis can occur as an isolated congenital anomaly and as a component of two different clinical entities: (1) as a nonfamilial syndrome resulting from fetal hypercalcemia and characterized by elfin facies (antiverted nostrils, patulous lips, and small chin), mental retardation, dental anomalies, and congenital supravalvular aortic stenosis;[61] and (2) a familial syndrome transmitted as an autosomal dominant trait and characterized by the presence of pulmonary and systemic arterial stenoses in the *absence* of mental retardation and elfin facies.[62–65] Although these two syndromes are often discussed in textbooks as representing a "spectrum of the same disease," they are clinically and genetically distinct disorders. Since the first syndrome is not transmitted by a single-gene mechanism but rather results from excessive exposure or excessive hypersensitivity of fetal tissues to vitamin D, it will not be discussed further.

Patients with familial supravalvular aortic stenosis can exhibit a wide range of arterial abnormalities. Although supravalvular aortic stenosis is the "typical" lesion, many affected individuals have stenosis of the pulmonary artery (peripheral or supravalvular), brachiocephalic arterial stenosis, hypoplasia or coarctation of the descending aorta, and dilatation and tortuosity of the coronary arteries. Like most dominant traits, the mutant gene is variably expressed even among affected persons in the same family.

Most patients initially come to attention because of an asymptomatic heart murmur. Clinical signs of dyspnea, angina pectoris, syncope, or claudication do not usually begin until after age 20 years. Those patients who manifest coarctation of the descending aorta may show signs of hypertension. Since affected individuals are at risk for bacterial endocarditis and should receive antibiotics at appropriate times, it is important to identify all affected relatives as early in life as possible.

KARTAGENER SYNDROME. Kartagener syndrome consists of the triad of sinusitis, bronchiectasis, and situs inversus with dextrocardia.[66–69] The disorder is inherited as an autosomal recessive trait; males and females are affected with equal frequency. In addition to the classic triad mentioned above, affected males are infertile as a result of immobile spermatozoa.

Since individuals with Kartagener syndrome are homozygous for a mutant gene, the clinical course is remarkably uniform among affected persons. These individuals initially come to attention as infants because of mucopurulent nasal discharge and repeated bouts of upper respiratory infections, otitis media, and pneumonia. By the preschool years, most patients exhibit persistent sinusitis, chronic bronchitis, and bronchiectasis. As many as 90 per cent of affected individuals have complete situs inversus, a mirror image reversal of internal organs due to a sinistral instead of a dextral rotation of the viscera occurring between days 10 and 15 of gestation.

In most affected individuals, dextrocardia is the only cardiac manifestation. Occasionally, one or more associated cardiac anomalies are present, such as transposition of the great arteries and trilocular or bilocular heart.

Kartagener syndrome occurs in about 1 person in 68,000. Of all persons with bronchiectasis, about 1.4 per cent have Kartagener syndrome, and of all persons with situs inversus, about 15 per cent have Kartagener syndrome.[70] The occurrence of this disorder in multiple siblings, male as well as female; the absence of any manifestations in the parents or in the children of affected individuals; and the presence of a higher than average frequency of consanguinity among the parents of affected individuals all support an autosomal recessive mode of inheritance.

The nature of the primary genetic defect in the Kartagener syndrome has recently been elucidated by electron microscopic investigation of a ciliated mucosal biopsy or of an ejaculate. These studies show that the nonmotile cilia and sperm obtained from affected individuals are structurally normal in most respects. However, the so-called dynein arms are abnormal.[66,70] Dynein arms are protein structures that normally form temporary cross bridges between adjacent microtubules in cilia and sperm tails (Fig. 47–4). The dynein arms play a role analogous to that of myosin in muscle in that they allow the sliding of the microtubules upon each other to generate movements of cilia and sperm.

Several different mutations can produce the Kartagener syndrome. In all cases the mutant gene disrupts the synthesis either of the dynein protein itself or of a protein that binds dynein to the microtubules,[66,70] causing any one of several types of morphological abnormalities in the ciliary axoneme: missing dynein arms (Fig. 47–4), abnormally short dynein arms, short spokes with no central sheath, missing central microtubules, or displacement of one of the nine peripheral microtubular doublets. The presence of any one of these abnormalities in the ciliary axoneme can presumably produce immobility of sperm and respiratory cilia, accounting for the clinical findings of infertility, sinusitis, and bronchiectasis. The molecular basis of the situs inversus is less certain, but it is reasonable to suppose that a malrotation of the visceral tissues occurs in the embryo when the ciliary movements of visceral epithelia do not occur.

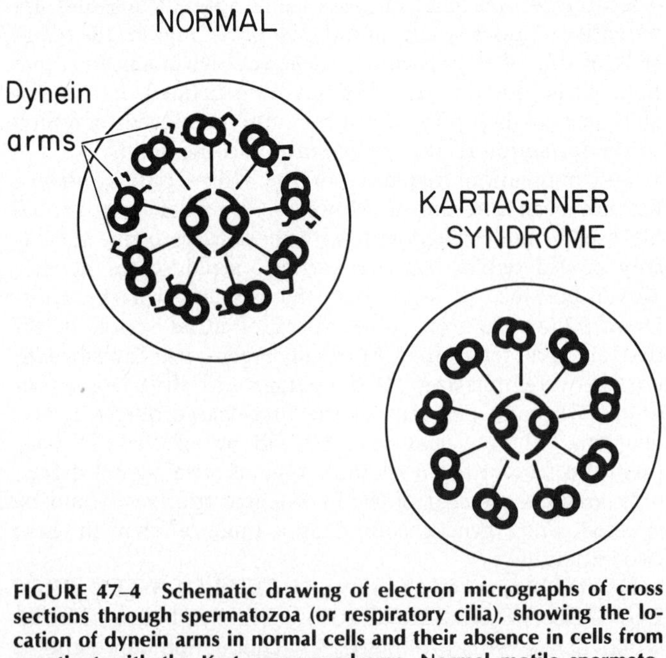

FIGURE 47–4 Schematic drawing of electron micrographs of cross sections through spermatozoa (or respiratory cilia), showing the location of dynein arms in normal cells and their absence in cells from a patient with the Kartagener syndrome. Normal motile spermatozoa and respiratory cilia possess nine micro-tubular doublets, each of which contains two dynein arms.

FAMILIAL PRIMARY PULMONARY HYPERTENSION (see also p. 839). Primary pulmonary hypertension is a disorder characterized by increased arterial pressure in the pulmonary circulation caused by changes that appear to be intrinsic to the pulmonary vasculature. Although most cases are sporadic, a familial form also occurs.[71-76] The mode of inheritance appears to be autosomal dominant. Many large pedigrees showing vertical transmission through three generations have been reported.[71-76] Onset of symptoms occurs from early childhood to middle age. Except for a history of family involvement, affected individuals show no unique clinical features that allow them to be distinguished from patients with nongenetic forms of primary pulmonary hypertension. However, the presence of the disorder in a man should be a clue to the familial form, since the nongenetic forms occur much more frequently in women than in men.

Multifactorial Disorders

The chromosomal abnormalities and single-gene disorders that produce congenital heart disease account for no more than 5 to 10 per cent of all cases of congenital heart disease.[10] The remaining "garden-variety" cases are believed to result from developmental defects involving multiple genes and possibly environmental factors. Hence, the genetic predisposition in most cases of congenital heart disease is multifactorial.[77-79]

In general, congenital heart defects produced by chromosomal errors (as in Down syndrome) and by single-gene mutations (as in Noonan syndrome and Kartagener syndrome) are a part of a multisystem disorder. On the other hand, congenital heart defects with multifactorial inheritance typically occur as discrete lesions that are not part of a multisystem disorder.

As in other disorders showing multifactorial inheritance, the recurrence risk to first-degree relatives of a patient with a "garden-variety" type of congenital heart disease is considerably less than the 25 to 50 per cent risk that occurs in single-gene disorders. Although the relative risk to the siblings and offspring of such a patient is 3 to 40 times the estimated population frequency, the overall absolute risk for these first-degree relatives is low, in the range of 1 to 4 per cent.[77,80] Table 47–3 lists the expected recurrence risk for siblings and offspring of patients with the 14 most common forms of congenital heart disease. Although these empirical data are useful in the genetic counseling of families that have had only one child with a congenital heart lesion, they do not apply in families with more than one affected person. When two first-degree relatives are affected, the recurrence risk is subsequent offspring doubles or triples; with three affected, the risks reach 10 to 20 per cent. When the first case is diagnosed in a given family, it is not possible to predict whether that family is at risk for multiple occurrences of congenital heart disease.

HEREDITARY DISORDERS OF CONNECTIVE TISSUE

Single-gene Disorders

The hereditary disorders of connective tissue are a group of diseases in which the predominant pathologic condition involves either the fibrous elements (such as collagen and elastin) or the nonfibrous elements (such as the mucopolysaccharide ground substance) of connective tissue throughout the body.[81] Since collagen, elastin, and mucopolysaccharides are all essential components of arteries and heart valves, it is not surprising that mutations affecting either the structure or the metabolism of these macromolecules would produce abnormalities in cardiac function. We now recognize 17 different hereditary connective tissue disorders in which cardiac involvement is a prominent feature. Each of these disorders is determined by a single-gene mechanism. The major clinical and genetic aspects of these disorders are summarized in Table 47–4.

As evident from this table, four types of cardiovascular disease—premature coronary artery disease, aortic regurgitation, mitral regurgitation, and abnormalities in the peripheral arteries—occur with high frequency in patients with the hereditary disorders of connective tissue. Of the 17 disorders listed in Table 47–4, 7 cause premature coronary artery disease (alkaptonuria, homocystinuria, pseudoxanthoma elasticum, idiopathic arterial calcification of infancy, Hurler syndrome, Hurler-Scheie compound, and Hunter syndrome), and 9 cause aortic or mitral regurgitation or both (Marfan syndrome, familial mitral valve prolapse syndrome, osteogenesis imperfecta, Hurler syndrome,

TABLE 47–3 EMPIRICAL RECURRENCE RISKS FOR SIBLINGS AND OFFSPRING OF PROBANDS WITH CONGENITAL HEART LESIONS

Abnormality in Proband	Risk to Siblings: *Number Affected/Total Number*	Risk to Siblings: *Per Cent*	Risk to Offspring: *Number Affected/Total Number*	Risk to Offspring: *Per Cent*
Ventricular septal defect	28/672	4.2	7/174	4.0
Patent ductus arteriosus	18/516	3.5	6/139	4.3
Tetralogy of Fallot	11/366	3.0	6/141	4.2
Atrial septal defect	11/380	2.9	5/199	2.7
Pulmonic stenosis	10/375	2.7	4/111	3.6
Aortic stenosis	8/361	2.2	4/103	3.9
Coarctation of aorta	5/281	1.8	7/253	2.7
Transposition of great vessels	4/229	1.7		
Atrioventricular canal	4/151	2.6		
Tricuspid atresia	1/98	1.0		
Ebstein anomaly	1/105	1.0		
Truncus arteriosus	1/86	1.2		
Pulmonic atresia	1/80	1.3		
Hypoplastic left heart	8/370	2.2		

(Modified from Nora, J. J., and Nora, A. H.: Circulation *57*:205–213, 1978; Nora, J. J., McGill, C. W., and McNamara, D. G.: Teratology *3*:325–330, 1970; and Nora, J. J., Dodd, P. F., Hattwick, M. A. W., et al.: J.A.M.A. *209*:2052–2053, 1969.)

TABLE 47–4 HEREDITARY DISORDERS OF CONNECTIVE TISSUE WITH CARDIOVASCULAR INVOLVEMENT

DISORDER	MAJOR CLINICAL MANIFESTATIONS *Cardiovascular*	*Noncardiovascular*	CARDIOVASCULAR INVOLVEMENT IN AFFECTED SUBJECTS *(Per Cent)*	TYPICAL AGE OF ONSET OF CARDIOVASCULAR ABNORMALITY	PRIMARY BIOCHEMICAL DEFECT	MECHANISM OF INHERITANCE	REFERENCES
Marfan syndrome	Aortic aneurysm and rupture, mitral regurgitation	Ectopia lentis, gracile habitus, arachnodactyly	50–70	Young adult	Not known	Dominant	81–83
Familial midsystolic click syndrome	Late systolic murmur, midsystolic clicks, abnormal EKG, mitral valve prolapse	None	100	Young adult	Not known	Dominant	84–87
Osteogenesis imperfecta	Aortic regurgitation	Multiple fractures, blue sclerae, otosclerosis, and deafness	Rare	Adult	Not known	Dominant	81
Ehlers-Danlos Type IV*	Rupture of aorta and other large arteries	Severe bruisability, rupture of bowel, minimal joint laxity	> 95	Young adult	Deficient synthesis of Type III collagen	Dominant	81, 88–91
Cutis laxa, recessive form	Peripheral pulmonic stenosis, arterial aneurysms	Pendulous skin, hernias, severe emphysema	50	Infancy	Not known	Recessive	92
Alkaptonuria	Calcific aortic stenosis, generalized atherosclerosis	Black urine, pigmentation of cartilage, degenerative joint changes	50–75	Adult	Deficiency of homogentisic acid oxidase	Recessive	81
Homocystinuria*	Arterial and venous thrombosis, myocardial infarction, pulmonary embolism	Ectopia lentis, osteoporosis, mental retardation	> 95	Young adult	Deficiency of cystathionine synthase	Recessive	81, 93–96
Pseudoxanthoma elasticum	Coronary artery disease, claudication, hypertension	Peau d'orange skin, retinal angioid streaks, gastrointestinal bleeding	50	Young adult	Not known	Dominant and recessive forms	81, 97–101
Idiopathic arterial calcification of infancy	Death from myocardial infarction in first 5 months of life, generalized calcification of peripheral arteries	None	100	Neonates	Not known	Recessive	102, 103
Mucopolysaccharidoses*					Abnormal degradation of mucopolysaccharidoses		81, 104, 105

Hurler-Scheie compound, Hunter syndrome, Morquio syndrome, Maroteaux-Lamy syndrome, and Type III mucolipidosis).

The Marfan syndrome and familial mitral valve prolapse syndrome are relatively common and are frequently encountered by cardiologists. Their genetic aspects are discussed here in detail. The 15 other inborn disorders listed in Table 47–4 are rare, each having a population frequency of 1 in 40,000 to 100,000 persons, and are not considered further in this chapter. Pertinent references in the literature are provided in the table.

MARFAN SYNDROME (see also p. 1665). Marfan syndrome is a generalized disorder of connective tissue that is inherited as an autosomal dominant trait. The cardinal manifestations consist of abnormalities of the eye (high-grade myopia and ectopia lentis), of the skeletal system (gangling habitus, arachnodactyly, pectus excavatum, and pectus carinatum), and of the cardiovascular system. In individual patients, all manifestations may not be present.[81]

Cardiac abnormalities occur in at least 60 per cent of affected adults.[81–83] The major cardiovascular lesion in adults is a dilatation of the aortic ring, the sinuses of Valsalva, and the ascending thoracic aorta. Stretching of the aortic valve leads ultimately to aortic regurgitation, aortic dissection (Chap. 44), or both.

Among 505 unselected cases of aortic dissection, 74 occurred in patients under age 40. Twelve of these younger patients (16 per cent) had Marfan syndrome.[108] Aortic dissection is the most serious complication. Together with the other aortic valve abnormalities, it represents the leading cause of death. Most of the patients are young (in the early 30's) and in good health when dissection occurs.[109] In patients with Marfan syndrome, it has been suggested that propranolol may be useful in preventing aortic dissection by reducing dP/dt to low-normal levels.[110] Pregnancy greatly increases the risk of aortic dissection and rupture and hence poses a serious risk to life.[111,112] Although the basic defect leading to the weakening of the aortic wall is unknown, histological studies show a striking loss of elastic fibers in the media of the damaged aortic segment.[81]

Mitral regurgitation is a frequently encountered cardiac abnormality in affected adults.[81–83] The mitral regurgitation is usually due to redundant cusps and chordae tendineae, producing a "floppy" prolapsed mitral valve (p. 1089). Cineangiography usually shows retroversion of a redun-

TABLE 47–4 HEREDITARY DISORDERS OF CONNECTIVE TISSUE WITH CARDIOVASCULAR INVOLVEMENT Continued

Disorder	Major Clinical Manifestations: Cardiovascular	Major Clinical Manifestations: Noncardiovascular	Cardiovascular Involvement in Affected Subjects (Per Cent)	Typical Age of Onset of Cardiovascular Abnormality	Primary Biochemical Defect	Mechanism of Inheritance	References
					due to:		
Type 1-H Hurler syndrome*	Aortic and mitral regurgitation, coronary artery disease, cardiomyopathy	Corneal clouding, coarse features, mental retardation, early death	50–75	Before age 2	Deficiency of α-L-iduronidase (I-H allele)	Recessive	81, 104, 105
Type I-S, Scheie syndrome	Aortic regurgitation	Stiff joints, normal intelligence, corneal clouding	> 95	Adult	Deficiency of α-L-iduronidase (I-S allele)	Recessive	81, 104, 105
Type I-H/S, Hurler-Scheie compound*	Aortic and mitral regurgitation	Phenotype intermediate between Hurler and Scheie syndromes	> 95	Young adult	Deficiency of α-L-iduronidase (I-H and I-S alleles)	Recessive; genetic compound of Type I-H and I-S alleles	81, 104, 105
Type II, Hunter syndrome (severe)*	Aortic and mitral regurgitation, coronary artery disease, cardiomyopathy	No corneal clouding; milder course than in Type I-H, but death before age 15	> 95	Childhood	Deficiency of sulfoiduronide sulfatase (severe allele)	X-linked	81, 104, 105
Type II, Hunter syndrome (mild)*	Aortic and mitral regurgitation, coronary artery disease	Survival to 30's and 50's, fair intelligence	> 95	Young adult	Deficiency of sulfoiduromide sulfatase (mild allele)	X-linked	81, 104, 105
Type IV, Morquio syndrome*	Aortic regurgitation	Severe bone changes with gibbus and dwarfism, corneal clouding, normal intelligence	> 75	Young adult	Deficiency of *N*-acetylhexosamine sulfate sulfatase	Recessive	81, 104, 105
Type VI, Maroteaux Lamy syndrome*	Aortic and mitral regurgitation	Corneal clouding, severe osseous changes, normal intelligence	> 95	Childhood	Deficiency of arylsulfatase B	Recessive	81, 104, 105
Mucolipidosis, Type III, (pseudo-Hurler polydystrophy)*	Aortic and mitral regurgitation	Claw hand and stiff joints, coarse facies, kyphoscoliosis, corneal clouding, carpal tunnel syndrome, low normal intelligence	> 95	Young adult	Deficiency of *N*-acetylglucosamine-1-phosphotransferase	Recessive	81, 106, 107

*Prenatal diagnosis is possible.

dant posterior mitral valve leaflet with regurgitation occurring in late systole. These patients typically manifest a late systolic murmur with or without mid- to late systolic clicks. In some patients the mitral regurgitation is severe and functionally significant. On the basis of echocardiographic findings, mitral prolapse may be more common than aortic regurgitation. Massive calcification of the mitral annulus is occasionally seen.[113] Less common complications include cystic disease of the lung, recurrent spontaneous pneumothorax, and bacterial endocarditis, which may be superimposed on minor changes of the heart valves.[81]

The cardiac manifestations of Marfan syndrome are more subtle and less severe in children than in adults.[83] The most common cardiac lesion in the pediatric age group is an isolated mitral regurgitation that is usually asymptomatic but can be very severe. In contrast to Marfan adults, affected children rarely manifest signs of aortic root disease. However, when aortic regurgitation is present, the patients show a rapidly deteriorating course. The overall mortality in one large study of children with Marfan syndrome was as high as 14 per cent.[83]

Although the basic defect has not been identified, the genetics of Marfan syndrome are well understood.[81] The disorder is inherited as an autosomal dominant trait with marked variability in clinical expression. In about 85 per cent of cases, one of the parents is affected. The other 15 per cent of cases occur sporadically and apparently represent new mutations occurring in the germ cells of one of the parents.[114] The average age of the fathers of those with sporadic cases is 7 years higher than that of the fathers of those having inherited cases. These data suggest that the new mutations occur in the father's germ cells and that their frequency increases with paternal age.[114]

Relatives at 50 per cent risk for having Marfan syndrome frequently request that studies be performed on them to determine whether they have it and are thus a risk of passing the mutant gene to their children. This may pose a problem for the physician, since some affected patients are asymptomatic and show no obvious features of the syndrome. Nevertheless, subtle manifestations can be detected in a high proportion of asymptomatic Marfan syndrome patients by performing three studies: echocardiography (looking for prolapse of the mitral valve and aortic root dilation), anthropometrical evaluation (measuring the upper and lower body segments), and ophthalmological examination (searching for ectopia lentis).[115,116]

FAMILIAL MITRAL VALVE PROLAPSE SYNDROME (see also p. 1089). Familial mitral valve prolapse syndrome is an autosomal dominant disorder characterized by ballooning or prolapse of the posterior mitral valve leaflet, which produces a midsystolic click and a late systolic murmur.[84-87] Since the initial delineation of the syndrome in 1963, myriad reports have appeared in the literature describing patients with this disorder. However, most of these reports have failed to take into account that prolapse of the mitral valve per se is etiologically a heterogeneous entity and that the dominantly inherited syndrome constitutes only one of its many causes.

A syndrome virtually identical to familial mitral valve prolapse syndrome has also been described in patients with Marfan syndrome, Turner syndrome, Ehlers-Danlos syndrome, hypertrophic obstructive cardiomyopathy, acute rheumatic fever, and coronary artery disease; following mitral commissurotomy; and in association with ruptured chordae tendineae and secundum atrial septal defect.[84,85] In these last-named disorders, prolapse of the mitral valve is considered a secondary phenomenon that results from a variety of abnormalities involving the mitral leaflets, chordae tendineae, papillary muscles, or mitral annulus. The clinical significance of the valvular dysfunction is usually subordinate to that of the primary disease process.

In contrast to the secondary causes of prolapse of the mitral valve, in familial mitral valve prolapse syndrome, the pathologic condition of the mitral valve almost always consists of a myxomatous degeneration.[84,85] Microscopy of involved leaflets shows replacement of the central fibrous tissue by metachromatically staining, loose, myxomatous material accompanied by fibroelastic thickening of the adjacent endocardium.[84]

A large degree of clinical variability appears in families affected with familial mitral valve prolapse syndrome. Affected females more often show clinical signs than do affected males. Symptoms of prolapse of the mitral valve can develop at any age and can range from mild to severe. Common presentations include palpitations, presyncope, syncope, chest pain, dyspnea, and/or fatigue.[84,85] The palpitations are usually due to atrial or ventricular arrhythmias. Sudden death is presumably due to ventricular arrhythmias. The major auscultatory findings typically consist of a nonejection click in midsystole or a late systolic murmur heard best at the cardiac apex or both.[84,85] Diagnosis can be confirmed by echocardiography or ventricular cineangiography. The major complications of the syndrome include bacterial endocarditis, severe mitral insufficiency, and life-threatening arrhythmias.[84,85]

The population frequency of the primary form of prolapse of the mitral valve has been reported to be as high as 6 to 17 per cent among apparently healthy young women.[117,118] These estimates, if correct, place prolapse of the mitral valve among the commonest of all cardiac abnormalities. Although an autosomal dominant mechanism appears to account for mitral valve prolapse in certain families,[84-87] the exact proportion of patients with the primary syndrome who owe their disease to a single mutant gene is unknown. Genetic studies designed to answer this question are made difficult by the presence of silent or asymptomatic prolapse in some subjects who are known to possess the abnormal gene.

CARDIOMYOPATHIES

Single-gene Disorders

At least ten single-gene–determined forms of cardiomyopathy are currently recognized. In some of these disorders, the myocardial disease dominates the clinical picture, as in Pompe disease, familial hypertrophic obstructive cardiomyopathy, and familial cardiomyopathy. In some, the cardiomyopathy occurs as part of a generalized metabolic disease, as in hemochromatosis and familial amyloidosis. In others, the cardiomyopathy occurs as part of a neuromyopathic syndrome, as in myotonic dystrophy, Duchenne muscular dystrophy, and Friedreich ataxia.

POMPE DISEASE (TYPE II GLYCOGEN STORAGE DISEASE) (see also p. 1051). Pompe disease is a rare inborn error of glycogen metabolism that results from an absence of the lysosomal enzyme acid α-1,4-glucosidase.[119] Once synthesized in cells, glycogen is degraded by several mechanisms, one of which involves a nonlysosomal phosphorylytic pathway that converts glycogen to glucose-6-phosphate. The other pathway involves hydrolysis of the glycogen to glucose within lysosomes. In the absence of the lysosomal acid maltase, large amounts of glycogen accumulate within lysosomes of tissues throughout the body including the heart. Since the nonlysosomal phosphorylytic pathway of glycogen breakdown is normal in Pompe disease, carbohydrate metabolism is normal and hypoglycemia does not occur.

The massive accumulation of glycogen in body tissues in Pompe disease leads to a characteristic clinical picture that becomes apparent within the first few months of life. Affected infants typically manifest feeding difficulty, inadequate weight gain, respiratory difficulty, hypotonia, atrophy of subcutaneous fat, enlarged tongue, and congestive heart failure.[119] Death from cardiac failure invariably occurs within the first year of life. The cardiomyopathy of Pompe disease is characterized by the absence of significant heart murmurs, the presence of massive cardiomegaly on chest roentgenograms, and the presence of several distinctive electrocardiographic findings. The latter include a short P-R interval (0.05 to 0.09 sec) and huge QRS complexes.[120]

Pompe disease is inherited as an autosomal recessive trait. The gene coding for lysosomal acid α-1,4-glucosidase is located on chromosome 17.[122] Because the disorder is quite rare (occurring with a population frequency of less than 1 in 100,000 persons[121]), about 20 per cent of affected cases are associated with parental consanguinity. As in most recessive disorders, the heterozygous parents manifest no detectable clinical abnormalities. Inasmuch as the lysosomal acid α-1,4-glucosidase enzyme is normally present in cultured amniotic fluid cells, prenatal diagnosis of homozygous affected fetuses is feasible and has successfully been carried out in couples who have a 25 per cent recurrence risk for having a second child with Pompe disease.[123]

FAMILIAL HYPERTROPHIC OBSTRUCTIVE CARDIOMYOPATHY (see also p. 1409). Familial hypertrophic obstructive cardiomyopathy is determined by an autosomal dominant mechanism. Recent studies of both the asymptomatic and the symptomatic relatives of patients with clinically apparent cases have demonstrated that asymmetrical septal hypertrophy, often without outflow obstruction, represents the most constant and characteristic feature of this disorder.[124,125] Asymmetrical septal hypertrophy is detected by echocardiography and is defined as the presence of a ventricular septum that is at least 30 per cent thicker than the posterobasal wall of the left ventricle.[124]

The mutant gene appears to be fully penetrant; that is, virtually all individuals who inherit the gene show asymmetrical septal hypertrophy. Nevertheless, the resulting clinical manifestations are variable from patient to patient.[124,125] In full-blown cases of hypertrophic obstructive cardiomyopathy, the asymmetrical septal hypertrophy progresses to ventricular outflow tract obstruction, and this, in turn, leads to the clinical findings of dyspnea, fatigability, angina, syncope, palpitations due to arrhythmias, and sudden death.[126] Patients with the complete syndrome, who typically come to medical attention between the ages of 20 and 30 years, probably represent no more than 20 per cent of all individuals affected with familial hypertrophic obstructive cardiomyopathy.[124] The other 80 per cent of subjects who have inherited the mutant gene show echocardiographic evidence of asymmetrical septal hypertrophy but manifest no clinical abnormalities (about 20 per cent of gene carriers) or show nonspecific electrocardiographic and auscultatory findings that are nondiagnostic (60 per cent of gene carriers).[124]

Many large pedigrees with familial hypertrophic obstructive cardiomyopathy have been reported in the literature, providing abundant evidence for autosomal dominant transmission.[126–129] The most impressive pedigree to date is that of a French-Canadian kindred in which the genealogical survey was extended to the original emigrant from France in the 1600's.[128] In family studies, echocardiography has demonstrated that 93 per cent of probands have an affected parent,[124] thus implying that no more than 7 per cent of cases of hypertrophic obstructive cardiomyopathy represent new mutations. This estimate agrees well with estimates of the limited extent to which this disorder reduces reproductive fitness.

A subgroup of families with unusually frequent premature deaths (termed "malignant" hypertrophic cardiomyopathy) has recently been identified.[129] Of the 69 first-degree relatives in these 8 families, 41 had clinical evidence of hypertrophic cardiomyopathy and 32 (78 per cent of those affected) died of heart disease before 50 years of age. Sudden and unexpected death occurred in 23 of the 32 patients.

The basic biochemical defect is unknown. Discovery of the mechanism of action of the mutant gene will undoubtedly provide insight into the biochemical and cellular basis of ventricular hypertrophy.

FAMILIAL CARDIOMYOPATHY (see also p. 1400). The designation familial cardiomyopathy is used to refer to an ill-defined and undoubtedly heterogeneous group of entities having the common denominators of cardiomegaly, congestive cardiomyopathy, and familial occurrence, suggestive of autosomal dominant inheritance. The major clinical manifestations of familial cardiomyopathy include cardiomegaly, congestive heart failure, arrhythmias, syncope, and sudden death. Angina pectoris and embolic episodes are also frequently noted. Electrocardiographic abnormalities, which include rhythm disturbances, left ventricular hypertrophy, intraventricular conduction defects, abnormal Q waves, and the Wolff-Parkinson-White pattern, are often present in affected individuals many years prior to signs of clinical deterioration.[130–135]

The prognosis is highly variable from person to person. Some affected individuals remain asymptomatic except for electrocardiographic abnormalities. Others die of intractable heart failure or of arrhythmias as young adults.[131] Histological examination of affected hearts typically reveals diffuse fibrosis with severe hypertrophy of the remaining muscle fibers.[130–135]

Although the autosomal dominant inheritance of familial cardiomyopathy is beyond doubt in certain pedigrees, there are no unique clinical manifestations of the mutant gene. Thus, in the patient who has a congestive cardiomyopathy and whose family history is not informative, it is difficult to know whether there is a 50 per cent risk of transmitting the disorder to children or whether the cardiomyopathy has a nongenetic etiology.

IDIOPATHIC HEMOCHROMATOSIS (see also p. 1425). Idiopathic hemochromatosis is a hereditary multisystem disorder characterized by the deposition of iron in the liver, pancreas, skin, and heart.[136,137] Clinical manifestations consist of cirrhosis, diabetes mellitus, hyperpigmentation, hypogonadism, cardiomyopathy, and a high incidence of hepatoma. The clinical manifestations are delayed for many years until iron overload has caused significant tissue damage and organ failure. The average diet in America allows a maximal routine iron balance of about 4 mg/per day in males.[137] The average age of overt clinical presentation is usually 40 years or older. Diagnosis is confirmed by the finding of an elevated serum iron concentration ($>$ 180 μg per cent), an elevated transferrin saturation ($>$ 80 per cent), an elevated serum ferritin level ($>$ 900 ng/ml), and an increase in the hepatic iron content ($>$ 600 μg/100 mg dry weight) in the absence of known causes of exogenous iron overload.

The major cardiac findings are rhythm and conduction disturbances and biventricular congestive heart failure, which occur separately or together.[136] The commonest arrhythmias are ventricular extrasystoles, paroxysmal atrial tachycardia and fibrillation, and atrioventricular block. The clinical manifestations of congestive failure include dyspnea, edema, ascites, and a large, globular cardiac silhouette on chest roentgenograms. Rarely, hemochromatosis simulates constrictive pericarditis (presumably because of the decrease in myocardial compliance caused by the iron infiltration of the myocardium), and in such patients a small or normal-sized heart is seen.

Cardiac manifestations are the presenting feature in only 15 per cent of cases, but approximately one-third of patients with hemochromatosis die from congestive heart failure.[137] Cardiac abnormalities are particularly prominent in young patients. Death usually follows within 1 year of onset. A program of repeated phlebotomy may alleviate congestive failure and increase survival in individual patients.

Idiopathic hemochromatosis has long been recognized to be an inherited disorder, yet its genetics remained, until recently, a controversial subject.[138,139] The difficulty in delineating the precise mode of inheritance arose for several reasons. First, the basic biochemical defect that causes excessive iron absorption from the intestine has not been de-

ally every type of cardiac arrhythmia and conduction defect, in most cases the available genetic data are insufficient to determine whether the defect in a given family results from a single-gene mutation or a multifactorial genetic mechanism. Evidence for a single-gene mechanism is compelling, however, in several distinct syndromes.

JERVELL AND LANGE-NIELSEN SYNDROME (see also p. 781). This disorder is characterized by congenital deafness, syncope, prolonged Q-T interval, and sudden death.[181–184] Affected individuals are seen typically in childhood with congenital high-tone perceptive deafness, which is bilateral and severe, and fainting spells precipitated by exertion or nervousness. The electrocardiogram shows a prolonged Q-T interval and large T waves. The syncopal attacks are believed due to episodic ventricular arrhythmias or Stokes-Adams attacks. Administration of digitalis can reduce the Q-T interval and diminish the frequency of syncopal attacks. Since syncopal attacks are usually provoked by exercise, fear, or anger, affected children should be protected from physical and mental stress. At autopsy, histological abnormalities in the artery to the sinus node and to the AV node have been demonstrated.

The cardiac and auditory abnormalities appear to represent a pleiotropic expression of a single gene abnormality, which is inherited by an autosomal recessive mechanism.[185] The incidence of consanguinity among the parents of affected subjects is increased.[182] Although the heterozygotes are clinically normal, their electrocardiograms may show a mildly prolonged Q-T interval.[182] The overall incidence of homozygous affected individuals among all deaf children is about 1 case in 100, whereas among the general population it is about 1 case in 300,000 persons.[182,185]

ROMANO-WARD SYNDROME (see also p. 781). Romano-Ward syndrome is similar to Jervell and Lange-Nielsen syndrome in that affected individuals show a prolonged Q-T interval and an abnormal configuration of T waves on their electrocardiograms and are prone to ventricular fibrillation and sudden death.[186–190] The two syndromes are clinically and genetically distinct: Deafness is not a feature of Romano-Ward syndrome, and Romano-Ward syndrome is inherited as an autosomal dominant trait.

Patients are usually healthy except for episodes which may take one of three forms: (1) transient attacks of palpitation, numbness, or anginal chest pain without loss of consciousness; (2) sudden loss of consciousness, usually precipitated by exertion or emotional stress; or (3) sudden death. The disorder is predominantly a childhood illness, with onset usually before age 3 years. However, as in most autosomal dominant disorders, a marked variation in the degree of clinical expression occurs, and some affected subjects do not show clinical signs until age 30 years. In general, the later the age of onset, the milder the disease and the less the threat of sudden death. The molecular basis for the underlying abnormality is not known.

FAMILIAL HEART BLOCK (see also page 1014). At least two genetically distinct causes of heart block are currently recognized—one with a congenital onset and one with an adult onset. The congenital disorder is seen either at the time of birth or in early childhood as severe bradycardia due to complete AV block. The prognosis for the congenital form of familial heart block is extremely poor. Most affected individuals die in the neonatal period. Autopsy of several cases has revealed an absence of the AV node as well as an absence of myocardial fibers in the lower part of the interatrial septum.[191,192]

Early studies suggested that congenital heart block was inherited as an autosomal recessive trait.[191,192] However, recent reports have shown that a large proportion of infants previously diagnosed as having the autosomal recessive form of congenital heart block are offspring of mothers who have systemic lupus erythematosus. The placental transfer of maternal immune complexes is presumed to cause damage to the fetal cardiac conduction system in utero.[193–195] In one study of congenital heart block, 14 of 22 affected children had been born to 11 mothers who had clinical or laboratory evidence of lupus.[194] Congenital heart block may thus represent a familial disease that is not genetic. The clinician should suspect the presence of lupus or a related collagen vascular disease in any mother who gives birth to an infant with congenital heart block.

Familial heart block of adult onset appears to be inherited as an autosomal dominant disorder with varying expressivity.[196–199] Affected individuals typically are seen between the ages of 30 and 50 years with one of the following conduction abnormalities: right bundle branch block alone, left-axis deviation alone, right bundle branch block and left-axis deviation, or complete heart block. Patients may also show atrial fibrillation, atrial flutter, or bidirectional tachycardia. It must be emphasized that affected individuals in the same family characteristically manifest different electrocardiographic patterns. The electrocardiogram in the adult form of familial heart block tends to show a wider QRS complex than is found in the congenital form of familial heart block. Left untreated without a pacemaker, most patients with the adult form of familial heart block ultimately develop syncopal episodes or die suddenly—hence the need for the physician to examine and treat asymptomatic relatives who are at 50 per cent genetic risk.

WOLFF-PARKINSON-WHITE SYNDROME (see also p. 712). The electrocardiographic features of this syndrome are the presence of a short P-R interval and a prolonged QRS, the latter being specifically characterized by a slurred upstroke of the R wave called a delta wave. Patients with Wolff-Parkinson-White (WPW) syndrome are especially prone to paroxysmal supraventricular tachycardia. Although the majority of patients with WPW syndrome do not have a familial disorder, a familial occurrence has been reported on numerous occasions.[200,201] In certain families, WPW syndrome occurs as a dominantly inherited disorder with no associated cardiac defects, whereas in other families it can occur in association with a dominantly inherited form of familial cardiomyopathy.[202]

CONSTRICTIVE PERICARDITIS

(See also Chap. 43)

MULIBREY NANISM. Mulibrey nanism is a rare autosomal recessive disorder in which constrictive pericarditis is one of the cardinal manifestations. Described for the first time in 1973, the syndrome was given the name mulibrey nanism to symbolize some of these protean features.

Mulibrey stands for *mu*scle, *li*ver, *br*ain, and *ey*es; nanism is derived from the Greek word for dwarf, *nanos*.[203,204] A more appropriate name would be "constrictive pericarditis with dwarfism" to emphasize the two most prominent and consistent features of the syndrome.

Growth failure is evident at the time of birth and is progressive. Affected infants show a triangular face often with hypocephaloid skull, muscular hypotonia, a peculiar squeaky voice, and yellowish dots and pigment dispersion in the ocular fundus. Of 28 patients described in the literature, 25 have shown clinical signs of pericardial constriction, as manifested by prominent neck veins, elevated right-heart pressures on cardiac catherization, and hepatomegaly.[203–208] About 30 per cent of the affected patients so far reported have had ascites, peripheral edema, and proven pericardial constriction necessitating treatment by pericardiotomy.[203–208] Microscopic examination shows a thickened pericardium with calcium deposits but without evidence of active inflammation.[208]

Twenty-four of the 28 reported cases have come from a sparsely settled area of Finland.[203,204] Two cases have been reported in Canadians,[206] one case in an American,[208] and one case in an Egyptian.[207] All the familial cases have been limited to siblings, and most of the single cases (three of the Finnish patients, the American patient, and the Egyptian patient) have been born to consanguineous parents. These observations strongly support autosomal recessive inheritance. The pathogenesis of this unique disorder is completely unknown.

CARDIAC TUMORS

(See also Chap. 42)

The two most common primary tumors of the heart, myxomas and rhabdomyomas, can occur with or without familial involvement. The nonfamilial cases could represent (1) the occurrence of nongenetic cases, (2) the sporadic occurrence of tumors owing to new single-gene mutations, or (3) the occurrence of only one homozygote in a sibship as in autosomal recessive inheritance. In general, patients with nonfamilial tumors tend to have a single tumor, whereas those with tumors of a genetic origin tend to have multiple tumors.

INTRACARDIAC MYXOMA (see also p. 1460). Most cases of intracardiac myxoma occur as sporadic cases without familial involvement. However, since 1971 at least five families with multiple affected members have been reported.[209–214] In three of the families, only siblings have been affected, suggesting autosomal recessive inheritance.[209–212] However, in two families autosomal dominant inheritance was suggested by the occurrence of myxomas in both a parent and one or more siblings.[213,214] Affected individuals typically come to attention between the ages of 20 and 40 years because of syncope or signs of systemic embolization. The unique feature of the familial myxoma syndrome, as distinct from the more common nonfamilial tumor, is the presence of multiple tumors that are frequently in atypical locations, such as the pulmonic valve and the right ventricle.

RHABDOMYOMA (see also p. 1461). At least 50 per cent of patients with a single rhabdomyoma of the heart and probably all patients with multiple cardiac rhabdomyomas have tuberous sclerosis.[215] This autosomal dominant disorder is characterized clinically by the following features: adenoma sebaceum of the skin, mental retardation, epilepsy, intracranial calcifications, cutaneous findings (shagreen patches, periungual fibromas, depigmented cutaneous areas), honeycomb lung, gliomas of the brain, retinal phakomas, mixed mesodermal tumors of the kidney, and multiple cardiac rhabdomyomas.[216,217] As in most autosomal dominant disorders, a wide range of variability in clinical expression from patient to patient occurs.

The most common clinical manifestations, present in at least 60 per cent of affected individuals, are adenoma sebaceum, epilepsy, mental retardation, shagreen patches, and depigmented cutaneous areas.[216,217] Multiple rhabdomyomas, although highly specific for tuberous sclerosis, are a relatively infrequent manifestation, with no more than 5 per cent of affected individuals developing clinically significant cardiac tumors. Although the rhabdomyomas can occur at any age, they typically come to clinical attention in the neonatal period.[215] The typical patient with rhabdomyomas either shows signs of cardiac failure in the first few days of life or has severe arrhythmias.[215] Some rhabdomyomas may undergo neoplastic change to rhabdomyosarcoma.

CORONARY ARTERY DISEASE

(See also Chap. 35)

Evidence that genetic factors contribute to the pathogenesis of coronary atherosclerosis is based on observations of four types: (1) differences in prevalence among genetically different groups living under similar environmental circumstances;[218] (2) familial aggregation in which first-degree relatives of index coronary patients less than 60 years of age show a five- to sevenfold increased risk of death from myocardial infarction, compared with controls;[219,220] (3) higher concordance for myocardial infarction in identical twins as opposed to fraternal twins (for female twin pairs: 44 per cent concordance for monozygotic twins and 14 per cent for dizygotic twins);[221] and (4) association with one or more genetically determined risk factors, such as hypercholesterolemia, hypertriglyceridemia, diabetes mellitus, hypertension, obesity, personality type, and distribution of coronary vasculature.[222–224,224a]

In most families that seem genetically predisposed to coronary artery disease by history, the nature of the genetic factors underlying this predisposition is obscure. Most patients with coronary artery disease have inherited multiple predisposing genes that interact with multiple environmental factors to produce the disease. In these patients atherosclerosis does not have a single cause. Yet treatment of one of the predisposing factors, such as mild hypertension, hypercholesterolemia, or smoking, will likely slow the progression of the disease.

TABLE 47–5 SINGLE GENE DISORDERS THAT PREDISPOSE TO PREMATURE CORONARY ARTERY DISEASE

Disorder	Typical Age for Myocardial Infarction	Primary Biochemical Defect	Mechanism of Inheritance	Estimated Population Frequency	References
Familial hypercholesterolemia		Defective cell surface receptor for plasma LDL	Dominant		7, 225–227
Heterozygous form	Adult			1 in 500	
Homozygous form*	Childhood			1 in 1,000,000	
Multiple lipoprotein-type hyperlipidemia (Familial combined hyperlipidemia	Adult	Not known	Dominant	1 in 200	225, 227
Familial hypertriglyceridemia	Adult	Not known	Dominant	1 in 300	225, 227
Familial dysbetalipoproteinemia	Adult	Deficiency of Apo E-III	Recessive	1 in 40,000	225, 227
Hurler syndrome, Type I-H mucopolysaccharidosis*	Childhood	Deficiency of α-L-iduronidase	Recessive	1 in 40,000	81,104
Hunter syndrome, Type II mucopolysaccharidosis*	Childhood	Deficiency of sulfoiduronide sulfatase	X-linked	1 in 30,000	81,104
Homocystinuria*	Young adult	Deficiency of cystathionine synthase	Recessive	1 in 75,000	81, 93–95
Pseudoxanthoma elasticum	Young adult	Not known	Dominant and recessive	1 in 100,000	81, 101
Alkaptonuria	Adult	Deficiency of homogentisic acid oxidase	Recessive	1 in 100,000	81
Werner syndrome	Adult	Not known	Recessive	1 in 500,000	228, 229
Fabry disease*	Young adult	Deficiency of α-galactosidase A	X-linked	1 in 40,000	230, 231
Cholesteryl ester storage disease*	Young adult	Deficiency of lysosomal acid lipase	Recessive	1 in 1,000,000	232
Arterial calcification of infancy	Neonates	Not known	Recessive	1 in 1,000,000	102, 103

*Prenatal diagnosis is possible.

In some patients coronary artery disease is produced by a single abnormal gene that has a major effect. At least 13 different single-gene disorders, and hence at least 13 different mutant genes, are known to predispose to premature coronary artery disease (Table 47–5). The most common of these single-gene disorders are those that produce hyperlipidemia. At least 20 per cent of consecutively studied survivors of acute myocardial infarction manifest one of these common autosomal dominant forms of familial hyperlipidemia: familial hypercholesterolemia, familial hypertriglyceridemia, or multiple lipoprotein–type hyperlipidemia.[225] The other monogenic hyperlipidemia that predisposes to coronary artery disease, familial dysbetalipoproteinemia (Type 3 hyperlipidemia), is much less common, occurring in only about 1 in 500 unselected survivors of myocardial infarction.[225] These four monogenic forms of hyperlipidemia are discussed in the next section.

In addition to the familial hyperlipidemias, at least nine inborn errors of metabolism are seen, in which coronary narrowing and occlusion are often part of the clinical syndrome, e.g., Hunter syndrome, Hurler syndrome, homocystinuria, alkaptonuria, pseudoxanthoma elasticum, Werner syndrome, idiopathic arterial calcification of infancy, cholesteryl ester storage disease, and Fabry disease (Table 47–5). The mechanism for the coronary occlusion differs for each disorder and is directly related to the action of the particular gene. For example, in the Hunter and Hurler syndromes (p. 1670), mucopolysaccharides accumulate in the coronary vessels, whereas in Fabry disease, glycolipids accumulate (p. 1425). Seven of these inborn errors are inherited as autosomal recessive traits (Table 47–5). Although the homozygous form of each condition occurs rarely, with incidences ranging from 1 to 40,000 (homocystinuria) to 1 in 500,000 (Werner syndrome), the estimated combined frequency for the heterozygous carriers of these seven genes is quite significant, involving somewhere between 1 in 30 and 1 in 100 persons in the population. It will therefore be important to determine whether any of the genes for these seven inborn errors can significantly predispose its heterozygous carriers to develop premature coronary atherosclerosis. No such data are currently available.

Single-gene Disorders Causing Hyperlipidemia and Premature Atherosclerosis

Four monogenic diseases exist in which hyperlipidemia results from a discrete inborn error of metabolism affecting the synthesis, degradation, or structure of a plasma lipoprotein. Each of these single-gene diseases predisposes to coronary atherosclerosis. Together, these diseases are responsible for about 20 per cent of myocardial infarctions that occur before the age of 60.[225] To provide a conceptual background for discussion of these disorders, a brief explanation of normal lipoprotein transport is necessary (for review, see references 233 and 234).

The plasma lipoproteins are globular particles of high molecular weight that transport triglycerides and cholesteryl esters. Each lipoprotein contains a nonpolar core in which cholesteryl ester and triglyceride molecules are packed to form an oil droplet (Fig. 47–5). Surrounding the core is a polar surface coat composed predominantly of phospholipids and unesterified cholesterol. Each lipoprotein also contains specific proteins (termed *apoproteins*) that bind to enzymes or transport proteins, directing the lipoprotein to its sites of metabolism.

The lipoproteins of human plasma can be divided into five major classes, which are discussed in detail in Chapter

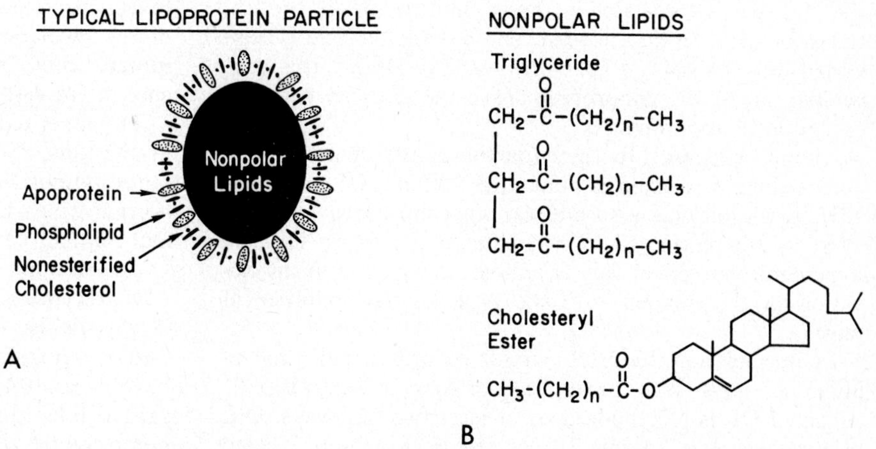

FIGURE 47–5 *A*, Diagrammatic representation of the structure of a typical plasma lipoprotein particle. The *core* of the spherical lipoprotein particle is composed of two nonpolar lipids, triglyceride and cholesteryl ester, which are present in different lipoproteins in varying amounts. The nonpolar core is surrounded by a *surface coat* composed primarily of phospholipids. Apoproteins are exposed at the surface and extend into the core. Variable amounts of unesterified cholesterol are interdigitated with the phospholipids of the surface coat. The quantitative composition of each of the different classes of lipoprotein particles in human plasma is discussed in Chapter 34 (see Fig. 34-3). *B*, Structures of the two nonpolar lipids, triglyceride and cholesteryl ester. In order for these nonpolar lipids to be assimilated into tissues, the ester bonds between the fatty acids and either glycerol (triglycerides) or cholesterol (cholesteryl esters) must be broken by lipoprotein lipase and the lysosomal cholesteryl esterase, respectively.

35. As shown in Table 35–3, p. 1210, each of these five lipoprotein classes differs from the others in the relative proportion of cholesteryl ester and triglyceride in the core, in the nature of its apoproteins, and in density, size, and electrophoretic mobility.[235]

A model showing the salient features of plasma lipoprotein transport is illustrated in Figure 47–6. Lipoproteins transport lipids that are absorbed from the intestine as well as those that are synthesized within the body.[233,234] Within the intestine, cholesterol and triglycerides are incorporated into large lipoprotein particles called *chylomicrons.* After they enter the bloodstream, the chylomicrons bind to an enzyme, *lipoprotein lipase,* which is adherent to capillary walls in adipose tissue and muscle. This enzyme hydrolyzes the triglycerides of the chylomicrons. The liberated fatty acids enter the underlying adipocytes or muscle cells, where they are either reesterified to triglycerides for storage or oxidized for energy.

After the triglycerides are removed, the remainder of the chylomicron dissociates from the capillary wall and reenters the circulation, where it is now designated as a *chylomicron remnant.* The chylomicron remnant is relatively poor in triglyceride and enriched in cholesteryl esters. It is also enriched in an important protein called *apoprotein E.* Chylomicron remnants travel to the liver, where they are taken up with great efficiency as a result of the binding of the apoprotein E to receptors on the surface of hepatocytes. Overall, the two-step pathway of chylomicron metabolism delivers dietary triglyceride to adipose tissue and muscle and dietary cholesterol to the liver.[233,234]

In the liver the metabolism of dietary fat and endogenously synthesized fat is coordinated to supply needed amounts of fuel and cholesterol to body tissues despite fluctuations in dietary intake. To supply cholesterol and trigylcerides to body tissues, the liver incorporates them into *very low-density lipoproteins (VLDL).*

VLDL particles are triglyceride-rich and thus resemble chylomicrons, although they are smaller in size. The triglycerides of VLDL are removed through interaction with lipoprotein lipase. The cholesteryl ester–rich remnant of VLDL metabolism is released from the endothelial wall and reenters the circulation, where it is designated *intermediate-density lipoprotein (IDL).* Although it is similar in structure to the chylomicron remnant, the IDL particle

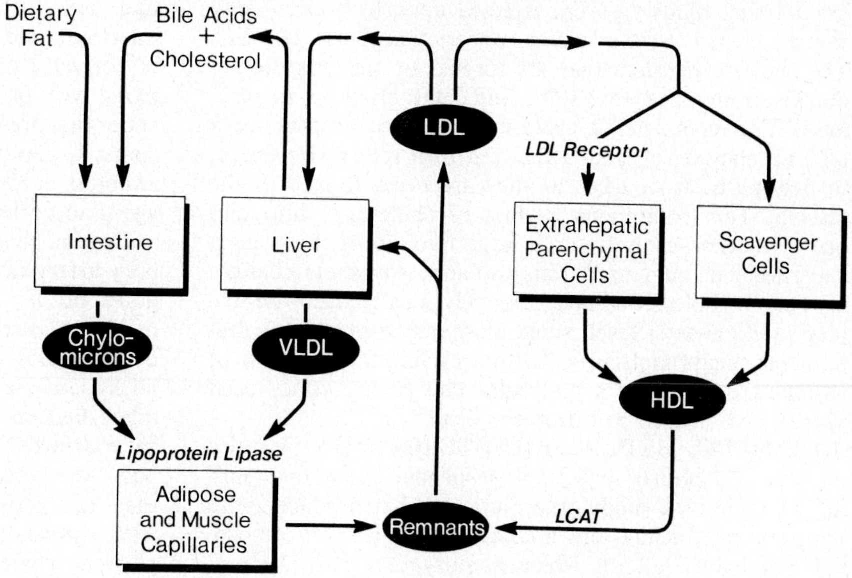

FIGURE 47–6 Model for plasma lipoprotein transport in humans. The details of this model are discussed in the text. VLDL=very low-density lipoprotein; LDL=low-density lipoprotein; HDL=high-density lipoprotein; LCAT=lecithin: cholesterol acyltransferase.

has a different fate. Instead of being taken up by the liver, the IDL particle remains in the circulation, where the last traces of triglyceride are removed, and the particle is converted into *low-density lipoprotein (LDL).* During this conversion, all of the apoproteins leave the particle, with the exception of apoprotein B.

About two-thirds to three-fourths of the cholesterol in normal human plasma is contained within LDL particles. LDL is the particle whose elevation is most frequently related to atherosclerosis. When patients are found to have hypercholesterolemia, this is almost always due to an elevation in the number of LDL particles per milliliter of plasma.

In normal humans LDL circulates with a half-time of about 1.5 days. It is metabolized in liver and extrahepatic tissues. LDL is metabolized by at least two pathways. One pathway involves specific *LDL receptors,* which are located on the surface of liver and extrahepatic cells. The receptor recognizes the *apoprotein B* component of LDL. Binding leads to the uptake and degradation of LDL through a process called *receptor-mediated endocytosis.* This process liberates cholesterol, which all cells need for synthesis of new plasma membranes and which specialized cells need for synthesis of steroid hormones and bile acids.[234]

In normal humans the LDL receptor mediates the degradation of one-third to two-thirds of the LDL particles that are metabolized each day. The remainder of LDL is degraded by receptor-independent pathways. Some of this degradation is believed to occur in macrophages and cells of the reticuloendothelial system, which degrade all plasma proteins. In contrast to the receptor-mediated pathway, which supplies cholesterol to cells for specific metabolic purposes, the *scavenger cell pathway* functions primarily to clear plasma of excess proteins.[233,234,236]

As the membranes of parenchymal cells and scavenger cells undergo turnover and as cells die and are renewed, cholesterol is released into the plasma, where it binds to *high-density lipoprotein (HDL).* When it leaves the tissues, cholesterol is in an unesterified form. For transport in plasma, the cholesterol must be esterified; that is, a fatty acid must be attached in ester linkage to the cholesterol. This esterification reaction occurs in the plasma. The cholesterol that binds to HDL is acted upon by a circulating enzyme called *lecithin:cholesterol acyltransferase (LCAT).* The cholesteryl esters that are formed by this enzyme are quickly transferred to VLDL and LDL particles in plasma.[237] This completes a cycle by which extrahepatic cells take up cholesterol from LDL and then return cholesterol to new particles of LDL as they are being formed in the plasma. This continuous cycling of cholesterol into and out of tissues accounts for a large fraction of the plasma cholesterol in humans.[234] This explains why acute changes in dietary cholesterol have relatively small effects on the plasma cholesterol level, since most of the plasma cholesterol represents molecules that are cycling into and out of various tissues and not molecules that have recently been synthesized or absorbed from the diet.[234]

FAMILIAL HYPERCHOLESTEROLEMIA (see also p. 1214). Familial hypercholesterolemia is the outstanding example of a single-gene mutation that produces both hypercholesterolemia and atherosclerosis. It is an autosomal dominant trait for which homozygotes exist. Heterozygotes for familial hypercholesterolemia number about 1 in 500 persons in the population, making this disease one of the most common disorders that is caused by a single mutant gene. Homozygotes for familial hypercholesterolemia are rare; they occur at a frequency of 1 in one million.[7,227]

The inherited defect in familial hypercholesterolemia lies in the gene for the cell-surface LDL receptor. Heterozygotes inherit one mutant gene for the receptor and one normal gene. Their cells are able to produce half the normal number of receptors. Homozygotes inherit two copies of the mutant gene. Their cells can produce few, if any, LDL receptors. The heterozygous and homozygous forms of the disease differ in severity. Heterozygotes have 2- to 3-fold elevations of plasma LDL, whereas homozygotes have 6- to 10-fold elevations. Heterozygotes develop myocardial infarctions typically in their 30's and 40's, whereas homozygotes usually develop mycardial infarctions before the age of 20.

Clinical Features

Heterozygous Familial Hypercholesterolemia. At the time of birth, these individuals have two- to three-fold elevation in the LDL-cholesterol level, which persists throughout life.[238] This hypercholesterolemia leads to cholesterol deposition in arteries (producing atheromas) and in tendons (producing xanthomas).

A number of studies have carefully documented the incidence of premature coronary artery disease in heterozygotes. In England, Slack found that the mean onset of coronary artery disease was 43 years for heterozygous men and 53 years for heterozygous women.[239] Eighty-five per cent of the affected males and 58 per cent of the affected females had sustained a myocardial infarction by age 60. In Denmark, Jensen et al. found that the incidence of coronary artery disease among heterozygotes over a 20-year period (32 per cent) was 25 times greater than among unaffected relatives (1.3 per cent).[240]

In the United States, familial hypercholesterolemia heterozygotes constitute about 5 per cent of all patients who have a myocardial infarction.[225] Stone et al. found that the cumulative probability of coronary artery disease by age 40 in male heterozygotes was 16 per cent.[241] By age 60 it had risen to 52 per cent, as opposed to 12.7 per cent in unaffected men. Female heterozygotes showed an incidence of coronary artery disease of 33 per cent by age 60, compared with only 9 per cent in unaffected females. Thus, despite the presence of the same genetic abnormality and similarly elevated plasma LDL levels, heterozygous women manifest coronary artery disease less often and at a later age than do heterozygous men.

Despite this marked increase in the frequency of coronary artery disease, familial hypercholesterolemia heterozygotes do *not* appear to have an increased frequency of cerebral vascular disease or of hypertension. The incidence of peripheral vascular disease is possibly elevated in familial hypercholesterolemia heterozygotes, but not in so striking a fashion as the incidence of coronary artery disease. In contrast, patients with familial dysbetalipoproteinemia have an increased incidence of both coronary artery disease and peripheral vascular disease (see below). Patients with dysbetalipoproteinemia accumulate IDL particles in plasma, whereas familial hypercholesterolemia patients ac-

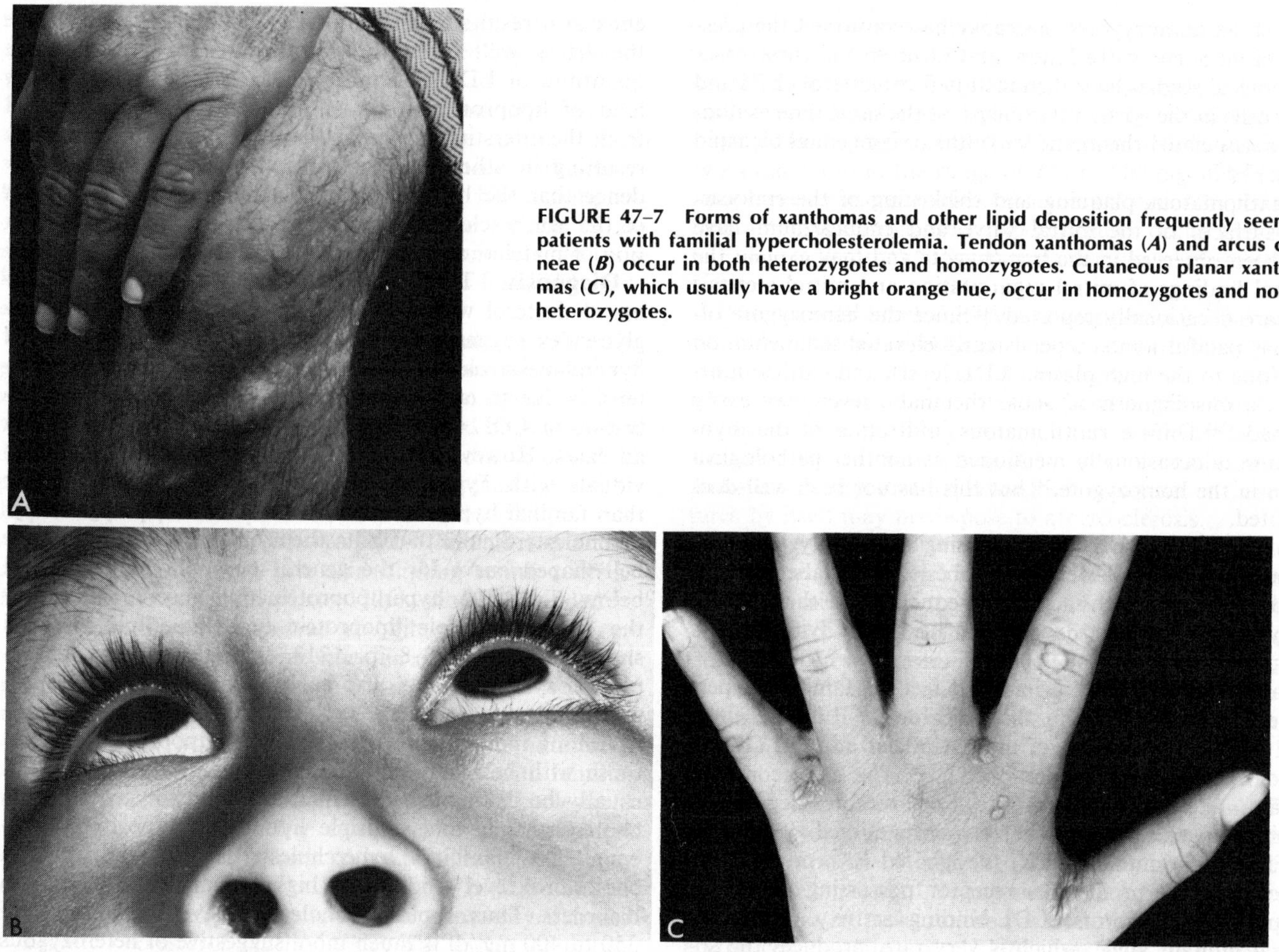

FIGURE 47–7 Forms of xanthomas and other lipid deposition frequently seen in patients with familial hypercholesterolemia. Tendon xanthomas (*A*) and arcus corneae (*B*) occur in both heterozygotes and homozygotes. Cutaneous planar xanthomas (*C*), which usually have a bright orange hue, occur in homozygotes and not in heterozygotes.

cumulate LDL particles. It is possible that the LDL particles have a greater toxicity for coronary arteries than for peripheral arteries, whereas IDL particles are equally toxic for both types of vessels.

Familial hypercholesterolemia heterozygotes also have tendon xanthomas, which are nodular swellings that may involve the Achilles tendon and various tendons about the knee, elbow, and dorsum of the hand (Fig. 47–7*A*). Like the atheromas, the xanthomas consist of massive deposits of cholesterol, apparently derived from the deposition of LDL particles. The cholesterol is located as amorphous extracellular deposits as well as vacuoles within scavenger cells (macrophages) that have invaded the lesion. The latter becomes so swollen with lipid droplets that they are termed foam cells.

In familial hypercholesterolemia heterozygotes, cholesterol deposits are also formed in the soft tissue of the eyelid, producing xanthelasma, and within the cornea, producing arcus cornae (Fig. 47–7*B*). Whereas tendon xanthomas are diagnostic of familial hypercholesterolemia, xanthelasma and arcus corneae are not specific. The latter also occur in many adults with normal plasma lipid levels. The incidence of tendon xanthomas in familial hypercholesterolemia increases with age, but no more than 75 per cent of affected heterozygotes display this sign.[227]

Homozygous Familial Hypercholesterolemia. Homozygotes have marked elevations in the plasma level of LDL from birth, the plasma cholesterol level usually being six- to eightfold above normal. A unique type of planar cutaneous xanthoma is often present at birth and always develops within the first 6 years of life.[227,242] These yellow xanthomas occur at points of trauma, such as over the knees, elbows, and buttocks. They almost always occur in the interdigital webs of the hands, particularly between the thumb and index finger (Fig. 46–7*C*). Tendon xanthomas, arcus corneae, and xanthelasma also occur in homozygotes.

Coronary artery atherosclerosis in homozygotes is rapidly progressive. Angina pectoris, myocardial infarction, or sudden death occur commonly in homozygotes between the ages of 5 and 30. One homozygote is even recorded as having had an acute myocardial infarction as early as 18 months of age. Very few homozygotes survive past age 30.[9,227]

In homozygotes, severe atherosclerosis occurs not only in the coronary arteries but also in the thoracic and abdominal aorta as well as in the major pulmonary arteries.[227,243] Microscopic examination of the coronary and pulmonary arterial lesions in these children and young adults shows typical atherosclerotic plaques as well as a striking intimal infiltration of xanthomatous foam cells and cholesterol clefts that are reminiscent of the histological appearance of a tendon xanthoma.[243,244] Atheromatous and xanthomatous involvement of the aortic valve is another characteristic cardiac manifestation observed in the homozygote. The deposition of cholesterol frequently produces significant aortic stenosis, which in turn causes congestive heart failure.[243,243a,245] In the administration of heparin is generally normal.

Diabetes and obesity tend to increase VLDL production and hence to exacerbate hypertriglyceridemia in this syndrome, but the increased prevalence of these conditions is believed to be fortuitous. There is evidence that hypertriglyceridemia and diabetes are inherited by independent mechanisms.[262] However, the hypertriglyceridemia is much more severe when an individual inherits both the gene or genes for diabetes and the gene for hypertriglyceridemia, and such a person is more likely to come to medical attention. Similarly, an individual of normal weight with familial hypertriglyceridemia will usually have mild hypertriglyceridemia and will be less likely to come to medical attention. However, if such an individual becomes obese, the hypertriglyceridemia will worsen, and a diagnosis is more likely to be made.[234]

Diagnosis. A moderate elevation in plasma triglyceride level, together with a normal cholesterol level, suggests the possibility of familial hypertriglyceridemia. Plasma electrophoresis shows an increase in the pre-beta fraction (Type IV lipoprotein pattern). In the occasional patient who exhibits severe hypertriglyceridemia with an elevation of chylomicrons and VLDL (Type V lipoprotein pattern), the plasma shows a creamy supernatant layer (chylomicrons) and a cloudy infranatant layer (VLDL) after overnight storage in the refrigerator.[234,260]

No simple test currently exists to determine whether an individual who has an elevation in VLDL levels with or without an elevation in chylomicrons has familial hypertriglyceridemia or hypertriglyceridemia due to some other genetic or acquired cause, such as multiple lipoprotein–type hyperlipidemia or sporadic hypertriglyceridemia. However, half of the first-degree relatives of patients with typical cases of familial hypertriglyceridemia exhibit hypertriglyceridemia, and no relatives with isolated hypercholesterolemia should be found. When the latter is present, the diagnosis of multiple lipoprotein–type hyperlipase is suggested.

Treatment. It is essential, first of all, to control all of the exacerbating conditions, including obesity. The diet should be restricted in calories, saturated fat, and alcohol. Diabetes mellitus and hypothyroidism, if present, should be treated vigorously; oral contraceptives should be avoided. However, if the above measures fail, clofibrate is usually effective[234,260] (p. 1226).

MULTIPLE LIPOPROTEIN–TYPE HYPERLIPIDEMIA (FAMILIAL COMBINED HYPERLIPIDEMIA). In this common disorder, inherited as an autosomal dominant trait, affected individuals in a single family characteristically show one of three different lipoprotein patterns: hypercholesterolemia (Type IIA), hypertriglyceridemia (Type IV), or both hypercholesterolemia and hypertriglyceridemia.[225,234] In this condition, hyperlipidemia is not usually present in affected patients in childhood but begins to appear at puberty and continues thereafter. The lipid elevations are often mild, and they change over time in affected individuals, often exhibiting a mildly elevated cholesterol level at one examination and/or a mildly elevated triglyceride level at another. An elevation in the incidence of myocardial infarction in affected women as well as men is characteristic, and there is usually a strong family history of premature coronary artery disease. Indeed, patients with multiple lipoprotein–type hyperlipidemia constitute about 10 per cent of all patients who have a myocardial infarction.[225] Xanthomas are not a feature of this condition. Although the incidence of obesity, hyperuricemia, and glucose intolerance is increased in affected individuals, especially those with hypertriglyceridemia, this association is not so striking as the one found with familial hypertriglyceridemia.

Pathogenesis. Since the disease is transmitted within families as an autosomal dominant trait, a mutation in a single gene is probably responsible. As would be expected with this mode of inheritance, about half of the first-degree relatives of an affected individual also have hyperlipidemia.[225,263–267] A key feature of this condition is the great variability of blood lipids among affected individuals in the same family and, as already pointed out, in the same individual at different times. About one-third of relatives of those individuals with hyperlipidemia will have hypercholesterolemia (Type IIA lipoprotein pattern), one-third will have hypertriglyceridemia (Type IV), and the remainder both hypercholesterolemia and hypertriglyceridemia (Type IIB). The plasma lipid levels tend to hover at the 95th percentile for the population. The variability of lipoprotein phenotypes that constitutes the characteristic feature of this condition is illustrated in Figure 47–8, which shows the pedigrees of four large families affected by this disorder.

It has been postulated that affected individuals have an elevated secretion rate for VLDL from the liver[225], and that this overproduction of VLDL may manifest itself alternatively as an elevation in plasma VLDL levels (hypertriglyceridemia), an elevation in LDL levels (hypercholesterolemia), or both, depending on the interplay of factors governing the efficiency of conversion of VLDL to LDL and the efficiency of catabolism of LDL. As in familial hypertriglyceridemia, the hyperlipidemia is worsened by diabetes, alcoholism, and hypothyroidism.

Diagnosis. There are no clinical or laboratory methods that indicate whether an individual with hyperlipidemia has the multiple lipoprotein–type disorder, since type IIA, IIB, and IV lipoprotein patterns can each occur in patients with several diseases (Table 35–8, p. 1213). However, this disorder should be suspected in any individual whose hyperlipoproteinemia is mild, whose lipoprotein type changes with time, and among whose relatives multiple abnormal lipoprotein types occur (Fig. 47–8). Tendon xanthomas in the patient or relatives or the finding of hypercholesterolemia in a relative under the age of 10 years, both of which suggest the diagnosis of heterozygous familial hypercholesterolemia , exclude the diagnosis of multiple lipoprotein–type hyperlipidemia.

Treatment. Weight reduction, restriction of dietary saturated fat and cholesterol, and avoidance of alcohol and oral contraceptives are useful general measures. In addition, clofibrate is effective when the triglyceride level is elevated with or without hypercholesterolemia, while a bile acid-binding resin usually lowers an elevated cholesterol level. However, the lowering of cholesterol levels with such a drug may be accompanied by an increase in triglyceride levels that tends to negate its beneficial effects.

FAMILIAL DYSBETALIPOPROTEINEMIA (TYPE III HYPERLIPOPROTEINEMIA) (see also p. 1215). The expression of this disorder, which is transmitted by a single-gene mechanism, requires the presence of contribu-

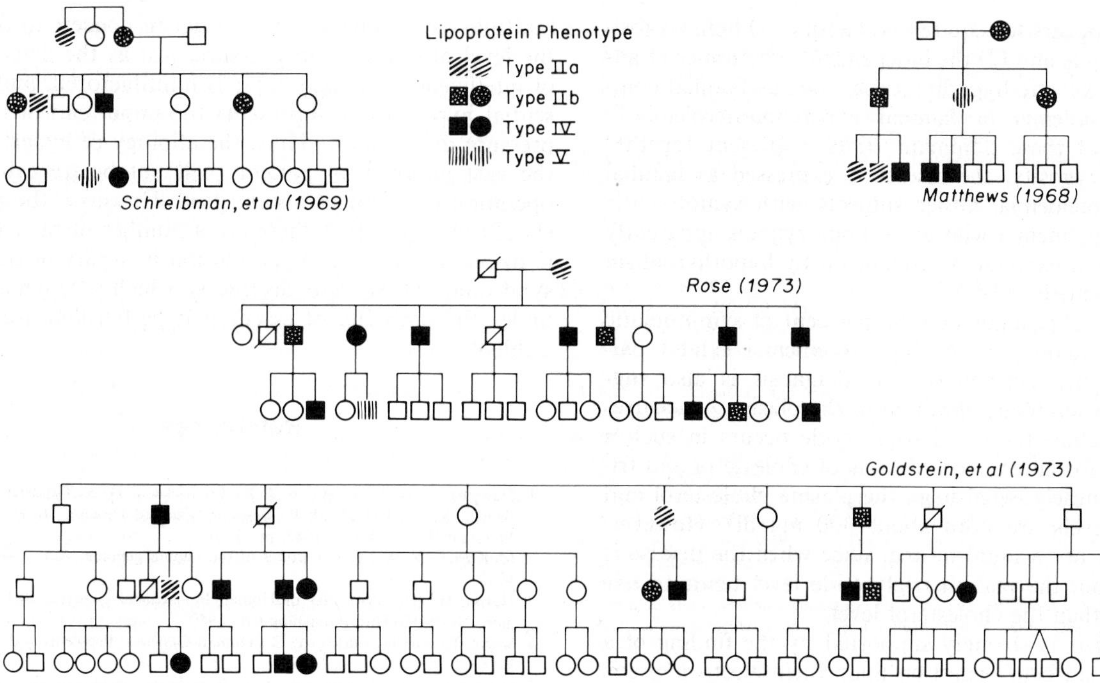

FIGURE 47–8 Pedigrees of four large families showing the characteristics of multiple lipoprotein-type hyperlipidemia. (Adapted from data contained in references 225 and 264 to 266.)

tory environmental or genetic factors.[234,268] The plasma concentrations of cholesterol and triglycerides are both elevated because of the accumulation in plasma of remnant-like particles derived from the partial catabolism of VLDL and chylomicrons.

Clinical Features. Hyperlipidemia or any of the other clinical features of the disease are usually not manifest until after the age of 20 years. Two types of cutaneous xanthomas are characteristic of familial dysbetalipoproteinemia: xanthomata striata palmaris, which appear as orange or yellow discolorations of the palmar and digital creases, and tuberous or tuberoeruptive xanthomas, which are bulbous cutaneous xanthomas that may vary from pea- to lemon-sized and are characteristically located over the elbows and knees. Xanthelasmas of the eyelids also occur, but these are not unique to this disorder (p. 16). Patients with clinical manifestations of dysbetalipoproteinemia are often found to have hypothyroidism, obesity, or diabetes mellitus.[234,268,269]

Clinically, this condition is characterized by severe atherosclerosis involving the coronary arteries, the internal carotids, and the abdominal aorta and its branches. Forty-three per cent of the nearly 50 patients described by Morganroth et al.[268] had detectable vascular disease, and in the one-third who had coronary artery disease the mean age of onset was 38 years in men and about a decade later in women. Peripheral vascular disease, manifest mainly as claudication, was also found in about one-third, again appearing earlier in men than in women; cerebrovascular disease occurred in 5 of their 47 patients. Except for homozygous familial hypercholesterolemia, familial dysbetalipoproteinemia probably results in as high a risk of premature vascular disease as any form of hyperlipidemia. This diagnosis should be considered in any patient who has hyperlipidemia and peripheral vascular disease.

Pathogenesis. This form of hyperlipidemia is caused by the accumulation of relatively large lipoprotein particles that contain both triglycerides and cholesteryl esters and that resemble the remnants that are normally produced from the catabolism of VLDL and chylomicrons through the action of lipoprotein lipase (Fig. 47–5). These remnant particles are rapidly taken up by the liver of normal subjects, and hence they are barely detectable in plasma. However, the uptake of remnants by the liver is blocked in patients with familial dysbetalipoproteinemia, leading to the accumulation of high levels of these lipoproteins in plasma and deposition in tissues, producing xanthomas and atherosclerosis.[234,268]

Patients with familial dysbetalipoproteinemia are homozygous for a mutant gene specifying apoprotein E, a normal constituent of VLDL and chylomicron remnants.[270] The normal function of apo E is to bind to hepatic lipoprotein receptors, an event which is necessary for the rapid hepatic uptake of IDL and chylomicron remnants.[235] The apo E gene is polymorphic in the population. The three common alleles are designated ϵ^2, ϵ^3, ϵ^4.[268,271] The ϵ^3 and ϵ^4 alleles code for proteins that function normally. The protein specified by the ϵ^2 allele is nonfunctional. It does not bind to hepatic receptors.[272]

About 1 per cent of Caucasian individuals are homozygous for the ϵ^2 allele. However, only 1 in 100 of these homozygous individuals (or 1 in 10,000 of the general population) has clear-cut familial dysbetalipoproteinemia.[268] The vast majority of ϵ^2 homozygotes are able to compensate somehow for their defective protein. They have very slight elevations in the concentration of IDL and chylomicron remnants in plasma and are asymptomatic. The reason why 1 per cent of the ϵ^2 homozygotes cannot compensate for their defect and develop severe dysbetalipoproteinemia is not known. In some families the expression of dysbetalipo-

102. Moran, J. J.: Idiopathic arterial calcification of infancy: A clinicopathologic study. Pathol. Annu. *10*:393, 1975.
103. Barson, A. J., Campbell, R. H. A., Langley, F. A., and Milner, R. D. G.: Idiopathic arterial calcification of infancy without intimal proliferation. Virchows Arch. Pathol. Anat. *372*:167, 1976.
104. Schieken, R. M., Kerber, R. E., Ionasescu, V. V., and Zellweger, H.: Cardiac manifestations of the mucopolysaccharidoses. Circulation *52*:700, 1975.
105. McKusick, V. A., and Neufeld, E. F.: The mucopolysaccharide storage diseases. *In* Stanbury, J. B., Wyngaarden, J. B., Fredrickson, D. S., Goldstein, J. L., and Brown, M. S. (eds.): The Metabolic Basis of Inherited Disease. 5th ed. New York, McGraw-Hill Book Co., 1983, p. 751.
106. Kelly, T. E., Thomas, G. H., Taylor, H. A., Jr., McKusick, V. A., Sly, W. S., Glaser, J. H., Robinow, M., Luzzatti, L., Espiritu, C., Feingold, M., Bull, M. J., Ashenhurst, E. M., and Ives, E. J.: Mucolipidosis III (pseudo-Hurler polydystrophy): Clinical and laboratory studies in a series of 12 patients. Johns Hopkins Med. J. *137*:156, 1975.
107. Neufeld, E. F., and McKusick, V. A.: Disorders of lysosomal enzyme synthesis and localization: I-cell disease and Pseudo-Hurler polydystrophy. *In* Stanbury, J. B., Wyngaarden, J. B., Fredrickson, D. S., Goldstein, J. L., and Brown, M. S. (eds.): The Metabolic Basis of Inherited Disease. 5th ed. New York, McGraw-Hill Book Co., 1983, p. 778.
108. Hirst, A. E., Jr., Johns, V. J., Jr., and Kime, S. W., Jr.: Dissecting aneurysm of the aorta: A review of 505 cases. Medicine *37*:217, 1958.
109. Murdoch, J. L., Walker, B. A., Halpern, B. L., Kuzma, J. W., and McKusick, V. A.: Life expectancy and causes of death in the Marfan syndrome. N. Engl. J. Med. *286*:804, 1972.
110. Halpern, B. L., Char, F., Murdoch, J. L., Horton, W. B., and McKusick, V. A.: A prospectus on the prevention of aortic rupture in the Marfan syndrome with data on survivorship without treatment. Johns Hopkins Med. J. *129*:123, 1971.
111. Elias, S., and Berkowitz, R. L.: The Marfan syndrome and pregnancy. Obstet. Gynecol. *47*:358, 1976.
112. Sutinen, S., and Piiroinen, O.: Marfan syndrome, pregnancy, and fatal dissection of aorta. Acta Obstet. Gynecol. Scand. *50*:295, 1971.
113. Grossman, M., Knott, A. P., Jr., and Jacoby, W. J., Jr.: Calcified annulus fibrosis with mitral insufficiency in the Marfan syndrome. Arch. Intern. Med. *121*:561, 1968.
114. Murdoch, J. L., Walker, B. A., and McKusick, V. A.: Parental age effects on the occurrence of new mutations for the Marfan syndrome. Ann. Hum. Genet. *35*:331, 1972.
115. Emanuel, R., Ng, R. A. L., Marcomichelakis, J., Moores, E. C., Jefferson, K. E., Macfaul, P. A., and Withers, R.: Formes frustes of Marfan's syndrome presenting with severe aortic regurgitation. Clinicogenetic study of 18 families. Br. Heart J. *39*:190, 1977.
116. Payvandi, M. N., Kerber, R. E., Phelps, C. D., Judisch, G. F., El-Khoury, G., and Schrott, H. G.: Cardiac, skeletal and ophthalmologic abnormalities in relatives of patients with the Marfan syndrome. Circulation *55*:797, 1977.
117. Procacci, P. M., Savran, S. V., Schreiter, S. L., and Bryson, A. L.: Prevalance of clinical mitral-valve prolapse in 1169 young women. N. Engl. J. Med. *294*:1086, 1976.
118. Markiewicz, W., Stoner, J., London, E., Hunt, S. A., and Popp, R. L.: Mitral valve prolapse in one hundred presumably healthy young females. Circulation *53*:464, 1976.

CARDIOMYOPATHIES

119. Howell, R. R., and Williams, J. C.: The glycogen storage diseases. *In* Stanbury, J. B., Wyngaarden, J. B., Fredrickson, D. S., Goldstein, J. L., and Brown, M. S. (eds.): The Metabolic Basis of Inherited Disease. 5th ed. New York, McGraw-Hill Book Co., 1983, p. 119.
120. Ehlers, K. H., Hagstrom, J. W. C., Lukas, D. S., Redo, S. F., and Engle, M. A.: Glycogen-storage disease of the myocardium with obstruction to left ventricular outflow. Circulation *25*:96, 1962.
121. Ockerman, P. A.: Incidence of glycogen storage disease in Sweden. Paediatr. Scand, *61*:533, 1972.
122. D'Ancona, G. G., Wurm, J., and Croce, C. M.: Genetics of type II glycogenesis: Assignment of the human gene for acid α-glucosidase to chromosome 17. Proc. Natl. Acad. Sci. USA. *76*:4526, 1979.
123. Butterworth, J., and Broadhead, D. M.: Diagnosis of Pompe's disease in cultured skin fibroblasts and primary amniotic fluid cells using 4-Methylumbelliferyl-α-D-glucopyranoside as substrate. Clin. Chim. Acta *78*: 335, 1977.
124. Clark, C. E., Henry, W L., and Epstein, S. E.: Familial prevalance and genetic transmission of idiopathic hypertrophic subaortic stenosis. N. Engl. J. Med. *289*:709, 1973.
125. Bjarnason, I., Jonsson, S., and Hardarson, T.: Mode of inheritance of hypertrophic cardiomyopathy in Iceland. Br. Heart J. *47*:122, 1982.
126. Braunwald, E., Lambrew, C. T., Rockoff, S. D., Ross, J., Jr., and Morrow, A. G.: Idiopathic hypertrophic subaortic stenosis. I. A description of the disease based on an analysis of 64 patients. Circulation *30*(Suppl. 4):3, 1964.
127. Horlick, L., Petkovich, N. J., and Bolton, C. F.: Idiopathic hypertrophic subvalvular stenosis. A study of a family involving four generations. Clinical, hemodynamic and pathologic observations. Am. J. Cardiol. *17*:411, 1966.
128. Pare, J. A. P., Fraser, R. G., Pirozynski, W. J., Shanks, J. A., and Stubington, D.: Hereditary cardiovascular dysplasia. A form of familial cardiomyopathy. Am. J. Med. *31*:37, 1961.
129. Maron, B. J., Lipson, L. C., Roberts, W. C., Savage, D. S., and Epstein, S. E.: "Malignant" hypertrophic cardiomyopathy: Identification of a subgroup of families with unusually frequent premature death. Am. J. Cardiol. *41*:1133, 1978.
130. Perloff, J. K.: The cardiomyopathies—current perspectives. Circulation *44*:942, 1971.
131. Kariv, I., Kreisler, B., Sherf, L., Feldman, S., and Rosenthal, T.: Familial cardiomyopathy. Am. J. Cardiol. *28*:693, 1971.
132. Whitfield, A. G. W.: Familial cardiomyopathy. Q. J. Med. *30*:119, 1961.
133. Ross, R. S., Bulkley, B. H., Hutchins, G. M., Harshey, J. S., Jones, R. A., Kraus, H., Liebman, J., Thorne, C. M., Weinberg, S. B., Weech, A. A., and Weech, A. A., Jr.: Idiopathic familial myocardiopathy in three generations: A clinical and pathologic study. Am. Heart J. *97*:170, 1978.
134. Csanady, M., and Szasz, K.: Familial cardiomyopathy. Cardiology *61*:122, 1976.
135. Boyd, D. L., Mishkin, M. E., Feigenbaum, H., and Genovese, P. D.: Three families with familial cardiomyopathy. Ann. Intern. Med. *63*:386, 1965.
136. Finch, S. C., and Finch, C. A.: Idiopathic hemochromatosis, an iron shortage disease. Medicine *34*:381, 1955.
137. Bothwell, T. H., Charlton, R. W., and Motulsky, A. G.: Idiopathic hemochromatosis. *In* Stanbury, J. B., Wyngaarden, J. B., Fredrickson, D. S., Goldstein, J. L., and Brown, M. S. (eds.): The Metabolic Basis of Inherited Disease. 5th ed. New York, McGraw-Hill Book Co., 1983, p. 1269.
138. Edwards, C. Q., Carroll, M., Bray, P., and Cartwright, G. E.: Hereditary hemochromatosis. N. Engl. J. Med. *297*:7, 1977.
139. Crosby, W. H.: Hemochromatosis: The unsolved problems. Semin. Hematol. *14*:135, 1977.
140. Saddi, R., and Feingold, J.: Idiopathic haemochromatosis: An autosomal recessive disease. Clin. Genet. *5*:234, 1974.
141. Simon, M., Alexandre, J-L., Bourel, M., le Marec, B., and Scordia, C.: Heredity of idiopathic haemochromatosis: A study of 106 families. Clin. Genet. *11*:327, 1977.
142. Rowe, J. W., Wands, J. R., Mexey, E., Waterbury, L. A., Wright, J. R., Tobin, J., and Andres, R.: Familial hemochromatosis: Characteristics of the precirrhotic stage in a large kindred. Medicine *56*:197, 1977.
143. Scheinberg, I. H.: The genetics of hemochromatosis. Arch. Intern. Med. *132*:126, 1973.
144. Simon, M., Bourel, M., Fauchet, R., and Genetet, B.: Association of HLA-A3 and HLA-B14 antigens with idiopathic haemochromatosis. Gut *17*:332, 1976.
145. Bomford, A., Eddleston, A. L. W. F., Kennedy, L. A., Batchelor, J. R., and Williams, R.: Histocompatibility antigens as markers of abnormal iron metabolism in patients with idiopathic haemochromatosis and their relatives. Lancet *1*:327, 1977.
146. Feller, E. R., Pont, A., Wands, J. R., Carter, E. A., Foster, G., Kourides, I. A., and Isselbacher, K. J.: Familial hemochromatosis. N. Engl. J. Med. *29*:1422, 1977.
147. Simon, M., Alexandre, J. L., Rauchet, R., Genetet, B., and Bourel, M.: The genetics of hemochromatosis, Prog. Med. Genet. *4*(new series):135, 1980.
148. Kyle, R. A., and Bayrd, E.D.: Amyloidosis: Review of 236 cases. Medicine *54*:271, 1975.
149. Andrade, C., Araki, S., Block, W. D., Cohen, A. S., Jackson, C. E., Kuroiwa, Y., McKusick, V. A., Nissism, J., Sohar, E., and Van Allen, M. W.: Hereditary amyloidosis. Arthritis Rheum. *13*:902, 1970.
150. Frederiksen, T., Gotzsche, H., Harboe, N., Kraer, W., and Mellemgaard, K.: Familial primary amyloidosis with severe amyloid heart disease. Am. J. Med. *33*:328, 1962.
151. Harrison, W. H., Jr., and Derrick, J. R.: Atrial standstill. A review and presentation of two new cases of familial and unusual nature with reference to epicardial pacing in one. Angiology *20*:610, 1969.
152. Harper, P. S.: Congenital myotonic dystrophy in Britain. Arch. Dis. Child. *50*:505, 1975.
153. Church, S. C.: The heart in myotonia atrophica. Arch. Intern. Med. *119*:176, 1967.
154. Griggs, R. C., David, R. J., Anderson, D. C., and Dove, J. T.: Cardiac conduction in myotonic dystrophy. Am. J. Med. *59*:37, 1975.
155. Salomon, J., and Easley, R. M.: Cardiovascular abnormalities in myotonic dystrophy. Chest *64*:135, 1973.
156. Tanaka, N., Tanaka, H., Takeda, M., Niimura, T., Kanehisa, T., and Terashi, S.: Cardiomyopathy in myotonic dystrophy. A light and electron microscopic study of the myocardium. Jpn. Heart J. *14*:202, 1973.
157. Bundey, S., Carter, C. O., and Soothill, J. F.: Early recognition of heterozygote for the gene for dystrophia myotonica. J. Neurol. Neurosurg. Psychiatry *33*:279, 1970.
158. Renwick, J. H., Bundey, S. E., Ferguson-Smith, M. A., and Izatt, M. M.: Confirmation of linkage of the loci for myotonic dystrophy and ABH secretion. J. Med. Genet. *8*:407, 1971.
159. Schrott, H. G., Karp, L., and Omenn, G. S.: Prenatal prediction in myotonic dystrophy: Guidelines for genetic counseling. Clin. Genet. *4*:38, 1973.
160. Zundel, W. S., and Tyler, F. H.: The muscular dystrophies. N. Engl. J. Med. *10*:537, 596, 1965.
161. Perloff, J. K., Roberts, W. C., De Leon, A. C., Jr., and O'Doherty, D.: The distinctive electrocardiogram of Duchenne's progressive muscular dystrophy. Am. J. Med. *42*:179, 1967.
162. Moser, H., and Emery, A. E. H.: The manifesting carrier in Duchenne muscular dystrophy. Clin. Genet. *5*:271, 1974.
163. Mann, O., DeLeon, A. C., Jr., Perloff, J. K., Simanis, J., and Horrigan, F. D.:

Duchenne's muscular dystrophy: The electrocardiogram in female relatives. Am. J. Med. Sci. *255*:376, 1968.
164. Emery, A. E. H.: Abnormalities of the electrocardiogram in female carriers of Duchenne muscular dystrophy. Br. Med. J. *2*:418, 1969.
165. Mahoney, M. J., Haseltine, F. P., Hobbins, J. C., Banker, B. Q., Caskey, C. T., and Golbus, M. S.: Prenatal diagnosis of Duchenne's muscular dystrophy. N. Engl. J. Med. *297*:968, 1977.
166. Boyer, S. H., IV, Chisholm, A. W., and McKusick, V. A.: Cardiac aspects of Friedreich's ataxia. Circulation *25*:493, 1962.
167. Thoren, C.: Cardiomyopathy in Friedreich's ataxia. Acta Paediatr. *153* (Suppl.):9, 1964.
168. Hewer, R. L.: Study of fatal cases of Friedreich's ataxia. Br. Med. J. *3*:649, 1968.
169. Perloff, J. K.: Cardiomyopathy associated with heredofamilial neuromyopathic diseases. Mod. Concepts Cardiovasc. Dis. *40*:23, 1971.
170. Smith, E. R., Sangalang, V. E., Heffernan, L. P., Welch, J. P., and Flemington, C. S.: Hypertrophic cardiomyopathy: The heart disease of Friedreich's ataxia. Am. Heart J. *94*:428, 1977.
171. Ruschhaupt, D. G., Thilenius, O. G., and Cassels, D. E.: Friedreich's ataxia associated with idiopathic hypertrophic subaortic stenosis. Am. Heart J. *84*:95, 1972.
172. Maione, S., Giunta, A., Mansi, D., Filla, A., Serino, A., Teti, G., de Falco, F. A., and Campanella, G.: Cardiac abnormalities in Friedreich's ataxia patients and first-degree relatives: Evidence of hypertrophic cardiomyopathy in obligate heterozygotes. Acta Neurol. (Naples) *35*:354, 1980.
173. Folger, G. M., Jr.: Endocardial fibroelastosis. Clin. Pediatr. *10*:246, 1971.
174. Mitchell, S. C., Froehlich, L. A., Banas, J. S., Jr., and Gilkeson, M. R.: An epidemiologic assessment of primary endocardial fibroelastosis. Am. J. Cardiol. *18*:859, 1966.
175. Vestermark, S.: Primary endocardial fibroelastosis in siblings. Acta Paediatr. *51*:94, 1962.
176. Hunter, A. S., and Keay, A. J.: Primary endocardial fibroelastosis. Arch. Dis. Child. *48*:66, 1973.
177. Westwood, M., Harris, R., Burn, J. L., and Barson, A. J.: Heredity in primary endocardial fibroelastosis. Br. Heart J. *37*:1077, 1975.
178. Chen, S., Thompson, M. W., and Rose, V.: Endocardial fibroelastosis: Family studies with special reference to counseling. J. Pediatr. *79*:385, 1971.
179. Tripp, M. E., Katcher, M. L., Peters, H. A., Gilbert, E. F., Arya, S., Hodach, R. J., and Shug, A. L.: Systemic carnitine deficiency presenting as familial endocardial fibroelastosis. N. Engl. J. Med. *305*:385, 1981.
180. Engel, A. G., and Angelini, C.: Carnitine deficiency of human skeletal muscle with associated lipid storage myopathy: A new syndrome. Science *179*:899,1973.
181. Jervell, A., and Lange-Nielsen, F.: Congenital deaf-mutism, functional heart disease with prolongation of Q-T interval and sudden death. Am. Heart J. *54*:59, 1957.
182. Jervell, A.: Surdocardiac and related syndromes in children. Adv. Intern. Med. *17*:425, 1971.
183. Schwartz, P. J., Periti, M., and Malliani, A.: The long Q-T syndrome. Am. Heart J. *89*:378, 1975.
184. Denes, P.: Congenital and acquired syndrome of a long Q-T interval. Chest *71*:126, 1977.
185. Fraser, G. R., Froggatt, P., and Murphy, T.: Genetical aspects of the cardioauditory syndrome of Jervell and Lange-Nielsen (congenital deafness and electrocardiographic abnormalities). Ann. Hum. Genet. *28*:133, 1964.
186. Romano, C.: Congenital cardiac arrhythmia. Lancet *1*:658, 1965.
187. Ward, O. C.: A new familial cardiac syndrome in children. J. Irish Med. Assoc. *54*:103, 1964.
188. Itoh, S., Munemura, S., and Satoh, H.: A study of the inheritance pattern of Romano-Ward syndrome. Clin. Pediatr. *21*:20, 1982.
189. Van Der Straaten, P. J. C., and Bruins, C. L. D.: A family with heritable electrocardiographic QT-prolongation. J. Med. Genet. *10*:158, 1973.
190. Moothart, R. W., Pryor, R., Hawley, R. L., Clifford, N. J., and Blount, S. G., Jr.: The heritable syndrome of prolonged Q-T interval, syncope, and sudden death. Chest *70*:263, 1976.
191. Sarachek, N. S., and Leonard, J. J.: Familial heart block and sinus bradycardia. Am. J. Cardiol. *29*:451, 1972.
192. Crittenden, I. H., Latta, H., and Ticinovich, D. A.: Familial congenital heart block. Am. J. Dis. Child. *108*:104, 1964.
193. Winkler, R. B., Nora, A. H., and Nora, J. J.: Familial congenital complete heart block and maternal systemic lupus erythematosus. Circulation *56*:1103, 1977.
194. McCue, C. M., Mantakas, M. E., Tingelstad, J. B., and Ruddy, S.: Congenital heart block in newborns of mothers with connective tissue disease. Circulation *56*:82, 1977.
195. Chameides, L., Truex, R. C., Vetter, V., Rashkind, W. J., Galioto, Jr., F. M., and Noonan, J. A.: Association of maternal systemic lupus erythematosus with congenital complete heart block. N. Engl. J. Med. *297*:1204, 1977.
196. Kennel, A. J., Callahan, J. A., Maloney, J. D., and Zajarilas, A.: Adult-onset familial infra-Hisian block. Am. Heart J. *102*:1447, 1981.
197. Vallianos, G., and Sideris, D. A.: Familial conduction defects. Cardiology *59*:190, 1974.
198. Amat-Y-Leon, F., Racki, A. J., Denes, P., Ten Eick, R. E., Singer, D. H., Bharati, S., Lev, M., and Rosen, K. M.: Familial atrial dysrhythmia with A-V block, Circulation *50*:1097, 1974.
199. Esscher, E., Hardell, L.-I., and Michaelsson, M.: Familial, isolated, complete right bundle-branch block. Br. Heart J. *37*:745, 1975.
200. Harnischfeger, W. W.: Hereditary occurrence of the pre-excitation (Wolff-Parkinson-White) syndrome with re-entry mechanism and concealed conduction. Circulation *19*:28, 1959.
201. Schneider, R. G.: Familial occurrence of Wolff-Parkinson-White syndrome. Am. Heart J. *78*:34, 1969.
202. Massumi, R. A.: Familial Wolff-Parkinson-White syndrome with cardiomyopathy. Am. J. Med. *43*:951, 1967.
203. Perheentupa, J., Autio, S., Leisti, S., Raitta, C., and Tuuteri, L.: Mulibrey nanism, an autosomal recessive syndrome with pericardial constriction. Lancet *2*:351, 1973.
204. Perheentupa, J., Autio, S., Leisti, S., Raitta, C., and Tuuteri, L.: Mulibrey nanism: Review of 23 cases of a new autosomal recessive syndrome. Birth Defects: Original Article Series *11*:3, 1975.
205. Tuuteri, L., Perheentupa, J., and Rapola, J.: The cardiopathy of mulibrey nanism, a new inherited syndrome. Chest *65*:628, 1974.
206. Cumming, G. R., Kerr, D., and Ferguson, C. C.: Constrictive pericarditis with dwarfism in two siblings (mulibrey nanism). J. Pediatr. *88*:569, 1976.
207. Thoren, C.: So-called mulibrey nanism with pericardial constriction. Lancet *2*:731, 1973.
208. Voorhess, M. L., Husson, G. S., and Blackman, M. S.: Growth failure with pericardial constriction. Am. J. Dis. Child. *130*:1146, 1976.
209. Krause, S., Adler, L. N., Reddy, P. S., and Magovern, G. J.: Intracardiac myxoma in siblings. Chest *60*:404, 1971.
210. Liebler, G. A., Magovern, G. J., Park, S. B., Cushing, W. J., Begg, F. R., and Joyner, C. R.: Familial myxomas in four siblings. J. Thorac. Cardiovasc. Surg. *71*:605, 1976.
211. Heydorn, W. H., Gomez, A. C., Kleid, J. J., and Haas, J. M.: Atrial myxoma in siblings. J. Thorac. Cardiovasc. Surg. *65*:484, 1973.
212. Farah, M. G.: Familial atrial myxoma. Ann. Intern. Med. *83*:358, 1975.
213. Siltanen, P., Tuuteri, L., Norio, R., Tala, P., Ahrenberg, P., and Halonen, P. I.: Atrial myxoma in a family. Am. J. Cardiol. *38*:252, 1976.
214. Powers, J. C., Falkoff, M., Heinle, R. A., Nanda, N. C., Ong, L. S., Weiner, R. S., and Barold, S. S.: Familial cardiac myxoma: Emphasis on unusual clinical manifestations. J. Thorac. Cardiovasc. Surg. *77*:782, 1979.
215. Tsakraklides, V., Burke, B., Mastri, A., Runge, W., Roe, E., and Anderson, R.: Rhabdomyomas of heart. Am. J. Dis. Child. *128*:639, 1974.
216. Lagos, J. C., and Gomez, M. R.: Tuberous sclerosis: Reappraisal of a clinical entity. Mayo Clin. Proc. *42*:26, 1967.
217. Nevin, N. C., and Pearce, W. G.: Diagnostic and genetical aspects of tuberous sclerosis. J. Med. Genet. *5*:273, 1968.

CORONARY ARTERY DISEASE

218. Epstein, F. H.: Risk factors in coronary heart disease—environmental and hereditary influences. Isr. J. Med. Sci. *3*:594, 1967.
219. Slack, J., and Evans, K. A.: The increased risk of death from ischaemic heart disease in first degree relatives of 121 men and 96 women with ischaemic heart disease. J. Med. Genet. *3*:239, 1966.
220. Rissanen, A. M., and Nikkila, E. A.: Coronary artery disease and its risk factors in families of young men with angina pectoris and in controls. Br. Heart J. *39*:875, 1977.
221. Harvald, B., and Hauge, M.: Coronary occlusion in twins. Acta. Genet. Med. Gemellol. (Roma) *19*:248, 1970.
222. Epstein, F. H., and Ostrander, L. D., Jr.: Detection of individual susceptibility toward coronary disease. Prog. Cardiovasc. Dis. *13*:324, 1971.
223. Kannel, W. B., Castelli, W. P., Gordon, T., and McNamara, P. M.: Serum cholesterol, lipoproteins, and the risk of coronary heart disease. Ann. Intern. Med. *74*:1, 1971.
224. Bloor, C. M.: Hereditary aspects of myocardial infarction. Circulation *39, 40* (Suppl. 4):130, 1969.
224a. Neufeld, H. N., and Goldbourt, U.: Coronary heart disease: Genetic aspects. Circulation *67*:943, 1983.
225. Goldstein, J. L., Schrott, H. G., Hazzard, W. R., Bierman, E. L., and Motulsky, A. G.: Hyperlipidemia in coronary heart disease. II. Genetic analysis of lipid levels in 176 families and delineation of a new inherited disorder, combined hyperlipidemia. J. Clin. Invest. *52*:1544, 1973.
226. Brown, M. S., and Goldstein, J. L.: Familial hypercholesterolemia: A genetic defect in the low-density lipoprotein receptor. N. Engl. J. Med. *294*:1386, 1976.
227. Goldstein, J. L., and Brown, M. S.: Familial hypercholesterolemia. *In* Stanbury, J. B., Wyngaarden, J. B., Fredrickson, D. S., Goldstein, J. L., and Brown, M. S. (eds.): The Metabolic Basis of Inherited Disease. 5th ed. New York, McGraw-Hill Book Co., 1983, p. 672.
228. Epstein, C. J., Martin, G. M., Schultz, A. L., and Motulsky, A. G.: Werner's syndrome: A review of its symptomatology, natural history, pathologic features, genetics and relationship to the natural aging process. Medicine *45*:177, 1966.
229. Zackai, A. H., Weber, D., and Noth, R.: Cardiac findings in Werner's syndrome. Geriatrics *29*:141, 1974.
230. Duncan, C., and McLeod, G. M.: Angiokeratoma corporis diffusum universale (Fabry's disease). Aust. Ann. Med. *1*:58, 1970.
231. Becker, A. E., Schoorl, R., Balk, A. G., and van der Heide, R. M.: Cardiac manifestations of Fabry's disease. Am. J. Cardiol. *36*:829, 1975.
232. Beaudet, A. L., Ferry, G. D., Nichols, B. L., Jr., and Rosenberg, H. S.: Cholesterol ester storage disease: Clinical, biochemical, and pathological studies. J. Pediatr. *90*:910, 1977.
233. Havel, R. J., Goldstein, J. L., and Brown, M. S.: Lipoproteins and lipid trans-

port. *In* Bondy, P. K., and Rosenberg, L. E. (eds.): Diseases of Metabolism. 8th ed. Philadelphia, W. B. Saunders Co., 1980, p. 393.
234. Brown, M. S., Kovanen, P. T., and Goldstein, J. L.: Regulation of plasma cholesterol by lipoprotein receptors. Science *212*:628–635, 1981.
235. Jackson, R. L., Morisett, J. D., and Gotto, A. M., Jr.: Lipoprotein structure and metabolism. Physiol. Rev. *56*:259, 1976.
236. Goldstein, J. L., and Brown, M. S.: Familial hypercholesterolemia: Pathogenesis of a receptor disease. Johns Hopkins Med. J. *143*:8, 1978.
237. Glomset, J. A., and Norum, K. R.: The metabolic role of lecithin-cholesterol acyltransferase: Perspectives from pathology. Adv. Lipid Res. *11*:1, 1973.
238. Kwiterovich, P. O., Jr., Levy, R. I., and Fredrickson, D. S.: Neonatal diagnosis of familial type-II hyperlipoproteinemia. Lancet *1*:118, 1973.
239. Slack, J.: Risks of ischaemic heart disease in familial hyperlipoproteinaemic states. Lancet *2*:1380, 1969.
240. Jensen, J., Blankenhorn, D. H., and Kornerup, V.: Coronary disease in familial hypercholesterolemia. Circulation *36*:77, 1967.
241. Stone, N. J., Levy, R. I., Fredrickson, D. S., and Verter, J.: Coronary artery disease in 116 kindred with familial type-II hyperlipoproteinemia. Circulation *49*:476, 1974.
242. Khachadurian, A. K., and Uthman, S. M.: Experiences with the homozygous cases of familial hypercholesterolemia. Nutr. Metab. *15*:132, 1973.
243. Goldstein, J. L.: The cardiac manifestations of the homozygous and heterozygous forms of familial type II hyperbetalipoproteinemia. Birth Defects: Original Article Series *8*:202, 1972.
243a. Forman, M. B., Kinsley, R. H., DuPlessis, J. P., Dansky, R., Milner, S., and Levin, S. E.: Surgical correction of combined supravalvular and valvular aortic stenosis in homozygous familial hypercholesterolaemia. S. Afr. Med. J. *61*:579, 1982.
244. Buja, L. M., Kovanen, P. T., and Bilheimer, D. W. : Cellular pathology of homozygous familial hypercholesterolemia. Am. J. Pathol. *97*:327, 1979.
245. Allen, J. M., Thompson, G. R., Myant, N. B., Steiner, R., and Oakley, C. M.: Cardiovascular complications of homozygous familial hypercholesterolaemia. Br. Heart J. *44*:361, 1980.
246. Glueck, C. J., Levy, R. I., and Fredrickson, D. S.: Acute tendinitis and arthritis: A presenting symptom of familial type II hyperlipoproteinemia. J.A.M.A. *206*:2895, 1969.
247. Goldstein, J. L., Brown, M. S., and Stone, J. J.: Genetics of the LDL receptor: Evidence that the mutations affecting binding and internalization are allelic. Cell. *12*:629, 1977.
248. Brown, M. S., and Goldstein, J. L.: Familial hypercholesterolemia: Model for genetic receptor disease. Harvey Lect. Vol. 73, 1977–78.
249. Goldstein, J. L., and Brown, M. S.: Atherosclerosis: The low density lipoprotein receptor hypothesis. Metabolism *26*:1257, 1977.
250. Bilheimer, D. W., Stone, N. J., and Grundy, S. M.: Metabolic studies in familial hypercholesterolemia: Evidence for a gene-dosage effect *in vivo.* J. Clin. Invest. *64*:524, 1979.
251. Bilheimer, D. W., Goldstein, J. L., Grundy, S. M., and Brown, M. S.: Reduction in cholesterol and low density lipoprotein synthesis after portavacal shunt surgery in a patient with homozygous familial hypercholesterolemia. J. Clin. Invest. *56*:1420, 1975.
252. Soutar, A. K., Myant, N. B., and Thompson, G. R.: Simultaneous measurement of apolipoprotein B turnover in very-low- and low-density lipoproteins in familial hypercholesterolaemia. Atherosclerosis *28*:247, 1977.
253. Ross, R., and Glomset, J. A.: The pathogenesis of atherosclerosis. N. Engl. J. Med. *295*:369, 420, 1976.
254. Bilheimer, D. W., Ho, Y. K., Brown, M. S., Anderson, R. G. W., and Goldstein, J. L.: Genetics of the low density lipoprotein receptor: Diminished receptor activity in lymphocytes from heterozygotes with familial hypercholesterolemia. J. Clin. Invest. *61*:678, 1978.
255. Brown, M. S., Kovanen, P. T., Goldstein, J. L., Vandenberghe, K., Pryns, J. P., Eeckels, R., Van Den Berghe, H., and Cassiman, J. J.: Prenatal diagnosis of homozygous familial hypercholesterolaemia. Lancet *1*:526, 1978.
256. Kane, J. P., and Malloy, M. J.: Treatment of hypercholesterolemia. Med. Clin. North Am. *66*:537, 1982.
257. Thompson, G. R., and Gotto, A. M.: Ileal bypass in the treatment of hyperlipoproteinaemia. Lancet *2*:35, 1973.
258. Starzl, T. E., Putnam, C. W., Chase, H. P., and Porter, K. A.: Portacaval shunt in hyperlipoproteinaemia. Lancet *2*:940, 1973.
259. Thompson, G. R., Lowenthal, R., and Myant, N. B.: Plasma exchange in the management of homozygous familial hypercholesterolaemia. Lancet *1*:1208, 1975.
260. Havel, R. J. (ed.): Symposium on lipid disorders. Med. Clin. North Am. Vol. 66, 1982, pp. 317–550.
261. Schonfeld, G., and Kudzma, D. J.: Type IV hyperlipoproteinemia. Arch. Intern. Med. *132*:55, 1973.
262. Brunzell, J. D., Schrott, H. H., Motulsky, A. G., and Bierman, E. L.: Myocardial infarction in the familial forms of hypertriglyceridemia. Metabolism *25*:313, 1976.
263. Nikkila, E. A., and Aro, A.: Family study of serum lipids and lipoproteins in coronary heart-disease. Lancet *1*:954, 1973.
264. Rose, H. G., Kranz, P., Weinstock, M., Juliano, J., and Haft, J. I.: Inheritance of combined hyperlipoproteinemia: Evidence for a new lipoprotein phenotype. Am. J. Med. *54*:148, 1973.
265. Matthews, R. J.: Type III and IV familial hyperlipoproteinemia: Evidence that these two syndromes are different phenotypic expressions of the same mutant gene(s). Am. J. Med. *44*:188, 1968.
266. Schriebman, P. H., Wilson, D. E., and Arky, R. A.: Familial type IV hyperlipoproteinemia. N. Engl. J. Med. *281*:981, 1969.
267. Glueck, C. J., Fallat, R., Buncher, C. R., Tsang, R., and Steiner, P.: Familial combined hyperlipoproteinemia: Studies in 91 adults and 95 children from 33 kindreds. Metabolism *22*:1403, 1973.
268. Brown, M. S., Goldstein, J. L., and Fredrickson, D. S.: Familial type 3 hypercholesterolemia (dysbetalipoproteinemia). *In* Stanbury, J. B., Wyngaarden, J. B., Fredrickson, D. S., Goldstein, J. L., and Brown, M. S. (eds.): The Metabolic Basis of Inherited Disease. 5th ed. New York, McGraw-Hill Book Co., 1983, p. 655.
269. Hazzard, W. R., and Bierman, E. L.: Aggravation of broad-beta disease (Type 3 hyperlipoproteinemia) by hypothyroidism. Arch. Intern. Med. *130*:822, 1972.
270. Utermann, G., Hees, M., and Steinnet, A.: Polymorphism of apolipoprotein E and occurrence of dysbetalipoproteinaemia in man. Nature *269*:604, 1977.
271. Zannis, V. I., and Breslow, J. L.: Human very low density lipoprotein apolipoprotein E isoprotein polymorphism is explained by genetic variation and posttranslational modification. Biochemistry *20*:1033, 1981.
272. Schneider, W. J., Kovanen, P. T., Brown, M. S., Goldstein, J. L., Utermann, G., Weber, W., Havel, R. J., Kotite, L., Kane, J. P., Innerarity, T. L., and Mahley, R. W.: Familial dysbetalipoproteinemia. Abnormal binding of mutant apoprotein E to low density lipoprotein receptors of human fibroblasts and membranes from liver and adrenal of rats, rabbits, and cows. J. Clin. Invest. *68*:1075, 1981.
273. Utermann, G., Vogelberg, K. H., Steinmetz, A., Schoenborn, W., Pruin, N., Jaeschke, M., Hees, M., and Canzler, H.: Polymorphism of apolipoprotein E. II. Genetics of hyperlipoproteinemia type III. Clin. Genet. *15*:37, 1979.

48 RHEUMATIC AND HERITABLE CONNECTIVE TISSUE DISEASES OF THE CARDIOVASCULAR SYSTEM

by Gene H. Stollerman, M.D.

Two groups of diseases that affect connective tissues are the so-called rheumatic diseases and the heritable disorders of connective tissues. *The rheumatic diseases* have many clinical features in common and are often classified together because they produce acute and/or chronic arthritis associated with a variety of systemic inflammatory manifestations. Pathologically, they are characterized by diffuse vascular lesions with varying degrees of exudation and fibrosis, and seem to be associated with hyperimmune phenomena. The etiologies of some of the syndromes have been established as complications of well-recognized infections; however, several of the rheumatic diseases remain obscure in regard to both etiology and pathogenesis. They all involve the heart differently and to varying degrees, as would be expected considering the variety of connective tissue structures that make up the heart's "skeleton"—its valve rings, valves, septa, and pericardial sac and the myocardial interstitium, through which courses its rich blood supply.

The *heritable disorders of connective tissue* are rare, genetically determined biochemical lesions of collagen, elastic tissue, or the mucopolysaccharides. In all, structural lesions are produced when the stresses of cardiac action "wear out" the defective cardiac skeleton.

RHEUMATIC DISEASES

RHEUMATIC FEVER (RF)

Rheumatic fever (RF) is frequently classified as a connective tissue disease because its anatomic hallmark is damage to collagen fibrils and to the ground substance of connective tissue (especially in the heart). Of major clinical importance is the presence of potentially lethal myocarditis during the acute attack or, more commonly, the fibrosis of the heart valves, which leads to the crippling hemodynamics of chronic rheumatic heart disease.

Epidemiology of Rheumatic Fever

The relation between the epidemiology of RF and that of streptococcal infection has been reviewed extensively.[1] The current confusion concerning the epidemiology of RF stems from the dramatic decline in incidence and prevalence of the disease despite the fact that group A streptococcal pharyngitis still appears to be common among populations in which RF has become rare.

THE CHANGING PATTERN OF RHEUMATIC FEVER: INCIDENCE, PREVALENCE AND MORTALITY

Since Halsey's study in 1921[2] virtually all those who study this disease have been impressed with the diminishing frequency and severity of acute rheumatic fever (ARF), particularly in the relatively affluent populations of North America and Europe (Fig. 48–1). Reasons for this decline are uncertain but are undoubtedly multiple. Certainly antibiotics for the treatment and prevention of streptococcal infection have been a factor, as demonstrated particularly in military populations.[3,4] However, the incidence and death rate from the disease were decreasing before the introduction of antibiotics. Changes in the virulence and serotypes of group A streptococci have been noteworthy (see below). Improved social conditions, such as better housing and slum clearance, have contributed to the decline, since crowding because of inadequate housing is probably the chief reason for the magnified risk of streptococcal infection and ARF in certain ethnic and disadvantaged populations. Improvement in the delivery of health care in defined populations may also be significant.[5]

The prevalence of rheumatic heart disease among American school children has dropped sharply in recent years, so that the number of cases of congenital heart disease now exceeds those of rheumatic heart disease in these populations.[6] When analyzed separately, the death rate from ARF has been noted to have fallen more sharply than that for rheumatic heart disease.[7] Notwithstanding its decline, rheumatic heart disease still constitutes the leading cause of death from heart disease in the 5-to 24-year-old age group in most parts of the world and continues to be a serious public health problem.[8]

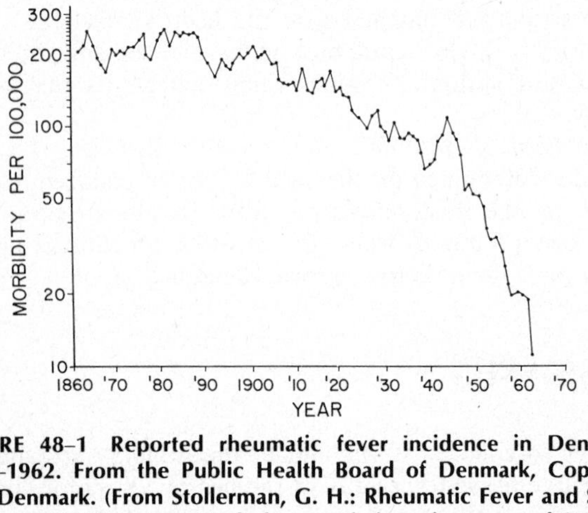

FIGURE 48–1 **Reported rheumatic fever incidence in Denmark, 1862–1962. From the Public Health Board of Denmark, Copenhagen, Denmark. (From Stollerman, G. H.: Rheumatic Fever and Streptococcal Infection. New York, by permission of Grune and Stratton, 1975.)**

FACTORS IN THE ATTACK RATE OF RHEUMATIC FEVER

Quantitative Factors. One factor is the severity of the antecedent pharyngeal streptococcal infection. The clearest relationship of group A streptococcal infection to RF is found in military populations subject to epidemic streptococcal sore throat. In patients with frank, exudative streptococcal pharyngitis caused by certain common prevalent pharyngeal strains of virulent group A streptococci, RF followed at a fairly predictable attack rate (approximately 3 per cent) regardless of the age, race, or ethnic group studied and regardless of the year or season in which the study was made.[3] The major variables which seem to be related to this attack rate in such studies are the magnitude of the immune response to the antecedent streptococcal infection[9] and the duration of convalescent carriage of the organism.[10] Weak antistreptolysin O (ASO) responses are associated with ARF attack rates considerably less than 1 per cent, whereas strong responses are associated with rates well in excess of 5 per cent. In fact, in some studies in which patients with still more vigorous responses are selected, the attack rate may equal 10 per cent.[3] If the infecting organism in the pharynx was not eradicated during convalescence, treatment of streptococcal pharyngitis failed to reduce the attack rate of rheumatic fever.

In contrast to the military studies, reports from civilian medical practice suggest that RF may occur less frequently following endemic, sporadic streptococcal disease.[11–14]

Qualitative Factors. Variations in the "rheumatogenicity" of group A streptococcal strains may constitute one factor influencing the attack rate of RF. In several laboratories where regular serotyping of group A streptococci isolated from pharyngeal infections is performed with available antisera prepared against known M-protein serotypes, the frequency of identification of such strains has decreased. Furthermore, the prevalence of several of the major M types notorious for causing epidemic RF (e.g., types 5, 14, and 24) has apparently declined,[13] and attention has shifted to the study of "new" M types among both pharyngeal strains and "skin" strains.[15] The issue of whether there are "nonrheumatogenic group A streptococci"[16] has been sharpened by the clear demonstration that group A streptococcal pyoderma, with or without complicating acute glomerulonephritis (AGN), does not cause ARF.[17] These skin infections are nonrheumatogenic.[18] Since the pharyngeal route of infection is now an accepted requirement for the pathogenesis of ARF (see below), the question of whether such pyoderma strains can cause RF when they produce pharyngitis is of particular interest. Studies in Memphis have clearly shown seasonal epidemiological separation of ARF and AGN.[19] Populations in the southern United States in which pyoderma and ARF both occur show large numbers of cases of AGN in summer when streptococcal pyoderma is prevalent and when ARF is virtually absent. In the fall, when school begins again, AGN and pyoderma decline rapidly and ARF appears abruptly. In Trinidad, where both AGN and ARF are concurrent in the same population with little seasonal variation, cyclical epidemics of AGN have been reported[20] but without parallel changes in the incidence of ARF. A study of the streptococcal strains in this population show a clear distinction between the serotypes associated with AGN and those associated with ARF.[21]

The studies of Widdowson et al. suggest that RF is associated with infections due to virulent strains capable of causing strong type-specific immune responses to M protein and other streptococcal antigens.[22] Such strains belong to the classic M serotypes known to cause ARF.[23,24]

GEOGRAPHY AND CLIMATE

The relationship of RF to the intensity and severity of streptococcal disease is the same in the tropics as in the temperate climates.[25] The clinical features of RF are also alleged to vary in different climates. In warm climates, there is a reported disparity between the high frequency of acute rheumatic carditis and the apparently low frequency of other manifestations of ARF. Sanyal et al. have recently reviewed the disparate studies from India which have emphasized, on the one hand, the absence or paucity of acute rheumatic manifestations in the population and, on the other, a very high incidence of severe carditis.[26] However, when *prospective* studies were made in a general pediatric department in which *all patients suspected of having ARF were admitted* and *recurrent attacks were excluded*, the frequency of the clinical manifestations of rheumatic fever were the same in New Delhi, India, as in the studies in the United States.

HOST FACTORS

Acquired Susceptibility Through Infections. Since ARF develops in a relatively small percentage of patients following even the most virulent streptococcal infection, the issue of host predisposition is often raised. Once RF is acquired, its activation following streptococcal infection is many times greater in rheumatic subjects than in the general population. The recurrence rate per infection, which is as high as 50 per cent during the first year, decreases sharply until 4 to 5 years after the attack, when it levels off at approximately 10 per cent[27,28] and never seems to fall much lower.[29] Although the persistently higher attack rate in individuals having had RF may suggest some degree of genetic predisposition,[30] the diminishing recurrence rate per infection appears to be acquired. An alternative explanation would be that an acquired sensitization persists virtually throughout life.

Age, Sex, and Race. Like streptococcal sore throat, ARF occurs most commonly in the young school-age child and very rarely in early infancy. It is estimated that 40 per cent of streptococcal infections in pediatric populations occur in children 2 to 6 years of age,[31] suggesting that repeated streptococcal infections and sensitization of the host are prerequisite to the development of RF.[32] No true differencs in sex, race, or ethnic group susceptibility have been established. Crowded living conditions account for whatever apparent increased susceptibility has been reported.

Etiology of Reumatic Fever

The four lines of evidence establishing the group A streptococcus as the sole agent causing initial and recurrent attacks of RF (described below) are of necessity indirect, because group A streptococci cannot be recovered from the lesions of RF and no satisfactory experimental model of the disease has been demonstrated.

Clinical Evidence. Although the frequency with which septic sore throat preceded ARF has been recognized for over 100 years, inconsistencies in this relationship have been pointed out repeatedly.[33,34] Almost one-third of patients with ARF deny the occurrence of antecedent sore throat. Throat and blood cultures in such patients show that the former is frequently negative and the latter virtually always sterile at the onset of the rheumatic attack. Recurrences of RF appeared even more mysterious when antecedent streptococcal sore throat was unrecognized and particularly when the chronicity of a rheumatic attack and the hemodynamic complications of rheumatic heart disease made it difficult to distinguish continued versus reactivated rheumatic carditis. On clinical grounds alone, therefore, it is difficult to establish the group A streptococcus as the sole etiological agent.

Epidemiological Evidence. The environmental, bacterial, and host factors which appear to play a role in the development of RF are important primarily because they are related to the incidence of preceding streptococcal infection. Thus, such factors as latitude, altitude, crowding, dampness, economic factors, and age all affect the incidence of RF because they are related to the incidence and severity of streptococcal infections in general (see above). Careful military epidemiological studies over a period of 20 years show a clear sequential relationship between outbreaks of streptococcal pharyngitis and RF.[35]

Immunological Evidence. Initial (primary) or recurrent (secondary) RF does not occur without a streptococcal antibody response.[36] Furthermore, the magnitude of the antibody response is a major variable determining the attack rate of RF following streptococcal pharyngitis.[9] This is true for both primary and secondary attacks.[27] Indeed, the streptococcal immune response is an important criterion for the diagnosis of RF (see below).

Prophylactic Evidence. The final and perhaps most convincing evidence is the prevention of both initial and recurrent attacks of RF by, in the former case, penicillin therapy and, in the latter, continuous chemoprophylaxis against streptococcal infections. Completely effective prophylaxis of streptococcal infections in rheumatic subjects allows us to conclude that RF cannot be reactivated by any other infection, illness, or trauma.[27,36]

Pathogenesis of Rheumatic Fever

Despite the elusiveness of the pathogenesis of RF, there are a few well-established requirements for the development of this postinfectious sequel: (1) the presence of the group A streptococcus, (2) a streptococcal antibody response indicative of actual recent infection, (3) persistence of the organism in the pharynx for a sufficient period of time, and (4) location of the infection in the throat.

Site of Infection. The possible role of lymphatic connections between the pharynx and the heart has been considered. The embryological derivation of the heart links it structurally with the neck in its vascular, lymphatic, and nervous supply. Impressive connections between tonsils and the heart in human beings have been demonstrated by injections of lymphatic channels in cadavers.[18]

Strain of Group A Streptococcus. The quantitative factor of severity of streptococcal infection bears a general relationship to the attack rate of RF. Although a constant attack rate of RF was shown to occur in military epidemics regardless of the M serotype of the infecting strain, these epidemics were caused by a relatively small number of M serotypes that are now well recognized as the most common and dangerous rheumatogenic pharyngeal strains but are not as commonly isolated as they were previously.

Direct Invasion by Group A Streptococci. Because of the sterility of joint and cerebrospinal fluid (in chorea), most attention has centered on a few reports of group A streptococci cultured from heart valves in acute rheumatic endocarditis.[37,38] Although repetition and extension of this work were hampered by the discovery of antibiotics, most investigators believe that these early reports were the results of either contamination at the time of autopsy or agonal or postmortem dissemination and proliferation of streptococci.[39] Attempts to cure RF by intensive antibiotic therapy have not been successful.

The Role of Toxins. Despite the popularity of the concepts of hyperimmunity and autoimmunity in the pathogenesis of RF (see below), none of the antibodies described to date, including those reactive with the heart, has been shown to be cytotoxic. A direct toxic effect, therefore, of some streptococcal product, particularly on the heart, has not yet been ruled out as a pathogenetic mechanism.[1,30]

IMMUNOLOGICAL THEORIES

The most popular pathogenic theory is that RF results from some type of hyperimmune reaction due either to bacterial allergy or autoimmunity. This view is supported by strong evidence, since RF patients are, in general, the population most intensively hyperimmune to all streptococcal products.

The mean antibody titer to virtually every streptococcal antigen that has been studied is increased in patients during the acute stage of RF. Yet no humoral mechanism of tissue injury has been defined. The latent period between streptococcal infection and the onset of RF resembles that of serum sickness, but several features of RF differentiate it from the immune complex diseases with their associated vascular lesions (see The Vasculitis Syndromes, below). The latent period of ARF does not decrease with repeated recurrences, as with repeated bouts of serum sickness. Angioneurotic edema and vasculitis rashes are not a feature of the disease. Complement levels are increased rather than decreased, and autoantibodies associated with immune complex disease (e.g., rheumatoid factor, anti-DNA, and others) are not present. Although low-grade microscopic hematuria may occur, frank lesions of glomerulonephritis are absent. Careful recent studies have identified circulating immune complexes, but they are of small size and not high titer and quickly disappear after the acute stage of polyarthritis.[40] Whether or not they actually cause arthritic inflammation is conjectural.

Much interest has been shown in the possible mechanism of cell-mediated cytotoxic reactions to various streptococcal antigens, particularly as a possible cause of rheumatic carditis. Although cell-mediated responses to some streptococcal antigens have been shown to be blunted during ARF, most reactions are normal or exaggerated. The specificity of these phenomena for the acute rheumatic process is uncertain, although a recent study suggests that some extracellular purified streptococcal products show diminished reactivity with lymphocytes of patients with rheumatic heart disease compared with those of control subjects.[41]

AUTOIMMUNITY. It has been known for many years that the serum of some patients with ARF contains autoantibodies to heart tissues, and numerous reports using a variety of techniques, mostly immunofluorescence, have confirmed this finding.[42–44] Anti-heart antibodies are gamma globulins with specificity for cardiac components reacting primarily with the sarcolemma. Their binding is also associated with deposition of large amounts of complement component C3. Anti-heart antibodies occur more frequently in RF patients who develop carditis than in those who escape it. The frequency of the appearance of such antibodies is very high in patients who have undergone mitral commissurotomy. These antibodies can be adsorbed by the patient's own atrial tissue and therefore are probably autoantibodies. Massive deposits of gamma globulin have also been identified in the hearts of children who died of rheumatic carditis. The role of such antibodies in the pathogenesis of rheumatic fever has been clouded by the growing understanding of autoantibody formation and complement activation as a general response to tissue injury. Cardiac damage by rheumatic, traumatic, or ischemic heart lesions leads to biochemical changes manifested by the production of autoantibody.[45] Thus, myocardial infarction and postpericardiotomy syndromes have been associated with the production of anti-heart antibodies and/or deposition of complement. It is therefore possible that anti-heart antibodies in rheumatic carditis are the *result* rather than the *cause* of tissue injury.

CROSS REACTIONS BETWEEN STREPTOCOCCI AND HUMAN HEART AND OTHER ORGANS. In the early 1960's Kaplan and his associates demonstrated that rabbit antisera against certain group A streptococci react with human heart preparations in the immunofluorescent test.[46,47] Since then, many additional immunological cross reactions have been described between streptococci and human tissues[48–62] (Fig. 48–2). The immunological details of these reactions and their possible relation to the pathogenesis of RF have been reported and reviewed in detail elsewhere.[1,30,53]

The relationship between anti-heart antibodies in RF and the development of rheumatic heart disease is not clear, and therefore there is no firm evidence for a causal relationship between such cross reactions and the development of rheumatic carditis, however attractive this hypothesis may be.

HOST FACTORS

Genetic Predisposition. The frequent observation of strong familial histories of RF despite the lack of evidence of clear genetic factors predisposing to RF has been puzzling. Only a few adequate studies in identical twins have shown a relatively low concordance of RF (less than 20 per cent), actually considerably lower than that found in some other infections, such as tuberculosis or poliomyelitis.[63] Furthermore, the incidence of ARF is remarkably similar in every human race or ethnic group exposed to rheumatogenic streptococcal disease. It has not been possible, therefore, to define any clear genetic predisposition to the disease, and familial clustering may reflect the factor of infection rather than host predisposition. Although haplotype distributions in rheumatic hosts have not been consistently correlated, there is a suggestion of prominence of HLA-B5, particularly in patients with polyarthritis who are found to have circulating immune complexes.[40]

Immune Response of RF Patients. All antibodies to streptococcal antigens that have been studied have been consistently increased in RF patients compared with patients who have uncomplicated streptococcal pharyngitis.[64] Patients with inactive rheumatic heart disease, however, have depressed cell-mediated responses to some purified streptococcal antigens.[41] RF patients respond normally to other antigens, such as diphtheria toxoid.[65] Conventional immunology would interpret the increased streptococcal immune response to mean that the antecedent streptococcal infection of RF must be of a greater magnitude antigenically than nonrheumatogenic streptococcal infections. Alternatively, or in addition, the rheumatic host may be hyperimmune because of more frequent or more severe streptococcal infections. The depressed cellular immune response to certain purified streptococcal antigens[41] is noteworthy, but the implications with regard to pathogenesis are not clear.

Pathology of Rheumatic Fever

There is often considerable disparity between the severity of the clinical manifestations of RF and the extent of the morbid anatomical changes it produces. Sydenham's chorea, cardiac atrioventricular conduction blocks, and erythema marginatum all appear to be related more to functional disturbances than to visible lesions. In contrast, the persistent focal inflammatory lesions of the myocardium, such as the *Aschoff nodule,* do not always correlate with clinical manifestations of active carditis and have led to differences between pathologists and clinicians with regard

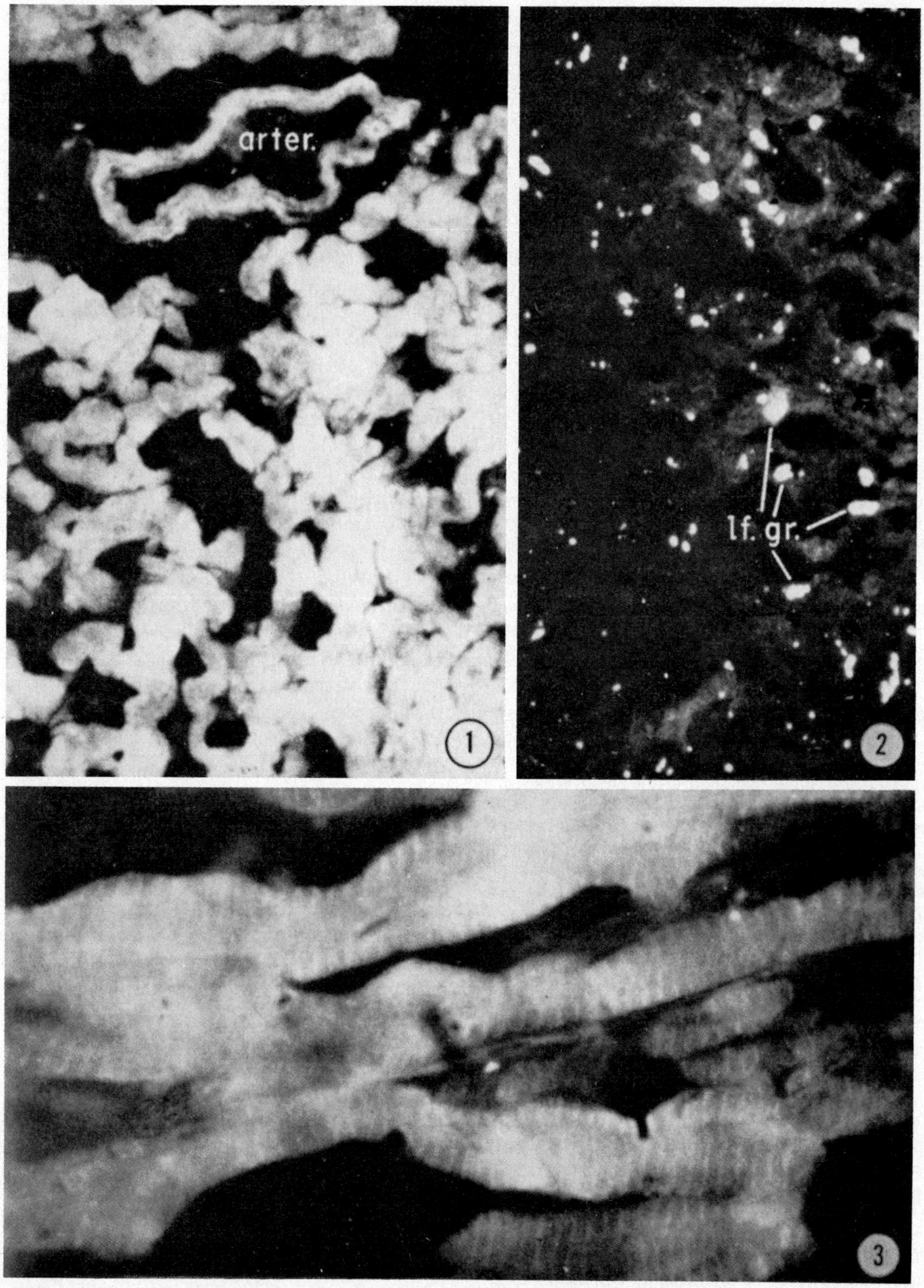

FIGURE 48–2 Immunofluorescent staining of cardiac tissue showing *1*, diffuse sarcoplasmic staining; *2*, absence of specific fluorescence in control section treated with rabbit antiserum free of heart antibody; and *3*, cross-striational staining pattern of left atrial muscle from a patient with rheumatic heart disease. (From Zabriskie, J. B., and Freimer, E. H.: An immunological relationship between the group A streptococcus and mammalian muscle. J. Exp. Med. *124*:661, 1966.)

to the definition of rheumatic activity. In general, however, the acute phase of RF is characterized by diffuse exudative and proliferative inflammatory reactions in the heart, joints, and skin. Small blood vessels and arterioles are commonly involved, but unlike the arteritis of some other connective tissue diseases, thrombotic lesions are not seen.

The term *fibrinoid degeneration* describes the basic structural changes in the collagen of connective tissues.[66,67] The fibrinoid substance resembles and stains like fibrin and is a feature of the earliest phase of the myocardial lesions. The collagen fibers in these mucoid areas become swollen and eosinophilic, forming a meshwork of rigid, waxlike fibers. This exudative-degenerative phase[68,69] lasts for 2 to 3 weeks, following which the most characteristic lesion of RF develops—the myocardial *Aschoff nodule*.[70] The proliferative and healing phase then follows and may persist for many months or even years.[71]

In the early stage of development of the Aschoff nodule,[72] lymphocytes collect around and between the eosinophilic material followed soon after by large and sometimes multinucleated cells with ragged basophilic cytoplasm.[72] Many of these cells have a characteristic *owl-*

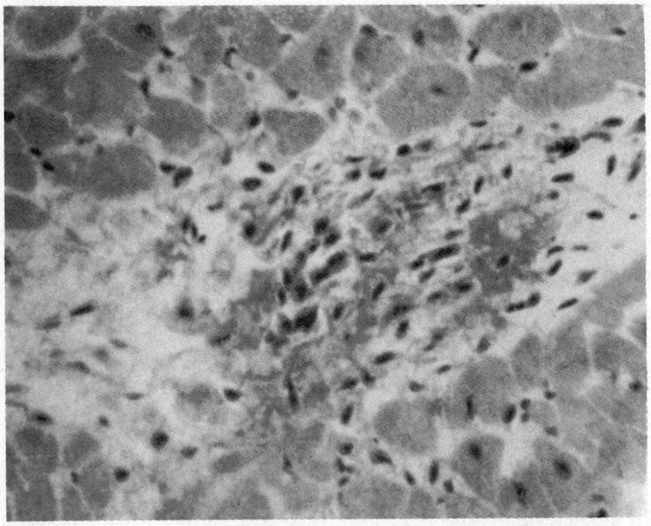

FIGURE 48–3 Early reticular Aschoff body. Note the rigid eosinophilic fibers and clumps of material. The cells are small and elongated (H and E, ×240). (From Lannigan, R.: Cardiac Pathology. London, Butterworth and Co., 1966.)

eye nucleus, which contains a heavy eccentric chromatin dot with fine fibrils radiating to the nuclear membrane (Fig. 48–3). Gradual healing of Aschoff nodules leaves a fibrous scar. Aschoff nodules are virtually pathognomonic of RF with or without collagen fibrinoid lesions.[76]

Ironically, the only lesion pathognomonic of RF is vague with regard to its origin, functional impact on the heart, and relation to the course and severity of the rheumatic attack.[72–78] Aschoff nodules do not seem to account for the acute dilatation of the heart in first attacks of severe carditis. The persistence of Aschoff nodules for many years after a rheumatic attack has been well recognized by pathologists. Biopsies of the left atrial appendage obtained during mitral valve surgery for mitral stenosis have shown persistence of Aschoff nodules in patients who no longer have clinical or laboratory evidence of rheumatic activity[79–81] and who have no recent evidence of streptococcal infection.[82] The persistence of Aschoff nodules seems to be correlated, however, with progressive fibrosis and stenosis of the mitral valve. One series[80,81] showed such lesions in 21 per cent of 191 surgically excised left atrial appendages in patients with mitral stenosis. In the same series, of 91 patients with pure mitral regurgitation, Aschoff nodules were present in the left atrial appendage of only 1 patient.

CARDIAC LESIONS

On gross inspection of the heart, a pancarditis is almost always evident, with fresh exudative pericardial lesions, dilatation of the heart, and verrucous endocardial lesions on the valves.[1,83]

Pericarditis (see also p. 1510). Both layers of the pericardium are thickened and covered with a fibrinous exudate, and serosanguineous pericardial fluid may be present. Mucoid edema occurs early. The deposition of eosinophilic, fibrin-staining material present in other layers of the heart is also seen in the pericardium. With healing, fibrosis and adhesions develop which partially or completely obliterate the pericardial sac, but constrictive pericarditis does *not* occur.

Myocarditis. In addition to the Aschoff bodies, a diffuse cellular infiltrate is present in interstitial tissues. The cells are usually lymphocytes, but polymorphonuclear leukocytes, histiocytes, and eosinophils may also be present. Exudate may be associated with damaged muscle. This interstitial myocarditis may be more important than the nodular Aschoff bodies in producing heart failure. Myocardial fibers are also damaged, and the greatest damage occurs in the vicinity of Aschoff nodules and around blood vessels,[84,85] leading to loss of striations, fatty degeneration, and vacuolation. Myocytolysis and complete loss of fibers may be noted in some areas,[72] and giant cell formation may occur in damaged fibers.

The Conduction System. Despite the high frequency of prolonged atrial ventricular conduction in ARF, visible changes in the bundle of His are seen in the minority of autopsy cases of ARF.[86] The evanescence of heart block and its easy reversibility in most cases by the administration of atropine fit the concept that a functional defect rather than a structural lesion is responsible for this conduction defect.

Endocarditis. The verrucous lesions at the valve edge appear as a mass of eosinophilic material staining as fibrin. At the base and edges of the valve, the cells line up in palisades at right angles to the base and often have elongated Aschoff-type nuclei. As the lesions progress, granulation tissue develops and vascularization and progressive fibrosis take place (Fig. 48–4). The changes involve the annulus as well as the cusps and chordae tendineae, which, as a result of scarring, thicken and shorten.

Arteritis in Coronary Arteries and Other Vessels. Coronary arteritis has been well described in RF for the past 80 years,[87,88] and many pathologists have considered these lesions important in producing myocardial damage in RF. Yet, despite such descriptions, thrombosis of large coronary vessels is very rare in ARF.

RHEUMATIC VALVULAR DEFORMITIES (See also Chap. 32)

Mitral Regurgitation. Incompetence or regurgitation may result from shortening of one or both cusps, from shortening and fusing of chordae and papillary muscles, or from dilatation of the valve ring. By far, the most common clinically apparent lesion of rheumatic heart disease is mitral regurgitation, and such lesions often occur subclinical-

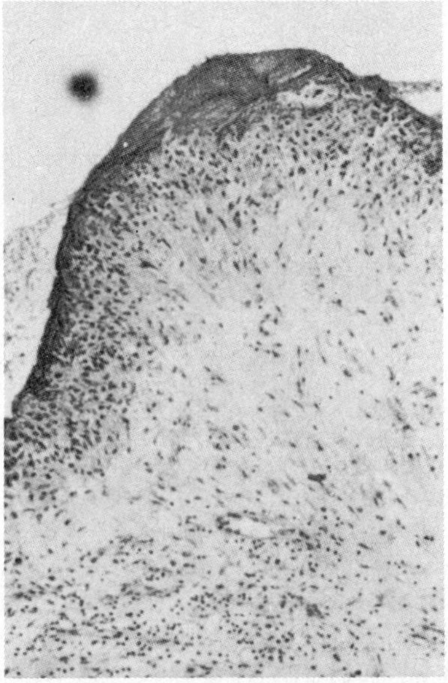

FIGURE 48–4 Rheumatic vegetation showing a layer of dense eosinophilic material and a cellular reaction beneath. The cusp also shows a diffuse cellular infiltrate (H and E, ×60). (From Lannigan, R.: Cardiac Pathology. London, Butterworth and Co., 1966.)

ly when extracardiac symptoms of ARF are absent. Dilatation of the valve ring occurs in active carditis more frequently as a result of acute dilatation of the left ventricle. Marked mitral regurgitation also occurs, however, without acute left ventricular dilatation when the valve cusps and the musculotendinous structures are severely swollen and disorganized by the rheumatic process without coexisting severe myocarditis. In cases of severe regurgitation the degree of stenosis is only moderate, but the same kinds of deformities may be seen in ring, cusps, chordae, and papillary muscles as those described for mitral stenosis. Characteristically, the posterior cusp of the mitral valve is most heavily involved (Fig. 48–5*A*).

Mitral Stenosis. This lesion occurs with varying degrees of mitral regurgitation. When stenosis is severe, regurgitation may be relatively unimportant, and the main hemodynamic problem is obstruction to blood flow during diastole. The gross changes in the mitral valve are variable. The cusps may fuse, leaving an ovoid opening, but the cusps themselves may remain thin and pliable. In other instances the cusps become thick, rigid, or even calcified. A "funnel-shaped valve" with its opening at the apex may result when fusion of the cusps occurs with shortening and thickening of the chordae tendineae and papillary muscles. A "buttonhole" mitral valve is formed when shortening of the chordae is less marked and a diaphragm effect, with an oval or slitlike opening, results. The degree of involvement of the chordae and papillary muscles is of great importance in determining the degree of valve dysfunction. The valve ring as well as the cusps contributes to the stenosis with thickening, rigidity, and calcification. Thus, the commissures, cusps, and chordae may all be involved in varying combinations, resulting in much variation in both hemodynamics and physical signs.

Aortic Valve Deformities. The most common aortic lesion is a combination of stenosis and regurgitation. Pure aortic stenosis is relatively uncommon, but a minimal degree of aortic regurgitation occurs frequently in mild rheumatic involvement. In most cases of symptomatic rheumatic aortic disease, both stenosis and regurgitation occur, but one or the other may be functionally predominant. Deformity of the valve results from fusion of the cusps at the commissures, rigidity and shortening of the cusps alone, or combinations of both processes with calcification superimposed (Fig. 48–5*B*).

Tricuspid Valve Deformities. These almost always exist in association with mitral and aortic lesions and occur in approximately 10 per cent of patients with chronic rheumatic heart disease.[83] Gross and Friedberg found that inflammatory lesions were common in the tricuspid and pulmonary valves in RF, but resulting deformities were uncommon.[86]

Pulmonary Valve Deformities. Pulmonary valve deformities are rarest of all. When they occur, stenosis is more usual than is incompetence. The pathological changes in the pulmonary valve are similar to those in the aortic valve.

Progressive Pathological Changes in Healed Rheumatic Heart Disease. There are manifestations of progressive changes and continued inflammation that seem unrelated to the original rheumatic process. Disruption of red blood cells ("cardiac hemolytic anemia") can result from valvular defects;[89] platelet turnover and destruction have recently been proved to be excessive in rheumatic heart disease,[90] and resultant thrombosis and fibrosis can occur along with calcification. Recurrent congestive heart failure may cause fatty changes in the myocardium and progressive fibrosis. The endocardium, especially the left atrium in mitral valvular deformity, is prone to develop organized thrombi, to stretch and dilate progressively, and to develop chronic inflammatory changes that are not exudative or clearly rheumatic at all.

EXTRACARDIAC LESIONS

Joints. Swelling and edema of the articular and periarticular structures with serous effusion into the joint space occur without ero-

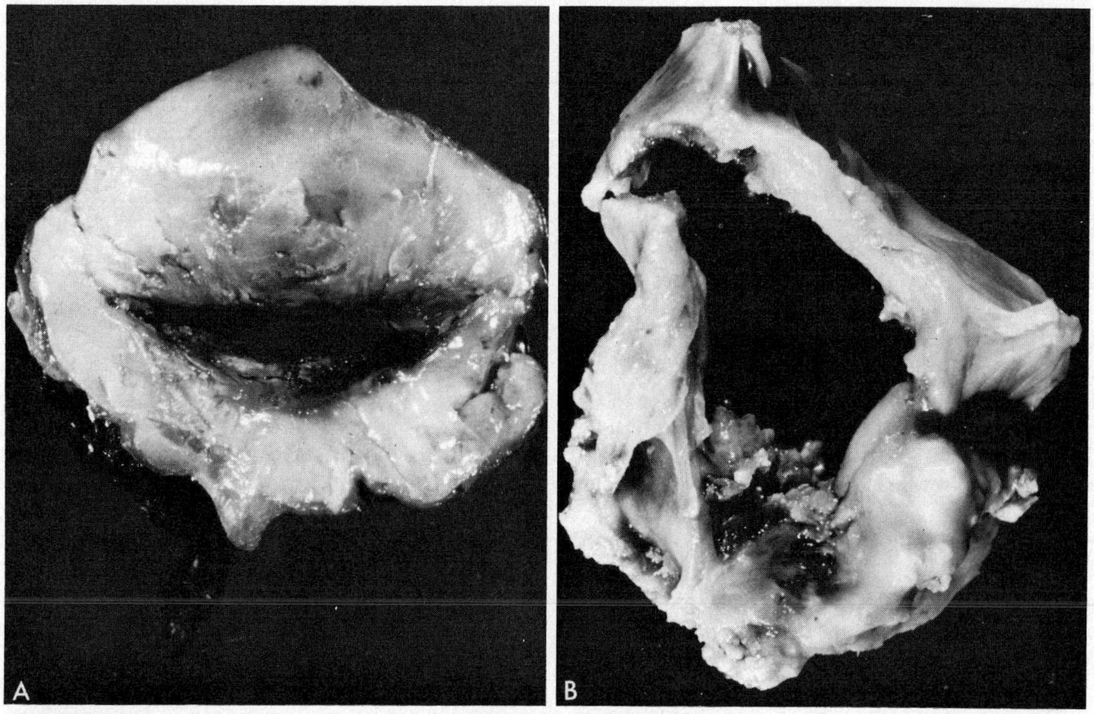

FIGURE 48–5 Excised rheumatic valve. *A*, "Fishmouth" mitral valve. *B*, Aortic valve fixed in open position. (Courtesy of Dr. James W. Pate. From Stollerman, G. H.: Rheumatic Fever and Streptococcal Infection. New York, by permission of Grune and Stratton, 1975.)

sion of the joint surface or pannus formation. The synovial membrane is reddened and thickened and covered with fibrinous exudate. Histologically there is marked edema, engorgement and dilation of blood vessels, and diffuse and focal infiltrates of lymphocytes and polymorphonuclear leukocytes, the latter more numerous initially. Later, focal fibrinoid lesions with histiocytic granulomas may appear,[69,91] but these lesions heal also without residua.

Subcutaneous Nodules. A central zone of fibrinoid necrotic material is surrounded by histiocytes and fibroblasts, and lymphocytes and polymorphonuclear leukocytes collect around small vessels. The structure resembles Aschoff bodies and may heal very rapidly, leaving no apparent scars.

Chorea. Considerable confusion exists concerning the pathology of Sydenham's chorea because (1) few patients die of "pure" chorea, (2) those who die of severe carditis may have inflammatory lesions of the central nervous system without chorea,[92] (3) no single site is consistently involved, (4) Aschoff bodies are not found in the brain,[93,94] and (5) it has not been possible to correlate clinical findings with pathologic changes. Changes found in the central nervous system include arteritis, cellular degeneration, perivascular round cell infiltration, and occasional petechial hemorrhages, but on the whole these are not impressive and are scattered throughout the cortex, cerebellum, and basal ganglia.[95,96]

Rheumatic Pneumonitis. Because this finding occurs with severe carditis only, there has been argument about whether the pulmonary lesion is a rheumatic manifestation or a complication of heart failure. The usual finding is a grossly hemorrhagic lung due to lesions that resemble small infarctions. Fibrin and hemosiderin are deposited in the alveoli, and a hyaline membrane is characteristic. Aschoff bodies are absent, but serous or serofibrinous pleural exudates may occur.

Clinical Manifestations of Rheumatic Fever

The signs and symptoms of ARF vary greatly and are determined by the systems involved, the severity of the lesions and when they appear in the course of the disease, and the stage of the disease when the patient is first observed by the physician. Certain manifestations that follow streptococcal infections (with a frequency far exceeding chance) occur simultaneously, in close succession, or singly. They have been called *major manifestations* and consist of carditis, arthritis, chorea, subcutaneous nodules, and erythema marginatum. The word "major" refers to their importance as diagnostic criteria and not to their importance in the severity of the process or its activity, or to the prognosis.

Minor manifestations of ARF are frequently present and helpful in recognizing the disease. They are too nonspecific, however, to be of major importance in diagnosis. Minor manifestations include such findings as fever, arthralgia, acute phase reactants in the blood, heart block, and a history of previous ARF or rheumatic heart disease.

Antecedent Streptococcal Infection. Evidence for an antecedent streptococcal infection may not be apparent. As many as one-third of patients do not remember having had any illness in the preceding month.[33] Furthermore, in patients with previous RF who were followed prospectively for recurrences, asymptomatic streptococcal infections accounted for 54[27] to 70 per cent[29] of recurrences of RF. The average interval between onset of symptoms of pharyngitis and the symptoms of RF (the latent period) was 18.6 days in one prospective study[97] but may be as short as 1 week or as long as 5 weeks. The latent period is no shorter in patients with previous RF than in those without.

Arthritis. This manifestation occurs in about three-fourths of patients during the acute stage of the disease. In general, joint involvement becomes more common with increasing age of the patient, a trend related to the concomitant decrease in the incidence of carditis and chorea.[98–101]

The arthritis of RF usually involves the large joints, particularly the knees, ankles, elbows, and wrists. Almost any joint, however, may be affected. In the classic attack, several joints are involved in quick succession, each for a brief period of time, resulting in the typical picture of migratory polyarthritis. Each joint remains inflamed for usually no more than a week before it begins to subside, and the inflammation usually abates spontaneously in 2 or 3 weeks. The course of the entire bout of polyarthritis is usually severe for a week in approximately two-thirds of patients and for an additional week or two in the remainder, but by the end of 4 weeks, it will have subsided, with rare exceptions. Flare-ups may occur, however, in a small percentage of patients treated with antirheumatic therapy for 4 to 6 weeks but rarely after a second 6-week course of antirheumatic treatment. Unlike rheumatoid arthritis, RF does not cause permanent joint deformities except for the so-called Jaccoud type of deformity of the metacarpophalaneal joints.[101–103,103a] Acute polyarthritis rarely occurs more than 35 days after the onset of the streptococcal infection, and for that reason, it is almost always associated with a rising or peak titer of streptococcal antibodies. This fact aids in identifying an isolated bout of polyarthritis as rheumatic or in *excluding* RF as an etiology for a given bout of polyarthritis when streptococcal antibodies are not increased.

CARDITIS

Variations in Onset and Course. The most important manifestation of ARF is carditis, which, in its most severe form, causes death from acute cardiac failure. More commonly, however, carditis is less intense, and the predominant effect is scarring of the heart valves. In contrast to the seriousness of its prognosis, rheumatic carditis most often causes no symptoms of its own and is usually diagnosed in the course of the examination of a patient with arthritis or chorea, which directs the physician's attention to the heart, where murmurs are detected. Carditis, therefore, does not come to medical attention if other symptoms of rheumatic fever are absent or if the carditis is not severe enough to cause heart failure, prolonged or severe fever, or the pain of pericarditis. Patients with undiagnosed carditis may later prove to have rheumatic heart disease and usually give no history of a previous rheumatic attack.

Cardiac involvement may often occur in the mildest form of the disease. The incidence of carditis in initial attacks of RF varies from 40 to 51 per cent in reports from the United States and Canada.[102–108] Murmurs indicative of carditis are usually present during the first week of the illness in about three-fourths of all patients in whom carditis is eventually diagnosed.[105] By the second or third week, murmurs will become manifest in 85 per cent of those in whom they will eventually develop.

In another form of its presentation, particularly in children under 6 years of age, carditis begins more insidiously, with only slight or no fever and with vague or absent joint pains. Constitutional symptoms are prominent, however, and anorexia, fatigue, and pallor may progress to shortness of breath and chest pain. The child will then appear wan and chronically ill. Signs of carditis are unequivocal and often include incipient or overt health failure. Such patients usually have serious cardiac involvement.

Acute heart failure in a young patient who has had rheumatic heart disease previously but who has been well compensated should always be suspected as a recurrence of acute rheumatic carditis. Young hearts with rheumatic disease rarely fail because of hemodynamic handicaps alone except when the latter are severe and protracted.

Clinical Signs and Criteria. The four major criteria for the clinical diagnosis of rheumatic carditis are (1) an organic heart murmur or murmurs not previously present, (2) enlargement of the heart, (3) congestive heart failure, and (4) pericardial friction rubs or signs of effusion. If any one of these is unequivocal in a patient with active RF, the diagnosis of carditis is justified.

Murmurs of Acute Rheumatic Carditis. Organic murmurs are almost invariably present. They may not be heard when the heart rate is too rapid, when cardiac output is very low in severe congestive heart failure, when they are obscured by a loud pericardial rub, or, rarely, when there is marked pericardial effusion. Otherwise, the signs of endocarditis are always associated with those of involvement of other layers of the heart.

Apical Systolic Murmur. The mitral valve is the most common site of rheumatic inflammation—about three times as frequently involved as the aortic valve. Inflammation ("valvulitis") causing edema, thickening, and verrucae leads to mitral regurgitation early in the course of the disease and often with mild cardiac involvement. The systolic murmur is heard best at the apex, usually grade 3 or more on a scale of 6 in intensity, and, most important, it has a high-pitched blowing quality.

The difference between functional or innocent apical murmurs and mitral regurgitation is difficult to describe, since it is based mainly on the subjective perception of what is the "pure blow" of regurgitation and what are the low-pitched musical overtones of the functional "vibratory" murmur. Moreover, some children will present with both kinds of murmurs. Furthermore, an unusually loud functional murmur accentuated by fear, pain, and excitement may be incorrectly interpreted as a "changing organic murmur" when antirheumatic treatment quiets the patient and reduces the intensity and quality of the murmur's overtones, whereas the organic blow under such conditions is still clearly heard. The latter may also disappear, but it does so gradually over a period of weeks or months.

Apical Mid-diastolic Murmur (Carey-Coombs Murmur). This murmur begins directly after the onset of the third heart sound and ends before the first heart sound. The mid-diastolic murmur is often transient, low-pitched, and easily missed. The presence of this murmur makes the diagnosis of "mitral valvulitis" more definite, confirms the significance of the apical systolic murmur, and adds to the seriousness of the prognosis for permanent valve injury. The mid-diastolic murmur is easy to confuse with the normal third heart sound heard so commonly in children, especially during increased cardiac output. It is, in fact, an extension and exaggeration of the third heart sound into a murmur and should not be mistaken for the rumbling murmur of mitral stenosis.

Aortic Diastolic Murmur. This murmur may appear early in the course of the disease as an expression of aortic valvulitis and may occur alone or with mitral valvulitis. The aortic diastolic blow may be audible only intermittently, depending, again, on cardiac output. The murmur is a soft, high-pitched, decrescendo blow heard immediately after the second heart sound. A diastolic cooing or crying "sea gull" murmur is rarely heard but can be present evanescently in the aortic valvulitis of acute carditis. Basal systolic murmurs, which are sometimes heard in children with first attacks of acute carditis, are physiologic sounds associated with the ejection of blood into the great vessels. They are functional murmurs of short ejection quality and should not be confused with aortic stenosis—a late sequel.

Cardiac Enlargement and Failure. The most reliable clinical expression of rheumatic myocarditis from the standpoint of diagnosis and prognosis is *dilatation,* particularly of the left atrium and ventricle. Heart size should be carefully measured both clinically and radiographically. In the presence of significant heart murmurs, the degree of enlargement generally reflects the severity of carditis. In two carefully performed cooperative studies designed to evaluate treatment of rheumatic carditis, cardiomegaly occurred in a little more than half the children who developed carditis.

Congestive heart failure is the least common but most serious manifestation of rheumatic carditis. It is reported in 5 to 10 per cent of first attacks of rheumatic carditis. It is more common, however, to encounter severe and fatal heart failure as a manifestation of a *rheumatic recurrence* than of a primary attack. S3 and S4 gallops often accompany congestive failure. Combined with mitral regurgitation due to the valvulitis, these may cause the rocking, chaotic apical impulses that are so characteristic on palpation and so ominous in significance. Chest x-ray evidence of vascular congestion and patchy edema may be more striking than the physical signs and almost always raises the suspicion of rheumatic pneumonitis or pulmonary arteriolar vasculitis and infarction as a differential diagnosis. It may be impossible to exclude the presence of all three complications, since all may occur in the severest forms of RF.

Signs of heart failure may occur during the course of any attack of active carditis, so that patients should be examined frequently and carefully for this complication. The tachypnea and hyperpnea caused by salicylism should not be mistaken for left ventricular failure, nor should enlargement of the liver, so commonly a consequence of the fatty infiltration caused by corticosteroids, be confused with right ventricular failure.

Pericarditis. Pericarditis occurs in approximately 5 to 10 per cent of most large series of ARF.[102,105] Occasionally, pericardial reaction and effusion will be more striking and prominent than the degree of myocarditis (Fig. 48–6). In such cases the regression in apparent heart size and the rate of healing of the attack can be rapid. Conversely, the pericarditis may be a relatively minor aspect of a profound case of heart failure due to severe myocardi tis. One rarely sees tamponade without severe heart failure as well.

Arrhythmias. Delayed atrioventricular (AV) conduction, as reflected in prolongation of the P-R interval, occurs with similar frequency to the polyarthritis of ARF,

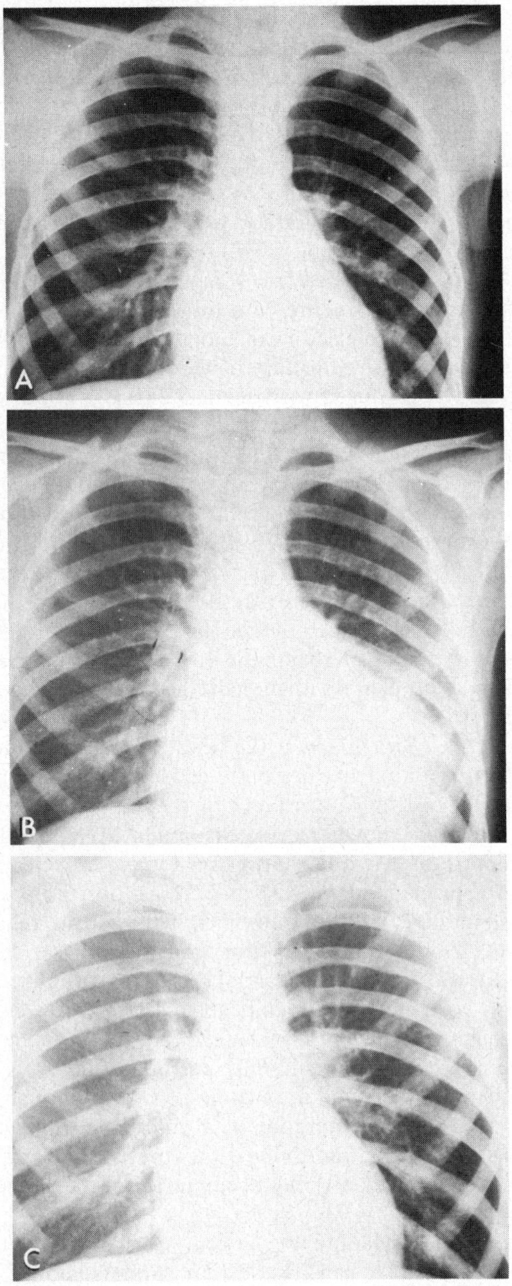

FIGURE 48–6 Pericarditis with effusion during acute rheumatic fever. *A*, Chest x-ray of a 9-year-old boy at onset of acute rheumatic polyarthritis and carditis. *B*, Chest x-ray one week later when a pericardial friction rub was heard. *C*, Chest x-ray about two weeks later when symptoms had subsided. (From Stollerman, G. H.: Rheumatic Fever and Streptococcal Infection. New York, by permission of Grune and Stratton, 1975.)

whether or not clear evidence of carditis is present. The prolongation of AV conduction is easily reversed with atropine,[109] suggesting that this feature is usually due to functional effects of the disease on AV conduction rather than to inflammation and fibrosis of the conduction system. Prolongation of AV conduction may lead to second-degree and, rarely, even third-degree block.[110] The latter is usually of brief duration and reverts spontaneously. Interference and dissociation phenomena are also characteristic of occasional nodal rhythms. Atrial fibrillation is rarely caused by acute rheumatic carditis in contrast to its frequency in patients with longstanding mitral valvular disease with atrial enlargement and chronic atrial subendocardial inflammation.

EXTRACARDIAC MANIFESTATIONS

Subcutaneous Nodules. These are a major manifestation of ARF.[111,112] However, they are not pathognomonic of RF, since they occur in rheumatoid arthritis and systemic lupus erythematosus as well. They rarely occur as an isolated manifestation and are associated most often with severe carditis, appearing usually several weeks after its onset.[113]

Nodules are round, firm, painless subcutaneous lesions varying in size from approximately 0.5 to 2.0 cm. The skin over them is freely movable and not inflamed. They are located over bony surfaces or prominences and over tendons, particularly the extensor of the fingers and toes and flexors of the wrists and ankles. They occur in crops and vary in number from one to usually three or four dozen; when numerous, they tend to be symmetrical (Fig. 48–7). Nodules are evanescent, disappearing sometimes within several days but usually lasting a week or two and rarely more than a month. They tend, therefore, to be much smaller and less persistent than rheumatoid nodules.

Erythema Marginatum. This is a less common feature of RF but is so characteristic that it has taken its rightful place among the five major diagnostic manifestations of the disease. However, it cannot be considered pathognomonic of ARF because it has been reported in sepsis, in drug reactions, in patients with glomerulonephritis, and in children in whom no etiological factor can be identified.[114]

Erythema marginatum appears as a bright-pink smoke ring spreading serpiginously through a pale skin. It is nonpruritic, nonpainful, and neither indurated nor raised. It blanches completely on pressure and is evanescent. The individual lesions usually appear on the trunk and the proximal parts of the extremities but not on the face (Fig. 48–8); they rarely extend distally beyond the elbows or knees. Erythema marginatum may recur intermittently for months, uninfluenced by antirheumatic agents, and when all other signs of rheumatic activity are gone, one can allow the patient to begin to ambulate without fear of a relapse.

Chorea (Sydenham's Chorea, St. Vitus' Dance). This neurological disorder characterized by involuntary, purposeless, rapid movements, muscular weakness, and emotional lability, may be associated with other manifestations of ARF, but it also may appear as the sole expression of the disease—so-called "pure chorea." After puberty it is present exclusively in women, and even in them it declines rapidly after adolescence. Chorea has decreased strikingly in frequency compared with arthritis and carditis.

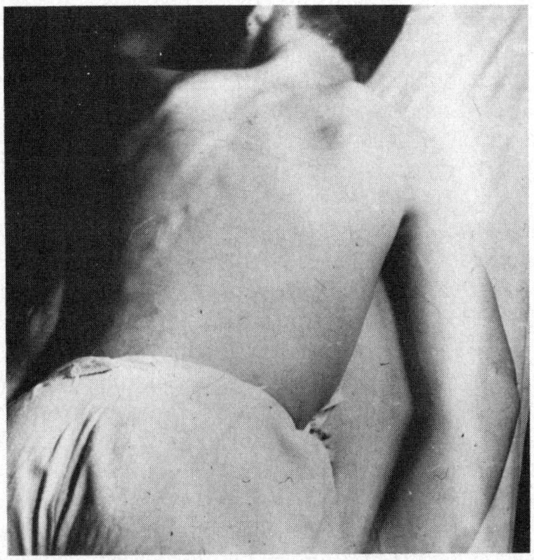

FIGURE 48–7 Subcutaneous nodules along the spinous processes. (From Stollerman, G. H.: Rheumatic Fever and Streptococcal Infection. New York, by permission of Grune and Stratton, 1975.)

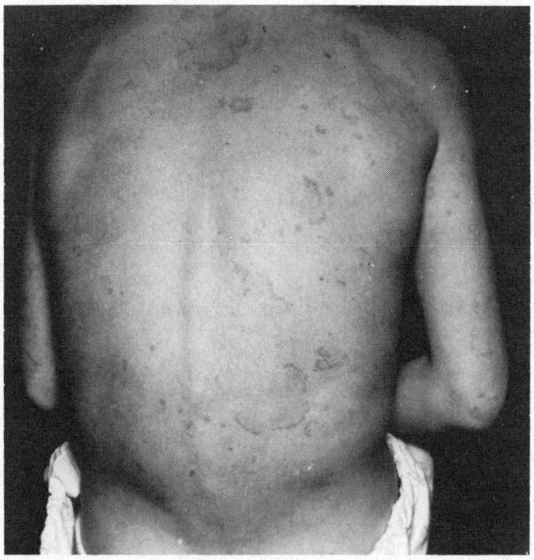

FIGURE 48–8 Erythema marginatum. (Courtesy of Dr. Benedict F. Massell.)

The movements of chorea are abrupt and erratic, not rhythmical or repetitive. In even the most violent attacks, all choreiform movements disappear during sleep and are less violent during rest and sedation. The patient cannot maintain a steady expression but grimaces, grins, frowns, and pouts in rapid succession. The tongue, when protruded, resembles "a bag of worms," may dart in and out, and may contribute to the typical choreiform speech, which is halting, staccato, explosive, and jerky. Handwriting may become clumsy or impossible to read and can be studied serially as a measure of healing; the muscular weakness may be severe enough to resemble a palsy. The electroencephalogram frequently shows abnormally slow waves.[115]

Emotional lability creates personality changes that often herald the onset of a bout of chorea. The patient may become fidgety, restless, cantankerous, and uncooperative.

Chorea may last from 1 week to more than 2 years but usually about 8 to 15 weeks, with a mean of 13.7.[116] Chorea is never seen simultaneously with arthritis but often coexists with carditis. When chorea appears alone, however, the other minor clinical and laboratory signs of ARF may be entirely absent. The erythrocyte sedimentation rate and C-reactive protein may be normal. Even more confusing, in such cases the ASO and other streptococcal antibody titers may not be increased because chorea appears only after a relatively long latent period (as long as 1 to 6 months) following the antecedent streptococcal infection, and after the longest latent period, both the acute phase reactants and the streptococcal antibody titers may have returned to normal.[117,118]

Fever. Some degree of fever accompanies almost all rheumatic attacks at their onset. Temperature usually ranges from 101° to 104°F (38.4° to 40°C), is rarely higher, and has no characteristic pattern. In the usual attack, fever decreases in approximately a week without antipyretic treatment and may become low-grade for another week or two. It rarely lasts for more than several weeks. When antirheumatic agents are used, however, a "rebound" of fever may occur after 4 to 6 weeks of treatment, but it usually subsides spontaneously within a few days except in unusually persistent attacks.

Abdominal Pain. The abdominal pain of RF, which occurs in fewer than 5 per cent of patients with ARF,[119] resembles that seen in other conditions in which acute microvascular mesenteric disease occurs, such as sickle cell crises, sepsis, endotoxin or anaphylactic shock, transfusion reactions, and anaphylactoid purpura.

Epistaxis. In the past, the incidence of epistaxis was reported from as high as 48 per cent in the early 1930's[120] to a low of 4 to 9 per cent in the late 1950's,[99] and perhaps it is even less frequent now.

Rheumatic Pneumonia. When the rheumatic process causes severe carditis, rheumatic inflammation also appears in the lung and cannot be distinguished from patchy pulmonary edema, segmental, platelike atelectatic lesions of pulmonary embolism, or thromboses from vasculitis.[121]

LABORATORY FINDINGS IN RHEUMATIC FEVER

Although there are no pathognomonic tests for RF, laboratory findings are helpful in two major ways: (1) in establishing the antecedent streptococcal infection and (2) in documenting the presence or persistence of an inflammatory process.

ANTECEDENT STREPTOCOCCAL INFECTION. The diagnosis of recent streptococcal infection can be made only tentatively by throat culture but definitely by antibody determinations. Throat cultures are usually negative by the time RF appears. When they are positive, one still cannot be certain whether the organism isolated represents convalescent carriage of the antecedent infection or an intercurrent acquisition of a different strain. Streptococcal antibodies are therefore more useful because they reach a peak titer shortly after the onset of ARF and indicate true infection rather than transient carriage.

ANTIBODIES. The specific antibodies used to diagnose streptococcal infections are primarily antistreptolysin O, antihyaluronidase, antistreptokinase, anti-NADase (anti-DPNase), and anti-DNAse B. Antistreptolysin O has been the most extensively used test and is generally available in hospitals in the United States.[122]

ASO titers vary with age, geographical area, and other factors influencing the frequency of streptococcal infection.[123] Titers of 200 to 300 units/ml are common in healthy children 6 to 14 years of age who live in crowded cities in the temperate zone of the United States.

The chances of detecting a significant antibody response is greatest 2 to 3 weeks after the onset of ARF, which is 4 to 5 weeks after the antecedent streptococcal infection. Thereafter, antibody titers fall off rapidly in the next few months, and after 6 months the decline levels off slowly. For this reason, evidence of increased streptococcal antibodies should be present in all patients at the onset of the rheumatic attack if such onset is well defined. Acute polyarthritis always occurs within a latent period of no more than 4 to 5 weeks after the antecedent streptococcal infection and therefore at or near the peak of the antibody response.

Anti-DNAse B,[124] together with the ASO, has become most generally recommended for diagnosis, with antihyaluronidase a useful third. Recently a product has been marketed which is a concentrate of a variety of extracellular streptococcal antigens made from supernates of broth cultures (antistreptozyme [ASTZ] test). Sheep cells sensitized with this concentrate will agglutinate in the presence of streptococcal antibodies that have not yet been defined. This slide agglutination test is a very sensitive measure of the streptococcal immune response.[125,126] The greatest value of the ASTZ test is in helping to rule out RF, particularly in the diagnosis of isolated polyarthritis when low titers reflect the absence of recent streptococcal disease.

ACUTE PHASE REACTANTS. Acute phase reactants include leukocyte counts, erythrocyte sedimentation rate (ESR), C-reactive protein (CRP), serum mucoprotein, serum hexosamine, serum protein electrophoresis, and several others. The two tests that have gained widest use are the CRP and the ESR. These tests are, of course, not specific for RF, but they are almost always abnormal during the active rheumatic process if it is not suppressed by antirheumatic drugs. "Pure" chorea and, occasionally, persistent erythema marginatum are exceptions. When rheumatic manifestations are obvious, as in the presence of fever and polyarthritis, CRP and ESR are of little value because inflammation is already apparent. During treatment, however, they are quite useful, particularly CRP, in measuring the effectiveness of suppression of the inflammatory process.[127] Particularly when treatment has been discontinued or dosages of antirheumatic agents have been reduced, CRP is very efficient in monitoring the patient for relapse of continued rheumatic inflammation ("rebounds") and in establishing when the active phase of rheumatic inflammation has abated. When ESR and CRP remain normal a few weeks after antirheumatic treatment has been discontinued, the attack will be over unless chorea appears. Even then, however, there will be no exacerbation of the systemic inflammatory component of the attack. Congestive heart failure may cause confusion with both tests. CRP may become positive in pulmonary edema or severe left heart failure of any cause, and the ESR may be slowed by cardiac decompensation.

ANEMIA. The anemia of RF is the normocytic normochromic anemia of chronic inflammation and is of mild to moderate degree.[128] Suppression of inflammation usually corrects the anemia partially or completely, and corticosteroids are particularly potent in this regard. Anemia is a good index of the severity and chronicity of RF.

ELECTROCARDIOGRAPHIC FINDINGS. The electrocardiogram in RF has no characteristic pattern, and the diagnosis of rheumatic carditis should never be made on the basis of electrocardiographic changes alone. Too often the diagnosis of carditis has been made incorrectly when a doubtful systolic murmur has been associated with a prolonged P-R interval or nonspecific ST-T changes. Neither the course of the acute rheumatic attack nor the subsequent development or valvular or myocardial damage can be predicted from the electrocardiographic changes.[104,129,130] Patients with ECG changes but with no other signs of carditis recover completely without the stigmata of rheumatic heart disease.[131]

Diagnosis of Rheumatic Fever

JONES CRITERIA. When T. Duckett Jones formulated his criteria for the diagnosis of ARF in 1944,[132] there was an immediate recognition of their value and considerable consensus about their use. These criteria were adopted in modified form in 1955 by the American Heart Association's Council on Rheumatic Fever and Congenital Heart Disease and were further revised by the same Council's committee in 1965.[133] The current criteria (Table 48–1) emphasize the importance of establishing the presence of the antecedent streptococcal infection by demonstration of increased streptococcal antibodies. If supported by such evidence, two major (or one major and two minor) manifestations indicate a high probability of ARF. However, because virtually all patients with Sydenham's chorea are rheumatic subjects, the diagnosis can be made even when chorea is the sole manifestation.

POLYARTHRITIS. Because of the numerous causes of polyarthritis, the diagnosis of RF is weakest when this manifestation appears alone, and particularly in the adolescent or adult population in which other arthritides are common.

TABLE 48–1 JONES CRITERIA (REVISED)

Major Manifestations	Minor Manifestations
Carditis	Fever
Polyarthritis	Arthralgia
Chorea	Previous rheumatic fever or rheumatic heart disease
Erythema marginatum	Elevated ESR or positive CRP
Subcutaneous nodules	Prolonged P-R interval

Plus supporting evidence of preceding streptococcal infection: history of recent scarlet fever; positive throat culture for group A streptococcus; increased ASO titer or other streptococcal antibodies.

From Jones Criteria (revised) for guidance in the diagnosis of rheumatic fever. Circulation *32*:664, 1965, by permission of the American Heart Association, Inc.

It is helpful to classify polyarthritis pathophysiologically and in the sequence of therapeutic priorities. For this reason, one should consider the following conditions in the differential diagnosis.

DIFFERENTIAL DIAGNOSIS OF POLYARTHRITIS

Bacteremias. In terms of the importance and urgency of diagnosis, it is essential to rule out bacterial infections in all cases of acute polyarthritis. Pneumococcal, meningococcal, gonococcal, streptococcal, and staphylococcal bacteremias should be excluded by obtaining blood for appropriate cultures before antibiotic therapy is initiated. When gonococcal polyarthritis cannot be excluded by cultures of the joints or blood (in the majority of cases), a therapeutic trial of penicillin should be used because a prompt response (within 24 to 48 hours) is almost invariable.[134,135]

Infective endocarditis must also be considered whenever a patient with rheumatic heart disease develops unexplained fever and arthritis[136,137] (Chap. 33).

Osteomyelitis. Especially when pain is referred to the hip, osteomyelitis can be difficult to exclude. Should the diagnosis be suspected, it is best to start treatment as soon as blood cultures are made and without waiting for the results.

Viremias. *Type B hepatitis* and other viruses that can cause rather prolonged viremias (Epstein-Barr virus and cytomegalovirus) can produce a serum sickness syndrome presumably by the formation of circulating immune complexes.

Rubella. The frequency with which rubella produces arthritis, particularly in adult women, has been increasingly appreciated,[138] especially where rubella vaccine is used extensively.[139] When the evanescent rash is either not noticed or not present and the characteristic suboccipital and retrocervical lymphadenopathy goes unnoticed, the presenting picture of arthritis can simulate RF closely.

Immune Complex Disease. A history of receiving animal sera may provide the necessary clue. When penicillin is given to treat streptococcal pharyngitis, however, the situation may be very confusing. Urticaria or angioneurotic edema points to *serum sickness*, as does evidence of acute glomerulonephritis and a fall in serum complement. Low levels of streptococcal antibodies may be the only reliable differential diagnostic feature if other clues of serum sickness are absent.

Sickle Cell Anemia and Other Hemoglobinopathies. Sickle cell disorders have many signs and symptoms that resemble ARF and other diffuse vascular diseases because they are, in fact, associated with microvascular thrombosis and inflammation (Chap. 49). Joint pain, abdominal pain, heart murmurs, cardiac enlargement, and fever all simulate ARF very closely.[140-142]

Rheumatoid Arthritis. When it begins with acute migratory polyarthritis involving the large joints, rheumatoid arthritis imitates ARF. Involvement of many small joints, particularly of the hands and feet, is more characteristic of rheumatoid arthritis, but such involvement may appear later in the course of the disease when it has become low-grade and chronic, with characteristic "morning stiffness" and fusiform swelling of the fingers. A macular rash, lymphadenopathy, and splenomegaly are also more characteristic of rheumatoid arthritis. The chronic course of rheumatoid arthritis may ultimately be the distinguishing features as well as the eventual joint deformities when granulation tissue develops to form the characteristic pannus in the synovia of rheumatoid joints. Streptococcal antibody titers are helpful in differential diagnosis only when they are not increased fortuitously in rheumatoid arthritis[143]

Lymphomas and Granulomas. Leukemia causes fever and acute polyarthritis quite often—10 per cent of cases in some series.[144] Confusion arises because arthritis can appear before the peripheral blood shows leukemic cells. Other lymphomas such as Hodgkin's disease and benign granulomas such as sarcoidosis can also cause hyperimmune phenomena and arthritis.

CARDITIS

Functional ("Innocent") Murmurs. When functional or organic murmurs are typical, there is little problem for the experienced physician. At times, however, a nondescript murmur, especially in an obese or heavy-chested person, may defy sharp distinctions, and repeated examinations and other studies may be required. Such murmurs are often classified as "doubtful" or "questionable" when no other decision can be made.

Myocarditis. In its severe and chronic form, myocarditis due to other diseases may be impossible to distinguish from chronic rheumatic carditis if the heart is dilated and mitral regurgitation is prominent. This situation occurs when patients with ARF have heart failure with no associated extracardiac manifestations to provide clues. In rheumatic carditis, as the patient recovers cardiac compensation, the valvular lesions persist, and the murmurs become, if anything, louder, whereas the reverse is true in viral and other forms of myocarditis.

Pericarditis. Although rheumatic carditis does not produce an isolated pericarditis, at the onset of RF, however, pericarditis may appear before valvulitis and myocarditis are evident. Although many causes of pericarditis can be listed (Chap. 43), primary viral pericarditis most often enters the differential diagnosis in children.[145,146]

Congenital Heart Disease. This is rarely a diagnostic problem except when the cardiac murmur is first discovered during a febrile illness, especially if the heart is overactive and early signs of congestive heart failure are present. Congenital defects of the mitral valve (p. 985) cause the greatest problem,[147] especially when it is an isolated defect. Children who have severe mitral regurgitation with a large failing heart and poor development may present a picture indistinguishable from chronic severe carditis.

Chorea. When chorea is the only manifestation of ARF, the diagnosis depends entirely on the clinician's ability to recognize this manifestation, and appropriate care must be taken to avoid misdiagnosis. Multiple tics or habit spasms in a hyperactive child may pose a problem.

Course, Prognosis, and Natural History of Rheumatic Fever

The clinical course of RF can be quite variable, but in general there is a characteristic sequence of the major manifestations and usually a predictable duration. The latent period between streptococcal infection and the onset of ARF is shortest in arthritis and erythema marginatum and longest in chorea, with that of carditis and subcutaneous nodules in between. The usual duration of a rheumatic attack is rarely longer than 3 months. When severe carditis is present, clinical rheumatic activity may continue for 6 months or more. In fewer than 5 per cent of patients, ARF may remain active for more than 6 months.[148] These cases are classified as "chronic" rheumatic fever.

Carditis. Of the patients in whom carditis develops, murmurs occur during the first week of illness in 76 per cent. In 93 per cent of patients there is evidence of carditis in the first 3 months. Age of onset and severity of carditis influence its chronicity. Before the age of 3 years, 92 per cent of patients in one study[149] and 90 per cent in another[150] had carditis. The incidence of carditis decreased to 50 per cent in the 3- to 6-year age group and to 32 per cent in the 14- to 17-year age group[99] in first attacks. Carditis occurs occasionally after the age of 25 in what are apparently first attacks of ARF. When carditis is mild or evidence for it is borderline, it usually disappears rapidly. Severe carditis prolongs the attack. When severe carditis subsides, low-grade fever and tachycardia often continue, cardiac enlargement usually persists, and new murmurs may appear. Congestive heart failure may occur at any time while carditis is still active.

The mean duration of rheumatic activity is shorter when no suppressive drugs are given.[151] Rheumatic activity appears prolonged when "rebounds" of activity occur after withdrawal of antirheumatic drugs. Suppressive therapy "masks" the inflammation but does not terminate the process and may actually prolong it. The majority of prolonged attacks occur in patients who have had one or more previous attacks, and the incidence of chronic RF increases with the number of recurrences. When antirheumatic therapy is withdrawn and no "rebound" of rheumatic activity is noted for 8 weeks or more, the attack is over and will not be reactivated without a new streptococcal infection.

PROGNOSIS. The data are now conclusive that RF does not recur when streptococcal disease is prevented. The prognosis is at present excellent for the rheumatic subject who escapes carditis during an initial attack of RF. In one 5-year follow-up, rheumatic heart disease did not develop when the acute attack was not accompanied by the appearance of organic heart murmurs.[130] In the United Kingdom–United States Cooperative Study on the treatment of RF,[103,104] similar patients without carditis (defined as the absence of organic murmurs) during the acute attack showed virtually no evidence of late or insidious development of rheumatic heart disease. The percentage of this group of patients with "no carditis" who subsequently had normal hearts was 96 at 5 years and 94 at 10 years. The prognoses become poorer with the increasing severity of initial carditis, so that the percentage of those with congestive heart failure during the acute attack showing complete healing was 30 at 5 years and 40 at 10 years. It is apparent that the healing rate of rheumatic carditis is remarkably high if recurrences are prevented.

Prospective cooperative studies[104] have shown, at 5 years, that the frequency of mitral stenosis was equally distributed between the sexes and was related to the severity of the initial attack of carditis. In fact, a large percentage of the deaths within 5 years were due to such severe mitral valvular deformity. The analysis at 10 years, however, showed the emergence of another group—those whose initial mitral lesion had been relatively mild and who showed slow, progressive obstruction without evidence of recurrent RF or streptococcal disease. This group consisted of predominantly female subjects. It is apparent, therefore, that host factors, as yet undefined, influence the course of valvular sclerosis once mitral deformity has occurred and that progression of rheumatic heart disease may be related to more than the rheumatic inflammation itself. In addition, the tendency of stenotic mitral valves that have been fractured or incised surgically to restenose without evidence of recurrent or active RF is quite apparent in several long-term follow-up studies.[152]

Recurrences of Rheumatic Fever. First attacks of RF in the general population following epidemic streptococcal pharyngitis average 3 per cent, whereas such infections in patients with a history of recent RF may produce a secondary attack rate as high as 65 per cent.[27] Two main explanations for this propensity to recurrences of the rheumatic host are (1) that patients who develop RF differ from the general population in a genetic, congenital, or constitutional manner and that this difference *antedates* the first attack of the disease; and (2) that the first attack *causes* the susceptibility of the patient to further attacks. In the Irvington House study,[153] rheumatic attack rate per infection (R/I) in children decreased from 23 to 11 per cent between the first and fifth year after a rheumatic attack.[28] In adults with rheumatic heart disease, this rate was 4.8 per cent 10 or more years after the last attack.[29] Recurrence rates decline, therefore, with the length of time elapsed since the last attack.

A second factor that clearly increases the chance that a streptococcal infection will be followed by a rheumatic attack is the presence of residual rheumatic heart disease. In the Irvington House studies, the recurrence rate in children with rheumatic heart disease and cardiomegaly was 43 per cent; in patients with rheumatic heart disease and no cardiomegaly, 27 per cent; and in patients without apparent residual heart disease, 10 per cent.[28]

A third factor influencing the R/I is the magnitude of the immune response to the antecedent streptococcal disease as reflected in the increase of ASO titer.

The natural history of RF can now be predicted rather accurately once an initial rheumatic attack abates and a period of convalescence enables an assessment of the degree of healing of carditis. If cardiac healing is complete, prevention of recurrences should guarantee freedom from rheumatic heart disease. Persistence of even a mild degree of mitral regurgitation, although usually quite compatible with normal longevity if rheumatic recurrences and infective endocarditis are avoided, must be observed continuously because of the small but significant percentage of patients in whom mitral stenosis evolves despite careful, continuous antistreptococcal prophylaxis. Such patients, however, constitute but a small percentage of the large numbers of patients with mild rheumatic heart disease whose lesions remain relatively static if rheumatic recurrences are prevented.[154,155] In patients with hemodynamically significant valvular lesions, prognosis should be related principally to the magnitude of the physiological defect. In such patients, of course, recurrent rheumatic carditis is most serious, and these hosts are at greatest risk if streptococcal reinfection is permitted to occur.

Treatment of Rheumatic Fever

GENERAL MANAGEMENT. In any given case of RF, this depends upon the manifestations and severity of the attack. Patients should remain in bed for the duration of the acute and febrile portion of the illness until clinical and laboratory evidence of inflammation abates.

The administration of antiinflammatory or suppressive therapy should ordinarily be delayed until the disease process is clearly expressed in order to establish the diagnosis. Aspirin or corticosteroids administered prematurely to a patient with arthralgia or early monoarticular arthritis and fever may mask the disease process and cause diagnostic confusion. Furthermore, in isolated polyarthritis a trial of penicillin therapy is often essential to eliminate the diagnosis of septic arthritis, especially gonococcemia (see above), and the therapeutic response to the antibiotic must be carefully evaluated.

Once the diagnosis is established, treatment can begin, usually with a *course of penicillin* adequate to eradicate residual group A streptococci that may be difficult to isolate. Massive penicillin treatment has been used by some investigators in an attempt to alter the frequency of cardiac damage but without success.[156] The usual course of penicillin consists of a single injection of 1.2 million units of benzathine penicillin intramuscularly, or 600,000 units of procaine penicillin intramuscularly, daily for 10 days. This is followed by continuous (secondary) prophylaxis (see below). The risk of contracting a new streptococcal infection may be especially high in hospital environments, and therefore prophylaxis should not be delayed until discharge from the hospital. Prophylaxis during hospitalization is a good way to observe patients for side effects from the medication and to educate them regarding its future use.

ANTIRHEUMATIC THERAPY. The selection of an antirheumatic agent is not critical to the outcome of most attacks of RF.[102-104,107,108,157,158] Corticosteroids and salicylates can be regarded as valuable symptomatic and supportive therapy, but they are not curative and may actually prolong the course of the disease. However, both steroids and salicylates control the toxic manifestations of the disease; contribute to the comfort of the patient; and combat anemia, anorexia, and other constitutional symptoms. In severe rheumatic carditis associated with heart failure, such nonspecific antiinflammatory effects may reduce the burden on the heart and occasionally may tilt the balance in favor of the survival of a critically ill patient. Corticosteroids are often more potent than salicylates in suppressing acute exudative inflammation, and some patients in whom salicylates fail to control the disease respond quickly to relatively large doses of corticosteroids. The effect of such doses on the course of chronic rheumatic carditis is disappointing, however, and their use in early cases of acute carditis has not been proved to decrease residual heart disease. Prolonged use of large doses beyond the period of time required to bring acute manifestations under control is not justified.

Patients with mild arthritis or arthralgia and no carditis may be treated with analgesics only, such as codeine, as needed. Two goals will be thus accomplished: First, the diagnosis may be made more certain by the appearance of definite arthritis in some of the initially questionable cases; and second, the duration of hospitalization or of close observation at home will be decreased because many of the patients will get well in 2 or 3 weeks; moreover, one will not have to worry about, and deal with, posttherapeutic rebounds.

Most current general policy is to administer salicylates when no clear evidence of carditis exists. If signs and symptoms are not adequately suppressed by salicylates, corticosteroids should be substituted. Patients with mild carditis are often given corticosteroids, but without the conviction that these are superior to salicylates. Those with severe carditis are usually treated promptly with corticosteroids, particularly if heart failure is evident, and with the precaution of adequate doses of diuretics and restriction of salt intake to combat sodium retention.

Since neither corticosteroids nor salicylates shorten the course of RF, the duration of therapy must be estimated according to the expected course of the attack. Approximately 75 to 80 per cent of most attacks will subside clinically within about 6 weeks. About 90 per cent will subside in about 12 weeks. Despite the form of therapy used, about 5 per cent of attacks will persist with clinically overt rheumatic manifestations for more than 6 months. The duration of treatment, therefore, can be tailored to the severity of the illness. For example, one might treat a mild attack for 4 weeks, tapering off the dosage of the antirheumatic agent during the ensuing 2 weeks.

It is important to reduce the dose of corticosteroids gradually over a period of about 2 weeks and to recognize that abrupt cessation of treatment leaves the patient in a state of temporary adrenal insufficiency resulting from suppression of endogenous adrenocortical activity during prolonged hormone therapy. For this reason the relapse of ARF following abrupt termination of hormone therapy may be more serious than the initial manifestation of the disease before treatment was started. It has been the policy of some to follow the gradual withdrawal of hormone therapy by administration of salicylates for several weeks or months to assure suppression of inflammation until recovery of normal adrenocortical function occurs.

When treatment of ARF is initiated with salicylates, a dose of 6 to 9 gm of acetylsalicylic acid per day is administered to patients weighing 70 kg or more, and proportionately smaller doses are given to patients weighing less. This is administered in divided doses every 4 hours. The initial doses of acetylsalicylic acid should be continued until a satisfactory clinical response is obtained, that is, until there is complete relief of symptoms and signs of arthritis and the temperature has returned to a normal range. Thereafter the dose may be reduced to two-thirds the initial value and may be maintained until all laboratory manifestations of inflammatory disease have returned to normal. For the remainder of the course of therapy, the dose may be reduced to half the initial daily dose. Should clinical or laboratory evidence of relapse occur when doses are reduced, it is advisable to return to the previous higher dose that suppressed the process.

Toxic manifestations are common with the use of larger doses of salicylates, and these may force a reduction in the dose before the response is adequate. If control of the inflammatory state is not sufficient with lower, subtoxic doses, substitution or addition of another agent should be considered.

An initial dose of prednisone of 40 to 60 mg/day in divided doses for adults and children alike may be started and varied according to the patient's response. With other analogs, such as triamcinolone and dexamethasone, the dose is based on their potency relative to prednisone.

Rebounds of Rheumatic Activity. Clinical or laboratory evidence of rheumatic activity may reappear when suppressive antirheumatic therapy is discontinued. Such reactivation has been termed a "rebound" and should clearly be distinguished from a recurrence. Spontaneous rebounds do not occur more than 5 weeks after complete cessation of all antirheumatic therapy; by far the majority occur within 2 seeks, but most occur within a few days or while reducing dosage.

Mild rebounds may be characterized only by fever, arthralgia, or mild arthritis; some patients may have only laboratory evidence of relapse, such as reappearance of C-reactive protein in blood and reelevation of erythrocyte sedimentation rate. Murmurs which had disappeared may again be heard. In patients with carditis, rebounds may be severe and a flare-up of pericarditis or congestive heart failure may occur—sometimes more severely than during the initial period of treatment. Mild rebounds subside spontaneously within a week or two and do not require medication.

Treatment of Chorea. This is nonspecific and consists of tranquilization and sedation. For complete details the reader is referred elsewhere.[1,159–161]

Prevention of Rheumatic Fever

The most effective preventive measures against RF are probably socioeconomic. The almost total absence of the disease in the affluent sections of the cities of the western world suggests that spacious housing and noncrowding are at least as important as good diagnosis and treatment of streptococcal sore throat in the prevention of rheumatic attacks. Nevertheless, the natural history of RF can be dramatically altered in several ways by the use of antimicrobials. Mass penicillin prophylaxis can halt epidemics of streptococcal sore throat. Adequate penicillin treatment of acute streptococcal sore throat will abort an initial attack and, less often, rheumatic recurrences. Continuous administration of sulfadiazine or penicillin will prevent recurrent attacks in rheumatic subjects.

SECONDARY PROPHYLAXIS. The term secondary prophylaxis is used to describe protection against rheumatic recurrences by means of continuous chemoprophylaxis.[162] After a diagnosis of RF is established, residual streptococci which may or may not be detectable on throat cultures should be eradicated by a therapeutic course of penicillin as described below for primary prevention.

The most effective form of continuous prophylaxis is a single monthly intramuscular injection of 1.2 million units of benzathine penicillin G.[163–165] An attack rate of less than 1 recurrence per 250 patient-years was documented in patients using this form of prophylaxis in the extensive studies reported by the Irvington House group.[164] This method does not depend upon the patient's fidelity to an oral regimen nor upon the vagaries of absorption from the gastrointestinal tract. It also imposes closer surveillance upon the patient by the managing physician. Studies on the use of intramuscular benzathine penicillin for mass prophylaxis in military populations have suggested that streptococcal infections rarely occur before 3 weeks after an injection of 1.2 million units of this respository penicillin salt. When they occur after this period in rheumatic subjects, the subsequent injection at 4 weeks probably serves as adequate therapy of the infection. Although the reaction rate is somewhat higher for all injectable forms of penicillin, regardless of kind,[166] than with oral penicillin, reactions are very rare after the first months of prophylaxis. In patients who are at highest risk to sustain rheumatic recurrences, especially those with rheumatic heart disease and recent RF, monthly injections of benzathine penicillin are undoubtedly the preferred form of prophylaxis.

Oral prophylaxis is less reliable than repository penicillin prophylaxis. In the Irvington House studies, a recurrence rate of almost 1 per 25 patient-years (10 times that of intramuscular benzathine penicillin) was observed in patients on oral medication.[164] The recommended dosages for oral sulfadiazine prophylaxis are 0.5 gm once daily for patients weighing less than 27 kg (60 lb) and 1 gm once a day for patients weighing more than 27 kg. For oral penicillin prophylaxis, the recommended dose is 200,000 to 250,000 units daily. Even when oral penicillin is administered twice daily no superiority over sulfadiazine has been demonstrated.[167]

Strains of streptococci resistant to sulfonamide have appeared with mass sulfonamide prophylaxis in military populations but have not been a problem in secondary prophylaxis of rheumatic subjects. Reaction rates are low with both oral medications and are rare after the first months of prophylaxis. For the rare patient who is sensitive to both sulfadiazine and penicillin, oral erythromycin may be substituted in a dose of 250 mg twice daily.[168]

It has been difficult to establish a general recommendation concerning the duration of prophylaxis because of the number of variables that influence the attack rate of recurrences following streptococcal infections (see Natural History, above). Although risks of recurrences decline with age and with increased interval from the last rheumatic attack, a relatively high recurrence rate per infection persists for a very long time—5 to 10 years or more. Exceptions to instituting or maintaining prophylaxis should be made in adults only and then only after assessing the risk of high exposure to streptococcal infection (e.g., working with school-age children, in military service, in medical or allied health positions). Patients with significant degrees of rheumatic heart disease or with a history of repeated recurrences (including chorea) or those having had a recent attack require most careful consideration before discontinuation of prophylaxis, a decision that must be regarded as a calculated risk.

Primary Prophylaxis. The term primary prophylaxis is applied to the prevention of first attacks of RF by treatment of the preceding streptococcal pharyngitis. In military populations with a high frequency of severe streptococcal pharyngitis, penicillin therapy reduced the attack rate of RF from 3.0 to 0.3 per cent.[169] The application of primary prevention to civilian populations, particularly children with sporadic or endemic streptococcal infections, has been more difficult because of the problem of differentiating viral pharyngitis in carriers of group A streptococci from current streptococcal infection and because frequent streptococcal exposure in children tends to keep streptococcal antibody titers elevated (see Epidemiology, above). Throat cultures are helpful, therefore, in eliminating the need for intensive penicillin therapy in patients with nonstreptococcal infection.

Effective therapy demands eradication of the infecting organism, which requires 10 days of consistent treatment if penicillin is administered orally. Many patients fail to extend such treatment beyond the first few days if acute symptoms of streptococcal pharyngitis subside. A single intramuscular injection of benzathine penicillin G (600,000 units in children under 27 kg [60 lb] and 1.2 million units in those over 27 kg) is the treatment of choice.[165] If given orally, penicillin G (200,000 or 250,000 units three to four times daily) is recommended. For those sensitive to penicillin, erythromycin (250 mg four times a day or 40 mg/kg per day in younger children) may be substituted.

Mass Antibiotic Prophylaxis. This type of prophylaxis is effective in populations in which streptococcal pharyngeal infections are epidemic.[170–173] This approach may be indicated occasionally in civilian or institutional epidemics, especially if several cases of RF occur within a few weeks. Mass intramuscular administration of 1.2 million units of benzathine penicillin G to all members of the affected population has been extremely effective.[4]

Immunization with Streptococcal Vaccines. Although no vaccine is currently available for general distribution, considerable progress has been made on the purification and immunology of streptococcal M proteins and holds promise for future streptococcal vaccine development.[24,174,175,176]

SERONEGATIVE SPONDYLOARTHROPATHIES

COMMON CLINICAL FEATURES AND NOSOLOGY. A group of rheumatological syndromes has been classified under the heading of seronegative spondyloarthropathies because they have clinical features in common and some pathological lesions, including those of the heart, that are identical.[177,178] They are distinguished from rheumatoid arthritis by the *absence of the characteristic serological changes* of the latter (e.g., increased rheumatoid factor); by the predilection of the arthritis for the sacroiliac, lumbosacral, and apophyseal joints of the spine; by the marked predominance in men over women; and by the extraarticular manifestations of iritis and of aortic regurgitation due to a characteristic lesion at the root of the aorta. The group of syndromes includes ankylosing spondylitis (AS), Reiter's disease (RD), psoriatic arthritis, the intestinal arthropathies, and Behçet's syndrome. Two of the major syndromes, AS and RD, have been associated with dysentery and urethritis. Although the causative agents are usually not apparent, dysentery due to specific bacteria (*Yersinia enterocolitica, Shigella,* and *Salmonella*) has produced most of the features of these syndromes.[178–180] Urethritis due to *Chlamydia trachomatis* has also been implicated as one of the causes of Reiter's syndrome,[181] but in most cases the etiological agent has not been identified.

HISTOCOMPATIBILITY ANTIGEN B27. The concept of a genetically determined aberrant host response to a variety of infectious agents that can invade the bowel or genitourinary tract has emerged from the demonstration of the striking association of the seronegative spondyloarthropathies with the histocompatibility antigen HLA-B27.[178,179] This membrane antigen occurs with a frequency of approximately 4 to 8 per cent in the normal population, whereas over 90 per cent of patients with either AS or Reiter's disease with spondyloarthropathy are B27-positive. When spondyloarthropathy complicates inflammatory bowel disease, the association with B27 is greater than 80 per cent, and 50 per cent of psoriatic patients with spondylitis are B27-positive. So far, 50 per cent of patients with anterior uveitis have this antigen. When an outbreak of a specific form of dysentery has permitted careful prospective studies, patients with the B27 antigen have had a much greater tendency to develop any form of arthritis than those lacking this antigen. The more specific features of the syndrome such as spondyloarthropathy, iritis, and cardiac involvement have been confined primarily to those who are B27-positive.

Ankylosing Spondylitis

CARDIAC PATHOLOGY. Several excellent prospective studies have documented the form of cardiac and aortic disease peculiar to ankylosing spondylitis (AS), consisting of the following: dilatation of the aortic valve ring; fibrous thickening, scarring, and variable focal inflammatory lesions of the aortic valve cusps, which sag into the ventricular cavity; dilatation of the sinuses of Valsalva; focal degenerative changes of elastic and muscle fibers of the aortic media; and patchy inflammatory lesions in all layers of the aorta, predominantly in the region adjacent to the aortic valve ring.[182–184] The lesions resemble those of syphilis except that in AS they remain close to the valve ring and do not affect the rest of the aorta. In addition, the basal rather than the distal portion of the aortic cusps is thickened in AS and the dense adventitial scarring extends into the endocardium in the immediate subaortic region. This extension may involve the base of the anterior mitral leaflet and the upper portion of the ventricular septum (Fig. 48–9*A*).

Aortic regurgitation results from thickening and shortening of the cusps and from their displacement caudally by the mass of fibrous tissue behind the commissures and by dilatation of the aortic valve root consequent to the destruction of elastic tissue (Fig. 48–9*B*). Mitral regurgitation is infrequent and usually insignificant but can result from dilatation of the left ventricle and from fibrous thickening of the basal portion of the anterior mitral leaflet.[185] The frequent heart block and conduction defects of AS are due to the extension of fibrosis into the muscular septum and destruction of the bundle of His and proximal bundle branches.[184–187]

The lesions of the myocardium are rather nonspecific, consisting of fibrosis, perivascular lymphocytic infiltration, and increased mucinous ground substance. Cardiac enlargement without any apparent cause and hypertrophy and dilatation of the left ventricle are often described, however, and the pathological findings are not commensurate with the clinical manifestations of cardiomyopathy noted in one report[188] nor with the frequency of the cardiac enlargement often described.[182]

Chronic fibrous obliteration of the pericardial cavity has been found at autopsy, but pericarditis is not a prominent clinical feature of the disease. Pericardial rubs and chest pain have been described, however, during more severe, acute, toxic episodes when there is active peripheral polyarthritis and in association with presumably early phases of the disease,[182] especially in association with early Reiter's syndrome or dysentery with polyarthritis.

CLINICAL FEATURES OF CARDIAC LESIONS. In many patients there is evidence of active carditis before aortic regurgitation appears. Precordial pain, pericardial friction rubs, marked tachycardia, cardiac enlargement not explained by hypertension, or other recognizable forms of heart disease and varying P-R intervals greater than 0.24 sec are frequently described, usually when patients have active peripheral arthritis and/or spondylitis with fever and increased erythrocyte sedimentation rates.[182] Remarkably few critical studies have been made of myocardial function in patients with AS before evidence of aortic insufficiency draws attention to cardiac involvement, but it is clear that cardiomyopathy may precede valvular involvement.[188] The usual cardiac features of AS are the gradual evolution of aortic regurgitation and varying degrees of atrioventricular block. The prevalence of the valve lesion is related to the duration of spondylitis and peripheral joint involvement, reaching an incidence in one series of 10 per cent in those with spondylitis for 30 years or more and of 18 per cent if peripheral joint involvement was also present. The prevalence of AV block in each of the above groups was 8.5 and 15.5 per cent, respectively.[182]

When aortic regurgitation is first recognized, the aortic second sound is characteristically accentuated as in syphilitic aortitis, and at this time systolic murmurs are trivial or absent. The aortic lesions tend to progress slowly, and free aortic regurgitation may not occur until as many as 7 years later, at which time the aortic second sound frequently disappears and loud harsh systolic murmurs are transmitted to the neck as the valve cusps become sclerosed. Austin Flint murmurs may also develop. Clinical and postmortem findings indicate that the cardiovascular lesions of some patients with AS may antedate articular disease and may regress spontaneously.[183,187] In one long follow-up of 97 patients with AS, of whom 14 had cardiovascular lesions, aortic regurgitation occurred in 10 patients. Mitral regurgitation and atrioventricular block

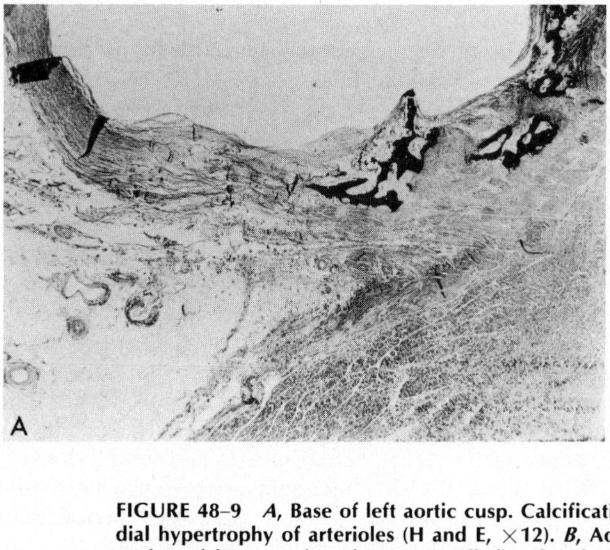

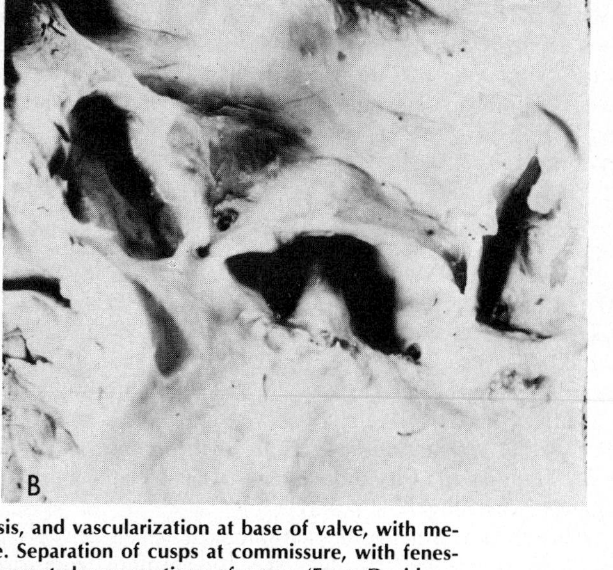

FIGURE 48–9 *A*, Base of left aortic cusp. Calcification, fibrosis, and vascularization at base of valve, with medial hypertrophy of arterioles (H and E, ×12). *B*, Aortic valve. Separation of cusps at commissure, with fenestration of free margins of cusps. Small, firm band of tissue connects lower portions of cusps. (From Davidson, P., et al.: Cardiac and aortic lesions in rheumatoid spondylitis. Mayo Clin. Proc. *38*:427, 1963.)

appeared as isolated findings in 1 and 3 patients, respectively. Nine of the 14 patients had peripheral arthritis, and 3 had iritis.[183] Anterior uveitis and extraspinal disease may also precede the articular lesions of AS by months or years. Hence the discovery of isolated aortic regurgitation in young or middle-aged men requires that AS be considered in the differential diagnosis. In addition, the aortic regurgitation of AS is now well documented to occur in so-called "secondary" forms of the disease such as spondylitis associated with psoriasis, regional enteritis,[183] ulcerative colitis,[189] and Reiter's disease.[190]

Aortic valve replacement (p. 1114) has been performed successfully in several centers, and patients with AS may be suitable candidates when such a procedure is indicated.[191] Cardiac pacemakers have been implanted for atrioventricular block.[183]

Reiter's Disease

Cardiac involvement in the acute stages of Reiter's disease has been described frequently and consists most commonly of acute pericarditis, apical systolic murmurs and gallops, prolongation of the P-R interval, and flattening of T waves. These changes disappear rapidly, and long-term follow-up of large series reveals only an occasional case of cardiac failure or third-degree atrioventricular block.[192] This acute form of Reiter's disease usually features nonspecific urethritis, nonsuppurative migratory polyarthritis, conjunctivitis, circinate balanitis, and keratoderma blenorrhagica. Initial attacks usually subside spontaneously, but second attacks occur in about 15 per cent of cases and chronic manifestations (almost always in B27-positive individuals[193]) may then ensue, with recurrent anterior uveitis, painful mutilating deformities of the feet, sacroiliitis, spondylitis, atrioventricular block, and an aortic valve lesion leading to aortic and occasionally to mitral regurgitation.[194–197]

Postmortem studies of the aortic valves have shown the cusps to be thickened, with rolled edges, and the aorta to incur changes similar if not identical to the lesions described in AS.[197,198]

The development of Reiter's disease in patients with *Yersinia* arthritis has prompted careful studies of the role of the B27 antigen in the frequency of expression of various clinical features of the syndrome.[199–203] In 5 of 49 patients who were B27-positive, carditis developed, two cases with "significant murmurs," one with friction rub, and two with transient cardiac enlargement, as evident on chest roentgenography.[180]

RHEUMATOID ARTHRITIS

PATHOLOGY. The heart is frequently involved in the inflammatory process of rheumatoid arthritis (RA), yet its function is seldom compromised by the lesions produced. The exudative type of rheumatoid inflammation affects the pericardial surfaces, producing a fibrinous pericarditis that is usually low-grade and subclinical. Pericardial inflammation becomes symptomatic and clinically significant in its more florid form, usually as part of a severe vasculitis (Chap. 43).

The most characteristic pathological lesion of RA, the nodular granuloma, involves the myocardium, endocardium, and valves of the heart.[204,205] The extent of this kind of involvement is generally proportionate to the severity of the disease and is almost always associated with diffusely distributed rheumatoid nodules, subcutaneously and elsewhere. These granulomas rarely compromise the function of the myocardium, however, nor do they often affect the function of the heart valves unless they become large and numerous enough to distort them (Fig. 48–10).

Diffuse arteritis, when present, affects small vessels, causing round cell infiltration, edema, fibrosis, and proliferation of the intima. Such involvement of the pericardial vessels may be extensive when it reflects an intense systemic form of RA, and the disease may begin in the pericardium before the joints become involved. Coronary arteritis is often observed at necropsy in severe RA, but it very rarely results in clinically apparent myocardial ischemia.

Although usually asymptomatic, the clinical syndromes of rheumatoid heart disease are well known and have been well described.[206–209] The more one keeps in mind the frequent participation of the connective tissues of the heart in the rheumatoid process, the more frequently will the alert clinician detect evidence of such involvement.

Clinical Features

PERICARDITIS (see also p. 1512). The frequency of rheumatoid pericarditis in necropsy studies ranges from 11 to 50 per cent, with an overall estimate of about 30 per cent.[209] Clinically, the diagnosis of pericarditis is made in about 2 per cent of cases in the adult form and in about 6 per cent in the juvenile form of RA. In careful studies of the more severe forms of the disease which require hospital admission, approximately 10 per cent of patients with RA have clinical evidence of rheumatoid pericarditis during the lifetime course of their disease. Part of the disparity between clinical and autopsy findings is due to the fact that the chest pain may be overshadowed by arthritic pains and may be masked by antirheumatic agents or mistaken for arthritic pain in neighboring joints. In addition, when symptoms of chest pain are lacking, careful and frequent auscultation for pericardial friction rubs is usually omitted. In controlled studies when signs of pericarditis have been actively sought, rubs have been detected in as many as 30 per cent of patients.[209]

The pathophysiology of the acute fibrinous pericarditis of RA is not clear, but in severe cases the pericardial fluid, like synovial fluid, shows decreased hemolytic complement (CH_{50}) and C3 levels. Immunofluorescence staining of the pericardium shows plasma cell infiltration and deposits of IgG, IgM, IgA, or C3 in the pericardial vessels.[210] Moreover, the polymorphonuclear leukocytes in the pericardial fluid may show cytoplasmic inclusions which stain for IgM, indicative of ingested immune complexes such as are also seen in the polymorphonuclear cells of synovial fluid in the same patients.[211] These findings are associated with extremely low levels of glucose, indicative of active phagocytosis, as observed in pleural and synovial rheumatoid fluids. About half the patients with overt rheumatoid pericarditis also have rheumatoid pleural and lung lesions.

With the availability of noninvasive cardiac procedures such as echocardiography, the diagnosis of pericardial involvement is being made earlier and more often.[212,213] In a

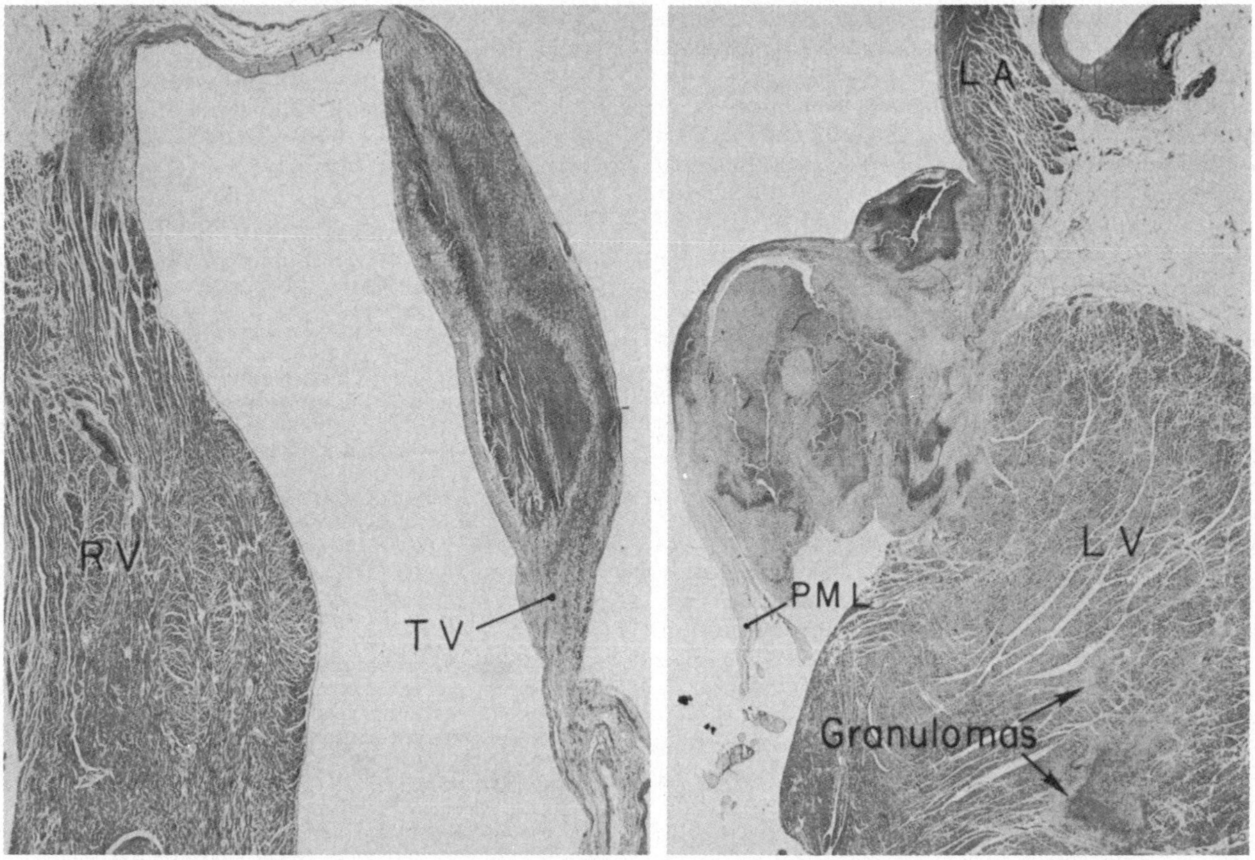

FIGURE 48–10 *Left,* Tricuspid value (TV) leaflet. Typical rheumatoid granuloma is located within substance of leaflet. RV indicates right ventricle (H and E, ×12). *Right,* Mitral valve. Section includes posterior mitral leaflet (PML) and adjacent portions of left atrial (LA) and left ventricular (LV) walls. Large rheumatoid granuloma is located within proximal three-fourths of posterior leaflet. Smaller nodule involves endocardium of left atrium as well. Two rheumatoid granulomas are located within the left ventricular wall (H and E, ×6.5). (From Roberts, W. C., et al.: Cardiac valvular lesions in rheumatoid arthritis. Arch. Intern. Med. *122*:141, 1968. Copyright 1968, American Medical Association.)

recent series of patients with RA studied by echocardiography, pericardial effusion was demonstrated in 30 per cent of all patients studied and in 50 per cent of those with subcutaneous nodules.[212] This incidence is as high as the reported frequency of postmortem findings of rheumatoid pericarditis.

Pericarditis may appear without relation to the duration of RA and sometimes may even be the harbinger of the onset of a severe form of the disease. It occurs most often in middle-aged men in whom arthritis was of acute onset. Most often, the clinical course is benign, and symptoms and signs will respond to moderate amounts of prednisone. Occasionally, however, the disease may be more protracted and severe, leading to cardiac tamponade and constrictive pericarditis.

In its florid form the disease has the usual symptoms and signs of pericarditis, and when persistent, it imitates closely tuberculous pericarditis, from which it must be carefully differentiated. Although some fatal cases have been described in which a true pancarditis was present,[214] such cases are exceptional, and even severe rheumatoid pericarditis usually spares myocardial and endocardial function.

Pericardial fluid is of considerable diagnostic value in cases in which the etiology of the pericarditis may be in doubt. The features of the pericardial fluid in RF have been noted above. In some cases, a high level of cholesterol has been found.[215] Such instances of so-called "cholesterol pericarditis" are probably due to poor absorption of lipid from pericardial effusions by the thickened pericardium in RA and in other forms of chronic pericarditis, which leads to the concentration and precipitation of cholesterol.

Treatment of rheumatoid pericarditis is the same as that for the arthritic disease. Although corticosteroids tend to be used more liberally in pericarditis to suppress inflammation, there is no evidence that such suppression will prevent adhesive or constrictive pericarditis. When tamponade occurs, surgical intervention is necessary, and pericardiectomy may be required. Needle pericardiocentesis is usually inadequate or difficult because of the thick, loculated nature of the effusion, and usually more vigorous procedures aimed at pericardial drainage by indwelling catheter or partial pericardiectomy are necessary.

RHEUMATOID MYOCARDITIS. Except for rare cases of myocarditis with diffuse granulomas or amyloid infiltration of the myocardium associated with very severe RA, myocarditis is mostly nonspecific and subclinical in the great majority of patients. The histological lesions may be focal or generalized infiltrations of lymphocytes, plasma cells, palisading histiocytes, and fibroblasts.[205] The incidence of myocarditis in autopsies of rheumatoid arthritis patients is reported as 19 per cent. Most of such cases are associated with severe arthritis, vasculitis, and endocarditis or pericarditis.

Whether drug toxicity, superimposed viral infection, or corticosteroid therapy may have caused some reported cases of severe myocarditis rather than primary rheumatoid disease cannot be determined with certainty. Although left ventricular function may be compromised by a variety of pathological processes in severe rheumatoid arthritis, the typical case is remarkable for its characteristic sparing of the myocardial musculature despite extensive involvement of the fibrous structures of the heart. Nevertheless, when there are unusually severe systemic manifestations of rheumatoid arthritis, rheumatoid pancarditis with congestive heart failure has been well described and confirmed by necropsy. Such patients exhibit the whole spectrum of rheumatoid inflammation of the heart.[214]

CORONARY ARTERY DISEASE. The incidence of coronary artery disease is higher in rheumatoid arthritis patients than in matched controls.[206,208] Clinicopathological correlation suggests that the nature of the coronary artery disease analyzed in some studies is probably rheumatoid rather than arteriosclerotic. Coronary arteritis is observed in about 20 per cent of rheumatoid arthritis patients at autopsy. This arteritis is probably a manifestation of generalized vasculitis often seen in RA. Inflammation with edema of the intima of the artery may lead to severe narrowing or occlusion of its lumen, to necrosis, and to angina or infarction. Nevertheless, myocardial necrosis secondary to this form of arteritis is rare.

VALVULAR AND ENDOCARDIAL LESIONS. As in myocarditis, the histological picture of the valves and adjacent endocardial areas of patients with RA shows nonspecific inflammation with fibrotic and sclerotic changes and infiltrations of histiocytes, plasma cells, lymphocytes, and occasional eosinophils.[204,205] The most characteristic lesions, however, are granulomas resembling rheumatoid nodules. Usually these do not interfere with valvular function unless they reach large enough proportions to produce frank valvular regurgitation by destroying the base of the valve and its cusps. Such regurgitation may be of sufficient magnitude and rapidity of onset to cause severe cardiac decompensation and death[216] (Chap. 32).

All valves may be involved, but the descending order of frequency is mitral, aortic, tricuspid, and pulmonary. Chronic endocarditis and valvular fibrosis was observed in 6 per cent of one series of hospitalized cases of severe RA.[208] Echocardiographic studies have shown a significant slowing of mitral valve movement in RA patients correlating with the duration of the disease and the extent of the formation of subcutaneous nodules.[213] It is not clear whether left ventricular disease can be excluded as a cause contributing to this finding or whether it is due entirely to intrinsic involvement of the mitral valve alone. At least in a few well-described cases, however, mitral and aortic valvular deformity with marked regurgitation due to rheumatoid nodules was the characteristic pathological picture.[214]

ELECTROCARDIOGRAPHIC ABNORMALITIES. Studies of the electrocardiogram in patients with RA and in matched controls show that first-degree atrioventricular block is the most significant finding in RA.[206] Complete heart block causing Adams-Stokes syndrome has been described, and other abnormalities include left bundle branch block, atrial fibrillation, and atrial and ventricular ectopic beats. Abnormal T waves, however, do not occur more frequently than in controls and are of little value in the diagnosis of rheumatoid heart disease despite the frequency of rheumatoid pericarditis.[209]

The Vasculitis Syndromes

Etiology. Most of the clinical manifestations of periarteritis nodosa, systemic lupus erythematosus (SLE), and several other forms of diffuse vasculitis may be produced by infections such as hepatitis B, in which massive and persistent antigenemia gives rise to circulating immune complexes, the qualitative and quantitative features of which determine the localization and character of the vascular lesions. It has also become clear that bacterial endocarditis, like hepatitis B, produces many of the varied glomerular lesions of SLE, produces large and small lesions of polyarteritis, and produces serological findings similar to those of SLE.[217-220]

In addition to infectious agents as a cause of immune complex disease, the prolonged administration of certain drugs can produce most, if not all, of the features of SLE (drug-induced lupus). Procainamide is the most notorious offender, but hydralazine, phenytoin (Dilantin), and several other anticonvulsants, isoniazide, sulfonamides, and several other drugs administered for prolonged periods may produce features of SLE.[221,222] Whereas true SLE nephritis is rare in drug-induced lupus, cases are now reported in which the entire syndrome has evolved when the drug has been given long enough and in sufficient doses. In one fatal case, a patient was reported to have ingested enormous amounts of procainamide during 9 years of continuous therapy; the full-blown syndrome was proved at autopsy, including lupus nephritis and Libman-Sacks endocarditis, and the serological features were characteristic.[223]

As in the case of the seronegative spondyloarthropathies (see above), only a small portion of the syndromes recognized can be shown to be due to specific infectious agents or drugs. Most cases of large-vessel polyarteritis, or the small-vessel and capillary diffuse vasculitis of SLE, must be considered idiopathic, but a careful search for known infectious agents capable of producing persistent antigenemia and for a history of drug therapy should be undertaken before one resorts to an idiopathic, descriptive diagnosis.

Systemic Lupus Erythematosus

Pathological Features. The hallmark of this disease is the presence of a number of antibodies to nuclear components, the antinuclear antibodies (ANA), which participate in the pathogenesis of SLE by forming antigen-antibody-complement complexes that are found in many of the lesions. These complexes tend to be trapped by vascular and glomerular basement membranes and to produce, through complement activation, lesions affecting small vessels and capillaries. In experimental immune complex disease in animals and in serum sickness in humans, inflammation of joints, skin, pleura, pericardium, brain, kidneys, and other systems occurs because of the persistent excess antigenemia and subsequent circulating immune complexes. These and probably other hyperimmune phenomena explain many of the protean clinical manifestations of SLE. Although anti-heart antibodies have been described in the sera of patients with SLE, they bear no clear relationship to the frequency and severity of cardiac lesions and may be a result rather than a cause of cardiac inflammation, presumably owing to release of myocardial antigens into the circulation.[224]

CARDIAC ABNORMALITIES. Because the basic anatomical lesion of SLE is a diffuse microvasculitis,[225,225a] the heart is almost always found to be involved at autopsy.[226] The clinical manifestations, however, are usually overshadowed by the symptoms and signs related to involvement of other organs, and attention is drawn to the heart only when the lesions of pericarditis, myocarditis, or endocarditis are florid. Clinical evidence of cardiac abnormalities has been observed, however, in as many as 50 to 60 per cent of cases in two large series.[227,228] As methodology becomes more sophisticated, detection of cardiac involvement begins to approach that found at necropsy (see below).

Pericarditis. This is found in approximately two-thirds to three-fourths of autopsies and is perhaps the commonest cardiac lesion of SLE (p. 1511).[226–231] The acute pericardial inflammation may extend into the sinoatrial and atrioventricular nodes, with destruction of conducting fibers.[232–235] Pericardial fluid may be clear or sanguineous and has a high protein content. Effusions may be voluminous and occasionally cause tamponade. Histologically, the pericardium shows fibrinoid degeneration, edema, and necrosis of connective tissue when the process is acute, and various stages of fibrosis with the formation of adhesions are found during the healing or chronic phase. Constrictive pericarditis occurs only rarely; however, pericardial tamponade and constrictive pericarditis both have been reported in cases of procainamide-induced lupus erythematosus.[236,237] Pericarditis, like arthritis, tends to be episodic and to heal well in remissions rather than to become chronic and sclerosing.[238]

Myocarditis. Subclinical myocarditis is common. Its severity is proportionate to the severity of the systemic disease process. The lesions observed at autopsy consist of fibrinoid necrosis involving interstitial tissues and blood vessels, and only rarely are the cardiac myofibrils destroyed. Small vessel changes include an arteriopathy of vessels 0.1 to 1.0 mm in diameter. The abnormal vessels are located in the conduction system of patients selected for study because of the presence of arrhythmias. Segmental arteritis and periarteritis with some occlusions of the arterial lumen and small areas of fibrosis distal to the obstruction are found. Involvement of the atrioventricular as well as the sinoatrial node in the inflammatory process of SLE has been shown at autopsy in a death due to arrhythmia in a 24-year-old man.[233] Rare cases of myocardial infarction, presumably due to arteritis of larger coronary vessels, have been reported.[239,240] Atherosclerotic coronary disease is being reported somewhat more frequently than might be expected in patients with SLE treated with corticosteroids, possibly related to worsening of hypertension in such patients.[241] Cardiac enlargement is frequent.[242]

Endocarditis. This is the most characteristic cardiac lesion of SLE.[225,226] The Libman-Sacks[243] verrucous valvular lesions are wartlike, varying from pinhead size to 3 to 4 mm. The lesions may be discrete or in clumps and are composed of degenerating valve tissue apparently extruded beyond the endothelium and accompanied by some fibrosis of the underlying leaflet. The lesions usually contain granular, basophilic masses of cellular debris, the characteristic so-called "hematoxylin bodies" composed of basophilic fragments in the cytoplasm of cells. They may be found anywhere on the endocardial surface of the heart but are most common in the angles of the atrioventricular valves and on the underside of the base of the mitral valve. They may also extend onto the chordae tendineae or papillary muscles. Generalized involvement of the entire thickness of the heart valves with inflammatory and fibrous changes may also occur. Aortic valve involvement is rare but has been well described.[244] Despite the frequency and extent of the endocardial lesions of SLE, they do not often profoundly affect the function of the valves and, unlike rheumatic fever, do not produce serious regurgitation during the acute phase of the disease. Only rarely do they lead to marked scarring and deformity during healing, requiring valve replacement.[245]

CLINICAL FEATURES. Although autopsy shows that at least two-thirds of patients have pericarditis at some time during the course of SLE, only one-third have recognizable symptoms and signs during life.[227–231] Typical pericardial pain may occur, but often the friction rubs, characteristic electrocardiographic changes, or enlargement of the cardiac silhouette on chest x-ray due to pericardial effusion may be found in the absence of symptoms, and therefore evidence of pericarditis should always be suspected and sought in *all* patients with SLE, even in those without clinical manifestations. Cardiac tamponade is rare but can occur, requiring repeated aspirations of fluid.[231] Systolic and diastolic murmurs at the mitral area, and less often at the aortic area, seem to come and go during the course of acute exacerbations of the disease and are presumably due to Libman-Sacks endocarditis. However, at autopsy the presence of these lesions is not always confirmed, and other factors such as anemia, tachycardia, fever, myocarditis, transient papillary muscle dysfunction, and the adventitious sounds of pleuropericarditis must be considered. Hemodynamically significant and permanent valvular regurgitation from lupus carditis is rare, but such cases have been reported and have even required valve replacement.[245]

Congestive heart failure due to SLE is also uncommon except when associated with hypertension secondary to renal disease. Heart failure may be mistakenly diagnosed in the presence of edema due to renal disease or pericardial effusion or both. Clinically apparent myocarditis, like that of rheumatic fever, producing tachycardia, gallop rhythm, and cardiac dilatation, is a feature of very toxic cases of SLE when high fever and other multisystem manifestations of acute vasculitis are present. Arrhythmias are also relatively uncommon and consist of atrial flutter and fibrillation with varying degrees of atrioventricular block.[232] Attention has been called to the development of congenital complete heart block, a "lupus-like syndrome," and pericarditis in infants born to mothers with active SLE.[246,247] The observation suggests that transplacental transfer of abnormal antibodies (or small immune complexes) may be of pathogenetic importance in these cases. During examination of a pregnant woman with SLE, fetal bradycardia should be recognized as a possible complication of lupus rather than fetal distress from other causes.

Echocardiography may be useful in SLE for demonstrating pericardial involvement and for evaluating valve function in the presence of various murmurs.[238,245,248] Extensive hemodynamic studies carried out on a group of five patients who had had SLE for 2½ to 7 years prior to heart catheterization and who had no obvious clinical findings of cardiac involvement showed considerable evidence of impairment of myocardial function.[249]

TREATMENT. To the extent that their antiinflammatory effect can control active myocarditis, corticosteroids may be necessary to manage severe cardiac involvement in SLE. Control of hypertension is also very helpful in the treatment and prevention of congestive heart failure. There is no evidence that corticosteroid treatment can prevent the rare cases of constrictive pericarditis or valvular deformity.[241] Although the inflammatory reaction may be dramatically suppressed, the basic disease process and tissue injury are not altered by corticosteroid therapy, which is at most supportive and sometimes causes problems (hypertension and fluid retention). Immunosuppressive therapy is usually reserved for the most severe, corticosteroid-resistant forms of the disease and especially for renal involvement. Death from the cardiac disease of SLE compared with other causes of fatality in this disease is rare, so that cardiac manifestations usually do not determine the choice of antiinflammatory therapy.

PERIARTERITIS NODOSA

As noted above, necrotizing inflammation of blood vessels is a common finding in immune complex diseases of known and unknown etiologies; however, because the origin and nature of the offending agent is unknown in most instances, the vasculitides continue to be classified on the basis of their histological and clinical features. These depend largely upon the size of the involved blood vessels, their anatomical sites, the stage of the inflammation, and the characteristics of the lesions.

The clinical features of most cases fit into one of the following five major categories: periarteritis nodosa, allergic granulomatosis, Wegener's granulomatosis, hypersensitivity vasculitis, and giant cell arteritis.[250]

Pathological Features. The muscular arteries, adjacent veins, and occasionally arterioles and venules (but not the capillaries) are involved in a necrotizing inflammation. Segments of vessels, at times only part of the circumference being affected, are involved in the lesions, especially at the bifurcation of arteries. Small aneurysms may form and rupture. In the acute stage of inflammation the lesions contain predominantly polymorphonuclear leukocytes, whereas in chronic lesions mononuclear cell infiltration and partial healing are apparent. However, both phases may be present at once, suggesting repeated or continuous insults.

The lesions are commonly found in the coronary arteries as well as kidneys, muscles, and vasa nervorum, but the lungs are usually spared. *Myocardial infarction* is therefore relatively common, and this leads to patchy myocardial fibrosis and left ventricular enlargement. The latter is also secondary to hypertension, frequently present owing to renal involvement. Hemorrhage into the pericardial sac with tamponade and death, inflammatory pericarditis, or uremic pericarditis are causes of pericardial involvement. Endocardial or valvular lesions do not occur unless the papillary muscle is injured by ischemia.

CLINICAL FEATURES. Periarteritis nodosa may occur at any age, produces fever and multisystem involvement, and may persist for months or years. Pericarditis may be clinically evident, frequently associated with pleuritis, but is not a prominent feature of the disease. Chest pain due to true angina pectoris is also relatively rare[251,252] despite the occurrence of myocardial infarction. In one series of 41 cases of periarteritis nodosa and myocardial infarction, only 3 were diagnosed clinically.[251] The most common form of heart involvement is congestive failure and hypertension due to renal disease, which causes most deaths.[251,252] Cardiac arrhythmias, most often atrial flutter and fibrillation, can occur. Death from ruptured aneurysms, particularly gastrointestinal bleeding, is not uncommon.

Kawasaki Disease (see also p. 1053). In recent years, Kawasaki and others have delineated a periarteritis-like vasculitis in Japanese infants. It is a complication of an acute febrile disease that they have called "mucocutaneous lymph node syndrome";[253,254] more recently this has become known as Kawasaki disease.[255] A polyarteritic syndrome occurs in approximately 2 per cent of infants following an acute mucocutaneous exanthematous febrile illness. Severe arteritis of the larger coronary arteries and of arteries of other organs results in rapid or sudden death from cardiac arrhythmias or massive myocardial infarction. Aneurysms of the coronary, brachial, iliac, and other vessels can be observed in the acute stage of the disease but may cause late-stage arterial aneurysms in children. The disease has been reported from Hawaii, continental United States, Canada, Greece, and Korea. Previously reported cases of "infantile periarteritis nodosa with coronary artery involvement" from the United States may be identical with Kawasaki disease.[255]

Laboratory Findings. Most helpful diagnostically is angiography when it reveals the characteristic multiple small aneurysms at branch points of mesenteric, renal, and other arteries (Fig. 48–11). The diagnosis may be quite difficult to establish in the absence of this finding, and biopsies of clinically involved tissues are usually necessary to establish the diagnosis. "Blind" muscle biopsy is positive in fewer than one-third of cases later confirmed. Hepatitis B soluble antigen is found in the blood of increasing numbers of patients with periarteritis nodosa in recently reported series, and this antigen has been identified in vascular lesions along with immunoglobulin and complement.[256,257] Other infectious diseases associated with prolonged antigenemia have been also identified as causes of polyarteritis, such as cytomegalovirus infections and trichinosis.[258,259]

COURSE AND TREATMENT. The prognosis of periarteritis nodosa is grave; one-half to two-thirds of patients die within a year when series comprised hospitalized cases. Treatment with corticosteroids is frequently followed by temporary improvement on doses of 40 to 60 mg of prednisone or prednisolone per day. Five-year survival of untreated patients is estimated at 13 per cent. Studies with immunosuppressive drugs have been encouraging in appar-

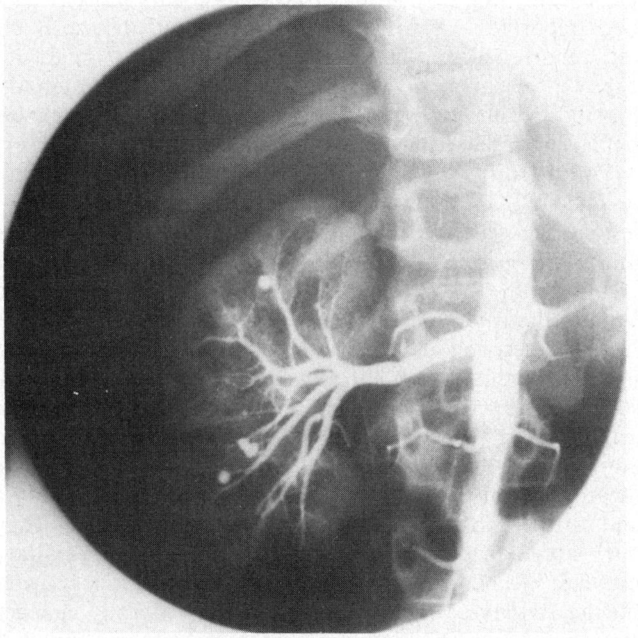

FIGURE 48–11 Renal artery angiogram in a 13-year-old boy with periarteritis nodosa. (From Stollerman, G. H.: Rheumatic Fever and Streptococcal Infection. New York, by permission of Grune and Stratton, 1975.)

ently prolonging the course in some cases, but adequate controlled studies have not been made.[260]

OTHER FORMS OF DIFFUSE VASCULITIS

Allergic Granulomatosis. This disease involves the vessels of the heart in the same way as periarteritis nodosa but eosinophils tend to be more abundant in the lesions, and granulomatous collections of epithelioid and giant cells are formed, accounting for the name of the condition.[260] Pulmonary involvement dominates the clinical picture, and patients tend to have a history of respiratory infection, asthma, and fever, often with a striking peripheral eosinophilia.

Wegener's Granulomatosis. This syndrome is distinguished by necrotizing granulomas of the upper respiratory tract, especially the destructive lesions of the nasopharynx and paranasal sinuses, middle ear, and bronchial tree. Necrotizing inflammation extends into the smaller pulmonary vessels of the lungs and other organs, particularly the kidneys. Pericardial and myocardial involvement is not uncommon, but the clinical picture is dominated by respiratory and renal involvement, without which the diagnosis cannot be made. The special feature of treatment is the encouraging response of this particular syndrome to cyclophosphamide therapy, resulting in dramatic remissions, often complete, and in prolonged survival.[260-262]

Hypersensitivity Vasculitis.[263] Hypersensitivity vasculitis is also called small-vessel vasculitis or angiitis and is characterized by involvement of arterioles, venules, and capillaries only. The presence of antigen-antibody complexes in the lesions all tend to be of the same age. It is difficult to tell at the inception of the disease whether it is part of a larger syndrome, such as SLE, subacute infective endocarditis, mixed cryoglobulinemia, Henoch-Schönlein purpura, or a drug reaction except by the course and distinguishing features of the other syndromes. Hypersensitivity vasculitis is the most common form of immune complex disease. Muscular and large arteries are spared, so that the tissue lesions are due to microinfarcts and hemorrhagic and exudative reactions at the capillary level rather than to thrombosis of large vessels with resulting ischemia and necrosis. The most common cardiac finding is pericarditis, but such involvement occurs along with that of many other organs, skin, mucous membranes, joints, and so on.

Giant Cell Arteritis.[260,264,265] Giant cell arteritis, also called cranial or temporal arteritis, affects predominantly older individuals. Large or medium-sized arteries, including the superficial temporal artery, are involved without small-vessel or capillary lesions. The lesions are usually cellular and granulomatous and contain multinucleated giant cells. Involvement of the arteries is spotty and segmented and tends to produce thrombosis at the site of involvement. The aorta is often involved, and aneurysms and dissection can result (p. 1560). External and internal carotids and vertebral arteries can be affected, and thrombosis of the ophthalmic or central retinal artery leads to blindness. Thrombosis of the coronary, iliac, femoral, or mesenteric arteries produces ischemia and infarctions.

Often the polymyalgia rheumatica syndrome is an associated finding. It is characterized by pain and stiffness in the neck and shoulders, upper arms, hips, and thighs. Joint and muscle pain and tenderness may be severe. Headache is characteristically associated with tender and thickened temporal arteries. The erythrocyte sedimentation rate is strikingly elevated owing primarily to a marked increase in the serum alpha-2 globulins. Myocarditis due to giant cell arteritis has been reported only rarely despite the frequently described association of this form of vasculitis with polymyalgia rheumatica.[264] Myocarditis may be present, however, even though clinically unsuspected, as was shown recently in an autopsy on a patient with giant cell arteritis involving primarily the aorta and lower extremities who died of a cerebral hemorrhage.[264] The lesions were difficult to distinguish from viral myocarditis, and, indeed, it is noteworthy that the polymyalgia rheumatica syndrome has been described in association with hepatitis B virus infection.[266] The dramatic response of all symptoms to relatively small doses of corticosteroids (15 to 20 mg per day of prednisone) is a good therapeutic test for the syndrome, and treatment with corticosteroids usually completely suppresses the symptoms and signs within a few days. After a few weeks the dose may be tapered to a maintenance dose of approximately 10 mg per day which will usually suffice to control the disease, and eventually treatment may be discontinued altogether in most patients.

PROGRESSIVE SYSTEMIC SCLEROSIS (DIFFUSE SCLERODERMA)

Progressive systemic sclerosis (PSS) is an insidious, chronic, fibrosing condition that presents as progressive tightening and thickening of the skin (scleroderma), developing over a period of many years. Raynaud's phenomena occur at some time in almost all patients. Visceral involvement may occur at any time during the course of the disease, affecting the gastrointestinal tract, lungs, heart or kidney. Much attention has been given to the classification of various subgroups of this syndrome that include patients with diffuse scleroderma, those without diffuse skin changes but with other shared features, such as calcinosis, Raynaud's phenomena, esophageal dyskinesia, sclerodactyly, and telangiectasia (the CREST syndrome), and those with features overlapping polymyositis or systemic lupus erythematosus or both. The implications of these classifications are dealt with elsewhere.[267-269]

Pathological Features and Pathogenesis. In contrast to the acute exudative forms of vasculitis associated with the necrotizing lesions described above, PSS seems to be a disease at the opposite end of the inflammatory scale, where very slow scarring and fibrosis results from gradual obliteration of small vessels. It is difficult to classify PSS pathophysiologically because the cause of the extensive fibrosis is not known. Hereditary factors have not been identified. Qualitative abnormalities of collagen are not documented. The disease apparently results from injury at the level of very small arteries, 150 to 500 μm in diameter, and capillaries are gradually obliterated.[270,271] Early in the course of the lesions, mononuclear cell infiltrates occur around small arteries and in the interstitium. The basement membrane of the capillaries appears thickened. Fibroblastic proliferation and overproduction of collagen result from the low-grade inflammatory process. Narrowing and obliteration of small arteries result in decreased vascularization of the skin, skeletal muscles, lung, and heart, followed by fibrosis. The interlobular arteries of the kidney are involved by intensive intimal proliferation, which causes the most serious complication of the disease, namely, rapid renal failure often with severe hypertension.

Biopsies of apparently unaffected muscles show basement membrane changes in capillaries with marked reduction in their numbers per unit area of muscle, suggesting that an early stage of involvement is at the level of the endothelial cell–fibroblast membrane.[271] Autopsy studies have shown pericarditis or pericardial effusions in about one-half of patients; the most common pathological lesions are fibrous adhesions resulting in obliteration of the pericardial sac.

CARDIAC LESIONS. The importance of primary cardiac involvement in the natural history of the disease has been repeatedly emphasized.[269,272,273] Heart involvement is a frequent cause of death and second only to involvement of the kidneys as a factor shortening the survival of patients with this disease.[274] Confusion concerning the question of primary involvement of the heart by the sclerosing process has been caused by the frequency of cor pulmonale resulting from pulmonary involvement of PSS and severe hypertension and hypertensive heart disease resulting from the renal involvement. Cardiac involvement without kidney involvement occurs in approximately 12 per cent of patients and shortens survival.

"Scleroderma heart" is primarily a myocardial disease, and the heart's small vessels are all vulnerable to the sclerosing process. Atherosclerosis of the major coronary arteries occurs to the same degree in patients with PSS as in age and sex-matched controls. PSS patients, however, have much more intimal sclerosis of the small coronary arteries than do controls,[275,276] and such involvement may lead to ischemia, small infarctions, and fibrosis. The combination of vascular insufficiency and fibrosis produces a cardiomyopathy with congestive heart failure and conduction system abnormalities.[277,278] Acute and chronic pericarditis, even in the absence of uremia, is common but usually asymptomatic. At times the resulting effusion can be large enough to cause tamponade,[279] although this degree of effusion is rare. Pericardial fluid, when obtainable, has the features of an exudate but lacks evidence of autoantibodies, immune complexes, or complement depletion, such as that seen in rheumatoid arthritis or SLE.[280] Endocardial involvement is rare, and the deformities of mitral and aortic valves that have been reported probably have little hemodynamic significance.

CLINICAL FEATURES. The primary clinical manifestations of scleroderma heart disease are those of pericarditis and congestive heart failure. In one series, pericarditis patients had a 7-year cumulative survival rate of 33 per cent, whereas none of the PSS patients with heart failure survived for 7 years.[281] Men have significantly worse survival rates than women, as do blacks and older patients. Although cardiac symptoms may appear months or even years before the skin is involved, as a rule overt heart disease is not a prominent part of the clinical picture of PSS until late in its course, when myocardial involvement and resultant heart failure indicate a grim prognosis. Pericarditis, however, may be intermittently symptomatic for long periods of time.

When dyspnea with exertion or at rest occurs in the patient with PSS, primary myocardial failure must be distinguished from myocardial failure secondary to hypertension from renal disease and pulmonary insufficiency from pulmonary fibrosis due to PSS. Cardiac murmurs are not usually due to valvular deformity but to cardiac dilatation and to anemia or to papillary weakness. Chest pain simulating ischemic heart disease as well as typical pericardial pain may occur. Right ventricular failure is a feature of pulmonary hypertension with or without myocardial involvement. Angina pectoris has been described in a patient who showed normal large coronary arteries on angiographic studies, and in another patient with anginal pain and scleroderma, the large coronary arteries were patent, but a slow flow velocity of the dye was observed in the vessels.[282] Such hemodynamic findings associated with biventricular dysfunction and with left ventricular hypokinesia are consistent with the small vessel involvement of PSS.

The *roentgenogram of the chest* may reveal cardiac enlargement from pericardial effusion, cardiomyopathy, or hypertension. The electrocardiographic findings are also nonspecific and may, indeed, be normal when the heart is seriously involved. All degrees of atrioventricular conduction blocks, right and left ventricular hypertrophy, and all varieties of arrhythmias have been described,[283,284] but conduction defects are found most often in patients with the primary cardiomyopathy of PSS.[278]

Echocardiographic studies revealed patterns consistent with a congestive cardiomyopathy or a restrictive cardiomyopathy (p. 128).[285] Echocardiographic abnormalities were reported in 37 (69 per cent) of a series of 54 patients with PSS, and in 22 of these, pericardial effusion was noted, although it was suspected clinically in only 7.[286]

TREATMENT. Many drugs have been used for the treatment of PSS but without significant or prolonged effect. The value of corticosteroids is limited to improvement of the early edematous phase of the disease, but this effect on the heart has not been systematically evaluated and probably will not influence the eventual course of the disease. Captopril has been observed to control the severe accelerated hypertension associated with the renovascular disease of scleroderma and to relieve the digital vasospasm of Raynaud's phenomena.[287]

POLYMYOSITIS AND DERMATOMYOSITIS

(See also p. 1715)

Polymyositis is a diffuse inflammatory disease of unknown cause affecting primarily proximal striated muscles and various connective tissues of the body, especially skin and joints.[288–292] When the disease involves the skin, it is called *dermatomyositis.* Polymyositis may be due to a pathological process common to several etiologies because it is seen in association with a variety of syndromes. It is grouped with the connective tissue or rheumatic diseases because of its overlapping clinical and laboratory features, especially when it is associated with rheumatoid arthritis and progressive systemic sclerosis but also with systemic lupus erythematosus or polyarteritis. Involvement of the heart in polymyositis has just begun to be fully appreciated in the past decade and was mentioned in earlier publications only as a rare finding, if at all.

Pathological Features. Polymyositis is either increasing in incidence or is being more frequently diagnosed, and it is now recognized as one of the most common myopathies.[293] The principal changes in muscle tissue consist of widespread destruction of muscle fibers with phagocytosis of destroyed cells. There may be focal infiltrates of inflammatory cells, such as lymphocytes, mononuclear leukocytes, plasma cells, and, only rarely, neutrophilic leukocytes. Regeneration of destroyed muscle in the form of proliferating sarcolemmal nuclei, basophilic sarcoplasm, and new myofibrils is a prominent feature. Residual muscle fibers may be small. In any given biopsy specimen, either degeneration of muscle fibers or infiltrations of inflammatory cells may predominate. In electron microscopic studies, the most significant changes, in addition to those in muscle fibers, are found in the endothelium and basement membrane of capillaries and small arterioles, much like those described in scleroderma and SLE. Inclusions in the cytoplasm of endothelial cells that are identical to those found in SLE and scleroderma have been described.[294]

PATHOLOGY OF THE HEART.[295–304] The cardiac lesions involve the conducting system predominantly but also can produce an extensive cardiomyopathy and pericarditis. The latter may appear far more often than would be suspected on clinical grounds. The cardiac valves and coronary arteries are spared except in overlap syndromes. The sinoatrial node shows conspicuous fibrosis, swelling and degeneration of collagen, and focal or complete replacement. The fibrosis extends into the adjacent myocardium of the right atrium. The atrioventricular node, bundle of His, and both bundle branches all may be involved in the degenerative and fibrotic process (Fig. 48–12). Cardiac muscle fibers in the atria and ventricles are replaced in scattered areas by fibrosis, and, in some cases, the pattern of focal myocardial necrosis and inflammation is the same as that seen in skeletal muscle.[296] Pericarditis is described more often clinically than pathologically.

CLINICAL FEATURES. Almost all authors comment on the rarity of cardiovascular manifestations in polymyositis, and, indeed, the best reported studies of survivorship do not relate death to cardiac causes but

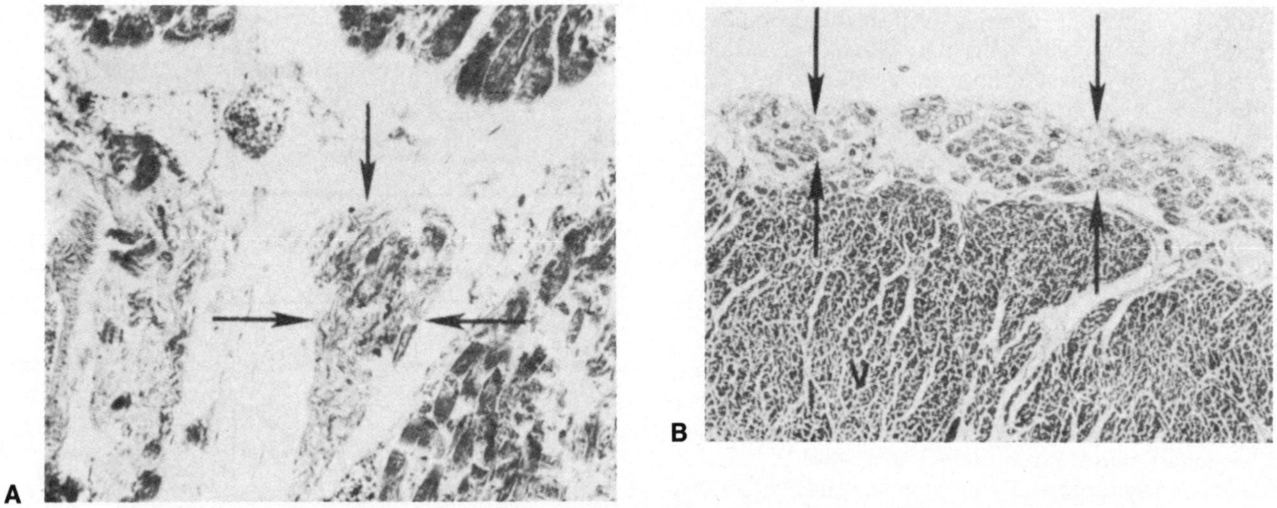

FIGURE 48–12 *A*, First part of right bundle branch (arrows). Note presence of only a few remaining cells in right bundle branch (Gomori's trichrome stain, original magnification ×150). *B*, Periphery of posterior fibers of left bundle branch (arrows), showing considerable fibrosis and loss of cells. V = ventricular myocardium (Gomori's trichrome stain, original magnification ×45). (From Lightfoot, P. R., et al.: Chronic dermatomyositis with intermittent trifascicular block. An electrophysiologic conduction system correlation. Chest *71*:413, 1977.)

rather to pneumonitis, which is relatively common from aspiration secondary to respiratory muscle weakness and dysphagia.[293] However, there have been informal reports indicating a much higher frequency of cardiac involvement in polymyositis than was previously appreciated. When standard 12-lead electrocardiograms are analyzed systematically, arrhythmias may be quite frequent;[304,305] these usually consist of supraventricular tachycardia, but ventricular tachycardia and advanced heart block associated with syncope or cardiac arrest have also been observed. Deaths have been attributed directly to cardiac failure or arrhythmias or both in some cases, and cardiac muscle histology has been found to be abnormal on autopsy.

TREATMENT. Corticosteroids and immunosuppressive drugs may be of benefit in the treatment of polymyositis-dermatomyositis,[290] but only a controlled prospective study can settle this issue. The course of the disease may not be truly modified by corticosteroids, but the complications of muscle weakness, especially of the respiratory and deglutitional muscles, which lead to pulmonary disease and death, might be diminished by the frequent improvement of muscle strength observed after this treatment.

In the absence of malignancy, survival statistics are favorable for all groups (87 to 91 per cent) in several studies. The leading causes of death, which in one series[290] were metastatic malignancy (24 per cent), sepsis (19 per cent), profound muscular weakness (9.5 per cent), and cardiovascular and cerebrovascular disorders (unspecified percentage), suggest that at least some of these may be modified by therapy and management to improve the prognosis.

HERITABLE DISORDERS OF CONNECTIVE TISSUE

The heritable disorders of connective tissue are characterized by a definable mode of inheritance and by the clinical expression of a generalized defect of some connective tissue element. This group of disorders includes Marfan syndrome, osteogenesis imperfecta, Ehlers-Danlos syndrome, and pseudoxanthoma elasticum, as well as Hurler syndrome and the other mucopolysaccharidoses.[305]

Involvement of the connective tissues of the large arteries, cardiac valves, and other cardiac connective tissue elements determines the cardiovascular manifestations of these disorders. The spectrum of cardiovascular involvement is broad and includes characteristic pathological changes of minimal clinical import as well as of major catastrophic valvular incompetence, aortic dissection, and death. In a number of these disorders, recent investigations of the metabolism and biochemistry of connective tissue have clarified the defects; in others, the basic abnormality remains obscure.[306]

In addition, there are some patients who manifest no or only subtle extracardiac changes of the generalized connective tissue disorders but who display pathological and clinical cardiovascular disease indistinguishable from the generalized disorders. Whether these patients represent a forme fruste of the generalized disease process or they express the limited response of the cardiovascular connective tissue to varied insults is not clear. Patients with myxomatous degeneration of connective tissue of the mitral and aortic valves and those with cystic medial necrosis with involvement of the aortic annulus are included in this group (Chap. 45).[307,308]

THE MARFAN SYNDROME[305]

The Marfan syndrome (also see p. 1620) is a generalized abnormality of connective tissue with major clinical features involving the skeletal, ocular, and cardiovascular systems. The typical skeletal manifestations include excessive limb length, arachnodactyly, loose-jointedness, kyphoscoliosis, and anterior chest deformity. Affected individuals are characteristically tall with long, thin extremities and show weakness of joint capsules, ligaments, tendons, and fascia that results in joint dislocation, hernia, and kyphoscoliosis. A sparsity of subcutaneous fat is a striking feature. The ocular manifestations include defective suspensory ligaments of the lens and subsequent ectopia lentis. The excessive length of the eyeball and involvement of the connective tissue of the retina contribute to the severe myopia and retinal detachment that is often found.

Involvement of the cardiovascular system includes aortic aneurysm with dissection, aortic insufficiency from dilation of both the aortic root and the annulus or from myxomatous involvement of the leaflets themselves and myxomatous degeneration of the mitral valve and its apparatus with secondary mitral incompetence (Fig. 48–13).

The Marfan syndrome exhibits simple mendelian autoso-

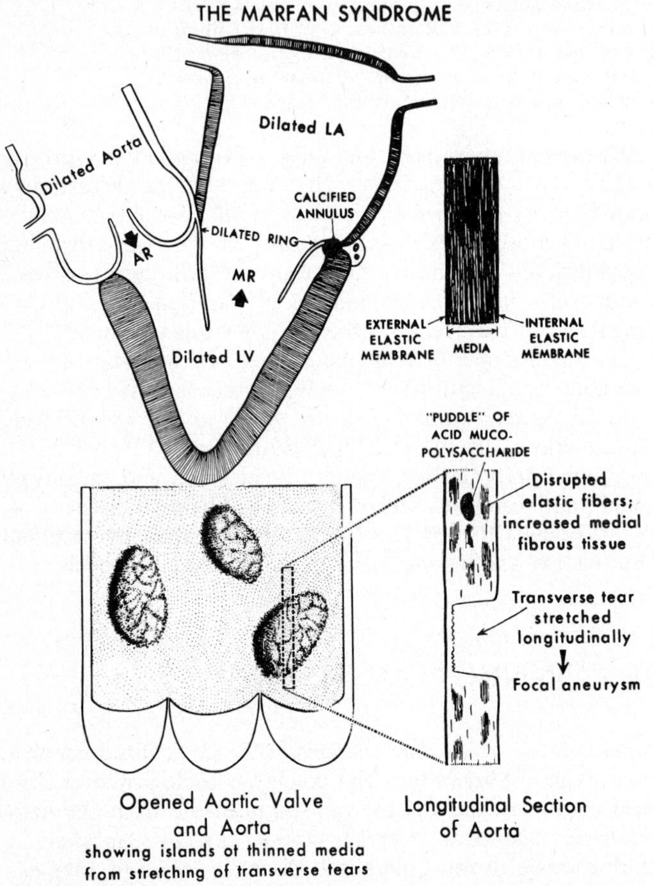

FIGURE 48–13 The various cardiovascular abnormalities found in Marfan's syndrome. The aortic regurgitation appears to be related primarily to dilatation of the aorta. The mitral regurgitation probably results from a combination of factors: dilatation of the left ventricular cavity, altering the papillary muscle–mitral leaflet angle; dilatation of the mitral annulus; calcification of the mitral annulus; and elongation of the mitral leaflets and chordae, allowing prolapse of the leaflets into the left atrium during ventricular systole. *Top right,* Longitudinal section of normal aorta. *Bottom right,* Longitudinal section in a patient with Marfan's syndrome. There is severe loss of elastic fibers, deposition of abnormal amounts of acid mucopolysaccharide material, and tears in the wall. The tears expand to cause the islands of thinning seen in the view of the opened aortic valve and aorta. (From Roberts, W. C., et al.: Nonrheumatic valvular cardiac disease. A clinicopathologic survey of 27 different conditions causing valvular dysfunction. *In* Likoff, W. (ed.): Valvular Heart Disease. Philadelphia, F. A. Davis Co., 1973, p. 368.)

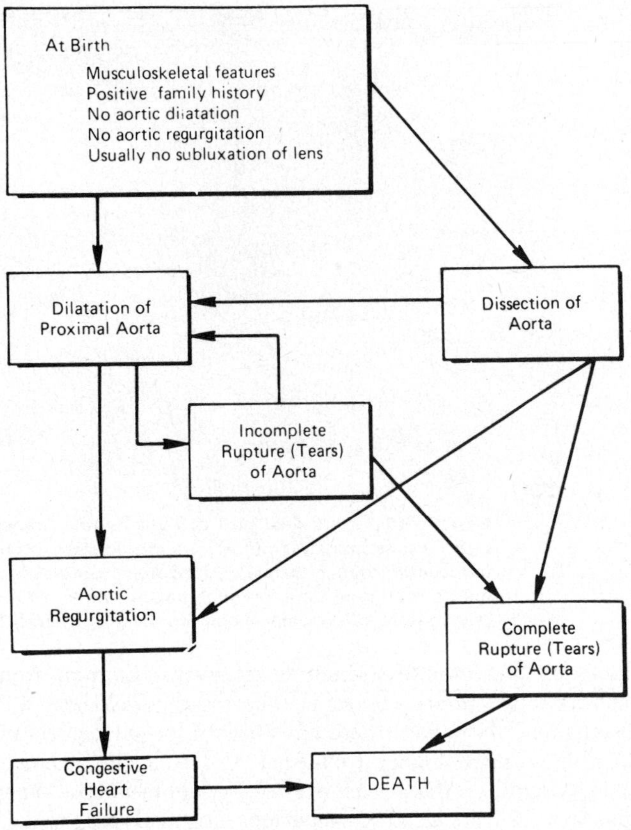

FIGURE 48–14 Schema of development of cardiovascular complications in the Marfan syndrome. (Reproduced with permission from Roberts, W. C.: Am. Heart J. *104*:115, 1982.)

mal dominant inheritance with variable phenotypic expression (Chap. 47). According to McKusick, 15 per cent of all cases are de novo mutations, and this likelihood increases with increasing paternal age.[305] The diagnosis of the Marfan syndrome is most secure when a positive family history of the disease is present or ectopia lentis is found in conjunction with the classic musculoskeletal or cardiovascular changes.[305,309,309a]

PATHOLOGICAL FEATURES. The pathological changes seen in patients with the Marfan syndrome[305,307,309–323] are most striking in the ascending aorta and annulus (p. 1556, Fig. 48–14). In patients with long-term aortic regurgitation, the proximal aorta is diffusely dilated along with the aortic annulus and sinuses of Valsalva. Dilatation of the pulmonary artery also occurs. Chronic aortic dissection and transverse tears without dissection are also found. Histologically, advanced changes include fragmented and sparse elastic tissue in the tunica media, with irregular whorls of smooth muscle and increased amounts of collagen. The vasa vasorum are dilated. The tunica media is interspersed with cystic vacuoles of metachromatically staining material, probably mucopolysaccharide. Inflammation is conspicuously absent. In patients succumbing to acute dissection, earlier changes in the aorta have been studied and reveal cystic medial necrosis and moderate degeneration of elastic elements with disorganization of the smooth muscle bundles. Faults in the media are seen that contain a mucopolysaccharide-rich ground substance. The left ventricle is often enlarged and hypertrophied, reflecting the

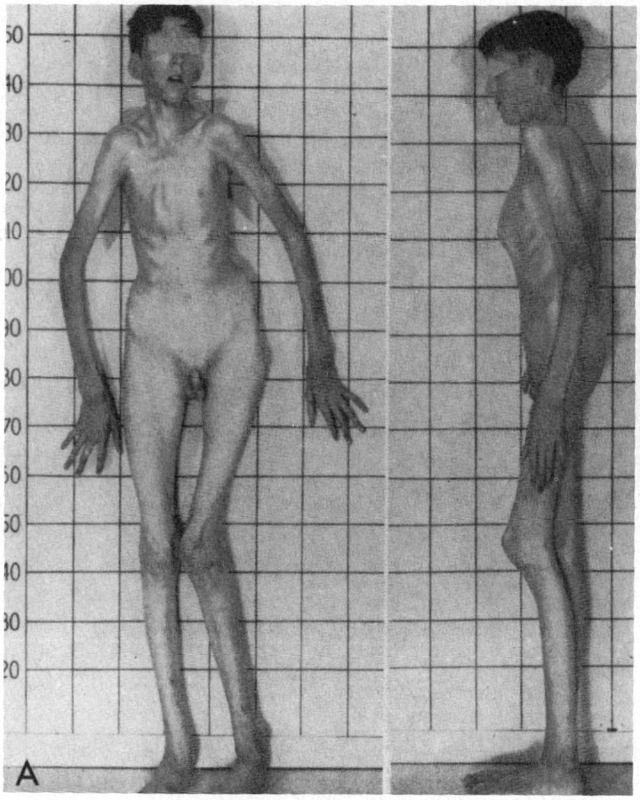

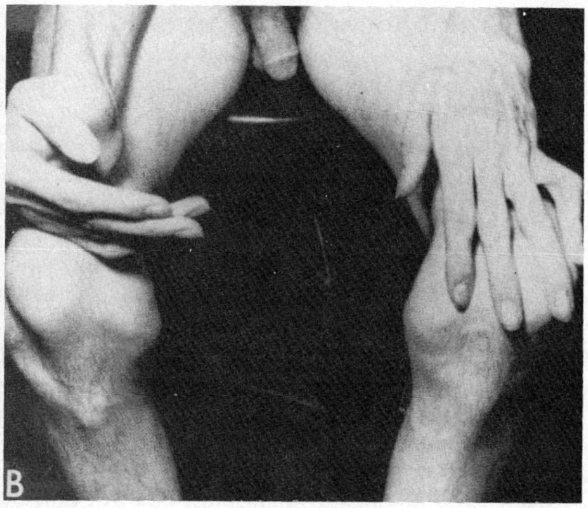

FIGURE 48–15 A, Eleven-year-old boy with Marfan's syndrome. Note excessive length of lower compared with upper segment; the extremities are very long. B, Arachnodactyly. (From McKusick, V.A.: Heritable Disorders of Connective Tissue, 4th ed. St. Louis, The C.V. Mosby Co., 1972.)

degree and duration of the hemodynamic burden imposed by aortic or mitral incompetence.

More recently, the pathological changes and clinical significance of primary valvular abnormalities of the Marfan syndrome have been recognized. Changes in the mitral valve have included ballooning and redundant cusps, fenestrations in the leaflets, elongated and thinned chordae tendineae, and occasionally ruptured and thickened valve cusps with rolled edges. Thin, shiny, diaphanous leaflets are also described. Similar changes in the aortic valve cusps have also been reported. The histological changes include disruption and loss of normal valvular architecture, increase in mucopolysaccharide ground substance, cystic degeneration, and loss of cellularity. These changes are similar to those found in cystic medial necrosis of the aorta. These valvular changes have been termed myxomatous degeneration.

James and coworkers studied the atrioventricular conduction system in two patients with the Marfan syndrome and clinical cardiac conduction abnormalities.[310] Medial degeneration, hyperplasia, and intimal proliferation with luminal narrowing were present in the nutrient arteries of the sinoatrial and atrioventricular nodes as well as in the intramyocardial arteries.

CLINICAL FEATURES. In this generalized disorder of connective tissue, there are ocular and skeletal as well as cardiovascular abnormalities. Weakness of the supporting tissues causes bilateral subluxation of the lens, minor degrees of which can be appreciated by slit-lamp examination. Increased length of the extremities, with an abnormally low ratio of the upper segment (crown to pubic symphysis) to the lower segment (lower than 0.84 in whites and 0.79 in blacks), very long "spider" fingers (arachnodactyly), long metacarpols, pectus carinatum, and pectus excavatum are other important features (Fig. 48–15).

Cardiovascular complications of the Marfan syndrome occur in 30 to 60 per cent of patients in different series. The poor prognosis in patients with the Marfan syndrome reflects the cardiovascular complications and the progressive nature of the lesions. Of 257 patients with the Marfan syndrome followed between 1939 and 1970, the average age at death of the 72 deceased patients was 32 years. Of 56 patients who died, the cause of death in 52 was cardiovascular complications, with aortic dilatation, rupture, and/or dissection accounting for 80 per cent of these.[311] In a study of the Marfan syndrome in infancy and childhood, 61 per cent of patients had cardiac abnormalities.[312,313] Mitral valve disease with mitral regurgitation was the most common lesion found (47 per cent). Mitral systolic clicks with late systolic murmurs were the most common signs. Generally the prognosis is good when isolated mitral valve involvement occurs. Severe mitral and aortic regurgitation may develop, however, requiring valve replacement.[313,314,314a]

During the course of the disease, the ascending aorta becomes dilated with worsening regurgitation, and the likelihood of rupture or dissection increases. In addition to signs and symptoms of left heart failure, chest pain with anginal features is often observed in the Marfan syndrome. This symptom may be secondary to aortic regurgitation, dilatation of the aorta, or coronary ostial involvement.

Systolic honks and musical murmurs may be heard. If chordae or leaflets rupture, loud thrills and longer murmurs may be heard. An echocardiographic study of 26 patients with clinical evidence of the Marfan syndrome showed 12 patients with isolated dysfunction of the mitral valve apparatus. Four patients demonstrated widening of the aortic root as well as abnormality of the mitral valve, and four patients showed abnormality of the aortic root alone.[315]

Infective endocarditis involving the mitral valve in patients with the Marfan syndrome is well documented, and this process has accounted for a significant number of deaths.[305,311,316,317]

PATHOGENESIS AND MANAGEMENT. The biochemical lesion of the Marfan syndrome remains undefined, but as emphasized by McKusick[305,305a] and Bowers[309] the cardiovascular manifestations most likely reflect the response of defective connective tissue to prolonged hemodynamic stresses. Theoretical considerations have prompted the use of the beta-adrenergic blocking agent propranolol in patients with the Marfan syndrome who manifest early signs of aortic dilatation. The murmur of aortic regurgitation, dilatation of the aorta on radiographic examination, and echocardiographic evidence of an enlarged aorta may serve as guides to the initiation and effectiveness of therapy.[315,319] Conclusive evidence of the efficacy of this therapy remains to be established.

The underlying connective tissue defect presents a considerable obstacle to surgical therapy. Although prosthetic valves are favored, not uncommonly they become dislodged. Aortic valve replacement and graft reconstruction of the ascending aorta have proved successful in the management of aortic regurgitation and congestive heart failure with and without aortic dissection.[320] Recurrent dissection, valvular incompetence, and progressive dilatation of any remaining native aorta have been late complications.[307] Elective prophylactic surgery of a greatly enlarged or enlarging aorta found on serial echocardiography in asymptomatic persons can be carried out at a relatively low risk and may prolong survival.[323]

The increasing recognition of mitral valve involvement in the Marfan syndrome that is morphologically indistinguishable from the mitral valve prolapse syndrome makes antibiotic prophylaxis of infective endocarditis appear to be warranted in these patients (p. 1094).

OSTEOGENESIS IMPERFECTA[324]

Osteogenesis imperfecta is a generalized disorder of connective tissue with major involvement of the bones, teeth, saliva, and inner ear. The disease involves other connective tissue elements as well, including fascia and tendons. The ascending aorta, the aortic valve and its annulus, and the mitral valve apparatus are the cardiovascular structures most commonly affected. The incidence of cardiovascular involvement is unknown but is probably low.

Osteogenesis imperfecta is inherited as an autosomal dominant trait with a wide range of phenotypic expression (Chap. 47). This variability has led to the clinical classifications of osteogenesis imperfecta congenita and tarda. In addition, there is most likely a second disorder presenting as osteogenesis imperfecta congenita inherited as an autosomal recessive.

Osteogenesis imperfecta congenita is characterized by extremely brittle bones and subsequent intrauterine fractures. The soft, membranous skull offers little protection at birth, and intracranial hemorrhage is common. The extremities are short and often bowed. Respiratory difficulty often occurs secondary to rib fractures and flail chest. All bones are poorly calcified, and the sclera is blue. Prolonged survival is rare.

In *osteogenesis imperfecta tarda*, a wide range of symptoms and signs is seen. In childhood, repeated fractures from trivial trauma are the hallmarks of the disease. Severe osteoporosis, lax ligaments and tendons, and repeated fractures lead to skeletal deformities, including small stature; bowed, misshapen long bones; and scolioses.

Involvement of the middle ear and petrous bone leads to early deafness. Blue sclera is the ocular hallmark of the disease, although it is not invariably present. The skin is thin and appears atrophic. A qualitative platelet abnormality and abnormal vessels may result in a bleeding diathesis. Although the basic defect in osteogenesis imperfecta is not clearly defined, recent investigations suggest that an abnormal ratio of molecular types of collagen is present. Fibroblasts from some patients synthesize decreased amounts of type I collagen, an important component of the osteoid matrix of bone.[322,323]

PATHOLOGICAL FEATURES. The connective tissues of the aorta, valve leaflets, and mitral apparatus are selectively involved in osteogenesis imperfecta as in Marfan's syndrome and probably for the same reasons.[305,323-326] Changes of cystic medial necrosis are seen in the aorta. The valve leaflets appear acellular, and cystic faults are present, containing metachromatically staining material—changes indistinguishable from myxomatous degeneration. Fenestrated aortic and mitral valve leaflets; ruptured chordae tendineae; and ballooning, torn, and redundant valve leaflets are described. The aorta and its annulus may be dilated, and aneurysms of the sinuses of Valsalva may be present.[325,326]

CLINICAL FEATURES. In adults the clinical features of cardiovascular involvement include aortic regurgitation, most often from dilatation of the aortic root and the annulus. The hemodynamic burden may be progressive, requiring valve replacement. Although cystic medial necrosis of the aorta is seen, aortic dissection has not been reported. Patients may present with sudden congestive heart failure secondary to chordal rupture and mitral regurgitation, or mitral regurgitation of less catastrophic onset may occur. The age at onset is variable and probably reflects the severity of the connective tissue disorder. Two cases of infective endocarditis in osteogenesis imperfecta have been reported.[305,324] Aortic dilatation may be conspicuous by chest roentgenogram without obvious valvular insufficiency.

MANAGEMENT. Management includes routine therapy of congestive heart failure. Successful prosthetic valve replacement is hampered by postoperative bleeding and by poor native connective tissue at the suture sites.[327,328] Prophylaxis for endocarditis appears warranted in clinically recognizable valvular disease.

EHLERS-DANLOS SYNDROME

The Ehlers-Danlos syndrome is a heterogeneous group of disorders of connective tissue that is characterized by hyperelasticity and fragility of the skin; hyperextensibility of the joints; easy bruisability; ocular abnormalities including blue sclera, microcornea, and ectopia lentis; and variable involvement of the respiratory, alimentary, and cardiovascular systems.

Recent biochemical studies have identified distinct abnormalities of collagen synthesis in Ehlers-Danlos syndrome. These findings have included abnormal ratios of collagen types and enzyme deficiencies that affect both normal collagen cross-linking and the conversion of collagen precursor to mature collagen fibers.[322] These studies have supported the clinical impression of distinct phenotypic patterns; seven types are recognized at present. The mode of inheritance is variable.

Histological studies of the cardiovascular lesions of the Ehlers-Danlos syndrome are scarce. Lesions similar to cystic medial necrosis have been described in the aorta in one case.[329] Although many congenital abnormalities of the cardiovascular system have been reported in this syndrome, including tetralogy of Fallot, atrial septal defect, and pulmonary artery and aortic arch anomalies, most authorities believe that these are coincidental and not reflections of the underlying disorder.[305]

CARDIOVASCULAR MANIFESTATIONS. Aortic dissection and spontaneous rupture and dissection of other large arteries with exsanguination are reported in the Ehlers-Danlos syndrome.[330] These episodes may be spontaneous or precipitated by minimal trauma, and significant morbidity secondary to arterial catheterization is reported. Dilatation of the aortic root and sinuses of Valsalva with aortic regurgitation occur.[331] Extensive reviews of patients with Ehlers-Danlos syndrome report various cardiovascular abnormalities, including atrioventricular conduction defects, mitral valve murmurs, nonspecific systolic murmurs, and aortic regurgitation.[332] Some of these findings have been attributed to the deformities of the chest wall found in this disorder.[333] More recently, however, reports of mitral valve murmurs and echocardiographic evidence of prolapse of the mitral valve have suggested widespread involvement of the cardiac connective tissue, and the occurrence of conduction abnormalities in Ehlers-Danlos syndrome has been emphasized. These include right bundle branch block, incomplete right bundle branch block, and left anterior hemiblock alone and with right bundle branch block.[334,335] The histological nature of the valvular and conduction tissue abnormalities remains unknown. Endocarditis prophylaxis in cases of mitral valve involvement is recommended.

PSEUDOXANTHOMA ELASTICUM[305]

Pseudoxanthoma elasticum is an inherited disorder of connective tissue with major involvement of the skin, eyes, and gastrointestinal and cardiovascular systems. The basic defect is thought to be a dysplasia or abiotrophy of elastic tissue. Although originally described as a disorder of the skin and the mesenchymal elements of the eye, involvement of the heart and the peripheral and visceral vasculature is responsible for the more serious manifestations of the disorder, including gastrointestinal hemorrhage, hypertension, congestive heart failure, premature myocardial infarction, peripheral vascular disease, and sudden death.

Pseudoxanthoma elasticum appears to be a heterogeneous group of disorders that Pope has divided into four types according to clinical patterns and modes of inheritance.[336,337] The basic biochemical lesion remains undefined, but in some types autosomal recessive inheritance suggests an enzymatic defect and in others with dominant inheritance, a structural defect.

PATHOLOGICAL FEATURES. Pathological studies of the cardiovascular system are not numerous, but distinctive lesions of the heart, arteries, and arterioles have been described. In the vessels the elastic membrane is often disrupted, and elastic fibers are increased, often shortened, wrinkled, and degenerated, and show an unusual propensity to calcify. Fibrous proliferation of media and intima may severely narrow the lumen.[338] Pathological studies of the heart reveal changes similar to those in the vessels.[339,340] The valve leaflets are also involved, and the cusps may be rolled or thickened; mitral valve prolapse is a common finding.[341] Endocardium of both the ventricle and the atrium is involved. Microscopically, the endocardium exhibits nodular plaques of altered and increased elastic tissue and collagen fibers. Involvement of conducting tissue is also described. Biopsy of the coronary artery has revealed changes indistinguishable from those of peripheral vessels.[342]

CLINICAL FEATURES. Clinically, pseudoxanthoma elasticum is characterized by thickened, coarse, and grooved skin having a leathery and "crepelike" appearance. The skin is lax and redundant with prominent folds. The face, neck, axillae, and inguinal folds are most commonly involved. Mucous membranes of the mouth and stomach may also show changes. The hallmarks of ocular involvement are angioid streaking and chorioretinitis with subsequent visual impairment. Skin changes may be obvious or evident only microscopically, and they usually appear in the second decade. Prominent visceral involvement, however, may occur despite trivial skin changes.

The clinical cardiovascular manifestations of pseudoxanthoma elasticum parallel the pathological changes described. The spectrum includes peripheral vascular disease, hypertension, coronary artery disease, restriction to filling due to subendocardial fibrosis with congestive heart failure, and the clinical manifestations of prolapse of the mitral valve.[341] Symptoms and physical findings appear in the second and third decades.

Intermittent claudication was present in 18 per cent of patients in one large study.[343] A distinctive feature of pseudoxanthoma elasticum is involvement of the arteries of the upper extremities, which distinguishes it from typical atherosclerosis. Physical examination reveals decreased pulses and atrophic changes. The pulse wave is often reduced in amplitude with a slow rise and plateau. Roentgenograms often show calcification of limb arteries.

Both the extraparenchymal and the intraparenchymal renal arteries may be involved in the vasculopathy of pseudoxanthoma elasticum, and the compromised renal blood flow is the most likely cause of the hypertension, often seen in adolescents and young adults.

The incidence of angina is quite variable in large studies of pseudoxanthoma elasticum. In a study of 200 cases, angina was reported in 29 per cent.[343] Acute myocardial infarction and sudden death are not common but are well-documented complications in the second and third decades.[344,345]

Congestive heart failure is an uncommon but recognized manifestation. Murmurs of mitral regurgitation, aortic stenosis, and aortic regurgitation are described.[346] Dilatation of the aorta or its annulus is not a feature of pseudoxanthoma elasticum. The congestive heart failure is probably multifactorial. The hemodynamic burdens imposed by the vascular lesions, combined with the endocardial fibroelastic changes,[345] may be the mechanism of congestive heart failure. However, the role of hypertension and coronary artery disease in cardiac pump function may also be significant. Recently, prolapse of the mitral valve has been described in one type of pseudoxanthoma elasticum.[336]

MANAGEMENT. There is no specific management for the cardiovascular complications of this disorder. Angina, hypertension, and congestive heart failure are managed conventionally. Intractable angina and the Leriche syndrome have been treated with vascular bypass surgery.[342]

HURLER SYNDROME AND OTHER MUCOPOLYSACCHARIDOSES

Hurler syndrome is the prototype of a group of disorders characterized by the abnormal metabolism of mucopolysaccharides. The accumulation of these moieties in mesenchymal cells and their excess urinary excretion serve to identify and classify the disorders. In several forms the enzymatic defect has been identified and the pathogenesis more clearly defined.

Pathological Features. The pathological hallmark of the disease is the presence of Hurler cells, connective tissue cells laden with the mucopolysaccharide moieties heparin sulfate and dermatan sulfate. These cells are found in the connective tissue stroma of many organs. Recently, cells containing intralysosomal collagen fibers have been described in the cardiac valves of patients with Hurler syndrome.[347]

The morphological changes in the heart are striking.[347–350] Grossly, the valves are thickened with fibrous nodules at the closure lines. Aneurysmal dilatations of the leaflets are also seen. The chordae tendineae are also thickened, resembling endocardial fibroelastosis. The cardiac chambers are enlarged. Microscopically, valve thickening is due to the presence of classic Hurler cells, cells with granular inclusions, and an increase in the extracellular collagenous matrix. Increased amounts of collagen and occasional clear cells are responsible for chordal and endocardial thickening. The myocardial cells are relatively spared, but the interstitium may contain Hurler cells. Narrowing of the coronary arteries is seen.

Clinical Features. Patients with classic Hurler syndrome are characterized by dwarfism, corneal clouding, mental retardation, skeletal malformations, hepatosplenomegaly, and cardiovascular lesions. Dermatan sulfate and heparin sulfate are excreted in the urine, and the activity of α-L-iduronidase, a lysosomal hydrolase, is decreased in the fibroblasts of these patients. The condition demonstrates autosomal recessive inheritance and results in early death, most often from respiratory and cardiovascular complications.

Cardiovascular Manifestations.[350–353] Clinically, symptoms of congestive heart failure and ischemic heart disease are most common and are important factors in the poor survival of individuals with Hurler syndrome. In one report 26 of 75 deaths were secondary to congestive heart failure, and 7 additional deaths were sudden. The morphological studies illustrating involvement of conduction tissue suggest arrhythmia as a possible cause of sudden death. Hypertension is also commonly seen, but the cause is unknown. The heart is enlarged on physical examination and chest roentgenogram. Murmurs of mitral regurgitation, aortic stenosis, and aortic regurgitation are often heard. The distorted and thickened mitral valve may produce hemodynamic stenosis. In 15 patients studied by cardiac catheterization,[351] only 1 of whom had clinical congestive heart failure, both systemic and pulmonary hypertension were common. Elevated left ventricular end-diastolic pressures were present in 5 of 9 patients. Angina pectoris occurs in children with Hurler syndrome.

Valvular lesions, thickened, noncompliant endocardium, hypertension, and severely compromised coronary circulation are the features that collectively produce congestive heart failure in Hurler syndrome and its variants. The four mucopolysaccharidoses that involve the cardiovascular system are Hurler syndrome, Hurler-Scheie syndrome, Hunter syndrome, and Morquio syndrome.[351]

Management. Treatment of these disorders with plasma in an effort to replace the deficient or defective enzyme has been reported. There is no specific treatment for the cardiovascular complications of the mucopolysaccharidoses, and early death has underscored the poor response to conventional therapy.

References

RHEUMATIC DISEASES

1. Stollerman, G. H.: Rheumatic Fever and Streptococcal Infection. New York, Grune and Stratton, 1975.
2. Halsey, R. H.: Heart disease in children of school age. J.A.M.A. *77*:672, 1921.
3. Rammelkamp. C. H., Denny, F. W., and Wannamaker, L. W.: Studies on the epidemiology of rheumatic fever in the armed services. *In* Thomas, L. (ed.): Rheumatic Fever. Minneapolis, University of Minnesota Press, 1952, pp. 72–89.
4. Frank, P. F., Stollerman, G. H., and Miller, L. F.: Protection of a military population from rheumatic fever. J.A.M.A. *193*:775, 1965.
5. Gordis, L.: Effectiveness of comprehensive-care programs in preventing rheumatic fever. N. Engl. J. Med. *289*:331, 1973.
6. Miller, R. A., Stamler, J., Smith, J. M., Milne, W. S., Paul, M. H., Abrams, I., Hastreiter, A. R., Restivo, R. M., and DeBoer, L.: The detection of heart disease in children. Results of mass field trials with use of tape-recorded heart sounds. II. The Michigan City study. Circulation *32*:956, 1965.
7. Stamler, J.: Cardiovascular diseases in the United States. Am. J. Cardiol. *10*: 319, 1962.
8. Argarwal, B. L.: Rheumatic heart disease unabated in developing countries. Lancet *2*:910, 1981.
9. Stetson, C. A.: The relation of antibody response to rheumatic fever. *In* McCarty, M. (ed.): Streptococcal Infections. New York, Columbia University Press, 1954, pp. 208–218.
10. Rammelkamp, C. H., Jr.: The Lewis A. Conner Memorial Lecture. Rheumatic heart disease—A challenge. Circulation *17*:842, 1958.
11. Siegel, A. C., Johnson, E. E., and Stollerman, G. H.: Controlled studies of streptococcal pharyngitis in a pediatric population. I. Factors related to the attack rate of rheumatic fever. N. Engl. J. Med. *265*:559, 1961.
12. Stollerman, G. H.: Factors determining the attack rate of rheumatic fever. J.A.M.A. *177*:823, 1961.
13. Stollerman, G. H., Siegel, A. C., and Johnson, E. E.: Variable epidemiology of streptococcal disease and the changing pattern of rheumatic fever. Mod. Concepts Cardiovasc. Dis. *34*:45, 1965.
14. Kaplan, E. L., Top, F. H., Dudding, B. A., and Wannamaker, L. W.: Diagnosis of streptococcal pharyngitis: Differentiation of active infection from the carrier state in the symptomatic child. J. Infect. Dis. *123*:490, 1971.
15. Top, F. H., Wannamaker, L. W., Maxted, W. R., and Anthony, G. V.: M antigens among group A streptococci isolated from skin lesions. J. Exp. Med. *126*:667, 1967.
16. Stollerman, G. H.: Nephritogenic and rheumatogenic group A streptococci. J. Infect. Dis. *120*:258, 1969.
17. Wannamaker, L. W.: Medical progress. Differences between streptococcal infections of the throat and of the skin. N. Engl. J. Med. *282*:23 and 78, 1970.
18. Wannamaker, L. W.: The chain that links the heart to the throat. Circulation *48*:9, 1973.
19. Bisno, A. L., Pearce, I. A., Wall, H. P., Moody, M. D. and Stollerman, G. H.: Contrasting epidemiology of acute rheumatic fever and acute glomerulonephritis. Nature of the antecedent streptococcal infection. N. Engl. J. Med. *283*:561, 1970.
20. Poon-King, T., Mohammed, I., Cox, R., Potter, E. V., Simon, N. M., Siegel, A. C., and Earle, D. P.: Recurrent epidemic nephritis in South Trinidad, N. Engl. J. Med. *277*:728, 1967.
21. Potter, E. V., Svartman, M., Poon-King, T., and Earle, D. P.: The families of patients with acute rheumatic fever or glomerulonephritis in Trinidad. Am. J. Epidemiol. *106*:130, 1977.
22. Widdowson, J.P., Maxted, W. R., Notley, C. M., and Pinney, A. M.: The antibody responses in man to infection with different serotypes of group A streptococci. J. Med. Microbiol. *7*:483, 1974.
23. Bisno, A. L.: The concept of rheumatogenic and nonrheumatogenic group A streptococci. *In* McCarty, M., and Zabriskie, J. B. (eds.): Streptococcal Diseases and the Immune reponse. New York, Academic Press, 1980, p. 789.
24. Stollerman, G. H.: Global changes in group A streptococcal diseases and strategies for their prevension. Adv. Intern. Med. *27*:373, 1982.
25. Stollerman, G. H.: The streptococcus, rheumatic fever and rheumatic heart disease. *In* Shaper, A. G., Hutt, M. S. R., and Fejfar, Z. (eds.): Cardiovascular Disease in the Tropics. London, British Medical Associates, 1974.
26. Sanyal, S. K., Thapar, M. K., Ahmed, S. H., Hooja, V., and Tewari, P.: The initial attack of acute rheumatic fever during childhood in North India. A prospective study of the clinical profile. Circulation *49*:7, 1974.
27. Taranta, A.: Rheumatic fever in children and adolescents. A long-term epidemiologic study of subsequent prophylaxis, streptococcal infections, and clinical sequelae. IV. Relation of the rheumatic fever recurrence rate per streptococcal infection to the titers of streptococcal antibodies. Ann. Intern. Med. *60*(Suppl. 5):47, 1964.
28. Taranta, A., Kleinberg, E., Feinstein, A. R., Wood, H. F., Tursky, E., and Simpson, R.: Rheumatic fever in children and adolescents. A long-term epidemiologic study of subsequent prophylaxis, streptococcal infections, and clinical sequelae. V. Relation of the rheumatic fever recurrence rate per streptococcal infection to pre-existing clinical features of the patients. Ann. Intern. Med. *60* (Suppl. 5):58, 1964.
29. Johnson, E. E., Stollerman, G. H., and Grossman, B. J.: Rheumatic recurrences in patients not receiving continuous prophylaxis. J.A.M.A. *190*:407, 1964.

30. Taranta, A.: Rheumatic fever made difficult. A critical review of pathogenetic theories. Paediatrician *5*:74, 1976.
31. Markowitz, M.: Cultures of the respiratory tract in pediatric practice. Am. J. Dis. Child. *105*:12, 1963.
32. Rantz, L. A., Boisvert, P. J., and Spink, W. W.: Etiology and pathogenesis of rheumatic fever. Arch. Intern. Med. *76*:131, 1945.
33. Zagala, J. G., and Feinstein, A. R.: The preceding illness of acute rheumatic fever. J.A.M.A. *179*:863, 1962.
34. Grossman, B. J., and Stamler, J.: Potential preventability of first attacks of acute rheumatic fever in children. J.A.M.A. *183*:985, 1963.
35. Rammelkamp, C. H., Jr.: Epidemiology of streptococcal infections. Harvey Lecture Series *51*:113, 1955–1956.
36. Stollerman, G. H.: The epidemiology of primary and secondary rheumatic fever. *In* Uhr, J. W. (ed.): The Streptococcus, Rheumatic Fever and Glomerulonephritis. Baltimore, Williams and Wilkins, 1964, pp. 311–337.
37. Green, C. A.: Researches into aetiology of acute rheumatism; rheumatic carditis. Postmortem investigation of nine consecutive cases. Ann. Rheum. Dis. *1*:86, 1939.
38. Collis, W. R. F.: Bacteriology of rheumatic fever. Lancet *2*:817, 1939.
39. Watson, R. F., Hirst, G. K., and Lancefield, R. C.: Bacteriological studies of cardiac tissues obtained at autopsy from eleven patients dying with rheumatic fever. Arthr. Rheum. *4*:74, 1961.
40. Yoshimoya, S., and Pope, R. M.: Detection of immune complexes in acute rheumatic fever and their relationship to HLA-B5. J. Clin. Invest. *65*:136, 1980.
41. Gray, E. D., Wannamaker, L. W., Ayoub, E. M., Kholy, A. E., and Abdin, Z. H.: Cellular immune responses to extracellular streptococcal products in rheumatic heart disease. J. Clin. Invest. *68*:665, 1982
42. Kaplan, M. H., Meyeserian, M., and Kushner, I.: Immunologic studies of heart tissue. IV. Serologic reactions with human heart tissue as revealed by immunofluorescent methods: Isoimmune, Wassermann, and auto-immune reactions. J. Exp. Med. *113*:17, 1961.
43. Burgio, G. R., Severi, F., Vaccaro, R., and Rossoni, R.: Antibodies reacting with heart tissue in the course of rheumatic fever in children. Schweiz. Med. Wschr. *96*:431, 1966.
44. Hess, E. V., Fink, C. W., Taranta, A., and Ziff, M.: Heart muscle antibodies in rheumatic fever and other diseases. J. Clin. Invest. *43*:886, 1964.
45. Ehrenfeld, E. N., Gery, I., and Davies, A. M.: Specific antibodies in heart disease. Lancet *1*:1138, 1961.
46. Kaplan, M. H.: Immunologic relation of streptococcal and tissue antigens. I. Properties of an antigen in certain strains of group A streptococci exhibiting an immunologic cross-reaction with human heart tissue. J. Immunol. *90*:595, 1963.
47. Kaplan, M. H., and Suchy, M. L.: Immunologic relation of streptococcal and tissue antigens. II. Cross reactions of antisera to mammalian heart tissue with a cell wall constituent of certain strains of group A streptococci. J. Exp. Med. *119*:643, 1964.
48. Zabriskie, J. B., and Freimer, E. H.: An immunological relationship between the group A streptococcus and mammalian muscle. J. Exp. Med. *124*:661, 1966.
49. Lyampert, I. M., Danilova, T. A., Borodyuk, N. A., and Beletskaya, L. V.: Mechanism of formation of antibodies to heart tissue in immunization with group A streptococci. Folia Biol. *12*:108, 1966.
50. Lyampert, I. M., Vvedenskaya, O. I., and Danilova, T. A.: Study on streptococcus group A antigens common with heart tissue elements. Immunology *11*: 313, 1966.
51. Goldstein, I., Halpern, B., and Robert, L.: Immunological relationship between streptococcus A polysaccharide and the structual glycoproteins of heart valves. Nature *213*:44, 1967.
52. Sandson, J., Hammerman, D., Janis, R., and Rojkind, M.: Immunologic and chemical similarities between the streptococcus and human connective tissue. Trans. Assoc. Am. Phys. *81*:249, 1968.
53. Bisno, A. L., Wood, J. W., Lawson, J., Roy, S., Beachey, E. H., and Stollerman, G. H.: Antigens in urine of patients with glomerulonephritis and in normal human serum which cross-react with group A streptococci: Identification and partial characterization. J. Lab. Clin. Med. *91*:500, 1978.
54. van de Rijn, I., Zabriskie, J. B., and McCarty, M.: Group A streptococcal antigens cross-reactive with myocardium. Purification of heart-reactive antibody and isolation and characterization of the streptococcal antigen. J. Exp. Med. *146*:579, 1977.
55. Beachey, E. H., Stollerman, G. H., Chiang, E. Y., Chiang, T. M., Seyer, J. M., and Kang, A. H.: Purification and properties of M protein extracted from group A streptococci with pepsin: Covalent structure of the amino terminal region of type 24 M antigen. J. Exp. Med. *145*:1469, 1977.
56. Stollerman, G. H.: Streptococcal vaccines revisited. J. Lab. Clin. Med. *91*:872, 1978.
57. Husby, G., van de Rijn, I., Zabriskie, J. B., Abdin, Z. H., and Williams, R. C.: Antibodies reacting with cytoplasm of subthalamic and caudate nuclei neurons in chorea and acute rheumatic fever. J. Exp. Med. *144*:1094, 1976.
58. Zabriskie, J. B., Hsu, K. C., and Seegal, B.C.: Heart-reactive antibody associated with rheumatic fever: Characterization and diagnostic significance. Clin. Exp. Immunol. *7*:147, 1970.
59. Yang, L. C., Soprey, P. R., Wittner, M. K., and Fox, E. N.: Streptococcal-induced cell-mediated immune destruction of cardiac myofibers in vitro. J. Exp. Med. *146*:344, 1977.
60. Beachey, E. H., and Stollerman, G. H.: Mediation of cytotoxic effects of streptococcal M protein by non-type-specific antibody in human sera. J. Clin. Invest. *52*:2563, 1973.
61. Zimmerman, R. A., Auernheimer, A. H., and Taranta, A.: Precipitating antibody to group A streptococcal polysaccharide in humans. J. Immunol. *107*: 832, 1971.
62. Ayoub, E. M., Taranta, A., and Bartley, T. D.: Effect of valvular surgery on antibody to the group A streptococcal carbohydrate. Circulation *50*:144, 1974.
63. Taranta, A., Torosdag, S., Metrakos, J., Jegier, W., and Uchida, I.: Rheumatic fever in monozygotic and dizygotic twins. *In* Proceedings of the Tenth International Congress of Rheumatology. Torino, Minerva Medica, 1961, pp. 96–98.
64. Stollerman, G. H.: Hypersensitivity and antibody responses in streptococcal disease. *In* Wannamaker, L. W., and Masten, J. M. (eds.): Streptococci and Streptococcal Diseases. Recognition, Understanding, and Management. New York, Academic Press, 1972, pp. 501–513.
65. Kuhns, W. J., and McCarty, M.: Studies of diphtheria antitoxin in rheumatic fever subjects. Analysis of reactions to the Schick test and of antitoxin responses following hyperimmunization with diphtheria toxoid. J. Clin. Invest. *33*:759, 1954.
66. Neumann, E.: Die Picrocarminfarbung und ihre Anwendung auf die Entzü ndungslehre. Arch. Mikr. Anat. (Bonn) *25*:130, 1880.
67. Neumann, E.: Zur Kenntnis der fibrinoiden Degeneration des Bindegewebes bei Entzündungen. Virchow Arch. Pathol. Anat. *144*:201, 1896.
68. Talalaev, V. T. (Talalajew, W. T.): Der akute Rheumatismus. Klin. Wochenschr. *8*:124, 1929.
69. Klinge, F.: Der Rheumatismus. Munich, J. Bergmann, 1933.
70. Aschoff, L.: Zur Myocarditisfrage. Verhandl. Dtsch. Pathol. Ges. *8*:46, 1904–1905.
71. Gross, L., and Ehrlich, J. C.: Studies on the myocardial Aschoff body. II. Life cycle, sites of predilection and relation to clinical course of rheumatic fever. Am. J. Pathol. *10*:489, 1934.
72. Murphy, G. E.: Nature of rheumatic heart disease with special reference to myocardial disease and heart failure. Medicine *39*:289, 1960.
73. Gitlin, D., Craig, J. M., and Janeway, J. A.: Studies on the nature of fibrinoid in the collagen diseases. Am. J. Pathol. *33*:55, 1957.
74. Vazquez, J. J., and Dixon, F. J.: Immunohistochemical analysis of lesions associated with "fibrinoid change." Arch. Pathol. *66*:504, 1958.
75. Wagner, B. M.: Studies in rheumatic fever. III. Histochemical reactivity of the Aschoff body. Ann. N.Y. Acad. Sci. *86*:992, 1960.
76. Aschoff, L.: The rheumatic nodules in the heart. Ann. Rheum. Dis. *1*:161, 1939.
77. Sokoloff, L.: The pathogenesis of rheumatic fever. *In* Mills, L. C., and Mayer, J. H. (eds.): Inflammation and Diseases of Connective Tissue. Philadelphia, W. B. Saunders Co., 1961, p. 135.
78. Pienaar, J. G., and Price, H. M.: Ultrastructure and origin of the Anitschkow cell. Am. J. Pathol. *51*:1063, 1967.
79. Kuschner, M., Ferrer, M. I., Harvey, R. M., and Wylie, R. H.: Rheumatic carditis in surgically removed appendages. Am. Heart J. *43*:286, 1952.
80. Virmani, R., and Roberts, W. C.: Aschoff bodies in operatively excised atrial appendages and in papillary muscles. Frequency and clinical significance. Circulation *55*:559, 1977.
81. Roberts, W. C., and Virmani, R.: Aschoff bodies at necropsy in valvular heart disease. Evidence from an analysis of 543 patients over 14 years of age that rheumatic heart disease, at least anatomically, is a disease of the mitral valve. Circulation *57*:803, 1978.
82. Stollerman, G. H., Lynch, W. F., Dolman, M. A., Young, D., and Schwedel, J. B.: Immunologic evidence of streptococcal infection in patients undergoing mitral commissurotomy. Circulation *15*:267, 1957.
83. Lanningan, R.: Cardiac Pathology. London, Butterworth and Co., 1966.
84. Coombs, C. F.: The myocardial lesions of the rheumatic infection. Br. Med. J. *2*:1513, 1907.
85. Reubner, B.: The relationship between muscle damage and the Aschoff cell in rheumatic carditis. J. Pathol Bacteriol. *68*:101, 1954.
86. Gross, L., and Friedberg, C. K.: Lesions of the cardiac valve rings in rheumatic fever. Am. J. Pathol. *12*:469, 1936.
87. Pappenheimer, A. M., and Von Glahn, W. C.: Studies on the pathology of rheumatic fever. Two cases presenting unusual cardiovascular lesions. Am. J. Pathol. *3*:583, 1927.
88. Gross, L., Kugel, M. A., and Epstein, E. Z.: Lesions of the coronary arteries and their branches in rheumatic fever. Am. J. Pathol. *11*:253, 1935.
89. Bayred, E. D.: Hematologic complications of cardiac surgery. Adv. Intern. Med. *19*:57, 1974.
90. Steele, P. P., Weily, H. S., Davies, H., and Genton, E.: Platelet survival in patients with rheumatic heart disease. N. Engl. J. Med. *290*:537, 1974.
91. Coombs, C. F.: The microscopic or "submiliary" nodules of active rheumatic carditis. J. Pathol. Bacteriol. *15*:489, 1910–1911.
92. Winkelman, N. W., and Eckel, J. L.: The brain in acute rheumatic fever. Nonsuppurative meningoencephalitis rheumatica. Arch. Neurol. Psychiatr. *28*:844, 1932.
93. Neubuerger, K. T.: The brain in rheumatic fever. Dis. Nerv. Syst. *8*:259, 1947.
94. Costero, I.: Cerebral lesions responsible for death of patients with active rheumatic fever. Arch. Neurol. Psychiatr. *62*:48, 1949.
95. Buchanan, D. N.: Pathologic changes in chorea. Am. J. Dis. Child. *62*:443, 1941.
96. Kernohan, J. W., Woltman, H. W., and Barnes, A. R.: Involvement of the

nervous system associated with endocarditis. Neuropsychiatric and neuropathologic observations in 42 cases of fatal outcome. Arch. Neurol. Psychiatr. *42*:789, 1939.
97. Rammelkamp, C. H., Jr., and Stolzer, B. L.: The latent period before the onset of acute rheumatic fever. Yale J. Biol. Med. *34*:386, 1961.
98. Deliee, E. M., Dodge, K. G., and McEwen, C.: The prognostic significance of age at onset in initial attacks of rheumatic fever. Am. Heart J. *26*:681, 1943.
99. Feinstein, A. R., and Spagnuolo, M.: The clinical patterns of acute rheumatic fever: A reappraisal. Medicine *41*:279, 1962.
100. Pader, E., and Elster, S. K.: Studies of acute rheumatic fever in the adult. I. Clinical and laboratory manifestations in thirty patients. Am. J. Med. *26*:424, 1959.
101. Ben-Dov, I., and Berry, E.: Acute rheumatic fever in adults over the age of 45 years: An analysis of 23 patients together with a review of the literature. Semin. Arthritis Rheum. *10*:100, 1980.
102. United Kingdom and United States Joint Report on Rheumatic Fever: The treatment of acute rheumatic fever in children. A cooperative clinical trial of ACTH, cortisone and aspirin. Circulation *11*:343, 1955.
103. United Kingdom and United States Joint Report on Rheumatic Heart Disease: The evolution of rheumatic heart disease in children. Five-year report of a cooperative clinical trial of ACTH, cortisone and aspirin. Circulation *22*:503, 1960.
103a. Bittl, J. A., and Perloff, J. K.: Chronic post-rheumatic fever arthropathy of Jaccoud. Am. Heart J. *105*:515, 1983.
104. United Kingdom and United States Joint Report on Rheumatic Heart Disease: The natural history of rheumatic fever and rheumatic heart disease. Ten-year report of a cooperative clinical trial of ACTH, cortisone and aspirin. Circulation *32*:457, 1965.
105. Massell, B. V., Fyler, D. C., and Roy, S. B.: The clinical picture of rheumatic fever. Diagnosis, immediate prognosis, course and therapeutic implications. Am. J. Cardiol. *1*:436, 1958.
106. Feinstein, A. R., and DiMassa, R.: The unheard diastolic murmur in acute rheumatic fever. N. Engl. J. Med. *260*:1331, 1959.
107. Combined Rheumatic Fever Study Group, 1960: A comparison of the effect of prednisone and acetylsalicylic acid on the incidence of residual rheumatic heart disease. N. Engl. J. Med. *262*:895, 1960.
108. Combined Rheumatic Fever Study Group, 1965: A comparison of the short-term, intensive prednisone and acetylsalicylic acid therapy in the treatment of acute rheumatic fever. N. Engl. J. Med. *272*:63, 1965.
109. Robinson, R. W.: Effect of atropine upon the prolongation of the P-R interval found in acute rheumatic fever and certain vagotonic persons. Am. Heart J. *29*:378, 1945.
110. Lenox, C. C., Zuberbuhler, J. R., Park, S. C., Neches, W. H., Mathews, R. A., and Zoltun, R.: Arrhythmias and Stokes-Adams attacks in acute rheumatic fever. Pediatrics *61*:599, 1979.
111. Meynet, P.: Rheumatisme articulaire subaigu avec production de tumeurs multiples dans les tissus fibreux periarticulaires et sur le perioste d'un grand numbre d'os. Lyons Med. *19*:495, 1875.
112. Cheadle, W. B.: Various Manifestations of the Rheumatic State as Exemplified in Childhood and Early Life. London, Smith, Elder, 1889.
113. Baldwin, J. S., Kerr, J. M., Kuttner, A. G., and Doyle, E. F.: Observations on rheumatic nodules over a 30-year period. J. Pediatr. *56*:465, 1960.
114. Burke, J. B.: Erythema marginatum. Arch. Dis. Child. *30*:359, 1955.
115. Diamond, E. F., and Tentler, R.: The electroencephalogram in rheumatic fever. J.A.M.A. *182*:685, 1962.
116. Lessof, M. H., and Bywaters, E. G. L.: The duration of chorea. Br. Med. J. *1*:1520, 1956.
117. Taranta, A., and Stollerman, G. H.: The relationship of Sydenham's chorea to infection with group A streptococci Am. J. Med. *20*:170, 1956.
118. Bland, E. F.: Chorea as a manifestation of rheumatic fever. A long-term perspective. Trans Am. Clin. Climatol. Assoc. *73*:209, 1961.
119. Doliopoulos, T.: Abdominal pain in rheumatic fever. Rheumatism *7*:42, 1951.
120. Coburn, A. F.: The Factor of Infection in the Rheumatic State. Baltimore, Williams and Wilkins, 1931.
121. Goldring, D., Behrer, M. R., Brown, G., and Elliott, G.: Rheumatic pneumonitis. Part II. Report on the clinical and laboratory findings in twenty-three patients. J. Pediatr. *53*:547, 1958.
122. Bisno, A. L., and Stollerman, G. H.: Streptococcal antibodies in the diagnosis of rheumatic fever. *In* Cohen, A. S. (ed.): Laboratory Diagnostic Procedures in the Rheumatic Diseases. 2nd ed. Boston, Little, Brown and Co., 1974.
123. Rantz, L. A., Randall, E., and Rantz, H. H.: Antistreptolysin "O." A study of this antibody in health and in hemolytic streptococcus respiratory disease in man. Am. J. Med. *5*:3, 1948.
124. Wannamaker, L. W.: Streptococcal deoxyribonucleases. *In* Uhr, J. W. (ed.): The Streptococcus, Rheumatic Fever and Glomerulonephritis. Baltimore, Williams and Wilkins, 1964, pp. 140–165.
125. Bergner-Rabinowitz, S., Ofek, I., Fleiderman, S., Zohar, M., Rabinowitz, K., and Ginsburg, I.: Evaluation of streptozyme and antistreptolysin O tests in streptococcal pyodermal nephritis. Appl. Microbiol. *26*:56, 1973.
126. Bisno, A. L., and Ofek, I.: Serologic diagnosis of streptococcal infection. Comparison of a rapid hemagglutination technique with conventional antibody tests. Am. J. Dis. Child. *127*:676, 1974.
127. Gewurz, H., Mold, C., Siegel, J., and Fiedel, B.: C-reactive protein and the acute phase response. Adv. Intern. Med. *27*:345, 1982.
128. Mauer, A. M.: The early anemia of acute rheumatic fever. Pediatrics *27*:707, 1961.
129. Mirowski, M., Rosenstein, B. J., and Markowitz, M.: A comparison of atrioventricular conduction in normal children and in patients with rheumatic fever, glomerulonephritis, and acute febrile illnesses. A quantitative study with determination of the P-R index. Pediatrics *33*:334, 1964.
130. Feinstein, A. R., and DiMassa, R.: Prognostic significance of valvular involvement in acute rheumatic fever. N. Engl. J. Med. *260*:1001, 1959.
131. Feinstein, A. R., Wood, H. F., Spagnuolo, M., Taranta, A., Jonas, S., Kleinberg, E., and Tursky, E.: Rheumatic fever in children and adolescents. VII. Cardiac changes and sequelae. Ann. Intern. Med. *60*(Suppl. 5):87, 1964.
132. Jones, T. D.: The diagnosis of rheumatic fever. J.A.M.A. *126*:481, 1944.
133. Jones Criteria (revised) for guidance in the diagnosis of rheumatic fever. Circulation *32*:664, 1965.
134. Trentham, D. E., McCravey, J. W., and Masi, A. T.: Low-dose penicillin for gonococcal arthritis. A comparative therapy trial. J.A.M.A. *236*:2410, 1976.
135. Stollerman, G. H.: Penicillin-sensitive gonococci and polyarthritis (editorial). J.A.M.A. *236*:2433, 1976.
136. Williams, R. C., Jr., and Kunkel, H. C.: Rheumatoid factor, complement and conglutinin aberrations in patients with subacute bacterial endocarditis. J. Clin. Invest. *41*:666, 1962.
137. Greenberg, M. S.: Ear lobe histiocytosis as a clue to the diagnosis of subacute bacterial endocarditis. Ann. Intern. Med. *61*:124, 1964.
138. Kantor, T. G., and Tanner, M.: Rubella arthritis and rheumatoid arthritis. Arthritis Rheum. *5*:378, 1962.
139. Dull, H. B.: Vaccinology and selected virus diseases. Adv. Intern. Med. *17*:143, 1971.
140. Uzsoy, N. K.: The coexistence of rheumatic heart disease and sickle cell anemia. Am. J. Med. Sci. *246*:462, 1963.
141. Wiernik, P. H.: Rheumatic heart disease occurring in sickle cell disease and trait. South. Med. J. *61*:404, 1968.
142. Mazzara, J. T., Burns, G. C., Mueller, H. S., and Ayres, S. M.: Coexistence of sickle cell anemia and rheumatic heart disease. N.Y. State J. Med. *71*:2426, 1971.
143. Calabro, J. J., and Marchesane, J. M.: Juvenile rheumatoid arthritis. N. Engl. J. Med. *277*:696, 1967.
144. Silverstein, M. N., and Kelly, P. J.: Bone and joint involvement in acute leukemia. Rheumatism *21*:67, 1965.
145. Brodie, H. R., and Marchessault, V.: Acute benign pericarditis caused by Coxsackie virus Group B. N. Engl. J. Med. *262*:1278, 1960.
146. Wolff, L., and Wolff, R.: Diseases of the pericardium. Ann. Rev. Med. *16*:21, 1965.
147. Keith, J. D.: Congenital mitral insufficiency. Progr. Cardiovasc. Dis. *5*:264, 1962.
148. Taranta, A., Spagnuolo, M., and Feinstein, A. R.: "Chronic" rheumatic fever. Ann. Intern. Med. *56*:367, 1962.
149. McIntosch, R., and Wood, C. L.: Rheumatic infections occurring in the first three years of life. Am. J. Dis. Child. *49*:835, 1935.
150. Rosenthal, A., Czoniczer, G., and Massell, B. F.: Rheumatic fever under three years of age. A report of ten cases. Pediatrics *41*:612, 1968.
151. Feinstein, A. R., and Spagnuolo, M.: The duration of activity in acute rheumatic fever. J.A.M.A. *175*:1117, 1961.
152. Ellis, L. B.: Recurrent mitral stenosis. Mod. Concepts Cardiovasc. Dis. *33*:851, 1964.
153. Wood, H. F., Simpson, R., Feinstein, A. R., Taranta, A., Tursky, E., and Stollerman, G. H.: Rheumatic fever in children and adolescents. I. Description of the investigative techniques and of the population studied. Ann. Intern. Med. *60*(Suppl. 5):6, 1964.
154. Stollerman, G. H.: Prognosis and treatment of acute rheumatic fever: The possible effect of treatment on subsequent cardiac disease. Progr. Cardiovasc. Dis. *3*:193, 1960.
155. Chen, S. C., Donahoe, J. R., and Fagan, L. F.: Rheumatic fever in children. A follow-up study with emphasis on cardiac sequelae. Jpn. Heart J. *22*:167, 1981.
156. Vaisman, S., Guasch, J., Vignau, A. Correa, E., Schuster, A., Mortimer, E. A., Jr., and Rammelkamp, C. H., Jr.: The failure of penicillin to alter acute rheumatic valvulitis. J.A.M.A. *194*:1284, 1965.
157. Stolzer, B. L., Houser, H. B., and Clark, E. J.: Therapeutic agents in rheumatic carditis. Comparative effects of acetylsalicylic acid, corticotropin, and cortisone. Arch. Intern. Med. *95*:677, 1955.
158. Czoniczer, G., Amezcua, F., Pelargonio, S., and Massell, B. F.: Therapy of severe rheumatic carditis. Comparison of adrenocortical steroids and aspirin. Circulation *29*:813, 1964.
159. Tierney, R. C., and Kaplan, S.: Treatment of Sydenham's chorea. Am. J. Dis. Child. *109*:408, 1965.
160. Lockman, L. A.: Movement disorders. *In* Swaiman, K., and Wright, F. (eds.): Practice of Pediatric Neurology. St. Louis, The C. V. Mosby Co., 1975.
161. Shields, W. D., and Bray, P. F.: A danger of haloperidol therapy in children. J. Pediatr. *88*:301, 1976.
162. Massell, B. F., Sturgis, G. P., Knobloch, J. D., Steeper, R. B., Hall, T. N., and Norcross, P.: Prevention of rheumatic fever by prompt penicillin therapy of hemolytic streptococci respiratory infections. J.A.M.A. *146*:1469, 1951.
163. Stollerman, G. H., Rusoff, J. H., and Hirschfeld, I.: Prophylaxis against group A streptococci in rheumatic fever. The use of single monthly injections of benzathine penicillin G. N. Engl. J. Med. *252*:787, 1955.
164. Albam, B., Epstein, J. A., Feinstein, A. R., Gavrin, J. B., Jonas, S., Kleinberg, E., Simpson, R., Spagnuolo, M., Stollerman, G. H., Taranta, A. Tursky, E., and Wood, H. F.: Rheumatic fever in children and adolescents. A long-term

epidemiologic study of subsequent prophylaxis, streptococcal infections, and clinical sequelae. Ann. Intern. Med. *60*(Suppl. 5): No. 2, Part II, 1964.

165. American Heart Association, Committee on Rheumatic Fever and Bacterial Endocarditis: Prevention of rheumatic fever. Circulation *55*:1, 1977.
166. Guthe, T., Idsoe, O., and Willcox, R. R.: Untoward penicillin reactions. Bull. WHO *19*:427, 1958.
167. Feinstein, A. R., Wood, H. F., Spagnuolo, M., Taranta, A., Tursky, E., and Kleinberg, E.: Oral prophylaxis of recurrent rheumatic fever: Sulfadiazine vs. a double daily dose of penicillin. J.A.M.A. *188*:489, 1964.
168. Stahlman, M. T., and Denny, F. W., Jr.: The prophylaxis of streptococcal infection in patients with rheumatic fever: A comparison between sulfadiazine and erythromycin. Am. J. Dis. Child. *98*:66, 1959.
169. Wannamaker, L. W., Rammelkamp, C. H., Jr., Denny, F. W., Brink, W. R., Houser, H. B., Hahn, E. O., and Dingle, J. H.: Prophylaxis of acute rheumatic fever by treatment of the preceding streptococcal infection with various amounts of depot penicillin. Am. J. Med. *10*:673, 1951.
170. Wannamaker, L. W., Denny, F. W., Perry, W. D., Rammelkamp, C. H., Jr., Eckhardt, G. C., Houser, H. B., and Hahn, E. O.: The effect of penicillin prophylaxis on streptococcal disease rates and the carrier state. N. Engl. J. Med. *249*:1, 1953.
171. Bernstein, S. H., Feldman, H. A., Harper, O. F., and Klingensmith, W. H.: Mass oral penicillin prophylaxis in control of streptococcal disease. Arch. Intern. Med. *93*:894, 1954.
172. Morris, A. J., and Rammelkamp, C. H., Jr.: Benzathine penicillin G in the prevention of streptococci infections. J.A.M.A. *165*:664, 1957.
173. Davis, J., and Schmidt, W. C.: Benzathine penicillin G. Its effectiveness in the prevention of streptococcal infections in a heavily exposed population. N. Engl. J. Med. *256*:339, 1957.
174. Beachey, E. H., Stollerman, G. H., Johnson, R. H., et al.: Human immune response to immunization with a structurally defined polypeptide fragment of streptococcal M protein. J. Exp. Med. *150*:862, 179.
175. Hasty, D. L., Beachey, E. H., Simpson, W. A., et al.: Hybridoma antibodies against protective and nonprotective antigenic determinants of a structurally defined polypeptide fragment of streptococcal M protein. J. Exp. Med. *155*: 1010, 1982.
176. Land, M. A., and Bisno, A. L. Acute rheumatic fever. A vanishing disease in suburbia. J.A.M.A. *249*:895, 1983.
177. Moll, J. M. H., Haslock, I., Macrae, I. F., and Wright, V.: Associations between ankylosing spondylitis, psoriatic arthritis, Reiter's disease, the intestinal arthropathies, and Behçet's syndrome. Medicine *53*:343, 1974.
178. Bluestone, R., and Pearson, C. M.: Ankylosing spondylitis and Reiter's syndrome: Their interrelationships and association with HLA B27. Adv. Intern. Med. *22*:1, 1977.
179. Khan, M. A., and Khan, M. K.: Diagnostic value of HLA-B27 testing in ankylosing spondylitis and Reiter's syndrome. Ann. Intern. Med. *96*:70, 1982.
180. Laitinen, O., Leirisalo, M., and Skylv, G.: Relation between HLA-B27 and clinical features in patients with Yersinia arthritis. Arthr. Rheum. *20*:1121, 1977.
181. Schachter, J.: Can chlamydial infections cause rheumatic disease? *In* Dumonde, D. C. (ed.): Infection and Immunology in Rheumatic Diseases. Oxford, Blackwell Scientific Publications, 1976, pp. 151–157.
182. Graham, D. C., and Smythe, H. A.: The carditis and aortitis of ankylosing spondylitis. Bull. Rheum. Dis. *9*:171, 1958.
183. Thomas, D., Hill, W., Geddes, R., Sheppard, M., Arnold, J., Fritzsche, J., and Brooks, P. M.: Early detection of aortic dilatation in ankylosing spondylitis using echocardiography. Aut. N.Z.J. Med. *12*:10, 1982.
184. Stewart, S. R., Robbins, D. L., and Castles, J. J.: Acute fulminant aortic and mitral insufficiency in ankylosing spondylitis. N. Engl. J. Med. *42*:901, 1978.
185. Roberts, W. C., Hollingsworth, J. F., Bulkley, B. H., Jaffe, R. B., Epstein, S. E., and Stinson, E. B.: Combined mitral and aortic regurgitation in ankylosing spondylitis. Angiographic and anatomic features. Am. J. Med. *56*:237, 1974.
186. Nitter-Hauge, S., and Otterstad, J. E.: Characteristics of atrioventricular conduction disturbances in ankylosing spondylitis (Mo. Bechterew). Acta Med. Scand. *210*:197, 200, 1981.
187. Bulkley, B. H., and Roberts, W. C.: Ankylosing spondylitis and aortic regurgitation. Description of the characteristic cardiovascular lesion from study of eight necropsy patients. Circulation *48*:1014, 1973.
188. Takkunen, J., Vuopala, U., and Isomaki, H.: Cardiomyopathy in ankylosing spondylitis. I. Medical history and results of clinical examination in a series of 55 patients. Ann. Clin. Res. *2*:106, 1970.
189. Cowan, G. O.: Aortic incompetence associated with ulcerative colitis and ankylosing spondylitis. Proc. Roy. Soc. Med. *63*:4, 1970.
190. Good, A. E.: Reiter's disease: A review with special attention to cardiovascular and neurologic sequelae. Semin. Arthr. Rheum. *3*:253, 1974.
191. Malette, W. G., Eiseman, B., Danielson, G. K., Mozzoleni, A., and Rams, J. J.: Rheumatoid spondylitis and aortic insufficiency. An operable combination. J. Thorac. Cardiovasc. Surg. *57*:471, 1969.
192. Sairanen, E., Paronen, I., and Mahonen, H.: Reiter's syndrome: A follow-up study. Acta Med. Scand. *185*:57, 1969.
193. Calin, A., and Fries, I. F.: An experimental epidemic of Reiter's syndrome revisited. Follow-up evidence on genetic and environmental factors. Ann. Intern. Med. *84*:564, 1976.
194. Cliff, J. M.: Spinal bony bridging and carditis in Reiter's disease. Ann. Rheum. Dis. *30*:171, 1971.
195. Rodnan, G. P., Benedek, T. G., Shaver, J. A., and Fennell, R. H., Jr.: Reiter's syndrome and aortic insufficiency. J.A.M.A. *189*:889, 1964.
196. Paulus, H. E., Pearson, C. M., and Pitts, W., Jr.: Aortic insufficiency in five patients with Reiter's syndrome: A detailed clinical and pathological study. Am. J. Med. *53*:464, 1972.
197. Collins, P.: Aortic incompetence and active myocarditis in Reiter's disease. Br. J. Vener. Dis. *48*:300, 1972.
198. Neu, L. T., Jr., Reider, R. A., and Mack, R. E.: Cardiac involvement in Reiter's disease: Report of a case with review of the literature. Ann. Intern. Med. *53*:215, 1960.
199. Arvastson, B., Damgaard, K., and Winblad, S.: Clinical symptoms of infection with *Yersinia enterocolitica*. Scand. J. Infect. Dis. *3*:37, 1971.
200. Ahvonen, P., Sievers, K., and Aho, K.: Arthritis associated with *Yersinia enterocolitica* infection. Acta Rheum. Scand. *15*:232, 1969.
201. Ahvonen, P., Hiisi-Brummer, L., and Aho, K.: Electrocardiographic abnormalities and arthritis in patients with *Yersinia enterocolitica* infection. Ann. Clin. Res. *3*:69, 1971.
202. Aho, K., Ahvonen, P., and Lassus, A.: HLA B27 in reactive arthritis. A study of Yersinia arthritis and Reiter's disease. Arthritis Rheum. *17*:521, 1974.
203. Hakansson, U., Eitrem, R., Löw, B., and Winblad, S. W.: HLA-antigen B27 in cases with joint affections in an outbreak in salmonellosis. Scand. J. Infect. Dis. *8*:245, 1976.
204. Cruickshank, B.: Heart lesions in rheumatoid disease. J. Pathol. Bacteriol. *76*: 223, 1958.
205. Lannigan, R.: Cardiac Pathology. London, Butterworth and Co., 1966.
206. Cathcart, E. S., and Spodick, D. H.: Rheumatoid heart disease. A study of the incidence and nature of cardiac lesions in rheumatoid arthritis. N. Engl. J. Med. *266*:959, 1962.
207. Bonfiglio, T., and Ativater, E. C.: Heart disease in patients with seropositive rheumatoid arthritis. A controlled autopsy study and review. Arch. Intern. Med. *124*:714, 1969.
208. Lebowitz, W. B.: The heart in rheumatoid arthritis (rheumatoid disease). A clinical and pathological study of sixty-two cases. Ann. Intern. Med. *58*:102, 1963.
209. Khan, A. H., Spodick, D. H.: Rheumatoid heart disease. Semin. Arthritis Rheum. *1*:327, 1972.
210. Butman, S., Espinoza, L. R., Del Carpio, J., and Osterland, C. K.: Rheumatoid pericarditis. Rapid deterioration with evidence of local vasculitis. J.A.M.A. *238*:2394, 1977.
211. Liss, J. P., and Bachmann, W. T.: Rheumatoid constrictive pericarditis, treated by pericardiectomy. Report of a case and review of the literature. Arthritis Rheum. *13*:869, 1970.
212. Bacon, P. A., and Gibson, D. G.: Cardiac involvement in rheumatoid arthritis. An echocardiographic study. Ann. Rheum. Dis. *33*:20, 1974.
213. MacDonald, W. J., Jr., Crawford, M. H., Klippel, J. H., Zvaifler, N. J., and O'Rourke, R. A.: Echocardiographic assessment of cardiac structure and function in patients with rheumatoid arthritis. Am. J. Med. *63*:890, 1977.
214. Roberts, W. C., Kehoe, J. A., and Carpenter, D. F.: Cardiac valvular lesions in rheumatoid arthritis. Arch. Intern. Med. *122*:141, 1968.
215. Kindred, L. H., Heilbrun, A., and Dunn, M.: Cholesterol pericarditis associated with rheumatoid arthritis. Treatment by pericardiectomy. Am. J. Cardiol. *23*:464, 1969.
216. Linch, D. C., Gillmer, D. J., Whimster, W. F., and Keates, J. R. W.: Rheumatoid aortic valve prolapse requiring emergency valve replacement. Br. Heart J. *43*:237, 1980.
217. Reed, W. P., and Williams, R. C.: Immune complexes in infectious diseases. Adv. Intern. Med. *22*:49, 1977.
218. Oldstone, M. B. A., and Dixon, F. J.: Immune complex disease in chronic viral infections. J. Exp. Med. *134*(Suppl.):32S, 1971.
219. Christian, C. L.: Systemic lupus erythematosus and type C RNA viruses (editorial). N. Engl. J. Med. *295*:501, 1976.
220. Agnello, V.: Complement deficiency states. Medicine *57*:1, 1978.
221. Lee, S. L., and Chase, P. H.: Drug-induced systemic lupus erythematosus: A critical review. Semin. Arthritis Rheum. *5*:83, 1975.
222. Stevens, M. B.: Procainamide-induced lupus. Johns Hopkins Med. J. *138*:289, 1976.
223. Levo, Y., Pick, A. I., Avidor, I., and Ben-Bassat, M.: Clinicopathological study of a patient with procainamide-induced systemic lupus erythematosus. Ann. Rheum. Dis. *35*:181, 1976.
224. Das, S. K., and Cassidy, J. T.: Antiheart antibodies in patients with systemic lupus erythematosus. Am. J. Med. Sci. *265*:275, 1973.
225. Klemperer, P., Pollack, A., and Baehr, G.: Pathology of disseminated lupus erythematosus. Arch. Pathol. *32*:569, 1941.
225a. Liberthson, R. R., Homcy, C., Fallon, J. T., Gross, S., Leppo, J., and Miller, L.: Systemic lupus erythematosus and heart disease. Primary Cardiol. *9*:77, 1983.
226. Gross, L.: Cardiac lesions in Libman-Sacks disease with consideration of its relationship to acute diffuse lupus erythematosus. Am. J. Pathol. *16*:375, 1940.
227. Harvey, A. M., Shulman, L. E., Tumulty, P. A., Conley, C. L., and Schoenrich, E. H.: Systemic lupus erythematosus: A review of the literature and clinical analyses of 138 cases. Medicine *33*:291, 1954.
228. Hejtmancik, M. R., Wright, J. C., Quint, R., and Jennings, F.: The cardiovascular manifestations of systemic lupus erythematosus. Am. Heart J. *68*:119, 1964.
229. Dubois, E. L.: Lupus Erythematosus; A Review of the Current Status of Discoid and Systemic Lupus Erythematosus and Their Variants. 2nd ed. Los Angeles, University of Southern California Press, 1974.
230. Brigden, W., Bywaters, E. G., Lessof, M. H., and Ross, I. P.: The heart in systemic lupus erythematosus. Br. Heart J. *22*:1, 1960.

231. Kong, T. Q., Kellum, R. E., and Haserick, J. R.: Clinical diagnosis of cardiac involvement in systemic lupus erythematosus. A correlation of clinical and autopsy findings in thirty patients. Circulation *26*:7, 1962.
232. James, T. N., Rupe, C. E., and Monto, R. W.: Pathology of the cardiac conduction system in systemic lupus erythematosus. Ann. Intern. Med. *63*: 402, 1965.
233. Ito, K., Yokoyama, N., Hashida, J., Kajiwara, N., and Okada, R.: A case of lupus erythematosus with arrhythmias. A complete morphological study of the conduction system. Jpn. Heart J. *15*:92, 1974.
234. Bharati, S., de la Fuente, D. J., Kallen, R. J., Freij, Y., and Lev, M.: Conduction system in systemic lupus erythematosus with atrioventricular block. Am. J. Cardiol. *35*:299, 1975.
235. Wray, R., and Iveson, M.: Complete heart block and systemic lupus erythematosus. Br. Heart J. *37*:982, 1975.
236. Sunder, S. K., and Shah, A.: Constrictive pericarditis in procainamide-induced lupus erythematosus syndrome. Am. J. Cardiol. *36*:960, 1975.
237. Ghose, M. K.: Pericardial tamponade. A presenting manifestation of procainamide-induced lupus erythematosus. Am. J. Med. *58*:581, 1975.
238. Elkayam, U., Weiss, S., and Laniado, S.: Pericardial effusion and mitral valve involvement in systemic lupus erythematosus: Echocardiographic study. Ann. Rheum. Dis. *36*:349, 1977.
239. Bonfiglio, T. A., Botti, R. E., and Hagstrom, J. W.: Coronary arteritis, occlusion and myocardial infarction due to lupus erythematosus. Am. Heart J. *83*: 153, 1972.
240. Benisch, B. M., and Pervez, N.: Coronary artery vasculitis and myocardial infarction with systemic lupus erythematosus. N.Y. State J. Med. *74*:873, 1974.
241. Bulkley, B. H., and Roberts, W. C.: The heart in systemic lupus erythematosus and the changes induced in it by corticosteroid therapy: A study of 36 necropsy patients. Am. J. Med. *58*:243, 1975.
242. del Rio, A., Vázquez, J. J., Sobrino, J. A., Gil, A., Barbado, J., Maté, I., and Ortiz-Vázquez, J.: Myocardial involvement in systemic lupus erythematosus: A noninvasive study of left ventricular function. Chest *74*:414, 1978.
243. Libman, E., and Sacks, B.: A hitherto undescribed form of valvular and mitral endocarditis. Arch. Intern. Med. *33*:701, 1924.
244. Rawsthorne, L., Ptacin, M. J., Choi, H., Olinger, G. N., and Bamrah, V. S.: Lupus valvulitis necessitating double valve replacement. Arthritis Rheum. *24*: 561, 1981.
245. Paget, S. A., Bulkley, B. H., Grauer, L. E., and Seningen, R.: Mitral valve disease os sytemic lupus erythematosus. A cause of severe congestive heart failure reversed by valve replacement. Am. J. Med. *59*:134, 1975.
246. McCue, C. M., Mantakus, M. E., Tingelstad, J. B., and Ruddy, S.: Congenital heart block in newborns of mothers with connective tissue disease. Circulation *56*:82, 1977.
247. Doshi, N., Smith, B., and Klionsky, B.: Congenital pericarditis due to maternal lupus erythematosus. J. Pediatr. *96*:699, 1980.
248. Maniscalco, B. S., Felner, J. M., McCans, J. L., and Chiapella, J. A.: Echocadiographic abnormalities in systemic lupus erythematosus. Circulation *52*(Suppl. 2):211, 1975.
249. Strauer, B. E., Brune, I., Schenk, H., Knoll, D., and Perings, E.: Lupus cardiomyopathy: Cardiac mechanics, hemodynamics, and coronary blood flow in uncomplicated systemic lupus erythematosus. Am. Heart J. *92*:715, 1976.
250. Zeek, P. M.: Periarteritis nodosa and other forms of necrotizing angiitis. N. Engl. J. Med. *148*:764, 1953.
251. Holsinger, D. R., Osmundsen, P. J., and Edwards, J. E.: The heart in periarteritis nodosa. Circulation *25*:610, 1962.
252. Griffith, G. C., and Vural, I. L.: Polyarteritis nodosa: Correlation of clinical and postmortem findings in 17 cases. Circulation *3*:481, 1951.
253. Kawasaki, T., Kosaki, F., Okawa, S., Shigematsu, I., and Yanagawa, H.: A new infantile acute febrile mucocutaneous lymph node syndrome (MLNS) prevailing in Japan. Pediatrics *54*:271, 1974.
254. Onouchi, Z., Tomizawa, N., Goto, M., Nakata, K., Fukuda, M., and Goto, M.: Cardiac involvement and prognosis in acute mucocutaneous lymph node syndrome. Chest *68*:297, 1975.
255. Landing, B. H., and Larson, E. J.: Are infantile periarteritis nodosa with coronary artery involvement and fatal mucocutaneous lymph node syndrome the same? Comparison of 20 patients from North America with patients from Hawaii and Japan. Pediatrics *59*:651, 1977.
256. Duffy, J., Lidsky, M. D., Sharp, J. T., Davis, J. S., Person, D. A., Hollinger, F. B., and Kyung-Whan, M.: Polyarthritis, polyarteritis and hepatitis B. Medicine *55*:19, 1976.
257. Michalak, T.: Immune complexes of hepatitis B surface antigen in the pathogenesis of periarteritis nodosa. A study of seven necropsy cases. Am. J. Pathol. *90*:619, 1978.
258. Doherty, M., and Bradfield, J. W.: Polyarteritis nodosa associated with acute cytomegalovirus infection. Ann. Rheum. Dis. *40*:419, 1981.
259. Frayha, R. A.: Trichinosis-related polyarteritis nodosa. Am. J. Med. *71*:307, 1981.
260. Cupps, T. R., and Fauci, A. S.: The vasculitis syndromes. Adv. Intern. Med. *27*:315, 1982.
261. Novack, S. N., and Pearson, C. M.: Cyclophosphamide therapy in Wegener's granulomatosis. N. Engl. J. Med. *284*:938, 1971.
262. Forstot, J. Z., Overlie, P. A., Neufeld, G. K., Harmon, C. E., and Forstot, S. L.: Cardiac complications of Wegener Granulomatosis: A case report of complete heart block and review of the literature. Semin. Arthritis Rheum. *10*: 148, 1980.
263. Sams, W. M., Jr., Claman, H. N., and Kohler, P. F.: Human necrotizing vasculitis: Immunoglobulins and complement in vessel walls of cutaneous lesions and normal skin. J. Invest. Derm. *64*:441, 1975.
264. Huston, K. A., and Hunder, G. G.: Giant cell (cranial) arteritis: A clinical review. Am. Heart J. *100*:99, 1980.
265. Klein, R. G., Hunder, G. G., Stanson, A. W., and Sheps, S. G.: Large artery involvement in giant cell (temporal) arteritis. Ann. Intern. Med. *83*:806, 1975.
266. Bacon, P. A., Doherty, S. M., and Zuckerman, A. J.: Hepatitis-B antibody in polymyalgia rheumatica. Lancet *2*:476, 1975.
267. Campbell, P. M., and LeRoy, E. C.: Pathogenesis of systemic sclerosis: A vascular hypothesis. Semin. Arthritis Rheum. *4*:351, 1975.
268. Masi, A. T., and Rodnan, G. P.: Preliminary criteria for the classification of systemic sclerosis (scleroderma). Bull. Rheum. Dis. *31*:1, 1981.
269. Botstein, G. R., and LeRoy, E. C.: Primary heart disease in systemic sclerosis (scleroderma): Advances in clinical and pathologic features, pathogenesis, and new therapeutic approaches. Am. Heart J. *102*:913, 1981.
270. Norton, W. L., and Nardo, J. M.: Vascular disease in progressive systemic sclerosis (scleroderma). Ann. Intern. Med. *73*:317, 1970.
271. Norton, W. L., Hurd, E. R., Lewis, D. C., and Ziff, M.: Evidence of microvascular injury in scleroderma and systemic lupus erythematosus: Quantitative study of the microvascular bed. J. Lab. Clin. Med. *71*:919, 1968.
272. Weiss, S., Stead, E., Warren, J., and Bailey, O.: Scleroderma heart disease. Arch. Intern. Med. *71*:749, 1943.
273. Oram, S., and Stokes, W.: The heart in scleroderma. Br. Heart J. *23*:243, 1961.
274. Medsger, T. A., Jr., Masi, A. T., Rodnan, G. P., Benedek, T. G., and Robinson, H.: Survival with systemic sclerosis (scleroderma). A life-table analysis of clinical and demographic factors in 309 patients. Ann. Intern. Med. *75*:369, 1971.
275. Bulkley, B. H., Ridolfi, R. L., Salyer, W. R., and Hutchins, G.: Myocardial lesions of progressive systemic sclerosis. A cause of cardiac dysfunction. Circulation *53*:483, 1976.
276. D'Angelo, W. A., Fries, J. F., Masi, A. T., and Shulman, L. E.: Pathologic observations in systemic sclerosis (scleroderma). A study of 58 autopsy cases and 58 matched controls. Am. J. Med. *46*:428, 1969.
277. James T. N.: De subitaneis mortibus. VIII. Coronary arteries and conduction system in scleroderma heart disease. Circulation *50*:844, 1974.
278. Roberts, N. K., Cabeen, W. R., Jr., Moss, J., Clements, P. J., and Furst, D. E.: The prevalence of conduction defects and cardiac arrhythmias in progressive systemic sclerosis. Ann. Intern. Med. *94*:38, 1981.
279. McWhorter, J. E., and LeRoy, E. C.: Pericardial disease in scleroderma (systemic sclerosis). Am. J. Med. *57*:566, 1974.
280. Gladman, D. D., Gordon, D. A., Urowitz, M. B., and Levy, H. L.: Pericardial fluid analysis in scleroderma (systemic sclerosis). Am. J. Med. *60*:1064, 1976.
281. Medsger, T. A., Jr., and Masi, A. T.: Survival with scleroderma. II. A life-table analysis of clinical and demographic factors in 358 male U.S. veteran patients. J. Chron. Dis. *26*:647, 1973.
282. Gupta, M. P., Zoneraich, S., Zeitlin, W., Zoneraich, O., and D'Angelo, W. A.: Scleroderma heart disease with slow flow velocity in coronary arteries. Chest *67*:116, 1975.
283. Ridolfi, R. L., Bulkley, B. H., and Hutchins, G. M.: The cardiac conduction system in progressive systemic sclerosis. Clinical and pathologic features of 35 patients. Am. J. Med. *61*:361, 1976.
284. Escudero, A., and McDevitt, E.: The electrocardiogram in scleroderma: Analysis of 60 cases and reviews of the literature. Am. Heart J. *56*:846, 1958.
285. Eggebrecht, R. F., and Kleiger, R. E.: Echocardiographic patterns in scleroderma. Chest *71*:47, 1977.
286. Smith, J. W., Clements, P. J., Levisman, J., Furst, D., and Ross, M.: Echocardiographic features of progressive systemic sclerosis (PSS). Correlation with hemodynamic and postmortem studies. Am. J. Med. *66*:28, 1979.
287. Whitman, H. H., Case, D. B., Laragh, J. H., Christian, C. C., Botstein, G., Marica, H., and Leroy, E. C.: Variable response to oral angiotensin-converting enzyme blocade in hypertensive scleroderma patients. Arthritis Rheum. *25*: 241, 1982.
288. Adams, R. D.: The pathological substratum of polymyositis. *In* Pearson, C. M., and Mostofi, F. K. (eds.): The Striated Muscle. Baltimore, Williams and Wilkins, 1973, p. 292.
289. Bohan, A., and Peter, J. B.: Polymyositis and dermatomyositis. N. Engl. J. Med. *292*:344 and 403, 1975.
290. Bohan, A., Peter, J. B., and Bowman, R. L., and Pearson, C. M.: A computer assisted analysis of 153 patients with polymyositis and dermatomyositis. Medicine *56*:255, 1977.
291. Bunch, T. W., Tancredi, R. G., and Lie, J. T.: Pulmonary hypertension in polymyositis. Chest *79*:105, 1981.
292. Singsen, B., Goldreyer, B., Stanton, R., and Hanson, V.: Childhood polymyositis with cardiac conduction defects. Am. J. Dis. Child. *130*:72, 1976.
293. Medsger, T. A., Jr., Robinson, H., and Masi, A. T.: Factors affecting survivorship in polymyositis. A life-table study of 124 patients. Arthritis Rheum. *14*: 249, 1971.
294. Norton, W. L., Velayos, E., and Robison, L.: Endothelial inclusions in dermatomyositis. Ann. Rheum. Dis. *29*:67, 1970.
295. Barnard, B. G., Rankin, A. M., and Robertson, J. H.: Polymyositis: Report on 3 cases from West Africa. Br. Med. J. *1*:1473, 1960.
296. Hill, D. L., and Barrows, H. S.: Identical skeletal and cardiac muscle involvement in a case of fatal polymyositis. Arch. Neurol. *19*:545, 1968.
297. Schaumburg, H. H., Melsen, S. L., and Yurchak, P. M.: Heart block in polymyositis. N. Engl. J. Med. *284*:480, 1971.
298. Lynch, P. G.: Cardiac involvement in chronic polymyositis. Br. Heart J. *33*: 416, 1971.

299. Lightfoot, P. R., Bharati, S., and Lev, M.: Chronic dermatomyositis with intermittent trifascicular block. An electrophysiologic conduction system correlation. Chest *71*:413, 1977.
300. Oppenheim, H.: Zur Dermatomyositis. Berlin. Klin. Wochenschr. *36*:805, 1899.
301. Sheard, C., Jr.: Dermatomyositis. Arch. Inter. Med. *88*:640, 1951.
302. Garcin, R., Lapresle, J., Gruner, J., and Scherrer, J.: Les polymyosites. Rev. Neurol. *92*:465, 1955.
303. Oka, M., and Raasakka, T.: Cardiac involvement in polymyositis. Scand J. Rheumatol. *7*:203, 1978.
304. Reid, J. M., and Murdoch, R.: Polymyositis and complete heart block. Br. Heart J. *41*:628, 1979.
305. McKusick, V. A.: Heritable Disorders of Connective Tissue. 4th ed. St. Louis, The C. V. Mosby Co., 1972.
305a. Pyeritz, R. E., and McKusick, V. A.: Basic defects in the Marfan syndrome. N. Engl. J. Med. *305*:1101, 1981.
306. Uitto, J., and Lichtenstein, J. R.: Defects in the biochemistry of collagen in diseases of connective tissue. J. Invest. Dermatol. *66*:59, 1976.
307. Roberts, W. C., and Honig, H. S.: The spectrum of cardiovascular disease in the Marfan syndrome: A clinico-morphologic study of 18 necropsy patients and comparison to 151 previously reported necropsy patients. Am. Heart J. *104*:115, 1982.
308. Chapman, D. W., Beazley, H. L., Petersen, P. K., et al.: Annulo-aortic ectasia with cystic medial necrosis. Diagnosis and surgical treatment. Am. J. Cardiol. *16*:679, 1965.
309. Bowers, D.: Pathogenesis of primary abnormalities of the mitral valve in the Marfan's syndrome. Br. Heart J. *31*:679, 1969.
309a. Missri, J. C., and Swett, D. D., Jr.: Marfan syndrome: A review Cardiovasc. Rev. Rep. *3*:1645, 1982.
310. James, T. N., Frame, B., and Schatz, I. J.: Pathology of cardiac conduction system in Marfan's syndrome. Arch. Intern. Med. *114*:339, 1964.
311. Murdoch, J. L., Walker, B. A., and Halpern, B. I., Kuzma, J. W., and McKusick, V. A.: Life expectancy and causes of death in the Marfan syndrome. N. Engl. J. Med. *286*:804, 1972.
312. Phornphutkul, C., Rosenthal, A., and Nadas, A.: Cardiac manifestation of Marfan syndrome in infancy and childhood. Circulation *47*:587, 1973.
313. Simpson, J. W., Nora, J. J., and McNamara, D. G.: Marfan syndrome and mitral valve disease: Acute surgical emergencies. Am. Heart J. *77*:96, 1969.
314. Nelson, R. M., and Vaughn, C. C.: Double valve replacement in Marfan's syndrome. J. Thorac. Cardiovasc. Surg. *57*:732, 1969.
314a. Pyeritz, R. E., and Wappel, M. A.: Mitral valve dysfunction in the Marfan syndrome. Clinical and echocardiographic study of prevalence and natural history. Am. J. Med. *74*:797, 1983.
315. Spangler, R. D., Nora, J. J., Lortscher, R. H., Wolfe, R. W., and Okin, J. T.: Echocardiography in Marfan's syndrome. Chest *69*:72, 1976.
316. Wunsch, C. M., Steinmetz, E. F., and Fisch, C.: Marfan's syndrome and subacute bacterial endocarditis. Am. J. Cardiol. *15*:102, 1965.
317. Dowling, J. N., Lee, W. S., Sacco, R. J., and Ho, H.: Endocarditis caused by Neisseria mucosa in Marfan syndrome. Ann. Intern. Med. *18*:641, 1974.
318. Prokop, E. K., Palmer, R. F., and Wheat, M. W., Jr.: Hydrodynamic forces in dissecting aneurysms. In-vitro studies in a Tygon model and in dog aortas. Circ. Res. *27*:121, 1970.
319. Halpern, B. L., Char, F., and Murdoch, J. L.: A prospectus on the prevention of aortic rupture in the Marfan syndrome with data on the survivorship without treatment. Johns Hopkins Med. J. *129*:123, 1971.
320. Symbas, P. N., Baldwin, B. J., and Silvermin, M. E.: Marfan's syndrome with aneurysms of ascending aorta and aortic regurgitation: Surgical treatment and new histochemical observations. Am. J. Cardiol. *25*:483, 1970.
321. Symbas, P. N., Raizner, A. E., and Tyras, D. A.: Aneurysms of all sinuses of Valsalva in patients with Marfan's syndrome: An unusual late complication following replacement of aortic valve and ascending aorta for aortic regurgitation and fusiform aneurysm of ascending aorta. Ann. Surg. *174*:902, 1971.
322. Hirst, A. E., and Gore, I.: Marfan's syndrome: A review. Prog. Cardiovasc. Dis. *16*:187, 1973.
323. Donaldson, R. M., Olsen, E. G. J., Emanuel, R. W., and Ross, D. N.: Management of cardiovascular complications in Marfan syndrome. Lancet *2*: 1178, 1980.
324. Remigio, P. A., and Grinvalsky, H. J.: Osteogenesis imperfecta congenita. Association with conspicuous extraskeletal connective tissue dysplasia. Am. J. Dis. Child. *119*:524, 1970.
325. Criscitello, M. G., Ronan, J. A., Jr., Besterman, E. M., and Schoenwetter, W.: Cardiovascular abnormalities in osteogenesis imperfecta. Circulation *31*:255, 1965.
326. Heppner, R., Babitt, H., Bianchine, J., and Warbasse, R.: Aortic regurgitation and aneurysm of sinus of Valsalva associated with osteogenesis imperfecta. Am. J. Cardiol. *31*:654, 1973.
327. Weisinger, B., Glassman, E., Spencer, F., and Bergner, A.: Successful aortic valve replacement for aortic regurgitation associated with osteogenesis imperfecta. Br. Heart J. *37*:475, 1975.
328. Wood, S. J., Thomas, J., and Braimbridge, M. V.: Mitral valve disease and open heart surgery in osteogenesis imperfecta tarda. Br. Heart J. *35*:103, 1973.
329. Madison, W. M., Bradley, E., and Castillo, A.: Ehlers-Danlos syndrome with cardiac involvement. Am. J. Cardiol. *11*:689, 1963.
330. McFarland, W., and Fuller, D.: Mortality in Ehlers-Danlos syndrome due to spontaneous rupture of large arteries. N. Engl. J. Med. *271*:1309, 1964.
331. Edmondson, P., Nellen, M., and Ross, D. N.: Aortic valve replacement in a case of Ehlers-Danlos syndrome. Br. Heart J. *42*:103, 1979.
332. Cupo, L. N., Pyeritz, R. E., Olson, J. L., McPhee, S. J., Hutchins, G. M., and McKusick, V. A.: Ehlers-Danlos syndrome with abnormal collagen fibrils, sinus of Valsalva aneurysms, myocardial infarction, panacinar emphysema and cerebral heterotopias. Am. J. Med. *72*:1051, 1981.
333. Antani, J., and Srinivas, H. V.: Ehlers-Danlos syndrome and cardiovascular abnormalities. Chest *63*:214, 1973.
334. Jaffe, A. S., Geltman, E. M., Rodey, G. E., and Vitto, J.: A consistent manifestation of type IV Ehlers-Danlos syndrome. The pathogenetic role of the abnormal production of type III collagen. Circulation *64*:121, 1981.
335. Come, P. C., Fortuin, N. J., White, R. K. Jr., and McKusick, V.A.: Echocardiographic assessment of cardiovascular abnormalities in the Marfan syndrome. Comparison with clinical findings and with roentgenographic estimation of aortic root size. Am. J. Med. *74*:465, 1983.
336. Pope, F. M.: Two types of autosomal recessive pseudoxanthoma elasticum. Arch. Dermatol. *110*:209, 1974.
337. Pope, F. M.: Two types of autosomal dominant pseudoxanthoma elasticum. J. Med. Genet. *11*:152, 1974.
338. Mendelsohn, G., Bulkley, B. H., and Hutchins, G. M.: Cardiovascular manifestations of pseudoxanthoma elasticum. Arch. Pathol. Lab. Med. *102*: 298, 1978.
339. Akhtar, M., and Brody, H.: Elastic tissue in pseudoxanthoma elasticum: Ultrastructural study of endocardial lesions. Arch. Pathol. *99*:667, 1975.
340. Huang, S. N., Steel, H. D., and Kumar, G.: Ultrastructural changes of elastic fibers in pseudoxanthoma elasticum: A study of histogenesis. Arch. Pathol. *83*: 108, 1967.
341. Lebwohl, M. G., Distefano, D., Prioleau, P. G., Uram, M., Yannuzi, L. A., and Fleischmajer, R.: Pseudoxanthoma elasticum and mitral valve prolapse. N. Engl. J. Med. *307*:228, 1982.
342. Bete, J., Banas, J., Jr., Moran, J., Pinn, V., and Levine, H. J.: Coronary artery disease in an 18-year-old girl with pseudoxanthoma elasticum: Successful surgical therapy. Am. J. Cardiol. *36*:515, 1975.
343. Eddy, D. D., and Farber, E. M.: Pseudoxanthoma elasticum: Internal manifestations. A report of cases and a statistical review of the literature. Arch. Dermatol. *86*:729, 1962.
344. Schachner, L., and Young, D.: Pseudoxanthoma elasticum with severe cardiovascular disease in a child. Am. J. Dis. Child. *127*:571, 1974.
345. Navarro-Lopez, F., Llorian, A., Ferrer-Roca, O., Betriu, A., and Sanz, G.: Restrictive cardiomyopathy in pseudoxanthoma elasticum. Chest *78*:113, 1980.
346. Coffman, J. D., and Sommers, S.: Familial pseudoxanthoma elasticum and valvular heart disease. Circulation *19*:242, 1959.
347. Renteria, V. G., and Ferrans, V. J.: Intracellular collagen fibrils in cardiac valves of patients with the Hurler syndrome. Lab. Invest. *34*:263, 1976.
348. Renteria, V. G., Ferrans, V. J., and Roberts, W. C.: The heart in the Hurler syndrome: Gross, histologic and ultrastructural observations in five necropsy cases. Am. J. Cardiol. *38*:487, 1976.
349. Okada, R., Rosenthal, I. M., Scaravelli, G., and Lev, M.: A histopathologic study of the heart in gargoylism. Arch. Pathol. *84*:20, 1967.
350. Krovetz, L. J., Lorincz, A. E., and Schiebler, G. L.: Cardiovascular manifestations of the Hurler syndrome: Hemodynamic and angiocardiographic observations in 15 patients. Circulation *31*:132, 1965.
351. Factor, S. M., Biempica, L., and Goldfischer, S.: Coronary intimal sclerosis in Morquio's syndrome. Virchows Arch. *379*:1, 1978.
352. Brosius, F. C., III, and Roberts, W. C.: Coronary artery disease in the Hurler syndrome. Qualitative and quantitative analysis of the extent of coronary narrowing at necropsy in six children. Am. J. Cardiol. *47*:649, 1981.
353. Johnson, G. L., Vine, D. L., Cottrill, C. M., and Noonan, J. A.: Echocardiographic mitral valve deformity in mucopolysaccharidosis. Pediatrics *67*:401, 1981.

49 HEMATOLOGIC-ONCOLOGIC DISORDERS AND HEART DISEASE

by David S. Rosenthal, M.D., Robert I. Handin, M.D., and Eugene Braunwald, M.D.

During the past two decades, the increased frequency of cardiovascular abnormalities in patients with hematologic and neoplastic disorders, as well as of hematologic disorders in patients treated for a variety of cardiovascular diseases, has led to more frequent interaction between these two specialties. Hematologist-oncologists frequently require the consultation of cardiologists for clinical problems ranging from the interpretation of abnormal physical, electrocardiographic, and echocardiographic changes in patients with neoplastic hematologic disorders to advise about the treatment of heart failure, pericardial effusion, or other cardiac complications that are frequent in patients with anemia and hematologic malignancies. Conversely, hematologic complications occur quite frequently in cardiac patients. Blood dyscrasias are rather common complications of cardiac medications, prosthetic heart valves, and cardiovascular surgery. The convergence of interests between these fields inspired an innovative monograph devoted to the hematologic complications of cardiac disorders.[1]

ANEMIA AND CARDIOVASCULAR DISORDERS

Anemia is one of the most common causes of increased cardiac output, sometimes resulting in high output failure. As discussed in Chapter 24, the combination of tissue hypoxia and reduced blood viscosity leads to decreased systemic vascular resistance, which is associated with an increase in cardiac output.[1-3] Acutely induced anemia reduces coronary vascular resistance (Fig. 24–2, p. 810), while chronic anemia enhances the growth of intercoronary collaterals.[4] All signs and symptoms of cardiovascular disease usually disappear when the hemoglobin concentration is restored to normal. The gradual development of anemia may lead to cardiac hypertrophy[3] and in experimental animals has been associated with high catecholamine levels in plasma and urine but decreased levels in myocardial tissue.[5]

CARDIAC SYMPTOMS OF ANEMIA. The symptoms of reduced cardiac reserve, fatigue, exertional dyspnea, and edema depend on the severity of the anemia and the presence of an underlying cardiovascular disorder such as myocardial or valvular heart disease. Castle and Minot[6] showed that severely anemic patients without heart disease have few if any symptoms. When hemoglobin values decline below 7 gm/dl, resting cardiac output increases.[2,7-9] There is general agreement that symptoms depend not only on the severity of the anemia but also on (1) the rapidity with which it develops, (2) the physical activity of the patient, and (3) the coexistence of underlying cardiac or coronary artery pathology. For example, in the presence of coronary artery disease, anemia lowers the threshold for development of angina pectoris, so that patients with mild anemia may have an increased frequency of anginal episodes. The following queries are usually posed by the clinician: (1) At what level does an individual become symptomatic with anemia? (2) Has the anemia developed acutely or chronically? (3) Are the cardiac symptoms due to the anemia alone or secondary to underlying heart disease? (4) Can the murmur and the electrocardiographic changes detected in the anemic patient be distinguished from those due to intrinsic cardiac disease?

If the anemia has developed gradually, patients with less than 7 gm Hb/dl may be able to compensate sufficiently to carry out all but the most strenuous activity. Although uncommon, severe congestive heart failure with pulmonary edema can occur solely on the basis of severe anemia (Hb less than 4 gm/dl in the absence of antecedent heart disease). It may be difficult to distinguish congestive heart failure secondary to chronic anemia from that related to myocardial infiltration with iron, i.e., to hemosiderosis resulting from multiple transfusions (p. 1682). However, the symptoms of reduced cardiac reserve secondary to anemia alone are usually relieved when the anemia is corrected and a normal red cell mass has been restored.

OXYGEN DISSOCIATION AND LEVELS OF 2,3-DIPHOSPHOGLYCERATE IN RED CELLS

To account for the circulatory adaptation that occurs in chronic anemia, it is important to realize that factors other than the hemoglobin concentration and blood flow play a role in the quantity of oxygen delivered to tissues. These include tissue oxygen tension and the position of the hemoglobin-oxygen dissociation curve (Fig. 49–1). Normally, 1 gm of hemoglobin binds 1.34 ml of O_2. With a hemoglobin concentration of 15 gm/dl, 100 ml of arterial blood contains 20 ml of O_2. As can be calculated from the hemoglobin-oxygen dissociation curve (Fig. 49–2), 100 ml of mixed venous blood having a pO_2 of 40 mm Hg will contain 15.5 ml of O_2. The difference, i.e., 4.5 ml of O_2 per 100 ml of arterial blood, would be available for delivery to tissues. If the body depended only upon the cardiac output to sustain oxygen delivery in the anemic state, blood flow would have to double in order to preserve tissue oxygenation when the hemoglobin declined from 15 to 7.5 gm/dl.

However, in most patients with anemia, the hemoglobin-oxygen dissociation curve is shifted to the right and more oxygen is released from hemoglobin as the pO_2 declines. The intracellular concentration of 2,3-diphosphoglycerate (2,3-DPG), which is known to vary in the red cells in a number of disease states,[10,11] profoundly affects the binding and release of oxygen by hemoglobin. Deoxygenated hemoglobin, which is more alkaline than oxyhemoglobin, stimulates increased production of 2,3-DPG, a by-product of glycolysis. As a consequence, the intraerythrocytic ratio of deoxy- to oxyhemoglobin serves as a critical regulator of 2,3-DPG concentration. For example, the decreased oxygen affinity seen in chronic anemia can be accounted for by this increase in red cell 2,3-DPG. As shown in Figure 49–1, at a normal arterial pO_2, arterial oxygen saturation remains high despite the reduction in oxygen affinity. However, at the lower

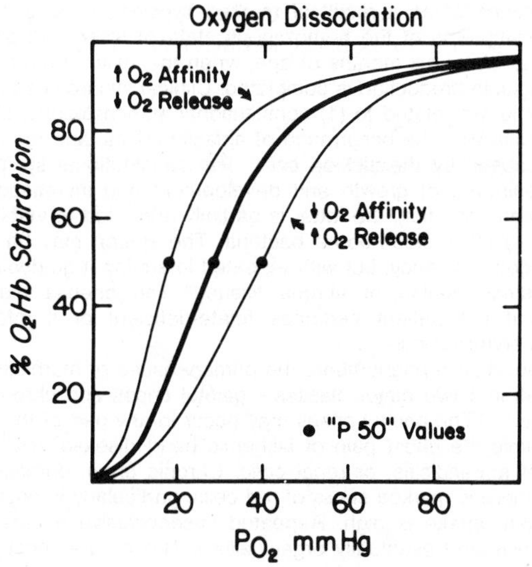

FIGURE 49–1 Oxygen dissociation curve of normal adult blood. P_{50} is the oxygen tension at 50 per cent oxygen saturation (normal = 27 mm Hg). With a shift to the right, oxygen affinity of hemoglobin decreases, releasing additional oxygen at a given tension. With a shift to the left, the opposite occurs. (From Oski, F.: The role of 2,3-DPG and oxygen delivery to tissues. *In* Jepson, J. H., and Frankl, W. (eds.): Haematological Complications in Cardiac Practice, Philadelphia, W. B. Saunders Co., 1975, p. 79.)

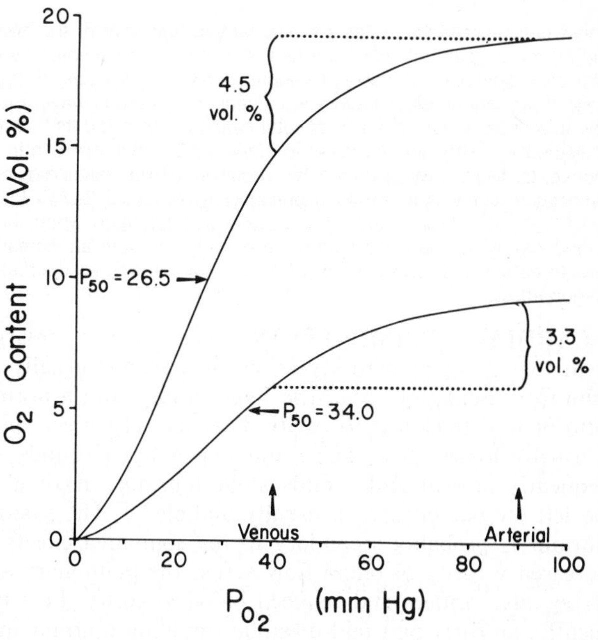

FIGURE 49–2 Enhancement of oxygen unloading by decreased red cell oxygen affinity in anemia with an increase in P_{50} from 26.5 to 34.0 (From Klocke, R. A.: Oxygen transport and 2,3-diphosphoglycerate. Chest *62*:795, 1972.)

pO_2 in the venous blood, elevated 2,3-DPG displaces the hemoglobin-oxygen dissociation curve to the right, enabling greater release of oxygen from the cells at any level of pO_2. Oski has calculated that decreased oxygen affinity mediated by increased red cell 2,3-DPG may compensate for up to half the oxygen deficit in anemia.[12] High levels of 2,3-DPG have also been found in subjects exposed to altitude[13] and in patients with pulmonary disease.[14]

The position of the oxygen-hemoglobin dissociation curve can be expressed by the P_{50}, i.e., the partial pressure of O_2 at which hemoglobin is 50 per cent saturated. A reduction of the oxygen affinity of hemoglobin, i.e., a shift to the right of the dissociation curve, is reflected in an elevation of the P_{50}. With a P_{50} of 34 mm Hg (instead of the normal P_{50} of 26.5 mm Hg), 3.3 ml of O_2 is unloaded per 100 ml of blood. As a consequence, an anemic individual with a 50 per cent reduction in red cell mass would suffer only a 27 per cent reduction in oxygen unloading (Fig. 49–2).

Figure 49–3 summarizes the factors responsible for oxygenation and response to hypoxia. Oxygen delivery to the metabolizing tissues depends directly on three principal factors: (1) blood flow, (2) hemo-

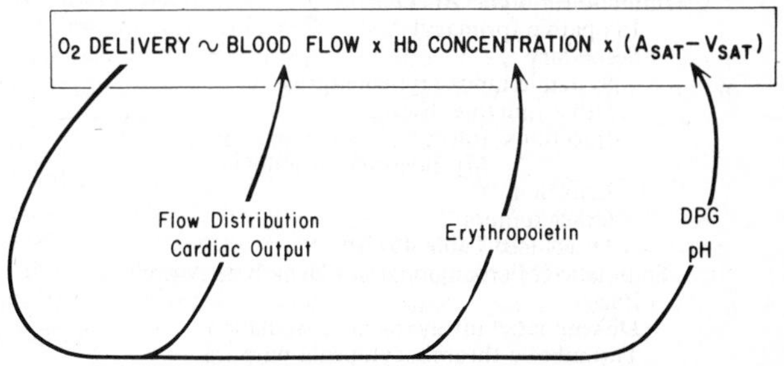

FIGURE 49–3 Oxygen delivery to an organ is directly proportional to (1) blood flow, (2) hemoglobin (Hb) concentration, and (3) the difference in oxygen saturation of the arterial and venous blood ($A_{sat} - V_{sat}$). Patients with various types of hypoxia may compensate in the following ways: (1) the distribution of blood flow may be altered to maintain oxygenation of vital organs; total cardiac output increases when hypoxia is severe; (2) increased erythropoietin production stimulates erythropoiesis; (3) oxygen unloading is enhanced by a shift to the right in the oxygen dissociation curve, mediated by red blood cell pH and 2,3-DPG. (From Bunn, H. F. in Petersdorf, R. L., et al. (eds.): *In* Harrison's Principles of Internal Medicine. 10th ed., McGraw-Hill Book Co., New York, 1983, p. 285.)

the cardiomegaly, iron overload of the heart is the most likely cause of myocardial damage.

Prior to the era of hypertransfusion and chelation therapy, patients with transfusion-dependent, chronic severe refractory thalassemia regularly manifested cardiac involvement, which was the most common cause of death, usually in the second decade of life. Congestive heart failure developed at an average age of 16 years. Death from heart failure occurred often within months. Occasional patients died suddenly, presumably of an arrhythmia. Intensive treatment of heart failure and antiarrhythmic therapy does not appear to have changed the natural history. At postmortem examination widespread iron deposition characteristic of hemochromatosis was found in all viscera, including the heart, which was hypertrophied and sometimes double the normal weight; it was stained a deep brown, with large amounts of iron in myocardial cells, demonstrated by staining with Prussian blue. The sinoatrial node is spared, but the A-V node is frequently involved. Cardiac dysfunction appeared to depend on the quantity of iron deposited in the ventricles. It has been suggested that myocardial damage results from iron-induced release of acid hydrolases from lysosomes.[14]

Pericarditis occurs in about half of all patients with thalassemia and is often recurrent and associated with fever, precordial pain and electrocardiographic changes characteristic of acute pericarditis[30] (p. 1474). Pericardial effusion is common; occasionally creation of a pericardial window is necessary for tamponade or recurrent pericardial effusion.

The electrocardiogram often shows left ventricular hypertrophy, nonspecific ST-T wave abnormalities, supraventricular or ventricular premature contractions, and first- or second-degree A-V block. The His bundle electrogram may show prolongation of the P-H interval, signifying an abnormality of conduction through the A-V node. The chest roentgenogram may show slight to moderate cardiac enlargement. The echocardiogram may disclose enlargement of left ventricular end-diastolic dimensions, left atrial and aortic root dimensions, and increased thickness of the left ventricular wall. A normal or elevated cardiac index with moderate elevations of the left ventricular end-diastolic pressure are the usual findings at cardiac catheterization. The ejection fraction may be reduced and the end-systolic volume increased.

There has been substantial interest in defining abnormalities of cardiac performance non-invasively in asymptomatic patients. Valdes-Cruz et al. have reported that in asymptomatic children with thalassemia major[36] the left ventricular posterior wall thinned more slowly than normal during diastole. Borow et al., utilizing a noninvasively determined index of left ventricular function that relates ventricular fractional shortening to end-systolic pressure (Fig. 14–15, p. 481, and Fig. 14–18, p. 482), identified preclinical left ventricular dysfunction (Fig. 49–5); this approach may be useful in the serial assessment of left ventricular contractility in response to chelation therapy (p. 1684).[37]

Supportive therapy, consisting primarily of an adequate transfusion program and even hypertransfusions, splenectomy, and early treatment of infections, has prolonged the life of patients with thalassemia. Roentgenographic evidence of cardiomegaly in children regresses with maintenance of the hemoglobin above 10 gm/dl.[35] Indeed, in one study, 4 of 7 patients with significant cardiomegaly had normal heart size one week after multiple transfusions had brought the hemoglobin level to near-normal levels. The use of chelating agents in both the treatment and prevention of iron overload is discussed on page 1684.

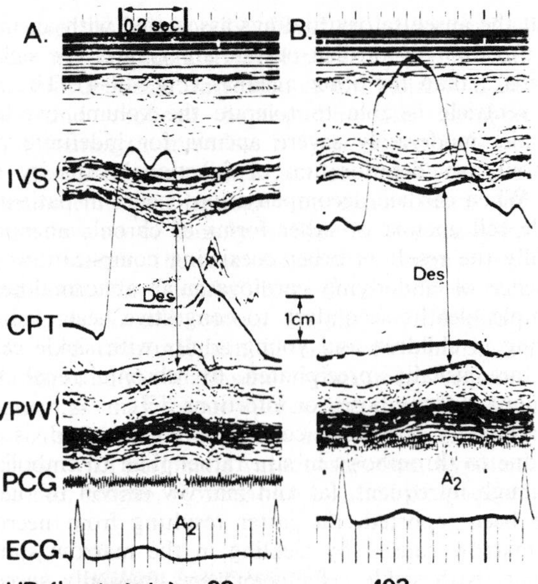

	A	B
HR (beats/min)	98	103
Pps/Pd (mmHg)	112/76	166/116
Pes (mmHg)	91	135
Des (cm)	3.30	4.10
Ded (cm)	4.60	4.90
%ΔD	28.3	16.3
m (mmHg/cm)	55	
m* (mmHg/cm*)	58	

FIGURE 49–5 Recordings from a 16-year old patient with thalassemia major during baseline conditions (*A*) and at peak methoxamine effect (*B*). Both the actual and corrected slope values (m and m*) were abnormal despite normal resting fractional shortening (%ΔD). The 44 mm Hg increase in end-systolic pressure (Pes) resulted in a 0.80-cm increase in end-systolic dimension (Des). For the control population, a comparable change in Pes resulted in a 0.40 ± 0.05-cm increase in Des. IVS = interventricular septum; LVPW = left ventricular posterior wall; A_2 = aortic component of the second heart sound; HR = heart rate; Pps = peak systolic pressure; Pd = aortic diastolic pressure; %ΔD = per cent fractional shortening; m = slope; m* = corrected slope. (Reproduced with permission from Borow, K. M., Propper, R., Bierman, F. Z., et al.: The left ventricular end-systolic pressure-dimensions relation in patients with thalassemia major. A new noninvasive method for assessing contractile state. Circulation *66*:980, 1982, by permission of the American Heart Association, Inc.)

HEMOLYTIC ANEMIA IN PATIENTS WITH VALVULAR HEART DISEASE

In 1964, Dameshek described a patient with aortic, mitral, and tricuspid stenosis and mitral regurgitation who had hemolytic anemia with distorted and fragmented red cells, including helmet cells, burr cells, and schistocytes.[38] At autopsy, numerous calcified excresences were present on the mitral valve and the free margins of the aortic valve. The presence of excess iron deposits in the kidney suggested intravascular hemolysis, but it could not be established whether the cardiac abnormalities were the cause. Subsequently, shortened red cell survival was demonstrated in other patients with aortic valve disease, some of whom had anemia.[39] In patients with rheumatic aortic valve disease, red cell survival may be significantly reduced during periods of exercise.[40] Although this form of hemolytic anemia is probably uncommon, it should be considered in patients with unexplained anemia and valvular heart disease.

Hemolytic Anemia During Cardiac Surgery. In the past, hemolysis frequently occurred as a consequence of extracorporeal circulation. When the blood of many donors must be transfused or is mixed in a pump-oxygenator, as may be the case in patients undergoing cardiac surgery, the question arises whether the samples should be cross-matched with each other as well as with the patient. The plasma of one donor may contain a potent antibody that might interact with cells from a donor who has the antigen specific for that antibody. Although infrequent, this phenomenon may explain some mild-to-moderate hemolysis and hemoglobinemia seen following cardiopulmonary bypass.

With the use of earlier heart-lung machines, red cells became damaged as they passed through the pump oxygenator, presumably as a result of shear forces leading to slight hemolysis and resulting in hemoglobinemia and hemoglobinuria. This problem has been largely obviated with newer machines, which also require little if any blood for priming. As a consequence, hemolytic complications have become far less frequent.[41] In addition, the use of autologous blood and blood aspirated and filtered for re-use during and following operation has been helpful in this regard.[42]

Hemolytic Anemia Following Cardiac Surgery. In 1954, following the surgical implantation of Hufnagel valves in the descending aorta for the treatment of aortic regurgitation, a significant number of patients developed anemia,[43] presumably on a hemolytic basis. When, in dogs, the Hufnagel valve was placed between the left ventricle and the aorta, red cell survival measured by chromium-51 was greatly reduced, and intravascular hemolysis commonly occurred. It was postulated that either red cells were traumatized by being forced between the rigid ball and valve casing or the red cell membrane was damaged, causing antigenic changes that could lead to antierythrocyte antibodies.[44]

The exact nature of the hemolytic anemia associated with intracardiac prostheses was not really appreciated until Sayed et al. noted the development of a chronic and severe hemolytic anemia characterized by microangiopathic red cell changes (consisting of fragmented cells, burr cells, and schistocytes) in a patient following a Teflon patch repair of an ostium primum atrial septal defect (Fig. 49–6).[45] Chromium-51 red cell survival studies confirmed that not only autologous red cells but also donor cells had a shortened half-life, indicating a defect *extrinsic* to the red cell. In keeping with intravascular hemolysis, high concentrations of hemoglobin in the plasma and urine were noted along with hemosiderinuria. At reoperation, the surgeons noted a jet of blood that regurgitated through a cleft in the mitral valve that had been impinging on the prosthetic interatrial Teflon patch. Part of the septum had become denuded of endothelium and had formed a small cul-de-sac in contact with a jet of blood. Repair of the cul-de-sac and re-endothelialization of the area were followed by cessation of the hemolysis. Microangiopathic hemolytic anemia has now been reported with many cardiac defects (Table 49–2).

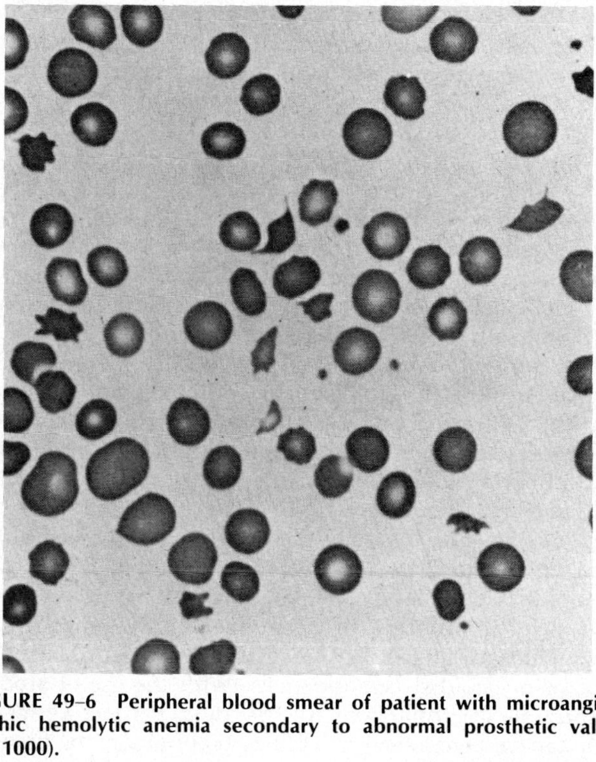

FIGURE 49–6 Peripheral blood smear of patient with microangiopathic hemolytic anemia secondary to abnormal prosthetic valve (× 1000).

TABLE 49–2 CARDIAC CAUSES OF MICROANGIOPATHIC HEMOLYTIC ANEMIA

Intracardiac and intravascular prostheses
Unsuccessful mitral valvuloplasty
Patch repairs for ostium primum defects
Repair of tetralogy of Fallot
Severe aortic valve disease
Ruptured aneurysms of sinus of Valsalva
Coarctation of aorta
Idiopathic hypertrophic subaortic stenosis

The incidence of microangiopathic hemolytic anemia following valvular surgery depends on many variables, including the specific operation, the surgical technique, and the tests used to determine hemolysis. The reported incidences vary from 4 per cent to 73 per cent.[46,47] In the latter study, red cell life span was determined in patients with aortic valve disease or valve replacement and the results compared with those in normal subjects. In many instances, diurnal variations occur with greater intravascular hemolysis during physical activity.[48]

The *clinical presentation* may be sudden or gradual. There is usually no associated splenomegaly. Rarely a vicious circle develops in a patient with a paravalvular leak: the resultant shear stress produces hemolytic anemia, which increases stroke volume and stress, which, in turn, intensifies the anemia. While it is agreed that direct mechanical trauma to the red cells is the cause of the hemolysis, the relative contributions of valve closure, denuded endothelium, turbulence, and the development of antierythrocyte autoantibodies is uncertain. Pirofsky et al. described seven patients with hemolytic anemia that developed within two weeks of aortic valve replacement.[49] Six had positive antiglobulin (Coombs') tests; the material that coated the erythrocyte was identified as an erythrocyte autoantibody; therapy with corticosteroids helped to correct the hemolysis in four patients. Although these and other studies raised the possibility of an immune reaction created by the artificial valve, the vast majority of patients have a negative antiglobulin test. It is likely that in some instances the hemolytic anemia observed in the early postoperative period is due simply to multiple transfusions during the operative procedure or to the lymphocyte-splenomegaly syndrome (post–pump-oxygenator syndrome) associated with cytomegaloviral infection.

Turbulence is the most common feature of all hemolytic anemias due to valvular disease and cardiac surgery. For example, following insertion of a prosthetic valve, paravalvular regurgitation will increase the stroke volume and therefore the turbulence through the narrowed orifice. Experiments in vitro have demonstrated that shearing stresses in excess of 3000 dynes/cm^2 can easily cause hemolysis and that such degrees of stress may readily develop in the presence of defects causing regurgitation from the aorta to the left ventricle.[50] This degree of shearing stress can also be seen in situations in which the lumen of the aortic valve prosthesis is small relative to the stroke volume or where the ball is relatively large for the diameter of the aorta. Although much less common, similar phenomena can occur with prosthetic mitral valves.

The definitive treatment of this hemolytic syndrome consists of surgical repair of the cardiac abnormality, i.e., either replacement or correction of the prosthesis or correction of the paravalvular leak. If a patient is not readily operable, rest will alleviate the condition; iron and folate replacement may be helpful. Treatment with corticosteroids is usually of no benefit.

Hemosiderosis and Hemochromatosis

(see also p. 1425)

A number of disease states are characterized by excessive iron stores in the body. The deposition of significant amounts of iron in the myocardium, liver, and pancreas may lead to varying degrees of dysfunction of these organs.[51] Insofar as the heart is concerned, myocardial deposits of iron may lead to congestive heart failure, conduction disturbances, and arrhythmias. Significant siderosis is most often encountered in patients with idiopathic hemochromatosis or in anemic patients with large and long-standing transfusion requirements.

Patients with *idiopathic hemochromatosis* absorb inappropriately large quantities of iron from the gastrointestinal tract. This inherited disorder with variable clinical expression develops slowly and depends, in part, upon environmental factors, such as the magnitude of dietary intake of iron, the quantity of alcohol intake, and the severity of any underlying liver disease. An association between hemochromatosis and HLA-A3 and HLA-B14 antigens has been described.[52] Prior to the histocompatibility studies, idiopathic hemochromatosis was thought to be autosomal-dominant. HLA subtyping has now suggested a recessive mode of transmission, has linked the disease with chromosome 6, and has helped to distinguish idiopathic hemochromatosis from iron overload secondary to liver disease.[53]

Clinical manifestations of hemochromatosis occur more frequently in men than in women. The disease rarely manifests itself before the age of 20 years and reaches its peak incidence in the fifth decade. Diabetes is the most common initial manifestation, occurring in half the patients. The classic clinical presentation includes increased pigmentation of the skin, hepatomegaly, and cardiac dysfunction. Loss of libido and other endocrinopathies, such as hypopituitarism, may also become apparent. Cellular damage results from iron-induced release of lysosomal acid hydrolases.[54]

The incidence of cardiac symptoms increases with time.[54,55] Dyspnea, edema, and ascites are noted early in the course in 15 to 20 per cent of the patients, but eventually about one third develop symptoms referable to the heart and approximately the same fraction eventually die of cardiac failure.[55] Arrhythmias are common and include paroxysmal atrial tachycardia and flutter, chronic atrial fibrillation, and frequent premature ventricular contractions; varying degrees of AV block have also been noted. Heart block and arrhythmias are often associated with iron deposits in the AV node[56] and supraventricular arrhythmias with iron deposition in the atria. Low voltage and nonspecific T wave changes are also frequently present.

Radiographic studies in symptomatic patients usually reveal a globular heart with biventricular enlargement and poor pulsations. Some patients may have elevated right ventricular and right atrial pressures[57] consequent to the restrictive cardiomyopathy secondary to iron deposition in the myocardium, as well as involvement of the pericardium itself.

TRANSFUSIONAL HEMOSIDEROSIS. This may become a clinical problem in patients with severe chronic anemia who survive long enough to accumulate toxic quantities of iron from transfused blood. For example, patients with thalassemia major, chronic refractory anemias, myeloid metaplasia, pure red cell aplasia, and aplastic anemia may accumulate 50 gm of iron from transfusions, resulting in a variety of clinical problems similar to those encountered in idiopathic hemochromatosis. Indeed, children with β-thalassemia major maintained on hypertransfusion programs, while spared the cardiac consequences of severe anemia, generally die of heart failure as a consequence of myocardial siderosis in their second decade of life.[31,33] In adults with chronic anemias, cardiac iron deposition secondary to transfusional hemosiderosis, may contribute to cardiovascular disability, which is often inappropriately attributed solely to high-output heart failure. Undoubtedly, the combination of impaired cardiac function secondary to iron deposition and the increased burden on the heart imposed by the persistent, partly treated anemia is responsible.

In a review of 135 hearts studied at autopsy, composed of 4 patients with hemochromatosis and 131 with chronic anemia requiring repeated transfusions, 19 were found to have cardiac iron deposits.[58] Among the patients with leukemia in this series, only 7 per cent lived long enough to develop cardiac iron deposits, whereas 30 per cent of those with refractory anemias who required repeated transfusions did so. Grossly visible iron deposits in the heart were always associated with a prior history of cardiac dysfunction and usually of chronic cardiac failure. The iron deposits were usually most extensive in idiopathic hemochromatosis and in patients who received more than 100 units of blood, without evidence of blood loss. In patients with cardiac hemosiderosis, histological examination revealed that the ventricular free walls and septum contained heavier deposits than did the atrial walls (Fig. 49–7). The quantity of iron in the various layers of the ventricular myocardium is quite variable. The epicardium and the papillary muscles contain the most iron, the subendocardium intermediate, and the midmyocardium and conduction tissue the least.

It is often difficult to determine whether myocardial dysfunction results from the chronic anemia or the presence of myocardial hemosiderosis. With the use of atomic absorption spectrophotometry, the exact concentrations of iron can be determined in various body organs or tissues.

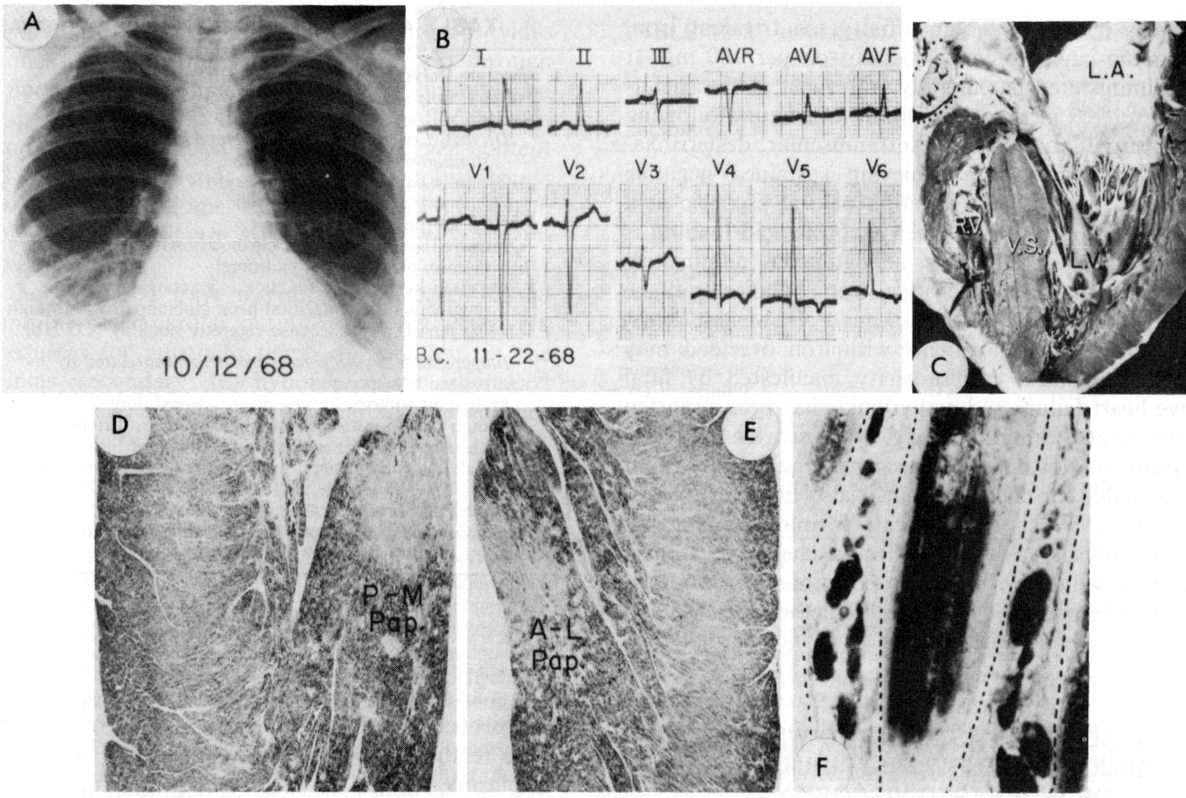

FIGURE 49–7 Observations in a 42-year-old woman with sickle cell anemia who developed congestive heart failure after cumulative transfusions of 260 units of blood. At the time of her death, she had received a total of 359 units of blood (90 gm iron). *A,* Chest roentgenogram two weeks prior to death, showing cardiomegaly. *B,* Ischemic ST and T wave changes can be seen on the electrocardiogram. *C,* At autopsy the walls of the right (R.V.) and left (L.V.) ventricles, left atrium (L.A.), and atrial and ventricular (V.S.) septa were rusty brown owing to extensive iron deposits. The right atrial wall (partially enclosed by dotted line), in contrast, was tan; only minute particles of iron were present on microscopic examination. *D* and *E,* Large areas of replacement fibrosis (pale areas) were present in both left ventricular papillary muscles. *F,* Severely degenerated myocardial fibers (enclosed by dotted lines) that also contained iron deposits were often found adjacent to viable myocardial fibers. (Prussian blue stains.) (From Buja, L. M., and Roberts, W. C.: Iron in the heart. Am. J. Med. *51*:209, 1971.)

Rarely is iron deposition found solely in the heart. Since the liver is easily accessible by biopsy and its iron concentration is closely related to that in the myocardium, liver biopsy appears to be a convenient way of confirming a diagnosis of myocardial siderosis. In some patients, it may be possible by echocardiography to detect early left ventricular dysfunction prior to the development of symptoms.[34,59] In a group of patients with severe β-thalassemia or transfusion-dependent anemias without clinical cardiac symptoms, left ventricular dysfunction measured by radionuclide cineangiography was demonstrated during exercise but not at rest.[59] Noninvasive assessment of the left ventricular end-systolic pressure-dimension relation (using a methoxamine challenge) can identify preclinical left ventricular dysfunction not evident from resting or dynamic exercise studies and not due to chronic anemia per se. This technique may be a very sensitive way of following therapies of iron overload diseases to prevent cardiac complications.

Since the "iron heart is not a strong heart, but a weak one,"[58] and the majority of patients with myocardial siderosis ultimately die of irreversible cardiac failure and arrhythmias, reversal of the iron overload should be attempted. In patients with idiopathic hemochromatosis, it is possible to mobilize iron stores by repeated phlebotomies, and this is the preferred mode of therapy.[60,61] Decrease in hepatic iron stores and fibrosis, improvement of liver function, amelioration of diabetes, and reversal of cardiomyopathy have all occurred. Since the average patient with idiopathic hemochromatosis has 20 to 40 gm of stored iron, a weekly to bimonthly phlebotomy schedule usually has to be continued for two to three years. Initially the hematocrit will drop but will then return toward normal despite repeated phlebotomies. Removal of excess body iron by phlebotomy has been possible even in patients with hematocrits as low as 30 per cent.

The distribution of tissue iron differs somewhat between individuals with idiopathic hematochromatosis and those with transfusion siderosis, who have relatively more iron stored in the reticuloendothelial cells. However, in the latter with repeated transfusions, organ dysfunction does occur in a pattern similar to that in idiopathic hemochromatosis.[62] Phlebotomy is, of course, not a therapeutic alternative in the management of iron overload due to the chronic administration of blood transfusions for the treatment of anemia. Chelation therapy, on the other hand, is the only available approach for the removal of iron in these anemic patients.[63,64]

Desferrioxamine B is the most widely studied iron chelator; this hydroxamic acid compound initially isolated from may be a higher incidence of ischemic episodes. In vitro studies suggest that white cells can contribute significantly to blood viscosity,[76] and, since leukocytosis is characteristic of polycythemia vera, white cells undoubtedly play a role in the elevated blood viscosity characteristic of this disease.

Cerebral blood flow is significantly reduced and is associated with cerebral symptoms in about half of patients with hematocrits averaging 53.6 per cent, confirming the relationship between cerebral vascular insufficiency and blood viscosity.[77,78] By lowering the hematocrit to 45.5 per cent, viscosity declines by 30 per cent and cerebral blood increases by 73 per cent. With hematocrit values ranging from 46 to 52 per cent, cerebral blood flow is still lower than normal, suggesting that even slight increases in red cell mass may interfere with cerebral perfusion. These studies suggest that patients with polycythemia vera should undergo phlebotomy until hematocrit levels reach the low 40s rather than the previously recommended level of approximately 45 per cent.

Secondary Polycythemias. The secondary polycythemias are logically divided into two subgroups: those in which the increased red cell mass compensates for a reduction in oxygen transport with appropriate stimulation by erythropoietin, and those in which erythrocytosis is associated with an inappropriate increase in erythropoietin production (Table 49–3). It has been suggested that with any hypoxic stimulus the production of an enzyme in the kidney, erythrogenin, becomes stimulated and generates erythropoietin by acting enzymatically on a proposed plasma protein substrate, which may be of hepatic origin.

If an individual living at sea level is transported to a high altitude, a rise in hemoglobin concentration occurs,[79] accompanied by an increase in urinary erythropoietin. Similarly, with severe degrees of chronic hypoxemia in chronic obstructive pulmonary disease, an arterial pO_2 less than 60 mm Hg usually leads to an increase in red cell mass. Although in some instances the hemoglobin has been reported to be as high as 24 gm/dl and the hematocrit as high as 75 per cent, in most patients with polycythemia secondary to chronic obstructive lung disease, the hematocrit does not exceed 57 per cent and the hemoglobin 17 gm/dl.[80] In cyanotic congenital heart disease, red cell mass increases as resting arterial oxygen saturation falls (p. 949). Hematocrits as high as 86 per cent may be seen with red blood cell masses almost three times normal.[81] Plasma volume may be diminished, but total blood volume remains significantly elevated because of the striking elevations of red cell mass. The most common congenital malformations producing these elevations include tetralogy of Fallot, transposition of the great arteries, and persistent truncus arteriosus.

Signs and symptoms of hyperviscosity will generally occur as the hematocrit increases above 60 per cent; cardiac function may be compromised because of both the constant volume load and the augmented vascular resistance secondary to the increased viscosity of the blood. Ruddy cyanosis, headache, dizziness, roaring in the ears, thrombotic episodes, and bleeding are major clinical findings and may be treated with phlebotomy.[82] Careful monitoring during phlebotomy is necessary, and acute reduction of blood volume may have to be overcome by replacement of volume with plasma expanders.[83] Following isovolemic phlebotomy, reducing the hematocrit from the 70s to the 60s, cardiac output rises, and, despite the fall in arterial oxygen content, systemic oxygen transport will usually increase. These favorable changes are attributed to the reduced blood viscosity and vascular resistance. Although the erythrocytosis is a homeostatic mechanism compensating for the chronic arterial hypoxemia, greatly increased hematocrits (with values exceeding 70 per cent) are generally undesirable.

The optimal level of hematocrit for patients with cyanotic congenital heart disease and other chronically hypoxemic states is poorly defined and presents an interesting and perplexing dilemma. The clinical presentation of the patient must be carefully considered. Reduction of cerebral blood flow occurs in secondary erythrocytosis as well as polycythemia vera and improves with phlebotomy.[84,85] If phlebotomy is deemed necessary, close monitoring of the patient's blood pressure, heart rate, arterial oxygen saturation, and general condition is necessary. As might be expected from the decreased oxygen transport associated with right-to-left shunts, the P_{50} and red cell 2,3-DPG are increased, but there is great variability in the relationship between decreased arterial oxygen tension and the rise in P_{50} and red cell 2,3-DPG.[86] Successful surgical correction of the cardiac defect will result in a normalization of the saturation and remove the necessity for the adaptive mechanism; hematocrit and blood volume will return to normal.

In 1966, it first became recognized that a hemoglobin variant with *increased* oxygen affinity could be associated with erythrocytosis.[87] These variants, which generally have amino acid substitutions at structural sites crucial to hemoglobin function, now number over 40. They are transmitted in an autosomal dominant fashion and cause a shift in the oxygen dissociation curve to the left with reduced level of P_{50}. The shift to the left of the oxygen-hemoglobin dissociation curve results in a marked reduction in the oxygen extraction by the tissues. Increased hemoglobin concentration and blood flow are available compensatory mechanisms to maintain oxygen delivery (Fig. 49–3). However, the primary response appears to be erythrocytosis mediated by increases in erythropoietin.[88] Cardiac output is usually normal.[89] Polycythemia constitutes the primary adjustment for oxygen delivery in patients with these hemoglobin variants. They do not have any increased incidence of myocardial ischemia or other forms of organ hypoxia.[90]

True erythrocytosis without demonstrable cause, other than excessive cigar and cigarette smoking, has also been noted in a significant number of individuals.[91] All had elevated levels of carboxyhemoglobin with shifts of the hemoglobin-oxygen dissociation curve to the left, resulting in the stimulation of erythropoiesis. In most cases of polycythemia secondary to inappropriate erythropoietin production, such as tumors, renal cysts, and hydronephrosis, and red cell mass, although increased, does not generally cause symptoms of hyperviscosity.

Relative Polycythemia. Relative polycythemia is a distinct and commonly encountered entity that is also referred to as spurious polycythemia, Gaisböck's syndrome, polycythemia hypertonica, pseudopolycythemia, and stress erythrocytosis. It is not a primary disease process and may be merely a physiological state in which the plasma volume is slightly reduced and the red cell mass slightly increased. The hematocrit rarely exceeds 60 per cent, and other blood constituents are normal. This disorder can be distinguished from polycythemia vera by measurement of red cell mass which, by definition, is normal in relative polycythemia and elevated in polycythemia vera. Patients are often hypertensive, prone to thromboembolic complications,[92] and obese. These complications appear to be unrelated to the hematological changes, and reduction of red cell mass by phlebotomy or chemotherapy is not appropriate. When present, the hypertension and thromboembolic complications should be treated in the usual manner.

NEOPLASTIC DISEASES

Primary tumors of the heart (Chap. 42) are quite rare, occurring at a frequency of 0.0017 to 0.1 per cent of autopsies. Metastatic tumors to the pericardium or heart are far more common, ranging from 1.5 to 20.6 per cent (average 6 per cent) in autopsies on patients with malignant diseases. Metastases usually occur to the pericardium (p. 1507) and myocardium and rarely involve the valves or endocardium; the right side of the heart appears to be affected more frequently than the left.[93,94] Solitary metastases to the heart are rare; co-existence with metastases to other organs is usual. Metastatic nodules in the heart are generally multiple (Figs. 49–10 and 49–11), but they may become diffuse and lead to the manifestations of a restrictive cardiomyopathy (p. 1422). The mode of spread may be by direct extension, as occurs in lung cancer; via the hematogenous route, as in malignant melanoma; or through lymphatic channels, as in lymphoma.

The most common primary tumor producing cardiac metastases is bronchogenic carcinoma (Fig. 49–10), with carcinoma of the breast, malignant melanoma, lymphomas, and leukemias next in order of frequency (Table 49–5).[93–97] At autopsy, 15 to 35 per cent of patients dying with primary lung cancer show cardiac involvement, while over 60 per cent of patients with melanoma will have cardiac metastases.[95] Hematological malignancies, especially lympho-

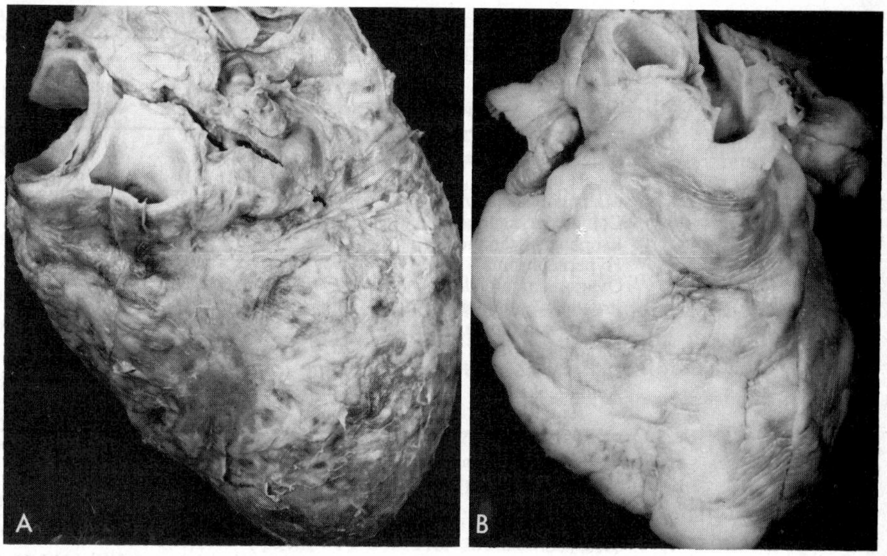

FIGURE 49–10 Metastatic carcinoma of the pericardium in two patients with bronchogenic carcinoma. *A*, The tumor nodules are obscured by fibrinous exudate. *B*, Extensive metastatic nodules. (From Edwards, J. E.: Effects of malignant noncardiac tumors upon the cardiovascular system. *In* Brest, A. N. (ed.): Cardiovascular Clinics. Vol. 4. Philadelphia, F. A. Davis, 1972, p. 282.)

mas, have been reported to account for 15 per cent of all metastases to the heart and pericardium.[96] Of patients dying of malignant lymphomas, approximately 15 per cent have cardiac involvement with tumor.

CLINICAL MANIFESTATIONS. Many metastatic cardiac lesions are clinically silent and are found only at necropsy.[97] For example, despite massive heart involvement with melanoma ("charcoal heart"), there may be little evidence of cardiac dysfunction.[98] The most common clinical manifestations result from pericardial effusion, tachyarrhythmias, AV block,[99] or congestive heart failure. Metastatic cardiac disease is rarely the presenting symptom of the primary tumor. The mode of spread may be by direct extension via the hematogenous route or through lymphatic channels. Routine chest radiographs, nuclide imaging with gallium or thallium, and/or echocardiography are sometimes helpful in diagnosis.[100–103] Osteogenic sarcoma, which may metastasize to the heart, is unique because the metastases contain bone and may be radiographically visible.[104]

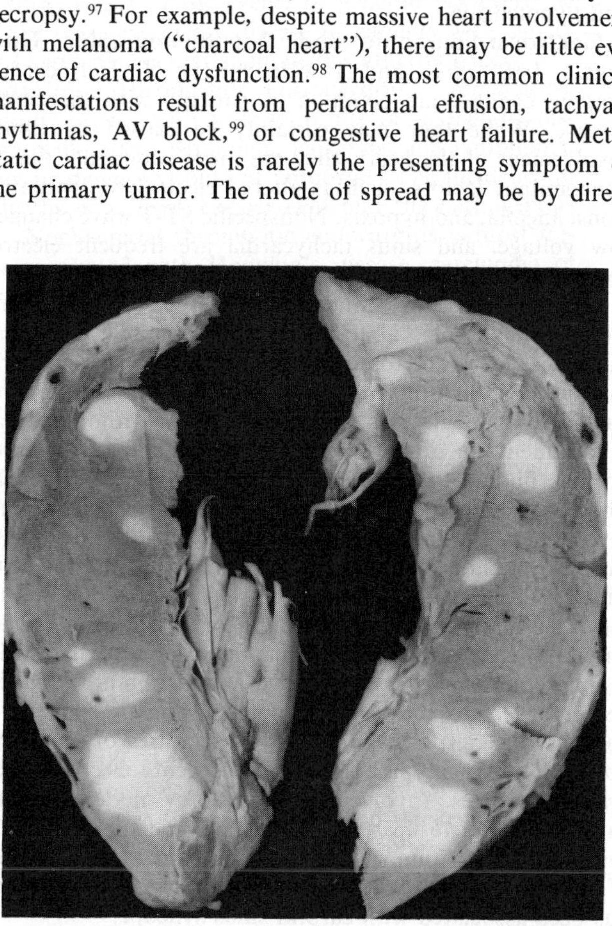

FIGURE 49–11 Sections of left ventricle showing metastatic nodules in the myocardium. Tumor was primary in a bronchus. (From Edwards, J. E.: Effects of malignant noncardiac tumors upon the cardiovascular system. *In* Brest, A. N. (ed.): Cardiovascular Clinics. Vol. 4. Philadelphia, F. A. Davis, 1972, p. 282.)

In recent years, aggressive chemotherapy and mega-voltage therapy have led to more favorable response rates in patients with various malignancies, such as Hodgkin's disease, non-Hodgkin's lymphoma, testicular tumors, and the leukemias. With the development of high remission rates and apparent cure, i.e., permanent remission in some instances, cardiac toxicity related to both forms of therapy has received significant attention. Anthracyclines and other therapeutic agents may cause a fatal cardiomyopathy (p. 1690), while irradiation of mediastinal structures may lead to pericarditis (p. 1689) and coronary artery obstruction. Cardiac metastases are usually a late phenomenon in most malignancies, but, in view of the prolonged remissions frequently obtained, it has become increasingly important to prevent, detect, and treat these cardiac complications.

Pericardial Involvement (see also p. 1507). The clinical syndromes of cardiovascular involvement in malignancies are listed in Table 49–6. Signs and symptoms of pericarditis with pericardial effusion and cardiac tamponade occur particularly in patients with carcinoma of the lung and breast, as well as in Hodgkin's disease, non-Hodgkin's lymphoma,[105] and the leukemias, particularly acute myelogenous, lymphoblastic leukemia and the blast crisis of chronic myelogenous leukemia.[106] Pericardial involvement is usually diagnosed premortem because of the resultant symptomatology and the radiographic picture. Clinically, the involvement takes the form of either cardiac tamponade or adhesive pericarditis, associated with extensive nodular tumor infiltration of the pericardium.[107] The finding of chylous pericardial effusion is usually characteristic of lymphomatous involvement.[108] Echocardiography is a key tool in the diagnosis of neoplastic involvement of the pericardium. With increased use of serial M-mode echocardiography in patients with advanced malignant disease, the incidence of pericardial effusions appears to be much rative forms of chemotherapy. It has been suggested that routine follow-up during the first year after irradiation should consist of frequent chest roentgenograms. If any evidence of increased cardiac diameter is noted, or if a patient develops clinical manifestations suggestive of pericarditis or pericardial effusion and there is no reason to suspect another cause of pericarditis, patients may be treated symptomatically but occasionally may require pericardiocentesis and/or pericardiectomy.[109,110,127] It is anticipated that, with current changes in radiotherapeutic techniques and available curative chemotherapy, the incidence of pericarditis will continue to decline.

Documented instances of clinical disease resulting from radiation damage to the myocardium and endocardium are quite rare.[124,128] Radiation-induced endocardial fibrosis may cause manifestations of a restrictive cardiomyopathy (p. 1422) and a variety of nonspecific electrocardiographic changes, as well as varying degrees of AV block,[129,] mitral regurgitation secondary to papillary muscle dysfunction, and aortic regurgitation as a consequence of endocardial valvular thickening. The onset of new murmurs occurring after radiation therapy should alert the physician to these possibilities. In an autopsy study of the cardiac effects of radiation exposure, three fourths of the patients exposed to more than 3500 rads, with a field resulting in more exposure of the anterior thorax, develop interstitial myocardial fibrosis, with more extensive involvement of the right than the left ventricle. Functional abnormalities demonstrated by echocardiography and radionuclide angiocardiography may occur 5 to 15 years after radiation but as with pericarditis should become less frequent with new techniques of radiotherapy.[129a]

Since the report by Cohn et al.[128] in 1967 of a 15-year-old boy suffering a fatal myocardial infarction 16 months after receiving 4000 rads to the heart for Hodgkin's disease, a number of similar occurrences have been reported.[110,129–131,131a] Although coronary artery disease is common, supportive evidence for radiation-induced coronary artery disease includes (1) its occurrence in subjects who are very young and without predisposing factors with disease limited to coronary vessels in the beam of radiation, (2) lack of atherosclerosis in arteries not exposed to irradiation, (3) reports of occlusive lesions in other arteries such as the carotid artery following irradiation,[132] (4) presence of distinctive pathological changes, and (5) production of similar lesions in experimental models.

Occlusive coronary and carotid artery disease following irradiation generally occurs from 6 to 12 years after exposure. In rabbits, 2500 rads has produced coronary atherosclerosis that is quite similar to human coronary artery disease.[133] Rabbits do not develop radiation-induced atherosclerosis unless they also receive a diet high in lipids and cholesterol, which by itself is insufficient to produce the atherosclerotic lesion. However, the coronary artery lesions presumably induced by radiotherapy appear to be distinct pathologically and contain severe medial and adventitial fibrosis in continuity with overlying epicardial fibrous tissue and a marked paucity of lipid in the intimal lesions.[130,134] In affected young patients examined at autopsy, the proximal portion of the arteries is significantly more narrowed than the distal. In addition, there is significant loss of smooth muscle cells from the media.[134]

Radiation-induced coronary artery or carotid artery occlusion may require surgical treatment. Because of the relatively low incidence of this complication and the concern that reduced radiation might impair chances of effective treatment of the neoplastic process requiring irradiation, no systematic attempts have been made to try to prevent this complication other than considering chemotherapeutic alternatives if whole-heart irradiation is deemed necessary to "cure" the disease.

CARDIOTOXICITY OF CHEMOTHERAPY FOR NEOPLASTIC DISEASE

For many years, the only notable cardiovascular complications of chemotherapy for neoplastic disease were the orthostatic hypotension[135] and the rare myocardial infarction[136] that occurred in the course of therapy with vincristine, a periwinkle alkaloid, and the interstitial disease and mild pulmonary hypertension secondary to the pulmonary fibrosis created by bleomycin or busulfan.[137] However, with the advent of the anthracycline group of drugs (doxorubicin, daunorubicin), the incidence of cardiac toxicity as a consequence of chemotherapy for neoplastic disease has increased greatly. Doxorubicin (Fig. 49–12) is a glycoside antibiotic, the potent antitumor effect of which is thought to be due to its ability to inhibit nucleic acid synthesis by binding to both strands of the DNA helix, intercalating between base pairs and thereby inhibiting the normal function of DNA and RNA polymerases. Doxorubicin has received more attention than the related compound daunorubicin because of its wider spectrum of antitumor activity in solid tumors and hematologic malignancies.[138] Complete remissions in 30 to 40 per cent of patients with Hodgkin's disease and non-Hodgkin's lymphoma and all types of acute leukemia have been reported with the single agent doxorubicin. Its effectiveness is enhanced by combination with other chemotherapeutic agents. Remission rates of 60 to 80 per cent are obtained in adults with leukemias when it is combined with cytosine arabinoside, and with lymphomas when used together with bleomycin, cyclophosphamide, vincristine, and corticosteroids.[139]

The majority of the toxic manifestations—alopecia, gastrointestinal distress, myelosuppression, and mucositis—produced by these drugs were predicted by animal studies.

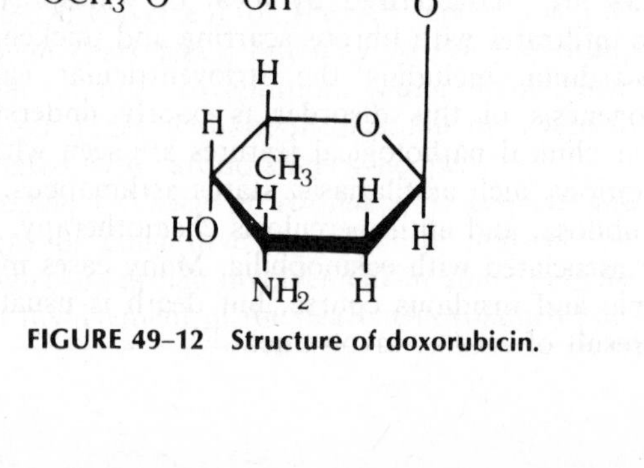

FIGURE 49–12 Structure of doxorubicin.

Not predicted, however, was the occurrence of cardiac toxicity and the interactions with radiation therapy. Arrhythmias, including supraventricular tachyarrhythmias, premature atrial and ventricular contractions, abnormalities of conduction such as left axis deviation, decreased QRS voltage, and a variety of nonspecific ST-segment and T-wave abnormalities, occur in approximately 11 per cent of patients, with a range from 0 to 41.2 per cent.[139,140] These electrocardiographic changes are usually transient, may occur even at low doses of doxorubicin, and usually are seen within several days after administration of the drug. Sudden death has been reported.[141]

Cardiomyopathy and congestive heart failure occurring during anthracycline therapy usually develop suddenly; the clinical manifestations consist of sinus tachycardia, tachypnea, cardiomegaly, peripheral and pulmonary edema, hepatomegaly, venous congestion, and pleural effusion. The cardiomyopathy is usually secondary to a cumulative effect of the drug, occurring with increasing frequency at higher doses of doxorubicin. Congestive heart failure occurs from 9 to 192 days, with a median of 34 days after the administration of the last dose. The congestive heart failure is refractory to therapy; when it is severe, survival is short, usually less than two weeks.[142] Pathological examination discloses enlarged, pale, flabby hearts with ventricular dilatation. Mural thrombi are occasionally found, but the coronary arteries and cardiac valves appear normal. Light microscopy reveals a severe cardiomyopathy with a reduction of the number of myocardial cells and the remaining cells showing degenerative changes. Electron microscopy shows extensive reduction in the number of myofibrillar bundles, myofibrillar lysis, and distortion and disruption of the Z-lines; the mitochondria are swollen with disrupted cristae and contain inclusion bodies[140,142] (Fig. 49–13).

The incidence of cardiomyopathy with doxorubicin administration is 1.7 per cent and with daunorubicin 4.4 per cent. It is fatal in over half the cases.[139] There is a clear

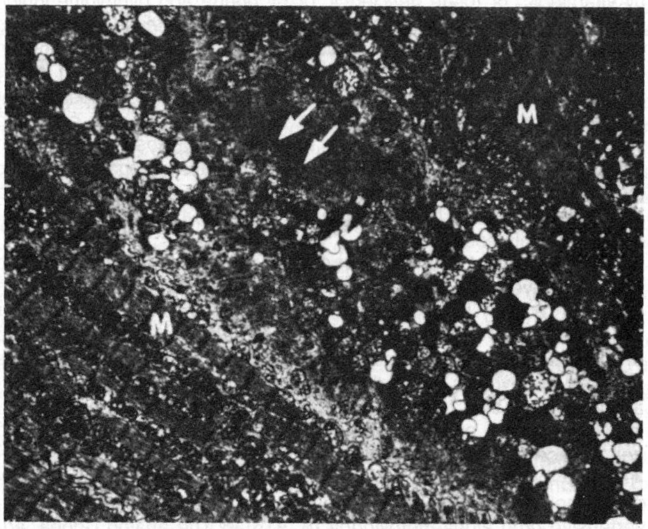

FIGURE 49–13 Myofibrillar loss (white arrows) and sarcotubular swelling (black arrows) are characteristic findings in patients who develop congestive heart failure during doxorubicin therapy. Juxtaposition of normal myocytes (M) and destroyed cells demonstrates microscopic focality of lesion. Histopathologic assessment may also be used to titrate dosage. (Reproduced with permission from Greene, H. L., Reich, S. D., and Dalen, J. E.: How to minimize doxorubicin toxicity. J. Cardiovasc. Med. *7*:306, 1982.)

TABLE 49–8 CORRELATION OF CARDIOMYOPATHY AND THE TOTAL DOSE OF ADRIAMYCIN IN ADULTS

Total Dose (*mg/M²*)	Patients at Risk	Patients with CMY	Frequency (*per cent*)
< 450	738	0	0
451–500	26	0	0
501–550	32	3	9
551–600	15	3	20
> 600	37	15	41
Total > 550	52	18	35
Total < 550	796	3	0.4

CMY = cardiomyopathy.

dose-related incidence of anthracycline cardiomyopathy. There were no cases of cardiomyopathy in 764 patients who received less than a cumulative dose of 500 mg/M^2, but a progressively increased frequency with higher doses was noted[142] (Table 49–8). It is therefore recommended that cumulative doses of doxorubicin be held to less than 450 to 500 mg/M^2 and 500 to 600 mg/M^2 of daunorubicin. However, with increasing frequency, cardiomyopathies are being reported with dosages less than 450 mg/M^2 of doxorubicin.[140,142,143] It has been suggested that the use of these agents in combination with other modalities of therapy, such as radiation or cyclophosphamide, may have been synergistic in the pathogenesis of the cardiomyopathy in some patients.[134,143–146] Both radiation and cyclophosphamide alone have been described as potentially cardiotoxic.

There is no established mechanism for doxorubicin cardiotoxicity, although numerous proposals have been put forward.[147] For example, lipid peroxidation may be caused by the binding of DNA by the drug, specifically bound to spectrin, actin, or cardiolipin.[148] Doxorubicin inhibits ATP production, interferes with the sarcolemmal sodium-potassium pump, inhibits oxidative phosphorylation, may provoke an autoimmune response, binds to DNA precursors, interferes with mitochondrial respiration by inhibiting coenzyme Q, and causes myocardial necrosis by allowing the build-up of high concentrations of calcium in myocardial cells.[149]

Because of the high incidence of toxicity, numerous approaches have been suggested for early detection of this complication and for predicting susceptible patients.[150,151] Noninvasive studies include serial follow-up of systolic time intervals, particularly the PEP/LVET ratio (p. 54) and radionuclide cineangiography (p. 360). The *PEP/LVET* was thought to be a sensitive parameter for monitoring toxicity. However, this has not held up in further study and, in fact, is criticized because false-positive changes may be responsible for the improper withholding of further doxorubicin therapy that is potentially life saving.[152,153] *Radionuclide angiography* appears to provide a sensitive and reproducible measurement of left ventricular dysfunction due to doxorubicin cardiotoxicity.[150] Sequential studies demonstrate the frequent presence of subclinical left ventricular abnormalities.[154] There may be, however, an increased incidence of abnormal results that may not be clinically significant if the studies are performed after exercise.[155] *Endomyocardial biopsy* (p. 297) appears at present to be more diagnostic of toxicity than any of the noninvasive evaluations. In the hands of trained personnel, it has become a safe procedure.[156] Administration of doxorunia persists well after the drug-antibody complex has been cleared. In this situation, some patients have had a gratifying elevation in platelet count.

The commonly used anticoagulant *heparin* is one of the most important causes of thrombocytopenia in cardiac patients. The incidence varies from 5 to 25 per cent of patients receiving heparin, is more common in patients receiving heparin derived from beef lung, and has been associated with all modes and doses of heparin administration.[172] Heparin has a direct platelet-aggregating effect that may contribute to thrombocytopenia. This property is most marked in those fractions with highest molecular weight and lowest affinity for antithrombin.[173] There is an increase in platelet-associated immunoglobulin in many of the cases, suggesting an immune etiology. However, the nature of the offending antigen in heparin and its relationship to the biologically active heparin fractions remain unclear. In addition, some patients with heparin-induced thrombocytopenia develop paradoxical thrombosis and disseminated intravascular coagulation. The development of thromboembolism in association with thrombocytopenia is unique to heparin.

Other Cardiac Drug Hematologic Abnormalities. Amyl nitrite, sodium nitrite, and nitroglycerin can oxidize hemoglobin to methemoglobin, which cannot effectively carry oxygen. The patient with methemoglobinemia has a cyanotic appearance but has a normal pO_2 and will not improve his color with oxygen therapy. Although normal adults can get symptomatic methemoglobinemia, most cases occur when children accidentally ingest medications prescribed for adults. Occasionally, adults with mild congenital methemoglobinemia will become markedly symptomatic when exposed to small doses of these same medications. With the current availability of intravenous nitroglycerin, this complication may become more frequent.[174] If venous blood is chocolate brown and the color remains after the blood is shaken in air, the diagnosis of methemoglobinemia is almost certain. The diagnosis is confirmed by the addition of a few drops of 10 per cent potassium cyanide, which results in the rapid production of the bright red cyanmethemoglobin. Symptoms are nonspecific and consist of dyspnea, headache, fatigue, and dizziness. They are usually self-limited if the responsible drugs are discontinued, since normal red cells can enzymatically reduce the methemoglobin. In severe cases or in patients with enzyme defects, methylene blue may be administered to stimulate reduction of the methemoglobin.

Other medications may interfere with oxygen delivery to tissues. For example, nitroprusside used in the treatment of hypertensive emergencies (Chap. 27) or for reduction of afterload in the management of heart failure (p. 537) may cause symptoms such as fatigue, nausea, abnormal behavior, and muscle spasm due to the reaction of the agent with oxyhemoglobin and the resultant production of cyanmethemoglobin and free cyanide ions.[175]

Hydralazine, procainamide, and rarely phenytoin can cause a lupus erythematosus–like syndrome, with urticaria, erythema multiforme, photosensitivity, delirium, and immune-mediated blood cell destruction. Although patients with drug-induced lupus have positive antinuclear antibody tests and many of the clinical manifestations of SLE, they do not usually have renal impairment, and all the symptoms remit within several months if the drugs are discontinued. The syndrome is of particular importance in cardiac patients, since the onset of chest pain, pleurisy, or pericardial effusion in the patient with heart disease could lead to an erroneous diagnosis unless drug-induced lupus is suspected.

THROMBOSIS, ANTICOAGULATION, AND BLEEDING IN HEART DISEASE

PATHOGENESIS OF THROMBOSIS

More than a century ago, Virchow proposed that thrombosis resulted from a combination of three factors: local vessel or tissue injury, circulatory stasis, and alterations in blood coagulability.[176] Since that time, both clinical observations on patients with thromboembolism and research on thrombosis have upheld these basic principles. The composition of thrombi varies with their anatomical site and depends upon the velocity of blood flow. In arteries, they consist of aggregated platelets with few fibrin strands, giving them a white appearance. Venous thrombi, which form in areas where the velocity of blood flow is slower, are made up of fibrin strands and entrapped red cells, giving them a red appearance. The role of platelets in venous thrombi is not clear, although platelets may provide the initial nidus for thrombus formation and can be seen at the head of thrombi, where they attach to damaged endothelium on venous valves.

To understand the development of thrombi, it is important to understand the normal hemostatic mechanism, its limiting reactions, and its inhibitors. Thrombosis has, in fact, been defined as blood coagulation occurring in the wrong place or at the wrong time. The sequence of events in clotting can be divided into: (1) formation of the platelet plug—platelet adhesion and aggregation; (2) the platelet release reaction; (3) the generation of thrombin; (4) the formation of the fibrin clot; and (5) dissolution of the fibrin clot through the fibrinolytic system.

Platelet Aggregation, Platelet Release, and Thrombin Generation. Following vascular injury, platelets adhere to exposed subendothelial collagen or to noncollagenous microfibrils (Fig. 49–14). Activated platelets release ADP and other mediators, which cause circulating platelets to be attracted to the traumatic site, beginning the formation of a "platelet plug."[175,178,179] As a result of endothelial cell

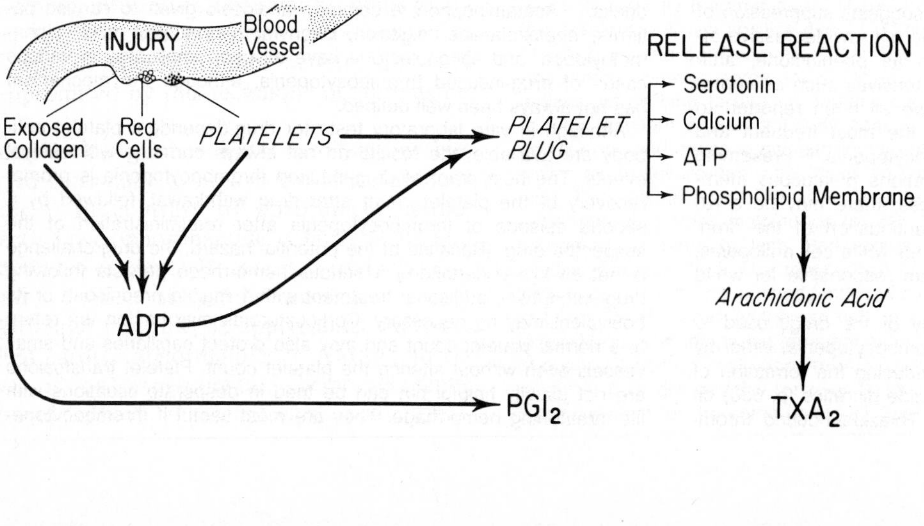

FIGURE 49–14 Diagram of the hemostatic reaction at the site of injury, showing the role of platelets. TXA_2 thromboxane; PGI_2 prostacyclin.

injury and platelet activation, metabolites of arachidonic acid—prostaglandins and thromboxanes—are formed that regulate platelet release and aggregation. Prostacyclin (PGI_2), produced by endothelial cells, is a potent inhibitor of platelet aggregation, while thromboxane (TXA_2), a product of arachidonic acid metabolism in the platelet, causes platelet release and aggregation.[179] In addition, platelets may serve as a site for the rapid activation of clotting factors.[177] There is evidence that prothrombin conversion to thrombin occurs several thousand times faster on platelets than in plasma.

As the platelet plug is being formed, exposed collagen and tissue thromboplastin from the damaged vessel activate the plasma coagulation system, leading to thrombin generation and fibrin formation (Fig. 49–15). There are two closely intertwined pathways for thrombin formation. They both involve the limited proteolysis of inactive precursors or proenzymes to produce active enzymes, which, in turn, proteolyze additional molecules in an enzymatic cascade. The reactions are carefully regulated by lipid and protein cofactors and plasma inhibitors so that sufficient thrombin is generated for local fibrin deposition without systemic coagulation. The intrinsic pathway is initiated by Hageman factor (Factor XII) contact with collagen. The activation of Factor XII is facilitated by two cofactors, high molecular weight kininogen and prekallikrein. Activated Hageman factor fragments then activate Factor XI, which, in concert with Factors IX and VIII, activates Factor X. In the extrinsic or tissue factor–dependent pathway, Factor VII forms a complex with tissue factor which can directly activate Factor X. Activated Factor X (X_a), in conjunction with Factor V, converts prothrombin to thrombin (Fig. 49–14). Formation of small amounts of thrombin accelerates further platelet aggregation and release and, eventually, more thrombin production.

Formation of Fibrin Clot. Once thrombin is formed, it attacks the fibrinogen molecule, converting it to fibrin with release of two fragments, fibrinopeptides A and B. As fibrin is laid down, the hemostatic plug is strengthened and stabilized by Factor XIII, which catalyzes covalent cross-links between polymerized fibrin molecules. The resultant clot becomes mechanically strong and able to withstand the trauma of collisional events within the vascular system.

Dissolution of the Fibrin Clot via the Fibrinolytic System. Plasminogen is normally incorporated into the fibrin clot and is ready to be activated to plasmin, an enzyme capable of fibrinolysis. Endothelial cells secrete a plasminogen activator that diffuses into the clot to initiate fibrinolysis. Fibrinolysis remains localized to the clot because of the high local concentration of plasminogen within the clot and the presence in plasma of the $alpha_2$ plasmin inhibitor,[180] which rapidly neutralizes any free plasmin. There has been a great deal of recent interest in the fibrinolytic system and its role in thrombosis, since patients have been described with recurrent thromboembolism who have either a deficiency of venous plasminogen activator or abnormal plasminogen molecules that resist activation and have reduced fibrinolytic potential.[181,182] In addition, pharmacologic agents that can activate the fibrinolytic system, such as urokinase or streptokinase, are under study for the treatment of venous and arterial thrombosis and embolism (see below).

Laboratory Tests—Hemostasis and Thrombosis. The integrity of the clotting mechanism can be evaluated by various laboratory studies. Platelet function can be screened by a simple bleeding time. In addition, studies of platelet aggregation and measurement of platelet release reactions after exposure to aggregating agents can serve as useful indicators of abnormal platelet physiology. Abnormalities of the intrinsic coagulation pathway can be detected by the partial thromboplastin time (PTT), while the extrinsic pathway is screened with the prothrombin time (PT). These tests are most useful for evaluating hemostatic failure and bleeding disorders and are of little help in the diagnosis of thromboembolism. Newer tests that can detect platelet secretion and activation of plasma coagulation and may be useful in patients with thromboembolism are discussed below.

THE HYPERCOAGULABLE STATE

In addition to tissue injury and changes in the vessel wall, a number of changes in the blood itself may predispose patients to thrombosis. These are collectively referred to as "the hypercoagulable state"[183] and include (1) abnormalities in blood flow, (2) decreased concentration of clotting inhibitors, (3) abnormal platelet release and aggregation, (4) delayed or impaired clearance of activated factors, and (5) defects in the fibrinolytic system (Table 49–11).

Abnormal Blood Flow. Although stasis alone does not ordinarily produce venous thrombosis, it is definitely a contributing factor. Many of the clinical disorders associated with abnormal blood flow and thrombosis have been previously discussed in this chapter and include sickle cell disease, the polycythemias, and hyperviscosity syndromes. In addition, the occurrence of thromboembolism in pregnancy or following the use of oral contraceptives may be related, in part, to changes in blood flow. There is increasing clinical evidence suggesting that exogenous estrogens used in contraception, in the therapy of prostatic carcinoma, in the treatment of endometriosis, or as prophylaxis for atherosclerosis may increase the incidence of thromboembolic disease.[184,185] In addition, during pregnancy, the frequency of thromboembolism increases slightly with each trimester but is highest during the early postpartum period, a time of maximal estrogen secretion.[186] Estrogen and progesterone have major effects on

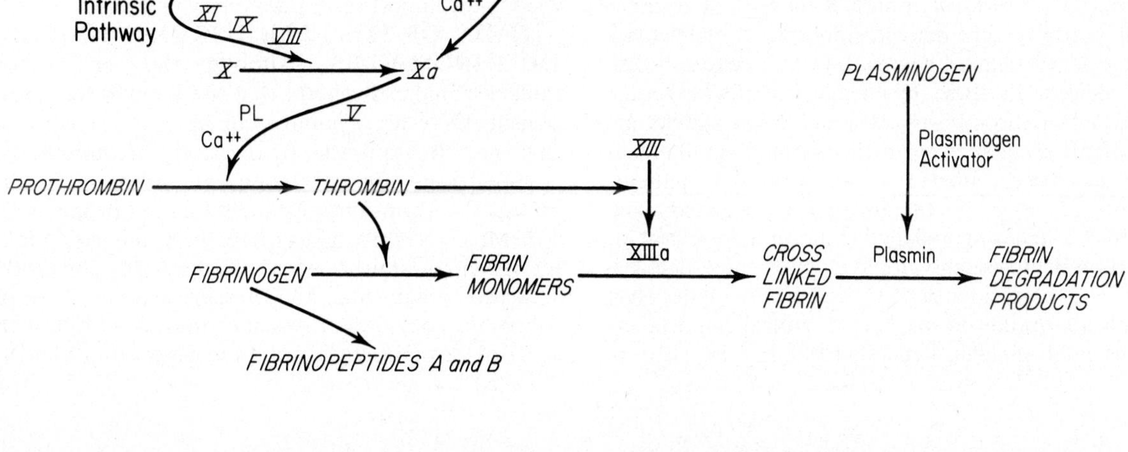

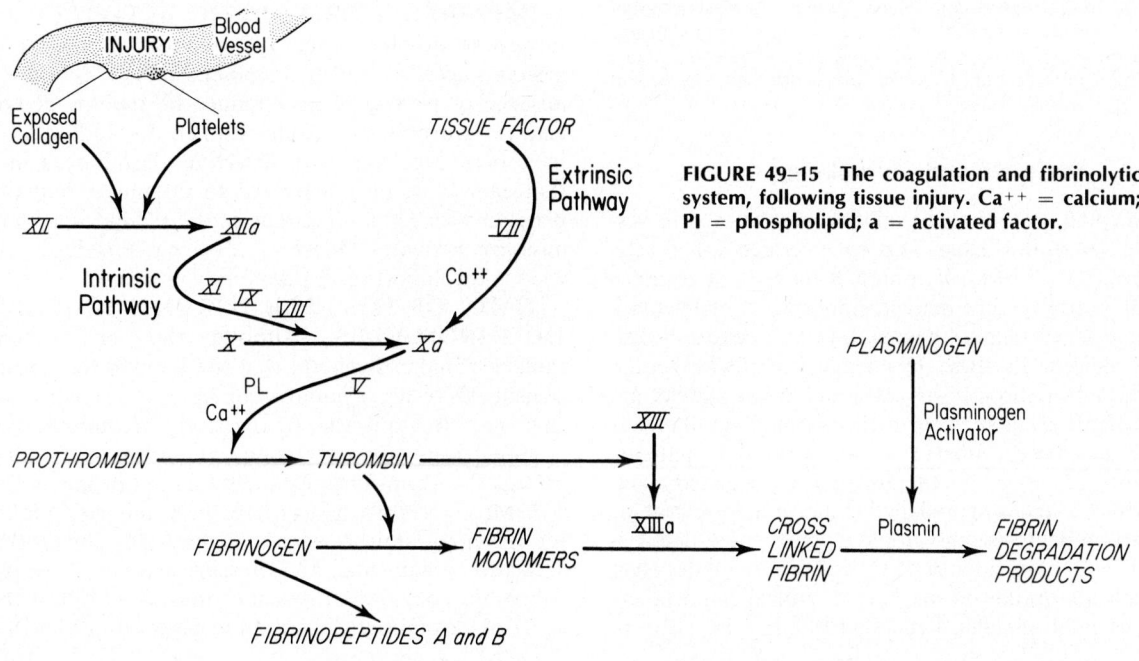

FIGURE 49–15 The coagulation and fibrinolytic system, following tissue injury. Ca++ = calcium; PI = phospholipid; a = activated factor.

TABLE 49–11 HEMATOLOGIC ABNORMALITIES THAT INCREASE THE RISK OF THROMBOEMBOLISM

Abnormal blood flow
Decreased levels of inhibitors
Antithrombin deficiency or dysfunction
Protein C deficiency
Impaired platelet release and aggregation
Thrombocytosis in myeloproliferative disorders
Impaired clearance of activated factors
Impaired fibrinolytic activity
Abnormal fibrinogen
Decreased vascular plasminogen activator content/release
Abnormal plasminogen

blood flow and rheology. For example, they reduce both venous flow velocity and distensibility in the lower limbs and red cell deformability, the latter leading to increased blood viscosity and increased pulmonary capillary blood volume as well as a minor increase in pulmonary artery pressure. As discussed below, oral contraceptives have multiple effects on the coagulation system that could account for their association with thromboembolism.

Decreased Level of Inhibitors. As previously pointed out, many coagulation proteins exist in the circulation as proenzymes, which are then cleaved to form the active clotting factors. There are several inhibitors in blood that can inactivate active clotting proteins by forming a stable but inactive complex (Table 49–13). The most well described is *antithrombin*, which binds to coagulation proteins such as thrombin, X_a, IX_a, XI_a, and XII_a. Its activity is markedly enhanced by the mucopolysaccharide heparin. In fact, the heparin cofactor activity of antithrombin is thought to account for the majority of heparin's anticoagulant activity. Deficient or biochemically abnormal antithrombin molecules have been reported in families with increased thrombosis.[186] The inheritance pattern is thought to be autosomal dominant with variable penetrance. Almost 70 per cent of patients with the deficiency have a thrombotic tendency. Levels of antithrombin III may fall slightly during active thrombosis, and it has been suggested that this reduction could perpetuate a thrombotic tendency. Heparin normally activates antithrombin activity, and markedly reduced levels of antithrombin III could explain rare cases of heparin resistance. It is still unclear, however, what activates antithrombin in vivo, although heparin-like molecules have been isolated from cell surfaces and vessel walls.

Recently, another clinically important inhibitor, *protein C*, has been discovered. Protein C is a vitamin K–dependent protease that is activated by thrombin after it is bound to an endothelial cell protein, thrombomodulin. Activated protein C can then inactivate Factors V and VIII and slow down coagulation reactions. Absence of this protein could lead to unchecked coagulation, by allowing excess thrombin generation and thrombosis.[187] At least one large family with this defect has been described to date.[188] Protein C also has some poorly understood profibrinolytic activity, which may help limit the size of thrombi.[189]

Platelets and Thrombosis

As noted, platelets adhere to microfibrils exposed in vessels denuded of endothelium and to ulcerated atherosclerotic plaques.[190] As previously noted, a number of complex biochemical pathways are activated following platelet adhesion that lead to platelet aggregation and release.[177] Imbalance or defects in these biochemical pathways could lead to bleeding or thrombosis. Although most platelet aggregation defects are associated with bleeding, spontaneous aggregation has been reported to occur in some patients with thrombotic states.[191] In disorders associated with thrombocytosis, including polycythemia vera, essential or primary thrombocytosis, and other myeloproliferative disorders in which the incidence of thrombosis is higher than normal, such abnormalities may be of clinical importance. Wu demonstrated platelet hyperaggregability in vitro in thrombocytosis due to myeloproliferative disorders but not in patients with reactive thrombocytosis.[192]

Assays for measuring components that are part of the "platelet release reaction" are now available.[193] Increased levels of two of these proteins, Platelet Factor four (PF-4) and beta-thromboglobulin (B-TG), have been reported in patients with disseminated intravascular coagulation and with venous or arterial thrombosis, pulmonary emboli, prosthetic cardiac valves, and severe cardiorespiratory failure. In addition, marked elevations are found in a significant number of patients with acute myocardial infarction, as well as in patients with angina pectoris or with exercise-induced ischemia.[194] In some studies, B-TG levels have been shown to correlate with the vascular complications that occur in diabetes.[195] While these studies of PF-4 and B-TG are of considerable interest and represent an important area for further investigation, at the present time it is unclear whether they represent the cause or the effect of thrombotic and vascular disease.

Platelets also serve as a potential link in supporting the concept that stress causes ischemic heart disease. Friedman and Rosenman observed that most of their myocardial infarction–prone patients were of the "type A" behavioral pattern (p. 1826) and exhibited accelerated clotting times and increased circulating catecholamines.[196] Epinephrine and norepinephrine are potent platelet-aggregating agents, making them more responsive to ADP and thrombin. Activation of the sympathoadrenal system might be implicated in the pathogenesis of coronary artery thrombosis by increasing arterial pressure, platelet aggregation, coronary vascular tone, and circulating free fatty acids, which all may act in concert to increase the severity of myocardial ischemia.

IMPAIRED CLEARANCE OF ACTIVATED FACTORS. The liver and reticuloendothelial systems normally remove activated clotting factors and plasminogen activators as well as soluble fibrin complexes from the circulation. Liver disease (cirrhosis, viral hepatitis, and so on) can impair the clearance mechanism and lead to widespread thrombosis and systemic fibrinolysis.

IMPAIRED FIBRINOLYTIC ACTIVITY. There is increasing evidence that abnormalities in the fibrinolytic system may also lead to thrombosis. As mentioned above, absence of protein C may reduce fibrinolytic activity and lead to thrombosis (Table 49–12). In addition, patients have been described with defective plasminogen molecules that cannot be fully activated to plasmin,[181] and there are patients with reduced venous content[180] and release of plasminogen activator. Most of these patients have recurrent venous thrombosis and pulmonary embolism.

TESTS OF POSSIBLE USE IN THE DIAGNOSIS OF THROMBOSIS. Although there are no firmly established diagnostic tests that are specific for thromboembolism, there are a number of blood coagulation changes that may be applicable to the study of thrombosis. These include fibrin monomer complexes, fibrinopeptides A and B, and the fibrin-fibrinogen degradation products (Fig. 49–15). More recently, assays have been reported for circulating thrombin-antithrombin complexes and for prothrombin activation fragments. The measurement of these products of various coagulation reactions may be useful in the diagnosis of thromboembolism and, when coupled with radio-

TABLE 49–12 CHARACTERISTICS OF THE COAGULATION PROTEIN INHIBITORS

Name	Mechanism of Action	Activator	Diagnostic Test	Clinical Disorder
Antithrombin III	Complexes with thrombin, X_a, and other serine proteases	Heparin	Immunoassay: Rate of thrombin neutralization ± heparin	Reduction or dysfunction causes recurrent venous arterial thrombosis
Protein C	Proteolyzes Factors V and VIII	Thrombin and thrombomodulin on the endothelial cell surface	Immunoassay	Decrease causes venous thromboembolism
α_2 plasmin inhibitor	Complexes with plasmin	None	Immunoassay	Absence causes rapid fibrinolysis, bleeding

isotope labeling studies utilizing coagulation proteins like fibrinogen or plasminogen, may localize the site of a thrombus. The fibrinopeptide A radioimmunoassay has been most widely employed and is elevated in patients with venous thrombosis and pulmonary embolism and promptly returns to normal following administration of heparin. Unfortunately, many nonspecific stimuli also raise the plasma fibrinopeptide A level, and the test is not yet clinically useful.[183]

EFFECTS OF ORAL CONTRACEPTIVES ON COAGULATION. Ingestion of oral contraceptives raises the risk of thromboembolism in young women and provides an interesting model for a drug-induced hypercoagulable state. Many of the blood changes discussed previously are induced by the use of oral contraceptives. In addition, the clinical and epidemiologic studies have firmly linked pill use to certain thrombotic and vascular complications. Venous thrombosis and embolism, myocardial infarction, and cerebrovascular disease, as well as other thromboembolic phenomena in young women, have all been attributed to oral contraceptives.[184,185] The presumed mechanisms include effects of the drug on the coagulation profile, i.e., high platelet counts, short partial thromboplastin times, elevation of the concentrations of various clotting factors, increased platelet adhesiveness, lowered levels of antithrombin III[183–186] (Table 49–12) and decreased clearance of activated clotting factors. In addition, since exogenous estrogens alter the endothelium of the cervix and endometrium, it is possible that similar changes may occur in vascular endothelium, causing an injury site—the first step in the formation of a thrombus. Thus, there is a definite hazard of vascular complications and thrombosis associated with the use of oral contraceptive agents. However, some of the risks, like venous thromboembolism, may be no greater than the risks associated with pregnancy itself.[186] Since the risks are not uniformly distributed among oral contraceptive users, attention must also be directed toward identifying the subpopulations that are especially prone to these thromboembolic complications. These include all women exceeding 35 years of age and women of any age with one of the other risk factors for atherosclerosis (i.e., cigarette smoking, hypertension, or hypercholesterolemia), or a history of a clotting disorder. In addition to their effect on the clotting system, oral contraceptives may enhance the risk of the development or exacerbation of hypertension (p. 873).

In conclusion, the following alterations in the blood have been shown to be associated with either an increased risk of thromboembolism or active thrombosis: (1) reduced antithrombin III, (2) reduced fibrinolytic activity, (3) increased platelet aggregation, (4) increased PF-4, (5) increased B-TG, (6) fibrin-monomer complexes, (7) fibrinopeptides, and (8) fibrin-fibrinogen degradation products.

Anticoagulants and Platelet Suppression

Anticoagulant therapy with heparin or warfarin is clearly of benefit in the treatment and prevention of venous thrombosis but is of limited value in patients at risk of arterial thrombosis. Parenteral heparin is effective in the treatment of thrombophlebitis and pulmonary embolism (p. 1588) and in prevention of thromboembolic events in bedridden or inactive patients, including those with heart failure (Chap. 16) and acute myocardial infarction (p. 1304). Warfarin and related coumarin drugs have the same spectrum of effects; however, their action is delayed and they are less potent than heparin. Advantages are their effectiveness following oral administration and their usefulness when long-term prophylaxis is needed, as in patients with artificial heart valves and vascular prostheses. Platelet-suppressive agents, aspirin, dipyridamole, and sulfinpyrazone, because of their ability to inhibit the platelet release reaction and aggregation, are useful to postoperative patients with prosthetic heart valves and in patients with coronary and cerebral artery disease.

HEPARIN. Heparin, a naturally occurring sulfated mucopolysaccharide, is a powerful anticoagulant acting at several sites in the clotting schema. Most important is the inhibition of activated Factor X and thrombin, accomplished by increasing the neutralizing effect of antithrombin III–heparin cofactors.[198] It is the most useful drug available for the prophylaxis and treatment of venous thromboembolism.[199] Mortality and morbidity rates have been markedly reduced in patients with acute pulmonary embolism (Chap. 46).

Studies in large numbers of postoperative patients have confirmed that low-dose prophylaxis reduces the incidence of deep-vein thrombosis and the mortality from subsequent pulmonary embolism.[200] The dosage required for the treatment of established thromboembolism is higher than that needed for prophylaxis because of the need to reduce the rate of thrombin generation. In addition, inhibitors like PF-4 released from activated platelets may partially neutralize heparin. The current recommended dose for treatment of patients with thromboembolism is 20,000 to 30,000 U/24 hr by continuous intravenous infusion or enough to keep the partial thromboplastin time at 1.5 to 2 times the control level.[201] Hemorrhagic complications are reduced with the use of continuous intravenous infusion of heparin.

Although prophylaxis of venous thrombosis with heparin has been widely employed in postoperative patients for over 40 years, not until 1970 was there any firm evidence to support its use.[198-201] Many clinical trials support the use of subcutaneous low-dose heparin in preventing postoperative deaths due to pulmonary embolism. In other clinical situations, such as following hip surgery or myocardial infarction, the regimen has been less successful. The dosage recommended in prophylaxis is approximately half that of the therapeutic dose—that is, 10,000 to 15,000 U/24 hr, given subcutaneously in two or three divided doses.

ORAL ANTICOAGULANTS. Warfarin and its derivatives prevent vitamin K–dependent carboxylation of glutamic acid residues on the prothrombin complex proteins in the liver. As a result, the activity of clotting Factors II, VII, IX, and X is markedly reduced, which impairs fibrin formation and the growth of thrombi. The primary indications for long-term therapy with these agents are venous thrombosis in the leg and pulmonary embolism after the patient has initially received intravenous heparin.[202] In patients with hemodynamically significant mitral stenosis, particularly those with transient or permanent atrial fibrillation and in those with prosthetic heart valves, embolic episodes are minimized by permanent treatment with oral anticoagulants (Chap. 32). In addition, oral anticoagulants are useful after an acute arterial embolic episode and after hip surgery. Their long-term use in cerebrovascular disease and after myocardial infarction is still controversial, and they may actually be dangerous in patients with completed strokes.

The starting dose of the commonly used agent warfarin is 10 mg/24 hr for three to four days, with a maintenance dose between 3 and 8 mg/24 hr, depending upon the individual patient. Prothrombin times are usually kept at 2 to 2.5 times those of control. Complications include significant bleeding, as with heparin, as well as failure of anticoagulation with rethrombosis. Both of these complications may occur because of the addition or omission of other medications that may potentiate or antagonize the effect of warfarin (Table 49–13). Prolonged prothrombin times and bleeding may also occur with infection, liver disease, cardiac failure, alcoholic excess, or radical alteration in the diet with resultant change in the microbial intestinal flora. Despite careful control of the prothrombin time, the incidence of serious hemorrhage is 5 to 10 per cent per patient-year at risk and the incidence of fatal complications 0.5 to 1 per cent per patient-year. Newer immunoassays that can monitor the concentration of normal and abnormal prothrombin and the assays that detect prothrombin activation fragments or thrombin-antithrombin complexes may provide better ways to monitor warfarin dose and both improve its efficacy as an antithrombotic agent and reduce the incidence of bleeding.

TABLE 49–13 INTERACTION OF COMMONLY USED DRUGS WITH COUMARIN DERIVATIVES

Potentiate	Antagonize
Phenylbutazone	Barbiturates
Salicylates	*Other*:
Thyroid	chronic alcohol
Other:	allopurinol
acute alcohol	cholestyramine
anabolic steroids	diuretics
antibiotics	glutethimide
antiplatelet drugs	nortriptyline
clofibrate	rifampin
phenytoin	
oral hypoglycemic agents	
quinidine sulfate	
sulfonamides	

THROMBOLYTIC THERAPY. Drugs that activate the fibrinolytic system can be administered to patients to hasten the resoultion of established thrombi. The mechanism of action of these drugs is outlined in Figure 49–16. Streptokinase (SK), a bacterial product, forms a complex with plasminogen which then activates additional plasminogen molecules. Urokinase (UK), derived from cultured kidney cells, directly activates plasminogen. Both of these agents have been used to treat patients with acute arterial thrombosis and massive pulmonary embolism. Since these drugs cause severe hypofibrinogenemia, bleeding is a potential complication. Intracoronary infusion of SK or UK is less hazardous and has been used to restore the patency of arteriovenous shunts or to reverse acute coronary occlusion (pp. 336 and 1324).

One potentially important new development is the successful commercial production of tissue plasminogen activator (TPA) using recombinant DNA technology. Since TPA must bind to fibrin to initiate fibrinolysis, it may selectively lyse thrombi without causing systemic fibrinogen depletion and bleeding. It is likely that systemic fibrinolytic therapy with TPA will become available for clinical studies.

PLATELET INHIBITORS. Because of the role of platelets in normal hemostasis and thrombosis, a number of drugs that interfere with platelet function in vitro have undergone clinical trials. Three agents have been shown to have some benefit: (1) aspirin, (2) sulfinpyrazone, and (3) dipyridamole (Table 49–14). Although the latter's precise

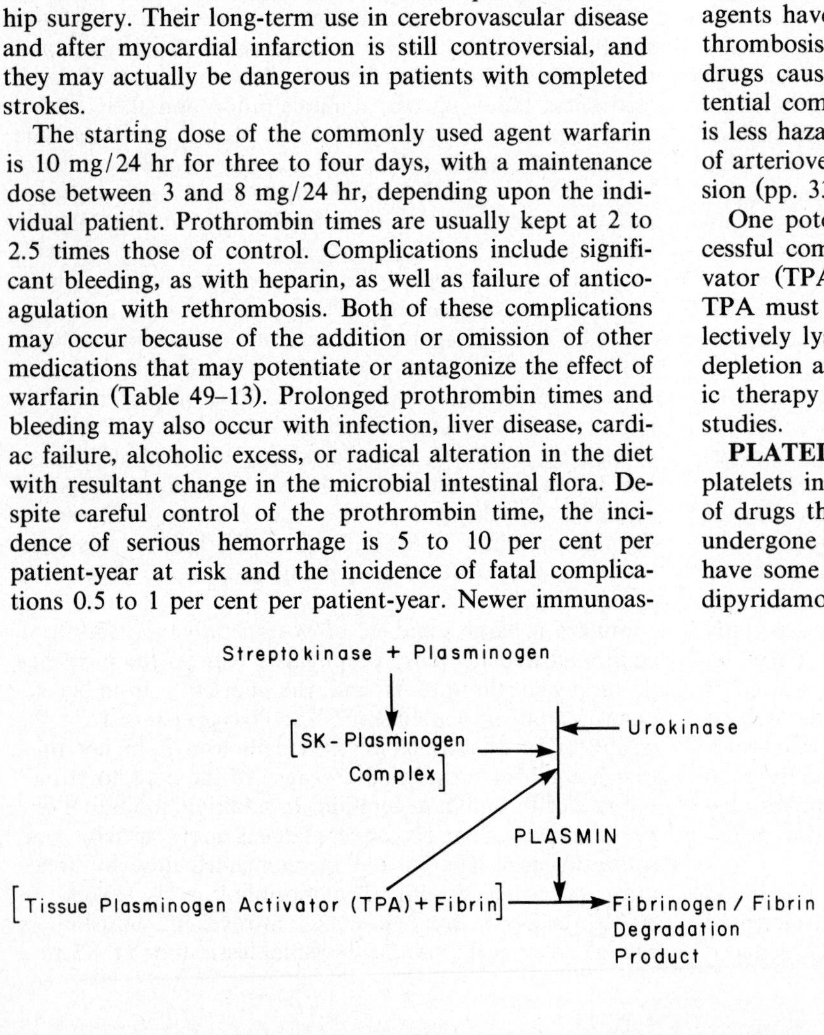

FIGURE 49–16 Mechanism of action of three fibrinolytic agents. Urokinase, which directly activates plasminogen; streptokinase (SK), which complexes to plasminogen; and tissue plasminogen activator (TPA), which requires fibrin to effectively activate plasminogen.

TABLE 49–14 ACTION OF ANTIPLATELET DRUGS

	ASPIRIN	DIPYRIDAMOLE	SULFINPYRAZONE
Mode of action	Irreversible acetylation of cyclooxygenase	Inhibition of platelet cAMP phosphodiesterase	Transient inhibition of cyclooxygenase (in vitro) ? effect on platelet-vessel wall interaction
Laboratory effects on platelets*			
Aggregation	$\downarrow$	0 (at clinical levels)	0
Adhesion	0	$\downarrow$	?
Survival	0	$\uparrow$	$\uparrow$
Bleeding time	$\uparrow$	0	0
Effects on clinical thromboembolism†			
Ischemia heart disease	−	−	+
Cerebrovascular disease	+	−	+/−
Venous thrombosis	+/−	−	+/−
Prosthetic surfaces			
Heart valves	− + with warfarin + with heparin	+ with warfarin	+ with warfarin
Shunts	+		+
Arterial prostheses			−
Coronary artery bypass‡ graft patency	+	+	

*($\downarrow$) diminished; ($\uparrow$) prolonged; (0) no effect
†(+) improved; (−) not improved; (+/−) conflicting data or positive trends without statistical significance
‡Combined therapy with aspirin and dipyridamole.
Modified from Schafer, A. I., and Handin, R. I.: The role of platelets in thrombotic and vascular disease. Prog. Cardiovasc. Dis. *22*:31–52, 1979.

site of action is still unclear, the first two agents interfere with normal platelet synthesis of prostaglandins and thromboxane[179] (Fig. 49–17). Platelet survival in patients with valvular heart disease and with prosthetic valves is significantly shortened, presumably because of platelet aggregation on, or consumption by, the abnormal surface. Antiplatelet medication may prevent these interactions that shorten platelet survival, and they are often given in addition to oral anticoagulants. Platelet survival is also shortened in cerebrovascular disease, and a recent study demonstrated aspirin's effectiveness in reducing complications of threatened strokes in men.[204]

Because of the postulated relationship between platelet aggregation and myocardial infarction, many studies are in progress to determine the benefit of platelet inhibition in coronary artery disease. One study using sulfinpyrazone claimed a reduction in mortality from sudden death in the first year after myocardial infarction, but the interpretation of the results has been disputed. The mechanism for this supposedly beneficial effect and the reproducibility of this finding are still unknown.[205] Dipyridamole appears to suppress experimentally induced arteriosclerosis in an animal model. Although there is no evidence for a similar effect in humans, the drug has been successful in reducing embolization from prosthetic valves, and the combination of aspirin and dipyridamole may improve coronary bypass graft patency.[206]

Bleeding Due to Platelet Dysfunction. Qualitative defects of platelet function, associated with normal platelet counts but prolonged bleeding time and decreased aggregation, are being noted with increasing frequency. The most common causes include abnormalities in platelet production or response to thromboxane A_2, or defects in the platelet packaging and storage of adenine nucleotides or other granule contents—storage pool disease. The most common cause of a decrease in TXA_2 production is the ingestion of nonsteroidal anti-inflammatory agents like aspirin, indomethacin, or ibuprofen. In fact, as discussed above, the antiplatelet effect of these drugs is being exploited as a means to prevent thromboembolism. One unavoidable side effect is the development of mild to moderate bleeding and the exacerbation of bleeding from organic lesions or at the

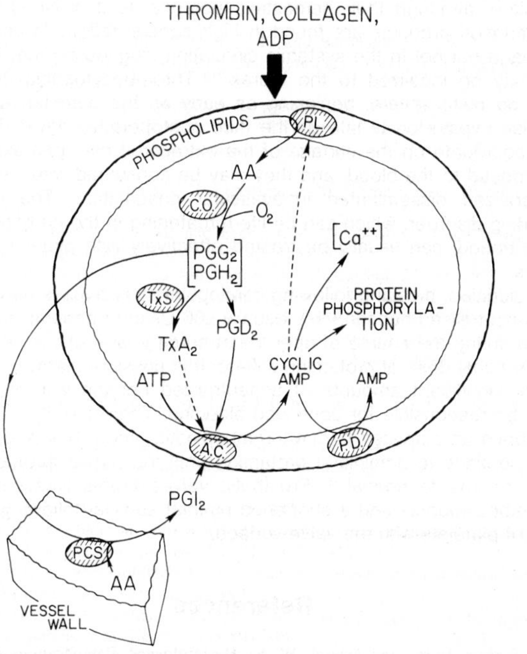

FIGURE 49–17 Prostaglandin and thromboxane metabolism in the platelet and vessel wall. The major platelet product is thromboxane A_2, a vasoconstrictor and platelet activator that inhibits adenylate cyclase, and the major vessel wall product PGI_2, a vasodilator and platelet inhibitor that stimulates adenylate cyclase and increases cyclic AMP. Hatched circles represent major control and synthetic enzymes. *PL* (phospholipase) releases the precursor arachidonic acid (AA) from membrane phospholipid. *CO* (cyclo-oxygenase) oxygenates AA to produce the prostaglandin intermediate PGG_2. *TxS* (thromboxane synthetase) converts PGG_2 to thromboxane A_2. *PCS* (prostacyclin synthetase) converts PGG_2 to PGI_2 in the endothelial cell. *AC* (adenylate cyclase) converts ATP to cyclic AMP, which inhibits platelet activation. *PD* (phosphodiesterase) breaks down cyclic AMP. Antiplatelet drugs exert their effects via these enzymes. Aspirin irreversibly inhibits CO and abolishes thromboxane production. Sulfinpyrazone also inhibits CO, although its effect is more short-lived. Dipyridamole (Persantine) blocks PD and prevents breakdown of cyclic AMP. Newer drugs which inhibit TxS or inhibit PL have not yet undergone extensive clinical testing.

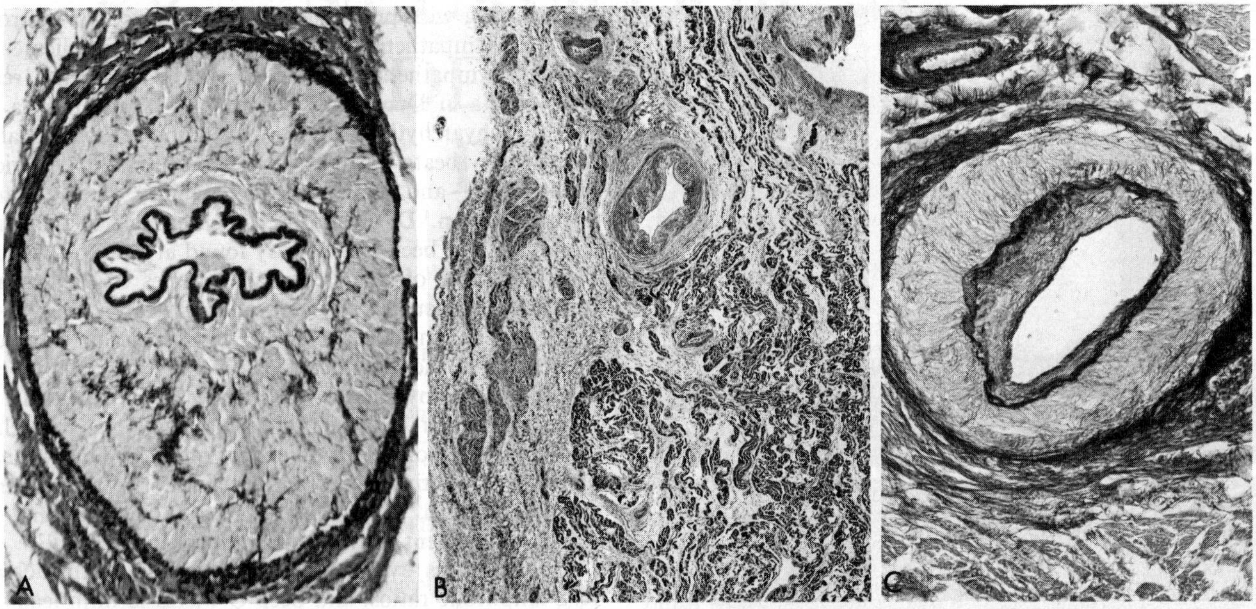

FIGURE 50–3 Small intramural coronary arteries in X-linked Duchenne's dystrophy. *A*, Small coronary artery from the left atrium of an 18-year-old boy. There is severe hypertrophy of the media with marked luminal narrowing (Verhoeff–van Gieson elastic tissue stains). *B*, Section from the right atrium in the region of the sinus node in the same patient. The neurogenic fibers of the sinus node are seen as well as an intramural coronary artery that has a thick wall and slightly narrowed lumen. Staining disclosed increased quantities of mucopolysaccharides in the vessel wall. *C*, Right atrial intramural coronary artery from a 12-year-old boy. The vessel exhibits a thick media and intima and a narrowed lumen (elastic tissue stain). (From Perloff, J. K., et al.: The distinctive electrocardiogram of Duchenne's muscular dystrophy. Am. J. Med. *42*:179, 1967.)

tered shapes of right precordial R waves (RSr'or polyphasic R waves). The electrocardiographic changes in Duchenne's dystrophy are *not* related to thoracic deformity, thoracic muscle atrophy, or pulmonary hypertension; to hypertrophy of the right ventricle, crista supraventricularis, or interventricular septum; or to abnormalities in right ventricular conduction.[1,4] Striking abnormalities have been found in small intramural coronary arteries (severe hypertrophy of the media with luminal narrowing) (Fig. 50–3), but the arteriopathy was not related to the electrocardiographic pattern or to the distribution of myocardial dystrophy[4,16] (see below). The occurrence of identical electrocardiograms in siblings with Duchenne's dystrophy implies a genetic determinant of the distinctive patterns.

The prominent anterior forces (anterior shift of the QRS vector loop) appear to represent a relative loss of

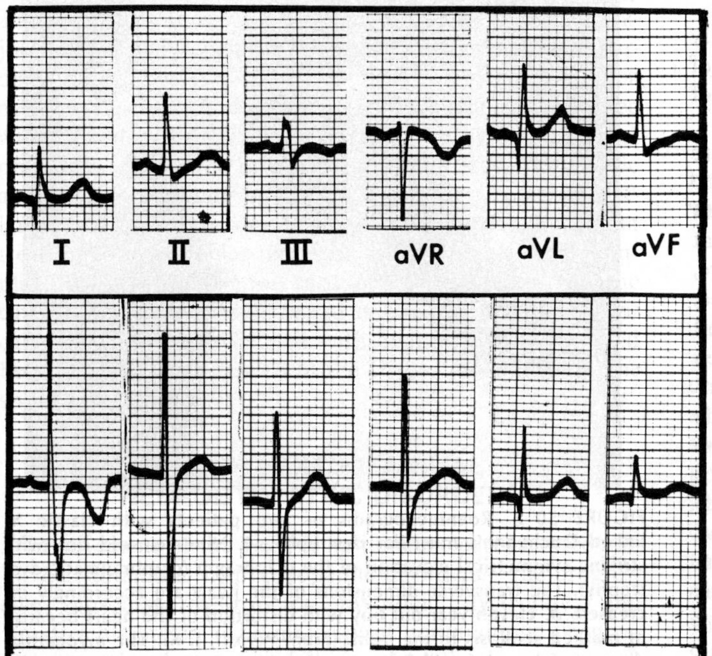

FIGURE 50–4 Electrocardiogram from a 12-year-old boy with classic Duchenne's progressive dystrophy. There is a tall R wave in lead V_1 in addition to deep Q waves in leads I and aVL. At necropsy myocardial dystrophy was found to be confined to the posterolateral left ventricular wall. (From Perloff, J. K.: The distinctive electrocardiogram of Duchenne's muscular dystrophy. Am. J. Med. *42*:179, 1967.)

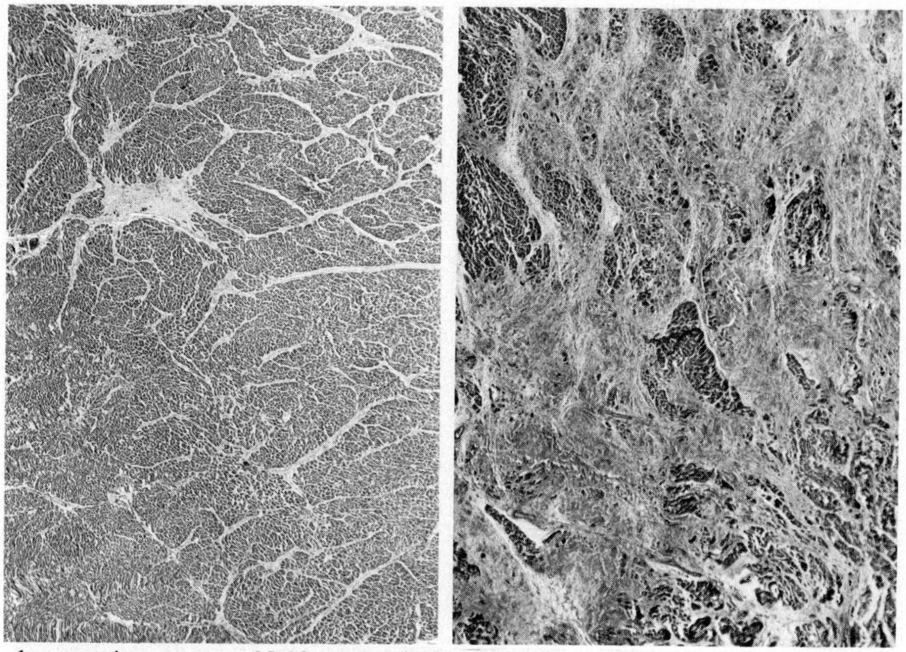

FIGURE 50–5 Photomicrographs from an 18-year-old boy who died of classic Duchenne's progressive muscular dystrophy. The ventricular septum (left) shows only a few microscopic scars, whereas the posterobasal left ventricular wall (right) is extensively scarred (hematoxylin and eosin stains). (From Perloff, J. K., et al.: The distinctive electrocardiogram of Duchenne's muscular dystrophy. Am. J. Med. *42*:179, 1967.)

posterobasal electrical activity, as in strictly posterior myocardial infarction,[1,4,13,17] and the Q waves may reflect lateral or diaphragmatic extension.[4,13] Necropsy studies have disclosed selective transmural scarring of the posterobasal left ventricle with or without lateral or inferior wall extension (Figs. 50–5 and 50–6), providing acceptable electrocardiographic/vectorcardiographic/necropsy correlations.[4,5,16] Positron computed tomography using F-18 deoxyglucose and N-13 ammonia has identified a regional metabolic abnormality in the posterior and posterolateral left ventricular wall.[18] Thus, the cardiomyopathy of Duchenne's dystrophy appears to be a unique form of heart disease in which a specific segment of ventricular myocardium is genetically labeled as the target site. Dystrophic involvement of the posterobasal left ventricle and contiguous posterior papillary muscle may cause mitral regurgitation (papillary muscle dysfunction),[4] sometimes with mitral prolapse seen on echocardiography.[5,19] Evaluation of left ventricular function by echocardiography provides additional information, especially on wall motion.[20]

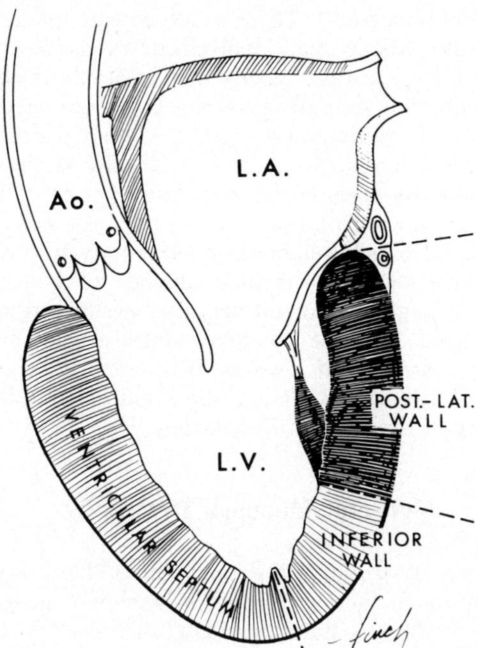

FIGURE 50–6 Diagram of the left side of the heart illustrating the location of myocardial dystrophy at necropsy. Scarring was limited to the posterolateral wall of the left ventricle. No significant scarring was observed in the inferior wall or in the ventricular septum. A papillary muscle was scarred in one patient who had clinical mitral regurgitation. (Courtesy of William C. Roberts, M.D., Pathology Branch, National Heart, Lung and Blood Institute, Bethesda, Maryland.)

Enzymes of skeletal muscle are copiously released into the plasma in Duchenne's dystrophy. This release, especially of creatine kinase, has been used to identify active systemic myopathy. However, the use of enzyme or isoenzyme quantification has not proved useful in detecting myocardial dystrophy.[1] It was hoped that distinctive isozyme profiles—both lactic dehydrogenase (LDH) and MB creatine phosphokinase (CPK)—might be used to identify active myocardial dystrophy, but these enzymes originate in dystrophic skeletal muscle and merely resemble those of cardiac muscle, compromising the specificity of the determinations.[2,21] Further, coronary sinus catheterization has not convincingly documented myocardial release of enzymes.[1] Measurement of creatine kinase has been established as a means of identifying "preclinical" systemic dystrophy in male siblings of propositi[22] and in female carriers in families with Duchenne's progressive muscular dystrophy.[14,15,23] The majority (about two-thirds) of female carriers of X-linked muscular dystrophy have elevated serum creatine kinase.[21] These female carriers sometimes manifest occult or overt muscle weakness and calf pseudohypertrophy[15,24] in addition to electrocardiographic evidence of cardiac involvement.[10,14,15]

SLOWLY PROGRESSIVE MUSCULAR DYSTROPHY OF EARLY ONSET.[25,26] Dystrophy with the phenotype of Duchenne may be slowly progressive and either early-onset, autosomal recessive, or late-onset, X-linked recessive (Becker's dystrophy) (Fig. 50–7). When family ped-

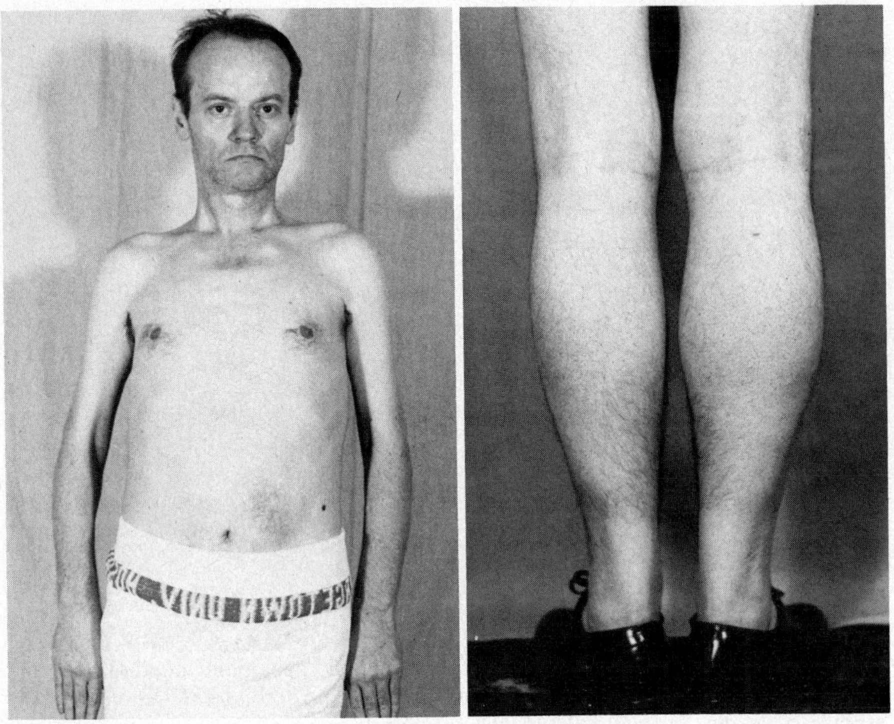

FIGURE 50–7 A 40-year-old man believed to have late-onset, slowly progressive Duchenne's muscular dystrophy (Becker's dystrophy). He died because of cardiomyopathy and complete heart block (see Fig. 49–12). Dystrophy of shoulder girdle, arms, pelvic girdle, and proximal leg muscle is seen, with mild asymmetrical pseudohypertrophy of the calves. (From Perloff, J. K., et al.: The cardiomyopathy of progressive muscular dystrophy. Circulation *33*:625, 1966, by permission of the American Heart Association, Inc.)

igrees are deficient, it is difficult to distinguish these two subvarieties from each other or from limb-girdle dystrophy of Erb with calf pseudohypertrophy.[1] Such patients may not only have cardiomyopathy[27] but stand a good chance of dying from it[1] (Fig. 50–8). The type of cardiac involvement differs from classic Duchenne's dystrophy.[1] The ventricles dilate and fail (biventricular dystrophy) with abnormalities of infranodal conduction (left bundle branch block and complete heart block) (Fig. 50–8).[1] In families with Becker's X-linked muscular dystrophy, congestive cardiomyopathy may appear in one member while other members are clinically spared.[27]

LIMB-GIRDLE DYSTROPHY OF ERB. Transmission is typically autosomal recessive, with insidious onset usually in the second decade.[28] Dystrophy of the hip girdle usually precedes involvement of the shoulders (Fig. 50–9*A*). Calf pseudohypertrophy occurs, but this is relatively late in onset and mild to moderate in degree[28] (Fig. 50–10). Progression is slow, but the majority of affected individuals are incapacitated within two decades. Although cardiac involvement is infrequent and seldom severe, it is expressed as (1) disturbances in rhythm and conduction, namely, sinus bradycardia (sick sinoatrial node), (2) atrial flutter (tachycardia), (3) first-degree heart block (abnormal atrioventricular node), and (4) complete right bundle branch block, QRS prolongation, and complete heart block (infranodal disease) (Table 50–1). Sporadic patients with limb-girdle dystrophy of Erb have both cardiomyopathy *and* extensive disease of the cardiac conducting system (sinus node, atrioventricular node, and infranodal tissue).[29,30]

TABLE 50–1 NEUROMUSCULAR DISEASES WITH COMPLETE HEART BLOCK

Myotonic muscular dystrophy
Kearns-Sayre syndrome
X-linked humeroperoneal dystrophy
Peroneal muscular atrophy
Limb-girdle dystrophy

FACIOSCAPULOHUMERAL DYSTROPHY (LANDOUZY-DÉJÉRINE). Transmission is autosomal dominant (equal incidence in males and females) with onset from the first to fourth decades. Dystrophy begins in the shoulder girdle (scapulohumeral) (Fig. 50–9*B*) with inevitable progression to the muscles of facial expression (thus "*facio*scapulohumeral"). There is subsequent spread to the pelvic girdle. Myocardial involvement in facioscapulohumeral dystrophy seldom occurs and as a rule is clinically unimportant,[1] but sporadic examples have been cited.[31,32]

The most dramatic and intriguing cardiac disorder associated with facioscapulohumeral dystrophy is permanent paralysis of the atria (atrial standstill).[33] It is of interest that the first documentation of atrial paralysis was in a patient with facioscapulohumeral muscular dystrophy.[34] Criteria for the diagnosis include absence of P waves on scalar, esophageal, and intracardiac electrocardiograms, lack of atrial response to direct (intracardiac) electrical stimulation, absence of *a* waves in the jugular venous and right atrial pressure pulses, a supraventricular QRS, and immobility of the atria on fluoroscopy.[33,35]

Myotonic Muscular Dystrophy

Myotonic dystrophy (dystrophia myotonica, myotonia atrophica, or Steinert's disease) is a slowly progressive, multisystem, autosomal dominant disorder.[36,37] Clinical manifestations characteristically appear in the third or fourth decade,[38] although occasional cases are seen in childhood and infancy. Myotonia (delayed relaxation after contraction) can be provoked by voluntary, mechanical, or electrical stimulation of muscles of the hands, forearms, tongue, and jaw. The myotonic response is typically elicited by tapping the thenar eminence (percussion myotonia), especially after the patient rapidly opens and closes the fist. Dystrophy (atrophy or wasting) is initially found

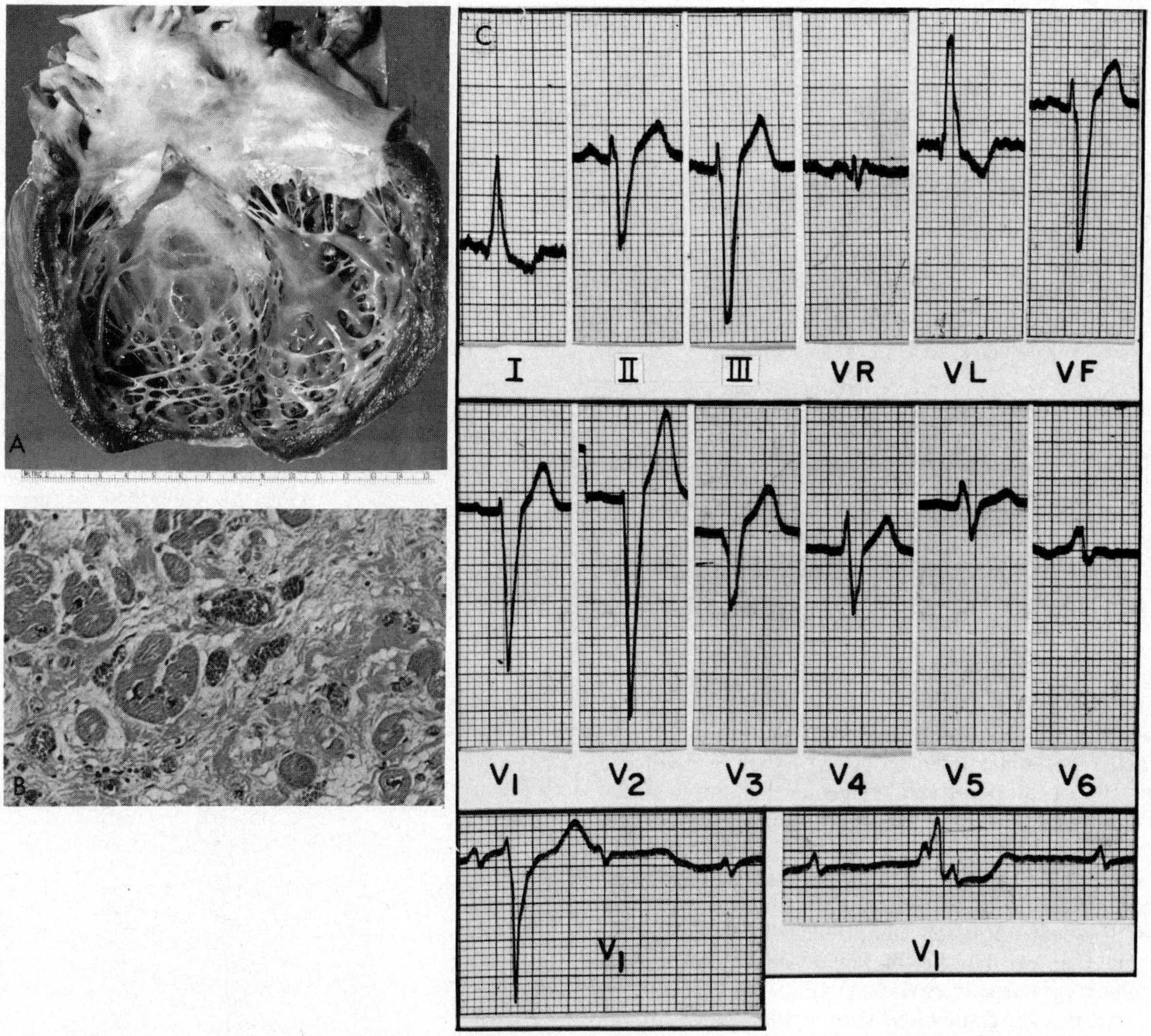

FIGURE 50–8 Gross and microscopic cardiac pathological specimens and the electrocardiogram from a 45-year-old man with late-onset, slowly progressive Becker's muscular dystrophy. *A*, Dilated, flabby left ventricle with focal endocardial thickening. The left atrium is also dilated. *B*, Microscopic section from the left ventricle shows marked confluent scarring with variations in fiber size; there was no significant coronary artery disease. *C*, Electrocardiogram recorded at age 40 years. The 12-lead tracing shows left-axis deviation, a QRS of 0.14 sec, small q waves in leads I and aVL and loss of R-wave amplitude in leads V_2 and V_3. The lower tracings, taken 4 years later (a year before death), show complete heart block with a variable QRS configuration. (From Perloff, J. K., et al.: The cardiomyopathy of progressive muscular dystrophy. Circulation *33*:625, 1966, by permission of the American Heart Association, Inc.)

in forearms, neck (especially sternocleidomastoid), and face (expressionless myopathic facies) (Fig. 50–11).[36,38] There is subsequent disturbance of the extensors of the knees and hips and dorsiflexors of the feet.[38] Myotonic dystrophy is a systemic disease that includes important nonmyotonic/nonmyopathic features: cataracts, gonadal atrophy, frontal baldness or thinning of hair (Fig. 50–11), and disease of muscles of the upper gastrointestinal tract.[36,38] Appropriate to this discussion is the cardiac involvement which has been known since the descriptions of Griffith in 1911.[39] Myotonia congenita (Thomsen's disease) with rare exception[40] does not involve the heart and is otherwise distinct from myotonic dystrophy.[41]

Apart from electrocardiographic abnormalities (see below), there is usually little overt clinical evidence of heart disease.[38,41–44] Even so, myotonic dystrophy may *present* as cardiac disease before the neuromuscular diagnosis has been established.[37,38,42,45–47] Cardiac involvement selectively disturbs impulse formation and conduction (Table 50–2).[37–39,41–44,46,48–57] Despite light microscopic[43,47,49,58] and ultrastructural abnormalities,[59,60] clinically detectable myocardi-

TABLE 50–2 ELECTROCARDIOGRAPHIC ABNORMALITIES IN MYOTONIC MUSCULAR DYSTROPHY

Disorders of impulse formation
- Sinus bradycardia
- Atrial flutter
- Atrial fibrillation
- Ventricular tachycardia

Disturbances in conduction
- AV nodal (P-R prolongation)
- Intra-His
- Infra-His (LAD, LBBB, RBBB, complete heart block)

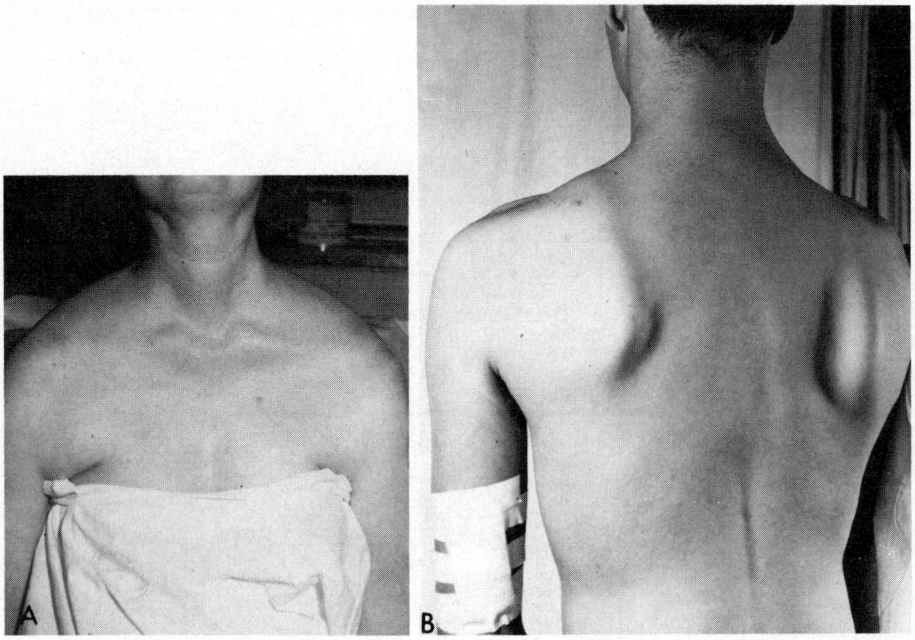

FIGURE 50–9 *A*, Woman with typical limb-girdle dystrophy (Erb's) showing involvement of the shoulder girdle. The proximal leg muscles and pelvic girdle were also involved, but her face was completely spared. *B*, Young man with facioscapulohumeral dystrophy (Landouzy-Déjérine) involving the shoulder girdle, proximal arm muscle (bandage at biopsy site), and face (not shown). (From Perloff, J. K., et al.: The cardiomyopathy of progressive muscular dystrophy. Circulation *33*:625, 1966, by permission of the American Heart Association, Inc.)

al disease is not a feature of myotonic dystrophy.[51] Nor is myocardial myotonia known to occur, either in myotonic dystrophy[49,61] or in myotonia congenita (Thomsen's disease). The earliest and most common electrocardiographic abnormalities are sinus bradycardia and prolongation of the P-R interval. Bradycardia[54] may be punctuated by episodes of tachycardia (atrial flutter or fibrillation).[37,38,41,47,62] The most frequent infranodal abnormality is defective conduction in the left bundle branch system (left bundle branch block or left-axis deviation) (Fig. 50–12),[37,41,42,44,51] and the vectorcardiogram often shows evidence of abnormal intraventricular conduction.[41,43,51,62] Left bundle branch block may initially be intermittent.[62] Both procainamide and phenytoin are used as antimyotonic agents.[46] However, it is preferable to use phenytoin, which shortens the atrioventricular nodal refractory period and has little or no effect on infranodal conduction; procainamide prolongs both AV nodal and infranodal conduction.[46] In addition to the disorders in rhythm and conduction listed in Table 50–2, low-voltage P waves, ST-segment abnormalities, and flattening or inversion of T waves occur.[37,42] Occasionally the electrocardiogram exhibits a pattern resembling myocardial infarction.[42]

Patients may manifest cardiomegaly without symptoms;[38,62] bradycardia may contribute to or be responsible for the enlargement.[49] There is a tendency for the systemic arterial pressure to be relatively low.[41,47] Recurrent syncope occurs because of complete heart block (Stokes-Adams attacks) or sinus bradycardia (Table 50–2),[38,45] and sudden death is a hazard.[36,42,47,50,58,62] Insertion of a transvenous right ventricular pacemaker is desirable in patients with serious bradyarrhythmias associated with this disease.[43,48,53]

In addition to intrinsic heart disease, patients with myotonic muscular dystrophy are at risk because of abnormalities of the neuromuscular apparatus of respiration.[36,38] Alveolar hypoventilation may result in hypercapnia and hypoxemia. There are several reports of prolapse of the mi-

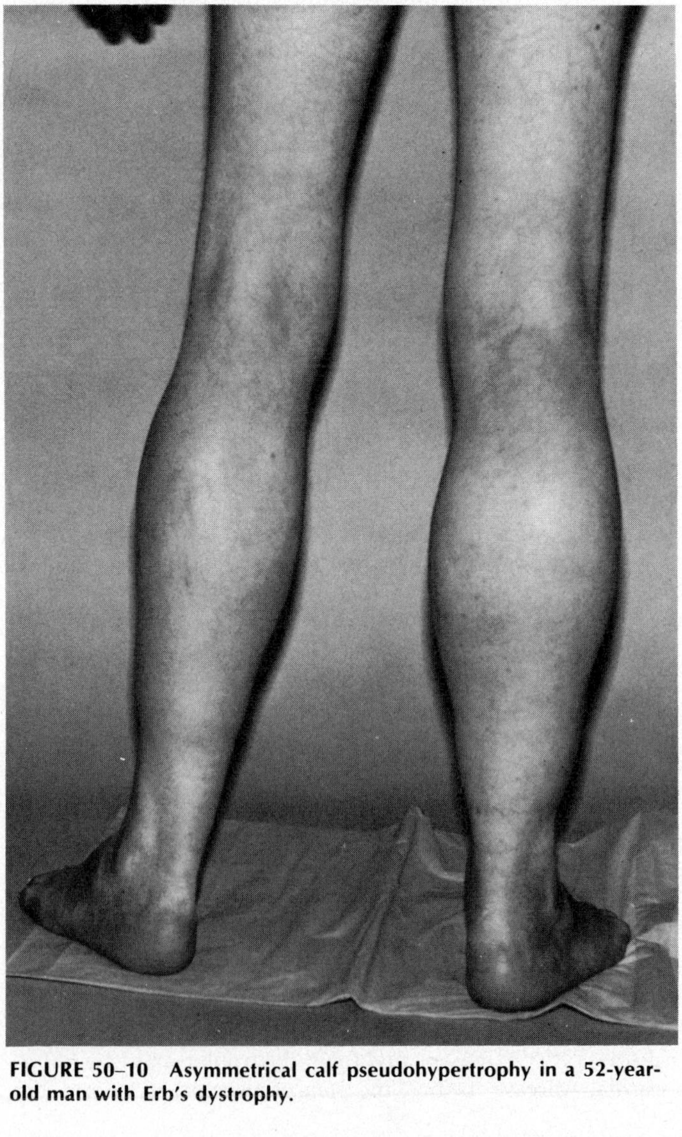

FIGURE 50–10 Asymmetrical calf pseudohypertrophy in a 52-year-old man with Erb's dystrophy.

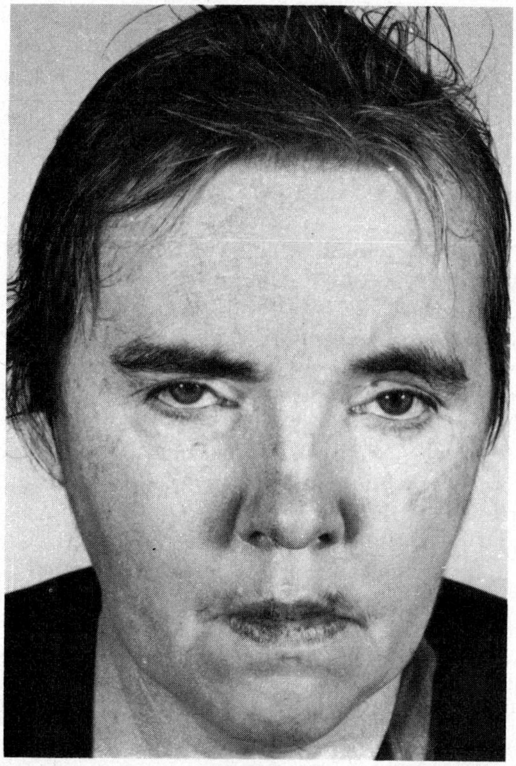

FIGURE 50–11 Fifty-year-old woman with myotonic muscular dystrophy, typical expressionless myopathic facies, and thinning of the frontal hair. (From Perloff, J. K., et al.: Uncommon or commonly unrecognized causes of heart failure. Prog. Cardiovasc. Dis. *12*:409, 1970, by permission of Grune and Stratton.)

tral valve in myotonic dystrophy, but it is unclear whether or not the relationship is coincidental.[18,63–65]

The combination of sinus bradycardia, tachycardia (atrial flutter/fibrillation), P-R interval prolongation, left/right bundle branch block, left-axis deviation, and complete heart block[65a] is an aggregate of related disorders of the sinus node, atrioventricular node, and infranodal conduction tissues analogous to the "sick sinus syndrome" in much older subjects. The heart disease of myotonic dystrophy may therefore take the form of premature aging of impulse regulation and conduction. Other features of premature aging occur in myotonic dystrophy, namely, a decrease in gonadal function, thinning of the hair, frontal baldness, and cataracts.

Friedreich's Ataxia

Friedreich's ataxia is a progressive heredofamilial disorder characterized by neurological disease and a cardiomyopathy.[66–70] Nicolaus Friedreich, in a series of five papers between 1863 and 1877, described a specific form of spinal degeneration with distinctive clinical and pathological features encountered in nine members of three sibships.[71] Despite a century of lively interest, Friedreich's ataxia has resisted precise clinical and biochemical definition,[70,72] and there is still disagreement on where this spinocerebellar degenerative disease fits within the complex framework of hereditary ataxias.[67] Phenotypically similar disorders (Charcot-Marie-Tooth disease,[73] cerebellar ataxia, Roussy-Levy syndrome,[74] and familial spastic paralysis) are sometimes found within the same family pedigree.[75] Charcot-Marie-Tooth disease, i.e., peroneal muscular atrophy, progresses more slowly than Friedreich's disease, has a better prognosis, is usually devoid of heart disease,[73] but occassionally is accompanied by high-degree heart block (p. 730). The ataxia of Marie is cerebellar rather than spinal and has no known association with heart disease.[75] Refsum's disease, an inborn error of lipid metabolism (phytanic acid), involves the heart and is occasionally mistaken for Friedreich's ataxia.[76]

The typical neuropathological findings identify Friedreich's disease principally as a spinal disorder with degeneration of posterior columns, spinocerebellar tracts, and pyramidal tracts.[67] The disease is inherited as an autosomal recessive trait. The onset is usually before the end of puberty and virtually never after age 20 years. Once the disorder begins, there are no remissions but, instead, relentlessly progressive ataxia of gait and muscle weakness, first of the lower limbs and then of all four extremities. Dysarthria is present very early. Pes cavus (Friedreich's foot) (Fig. 50–13) and kyphoscoliosis develop within 2 years of onset. In addition, somewhat fewer than half the

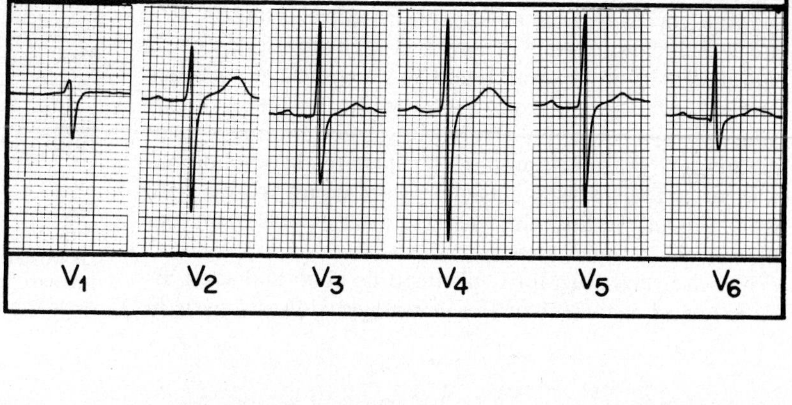

FIGURE 50–12 Electrocardiogram from a 41-year-old woman with myotonic muscular dystrophy. The P-R interval is 0.28 sec. The QRS complex exhibits left-axis deviation (left anterior hemiblock).

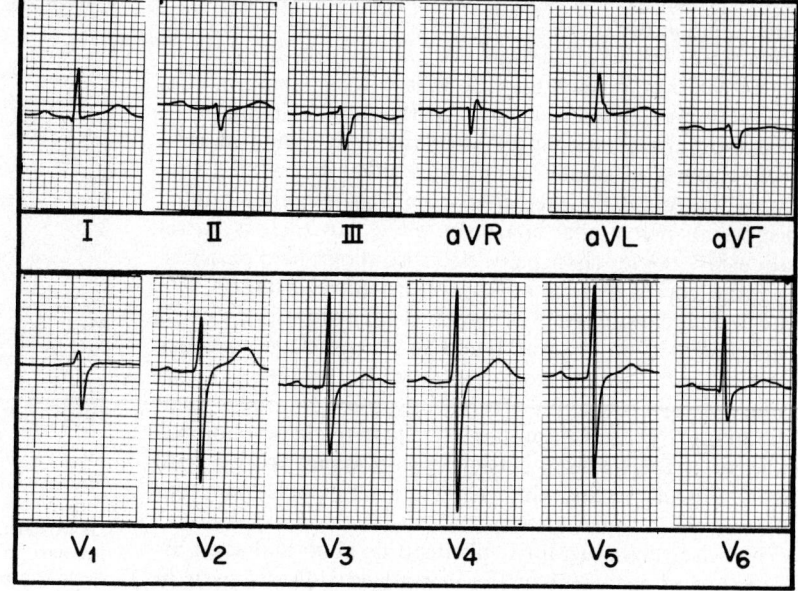

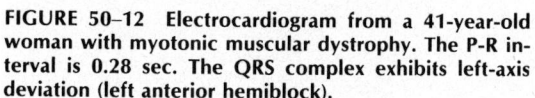

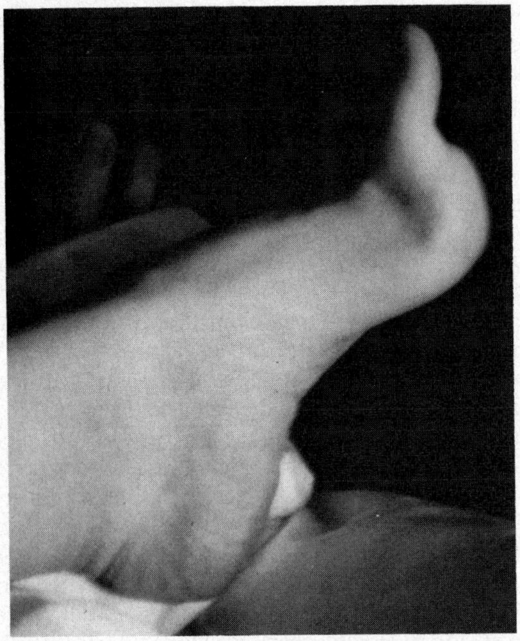

FIGURE 50–13 Typical "Friedreich's foot" showing pes cavus and hammer toe. (From Perloff, J. K., et al.: Uncommon or commonly unrecognized causes of heart failure. Prog. Cardiovasc. Dis. *12*:409, 1970, by permission of Grune and Stratton.)

patients have nystagmus.[77] Abnormal amounts of skeletal muscle enzymes are not consistently released into the circulation because the disorder is essentially neurological rather than myopathic.[78]

It is now estimated that 10 to 50 per cent of patients have cardiac symptoms,[79,80] nearly 100 per cent have abnormalities of electrocardiogram, vectorcardiogram, or echocardiogram (Fig. 50–14), one-half to two-thirds die of cardiac disorders,[80] and virtually all cases studied at necropsy have involvement of the heart.[80,82] In the usual clinical pattern, progressively severe ataxia occurs long before symptomatic heart disease.[83] Rarely, however, evidence of cardiac disease precedes the neurological manifestations.[75,84,85] There is no necessary relationship between the severity of cardiac involvement and the degree of neurological impairment.[84] Severe scoliosis, together with neuromuscular impairment of respiratory muscles, leads to impairment of lung function that varies from mild to severe.[86] It is of further interest that cardiac abnormalities are sometimes found in neurologically normal siblings.[75]

Inappropriate tachycardia is relatively common at rest, with changes in position, and with slight stress.[75,87] Occasional patients experience chest pain that resembles angina pectoris or myocardial infarction,[75,81,82,88] but there is no relationship among chest pain, electrocardiographic patterns, and the coronary arteriopathy of Friedreich's ataxia (see later). One child 6 years of age died following severe chest pain and at necropsy was found to have normal coronary arteries and no infarction. Symptomatic congestive heart failure is rare before puberty.[80] Midsystolic murmurs, usually grade 2 or 3 of 6, may relate either to the kyphoscoliosis or hypertrophic obstructive cardiomyopathy (see later). In this regard, the systemic arterial pulse may exhibit a typical rapid upstroke.[87]

The electrocardiogram is likely to be abnormal soon after if not at the onset of the neurological disease even in young children. Electrocardiographic alterations fall into two categories: (1) disturbances in rhythm, and (2) abnormalities in QRS-T patterns. Inappropriate sinus tachycardia[75,81,83,89,90] has been attributed to increased stimulation by the sympathetic nervous system.[75] Other rhythm disturbances include supraventricular and ventricular ectopic beats, paroxysmal atrial tachycardia, atrial fibrillation, and atrial flutter.[75,81,83,89,90] The commonest abnormality of the QRS-T in the standard scalar electrocardiogram is left ventricular hypertrophy (both voltage and repolarization criteria) or nonspecific ST–T-wave changes.[75,81,83,88–90] Occasionally there are electrocardiographic signs of right ventricular or biventricular hypertrophy, despite little or no necropsy evidence of right ventricular involvement.[90] Vectorcardiographic studies support these conclusions and in addition display QRS vector loops that are often irregular and altered by continuous abnormalities during the course of inscription.[88]

It is no mere coincidence that left ventricular hypertrophy is a common feature of the electrocardiogram. There is now substantial evidence that the cardiomyopathy of Friedreich's ataxia *is* hypertrophic, usually symmetrical (concentric) (Fig. 50–14*B*) and less commonly asymmetrical (disproportionate septal thickness) (Figs. 50–15, 50–16).[66,67,69,84,87,91–98] Obstruction to left ventricular outflow can be present, absent, or provocable.[66,67,84] The echocardiogram in Friedreich's ataxia identifies cardiac abnormalities in a high percentage of patients (upwards of 90 per

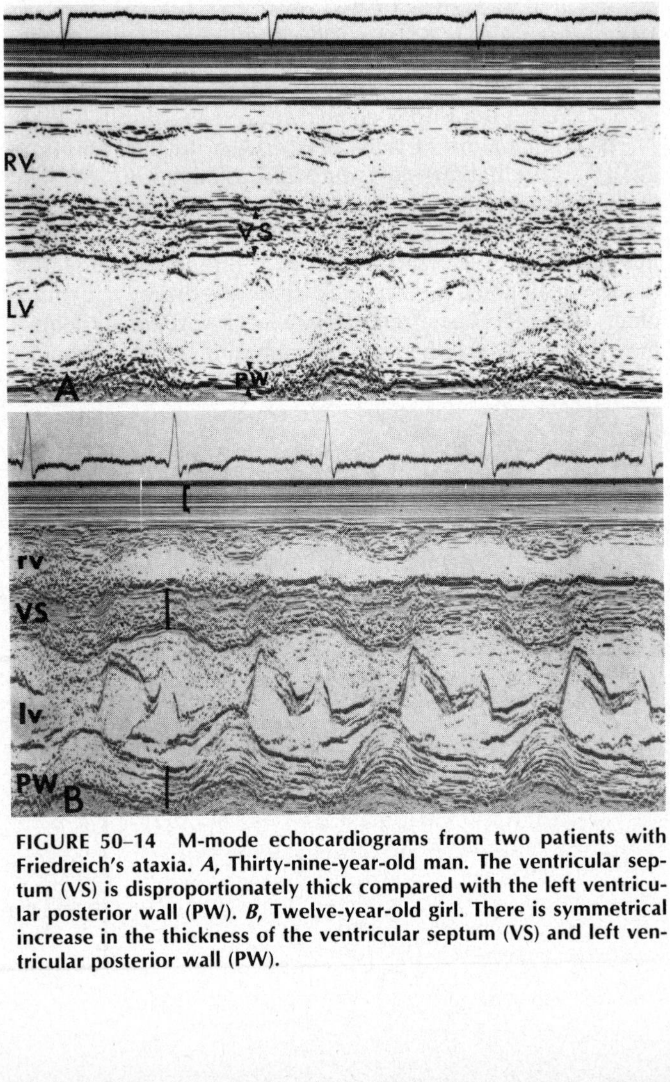

FIGURE 50–14 M-mode echocardiograms from two patients with Friedreich's ataxia. *A*, Thirty-nine-year-old man. The ventricular septum (VS) is disproportionately thick compared with the left ventricular posterior wall (PW). *B*, Twelve-year-old girl. There is symmetrical increase in the thickness of the ventricular septum (VS) and left ventricular posterior wall (PW).

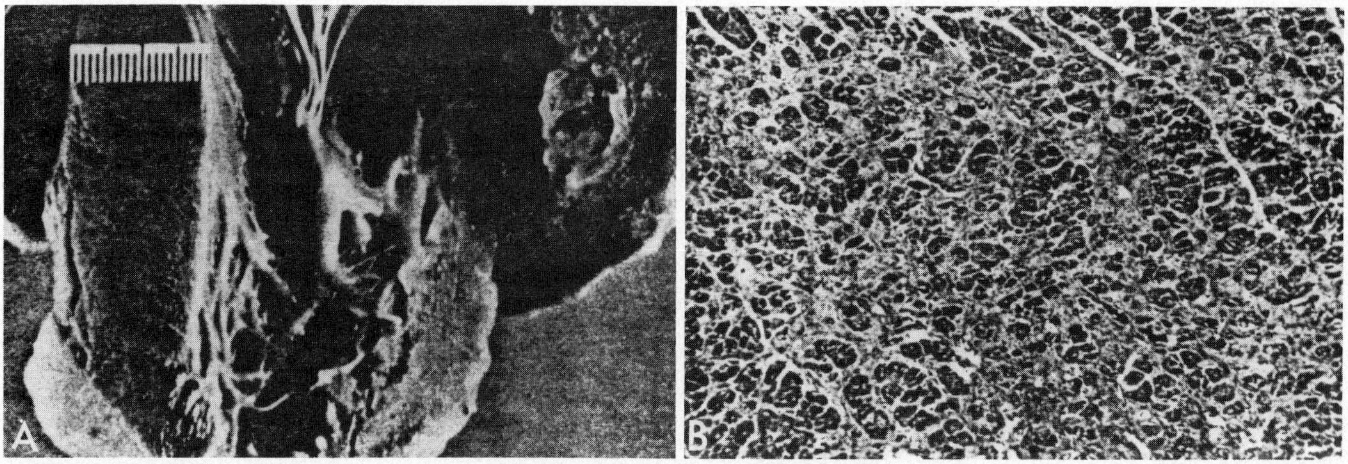

FIGURE 50–15 A. Heart of patient with Friedreich's ataxia showing the hypertrophy of the septum (ruler), which measures 2 cm in thickness. The left ventricular free wall, to the right side of the septum, is 1.4 cm thick. B, Left ventricle showing marked interstitial fibrosis and the hypertrophy of the myocardial fibers. (Mason's trichrome ×33.) (Reproduced with permission from Lamarche, J. B., Cote, M., and Lemieux, B.: The cardiomyopathy of Friedreich's ataxia. Neurology *7*:389, 1980.)

cent)[66,67,95,97–99] (Fig. 50–14). The tracings are characterized by ventricular septal hypertrophy, hypertrophy of the left ventricular free wall, and occasionally an abnormal ratio of septal to posterior wall thickness.[67,91,95] The echocardiograms may exhibit all of the typical features of hypertrophic obstructive cardiomyopathy (p. 1415), that is, asymmetrical septal hypertrophy, hypokinetic septum, and systolic anterior motion of the anterior mitral leaflet.[66,91,95,97,98] However, the extensive septal cellular disarray that is a hallmark of typical genetic hypertrophic cardiomyopathy has not been described in necropsy reports.[75,80,81,100–102]

If the cardiac involvement in Friedreich's ataxia is hypertrophic, what is the connection between this form of cardiomyopathy and the neurological disease? The sympathetic nervous system may be the link. Increased sympathetic activity (catecholamines)[103] or an abnormal response by developing myocardium (receptor sites) has been proposed as a pathogenetic mechanism in genetic hypertrophic cardiomyopathy with asymmetrical septal hypertrophy and septal cellular disarray.[104] In Friedreich's ataxia, the sympathetic nervous system has been implicated in the pathogenesis of the cardiac involvement since 1938,[100] and more recently increased sympathetic stimulation has been held responsible for the inappropriate sinus tachycardia.[75]

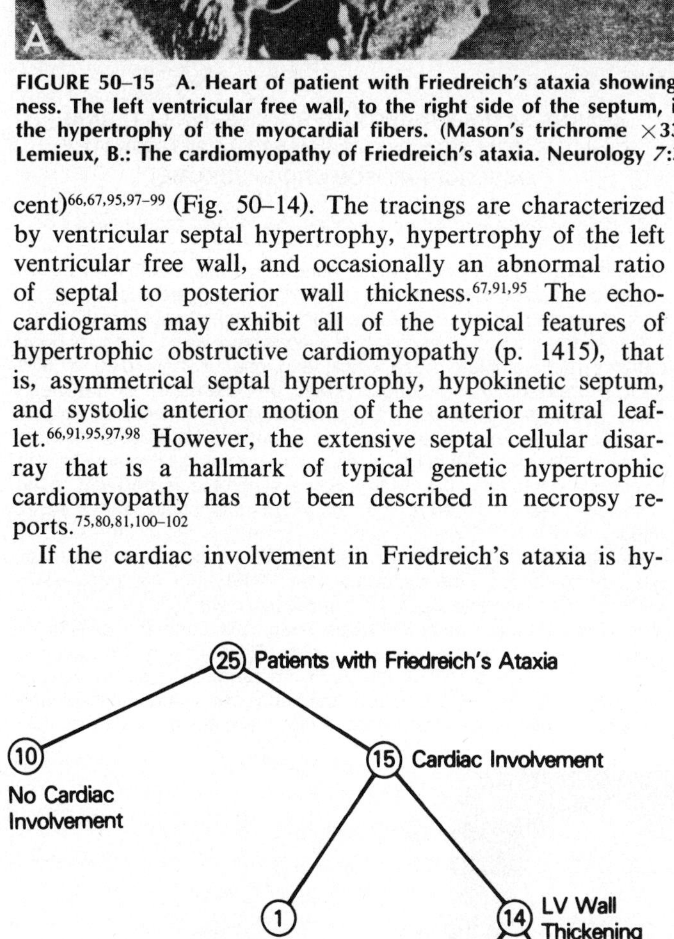

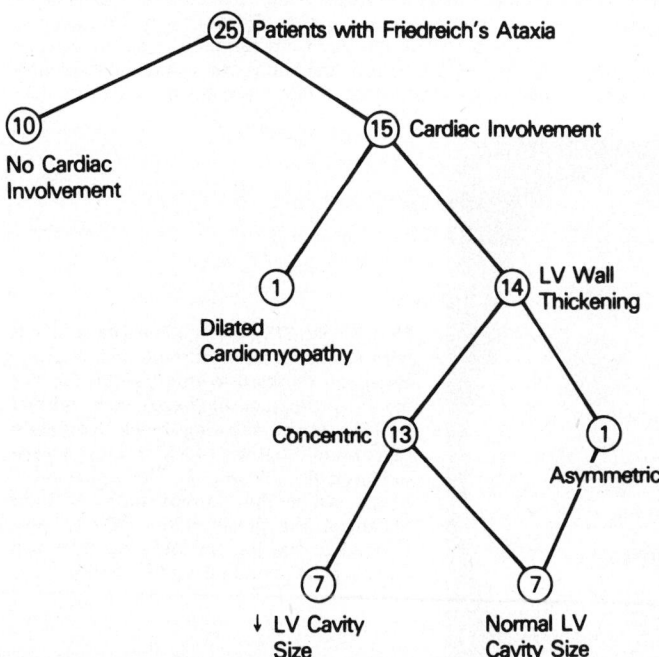

FIGURE 50–16 Flow diagram summarizing echocardiographic data in 25 patients with Friedreich's ataxia. LV, left ventricular; ↓, decreased. (Reproduced with permission from Gottdiener, J. S., Hawley, R. J., Maron, B. J., et al.: Characteristics of the cardiac hypertrophy in Friedreich's ataxia. Am. Heart J. *103*:525, 1982.)

In addition to disease of the myocardium, attention has been called to abnormalities of coronary arteries that may show all stages of luminal narrowing, from trivial intimal proliferation to complete obliteration.[75,80–83,105] Particular attention has been paid to involvement of small intramural coronary arteries,[105] but large and medium-sized branches can also be affected.[75,80] The vessels exhibit neither thrombi nor atheroma,[75,80,81] and a relationship between coronary arteriopathy and the diabetes mellitus that sometimes occurs with Friedreich's ataxia is unsubstantiated.[75,81,106] Although no theory can ignore the striking coronary arteriopathy, the coronary disorder does not appear to be the cause of the myocardial disease.

SPORADIC NEUROMUSCULAR DISEASES SOMETIMES ASSOCIATED WITH CARDIAC DISORDERS

PERONEAL MUSCULAR ATROPHY (CHARCOT-MARIE-TOOTH DISEASE)

Peroneal muscular atrophy, which is believed to be related to Friedreich's ataxia, is a slowly progressive neurogenic disorder principally affecting distal muscles of the legs and, occasionally, intrinsic muscles of the hands.[107–109] Although cardiac disease is commonly associated with Friedreich's ataxia, as noted, peroneal muscular atrophy seldom involves the heart.[74] In 1961 a single case was identified, with atrial flutter and heart failure.[108] A decade then passed before additional reports appeared of a family with peroneal muscular atrophy and disturbances of cardiac impulse formation and conduction.[110,111] The propositus in these latter reports, a man of 41 years, had experienced dizziness for 2 years and was found to have sinus bradycardia, complete right bundle branch block, and left-axis deviation. Admission to hospital was preceded by a Stokes-Adams attack caused by complete heart block (Table 50–1). The patient had a sick sinus node (sinus bradycardia) with infranodal disease (right bundle branch block and left-axis deviation), culminating in complete (infranodal) heart block. It is of interest that 10 members of three generations were affected; in some, heart block and peroneal muscular atrophy coexisted; in others, right bundle branch block occurred alone; and in one, peroneal muscular atrophy occurred without a conduction defect.[110] If this family represents an example of heredofamilial neuromuscular disease with involvement of the heart, the cardiac disorder seems to have been confined to the sinus node and conduction system, leaving the myocardium clinically uninvolved.

X-LINKED HUMEROPERONEAL DYSTROPHY

This disorder is characterized by slowly progressive muscle weakness most marked in the humeral muscles (less in peroneals), with heel cord and elbow contractures developing in the first decade of life and stabilizing near the end of the second decade.[112,113] The X-linked scapuloperoneal syndrome is believed to be nosologically similar if not identical,[113–115] but an autosomal dominant scapuloperoneal syndrome has also been described with a high incidence of cardiomyopathy.[114] Characteristic cardiac involvement takes the form of atrial arrhythmias, atrial paralysis (standstill), and profound bradycardia and high-degree heart block (Table 49–1).[112,113,115–117] Electrocardiograms show abnormally small P waves, P-R interval prolongation (atrioventricular node), atrial fibrillation, atrial flutter, permanent atrial paralysis with slow junctional pacemaker, and complete atrioventricular block (infranodal).[112] H-V intervals are prolonged. Exploration of the right atrium with an electrode catheter revealed no atrial electrical activity, and stimulation of the right atrium induced no electrical response.[112] It is of interest that ventricular function appears to be normal. Accordingly, cardiac involvement in this X-linked form of muscular dystrophy seems to represent primarily disease of atrial muscle (atrial standstill) with sinus bradycardia, atrial fibrillation, and atrial flutter, together with evidence of fibroskeletal disease (AV node disease represented by P-R interval prolongation and infranodal disease represented by H-V prolongation or heart block).

CENTRONUCLEAR MYOPATHY

In 1966 the first description was published of a congenital myopathy histologically characterized by central nuclei in 85 per cent of skeletal muscle fibers.[118] A number of identical cases have subsequently been reported.[119–121] Centronuclear myopathy typically exhibits a slow but progressive wasting and weakness of skeletal muscle, beginning at birth. Ptosis of the eyelids is the rule, and patients are hyporeflexic or areflexic. Serum creatine kinase is released from diseased skeletal muscle. The electroencephalogram is usually abnormal, and seizures have been described. The central or internal location of nuclei in a high percentage of skeletal muscle fibers is the dominant histological abnormality, giving the disease its name. In addition, pronounced variation of diameter of muscle fibers is often found. Familial occurrence is known, but the mode of inheritance is unclear because pedigree data are insufficient. Two brothers with centronuclear myopathy were reported; both had cardiomyopathy, which caused death in one.[119] At necropsy there was diffuse cardiac dilatation and extensive fibrosis. Even though the total number of cases is small, there is presumptive evidence that centronuclear myopathy may be associated with a cardiomyopathy that can cause death at an early age. It is a point of interest that in one study on skeletal muscle in patients with idiopathic cardiomyopathy, numerous internal nuclei were visible in an illustrated figure;[121] apparently, centronuclear myopathy had occurred as cardiomyopathy before the neuromuscular disease was diagnosed.

KEARNS-SAYRE SYNDROME (PROGRESSIVE EXTERNAL OPHTHALMOPLEGIA WITH PIGMENTARY RETINOPATHY; OCULOCRANIOSOMATIC SYNDROME)

In 1958, Kearns and Sayre identified the triad of progressive external ophthalmoplegia, atypical pigmentary retinopathy, and heart block.[122] Subsequent observations established the Kearns-Sayre syndrome as nosologically distinct among the many neuromuscular disorders characterized by progressive external ophthalmoplegia (Fig. 50–17).[123] In the original description of Kearns and Sayre, both reported patients had complete heart block, and one of them died of it.[122] Kearns predicted that prognosis would be determined by the heart block and was proved correct (Table 50–1),[29,124,125] but with notable exceptions.[126] In many cases, there is evidence of a widespread neurological disorder. Although multisystem neurological diseases are frequently hereditary, the Kearns-Sayre syndrome is believed to be acquired, beginning before age 20 years and involving the sexes equally.[123]

Morphological alterations in skeletal muscle are characterized by ragged-red fibers in the trichrome stain.[123] Whether the progressive external ophthalmoplegia is neurogenic or myopathic in origin has long been debated, and doubt has been cast upon the criteria for making this distinction in ocular muscles. Similarly, it is necessary to ask whether involvement of the heart represents a neural or muscle disorder.[127] Even though the term "cardiomyopathy" has been loosely applied,[123] there is reason to believe that the cardiac disease primari-

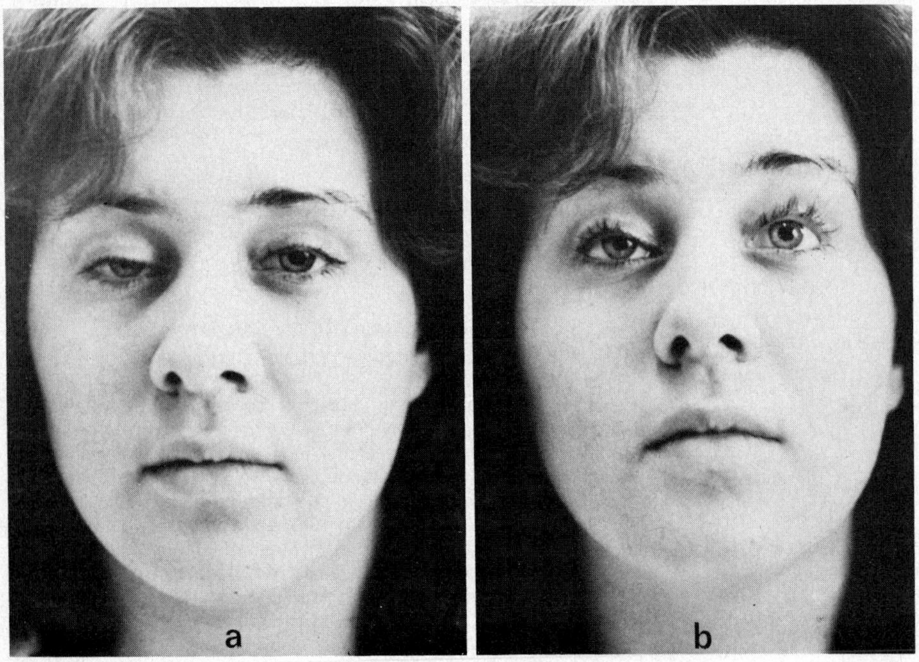

FIGURE 50–17 An eighteen-year-old girl with Kearns-Sayre syndrome and bilateral asymmetric ptosis. Within 24 months, her electrocardiogram changed from normal to bifascicular showing block (complete right bundle branch block and left anterior fascicular block). *A,* The asymmetric ptosis when the patient looks straight ahead. *B,* The ptosis of the right lid persists when the patient looks up. She also had atypical pigmentary retinopathy.

ly, if not exclusively, afflicts the specialized conduction pathways rather than the myocardium.[127] Despite ultrastructural changes, clinically detectable myocardial disease is not a feature of the Kearns-Sayre syndrome.[125] All signs thus far support the view that cardiac involvement in this disorder is "neurogenic" rather than myopathic and that two alterations in cardiac conduction coexist: a gradual progressive impairment of infranodal conduction (left anterior hemiblock, right bundle branch block, complete heart block) and a concomitant enhancement of AV nodal conduction.[127,128]

A convincing morphological basis for impaired infranodal conduction in Kearns-Sayre syndrome was demonstrated in a patient whose electrophysiological study had shown trifascicular block (right bundle branch block, left anterior hemiblock, and a very prolonged H-V interval).[128] At necropsy, there were extensive changes in the distal portion of the bundle of His, extending to the origins of the bundle branches.[128] Recently, evidence of enhanced AV nodal conduction was identified with bundle of His electrocardiography.[127] A short or relatively short P-R interval should therefore not be taken as evidence against the risk inherent in trifascicular disease in patients with Kearns-Sayre syndrome with right bundle branch block and left anterior hemiblock.[127]

Myasthenia Gravis. The association of myocardial disease with thymoma, especially malignant thymoma, is generally accepted. The association of myasthenia gravis with heart disease is less clear, despite a considerable body of suggestive information.[129] A specific cardiac pathological condition for this neuromuscular disorder is unproven in spite of clinical, electrocardiographic, vectorcardiographic, and necropsy data implicating the myocardium.[129]

McArdle's Syndrome. This condition is a metabolic myopathy (muscle phosphorylase deficiency) resulting in inadequate skeletal muscle glycolysis.[130] The disease is clinically manifested by exercise intolerance due to muscle cramps. The electrocardiogram may reveal sinus bradycardia, increased QRS voltage, and P-R interval prolongation.[130] The disorder differs from another metabolic myopathy characterized by mitochondrial myopathy of skeletal and cardiac muscle with storage of glycogen and lipid and exercise-induced lactic acidemia.[131]

GUILLAIN-BARRÉ SYNDROME

The Guillain-Barré syndrome, or Landry's ascending paralysis, is characterized by an elevated cerebrospinal fluid protein concentration without increase in the number of white blood cells at a normal pressure. The protein-cell dissociation in the spinal fluid is necessary for the diagnosis. The motor paralysis is flaccid and has a considerable tendency to ascend, hence the eponym of Landry. Involvement of thoracic muscle makes assisted ventilation necessary. Despite the use of mechanical ventilation, the Guillain-Barré syndrome is fatal in approximately 20 per cent of children who manifest significant involvement of trunk muscles and who develop respiratory insufficiency.[132]

When sudden death occurs, postmortem studies have shed no light on the cause. There is evidence, however, that deaths are often related to arrhythmias.[132-135] Bradyarrhythmias (sinus arrest, complete heart block), tachyarrhythmias (supraventricular and ventricular), as well as premature atrial and ventricular beats, are relatively frequent and are enhanced by use of a respirator.[134,135] Pacemaker support has been required because of recurrent asystole.[135] In one patient, tracheal aspiration (tracheostomy) produced an idioventricular rhythm of 40 beats/min, which reverted to sinus rhythm when aspiration was stopped.[132] Cardiac monitoring is wise, especially when the Guillain-Barré syndrome is sufficiently severe to warrant assisted ventilation.[132,134]

NEUROMUSCULAR DISORDERS PRESENTING AS CARDIOMYOPATHY

Heart block (selective involvement of the specialized conduction system) is occasionally the presenting problem in patients subsequently found to have neuromuscular disorders, such as Kearns-Sayre syndrome, myotonic muscular dystrophy, or the X-linked humeroperoneal syndrome (previously discussed) (Table 50–1).[29,116,122] Other patients are seen with disease of the cardiac conduction system *plus* cardiomyopathy and are found to have neuromuscular disorders such as limb-girdle dystrophy of Erb.[30] Still others show cardiomyopathy alone and are found to have skeletal muscle disease either on careful study or with subsequent development of clinical disease.[85] Thus, occasional patients with little or no clinical evidence of a systemic neuromuscular disorder come to attention initially because of overt cardiac disease.[136]

Evans commented on skeletal muscle involvement in idiopathic cardiomyopathy more than 30 years ago.[137] Patients with idiopathic congestive cardiomyopathy have been found to exhibit histological evidence of centronuclear myopathy.[120,121] In addition, occasionally mothers of patients with classic X-linked Duchenne's muscular dystrophy have cardiomyopathy with mild or occult clinical evidence of systemic muscle involvement.[2,10,14,15] Hypertrophic cardiomyopathy is a primary disease of cardiac muscle. Nevertheless, abnormalities of skeletal muscle have been found on electromyography and on both light and electron microscopic studies of biopsy material.[138,139] The conclusion should not be overstated, but occasionally it might prove useful to consider coexisting neuromuscular disease as the underlying cause in relatively young patients with sinoatrial or atrioventricular conduction disease or with idiopathic congestive cardiomyopathy.

Polymyositis (also see p. 1664)

Polymyositis occurs in both adults and children and, when accompanied by the characteristic skin rash, is designated *dermatomyositis* because the muscle disease appears to be the same in either case.[140,141] Patients develop symmetrical muscle weakness, especially in the limb-girdle and anterior neck flexors.[140] When the disorder occurs without rash, a mistaken diagnosis of muscular dystrophy may be made, especially in children. On muscle biopsy and at necropsy, diffuse interstitial and perivascular mononuclear cell infiltration and fiber necrosis, usually with multivacuolated fibers showing regeneration, degeneration, and fibrosis, are seen.[140] Electromyography discloses fractionation of the motor unit (small amplitude, excessive motor action potentials on slight voluntary effort, and fibrillations).[140] Cardiac involvement is believed to occur only rarely in childhood polymyositis but may merely be clinically occult.[141] In adults, the frequency of symptomatic involvement of the heart contrasts with a relatively high incidence of electrocardiographic abnormalities, especially rhythm and conduction disturbances,[140] that take the form of atrial fibrillation or flutter, premature beats (atrial and ventricular), multifocal atrial tachycardia, impaired AV conduction (first-, second-, and third-degree heart block), and abnormalities of infranodal conduction (left-axis deviation and bundle branch block).[140,141]

At necropsy, infiltration, degeneration, and fibrous replacement of sinoatrial node, distal bundle of His, and left and right bundle branches wholly or in part underlie the conduction defects.[140,141] In addition to the occasional occurrence of fibrinous pericarditis, pathological changes in the myocardium are usually similar to those in skeletal muscle, including diffuse mononuclear cell infiltration and myofiber degeneration, regeneration, and fibrosis.[140] It would seem that these abnormalities should manifest themselves clinically as congestive heart failure—and this may be so—but recent echocardiographic studies have identified a high incidence of *enhanced* left ventricular function.[140] If these puzzling observations are correct, the mechanism is not known. Prolapse of the mitral valve has also been recorded,[140] but it is unclear whether polymyositis is causal or coincidental.

Periodic Paralysis

This disorder, characterized by recurrent attacks of flaccid weakness, is accompanied by either abnormally high or abnormally low levels of serum potassium.[142] In the hypokalemic type,[143] attacks typically begin in late childhood or adolescence, usually occur at night,

51 ENDOCRINE AND NUTRITIONAL DISORDERS AND HEART DISEASE

by Gordon H. Williams, M.D., and Eugene Braunwald, M.D.

In 1835, Robert Graves described "three cases of violent and long-continued palpitation in females" with thyrotoxicosis.[1] Twenty years later, Thomas Addison reported that patients with disease of the "suprarenal capsules" had a "pulse, small and feeble . . . excessively soft and compressible." As the disease progressed "the body wastes . . . the pulse becomes smaller and weaker, and . . . the patient at length gradually sinks and expires."[2] Thus, since the mid-19th century, it has been known that deranged hormonal secretion can significantly alter cardiovascular function. However, only in the last few decades with the advent of techniques to measure the concentration of circulating hormones has the magnitude of the endocrine system's influence on cardiovascular function been generally appreciated. The purpose of this chapter is to summarize the more important cardiovascular manifestations of endocrine and nutritional diseases.

ACROMEGALY

The anterior pituitary gland secretes at least seven polypeptide hormones. Four (ACTH, FSH, LH, and TSH) primarily produce their biological effect indirectly by altering hormonal secretion from a specific target gland (adrenal cortex, gonad, and thyroid). Thus, the pathophysiological manifestations of a derangement in their secretion are the same as those of their target organs and will be discussed later. There are no cardiovascular manifestations of altered prolactin secretion or growth hormone deficiency; however, acromegaly (growth hormone excess) is associated with a number of clinical signs and symptoms related to the cardiovascular system.

Action of Growth Hormone. Growth hormone influences many metabolic processes, but its net effect is anabolic. Thus, when growth hormone is administered to a growth hormone–deficient individual, positive nitrogen balance, accompanied by retention of calcium, sodium, potassium, magnesium, and chloride, is manifest within days.[3,4] While many facets of nitrogen metabolism following administration of growth hormone have been studied, its primary effect has not been assessed definitively. Growth hormone increases the synthesis of both transfer and messenger RNA.[5] It reduces the breakdown of amino acids to urea and increases the transport of amino acids into skeletal and cardiac muscle, thus augmenting the substrate available for protein synthesis.[6] However, direct measurement of intracellular amino acid content has not documented the increase expected if these actions were the only ones responsible for the increased protein synthesis.

Growth hormone also induces changes in both fat and carbohydrate metabolism.[7,8] When administered acutely, it increases the uptake and utilization of glucose by fat cells, thus increasing lipogenesis. However, when administered chronically, it promotes lipolysis, thus increasing plasma free fatty acid levels and their oxidation and promoting ketogenesis, particularly in diabetic patients or animals. Growth hormone reduces glucose uptake by fat and muscle cells, increases gluconeogenesis, and increases peripheral resistance to insulin; as a consequence, plasma glucose levels rise. Because of this reduced tissue uptake of glucose and the increased blood levels of free fatty acids and ketones, those tissues, like the myocardium, that are able to use these latter compounds as energy substrates, do so.[9] Growth hormone can also increase the synthesis and/or accumulation of sulfated mucopolysaccharides in connective tissue.

Clinical and Biochemical Manifestations. Acromegaly is almost invariably the result of a growth hormone–producing chromophobic or eosinophilic pituitary adenoma. Characteristically, the disease is a slowly progressive one with signs and symptoms often predating diagnosis by more than 10 years. The striking physical findings (broad, spadelike hands and feet) are the result of growth hormone's effect on bone, muscle, and connective tissue. Osteoarthritis is common, as is organomegaly, hypertrichosis, hyperhidrosis, and modest weight gain.[4]

A derangement in carbohydrate metabolism is the most common metabolic consequence of chronic overproduction of growth hormone. Impaired glucose tolerance is found in half the patients, and hyperinsulinism is present in nearly all; thus, a state of insulin resistance exists. However, clinical diabetes mellitus is present in only 10 per cent of patients, which suggests that only those who are predisposed and have limited insulin reserve actually develop overt disease.[10] While it might be anticipated that hyperlipidemia would be common in acromegaly, it is in fact infrequently observed except in patients with clinical diabetes mellitus.[10,11] Even in these patients, it is probably secondary to the decreased secretion of insulin rather than to the increased secretion of growth hormone.

Cardiovascular Manifestations

The cardiac manifestations of acromegaly include cardiac enlargement which is greater than would be anticipated for the generalized organomegaly. In addition, the frequency of a number of other cardiovascular disorders is increased in acromegaly: hypertension, premature coronary artery disease, congestive heart failure, and cardiac arrhythmias, particularly frequent ventricular premature beats and intraventricular conduction defects.[12–14] Indeed, because of the frequent occurrence of congestive heart failure and cardiac arrhythmias in patients who otherwise have no predisposing factors (e.g., no hypertension or arteriosclerosis), it has been suggested that a specific acromegalic cardiomyopathy exists[15] (see below).

CARDIOMEGALY. Nearly all patients with acromegaly have cardiomegaly (Fig. 51–1), particularly after the fifth decade.[16] Echocardiographic assessment suggests that frequently there is an increase in cardiac mass with little other evidence of cardiac disease.[17,17a] Although the cardiomegaly may be related to the generalized effect of growth hormone on protein synthesis, some data suggest that other factors may also be important. For example, enlargement of the heart is often greater than that of other organs. Furthermore, there is no direct relationship between the degree of cardiomegaly and the level of circulating growth hormone.[14] While there is a correlation between the duration of acromegaly and cardiac hypertrophy,[15] other factors which may be important in the genesis of cardiomegaly include hypertension and atherosclerosis, both of which occur with increased frequency in acromegaly. Focal cardiac interstitial fibrosis and a myocarditis with lymphocytic infiltrate also have been reported in the majority of cases.[15,18] The former is probably due to the effect of growth hormone on collagen synthesis. Recently, it has

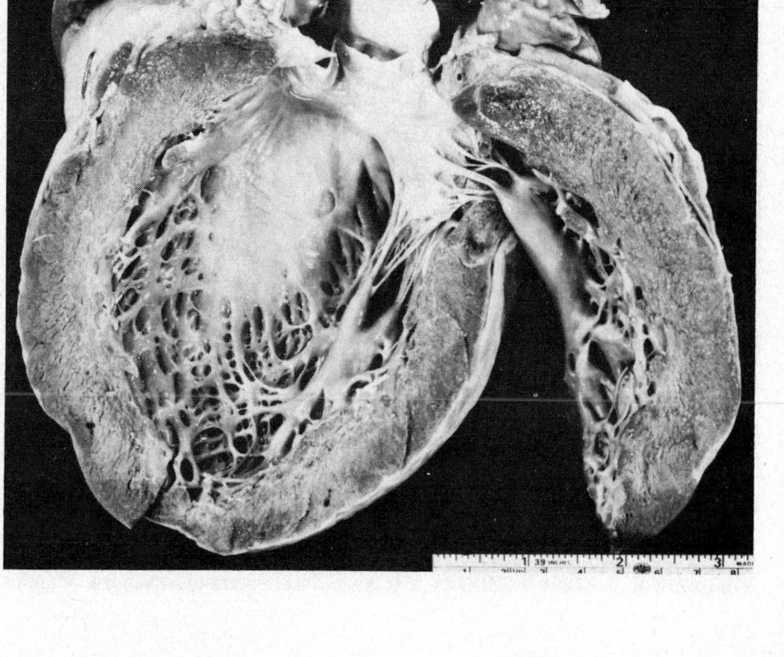

FIGURE 51–1 Opened left ventricle of the heart, showing the marked dilatation and hypertrophy, with fibrosis in the left septal endocardium. (From Rossi, L., et al.: Dysrhythmias and sudden death in acromegalic heart disease. A clinicopathologic study. Chest *72*:496, 1977.)

been reported that small vessel disease of the myocardium occasionally may be present.[15] The resultant dysfunction in cardiac contraction secondary to any of these pathological changes could also contribute to the cardiac hypertrophy. Finally, cardiomyopathy characteristic of acromegaly may also contribute to the cardiomegaly.

HYPERTENSION. Hypertension is the most common cardiovascular manifestation of acromegaly, occurring in 15 to 50 per cent of patients if individuals with hypopituitarism are excluded. Hypertensive acromegalic patients tend to be older and to have had their acromegaly longer than nonhypertensive acromegalic patients. The underlying pathophysiology is uncertain. Most investigators either have searched for factors other than growth hormone that could cause hypertension or have attempted to determine how growth hormone itself may produce hypertension. Early studies suggested that the urine of patients with hypertension and acromegaly contains a specific pressor substance that was not derived from the pituitary gland and that was not a catecholamine;[19] however, these findings have not been confirmed. In many respects patients with acromegaly appear to be volume-expanded; the presence of an increase in glomerular filtration rate, renal plasma flow, extracellular fluid volume and sodium space, and reduction in plasma renin activity all support this hypothesis.[20–22] Thus, several studies have assessed the secretion of aldosterone in acromegaly; while increased secretion has been reported, this is an uncommon finding.[21–23] What does appear to occur frequently in acromegalics, however, is a change in tissue responsiveness to angiotensin II. Thus, on a sodium-restricted intake the response of aldosterone production to angiotensin II is decreased, but the vasoconstrictor response is increased when compared to normal subjects. This abnormality is present in both hypertensive and normotensive acromegalics.[24] Whether this is related to the pathogenesis of the elevated arterial pressure or simply a reflection of an expanded extracellular fluid volume is unclear.

A number of studies have suggested that growth hormone itself may be responsible for the hypertension. Thus, pituitary irradiation or hypophysectomy significantly reduces arterial pressure in hypertensive acromegalic patients, even when full glucocorticoid replacement is carried out.[24] Indeed, the apparent volume expansion may be directly related to the elevated growth hormone levels, since administration of growth hormone can produce retention of sodium and expansion of extracellular fluid volume.[25] It has been proposed that the pathophysiology of the hypertension in acromegaly may be similar to that in essential hypertension. In both conditions, initially there may be an elevation of cardiac output secondary to an expansion of extracellular fluid volume (Chap. 26). This could lead to a rise in arterial pressure and, finally, to changes in the peripheral vasculature producing fixed hypertension.

Early studies suggested that the presence of hypertension was a poor prognostic sign in acromegalic patients. Recent observations, however, are that the hypertension usually is mild, uncomplicated, and readily responsive to drugs.[14] This discrepancy may reflect the greater severity of the acromegalic process in earlier studies and the recognition now of the disorder at an earlier stage, rather than a change in the course of the disease.

ATHEROSCLEROSIS. Since growth hormone produces significant alterations in carbohydrate and lipid metabolism as well as hypertension, it is not surprising that premature atherosclerosis occurs in patients with acromegaly. What is uncertain is its frequency. One recent report suggests that major coronary disease may be present in only 10 per cent of acromegalics.[15] Coronary atherosclerosis could also contribute to the cardiomegaly observed in these patients.

ACROMEGALIC CARDIOMYOPATHY. Some patients with acromegaly without evidence of hypertension or atherosclerosis have significant cardiac dysfunction.[15] They primarily have either cardiomegaly, congestive heart failure, and/or cardiac dysrhythmias;[18] the congestive heart

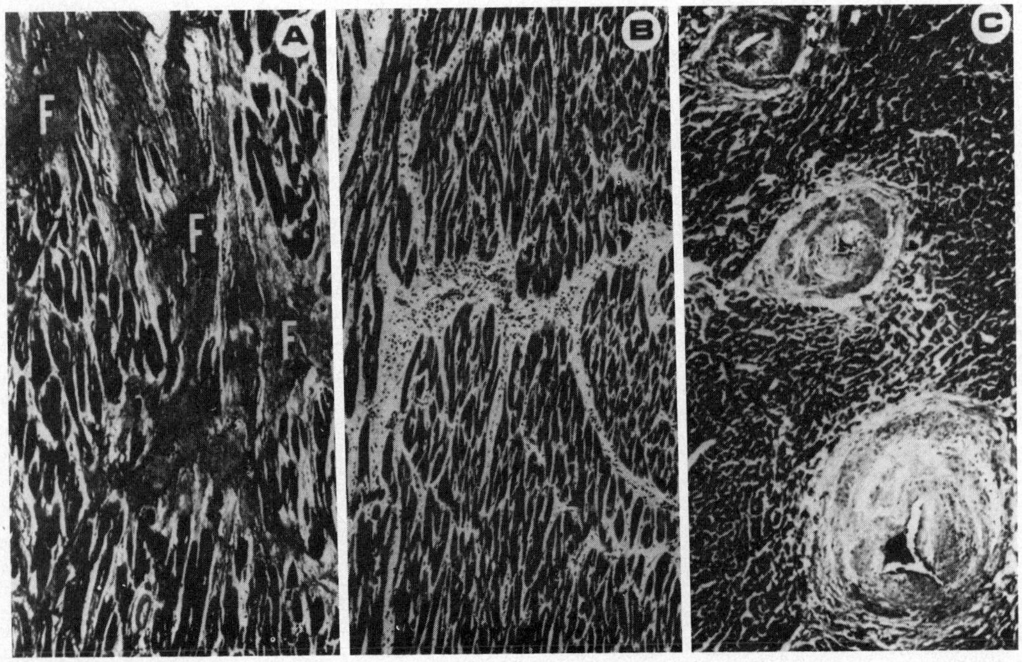

FIGURE 51–2 Histopathological features of acromegalic heart disease. *A,* Nonspecific myocardial hypertrophy and interstitial fibrosis (F). *B,* Myocarditis with predominantly lymphomononuclear cell infiltrate. *C,* Small vessel disease (proliferative fibrous wall thickening) of intramural coronary artery branches. (Reproduced with permission from Lie, J.T.: Acromegaly and heart disease. Primary Cardiol. *7*:53, 1981. Copyright PW Communications, Inc.)

failure is particularly resistant to conventional therapy. It has been suggested that these are manifestations of an acromegalic cardiomyopathy which is related to the higher collagen content per gram of heart than in normal myocardium.[27] Histological observations show cellular hypertrophy, patchy fibrosis, and myofibrillar degeneration (Fig. 51–2). Sudden death has been associated with inflammatory and degenerative damage to the sinoatrial perinodal nerve plexus and degeneration of the AV node.[18]

It is not clear whether acromegalic cardiomyopathy is a specific entity. The evidence in favor of this position is indirect and comes from four types of observations: (1) Nearly 50 per cent of acromegalic patients have electrocardiographic abnormalities.[12,13,28] The most common findings are ST-segment depression with or without T-wave abnormalities, patterns consistent with left ventricular hypertrophy, intraventricular conduction disturbances—specifically, bundle branch block—and, infrequently, supraventricular or ventricular ectopic rhythms. While hypertension or other signs of atherosclerosis are present in many, 10 to 20 per cent of patients with acromegaly and electrocardiographic changes have no evidence of these conditions. (2) Ten to 20 per cent of acromegalics have overt congestive heart failure. In perhaps a fourth of these there is no known predisposing cause. (3) The majority of patients with acromegaly but without hypertension or atherosclerosis have subclinical evidence for cardiac dysfunction, as manifested by a shortening of the left ventricular ejection time (LVET), prolongation of the preejection period (PEP), and an elevation of the PEP/LVET ratio[29] (p. 54).[4] Approximately half of all patients with acromegaly, including patients without hypertension, have echocardiographic evidence of left ventricular hypertrophy.[30] These patients have growth hormone levels that are significantly higher than those of patients without left ventricular hypertrophy. Half of the patients with left ventricular hypertrophy exhibit asymmetrical septal hypertrophy, and these patients have a significantly greater percentage of internal dimensional shortening during systole than either the patients with concentric hypertrophy or those without left ventricular hypertrophy.

Diagnosis and Treatment

The *diagnosis* of acromegaly is established by documenting the nonsuppressibility of serum growth hormone levels following glucose loading.[4] In most laboratories, growth hormone concentrations in normal subjects are less than 2 ng/ml 120 minutes after the oral administration of 100 gm of glucose. It is also important to evaluate the integrity of the other pituitary hormones and, in hypertensive patients, to rule out an associated pheochromocytoma or aldosteronoma. The presence of sinus tachycardia or atrial fibrillation in a patient with acromegaly warrants a careful search for co-existing hyperthyroidism.

Surgery and irradiation remain the mainstays of treatment. The surgical approach is more often transsphenoidal[31] rather than transfrontal; heavy particle (proton beam) instead of conventional irradiation is being used with increasing frequency.[32] Preliminary studies suggest that growth hormone can be suppressed in some acromegalics with the dopamine agonist, bromocriptine. Whether this agent has any effect on tumor growth, however, is unclear.

Acromegalic patients with cardiovascular abnormalities usually respond to conventional therapeutic measures for hypertension, heart failure, or arrhythmias. Two caveats: (1) those with hypertension appear to be particularly responsive to volume-depleting maneuvers, i.e., diuretics and sodium restriction, perhaps even more so than patients with essential hypertension; and (2) some patients with congestive heart failure, primarily those *without* underlying hypertensive heart disease (i.e., those who are considered to have acromegalic cardiomyopathy), appear to be particularly resistant to therapy.

THYROID DISEASE

Thyroid hormone has a profound effect on a number of metabolic processes in virtually all tissues, with the heart being particularly sensitive to its effects. Therefore, it is not surprising that thyroid dysfunction can produce dramatic cardiovascular effects, often mimicking primary cardiac disease.

Action of Thyroid Hormone. Two biologically active hormones are secreted by the thyroid: thyroxine (T4) and triiodothyronine (T3). The relative importance of T4 and T3 in mediating the effects of thyroid hormone is being actively investigated. The question is not completely resolved, though most studies support the hypothesis that T3 is the final mediator and that T4 is a prohormone.[33] Major support for this position comes from the universal presence of T3 but not T4 nuclear receptors in tissues responsive to thyroid hormones.[34]

Even though the mechanism of action of thyroid hormone has been intensively investigated over the past three decades, uncertainty still exists about its principal effects. Most studies have provided data to support one of two general hypotheses. The older hypothesis suggests that thyroid hormone alters cellular metabolism by a direct action on mitochondria and is supported by studies showing (1) uncoupling of oxidative phosphorylation in isolated mitochondria by thyroxine; (2) increased total body oxygen consumption by thyroid hormone; and (3) increased substrate utilization with little generation of high-energy phosphate by thyroid hormone.[35] However, the following findings oppose this hypothesis: (1) the dose of thyroxine necessary to produce uncoupling of oxidative phosphorylation is more than 100 times the physiological dose; (2) the administration of dinitrophenol, a compound that also uncouples oxidative phosphorylation, does not induce a euthyroid state in hypothyroid animals[36]; and (3) it is possible that the uncoupling of oxidative phosphorylation may actually be an artifact of the in vitro systems.[37]

The second hypothesis, which has gained increasing support and is more likely to be correct, proposes that the major site of initiation of action of thyroid hormone is on the cell nucleus.[38] It has been observed that thyroid hormone is specifically bound to a chromatin-bound nonhistone nucleoprotein in the nucleus. As a result of that binding, alterations occur in protein synthesis, leading to many of the biochemical and metabolic effects observed with thyroxine administration. According to this hypothesis, the increased oxygen consumption results not from a direct interaction between thyroid hormone and mitochondria but rather indirectly via an increase in mitochondrial protein synthesis secondary to the effect of the thyroid hormone on the nucleus. Support for this hypothesis comes from several sources: (1) specific binding of T3 and, much less strongly, of T4 to nuclear receptor sites has been documented; (2) those tissues sensitive to thyroid hormone have nuclear binding sites; (3) the addition of thyroid hormone in vitro produces an increase in O_2 consumption only after a significant time lag; (4) an early metabolic effect of thyroxine is an increased rate of incorporation of a labeled precursor into nuclear RNA; (5) inhibitors of protein synthesis prevent many, if not most, of thyroid hormone's effects; and (6) treatment of hypothyroid animals with T3 causes increases in in vivo synthesis of specific messenger RNA's in several tissues including the heart.[39]

Edelman and Ismail-Beigi have extended this hypothesis one step further.[40] They postulated that not only does thyroid hormone enhance protein synthesis, but it specifically increases the activity of Na^+-K^+-ATPase. Thus, the augmented hydrolysis of ATP at the site of the sodium pump in the sarcolemma stimulates cellular (mitochondrial) oxygen consumption. Support for this hypothesis includes the observations that (1) hypothyroid rats treated with T3 exhibit a reduction in active sodium transport in crude homogenates and membrane-rich fractions and a decrease in intracellular Na^+/K^+ ratio in liver, diaphragm, and kidney,[41–42] and (2) the number of renal Na^+ pump sites and the incorporation of radiolabeled methionine into renal cortical Na^+-K^+-ATPase are both increased, suggesting an increase in protein synthesis as the primary event.[41,42] Some reports, however, have suggested that the effect of thyroid hormone on cellular respiration cannot be entirely secondary to a change in the activity of this enzyme[44,45]

RELATION BETWEEN THE THYROID AND THE SYMPATHETIC NERVOUS SYSTEM

While the effects of thyroid hormone on the heart are varied and complex, it has been proposed that some of them are indirect, being secondary to changes in the activity of the sympathetic nervous system (Table 51–1). For example, many of the cardiovascular effects of hyperthyroidism, i.e., tachycardia, systolic hypertension, increased cardiac output, and myocardial contractility, can be abolished or reduced by blocking the activity of the sympathetic nervous system.[46] It has been proposed that thyroid hormone may alter the relationship between the sympathetic nervous and cardiovascular systems, either by increasing the activity of the sympathoadrenal system, or enhancing the response of cardiac tissue to normal sympathetic stimulation. Also, it has been suggested that sympathetic stimuli merely exert a direct additive effect on cardiovascular function above that produced by thyroid hormone. On the other hand, there is also evidence that hyperthyroidism reduces the sensitivity of cardiac tissue to sympathetic stimuli.[47]

Thus, the results of experiments on the relationship between the sympathoadrenal system and hyperthyroidism have evoked considerable controversy. On one hand, the plasma and urine levels of norepinephrine, epinephrine, and dopamine-β-hydroxylase are either low or normal in hyperthyroidism and either normal or elevated in hypothyroidism,[48–50] which suggests that the sympathomimetic features of hyperthyroidism cannot be explained by a simple change in adrenergic activity. On the other hand, we observed in a study on conscious, instrumented dogs rendered hyperthyroid that the reductions of heart rate and myocardial contractility induced by propranolol were greater than they were in the euthyroid state, a finding which indicates that the contribution of adrenergic stimulation to heart rate and myocardial contractility is greater in the hyperthyroid than the euthyroid state. However, the levels of heart rate and contractility following beta blockade were still greater when the dogs were hyperthyroid than when they were euthyroid, providing support for the concept that thyroid hormone exerts a direct effect on cardiac function, independent of any effect on the sympathoadrenal system.[51]

TABLE 51–1 CLINICAL FEATURES OF HYPERTHYROIDISM*

DIRECT THYROID HORMONE EFFECT†	BETA-ADRENERGIC-LIKE EFFECT†
Resting heart rate > 90/min (90%)	**Resting heart rate > 90/min (90%)**
Palpitations (85%)	**Palpitations (85%)**
Atrial fibrillation (10%)	**Exertional dyspnea (80%)**
Pedal edema (30%)	**Increased pulse pressure (systolic hypertension)**
Increased oxygen consumption (basal metabolism)	**Active apical impulse**
Weight loss	**Loud first heart sound and pulmonic component of second heart sound**
Skeletal muscle myopathy	**Midsystolic murmur, usually basal**
Increased bone turnover (occasional osteoporosis or hypercalcemia)	**Third heart sound (occasional)**
Fine skin	**Means-Lerman scratch (rare)‡**
Fine brittle hair	Tremor
Brittle nails	Brisk reflexes
Oligo- or amenorrhea	Increased perspiration
Increased bowel frequency	Heat intolerance
	Insomnia
	Anxiety
	Stare, lid lag§

*Cardiac response to hyperthyroidism and symptoms of hyperthyroidism that mimic those of heart disease are shown in boldface type. The numbers in parentheses are approximate prevalences of the findings, compiled from several large series. Goiter is almost always present, though in elderly patients the thyroid enlargement may be minimal or absent.

†Both types of effects contribute to the tachycardia and palpitations.

‡A systolic scratch or click in the second left intercostal space that is probably generated by the pleura and pericardium rubbing together.

§These reflect upper-lid retraction. Infiltrative ophthalmyopathy with exophthalmos is found only when Graves' disease is the cause of the hyperthyroidism and is not related to the hyperthyroid state per se.

Reproduced with permission from Kaplan, M. M.: The thyroid and the heart: How do they interact? J. Cardiovasc. Med. 7:893, 1982.

After 50 years of investigation, disagreement still exists regarding a possible role for thyroid hormone in enhancing cardiac responses to catecholamines. Early studies reported an augmented sensitivity,[52] but later investigations suggested no significant displacement of the dose-response relationship.[53] In a study using fetal mouse hearts in tissue culture to avoid the problems of the delayed effect of thyroid hormone and the difficulty of interpreting the results using tissue obtained from animals with experimental hyperthyroidism, it was shown that T3 shifts the catecholamine dose-response curve to the left and that this increase in sensitivity is specific for those agents which stimulate beta receptors.[54,55] In support of this finding are the observations that there is an increase in either the number or the affinity of cardiac beta receptors after administration of thyroid hormone.[56–59] Further support comes from the study by Guarnieri et al., who showed that hyperthyroid rats have an enhanced activation of protein kinase and contractile response following administration of threshold doses of the beta-adrenergic agonist, isoproterenol.[60] In the aforementioned study on conscious hyperthyroid dogs,[51] however, we found no alteration in the sensitivity of the inotropic response to isoproterenol and norepinephrine.

The reasons for the conflicting results in this area may be related to the specificity of the technique used to assess beta-receptor activity, since it has been postulated that thyroid hormone influences the interconversion of alpha and beta receptors. Thus, rat atria obtained from hypothyroid animals have increased alpha and decreased beta receptor activity,[61] and there is evidence that hyperthyroidism produces the opposite effect.[56] Thus, if the agent used to determine adrenergic receptor activity were not highly specific for beta receptors, incorrect conclusions could be drawn.

EFFECT OF THYROID HORMONE ON THE HEART

There is evidence that thyroid hormone may alter cardiac function directly. Thus, the addition of thyroid to fragments of chick embryonic heart increases the rate of beating of the cells.[62] Additionally, the increased heart rate and myocardial contractility observed in experimental hyperthyroidism are not completely reversed by either sympathetic or parasympathetic blockade.[47,51] Finally, thyroxine enhances the rate of contraction of cardiac muscle even in the presence of adrenergic blockade.[63] Right ventricular papillary muscles isolated from cats rendered hyperthyroid exhibited augmented myocardial contractility, as reflected in an upward shift of the myocardial force-velocity curve,[47] with a greatly increased velocity of myocardial fiber shortening, a reduced time to peak tension during isometric contraction, and an augmented peak tension development (Fig. 51–3). Prior catecholamine depletion by pretreatment of the hyperthyroid cats with reserpine did not alter this inotropic effect of hyperthyroidism, providing further evidence for a direct cardiac effect.[47] Assessment of this hypothesis in the intact conscious calf recently has been performed. The results suggest that the major actions of thyroxine on the left ventricle are (1) a direct positive inotropic effect and (2) an increase in the size of the ventricular cavity without a change in the end-diastolic pressure or length of the sarcomere in diastole.[64]

The available data suggest that the direct effect of thyroid hormone on the heart is mediated via a change in protein synthesis.[64a,64b] Thyroid hormone increases the activity of the sodium pump in myocardial cells as it does in other tissues. Philipson and Edelman have documented that the activity of both the Na^+-K^+-ATPase and the K^+-dependent *p*-nitrophenyl phosphatase in the heart is increased by more than 50 per cent when T3 is administered to hypothyroid rats.[65] The hearts of euthyroid rabbits rendered hyperthyroid exhibited a doubling of myofibrillar ATPase activity.[66] Reverse T3 (a biologically inactive analog) has no effect. Curfman et al. have suggested that this increased activity is the result of an increase in the number of functional enzyme complexes.[67] There is evidence that thyroid hormone both increases the synthesis of myosin and alters its structure, increasing its contractile properties,[68] particularly by increasing the more mobile myosin isoenzyme as determined by polyacrylamide gel electrophoresis.[68–70] The heart appears to respond to thyrotoxicosis by enhancing synthesis of a myosin isoenzyme with a fast ATPase activity.[66,69] The augmented myosin ATPase activity appears to contribute to the enhanced contractile response of the hyperthyroid heart, since the activity level of this enzyme is thought to regulate the rate of turnover of actin-myosin cross-bridge links in cardiac muscle. However, this is probably not the principal cause, since administration of exogenous thyroid can stimulate contractility before any change in the myosin ATPase activity occurs.[71] The sarcoplasmic reticulum isolated from hyperthyroid dogs and rabbits accumulates and exchanges calcium at an increased rate,[72] resulting in increased availability of calcium to the myofibrils during activation, as well as an enhanced rate of myofibrillar relaxation.

The tachycardia observed in hyperthyroidism appears to be due to a combination of an increased rate of diastolic depolarization and a decreased duration of the action potential in the sinoatrial node cells.[73] The propensity for the development of atrial fibrillation may be due to the shortened refractory period of atrial cells.[74]

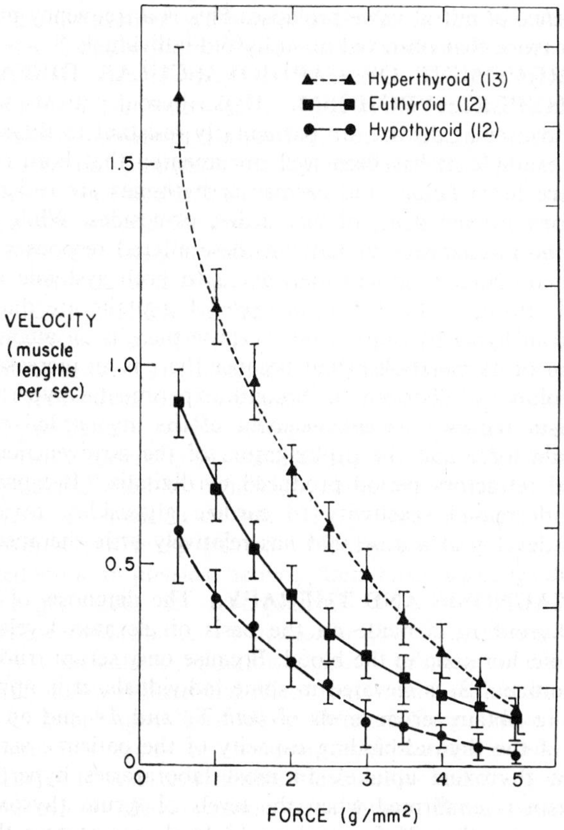

FIGURE 51–3 The average force-velocity relationship for papillary muscles from hyperthyroid, euthyroid, and hypothyroid cats. Initial velocity of shortening is normalized in terms of muscle lengths per second; load, corrected for cross-sectional area of individual muscles is expressed in gm/mm². Brackets represent ± SEM. (From Buccino, R. A., Spann, J. F., Poole, P. E., and Braunwald, E.: Influence of the thyroid state on the intrinsic contractile properties and the energy stores of the myocardium. J. Clin. Invest. *46*:1669, 1967.)

Hyperthyroidism

Hyperthyroidism is the clinical state resulting from the excess production of triiodothyronine, thyroxine, or both. The most common cause is a diffuse toxic goiter (Graves' disease). Although the etiology of this condition is still unkown, the hyperproduction of T4 and T3 are thought to result from circulating IgG autoantibodies that bind to the thyrotropin receptor on the thyroid gland. The second most common form of hyperthyroidism is nodular toxic goiter, a condition in which localized areas of the gland function excessively and autonomously. Less common causes include a single toxic adenoma, ingestion of excessive amounts of thyroid hormone, and subacute thyroiditis, in which there may be a self-limited phase of hyperthyroidism. Rarely, hyperthyroidism may also occur as a result of the production of thyroid hormone by a thyroid carcinoma or production of a thyrotropic substance (probably HCG) by a hydatidiform mole or choriocarcinoma.

Hyperthyroidism is a relatively common disease, occurring four to eight times more commonly in women than in men, with a peak incidence in the third and fourth decades. The commonly associated signs and symptoms include fatigue, hyperactivity, insomnia, heat intolerance, palpitations, dyspnea, increased appetite with weight loss, nocturia, diarrhea, oligomenorrhea, muscle weakness, tremor, emotional lability, increased heart rate, systolic hypertension, hyperthermia, warm moist skin, lid lag, stare, and brisk reflexes. In the vast majority of cases a goiter can be palpated. Hyperthyroidism in childhood occurs most frequently just before or during adolescence. It is usually associated with a diffuse goiter. The most common early manifestations of juvenile hyperthyroid patients are excessive movements and emotional lability.

T3 levels are invariably elevated and serum T4 levels are usually increased as well. In addition to the signs and symptoms directly related to increased production of thyroid hormone, patients with Graves' disease often have exophthalmos and occasionally circumscribed areas of thickening of the skin, particularly of the lower extremities; presumably these are related to the immunological aspects of the disease.

There are three well-defined control mechanisms for aldosterone release.[121]

1. The renin-angiotensin system is the major system for the control of extracellular fluid volume by regulating aldosterone secretion. Aldosterone is linked in a negative feedback loop with the renin-angiotensin system. Thus, during periods registered as volume deficiency there is an increased release of the enzyme renin from the juxtaglomerular cells of the kidney. Renin then increases the production of angiotensin I from its substrate. Angiotensin I is rapidly converted into the biologically active angiotensin II, which increases aldosterone secretion. Angiotensin II also produces vasoconstriction, thereby raising blood pressure and reducing blood flow to a variety of tissues, especially the kidney.

2. Potassium ion also regulates aldosterone secretion independent of the renin-angiotensin system; elevation of potassium concentration increases aldosterone secretion and vice versa. The adrenal cortex is very sensitive to changes in potassium concentration with as little as a 0.1 mEq/l increment producing significant changes in the plasma aldosterone levels.

3. ACTH also has been documented to affect aldosterone secretion profoundly. However, because the control of aldosterone release is not appreciably altered in patients who have been on long-term steroid therapy, ACTH probably has a smaller role than the other two factors in maintaining normal aldosterone secretion. Finally, the prior dietary intake of both sodium and potassium alters the magnitude of the aldosterone response to acute stimulation, sodium restriction, and potassium loading, both enhancing the response of the adrenal.

Diseases of the adrenal cortex, therefore, primarily affect the cardiovascular system via changes in blood pressure or volume homeostasis. Three specific conditions will be discussed next: glucocorticoid excess (Cushing's syndrome), mineralocorticoid excess (primary aldosteronism), and adrenal insufficiency (Addison's disease).

Cushing's Syndrome (See also p. 885)

In 1932 Harvey Cushing reported a syndrome characterized by truncal obesity, hypertension, fatigue, weakness, amenorrhea, hirsutism, purple abdominal striae, glucosuria, edema, and osteoporosis.[122] Since his original description, a number of specific causes for this syndrome have been described. However, the majority are secondary to bilateral adrenal hyperplasia, with the predominant feature being excess production of glucocorticoids and androgens.[123] Some cases are due to ACTH-producing tumors, of either the pituitary gland (Cushing's disease) or nonendocrine tissue (ectopic ACTH production). Fifteen to 20 per cent of the cases are due to primary adrenal neoplasia, either adenoma or carcinoma. Three times as many women as men are afflicted and the onset is usually in the third or fourth decade of life. Most patients have the typical body habitus: central obesity and slender extremities with proximal muscle weakness. Hypertension is present in 80 to 90 per cent of patients and diabetes occurs in 20 per cent, probably in those individuals with a predisposition.[121,123] Evidence of androgen excess may also be present including hirsutism, amenorrhea, clitoromegaly, and, in some cases, deepening of the voice. The majority of patients also have significant emotional changes ranging from lability of mood to severe depression, confusion, or even frank psychosis.

Laboratory tests disclose evidence of excess production of both glucocorticoids and androgens in the majority of cases. Thus, urinary metabolites of these steroids, 17-ketosteroids and 17-hydroxy-steroids, are characteristically elevated. Most patients show some evidence of glycosuria or hyperglycemia. There is usually generalized osteoporosis, most marked in the spine and pelvis; polycythemia is frequently encountered. In severe cases, hypokalemia, a mineralocorticoid manifestation, may also occur.

CARDIOVASCULAR MANIFESTATIONS. Prior to the development of effective treatment for Cushing's syndrome, accelerated atherosclerosis was a common finding. Early death from either myocardial infarction, congestive heart failure, or stroke usually occurred. While the pathophysiology of the accelerated atherosclerosis is not clear, the hypertensive process probably contributes. However, it is unlikely to be the sole reason, since the hypertension of patients with primary aldosteronism may be as significant and yet atherosclerosis is unusual. Part of the atherosclerotic changes may be mediated by the lipid-mobilizing effect of cortisol. Chronic excess production of cortisol leads to hyperlipidemia and hypercholesterolemia, both of which may promote the development of atherosclerosis.[124]

The pathophysiology of the hypertension in Cushing's syndrome has been much debated. Early studies suggested that it was secondary to volume expansion due to cortisol's mineralocorticoid properties. However, recent studies have not supported this hypothesis. Alternative hypotheses include glucocorticoid potentiation of response of vascular smooth muscle to vasoconstrictive agents[125] and ACTH- or cortisol-induced increases in renin substrate.[126] The latter thesis suggests that the increased blood pressure is secondary to increased generation of angiotensin II. Thus, the pathophysiology of the hypertension may be multifactoral, being related to volume expansion, increased production of vasoactive agents, e.g., angiotensin II, and increased sensitivity of vascular smooth muscle to vasoactive agents.

Hemodynamic, electrocardiographic, and roentgenographic studies of patients with Cushing's syndrome have revealed no specific abnormalities except those that are, in general, associated with either hypertension or hypokalemia. The P-R interval tends to be shorter than normal.

DIAGNOSIS AND TREATMENT. The diagnosis of Cushing's syndrome is established by the lack of appropriate suppression of cortisol secretion by dexamethasone. The best screening test is the administration of 1 mg of dexamethasone at bedtime with measurement of plasma cortisol between 7 and 10 A.M. the next morning. In normal subjects cortisol levels will be less than 5 μg/dl. Some patients, particularly the obese, may have false-positive responses, but false-negative responses occur only rarely. The definitive diagnosis of Cushing's syndrome is made by administration of 0.5 mg of dexamethasone every 6 hours for two days with measurement either of plasma cortisol levels at the end of the second day (normal $< 5 \mu$g/dl) or of the 24 hour 17-OH excretory rate on the second day of dexamethasone supression (normal < 3 mg/24 hr).[127]

Therapy of Cushing's syndrome is usually directed at the specific cause. Thus, patients with adrenal carcinoma or adenoma are treated surgically. In some cases, patients with adrenal carcinoma have nonresectable lesions and therefore surgery is combined with chemotherapy. The treatment of patients with bilateral hyperplasia is controversial, since the etiology is often unknown. In some centers, bilateral adrenalectomy is the treatment of choice, while in others, therapy directed at the pituitary (either surgery or irradiation) is used.[128]

The treatment of cardiovascular abnormalities associated with Cushing's syndrome is directed at lowering blood pressure and correcting the hypokalemia if present. Caution should be exercised in treating the hypertension with potassium-losing diuretics because of the tendency for these patients to develop hypokalemia. Thus, potassium-sparing diuretics or potassium supplements should be administered. In many cases, the hypertension may be more specifically treated with agents that block the action or production of renin, such as beta blockers (e.g., propranolol) or converting enzyme inhibitors (e.g., captopril). As in all clinical conditions in which hypokalemia may be present, cardiac glycosides should be used with caution in patients with Cushing's syndrome.

Hyperaldosteronism

(See also p. 883)

Clinical and Biochemical Manifestations. Aldosteronism is a syndrome associated with hypersecretion of aldosterone. Primary aldosteronism signifies that the stimulus for the excess aldosterone production resides within the adrenal. In secondary aldosteronism, the stimulus is of extra-adrenal origin. These two conditions have similar effects on potassium metabolism.

In patients with primary aldosteronism, which most commonly is due to an aldosterone-producing adrenal adenoma, hypertension, hypokalemia, and metabolic alkalosis are common.[129,130] Polyuria may exist because of the hypokalemia, and glucose intolerance is increased in frequency. Muscle cramps due to the hypokalemia may be present, but little else distinguishes this from other forms of hypertension. Laboratory studies confirm the presence of hypokalemic alkalosis with a low specific gravity of urine and normal levels of adrenal glucocorticoids. The incidence of primary aldosteronism is between 0.5 and 2 per cent of the hypertensive population and occurs twice as frequently in females as in males, with an initial presentation usually between the ages of 30 and 50 years.[121]

CARDIOVASCULAR MANIFESTATIONS. Many of the cardiovascular effects of aldosteronism are nonspecific, being related to aldosterone's effect on atrial pressure and potassium balance. Thus, T wave flattening or U wave prominence on the electrocardiogram (p. 236) and the presence of premature ventricular contractions and other arrhythmias due to hypokalemia are observed.[28] Evidence of left ventricular hypertrophy, either on the electrocardiogram or on the chest roentgenogram, may also be present in patients with long-standing hypertension and hyperaldosteronism. Malignant hypertension and changes in renal function secondary to severe hypertensive angiopathy are infrequent.

DIAGNOSIS AND TREATMENT. The diagnosis of primary aldosteronism is made by the presence of diastolic hypertension without edema, hypersecretion of aldosterone that fails to suppress appropriately during volume expansion, hyposecretion of renin, and hypokalemia with inappropriate urinary potassium loss during salt loading. The state of the renin-angiotensin system is often used to distinguish primary aldosteronism from other conditions that produce hypertension and hypokalemia. For example, hypertension and hypokalemia may be part of the clinical picture of secondary aldosteronism that accompanies malignant or accelerated hypertension or is associated with renal artery stenosis. Secondary aldosteronism can be readily distinguished from primary aldosteronism by the plasma renin activity, which is elevated in the former and reduced in the latter. However, the combination of hypertension and a low plasma renin activity does not necessarily mean primary aldosteronism. Between 15 and 30 per cent of patients with essential hypertension have low renin levels, so-called "low renin" essential hypertension.[131] These patients have been extensively evaluated for excess mineralocorticoid secretion; however, no definitive evidence for such exists (Chap. 26).

The principal treatment for primary aldosteronism is surgical removal of the aldosterone-producing adenoma. In some cases, this is not possible because of the excessive risk imposed by the general physical status of the patient; then, spironolactone, which pharmacologically blocks the effects of aldosterone, is used long-term. This form of therapy may be of limited benefit in males, since compliance is reduced by the undesirable side effects of gynecomastia and impotency, particularly when doses greater than 200 mg per day are required.[132]

Although congestive heart failure occurs infrequently in patients with primary aldosteronism, treatment of patients with this condition with cardiac glycosides must be cautious because of the hypokalemia.

In some patients, primary aldosteronism is not due to a solitary adenoma but to bilateral hyperplasia.[121] While the clinical characteristics of these two conditions are similar, their responses to surgery are different. In both cases hypokalemia is corrected, but patients with bilateral hyperplasia often do not exhibit reduction in arterial pressure. Patients with bilateral hyperplasia are best treated with spironolactone and other antihypertensive agents. Thus, preoperative distinction between bilateral hyperplasia and an adrenal adenoma using adrenal venography or adrenal scanning is important.

Adrenal Insufficiency

Hypofunction of the adrenal cortex includes all conditions in which the level of secretion of adrenal steroids is less than the needs of the body. There are two major categories: those associated with primary damage to the adrenal cortex, and those associated with secondary failure due to the lack of a stimulator such as ACTH. Clinically, patients with adrenal insufficiency can be divided into four types:[121] (1) the most common, primary insufficiency (Addison's disease); (2) secondary insufficiency due to a lack of ACTH; (3) selective hypoaldosteronism; and (4) enzyme deficiency (congenital adrenal hyperplasia).

Clinical and Biochemical Manifestations. Addison's disease may occur at any age and affects both sexes equally. It is commonly due to a destructive process involving both adrenal glands, sometimes infectious, but most often idiopathic atrophy, probably autoimmune in nature. Nearly all patients with primary adrenal insufficiency have weakness, increased skin pigmentation, significant weight loss, anorexia, nausea, vomiting, and hypotension, particularly postural. A significant minority also complain of abdominal pain, salt craving, and diarrhea or constipation. In mild forms, baseline laboratory studies are usually within normal limits. However, as the disease progresses, there is a gradual reduction in serum levels of sodium, chloride, and bicarbonate and an increase in potassium. The hyponatremia is due to extravascular loss of sodium, both into the urine (because of aldosterone deficiency) and into the intracellular compartment. The hyperkalemia is due both to the deficiency of aldosterone and to the impaired glomerular filtration rate and acidosis present in these patients. Other nonspecific findings include a reduction in basal metabolic rate with normal thyroid function and a normocytic anemia with relative lymphocytosis. While Addison's disease is often thought of as a common cause of significant eosinophilia, this is observed only occasionally.

Cardiovascular Manifestations. The most common cardiovascular finding in adrenal insufficiency is arterial hypotension. In severe cases, the pressure may be in the range of 80/50 mm Hg, with postural accentuation. Indeed, syncope occurs in a significant percentage of patients. In severe cases, heart size and peripheral pulses decrease. The electrocardiogram is abnormal in the majority of patients with Addison's disease.[28] The most common abnormalities are low or inverted T waves, sinus bradycardia, prolonged $Q\text{-}T_c$ interval, and low voltage. Conduction defects also occur, with first-degree block present in 20 per cent of patients. Changes secondary to the hyperkalemia are not common even though the serum potassium levels may be elevated. It is of interest that the electrocardiographic abnormalities, other than those secondary to hyperkalemia, do not respond to mineralocorticoids but require glucocorticoid replacement. Cardiac failure in prolonged adrenocortical insufficiency has also been reported.[28a]

Diagnosis and Treatment. Decreased response of the adrenal cortex to ACTH establishes the diagnosis of Addison's disease. The best screening test is the administration of synthetic ACTH (cosyntropin), 0.25 mg IM or IV, with measurement of plasma cortisol levels 30 and 60 minutes later. Cortisol levels double or increase by 10 μg/dl in normal subjects. Definitive evaluation is by prolonged (usually 24-hour) infusion of ACTH with assessment of either plasma cortisol or excretion of 17-hydroxysteroids or both.[121]

It is possible to differentiate primary adrenal insufficiency from secondary adrenal insufficiency, isolated hypoaldosteronism, or congenital adrenal hyperplasia because one of the adrenal hormonal functions is normal in each of the latter three conditions. Thus, in secondary adrenal insufficiency due to ACTH deficiency, aldosterone secretion is normal and the biochemical effects of mineralocorticoid deficiency, i.e., hyperkalemia, are not present. In isolated hypoaldosteronism, glucocorticoid function is normal. Female patients with congenital adrenal hyperplasia have evidence of androgen excess, such as virilization and hirsutism, and hypertension may also be present with a deficiency of 11-hydroxylase[133] (p. 887).

An increasingly common form of hypoaldosteronism is that associated with hyporeninism. Most commonly, this syndrome is observed in older diabetic patients with a mild degree of renal impairment and hypertension; acidosis is also common. Usually, these patients present with unexplained hyperkalemia. The cause is unknown but may be secondary to damage to the juxtaglomerular apparatus and/or reduced conversion of a renin precursor into the active enzyme.[134]

The treatment of adrenal insufficiency is accomplished by replacement of the deficient steroid. In adults with primary or secondary insufficiency, hydrocortisone, 20 to 30 mg daily, is administered in divided doses, usually two thirds in the morning and one third in midafternoon. In those patients with associated aldosterone deficiency, 9-α-fluorohydrocortisone, 0.05 to 0.10 mg daily, is given. During periods of significant stress (surgery, infection, or trauma), the dose of glucocorticoids should be increased. Occasionally, acute adrenal insufficiency in patients who previously had apparently normal adrenal function, is precipitated by the stress of cardiac surgery.[135]

PHEOCHROMOCYTOMA

(Also see p. 885)

In 1859, Oliver and Shafer demonstrated that adrenal extract raised blood pressure when injected into experimental animals. In 1901, one active ingredient, epinephrine, was isolated and characterized and in 1922 a syndrome of paroxysmal hypertension associated with an adrenal medullary tumor, pheochromocytoma, was reported.

EFFECTS OF CATECHOLAMINES ON THE CARDIOVASCULAR SYSTEM

The adrenal medulla and sympathetic nervous system are linked morphologically, biochemically, and physiologically and are often referred to as the sympathoadrenal system.[136] The sympathoadrenal system differs from other endocrine systems in several respects, including the fact that plasma levels of the secretory product, catecholamines, are not regulated by a direct feedback mechanism. Instead, catecholamine secretion is the efferent branch of a reflex arc involving centers in the brain stem, the hypothalamus, and perhaps the cerebral cortex as well. The human adrenal medulla contains about 1 mg of catecholamine per gram of tissue, approximately 85 per cent of which is epinephrine. The strategic location of the adrenal medullary cells within the cortex is associated with their capacity to form epinephrine, since high-dose glucocorticoids induce the formation of phenylethanolamine-N-methyl-transferase, the enzyme needed to convert norepinephrine into epinephrine.[137]

In addition to their important effects on the cardiovascular system, catecholamines also have significant metabolic effects, stimulating glycogenolysis and gluconeogenesis, that is, increasing the production of glucose from glycogen and amino acid precursors and stimulating lipolysis, thereby mobilizing free fatty acids and inhibiting secretion of insulin. The absence of the adrenal medulla does not produce definable disease in humans. However, the presence of a hormonally active adrenal medullary tumor produces a number of significant findings.

Clinical and Biochemical Manifestations. A pheochromocytoma is a catecholamine-producing tumor derived from chromaffin cells. Those arising from extra-adrenal chromaffin cells are called nonadrenal pheochromocytomas or paraganglionomas. Probably less than 0.1 per cent of patients with hypertension have a pheochromocytoma. Despite the fact that it is an uncommon disease, pheochromocytomas generate a great deal of interest, largely because the morbidity and mortality associated with these tumors are significant, with detection often resulting in cure. Pheochromocytomas are highly vascular tumors; less than 10 per cent are malignant as indicated by local invasion or metastasis, but, as with other endocrine tumors, malignancy cannot always be determined by microscopic appearance alone.

While the vast majority of tumors occur sporadically, approximately 5 per cent are inherited as an autosomal trait, of which they are often part of a pluriglandular neoplastic syndrome[138] which, in addition to pheochromocytoma, may consist of medullary carcinoma of the thyroid, parathyroidadenoma, and retinal or cerebellar hemangioblastomas. Most pheochromocytomas are solitary adrenal tumors, with 10 per cent being bilateral and 10 per cent nonadrenal. However, in the familial form of pheochromocytoma nearly half the patients have bilateral adrenal tumors.

The features that suggest pheochromocytoma in hypertensive patients are (1) paroxysmal attacks of any kind, (2) headaches, (3) excessive sweating, (4) signs of hypermetabolism, (5) orthostatic hypotension, and (6) unusual blood pressure elevations to trauma or operation.[136,139] Many of the features are similar to those of hyperthyroidism. While paroxysmal attacks are the hallmark of pheochromocytoma, more than half the patients have fixed hypertension and nearly 10 per cent are normotensive.

CARDIOVASCULAR MANIFESTATIONS. Hypertension is the major cardiovascular manifestation of pheochromocytoma. Its lability sometimes distinguishes it from other forms of hypertension; however, only clinical awareness of the entity and specific laboratory testing permit establishment of the proper diagnosis. The lability of blood pressure in patients with pheochromocytoma has been suggested to be due not only to episodic discharge of catecholamines but also to a reduction in plasma volume, as well as to impaired sympathetic reflexes. Recent studies have indicated that an absolute reduction of plasma volume exists in only a minority of cases,[140,141] but a number of observations suggest that chronic volume depletion is present. For example, alpha-adrenergic blockade or removal of the tumor produces severe hypotension, which is correctable by volume expansion.[136,142] Cardiac output has been reported to be normal, whereas heart rate is increased and orthostatic hypotension is accompanied by decreased stroke volume and inadequate adjustments in peripheral resistance indicative of impaired peripheral vascular reflexes.[141]

The electrocardiogram is abnormal in as many as 75 per cent of the patients with pheochromocytoma.[28] The changes consist of T-wave inversion, left ventricular hypertro-

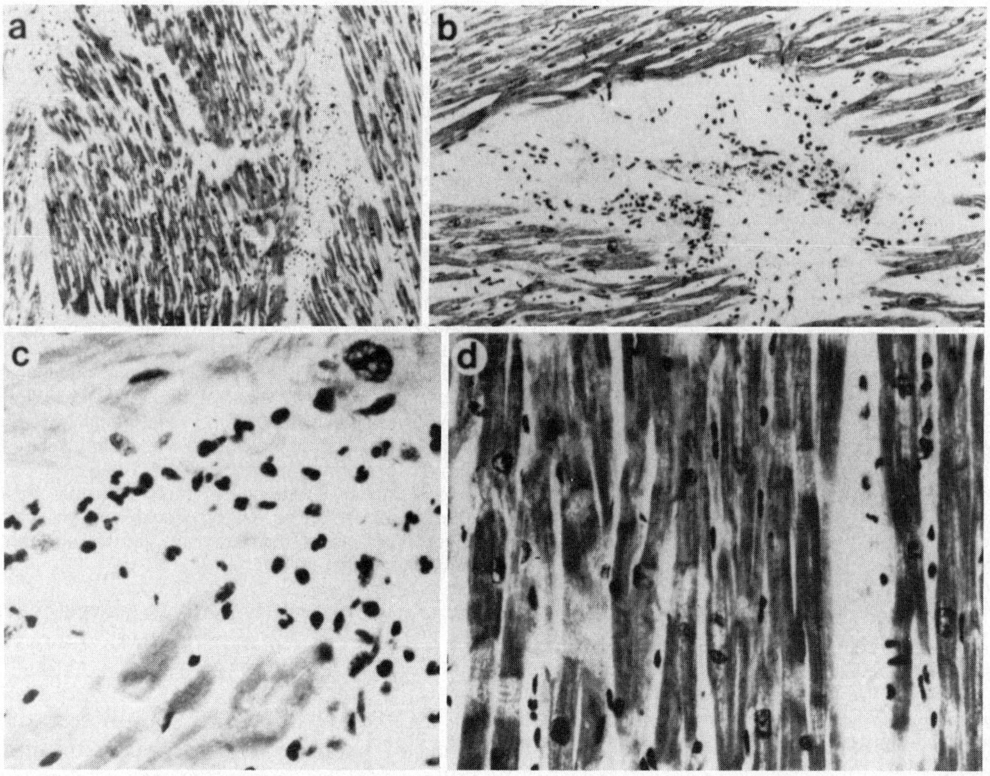

FIGURE 51–4 Left ventricular myocardium with acute myocarditis and contraction band necrosis in a patient with pheochromocytoma dying of catecholamine crisis. *a,* Diffuse infiltration by inflammatory cells through myocardium. *b,* Perivascular inflammation. *c,* Close-up of the inflammatory infiltrate. *d,* Contraction-band necrosis of myocytes. (Hematoxylin and eosin stains; original magnification × 20 (a), × 45 (b), × 540 (c), × 330 (d)). (Reproduced with permission from McManus, B. M., Fleury, T. A., and Roberts, W. C.: Fatal catecholamine crisis in pheochromocytoma: Curable cause of cardiac arrest. Am. Heart J. *102*:930, 1981.)

phy, sinus tachycardia, and, in some cases, other alterations in rhythm, such as frequent supraventricular ectopic beats or paroxysmal supraventricular tachycardia. When arterial pressure increases markedly, changes suggestive of myocardial damage, including transient ST-segment elevations, marked diffuse T-wave inversions, and depression of ST-segments are present. These changes are usually transient, and the electrocardiographic pattern reverts to normal after removal of the tumor or pharmacological blockade.[143] Some of the electrocardiographic abnormalities are presumably due to hypertensive heart disease or myocardial ischemia. However, a specific catecholamine-induced myocarditis has also been suggested.[144]

The echocardiogram during a hypertensive crisis may show systolic anterior involvement of the anterior mitral leaflet, paradoxical septal motion and proximal exclusion of the posterior wall.[145]

Myocarditis. Pathologically, the myocarditis consists of focal necrosis with infiltration of inflammatory cells, perivascular inflammation, and contraction band necrosis[146] (Fig. 51–4), finally resulting in fibrosis. In one study, 50 per cent of patients who died from pheochromocytoma had myocarditis,[140] usually accompanied by left ventricular failure and pulmonary edema. Although coronary atherosclerosis is usually present, medial thickening is the most characteristic lesion of the coronary arteries. The high catecholamine levels may have been the cause, since similar lesions were found in rats exposed to high levels of norepinephrine.

DIAGNOSIS AND TREATMENT. The diagnosis of pheochromocytoma is established by documenting increased urinary, blood, or platelet levels of catecholamines or one of their metabolites.[142,147–149] Three tests are commonly employed: (1) total catecholamines, (2) vanillylmandelic acid (VMA); and (3) metanephrine. The latter two are metabolites of catecholamine and were first used to screen for pheochromocytoma because they are present in greater quantities. When reliably performed, these tests are probably equivalent in accuracy. The probability of a pheochromocytoma being present in a hypertensive patient with a single normal urine level is less than 5 per cent. It is most desirable to measure both the catecholamines and one of the two metabolites, preferably metanephrine, in screening for pheochromocytoma. If the blood pressure fluctuates it is particularly important to collect the urine at a time the pressure is elevated. Specific pharmacological tests to screen for pheochromocytoma are of limited benefit, usually hazardous, and therefore warranted only in unusual circumstances. Recently, clonidine has been proposed as a useful definitive test for pheochromocytoma. Normal subjects suppress catecholamine levels following clonidine administration via stimulation of central alpha-adrenergic receptors; patients with pheochromocytoma do not[150] (Fig. 51–5). Unfortunately, profound and prolonged hypotension has been reported in some patients during the course of this test.

Once the diagnosis of pheochromocytoma is established, specific pharmacological blockade should be initiated.[151] Phenoxybenzamine hydrochloride should be begun, with the initial dose 10 mg q 12 hr; the dose is then gradually increased every two to three days until the arterial pressure is restored to normal. However, it should be noted that alpha-adrenergic blockade may induce a decline in ar-

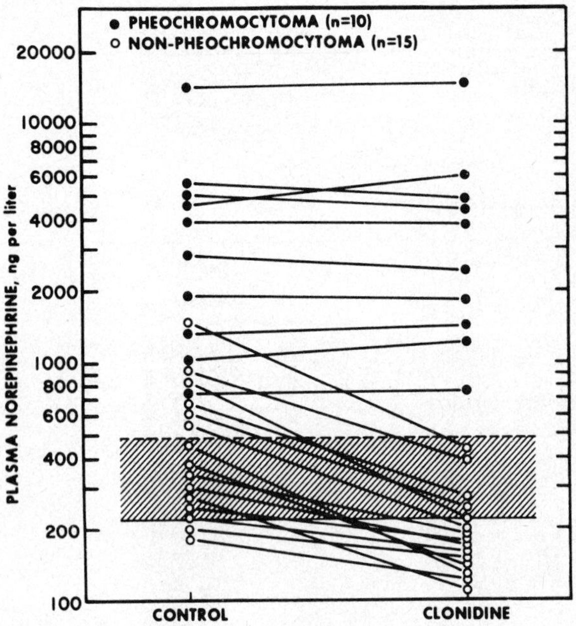

FIGURE 51–5 Plasma norepinephrine values in individual patients before and three hours after a single oral dose of clonidine (0.3 mg). The hatched area represents the mean of values obtained from 60 adult healthy subjects (+3 S.D.). To convert norepinephrine values to nanomoles per liter, multiply by 0.006. (Reproduced with permission from Bravo, E. L., Tarazi, R. C., Fouad, F. M.,et al: Clonidine-suppression test: A useful aid in the diagnosis of pheochromocytoma. N. Engl. J. Med. *305*:623, 1981.)

terial pressure accompanied by serious postural hypotension, presumably because of the vasodilatation occurring in the presence of hypovolemia. This hypotensive response can be prevented by adequate sodium intake; if it is very striking, the infusion of saline may be required. Adequate control of arterial pressure is essential prior to any arteriographic procedure, before initiating beta-receptor blockade, and before operation.

Beta-adrenergic blockade is useful in patients with pheochromocytoma who have significant tachycardia, palpitations, and catecholamine-induced arrhythmias. However, beta blockade with a drug affecting beta-2 receptors must *not* be initiated prior to adequate alpha blockade, since severe *hypertension* may occur as a result of the unopposed alpha-stimulating activity of the circulating catecholamines.

Definitive treatment is surgical removal of the tumor, usually after localization with CAT scan, arteriography, or scanning using an ^{131}I-derivative of guanethidine as the scanning agent.[152] In those patients with inoperable lesions, long-term use of the combination of alpha- and beta-adrenergic blockers has been helpful. Drugs that inhibit the biosynthesis of catecholamines, such as alpha-methyltyrosine, have also been used in patients with malignant pheochromocytoma.[142,153]

PARATHYROID DISEASE

Disordered parathyroid secretion is associated with two cardiovascular disturbances, cardiac arrythmias and hypertension. Changes in calcium metabolism as well as a direct effect of parathyroid hormone on the heart appear to be responsible.

Clinical and Biochemical Manifestations. Parathyroid hormone (PTH) is a single-chain polypeptide of 84 amino acids. Its major biological effect is to increase mobilization of calcium into the extracellular fluid from a variety of tissues; this action is linked in a negative feedback loop with serum unbound calcium concentration. Thus, an increase in serum calcium concentration reduces parathyroid hormone release and vice versa.[154] PTH also increases urinary excretion of phosphate, augments bone resorption and reduces the urinary excretion of calcium. It also indirectly increases the absorption of calcium from the gastrointestinal tract by increasing the rate of conversion of 25-hydroxy vitamin D into the biologically active 1,25-dihydroxy vitamin D.[155]

Hyperparathyroidism, the excess production of parathyroid hormone, is usually secondary to a solitary parathyroid adenoma. Occasionally, generalized parathyroid hyperplasia exists, and, infrequently, carcinoma of the parathyroid gland is found. In many cases, hyperparathyroidism is asymptomatic; 10 to 20 per cent of patients are first diagnosed as the result of a routine chemical screening test.[156]

The signs and symptoms of hyperparathyroidism are related to direct effects of PTH on kidney or bone or those associated with the hypercalcemia. Nearly half the patients have signs and symptoms of renal dysfunction, such as polyuria, nocturia, renal stones, and, in severe cases, nephrocalcinosis and renal failure. In many patients, there are also nonspecific joint and back symptoms, and in unusual circumstances spontaneous fractures occur. Hypercalcemia reduces the excitability of the neuromuscular system, which can lead to such diverse effects as significant myocardial dysfunction and decreased auditory acuity.

CARDIOVASCULAR MANIFESTATIONS OF HYPERPARATHYROIDISM

(See also page 887)

CARDIAC EFFECTS. Until recently, most of the effects of parathyroid hormone on the heart have been assumed to be secondary to a change in extracellular calcium. It has now been documented that PTH also has a direct effect on the heart resulting in an increased beating rate of isolated heart cells and a positive inotropic action.[157,158] These effects are probably mediated by PTH binding to specific receptors, leading to an increased entry of calcium into the heart cell and by PTH increasing the release of endogenous myocardial norepinephrine. The direct effect of PTH may be deleterious, since it causes early death in rat heart cells and may be directly responsible for the increased accumulation of calcium in dystrophic muscles and for the heart damage found in uremia.[157,159] On the other hand, hypoparathyroidism may cause a dilated cardiomyopathy, caused presumably by hypocalcemia, but perhaps also by hypomagnesemia and reduced circulating PTH.[160]

In addition to any direct action of PTH on the heart, hypercalcemia also has an adverse effect. Chronic hypercalcemia from a variety of causes is associated with increased deposition of calcium in the fibrous skeleton of the heart and valvular cusps as well as in coronary arteries and in myocardial fibers[161] (Figs. 51–6 and 51–7).

The plateau of the action potential of cardiac fibers is prolonged by low and shortened by high extracellular calcium concentrations (Chap. 19). Lengthening of the plateau prolongs the duration of the action potential, whereas shortening of the plateau has the opposite effect. These changes in duration of action potential are accompanied by corresponding changes in the duration of the refractory period, of the ST segment, and of the Q-T interval.[28,162] Thus, the major electrocardiographic change in hypercalcemia is shortening of the Q-T interval. Less frequently, disorders of intraventricular conduction have been reported with shortening of the P-R interval.[28] Complete heart block occurs only rarely.

HYPERTENSION. Hypercalcemic patients detected by routine serum calcium screening techniques have higher

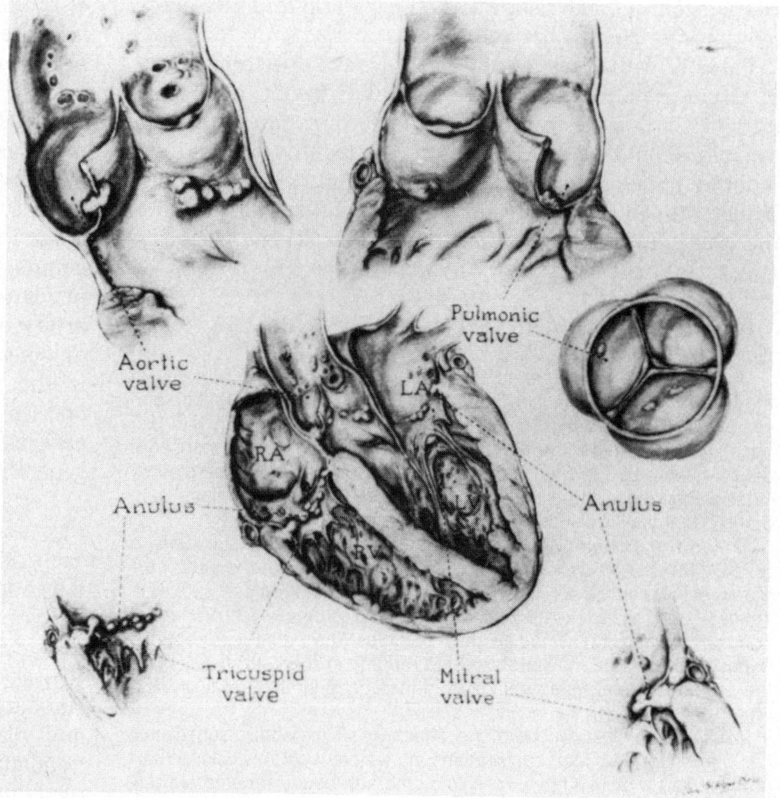

FIGURE 51–6 Drawing of heart showing distribution of calcific deposits in the tricuspid and mitral valve anuli and at the bases of both pulmonic and aortic valve cusps in a 43-year-old woman with hypercalcemia secondary to primary hyperparathyroidism. (Reproduced with permission from Roberts, W. C., and Waller, B. F.: Effect of chronic hypercalcemia on the heart: An analysis of 18 necropsy patients. Am. J. Med. *71*:371, 1981.)

arterial pressure than do matched normocalcemic subjects;[163,164] the pathophysiology of the hypertension may be related to one or more factors. For example, hypercalcemia produces nephrocalcinosis, which may lead to renal failure and hypertension. Thus, reversal of hypertension after successful parathyroid surgery is more likely to occur when renal function is normal. Elevated serum calcium also increases myocardial contractility, peripheral resistance, and release of or vascular sensitivity to vasoconstrictor agents, such as angiotensin II and norepinephrine.[165] While hypercalcemia can increase cardiac contractility and arterial pressure acutely,[166] it is unlikely that this action produces a significant alteration in cardiac output or performance in the absence of PTH on a chronic basis. Thus, an elevation of peripheral resistance is the most likely cause of the hypertension associated with hyperparathyroidism. Resnick has concluded that primary hyperparathyroidism is frequently associated with hypertension. While the mechanism of hypertension in these patients remains to be elucidated, it (1) may be renin-dependent, (2) is associated with and apparently caused by increased circulating PTH rather than hypercalciuria, and (3) is curable surgically in a significant number of patients.[167]

DIAGNOSIS AND TREATMENT

If hypercalcemia is *not* due to primary hyperparathyroidism, circulating concentration of parathyroid hormone should be suppressed. Thus, an elevated or even a normal concentration of parathyroid hormone in the presence of hypercalcemia establishes the diagnosis of hyperparathyroidism; many patients with this condition manifest hypercalcemia for the first time after starting thiazide therapy for treatment of the associated hypertension. Treatment

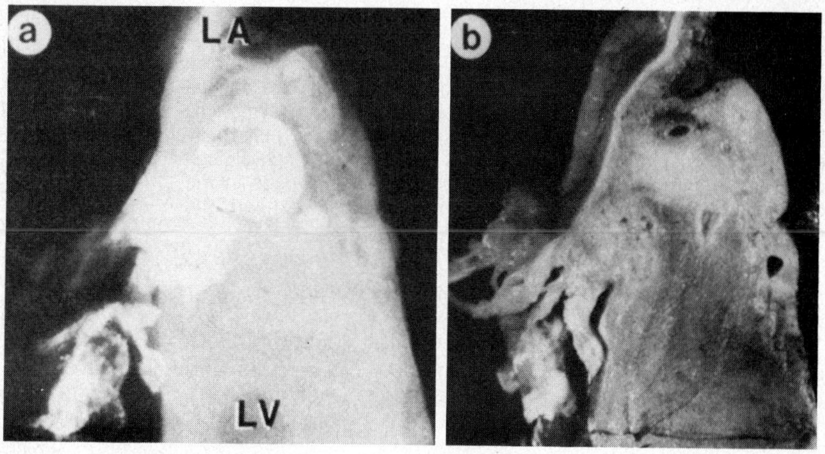

FIGURE 51–7 Longitudinal section of wall of left atrium (LA) and left ventricle (LV) showing heavy calcific deposits in the mitral anular region and also some deposits in the adjacent coronary artery. *a*, radiography; *b*, gross photograph of same area. (Reproduced with permission from Roberts, W. C., and Waller, B. F.: Effect of chronic hypercalcemia on the heart: An analysis of 18 necropsy patients. Am. J. Med. *71*:371, 1981.)

consists of surgical removal of the parathyroid tumor or hyperplastic glands.

Patients with hypertension should have a determination of serum calcium levels before therapy is begun. If thiazide diuretics are used in treatment, determination of serum calcium should be repeated every six months. If thiazide-induced hypercalcemia occurs, the serum calcium should be determined for two to three months after discontinuing the thiazides. Persistence of the hypercalcemia suggests that the patient has primary hyperparathyroidism.[163]

DIABETES MELLITUS

Diabetes mellitus is one of the leading public health problems in the industrialized world, and it has a profound effect on the cardiovascular system. Nearly 10 million people are afflicted with this disease in the United States; it is the eighth health-related cause of death. Nearly all the morbidity from diabetes is related to cardiovascular dysfunction, either coronary artery disease or renal failure secondary to vascular disease.

Actions of Insulin. Insulin is a double-chain polypeptide derived from proinsulin, which is synthesized in the islet cells of the pancreas. Many stimuli, such as glucose, glucagon, amino acids, catecholamines, and gastrointestinal hormones, can promote insulin secretion, which usually occurs in two phases. The rapid early phase releases preformed insulin stored in granules in the beta cells, while the prolonged late phase results from increased biosynthesis of insulin.[168,169]

Insulin is an anabolic hormone affecting all metabolic substrates, i.e., carbohydrates, fats, and proteins, as well as nucleic acids. All target tissues for insulin have specific membrane-bound receptors; thus, binding to the receptor is the first step in initiating its metabolic effect. Cahill and his colleagues have popularized the concept that insulin is the "fed" hormone.[170] Thus, the ingestion of fuel substances provokes a rapid rise in the concentration of circulating insulin, which then facilitates the transfer of these substances into their respective depots. According to this theory, in the fasted state insulin levels are low; as a result, there is increased gluconeogenesis by the liver, decreased lipogenesis with lipolysis and fatty acid release from fat tissue, and decreased glucose uptake in cardiac and skeletal muscle. On the other hand, in the fed state insulin levels are high; gluconeogenesis by the liver is reduced; and in cardiac and skeletal muscle, there is increased glucose and amino acid uptake and increased protein synthesis. In adipose tissue, there is increased glucose and triglyceride uptake, lipogenesis, and absence of release of fatty acids.

In the patient with diabetes, because there is decreased insulin release in response to the ingested fuel, there is a delay in the uptake and the disposal of these fuels into their respective depots, which leads to abnormal circulating levels of the substrates. The increased concentrations of lipids in the circulation may be the underlying pathophysiological effect producing a number of the clinical complications of diabetes mellitus.

Clinical and Biochemical Manifestations. In the past several years, our understanding of the pathogenesis of diabetes mellitus has been significantly altered. Several lines of evidence suggest that in many instances the juvenile form may be infectious in origin, while in most cases the adult onset is probably the result of a genetic predisposition.[171]

Most of the signs and symptoms of this disease either are related to the increased levels of blood glucose or are secondary to changes in the cardiovascular system. Thus, the classic presenting symptoms (observed in about 25 per cent of patients) are polyuria, polydipsia, and polyphagia, all due to the glucosuria. The major pathophysiological consequence of diabetes mellitus is related to changes in the vascular system. The specific target organs include the heart, the eye, the kidney, and the peripheral vasculature.

Cardiovascular Changes in Diabetes

PATHOLOGY. The vascular disease associated with diabetes mellitus can be nonspecific (atherosclerosis and arteriosclerosis) or specific (microangiopathic or endothelial proliferative changes of arterioles). The former primarily involves large vessels (especially in the lower extremities), heart, and brain of older patients, while the latter is localized to small vessels and may be seen in patients of all ages. The atherosclerosis tends to be more extensive and more severe than in nondiabetics, resulting in an increased frequency of myocardial infarction and cerebral and peripheral vascular disease.[172] Indeed, coronary heart disease is the leading cause of death among adult diabetics and accounts for about three times as many deaths among diabetics as among nondiabetics. The incidence of coronary artery disease correlates more closely with the duration of diabetes than with the severity of the diabetes. Of interest is the recent documentation that diabetics have an increased mortality for noncardiovascular diseases (e.g., cancer) as well.[173] The mechanism(s) responsible for this generalized increased mortality is unclear.

Certainly, diabetes should be considered to be a separate risk factor for coronary heart disease[174] (p. 1217). Since each risk factor for vascular disease is thought to add independently (though not equally) to the likelihood for the development of ischemic disease, the diabetic should be considered a high-risk patient in whom all correctable factors should be managed. It is logical to approach cigarette smoking and even moderate elevation of blood pressure and plasma lipids more intensively in diabetic than in nondiabetic patients. Contraceptive drugs that suppress ovulation probably should be avoided, since they may contribute to the metabolic abnormalities that underlie their increased risk for vascular disease. The obese diabetic patient should lose weight; this is often accompanied by gratifying improvement of hypertension, hyperglycemia, hyperinsulinemia, and hypertriglyceridemia.[174]

The microangiopathy produces a characteristic thickening of the basement membrane of the capillaries in the retina, conjunctiva, glomerulus, brain, pancreas, and myocardium.[175] In some cases, there is also proliferation of the epithelial cells leading to occlusion of small arterioles, similar to that observed in immune arteritis.

CARDIAC INVOLVEMENT. Not only is the frequency of acute myocardial infarction increased in diabetic patients,[176] but also the treatment of the infarct is more complicated than in the nondiabetic patient. Patients with acute myocardial infarction and with poor control of the diabetes before hospital admission exhibit a significantly higher mortality than those with good control, but there appears to be no significant difference in mortality between well-controlled diabetics and nondiabetics. Thus, these patients' precarious metabolic status and the difficulty of adjusting insulin therapy to prevent ketoacidosis while not precipitating hypoglycemia probably contribute to the increased mortality from acute myocardial infarction.[177]

The occurrence of a myocardial infarction has a distinctly adverse effect on carbohydrate and fat metabolism[178] and often leads to stimulation of the sympathetic nervous system and increased catecholamine concentration (p. 1276). Subsequent increases in circulating free fatty acid levels and reductions in glucose tolerance appear to be related to a number of physiological functions—adipose tissue lipolysis, hepatic and muscle glycogenolysis, catecholamine-induced suppression of insulin release, and increased circulating concentrations of growth hormone and cortisol. The net result is that carbohydrate intolerance is common following a myocardial infarction, even in nondiabetics. Also, the high concentrations of free fatty acid in the acute phases of a myocardial infarction may lead to ventricular arrhythmias.[179] The suppression of insulin release as a consequence of increased catecholamine activity may decrease glucose utilization by a myocardium that may require this fuel for glycolytic activity.[180]

Diabetic patients with acute myocardial infarction differ from nondiabetics in that their pain patterns are more variable, and infarction may actually occur without pain. Also, survival after infarction is more limited than in the nondiabetics.[181]

Peripheral somatic neuropathy is a common complication of diabetes mellitus; also, diabetic autonomic neuropathy leading to diarrhea, vomiting, and other gastrointestinal disturbances is well known in this disease. Cardiac autonomic dysfunction also exists in many diabetic patients.[182] Occasionally, it may be present before clinical symptoms of generalized autonomic neuropathy are demonstrable.[183] Furthermore, the neuropathy may involve the sympathetic nervous system and/or the parasympathetic nervous system. Indeed, it may become so severe as to lead to total cardiac denervation.[184] These changes in adrenergic nervous system function result in tachycardia and a fixed, rapid heart rate that barely responds to physiological stimuli, such as the Valsalva maneuver, carotid sinus pressure, or tilting, or to drugs, such as phenylephrine, atropine, or propranolol. Rarely, these denervated hearts develop arrhythmias.

Congestive Heart Failure. Insulin-dependent diabetes mellitus appears to increase the likelihood of the development of congestive heart failure from all causes. The role of diabetes in congestive heart failure in the Framingham study was analyzed,[185] and the risk of developing heart failure was found to be increased substantially. Even when patients with prior coronary or rheumatic heart disease were excluded, diabetic subjects had a four- to five-fold increased risk of congestive heart failure. Furthermore, this increased risk persisted after age, blood pressure, weight, and cholesterol values, as well as coronary heart disease, were taken into account. On the basis of these findings it appeared that the excessive risk of heart failure in diabetic patients is caused by factors other than accelerated atherogenesis and coronary heart disease. One suggested possibility is a diabetes-induced cardiomyopathy.[184a]

A statistically significant increase in the frequency of diabetes in patients with idiopathic cardiomyopathy has been reported.[174,186] These patients had serious congestive heart failure, which was difficult to control and invariably at autopsy showed patent large coronary arteries but abnormalities in the small intramural coronary vessels, including intimal fibroblastic thickening and hyaline deposits, as well as inflammatory changes. In contrast, small vessel disease was rare in patients with cardiomyopathy without diabetes. In addition, significant extravascular deposition was noted of collagen, triglyceride, and cholesterol, which may have contributed to the cardiomyopathy. These findings further supported the idea that diabetic patients can develop myocardial disease without large coronary artery involvement, possibly owing to pathological changes in small coronary vessels, but there is considerable dispute concerning the role, if any, of involvement of the latter.

Further clinical evidence for a diabetic cardiomyopathy came from the observations of Regan et al.[187] They studied a group of diabetic patients without evident heart failure who exhibited an elevation of left ventricular end-diastolic pressure and of the left ventricular end-diastolic pressure/volume ratio. Increments of afterload effected an abnormal increase of filling pressure without an increase in stroke volume, compared to normal subjects, consistent with a preclinical cardiomyopathy. Left ventricular biopsy in two patients without ventricular decompensation showed interstitial deposition of collagen with relatively normal muscle cells. These findings suggest a nonischemic myopathic process.

An abnormality of left ventricular function in diabetes is also reflected in the shortening of the left ventricular ejection time, the prolongation of the preejection period, and the elevation of the ratio of the preejection period to the left ventricular ejection time (PEP/LVET).[188] Left ventricular function has also been assessed by echocardiography in diabetic patients with microangiopathy, defined as proteinuria exceeding 3 gm/24 hr, or proliferative retinopathy, but without angina, previous myocardial infarction, hypertension, or alcoholism and with normal electrocardiograms and chest radiographs.[189] Diabetics with microangiopathy had impaired left ventricular function, whereas those with uncomplicated diabetes exhibited normal function. This finding supports the existence of a specific diabetic cardiomyopathy associated with microangiopathy rather than secondary to a metabolic defect.[190] This association between microangiopathy and impaired left ventricular function may help to explain the high incidence of cardiogenic shock, congestive heart failure, and mortality which has been reported in some series of myocardial infarction in diabetics. There is also now accumulated a large body of evidence that impaired left ventricular diastolic function, reflected in a reduced rate of left ventricular wall thinning and dimension increase, may be present in many asymptomatic diabetic patients,[191] particularly those with severe microvascular complications.[192]

In postmortem studies of 11 diabetic patients, of whom 9 were without significant obstructive disease of the proximal coronary arteries and who had died of cardiac failure, all exhibited positive periodic acid–Schiff staining material in the interstitium, but none had luminal narrowing of the intramural vessels. Collagen accumulation was present in perivascular loci, between the myofibers, or as replacement fibrosis. Multiple samples of left ventricle and septum revealed abnormally increased deposits of triglyceride and cholesterol.[187] Thus these observations, taken in toto, suggest that a diffuse abnormality, either extravascular or involving the microvasculature, may be the basis for the cardiomyopathic features of diabetes. Hypertension appears to accelerate this process, as severe interstitial fibrosis, focal scars, and myocytolytic activity were significantly more frequent in hypertensive diabetics with chronic heart failure examined at postmortem than in normotensive diabetics[193] (Fig. 51–8).

In order to gain a better understanding of diabetic cardiomyopathy, a mild, noninsulin-requiring, alloxan diabetes was produced in dogs.[194] Despite similar end-diastolic

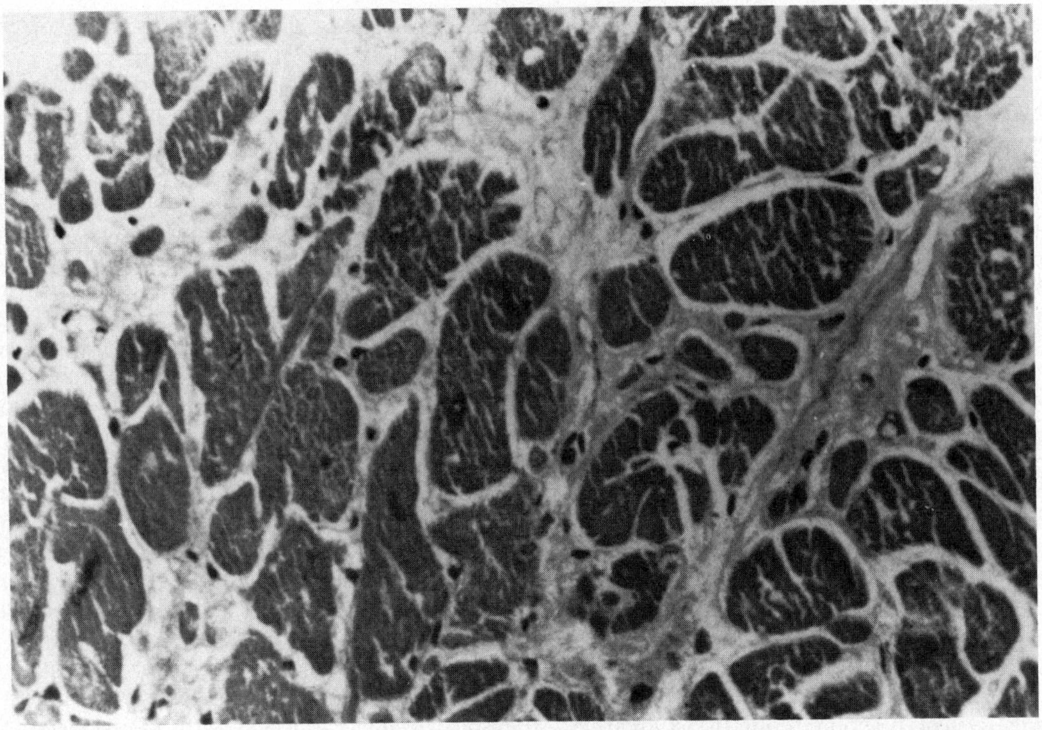

FIGURE 51–8 This section of left ventricular myocardium from a 46-year-old white male (at death) who had insulin-dependent diabetes for 20 years. It demonstrates diffuse interstitial fibrosis. There is marked variability of myocardial cell size, with virtually every cell surrounded by dense collagen. This abnormality is a characteristic feature of the hypertensive-diabetic heart (hematoxylin-eosin; original magnification × 250). (Reproduced with permission from Factor, S. M., Minase, T., and Sonnenblick, E. H.: Clinical and morphological features of human hypertensive-diabetic cardiomyopathy. Am. Heart J. *99*:446, 1980.)

pressures, the end-diastolic volume and stroke volume were significantly less than in control dogs. During acute volume expansion of the ventricle with saline, the end-diastolic pressure increment in diabetic dogs was twice that observed in control dogs. These responses were attributed to an increased stiffness of the left ventricle that was apparently due to accumulation of glycoproteins in the interstitium, measured by periodic acid–Schiff staining. Similar abnormalities were observed in dogs with diabetes that occurred spontaneously. During infusion of ^{14}C-l-oleic acid, fatty acid incorporation, which was predominantly into phospholipid in the control dogs, was diverted to triglyceride in the diabetic dogs; analysis of lipids in the left ventricle revealed elevated concentrations of triglyceride and cholesterol despite normal plasma levels. Thus, these experimental observations support the hypothesis that chronic diabetes mellitus can alter myocardial composition and function independent of its vascular and acute metabolic effects. In this model, therapy with insulin for one year did not reverse all of the myocardial abnormalities.[195] Additional experimental studies suggest, however, that adequate control of the hyperglycemia may reverse the process. In the streptozotocin-induced diabetic rat, there is a significant decrease in contractile protein ATPase activity, resulting in a slowing of relaxation and a depression of shortening velocity.[196] Treatment with insulin acutely—less than one week—did not modify these abnormalities. However, treatment for one month completely reversed them.[197] Whether the different effect of insulin therapy in these studies is related to species differences or differing methods to induce the diabetic state is uncertain.

Other (nondiabetic) cardiomyopathies may exhibit similar hemodynamic abnormalities; an abnormal rise of ventricular filling pressure without a stroke volume increase in response to afterload increments has also been observed in the preclinical phase of alcoholic cardiomyopathy,[198] in which the interstitium is also altered.[199] More severely altered interstitial changes may be the predominant lesion in the incipient stages of amyloid heart disease.[199]

Diabetes mellitus is associated with another form of cardiomyopathy. Approximately half the infants of diabetic mothers have either radiographic cardiomegaly or clinical features suggesting congestive heart failure.[200] The cardiomyopathy in these infants may be transient and secondary to hematological, respiratory, and metabolic problems or a more protracted form of nonobstructive or obstructive hypertrophic cardiomyopathy, which appears to be secondary to maternal hormonal influences and to be reversible.

Electrocardiographic changes are commonly observed in patients with diabetes.[28] While many of the changes are predictable on the basis of the associated hypertension or coronary artery disease, in some there is an unexplained diffuse T-wave abnormality that may be related to the cardiomyopathy.

VASCULAR DISEASE. Peripheral vascular disease is a frequent and significant manifestation of diabetes mellitus, often leading to gangrene and amputation of the lower extremity. The smaller arteries below the knee are more likely to be involved in patients with diabetes in contrast to iliac or femoral artery disease in nondiabetic patients. Cerebral vascular disease is also more frequent, with a greater incidence of cerebral infarction though not cerebral hemorrhage. The increased atherosclerosis of the cerebral vessels and the proliferative changes in the cerebral arterioles both contribute to this increased rate of infarction.

The renal vasculature is affected in a number of ways: atherosclerosis is common in the larger vessels, with proliferative endothelial changes occurring in small vessels. Third, capillary basement membrane thickening is common, particularly in the glomerular tuft where a pathognomonic change—nodular glomerulosclerosis—is often found. These vascular changes, in concert with parenchymal changes secondary to pyelonephritis, lead to a variety of renal disorders, including the nephrotic syndrome, hypertension, and renal failure.

Most studies have reported an increased incidence of hypertension in diabetes, in part related to renal disease. Volume overload may be an additional factor contributing to the hypertension, since many diabetic patients have low renin levels; often the hypertension is best managed by diuretics and sodium restriction. Indeed, more than one third of diabetic patients have hypertension, an incidence that is higher than that of the general population. It is possible to explain the increased susceptibility of diabetics to arteriosclerotic cardiovascular disease in large measure by the increased incidence of hypertension.

DIAGNOSIS AND TREATMENT OF DIABETES MELLITUS

It is generally agreed that therapy directed at the control of excessive fatty acid mobilization and oxidation and protein catabolism is essential in the treatment of diabetes mellitus. On the other hand, disagreement still exists regarding the usefulness of treating asymptomatic hyperglycemia. Recently, it has been documented that the synthesis of polyols and basement membrane glycoproteins is increased by hyperglycemia.[175,201] Thus, "tight control" of blood glucose may be important if the long-term complications of diabetes mellitus are to be reduced.

Diet, insulin, and oral hypoglycemic agents have been the mainstays of treatment. However, a controversy has arisen concerning the efficacy of oral hypoglycemic agents, such as the sulfonylureas.[202,203] While hyperglycemia is better controlled with these agents than it is with diet alone, an increased frequency of myocardial infarction has been reported. Although the interpretation and implications of these findings are still controversial, there is some experimental evidence suggesting that sulfonylureas may have an adverse effect on the myocardium. Wu and colleagues have reported increased "stiffness" of the myocardium secondary to interstitial accumulation of periodic acid–Schiff staining material which reduced left ventricular function in dogs treated with tolbutamide.[204]

On the basis of available information, in our judgment the only patients with diabetes who should use oral hypoglycemic agents are those who are not ketosis-prone, whose hyperglycemia cannot be controlled with diet alone, and who are unwilling or unable to receive insulin injections. It should also be recognized that beta-adrenergic blockers reduce the hyperglycemic reaction to stress, and it is possible that beta-adrenergic blocker therapy may require a downward adjustment of insulin dosage, since patients receiving beta blockers may be more susceptible to hypoglycemia. Since many of the symptoms of which the hypoglycemic patient is aware are due to the effects of the epinephrine which is released, both physician and patient must be alert to the possibility that hypoglycemia occurring in the beta blocker–treated diabetic may be relatively asymptomatic. Since certain diuretics, such as the thiazides and furosemide, may result in hypokalemia, and because hypokalemia can inhibit insulin release, these drugs may intensify the glucose intolerance of diabetic patients.

In patients with diabetes mellitus and impairment of left ventricular function, a sudden increase in the glucose concentration of extracellular fluid, as occurs with the development of insulin deficiency, may result in the movement of fluid from the intracellular to the extracellular space and an intensification of heart failure. This responds to the lowering of blood glucose concentration by insulin.[205]

OBESITY

There are two types of obesity: adult-onset and lifelong. Adult-onset obesity is extremely common, probably occurring to a varying extent in nearly all individuals in developed countries. Its clinical course consists of normal weight patterns during childhood and adolescence, with a gradual increase in weight beginning between 20 and 40 years of age; it reflects an imbalance between caloric intake and utilization.[206] Much less frequent is lifelong obesity, characterized by the development of obesity early in childhood, with significant increase in weight during adolescence and, in the female, during and after pregnancy. These individuals are usually grossly obese, weighing more than 150 per cent of their ideal weight as adults.

Hirsch and coworkers have documented an increase both in the size and the number of adipose cells in individuals with lifelong obesity, while in adult-onset obesity, only an increase in cell size occurs.[207] With weight reduction the size of the adipose cells decreases in both conditions; however, the number does not change in either. Whether in lifelong obesity the increased number of adipose cells is determined by genetic or environmental factors is uncertain. However, it has been documented that there is no significant change in the number of adipose cells when obesity develops after late childhood in both experimental animals and humans. On the other hand, some evidence suggests that early infant feeding habits may significantly alter their number.[208] The metabolic consequences of obesity include decreased sensitivity to insulin, with resultant hyperinsulinemia, glucose intolerance, hypercholesterolemia, hypertriglyceridemia, and hyperaminoacidemia.

CARDIOVASCULAR CONSEQUENCES OF SEVERE OBESITY

It is well known from a variety of statistical data that marked obesity is accompanied by an increased morbidity and excessive mortality, a large portion of which is related to cardiovascular abnormalities. *Hypertension* is common in the grossly obese,[208a] although it must be recognized that indirect measurement of blood pressure frequently leads to overestimation of the arterial pressure by the standard cuff method (p. 22). Nonetheless, direct measurement of arterial pressure frequently shows moderate elevations that can usually be promptly restored to normal by means of weight reduction and salt restriction.

Evidence of circulatory dysfunction in the massively obese, associated with cardiac enlargement during life and at autopsy, was first described by Smith and Willius in 1933.[209] It is now widely appreciated that massive obesity is accompanied by a marked increase in blood volume and cardiac output, which are proportional to the excess of body weight;[210–212] the hematocrit is often slightly elevated as well. The elevated cardiac output is secondary to an increased stroke volume, since heart rate is normal; the cardiac output rises normally during exercise. Left ventricular filling pressures are at or close to the upper limits of normal in the supine position in the basal state, but increase with passive leg raising, and reach strikingly elevated levels during exercise. These increases in ventricular filling pressure are associated with a high resting central blood volume, which also increases significantly with exertion. The maximum velocity of myocardial fiber shortening and the ratio of stroke work index to left ventricular end-diastolic pressure were reduced, even in relatively young obese persons, without any other evidence of heart disease[211] (Fig. 51–9). Massive edema may occur as a consequence of the elevated ventricular filling pressure, despite elevation of the cardiac output.

Examination of the gross and microscopic anatomy of the heart in patients with marked chronic obesity showed heart weight to be considerably greater than predicted for

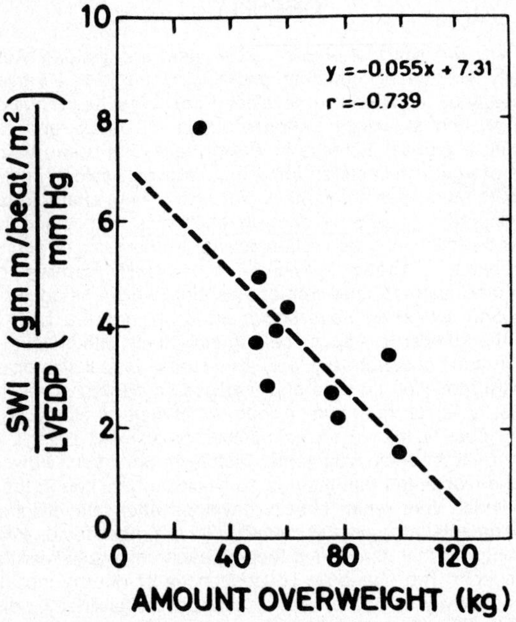

FIGURE 51–9 The significant negative correlation between the ratio of the stroke work index (SWI) to the left ventricular end-diastolic pressure (LVEDP) and the amounts of overweight shows that the higher the degree of obesity, the greater the impairment of left ventricular function. (Reproduced with permission from Divitiis, O., Fazio, S., Petitto, M., et al: Obesity and cardiac function. Circulation *64*:477, 1981, by permission of the American Heart Association, Inc.)

ideal body weight, with marked left ventricular hypertrophy and, in a few instances, right ventricular hypertrophy as well.[212a] This increase in cardiac weight is not due to excess epicardial fat and fatty infiltration of the myocardium, which were previously considered to be the principal features of the obese heart.[213] Thus, when these clinical, hemodynamic, and pathological observations are taken together, it appears that manifestations of myocardial dysfunction occur in very obese subjects without evidence of other heart disease and that in the absence of the obesity hypoventilation syndrome (p. 1596), cor pulmonale is not a presenting feature.

Heart failure in the markedly obese is usually chronic. The pulmonary and systemic congestion with symptoms of dyspnea and edema are, at first, simply related to the reductions in ventricular compliance and elevations of filling pressures. Later, these symptoms are related also to increases in ventricular end-diastolic volume and the reduction of myocardial contractility. Thus, the marked chronic elevation of cardiac work, i.e., of cardiac output and arterial pressure, ultimately leads to heart failure.

Fortunately, weight reduction is beneficial in the majority of patients, even those with heart failure. It usually improves the exercise capacity of patients with chronic exogenous obesity and decreases total body oxygen uptake, the cardiothoracic ratio on chest roentgenogram, systemic arterial pressure, blood volume, cardiac output, arteriovenous oxygen difference, and left ventricular filling pressure at rest.[210] However, evidence of left ventricular dysfunction persists, as reflected in the elevation of left ventricular filling pressure with exercise.[214,215]

Treatment of heart failure in these patients consists of maintenance of the reduced body weight, dietary sodium restriction, cardiac glycosides, and diuretics. Often, patients with massive obesity have associated arteriosclerotic coronary artery disease and the salutary results of weight reduction may be particularly striking in them.

TREATMENT

Most cases of adult-onset obesity are the result of imbalance between intake and output. Thus, reduction of intake is the most significant factor in treating this disease. While abnormalities in endocrine function, particularly of the thyroid or adrenal, have often been implicated in the pathophysiology of obesity, this thesis is rarely substantiated by detailed evaluation. The amount and rate of weight loss with a given level of caloric restrictions depends on the degree of energy expenditure. Energy expenditure depends on both the physical activity and mass of the individual. Thus, with a fixed level of intake and activity, the rate of weight loss decreases as the total weight decreases. There is no evidence that a specific type of diet has any intrinsic benefit except as it is related to its caloric content. Thus, the claim that high protein diets are more efficacious is related not to their caloric content but rather to the accompanying ketosis that suppresses appetite.

MALNUTRITION

Malnutrition, particularly protein-calorie deficiency, is prevalent in many underdeveloped areas of the world. However, in recent years, it has also become a concern in developed countries in those individuals who have chronic diseases, in whom it exists as a result of both anorexia and hypermetabolism. The clinical picture is similar to adult kwashiorkor reported from underdeveloped countries, described below.

Protein-calorie malnutrition of childhood refers to syndromes of nutritional deficiency, which range from marasmus to kwashiorkor and which result from a stress like a serious infection superimposed upon an inadequate diet.[93] *Marasmus* is a state of malnutrition in an infant who has been weaned early and fed a diet grossly deficient in calories, protein, and other essential nutrients. *Kwashiorkor* usually occurs in children 1 to 4 years of age and is due to deficiency of protein relative to calories.

The circulatory status of patients with severe nutritional depletion and electrolyte imbalance is precarious; the cardiac output, systolic pressure, and pulse pressure are abnormally low and there may be massive, generalized edema; the P-R interval may be shortened. There is loss of subcutaneous fat and general wasting and atrophy of most organs, including the heart, which is thin-walled, pale, and flabby on gross examination. Histological study reveals atrophy of the muscle fibers, sometimes with interstitial edema. In experimental chronic protein-calorie undernutrition, not only is the heart atrophic, but also left ventricular function may be abnormal. In the dog, there are reductions in left ventricular compliance and contractility,[216] whereas in the rat this apparently does not occur, although there is striking atrophy of the heart.[217] The treatment of the dehydrated or severely anemic patient with protein-calorie malnutrition involves correction of hematological, fluid, and electrolyte imbalance and the treatment of infection. Congestive failure can be avoided if care is taken to avoid overloading with sodium, water, or blood. Digitalis must be given cautiously when these patients are in heart failure because of their sensitivity to glycosides.

In parts of the world where pediatric kwashiorkor is common, there are also cases of adults with similar clinical features.[218] These features include loss of subcutaneous fat and muscle with edema, weakness, depression, anorexia, diarrhea, abdominal distention, hair loss, and thinning of the skin. Classically, plasma albumin and amino acid levels are low, as are serum concentrations of sodium, magnesium, and phosphorus. Urinary excretion of nitrogen is reduced, as is total body potassium. On the other hand, total body and extracellular water and plasma volume are usually increased. The primary pathophysiological event is protein malnutrition. All the clinical signs and symptoms are related to this basic defect.

MALNUTRITION IN CARDIAC DISEASE

Assessment of protein-calorie nutritional status in cardiac patients has not been extensively evaluated. However, during the last two decades there has been an increasing awareness that some patients with cardiovascular disease have clinical features similar to those described above. In these cases, instead of involuntary protein deprivation, anorexia plays a significant role. For example, chronic congestive heart failure leads to cellular hypoxia as well as hypermetabolism. Gastrointestinal hypoxia produces anorexia, which then initiates a vicious circle. Decreased protein intake produces cardiac atrophy and increasing congestive heart failure, which produces more cellular hypoxia, greater anorexia, and finally death.[219]

A similar condition has been described in some patients undergoing open heart surgery for correction of rheumatic valvular disease. In some malnourished patients, the mortality reaches 20 per cent, significantly greater than the 1 to 2 per cent in normally nourished patients undergoing the same procedure. The underlying pathophysiology is uncertain but probably includes (1) decreased cardiac mass, (2) reduction of biosynthetic activity of liver, (3) poor healing due to reduced levels of substrate, and (4) impairment of cell-mediated immunity.[219,220] As a result, wound healing is retarded, skin ulcers occur, and requirements for artificial ventilation are prolonged. Abel and colleagues have suggested that hyperalimentation in the immediate postoperative period does not significantly alter the increased morbidity.[219] This has led Blackburn et al. to suggest that both preoperative and concurrent nutritional support is necessary[220] (Fig. 51–10). However, definitive studies to distinguish between nutritional status and severity of the cardiovascular disease as the cause for the increased morbidity have not been reported.

CARDIOVASCULAR MANIFESTATIONS OF VITAMIN DEFICIENCY

Thiamine Deficiency (see p. 814)

Other Vitamin Deficiencies. Deficiencies of other vitamins have not led to specifically definable cardiovascular abnormalities, except for the hypocalcemia-accompanied vitamin D deficiency. However, vitamin deficiencies, particularly of the B group and folic acid, have been diagnosed with increasing frequency in patients with cardiovascular disease. For example, nearly a third of infants and children with congenital heart disease have been reported to be deficient in a number of the B vitamins.[221] Folic acid deficiency has been documented in a significant number of patients with congestive heart failure. Whiie the deficient state may simply be related to decreased intake, abnormal intestinal absorption or increased rates of excretion may also contribute.

ALTERATIONS IN GONADAL HORMONE SECRETION

There are no specific cardiovascular abnormalities associated with altered gonadal function even though the heart does contain androgen receptors, whose function has not been defined.[222] However, the effect of sex steroids on the development of atherosclerosis has been the subject of intensive investigation over the past decade.

GONADAL FUNCTION AND CARDIOVASCULAR DISEASE

Middle-aged men are at a higher risk for developing cardiovascular disease than age-matched women. Because the discrepancy between male and female mortality disappears in older, postmenopausal women, some investigators have suggested that estrogen reduces the rate of development of coronary atherosclerosis. Support for this thesis includes the observation that total cholesterol is lower and HDL cholesterol is higher in postmenopausal women who are taking estrogens than in those who are not.[223,224] Additionally, the risk ratio for coronary artery disease death is only 0.43 in postmenopausal estrogen users compared to nonusers[225] (p. 1218). Several studies, however, have provided evidence against this thesis. First, it has been documented that the development of coronary artery disease in women who underwent hysterectomies and were also castrated is no different than in age-matched noncastrated women.[226] Second, widespread use of oral contraceptives, most of which contain estrogen, has proved that estrogen administration is not without cardiovascular risk, since it can increase total cholesterol and beta-lipoprotein (LDL) cholesterol and decrease alpha-lipoprotein (HDL) cholesterol in premenopausal females.[227,228] Additionally, it has been

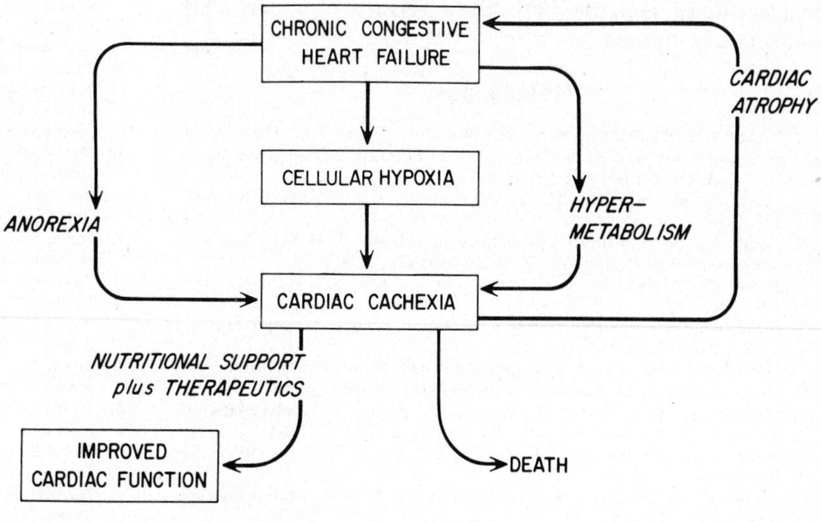

FIGURE 51–10 Pathogenesis of cardiac cachexia. A positive feedback loop forms a vicious circle that leads to irreversible protein malnutrition. Heart failure therapy must begin and forced feeding must be initiated to reduce morbidity and mortality. (From Blackburn, G. L., et al.: Nutritional support in cardiac cachexia. J. Thorac. Cardiovasc. Surg. *73*:494, 1977.)

shown to increase the degree of abnormality in post-exercise electrocardiograms in those individuals who had abnormal tests prior to estrogen therapy.[229]

This has led some investigators to suggest that it is not the increased estrogen but the decreased testosterone that is protective to women. They base this theory on the documented reduction in serum cholesterol levels and incidence of atherosclerosis in castrated men and the positive correlation between plasma testosterone and high density lipoprotein cholesterol levels.[230] However, the similar frequency of coronary artery disease in postmenopausal women and men of similar age with significantly different testosterone levels is unexplained.

CARDIOVASCULAR EFFECTS OF ORAL CONTRACEPTIVES

Within the last decade, several studies have documented that in some patients the use of oral contraceptives is accompanied by an increased risk of cardiovascular morbidity and mortality in premenopausal females.[227–229,231] Specifically, there is an increased frequency of diabetes mellitus, hypertension, and thromboembolic disease. While the increased risk is small, nevertheless caution in the use of oral contraceptive agents by individuals who may be predisposed to the development of these diseases is warranted.

HYPERTENSION (see also p. 873). The hypertension associated with estrogen administration is probably related to its effect in modifying the production of renin substrate by the liver.[232] It has been clearly documented that oral contraceptives increase the concentration of renin substrate and blood angiotensin II.[233] However, most individuals do not develop clinical hypertension, which suggests that a counter-regulatory mechanism(s) is activated, reducing the vascular effect of angiotensin II. Alternatively, blood pressure may increase in all patients, but only the predisposed will develop hypertension. Thus, individuals who have a personal or family history of renal disease are more likely to develop hypertension with estrogen administration.

THROMBOEMBOLIC DISEASE. At least two clearly defined alterations in the clotting system are produced by oral contraceptive agents; either or both could be responsible for the increased frequency of thromboembolic disease.[231] First, estrogen enhances the biosynthesis of a number of the clotting factors by the liver. Second, oral contraceptives increase both the viscosity of blood and platelet adhesiveness.

References

1. Graves, R. J.: Clinical lectures. London Med. Surg. J. (Part II):7, 516, 1835.
2. Addison, T.: On the Constitutional and Local Effects of Disease of the Supra-renal Capsules. London, Highley, 1855.
3. Sonenberg, M., and Cohen, H.: Growth hormone. Ann. N.Y. Acad. Sci. *148*: 291, 1968.
4. Daughaday, W. H.: The adenohypophysis. *In* Williams, R. H. (ed.): Textbook of Endocrinology, Philadelphia, W. B. Saunders Co., 1974, p. 31.
5. Korner, A.: Anabolic action of growth hormone. Ann. N.Y. Acad. Sci. *148*: 408, 1968.
6. Frelin, C.: The regulation of protein turnover in newborn rat heart cell cultures. J. Biol. Chem. *255*:11149, 1980.
7. Goodman, H. M.: Growth hormone and the metabolism of carbohydrate and lipid in adipose tissue. Ann. N.Y. Acad. Sci. *148*:419, 1968.
8. Mautalen, C. A., Mellinger, R. C., and Smith, R. W., Jr.: Lipolytic effect of growth hormone in acromegaly. J. Clin. Endocrinol. *28*:1031, 1968.
9. Randle, P. J., and Morgan, H. E.: Regulation of glucose uptake by muscle. Vitam. Horm. *20*:199, 249, 1962.
10. Coggeshall, C., and Root, H. F.: Acromegaly and diabetes mellitus. Endocrinology *26*:1, 1940.
11. Aloia, J. F., Roginsky, M. D., and Field, R. A.: Absence of hyperlipidemia in acromegaly. J. Clin. Endocrinol. *35*:921, 1972.
12. Courville, C., and Mason, V. R.: The heart in acromegaly. Arch. Intern. Med. *61*:704, 1938.
13. Hejtmancik, M. R., Bradfield, J. Y., and Hermann, G. R.: Acromegaly and the heart: A clinical and pathologic study. Ann. Intern. Med. *34*:1445, 1951.
14. McGuffin, W. L., Sherman, B. M., Roth, J., Gorden, P., Kahn, C. R., Roberts, W. C., and Frommer, P. L.: Acromegaly and cardiovascular disorders. Ann. Intern. Med. *81*:11, 1974.
15. Lie, J. T., and Grossman, S. J.: Pathology of the heart in acromegaly: Anatomic findings in 27 autopsied patients. Am. Heart J. *100*:41, 1980.
16. Mather, H. M., Boyd, M. J., and Jenkins, J. S.: Heart size and function in acromegaly. Br. Heart J. *41*:697, 1979.
17. Savage, D. D., Henry, W. L., Eastman, R. C., Borer, J. S., and Gorden, P.: Echocardiographic assessment of cardiac anatomy and function in acromegalic patients. Am. J. Med. *67*:823, 1979.
17a. Csanady, M., Gaspar, L., Hogye, M., Hogye, M., and Gruber, N.: The heart in acromegaly: An echocardiographic study. Intern. J. Cardiol. *2*:349, 1983.
18. Rossi, L., Thiene, G., Caregaro, L., Giordano, R., and Lauro, S.: Dysrhythmias and sudden death in acromegalic heart disease. A clinicopathologic study. Chest *72*:495, 1977.
19. Hamwi, G. J., Skillman, T. G., and Tufts, K. C., Jr.: Acromegaly. Am. J. Med. *29*:690, 1960.
20. Falkheden, T., and Sjögren, B.: Extracellular fluid volume and renal function in pituitary insufficiency and acromegaly. Acta Endocrinol. *46*:80, 1964.
21. Cain, J. P., Williams, G. H., and Dluhy, R. G.: Plasma renin activity and aldosterone secretion in patients with acromegaly, J. Clin. Endocrinol. *34*:73, 1972.
22. Strauch, G., Vallotton, M. B., and Touitou, Y.: The renin-angiotensin-aldosterone system in normotensive and hypertensive patients with acromegaly. N. Engl. J. Med. *287*:795, 1972.
23. Dluhy, R. G., and Williams, G. H.: Primary aldosteronism in a hypertensive acromegalic patient. J. Clin. Endocrinol. *29*:1319, 1969.
24. Moore, T. J., Thein-Wai, W., Dluhy, R. G., Dawson-Hughes, B. F., Hollenberg, N. K., and Williams, G. H.: Abnormal adrenal and vascular responses to angiotensin II and an angiotensin antagonist in acromegaly. J. Clin. Endocrinol. Metab. *51*:215, 1980.
25. Souadjian, J. V., and Schirger, A.: Hypertension in acromegaly. Am. J. Med. Sci. *254*:629, 1967.
26. Biglieri, E. G., Watlington, C. O., and Forsham, P. H.: Sodium retention with human growth hormone and its subfractions. J. Clin. Endocrinol. *21*:361, 1961.
27. Kellgron, J. A., Ball, J., and Tutton, G. K.: The articular and other limb changes in acromegaly. Q. J. Med. *21*:405, 1952.
28. Surawicz, B., and Mangiardi, M. L.: Electrocardiogram in endocrine and metabolic disorders. *In* Rios, J. C. (ed.): Clinical Electrocardiographic Correlations. Philadelphia, F. A. Davis, 1977, p. 243.
28a. Knowlton, A. I., and Baer, L.: Cardiac failure in Addison's disease. Am. J. Med. *74*:829, 1983.
29. Jonas, E. A., Aloia, J. F., and Lane, F. J.: Evidence of subclinical heart muscle dysfunction in acromegaly. Chest *67*:190, 1975.
30. Smallridge, R. C., Rajfer, S., Davis, J., and Schaaf, M.: Acromegaly and the heart. Am. J. Med. *66*:22, 1979.
31. Hardy, J.: Trans-sphenoidal microsurgical removal of pituitary microadenoma. Progr. Neurol. Surg. *6*:200, 1975.
32. Kjellberg, R. M. Proton-beam therapy in acromegaly. N. Engl. J. Med. *278*: 689, 1968.
33. Schimmel, M., and Utiger, R. D.: Thyroidal and peripheral production of thyroid hormones. Review of recent findings and their clinical implications. Ann. Intern. Med. *87*:760, 1977.
34. Kaplan, M. M.: The thyroid and the heart; how do they interact? J. Cardiovasc. Med., *7*:893, 1982.
35. Lardy, H. A., and Feldott, H. G.: Metabolic effects of thyroxine *in vitro*. Ann. N.Y. Acad. Sci. *54*:636, 1951.
36. Tata, J., Ernster, L., and Lindberg, O.: The action of thyroid hormones at the cell level. Biochem. J. *86*:408, 1963.
37. Stocker, W. W., Samaha, F. J., and Degroot, L. J.: Coupled oxidative phosphorylation in muscle of thyrotoxic patients. Am. J. Med. *44*:900, 1968.
38. Oppenheimer, J. H., Schwartz, H. L., Surks, M. I., Koerner, D., and Dillmann, W. H.: Nuclear receptors and the initiation of thyroid hormone action. *In* Greep, R. O. (ed.): Recent Progress in Hormone Research. New York, Academic Press, 1976, p. 529.
39. Seelig, S., Liaw, C., Towle, H. C., and Oppenheimer, J. H.: Thyroid hormone attenuates and augments hepatic gene expression at a pretranslational level. Proc. Natl. Acad. Sci. USA *78*:4733–4737, 1981.
40. Edelman, I. S., and Ismail-Beigi, F.: Thyroid thermogenesis and active sodium transport. Recent Progr. Horm. Res. *30*:235, 1974.
41. Asano, Y., Liberman, U. A., and Edelman, I. S.: Thyroid thermogenesis: Relationships between Na^+-dependent respiration and Na^{++}-K^+-adenosine triphosphatase activity in rat skeletal muscle. J. Clin. Invest. *57*:368, 1976.
42. Lo, C. S., August, T. R., Liberman, U. A., and Edelman, I. S.: Dependence of renal ($Na^+ + K^+$) adenosine triphosphatase activity on thyroid status. J. Biol. Chem. *251*:7826, 1976.
43. Lo, C. S., and Edelman, I. S.: Effect of triiodothyronine on the synthesis and degradation of renal cortical ($Na^+ + K^+$) adenosine triphosphatase. J. Biol. Chem. *251*:7834, 1976.

44. Fain, J. N., and Rosenthal, J. W.: Calorigenic action of triiodothyronine on white cells: Effects of ouabain, oligomycin, and cathecholamines. Endocrinology *89*:1205, 1971.
45. Primack, M. P., and Buchanan, J. L.: Control of oxygen consumption in liver slices from normal and T4-treated rats. Endocrinology *95*:619, 1974.
46. Knight, R. A.: The use of spinal anesthesia to control sympathetic overactivity in hyperthyroidism. Anesthesiology *6*:225, 1945.
47. Buccino, R. A., Spann, J. F., Pool, P. E., and Braunwald, E.: Influence of the thyroid state on the intrinsic contractile properties and the energy stores of the myocardium. J. Clin. Invest. *46*:1669, 1967.
48. Bayliss, R. I. S., and Edwards, O. M.: Urinary excretion of free catecholamines in Graves' disease. Endocrinology *49*:167, 1971.
49. Christensen, H. J.: Plasma noradrenaline and adrenaline in patients with thyrotoxicosis and myxoedema. Clin. Sci. Molec. Med. *45*:163, 1973.
50. Nishizawa, Y., Hamada, N., Fujii, S., Morii, H., Okuda, K., and Wada, M.: Serum dopamine-beta-hydroxylase activity in thyroid disorders. J. Clin. Endocrinol. Metab. *39*:599, 1974.
51. Rutherford, J. P., Vatner, S. F., and Braunwald, E.: Adrenergic control of myocardial contractility in conscious hypertrophied dogs. Am. J. Physiol. *237*: 590, 1980.
52. Brester, W. R., Isaacs, J. R., and Osgood, P. F.: The hemodynamic and metabolic interrelationships in the activity of epinephrine, norepinephrine, and the thyroid hormones. Circulation *13*:1, 1956.
53. Van Der Schoot, J. B., and Moran, N. C.: An experimental evaluation of the reported influence of thyroxine on the cardiovascular effects of catecholamines. J. Pharmacol. Exp. Ther. *149*:336, 1965.
54. Wildenthal, K.: Studies of isolated fetal mouse hearts in organ culture: Evidence for a direct effect of triiodothyronine in enhancing cardiac responsiveness to norepinephrine. J. Clin. Invest. *51*:2702, 1972.
55. Wildenthal, K.: Studies on fetal mouse hearts in organ culture: Influence of prolonged exposure to triiodothyronine on cardiac responsiveness to isoproterenol, glucagon, theophylline, acetylcholine, and dibutyryl cyclic 3', 5'-adenosine monophosphate. J. Pharmacol. Exp. Ther. *109*:272, 1974.
56. Williams, L. T., Lefkowitz, R. J., Watanbe, A. M., Hathaway, D. R., and Besch, H. R.: Thyroid hormone regulation of beta-adrenergic receptor number. J. Biol. Chem. *252*:2787, 1977.
57. Scarpace, P. J., and Abrass, I. B.: Thyroid hormone regulation of rat heart, lymphocyte, and lung beta-adrenergic receptors. Endocrinology *108*:1007, 1981.
58. Whitsett, J. A., Pollinger, J., and Matz, S.: β-adrenergic receptors and catecholamine sensitive adenylate cyclase in developing rat ventricular myocardium: Effect of thyroid status. Pediatr. Res. *16*:463, 1982.
59. Tse, J., Wrenn, R. W., and Kuo, J. F.: Thyroxine-induced changes in characteristics and activities of beta-adrenergic receptors and adenosine 3', 5'-monophosphate and guanosine 3', 5'-monophosphate systems in the heart may be related to reputed catecholamine supersensitivity in hyperthyroidism. Endocrinology *107*:6, 1980.
60. Guarnieri, T., Filburn, C. R., Beard, E. S., and Lakatta, E. G.: Enhanced contractile response and protein kinase activation to threshold levels of β-adrenergic stimulation in hyperthyroid rat heart. J. Clin. Invest. *65*:861, 1980.
61. Kunos, G., Vermes-Kunos, I., and Nickerson, M.: Effects of thyroid state on adrenoreceptor properties. Nature *250*:779, 1974.
62. Markowitz, C., and Yater, W. M.: Response of explanted cardiac muscle to thyroxine. Am. J. Physiol. *100*:162, 1932.
63. Murayama, M., and Goodkind, M. J.: Effect of thyroid hormone on the frequency-force relationship of atrial myocardium from the guinea pig. Circ. Res. *23*:743, 1968.
64. Goldman, S., Olajos, M., Friedman, H., Roeske, W. R., and Morkin, E.: Left ventricular performance in conscious thyrotoxic calves. Am. J. Physiol. *242*: H113, 1982.
64a. Morkin, E., Flink, I. L., and Goldman, S.: Biochemical and physiologic effects of thyroid hormone on cardiac performance. Prog. Cardiovasc. Dis. *25*:435, 1983.
64b. Banerjee, S. K.: Comparative studies of atrial and ventricular myosin from normal, thyrotoxic, and thyroidectomized rabbits. Circ. Res. *52*:131, 1983.
65. Philipson, K. D., and Edelman, I. S.: Thyroid hormone control of Na^+-K^+-ATPase and K^+-dependent phosphatase in rat heart. Am. J. Physiol. *232*: C196, 1977.
66. Litten, R. Z., Martin, B. J., Howe, E. R., Alpert, N. R., and Solaro, R. J.: Phosphorylation and adenosine triphosphate activity of myofibrils from thyrotoxic rabbit hearts. Circ. Res. *48*:498, 1981.
67. Curfman, G. D., Crowley, T. J., and Smith, T. W.: Thyroid-induced alterations in myocardial sodium- and potassium-activated adenosine triphosphatase, monovalent cation active transport and cardiac glycoside binding. J. Clin. Invest. *59*:586, 1977.
68. Banerjee, S. K., Flink, I. L., and Morkin, E.: Enzymatic properties of native and *N*-ethylmaleimide-modified cardiac myosin from normal and thyrotoxic rabbits. Circ. Res. *39*:319, 1976.
69. Litten, R. Z., III, Martin, B. J., Low, R. B., and Alpert, N. R.: Altered myosin isozyme patterns from pressure-overloaded and thyrotoxic hypertrophied rabbit hearts. Circ. Res. *50*:856, 1982.
70. Chizzonite, R. A., Everett, A. W., Clark, W. A., Jakovcic, S., Rabinowitz, M., and Zak, R.: Isolation and characterization of two molecular variants of myosin heavy chain from rabbit ventricle. Change in their content during normal growth and after treatment with thyroid hormone. J. Biol. Chem. *257*:2056, 1982.
71. Goodkind, M. J., Dambach, G. E., Thyrum, P. T., and Luchi, R. J.: Effect of thyroxine on ventricular myocardial contractility of ATPase activity in guinea pigs. Am. J. Physiol. *226*:66, 1974.
72. Suko, J.: The calcium pump of cardiac sarcoplasmic reticulum. Functional alterations at different levels of thyroid state in rabbits. J. Physiol. (Lond.) *228*:563, 1973.
73. Johnson, P. N., Freedberg, A. S., and Marshall, J. M.: Action of thyroid hormone on the transmembrane potentials from sinoatrial cells and atrial muscle cells in isolated atria of rabbits. Cardiology *58*:273, 1973.
74. Arnsdorf, M. D., and Childers, R. W.: Atrial electrophysiology in experimental hyperthyroidism in rabbits. Circ. Res. *26*:575, 1970.
75. Davis, P. J., and Davis, F. B.: Hyperthyroidism in patients over the age of 60 years. Medicine *53*:161, 1974.
75a. Talafih, K., Briden, K. L., and Weiss, H. R.: Thyroxine-induced hypertrophy of the rabbit heart. Effect on regional oxygen extraction, flow, and oxygen consumption. Circ. Res. *52*:272, 1983.
76. Hillis, W. S., Bremmer, W. F., Lawrie, T. D. V., and Thomson, J. A.: Systolic time intervals in thyroid disease. Clin. Endocrinol. *4*:617, 1975.
77. Cohen, M. V., Schulman, I. C., Spenillo, A., and Surks, M. I.: Effects of thyroid hormone on left ventricular function in patients treated for thyrotoxicosis. Am. J. Cardiol. *48*:33, 1981.
78. Hoffman, I., and Lowrey, R. D.: The electrocardiogram in thyrotoxicosis. Am. J. Cardiol. *6*:893, 1960.
79. Goel, B. G., Hanson, C. S., and Han, J.: A-V conduction in hyper- and hypothyroid dogs. Am. Heart J. *83*:504, 1972.
80. Miller, R. H., Corcoran, F. H., and Baker, W. P.: Second and third degree atrioventricular block with Graves' disease: A case report and review of the literature. PACE *3*:702, 1980.
81. Benker, V. G., Preiss, H., and Kreuser, H.: EKG—Veranderungen Hyperthyreose. Untersuchungen an 542 Patienten. Z. Kardiol. *63*:799, 1974.
82. Shapiro, S., Steier, M., and Dimich, I.: Congestive heart failure in neonatal thyrotoxicosis. A curable cause of heart failure in the newborn. Clin. Pediatr. *14*:1155, 1975.
83. Forfar, J. C., Muir, A. L., Sawers, S. A., and Toft, A. D.: Abnormal left ventricular function in hyperthyroidism: Evidence for a possible reversible cardiomyopathy. N. Engl. J. Med. *307*:1165, 1982.
84. Channick, B. J., Adlin, E. V., Marks, A. D., Denenberg, B. S., McDonough, M. T., Chakko, C. S., and Spann, J. F.: Hyperthyroidism and mitral-valve prolapse. N. Engl. J. Med. *305*:497, 1981.
85. Doherty, J. E., and Perkins, W. H.: Digoxin metabolism in hypo- and hyperthyroidism. Studies with tritiated digoxin in thyroid disease. Ann. Intern. Med. *64*:489, 1966.
86. Morrow, D. H., Gaffney, T. E., and Braunwald, E.: Studies on digitalis. VIII. Effect of autonomic innervation and of myocardial catecholamine stores upon the cardiac action of ouabain. J. Pharmacol. Exp. Ther. *140*:236, 1963.
87. Forfar, J. C., Feek, C. M., Miller, H. C., and Toft, A. D.: Atrial fibrillation and isolated suppression of the pituitary-thyroid axis: Response to specific antithyroid therapy. Int. J. Cardiol. *1*:43, 1981.
88. Sandler, G., and Wilson, G. M.: The nature and prognosis of heart disease in thyrotoxicosis. A review of 150 patients treated with ^{131}I. Q. J. Med. *28*:347, 1959.
89. Nakazawa, H. K., Sakurai, K., Hamada, N., Momotani, N., and Ito, K.: Management of atrial fibrillation in the post-thyrotoxic state. Am. J. Med. *72*:903–906, 1982.
90. Staffurth, J. S., Gibberd, M. C., and Fui, S. T.: Arterial embolism in thyrotoxicosis with atrial fibrillation. Br. Med. J. *2*:688, 1977.
91. Ingbar, S. H.: The role of antiadrenergic agents in the management of thyrotoxicosis. Cardiovasc. Rev. Rep. *2*:683, 1981.
92. Grossman, W., Robin, N. I., Johnson, L. W., Brooks, H., Selenkow, H. A., and Dexter, L.: Effects of beta blockade on the peripheral manifestations of thyrotoxicosis. Ann. Intern. Med. *74*:875, 1971.
93. Whittemore, R., and Caddell, J. L.: Metabolic and nutritional diseases. *In* Moss, A., et al. (eds.): Heart Disease in Infants, Children and Adolescents. Baltimore, Williams and Wilkins, 1977, p. 887.
94. Skelton, C. L., and Sonnenblick, E. H.: Cardiovascular system in hypothyroidism. *In* Werner, S. C., and Ingbar, S. H. (eds.): The Thyroid. 2nd Ed. New York, Harper and Row, 1962, p. 873.
95. Kerber, R. E., and Sherman, B.: Echocardiographic evaluation of pericardial effusion in myxedema. Incidence and biochemical and clinical correlations. Circulation *52*:823, 1975.
96. Smolar, E. N., Rubin, J. E., Avramides, A., and Carter, A. C.: Cardiac tamponade in primary myxedema and review of the literature. Am. J. Med. Sci. *272*:345, 1976.
97. Khaleeli, A. A., and Memon, N.: Factors affecting resolution of pericardial effusions in primary hypothyroidism: A clinical, biochemical and echocardiographic study. Postgrad. Med. J. *58*:1073, 1982.
98. Vanhaelst, I., and Neve, P.: Coronary artery disease in hypothyroidism. Lancet *2*:800, 1967.
99. Aber, C. P., and Thompson, G. S.: Factors associated with cardiac enlargement in myxedema. Br. Heart J. *25*:421, 1963.
100. Fouron, J. C., Bourgin, J. H., Letarte, J., Dussault, J. H., Ducharme, G., and Davignon, A.: Cardiac dimensions and myocardial function of infants with congential hypothyroidism: An echocardiographic study. Br. Heart J. *47*:584, 1982.
101. Graettinger, J. S., Muenster, J. J., and Checchia, C.: A correlation of clinical and hemodynamic studies in patients with hypothyroidism. J. Clin. Invest. *37*:502, 1958.

102. Stewart, J. H., and Evans, W. F.: Peripheral blood flow in myxedema. Arch. Intern. Med. *69*:808, 1942.
103. Manns, J. J., Shepherd, A. M. M., Crooks, J., and Adamson, D. B.: Measurement of cardiac muscle relaxation in hypothyroidism. Br. Med. J. *1*:1366, 1976.
104. Hillis, W. S., Bremner, W. F., Lawrie, T. D. V., and Thomson, J. A.: Systolic time intervals in thyroid disease. Clin. Endocrinol. *4*:617, 1975.
105. Aber, C. P., and Thompson, G. S.: The heart in hypothyroidism. Am. Heart J. *68*:429, 1964.
106. McBrion, D. J., and Hindle, W.: Myxoedema and heart failure. Lancet *1*:1065, 1963.
107. Margolius, H. S., and Gaffney, T. E.: Effects of injected norepinephrine and sympathetic nerve stimulation in hypothyroid and hyperthyroid dogs. J. Pharmacol. Exp. Ther. *149*:329, 1965.
108. Levey, G. S., Skelton, C. L., and Epstein, S. E.: Decreased myocardial adenyl cyclase activity in hypothyroidism. J. Clin. Invest. *48*:2244, 1969.
109. Rovetto, M. J., Hjarmarson, A. C., and Morgan, H. E.: Hormonal control of cardiac myosin adenosine triphosphate in the rat. Circ. Res. *31*:397, 1972.
110. Steinberg, A. D.: Myxedema and coronary artery disease—a comparative autopsy study. Ann. Intern. Med. *68*:338, 1968.
111. Myasnikov, A. L., and Zaitzev, V. F.: The influence of thyroid hormones on cholesterol metabolism in experimental atherosclerosis in rabbits. J. Atheroscler. Res. *3*:295, 1963.
112. Vanhaelst, L., Neve, P., Chailly, P., and Bastenie, P. A.: Coronary-artery disease in hypothyroidism. Lancet *2*:800, 1967.
113. Karlsberg, R. P., Friscia, D. A., Aronow, W. S., and Sekhon, S. S.: Deleterious influence of hypothyroidism on evolving myocardial infarction in conscious dogs. J. Clin. Invest. *67*:1024, 1981.
114. Littman, D. S., Jeffers, W. A., and Rose, E.: The infrequency of myocardial infarction in patients with thyrotoxicosis. Am. J. Med. Sci. *233*:10, 1957.
115. Keating, F. R., Parkin, T. W., Selby, J. B., and Dickinson, L. S.: Treatment of heart disease associated with myxedema. Progr. Cardiovasc. Dis. *3*:364, 1960.
116. Griffiths, P. D.: Serum enzymes in diseases of the thyroid gland. J. Clin. Pathol. *18*:660, 1965.
117. Morrow, D. H., Gaffney, T. E., and Braunwald, E.: Studies on digitalis. VII. Influence of hyper- and hypothyroidism in the myocardial response to ouabain. J. Pharmacol. Exp. Ther. *140*:324, 1963.
118. Paino, T. D., Rogers, W. J., Baxley, W. A., and Russell, R. O.: Coronary arterial surgery in patients with incapacitating angina pectoris and myxedema. Am. J. Cardiol. *40*:226, 1977.
119. Hay, I. D., Duick, D. S., Vlietstra, R. E., Maloney, J. D., and Pluth, J. R.: Thyroxine therapy in hypothyroid patients undergoing coronary revascularization: A retrospective analysis. Ann. Intern. Med. *95*:456, 1981.
120. Kaplan, M. M., Larsen, P. R., Crantz, F. R., Dzau, V. J., and Rossing, T. H.: Prevalence of abnormal thyroid function test results in patients with acute medical illnesses. Am. J. Med. *72*:9, 1982.
121. Williams, G. H., and Dluhy, R. G.: Diseases of the adrenal cortex. *In* Thorn, G. W., Adams, R. D., Braunwald, E., Isselbacher, K. J., and Petersdorf, R. G. (eds.): Harrison's Principles of Internal Medicine, 10th ed. New York, McGraw-Hill Book Co., 1983 (in press).
122. Cushing, H.: The basophil adenomas of the pituitary body and their clinical manifestations (pituitary basophilism). Bull. Johns Hopkins Hosp. *50*:137, 1932.
123. Liddle, G. W.: Pathogenesis of glucocorticoid disorders. Am. J. Med. *53*:638, 1972.
124. Soffer, L. J., Iannaecone, A., and Gabrilove, J. L.: Cushing's syndrome (study of 50 patients). Am. J. Med. *45*:116, 1961.
125. Kalsner, S.: Mechanism of hydrocortisone potentiation of response to epinephrine and norepinephrine in rabbit aorta. Circ. Res. *24*:383, 1969.
126. Krakoff, L., Nicolis, G., and Amsel, B.: Pathogenesis of hypertension in Cushing's syndrome. Am. J. Med. *58*:216, 1975.
127. Liddle, C. W.: Tests of pituitary-adrenal suppressibility in the diagnosis of Cushing's syndrome. J. Clin. Endocrinol. *20*:1539, 1960.
128. Tyrrel, J. B., Brooks, R. M., Fitzgerald, P. A., Cofoid, P. B., Forsham, P. H., and Wilson, C. B.: Cushing's disease: Selective transsphenoidal resection of pituitary microadenomas. N. Engl. J. Med. *298*:753, 1978.
129. Conn, J. W.: Primary aldosteronism, a new clinical syndrome. J. Lab. Clin. Med. *45*:3, 1955.
130. Cain, J. P., Tuck, M. L., Williams, G. H., Dluhy, R. G., and Rosenoff, S. H.: The regulation of aldosterone secretion in primary aldosteronism. Am. J. Med. *53*:637, 1972.
131. Tuck, M. L., Williams, G. H., Cain, J. P., Sullivan, J. M., and Dluhy, R. G.: The relationship of age, diastolic blood pressure, and known duration of hypertension to the presence of low-renin essential hypertension. Am. J. Cardiol. *22*:637, 1973.
132. Rose, L. I., Underwood, R. H., Newmark, S. R., Kisch, E. S., and Williams, G. H.: Pathophysiology of spironolactone-induced gynecomastia. Ann. Intern. Med. *87*:398, 1977.
133. Bongiovanni, A. M., and Eberlein, W. R.: Disorders of adrenal steroid biogenesis. Recent Prog. Horm. Res. *23*:375, 1967.
134. Schambelan, M., Sebastian, A., and Biglieri, E. G.: Prevalence, pathogenesis and functional significance of aldosterone deficiency in hyperkalemic patients with chronic renal insufficiency. Kidney Int. *17*:89, 1980.
135. Alford, W. C., Meador, C. K., Mihalevich, J., Burrus, G. R., Glassford, D. M., Stoney, W. S., and Thomas, C. S.: Acute adrenal insufficiency following cardiac surgical procedures. J. Thorac. Cardiovasc. Surg. *78*:489, 1979.
136. Levine, R. J., and Landsberg, L.: Catecholamine and the adrenal medulla. *In* Bondy, P. K. (ed.): Duncan's Diseases of Metabolism. Philadelphia, W. B. Saunders Co., 1974, p. 1181.
137. Wurtman, R. J., and Axelrod, J.: Control of enzymatic synthesis of adrenaline in the adrenal medulla by adrenal cortical steroids. J. Biol. Chem. *241*:2301, 1966.
138. Goldsmith, R. E.: Polyendocrine syndromes and the heart. Primary Cardiol. *7*: 153, 1981.
139. DeLarue, N. C., Morrow, J. D., Kerr, J. H., and Colapinto, R. F.: Pheochromocytoma in the modern context. Can. J. Surg. *21*:387, 1978.
140. Sjoerdsma, A., Engelman, K., and Waldmann, T. A.: Pheochromocytoma: Current concepts of diagnosis and treatment. Ann. Intern. Med. *65*:1302,1966.
141. Levenson, J. A., Safar, M. E., London, G. M., and Simon, A. C.: Haemodynamics in patients with phaeochromocytoma. Clin. Sci. *58*:349, 1980.
142. Melmon, K. L.: The adrenals: Catecholamines and adrenal medulla. *In* Williams, R. H. (ed.): Textbook of Endocrinology. Philadelphia, W. B. Saunders Co., 1974, p. 283.
143. Cheng, T. O., and Bashour, T. T.: Striking electrocardiographic changes associated with pheochromocytoma. N. Engl. J. Med. *274*:1102, 1966.
144. Van Vliet, P. D., Burchell, H. B., and Titus, J. L.: Myocarditis associated with pheochromocytoma. N. Engl. J. Med. *274*:1102, 1966.
145. Cueto, L., Arriaga, J., and Zinser, J.: Echocardiographic changes in pheochromocytoma. Chest *76*:600, 1979.
146. McManus, B. M., Fleury, T. A., and Roberts, W. C.: Fatal catecholamine crisis in pheochromocytoma: Curable form of cardiac arrest. Am. Heart J. *102*:930, 1981.
147. Jones, D. H., Allison, D. J., Hamilton, C. A., and Reid, J. L.: Selective venous sampling in the diagnosis and localization of phaeochromocytoma. Clin. Endocrinol. *10*:179, 1979.
148. Bravo, E. L., Tarazi, R. C., Gifford, R. W., and Stewart, B. H.: Circulating and urinary catecholamines in pheochromocytoma: Diagnostic and pathophysiologic implications. N. Engl. J. Med. *301*:682, 1979.
149. Zweifler, A. J., and Julius, S.: Increased platelet catecholamine content in pheochromocytoma: A diagnostic test in patients with elevated plasma catecholamines. N. Engl. J. Med. *306*:890, 1982.
150. Bravo, E. L., Tarazi, R. C., Fouad, F. M., Vidt, D. G., and Gifford, Jr., R. W.: Clonidine-suppression test: A useful aid in the diagnosis of pheochromocytoma. N. Engl. J. Med. *305*:623, 1981.
151. Crago, R. M., Eckholdt, J. W., and Wiswell, J. G.: Pheochromocytoma: Treatment with alpha and beta adrenergic blocking drugs. J.A.M.A. *202*:870, 1967.
152. Sisson, J. C., Frager, M. S., Valk, T. W., Gross, M. D., Swanson, D. P., Wieland, D. M., Tobes, M. C., Beierwaltes, W. H., and Thompson, N. W.: Scintigraphic localization of pheochromocytoma. N. Engl. J. Med. *305*:12,1981.
153. Hengstmann, J. H., Gugler, R., and Dengler, H. J.: Malignant pheochromocytoma. Effect of oral α-methyl-p-tyrosine upon catecholamine metabolism. Klin. Wochenschr. *57*:351, 1979.
154. Keutmann, H. T., Dawson, B. F., and Aurbach, G. D.: Structure, synthesis, and mechanism of action of parathyroid hormone. Recent Prog. Horm. Res. *28*:353, 1972.
155. Rasmussen, H., and Wong, M.: Hormonal control of the renal conversion of 25-hydroxycholecalciferol to 1,25-dihydroxycholecalciferol. J. Clin. Invest. *51*: 2502, 1972.
156. Habener, J. F., and Potts, J. T.: Parathyroid physiology and primary hyperparathyroidism . *In* Avioli, L. V., and Krane, S. M. (eds.): Metabolic Bone Disease. Vol. 2. New York, Academic Press, 1978.
157. Bogin, E., Massry, S. G., and Harary, I.: Effect of parathyroid hormone on rat heart cells. J. Clin. Invest. *67*:1215, 1981.
158. Katoh, Y., Klein, K. L., Kaplan, R. A., Sanborn, W. G., and Kurokawa, K.: Parathyroid hormone has a positive inotropic action in the rat. Endocrinology *109*:2252, 1981.
159. Palmieri, G. M., Nutting, D. F., Bhattacharya, S. K., Bertorini, T. E., and Williams, J. C.: Parathyroid ablation in dystrophic hamsters: Effects of Ca content and histology of heart, diaphragm, and rectus femoris. J. Clin. Invest. *68*:646, 1981.
160. Giles, T. D., Iteld, B. J., and Rires, K. L.: The cardiomyopathy of hypoparathyroidism. Chest *79*:225, 1981.
161. Roberts, W. C., and Waller, B. F.: Effect of chronic hypercalcemia on the heart: An analysis of 18 necropsy patients. Am. J. Med. *71*:371, 1981.
162. Surawicz, B.: Relationship between electrocardiogram and electrolytes. Am. Heart J. *73*:814, 1967.
163. Kleerekoper, M., Rao, D. S., and Frame, B.: Hypercalcemia, hyperparathyroidism and hypertension. Cardiovasc. Med. *3*:1283, 1978.
164. Christensson, T., Hellstrom, K., and Wengle, B.: Blood pressure in subjects with hypercalcemia and primary hyperparathyroidism detected in a health screening program. Eur. J. Clin. Invest. *7*:109, 1977.
165. Weidmann, P., Massry, S. G., and Coburn, J. W.: Blood pressure effects of acute hypercalcemia. Ann. Intern. Med. *76*:741, 1972.
166. Sialer, S., McKenna, D. H., Corliss, R. J., et al.: Systemic and coronary hemodynamic effects of intravenous administration of calcium chloride. Arch. Int. Pharmacodyn. *169*:177, 1967.
167. Resnick, L. M.: Calcium, parathyroid disease, and hypertension. Cardiovasc. Rev. Rep. *3*:1341, 1982.
168. Grodsky, G. M., Curry, D. L., Landahl, H., and Bennett, L.: Further studies on the dynamic aspects of insulin release in vitro with evidence for a two-compartmental storage system. Acta Diabetol. Lat. *1* (Suppl.):554, 1969.
169. Cerasi, E.: An analogue computer model for the insulin response to glucose infusion. Acta Endocrinol. (Kbh.)*55*:163, 1967.
170. Cahill, G. F., Jr.: Physiology of insulin in man. Diabetes *20*:785, 1971.

171. Rimoin, D. L.: Inheritance in diabetes mellitus. Med. Clin. North Am. *55*:807, 1971.
172. Waller, B. F., Palumbo, P. J., Lie, J. T., and Roberts, W. C.: Status of the coronary arteries at necropsy in diabetes mellitus with onset after age 30 years: Analysis of 229 diabetic patients with and without clinical evidence of coronary heart disease and comparison to 183 control subjects. Am. J. Med. *69*: 498, 1980.
173. Yano, K., Kagan, A., McGee, D., and Rhoads, G. G.: Glucose intolerance and nine-year mortality in Japanese men in Hawaii. Am. J. Med. *72*:71, 1982.
174. Zoneraich, S.: Diabetes and the Heart. Springfield, Ill., Charles C. Thomas, 1978, p. 303.
175. Factor, S. M., Okun, E. M., and Minase, T.: Capillary microaneurysms in the human heart. N. Engl. J. Med. *302*:384, 1980.
176. Bryfogle, J. W., and Bradley, R. F.: The vascular complications of diabetes mellitus. A clinical study. Diabetes *6*:159, 1957.
177. Harrower, A. D. B., and Clarke, B. F.: Experience of coronary care in diabetes. Br. Med. J. *1*:126, 1976.
178. Oliver, M. F.: Metabolic response during impending myocardial infarction. II. Clinical implications. Circulation *42*:981, 1970.
179. Oliver, M. F., Rowe, M. J., Luxton, M. R., Miller, N. E., and Neilson, J. M.: Effect of reducing circulating free fatty acids on ventricular arrhythmias during myocardial infarction and on ST-segment depression during exercise-induced ischemia. *In* Braunwald, E. (ed.): Protection of the Ischemic Myocardium. American Heart Association Monograph No. 48, 1976, p. 210.
180. Opie, L. H., Tansey, M. J., and Kennelly, B. M.: The heart in diabetes melli-tus. Acute myocardial infarction and diabetes. II. S. Afr. Med. J. *56*:256, 1979.
181. Beard, O. W., Hipp, H. R., Robins, M., and Verzolini, V. R.: Survival in myocardial infarction. Am. Heart J. *73*:317, 1967.
182. Smith, S. E., Smith, S. A., and Brown, P. M.: Cardiac autonomic dysfunction in patients with diabetic retinopathy. Diabetologia *21*:525, 1981.
183. Pfeifer, M. A., Cook, D., Brodsky, J., Tice, D., Reenan, A., Swedine, S., Halter, J. B., and Porte, J. R.: Quantitative evaluation of cardiac parasympathetic activity in normal and diabetic man. Diabetes *31*:339, 1982.
184. Lloyd-Mostyn, R. H., and Watkins, P. J.: Total cardiac denervation in diabetic autonomic neuropathy. Diabetes *25*:748, 1976.
184a. Vered, Z., Battler, A., Segal, P., Liberman, D., Yerushalmi, Y., Berezlin, M., and Neufeld, H. N.: Exercise induced left ventricular dysfunction in young asymptomatic male diabetic patients. A diabetic cardiomyopathy. J. Am. Coll. Cardiol. *1*:723, 1983.
185. Kannel, W. B., Hjortland, M., and Castelli, W. P.: The role of diabetes in congestive heart failure: the Framingham study. Am. J. Cardiol. *34*:29, 1974.
186. Hamby, R. I., Zoneraich, S., and Sherman, L.: Diabetic cardiomyopathy. J.A.M.A. *229*:1749, 1974.
187. Regan, T. J., Lyons, M. M., Ahmed, S. S., Levinson, G. E., Oldewurtel, H. A., Ahman, M. R., and Haider, B.: Evidence for cardiomyopathy in familial diabetes mellitus. J. Clin. Invest. *60*:885, 1977.
188. Ahmed, S. S., Jaferi, G. A., Narang, R. M., and Regan, T. J.: Preclinical abnormality of left ventricular function in diabetes mellitus. Am. Heart J. *89*: 153, 1975.
189. Seneviratne, B. I. B.: Diabetic cardiomyopathy: The preclinical phase. Br. Med. J. *1*:1444, 1977.
190. A. D'Elia, J. A., Weinrauch, L. A., Healy, R. W., Libertino, T. A., Bradley, R. F., and Leland, O. S.: Myocardial dysfunction without coronary artery disease in diabetic renal failure. Am. J. Cardiol. *43*:193, 1979.
191. Shapiro, L. M., Howat, A. P., and Calter, M. M.: Left ventricular function in diabetes mellitus. I: Methodology, and prevalence and spectrum of abnormalities. Br. Heart J. *45*:122, 1981.
192. Shapiro, L. M.: Echocardiographic features of impaired ventricular function in diabetes mellitus. Br. Heart J. *47*:439, 1982.
193. Factor, S. M., Minase, T., and Sonnenblick, E. H.: Clinical and morphological features of human hypertensive-diabetic cardiomyopathy. Am. Heart J. *99*:446, 1980.
194. Regan, T. J., Ettinger, P. O., Khan, M. I., Jesrani, M. U., Lyons, M. M., Oldewurtel, H. A., and Weber, M.: Altered myocardial function and metabolism in chronic diabetes mellitus without ischemia in dogs. Circ. Res. *35*:222, 1974.
195. Regan, T. J., Wu, C. F., Yeh, C. K., Oldewurtel, H. A., and Haider, B.: Myocardial composition and function in diabetes: The effects of chronic insulin use. Circ. Res. *49*:1268, 1981.
196. Malhotra, A., Penpargkul, S., Fein, F. S., Sonnenblick, E. H., and Scheuer, J.: The effect of streptozotocin-induced diabetes in rats on cardiac contractile proteins. Circ. Res. *49*:1243, 1981.
197. Fein, F. S., Strobeck, J. E., Malhotra, A., Scheuer, J., and Sonnenblick, E. H.: Reversibility of diabetic cardiomyopathy with insulin in rats. Circ. Res. *49*:1251, 1981.
198. Regan, T. J., Levinson, G. E., Oldewurtel, H. A., Frank, M. J., Weisse, A. B., and Moschos, C. B.: Ventricular function in noncardiacs with alcohol fatty liver. The role of ethanol in the production of cardiomyopathy. J. Clin. Invest. *48*:397, 1969.
199. Regan, T. J., Wu, C. F., Weisse, A. B., Moschos, C. B., Haider, B., Ahmed, S. S., and Lyons, M. M.: Acute myocardial infarction in toxic cardiomyopathy without coronary obstruction. Circulation *51*:453, 1975.
200. Wolfe, R. R., and Way, G. L.: Cardiomyopathies in infants of diabetic mothers. Johns Hopkins Med. J. *140*:177, 1977.
201. Gabbay, K. H., and O'Sullivan, J. B.: The sorbitol pathway. Enzyme localization and content in normal and diabetic nerve and cord. Diabetes *17*:239, 1968.
202. University Group Diabetes Program: A study of the effect of hypoglycemic agents on vascular complications in patients with adult-onset diabetes. Diabetes *19* (Suppl. II):474, 1970.
203. University Group Diabetes Program: A study of the effects of hypoglycemic agents on vascular complications in patients with adult-onset diabetes. V. Evaluation of phenformin therapy. Diabetes *24*(Suppl. I):65, 1975.
204. Wu, C. F., Haider, B., Ahmed, S. S., Oldewurtel, H. A., Lyons, M. M., and Regan, T. J.: The effects of tolbutamide on the myocardium in experimental diabetes. Circulation *55*:200, 1977.
205. Axelrod, L.: Response of congestive heart failure to correction of hyperglycemia in the presence of diabetic nephropathy. N. Engl. J. Med. *293*:1243, 1975.
206. Salans, L. B.: Obesity and the adipose cell. *In* Bondy, P. K., and Rosenberg, L. E. (eds.): Metabolic Control and Disease. 9th ed. Philadelphia, W. B. Saunders Co., 1980, p. 510.
207. Hirsch, J., and Knittle, J.: Cell lipid content and cell number in obese and nonobese human adipose tissue. J. Clin. Invest. *45*:1023, 1966.
208. Hirsch, J., and Knittle, J. L.: Cellularity of obese and nonobese human adipose tissue. Fed. Proc. *29*:1516, 1970.
208a. Messerli, F. H., Sundgaard-Riise, K., Reisin, E., Dreslinski, G., Dunn, F. G., and Frohlich, E.: Disparate cardiovascular effects of obesity and arterial hypertension. Am. J. Med. *74*:808, 1983.
209. Smith, H. L., and Willius, R. A.: Adiposity of the heart. A clinical and pathologic study of one hundred and thirty-six obese patients. Arch. Intern. Med. *52*:911, 1933.
210. Kaltman, A. J., and Goldring, R. M.: Role of circulatory congestion in the cardiorespiratory failure of obesity. Am. J. Med. *60*:645, 1976.
211. De Divitiis, O., Fazio, S., Petitto, M., Maddalena, G., Contaldo, F., and Mancini, M.: Obesity and cardiac function. Circulation *64*:477, 1981.
212. Messerli, F. H., Ventura, H. O., Reisin, E., Dreslinski, G. R., Dunn, F. G., MacPhee, A. A., and Frohlich, E. D.: Borderline hypertension and obesity: Two prehypertensive states with elevated cardiac output. Circulation *66*:55, 1982.
212a. Ventura, H. O., Messerli, F. H., Dunn, F. G., and Frohlich, E. D.: Left ventricular hypertrophy in obesity: Discrepancy between echo and electrocardiogram. J. Am. Coll. Cardiol. *1*:682, 1983.
213. Amad, K. H., Brennan, J. C., and Alexander, J. K.: The cardiac pathology of chronic exogeneous obesity. Circulation *32*:740, 1965.
214. Alexander, J. K., and Peterson, K. L.: Cardiovascular effects of weight reduction. Circulation *40*:310, 1972.
215. Backman, L., Freyschuss, U., Hallberg, D., and Melcher, A.: Reversibility of cardiovascular changes in extreme obesity: Effects of weight reduction through jejunoileostomy. Acta Med. Scand. *205*:367, 1979.
216. Abel, R. M., Grimes, J. B., Alonso, D., Alonso, M., and Gay, W. A., Jr.: Adverse hemodynamic and ultrastructural changes in dog hearts subjected to protein-calorie malnutrition. Am. Heart J. *97*:733, 1979.
217. Nutter, D. O., Murray, T. G., Heymsfield, S. T., and Fuller, E. O.: The effect of chronic protein-calorie undernutrition in the rat on myocardial function and cardiac function. Cir. Res. *45*:144, 1979.
218. Gillanders, A. D.: Nutritional heart disease. Br. Heart J. *13*:177, 1951.
219. Abel, R. M., Fischer, J. E., Buckley, M. J., Barnett, G. O., and Austen, W. G.: Malnutrition in cardiac surgical patients. Arch. Surg. *111*:45, 1976.
220. Blackburn, G. L., Gibbons, G. W., Bothe, A., Benotti, P. N., Harken, D. E., and McEnany, T. M.: Nutritional support in cardiac cachexia. J. Thorac. Cardiovasc. Surg. *73*:489, 1977.
221. Steier, M., Lopez, R., and Cooperman, J. M.: Riboflavin deficiency in infants and children with heart disease. Am. Heart J. *92*:139, 1976.
222. McGill, Jr., H. C., Anselmo, V. C., Buchanan, J. M., and Sheridan, P. J.: The heart is a target organ for androgen. Science *207*:775, 1980.
223. Barrett-Connor, E., Brown, W. V., Turner, J., Austin, M., and Criqui, M. H.: Heart disease risk factors and hormone use in postmenopausal women. J.A.M.A. *241*:2167, 1979.
224. Wallace, R. B., Hoover, J., Barrett-Conner, E., Rifkind, B. M., Hunninghake, D. B., MacKenthun, A., and Heiss, G.: Altered plasma lipid and lipo-protein levels associated with oral contraceptive and estrogen use. Lancet *2*:112, 1979.
225. Ross, R. K., Paganini-Hill, A., Mack, T. M., and Arthur, M., and Henderson, B. E.: Menopausal oestrogen therapy and protection from death from ischaemic heart disease. Lancet *1*:858, 1981.
226. Ritterband, A. B., Jaffee, I. A., and Densen, P. M.: Gonadal function and the development of coronary heart disease. Circulation *27*:237, 1963.
227. The Coronary Drug Project: Initial findings leading to modifications of its research protocol. J.A.M.A. *214*:1303, 1970.
228. Webber, L. S., Hunter, S. M., Baugh, J. G., Srinivasan, S. R., Sklov, M. C., and Berenson, G. S.: The interaction of cigarette smoking, oral contraceptive use, and cardiovascular risk factor variables in children: The Bogalusa Heart Study. Am. J. Publ. Health *72*:266, 1982.
229. Jaffe, M. D.: Effect of oestrogens on postexercise electrocardiogram. Br. Heart J. *38*:1299, 1976.
230. Gutai, J., LaPorte, R., Kuller, L., Dai, W., Falvo-Gerard, L., and Caggiula, A.: Plasma testosterone, high density lipoprotein cholesterol and other lipoprotein fractions. Am. J. Cardiol. *48*:897, 1981.
231. Wood, J. E.: The cardiovascular effects of oral contraceptives. Mod. Concepts Cardiovasc. Dis. *41*:37, 1972.
232. Boyd, W. N., Burden, R. P., and Aber, G. M.: Intrarenal vascular changes in patients receiving estrogen-containing compounds—A clinical, histological and angiographic study. Q. J. Med. *44*:415, 1975.
233. Hollenberg, N. K., Williams, G. H., Burger, B., Chenitz, W., Hooshmand, I., and Adams, D. F.: Renal blood flow and its response to A II: An interaction between oral contraceptive agents, sodium intake and the renin-angiotensin system in healthy young women. Circ. Res. *38*:35, 1976.

52 RENAL DISORDERS AND HEART DISEASE

by Eugene Braunwald, M.D., and Michael N. Gottlieb, M.D.

There is an intimate relation between disorders of the heart and of the kidneys. Some of the principal clinical manifestations of impairment of the heart's performance as a pump result from the renal retention of sodium and water; a number of diseases of the heart, such as infective endocarditis and cardiogenic shock, may result in serious renal disease. Conversely, chronic renal failure frequently results in hypertension and lipid abnormalities, which often lead to accelerated atherosclerosis so that coronary artery disease is a common cause of death in patients being treated for chronic renal insufficiency. Also, uremia may result in pericarditis and thereby lead to cardiac tamponade or constrictive pericarditis; renal failure may also cause secondary hyperparathyroidism, which can produce cardiac calcification with a variety of disturbances of cardiac function.

EFFECTS OF CARDIAC DISEASE ON RENAL FUNCTION

Changes in Renal Function and Electrolyte Balance in Heart Failure

The pathophysiology of congestive heart failure is described in Chapters 13 and 15; and the use of diuretics in treating heart failure is discussed in Chapter 16; the alterations in renal function are reviewed here. J. P. Peters at Yale is credited with the concept that the kidney in heart failure is physiologically similar to the kidney in hypovolemia, both states a consequence of inadequate cardiac output. Retention of salt and water occurs in an attempt to restore the effective arterial blood volume, an as yet poorly defined parameter of the filling of the arterial tree, related in some manner to the ratio of the arterial blood volume to the capacity of the vascular bed.

Modulation of the tubular transport of sodium provides the most important mechanism for regulation of sodium excretion. The proximal tubule is the primary site for sodium reabsorption in the nephron, with approximately 60 per cent of filtered sodium being reabsorbed isotonically at this site. As shown in Figure 52–1, blood enters the nephron at the afferent arteriole, passes through the glomerulus to the efferent arteriole, and moves on to a network of peritubular capillaries. The current concepts of the forces governing the proximal tubular reabsorption of sodium in the normal state and in heart failure are shown in Figure 52–2. As cardiac output falls, several stimuli—including augmented alpha-adrenergic neural activity, circulating catecholamines, and increased circulating and locally produced angiotensin II—cause renal vasoconstriction, particularly of the efferent arterioles (Fig. 52–3). As a consequence, the glomerular filtration rate declines, but there is a proportionately greater fall in renal blood flow, and, therefore, filtration fraction—i.e., the ratio of glomerular filtration rate to renal blood flow—rises. This results in an elevation of the protein concentration in the peritubular capillaries and a decline in the postglomerular capillary hydrostatic pressure; thus, the transcapillary hydraulic pressure gradient falls.

The combination of these two events, i.e., the reduction of peritubular capillary hydrostatic pressure and an elevation of peritubular oncotic pressure, enhances the peritubular capillary uptake of proximal tubular fluid and thereby increases the absolute quantity of sodium reabsorbed by the proximal tubule.[1,2] An additional proposed mechanism for sodium retention in heart failure is the redistribution of blood flow from cortical to juxtamedullary nephrons that have longer loops of Henle and that, therefore, are capable of greater sodium reabsorption.

In addition to the more avid sodium reabsorption in the proximal convoluted tubule, increased sodium reabsorption also occurs in distal nephron sites, including the collecting duct segments. This results from the operation of Starling forces, i.e., a lowering of capillary hydrostatic pressure and an elevation of oncotic pressure, such as those described for the proximal tubule; in addition, the action of aldosterone, whose sodium reabsorption action is limited to the

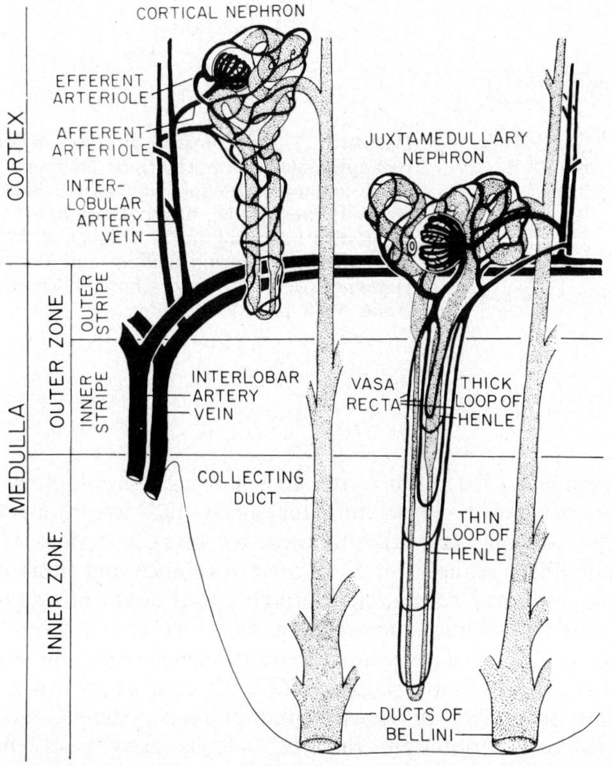

FIGURE 52–1 **Anatomy of the kidney, emphasizing comparison of the blood supplies of cortical and juxtamedullary nephrons. (Reproduced with permission from Pitts, R. F.: Physiology of the Kidney and Body Fluids. 3rd ed. Copyright 1974 by Year Book Medical Publishers, Inc., Chicago.)**

terminal segment of the nephron, the distal tubule, and the collecting duct system, has been recognized as an important factor in the sodium retention associated with congestive heart failure. The absolute concentration of circulating aldosterone is increased in some patients with congestive heart failure because of a combination of the stimulation of production by the renin-angiotensin axis and the diminished metabolism of aldosterone. In acute heart failure, decreased renal perfusion (whether caused by a reduction in total cardiac output or by a decrease in the renal fraction of the cardiac output) activates the juxtaglomerular apparatus to enhance renin release, which in turn augments the generation of angiotensin II, the stimulus for aldosterone secretion and thus for retention of sodium[3] (Figure 26–21, p. 868). Angiotensin II, both circulating and locally produced, also plays a role in the constriction of efferent arterioles and the resultant elevation in the filtration fraction, discussed above. Indeed, the administration of angiotensin II–converting enzy me inhibitor in heart failure markedly increases renal blood flow and glomerular filtration with return of filtration fraction toward normal and usually induces a natriuresis. The impairment in aldosterone biodegradation that sometimes occurs in heart failure is consequent to hepatic congestion, as well as reduced splanchnic blood flow secondary to reduced cardiac output and splanchnic vasoconstriction.[4]

The renal retention of sodium expands extracellular fluid volume and tends to return the renin-angiotensin-aldosterone system toward normal. For that reason, circulating angiotensin II and aldosterone concentrations are frequently normal in chronic stable heart failure, although they tend to be high relative to the expanded extracellular fluid volume (Figs. 52–4 and 52–5). In terminal heart failure, however, with further impairment of renal perfusion, the production of renin is again enhanced, despite the expansion of extracellular fluid volume.

The role of other vasoactive substances, such as prostaglandins, kallikreins, and kinins, has yet to be determined, but they have also been implicated as factors in sodium balance.[5,6] Intrarenal prostaglandins act to oppose the actions of angiotensin II on the renal vascular bed.[7] In heart failure, infusion of prostaglandin A_2 may enhance sodium excretion,[8] whereas inhibition of prostaglandin synthesis by means of prostaglandin synthesis inhibitors such as indomethacin may enhance arteriolar resistance, depress glomerular filtration rate, and increase sodium retention.[9]

The mechanisms for *water retention* in congestive heart failure are outlined in Figure 52–6. Enhanced proximal reabsorption, together with a decline in glomerular filtration rate, results in a fall in the delivery of tubular fluid to the diluting segments of the nephron;[10] in addition, with a reduction in renal blood flow, renal medullary blood flow is diminished, which also results in a decreased capacity of the nephron to excrete water.[1] The lowered effective arteri-

FIGURE 52–2 **Peritubular control of proximal tubule fluid reabsorption. Current concept of the role of peritubular capillary physical forces in the regulation of proximal tubule fluid reabsorption in the normal state (*left*) and in the patient with congestive heart failure (*right*). ΔP and Δπ are, respectively, the transcapillary hydraulic and oncotic pressure differences operating across the peritubular capillary. The increase in filtration fraction causes Δπ to rise in heart failure. The increase in renal vascular resistance in CHF is thought to reduce ΔP. Both the increase in Δπ and the fall in ΔP serve to enhance peritubular capillary uptake of proximal reabsorbate and thus increase absolute sodium reabsorption by the proximal tubule. (From Humes, H. D., et al.: The kidney in congestive heart failure. *In* Brenner, B. M., and Stein, J. H. [eds.]: Sodium and Water Homeostasis. New York, Churchill Livingstone, 1978, p. 51.)**

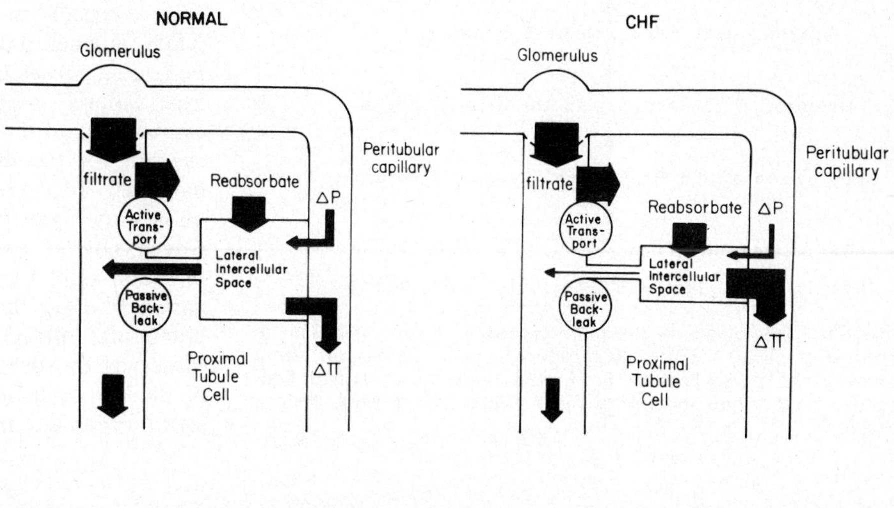

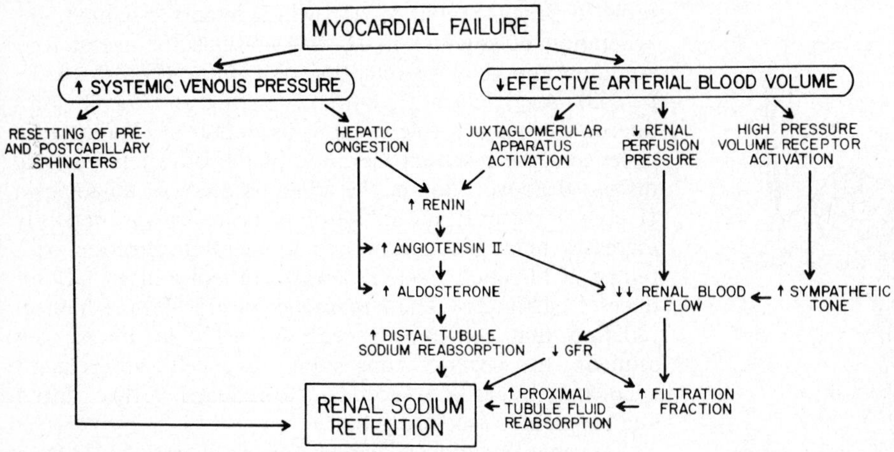

FIGURE 52-3 Summary of the major pathophysiological mechanisms leading to renal sodium retention in heart failure. (From Humes, H. D., et al.: The kidney in congestive heart failure. *In* Brenner, B. M., and Stein, J. H. [eds.]: Sodium and Water Homeostasis. New York, Churchill Livingstone, 1978, p. 51.)

al blood volume serves as a nonosmotic stimulus to enhanced release of antidiuretic hormone, which favors water retention. Furthermore, heart failure stimulates the sensation of thirst;[11] angiotensin II, acting centrally, may also be responsible for stimulating the thirst mechanism.[12] A number of nonosmotic stimuli for release of antidiuretic hormone (ADH), such as discomfort, anxiety, beta-adrenergic agonists, and central nervous system depressants, including barbiturates and narcotics, are commonly present in congestive heart failure. There is a high incidence of inappropriately elevated ADH secretion, which plays an important role in the dilutional hypoosmolality present in many patients with heart failure.[13,14]

The elevated peripheral venous pressure characteristic of heart failure also causes a reflex resetting of pre- and postcapillary resistance in the systemic vascular bed, so that the transudation of fluid into the interstitial space is favored,[15] which tends to lower blood volume and thereby enhances sodium retention. Elevated systemic venous pressure transmitted to the ostium of the thoracic duct impedes lymphatic drainage, enhancing the formation of edema and decreasing intravascular volume. In short-term experiments, distention of the atria activates receptors that may be considered to monitor atrial and intrathoracic blood volume. Activation of these receptors and vagal afferent fibers reduces renal vascular resistance and inhibits the secretion of antidiuretic hormone, thus augmenting the excretion of sodium and water (p. 462).[16] However, a resetting of the atrial pressure receptors occurs with chronic cardiac failure and atrial distention. In animals with heart failure secondary to experimental pulmonic stenosis and tricuspid regurgitation, the spontaneous activity of the atrial receptors was found to be depressed,[17,18] and in dogs with heart failure caused by an aortocaval fistula, the water diuretic response to left atrial distention is blunted.[19] This attenuated sensitivity of venous and atrial pressure receptors may be responsible for reduced renal vasodilatation (i.e., a higher renal vascular resistance), which, in turn, contributes to salt and water retention in heart failure by mitigating the diuresis and natriuresis that would otherwise accompany the volume expansion and atrial distention characteristic of heart failure.

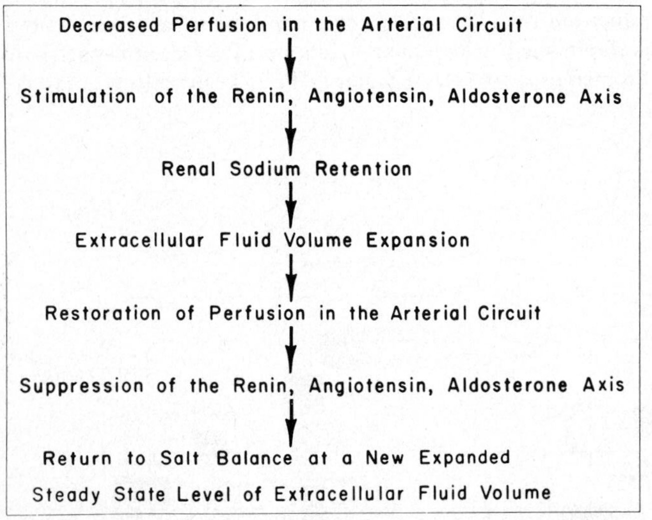

FIGURE 52-4 Stages in the pathogenesis of sodium retention in congestive heart failure. (Reproduced with permission from Skorecki, K. L., and Brenner, B. M.: Body fluid homeostasis in congestive heart failure and cirrhosis with ascites. Am. J. Med. *72*:323, 1982.)

Total body *sodium* is uniformly elevated in edematous patients with congestive heart failure[20] and total body water is usually increased to an even greater extent. The serum concentration is thus usually slightly reduced in heart failure; in some patients with severe heart failure, it is greatly reduced. Furthermore, sodium may become osmotically inactivated in edema,[21] perhaps by binding to chondroitin sulfate[22] as well as to other polyelectrolytes.

PRERENAL AZOTEMIA IN HEART FAILURE. Azotemia is a common finding in severe congestive heart failure.[23] The enhanced water reabsorption in the collecting duct, especially in the presence of inappropriately elevated ADH, augments the passive reabsorption of urea. In addition, urea production may be enhanced in some forms of heart failure[24]—especially in acute myocardial infarction; a catabolic state induced by the stress of heart failure may account for the increased urea load. The combination of increased urea production and decreased excretion (secondary to augmented reabsorption) elevates blood urea nitrogen (BUN) even prior to a reduction of glomerular filtration rate. However, the principal mechanism for elevation of BUN and serum creatinine is reduction of the glomerular filtration rate. As already noted, the latter is preserved by efferent arteriolar constriction in the presence of modest reductions in renal plasma flow, and therefore serum creatinine may remain normal until, in severe heart

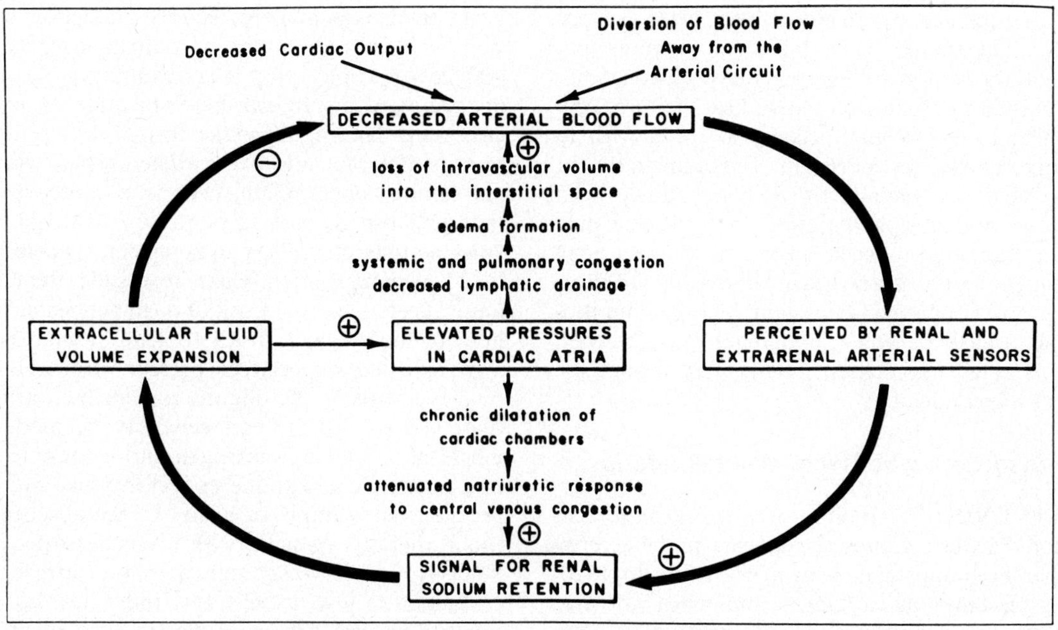

FIGURE 52–5 Sensing mechanisms that initiate and maintain renal sodium retention in congestive heart failure. (Reproduced with permission from Skorecki, K. L., and Brenner, B. M.: Body fluid homeostasis in congestive heart failure and cirrhosis with ascites. Am. J. Med. *72*:323, 1982.)

failure, there are marked reductions in renal plasma flow, constriction of afferent arterioles, and reduction of glomerular filtration rate. Thus, an elevation of serum creatinine is usually a sign of advanced heart failure. It is not uncommon in heart failure for the BUN/creatinine ratio to exceed 10 to 1. In severe heart failure, when glomerular filtration rate declines, the BUN may exceed 100 mg/dl and the serum creatinine, 4 mg/dl.

Prerenal azotemia of this degree is a poor prognostic sign in heart failure. Treatment should be directed at improvement of cardiac function, as outlined in Chapter 16.

HEART FAILURE IN PATIENTS WITH RENAL DISEASE. The improved therapy of heart failure (Chap. 16) has prolonged the life of many patients with the combination of cardiac failure and chronic renal disease. In many such patients, the intrinsic renal disease is not severe enough to cause salt, water, or nitrogen retention in the presence of a normal cardiac output. However, when heart failure and the attendant alterations in renal hemodynamics described above are superimposed on intrinsic renal disease, serious problems in salt, water, and nitrogen retention readily occur. Hemodialysis with ultrafiltration or peritoneal dialysis can be effective in the management of this combination of disorders.

POTASSIUM BALANCE IN HEART FAILURE. Mild hypokalemia is a relatively common finding in patients with congestive heart failure, as a consequence of the distal tubular exchange of sodium for potassium and hydrogen under the influence of excess aldosterone. In addition, since all of the major diuretics (other than spironolactone, triamterene, and amiloride) inhibit sodium chloride reabsorption proximal to the site of action of aldosterone in the distal tubule, they increase the delivery of sodium to the distal tubule, enhancing the likelihood of the exchange of sodium for hydrogen and potassium (p. 531). Therefore, serum potassium should be monitored in patients with congestive heart failure to ascertain the need for potassium replacement therapy. Since potassium excretion is aug-

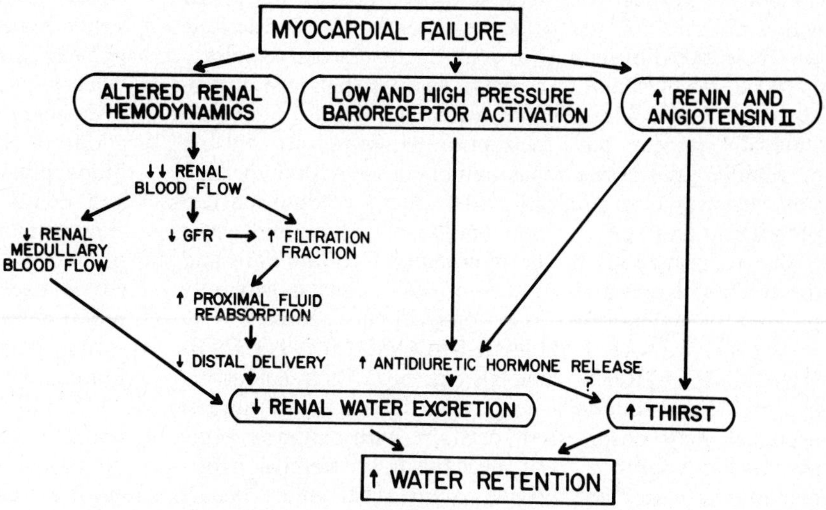

FIGURE 52–6 Summary of the major pathophysiological mechanisms leading to water retention in congestive heart failure. (From Humes, H. D., et al.: The kidney in congestive heart failure. *In* Brenner, B. M., and Stein, J. H. [eds.]: Sodium and Water Homeostasis. New York, Churchill Livingstone, 1978, p. 51.)

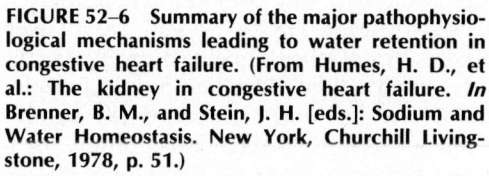

mented and accompanied by alkalosis, any necessary potassium replacement should be in the form of potassium chloride rather than potassium bicarbonate or gluconate.

In the end stage of chronic congestive heart failure, prerenal azotemia and oliguria may become severe enough to limit the ability to excrete potassium. Fundamentally, at this stage the delivery of sodium to the distal tubule is so low, even in the presence of diuretics, that its exchange with potassium becomes reduced and hyperkalemia may develop. In patients with severe heart failure and progressive azotemia and oliguria, potassium-sparing diuretics (spironolactone, amiloride, and triamterene) must be used with caution, if at all, since these agents may hasten the development of hyperkalemia.

Cardiac Disorders with Renal Manifestations

INFECTIVE ENDOCARDITIS (see also Chap. 33.) The association between glomerulonephritis and bacterial endocarditis has been appreciated for many years. In 1920, prior to the availability of antibiotics and when infective endocarditis was uniformly fatal, 11 per cent of patients with this infection ultimately died of renal failure.[25] It was initially thought that the glomerular lesion was secondary to septic embolization to the kidneys from infected valvular vegetations, but little firm evidence supports this theory. Instead, the pathogenesis of the renal lesions appears to be more in keeping with the generally accepted pathogenesis of most types of glomerulonephritis.[26] Soluble antigenic components of the infecting organism and antibody directed against these antigens have been demonstrated in the glomeruli.[27] As indicated in Chapter 33, many organisms have been responsible for the infective endocarditis that may be associated with glomerulonephritis. By immunofluorescence, the presence of immune complexes and the third component of complement (C3) can be demonstrated in the glomeruli of patients with endocarditis and glomerulonephritis;[27] early in the course, there is a decline in the serum level of C3 and of another component of the complement system, C1q. It now appears that the glomerular lesion of endocarditis results from the deposition of immune complexes along the glomerular basement membrane and in the mesangium.

The most commonly observed abnormality by light microscopy is a focal, proliferative glomerulonephritis, often with focal fibrinoid necrosis. Less commonly, the lesions may be more diffuse, and in some instances extracapillary epithelial proliferation (crescents), such as that seen in rapidly progressive glomerulonephritis, has been observed.[27] Clinically, patients have the typical manifestations of acute or rapidly progressive renal failure, often with hypertension, hematuria, and red cell casts, usually without marked proteinuria and edema. The retention of sodium and water is due to reductions in the glomerular filtration rate and the fractional excretion of sodium.[28] Azotemia is generally progressive, unless rapid bacteriological cure occurs.

ACUTE RENAL FAILURE SECONDARY TO CARDIOGENIC SHOCK (see also p. 587). Prerenal azotemia and, less commonly, acute renal failure (acute tubular necrosis) may occur in association with massive acute myocardial infarction. The mechanism of prerenal azotemia has been discussed above. Acute renal failure occurs when there is a marked, sudden reduction of renal perfusion.[29] The myoglobinuria accompanying excessive myocardial necrosis may play a contributory role. It is critically important to distinguish between prerenal azotemia and acute renal failure, since the former will generally respond to measures that improve cardiac output, whereas acute renal failure, once established, is a more serious problem that will usually not respond to extrarenal manipulation. Brief periods of modest hypotension (generally lasting less than an hour) often elicit reversible derangements, but more prolonged or profound hypotension lasting for 1 hour or more usually leads to acute tubular necrosis.

The distinction between prerenal azotemia and acute tubular necrosis in the oliguric patient (i.e., urine output less than 400 ml/24 hr) can generally be made by measurements of serum urea nitrogen and creatinine and the sodium, urea, and creatinine concentrations and osmolality of a concurrent sample of urine. In the absence of recent diuretic therapy, patients with prerenal azotemia retain their ability to conserve sodium; therefore, urinary sodium concentration is low, usually less than 20 mEq/liter. Tubular function is well preserved, as reflected in urine osmolality exceeding 500 mOsm, and the urinary/plasma ratios for urea and creatinine exceed 8 and 40, respectively. The BUN is more than 10 times the serum creatinine concentration.

In acute tubular necrosis, tubular function is impaired and the urinary sodium concentration generally exceeds 40 mEq/liter; the impairment of tubular function is also reflected in a urine osmolality less than 350 mOsm; the urinary/plasma values for urea and creatinine are below 2 and 20, respectively; and the BUN exceeds the serum creatinine by a ratio of less than 10 to 1. The urinary sediment may also be helpful in the differential diagnosis; patients with prerenal azotemia usually have a relatively clear sediment with a few granular or hyaline casts, whereas those with acute tubular necrosis have many tubular cells and casts in the urine.

As in patients with other causes of acute renal failure, the treatment of acute renal failure secondary to myocardial infarction and pump failure consists of controlling fluid intake to levels in accord with urinary output and insensible losses, as well as modifying the dosages of medications that are excreted by the kidneys, observing the patient closely for hyperkalemia, and intervening with dialysis for severe hyperkalemia or azotemia. In general, dialytic therapy, either hemodialysis or peritoneal dialysis, is initiated when serum creatinine levels reach 8 to 10 mg/dl and no reversible component for the renal failure is apparent. In addition, efforts must be made to maintain left ventricular filling pressure at levels that will optimize cardiac output and therefore renal perfusion (18 to 22 mm Hg). Given sufficient time and with no other associated problems, the prognosis for acute renal failure, when appropriately treated, is excellent.[29] However, when failure of the cardiac pump is severe enough to lead to acute renal failure, myocardial insufficiency rather than the renal failure is the determinant of the patient's poor prognosis.

ATHEROEMBOLIC DISEASE. Atheromatous embolization to the kidneys, which results in chronic, fibrotic, interstitial disease, is relatively uncommon.[30,31] It may occur spontaneously but more commonly follows operation on the aorta and renal arteries and catheter manipulation and aortography in patients with severe atheromatous disease of the aorta (p. 1566). Patchy areas of necrosis develop, followed by fibrosis with cholesterol clefts, as well as the response of a foreign body containing multinucleated giant cells. The disorder may be suspected if there has been some manipulation of the atheromatous aorta preceding the onset of progressive renal insufficiency. Examination of the urine is sometimes helpful in confirming the diagnosis; when it is allowed to sediment, fat will be found floating at the top. Treatment consists of avoiding further arterial and aortic manipulation, but progressive destruction of renal tissue occurs with subsequent renal insufficiency; the prognosis for improvement of renal function is guarded.

EFFECTS OF RENAL DISEASE ON THE CARDIOVASCULAR SYSTEM

The successful treatment of end-stage renal disease by dialysis and transplantation is widely considered to be one of the major advances of modern medicine. However, the mortality rate for patients treated by chronic hemodialysis still remains approximately 10 per cent per year.[32] Cardiovascular disease is the principal cause of mortality in these patients, accounting for 50 to 60 per cent of deaths,[33] compared with less than 15 per cent of deaths in age-corrected control populations. Myocardial infarction accounts for 25 to 30 per cent of deaths,[34] and cerebrovascular disease, for 10 to 15 per cent.

As shown in Figure 52–7 and Table 52–1, numerous risk factors for atherosclerosis have been identified in patients with end-stage renal disease.[35] These patients have a high incidence of complex premature ventricular contractions,[36] and in those with angina pectoris that is refractory to medical therapy, coronary bypass surgery has been carried out successfully.[37,38] In addition, angina unassociated with coronary atherosclerosis, presumably related to the combination of severe hypertension, left ventricular hypertrophy, and anemia, has been reported in chronic renal failure.[39]

TABLE 52–1 POSSIBLE CAUSES OF HEART FAILURE IN RENAL INSUFFICIENCY

Hypertension	Increased ventricular afterload
Hypervolemia	Increased ventricular preload
Anemia	Increased cardiac work (high output state)
Lipid abnormalities	Increased atherogenesis
Pericarditis	Restriction of ventricular filling
Ionic alterations	Negative inotropic effect
Hyperkalemia	
Hypocalcemia	
Hypermagnesemia	
Metabolic acidosis	
Disordered calcium and vitamin D metabolism	(A) Metastatic calcification (cardiac and vascular) (B) ? Vitamin D deficiency cardiomyopathy
Arteriovenous shunt for hemodialysis	Increased cardiac work (high output state)
Thiamine depletion by dialysis	Increased cardiac work (high output state)
Beriberi (?)	
Uremic toxins (?)	Depressed contractility; ? cardiomyopathy

Hypertension (See also Chap. 26)

Few patients develop chronic renal failure requiring dialysis without experiencing hypertension, which is probably the most important risk factor in the development of atherosclerotic cardiovascular disease. Hemodynamic studies in patients with end-stage renal disease have shown an elevated cardiac index and mean arterial pressure but a normal systemic vascular resistance.[40] The elevated cardiac index and normal systemic vascular resistance are related to the anemia; when the anemia is corrected, the cardiac index falls, and both arterial pressure and systemic vascular resistance rise.[41] The majority of patients with end-stage renal failure who develop hypertension have so-called *volume-dependent hypertension* (Chap. 26). Many studies in patients with end-stage renal failure have shown that arterial pressure is exquisitely dependent on blood volume[42–45] and that blood pressure control may be achieved by ultrafiltration during dialysis and control of salt and water intake in the interdialytic interval[42] (Fig. 52–8). However, a minority of patients with chronic renal failure have hyper-

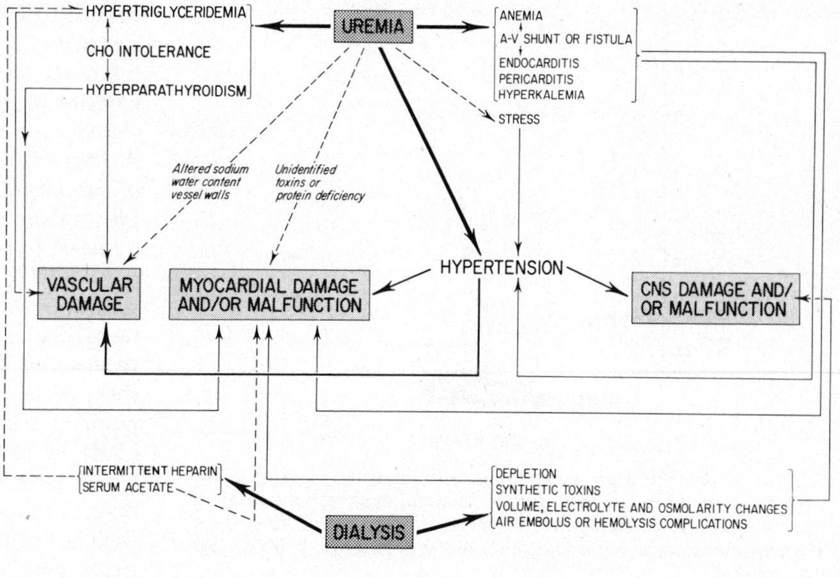

FIGURE 52–7 Risk factors for cardiovascular disease associated with chronic renal failure. CHO = carbohydrate; CNS = central nervous system. (From Lazarus, J. M., and Kjellstrand, C. M.: Dialysis: Medical aspects. *In* Brenner, B. M., and Rector, F. C. (eds.): The Kidney. Philadelphia, W. B. Saunders Co., 1980.)

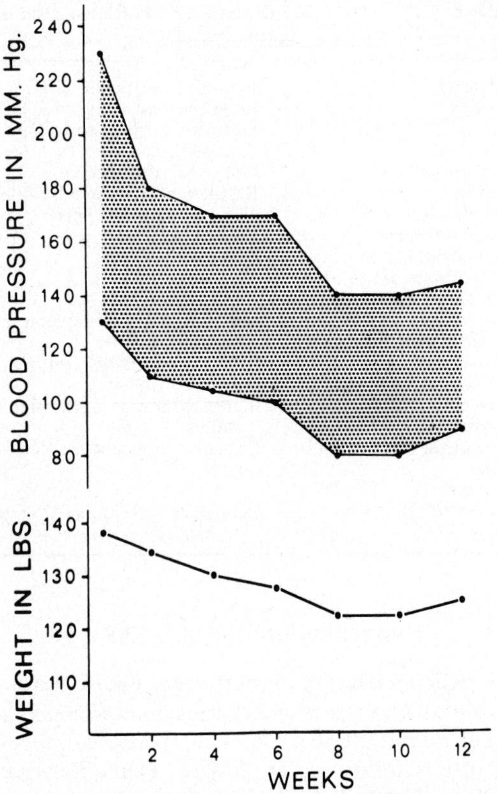

FIGURE 52–8 Blood pressure response to achievement of dry weight in a typical patient with volume-mediated hypertension. (From Vertes, V., et al.: Hypertension in end-stage renal disease. N. Engl. J. Med. *280*:978, 1969.)

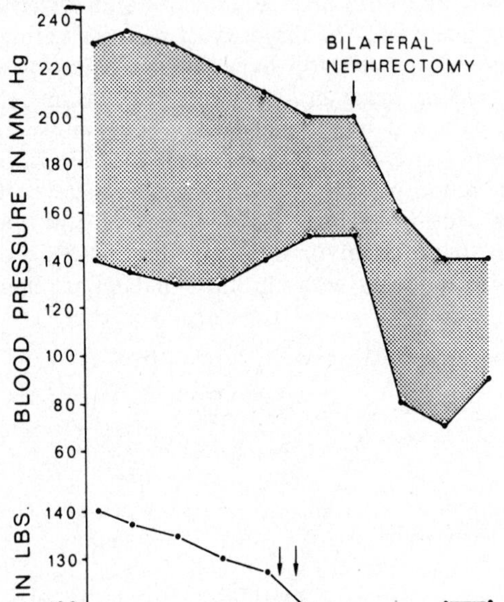

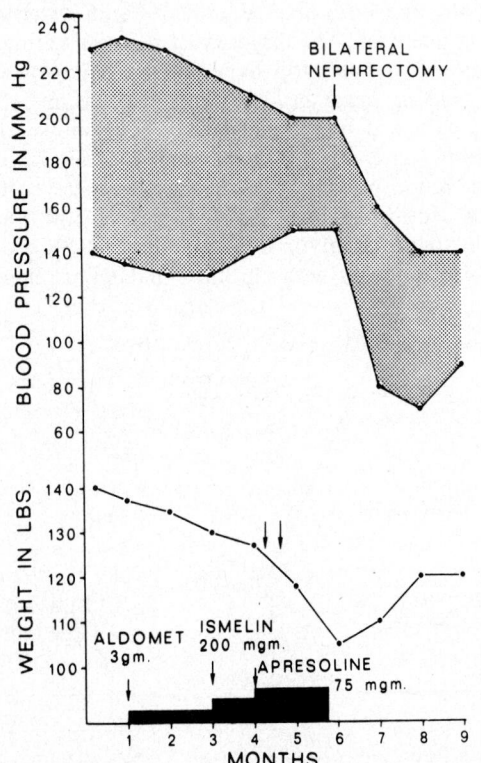

FIGURE 52–9 Blood pressure response to intensive dialysis, antihypertensive drug therapy, and, finally, bilateral nephrectomy in a typical patient with renin-mediated hypertension. (From Vertes, V., et al.: Hypertension in end-stage renal disease. N. Engl. J. Med. *280*: 978, 1969.)

tension that is not volume-related but instead is secondary to elevation of plasma renin activity; the hypertension is uncontrollable by lowering blood volume but does respond to bilateral nephrectomy with consequent reduction in plasma renin activity (Fig. 52–9). Dustan and Page demonstrated the volume-dependent nature of hypertension but also showed that arterial pressure was higher for any given volume when the kidneys were present than after they had been removed.[42] Subsequently, a significant correlation between *plasma renin* levels and arterial pressure was demonstrated.[46] The importance of plasma renin is reflected also in observations on patients with renal failure, hypertension, and expanded blood volume who exhibited renin values which, although normal, were higher than expected for the expanded state of their extracellular volume and which therefore may have contributed to the maintenance of hypertension.[47]

A third mechanism, which operates in patients whose blood pressure cannot be controlled either by volume reduction or bilateral nephrectomy or explained by elevations in plasma renin activity, may be related to *sympathetically mediated vasoconstriction.* Reduced baroreceptor activity has been demonstrated in patients with chronic renal failure by their response to the inhalation of amyl nitrite and the Valsalva maneuver.[48,49] Inhalation of amyl nitrite results in peripheral vasodilation and therefore a fall in blood pressure, which normally results in reflex vasoconstriction and tachycardia. A blunted response in heart rate elevation is taken as evidence of reduced baroreceptor function. Autonomic insufficiency, as evidenced by an inadequate response to the Valsalva maneuver, is said to be present if both bradycardia and arterial pressure overshoot are absent after release of forced expiration against a standard pressure (40 mm Hg) for a set time (12 sec). Many patients with renal insufficiency whose hypertension is caused by sympathetically mediated vasoconstriction exhibit an exaggerated response to the cold pressor test and elevated plasma levels of dopamine beta-hydroxylase as indices of increased adrenergic function but become hypotensive during dialysis.

A fourth possible mechanism of hypertension in patients with renal failure is the *secretion of pressor substances not related to the renin-angiotensin system.* A pressor substance that differs from and is a more potent constrictor than angiotensin II has been isolated from the blood of dogs with bilateral, surgically induced renal artery stenosis.[50] The identity of this substance and its role in hypertension associated with human renal disease remains to be elucidated. A fifth mechanism that has been proposed is the *absence of vasodepressor substances* of renal origin, such as the prostaglandins, which may play a role in the genesis of renoprival hypertension.[51,52]

TREATMENT. Since volume-dependent hypertension is the most common mechanism in patients with chronic renal disease, the reduction of plasma volume should be the central theme in the management of hypertension in these patients. Before renal function has deteriorated to the point at which dialysis is required, an attempt should be made to reduce plasma volume, but not to the point at which glomerular filtration will decline further; dietary sodium should be restricted to the lowest level consistent with a normal sodium balance. However, since many patients may have difficulty with this degree of sodium restriction on a long-term basis, and since they may have an inability to excrete even this low quantity of sodium, it is often necessary to add diuretics. Generally, for patients with creatinine clearances exceeding 40 ml/min, thiazide diuretics are effective. However, when the glomerular filtration rate falls below this level, furosemide is required, sometimes in very high doses.

If the arterial pressure remains elevated despite sodium restriction and diuretic agents, antihypertensive agents are generally effective. These include clonidine, alpha-methyldopa, propranolol, hydralazine, prazosin (and, for the patient refractory to these agents, minoxidil). Sympatholytic agents such as guanethidine are not advisable, since they may be associated with particularly profound postural changes in blood pressure in patients with renal failure.

The problem of the control of hypertension is simpler in patients with chronic renal failure who are maintained on intermittent hemodialysis. In addition to dietary restriction of sodium intake, lowering of blood volume by ultrafiltration during hemodialysis may be employed (Fig. 52–8). In patients in whom volume reduction does not control blood pressure, pharmacological treatment is indicated. Agents such as alpha-methyldopa and propranolol lower plasma renin activity, but vasodilators (hydralazine and minoxidil) may have to be added;[53,54] it is unusual to encounter patients with renal insufficiency who do not respond to a combination of minoxidil and propranolol. However, minoxidil may induce a pericardial effusion, and patients receiving this medication should be monitored by echocardiography to determine the presence of free pericardial fluid that may develop during therapy; it generally resolves within 1 month after withdrawal of the drug.[55]

Angiotensin-converting enzyme inhibitors appear to be particularly useful antihypertensive agents in patients with renal insufficiency (p. 921). Bilateral nephrectomy[56] is employed only in those patients who do not respond to antihypertensive drugs, cannot comply with antihypertensive regimens, or have intolerable side effects of antihypertensive medication. Although aggressive therapy of hypertension for the patient with renin-mediated malignant hypertension may transiently compromise renal function to the point at which dialysis is required, the increased survival associated with control of the hypertension[57] outweighs the risks attending maintenance hemodialysis.

HYPERTENSION FOLLOWING RENAL TRANSPLANTATION. Hypertension occurs in 30 to 80 per cent of patients in the post-transplant period.[58] Multiple factors have been implicated in its etiology, including acute and chronic rejection,[59] recurrent disease in the transplanted kidney,[60] stenosis of the transplanted renal artery,[61] and large doses of steroids.[59] During acute rejection episodes, the levels of renin and angiotensin are markedly elevated. In addition, the renin-angiotensin-aldosterone system appears to be of pathogenic importance in the hypertension associated with stenosis of the artery to the transplanted kidney, a complication that occurs in 10 per cent of the transplant population,[61] as well as in some patients in whom the diseased native kidneys release renin.

The treatment of hypertension in the post-transplant period depends on elucidating the underlying mechanisms of the disorder. In patients with severe refractory hypertension that cannot be ascribed to rejection, angiography and determination of renin activity in venous blood both from the native and the transplanted kidneys are indicated. Surgical revision of a stenosed renal artery or nephrectomy of the native kidney may be in order.

Whereas hypertriglyceridemia is the predominant lipid abnormality in patients with chronic renal failure (see below), hypercholesterolemia Types IIA and B tend to predominate following renal allotransplantation, although in some transplanted patients hypertriglyceridemia persists.[62] The etiology of these lipid abnormalities in the post-transplant period is unclear, but they may be related to the large doses of glucocorticoids administered to these patients.[62] In view of the combination of hypertension and lipid abnormalities in a substantial fraction of patients following transplantation, it is not surprising that coronary atherosclerosis accounts for more deaths than any disease process other than infection.[63]

Lipid Abnormalities

Hypertriglyceridemia with elevations of very low density lipoproteins (VLDL), i.e., Type IV hyperlipoproteinemia (p. 1215), is common in patients with chronic renal failure. Bagdade et al. studied both undialyzed and dialyzed patients with uremia not associated with the nephrotic syndrome and found the plasma triglyceride concentrations to be elevated in both groups.[64] There appears to be no relation between the duration of dialysis or the etiology of the renal disease and the severity of the hyperlipidemia. A second abnormality in lipid metabolism, *reduced concentration of high density lipoprotein (HDL) cholesterol,* has also been documented in chronic renal failure,[64,65] a finding of potential importance in view of the strong negative correlation between HDL concentration and the risk of the development of ischemic heart disease (p. 1211). An inverse correlation has been noted between plasma triglyceride and HDL cholesterol levels in both uremic and nonuremic subjects.[65]

Several suggestions have been proposed to explain the elevation of plasma triglycerides in chronic renal failure. The first is that the increased hepatic synthesis of triglycerides, presumably secondary to insulin resistance and the resultant elevated levels of plasma insulin, and/or of abnormally high levels of growth hormone—both of which occur in renal failure—causes increased release of fatty acids from adipose tissue. A second possibility, for which there is increasing evidence,[66,67] centers on deficiencies in lipoprotein lipase and hepatic triglyceride lipase, known to be necessary for the removal of triglycerides from plasma and their ultimate catabolism; this deficiency may also result from elevated insulin levels, from direct inhibition of these lipases by a nondialyzable factor in uremic serum,[67] or from a deficiency of apoprotein CII in both HDL and VLDL.[68] The reduction of hepatic triglyceride lipase[69] and lipoprotein lipase[70] causes a defect in the catabolism of triglyceride-rich lipoproteins, which in turn leads to the accumulation of VLDL[71] and of enrichment of intermediate-density lipoprotein and low-density lipoproteins with triglyceride; it is also associated with the appearance of apoprotein B48, an increased concentration of apoprotein AIV, and the presence in LDL of apoproteins C and E (proteins not normally found in LDL). It has been suggested that these abnormal substances may be atherogenic.[67]

In one study, HDL cholesterol was significantly reduced in patients with renal failure on chronic hemodialysis (average, 26 mg/dl) compared with normal persons (average, 52 mg/dl).[66] This reduction of HDL was due to a reduced protein content of all its subfractions. Apoprotein electrophoresis showed an increase in "arginine-rich" peptide in the VLDL and the HDL fraction and, as noted, a reduction of apoprotein CII, which is transferred to VLDL from HDL[72] and which functions as an activator of the enzyme lipoprotein lipase.[73]

Treatment. The standard dietary therapy of patients with Type IV hyperlipoproteinemia in the absence of renal failure consists of weight reduction, limitation of alcohol intake, a reduction in carbohydrate consumption, and, if these measures are inadequate, the administration of clofibrate (p. 1226).[74] In patients with chronic renal failure, the lipid abnormality is not usually associated with excessive body weight or alcohol consumption, and reduction in carbohydrate intake is somewhat difficult to achieve owing to the limitations imposed on the patient's diet by virtue of the reduced protein intake. A reasonable therapeutic approach is to provide caloric replacement through increases in polyunsaturated fat in the diet.[75] With this diet, a significant reduction in plasma triglyceride levels has been observed, both in conservatively treated patients with chronic renal failure and in patients on dialysis.[76]

Clofibrate is normally metabolized by the kidney, and active metabolites can accumulate in patients with severely compromised renal function; patients with renal failure may develop severe myositis in association with the ingestion of the usual doses of this drug.[77] A reduction in total dosage of clofibrate to 1.5 gm per week may lead to a lowering of plasma triglyceride concentration without producing myositis. However, even with this reduced dosage, an increase in serum creatine kinase levels has been reported, presumably as a consequence of damage to skeletal muscle.[77]

Hemodialysis

Technical Considerations. Hemodialysis may accomplish three objectives. It may (1) remove solutes, (2) alter the electrolyte concentration of the patient's extracellular fluid, and (3) remove as much as 1 liter of extracellular fluid per hour. These three processes should be viewed as being essentially independent of one another, and it is often desirable, in the course of a single dialysis, to carry out only one or two of these three functions.

Patients with heart failure, circulatory congestion, or hypertension often derive benefit from removal of fluid by ultrafiltration during the course of hemodialysis. This must be carefully done, since normotensive patients may become hypotensive with removal of excess fluid.[78] Echocardiography is a useful noninvasive method for evaluating left ventricular function serially during hemodialysis; it can distinguish between left ventricular failure, decreased left ventricular compliance, and fluid overload.[79–81]

Electrolyte Shifts. In manipulating electrolyte concentrations, it is important to appreciate that most dialysates contain 1.5 to 3.0 mEq/liter of potassium and 3 to 3.5 mEq/liter of calcium (6 to 7 mg/dl of ionized Ca^{++}). Since most patients commence dialysis with some elevation of serum potassium, the serum potassium may fall precipitously when dialysis begins, whereas the concentration of ionized calcium rises, setting the stage for digitalis intoxication in digitalized patients (p. 523). The likelihood of this complication is enhanced by any digoxin excess, which might come about if the dosage has not been adjusted downward to take into consideration the markedly prolonged half-life of this drug in patients with renal failure (p. 514). In patients on hemodialysis who are not hypoxemic, myocardial performance, as reflected in the echocardiogram, often improves; this may be related to a reduction in serum potassium and an elevation of calcium.[80]

Arteriovenous Fistulas. To achieve vascular access to dialysis, an arteriovenous fistula must be created. These shunts have a flow rate of 250 to 750 ml/minute and thereby add to the cardiac workload. As discussed on page 814, in association with the anemia characteristic of chronic renal failure, this may contribute to the development of high-output heart failure.[82] In our experience, this form of heart failure can be readily controlled if any excess fluid accumulation is prevented by ultrafiltration during dialysis and if the anemia is partially treated by transfusion. Obviously, it is desirable to have only a single vascular access site present in a patient at any one time and to limit the size of the anastomosis to the smallest required for successful dialysis. The contribution of the fistula to the heart failure state can be determined by studying the effect of occlusion of the fistula on left ventricular function, as assessed by echocardiography or radionuclide ventriculography.[78]

Infection is a major complication of arteriovenous shunts and may become metastatic. Septic pulmonary emboli and infective endocarditis, most often staphylococcal, have been reported.[83] Since patients on hemodialysis often have functional systolic and occasionally even diastolic murmurs, which may change with the patient's altered hemodynamic status, the diagnosis of endocarditis may be missed. Therefore, the *early* diagnosis of endocarditis in patients with infected vascular access sites depends on a high index of clinical suspicion and the immediate obtaining of blood cultures. However, the diagnosis of infective endocarditis may be difficult, since an infected vascular access site without infection of the endocardium can also give rise to positive blood cultures.

Hypoxemia. A fall in arterial oxygen tension of 10 to 15 mm Hg occurs frequently within the first 30 minutes of hemodialysis and persists throughout the procedure.[84] This event is obviously undesirable in patients with heart or lung disease and may lead to serious hypoxemia in patients with even mild arterial desaturation at the commencement of the hemodialysis. Together with the electrolyte changes which occur during hemodialysis referred to above, it may lower the threshold for the development of arrhythmias. Also, the PEP/LVET ratio (p. 54) may increase significantly during dialysis,[85,86] an increase which correlates significantly with the fall in arterial oxygen tension, suggesting that the latter actually impairs left ventricular function.

The mechanism responsible for the decline in arterial pO_2 is in some dispute. It has been reported that activation of complement leads to aggregation of neutrophils in the lungs that interfere with normal oxygenation.[87] An alternative explanation is that it is due to physiological hypoventilation secondary to the diffusion of carbon dioxide across the dialyzer.[85] Whatever the mechanism, patients with impaired pulmonary function and severe heart disease should be monitored for arterial hypoxemia during the early phase of dialysis and may require inhalation of oxygen-enriched mixtures during the procedure.

Potassium Balance

Life-threatening hyperkalemia may occur in acute oliguric renal failure, in end-stage chronic renal failure, and, rarely, in terminal heart failure (p. 500). The principal detrimental effect of hyperkalemia is in its electrical effect on the heart. The progressive electrocardiographic abnormalities associated with hyperkalemia are illustrated in Figures 7–43 (p. 236). Generally, the earliest electrocardiographic sign of hyperkalemia is peaking of the T waves, followed progressively by an increase in T-wave amplitude, a widening of the QRS complex, and loss of atrial activity. Finally, with extreme hyperkalemia, a sine wave pattern is noted on the electrocardiogram, followed by cardiac arrest.[88] Unfortunately, however, only a rough correlation exists between the level of serum potassium and the electrocardiographic changes, although in any given patient, directional changes in the serum potassium can be estimated from the electrocardiogram. Even severe hyperkalemia per se produces few if any symptoms; occasionally, weakness of skeletal muscles or dyspnea presumably secondary to paralysis of respiratory muscles may be noted.

TREATMENT. Severe hyperkalemia is a medical emergency, and its treatment can generally be divided into acute and chronic phases. The most rapid means of counteracting the toxic cardiac effects of potassium is with the administration of intravenous calcium, given in the form of 10 to 20 ml of 10 per cent *calcium chloride* with electrocardiographic monitoring to assure that the electrocardiographic signs of hyperkalemia have been reversed. While administration of calcium chloride is an effective emergency measure, it does not lower the elevated serum potassium concentration.

The second aspect of therapy relies upon lowering the serum potassium. In patients with hyperkalemia and acidosis, *sodium bicarbonate* causes a fall in serum potassium; the usual dose is 1 to 2 ampoules (44 to 88 mEq) administered intravenously. The combination of *glucose and insulin* will also result in a redistribution of potassium from the extracellular to the intracellular space; the usual dose is 50 ml of 50 per cent glucose with 10 units of regular insulin, intravenously. The effects of alkalinization or glucose and insulin administration can be observed within 15 to 30 minutes and may last for several hours. Although these forms of therapy are useful for rapidly lowering the serum potassium concentration, they do *not* lower total body potassium stores.

Further treatment of hyperkalemia involves removal of potassium from the body, which can be accomplished by the administration of *cation exchange resins* by mouth or enema. The resin most commonly employed is sodium polystyrene sulfonate (Kayexalate), 1 gm of which exchanges approximately 1 mEq of sodium for potassium. The usual dose is 50 gm two or three times daily. When administered by mouth, it is desirable to accompany it with an osmotic cathartic to prevent intestinal obstruction as a consequence of inspissation of the resin in the gut.

The most effective means of reducing the body's potassium stores is by means of *dialysis*, either hemodialysis or peritoneal dialysis. However, when using these modalities care must be exercised not to lower the serum potassium too precipitously, especially in those patients who are receiving cardiac glycosides. This can be accomplished by beginning with a dialysis solution having a potassium concentration of approximately 4 mEq/liter and then progressively lowering it as the serum potassium declines.

Secondary Hyperparathyroidism

Ectopic calcification in a variety of tissues, including the heart and arterial bed, is a common manifestation of secondary hyperparathyroidism, which is a frequent complication of chronic renal failure. Involvement of the sinoatrial and atrioventricular nodes, the valvular annuli and cusps (particularly the mitral annulus,[88a,88b]), the intima and media of epicardial coronary arteries, the interventricular septum, and the ventricular myocardium similar to that illustrated in Figures 51–6 and 51–7 (p. 1737)[89–91] has been described; clinical and electrocardiographic changes include left ventricular failure and varying degrees of atrioventricular block.[92,93] As many as half the patients on maintenance hemodialysis have been reported to have radiological evidence of arterial calcification;[94,95] calcium deposition is generally in the media, leading to Mönckeberg sclerosis.[96] Calcium deposition may be associated with almost complete obliteration of the vascular lumen and may result in ischemia and, ultimately, gangrene of tissue distal to the involved vessels.[94–97]

The most effective *treatment* of secondary hyperparathyroidism consists of renal transplantation or subtotal parathyroidectomy. The latter procedure has been shown to improve cardiac contractility.[97] For patients maintained on dialysis, dietary phosphate restriction, the use of nonabsorbable aluminum-containing antacids and the use of dihydrotachysterol (DHT), a synthetic analog of vitamin D, given in doses of 0.125 to 0.5 mg/24 hr, are also useful measures.[98] Recently, the active form of vitamin D, 1,25-dihydroxycholecalciferol, has become available commercially.

Uremic Pericarditis (See also p. 1505)

Pericarditis is a common complication of both acute and chronic renal failure. Prior to the era of dialysis, the appearance of pericarditis in the uremic patient was generally taken as a sign of limited life expectancy.[99] Its incidence varies among different series, but it has been reported to occur in up to 50 per cent of patients at the initiation of dialysis;[100] its incidence appears to be declining with the increasing use of early dialysis prior to the development of advanced uremia. The mechanism of development of pericarditis is not clear, but it is probably related to the accumulation of uremic toxin(s), which is responsible for an inflammatory serositis. The serositis most commonly involves the pericardium but can also involve the pleura.[101] Fibrinous pleuritis, pleural friction rubs,[102] hemorrhagic pleural effusion,[103] and pneumonitis[101] have also been reported to occur in uremia.

Three and a half per cent of the patients accepted for dialysis at the Brigham and Women's Hospital during a 5-year period developed clinical evidence of pericarditis and pericardial effusion while on dialytic therapy.[104] Pericarditis occurring in patients with stable chronic dialysis may be related to inadequate dialysis or to an intercurrent illness, such as a viral infection. In patients with renal failure, pericarditis is frequently preceded by an otherwise benign respiratory tract infection; infection with cytomegalovirus and other conditions such as systemic lupus erythematosus and acute myocardial infarction have also been implicated as causes.[105]

The clinical features of uremic pericarditis are summarized in Table 52–2. The diagnosis is made by the same clinical criteria used for other forms of pericarditis, i.e., chest pain generally ameliorated by sitting up and leaning forward, typical electrocardiographic and echocardiographic changes, increases in heart size on chest roentgenogram, and evidence of circulatory embarrassment with severe pericarditis. With echocardiography, a surprisingly high incidence (32 per cent) of small, asymptomatic, pericardial effusions was found in our institution in patients on chronic maintenance hemodialysis,[110] a finding in concert with those of other observers.[111] The development of hypotension during dialysis, which cannot be readily attributed to changes in intravascular volume, is a useful clue to the presence of significant pericardial effusion. However, the diagnosis of pericarditis may sometimes be made in error. Uremic patients frequently develop a systolic ejection murmur, most probably related to the high-output state secondary to chronic anemia. Occasionally, patients with chronic renal failure and hypertension develop diastolic blowing murmurs of aortic regurgitation, and the combination of these two murmurs may be mistaken for a to-and-fro pericardial friction rub.

Cardiac tamponade is the major and a potentially lethal complication of pericarditis. Pericardial fluid is generally exudative and bloody,[100,101] and the heparinization required for hemodialysis may cause serious bleeding into the pericardial cavity in patients with pericarditis. Therefore, it is important to avoid systemic heparinization during hemodialysis in the presence of active pericarditis and large effusions. However, systemic heparinization can be used safely in patients with small pericardial effusions without associated physical signs and symptoms of active pericarditis. The development of *chronic constrictive pericarditis* is an unusual complication of uremic pericarditis. It developed in 2 of 25 patients at the Brigham and Women's Hospital with prior severe effusions;[104] other centers report a similarly low incidence.

TABLE 52–2 CLINICAL FEATURES OF UREMIC PERICARDITIS*

FEATURE	FREQUENCY (%)
Pain	66
Pericardial friction rub	93
Fever	84
Leukocytosis	56
Arrhythmias	23
Hypotension	56
Hepatomegaly	60
Elevated venous pressure	71
Abnormal electrocardiogram	90
Enlarged cardiac silhouette	96

*Adapted from Lowenthal,[106] Comty et al.,[107] Ribot,[108] and Silverberg et al.[109]

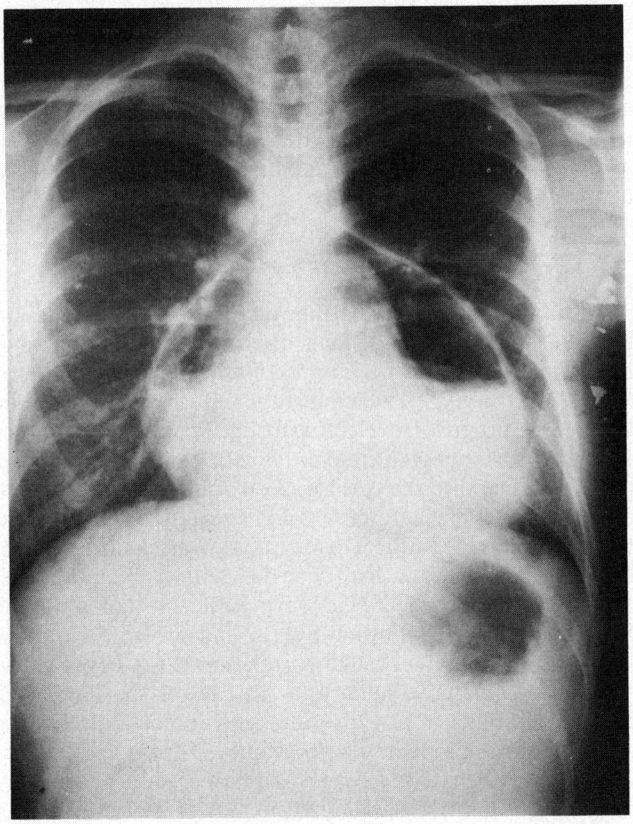

FIGURE 52–10 Chest roentgenogram showing air-fluid level in the pericardial space of a patient with a uremic pericardial effusion, following instillation of air and removal of pericardial fluid.

Treatment. Management of the patient with asymptomatic pericardial effusion should consist of vigorous hemodialysis and the use of regional heparinization (see below). Uremic pericarditis complicated by tamponade or persistent large effusion should be treated with immediate pericardiocentesis, coupled with vigorous hemodialysis; this results in a very high rate of resolution.[100,104] The placement of air into the pericardial space has the advantage of limiting the apposition of visceral and parietal pericardial surfaces and providing an air-fluid level, thereby allowing the rate of reaccumulation of fluid to be followed readily on a routine chest roentgenogram (Fig. 52–10). The instillation of corticosteroids into the pericardial cavity,[112] the use of oral indomethacin, catheter drainage of the pericardial effusion,[113] and the construction of a pericardial window have all been advocated. The early use of pericardial stripping for the treatment of uremic pericardial effusion has been suggested.[114] However, because of the rarity of the development of constrictive pericarditis, we believe that *prophylactic* pericardiectomy is not justified.

It is our practice to treat uremic pericarditis by vigorous dialysis and catheter drainage of the pericardial space with the instillation of air. However, placement of the catheter into the pericardial cavity should be attempted only by persons experienced in this technique, and in our institution it is performed by cardiothoracic surgeons. The use of the local instillation of nonabsorbable steroids or the systemic use of indomethacin or both may be of additional benefit, but more experience with these modalities is required. Pericardial stripping is the treatment of choice in patients with subacute or chronic constrictive pericarditis secondary to uremia.[104,106,115]

Cardiac Infections in Renal Failure. Patients with chronic renal failure on hemodialysis are compromised hosts with impairment of most immunological defense mechanisms. Infections are responsible for about one-fifth of all deaths in these patients. Arteriovenous shunts and fistulas are particularly susceptible to bacterial infections and, as already pointed out, may result in septicemia and infective endocarditis. Viral or purulent pericarditis is another common infection in patients with chronic renal failure and may be confused with uremic pericarditis. Patients with transplanted kidneys on immunosuppressive therapy have a particularly high risk of infection.

MANAGEMENT OF PATIENTS WITH CARDIAC DISEASE IN RENAL FAILURE

The generally greater availability of dialysis facilities and the broadened criteria for acceptance of patients into treatment programs for end-stage renal disease have resulted in a patient population in whom other diseases, including cardiac disease which may require surgical treatment, may be present. The high frequency of coronary artery disease that develops among patients with renal failure and the occasional presence of coexisting valvular heart disease often lead to a consideration of cardiopulmonary bypass among these patients. Patients on maintenance hemodialysis can undergo major operations without a great excess of mortality or morbidity,[116] and several series have been published documenting the ability of patients with renal failure to tolerate open heart surgery, both coronary renovascularization and valve replacement.[117,118] It has been our experience that among patients with end-stage renal disease, cardiac operations may be performed with equal success regardless of whether the renal failure has been treated by dialysis or transplantation.[119,120]

The major problems associated with operation in patients with chronic renal failure include the development of hyperkalemia, fluid overload, and arrhythmias. However, with the appropriate use of hemodialysis both before and after operation and careful monitoring of the patient's hemodynamic status and electrolytes, the excess risks of operation have been contained. Although many observers feel that patients who have severely impaired renal failure but who do not yet require hemodialysis may undergo cardiac surgery without hemodialysis, it is our policy to dialyze patients with less than 20 per cent of normal glomerular filtration rate on several occasions on the days preceding and following such operations.

The management of patients with hypertrophic obstructive cardiomyopathy (p. 1409) and chronic renal failure presents a unique problem. It is well established that these patients are particularly sensitive to acute changes in blood volume and to tachyarrhythmias. During hemodialysis, blood volume is ordinarily reduced. Although most patients tolerate this volume depletion without difficulty, those with hypertrophic cardiomyopathy often develop an acute increase in obstruction to left ventricular outflow. In our experience, this complication can be avoided by using dialysis apparatus requiring a low extracorporeal volume and having precise control of ultrafiltration. In addition, these patients are treated with propranolol and transfused to maintain the hematocrit in the range of 30 per cent.

Modification of Common Cardiac Medications in Patients with Renal Failure

Since many drugs (and/or their active metabolites) used in the treatment of heart disease are excreted by the kidney, renal failure affects the pharmacokinetics of many agents, including those commonly used to treat heart disease.

CARDIAC GLYCOSIDES (also see p. 514). *Digoxin* is filtered in the glomeruli, and the excretion of digoxin by the kidneys is directly proportional to the glomerular filtration rate. It is not altered by the rate of urine flow and therefore by the administration of diuretics;[121] only very small quantities of digoxin may be secreted by the distal convoluted tubule.[122] The ratio of the clearance of digoxin to endogenous creatine is 0.8 and the percentage of the body's total stores of digoxin lost per day can be calculated as $14 + 0.2 \times$ creatinine clearance in milliliters per minute. Thus, 85 per cent of administered digoxin is normally excreted in the urine, most in unchanged form, and only 10 to 15 per cent is eliminated in the stool through biliary excretion. Normally, 38 per cent of the body's stores of digoxin are either metabolized or excreted per day,[123] whereas in anephric patients, 14 per cent of total body digoxin stores are eliminated per day via the biliary tree. Therefore, in the patient without significant renal function, digoxin elimination is reduced to approximately 37 per cent of normal, and digoxin dosage should be modified accordingly.

In patients with end-stage renal disease requiring treatment with digoxin, it is our policy to use a loading dose of 0.25 mg and maintenance doses of 0.125 mg every other day. Digoxin levels are determined 1 week later, and, depending on the clinical response, the dose is modified, often upward, to 0.125 mg orally daily. In contrast to digoxin, the half-life of *digitoxin* is not greatly affected by impaired renal function,[124] and therefore the dosage does not need to be altered in patients with renal failure. Because of high tissue and protein binding of both digoxin and digitoxin, little removal occurs with either hemo- or peritoneal dialysis.[125] Therefore, these methods are ineffective in the treatment of digitalis intoxication.

ANTIARRHYTHMIC DRUGS (see also Chap. 21). The dose of *procainamide* must be modified in patients with end-stage renal disease because this drug is normally eliminated by both renal excretion and hepatic metabolism. Procainamide is readily dialyzable.[126]

Quinidine is metabolized by a variety of tissues, including the liver, mostly to hydroxy derivatives; no specific modification of the dose is necessary in patients with impaired renal function. Since quinidine is 80 per cent protein-bound[127] and is widely distributed in tissue, clearance by dialysis would be expected to be quite poor; indeed, clearances by peritoneal dialysis have been measured and found to be less than 10 ml/min.[128]

The half-life of *lidocaine* is about 1 hour, and its deactivation depends largely on hepatic metabolism; no dosage modification is necessary in patients with renal failure.[129]

No data are available on its dialyzability, but, because of a high degree of protein-binding (approximately 60 per cent),[130] it is probably poor.

The liver is also the principal site of inactivation of *phenytoin.*[131] Because of the diminished protein-binding of the drug in patients with renal failure, therapeutic and toxic levels may be achieved at lower doses than those used in patients with renal function.[132] Therefore, the usual dosage should be reduced by one third in patients with creatinine clearance below 30 ml/min. As is the case for most of the antiarrhythmic agents, phenytoin is poorly dialyzed.[133]

Propranolol is used extensively in patients with renal failure for its effects on arterial pressure, angina pectoris, and, less commonly, cardiac arrhythmias. Since it is metabolized primarily by the liver, its half-life is not altered by renal failure.[134,135] It is largely (90 per cent) protein-bound and has a large volume of distribution;[136] therefore, it is not surprising that it is poorly dialyzed.

Heart Failure Secondary to Renal Failure

Chronic renal failure can impair cardiac performance by a variety of mechanisms, many of which result from an augmentation of cardiac work (Table 52–1). It has been found that there is an increased left ventricular stroke work index and left ventricular end-diastolic pressure and size in many patients with end-stage renal disease.[79,137,138] In addition, an increase in pulmonary capillary permeability tending to lead to pulmonary edema, even in the absence of elevation of pulmonary capillary wedge pressure, has been reported in renal insufficiency as well.[139] Impairment of cardiac performance also occurs secondary to ischemic heart disease as a consequence of the accelerated atherogenesis referred to earlier (p. 1753). The possibility must be considered that dialysis results in the depletion of essential substances; thus, the water-soluble vitamins are dialyzable, and it has been suggested that their loss can lead to beriberi heart disease.[140] Therefore, it seems desirable to provide supplements of these vitamins for patients who are on maintenance hemodialysis. It is possible that long-term dialysis leads to depletion of other, as yet unidentified substances necessary for normal cardiac performance, but this has not been established.

The possibility that the uremic state depresses myocardial function is intriguing. As early as 1944, Raab suggested that specific myocardial toxins might be present in uremia.[141] Recently, depression of cardiac function in isolated rat heart preparations perfused with urea, creatinine, guanidinosuccinic acid, and methyl-guanidine, singly and in combination, has been reported.[142] Similarly, a depression of myocardial contractility has been demonstrated in a guinea pig model of uremia secondary to acute obstructive renal failure.[143]

Uremia produces serious disturbances in monovalent cation transport. Red blood cells, leukocytes, lung, and bone from patients with renal insufficiency have an elevated sodium content and a reduction in ouabain-sensitive Na-K–activated ATPase activity.[144,145] It is possible that this same fundamental abnormality is responsible for the observed reduction in human skeletal muscle transmembrane potential, which returns toward normal with vigorous hemodialysis.

The presence of a *cardiomyopathy* in uremic patients has been suggested, but its existence as a specific entity has been difficult to document in view of the many other possible causes of abnormal cardiac function in such patients.[146,147] Although reversibility of myocardial dysfunction with treatment of uremia is not clear,[148] there is suggestive evidence that it can occur. In one study, patients with severe cardiomyopathy and uremia were reported to have developed their cardiac disease while on low-protein diets prior to initiation of hemodialysis, and all had striking clinical improvement with dialysis.[149] In another, hemodialysis raised the left ventricular ejection fraction, both acutely and chronically,[150] whereas in a third, left ventricular function improved following renal transplantation.[137]

References

1. Skorecki, K. L., and Brenner, B. M.: Body fluid homeostasis in congestive heart failure and cirrhosis with ascites. Am. J. Med. *72*:323, 1982.
2. Hostetter, T. H., Pfeffer, J. M., Pfeffer, M. A., Braunwald, E., and Brenner, B. M.: Cardiorenal hemodynamics and sodium excretion in rats with myocardial infarction. Am. J. Physiol. 1983, in press.
3. Watkins, L., Burton, J. A., Cant, J. R., Smith, F. W., and Barger, A. C.: The renin-angiotensin-aldosterone system in congestive heart failure in conscious dogs. J. Clin. Invest. *57*:1606, 1976.
4. Higgins, C. B., Vatner, S. F., Franklin, D., and Braunwald, E.: Effects of experimentally produced heart failure on the peripheral vascular response to severe exercise in conscious dogs. Circ. Res. *31*:186, 1972.
5. McGiff, J., and Itskovitz, H. D.: Prostaglandin and the kidney. Circ. Res. *33*:479, 1973.
6. Mills, I. H., MacFarlane, N. A. A., Ward, P. E., and Obika, L. F. O.: The renal kallikrein-kinin system and the regulation of salt and water excretion. Fed. Proc. *35*:181, 1976.
7. Ichikawa, I., Pfeffer, J. M., Pfeffer, M. A., Hostetter, T. H., Braunwald, E., and Brenner, B. M.: Glomerular response to severe congestive heart failure in the rat. Proceedings, 15th Annual Meeting of the American Society of Nephrology, 152a, 1982.
8. DiPerri, T., Forconi, S., Puccetti, F., Vittoria, A., and Guerrini, M.: Effects of prostaglandin A_1 on renal handling of salt and water in congestive heart failure. J. Cardiovasc. Pharm. *2*:215, 1980.
9. Boudreau, R. J., and Mandin, H.: The role of prostaglandins in the regulation of renal function during chronic pericardial tamponade. Effect of indomethacin and arachidonic acid on renal function in cardiac edema. Circ. Res. *26*:867A, 1978.
10. Berliner, R. W., and Davidson, P. G.: Production of hypertonic urine in the absence of pituitary antidiuretic hormone. J. Clin. Invest. *36*:1416, 1957.
11. Fitzsimmons, J. T.: Thirst. Physiol. Rev. *52*:468, 1972.
12. Fitzsimmons, J. T., and Simons, B. J.: The effect on drinking in the rat of intravenous infusion of angiotensin given alone or in combination with other stimuli of thirst. J. Physiol. (Lond.) *203*:45, 1969.
13. Riegger, G. A. J., Liebau, G., and Kochsiek, K.: Antidiuretic hormone in congestive heart failure. Am. J. Med. *72*:49, 1982.
14. Szatalowicz, V. L., Arnold, P. E., Chaimovitz, C., Bichet, D., Bert, T., and Schrier, R. W.: Radioimmunoassay of plasma arginine vasopressin in hyponatremic patients with congestive heart failure. N. Engl. J. Med. *305*:263, 1981.
15. Oberg, B.: Effects of cardiovascular reflexes on net capillary fluid transfer. Acta Physiol. Scand. (Suppl.) *62*:229, 1964.
16. Braunwald, E., Ross, J., Jr., and Sonnenblick, E. H.: Mechanisms of Contraction in the Normal and Failing Heart. 2nd ed. Boston, Little, Brown, 1976, pp. 250–254.
17. Greenberg, T. T., Richmond, W. H., Stocking, R. A., Gupta, P. D., Meehan, J. P., and Henry, J. P.: Impaired arterial stretch receptor responses in dogs with heart failure due to tricuspid insufficiency and pulmonary artery stenosis. Circ. Res. *32*:424, 1973.
18. Zucker, I. H., Earle, A. M., and Gilmore, J. P.: The mechanism of adaptation of left atrial stretch receptors in dogs with chronic congestive heart failure. J. Clin. Invest. *60*:323, 1977.
19. Zucker, I. H., Share, L., and Gilmore, J. P.: Renal effects of left atrial distention in dogs with chronic congestive heart failure. Am. J. Physiol. *236*:H554, 1979.
20. Birkenfeld, L. W., Liebman, J., O'Meara, M. P., and Edelman, I. S.: Total exchangeable sodium, total exchangeable potassium, and total body water in edematous patients with cirrhosis of the liver and congestive heart failure. J. Clin. Invest. *37*:687, 1958.
21. Carroll, H. J., Gotterer, R., and Altshuler, B.: Exchangeable sodium, body potassium, and body water in previously edematous cardiac patients. Evidence for osmotic inactivation of cation. Circulation *32*:185, 1965.
22. Farber, S. J., and Schubert, M.: The binding of cations by chondroitin sulfate. J. Clin. Invest. *36*:1715, 1957.

23. Hricik, D. E., and Kassirer, J. P.: Azotemia in cardiac failure. J. Cardiovasc. Med. *8*:397, 1983.
24. Domenet, J. G., and Evans, D. W.: Uremia in congestive heart failure. Q. J. Med. *38*:117, 1969.
25. Baehr, G., and Laude, H.: Glomerulonephritis as a complication of subacute streptococcus endocarditis. J.A.M.A. *75*:789, 1920.
26. Glassock, R. J.: Pathophysiology of glomerular diseases. *In* Brenner, B. M., and Rector, F. C. (eds.): The Kidney. 2nd ed. Philadelphia, W. B. Saunders Co., 1980.
27. Gutman, R. A., Striker, G. E., Gilliland, B. C., and Cutler, R. E.: The immune complex glomerulonephritis of bacterial endocarditis. Medicine *51*:1, 1972.
28. Coggins, C. H.: Nephrotic and nephritic edema. *In* Brenner, B. M., and Stein, J. H. (eds.): Sodium and Water Homeostasis. New York, Churchill Livingstone, 1978, p. 117.
29. Levinsky, N. G., Alexander, E. A., and Venkatachalam, M. A.: Acute renal failure. *In* Brenner, B. M., and Rector, F. C. (eds.): The Kidney. 2nd ed. Philadelphia, W. B. Saunders Co., 1980.
30. Harrington, J. T., Sommers, S. C., and Kassirer, J. P.: Atheromatous emboli with progressive renal failure. Renal arteriography as the probable inciting factor. Ann. Intern. Med. *68*:152, 1968.
31. Kassirer, J. P.: Atheroembolic renal disease. N. Engl. J. Med. *280*:812, 1969.
32. Strange, P. V., and Sumner, A. T.: Predicting treatment costs and life expectancy for end-stage renal disease. N. Engl. J. Med. *298*:372, 1978.
33. Lindner, A., Charra, B., Sherrard, D. J., and Scribner, B. H.: Accelerated atherosclerosis in prolonged maintenance hemodialysis. N. Engl. J. Med. *290*: 697, 1974.
34. Lazarus, J. M., Lowrie, E. G., Hampers, C. L., and Merrill, J. P.: Cardiovascular disease in uremic patients on hemodialysis. Kidney Int. *7* (Suppl. 2): S167, 1975.
35. Friedman, H. S., Shah, B. N., Kim, H. J. G., Bove, L. A., Del Monte, M. M., and Smith, A. J.: Clinical study of the cardiac findings in patients with chronic maintenance hemodialysis: The relationship to coronary risk factors. Clin. Nephrol. *16*:75, 1981.
36. deMello, V. R., Malone, D., Thanovaro, S., Kleiger, R. E., Kessler, G., and Oliver, G. C.: Cardiac arrhythmias in end-stage renal disease. South. Med. J. *74*:178, 1981.
37. Zawada, E. T., Jr., Stinson, J. B., and Done, G.: New perspectives on coronary artery disease in hemodialysis patients. South. Med. J. *75*:694, 1982.
38. Francis, G. S., Conty, C. M., Sharma, B., and Helseth, H. K.: Myocardial revascularization in chronic renal disease patients. *In* Love, J. (ed.): Cardiac Surgery in Patients with Chronic Renal Disease. Mt. Kisco, N.Y., Futura Publishing Co., 1982, pp. 115–134.
39. Roig, E., Betriu, A., Castaner, A., Magrina, J., Sanz, G., and Navarrlo-Lopez, F.: Disabling angina pectoris with normal coronary arteries in patients undergoing long-term hemodialysis. Am. J. Med. *71*:431, 1981.
40. Kim, K. E., Onesti, G., and Schwartz, A. B.: Hemodynamics of hypertension in chronic end-stage renal disease. Circulation *467*:456, 1972.
41. Kim, K. E., Onesti, G., and Schwartz, A. B.: Hemodynamic alterations in hypertension of chronic end-stage renal disease. *In* Onesti, G., Kim, K. E., and Moyer, J. H. (eds.): Hypertension: Mechanisms and Management. New York, Grune and Stratton, 1973, p. 609.
42. Dustan, H. P., and Page, I. H.: Some factors in renal and renoprival hypertension. J. Lab. Clin. Med. *64*:948, 1964.
43. Vertes, V., Cangiano, J. L., Berman, L. B., and Gould, A.: Hypertension in end-stage renal disease. N. Engl. J. Med. *280*:978, 1969.
44. DePlanque, B. A., Mulder, E., and Mees, E. J. D.: The behavior of blood and extracellular volume in hypertensive patients with renal insufficiency. Acta Med. Scand. *186*:75, 1969.
45. Lazarus, J. M., Hampers, C. L., and Merrill, J. P.: Hypertension and chronic renal failure. Treatment with hemodialysis and nephrectomy. Arch. Intern. Med. *133*:1059, 1974.
46. Wilkinson, R., Scott, D. F., Uldall, P. R., Kerr, D. N. S., and Swinney, J.: Plasma renin and exchangeable sodium in the hypertension of chronic renal failure. The effect of bilateral nephrectomy. Q. J. Med. *39*:377, 1970.
47. Cangiano, J. L., Ramirez-Muxo, O., Ramirez-Gonzalez, R., Trevino, A., and Campos, J. A.: Normal renin uremic hypertension. Arch. Intern. med. *136*:17, 1976.
48. Lazarus, J. M., Hampers, C. L., Lowrie, E. G., and Merrill, J. P.: Baroreceptor activity in normotensive and hypertensive uremic patients. Circulation *47*: 1015, 1973.
49. Lilley, J. J., Golden, J., and Stone, R. A.: Adrenergic regulation of blood pressure in chronic renal failure. J. Clin. Invest. *57*:1190, 1976.
50. Grollman, A., and Krishnamurty, V. S. R.: A new pressor agent of renal origin: Its differentiation from renin and angiotensin. Am. J. Physiol. *221*: 1499, 1971.
51. Muirhead, E. E., Brown, G. B., Germain, G. S., and Leach, B. E.: The renal medulla as an antihypertensive organ. J. Lab. Clin. med. *76*:641, 1970.
52. Lee, J. B., and Mookerjee, B. K.: The renal prostaglandins as etiologic factors in human essential hypertension. Fact or fantasy? Cardiovasc. Med. *1*:302, 1976.
53. Hull, A. R., Long, D. L., Prati, R. C., Pettinger, W. A., and Parker, T. F., III: The control of hypertension in patients undergoing regular maintenance dialysis. Kidney Int. *7* (Suppl. 2):S184, 1975.
54. Briggs, W. A., Lowenthal, D. T., Cirksina, W. J., Price, W. E., Gibson, T. P., and Flamenbaum, W.: Propranolol in hypertensive dialysis patients: Efficacy and compliance. Clin. Pharmacol. Ther. *18*:606, 1975.
55. Gelfand, M. C., Horton, J., Gottlieb, M., Winchester, J. F., Lowrie, E. G., Farate, A., Miller, D., Lazarus, J. M., and Schreiner, G. E.: Asymptomatic pericardial effusion—A possible complication of minoxidil therapy in patients with chronic renal failure. Abstracts, Sixth International Congress of Nephrology, Montreal, 1978, p. B23.
56. Lazarus, J. M., Hampers, C. L., Bennett, A. H., VanDam, L. D., and Merrill, J. P.: Urgent bilateral nephrectomy for severe hypertension. Ann. Intern. Med. *76*:733, 1972.
57. Woods, T. W., Blythe, W. B., and Huffines, W. D.: Malignant hypertension and renal insufficiency. N. Engl. J. Med. *291*:10, 1974.
58. Bachy, C., Alexandre, G. P. J., and van Ypersele de Strihou, C.: Hypertension after renal transplantation. Br. Med. J. *2*:1287, 1976.
59. Popovtzer, M. M., Pinnggera, W., Katz, F. H., Corman, J. L., Robinette, J., Lanois, B., Halgrimson, C. G., and Starzl, T. E.: Variations in arterial blood pressure after kidney transplantation: Relation to renal function, plasma renin activity and the dose of prednisone. Circulation *47*:1297, 1973.
60. McPhaul, J. J., Jr., Thompson, A. L., Jr., Lordon, R. E., Klebanoff, G., Cosimi, A. B., de Lemos, R., and Smith, R. B.: Evidence suggesting persistence of nephritogenic immunopathologic mechanisms in patients receiving renal allografts. J. Clin. Invest. *52*:1059, 1973.
61. Lacombe, M.: Arterial stenosis complicating allotransplantation in man. Ann. Surg. *181*:283, 1975.
62. Ibels, L. S., Alfrey, A. C., and Weil, R., III: Hyperlipidemia in adult, pediatric and diabetic transplant recipients. Am. J. Med. *64*:634, 1978.
63. Matas, A. J., Simmons, R. L., Buselmeier, T. J., Kjellstrand, C. M., and Najarian, J. S.: The fate of patients surviving three years after renal transplantation. Surgery *80*:390, 1976.
64. Bagdade, J., Casaretto, A., and Albers, J.: Effects of chronic uremia, hemodialysis and renal transplantation on plasma lipids and lipoproteins in man. J. Lab. Clin. Med. *87*:37, 1976.
65. Brunzell, J. D., Albers, J. J., Haas, L. B., Goldberg, A. P., Agode, L., and Sherrard, D. J.: Prevalence of serum lipid abnormalities in chronic hemodialysis. Metabolism *26*:903, 1977.
66. Rapoport, J., Aviram, M., Chaimovitz, C., and Brook, J. G.: Defective high density lipoprotein composition in patients on chronic hemodialysis. N. Engl. J. Med. *299*:1326, 1978.
67. Nestel, P. J., Fidge, N. H., and Tan, M. H.: Increased lipoprotein-remnant formation in chronic renal failure. N. Engl. J. Med. *307*:329, 1982.
68. Murase, T., Cattran, D. C., Pakenstein, B., and Steiner, G.: Inhibition of lipoprotein lipase by uremic serum. A possible cause of hypertriglyceridemia. Metabolism *24*:1279, 1975.
69. Mordasini, R., Frey, F., Flury, W., Klose, G., and Greten, H.: Selective deficiency of hepatic triglyceride lipase in uremia patients. N. Engl. J. Med. *297*:1362, 1977.
70. Goldberg, A. P., Sherrard, D. J., and Brunzell, J.: Hypertriglyceridemia in hemodialysis patients; dual defect of adipose tissue lipoprotein lipase. Clin. Res. *24*:361A, 1976.
71. Cattran, D. C., Fenton, S. S. A., Wilson, D. R., and Steiner, G.: Defective triglyceride removal in lipemia associated with peritoneal dialysis and haemodialysis. Ann. Intern. Med. *85*:29, 1976.
72. Havel, R. J., Kane, J. P., and Kashyap, M. L.: Interchange of apolipoproteins between chylomicrons and high density lipoproteins during alimentary lipemia in man. J. Clin. Invest. *52*:32, 1973.
73. LaRosa, J. C., Levy, R. I., Herbert, P., Lux, S. E., and Fredrickson, D. S.: A specific apoprotein activator for lipoprotein lipase. Biochem. Biophys. Res. Commun. *41*:57, 1970.
74. Fisher, W. R., and Truitt, D. H.: The common hyperlipoproteinemias. Ann. Intern. Med. *85*:497, 1976.
75. Uraemia, lipoproteins and atherosclerosis. Lancet *2*:1151, 1981.
76. Sanfelippo, M. L., Swensen, R. S., and Reaven, G. M.: Reduction of plasma triglycerides by diet in subjects with chronic renal failure. Kidney Int. *11*:54, 1977.
77. Goldberg, A. P., Sherrard, D. J., Haas, L. B., and Brunzell, J. D.: Control of clofibrate toxicity in uremic hypertriglyceridemia. Clin. Pharmacol. Ther. *21*: 317, 1977.
78. Eiser, A. R., and Swartz, C. E.: Hemodialysis and peritoneal dialysis in patients with cardiac disease. *In* Lowenthal, D. T. (ed.): Management of the Cardiac Patient with Renal Failure. Philadelphia, F. A., Davis Co., 1981, pp. 78–80.
79. Kleiger, R. E., deMello, V. R., Malone, D., Fernandes, J., Thanavaro, S., Connors, J. P., and Oliver G. C.: Left ventricular function in end-stage renal disease. Echocardiographic classification. South. Med. J. *74*:819, 1981.
80. Chaignon, M., Chen, W.-T., Tarazi, R. C., Nakamoto, S., and Salcedo, E.: Acute effects of hemodialysis on echographic-determined cardiac performance: Improved contractility resulting with serum increased calcium with reduced potassium despite hypovolemic-reduced cardiac output. Am. Heart J. *103*:374, 1982.
81. Cini, G., Camici, M., Pentimone, F., and Palla, R.: Echocardiographic hemodynamic study during ultrafiltration sequential dialysis. Nephron *30*:124, 1982.
82. Arduson, C. B., Codd, J. R., Graff, R. A., Grace, M. A., Harter, H. R., and Newton, W. T.: Cardiac failure in upper extremity arteriovenous dialysis fistulae. Arch. Intern. Med. *136*:292, 1976.
83. Nsouli, K. A., Lazarus, J. M., Schoenbaum, S. C., Gottlieb, M. N., Lowrie, E. G., and Shocair, M.: Bacteremic infection in hemodialysis. Arch. Intern. Med. *139*:1255, 1979.
84. Aurigemma, N. M., Feldman, N. T., Gottlieb, M. N., Ingram, R. H., Lazarus, J. M., and Lowrie, E. G.: Arterial oxygenation during hemodialysis. N. Engl. J. Med. *297*:871, 1977.

85. Mahajan, S., Kinhal, V., Gardiner, H., Briggs, W., and McDonald, F.: Cardiac functional changes during hemodialysis. Proc. Clin. Dial. Transplant Forum *7*:99, 1977.
86. Thayssen, P., Anderson, K. H., and Pindborg, T.: Non-invasive monitoring of cardiac function during haemodialysis. Scand. J. Urol. Nephrol. *15*:313, 1981.
87. Craddock, P. R., Fehr, J., Brigham, K. L., Dronenberg, R. S., and Jacob, H. S.: Complement and leukocyte mediated pulmonary dysfunction in hemodialysis. N. Engl. J. Med. *296*:769, 1977.
88. Fisch, C.: Relation of electrolyte disturbances to cardiac arrhythmias. Circulation *47*:408, 1973.
88a. D'Cruz, I. A., Jain, M., Fishman, S., Abrahams, C., and Kathpalia, S.: Calcification of the mitral region in patients with chronic renal failure: 2-D echocardiographic, hormonal and autopsy correlation. J. Am. Coll. Cardiol. *1*:625, 1983.
88b. Nestico, P. F., DePace, N. L., Kotler, M. N., Rose, L. I., Brezin, J. H., Swartz, C., Mintz, G., and Schwartz, A. B.: Calcium and phosphorus metabolism in dialysis patients with and without mitral anular calcium. Analysis of 30 patients. Am. J. Cardiol. *51*:497, 1983.
89. Roberts, W. C., and Waller, B. F.: Effect of chronic hypercalcemia on the heart. An analysis of 18 necropsy patients. Am. J. Med. *71*:371, 1981.
90. Depace, N. L., Rohrer, A. H., Kotler, M. N., Brezin, J. H., and Parry, W. R.: Rapidly progressing, massive mitral annular calcification. Arch. Intern. Med. *141*:1663, 1981.
91. Jain, M. C., D'Cruz, I., and Kathpalia, S.: Chronic renal failure: Intracardiac calcification. Primary Cardiol. Clin. *4*:27, 1981.
92. Terman, D. S., Alfrey, A. C., Hammond, W. S., Donndelinger, T., Ogden, D. A., and Holmes, J. H.: Cardiac calcification in uremia. A clinical, biochemical and pathologic study. Am. J. Med. *50*:744, 1971.
93. Arora, K., Lacy, J. P., Schacht, R. A., Martin, D. G., and Gutch, C. F.: Calcific cardiomyopathy in advanced renal failure. Arch. Intern. Med. *135*:603, 1975.
94. Friedman, S. A., Novak, S., and Thompson, G. E.: Arterial calcification and gangrene in uremia. N. Engl. J. Med. *280*:1392, 1969.
95. Rosen, H., Friedman, S. A., Raizner, A. E., and Gerstmann, K.: Azotemic arteriopathy. Am. Heart J. *84*:250, 1972.
96. Ejerblad, S., Ericsson, J. L. E., and Eriksson, I.: Arterial lesions of the radial artery in uraemic patients. Acta. Chir. Scand. *145*:415, 1979.
97. Drueke, T., Fleury, J., Toure, Y., deVernejoul, P., Fauchet, M., Lesourd, P., LePailleur, C., and Crosnier, J.: Effect of parathyroidectomy on left ventricular function in haemodialysis patients. Lancet *1*:112, 1980.
98. Verberckmoes, R., Bouillon, R., and Krempien, B.: Disappearance of vascular calcifications during treatment of renal osteodystrophy. Ann. Intern. Med. *82*: 529, 1975.
99. Wacker, W., and Merrill, J. P.: Uremic pericarditis in acute and chronic renal failure. J.A.M.A. *156*:764, 1954.
100. Bailey, G. L., Hampers, C. L., Hager, E. B., and Merrill, J. P.: Uremic pericarditis: Clinical features and management. Circulation *38*:582, 1968.
101. Hoops, H. C., and Wissler, R. W.: Uremic pneumonitis. Am. J. Pathol. *31*: 361, 1955.
102. Nidus, B. D., Matalon, R., Cantazino, D., and Eisinger, R. P.: Uremic pleuritis—A clinicopathological entity. N. Engl. J. Med. *281*:255, 1969.
103. Galen, M. A., Steinberg, S. M., Lowrie, E. G., Lazarus, J. M., Hampers, C. L., and Merrill, J. P.: Hemorrhagic pleural effusions in patients undergoing chronic hemodialysis. Ann. Intern. Med. *82*:359, 1975.
104. Goldberg, M., Lazarus, J. M., Gottlieb, M. N., Lowrie, E. G., and Merrill, J. P.: Treatment of uremic pericardial effusion. Proc. Clin. Dial. Transplant Forum *5*:20, 1975.
105. Hampers, C. L., Schupak, E., Lowrie, E. G., and Lazarus, J. M.: Long Term Hemodialysis. 2nd ed. New York, Grune and Stratton, 1973, p. 80.
106. Kotler, M. N., and Parry, W. R.: Pericardial disease in chronic renal failure. *In* Lowenthal, D. T. (ed.): Management of the Cardiac Patient in Renal Failure. Philadelphia, F. A. Davis Co., 1981, pp. 78–80.
107. Comty, C. M., Cohen, S. L., and Shapiro, F. L.: Pericarditis in chronic uremia and its sequels. Ann. Intern. Med. *75*:173, 1971.
108. Ribot, S., Frankel, H. J., and Gielchinsky, I.: Treatment of uremic pericarditis. Clin. Nephrol. *2*:127, 1974.
109. Silverberg, S., Oreopoulos, D. G., and Wise, D. J.: Pericarditis in patients undergoing long-term hemodialysis and peritoneal dialysis. Incidence, complications and management. Am. J. Med. *63*:874, 1977.
110. Lazarus, J. M., Gottlieb, M. N., Lowrie, E. G., Teicholtz, L., and Merrill, J. P.: Echocardiographic findings in stable hemodialysis patients. Proc. Clin. Dial. Transplant Forum *6*:53, 1976.
111. Kleiman, J. H., Motta, J., London, E., Pennell, J. P., and Popp, R. L.: Pericardial effusions in patients with end-stage renal disease. Br. Heart J. *40*:190, 1978.
112. Fuller, T. J., Knochel, J. P., Brennan, J. P., Tetnu, C. D., and White, M. G.: Reversal of intractable uremic pericarditis by triamcinolone hexacetonide. Arch. Intern. Med. *136*:979, 1976.
113. Buselmeier, T. J., Simmons, R. L., Najarian, J. S., Mauer, S. M., Matas, A. J., and Kjellstrand, C. M.: Uremic pericardial effusion: Treatment by catheter drainage and local nonabsorbable steroid administration. Nephron *16*:371, 1976.
114. Connors, J. P., Kleiger, R. E., Shaw, R. C., Voiles, J. D., Clark, R. E., Harter, H., and Roper, C. L.: The indications for pericardiectomy in the uremic pericardial effusion. Surgery *80*:689, 1976.
115. Pillay, V. K. G., Sarpel, S. C., and Kurtzman, N. A.: Subacute constrictive uremic pericarditis: Survival after pericardiectomy. J.A.M.A. *235*:1351, 1976.
116. Hampers, C. L., Bailey, G. L., Hager, E. B., VanDam, L. D., and Merrill, J. P.: Major surgery in patients on maintenance hemodialysis. Am. J. Surg. *115*: 747, 1968.
117. Crawford, F. A., Jr., Selby, J. H., Jr., Bower, J. D., and Lehan, D. H.: Coronary revascularization in patients maintained on chronic hemodialysis. Circulation *56*:684, 1977.
118. Connors, J. P., and Shaw, R. C.: Considerations in the management of open-heart surgery in uremic patients. J. Thorac. Cardiovasc. Surg. *75*:400, 1978.
119. Lamberti, J. J., Jr., Cohn, L. H., and Collins, J. J., Jr.: Cardiac surgery in patients undergoing renal dialysis or transplantation. Ann. Thorac. Surg. *19*:135, 1975.
120. Chawla, R., Gailiunas, P., Jr., Lazarus, J. M., Gottlieb, M. N., Lowrie, E. G., Collins, J. J., and Merrill, J. P.: Cardiopulmonary bypass surgery in chronic hemodialysis and transplant patients. Trans. Am. Soc. Artif. Intern. Organs *23*:694, 1977.
121. Falch, D.: The influence of kidney function, body size and age on plasma concentration and urinary excretion of digoxin. Acta Med. Scand. *194*:251, 1973.
122. Steiness, E.: Renal tubular secretion of digoxin. Circulation *50*:103, 1974.
123. Jelliffe, R. W.: An improved method of digoxin therapy. Ann. Intern. Med. *69*:703, 1968.
124. Rasmussen, K., Jervell, J., Storstein, L., and Gjerdrum, K.: Digitoxin kinetics in patients with impaired renal function. Clin. Pharmacol. Ther. *13*:6, 1972.
125. Ackerman, G. L., Doherty, J. F., and Flanigan, W. J.: Peritoneal dialysis and hemodialysis of tritiated digoxin. Ann. Intern. Med. *67*:718, 1967.
126. Gibson, T. P., Lowenthal, D. T., Nelson, H. A., and Briggs, W. A.: Elimination of procainamide in end-stage renal failure. Clin. Pharmacol. Ther. *17*:321, 1975.
127. Conn, H. L., and Luchi, R. J.: Some quantitative aspects of the binding of quinidine and related quinolone compounds by human serum albumin. J. Clin. Invest. *40*:509, 1961.
128. Donadu, J. V., Whelton, A., and Kazyak, I.: Quinidine therapy and peritoneal dialysis in acute renal failure. Lancet *1*:375, 1968.
129. Thompson, P. D., Melmon, K. L., Richardson, J. A., Cohn, K., Steinbrunn, W., Cudikee, R., and Rowland, M.: Lidocaine pharmacokinetics in advanced heart failure, liver disease and renal failure in humans. Ann. Intern. Med. *78*: 499, 1973.
130. Eriksson, E., Granberg, P., and Ortengren, B.: Study of renal excretion of prilocaine and lidocaine. Acta Chir. Scand. *358*(Suppl):55, 1966.
131. Letteri, J. M., Mellk, H., Louis, S., Kutti, H., Durante, P., and Glazko, A.: Diphenylhydantoin metabolism in uremia. N. Engl. J. Med. *285*:648, 1971.
132. Reidenberg, M. M., Odar-Cederlof, I., VonBahr, C., Borga, M. L., and Sjoqvist, F.: Protein binding of diphenylhydantoin and dimethylimipramine in plasma from patients with poor renal function. N. Engl. J. Med. *285*:264, 1971.
133. Anderson, R. J., Gambertoglio, J. G., and Schrier, R. W.: Clinical Use of Drugs in Renal Failure. Springfield, Ill., Charles C Thomas, 1976, p. 251.
134. Evans, G. H., Nies, A. S., and Shand, D. G.: The disposition of propranolol. J. Pharmacol. Exp. Ther. *186*:114, 1973.
135. Thompson, P. D., Joekes A. M., and Foulkes, D. M.: Pharmacodynamics of propranolol in renal failure. Br. Med. J. *2*:434, 1972.
136. Shand, D. G., Wed, A. J. J., Vestal, R. E., Wilkinson, G. R., and Branch, R. A.: Pharmacokinetic and pharmacodynamic factors determining variations in propranolol responsiveness. *In* Braunwald, E. (ed.): Beta-Adrenergic Blockade. New York, Elsevier, 1978, pp. 74–80.
137. Lai, K. N., Barnden, L., and Mathew, T. H.: Effect of renal transplantation on left ventricular function in hemodialysis patients. Clin. Nephrol. *18*:74, 1982.
138. Capelli, J. P., and Kasparian, H.: Cardiac work demands and left ventricular function in end-stage renal disease. Ann. Intern. Med. *86*:261, 1977.
139. Crosbie, W. A., Snowden, S., and Parsons, V.: Changes in lung capillary permeability in renal failure. Br. Med. J. *4*:388, 1972.
140. Gotloib, L., and Servadio, C.: A possible case of beriberi heart failure in a chronic hemodialysis patient. Nephron *14*:293, 1975.
141. Raab, W.: Cardiotoxic substances in the blood and heart muscle in uremia. J. Lab. Clin. Med. *29*:715, 1944.
142. Scheuer, J., and Stezoski, S. W.: The effects of uremic components on cardiac function and metabolism. J. Mol. Cell. Cardiol. *5*:287, 1973.
143. Reicker, G., Velker, W., and Strauer, B. E.: Cardiac and circulatory disorders in renal insufficiency. *In* Uraemia: An International Conference on Pathogenesis, Diagnosis and Therapy. London, Churchill Livingstone, 1971, pp. 72–78.
144. Welt, L. G., Smith, E. K. M., Dunn, M. J., Czerwinski, A., Proctor, H., Cole, C., Balfo, J. W., and Gitelman, H. J.: Membrane transport defect: The sick cell. Tr. Assoc. Am. Physicians *80*:217, 1967.
145. Patrick, J., and Jones, N. F.: Cell sodium, potassium and water in uremia and the effects of regular dialysis as studied in the leukocyte. Clin. Sci. Mol. Med. *46*:583, 1974.
146. Prosser, D., and Parsons, V.: The case for a specific uremic myocardiopathy. Nephron *15*:4, 1975.
147. Gueron, M., Berlyne, C. M., Nord, E., and BenAri, J.: The case against the existence of a specific uraemic myocardiopathy. Nephron *15*:2, 1975.
148. Drüeke, T., Le Pailleur, C., Meilhac, B., Kontoudis, C., Zingraff, J., DiMatteo, J., and Crosnier, J.: Congestive cardiomyopathy in uremic patients on long-term haemodialysis. Br. Med. J. *1*:350, 1977.
149. Bailey, G. L., Hampers, C. L., and Merrill, J. P.: Reversible cardiomyopathy in uremia. Tr. Am. Soc. Artif. Intern. Organs *13*:263, 1967.
150. Hung, J., Harris, P. J., Uren, R. F., Tiller, D. J., and Kelly, D. T.: Uremic cardiomyopathy—Effect of hemodialysis on left ventricular function in end-stage renal failure. N. Engl. J. Med. *302*:547, 1980.

53 PREGNANCY AND CARDIOVASCULAR DISEASE

by Joseph K. Perloff, M.D.

IMPORTANCE OF THE PROBLEM

For statistical information to be meaningful it must take into consideration the population under study, since figures vary widely, especially in comparisons between populations of developed and underdeveloped countries. In India, for example, acute and chronic rheumatic heart disease still constitute a major health problem in the pregnant woman. In Venezuela and Argentina, the relatively high prevalence of Chagas' disease materially increases the probability of Chagasic cardiomyopathy among pregnant women.[1] In Western Europe and North America, maternal mortality from all causes has been steadily decreasing for decades. This favorable trend has resulted mainly from control of noncardiac causes of maternal death, especially preeclampsia, hemorrhage, and infection. During the first half of this century, approximately 1 to 4 per cent of pregnancies in the United States and Western Europe were complicated by cardiac disease, 90 per cent of which was rheumatic.[2] As a consequence of the decline in incidence of chronic rheumatic heart disease among pregnant patients, this condition now represents no more than 75 per cent of the cardiac disorders complicating pregnancy.[2]

Congenital heart disease previously constituted most of the 10 per cent of nonrheumatic heart disease complicating pregnancy. In recent years, the relative frequency of rheumatic and congenital heart disease in childbearing women has undergone a change. Although the number of pregnant women with rheumatic heart disease has declined, as pointed out above, the number of pregnant women with congenital heart disease has increased, because the natural rate of occurrence of congenital heart disease remains relatively constant at 0.8 per cent of live births and because, in addition, successful cardiac surgery has produced a new population of patients—the postoperative cardiac patient.[3, 3a] Operative intervention in childhood has permitted increasing numbers of women with congenital heart disease to reach childbearing age, including those with anomalies that heretofore would not have permitted survival beyond childhood.[3] Systemic hypertension, apart from coarctation of the aorta, may antedate pregnancy or appear for the first time during gestation. Preeclampsia is more frequent in pregnant patients with preexisting hypertension than in initially normotensive pregnant women.[4] Cardiomyopathy complicating pregnancy chiefly takes the form of postpartum or peripartum inflammatory disease of the myocardium.[5–7]

CARDIOPULMONARY CHANGES IN NORMAL PREGNANCY

Rational management of heart disease in pregnancy presupposes an understanding of the circulatory adaptations to the normal gravid state (Table 53–1).[8–11a] To describe these adaptive responses, four variables must be characterized: the time of onset of the adaptive change, the magnitude of the change, the time when the change reaches its peak, and the behavior of the adaptive response after it has reached its maximum deviation from the nonpregnant state. These data should be based upon serial studies in the same patients in order to circumvent the problem of variation among individuals.[12–14]

Cardiac Output

It is generally agreed that a rise in cardiac output is well under way by the end of the first trimester.[2,12–17] The peak increment—on the order of 30 to 50 per cent—is reached by the twentieth to twenty-fourth week of gestation.[2,12–14,16] Up to the twentieth week, an increase in heart rate is responsible for the augmented cardiac output, but thereafter an increase in stroke volume contributes.[14] Once the maximum cardiac output is achieved, the level is maintained

TABLE 53–1 CIRCULATORY CHANGES IN NORMAL PREGNANCY

Cardiac output	↑ 30 to 50%
Stroke volume	↑
Heart rate	↑ Average 10 beats/min
Blood volume	↑ 40 to 50%
Systemic blood pressure	↓ Slightly until term
Systemic vascular resistance	↓
Pulmonary vascular resistance	↓

throughout the course of pregnancy[2,12,16] when output is measured with the patient in the lateral recumbent but not in the supine position. The older belief that the elevated cardiac output declined toward the end of gestation[18] has been resolved by taking into account the position of the patient (supine or lateral) and the mechanical effects of the gravid uterus.[2,13,14,17,19–25] Early studies showing a late fall in cardiac output were performed with patients in the supine position.

It has long been known that the gravid uterus can exert profound mechanical effects simply by virtue of its weight and size and the position of the patient. When the uterus is manually lifted away from the inferior cava during cesarean section, the caval pressure falls dramatically, as it does when the patient turns on her side (Fig. 53–1).[19] When the cava is manually compressed under direct vision, complete occlusion produces a pressure equal to but not greater than that found in the supine position before delivery. These observations imply that complete caval occlusion occurs in supine patients late in pregnancy. Predelivery caval angiograms confirm complete occlusion in the majority of patients studied while supine and caval patency when patients were restudied in the lateral position. Venous return during caval occlusion is channeled via the azygous, lumbar, and paraspinal veins. The fall in caval pressure that occurs when the position is changed from supine to lateral is consistently accompanied by a reciprocal rise in cardiac output. Echocardiographic determinations of cardiac output at term have confirmed that when patients turn from supine to lateral recumbence, the output rises appreciably.[13,14,17] Interestingly, these postural hemodynamic changes appear to be attenuated when the fetal head is engaged in the pelvis, thus rendering the uterus less mobile.[19] In addition to its effect on the cava, the gravid uterus partially compresses the abdominal aorta and displaces it laterally.[24]

As a rule, the normal fall in cardiac output in the supine position is not associated with a decline in systemic blood pressure, implying that peripheral vascular resistance rises appropriately.[2,19] In fact, brachial arterial pressure in the left lateral position may be lower than in the supine position, even after the twenty-eighth week.[20,21] However, there is a tendency for a supine related fall in femoral arterial pressure.[22] An occasional patient experiences lightheadedness or frank syncope when supine; arterial pressure becomes depressed, and the heart rate slows, i.e., bradycardiac syncope occurs.[2,19,26] This is the most dramatic form of the so-called supine hypotensive syndrome of pregnancy, which can be promptly relieved simply by turning the patient on her side. Postural shock is a special problem when it manifests itself under anesthesia, which sometimes abolishes the compensatory peripheral vasoconstriction required to maintain systemic blood pressure in the supine position.[19]

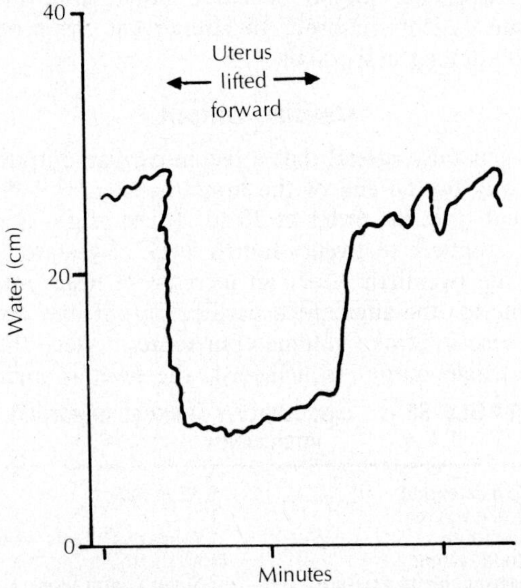

FIGURE 53–1 Effect on the inferior cava pressure of lifting the gravid uterus forward before opening the uterus at cesarean section. (From Kerr, M. G.: The mechanical effects of the gravid uterus in late pregnancy. J. Obstet. Gynecol. Br. Comm. *72*:513, 1965.)

The 30 to 50 per cent rise in resting cardiac output which occurs during pregnancy is accompanied by increments in stroke volume[2,13,14,16,17] but not necessarily in ejection fraction and mean velocity of circumferential fiber shortening.[13,17] An adaptive increase in left ventricular mass accompanies an increase in end-diastolic volume.[13] The magnitude and time course of these variables generally approximate the changes in cardiac output.[13,14,17] In addition, there is a rise in resting heart rate (average 10 beats per minute), which remains relatively constant in both supine and lateral recumbency, even at term.[2,13,19] Despite supine caval compression and a fall in cardiac output, the heart rate does not usually accelerate in this position. Failure to accelerate appears to be a feature of caval occlusion and has been demonstrated in nonpregnant patients undergoing laparotomy.[19]

Blood Volume and Intravascular Pressures

Blood volume is consistently elevated in normal pregnancy; plasma volume begins to rise as early as 6 weeks of gestation and increases rapidly until about midpregnancy and then more slowly until term. Total red cell volume, in contrast, increases steadily throughout pregnancy.[27] The relative difference between the increment in plasma volume (50 per cent) and that of red cell mass (20 to 40 per cent) accounts for the "physiologic anemia" of pregnancy. The increase in total blood volume is on the order of 40 to 50 per cent. The increment is higher in twin pregnancy than in single pregnancy and greater in multigravidas than in primigravidas.[2,28] Importantly, the time course of the changes in blood volume does not parallel the variations in cardiac output.[16] The average increase in exchangeable sodium is about 500 to 600 mEq, and in the average pregnant woman total body water increases by about 8.5 liters.[2]

Systemic arterial blood pressure declines slightly in early pregnancy. Systolic pressure falls from the nonpregnant level, and there is a somewhat greater reduction in diastolic pressure, resulting in a slight increase in pulse pressure that reflects the augmentation of stroke volume.[13,14] Both systolic and diastolic pressures tend to return toward nonpregnant levels before term.[2,29] Peripheral vascular resistance and mean arterial pressure appear to be lowest when cardiac output is maximal. Both maternal age and parity affect blood pressure during pregnancy. Systolic and diastolic pressures within a given age group decrease as parity increases, with the greatest difference observed between primiparas and multiparas; within each parity level, arterial pressures increase in older gravidas.[29] The effect of cigarette smoking on blood pressure is noteworthy. Smoking one to two cigarettes causes a prompt, short-term elevation in blood pressure and, in late pregnancy, a significant increase in fetal heart rate and a reduction in fetal breathing movements (see below).[30,31]

Pulmonary arterial systolic, diastolic, and mean pressures remain unchanged during the course of normal pregnancy despite the increased cardiac output, implying a reciprocal decline in pulmonary vascular resistance.[2,18] Thus, the right ventricle, like the left, handles an augmented volume but ejects this load at a normal systolic pressure. The increased work performed by both ventricles thus represents pure volume overload.[18]

Peripheral edema is a normal occurrence in uncomplicated pregnancy and can occur in the absence of either cardiac or renal disease.[2] Increased tissue hydration is considered universal in normal pregnancy, and clinical edema is found in 50 to 80 per cent of healthy gravid women.[32] The frequency of peripheral edema increases with maternal age, especially over 30 years. The presence and degree of edema are chiefly attributable to the increase in body water and total exchangeable sodium. In the third trimester there is the additive effect of increased venous pressure in the lower extremities in the supine and especially in the standing posture;[2] this is produced by compression of the inferior vena cava by the gravid uterus, particularly in the face of increased uterine blood flow draining into the inferior cava (see below). Varicosities are not normal features of pregnancy, but the above factors predispose to them.

Light to moderate exercise during uncomplicated pregnancy provokes an appropriate rise in cardiac output. The increments in cardiac output relative to oxygen consumption are normal and constant in all stages of pregnancy.[33] However, since the resting cardiac output is increased, the circulatory demands of exercise for any given workload are additive, implying that maximum cardiac output is reached at a correspondingly lower work level in pregnancy than in the nonpregnant state.[34]

Effects of Labor and Delivery

Labor and delivery initiate circulatory responses that are best understood when consideration is given to the method of delivery, the maternal posture, and the type and amount of sedation and anesthesia. In lightly sedated but unanesthetized women who deliver vaginally, maternal hemodynamics vary at different stages of labor according to the intensity and frequency of uterine contractions. The contracting uterus finds its support in the retrouterine fulcrum formed by the most protruding segment of lumbar lordosis (L_4-L_5).[24] During major uterine contractions, mean systemic arterial pressure rises approximately 10 per cent, and a significant amount of blood (estimated at 300 to 500 ml) is expressed into the maternal circulation.[23] The increment in venous return and the transient increase in heart rate result in augmentation of cardiac output (15 to 20 per cent) followed by reflex bradycardia.[2,23]

Contraction of the uterus also results in extrinsic compression of the aorta, particularly in the supine position.[23] This, combined with compression of the uterine vasculature within the contracting wall, transiently diverts cardiac output from the uterus and lower extremities with each contraction.[18] The rises in cardiac output and systemic arterial pressure indicate an increase in cardiac work. Caudal anesthesia does not affect the hemodynamic changes caused by uterine contraction per se, but the elevation of cardiac output during periods of uterine quiescence is abolished, since that rise is largely a response to pain and apprehension.[2]

The circulatory changes immediately following delivery are necessarily influenced by the amount of blood loss, which averages 500 ml or more with vaginal delivery and approximates 1000 ml with cesarean section. The pregnant woman tolerates such losses without ill effect, which is understandable, since the loss is in large part a desirable corrective for the increased blood volume accumulated during pregnancy. Accordingly, gestational hypervolemia can be looked upon as a safeguard against maternal blood loss at delivery, and normal maternal blood loss can be looked on as a corrective against the no longer needed gestational hypervolemia.[18] Nevertheless, the early puerperium is generally characterized by bradycardia, regardless of anesthetic technique, and a rise in cardiac output of about 10 to 20 per cent above predelivery levels.[2,35] Cardiac output begins to increase immediately after delivery as a consequence of the relief of inferior vena cava compression by the gravid uterus, and, along with puerperal bradycardia, this increase may persist for 2 weeks. A transient postpartal increase in blood volume has been attributed to both the autotransfusion from the contracting uterus and the absorption into the circulation of extracellular fluid accumulated during gestation. Puerperal diuresis then reduces total body water, and nongravid blood volume is restored 4 to 6 weeks after delivery.[2] However, this transient rise in blood volume is not a necessary feature of the early puerperium. Apart from blood loss during delivery, good renal function appears to be capable of rapid clearance of excess extracellular fluid without a detectable rise in blood volume.[28]

MECHANISM OF CIRCULATORY CHANGES

The circulatory changes of normal pregnancy described above can be looked upon from two points of view: either as responses that precede and therefore anticipate the needs of the growing fetus or as adaptive responses to the metabolic and nutritional needs of the fetus.[16] The increases in body water, blood volume, cardiac output, heart rate, and stroke volume and the fall in peripheral vascular resistance begin by the end of the first trimester, i.e., before fetal metabolic demands are fully evident.[2,12-17,36] Further, the time courses of changes in cardiac output and in blood volume are not parallel, so the former does not depend entirely upon the latter.[16] The timing and magnitude of the hemodynamic changes of normal pregnancy therefore precede and for a time exceed the demands of the fetus, whose needs are nicely anticipated. Similarly, the hypothesis that the placenta acts as a large arteriovenous fistula provoking most if not all of the above circulatory responses is not borne out, because hemodynamic changes begin before the placenta is well enough developed to function as a fistula.[16] If neither the metabolic and nutritional needs of the fetus nor the effect of the placenta as a fistula initiates the cardiocirculatory changes of pregnancy, what are the alternatives? Ovarian and/or placental sex steroids may play pivotal roles. Estrogen administration to pregnant ewes causes an increase in heart rate, cardiac output, and blood flow to the breast, uterus, and skin, whereas peripheral vascular resistance declines.[37,38] Moreover, estrogens have been found to increase myocardial contractility by what may be a direct effect on the contractile proteins.[39] Estrogen and progesterone concentrations rise progressively during gestation, and, by stimulating an increase in circulating levels of aldosterone, serve to promote retention of sodium and an increase of total body water.[40] Progesterone also causes venous relaxation, thereby increasing vascular capacity and promoting fluid retention.[41]

The importance of hormonal effects on circulatory physiology early in the course of normal pregnancy should not obscure the roles of a host of other factors that contribute in varying degrees as pregnancy proceeds into the second and third trimesters. Growth of the uterus, placenta, and breasts is associated with an increase in vascular capacity and in total circulating blood volume.[16] There is a general correlation between total blood volume and the weight of the products of conception.[28] Moreover, in the supine position in late pregnancy, the ability to excrete large water loads is limited.[19]

THE AORTA IN PREGNANCY

The morphology of the aorta in normal pregnancy has been the subject of several studies but with conflicting results. Significant and specific changes were found in the aortic media of pregnant rabbits, and similar alterations have been described in the aorta of gravid women. Histochemical changes varied according to the duration of pregnancy and included fragmentation of reticular fibers, decrease in acid mucopolysaccharides, loss of the normal corrugation (wavy pattern) of elastic fibers, and both hypertrophy and hyperplasia of smooth muscle cells. These biochemical and morphological alterations in the aortic wall have been attributed to hormonal effects,[42] but the findings have not been confirmed.[43]

RESPIRATORY CHANGES IN NORMAL PREGNANCY

Changes in the control of respiration, in lung volumes and mechanics, and in acid-base balance normally occur during pregnancy (Table 53–2). In addition, the placenta provides the means for the critical interplay between maternal and fetal gas exchange. Thus, respiratory physiology of the normal pregnant state may be appropriately considered from two points of view, namely, changes in maternal respiration and maternal/fetal respiratory interactions.[34,44]

Resting oxygen consumption rises progressively during the course of normal pregnancy, reaching a maximum of about 30 per cent near term.[44] Hyperventilation, which is consistently present, is manifested by an increase in minute ventilation that both precedes the rise in oxygen consumption and is approximately twice its magnitude. The increase in resting minute ventilation begins early in pregnancy and reaches a maximum of approximately 40 to 50 per cent in the last 4 weeks of gestation. Hyperventilation is believed to be mediated primarily by progesterone. The hormonally mediated hyperventilation and hypocapnia of pregnancy are associated with renal excretion of HCO_3, so that pH is maintained within the normal range. Thus, compensated respiratory alkalosis is the principal acid-base pattern of normal pregnancy.[44]

During mild to moderate exercise in the first two trimesters, the ventilatory response is similar to that occurring in the nonpregnant state.[34,44] In the last trimester, however, exercise-induced increments in minute ventilation and oxygen consumption are greater in magnitude.[45]

The functional residual capacity (lung volume at the end of quiet expiration) falls as the gravid uterus elevates the diaphragm. However, this fall is accompanied by an increase in inspiratory capacity, so that total lung capacity is reduced little, if at all.[44,46,47] Pulmonary capillary blood volume is not increased in normal pregnant women,[46] and pulmonary compliance remains normal.[44]

There is a decrease in *total* pulmonary respiratory resistance to approximately one-half that in the nongravid state.[44] This reduction is almost entirely the result of diminished airway resistance per se, suggesting a hormonally mediated effect on tracheobronchial smooth muscle tone and an increase in airway cross-sectional area.[44]

Although pulmonary compliance remains normal during pregnancy, the work of breathing increases,[48] owing partly to hyperventilation and partly to the extra work required to displace the diaphragm as the uterus enlarges. Because of the reduction in airway resistance, only a small increase in the work of quiet breathing occurs during normal gestation.[44]

Placental production of progesterone contributes to maternal hyperventilation, favoring the transfer of carbon dioxide from fetal to maternal blood. The placenta has sometimes been considered functionally analogous to the lung,[49] but there are significant differences. Placental oxygen transfer is facilitated by the relatively higher affinity of fetal hemoglobin for oxygen. However, hemoglobin concentration and the rates of uterine and umbilical blood flow are more important determinants of the rate of placental oxygen transfer.

Cardiorespiratory Symptoms and Signs in Normal Pregnancy

Normal uncomplicated pregnancy is accompanied by symptoms, physical signs, and electrocardiographic, roentgenographic, and echocardiographic changes that simulate heart disease and can be erroneously attributed to it (Table 53–3). The circulatory and respiratory changes occurring during normal pregnancy described above provide an explanation for these findings.

TABLE 53–2 RESPIRATORY CHANGES IN NORMAL PREGNANCY

O_2 consumption	↑
Minute ventilation	↑
Functional residual capacity	↓
Inspiratory capacity	↑
Vital capacity	Unchanged
Total lung capacity	Unchanged
Pulmonary compliance	Unchanged
Airway resistance	↓
Compensated respiratory alkalosis	

TABLE 53–3 CARDIORESPIRATORY SYMPTOMS AND SIGNS IN NORMAL PREGNANCY

Dyspnea
Hyperventilation
Easy fatigability
Decreased exercise tolerance
Lightheadedness
Syncope
Peripheral edema
Basilar rales
Small waterhammer pulse
Prominent jugular venous *a-v* crests and *x-y* troughs
Brisk, displaced left ventricular impulse
Right ventricular impulse
Increased first heart sound
Persistently split second heart sound
Third heart sound
Pulmonic midsystolic murmur
Supraclavicular systolic murmur
Continuous murmurs
ECG changes in rhythm, axis, and repolarization
X-ray—lateral displacement of apex, increased lung markings

Dyspnea, easy fatigability, and a reduction in exercise tolerance are relatively common.[12] In late pregnancy, the supine hypotensive syndrome (see above) occasionally causes lightheadedness or even syncope.[19] On physical examination, the combination of basilar rales (that disappear after coughing or deep breathing) and peripheral edema may be misleading. The systemic arterial pulse often exhibits a brisk rise and collapse (small waterhammer) beginning as early as the end of the first trimester,[50] findings in accord with augmented stroke volume, and echocardiographic registration of increased systolic motion of the aortic root.[17] Arterial pulsations can sometimes be palpated in the fingertips.

On *precordial palpation* (p. 26) there is generally a brisk, nonsustained left ventricular impulse that may be displaced to the left and often also an impulse over the right ventricle (mid to lower left sternal edge) and pulmonary trunk (second left intercostal space).[50] However, as pregnancy progresses, enlargement of the breasts and abdomen makes these signs difficult to elicit.

The *jugular venous pulse* (p. 20) is more easily seen during pregnancy, with clearly defined and relatively prominent *a* and *v* peaks and brisk *x* and *y* descents. The mean jugular venous pressure, as estimated from the superficial jugular vein, remains normal.

AUSCULTATORY FINDINGS. During normal gestation these start at the end of the first trimester, disappear (with few exceptions) a week after delivery, and include variations in heart sounds and the presence of systolic and continuous murmurs.[50,51] The *first heart sound* is increased in intensity (tachycardia and increased left ventricular contractility) and is often prominently split. The *second heart sound,* at least toward the end of pregnancy, tends to exhibit persistent expiratory splitting, especially when patients are examined in the lateral position. However, the supine position may restore the splitting to normal, owing to decreased venous return caused by uterine compression of the inferior vena cava. Since *third heart sounds* are common in normal young nonpregnant women, it is not surprising that the increased rate of atrioventricular flow during pregnancy would augment the intensity of these sounds.[50] Occasionally, a prominent third heart sound is followed by brief, soft, low-frequency after-vibrations that can be mistaken for a short mid-diastolic murmur. With this exception, diastolic murmurs are not features of uncomplicated pregnancy. Fourth heart sounds seldom occur in healthy young persons, male or female, and should not occur during normal pregnancy. Low-frequency oscillations with the timing of fourth heart sounds are occasionally recorded with appropriate phonocardiographic filters, but these vibrations are seldom audible.[50]

Murmurs. Two types of functional (innocent) *systolic murmurs* occur in healthy nonpregnant women, and these murmurs increase in intensity and prevalence during pregnancy.[52] The innocent or normal pulmonic midsystolic murmur (maximal in the second left intercostal space) represents audible vibrations caused by right ventricular ejection into the pulmonary trunk; innocent or normal supraclavicular systolic murmurs originate in brachiocephalic arteries at their points of branching from the aortic arch.[53] Both these murmurs are midsystolic, beginning after the first heart sound and terminating before the second, and both are understandably augmented by the increased cardiac output and stroke volume during pregnancy. The pulmonic midsystolic murmur seldom exceeds grade 3 (of six), but the supraclavicular systolic murmur may exceed grade 4 and occasionally radiates, with attenuation, below the clavicles. A third innocent murmur, this one peculiar to pregnancy—the *mammary souffle*—can be either systolic or continuous. The mammary souffle, like all arterial murmurs, is louder in systole whether or not it is continuous, and at times it is confined to systole.[53,54] This murmur is heard over the breasts late in pregnancy, but especially in the postpartum period in lactating women. There is a tendency for the murmur to be loudest in the second or third right or left intercostal spaces bilaterally. The souffle is best heard with the patient supine and may vanish altogether in the upright position, with firm pressure of the stethoscope or with digital compression adjacent to the site of auscultation. In addition, the day-to-day or cycle-to-cycle variation of the murmur and its permanent disappearance following termination of lactation are reassuring features of normality. A second and far more common continuous murmur is the *venous hum* (p. 30). The hum is relatively frequent in nonpregnant young women and, if properly sought, is almost universal during gestation. Rarely, the hum is loud enough to radiate beneath the clavicle, but wherever heard, it promptly vanishes with compression of the ipsilateral deep jugular vein.

Some murmurs caused by organic heart disease increase in intensity during pregnancy owing to the increase in cardiac output and stroke volume associated with the gravid state. The murmurs of pulmonic stenosis and aortic stenosis fall into this category; the murmur of mitral stenosis is especially accentuated because the increased blood flow and the shortening of diastolic filling time as the heart rate increases combine to augment the rate of flow across the mitral valve.

The diminution or disappearance of organic murmurs during pregnancy is less well-known but equally important.[51] The decrease in peripheral vascular resistance that accompanies pregnancy may cause the murmurs of aortic regurgitation or mitral regurgitation to soften or even disappear.[55] Prolapse of the mitral valve is relatively common in healthy young women (p. 1089), and the auscultatory hallmarks—the systolic click(s) and late systolic murmur—vary with alterations in left ventricular volume and shape.[56] The increase in left ventricular internal dimensions and volume at end diastole during pregnancy[17] may be enough to attenuate or abolish both the click(s) and late systolic murmur.[57] Similarly, the systolic murmur of hypertrophic obstructive cardiomyopathy may decrease or vanish as the left ventricle handles a larger volume during gestation (p. 1409).[58]

ELECTROCARDIOGRAPHIC CHANGES. The electrocardiogram in normal pregnant women may exhibit changes in rate, rhythm, P-R interval, QRS axis, ST segment, T wave, and Q-T interval.[59] Heart rate increases (see above), accounting for a slight decrease in PR interval and QT interval.[60] Premature atrial and ventricular beats are relatively frequent, and apparently innocent ventricular bigeminy sometimes occurs. Reentrant supraventricular tachycardia is most common in normal young women, and pregnancy lowers the threshold for recurrences in susceptible patients.[2] The P wave exhibits no change in amplitude, duration, or axis. The QRS amplitude and duration remain unaltered but not the axis, which may undergo a leftward shift averaging 40 degress in the third trimester.[60] The axis sometimes becomes more vertical somewhat near term as the fetus descends into the pelvis. A small Q wave may accompany T-wave inversions in lead III; deep inspiration tends to decrease or abolish both these changes.[2] Apart from this slight leftward shift of the T axis in the third trimester, there are no significant changes in amplitude, duration, or axis of the T wave,[60] with the following exception. Occasionally, slight, transient ST-segment depressions and T-wave inversions occur in limb and precordial leads and may recur during subsequent pregnancies in the same patient.[61] The mechanism is unknown. Atrioventricular conduction is seldom altered in normal pregnancy except for the slight decrease in P-R interval. In a study of 26,000 electrocardiograms in pregnant women with no other demonstrable heart disease, there were six examples of second-degree atrioventricular block of the Wenckebach type[62] (p. 731). An early report of paroxysmal ventricular tachycardia in a normal young pregnant woman probably represented a misdiagnosis of the Wolff-Parkinson-White syndrome.[63,64]

CHEST X-RAY. Radiation exposure is avoided in pregnant women, so there is relatively little information on plain film radiography. As pregnancy advances, elevation of the diaphragm results in a relatively horizontal cardiac position (upward and lateral displacement of the apex), with an increase in the cardiothoracic ratio.[2] The left cardiac silhouette straightens, and the vascular soft-tissue densities increase slightly.[2] Straightening of the left heart border as well as radiographic prominence of the main pulmonary artery is usually attributable to the hyperlordosis of pregnancy.[65]

ECHOCARDIOGRAM. Since echocardiography can be used with impunity during pregnancy, it is important to recognize that increases in stroke volume, cardiac output, ventricular volumes, and internal dimensions at end diastole are normal and expected (see above).

HEART DISEASE IN WOMEN OF CHILDBEARING AGE

The cardiocirculatory and respiratory changes and the symptoms and signs that accompany normal pregnancy set the stage for discussing the clinical manifestations of heart disease in the gravid woman. Cardiac disease can preexist the pregnancy or be induced by the gravid state (preclampsia/eclampsia, thromboembolic disease, possibly peripartum cardiomyopathy, and rarely, dissecting aneurysm). The types of cardiac disorders—acquired, congenital, or developmental—that are of the greatest clinical importance during pregnancy are obviously those most likely to occur in young women.[66] In addition, as has already been pointed out, cardiac surgery has produced a new and increasing patient population—the postoperative cardiac patient of childbearing age.[3] The prevailing patterns of heart disease vary geographically and socioeconomically and have changed during the course of time, especially in the last two decades.[2,67,68] It was long considered a truism that rheumatic mitral stenosis constituted the principle cardiac threat in pregnancy, since the most common form of heart disease in young women was the result of rheumatic fever, and its most common morphological expression, mitral stenosis, is a condition in which the female:male ratio of incidence is 4:1. However, although mitral stenosis is still the most frequent valvular abnormality in pregnancy, there has been a progressive decline since the early 1960's in both the incidence and the severity of rheumatic heart disease in prenatal clinics.[69]

Acute Rheumatic Fever (see p. 1641)

Acute rheumatic fever, especially the first episode, has its peak incidence before puberty, but because of recurrence, an occasional young woman conceives during the active phase of the rheumatic disease. Although there is no acceptable evidence that pregnancy per se predisposes to active rheumatic fever, evidence of recurrence is sometimes found during gestation.[70]

Chorea as a manifestation of active rheumatic fever has been reported during pregnancy,[70] and about two-thirds of women with chorea gravidarum have histories of prior chorea or rheumatic fever.[72] However, there are reports of women who manifest chorea during consecutive pregnancies but are otherwise free of it and, rarely, free of clinical evidence of rheumatic heart disease.[71] Chorea is more likely to occur in primigravidas, and in about half the instances it begins in the first trimester. Chorea remits prior to delivery in approximately one-third of the patients and shortly thereafter in the remainder.[72] Severe chorea has been accompanied by spontaneous abortion, premature labor, intrauterine fetal death, maternal heart failure, hyperpyrexia, and profound exhaustion. Termination of pregnancy is indicated when severe chorea is accompanied by violent, uncontrollable movements, agitation, and psychiatric disturbances.[72]

Active rheumatic carditis is a serious complication of pregnancy. Patients may die suddenly during labor or shortly after delivery, and a number of fatal cases have been reported without preexisting rheumatic valvular heart disease.[2] Conversely, active rheumatic carditis may initiate or aggravate heart failure in patients with established rheumatic valvular disease.

Chronic Rheumatic Valvular Disease
(See also Chap. 32)

MITRAL STENOSIS. Chronic rheumatic valvular heart disease in pregnancy is represented by pure or predominant mitral stenosis in 90 per cent of cases, by mitral regurgitation in about 6 to 7 per cent, and by aortic regurgitation/stenosis in the remainder.[2] In most cases women with rheumatic valvular disease—mild, moderate, and even severe—can be managed through relatively uneventful pregnancy and delivery. Nevertheless, these patients run the risk of complications, the majority relating to mitral stenosis and taking the form of pulmonary venous congestion (cough, breathlessness, orthopnea, paroxysmal nocturnal dyspnea, or pulmonary edema); sudden brisk hemoptysis (hemorrhage from varicosed bronchial veins); and, less commonly, atrial fibrillation, systemic or pulmonary emboli, and infective endocarditis.[2,73] One or more of these complications occur in about one-fourth of pregnant women with chronic rheumatic heart disease, but the incidence has declined in the past decade.[67,68]

The basic hemodynamic defect in mitral stenosis is the impediment to effective emptying of the left atrium. This defect is aggravated by at least two of the normal cardiocirculatory responses to pregnancy, namely, the increased cardiac output and the increase in heart rate, both of which augment the left atrioventricular pressure gradient and increase left atrial, pulmonary venous, and capillary pressures. Should atrial fibrillation supervene, the hemodynamic burden is compounded by the loss of left atrial contraction and often by a further acceleration of heart rate (and consequent reduction in the duration of diastole). Generally, the smaller the stenotic mitral orifice, the more likely symptomatic pulmonary venous congestion and its sequelae.

The woman with mitral stenosis faces hazards during pregnancy in addition to those of pulmonary congestion. These include right ventricular failure, thromboembolism, and pulmonary arterial hypertension. Right ventricular failure is, of course, undesirable in its own right, but especially during gestation because of the tendency of the pregnant woman to develop peripheral edema and varicose veins. Moreover, chronic peripheral venous stasis increases the risk of pulmonary embolism. Severe pulmonary hypertension—or, more precisely, high pulmonary vascular resistance—exposes the gravid female to special risks.[53,74] Physiological adaptations to fluctuations in cardiac output are limited; an increase in venous return is accompanied by a rise in pulmonary arterial pressure and/or further right ventricular failure; physical effort, stress, or excitement may provoke syncope due to acute right ventricular failure and little or no increase in cardiac output in the face of a fall in systemic vascular resistance. Pulmonary emboli are more likely to occur and more apt to be serious, if not lethal.

OTHER VALVULAR LESIONS. Patients with pure or predominant *rheumatic mitral regurgitation,* especially those with sinus rhythm, usually accommodate to the increased cardiac output and tachycardia of normal pregnancy. The left ventricle copes comparatively well with the increment in volume; the increase in heart rate is little or no handicap, and pulmonary hypertension is uncommon, but infective endocarditis is a real risk. Acute augmentation of mitral regurgitation due to rupture of chordae tendineae in the setting of rheumatic mitral valve disease is almost always a sequel of infective endocarditis.[75,76] As described below, spontaneous chordal rupture occurs in a different setting.[77,78]

Rheumatic aortic valve disease is usually accompanied by mitral valve disease, and the hemodynamic consequences of pregnancy must be considered in this light. The responses to isolated pure aortic regurgitation or aortic stenosis are discussed later.

Rheumatic tricuspid stenosis seldom occurs without associated mitral stenosis.[79] In this setting the aortic valve can be purely incompetent, can be purely stenotic, or can have varying combinations of each, but it is seldom normal. Obstruction of the tricuspid orifice serves to increase systemic venous pressure, promote peripheral edema, aggravate varices, and limit cardiac output, both at rest and with effort or stress.

The *time course of symptoms* complicating chronic rheumatic valvular disease, especially mitral stenosis, is noteworthy. Heart failure can occur at any stage, but the incidence rises as pregnancy progresses;[80] this trend continues to term because, as already discussed, cardiac output does not fall prior to delivery. The frequency of pulmonary venous congestion in patients with mitral stenosis increases with maternal age and parity, doubling when women over 30 years of age are compared with those younger than 20 years of age, especially during or after the third pregnancy.[2] It is important to emphasize, however, that previously asymptomatic women with rheumatic mitral stenosis and less than 30 years of age may also develop unanticipated acute pulmonary edema during pregnancy. This is usually provoked by undue effort or emotional stress, paroxysms of sinus or atrial tachycardia, or upper respiratory infections, but sometimes no apparent precipitating cause can be identified.[2]

Labor can also aggravate preexisting heart failure, but heart failure seldom has its onset during labor, especially if the pregnancy has been well managed. Therefore, the patient whose rheumatic valvular heart disease is well compensated at term can anticipate labor with little fear. However, the rapidly changing physiological adjustments during the puerperium (see above) are not without risk.

Congenital Heart Disease (See also Chap. 30)

Survival to adulthood of patients with congenital heart disease occurs as a result of natural selection or because of surgical intervention. Operation not only increases the life span of patients with anomalies in which there is an inherent tendency toward survival to adulthood but also permits increasing numbers of patients with disorders that were previously fatal in childhood to reach adult life.[3,81,82]

COMMON CONGENITAL DEFECTS. Common congenital cardiac defects in which adult survival can be anticipated, in order of female prevalence, are ostium secundum atrial septal defect, patent ductus arteriosus, valvular pulmonic stenosis, ventricular septal defect with pulmonic stenosis, functionally normal bicuspid aortic valve, valvular aortic stenosis, aortic regurgitation, and coarctation of the aorta.

Ostium secundum atrial septal defect (p. 1027) remains one of the most common forms of congenital heart disease found in adults. Since the natural history spans the childbearing age, and since the majority of patients are female,[53] the anomaly is of special importance in any consideration of congenital heart disease and pregnancy.[53,81,83] The great majority of women with uncomplicated ostium secundum atrial septal defects endure the hemodynamic burden of pregnancy—even multiple pregnancies—with relatively little difficulty.[2,53] Infective endocarditis poses little or no threat unless there is associated prolapse of the mitral valve with incompetence.[56]

The most important practical concerns in pregnant women with atrial septal defect are pulmonary hypertension, right ventricular failure, and atrial arrhythmias. After the fourth decade, atrial arrhythmias—fibrillation, flutter, or paroxysmal supraventricular tachycardia—increase in frequency and represent serious complications leading to disability and cardiac failure.[53,83] Peripheral edema predisposes to thromboembolism, which may enter the systemic circulation as a paradoxical embolus; death has occurred in this setting, even during the puerperium.[2] Pulmonary hypertension is a relatively late occurrence in ostium secundum atrial septal defect and is seldom a complicating issue in pregnant women below age 30 years. A much higher incidence and earlier onset occur among patients with atrial septal defect who are born at high altitudes.[84] Although an occasional woman with pulmonary hypertension complicating ostium secundum atrial septal defect tolerates pregnancy with surprisingly little difficulty, this is the exception and not the rule.[85]

Patent ductus arteriosus (p. 1038) also predominates in females.[41,53] Beginning with the third decade, an increasing number of patients with large shunts develop cardiac failure, whereas those with small communications remain asymptomatic.[53] The incidence of large patent ductus arteriosus with suprasystemic pulmonary vascular resistance and right-to-left shunt is relatively infrequent. Happily, the combination of patent ductus arteriosus and pregnancy is becoming of less and less practical importance, since the clinical diagnosis of patent ductus is simple, and surgical division is safe, routine, and curative in childhood.

The response to pregnancy in patients with patent ductus arteriosus depends in large part upon where in the spectrum of the lesion gestation occurs. The asymptomatic young woman with a small or moderate-sized patent ductus arteriosus and normal pulmonary arterial pressure experiences uncomplicated pregnancy,[2] although such patients are at risk to develop infective endocarditis (see below). Left ventricular failure may occur or be aggravated during pregnancy in the presence of a large ductus and left-to-right shunt. In patients with large patent ductus arteriosus, pulmonary hypertension, and reversed shunts, right ventricular failure and maternal mortality are distinct threats. Rarely, such patients experience uneventful pregnancies.[2]

Isolated *valvular pulmonic stensosis* (p. 1037) is a relatively common congenital cardiac defect occurring with equal frequency in males and females. Survival into adulthood is comparatively frequent, even though signs of the anomaly are usually present from infancy. In one review of 69 anatomically proven unoperated cases, the average age of death was 26 years.[53] The tendency for the pulmonary valve to grow in proportion to the increase in body size may in part account for this. The majority of patients with pulmonic stenosis proceed through infancy and childhood with little handicap. The increased cardiac output of pregnancy augments the burden on an already pressure-loaded right ventricle, but in young asymptomatic women with mild to moderate and occasionally even severe pulmonic stenosis, pregnancy is, as a rule, satisfactorily tolerated.[2] In view of the relatively conspicuous murmur, the safety and simplicity of diagnostic confirmation, and the low risk of surgical correction, patients with moderate to severe pulmonic stenosis should, and now usually do, undergo operation long before pregnancy, preferably in childhood.

Isolated *ventricular septal defect* (p. 1033) is one of the most common congenital cardiac malformations, occurring with equal prevalence in males and females, although in one series, the majority of patients over age 20 years were women.[53] However, this anomaly is of relatively little importance as a potential complication of pregnancy because of its infrequency in adults. As many as 45 per cent of ventricular septal defects close spontaneously; in patients with large nonrestrictive defects not surgically corrected, either congestive heart failure causes death in infancy or the left-to-right shunts become reduced because of a decrease in ventricular septal defect size, a rise in pulmonary vascular resistance, or the development of obstruction to right ventricular outflow (see below). The occasional acyanotic adult survivor with little or no pulmonary hypertension will tolerate pregnancy in accordance with the magnitude of the left-to-right shunt and the functional state of the left ventricle. In women with relatively large shunts, the added volume load of pregnancy can cause heart failure, and sporadic deaths have been reported as a result of antepartum cardiac failure and postpartum paradoxical embolism.[2] There is a risk of infective endocarditis in patients with this anomaly.

Although isolated ventricular septal defects, irrespective of size, are seldom seen in adults, when large ventricular septal defects are associated with appropriate degrees of pulmonic stenosis, prolonged survival is relatively frequent. Thus, a number of patients with ventricular septal defect and pulmonic stenosis reach childbearing age.

A large ventricular septal defect with obstruction to right ventricular outflow that offers resistance at or above systemic levels, i.e., *tetralogy of Fallot* is the most common congenital anomaly associated with cyanosis in adults with congenital heart disease[53] (p. 1034). Adult survival with this combination of lesions implies a degree of obstruction to right ventricular outflow that permits pulmonary blood flow that is adequate for oxygenation but is not enough to overload the left ventricle. Despite an increased tendency for adult survival, women with cyanotic tetralogy of Fallot seldom have normal full-term pregnancies; their offspring have low birth weights, an observation in accord with the generalization (discussed below) that infants born of cyanotic mothers are typically small for gestational age (see later).[53,86–88] The magnitude of the right-to-left shunt varies inversely with the systemic vascular resistance in patients with tetralogy of Fallot. In pregnancy, the decrease in peripheral vascular resistance coupled with the increase in cardiac output (and venous return to the obstructed right ventricle) results in a larger right-to-left shunt, a fall in systemic arterial oxygen saturation, deeper cyanosis, and a rising hematocrit. Although full-term pregnancies occur occasionally, the risk to both mother and child is considerable, as discussed below. The labile hemodynamic adjustments during the immediate postpartum period place the patient at further risk. A sudden reduction in systemic vascular resistance may provoke intense, and occasionally fatal, cyanosis and syncope.[2] In addition, there is the risk of infective endocarditis.

In women with pulmonary vascular obstructive disease associated with *Eisenmenger's complex*, i.e., large, nonrestrictive ventricular septal defects with pulmonary vascular resistance at or above systemic levels,[53] (p. 832) hemoptysis may recur or first appear during gestation.[89] The level of the pulmonary vascular resistance is the chief determinant of the risk of pregnancy.[90,91] Maternal mortality has been estimated at 30 to 70 per cent, and death may occur during either the gestational period or the puerperium.[91,92] A number of physiological changes in pregnancy conspire as potential threats. A fall in systemic vascular resistance augments the right-to-left shunt, reduces the arterial oxygen saturation, and increases the hematocrit, just as in the case of tetralogy of Fallot. Conversely, bearing down during labor, by increasing systemic vascular resistance, can suddenly depress cardiac output and provoke syncope with dangerous sequelae. Thus, fluctuations in systemic vascular resistance, cardiac output, and blood volume are tolerated poorly, since the fixed pulmonary resistance permits little or no circulatory reserve. It has further been proposed that widespread thromboses in already compromised small pulmonary arteries and arterioles sometimes result in a rapid postpartum increase in pulmonary vascular obstruction.[91]

Congenital aortic valve disease—Functionally normal bicuspid aortic valve, aortic stenosis, or aortic regurgitation—predominates in males, but this does not reduce the importance of these lesions when they occur in individual pregnant females. A *functionally normal bicuspid aortic valve* is perhaps the most common congenital anomaly of the heart or great arteries.[93] The high susceptibility to infective endocarditis poses a constant threat. Since it is unlikely that an isolated, functionally normal, congenital bicuspid aortic valve would be identified in a young woman before or during pregnancy, the presence of the anomaly may rarely announce itself after delivery because of infective endocarditis which may be accompanied by the sudden appearance of aortic regurgitation.[94]

Congenital valvular aortic stenosis (p. 1026) results from progressive fibrosis and calcification of an initially functionally normal bicuspid valve or from a valve that is inherently obstructed from birth.[53] The fixed obstruction to left ventricular outflow resulting from aortic stenosis imposes a pressure load upon the left ventricle. Pregnancy, by adding the stress of increased cardiac output to an already pressure-loaded left ventricle, increases the transaortic gradient and the left ventricular systolic pressure and work. Patients with mild to moderate aortic stenosis tolerate pregnancy relatively well, but infective endocarditis following delivery remains a risk irrespective of severity. An occasional patient who has asymptomatic severe aortic stenosis prior to conception remains symptom-free throughout pregnancy,[2] but the risk is ever-present, reserve is limited, and syncope, especially after effort or excitement, may first appear during gestation. Should cerebral symptoms, dyspnea, or angina precede conception or develop during early pregnancy, serious sequelae can be anticipated. In any event, abrupt, strenuous, or isometric exercise should be scrupulously avoided.

Like aortic valve lesions, *coarctation of the aortic isthmus* (p. 1038), with or without a coexisting bicuspid aortic valve, occurs predominantly in males.[53] The majority of patients without surgical correction live to adulthood, but only a minority reach 40 years of age. Major symptoms in uncorrected coarctation derive from four complications: congestive heart failure, rupture of the aorta or dissecting aneurysm, infective endocarditis (usually at the site of a bicuspid valve), and cerebral hemorrhage. Beyond infancy, the incidence of cardiac failure peaks after the second decade. Rupture of the aorta or dissecting aneurysm is a dramatic complication that occurs most frequently in the third and fourth decades, whereas cerebral hemorrhage is most common in the second and third decades. Intracranial hemorrhage is usually due to rupture of an aneurysm of the circle of Willis. The behavior of the arterial pressure in pregnancy complicating coarctation of the aorta is analogous to that occurring in normal pregnancy, i.e., the directional changes are similar but from an initially higher level.[53] The risk of complications increases in pregnant women with uncorrected coarctation, and, not surprisingly, death has been reported from rupture of the aorta, cerebrovascular accidents, congestive heart failure, pulmonary edema, and infective endocarditis of a bicuspid aortic valve.[2,95] Overall maternal mortality is estimated at 3.5 per cent[2,96] and morbidity, i.e., cardiovascular complications without death, at 90 per cent.[97,98]

Surgical correction of coarctation of the aorta is now generally performed in children around the age of 4 years, so that more and more patients born with this anomaly are reaching childbearing age *after* having undergone operative repair. Even so, there is the persistent risk of the coexisting bicuspid aortic valve and of late recurrence of systemic hypertension. Also, it is not likely that the threat of rupture of an aneurysm of the circle of Willis is abolished by surgical repair of coarctation.[3]

UNCOMMON CONGENITAL DEFECTS

Some uncommon congenital cardiac defects with expected survival to adulthood are listed in Table 53–4. Pure *congenital aortic regurgitation* (p. 1105), generally due to a bicuspid aortic valve, varies from the trivial to the severe, with all gradations in between. Although the risk of infective endocarditis is present irrespective of severity, pregnancy is otherwise tolerated well, especially in women with mild to moderate regurgitation but also in those with severe incompetence, in whom symptoms are absent prior to pregnancy and in whom left ventricular end-diastolic pressure is normal. The increase in cardiac output during gestation is generally handled well, and its effects are in part corrected by both the fall in systemic vascular resistance and the acceleration in heart rate accompanied by an abbreviation of diastole, which serve to decrease the volume of regurgitant flow. However, in patients with free aortic regurgitation who are symptomatic before conception, especially if the left ventricular end-diastolic pressure is elevated, progressive left ventricular failure can be anticipated during the course of gestation. Similar considerations apply to rheumatic aortic regurgitation.

Uncomplicated *situs inversus* carries no risk, since the heart and circulation are otherwise anatomically and physiologically normal.

TABLE 53–4 UNCOMMON CONGENITAL CARDIAC DEFECTS IN WHICH ADULT SURVIVAL IS EXPECTED

Aortic regurgitation
Situs inversus (mirror-image dextrocardia)
Situs solitus with right thoracic heart
Congenital complete heart block
Congenitally corrected transposition of the great arteries
Idiopathic dilatation of the pulmonary trunk
Congenital pulmonary valve regurgitation
Ebstein's anomaly of the tricuspid valve
Primary pulmonary hypertension
Congenital pulmonary arteriovenous fistula
Lutembacher's syndrome
Coronary arteriovenous fistula

Situs solitus with a right cardiac apex is almost invariably complicated by additional congenital cardiac malformations, the presence and degree of which determine the response to pregnancy. The commonest coexisting anomalies are congenitally corrected transposition of the great arteries, pulmonic stenosis, and ventricular septal defect.[53] The isolated association of corrected transposition, mild pulmonic stenosis, small ventricular septal defect, or a left-to-right interatrial shunt poses little or no problem, but severe pulmonic stenosis with reversed ventricular or atrial shunts involves the risks of anomalies producing cyanosis cited above.

Congenital complete heart block (p. 1043) has no sex predilection, and the natural history generally justifies cautious optimism;[53,99] pregnancy is usually uneventful in otherwise normal women with congenital complete heart block, although there are a few reports of women in whom Stokes-Adams attacks first appeared during gestation.[2,53] It is noteworthy that the functional state of the heart can apparently remain unimpaired when a pregnant woman has an artificial fixed-rate pacemaker.[100]

In *congenitally corrected transposition of the great arteries* (p. 1003), the response to pregnancy is determined by the type and degree of coexisting anomalies that are usually present and most commonly consist of prolonged atrioventricular conduction, incompetence of the systemic atrioventricular valve, ventricular septal defect, and pulmonic stenosis.[53]

Ebstein's anomaly of the tricuspid valve (p. 1040) involves males and females equally and is sometimes compatible with a relatively long and active life;[53] successful pregnancies have been reported in women with Ebstein's anomaly,[101] but gestation poses a number of potential hazards. The functionally inadequate right ventricle, already burdened by tricuspid regurgitation, copes poorly with the increased cardiac output of pregnancy. Recurrent episodes of supraventricular tachycardia, atrial fibrillation, or atrial flutter occur in about one-third of nongravid patients with Ebstein's anomaly and are not likely to be well tolerated during pregnancy, especially when preexcitation (Wolff-Parkinson-White bypass tracts) permits very rapid ventricular rates.[53,64] Cyanosis due to reversed interatrial shunting may first appear in pregnancy during an episode of rapid heart action, especially when acute right ventricular failure is provoked.[53] Chronic cyanosis diminishes the probability of successful gestation and introduces the risk of paradoxical embolism.

The risks of pregnancy in *primary pulmonary hypertension* are formidable,[74] and the disorder is most frequent in young women, with a female:male ratio of 5:1 (p. 836).[53] Sudden death can be precipitated by a variety of stresses that would ordinarily be considered innocuous, and maternal mortality is about 50 per cent.[2,53,74] Effort syncope, chest pain, dyspnea, weakness, and fatigue may first appear during pregnancy, and, as expected, mortality is highest in symptomatic women.[53] The increase in cardiac output and fall in systemic vascular resistance are badly tolerated in the face of the high fixed pulmonary vascular resistance. Labor and the puerperium are even more critical times.

Developmental Defects

Two cardiac disorders that might be called "developmental"—prolapse of the mitral valve and Marfan's syndrome—may complicate pregnancy. About 6 per cent of echocardiograms in presumably normal young females reveal *prolapse of the mitral valve* (p. 1089).[56] These estimates place prolapse of the mitral valve among the commonest clinical cardiac abnormalities (if, in fact, all gradations of echocardiographic prolapse can be called abnormal). The increased cardiac output and reduced systemic vascular resistance characteristic of normal pregnancy serve to diminish leaflet/chordal redundancy and attenuate prolapse; the late systolic murmur may soften or disappear, and the clicks may soften or disappear altogether. Under these circumstances, a diagnosis of mitral prolapse may be clinically impossible (or at least impractical). Yet prolapse is susceptible to infective endocarditis, certainly when accompanied by mitral regurgitation, and bacteremia may occur during labor and delivery. Spontaneous, i.e., noninfectious, rupture of chordae tendineae occasionally complicates mitral prolapse,[56] but it is not yet clear whether the presumed connective tissue changes in pregnancy or the stress of labor and delivery or both increase susceptibility to this complication.[78] A more practical issue is the frequency of disturbances in cardiac rhythm. The commonest sustained tachyarrhythmia is supraventricular tachycardia,[56] an undesirable occurrence during pregnancy, especially toward term, labor, or delivery.

Classic *Marfan syndrome* (p. 1665) has been reported in approximately 4 per cent of patients with prolapse of the mitral valve;[56] conversely, nearly all patients with Marfan syndrome have prolapse of the mitral valve. Myxomatous degeneration of both the aortic and the mitral valves is associated with diaphanous thinning of elongated chordae tendineae. The mitral annulus may be remarkably dilated as a part of the connective tissue defect, and the aortic sinuses and aortic root share in this disorder. Dissection of the aorta is uncommon in nonhypertensive women of childbearing age, but when it does occur it is associated with pregnancy at least half the time;[102,103] structural alterations in the aortic wall during gestation are believed to be responsible,[2,102] and Marfan syndrome, with its inherent abnormality of the aortic media, predisposes to aortic dissection.

Accordingly, the pregnant female with Marfan syndrome is at increased risk,[104] apart from and in addition to the complications associated with the abnormality of the mitral and aortic valves (regurgitation and infective endocarditis). Importantly, the strain of labor and delivery is not necessarily a precipitating factor in aortic dissection, since rupture occurs most commonly in the third trimester or in the first stage of labor.[102]

Cardiomyopathies

The cardiomyopathies are important in pregnancy chiefly with respect to *postpartum* or *peripartum cardiomyopathy,* the term applied to a form of idiopathic congestive cardiomyopathy (p. 1400) beginning in the last month of gestation or the first few months after delivery.[1,5–7,104a] The incidence is low, but the maternal consequences can be dire. At necropsy, cardiac enlargement and mural thrombi have been found with histologic evidence of degeneration and fibrosis of myocardial fibers.[5,6] The etiology of the disorder is unknown, but the probability of its occurrence is increased if a gravid woman of age 30 years or more is experiencing her third or subsequent pregnancy, is pregnant with twins, or has toxemia.[2,5,6] Malnutrition can aggravate the disease but is not a necessary ingredient in its cause or progression. The current consensus is that patients presenting with idiopathic heart failure in the last trimester or in the puerperium are probably examples of dilated preexisting cardiomyopathy that was unrecognized before pregnancy. Even so, the precipitating causes of overt heart failure are unknown. However, in Nigeria, a uniquely high incidence of peripartum heart failure has been related to the custom of ingesting an excessive amount of local lake salt for 40 days postpartum under conditions which diminish evaporative water loss.[105] The long-term prognosis in peripartum cardiomyopathy relates to the rapidity and degree with which heart size returns to normal in response to conventional treatment (Fig. 53–2).[5,6] Patients who maintain cardiomegaly for 6 months or more have an extremely poor prognosis.[5,6] There is a tendency for recurrence of the syndrome in subsequent pregnancies, especially in patients with persistent cardiomegaly.[5,6]

Hypertrophic obstructive cardiomyopathy (p. 1409) is affected by a number of hemodynamic variables that exist during the course of normal pregnancy, labor, and delivery.[2,106] As a rule, gestation is tolerated well.[107] As discussed in Chapter 40, the degree of obstruction to left ventricular outflow is determined chiefly by the interplay among three variables—the left ventricular end-diastolic dimensions (volume), the systemic vascular resistance, and the inotropic state of the left ventricle. During pregnancy, the increase in cardiac output (and left ventricular diastolic volume) should reduce the obstruction, but the fall in systemic vascular resistance counteracts this effect.[106] When mitral regurgitation complicates the syndrome, the hemodynamic effects of pregnancy may dramatically increase its severity, so that pulmonary congestion supervenes.[106] In

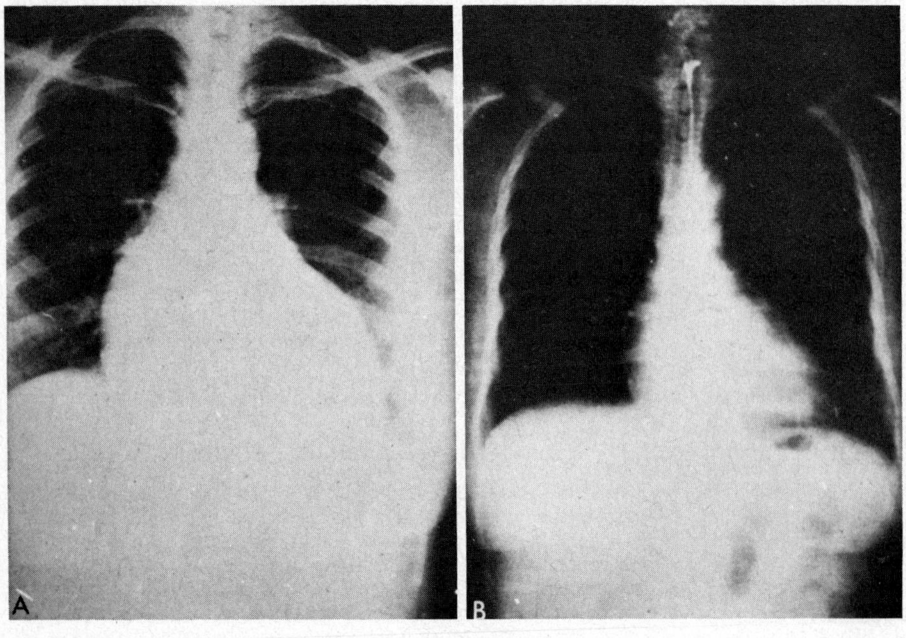

FIGURE 53–2 *A,* Admission chest roentgenogram showing cardiomegaly in a patient with peripartum cardiomyopathy, *B,* Normal heart size in same patient 6 months later. (From Demakis, J. G., et al.: Natural course of peripartum cardiomyopathy. Circulation *44*:1053, 1971, by permission of the American Heart Association, Inc.)

later pregnancy, compression of the inferior vena cava in the supine position by the gravid uterus decreases venous return and left ventricular volume and accordingly augments the obstruction of left ventricular outflow; patients are therefore well advised to avoid the supine position. A number of opposing variables came into play during labor. The adrenergic stimulation associated with pain and emotional stress, together with the Valsalva maneuver (bearing down), serves to increase outflow obstruction, but the rise in central blood volume during active uterine contraction has the opposite effect.[106] Moreover, the rapid decline in blood volume in the puerperium[29] can reduce left ventricular internal dimensions and intensify the obstruction. In addition, the frequency of coexisting mitral regurgitation exposes patients to the risk of infective endocarditis.

Hypertension (See also p. 888)

Central to the issue of hypertension during gestation are the problems of the previously hypertensive woman who becomes pregnant, the problem of the hypertension of preeclampsia in women who were previously normotensive, and the occurrence of preeclampsia in previously hypertensive women.[108] The incidence of hypertension during pregnancy from all causes has been estimated at 6 per cent, and in about one-fourth of these, elevated blood pressure preceded pregnancy.[2,109] Untoward events related to hypertension in pregnancy are greater in black than in white women.[110,111] The changes in systemic blood pressure that characterize normotensive pregnancy also occur in a significant number of pregnant women with essential hypertension.[2] Thus, the systolic pressure may fall 20 to 30 mm Hg, and the diastolic may decline 10 to 15 mm Hg in the first trimester. There are important variations, however. In some patients, the blood pressure remains unchanged, in others it increases, and in still others blood pressure normalizes during gestation but returns to the preexisting hypertensive levels in the third trimester or after delivery.[112] Gravid women with labile blood pressure generally experience uncomplicated pregnancies, but some develop sustained hypertension late in gestation.[2] Although this labile elevation of pressure is likely to normalize following delivery, a substantial portion of such patients manifest persistent hypertension years later. Criteria for the diagnosis of hypertension usually include a consistent rise in blood pressure of 30/15 mm Hg or an absolute level of greater than 140/90 mm Hg or both (Chap. 26).

As a general rule, maternal prognosis is excellent in women whose arterial pressure is below 160/100 mm Hg during the first 20 weeks of pregnancy,[2] provided renal and cardiac functions are good and preeclampsia does not develop. Conversely, more severe hypertension early in gestation exposes both mother and fetus to increasing risk and requires special medical and obstetrical care.

Treatment. Physical activity should be restricted; anxiety should be controlled with sedatives; long periods of bed rest should be imposed; and sodium restriction, diuretics, and antihypertensive agents (hydralazine, beta blockade, or methyl dopa) should be employed.[2,112] Successful pregnancy is possible even in women who have experienced malignant hypertension, provided that blood pressure is controlled during gestation.[114] However, even mild hypertension is a risk to the fetus (see below).[115] In selecting appropriate pharmacological treatment, it should be borne in mind that there is evidence of a significant deficit in intravascular volume in many hypertensive pregnant women, especially those with severe preeclampsia or with preeclampsia superimposed upon chronic hypertension.[116] Accordingly, diuretics must be used judiciously because of the risk of decreased plasma volume and uterine (placental) blood flow.[112,113] Unless the hypertension is severe, it is advisable to decrease or discontinue treatment 2 to 3 days before delivery. One major objective of early vigorous treatment of hypertension is the prevention of preeclampsia, which puts the fetus at serious risk, even if the high blood pressure is subsequently reduced.

Preeclampsia

This condition is characterized by normal blood pressure before pregnancy and during the first half of gestation but a rise in blood pressure in the second half, especially during the third trimester. The earlier preeclampsia occurs in the pregnancy, the greater the risk to both mother and fetus.[109] Preeclampsia is more frequent in primiparas, in twin pregnancies, and in women with a history of toxemia or hypertension. Indeed, preexisting moderate essential hypertension is complicated by preeclampsia in 10 to 20 per cent of cases; in this situation, blood pressure is elevated early in pregnancy with a substantial increase in the third trimester. Progression to eclampsia is ominous, with a 5 to 10 per cent maternal mortality and a 20 to 25 per cent fetal mortality. If preeclampsia does not subside within a few days of hospitalization (during which bed rest, sedation, sodium restriction, and pharmacological control of blood pressure are prescribed), the pregnancy should be interrupted as soon as possible by cesarean section unless term is sufficiently near for induction of labor. It has been emphasized that the premature infant of a preeclamptic mother has a better chance in a neonatal intensive care unit than in utero.

It is important to distinguish between edema of the lower extremities of normal pregnancy and the periorbital and hand edema of toxemia (preeclampsia and eclampsia).[112] Similarly, *proteinuria* must be properly interpreted; it usually appears in toxemia *after* the rise in systemic arterial pressure and the development of edema.[112] In a normotensive pregnant woman without edema, proteinuria is more likely due to genitourinary tract infection.[112] Thus, the proteinuria of toxemia must be distinguished from pyelonephritis, and the edema of pregnancy must be separated from the edema of toxemia.

Considerable attention has been focused on the important questions of whether pregnancy permanently aggravates systemic hypertension and whether preeclampsia in previously normotensive women predisposes to the late postpartum development of sustained hypertension. It is current consensus that essential hypertension, at least in white women, is not generally aggravated by pregnancy unless there is superimposed toxemia.[2] The long-term effects of toxemia are more controversial. White women with a history of documented preeclampsia in their first pregnancy have the same prognosis for sustained hypertension or for survival as white women of the same age with no history of preeclampsia. On the other hand, there is a significant increase in the prevalence of sustained hypertension among black women who had preeclampsia as primiparas and among both black and white women who had preeclampsia as multiparas. These observations suggest that toxemia of pregnancy, when it occurs in black women in any pregnancy or in white women after their first pregnancy, marks a tendency for the development of chronic sustained hypertension in later life.[117] Toxemia *per se*, i.e., independent of the presence and degree of systemic hypertension, can result in acute pulmonary edema and T-wave inversions in the electrocardiogram.[2] Cardiac size is not significantly increased in these patients, and the pulmonary edema has been ascribed to retention of fluid and perhaps to effects on pulmonary capillary permeability.[2]

Vascular spasm is an important component of the toxemic state. Approximately one-third of patients with fatal eclampsia (hypertension, edema, proteinuria, and convulsions) were found at autopsy to have contraction band necrosis, a lesion secondary to coronary reflow after periods of no flow.[118] This finding suggests that coronary spasm may be common in patients who die of eclampsia.[118]

Arrhythmias

During pregnancy arrhythmias fall into two general categories: (1) those occurring in the course of an otherwise normal, uncomplicated gestation and (2) those associated with certain cardiac diseases that are likely to be found in women of childbearing age. The type and prevalence of rhythm disturbances are yet to be firmly identified by continuous monitoring of gravid females at different stages of gestation, labor, and the puerperium. Nevertheless, routine electrocardiographic and clinical examination has disclosed a number of arrhythmias in healthy pregnant women. Palpitations caused by premature beats are relatively common during gestation and the puerperium.[59] The premature beats may arise in the atria, the atrioventricular junction, or infranodal sites (ventricular) and occasionally produce bigeminy or trigeminy.

The sporadic occurrence of premature beats is of no clinical importance, especially if they are not subjectively disturbing and if the patient is reassured of their innocence. The most likely sustained arrhythmia in pregnancy is reentrant paroxysmal supraventricular tachycardia, since this rhythm disturbance is relatively common and has its peak incidence in young women. During the obstetrical history, the physician should inquire about prior paroxysmal rapid heart action, since reentrant supraventricular tachycardia often begins in the teens or earlier, forewarning of potential recurrences to which pregnancy predisposes, especially in the third trimester.[59,119] As a rule, the clinical manifestations, pharmacological management, and response to therapy are similar to conventional experience in nonpregnant women, but occurrences close to term, during labor, or in the puerperium are potentially hazardous. Rarely, supraventricular tachycardia is refractory to standard drug therapy. In one such instance, the patient underwent cardioversion seven times during three successive pregnancies with no apparent ill effect on the fetus.[119]

Occasional premature ventricular beats, even with bigeminy or trigeminy, are generally unimportant in the pregnant woman without evident organic heart disease, but multiform beats or repetitive firing—especially toward term or in the puerperium—should arouse suspicion of peripartum cardiomyopathy. Atrial flutter or atrial fibrillation is for all practical purposes evidence of coexisting organic heart disease, either acquired (most commonly rheumatic mitral stenosis) or congenital (especially ostium secundum atrial septal defect, or Ebstein's anomaly of the tricuspid valve). The Wolff-Parkinson-White syndrome with attacks of paroxysmal supraventricular tachycardia or atrial fibrillation at a very rapid ventricular rate (p. 712) may occur during pregnancy.[120]

Venous Disease

The gravid state, and especially repeated pregnancies, predisposes to peripheral venous disease and thromboembolism. If short-term anticoagulants are required, heparin is the drug of choice. The problems of long-term anticoagulant therapy are dealt with below. Increased venous pressure in the lower extremities is an important factor in the development of varicosities. In addition, a prolonged and difficult labor has been implicated as a cause of pelvic vein thrombosis.[2] In either case, overt or occult pulmonary emboli are potential threats. Multiple recurrent pulmonary emboli—insidious or overt—can result in a clinical picture closely resembling if not indistinguishable from primary pulmonary hypertension (pp. 836 and 1597).[121] Symptoms of venous disease or of pulmonary embolism or of both may begin within a few months after delivery or may be delayed for years.[2] In fact, there is a significant increase in the incidence of superficial and deep phlebitis of leg veins during the first four postpartum weeks. Oral contraceptives in the postpartum period should be avoided, not only because of the added risk of venous thrombosis and pulmonary embolism, but because of evidence that an already elevated pulmonary vascular resistance may rapidly increase in women on anovulatory pills even in the absence of identifiable thromboembolism.[122]

Pregnancy After Cardiac Surgery

One of the most important relationships between pregnancy and heart disease involves a new and increasing population—the postoperative cardiac patient.[3] Those who previously would not have reached childbearing age or who might have done so physiologically ill equipped for pregnancy are now presenting postoperatively for obstetrical and cardiological care.

Although cardiac surgery can be performed *during* gestation (see below), the objective of operative intervention should be anticipatory, i.e., to increase the safety and success of pregnancy and the subsequent health of both mother and child.[96] However, it is important to bear in mind that with few exceptions cardiac surgery is not curative, and both the patient and the physician must recognize the need for continuing medical care. The form of management is determined by the presence, type, and degree of postoperative cardiac and vascular residua and sequelae. On the other hand, serious cardiovascular disease can appreciably reduce sexual and ovarian function, and successful cardiac surgery may increase fertility.[96] Relief of cyanosis may not only permit a woman to conceive but substantially improves stability of the pregnancy and the probability of delivery at or near term.[96] Thus, there is general agreement that cardiac surgery *prior* to pregnancy may be enormously beneficial. For example, the complication rate during pregnancy in surgically treated women with previously symptomatic mitral stenosis is reduced significantly.[2,96,124] Uncomplicated gestation has followed intracardiac repair of tetralogy of Fallot, one woman sustaining five pregnancies without incident.[125]

There are special problems in the management of pregnant women with *prosthetic cardiac valves,* namely the risk of infective endocarditis from potential bacteremia during labor and delivery, the risk to the mother of thromboembolism, and the risk to the fetus of anticoagulants, both coumarin-related vitamin K antagonists and heparin.[124–137] The methods of prophylaxis for infective endocarditis are conventional (see below), but anticoagulants pose serious problems that require refined judgment and meticulous care (p. 1778). In pregnant women with rigid prosthetic valves, omission of anticoagulants substantially increases the probability of systemic embolism.[126–128,131] Although anticoagulants do not eliminate thromboembolic complications, the risk is higher in pregnant women with prosthetic valves in whom anticoagulants are discontinued than in those who continue to take the drugs or who have never received them.[131,136] The responses may in part be affected by the relative state of hypercoagulability believed to exist during pregnancy.[126,128] Although the use of oral anticoagulants benefits the mother, the drugs readily cross the placental barrier and expose the fetus to appreciable risks.[126,128,131,134,135,137–139]

Of nearly 450 reported pregnancies in which coumarin derivatives were used, at most two-thirds resulted in apparently normal infants.[139] When coumadin was given in the first trimester, the commonest disorder was what has been called "warfarin embryopathy" or chondrodysplasia punctata[137–139]. Features include saddle nose, hypoplasia of nares and air passages resulting in upper airway obstruction and neonatal respiratory distress, hypertelorism, frontal bossing, short neck, short stature, and stippled epiphyses (punctata).[137–139] Even in the second and the third trimesters, coumadin administration is hardly devoid of fetal risks, which consist of spontaneous abortion, stillbirth, or live offspring with significant abnormalities in one-third of cases.[139] In addition to the ongoing risk of hemorrhagic complications, malformations include optic atrophy, microphthalmia, deafness, malformed ears, low weight for gestational age, dwarfism, dystrophic nails with short fingers, and central nervous system defects, especially mental retardation, microcephaly, hydrocephalus, mengingocele, and cerebral atrophy.[139]

With the hope of circumventing these risks, heparin, which does not cross the placenta, has been proposed during the first or first and second trimesters.[126,135] However, the drug is relatively cumbersome to administer and control, the incidence of maternal hemorrhagic complications is not greater than with coumadin,[139a] but isolated use in the first trimester still results in an overall neonatal morbidity and mortality of 36 per cent—prematurity, death with prematurity, or stillbirth.[139] Apart from the risks of placental or fetal hemorrhage, the chelating effects of heparin (calcium and other cations) with intrauterine deficiencies have been proposed as causes of fetal injury.[139]

Despite the Scylla of maternal thromboembolism and the Charybdis of fetal death or malformation, anticoagulants are routinely employed in the pregnant woman with rigid prosthetic cardiac valves. Heparin in the first trimester does not appear to be superior to coumadin throughout.[139] When coumadin is used, meticulous regulation should maintain the prothrombin time at one and one half times and certainly less than twice the control time.

Management of anticoagulants at the end of pregnancy is much clearer than at the beginning. The hazard of fetal hemorrhage is increased by the obligatory trauma of labor and delivery. During the last 2 weeks of pregnancy, coumadin should be replaced by heparin.[132,133] At the earliest onset of labor or in anticipation of it, and through delivery, protamine is administered and heparin is discontinued. The timing of these events is more readily controlled if labor is induced electively. Should spontaneous labor begin in a patient receiving oral anticoagulants, administration of fresh frozen plasma is desirable.[132] Under these circumstances, birth by cesarean section is said to be associated with a lower risk of fetal death than that by vaginal delivery.[126] If elective cesarean section is planned for any reason, anticoagulants are discontinued 2 to 3 days before delivery.[128] Twenty-four hours after delivery, anticoagulants should be resumed, some clinicians recommending resumption with heparin and gradual replacement by oral anticoagulants.[130,133] In any event, breast feeding should be avoided because oral anticoagulants are secreted in the milk.[2] Antiplatelet agents have been suggested instead of oral anticoagulants in pregnant women with prosthetic heart valves, but the safety and effectiveness of these agents are unproved.[126,127] The availability and value of porcine and human cadaver tissue valves which are nonthrombogenic and which do not require anticoagulant treatment should largely obviate this problem. Although many surgeons continue to prefer rigid prostheses, these devices should, if at all possible, be avoided in women of childbearing age (p. 1086).

The interaction between pregnancy and maternal heart disease—preoperative or postoperative—has thus far focused on gestation, delivery, and the puerperium (see above), and there is general agreement that each of these periods entails an added risk in patients with certain types of organic heart disease. It is also important to ask whether pregnancy, once successfully concluded, alters the subsequent course of maternal heart disease. It has been stated without apparent irony that ". . . most physicians have believed that a woman's impaired cardiac reserve is like a bank account that is irreversibly depleted by the cost of pregnancy."[140] Current opinion does not support this view, at least for rheumatic heart disease.[141] Women with significant impairment of cardiac reserve are at higher risk *during* their pregnancies, but if they survive, no long-term harmful effects have been identified except those attendant on the postpartum exertion necessary for the care of another child.[140] Studies have not provided convincing evidence of a remote adverse effect of pregnancy on the course of chronic rheumatic valvular disease[2,141–143], except in certain underdeveloped countries.[144]

Other Forms of Heart Disease

Atherosclerosis of the large extramural coronary arteries is rare in young menstruating women who have no major risk factors. However, there are a number of reports of postpartum myocardial infarction secondary to coronary thrombosis, but with otherwise normal coronary arteries.[145,146] Occasional examples have been reported of pregnancy complicated by still other forms of heart disease, e.g., luetic heart disease, acute or chronic pericarditis,[2] and Takayasu's disease.[147] These and other sporadic disorders, while individually important, have little collective impact and will not be dealt with further here.

MANAGEMENT OF THE MOTHER WITH HEART DISEASE

Care of the expectant mother with heart disease is based upon a number of simple principles. Maternal mortality varies directly with functional class (Table 53–5). The mother's cardiac reserve is inherently limited by her heart disease and is called upon to meet the additional circulatory demands of pregnancy. This challenge can almost always be met by minimizing unnecessary demands upon the circulation and by meticulous medical management of the cardiovascular disease per se. In so doing, a place can be made for pregnancy within the framework of a limited cardiovascular reserve. Conversely, interruption of pregnancy as a means of preserving or restoring cardiac compensation is seldom warranted. If the decision is made to terminate pregnancy on other grounds, the interruption should be done when safest, i.e., during the first trimester. However, in the presence of a few cardiovascular lesions, child-bearing imposes such a significant threat to maternal survival that interruption of pregnancy is recommended. These include women whose pulmonary vascular resistance is at or above systemic resistance, women with Marfan's syndrome, and women with persistent cardiomegaly following peripartum cardiomyopathy.

Factors that serve to aggravate the heart disease and needlessly encroach on cardiac reserve should be identified, removed, or at least minimized (Table 53–6). Anxiety is a tangible source of stress, especially in the primipara who anticipates the new experience of pregnancy in the face of her heart disease. Reassurance begins with a frank, clear, but euphemistic appraisal designed to remove fear of the unknown. The expectant mother should be told what to expect during each stage of pregnancy through labor, delivery, and the puerperium. Coordination between obstetrician and cardiologist is obligatory to provide intelligent care and to assure that the patient does not receive conflicting and therefore disturbing information. Acute and often unnecessary anxiety can provoke pulmonary edema in young women with mitral stenosis whether or not they are pregnant. The reassurance that the pain of labor and delivery will be relieved is especially important. Thus, "natural childbirth" should be discouraged.

TABLE 53–5

MATERNAL MORTALITY ACCORDING TO FUNCTIONAL CLASS[2,52]	
Classes I and II	*Classes III and IV*
0.4%	6.8%
FETAL MORTALITY ACCORDING TO FUNCTIONAL CLASS[2]	
Class I	*Class IV*
NIL	30%

TABLE 53–6 FACTORS THAT AGGRAVATE MATERNAL HEART DISEASE

Anxiety
Retention of sodium and water
Sudden, strenuous, or isometric exercise
Heat and humidity
Anemia
Pyelonephritis
Lower respiratory infection
Hyperthyroidism
Arrhythmias
Thromboembolism

The tendency for body water and total exchangeable sodium to increase in the normal gravid woman must be reckoned with in the pregnant cardiac patient; initial restriction of sodium followed by judicious use of diuretics prevents these increases from reaching undesirable proportions. Body weight should be carefully recorded each morning before breakfast. Not only is weight an important means to detect excess sodium and water retention, but excess dry body weight (obesity) is also a cardiocirculatory burden that is best minimized. Since exercise augments an already increased basal cardiac output, the pregnant cardiac patient should avoid abrupt, strenuous, or isometric effort; should rest an hour or two during the day, preferably in the early afternoon; and should be assured of a restful night even if sedatives are required. Gradations clearly exist. The asymptomatic patient with physiologically mild cardiac disease, e.g., mild isolated mitral regurgitation, needs little or no restriction, whereas the symptomatic pregnant patient with serious cardiac compromise may require prolonged hospitalization with complete bed rest.[78] The psychological impact of hospitalization for this purpose must, of course, be balanced against the anticipated benefits.

Certain environmental conditions exert important effects on the heart and circulation and may initiate or intensify heart failure in susceptible individuals. The combination of heat and humidity increases the hemodynamic burden,[148] and may serve as an important aggravating cause of heart failure in an otherwise stable pregnant cardiac patient.[1] Since gestation is normally accompanied by a high–cardiac output state (p. 1763) and greater heat production owing to the metabolic activity of the products of conception, increased skin blood flow and a cool, dry environment are required for dissipation of heat and proper regulation of body temperature. Pregnancy, heat, and humidity independently increase resting cardiac output;[148] the additive effects decrease cardiac reserve, so an air-conditioned environment can be therapeutic.

Alcohol decreases cardiac output in patients with heart disease.[149] When used in moderation, it may be helpful in the relief of anxiety, but excessive use must be avoided. Alcohol solutions are sometimes used intravenously to stop premature labor. In addition to the deleterious effect on cardiac performance which may result (p. 1406), large volumes of hypertonic solution are occasionally administered for this purpose, a practice hazardous to the patient with heart disease. Coexisting noncardiac diseases may also exert undesirable circulatory effects, especially in the pregnant cardiac patient. *Anemia* is a case in point and with rare exception can be corrected by oral iron. Pathological anemia must be distinguished from the "physiologic" anemia of pregnancy (see above), but even the latter can be deleterious in patients with marginal ventricular function. *Infection*, especially pyelonephritis, is relatively common during pregnancy and the postpartum period, so the index of suspicion should be appropriately high.[112] *Lower respiratory infection*, though coincidental, poses special problems in the pregnant cardiac patient with marginally elevated or increased pulmonary venous pressure. Epidemic *influenza* is associated with greater morbidity and mortality during pregnancy and is especially dangerous to women with mitral stenosis.[150] Vaccination with a killed vaccine is recommended for these patients.

Hyperthyroidism may not be as readily suspected because of the hyperkinetic circulation of pregnancy, but the effect is no less harmful, since the two hypermetabolic states (Chap. 24) conspire to reduce cardiac reserve. *Arrhythmias* should be anticipated and appropriate drugs used prophylactically. A history of recurrent supraventricular tachycardia in a previously healthy woman or reports of recurrent atrial fibrillation in a pregnant patient with mitral stenosis dictate the use of digoxin. Quinidine has been incriminated as a cause of premature labor,[59] but the drug has only minimal oxytocic effect and then not until spontaneous uterine contractions have begun.[2] The inherent tendency for stasis in leg veins and the attendant risk of thromboembolism can be minimized in a number of relatively simple ways. Aside from judicious use of sodium restriction and diuretics, the patient should be given detailed instructions on leg care, i.e., passive standing should be avoided, the supine position should be minimized (supine vena caval compression), the knees should be straightened when sitting (the legs need not be uncomfortably elevated), and ambulation should begin as soon as practical after delivery. In high-risk cases in which there is a history of thromboembolism, administration of prophylactic heparin within 24 hours after delivery has been advised.[151] The risks of oral anticoagulants, especially to the fetus, were discussed above.

Medical Management

With this background, let us now turn to the medical (i.e., nonsurgical) management of heart disease per se during pregnancy, labor, delivery, and the puerperium. Because of the hazards of radiation, chest roentgenography, cardiac catheterization, and angiography are usually deferred until after the completion of pregnancy. Treatment of occult congestive heart failure is important, but the management of acute pulmonary edema is pivotal, since this complication ranks as the greatest single cause of maternal cardiac mortality, accounting for 50 per cent of deaths in pregnant women with rheumatic heart disease.[2,144] The detection of incipient pulmonary congestion in the pregnant cardiac patient is essential. At each visit evidence must be sought by means of history and physical examination for developing pulmonary and peripheral venous congestion. A change in exercise tolerance or a sudden gain in weight requires explanation. Since the basal circulatory burden is elevated beginning in the first trimester, symptoms of reduced cardiac reserve can become manifest early in women with severe heart disease. Cardiac failure is best treated promptly and vigorously with marked restriction of physical activity, even bed rest, in addition to digitalis, diuretics, and salt restriction. Aggravating or precipitating causes should be diligently sought and corrected,[80] as emphasized earlier.

Comment was made (see above) on elective induction of labor near term in preeclampsia and in order to provide controlled timing when anticoagulants are administered to pregnant women with prosthetic valves. However, induction of labor well before term is not an appropriate method of delivery for the pregnant cardiac patient and, in fact, may increase the risk of heart failure. It is still the consensus that a spontaneous term vaginal delivery with adequate relief of pain and apprehension, performed with the aid of an experienced obstetrical anesthesiologist, is the method of choice in the pregnant woman with heart disease. The importance of the relief of pain and anxiety should be underscored. Cesarean section using epidural anesthesia[92] or thiopental, nitrous oxide, and succinylcholine anesthesia has been proposed for selected seriously ill pregnant cardiac patients.[152]

Infective endocarditis following uncomplicated vaginal delivery is rare.[153] Blood cultures taken at intervals during labor and delivery have not confirmed that bacteremia is a natural or necessary occurrence,[2] and some authorities have indicated that antibiotic prophylaxis is not necessary at the time of delivery in cardiac patients.[153] However, in pregnant women with cardiac lesions susceptible to infective endocarditis, it is not prudent to assume that delivery will be uncomplicated. Accordingly, prophylactic antibiotics (p. 1175) are recommended from the onset of labor through the fourth to sixth postpartum day.[2]

Cardiac Surgery

Fortunately, the issue of whether or not cardiac surgery is required in the pregnant cardiac patient seldom arises. When the problem is posed, it is almost always in women with rheumatic mitral stenosis[2,68,154,155] and only rarely in those with congenital heart disease.[83,96] Mitral valvotomy (without use of extracorporeal circulation) probably has a role, albeit a limited one. The most defensible indications are intractable (medically refractory) pulmonary edema and persistent massive hemoptysis in a patient with proven severe mitral stenosis.[2,68] Many cardiologists and obstetricians agree that, whenever possible, premature termination of pregnancy is preferable to cardiac surgery in patients with life-threatening heart failure that is unresponsive to medical management. Although valvotomy has been carried out at various stages in pregnancy, it is desirable to proceed as early as possible. The use of a pump oxygenator and extracorporeal circulation introduces a major variable of a completely different order of magnitude—the high risk of fetal mortality, which is greater than 30 per cent.[68,83,155] Moreover, even if the fetus survives, it may be born deformed.[93] Sporadic reports exist, however, of patients with mitral stenosis and intractable pulmonary edema responding to emergency open mitral valvotomy during the third trimester and subsequently delivering a normal infant at term.[155] On one occasion, cesarean section was successfully performed while the mother was on cardiopulmonary bypass.[156] When confronted with the rare catastrophe of sudden maternal death, consideration must be given to immediate postmortem cesarean section. About 150 postmortem cesarean sections have been reported, with an infant survival of approximately 15 per cent.[157]

EFFECTS OF MATERNAL HEART DISEASE ON THE FETUS

In the pregnant woman with heart disease, the lives of both the mother and the fetus are at stake, and it is now appropriate to summarize the effects of maternal cardiac disease on the fetus,[11a] even though a number of points have already been made. The fetus is exposed both to immediate risks that threaten its viability and to remote risks that express themselves as congenital malformations. Normal uterine blood flow and normal placental function are fundamental determinants of the intrauterine milieu upon which fetal integrity largely depends. Maternal heart disease, by reducing uterine blood flow and by altering the physiology of the placenta, threatens the growth, development, and viability of the fetus. Moreover, the fetus is at independent risk of congenital malformations which can result from genetic transmission of certain types of maternal heart disease or from transplacental transfer of teratogens, often in the form of drugs used in treating the pregnant cardiac patient.

In addition, certain factors unrelated to heart disease per se threaten the fetus and should not be disregarded. The fetal alcohol syndrome is a major risk in pregnant women who consume the equivalent of 90 ml or more of absolute alcohol per day, but lower levels of consumption may impose some risk.[158] Cigarette smoking throughout pregnancy can damage the umbilical artery and vein and the vessels of placental villi.[159] The placentas are relatively small and poorly vascularized, birth weights are low for gestational age, and there is increased risk of first trimester abortion, stillbirth, prematurity, and perinatal mortality.[29,159,160] Occasionally, supine vena caval obstruction results in a reduction in cardiac output sufficient to cause fetal hypoxia, but this effect is transient and readily reversed merely by having the mother turn on her side.[19]

The effects of maternal heart disease itself and the effects of the medical and surgical interventions employed to treat the cardiac disorder are of the greatest importance for fetal survival. The functional class of the mother materially influences fetal mortality; the risk varies from virtually nil in the asymptomatic pregnant woman with heart disease (Class I) to nearly 30 per cent in gravid women who are symptomatic at rest (Class IV) (Table 53–5).[2,52] There is no evidence, however, that live offspring of such women have a higher incidence of congenital malformations.

Certain types of heart disease pose greater threats than others to the fetus. *Systemic hypertension,* independent of the high risk of preeclampsia,[2,161] is associated with intrauterine growth retardation and an increased incidence of stillbirths and perinatal mortality.[2,108,110,162] The absolute level of blood pressure need not be great to increase fetal mortality. If the diastolic level exceeds 84 mm Hg at any time during gestation, the risk to the fetus increases, even more so when proteinuria is present.[163] In the United States, annual fetal attrition due to maternal hypertension is about 10,000.[164] *Maternal congenital heart disease* threatens the fetus in a number of respects. Aside from its effect on the functional class of the mother (see above), there is a material risk of genetic transmission (Chap. 47). Congenital cardiac defects have been found in 13.8 per cent of infants born of mothers with congenital heart disease, regardless of whether or not they had been operated upon.[165] Surgical correction, by permitting more patients to reach maturity, necessarily increases the number of women who will produce children at increased risk of congenital cardiac anomalies.[3]

Maternal cyanosis substantially increases fetal risk, even though in cyanotic forms of congenital heart disease, certain responses serve to facilitate delivery of oxygen to the fetus.[165,166] Systemic arterial hypoxemia increases red cell mass and oxygen-carrying capacity of the blood and displaces the whole blood–oxyhemoglobin dissociation curve to the right.[166] The placenta is proportionately larger in infants of hypoxic mothers, and it has been shown that the fetus responds to severe maternal hypoxemia by increasing 2, 3-DPG, and decreasing red cell oxygen affinity, thus facilitating the release of oxygen to the tissues.[165]

Despite these compensatory mechanisms, the vast majority of infants born to mothers with cyanosis are dysmature (small for gestational age)[96] or premature (gestation less than 37 weeks). In addition, there is a high rate of spontaneous abortion, the incidence of which increases in parallel with the mother's hematocrit; however, even in the presence of relatively mild cyanosis, the spontaneous abortion rate exceeds 50 per cent.[96]

Cardiovascular Drugs in Pregnancy

The response of the pregnant patient to cardiovascular drugs is important in a number of respects, especially the effect on uteroplacental blood flow, the effect on the tone of uterine muscle (and therefore on labor), and the effect on the fetus.[167] Transplacental transfer of drugs such as oral anticoagulants, together with the ill effects on the fetus of heparin, even though it does not cross the placental barrier, have already been discussed (p. 1775). The breast-fed neonate is also vulnerable to the drugs that the mother is taking, since a number of potentially harmful drugs are excreted in the milk.[2] As a matter of principle, it is desirable to minimize or avoid drug administration in the first trimester of pregnancy during fetal organogenesis.

Alpha-adrenergic stimulants, beta-adrenergic agonists, and drugs with combined alpha and beta effects influence both uterine blood flow and contraction. A vasoconstrictor given to a hypotensive pregnant patient is likely to increase uteroplacental blood flow by raising perfusion pressure, whereas the converse is the case when vasoconstriction is induced by administering such a drug to a normotensive subject. Beta-adrenergic agonists such as isoproterenol inhibit contraction of smooth muscle and accordingly depress both spontaneous and oxytocin-stimulated uterine contraction.[167] The unstressed heart rate of the fetus and neonate are under minimal beta-adrenergic control,[168] and offspring of propranolol-treated mothers have not manifested cardiac effects attributable to beta blockade.[167] Nevertheless, blockade of the humoral stimulation of beta-adrenergic receptor sites removes a potentially important reserve response to acute fetal stress and therefore seems undesirable under certain circumstances of fetal adaptation.[167] Propranolol increases uterine activity, an effect more pronounced in nonpregnant than in pregnant women.[169] The drug also crosses the placenta and is secreted in breast milk, thus potentially affecting fetal and neonatal heart rate and respiration.

Blood concentrations of *digitalis* are significantly lower in pregnant women than in nonpregnant patients receiving the same dose.[167] The glycosides freely cross the placental barrier, but there is no evidence of a harmful effect on the fetus.[170,171] Interestingly, digitalis not only increases the force of myocardial contraction but also may have a similar effect on the myomentrium.[172] It is not yet clear whether this effect accounts for the clinical impression that digitalized patients have shorter labors.

Inhibitors of prostaglandin synthesis—aspirin, indomethacin, and naproxen—are sometimes recommended for delaying premature labor.[173] These drugs interfere with uterine contractility and with maternal, fetal, and neonatal platelet function and are capable of constricting the fetal ductus with significant elevation of pulmonary arterial pressure.[173]

Diuretics administered in late pregnancy produce no apparent ill effects. However, in early gestation, care should be taken not to give diuretics injudiciously merely because of the presence of the mild ankle edema so common in normal pregnancy. An inappropriate reduction in maternal plasma volume is undesirable and potentially harmful to the fetus.[113] Antiarrhythmic agents such as quinidine, procainamide, lidocaine, and phenytoin have not been found to have adverse effects on the fetus but are best avoided during the first trimester as a matter of principle.[2] Disopyramide has been reported to initiate uterine contractions in the thirty-second week of pregnancy.[174] Antibiotics cross the placenta but are apparently not teratogenic, although tetracyclines given in late pregnancy can cause discoloration of the infant's teeth, and prolonged administration of streptomycin increases the risk of damage to the eighth cranial nerve of the fetus.[2] Morphine significantly reduces fetal heart rate and causes respiratory depression in the newborn. Prednisone has been held responsible for depressing placental function.[2] The high risk to the fetus of oral anticoagulants and heparin has been discussed and includes both the risk to fetal viability (fatal hemorrhage) and the teratogenic hazard.[130,131,137-139] Oral anticoagulants are secreted in the milk, but heparin is not. Open heart surgery carried out on the mother imposes a substantial risk to the life and normal development of the fetus.

References

1. Perloff, J. K., Lindgren, K. M., and Groves, B. M.: Uncommon or commonly unrecognized causes of heart failure. Prog. Cardiovasc. Dis. *12*:409, 1970.
2. Szekely, P., and Snaith, L.: Heart Disease and Pregnancy. Edinburgh and London, Churchill-Livingstone, 1974.
3. Perloff, J. K.: Late postoperative concerns in adults with congenital heart disease. *In* Pediatric Cardiovascular Disease. Philadelphia, F.A. Davis Co., 1981.
3a. Engle, M. A., and Perloff, J. K. (eds.): Symposium on postoperative congenital heart disease in adults. Am. J. Cardiol. *50*:541, 1982.
4. Chesley, L. C., Cosgrove, R. A., and Annito, J. E.: A follow-up study of eclamptic women. Am. J. Obstet. Gynecol. *83*:1360, 1962.
5. Demakis, J. G., and Rahimtoola, S. H.: Peripartum cardiomyopathy. Circulation *44*:964, 1971.
6. Demakis, J. G., Rahimtoola, S. H., Sutton, G. C., Meadows, W. R., Szanto, P. B., Tobin, J. R., and Gunnar, R. M.: Natural course of peripartum cardiomyopathy. Circulation *44*:1053, 1971.
7. Burch, G. E.: Heart disease and pregnancy. Am. Heart J. *93*:104, 1977.
8. Metcalf, J., and Ueland, K.: Maternal cardiovascular adjustments to pregnancy. Prog. Cardiovasc. Dis. *16*:363, 1974.
9. Lees, M. M.: Central circulatory responses in normotensive and hypertensive pregnancy. Postgrad. Med. J. *55*:311, 1979.
10. Spielman, F. J., and Popio, K. A.: Pregnancy and heart disease (key references). Circulation *65*:831, 1982.
11. Leman, R. B., and Assey, M. E.: Heart disease and pregnancy. South. Med. J. *74*:944, 1981.
11a. Elkayam, U., and Gleicher, N.: Cardiac Problems in Pregnancy. New York, Alan R. Liss, Inc., 1982.
12. Ueland, K., Novy, M. J., Peterson, E. N., and Metcalfe, J.: Maternal cardiovascular dynamics. IV. The influence of gestational age on the maternal cardiovascular response to posture and exercise. Am. J. Obstet. Gynecol. *104*: 856, 1969.
13. Katz, R., Karliner, J. S., and Resnik, R.: Effects of a natural volume overload state (pregnancy) on left ventricular performance in normal human subjects. Circulation *58*:434, 1978.
14. Lavid-Meeter, K., van de Ley, G., Bom T. H., Wladimiroff, J. W., and Roelandt, J.: Cardiocirculatory adjustments during pregnancy—An echocardiographic study. Clin. Cardiol. *2*:328, 1979.
15. Atkins, H. J., Watt, J. M., Milan, P., Davies, P., and Crawford, J. S.: A longitudinal study of cardiovascular dynamic changes throughout pregnancy. Eur. J. Obstet. Gynaecol. Reprod. Biol. *12*:215, 1981.
16. Lees, M. M., Taylor, S. H., Scott, D. B., and Kerr, M. G.: A study of cardiac output at rest throughout pregnancy. J. Obstet. Gynec. Br. Comm. *74*:319, 1967.
17. Rubler, S., Damani, P. M., and Pinto, E. R.: Cardiac size and performance during pregnancy estimated with echocardiography. Am. J. Cardiol. *40*:534, 1977.
18. Rose, D. J., Bader, M. E., Bader, R. A., and Braunwald, E.: Catheterization studies of cardiac hemodynamics in normal pregnant women with reference to left ventricular work. Am. J. Obstet. Gynecol. *72*:233, 1956.
19. Kerr, M. G.: The mechanical effects of the gravid uterus in late pregnancy. J. Obstet. Gynecol. Br. Comm. *72*:513, 1965.
20. Van Donsen, P. W., Eskes, T. K., Martin, D. B., and Van Hof, M. A.: Postural blood pressure differences in pregnancy. Am. J. Obstet. Gynecol. *138*: 1, 1980.
21. Atkins, H. J., Watt, J. M., Milan, P., Davies, P., and Crawford, J. S.: The influence of posture upon cardiovascular dynamics throughout pregnancy. Eur. J. Obstet. Gynaecol. Reprod. Biol. *12*:357, 1981.
22. Marx, G. F., Husain, F. J., and Shian, H. F.: Brachial and femoral blood pressures during the prenatal period. Am. J. Obstet. Gynecol. *136*:11, 1980.
23. Ueland, K., and Hansen, J. M.: Maternal cardiovascular dynamics. II. Posture and uterine contractions. Am. J. Obstet. Gynecol. *103*:1, 1969.
24. Bieniarz, J., Crottogini, J. K., Curuchet, E., Romero-Salinas, G., Yoshida, T., Poseiro, J. J., and Caldeyro-Barcia, R.: Aortocaval compression by the uterus in late human pregnancy. II. An arteriographic study. Am. J. Obstet. Gynecol. *100*:203, 1968.
25. Blake, S., O'Neill, H., and MacDonald, D.: Haemodynamic effects of pregnancy in patients with heart failure. Br. Heart J. *47*:495, 1982.
26. Kim, Y. I., Chandra, P., and Marx, G. F.: Successful management of severe aortocaval compression in twin pregnancy. Obstet. Gynecol. *46*:362, 1975.
27. Lund, C. J., and Donovan, J. C.: Blood volume during pregnancy. Significance of plasma and red cell volume. Am. J. Obstet. Gynecol. *98*:393, 1967.
28. Ueland, K.: Maternal cardiovascular dynamics. VII. Intrapartum blood volume changes. Am. J. Obstet. Gynecol. *126*:671, 1976.
29. Christianson, R. E.: Studies on blood pressure during pregnancy. I. Influence of parity and age. Am. J. Obstet. Gynecol. *125*:509, 1976.
30. Biggs, J. S. G.: Blood pressure changes following smoking in pregnancy. Aust. N. Z. J. Obstet. Gynaecol. *15*:204, 1975.
31. Ritchie, K.: The fetal response to changes in the composition of maternal inspired air in human pregnancy. Semin. Perinatol. *4*:295, 1980.
32. Robertson, E. G.: The natural history of oedema during pregnancy. J. Obstet Gynecol. Br. Comm. *78*:520, 1971.
33. Artal, R., Platt, L. D., Sperling, M., Kammula, R. K., Jilek, J., and Nakamura, R.: Maternal cardiovascular and metabolic responses in normal pregnancy. Am. J. Obstet. Gynecol. *140*:123, 1981.
34. Guzman, C. A., and Caplan, R.: Cardiorespiratory response to exercise during pregnancy. Am. J. Obstet. Gynecol. *108*:600, 1970.
35. Ueland, K., and Hansen, J. M.: Maternal cardiovascular dynamics. III. Labor and delivery under local and caudal analgesia. Am. J. Obstet. Gynecol. *103*:8, 1969.
36. Liebson, P. R., Mann, L. I., Evans, M. I., Duchin, S., and Arditi, L.: Cardiac performance during pregnancy. Serial evaluation using external systolic time intervals. Am. J. Obstet. Gynecol. *122*:1, 1975.
37. King, T. M., Whitehorn, W. V., and Reeves, B.: Effects of estrogen on composition and function of cardiac muscle. Am. J. Physiol. *196*:1282, 1959.
38. Ueland K., and Parer, J. T.: Effects of estrogens on the cardiovascular system of the ewe. Am. J. Obstet. Gynecol. *96*:400, 1966.
39. Csapo, A.: Actomyosin formation by estrogen action. Am. J. Physiol. *162*:406, 1950.
40. Hytten, F. E., and Thompson, A. M.: Water and electrolytes in pregnancy. Br. Med. Bull. *24*:15, 1958.
41. Wood, J. E.: The cardiovascular effects of oral contraceptives. Mod. Concepts Cardiovasc. Dis. *41*:37, 1972.
42. Manalo-Estrella, P., and Barker, A. E.: Histopathologic findings in human aortic media associated with pregnancy. A study of 16 cases. Arch. Pathol. *83*: 336, 1967.
43. Cavanzo, F. J., and Taylor, H. B.: Effect of pregnancy on the human aorta and its relationship to dissecting aneurysms. Am. J. Obstet. Gynecol. *105*:567, 1969.
44. Novy, M. J., and Edwards, M. J.: Respiratory problems in pregnancy. Am. J. Obstet. Gynecol. *99*:1024, 1967.
45. Pernoll, M. L., Metcalfe, J., Schlenker, T. L., Welch, J. E., and Matsumoto, J. A.: Oxygen consumption at rest and during exercise in pregnancy. Respir. Physiol. *25*:285, 1975.
46. Gazioglu, K., Kaltreider, N. L., Rosen, M., and Yu, P. N.: Pulmonary function during pregnancy in normal women and in patients with cardiopulmonary disease. Thorax *25*:445, 1970.
47. Pernoll, M. L., Metcalfe, J., Kovach, P. A., Wachtel, R., and Dunham, M. J.: Ventilation during rest and exercise in pregnancy and postpartum. Respir. Physiol. *25*:295, 1975.
48. Bader, R. A., Bader, M. E., and Rose, D. J.: The oxygen cost of breathing in dyspnoeic subjects as studied in normal pregnant women. Clin. Sci. *18*:223, 1959.
49. Burwell, C. S., and Metcalfe, J.: Heart Disease and Pregnancy. Physiology and Management. Boston, Little, Brown & Co., 1958.
50. Cutforth, R., and MacDonald, C. B.: Heart sounds and murmurs in pregnancy. Am. Heart J. *71*:741, 1966.
51. Goldberg, L. M., and Uhland, H.: Heart murmurs in pregnancy: A phonocardiographic study of their development, progression, and regression. Dis. Chest *52*:381, 1967.
52. Selzer, A.: Risks of pregnancy in women with cardiac disease. J.A.M.A. *238*: 892, 1977.
53. Perloff, J. K.: The Clinical Recognition of Congenital Heart Disease. 2nd ed. Philadelphia, W. B. Saunders Co., 1978.

54. Tabatznik, B., Randall, T. W., and Hersch, C.: The mammary souffle of pregnancy and lactation. Circulation *22*:1069, 1960.
55. Marcus, F. I., Ewy, F. A., O'Rourke, R. A., Walsh, B., and Bleich, A. C.: The effect of pregnancy on murmurs of mitral and aortic regurgitation. Circulation *41*:795, 1970.
56. Devereux, R. B., Perloff, J. K., Reichek, N., and Josephson, M. E.: Mitral valve prolapse. Circulation *54*:3, 1976.
57. Haas, J. M.: The effect of pregnancy on the midsystolic click and murmur of the prolapsing posterior leaflet of the mitral valve. Am. Heart J. *92*:407, 1976.
58. Kolibash, A. J., Ruiz, D. E., and Lewis, R. P.: Idiopathic hypertrophic subaortic stenosis in pregnancy. Ann. Intern. Med. *82*:791, 1975.
59. Bellet, S.: Essentials of Cardiac Arrhythmias. Diagnosis and Management. Philadelphia, W. B. Saunders Co., 1972.
60. Carruth, J. E., Mirvis, S. B., Brogan, D. R., and Wenger, N. K.: The electrocardiogram in normal pregnancy. Am. Heart J. *102*:1075, 1981.
61. Boyle, D. M., and Lloyd-Jones, L. L.: The electrocardiographic ST segment in pregnancy. J. Obstet. Gynecol. Br. Comm. *73*:986, 1966.
62. Copeland, G. D., and Stern, T. N.: Wenckebach periods in pregnancy and puerperium. Am. Heart J. *56*:291, 1958.
63. McMillan, T. M., and Bellet, S.: Ventricular paroxysmal tachycardia: Report of a case in a pregnant girl of 16 years with apparently normal heart. Am. Heart J. *7*:70, 1931.
64. Gallagher, J. J., Gilbert M., and Sverson, R. H.: Wolff-Parkinson-White syndrome. The problems, evaluation and surgical correction. Circulation *51*: 767, 1975.
65. Turner, A. F.: The chest radiograph in pregnancy. Clin. Obstet. Gynecol. *18*: 65, 1975.
66. Petch, M. C.: Cardiac disease in pregnancy. Postgrad. Med. J. *55*:315, 1979.
67. Besterman, E.: The changing face of acute rheumatic fever. Br. Heart J. *32*: 579, 1970.
68. Szekely, P., Turner, R., and Snaith, L.: Pregnancy and the changing pattern of rheumatic heart disease. Brit. Heart J. *35*:1293, 1973.
69. Chesley, L. C.: Severe rheumatic cardiac disease and pregnancy: The ultimate prognosis. Am. J. Obstet. Gynecol. *136*:552, 1980.
70. Ueland, K., and Metcalfe, J.: Acute rheumatic fever in pregnancy. Am. J. Obstet. Gynecol. *95*:586, 1966.
71. Lewis, B. V., and Parsons, M.: Chorea gravidarum. Lancet *1*:284, 1966.
72. Barnes, C. C.: Medical Disorders in Obstetric Practice. 3rd ed. Oxford, Blackwell Scientific Publishers, 1970.
73. Wood, P.: An appreciation of mitral stenosis. Br. Med. J. *1*:1051, 1113, 1954.
74. Nielsen, N. C., and Fabricius, J.: Primary pulmonary hypertension with special reference to prognosis. Acta Med. Scand. *170*:731, 1961.
75. Ronan, J. A., Steelman, R. B., DeLeon, A. C., Waters, T. J., Perloff, J. K., and Harvey, W. P.: The clinical diagnosis of acute severe mitral insufficiency. Am. J. Cardiol. *27*:284, 1971.
76. Reichek, N., Shelburne, J. C., and Perloff, J. K.: Clinical aspects of rheumatic valvular disease. Prog. Cardiovasc. Dis. *15*:491, 1973.
77. Roberts, W. C., and Perloff, J. K.: Mitral valvular disease. A clinicopathologic survey of the conditions causing the mitral valve to function abnormally. Ann. Intern. Med. *77*:939, 1972.
78. Caves, P. K., and Paneth, M.: Acute mitral regurgitation in pregnancy due to ruptured chordae tendineae. Br. Heart J. *34*:541, 1972.
79. Perloff, J. K., and Harvey, W. P.: Clinical recognition of tricuspid stenosis. Circulation *22*:346, 1960.
80. Selzer, A.: When is cardiac surgery necessary during pregnancy? J. Cardiovasc. Med. *7*:1332, 1982.
81. Perloff, J. K.: Congenital heart disease. *In* Beeson, P. B., and McDermott, W.: Textbook of Medicine. 16th ed. Philadelphia, W. B. Saunders Co., 1982.
82. Perloff, J. K., and Lindgren, K. M.: Adult survival in congenital heart disease. Geriatrics *29*:93, 94, 99, 1974.
83. Cannell, D. E., and Vernon, C. P.: Congenital heart disease and pregnancy. Am. J. Obstet. Gynecol. *85*:744, 1963.
84. Khoury, G. H., and Hawes, C. R.: Atrial septal defect associated with pulmonary hypertension in children living at high altitudes. J. Pediat. *70*:432, 1967.
85. Arias, F.: Maternal death in a patient with Eisenmenger's syndrome. Obstet. Gynecol. *50*:76, 1977.
86. Meyer, E. C., Tulsky, A. S., Sigmann, P., and Siber, E. N.: Pregnancy in the presence of tetralogy of Fallot. Am. J. Cardiol. *14*:874, 1964.
87. Jacoby, W. J.: Pregnancy with tetralogy and pentalogy of Fallot. Am. J. Cardiol. *14*:866, 1964.
88. Leibbrandt, G., Münch, U., and Gander, M.: Two successful pregnancies in a patient with single ventricle and transposition of the great arteries. Intl. J. Cardiol. *1*:257, 1982.
89. Haroutunian, L. M., and Neill, C. A.: Pulmonary complications of congenital heart disease: Hemoptysis. Am. Heart J. *84*:540, 1972.
90. Naeye, R. L., Hagstrom, J. W. C., and Talmadge, B. R.: Postpartum death with maternal congenital heart disease. Circulation *36*:304, 1967.
91. Pitts, J. A., Crosby, W. M., and Basta, L. L.: Eisenmenger's syndrome in pregnancy: Does heparin prophylaxis improve the maternal mortality rate? Am. Heart J. *93*:321, 1977.
92. Spinnato, J. A., Kraynak, B. J., and Cooper, M. W.: Eisenmenger's syndrome in pregnancy. New Engl. J. Med. *304*:1215, 1981.
93. Roberts, W. C.: The congenitally bicuspid aortic valve. Am. J. Cardiol. *26*:72, 1970.
94. Morganroth, J., Perloff, J. K., Zeldis, S. M., and Dunkman, W. V.: Acute severe aortic regurgitation. Ann. Intern. Med. *87*:223, 1977.
95. Deal, K., and Wooley, C. F.: Coarctation of aorta and pregnancy. Ann. Intern. Med. *78*:706, 1973.
96. Ueland, K.: Cardiac surgery and pregnancy. Am. J. Obstet. Gynecol. *92*:148, 1965.
97. Barash, P. G., Hobbins, J. C., Hook, R., Stansel, H. C., Whittmore, R., and Hehre, F. W.: Management of coarctation of the aorta during pregnancy. J. Thorac. Cardiovasc. Surg. *69*:781, 1975.
98. Mortensen, J. D., and Joelsson, I.: Coarctation of the aorta in pregnancy. J.A.M.A. *191*:596, 1965.
99. Kenmure, A. C. F., and Cameron, A. J. V.: Congenital complete heart block in pregnancy. Br. Heart J. *29*:910, 1967.
100. Shouse, E. E., and Acker, G. E.: Pregnancy and delivery in a patient with external-internal cardiac pacemaker. Obstet. Gynecol. *24*:817, 1964.
101. Littler, W. A.: Successful pregnancy in a patient with Ebstein's anomaly. Br. Heart J. *32*:711, 1970.
102. Anagnostopoulos, C. E., Prabhakar, M., and Kittle, C. F.: Aortic dissections and dissecting aneurysms. Am. J. Cardiol. *30*:263, 1972.
103. Wilson, S. K., and Hutchins, G. M.: Aortic dissecting aneurysms: Causative factors in 204 subjects. Arch. Pathol. Lab. Med. *106*:175, 1982.
104. Huseybe, K. O., Wolff, H. J., and Friedman, L.: Aortic dissection in pregnancy: A case of Marfan's syndrome. Am. Heart J. *55*:662, 1958.
104a. Cepin, D., James, F., and Carabello, B. A.: Left ventricular function in peripartum cardiomyopathy. Chest *83*:701, 1983.
105. Fillmore, S. J., and Parry, E. H. O.: The evolution of peripartal heart failure in Zaria, Nigeria. Circulation *56*:1058, 1977.
106. Kolibash, A. J., Ruiz, D. E., and Lewis, R. P.: Idiopathic hypertrophic subaortic stenosis in pregnancy. Ann. Intern. Med. *82*:791, 1975.
107. Oakley, G. D. G., McGarry, K., Limb, D. G., and Oakley, C. M.: Management of pregnancy in patients with hypertrophic cardiomyopathy. Br. Med. J. *1*:1749, 1979.
108. Gant, N. F., and Worley, R. J.: Hypertension in Pregnancy: Concepts and Management. New York, Appleton-Century-Crofts, 1980.
109. Lin, C. C., Lindheimer, M. D., River, P., and Moawad, A. H.: Fetal outcome in hypertensive disorders of pregnancy. Am. J. Obstet. Gynecol. *142*:255, 1982.
110. Page, E. W., and Christianson, R.: Influence of blood pressure changes with and without proteinuria upon outcome of pregnancy. Am. J. Obstet. Gynecol. *126*:821, 1976.
111. Finnerty, F. A.: Hypertension is different in blacks. J.A.M.A. *216*:1634, 1971.
112. Finnerty, F. A.: Hypertension and pregnancy. J. Cardiovasc. Med. *5*:559, 1980.
113. Lindheimer, M. D., and Katz, A. I.: Sodium and diuretics in pregnancy. N. Engl. J. Med. *288*:891, 1973.
114. Weir, R. J., and Willocks, J.: A successful pregnancy following malignant phase hypertension. Brit. J. Obstet. Gynecol. *83*:584, 1976.
115. Silverstone, A., Trudinger, B. J., Lewis, P. J., and Bulpitt, C. J.: Maternal hypertension and intrauterine fetal death in midpregnancy. Br. J. Obstet. Gynaecol. *87*:457, 1980.
116. Soffronoff, E. C., Kaufmann, B. M., and Connaughton, J. F.: Intravascular volume determinations and fetal outcome in hypertensive diseases of pregnancy. Am. J. Obstet. Gynecol. *127*:4, 1977.
117. Chesley, L. C., Annitto, J. E., and Cosgrove, R. A.: The remote prognosis of eclamptic women: Sixth periodic report. Am. J. Obstet. Gynecol. *124*:446, 1976.
118. Bauer, T. W., Moore, G. W., and Hutchins, G. M.: Morphologic evidence for coronary artery spasm in eclampsia. Circulation *65*:255, 1982.
119. Schroeder, J. S., and Harrison, D. C.: Repeated cardioversion during pregnancy. Am. J. Cardiol. *27*:445, 1971.
120. Gleicher, N., Meller, J., Sandler, R. Z., and Sullum, S.: Wolf-Parkinson-White syndrome in pregnancy. Obstet. Gynecol. *58*:748, 1981.
121. Perloff, J. K.: Auscultatory and phonocardiographic manifestations of pulmonary hypertension. Prog. Cardiovasc. Dis. *9*:303, 1967.
122. Oakley, C., and Somerville, J.: Oral contraceptives and progressive pulmonary vascular disease. Lancet *1*:890, 1968.
123. Mendelson, C. L.: Medical care, cardiovascular surgery and obstetric management as related to maternal and fetal welfare. *In* Mendelson, C. L.: Cardiac Disease in Pregnancy. Philadelphia, F. A. Davis Co., 1960, pp. 218–255.
124. Wallace, W. A., Harken, D. E., and Ellis, L. B.: Pregnancy following closed mitral valvuloplasty. J.A.M.A. *217*:297, 1971.
125. Ralstin, J. H., and Dunn, M.: Pregnancies after surgical correction of tetralogy of Fallot. J.A.M.A. *235*:2627, 1976.
126. Limet R., and Grondin, C. M.: Cardiac valve prostheses, anticoagulation, and pregnancy. Ann. Thorac. Surg. *23*:337, 1977.
127. Taguchi, K.: Pregnancy in patients with a prosthetic heart valve. Surg. Gynecol. Obstet. *145*:206, 1977.
128. Ibarra-Perez, C., Arevalo-Toledo, N., Cadena, O. A., and Noriega-Guerra, L.: The course of pregnancy in patients with artificial heart valves. Am. J. Med. *61*:504, 1976.
129. Ibarra-Perez, C., and Bosque-Ruiz, M.: Pregnancy in six patients with Starr-Edwards heart valve prostheses. Am. J. Cardiol. *30*:565, 1972.
130. Chew, P. C. T., and Ratnam, S. S.: Pregnancies in patients with prosthetic heart valves: A review and report of two further cases. Aust. N. Z. J. Obstet. Gynaecol. *15*:150, 1975.
131. Buxbaum, A., Aygen, M. M., Sajhin, W., Levy, M. J., and Ekerling, B.: Pregnancy in patients with prosthetic heart valves. Chest *59*:639, 1971.
132. McCans, J. L., and Wenger, N. K.: Problems in management of the pregnant

patient with rheumatic heart disease and valve prosthesis. South. Med. J. *69*: 1007, 1976.
133. Saka, D. M., and Marx, G. F.: Management of a patient with cardiac valve prosthesis. Anesth. Analg. Curr. Res. *55*:214, 1976.
134. Palacios-Macedo, X., Diaz-Devis, C., and Escudero, J.: Fetal risk with the use of coumarin anticoagulant agent in pregnant patients with intracardiac ball valve prosthesis. Am. J. Cardiol. *24*:853, 1969.
135. Hirsh, J., Cade, J. K., and Gallus, A. S.: Anticoagulants in pregnancy: A review of indications and complications. Am. Heart J. *83*:301, 1972.
136. Casanegra, P., Aviles, G., Maturana, G., and Dubernet, J.: Cardiovascular management of pregnant women with a heart valve prosthesis. Am. J. Cardiol. *36*:802, 1975.
137. Pettifor, J. M., and Benson, R.: Congenital malformations associated with the administration of oral anticoagulants during pregnancy. J. Pediatr. *86*:459, 1975.
138. Shaul, W. L., Emery, H., and Hall, J. G.: Chondrodysplasia punctata and maternal warfarin use during pregnancy. Am. J. Dis. Child. *129*:360, 1975.
139. Hall, J. G., Pauli, R. M., and Wilson, K. M.: Maternal and fetal sequelae of anticoagulation during pregnancy. Am. J. Med. *68*:122, 1980.
139a. Hull, R., Delmore, T., Carter, C., Hirsh, J., Genton, E., Gent, M., Turpie, G., and McLaughlin, D.: Adjusted subcutaneous heparin versus warfarin sodium in the long-term treatment of venous thrombosis. N. Engl. J. Med. *306*:189, 1982.
140. Chesley, L. C.: Rheumatic cardiac disease in pregnancy. Obstet. Gynecol. *46*: 699, 1975.
141. Chesley, L. C.: Severe rheumatic cardiac disease and pregnancy. Am. J. Obstet. Gynecol. *136*:552, 1979.
142. Boyer, N. H., and Nadas, A. S.: The ultimate effect of pregnancy on rheumatic heart disease. Ann. Intern. Med. *20*:99, 1944.
143. Maynard, E. P., and Grover, Z.: The effect of childbearing on the course of rheumatic heart disease: A 25-year study. Ann. Intern. Med. *52*:163, 1960.
144. Cole, T. O., and Adaleye, J. A.: Rheumatic heart disease and pregnancy in Nigerian women. Clin. Cardiol. *5*:280, 1982.
145. Henion, W. A., Hilal, A., Matthew, P. K., Lazarus, A., and Cohen, J.: Postpartum myocardial infarction. N. Y. State J. Med. *82*:57, 1982.
146. Ciraulo, D. A., and Markovitz, A.: Myocardial infarction in pregnancy associated with a coronary artery thrombus. Arch. Intern. Med. *139*:1046, 1979.
147. Hauth, J. C., Cunningham, F. G., and Young, P. K.: Takayasu's syndrome in pregnancy. Obstet. Gynecol. *50*:373, 1977.
148. Burch, G. E., and Giles, T. D.: The burden of a hot humid environment on the heart. Mod. Concepts Cardiovasc. Dis. *39*:115, 1970.
149. Gould, L., Zahir, M., DeMartino, A., and Gomprecht, R. F.: Cardiac effects of a cocktail. J.A.M.A. *218*:1799, 1971.
150. Stevens, K. M.: Cardiac stroke volume as a determinant of influenzal fatality. N. Engl. J. Med. *295*:1363, 1976.
151. Jackson, P.: Puerperal thromboembolic disease in high risk cases. Br. Med. J. *1*:263, 1973.
152. Ueland, K., Hansen, J., Eng, M., Kaloppa, R., and Parer, J. T.: Maternal cardiovascular dynamics. V. Cesarean section under thiopental, nitrous oxide and succinylcholine anesthesia. Am. J. Obstet. Gynecol. *108*:615, 1970.
153. Kaplan, E. L., Anthony, B. F., Bisno, A., Durack, D., Hauser, H., Millard, H. D., Sanford, J., Shulman, S. T., Stillerman, M., Taranta, A., and Wenger, N.: Prevention of bacterial endocarditis. Circulation *56*:139A, 1977.
154. Kay, C. F., and Smith, K.: Surgery in the pregnant cardiac patient. Am. J. Cardiol. *12*:293, 1963.
155. Salomon, J., Yortner, R., and Levy, M. J.: Open heart surgery during pregnancy—Case report. Vasc. Surg. *9*:257, 1975.
156. Martin, M. C., Pernoll, M. L., Boruszak, A. N., Jones, J. W., and Lo Cicero, J.: Cesarian section while on cardiac bypass. Obstet. Gynecol. *57*:41-S, 1981.
157. Wever, C. E.: Postmortem cesarean section: Review of the literature and case reports. Am. J. Obstet. Gynecol. *110*:158, 1971.
158. Clarren, S. K., and Smith, D. W.: The fetal alcohol syndrome. N. Engl. J. Med. *298*:1063, 1978.
159. Amussen, I.: Fetal cardiovascular system as influenced by maternal smoking. Clin. Cardiol. *2*:246, 1979.
160. Meyer, M. B., and Tonascia, J. A.: Maternal smoking, pregnancy complications and perinatal mortality. Am. J. Obstet. Gynecol. *128*:494, 1977.
161. Valentine, B. H., and Baker, J. L.: Treatment of recurrent pregnancy hypertension by prophylactic anticoagulation. Br. J. Obstet. Gynecol. *84*:309, 1977.
162. Redman, C. W. G., Beilin, L. J., Bonnar, J., and Ounsted, M. K.: Fetal outcome in trial of antihypertensive treatment in pregnancy. Lancet *2*:753, 1976.
163. Friedman, E. A., and Neff, R. K.: Hypertension-hypotension in pregnancy. Correlation with fetal outcome. J.A.M.A. *239*:2249, 1978.
164. Chesley, L. C.: Hypertensive Disorders in Pregnancy. New York, Appleton-Century-Crofts. 1978.
165. Whittemore, R., Hobbins, J. C. and Engle, M. A.: Pregnancy and its outcome in women with and without surgical treatment of congenital heart disease. Am. J. Cardiol. *50*:641, 1982.
166. Novy, M. J., Peterson, E. N., and Metcalfe, J.: Respiratory characteristics of maternal and fetal blood in cyanotic congenital heart disease. Am. J. Obstet. Gynecol. *100*:821, 1968.
167. Brinkman, C. R., and Woods, J. R.: Effects of cardiovascular drugs during pregnancy. Cardiovasc. Med. *1*:231, 1976.
168. Nuwayhid, B., Brinkman, C. R., Su, C., Bevan, J. A., and Assali, N. S.: Development of autonomic control of fetal circulation. Am J. Physiol. *228*: 337, 1975.
169. Pruyn, C. S., Phelan, J. P., and Buchanan, G. C.: Long-term propranalol therapy in pregnancy: Maternal and fetal outcome. Am. J. Obstet. Gynecol. *135* :485, 1979.
170. Okita, G. T., Plotz, E. J., and Davis, M. E.: Placental transfer of radioactive digitoxin in pregnant women and its fetal distribution. Circ. Res. *4*:376, 1956.
171. Rogers, M. C., Willerson, J. T., Goldblatt, A., and Smith, T. W.: Serum digoxin concentrations in the human fetus, neonate and infant. N. Engl. J. Med. *287*:1010, 1972.
172. Norris, P. R.: The action of cardiac glycosides on the human uterus. J. Obstet. Gynecol. Br. Comm. *68*:916, 1961.
173. Rudolph, A. M.: Effects of aspirin and acetaminophen in pregnancy and in the newborn. Arch. Intern. Med. *141*:358, 1981.
174. Leonard, R. F., Braun, T. E., and Levy, A. M.: Initiation of uterine contractions by disopyramide during pregnancy. N. Engl. J. Med. *299*:84, 1978.

54 RELATIONSHIP BETWEEN DISEASES OF THE HEART AND LUNGS

by E. Regis McFadden, Jr., M.D., and Roland H. Ingram, Jr., M.D.

Because of the integrated nature of the function of the heart and lungs, it is difficult for one component to be compromised without altering the physiology of the other. In fact, with chronic disease originating in either the heart or the lungs, there is both subjective and objective evidence of dysfunction in both systems. While a great deal is known about right ventricular hypertrophy or dilatation secondary to lung disease (e.g., cor pulmonale, Chapter 46) and pulmonary malfunction in acute left ventricular failure (e.g., pulmonary edema, Chapter 17), many other pathophysiological interfaces between the cardiovascular and pulmonary systems exist clinically. The purposes of this chapter are to explore these interactions and to detail their mechanisms as far as they are known.

MECHANISMS BY WHICH HEART DISEASE LEADS TO LUNG DYSFUNCTION

Cardiac disease can alter lung function or induce pulmonary disease through the effects of (1) pulmonary venous hypertension from elevated left ventricular end-diastolic and/or left atrial pressures[1–15]; (2) compression of mediastinal structures, airways, or lung by global cardiomegaly, pericardial and pleural effusions, and specific chamber enlargement[16–20]; (3) pharmacological agents used to treat cardiac disease, such as beta antagonists, diuretics, nitrates, and others[21–26]; and (4) miscellaneous phenomena such as hemoptysis due to cardiac disease giving rise to blood pneumonias. Of these, the most important factor is pulmonary venous hypertension.

Increased Pulmonary Venous Pressure

Physiologically significant increases in left ventricular end-diastolic or left atrial pressures are invariably transmitted retrogradely to the pulmonary vasculature and, in addition to producing pulmonary arterial hypertension, evoke one or more of the stages of pulmonary edema formation, i.e., increased lymph flow, interstitial edema, or alveolar edema (Chapter 17). The magnitude and duration of the pulmonary venous hypertension then determines the extent to which the lung is affected. If the changes in pressure are acute and modest in degree, then vascular engorgement and perivascular and interstitial edema predominate. In these circumstances the effects on the lung tend to be subtle. If the venous pressure changes are chronic, then the changes in lung function are more easily measured because, in addition to the above, anatomical changes such as fibrosis, medial hypertrophy, and intimal thickening may develop in the arteries and veins, airways narrow from peribronchiolar and mucosal edema, and the interstitial edema within the parenchyma may eventually be replaced by fibrosis.[27,28] In rare instances, the last can be so severe that dense calcification and actual bone formation can develop.[29] Thus, it is not possible to elevate pulmonary venous pressures without altering lung function. The *lung* is the organ that undergoes the anatomical and physiological disturbances responsible for dyspnea, chest tightness, and cough.

ALTERATIONS IN PULMONARY MECHANICS. From a mechanical standpoint, patients with chronically elevated pulmonary venous pressure can be characterized as having "restrictive ventilatory defects," i.e., loss of lung volume. Typically, vital capacity is reduced, residual volume and functional residual capacity are normal or nearly so, and total lung capacity is less than predicted.[6–10,30,31] The reduction in total lung capacity results from replacement of the air in the lung with either blood or interstitial fluid, with resulting changes in the elastic properties of the pulmonary parenchyma. As pulmonary venous hypertension (hence, interstitial and alveolar wall edema) advances, the lung becomes stiffer or less compliant. As this process worsens, air trapping can occur because of earlier than normal closure of dependent airways, and residual volume may actually increase as total lung capacity decreases.[5]

The progressive changes in lung size and recoil tend to increase the pleural pressures required to efffect respiration, thus elevating the work of breathing[8] and thereby leading to tachypnea with a low tidal volume and high respiratory frequency (Fig. 15–2. p. 493).[32]

In addition to volume loss, there is evidence that pulmonary vascular congestion and edema can interfere with peripheral airway function.[5,33–39] Studies in animals have shown that the resistance in distal airways increases to a greater degree in response to elevations of left atrial pressure than does total airway resistance and that with sustained increases of pressure pulmonary changes are slow to resolve. These findings suggest that engorgement of the blood vessels within the confines of the bronchovascular sheath can encroach upon the lumina of the airways and promote edema formation, which can persist for considerable periods. Such observations provide the basis for understanding disturbances in ventilation-perfusion relationships that can often be profound in pulmonary congestion or edema.

ALTERATIONS IN THE DISTRIBUTION OF VENTILATION AND PERFUSION. The mechanical factor that determines the distribution of ventilation within the lung is the product of the resistance of the bronchi and the compliance of the alveolar units subtended to them. This product is called a time constant ($R \times C = \tau$), and in the normal lung the regional values for τ are nearly equal so that all the alveoli fill and empty synchronously when respiration is initiated at functional residual capacity.[40] However, because of the above derangements in compliance and resistance, in heart disease inter- and intraregional nonhomogeneities develop and result in maldistribution of inspired air. Regional alveolar hypoxia then ensues with its attendant sequelae.[41] The maldistribution becomes more severe with increases in respiratory frequency,[41,42] thus the exercise performance of affected patients is also altered.

The disease in the pulmonary vessels gives rise to abnormal distribution of perfusion, with a reversal of the normal apex-to-base gradient (Fig. 46–5, p. 1576), i.e., the apical lung zones are perfused more than the basilar lung zones.[11–15] The extent of reversal correlates well with increases in pulmonary capillary wedge pressure.[11,12,14] Although there is evidence that the arterioles in the basilar zones of the lung are more responsive to hypoxia than are their apical counterparts in normal subjects,[43] breathing 100 per cent oxygen in mitral stenosis does not completely correct the abnormal distribution of blood flow,[44] suggesting that hypoxic vasoconstriction is not the sole cause for the reversed flow pattern. Acute perivascular edema probably accounts for some of the changes in the flow pattern, but, in chronic pulmonary venous hypertension, structural vascular alterations develop (p. 829) and play a prominent role. These pathological changes tend to be more severe in the basilar zones.[44,45] The overall physiological consequences of all these abnormalities are mismatched ventilation-perfusion relationships that result in widened alveolar-arterial differences for oxygen, arterial hypoxemia, and enlarged dead space-tidal volume ratios.[30]

An additional factor often considered to *cause* the reductions in arterial oxygen content and partial pressure seen in heart disease is a depressed partial pressure of oxygen in the mixed venous blood.[46,47] However, for several reasons, consideration of this factor as a cause of arterial hypoxemia leads to circular and nonproductive reasoning. In normal subjects engaging in heavy exercise at sea level while breathing air, the mixed venous oxygen content diminishes to extremely low values, yet the arterial content remains normal. Hence low values for mixed venous oxygen do not a priori cause a lower than normal arterial value. However, when there is abnormal gas exchange in the lung, whether due to ventilation-perfusion abnormalities or shunt, low arterial oxygen contents result in lower mixed venous values at any given oxygen consumption and cardiac output. Basically, then, the values for mixed venous oxygen are the most dependent of the variables affecting heart-lung interrelations and are the result of oxygen transfer in the lung, cardiac output, and peripheral tissue metabolic consumption of oxygen. Therefore, this factor should always be considered as a *consequence* of hypoxemia rather than as a principal cause.

ALTERATIONS IN ARTERIAL BLOOD GASES. The extent to which arterial blood gases are disturbed depends upon the severity and suddenness of the rise in left-side pressures. In acute pulmonary edema secondary to left ventricular decompensation, gas exchange can be so severely compromised that frank respiratory failure can result. Aberman and Fulop, in a prospective study of 50 consecutive cases of pulmonary edema, demonstrated that, prior to treatment, affected patients as a group had severe hypoxemia and either metabolic or combined metabolic and respiratory acidosis.[48] In this study, 58 per cent of the patients had values for arterial pO_2 that were less than 50 mm Hg, and 83 per cent had acidemia with a pH less than 7.36. Hypoxemia was most severe in the patients with the greatest acidosis. Twenty-three patients had hypocapnia, 12 were eucapnic, and 11 had arterial CO_2 tensions in excess of 45 mm Hg. The hypercapnic patients did not have a greater incidence of underlying chronic airway obstruction than those without CO_2 retention. The arterial CO_2 tensions and pH rapidly returned to normal, with resolution of alveolar hypoventilation resulting from alveolar flooding and interstitial edema, and with the disappearance of the lactic acidosis secondary to the low cardiac output state.

RESPIRATORY RESPONSE TO EXERCISE. The abnormalities in mechanics and gas-exchanging function of the lung described thus far are related to the degree and chronicity of the elevated pulmonary capillary pressures.

Since there are further increases in pulmonary venous hypertension with exercise in congestive heart failure, one would anticipate that the degree of pulmonary dysfunction would increase in direct proportion to the degree of acute change.[49]

With physical exertion in patients with pulmonary venous hypertension, left atrial and pulmonary artery pressures rise, causing transudation of fluid from the intravascular space so that pulmonary extravascular fluid volume increases.[4] Concomitantly, the lung becomes stiffer, and the work of breathing and resistance to air flow greatly increase.[50,51] Presumably as a result of these factors, these patients ventilate at higher frequencies for any given level of oxygen consumption, so the ventilation equivalent $\dot{V}_E/VO_2$ is abnormal,[52] and maximal oxygen uptakes reduced.[53] Some studies have demonstrated that dead space ventilation in patients with mitral stenosis is greater both at rest and with exercise than in normal subjects.[30,54]

The effects of exercise on arterial O_2 tensions in patients with pulmonary venous hypertension are inconsistent. Some investigators have noted decreases,[55] while others have reported no change.[52] These discrepancies result in part from the fact that a change in pulmonary blood flow distribution occurs that could possibly offset the effect of an increase in wasted ventilation with exercise. The previously described resting reversal of the normal pulmonary blood flow distribution pattern can return toward normal during physical exertion in some patients, resulting in relative increases in basilar perfusion.[56] Under these circumstances one would expect to find an improvement in gas exchange to the extent that basilar lung units are ventilated. Despite the above derangements, exercise limitations per se in patients with congestive heart failure or mitral stenosis do not appear to be related simply to the level of the pulmonary venous pressure that is reached. Rather, it seems that a complex interaction of respiratory, cardiac, and peripheral mechanisms is involved.

INTRATHORACIC SPACE-OCCUPYING EFFECTS

Heart disease can alter lung function or produce pulmonary symptoms directly, by compression of mediastinal structures such as the trachea, major bronchi, and esophagus, and indirectly, through the effects of pleural effusions. Partial obstruction of the esophagus can occasionally interfere with deglutition and give rise to aspiration pneumonias. The consequences of compressive effects of major airways are much more severe in infants, compared with older children and adults.

In infants, vascular abnormalities such as vascular ring (p. 1013) can produce tracheal obstruction with dyspnea, wheezing, use of accessory muscles of respiration, and a crowing stridor on both inspiration and expiration.[16] There is commonly a history of recurrent pulmonary infections and the condition is frequently misdiagnosed as croup, bronchitis, or asthma. Bronchial obstruction may occur as a result of any cardiac condition in which there is a large left-to-right shunt, but it is most commonly due to a ventricular septal defect or to a large patent ductus arteriosus.[17,18] Also, any condition associated with massive cardiomegaly, particularly a greatly enlarged left atrium, as occurs in some patients with severe mitral regurgitation (p. 1083), may compress the bronchi. With large left-to-right shunts, the dilated pulmonary artery and the distended left atrium can cause atelectasis or hyperinflation, depending upon the degree of obstruction.[17] Sites of predilection are the left main, left upper, and right middle lobe bronchi.[17] With massive cardiomegaly, the left main bronchus may be completely obstructed, with resulting atelectasis of the left lung.[17]

Because the magnitude of the left-to-right shunt is limited by the high pulmonary vascular resistance in the neonatal period, bronchial obstruction from this mechanism is rare in this age period. The peak incidence of bronchial obstruction occurs between two and nine months of age when pulmonary artery pressure tends to rise. Other cardiac abnormalities that cause compression of major airways via large pulmonary arteries and distended left atria, with or without left ventricular decompensation, are anomalous pulmonary venous drainage, cor triatriatum, and left atrial obstruction due to a supravalvular mitral ring or congenital mitral stenosis.[19] In adults it has long been recognized that massive cardiomegaly or pericardial effusions can compress the left lower lobe and so give rise to Ewart's sign (dullness, bronchial breathing, and increased tactile fremitus near the angle of the scapula). Hypoventilation of the entire left lung has also been reported.

Lung function in patients with pleural effusion has not been extensively studied, but the available data suggest that effusions, if large enough, can act as space-occupying lesions that limit lung volume and gas exchange.[57,58] In pleuritis regional lung function deteriorates as the result of resolved pleural effusions. Both blood flow and ventilation are shifted away from the lung base on the involved side.[59]

EFFECTS ON LUNG FUNCTION OF DRUGS USED TO TREAT HEART DISEASE

Of all the agents in use for the treatment of cardiac disease, the ones that have received the most attention for their potentially harmful pulmonary effects are the beta-antagonists. While there is no doubt that beta-adrenergic receptor blockade in asthmatic subjects may cause precipitous and prolonged airway narrowing and an increased sensitivity of the tracheobronchial tree to other constrictor stimuli,[21,60,61] responses in normal subjects and in patients with other forms of obstructive airway disease have been conflicting. Recent evidence based upon an extensive evaluation of the pressure-flow-volume interrelationships of the lung demonstrates that the intravenous administration of 20 mg of propranolol is entirely innocuous in normal subjects.[62] This is not true in patients with hay fever or chronic obstructive lung disease.

For reasons not completely understood, some patients with chronic bronchitis are hyperresponsive to constrictor stimuli and, when given beta blockers, develop severe bronchoconstriction.[61,63,64] Similarly, asymptomatic nonasthmatic first-degree relatives of asthmatics and individuals with atopic histories but without asthma may behave similarly.[61] These effects are also seen with agents purported to be more selective beta blockers. Unfortunately, in the doses required for treatment of angina in the majority of patients, the so-called cardioselective beta blockers ($beta_1$) produce sufficient $beta_2$ blockade that bronchoconstriction may still be a troublesome side effect in susceptible patients. Thus, the advantages of the "cardioselective" beta blockers exist only when very small doses of these agents are employed.

Beta-adrenergic blockers, in addition to producing acute bronchospasm in asthmatics, have also been found to worsen airway function in individuals with nonspecific chronic obstructive lung disease.[63–65] In fact, even small quantities of these drugs absorbed from remote sites can have adverse effects; for example, the conjunctival instillation of timolol has been reported to worsen lung function in susceptible individuals.[65] Therefore, these drugs should be used with care, and careful pulmonary and allergic histories should be routinely sought before one prescribes these agents. The *calcium-channel blocking agents* have not been shown to have any adverse pulmonary effects.[66] Hence, these drugs may be the treatment of choice for myocardial ischemia in patients with coexisting primary airway disease who otherwise would receive beta blockers.

Sodium nitroprusside, nitroglycerin, dopamine, and *hydralazine* can all have adverse effects on gas exchange in patients with left-sided heart disease.[23,25,67–69] These agents have been shown to cause a fall in arterial oxygen tension despite improving cardiac hemodynamics. Usually, the depression in O_2 is modest ($\leq$ 10 mm Hg) and is believed to be secondary to alterations in ventilation-perfusion relationships, i.e., it is caused by improved perfusion of poorly ventilated alveoli.

Compensatory alveolar hypoventilation with CO_2 retention has been reported to occur rarely in patients with cardiac disease who have developed severe metabolic alkalosis secondary to diuretics that increase potassium excretion.[70] Severe H^+ and Cl^- depletion, together with dehydration, appears to be responsible.

The effects of therapeutic doses of morphine on lung function are controversial. Some authors have warned against the use of this drug in patients with myocardial infarction or acute pulmonary edema because of its tendency to interfere with gas exchange by ventilatory depression.[71] While there is little doubt that this does occur in some individuals, it has been shown that 15 mg of morphine administered by intramuscular injection are well tolerated in both groups of patients.[24,72] Arterial pO_2 falls 2 to 3 mm Hg and CO_2 increases 4 to 5 mm Hg within an hour of receiving an intramuscular injection.[24,72] However, it should be noted that the respiratory depression produced by morphine may be potentiated by lidocaine, and the adverse effects of morphine on gas exchange in patients with preexisting chronic obstructive lung disease who develop an acute myocardial infarction can be dramatic.

PULMONARY EFFECTS SECONDARY TO SPECIFIC CARDIAC DISORDERS

MITRAL STENOSIS AND CONGESTIVE HEART FAILURE

In view of the similarity of the effects of mitral stenosis and left ventricular failure on pulmonary vascular pressures, they are discussed together. Because much of the general information regarding the pulmonary alterations in these conditions is presented elsewhere (pp. 492 and 1066), this section will focus primarily on the degree and kinds of lung dysfunction that occur in relation to the functional cardiac classification.[30,31]

When the underlying condition is mild with no limitation on ordinary activity (Class I), then, generally speaking, lung function tends to be relatively normal at rest (Figs. 54–1 and 54–2). Vital capacity may be slightly reduced and the alveolar-arterial gradient for O_2 may be increased. As the disease process worsens, and the patient's symptomatic disability increases, virtually all aspects of lung function deteriorate. Vital capacity, forced expiratory flow rates and volumes, maximum breathing capacity, dynamic compliance, resting diffusing capacities, and arterial oxygen tensions all fall progressively, while airway resistance and alveolar-arterial gradients for O_2 rise.[30,31] These measurements correlate well with the increase in pulmonary artery pressure and pulmonary vascular resistance.

Patients with Class IV disability generally have severely compromised lung function.[72a] Mean values for vital capacity are 60 to 70 per cent of predicted values, while flow rates in the midvital capacity tend to be around 30 per cent of expected normal. Diffusing capacity tends to be abnormally low and about one-half that observed in Class I, while dynamic compliance is severely reduced, being only one-third of its previous value. Arterial oxygen tensions range between 58 and 75 mm Hg (normal = 95 ± 5 mm Hg), and the alveolar-arterial gradients for O_2 lie between 30 and 41 mm Hg (normal ≤ 20 mm Hg).

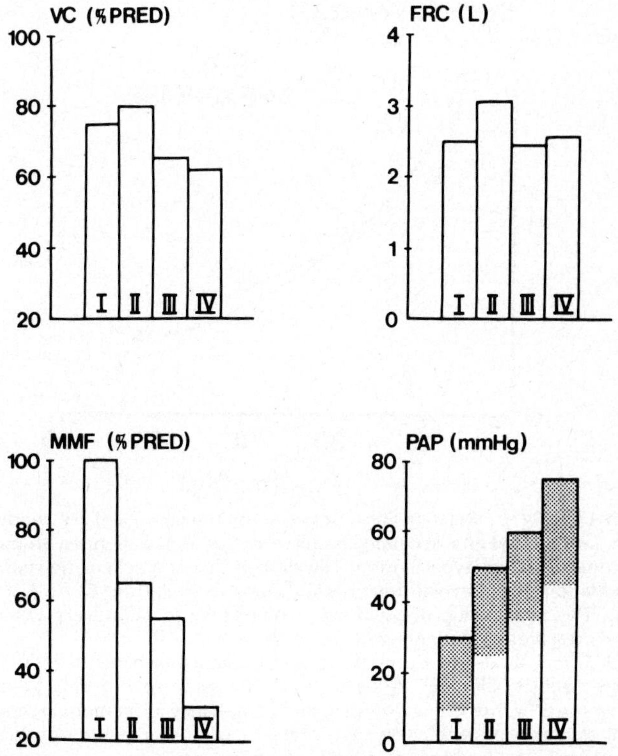

FIGURE 54–1 Alterations in pulmonary mechanics and pulmonary artery pressures observed in the various clinical stages of mitral stenosis. The heights of the bars represent mean values. VC = vital capacity; FRC = functional residual capacity; MMF = maximum midexpiratory flow rate; PAP = pulmonary artery pressure. In the PAP graph the top of the shaded area represents the systolic pressure and the bottom, the diastolic pressure. Roman numerals represent stages of increasing clinical disability. (Data redrawn from Palmer, W. H., et al.: Disturbances of pulmonary function in mitral valve disease. Canad. Med. Assoc. J. *89*:744, 1963.)

The changes in dynamic compliance (i.e., compliance measured during tidal respiration) vary inversely with pulmonary capillary wedge pressures.[9,10] When compliance is normal at rest, as it tends to be in patients with Class I and II disability, pulmonary wedge pressure tends to be normal; as wedge pressure rises with progression of the disease, or with exercise, dynamic compliance falls (Fig. 54–3).

Measurements of the static pressure-volume (recoil) properties have shown that the lungs of patients with mitral stenosis are altered in a distinct manner.[7,73] As can be seen in Figure 54–4*A*, elastic recoil is increased at high lung volumes, is normal at functional residual capacity, and then becomes abnormally low as residual volume is

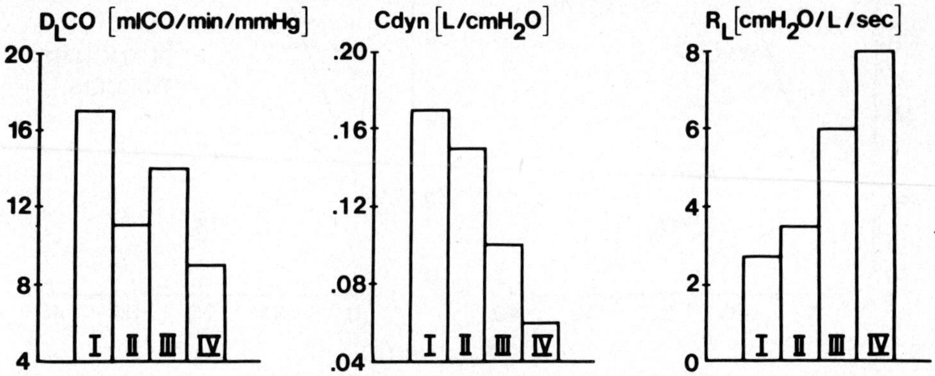

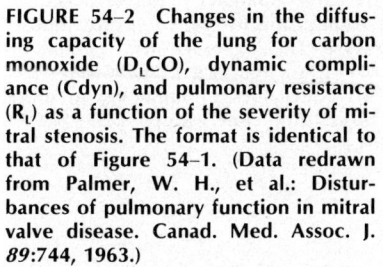

FIGURE 54–2 Changes in the diffusing capacity of the lung for carbon monoxide (D_LCO), dynamic compliance (Cdyn), and pulmonary resistance (R_L) as a function of the severity of mitral stenosis. The format is identical to that of Figure 54–1. (Data redrawn from Palmer, W. H., et al.: Disturbances of pulmonary function in mitral valve disease. Canad. Med. Assoc. J. *89*:744, 1963.)

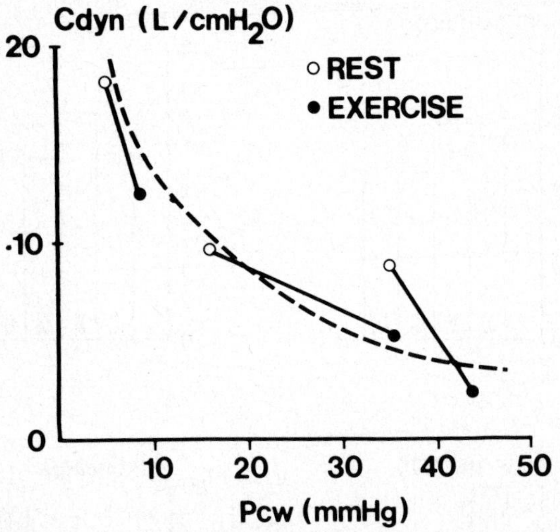

FIGURE 54–3 Relationships between pulmonary capillary wedge pressure (Pcw) and dynamic compliance (Cdyn) in patients with pulmonary venous hypertension. The dashed line is a schematic representation of the overall relationship. (Data from Saxton, G. A., Jr., et al.: The relationship of pulmonary compliance to pulmonary vascular pressures in patients with heart disease. J. Clin. Invest. *35*:611, 1965, and White, H. C., et al.: Lung compliance in patients with mitral stenosis. Clin. Sci. *17*:667, 1958.) The three sets of data points demonstrate the effects on dynamic compliance of acutely increasing pulmonary capillary wedge pressure with exercise. (Data from Saxton, G. A., Jr., et al., as cited.)

approached. This is unlike the situation seen in either atrial septal defect or pulmonary fibrosis (Fig. 54–4*B*). It has been suggested that vascular plethora accounts for the loss of recoil at small lung volumes and that pulmonary fibrosis produces the increased retractive forces at the larger volumes. Regardless of the mechanism involved, this type of change in elastic properties helps to explain why functional residual capacity and residual volume can remain normal in the presence of a reduced total lung capacity. In the case of functional residual capacity, the resting mechanical balance of the respiratory system, set by the tendency of the lung to recoil and the chest wall to spring outward, appears intact. With respect to residual volume, it can be seen that two forces (airway compression from engorgement or edema of the vascular sheath and loss of recoil with resultant loss of radial traction of the airways) combine to promote early airway closure with air trapping.[5] In addition to these functional abnormalities it has been suggested that there is a disturbance of respiratory muscle function in patients with mitral valve disease.[73]

Collins and colleagues evaluated airway function in 72 patients with left-sided valvular and ischemic heart disease who were free of symptoms and demonstrated that, as a group, these individuals had lower values for standard spirometric indices (forced vital capacity [FVC] and one-second forced expiratory volumes [FEV_1]) than did healthy subjects. These findings were taken as evidence of airway obstruction, but the FEV_1/FVC ratio averaged 0.75. This value is within normal limits for a population of this age and implies that the lungs were emptying normally but from a lower volume. The significance of these findings is that they are consistent with the observations of the Framingham study[74] that reductions in vital capacity can predict the development of congestive heart failure. In 5209 persons evaluated over an 18-year period, the risk of congestive heart failure varied in inverse proportion to vital capacity. Both a persistently low and a recent fall in vital capacity were associated with increased risk. Among persons with ischemic heart disease, hypertension, or rheumatic heart disease, chances of developing congestive failure were doubled in men and tripled in women with low vital capacities. It is possible that a reduction of vital capacity is not a "risk factor" for heart failure in the classic sense that cigarette smoking is a risk factor for ischemic heart disease, but actually represents a manifestation of heart failure that is not otherwise evident clinically.

MYOCARDIAL INFARCTION (See also page 1276)

Arterial hypoxemia and abnormalities in regional ventilation-perfusion relations and pulmonary mechanics regularly occur in patients with acute myocardial infarction and unstable angina as well as in experimentally provoked coronary insufficiency.[34–39,75–77] The sequence of events is believed to be left ventricular dysfunction from either left ventricular failure and/or a reduction in ventricular com-

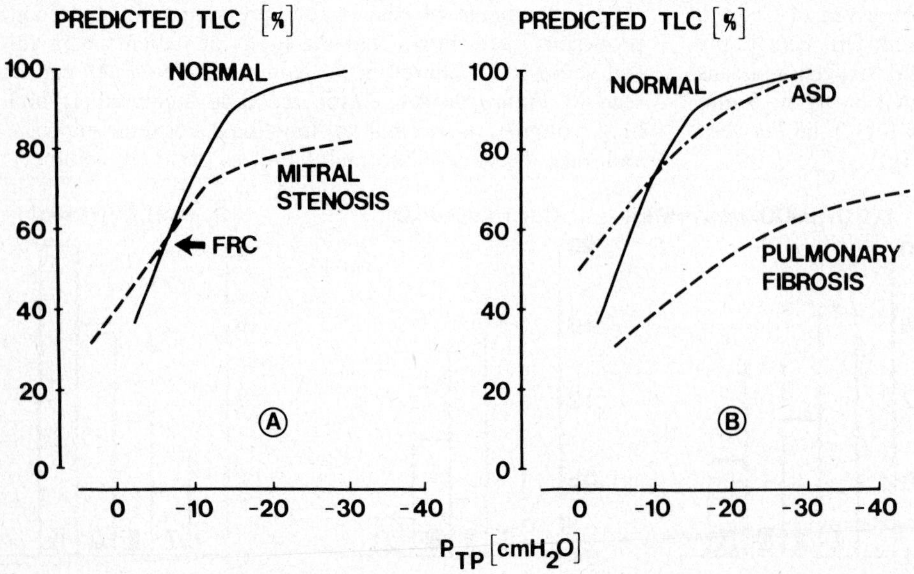

FIGURE 54–4 Comparison of the static pressure-volume relationships of the lung in normal subjects and in patients with (*A*) mitral stenosis and (*B*) atrial septal defects (ASD) and pulmonary fibrosis. TLC = total lung capacity; P_{TP} = transpulmonary pressure; FRC = functional residual capacity. (Data redrawn from Wood, T. E., et al.: Mechanics of breathing in mitral stenosis. Am. Rev. Resp. Dis. *104*:52, 1971.)

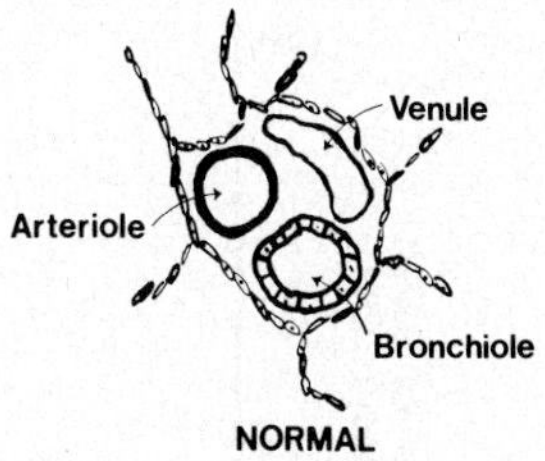

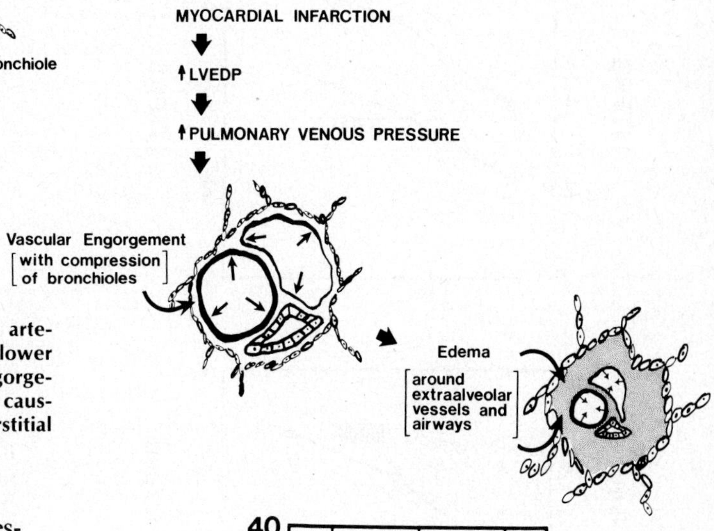

FIGURE 54–5 Normally the loose interstitial space containing arterioles, venules, and bronchioles allows the bronchiole, despite its lower intraluminal pressure, to remain widely open. With vascular engorgement, the dilated venules and arterioles compress the bronchiole, causing an increase in the resistance of these airways. With interstitial edema, the lumina of all structures are compromised.

pliance, leading to acute elevations in end-diastolic pressure with subsequent development of pulmonary vascular congestion and edema that lasts for hours or up to two days in uncomplicated cases. With the onset of edema, the arterioles and bronchioles become compressed, causing the pathogenetic sequence discussed earlier. As this occurs, there is widespread closure of dependent airways with resultant arterial hypoxemia[39,75] (Fig. 54–5). Several studies have demonstrated that after a myocardial infarction or during an episode of prolonged myocardial ischemia, the lung volume at which airway closure begins can encroach upon, or even exceed, functional residual capacity.[39,75] Therefore, during normal respiration, some alveoli are not ventilated and act as anatomical shunts. More severe elevation of pulmonary capillary pressure results in alveolar flooding (Chap. 17).

In addition to alterations in gas exchange, myocardial ischemia and/or infarction may cause acute elevations in airway resistance and reductions in pulmonary compliance[36,37] (Figs. 54–6 and 54–7). A schematic representation of the pulmonary consequences of vascular engorgement, interstitial edema, and alveolar flooding is contained in Figure 54–8. Many patients with coronary artery disease are cigarette smokers and frequently show the changes in pulmonary function resulting therefrom, including elevated residual volume, reduced air flow rates, and increasingly abnormal dynamic compliance with increasing respiratory frequency. In most patients with acute myocardial ischemia it is difficult to distinguish between the various causes of impaired lung function, but the contribution of acute myocardial ischemia can be assessed by repeating the measurements after the cessation of the acute episode and return of the hemodynamics to the baseline state. It is also difficult to determine whether the changes in mechanics and gas exchange are secondary to left ventricular dysfunction or to other factors, such as smoking. One method is to observe whether acute improvement follows the administration of diuretics.[75]

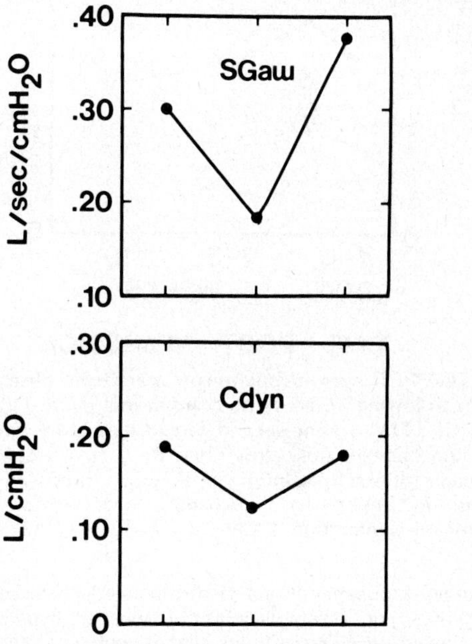

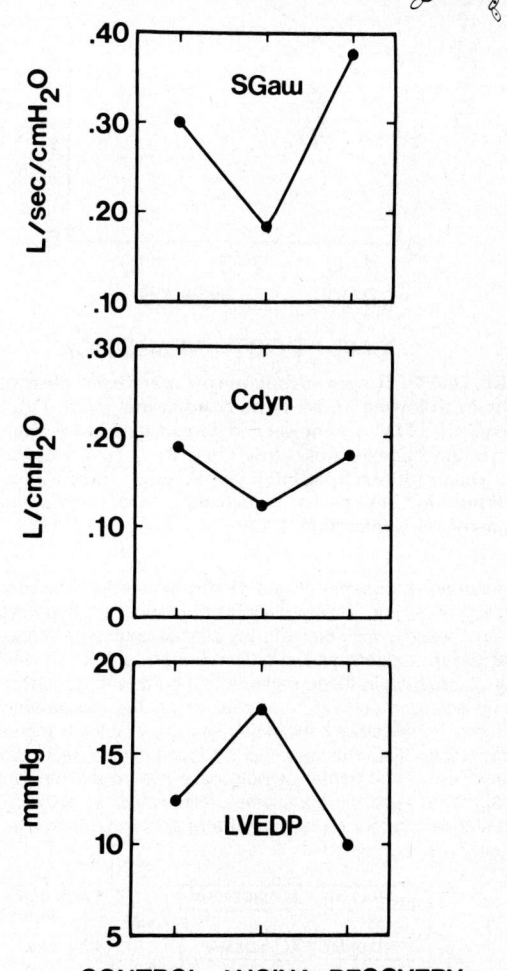

FIGURE 54–6 Interrelationships between heart and lung function during induced myocardial ischemia. SGaw = specific conductance (the reciprocal of airway resistance corrected for the volume at which it was measured); Cdyn = dynamic compliance; LVEDP = left ventricular end-diastolic pressure. The data points are mean values during a control period (left), during the induction of angina (center), and during recovery (right). (Data redrawn from Pepine, C. J., and Wiener, L.: Relationship of anginal symptoms to lung mechanisms during myocardial ischemia. Circulation *46*:863, 1972, by permission of the American Heart Association, Inc.)

CONGENITAL HEART DISEASE

It is convenient to discuss congenital heart disease in terms of the effects of left-to-right and right-to-left intracardiac shunts on pulmo-

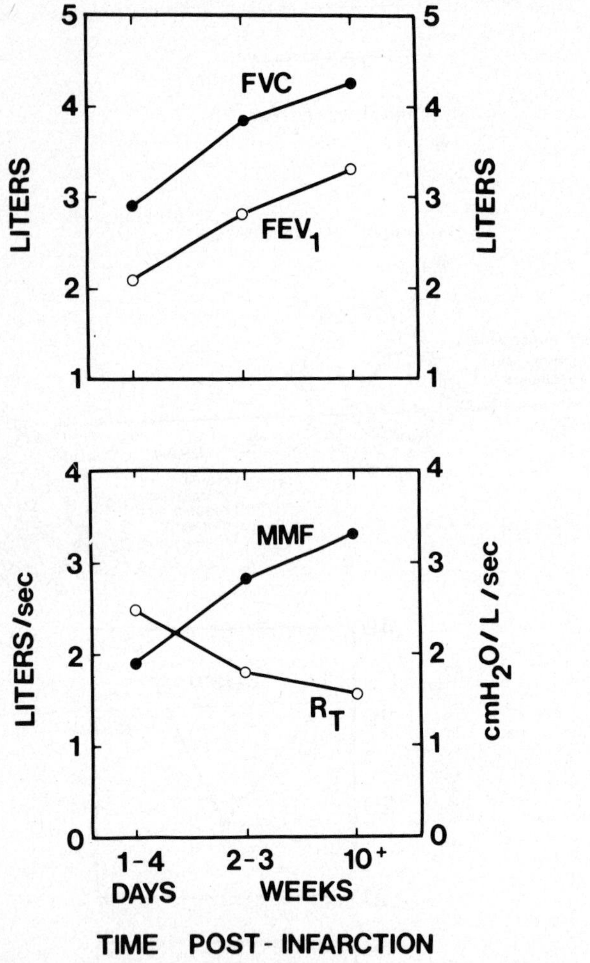

FIGURE 54–7 Changes in pulmonary mechanics observed at various times following an acute myocardial infarction. FVC = forced vital capacity; FEV_1 = one-second forced expiratory volume; MMF = maximum midexpiratory flow rates; R_T = total respiratory resistance. (Data redrawn from Interiano, B., et al.: Interrelation between alterations in pulmonary mechanics and hemodynamics in acute myocardial infarction. J. Clin. Invest. *52*:1994, 1973.)

nary function. Frequently, signs of obstructive lung disease such as wheezing, use of accessory muscles of respiration, hyperinflation, and lobar emphysema will dominate the clinical course of infants with ventricular septal defects and large left-to-right shunts (p. 963).[78,79] The airway obstruction in these patients can be due to compression of airways by enlarged pulmonary arteries or cardiac chambers, and to an increase in small airway resistance as the result of accumulation of peribronchiolar fluid. Pulmonary compliance is also decreased.[80]

Infants with atrial septal defects have also been reported to have low values for dynamic compliance.[80] However, in older children and adults the respiratory consequences of a chronic increase in pulmo-

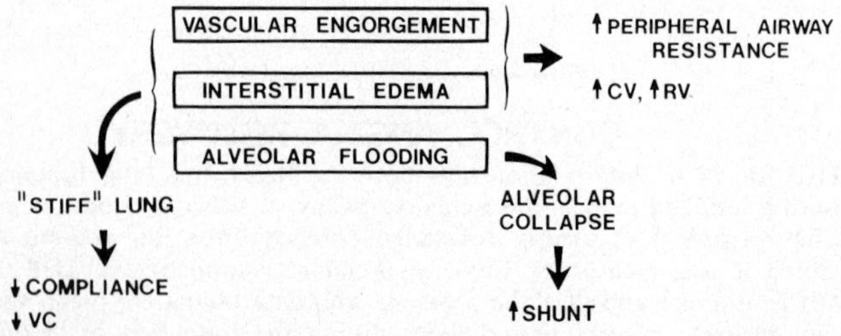

FIGURE 54–8 The functional alterations resulting from vascular engorgement, interstitial edema, and alveolar flooding are shown schematically.

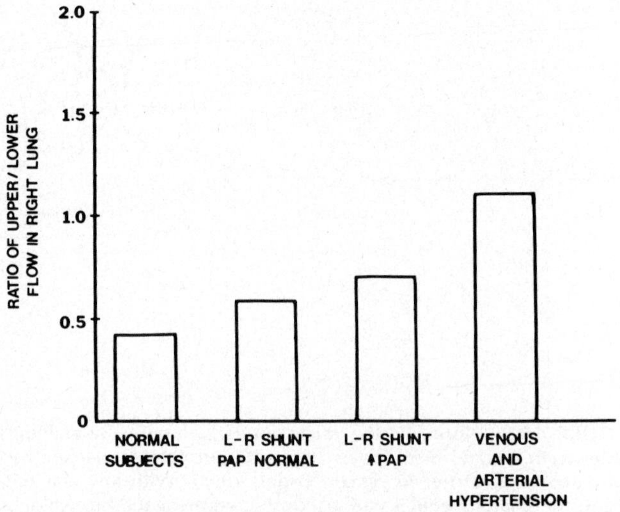

FIGURE 54–9 Alterations in regional pulmonary blood flow in patients with congenital heart disease. PAP = pulmonary artery pressure. (Redrawn from Friedman, W. F., Braunwald, E., and Morrow, A. G.: Alterations in regional pulmonary blood flow in patients with congenital heart disease studied by radioisotope scanning. Circulation *37*:747, 1968, by permission of the American Heart Association, Inc.)

nary blood flow from atrial septal defects are more extensive and can be related to the level of pulmonary hypertension.[81] In those patients in whom the mean pulmonary artery pressure is normal, the only change observed is an increase in diffusing capacity. Thus when pulmonary blood flow is abnormally high but vascular pressures are normal, pulmonary mechanics are normal. However, when both blood flow and pressures are increased, lung function deteriorates. Consequently, in those patients with modest pulmonary hypertension, there is an overt decrease in maximum expiratory flows at all lung volumes and some reduction in static compliance, in addition to the increased diffusing capacity (Fig. 54–4*B*). However, when pulmonary hypertension becomes severe, air flow rates are markedly depressed, elastic recoil and lung volumes are sharply reduced, airway resistance is elevated, and diffusing capacity becomes normal.

Alterations in regional pulmonary blood flow have been recorded in patients with both atrial and ventricular septal defects.[82,83] Typically, abnormalities characterized by increased pulmonary blood flow or elevated pulmonary arterial pressures, or both, increase the ratio of pulmonary blood flow in the lung apices relative to that in the dependent lung zones (Fig. 54–9). Studies of regional lung function in patients with ventricular septal defect have demonstrated mildly abnormal ventilation-perfusion relationships. Ventilation to the left lung tends to be depressed slightly while perfusion is slightly increased.[83] These changes improve with closure of the defect.

Patients with right-to-left intracardiac shunts tend to have normal pulmonary mechanics.[84] However, there are abnormalities in regional lung function and ventilatory control mechanisms.[85,86] Individuals with tetralogy of Fallot have been reported to have a high incidence of hyperperfusion of one lung relative to the other.[85] The significance of this observation with respect to regional gas exchange has not been evaluated, but it is known that children with this condition lack carotid body sensitivity to arterial hypoxemia.[86] As a result, the superimposition of alveolar hypoxia from lung disease or anesthesia may threaten life by aggravating systemic hypoxia to intolerable levels. The mechanism responsible for the blunting of the ventilatory responses to hypoxia in patients with congenital cyanotic heart disease is not clear, but recent evidence suggests it may represent an acquired adaptation to prolonged hypoxemia, because the defect disappears with surgical correction of the cardiac abnormalities.[86]

CARDIOGENIC SHOCK (See page 583)

As noted previously, respiratory insufficiency with abnormal gas exchange frequently develops in conjunction with acute myocardial infarction or pulmonary edema. Usually the mechanisms are related to

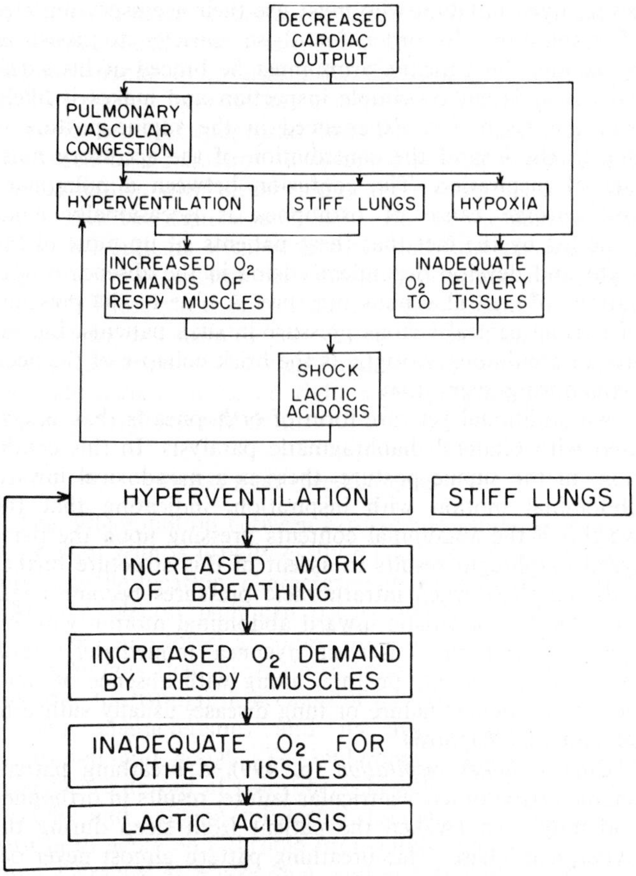

FIGURE 54–10 *Top,* Schema showing how oxygen demands of respiratory muscles can contribute to cardiogenic shock in the face of decreased cardiac output. *Bottom,* Vicious circle whereby hyperventilation and increased work of breathing contribute to O_2 lack and lactic acidosis, which in turn further increases ventilation and respiratory work. (From Macklem, P. T.: Respiratory muscles: The vital pump. Chest *78*:753, 1980.)

alterations in ventilation-perfusion relationships from interstitial edema and alveolar flooding, but new evidence suggests that other factors may also play a role.[87] In situations in which the cardiac output is low, the work of breathing increases substantially because of the hyperventilation induced by hypoxemia and acidemia and because of the mechanical alterations secondary to pulmonary vascular congestion. However, despite the increase in energy demands and expenditure, the blood supply to the respiratory muscles may be reduced because of the very low cardiac output, thus limiting their perfusion. Respiratory muscle fatigue may then occur, leading to respiratory failure. This train of events is shown schematically in Figure 54–10.

CARDINAL MANIFESTATIONS OF HEART VERSUS LUNG DISEASE

Because of the functional interrelations of the heart and lungs, it is not surprising that the cardinal symptoms of heart and lung disease are similar: dyspnea, cough, chest pain, and hemoptysis. It is likely that cough and dyspnea appear only with lung dysfunction, whether it is primary or solely secondary to cardiac dysfunction. Hence, their etiology cannot be clearly distinguished in many instances. In contrast, chest pain and hemoptysis have features characteristic enough to provide a better idea of the primary process.

DYSPNEA (See also pp. 4 and 493)

It is frequently difficult to differentiate cardiac from pulmonary causes of dyspnea.[72a,87a] In actual practice the major functional classifications of patients with either heart or lung disease are based largely upon the degree of exertion necessary to produce breathlessness (p. 12). Such classifications provide no differentiation between primary heart and lung disease. Furthermore, they cannot be rigidly applied as quantitators of disease in either system. For example, a conditioned athlete who begins to develop dyspnea during previously tolerated activity may have a more serious disturbance than a sedentary person who complains of greater breathlessness with much less exertion. On the other hand, other diseases, such as musculoskeletal disorders, may prevent a level of activity that would be necessary to produce dyspnea.

Lest all appear hopeless, in most patients the cause of dyspnea can usually be clearly identified. Thus, a patient with systemic hypertension, an enlarged left ventricle, an S_3 gallop, and bilateral inspiratory rales should not present a problem in identification of left ventricular failure as the cause of dyspnea. In like manner, a long-term smoker with chronic bronchitis, a normal cardiac silhouette, severe hyperinflation, and airway obstruction undoubtedly has sufficient lung disease to account for the shortness of breath. Any number of such clear-cut examples could be cited by a physician with only limited clinical experience.

However, an overweight, middle-aged, male cigarette smoker, with mild chronic bronchitis and mild systemic hypertension, who begins to complain of dyspnea during previously tolerated activity presents a challenging problem. Neither history nor physical examination may reveal sufficient abnormalities to account for symptoms, and laboratory results may be within normal limits. In such an instance complete pulmonary function testing, including arterial blood gas determinations before, during, and after exercise, electrocardiographic stress testing, and cardiac catheterization at rest and during exercise, may be needed in order to identify the process accounting for his exertional dyspnea. Usually, however, such an extensive work-up is not necessary and utilization of simple tests and therapeutic trials will suffice.

For example, mild airway obstruction that responds briskly to bronchodilators would justify a trial of sympathomimetic bronchodilators. If this treatment, along with smoking cessation, controlled symptoms, it would seem likely that lung disease predominated. If pulmonary function testing showed no response to the short-term administration of bronchodilators, it would seem reasonable to administer diuretics with or without cardiac glycosides in a therapeutic trial. Regression of symptoms with this treatment would point toward congestive failure as the cause for his complaints. Given the age and risk factors for the patient in question, an electrocardiographic stress test would be reasonable to perform, either before or after the therapeutic trials. If positive, the question would be whether painless myocardial ischemia were leading to transient elevation of left ventricular diastolic pressure during exertion. In the latter instance, pretreatment with nitroglycerin and repeat of the exercise challenge might help to indicate whether myocardial ischemia were accounting for his exertional dyspnea.

multifocal atrial tachycardia, and atrioventricular junctional tachycardia, have been reported. In addition, ventricular arrhythmias such as bigeminy, atrioventricular dissociation, idioventricular rhythm, ventricular tachycardia, and fibrillation have been observed as well. These arrhythmias usually develop in association with episodes of increasing hypoxemia with or without hypercapnia, particularly during sleep. The nocturnal hypoxia that develops in patients with chronic airway obstruction predisposes them to atrial and ventricular arrhythmias.[114] Similar problems occur in patients with sleep apnea; arrhythmias can be prevented or diminished by nocturnal oxygen therapy. Cardiac arrhythmias may also be provoked by reducing arterial CO_2 tension during ventilatory support, particularly in patients with renal compensation for chronic hypercapnia.[109]

The precise cause of the arrhythmias is not known. It has been suggested that the severe hypoxemia, hypercapnia, and changes in pH common in respiratory failure alter the automaticity of the cardiac conducting tissue or permit the development of reentry circuits. Other factors, such as the catecholamines, theophylline, glucocorticoids, and diuretics used to treat the respiratory symptoms and right heart failure, alone or in combination with the blood gas abnormalities, can also reduce electrical stability either directly or secondarily through their effects on cellular ion transport. In addition some evidence indicates that the sinus node may be damaged in patients with cor pulmonale.[115]

Although the use of cardiac glycosides to control atrial arrhythmias is well established, their role in the treatment of cor pulmonale is ambiguous and controversial. A review of the literature suggests that patients with pulmonary disease may be more susceptible to the toxic effects of cardiac glycosides than patients without primary airway or parenchymal disease (p. 521).[116] However, few studies correlating the effects of digitalis with pulmonary status have characterized the type of respiratory illness present or controlled for concurrent unrelated left ventricular disease. Thus, our current state of knowledge suggests that digitalis be used with caution in patients with respiratory failure; to minimize the risk of toxicity, the specific therapeutic goal should be defined as clearly as possible. Frequent observation and regulation of dosage must be undertaken.

CARDIAC EFFECTS OF DRUGS AND OTHER MODALITIES USED TO TREAT LUNG DISORDERS

Of the various agents currently in use in the treatment of obstructive lung disease, only two classes (adrenergic stimulants and methylxanthines) have significant cardiovascular effects.

ADRENERGIC STIMULANTS

This class of compounds consists of catecholamines (norepinephrine, epinephrine, isoproterenol, and isoetharine), resorcinols (metaproterenol and terbutaline), saligenins (albuterol), and ephedrine which act through stimulation of adrenergic receptors.[117] In 1948, Ahlquist demonstrated that the response to adrenergic drugs appears to be mediated through at least two receptor systems (α and β).[118] Stimulation of α receptors is associated with vasoconstriction, increased uterine activity, and relaxation of intestinal muscle, while stimulation of the β receptors results in inhibition of smooth muscle contraction in the respiratory tract, uterus, and blood vessels and positive inotropic and chronotropic cardiac stimulation. Later, Lands and colleagues demonstrated that beta-adrenergic effects could be differentiated further into β_1 and β_2: β_1 agonists cause cardiac stimulation and β_2 agonists produce bronchodilatation and vasodilation.[119]

Given this information, one can easily appreciate that the perfect agent in this class would be one with pure β_2 activity. Unfortunately, no such compound exists. However, isoetharine, terbutaline, metaproterenol, and albuterol have more β_2 selectivity than the others.[117]

In isolated cardiac tissues, albuterol and terbutaline are much less active than isoproterenol and metaproterenol. The available data indicate that albuterol has minimal cardiac effects, irrespective of the route of administration, whereas terbutaline by intravenous injection may produce a reflex increase in heart rate secondary to its vasodilator activity. Metaproterenol has little cardiac-sparing effect when given orally, but it is usually well tolerated by inhalation. It is of interest that albuterol has been shown to be useful in the treatment of chronic heart failure presumably by reducing afterload by vasodilatation.[120]

In patients with symptomatic obstructive lung disease coexistent with an ischemic or hypertensive cardiomyopathy, aerosols of selective β_2 agonists such as albuterol can be used with safety, and this is the preferred mode of therapy. We have yet to observe the precipitation of an arrhythmia or worsening of hypertension or angina with albuterol aerosols, although this has occurred with the oral use of such agents. Since only micrograms of these drugs are nebulized and milligrams are ingested, presumably this behavior reflects the substantial differences in the quantity of medication absorbed systemically between the two routes.

A particularly difficult clinical problem is posed by the patient with the combination of reactive airways and severely symptomatic angina with or without arrhythmias. One solution is to employ a β_1 antagonist to control the cardiac symptoms and a β_2 agonist to treat the airways in an effort to avoid the undesirable β_1-induced cardiac stimulation and β_2-blockade–induced bronchoconstriction. A word of caution should be interjected, however; this course of action is not without the potential hazards of excessive cardiac stimulation and bronchoconstriction initially, so that the patient's cardiac and pulmonary status should be carefully monitored until the safety and efficacy of the final dosage of both drugs have been determined. Any change in dose of either agent should also be followed objectively.

Another potential solution is to treat the angina pectoris with a calcium-channel blocker. Although these drugs can attenuate the airway obstruction that follows certain constrictor stimuli in asthmatics,[66] they have no effect on resting airway tone and are not bronchodilators. Hence, should there be an acute exacerbation of airway obstruction, a bronchodilator would be required. It has not yet been determined whether the calcium-channel blocker would protect against any cardiac stimulation that might occur as a consequence of the administration of beta-adrenergic agonists. Further, it is not known how this class of compounds interacts with the effects of sympathomimetics and/or methylxanthines on airway smooth muscle.

The toxicity of *halogenated hydrocarbon propellants* has been extensively studied and it has become clear that these agents are not "inert" as was once believed, but neither do they appear to be potentially fatal in patients with lung disease.[120–124] In experimental animals these compounds can sensitize the myocardium to the arrhythmogenic effects of sympathomimetics, but data from many studies in humans indicate that extremely high levels of these compounds are required.[120–122,125] Hence, it appears that only the most flagrant abuse of pressurized aerosols will result in blood concentrations high enough to have this effect.

METHYLXANTHINES

In general, theophylline is safer than the catecholamines and has been shown to improve the performance of both ventricles in patients with obstructive lung disease.[126] However, it also has potentially serious side effects. Like the catecholamines, methylxanthines increase left ventricular work, and relative myocardial ischemia may be produced even though mild coronary artery dilation may also occur. Because theophylline is typically well tolerated, its potential for abuse is high. Until measurements of serum levels became widely available, aminophylline was usually administered in a fixed amount, and if the desired effect was not forthcoming, the dose was increased until toxic side effects were observed. The hazard of this approach can be readily appreciated, and it is not surprising that aminophylline administration has been implicated as a predisposing factor in 60 per cent of the cases of cardiac arrest in one study involving patients in intensive care units.[127]

The therapeutic range for theophylline lies between 10 and 20 μg/ml, and this can be readily achieved in most patients with an intravenous infusion of aminophylline, 5 to 6 mg/kg. However, there is great variability among patients in the metabolism of this drug and the half-life is markedly prolonged in patients with congestive heart failure, acute pulmonary edema, chronic obstructive lung disease, or liver disease. Thus, therapy must be individualized and frequent assessment of serum concentration is required.

POSITIVE END-EXPIRATORY PRESSURE

It has long been noted that high inflation pressures during mechanical ventilation with or without positive end-expiratory pressure (PEEP) are associated with a fall in blood pressure. Changes in each of the two determinants of blood pressure (cardiac output and peripheral vascular resistance) have been considered to be responsible.

Of the two possible causes, much more attention has appropriately been focused upon the diminution in cardiac output. Several reasons have been proposed for a fall in cardiac output during mechanical ventilation with PEEP, one of which is that the positive airway pressure, with secondary increases in pleural pressure, simply increases the impedance to venous return (p. 435). While this is undoubtedly a contributory factor, a surprising experimental finding was an increase in left-sided filling pressures (mean left atrial and left ventricular end-diastolic).[128] Higher filling pressures and decreased cardiac output indicated an alteration in left ventricular function. With positive intrapleural pressures it was important that cardiac chamber pressures be analyzed in terms of true, transmural (i.e., inside minus outside) distending forces. Earlier experimental studies assumed that intrapleural pressure was a reasonable estimate of the pressure surrounding the heart. Based on this assumption, the following sequence evolved: (1) increases in lung volume with PEEP increase pulmonary vascular resistance; (2) this results in an increase in right ventricular pressures which, in turn, displaces the interventricular septum to encroach upon the left ventricular cavity; (3) left ventricular diastolic filling thus becomes impaired, leading to a smaller end-diastolic volume at higher pressures[129]; (4) the subsequent stroke volume is smaller and contributes to the decrease in cardiac output. Previous considerations of humoral factors that might impair cardiac contractility were eliminated by the appropriate experiments. These experimental results in animals have now been supported by clinical studies.[130] Thus the idea of "ventricular interdependence" as a contributor to diminution in cardiac output and the hypotension seen with PEEP appears to be supported in a clinical setting.

As attractive as these ideas may be, further experimental evidence has been obtained that indicates that pericardial pressures are much greater than pleural pressures, leading to the view that the heart is directly compressed[131,132] by the hyperinflated lung to impair filling without alteration of the left ventricular volume versus transmural pressure relationship. This controversy is not yet settled and may revolve around the validity of any technique to assess pericardial pressure with accuracy. Nonetheless, despite lack of unanimity concerning transmural pressure, it is agreed that diastolic filling of the left ventricle is impaired; thus, stroke volume is diminished with PEEP.

Experimental studies of the decrease in peripheral vascular resistance with lung hyperinflation have suggested that humoral agents are released to account for this finding, but vascularly isolated and perfused limbs and muscles also decrease their resistance. Hence, humoral factors alone cannot account for the hypotension. When the vagus nerves from the lung are interrupted, hyperinflation of the lung no longer results in a diminution in peripheral vascular tone.[133] Thus, a reflex mechanism is also a likely contributor. With regard to the clinical relevance of these experiments, however, the very large alveolar pressures required to produce this change are greater than those likely to be seen during mechanical ventilation.

PREOPERATIVE PULMONARY EVALUATION FOR CARDIAC SURGERY

Although pulmonary complications in the postoperative period are more common in patients with preexisting lung disease,[134] it is not possible to predict the risk precisely based upon preoperative pulmonary function testing. An additional concern arises when pulmonary resection is contemplated. Here the issue is whether sufficient pulmonary reserve will be left following surgery; rather elaborate preoperative assessments have been proposed.[135,136] Despite these recommendations, most surgeons simply observe the patient's tolerance to climb two flights of stairs.

This empirical assessment of integrated heart-lung function clearly has no place in the evaluation of most candidates for cardiac surgery, since such patients usually have sufficient cardiac embarrassment that angina or dyspnea during exercise is a problem that will likely be alleviated by the surgical procedure. Even extensive pulmonary function testing may be of little help, since, as already discussed, the effects of heart disease on pulmonary function can be prominent enough to mimic primary lung disease. This is particularly true in patients with longstanding pulmonary venous hypertension.

The major issues, then, are whether there is coexisting primary lung disease that will not be improved by surgery and whether the lung dysfunction will contribute to the likelihood of postoperative mortality and morbidity. There are no prospective studies to provide guidelines in the resolution of this issue. Usually, however, complete clinical assessment, including pulmonary function testing and blood gas determinations at rest and during exercise, suffices in discovering whether there is coexisting lung disease. For example, marked air trapping, severe hypoxemia, and hypercapnia in a patient at rest point toward primary lung dysfunction. Alternatively, the development, or worsening, of pulmonary mechanical and gas-exchange abnormalities during exercise in a patient with a surgically correctable heart disease, who shows only subtle changes in lung function at rest, implicates heart disease as the primary problem. In the latter circumstance, cardiac surgery would be expected to improve lung function to the extent that cardiac function improved; in the former case, surgery is particularly hazardous.

In general, if there is primary lung disease, pulmonary function testing gives a good quantitative assessment of its severity, and this information has some value in predicting whether a patient is likely to tolerate cardiac surgery. When the vital capacity and flow rates are 80 per cent or more of their predicted values, there is little cause for concern from the point of view of pulmonary function.[137] On the other hand, if the values for these indices fall below 50 per cent of predicted values, the possibility of postoperative respiratory insufficiency and death increases.[137] However, since the approach to postoperative intensive care for the pulmonary complications of cardiac surgery is improving dramatically, it is likely that the risk of cardiac surgery in patients with impaired pulmonary function will diminish in the future.

RESPIRATORY CARE AFTER CARDIAC SURGERY

The major respiratory problems that arise in the period immediately after cardiac surgery are related to (1) the thoracotomy itself; (2) the use of drugs in the postoperative period; (3) the effects of cardiopulmonary bypass on the lungs; (4) the effects of coexisting morbid processes, such as chronic airway obstruction; and (5) the transitory effects on the heart of the surgical intervention.

Certainly the disruption of the chest wall by either a lateral thoracotomy or a median sternotomy interferes with its movement; a clouded sensorium caused by medications and self-imposed restriction of movement to avoid pain further contribute to impairment of chest wall motion and may lead to atelectasis. Perhaps even more important, the pain, sedatives, and mechanical restriction lead to an impaired coughing mechanism and the patient's reluctance even to try coughing, and as a consequence, secretions accumulate. These problems are often managed by leaving the endotracheal tube in place and providing mechanical ventilatory assistance in the first few postoperative hours. During this time the tracheobronchial tree is periodically suctioned to remove secretions, and sufficient tidal volumes are provided to prevent atelectasis.

Some patients develop the adult respiratory distress syndrome (Chapters 17 and 18), characterized by increasing intrapulmonary shunting, decreasing lung compliance, and diffuse alveolar infiltrates. This syndrome, which may not develop fully until 24 hours after operation, has been attributed to the use of the extracorporeal membrane oxygenator and perfusion pump and has therefore been referred to as "pump lung." Many theories have been proposed regarding the pathogenesis, yet no single factor has been firmly identified. It is our impression that the incidence of this syndrome has diminished in recent years, perhaps related to shorter bypass times. The pathophysiology and management are detailed in Chapter 18.

Extra attention and effort should be directed toward the postoperative management of the patient with chronic obstruction of the airways by using bronchodilators, by encouraging cough, and, when possible, by the application of physical therapy techniques for mobilization of secretions.

References

1. Glauser, F. L., Hoshiko, M., Watanabe, M., and Wilson, A. F.: Physiologic changes associated with increasing pulmonary wedge pressures in the dog. Respiratory *31*:459, 1974.
2. Gump, F. E., Zikria, B. A., and Mashima, Y.: The effect of interstitial edema on pulmonary function in the dog. J. Trauma *12*:764, 1972.
3. Hauge, A., Bø, G., and Waaler, B. A.: Interrelations between pulmonary liquid volumes and lung compliance. J. Appl. Physiol. *38*:608, 1975.
4. Luepker, R., Liander, B., Korsgren, M., and Varnauskas, E.: Pulmonary intravascular and extravascular fluid volumes in exercising cardiac patients. Circulation *44*:626, 1971.
5. Collins, J. V., Clark, T. J. H., and Brown, D. J.: Airway function in healthy subjects and in patients with left heart disease. Clin. Sci. Molec. Med. *49*:217, 1975.
6. Frank, N. R., Lyons, H. A., Siebens, A. A., and Nealon, T. F.: Pulmonary compliance in patients with cardiac disease. Am. J. Med. *22*:516, 1957.
7. Wood, T. E., McLeod, P., Anthonisen, N. R., and Macklem, P. T.: Mechanics of breathing in mitral stenosis. Am. Rev. Resp. Dis. *104*:52, 1971.
8. Marshall, R., McIlroy, M. B., and Christie, R. V.: The work of breathing in mitral stenosis. Clin. Sci. *13*:137, 1954.
9. White, H. C., Butler, J., and Donald, K. W.: Lung compliance in patients with mitral stenosis. Clin. Sci. *17*:667, 1958.
10. Saxton, G. A., Jr., Rabinowitz, M., Dexter, L., and Haynes, F.: The relationship of pulmonary compliance to pulmonary vascular pressures in patients with heart disease. J. Clin. Invest. *35*:611, 1965.
11. James, A. E., Jr., Cooper, M., White, R. I., and Wagner, H. N., Jr.: Perfusion changes on lungs in patients with congestive heart failure. Radiology *100*:99, 1971.
12. Giuntini, C., Mariani, M., Barsotti, A., Fazio, F., and Santolicandro, A.: Factors affecting regional pulmonary blood flow in left heart valvular disease. Am. J. Med. *57*:421, 1974.
13. Dawson, A., Rocamora, J. M., and Morgan, J. R.: Regional lung function in chronic pulmonary congestion with and without mitral stenosis. Am. Rev. Resp. Dis. *113*:51, 1976.
14. Pain, M. C. F., Bucens, D., Cade, J. F., and Sloman, J. G.: Regional lung function in patients with mitral stenosis. Aust. N.Z. J. Med. *3*:228, 1972.
15. Hughes, J. M. B., Glazier, J. B., Rosenzweig, D. Y., and West, J. B.: Factors determining the distribution of pulmonary blood flow in patients with raised pulmonary venous pressure. Clin. Sci. *37*:847, 1969.
16. Blumenthal, S., and Ravitch, M. M.: Seminar on aortic vascular rings and other anomalies of the aortic arch. Pediatrics *20*:896, 1957.
17. Stranger, P., Lucas, R. V., Jr., and Edwards, J. E.: Anatomic factors causing respiratory distress in acyanotic congenital cardiac disease: Special reference to bronchial obstruction. Pediatrics *43*:760, 1969.
18. Bryk, D.: Atelectasis, emphysema, and heart disease. Am. J. Dis. Child. *110*: 100, 1965.
19. Moss, A. J., and McDonald, L. V.: Cardiac disease in the wheezing child. Chest *71*:187, 1977.
20. Spellberg, R. D., Surprenant, E. L., and O'Reilly, R. J.: Hypoventilation of left lung in acquired heart disease. Am. J. Roentgenol. Radium Ther. Nucl. Med. *118*:785, 1973.
21. Ryo, U. Y., and Townley, R. G.: Comparison of respiratory and cardiovascular effects of isoproterenol, propranolol, and practolol in asthmatic and normal subjects. J. Allergy Clin. Immunol. *57*:12, 1976.
22. Nordstrom, L. A., MacDonald, F., and Gobel, F. L.: Effect of propranolol on respiratory function and exercise tolerance in patients with chronic obstructive lung disease. Chest *67*:287, 1975.
23. Mookherjee, S., Fuleihan, D., Warner, R. A., Vardan, S., and Obeid, A. I.: Effects of sublingual nitroglycerine on resting pulmonary gas exchange and hemodynamics in man. Circulation *57*:106, 1978.
24. Hoel, B. L., Bay, G., and Refsum, H. E.: The effects of morphine on the arterial and mixed venous blood gas state and on the hemodynamics in patients with clinical pulmonary congestion. Acta Med. Scand. *190*:549, 1971.
25. Huckauf, H., Ramdohr, B., and Schroder, R.: Dopamine induced hypoxemia in patients with left heart failure. Int. J. Clin. Pharmacol. *14*:217, 1976.
26. Goldring, R. M., Cannon, P. J., Heinemann, H. O., and Fishman, A. P.: Respiratory adjustment to chronic metabolic alkalosis in man. J. Clin. Invest. *47*: 118, 1968.
27. Turino, G. M., and Fishman, A. P.: The congested lung. J. Chron. Dis. *9*:510, 1959.
28. Heard, B. E., Steiner, R. E., Herdon, A., and Gleason, D.: Oedema and fibrosis of the lungs in left ventricular failure. Br. J. Radiol. *41*:161, 1968.
29. Galloway, R. W., Epstein, E. J., and Coulshed, N.: Pulmonary ossific nodules in mitral valve disease. Br. Heart J. *23*:297, 1961.
30. Friedman, B. L., Macias, D. J., and Yu, P. N.: Pulmonary function studies in patients with mitral stenosis. Am. Rev. Tuberc. *79*:265, 1959.
31. Palmer, W. H., Gee, J. B. L., and Bates, D. V.: Disturbances of pulmonary function in mitral valve disease. Canad. Med. Assoc. J. *89*:744, 1963.
32. Milic-Emili, J., and Petit, J. M.: Mechanical efficiency of breathing. J. Appl. Physiol. *15*:359, 1960.
33. Hogg, J. C., Agarawal, J. B., Gardiner, A. J. S., Palmer, W. H., and Macklem, P. T.: Distribution of airway resistance with developing pulmonary edema in dogs. J. Appl. Physiol. *32*:20, 1972.
34. Sutherland, P. W., Cade, J. F., and Pain, M. C. F.: Pulmonary extravascular fluid volume and hypoxaemia in myocardial infarction. Aust. N.Z. J. Med. *1*: 141, 1971.
35. Tattersfield, A. E., McNicol, M. W., and Sillett, R. W.: Relationship between haemodynamic and respiratory function in patients with myocardial infarction and left ventricular failure. Clin. Sci. *42*:751, 1972.
36. Pepine, C. J., and Wiener, L.: Relationship of anginal symptoms to lung mechanics during myocardial ischemia. Circulation *46*:863, 1972.
37. Interiano, B., Hyde, R., Hodges, M., and Yu, P. N.: Interrelation between alterations in pulmonary mechanics and hemodynamics in acute myocardial infarction. J. Clin. Invest. *52*:1994, 1973.
38. Al Bazzar, F. J., and Kazemi, H.: Arterial hypoxemia and distribution of perfusion after uncomplicated myocardial infarction. Am. Rev. Resp. Dis. *106*: 721, 1972.
39. Demedts, M., Sniderman, A., Utz, G., Palmer, W. H., and Becklake, M. R.: Lung volumes including closing volume and arterial blood gas measurements in acute ischaemic left heart failure. Bull. Physiopathol. Resp. *10*:11, 1974.
40. Otis, A. B., McKerrow, C. B., Bartlett, R. A., Mead, J., McIlroy, M. B., Silverstone, N. J., and Radford, E. P., Jr.: Mechanical factors in distribution of pulmonary ventilation. J. Appl. Physiol. *8*:427, 1956.
41. Raine, J., and Bishop, J. M.: The distribution of alveolar ventilation in mitral stenosis at rest and after exercise. Clin. Sci. *24*:63, 1963.
42. Ingram, R. H., Jr., and Schilder, D. P.: Association of a decrease in dynamic compliance with a change in gas distribution. J. Appl. Physiol. *23*:911, 1967.
43. Dawson, A.: Regional pulmonary blood flow in sitting and supine man during and after acute hypoxia. J. Clin. Invest. *48*:301, 1969.

44. Dawson, A., Kaneko, K., and McGregor, M.: Regional lung function in patients with mitral stenosis studied with xenon[133] during air and oxygen breathing. J. Clin. Invest. *44*:999, 1965.
45. Wagenvoort, C. A., Heath, D., and Edwards, J. E.: The Pathology of the Pulmonary Vasculature, Springfield, Ill., Charles C Thomas, 1964, p. 186.
46. Kelman, G. R., Nunn, J. F., Prys-Roberts, C., and Greenbaum, R.: The influence of cardiac output on arterial oxygenation: A theoretical study. Br. J. Anaesthesiol. *39*:450, 1967.
47. Tenny, S. M.: A theoretical analysis of the relationship between venous blood and mean tissue oxygen pressures. Resp. Physiol. *20*:283, 1974.
48. Aberman, A., and Fulop, M.: The metabolic and respiratory acidosis of acute pulmonary edema. Ann. Intern. Med. *76*:173, 1972.
49. Ingram, R. H., Jr., and McFadden, E. R., Jr.: Respiratory changes during exercise in patients with pulmonary venous hypertension. Progr. Cardiovasc. Dis. *19*:109, 1976.
50. Hayward, G. W., and Knotts, J. M. S.: The effect of exercise on lung distensibility and respiratory work in mitral stenosis. Br. Heart J. *17*:303, 1955.
51. Gilbert, R., and Auchincloss, J. H., Jr.: Cardiac and pulmonary function at the exercise breaking point in cardiac patients. Am. J. Med. Sci. *257*:370, 1969.
52. Jebavy, P., Widimsky, J., and Stanek, V.: Distribution of inspired gas and pulmonary diffusing capacity at rest and during graded exercise in patients with mitral stenosis. Respiration *28*:216, 1971.
53. Auchincloss, J. H., Jr., Gilbert, R., and Baule, G. H.: Unsteady state measurement of oxygen transfer in patients with rheumatic heart disease. Clin. Sci. *39*:21, 1970.
54. Goodenday, L. S., Simon, G., Craig, H., and Dalby, L.: Abnormal distribution of pulmonary blood flow in aortic valve disease. Relation between pulmonary function and chest radiograph. Br. Heart J. *32*:406, 1970.
55. Hurych, J., Widimsky, J., and Kasalicky, J.: Pulmonary gas exchange at rest and during exercise in patients with mitral stenosis. Bull. Physiopathol. Resp. *2*:472, 1966.
56. Bjure, J., Liander, B., and Widimsky, J.: Effect of exercise on distribution of pulmonary blood flow in patients with mitral stenosis. Br. Heart J. *33*:438, 1971.
57. Yoo, O. H., and Ting, E. Y.: The effect of pleural effusions on lung function. Am. Rev. Resp. Dis. *89*:55, 1964.
58. Anthonisen, N. R., and Martin, R. R.: Regional lung function in pleural effusion. Am. Rev. Resp. Dis. *116*:201, 1977.
59. Davidson, F. F., and Glazier, J. B.: Unilateral pleuritis and regional lung function. Ann. Intern. Med. *77*:37, 1972.
60. MacDonald, A. J., Ingram, C. G., and McNeil, R. S.: The effect of propranolol on airway resistance. Br. J. Anaesthesiol. *39*:919, 1967.
61. Zaid, G., and Beall, G. N.: Bronchial response to beta-adrenergic blockade. N. Engl. J. Med. *275*:580, 1966.
62. Tattersfield, R. E., Leaver, D. G., and Pride, N. B.: Effects of β-adrenergic blockade and stimulation on normal human airways. J. Appl. Physiol. *35*:613, 1973.
63. Wunderlich, J., Macha, H. N., Wudicke, H., and Huckauf, H.: Beta adrenergic blockers and terbutaline in patients with chronic obstructive lung disease. Chest *78*:714, 1980.
64. Tivenius, L.: Effects of multiple doses of metoprolol and propranolol on ventilatory function in patients with chronic obstructive lung disease. Scand. J. Resp. Dis. *57*:190, 1976.
65. McMahon, C. D., Shaffer, R. N., Hoskins, H. D., and Hetherington, J.: Adverse effects experienced by patients taking timolol. Am. J. Ophthalmol. *88*:736, 1979.
66. McFadden, E. R.: Calcium-channel blocking agents and asthma. Ann. Intern. Med. *95*:232, 1981.
67. Mookherjee, S., Warner, R., Keighley, J., and Obeid, A.: Worsening of ventilation perfusion relationship in the lungs in the face of hemodynamic improvement during nitroprusside infusion. Am. J. Cardiol. *39*:282, 1977.
68. Pierpont, G., Hale, K. A., Franciosa, J. A., and Cohn, J. N.: Effects of vasodilators on pulmonary hemodynamics and gas exchange in left ventricular failure. Am. Heart J. *49*:208, 1980.
69. Chick, J. W., Kochukoshy, K. N., Matsumoto, S., and Leach, J. K.: The effect of nitroglycerine on gas exchange, hemodynamics, and oxygen transport in patients with chronic obstructive pulmonary disease. Am. J. Med. Sci. *276*:105, 1978.
70. Tuller, M. A., and Mehdi, F.: Compensatory hypoventilation and hypercapnia in primary metabolic alkalosis. Am. J. Med. *501*:281, 1971.
71. Nagle, R. E., and Pilcher, J.: Respiratory and circulatory effects of pentazocine. Review of analgesics used after myocardial infarction. Br. Heart J. *34*:244, 1972.
72. Hoel, B. L., and Refsum, H. E.: The effect of morphine on arterial blood gases in patients with acute myocardial infarction. Acta Med. Scand. *186*:511, 1969.
72a. Nery, L. E., Wasserman, K., French, W., Oren, A., and Davis, J. A.: Contrasting cardiovascular and respiratory responses to exercise in mitral valve and chronic obstructive pulmonary diseases. Chest *83*:446, 1983.
73. DeTroyer, A., Estenne, M., and Yernault, J. C.: Disturbance of respiratory muscle function in patients with mitral valve disease. Am. J. Med. *69*:867, 1980.
74. Kannel, W. B., Seidman, J. M., Fercho, W., and Castelli, W. P.: Vital capacity and congestive heart failure. The Framingham study. Circulation *49*:1160, 1974.
75. Hales, C. A., and Kazemi, H.: Small-airways function in myocardial infarction. N. Engl. Med. *290*:761, 1974.
76. Rotsztain, A., Shugoll, G. I., and Lloyd, R. A.: Hypoxemia in acute myocardial infarction and in coronary insufficiency. Am. J. Med. Sci. *266*:255, 1973.
77. Biddle, T. L., Khanna, P., Yu, P. N., Hodges, M., and Shah, P. M.: Lung water in patients with acute myocardial infarction. Circulation *49*:115, 1974.
78. Hordof, A. J., Mellins, R. B., Gersony, W. M., and Steeg, C. N.: Reversibility of chronic obstructive lung disease in infants following repair of ventricular septal defect. J. Pediatr. *90*:187, 1977.
79. Howlett, G.: Lung mechanics in normal infants and infants with congenital heart disease. Arch. Dis. Child. *471*:707, 1972.
80. Bancalari, E., Jesse, M. J., Gelband, H., and Garcia, O.: Lung mechanics in congenital heart disease with increased and decreased pulmonary blood flow. J. Pediatr. *90*:192, 1977.
81. De Troyer, A., Yernault, J. C., and Englert, M.: Mechanics of breathing in patients with atrial septal defect. Am. Rev. Resp. Dis. *115*:413, 1977.
82. Friedman, W. F., Braunwald, E., and Morrow, A. G.: Alterations in regional pulmonary blood flow in patients with congenital heart disease studied by radioisotope scanning. Circulation *37*:747, 1968.
83. Sade, R. M., Williams, R. G., Castaneda, A. R., and Treves, S.: Abnormalities of regional lung function associated with ventricular septal defect and pulmonary artery band. J. Thorac. Cardiovasc. Surg. *71*:572, 1976.
84. Bates, D. V., Macklem, P. T., and Christie, R. V.: Respiratory function in disease. 2nd ed. Philadelphia, W. B. Saunders Co., 1971, p. 351.
85. Gates, G. F., Orme, H. W., and Dore, E. K.: The hyperperfused lung. Detection in congenital heart disease. J.A.M.A. *233*:782, 1975.
86. Edelman, N. H., Lahiri, S., Braudo, L., Cherniack, N. S., and Fishman, A. P.: The blunted ventilatory response to hypoxia in cyanotic congenital heart disease. N. Engl. J. Med. *282*:405, 1970.
87. Aubier, M., Trippenbach, T., and Roussos, C.: Respiratory muscle fatigue during cardiogenic shock. J. Appl. Physiol. Resp. Environ. Exercise Physiol. *51*:499, 1981.
87a. Loke, J.: Distinguishing cardiac versus pulmonary limitation in exercise performance. Chest *83*:441, 1983.
88. De Vries, K., Goei, J. T., Booy-Noord, H., and Orie, N. G. M.: Changes during 24 hours in the lung function and histamine hyperreactivity of the bronchial tree in asthmatic and bronchitic patients. Int. Arch. Allergy *20*:93, 1962.
89. Rees, P. J., and Clark, T. J. H.: Paroxysmal nocturnal dyspnea and periodic respiration. Lancet *2*:1315, 1979.
90. Zorck, M. B., Pontoppidan, H., and Kazemi, H.: The effect of lateral positions on gas exchange in pulmonary disease. Am. Rev. Resp. Dis. *110*:49, 1974.
91. Altman, M., and Robin, E. D.: Platypnea: Diffuse zone I phenomenon? N. Engl. J. Med. *281*:1347, 1969.
92. Robin, E. D., and Altman, M.: By a waterfall: "Zone I and Zone II phenomena" in obstructive lung disease. Am. J. Med. Sci. *258*:219, 1969.
93. Montgomery, G. E., Geraci, J. E., Parker, R. L., and Wood, E. H.: The arterial oxygen saturation in cyanotic types of congenital heart disease. Proc. Staff Meet. Mayo Clin. *23*:169, 1948.
94. Lurie, P. R.: Postural effects in tetralogy of Fallot. Am. J. Med. *10*:297, 1953.
95. Schnabel, T. G., Jr., Ratto, O., Kirby, C. K., Johnson, J., and Comroe, J. H., Jr.: Postural cyanosis and angina pectoris following pneumonectomy: Relief by closure of an interatrial septal defect. J. Thorac. Surg. *32*:246, 1956.
96. Begin, R.: Platypnea after pneumonectomy. N. Engl. J. Med. *293*:342, 1975.
97. Munsell, W. P.: Pneumomediastinum. J.A.M.A. *202*:689, 1967.
98. Copeland, R. B., and Omenn, G. S.: Electrocardiograms suggestive of coronary artery disease in pneumothorax. Arch. Intern. Med. *25*:151, 1970.
99. Littmann, D.: Electrocardiographic phenomena associated with spontaneous pneumothorax and mediastinal emphysema. J. Med. Sci. *212*:682, 1946.
100. Millard, C. E.: Pneumomediastinum. Dis. Chest *56*:297, 1969.
101. Heller, R.: The significance of hemoptysis. Tubercle *27*:70, 1946.
102. Abbott, D. A.: The clinical significance of pulmonary hemorrhage: A study of 1,316 patients with chest disease. Dis. Chest *14*:824, 1948.
103. Levitt, N.: Clinical significance of hemoptysis. J. Mich. State Med. Soc. *50*:606, 1951.
104. Souders, C. R., and Smith, A. T.: The clinical significance of hemoptysis. J.A.M.A. *150*:746, 1952.
105. Haroutunian, L. M., and Neill, C. A.: Pulmonary complications of congenital heart disease: Hemoptysis. Am. Heart J. *84*:540, 1972.
106. Finley, T. N., Aronow, A., Cosentino, A. M., and Golde, D. W.: Occult pulmonary hemorrhage in anticoagulated patients. Am. Rev. Resp. Dis. *112*:23, 1975.
107. Corazza, L. J., and Pastor, B. H.: Cardiac arrhythmias in chronic cor pulmonale. N. Engl. J. Med. *259*:862, 1958.
108. Shine, K. I., Kastor, J. A., and Yurchak, P. M.: Multifocal atrial tachycardia. Clinical and electrocardiographic features in 32 patients. N. Engl. J. Med. *279*:344, 1968.
109. Ayres, S. M., and Grace, W. J.: Inappropriate ventilation and hypoxemia as causes of cardiac arrhythmias. The control of arrhythmias without antiarrhythmic drugs. Am. J. Med. *46*:495, 1969.
110. Kleiger, R. E., and Senior, R. M.: Long-term electrocardiographic monitoring of ambulatory patients with chronic airway obstruction. Chest *65*:483, 1974.
111. Hudson, L. D., Kurt, T. L., Petty, T. L., and Genton, E.: Arrhythmias associated with acute respiratory failure in patients with chronic airway obstruction. Chest *63*:661, 1973.
112. Holford, F. D., and Mithoefer, J. C.: Cardiac arrhythmias in hospitalized pa-

tients with chronic obstructive pulmonary disease. Am. Rev. Resp. Dis. *108*: 979, 1973.

113. Sideris, D. A., Katsadoros, D. P., Valianos, G., and Assioura, A.: Type of cardiac dysrhythmias in respiratory failure. Am. Heart J. *89*:32, 1975.
114. Tirlapur, V. G., and Mir, M. A.: Nocturnal hypoxemia and associated electrocardiographic changes in patients with chronic obstructive airway disease. N. Engl. J. Med. *306*:125, 1982.
115. Thomas, M. A., and Wee, A. S. T.: The sinus node in cor pulmonale. Isr. J. Med. Sci. *5*:831, 1969.
116. Green, L. H., and Smith, T. W.: The use of digitalis in patients with pulmonary disease. Ann. Intern. Med. *87*:459, 1977.
117. McFadden, E. R., Jr.: Beta 2 receptor agonists: Metabolism and pharmacology. J. Allergy Clin. Immunol. *68*:91, 1981.
118. Ahlquist, R. P.: A study of the adrenotropic receptors. Am. J. Physiol. *153*: 586, 1948.
119. Lands, A. M., Arnold, A., McAuliff, J. P., Luduena, F. P., and Brown, T. G.: Differentiation of receptor systems activated by sympathomimetic amines. Nature *214*:597, 1967.
120. Bourdillon, P. D. V., Dawson, J. R., Foale, R. A., Timmis, A. D., Poole-Wilson, P. A., and Sutton, J. C.: Salbutamol in treatment of heart failure. Br. Heart J. *43*:206, 1980.
121. Brooks, S. M., Mintz, S., and Weiss, E.: Changes occurring after freon inhalation. Am. Rev. Resp. Dis. *105*:640, 1972.
122. Clark, D. G., and Tinston, D. J.: Cardiac effects of isoproterenol, hypoxia, hypercapnia, and fluorocarbon propellents and their use in asthma inhalers. Ann. Allergy *30*:536, 1972.
123. Fabel, H., Wettengel, R., and Hartmann, W.: Myokardischamie und Arrhythmien durch den Gebrauch von Dosieraerosolen beim Menschen? Dtsch. Med. Wschr. *97*:428, 1972.
124. Silverglade, A.: Cardiac toxicity of aerosol propellents. J.A.M.A. *222*:827, 1972.
125. Speizer, F. E., Wegman, D. H., and Ramirez, A.: Palpitation rates associated with fluorocarbon exposure in a hospital setting. New Engl. J. Med. *292*:624, 1975.
126. Matthay, R. A., Berger, H. J., Loke, J., Gottschalk, A., and Zaret, B. L.: Effect of aminophylline upon right and left ventricular performance in chronic obstructive pulmonary disease. Am. J. Med. *65*:903, 1978.
127. Camarata, S. J., Weil, M. H., and Hanashiro, D. K.: Cardiac arrest in the critically ill. A study of predisposing causes in 132 patients. Circulation *44*: 688, 1971.
128. Scharf, S. M., Caldini, P., and Ingram, R. H., Jr.: Cardiovascular effects of increasing airway pressure in the dog. Am. J. Physiol. *232*:435, 1977.
129. Haynes, J. B., Carson, S. D., Whitney, W. P., Zerbe, G. O., Hyers, T. M., and Steele, P.: Positive end-expiratory pressure shifts and left ventricular diastolic pressure-area curves. J. Appl. Physiol. Resp. Environ. Exercise Physiol. *48*: 670, 1980.
130. Jardin, F., Farcot, J. C., Boisante, L., Curien, N., Margairaz, A., and Bourdarias, J. P.: Influence of positive end-expiratory pressures on left ventricular performance. N. Engl. J. Med. *304*:387, 1981.
131. Wise, R. A., Robotham, J. L., Bromberger-Barnea, B., and Permutt, S.: Effect of PEEP on left ventricular function in right-heart–bypassed dogs. J. Appl. Physiol. Resp. Environ. Exercise Physiol. *51*:541, 1981.
132. Fewell, J. E., Abendschein, D. R., Carlson, C. J., Rapaport, E., and Murray, J.: Mechanism of decreased right and left ventricular end-diastolic volumes during continuous positive-pressure ventilation in dogs. Circ. Res. *47*:467, 1980.
133. Cassidy, S. S., Eschenbacher, W. L., and Johnson, R. L., Jr.: Reflex cardiovascular depression during unilateral lung hyperinflation in the dog. J. Clin. Invest. *64*:620, 1979.
134. Gaensler, E. A., and Weisel, R. D.: The risks of abdominal and thoracic surgery in COPD. Postgrad. Med. *54*:183, 1973.
135. Olsen, G. N., Block, A. J., and Tobias, J. A.: Prediction of postpneumonectomy pulmonary function using quantitative macroaggregate lung scanning. Chest *66*:13, 1974.
136. Tisi, G. M.: Preoperative evaluation of pulmonary function. *In* Isselbacher, K. J., et al. (eds.): Principles of Internal Medicine, Update III. New York, McGraw-Hill Book Co., 1982, p. 101.
137. Mittman, C.: Assessment of operative risk in thoracic surgery. Am. Rev. Resp. Dis. *84*:197, 1961.

55 GENERAL PRINCIPLES OF CARDIAC SURGERY

by John W. Kirklin, M.D., Eugene H. Blackstone, M.D., and James K. Kirklin, M.D.

Cardiac surgery, like other forms of surgery, is advised for any given patient when the surgical risks to survival and useful life are fewer than those of nonsurgical treatment. Ideally, cardiac surgery should have a *hospital mortality* rate *approaching zero** and should prevent *premature late death.*** When these criteria are associated with full functional capacity, the operation is considered *curative.* In some patients, cure may be unattainable, and for them a life expectancy and a functional capacity better than that imposed by the disease itself are sought (*palliative* operation).

The purpose of this chapter is to describe the general aspects of cardiac surgery that affect early and late results and to provide insight into some of the mechanisms underlying its current problems.

PREOPERATIVE CONDITIONS AFFECTING EARLY AND LATE RESULTS OF CARDIAC SURGERY

The Lesion

The early and late results of cardiac surgery depend significantly upon the specific cardiac lesion being treated. For example, hospital mortality approaches zero for the repair of uncomplicated atrial septal defects (hospital mortality, 0.9 per cent; 70 per cent CL, 0.4 to 1.8 per cent*) and for coronary artery bypass grafting (0.7 per cent; 70 per cent CL, 0.6 to 0.9 per cent), whereas that for primary combined aortic and mitral valve replacement is 4 per cent (70 per cent CL, 3 to 7 per cent) and that for an operation such as the modified Fontan procedure for single ventricle and other types of complex congenital heart disease other than tricuspid atresia is 29 per cent (70 per cent CL, 17 to 49 per cent).

The early and late risks of cardiac surgery may, in the case of some lesions, result from the noncorrectable (by current techniques) aspects of their morphology or from morphology that is manageable only by methods that themselves have important risks. For example, extensive three-vessel coronary artery disease with a left ventricular ejection fraction of 0.2 or less results in a significant risk for premature late death in the postoperative period because of surgically untreatable left ventricular scarring. Similarly, survival and salvage of left ventricular function after acute revascularization following acute myocardial infarction with cardiogenic shock may be limited by the amount of irreversible myocardial injury. Atrioventricular (AV) septal (canal) defects with severe left AV valve regur-

*By this is meant a hospital mortality rate whose lower 70 per cent confidence limit (CL) is less than 1 per cent and whose upper one is less than 5 per cent.

**By this is meant an actuarial survival rate whose upper 70 per cent CL or 1 standard deviation overlaps the survival rate of an age-sex-race–matched general population.

*70 per cent CL = 70 per cent confidence limit, analogous to 1 standard deviation. The representative hospital mortalities presented are from the Department of Surgery, University of Alabama in Birmingham (UAB), unless otherwise stated.

gitation may continue to have severe left AV valve regurgitation after repair because of leaflet deficiency. Tetralogy of Fallot with a very small pulmonary annulus requires either a transannular patch with its resultant pulmonary valvular regurgitation and consequent damaging effect on the right ventricle or an orthotopic or bypassing pulmonary valve replacement with its long-term uncertainties.

However, it is not only the complexity of the cardiac condition itself that increases the risks. It also may be that patients with a particular lesion have come to operation unusually ill, especially young, or with other major associated cardiac conditions. In the case of some lesions (for example, mitral and aortic regurgitation), the apparently unfavorable effect of the lesion on late mortality may be related in large part to the lesion's damaging influence on ventricular structure and function. The increased risks of operation for some lesions may be related to the complexity of the operation required or to lack of knowledge about some particular aspect of postoperative care, rather than to risk factors within the patient. All of these considerations make multivariate analysis necessary to the development of an understanding of the lesion's effect on the results of operation.

Ventricular Structure and Function

THE SECONDARY CARDIOMYOPATHIES. One of the most important limitations of the surgical treatment of heart disease may be the damage already sustained by the ventricles by the time the operation is undertaken. This *secondary cardiomyopathy* is produced by a chronic pressure or volume overload (p. 449) or by acute or chronic myocardial ischemia. It is sometimes forgotten that the *right,* as well as the left ventricle is subject to these damaging effects; the time required for the development of secondary right ventricular cardiomyopathy, however, seems to be somewhat longer than in the case of the left ventricle.

An early response to volume or pressure overload or to myocardial scarring is increased ventricular mass. This results initially from myocardial cell hypertrophy. In the case of volume overload, the increased ventricular mass is primarily associated with greater ventricular volume at any given diastolic pressure. In the case of pressure overload, it is mainly linked with increased ventricular wall thickness. When the volume or pressure overload or ischemic damage is inordinate or prolonged, mitochondrial changes occur as well as disruption of sarcomeres and fiber disarray.

Modest increase in ventricular mass may not impair ventricular systolic or diastolic function. In fact, it may be compensatory and preserve function, such as occurs in aortic stenosis when the increased left ventricular wall thickness maintains nearly normal systolic wall stress (and thus afterload) despite elevated left ventricular systolic pressure (p. 453).[1] When the hypertrophy no longer keeps pace with the ventricular overload, such as in the afterload mismatch of long-standing aortic stenosis, ventricular systolic and diastolic functions are adversely affected even though degenerative myocardial changes are not present. When myocardial degenerative changes are present, contractility is usually impaired in proportion to the extent and severity of the degenerative changes.

All of these factors are of great surgical importance because of the tendency of the secondary cardiomyopathy to become irreversible. If only hypertrophy is present, the ventricular mass regresses toward but not *to* a normal state, and systolic and diastolic functions are improved and may become normal. Degenerative changes are irreversible, and in their presence the regression of ventricular mass toward a normal state is more limited. When degenerative changes are extensive, little regression of mass occurs, contractility remains impaired postoperatively, and symptomatic improvement is limited. Several months or years after operation, extreme secondary cardiomyopathy may worsen in spite of mechanical relief of the defect, resulting in further impairment of systolic and diastolic function, increasing symptoms, increasing ventricular electrical instability, and premature late death.

These phenomena must be taken into consideration in choosing the time of operation for many forms of congenital and acquired heart disease. In delaying operation, the disadvantages of the progression of the secondary cardiomyopathy must be weighed against the advantages of continued medical therapy or of awaiting improved surgical methods.

VOLUME OVERLOAD (see also p. 453). Ventricular volume overload, in surgically treatable states, exists when the ventricular stroke volume is greater than net forward systemic blood flow. The return toward but not to normal ventricular mass when volume overload has been of brief duration ($\pm$ 30 days) was demonstrated experimentally by Papadimitriou and colleagues[2] (Table 55–1). When this kind of regression occurs in humans after an operation, premature late death is infrequent and the functional results are good. When regression of the secondary cardiomyopathy does not take place, or particularly when the cardiomyopathy increases postoperatively, premature late death is common.

Since myocardial biopsies are rarely performed in surgical patients, and death followed by autopsies is rather infrequent, much of the evidence for a cardiomyopathy secondary to chronic volume overload is circumstantial and is based upon the observation of depressed ventricular systolic function and advanced functional disability in patients with volume-overloaded ventricles. In this regard, it is noteworthy that patients with depressed left ventricular systolic function in whom aortic valve replacement has been carried out for aortic regurgitation have a lower 5-year survival rate after hospital dismissal than do patients whose systolic function is normal preoperatively (Fig. 55–1A).[3] In such patients, depressed preoperative exercise capacity (or increased NYHA Functional Class) still further depresses the late survival rate (Figs. 55–1B, 55–2, and 55–3).[3,4,5] Poor functional capacity or depressed systolic function in the preoperative period also predisposes to lack of improvement of ventricular diastolic function late in the postoperative period (Fig. 55–4)[5,6] (see also p. 454).

Patients with *atrial septal defect* (ASD) have a *volume overload* of the *right ventricle,* and the same type of *secondary* cardiomyopathy slowly develops in time. Thus, older patients with ASD have more severe symptoms preoperatively than younger ones (Table 55–2), symptomatic patients undergoing repair of their ASD are older than asymptomatic ones, and the right ventricular systolic func-

TABLE 55–1 MEASUREMENTS IN NORMAL DOGS; IN DOGS WITH SURGICALLY CREATED LARGE AORTOCAVAL FISTULA OF ±30 DAYS' DURATION; AND IN DOGS 3 MONTHS AND 6 MONTHS AFTER FISTULA CLOSURE

	Body Weight (kg)	Heart Rate (beats/min)	Left Ventricular End-Diastolic Pressure (mm Hg)	Cardiac Index (ml/min/kg)	Left Ventricle Weight (gm/kg)
Normal (8)	21.3 ± 3.3	88 ± 27	5 ± 3	134 ± 41	4.19 ± 0.47
Patent fistula (7)	21.1 ± 2.9	124 ± 18	31 ± 7	459 ± 135	5.34 ± 0.34
p value compared with normal dogs	NS	<0.01	<0.001	<0.001	<0.001
Fistula closed at 3 mos (5)	20.6 ± 1.3	67 ± 10	6 ± 2	130 ± 26	5.25 ± 0.16
p value compared with normal dogs	NS	NS	NS	NS	<0.001
p value compared with dogs with patent fistulas	NS	<0.001	<0.001	<0.001	NS
Fistula closed at 6 mos (6)	22.5 ± 2.4	82 ± 29	7 ± 1.4	186 ± 64	4.82 ± 0.54
p value compared with normal dogs	NS	NS	NS	NS	<0.05
p value compared with dogs with patent fistulas	NS	<0.01	<0.001	<0.001	NS

All values are means ± SD. The number of dogs studied is given in parentheses. NS = nonsignificant; SD = standard deviation; mos = months. (Modified from Papadimitriou, J. M., et al.: Regression of left ventricular dilation and hypertrophy after removal of volume overload. Circ. Res. *35*:127, 1974.)

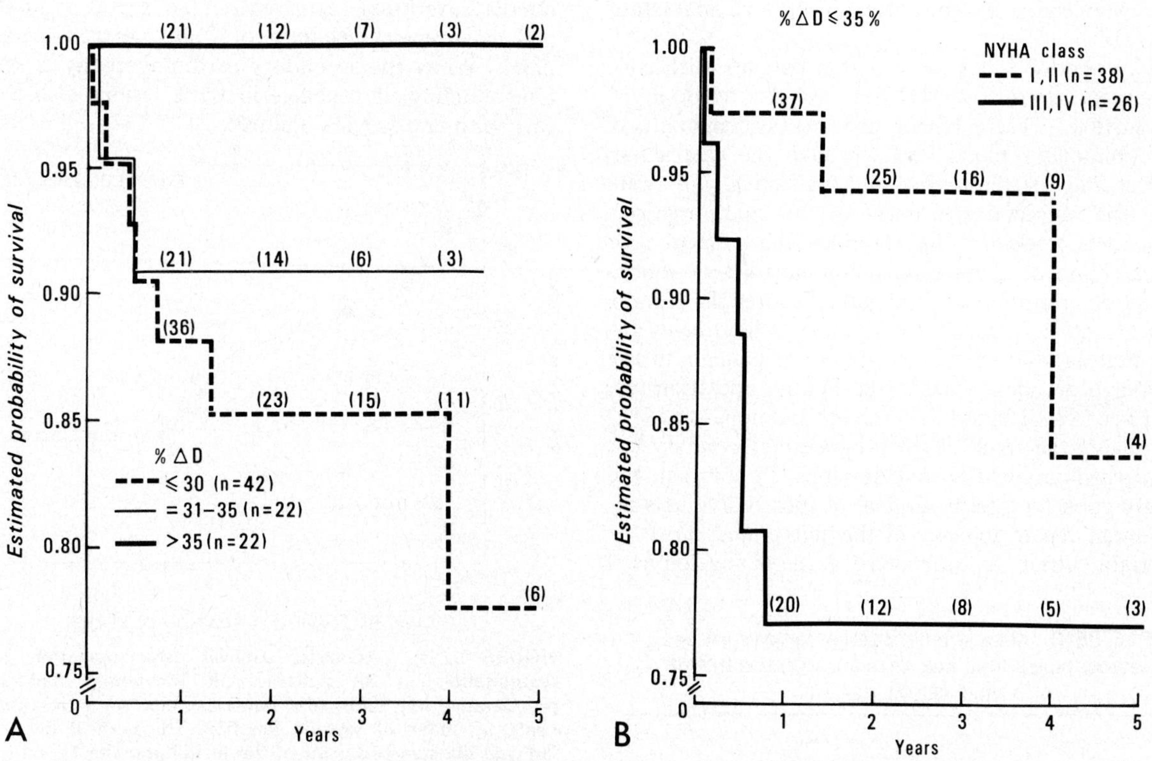

FIGURE 55–1 *A*, Relation between probability of survival after valve replacement for aortic insufficiency and preoperative per cent change of left ventricular dimension (% Δ D), an index of systolic function. Patients with low values, and thus diminished systolic function, have significantly decreased probability of survival ($p < 0.05$). (Numbers in parentheses are numbers of patients at risk at each interval.) *B*, Relation between preoperative NYHA functional classification and probability of survival after valve replacement for aortic insufficiency in patients with preoperatively depressed left ventricular systolic function. Patients in Functional Class I or II had longer survival than those in Class III or IV ($p = 0.05$). (From Cunha, C. L. P., Giuliani, E. R., Fuster, V., Seward, J. B., Brandenburg, R. O., and McGoon, D. C.: Preoperative M-mode echocardiography as a predictor of surgical results in chronic aortic insufficiency. J. Thorac. Cardiovasc. Surg. *79*:256, 1980.)

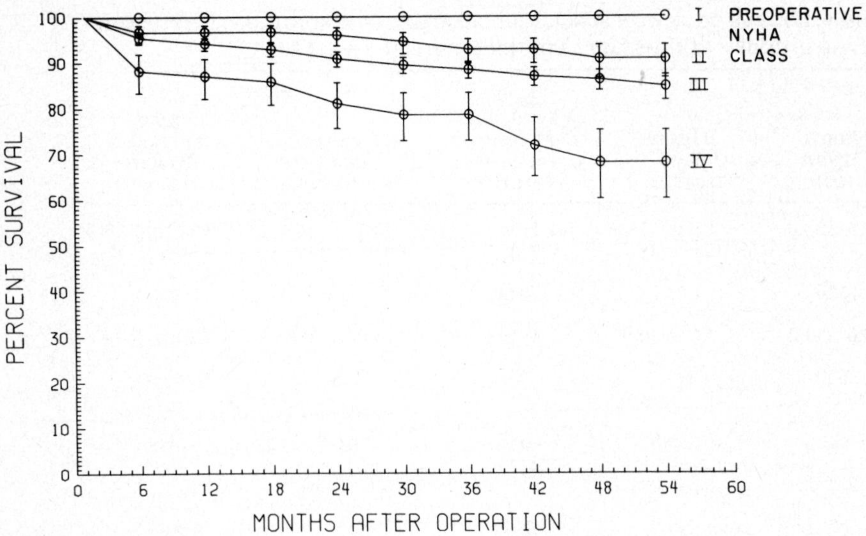

FIGURE 55–2 Actuarial survival of hospital survivors after aortic, mitral, or aortic and mitral valve replacement, according to the preoperative NYHA Functional Class. These relations hold for any of these subgroups. The vertical bars enclose the 70 per cent confidence limits (1 standard deviation). (From Karp, R. B., Cyrus, R. J., Blackstone, E. H., Kirklin, J. W., Kouchoukos, N. T., and Pacifico, A. D.: The Bjork-Shiley valve. J. Thorac. Cardiovasc. Surg. *81*:602, 1981.)

tion is less efficient in the older patient (Table 55–3).[7] When this secondary right ventricular cardiomyopathy is long-standing, it is apt to be irreversible, as it is in other types of secondary cardiomyopathy. Thus, only about 20 per cent of older patients have nearly normal right ventricular end-diastolic volume late after repair of their ASD, and only about 60 per cent of patients aged 10 years at operation experienced a return to a nearly normal state (Table 55–4).[8]

Sometimes overlooked is the fact that patients with *congenital tricuspid atresia* (p. 984) have volume overload of the left ventricle. This chamber provides systemic blood flow plus pulmonary blood flow (through the ventricular septal defect and the diminutive and ineffective right ventricle into the pulmonary arteries) in this malformation. The overload is frequently increased by the surgical creation in early life of a systemic–pulmonary artery shunt. The gradual deterioration of these patients after the second decade of life, their frequent development of increasing mitral regurgitation, and the poor response of patients in the third or fourth decades of life to the Fontan operation (diversion of vena caval blood into the left pulmonary artery) are all probably the result of the progressing secondary left ventricular cardiomyopathy that develops. In contrast, the surprisingly good long-term survival of such individuals after the Fontan repair[9] (closure of the shunts and direct or indirect right atrial to pulmonary artery anastomosis) when it is done in the first decade of life is probably due as much to the relief of the left ventricular volume overload as to the ablation of cyanosis.

Other lesions resulting in chronic left or right ventricular volume overload, with all its implications for the development of a secondary cardiomyopathy, include ventricular septal defect, aortopulmonary window, large patent ductus arteriosus, atrioventricular septal (canal) defect, and post-repair tetralogy of Fallot with a transannular patch. When the secondary cardiomyopathy is severe and long-standing, it becomes in these lesions also a cause of early and late surgical failures.

TABLE 55–2 RELATION BETWEEN SYMPTOMS (NYHA FUNCTIONAL CLASS) AND AGE AT OPERATION FOR REPAIR OF ATRIAL SEPTAL DEFECT

NYHA Functional Class at Time of Operation	Age (yrs) at Operation Mean	Median	Range
I	16	12	3.3–63
II	32	30	4.2–72
III	50	54	0.9–68
IV	51	57	2.2–66

From Kirklin, J. W.: Unpublished data, 1967–1979, n = 340.

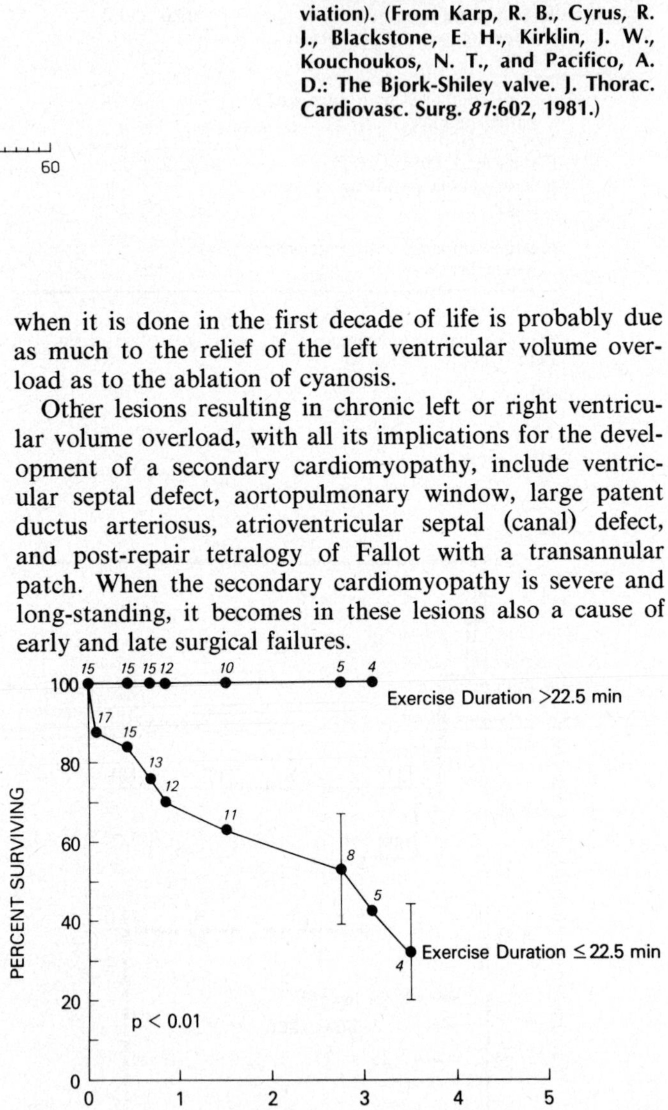

FIGURE 55–3 Actuarial survival after operation for aortic regurgitation in 32 patients, all of whom had subnormal preoperative left ventricular fractional shortening (less than 29 per cent), an index of systolic function. The vertical lines with bars indicate the standard error of the technique. The 15 patients whose exercise duration was greater than 22.5 minutes had significantly preoperative better survival than the 17 patients whose exercise duration was 22.5 minutes or less. The number of patients at risk is indicated at each interval. (From Bonow, R. O., Borer, J. S., Rosing, D. R., Henry, W. L., Pearlman, A. S., McIntosh, C. L., Morrow, A. G., and Epstein, S. E.: Preoperative exercise capacity in symptomatic patients with aortic regurgitation as a predictor of postoperative left ventricular function and long-term prognosis. Circulation *62*:1280, 1980, by permission of the American Heart Association, Inc.)

A special situation exists when the ventricular volume overload is from mitral or tricuspid valve regurgitation, because of the favorable effect on afterload of the abnormally rapid decrease in ventricular volume and increase in wall thickness during each systole (Fig. 55–5).[10] This masks the developing left ventricular secondary cardiomyopathy until very late in the natural history of the disease by improving apparent left ventricular systolic function. Surgical correction of the AV valve regurgitation may unmask the secondary cardiomyopathy and show it to be more advanced than suspected preoperatively (Fig. 55–6.)[11] As in other situations, the cardiomyopathy may then progress and may result in worsening left ventricular systolic

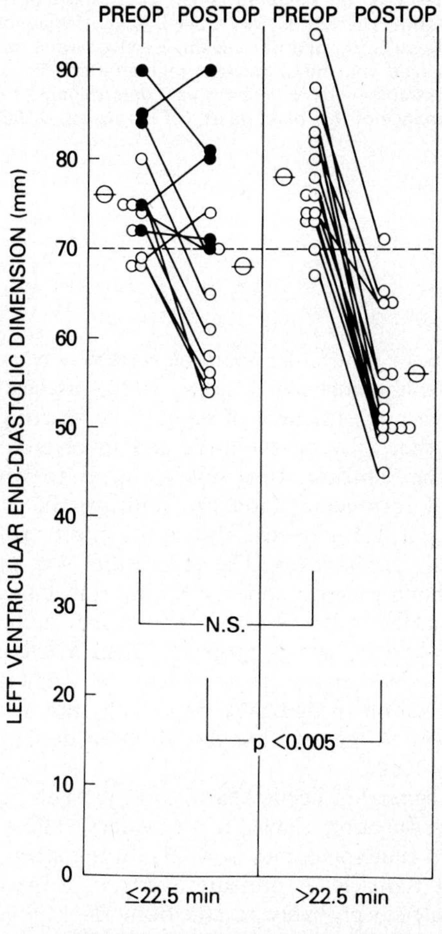

FIGURE 55–4 Changes in echocardiographic left ventricular end-diastolic dimension (an index of diastolic function) as a result of operation in symptomatic patients undergoing valve replacement for aortic regurgitation, according to preoperative exercise duration. Patients who completed Stage I before operation (more than 22.5 minutes) had a greater decrease in diastolic size late in the postoperative period than patients who could not complete Stage I (22.5 minutes or less). The dashed line at 70 mm indicates the value of postoperative diastolic dimension above which patients have been shown to be at high risk of subsequent death from congestive heart failure. ○-alive; ●-late death from congestive heart failure: N.S.-not significant. (From Bonow, R. O., Borer, J. S., Rosing, D. R., Henry, W. L., Pearlman, A. S., McIntosh, C. L., Morrow, A. G., and Epstein, S. E.: Preoperative exercise capacity in symptomatic patients with aortic regurgitation as a predictor of postoperative left ventricular function and long-term prognosis. Circulation *62*:1280, 1980, by permission of the American Heart Association, Inc.)

TABLE 55–3 OLDER AGE AND DECREASED RIGHT VENTRICULAR SYSTOLIC FUNCTION IN SYMPTOMATIC PATIENTS WITH ATRIAL SEPTAL DEFECTS

Group	Age, Years (Mean Value)	Right Ventricular Ejection Fraction (Mean Value)
Asymptomatic	25	64%
Symptomatic	52	36%

From Liberthson, R. R., Boucher, C. A., Strauss, H. W., Dinsmore, R. E., McKusick, K. A., and Pohost, G. M.: Right ventricular function in adult atrial septal defect. Am. J. Cardiol. *47*:56, 1981.

and diastolic function late in the postoperative period and in premature late death.

PRESSURE OVERLOAD. The chronic pressure overload of abnormally high intraventricular systolic pressure initially produces hypertrophy of myocardial cells and increased ventricular mass and wall thickness. Initially, the increase in wall thickness results in continued normal left ventricular afterload, a process called *afterload matching* (p. 452).[1] In this situation, the systolic function returns toward normal after surgical relief of the pressure overload.

Late in the course of a chronic pressure overload (Fig. 13–9, p. 453), or at birth in the case of the pressure overload produced by some kinds of congenital heart disease (Table 55–5), the increase in wall thickness may be insufficient to normalize ventricular afterload, a condition of *afterload* mismatch.[12,13] Ventricular systolic function is thereby reduced. When the afterload mismatch is a long-standing phenomenon, secondary cardiomyopathy develops. In such situations, the advanced cardiomyopathy is associated with degenerative myocardial structural changes[14] and reduced *myocardial contractility*. These may *not* regress after surgical relief of the pressure overload.

Chronic left ventricular pressure overload is present in all forms of left ventricular outflow tract obstruction (subaortic, valvular, and supravalvular aortic stenosis), in aortic coarctation, and in systemic arterial hypertension. Chronic right ventricular pressure overload occurs in all forms of right ventricular outflow obstruction, including tetralogy of Fallot and pulmonary stenosis with intact septum. It is also present in pulmonary hypertension from any cause.

ISCHEMIC CARDIOMYOPATHY (see also p. 1364). Myocardial infarction in patients with ischemic heart dis-

TABLE 55–4 LATE POSTOPERATIVE RIGHT VENTRICULAR FUNCTION AFTER REPAIR OF ATRIAL SEPTAL DEFECT

Age at Operation (Years)	n	Proportion with Near Normal RV End-diastolic Volume
< 10	11	64% (CL, 44%–81%)
> 25	14	21% (CL, 10%–38%)

p = 0.04;
CL = 70% confidence limits;
RV = right ventricular.
(From Pearlman, A. S., Borer, J. S., Clark, C. E., Henry, W. L., Redwood, D. R., Morrow, A. G., Epstein, S. E., Burn, C., Cohen, E., and McKay, F. J.: Abnormal right ventricular size and ventricular septal motion after atrial septal defect closure. Am. J. Cardiol. *41*:295, 1978.)

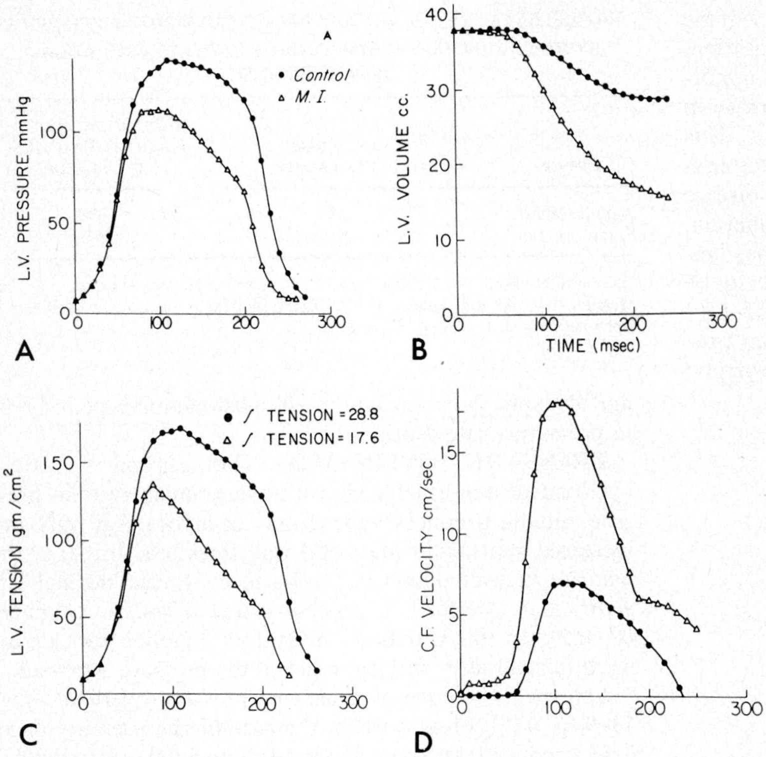

FIGURE 55–5 *A*, Experimental demonstration of the effect of mitral regurgitation on left ventricular (LV) afterload by the rapid reduction of volume during systole, *B*, and by decrease in wall tension, *C*. The result is an increase in systolic function as expressed by the mean velocity of circumferential fiber shortening (CF), *D*. (From Urschel, C. W., Covell, J. W., Sonnenblick, E. H., Ross, J., Jr., and Braunwald, E.: Myocardial mechanics in aortic and mitral valvular regurgitation: The concept of instantaneous impedance as a determinant of the performance of the intact heart. J. Clin. Invest. *47*:867, 1968.)

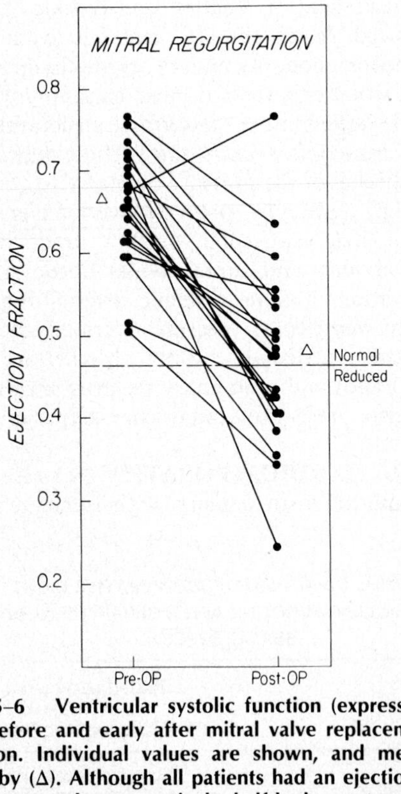

FIGURE 55–6 Ventricular systolic function (expressed as ejection fraction) before and early after mitral valve replacement for mitral regurgitation. Individual values are shown, and mean values are expressed by (Δ). Although all patients had an ejection fraction that was at least normal preoperatively, half had a postoperative ejection fraction below normal. (The lower limit of normal [0.50] is represented by a broken line.) All but one had a decrease in ejection fraction after operation. (From Boucher, C. A., Bingham, J. B., Osbakken, M. D., Okada, R. D., Strauss, H. W., Black, P. C., Levine, F. H., Phillips, H. R., and Pohost, G. M.: Early changes in left ventricular size and function after correction of left ventricular volume overload. Am. J. Cardiol. *47*:991, 1981.)

ease results in ventricular scars of variable size and homogeneity. Nonhomogeneous scars (viable myocardial cells scattered through the area of myocardial scarring) may be small, or they may be extensive and involve a large segment of the ventricle. It is not yet clear to what extent myocardial revascularization can improve the function in such areas of ischemic scarring, by its effect on the viable muscle cells in the areas. The myocardial scar may be essentially homogeneous and transmural and devoid of viable myocardial cells. When such a scar is large, it is usually dyskinetic and is properly called a *left ventricular aneurysm*. Not only is recovery of function after revascularization theoretically impossible, but also the coronary artery to the area has usually been destroyed in the necrotic process.

These regional ischemic changes in left ventricular structure and function have a secondary effect on the nonscarred (but sometimes ischemic during stress) portions of the left ventricle. A pressure overload of the remainder of the ventricle probably results from the regional abnormalities in the scarred areas and their effect on the geometry of the ventricle (an increase in ventricular volume and a resulting augmentation of wall tension, according to the Law of Laplace, p. 431), with the same opportunities for development and progression of the secondary cardiomyopathy as exists in general for pressure-overloaded ventricles.

Secondary Subsystem Abnormalities of Structure and Function

The Lungs. Abnormalities in structure and function of the lungs are commonly involved in early and late deaths after cardiac surgery. This involvement results in part from the vulnerability of the lungs to the damaging effects of cardiopulmonary bypass (see below) and in part from the

TABLE 55–5 LEFT VENTRICULAR SYSTOLIC FUNCTION (EJECTION FRACTION) IN COARCTATION OF THE AORTA

AGE (WEEKS)	LV MASS	LV EJECTION FRACTION	COMMENT
<2	Normal	Severely depressed	Afterload mismatch
4 < 24	Increased	Mildly depressed	Afterload match

LV = left ventricular. (From Graham, T. P., Jr., Atwood, G. F., Boerth, R. C., Boucek, R. J., Jr., and Smith, C. W.: Right and left heart size and function in infants with symptomatic coarctation. Circulation *56*:641, 1977, by permission of the American Heart Association, Inc.)

frequency with which they have preoperative abnormalities of structure and function.

Hypertensive pulmonary vascular disease complicates many kinds of congenital heart disease (pp. 832 and 950). It is reversible in infants after correction of the underlying congenital cardiac malformation under many circumstances[15,16] (p. 950) (Fig. 55–7), but in older patients, when advanced, it persists after operation and may progress to cause premature late death. The classic description of the various stages of this kind of pulmonary vascular disease by Heath and Edwards,[17] supplemented by the more recent morphometric studies by Reid and colleagues,[18] has provided an excellent morphological understanding of the condition. Although there is a correlation between this morphology and the calculated pulmonary vascular resistance, it is not sufficiently strong to allow exact prediction of one from the other.[19]

When hypertensive pulmonary vascular disease becomes severe, the reactivity of the pulmonary vascular bed to physiological stimuli such as exercise disappears. In this situation, characterized by moderate or severe elevation of pulmonary vascular resistance, an increase in pulmonary blood flow in response to exercise cannot occur. As long as there is a defect or communication between the pulmonary and systemic circulations, systemic blood flow can be augmented during exercise by right-to-left shunting, although arterial desaturation results. If the defect is closed, the opportunity for augmentation of systemic blood flow by right-to-left shunting is lost, and there is a risk of sudden death during exercise or stress resulting from an inability to increase systemic and thus coronary blood flow because of the high, nonyielding ("fixed") pulmonary vascular resistance. Therefore, pulmonary vascular disease of such severity is a contraindication to repair of the defect.

A similar but usually less severe type of pulmonary vascular disease develops gradually in patients with *chronically elevated left atrial pressure,* generally from mitral stenosis (p. 830). Although in unusual cases advanced morphological changes are present, more commonly a large element of arteriolar spasm is present. This is evident from the fact that pulmonary arteriolar resistance usually falls immediately after left atrial pressure is reduced by mitral valvotomy or replacement.[5,20]

Pulmonary vascular disease of a different type may be present in patients with *cyanotic congenital heart disease.* Although it has some of the features of hypertensive pulmonary vascular disease, thrombotic occlusive lesions are a major component of this abnormality and tend to be more extensive the more advanced the cyanotic congenital heart disease and its accompanying polycythemia.[21] In some patients, particularly those in whom congenital pulmonary atresia is a part of the malformation, congenital stenoses in the small and large branches of the pulmonary arterial tree, as well as hypertrophy of the distal pulmonary arteriolar walls, add to the hypertensive effect of the pulmonary vasculature.[22] These changes, *in toto,* must be evaluated and considered preoperatively in deciding upon the probable early and late results of cardiac surgery in an individual patient with cyanotic congenital heart disease.

Pulmonary disease unrelated to the cardiac disease may

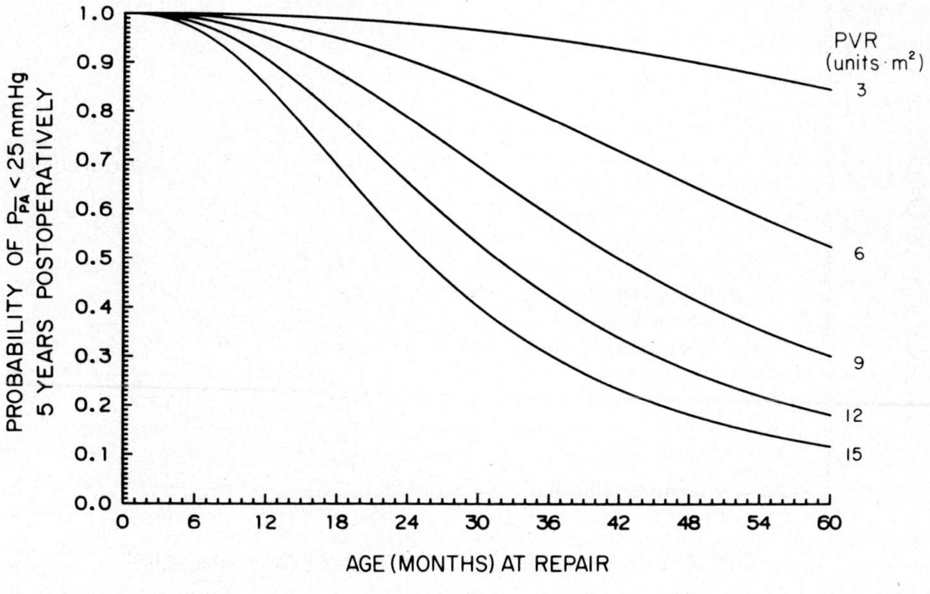

FIGURE 55–7 Probability of mean pulmonary artery pressure less than 25 mm Hg, 5 or more years after repair of ventricular septal defect. Age at operation is along the horizontal axis. The family of curves represents levels of preoperative pulmonary vascular resistance (units · meter²). Note the high probability in infants, even when PVR is high, and the low probability when PVR is high in older patients. (Nomogram from Blackstone, E. H., Kirklin, J. W., Bradley, E. L., DuShane, J. W., and Appelbaum, A.: Optimal age and results in repair of large ventricular septal defects. J. Thorac. Cardiovasc. Surg. *72*:661, 1976.)

also be present and may complicate the early and late postoperative period. The most common of these is *chronic obstructive pulmonary disease.* Its presence affects not only the risk of cardiac surgery, and thus the indications for it, but also the postoperative management of the patient.

The Kidneys (see also Chap. 52). Preexisting *chronic renal disease* increases the risk of developing acute renal dysfunction and renal failure early in the postoperative period and thus affects patient management in this period and the risk of the operation.[23,24] *Cyanotic congenital heart disease* predisposes the patient to acute renal failure early postoperatively, probably because such a patient gradually develops morphological renal abnormalities.[25] *Preoperative chronic congestive heart failure* likewise predisposes to acute renal failure soon after operation, most likely because of the abnormalities of renal function and structure that result from this state.

The Blood. The *polycythemia* secondary to cyanotic congenital heart disease (pp. 949 and 1686) is overcome immediately at the start of cardiopulmonary bypass by the hemodilution that is used. However, most patients who were polycythemic preoperatively have a greater than usual tendency to bleed in the perioperative period. Special preventive measures are required.

Long-standing *congestive heart failure* with hepatic congestion may reduce hepatic synthesis of normal clotting factors and thereby increase the tendency for bleeding after cardiopulmonary bypass. Because of the current prevalence of *aspirin ingestion* and the use of other drugs that affect platelet function, preoperative laboratory determination of bleeding time is advisable in most patients.

The Liver. Even mild preexisting liver disease increases the risk of acute hepatic failure early after cardiac surgery. Thus, its presence must be taken into account in planning the conduct of the operation and management in the early postoperative period.

The Brain. Patients who have recovered virtually completely from a hemiplegic episode prior to their cardiac surgery may have a temporary reappearance of the hemiplegic signs and symptoms immediately after cardiac surgery using cardiopulmonary bypass. This does not necessarily indicate that a new neurological injury has occurred, and recovery from this temporary relapse is usually rapid.

Because of the largely nonpulsatile nature of perfusion during cardiopulmonary bypass, patients with significant carotid artery stenosis may be at increased risk for ischemic neurological injury during and after operation. Thus, signs and symptoms of cerebrovascular insufficiency should be sought in adult patients with generalized atherosclerosis so that proper preoperative evaluation and intraoperative management may be employed to minimize the risk of neurological injury.

Other Factors Affecting The Outcome of Surgery

Preoperative Symptomatic State. Advanced preoperative symptoms affect the early results of cardiac surgery because they are usually associated with impaired ventricular systolic and diastolic performance, as well as other organ dysfunction. They affect late results because of their implications with regard to the secondary cardiomyopathy.

As an example of the effect on early results, in infants less than 3 months old, at least between 1967 and 1978, the hospital mortality was directly related to the preoperative symptomatic state[26] (Table 55–6). As another instance, the preoperative symptomatic state of the patient undergoing aortic valve replacement (isolated or combined with mitral valve replacement) affects the probability of early postoperative death from cardiac causes (Fig. 55–8). Aortic valve replacement, isolated or combined with mitral valve replacement, exemplifies the effect of preoperative symptoms on late results as well (Fig. 55–2).

Age of the Patient. Very young age and very old age are incremental risks for hospital death under many circumstances. This does not mean that hospital mortality is necessarily higher in the very young and the very old. It

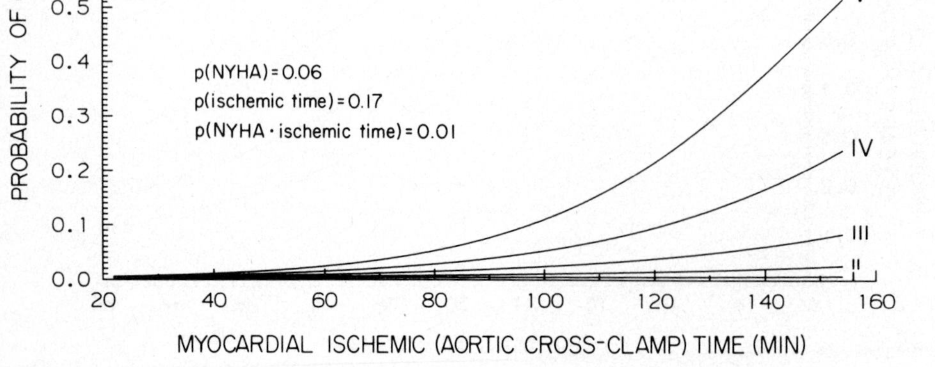

FIGURE 55–8 Relation of preoperative clinical status and myocardial ischemic (aortic cross-clamp) time to probability of cardiac death after primary or secondary, isolated or combined, aortic valve replacement, UAB[19] (n = 1,042, 1975 to July 1979).

TABLE 55–6 THE RELATION OF PREOPERATIVE SYMPTOMATIC CLASS TO HOSPITAL DEATH AFTER INTRACARDIAC OPERATION IN THE FIRST 3 MONTHS OF LIFE

Preoperative Class	*n*	Hospital Deaths		
		n	%	70% CL (%)
II	15	3	20	9–36
III	68	15	22	17–28
IV	68	37	54	47–94
V	23	20	87	75–94
Total	174	75	43	39–47

p(chi-square) for table < 0.0001.
CL = confidence limits.
UAB, 1967 to July 1981. Classes II, III, IV correspond to the NYHA Class, and Class V indicates preoperative shock or metabolic acidosis.
(From Kirklin, J. K., Blackstone, E. H., Kirklin, J. W., McKay, R., Pacifico, A. D., and Bargeron, L. M., Jr.: Intracardiac surgery in infants under age 3 months: Incremental risk factors for hospital mortality. Am. J. Cardiol. *48*:500, 1981.)

means only that it is *more difficult* to obtain very low hospital mortality rates in these two groups.

The incremental risk of very young age (less than about 6 months) is probably related to the very young patient's increased sensitivity to the damaging effects of cardiopulmonary bypass (see below). For many lesions, however, appropriate knowledge and experience can neutralize this incremental risk (Fig. 55–9).[27]

Date of Operation. The knowledge and techniques of cardiac surgery continue to improve. As a result, both the early and the late results of cardiac surgery improve with time (Fig. 55–9).[28] This makes comparisons between nonconcurrent clinical studies hazardous, unless a specific effort is made to take into account these changes with time.

Institution of Operation. There are true institutional (and surgeon-to-surgeon) differences in the early and late results of cardiac surgery. These are related to variations in knowledge, technique, and experience. Since these differences are generally identified by comparisons between two or more prospective but not necessarily concurrent clinical studies involving a more or less heterogeneous population, the comparisons must be done with great care and full knowledge of the multivariate nature of the determinants of these results. For example, a preliminary comparison of the results of coronary artery bypass grafting in hospital A and in hospital B may indicate that the hospital mortality rate is the same in the two institutions. The conclusion might be drawn that the quality of work in the two hospitals is similar. However, analysis of the two patient populations may show a much higher proportion of patients with moderately or severely depressed left ventricular function in hospital B, which is an incremental risk factor for hospital death even when the patient is in highly knowledgeable and experienced hands. The conclusion would be that the quality of the work in hospital B was in fact superior.

Comments. It is evident that a very large number of preoperative variables affect the results of cardiac surgery. This must be taken into account in estimating the risks, and thus the advisability of, surgical treatment for an individual patient. In addition, the complexities of *comparative* analysis of results are apparent from this and from the large number of intraoperative variables that also affect results (see below). Such comparative studies must therefore be based upon precise and extensive data gathering, sophisticated and multivariate statistical methods, and a contemplative analysis of the results.

INTRAOPERATIVE CONDITIONS AFFECTING EARLY AND LATE RESULTS

Cardiopulmonary Bypass (CPB)

CPB could be considered a safe support system for clinical cardiac surgery, judging from the fact that the hospital mortality for coronary artery bypass grafting (CABG) in recent years approaches zero. However, there are important damaging effects of CPB that contribute to in-hospital morbidity and mortality and must be considered in early postoperative management.

The manifestations of the damaging effects of CPB include an abnormal tendency to bleed externally and into tissues; a diffuse or whole-body "inflammatory reaction," characterized by increased capillary permeability with con-

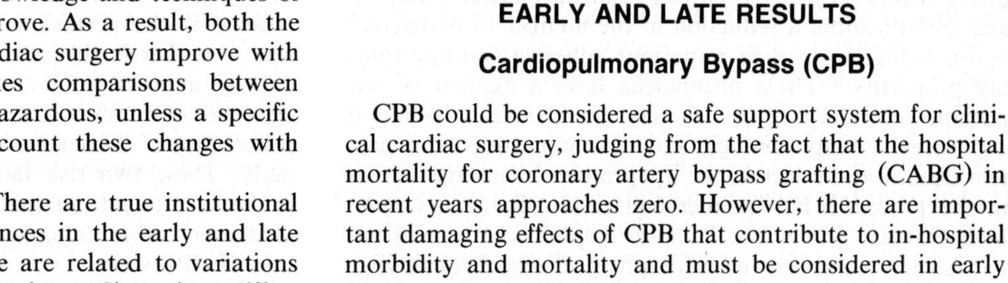

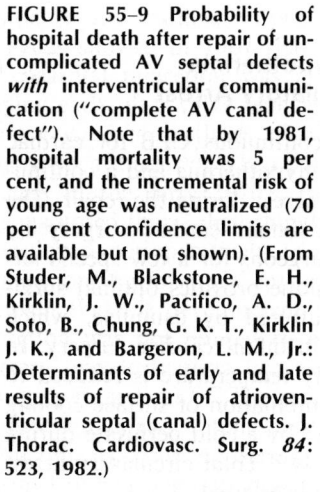

FIGURE 55–9 Probability of hospital death after repair of uncomplicated AV septal defects *with* interventricular communication ("complete AV canal defect"). Note that by 1981, hospital mortality was 5 per cent, and the incremental risk of young age was neutralized (70 per cent confidence limits are available but not shown). (From Studer, M., Blackstone, E. H., Kirklin, J. W., Pacifico, A. D., Soto, B., Chung, G. K. T., Kirklin J. K., and Bargeron, L. M., Jr.: Determinants of early and late results of repair of atrioventricular septal (canal) defects. J. Thorac. Cardiovasc. Surg. *84*: 523, 1982.)

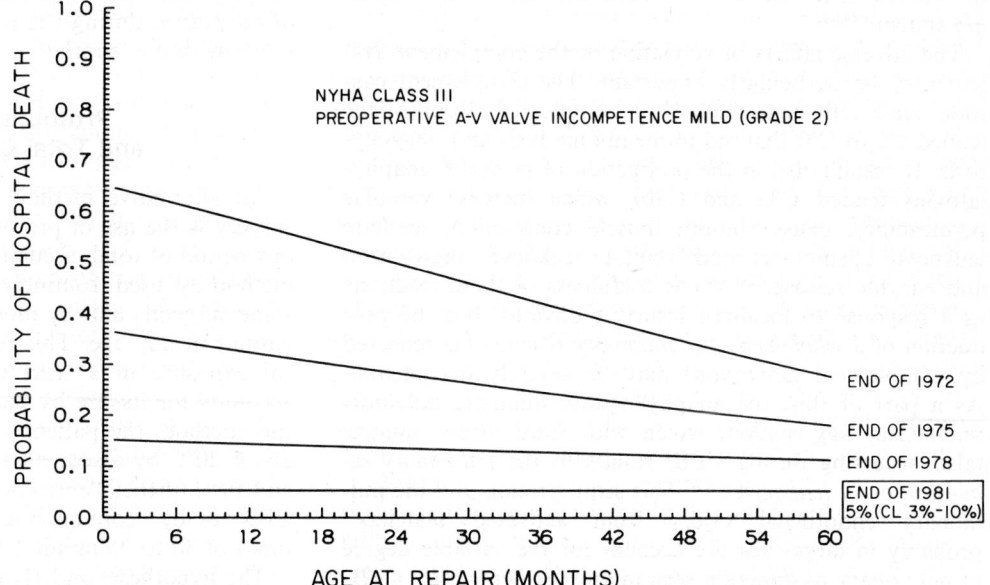

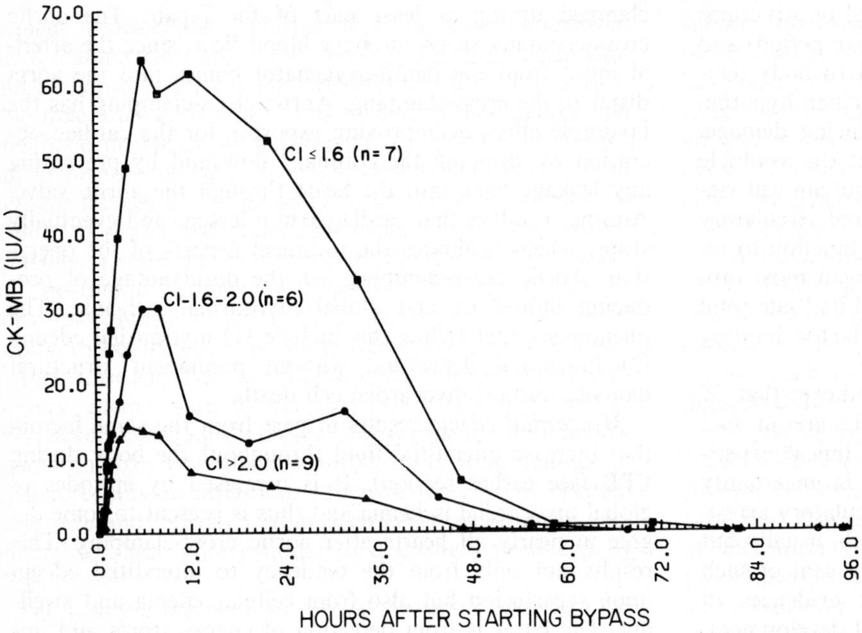

FIGURE 55–10 The relation of extent of perioperative myocardial necrosis (reflected in the blood CK-MB isoenzyme values along the vertical axis) and the early postoperative cardiac index (CI in liters · min^{-1} · $meter^{-2}$) in 22 consecutive patients undergoing mitral valve replacement at UAB in 1975, using simple cold ischemic arrest. Geometric mean values are portrayed. Note the very high levels of CK-MB in patients with low cardiac output (1.6 or less) and the low levels in patients with large cardiac output (more than 2.0). The overall correlation of CK-MB (duration, peak, and integrated area) and cardiac index is $r = -0.4$ and $p = 0.04$. (From Kirklin, J. W., and Barratt-Boyes, B. G.: Textbook of Cardiac Surgery. New York, John Wiley and Sons [in preparation].)

(the prerequisite of which is cell death). During cardiac surgery, reperfusion of a heart that has been severely damaged by ischemia may produce a sudden massive palpable *contracture*[74,75,76] (localized or global "stone heart"), which may seem to the surgeon to be simply ventricular fibrillation but which is not. This is *not* the true contracture (or rigor) of ischemia[84] but is a phenomenon of reperfusion of a ventricle that has experienced severe ischemic damage. This may be the gross analogue of the contraction bands observed microscopically. With reperfusion, calcium accumulations become abnormally high in the mitochondria,[88,89] secondary to an accelerated entry of calcium ions into the cells. This accelerated entry results from loss of membrane selective permeability properties in the presence of a reduced capacity for the control of cytoplasmic calcium concentration by the sodium-calcium pump, believed to be the result of low levels of ATP[90] (p. 1253).

The incidence and extent of perioperative ischemic myocardial necrosis are significantly related to the *duration of the global myocardial ischemia,* no matter what method of myocardial protection is used.[91] When the myocardium is hypothermic during the ischemic period, the proportion of cells dying in any given ischemic time is less, such that the degree of damage is directly related to myocardial temperature during the period of global ischemia.[92] When the heart's electromechanical activity is stopped shortly after the start of global ischemia ("cardioplegia"), myocardial necrosis is still further reduced.

Myocardial Protection. A number of methods for *myocardial protection* during cardiac surgery have been used, but in recent years most surgeons have turned to the technique of myocardial preservation with cold and cardioplegia. This method takes advantage of the protective effect of cold and of sudden cessation of electromechanical activity. It greatly extends the "safe" time of global myocardial ischemia (ischemia without myocardial necrosis). The data on humans indicate that with this method no significant myocardial necrosis or permanent functional damage results from total myocardial ischemia for up to 120 minutes, if the preoperative myocardial reserves are good (i.e., NYHA Functional Class I or II). However, decreased preoperative myocardial reserves (presumably present in patients in NYHA Functional Classes III and IV) appear to lower the safe time limits of cold cardioplegia, and the data suggest that only about 80 minutes are allowed in patients with advanced heart failure (Fig. 55–8).

The most commonly used cardioplegic agent at present is potassium, in concentrations of 15 to 35 mEq. Potassium in this concentration blocks the initial "fast" (inward sodium current) phase of myocardial cellular depolarization. Even with this concentration of potassium, electromechanical activity can persist or return in the presence of agents such as catecholamines, which "open" the latter "slow" (inward calcium and sodium current) phase of myocardial cellular depolarization on which potassium has no effect, and when noncoronary collateral flow is large. Proper methodology overcomes these potential problems. The cardioplegic vehicle is either asanguineous (some type of buffered electrolyte solution usually containing mannitol) or sanguineous (made up of blood from the pump-oxygenator). It is delivered into the aortic root, or directly into the coronary ostia, at a temperature of about 4°C. Infusions are repeated about every 30 minutes during the ischemic period.

Completeness of Repair

It is sometimes forgotten that a poor hemodynamic state early in the postoperative period may be related, in part at least, to an incomplete surgical procedure (such as replacement of only one valve when two are significantly abnormal in function, very incomplete myocardial revascularization, incomplete repair of a large ventricular septal defect, the leaving of important right ventricular outflow tract obstruction in the repair of tetralogy of Fallot, and so forth). This emphasizes the need for complete knowledge of the preoperative cardiac conditions, a wise assessment of the surgical procedures needed to correct them, and a skillful and determined surgical effort to carry out a completely corrective procedure.

CONVALESCENCE AND CARE AFTER CARDIAC SURGERY

The primary determinants of the success of a cardiac operation are events in the operating room. However, every cardiac surgical patient requires postoperative care. Unfortunately, all invasive monitoring and some that is noninvasive (for example, the recording of an electrocardiogram without proper grounding), as well as all interventions, involve risks of varying magnitude to the patient. They should, therefore, be used only when the probability of postoperative problems is greater than their inherent risks.

After cardiac operations, the combination of the basic cardiac disease, the cardiac trauma of the operation, and the whole-body response to cardiopulmonary bypass (CPB) creates special problems. The problems related to CPB are particularly complex (see earlier section). Many conceptual, scientific, and management errors are made by failing to realize that humans during and for a time after CPB are in a special biological situation to which the knowledge and rules derived for "intact" humans may or *may not* apply. Fortunately, in spite of these problems, many cardiac operations are now almost without risk (risk approaches zero). Postoperative care can be quite simple for patients undergoing these operations. Yet certain situations still have an appreciable probability of hospital death or morbidity, and in them more extensive monitoring and interventions are needed.

The patient may be considered as a complex integrated system composed of a number of separate but interrelated subsystems (i.e., cardiovascular, pulmonary, renal, nervous, and alimentary). The care of such a patient can be accomplished effectively utilizing a "subsystems analysis" approach.[93] This commences in the operating room as CPB is discontinued and continues into the early and late postoperative period.

An *uncomplicated or normal convalescence* is one devoid of any findings or events that increase the probability of hospital death or of important complications or of a suboptimal late result. As long as this pattern of normal convalescence continues, monitoring, testing, and interventions can safely be minimized. Alertness to deviations from the pattern of an uncomplicated convalescence is required, as these are an indication for greater intensity of observation and treatment.

Cardiovascular Subsystem

Most perioperative complications, hospital deaths, and late failures after cardiac surgery are in some way a failure of the cardiovascular subsystem. An understanding of its function and postoperative management is therefore necessary.

Convalescence can be considered normal with regard to the cardiovascular subsystem when the cardiac output is adequate for the metabolic needs of the organism. The output can be evaluated either by measuring the cardiac output or by assessing its adequacy, or by both methods. Cardiac output may be measured by indocyanine green indicator dilution techniques or by thermodilution. The former has the advantage that residual intracardiac shunts can be detected by the contour of the indicator dilution curve or by double sampling techniques. The adequacy of cardiac output is assessed by evaluation of the pedal pulses and skin temperature, urine flow, and mixed venous oxygen levels, and these methods are generally highly reliable. Arterial blood pressure is ordinarily an insensitive guide to cardiac performance early in the postoperative period, chiefly because the systemic vascular resistance is unusually high. However, arterial hypotension is always an indication for intense evaluation, and the patient cannot be considered to be convalescing normally when mean arterial blood pressure is less than 10 per cent below normal for age.

The treatment of *inadequate cardiac output* is directed at increasing the output by manipulation of preload, afterload, the contractile state, and heart rate and at improving tissue oxygen levels by other means as well. When cardiac output is low, preload is made appropriate by increasing blood volume until the higher of the two atrial pressures is approximately 15 mm Hg. If the wall thickness of the left ventricle is unusually great, or its contractility or compliance or both are decreased, it may be helpful to take mean left atrial pressure to 20 mm Hg. When the right ventricle is the limiting one, right atrial pressure usually can advantageously be taken only to approximately 18 mm Hg. Above these levels, a fall in cardiac output may occur.

Afterload reduction (p. 534) can often be used to improve cardiac performance early after cardiac surgery. When the left ventricular performance is the limiting one, and systemic arterial blood pressure is more than approximately 10 per cent above normal, its afterload should be reduced by lowering arterial blood pressure to between normal and 10 per cent above normal, generally with nitroprusside. However, vasodilator therapy, which results in a mean arterial blood pressure lower than normal, often is associated with a reduction in cardiac output and is dangerous.[94] Rarely, in patients with severe long-standing mitral valve disease or congenital heart disease with pulmonary vascular obstructive changes, right ventricular dysfunction associated with elevated pulmonary artery pressure may limit cardiac performance, and reduction of right ventricular afterload with vasodilator agents is indicated.

Heart rate is optimized as necessary. For patients in sinus or junctional rhythm, atrial pacing is used; if atrial fibrillation is present, ventricular pacing is used; and if AV dissociation is the rhythm, AV sequential pacing is used. If tachyarrhythmias are present, control is usually obtained by pharmacological means or by specialized pacing methods.[95]

If these relatively simple measures do not bring cardiac output to an adequate level, administration of catecholamines or intraaortic balloon pumping (IABP) is used. The former is chosen in infants and children, in adults without major myocardial necrosis and with only mild or moderate impairments, and in those with a contraindication to IABP. If catecholamines are indicated, dopamine (p. 542) is begun at low doses, which can be increased up to 15 $\mu g \cdot kg^{-1} \cdot min^{-1}$ if needed. When dopamine is not effective, dobutamine (p. 543) is added, and the dosages are similar. Dobutamine is a potent inotropic agent that usually does not increase systemic or pulmonary vascular resistance and has less tendency to produce tachycardia.

Epinephrine, isoproterenol, and norepinephrine are now rarely used. However, in the presence of predominantly right ventricular dysfunction and decreased or normal heart rate, isoproterenol may be the preferred drug because of its favorable effect on pulmonary vascular resistance. When catecholamines are administered, and a satisfactory response obtained, 8 to 12 hours later an aggressive and persistent effort is begun *gradually* to reduce and finally discontinue them.

In adults, if adjustment of preload, afterload, and heart rate and modest doses (2.5 to 5 $\mu g \cdot kg^{-1} \cdot min^{-1}$) of dopamine do not result in adequate cardiac performance, intraaortic balloon pumping (IABP) (p. 593) is considered. If a strong suspicion of myocardial necrosis exists or if ventricular electrical instability is present, IABP is preferable to catecholamines as *initial* treatment.

While efforts are being made to increase cardiac output, the tissue and mixed venous oxygen levels should also be raised by attention to the other variables represented in the Fick equation. The blood hemoglobin is kept above 10 to 12 $gm \cdot dl^{-1}$ by administration of packed red blood cells or whole blood, and the PaO_2 is maintained at 100 to 200 mm Hg by increasing the fractional concentration of oxygen in the inspired air. Unduly high oxygen consumption ($\dot{V}O_2$) is prevented while the patient is on a ventilator, by use of sedation or paralyzing drugs, to prevent restlessness or agitation. Hyperthermia (rectal or central temperature $\geq$ 39.7°C, or 103.5°F) is treated vigorously.

Postoperative morbidity and mortality can result from *cardiac arrhythmias.* These may occur when the cardiac subsystem has been otherwise functioning normally or as a complication of low cardiac output. They may be the manifestation of a severe secondary cardiomyopathy. Atrial and ventricular pacing wires, routinely placed at operation and left for 5 to 10 postoperative days, are of utmost importance in the diagnosis[96] and treatment[97,98] of postoperative arrhythmias.[95]

Ventricular electrical instability, which includes *premature ventricular contractions* (PVC's) and *ventricular tachycardia,* is an extremely important arrhythmia. Although controversy exists concerning the proportion of patients with PVC's who develop ventricular fibrillation, it may be that this potential exists in any patient who has significant intermittent or continuous ventricular electrical instability. Therefore, the electrocardiogram is monitored continuously for at least 48 hours in all patients, and ventricular electrical instability is treated vigorously by the methods generally used in other settings (p. 720).

Various *atrial arrhythmias* may complicate the postoperative period. *Atrial fibrillation* (p. 699) is treated initially with digitalis. If it persists until the seventh postoperative day in patients who have not been in atrial fibrillation preoperatively, electroversion should usually be carried out. *Atrial flutter* (p. 697), formerly a difficult arrhythmia to manage postoperatively, is now usually converted to sinus rhythm by rapid atrial pacing (via the two implanted atrial wires) at the so-called critical pacing rate with sudden cessation of pacing after about 20 seconds.[95] Digoxin is begun and continued for 6 weeks. Procainamide is begun and continued for 8 weeks, with a switch to quinidine if long-term drug therapy is indicated. *Paroxysmal atrial contractions* (PAC's) (p. 694) may trigger or lead to atrial fibrillation, and, therefore, an attempt is made to suppress them with atrial pacing, digoxin, procainamide (Pronestyl), or quinidine. *Paroxysmal atrial tachycardia* (PAT) (p. 702) is usually first treated by rapid atrial pacing and then sudden cessation.[95] If this is unsuccessful, intravenous propranolol, verapamil, or digoxin is usually successful. If PAT is recurrent or refractory to treatment, continuous rapid atrial pacing at approximately 100 beats faster than the intrinsic atrial rate is employed to produce and sustain a 2:1 block. Patients who have had PAT generally should receive digoxin for about 6 weeks.

When the onset of a supraventricular tachyarrhythmia is accompanied by significant hemodynamic deterioration, prompt cardioversion (p. 669) is indicated if atrial wires are not in place.

Renal Subsystem

Convalescence after cardiac surgery can be considered uncomplicated when urine volume is "adequate". Useful but somewhat arbitrary criteria are that it be greater than 500 $ml \cdot 24\ hours^{-1} \cdot meter^{-2}$ or 167 $ml \cdot 8\ hours^{-1} \cdot meter^{-2}$ or 20 $ml \cdot hr^{-1} \cdot meter^{-2}$. Solute excretion must also be "adequate," and the convalescence is abnormal when solute excretion is insufficient to keep serum potassium levels below 5 $mEq \cdot liter^{-1}$, blood urea nitrogen (BUN) levels below 40 $mg \cdot dl^{-1}$, and creatinine levels below 1.5 $mg \cdot dl^{-1}$. Others use different criteria. Convalescence cannot be considered normal when the urine is pink but without red blood cells early in the postoperative period, for this indicates an inordinate and potentially dangerous amount of hemolysis (free plasma hemoglobin levels >40 $mg \cdot dl^{-1}$).

As a guide to the continuing evaluation of the renal subsystem, a urinary catheter is inserted in the operating room preoperatively and left for 24 to 48 hours to monitor urine flow. Serum potassium is measured every 4 hours during the first 24 postoperative hours, and if convalescence is not normal, every 8 hours for at least the next 48 hours. Serum creatinine and BUN are measured each morning for at least the first 48 hours.

Acute renal failure after cardiac surgery is rare in adults, occurring in fewer than 0.1 per cent of patients undergoing operations such as coronary artery bypass grafting, but may occur in 8 to 10 per cent of infants undergoing open intracardiac operations.[99,100] It is usually associated with low cardiac output initially, but rarely may happen when the other criteria of cardiac subsystem performance are satisfactory.[24,100,101]

The probability of acute renal failure after surgery with CPB is also influenced by certain incremental risk factors other than low cardiac output:

1. *Young age*: One reason for the apparently increased incidence in infants (noted above) is the higher proportion in this age group of seriously ill patients with low cardiac output early in the postoperative period. The immaturity of the kidney in infants and young children, resulting in less ability to concentrate the urine, may also predispose them to acute renal failure. Infants may develop more tissue hypoxia during and early after CPB than do older patients, with a resultant increased production of potassium, urea nitrogen, and other substances, some of which may be nephrotoxic.

2. *Cyanotic heart disease*: Acute renal failure is more likely to occur after operations for cyanotic heart disease.[25] A renal lesion is known to exist in many such patients preoperatively.

3. *Preoperative impairment of renal function* considerably increases the risk of acute renal failure early in the postoperative period.[23,101] Therefore, a part of the preoperative evaluation should be the determination of renal function.

4. A *long period* of *CPB* (> 180 minutes in adults, less than this in infants and small children) probably increases the risk of acute renal failure.

5. The additional risk from *profound hypothermia and total circulatory arrest* is not known, nor is that of long periods of *reduced flow* during *hypothermic CPB*. However, flows 1.6 liter · min^{-1} · m^{-2} or more at 28°C and mean arterial blood pressure 30 mm Hg or more during CPB at moderate hypothermia seem adequate to minimize acute renal failure.[24]

6. A *high plasma hemoglobin level* (> 40 mg · dl^{-1}) during and early after CPB probably increases the risk of acute renal failure.

7. The suggestion that a *whole blood prime* is an incremental risk is supported by several studies.[102,103]

8. *Aminoglycosides* (gentamicin) and some other antibiotics may increase the risk of acute renal failure after CPB.

Acute renal failure may develop within 12 to 48 hours after operation. Its first effect is resistant oliguria of increasing severity, resulting in very rapidly rising serum potassium levels (probably because of the acute loss of potassium from hemolyzing red blood cells and from the whole-body loss of intracellular potassium that characterizes the perioperative period in patients who have been on CPB) and more slowly rising BUN and creatinine levels. Although this form of acute renal failure is rarely the primary mode of death, it complicates recovery in a major way unless effective interventions are promptly made. It is the type usually seen in infants. A less lethal form becomes apparent on the third or fourth postoperative day. This manifests itself by a progressive rise in BUN and creatinine levels, which peak at 80 to 120 and 5 to 8 mg · dl^{-1}, respectively, about 7 to 10 days postoperatively. There is often little or no oliguria, and hyperkalemia greater than 5 mEq · $liter^{-1}$ does not usually develop. Spontaneous resolution usually follows, and as long as the patient's clinical condition is satisfactory, urine flow is adequate, and BUN and creatinine levels eventually begin to fall, dialysis is not indicated.

When *oliguria* occurs early postoperatively, *cardiac preload performance* should be optimized (see above). Intravenous *furosemide* (1 mg · kg^{-1}) is sometimes administered. If a good response is obtained, this is repeated every 6 hours for 3 days. If a response to furosemide is not obtained, the dose is doubled, and then quadrupled, and then 8 mg · kg^{-1} is given. When the *serum potassium* level rises above *5.5 mEq* · l^{-1}, *glucose-insulin solution* is given *intravenously* and *sodium polystyrene sulfonate (Kayexalate) enemas* are used.

Unless oliguria and hyperkalemia respond to treatment within a few hours, and especially in infants, the nephrologist should proceed immediately with dialysis. Usually, peritoneal dialysis is used early postoperatively, particularly in infants.[104] In older patients hemodialysis may be substituted for peritoneal dialysis after a few days if acute renal failure persists. With these measures many patients can be maintained in good condition until cardiac and renal functions improve and ultimately recover fully.[100]

Pulmonary Subsystem

Patients are extubated early after cardiac surgery, as soon as the effects of the anesthetic agents have disappeared, when normal convalescence is likely. In patients undergoing *closed* operations, including infants, this usually means extubation in the operating room. After *open* operations of an uncomplicated nature, such as repair of simple congenital lesions, coronary artery bypass grafting, or isolated valve replacement or valvotomy, patients, including infants, are usually extubated within 4 to 8 hours postoperatively. Following complex open operations, ventilation is continued at least overnight, and the patient is not extubated until the appropriate criteria are met.

While intubated, the patient is ventilated with a volume-controlled respirator that provides *intermittent positive pressure breathing* (IPPB). It should be equipped with valves that allow the patient to breathe himself, when he will, in between the *intermittent mandatory ventilation* (IMV) from the ventilator. The IMV is reduced gradually as soon as spontaneous breathing is sufficient, to accustom the patient to breathing again and to gain the hemodynamic advantages of the negative intrapleural pressures that develop during spontaneous inspiration. *Positive end-expiratory pressure* (PEEP) should be used in most patients. PEEP is preferred because of the studies that suggest larger lung volumes and fewer perfused but nonventilated alveoli during ventilation and smaller alveolar-arterial oxygen differences (A-a) pO_2 after extubation when it is used.[105] PEEP is not used in patients with chronic obstructive lung disease (for fear of air-trapping and rupturing a bulla with consequent pneumothorax), in infants who have undergone interatrial transposition of venous return, Fontan's operation, or a superior vena caval–right atrial anastomosis (to avoid still further elevation of jugular venous pressure). While the patient is intubated and ventilated, the inspired gases are warmed and humidified. Appropriate aspiration of the trachea, turning of the patient, and chest physiotherapy are carried out. After extubation, which should be done as soon as possible, *reintubation* is usually not necessary when the patient truly meets the criteria for extubation. However, when the work of breathing is excessive, when CO_2 retention is enough to produce significant respiratory acidosis, or when the patient is becoming exhausted by ventilatory efforts, reintubation is indicated. When the situation is borderline, careful observation by senior members of the team is required for proper decision-making.

Other Subsystems

Abnormalities of the other subsystems are infrequent during convalescence from cardiac surgery using a pump-oxygenator. Therefore, management of them is relatively straightforward.

Because of the increase in extracellular fluid and total exchangeable sodium and the decrease in exchangeable potassium that develop during CPB, early postoperative *fluid*

80. Neely, J. R., Liedtke, A. J., Whitman, J. T., and Rovelto, M. J.: Relationship between coronary flow and adenosine triphosphate production from glycolysis and oxidative metabolism. *In* Roy, D. C., and Harris, P. (eds.): The Cardiac Sarcoplasm. Vol 8. Baltimore, University Park Press, 1975, p. 301.
81. Hearse, D. J., Garlick, P. B., and Humphrey, S. M.: Ischemic contracture of the myocardium: Mechanisms and prevention. Am. J. Cardiol. *39*:986, 1977.
82. Schaper, J., Mulch, J., Winkler, B., and Shaper, W.: Ultrastructural, functional, and biochemical criteria for estimation of reversibility of ischemic injury: A study on the effects of global ischemia on the isolated dog heart. J. Mol. Cell. Cardiol. *11*:521, 1979.
83. Chance, B.: The energy-linked reactions of calcium with mitochrondria. J. Biol. Chem. *240*:2729, 1965.
84. Sapsford, R. N., Blackstone, E. H., Kirklin, J. W., Karp, R. B., Kouchoukos, N. T., Pacifico, A. D., Roe, C. R., and Bradley, E. L.: Coronary perfusion versus cold ischemic arrest during aortic valve surgery; a randomized study. Circulation *49*:1190, 1974.
85. Jennings, R. B., Sommer, H. M., Herdson, P. B., and Kaltenback, J. P.: Ischemic injury of myocardium. Ann. N. Y. Acad. Sci. *156*:61, 1969.
86. Moulder, P. V., Blackstone, E. H., Eckner, F. A. O., and Lev, M.: Pressure derivative loop for left ventricular resuscitation. Arch. Surg. *96*:323, 1968.
87. Martin, A. M., Jr., and Hackel, D. B.: An electron microscopic study of the progression of myocardial lesions in the dog after hemorrhage shock. Lab. Invest. *15*:243, 1966.
88. Isom, O. W., Kutin, W. D., Falk, E. A., and Spencer, F. C.: Patterns of myocardial metabolism during cardiopulmonary bypass and coronary perfusion. J. Thorac. Cardiovasc. Surg. *66*:705, 1973.
89. Shen, A. C., and Jennings, R. B.: Myocardial calcium and magnesium in acute ischemic injury. Am. J. Pathol. *67*:417, 1972.
90. Nayler, W. G., Poole-Wilson, P. A., and Williams, A.: Hypoxia and calcium J. Mol. Cell. Cardiol. *11*:683, 1979.
91. Jennings, R. B., Sommers, H. M., Smyth, G. A., Flack, H. A., and Linn, H.: Myocardial necrosis induced by temporary occlusion of a coronary artery in the dog. Arch. Pathol. *70*:82, 1960.
92. Hearse, D. J., Stewart, D. A., and Braimbridge, M. V.: Cellular protection during myocardial ischemia. The development and characterization of a procedure for the induction of reversible ischemic arrest. Circulation *54*:193, 1976.
93. Kirklin, J. W.: Systems Analysis in Surgical Patients with Particular Attention to the Cardiac and Pulmonary Subsystems (Macewen Memorial Lecture). Glasgow, University of Glasgow Press, 1970.
94. Stinson, E. B., Holloway, E. L., and Derby, G. C.: Control of myocardial performance early after open-heart operations by vasodilator treatment. J. Thorac. Cardiovasc. Surg. *73*:523, 1977.
95. Waldo, A. L., and MacLean, W. A. H.: Diagnosis and Treatment of Cardiac Arrhythmias following Open Heart Surgery. Emphasis on the Use of Atrial and Ventricular Epicardial Wire Electrodes. New York, Futura Publishing Company, 1980.
96. Waldo, A. L., Ross, S. M., and Kaiser, G. A.: The epicardial electrogram in the diagnosis of cardiac arrhythmias following cardiac surgery. Geriatrics *26*:108, 1971.
97. Friesen, W. G., Woodson, R. D., Ames, A. W., Herr, R. H., Starr, A., and Kassebaum, D. G.: A hemodynamic comparison of atrial and ventricular pacing in postoperative cardiac surgical patients. J. Thorac. Cardiovasc. Surg. *55*:271, 1968.
98. Waldo, A. L., MacLean, W. A. H., Karp, R. B., Kouchoukos, N. T., and James, T. N.: Sustained rapid atrial pacing to control supraventricular tachycardias following open heart surgery. Circulation *51* and *52* (Suppl. II):II–13, 1975.
99. Chesney, R. W., Kaplan, B. S., Freedom, R. M., Haller, J. A., and Drummond, K. N.: Acute renal failure: An important complication of cardiac surgery in infants. J. Pediatr. *87*:381, 1975.
100. Srinivasan, V., Levinsky, L., Choh, J. H., Baliah, T., and Subramanian, S.: Renal failure following intracardiac surgery in infants — Improved survival with early dialysis: Indications and results. J. Pediatr. (in press).
101. Bourgeois, B. F. D., Donath, A., Paunier, L., and Rouge, J.-C.: Effects of cardiac surgery on renal functions in children. J. Thorac. Cardiovasc. Surg. *77*:283, 1979.
102. German, J. C., Chalmers, G. S., Hirai, J., Nrisingha, M. D., Wakabayashi, A., and Connolly, J. E.: Comparison of nonpulsatile and pulsatile extracorporeal circulation on renal tissue perfusion. Chest *61*:65, 1972.
103. Williams, G. D., Seifen, A. B., Lawson, N. W., Norton, J. B., Readinger, R. I., Dungan, T. W., and Callaway, J. K.: Pulsatile perfusion versus conventional high-flow nonpulsatile perfusion for rapid core cooling and rewarming of infants for circulatory arrest in cardiac operation. J. Thorac. Cardiovasc. Surg. *78*:667, 1979.
104. Norman, J. C., McDonald, H. P., and Sloan, H.: The early and aggressive treatment of acute renal failure following cardiopulmonary bypass with continuous peritoneal dialysis. Surgery *56*:240, 1964.
105. Ashbaugh, D. G., and Petty, T. L.: Positive end-expiratory pressure. J. Thorac. Cardiovasc. Surg. *65*:165, 1979.
106. Sturtz, G. S., Kirklin, J. W., Burke, E. C., and Power, M. H.: Water metabolism after cardiac operations involving a Gibbon-type pump-oxygenator. I. Daily water metabolism, obligatory water losses, and requirements. Circulation. *16*:988, 1957.
107. Astrup, P., Andersen, O. S., Jorgenson, K., and Engel, K.: The acid-base metabolism. A new approach. Lancet *1*:1035, 1960.
108. Livelli, F. D., Jr., Johnson, R. A., McEnany, M. T., Sherman, E., Newell, J., Block, P. C., and DeSanctis, R. W.: Unexplained in-hospital fever following cardiac surgery. Circulation *57*:968, 1978.

56 GENERAL ANESTHESIA AND NONCARDIAC SURGERY IN PATIENTS WITH HEART DISEASE

by Marshall A. Wolf, M.D., and Eugene Braunwald, M.D.

The cardiovascular system of patients undergoing general anesthesia and noncardiac surgical procedures is subject to multiple stresses due to depression of myocardial contractility and respiration as well as fluctuations in temperature, arterial pressure, ventricular filling pressure, blood volume and activity of the autonomic nervous system. Complications of anesthesia and operation, such as hemorrhage, infection, fever, pulmonary embolism, and myocardial infarction, impose additional burdens on the cardiovascular system. The patient with cardiac disease who is compensated preoperatively may be unable to meet these increased demands during the perioperative period, in which case heart failure, myocardial ischemia, and/or arrhythmias may develop.[1,1a] As a consequence, one-fourth to one-half of all deaths in most series of noncardiac operations result from cardiovascular complications.

Since both the frequency and seriousness of cardiovascular complications of anesthesia and operation are considerably increased in the patient with known cardiovascular disease, one must appreciate the magnitude of these risks in order to reduce cardiovascular morbidity and mortality. In addition, both the life expectancy and quality of life of the patient must be taken into account. For instance, a high surgical risk may be difficult to justify if the cardiac condition precludes a survival period sufficient to allow the patient to reap the benefits of the surgical procedure, should the outcome be successful. In addition, the dangers and disability of the disease for which an operation is being proposed must also be balanced against the risk of the operation itself. In assessing the latter, the skills of the surgical and anesthesia teams must be taken into account.

ANESTHESIA

Changes in cardiovascular function during general anesthesia are due to many factors, including direct effects of the anesthetic agent(s) on the heart and indirect effects mediated primarily through the autonomic nervous system. In addition, if respiration is inadequately maintained, the resulting hypoxia, hypercarbia, and acidosis may further depress myocardial contractility and increase cardiac irritability. The interplay of all these variables may produce changes in arterial and central venous pressures, cardiac output, and rate and rhythm. To minimize the risk of operation in the patient with a compromised cardiovascular system, it is essential to minimize these fluctuations.[2]

CARDIOVASCULAR EFFECTS OF ANESTHESIA. Most general anesthetic agents depress myocardial contractility (Table 56–1). Studies on isolated cardiac muscle demonstrate a range of depressant effects, with agents such as halothane and methoxyflurane being the most depressant[3] and diethyl ether, nitrous oxide, and cyclopropane having the least effect on cardiac contractility. Superimposed on this direct myocardial depression, however, are alterations of the sympathetic nervous system, which may change the degree of depression observed in vivo. Thus, halothane, which produces minimal stimulation of sympathetic activity, may cause hypotension when administered

THE NATURE OF THE OPERATION. The extent to which cardiovascular disease contributes to a patient's risk varies greatly depending on the nature of the surgical procedure.[11,15,27] For example, Skinner and Pearce demonstrated minimal and equal mortality in patients with and without cardiac disease subjected to herniorrhaphy or transurethral prostatic resection (Fig. 56–1).[27] In contrast, mortality among cardiac patients subjected to cholecystectomy, subtotal gastrectomy, or bowel resection was twice that of patients without heart disease. Among patients who have had previous myocardial infarctions,[11,14] major vascular surgery is associated with a two- to threefold increase in risk, while results of surgery involving the extremities do not appear to be affected.

Emergency operation is associated with a greatly increased mortality in patients with cardiovascular disease. Skinner and Pearce[27] noted that mortality from cholecystectomy among cardiac patients was 10 per cent for an elective procedure versus 29 per cent when it was carried out on an emergency basis. Similar differences were noted for bowel resections (18 vs. 50 per cent) and other intraperitoneal operations (21 vs. 47 per cent). In Goldman's series[10] patients over 40 years of age who underwent emergency major surgery experienced a fourfold greater incidence of postoperative infarction or cardiac death—an increased risk that remains highly significant after multivariate analysis.[24] Obviously, while it is always desirable to avoid emergency operation, this is especially important in the patient with cardiac disease.

THE DURATION OF OPERATION. The relationship between the duration of anesthesia and the risk of cardiovascular mortality and morbidity is uncertain. Although it is generally assumed that the longer the operation, the greater the hazard to the patient with cardiovascular disease, this relation is, in part, confounded by the fact that more serious operations frequently take longer. It is of interest that in Skinner and Pearce's study, when the influence of the duration of operation was examined for the same surgical procedure, there was actually an inverse relationship between mortality and duration.[27] Tarhan et al. also noted no greater incidence of reinfarction as duration of anesthesia increased.[14] On the other hand, Steen and associates, who limited their analysis to patients with previous myocardial infarction, found that in procedures involving the aorta, thorax, and upper abdomen, mortality was a function of the duration of anesthesia.[11] Goldman et al. noted an increased risk of heart failure but not infarction or cardiac death when surgery lasted more than 5 hours.[10]

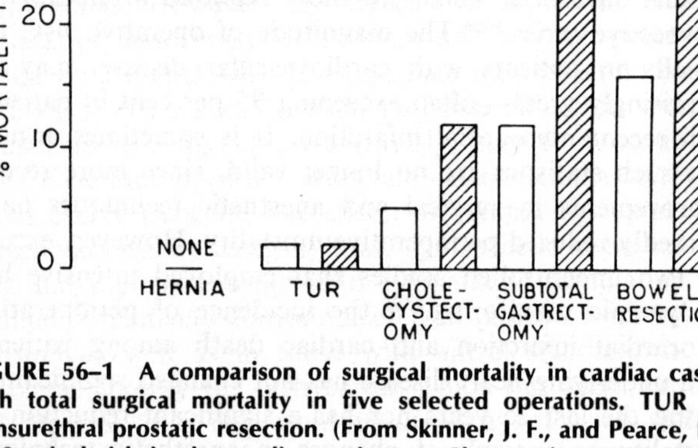

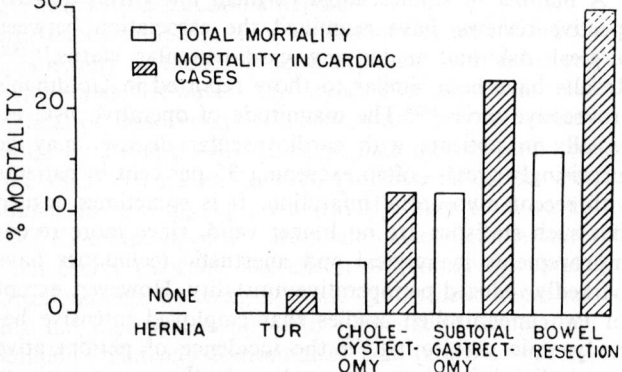

FIGURE 56–1 A comparison of surgical mortality in cardiac cases with total surgical mortality in five selected operations. TUR = transurethral prostatic resection. (From Skinner, J. F., and Pearce, M. L.: Surgical risk in the cardiac patient. J. Chron. Dis. *17*:57, 1964. Copyright 1964, Pergamon Press, Ltd.)

UNDERLYING CARDIOVASCULAR DISEASE

ISCHEMIC HEART DISEASE

Ischemic heart disease is a major determinant of perioperative morbidity and mortality. The incidence of perioperative myocardial infarction is increased 10- to 50-fold in patients who have previously suffered infarcts.[15] Patients undergoing general anesthesia soon after myocardial infarction are at particularly high risk of reinfarction. Tarhan et al. noted a 37 per cent reinfarction rate in patients operated on within 3 months of a previous myocardial infarction; this rate fell to 16 per cent when the operation was performed 3 to 6 months after the prior attack, and to 5 per cent when surgery was performed more than 6 months after the initial infarct.[14] Several other studies have confirmed a similar high risk when operation is performed within the first 6 months after myocardial infarction.[10–13,15] Obviously, whenever possible, elective surgery should be avoided during this period.

Innovations in anesthetic techniques during the last two decades may have reduced the risk of intraoperative infarction, but they have had little effect on postoperative infarction and the overall incidence of perioperative events. In 1978, Steen et al. documented new, perioperative infarctions in 36 of 587 patients (6.1 per cent) who had previous infarctions[11]; a similar study from the same institution carried out seven years earlier noted perioperative reinfarctions in 28 of 422 patients (6.6 per cent)[14] (Table 56–2).

Myocardial infarction occurring in the perioperative period is often painless[14,28]; indeed, half of Goldman's patients described no chest discomfort in association with their infarctions,[10] and only 11 of the 28 patients in Steen's series who experienced postoperative reinfarction gave a history of chest pain.[11] Obviously, then, the incidence of perioperative infarction will be underestimated if electrocardiograms are not obtained routinely during the postoperative period. Furthermore, the electrocardiogram detects only a fraction of infarcts, and it is likely that if the incidence of infarction were determined by more sensitive methods, such as serial estimations of serum creatine kinase (MB fraction), it would be even higher. Seventy per cent of perioperative infarcts occur within the first six days, with the peak incidence on the third day.[29]

While the mortality for patients experiencing an initial infarction during the perioperative period is similar to that for the general population with a first infarction, the risk of a second infarction occurring in the perioperative period is substantially greater.[14,30] Mortality among patients suffering a postoperative myocardial infarction *without* a prior infarction was 26.6 per cent, whereas mortality among those *with* a prior infarction was 2.5 times higher (64.1 per cent). It is discouraging that the management of patients experiencing a second infarct in an intensive care setting, who are presumably receiving excellent care, does not appear to have reduced this high mortality significantly.[11]

Two recent studies utilizing intensive intraoperative and

TABLE 56–2 EFFECT OF A PREVIOUS MYOCARDIAL INFARCTION ON INCIDENCE OF PERIOPERATIVE MYOCARDIAL INFARCTION AND ON MORTALITY

		No. of Patients		Patients with New Postoperative Infarction		
Author	Year of Study	*Previous Infarction*	*No Previous Infarction*	*History of Previous Infarction(%)*	*No History of Previous Infarction(%)*	Mortality (%)
Knapp[23]	1962	427	8,557	6.0	0.7	58
Topkins[13]	1964	658	12,054	6.5	0.7	70
Tarhan[14]	1972	422	32,455	6.6	0.1	54
Steen[11]	1978	587	—	6.1	—	69
Averages				6.4	0.4	63

postoperative hemodynamic monitoring have reported a much lower incidence of perioperative myocardial infarction. Wells and Kaplan reported a series of 48 patients who underwent noncardiac surgery 3 months after infarction; there were no reinfarctions, although 15 per cent of the patients experienced significant arrhythmias.[25] In Rao and El-Etr's series, only 7.8 per cent of 38 patients operated within 3 months of a previous infarct experienced reinfarction; the 59 patients who underwent surgery 3 to 6 months after their previous infarction experienced an infarction rate of 3.4 per cent.[26]

Patients with ischemic heart disease tolerate unplanned, sustained intraoperative hypotension poorly, presumably because it intensifies ischemia in marginally perfused tissue. Conversely, patients suffering an intraoperative infarction may experience unexplained hypotension. Mauney et al. described a fourfold greater incidence of intraoperative hypotension in those patients who suffered a perioperative infarction.[30] Steen et al. noted a 15.2 per cent infarction rate in patients in whom systolic pressure decreased by at least 30 per cent for at least 10 minutes or more during anesthesia vs. a 3.2 per cent infarction rate in patients who did not experience such a pressure drop.[11] While it has been presumed that hypotension was the inciting event for the infarction in these patients, the possibility that it was the *consequence* of the infarct has not been excluded.

The role of coronary artery bypass grafting in altering the mortality and morbidity from general anesthesia and surgery in the patient with manifest coronary artery disease is still unclear. Several studies have suggested that patients who had coronary artery bypass surgery may be at reduced risk from subsequent major noncardiac surgery[31–36]; however, controlled studies are needed to establish the validity of these observations.

HYPERTENSION

Patients with mild to moderate essential hypertension, uncomplicated by congestive heart failure, renal failure, or coronary artery disease, can be expected to tolerate the stresses of general anesthesia and operation as well as normotensive patients.[37–39] However, hypertensive patients are subject to more frequent and wider swings of pressure during anesthesia and operation.[40] Hypertensive episodes are more likely to occur during induction and intubation but can be minimized with careful technique,[41] while hypotensive episodes may result from the hypovolemia that is common among hypertensive patients treated with diuretics.[42] Halothane anesthesia, which causes vasodilation as well as myocardial depression, is particularly likely to elicit intraoperative hypotension in these patients.

Controversy continues concerning management with antihypertensive medications during the perioperative period. Early studies, emphasizing the hazards of hypotension that occur during general anesthesia,[43,44] suggested that this tendency was increased by treatment with *reserpine* and led to the recommendation that reserpine be discontinued about 10 days prior to planned general anesthesia. However, several investigators have shown that the fluctuations of arterial pressure are *not* greater in hypertensive patients who received reserpine than in those who did not.[45–47] Indeed, Prys-Roberts et al. have demonstrated that patients with well-controlled hypertension whose drug therapy was maintained up to and including the day of operation were more stable during anesthesia than were patients with untreated hypertension.[47,48]

More recently, a controversy reminiscent of that engendered by reserpine has developed concerning the maintenance of *propranolol* therapy in the immediate preoperative period. On the basis of several case reports, Viljoen et al. suggested that propranolol might significantly increase the myocardial depression produced by most anesthetic agents and recommended that the drug be withdrawn at least 2 weeks before operation.[49] However, subsequent studies have documented no adverse reactions in patients undergoing cardiopulmonary bypass while receiving propranolol.[50–52] Actually, it has been suggested that beta-adrenergic blocking agents reduce the incidence of intraoperative arrhythmias and myocardial ischemia.[41] Patients taking propranolol had no adverse reactions during anesthesia and vascular surgery, and Prys-Roberts concluded that "for patients with hypertension or ischemic heart disease, maintenance of beta receptor blocking therapy through the period of anesthesia and surgery, far from causing adverse reactions, may be beneficial."[48] Indeed, sudden withdrawal of beta-adrenergic blockers in patients with ischemic heart disease who have been receiving these drugs on a chronic basis may cause a rebound effect, with intensification of the severity of ischemia; for this reason it now seems most unwise to withdraw these agents during the preoperative period,[50–54] and it is our policy not to do so.

VALVULAR HEART DISEASE

Patients with valvular heart disease undergoing anesthesia and operation are subject to many potential hazards:

ventricular dysfunction, nor should it be given only for the purpose of counteracting the cardiac depression caused by anesthetics.[74] Careful postoperative monitoring and prompt digitalization when failure or arrhythmias develop is recommended for patients with less severe cardiac disease.

Postoperative Arrhythmias

Arrhythmias are very common after operation and are often a manifestation of a noncardiac complication such as bleeding, infection, or an acid-base or electrolyte imbalance occurring in a patient with heart disease. Management of these arrhythmias often requires recognition and correction of these extracardiac factors.

To assess the clinical correlates and therapeutic outcome of new postoperative supraventricular tachyarrhythmias, Goldman prospectively followed 916 patients who were in sinus rhythm throughout the course of major noncardiac surgery.[75] The 35 patients who developed new postoperative supraventricular tachyarrhythmias (4 per cent of the 916) frequently had concurrent medical problems: 46 per cent had acute cardiac conditions, 31 per cent had major infections, 29 per cent had preexisting hypotension, 26 per cent had anemia, 23 per cent had metabolic derangements, 23 per cent had received parenteral drug therapy, and 20 per cent were hypoxic. Forty per cent of the patients required no new therapy with cardiac medications, and only two required electrical cardioverson; the arrhythmias of all treated patients reverted to sinus rhythm. No deaths were related to the supraventricular tachyarrhythmias per se, but half the patients in whom these arrhythmias occurred died as a result of the concurrent medical problems. Goldman concluded that the onset of a new postoperative supraventricular tachyarrhythmia should prompt a search for remediable medical problems. Direct antiarrhythmic therapy is often unnecessary and is usually secondary in importance to correction of the underlying cause of the arrhythmia.

Sinus tachycardia is the most common rhythm disturbance in the postoperative patient. Multiple noncardiac etiologies have been identified, including hypo- or hypervolemia, fever, anemia, hypoxemia, pulmonary emboli, pain, anxiety, infection, hypotension, and electrolyte abnormalities (especially hypokalemia). These noncardiac etiologies are much more common causes of sinus tachycardia in the postoperative cardiac patient than is either myocardial infarction or heart failure. Sinus tachycardia not due to congestive heart failure will not slow with cardiac glycosides. The therapeutic/toxic ratio of these drugs is actually reduced by most of the above-mentioned noncardiac causes of sinus tachycardia and therefore, digitalis drugs are not considered appropriate therapeutic agents for postoperative patients unless the sinus tachycardia is likely to be caused by impaired cardiac function.

Atrial fibrillation is also a common postoperative arrhythmia. Atrial dilatation, which lowers the threshold for development of this arrhythmia, may result from heart failure, mitral valve disease, and/or hypervolemia. Noncardiac precipitant causes include pneumonia, atelectasis, and pulmonary emboli. Mowry and Reynolds observed atrial fibrillation in 19 per cent of all patients after pneumonectomy; it occurred in 23 per cent of patients after left pneumonectomy, in 14 per cent after right pneumonectomy, and in 28 per cent of patients 50 years of age or over.[76] Initially, treatment of the postoperative patient with atrial fibrillation should be a digitalis glycoside; in addition, a beta-adrenergic blocker or verapamil can be used to help gain rapid control of the ventricular rate. Cardioversion is usually delayed until the precipitating factors have been eliminated, since the patient who is cardioverted prior to clearing the atelectasis or pneumonia frequently reverts to atrial fibrillation, while the patient whose pulmonary problem or congestive heart failure is adequately treated often reverts spontaneously to sinus rhythm.

Atrial flutter, which may be the initial manifestation of pulmonary embolism,[77] is often poorly tolerated because of the rapid ventricular rate and the difficult pharmacological management. Cardioversion is usually the treatment of choice, along with quinidine or procainamide administered to prevent recurrences (p. 698).

THE ROLE OF THE MEDICAL CONSULTANT

The physician called upon to evaluate a patient with suspected or overt cardiac disease prior to elective or emergency noncardiac surgery must first determine whether cardiovascular disease is present and, if it is, must identify those factors that may increase the risk of operation. It may be necessary to invest considerable time and effort to prepare the patient for operation. In addition, the patient must be followed carefully after operation to detect and manage the cardiac problems that frequently complicate the postoperative period.

ESTIMATION OF RISK. A few patients have such compelling reasons for operation, e.g., rupturing aortic aneurysm, perforated or necrotic bowel, life-threatening hemorrhage, or some forms of intestinal obstruction, that estimation of operative risk is an academic exercise, since failure to operate almost certainly dooms the patient. Often, however, the timing or even the performance of an operation is elective, and under these circumstances estimation of risk is an important aspect of the medical consultant's role. Certain cardiovascular problems such as recent myocardial infarction (less than 3 months), overt congestive heart failure, and severe mitral or aortic stenosis are absolute contraindications to truly *elective* surgery. Relative contraindications include more remote myocardial infarction (3 to 6 months earlier), angina pectoris, mild heart failure, cyanotic congenital heart disease with severe polycythemia and a coagulation abnormality. Several other problems should be recognized and treated prior to operation: anemia, hypovolemia, polycythemia, pulmonary disease causing hypoxemia, adrenal hyporesponsiveness secondary to chronic administration of adrenal steroids, hypertension, electrolyte abnormalities, as well as the entire gamut of cardiac arrhythmias. Considerable judgment must be exercised when one or more of the above-mentioned contraindications are present and when a patient requires prompt surgical treatment but the situation is not a true emergency, as for neoplastic disease.

To identify those preoperative factors associated with the development of cardiac complications after major noncardiac operation, Goldman et al. prospectively studied

TABLE 56–3 CARDIAC RISK FACTORS AND CARDIAC RISK CLASSES DERIVED BY SUMMATING TOTAL POINTS FOR CARDIAC RISK FACTORS*

MEANS OF EVALUATION	FINDING	NO. OF POINTS
History	Myocardial infarction < 6 months prior to surgery	10
	Age > 70	5
Physical examination	S_3 gallop or jugular venous distention	11
	Signs of aortic stenosis	3
ECG	*Any* rhythm other than sinus rhythm or Premature atrial contractions on last preoperative ECG	7
	More then 5 premature contractions per minute on *any* previous ECG	7
Laboratory data	Po_2 < 60; Pco_2 > 50; K^+ < 3.0; HCO_3 > 20; BUN > 50; creatinine >; 3.0. Abnormal SGOT or signs of chronic liver disease	3
Operation	Emergency	4
	Intraperitoneal, thoracic, or major vascular procedure	3
	TOTAL	53

CLASS	NO. OF POINTS	NO OR MINOR COMPLICATIONS (%)	LIFE-THREATENING COMPLICATIONS† (%)	CARDIAC DEATH (%)
I	0–5	99	0.7	0.2
II	6–12	93	5	2
III	13–25	86	11	2
IV	26	22	22	56

*Data from Goldman, L., et al.: N. Engl. J. Med. *297*:845, 1977, and Goldman, L., et al.: Medicine *57*:357, 1978.

†Myocardial infarction, ventricular tachycardia, pulmonary edema.

1001 patients over 40 years of age.[24] Using multivariate discriminant analysis, they identified nine independent significant correlates of life-threatening and fatal cardiac complications, weighed these factors based on their relative significance as predictors of cardiac outcome, and devised a scale for predicting perioperative risk (Table 56–3). They then separated patients into four classes of varying risk and found that 10 of the 19 postoperative cardiac fatalities occurred in the 118 patients at highest risk. Notably, *unimportant* factors included smoking, glucose intolerance, hyperlipidemia, hypertension, peripheral atherosclerotic vascular disease, angina, and remote myocardial infarction. The predictive value of the Goldman index was confirmed by Weathers and Paine; 20 of the 23 perioperative cardiovascular deaths occurred in patients in Goldman Classes III and IV.[78]

Several of the factors involved in determining the cardiac risk index are potentially controllable, such as the third heart sound, jugular venous distention, recent myocardial infarction, and poor general medical condition. Thus, elective surgery should be delayed until congestive heart failure has been treated, the patient's general medical condition has improved, and (if possible) 6 months have elapsed since a previous myocardial infarction. Several studies have suggested that preoperative cardiac catheterization in high-risk patients allows the adjustment of preload, afterload, and inotropic state to optimize cardiac performance.[79,80] Coronary arteriography might be advisable to distinguish patients with ischemic heart disease from those without clinical evidence of heart disease but with positive exercise tests and/or evidence of other vascular disease who are to undergo major elective noncardiac surgery. Such an approach would allow identification of high-risk patients, and performing coronary revascularization first and/or careful hemodynamic monitoring during the noncardiac surgery in these patients might reduce operative mortality[36,79;–82] however, the value of this more aggressive approach has not yet been established.[83]

PREPARATION OF THE PATIENT FOR ANESTHESIA AND OPERATION

Careful preparation of the cardiac patient for operation may diminish the frequency and seriousness of intraoperative and postoperative complications.[84] Since many of these complications are the result of hypotension, hypoxemia, or both, every effort should be made to diminish the incidence, duration, and severity of these stresses. Adequate preparation for an elective operation may require days to weeks. The medical consultant should not hesitate to urge postponement or cancellation of an elective operation in order to have sufficient time to institute measures necessary to minimize the risk. In addition to providing a detailed general medical assessment, the consultant physician should take the following steps during this preoperative period:

1. Obtain a careful medication history. This should include current medications in order to identify those drugs which might interact with anesthetic agents. In particular, the patient's experiences during prior surgery, especially adverse reactions to previously employed anesthetic techniques and agents should be identified as should allergies and drug reactions.

2. Treat congestive heart failure without inducing hypovolemia or electrolyte imbalance.

3. Correct anemia or polycythemia. When anemia is severe in the patient with heart failure or cardiomegaly, packed red cells should be given in place of whole blood. Phlebotomy may be helpful in minimizing the hemorrhagic and thrombotic complications of polycythemia. Particular

care must be taken to avoid dehydration in polycythemic patients.

4. Control arrhythmias.

5. Check or insert pacemaker.

6. Adjust antihypertensive medications to achieve good control.

7. Correct acid-base and electrolyte disturbances. Hypokalemia predisposes to arrhythmias and sensitizes the myocardium to the toxic effects of digitalis, while hyponatremia may predispose to hypotension.

8. Adjust anticoagulant therapy for patients with prosthetic valves.

9. Estimate and, if necessary, improve pulmonary function.

10. Provide appropriate antibiotic coverage for the patient with valvular or congenital heart disease.

11. In consultation with the anesthetist and the surgeon, determine the variables to be monitored intraoperatively and discuss the choice of anesthetic agents.

POSTOPERATIVE MEDICAL COMPLICATIONS

Cardiac complications occur much more frequently during the postoperative period than during the intraoperative period. Peak incidence of myocardial infarction is on the third postoperative day, and electrocardiograms should be obtained daily for the first 4 to 5 days after operation in patients with previous myocardial infarction or who have experienced intraoperative hypotension. Because anemia, hypo- and hypervolemia, hypoxemia, fever, and electrolyte abnormalities may be poorly tolerated by patients with a compromised cardiovascular system, these abnormalities should be watched for and corrected if present. Arrhythmias require prompt recognition and management. Agitation and psychosis are common in patients with life-threatening illnesses who undergo general anesthesia and major surgery (particularly the elderly) and may impose an additional cardiovascular stress. Postoperative thromboembolic disease is more frequent and often of greater clinical severity in patients with heart disease. Measures to minimize thromboembolic complications include early ambulation, exercise of the lower extremities while the patient is in bed, use of elastic stockings, and small (mini) doses of heparin (Chap. 46).

Pulmonary parenchymal complications also occur more frequently in cardiac than in noncardiac patients, perhaps because of the chronic pulmonary congestion characterizing the former. Thoracic operations add to the risk of ventilatory disturbances because they interfere with movements of the chest wall and impair the patient's ability to cough and eliminate secretions. Postoperative pulmonary complications may be diminished by postural drainage, by the inspiration of humidified air, and by the use of bronchodilators in patients with postoperative bronchospasm; the value of the routine use of antibiotics is controversial. In patients with suspected respiratory failure, measurements of ventilation and arterial blood gases are mandatory as a guide to therapy.

Prompt recognition and management of the multiple problems that may complicate the postoperative period are possible only if the physician closely follows the patient throughout convalescence. All too often the patient with heart disease is appropriately prepared for a noncardiac operation and survives the procedure but is not followed adequately during the early postoperative period, when the risk of serious complications still exists.

References

1. Glasser, S. P. (ed.): Noncardiac Surgery in the Cardiac Patient. Mt. Kisco, N.Y., Futura Publishing Co., 1983.

1a. Hillis, L. D., and Cohn, P. F.: Noncardiac surgery in patients with coronary artery disease: Risks, precautions and perioperative management. Arch. Intern. Med. *138*:972, 1978.

2. Kaplan, J. A. (ed.): Cardiac Anesthesia. New York, Grune and Stratton, 1979.

3. Sorensen, B., Rasmussen, J. P., Dauchot, P. J., and Regula, G.: Cardiac function during induction and early anesthesia with methoxyflurane. An evaluation using systolic time intervals and pressure time indices. Acta Anaesth. Scand. *22*:615, 1978.

4. Ngai, S. H.: Current concepts in anesthesiology. Effects of anesthetics on various organs. N. Engl. J. Med. *302*:564, 1980.

5. Christensen, V., Sorensen, M. B., Klauber, P. V., and Skovsted, P.: Haemodynamic effects of enflurane in patients with valvular heart disease. Acta Anaesth. Scand. *67*:34, 1978.

6. Bille-Brahe, N. E., Sorensen, M. B., Mondorf, T., and Engell, H. C.: Central haemodynamics during induction of neurolept anaesthesia in patients with arteriosclerotic heart disease. Acta Anaesth. Scand. Suppl. *67*:47, 1978.

7. Friedberg, C. K.: Surgical procedures in the cardiac patient (Chap. 49). *In* Diseases of the Heart. 3rd ed. Philadelphia, W. B. Saunders Co., 1966.

8. Radney, P. A., Arai, T., and Nagashima, H.: Ketamine-gallamine anesthesia for great-vessel operations in infants. Anesth. Analg. *53*:365, 1974.

9. Hug, C. C., Jr.: Pharmacology—anesthetic drugs. *In* Kaplan, J. A. (ed.): Cardiac Anesthesia. New York, Grune and Stratton, 1979, p. 3.

10. Goldman, L., Caldera, D. L., Southwick, F. S., Nussbaum, S. R., Murray, B., O'Malley, T. A., Goroll, A. H., Caplan, C. H., Nolan, J., Burke, D. S., Krogstad, D., Carabello, B., and Slater, E. E.: Cardiac risk factors and complications in non-cardiac surgery. Medicine *57*:357, 1978.

11. Steen, P. A., Tinker, J. H., and Tarhan, S.: Myocardial reinfarction after anesthesia and surgery. J.A.M.A. *239*:2566, 1978.

12. Arkins, R., Smessaert, A. A., and Hicks, R. G.: Mortality and morbidity in surgical patients with coronary heart disease. J.A.M.A. *190*:485, 1964.

13. Topkins, M. J., and Artusio, J. F., Jr.: Myocardial infarction and surgery: A five year study. Anesth. Analg. *43*:716, 1964.

14. Tarhan, S., Moffitt, E. A., Taylor, W. F., and Giulioni, E. R.: Myocardial infarction after general anesthesia. J.A.M.A. *220*:1451, 1972.

15. Knorring, J.: Postoperative myocardial infarction: A prospective study in a high-risk group of surgical patients. Surgery *90*:55, 1981.

16. Tinker, J. H., Noback, C. R., Vlietstra, R. E., and Frye, R. L.: Management of patients with heart disease for noncardiac surgery. J.A.M.A. *246*:1348, 1981.

17. Kaplan, J. A., and Dunbar, R. W.: Anesthesia for noncardiac surgery in patients with cardiac disease. *In* Kaplan, J. A. (ed.): Cardiac Anesthesia. New York, Grune and Stratton, 1979, p. 377.

18. Katz, R. L., and Bigger, J. T., Jr.: Cardiac arrhythmias during anesthesia and operation. Anesthesiology *33*:193, 1970.

19. Vanik, P. E., and Davis, H. S.: Cardiac arrhythmias during halothane anesthesia. Anesth. Analg. *47*:299, 1968.

20. Walton, H. J., Cross, P., and Pollack, E. W.: Ventricular cardiac arrhythmias during anesthesia: Feasibility of preoperative recognition. South Med. J. *75*:27, 1982.

21. Joas, T. A., and Stevens, W. C.: Comparison of the arrhythmic doses of epinephrine during forane, halothane and fluroxene anesthesia in dogs. Anesthesiology *35*:48, 1971.

22. Narahara, K. A., and Blettel, M. L.: Effect of rate on left ventricular volumes and ejection fraction during chronic ventricular pacing. Circulation *67*:323, 1983.

23. Knapp, R. B., Topkins, M. J., and Artusio, J. F., Jr.: The cerebrovascular accident and coronary occlusion in anesthesia. J.A.M.A. *182*:332, 1962.

24. Goldman, L., Caldera, D. L., Nussbaum, S. R., Southwick, F. S., Krogstad, D., Murray, B., Burke, D. S., O'Malley, T. A., Goroll, A. H., Caplan, C. H., Nolan, J., Carabello, B., and Slater, E. E.: Multifactorial index of cardiac risk in noncardiac surgical procedures. N. Engl. J. Med. *297*:845, 1977.

25. Wells, P. H., and Kaplan, J. A.: Optimal management of patients with ischemic heart disease for noncardiac surgery by complementary anesthesiologist and cardiologist interaction. Am. Heart J. *102*:1029, 1981.

26. Rao, T. L. K., and El-Etr, A. A.: Myocardial reinfarction following anesthesia in patients with recent infarction. Anesth. Analg. *60*:271, 1981.

27. Skinner, J. F., and Pearce, M. L.: Surgical risk in the cardiac patient. J. Chron. Dis. *17*:57, 1964.

28. Driscoll, A. C., Hobika, J. H., Etsten, B. E., and Proger, S.: Clinically unrecognized myocardial infarction following surgery. N. Engl. J. Med. *264*:633, 1961.

29. Salem, D. N., Homans, D. C., and Isner, J. M.: Management of cardiac disease in the general surgical patient. *In* Harvey, W. P. (ed.): Current Problems in Cardiology Vol. 5. Chicago, Year Book Medical Publishers, Inc., 1980.

30. Mauney, F. M., Jr., Ebert, P. A., and Sabiston, D. C., Jr.: Postoperative myocardial infarction: A study of predisposing factors, diagnosis and mortality in a high risk group of surgical patients. Ann. Surg. *172*:497, 1970.
31. McCollum, C. H., Garcia-Rinaldi, R., Graham, J. M., and DeBakey, M. E.: Myocardial revascularization prior to subsequent major surgery in patients with coronary artery disease. Surgery *81*:302, 1977.
32. Mahar, L. J., Steen, P. A., Tinker, H. H., Vlietstra, R. E., Smith, H. C., and Pluth, J. R.: Perioperative myocardial infarction in patients with coronary artery disease with and without aorta-coronary artery bypass grafts. J. Thorac. Cardiovasc. Surg. *76*:533, 1978.
33. Scher, K., and Tice, D. A.: Operative risk in patients with previous coronary bypass. Arch. Surg. *111*:807, 1976.
34. Edwards, W. H., Mulhern, J. L., and Wolher, W. E.: Vascular reconstructive surgery following myocardial revascularization. Ann. Surg. *187*:653, 1978.
35. Crawford, E. S., Morris, G. C., Howell J. F., et al.: Operative risk in patients with previous coronary artery bypass. Ann. Thorac. Surg. *26*:215, 1978.
36. Fudge, T. L., McKinnon, W. M. P., Schoettle, P., Ochsner, J. L., and Mills, N. L.: Improve operative risk after myocardial revascularization. South. Med. J. *74*:799, 1981.
37. Goldman, L., and Caldera, D. L.: Risks of general anesthesia and elective surgery in the hypertensive patient. Anesthesiology *50*:285, 1979.
38. Chamberlain, D. A., and Edmunds-Seal, J.: Effects of surgery under general anesthesia on the electrocardiogram in ischemic heart disease and hypertension. Br. Med. J. *2*:784, 1964.
39. Rosen, M., Mushin, W. W., Kilpatrick, G. S., Campbell, H., Davies, L. G. G., and Harrison, E.: Study of myocardial ischemia in surgical patients. Br. Med. J. *2*:1415, 1966.
40. Seltzer, J. L., Gerson, J. I., and Grogono, A. W.: Hypertension in the perioperative period. N. Y. State J. Med. *80*:29, 1980.
41. Prys-Roberts, C., Greene, L. T., Meloche, R., and Foex, P.: Studies of anesthesia in relation to hypertension. II: Hemodynamic consequences of induction and endotracheal intubation. Br. J. Anesth. *43*:531, 1971.
42. Tarazi, R. C., Frohlich, E. D., and Dustan, H. P.: Plasma volume in man with essential hypertension. N. Engl. J. Med. *278*:762, 1968.
43. Foster, M. W., Jr., and Gayle, R. F., Jr.: Dangers in combining reserpine with electroconvulsive therapy. J.A.M.A. *159*:1520, 1955.
44. Ziegler, C. H., and Lovette, J. B.: Operative complications after therapy with reserpine and reserpine compounds. J.A.M.A. *176*:916, 1961.
45. Katz, R. L., Weintraub, H. D., and Papper, E. M.: Anesthesia, surgery and rauwolfia. Anesthesiology *25*:142, 1964.
46. Munson, W. M., and Jenicek, J. A.: Effect of anesthetic agents on patients receiving reserpine therapy. Anesthesiology *23*:741, 1962.
47. Prys-Roberts, C., Meloche, R., and Foex, P.: Studies of anesthesia in relation to hypertension. 1. Cardiovascular responses of treated and untreated patients. Br. J. Anesth. *43*:122, 1971.
48. Prys-Roberts, C.: Medical problems of surgical patients. Hypertension and ischaemic heart disease. Ann. R. Coll. Surg. Engl. *58*:465, 1976.
49. Viljoen, J. F., Estafanous, G., and Kellner, G. A.: Propranolol and cardiac surgery. J. Thorac. Cardiovasc. Surg. *64*:826, 1972.
50. Caralps, J. M., Mulet, J., Wienke, H. R., Moran, J. M., and Pifarre, R.: Results of coronary artery surgery in patients receiving propranolol. J. Thorac. Cardiovasc. Surg. *67*:526, 1974.
51. Kaplan, J. A., Dunbar, R. W., Bland, J. W., Sumpter, R., and Jones, E. L.: Propranolol and cardiac surgery: A problem for the anesthesiologist. Anesth. Analg. *54*:571, 1975.
52. Should propranolol be stopped before surgery? Med. Lett. *18*:41, 1976.
53. Goldman, L.: Noncardiac surgery in patients receiving propranolol. Case reports and a recommended approach. Arch. Intern. Med. *141*:193, 1981.
54. Goldman, L.: Noncardiac surgery in patients receiving propranol. Arch. Intern. Med. *141*:193, 1981.
55. Stone, J. G., Hoar, P. F., Calabro, J. R., DePetrillo, M. A., and Bendixen, H. H.: Afterload reduction and preload augmentation improve the anesthetic management of patients with cardiac failure and valvular regurgitation. Anesth. Analg. *59*:737, 1980.
56. Tinker, J. H., and Tarhan, S.: Discontinuing anticoagulant therapy in surgical patients with cardiac valve prostheses. J.A.M.A. *239*:738, 1978.
57. Katholi, R. E., Nolan, S. P., and McGuire, L. B.: Living with prosthetic heart valves. Subsequent noncardiac operations and the risk of thromboembolism or hemorrhage. Am. Heart J. *92*:162, 1976.
58. Kaplan, E. L., Anthony, B. F., and Bishop, A.: Prevention of bacterial endocarditis. Circulation *56*:139A, 1977.
59. Sommerville, J., McDonald, L., and Edgill, M.: Postoperative haemorrhage and related abnormalities of blood coagulation in cyanotic congenital heart disease. Br. Heart J. *27*:440, 1965.
60. Berg, G. R., and Kotler, M. N.: The significance of bilateral bundle branch block in the preoperative patient. Chest *59*:62, 1971.
61. Kunstadt, D., Punja, M., Cagin, N., Fernandez, P., Levitt, B., and Yuceoglu, Y. Z.: Bifascicular block: A clinical and electrophysiologic study. Am. Heart J. *86*:173, 1973.
62. Rooney, S. M., Goldiner, P. L., and Muss, E.: Relationship of right bundle branch block and marked left axis deviation to complete heart block during general anesthesia. Anesthesiology *44*:64, 1976.
63. Simon, A. B.: Perioperative management of the pacemaker patient. Anesthesiology *46*:127, 1977.
64. Logue, R. B., and Kaplan, J. A.: The cardiac patient and noncardiac surgery. *In* Harvey, W. P. (ed.): Current Problems in Cardiology. Vol. 7. Chicago, Year Book Medical Publishers, Inc., 1982.
65. Deutsch, S., and Dalen, J. E.: Indications for prophylactic digitalization. Anesthesiology *30*:648, 1969.
66. Dalen, J. E., and Dexter, L.: Operation in the patient with heart disease. *In* Conn, H. L. (ed.): Cardiovascular Diseases. Philadelphia, Lea & Febiger Co., 1971.
67. Perlroth, M. G., and Hultgren, H. N.: The cardiac patient and general surgery. J.A.M.A. *233*:1279, 1979.
68. Wheat, M. W., Jr., and Burford, T. H.: Digitalis in surgery: Extension of classical indications. J. Thorac. Cardiovasc. Surg. *41*:162, 1961.
69. Goldberg, A. H., Maling, H. M., and Gaffney, T. E.: The effect of digoxin pretreatment in heart contractile force during thiopental infusion in dogs. Anesthesiology *22*:974, 1961.
70. Goldberg, A. H., Maling, H. M., and Gaffney, T. E.: The value of prophylactic digitalization in halothane anesthesia. Anesthesiology *23*:207, 1962.
71. Shimosato, S. A., and Etsten, B.: Performance of digitalized heart during halothane anesthesia. Anesthesiology *24*:41, 1963.
72. Bille-Brahe, N. E.: Digitalization of surgical patients with impaired left ventricular function. Danish Med. Bull. *29*:45, 1982.
73. Selzer, A., and Cohn, K. E.: Some thoughts concerning the prophylactic use of digitalis. Am. J. Cardiol. *26*sf,1 :214, 1970.
74. Foex, P.: Preoperative assessment of the patient with cardiovascular disease. Br. J. Anaesth. *53*:731, 1981.
75. Goldman, L.: Supraventricular tachyarrhythmias in hospitalized adults after surgery. Chest *73*:450, 1978.
76. Mowry, F. M., and Reynolds, E. W.: Cardiac rhythm disturbances complicating resectional surgery of the lung. Ann. Intern. Med. *61*:688, 1964.
77. Johnson, J. C., Flowers, N. C., and Horan, L. G.: Unexplained atrial flutter: A frequent herald of pulmonary embolism. Chest *60*:29, 1971.
78. Weathers, L. W., and Paine, R.: The risk of surgery in cardiac patients. Ann. Intern. Med. *2*:57, 1981.
79. DelGuercio, L. R. M., and Cohn, J. D.: Monitoring operative risk in the elderly. J.A.M.A. *243*:1350, 1980.
80. Babu, S. C., Sharma, P. V. P., and Raciti, A.: Operability with safety is increased in patients with peripheral vascular disease. Arch. Surg. *115*:1384, 1980.
81. Gage, A. A., Bhayana, J. N., Balu, V., and Hook, N.: Assessment of cardiac risk in surgical patients. Arch. Surg. *112*:1488, 1977.
82. Hertzer, N. R., Young, J. R., Kramer, J. R., Phillips, D. F., deWolfe, V. G., Ruschhaupt, W. F., and Beven, E. G.: Routine coronary angiography prior to elective aortic reconstruction. Arch. Surg. *114*:1336, 1979.
83. Bille-Brahe, N. E., and Eickhoff, J. H.: Measurement of central haemodynamic parameters during preoperative exercise testing in patients suspected of arteriosclerotic heart disease. Acta Chir. Scand. *502*:38, 1980.
84. Abrams, L. M., and Chambers, D. A.: Preoperative management. *In* Kaplan, J. A. (ed.): Cardiac Anesthesia, New York, Grune and Stratton, 1979, p. 169.

57 EMOTION, PSYCHIATRIC DISORDERS, AND THE HEART

by Thomas P. Hackett, M.D., and Jerrold F. Rosenbaum, M.D.

"Every affection of the mind that is attended with either pain or pleasure, hope or fear, is the cause of an agitation whose influence extends to the heart."

WILLIAM HARVEY, EXERCITATIO DE MOTU CORDIS ET SANGUINIS, 1628[1]

Although few would disclaim Harvey's sentiment, the precise nature of the link between the mind and heart disease remains to be defined. Substantial evidence exists to indicate associations between psychosocial stresses and coronary artery disease, hypertension, arrhythmia, and sudden death, but the intervening variables that mediate pathological changes have yet to be subjected to rigorous, prospective study. In this chapter these and other issues relevant to the interface between cardiology and psychiatry are discussed.

PSYCHIATRIC ASPECTS OF CORONARY ARTERY DISEASE

Psychosocial Factors

Clinicians have long suspected that the accumulation of small stresses from longstanding conflicts can augment the development of cardiovascular disease, most especially of essential hypertension and coronary atherosclerosis. In the 1910 Lumleian lecture, Sir William Osler, commenting on physicians with angina pectoris, said, ". . . the outstanding feature was the incessant treadmill of practice; and yet if hard work—that 'badge of our tribe'—was alone responsible, would there not be a great many more cases? Every one of these men had an additional factor—worry; in not a single case under fifty years of age was this feature absent. . . ."[2] Three decades later, Flanders Dunbar gave the following capsule description of patients with coronary artery disease: "They are compulsive, have a tendency to work long hours and not take vacations, a tendency to seize authority; dislike of sharing responsibility, . . . articulate, . . . few neurotic traits, . . . a tendency to depression which is rarely admitted to, . . . a tendency to minimize symptoms, . . . self-neglect. . . ."[3] This sketch of the coronary patient, consumed in work and beset by worry, has been recognized and redrawn by many clinicians.

Although researchers have examined the roles of life dissatisfaction, acute stress, personal loss, sociological factors, and personality traits in coronary artery disease, much time and effort have also been devoted to describing a personality behavior pattern characteristic of the overworked and anxious coronary patient. Friedman and Rosenman developed the concept of a "coronary-prone behavior pattern," which they termed *Type A behavior*.[4] Over the last two decades they have relentlessly investigated the association between Type A behavior and coronary artery disease and have concluded that Type A behavior is as significant as any of the major risk factors of coronary artery disease, such as cigarette smoking, hypercholesterolemia, and hypertension; Friedman defines Type A behavior as "a characteristic action-emotion complex" found in people who are constantly struggling to reach poorly defined goals in the shortest time possible.[4] In his opinion, the most critical aspects of Type A behavior patterns are excesses of competitiveness, pace, and aggression. Diagnostic indicators of Type A behavior are listed in Table 57–1. Type B individuals exhibit the opposite type of behavior; they are relaxed, unhurried, and less aggressive. Although they may be interested in success, and may indeed be successful, in most instances they do not struggle so vigorously as Type A individuals in pursuit of this goal.

In the Western Collaborative Group Study (WCGS)[5] male subjects were sorted into groups on the basis of the prominence of Type A behavior patterns, measured in an interview designed to test the behavior of each subject. The study was conducted in double-blind fashion; neither the rating team nor the medical examiner had knowledge of all risk factors. Follow-up at 4½, 6½, and 8½ years revealed that men with coronary-prone Type A behavior at entry experienced 1.7 to 4.5 times the rate of new coronary diseases as did Type B men (Fig. 57–1).

Research data from various other demographical and geographical settings consistently relate Type A behavior to coronary artery disease.[6] Investigations in Europe, Australia, and Israel point to the cross-cultural relevance of some aspects of such behavior.[7] Other studies have shown that the Type A pattern appears to be specifically related to atherosclerosis. Individuals with other diseases, such as lung disease and cancer, tend to include an equal distribution of Types A and B.[7,8] Jenkins feels that there is a strong link between Type A behavior and the clinical emergence of myocardial infarction and coronary artery disease and that Type A behavior has "about the same strength of associations with coronary artery disease prevalence and incidence as do other standard risk factors."[7] This point of view is now shared by a number of experienced cardiologists.[9] Some studies have attempted to correlate anxiety and neuroticism with coronary artery disease.[6] These studies are all retrospective and tend to indicate that these variables are more predictive of angina pectoris than of myocardial infarction. Friedman and his associates provided advice and instructions designed to diminish Type A behavior to 600 patients who had suffered a myocardial infarction. After 1 year the rate of nonfatal infarction was significantly lower among subjects who received behavioral and cardiological counseling than among those who received cardiological counseling on the usually accepted risk factors alone.[10]

Stress and life change have largely been investigated by means of the Holmes and Rahe Schedule of Recent Experience.[11-13] A number of studies[7,12-14] have shown that the Holmes-Rahe scores for myocardial infarction victims in a 6-month period prior to infarction were two to three times greater than those for a control group. This association of life change with the presence of coronary artery disease supports the findings reported in the admirable studies in England by Rees and Lutkins[15] and by Parkes and colleagues,[16] which indicate increased mortality during the first year of bereavement among widowers, widows, and other relatives close to the deceased, and of Engel[17,18] and Greene et al.[19] of loss preceding sudden death from coronary artery disease. However, many of these studies may be challenged because of their retrospective nature. One prospective study by Theorell et al.[20] showed no connection between a high life change score and the incidence of acute myocardial infarction.

Attempts have also been made to correlate coronary artery disease with *life or work dissatisfaction.* Wolf described a Sisyphean pattern, in which the individual "strives without joy."[21] Rarely is this individual rewarded by the satisfaction of accomplishment. Instead he doggedly toils on to

TABLE 57–1 DIAGNOSTIC INDICATORS OF TYPE A BEHAVIOR

Time Urgency

A. Psychomotor manifestations
  1. Characteristic facial tautness expressing tension
  2. Rapid horizontal eyeball movements during ordinary conversation
  3. Rapid eye blinking (over 40 blinks/min)
  4. Knee jiggling or rapid vigorous tapping of fingers
  5. Rapid, frequently dysrhythmic speech involving elimination of terminal words of sentences
  6. Lip clicking during ordinary speaking
  7. Rapid ticlike eyebrow lifting
  8. Head nodding when speaking
  9. Sucking in of air during speech
  10. Humming (tuneless)
  11. Speech hurrying
  12. Tense posture
  13. Motorization accompanying responses
  14. Expiratory sighing
  15. Rapid body movements
B. Direct behavioral tests
  1. The interviewer, in posing a question whose answer is already clear from its contents, hesitates, becomes laboriously tedious or repetitive, and then stammers. The subject interrupts the stammering with his answer.
C. Physiological indicators
  1. Periorbital pigmentation
  2. Excessive forehead and upper lip perspiration
D. Significant biographical content
  1. Self-awareness of presence of Type A behavior
  2. Polyphasic activities (e.g., reads while driving, reads while using electric shaver, and thinks of other matters during conversation with others)
  3. Walks fast, eats fast, and does not dawdle at table
  4. Subject makes fetish of always being on time under all circumstances
  5. Has been told by spouse to slow down in working and living habits
  6. Difficulty in sitting and doing nothing
  7. Subject habitually substitutes numerals for metaphors in his speech

Excessive Competitiveness and Hostility

A. Psychomotor manifestations
  1. Characteristic facial set exhibiting aggression and hostility (eye and jaw muscles)
  2. Characteristic ticlike drawing back of corner of lips, almost exposing teeth
  3. Hostile, jarring laugh
  4. Use of clenched fist and table pounding or excessively forceful use of hands and fingers
  5. Explosive, staccato, frequently unpleasant-sounding voice
  6. Frequent use of obscenity
  7. Subject exhibits irritation and rage when asked about some past events in which he became angered
B. Direct behavioral tests
  1. The interviewer directly challenges the validity of some comment or behavior that the subject has reported. The subject reacts in a hostile or unpleasant manner.
  2. The interviewer questions the subject about his views on politics, races, women, or competitors. The subject responds with absolute, almost angry generalizations.
C. Significant biographical content
  1. The subject reports that he is irritated if kept waiting for any reason or if driving behind a car moving too slowly in his view
  2. The subject expresses general distrust of other people's motives (e.g., distrust of altruism)
  3. The subject reports that he almost always plays any type of game to win (even with young children)

Modified from Friedman, M., et al.: Circulation *66*:83, 1982, by permission of the American Heart Association, Inc.

tery disease were monitored.[65] Heart rates of up to 180 beats/min, as well as elevations of plasma catecholamine and free fatty acid concentration were observed in both groups. Ischemic ST-segment depression occurred in six of the seven coronary subjects. More than six ectopic beats per minute were recorded in six of the normal subjects while they were speaking. Five of the seven coronary subjects had multiple or multifocal ventricular ectopic beats. A beta-blocking agent suppressed the tachycardia and electrocardiographic changes in both groups. Lown and colleagues studied a man with normal coronary arteries and cardiac function in whom ventricular fibrillation and cardiac arrest and, following recovery, ventricular premature beats were provoked by psychophysiological stress.[62] Beta blockade and other measures to reduce sympathetic activity attenuated the arrhythmia.

Despite the apparent importance of peripheral sympathetic activity in emotionally induced arrhythmia, Lown and coworkers have reported data implicating central neural mechanisms as primary in triggering, via sympathetic efferents, the aberrant electrical activity.[66] In animals, hypothalamic and stellate ganglion stimulation has produced ventricular fibrillation that was abolished with beta-adrenergic blockade.[67] In the presence of an electrically unstable heart, a diseased myocardium, or coronary artery disease, psychological distress is a potentially lethal stimulus.

In addition to the sympathetically mediated ventricular irritability and increased oxygen demand, life-threatening "vagal reaction" leading to bradycardia and circulatory collapse has been reported.[68] The parasympathetic or vagal response to emotional stimuli producing decreased heart rate, fall in arterial pressure, and syncope in some individuals is a familiar syndrome, although not in itself as a cause of sudden death.

Although a major stressful life event, such as hearing of a loved one's demise, could be the proximal "cause" of death, more often the terminal stress is not in itself extraordinary; rather, as reported by Greene and coworkers, the scenario in the weeks preceding the final stressful event is one of increased emotionally vulnerability, often following a series of losses, with chronic depression, fatigue, frustration, or disappointment.[19] This observation is reminiscent of other theories of the emotional vulnerability to serious illness resulting from feelings of hopelessness and the "giving-up–given-up" response.[69] For example, a patient with a perceived loss in professional or job status, possibly having had a prior myocardial infarction, feeling sad and discouraged, becomes angry or anxious while performing an ordinary stressful task, such as income tax preparation, triggering a fatal arrhythmia. The notion that preceding stressful life events, whether losses or positive life changes, lays the physiological foundation for sudden death is supported by Rahe's data measuring accumulated life change units (Table 57–2).[70]

One implication of the foregoing for the clinical management of the cardiac patient is the necessity to be alert for signs of depression and fatigue, for reports of recent major life events, and for indications of anxiety-provoking circumstances in the patient's life. In addition, the physician can counsel the patient to avoid stressful settings when possible and encourage conscious control over emotional arousal ("Is this worth dying for?") when necessary. Other strategies to diminish the impact of emotional stress include relaxation training, anxiolytics (e.g., the benzodiazepines) in small doses as needed, and in the absence of contraindications, administration of beta-adrenergic blocking drugs. The cardiac patient who manifests sustained depression should be referred for psychiatric consultation as a prophylactic and therapeutic measure.

TABLE 57–2 LIFE CHANGE EVENTS IN MEN AND THEIR WEIGHTS IN LIFE CHANGE UNITS (LCU) SCALED FOR FINLAND

Event	Finnish LCU Weight
Health	
Recent illness (in bed for a week or hospitalization)	62
Change in heavy physical work or exercise	19
Change in sleeping habits	15
Change in eating habits	11
Work	
Recently out of work	50
Recently fired from work	50
Retirement from farming, forestry, or industry	40
Change to new type of work	36
Change in work responsibilities	29
Troubles with boss	22
Work or life going well (awards, achievements, etc.)	20
Correspondence courses (home study)	17
Change in hours of work a day	13
Home and Family	
Concern over health of family member	54
Recently married	50
Separation from wife due to marital problems	48
Gaining a new family member (in the home)	39
Separation from wife due to work	34
Engaged to be married	32
New home improvements	26
Son or daughter leaving home	23
Wife began or ended work	23
Troubles with in-laws	22
Change in get-togethers with friends	21
Change to a new residence	15
Change in get-togethers with relatives	13
Vacation	11
Personal and Social	
Death of wife	105
Divorce	80
Held in jail	64
Sexual difficulties	41
Change in number of arguments with wife	40
Death of a close relative	39
Financial difficulties	38
Major decisions regarding the future	38
Death of a close friend	34
Unpaid bills leading to threatened legal action	26
Recent purchases worth more than 8000 Fmk ($2000)	22
Change in religious or political convictions	20
Change in personal habits	12
Recent purchases worth less than 8000 Fmk	11
Minor violations of the law	7

Rahe, R. H., et al.: Subjects' recent life changes and coronary heart disease in Finland. Am. J. Psychiatry *130*:1223, 1973.

PSYCHIATRIC ISSUES IN HYPERTENSION

EMOTIONAL FACTORS IN ESSENTIAL HYPERTENSION. Though definitive study of the causes of hypertension remains to be done, reports so far indicate associations between elevated arterial pressure and a variety of environmental and psychological conditions. Environmental factors, including diet (salt), social conditions, life changes, psychological conflicts, and psychophysiological mechanisms, have been estimated as contributing substantially to the etiology of essential hypertension.[71] These factors are also discussed in Chapter 26.

SOCIOCULTURAL FACTORS. Henry and Cassel observed that blood pressure levels were lower in groups or societies based on firm traditions and stable social structures.[72] In societies in which traditions were disintegrating or in those in transition, arterial pressures for the populations rose (e.g., southern Black society in the late 1950's). Blood pressure has been reported as higher in city than in rural dwellers.[73] Harburg et al. described one city in which citizens in the higher crime and lower socioeconomic district had significantly elevated levels of blood pressure,[74] apparently confirming earlier cross-cultural observations that hypertension was more prevalent in societies dominated by social stress and conflict.[75]

In the most intriguing animal study of social factors involved in elevated arterial pressure, Henry et al. manipulated social interactions of mice by crowding them into small boxes, building a system of tunnel-connected cages that forced frequent confrontations, exposing the mice to a cat for 6 to 12 months, and introducing isolation-reared mice into the regular population. The resultant territorial conflict and concomitant constant defensive vigilance resulted in relatively sustained increases in blood pressure.[76]

PSYCHOLOGICAL FACTORS. Life changes and traumatic life events have been associated with the onset of sustained hypertension[77] and with the shift from the benign to the malignant form of the disease.[78] In addition, specific personality traits have been implicated as contributory to essential hypertension. Despite the subjective and anecdotal nature of descriptions of hypertensive individuals, the following characteristics are consistently noted: The hypertensive person manifests a desire to please, a wish to be liked; however, while outwardly calm, the internal stance is that of suppressed anger, tension, and suspicion.[79–81] Presumably these traits derive from early experience with individuals (parents) on whom the person depended and toward whom anger and hostility could not be expressed, because of the real or imagined threat of loss of love. The desire to please and be approved of by authority figures, combined with a rebellious "ready-to-fight" unconscious posture, was felt to be characteristic of many individuals with essential hypertension.

Wolf and Wolff found that in subjects with restrained hostility or anxiety, peripheral vascular resistance rises without change in cardiac output.[82] These individuals were thought to be blood pressure "responders," especially in situations that triggered repressed hostile feelings. Hypertension, therefore, had an adaptive quality, in that a rise in blood pressure could be seen as a preparation to deal with a threat. Alexander, describing the conflict between aggressive feelings and dependence on the object of the aggression, viewed sustained hypertension as a permanent "emergency state," emotionally triggered and physically expressed.[79] Several studies have demonstrated increases in diastolic pressure with inhibited anger[83,84] or with deferential behavior.[85]

Most data indicate that certain traits may be associated with hypertension, but their role in etiology is unclear; certainly many individuals with similar characteristics never become hypertensive. Ostfeld and Lebovitz[86] failed to show personality differences between renovascular and essential hypertensives and have criticized the "specific conflict" notion of a hypertensive personality.[87] Another difficulty with studies of psychological aspects of hypertension is their failure to differentiate labile from sustained hypertensives. The labile group may experience transient rises in stressful situations (e.g., blood pressure–taking by a physician) but are normotensive in other settings. As a result, repeated readings of blood pressure are necessary for the diagnosis of essential hypertension.

PSYCHOPHYSIOLOGICAL FACTORS. Many environmental and psychological factors can cause acute elevations of baseline blood pressure in both normotensive and hypertensive individuals. It is normal for arterial pressure to fluctuate during the course of a day[88]; however, elevated blood pressure is more prevalent, for example, in generally stressful occupations such as air traffic controllers.[89] The common denominator in cases of hypertension may be "stress" in a nonspecific sense, since stressful events (often idiosyncratic in impact, such as life trauma, social and interpersonal conflicts, and unacknowledged and unexpressed emotion) generate sympathetically mediated vasoconstriction and other autonomic responses that may well have a greater and more sustained impact on blood pressure in individuals predisposed to hypertension. Brod and colleagues have found that the vasoconstrictive response to stress is more prolonged in hypertensive than in normotensive subjects.[90,91] Lacy's notion of an "autonomic response specificity" suggests that constitutionally predisposed individuals respond to specific and general stress with acute and sustained elevations of arterial pressure.[92] The finding that normotensive sons of essential hypertensives react more readily to stress with elevations of blood pressure is of interest in this regard.[93]

Cardiovascular reaction patterns to stress vary in animals and humans, but operant conditioning studies have demonstrated that animals can be conditioned to experience blood pressure elevations in response to specific and general stimuli.[94] For humans as well, Shapiro et al. have reported that subjects in the laboratory could learn to elevate their blood pressure without changes in heart rate.[95]

BEHAVIORAL THERAPY. Since psychophysiological data implicate stress, autonomic arousal, and conditioned learning as causes of blood pressure elevation, various types of behavioral therapy—relaxation, meditation, and biofeedback—have been applied to hypertensives.[96–98] Although it would be of great benefit if these nonpharmacological treatments were effective, especially for the borderline hypertensive, clinical studies suggest only a minor role for behavioral regimens at this time. However, the fact that these treatments are without risk and are associated with an increased sense of well-being renders them appropriate adjunctive modalities despite the modest claims of the data so far reported.

Benson has hypothesized that a variety of techniques, including relaxation exercises, meditation, yoga, and hypnosis, have the ability to evoke an integrated hypothalamic "relaxation response" that results in reduced heart rate, blood pressure, and respiratory rate as well as the subjective feeling of relaxation.[49] Shapiro et al. have noted that relaxation-induced blood pressure changes are small but statistically significant, ranging from 7/4 to 37/22 mm Hg; the higher the pretreatment pressure, the greater the decrease with relaxation. If subjects discontinued the regimen, values returned to baseline levels.[98] A fall in adrenergic activity, as reflected in lower dopamine beta-hydroxylase levels, in patients performing an Eastern meditation exercise has been reported.[99] One well-constructed series of studies, including some 12-month follow-ups, control groups, and cross-over treatment of controls, and based on a program of relaxation and galvanic skin response biofeedback, demonstrated an average decrease in blood pressure of 27/15 mm Hg and decreased requirements for medication.[100,101] Using an ambulatory monitoring device, one group has demonstrated sustained blood pressure decreases during the work day for essential hypertensives trained in relaxation.[102]

When an individual is made aware of changes in blood pressure by means of visual or auditory biofeedback, he becomes able, through unknown mechanisms, to use this sensory input to alter his own blood pressure. The results of blood pressure biofeedback also vary, ranging from virtually no change to sustained decreases of 18/8 mm Hg.[103]

PSYCHOTHERAPY. Before the era of antihypertensive medication, Reiser et al. reported decreased arterial pressure and symptomatic improvement in a group of 98 hypertensive patients receiving varying degrees of supportive psychotherapy.[77] This salutary effect of a constant, supportive relationship with the physician should not be discounted.

PATIENT COMPLIANCE WITH ANTIHYPERTENSIVE TREATMENT. Reviews of the issue of noncompliance underscore the significance, magnitude, and complexity of this problem.[104–107] Sackett has noted over 200 reported determinants of noncompliance, including educational, demographic, personality, and prescribing factors.[108] Patients with relatively high levels of physical complaints and those with attitudes of suspiciousness have a high incidence of poor compliance.[109] Surveys consistently estimate that 30 to 50 per cent of hypertensive patients neglect their treatment, even as public awareness of the dangers of "high blood pressure" increases.[106,109a] Physicians are generally unable to predict and recognize those who do not follow instructions[110] and too often attribute the cause of the problem to the patient's lack of responsibility.

Attempts to understand adherence to medical regimens using the sociobehavioral "health belief model" emphasize the patient's (1) estimate of personal vulnerability to and seriousness of the disease; (2) perception of the efficacy and feasibility of the treatment; and (3) internal and external motivations to treatment, such as the desire to relieve symptoms or to avoid the sick role (internal), or as a response to public health campaigns (external).[104] Although all these factors were deemed relevant when studied retrospectively, recent prospective work has confirmed only the "attitude toward the sick role" as predictive of compliance —those who perceive social and interpersonal consequences of illness as negative are likely to comply with treatment.[108]

Efforts to indict any one factor as the "cause" of noncompliance will be inadequate given the individual variability of patients' personalities and manners of coping with adversity. Some patients do not follow directions because of lack of concern or low anxiety levels, whereas others manifest a denial and rationalization response because of high levels of anxiety. Engendering increased concern is to no avail in the latter type of patient. A sufficiently independent patient will appreciate the opportunity to monitor his own blood pressure and be "responsible" for his treatment, whereas dependent patients will require more nurturing and didactic care and frequent follow-up visits.

The following factors are generally acknowledged as useful in maintaining patient compliance with treatment programs:

1. Creating a doctor-patient relationship characterized by mutual trust and a sense of alliance or working together to solve the problem.[109a,111]
2. Providing sufficient time with a care-giver (whether physician, physician's assistant, or nurse clinician).[112,113]
3. Prescribing an effective yet simple treatment regimen and making sure the patient understands the regimen before he leaves the office or clinic.[106]
4. Adapting dosage schedules to the patient's daily routine or habits.[114]
5. Educating and enlisting the help of family members, especially spouses (who may also deny the importance of treatment).
6. Anticipating with the patient possible side effects of medications and how these will be handled.
7. Offering assistance on follow-up visits to the patient who has had difficulty adhering to the treatment program.
8. Monitoring compliance (e.g., pill counts) and attempting to adapt the interpersonal approach to the noncompliant patient's needs and fears.

PSYCHIATRIC COMPLICATIONS OF ANTIHYPERTENSIVE MEDICATIONS (see also Chap. 27). Medications used to treat hypertension have neuropsychiatric effects, primarily depression. Rauwolfia alkaloids such as reserpine, which deplete central intraneuronal stores of catecholamines, can result in severe depressive illness that may endure well beyond withdrawal from the medication.[115] These agents are rarely used at present, but when the physician does wish to prescribe one of them, patients having suffered prior depressions should be screened, because of their increased vulnerability to this drug-induced affective illness. Alpha-methyldopa has also been associated with depression and other psychiatric symptoms (lethargy, insomnia, decreased mental acuity)[116–118] as well as confusional states in conjunction with haloperidol[119] and lithium.[120] Patients on alpha-methyldopa are at greater risk for lithium toxicity. Those taking propranolol may experience increased lethargy, mental slowing, and occasionally clinical depression. Hydralazine also induces lethargy and drowsiness. Drugs that cause impotence such as guanethidine or alpha-methyldopa may secondarily precipitate depression in the emotionally vulnerable patient. Diuretics are associated with mental changes, primarily as the result of electrolyte disturbances.

A variety of interactions with psychotropic medication may occur with antihypertensive agents.[121] The antipsychotics potentiate the hypotensive effects of reserpine, alpha-methyldopa, hydralazine, and propranolol, and, except for molindone, antagonize guanethidine.

The tricyclic antidepressants generally interfere with drugs that require uptake into adrenergic nerve terminals, blocking the action, for example, of guanethidine with the possibility of causing severe withdrawal hypotension and impeding the efficacy of clonidine.[123] These antidepressants may also interact centrally with alpha-methyldopa, reserpine, and propranolol, resulting in diminished blood pressure control.[124] The newer agent, mianserin, is reported at this early date to be free of the above interactions.[125] Initially, the tricyclics may cause hypertension when reserpine is administered. The monoamine oxidase inhibitors increase the hypotensive effects of diuretics and hydralazine but can lead to acute hypertension when administered with guanethidine, alpha-methyldopa, or reserpine.

For patients taking lithium and such diuretics as the thiazides, which act on the distal tubule, sodium loss in the distal tubule results in the reabsorption of lithium proximally and hence in elevated lithium levels.[126] Higher blood lithium levels increase the risk of side effects and toxicity. When such a combination is necessary, lithium dosages must be lowered and levels must be monitored. In addition, increased vigilance must be kept concerning other potential causes of additional sodium loss, such as sweating or diarrhea.

PSYCHOPATHOLOGY AND CARDIAC SYMPTOMS

Patients with any of a number of psychiatric disorders may attribute their distress to alterations of body function and may seek treatment from the nonpsychiatric physician; furthermore, objective physical symptoms may derive from specific functional conditions, as in the case of bursts of tachycardia from attacks of panic or anxiety. Estimates of the prevalence in cardiological practices of patients with anxiety-derived complaints range from 10 to 14 per cent.[127] The heart is a frequent focus of emotionally based complaints, not only because of its actual response to psychological stress but also because of its psychological and symbolic importance. Recognition of the psychiatric component of patients' complaints is a crucial task for the physician. The anxious and depressed patient suffers no less than the patient with a primary physical illness, and many of the psychiatric conditions underlying the distress can respond dramatically to prompt treatment; for others, proper management can greatly improve the quality of life. Finally, diagnosis of relevant psychological factors may obviate medical or surgical interventions and their attendant morbidity.

Anxiety Disorders

Anxiety may be defined as a psychological and physiological response similar to fear but in response to internal stimuli or inappropriate to the reality of external stimuli; it may be a life-long constant *trait* or a transient *state* relative to specific life events. The psychological component of the anxiety experience includes such descriptors as dread, edginess, nervousness, tension, or worry. Among the physical signs and symptoms, generally consequent to sympathetic arousal, are chest pain or tightness, diaphoresis, dyspnea, faintness, fatigue, flushing, muscle tension, palpitations, queasy stomach, tachycardia, tachypnea, and tremulousness.

Although the experience of anxiety is universal, pathological anxiety—an anxiety disorder capable of significantly impairing or restricting the life of a patient—is estimated to afflict between 2 and 4 per cent of the general population.[128] Anxiety symptoms are a particularly prominent component of phobic disorders such as agoraphobia (fear of being alone or in public), social phobia (fear of scrutiny by others), and simple phobias (e.g., insects, elevators), as well as post-traumatic stress disorder (e.g., following military combat) and obsessive-compulsive disorder. For patients seeking treatment from the nonpsychiatric physician, the more common syndromes encountered, however, are generalized anxiety disorder and panic disorder.

Generalized Anxiety Disorder. The patient with generalized anxiety manifests such persistent anxiety symptoms as ubiquitous uneasiness, moist palms, a worried look, and difficulty in falling asleep. Although often chronic or life-long, the signs of motor tension, autonomic hyperactivity, and apprehension may emerge only during discrete periods or be of clinical significance only during times of relative exacerbation. The variety of bodily symptoms, particularly in the cardiovascular system, lead many sufferers to seek a primary medical cause.

Panic Disorder. Patients with panic disorder experience recurrent panic (anxiety) attacks—the sudden, often spontaneous onset of massive autonomic, particularly sympathetic, arousal accompanied by a feeling of terror or impending doom. Although the predominant symptom may vary, the usual bodily response to panic includes symptoms suggestive of heart disease, such as dyspnea, hyperventilation, chest pain, tachycardia, palpitations, tremulousness, dizziness, faintness, hot and cold flashes, and diaphoresis. The typical behavioral response is to flee home or to a safe or familiar place.

Patients having panic attacks have little if any conscious control over the experience. Those unfamiliar with the syndrome believe they are stricken with a myocardial infarction, stroke, or other life-threatening condition. For patients with ischemic heart disease or myocardial electrical instability, the sympathetic arousal is indeed life-threatening. In addition to the exceptional distress of the condition, untreated panic disorder often leads to agoraphobia. After a period of avoiding places with restricted escape (in the event of an attack), such as public transportation, tunnels, traffic congestion, and crowded stores, sufferers may become homebound. A secondary generalized or anticipatory anxiety may follow the onset of panic attacks, and depressive signs and symptoms also can occur.

Panic disorder occurs twice as frequently in women as men,[129] often has its onset in early adulthood, is more common in family members of patients with the disorder,[129] and is associated with an excess mortality,[130] particularly in men. As with affective illness, the disorder may be recurrent or chronic, mild or severe.

Early attempts to elucidate the physiology of panic attacks have drawn on the work of Pitts and McClure,[131,132] who, by infusing intravenous sodium lactate, provoked attacks in those with the disorder, and on the report by Frohlich[133] of patients with hyperdynamic beta-adrenergic circulatory state who experienced dramatic emotional responses to isoproterenol. A more recent hypothesis based on neurophysiological studies and effects of psychotropic drugs implicates a central site, possibly the locus ceruleus,[134] as the "trigger" mechanism generating sympathetic arousal peripherally and a cortical response of terror or need to flee.

Differential Diagnosis of Anxiety Disorders. Patients with anxiety disorders account for a significant percentage of general medical and cardiological practices.[127] The list of possible medical illnesses producing symptoms mimicking anxiety or panic is extensive. Any condition that leads to sympathetic discharge or causes such symptoms as tremors, dizziness, respiratory distress, tachycardia, or restlessness may resemble an anxiety state.

A thorough yet efficient medical evaluation includes the following considerations.[135] In a patient with a known medical illness, that ailment (including its possible symptoms, complications, and treatment) should be suspect. For the apparently well patient, beyond a general review of symptoms and physical examination, particular scrutiny should be directed at conditions commonly associated with anxiety: arrhythmias, excessive ingestion of caffeine or other stimulants, drug or alcohol withdrawal, thyroid abnormalities (especially hyperthyroidism), and hypoglycemia. Additional evaluation directed toward the patient's "somatic locus"[136] of anxiety—the system most prominently affected (e.g., cardiovascular, respiratory, gastrointestinal)—affords the greatest yield from investigations.

The mitral valve prolapse syndrome (p. 1089) appears to be approximately twice as prevalent in patients with panic disorder compared with the normal population.[129,137] Whether this association represents a cause and effect relationship is unclear, since patients with prolapse of the mitral valve and panic disorder cannot be distinguished from those with panic disorder alone by family history studies,[129] response to lactate infusion,[138] or efficacy of psychotropic drug treatment.[138] On the other hand, patients with prolapse of the mitral valve alone are significantly affected, with increased arrhythmias, by psychological stress and anxiety.[139]

TREATMENT. For patients with emergence of anxiety symptoms during or following a life crisis, explanation and reassurance of their physical well-being and a sympathetic attitude are important, with referral for supportive or brief psychotherapeutic intervention when necessary. Generalized anxiety symptoms abate and become more tolerable with the use of anxiolytics, preferably the benzodiazepines, since others such as barbiturates are more sedative, more lethal in overdose, and more physically addicting. The dose should be titrated to help the patient to manage, not eliminate, his symptoms and should be administered on an as-needed basis with daily limits. Some evidence indicates that patients with more prominent "somatic" or bodily symptoms from anxiety do well with varying doses of a beta-adrenergic blocker.[140] Relaxation training is helpful for many anxious patients. Psychodynamic and behavioral therapy offers relief for patients with specific conflicts associated with their symptoms.

Panic attacks are only partially attenuated by anxiolytics, but these agents often will not prevent attacks. Certain antidepressants, however, especially the tricyclic imipramine and the monoamine oxidase inhibitor phenelzine, usually at full antidepressant dosages, are frequently successful in abolishing anxiety attacks after 2 to 4 weeks of treatment.[141] A beta-adrenergic blocker may serve some patients as a second-line treatment of panic disorder.[140]

Depression

Sadness and grief, the normal human emotional responses to loss, are distinct from clinical depressive illness. Depression may be associated with an antecedent loss but constitutes a unique constellation of psychological and vegetative features. The cardiologist should be familiar with the presentation of depression, not only because it frequently coexists with chronic or serious illness but also because depressed patients, particularly older ones, experience an increase in physical symptoms which they attribute to bodily illness. A depressed patient, feeling fatigue or chest pain, not infrequently presents with cardiac complaints.

The following signs and symptoms are the most sensitive indicators of the presence of a clinical depressive illness: early morning awakening and disturbance of sleep continuity (or hypersomnia); tearfulness, sadness, or crying spells; loss of appetite and weight; loss of energy, ability to concentrate, and sexual interest; and loss of interest in usually pleasurable activities. Psychomotor retardation with prolonged response latency to questions and immobile or sad facies, may be observed in some, whereas a hand-wringing motor restlessness or agitation is prominent in others. The psychological state is one of despair, hopelessness, and helplessness, with marked loss of self-esteem and feelings of guilt and worthlessness.

TREATMENT. For patients suffering sadness or grief, the sense of personal injury and loss following the death of a loved one, job loss, or convalescence from myocardial infarction often will resolve with support, understanding, and time. Depressive illness, unlike grief, generally requires biological therapy. In most cases (80 to 90 per cent), depression will respond to antidepressant medication or, in severe or refractory cases, electroconvulsive therapy.[121]

Hypochondriasis

The cardiologist will most certainly be faced with the patient whose anxious overconcern extends to a morbid preoccupation with bodily functions and fear of illness. The hypochondriac often firmly believes that he is sick and that the physician has overlooked the urgency of his complaints, which may be monosymptomatic or may include multiple organ systems with minimal physical findings. Kenyon estimates that 85 per cent of cases of hypochondriasis are secondary to anxiety states, depressive illness, and other emotional disorders.[142] Reports of pain, the most frequent hypochondriacal symptom, may resolve if any underlying affective illness is treated. Cardiac symptoms often reflect an unrecognized anxiety disorder with tachycardia, palpitations, pain, and increased cardiac awareness.

Cardiac neurosis refers to hypochondriacal concern, usually in the setting of recovery from myocardial infarction or other cardiac illness, with obsessive focus on heart symptoms and exaggerated restriction of daily functioning. The syndrome may be iatrogenic, deriving from incomplete explanation to the patient of his condition. Signs and symptoms of depressive illness should be reviewed, since cardiac neurosis may be a "depressive equivalent," that is, the somatic expression of an underlying change of mood. A treatable anxiety disorder, causing cardiac symptoms, may have been overlooked in the patient with a cardiac neurotic behavior pattern. When the patient's symptoms and disability are not secondary to misunderstanding, depression, or anxiety, the physician should seek to enhance the patient's ability to cope by *prescribing* graduated tasks or stepwise goals to achieve the appropriate level of activity.

Cardiac neurosis should not be taken lightly at its onset, since it may herald a chronic pattern of hypochondriacal behavior and unwarranted invalidism. The likelihood that the syndrome reflects a massive defensive effort to deal with underlying inadequacies emphasizes the value of early psychiatric referral.

A *conversion (hysterical) symptom* is an unexplained medical symptom involving motor function or sensation. This condition arises for a variety of psychological and interpersonal reasons which must be discovered on psychiatric examination. Prominent in medical and psychiatric lore is the concept of an anniversary reaction, the development of a conversion symptom (e.g., chest pain) at the same time of year as a prior traumatic event, such as death of a loved one from myocardial infarction.

CARDIOVASCULAR EFFECTS OF PSYCHOTROPIC AGENTS

Psychotropic medications, frequently administered to the elderly and those with or at risk for heart disease, have a significant impact on the cardiovascular system. Since untreated psychiatric illness carries its own morbidity and mortality and can also exacerbate cardiac illness (e.g., exhaustion from mania), the risks and benefits of medication must be carefully weighed. The following section describes the important cardiovascular effects of psychotropic drugs.

Antidepressants

In the late 1950's, the development of effective antidepressant pharmacotherapy heralded a significantly improved quality of life for those suffering from clinical depressive syndromes. The monoamine oxidase inhibitors (MAOI) and a few years later the tricyclic antidepressants (TCA) were the first consistently effective pharmacological interventions in the treatment of mood disorders. More recently, a number of agents with chemical structures distinct from TCA are being explored and introduced in hopes of achieving therapeutic benefits without such adverse effects as cardiotoxicity. Current hypotheses suggest that TCA and the newer antidepressants combat depression by increasing the activity of such central neurotransmitters as norepinephrine and serotonin either by blocking re-uptake from synaptic clefts or by binding to presynaptic (α_2) receptors.

TRICYCLIC ANTIDEPRESSANTS. Of significant benefit in 60 to 80 per cent of severe depressions,[121] TCA remain in wide use as acute and maintenance treatment for mood disorders. Their pharmacological effects are wide-ranging, acting on many systems in addition to the central nervous system. Their impact on the cardiovascular system has been viewed as a major limitation on the use of these medications, especially in patients with cardiac illness and depression.[143–145] For example, a higher than expected incidence of sudden death had been noted in patients with acute cardiovascular disorders who received these drugs, especially amitriptyline.[146–148] In clinical and laboratory studies, TCA have a variety of pharmacological actions beside their effect on catecholamine reabsorption by the adrenergic neuron. These include anticholinergic activity, quinidine-like effects (depressing conduction velocity and myocardial contractility) and alpha-adrenergic blocking properties, and it is clinically relevant that these actions vary among the TCA.

Electrocardiographic Changes. Electrocardiographic abnormalities with TCA include widened QRS complexes, increased P-R and Q-T intervals, ST-segment and T-wave changes, atrioventricular (Fig. 57–4) and intraventricular conduction defects, and tachycardia and bradycardia.[149–151] The most common changes at therapeutic doses (75 to 250 mg/day for imipramine) in healthy individuals are reversible T-wave changes and tachycardia. The latter occurred in 30 per cent of individuals on amitriptyline in one study.[152] Some increase in heart rate probably occurs and remains for the duration of treatment in every patient receiving these medications. At toxic levels, which can last for 3 to 4 days after overdose,[153] any and all types of arrhythmias may occur.[154] Although the reported frequency of serious TCA-induced electrocardiographic change varies with the population and the specific drug, for older patients with cardiac disease, in one report, the risk involved is up to 10 times greater than in young, healthy individuals.[147]

The pharmacological properties responsible for the electrocardiographic changes are principally anticholinergic effects and Type I antiarrhythmic activity (quinidine-like effects, p. 652). The former is probably the main direct factor in the drug-induced tachycardia. TCA have atropine-like effects that cause partial vagal blockade and tachycardia, of particular concern in patients with ischemic heart disease and congestive heart failure. Amitriptyline is the most anticholinergic TCA, followed in order by doxepin, nortriptyline, imipramine, and desipramine,[155] the last being the TCA of choice in patients requiring a minimum of anticholinergic effects. In cases of TCA toxicity, temporary inprovement in tachycardia is attained with physostigmine,[156] the drug of choice to reverse the central nervous system "atropine psychosis."[157] Propranolol has also been suggested as useful in modifying TCA-induced tachycardia.[152]

TCA resemble quinidine in the capacity to delay cardiac conduction.[149,158,159] His bundle electrocardiography has demonstrated prolonged distal (H-V) conduction time for imipramine, nortriptyline, and amitriptyline.[160]

For the majority of patients at therapeutic, not toxic, doses and plasma levels of TCA, the quinidine-like side effects are of little clinical consequence. Bigger and colleagues have suggested that imipramine could actually be effective as an antiarrhythmic, like quinidine or procainamide, since it is a potent antiarrhythmic drug with a long duration of action and relatively few major adverse effects.[158,159,161,161a] Certainly, for patients on TCA, dosage levels of these antiarrhythmics should be lowered. For patients with preexisting conduction delay, institution of TCA treatment should be approached with caution, given the risk of increased or complete heart block and subsequent ventricular arrhythmia. Therefore, in patients over 40, a pretreatment electrocardiogram should be obtained with particular attention to the presence of intraventricular or atrioventricular block; on repeat study after treatment is initiated, one should be alert for a prolonged Q-T interval corrected for rate ($Q\text{-}T_c$).[162] In the event of TCA overdose, cardiac arrhythmias should be managed in a manner similar to quinidine toxicity.

Doxepin has been touted as the TCA of choice for treatment of depression in patients with intraventricular or

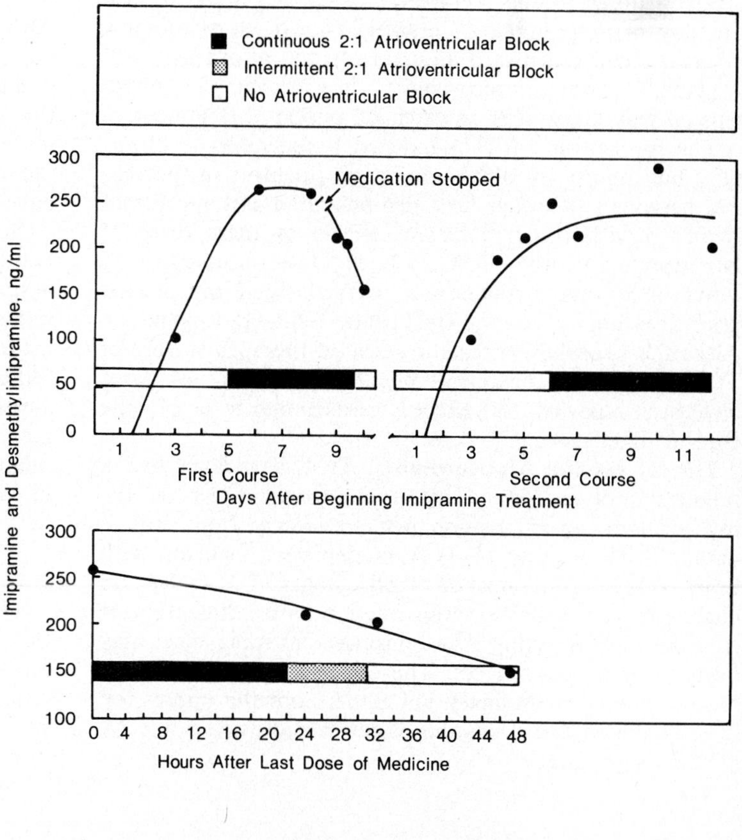

FIGURE 57–4 ***Top,*** **Concentration of imipramine and its psychoactive metabolite desmethylimipramine plotted against days after beginning drug administration during two separate treatment courses. Solid bars indicate the occurrence of 2:1 atrioventricular block.** ***Bottom,*** **Concentration of imipramine and desmethylimipramine plotted against hours after discontinuation of drug treatment. Solid bars indicate the period of continuous 2:1 atrioventricular block. Stippled bars indicate intermittent periods of 2:1 atrioventricular block. (From Kantor, S. J., et al.: Imipramine-induced heart block. J.A.M.A.,** ***231*****:1364, 1975. Copyright 1975, American Medical Association.)**

atrioventricular conduction disturbances. This claim is controversial, resting in part on poorly controlled data that may primarily reflect the propensity of doxepin to achieve lower plasma levels than other TCA at similar oral doses. Despite this and other evidence that doxepin does indeed have some impact on cardiac conduction,[163] a number of reports of a relative advantage lend support to the practice of selecting doxepin as the TCA of choice for these patients. The argument may become moot with the introduction of newer agents without these effects.

Despite the general safety of TCA for most patients, idiosyncratic vulnerability to serious (ventricular) arrhythmia may be encountered.[164] In patients receiving TCA (or other psychotropic drugs) who experience a life-threatening arrhythmia, administration of the suspected drug in the course of electrophysiological study may identify those in whom administration of the agent may be fatal or in whom it may be unrelated to the arrhythmia that was experienced.[165]

Effects on Blood Pressure. Postural hypotension is a common complication of TCA treatment.[152,166] Although the postural decrease in pressure does not differ significantly according to age, the experience of symptoms and such untoward consequences as fractures and lacerations from falling is greater among the elderly.[167,168] Although up to 20 per cent of patients on TCA may suffer postural hypotension, there is a markedly increased prevalence among those with left ventricular impairment or those on cardiovascular medication.[167]

For most patients who experience a postural change upon initiation of TCA treatment, the *symptoms* of orthostatic hypotension usually improve or disappear over days to weeks, despite persistence of a measurable postural drop in pressure.[168] The dosages at which orthostatic changes occur are usually well below therapeutic levels, and increasing doses to the therapeutic range (e.g., 100 to 200 mg/day of imipramine) is unlikely to worsen symptoms, whereas small downward adjustments will afford little advantage.[168] Some improvement in measurable hypotension may occur after an extended period of treatment.

The mechanism of TCA-induced hypotension is uncertain, but affinity for alpha-adrenergic receptors in the central nervous system has been demonstrated and appears to correlate with the hypotensive effects of these drugs.[169] Nortriptyline is the TCA with the least propensity to cause orthostatic hypotension, particularly if the plasma level does not exceed the therapeutic limit (150 ng/ml).[168] Although *hypertension* resulting from a therapeutic dose of TCA alone is a theoretical possibility, and a few cases have been reported, this effect is rare enough to be of little clinical significance.[152]

Effects on the Myocardium. TCA have long had a reputation of exerting a direct depressant effect on the myocardium, an impression derived largely from animal data.[144,152] In a study of TCA in depressed patients with heart disease, radionuclide ventriculograms revealed no change in ventricular ejection fraction with antidepressant treatment,[170] suggesting that a negative inotropic effect may occur only at toxic doses. The conclusions of this study are considered preliminary but underscore the impression of exaggerated early concerns about cardiotoxicity of TCA at therapeutic doses.

MONOAMINE OXIDASE INHIBITORS (MAOI). The renewed popularity of these medications, which block the oxidative deamination of norepinephrine, epinephrine, serotonin, and other amines by the enzyme monoamine oxidase, derives from their efficacy in treating panic disorder, atypical depressions, and some TCA-refractory depressed patients. A cardiovascular limitation to their use is their ability to cause severe orthostatic hypotension. Presumably, this is related to a "false neurotransmitter" effect, either from the drug itself or from the buildup of other nonvasoactive amines. Because of this property, pargyline has found a place in the treatment of hypertension.

The greatest risk of MAOI (e.g., phenelzine, tranylcypromine, and isocarboxazid), especially for cardiac patients, is the acute hypertensive crisis and the complications concomitant with ingestion of tyramine-containing foods and beverages or the administration of sympathomimetic medications. The failure of liver and intestinal MAO to deaminate tyramine in such foods as cheeses, red wine, yogurt, and chicken liver leads to a tyramine-induced release of adrenergic neurotransmitters. Arrhythmias may occur in addition to hypertension. These reactions, although rare, justify caution in prescribing MAOI to patients with serious cardiac disease. This is unfortunate, because they lack the anticholinergic and other cardiotoxic properties of TCA.[121]

Antihypertensive agents such as reserpine and guanethidine, which acutely release vasoactive amines, and alpha-methyldopa, which is converted to sympathomimetic amines, should also be avoided by patients receiving MAOI. In the event of hypertensive crisis with MAOI, an alpha-adrenergic blocking drug, such as phentolamine, should be administered.

NEWER ANTIDEPRESSANTS. A number of new antidepressant compounds with a variety of chemical structures are available for clinical and experimental use. Although none are more effective than TCA in treating depression, their main attraction is the possibility of diminished side effects, particularly cardiotoxic ones. Although the claims of relative cardiac safety appear justified for many of these agents, they have not been subjected to the extensive clinical and laboratory scrutiny that the TCA have.

Maprotiline and amoxapine, for example, although heralded as producing low cardiotoxicity, have anticholinergic and other effects similar to those of TCA. Trazodone, however, is virtually devoid of anticholinergic properties but does pose some risk of postural hypotension. Other compounds without anticholinergic effects are zimelidine, fluvoxamine, and bupropion; those with minimal anticholinergic effects include nomifensine and mianserin. These agents appear to present a very low risk of cardiotoxicity.[171]

The Antipsychotics

This group of psychotropic agents includes the phenothiazines, thioxanthenes, butyrophenones, dibenzepins, and indolones. They are often dramatically effective in abating the severity of symptoms in psychotic episodes. Their action is presumed to be related to their common property of blocking central dopamine receptors.

With the widespread use of the phenothiazines have come reports of sudden death. Since some of the fatalities occurred in young and apparently healthy individuals, cardiovascular effects, especially arrhythmias, have been implicated.[150,172,173] Nearly all such reports were of patients taking either thioridazine or chlorpromazine. Other cardiovascular complications of the antipsychotics derive from central and peripheral alpha-blocking and anticholinergic effects, producing orthostatic hypotension and tachycardia.

Electrocardiographic Changes. The phenothiazines have been associated with a variety of electrocardiographic changes,[150,174] including prolongation of P-R and Q-T intervals, widened QRS complex, ST-segment depression, T-wave changes (usually blunting and widening), variable degrees of heart block, and serious ventricular arrhythmias.[150] The T-wave alterations, benign and reversible, are the most common ECG changes. Accentuated U waves occur with thioridazine. Electrocardiographic changes in general are associated with the phenothiazines of the aliphatic (chlorpromazine) and piperidine (thioridazine) types.

Alpha-adrenergic Blocking Effects. The antipsychotics, especially the aliphatic and piperidine phenothiazines, have both central and peripheral alpha-adrenergic blocking properties[175] in addition to their ability to block dopamine. This property correlates with the degree of hypotension and sedation associated with the specific agent and is of a greater degree than the mild alpha-blocking properties of the TCA but is minimal in the butyrophenone haloperidol. Severe hypotension, which occurs with an overdose, should not be treated with epinephrine or with agents having both alpha and beta effects, since increased hypotension can result; instead, alpha-adrenergic pressors such as norepinephrine should be employed.

Anticholinergic Activity. With the exception of thioridazine, the antipsychotics have less anticholinergic activity than TCA.[176] Nonetheless, they produce sufficient vagal blockade, especially in overdose, to be of clinical significance. This effect is often compounded by the administration of antiparkinsonian agents, such as benztropine or trihexyphenidyl, which also inhibit cholinergic activity.

Other Cardiovascular Effects. Quinidine-like activity has been reported for some of the phenothiazines.[150,174] A toxic cardiomyopathy has been associated with phenothiazine administration,[172,173] and congestive heart failure may be exacerbated by a negative inotropic effect. Changes in intracellular potassium ion concentration have been proposed to explain some phenothiazine-induced electrocardiographic changes.[174] Depression of autonomic midbrain centers and alterations in adrenal medulla secretion have also been implicated in phenothiazine-induced hypotension.[172]

Choice of Antipsychotic. The incidence of adverse cardiac effects of antipsychotics is increased in patients with cardiovascular disease, in the elderly, in higher doses, in synergy with other drugs (especially TCA), and with intramuscular administration. The nonphenothiazines such as haloperidol, molindone, loxapine, and thiothixene have not been shown to have cardiotoxic effects. The high-potency phenothiazines of the piperazine type (e.g., fluphenazine) induce minimal adverse cardiac reactions. Haloperidol, a very high-potency antipsychotic with low anticholinergic[176] and alpha-blocking properties,[169] is often the drug of choice for treating the psychotic or severely agitated cardiac patient; recent reports describe successful intravenous administration in life-threatening states of delirium.[177] Thioridazine, on the other hand, should be avoided in the treatment of cardiac patients.

Lithium

Lithium carbonate is valuable in the management of patients with mood disorders, especially manic-depressive illness. The major toxic effects are neurological and require frequent monitoring of plasma levels. Although prescribing information has generally implied that lithium is cardiotoxic, a variety of reports have indicated its relative cardiac safety.[178,179] The negative response to this drug derives in part from its unrestricted use as a salt substitute in the 1940's, with subsequent morbidity and mortality from lithium poisoning. Reported cardiovascular complications—hypotension, circulatory collapse, and arrhythmia—were agonal events in patients in prolonged coma.[180] In the majority of patients receiving lithium, the drug appears to cause minimal cardiotoxicity and is not associated with blood pressure changes. Congestive heart failure and myocarditis are rare. Instances of syncope secondary to sinus node dysfunction have been reported consequent to lithium treatment.[181]

Electrocardiographic Changes. T-wave changes, similar to those in hypokalemia and possibly related to displacement of intracellular potassium by lithium ions, occurs in virtually all patients treated with this drug.[182] Decreased amplitude, flattening, and even inversion of T waves are considered to be benign and reversible effects that generally do not constitute a reason to discontinue treatment. Individual case reports of arrhythmias, including conduction defects and increased frequency of extrasystoles, suggest that some patients may show idiosyncratic sensitivity to lithium.[178,183] Cases of disordered sinus node function in patients receiving lithium have also been registered.[178,184]

Toxic Effects. The primary concern for cardiac patients is the development of lithium toxicity—nausea, vomiting, diarrhea, ataxia, slurred speech, convulsions, coma, and death—resulting from failure to maintain adequate renal clearance. The patient with congestive heart failure is particularly vulnerable, because of decreased glomerular filtration rate, dietary restriction of sodium chloride, and use of diuretics. The thiazide diuretics elevate plasma lithium significantly and necessitate downward adjustment of daily doses and close monitoring of drug levels.[126] It is good practice to evaluate cardiac parameters carefully before and after initiating lithium treatment for patients with cardiac disease.[184]

Electroconvulsive Therapy (ECT)

Because it is the most consistently effective treatment for severe depression and does not have the cardiotoxic effects of TCA, electroconvulsive therapy has been advocated as the antidepressant therapy of choice for cardiac patients. It should be remembered, however, that ECT is not an entirely benign treatment. Enhanced sympathetic activity following induction of the seizure leads to brief periods of occasionally serious hypertension and arrhythmias.[185–187] Myocardial infarctions following ECT have been reported.[188] The type of barbiturate anesthesia used is also a factor in cardiac morbidity.[189] Careful monitoring and the use of a rapid-acting antihypertensive, such as nitroprusside, can help avert the complications of hypertension. Since the general mortality from ECT is quite low (0.2 to 0.3 per cent)[190] and since depression carries its own mortality, ECT should be considered in treating the severely depressed cardiac patient.

References

1. Harvey, W.: Exercitatio de motu cordis et sanguinis. Cited in Jenkins, C. D.: Behavioral risk factors in coronary artery disease. Ann. Rev. Med. *29*:543, 1978.
2. Osler, W.: The Lumleian lectures on angina pectoris. Delivered before the Royal College of Physicians of London. Lancet *1*:939, 1910.
3. Dunbar, F.: Psychosomatic Diagnosis. New York, Paul B. Hoeber, Inc., 1943, p. 309.
4. Friedman, M.: Pathogenesis of Coronary Artery Disease. New York, McGraw-Hill Book Co., 1969.
5. Rosenman, R. H., Brand, R. J., Jenkins, C. D., Friedman, M., Straus, R., and Wurm, M.: Coronary heart disease in the Western Collaborative Group Study: Final follow-up experience of 8½ years. J.A.M.A. *233*:872, 1975.
6. Jenkins, C. D.: Recent evidence supporting psychologic and social risk factors for coronary disease. N. Engl. J. Med. *294*:987, 1976.
7. Jenkins, C. D.: Behavioral risk factors in coronary artery disease. Ann. Rev. Med. *29*:543, 1978.
8. Kenigsberg, D., Zyzanski, S. J., Jenkins, C. D., Wardwell, W. I., and Licciardello, A. T.: The coronary prone behavior pattern in hospitalized patients with and without coronary heart disease. Psychosom. Med. *36*:344, 1974.
9. Review Panel on Coronary-Prone Behavior and Coronary Heart Disease: Coronary-prone behavior and coronary heart disease: A critical study. Circulation *63*:1199, 1981.
10. Friedman, M., Thoresen, C. E., Gill, J. J., Ulmer, D., Thompson, L., Powell, L., Price, V., Elek, S. R., Rabin, D. D., Breall, W. S., Piaget, G., Dixon, T., Bourg, E., Levy, R. A., and Tasto, D. L.: Feasibility of altering Type A behavior pattern after myocardial infarction. Recurrent coronary prevention project study: Methods, baseline results and preliminary findings. Circulation *66*:83, 1982.
11. Holmes, T. H., and Rahe, R. H.: The social readjustment rating scale. J. Psychosom. Res. *11*:213, 1967.
12. Rahe, R. H., and Lind, E.: Psychosocial factors and sudden cardiac death: A pilot study. J. Psychosom. Res. *15*:19, 1971.
13. Rahe, R. H., and Paasikivi, J.: Psychosocial factors and myocardial infarction: An outpatient study in Sweden. J. Psychosom. Res. *15*:33, 1971.
14. Rahe, R. H., Bennett, L., Romo, M., Siltanen, P., and Arthur, R. J.: Subjects' recent life changes and coronary heart disease in Finland. Am. J. Psychiatr. *130*:1222, 1973.
15. Rees, W. D., and Lutkins, S. G.: Mortality of bereavement. Br. Med. J. *4*:13, 1967.
16. Parkes, C. M., Benjamin, B., and Fitzgerald, R. G.: Broken heart: A statistical study of increased mortality among widowers. Br. Med. J. *1*:740, 1969.
17. Engel, G. L.: Sudden death and the medical model in psychiatry. Can. Psychiatr. Assoc. J. *15*:527, 1970.
18. Engel, G. L.: Sudden and rapid death during psychological stress—folklore or folk wisdom? Ann. Intern. Med. *74*:771, 1971.
19. Greene, W. A., Goldstein, S., and Moss, A. J.: Psychosocial aspects of sudden death—a preliminary report. Arch. Int. Med. *129*:725, 1972.
20. Theorell, T., Lind, E., and Floderus, B.: The relationship of disturbing life changes and emotions to the early development of myocardial infarction and other serious illnesses. Int. J. Epidemiol. *4*:281, 1975.
21. Wolf, S.: The end of the rope: The role of the brain in cardiac death. Can. Med. Assoc. J. *97*:1022, 1967.
22. Bruhn, J. G., Paredes, A., Adsett, C. A., and Wolf, S.: Psychological predictors of sudden death in myocardial infarction. J. Psychosom. Res. *18*:187, 1974.
23. Hackett, T. P., and Cassem, N. H.: Factors contributing to delay in responding to the signs and symptoms of acute myocardial infarction. Am. J. Cardiol. *24*:651, 1969.
24. Moss, A. J., and Goldstein, S.: The pre-hospital phase of acute myocardial infarction. Circulation *41*:737, 1970.
25. Simon, A. B., Feinleib, M., and Thompson, H. K.: Components of delay in the pre-hospital phase of acute myocardial infarction. Am. J. Cardiol. *30*:476, 1972.
26. Wallace, W. A., and Yu, P. N.: Sudden death and the pre-hospital phase of acute myocardial infarction. Ann. Rev. Med. *26*:1, 1975.
27. Sjögren, A., Erhardt, L. R., and Theorell, T.: Circumstances around the onset of a myocardial infarction. Acta Med. Scand. *205*:287, 1979.
28. Hamburg, D. A., Coelho, G. V., and Adams, J. E.: Coping and Adaptation. New York, Basic Books, Inc., 1974.
29. Weisman, A. D., and Hackett, T. P.: The predilection to death. Psychosom. Med. *23*:232, 1961.
30. Cassem, N. H., Wishnie, H. A., and Hackett, T. P.: How coronary patients respond to last rites. Postgrad. Med. *45*:147, 1969.
31. Hackett, T. P., Cassem, N. H., and Wishnie, H. A.: The coronary care unit: An appraisal of its psychological hazards. New Engl. J. Med. *279*:1365, 1968.
32. Cay, E. L., Vetter, N., Philip, A. E., and Dugard, P.: Psychological reactions to a coronary care unit. J. Psychosom. Res. *16*:425, 1972.
33. Dominian, J., and Dobson, M.: Study of patients' psychological attitudes to a coronary care unit. Br. Med. J. *4*:795, 1969.
34. Bruhn, J. G., Thurman, A. E., Jr., Chandler, B. C., and Bruce, T. A.: Patients' reactions to death in a coronary care unit. J. Psychosom. Res. *14*:65, 1970.
35. Kübler-Ross, E.: Death does not exist. J. Holistic Health *2*:60, 1977.
36. Druss, R. G., and Kornfeld, D. S.: Survivors of cardiac arrest: Psychiatric study. J.A.M.A. *201*:291, 1967.
37. Hackett, T. P.: The Lazarus complex revisited. Ann. Intern. Med. *76*:135, 1972.
38. Dobson, M., Tattersfield, A. E., Adler, M. M., and McNicol, M. W.: Attitudes and long-term adjustment of patients surviving cardiac arrest. Br. Med. J. *3*:207, 1971.
39. Parker, D. L., and Hodge, J. R.: Delirium in the coronary care unit. J.A.M.A. *201*:702, 1967.
40. Farber, I. J.: Hospitalized cardiac patient: Some psychological aspects. N.Y. State J. Med. *78*:2045, 1978.
41. Klein, R. F., Kliner, V. A., Zipes, D. P., Troyer, W. G., Jr., and Wallace, A. G.: Transfer from a coronary care unit. Arch. Intern. Med. *122*:104, 1968.
42. Wishnie, H. A., Hackett, T. P., and Cassem, N. H.: Psychological hazards of convalescence following myocardial infarction. J.A.M.A. *215*:1292, 1971.
43. Cassem, N. H., and Hackett, T. P.: Psychological rehabilitation of myocardial infarction patients in the acute phase. Heart Lung *2*:383, 1973.
44. Ueno, M.: The so-called coition death. Jap. J. Leg. Med. *17*:330, 1963.
45. Hellerstein, H. K., and Friedman, E. H.: Sexual activity and the post-coronary patient. Arch. Intern. Med. *125*:987, 1970.
46. Naughton, J.: The effects of acute and chronic exercise on cardiac patients. *In* Naughton, J. P., and Hellerstein, H. K. (eds.): Exercise Testing and Exercise Training in Coronary Heart Disease. New York, Academic Press, 1973.
47. Hackett, T. P., and Cassem, N. H.: Psychological adaptation to convalescence in myocardial infarction patients. *In* Naughton, J. P., and Hellerstein, H. K. (eds.): Exercise Testing and Exercise Training in Coronary Heart Disease. New York, Academic Press, 1973.
48. Bilodeau, C. J., and Hackett, T. P.: Issues raised in a group setting by patients recovering from initial myocardial infarction. Am. J. Psychiatry *128*:73, 1971.
49. Benson, H.: The Relaxation Response. New York, William Morrow and Co.. 1975.
50. Gilberstadt, H., and Sako, Y.: Intellectual and personality changes following open-heart surgery. Arch. Gen. Psychiatry *16*:210, 1967.
51. Kimball, C. P.: Psychological responses to the experience of open-heart surgery. Am. J. Psychiatry *126*:348, 1969.
52. Heller, S. S., Frank, K. S., Malm, J. R., Bowman, F. O., Harris, P. D., Charlton, M. H., and Kornfeld, D. S.: Psychiatric complications of open-heart surgery: A re-examination. N. Engl. J. Med. *283*:1015, 1970.
53. Surman, O. S.: The surgical patient. *In* Hackett, T. P., and Cassem, E. H. (eds.): MGH Handbook of General Hospital Psychiatry. St. Louis, C. V. Mosby Co., 1978.
54. Abram, H. S.: Psychological reaction to cardiac operation: A historical perspective. Int. J. Psychiat. Med. *1*:277, 1970.
55. Kimball, C. P.: Psychological responses to the experience of open-heart surgery. Am. J. Psychiatry *126*:348, 1969.
56. Kimball, C. P.: The experience of cardiac surgery: Psychological patterns and predictions of outcome. Presented at the 9th European Conference on Psychosomatic Research. Vienna, April 30, 1972.
57. Bove, A. A.: The cardiovascular response to stress. Psychosomatics *18*:13, 1977.
58. Chambers, W. N., and Reiser, M. F.: Emotional stress and the precipitation of congestive heart failure. Psychosom. Med. *15*:38, 1953.
59. Klein, R. F., Garrity, T. F., and Gelein, J.: Emotional adjustment and catecholamine excretion during early recovery from myocardial infarction. J. Psychosom. Res. *18*:425, 1974.
60. Bishop, L. F., and Reichert, P.: Emotion and heart failure. Psychosomatics *12*: 412, 1971.
61. Regestein, Q. R.: Relationships between psychological factors and cardiac rhythm and electrical disturbances. Compr. Psychiatry *16*:137, 1975.
62. Lown, B., Temte, J. V., Reich, P., Gaughan, C., Regestein, Q. R., and Hai, H.: Basis for recurring ventricular fibrillation in the absence of coronary heart disease and its management. N. Engl. J. Med. *294*:623, 1976.
63. Reich, P., DeSilva, R. A., Lown, B., and Murawski, B. J.: Acute psychological disturbance preceding life-threatening arrhythmias. J.A.M.A. *246*:233, 1981.
64. Taggart, P., Gibbons, D., and Somerville, W.: Some effects of motor-car driving on the normal and abnormal heart. Br. Med. J. *4*:130, 1969.
65. Taggart, P., Carruthers, M., and Somerville, W.: Electrocardiogram, plasma catecholamines, and lipids, and their modification by oxyprenolol when speaking before an audience. Lancet *2*:341, 1973.
66. Lown, B., and DeSilva, R. A.: Roles of psychologic stress and autonomic ner-

vous system changes in provocation of ventricular premature complexes. Am. J. Cardiol. *41*:979, 1978.
67. Verrier, R. L., Calvert, A., and Lown, B.: The effect of posterior hypothalamic stimulation on ventricular fibrillation threshold. Am. J. Physiol. *228*:923, 1975.
68. Schlesinger, Z., Barzilay, J., Stryjer, D., and Almog, C. H.: Life-threatening "vagal reaction" to emotional stimuli. Isr. J. Med. Sci. *13*:59, 1977.
69. Engel, G.: A life setting conducive to illness: The giving-up—given-up complex. Ann. Intern. Med. *69*:293, 1968.
70. Rahe, R., and Romo, M.: Recent life changes and the onset of myocardial infarction and sudden death in Helsinki. *In* Gunderson, E. K., and Rahe, R. (eds.): Life Stress and Illness. Springfield, Ill., Charles C Thomas, 1974, p. 105.
71. Weiner, H.: Essential hypertension. *In* Weiner, H.: Psychobiology and Human Disease. New York, Elsevier-North Holland, Inc., 1977, p. 116.
72. Henry, J. P., and Cassel, J. C.: Psychological factors in essential hypertension. Recent epidemiologic and animal experimental evidence. Am. J. Epidemiol. *90*:171, 1969.
73. Stamler, J., Stamler, R., and Pullman, T.: The Epidemiology of Essential Hypertension. New York, Grune and Stratton, 1967.
74. Harburg, E., Erfurt, J. C., Hauenstein, L. S., Chape, C., Schull, W. J., and Schork, M. A.: Socio-ecological stress, suppressed hostility, skin color, and black-white male blood pressure: Detroit. Psychosom. Med. *35*:276, 1973.
75. Donnison, C. P.: Blood pressure in the African native, its bearing on the etiology of hyperpiesia and arteriosclerosis. Lancet *1*:6, 1929.
76. Henry, J. P., Meehan, J. P., and Stephens, P. M.: The use of psychosocial stimuli to induce prolonged hypertension in mice. Psychosom. Med. *29*:408, 1967.
77. Reiser, M. F., Brust, A. A., and Ferris, E. B., Jr.: Life situations, emotions and the course of patients with arterial hypertension. Psychosom. Med. *13*:133, 1951.
78. Reiser, M. F., Rosenbaum, M., and Ferris, E. B., Jr.: Psychological mechanisms in malignant hypertension. Psychosom. Med. *13*:147, 1951.
79. Alexander, F.: Psychosomatic Medicine. New York, W. W. Norton, 1950.
80. Binger, C. A., Ackerman, N. W., Cohn, A. E., Chroeder, H. A., and Steele, J. M.: Personality in Arterial Hypertension. New York, Brunner, 1945.
81. Weiss, E.: Psychosomatic aspects of hypertension. J.A.M.A. *120*:1081, 1942.
82. Wolf, S., and Wolff, H. G.: A summary of experimental evidence relating life stress to the pathogenesis of essential hypertension in man. *In* Bell, E. T. (ed.): Hypertension. Minneapolis, University of Minnesota Press, 1951.
83. Oken, D.: An experimental study of suppressed anger and blood pressure. Arch. Gen. Psychiatry *2*:441, 1960.
84. Wolff, H. G.: Stress and Disease. Springfield, Ill., Charles C Thomas, 1953.
85. Pilowsky, I., Spalding, D., Shaw, J., and Korner, P. I.: Hypertension and personality. Psychosom. Med. *35*:15, 1973.
86. Ostfeld, A. M., and Lebovitz, B. Z.: Personality factors and pressor mechanisms in renal and essential hypertension. Arch. Intern. Med. *104*:497, 1959.
87. Ostfeld, A. M.: Editorial: What's the payoff in hypertension research? Psychosom. Med. *35*:1, 1973.
88. Sokolow, M., Werdegar, D., Perloff, D. B., Cowan, R. M., and Brenenstuhl, H.: Preliminary studies relating portably recorded blood pressures to daily life events in patients with essential hypertension. Bibl. Psychiatr. *144*:164, 1970.
89. Cobb, S., and Rose, R. M.: Hypertension, peptic ulcer and diabetes in air traffic controllers. J.A.M.A. *224*:489, 1973.
90. Brod, J., Fencl, V., Hejl, Z., and Jirka, J.: Circulatory changes underlying blood pressure elevation during acute emotional stress (mental arithmetic) in normotensive and hypertensive subjects. Clin. Sci. *18*:269, 1959.
91. Brod, J.: Hemodynamics and emotional stress. Bibl. Psychiatr. *144*:13, 1970.
92. Lacey, J. I., Bateman, D. E., and Van Lehn, R.: Autonomic response specificity: An experimental study. Psychosom. Med. *15*:8, 1953.
93. Doyle, A. E., and Fraser, J. R. E.: Essential hypertension and inheritance of vascular reactivity. Lancet *2*:509, 1961.
94. Gantt, W. H.: Cardiovascular component of the conditioned reflex to pain, food and other stimuli. Physiol. Rev. *40*(Suppl. 4):266, 1960.
95. Shapiro, D., Tursky, B., and Schwartz, G. E.: Differentiation of heart rate and blood pressure in man by operant conditioning. Psychosom. Med. *32*:417, 1970.
96. Blanchard, E. B., and Miller, S. T.: Psychological treatment of cardiovascular disease. Arch. Gen. Psychiatry *34*:1402, 1977.
97. Jacob, R. G., Kraemer, H. C., and Agras, S.: Relaxation therapy in the treatment of hypertension: A review. Arch. Gen. Psychiatry *34*:1417, 1977.
98. Shapiro, A. P., Schwartz, G. E., Ferguson, D. C. E., Redmond, D. P., and Weiss, S. M.: Behavioral methods in the treatment of hypertension: A review of their clinical status. Ann. Intern. Med. *86*:626, 1977.
99. Stone, R. A., and DeLeo, J.: Psychotherapeutic control of hypertension. N. Engl. J. Med. *294*:80, 1976.
100. Patel, C. H.: 12 month follow-up of yoga and bio-feedback in the management of hypertension. Lancet *1*:62, 1975.
101. Patel, C. H., and North, W. R. S.: Randomized controlled trial of yoga and bio-feedback in management of hypertension. Lancet *2*:93, 1975.
102. Southam, M. A., Agras, W. S., Taylor, C. B., and Kraemer, H. C.: Relaxation training, blood pressure lowering during the working day. Arch. Gen. Psychiatry *39*:715, 1982.
103. Kristt, D. A., and Engel, B. T.: Learned control of blood pressure in patients with high blood pressure. Circulation *51*:370, 1975.
104. Becker, M. H., and Maiman, L. A.: Sociobehavioral determinants of compliance with health and medical care recommendations. Med. Care *13*:10, 1975.
105. Blackwell, B.: Drug therapy: Patient compliance. New Engl. J. Med. *289*:249, 1973.
106. Gillum, R. F., and Barsky, A. J.: Diagnosis and management of patient noncompliance. J.A.M.A. *228*:1563, 1974.
107. Haynes, R. B.: A critical review of the "determinants" of patient compliance with therapeutic regimens. *In* Sackett, D. L., and Haynes, R. B. (eds.): Compliance with Therapeutic Regimens. Baltimore, Johns Hopkins University Press, 1976, p. 26.
108. Sackett, D. L.: Patients and therapies: Getting the two together. N. Engl. J. Med. *298*:278, 1978.
109. Zacest, R., Barrow, C. G., O'Halloran, M. W., and Wilson, L. L: Relationship of psychological factors to failure of antihypertensive drug treatment. Aust. N. Z. J. Med. *11*:501, 1981.
109a. National Heart and Lung Institute: National Heart and Lung Institute's hypertension detection and follow-up study. Cited in Hypertension: Getting—and keeping—it under control. Med. World News *17*:52, 1976.
110. Mushlin, A. I., and Appel, F. A.: Diagnosing potential noncompliance: Physicians' ability in a behavioral dimension of medical care. Arch. Intern. Med. *137*:318, 1977.
111. Schmidt, D. D.: Patient compliance: The effect of the doctor as a therapeutic agent. J. Fam. Pract. *4*:853, 1977.
112. Finnerty, F. A., Jr., Mattie, E. C., and Finnerty, F. A., III: Hypertension in the inner city. I. Analysis of clinic dropouts. Circulation *47*:73, 1973.
113. Finnerty, F. A., Jr., Shaw, L. W., and Himmelsbach, C. K.: Hypertension in the inner city, II. Detection and follow-up. Circulation *47*:76, 1973.
114. Haynes, R. B., Sackett, D. L., Gibson, E. S., Taylor, D. W., Hackett, B. C., Roberts, R. S., and Johnson, A. L.: Improvement of medication compliance in uncontrolled hypertension. Lancet *1*:1265, 1976.
115. Goodwin, F. K., and Bunney, W. E.: Depressions following reserpine: A reevaluation. Semin. Psychiatry *3*:435, 1971.
116. Hamilton, M., and Kopelman, H.: Treatment of severe hypertension with methyldopa. Br. Med. J. *1*:151, 1963.
117. Smirk, H.: Hypotensive action of methyldopa. Br. Med. J. *1*:146, 1963.
118. Alder, S.: Methyldopa-induced decrease in mental activity. J.A.M.A. *230*:1428, 1974.
119. Thornton, W. E.: Dementia induced by methyldopa with haloperidol. N. Engl. J. Med. *294*:1222, 1976.
120. O'Regan, J. B.: Adverse interaction of lithium carbonate and methyldopa. Can. Med. Assoc. J. *115*:385, 1976.
121. Baldessarini, R. J.: Chemotherapy in Psychiatry. Cambridge, Harvard University Press, 1977.
122. Simpson, L. L.: Combined use of molindone and guanethidine in patients with schizophrenia and hypertension. Am. J. Psychiatry *136*:1410, 1979.
123. Von Zwieten, P. A.: Interaction between centrally acting hypotensive drugs and tricyclic antidepressants. Arch. Int. Pharmacodyn. Ther. *214*:12, 1975.
124. Risch, C. S., Groom, G. P., and Janowsky, D. S.: The effects of psychotropic drugs on the cardiovascular system. J. Clin. Psychiatry *43*:16, 1982.
125. Burgess, C. D., Turner, P., Wadsworth, J.: Cardiovascular responses to mianserin hydrochloride: A comparison with tricyclic antidepressant drugs. Br. J. Clin. Pharmacol. *5*(Suppl. 1):215, 1978.
126. Himmelhoch, J. M., Poust, R. I., Mallinger, A. G., Hanin, I., and Neil, J. F.: Adjustment of lithium dose during lithium-chlorothiazide therapy. Clin. Pharmacol. Ther. *22*:225, 1977.
127. Marks, I., and Lader, M.: Anxiety states (anxiety neurosis): A review. J. Nerv. Ment. Dis. *156*:3, 1973.
128. Diagnostic and Statistical Manual of Mental Disorders. (3rd ed.) Washington, D.C., American Psychiatric Association, 1980.
129. Crowe, R. R., Pauls, D. L., Slymen, D. J., and Noyes, R.: A family study of anxiety neurosis: Morbidity risk in families with and without mitral valve prolapse. Arch. Gen. Psychiatry *37*:701, 1982.
130. Coryell, W., Noyes, R., and Clancy, J.: Excess mortality in panic disorder. Arch. Gen. Psychiatry *39*:701, 1982.
131. Pitts, F. N., and McClure, J. N.: Lactate metabolism in anxiety neurosis. N. Engl. J. Med. *277*:1329, 1967.
132. Pitts, F. N.: Biochemical factors in anxiety neurosis. Behav. Sci. *16*:82, 1971.
133. Frohlich, E. D., Tarazi, R. C., and Dustan, H. P.: Hyperdynamic β-adrenergic circulatory state: Increased beta receptor responsiveness. Arch. Intern. Med. *123*:1, 1969.
134. Hoehn-Saric, R.: Neurotransmitters in anxiety. Arch. Gen. Psychiatry *39*:735, 1982.
135. Rosenbaum, J. F.: The drug treatment of anxiety. N. Engl. J. Med. *306*:401, 1982.
136. Rosenbaum, J. F.: Anxiety. *In* Lazare, A. (ed.): Outpatient Psychiatry: Diagnosis and Treatment. Baltimore, Williams and Wilkins Co., 1979, pp. 252–256.
137. Weinstein, G., Allen, G., and Ford, C. V.: Anxiety and mitral valve prolapse syndrome. J. Clin. Psychiatry *43*:33, 1982.
138. Gorman, J. M., Fyer, A. F., Gliklich, J., King, D., and Klein, D. F.: Effect of sodium lactate on patients with panic disorder and mitral valve prolapse. Am. J. Psychiatry *138*:247, 1981.
139. Combs, R. L., Shah, P. M., Klorman, R. S., and Klorman, R.: Effects of psychological stress on click and rhythm in mitral valve prolapse. Am. Heart J. *99*:714, 1980.
140. Schuckit, M. A.: Current therapeutic options in the management of typical anxiety. J. Clin. Psychiatry *42*:15, 1981.
141. Sheehan, D. V., Ballenger, J., and Jacobsen, G.: Treatment of endogenous anx-

iety with phobic, hysterical, and hypochondriacal symptoms. Arch. Gen. Psychiatry *37*:51, 1980.
142. Kenyon, F. E.: Hypochondriacal states. Br. J. Psychiatry *129*:1, 1976.
143. Muller, O. F., Goodman, N., and Bellet, S.: The hypotensive effect of imipramine hydrochloride in patients with cardiovascular disease. Clin. Pharmacol. Ther. *2*:300, 1961.
144. Robinson, D. S., and Barker, E: Tricyclic antidepressant cardiotoxicity. J.A.M.A. *236*:2089, 1976.
145. Carlsson, A.: Pharmacological depletion of catecholamine stores. Pharmacol. Rev. *18*:541, 1966.
146. Coull, D. C., Crooks, J., Dingwall-Fordyce, I., Scott, A. M., and Weir, R. D.: Amitriptyline and cardiac disease, risk of sudden death identified by monitoring system. Lancet *2*:590, 1970.
147. Swett, C. P., Jr., and Shader, R. I.: Cardiac side effects and sudden death in hospitalized psychiatric patients. Dis. Nerv. Syst. *38*:69, 1977.
148. Moir, D. C., Crooks, J., Cornwell, W. B., O'Malley, K., Dingwall-Fordyce, I., Turnbull, M. J., and Weir, R. D.: Cardiotoxicity of amitriptyline. Lancet *2*: 561, 1972.
149. Ziegler, V. E., Co, B. T., and Biggs, J. T.: Electrocardiographic findings in patients undergoing amitriptyline treatment. Dis. Nerv. Syst. *38*:697, 1977.
150. Fowler, N. O., McCall, D., Chou, T., Holmes, J. C., and Hanenson, I. B.: Electrocardiographic changes and cardiac arrhythmias in patients receiving psychotropic drugs. Am. J. Cardiol. *37*:223, 1976.
151. Marshall, J. B., and Forker, A. D.: Cardiovascular effects of tricyclic antidepressant drugs: Therapeutic usage, overdose, and management of complications. Am. Heart J. *103*:401, 1982.
152. Jefferson, J. W.: A review of the cardiovascular effects and toxicity of tricyclic antidepressants. Psychosom. Med. *37*:160, 1975.
153. Spiker, D. G., and Biggs, J. T.: Tricyclic antidepressants: Prolonged plasma levels after overdose. J.A.M.A. *236*:1711, 1976.
154. Siddiqui, J. H., Vakassi, M. M., and Ghani, M. F.: Cardiac effects of amitriptyline overdosage. Curr. Ther. Res. *22*:321, 1977.
155. Snyder, S., and Yamamura, H.: Antidepressants and the muscarinic acetylcholine receptor. Arch. Gen. Psychiatry *34*:236, 1977.
156. Tobis, J., and Das, B.: Cardiac complications in amitriptyline poisoning: Successful treatment with physostigmine. J.A.M.A. *235*:1474, 1976.
157. Granacher, R. P., and Baldessarini, R. J.: Physostigmine: Its use in acute anticholinergic syndrome with antidepressant and antiparkinson drugs. Arch. Gen. Psychiatry *32*:375, 1975.
158. Bigger, J. T., Jr., Giardina, E. G. V., Perel, J. M., Kantor, S. J., and Glassman, A. H.: Cardiac antiarrhythmic effect of imipramine hydrochloride. N. Engl. J. Med. *296*:206, 1977.
159. Giardina, E.-G. V., Bigger, J. T., Jr., Glassman, A. H., Perel, J. M., and Kantor, S. J.: The electrocardiographic and antiarrhythmic effects of imipramine hydrochloride at therapeutic plasma concentrations. Circulation *60*:1045, 1979.
160. Burrows, G. D., Vohra, J., Hunt, D., Sloman, J. G., Scoggins, B. A., and Davies, B.: Cardiac effects of different tricyclic antidepressant drugs. Br. J. Psychiatry *129*:335, 1976.
161. Giardina, E.-G. V., and Bigger, J. T.: Antiarrhythmic effect of imipramine hydrochloride in patients with ventricular premature complexes without psychological depression. Am. J. Cardiol. *50*:172, 1982.
161a. Veith, R. C., Raskind, M. A., Caldwell, J. H., Barns, R. F., Gumbrecht, G., and Ritchie, J. L.: Cardiovascular effects of tricyclic antidepressants in depressed patients with chronic heart failure. N. Engl. J. Med. *306*:954, 1982.
162. Rainey, J. M., Pohl, R. B., and Bilolikar, S. G.: The QT interval in drug-free depressed patients. J. Clin. Psychiatry *43*:39, 1982.
163. Brennan, F. J.: Electrophysiologic effects of imipramine and doxepin on normal and depressed cardiac Purkinje fibers. Am. J. Cardiol. *46*:599, 1980.
164. Marshall, J. B., and Forker, A. D.: Cardiovascular effects of tricyclic antidepressant drugs: Therapeutic usage, overdose, and management of complications. Am. Heart J. *103*:401, 1982.
165. Magorien, R. D., Jewell, G. M., Schaal, S. F., and Leier, C. V.: Electrophysiologic studies of perphenazine and protriptyline in a patient with psychotropic drug-induced ventricular fibrillation. Am. J. Med. *67*:353, 1979.
166. Burckhardt, D., Raeder, E., Müller, V., Imhof, P., and Neubauer, H.: Cardiovascular effects of tricyclic and tetracyclic antidepressants. J.A.M.A. *239*:213, 1978.
167. Glassman, A. H., Walsh, T. W., Roose, S. P., Rosenfeld, M. A., Bruno, R. L., Bigger, J. T., Jr., and Giardina, E. V.: Factors related to orthostatic hypotension associated with tricyclic antidepressants. J. Clin. Psychiatry *43*:35, 1982.
168. Glassman, A. H., and Bigger, T., Jr.: Cardiovascular effects of therapeutic doses of tricyclic antidepressants. Arch. Gen. Psychiatry *38*:815, 1981.
169. U'Prichard, D. C., Greenberg, D. A., Sheehan, P. P., and Snyder, S. H.: Tricyclic antidepressants: Therapeutic properties and affinity for alpha-noradrenergic receptor binding sites in the brain. Science *199*:197, 1978.
170. Veith, R. C., Raskind, M. A., Caldwell, J. H., Barnes, R. F., Gumbrecht, G., and Ritchie, J. L.: Cardiovascular effects of tricyclic antidepressants in depressed patients with chronic heart disease. N. Engl. J. Med. *306*:954, 1982.
171. Feighner, J. P.: Clinical efficacy of the newer antidepressants. J. Clin. Psychopharm. *1*:23, 1981.
172. Leestma, J. E., and Koenig, K. L.: Sudden death and phenothiazines: A current controversy. Arch. Gen. Psychiatry *18*:137, 1968.
173. Alexander, C. S., and Niño, A.: Cardiovascular complications in young patients taking psychotropic drugs: A preliminary report. Am. Heart J. *78*:757, 1969.
174. Chouinard, G., and Annable, L.: Phenothiazine-induced ECG abnormalities: Effect of a glucose load. Arch. Gen. Psychiatry *34*:951, 1977.
175. Peroutka, S. J., U'Prichard, D. C., Greenberg, D. A., and Snyder, S. H.: Neuroleptic drug interactions with norepinephrine alpha receptor binding-sites in rat brain. Neuropharmacology *16*:549, 1977.
176. Snyder, S., Greenberg, D., and Yamamura, H. I.: Anti-schizophrenic drugs and brain cholinergic receptors. Arch. Gen. Psychiatry *31*:58, 1974.
177. Sos, J., and Cassem, N. H.: The intravenous use of haloperidol for acute delirium in intensive care settings. *In* Speidel, H., and Rodewald, G. (eds.): Psychic and Neurologic Dysfunctions after Open Heart Surgery. Stuttgart, Georg Thieme Verlag, 1980.
178. Tilkian, A. G., Schroeder, J. S., Kao, J. J., and Hultgren, H. N.: The cardiovascular effects of lithium in man: Review of the literature. Am. J. Med. *61*: 665, 1976.
179. Jefferson, J. W., and Greist, J. H.: Primer of Lithium Therapy. Baltimore, Williams and Wilkins Co., 1977.
180. Gershon, S., and Shopsin, B.: Lithium: Its Role in Psychiatric Research and Treatment. New York, Plenum Press, 1973, P. 108.
181. Hagman, A., Arnman, K., and Rydén, L.: Syncope caused by lithium treatment: Report on two cases and a prospective investigation of the prevalence of lithium-induced sinus node dysfunction. Acta Med. Scand. *205*:467, 1979.
182. Demers, R. G., and Heninger, G. R.: Electrocardiographic T-wave changes during lithium carbonate treatment. J.A.M.A. *218*:381, 1971.
183. Tilkian, A. G., Schroeder, J. S., Kao, J., and Hultgren, H.: Effect of lithium on cardiovascular performance: Report on extended ambulatory monitoring and exercise testing before and during lithium therapy. Am. J. Cardiol. *38*:701, 1976.
184. Mitchell, J. E., and MacKenzie, T.: Cardiac effects of lithium in man: a review. J. Clin. Psychiatry *43*:47, 1982.
185. Anton, A. H., Uy, D. S., and Redderson, C. L.: Autonomic blockade and the cardiovascular and catecholamine response to electroshock. Anesth. Analg. *56*: 46, 1977.
186. Arneson, G. A., and Butler, T.: Cardiac arrest and electroshock therapy. Am. J. Psychiatry *117*:1020, 1961.
187. McKenna, G., Engle, R. P., Jr., Brooks, H. N., and Dolen, J.: Cardiac arrhythmias during electroshock therapy: Significance, prevention, and treatment. Am. J. Psychiatry *127*:530, 1970.
188. Hussar, A. E., and Pachter, M.: Myocardial infarction and fatal coronary insufficiency during electroconvulsive therapy. J.A.M.A. *204*:1004, 1968.
189. Pitts, F. N., Jr., Desmarais, G. M., Stewart, W., and Schaberg, W.: Induction of anesthesia with methohexital and thiopental in electroconvulsive therapy. N. Engl. J. Med. *273*:353, 1965.
190. Kalinowsky, L. B.: The convulsive therapies. *In* Freedman, A. M., Kaplan, H. I., and Saddock, B. J. (eds.): Comprehensive Textbook of Psychiatry/II. Baltimore, Williams and Wilkins Co., 1975.

INDEX

Pages in *italics* indicate illustrations. Page numbers followed by t indicate tables.